TABLE OF CONTENTS

REF
RM
301.12
.D78
2016/17

DRUG INFORMATION HANDBOOK EDITORIAL ADVISORY PANEL

Amanda H. Corbett, PharmD, BCPS, FCCP, AAHIVE
Clinical Assistant Professor
Eshelman School of Pharmacy, University of North Carolina

William J. Dana, PharmD, FASHP
Pharmacotherapy Contributor
Houston, Texas

Julie A. Golembiewski, PharmD
Clinical Associate Professor and *Clinical Pharmacist, Anesthesia/Pain*
Colleges of Pharmacy and Medicine, University of Illinois

Jeffrey P. Gonzales, PharmD, BCPS
Critical Care Clinical Pharmacy Specialist
University of Maryland Medical Center

Sallie Johnson, PharmD, BCPS, AQ Cardiology
Clinical Pharmacy Specialist, Cardiology
Penn State Milton S. Hershey Medical Center

Jennifer Fisher Lowe, PharmD, BCOP
Pharmacotherapy Contributor
Zionsville, Indiana

Amy Rybarczyk, PharmD, BCPS
Pharmacotherapy Specialist, Internal Medicine
Akron General Medical Center

Joseph Snoke, RPh, BCPS
Director, Core Pharmacology Group
Wolters Kluwer

DRUG INTERACTIONS EDITORIAL ADVISORY PANEL

Kay Burke, PharmD
Senior Clinical Editor
Wolters Kluwer

Jamie Hoffman, PharmD, BCPS
Senior Clinical Editor
Wolters Kluwer

Carrie Nemerovski, PharmD, BCPS
Senior Clinical Content Specialist
Wolters Kluwer

Steve Sklar, PharmD
Senior Clinical Manager
Wolters Kluwer

Stephen Marc Stout, PharmD, MS, BCPS
Director, Clinical Content
Wolters Kluwer

Dan Streetman, PharmD, RPh
Clinical Manager, Metabolism, Interactions, & Genomics Group
Wolters Kluwer

David M. Weinstein, PhD, RPh
Senior Director, Clinical Content
Wolters Kluwer

EDITORIAL ADVISORY PANEL

Joseph F. Alexander Jr., MD
Clinical Professor of Internal Medicine
Northeast Ohio Medical University (NEOMED)
Allergist/Immunologist
Summa Health System

Roaa Al-Gain, PharmD, BCPS, BCACP
Drug Information Pharmacist and *Clinical Pharmacist, Anticoagulation*
King Faisal Specialist Hospital & Research Center

Abdulrazaq Al-Jazairi, PharmD, FCCP, BCPS, AQ Cardiology
Head, Medical/Critical Care Pharmacy Services and *Clinical Pharmacist, Cardiology*
Department of Pharmacy Services, King Faisal Specialist Hospital & Research Center

Nada Alqadheeb, PharmD, BCPS, FCCP
Clinical Pharmacy Consultant, Critical Care
King Faisal Specialist Hospital & Research Center

Aljohara Al-Sakran, PharmD, BCPS
Clinical Pharmacy Specialist, Pediatrics
King Faisal Specialist Hospital & Research Center

William Alvarez Jr., BS, PharmD, BCPS
Clinical Manager, Core Pharmacology
Wolters Kluwer

Tracy Anderson-Haag, PharmD, BCPS
Clinical Pharmacy Specialist, Kidney Transplantation
Hennepin County Medical Center

Christina L. Aquilante, PharmD, FCCP
Associate Professor
Department of Pharmaceutical Sciences
Co-Director
Center for Translational Pharmacokinetics & Pharmacogenomics, University of Colorado Denver School of Pharmacy

Aaron Ballensky, PharmD
Inpatient and Informatics Pharmacist
Mercy Medical Center

Kylie Barnes, PharmD, BCPS
Clinical Pharmacist
Kansas City Care Clinic
Clinical Assistant Professor
Department of Pharmacy Practice,
University of Missouri Kansas City, School of Pharmacy

Elizabeth A. Bartis, RN, MSN, FNP
Family Nurse Practitioner
Charlotte, North Carolina

Verna L. Baughman, MD
Professor
Anesthesiology and Neurosurgery, University of Illinois

Elizabeth Beckman, PharmD, BCPS
Clinical Pharmacist Specialist, Pediatric Cardiovascular ICU
Indiana University Health Riley Hospital for Children

Judith L. Beizer, PharmD, CGP, FASCP, AGSF
Clinical Professor
Department of Clinical Pharmacy Practice, St John's University College of Pharmacy and Health Sciences

Jeffrey R. Bishop, PharmD, MS, BCPP
Assistant Professor
Department of Pharmacy Practice, University of Illinois at Chicago

Mark F. Bonfiglio, BS, PharmD, RPh
Vice President, Content Operations
Wolters Kluwer

Diedra L. Bragalone, PharmD, MBA, BCOP, BCPS
Senior Clinical Content Specialist
Wolters Kluwer

Lee Bragg, PharmD
Senior Clinical Content Specialist
Wolters Kluwer

Leslie A. Briscoe, MSN, PMHNP-BC
Certified Nurse Practitioner – Psychiatry
Louis Stokes Cleveland VA Medical Center, US Department of Veterans Affairs

Susan P. Bruce, PharmD, BCPS
Chair and Associate Professor
Department of Pharmacy Practice, Northeast Ohio Medical University (NEOMED)

Gretchen L. Brummel, PharmD, BCPS
Pharmacotherapy Contributor
Wausau, Wisconsin

William F. Buss, PharmD
Clinical Pharmacist
Neonatal Intensive Care Unit, Indiana University Health, James Whitcomb Riley Hospital for Children

Katie Carls, PharmD, BCPP
Clinical Manager, International Content
Wolters Kluwer

Corey A. Carter, MD
Chief of Thoracic Oncology
John P. Murtha Cancer Center, Walter Reed National Military Medical Center

Regine L. Caruthers, PharmD, RPh
Clinical Pharmacist
University of Michigan Health System

Romulo Carvalho
Pharmacotherapy Contributor
Rio de Janeiro, Brazil

Jared Cash, PharmD, BCPS
Director, Pharmacy
Primary Children's Hospital, Intermountain Healthcare

Larisa H. Cavallari, PharmD, BCPS
Assistant Professor
Department of Pharmacy Practice, University of Illinois

Alexandre Chan, PharmD, MPH, BCPS, BCOP
Associate Professor
National University of Singapore
Associate Consultant Clinical Pharmacist
National Cancer Centre Singapore

Kyung H. Choi, PharmD, PhD
Senior Clinical Content Specialist
Wolters Kluwer

Angela Clark, PharmD, BCPS
Clinical Pharmacy Specialist, Cardiothoracic Intensive Care Unit and *Cardiology Team Lead*
University of Michigan Health System

M. Petrea Cober, PharmD, BCNSP
Clinical Pharmacy Coordinator
Neonatal Intensive Care Unit, Children's Hospital of Akron
Assistant Professor of Pharmacy Practice
Northeast Ohio Medical University (NEOMED)

Christine M. Cohn, PharmD, BCPS
Senior Clinical Content Specialist
Wolters Kluwer

Jessica Connell, RN, BSN
Pharmacotherapy Contributor
Tifton, Georgia

Kim Connell, PharmD
Pharmacotherapy Contributor
Thomasville, Georgia

Amanda H. Corbett, PharmD, BCPS, FCCP, AAHIVE
Clinical Assistant Professor
Eshelman School of Pharmacy, University of North Carolina

Susan Cornell, PharmD, CDE, FAPhA, FAADE
Associate Professor
Department of Pharmacy Practice
Assistant Director of Experimental Education
Midwestern University, Chicago College of Pharmacy

Marilyn Cortell, RDH, MS, FAADH
Associate Professor
New York City College of Technology, City University of New York

Harold L. Crossley, DDS, MS, PhD
Professor Emeritus
Baltimore College of Dental Surgery, University of Maryland Baltimore

Melanie W. Cucchi, BS, PharmD, RPh
Clinical Manager, Pediatric & Neonatal Content
Wolters Kluwer

Laura Cummings, PharmD, BCPS
Senior Clinical Content Specialist
Wolters Kluwer

William J. Dana, PharmD, FASHP
Pharmacotherapy Contributor
Houston, Texas

Lacey Davis, PharmD, BCPS
Clinical Pharmacist – Hospice, Palliative Care,
and Post-Acute Care
Aultman Hospital

Beth Deen, PharmD, BDNSP
Senior Pediatric Clinical Pharmacy Specialist
Cook Children's Medical Center

Jodi Dreiling, PharmD, BCPS
Pharmacotherapy Specialist in Critical Care
Akron General Medical Center

Kim S. Dufner, PharmD
Clinical Content Specialist
Wolters Kluwer

Teri Dunsworth, PharmD, FCCP, BCPS
Senior Clinical Content Specialist
Wolters Kluwer

Michael S. Edwards, PharmD, MBA, BCOP
Pharmacotherapy Contributor
Chevy Chase, Maryland

Vicki L. Ellingrod, PharmD, BCPP
Head, Clinical Pharmacogenomics Laboratory
and Associate Professor
Department of Psychiatry, Colleges of Pharmacy
and Medicine, University of Michigan

Kelley K. Engle, BSPharm
Pharmacotherapy Contributor
Stow, Ohio

Christopher Ensor, PharmD, BCPS (AQ-CV)
Clinical Pharmacy Specialist, Thoracic Transplantation
University of Pittsburgh Medical Center

Erin Fabian, PharmD, RPh, BCPS
Senior Clinical Content Specialist
Wolters Kluwer

Elizabeth A. Farrington, PharmD, FCCP,
FCCM, FPPAG, BCPS
Pharmacist III - Pediatrics
New Hanover Regional Medical Center

Margaret A. Fitzgerald, MS, APRN, BC,
NP-C, FAANP
President
Fitzgerald Health Education Associates, Inc.
Family Nurse Practitioner
Greater Lawrence Family Health Center

Carole W. Fuseck, MSN, RN,
ACCNS-AG, VA-BC
Clinical Nurse Specialist, Critical Care
Louis Stokes Cleveland Department of
Veteran Affairs Medical Center

Joyce Generali, RPh, MS, FASHP
Senior Clinical Manager, In-depth Content
Wolters Kluwer

Heather L. Girand, PharmD
Professor of Pharmacy, Pediatrics
Pharmacy Practice, Ferris State University
College of Pharmacy

Morton P. Goldman, RPh, PharmD,
BCPS, FCCP
Health Care Consultant
American Pharmacotherapy, Inc

Julie A. Golembiewski, PharmD
Clinical Associate Professor and Clinical Pharmacist,
Anesthesia/Pain
Colleges of Pharmacy and Medicine, University of Illinois

Jeffrey P. Gonzales, PharmD, BCPS
Critical Care Clinical Pharmacy Specialist
University of Maryland Medical Center

John Grabenstein, RPh, PhD, FAPhA
Pharmacotherapy Contributor
West Point, Pennsylvania

Larry D. Gray, PhD, ABMM
Pharmacotherapy Contributor
Cincinnati, Ohio

Tracy Hagemann, PharmD
Associate Dean and Professor of Clinical Pharmacy
University of Tennessee College of Pharmacy

JoEllen L. Hanigosky, PharmD
Clinical Coordinator
Department of Hematology/Oncology/Bone Marrow
Transplant, Children's Hospital of Akron

Martin D. Higbee, PharmD
Associate Professor
Department of Pharmacy Practice and Science,
The University of Arizona

Mark T. Holdsworth, PharmD
Associate Professor of Pharmacy & Pediatrics and
Pharmacy Practice Area Head
College of Pharmacy, The University of New Mexico

Edward Horn, PharmD, BCPS
Clinical Specialist, Transplant Surgery
Allegheny General Hospital

Collin A. Hovinga, PharmD
Director of Research and Associate Professor
Dell Children's Medical Center, UT Austin School of Pharmacy

Jane Hurlburt Hodding, PharmD
Executive Director, Inpatient Pharmacy
Services and Clinical Nutrition Services
Long Beach Memorial Medical Center and
Miller Children's Hospital

Makiko Iwasawa, PharmD, BCPS
Chief Pharmacist, Drug Information Center
National Cerebral and Cardiovascular Center

Adam B. Jackson, PharmD, BCPS
Clinical Pharmacy Specialist in Infectious Diseases
Kaiser Permanente

Douglas L. Jennings, PharmD, AACC, BCPS-AQ
Cardiology, FCCP
Clinical Pharmacy Manager, Heart Transplant and
Mechanical Circulatory Support
New York Presbyterian Columbia Medical Center

Sallie Johnson, PharmD, BCPS, AQ Cardiology
Clinical Pharmacy Specialist, Cardiology
Penn State Milton S. Hershey Medical Center

Michael A. Kahn, DDS
Professor and Chairman
Department of Oral and Maxillofacial Pathology,
Tufts University School of Dental Medicine

Julie J. Kelsey, PharmD
Clinical Specialist
Women's Health and Family Medicine, Department of
Pharmacy Services, University of Virginia Health System

Patrick J. Kiel, PharmD, BCPS, BCOP
Clinical Pharmacy Specialist
Hematology and Stem Cell Transplant, Indiana University
Simon Cancer Center

Polly E. Kintzel, PharmD, BCPS, BCOP
Clinical Pharmacy Specialist – Oncology
Spectrum Health

Michael Klepser, PharmD, FCCP
Professor of Pharmacy
Department of Pharmacy Practice, Ferris State University

Sandra Knowles, RPh, BScPhm
Drug Policy Research Specialist
Li Ka Shing Institute, St. Michael's Hospital

Omer N. Koc, MD
Staff Physician
Hematology and Medical Oncology Department,
Cleveland Clinic

Jill M. Kolesar, PharmD, FCCP, BCPS
Associate Professor
School of Pharmacy, University of Wisconsin Paul P. Carbone
Comprehensive Cancer Center

EDITORIAL ADVISORY PANEL

Susannah E. Koontz, PharmD, BCOP
Principal and Consultant
Pediatric Hematology/Oncology and Stem Cell
Transplantation/Cellular Therapy, Koontz
Oncology Consulting, LLC

Donna M. Kraus, PharmD, FAPhA, FPPAG, FCCP
Associate Professor of Pharmacy Practice and
Pediatric Clinical Pharmacist
Departments of Pharmacy Practice and Pediatrics,
University of Illinois

Daniel L. Krinsky, RPh, MS
Manager, MTM Services
Giant Eagle Pharmacy
Assistant Professor
Department of Pharmacy Practice,
Northeast Ohio Medical University (NEOMED)

Tim T.Y. Lau, PharmD, ACPR, FCSHP
Pharmacotherapeutic Specialist in Infectious Diseases
Pharmaceutical Sciences, Vancouver General Hospital

Lisiane Leal
Pharmacotherapy Contributor
Porto Alegre, Brazil

Mandy C. Leonard, PharmD, BCPS
Assistant Professor
Cleveland Clinic Lerner College of Medicine of
Case Western University
Assistant Director, Drug Information Services
Cleveland Clinic

Jonathan Leung, PharmD, BCPS, BCPP
Neuropsychiatric Clinical Pharmacist
Mayo Clinic

John J. Lewin III, PharmD, BCPS
Clinical Specialist, Neurosciences Critical Care
The Johns Hopkins Hospital

Jeffrey D. Lewis, PharmD, MACM
*Associate Dean and Associate Professor of
Pharmacy Practice*
Cedarville University School of Pharmacy

John Lindsley, PharmD, BCPS
Cardiology Clinical Pharmacy Specialist
The Johns Hopkins Hospital

Nicholas A. Link, PharmD, BCOP
Clinical Specialist, Oncology
Hillcrest Hospital

Jennifer Loucks, PharmD, BCPS
Solid Organ Transplant Clinical Pharmacist
The University of Kansas Hospital

Jennifer Fisher Lowe, PharmD, BCOP
Pharmacotherapy Contributor
Zionsville, Indiana

Sherry Luedtke, PharmD
Associate Professor
Department of Pharmacy Practice,
Texas Tech University HSC School of Pharmacy

Shannon N. Lukez, RN, MSN, ANP-BC
Adult Nurse Practitioner – Orthopedics
Mountaineer Orthopedic Specialists

Janis MacKichan, PharmD, FAPhA
Professor and Vice Chair
Department of Pharmacy Practice,
Northeast Ohio Medical University (NEOMED)

Jason Makii, PharmD, BCPS
Clinical Pharmacy Specialist, Neurosciences Critical Care
University Hospitals Case Medical Center

Melissa Makii, PharmD, BCPS
Clinical Pharmacy Specialist
Pediatric Oncology,
Rainbow Babies & Children's Hospital

Vincent F. Mauro, BS, PharmD, FCCP
Professor of Clinical Pharmacy and
Adjunct Professor of Medicine
Colleges of Pharmacy and Medicine,
The University of Toledo

Joseph McGraw, PharmD, MPH, PhD, BCPS
Assistant Professor of Pharmaceutical Science and
Metabolism Laboratory Director
Concordia University Wisconsin, School of Pharmacy

Ann Marie McMullin, MD
Associate Staff
Emergency Services Institute, Cleveland Clinic

Christopher McPherson, PharmD
Clinical Pharmacy Practice Manager
Neonatal Intensive Care Unit, Brigham and Women's Hospital
Instructor
Department of Pediatric Newborn Medicine,
Harvard Medical School

Timothy F. Meiller, DDS, PhD
Professor
Oncology and Diagnostic Sciences, Baltimore College of
Dental Surgery
Professor of Oncology
Marlene and Stewart Greenebaum Cancer Center, University
of Maryland Medical System

Micheline Meiners, MSc, PhD
Pharmacotherapy Contributor
Lago Norte, Brazil

Cathy A. Meives, PharmD
Clinical Manager, Core Pharmacology
Wolters Kluwer

Megan Menon, PharmD, BCOP
Clinical Pharmacy Specialist
Roswell Park Cancer Institute

Charla E. Miller Nowak, RPh, PharmD
Neonatal Clinical Pharmacy Specialist
Wolfson Children's Hospital

Julie Miller, PharmD
Pharmacy Clinical Specialist, Cardiology
Columbus Children's Hospital

Stacy E. Miller, PharmD, BCPS, BCPP
Senior Clinical Content Specialist
Wolters Kluwer

Katherine Mills, PharmD
Pharmacotherapy Contributor
Bristow, Virginia

Stephanie S. Minich, PharmD, BCOP
Senior Clinical Content Specialist
Wolters Kluwer

Lauri Moore, RPh, MBA
Vice President, Content Development
Wolters Kluwer

Kara M. Morris, DDS, MS
Pediatric Dentist
Olentangy Pediatric Dentistry

Kevin M. Mulieri, BS, PharmD
Pediatric Hematology/Oncology Clinical Specialist
Penn State Milton S. Hershey Medical Center
Instructor of Pharmacology
Penn State College of Medicine

Naoto Nakagawa, PharmD, PhD
Chief Pharmacist
Drug Information Center, Japan

Lynne Nakashima, PharmD
Professional Practice Leader, Clinical Professor
B.C. Cancer Agency, Vancouver Centre, University of BC

Carrie Nemerovski, PharmD, BCPS
Senior Clinical Content Specialist
Wolters Kluwer

Elizabeth A. Neuner, PharmD, BCPS
Infectious Diseases Clinical Specialist
Cleveland Clinic

Kimberly Novack, PharmD, BCPS
Clinical Pharmacy Specialist, Cystic Fibrosis and *Pharmacy
Clinical Coordinator*
Nationwide Children's Hospital

Carlene N. Oliverio, PharmD, BCPS
Clinical Content Specialist
Wolters Kluwer

Neeta O'Mara, PharmD, BCPS
Clinical Pharmacist
Dialysis Clinic

Tom Palma, MS, RPh
Clinical Content Specialist
Wolters Kluwer

Susie H. Park, PharmD, BCPP
Assistant Professor of Clinical Pharmacy
University of Southern California

Nicole Passerrello, PharmD, BCPPS, BCPS
Senior Clinical Content Specialist
Wolters Kluwer

Rebecca Pettit, PharmD, MBA, BCPS
Pediatric Pulmonary Clinical Pharmacy Specialist
Riley Hospital for Children, Indiana University Health,
Department of Pharmacy

Jennifer L. Placencia, PharmD
Neonatal Clinical Pharmacy Specialist
Texas Children's Hospital

Amy L. Potts, PharmD, BCPS
Assistant Director
Department of Pharmacy
PGY1 & PGY2 Residency Program Director
Monroe Carell Jr. Children's Hospital at Vanderbilt

Sally Rafie, PharmD, BCPS
Medical Safety Pharmacist
UC San Diego Health System

Esta Razavi, PharmD
Clinical Content Specialist
Wolters Kluwer

James Reissig, PharmD, BCPS
Assistant Director, Clinical Services
Akron General Medical Center

A.J. (Fred) Remillard, PharmD
Assistant Dean, Research and Graduate Affairs
College of Pharmacy and Nutrition,
University of Saskatchewan

Elizabeth Rich, RN, BSN, BA
Registered Nurse – Medical Intensive Care Unit
Cleveland Clinic

P. David Rogers, PharmD, PhD, FCCP
Director, Clinical and Translational Therapeutics
University of Tennessee College of Pharmacy

Amy Rybarczyk, PharmD, BCPS
Pharmacotherapy Specialist, Internal Medicine
Akron General Medical Center

Todd P. Semla, MS, PharmD, BCPS, FCCP, AGSF
*National PBM Clinical Program Manager –
Mental Health & Geriatrics*
Department of Veterans Affairs, Pharmacy Benefits
Management Services
Associate Professor, Clinical
Department of Medicine, Psychiatry and
Behavioral Health, Feinberg School of Medicine,
Northwestern University

Karen Shalaby, PharmD
Pharmacotherapy Contributor
Ford, Pennsylvania

Chasity M. Shelton, PharmD, BCPS, BCNSP
Assistant Professor of Clinical Pharmacy
Department of Clinical Pharmacy
Neonatal Clinical Pharmacy Specialist
University of Tennessee Health Science Center

Pamela J. Sims, PharmD, PhD
Professor
Department of Pharmaceutical, Social, and
Administrative Sciences, McWhorter
School of Pharmacy, Samford University

Grant Sklar, PharmD, BCPS
*Assistant Professor, Department of Pharmacy and
Principal Clinical Pharmacist, General Medicine*
National University Hospital of Singapore

Michael Smith, PharmD, BCPS
Assistant Professor of Clinical Pharmacy
Department of Pharmacy Practice and Pharmacy
Administration, University of the Sciences in Philadelphia

Joseph Snoke, RPh, BCPS
Director, Core Pharmacology Group
Wolters Kluwer

Patricia L. Spenard, PharmD
Clinical Content Specialist
Wolters Kluwer

Joni Lombardi Stahura, BS, PharmD, RPh
Senior Clinical Content Specialist
Wolters Kluwer

Kim Stevens, RN
Home Care
Samaritan Regional Health System

Stephen Marc Stout, PharmD, MS, BCPS
Director, Clinical Content
Wolters Kluwer

Dan Streetman, PharmD, RPh
*Clinical Manager, Metabolism,
Interactions, & Genomics Group*
Wolters Kluwer

Darcie-Ann Streetman, PharmD, RPh
Senior Clinical Content Specialist
Wolters Kluwer

Carol K. Taketomo, PharmD
Director of Pharmacy and Nutrition Services
Children's Hospital Los Angeles

Mary Temple-Cooper, PharmD
Pediatric Clinical Research Specialist
Hillcrest Hospital

Jennifer Thackray, PharmD, BCPS
Pediatric Oncology Clinical Pharmacist
Memorial Sloan-Kettering Cancer Center

Christopher Thomas, PharmD
Clinical Pharmacy Specialist, Pediatric CVICU
Riley Hospital for Children, Indiana University Health

Kelan Thomas, PharmD, MS, BCPS, BCPP
Assistant Professor of Pharmacy Practice
Touro University California, College of Pharmacy
Clinical Pharmacist
St. Helena Hospital Center for Behavioral Health Office

Elizabeth A. Tomsik, PharmD, BCPS
Senior Clinical Director, Drug Content
Wolters Kluwer

Leslye Trachte, PharmD
Pharmacotherapy Contributor
Lawton, Oklahoma

Dana Travis, RPh
Clnical Content Specialist
Wolters Kluwer

Heidi Trinkman, PharmD
Pediatric Hematology/Oncology Clinical Pharmacy Specialist
Cook Children's Medical Center

Jennifer Trofe-Clark, PharmD
Clinical Transplant Pharmacist
Hospital of The University of Pennsylvania

Amy Van Orman, PharmD, BCPS
Senior Clinical Content Specialist
Wolters Kluwer

Carlos Vidotti
Pharmacotherapy Contributor
Brasilia DF, Brazil

Geoffrey Wall, RPh, PharmD, FCCP, BCPS, CGP
*Professor of Clinical Sciences and Associate Professor of
Pharmacy Practice*
Drake University

Kristin Watson, PharmD, BCPS
*Assistant Professor, Cardiology and Clinical Pharmacist,
Cardiology Service*
Heart Failure Clinic, University of Maryland Medical Center

David M. Weinstein, PhD, RPh
Senior Director, Clinical Content
Wolters Kluwer

Sarah White, PharmD, BCPS
Pharmacotherapy Contributor
Medford, Oregon

EDITORIAL ADVISORY PANEL

Greg Wiggers, PharmD, PhD
Clinical Content Specialist
Wolters Kluwer

Sherri J. Willard Argyres, MA, PharmD
Senior Clinical Content Specialist
Wolters Kluwer

Andrea Williams, RPh
Senior Clinical Content Specialist
Wolters Kluwer

John C. Williamson, PharmD, BCPS
Pharmacy Clinical Coordinator, Infectious Diseases
Wake Forest Baptist Health

Nathan Wirick, PharmD, BCPS
Clinical Specialist in Infectious Diseases and Antibiotic Management
Hillcrest Hospital

Wende Wood, RPh, BSPharm, BCPP
Pharmacotherapy Contributor
Toronto, Ontario, Canada

Richard L. Wynn, BSPharm, PhD
Professor of Pharmacology
Baltimore College of Dental Surgery, University of Maryland

Jessica Zatroch, DDS
Private Practice Dentist
Willoughby Hills, OH

DESCRIPTION OF SECTIONS AND FIELDS USED IN THIS HANDBOOK

The *Drug Information Handbook, 25th Edition* is divided into four sections.

The first section is a compilation of introductory text pertinent to the use of this book.

The drug information section of the handbook, in which all drugs are listed alphabetically, details information pertinent to each drug. Extensive cross-referencing is provided by US brand names, Canadian brand names, and index terms.

The third section is an invaluable appendix which offers a compilation of tables, guidelines, nomograms, and algorithms which can be helpful when considering patient care.

The last section of this handbook contains a Pharmacologic Category Index which lists all drugs in this handbook in their unique pharmacologic class.

The **Alphabetical Listing of Drugs** is presented in a consistent format and provides the following fields of information:

Generic Name	US adopted name
Pronunciation	Phonetic pronunciation guide
Brand Names: US	Trade names (manufacturer-specific) found in the United States. The symbol [DSC] appears after trade names that have been recently discontinued.
Brand Names: Canada	Trade names found in Canada
Index Terms	Other names or accepted abbreviations of the generic drug. May also include common brand names no longer available; this field is used to create cross-references to monographs.
Pharmacologic Category	Unique systematic classification of medications
Additional Appendix Information	Cross-reference to other pertinent drug information found in the appendix section of this handbook
Use	Information pertaining to FDA- or Canadian-approved indications for the drug
Pregnancy Considerations	A summary of human and/or animal information pertinent to or associated with the use of the drug as it relates to clinical effects on the fetus, newborn, or pregnant women
Breast-Feeding Considerations	Information pertinent to or associated with the human use of the drug as it relates to clinical effects on the nursing infant or postpartum woman
Prescribing and Access Restrictions	Provides information on any special requirements regarding the prescribing, obtaining or dispensing of drugs, including access restrictions pertaining to drugs with REMS elements and those drugs with access restrictions that are not REMS-related
Medication Guide Available	Identifies drugs that have an FDA-approved Medication Guide
Contraindications	Information pertaining to inappropriate use of the drug as dictated by approved labeling
Warnings/Precautions	Precautionary considerations, hazardous conditions related to use of the drug, and disease states or patient populations in which the drug should be cautiously used. Boxed warnings, when present, are clearly identified and are adapted from the FDA-approved labeling. Consult the product labeling for the exact black box warning through the manufacturer's or the FDA website.
Adverse Reactions	Side effects are grouped by percentage of incidence (if known) and/or body system; in the interest of saving space, <1% effects are grouped only by percentage.
Drug Interactions	
Metabolism/Transport Effects	If a drug has demonstrated involvement with cytochrome P450 enzymes, or other metabolism or transport proteins, this field will identify the drug as an inhibitor, inducer, or substrate of the specific enzyme(s) (eg, CYP1A2 or UGT1A1). CYP450 isoenzymes are identified as substrates (minor or major), inhibitors (weak, moderate, or strong), and inducers (weak or strong).
Avoid Concomitant Use	Designates drug combinations which should not be used concomitantly, due to an unacceptable risk:benefit assessment. Frequently, the concurrent use of the agents is explicitly prohibited or contraindicated by the product labeling
Increased Effect/Toxicity	Drug combinations that result in a increased or toxic therapeutic effect between the drug listed in the monograph and other drugs or drug classes
Decreased Effect	Drug combinations that result in a decreased therapeutic effect between the drug listed in the monograph and other drugs or drug classes
Food Interactions	Possible important interactions between the drug listed in the monograph and food, alcohol, or other beverages
Preparation for Administration	Provides information regarding the preparation of drug products prior to administration, including dilution, reconstitution, etc.
Storage/Stability	Information regarding storage and stability of commercially available products and products that have been reconstituted, diluted or otherwise prepared. Provides the time and conditions for which a solution or mixture will maintain potency.
Mechanism of Action	How the drug works in the body to elicit a response
Pharmacodynamics/Kinetics	The magnitude of a drug's effect depends on the drug concentration at the site of action. The pharmacodynamics are expressed in terms of onset of action and duration of action. Pharmacokinetics are expressed in terms of absorption, distribution, protein binding, metabolism, bioavailability, half-life, time to peak serum concentration, and elimination.

◄ **Dosing**	The amount of drug to be typically given or taken during therapy; may include the following:
Adult	The recommended amount of drug to be given to adult patients
Adult & Geriatric	This combined field is only used to indicate that no specific adjustments for elderly patients were identified. However, other issues should be considered (eg, renal or hepatic impairment).
Geriatric	A suggested amount of drug to be given to elderly patients; may include adjustments from adult dosing (lack of information in the monograph may imply that the drug is not used in the elderly patient or no specific adjustments could be identified)
Pediatric	Suggested amount of drug to be given to neonates, infants, and children. The following age group definitions are utilized to characterize age-related dosing unless otherwise specified in the monograph: Neonate (0 to 28 days of age), infant (>28 days to 1 year of age), children (1 to 12 years of age), and adolescent (13 to 18 years of age).
Renal Impairment	Suggested dosage adjustments based on compromised renal function; may include dosing instructions for patients on dialysis
Hepatic Impairment	Suggested dosage adjustments based on compromised liver function
Obesity	Dosing adjustment or dosing considerations for the obese adult patient. Obesity is defined as a BMI ≥ 30 kg/m^2 (based on the World Health Organization [WHO]).
Adjustment for Toxicity	Suggested dosage adjustments in the event specific toxicities related to therapy are noted, such as hematologic toxicities related to cancer chemotherapy
Dietary Considerations	Specific dietary modifications and/or restrictions (eg, information about sodium content)
Usual Infusion Concentrations	Information describing the usual concentrations of drugs for continuous infusion administration in the pediatric and adult populations as appropriate. Concentrations are derived from the literature, manufacturer recommendation, or organizational recommendations (eg, the Institute for Safe Medication Practices [ISMP]) and are universally established. Institution-specific standard concentrations may differ from those listed.
Administration	Information regarding the recommended final concentrations, rates of administration for parenteral drugs, or other guidelines or relevant information to properly administer medications
Monitoring Parameters	Laboratory tests and patient physical parameters that should be monitored for safety and efficacy of drug therapy
Reference Range	Therapeutic and toxic serum concentrations listed including peak and trough levels
Test Interactions	Listing of assay interferences when relevant; (B) = Blood; (S) = Serum; (U) = Urine
Additional Information	Information about sodium content and/or pertinent information about specific brands
Product Availability	Provides availability information on products that have been approved by the FDA, but not yet available for use. Estimates for when a product may be available are included, when this information is known. May also provide any unique or critical drug availability issues.
Dosage Forms Considerations	More specific information regarding product concentrations, ingredients, package sizes, amount of doses per container, and other important details pertaining to various formulations of medications
Dosage Forms	Information with regard to form, strength, and availability of the drug in the United States. **Note:** Additional formulation information (eg, excipients, preservatives) is included when available. Please consult labeling for further information.
Dosage Forms: Canada	Information with regard to form, strength, and availability of products that are uniquely available in Canada but currently are not available in the United States
Controlled Substance	Contains controlled substance schedule information as assigned by the United States Drug Enforcement Administration (DEA) or Canada's Controlled Drugs and Substance Act (CDSA). CDSA information is only provided for drugs available in Canada and not available in the US.
Extemporaneous Preparations	Directions for preparing liquid formulations from solid drug products. May include stability information and references.

PREVENTING PRESCRIBING ERRORS

Prescribing errors account for the majority of reported medication errors and have prompted health care professionals to focus on the development of steps to make the prescribing process safer. Prescription legibility has been attributed to a portion of these errors and legislation has been enacted in several states to address prescription legibility. However, eliminating handwritten prescriptions and ordering medications through the use of technology [eg, computerized prescriber order entry (CPOE)] has been the primary recommendation. Whether a prescription is electronic, typed, or hand-printed, additional safe practices should be considered for implementation to maximize the safety of the prescribing process. Listed below are suggestions for safer prescribing:

- Ensure correct patient by using at least 2 patient identifiers on the prescription (eg, full name, birth date, or address). Review prescription with the patient or patient's caregiver.

- If pediatric patient, document patient's birth date or age and most recent weight. If geriatric patient, document patient's birth date or age.

- Prevent drug name confusion: For more information, see http://www.ismp.org/tools/confuseddrugnames.pdf.

  - Use TALLman lettering (eg, buPROPion, busPIRone, predniSONE, prednisoLONE). For more information, see http://www.fda.gov/drugs/drugsafety/medicationerrors/default.htm.

  - Avoid abbreviated drug names (eg, MSO_4, $MgSO_4$, MS, HCT, 6MP, MTX), as they may be misinterpreted and cause error.

  - Avoid investigational names for drugs with FDA approval (eg, FK-506, CBDCA).

  - Avoid chemical names such as 6-mercaptopurine or 6-thioguanine, as sixfold overdoses have been given when these were not recognized as chemical names. The proper names of these drugs are mercaptopurine or thioguanine.

  - Use care when prescribing drugs that look or sound similar (eg, look-alike, sound-alike drugs). Common examples include: Celebrex vs Celexa, hydroxyzine vs hydralazine, Zyprexa vs Zyrtec.

- Avoid dangerous, error-prone abbreviations (eg, regardless of letter-case: U, IU, QD, QOD, µg, cc, @). Do not use apothecary system or symbols. Additionally, text messaging abbreviations (eg, "2Day") should never be used.

  - For more information, see http://www.ismp.org/tools/errorproneabbreviations.pdf.

- Always use a leading zero for numbers <1 (0.5 mg is correct and .5 mg is **incorrect**) and never use a trailing zero for whole numbers (2 mg is correct and 2.0 mg is **incorrect**).

- Always use a space between a number and its units as it is easier to read. There should be no periods after the abbreviations mg or mL (10 mg is correct and 10mg is **incorrect**).

- For doses that are ≥1,000 dosing units, use properly placed commas to prevent 10-fold errors (100,000 units is correct and 100000 units is **incorrect**).

- Do not prescribe drug dosage by the type of container in which the drug is available (eg, do not prescribe "1 amp", "2 vials", etc).

- Do not write vague or ambiguous orders which have the potential for misinterpretation by other health care providers. Examples of vague orders to avoid: "Resume pre-op medications," "give drug per protocol," or "continue home medications."

- Review each prescription with patient (or patient's caregiver) including the medication name, indication, and directions for use.

- Take extra precautions when prescribing *high alert drugs* (drugs that can cause significant patient harm when prescribed in error). Common examples of these drugs include: Anticoagulants, chemotherapy, insulins, opioids, and sedatives.

  - For more information, see http://www.ismp.org/tools/institutionalhighalert.asp or http://www.ismp.org/communityRx/tools/ambulatoryhighalert.asp.

To Err Is Human: Building a Safer Health System, Kohn LT, Corrigan JM, Donaldson MS, eds. Washington, D.C.: National Academy Press. 2000.

A Complete Outpatient Prescription[1]

A complete outpatient prescription can prevent the prescriber, the pharmacist, and/or the patient from making a mistake and can eliminate the need for further clarification. The complete outpatient prescription should contain:

- Patient's full name

- Medication indication

- Allergies

- Prescriber name and telephone or pager number

- For pediatric patients: Their birth date or age and current weight

- For geriatric patients: Their birth date or age

- Drug name, dosage form and strength

- For pediatric patients: Intended daily weight-based dose so that calculations can be checked by the pharmacist (ie, mg/kg/day or units/kg/day)

- Number or amount to be dispensed

- Complete instructions for the patient or caregiver, including the purpose of the medication, directions for use (including dose), dosing frequency, route of administration, duration of therapy, and number of refills.

- Dose should be expressed in convenient units of measure.

- When there are recognized contraindications for a prescribed drug, the prescriber should indicate knowledge of this fact to the pharmacist (ie, when prescribing a potassium salt for a patient receiving an ACE inhibitor, the prescriber should write "K serum leveling being monitored").

Upon dispensing of the final product, the pharmacist should ensure that the patient or caregiver can effectively demonstrate the appropriate administration technique. An appropriate measuring device should be provided or recommended. Household teaspoons and tablespoons should not be used to measure liquid medications due to their variability and inaccuracies in measurement; oral medication syringes are recommended.

For additional information, see http://www.ismp.org/Newsletters/acutecare/articles/20020601.asp

[1]Levine SR, Cohen MR, Blanchard NR, et al. Guidelines for preventing medication errors in pediatrics. *J Pediatr Pharmacol Ther.* 2001;6:426-442.

FDA NAME DIFFERENTIATION PROJECT: THE USE OF TALL-MAN LETTERS

Confusion between similar drug names is an important cause of medication errors. For years, The Institute For Safe Medication Practices (ISMP), has urged generic manufacturers to use a combination of large and small letters as well as bolding (ie, chlorpro**MAZINE** and chlorpro**PAMIDE**) to help distinguish drugs with look-alike names, especially when they share similar strengths. Recently the FDA's Division of Generic Drugs began to issue recommendation letters to manufacturers suggesting this novel way to label their products to help reduce this drug name confusion. Although this project has had marginal success, the method has successfully eliminated problems with products such as diphenhydr**AMINE** and dimenhy**DRINATE**. Hospitals should also follow suit by making similar changes in their own labels, preprinted order forms, computer screens and printouts, and drug storage location labels.

Lexi-Comp, Inc. Medical Publishing will use "Tall-Man" letters for the drugs suggested by the FDA or recommended by ISMP.

The following is a list of generic and brand name product names and recommended revisions.

Drug Product	Recommended Revision
acetazolamide	aceta**ZOLAMIDE**
alprazolam	**ALPRAZ**olam
amiloride	a**MIL**oride
amlodipine	am**LODIP**ine
aripiprazole	**ARIP**iprazole
atomoxetine	ato**MOX**etine
atorvastatin	atorva**STAT**in
Avinza	**AVIN**za
azacitidine	aza**CITID**ine
azathioprine	aza**THIO**prine
bupropion	bu**PROP**ion
buspirone	bus**PIR**one
carbamazepine	car**BAM**azepine
carboplatin	**CARBO**platin
cefazolin	ce**FAZ**olin
cefotetan	cefo**TE**tan
cefoxitin	cef**OX**itin
ceftazidime	cef**TAZ**idime
ceftriaxone	cef**TRIAX**one
Celebrex	Cele**BREX**
Celexa	Cele**XA**
chlordiazepoxide	chlordiaze**POXIDE**
chlorpromazine	chlorpro**MAZINE**
chlorpropamide	chlorpro**PAMIDE**
cisplatin	**CIS**platin
clobazam	clo**BAZ**am
clomiphene	clomi**PHENE**
clomipramine	clomi**PRAMINE**
clonazepam	clonaze**PAM**
clonidine	clo**NID**ine
clozapine	clo**ZAP**ine
cycloserine	cyclo**SERINE**
cyclosporine	cyclo**SPORINE**
dactinomycin	**DACTIN**omycin
daptomycin	**DAPTO**mycin
daunorubicin	**DAUNO**rubicin
dimenhydrinate	dimenhy**DRINATE**
diphenhydramine	diphenhydr**AMINE**
dobutamine	**DOBUT**amine
docetaxel	**DOCE**taxel
dopamine	**DOP**amine
doxorubicin	**DOXO**rubicin
duloxetine	**DUL**oxetine
ephedrine	e**PHED**rine
epinephrine	**EPINEPH**rine
epirubicin	**EPI**rubicin
eribulin	eri**BUL**in
fentanyl	fenta**NYL**
flavoxate	flavox**ATE**
fluoxetine	**FLU**oxetine
fluphenazine	flu**PHENAZ**ine
fluvoxamine	fluvoxa**MINE**
glipizide	glipi**ZIDE**
glyburide	gly**BURIDE**
guaifenesin	guai**FEN**esin
guanfacine	guan**FACINE**
Humalog	Huma**LOG**
Humulin	Humu**LIN**
hydralazine	hydr**ALAZINE**

Drug Product	Recommended Revision
hydrocodone	**HYDRO**codone
hydromorphone	**HYDRO**morphone
hydroxyzine	hydr**OXY**zine
idarubicin	**IDA**rubicin
idarucizumab	idaru**CIZUMAB**
infliximab	in**FLIX**imab
Invanz	**INV**anz
isotretinoin	**ISO**tretinoin
Klonopin	Klono**PIN**
Lamictal	La**MIC**tal
Lamisil	Lam**ISIL**
lamivudine	lami**VUD**ine
lamotrigine	lamo**TRI**gine
levetiracetam	Lev**ETIRA**cetam
levocarnitine	lev**OCARN**itine
lorazepam	**LOR**azepam
medroxyprogesterone	medroxy**PROGESTER**one
metformin	met**FORMIN**
methylprednisolone	methyl**PREDNIS**olone
methyltestosterone	methyl**TESTOSTER**one
metronidazole	metro**NIDAZOLE**
mitomycin	mito**MY**cin
mitoxantrone	Mito**XAN**trone
Nexavar	Nex**AVAR**
Nexium	Nex**IUM**
nicardipine	ni**CAR**dipine
nifedipine	**NIFE**dipine
nimodipine	ni**MOD**ipine
Novolin	Novo**LIN**
Novolog	Novo**LOG**
olanzapine	**OLANZ**apine
oxcarbazepine	**OX**carbazepine
oxycodone	oxy**CODONE**
Oxycontin	Oxy**CONTIN**
paclitaxel	**PACL**itaxel
paroxetine	**PAR**oxetine
pazopanib	**PAZOP**anib
pemetrexed	**PEME**trexed
penicillamine	penicill**AMINE**
pentobarbital	**PENT**obarbital
phenobarbital	**PHEN**obarbital
ponatinib	**PONAT**inib
pralatrexate	**PRALA**trexate
prednisolone	predniso**LONE**
prednisone	predni**SONE**
Prilosec	Pri**LOSEC**
Prozac	**PRO**zac
quetiapine	**QUE**tiapine
quinidine	qui**NID**ine
quinine	qui**NINE**
rabeprazole	**RABE**prazole
Risperdal	Risper**DAL**
risperidone	risperi**DONE**
rituximab	ri**TUX**imab
romidepsin	romi**DEP**sin
romiplostim	romi**PLOS**tim
ropinirole	r**OPINIR**ole
Sandimmune	sand**IMMUNE**
Sandostatin	Sando**STATIN**
Seroquel	**SERO**quel
Sinequan	**SINE**quan
sitagliptin	sita**GLIP**tin
Solu-Cortef	Solu-**CORTEF**
Solu-Medrol	Solu-**MEDROL**
sorafenib	**SORA**fenib
sufentanil	**SUF**entanil
sulfadiazine	sulf**ADIAZINE**
sulfasalazine	sulfa**SALA**zine
sumatriptan	**SUMA**triptan
sunitinib	**SUNI**tinib
Tegretol	**TEG**retol
tiagabine	tia**GAB**ine
tizanidine	ti**ZAN**idine
tolazamide	**TOLAZ**amide

Drug Product	Recommended Revision
tolbutamide	**TOLBUT**amide
tramadol	tra**MAD**ol
trazodone	tra**ZOD**one
Trental	**TREN**tal
valacyclovir	val**ACY**clovir
valganciclovir	val**GAN**ciclovir
vinblastine	vin**BLAS**tine
vincristine	vin**CRIS**tine
zolmitriptan	**ZOLM**itriptan
Zyprexa	Zy**PREXA**
Zyrtec	Zyr**TEC**

FDA and ISMP lists of look-alike drug names with recommended tall man letter. http://www.ismp.org/tools/tallmanletters.pdf. Accessed January 6, 2011.
Name differentiation project. http://www.fda.gov/Drugs/DrugSafety/MedicationErrors/ucm164587.htm. Accessed January 6, 2011.
U.S. Pharmacopeia. USP quality review: use caution − avoid confusion. March 2001, No. 76. http://www.usp.org

ALPHABETICAL LISTING OF DRUGS

Abacavir (a BAK a veer)

Brand Names: US Ziagen
Brand Names: Canada Ziagen
Index Terms Abacavir Sulfate; ABC
Pharmacologic Category Antiretroviral, Reverse Transcriptase Inhibitor, Nucleoside (Anti-HIV)
Use HIV-1 infection: Treatment of HIV-1 infection in combination with other antiretroviral agents

Pregnancy Considerations Abacavir has a high level of transfer across the human placenta. No increased risk of overall birth defects has been observed following first trimester exposure according to data collected by the antiretroviral pregnancy registry. Cases of lactic acidosis/hepatic steatosis syndrome related to mitochondrial toxicity have been reported in pregnant women with prolonged use of nucleoside analogues. It is not known if pregnancy itself potentiates this known side effect; however, women may be at increased risk of lactic acidosis and liver damage. In addition, these adverse events are similar to other rare but life-threatening syndromes which occur during pregnancy (eg, HELLP syndrome). Hepatic enzymes and electrolytes should be monitored in women receiving nucleoside analogues and clinicians should watch for early signs of the syndrome. In addition, mitochondrial dysfunction may develop in infants following in utero exposure. The pharmacokinetics of abacavir are not significantly changed by pregnancy and dose adjustment is not needed for pregnant women. The DHHS Perinatal HIV Guidelines consider abacavir in combination with lamivudine to be a preferred NRTI backbone for use in antiretroviral-naive pregnant women.

Regardless of CD4 count or HIV RNA copy number, all HIV-infected pregnant women should receive a combination antiretroviral (ARV) drug regimen. A combination of antepartum, intrapartum, and infant ARV prophylaxis is recommended. ARV therapy should be started as soon as possible in women with symptomatic infection. Although earlier initiation may be more effective in reducing the perinatal transmission of HIV, initiation may be delayed until after 12 weeks gestation in women who do not require immediate treatment after careful consideration of maternal conditions (eg, nausea and vomiting) and the potential risks of first trimester fetal exposure for specific agents. A scheduled cesarean delivery at 38 weeks gestation is recommended for all women with HIV RNA >1000 copies/mL or unknown concentrations near delivery in order to decrease transmission. If ARV therapy must be interrupted for <24 hours during the peripartum period, stop then restart all medications simultaneously in order to decrease the chance of developing resistance. Long-term follow-up is recommended for all infants exposed to ARV medications. In couples who want to conceive, the HIV-infected partner should attain maximum viral suppression prior to conception.

Healthcare providers are encouraged to enroll pregnant women exposed to antiretroviral medications in the Antiretroviral Pregnancy Registry (1-800-258-4263 or www.-APRegistry.com). Healthcare providers caring for HIV-infected women and their infants may contact the National Perinatal HIV Hotline (888-448-8765) for clinical consultation (HHS [perinatal] 2014).

Breast-Feeding Considerations Abacavir is excreted into breast milk. Maternal or infant antiretroviral therapy does not completely eliminate the risk of postnatal HIV transmission. In addition, multiclass-resistant virus has been detected in breast-feeding infants despite maternal therapy. Therefore, in the United States, where formula is accessible, affordable, safe, and sustainable, and the risk of infant mortality due to diarrhea and respiratory infections is low, complete avoidance of breast-feeding by HIV-infected women is recommended to decrease potential transmission of HIV (HHS [perinatal] 2014).

Medication Guide Available Yes

Contraindications Hypersensitivity to abacavir or any component of the formulation; patients who are positive for the HLA-B*5701 allele; moderate to severe hepatic impairment

Warnings/Precautions Hazardous agent; use appropriate precautions for handling and disposal (NIOSH 2014 [group 2]).

Abacavir should always be used as a component of a multidrug regimen; concomitant use with other abacavir-containing products is not recommended. Do not use abacavir/lamivudine (plus efavirenz or plus atazanavir/ritonavir) in adolescent and adult HIV-1 patients with a pre-ART HIV RNA >100,000 copies/mL (HHS [adult] 2015). **[US Boxed Warning]: Serious and sometimes fatal hypersensitivity reactions have occurred. Patients who carry the HLA-B*5701 allele are at a higher risk for a hypersensitivity reaction to abacavir, although hypersensitivity reactions have occurred in patients who do not carry the HLA-B*5701 allele. All patients should be screened for the HLA-B*5701 allele prior to initiating or reinitiation of therapy unless patients have had a previously documented HLA-B*5701 allele assessment. Discontinue abacavir if a hypersensitivity reaction is suspected. Abacavir is contraindicated in patients who have the HLA-B*5701 allele or in patients with a prior hypersensitivity reaction to abacavir. Reintroduction of any abacavir-containing product can result in life-threatening or fatal hypersensitivity reactions, even in patients who have no history of hypersensitivity to abacavir therapy. Such reactions can occur within hours.** An allergy to abacavir should be documented in the medical record of allele-positive patients. Reactions usually occur within 9 days of starting abacavir; ~90% occur within 6 weeks, although these reactions may occur at any time during therapy (HHS [adult] 2015). These reactions usually include signs or symptoms from two or more of the following: Fever, skin rash, constitutional symptoms (malaise, fatigue, aches), respiratory symptoms (eg, pharyngitis, dyspnea, cough), and GI symptoms (eg, abdominal pain, diarrhea, nausea, vomiting). Other signs and symptoms include lethargy, headache, myalgia, edema, abnormal chest x-ray findings, arthralgia and paresthesia. Anaphylaxis, liver failure, renal failure, hypotension, adult respiratory distress syndrome, respiratory failure, myolysis, and death have occurred in association with hypersensitivity reactions. Physical findings (lymphadenopathy, mucous membrane lesions, and rash [maculopapular, urticarial or variable]) may occur. Erythema multiforme has also been reported. Laboratory abnormalities (eg, elevated liver function tests, elevated creatine phosphokinase, elevated creatinine, and lymphopenia) may occur. Abacavir should be permanently discontinued if hypersensitivity cannot be ruled out, even when other diagnoses are possible and regardless of HLA-B*5701 status. Abacavir SHOULD NOT be restarted because more severe symptoms may occur within hours, including LIFE-THREATENING HYPOTENSION AND DEATH. If abacavir is restarted following an interruption in therapy not associated with symptoms of a hypersensitivity reaction, carefully evaluate the patient for previously unsuspected symptoms of hypersensitivity. Do not restart if hypersensitivity is suspected or cannot be ruled out regardless of HLA-B*5701 status. If abacavir is restarted, continually monitor for symptoms of a hypersensitivity reaction. Make the patient aware that reintroduction should only take place if medical care is readily accessible.

[US Boxed Warning]: Lactic acidosis and severe hepatomegaly with steatosis (sometimes fatal) have occurred with antiretroviral nucleoside analogues. Female gender, prior liver disease, obesity, and prolonged treatment may increase the risk of hepatotoxicity. May be associated with fat redistribution (eg, buffalo hump, peripheral wasting with increased abdominal girth, cushingoid appearance). Immune reconstitution syndrome may develop, resulting in the occurrence of an inflammatory response to an indolent or residual opportunistic infection during initial HIV treatment or activation of autoimmune disorders (eg, Graves disease, polymyositis, Guillain-Barré syndrome) later in therapy; further evaluation and treatment may be required. Use with caution and adjust dosage in patients with mild hepatic impairment (contraindicated in moderate to severe impairment).

Use has been associated with an increased risk of myocardial infarction (MI) in observational studies; however, based on a meta-analysis of 26 randomized trials, the FDA has concluded there is not an increased risk. Consider using with caution in patients with risks for coronary heart disease and minimizing modifiable risk factors (eg, hypertension, hyperlipidemia, diabetes mellitus, and smoking) prior to use. Potentially significant drug-drug interactions may exist, requiring dose or frequency adjustment, additional monitoring, and/or selection of alternative therapy. Some dosage forms may contain propylene glycol; large amounts are potentially toxic and have been associated

with hyperosmolality, lactic acidosis, seizures and respiratory depression; use caution (AAP, 1997; Zar, 2007). Oral solution contains sorbitol. Use oral solution with caution in patients who are fructose intolerant; may experience abdominal discomfort and/or diarrhea with administration of the oral solution.

Adverse Reactions Hypersensitivity reactions (which may be fatal) occur in ~5% of patients. Symptoms may include anaphylaxis, fever, rash (including erythema multiforme), fatigue, diarrhea, abdominal pain; respiratory symptoms (eg, pharyngitis, dyspnea, cough, adult respiratory distress syndrome, or respiratory failure); headache, malaise, lethargy, myalgia, myolysis, arthralgia, edema, paresthesia, nausea and vomiting, mouth ulcerations, conjunctivitis, lymphadenopathy, hepatic failure, and renal failure.

Note: Rates of adverse reactions were defined during combination therapy with other antiretrovirals (lamivudine and efavirenz **or** lamivudine and zidovudine). Only reactions which occurred at a higher frequency in adults (except where noted) than in the comparator group are noted. Adverse reaction rates attributable to abacavir alone are not available.

>10%:
  Central nervous system: Headache (7% to 13%)
  Gastrointestinal: Nausea (7% to 19%, children 9%)
1% to 10%:
  Central nervous system: Depression (6%), fever/chills (6%, children 9%), anxiety (5%)
  Dermatologic: Rash (5% to 6%, children 7%)
  Endocrine & metabolic: Triglycerides increased (2% to 6%)
  Gastrointestinal: Diarrhea (7%), vomiting (children 9%), amylase increased (2%)
  Hematologic: Thrombocytopenia (1%)
  Hepatic: AST increased (6%)
  Neuromuscular & skeletal: Musculoskeletal pain (5% to 6%)
  Miscellaneous: Hypersensitivity reactions (2% to 9%; may include reactions to other components of antiretroviral regimen), infection (ENT 5%)
<1% (Limited to important or life-threatening): Erythema multiforme, fat redistribution, GGT increased, hepatic steatosis, hepatomegaly, hepatotoxicity, immune reconstitution syndrome, lactic acidosis, MI, pancreatitis, Stevens-Johnson syndrome, toxic epidermal necrolysis

Drug Interactions
  Metabolism/Transport Effects None known.
  Avoid Concomitant Use There are no known interactions where it is recommended to avoid concomitant use.
  Increased Effect/Toxicity
    The levels/effects of Abacavir may be increased by: Ganciclovir-Valganciclovir; Ribavirin (Oral Inhalation); Ribavirin (Systemic)
  Decreased Effect
    Abacavir may decrease the levels/effects of: Methadone

    The levels/effects of Abacavir may be decreased by: Methadone; Protease Inhibitors

Food Interactions Ethanol decreases the elimination of abacavir and may increase the risk of toxicity. Management: Avoid ethanol during therapy; if ethanol is consumed during therapy, monitor for signs/symptoms of abacavir toxicity.

Storage/Stability Store at 20°C to 25°C (68°F to 77°F). Oral solution may be refrigerated; do not freeze.

Mechanism of Action Nucleoside reverse transcriptase inhibitor. Abacavir is a guanosine analogue which is phosphorylated to carbovir triphosphate which interferes with HIV viral RNA-dependent DNA polymerase resulting in inhibition of viral replication.

Pharmacodynamics/Kinetics
  Absorption: Rapid and extensive absorption
  Distribution: V_d: 0.86 ± 0.15 L/kg
    CSF to plasma AUC ratio: 27% to 33%
  Protein binding: 50%
  Metabolism: Hepatic via alcohol dehydrogenase and glucuronyl transferase to inactive carboxylate and glucuronide metabolites; not significantly metabolized by cytochrome P450 enzymes; intracellularly metabolized to carbovir triphosphate.
  Bioavailability: Tablet: 83%; Solution and tablet provide comparable AUCs
  Half-life elimination (serum):
    Pediatric patients ≥3 months to ≤13 years: 1 to 1.5 hours (Hughes 1999; Kline 1999)
    Adults: 1.54 ± 0.63 hours
    Hepatic impairment (mild): Increases half-life by 58%
  Half-life, intracellular: 12 to 26 hours

Time to peak:
  Pediatric patients ≥3 months to ≤13 years: Within 1.5 hours (Hughes 1999)
  Adults: 0.7 to 1.7 hours
Excretion: Urine: ~83% (1.2% as unchanged drug, 30% as 5'-carboxylic acid metabolite, 36% as the glucuronide, and 15% as other metabolites); feces (16% total dose)
Clearance (apparent): Single dose 8 mg/kg (Hughes 1999):
  Pediatric patients ≥3 months to ≤13 years: 17.84 mL/minute/kg
  Adults: 10.14 mL/minute/kg

Dosing
  Adult & Geriatric
    HIV-1 treatment: Oral: 300 mg twice daily or 600 mg once daily in combination with other antiretroviral agents. **Note:** Abacavir is a component of a recommended initial regimen with dolutegravir plus lamivudine (or emtricitabine) for ART-naïve patients who are HLA-B*5701 negative (HHS [adult] 2015).
  Pediatric
    HIV-1 treatment: Oral:
      Infants ≥3 months, Children, and Adolescents (US labeling) or Infants ≥3 months, Children and Adolescents (<25 kg) (Canadian labeling): 16 mg/kg/day in 1 or 2 divided doses (maximum: 600 mg/day) in combination with other antiretroviral agents. **Note:** May consider up to 20 mg/kg once-daily dosing (maximum: 600 mg/day) in stable patients with undetectable viral load and stable CD4 count for more than 6 months (HHS [pediatric] 2014)
      Alternative dosing to be considered for pediatric patients ≥14 kg who are able to swallow tablets: **Note:** In clinical studies, data with once-daily dosing are limited to subjects transitioned from twice-daily dosing to once-daily dosing after 36 weeks of treatment.
        14 to <20 kg: 300 mg once daily or 150 mg twice daily
        ≥20 to <25 kg: 450 mg once daily or 150 mg in the morning and 300 mg in the evening
        ≥25 kg: 600 mg once daily or 300 mg twice daily
      Children and Adolescents (≥25 kg) (Canadian labeling): Refer to adult dosing.
  Renal Impairment
    US labeling: There are no dosage adjustments provided in the manufacturer's labeling (has not been studied).
    Canadian labeling: No dosage adjustment necessary. Use of 600 mg once daily dosing has not been studied.
  Hepatic Impairment
    Mild impairment (Child-Pugh class A): 200 mg twice daily (oral solution is recommended).
    Moderate to severe impairment (Child-Pugh class B or C): Use is contraindicated (has not been studied).

Administration May be administered with or without food.

Hazardous agent; use appropriate precautions for handling and disposal (NIOSH 2014 [group 2]).

Monitoring Parameters CBC with differential, serum creatine kinase, CD4 count, HIV RNA plasma levels, serum transaminases, triglycerides, serum amylase; HLA-B*5701 genotype status prior to initiation of therapy and prior to reinitiation of therapy in patients of unknown HLA-B*5701 status; signs and symptoms of hypersensitivity

Additional Information Use regimens of abacavir and nevirapine with caution; both agents cause hypersensitivity reactions early in therapy (HHS [adult] 2015).

Hypersensitivity testing (*HLA-B*5701*): Prevalence of hypersensitivity reactions has been estimated at 5% to 8% in Caucasians and 2% to 3% in African-Americans. Pretherapy identification of *HLA-B*5701-positive patients, and subsequent avoidance of abacavir therapy in these patients has been shown to reduce the occurrence of abacavir-mediated hypersensitivity reactions. An allergy to abacavir should be reported in the patient's medical record (HHS [adult] 2015). A skin patch test is in development for clinical screening purposes; however, only PCR-mediated genotyping methods are currently in clinical practice use for documentation of this susceptibility marker.

Dosage Forms Excipient information presented when available (limited, particularly for generics); consult specific product labeling.
  Solution, Oral:
    Ziagen: 20 mg/mL (240 mL) [contains methylparaben, propylene glycol, propylparaben, saccharin sodium; strawberry-banana flavor]
  Tablet, Oral:
    Ziagen: 300 mg [scored]
    Generic: 300 mg

Abacavir and Lamivudine
(a BAK a veer & la MI vyoo deen)

Brand Names: US Epzicom
Brand Names: Canada Kivexa
Index Terms Abacavir Sulfate and Lamivudine; Lamivudine and Abacavir
Pharmacologic Category Antiretroviral, Reverse Transcriptase Inhibitor, Nucleoside (Anti-HIV)
Use HIV-1 infection: Treatment of HIV infection in combination with other antiretroviral agents
Medication Guide Available Yes
Dosing
Adult
HIV-1 treatment: Oral: One tablet (abacavir 600 mg and lamivudine 300 mg) once daily. **Note:** Abacavir/lamivudine is a component of a recommended initial regimen with dolutegravir for ART treatment-naive patients who are HLA B*5701 negative (HHS [adult] 2015).
Pediatric
HIV-1 treatment: Children and Adolescents weighing ≥25 kg: Oral: One tablet (abacavir 600 mg and lamivudine 300 mg) once daily. **Note:** For patients who are HLA-B*5701 negative, abacavir plus lamivudine is a component of a recommended regimen (with dolutegravir) for all treatment-naive patients and a component of a recommended regimen (with efavirenz or ritonavir boosted atazanavir) for patients with pre-ART plasma HIV RNA <100,000 copies/mL (HHS [pediatric] 2014)
Renal Impairment
CrCl ≥50 mL/minute: No dosage adjustment necessary.
CrCl <50 mL/minute: Use is not recommended.
Hepatic Impairment
US labeling:
Mild impairment (Child-Pugh class A): Use is not recommended.
Moderate and severe impairment (Child-Pugh class B or C): Use is contraindicated.
Canadian labeling: Use is contraindicated (regardless of severity).
Additional Information Complete prescribing information should be consulted for additional detail.
Dosage Forms Excipient information presented when available (limited, particularly for generics); consult specific product labeling.
Tablet, Oral:
Epzicom: Abacavir 600 mg and lamivudine 300 mg [contains fd&c yellow #6 (sunset yellow)]

Abacavir, Dolutegravir, and Lamivudine
(a BAK a veer, doe loo TEG ra vir, & la MI vyoo deen)

Brand Names: US Triumeq
Brand Names: Canada Triumeq
Index Terms Abacavir Sulfate, Dolutegravir, and Lamivudine; Dolutegravir, Lamivudine, and Abacavir; Lamivudine, Abacavir, and Dolutegravir
Pharmacologic Category Antiretroviral, Integrase Inhibitor (Anti-HIV); Antiretroviral, Reverse Transcriptase Inhibitor, Nucleoside (Anti-HIV)
Use
HIV infection: Treatment of human immunodeficiency virus type 1 (HIV-1) infection
Limitations of use: Not recommended for use in patients with current or past history of resistance to abacavir, dolutegravir, or lamivudine; not recommended in patients with resistance-associated integrase substitutions or clinically suspected integrase strand transfer inhibitor resistance because the dose of dolutegravir is insufficient in these subpopulations.
Medication Guide Available Yes
Dosing
Adult & Geriatric
HIV treatment: Oral: One tablet daily
Dosage adjustment for concomitant therapy:
US labeling: With efavirenz, fosamprenavir/ritonavir, tipranavir/ritonavir, carbamazepine, or rifampin: One tablet daily, with an additional dolutegravir 50 mg tablet daily administered 12 hours after Triumeq
Canadian labeling: With efavirenz, etravirine (in addition to atazanavir/ritonavir, darunavir/ritonavir, or lopinavir/ritonavir in INI-resistant patients), fosamprenavir/ritonavir, tipranavir/ritonavir, oxcarbazepine, carbamazepine, phenytoin, phenobarbital, St. John's wort or rifampin: One tablet daily, with an additional single-component dolutegravir 50 mg tablet administered daily 12 hours after Triumeq
Renal Impairment
CrCl ≥50 mL/minute: No dosage adjustment necessary.
CrCl <50 mL/minute: Use is not recommended (use dose-adjusted individual component drugs).

Hepatic Impairment
Mild impairment (Child-Pugh class A): Use is not recommended (use dose-adjusted individual component drugs).
Moderate to severe impairment (Child-Pugh class B or C):
U.S. labeling: Use is contraindicated.
Canadian labeling: Use is not recommended.
Additional Information Complete prescribing information should be consulted for additional detail.
Dosage Forms Excipient information presented when available (limited, particularly for generics); consult specific product labeling.
Tablet, Oral:
Triumeq: Abacavir 600 mg, dolutegravir 50 mg, and lamivudine 300 mg

Abacavir, Lamivudine, and Zidovudine
(a BAK a veer, la MI vyoo deen, & zye DOE vyoo deen)

Brand Names: US Trizivir
Brand Names: Canada Trizivir
Index Terms 3TC, Abacavir, and Zidovudine; Azidothymidine, Abacavir, and Lamivudine; AZT, Abacavir, and Lamivudine; Compound S, Abacavir, and Lamivudine; Lamivudine, Abacavir, and Zidovudine; ZDV, Abacavir, and Lamivudine; Zidovudine, Abacavir, and Lamivudine
Pharmacologic Category Antiretroviral, Reverse Transcriptase Inhibitor, Nucleoside (Anti-HIV)
Use
HIV infection: Treatment of HIV-1 infection alone or in combination with other antiretroviral agents.
Limitations of use: Limited data exist on use alone in patients with higher baseline viral load levels (>100,000 copies/mL).
Medication Guide Available Yes
Dosing
Adult & Geriatric
HIV treatment: Oral:
US labeling: One tablet twice daily.
Canadian labeling: ≥40 kg: One tablet twice daily. **Note:** Not recommended for patients <40 kg.
Pediatric HIV treatment: Children and Adolescents ≥40 kg: Refer to adult dosing. **Note:** Not recommended for pediatric patients <40 kg. The Canadian labeling does not include an indication for use in patients <18 years.
Renal Impairment
CrCl ≥50 mL/minute: No dosage adjustment necessary.
CrCl <50 mL/minute: Use is not recommended (use dose-adjusted individual components).
Hepatic Impairment
US labeling:
Mild impairment (Child-Pugh class A): Use is not recommended (use dose-adjusted individual components).
Moderate to severe hepatic impairment (Child-Pugh Class B or C): Use is contraindicated.
Canadian labeling: Use is contraindicated (regardless of severity of impairment).
Additional Information Complete prescribing information should be consulted for additional detail.
Dosage Forms Excipient information presented when available (limited, particularly for generics); consult specific product labeling.
Tablet, Oral:
Trizivir: Abacavir sulfate 300 mg, lamivudine 150 mg, and zidovudine 300 mg [contains fd&c blue #2 (indigotine)]
Generic: Abacavir sulfate 300 mg, lamivudine 150 mg, and zidovudine 300 mg

◆ Abacavir Sulfate *see* Abacavir *on page 16*
◆ Abacavir Sulfate and Lamivudine *see* Abacavir and Lamivudine *on page 18*
◆ Abacavir Sulfate, Dolutegravir, and Lamivudine *see* Abacavir, Dolutegravir, and Lamivudine *on page 18*

Abatacept (ab a TA sept)

Brand Names: US Orencia
Brand Names: Canada Orencia
Index Terms BMS-188667; CTLA-4Ig
Pharmacologic Category Antirheumatic, Disease Modifying; Selective T-Cell Costimulation Blocker
Use
Rheumatoid arthritis: Treatment of moderately to severely active adult rheumatoid arthritis (RA); may be used as monotherapy or in combination with other DMARDs

Juvenile idiopathic arthritis: Treatment of moderately to severely active polyarticular juvenile idiopathic arthritis (JIA); may be used as monotherapy or in combination with methotrexate

Note: Abatacept should **not** be used in combination with anakinra or TNF-blocking agents

Pregnancy Considerations Adverse effects were not observed in animal studies. Due to the potential risk for development of autoimmune disease in the fetus, use during pregnancy only if clearly needed. A pregnancy registry has been established to monitor outcomes of women exposed to abatacept during pregnancy (1-877-311-8972).

Breast-Feeding Considerations It is not known if abatacept is excreted into human milk. Due to the potential for serious adverse reactions in the nursing infant, a decision should be made to discontinue nursing or to discontinue the drug, taking into account the importance of treatment to the mother.

Contraindications There are no contraindications listed within the manufacturer's U.S. labeling.

Canadian labeling: Hypersensitivity to abatacept or any component of the formulation; patients with, or at risk of sepsis syndrome (eg, immunocompromised, HIV positive)

Warnings/Precautions Serious and potentially fatal infections (including tuberculosis and sepsis) have been reported, particularly in patients receiving concomitant immunosuppressive therapy. RA patients receiving a concomitant TNF antagonist experienced an even higher rate of serious infection. Caution should be exercised when considering the use of abatacept in any patient with a history of recurrent infections, with conditions that predispose them to infections, or with chronic, latent, or localized infections. Patients who develop a new infection while undergoing treatment should be monitored closely. If a patient develops a serious infection, abatacept should be discontinued. Screen patients for latent tuberculosis infection prior to initiating abatacept; safety in tuberculosis-positive patients has not been established. Treat patients testing positive according to standard therapy prior to initiating abatacept. Adult patients receiving abatacept in combination with TNF-blocking agents had higher rates of infections (including serious infections) than patients on TNF-blocking agents alone. Potentially significant drug-drug interactions may exist, requiring dose or frequency adjustment, additional monitoring, and/or selection of alternative therapy. The manufacturer does not recommend concurrent use with anakinra or TNF-blocking agents. Monitor for signs and symptoms of infection when transitioning from TNF-blocking agents to abatacept. Due to the effect of T-cell inhibition on host defenses, abatacept may affect immune responses against infections and malignancies; impact on the development and course of malignancies is not fully defined.

Use caution with chronic obstructive pulmonary disease (COPD), higher incidences of adverse effects (COPD exacerbation, cough, rhonchi, dyspnea) have been observed; monitor closely. Rare cases of hypersensitivity, anaphylaxis, or anaphylactoid reactions have been reported with intravenous administration; may occur with first infusion. Some reactions (hypotension, urticaria, dyspnea) occurred within 24 hours of infusion. Discontinue treatment if anaphylaxis or other serious allergic reaction occurs; medications for the treatment of hypersensitivity reactions should be available for immediate use. Patients should be screened for viral hepatitis prior to use; antirheumatic therapy may cause reactivation of hepatitis B. Patients should be brought up to date with all immunizations before initiating therapy. Live vaccines should not be given concurrently or within 3 months of discontinuation of therapy; there is no data available concerning secondary transmission of live vaccines in patients receiving therapy. Powder for injection may contain maltose, which may result in falsely-elevated serum glucose readings on the day of infusion. Higher incidences of infection and malignancy were observed in the elderly; use with caution.

Adverse Reactions Note: Percentages not always reported; COPD patients experienced a higher frequency of COPD-related adverse reactions (COPD exacerbation, cough, dyspnea, pneumonia, rhonchi)

>10%:
Central nervous system: Headache (≤18%)
Gastrointestinal: Nausea
Respiratory: Nasopharyngitis (12%), upper respiratory tract infection
Miscellaneous: Infection (adults 54%; children 36%), antibody development (2% to 41%)

1% to 10%:
Cardiovascular: Hypertension (7%)
Central nervous system: Dizziness (9%)

Dermatologic: Skin rash (4%)
Gastrointestinal: Dyspepsia (6%), abdominal pain, diarrhea
Genitourinary: Urinary tract infection (6%)
Immunologic: Immunogenicity (1% to 2%)
Infection: Herpes simplex infection, influenza
Local: Injection site reaction (3%)
Neuromuscular & skeletal: Back pain (7%), limb pain (3%)
Respiratory: Cough (8%), bronchitis, pneumonia, rhinitis, sinusitis
Miscellaneous: Infusion-related reaction (≤9%), fever
<1% (Limited to important or life-threatening): Acute lymphocytic leukemia, anaphylactoid reaction, anaphylaxis, cellulitis, diverticulitis, dyspnea, exacerbation of arthritis, exacerbation of chronic obstructive pulmonary disease, hypersensitivity, hypotension, joint wear, malignant neoplasm (including malignant melanoma, malignant neoplasm of the bile duct, malignant neoplasm of bladder, malignant neoplasm of breast, malignant neoplasm of cervix, malignant neoplasm of kidney, malignant neoplasm of prostate, malignant neoplasm of skin, malignant neoplasm of thyroid, myelodysplastic syndrome, and uterine neoplasm), malignant neoplasm of lung, ovarian cyst, pruritus, pyelonephritis, rhonchi, urticaria, varicella, vasculitis (including hypersensitivity angiitis [cutaneous vasculitis and leukocytoclastic vasculitis]), wheezing

Drug Interactions

Metabolism/Transport Effects None known.

Avoid Concomitant Use

Avoid concomitant use of Abatacept with any of the following: Anakinra; Anti-TNF Agents; BCG (Intravesical); Belimumab; Natalizumab; Pimecrolimus; RiTUXimab; Tacrolimus (Topical); Tocilizumab; Tofacitinib; Vaccines (Live)

Increased Effect/Toxicity

Abatacept may increase the levels/effects of: Belimumab; Fingolimod; Leflunomide; Natalizumab; Tofacitinib; Vaccines (Live)

The levels/effects of Abatacept may be increased by: Anakinra; Anti-TNF Agents; Denosumab; Pimecrolimus; RiTUXimab; Roflumilast; Tacrolimus (Topical); Tocilizumab; Trastuzumab

Decreased Effect

Abatacept may decrease the levels/effects of: BCG (Intravesical); Coccidioides immitis Skin Test; Sipuleucel-T; Vaccines (Inactivated); Vaccines (Live)

The levels/effects of Abatacept may be decreased by: Echinacea

Preparation for Administration

IV: Reconstitute each vial with 10 mL SWFI using the provided silicone-free disposable syringe (discard solutions accidentally reconstituted with siliconized syringe as they may develop translucent particles). Inject SWFI down the side of the vial to avoid foaming. The reconstituted solution contains 25 mg/mL abatacept. Further dilute (using a silicone-free syringe) in 100 mL NS to a final concentration of ≤10 mg/mL. Prior to adding abatacept to the 100 mL bag, the manufacturer recommends withdrawing a volume of NS equal to the abatacept volume required, resulting in a final volume of 100 mL. Mix gently; do not shake.

SubQ: Allow prefilled syringe to reach room temperature prior to administration by removing from refrigerator 30-60 minutes prior to administration.

Storage/Stability

Prefilled syringe: Store at 2°C to 8°C (36°F to 46°F); do not freeze. Protect from light.

Powder for injection: Prior to reconstitution, store at 2°C to 8°C (36°F to 46°F); do not freeze. Protect from light. After dilution, may be stored for up to 24 hours at room temperature or refrigerated at 2°C to 8°C (36°F to 46°F). Must be used within 24 hours of reconstitution.

Mechanism of Action Selective costimulation modulator; inhibits T-cell (T-lymphocyte) activation by binding to CD80 and CD86 on antigen presenting cells (APC), thus blocking the required CD28 interaction between APCs and T cells. Activated T lymphocytes are found in the synovium of rheumatoid arthritis patients.

Pharmacodynamics/Kinetics

Distribution: V_{ss}: 0.07 L/kg (range: 0.02 to 0.13 L/kg)
Bioavailability: SubQ: 78.6% (relative to IV administration)
Half-life elimination: RA: 13.1 days (range: 8 to 25 days)
Clearance: 0.22 to 0.23 mL/hour/kg; Children 6 to 17 years: JIA: 0.4 mL/hour/kg (increases with baseline body weight)

Dosing

Adult

Rheumatoid arthritis (RA):
IV: Dosing is according to body weight. Following the initial IV infusion (using the weight-based dosing), ▶

repeat IV infusion (using the same weight-based dosing) at 2 weeks and 4 weeks after the initial infusion, and every 4 weeks thereafter.

<60 kg: 500 mg
60-100 kg: 750 mg
>100 kg: 1000 mg

SubQ: 125 mg subcutaneously once weekly. **Note:** SubQ dosing may be initiated with or without an IV loading dose.

If initiating with an IV loading dose, administer the initial IV infusion (using the weight-based dosing), then administer 125 mg subcutaneously within 24 hours of the infusion, followed by 125 mg subcutaneously once weekly thereafter.

If transitioning from IV therapy to SubQ therapy, administer the first SubQ dose instead of the next scheduled IV dose.

Geriatric Refer to adult dosing. Due to potential for higher rates of infections and malignancies, use caution.

Pediatric Juvenile idiopathic arthritis (JIA): IV:
Children ≥6 years and <75 kg: 10 mg/kg (based on body weight at each administration), repeat dose at 2 weeks and 4 weeks after initial infusion, and every 4 weeks thereafter.

Children ≥6 years and ≥75 kg: **Note:** Dosage is according to body weight. Repeat dose at 2 weeks and 4 weeks after initial dose and every 4 weeks thereafter:
75-100 kg: 750 mg
>100 kg: 1000 mg

Renal Impairment No dosage adjustment provided in manufacturer's labeling (has not been studied).

Hepatic Impairment No dosage adjustment provided in manufacturer's labeling (has not been studied).

Adjustment for Toxicity Discontinue in patients who develop a serious infection.

Administration
IV: Infuse over 30 minutes. Administer through a 0.2-1.2 micron low protein-binding filter

SubQ: Allow prefilled syringe to warm to room temperature (for 30-60 minutes) prior to administration. Inject into the front of the thigh (preferred), abdomen (except for 2-inch area around the navel), or the outer area of the upper arms (if administered by a caregiver). Rotate injection sites (≥1 inch apart); do not administer into tender, bruised, red, or hard skin.

Monitoring Parameters Signs and symptoms of infection, signs and symptoms of hypersensitivity reaction; hepatitis and TB screening prior to therapy initiation

Test Interactions Contains maltose; may result in falsely elevated blood glucose levels with dehydrogenase pyrroloquinolinequinone or glucose-dye-oxidoreductase testing methods on the day of infusion. Glucose monitoring methods which utilize glucose dehydrogenase nicotine adenine dinucleotide (GDH-NAD), glucose oxidase, or glucose hexokinase are recommended.

Dosage Forms Excipient information presented when available (limited, particularly for generics); consult specific product labeling.

Solution Prefilled Syringe, Subcutaneous [preservative free]:
Orencia: 125 mg/mL (1 mL)

Solution Reconstituted, Intravenous [preservative free]:
Orencia: 250 mg (1 ea)

Abciximab (ab SIK si mab)

Brand Names: US ReoPro
Brand Names: Canada ReoPro
Index Terms 7E3; C7E3
Pharmacologic Category Antiplatelet Agent, Glycoprotein IIb/IIIa Inhibitor

Use Prevention of cardiac ischemic complications in patients undergoing percutaneous coronary intervention (PCI); prevention of cardiac ischemic complications in patients with unstable angina (UA)/non-ST-elevation myocardial infarction (NSTEMI) unresponsive to conventional therapy when PCI is scheduled within 24 hours

Note: Intended for use with aspirin and heparin, at a minimum.

Pregnancy Considerations Animal reproduction studies have not been conducted. *In vitro* studies have shown only small amounts of abciximab to cross the placenta. It is not known whether abciximab can cause fetal harm when administered to a pregnant woman or can affect reproduction capacity.

Breast-Feeding Considerations It is not known if abciximab is excreted in breast milk. The manufacturer recommends that caution be exercised when administering abciximab to nursing women.

Contraindications Hypersensitivity to abciximab, murine proteins, or any component of the formulation; active internal hemorrhage or recent (within 6 weeks) clinically-significant GI or GU bleeding; history of cerebrovascular accident within 2 years or with significant neurological deficit; clotting abnormalities or administration of oral anticoagulants within 7 days unless prothrombin time (PT) is ≤1.2 times control PT value; thrombocytopenia (<100,000 cells/µL); recent (within 6 weeks) major surgery or trauma; intracranial tumor, arteriovenous malformation, or aneurysm; severe uncontrolled hypertension; history of vasculitis; use of dextran before PTCA or intent to use dextran during PTCA; concomitant use of another parenteral GP IIb/IIIa inhibitor

Warnings/Precautions Administration of abciximab is associated with increased frequency of major bleeding complications, including retroperitoneal bleeding, pulmonary bleeding, spontaneous GI or GU bleeding, and bleeding at the arterial access. Risk may be increased with patients weighing <75 kg, elderly patients (>65 years of age), history of previous GI disease, and recent thrombolytic therapy. When attempting IV access, avoid noncompressible sites (eg, subclavian or jugular veins).

The risk of major bleeds may increase with concurrent use of thrombolytics. Anticoagulation, such as with heparin, may contribute to the risk of bleeding. In serious, uncontrolled bleeding, abciximab and heparin should be stopped. Increased risk of hemorrhage during or following angioplasty is associated with unsuccessful PTCA, PTCA procedure >70 minutes duration, or PTCA performed within 12 hours of symptom onset for acute myocardial infarction. Prior to pulling the sheath, heparin should be discontinued for 3-4 hours and ACT ≤175 seconds or aPTT ≤50 seconds. Use standard compression techniques after sheath removal. Watch the site closely afterwards for further bleeding.

Administration of abciximab may result in human antichimeric antibody formation that can cause hypersensitivity reactions (including anaphylaxis), thrombocytopenia, or diminished efficacy. Readministration of abciximab within 30 days or in patients with human antichimeric antibodies (HACA) increases the incidence and severity of thrombocytopenia.

Adverse Reactions As with all drugs which may affect hemostasis, bleeding is associated with abciximab. Hemorrhage may occur at virtually any site. Risk is dependent on multiple variables, including the concurrent use of multiple agents which alter hemostasis and patient susceptibility.

>10%:
Cardiovascular: Hypotension (14%), chest pain (11%)
Gastrointestinal: Nausea (14%)
Hematologic & oncologic: Minor hemorrhage (4% to 17%), major hemorrhage (1% to 14%)
Neuromuscular & skeletal: Back pain (18%)
Miscellaneous: Antibody development (HACA, first exposure: 6%; readministration: 27%; four or more exposures: 44%)

1% to 10%:
Cardiovascular: Bradycardia (5%), peripheral edema (2%)
Gastrointestinal: Abdominal pain (3%)
Hematologic & oncologic: Thrombocytopenia: <100,000 cells/mm³ (3% to 6%); <50,000 cells/mm³ (0.4% to 2%)
Local: Pain at injection site (4%)

<1% (Limited to important or life-threatening): Abnormality in thinking, abscess, allergic reaction (possible), anaphylaxis (possible), arteriovenous fistula, bronchitis, bullous skin disease, cellulitis, cerebrovascular accident, coma, complete atrioventricular block, confusion, diabetes mellitus, edema, embolism, gastroesophageal reflux disease, hyperkalemia, hypertonia, incomplete atrioventricular block, inflammation, intestinal obstruction, intracranial hemorrhage, leukocytosis, nodal arrhythmia, pleural effusion, pleurisy, pneumonia, prostatitis,

pseudoaneurysm, pulmonary alveolar hemorrhage, pulmonary embolism, renal insufficiency, thrombophlebitis, urinary retention, ventricular tachycardia

Drug Interactions

Metabolism/Transport Effects None known.

Avoid Concomitant Use

Avoid concomitant use of Abciximab with any of the following: Belimumab; Dextran; Urokinase

Increased Effect/Toxicity

Abciximab may increase the levels/effects of: Agents with Antiplatelet Properties; Anticoagulants; Apixaban; Belimumab; Collagenase (Systemic); Dabigatran Etexilate; Deoxycholic Acid; Edoxaban; Ibritumomab; Obinutuzumab; Rivaroxaban; Salicylates; Thrombolytic Agents; Tositumomab and Iodine I 131 Tositumomab; Urokinase

The levels/effects of Abciximab may be increased by: Dasatinib; Dextran; Glucosamine; Herbs (Anticoagulant/Antiplatelet Properties); Ibrutinib; Limaprost; Multivitamins/Fluoride (with ADE); Multivitamins/Minerals (with ADEK, Folate, Iron); Multivitamins/Minerals (with AE, No Iron); Omega-3 Fatty Acids; Pentosan Polysulfate Sodium; Pentoxifylline; Prostacyclin Analogues; Tipranavir; Vitamin E; Vitamin E (Oral)

Decreased Effect There are no known significant interactions involving a decrease in effect.

Preparation for Administration Bolus dose: Aseptically withdraw the necessary amount of abciximab for the bolus dose into a syringe using a 0.2 or 5 micron low protein-binding syringe filter (or equivalent); the bolus should be administered 10-60 minutes before the procedure.

Continuous infusion: Aseptically withdraw amount required of abciximab for the infusion through a 0.2 or 5 micron low protein-binding syringe filter into a syringe; inject this into 250 mL of NS or D$_5$W to make solution. If a syringe filter was not used when preparing the infusion, administer using an in-line 0.2 or 0.22 micron low protein-binding filter.

Note: A standard concentration of 7.2 mg in 250 mL of NS or D$_5$W may also be prepared for all patients and administered at the standard dose (0.125 mcg/kg/minute; maximum: 10 mcg/minute) with a variable rate in mL/hour. Infuse for 12-24 hours via pump after bolus dose; length of therapy dependent on indication. Some institutions use a standard concentration of 9 mg in 250 mL of D$_5$W or NS.

Storage/Stability Vials should be stored at 2°C to 8°C (36°F to 46°F). Do not freeze or shake. After admixture, the prepared solution is stable for 12 hours.

The following stability information has also been reported: May store intact vials at 24°C to 28°C (76°F to 82°F) for up to 8 days (data on file [Eli Lilly, 2011]). However, the manufacturer recommends storage under refrigeration. Room temperature stability information should only be utilized in situations where the drug has been inadvertently exposed to prolonged room temperature.

Mechanism of Action Fab antibody fragment of the chimeric human-murine monoclonal antibody 7E3; this agent binds to platelet IIb/IIIa receptors, resulting in steric hindrance, thus inhibiting platelet aggregation

Pharmacodynamics/Kinetics

Onset: Rapid; platelet aggregation reduced to <20% of baseline at 10 minutes

Duration: Up to 72 hours for restoration of normal hemostasis (Schror, 2003)

Distribution: V$_d$: 0.07 L/kg (Schror, 2003)

Protein binding: Mostly bound to GP IIb/IIIa receptors on platelet surface

Metabolism: Unbound abciximab metabolized via proteolytic cleavage (Schror, 2003)

Half-life elimination: Plasma: ~30 minutes; dissociation half-life from GP IIb/IIIa receptors: up to 4 hours (Schror, 2003). **Note:** 29% and 13% of abciximab estimated to remain on GP IIb/IIIa receptors at 8 and 15 days, respectively (Mascelli, 1998). Platelet function may remain abnormal for up to 7 days post infusion (Osende, 2001).

Time to peak: Platelet inhibition: ~30 minutes (Mascelli, 1998)

Dosing

Adult & Geriatric

Percutaneous coronary intervention (PCI): IV: 0.25 mg/kg bolus administered 10-60 minutes prior to start of PCI followed by an infusion of 0.125 mcg/kg/minute (maximum: 10 mcg/minute) for 12 hours

Unstable angina/non-ST-elevation MI (UA/NSTEMI) unresponsive to conventional medical therapy with planned PCI within 24 hours: IV: 0.25 mg/kg bolus followed by an 18- to 24-hour infusion of 10 mcg/minute, concluding 1 hour after PCI.

ST-elevation myocardial infarction (STEMI) undergoing primary percutaneous coronary intervention (PCI) (off-label use) (ACCF/AHA [O'Gara, 2013]): IV:

Loading dose: 0.25 mg/kg bolus administered at the time of PCI

Maintenance infusion: 0.125 mcg/kg/minute (maximum: 10 mcg/minute) continued for up to 12 hours

Intracoronary (off-label route): 0.25 mg/kg bolus administered directly to the site of the infarct lesion; may be followed with an intravenous maintenance infusion if refractory intraprocedural thrombotic complications occur (Stone, 2012)

Renal Impairment There are no dosage adjustments provided in the manufacturer's labeling.

Hepatic Impairment There are no dosage adjustments provided in the manufacturer's labeling.

Usual Infusion Concentrations: Adult IV infusion: 7.2 mg in 250 mL (concentration: 28.8 **mcg**/mL) **or** 9 mg in 250 mL (concentration: 36 **mcg**/mL) of D$_5$W or NS

Administration

Abciximab is intended for coadministration with aspirin postangioplasty and heparin infused and weight adjusted to maintain a therapeutic bleeding time (eg, ACT 300 to 500 seconds). Solution must be filtered prior to administration. Do not shake the vial.

Intracoronary administration (off-label route): In select STEMI cases (eg, anterior STEMI), abciximab bolus may be administered through the guiding catheter directly to the culprit lesion site (Stone, 2012; Thiele, 2012)

Monitoring Parameters Prothrombin time, activated partial thromboplastin time (aPTT), hemoglobin, hematocrit, platelet count, fibrinogen, fibrin split products, transfusion requirements, signs of hypersensitivity reactions, guaiac stools, Hemastix® urine. Platelet count should be monitored at baseline, 2-4 hours following bolus infusion, and at 24 hours (or prior to discharge, if before 24 hours). To minimize risk of bleeding:

Abciximab initiated 18-24 hours prior to PCI: Maintain aPTT between 60-85 seconds during the heparin/abciximab infusion period

During PCI: Maintain ACT between 200-300 seconds

Following PCI (if anticoagulation is maintained): Maintain aPTT between 50-75 seconds

Sheath removal should not occur until aPTT is ≤50 seconds or ACT ≤175 seconds.

Maintain bleeding precautions, avoid unnecessary arterial and venous punctures, use saline or heparin lock for blood drawing, assess sheath insertion site and distal pulses of affected leg every 15 minutes for the first hour and then every 1 hour for the next 6 hours. Arterial access site care is important to prevent bleeding. Care should be taken when attempting vascular access that only the anterior wall of the femoral artery is punctured, avoiding a Seldinger (through and through) technique for obtaining sheath access. Femoral vein sheath placement should be avoided unless needed. While the vascular sheath is in place, patients should be maintained on complete bedrest with the head of the bed at a 30° angle and the affected limb restrained in a straight position.

Observe patient for mental status changes, hemorrhage; assess nose and mouth mucous membranes, puncture sites for oozing, ecchymosis, and hematoma formation; and examine urine, stool, and emesis for presence of occult or frank blood; gentle care should be provided when removing dressings.

Dosage Forms Excipient information presented when available (limited, particularly for generics); consult specific product labeling.

Solution, Intravenous:

ReoPro: 2 mg/mL (5 mL)

Abiraterone Acetate (a bir A ter one AS e tate)

Brand Names: US Zytiga

Brand Names: Canada Zytiga

Index Terms Abiraterone; CB7630

Pharmacologic Category Antiandrogen; Antineoplastic Agent, Antiandrogen

Use Prostate cancer: Treatment of metastatic, castration-resistant prostate cancer (in combination with prednisone) ▶

Pregnancy Considerations Adverse effects were observed in animal reproduction studies at doses resulting in less systemic exposure than in humans. Adverse effects were also observed in the reproductive system of animals during toxicology and pharmacology studies. Based on the mechanism of action, abiraterone may cause fetal harm or fetal loss if administered during pregnancy. Abiraterone is not indicated for use in women and is specifically contra-indicated in women who are or may become pregnant. It is not known if abiraterone is excreted in semen, therefore, men should use a condom and another method of birth control during treatment and for 1 week following therapy if having intercourse with a woman of reproductive age. Women who are or may become pregnant should wear gloves if contact with tablets may occur.

Breast-Feeding Considerations Not indicated for use in women

Contraindications Women who are or may become pregnant

Canadian labeling: Additional contraindication (not in U.S. labeling): Hypersensitivity to abiraterone acetate or any component of the formulation or container

Warnings/Precautions Hazardous agent - use appropriate precautions for handling and disposal (NIOSH 2014 [group 1]). Significant increases in liver enzymes have been reported (higher likelihood in patients with baseline elevations), generally occurring in the first 3 months of treatment. May require dosage reduction, treatment interruption, and/or discontinuation. ALT, AST, and bilirubin should be monitored prior to treatment, every 2 weeks for 3 months and monthly thereafter; patients with hepatic impairment, elevations in liver function tests, or experiencing hepatotoxicity require more frequent monitoring (see Dosage Adjustment for Hepatic Impairment and Monitoring Parameters). Evaluate liver function promptly with signs or symptoms of hepatotoxicity. The safety of retreatment after significant elevations (ALT or AST >20 times the upper limit of normal [ULN] and/or total bilirubin >10 times ULN) has not been evaluated. Do not use in patients with preexisting severe hepatic impairment (Child-Pugh class C); dosage reduction is recommended in patients with baseline moderate impairment. Canadian labeling (not in U.S. labeling) also recommends avoiding use in patients with preexisting moderate hepatic impairment.

Concurrent infection, stress, or interruption of daily corticosteroids is associated with reports of adrenocortical insufficiency. Monitor closely for signs and symptoms of adrenocorticoid insufficiency, which could be masked by adverse events associated with mineralocorticoid excess. Diagnostic testing for adrenal insufficiency may be clinically indicated. Increased corticosteroid doses may be required before, during, and after stress. May cause increased mineralocorticoid levels, which may result in hypertension, hypokalemia and fluid retention (including grades 3 and 4 events). Concomitant administration with corticosteroids reduces the incidence and severity of these adverse events. Control hypertension and correct hypokalemia prior to and during treatment. Use with caution in patients with cardiovascular disease (particularly heart failure, recent MI, or ventricular arrhythmia); patients with left ventricular ejection fraction (LVEF) <50% or NYHA class III or IV heart failure were excluded from clinical trials. Monitor at least monthly for hypertension, hypokalemia, and fluid retention.

Abiraterone must be administered on an empty stomach (administer at least 1 hour before and 2 hours after any food); abiraterone AUC (exposure) may be increased up to 10-fold if administered with a meal. Potentially significant drug-drug interactions may exist, requiring dose or frequency adjustment, additional monitoring, and/or selection of alternative therapy.

Adverse Reactions Note: Adverse reactions reported for use in combination with prednisone.

>10%:
Cardiovascular: Edema (25% to 27%; grades 3/4: ≤2%; includes anasarca, peripheral edema, pitting edema), hypertension (9% to 22%; grades 3/4: 1% to 4%)
Central nervous system: Fatigue (39%), insomnia (14%)
Dermatologic: Bruise (13%)
Endocrine & metabolic: Hypertriglyceridemia (63%), hyperglycemia (57%), hypernatremia (33%), hypokalemia (17% to 28%; grades 3/4: 3% to 5%), hypophosphatemia (24%; grades 3/4: 7%), hot flash (19% to 22%)
Gastrointestinal: Constipation (23%), diarrhea (18% to 22%), dyspepsia (6% to 11%)
Genitourinary: Urinary tract infection (12%)
Hematologic & oncologic: Lymphocytopenia (38%; grades 3/4: 9%)

Hepatic: Increased serum ALT (11% to 42%; grades 3/4: 1% to 6%), increased serum AST (37%; grades 3/4: 3%)
Neuromuscular & skeletal: Joint swelling (30%, includes arthralgia, arthritis, joint discomfort, joint stiffness), myalgia (26%; includes muscle rigidity, muscle spasm, musculoskeletal discomfort, musculoskeletal pain)
Respiratory: Cough (11% to 17%), upper respiratory infection (5% to 13%), dyspnea (12%), nasopharyngitis (11%)
1% to 10%:
Cardiovascular: Cardiac arrhythmia (7%; includes atrial fibrillation, atrial tachycardia, bradycardia, cardiac conduction disturbance, complete atrioventricular block, supraventricular tachycardia, tachycardia), chest pain (4%; includes angina pectoris, chest discomfort, unstable angina pectoris); cardiac failure (2%; includes cardiogenic shock, cardiomegaly, cardiomyopathy, congestive heart failure, left ventricular dysfunction, reduced ejection fraction)
Central nervous system: Falling (6%)
Dermatologic: Skin rash (8%)
Genitourinary: Hematuria (10%), groin pain (7%), urinary frequency (7%), nocturia (6%)
Hepatic: Increased serum bilirubin (7%; grades 3/4: <1%)
Neuromuscular & skeletal: Bone fracture (6%)
Miscellaneous: Fever (9%)
<1% (Limited to important or life-threatening): Adrenocortical insufficiency, myopathy (includes rhabdomyolysis), noninfectious pneumonitis

Drug Interactions

Metabolism/Transport Effects Substrate of CYP3A4 (major); **Note:** Assignment of Major/Minor substrate status based on clinically relevant drug interaction potential; **Inhibits** CYP1A2 (weak), CYP2C19 (moderate), CYP2C8 (weak), CYP2C9 (moderate), CYP2D6 (moderate), P-glycoprotein, SLCO1B1

Avoid Concomitant Use
Avoid concomitant use of Abiraterone Acetate with any of the following: Amodiaquine; Bosutinib; CYP3A4 Inducers (Strong); Indium 111 Capromab Pendetide; PAZOPanib; Silodosin; Thioridazine; Topotecan; VinCRIStine (Liposomal)

Increased Effect/Toxicity
Abiraterone Acetate may increase the levels/effects of: Afatinib; Amodiaquine; Bosentan; Bosutinib; Brentuximab Vedotin; Cannabis; Cilostazol; Citalopram; Colchicine; CYP1A2 Substrates; CYP2C19 Substrates; CYP2C8 Substrates; CYP2C9 Substrates; CYP2D6 Substrates; Dabigatran Etexilate; DOXOrubicin (Conventional); Dronabinol; Edoxaban; Eliglustat; Everolimus; Fesoterodine; Ledipasvir; Metoprolol; Naloxegol; Nebivolol; PAZOPanib; P-glycoprotein/ABCB1 Substrates; Prucalopride; Ranolazine; Rifaximin; Silodosin; Tetrahydrocannabinol; Thioridazine; TiZANidine; Topotecan; VinCRIStine (Liposomal)

The levels/effects of Abiraterone Acetate may be increased by: Osimertinib; Propafenone

Decreased Effect
Abiraterone Acetate may decrease the levels/effects of: Choline C 11; Clopidogrel; Codeine; Indium 111 Capromab Pendetide; Tamoxifen; TraMADol

The levels/effects of Abiraterone Acetate may be decreased by: Bosentan; CYP3A4 Inducers (Moderate); CYP3A4 Inducers (Strong); Dabrafenib; Deferasirox; Osimertinib; Siltuximab; Spironolactone; St Johns Wort; Tocilizumab

Food Interactions Taking abiraterone with food will increase systemic exposure (up to 10-fold). Management: Do not administer with food. Abiraterone must be taken on an empty stomach, at least 1 hour before and 2 hours after food.

Storage/Stability Store at 20°C to 25°C (68°F to 77°F); excursions are permitted between 15°C and 30°C (59°F and 86°F).

Mechanism of Action Selectively and irreversibly inhibits CYP17 (17 alpha-hydroxylase/C17,20-lyase), an enzyme required for androgen biosynthesis which is expressed in testicular, adrenal, and prostatic tumor tissues. Inhibits the formation of the testosterone precursors dehydroepiandrosterone (DHEA) and androstenedione.

Pharmacodynamics/Kinetics
Distribution: V_{dss}: 19,669 ± 13,358 L
Protein binding: >99%; to albumin and alpha$_1$-acid glycoprotein
Metabolism: Abiraterone acetate is hydrolyzed to the active metabolite abiraterone; further metabolized to inactive metabolites abiraterone sulphate and N-oxide abiraterone sulphate via CYP3A4 and SULT2A1
Bioavailability: Systemic exposure is increased by food
Half-life elimination: 14.4 to 16.5 hours (Acharya 2012)

Time to peak: 2 hours (Acharya 2012)

Excretion: Feces (~88%); urine (~5%)

Dosing

Adult & Geriatric Prostate cancer, metastatic, castration-resistant: Oral: 1000 mg once daily (in combination with prednisone 5 mg twice daily)

Dosage adjustment for concomitant strong CYP3A4 inducers: Avoid concomitant strong CYP3A4 inducers; if a strong CYP3A4 inducer must be administered concurrently, increase the abiraterone frequency to twice daily (eg, from 1000 mg once daily to 1000 mg twice daily). Upon discontinuation of the strong CYP3A4 inducer, reduce abiraterone back to the prior dose and frequency.

Renal Impairment No dosage adjustment necessary.

Hepatic Impairment

Hepatic impairment *prior to* treatment initiation:

Mild (Child-Pugh class A): No dosage adjustment necessary.

Moderate (Child-Pugh class B):

U.S. labeling: 250 mg once daily. Permanently discontinue if ALT and/or AST >5 times the upper limit of normal (ULN) or total bilirubin >3 times ULN during treatment.

Canadian labeling: Use is not recommended.

Severe (Child-Pugh class C): Do not use.

Hepatotoxicity *during* treatment:

U.S. labeling:

ALT and/or AST >5 times ULN or total bilirubin >3 times ULN: Withhold treatment until liver function tests return to baseline or ALT and AST ≤2.5 times ULN and total bilirubin ≤1.5 times ULN, then reinitiate at 750 mg once daily.

Recurrent hepatotoxicity on 750 mg/day: Withhold treatment until liver function tests return to baseline or ALT and AST ≤2.5 times ULN and total bilirubin ≤1.5 times ULN, then reinitiate at 500 mg once daily.

Recurrent hepatotoxicity on 500 mg once daily: Discontinue treatment

Canadian labeling:

ALT or AST >5 times ULN or total bilirubin >3 times ULN:

Withhold treatment until liver function tests normalize, then (when hepatic function returns to baseline) reinitiate at 500 mg once daily

Recurrent hepatotoxicity on 500 mg once daily: Discontinue treatment

ALT >20 times ULN (any time during treatment): Discontinue permanently.

Adjustment for Toxicity Hepatotoxicity: Refer to Dosing: Hepatic Impairment.

Administration Administer abiraterone orally on an empty stomach, at least 1 hour before and 2 hours after food.

Note: The prescribing information describes when to give food with respect to abiraterone; no food should be consumed for at least 2 hours before or for at least 1 hour after the abiraterone dose. Swallow tablets whole with water. Do not crush or chew.

Hazardous agent; use appropriate precautions for handling and disposal (NIOSH 2014 [group 1]). Women who are or may become pregnant should wear gloves if handling the tablets.

Monitoring Parameters ALT, AST, and bilirubin prior to treatment, every 2 weeks for 3 months and monthly thereafter; if baseline moderate hepatic impairment (Child-Pugh class B), monitor ALT, AST, and bilirubin prior to treatment, weekly for the first month, every 2 weeks for 2 months then monthly thereafter. If hepatotoxicity develops during treatment (and only after therapy is interrupted and liver function tests have returned to safe levels), monitor ALT, AST, and bilirubin every 2 weeks for 3 months and monthly thereafter. Monitoring of testosterone levels is not necessary. Serum potassium (prior to treatment and at least monthly).

Monitor for signs and symptoms of adrenocorticoid insufficiency; if clinically indicated, consider appropriate diagnostics to confirm adrenal insufficiency. Monitor blood pressure and for fluid retention (prior to treatment and at least monthly).

Dosage Forms Excipient information presented when available (limited, particularly for generics); consult specific product labeling.

Tablet, Oral:

Zytiga: 250 mg

AbobotulinumtoxinA

(aye bo BOT yoo lin num TOKS in aye)

Brand Names: US Dysport; Dysport (Glabellar Lines)

Index Terms Botulinum Toxin Type A

Pharmacologic Category Neuromuscular Blocker Agent, Toxin

Use

Cervical dystonia: Treatment of adult patients with cervical dystonia.

Glabellar lines: Temporary improvement in the appearance of moderate to severe glabellar lines associated with corrugator and procerus muscle activity in adults <65 years.

Upper limb spasticity: Treatment of upper limb spasticity in adult patients, to decrease the severity of increased muscle tone in elbow flexors, wrist flexors, and finger flexors

Medication Guide Available Yes

Dosing

Adult

Cervical dystonia: IM: Initial: 500 units divided among affected muscles in toxin-naïve or toxin-experienced patients. May re-treat at intervals of ≥12 weeks

Dosage adjustments: Adjust dosage in 250-unit increments; do not administer at intervals <12 weeks; dosage range used in studies: 250 to 1,000 units

Glabellar lines: Adults <65 years: IM: Inject 10 units into each of 5 sites (2 injections in each corrugator muscle and 1 injection in the procerus muscle) for a total dose of 50 units; do not administer at intervals <3 months; efficacy has been demonstrated with up to 4 repeated administrations

Upper limb spasticity: IM: Individualize dose based on patient size, number and location of muscle involvement, severity of spasticity, local muscle weakness, response to prior treatment, and/or adverse reaction history. May repeat therapy at intervals ≥12 weeks; in clinical studies, the majority of patients were re-treated between 12 to 16 weeks; however, some patients had a longer duration of response (eg, 20 weeks). Total doses of 500 and 1,000 units divided among selected muscles were used in clinical trials.

Brachialis: 200 to 400 units (1 to 2 injections per muscle)

Brachioradialis: 100 to 200 units (1 to 2 injections per muscle)

Biceps brachii: 200 to 400 units (1 to 2 injections per muscle)

Flexor carpi radialis: 100 to 200 units (1 to 2 injections per muscle)

Flexor carpi ulnaris: 100 to 200 units (1 to 2 injections per muscle)

Flexor digitorum profundus: 100 to 200 units (1 to 2 injections per muscle)

Flexor digitorum superficialis: 100 to 200 units (1 to 2 injections per muscle)

Pronator teres: 100 to 200 units (1 injection per muscle)

Geriatric

Cervical dystonia: Refer to adult dosing. No specific adjustment recommended.

Glabellar lines: Not recommended in patients ≥65 years of age.

Upper limb spasticity: Refer to adult dosing.

Renal Impairment There are no dosage adjustments provided in the manufacturer's labeling; however, dosage adjustment unlikely as abobotulinumtoxin A is not expected to be present in peripheral blood at recommended doses following intramuscular (IM) injection.

Hepatic Impairment There are no dosage adjustments provided in the manufacturer's labeling; however, dosage adjustment unlikely as abobotulinumtoxin A is not expected to be present in peripheral blood at recommended doses following intramuscular (IM) injection.

Additional Information Complete prescribing information should be consulted for additional detail.

Dosage Forms Excipient information presented when available (limited, particularly for generics); consult specific product labeling.

Solution Reconstituted, Intramuscular:

Dysport: 300 units (1 ea); 500 units (1 ea) [contains milk protein]

Dysport (Glabellar Lines): 300 units (1 ea) [contains albumin human, milk protein]

◆ AC 2993 *see* Exenatide *on page 727*

◆ ACAM2000 *see* Smallpox Vaccine *on page 1668*

Acamprosate (a kam PROE sate)

Brand Names: US Campral [DSC]
Brand Names: Canada Campral®
Index Terms Acamprosate Calcium; Calcium Acetylhomotaurinate; Campral
Pharmacologic Category GABA Agonist/Glutamate Antagonist
Use
Alcohol abstinence: Maintenance of abstinence from alcohol in patients with alcohol dependence who are abstinent at treatment initiation, as part of a comprehensive management program
Limitations of use: Efficacy has not been demonstrated in subjects who have not undergone detoxification and not achieved alcohol abstinence prior to beginning treatment. Efficacy in promoting abstinence from alcohol in polysubstance abusers has not been adequately assessed.
Dosing
Adult & Geriatric Alcohol abstinence: Oral: 666 mg 3 times daily (a lower dose may be effective in some patients). **Note:** Treatment should be initiated as soon as possible following the period of alcohol withdrawal when the patient has achieved abstinence and should be maintained if patient relapses.
Renal Impairment
CrCl 30 to 50 mL/minute: Initial dose: 333 mg 3 times daily
CrCl ≤30 mL/minute: Use is contraindicated.
Hepatic Impairment
Mild to moderate impairment (Child-Pugh class A or B): No dosage adjustment necessary.
Severe impairment (Child-Pugh class C): There are no dosage adjustments provided in manufacturer's labeling.
Additional Information Complete prescribing information should be consulted for additional detail.
Dosage Forms Excipient information presented when available (limited, particularly for generics); consult specific product labeling. [DSC] = Discontinued product
Tablet Delayed Release, Oral, as calcium:
Campral: 333 mg [DSC]
Generic: 333 mg

◆ Acamprosate Calcium *see* Acamprosate *on page 24*

Acarbose (AY car bose)

Brand Names: US Precose
Brand Names: Canada Glucobay
Pharmacologic Category Antidiabetic Agent, Alpha-Glucosidase Inhibitor
Use Diabetes mellitus, type 2: Adjunct to diet and exercise to improve glycemic control in adults with type 2 diabetes mellitus (noninsulin dependent, NIDDM)
Dosing
Adult & Geriatric
Diabetes mellitus, type 2: Oral: **Note:** Dosage must be individualized on the basis of effectiveness and tolerance.
US labeling: Initial dose: 25 mg 3 times daily with the first bite of each main meal (may also initiate at 25 mg once daily with gradual titration to 25 mg 3 times daily as tolerated); increase dose at 4- to 8-week intervals based on 1-hour postprandial glucose or glycosylated hemoglobin levels and tolerance until maintenance dose of 50 to 100 mg 3 times daily is reached (maximum dose: ≤60 kg: 50 mg 3 times daily; >60 kg: 100 mg 3 times daily)
Canadian labeling: Initial dose: 50 mg once daily with the first bite of a main meal; increase dosage to 50 mg twice daily after 1 to 2 weeks, with a subsequent increase to 50 mg 3 times daily after an additional 1 to 2 weeks. Adjust dose at 4- to 8-week intervals based on 2-hour postprandial glucose and tolerance; maintenance dose: 50 to 100 mg 3 times daily (maximum dose: 100 mg 3 times daily)
Renal Impairment
US labeling:
Serum creatinine ≤2 mg/dL: There are no dosage adjustments provided in the manufacturer's labeling.
Serum creatinine >2 mg/dL: Use not recommended (has not been studied).
Canadian labeling:
CrCl ≥25 mL/minute: There are no dosage adjustments provided in the manufacturer's labeling.
CrCl <25 mL/minute: Use is not recommended.

Hepatic Impairment There are no dosage adjustments provided in the manufacturer's labeling; contraindicated in patients with cirrhosis.
Additional Information Complete prescribing information should be consulted for additional detail.
Dosage Forms Excipient information presented when available (limited, particularly for generics); consult specific product labeling.
Tablet, Oral:
Precose: 25 mg, 50 mg, 100 mg
Generic: 25 mg, 50 mg, 100 mg

◆ A-Caro-25 [OTC] *see* Beta-Carotene *on page 221*

◆ Accel-Amlodipine (Can) *see* AmLODIPine *on page 101*

◆ ACCEL-Celecoxib (Can) *see* Celecoxib *on page 355*

◆ Accel-Clarithromycin (Can) *see* Clarithromycin *on page 401*

◆ Accel-Clopidogrel (Can) *see* Clopidogrel *on page 424*

◆ Accel-Donepezil (Can) *see* Donepezil *on page 583*

◆ Accell-Citalopram (Can) *see* Citalopram *on page 398*

◆ Accel-Olanzapine (Can) *see* OLANZapine *on page 1314*

◆ Accel-Pioglitazone (Can) *see* Pioglitazone *on page 1454*

◆ Accolate *see* Zafirlukast *on page 1922*

◆ AccuHist Drops [OTC] [DSC] *see* Chlorpheniramine and Phenylephrine *on page 376*

◆ AccuNeb *see* Albuterol *on page 57*

◆ AccuNeb [DSC] *see* Albuterol *on page 57*

◆ Accupril *see* Quinapril *on page 1540*

◆ Accutane *see* ISOtretinoin *on page 996*

Acebutolol (a se BYOO toe lole)

Brand Names: US Sectral
Brand Names: Canada Apo-Acebutolol®; Ava-Acebutolol; Mylan-Acebutolol; Mylan-Acebutolol (Type S); Nu-Acebutolol; Rhotral; Sandoz-Acebutolol; Sectral®; Teva-Acebutolol
Index Terms Acebutolol Hydrochloride
Pharmacologic Category Antiarrhythmic Agent, Class II; Antihypertensive; Beta-Blocker With Intrinsic Sympathomimetic Activity
Use Treatment of hypertension; management of ventricular arrhythmias
The 2014 guideline for the management of high blood pressure in adults (Eighth Joint National Committee [JNC 8; James, 2013]) recommends initiation of pharmacologic treatment to lower blood pressure for the following patients:
• Patients ≥60 years of age with systolic blood pressure (SBP) ≥150 mm Hg or diastolic blood pressure (DBP) ≥90 mm Hg. Goal of therapy is SBP <150 mm Hg and DBP <90 mm Hg.
• Patients <60 years of age with SBP ≥140 mm Hg or DBP ≥90 mm Hg. Goal of therapy is SBP <140 mm Hg and DBP <90 mm Hg.
• Patients ≥18 years of age with diabetes and SBP ≥140 mm Hg or DBP ≥90 mm Hg. Goal of therapy is SBP <140 mm Hg and DBP <90 mm Hg.
• Patients ≥18 years of age with chronic kidney disease (CKD) and SBP ≥140 mm Hg or DBP ≥90 mm Hg. Goal of therapy is SBP <140 mm Hg and DBP <90 mm Hg.
In patients with CKD, regardless of race or diabetes status, the use of an ACE inhibitor (ACEI) or angiotensin receptor blocker (ARB) as initial therapy is recommended to improve kidney outcomes. In the general nonblack population (without CKD), including those with diabetes, initial antihypertensive treatment should consist of a thiazide-type diuretic, calcium channel blocker, ACEI, or ARB. In the general black population (without CKD), including those with diabetes, initial antihypertensive treatment should consist of a thiazide-type diuretic or a calcium channel blocker instead of an ACEI or ARB.
Dosing
Adult
Angina, ventricular arrhythmia: Oral: 400 mg/day in 2 divided doses; maintenance: 600 to 1200 mg/day in divided doses; maximum: 1200 mg/day
Hypertension: Oral: Initial: 400 mg in 1 to 2 divided doses; optimal response usually seen at 400 to 800 mg daily (larger doses may be divided) although some patients may respond to as little as 200 mg daily; usual dose range (ASH/ISH [Weber, 2014]): 200 to 400 mg daily; maximum dose: 1200 mg in 2 divided doses

Chronic stable angina (off-label use): Oral: Usual dose: 400 to 1200 mg/day in 2 divided doses (Gibbons, 2003); low doses (ie, 400 mg/day) may also be given as once daily (Pina, 1988)

Geriatric Refer to adult dosing. Consider dose reduction due to age-related increase in bioavailability; do not exceed 800 mg/day. In the management of hypertension, consider lower initial dose (eg, 200 to 400 mg/day) and titrate to response (Aronow, 2011).

Renal Impairment
CrCl 25 to 49 mL/minute: Reduce dose by 50%.
CrCl <25 mL/minute: Reduce dose by 75%.

Hepatic Impairment There are no dosage adjustments provided in manufacturer's labeling; use with caution.

Additional Information Complete prescribing information should be consulted for additional detail.

Dosage Forms Excipient information presented when available (limited, particularly for generics); consult specific product labeling.

Capsule, Oral, as hydrochloride:
Sectral: 200 mg [contains brilliant blue fcf (fd&c blue #1), fd&c yellow #6 (sunset yellow)]
Sectral: 400 mg [contains brilliant blue fcf (fd&c blue #1), fd&c red #40, fd&c yellow #6 (sunset yellow)]
Generic: 200 mg, 400 mg

Dosage Forms: Canada Excipient information presented when available (limited, particularly for generics); consult specific product labeling.

Tablet, Oral, as hydrochloride:
Sectral: 100 mg, 200 mg, 400 mg

- ◆ Acebutolol Hydrochloride *see* Acebutolol *on page* 24
- ◆ Aceon *see* Perindopril *on page* 1430
- ◆ Acephen [OTC] *see* Acetaminophen *on page* 25
- ◆ Acerola C 500 [OTC] *see* Ascorbic Acid *on page* 155
- ◆ Acetadote *see* Acetylcysteine *on page* 31
- ◆ Aceta-Gesic® *see* Acetaminophen and Diphenhydramine *on page* 29

Acetaminophen (a seet a MIN oh fen)

Brand Names: US Acephen [OTC]; Aspirin Free Anacin Extra Strength [OTC]; Cetafen Extra [OTC]; Cetafen [OTC]; FeverAll Adult [OTC]; FeverAll Childrens [OTC]; FeverAll Infants [OTC]; FeverAll Junior Strength [OTC]; Little Fevers [OTC]; Mapap Arthritis Pain [OTC]; Mapap Children's [OTC]; Mapap Extra Strength [OTC]; Mapap Infant's [OTC]; Mapap [OTC]; Non-Aspirin Pain Reliever [OTC]; Nortemp Children's [OTC]; Ofirmev; Pain & Fever Children's [OTC]; Pain Eze [OTC]; Pharbetol Extra Strength [OTC]; Pharbetol [OTC]; Q-Pap Children's [OTC]; Q-Pap Extra Strength [OTC]; Q-Pap Infant's [OTC]; Q-Pap [OTC]; Silapap Children's [OTC]; Silapap Infant's [OTC]; Triaminic Children's Fever Reducer Pain Reliever [OTC]; Tylenol 8 Hour [OTC]; Tylenol Arthritis Pain [OTC]; Tylenol Children's Meltaways [OTC] [DSC]; Tylenol Children's [OTC]; Tylenol Extra Strength [OTC]; Tylenol Jr. Meltaways [OTC]; Tylenol [OTC]; Valorin Extra [OTC]; Valorin [OTC]

Brand Names: Canada Abenol; Apo-Acetaminophen; Atasol; Novo-Gesic; Pediatrix; Tempra; Tylenol

Index Terms APAP (abbreviation is not recommended); N-Acetyl-P-Aminophenol; Paracetamol

Pharmacologic Category Analgesic, Miscellaneous

Use

Pain management:
Injection: Treatment of mild to moderate pain; treatment of moderate to severe pain when combined with opioid analgesia
Oral/Rectal: Temporary relief of minor aches, pains, and headache

Fever: Temporary reduction of fever

Pregnancy Considerations Adverse events were observed in some animal reproduction studies. Acetaminophen crosses the placenta and can be detected in cord blood, newborn serum, and urine immediately after delivery (Levy, 1975; Naga Rani, 1989; Wang, 1997). An increased risk of teratogenic effects has not been observed following maternal use of acetaminophen during pregnancy. Prenatal constriction of the ductus arteriosus has been noted in case reports following maternal use during the third trimester (Suhag, 2008; Wood, 2005). The use of acetaminophen in normal doses during pregnancy is not associated with an increased risk of miscarriage or still birth; however, an increase in fetal death or spontaneous abortion may be seen following maternal overdose if treatment is delayed (Li, 2003; Rebordosa, 2009; Riggs, 1989). Frequent maternal use of acetaminophen during pregnancy may be associated with wheezing and asthma in early childhood (Perzanowki, 2010).

Breast-Feeding Considerations Low concentrations of acetaminophen are excreted into breast milk and can be detected in the urine of nursing infants (Notarianni, 1987). Adverse reactions have generally not been observed; however, a rash caused by acetaminophen exposure was reported in one breast-feeding infant (Matheson, 1985). The manufacturer recommends that caution be used if administered to a nursing woman.

Contraindications

Injection: Hypersensitivity to acetaminophen or any component of the formulation; severe hepatic impairment or severe active liver disease

OTC labeling: When used for self-medication, do not use with other drug products containing acetaminophen or if allergic to acetaminophen or any of the inactive ingredients

Warnings/Precautions [Injection: US Boxed Warning]: Acetaminophen has been associated with acute liver failure, at times resulting in liver transplant and death. Hepatotoxicity is usually associated with excessive acetaminophen intake and often involves more than one product that contains acetaminophen. Do not exceed the maximum recommended daily dose (>4 g daily in adults). In addition, chronic daily dosing may also result in liver damage in some patients. Limit acetaminophen dose from all sources (prescription, OTC, combination products) and all routes of administration (IV, oral, rectal) to ≤4 g/day (adults). Use with caution in patients with alcoholic liver disease; consuming ≥3 alcoholic drinks/day may increase the risk of liver damage. Use caution in patients with hepatic impairment or active liver disease; use of IV formulation is contraindicated in patients with severe hepatic impairment or severe active liver disease.

[Injection: US Boxed Warning]: Take care to avoid dosing errors with acetaminophen injection, which could result in accidental overdose and death; ensure that the dose in mg is not confused with mL, dosing in patients <50 kg is based on body weight, infusion pumps are properly programmed, and total daily dose of acetaminophen from all sources does not exceed the maximum daily limits.

Hypersensitivity and anaphylactic reactions have been reported including life-threatening anaphylaxis; discontinue immediately if symptoms occur. Serious and potentially fatal skin reactions, including acute generalized exanthematous pustulosis (AGEP), Stevens-Johnson syndrome (SJS), and toxic epidermal necrolysis (TEN), have occurred rarely with acetaminophen use. Discontinue therapy at the first appearance of skin rash.

Benzyl alcohol and derivatives: Some dosage forms may contain benzyl alcohol and/or sodium benzoate/benzoic acid; benzoic acid (benzoate) is a metabolite of benzyl alcohol; large amounts of benzyl alcohol (≥99 mg/kg/day) have been associated with a potentially fatal toxicity ("gasping syndrome") in neonates; the "gasping syndrome" consists of metabolic acidosis, respiratory distress, gasping respirations, CNS dysfunction (including convulsions, intracranial hemorrhage), hypotension and cardiovascular collapse (AAP ["Inactive" 1997]; CDC, 1982); some data suggests that benzoate displaces bilirubin from protein binding sites (Ahlfors, 2001); avoid or use dosage forms containing benzyl alcohol and/or benzyl alcohol derivative with caution in neonates. See manufacturer's labeling.

Polysorbate 80: Some dosage forms may contain polysorbate 80 (also known as Tweens). Hypersensitivity reactions, usually a delayed reaction, have been reported following exposure to pharmaceutical products containing polysorbate 80 in certain individuals (Isaksson, 2002; Lucente 2000; Shelley, 1995). Thrombocytopenia, ascites, pulmonary deterioration, and renal and hepatic failure have been reported in premature neonates after receiving parenteral products containing polysorbate 80 (Alade, 1986; CDC, 1984). See manufacturer's labeling. Some products may contain aspartame which is metabolized to phenylalanine and must be avoided (or used with caution) in patients with phenylketonuria.

Propylene glycol: Some dosage forms may contain propylene glycol; large amounts are potentially toxic and have been associated hyperosmolality, lactic acidosis, seizures, and respiratory depression; use caution (AAP ["Inactive" 1997]; Zar, 2007).

When used for self-medication (OTC), patients should be instructed to contact healthcare provider if symptoms get worse or new symptoms appear, redness or swelling is present in the painful area, fever lasts >3 days (all ages), or pain (excluding sore throat) lasts longer than: Adults: 10 days, Children and Adolescents: 5 days, Infants: 3 days. When treating children with sore throat, if sore throat is ▶

severe, persists for >2 days, or is followed by fever, rash, headache, nausea, or vomiting, consult health care provider immediately.

Use with caution in patients with chronic malnutrition or severe renal impairment; use intravenous formulation with caution in patients with severe hypovolemia. Use with caution in patients with known G6PD deficiency.

Adverse Reactions

Oral, Rectal: Frequency not defined:

Dermatologic: Skin rash

Endocrine & metabolic: Decreased serum bicarbonate, decreased serum calcium, decreased serum sodium, hyperchloremia, hyperuricemia, increased serum glucose

Genitourinary: Nephrotoxicity (with chronic overdose)

Hematologic & oncologic: Anemia, leukopenia, neutropenia, pancytopenia

Hepatic: Increased serum alkaline phosphatase, increased serum bilirubin

Hypersensitivity: Hypersensitivity reaction (rare)

Renal: Hyperammonemia, renal disease (analgesic)

IV:

>10%: Gastrointestinal: Nausea (adults 34%; children ≥5%), vomiting (adults 15%; children ≥5%)

1% to 10%:

Cardiovascular: Hypertension, hypotension, peripheral edema, tachycardia

Central nervous system: Headache (adults 10%; children ≥1%), insomnia (adults 7%; children ≥1%), agitation (children ≥5%), anxiety, fatigue, trismus

Dermatologic: Pruritus (children ≥5%), skin rash

Endocrine & metabolic: Hypervolemia, hypoalbuminemia, hypokalemia, hypomagnesemia, hypophosphatemia

Gastrointestinal: Constipation (children ≥5%), abdominal pain, diarrhea

Genitourinary: Oliguria (children ≥1%)

Hematologic & oncologic: Anemia

Hepatic: Increased serum transaminases

Local: Infusion site reaction (pain)

Neuromuscular & skeletal: Limb pain, muscle spasm

Ophthalmic: Periorbital edema

Respiratory: Atelectasis (children ≥5%), abnormal breath sounds, dyspnea, hypoxia, pleural effusion, pulmonary edema, stridor, wheezing

Miscellaneous: Fever (children ≥1%)

All formulations: <1% (Limited to important or life-threatening): Anaphylaxis, hepatic injury (dose-related), hypersensitivity reaction, severe dermatological reaction (acute generalized exanthematous pustulosis, Stevens-Johnson syndrome, toxic epidermal necrolysis)

Drug Interactions

Metabolism/Transport Effects Substrate of CYP1A2 (minor), CYP2A6 (minor), CYP2C9 (minor), CYP2D6 (minor), CYP2E1 (minor), CYP3A4 (minor); **Note:** Assignment of Major/Minor substrate status based on clinically relevant drug interaction potential

Avoid Concomitant Use There are no known interactions where it is recommended to avoid concomitant use.

Increased Effect/Toxicity

Acetaminophen may increase the levels/effects of: Busulfan; Dasatinib; Imatinib; Mipomersen; Phenylephrine (Systemic); Prilocaine; Sodium Nitrite; SORAfenib; Vitamin K Antagonists

The levels/effects of Acetaminophen may be increased by: Alcohol (Ethyl); Dapsone (Topical); Dasatinib; Isoniazid; Metyrapone; Nitric Oxide; Probenecid; SORAfenib

Decreased Effect

The levels/effects of Acetaminophen may be decreased by: Barbiturates; CarBAMazepine; Cholestyramine Resin; Fosphenytoin-Phenytoin

Food Interactions Rate of absorption may be decreased when given with food. Management: Administer without regard to food.

Preparation for Administration Injectable solution may be administered directly from the vial without further dilution.

Doses <1000 mg (<50 kg): Withdraw appropriate dose from vial and transfer to a separate sterile container (eg, glass bottle, plastic IV container, syringe) for administration. Small volume pediatric doses (up to 600 mg [60 mL]) may be placed in a syringe and infused over 15 minutes via syringe pump.

Doses of 1000 mg (≥50 kg): Insert vented IV set through vial stopper.

Storage/Stability

Injection: Store intact vials at 20°C to 25°C (68°F to 77°F); do not refrigerate or freeze. Use within 6 hours of opening vial or transferring to another container. Discard any unused portion.

Oral formulations: Store at 20°C to 25°C (68°F to 77°F); avoid excessive heat (20°C [104°F]). Avoid high humidity (chewable tablets).

Suppositories: Store at 2°C to 27°C (25°F to 80°F); do not freeze.

Mechanism of Action Although not fully elucidated, believed to inhibit the synthesis of prostaglandins in the central nervous system and work peripherally to block pain impulse generation; produces antipyresis from inhibition of hypothalamic heat-regulating center

Pharmacodynamics/Kinetics

Onset of action:

Oral: <1 hour

IV: Analgesia: 5 to 10 minutes; Antipyretic: Within 30 minutes

Peak effect: IV: Analgesic: 1 hour

Duration:

IV, Oral: Analgesia: 4 to 6 hours

IV: Antipyretic: ≥6 hours

Absorption: Primarily absorbed in small intestine (rate of absorption dependent upon gastric emptying); minimal absorption from stomach; varies by dosage form

Distribution: ~1 L/kg at therapeutic doses

Protein binding: 10% to 25% at therapeutic concentrations; 8% to 43% at toxic concentrations

Metabolism: At normal therapeutic dosages, primarily hepatic metabolism to sulfate and glucuronide conjugates, while a small amount is metabolized by CYP2E1 to a highly reactive intermediate, N-acetyl-p-benzoquinone imine (NAPQI), which is conjugated rapidly with glutathione and inactivated to nontoxic cysteine and mercapturic acid conjugates. At toxic doses (as little as 4 g daily) glutathione conjugation becomes insufficient to meet the metabolic demand causing an increase in NAPQI concentrations, which may cause hepatic cell necrosis. Oral administration is subject to first pass metabolism.

Half-life elimination: Prolonged following toxic doses

Neonates: 7 hours (range: 4 to 10 hours)

Infants: ~4 hours (range: 1 to 7 hours)

Children: 3 hours (range: 2 to 5 hours)

Adolescents: ~3 hours (range: 2 to 4 hours)

Adults: ~2 hours (range: 2 to 3 hours); may be slightly prolonged in severe renal insufficiency (CrCl <30 mL/minute): 2 to 5.3 hours

Time to peak, serum: Oral: Immediate release: 10 to 60 minutes (may be delayed in acute overdoses); IV: 15 minutes

Excretion: Urine (<5% unchanged; 60% to 80% as glucuronide metabolites; 20% to 30% as sulphate metabolites; ~8% cysteine and mercapuric acid metabolites)

Dosing

Adult & Geriatric Note: In 2011, McNeil Consumer Healthcare reduced the maximum doses and increased the dosing interval on the labeling of some of their acetaminophen OTC products used in older pediatric patients (usually children ≥12 years and adolescents) and adults in an attempt to protect consumers from inadvertent overdoses. For example, the maximum daily dose of Tylenol Extra Strength and Tylenol Regular Strength was decreased and the dosing interval for Tylenol Extra Strength was increased. Health care professionals may still prescribe or recommend the 4 g daily maximum to patients (but are advised to use their own discretion and clinical judgment) (McNeil Consumer Healthcare, 2014).

Pain or fever:

Oral: **Note:** OTC dosing recommendations may vary by product and/or manufacturer. When calculating the maximum daily dose, consider all sources of acetaminophen (prescription and OTC) and all routes of administration. Do not exceed the maximum recommended daily dose. No dose adjustment required when converting between different acetaminophen formulations.

Immediate-release:

Regular strength: 650 mg every 4 to 6 hours; maximum daily dose: 3250 mg **daily** unless directed by health care provider; under health care provider supervision, daily doses ≤4 g may be used

Extra strength: 1000 mg every 6 hours; maximum daily dose: 3000 mg **daily** unless directed by a health care provider; under health care provider supervision, daily doses ≤4 g may be used

Extended-release: 1300 mg every 8 hours; maximum daily dose: 3900 mg **daily**

Rectal: 650 mg every 4 to 6 hours; maximum daily dose: 3900 mg **daily**

IV:

<50 kg: 15 mg/kg every 6 hours or 12.5 mg/kg every 4 hours; maximum single dose: 15 mg/kg/dose (≤750 mg/dose); maximum daily dose: 75 mg/kg/day (≤3.75 g daily)

≥50 kg: 650 mg every 4 hours or 1000 mg every 6 hours; maximum single dose: 1000 mg/dose; maximum daily dose: 4 g daily

Pediatric Note: In 2011, McNeil Consumer Healthcare reduced the maximum doses and increased the dosing interval on the labeling of some of their acetaminophen OTC products used in older pediatric patients (usually children ≥12 years and adolescents) in an attempt to protect consumers from inadvertent overdoses. For example, the maximum daily dose of Tylenol Extra Strength OTC and Tylenol Regular Strength OTC was decreased and the dosing interval for Tylenol Extra Strength OTC was increased. Health care professionals may still prescribe or recommend the 4 g daily maximum to patients (but are advised to use their own discretion and clinical judgment) (McNeil Consumer Healthcare, 2014).

Pain or fever:
Oral: **Note:** When calculating the maximum daily dose, consider all sources of acetaminophen (prescription and OTC) and all routes of administration. Do not exceed the maximum recommended daily dose (see dosing information for further detail).

Weight-based dosing: Infants, Children, and Adolescents: 10 to 15 mg/kg/dose every 4 to 6 hours as needed (APS, 2008; Sullivan, 2011); do **not** exceed 5 doses in 24 hours; maximum daily dose: 75 mg/kg/day not to exceed 4 g daily.

Fixed dosing: Oral suspension, chewable tablets: Infants and Children <12 years: Consult specific product formulations for appropriate age groups. See table; use of weight to select dose is preferred; if weight is not available, then use age; doses may be repeated every 4 hours; maximum: 5 doses daily.

Acetaminophen Pediatric Dosing (Oral)[1]

Weight (kg)	Weight (lbs)	Age	Dosage (mg)
2.7-5.3	6-11	0-3 mo	40
5.4-8.1	12-17	4-11 mo	80
8.2-10.8	18-23	1-2 y	120
10.9-16.3	24-35	2-3 y	160
16.4-21.7	36-47	4-5 y	240
21.8-27.2	48-59	6-8 y	320
27.3-32.6	60-71	9-10 y	400
32.7-43.2	72-95	11 y	480

[1]Manufacturer's recommendations are based on weight in pounds (OTC labeling); weight in kg listed here is derived from pounds and rounded; kg weight listed also is adjusted to allow for continuous weight ranges in kg. OTC labeling instructs consumer to consult with health care provider for dosing instructions in infants and children under 2 years of age.

Immediate release solid dosage formulations: **Note:** Actual OTC dosing recommendations may vary by product and/or manufacturer:

Children 6 to 11 years: 325 mg every 4 to 6 hours; maximum daily dose: 1625 mg **daily**; Note: Do not use for more than 5 days unless directed by a health care provider

Children ≥12 years and Adolescents: Refer to adult dosing.

Extended release: Children ≥12 years and Adolescents: Refer to adult dosing.

Rectal:
Infants 6 to 11 months: 80 mg every 6 hours; maximum daily dose: 320 mg **daily**

Infants and Children 12 to 36 months: 80 mg every 4 to 6 hours; maximum daily dose: 400 mg **daily**

Children >3 to 6 years: 120 mg every 4 to 6 hours; maximum daily dose: 600 mg **daily**

Children >6 up to 12 years: 325 mg every 4 to 6 hours; maximum daily dose: 1625 mg **daily**

Children ≥12 years and Adolescents: Refer to adult dosing.

IV:
Children 2 to 12 years: 15 mg/kg every 6 hours **or** 12.5 mg/kg every 4 hours; maximum single dose: 15 mg/kg/dose (≤750 mg/dose); maximum daily dose: 75 mg/kg/day (≤3.75 g daily)

Adolescents: Refer to adult dosing.

Renal Impairment
Oral (Aronoff, 2007):
Adults:
GFR ≥50 mL/minute/1.73 m^2: No dosage adjustment necessary.
GFR 10 to 50 mL/minute/1.73 m^2: Administer every 6 hours.

GFR <10 mL/minute/1.73 m^2: Administer every 8 hours.
CRRT: Administer every 6 hours.
Infants, Children, and Adolescents:
GFR ≥10 mL/minute/1.73 m^2: No dosage adjustment necessary.
GFR <10 mL/minute/1.73 m^2: Administer every 8 hours.
Intermittent hemodialysis or peritoneal dialysis: Administer every 8 hours.
CRRT: No dosage adjustment necessary.
IV: Children, Adolescents, and Adults: CrCl ≤30 mL/minute: Use with caution; consider decreasing daily dose and extending dosing interval.

Hepatic Impairment
Oral: Use with caution. Limited, low-dose therapy is usually well tolerated in hepatic disease/cirrhosis. However, cases of hepatotoxicity at daily acetaminophen dosages <4 g daily have been reported.
IV:
Mild to moderate impairment: Use with caution in hepatic impairment or active liver disease; manufacturer's labeling suggests a reduced total daily dosage may be warranted, although no specific dosage adjustments are provided.
Severe impairment: Use is contraindicated.

Dietary Considerations Some products may contain phenylalanine and/or sodium.

Administration
Oral: May administer without regard to food; may administer with food to decrease possible GI upset; shake drops and suspension well before use; do not crush or chew extended release products

Injection: For IV infusion only. Administer undiluted over 15 minutes. Use within 6 hours of opening vial or transferring to another container.
For doses <1000 mg (<50 kg): Withdraw appropriate dose from vial and place into separate empty, sterile container prior to administration.
For doses ≥1000 mg (≥50 kg): Insert vented IV set through vial stopper

Rectal: Remove wrapper; insert suppository well up into the rectum

Monitoring Parameters Serum acetaminophen levels: Where acute overdose suspected and with long-term use in patients with hepatic disease; relief of pain or fever

Test Interactions Acetaminophen may cause false-positive urinary 5-hydroxyindoleacetic acid.

Dosage Forms Excipient information presented when available (limited, particularly for generics); consult specific product labeling. [DSC] = Discontinued product
Caplet, oral: 500 mg
Cetafen Extra: 500 mg
Mapap Extra Strength: 500 mg
Mapap Extra Strength: 500 mg [scored]
Pain Eze: 650 mg
Tylenol: 325 mg
Tylenol Extra Strength: 500 mg
Caplet, extended release, oral:
Mapap Arthritis Pain: 650 mg
Tylenol 8 Hour: 650 mg
Tylenol Arthritis Pain: 650 mg
Capsule, oral:
Mapap Extra Strength: 500 mg
Elixir, oral:
Mapap Children's: 160 mg/5 mL (118 mL, 480 mL) [ethanol free; contains benzoic acid, propylene glycol, sodium benzoate; cherry flavor]
Injection, solution [preservative free]:
Ofirmev: 10 mg/mL (100 mL)
Liquid, oral: 160 mg/5 mL (120 mL, 473 mL); 500 mg/5 mL (240 mL)
Mapap Extra Strength: 500 mg/5 mL (237 mL) [contains propylene glycol, sodium 9 mg/15 mL, sodium benzoate; cherry flavor]
Q-Pap Children's: 160 mg/5 mL (118 mL, 473 mL) [ethanol free; contains propylene glycol, sodium 2 mg/5 mL, sodium benzoate; cherry flavor]
Q-Pap Children's: 160 mg/5 mL (118 mL) [ethanol free; contains propylene glycol, sodium 2 mg/5 mL, sodium benzoate; grape flavor]
Silapap Children's: 160 mg/5 mL (118 mL, 237 mL, 473 mL) [ethanol free, sugar free; contains propylene glycol, sodium benzoate; cherry flavor]
Tylenol Extra Strength: 500 mg/15 mL (240 mL) [ethanol free; contains propylene glycol, sodium benzoate; cherry flavor]
Solution, oral: 160 mg/5 mL (5 mL, 10 mL, 20 mL)
Pain & Fever Children's: 160 mg/5 mL (118 mL, 473 mL) [ethanol free, sugar free; contains propylene glycol, sodium 1 mg/5 mL, sodium benzoate; cherry flavor]

◀ Solution, oral [drops]: 80 mg/0.8 mL (15 mL [DSC])
  Little Fevers: 80 mg/mL (30 mL [DSC]) [dye free, ethanol free, gluten free; contains propylene glycol, sodium benzoate; berry flavor]
  Q-Pap Infant's: 80 mg/0.8 mL (15 mL) [ethanol free; contains propylene glycol; fruit flavor]
  Silapap Infant's: 80 mg/0.8 mL (15 mL, 30 mL) [ethanol free; contains propylene glycol, sodium benzoate; cherry flavor]
Suppository, rectal: 120 mg (12s); 325 mg (12s); 650 mg (12s)
  Acephen: 120 mg (12s, 50s, 100s); 325 mg (6s, 12s, 50s, 100s); 650 mg (12s, 50s, 100s)
  FeverAll Adults: 650 mg (50s)
  FeverAll Childrens: 120 mg (6s, 50s)
  FeverAll Infants: 80 mg (6s, 50s)
  FeverAll Junior Strength: 325 mg (6s, 50s)
Suspension, oral: 160 mg/5 mL (5 mL, 10.15 mL, 20.3 mL)
  Mapap Children's: 160 mg/5 mL (118 mL) [ethanol free; contains propylene glycol, sodium benzoate; cherry flavor]
  Mapap Infant's: 160 mg/5 mL (59 mL) [dye free, ethanol free; contains propylene glycol, sodium benzoate; cherry flavor]
  Nortemp Children's: 160 mg/5 mL (118 mL) [ethanol free; contains propylene glycol, sodium benzoate; cotton candy flavor]
  Pain & Fever Children's: 160 mg/5 mL (60 mL) [ethanol free; contains propylene glycol, sodium benzoate; cherry flavor]
  Q-Pap Children's: 160 mg/5 mL (118 mL) [ethanol free; contains sodium 2 mg/5 mL, sodium benzoate; bubble-gum flavor]
  Q-Pap Children's: 160 mg/5 mL (118 mL) [ethanol free; contains sodium 2 mg/5 mL, sodium benzoate; cherry flavor]
  Q-Pap Children's: 160 mg/5 mL (118 mL) [ethanol free; contains sodium 2 mg/5 mL, sodium benzoate; grape flavor]
  Tylenol Children's: 160 mg/5 mL (120 mL) [dye free, ethanol free; contains propylene glycol, sodium benzoate; cherry flavor]
  Tylenol Children's: 160 mg/5 mL (120 mL) [ethanol free; contains propylene glycol, sodium 2 mg/5 mL, sodium benzoate; bubblegum flavor]
  Tylenol Children's: 160 mg/5 mL (60 mL, 120 mL) [ethanol free; contains propylene glycol, sodium 2 mg/5 mL, sodium benzoate; cherry flavor]
  Tylenol Children's: 160 mg/5 mL (120 mL) [ethanol free; contains propylene glycol, sodium 2 mg/5 mL, sodium benzoate; grape flavor]
  Tylenol Children's: 160 mg/5 mL (120 mL) [ethanol free; contains propylene glycol, sodium 2 mg/5 mL, sodium benzoate; strawberry flavor]
Syrup, oral:
  Triaminic Children's Fever Reducer Pain Reliever: 160 mg/5 mL (118 mL) [contains benzoic acid, sodium 6 mg/5 mL; bubblegum flavor]
  Triaminic Children's Fever Reducer Pain Reliever: 160 mg/5 mL (118 mL) [contains sodium 5 mg/5 mL, sodium benzoate; grape flavor]
Tablet, oral: 325 mg, 500 mg
  Aspirin Free Anacin Extra Strength: 500 mg
  Cetafen: 325 mg
  Mapap: 325 mg
  Mapap Extra Strength: 500 mg
  Non-Aspirin Pain Reliever: 325 mg
  Pharbetol: 325 mg
  Pharbetol Extra Strength: 500 mg
  Q-Pap: 325 mg [scored]
  Q-Pap Extra Strength: 500 mg [scored]
  Tylenol: 325 mg
  Tylenol Extra Strength: 500 mg
  Valorin: 325 mg [sugar free]
  Valorin Extra: 500 mg [sugar free]
Tablet, chewable, oral: 80 mg
  Mapap Children's: 80 mg [fruit flavor]
Tablet, dispersible, oral: 80 mg, 160 mg
  Mapap Children's: 80 mg [bubblegum flavor]
  Mapap Children's: 80 mg [grape flavor]
  Tylenol Children's Meltaways: 80 mg [scored; bubblegum flavor] [DSC]
  Tylenol Children's Meltaways: 80 mg [scored; grape flavor] [DSC]
  Tylenol Jr. Meltaways: 160 mg [bubblegum flavor]
  Tylenol Jr. Meltaways: 160 mg [grape flavor]

◆ **Acetaminophen and Butalbital** see Butalbital and Acetaminophen on page 275
◆ **Acetaminophen and Chlorpheniramine** see Chlorpheniramine and Acetaminophen on page 376

Acetaminophen and Codeine
(a seet a MIN oh fen & KOE deen)

Brand Names: US Capital/Codeine; Tylenol with Codeine #3; Tylenol with Codeine #4
Brand Names: Canada Acet-Codeine; PHL-Acet-Codeine; PMS-Acetaminophen with Codeine Elixir; Procet-30; ratio-Emtec-30; ratio-Lenoltec No. 4
Index Terms Codeine and Acetaminophen; Emtec; Tylenol #2; Tylenol #3; Tylenol Codeine
Pharmacologic Category Analgesic Combination (Opioid); Analgesic, Opioid
Use Mild to moderate pain: Relief of mild to moderate pain
Dosing
Adult Note: Doses should be adjusted according to severity of pain and response of the patient. Adult doses ≥60 mg codeine fail to give commensurate relief of pain but merely prolong analgesia and are associated with an appreciably increased incidence of side effects.

US labeling:
  Mild to moderate pain: Oral:
    Solution or suspension: Acetaminophen 120 mg and codeine 12 mg per 5 mL: 15 mL every 4 hours as needed.
    Tablets: Acetaminophen (300 to 1,000 mg/dose) and codeine (15 to 60 mg/dose) every 4 hours as needed (maximum: Acetaminophen 4,000 mg and codeine 360 mg per 24 hours)
Canadian labeling:
  Mild to moderate pain: Oral: Solution: Acetaminophen 160 mg and codeine 8 mg per 5 mL: 10 to 20 mL every 4 hours as needed (maximum: 100 mL [acetaminophen 3,200 mg and codeine 160 mg] per 24 hours)
  Mild to severe pain: Oral: Tablets: Acetaminophen (300 to 600 mg/dose) and codeine (30 to 60 mg/dose) every 4 to 6 hours as needed (maximum: Acetaminophen 3,600 mg and codeine 360 mg per 24 hours)
Geriatric Refer to adult dosing. Doses should be titrated to appropriate analgesic effect.
Pediatric
US labeling: **Mild to moderate pain:** Oral: Acetaminophen 120 mg and codeine 12 mg per 5 mL (solution or suspension):
  Children 3 to 6 years: 5 mL 3 to 4 times daily as needed
  Children 7 to 12 years: 10 mL 3 to 4 times daily as needed
  Children >12 years and Adolescents: 15 mL every 4 hours as needed
Canadian labeling: Children ≥12 years and Adolescents: Refer to adult dosing.
Renal Impairment There are no dosage adjustments provided in the manufacturer's labeling; use with caution in severe renal impairment.
Hepatic Impairment There are no dosage adjustments provided in the manufacturer's labeling; use with caution in severe renal impairment; use with caution; hepatotoxicity with daily acetaminophen dosages <4 g/day have been reported.
Additional Information Complete prescribing information should be consulted for additional detail.
Dosage Forms Excipient information presented when available (limited, particularly for generics); consult specific product labeling. [DSC] = Discontinued product
Solution, Oral:
  Generic: Acetaminophen 120 mg and codeine phosphate 12 mg per 5 mL (5 mL, 10 mL [DSC], 12.5 mL, 15 mL [DSC], 118 mL, 120 mL, 473 mL)
Suspension, Oral:
  Capital/Codeine: Acetaminophen 120 mg and codeine phosphate 12 mg per 5 mL (473 mL) [fruit punch flavor]
Tablet, Oral:
  Tylenol with Codeine #3: Acetaminophen 300 mg and codeine phosphate 30 mg [contains sodium metabisulfite]
  Tylenol with Codeine #4: Acetaminophen 300 mg and codeine phosphate 60 mg [contains sodium metabisulfite]
  Generic: Acetaminophen 300 mg and codeine phosphate 15 mg, Acetaminophen 300 mg and codeine phosphate 30 mg, Acetaminophen 300 mg and codeine phosphate 60 mg
Dosage Forms: Canada Excipient information presented when available (limited, particularly for generics); consult specific product labeling. **Note:** In countries outside of the US, some formulations of Tylenol with Codeine include caffeine.

Caplet:
ratio-Lenoltec No. 1, Tylenol No. 1: Acetaminophen 300 mg, codeine phosphate 8 mg, and caffeine 15 mg
Tylenol No. 1 Forte: Acetaminophen 500 mg, codeine phosphate 8 mg, and caffeine 15 mg
Solution, Oral:
pms-Acetaminophen with Codeine Elixir: Acetaminophen 160 mg and codeine phosphate 8 mg per 5 mL
Tablet:
Acet-Codeine, Procet-30, ratio-Emtec-30, Triatec-30: Acetaminophen 300 mg and codeine phosphate 30 mg
Acet-Codeine, ratio-Lenoltec No. 4, Tylenol No. 4 with Codeine: Acetaminophen 300 mg and codeine phosphate 60 mg
ratio-Lenoltec No. 1: Acetaminophen 300 mg, codeine phosphate 8 mg, and caffeine 15 mg
ratio-Lenoltec No. 2, Tylenol No. 2 with Codeine: Acetaminophen 300 mg, codeine phosphate 15 mg, and caffeine 15 mg
ratio-Lenoltec No. 3, Tylenol No. 3 with Codeine: Acetaminophen 300 mg, codeine phosphate 30 mg, and caffeine 15 mg
Triatec-8: Acetaminophen 325 mg, codeine phosphate 8 mg, and caffeine 30 mg
Triatec-8 Forte: Acetaminophen 500 mg, codeine phosphate 8 mg, and caffeine 30 mg
Controlled Substance Liquid products: C-V; Tablet: C-III

Acetaminophen and Diphenhydramine
(a seet a MIN oh fen & dye fen HYE dra meen)

Brand Names: US Aceta-Gesic®; Excedrin PM® [OTC]; Goody's PM® [OTC]; Legatrin PM® [OTC]; Mapap PM [OTC]; Percogesic® Extra Strength [OTC]; TopCare® Pain Relief PM [OTC]; Tylenol® PM [OTC]; Tylenol® Severe Allergy [OTC]
Index Terms Diphenhydramine and Acetaminophen
Pharmacologic Category Analgesic, Miscellaneous
Use Aid in the relief of insomnia accompanied by minor pain
Dosing
Adult & Geriatric Insomnia and pain: Oral: Adults: 50 mg of diphenhydramine HCl (76 mg diphenhydramine citrate) at bedtime or as directed by physician; do not exceed recommended dosage
Pediatric Not for use in children <12 years of age.
Hepatic Impairment Use with caution. Limited, low-dose therapy is usually well tolerated in hepatic disease/cirrhosis; however, cases of hepatotoxicity at daily acetaminophen dosages <4 g/day have been reported. Avoid chronic use in hepatic impairment.
Additional Information Complete prescribing information should be consulted for additional detail.
Dosage Forms Excipient information presented when available (limited, particularly for generics); consult specific product labeling.
Caplet, oral:
Excedrin PM®: Acetaminophen 500 mg and diphenhydramine citrate 38 mg
Legatrin PM®: Acetaminophen 500 mg and diphenhydramine hydrochloride 50 mg
Mapap PM: Acetaminophen 500 mg and diphenhydramine hydrochloride 25 mg
Percogesic® Extra Strength: Acetaminophen 500 mg and diphenhydramine hydrochloride 12.5 mg
TopCare® Pain Relief PM: Acetaminophen 500 mg and diphenhydramine citrate 25 mg
Tylenol® PM: Acetaminophen 500 mg and diphenhydramine hydrochloride 25 mg
Tylenol® Severe Allergy: Acetaminophen 500 mg and diphenhydramine hydrochloride 12.5 mg
Liquid, oral:
Tylenol® PM: Acetaminophen 500 mg and diphenhydramine hydrochloride 25 mg per 15 mL (240 mL) [contains sodium benzoate; vanilla flavor]
Powder for solution, oral:
Goody's PM®: Acetaminophen 500 mg and diphenhydramine citrate 38 mg [contains potassium 41.9 mg and sodium 3.15 mg per powder]
Tablet, oral:
Aceta-Gesic®: Acetaminophen 325 mg and diphenhydramine hydrochloride 12.5 mg
Excedrin PM: Acetaminophen 500 mg and diphenhydramine citrate 38 mg
Generic: Acetaminophen 500 mg and diphenhydramine hydrochloride 25 mg

◆ **Acetaminophen and Hydrocodone** see Hydrocodone and Acetaminophen on page 884
◆ **Acetaminophen and Oxycodone** see Oxycodone and Acetaminophen on page 1361

Acetaminophen and Tramadol
(a seet a MIN oh fen & TRA ma dole)

Brand Names: US Ultracet
Brand Names: Canada ACT Tramadol/Acet; Apo-Tramadol/Acet; JAMP-ACET-Tramadol; Mar-Tramadol/Acet; Mint-Tramadol/Acet; PMS-Tramadol/Acet; Priva-Tramadol/Acet; RAN-Tramadol/Acet; TEVA-Tramadol/Acetaminophen; Tramacet
Index Terms Tramadol Hydrochloride and Acetaminophen
Pharmacologic Category Analgesic Combination (Opioid); Analgesic, Miscellaneous
Use
US labeling: Short-term (≤5 days) management of acute pain
Canadian labeling: Management of moderate to moderately severe pain
Dosing
Adult
Acute pain: Oral:
US labeling: Two tablets every 4 to 6 hours as needed for pain relief (maximum: 8 tablets daily); treatment should not exceed 5 days
Canadian labeling: 1 to 2 tablets every 4 to 6 hours as needed for pain relief (maximum: 8 tablets daily)
Geriatric Refer to adult dosing. Use with caution due to increased risk of renal or hepatic impairment in elderly patients.
Renal Impairment
CrCl ≥30 mL/minute: No dosage adjustment necessary. US labeling recommends treatment not exceed 5 days.
CrCl <30 mL/minute: Maximum of 2 tablets every 12 hours; US labeling recommends treatment not exceed 5 days.
Hepatic Impairment
US labeling: Mild to severe impairment: There are no dosage adjustments provided in the manufacturer's labeling (has not been studied); use is not recommended.
Canadian labeling:
Mild or moderate impairment: There are no dosage adjustments provided in the manufacturer's labeling (has not been studied); use caution as both acetaminophen and tramadol undergo extensive hepatic metabolism.
Severe impairment: Use is not recommended.
Additional Information Complete prescribing information should be consulted for additional detail.
Dosage Forms Excipient information presented when available (limited, particularly for generics); consult specific product labeling.
Tablet, oral: Acetaminophen 325 mg and tramadol hydrochloride 37.5 mg
Ultracet: Acetaminophen 325 mg and tramadol hydrochloride 37.5 mg
Controlled Substance C-IV

Acetaminophen, Aspirin, and Caffeine
(a seet a MIN oh fen, AS pir in, & KAF een)

Brand Names: US Anacin Advanced Headache Formula [OTC]; Excedrin Extra Strength [OTC]; Excedrin Migraine [OTC]; Fem-Prin [OTC]; Goody's Extra Strength Headache Powder [OTC]; Goody's Extra Strength Pain Relief [OTC]; Pain-Off [OTC]; Vanquish Extra Strength Pain Reliever [OTC]
Index Terms Aspirin, Acetaminophen, and Caffeine; Aspirin, Caffeine and Acetaminophen; Caffeine, Acetaminophen, and Aspirin; Caffeine, Aspirin, and Acetaminophen
Pharmacologic Category Analgesic, Miscellaneous
Use
Migraine: Relief of migraine headache
Pain: Relief of minor aches and pain
Dosing
Adult & Geriatric
Minor aches and pain: Oral:
Acetaminophen 194 mg/aspirin 227 mg/caffeine 33 mg: Two tablets every 6 hours as needed (maximum: 8 tablets per 24 hours)
Acetaminophen 250 mg/aspirin 250 mg/caffeine 65 mg: Two tablets every 6 hours as needed (maximum: 8 tablets per 24 hours)
Acetaminophen 260 mg/aspirin 520 mg/caffeine 32.5 mg: Contents of 1 powder packet, placed on tongue or dissolved in water or other liquid, every 6 hours as needed (maximum: 4 powder packets per 24 hours)

Acetaminophen 325 mg/aspirin 500 mg/caffeine 65 mg: Contents of 1 powder packet, placed on tongue or dissolved in water or other liquid, every 6 hours as needed (maximum: 4 powder packets per 24 hours)

Migraine headache: Oral: Acetaminophen 250 mg/ aspirin 250 mg/caffeine 65 mg: Two tablets once every 24 hours (maximum: 2 tablets per 24 hours)

Pediatric Minor aches and pain: Children >12 years and Adolescents: Oral: Refer to adult dosing

Renal Impairment There are no dosage adjustments provided in the manufacturer's labeling.

Hepatic Impairment There are no dosage adjustments provided in the manufacturer's labeling.

Additional Information Complete prescribing information should be consulted for additional detail.

Dosage Forms Excipient information presented when available (limited, particularly for generics); consult specific product labeling.

Caplet, oral:
Excedrin Extra Strength, Excedrin® Migraine: Acetaminophen 250 mg, aspirin 250 mg, and caffeine 65 mg
Vanquish Extra Strength Pain Reliever: Acetaminophen 194 mg, aspirin 227 mg, and caffeine 33 mg

Powder, oral:
Goody's Extra Strength Headache Powder: Acetaminophen 260 mg, aspirin 520 mg, and caffeine 32.5 mg [contains lactose]

Tablet, oral:
Anacin Advanced Headache Formula: Acetaminophen 250 mg, aspirin 250 mg, and caffeine 65 mg
Excedrin Extra Strength, Excedrin® Migraine, Pain-Off: Acetaminophen 250 mg, aspirin 250 mg, and caffeine 65 mg
Fem-Prin: Acetaminophen 194.4 mg, aspirin 226.8 mg, and caffeine 32.4 mg
Goody's Extra Strength Pain Relief: Acetaminophen 130 mg, aspirin 260 mg, and caffeine 16.25 mg

♦ **Acetaminophen, Butalbital, and Caffeine** see Butalbital, Acetaminophen, and Caffeine on page 275

♦ **Acetasol HC** see Acetic Acid, Propylene Glycol Diacetate, and Hydrocortisone on page 31

♦ **Acetazolam (Can)** see AcetaZOLAMIDE on page 30

AcetaZOLAMIDE (a set a ZOLE a mide)

Brand Names: US Diamox Sequels
Brand Names: Canada Acetazolam; Diamox®
Pharmacologic Category Anticonvulsant, Miscellaneous; Carbonic Anhydrase Inhibitor; Diuretic, Carbonic Anhydrase Inhibitor; Ophthalmic Agent, Antiglaucoma
Use Treatment of glaucoma (chronic simple open-angle, secondary glaucoma, preoperatively in acute angle-closure); drug-induced edema or edema due to congestive heart failure (adjunctive therapy; IV and immediate release dosage forms); centrencephalic epilepsies (IV and immediate release dosage forms); prevention or amelioration of symptoms associated with acute mountain sickness (immediate and extended release dosage forms)
Dosing
Adult Note: IM administration is not recommended because of pain secondary to the alkaline pH.
Altitude illness: Oral: Manufacturer's labeling: 500-1000 mg/day in divided doses every 8-12 hours (immediate release tablets) or divided every 12-24 hours (extended release capsules). These doses are associated with more frequent and/or increased side effects. Alternative dosing has been recommended:
Prevention: 125 mg twice daily; beginning either the day before (preferred) or on the day of ascent; may be discontinued after staying at the same elevation for 2-3 days or if descent initiated (Basnyat, 2006; Luks, 2010). **Note:** In situations of rapid ascent (such as rescue or military operations), 1000 mg/day is recommended by the manufacturer. The Wilderness Medical Society recommends consideration of using dexamethasone in addition to acetazolamide in these situations (Luks, 2010).
Treatment: 250 mg twice daily. **Note:** With high altitude cerebral edema, dexamethasone is the primary treatment; however, acetazolamide may be used adjunctively with the same treatment dose (Luks, 2010).
Edema: Oral, IV: 250-375 mg once daily
Epilepsy: Oral: 8-30 mg/kg/day in divided doses. A lower dosing range of 4-16 mg/kg/day in 1-4 divided doses has also been recommended; maximum dose: 30 mg/kg/day or 1 g/day (Oles, 1989; Reiss, 1996). **Note:** Minimal additional benefit with doses >16 mg/kg/day. **Extended release capsule is not recommended for treatment of epilepsy.**

Glaucoma: Oral, IV:
Chronic simple (open-angle): 250 mg 1-4 times/day or 500 mg extended release capsule twice daily
Secondary or acute (closed-angle): Initial: 250-500 mg; maintenance: 125-250 mg every 4 hours (250 mg every 12 hours has been effective in short-term treatment of some patients)
Metabolic alkalosis (off-label use): IV: 500 mg as a single dose; reassess need based upon acid-base status (Marik, 1991; Mazur, 1999)
Respiratory stimulant in stable hypercapnic COPD (off-label use): Oral: 250 mg twice daily (Wagenaar, 2003)
Geriatric Refer to adult dosing. Oral: Initial doses should begin at the low end of the dosage range.
Pediatric Note: IM administration is not recommended because of pain secondary to the alkaline pH.
Epilepsy: Oral: Refer to adult dosing.
Altitude illness: Oral:
Prevention: 2.5 mg/kg/dose every 12 hours started either the day before (preferred) or on the day of ascent and may be discontinued after staying at the same elevation for 2-3 days or if descent initiated; maximum dose: 125 mg/dose (Luks, 2010). **Note:** The International Society for Mountain Medicine does not recommend prophylaxis in children except in the rare circumstance of unavoidable rapid ascent or in children with known previous susceptibility to acute mountain sickness (Pollard, 2001).
Treatment: 2.5 mg/kg/dose every 8-12 hours; maximum dose: 250 mg/dose. **Note:** With high altitude cerebral edema, dexamethasone is the primary treatment; however, acetazolamide may be used adjunctively with the same treatment dose (Luks, 2010; Pollard, 2001).
Renal Impairment Note: Use is contraindicated in marked renal impairment; creatinine clearance cutoff not specified in manufacturer's labeling.
CrCl 10-50 mL/minute: Administer every 12 hours.
CrCl <10 mL/minute: Avoid use.
Hemodialysis: Moderately dialyzable (20% to 50%).
Peritoneal dialysis: Supplemental dose is not necessary (Schwenk, 1994).
Hepatic Impairment Use contraindicated in patients with cirrhosis or marked liver disease or dysfunction.
Additional Information Complete prescribing information should be consulted for additional detail.
Dosage Forms Excipient information presented when available (limited, particularly for generics); consult specific product labeling.
Capsule Extended Release 12 Hour, Oral:
Diamox Sequels: 500 mg
Generic: 500 mg
Solution Reconstituted, Injection [preservative free]:
Generic: 500 mg (1 ea)
Tablet, Oral:
Generic: 125 mg, 250 mg

♦ **Acet-Codeine (Can)** see Acetaminophen and Codeine on page 28

Acetic Acid (Otic) (a SEE tik AS id)

Index Terms Ethanoic Acid
Pharmacologic Category Otic Agent, Anti-infective
Use Treatment of superficial bacterial infections of the external auditory canal
Dosing
Adult & Geriatric Otitis externa: Otic: Insert saturated wick; keep moist 24 hours by adding 3 to 5 drops every 4 to 6 hours; remove wick after 24 hours and instill 5 drops 3 to 4 times/day
Pediatric
Otitis externa: Children ≥3 years and Adolescents: Otic: Insert saturated wick; keep moist 24 hours by adding 3 to 5 drops every 4 to 6 hours; remove wick after 24 hours and instill 5 drops 3 to 4 times/day. **Note:** 3 to 4 drops may be sufficient in children due to the smaller capacity of the ear canal.
Renal Impairment There are no dosage adjustments provided in the manufacturer's labeling. However, dosage adjustment unlikely due to low systemic absorption.
Hepatic Impairment There are no dosage adjustments provided in the manufacturer's labeling. However, dosage adjustment unlikely due to low systemic absorption.
Additional Information Complete prescribing information should be consulted for additional detail.
Dosage Forms Excipient information presented when available (limited, particularly for generics); consult specific product labeling.
Solution, Otic:
Generic: 2% (15 mL, 60 mL)

Acetic Acid (Topical) (a SEE tik AS id)

Index Terms Ethanoic Acid
Pharmacologic Category Topical Skin Product
Use Irrigation of the bladder; periodic irrigation of indwelling catheters
Dosing
Adult & Geriatric
Irrigation (**Note:** Dosage of an irrigating solution depends on the capacity or surface area of the structure being irrigated):
For continuous irrigation of the urinary bladder with 0.25% acetic acid irrigation, the rate of administration will approximate the rate of urine flow; usually 500 to 1,500 mL/24 hours
For periodic irrigation of an indwelling urinary catheter to maintain patency, about 50 mL of 0.25% acetic acid irrigation is required.
Renal Impairment There are no dosage adjustments provided in the manufacturer's labeling.
Hepatic Impairment There are no dosage adjustments provided in the manufacturer's labeling.
Additional Information Complete prescribing information should be consulted for additional detail.
Dosage Forms Excipient information presented when available (limited, particularly for generics); consult specific product labeling.
Solution, Irrigation:
Generic: 0.25% (250 mL, 500 mL, 1000 mL)

◆ Acetic Acid, Hydrocortisone, and Propylene Glycol Diacetate *see* Acetic Acid, Propylene Glycol Diacetate, and Hydrocortisone *on page 31*

Acetic Acid, Propylene Glycol Diacetate, and Hydrocortisone
(a SEE tik AS id, PRO pa leen GLY kole dye AS e tate, & hye droe KOR ti sone)

Brand Names: US Acetasol HC; VoSolHC [DSC]
Index Terms Acetic Acid, Hydrocortisone, and Propylene Glycol Diacetate; Hydrocortisone, Acetic Acid, and Propylene Glycol Diacetate; Propylene Glycol Diacetate, Acetic Acid, and Hydrocortisone
Pharmacologic Category Otic Agent, Anti-infective
Use Treatment of superficial infections of the external auditory canal caused by organisms susceptible to the action of the antimicrobial, complicated by swelling
Dosing
Adult & Geriatric Otitis externa (superficial): Otic: Instill 3 to 5 drops in affected ear(s) every 4 to 6 hours while cotton wick inserted; after cotton wick removed, instill 5 drops in affected ear(s) 3 or 4 times daily. **Note:** Use of 3 to 4 drops may be sufficient in children due to smaller ear canal capacity.
Pediatric Otitis externa (superficial): Children ≥3 years and Adolescents: Otic: Refer to adult dosing.
Renal Impairment There are no dosage adjustments provided in the manufacturer's labeling. However, dosage adjustment unlikely due to low systemic absorption.
Hepatic Impairment There are no dosage adjustments provided in the manufacturer's labeling. However, dosage adjustment unlikely due to low systemic absorption.
Additional Information Complete prescribing information should be consulted for additional detail.
Dosage Forms Excipient information presented when available (limited, particularly for generics); consult specific product labeling. [DSC] = Discontinued product
Solution, otic [drops]: Acetic acid 2%, propylene glycol diacetate 3%, and hydrocortisone 1% (10 mL)
Acetasol HC: Acetic acid 2%, propylene glycol diacetate 3%, and hydrocortisone 1% (10 mL) [contains benzethonium chloride]
VoSol HC: Acetic acid 2%, propylene glycol diacetate 3%, and hydrocortisone 1% (10 mL [DSC]) [contains benzethonium chloride]

◆ Acetoxymethylprogesterone *see* MedroxyPROGESTERone *on page 1131*

Acetylcholine (a se teel KOE leen)

Brand Names: US Miochol-E
Brand Names: Canada Miochol®-E
Index Terms Acetylcholine Chloride
Pharmacologic Category Cholinergic Agonist; Ophthalmic Agent, Miotic
Use Produces complete miosis in cataract surgery, keratoplasty, iridectomy, and other anterior segment surgery where rapid miosis is required

Dosing
Adult & Geriatric To produce miosis: Intraocular: 0.5-2 mL of 1% injection (5-20 mg) instilled into anterior chamber before or after securing one or more sutures
Renal Impairment No dosage adjustment provided in manufacturer's labeling.
Hepatic Impairment No dosage adjustment provided in manufacturer's labeling.
Additional Information Complete prescribing information should be consulted for additional detail.
Dosage Forms Excipient information presented when available (limited, particularly for generics); consult specific product labeling.
Solution Reconstituted, Intraocular, as chloride:
Miochol-E: 20 mg (1 ea) [contains mannitol]

◆ Acetylcholine Chloride *see* Acetylcholine *on page 31*

Acetylcysteine (a se teel SIS teen)

Brand Names: US Acetadote
Brand Names: Canada Acetylcysteine Injection; Acetylcysteine Solution; Mucomyst; Parvolex
Index Terms N Acetylcysteine; N-Acetyl-L-cysteine; N-Acetylcysteine; Acetylcysteine Sodium; Mercapturic Acid; Mucomyst; NAC
Pharmacologic Category Antidote; Mucolytic Agent
Use Antidote for acute acetaminophen poisoning; repeated supratherapeutic ingestion (RSTI) of acetaminophen; adjunctive mucolytic therapy in patients with abnormal or viscid mucous secretions in acute and chronic bronchopulmonary diseases; pulmonary complications of surgery and cystic fibrosis; diagnostic bronchial studies
Pregnancy Considerations Adverse events have not been observed in animal reproduction studies. Based on limited reports using acetylcysteine to treat acetaminophen poisoning in pregnant women, acetylcysteine has been shown to cross the placenta and may provide protective levels in the fetus.

Acetylcysteine may be used to treat acetaminophen overdose in during pregnancy (Wilkes, 2005). In general, medications used as antidotes should take into consideration the health and prognosis of the mother; antidotes should be administered to pregnant women if there is a clear indication for use and should not be withheld because of fears of teratogenicity (Bailey, 2003).
Breast-Feeding Considerations It is not known if acetylcysteine is excreted in breast milk. The manufacturer recommends that caution be exercised when administering acetylcysteine to nursing women. Based on its pharmacokinetics, acetylcysteine should be nearly completely cleared 30 hours after administration; therefore, nursing women may consider resuming nursing 30 hours after dosing is complete.
Contraindications Hypersensitivity to acetylcysteine or any component of the formulation
Warnings/Precautions
Inhalation: Since increased bronchial secretions may develop after inhalation, percussion, postural drainage, and suctioning should follow. If bronchospasm occurs, administer a bronchodilator; discontinue acetylcysteine if bronchospasm progresses.
Intravenous: Acute flushing and erythema have been reported; usually occurs within 30-60 minutes and may resolve spontaneously. Serious anaphylactoid reactions have also been reported and are more commonly associated with IV administration, but may also occur with oral administration (Mroz, 1997). When used for acetaminophen poisoning, the incidence is reduced when the initial loading dose is administered over 60 minutes. The acetylcysteine infusion may be interrupted until treatment of allergic symptoms is initiated; the infusion can then be carefully restarted. Treatment for anaphylactoid reactions should be immediately available. Use caution in patients with asthma or history of bronchospasm as these patients may be at increased risk. Conversely, patients with high acetaminophen levels (>150 mg/L) may be at a reduced risk for anaphylactoid reactions (Pakravan, 2008; Sandilands, 2009; Waring, 2008).
Acute acetaminophen poisoning: Acetylcysteine is indicated in patients with a serum acetaminophen level that indicates they are at "possible" risk or greater for hepatotoxicity when plotted on the Rumack-Matthew nomogram. There are several situations where the nomogram is of limited use. Serum acetaminophen levels obtained <4 hours postingestion are not interpretable; patients presenting late may have undetectable serum concentrations, despite having received a toxic dose. The nomogram is less predictive of hepatic injury following an acute overdose with an extended release acetaminophen product. The nomogram also does not take into account ▶

patients who may be at higher risk of acetaminophen toxicity (eg, alcoholics, malnourished patients, concurrent use of CYP2E1 enzyme-inducing agents [eg, isoniazid]). Nevertheless, acetylcysteine should be administered to any patient with signs of hepatotoxicity, even if the serum acetaminophen level is low or undetectable. Patients who present >24 hours after an acute ingestion or patients who present following an acute ingestion at an unknown time may be candidates for acetylcysteine therapy; consultation with a poison control center or clinical toxicologist is highly recommended.

Repeated supratherapeutic ingestion (RSTI) of acetaminophen: The Rumack-Matthew nomogram is not designed to be used following RSTIs. In general, an accurate past medical history, including a comprehensive acetaminophen ingestion history, in conjunction with AST concentrations and serum acetaminophen levels, may give the clinician insight as to the patient's risk of acetaminophen toxicity. Some experts recommend that acetylcysteine be administered to any patient with "higher than expected" serum acetaminophen levels or serum acetaminophen level >10 mcg/mL, even in the absence of hepatic injury; others recommend treatment for patients with laboratory evidence and/or signs and symptoms of hepatotoxicity (Hendrickson, 2006; Jones, 2000). Consultation with a poison control center or a clinical toxicologist is highly recommended.

Adverse Reactions

Inhalation: Frequency not defined.

Central nervous system: Drowsiness, chills, fever

Gastrointestinal: Vomiting, nausea, stomatitis

Local: Irritation, stickiness on face following nebulization

Respiratory: Bronchospasm, rhinorrhea, hemoptysis

Miscellaneous: Acquired sensitization (rare), clamminess, unpleasant odor during administration

Intravenous:

>10%: Miscellaneous: Anaphylactoid reaction (8% to 18%; shorter infusion periods [eg, <60 minutes] associated with increased incidence)

1% to 10%:

Cardiovascular: Flushing (1% to 8%), tachycardia (1% to 4%), edema (1% to 2%)

Dermatologic: Urticaria (6% to 8%), rash (2% to 4%), pruritus (1% to 4%)

Gastrointestinal: Vomiting (2% to 10%), nausea (1% to 6%)

Respiratory: Pharyngitis (≤1%), rhinorrhea (≤1%), rhonchi (≤1%), throat tightness (≤1%)

<1% (Limited to important or life-threatening): Anaphylaxis, angioedema, bronchospasm, chest tightness, cough, dizziness, dyspnea, headache, hypotension, respiratory distress, stridor, wheezing

Oral (Bebarta, 2010; Mroz, 1997):

Cardiovascular: Hypotension, tachycardia

Dermatologic: Angioedema, pruritus, urticaria

Gastrointestinal: Nausea, vomiting

Respiratory: Bronchospasm

Drug Interactions

Metabolism/Transport Effects None known.

Avoid Concomitant Use There are no known interactions where it is recommended to avoid concomitant use.

Increased Effect/Toxicity There are no known significant interactions involving an increase in effect.

Decreased Effect There are no known significant interactions involving a decrease in effect.

Preparation for Administration

Oral: Treatment of acetaminophen poisoning: Dilute the 20% solution 1:3 with a cola, orange juice, or other soft drink to prepare a 5% solution. Use within 1 hour of preparation.

Solution for injection (Acetadote): Acetaminophen poisoning: IV:

Loading dose: Dilute 150 mg/kg (maximum: 15 **g**) in D$_5$W 200 mL.

Second dose: Dilute 50 mg/kg (maximum: 5 **g**) in D$_5$W 500 mL

Third dose: Dilute 100 mg/kg (maximum: 10 **g**) in D$_5$W 1000 mL

Note: To avoid fluid overload in patients <40 kg and those requiring fluid restriction, decrease volume of D$_5$W proportionally (see table in Dosing). Discard unused portion.

Solution for inhalation: The 20% solution may be diluted with sodium chloride or sterile water; the 10% solution may be used undiluted.

Intravenous administration of solution for inhalation (off-label route): Using D$_5$W, dilute acetylcysteine 20% oral solution to a 3% solution.

Storage/Stability

Solution for injection (Acetadote): Store unopened vials at room temperature, 20°C to 25°C (68°F to 77°F). Following reconstitution with D$_5$W, solution is stable for 24 hours at room temperature. A color change may occur in opened vials (light pink or purple) and does not affect the safety or efficacy.

Solution for inhalation: Store unopened vials at room temperature; once opened, store under refrigeration and use within 96 hours. A color change may occur in opened vials (light purple) and does not affect the safety or efficacy.

Mechanism of Action Exerts mucolytic action through its free sulfhydryl group which opens up the disulfide bonds in the mucoproteins thus lowering mucous viscosity.

In patients with acetaminophen toxicity, acetylcysteine acts as a hepatoprotective agent by restoring hepatic glutathione, serving as a glutathione substitute, and enhancing the nontoxic sulfate conjugation of acetaminophen.

The presumed mechanism in preventing contrast-induced nephropathy is its ability to scavenge oxygen-derived free radicals and improve endothelium-dependent vasodilation.

Pharmacodynamics/Kinetics

Onset of action: Inhalation: 5-10 minutes

Duration: Inhalation: >1 hour

Distribution: 0.47 L/kg

Protein binding: 83%

Half-life elimination:

Reduced acetylcysteine: 2 hours

Total acetylcysteine: Adults: 5.6 hours; Newborns: 11 hours

Time to peak, plasma: Oral: 1-2 hours

Excretion: Urine

Dosing

Adult & Geriatric

Acetaminophen poisoning: Only the 72-hour oral and 21-hour IV regimens are FDA-approved. Ideally, in patients with an acute acetaminophen ingestion, treatment should begin within 8 hours of ingestion or as soon as possible after ingestion. In patients who present following RSTI and treatment is deemed appropriate, acetylcysteine should be initiated immediately. Regardless of the treatment regimen selected, serum acetaminophen levels, liver function, and clinical status should be evaluated during and prior to the end of the treatment regimen to determine if treatment discontinuation is appropriate. In patients who continue to experience symptoms of hepatotoxicity or elevated liver function tests at the conclusion of a 72-hour oral or 21-hour IV regimen, extending the treatment course may be appropriate; however, when and to which patients additional doses should be administered is unclear. Possible candidates for extended therapy include patients with a suspected massive overdose, concomitant ingestion of other substances, or patients with preexisting liver disease. In patients with persistently elevated acetaminophen levels, persistently elevated liver function tests, or an elevated INR, additional acetylcysteine should be administered. Typically, an additional "third dose" or "third bag" (IV: 100 mg/kg [maximum: 10 g] infused over 16 hours) is administered; however, this dose may be inadequate in some patients (Rumack, 2012). Consultation with a poison control center or clinical toxicologist is highly recommended to determine optimal patient care.

Oral: **Note:** Consultation with a poison control center or clinical toxicologist is highly recommended when considering the discontinuation of oral acetylcysteine prior to the conclusion of a full 18-dose course of therapy.

72-hour regimen: Consists of 18 doses; total dose delivered: 1330 mg/kg

Loading dose: 140 mg/kg

Maintenance dose: 70 mg/kg every 4 hours; repeat dose if emesis occurs within 1 hour of administration

IV (Acetadote):

21-hour regimen: Consists of 3 doses; total dose delivered: 300 mg/kg

Loading dose: 150 mg/kg (maximum: 15 **g**) infused over 60 minutes

Second dose: 50 mg/kg (maximum: 5 **g**) infused over 4 hours

Third dose: 100 mg/kg (maximum: 10 **g**) infused over 16 hours

Note: The fluid volume should be reduced in patients weighing <40 kg according to the following table:

Acetadote Dosing / Fluid Volume Guidelines for Patients ≤40 kg

Body Weight (kg)	Loading Dose 150 mg/kg over 1 h		Second Dose 50 mg/kg over 4 h		Third Dose 100 mg/kg over 16 h	
	Acetadote (mL)	D₅W (mL)	Acetadote (mL)	D₅W (mL)	Acetadote (mL)	D₅W (mL)
40	30	100	10	250	20	500
30	22.5	100	7.5	250	15	500
21	15.75	100	5.25	250	10.5	500
20	15	60	5	140	10	280
15	11.25	45	3.75	105	7.5	210
10	7.5	30	2.5	70	5	140
5	3.75	15	1.25	35	2.5	70

Obesity: In patients who weigh >100 kg, the following dosing regimen is recommended: IV (Acetadote): 21-hour regimen: Consists of 3 doses; total dose delivered: 30 **g**
Loading dose: 15 **g** infused over 60 minutes
Second dose: 5 **g** infused over 4 hours
Third dose: 10 **g** infused over 16 hours

Adjuvant therapy in respiratory conditions:
Note: Patients should receive an aerosolized bronchodilator 10-15 minutes prior to dose.
Inhalation, nebulization (face mask, mouth piece, tracheostomy): Acetylcysteine 10% and 20% solution (dilute 20% solution with sodium chloride or sterile water for inhalation); 10% solution may be used undiluted: 3-5 mL of 20% solution or 6-10 mL of 10% solution until nebulized given 3-4 times/day; dosing range: 1-10 mL of 20% solution or 2-20 mL of 10% solution every 2-6 hours
Inhalation, nebulization (tent, croupette): Dose must be individualized; may require up to 300 mL solution/treatment
Direct instillation:
Into tracheostomy: 1-2 mL of 10% to 20% solution every 1-4 hours
Through percutaneous intratracheal catheter: 1-2 mL of 20% or 2-4 mL of 10% solution every 1-4 hours via syringe attached to catheter

Diagnostic bronchogram: Nebulization or intratracheal: 1-2 mL of 20% solution or 2-4 mL of 10% solution administered 2-3 times prior to procedure

Prevention of contrast-induced nephropathy (CIN) (off-label use): Oral: 600-1200 mg twice daily for 2 days (beginning the day before the procedure); may be given as powder in capsules (some centers use solution, diluted in cola beverage or juice). **Note:** No longer recommended for use prior to percutaneous coronary intervention; instead adequate hydration is preferred (Levine, 2011).

Pediatric
Acetaminophen poisoning: Refer to adult dosing.
Adjuvant therapy in respiratory conditions:
Note: Patients should receive an aerosolized bronchodilator 10-15 minutes prior to acetylcysteine
Inhalation, nebulization (face mask, mouth piece, tracheostomy): Acetylcysteine 10% and 20% solution (dilute 20% solution with sodium chloride or sterile water for inhalation); 10% solution may be used undiluted.
Infants: 1-2 mL of 20% solution or 2-4 mL 10% solution until nebulized given 3-4 times/day
Children: Refer to adult dosing.
Inhalation, nebulization (tent, croupette): Children: Refer to adult dosing.
Renal Impairment Oral, IV: No dosage adjustment provided in manufacturer's labeling.
Hepatic Impairment Oral: No dosage adjustment provided in manufacturer's labeling.
IV: No dosage adjustment required.
Obesity Refer to indication-specific dosing for obesity-related information (may not be available for all indications).

Administration
Inhalation: Acetylcysteine is incompatible with tetracyclines, erythromycin, amphotericin B, iodized oil, chymotrypsin, trypsin, and hydrogen peroxide. Administer separately. Intermittent aerosol treatments are commonly given when patient arises, before meals, and just before retiring at bedtime.
Oral: Treatment of acetaminophen poisoning, administer orally as a 5% solution. Use within 1 hour of preparation.

The unpleasant odor (sulfur-like) becomes less noticeable as treatment progresses. If patient vomits within 1 hour of dose, readminister. (**Note:** It is helpful to put the acetylcysteine on ice, in a cup with a cover, and drink through a straw; alternatively, administer via an NG tube).
IV (Acetadote): Acetaminophen poisoning:
Loading dose: Administer over 60 minutes.
Second dose: Administer over 4 hours.
Third dose: Administer over 16 hours.
If the commercial IV form is unavailable, the solution for inhalation has been used; each dose should be infused through a 0.2 micron Millipore filter (in-line) over 60 minutes (Yip, 1998); intravenous administration of the solution for inhalation is not USP 797-compliant.
Note: Undiluted injection, solution (Acetadote) is hyperosmolar (2600 mOsmol/L); when the diluent volume is decreased for patients <40 kg or requiring fluid restriction, the osmolarity of the solution may remain higher than desirable for intravenous infusion. To ensure tolerance of the infusion, osmolarity should be adjusted to a physiologically safe level (eg, ≥150 mOsmol/L in children).
Acetadote concentration: 7 mg/mL
Osmolarity in D₅W: 343 mOsmol/L
Osmolarity in ½NS: 245 mOsmol/L
Osmolarity in SWFI: 91 mOsmol/L
Acetadote concentration: 24 mg/mL
Osmolarity in D₅W: 564 mOsmol/L
Osmolarity in ½NS: 466 mOsmol/L
Osmolarity in SWFI: 312 mOsmol/L

Monitoring Parameters Acetaminophen poisoning: Monitor patient for the development of anaphylaxis or anaphylactoid reactions; monitor serum acetaminophen levels, AST, ALT, bilirubin, PT, INR, serum creatinine, BUN, serum glucose, hemoglobin, hematocrit, and electrolytes. Assess patient for nausea, vomiting, and skin rash following oral administration. Reassess LFTs for possible hepatotoxicity every 4-6 hours. An early elevation in the INR may be related to acetylcysteine therapy (Schmidt, 2002).
Acute ingestion: Obtain the first acetaminophen level 4 hours postingestion (or as soon as possible thereafter); plot on the Rumack-Matthew nomogram. In patients who have ingested an extended release formulation of acetaminophen or have coingested an agent known to delay gastric emptying, obtain a repeat serum acetaminophen measurement 4-6 hours following the first measurement if the original level (taken at 4-8 hours postingestion) when plotted on the Rumack-Matthew nomogram indicated that treatment was not necessary.

Dosage Forms Excipient information presented when available (limited, particularly for generics); consult specific product labeling.
Injection, solution [preservative free]: 20% (30 mL)
Acetadote: 20% [200 mg/mL] (30 mL)
Solution, for inhalation/oral: 10% [100 mg/mL] (10 mL, 30 mL); 20% [200 mg/mL] (10 mL, 30 mL)
Solution, for inhalation/oral [preservative free]: 10% [100 mg/mL] (4 mL, 10 mL, 30 mL); 20% [200 mg/mL] (4 mL, 10 mL, 30 mL)

Acitretin (a si TRE tin)

Brand Names: US Soriatane
Brand Names: Canada Soriatane
Pharmacologic Category Retinoid-Like Compound
Use

Psoriasis: Treatment of severe psoriasis in adults.
Limitations of use: Not for the treatment of acne.
Canadian labeling: Additional uses (not in U.S. labeling): Other disorders of keratinization

Pregnancy Considerations [US Boxed Warning]: Acitretin is a known teratogen and use is contraindicated in females who are or may become pregnant. Birth defects (including facial, ear, central nervous system, cardiovascular, limb, bone, and joint) have been noted following acitretin exposure during pregnancy. Use only in women with severe psoriasis that is unresponsive to other therapies or with contraindications to the use of alternative treatments. Pregnancy must be avoided for at least 3 years after treatment discontinuation. Two reliable forms of contraception must be used simultaneously for 1 month prior to initiating therapy, during therapy, and for 3 years after discontinuation. Two negative pregnancy tests (sensitivity at least 25 milliunits/mL) are required prior to initiating therapy; pregnancy tests must be repeated every month during treatment. In addition, because ethanol forms a teratogenic metabolite and would increase the duration of teratogenic potential, ethanol should not be consumed during treatment or for 2 months after discontinuation.

Only physicians experienced with the diagnosis and treatment of severe psoriasis, including the use of retinoid treatment, and physicians who understand the risk of teratogenicity should prescribe acitretin. Females of childbearing potential must be able to fulfill all conditions for use prior to initiating therapy, including a Patient Agreement/Informed Consent (consult manufacturer's labeling for further detail). Prescriptions should be written for a monthly supply. The Do Your P.A.R.T. (Pregnancy Prevention Actively Required During and After Treatment) program explains teratogenic risks and requirements expected of females of childbearing potential to prevent pregnancies from occurring during use and 3 years following discontinuation; this should be used to educate patients and healthcare providers. Information for the Do Your P.A.R.T. program is available at www.soriatane.com/doyour-part-Program.html or by calling 1-888-784-3335.

Limited amounts of acitretin are found in seminal fluid; although it appears this poses little risk to a fetus, the actual risk of teratogenicity is not known.

Any pregnancy which occurs during treatment, or within 3 years after treatment is discontinued, should be reported to the manufacturer at 1-888-784-3335 or to the FDA at 1-800-FDA-1088.

Breast-Feeding Considerations Acitretin is excreted in breast milk. Due to the potential for serious adverse reactions in the nursing infant, the manufacturer does not recommend acitretin prior to or during nursing (Canadian labeling recommends that women should avoid breast-feeding for at least 3 years after acitretin is discontinued).

Information is available from a woman who started acitretin 40 mg per day, 8 months postpartum. The woman discontinued nursing prior to the study. Milk samples were collected prior to the first dose and twice daily for 9 days; maternal serum samples were also collected. Acitretin and its metabolite were detected in breast milk. Total concentrations of acitretin + metabolite remained relatively stable over the study period (30 to 40 ng/mL) showing no diurnal variation. Because acitretin is primarily distributed into milk fat, actual concentrations in breast milk may vary depending upon the lipid and fat content of the milk (Rollman, 1990).

Current guidelines do not recommend use during lactation due to the potential for cumulative toxicity in a nursing infant (Butler, 2014).

Medication Guide Available Yes
Contraindications

Hypersensitivity (eg, angioedema, urticaria) to acitretin, other retinoids, or any component of the formulation; patients who are pregnant or intend on becoming pregnant during therapy or within 3 years after treatment discontinuation; severe hepatic or renal dysfunction; chronic abnormally elevated blood lipid levels; concomitant use with methotrexate or tetracyclines

Acitretin is contraindicated in females of childbearing potential unless all of the following conditions apply.
1) Patient has severe psoriasis unresponsive to other therapy or if clinical condition contraindicates other treatments.
2) Patient must have two negative urine or serum pregnancy tests prior to therapy.
3) Patient must have pregnancy test repeated monthly during therapy. After discontinuation of therapy, a pregnancy test must be repeated every 3 months for at least 3 years.
4) Patient must commit to using two effective forms of birth control starting 1 month prior to acitretin treatment and for 3 years after discontinuation. Prescriber must counsel patient about contraception every month during therapy and every 3 months following discontinuation for at least 3 years.
5) Patient is reliable in understanding and carrying out instructions.
6) Patient has received, and acknowledged, understanding of a careful oral and printed explanation of the hazards of fetal exposure to acitretin and the risk of possible contraception failure. Patient must sign an agreement/informed consent document stating that she understands these risks and that she should not consume ethanol during therapy or for 2 months after discontinuation.

Canadian labeling: Additional contraindications (not in U.S. labeling): Breast-feeding; concomitant use with Vitamin A or other retinoids

Warnings/Precautions Hazardous agent - use appropriate precautions for handling and disposal (NIOSH 2014 [group 3]).

[US Boxed Warning]: Acitretin is a known teratogen and contraindicated in females who are or may become pregnant. Birth defects (including facial, ear, central nervous system, cardiovascular, limb, bone, and joint) have been noted following acitretin exposure during pregnancy. Use only in women with severe psoriasis that is unresponsive to other therapies or with contraindications to the use of alternative treatments. Pregnancy must be avoided for at least 3 years after treatment discontinuation. Two reliable forms of contraception must be used simultaneously for 1 month prior to initiating therapy, during therapy, and for 3 years after discontinuation. Two negative pregnancy tests (sensitivity at least 25 milliunits/mL) are required prior to initiating therapy; pregnancy tests must be repeated every month during treatment. In addition, because ethanol forms a teratogenic metabolite and would increase the duration of teratogenic potential, ethanol should not be consumed during treatment or for 2 months after discontinuation. Any pregnancy which occurs during treatment, or within 3 years after treatment is discontinued, should be reported to the manufacturer at 1-888-784-3335 or to the FDA at 1-800-FDA-1088.

[US Boxed Warning]: Females of childbearing potential must be able to fulfill all conditions for use prior to initiating therapy, including a Patient Agreement/Informed Consent (consult manufacturer's labeling for further detail). Prescriptions should be written for a monthly supply. The Do Your P.A.R.T. (Pregnancy Prevention Actively Required During and After Treatment) program explains teratogenic risks and requirements expected of females of childbearing potential to

prevent pregnancies from occurring during use and 3 years following discontinuation; this should be used to educate patients and healthcare providers. Information for the Do Your P.A.R.T. program is available at www.soriatane.com/doyour-part-Program.html or by calling 1-888-784-3335.

[US Boxed Warning]: Female patients should abstain from ethanol or ethanol-containing products during therapy and for 2 months after discontinuation. [US Boxed Warning]: All patients should be advised not to donate blood during therapy or for 3 years following completion of therapy. [US Boxed Warning]: Changes in transaminases have occurred in up to 1/3 of patients, which generally returned to normal after discontinuation of treatment. Monitor for hepatotoxicity; discontinue if hepatotoxicity is suspected. [US Boxed Warning]: Hepatitis has been reported (including fatalities); some patients received etretinate for ≤1 month before presenting with hepatic signs or symptoms.

Use with caution in patients at risk of hypertriglyceridemias (eg, patients with lipid metabolism disturbances, diabetes mellitus, obesity, increased alcohol intake, or a familial history of these conditions). Lipid changes including, increased triglycerides, increased cholesterol, and decreased HDL are common (up to 66%), which were reversible upon discontinuation of treatment; increased triglycerides may lead to pancreatitis. Fatal fulminant pancreatitis has been reported. Consider discontinuation if hypertriglyceridemia and decreased HDL persist. Use is contraindicated in patients with chronic abnormally elevated blood lipid values. Retinoids, including acitretin, have been associated with pseudotumor cerebri (benign intracranial hypertension). Concurrent use of other drugs associated with this effect (eg, tetracyclines) may increase risk; pseudotumor cerebri has been reported with use of tetracyclines and acitretin independently. Early signs and symptoms include papilledema, headache, nausea, vomiting, and visual disturbances. Discontinue use in patients experiencing papilledema. Impaired glucose control has been reported with retinoid use. Use with caution in patients with diabetes mellitus; new cases of diabetes have been diagnosed. Discontinue if visual changes occur. May cause adverse effects to the eyes and vision, including a decrease in night vision or decreased tolerance to contact lenses. Use caution when operating vehicles at night; discontinue if visual changes occur. Tinnitus and impaired hearing have been reported with use; consider therapy discontinuation and further evaluation if clinically indicated. Patients receiving long-term treatment should be periodically examined for bony abnormalities; risk versus benefit of therapy should be considered if abnormalities occur. Depression, including aggressive behavior and thoughts of self-harm have been reported; use with caution in patients with a history of mental illness. May be photosensitizing; minimize sun or other UV exposure to treated areas. The risk of burning is increased with phototherapy; decreased doses are required. Capillary leak syndrome, a potential manifestation of retinoic acid syndrome (differentiation syndrome) has been reported with acitretin use. Capillary leak syndrome features may include localized or generalized edema with secondary weight gain, fever, and hypotension; rhabdomyolysis and myalgias have also been reported. Laboratory tests may show neutrophilia, hypoalbuminemia, and an elevated hematocrit. Discontinue use if capillary leak syndrome develops during therapy. Exfoliative dermatitis has been reported with acitretin use; discontinue use if exfoliative dermatitis occurs during therapy. Transient worsening of psoriasis may initially occur; patients should be advised that it may take 2 to 3 months to achieve the full benefits of treatment. Most patients experience relapse of psoriasis after discontinuing therapy. Subsequent courses, when clinically indicated, have produced results similar to the initial course of therapy.

[US Boxed Warning]: All patients must be provided with a medication guide each time acitretin is dispensed. Female patients must also sign an informed consent prior to therapy. [US Boxed Warning]: Only physicians experienced with the diagnosis and treatment of severe psoriasis, including the use of retinoid treatment, and physicians who understand the risk of teratogenicity should prescribe acitretin. Safety and efficacy for pediatric patients have not been established; growth potential may be affected. Potentially significant drug-drug interactions may exist, requiring dose or frequency adjustment, additional monitoring, and/or selection of alternative therapy.

Adverse Reactions

>10%:

Central nervous system: Hyperesthesia (10% to 25%), paresthesia (10% to 25%), rigors (10% to 25%)

Dermatologic: Cheilitis (>75%), alopecia (50% to 75%), exfoliation of skin (50% to 75%), xeroderma (25% to 50%), nail disease (25% to 50%), pruritus (25% to 50%), erythematous rash (10% to 25%), paronychia (10% to 25%), skin atrophy (10% to 25%), acquired cutaneous adherence (10% to 25%)

Endocrine & metabolic: Hypertriglyceridemia (50% to 75%), increased serum glucose (fasting; 25% to 50%), decreased HDL cholesterol (25% to 50%), hypercholesterolemia (25% to 50%), acetonuria (10% to 25%), decreased serum glucose (fasting; 10% to 25%), decreased serum magnesium (10% to 25%), hypermagnesemia (10% to 25%), hyperphospheremia (10% to 25%), increased gamma-glutamyl transferase (10% to 25%), increased serum potassium (10% to 25%), increased serum sodium (10% to 25%), increased uric acid (10% to 25%)

Gastrointestinal: Xerostomia (10% to 25%)

Genitourinary: Erythrocyturia (10% to 25%), hematuria (10% to 25%)

Hematologic & oncologic: Leukocyturia (25% to 50%), reticulocytosis (25% to 50%), increased haptoglobin (10% to 25%), decreased hematocrit (10% to 25%), decreased hemoglobin (10% to 25%), increased neutrophils (10% to 25%), change in WBC count (10% to 25%)

Hepatic: Increased liver enzymes (25% to 50%), increased serum alkaline phosphatase (10% to 25%), increased direct serum bilirubin (10% to 25%)

Neuromuscular & skeletal: Increased creatine phosphokinase (25% to 50%), arthralgia (10% to 25%), spinal hyperostosis (progression; 10% to 25%)

Ophthalmic: Xerophthalmia (10% to 25%)

Respiratory: Rhinitis (25% to 50%), epistaxis (10% to 25%)

1% to 10%:

Cardiovascular: Edema, flushing

Central nervous system: Bell's palsy, depression, drowsiness, fatigue, headache, hypertonia, insomnia, pain

Dermatologic: Abnormal hair texture, abnormal skin odor, Bullous skin disease, cold and clammy skin, dermatitis, diaphoresis (increased), madarosis, psoriasiform eruption, pyogenic granuloma, seborrhea, skin fissure, skin rash, sunburn

Endocrine & metabolic: Decreased haptoglobins, decreased serum albumin, decreased serum calcium, decreased serum iron, decreased serum potassium, decreased serum sodium, diaphoresis (increased), glycosuria, hot flash, hyperchloremia, hypochloremia, hypophosphatemia, increased serum albumin, increased serum calcium, increased serum iron, increased thirst

Gastrointestinal: Abdominal pain, anorexia, aphthous stomatitis, diarrhea, dysgeusia, gingival hemorrhage, gingivitis, increased appetite, nausea, sialorrhea, stomatitis, tongue disease

Genitourinary: Proteinuria

Hematologic & oncologic: Change in RBC count, decreased neutrophils, increased hematocrit, increased hemoglobin, reticulocytopenia, purpura

Hepatic: Increased serum bilirubin

Neuromuscular & skeletal: Arthritis, back pain, myalgia, ostealgia, osteoarthritis, peripheral joint hyperostosis

Ophthalmic: Blepharitis, blurred vision, cataract, conjunctivitis, diplopia, epithelial keratopathy, eye pain, nocturnal amblyopia, photophobia

Otic: Otalgia, tinnitus

Renal: Increased blood urea nitrogen, increased serum creatinine

Respiratory: Sinusitis

Miscellaneous: Ulcer

<1% (Limited to important or life-threatening): Abnormal gait, abnormal lacrimation, acne vulgaris, ageusia, aggressive behavior, alcohol intolerance, anal disease, bone disease, bursitis (olecranon), candidiasis, capillary leak syndrome, cerebrovascular accident, chalazion, conjunctival hemorrhage, constipation, corneal lesion, corneal ulcer, cutaneous nodule, cyanosis, cyst, deafness, decreased libido, dyspepsia, dysuria, ectropion, epidermal thinning, exfoliative dermatitis, flu-like symptoms, fungal infection, furunculosis, gastritis, gingival hyperplasia, glossitis, hair discoloration, hepatic cirrhosis, hepatic dysfunction, hepatitis, herpes simplex infection, hordeolum (recurrent), hyperkeratosis, hypersensitivity reaction, hypertrichosis, hypoesthesia, increased bronchial secretions, increased cerumen production, intermittent claudication, laryngitis, leukorrhea, mastalgia, melena, migraine, myasthenia, myocardial infarction, myopathy (with peripheral neuropathy), nail disease (fragility), neuritis, otitis media, pancreatitis, papilledema, peripheral ischemia, pharyngitis, prolonged bleeding time, pseudotumor cerebri, skin hypertrophy,

skin photosensitivity, spinal hyperostosis (new lesion), suicidal ideation, tendonitis, tenesmus, thromboembolism, tongue ulcer, vaginitis, voice disorder, warts, weight gain, wound healing impairment

Drug Interactions

Metabolism/Transport Effects None known.

Avoid Concomitant Use

Avoid concomitant use of Acitretin with any of the following: Alcohol (Ethyl); Methotrexate; Multivitamins/Fluoride (with ADE); Multivitamins/Minerals (with ADEK, Folate, Iron); Multivitamins/Minerals (with AE, No Iron); Tetracycline Derivatives; Vitamin A

Increased Effect/Toxicity

Acitretin may increase the levels/effects of: Methotrexate; Porfimer; Verteporfin

The levels/effects of Acitretin may be increased by: Alcohol (Ethyl); Multivitamins/Fluoride (with ADE); Multivitamins/Minerals (with ADEK, Folate, Iron); Multivitamins/Minerals (with AE, No Iron); Tetracycline Derivatives; Vitamin A

Decreased Effect

Acitretin may decrease the levels/effects of: Contraceptives (Estrogens); Contraceptives (Progestins)

Food Interactions

Ethanol: Use leads to formation of etretinate, a teratogenic metabolite with a prolonged half-life. Management: Female patients must avoid ethanol or ethanol-containing products concomitantly or within 2 months after discontinuing acitretin.

Food: Absorption increased when administered with food. Management: Take with food; avoid ingestion of additional sources of vitamin A (in excess of RDA).

Storage/Stability Store between 15°C to 25°C (59°F to 77°F). Avoid high temperatures and humidity. Protect from light.

Mechanism of Action Binds to and activates all nuclear subtypes (alpha, beta, and gamma) of retinoid X receptors (RXR) and retinoic acid receptors (RAR) to inhibit the expression of the proinflammatory cytokines interleukin-6 (IL-6), migration inhibitory factor-related protein-8 (MRP-8), and interferon-gamma (markers of hyperproliferation and abnormal keratinocyte differentiation). Resulting actions are anti-inflammatory and antiproliferative, and keratinocyte differentiation is normalized in the epithelium.

Pharmacodynamics/Kinetics Etretinate has been detected in serum for up to 3 years following therapy, possibly due to storage in adipose tissue.

Onset of action: May take 2 to 3 months for full effect; improvement may be seen within 8 weeks.

Absorption: Oral: ~72% absorbed when given with food

Protein binding: >99% bound, primarily to albumin

Metabolism: Metabolized to *cis*-acitretin; both compounds are further metabolized. Concomitant ethanol use leads to the formation of etretinate (active).

Half-life elimination: Acitretin: 49 hours (range: 33 to 96); *cis*-acitretin: 63 hours (range: 28 to 157); etretinate: 120 days (range: Up to 168 days)

Time to peak: 2 to 5 hours

Excretion: Feces (34% to 54%); urine (16% to 53%)

Dosing

Adult & Geriatric

US labeling:

Psoriasis: Oral: Individualization of dosage is required to achieve maximum therapeutic response while minimizing side effects

Initial: 25 to 50 mg daily, given as a single dose with the main meal

Maintenance: 25 to 50 mg daily may be given after initial response to treatment; the maintenance dose should be based on clinical efficacy and tolerability

American Academy of Dermatology recommendations: 10 to 50 mg daily as a single dose; doses ≤25 mg daily are used to decrease side effects (Menter, 2009)

Canadian labeling:

Psoriasis: Oral:

Initial: 25 mg daily, given as a single dose with the main meal. If response is inadequate after 4 weeks of therapy, the dose may be gradually increased (as tolerated) up to a maximum of 75 mg daily. Reduce dose if necessary to minimize side effects.

Maintenance: 25 to 50 mg daily may be given after initial response to treatment; the maintenance dose should be based on clinical efficacy and tolerability. Maximum: 75 mg daily

Other keratinization disorders: Adults: Oral: 10 to 50 mg daily; maximum: 50 mg daily

Renal Impairment There are no dosage adjustments provided in manufacturer's labeling; use is contraindicated in patients with severely impaired renal function.

Hemodialysis: Not removed by hemodialysis

Hepatic Impairment There are no dosage adjustments provided in manufacturer's labeling; use is contraindicated in patients with severely impaired liver function.

Dietary Considerations Take with food. Avoid ingestion of additional sources of exogenous vitamin A (in excess of RDA); use of ethanol and ethanol-containing products is contraindicated.

Administration Administer with food, preferably with the main meal of the day.

Hazardous agent; use appropriate precautions for handling and disposal (NIOSH 2014 [group 3]).

Monitoring Parameters Lipid profile (baseline and at 1- to 2-week intervals for 4 to 8 weeks, then as clinically indicated); liver function tests (baseline, and at 1- to 2-week intervals until stable, then as clinically indicated); blood glucose in patients with diabetes; evaluate for bone abnormalities (with long-term use); pregnancy tests (2 negative tests prior to therapy initiation, monthly during treatment, and every 3 months for ≥3 years after discontinuation of therapy)

The American Academy of Dermatology recommends: CBC and renal function tests (baseline and then every 12 weeks); liver function tests (every 2 weeks for the first 8 weeks, then every 6 to 12 weeks thereafter) (Menter, 2009)

Dosage Forms Excipient information presented when available (limited, particularly for generics); consult specific product labeling.

Capsule, Oral:

Soriatane: 10 mg, 17.5 mg, 25 mg [contains edetate calcium disodium]

Generic: 10 mg, 17.5 mg, 25 mg

- ◆ Aclaro *see* Hydroquinone *on page 893*
- ◆ Aclaro PD *see* Hydroquinone *on page 893*
- ◆ Aclasta (Can) *see* Zoledronic Acid *on page 1934*
- ◆ Aclovate *see* Alclometasone *on page 59*

Acrivastine and Pseudoephedrine
(AK ri vas teen & soo doe e FED rin)

Brand Names: US Semprex®-D

Index Terms Pseudoephedrine Hydrochloride and Acrivastine

Pharmacologic Category Alkylamine Derivative; Alpha/Beta Agonist; Decongestant; Histamine H_1 Antagonist; Histamine H_1 Antagonist, Second Generation

Use Relief of symptoms associated with seasonal allergic rhinitis

Dosing

Adult & Geriatric Rhinitis, nasal congestion, allergic symptoms: Oral: One capsule every 4-6 hours (maximum: 4 doses/24 hours); treatment for >14 days has not been evaluated

Pediatric Children ≥12 years: Refer to adult dosing.

Renal Impairment Avoid use in patients with CrCl ≤48 mL/minute.

Hepatic Impairment There are no dosage adjustments recommended in manufacturer's labeling.

Additional Information Complete prescribing information should be consulted for additional detail.

Dosage Forms Excipient information presented when available (limited, particularly for generics); consult specific product labeling.

Capsule:

Semprex®-D: Acrivastine 8 mg and pseudoephedrine hydrochloride 60 mg

- ◆ Act [OTC] *see* Fluoride *on page 782*
- ◆ ACT-D *see* DACTINomycin *on page 481*
- ◆ ACT-293987 *see* Selexipag *on page 1647*
- ◆ ACT-Amlodipine (Can) *see* AmLODIPine *on page 101*
- ◆ ACT-Anastrozole (Can) *see* Anastrozole *on page 128*
- ◆ ACT Atorvastatin (Can) *see* AtorvaSTATin *on page 169*
- ◆ ACT-Azithromycin (Can) *see* Azithromycin (Systemic) *on page 190*
- ◆ ACT Bicalutamide (Can) *see* Bicalutamide *on page 230*
- ◆ ACT Bosentan (Can) *see* Bosentan *on page 246*
- ◆ ACT Cabergoline (Can) *see* Cabergoline *on page 279*
- ◆ ACT Celecoxib (Can) *see* Celecoxib *on page 355*
- ◆ ACT Ciprofloxacin (Can) *see* Ciprofloxacin (Systemic) *on page 388*
- ◆ ACT Citalopram (Can) *see* Citalopram *on page 398*
- ◆ ACT Clopidogrel (Can) *see* Clopidogrel *on page 424*
- ◆ ACT Diclo-Miso (Can) *see* Diclofenac and Misoprostol *on page 544*
- ◆ ACT Diltiazem CD (Can) *see* Diltiazem *on page 553*

Acyclovir (Systemic) (ay SYE kloe veer)

Brand Names: US Zovirax
Brand Names: Canada Acyclovir Sodium for Injection; Acyclovir Sodium Injection; Apo-Acyclovir; Mylan-Acyclovir; ratio-Acyclovir; Teva-Acyclovir; Zovirax
Index Terms Aciclovir; ACV; Acycloguanosine; Zovirax
Pharmacologic Category Antiviral Agent
Use

Oral:
Herpes zoster (shingles): Acute treatment of herpes zoster (shingles).
Herpes simplex virus (HSV), genital: Treatment of initial episodes and the management of recurrent episodes of genital herpes.
Varicella (chickenpox): Treatment of varicella (chickenpox).

Injection:
Herpes simplex virus (HSV), mucocutaneous infection in immunocompromised patients: Treatment of initial and recurrent mucosal and cutaneous herpes simplex (HSV-1 and HSV-2) in immunocompromised patients.

Herpes simplex virus (HSV), genital infection (severe): Treatment of severe initial clinical episodes of genital herpes in immunocompetent patients.

Herpes simplex encephalitis: Treatment of herpes simplex encephalitis.

Herpes simplex virus (HSV), neonatal: Treatment of neonatal herpes infections.

Herpes zoster (shingles) in immunocompromised patients: Treatment of herpes zoster (shingles) in immunocompromised patients.

Pregnancy Considerations Teratogenic effects were not observed in animal reproduction studies. Acyclovir has been shown to cross the human placenta (Henderson 1992). Results from a pregnancy registry, established in 1984 and closed in 1999, did not find an increase in the number of birth defects with exposure to acyclovir when compared to those expected in the general population. However, due to the small size of the registry and lack of long-term data, the manufacturer recommends using during pregnancy with caution and only when clearly needed. Acyclovir may be appropriate for the treatment of genital herpes in pregnant women (CDC 2010).

Breast-Feeding Considerations Acyclovir is excreted in breast milk. The manufacturer recommends that caution be exercised when administering acyclovir to nursing women. Limited data suggest exposure to the nursing infant of ~0.3 mg/kg/day following oral administration of acyclovir to the mother. Nursing mothers with herpetic lesions near or on the breast should avoid breast-feeding (Gartner 2005).

Contraindications Hypersensitivity to acyclovir, valacyclovir, or any component of the formulation

Warnings/Precautions Use with caution in immunocompromised patients; thrombocytopenic purpura/hemolytic uremic syndrome (TTP/HUS) has been reported. Use caution in the elderly, preexisting renal disease (may require dosage modification), or in those receiving other nephrotoxic drugs. Renal failure (sometimes fatal) has been reported. Maintain adequate hydration during oral or intravenous therapy. Use IV preparation with caution in patients with underlying neurologic abnormalities, serious hepatic or electrolyte abnormalities, or substantial hypoxia.

Varicella-zoster: Treatment should begin within 24 hours of appearance of rash; oral route not recommended for routine use in otherwise healthy children with varicella, but may be effective in patients at increased risk of moderate-to-severe infection (>12 years of age, chronic cutaneous or pulmonary disorders, long-term salicylate therapy, corticosteroid therapy).

Adverse Reactions

Oral:

>10%: Central nervous system: Malaise (≤12%)

1% to 10%:

Central nervous system: Headache (≤2%)

Gastrointestinal: Nausea (2% to 5%), vomiting (≤3%), diarrhea (2% to 3%)

Parenteral:

1% to 10%:

Dermatologic: Hives (2%), itching (2%), rash (2%)

Gastrointestinal: Nausea/vomiting (7%)

Hepatic: Liver function tests increased (1% to 2%)

Local: Inflammation at injection site or phlebitis (9%)

Renal: BUN increased (5% to 10%), creatinine increased (5% to 10%), acute renal failure

All forms: <1% (Limited to important or life-threatening): Abdominal pain, aggression, agitation, anemia, anorexia, ataxia, coma, confusion, consciousness decreased, delirium, desquamation, disseminated intravascular coagulopathy (DIC), dizziness, dysarthria, encephalopathy, fatigue, fever, gastrointestinal distress, hallucinations, hematuria, hemolysis, hepatitis, hyperbilirubinemia, hypotension, insomnia, jaundice, leukocytoclastic vasculitis, leukocytosis, leukopenia, lymphadenopathy, mental depression, myalgia, neutrophilia, pain, psychosis, renal failure, renal pain, seizure, somnolence, sore throat, thrombocytopenia, thrombocytopenic purpura/hemolytic uremic syndrome (TTP/HUS), thrombocytosis, visual disturbances

Drug Interactions

Metabolism/Transport Effects None known.

Avoid Concomitant Use

Avoid concomitant use of Acyclovir (Systemic) with any of the following: Foscarnet; Varicella Virus Vaccine; Zoster Vaccine

Increased Effect/Toxicity

Acyclovir (Systemic) may increase the levels/effects of: Mycophenolate; Tenofovir Products; Zidovudine

The levels/effects of Acyclovir (Systemic) may be increased by: Foscarnet; Mycophenolate; Tenofovir Products

Decreased Effect

Acyclovir (Systemic) may decrease the levels/effects of: Talimogene Laherparepvec; Varicella Virus Vaccine; Zoster Vaccine

Food Interactions Food does not affect absorption of oral acyclovir.

Preparation for Administration Powder for injection: Reconstitute acyclovir 500 mg powder with SWFI 10 mL; do not use bacteriostatic water containing benzyl alcohol or parabens. For intravenous infusion, dilute in D_5W, D_5NS, $D_5^{1}/4NS$, $D_5^{1}/2NS$, LR, or NS to a final concentration ≤7 mg/mL. Concentrations >10 mg/mL increase the risk of phlebitis.

Storage/Stability

Capsule, oral suspension, tablet: Store at controlled room temperature of 15°C to 25°C (59°F to 77°F); protect from capsule and tablet from moisture.

Injection: Store powder at controlled room temperature of 15°C to 25°C (59°F to 77°F). Reconstituted solutions remain stable for 12 hours at room temperature. Do not refrigerate reconstituted solutions or solutions diluted for infusion as they may precipitate. Once diluted for infusion, use within 24 hours.

Mechanism of Action Acyclovir is converted to acyclovir monophosphate by virus-specific thymidine kinase then further converted to acyclovir triphosphate by other cellular enzymes. Acyclovir triphosphate inhibits DNA synthesis and viral replication by competing with deoxyguanosine triphosphate for viral DNA polymerase and being incorporated into viral DNA.

Pharmacodynamics/Kinetics

Absorption: Oral: 15% to 30%

Distribution: Widely (eg, brain, kidney, lungs, liver, spleen, muscle, uterus, vagina, CSF); CSF acyclovir concentration is 50% of serum

V_d:

Neonates to 3 months of age: 28.8 L/1.73 m^2

Children 1 to 2 years: 31.6 L/1.73 m^2

Children 2 to 7 years: 42 L/1.73 m^2

Adults: 0.8 L/kg (63.6 L)

Protein binding: <9% to 33%

Metabolism: Converted by viral enzymes to acyclovir monophosphate, and further converted to diphosphate then triphosphate (active form) by cellular enzymes

Bioavailability: Oral: 10% to 20% with normal renal function (bioavailability decreases with increased dose)

Half-life elimination: Terminal: Neonates: 4 hours; Children 1 to 12 years: 2 to 3 hours; Adults: 2 to 3.5 hours (with normal renal function); hemodialysis: ~5 hours

Time to peak, serum: Oral: Within 1.5 to 2 hours

Excretion: Urine (62% to 90% as unchanged drug and metabolite)

Dosing

Adult & Geriatric

Herpes simplex virus (HSV), genital infection:

Immunocompetent:

IV: Initial episode, severe: 5 mg/kg/dose every 8 hours for 5 to 7 days **or** 5 to 10 mg/kg/dose every 8 hours for 2 to 7 days, follow with oral therapy to complete at least 10 days of therapy (CDC 2010)

Oral:

Initial episode: 200 mg 5 times daily while awake for 10 days **or** 400 mg 3 times daily for 7 to 10 days (CDC 2010)

Recurrence:

Manufacturer's labeling: **Note:** begin at earliest signs of disease: 200 mg 5 times daily while awake for 5 days

Alternate recommendation: 400 mg 3 times daily for 5 days **or** 800 mg twice daily for 5 days **or** 800 mg 3 times daily for 2 days (CDC 2010)

Chronic suppression: 400 mg twice daily or 200 mg 3 to 5 times daily, for up to 12 months followed by re-evaluation

HIV-infected patients (off-label use) (HHS [OI adult 2015]): Oral:

Initial or recurrent episodes: 400 mg 3 times daily for 5 to 14 days

Chronic suppressive therapy: 400 mg twice daily; continue indefinitely regardless of CD4 count in patients with severe recurrences of genital herpes or in patients who want to minimize frequency of recurrences

HSV encephalitis: IV: Independent of HIV status:

Manufacturer's labeling: 10 mg/kg/dose every 8 hours for 10 days

Alternate recommendation: 10 mg/kg/dose every 8 hours for 14 to 21 days (*Red Book* [AAP 2012])

HSV, mucocutaneous treatment:
Immunocompromised:
IV:
Manufacturer's labeling: 5 mg/kg/dose every 8 hours for 7 days
Alternate recommendations: 5 to 10 mg/kg/dose every 8 hours for 7 days (Leflore 2000)
Oral (off-label use): 400 mg 5 times daily for 7 days (Leflore 2000)
HIV-infected patients: (off-label use)
IV: 5 mg/kg/dose every 8 hours; may switch to oral after lesions begin to heal (HHS [OI adult 2015])
Oral: After initial IV therapy, may switch to 400 mg 3 times daily; continue until lesions are completely healed (HHS [OI adult 2015])

HSV, orolabial (cold sores) (off-label use): Oral:
Immunocompetent:
Treatment: (episodic/recurrent): 200 to 400 mg 5 times daily for 5 days (Cernik 2008; Leflore 2000; Spruance 1990).
Chronic suppression: 400 mg 2 times daily (has been clinically evaluated for up to 1 year) (Cernik 2008; Rooney 1993)
HIV-infected patients: Treatment: 400 mg 3 times daily for 5 to 10 days (HHS [OI adult 2015])

Herpes zoster (shingles), treatment:
Manufacturer's labeling:
IV: Immunocompromised: 10 mg/kg/dose every 8 hours for 7 days
Oral: Immunocompetent: 800 mg 5 times daily for 7 to 10 day
Alternate recommendations: HIV-infected patients (HHS [OI adult 2015]):
IV: Extensive cutaneous lesions or visceral involvement: 10 to 15 mg/kg/dose every 8 hours until clinical improvement; switch to oral famciclovir or valacyclovir (preferred) or acyclovir (alternative) to complete a 10 to 14 day course when formation of new lesions has ceased and signs/symptoms of visceral infection are improving
Oral (off-label use): Acute localized infection (as an alternative to valacyclovir or famciclovir): 800 mg 5 times daily for 7 to 10 days; consider longer duration if lesions resolve slowly

Prevention of early HSV reactivation in seropositive hematopoietic stem cell transplant (HSCT) recipients (off-label use): Note: Start at the beginning of conditioning therapy and continue until engraftment or until mucositis resolves (~30 days) (Tomblyn 2009)
Oral: 400 to 800 mg twice daily
IV: 250 mg/m^2 every 12 hours

Prevention of late HSV reactivation in seropositive HSCT recipients (off-label use): Oral: 800 mg twice daily; continue therapy for 1 year after HSCT (Tomblyn 2009).

Prevention of HSV reactivation in seropositive patients undergoing acute myeloid leukemia induction or reinduction (off-label use): Oral: 400 mg twice daily; continue during active therapy and throughout periods of neutropenia (Bergmann 1995; Freifeld 2011)

Prevention of VZV reactivation in HSCT recipients (off-label use): Oral: 800 mg twice daily; continue therapy for 1 year after HSCT (Tomblyn 2009).

Prophylaxis of CMV in low-risk allogeneic HSCT (off-label use; alternate therapy): Note: Begin at engraftment and continue to day 100; requires close monitoring for CMV reactivation (due to weak activity); not for use in patients at high risk for CMV disease (Tomblyn 2009)
Oral: 800 mg 4 times daily
IV: 500 mg/m^2 every 8 hours

Varicella (chickenpox), treatment: Begin treatment within the first 24 hours of rash onset:
Oral:
Immunocompetent (>40 kg): 800 mg 4 times daily for 5 days
HIV-infected patients (off-label use): Uncomplicated cases (as an alternative to valacyclovir or famciclovir): 800 mg 5 times daily for 5 to 7 days (HHS [OI adult 2015])
IV: HIV-infected patients (off-label use): Severe or complicated cases: 10 to 15 mg/kg/dose every 8 hours for 7 to 10 days; may switch to oral famciclovir or valacyclovir (preferred) or acyclovir (alternative) after defervescence if no evidence of visceral involvement (HHS [OI adult 2015])

Varicella-zoster virus acute retinal necrosis (ARN) in HIV-infected patients (off-label use): IV: 10 to 15 mg/kg/dose every 8 hours for 10 to 14 days, followed by valacyclovir for 6 weeks plus intravitreal ganciclovir twice weekly for 1 to 2 doses (HHS [OI adult 2015])

Pediatric

Herpes simplex virus (HSV), genital infection:
IV: Children ≥12 years and Adolescents: Immunocompetent: Initial episode, severe: 5 mg/kg/dose every 8 hours for 5 to 7 days or 5 to 10 mg/kg/dose every 8 hours for 2 to 7 days, follow with oral therapy to complete at least 10 days of therapy (CDC 2010)
Oral:
Infants and Children <12 years: Immunocompetent (off-label use):
Initial episode: 40 to 80 mg/kg/day divided into 3 to 4 doses for 5-10 days (maximum: 1,000 mg daily) (Red Book [AAP 2012])
Chronic suppression: 40 to 80 mg/kg/day in 3 divided doses for ≤12 months; (maximum: 1,000 mg daily) (Red Book [AAP 2009])
Children ≥12 years and Adolescents: Immunocompetent (off-label use):
Initial episode: 200 mg every 4 hours while awake (5 times daily) or 400 mg 3 times daily for 7 to 10 days; treatment can be extended beyond 10 days if healing is not complete (CDC 2010; Red Book [AAP 2012])
Chronic suppression: 800 mg daily in 2 divided doses for ≤12 continuous months (Red Book [AAP 2012])
Children: HIV-exposed/-positive (off-label use):
Children <45 kg:
Initial episode: 60 mg/kg/day divided into 3 doses daily for 5 to 14 days (maximum: 1,200 mg daily) (CDC 2009)
Chronic suppression: 20 mg/kg/dose twice daily (maximum dose: 400 mg) (CDC 2009)
Children ≥45 kg:
Initial episode: 400 mg twice daily for 5 to 14 days (CDC 2009)
Chronic suppression: 20 mg/kg/dose twice daily (maximum dose: 400 mg) (CDC 2009)
Children <12 years: Recurrent infection: Non-HIV-exposed/-positive: Oral: 20 to 25 mg/kg/dose twice daily; maximum dose: 400 mg (Bradley 2011)
Children ≥12 years: Recurrent infection: Non-HIV-exposed/-positive: 200 mg every 4 hours while awake (5 times daily) for 5 days or 800 mg twice daily for 5 days or 800 mg 3 times daily for 2 days (CDC 2010; Red Book [AAP 2012])
Adolescents: HIV-positive patients: (off-label use): Refer to adult dosing.

HSV encephalitis: IV:
Infants and Children 3 months to <12 years:
Immunocompetent:
Manufacturer's labeling: 20 mg/kg/dose every 8 hours for 10 days. **Note:** Doses ≥20 mg/kg may be associated with a higher incidence of nephrotoxicity (Red Book [AAP 2012])
Alternate recommendation: 10 to 15 mg/kg/dose every 8 hours for 14 to 21 days (Red Book [AAP 2012])
HIV-exposed/-positive: 10 mg/kg/dose every 8 hours for 21 days; do not discontinue therapy until a repeat HSV DNA PCR assay of the cerebrospinal fluid is negative (CDC 2009)
Children ≥12 years and Adolescents: Independent of HIV status:
Manufacturer's labeling: 10 mg/kg/dose every 8 hours for 10 days
Alternate recommendation: 10 mg/kg/dose every 8 hours for 14 to 21 days (Red Book [AAP 2012])

HSV gingivostomatitis (off-label use): HIV-exposed/-positive:
Mild, symptomatic: Oral: Infants and Children: 20 mg/kg/dose 3 times daily for 5 to 10 days (maximum dose: 400 mg) (CDC 2009)
Moderate to severe, symptomatic: IV: Infants and Children: 5 to 10 mg/kg/dose every 8 hours; **Note:** switch to oral therapy once lesions begin to regress (CDC 2009)

HSV, mucocutaneous treatment:
Immunocompromised:
IV:
Infants, Children, and Adolescents: 10 mg/kg/dose every 8 hours for 7 to 14 days (Red Book [AAP 2012])

Oral (off-label use):

Children ≥2 years and Adolescents: 1,000 mg daily in 3 to 5 divided doses for 7 to 14 days; some suggest the maximum daily dose should not exceed 80 mg/kg/day (*Red Book* [AAP 2009]; Red Book [AAP 2012])

HIV-infected patients (off-label use): Adolescents: IV, Oral: Refer to adult dosing.

Suppression, chronic (cutaneous, ocular) episodes: Immunocompromised: Oral:

Infants and Children (HIV-exposed/-positive): 20 mg/kg/dose twice daily for 5 to 14 days; maximum dose: 400 mg (CDC 2009)

Children and Adolescents ≥12 years (independent of HIV status): 400 mg twice daily for up to 12 months (*Red Book* [AAP 2012])

HSV, neonatal: IV: Infants: Birth to 3 months: Treatment: *Manufacturer's labeling:* 10 mg/kg/dose every 8 hours for 10 days

Alternate recommendations: 20 mg/kg/dose every 8 hours for 14 days (skin and mucous membrane disease) to 21 days (CNS disease) (CDC 2010; Kimberlin 2013; *Red Book* [AAP 2012])

HSV, orolabial (cold sores) (off-label use): Oral:

Immunocompetent: Chronic suppression: Children: 30 mg/kg/day in 3 divided doses for up to 12 months (maximum: 1,000 mg/day). **Note:** Re-evaluate after 12 months (*Red Book* [AAP 2012])

HIV-infected patients: Treatment: Adolescents: Refer to adult dosing.

Herpes zoster (shingles), treatment:
IV:

Immunocompetent (off-label use):

Infants: 10 mg/kg/dose every 8 hours for 7 to 10 days (*Red Book* [AAP 2012])

Children ≥1 year and Adolescents: 500 mg/m²/dose every 8 hours for 7 to 10 days; some experts recommend 10 mg/kg/dose every 8 hours (*Red Book* [AAP 2012])

Immunocompromised:

Children <12 years: (off-label dose): 10 mg/kg/dose every 8 hours for 7 to 10 days (*Red Book* [AAP 2012])

Children ≥12 years and Adolescents: Manufacturer's labeling: Refer to adult dosing.

HIV-infected patients: Adolescents (off-label dose): *Extensive cutaneous lesions or visceral involvement:* Refer to adult dosing.

Oral:

Immunocompetent:

Manufacturer's labeling: Children ≥2 years and Adolescents: Refer to adult dosing.

Alternate recommendations: Children ≥12 years and Adolescents: 800 mg 5 times daily for 5 to 7 days (*Red Book* [AAP 2012])

Immunocompromised: HIV-infected patients (off-label use): *Acute localized infection (as an alternative to valacyclovir or famciclovir):* Adolescents: Refer to adult dosing.

Prevention of HSV reactivation in HIV-exposed/-positive patients (off-label use): Oral: Children: 20 mg/kg/dose twice daily (maximum: 400 mg per dose) (CDC 2009)

Prevention of early HSV reactivation in seropositive hematopoietic stem cell transplant (HSCT) recipients (off-label use): Note: Start at the beginning of conditioning therapy and continue until engraftment or until mucositis resolves (~30 days) (Tomblyn 2009):
Oral:

Infants, Children, and Adolescents <40 kg (alternate therapy): 60 to 90 mg/kg/day in 2 to 3 divided doses

Children and Adolescents ≥40 kg: 400 to 800 mg twice daily

IV:

Infants, Children, and Adolescents <40 kg: 250 mg/m² every 8 hours or 125 mg/m² every 6 hours (maximum daily dose: 80 mg/kg/day)

Children and Adolescents ≥40 kg: 250 mg/m² every 12 hours

Prevention of late HSV reactivation in seropositive HSCT recipients (off-label use): Note: Continue therapy for 1 year after HSCT (Tomblyn 2009).

Infants, Children, and Adolescents <40 kg: Oral: 60 to 90 mg/kg/day in 2 to 3 divided doses (maximum dose: 800 mg twice daily)

Children and Adolescents ≥40 kg: Oral: 800 mg twice daily

Prevention of VZV reactivation in HSCT recipients (off-label use): Note: Continue therapy for 1 year after HSCT (Tomblyn 2009)

Infants, Children, and Adolescents <40 kg: Oral: 60 to 80 mg/kg/day in 2 to 3 divided doses

Children and Adolescents ≥40 kg: Oral: 800 mg twice daily

Prophylaxis of CMV in low-risk allogeneic HSCT (off-label use; alternate therapy): Note: Begin at engraftment and continue to day 100; requires close monitoring for CMV reactivation (due to weak activity); not for use in patients at high risk for CMV disease (Tomblyn 2009)

Oral:

Infants, Children, and Adolescents <40 kg: 600 mg/m² 4 times daily

Children and Adolescents ≥40 kg: 800 mg 4 times daily

IV: Infants, Children, and Adolescents: 500 mg/m² every 8 hours

Varicella (chickenpox), treatment: Begin treatment within the first 24 hours of rash onset:
Oral:

Immunocompetent:

Children ≥2 years and ≤40 kg: 20 mg/kg/dose (maximum: 800 mg per dose) 4 times daily for 5 days

Children >40 kg: Refer to adult dosing.

HIV-infected patients (off-label use):

Infants and Children: Mild, uncomplicated disease and no or moderate immune suppression: 20 mg/kg/dose (maximum dose: 800 mg) 4 times daily for 7 to 10 days or until no new lesions for 48 hours (CDC 2009)

Adolescents: Uncomplicated cases (as an alternative to valacyclovir or famciclovir): Refer to adult dosing.

IV:

Immunocompetent (off-label use): Children ≥2 years: 10 mg/kg/dose or 500 mg/m²/dose every 8 hours for 7 to 10 days (CDC 2009; *Red Book* [AAP 2012])

Immunocompromised (off-label use):

Infants (off-label dose): 10 mg/kg/dose every 8 hours for 7 to 10 days (*Red Book* [AAP 2012])

Children and Adolescents (off-label dose): 500 mg/m²/dose every 8 hours for 7 to 10 days; some experts recommend 10 mg/kg/dose every 8 hours (*Red Book* [AAP 2012])

HIV-exposed/-positive (off-label use):

Infants: 10 mg/kg/dose every 8 hours for 7 to 10 days or until no new lesions for 48 hours (CDC 2009)

Children ≥1 year: 10 mg/kg/dose or 500 mg/m²/dose every 8 hours for 7 to 10 days or until no new lesions for 48 hours (CDC 2009)

Adolescents: Refer to adult dosing.

Varicella-zoster virus acute retinal necrosis in HIV-exposed/-positive patients (off-label use): IV:

Infants and Children: 10 to 15 mg/kg/dose every 8 hours for 10 to 14 days, followed by oral acyclovir or valacyclovir for 4 to 6 weeks (CDC 2009)

Adolescents: Refer to adult dosing.

Renal Impairment
Oral:

CrCl 10-25 mL/minute/1.73 m²: Normal dosing regimen 800 mg 5 times daily: Administer 800 mg every 8 hours

CrCl <10 mL/minute/1.73 m²:

Normal dosing regimen 200 mg 5 times daily or 400 mg every 12 hours: Administer 200 mg every 12 hours

Normal dosing regimen 800 mg 5 times daily: Administer 800 mg every 12 hours

Intermittent hemodialysis (IHD): Dialyzable (60% reduction following a 6-hour session):

Normal dosing regimen 200 mg 5 times daily or 400 mg every 12 hours: Administer 200 mg every 12 hours; administer after hemodialysis on dialysis days

Normal dosing regimen 800 mg 5 times daily: Administer 800 mg every 12 hours; administer after hemodialysis on dialysis days

IV:

CrCl 25-50 mL/minute/1.73 m²: Administer recommended dose every 12 hours

CrCl 10-25 mL/minute/1.73 m²: Administer recommended dose every 24 hours

CrCl <10 mL/minute/1.73 m²: Administer 50% of recommended dose every 24 hours

Intermittent hemodialysis (IHD) (administer after hemodialysis on dialysis days): Dialyzable (60% reduction following a 6-hour session): 2.5-5 mg/kg every 24 hours (Heintz 2009). **Note:** Dosing dependent on the assumption of 3 times weekly, complete IHD sessions.

Peritoneal dialysis (PD): Administer 50% of normal dose once daily; no supplemental dose needed (Aronoff 2007)

Continuous renal replacement therapy (CRRT) (Heintz 2009; Trotman 2005): Drug clearance is highly dependent on the method of renal replacement, filter type, and flow rate. Appropriate dosing requires close monitoring of pharmacologic response, signs of adverse reactions due to drug accumulation, as well as drug concentrations in relation to target trough (if appropriate). The following are general recommendations only (based on dialysate flow/ultrafiltration rates of 1-2 L/hour and minimal residual renal function) and should not supersede clinical judgment:

CVVH: 5-10 mg/kg every 24 hours

CVVHD/CVVHDF: 5-10 mg/kg every 12-24 hours

Note: The higher end of dosage range (eg, 10 mg/kg every 12 hours for CVVHDF) is recommended for viral meningoencephalitis and varicella-zoster virus infections.

Hepatic Impairment Oral, IV: There are no dosage adjustments provided in the manufacturer's labeling; use caution in patients with severe impairment.

Obesity Obese patients should be dosed using ideal body weight.

Dietary Considerations May be taken with or without food. Some products may contain sodium.

Administration

Oral: May be administered with or without food.

IV: Avoid rapid infusion; infuse over 1 hour to prevent renal damage; maintain adequate hydration of patient; check for phlebitis and rotate infusion sites. Avoid IM or SubQ administration.

Monitoring Parameters Urinalysis, BUN, serum creatinine, liver enzymes, CBC

Dosage Forms Excipient information presented when available (limited, particularly for generics); consult specific product labeling.

Capsule, Oral:

Zovirax: 200 mg [contains fd&c blue #2 (indigotine), parabens]

Generic: 200 mg

Solution, Intravenous, as sodium [strength expressed as base]:

Generic: 50 mg/mL (10 mL, 20 mL)

Solution Reconstituted, Intravenous, as sodium [strength expressed as base]:

Generic: 500 mg (1 ea); 1000 mg (1 ea)

Suspension, Oral:

Zovirax: 200 mg/5 mL (473 mL) [contains methylparaben, propylparaben; banana flavor]

Generic: 200 mg/5 mL (473 mL)

Tablet, Oral:

Zovirax: 400 mg

Zovirax: 800 mg [contains fd&c blue #2 (indigotine)]

Generic: 400 mg, 800 mg

Acyclovir (Topical) (ay SYE kloe veer)

Brand Names: US Sitavig; Zovirax

Brand Names: Canada Zovirax

Index Terms Aciclovir; ACV; Acycloguanosine

Pharmacologic Category Antiviral Agent, Topical

Use Herpes virus:

Buccal tablet: Treatment of recurrent herpes labialis (cold sores) in immunocompetent adults.

Cream: Treatment of recurrent herpes labialis (cold sores) in immunocompetent children ≥12 years of age, adolescents, and adults.

Ointment: Management of initial genital herpes and in limited non-life-threatening mucocutaneous herpes simplex virus infections in immunocompromised patients.

Dosing

Adult & Geriatric

Genital HSV: Topical ointment: Initial episode: 1/2" ribbon of ointment for a 4" square surface area every 3 hours (6 times daily) for 7 days

Herpes labialis (cold sores):

Topical cream: Apply 5 times daily for 4 days

Buccal tablet: Apply one 50 mg tablet as a single dose to the upper gum region (canine fossa).

Mucocutaneous HSV (non-life-threatening, immunocompromised): Topical ointment: 1/2" ribbon of ointment for a 4" square surface area every 3 hours (6 times daily) for 7 days

Pediatric Herpes labialis (cold sores): Children ≥12 years and Adolescents: Topical cream: Refer to adult dosing.

Renal Impairment There are no dosage adjustments provided in the manufacturer's labeling. However, dosage adjustment is unlikely due to low systemic absorption.

Hepatic Impairment There are no dosage adjustments provided in the manufacturer's labeling. However, dosage adjustment is unlikely due to low systemic absorption.

Additional Information Complete prescribing information should be consulted for additional detail.

Dosage Forms Excipient information presented when available (limited, particularly for generics); consult specific product labeling. [DSC] = Discontinued product

Cream, External:

Zovirax: 5% (2 g [DSC], 5 g) [contains cetostearyl alcohol, propylene glycol]

Ointment, External:

Zovirax: 5% (30 g)

Generic: 5% (5 g, 15 g, 30 g)

Tablet, Buccal:

Sitavig: 50 mg [contains milk protein concentrate]

◆ **Acyclovir Sodium for Injection (Can)** see Acyclovir (Systemic) on page 37

◆ **Acyclovir Sodium Injection (Can)** see Acyclovir (Systemic) on page 37

◆ **ACZ885** see Canakinumab on page 293

◆ **AD32** see Valrubicin on page 1865

◆ **aDabi-Fab** see IdaruCIZUMAB on page 910

◆ **Adacel** see Diphtheria and Tetanus Toxoids, and Acellular Pertussis Vaccine on page 567

◆ **Adacel-Polio (Can)** see Diphtheria and Tetanus Toxoids, Acellular Pertussis, and Poliovirus Vaccine on page 566

◆ **Adagen** see Pegademase Bovine on page 1406

◆ **Adalat XL (Can)** see NIFEdipine on page 1279

◆ **Adalat CC** see NIFEdipine on page 1279

Adalimumab (a da LIM yoo mab)

Brand Names: US Humira; Humira Pediatric Crohns Start; Humira Pen; Humira Pen-Crohns Starter; Humira Pen-Psoriasis Starter

Brand Names: Canada Humira

Index Terms Antitumor Necrosis Factor Alpha (Human); D2E7; Human Antitumor Necrosis Factor Alpha

Pharmacologic Category Antirheumatic, Disease Modifying; Gastrointestinal Agent, Miscellaneous; Monoclonal Antibody; Tumor Necrosis Factor (TNF) Blocking Agent

Use

Ankylosing spondylitis: Treatment (to reduce signs/symptoms) of ankylosing spondylitis in adult patients

Crohn disease: Treatment (to reduce signs/symptoms and to induce and maintain clinical remission) of active Crohn disease (moderate to severe) in adult patients with inadequate response to conventional treatment or who have lost response to or are intolerant of infliximab and in pediatric patients (≥6 years of age [US labeling] or ≥13 years of age [Canadian labeling]) who have had an inadequate response to corticosteroids or immunomodulators (such as azathioprine, 6-mercaptopurine, or methotrexate.

Hidradenitis suppurativa: Treatment of moderate to severe hidradenitis suppurativa

Juvenile idiopathic arthritis: Treatment (to reduce signs/symptoms) of active polyarticular juvenile idiopathic arthritis (moderate to severe) in patients ≥2 years of age; may be used alone or in combination with methotrexate

Plaque psoriasis: Treatment of chronic plaque psoriasis (moderate to severe) in adult patients who are candidates for systemic therapy or phototherapy and when other agents are less appropriate (with close monitoring and regular follow-up)

Psoriatic arthritis: Treatment (to reduce signs/symptoms, inhibit progression of structural damage, and improve physical function) of active psoriatic arthritis in adult patients; may be used alone or in combination with methotrexate or other nonbiologic DMARDs

Rheumatoid arthritis: Treatment (to reduce signs/symptoms, to induce major clinical response, inhibit progression of structural damage, and improve physical function) of active rheumatoid arthritis (moderate to severe) in adult patients; may be used alone or in combination with methotrexate or other nonbiologic DMARDs

Ulcerative colitis: Treatment (to induce and sustain clinical remission) of active ulcerative colitis (moderate to severe) in adult patients unresponsive to immunosuppressants (**Note:** Efficacy in patients that are intolerant to or no longer responsive to other TNF blockers has not been established.)

Pregnancy Considerations Adverse events were not observed in animal reproduction studies. Adalimumab crosses the placenta and can be detected in cord blood at birth at concentrations higher than those in the maternal serum. In one study of pregnant women with inflammatory bowel disease, adalimumab was found to be measurable in a newborn for up to 11 weeks following delivery. Maternal doses of adalimumab were 40 mg every other week (n=9) or 40 mg weekly (n=1) and the last dose was administered 0.14-8 weeks prior to delivery (median 5.5 weeks) (Mahadevan 2013). If therapy for inflammatory bowel disease is needed during pregnancy, adalimumab should be discontinued before 30 weeks gestation in order to decrease exposure to the newborn. In addition, the administration of live vaccines should be postponed until anti-TNF concentrations in the infant are negative (Habal 2012; Mahadeven 2013; Zelinkova 2013).

Women exposed to adalimumab during pregnancy for the treatment of an autoimmune disease (eg, inflammatory bowel disease) may contact the OTIS Autoimmune Diseases Study at 877-311-8972.

Breast-Feeding Considerations Low concentrations of adalimumab may be detected in breast milk but are unlikely to be absorbed by a nursing infant. The US labeling recommends caution be used if administered to a nursing woman. The Canadian labeling recommends a decision be made to discontinue nursing or to discontinue the drug, taking into account the importance of treatment to the mother and to avoid nursing for at least 5 months after the last dose of adalimumab.

Medication Guide Available Yes

Contraindications

There are no contraindications listed in the manufacturer's US labeling.

Canadian labeling: Hypersensitivity to adalimumab or any component of the formulation; severe infection (eg, sepsis, tuberculosis, opportunistic infection); moderate-to-severe heart failure (NYHA class III/IV)

Warnings/Precautions [US Boxed Warnings]: Patients should be evaluated for latent tuberculosis infection with a tuberculin skin test prior to therapy. Treatment of latent tuberculosis should be initiated before adalimumab is used. Tuberculosis (disseminated or extrapulmonary) has been reactivated while on adalimumab. Most cases have been reported within the first 8 months of treatment. **Patients with initial negative tuberculin skin tests should receive continued monitoring for tuberculosis throughout treatment; active tuberculosis has developed in this population during treatment.** An induration of ≥5 mm should be considered a positive skin test result, even for patients previously vaccinated with BCG vaccine. Rare reactivation of hepatitis B virus (HBV) has occurred in chronic virus carriers; use with caution; evaluate prior to initiation and during treatment.

[US Boxed Warning]: Patients receiving adalimumab are at increased risk for serious infections which may result in hospitalization and/or fatality; infections usually developed in patients receiving concomitant immunosuppressive agents (eg, methotrexate or corticosteroids) and may present as disseminated (rather than local) disease. Active tuberculosis (or reactivation of latent tuberculosis), invasive fungal (including aspergillosis, blastomycosis, candidiasis, coccidioidomycosis, histoplasmosis, and pneumocystosis) and bacterial, viral or other opportunistic infections (including legionellosis and listeriosis) have been reported in patients receiving TNF-blocking agents, including adalimumab. Monitor closely for signs/symptoms of infection. Discontinue for serious infection or sepsis. Consider risks versus benefits prior to use in patients with a history of chronic or recurrent infection. Consider empiric antifungal therapy in patients who are at risk for invasive fungal infection and develop severe systemic illness. Caution should be exercised when considering use in the elderly or in patients with conditions that predispose them to infections (eg, diabetes) or residence/travel from areas of endemic mycoses (blastomycosis, coccidioidomycosis, histoplasmosis), or with latent or localized infections. Do not initiate adalimumab therapy with clinically important active infection. Patients who develop a new infection while undergoing treatment should be monitored closely. There is limited experience with patients undergoing surgical procedures while on therapy; consider long half-life with planned procedures and monitor closely for infection.

[US Boxed Warning]: Lymphoma and other malignancies (some fatal) have been reported in children and adolescent patients receiving TNF-blocking agents, including adalimumab. Half the cases are lymphomas (Hodgkin and non-Hodgkin) and the other cases are varied, but include malignancies not typically observed in this population. Most patients were receiving concomitant immunosuppressants. **[US Boxed Warning]: Hepatosplenic T-cell lymphoma (HSTCL), a rare T-cell lymphoma, has also been reported primarily in patients with Crohn disease or ulcerative colitis treated with adalimumab and who received concomitant azathioprine or mercaptopurine; reports occurred predominantly in adolescent and young adult males.** Rare cases of lymphoma have also been reported in association with adalimumab. A higher incidence of nonmelanoma skin cancers was noted in adalimumab treated patients, when compared to the control group. Impact on the development and course of malignancies is not fully defined. May exacerbate preexisting or recent-onset central or peripheral nervous system demyelinating disorders. Consider discontinuing use in patients who develop peripheral or central nervous system demyelinating disorders during treatment.

May exacerbate preexisting or recent-onset demyelinating CNS disorders. Worsening and new-onset heart failure (HF) has been reported; use caution in patients with decreased left ventricular function. Use caution in patients with HF (Canadian labeling contraindicates use in NYHA III/IV). Patients should be brought up to date with all immunizations before initiating therapy. No data are available concerning the effects of adalimumab on vaccination. Live vaccines should not be given concurrently. No data are available concerning secondary transmission of live vaccines in patients receiving adalimumab. Rare cases of pancytopenia (including aplastic anemia) have been reported with TNF-blocking agents; with significant hematologic abnormalities, consider discontinuing therapy. Positive antinuclear antibody titers have been detected in patients (with negative baselines) treated with adalimumab. Rare cases of autoimmune disorder, including lupus-like syndrome, have been reported; monitor and discontinue adalimumab if symptoms develop. May cause hypersensitivity reactions, including anaphylaxis; monitor. Infection and malignancy has been reported at a higher incidence in elderly patients compared to younger adults; use caution in elderly patients. Potentially significant drug-drug interactions may exist, requiring dose or frequency adjustment, additional monitoring, and/or selection of alternative therapy.

The packaging (needle cover of prefilled syringe) may contain latex. Some dosage forms may contain polysorbate 80 (also known as Tweens). Hypersensitivity reactions, usually a delayed reaction, have been reported following exposure to pharmaceutical products containing polysorbate 80 in certain individuals (Isaksson 2002; Lucente 2000; Shelley, 1995). Thrombocytopenia, ascites, pulmonary deterioration, and renal and hepatic failure have been reported in premature neonates after receiving parenteral products containing polysorbate 80 (Alade, 1986; CDC, 1984). See manufacturer's labeling. According to the Centers for Disease Control and Prevention (CDC), pen-shaped injection devices should never be used for more than one person (even when the needle is changed) because of the risk of infection. The injection device should be clearly labeled with individual patient information to ensure that the correct pen is used (CDC 2012).

Adverse Reactions

>10%:

Central nervous system: Headache (12%)

Dermatologic: Skin rash (6% to 12%)

Hematologic & oncologic: Positive ANA titer (12%)

Immunologic: Antibody development (3% to 26%; significance unknown)

Local: Injection site reaction (12% to 20%; includes erythema, itching, hemorrhage, pain, swelling)

Neuromuscular & skeletal: Increased creatine phosphokinase (15%)

Respiratory: Upper respiratory tract infection (17%), sinusitis (11%)

1% to 10%:

Cardiovascular: Hypertension (5%), atrial fibrillation (<5%), cardiac arrest (<5%), cardiac arrhythmia (<5%), chest pain (<5%), coronary artery disease (<5%), deep vein thrombosis (<5%), hypertensive encephalopathy (<5%), myocardial infarction (<5%), palpitations (<5%), pericardial effusion (<5%), pericarditis (<5%), peripheral edema (<5%), subdural hematoma (<5%), syncope (<5%), tachycardia (<5%)

Central nervous system: Confusion (<5%), myasthenia (<5%), paresthesia (<5%), thorax pain (<5%)

Dermatologic: Cellulitis, erysipelas

Endocrine & metabolic: Hyperlipidemia (7%), hypercholesterolemia (6%), dehydration (<5%), ketosis (<5%), menstrual disease (<5%), parathyroid disease (<5%)

Gastrointestinal: Nausea (9%), dental caries (≤9%), gastroenteritis (≤9%), rotavirus (≤9%), varicella (≤9%), abdominal pain (7%), cholecystitis (<5%), cholelithiasis (<5%), esophagitis (<5%), gastrointestinal hemorrhage (<5%), vomiting (<5%), diverticulitis

Genitourinary: Urinary tract infection (≤8%), hematuria (5%), cystitis (<5%), pelvic pain (<5%)

Hematologic & oncologic: Adenoma (<5%), agranulocytosis (<5%), paraproteinemia (<5%), polycythemia (<5%), carcinoma (including breast, gastrointestinal, skin, urogenital), malignant lymphoma, malignant melanoma

Hepatic: Increased serum alkaline phosphatase (5%), hepatic necrosis (<5%)

Hypersensitivity: Hypersensitivity reaction (children 6%; adults 1%)

Infection: Herpes simplex infection (≤4%), herpes zoster (≤4%), sepsis

Local: Injection site reaction (8%; other than erythema, itching, hemorrhage, pain, swelling)

Neuromuscular & skeletal: Back pain (6%), arthritis (<5%), arthropathy (<5%), bone disease (<5%), bone fracture (<5%), limb pain (<5%), muscle cramps (<5%), myasthenia (<5%), osteonecrosis (<5%), septic arthritis (<5%), synovitis (<5%), tendon disease (<5%), tremor (<5%), arthralgia (3%; plaque psoriasis)

Ophthalmic: Cataract (<5%)

Renal: Nephrolithiasis (<5%), pyelonephritis

Respiratory: Flu-like symptoms (7%), asthma (<5%), bronchospasm (<5%), dyspnea (<5%), pleural effusion (<5%), respiratory depression (<5%), pharyngitis (juvenile idiopathic arthritis: ≤4%), pneumonia (≤4%), tuberculosis (including reactivation of latent infection; disseminated, miliary, lymphatic, peritoneal, and pulmonary)

Miscellaneous: Accidental injury (10%), abnormal healing (<5%), postoperative complication (infection)

<1% (Limited to important or life-threatening): Abscess (limb, perianal), alopecia, anal fissure, anaphylactoid reaction, anaphylaxis, angioedema, aplastic anemia, appendicitis, bacterial infection, basal cell carcinoma, cardiac failure, cerebrovascular accident, cervical dysplasia, circulatory shock, cytopenia, dermal ulcer, endometrial hyperplasia, erythema multiforme, fixed drug eruption, fulminant necrotizing fasciitis, fungal infection, Guillain-Barré syndrome, hepatic failure, hepatitis B (reactivation), hepatosplenic T-cell lymphomas (children, adolescents, and young adults), hepatotoxicity (idiosyncratic) (Chalasani 2014), histoplasmosis, hypersensitivity angiitis, increased serum transaminases, interstitial pulmonary disease (eg, pulmonary fibrosis), intestinal obstruction, intestinal perforation, leukemia, leukopenia, liver metastases, lupus-like syndrome, lymphadenopathy, lymphocytosis, malignant neoplasm of ovary, meningitis (viral), Merkel cell carcinoma, multiple sclerosis, mycobacterium avium complex, myositis (children and adolescents), neutropenia, optic neuritis, pancreatitis, pancytopenia, protozoal infection, psoriasis (including new onset, palmoplantar, pustular, or exacerbation), pulmonary embolism, respiratory failure, sarcoidosis, septic shock, skin granuloma (annulare; children and adolescents), Stevens-Johnson syndrome, streptococcal pharyngitis (children and adolescents), systemic lupus erythematosus, testicular neoplasm, thrombocytopenia, vasculitis (systemic), viral infection

Drug Interactions

Metabolism/Transport Effects None known.

Avoid Concomitant Use

Avoid concomitant use of Adalimumab with any of the following: Abatacept; Anakinra; BCG (Intravesical); Belimumab; Canakinumab; Certolizumab Pegol; InFLIXimab; Natalizumab; Pimecrolimus; Rilonacept; Tacrolimus (Topical); Tocilizumab; Tofacitinib; Vaccines (Live); Vedolizumab

Increased Effect/Toxicity

Adalimumab may increase the levels/effects of: Abatacept; Anakinra; Belimumab; Canakinumab; Certolizumab Pegol; Fingolimod; InFLIXimab; Leflunomide; Natalizumab; Rilonacept; Tofacitinib; Vaccines (Live); Vedolizumab

The levels/effects of Adalimumab may be increased by: Denosumab; Pimecrolimus; Roflumilast; Tacrolimus (Topical); Tocilizumab; Trastuzumab

Decreased Effect

Adalimumab may decrease the levels/effects of: BCG (Intravesical); Coccidioides immitis Skin Test; CycloSPORINE (Systemic); Sipuleucel-T; Theophylline Derivatives; Vaccines (Inactivated); Vaccines (Live); Warfarin

The levels/effects of Adalimumab may be decreased by: Echinacea

Storage/Stability Store at 2°C to 8°C (36°F to 46°F) in original container; do not freeze. Do not use if frozen even if it has been thawed. Do not store in extreme heat or cold. Protect from light. Allow to reach room temperature for 15 to 30 minutes prior to administration. If needed, may be stored at room temperature up to a maximum of 25°C (77°F) for up to 14 days; discard if not used within 14 days.

Mechanism of Action Adalimumab is a recombinant monoclonal antibody that binds to human tumor necrosis factor alpha (TNF-alpha), thereby interfering with binding to TNFα receptor sites and subsequent cytokine-driven inflammatory processes. Elevated TNF levels in the synovial fluid are involved in the pathologic pain and joint destruction in immune-mediated arthritis. Adalimumab decreases signs and symptoms of psoriatic arthritis, rheumatoid arthritis, and ankylosing spondylitis. It inhibits progression of structural damage of rheumatoid and psoriatic arthritis. Reduces signs and symptoms and maintains clinical remission in Crohn disease and ulcerative colitis; reduces epidermal thickness and inflammatory cell infiltration in plaque psoriasis.

Pharmacodynamics/Kinetics

Distribution: V_d: 4.7 to 6 L; Synovial fluid concentrations: 31% to 96% of serum

Bioavailability: Absolute: 64%

Half-life elimination: Terminal: ~2 weeks (range: 10 to 20 days)

Time to peak, serum: SubQ: 131 ± 56 hours

Dosing

Adult & Geriatric

Ankylosing spondylitis: SubQ: 40 mg every other week (may continue methotrexate, other nonbiologic DMARDS, corticosteroids, NSAIDs and/or analgesics)

Crohn disease: SubQ (may continue aminosalicylates and/or corticosteroids; if necessary, azathioprine, mercaptopurine, or methotrexate may also be continued):

Initial: 160 mg (given as four 40 mg injections on day 1 **or** given as two 40 mg injections per day over 2 consecutive days), then 80 mg 2 weeks later (day 15).

Maintenance: 40 mg every other week beginning day 29. **Note:** Some patients may require 40 mg every week as maintenance therapy (Lichtenstein 2009).

Hidradenitis suppurativa: SubQ:

Initial: 160 mg (given as four 40 mg injections on day 1 **or** given as two 40 mg injections per day over 2 consecutive days), then 80 mg 2 weeks later (day 15).

Maintenance: 40 mg every week beginning day 29.

Plaque psoriasis: SubQ:

Initial: 80 mg as a single dose

Maintenance: 40 mg every other week beginning 1 week after initial dose

Psoriatic arthritis: SubQ: 40 mg every other week (may continue methotrexate, other nonbiologic DMARDS, corticosteroids, NSAIDs and/or analgesics)

Rheumatoid arthritis: SubQ: 40 mg every other week (may continue methotrexate, other nonbiologic DMARDS, corticosteroids, NSAIDs, and/or analgesics); patients not taking concomitant methotrexate may increase adalimumab dose to 40 mg every week

Ulcerative colitis: SubQ (may continue aminosalicylates and/or corticosteroids; if necessary, azathioprine, or mercaptopurine may also be continued):

Initial: 160 mg (given as four 40 mg injections on day 1 **or** given as two 40 mg injections per day over 2 consecutive days), then 80 mg 2 weeks later (day 15).

Maintenance: 40 mg every other week beginning day 29. **Note:** Only continue maintenance dose in patients demonstrating clinical remission by 8 weeks (day 57) of therapy.

Pediatric

Crohn disease: SubQ:

Children ≥6 years and Adolescents:

US labeling:

17 kg to <40 kg:

Initial: 80 mg (administered as two 40 mg injections on day 1), then 40 mg 2 weeks later (day 15).

Maintenance: 20 mg every other week beginning week 4 (day 29).

≥40 kg:

Initial: 160 mg (administered as four 40 mg injections on day 1 **or** as two 40 mg injections per day over 2 consecutive days), then 80 mg 2 weeks later (day 15; given as two 40 mg injections on the same day).

Maintenance: 40 mg every other week beginning week 4 (day 29).

Adolescents ≥13 years and ≥40 kg:

Canadian labeling:

Initial: 160 mg (given as four 40 mg injections on day 1 **or** given as two 40 mg injections per day over 2 consecutive days), then 80 mg 2 weeks later (day 15; given as two 40 mg injections on the same day).

Maintenance: 20 mg every other week beginning week 4 (day 29); may consider increasing dose to 40 mg every other week for disease flare or inadequate response. Potential benefits of continued therapy should be reassessed if inadequate response at 12 weeks.

Juvenile idiopathic arthritis (JIA): SubQ:

Children ≥2 years and Adolescents:

US labeling:

10 to <15 kg: 10 mg every other week

15 kg to <30 kg: 20 mg every other week

≥30 kg: 40 mg every other week

Canadian labeling:

2 to <4 years (≥10 kg): 24 mg/m²/dose (maximum: 20 mg/dose) every other week

4 to 17 years (≥10 kg): 24 mg/m²/dose (maximum: 40 mg/dose) every other week

Renal Impairment There are no dosage adjustments provided in the manufacturer's labeling (has not been studied).

Hepatic Impairment There are no dosage adjustments provided in the manufacturer's labeling (has not been studied).

Administration For SubQ injection at separate sites in the thigh or lower abdomen (avoiding areas within 2 inches of navel); rotate injection sites. May leave at room temperature for ~15 to 30 minutes prior to use; do not remove cap or cover while allowing product to reach room temperature. Do not use if solution is discolored or contains particulate matter. Do not administer to skin which is red, tender, bruised, or hard. Needle cap of the prefilled syringe or needle cover for the adalimumab pen may contain latex. Prefilled pens and syringes are available for use by patients and the full amount of the syringe should be injected (self-administration); the vial is intended for institutional use only. Vials do not contain a preservative; discard unused portion.

Monitoring Parameters Monitor improvement of symptoms and physical function assessments. Latent TB screening prior to initiating and during therapy; signs/symptoms of active infection, including tuberculosis (prior to, during, and following therapy); CBC with differential; signs/symptoms/worsening of heart failure; HBV screening prior to initiating (all patients), HBV carriers (during and for several months following therapy); signs and symptoms of hypersensitivity reaction; symptoms of lupus-like syndrome; signs/symptoms of malignancy (eg, splenomegaly, hepatomegaly, abdominal pain, persistent fever, night sweats, weight loss), including periodic skin examination.

Dosage Forms Excipient information presented when available (limited, particularly for generics); consult specific product labeling.

Pen-injector Kit, Subcutaneous [preservative free]:

Humira Pen: 40 mg/0.8 mL (1 ea) [contains polysorbate 80]

Humira Pen-Crohns Starter: 40 mg/0.8 mL (1 ea) [contains polysorbate 80]

Humira Pen-Psoriasis Starter: 40 mg/0.8 mL (1 ea) [contains polysorbate 80]

Prefilled Syringe Kit, Subcutaneous [preservative free]:

Humira: 10 mg/0.2 mL (1 ea); 20 mg/0.4 mL (1 ea); 40 mg/0.8 mL (1 ea) [contains polysorbate 80]

Humira Pediatric Crohns Start: 40 mg/0.8 mL (1 ea) [contains polysorbate 80]

Dosage Forms: Canada Also refer to Dosage Forms. Excipient information presented when available (limited, particularly for generics); consult specific product labeling.

Injection, solution [pediatric, preservative free]:

Humira: 40 mg/0.8 mL (0.8 mL) [vial] [contains polysorbate 80]

◆ **Adamantanamine Hydrochloride** *see* Amantadine *on page 86*

Adapalene (a DAP a leen)

Brand Names: US Differin

Brand Names: Canada Differin®; Differin® XP

Pharmacologic Category Acne Products; Topical Skin Product, Acne

Use Acne vulgaris: Treatment of acne vulgaris.

Dosing

Adult & Geriatric Acne vulgaris: Topical: Apply once daily; use cream and gel in the evening before bedtime

Pediatric Acne vulgaris: Children ≥12 years and Adolescents: Refer to adult dosing.

Renal Impairment There are no dosage adjustments provided in manufacturer's labeling; however, systemic absorption is not extensive, making the need for a dose adjustment unlikely.

Hepatic Impairment There are no dosage adjustments provided in manufacturer's labeling; however, systemic absorption is not extensive, making the need for a dose adjustment unlikely.

Additional Information Complete prescribing information should be consulted for additional detail.

Dosage Forms Excipient information presented when available (limited, particularly for generics); consult specific product labeling.

Cream, External:

Differin: 0.1% (45 g)

Generic: 0.1% (45 g)

Gel, External:

Differin: 0.1% (45 g)

Differin: 0.3% (45 g) [contains edetate disodium, methylparaben, propylene glycol]

Generic: 0.1% (45 g); 0.3% (45 g)

Lotion, External:

Differin: 0.1% (59 mL) [contains methylparaben, propylene glycol, propylparaben]

Generic: 0.1% (59 mL)

Adapalene and Benzoyl Peroxide
(a DAP a leen & BEN zoe il peer OKS ide)

Brand Names: US Epiduo; Epiduo Forte

Brand Names: Canada Tactupump; Tactupump Plus

Index Terms Benzoyl Peroxide and Adapalene; Epiduo Forte

Pharmacologic Category Acne Products; Topical Skin Product; Topical Skin Product, Acne

Use Acne vulgaris:

US labeling: Topical treatment of acne vulgaris in patients 9 years and older (Epiduo) or 12 years and older (Epiduo Forte).

Canadian labeling: Topical treatment of mild and moderate acne vulgaris, characterized by comedones, inflammatory papules/pustules in patients 9 years and older (Tactupump) or treatment of moderate and severe acne vulgaris characterized by comedones, inflammatory papules/pustules with or without occasional nodules in patients 12 years and older (Tactupump Plus).

Dosing

Adult & Geriatric

Acne vulgaris: Adapalene 0.1%/benzoyl peroxide 2.5% or Adapalene 0.3%/benzoyl peroxide 2.5%: Topical: Apply to affected areas of skin once daily.

Pediatric

Acne vulgaris:

Adapalene 0.1%/benzoyl peroxide 2.5%: Children ≥9 years and Adolescents: Topical: Refer to adult dosing.

Adapalene 0.3%/benzoyl peroxide 2.5%: Children ≥12 years and Adolescents: Topical: Refer to adult dosing.

Renal Impairment There are no dosage adjustments provided in manufacturer's labeling; however, systemic absorption is not extensive making the need for a dose adjustment unlikely.

Hepatic Impairment There are no dosage adjustments provided in manufacturer's labeling; however, systemic absorption is not extensive making the need for a dose adjustment unlikely.

Additional Information Complete prescribing information should be consulted for additional detail.

Dosage Forms Excipient information presented when available (limited, particularly for generics); consult specific product labeling.

Gel, topical:

Epiduo: Adapalene 0.1% and benzoyl peroxide 2.5% (45 g)

Epiduo Forte: Adapalene 0.3% and benzoyl peroxide 2.5% (45 g)

Dosage Forms: Canada Excipient information presented when available (limited, particularly for generics); consult specific product labeling.

Gel, topical:

Tactupump: Adapalene 0.1% and benzoyl peroxide 2.5% (70 g)

Tactupump Plus: Adapalene 0.3% and benzoyl peroxide 2.5% (70 g)

◆ **Adasuve** *see* Loxapine *on page 1113*

◆ **Adcetris** *see* Brentuximab Vedotin *on page 250*

- Adcirca *see* Tadalafil *on page 1730*
- ADD 234037 *see* Lacosamide *on page 1021*
- Addaprin [OTC] *see* Ibuprofen *on page 905*
- Adderall *see* Dextroamphetamine and Amphetamine *on page 533*
- Adderall XR *see* Dextroamphetamine and Amphetamine *on page 533*
- Addyi *see* Flibanserin *on page 774*

Adefovir (a DEF o veer)

Brand Names: US Hepsera
Brand Names: Canada Hepsera
Index Terms Adefovir Dipivoxil; Bis-POM PMEA
Pharmacologic Category Antihepadnaviral, Reverse Transcriptase Inhibitor, Nucleotide (Anti-HBV)
Use Treatment of chronic hepatitis B with evidence of active viral replication (based on persistent elevation of ALT/AST or histologic evidence), including patients with lamivudine-resistant hepatitis B
Pregnancy Considerations Adverse events have been observed in animal reproduction studies.

Health care providers are encouraged to enroll women exposed to adefovir during pregnancy in the Hepsera pregnancy registry (800-258-4263).

Breast-Feeding Considerations It is not known if adefovir is excreted in breast milk. Due to the potential for serious adverse reactions in the nursing infant, the manufacturer recommends a decision be made whether to discontinue nursing or to discontinue the drug, taking into account the importance of treatment to the mother.

Contraindications Hypersensitivity to adefovir or any component of the formulation

Warnings/Precautions [U.S. Boxed Warning]: Use with caution in patients with renal dysfunction or in patients at risk of renal toxicity (including concurrent nephrotoxic agents or NSAIDs). Chronic administration may result in nephrotoxicity. Dosage adjustment is required in adult patients with renal dysfunction or in patients who develop renal dysfunction during therapy; no data available for use in children ≥12 years or adolescents with renal impairment. Not recommended as first line therapy of chronic HBV due to weak antiviral activity and high rate of resistance after first year. May be more appropriate as second-line agent in treatment-naïve patients. Combination therapy with lamivudine in nucleoside-naïve patients has not been shown to provide synergistic antiviral effects. In patients with lamivudine-resistant HBV, switching to adefovir monotherapy was associated with a higher risk of adefovir resistance compared to adding adefovir to lamivudine therapy (Lok, 2009).

Calculate creatinine clearance before initiation of therapy. Consider alternative therapy in patients who do not respond to adefovir monotherapy treatment. **[U.S. Boxed Warning]: May cause the development of HIV resistance in patients with unrecognized or untreated HIV infection.** Determine HIV status prior to initiating treatment with adefovir. **[U.S. Boxed Warning]: Fatal cases of lactic acidosis and severe hepatomegaly with steatosis have been reported with the use of nucleoside analogues alone or in combination with other antiretrovirals.** Female gender, obesity, and prolonged treatment may increase the risk of hepatotoxicity. Treatment should be discontinued in patients with lactic acidosis or signs/symptoms of hepatotoxicity (which may occur without marked transaminase elevations). **[U.S. Boxed Warning]: Acute exacerbations of hepatitis may occur (in up to 25% of patients) when antihepatitis therapy is discontinued.** Exacerbations typically occur within 12 weeks and may be self-limited or resolve upon resuming treatment; risk may be increased with advanced liver disease or cirrhosis. Monitor patients following discontinuation of therapy. Ethanol should be avoided in hepatitis B infection due to potential hepatic toxicity. Do not use concurrently with tenofovir (Viread®) or any product containing tenofovir (eg, Truvada®, Atripla®, Complera®).

Adverse Reactions
>10%:
Central nervous system: Headache (24% to 25%)
Gastrointestinal: Abdominal pain (15%), diarrhea (up to 13%)
Hepatic: Hepatitis exacerbation (up to 25% within 12 weeks of adefovir discontinuation)
Neuromuscular & skeletal: Weakness (up to 25%)
Renal: Hematuria (grade ≥3: 11%)

1% to 10%:
Dermatologic: Rash, pruritus
Endocrine & metabolic: Hypophosphatemia (<2 mg/dL; 1% and 3% in pre-/post-liver transplant patients, respectively)
Gastrointestinal: Flatulence (up to 8%), dyspepsia (5% to 9%), nausea, vomiting
Neuromuscular & skeletal: Back pain (up to 10%)
Renal: Serum creatinine increased (≥0.5 mg/dL: 2% to 3% in compensated liver disease; incidence may be higher in patients with decompensated cirrhosis or in liver transplant recipients), renal failure
Note: In liver transplant patients with baseline renal dysfunction, frequency of increased serum creatinine has been observed to be as high as 32% to 51% at 48 and 96 weeks post-transplantation, respectively; considering the concomitant use of other potentially nephrotoxic medications, baseline renal insufficiency, and predisposing comorbidities, the role of adefovir in these changes could not be established.
Respiratory: Cough (6% to 8%), rhinitis (up to 5%)
Postmarketing and/or case reports: Fanconi syndrome, hepatitis, myopathy, nephrotoxicity, osteomalacia, pancreatitis, proximal renal tubulopathy

Drug Interactions
Metabolism/Transport Effects None known.
Avoid Concomitant Use
Avoid concomitant use of Adefovir with any of the following: Tenofovir Products
Increased Effect/Toxicity
Adefovir may increase the levels/effects of: Tenofovir Products

The levels/effects of Adefovir may be increased by: Ganciclovir-Valganciclovir; Ribavirin (Oral Inhalation); Ribavirin (Systemic); Tenofovir Products
Decreased Effect
Adefovir may decrease the levels/effects of: Tenofovir Products
Food Interactions Food does not have a significant effect on adefovir absorption. Management: Administer without regard to meals.
Storage/Stability Store controlled room temperature of 25°C (77°F); excursions permitted between 15°C to 30°C (59°F to 86°F).
Mechanism of Action Acyclic nucleotide reverse transcriptase inhibitor (adenosine analog) which interferes with HBV viral RNA-dependent DNA polymerase resulting in inhibition of viral replication.
Pharmacodynamics/Kinetics
Distribution: 0.35 to 0.39 L/kg
Protein binding: ≤4%
Metabolism: Prodrug; rapidly converted to adefovir (active metabolite) in intestine
Bioavailability: 59%
Half-life elimination: 7.5 hours; prolonged in renal impairment
Time to peak: Median: 1.75 hours (range: 0.58 to 4 hours)
Excretion: Urine (45% as active metabolite within 24 hours); Dialysis: ~35% of dose (10 mg) removed during 4 hours hemodialysis session
Dosing
Adult & Geriatric Hepatitis B (chronic): Oral: 10 mg once daily
Treatment duration (AASLD practice guidelines): Adults:
Hepatitis Be antigen (HBeAg) positive chronic hepatitis: Treat ≥1 year until HBeAg seroconversion and undetectable serum HBV DNA; continue therapy for ≥6 months after HBeAg seroconversion
HBeAg negative chronic hepatitis: Treat >1 year until hepatitis B surface antigen (HBsAg) clearance
Note: Patients not achieving a <2 log decrease in serum HBV DNA after at least 6 months of therapy should either receive additional treatment or be switched to an alternative therapy (Lok, 2009).
Pediatric Hepatitis B (chronic): Children ≥12 years: Oral: 10 mg once daily
Renal Impairment Adult recommendations only (no dosage adjustment recommendations available for patients <18 years with renal impairment):
CrCl ≥50 mL/minute: No dosage adjustment necessary
CrCl 20-49 mL/minute: 10 mg every 48 hours
CrCl 10-19 mL/minute: 10 mg every 72 hours
Hemodialysis: 10 mg every 7 days (following dialysis)
Hepatic Impairment No adjustment required.
Dietary Considerations May be taken without regard to food.
Administration May be administered without regard to food.

Monitoring Parameters HIV status (prior to initiation of therapy); serum creatinine (prior to initiation and during therapy; every 3 months in patients with medical conditions which predispose to renal insufficiency and in all patients treated for >1 year; more frequent monitoring required if preexisting real insufficiency detected [Lok, 2009]); LFTs for several months following discontinuation of adefovir; HBV DNA (every 3-6 months during therapy); HBeAg and anti-HBe

Additional Information Adefovir dipivoxil is a prodrug, rapidly converted to the active component (adefovir). It was previously investigated as a treatment for HIV infections (at dosages substantially higher than the approved dose for hepatitis B). The NDA was withdrawn, and no further studies in the treatment of HIV are anticipated (per manufacturer).

Dosage Forms Excipient information presented when available (limited, particularly for generics); consult specific product labeling.
Tablet, Oral, as dipivoxil:
Hepsera: 10 mg
Generic: 10 mg

Adenosine (a DEN oh seen)

Brand Names: US Adenocard; Adenoscan
Brand Names: Canada Adenocard; Adenosine Injection, USP; PMS-Adenosine
Index Terms 9-Beta-D-Ribofuranosyladenine
Pharmacologic Category Antiarrhythmic Agent, Miscellaneous; Diagnostic Agent
Additional Appendix Information
Adult ACLS Algorithms on page 1993
Pediatric ALS (PALS) Algorithms on page 1990
Use
Adenocard: Treatment of paroxysmal supraventricular tachycardia (PSVT) including that associated with accessory bypass tracts (Wolff-Parkinson-White syndrome); when clinically advisable, appropriate vagal maneuvers should be attempted prior to adenosine administration; **not effective for conversion of atrial fibrillation, atrial flutter, or ventricular tachycardia**

Note: While adenosine will not convert atrial fibrillation or atrial flutter, the transient AV-nodal block may aid in the identification of the arrhythmia by exposing the underlying atrial fibrillation or flutter electrocardiographic morphology.

Adenoscan: Pharmacologic stress agent used in myocardial perfusion thallium-201 scintigraphy

Pregnancy Considerations Animal reproduction studies have not been conducted. Adenosine is an endogenous substance and adverse fetal effects would not be anticipated. Case reports of administration during pregnancy have indicated no adverse effects on fetus or newborn attributable to adenosine (Blomström-Lundqvist 2003). ACLS guidelines suggest use is safe and effective in pregnancy (ACLS [Neumar 2010]).

Breast-Feeding Considerations It is not known if adenosine is excreted in breast milk following maternal administration. Adenosine is endogenous in breast milk (Sugawara 1995). Due to the potential for adverse reactions in the nursing infant, the manufacturer recommends a decision be made to interrupt nursing or not administer adenosine taking into account the importance of treatment to the mother.

Contraindications Hypersensitivity to adenosine or any component of the formulation; second- or third-degree AV block, sick sinus syndrome, or symptomatic bradycardia (except in patients with a functioning artificial pacemaker); known or suspected bronchoconstrictive or bronchospastic lung disease (Adenoscan), asthma (ACLS [Neumar, 2010]; Adenoscan prescribing information, 2014)

Warnings/Precautions ECG monitoring required during use. Equipment for resuscitation and trained personnel experienced in handling medical emergencies should always be immediately available. Adenosine decreases conduction through the AV node and may produce first-, second-, or third-degree heart block. Patients with preexisting S-A nodal dysfunction may experience prolonged sinus pauses after adenosine; use caution in patients with first-degree AV block or bundle branch block. Use is contraindicated in patients with high-grade AV block, sinus node dysfunction or symptomatic bradycardia (unless a functional artificial pacemaker is in place). Rare, prolonged episodes of asystole have been reported, with fatal

outcomes in some cases. Discontinue adenosine in any patient who develops persistent or symptomatic high-grade AV block. Use caution in patients receiving other drugs which slow AV node conduction (eg, digoxin, verapamil). Potentially significant interactions may exist, requiring dose or frequency adjustment, additional monitoring, and/or selection of alternative therapy.

There have been reports of atrial fibrillation/flutter after adenosine administration in patients with PSVT associated with accessory conduction pathways; has also been reported in patients with or without a history of atrial fibrillation undergoing myocardial perfusion imaging with adenosine infusion. Adenosine may also produce profound vasodilation with subsequent hypotension. When used as a bolus dose (PSVT), effects are generally self-limiting (due to the short half-life of adenosine). However, when used as a continuous infusion (pharmacologic stress testing), effects may be more pronounced and persistent, corresponding to continued exposure; discontinue infusion in patients who develop persistent or symptomatic hypotension. Adenosine infusions should be used with caution in patients with autonomic dysfunction, stenotic valvular heart disease, pericarditis, pleural effusion, carotid stenosis (with cerebrovascular insufficiency), or uncorrected hypovolemia. Use caution in elderly patients; may be at increased risk of hemodynamic effects, bradycardia, and/or AV block.

Avoid use in patients with bronchoconstriction or bronchospasm (eg, asthma); dyspnea, bronchoconstriction, and respiratory compromise have occurred during use. Per the ACLS guidelines and the manufacturer of Adenoscan, use considered contraindicated in patients with asthma. Use caution in patients with obstructive lung disease not associated with bronchoconstriction (eg, emphysema, bronchitis). Immediately discontinue therapy if severe respiratory difficulty is observed. Appropriate measures for resuscitation should be available during use.

Adenocard: Transient AV block is expected. Administer as a rapid bolus, either directly into a vein or (if administered into an IV line), as close to the patient as possible (followed by saline flush). Dose reduction recommended when administered via central line (ACLS, 2010). When used in PSVT, at the time of conversion to normal sinus rhythm, a variety of new rhythms may appear on the ECG. Watch for proarrhythmic effects (eg, polymorphic ventricular tachycardia) during and shortly after administration/termination of arrhythmia. Benign transient occurrence of atrial and ventricular ectopy is common upon termination of arrhythmia. Adenosine does not convert atrial fibrillation/flutter to normal sinus rhythm; however, may be used diagnostically in these settings if the underlying rhythm is not apparent. Adenosine should not be used in patients with Wolff-Parkinson-White (WPW) syndrome and preexcited atrial fibrillation/flutter since ventricular fibrillation may result (AHA/ACC/HRS [January, 2014]). Use with extreme caution in heart transplant recipients; adenosine may cause prolonged asystole; reduction of initial adenosine dose is recommended (ACLS, 2010); considered by some to be contraindicated in this setting (Delacrétaz, 2006). Avoid use in irregular or polymorphic wide-complex tachycardias; may cause degeneration to ventricular fibrillation (ACLS, 2010). When used for PSVT, dosage reduction recommended when used with concomitant drugs which potentiate the effects of adenosine (carbamazepine, dipyridamole)

Adenoscan: Hypersensitivity reactions (including dyspnea, pharyngeal edema, erythema, flushing, rash, or chest discomfort) have been reported following Adenoscan administration. Seizures (new-onset or recurrent) have been reported following Adenoscan administration; risk may be increased with concurrent use of aminophylline. Use of any methylxanthine (eg, aminophylline, caffeine, theophylline) is not recommended in patients experiencing seizures associated with Adenoscan administration. Drugs which antagonize adenosine (theophylline [includes aminophylline], caffeine) should be withheld for five half-lives prior to adenosine use. Avoid dietary caffeine for at least 12 hours prior to pharmacologic stress testing (Henzlova, 2006). Withhold dipyridamole-containing medications for at least 24 hours prior to pharmacologic stress testing (Henzlova, 2006).

Cardiovascular events: Cardiac arrest (fatal and nonfatal), myocardial infarction (MI), cerebrovascular accident (hemorrhagic and ischemic), and sustained ventricular tachycardia (requiring resuscitation) have occurred following Adenoscan use. Avoid use in patients with signs or symptoms of unstable angina, acute myocardial ischemia, or cardiovascular instability due to possible increased risk of significant cardiovascular consequences. Appropriate measures for resuscitation should be available during

use. In addition, systolic and diastolic pressure increases have been observed with Adenoscan infusion. In most instances, blood pressure increases resolved spontaneously within several minutes; occasionally, hypertension lasted for several hours.

Pulmonary artery hypertension: Acute vasodilator testing (not an approved use): Use with extreme caution in patients with concomitant heart failure (LV systolic dysfunction with significantly elevated left heart filling pressures) or pulmonary veno-occlusive disease/pulmonary capillary hemangiomatosis; significant decompensation has occurred with other highly selective pulmonary vasodilators resulting in acute pulmonary edema.

Adverse Reactions Note: Frequency varies based on use and is not always defined; higher frequency of infusion-related effects, such as flushing and lightheadedness/dizziness, were reported with continuous infusion (Adenoscan).

>10%:
Cardiovascular: Cardiac arrhythmia (transient and new arrhythmia after cardioversion; eg, atrial premature contractions, atrial fibrillation, premature ventricular contractions; 55%), chest pressure (and discomfort; 7% to 40%)
Central nervous system: Headache (2% to 18%), dizziness (≤12%)
Dermatologic: Facial flushing (18% to 44%)
Gastrointestinal: Gastrointestinal distress (13%)
Neuromuscular & skeletal: Neck discomfort (includes throat, jaw; <1% to 15%)
Respiratory: Dyspnea (12% to 28%)
1% to 10%:
Cardiovascular: Atrioventricular block (infusion 6%; third-degree <1%), depression of ST segment on ECG (3%), hypotension (<1% to 2%), chest pain, palpitations
Central nervous system: Nervousness (2%), paresthesia (≤2%), numbness (1%), apprehension
Dermatologic: Diaphoresis
Gastrointestinal: Nausea (3%)
Neuromuscular & skeletal: Upper extremity discomfort (≤4%)
Respiratory: Hyperventilation
<1% (Limited to important or life-threatening): Atrial fibrillation, blurred vision, bradycardia, bronchospasm, cardiac arrest, increased intracranial pressure, injection site reaction, myocardial infarction, respiratory arrest, torsades de pointes, transient hypertension, ventricular arrhythmia, ventricular fibrillation, ventricular tachycardia

Drug Interactions
Metabolism/Transport Effects None known.
Avoid Concomitant Use There are no known interactions where it is recommended to avoid concomitant use.
Increased Effect/Toxicity
The levels/effects of Adenosine may be increased by: CarBAMazepine; Digoxin; Dipyridamole; Nicotine
Decreased Effect
The levels/effects of Adenosine may be decreased by: Caffeine and Caffeine Containing Products; Theophylline Derivatives

Storage/Stability Store between 15°C and 30°C (59°F and 86°F). Do **not** refrigerate; crystallization may occur (may dissolve by warming to room temperature).

Mechanism of Action
Antiarrhythmic actions: Slows conduction time through the AV node, interrupting the re-entry pathways through the AV node, restoring normal sinus rhythm
Myocardial perfusion scintigraphy: Adenosine also causes coronary vasodilation and increases blood flow in normal coronary arteries with little to no increase in stenotic coronary arteries; thallium-201 uptake into the stenotic coronary arteries will be less than that of normal coronary arteries revealing areas of insufficient blood flow.

Pharmacodynamics/Kinetics
Onset of action: Rapid
Duration: Very brief
Metabolism: Removed from systemic circulation primarily by vascular endothelial cells and erythrocytes (by cellular uptake); rapidly metabolized intracellularly; phosphorylated by adenosine kinase to adenosine monophosphate (AMP) which is then incorporated into high-energy pool; intracellular adenosine is also deaminated by adenosine deaminase to inosine; inosine can be metabolized to hypoxanthine, then xanthine and finally to uric acid.
Half-life elimination: <10 seconds

Dosing
Adult
Paroxysmal supraventricular tachycardia (Adenocard): IV (rapid, over 1 to 2 seconds, via peripheral line; see **Note**): Initial: 6 mg; if not effective within 1 to 2 minutes, 12 mg may be given; may repeat 12 mg bolus

if needed (maximum single dose: 12 mg). Follow each dose with 20 mL normal saline flush. **Note:** Initial dose of adenosine should be reduced to 3 mg if patient is currently receiving carbamazepine or dipyridamole, has a transplanted heart or if adenosine is administered via central line (ACLS 2010; Chang 2002).

Pharmacologic stress testing (Adenoscan): IV: Continuous IV infusion via peripheral line: 140 mcg/kg/minute for 6 minutes using syringe or volumetric infusion pump; total dose: 840 mcg/kg. Thallium-201 is injected at midpoint (3 minutes) of infusion.

Acute vasodilator testing in pulmonary artery hypertension (off-label use) (Adenoscan): IV: Initial: 50 mcg/kg/minute increased by 50 mcg/kg/minute every 2 minutes to a maximum dose of 500 mcg/kg/minute (Schrader, 1992) or to a maximum dose of 350 mcg/kg/minute(ACCF/AHA [McLaughlin, 2009]; ESC/ERS/ISHLT [Galie 2009]; Zuo 2012); acutely assess vasodilator response

Geriatric Refer to adult dosing. Elderly may be more sensitive to effects of adenosine.

Pediatric Rapid IV push (over 1 to 2 seconds) via peripheral line, followed by a normal saline flush: Paroxysmal supraventricular tachycardia (Adenocard): Infants and Children: IV:
Manufacturer's labeling:
Children <50 kg: Initial: 0.05 to 0.1 mg/kg (maximum initial dose: 6 mg). If conversion of PSVT does not occur within 1 to 2 minutes, may increase dose by 0.05 to 0.1 mg/kg. May repeat until sinus rhythm is established or to a maximum single dose of 0.3 mg/kg or 12 mg. Follow each dose with normal saline flush.
Children ≥50 kg: Refer to adult dosing.
Pediatric advanced life support (PALS, 2010): Treatment of SVT: IV, I.O.: Initial: 0.1 mg/kg (maximum initial dose: 6 mg); if not effective within 1 to 2 minutes, administer 0.2 mg/kg (maximum single dose: 12 mg). Follow each dose with ≥5 mL normal saline flush.

Renal Impairment There are no dosage adjustments provided in the manufacturer's labeling. However, adenosine is not renally eliminated.

Hepatic Impairment There are no dosage adjustments provided in the manufacturer's labeling. However, adenosine is not hepatically eliminated.

Dietary Considerations Avoid dietary caffeine for at least 12 hours prior to pharmacologic stress testing.

Administration
Adenocard: For rapid bolus IV use only; administer IV push over 1 to 2 seconds at a peripheral IV site as proximal as possible to trunk (not in lower arm, hand, lower leg, or foot); follow each bolus with a rapid normal saline flush (infants and children ≥5 mL; adults 20 mL). Use of 2 syringes (one with adenosine dose and the other with NS flush) connected to a T-connector or stopcock is recommended. If administered via **central line** in adults, reduce initial dose to 3 mg (ACLS 2010; Chang 2002).
Adenoscan: For IV infusion only via peripheral line

Monitoring Parameters ECG, heart rate, blood pressure; consult individual institutional policies and procedures

Dosage Forms Excipient information presented when available (limited, particularly for generics); consult specific product labeling.
Solution, Intravenous:
Adenocard: 6 mg/2 mL (2 mL); 12 mg/4 mL (4 mL)
Adenoscan: 3 mg/mL (20 mL, 30 mL)
Generic: 3 mg/mL (20 mL, 30 mL); 6 mg/2 mL (2 mL)
Solution, Intravenous [preservative free]:
Generic: 3 mg/mL (20 mL, 30 mL); 6 mg/2 mL (2 mL); 12 mg/4 mL (4 mL)

◆ Adenosine Injection, USP (Can) *see* Adenosine *on page 46*

◆ Adept *see* Icodextrin *on page 910*

◆ ADH *see* Vasopressin *on page 1879*

◆ Adipex-P *see* Phentermine *on page 1440*

◆ A&D Jr. [OTC] *see* Vitamin A and Vitamin D (Systemic) *on page 1906*

◆ ADL-2698 *see* Alvimopan *on page 86*

◆ Ado Trastuzumab *see* Ado-Trastuzumab Emtansine *on page 47*

Ado-Trastuzumab Emtansine
(a do tras TU zoo mab em TAN seen)

Brand Names: US Kadcyla
Brand Names: Canada Kadcyla
Index Terms Ado Trastuzumab; Adotrastuzumab; T-DM1; Trastuzumab Emtansine; Trastuzumab-DM1; Trastuzumab-MCC-DM1

Pharmacologic Category Antineoplastic Agent, Anti-HER2; Antineoplastic Agent, Antibody Drug Conjugate; Antineoplastic Agent, Antimicrotubular; Antineoplastic Agent, Monoclonal Antibody

Use Breast cancer, metastatic: Treatment (single-agent) of HER2-positive, metastatic breast cancer in patients who previously received trastuzumab and a taxane, separately or in combination, and have either received prior therapy for metastatic disease or developed disease recurrence during or within 6 months of completing adjuvant therapy.

Pregnancy Considerations Animal reproduction studies have not been conducted. **[US Boxed Warning]: Exposure to ado-trastuzumab emtansine may cause embryo-fetal death or birth defects. Effective contraception must be used in women of reproductive potential.** Oligohydramnios, pulmonary hypoplasia, skeletal malformations and neonatal death were observed following trastuzumab exposure during pregnancy (trastuzumab is the antibody component of ado-trastuzumab emtansine). The DM1 component of the ado-trastuzumab emtansine formulation is toxic to rapidly dividing cells and is also expected to cause fetal harm. Pregnancy status should be verified prior to therapy. Effective contraception is recommended during therapy and for 7 months after the last dose for women of childbearing potential.

If ado-trastuzumab emtansine exposure occurs during pregnancy or within 7 months prior to conception, healthcare providers should report the exposure to the Genentech Adverse Event Line (888-835-2555). Women exposed to ado-trastuzumab emtansine during pregnancy or within 7 months prior to conception are encouraged to enroll in MotHER Pregnancy Registry (1-800-690-6720).

European Society for Medical Oncology (ESMO) guidelines for cancer during pregnancy recommend delaying treatment with HER-2 targeted agents until after delivery in pregnant patients with HER-2 positive disease (Peccatori 2013).

Breast-Feeding Considerations It is not known if ado-trastuzumab emtansine is excreted into breast milk. Endogenous immunoglobulins are found in breast milk. Due to the potential for serious adverse reactions in the nursing infant, the decision to discontinue ado-trastuzumab emtansine or discontinue breast-feeding during treatment should take in account the wash-out period for the trastuzumab component and the benefits of treatment to the mother. Canadian labeling recommends avoiding breast-feeding for 7 months after completion of therapy.

Contraindications

US labeling: There are no contraindications in the manufacturer's labeling.

Canadian labeling: Hypersensitivity to trastuzumab emtansine or any component of the formulation.

Warnings/Precautions Hazardous agent - use appropriate precautions for handling and disposal (NIOSH 2014 [group 1]).

[US Boxed Warning]: May result in left ventricular ejection fraction (LVEF) reductions. Evaluate left ventricular function (in all patients) prior to and at least every 3 months during treatment; withhold for clinically significant left ventricular function decreases. Treatment interruption or dosage reductions are required inpatients who develop decreased LVEF. Use has not been studied in patients with LVEF <50% at baseline, with a history of symptomatic CHF, serious arrhythmia, or recent history (within 6 months) of MI or unstable angina.

[US Boxed Warning]: Serious hepatotoxicity, including liver failure and death, has been reported. Monitor transaminases and bilirubin at baseline and prior to each dose. Increases (transaminases or total bilirubin) may require dose reductions or discontinuation. Hepatotoxicity is typically manifested by asymptomatic and transient increases in transaminases, although fatal cases of drug induced liver injury and hepatic encephalopathy have occurred; may be confounded by comorbidities or concomitant hepatotoxic medications. Use has not been studied in patients with baseline serum transaminases >2.5 times ULN or bilirubin >1.5 times ULN, or in patients with active hepatitis B or C virus. Cases of nodular regenerative hyperplasia (NRH), a rare liver disorder characterized by widespread benign transformation of hepatic parenchyma into small regenerative nodules, have been observed (by biopsy). NRH may develop into noncirrhotic portal hypertension. Consider NRH in patients with clinical symptoms of portal hypertension and/or cirrhosis-like pattern seen on liver CT scan, although without associated transaminase elevations or other manifestations of cirrhosis. Diagnosis of NRH is confirmed by histopathology; permanently discontinue if histopathology confirms NRH.

[US Boxed Warning]: Exposure to ado-trastuzumab emtansine may cause embryo-fetal death or birth defects. Effective contraception must be used in women of reproductive potential. Pregnancy status should be verified prior to therapy; effective contraception is recommended during therapy and for 7 months after the last dose for women of childbearing potential.

Infusion reactions (flushing, chills, fever, bronchospasm, dyspnea, wheezing, hypotension, and/or tachycardia) have been reported. After termination of infusion, these reactions generally resolved within several hours to a day. Medications for the treatment of reactions should be available for immediate use. Monitor closely for infusion reactions, especially during initial infusion. If reaction occurs, decrease infusion rate; for severe infusion reactions, interrupt infusion; permanently discontinue for life-threatening reactions. Serious allergic/anaphylactic reaction was observed (rare). Use is not recommended in patients who had trastuzumab permanently discontinued due to infusion reaction or hypersensitivity (has not been evaluated).

Thrombocytopenia may occur (nadir achieved: by day 8; generally resolves to ≤ grade 1 by the next scheduled dose); the incidence of thrombocytopenia may be higher in patients of Asian ancestry; monitor platelet count at baseline and prior to each dose; may require treatment interruption or dose reduction. Monitor closely if at bleeding risk due to thrombocytopenia and/or concomitant anticoagulant use. Has not been studied in patients with platelets <100,000/mm^3 at treatment initiation. Neutropenia and anemia have also occurred. Hemorrhagic events, including central nervous system, respiratory, and gastrointestinal hemorrhage, have been observed; some hemorrhages were fatal. Some events occurred in patients who were receiving anticoagulation or antiplatelet therapy, or in patients with thrombocytopenia, although bleeding also occurred in patients without additional risk factors. Use caution when administering with antiplatelet agents or anticoagulants; consider additional monitoring when indicated. Local reactions (erythema, irritation, pain, swelling, or tenderness) secondary to extravasation have been noted; these were generally mild and typically occurred within 24 hours of infusion; monitor infusion site during infusion for possible infiltration. Sensory peripheral neuropathy has been reported, usually grade 1, although grade 3 peripheral neuropathy was also described; monitor for signs and symptoms of neuropathy; may require treatment interruption and/or dose reduction. Interstitial lung disease (ILD), including pneumonitis has been reported; some cases resulted in acute respiratory distress syndrome and/or fatalities; permanently discontinue with diagnosis of ILD or pneumonitis. Signs and symptoms of pneumonitis include dyspnea, cough, fatigue, and pulmonary infiltrates; may or may not occur in correlation with infusion reaction. Patients with dyspnea at rest (due to advance malignancy complications or comorbidity) may be at increased risk for pulmonary toxicity.

[US Boxed Warning]: Ado-trastuzumab emtansine and conventional trastuzumab are NOT interchangeable. Do not substitute. In Canada, the generic name for Kadcyla is trastuzumab emtansine (ie, lacks Ado- prefix) and may be confused with conventional trastuzumab. Verify product label prior to reconstitution and administration to prevent medication errors. Potentially significant drug-drug or drug-food interactions may exist, requiring dose or frequency adjustment, additional monitoring, and/or selection of alternative therapy. Establish HER2 overexpression or gene amplification status prior to treatment; has only been studied in patients with evidence of HER2 overexpression, either as 3+ IHC (Dako Herceptest™) or FISH amplification ratio ≥2 (Dako *HER2* FISH pharmDx™ test); there is only limited data on patients with breast cancer positive by FISH and 0 or 1+ by IHC.

Adverse Reactions

>10%:

Central nervous system: Fatigue (36%), headache (28%), peripheral neuropathy (21%; grades 3/4: 2%), insomnia (12%)

Dermatologic: Skin rash (12%)

Endocrine & metabolic: Decreased serum potassium (33%; grade 3: 3%)

Gastrointestinal: Nausea (40%), constipation (27%), diarrhea (24%), abdominal pain (19%), vomiting (19%), xerostomia (17%), stomatitis (14%)

Hematologic & oncologic: Decreased platelet count (83% [nadir by day 8]; grade 3: 14%; grade 4: 3%), decreased hemoglobin (60%; grade 3: 4%; grade 4: 1%), decreased neutrophils (39%; grade 3: 3%; grade 4: <1%), hemorrhage (32%; grades 3/4: 2%), thrombocytopenia (31%; grades 3/4: 15%; Asians grades 3/4: 45%), anemia (14%; grades 3/4: 4%)

Hepatic: Increased serum AST (98%; grades 3/4: <8%), increased serum ALT (82%; grades 3/4: <6%), increased serum transaminases (29%), increased serum bilirubin (17%)

Neuromuscular & skeletal: Musculoskeletal pain (36%), arthralgia (19%), weakness (18%), myalgia (14%)

Respiratory: Epistaxis (23%), cough (18%), dyspnea (12%)

Miscellaneous: Fever (19%)

1% to 10%:

Cardiovascular: Peripheral edema (7%), hypertension (5%; grades 3/4: 1%), left ventricular dysfunction (2%; grades 3/4: <1%)

Central nervous system: Dizziness (10%), chills (8%)

Dermatologic: Pruritus (6%)

Endocrine & metabolic: Hypokalemia (10%; grades 3/4: 3%)

Gastrointestinal: Dyspepsia (9%), dysgeusia (8%)

Genitourinary: Urinary tract infection (9%)

Hematologic & oncologic: Neutropenia (7%; grades 3/4: 2%)

Hepatic: Increased serum alkaline phosphatase (5%)

Hypersensitivity: Hypersensitivity (2%)

Immunologic: Antibody development (5%)

Ophthalmic: Blurred vision (5%), conjunctivitis (4%), dry eye syndrome (4%), increased lacrimation (3%)

Respiratory: Pneumonitis (≤1%)

Miscellaneous: Infusion related reaction (1%)

<1% (Limited to important or life-threatening): Anaphylactoid reaction, hepatic encephalopathy, hepatotoxicity, nodular regenerative hyperplasia, portal hypertension

Drug Interactions

Metabolism/Transport Effects Substrate of CYP3A4 (major); **Note:** Assignment of Major/Minor substrate status based on clinically relevant drug interaction potential

Avoid Concomitant Use

Avoid concomitant use of Ado-Trastuzumab Emtansine with any of the following: BCG (Intravesical); Belimumab; Conivaptan; CYP3A4 Inhibitors (Strong); Deferiprone; Dipyrone; Fusidic Acid (Systemic); Idelalisib; Natalizumab; Pimecrolimus; Tacrolimus (Topical); Tofacitinib; Vaccines (Live)

Increased Effect/Toxicity

Ado-Trastuzumab Emtansine may increase the levels/effects of: Belimumab; CloZAPine; Deferiprone; Fingolimod; Leflunomide; Natalizumab; Tofacitinib; Vaccines (Live)

The levels/effects of Ado-Trastuzumab Emtansine may be increased by: Aprepitant; Conivaptan; CYP3A4 Inhibitors (Moderate); CYP3A4 Inhibitors (Strong); Dasatinib; Denosumab; Dipyrone; Fosaprepitant; Fusidic Acid (Systemic); Idelalisib; Ivacaftor; Luliconazole; Mifepristone; Netupitant; Osimertinib; Palbociclib; Pimecrolimus; Roflumilast; Simeprevir; Stiripentol; Tacrolimus (Topical); Trastuzumab

Decreased Effect

Ado-Trastuzumab Emtansine may decrease the levels/effects of: BCG (Intravesical); Coccidioides immitis Skin Test; Sipuleucel-T; Vaccines (Inactivated); Vaccines (Live)

The levels/effects of Ado-Trastuzumab Emtansine may be decreased by: Echinacea; Osimertinib

Preparation for Administration Hazardous agent; use appropriate precautions for handling and disposal (NIOSH 2014 [group 1]). Check vial labels to assure appropriate product is being reconstituted (ado-trastuzumab emtansine and conventional trastuzumab are different products and are **NOT** interchangeable).

Slowly inject sterile water for injection into the vial (5 mL for 100 mg vial or 8 mL for 160 mg vial) to a reconstituted concentration of 20 mg/mL. Gently swirl vial until completely dissolved. Reconstituted solution will be clear or slightly opalescent (there should be no visible particles) and colorless to pale brown. Dilute for infusion by adding to 250 mL sodium chloride 0.9%; gently invert bag to mix (do not shake).

Storage/Stability Store intact vials at 2°C to 8°C (36°F to 46°F). Do not freeze or shake intact vials, reconstituted solution, or solutions diluted for infusion. Reconstituted vials do not contain preservative and should be used immediately, although may be stored for up to 24 hours at 2°C to 8°C (36°F to 46°F). Solutions diluted for infusion should be used immediately, although may be stored at 2°C to 8°C (36°F to 46°F) for up to 24 hours prior to use. This storage time is additional to the time allowed for the reconstituted vials.

Mechanism of Action Ado-trastuzumab emtansine is a HER2-antibody drug conjugate which incorporates the HER2 targeted actions of trastuzumab with the microtubule inhibitor DM1 (a maytansine derivative). The conjugate, which is linked via a stable thioether linker, allows for selective delivery into HER2 overexpressing cells, resulting in cell cycle arrest and apoptosis.

Pharmacodynamics/Kinetics

Distribution: V_d: 3.13 L

Protein binding: DM1: 93%

Metabolism: DM1 undergoes hepatic metabolism via CYP3A4/5

Half-life elimination: ~4 days

Time to peak: Near the end of the infusion

Dosing

Adult & Geriatric Note: Do not substitute ado-trastuzumab emtansine (US) or trastuzumab emtansine (Canada) for or with conventional trastuzumab; products are different and are **NOT** interchangeable.

Breast cancer, metastatic, HER2+: IV: 3.6 mg/kg every 3 weeks until disease progression or unacceptable toxicity; Maximum dose: 3.6 mg/kg

Missed or delayed doses: If a planned dose is missed or delayed, administer as soon as possible (at the dose and rate most recently tolerated), do not wait until the next planned cycle. Then adjust schedule to maintain a 3-week interval between doses.

Renal Impairment

CrCl ≥30 mL/minute: No dosage adjustment necessary.

CrCl <30 mL/minute: There are no dosage adjustments provided in the manufacturer's labeling (has not been studied).

Hepatic Impairment

Hepatic impairment prior to treatment initiation: There are no dosage adjustments provided in the manufacturer's labeling (has not been studied).

Hepatotoxicity during treatment: Refer to Dosage Adjustment for Toxicity.

Adjustment for Toxicity Note: After a dose reduction is implemented, do not re-escalate dose.

Infusion-related reaction: Slow infusion rate or interrupt infusion. Permanently discontinue if life-threatening infusion reactions occur.

Dose levels for dosage reductions and/or discontinuation:

Starting dose: 3.6 mg/kg

First dose reduction: Reduce dose to 3 mg/kg

Second dose reduction: Reduce dose to 2.4 mg/kg

Further reductions necessary: Discontinue treatment.

Hematologic toxicity:

Grade 3 thrombocytopenia (platelets 25,000/mm³ to <50,000/mm³): Withhold treatment until platelet count recovers to ≤ grade 1 (platelets ≥75,000/mm³), then resume treatment at the same dose level.

Grade 4 thrombocytopenia (platelets <25,000/mm³): Withhold treatment until platelet count recovers to ≤ grade 1 (platelets ≥75,000/mm³), then resume treatment with one dose level reduction.

Cardiotoxicity:

LVEF >45%: Continue treatment.

LVEF 40% to ≤45% and decrease is <10% points from baseline: Continue treatment and repeat LVEF assessment within 3 weeks.

LVEF 40% to ≤45% and decrease is ≥10% points from baseline: Withhold treatment and repeat LVEF assessment within 3 weeks; if repeat LVEF has not recovered to within 10% points from baseline, discontinue treatment.

LVEF <40%: Withhold treatment and repeat LVEF assessment within 3 weeks; if repeat LVEF is confirmed <40%, discontinue treatment.

HF (symptomatic): Discontinue treatment.

Hepatotoxicity:

Grade 2 ALT, AST elevations (>2.5 to ≤5 times ULN): Continue at same dose level.

Grade 3 ALT, AST elevations (>5 to ≤20 times ULN): Withhold until ALT, AST recover to ≤ grade 2, then resume with one dose level reduction.

Grade 4 ALT, AST elevations (>20 times ULN): Permanently discontinue treatment.

Grade 2 hyperbilirubinemia (>1.5 to ≤3 times ULN): Withhold until bilirubin recovers to ≤ grade 1 (≤1.5 times ULN), then resume at the same dose level.

Grade 3 hyperbilirubinemia (>3 to ≤10 times ULN): Withhold until bilirubin recovers to ≤ grade 1, then resume with one dose level reduction.

Grade 4 hyperbilirubinemia (>10 times ULN): Permanently discontinue treatment.

Concomitant ALT, AST >3 times ULN and total bilirubin >2 times ULN: Permanently discontinue treatment.

Nodular regenerative hyperplasia: Permanently discontinue treatment.

Peripheral neuropathy, grade 3 or 4: Temporarily discontinue until resolves to ≤ grade 2.

Pulmonary toxicity: Interstitial lung disease or pneumonitis: Permanently discontinue.

Administration Check label to ensure appropriate product is being administered (ado-trastuzumab emtansine [US] or trastuzumab emtansine [Canada] and conventional trastuzumab are different products and are **NOT** interchangeable).

Infuse over 90 minutes (first infusion) or over 30 minutes (subsequent infusions if prior infusions were well tolerated) through a 0.2 or 0.22 micron inline nonprotein adsorptive polyethersulfone filter. Do not administer IV push or bolus. Do not administer with other medications.

Closely monitor infusion site during administration. Monitor patient during infusion for signs of infusion-related reactions (eg, fever, chills); monitor for at least 90 minutes following initial infusion and (if tolerated) for at least 30 minutes following subsequent infusions.

Hazardous agent; use appropriate precautions for handling and disposal (NIOSH 2014 [group 1]).

Monitoring Parameters Platelet count (at baseline and prior to each dose), transaminases and bilirubin (at baseline and prior to each dose); verify pregnancy status prior to treatment initiation; HER2 expression status. Evaluate left ventricular function (prior to and at least every 3 months during treatment; for LVEF <40% or 40% to 45% with ≥10% absolute decrease below baseline value, reassess within 3 weeks. Monitor infusion site during infusion for possible infiltration; monitor for infusion reactions (during infusion and for 90 minutes after initial infusion and for 30 minutes after subsequent infusions); signs and symptoms of bleeding, neuropathy, and/or pulmonary toxicity

Dosage Forms Excipient information presented when available (limited, particularly for generics); consult specific product labeling.

Solution Reconstituted, Intravenous [preservative free]:
Kadcyla: 100 mg (1 ea); 160 mg (1 ea) [contains mouse protein (murine) (hamster)]

Afatinib (a FA ti nib)

Brand Names: US Gilotrif
Brand Names: Canada Giotrif
Index Terms Afatinib Dimaleate; BIBW 2992
Pharmacologic Category Antineoplastic Agent, Epidermal Growth Factor Receptor (EGFR) Inhibitor; Antineoplastic Agent, Tyrosine Kinase Inhibitor

Use
Non-small cell lung cancer, metastatic: First-line treatment of metastatic non-small cell lung cancer (NSCLC) in patients whose tumors have epidermal growth factor receptor (EGFR) exon 19 deletions or exon 21 (L858R) substitution mutations as detected by an approved test.
Limitations of use: Safety and efficacy have not been established in patients whose tumors express EGFR mutations other than exon 19 deletion or exon 21 (L858R) substitution.

Pregnancy Considerations Adverse events were observed in animal reproduction studies. Based on its mechanism of action, afatinib is expected to cause fetal harm if used during pregnancy. Women of reproductive potential should use highly-effective contraception during therapy and for at least 2 weeks after treatment has been discontinued.

Breast-Feeding Considerations It is not known if afatinib is excreted into breast milk. Due to the potential for serious adverse reactions in the nursing infant, the U.S. manufacturer's labeling recommends a decision be made whether to discontinue nursing or to discontinue the drug, taking into account the importance of treatment to the mother. The Canadian labeling recommends avoiding breast-feeding during therapy and for at least 2 weeks after treatment has been discontinued.

Contraindications
U.S. labeling: There are no contraindications listed in the manufacturer's labeling.
Canadian labeling: Hypersensitivity to afatinib or any component of the formulation.

Warnings/Precautions Hazardous agent – use appropriate precautions for handling and disposal (meets NIOSH 2014 criteria). Cutaneous reactions (eg, acneiform rash, erythema, and rash) are common; grade 3 reactions (characterized by bullous, blistering, and exfoliating lesions) and palmar-plantar erythrodysesthesia syndrome were also seen in clinical trials. May require therapy interruption and dosage reduction; discontinue if life-threatening cutaneous lesions occur. Patients should be cautioned to avoid sun exposure and/or utilize adequate sun protection. Paronychia requiring dose reduction and discontinuation of therapy has been observed. In clinical trials, diarrhea and stomatitis frequently occurred in patients treated with afatinib; diarrhea was observed in the majority of patients and typically appeared within the first 6 weeks of therapy. Dehydration and renal impairment may occur as a consequence of diarrhea; monitor closely. Patients may require antidiarrheal therapy (eg, loperamide); initiate at the onset of diarrhea and continue until free of loose bowel movements for 12 hours. May necessitate therapy interruption and dosage reduction. The Canadian labeling recommends avoiding use in patients with GI disorders associated with diarrhea (eg, Crohn disease, malabsorption).

Decreases from baseline in left ventricular ejection fraction (LVEF) were noted in some patients receiving afatinib. Patients with abnormal LVEF or a significant cardiac history were excluded from clinical trials; use with caution in patients with cardiac risk factors and/or decreased LVEF. Keratitis was reported rarely in clinical trials; monitor for signs/symptoms of keratitis (eg, acute or worsening eye inflammation, blurred vision, eye pain, lacrimation, light sensitivity, red eye). Interrupt therapy in patients with suspected keratitis and consider discontinuation if diagnosis of ulcerative keratitis is confirmed (permanently discontinue for persistent ulcerative keratitis). Use with caution in patients with a history of keratitis, severe dry eye, ulcerative keratitis, or who wear contact lens (risk factor for keratitis and ulceration). Interstitial lung disease (ILD) or ILD-like reactions occurred in a small percentage of patients treated with afatinib (some fatal). ILD incidence appeared to be higher in Asian as compared to non-Asian patients. Monitor closely for signs/symptoms of ILD (eg, acute respiratory distress syndrome, allergic alveolitis, lung infiltration, pneumonitis). Interrupt therapy for suspected ILD; discontinue therapy with confirmed diagnosis.

Hepatic function test abnormalities (some fatal) were observed in clinical trials. Monitor liver function tests periodically; may require therapy interruption and dosage reduction. Discontinue if severe hepatic impairment occurs during therapy. Closely monitor patients with moderate-to-severe renal impairment, may require dosage adjustments if not tolerated. The Canadian labeling does not recommend use in severe hepatic or severe renal impairment. Potentially significant drug-drug interactions may exist, requiring dose or frequency adjustment, additional monitoring, and/or selection of alternative therapy. Safety and efficacy have not been established in patients with non-small cell lung cancer whose tumors express EGFR mutations other than exon 19 deletion or exon 21 (L858R) substitution. Increased mortality has been observed in a clinical trial evaluating afatinib in combination with vinorelbine for HER2-positive metastatic breast cancer (not an approved use). This combination was also associated with a higher incidence of adverse events (eg, diarrhea, rash), as well as fatalities due to infection and cancer progression. Afatinib should not be used in combination with vinorelbine for the treatment of HER2-positive metastatic breast cancer. Contains lactose; Canadian labeling recommends avoiding use in patients with hereditary conditions of galactose intolerance, Lapp lactase deficiency, or glucose-galactose malabsorption.

Adverse Reactions

>10%:
Dermatologic: Acneiform eruption (90%; grade 3: 16%), paronychia (58%; grade 3: 11%), xeroderma (31%), pruritus (21%), cheilitis (12%)
Endocrine & metabolic: Weight loss (17%; grade 3: 1%), hypokalemia (11%; grades 3/4: 4%)
Gastrointestinal: Diarrhea (96%; grade 3: 15%), stomatitis (71%; grade 3: 9%), decreased appetite (29%; grade 3: 4%), vomiting (23%)
Genitourinary: Cystitis (13%; grade 3: 1%)
Hepatic: Increased serum ALT (11%; grades 3/4: 2%), increased serum AST (8%; grades 3/4: 2%)
Ophthalmic: Conjunctivitis (11%)
Respiratory: Epistaxis (17%), rhinorrhea (11%)
Miscellaneous: Fever (12%)
1% to 10%:
Central nervous system: Fatigue (<2%)
Dermatologic: Palmar-plantar erythrodysesthesia (7%)
Ophthalmic: Keratitis (2%; grade 3: <1%)
Renal: Renal insufficiency (6%; grade 3: >1%)
Respiratory: Pneumonitis (>1%; Asian descent: 2%)
<1% (Limited to important or life-threatening): Pancreatitis, pneumonia, sepsis

Drug Interactions

Metabolism/Transport Effects Substrate of BCRP, P-glycoprotein; **Inhibits** BCRP, P-glycoprotein

Avoid Concomitant Use There are no known interactions where it is recommended to avoid concomitant use.

Increased Effect/Toxicity
Afatinib may increase the levels/effects of: Porfimer; Verteporfin

The levels/effects of Afatinib may be increased by: Lumacaftor; P-glycoprotein/ABCB1 Inhibitors

Decreased Effect
The levels/effects of Afatinib may be decreased by: Lumacaftor; P-glycoprotein/ABCB1 Inducers

Food Interactions Administration with a high-fat meal decreases C_{max} by 50% and AUC by 39% as compared to the fasted state. Management: Take at least 1 hour before or 2 hours (U.S. labeling) or 3 hours (Canadian labeling) after a meal.

Storage/Stability Store at 25°C (77°F); excursions are permitted between 15°C and 30°C (59°F and 86°F). Dispense in original bottle; protect from high humidity and light.

Mechanism of Action Highly selective blocker of the ErbB family, including EGFR (ErbB1), HER2 (ErbB2), and HER4 (ErbB4); covalently and irreversibly binds to the intracellular tyrosine kinase domain, resulting in tumor growth inhibition and tumor regression

Pharmacodynamics/Kinetics

Absorption: Decreased with high-fat meals
Protein binding: ~95%
Metabolism: Covalently adducted to proteins and nucleophilic small molecules (minimal enzymatic metabolism) (Wind, 2013)
Bioavailability: Tablets: 92% (as compared to an oral solution)
Half-life elimination: 37 hours
Time to peak: 2 to 5 hours
Excretion: Feces (85%); urine (4%); primarily as unchanged drug

Dosing

Adult & Geriatric Non-small cell lung cancer (NSCLC), metastatic, with EGFR exon 19 deletions or exon 21 (L858R) substitution mutations: Oral: 40 mg once daily until disease progression or unacceptable toxicity
Missed doses:
U.S. labeling: Do not take a missed dose within 12 hours of next dose
Canadian labeling: Do not take a missed dose within 8 hours of next dose

Dosage adjustment for concomitant therapy:
U.S. labeling:
P-gp inhibitors: If concomitant therapy is not tolerated, reduce afatinib daily dose by 10 mg. Upon discontinuation of the P-gp inhibitor, resume previous dose as tolerated.
P-gp inducers: Increase afatinib daily dose by 10 mg if on chronic concomitant therapy with a P-gp inducer. Resume previous dose 2 to 3 days after discontinuation of P-gp inducer.
Canadian labeling: Avoid concurrent use with strong P-gp inhibitors or inducers. If concurrent use with a P-gp inhibitor is necessary, administer simultaneously with or after afatinib; monitor closely for adverse effects. The manufacturer labeling does not provide specific recommendations when concurrent use of a P-gp inducer is necessary.

Renal Impairment

Preexisting mild impairment (CrCl ≥60 mL/minute): No dosage adjustment is necessary.
Preexisting moderate-to-severe impairment (CrCl <60 mL/minute): There are no dosage adjustments provided in the manufacturer's labeling (has not been studied in patients with severe impairment [CrCl <30 mL/minute]); closely monitor and adjust dose if necessary. The Canadian labeling recommends avoiding use if CrCl <30 mL/minute.
Renal toxicity during treatment: If ≥ grade 2 renal toxicity occurs, withhold therapy. Upon improvement to baseline or ≤ grade 1, resume therapy at 10 mg per day less than previous dose.

Hepatic Impairment

Preexisting mild-to-moderate impairment (Child-Pugh class A or B): No dosage adjustment is necessary.
Preexisting severe impairment (Child-Pugh class C):
U.S. labeling: There are no dosage adjustments provided in the manufacturer's labeling (has not been studied); closely monitor and adjust dose if necessary.
Canadian labeling: Avoid use.
Hepatotoxicity during treatment: Withhold therapy for ≥ grade 3 hepatic dysfunction. Upon improvement to baseline or ≤ grade 1, resume therapy at 10 mg per day less than previous dose. Permanently discontinue for severe afatinib-induced hepatic impairment.

Adjustment for Toxicity Note: Permanently discontinue for intolerability or severe reaction occurring at a dose of 20 mg daily. The Canadian labeling recommends permanently discontinuing therapy for toxicities that do not resolve to ≤ grade 1 within 14 days of therapy interruption.
Cardiovascular: Permanently discontinue for symptomatic left ventricular dysfunction.
Dermatologic: Withhold therapy for prolonged (>7 days) or intolerable grade 2 or higher cutaneous reactions. Upon improvement to baseline or ≤ grade 1, resume therapy at 10 mg per day less than previous dose. Discontinue permanently for life-threatening bullous, blistering, or exfoliative skin lesions.
Gastrointestinal:
Diarrhea: Greater than or equal to grade 2 diarrhea that persists for ≥2 consecutive days despite antidiarrheal therapy: Interrupt therapy until resolution to ≤ grade 1, then resume at 10 mg per day less than previous dose.
Nausea/vomiting: Canadian labeling (not in U.S. labeling): Intolerable grade 2 or persistent (≥7 days) nausea/vomiting despite antiemetic therapy: Interrupt therapy until resolution to ≤ grade 1, then resume at 10 mg per day less than previous dose.
Ocular: Interrupt therapy for suspected keratitis; consider discontinuation if diagnosis of ulcerative keratitis is confirmed. Permanently discontinue for persistent ulcerative keratitis.
Pulmonary: Interrupt therapy for suspected interstitial lung disease (ILD); permanently discontinue if diagnosis is confirmed.

Other toxicity:
Greater than or equal to grade 3 adverse reactions: Withhold therapy for ≥ grade 3 adverse reactions. Upon improvement to baseline or ≤ grade 1, resume therapy at 10 mg per day less than previous dose.

Other poorly tolerated grade 2 adverse reactions persisting ≥7 days: Canadian labeling (not in U.S. labeling): Interrupt therapy until resolution to ≤ grade 1, then resume at 10 mg per day less than previous dose.

Dietary Considerations Take at least 1 hour before or 2 hours (U.S. labeling) or 3 hours (Canadian labeling) after a meal.

Administration
U.S. labeling: Administer orally at least 1 hour before or 2 hours after a meal. Do not take a missed dose within 12 hours of the next dose. Hazardous agent; use appropriate precautions for handling and disposal (meets NIOSH 2014 criteria).

Canadian labeling: Administer orally at least 1 hour before or 3 hours after a meal. Do not take a missed dose within 8 hours of the next dose. Swallow whole with water.

Monitoring Parameters EGFR mutation status; liver and renal function (periodically); monitor for skin toxicity, diarrhea, signs/symptoms of dehydration; monitor for signs/ symptoms of interstitial lung disease (eg, acute respiratory distress syndrome, allergic alveolitis, lung infiltration, pneumonitis) and keratitis (eg, acute or worsening eye inflammation, blurred vision, eye pain, lacrimation, light sensitivity, red eye). Consider left ventricular ejection fraction assessment prior to and during therapy in patients with cardiac risk factors or conditions that may impair left ventricular function.

Dosage Forms Excipient information presented when available (limited, particularly for generics); consult specific product labeling.
Tablet, Oral:
Gilotrif: 20 mg
Gilotrif: 30 mg, 40 mg [contains fd&c blue #2 (indigotine)]

Dosage Forms: Canada Excipient information presented when available (limited, particularly for generics); consult specific product labeling.
Tablet, Oral:
Giotrif: 20 mg, 30 mg, 40 mg

Aflibercept (Ophthalmic) (a FLIB er sept)

Brand Names: US Eylea
Brand Names: Canada Eylea
Index Terms AVE 0005; AVE 005; AVE-0005; VEGF Trap; VEGF Trap-Eye
Pharmacologic Category Ophthalmic Agent; Vascular Endothelial Growth Factor (VEGF) Inhibitor
Use
Diabetic retinopathy: Treatment of diabetic retinopathy in patients with diabetic macular edema
Macular degeneration: Treatment of neovascular (wet) age-related macular degeneration (AMD)
Macular edema: Treatment of macular edema following retinal vein occlusion (RVO) and diabetic macular edema
Dosing
Adult & Geriatric
Age-related macular degeneration (AMD): Intravitreal: 2 mg (0.05 mL) once every 4 weeks (monthly) for the first 12 weeks (every 3 months), followed by 2 mg (0.05 mL) once every 8 weeks (every 2 months) thereafter. Although may be administered every 4 weeks, additional efficacy has not been demonstrated (compared with every 8 week administration).

Diabetic macular edema (DME): Intravitreal: 2 mg (0.05 mL) once every 4 weeks (monthly) for the first 5 injections, followed by 2 mg (0.05 mL) once every 8 weeks (every 2 months). Although may be administered every 4 weeks, additional efficacy has not been demonstrated (compared with every 8 week administration).

Diabetic retinopathy (DR) in patients with DME: Intravitreal: 2 mg (0.05 mL) once every 4 weeks (monthly) for the first 5 injections, followed by 2 mg (0.05 mL) once every 8 weeks (every 2 months). Although may be administered every 4 weeks, additional efficacy has not been demonstrated (compared with every 8 week administration).

Macular edema following retinal vein occlusion (RVO): Intravitreal: 2 mg (0.05 mL) once every 4 weeks (monthly)
Renal Impairment No dosage adjustment necessary.
Hepatic Impairment There are no dosage adjustments provided in the manufacturer's labeling (has not been studied); however, no adjustment expected due to minimal systemic absorption.
Additional Information Complete prescribing information should be consulted for additional detail.
Dosage Forms Excipient information presented when available (limited, particularly for generics); consult specific product labeling.
Solution, Intraocular [preservative free]:
Eylea: 2 mg/0.05 mL (0.05 mL) [contains mouse protein (murine) (hamster)]

Agalsidase Beta (aye GAL si days BAY ta)

Brand Names: US Fabrazyme
Brand Names: Canada Fabrazyme
Index Terms Alpha-Galactosidase-A (Recombinant); r-h α-GAL
Pharmacologic Category Enzyme
Use Replacement therapy for Fabry disease
Dosing
Adult & Geriatric Fabry disease: IV: 1 mg/kg every 2 weeks
Pediatric Fabry disease: Children ≥8 years: IV: 1 mg/kg every 2 weeks
Renal Impairment No dosage adjustment required.
Hepatic Impairment No dosage adjustment provided in manufacturer's labeling.
Adjustment for Toxicity Patient with IgE antibodies to agalsidase beta (rechallenge): 0.5 mg/kg every 2 weeks at an initial maximum infusion rate of 0.01 mg/minute; may gradually escalate dose (to maximum of 1 mg/kg every 2 weeks) and/or infusion rate (doubling the infusion rate every 30 minutes to a maximum rate of 0.25 mg/minute) as tolerated.
Additional Information Complete prescribing information should be consulted for additional detail.
Dosage Forms Excipient information presented when available (limited, particularly for generics); consult specific product labeling.
Solution Reconstituted, Intravenous:
Fabrazyme: 5 mg (1 ea); 35 mg (1 ea) [contains mouse protein (murine) (hamster)]

- Airavite *see* Folic Acid, Cyanocobalamin, and Pyridoxine *on page 805*
- Airomir (Can) *see* Albuterol *on page 57*
- AJ-PIP/TAZ (Can) *see* Piperacillin and Tazobactam *on page 1456*
- AK Cide Oph (Can) *see* Sulfacetamide and Prednisolone *on page 1708*
- AK-Fluor *see* Fluorescein *on page 782*
- Akne-Mycin [DSC] *see* Erythromycin (Topical) *on page 672*
- AK-Pentolate [DSC] *see* Cyclopentolate *on page 455*
- AK Pentolate Oph Soln (Can) *see* Cyclopentolate *on page 455*
- AK-Poly-Bac *see* Bacitracin and Polymyxin B (Ophthalmic) *on page 196*
- AK Sulf Liq (Can) *see* Sulfacetamide (Ophthalmic) *on page 1707*
- Akynzeo *see* Netupitant and Palonosetron *on page 1269*
- ALA *see* Aminolevulinic Acid *on page 94*
- 5-ALA *see* Aminolevulinic Acid *on page 94*
- Ala Cort *see* Hydrocortisone (Topical) *on page 886*
- Alagesic LQ *see* Butalbital, Acetaminophen, and Caffeine *on page 275*
- Alamag Plus [OTC] *see* Aluminum Hydroxide, Magnesium Hydroxide, and Simethicone *on page 85*
- Ala Scalp *see* Hydrocortisone (Topical) *on page 886*
- Alavert [OTC] *see* Loratadine *on page 1101*
- Alavert™ Allergy and Sinus [OTC] *see* Loratadine and Pseudoephedrine *on page 1102*
- Alaway [OTC] *see* Ketotifen (Ophthalmic) *on page 1018*
- Alaway Childrens Allergy [OTC] *see* Ketotifen (Ophthalmic) *on page 1018*
- Albalon (Can) *see* Naphazoline (Ophthalmic) *on page 1256*

Albendazole (al BEN da zole)

Brand Names: US Albenza
Pharmacologic Category Anthelmintic
Use Treatment of parenchymal neurocysticercosis caused by *Taenia solium* and cystic hydatid disease of the liver, lung, and peritoneum caused by *Echinococcus granulosus*
Pregnancy Considerations Adverse events were observed in animal reproduction studies. Albendazole should not be used during pregnancy, if at all possible. The manufacturer recommends a pregnancy test prior to therapy in women of reproductive potential. Women should be advised to avoid pregnancy for at least 1 month following therapy. Discontinue if pregnancy occurs during treatment.

Breast-Feeding Considerations Albendazole excretion into breast milk was studied following a single oral 400 mg dose in breast-feeding women 2 weeks to 6 months postpartum (n=33). Mean albendazole concentrations 6 hours after the dose were 63.7 ± 11.9 ng/mL (maternal serum) and 31.9 ± 9.2 ng/mL (milk). An active and inactive metabolite was also detected in breast milk (Abdel-tawab, 2009). The manufacturer recommends that caution be exercised when administering albendazole to nursing women.

Contraindications Hypersensitivity to albendazole, benzimidazoles, or any component of the formulation
Warnings/Precautions Reversible elevations in hepatic enzymes have been reported; patients with abnormal LFTs and hepatic echinococcosis are at an increased risk of hepatotoxicity. Discontinue therapy if LFT elevations are >2 times the upper limit of normal; may consider restarting treatment with frequent monitoring of LFTs when hepatic enzymes return to pretreatment values. Agranulocytosis, aplastic anemia, granulocytopenia, leukopenia, and pancytopenia have occurred leading to fatalities (rare); use with caution in patients with hepatic impairment (more susceptible to hematologic toxicity). Discontinue therapy in all patients who develop clinically significant decreases in blood cell counts.

Neurocysticercosis: Corticosteroids (eg, dexamethasone or prednisolone) should be administered before or upon initiation of albendazole therapy to minimize inflammatory reactions and prevent cerebral hypertension. Anticonvulsant therapy should be used concurrently during the first week of therapy to prevent seizures. These measures are important to minimize neurological symptoms which may result from uncovering of preexisting neurocysticercosis when using albendazole to treat other conditions. If retinal lesions exist, weigh risk of further retinal damage due to

albendazole-induced changes to the retinal lesion vs benefit of disease treatment.
Adverse Reactions
>10%:
Central nervous system: Headache (11% neurocysticercosis; 1% hydatid)
Hepatic: LFTs increased (16% hydatid; <1% neurocysticercosis)
1% to 10%:
Central nervous system: Intracranial pressure increased (≤2%), dizziness (≤1%), fever (≤1%), vertigo (≤1%), meningeal signs (1%)
Dermatologic: Alopecia (<1% to 2%)
Gastrointestinal: Abdominal pain (≤6%), nausea/vomiting (4% to 6%)
<1% (Limited to important or life-threatening symptoms): Acute liver failure, acute renal failure, aplastic anemia, agranulocytosis, erythema multiforme, granulocytopenia, hepatitis, hypersensitivity reaction, leukopenia, neutropenia, pancytopenia, rash, Stevens-Johnson syndrome, thrombocytopenia, urticaria
Drug Interactions
Metabolism/Transport Effects Substrate of CYP1A2 (minor), CYP3A4 (minor); **Note:** Assignment of Major/Minor substrate status based on clinically relevant drug interaction potential
Avoid Concomitant Use There are no known interactions where it is recommended to avoid concomitant use.
Increased Effect/Toxicity
The levels/effects of Albendazole may be increased by: Grapefruit Juice
Decreased Effect
The levels/effects of Albendazole may be decreased by: Aminoquinolines (Antimalarial); CarBAMazepine; PHENobarbital; Phenytoin
Food Interactions Albendazole serum levels may be increased if taken with a fatty meal (increases the oral bioavailability by up to 5 times). Management: Should be administered with a high-fat meal (peanuts or ice cream).
Storage/Stability Store between 20°C and 25°C (68°F to 77°F)
Mechanism of Action Active metabolite, albendazole sulfoxide, causes selective degeneration of cytoplasmic microtubules in intestinal and tegmental cells of intestinal helminths and larvae; glycogen is depleted, glucose uptake and cholinesterase secretion are impaired, and desecratory substances accumulate intracellulary. ATP production decreases causing energy depletion, immobilization, and worm death.
Pharmacodynamics/Kinetics
Absorption: Poor from the GI tract; may increase up to 5 times when administered with a fatty meal
Distribution: Widely distributed throughout the body including urine, bile, liver, cyst wall, cyst fluid, and CSF
Protein binding: 70%
Metabolism: Hepatic; extensive first-pass effect; pathways include rapid sulfoxidation to active metabolite (albendazole sulfoxide [major]), hydrolysis, and oxidation
Half-life elimination: 8 to 12 hours (albendazole sulfoxide)
Time to peak, serum: 2 to 5 hours for the metabolite
Excretion: Urine (<1% as active metabolite); feces
Dosing
Adult & Geriatric
Neurocysticercosis: Oral:
<60 kg: 15 mg/kg/day in 2 divided doses (maximum: 800 mg/day) for 8-30 days
≥60 kg: 800 mg/day in 2 divided doses for 8-30 days
Note: Give concurrent anticonvulsant and corticosteroid (eg, dexamethasone or prednisolone) therapy during first week.
Hydatid: Oral:
<60 kg: 15 mg/kg/day in 2 divided doses (maximum: 800 mg/day)
≥60 kg: 800 mg/day in 2 divided doses
Note: Administer dose for three 28-day cycles with a 14-day drug-free interval in between each cycle.
Ancylostoma caninum, Ascaris lumbricoides (**roundworm**), *Ancylostoma duodenale* (**hookworm**), **and** *Necator americanus* (**hookworm**) (off-label use): Oral: 400 mg as a single dose
Clonorchis sinensis (**Chinese liver fluke**) (**off-label use**): Oral: 10 mg/kg/day for 7 days
Cutaneous larva migrans (off-label use): Oral: 400 mg once daily for 3 days
Enterobius vermicularis (**pinworm**) (**off-label use**): Oral: 400 mg as a single dose; repeat in 2 weeks
Giardia duodenalis (**giardiasis**) (**off-label use**): Oral: 400 mg once daily for 5 days
Gnathostoma spinigerum (**off-label use**): Oral: 800 mg/day in 2 divided doses for 21 days
Gongylonemiasis (off-label use): Oral: 400 mg once daily for 3 days

Mansonella perstans (off-label use): Oral: 800 mg/day in 2 divided doses for 10 days

Oesophagostomum bifurcum (off-label use): Oral: 400 mg as a single dose (Ziem, 2004)

Trichinella spiralis (Trichinellosis) (off-label use): Oral: 800 mg/day in 2 divided doses for 8-14 days plus corticosteroids for severe symptoms

Visceral larva migrans (toxocariasis) (off-label use): Oral: 800 mg/day in 2 divided doses for 5 days

Cysticercus cellulosae (off-label use): Oral: 800 mg/day in 2 divided doses for 8-30 days; may be repeated as necessary

Echinococcus granulosus (tapeworm) (off-label use): Oral: 800 mg/day in 2 divided doses for 1-6 months

Microsporidiosis (not limited to the HIV-infected patient) (off-label use; Anon 2007): Oral:

Disseminated microsporidiosis: 800 mg/day in 2 divided doses

Intestinal microsporidiosis (*E. intestinalis*): 800 mg/day in 2 divided doses for 21 days

Ocular microsporidiosis: 800 mg/day in 2 divided doses, in combination with fumagillin

Microsporidiosis in HIV-infected patients (off-label use; HHS [OI adult 2015]): Oral:

Disseminated microsporidiosis (caused by *Trachipleistophora* or *Anncaliia*): 800 mg/day in 2 divided doses in combination with itraconazole

Disseminated or intestinal microsporidiosis (caused by microsporidiosis other than *E. bieneusi* and *V. corneae*): 800 mg/day in 2 divided doses; continue until CD4 count >200 cells/mm³ for >6 months after ART initiation

Ocular microsporidiosis: 800 mg/day in 2 divided doses, in combination with fumagillin; discontinue therapy after ocular infection resolution if CD4 count >200 cells/mm³; continue therapy until ocular infection resolution and increase in CD4 count to >200 cells/mm³ for at least 6 months in response to ART if CD4 count ≤200 cells/mm³

Pediatric

Neurocysticercosis: Oral: Refer to adult dosing.

Hydatid: Oral: Refer to adult dosing.

Cysticercus cellulosae (off-label use): Oral: 15 mg/kg/day (maximum: 800 mg/day) in 2 divided doses for 8-30 days; may be repeated as necessary

Echinococcus granulosus (tapeworm) (off-label use): Oral: 15 mg/kg/day (maximum: 800 mg) divided twice daily for 1-6 months

Giardia duodenalis (giardiasis) (off-label use): Oral: 10 mg/kg/day for 5 days (Yereli, 2004)

Microsporidiosis in HIV-exposed/-infected patients (off-label use): Oral:

Disseminated or intestinal infection (caused by microsporidiosis other than *E. bieneusi* or *V. corneae*):

Infants and Children: 15 mg/kg/day (maximum: 800 mg/day) in 2 divided doses continued until immune reconstitution after HAART initiation (CDC, 2009)

Adolescents: Refer to adult dosing.

Disseminated microsporidiosis (caused by *Trachipleistophora* or *Anncaliia*): Adolescents: Refer to adult dosing.

Ocular microsporidiosis: Adolescents: Refer to adult dosing.

For the following off-label uses, refer to adult dosing:

Ancylostoma caninum, Ascaris lumbricoides (roundworm), *Ancylostoma duodenale* (hookworm), *Clonorchis sinensis*, (Chinese liver fluke), cutaneous larva migrans, *Enterobius vermicularis* (pinworm), *Gnathostoma spinigerum*, gongylonemiasis, *Mansonella perstans, Necator americanus* (hookworm), *Oesophagostomum bifurcum, Trichinella spiralis* (Trichinellosis), visceral larva migrans (toxocariasis)

Renal Impairment No dosage adjustment provided in the manufacturer's labeling (has not been studied). However, the need for adjustment not likely since albendazole is primarily eliminated by hepatic metabolism.

Hepatic Impairment No dosage adjustment provided in manufacturer's labeling. However, patients with underlying liver disease may be more at risk for adverse effects.

Dietary Considerations Should be taken with a high-fat meal.

Administration Should be administered with a high-fat meal. Administer anticonvulsant and corticosteroid therapy during first week of neurocysticercosis therapy. If patients have difficulty swallowing, tablets may be crushed or chewed, then swallowed with a drink of water.

Monitoring Parameters Monitor fecal specimens for ova and parasites for 3 weeks after treatment; if positive, retreat; LFTs and CBC with differential at start of each 28-day cycle and every 2 weeks during therapy (more frequent monitoring for patients with liver disease); ophthalmic exam (patients with neurocysticercosis); pregnancy test

Dosage Forms Excipient information presented when available (limited, particularly for generics); consult specific product labeling.

Tablet, Oral:

Albenza: 200 mg [contains saccharin sodium]

◆ **Albenza** see Albendazole *on page 53*

Albiglutide (al bi GLOO tide)

Brand Names: US Tanzeum

Index Terms Tanzeum

Pharmacologic Category Antidiabetic Agent, Glucagon-Like Peptide-1 (GLP-1) Receptor Agonist

Use Diabetes mellitus, type 2: Adjunct to diet and exercise to improve glycemic control in the treatment of type 2 diabetes mellitus (noninsulin dependent, NIDDM)

Pregnancy Considerations Adverse events have been observed in some animal reproduction studies. Because of the long washout period, consider stopping albiglutide at least 1 month before a planned pregnancy.

In women with diabetes, maternal hyperglycemia can be associated with congenital malformations as well as adverse effects in the fetus, neonate, and the mother (ACOG 2005; ADA 2015; Kitzmiller 2008; Metzger 2007). To prevent adverse outcomes, prior to conception and throughout pregnancy maternal blood glucose and HbA$_{1c}$ should be kept as close to target goals as possible but without causing significant hypoglycemia (ACOG 2013; ADA 2015; Blumer 2013; Kitzmiller 2008). Prior to pregnancy, effective contraception should be used until glycemic control is achieved (Kitzmiller 2008). Other agents are currently recommended to treat diabetes in pregnant women (ACOG 2013; Blumer 2013).

Breast-Feeding Considerations It is not known if albiglutide is excreted in breast milk. The manufacturer recommends a decision be made whether to discontinue nursing or to discontinue the drug, taking into account the importance of treatment to the mother.

Medication Guide Available Yes

Contraindications Severe hypersensitivity to albiglutide or any component of the formulation; history of or family history of medullary thyroid carcinoma (MTC); patients with multiple endocrine neoplasia syndrome type 2 (MEN2)

Warnings/Precautions [US Boxed Warning] Thyroid C-cell tumors have developed in animal studies with glucagon-like peptide-1 (GLP-1) receptor agonists; it is not known if albiglutide causes thyroid C-cell tumor, including medullary thyroid carcinoma (MTC) in humans. Routine monitoring of serum calcitonin or using thyroid ultrasound monitoring is of uncertain value for early detection of MTC in patients treated with albiglutide. Patients should be counseled on the potential risk of MTC with the use of albiglutide and informed of symptoms of thyroid tumors (eg, neck mass, dysphagia, dyspnea, persistent hoarseness). Use is contraindicated in patients with a personal or a family history of MTC and in patients with multiple endocrine neoplasia syndrome type 2 (MEN2). Consultation with an endocrinologist is recommended in patients with thyroid nodules on physical examination or neck imaging and patients who develop elevated calcitonin concentrations. Serious hypersensitivity reactions (including pruritus, rash, and dyspnea) have been reported with use; discontinue therapy in the event of a hypersensitivity reaction; treat appropriately and monitor patients until signs and symptoms resolve. Cases of acute pancreatitis have been reported; monitor for signs and symptoms of pancreatitis (eg, persistent severe abdominal pain which may radiate to the back and which may or may not be accompanied by vomiting). If pancreatitis is suspected, discontinue use. Do not resume unless an alternative etiology of pancreatitis is confirmed. Consider antidiabetic therapies other than albiglutide in patients with a history of pancreatitis.

Not recommended for first-line therapy of type 2 diabetes mellitus in patients inadequately controlled on diet and exercise alone. Do not use in patients with type 1 diabetes mellitus or for the treatment of diabetic ketoacidosis; not a substitute for insulin. Diabetes self-management education (DSME) is essential to maximize the effectiveness of therapy. Use with caution in patients with renal impairment, particularly during initiation of therapy and dose escalation. Acute renal failure and chronic renal failure exacerbation (sometimes requiring hemodialysis) have been reported; some cases have been reported in patients with no known preexisting renal disease. Reports primarily occurred in patients with nausea/vomiting/diarrhea or dehydration.

Use is not recommended in patients with preexisting severe gastrointestinal disease. Potentially significant drug-drug interactions may exist, requiring dose or frequency adjustment, additional monitoring, and/or selection of alternative therapy. Concomitant use of insulin or insulin secretagogues (eg, sulfonylureas) may increase the risk of hypoglycemia; dosage reduction of insulin or insulin secretagogues may be required. Concurrent use with prandial insulin therapy has not been evaluated. Due to its effects on gastric emptying, albiglutide may reduce the rate and extent of absorption of orally-administered drugs; use with caution in patients receiving medications with a narrow therapeutic window or that require rapid absorption from the GI tract.

Adverse Reactions Reactions reported from monotherapy and combination therapy.

>10%:
Endocrine & metabolic: Hypoglycemia (combination therapy; 3% to 17%)
Gastrointestinal: Diarrhea (13%), nausea (11%)
Local: Injection site reaction (11% to 18%, including erythema at injection site [2%], hypersensitivity reaction at injection site [1%], rash at injection site [1%], itching at injection site)
Respiratory: Upper respiratory tract infection (14%)

1% to 10%:
Cardiovascular: Atrial fibrillation (1%)
Endocrine & metabolic: Increased gamma-glutamyl transferase (2%)
Gastrointestinal: Gastroesophageal reflux disease (4%), vomiting (4%)
Immunologic: Antibody development (non-neutralizing; 6%)
Infection: Influenza (5%)
Neuromuscular & skeletal: Arthralgia (7%), back pain (7%)
Respiratory: Cough (7%), pneumonia (2%)

<1% (Limited to important or life-threatening): Appendicitis, atrial flutter, hypersensitivity, increased serum ALT, increased serum bilirubin, pancreatitis

Drug Interactions
Metabolism/Transport Effects None known.
Avoid Concomitant Use There are no known interactions where it is recommended to avoid concomitant use.
Increased Effect/Toxicity
Albiglutide may increase the levels/effects of: Hypoglycemia-Associated Agents; Insulin; Sulfonylureas

The levels/effects of Albiglutide may be increased by: Alpha-Lipoic Acid; Androgens; MAO Inhibitors; Pegvisomant; Quinolone Antibiotics; Salicylates; Selective Serotonin Reuptake Inhibitors

Decreased Effect
The levels/effects of Albiglutide may be decreased by: Hyperglycemia-Associated Agents; Quinolone Antibiotics; Thiazide Diuretics

Preparation for Administration Reconstitute powder with the diluent contained in the pen device. Refer to manufacturer's product labeling for full reconstitution instructions. Administer within 8 hours of reconstitution.

Storage/Stability Store unused pens at 2°C to 8°C (36°F to 46°F); may be stored at room temperature (≤30°C [86°F]) for ≤4 weeks prior to reconstitution. Do not freeze. Use within 8 hours of reconstitution.

Mechanism of Action Albiglutide is an agonist of human glucagon-like peptide-1 (GLP-1) receptor and augments glucose-dependent insulin secretion and slows gastric emptying.

Pharmacodynamics/Kinetics
Distribution: V_d: 11 L
Metabolism: Degradation to small peptides and individual amino acids by proteolytic enzymes.
Half-life elimination: ~5 days
Time to peak, plasma: 3 to 5 days

Dosing
Adult & Geriatric
Diabetes mellitus, type 2: SubQ: 30 mg once weekly; may increase to 50 mg once weekly if inadequate glycemic response. Titration to 50 mg once weekly occurred at week 12 in a monotherapy trial and after a minimum of 4 weeks in combination therapy trials.
Missed doses: If a dose is missed, administer as soon as possible within 3 days after the missed dose; dosing can then be resumed on the usual day of administration. If more than 3 days have passed since the dose was missed, omit the missed dose and resume administration at the next regularly scheduled weekly dose.

Renal Impairment No dosage adjustment necessary; use caution when initiating or escalating doses.

Hepatic Impairment There are no dosage adjustments provided in the manufacturer's labeling (has not been studied); however, changes in hepatic function are not likely to have an effect on elimination.

Dietary Considerations Individualized medical nutrition therapy (MNT) based on ADA recommendations is an integral part of therapy.

Administration Do not inject intravenously or intramuscularly. Inject subcutaneously into the upper arm, thigh, or abdomen; when administering within the same body region, use a different injection site each week. Administer once weekly on the same day each week, without regard to meals or time of day. The day of weekly administration may be changed, as long as the last dose was administered ≥4 days before. Use immediately after attaching and priming the needle; solution can clog the needle if allowed to dry in the primed needle. If using concomitantly with insulin, administer as separate injections (do not mix); may inject in the same body region as insulin, but not adjacent to one another.

Monitoring Parameters Plasma glucose, HbA$_{1c}$, renal function, signs/symptoms of pancreatitis

Reference Range
Recommendations for glycemic control in nonpregnant adults with diabetes (ADA, 2015):
HbA$_{1c}$: <7% (a more aggressive [<6.5%] or less aggressive [<8%] HbA$_{1c}$ goal may be targeted based on patient-specific characteristics)
Preprandial capillary plasma glucose: 80 to 130 mg/dL
Peak postprandial capillary blood glucose: <180 mg/dL

Recommendations for glycemic control in pediatric (all age groups) patients with type 1 diabetes (ADA, 2015):
HbA$_{1c}$: <7.5% (individualization may be appropriate based on patient-specific characteristics; <7% is reasonable if it can be achieved without excessive hypoglycemia)
Preprandial capillary plasma glucose: 90 to 130 mg/dL
Bedtime and overnight capillary blood glucose: 90 to 150 mg/dL

Dosage Forms Excipient information presented when available (limited, particularly for generics); consult specific product labeling.
Pen-injector, Subcutaneous [preservative free]:
Tanzeum: 30 mg (1 ea); 50 mg (1 ea) [contains polysorbate 80]

◆ Albuked 5 *see* Albumin *on page* 55
◆ Albuked 25 *see* Albumin *on page* 55

Albumin (al BYOO min)

Brand Names: US Albuked 25; Albuked 5; Albumin-ZLB; Albuminar-25; Albuminar-5; AlbuRx; Albutein; Buminate; Flexbumin; Human Albumin Grifols; Kedbumin; Plasbumin-25; Plasbumin-5

Brand Names: Canada Alburex 25; Alburex 5; Albutein 25%; Albutein 5%; Buminate-25%; Buminate-5%; Plasbumin-25; Plasbumin-5

Index Terms Albumin (Human); Normal Human Serum Albumin; Normal Serum Albumin (Human); Salt Poor Albumin; SPA

Pharmacologic Category Blood Product Derivative; Plasma Volume Expander, Colloid

Use Hypovolemia: Plasma volume expansion and maintenance of cardiac output in the treatment of certain types of shock or impending shock; may be useful for burn patients, ARDS, severe nephrosis, hemolytic disease of the newborn, and cardiopulmonary bypass; unless the condition responsible for hypoproteinemia can be corrected, albumin can provide only symptomatic relief or supportive treatment

Note: Nutritional supplementation is not an appropriate indication.

Pregnancy Considerations Animal reproduction studies have not been conducted. Albumin is used for the treatment of ovarian hyperstimulation syndrome (ASRM, 2008). Use for other indications may be considered in pregnant women when contraindications to nonprotein colloids exist (Liumbruno, 2009).

Breast-Feeding Considerations Endogenous albumin is found in breast milk. The manufacturer recommends that caution be exercised when administering albumin to nursing women.

Contraindications Hypersensitivity to albumin or any component of the formulation; patients at risk of volume overload (eg, patients with renal impairment, severe anemia, or heart failure); dilution with sterile water for injection ▶

Warnings/Precautions Anaphylaxis may occur; discontinue immediately if allergic or anaphylactic reactions are suspected. Cardiac or respiratory failure, renal failure, or increasing intracranial pressure can occur; closely monitor hemodynamic parameters in all patients. Use with caution in conditions where hypervolemia and its consequences or hemodilution may increase the risk of adverse effects (eg, heart failure, pulmonary edema, hypertension, hemorrhagic diathesis, esophageal varices). Adjust rate of administration per hemodynamic status and solution concentration; monitor closely with rapid infusions. Avoid rapid infusions in patients with a history of cardiovascular disease (may cause circulatory overload and pulmonary edema). Discontinue at the first signs of cardiovascular overload (eg, headache, dyspnea, jugular venous distention, rales, abnormal elevations in systemic or central venous blood pressure). All patients should be observed for signs of hypervolemia such as pulmonary edema.

Use with caution in patients with hepatic or renal impairment because of added protein load. Use with caution in those patients for whom sodium restriction is necessary. The parenteral product may contain aluminum (Kelly, 1989); toxic aluminum concentrations may be seen with high doses, prolonged use, or renal dysfunction. Premature neonates are at higher risk due to immature renal function and aluminum intake from other parenteral sources. Parenteral aluminum exposure of >4 to 5 mcg/kg/day is associated with CNS and bone toxicity; tissue loading may occur at lower doses (Federal Register, 2002). See manufacturer's labeling. Albumin is a product of human plasma, may potentially contain infectious agents which could transmit disease. Screening of donors, as well as testing and/or inactivation or removal of certain viruses, reduces the risk. Infections thought to be transmitted by this product should be reported to the manufacturer. Packaging may contain natural latex rubber. Patients with chronic renal insufficiency receiving albumin solution may be at risk for accumulation of aluminum and potential toxicities (eg, hypercalcemia, vitamin D refractory osteodystrophy, anemia, and severe progressive encephalopathy). In patients with increased microvascular permeability (eg, sepsis, trauma, burn), the translocation of fluid from the interstitial compartment to the intravascular compartment may decrease due to increased albumin in the interstitial space. Furthermore, in extreme microvascular permeability states, administration of albumin (or other colloids) may increase the net flux of fluid into the interstitial space reducing intravascular volume and precipitating edematous states (eg, pulmonary edema) (Roberts, 1998).

Adverse Reactions Frequency not defined.
Cardiovascular: Congestive heart failure (precipitation), edema, hypertension, hypotension, tachycardia
Central nervous system: Chills, headache
Dermatologic: Pruritus, skin rash, urticaria
Endocrine & metabolic: Hypervolemia
Gastrointestinal: Nausea, vomiting
Hypersensitivity: Anaphylaxis
Respiratory: Bronchospasm, pulmonary edema
Miscellaneous: Fever

Drug Interactions
Metabolism/Transport Effects None known.
Avoid Concomitant Use There are no known interactions where it is recommended to avoid concomitant use.
Increased Effect/Toxicity There are no known significant interactions involving an increase in effect.
Decreased Effect There are no known significant interactions involving a decrease in effect.

Preparation for Administration May dilute 25% albumin solutions with NS or D_5W. Do not use sterile water to dilute albumin solutions, as this has been associated with hypotonic-associated hemolysis. If 5% human albumin is unavailable, it may be prepared by diluting 25% human albumin with 0.9% sodium chloride or 5% dextrose in water.

Storage/Stability Store at ≤30°C (86°F); do not freeze. Do not use solution if it is turbid or contains a deposit; use within 4 hours after opening vial; discard unused portion.

Mechanism of Action Provides increase in intravascular oncotic pressure and causes mobilization of fluids from interstitial into intravascular space

Pharmacodynamics/Kinetics Half-life: 15 to 20 days

Dosing
Adult & Geriatric Note: Use **5%** solution in hypovolemic patients or intravascularly-depleted patients. Use **25%** solution in patients in whom fluid and sodium intake is restricted.
Usual dose: 25 g; initial dose may be repeated in 15 to 30 minutes if response is inadequate.

Hypovolemia: 5% albumin: 12.5 to 25 g (250 to 500 mL); repeat as needed. **Note:** May be considered after inadequate response to crystalloid therapy and when nonprotein colloids are contraindicated. The volume administered and the speed of infusion should be adapted to individual response.

Large-volume paracentesis (>5 L) (off-label use): 25% albumin: 5 to 8 g for every liter removed (Garcia-Compeán, 1993; Moore, 2003) **or** 50 g total for paracentesis >5 L (ATS, 2004). **Note:** Administer soon after the procedure to avoid postprocedural complications (eg, hypovolemia, hyponatremia, renal impairment) (Moore, 2003).

Spontaneous bacterial peritonitis (treatment) (off-label use): 25% albumin: Initial: 1.5 g/kg within 6 hours of diagnosis (in conjunction with appropriate antimicrobial therapy), followed by 1 g/kg on day 3 (Abd, 2012; Runyon, 2012; Sort, 1999). **Note:** Clinical trials used albumin 20%; the difference in concentration compared with 25% albumin is deemed to be clinically inconsequential.

Pediatric Note: 5% should be used in hypovolemic patients or intravascularly-depleted patients. 25% should be used in patients in whom fluid and sodium intake must be minimized.

Hemolytic disease of the newborn: Infants: IV: 1 g/kg/dose of 25% albumin prior to or during exchange transfusion

Hypovolemia:
Infants and Younger Children: IV: 0.5 to 1 g/kg/dose (10 to 20 mL/kg/dose of albumin 5%); repeat in 30 minute intervals as needed
Older Children and Adolescents: IV: 12.5 to 25 g (250 to 500 mL of albumin 5%); repeat in 30 minute intervals as needed.

Renal Impairment There are no dosage adjustments provided in the manufacturer's labeling; use with caution.

Hepatic Impairment There are no dosage adjustments provided in the manufacturer's labeling; use with caution.

Dietary Considerations Some products may contain potassium and/or sodium.

Administration
For IV administration only. Use within 4 hours after entering package; discard unused portion. In emergencies, may administer as rapidly as necessary to improve clinical condition. After initial volume replacement:
5%: Do not exceed 2 to 4 mL/minute in patients with normal plasma volume; 5 to 10 mL/minute in patients with hypoproteinemia
25%: Do not exceed 1 mL/minute in patients with normal plasma volume; 2 to 3 mL/minute in patients with hypoproteinemia

Rapid infusion may cause vascular overload. Albumin 25% may be given undiluted or diluted in normal saline. May give in combination or through the same administration set as saline or carbohydrates. Do not use with ethanol or protein hydrolysates (precipitation may form).

Monitoring Parameters Hemodynamic parameters, blood pressure, pulmonary edema, hematocrit, electrolytes, infusion rate

Additional Information Albumin 5% and 25% solutions contain 130-160 mEq/L sodium and are considered isotonic with plasma. Dilution of albumin 25% solution with sterile water produces a hypotonic solution; administration of such can cause hemolysis and/or renal failure. An albumin 5% solution is osmotically equivalent to an equal volume of plasma, whereas a 25% solution is osmotically equivalent to 5 times its volume of plasma. Albumin solutions are heated to 60°C for 10 hours, decreasing any possible risk of viral hepatitis transmission. To date, there have been no reports of viral transmission using these products.

Dosage Forms Excipient information presented when available (limited, particularly for generics); consult specific product labeling. [DSC] = Discontinued product
Solution, Intravenous:
Albumin-ZLB: 5% (250 mL, 500 mL); 25% (50 mL, 100 mL)
Albuminar-5: 5% (250 mL, 500 mL)
Albuminar-25: 25% (50 mL, 100 mL)
AlbuRx: 5% (250 mL, 500 mL)
Albutein: 25% (50 mL, 100 mL)
Buminate: 5% (250 mL, 500 mL); 25% (20 mL)
Plasbumin-5: 5% (50 mL, 250 mL)
Plasbumin-25: 25% (20 mL, 50 mL, 100 mL)
Generic: 5% (50 mL [DSC]); 25% (50 mL, 100 mL)

Solution, Intravenous [preservative free]:
Albuked 5: 5% (50 mL [DSC], 250 mL)
Albuked 25: 25% (50 mL, 100 mL)
Albutein: 5% (50 mL, 500 mL); 25% (50 mL, 100 mL)
Flexbumin: 5% (250 mL); 25% (50 mL, 100 mL)
Human Albumin Grifols: 25% (50 mL, 100 mL)
Kedbumin: 25% (50 mL, 100 mL)
Plasbumin-5: 5% (50 mL, 250 mL)
Plasbumin-25: 25% (20 mL, 50 mL, 100 mL)
Generic: 5% (100 mL, 250 mL, 500 mL); 25% (50 mL, 100 mL)

- ◆ Albuminar-5 *see Albumin on page 55*
- ◆ Albuminar-25 *see Albumin on page 55*
- ◆ Albumin-Bound Paclitaxel *see PACLitaxel (Protein Bound) on page 1371*
- ◆ Albumin (Human) *see Albumin on page 55*
- ◆ Albumin-Stabilized Nanoparticle Paclitaxel *see PACLitaxel (Protein Bound) on page 1371*
- ◆ Albumin-ZLB *see Albumin on page 55*
- ◆ Alburex 5 (Can) *see Albumin on page 55*
- ◆ Alburex 25 (Can) *see Albumin on page 55*
- ◆ AlbuRx *see Albumin on page 55*
- ◆ Albutein *see Albumin on page 55*
- ◆ Albutein 5% (Can) *see Albumin on page 55*
- ◆ Albutein 25% (Can) *see Albumin on page 55*

Albuterol (al BYOO ter ole)

Brand Names: US AccuNeb [DSC]; ProAir HFA; ProAir RespiClick; Proventil HFA; Ventolin HFA; VoSpire ER
Brand Names: Canada Airomir; Apo-Salvent; Apo-Salvent AEM; Apo-Salvent CFC Free; Apo-Salvent Sterules; Dom-Salbutamol; Novo-Salbutamol HFA; PHL-Salbutamol; PMS-Salbutamol; ratio-Ipra-Sal; ratio-Salbutamol; Salbutamol HFA; Sandoz-Salbutamol; Teva-Salbutamol Sterinebs P.F.; Ventolin Diskus; Ventolin HFA; Ventolin I.V. Infusion; Ventolin Nebules P.F.; Ventolin Respirator
Index Terms AccuNeb; Albuterol Sulfate; ProAir RespiClick; Salbutamol; Salbutamol Sulphate; Volmax
Pharmacologic Category Beta$_2$ Agonist
Use Treatment or prevention of bronchospasm in patients with reversible obstructive airway disease; prevention of exercise-induced bronchospasm
Pregnancy Considerations Adverse events have been observed in some animal reproduction studies. Albuterol crosses the placenta (Boulton, 1997). Congenital anomalies (cleft palate, limb defects) have rarely been reported following maternal use during pregnancy. Multiple medications were used in most cases, no specific pattern of defects has been reported, and no relationship to albuterol has been established. The amount of albuterol available systemically following inhalation is significantly less in comparison to oral doses.

Uncontrolled asthma is associated with adverse events on pregnancy (increased risk of perinatal mortality, preeclampsia, preterm birth, low birth weight infants). Albuterol is the preferred short acting beta agonist when treatment for asthma is needed during pregnancy (NAEPP, 2005; NAEPP, 2007).

Albuterol may affect uterine contractility. Maternal pulmonary edema and other adverse events have been reported when albuterol was used for tocolysis. Albuterol is not approved for use as a tocolytic; use caution when needed to treat bronchospasm in pregnant women. Use of the injection (Canadian product; not available in the U.S.) is specifically contraindicated in women during the first or second trimester who may be at risk of threatened abortion.
Breast-Feeding Considerations It is not known if albuterol is excreted in breast milk. The amount of albuterol available systemically following inhalation is significantly less in comparison to oral doses. According to the manufacturer, the decision to continue or discontinue breast-feeding during therapy should take into account the risk of exposure to the infant and the benefits of treatment to the mother. The use of beta-2-receptor agonists are not considered a contraindication to breast-feeding (NAEPP, 2005).
Contraindications
Inhalation, Oral: Hypersensitivity to albuterol or any component of the formulation; severe hypersensitivity to milk proteins (powder for inhalation).
Injection [Canadian product]: Hypersensitivity to albuterol or any component of the formulation; tachyarrhythmias; risk of abortion during first or second trimester
Warnings/Precautions Albuterol is a short-acting beta$_2$-agonist (SABA) that should be used as needed for quick relief of asthma symptoms. Based on a step-wise treatment approach using asthma guidelines, monotherapy without concurrent use of a long-term controller medication should only be reserved for patients with mild, intermittent forms of asthma without the presence of risk factors (Step 1 and/or exercise-induced) (GINA, 2015; NAEPP, 2007). Patient must be instructed to seek medical attention in cases where acute symptoms are not relieved or a previous level of response is diminished. The need to increase frequency of use may indicate deterioration of asthma, and treatment must not be delayed.

Use with caution in patients with cardiovascular disease (arrhythmia, coronary insufficiency, or hypertension, or HF heart failure); beta-agonists may produce ECG changes (flattening of the T wave, prolongation of the QTc interval, ST segment depression) and/or cause elevation in blood pressure, heart rate and result in CNS stimulation/excitation. Beta$_2$-agonists may increase risk of arrhythmia, increase serum glucose (and aggravate preexisting diabetes and ketoacidosis), or decrease serum potassium. Use with caution in patients with renal impairment.

Immediate hypersensitivity reactions (urticaria, angioedema, rash, bronchospasm), including anaphylaxis, have been reported. Do not exceed recommended dose; serious adverse events, including fatalities, have been associated with excessive use of inhaled sympathomimetics. Rarely, paradoxical bronchospasm may occur with use of inhaled bronchodilating agents (may be fatal); this should be distinguished from inadequate response. All patients should utilize a spacer device or valved holding chamber when using a metered-dose inhaler; in addition, use spacer for children <5 years of age and consider adding a face mask for infants and children <4 years of age. Powder for oral inhalation contains lactose; hypersensitivity reactions (eg, anaphylaxis, angioedema, pruritus, and rash) have been reported in patients with milk protein allergy. Potentially significant interactions may exist, requiring dose or frequency adjustment, additional monitoring, and/or selection of alternative therapy.
Adverse Reactions Incidence of adverse effects is dependent upon age of patient, dose, and route of administration. Frequency not always defined.
>10%:
Central nervous system: Excitement (children and adolescents 2 to 14 years: 20%), nervousness (4% to 15%)
Neuromuscular & skeletal: Tremor (≥5% to 38%; frequency increases with age)
Respiratory: Upper respiratory tract infection (≥5% or 21%), rhinitis (5% to 16%), bronchospasm (8% to 15%; exacerbation of underlying pulmonary disease), pharyngitis (14%), exacerbation of asthma (11% to 13%)
1% to 10%:
Cardiovascular: Tachycardia (≤7%), hypertension (1% to 3%), chest pain (<3%), edema (<3%), extrasystoles (<3%), chest discomfort, flushing, palpitations
Central nervous system: Shakiness (children and adolescents 6 to 14 years: 9%), headache (3% to 7%), dizziness (<7%), insomnia (1% to 3%), anxiety (<3%), ataxia (<3%), depression (<3%), drowsiness (<3%), rigors (<3%), voice disorder (<3%), hyperactivity (children and adolescents 6 to 14 years: 2%), malaise (2%), pain (2%), migraine (≤2%), emotional lability (1%), fatigue (1%), restlessness, vertigo
Dermatologic: Diaphoresis (<3%), skin rash (<3%), urticaria (≤2%), pallor (children 2 to 6 years: 1%)
Endocrine & metabolic: Increased serum glucose (10%), diabetes mellitus (<3%)
Gastrointestinal: Nausea (2% to 10%), vomiting (7%), unpleasant taste (inhalation site, 4%), gastroenteritis (3%), increased appetite (children and adolescents 6 to 14 years: 3%), diarrhea (<3%), eructation (<3%), flatulence (<3%), glossitis (<3%), xerostomia (<3%), gastrointestinal symptoms (children 2 to 6 years: 2%), dyspepsia (1% to 2%), viral gastroenteritis (1% to 3%), anorexia (children 2 to 6 years: 1%)
Genitourinary: Urinary tract infection (≤3%), difficulty in micturition
Hematologic & oncologic: Decreased hematocrit (7%), decreased hemoglobin (7%), decreased white blood cell count (4%), lymphadenopathy (3%)
Hepatic: Increased serum ALT (5%), increased serum AST (4%)
Hypersensitivity: Hypersensitivity reaction (3% to 6%)
Infection: Cold symptoms (3%), infection (<3%; skin/appendage: ≤2%)
Local: Application site reaction (HFA inhaler: 6%)
Neuromuscular & skeletal: Muscle cramps (1% to 7%; frequency increases with age), musculoskeletal pain (3% to 5%), back pain (2% to 4%), hyperkinesia (≤4%), leg cramps (<3%)

Ophthalmic: Conjunctivitis (children 2 to 6 years: 1%)

Otic: Otitis media (≤4%), ear disease (<3%), otalgia (<3%), tinnitus (<3%)

Respiratory: Throat irritation (10%), viral upper respiratory tract infection (7%), respiratory tract disease (6%), nasopharyngitis (≥5%), oropharyngeal pain (≥5%), sinusitis (≥5%), upper respiratory tract inflammation (5%), cough (≥3%), flu-like symptoms (3%), dyspnea (<3%), laryngitis (<3%), oropharyngeal edema (<3%), pulmonary disease (<3%), bronchitis (≥2%), increased bronchial secretions (2%), wheezing (1% to 2%), epistaxis (children and adolescents 6 to 14 years: 1%), nasal congestion (1%), sinus headache (1%)

Miscellaneous: Fever (≥5% to 6%), accidental injury (<3%)

<1% (Limited to important or life-threatening): Anaphylaxis, atrial fibrillation, exacerbation of diabetes mellitus, gag reflex, glossitis, hyperglycemia, hypokalemia, hypotension, ketoacidosis, lactic acidosis, paradoxical bronchospasm, peripheral vasodilation, supraventricular tachycardia, tongue ulcer

Drug Interactions

Metabolism/Transport Effects None known.

Avoid Concomitant Use

Avoid concomitant use of Albuterol with any of the following: Beta-Blockers (Nonselective); Iobenguane I 123; Loxapine

Increased Effect/Toxicity

Albuterol may increase the levels/effects of: Atosiban; Doxofylline; Highest Risk QTc-Prolonging Agents; Loop Diuretics; Loxapine; Moderate Risk QTc-Prolonging Agents; Sympathomimetics; Thiazide Diuretics

The levels/effects of Albuterol may be increased by: AtoMOXetine; Cannabinoid-Containing Products; Linezolid; MAO Inhibitors; Mifepristone; Tedizolid; Tricyclic Antidepressants

Decreased Effect

Albuterol may decrease the levels/effects of: Iobenguane I 123

The levels/effects of Albuterol may be decreased by: Beta-Blockers (Beta1 Selective); Beta-Blockers (Nonselective); Betahistine

Preparation for Administration

Solution for nebulization: To prepare a 2.5 mg dose, dilute 0.5 mL of solution to a total of 3 mL with normal saline; also compatible with cromolyn or ipratropium nebulizer solutions.

IV [Canadian product]: Dilute 5 mg/ 5 mL ampul in 500 mL of a compatible solution (final concentration: 10 mcg/mL). Use within 24 hours.

Storage/Stability

HFA aerosols: Store at 15°C to 25°C (59°F to 77°F). Do not store at temperature >120°F. Do not puncture. Do not use or store near heat or open flame.

Ventolin HFA: Discard when counter reads 000 or 12 months after removal from protective pouch, whichever comes first. Store with mouthpiece down.

Infusion solution [Canadian product]: Ventolin IV: Store at 15°C to 30°C (59°F to 86°F). Protect from light. After dilution, discard unused portion after 24 hours.

Inhalation powder: Store between 15°C and 25°C (59°F and 77°F). Avoid exposure to extreme heat, cold, or humidity. Discard 13 months after opening the foil pouch, or when the counter displays 0, whichever comes first.

Solution for nebulization: Store at 2°C to 25°C (36°F to 77°F). Do not use if solution changes color or becomes cloudy. Products packaged in foil should be used within 1 week (or according to the manufacturer's recommendations) if removed from foil pouch.

Syrup: Store at 20°C to 25°C (68°F to 77°F).

Tablet: Store at 20°C to 25°C (68°F to 77°F).

Tablet, extended release: Store at 20°C to 25°C (68°F to 77°F)

Mechanism of Action
Relaxes bronchial smooth muscle by action on beta$_2$-receptors with little effect on heart rate

Pharmacodynamics/Kinetics

Onset of action: Peak effect:

Nebulization/oral inhalation: 0.5 to 2 hours

CFC-propelled albuterol: 10 minutes

Inhalation powder: 30 minutes

Ventolin HFA: 25 minutes

Oral: Immediate release: 2 to 3 hours

Duration: Nebulization/oral inhalation: 2 to 5 hours; Oral: Immediate release: 4 to 6 hours; extended release tablets: Up to 12 hours

Protein binding: 10%

Metabolism: Hepatic to an inactive sulfate

Half-life elimination: Inhalation: 3.8 hours; Oral: 3.7 to 5 hours

Excretion: Urine (30% as unchanged drug); feces (<20%)

Dosing

Adult

Bronchospasm:

Metered-dose inhaler (90 mcg/actuation): Inhalation aerosol or powder: 2 inhalations every 4 to 6 hours as needed (NAEPP 2007):

Metered-dose inhaler (100 mcg/actuation): Airomir [Canadian product]: Inhalation aerosol:

Acute treatment: 1 to 2 inhalations; additional inhalations may be necessary if inadequate relief however patients should be advised to promptly consult health care provider or seek medical attention if no relief from acute treatment

Maintenance: 1 to 2 inhalations 3 to 4 times daily (maximum: 8 inhalations daily)

Nebulization solution: 2.5 mg 3 to 4 times daily as needed; Quick relief: 1.25 to 5 mg every 4 to 8 hours as needed (NAEPP 2007)

Oral: **Note:** Oral is not the preferred route for treatment of asthma; inhalation via nebulization or MDI is preferred (NAEPP 2007).

Regular release: 2 to 4 mg/dose 3 to 4 times daily; maximum dose not to exceed 32 mg daily (divided doses)

Extended release: 8 mg every 12 hours; maximum dose not to exceed 32 mg/day (divided doses). A 4 mg dose every 12 hours may be sufficient in some patients, such as adults of low body weight.

IV continuous infusion [Canadian product]: Severe bronchospasm and status asthmaticus: Initial: 5 mcg/minute; may increase up to 10 to 20 mcg/minute at 15- to 30-minute intervals if needed

Exacerbation of asthma (acute, severe) (NAEPP 2007):

Metered-dose inhaler (90 mcg/actuation): Inhalation aerosol or powder: 4 to 8 inhalations every 20 minutes for up to 4 hours, then every 1 to 4 hours as needed

Nebulization solution: 2.5 to 5 mg every 20 minutes for 3 doses, then 2.5 to 10 mg every 1 to 4 hours as needed, **or** 10 to 15 mg/hour by continuous nebulization

Exercise-induced bronchospasm (prevention):

Metered-dose inhaler (90 mcg/actuation): Inhalation aerosol or powder: 2 inhalations 5 minutes prior to exercise

Metered-dose inhaler (100 mcg/actuation): Airomir [Canadian product]: Inhalation aerosol: 2 inhalations 30 minutes prior to exercise

Geriatric

Inhalation: Refer to adult dosing.

Bronchospasm (treatment): *Oral, regular release:* 2 mg 3 to 4 times daily; maximum: 8 mg 4 times daily

Pediatric

Bronchospasm:

Metered-dose inhaler (90 mcg/actuation) (NAEPP 2007): Inhalation aerosol or powder: Quick relief:

Children ≤4 years: 2 inhalations every 4 to 6 hours as needed

Children 5 to 11 years: 2 inhalations every 4 to 6 hours as needed

Children ≥12 years and Adolescents: 2 inhalations every 4 to 6 hours as needed

Metered-dose inhaler (100 mcg/actuation): Airomir [Canadian product]: Inhalation aerosol:

Children 6 to 11 years:

Acute treatment: 1 inhalation; additional inhalations may be necessary if inadequate relief; however, patients should be advised to promptly consult health care provider or seek medical attention if no relief from acute treatment

Maintenance: 1 inhalation; may increase to maximum of 1 inhalation 4 times daily

Children ≥12 years and Adolescents: Refer to adult dosing.

Nebulization solution:

Manufacturer's recommendations:

Children 2 to 12 years: 0.63 to 1.25 mg 3 to 4 times daily as needed

Children ≥12 years and Adolescents: 2.5 mg 3 to 4 times daily as needed

NIH Guidelines 2007: Quick relief:

Children ≤4 years: 0.63 to 2.5 mg every 4 to 6 hours as needed

Children 5 to 11 years: 1.25 to 5 mg every 4 to 8 hours as needed

Children ≥12 years and Adolescents: Refer to adult dosing.

Oral: **Note:** Oral is not the preferred route for treatment of asthma; inhalation via nebulization or MDI is preferred (NAEPP 2007).

Regular release:

Children 2 to 6 years: 0.1 to 0.2 mg/kg/dose 3 times daily (maximum: 12 mg daily)

Children 6 to 12 years: 2 mg/dose 3 to 4 times daily (maximum: 24 mg daily)

Children >12 years and Adolescents: 2 to 4 mg/dose 3 to 4 times daily (maximum: 32 mg daily)

Extended release:

Children 6 to 12 years: 4 mg every 12 hours (maximum: 24 mg daily)

Children >12 years and Adolescents: 8 mg every 12 hours (maximum: 32 mg daily)

Exacerbation of asthma (acute, severe) (NAEPP 2007):

Metered-dose inhaler (90 mcg/actuation): Inhalation aerosol or powder:

Children <12 years: 4 to 8 inhalations every 20 minutes for 3 doses, then every 1 to 4 hours as needed

Children ≥12 years and Adolescents: 4 to 8 inhalations every 20 minutes for up to 4 hours, then every 1 to 4 hours as needed

Nebulization solution:

Children <12 years: 0.15 mg/kg (minimum: 2.5 mg) every 20 minutes for 3 doses, then 0.15 to 0.3 mg/kg (maximum: 10 mg) every 1 to 4 hours as needed, **or** 0.5 mg/kg/hour by continuous nebulization

Children ≥12 years and Adolescents: 2.5 to 5 mg every 20 minutes for 3 doses, then 2.5 to 10 mg every 1 to 4 hours as needed, **or** 10 to 15 mg/hour by continuous nebulization

Exercise-induced bronchospasm (prevention):

Metered-dose inhaler (90 mcg/actuation): Inhalation aerosol or powder:

Children ≤4 years: 1 to 2 inhalations 5 minutes prior to exercise (NAEPP 2007):

Children >4 years and Adolescents: 2 inhalations 5 minutes prior to exercise

Metered-dose inhaler (100 mcg/actuation): Airomir [Canadian product]: Inhalation aerosol:

Children 6 to 11 years: 1 inhalation 30 minutes prior to exercise

Children ≥12 years and Adolescents: Refer to adult dosing.

Renal Impairment There are no dosage adjustments provided in the manufacturer's labeling; use with caution. No dosage adjustment required in patients on hemodialysis, peritoneal dialysis, or CRRT (Aronoff 2007).

Hepatic Impairment There are no dosage adjustments provided in the manufacturer's labeling.

Administration

Infusion solution [Canadian product]: Do not inject undiluted. Reduce concentration by at least 50% before infusing. Administer as a continuous infusion via infusion pump.

Inhalation powder: Inhaler device is breath-actuated; does not require priming. Do not use with spacer or volume holding chamber. Keep inhaler clean and dry by wiping with dry cloth or tissue as needed; do not wash or put any part of inhaler in water.

Metered-dose inhalers:

Inhalation aerosol: Shake well before use; prime prior to first use, and whenever inhaler has not been used for >2 weeks or when it has been dropped, by releasing 3 to 4 test sprays into the air (away from face). Airomir Canadian product labeling recommends releasing a minimum of 4 test sprays when priming. HFA inhalers should be cleaned with warm water at least once per week; allow to air dry completely prior to use. A spacer device or valved holding chamber is recommended for use with metered-dose inhalers.

Inhalation powder: Inhaler device is breath-actuated; does not require priming. Do not use with spacer or volume holding chamber. Keep inhaler clean and dry by wiping with dry cloth or tissue as needed; do not wash or put any part of inhaler in water.

Nebulization solution: Concentrated solution should be diluted prior to use. Blow-by administration is not recommended, use a mask device if patient unable to hold mouthpiece in mouth for administration.

Oral: Do not crush or chew extended release tablets.

Monitoring Parameters FEV_1, peak flow, and/or other pulmonary function tests; blood pressure, heart rate; CNS stimulation; serum glucose, serum potassium; asthma symptoms; arterial or capillary blood gases (if patients condition warrants)

Test Interactions Increased renin (S), increased aldosterone (S)

Additional Information The 2007 National Heart, Lung, and Blood Institute Guidelines for the Diagnosis and Management of Asthma do not recommend the use of oral systemic albuterol as a quick-relief medication and do not recommend regularly scheduled daily, chronic use of inhaled beta-agonists for long-term control of asthma.

Dosage Forms Considerations

ProAir HFA 8.5 g canisters and Proventil HFA 6.7 g canisters contain 200 inhalations.

Ventolin HFA 18 g canisters contain 200 inhalations and the 8 g canisters contain 60 inhalations.

Dosage Forms Excipient information presented when available (limited, particularly for generics); consult specific product labeling. [DSC] = Discontinued product

Aerosol Powder Breath Activated, Inhalation:

ProAir RespiClick: 90 mcg/actuation (1 ea) [contains milk protein]

Aerosol Solution, Inhalation:

ProAir HFA: 90 mcg/actuation (8.5 g)

Proventil HFA: 90 mcg/actuation (6.7 g)

Ventolin HFA: 90 mcg/actuation (8 g, 18 g)

Nebulization Solution, Inhalation:

Generic: 0.63 mg/3 mL (3 mL); 0.083% [2.5 mg/3 mL] (3 mL); 0.5% [2.5 mg/0.5 mL] (20 mL)

Nebulization Solution, Inhalation [preservative free]:

AccuNeb: 0.63 mg/3 mL (3 mL [DSC]); 1.25 mg/3 mL (3 mL [DSC])

Generic: 0.63 mg/3 mL (3 mL); 1.25 mg/3 mL (3 mL); 0.083% [2.5 mg/3 mL] (3 mL); 0.5% [2.5 mg/0.5 mL] (1 ea)

Syrup, Oral:

Generic: 2 mg/5 mL (473 mL)

Tablet, Oral:

Generic: 2 mg, 4 mg

Tablet Extended Release 12 Hour, Oral:

VoSpire ER: 4 mg [contains fd&c blue #1 aluminum lake, fd&c yellow #10 aluminum lake]

VoSpire ER: 8 mg

Generic: 4 mg, 8 mg

Dosage Forms: Canada Excipient information presented when available (limited, particularly for generics); consult specific product labeling.

Aerosol Solution, inhalation:

Airomir: 100 mcg/inhalation (3.7 g) [chlorofluorocarbon free; 100 metered actuations]

Airomir: 100 mcg/inhalation (6.7 g) [chlorofluorocarbon free; 200 metered actuations]

Solution, Injection, as sulphate:

Ventolin I.V.: 1 mg/1mL (5 mL)

◆ Albuterol and Ipratropium *see* Ipratropium and Albuterol *on page 978*

◆ Albuterol Sulfate *see* Albuterol *on page 57*

◆ Alcaine *see* Proparacaine *on page 1515*

◆ Alcaine® (Can) *see* Proparacaine *on page 1515*

◆ Alcalak [OTC] *see* Calcium Carbonate *on page 287*

Alclometasone (al kloe MET a sone)

Brand Names: US Aclovate

Index Terms Alclometasone Dipropionate

Pharmacologic Category Corticosteroid, Topical

Additional Appendix Information

Topical Corticosteroids *on page 1952*

Use Treatment of inflammation of corticosteroid-responsive dermatosis (low to medium potency topical corticosteroid)

Dosing

Adult & Geriatric Steroid-responsive dermatoses: Topical: Apply a thin film to the affected area 2-3 times/day. **Note:** Therapy should be discontinued when control is achieved; if no improvement is seen within 2 weeks, reassessment of diagnosis may be necessary.

Pediatric Steroid-responsive dermatoses: Topical: Children ≥1 year: Apply thin film to affected area 2-3 times/day. **Note:** Therapy should be discontinued when control is achieved; if no improvement is seen within 2 weeks, reassessment of diagnosis may be necessary. Do not use for >3 weeks.

Additional Information Complete prescribing information should be consulted for additional detail.

Dosage Forms Excipient information presented when available (limited, particularly for generics); consult specific product labeling.

Cream, External, as dipropionate:

Aclovate: 0.05% (15 g, 60 g) [contains cetearyl alcohol, propylene glycol]

Generic: 0.05% (15 g, 45 g, 60 g)

Ointment, External, as dipropionate:

Generic: 0.05% (15 g, 45 g, 60 g)

◆ Alclometasone Dipropionate *see* Alclometasone *on page 59*

◆ Alcortin A *see* Iodoquinol and Hydrocortisone *on page 974*

◆ Aldactone *see* Spironolactone *on page 1697*
◆ Aldara *see* Imiquimod *on page 926*
◆ Aldara P (Can) *see* Imiquimod *on page 926*

Aldesleukin (al des LOO kin)

Brand Names: US Proleukin
Brand Names: Canada Proleukin
Index Terms IL-2; Interleukin 2; Interleukin-2; Lymphocyte Mitogenic Factor; Recombinant Human Interleukin-2; T-Cell Growth Factor; TCGF; Thymocyte Stimulating Factor
Pharmacologic Category Antineoplastic Agent, Biological Response Modulator; Antineoplastic Agent, Miscellaneous

Use
Melanoma, metastatic: Treatment of metastatic melanoma
Renal cell cancer, metastatic: Treatment of metastatic renal cell cancer
Limitations of use: Careful patient selection is necessary. Assess performance status (PS); patients with a more favorable PS (Eastern Cooperative Oncology Group [ECOG] PS 0) at treatment initiation respond better to aldesleukin (higher response rate and lower toxicity). Experience in patients with ECOG PS >1 is limited.

Pregnancy Considerations Adverse events were observed in animal reproduction studies. Use during pregnancy only if benefits to the mother outweigh potential risk to the fetus. Effective contraception is recommended for fertile males and/or females using this medication.

Breast-Feeding Considerations It is not known if aldesleukin is excreted in breast milk. Due to the potential for serious adverse reactions in the breast-feeding infant, a decision should be made to discontinue breast-feeding or to discontinue the drug, taking into account the importance of treatment to the mother.

Contraindications Hypersensitivity to aldesleukin or any component of the formulation; patients with abnormal thallium stress or pulmonary function tests; patients who have had an organ allograft. **Re-treatment is contraindicated** in patients who have experienced sustained ventricular tachycardia (≥5 beats), uncontrolled or unresponsive cardiac arrhythmias, chest pain with ECG changes consistent with angina or MI, cardiac tamponade, intubation >72 hours, renal failure requiring dialysis for >72 hours, coma or toxic psychosis lasting >48 hours, repetitive or refractory seizures, bowel ischemia/perforation, or GI bleeding requiring surgery.

Warnings/Precautions [U.S. Boxed Warning]: Aldesleukin therapy has been associated with capillary leak syndrome (CLS), characterized by vascular tone loss and extravasation of plasma proteins and fluid into extravascular space. CLS results in hypotension and reduced organ perfusion, which may be severe and can result in death. Cardiac arrhythmia, angina, myocardial infarction, respiratory insufficiency (requiring intubation), gastrointestinal bleeding or infarction, renal insufficiency, edema and mental status changes are also associated with CLS. CLS onset is immediately after treatment initiation. Monitor fluid status and organ perfusion status carefully; consider fluids and/or pressor agents to maintain organ perfusion. **[U.S. Boxed Warning]: Therapy should be restricted to patients with normal cardiac and pulmonary functions as defined by thallium stress and formal pulmonary function testing. Extreme caution should be used in patients with a history of prior cardiac or pulmonary disease** and in patients who are fluid-restricted or where edema may be poorly tolerated. Withhold treatment for signs of organ hypoperfusion, including altered mental status, reduced urine output, systolic BP <90 mm Hg or cardiac arrhythmia. Once blood pressure is normalized, may consider diuretics for excessive weight gain/edema. Recovery from CLS generally begins soon after treatment cessation. Perform a thorough clinical evaluation prior to treatment initiation; exclude patients with significant cardiac, pulmonary, renal, hepatic, or central nervous system impairment from treatment. Patients with a more favorable performance status prior to treatment initiation are more likely to respond to aldesleukin treatment, with a higher response rate and generally lower toxicity.

[U.S. Boxed Warning]: Should be administered under the supervision of an experienced cancer chemotherapy physician in a facility with cardiopulmonary or intensive specialists and intensive care facilities available. Adverse effects are frequent and sometimes fatal. May exacerbate preexisting or initial presentation of autoimmune diseases and inflammatory disorders; exacerbation and/or new onset have been reported with aldesleukin and interferon alfa combination therapy. Thyroid disease (hypothyroidism, biphasic thyroiditis, and thyrotoxicosis) may occur; the onset of hypothyroidism is usually 4 to 17 weeks after treatment initiation; may be reversible upon treatment discontinuation (Hamnvik, 2011). Patients should be evaluated and treated for CNS metastases and have a negative scan prior to treatment; new neurologic symptoms and lesions have been reported in patients without preexisting evidence of CNS metastases (symptoms generally improve upon discontinuation, however, cases with permanent damage have been reported). Mental status changes (irritability, confusion, depression) can occur and may indicate bacteremia, sepsis, hypoperfusion, CNS malignancy, or CNS toxicity. May cause seizure; use with caution in patients with seizure disorder. Ethanol use may increase CNS adverse effects.

[U.S. Boxed Warning]: Impaired neutrophil function is associated with treatment; patients are at risk for disseminated infection (including sepsis and bacterial endocarditis), and central line-related gram-positive infections. Treat preexisting bacterial infection appropriately prior to treatment initiation. Antibiotic prophylaxis that has been associated with a reduced incidence of staphylococcal infections in aldesleukin studies includes the use of oxacillin, nafcillin, ciprofloxacin, or vancomycin. Monitor for signs of infection or sepsis during treatment.

[U.S. Boxed Warning]: Withhold treatment for patients developing moderate-to-severe lethargy or somnolence; continued treatment may result in coma. Standard prophylactic supportive care during high-dose aldesleukin treatment includes acetaminophen to relieve constitutional symptoms and an H_2 antagonist to reduce the risk of GI ulceration and/or bleeding. May impair renal or hepatic function; patients must have a serum creatinine ≤1.5 mg/dL prior to treatment. Concomitant nephrotoxic or hepatotoxic agents may increase the risk of renal or hepatic toxicity. Potentially significant drug-drug interactions may exist, requiring dose or frequency adjustment, additional monitoring, and/or selection of alternative therapy. Enhancement of cellular immune function may increase the risk of allograft rejection in transplant patients. An acute array of symptoms resembling aldesleukin adverse reactions (fever, chills, nausea, rash, pruritus, diarrhea, hypotension, edema, and oliguria) were observed within 1 to 4 hours after iodinated contrast media administration, usually when given within 4 weeks after aldesleukin treatment, although has been reported several months after aldesleukin treatment. The incidence of dyspnea and severe urogenital toxicities is potentially increased in elderly patients. Aldesleukin doses >12 to 15 million units/m^2 are associated with a moderate emetic potential; antiemetics are recommended to prevent nausea and vomiting (Dupuis, 2011).

Adverse Reactions
>10%:
Cardiovascular: Hypotension (71%; grade 4: 3%), peripheral edema (28%), tachycardia (23%), edema (15%), vasodilation (13%), supraventricular tachycardia (12%; grade 4: 1%), cardiovascular disorder (11%; includes blood pressure changes, HF and ECG changes)
Central nervous system: Chills (52%), confusion (34%; grade 4: 1%), fever (29%; grade 4: 1%), malaise (27%), somnolence (22%), anxiety (12%), pain (12%), dizziness (11%)
Dermatologic: Rash (42%), pruritus (24%), exfoliative dermatitis (18%)
Endocrine & metabolic: Acidosis (12%; grade 4: 1%), hypomagnesemia (12%), hypocalcemia (11%)
Gastrointestinal: Diarrhea (67%; grade 4: 2%), vomiting (19% to 50%; grade 4: 1%), nausea (19% to 35%), stomatitis (22%), anorexia (20%), weight gain (16%), abdominal pain (11%)
Hematologic: Thrombocytopenia (37%; grade 4: 1%), anemia (29%), leukopenia (16%)
Hepatic: Hyperbilirubinemia (40%; grade 4: 2%), AST increased (23%; grade 4: 1%)
Neuromuscular & skeletal: Weakness (23%)
Renal: Oliguria (63%; grade 4: 6%), creatinine increased (33%; grade 4: 1%)
Respiratory: Dyspnea (43%; grade 4: 1%), lung disorder (24%; includes pulmonary congestion, rales, and rhonchi), cough (11%), respiratory disorder (11%; includes acute respiratory distress syndrome, infiltrates and pulmonary changes)
Miscellaneous: Antibody formation (66% to 74%), infection (13%; grade 4: 1%)
1% to 10%:
Cardiovascular: Arrhythmia (10%), cardiac arrest (grade 4: 1%), MI (grade 4: 1%), ventricular tachycardia (grade 4: 1%)

Central nervous system: Coma (grade 4: 2%), stupor (grade 4: 1%), psychosis (grade 4: 1%)

Gastrointestinal: Abdomen enlarged (10%)

Hematologic: Coagulation disorder (grade 4: 1%; includes intravascular coagulopathy)

Hepatic: Alkaline phosphatase increased (10%)

Renal: Anuria (grade 4: 5%), acute renal failure (grade 4: 1%)

Respiratory: Rhinitis (10%), apnea (grade 4: 1%)

Miscellaneous: Sepsis (grade 4: 1%)

<1% (Limited to important or life-threatening): Allergic interstitial nephritis, anaphylaxis, angioedema, asthma, atrial arrhythmia, AV block, blindness (transient or permanent), bowel infarction/necrosis/perforation, bradycardia, bullous pemphigoid, capillary leak syndrome, cardiomyopathy, cellulitis, cerebral edema, cerebral lesions, cerebral vasculitis, cholecystitis, colitis, crescentic IgA glomerulonephritis, Crohn's disease exacerbation, delirium, depression (severe; leading to suicide), diabetes mellitus, duodenal ulcer, encephalopathy, endocarditis, extrapyramidal syndrome, hemorrhage (including cerebral, gastrointestinal, retroperitoneal, subarachnoid, subdural), hepatic failure, hepatitis, hepatosplenomegaly, hypertension, hyperuricemia, hypothermia, hyperthyroidism, inflammatory arthritis, injection site necrosis, insomnia, intestinal obstruction, intestinal perforation, leukocytosis, malignant hyperthermia, meningitis, myocardial ischemia, myocarditis, myopathy, myositis, neuralgia, neuritis, neuropathy, neutropenia, NPN increased, oculobulbar myasthenia gravis, optic neuritis, organ perfusion decreased, pancreatitis, pericardial effusion, pericarditis, peripheral gangrene, phlebitis, pneumonia, pneumothorax, pulmonary edema, pulmonary embolus, respiratory acidosis, respiratory arrest, respiratory failure, rhabdomyolysis, scleroderma, seizure, Stevens-Johnson syndrome, stroke, syncope, thrombosis, thyroiditis, tracheoesophageal fistula, transient ischemic attack, tubular necrosis, ventricular extrasystoles

Drug Interactions

Metabolism/Transport Effects None known.

Avoid Concomitant Use

Avoid concomitant use of Aldesleukin with any of the following: BCG (Intravesical); Corticosteroids; Deferiprone; Dipyrone

Increased Effect/Toxicity

Aldesleukin may increase the levels/effects of: Amifostine; Antipsychotic Agents (Second Generation [Atypical]); CloZAPine; Deferiprone; DULoxetine; Iodinated Contrast Agents; Levodopa

The levels/effects of Aldesleukin may be increased by: Alfuzosin; Barbiturates; Blood Pressure Lowering Agents; Brimonidine (Topical); Diazoxide; Dipyrone; Herbs (Hypotensive Properties); Interferons (Alfa); Molsidomine; Nicorandil; Obinutuzumab; Pentoxifylline; Phosphodiesterase 5 Inhibitors; Prostacyclin Analogues

Decreased Effect

Aldesleukin may decrease the levels/effects of: BCG (Intravesical)

The levels/effects of Aldesleukin may be decreased by: Corticosteroids

Preparation for Administration Reconstitute vials with 1.2 mL SWFI (preservative free) to a concentration of 18 million units (1.1 mg)/1 mL (sterile water should be injected towards the side of the vial). Gently swirl; do not shake. Further dilute with 50 mL of D₅W. Smaller volumes of D₅W should be used for doses ≤1.5 mg; avoid concentrations <30 mcg/mL and >70 mcg/mL (an increased variability in drug delivery has been seen). Plastic (polyvinyl chloride) bags result in more consistent drug delivery and are recommended. Filtration may result in loss of bioactivity. Addition of 0.1% albumin has been used to increase stability and decrease the extent of sorption if low final concentrations cannot be avoided.

Avoid bacteriostatic water for injection and NS for reconstitution or dilution; increased aggregation may occur.

Storage/Stability Store intact vials under refrigeration at 2°C to 8°C (36°F to 46°F). Protect from light. Plastic (polyvinyl chloride) bags result in more consistent drug delivery and are recommended. According to the manufacturer, reconstituted vials and solutions diluted for infusion are stable for 48 hours at room temperature or refrigerated although refrigeration is preferred because they do not contain preservatives. Do not freeze.

Mechanism of Action Aldesleukin is a human recombinant interleukin-2 product which promotes proliferation, differentiation, and recruitment of T and B cells, natural killer (NK) cells, and thymocytes; causes cytolytic activity in a subset of lymphocytes and subsequent interactions between the immune system and malignant cells; can stimulate lymphokine-activated killer (LAK) cells and tumor-infiltrating lymphocytes (TIL) cells.

Pharmacodynamics/Kinetics

Absorption: Oral: Not absorbed

Distribution: Primarily into plasma, lymphocytes, lungs, liver, kidney, and spleen; V_d: 6.3 to 7.9 L (Whittington 1993)

Metabolism: Renal (metabolized to amino acids in the cells lining the proximal convoluted tubules of the kidney)

Half-life elimination: IV:

Children: Distribution: 14 ± 6 minutes; Elimination: 51 ± 11 minutes

Adults: Distribution: 13 minutes; Terminal: 85 minutes

Excretion: Urine (primarily as metabolites)

Dosing

Adult & Geriatric Consider premedication with an antipyretic to reduce fever, an H_2 antagonist for prophylaxis of gastrointestinal irritation/bleeding, antiemetics, and antidiarrheals; continue for 12 hours after the last aldesleukin dose. Antibiotic prophylaxis is recommended to reduce the incidence of infection. Aldesleukin doses >12 to 15 million units/m² are associated with a moderate emetic potential; antiemetics are recommended to prevent nausea and vomiting.

Renal cell carcinoma, metastatic: IV: 600,000 units/kg every 8 hours for a maximum of 14 doses; repeat after 9 days for a total of 28 doses per course; re-treat if tumor shrinkage observed (and if no contraindications) at least 7 weeks after hospital discharge date

or

Off-label dosing: 720,000 units/kg every 8 hours for up to 12 doses; repeat with a second cycle 10 to 15 days later (Klapper, 2008)

Melanoma, metastatic: IV:

Single-agent use: 600,000 units/kg every 8 hours for a maximum of 14 doses; repeat after 9 days for a total of 28 doses per course; re-treat if tumor shrinkage observed (and if no contraindications) at least 7 weeks after hospital discharge date

or

Off-label dosing: 720,000 units/kg every 8 hours for 12 to 15 doses; repeat with a second cycle ~14 days after the first dose of the initial cycle (Smith, 2008)

Combination biochemotherapy (off-label use): 9 million units/m²/day continuous infusion over 24 hours for 4 days every 3 weeks for up to 4 cycles (Atkins, 2008) or 9 million units/m²/day continuous infusion over 24 hours days 5 to 8, 17 to 20, and 26 to 29 every 42 days for up to 5 cycles (Eton, 2002) or 9 million units/m²/day continuous infusion over 24 hours for 4 days every 3 weeks for 6 cycles (Legha, 1998)

Pediatric Consider premedication with an antipyretic to reduce fever, an H_2 antagonist for prophylaxis of gastrointestinal irritation/bleeding, antiemetics, and antidiarrheals; continue for 12 hours after the last aldesleukin dose. Antibiotic prophylaxis is recommended to reduce the incidence of infection. Aldesleukin doses >12 to 15 million units/m² are associated with a moderate emetic potential; antiemetics are recommended to prevent nausea and vomiting (Dupuis, 2011).

Neuroblastoma (off-label use): IV: 3 million units/m²/day continuous infusion over 24 hours daily for 4 days during week 1 and 4.5 million units/m²/day continuous infusion over 24 hours daily for 4 days during week 2 of cycles 2 and 4 (regimen also includes isotretinoin, dinutuximab, and sargramostim) (Yu, 2010).

Renal Impairment Adults:

Renal impairment prior to treatment initiation:

Serum creatinine ≤1.5 mg/dL: There are no dosage adjustments provided in the manufacturer's labeling.

Serum creatinine >1.5 mg/dL: Do not initiate treatment.

Renal toxicity during treatment:

Serum creatinine >4.5 mg/dL (or ≥4 mg/dL with severe volume overload, acidosis, or hyperkalemia): Withhold dose; may resume when <4 mg/dL and fluid/electrolyte status is stable.

Persistent oliguria or urine output <10 mL/hour for 16 to 24 hours with rising serum creatinine: Withhold dose; may resume when urine output >10 mL/hour with serum creatinine decrease of >1.5 mg/dL or normalization.

Hemodialysis: Re-treatment is contraindicated in patients with renal failure requiring dialysis for >72 hours.

Hepatic Impairment Adults:

Hepatic impairment prior to treatment initiation: There are no dosage adjustments provided in the manufacturer's labeling.

Hepatotoxicity during treatment: Signs of hepatic failure (encephalopathy, increasing ascites, liver pain, hypoglycemia): Withhold dose and discontinue treatment for

balance of cycle; may initiate a new course if indicated only after at least 7 weeks past resolution of all signs of hepatic failure (including hospital discharge).

Adjustment for Toxicity Withhold or interrupt a dose for toxicity; do not reduce the dose.

Cardiovascular toxicity:

Atrial fibrillation, supraventricular tachycardia, or bradycardia that is persistent, recurrent, or requires treatment: Withhold dose; may resume when asymptomatic with full recovery to normal sinus rhythm.

Systolic BP <90 mm Hg (with increasing pressor requirements): Withhold dose; may resume treatment when systolic BP ≥90 mm Hg and stable or pressor requirements improve.

Any ECG change consistent with MI, ischemia or myocarditis (with or without chest pain), or suspected cardiac ischemia: Withhold dose; may resume when asymptomatic, MI/myocarditis have been ruled out, suspicion of angina is low, or there is no evidence of ventricular hypokinesia.

CNS toxicity: Mental status change, including moderate confusion or agitation: Withhold dose; may resume when resolved completely.

Dermatologic toxicity: Bullous dermatitis or marked worsening of preexisting skin condition: Withhold dose; may treat with antihistamines or topical products (do not use topical steroids); may resume with resolution of all signs of bullous dermatitis.

Gastrointestinal: Stool guaiac repeatedly >3-4+: Withhold dose; may resume with negative stool guaiac.

Infection: Sepsis syndrome, clinically unstable: Withhold dose; may resume when sepsis syndrome has resolved, patient is clinically stable, and infection is under treatment.

Respiratory toxicity: Oxygen saturation <90%: Withhold dose; may resume when >90%.

Re-treatment with aldesleukin is contraindicated with the following toxicities: Sustained ventricular tachycardia (≥5 beats), uncontrolled or unresponsive cardiac arrhythmias, chest pain with ECG changes consistent with angina or MI, cardiac tamponade, intubation >72 hours, renal failure requiring dialysis for >72 hours, coma or toxic psychosis lasting >48 hours, repetitive or refractory seizures, bowel ischemia/perforation, or GI bleeding requiring surgery

Administration Aldesleukin doses >12 to 15 million units/m² are associated with a moderate emetic potential; antiemetics are recommended to prevent nausea and vomiting (Dupuis, 2011).

Administer as IV infusion over 15 minutes (do not administer with an inline filter). Allow solution to reach room temperature prior to administration. Flush before and after with D₅W, particularly if maintenance IV line contains sodium chloride. Some off-label uses/doses are infused as a continuous infusion (Legha, 1998; Yu, 2010). Has also been administered by SubQ injection (off-label route).

Monitoring Parameters

Baseline and periodic: CBC with differential and platelets, blood chemistries including electrolytes, renal and hepatic function tests, and chest x-ray; pulmonary function tests and arterial blood gases (baseline), thallium stress test (prior to treatment). Monitor thyroid function tests (TSH at baseline then every 2-3 months during aldesleukin treatment [Hamnvik, 2011]).

Monitoring during therapy should include daily (hourly if hypotensive) vital signs (temperature, pulse, blood pressure, and respiration rate), weight and fluid intake and output; in a patient with a decreased blood pressure, especially systolic BP <90 mm Hg, cardiac monitoring for rhythm should be conducted. If an abnormal complex or rhythm is seen, an ECG should be performed; vital signs in these hypotension patients should be taken hourly and central venous pressure (CVP) checked; monitor for change in mental status, and for signs of infection.

Additional Information 18 x 10⁶ units = 1.1 mg protein

Dosage Forms Excipient information presented when available (limited, particularly for generics); consult specific product labeling.

Solution Reconstituted, Intravenous [preservative free]:
Proleukin: 22,000,000 units (1 ea)

- ◆ Aldex® CT [DSC] *see* Diphenhydramine and Phenylephrine *on page 564*
- ◆ Aldex GS DM *see* Guaifenesin, Pseudoephedrine, and Dextromethorphan *on page 864*
- ◆ Aldomet *see* Methyldopa *on page 1177*
- ◆ Aldroxicon I [OTC] *see* Aluminum Hydroxide, Magnesium Hydroxide, and Simethicone *on page 85*
- ◆ Aldroxicon II [OTC] *see* Aluminum Hydroxide, Magnesium Hydroxide, and Simethicone *on page 85*
- ◆ Aldurazyme *see* Laronidase *on page 1037*
- ◆ Aldurazyme® (Can) *see* Laronidase *on page 1037*

Alemtuzumab (ay lem TU zoo mab)

Brand Names: US Campath; Lemtrada

Brand Names: Canada Lemtrada; MabCampath

Index Terms Anti-CD52 Monoclonal Antibody; Campath; Campath-1H; Humanized IgG1 Anti-CD52 Monoclonal Antibody; MoAb CD52; Monoclonal Antibody Campath-1H; Monoclonal Antibody CD52

Pharmacologic Category Antineoplastic Agent, Anti-CD52; Antineoplastic Agent, Monoclonal Antibody; Monoclonal Antibody

Use

B-cell chronic lymphocytic leukemia: Campath or MabCampath [Canadian product]: Treatment (as a single agent) of B-cell chronic lymphocytic leukemia (B-CLL)

Multiple sclerosis, relapsing: Lemtrada: Treatment of patients with relapsing forms of multiple sclerosis (MS), generally who have had an inadequate response to 2 or more medications indicated for the treatment of MS.

Pregnancy Considerations Adverse events were observed in animal reproduction studies. Human IgG is known to cross the placental barrier; therefore, alemtuzumab may also cross the barrier and cause fetal B- and T-lymphocyte depletion. Use during pregnancy only if the benefit to the mother outweighs the potential risk to the fetus. Effective contraception is recommended during and for at least 6 months (Campath) or 4 months (Lemtrada) after treatment for women of childbearing potential and men of reproductive potential.

Breast-Feeding Considerations Human IgG is excreted in breast milk; therefore, alemtuzumab may also be excreted in milk. Due to the potential for serious adverse reactions in the nursing infant, the decision to discontinue alemtuzumab or to discontinue breast-feeding should take into account the importance of treatment to the mother and the half-life of alemtuzumab. The Canadian labeling recommends discontinuing nursing during treatment and for at least 3 months (MabCampath) or 4 months (Lemtrada) after completing treatment course.

Prescribing and Access Restrictions As of September 4, 2012, alemtuzumab (Campath) is no longer commercially available in the United States (or Europe); a restricted distribution program will allow access (free of charge) for appropriate patients. Information on necessary documentation and requirements is available at Campath Distribution Program (1-877-422-6728) or Genzyme Medical Information (1-800-745-4447, option 2).

Medication Guide Available Yes

Contraindications

U.S. labeling: There are no contraindications listed in the manufacturer's Campath labeling. Lemtrada is contraindicated in patients infected with HIV (due to prolonged reduction in CD4+ lymphocytes).

Canadian labeling:

Lemtrada: Hypersensitivity to alemtuzumab or any component of the formulation; HIV infection; active or latent tuberculosis; severe active infections; active malignancies; concurrent antineoplastic or immunosuppressive therapy; history of progressive multifocal leukoencephalopathy (PML)

MabCampath: Known type 1 hypersensitivity or anaphylactic reactions to alemtuzumab or any component of the formulation; active infections; underlying immunodeficiency (eg, seropositive for HIV); active secondary malignancies; current or history of progressive multifocal leukoencephalopathy (PML)

Warnings/Precautions [U.S. Boxed Warning (Lemtrada)]: Alemtuzumab causes serious, sometimes fatal, autoimmune conditions, such as immune thrombocytopenia and antiglomerular basement membrane disease, in patients receiving alemtuzumab for the treatment of multiple sclerosis (MS). Monitor complete blood counts with differential, serum creatinine levels, and urinalysis with urine cell counts at periodic intervals for 48 months after the last dose of alemtuzumab. Monitor for symptoms of immune thrombocytopenia (easy bruising, petechiae, spontaneous mucocutaneous bleeding, heavy menstrual bleeding) in patients receiving alemtuzumab for MS. Monitor for nephropathy symptoms (eg, elevated serum creatinine, hematuria, proteinuria). Alveolar hemorrhage manifesting as hemoptysis may be present in antiglomerular basement membrane disease. Glomerular nephropathies require urgent evaluation; may lead to renal failure if not treated. Prompt intervention is necessary for autoimmune cytopenias. Idiopathic thrombocytopenic purpura, thyroid disorders, autoimmune hemolytic anemia,

autoimmune pancytopenia, undifferentiated connective tissue disorders, acquired hemophilia A, rheumatoid arthritis, vitiligo, retinal pigment epitheliopathy have been reported in patients receiving alemtuzumab for MS. Guillain-Barre syndrome and chronic inflammatory demyelinating polyradiculoneuropathy have been reported in patients receiving alemtuzumab for other uses. Alemtuzumab may increase the risk for other autoimmune conditions. Autoimmune thyroid disorders occurred in over one-third of patients receiving alemtuzumab for MS. In a trial evaluating alemtuzumab versus interferon beta-1a in patients with MS, thyroid dysfunction occurred more frequently in patients taking alemtuzumab (34% versus 6.5%) (Daniels, 2014). The incidence of the first episode of thyroid dysfunction increased annually the first 3 years (year 1: 4.6%; year 2: 13.3%; year 3: 16.1%) then gradually decreased thereafter. Among patients with alemtuzumab-related thyroid dysfunction, Graves' hyperthyroidism occurred most commonly (23%), followed by hypothyroidism and subacute thyroiditis (7% and 4%, respectively). Thyroid dysfunction (thyroiditis, Graves' disease) has also been reported with alemtuzumab use for the treatment of other conditions. For B-CLL treatment, TSH monitoring is recommended; monitor TSH at baseline and every 2 to 3 months during alemtuzumab treatment (Hamnvik, 2011). For MS, monitor TSH at baseline and every 3 months until 48 months after last infusion or longer or at any time during therapy if clinically indicated.

[U.S. Boxed Warning]: Serious and potentially fatal infusion-related reactions may occur; monitor for infusion reaction; carefully monitor during infusion; withhold treatment for serious or grade 3 or 4 infusion reactions. For B-cell chronic lymphocytic leukemia (B-CLL), gradual escalation to the recommended maintenance dose is required at initiation and with treatment interruptions (for ≥7 days) to minimize infusion-related reactions. For multiple sclerosis, must be administered in a setting with appropriate equipment and personnel to manage anaphylaxis or serious infusion reaction; monitor for 2 hours after each infusion; inform patients that serious infusion reactions may also occur after the 2-hour monitoring period. Infusion reactions have been reported more than 24 hours after infusion. In patients treated for B-CLL, infusion reaction symptoms may include acute respiratory distress syndrome, anaphylactic shock, angioedema, bronchospasm, cardiac arrest, cardiac arrhythmias, chills, dyspnea, fever, hypotension, myocardial infarction, pulmonary infiltrates, rash, rigors, syncope, or urticaria. The incidence of infusion reaction is highest during the first week of B-CLL treatment. Premedicate with acetaminophen and an oral antihistamine. Medications for the treatment of reactions should be available for immediate use. Use caution and carefully monitor blood pressure in patients with ischemic heart disease and patients on antihypertensive therapy. For B-CLL, reinitiate with gradual dose escalation if treatment is withheld ≥7 days. Similar infusion reactions have been observed with use in the treatment of multiple sclerosis; premedication with corticosteroids for initial 3 days of each treatment course is recommended. Antihistamines and/or antipyretics may also be considered. Consider additional monitoring in patients with existing cardiovascular or respiratory compromise (the Canadian labeling recommends obtaining an ECG prior to each treatment course). Observe for infusion-related reactions; advise patients to monitor for signs/symptoms of infusion reaction, particularly during the 24 hours following infusion.

[U.S. Boxed Warning (Campath): Serious and fatal cytopenias (including pancytopenia, bone marrow hypoplasia, autoimmune hemolytic anemia, and autoimmune idiopathic thrombocytopenia) have occurred. Single doses >30 mg or cumulative weekly doses >90 mg are associated with an increased incidence of pancytopenia. Severe prolonged myelosuppression, hemolytic anemia, pure red cell aplasia, bone marrow aplasia, and bone marrow hypoplasia have also been reported with use at the normal dose for the treatment of B-CLL. Discontinue for serious hematologic or other serious toxicity (except lymphopenia) until the event resolves. Permanently discontinue if autoimmune anemia or autoimmune thrombocytopenia occurs. Patients receiving blood products should only receive irradiated blood products due to the potential for transfusion-associated GVHD during lymphopenia.

[U.S. Boxed Warning (Campath): Serious and potentially fatal infections (bacterial, viral, fungal, and protozoan) have been reported. Administer prophylactic medications against PCP pneumonia and herpes viral infections during treatment and for at least 2 months following last dose or until CD4+ counts are ≥200 cells/mm^3 (whichever is later). Severe and prolonged

lymphopenia may occur; CD4+ counts usually return to ≥200 cells/mm^3 within 2 to 6 months; however, CD4+ and CD8+ lymphocyte counts may not return to baseline levels for more than 1 year. Withhold treatment during serious infections; may be reinitiated upon resolution of infection. Monitor for CMV infection (during and for at least 2 months after completion of therapy); initiate appropriate antiviral treatment and withhold alemtuzumab for CMV infection or confirmed CMV viremia (withhold alemtuzumab during CMV antiviral treatment). For patients being treated for MS, initiate antiviral prophylaxis (for herpetic viral infections) beginning on the first day of treatment and continue for at least 2 months or until CD4+ lymphocyte count is ≥200/mm^3. In clinical trials for MS, infections seen more commonly in alemtuzumab-treated patients included nasopharyngitis, urinary tract infection, upper respiratory tract infection, sinusitis, herpetic infections, influenza, and bronchitis; serious cases of appendicitis, gastroenteritis, pneumonia, herpes zoster, and tooth infection also occurred. Consider delaying treatment in patients with active infection until infection is controlled. Patients should be screened for human papilloma virus (HPV) and tuberculosis as clinically necessary. Progressive multifocal leukoencephalopathy (PML) been reported with use (rarely); withhold therapy immediately for signs/symptoms suggestive of PML. According to the Canadian labeling, alemtuzumab is contraindicated in patients with a history of PML.

[U.S. Boxed Warning (Lemtrada): Alemtuzumab may cause an increased risk of malignancies, including thyroid cancer, melanoma, and lymphoproliferative disorders, Perform baseline and yearly skin exams. Other malignant neoplasm (breast cancer or basal cell carcinoma) has been observed (rarely) in patients receiving treatment for MS. Use of Lemtrada in patients with active malignancies is contraindicated; use caution if initiating treatment in patients with preexisting malignancy (Canadian labeling).

Pneumonitis (hypersensitivity or fibrosis) has been reported. Monitor for symptoms (dyspnea, cough, wheezing, hemoptysis, chest pain/tightness). Alemtuzumab is associated with a moderate emetic potential in the oncology setting; antiemetics may be recommended to prevent nausea and vomiting (Basch, 2011; Roila, 2010). Potentially significant drug-drug interactions may exist, requiring dose or frequency adjustment, additional monitoring, and/or selection of alternative therapy. If considering Lemtrada treatment for use in a patient who has previously received Campath/MabCampath, consider the additive and long-lasting immune system effects. Patients should not be immunized with live, viral vaccines during or recently after treatment. The ability to respond to any vaccine following therapy is unknown. Testing for antibodies to varicella zoster virus (VZV) is recommended prior to initiation of Lemtrada if history of chickenpox or VZV vaccination status is unknown. When using for the treatment of multiple sclerosis, complete necessary immunizations at least 6 weeks prior to initiating alemtuzumab. Determine if patient has a history varicella or vaccination for VZV; if not, test for VZV antibodies and consider vaccinations for antibody-negative patients; postpone alemtuzumab treatment for 6 weeks following VZV vaccination.

Alemtuzumab is not recommended for use in MS patients with inactive disease or who are stable on other treatment. Patients should commit to at least 48 months of follow-up after the last infusion. Alemtuzumab has not been studied in MS patients infected with HBV or HCV; consider screening patients at increased risk of infection prior to initiating treatment. Use with caution in HBV or HCV carriers; patients may be at risk for viral reactivation. **[U.S. Boxed Warning (Lemtrada): Due to the risk of autoimmunity, infusion reactions, and malignancies, alemtuzumab is available only through restricted distribution under a Risk Evaluation Mitigation Strategy (REMS) Program when used for the treatment of MS. Contact 1-855-676-6326 to enroll in the Lemtrada REMS program.** Prescribers and pharmacies must be certified with the REMS program, and patients and healthcare facilities must be enrolled and comply with ongoing monitoring.

Adverse Reactions Adverse reactions listed below are reflective of both the U.S. and Canadian product information.

>10%:
  Central nervous system: Headache (44% to 52%), fatigue (8% to 21%), insomnia (11% to 17%), paresthesia (10% to 12%)
  Dermatologic: Skin rash (43% to 53%), urticaria (15% to 17%), pruritus (13% to 17%)
  Endocrine & metabolic: Thyroid disease (13% to 34%)
  Gastrointestinal: Nausea (16% to 22%), diarrhea (12%), oral candidiasis (3% to 12%)

Genitourinary: Urinary tract infection (18% to 19%), vulvovaginal candidiasis (3% to 12%)

Hematologic & oncologic: Lymphocytopenia (6% to 100%)

Immunologic: Antibody development (8% to 85%; no effect on drug efficacy; anti-alemtuzumab: 2%)

Infection: Infection (71%), herpes virus infection (16%), fungal infection (12% to 13%)

Local: Infusion related reaction (92%)

Neuromuscular & skeletal: Arthralgia (12% to 13%), limb pain (13%), back pain (12%)

Respiratory: Nasopharyngitis (24% to 25%), upper respiratory tract infection (15% to 16%), oropharyngeal pain (11%), sinusitis (11%)

Miscellaneous: Fever (26% to 30%)

1% to 10%:

Cardiovascular: Flushing (10%), chest discomfort (7% to 8%), tachycardia (6% to 8%), peripheral edema (5%), palpitations (4%), bradycardia (3%), hypotension (3%), chest pain (2%), cold extremities (1%)

Central nervous system: Chills (9% to 10%), dizziness (10%), anxiety (7%), pain (5% to 7%), vertigo (4%), equilibrium disturbance (3%), hyperthermia (3%), increased body temperature (3%), drowsiness (2%), facial hypoesthesia (2%), hypertonia (2%)

Dermatologic: Skin rash (generalized; 7% to 8%), erythema (6%), acne vulgaris (3%), allergic dermatitis (3%), alopecia (3%), erythematous rash (3%), hyperhidrosis (3%), pruritic rash (3%), papular rash (2%), pruritus (generalized; 2%), skin blister (1%), xeroderma (1%)

Endocrine & metabolic: Hypothyroidism (5%), hypermenorrhea (4%), hyperthyroidism (4%), chronic lymphocytic thyroiditis (2%), Graves' disease (2%), thyroid stimulating hormone suppression (2%), goiter (1%)

Gastrointestinal: Vomiting (10%), abdominal pain (5% to 10%), oral herpes (9%), dyspepsia (6% to 9%), dysgeusia (8%), gastroenteritis (4%), upper abdominal pain (4%), abdominal distention (2%), oral mucosa ulcer (1%)

Genitourinary: Occult blood in urine (4% to 8%), uterine hemorrhage (5%), hematuria (3%), cystitis (2%), fungal vaginosis (2%), increase in urinary protein (2%), irregular menses (2%), proteinuria (2%), abnormal urinalysis (1%), herpes genitalis (1%), vaginal hemorrhage (1%)

Hematologic & oncologic: Bruise (10%), decreased CD-4 cell count (5% to 6%), decreased CD-8 cell counts (5% to 6%), decreased absolute lymphocyte count (4% to 5%), decreased T cell lymphocytes (4%), reduction of B-cells (4%), abnormal white blood cell differential (lymphocyte percentage decreased: 3%; lymphocyte percentage increased: 2%), immune thrombocytopenia (2%), nonthrombocytopenic purpura (2%), hematoma (1%), petechia (1%)

Hypersensitivity: Cytokine release syndrome (2%)

Infection: Influenza (8%), herpes zoster (4%), bacterial infection (3%), herpes simplex infection (2%), human papilloma virus infection (2%)

Local: Catheter pain (1%), infusion related reaction

Neuromuscular & skeletal: Myalgia (6% to 7%), myasthenia (7%), muscle spasm (6%), weakness (5% to 6%), neck pain (5%), joint sprain (2%), joint swelling (2%), musculoskeletal chest pain (2%)

Ophthalmic: Blurred vision (5%), conjunctivitis (2%), Graves' ophthalmopathy (1%)

Otic: Otalgia (3%), otic infection (3%)

Respiratory: Cough (9%), dyspnea (8% to 9%), bronchitis (7%), epistaxis (5%), pharyngitis (4%), rhinitis (4%), sinus congestion (3%), nasal congestion (2%), wheezing (2%), bronchospasm (1%)

<1% (Limited to important or life-threatening): Abnormal hepatic function tests, acquired blood coagulation disorder, allodynia, altered blood pressure, amenorrhea, anemia, anti-GBM disease, antithyroid antibody positive, aphthous stomatitis, asthma, ataxia, atrial fibrillation, autoimmune hemolytic anemia, autoimmune thrombocytopenia, bacterial vaginosis, candidiasis, cardiac failure, cellulitis, cervical dysplasia, cervicitis, chronic inflammatory demyelinating polyradiculoneuropathy, connective tissue disease (undifferentiated), decreased hematocrit, decreased hemoglobin, decreased monocytes, decreased neutrophils, dehydration, depression, desquamation, eosinopenia, eosinophilia, Epstein-Barr-associated lymphoproliferative disorder, Epstein-Barr infection, esophagitis, furuncle, gastroesophageal reflux disease, gastrointestinal disease, gingival hemorrhage, glycosuria, graft versus host disease (transfusion associated), Guillain-Barre syndrome, hemiparesis, hemophilia A (acquired [anti-Factor VIII antibodies]), hyperemia, hypersensitivity reaction, increased monocytes, infusion site reaction, labyrinthitis, leukocytosis, lymphoproliferative disorder, maculopapular rash, major hemorrhage, malignant lymphoma, malignant melanoma, malignant neoplasm of thyroid, membranous glomerulonephritis, memory impairment, meningitis due to listeria monocytogenes, meningitis (herpes), migraine, mucosal inflammation, multiple sclerosis, muscle spasticity, natural killer cell count increased, neutropenia, night sweats, onychomycosis, optic neuropathy, ostealgia, ovarian cyst, pancytopenia, papule, peripheral neuropathy, photophobia, pleurisy, pneumonia, pneumonitis, positive direct Coombs test, postherpetic neuralgia, progressive multifocal leukoencephalopathy, protozoal infection, psychomotor agitation, pyelonephritis, reactivation of disease, reduced ejection fraction, restless leg syndrome, retinal pigment changes (epitheliopathy), rheumatoid arthritis, serum sickness, skin hyperpigmentation, skin lesion, streptococcal pharyngitis, subacute thyroiditis, suicidal ideation, suicidal tendencies, syncope, tachypnea, thrombocytopenia, tongue discoloration, tonsillitis, tooth abscess, tracheobronchitis, tuberculosis, tumor lysis syndrome, type 1 diabetes mellitus, upper airway symptoms (cough syndrome), urethritis, urinary incontinence, varicella, viral infection, vitiligo, voice disorder, weight gain, weight loss

Drug Interactions

Metabolism/Transport Effects None known.

Avoid Concomitant Use

Avoid concomitant use of Alemtuzumab with any of the following: BCG (Intravesical); Belimumab; Deferiprone; Dipyrone; Natalizumab; Pimecrolimus; Tacrolimus (Topical); Tofacitinib; Vaccines (Live)

Increased Effect/Toxicity

Alemtuzumab may increase the levels/effects of: Belimumab; CloZAPine; Deferiprone; Fingolimod; Leflunomide; Natalizumab; Tofacitinib; Vaccines (Live)

The levels/effects of Alemtuzumab may be increased by: Denosumab; Dipyrone; Pimecrolimus; Roflumilast; Tacrolimus (Topical); Trastuzumab

Decreased Effect

Alemtuzumab may decrease the levels/effects of: BCG (Intravesical); Coccidioides immitis Skin Test; Sipuleucel-T; Vaccines (Inactivated); Vaccines (Live)

The levels/effects of Alemtuzumab may be decreased by: Echinacea

Preparation for Administration

Campath, MabCampath [Canadian product]: Dilute for infusion in 100 mL NS or D$_5$W. Compatible in polyvinyl-chloride (PVC) bags. Gently invert the bag to mix the solution. Do not shake prior to use.

Lemtrada: Withdraw 12 mg (1.2 mL) from vial and add to 100 mL bag of NS or D$_5$W. Gently invert the bag to mix the solution.

Storage/Stability

Campath: Prior to dilution, store intact (30 mg/1 mL) vials at 2°C to 8°C (36°F to 46°F); do not freeze (if accidentally frozen, thaw in refrigerator prior to administration). Do not shake; protect from light. Following dilution, store at room temperature or refrigerate; protect from light; use within 8 hours. Discard unused portion in the vial.

Lemtrada: Prior to dilution, store intact vials at 2°C to 8°C (36°F to 46°F). Do not freeze. Do not shake; protect from light. Following dilution, store at room temperature or refrigerate; use within 8 hours.

MabCampath [Canadian product]: Prior to dilution, store vials at 2°C to 8°C (36°F to 46°F). Do not freeze (discard vial if frozen). Do not shake. Protect from light. Following dilution, store at room temperature or refrigerate; use within 8 hours.

Mechanism of Action Binds to CD52, a nonmodulating antigen present on the surface of B and T lymphocytes, a majority of monocytes, macrophages, NK cells, and a subpopulation of granulocytes. After binding to CD52⁺ cells, an antibody-dependent lysis of malignant cells occurs. In multiple sclerosis, alemtuzumab immunomodulatory effects may include alteration in the number, proportions, and properties of some lymphocyte subsets following treatment.

Pharmacodynamics/Kinetics

Distribution: V$_d$: IV: Campath: 0.18 L/kg (range: 0.1 to 0.4 L/kg); Lemtrada: 14.1 L

Metabolism: Campath: Clearance decreases with repeated dosing (due to loss of CD52 receptors in periphery), resulting in a sevenfold increase in AUC after 12 weeks of therapy.

Half-life elimination: IV: Campath: 11 hours (following first 30 mg dose; range: 2 to 32 hours); 6 days (following the last 30 mg dose; range: 1 to 14 days); Lemtrada: ~2 weeks

Dosing

Adult & Geriatric

B-cell chronic lymphocytic leukemia (B-CLL): Campath: IV: Gradually escalate to a maintenance of 30 mg per dose 3 times weekly on alternate days for a total duration of therapy of up to 12 weeks (Hillmen, 2007; Keating, 2002)

Note: Dose escalation is required; usually accomplished in 3 to 7 days. Single doses >30 mg or cumulative doses >90 mg/week increase the incidence of pancytopenia. Pretreatment (with acetaminophen 500 to 1,000 mg and diphenhydramine 50 mg) is recommended prior to the first dose, with dose escalations, and as clinically indicated; IV glucocorticoids may be used for severe infusion-related reactions. Administer antiviral prophylaxis (for herpetic viral infections) and *Pneumocystis jiroveci* pneumonia (PCP) prophylaxis; continue for at least 2 months after completion of alemtuzumab and until CD4+ lymphocyte count is ≥200/mm^3. Reinitiate with gradual dose escalation if treatment is withheld ≥7 days. Alemtuzumab is associated with a moderate emetic potential in the oncology setting; antiemetics may be recommended to prevent nausea and vomiting (Basch, 2011; Roila, 2010).

Dose escalation: Initial: 3 mg daily beginning on day 1; if tolerated (infusion reaction ≤ grade 2), increase to 10 mg daily; if tolerated (infusion reaction ≤ grade 2), may increase to maintenance of 30 mg per dose 3 times weekly if required.

B-CLL (off-label route): SubQ: Initial: 3 mg on day 1; if tolerated 10 mg on day 3; if tolerated increase to 30 mg on day 5; maintenance: 30 mg per dose 3 times weekly for a maximum of 18 weeks (Lundin, 2002) **or** 3 mg on day 1; if tolerated 10 mg on day 2; if tolerated 30 mg on day 3, followed by 30 mg per dose 3 times weekly for 4 to 12 weeks (Stilgenbauer, 2009)

Multiple sclerosis, relapsing: Lemtrada: IV: 12 mg daily for 5 consecutive days (total 60 mg), followed 12 months later by 12 mg daily for 3 consecutive days (total 36 mg); total duration of therapy: 24 months.

Note: Premedicate with corticosteroids (methylprednisolone 1,000 mg or equivalent) immediately prior to alemtuzumab for the first 3 days of each treatment course. Antihistamines and/or antipyretics may also be considered. Administer antiviral prophylaxis (for herpetic viral infections) beginning on the first day of treatment and continue for at least 2 months after completion of alemtuzumab and until CD4+ lymphocyte count is ≥200/mm^3. In some clinical trials patients received an additional 12 mg daily for 3 consecutive days 12 months later (total duration of 36 months) (CAMMS223, 2008; Coles, 2012).

Autoimmune cytopenias, CLL-induced, refractory (off-label use): IV, SubQ: Gradually escalate to a maintenance of 10 to 30 mg per dose 3 times weekly for 4 to 12 weeks (Karlsson, 2007; Osterborg, 2009)

Graft versus host disease (GVHD), acute, steroid refractory, treatment (off-label use): IV: 10 mg daily for 5 consecutive days, then 10 mg weekly on days 8, 15, and 22 if CR not achieved (Martinez, 2009) **or** 10 mg weekly until symptom resolution (Schnitzler, 2009)

Renal transplant, induction (off-label use): IV: 30 mg as a single dose at the time of transplant (Hanaway, 2011)

Stem cell transplant (allogeneic) conditioning regimen (off-label use): IV: 20 mg daily for 5 days (in combination with fludarabine and melphalan) beginning 8 days prior to transplant (Mead, 2010) **or** beginning 7 days prior to transplant (Van Besien, 2009)

T-cell prolymphocytic leukemia (T-PLL; off-label use): IV: Initial test dose 3 mg or 10 mg, followed by dose escalation to 30 mg per dose 3 times weekly as tolerated until maximum response (Dearden, 2001) **or** Initial dose: 3 mg day 1, if tolerated increase to 10 mg day 2, if tolerated increase to 30 mg on day 3 (days 1, 2, and 3 are consecutive days), followed by 30 mg per dose every Monday, Wednesday, Friday for a total of 4 to 12 weeks (Keating, 2002)

Renal Impairment There are no dosage adjustments provided in the manufacturer's labeling (has not been studied).

Hepatic Impairment There are no dosage adjustments provided in the manufacturer's labeling (has not been studied).

Obesity *American Society for Blood and Marrow Transplantation (ASBMT) practice guideline committee position statement on chemotherapy dosing in obesity:* Utilize a flat dose based on the regimen selected for hematopoietic stem cell transplant conditioning in adults (Bubalo, 2014).

Adjustment for Toxicity

Dosage adjustment for nonhematologic toxicity:

Treatment of B-CLL: Campath:

Note: If treatment is withheld ≥7 days, reinitiate at 3 mg with re-escalation to 10 mg and then 30 mg.

Grade 3 or 4 infusion reaction: Withhold infusion

Serious infection or other serious adverse reaction: Withhold alemtuzumab until resolution

Autoimmune anemia or autoimmune thrombocytopenia: Discontinue alemtuzumab

Treatment of MS: Lemtrada: Serious infusion reaction: Consider immediate discontinuation

Dosage adjustment for hematologic toxicity (severe neutropenia or thrombocytopenia, not autoimmune): Treatment of B-CLL: Campath:

Note: If treatment is withheld ≥7 days, reinitiate at 3 mg with re-escalation to 10 mg and then 30 mg.

ANC <250/mm^3 and/or platelet count ≤25,000/mm^3:

First occurrence: Withhold treatment; resume at 30 mg per dose when ANC ≥500/mm^3 and platelet count ≥50,000/mm^3

Second occurrence: Withhold treatment; resume at 10 mg per dose when ANC ≥500/mm^3 and platelet count ≥50,000/mm^3

Third occurrence: Discontinue alemtuzumab.

Patients with a baseline ANC ≤250/mm^3 and/or a baseline platelet count ≤25,000/mm^3 at initiation of therapy: If ANC and/or platelet counts decrease to ≤50% of the baseline value:

First occurrence: Withhold treatment; resume at 30 mg per dose upon return to baseline values

Second occurrence: Withhold treatment; resume at 10 mg per dose upon return to baseline values

Third occurrence: Discontinue alemtuzumab.

Administration

Campath or MabCampath [Canadian product]: Administer by IV infusion over 2 hours. Premedicate with diphenhydramine 50 mg and acetaminophen 500 to 1000 mg 30 minutes before each infusion. IV glucocorticoids have been effective in decreasing severe infusion-related events. Start anti-infective prophylaxis. Other drugs should not be added to or simultaneously infused through the same IV line. Do not give IV push or bolus. Compatible in polyvinylchloride (PVC) or polyethylene lined administration sets or low protein binding filters.

Campath: SubQ (off-label route): SubQ administration has been studied (Lundin, 2002; Stilgenbauer, 2009); an increased rate of injection site reactions has been observed, with only rare incidences of chills or infusion-like reactions typically observed with IV infusion. A longer dose escalation time (1 to 2 weeks) may be needed due to injection site reactions (Lundin, 2002). Premedicate with diphenhydramine 50 mg and acetaminophen 500 to 1000 mg 30 minutes before dose. The subQ route should **NOT** be used for the treatment of T-PLL (Deardon, 2011). Alemtuzumab is associated with a moderate emetic potential in the oncology setting; antiemetics may be recommended to prevent nausea and vomiting (Basch, 2011; Roila, 2010).

Lemtrada: Administer by IV infusion over 4 hours (beginning within 8 hours after dilution); do not administer by IV push or bolus. Do not infuse other medications through the same IV line. Premedicate with corticosteroids (methylprednisolone 1,000 mg or equivalent) for first 3 days of each treatment course. Administer in a setting with personnel and equipment appropriate to manage infusion reactions. Monitor vital signs prior to and periodically during the infusion. Infusion reactions should be managed symptomatically; consider discontinuing immediately for severe infusion reaction. Observe for at least 2 hours after each infusion, longer if clinically indicated.

Monitoring Parameters Campath: CBC with differential and platelets (weekly, more frequent if worsening); signs and symptoms of infection; CD4+ lymphocyte counts (after treatment until recovery); CMV antigen (routinely during and for 2 months after treatment); consider TSH at baseline and then every 2 to 3 months during alemtuzumab treatment (Hamnvik, 2011). Monitor closely for infusion reactions (including hypotension, rigors, fever, shortness of breath, bronchospasm, chills, and/or rash); vital signs (prior to and during infusion); carefully monitor BP especially in patients with ischemic heart disease or on antihypertensive medications;

Lemtrada: CBC with differential prior to initiation then monthly until 48 months after last infusion; serum creatinine prior to initiation then monthly until 48 months after last infusion or at any time during therapy if clinically indicated; urinalysis with urine cell counts (prior to initiation then monthly); signs/symptoms of infection; TSH at baseline and every 3 months until 48 months after last infusion or longer or at any time during therapy if clinically

indicated; observe for at least 2 hours after each infusion, longer if clinically indicated; ECG prior to each treatment course; annual HPV screening; signs/symptoms of PML; baseline and annual skin exams (for melanoma).

Test Interactions May interfere with diagnostic serum tests that utilize antibodies.

Dosage Forms Excipient information presented when available (limited, particularly for generics); consult specific product labeling.

Solution, Intravenous [preservative free]:

Campath: 30 mg/mL (1 mL) [contains edetate disodium dihydrate, mouse protein (murine) (hamster), polysorbate 80]

Lemtrada: 12 mg/1.2 mL (1.2 mL) [contains edetate disodium dihydrate, mouse protein (murine) (hamster), polysorbate 80]

Dosage Forms: Canada Excipient information presented when available (limited, particularly for generics); consult specific product labeling.

Injection, solution [preservative free]:

MabCampath: 30 mg/mL (1 mL) [contains edetate disodium, polysorbate 80]

Injection, solution [preservative free]:

Lemtrada: 10 mg/mL (1.2 mL) [contains edetate disodium, polysorbate 80]

Alendronate (a LEN droe nate)

Brand Names: US Binosto; Fosamax

Brand Names: Canada ACH-Alendronate; Alendronate-70; Alendronate-FC; Apo-Alendronate; Auro-Alendronate; CO Alendronate; Dom-Alendronate; Fosamax; JAMP-Alendronate; Mint-Alendronate; Mylan-Alendronate; PHL-Alendronate; PMS-Alendronate; PMS-Alendronate-FC; Q-Alendronate; Ran-Alendronate; ratio-Alendronate; Riva-Alendronate; Sandoz-Alendronate; Teva-Alendronate

Index Terms Alendronate Sodium; Alendronic Acid Monosodium Salt Trihydrate; MK-217

Pharmacologic Category Bisphosphonate Derivative

Use

Osteoporosis: Treatment of osteoporosis in postmenopausal females (Fosamax, Binosto); prevention of osteoporosis in postmenopausal females (Fosamax); treatment of osteoporosis in males (Fosamax, Binosto); treatment of Paget disease of the bone in patients who are symptomatic, at risk for future complications, or with alkaline phosphatase ≥2 times the upper limit of normal (Fosamax); treatment of glucocorticoid-induced osteoporosis in males and females with low bone mineral density who are receiving a daily dosage ≥7.5 mg of prednisone (or equivalent) (Fosamax)

Canadian labeling: Additional use (not in US labeling): Prevention of glucocorticoid-induced osteoporosis in males and females

Pregnancy Considerations Adverse events were observed in animal reproduction studies. It is not known if bisphosphonates cross the placenta, but fetal exposure is expected (Djokanovic 2008; Stathopoulos 2011). Bisphosphonates are incorporated into the bone matrix and gradually released over time. The amount available in the systemic circulation varies by dose and duration of therapy. Theoretically, there may be a risk of fetal harm when pregnancy follows the completion of therapy; however, available data have not shown that exposure to bisphosphonates during pregnancy significantly increases the risk of adverse fetal events (Djokanovic 2008; Levy 2009; Stathopoulos 2011). Until additional data is available, most sources recommend discontinuing bisphosphonate therapy in women of reproductive potential as early as possible prior to a planned pregnancy; use in premenopausal women should be reserved for special circumstances when rapid bone loss is occurring (Bhalla 2010; Pereira 2012; Stathopoulos 2011). Because hypocalcemia has been described following *in utero* bisphosphonate exposure, exposed infants should be monitored for hypocalcemia after birth (Djokanovic 2008; Stathopoulos 2011).

Breast-Feeding Considerations It is not known if alendronate is excreted into breast milk. The manufacturer recommends that caution be exercised when administering alendronate to nursing women.

Medication Guide Available Yes

Contraindications

Hypersensitivity to alendronate, other bisphosphonates, or any component of the formulation; hypocalcemia; abnormalities of the esophagus (eg, stricture, achalasia) which delay esophageal emptying; inability to stand or sit upright for at least 30 minutes; increased risk of aspiration (effervescent tablets; oral solution)

Canadian labeling: Additional contraindications (not in US labeling): Renal insufficiency with creatinine clearance <35 mL/minute

Warnings/Precautions Use caution in patients with renal impairment (not recommended for use in patients with CrCl <35 mL/minute); hypocalcemia must be corrected before therapy initiation; ensure adequate calcium and vitamin D intake. May cause irritation to upper gastrointestinal mucosa. Esophagitis, dysphagia, esophageal ulcers, esophageal erosions, and esophageal stricture (rare) have been reported; risk increases in patients unable to comply with dosing instructions. Use with caution in patients with dysphagia, esophageal disease, gastritis, duodenitis, or ulcers (may worsen underlying condition). Discontinue use if new or worsening symptoms develop.

Osteonecrosis of the jaw (ONJ) has been reported in patients receiving bisphosphonates. Risk factors include invasive dental procedures (eg, tooth extraction, dental implants, boney surgery); a diagnosis of cancer, with concomitant chemotherapy or corticosteroids; poor oral hygiene, ill-fitting dentures; and comorbid disorders (anemia, coagulopathy, infection, preexisting dental disease); risk may increase with duration of bisphosphonate use. Most reported cases occurred after IV bisphosphonate therapy; however, cases have been reported following oral therapy. A dental exam and preventive dentistry should be performed prior to placing patients with risk factors on chronic bisphosphonate therapy. The manufacturer's labeling states that discontinuing bisphosphonates in patients requiring invasive dental procedures may reduce the risk of ONJ. However, other experts suggest that there is no evidence that discontinuing therapy reduces the risk of developing ONJ (Assael 2009). The risk:benefit must be assessed by the treating physician and/or dentist/surgeon prior to any invasive dental procedure. Patients developing ONJ while on bisphosphonates should receive care by an oral surgeon.

Atypical femur fractures have been reported in patients receiving bisphosphonates for treatment/prevention of osteoporosis. The fractures include subtrochanteric femur (bone just below the hip joint) and diaphyseal femur (long segment of the thigh bone). Some patients experience prodromal pain weeks or months before the fracture occurs. It is unclear if bisphosphonate therapy is the cause for these fractures, although the majority of cases have been reported in patients taking bisphosphonates. Patients receiving long-term (>3 to 5 years) therapy may be at an increased risk. Discontinue bisphosphonate therapy in patients who develop a femoral shaft fracture.

Severe (and occasionally debilitating) bone, joint, and/or muscle pain have been reported during bisphosphonate treatment. The onset of pain ranged from a single day to several months. Consider discontinuing therapy in patients who experience severe symptoms; symptoms usually resolve upon discontinuation. Some patients experienced recurrence when rechallenged with same drug or another bisphosphonate; avoid use in patients with a history of these symptoms in association with bisphosphonate therapy. In the management of osteoporosis, re-evaluate the need for continued therapy periodically; the optimal duration of treatment has not yet been determined. Consider discontinuing after 3 to 5 years of use in patients at low-risk for fracture; following discontinuation, re-evaluate fracture risk periodically.

Potentially significant drug-drug interactions may exist, requiring dose or frequency adjustment, additional monitoring, and/or selection of alternative therapy. Consult drug interactions database for more detailed information. Each effervescent tablet contains 650 mg of sodium (NaCl 1650 mg); use with caution in patients following a sodium-restricted diet.

Adverse Reactions Note: Incidence of adverse effects (mostly GI) increases significantly in patients treated for Paget's disease at 40 mg/day.

>10%: Endocrine & metabolic: Decreased serum calcium (18%; transient, mild)

1% to 10%:

Central nervous system: Headache (3%)

Endocrine & metabolic: Decreased serum phosphate (10%; transient, mild)

Gastrointestinal: Abdominal pain (2% to 7%), acid regurgitation (1% to 5%), flatulence (≤4%), gastroesophageal reflux disease (3%), constipation (≤3%), diarrhea (≤3%), dyspepsia (1% to 3%), nausea (1% to 3%), esophageal ulcer (2%), dysphagia (1%), melena (1%), abdominal distension (≤1%), gastric ulcer (≤1%; may be severe with complications), gastritis (≤1%)

Neuromuscular & skeletal: Musculoskeletal pain (≤6%; includes bone pain, joint pain, and muscle pain), muscle cramps (≤1%)

<1% (Limited to important or life-threatening): Alopecia, cholesteatoma, duodenal ulcer (may be severe with complications), dysgeusia, episcleritis, erythema, erosive

esophagitis, esophageal perforation, esophageal stenosis, esophageal ulcer, esophagitis, exacerbation of asthma, femur fracture (low energy fractures, including subtrochanteric and diaphyseal), hypersensitivity reaction (includes angioedema and urticaria), hypocalcemia (symptomatic), joint swelling, malaise, oropharyngeal ulcer, osteonecrosis of the jaw (generally associated with tooth extraction and/or local infection with delayed healing), peripheral edema, scleritis, skin rash (occasionally with photosensitivity), Stevens-Johnson syndrome, toxic epidermal necrolysis, uveitis, vertigo, weakness

Drug Interactions

Metabolism/Transport Effects None known.

Avoid Concomitant Use

Avoid concomitant use of Alendronate with any of the following: Parathyroid Hormone

Increased Effect/Toxicity

Alendronate may increase the levels/effects of: Deferasirox

The levels/effects of Alendronate may be increased by: Aminoglycosides; Aspirin; Nonsteroidal Anti-Inflammatory Agents; Systemic Angiogenesis Inhibitors

Decreased Effect

Alendronate may decrease the levels/effects of: Parathyroid Hormone

The levels/effects of Alendronate may be decreased by: Antacids; Calcium Salts; Iron Salts; Magnesium Salts; Multivitamins/Minerals (with ADEK, Folate, Iron); Multivitamins/Minerals (with AE, No Iron); Proton Pump Inhibitors

Food Interactions All food and beverages interfere with absorption. Coadministration with dairy products may decrease alendronate absorption. Beverages (especially orange juice, coffee, and mineral water) and food may reduce the absorption of alendronate as much as 60%. Management: Alendronate must be taken first thing in the morning and ≥30 minutes before the first food, beverage (except plain water), or other medication of the day.

Preparation for Administration Tablet, effervescent (Binosto): Dissolve effervescent tablet in 120 mL of room temperature plain water (not mineral water or flavored water); wait ≥5 minutes after effervescence stops, then stir for 10 seconds and administer.

Storage/Stability

Oral solution: Store at 25°C (77°F), excursions permitted to 15°C to 30°C (59°F to 86°F). Do not freeze.

Tablet (Fosamax): Store at room temperature of 15°C to 30°C (59°F to 86°F). Keep in well-closed container.

Tablet, effervescent (Binosto): Store at 20°C to 25°C (68°F to 77°F), excursions permitted to 15°C to 30°C (59°F to 86°F). Protect from moisture. Store in original blister package until use.

Mechanism of Action A bisphosphonate which inhibits bone resorption via actions on osteoclasts or on osteoclast precursors; decreases the rate of bone resorption, leading to an indirect increase in bone mineral density. In Paget's disease, characterized by disordered resorption and formation of bone, inhibition of resorption leads to an indirect decrease in bone formation; but the newly-formed bone has a more normal architecture.

Pharmacodynamics/Kinetics

Distribution: 28 L (exclusive of bone)

Protein binding: ~78%

Metabolism: None

Bioavailability: Fasting: 0.6%; reduced up to 60% with coffee or orange juice

Half-life elimination: Exceeds 10 years

Excretion: Urine; feces (as unabsorbed drug)

Dosing

Adult & Geriatric Note: Consider discontinuing after 3 to 5 years of use for osteoporosis in patients at low-risk for fracture. Patients should receive supplemental calcium and vitamin D if dietary intake is inadequate.

Osteoporosis in postmenopausal females: Oral:
Prophylaxis: 5 mg once daily **or** 35 mg once weekly
Treatment: 10 mg once daily **or** 70 mg once weekly

Osteoporosis in males: Oral: Treatment: 10 mg once daily **or** 70 mg once weekly

Osteoporosis secondary to glucocorticoids in males and females: Oral: Treatment (US labeling) or Treatment and prevention (Canadian labeling): 5 mg once daily; a dose of 10 mg once daily should be used in postmenopausal females who are not receiving estrogen

Paget disease of bone in males and females: Oral: 40 mg once daily for 6 months
Re-treatment: Following a 6-month post-treatment evaluation period, treatment with alendronate may be considered in patients who have relapsed based on increases in serum alkaline phosphatase, which should be measured periodically. Re-treatment may

also be considered in those who failed to normalize their serum alkaline phosphatase. The Endocrine Society guidelines suggest re-treatment may be required between 2 and 6 years (Singer 2014).

Missed doses (once weekly): If a once-weekly dose is missed, it should be given the next morning after remembered; may then return to the original once-weekly schedule (original scheduled day of the week), however, do not give 2 doses on the same day.

Renal Impairment

CrCl ≥35 mL/minute: No dosage adjustment necessary.

CrCl <35 mL/minute: Use not recommended.

Hepatic Impairment No dosage adjustment necessary.

Dietary Considerations Ensure adequate calcium and vitamin D intake; if dietary intake is inadequate, dietary supplementation is recommended. Women and men should consume:

Calcium: 1,000 mg/day (men: 50 to 70 years) **or** 1,200 mg/day (women ≥51 years and men ≥71 years) (IOM 2011; NOF [Cosman 2014])

Vitamin D: 800 to 1,000 int. units/day (men and women ≥50 years) (NOF [Cosman 2014]). Recommended Dietary Allowance (RDA): 600 int. units daily (men and women ≤70 years) **or** 800 int. units/day (men and women ≥71 years) (IOM 2011).

Administration Administer first thing in the morning and ≥30 minutes before the first food, beverage (except plain water), or other medication(s) of the day. Do not take with mineral water or with other beverages. Patients should be instructed to stay upright (not to lie down) for at least 30 minutes **and** until after first food of the day (to reduce esophageal irritation).

Oral solution: Administer oral solution, followed with at least 2 oz of plain water.

Tablet (Fosamax): Must be taken with 6 to 8 oz of plain water. The tablet should be swallowed whole; do not chew or suck.

Tablet, effervescent (Binosto): Dissolve one tablet in 4 oz of room temperature plain water only; once effervescence stops, wait ≥5 minutes and stir the solution for ~10 seconds and then drink.

Monitoring Parameters

Osteoporosis: Bone mineral density (BMD) should be evaluated 1 to 2 years after initiating therapy and every 2 years thereafter (NOF [Cosman 2014]); in patients with combined alendronate and glucocorticoid treatment, BMD should be made at initiation and repeated after 6 to 12 months; annual measurements of height and weight, assessment of chronic back pain; serum calcium and 25(OH)D; may consider monitoring biochemical markers of bone turnover

Paget disease: Alkaline phosphatase at 6 to 12 weeks for initial response to treatment (when bone turnover will have shown a substantial decline) and potentially at 6 months (maximal suppression of high bone turnover); following treatment completion, monitor at ~6- to 12-month intervals (Singer 2014); monitoring more specific biochemical markers of bone turnover (eg, serum P1NP, NTX, serum beta-CTx) is generally only warranted in patients with Paget disease who have abnormal liver or biliary tract function or when early assessment of response to treatment is needed (eg, spinal compression, very active disease) (Singer 2014); pain; serum calcium and 25(OH)D

Reference Range

Calcium (total): Adults: 9.0 to 11.0 mg/dL (2.05 to 2.54 mmol/L), may slightly decrease with aging

Phosphorus: 2.5 to 4.5 mg/dL (0.81 to 1.45 mmol/L)

Vitamin D: There is no clear consensus on a reference range for total serum 25(OH)D concentrations or the validity of this level as it relates clinically to bone health. In addition, there is significant variability in the reporting of serum 25(OH)D levels as a result of different assay types in use; however, the following ranges have been suggested:

Adults (IOM 2011): Sufficient levels in practically all persons: ≥20 ng/mL (50 nmol/L); concern for risk of toxicity: >50 ng/mL (125 nmol/L)

Osteoporosis patients (NOF [Cosman 2014]): Recommended level to reach and maintain: ~30 ng/mL (75 nmol/L)

Test Interactions Bisphosphonates may interfere with diagnostic imaging agents such as technetium-99m-diphosphonate in bone scans.

Dosage Forms Excipient information presented when available (limited, particularly for generics); consult specific product labeling.

Solution, Oral:
Generic: 70 mg/75 mL (75 mL)

Tablet, Oral:
Fosamax: 70 mg
Generic: 5 mg, 10 mg, 35 mg, 40 mg, 70 mg

Tablet Effervescent, Oral:
Binosto: 70 mg

Dosage Forms: Canada Refer to Dosage Forms. **Note:** Effervescent tablet and oral solution are not available in Canada.

◆ Alendronate-70 (Can) *see* Alendronate *on page 66*

Alendronate and Cholecalciferol
(a LEN droe nate & kole e kal SI fer ole)

Brand Names: US Fosamax Plus D®
Brand Names: Canada Fosavance
Index Terms Alendronate Sodium and Cholecalciferol; Cholecalciferol and Alendronate; Vitamin D_3 and Alendronate
Pharmacologic Category Bisphosphonate Derivative; Vitamin D Analog
Use Treatment of osteoporosis in postmenopausal females; increase bone mass in males with osteoporosis
Medication Guide Available Yes
Dosing

Adult & Geriatric Osteoporosis: Oral: One tablet (alendronate 70 mg/cholecalciferol 2800 units **or** alendronate 70 mg/cholecalciferol 5600 units) once weekly. Consider discontinuing after 3-5 years of use for osteoporosis in patients at low-risk for fracture. Supplemental calcium and vitamin D may be necessary if dietary intake is inadequate.

Missed doses: If a once-weekly dose is missed, it should be given the next morning after remembered; may then return to the original once-weekly schedule (original scheduled day of the week), however, do not give 2 doses on the same day.

Renal Impairment
CrCl ≥35 mL/minute: No dosage adjustment necessary.
CrCl <35 mL/minute: Use is not recommended.

Hepatic Impairment Alendronate: No dosage adjustment necessary. Cholecalciferol: May not be adequately absorbed in patients who have malabsorption due to inadequate bile production.

Additional Information Complete prescribing information should be consulted for additional detail.

Dosage Forms Excipient information presented when available (limited, particularly for generics); consult specific product labeling.
Tablet:
Fosamax Plus D® 70/2800: Alendronate 70 mg and cholecalciferol 2800 units
Fosamax Plus D® 70/5600: Alendronate 70 mg and cholecalciferol 5600 units

◆ Alendronate-FC (Can) *see* Alendronate *on page 66*
◆ Alendronate Sodium *see* Alendronate *on page 66*
◆ Alendronate Sodium and Cholecalciferol *see* Alendronate and Cholecalciferol *on page 68*
◆ Alendronic Acid Monosodium Salt Trihydrate *see* Alendronate *on page 66*
◆ Aler-Dryl [OTC] *see* DiphenhydrAMINE (Systemic) *on page 561*
◆ Alertec (Can) *see* Modafinil *on page 1222*
◆ Alesse (Can) *see* Ethinyl Estradiol and Levonorgestrel *on page 703*
◆ Alevazol [OTC] *see* Clotrimazole (Topical) *on page 428*
◆ Aleve [OTC] *see* Naproxen *on page 1256*
◆ Aleve (Can) *see* Naproxen *on page 1256*
◆ Alfenta *see* Alfentanil *on page 68*

Alfentanil (al FEN ta nil)

Brand Names: US Alfenta
Brand Names: Canada Alfenta; Alfentanil Injection, USP
Index Terms Alfentanil Hydrochloride
Pharmacologic Category Analgesic, Opioid; Anilidopiperidine Opioid
Use

Analgesia: Analgesic adjunct for the maintenance of anesthesia with barbiturate/nitrous oxide/oxygen; analgesic with nitrous oxide/oxygen in the maintenance of general anesthesia; analgesic component for monitored anesthesia care

Anesthetic: Primary anesthetic for induction of anesthesia in general surgery when endotracheal intubation and mechanical ventilation are required

Dosing

Adult Doses should be titrated to appropriate effects; wide range of doses is dependent upon desired degree of analgesia/anesthesia

Anesthesia: Base dose on actual body weight unless >20% above ideal body weight, then base dose on lean body weight.

Alfentanil

Indication	Approx Duration of Anesthesia (min)	Induction Period (Initial Dose) (mcg/kg)	Maintenance Period (increments/ Infusion)	Total Dose (mcg/kg)	Effects
Incremental injection	≤30	8-20	3-5 mcg/kg every 5-20 minutes or 0.5-1 mcg/kg/min	8-40	Spontaneously breathing or assisted ventilation when required.
	30-60	20-50	5-15 mcg/kg every 5-20 minutes	Up to 75	Assisted or controlled ventilation required. Attenuation of response to laryngoscopy and intubation.
Continuous infusion	>45	50-75	0.5-3 mcg/kg/min; average infusion rate 1-1.5 mcg/kg/min	Dependent on duration of procedure	Assisted or controlled ventilation required. Some attenuation of response to intubation and incision, with intraoperative stability.
Anesthetic induction	>45	130-245	0.5-1.5 mcg/kg/min or general anesthetic	Dependent on duration of procedure	Assisted or controlled ventilation required. Administer induction dose slowly (over 3 minutes). Concentration of inhalation agents reduced by 30% to 50% for initial hour.
Monitored Anesthesia Care (MAC)	3-8		3-5 mcg/kg every 5-20 minutes or 0.25-1 mcg/kg/min	3-40	Sedation, responsiveness, spontaneous breathing

Geriatric Refer to adult dosing. Appropriately reduce the initial dose in elderly patients; consider the effect of the initial dose in determining supplemental doses.

Pediatric
Children <12 years: Dose has not been established.
Children ≥12 years: Refer to adult dosing.

Renal Impairment There are no dosage adjustments provided in the manufacturer's labeling; use with caution. The pharmacokinetics of alfentanil were evaluated in adult patients with chronic renal failure and compared to patients with normal renal function. Although V_{dss} was increased in patients with renal failure, elimination half-life was similar between the 2 groups (Chauvin, 1987). Therefore, prolongation of alfentanil duration of action is not expected and dosage adjustment is not necessary.

Hepatic Impairment There are no dosage adjustments provided in the manufacturer's labeling; use with caution.

Obesity In patients weighing >20% above ideal body weight, determine dose based on lean body weight.

Additional Information Complete prescribing information should be consulted for additional detail.

Dosage Forms Excipient information presented when available (limited, particularly for generics); consult specific product labeling.
Injectable, Injection [preservative free]:
Alfenta: 500 mcg/mL (2 mL, 5 mL)
Generic: 500 mcg/mL (2 mL, 5 mL)

Controlled Substance C-II

◆ Alfentanil Hydrochloride *see* Alfentanil *on page 68*
◆ Alfentanil Injection, USP (Can) *see* Alfentanil *on page 68*
◆ Alferon N *see* Interferon Alfa-n3 *on page 969*

Alfuzosin (al FYOO zoe sin)

Brand Names: US Uroxatral
Brand Names: Canada Apo-Alfuzosin®; Sandoz-Alfuzosin; Teva-Alfuzosin PR; Xatral
Index Terms Alfuzosin Hydrochloride
Pharmacologic Category Alpha$_1$ Blocker
Use Benign prostatic hyperplasia: Treatment of signs and symptoms of benign prostatic hyperplasia (BPH)
Pregnancy Considerations Adverse events have not been observed in animal reproduction studies.
Breast-Feeding Considerations It is not known if alfuzosin is excreted in breast milk.

Contraindications

Hypersensitivity to alfuzosin or any component of the formulation; moderate or severe hepatic impairment (Child-Pugh class B and C); concurrent use with potent CYP3A4 inhibitors (eg, itraconazole, ketoconazole, ritonavir)

Canadian labeling: Additional contraindications (not in US labeling): Concurrent use with other alpha1-blockers

Warnings/Precautions

Not intended for use as an antihypertensive drug. May cause orthostatic hypotension and syncope within a few hours following administration; anticipate a similar effect if therapy is interrupted for a few days, if dosage is rapidly increased, or if another antihypertensive drug, PDE-5 inhibitors, or nitrates is introduced. Use with caution in patients with symptomatic orthostatic hypotension. Discontinue if symptoms of angina occur or worsen. Alfuzosin has been shown to prolong the QT interval alone (minimal) and with other drugs with comparable effects on the QT interval (additive); use with caution in patients with known QT prolongation (congenital or acquired). Rule out prostatic carcinoma before beginning therapy. Use caution with severe renal or mild hepatic impairment; contraindicated in moderate-to-severe hepatic impairment. Intraoperative floppy iris syndrome has been observed in cataract surgery patients who were on or were previously treated with alpha₁-blockers; there appears to be no benefit in discontinuing alpha-blocker therapy prior to surgery. May require modifications to surgical technique. May cause priapism; seek immediate medical assistance for erections lasting longer than 4 hours. Use with caution in patients with histories of tachyarrhythmia or with certain cardiovascular conditions, such as myocardial ischemia. May cause CNS depression, which may impair physical or mental abilities; patients must be cautioned about performing tasks that require mental alertness (eg, operating machinery or driving). Potentially significant interactions may exist, requiring dose or frequency adjustment, additional monitoring, and/or selection of alternative therapy.

Adverse Reactions

1% to 10%:

Central nervous system: Dizziness (6%), fatigue (3%), headache (3%), pain (1% to 2%)

Gastrointestinal: Abdominal pain (1% to 2%), constipation (1% to 2%), dyspepsia (1% to 2%), nausea (1% to 2%)

Genitourinary: Impotence (1% to 2%)

Respiratory: Upper respiratory tract infection (3%), bronchitis (1% to 2%), pharyngitis (1% to 2%), sinusitis (1% to 2%)

<1% (Limited to important or life-threatening): Angioedema, atrial fibrillation, chest pain, edema, hepatic injury (including cholestatic), hypotension, intraoperative floppy iris syndrome (with cataract surgery), priapism, pruritus, thrombocytopenia, toxic epidermal necrolysis

Drug Interactions

Metabolism/Transport Effects Substrate of CYP3A4 (major); **Note:** Assignment of Major/Minor substrate status based on clinically relevant drug interaction potential

Avoid Concomitant Use

Avoid concomitant use of Alfuzosin with any of the following: Alpha1-Blockers; Conivaptan; CYP3A4 Inhibitors (Strong); Fusidic Acid (Systemic); Idelalisib; Protease Inhibitors; Telaprevir

Increased Effect/Toxicity

Alfuzosin may increase the levels/effects of: Alpha1-Blockers; Blood Pressure Lowering Agents; Highest Risk QTc-Prolonging Agents; Moderate Risk QTc-Prolonging Agents; Nitroglycerin

The levels/effects of Alfuzosin may be increased by: Aprepitant; Beta-Blockers; Conivaptan; CYP3A4 Inhibitors (Moderate); CYP3A4 Inhibitors (Strong); Dapoxetine; Dasatinib; Fosaprepitant; Fusidic Acid (Systemic); Idelalisib; Ivacaftor; Luliconazole; Mifepristone; Netupitant; Osimertinib; Palbociclib; Phosphodiesterase 5 Inhibitors; Protease Inhibitors; Simeprevir; Stiripentol; Telaprevir

Decreased Effect

Alfuzosin may decrease the levels/effects of: Alpha-/Beta-Agonists; Alpha1-Agonists

The levels/effects of Alfuzosin may be decreased by: Bosentan; CYP3A4 Inducers (Moderate); CYP3A4 Inducers (Strong); Dabrafenib; Deferasirox; Enzalutamide; Mitotane; Osimertinib; Siltuximab; St Johns Wort; Tocilizumab

Food Interactions Food increases the extent of absorption. Management: Administer immediately following a meal at the same time each day.

Storage/Stability Store at 25°C (77°F); excursions permitted to 15°C to 30°C (59°F to 86°F). Protect from light and moisture.

Mechanism of Action

An antagonist of alpha₁-adrenoreceptors in the lower urinary tract. Smooth muscle tone is mediated by the sympathetic nervous stimulation of alpha₁-adrenoreceptors, which are abundant in the prostate, prostatic capsule, prostatic urethra, and bladder neck. Blockade of these adrenoreceptors can cause smooth muscles in the bladder neck and prostate to relax, resulting in an improvement in urine flow rate and a reduction in BPH symptoms.

Pharmacodynamics/Kinetics

Absorption: Decreased 50% under fasting conditions

Distribution: V_d: 3.2 L/kg

Protein binding: 82% to 90%

Metabolism: Hepatic, primarily via CYP3A4; metabolism includes oxidation, O-demethylation, and N-dealkylation; forms metabolites (inactive)

Bioavailability: 49% following a meal

Half-life elimination: 10 hours

Time to peak, plasma: 8 hours following a meal

Excretion: Feces (69%); urine (24%; 11% as unchanged drug)

Dosing

Adult & Geriatric

Benign prostatic hyperplasia (BPH): Oral: 10 mg once daily

Ureteral stones, expulsion (off-label use): Oral: 10 mg once daily, discontinue after successful expulsion (average time to expulsion 1-2 weeks) (Agrawal, 2009; Ahmed, 2010; Gurbuz, 2011). **Note:** Patients with stones >10 mm were excluded from studies.

Renal Impairment There are no dosage adjustments provided in the manufacturer's labeling; use with caution in severe renal impairment (CrCl <30 mL/minute).

Hepatic Impairment

Mild hepatic impairment (Child-Pugh class A): There are no dosage adjustments provided in the manufacturer's labeling (has not been studied); use with caution.

Moderate or severe hepatic impairment (Child-Pugh class B or C): Use is contraindicated.

Dietary Considerations Take immediately following a meal.

Administration Administer immediately following a meal at the same time each day. Swallow tablet whole; do not crush or chew.

Monitoring Parameters Urine flow, blood pressure, PSA

Dosage Forms Excipient information presented when available (limited, particularly for generics); consult specific product labeling.

Tablet Extended Release 24 Hour, Oral, as hydrochloride:

Uroxatral: 10 mg [contains hydrogenated castor oil]

Generic: 10 mg

◆ Alfuzosin Hydrochloride *see* Alfuzosin *on page 68*

◆ Alglucosidase *see* Alglucosidase Alfa *on page 69*

Alglucosidase Alfa (al gloo KOSE i dase AL fa)

Brand Names: US Lumizyme; Myozyme

Brand Names: Canada Myozyme

Index Terms Alglucosidase; GAA; rhGAA

Pharmacologic Category Enzyme

Use

Pompe disease: For use in patients with Pompe disease (acid alpha-glucosidase [GAA] deficiency).

Limitations of use: Myozyme: Improves ventilator-free survival in patients with infantile-onset Pompe disease compared with an untreated historical control, whereas use of Myozyme in patients with other forms of Pompe disease has not been adequately studied to ensure safety and efficacy.

Prescribing and Access Restrictions Access to Myozyme is restricted by the manufacturer and allowed only to patients with infantile-onset Pompe disease. To obtain Myozyme, call 1-800-745-4447; no formal distribution program is established, but availability is controlled by Genzyme.

Dosing

Adult

Pompe disease: *Noninfantile, late-onset (Lumizyme):* IV: 20 mg/kg every 2 weeks

Pediatric

Pompe disease: IV:

Infantile-onset (Lumizyme, Myozyme): Infants ≥1 month, Children, and Adolescents: 20 mg/kg every 2 weeks

Noninfantile, late-onset (Lumizyme): Infants ≥1 month, Children, and Adolescents: Refer to adult dosing.

Renal Impairment There are no dosage adjustments provided in the manufacturer's labeling.

Hepatic Impairment There are no dosage adjustments provided in the manufacturer's labeling.

Additional Information Complete prescribing information should be consulted for additional detail.

Dosage Forms Excipient information presented when available (limited, particularly for generics); consult specific product labeling.

Solution Reconstituted, Intravenous [preservative free]:
Lumizyme: 50 mg (1 ea) [contains polysorbate 80]
Myozyme: 50 mg (1 ea)

- ◆ Alimta see PEMEtrexed *on page 1416*
- ◆ Alinia see Nitazoxanide *on page 1287*

Alirocumab (al i ROK ue mab)

Brand Names: US Praluent
Index Terms REGN727; SAR236553
Pharmacologic Category Antilipemic Agent, PCSK9 Inhibitor; Monoclonal Antibody
Use

Hyperlipidemia, primary: Adjunct to diet and maximally tolerated statin therapy for the treatment of adults with heterozygous familial hypercholesterolemia or clinical atherosclerotic cardiovascular disease, who require additional lowering of LDL-cholesterol (LDL-C).

Limitation of use: The effect of alirocumab on cardiovascular morbidity and mortality has not been determined.

Pregnancy Considerations Adverse events were not observed in animal reproduction studies. Information specific to alirocumab in pregnancy is not available. However, IgG molecules are known to cross the placenta, with increasing amounts during the second and third trimesters of pregnancy.

Breast-Feeding Considerations Information specific to alirocumab is not available, however, IgG molecules are known to be present in breast milk. Serum concentrations to a nursing infant are not expected to be substantial. According to the manufacturer, the decision to breastfeed during therapy should take into account the risk of exposure to the nursing to the infant, and the benefits of treatment to the mother.

Prescribing and Access Restrictions Only available via specialty pharmacies. Call 844-772-5836 or visit https://www.praluenthcp.com/support for additional information..

Contraindications

Serious hypersensitivity to alirocumab or any component of the formulation.

Documentation of allergenic cross-reactivity for PCSK9 inhibitors is limited. However, because of similarities in chemical structure and/or pharmacologic actions, the possibility of cross-sensitivity cannot be ruled out with certainty.

Warnings/Precautions Hypersensitivity reactions, including some severe reactions requiring hospitalization (eg, hypersensitivity vasculitis), have been reported. Discontinue treatment and initiate supportive treatment in patients who develop serious allergic reactions. Other hypersensitivity reactions including pruritus, rash and urticaria have been reported.

Adverse Reactions Frequency not always defined.

Gastrointestinal: Diarrhea (5%)
Hepatic: Liver enzyme disorder (3%), increased serum transaminases (>3X ULN; 2%)
Hypersensitivity: Hypersensitivity reaction
Infection: Influenza (6%)
Local: Injection site reaction (7%)
Neuromuscular & skeletal: Myalgia (4%), muscle spasm (3%)
Respiratory: Cough (3%)
<1% (Limited to important or life-threatening): Confusion, memory impairment

Drug Interactions

Metabolism/Transport Effects None known.

Avoid Concomitant Use

Avoid concomitant use of Alirocumab with any of the following: Belimumab

Increased Effect/Toxicity

Alirocumab may increase the levels/effects of: Belimumab

Decreased Effect There are no known significant interactions involving a decrease in effect.

Preparation for Administration Warm prefilled pen or syringe to room temperature for 30 to 40 minutes prior to use; use as soon as possible after it has been warmed.

Storage/Stability Store at 2°C to 8°C (36°F to 46°F) in the outer carton to protect from light. Time out of refrigeration should not exceed 24 hours at 25°C (77°F). Do not freeze. Do not expose to extreme heat. Do not shake.

Mechanism of Action Alirocumab is a human monoclonal antibody (IgG1 isotype) that binds to proprotein convertase subtilisin kexin type 9 (PCSK9). PCSK9 binds to the low-density lipoprotein receptors (LDLR) on hepatocyte surfaces to promote LDLR degradation within the liver. LDLR is the primary receptor that clears circulating LDL; therefore, the decrease in LDLR levels by PCSK9 results in higher blood levels of LDL-cholesterol (LDL-C). By inhibiting the binding of PCSK9 to LDLR, alirocumab increases the number of LDLRs available to clear LDL, thereby lowering LDL-C levels.

Pharmacodynamics/Kinetics

Onset: Peak effect: Proprotein convertase subtilisin kexin type 9 (PCSK9) suppression: 4 to 8 hours
Distribution: IV: V_d: ~0.04 to 0.05 L/kg
Metabolism: Expected to undergo proteolysis and be degraded to small peptides and amino acids
Bioavailability: SubQ: ~85%
Half-life elimination: SubQ: Steady-state: 17 to 20 days; reduced to 12 days when administered with a statin
Time to peak: SubQ: 3 to 7 days

Dosing

Adult & Geriatric

Hyperlipidemia: SubQ: 75 mg once every 2 weeks; may increase to 150 mg once every 2 weeks if an adequate response is not achieved within 4 to 8 weeks.

Missed dose: If a dose is missed ≤7 days from the usual day of administration, administer the dose as soon as possible and then resume the original schedule; otherwise, if beyond 7 days, skip the missed dose and resume the normal dosing schedule.

Renal Impairment

Mild to moderate impairment: No dosage adjustment necessary.

Severe impairment: There are no dosage adjustments provided in the manufacturer's labeling (has not been studied); however, dosage adjustment is unlikely to be required as monoclonal antibodies are not known to be renally eliminated.

Hepatic Impairment

Mild to moderate impairment: No dosage adjustment necessary.

Severe impairment: There are no dosage adjustments provided in the manufacturer's labeling (has not been studied).

Administration SubQ: Allow solution to come to room temperature for 30 to 40 minutes prior to administration. Do not shake. Administer by subcutaneous injection into the thigh, abdomen, or upper arm; rotate injection site with each injection. Do not injection into areas of active skin disease or injury (eg, sunburns, skin rashes, inflammation, skin infections). Do not coadminister with other injectable drugs at the same injection site.

Monitoring Parameters LDL cholesterol (LDL-C; within 4 to 8 weeks of initiation or dose titrations). Monitor for hypersensitivity reactions.

Dosage Forms Excipient information presented when available (limited, particularly for generics); consult specific product labeling.

Solution Pen-injector, Subcutaneous [preservative free]:
Praluent: 75 mg/mL (1 mL); 150 mg/mL (1 mL) [contains mouse protein (murine) (hamster)]
Solution Prefilled Syringe, Subcutaneous [preservative free]:
Praluent: 75 mg/mL (1 mL); 150 mg/mL (1 mL) [contains mouse protein (murine) (hamster)]

Aliskiren (a lis KYE ren)

Brand Names: US Tekturna
Brand Names: Canada Rasilez
Index Terms Aliskiren Hemifumarate; SPP100
Pharmacologic Category Renin Inhibitor
Use

Hypertension: Treatment of hypertension, alone or in combination with other antihypertensive agents

Note: According to the Eighth Joint National Committee (JNC 8) guidelines, aliskiren is **not** recommended for the initial treatment of hypertension (James, 2013).

Pregnancy Considerations [US Boxed Warning]: Drugs that act on the renin-angiotensin system can cause injury and death to the developing fetus. Discontinue as soon as possible once pregnancy is detected. The use of drugs which act on the renin-angiotensin system are associated with oligohydramnios. Oligohydramnios, due to decreased fetal renal function, may lead to fetal lung hypoplasia and skeletal malformations. Use is also associated with anuria, hypotension, renal failure, skull hypoplasia, and death in the fetus/neonate. The exposed fetus should be monitored for fetal growth, amniotic fluid volume, and organ formation. Infants

exposed *in utero* should be monitored for hyperkalemia, hypotension, and oliguria.

Breast-Feeding Considerations It is not known if aliskiren is excreted in breast milk. Due to the potential for serious adverse reactions in the nursing infant, a decision should be made whether to discontinue nursing or to discontinue the drug, taking into account the importance of treatment to the mother.

Contraindications

US labeling: Hypersensitivity to aliskiren or any component of the formulation; concomitant use with an ACE inhibitor or ARB in patients with diabetes mellitus

Canadian labeling: Additional contraindications (not in US labeling): History of angioedema with aliskiren, ACE inhibitors, or ARBs; hereditary or idiopathic angioedema; pregnancy; breast-feeding; concomitant use with ACE inhibitors or ARBs in patients with GFR <60 mL/minute/ 1.73 m²; patients <2 years of age.

Warnings/Precautions [US Boxed Warning]: Drugs that act on the renin-angiotensin system can cause injury and death to the developing fetus. Discontinue as soon as possible once pregnancy is detected. Hypersensitivity reactions, including anaphylaxis and angioedema have been reported; since the effect of aliskiren on bradykinin levels is unknown, the risk of kinin-mediated etiologies of angioedema occurring is also unknown. Use with caution in any patient with a history of angioedema (of any etiology) as angioedema, some cases necessitating hospitalization and intubation, has been observed (rarely) with aliskiren use. Discontinue immediately following the occurrence of anaphylaxis or angioedema; do not readminister. Prolonged frequent monitoring may be required especially if tongue, glottis, or larynx are involved as they are associated with airway obstruction. Patients with a history of airway surgery may have a higher risk of airway obstruction. Early, aggressive, and appropriate management is critical. Hyperkalemia may occur (rarely) during monotherapy; risk may increase in patients with predisposing factors (eg, renal dysfunction, diabetes mellitus, or concomitant use with ACE inhibitors, ARBs, NSAIDS including COX-2 inhibitors, potassium-sparing diuretics, potassium supplements, and/or potassium-containing salts). Symptomatic hypotension may occur (rarely) during the initiation of therapy, particularly in volume or salt-depleted patients or with concomitant use of other agents acting on the renin-angiotensin-aldosterone system. If hypotension does occur, this is not a contraindication for further use; once blood pressure has been stabilized, aliskiren usually can be continued without difficulty. Use with caution or avoid in patients with deteriorating renal function or low renal blood flow (eg, renal artery stenosis, severe heart failure, post-MI, volume depletion); may increase risk of developing acute renal failure and hyperkalemia. Concomitant use with an ACE inhibitor, ARB, or NSAID (including COX-2 inhibitors) may increase risk of developing acute renal failure; concomitant use with an ACE inhibitor or ARB should be avoided in patient with GFR <60 mL/minute. Use (monotherapy or combined with ACE inhibitors or ARBs) in patients with type 2 diabetes mellitus has demonstrated an increased incidence of renal impairment, hypotension, and hyperkalemia; use is contraindicated in patients with diabetes mellitus who are taking an ACE inhibitor or ARB. Potentially significant drug-drug interactions may exist, requiring dose or frequency adjustment, additional monitoring, and/ or selection of alternative therapy. Serious skins reactions including Stevens Johnson syndrome and toxic epidermal necrolysis (TEN) have been reported.

Adverse Reactions

1% to 10%:

Dermatologic: Skin rash (1%)

Gastrointestinal: Diarrhea (2%)

Neuromuscular & skeletal: Increased creatine phosphokinase (>300% increase: 1%)

Renal: Increased blood urea nitrogen (≤7%), increased serum creatinine (≤7%)

Respiratory: Cough (1%)

<1% (Limited to important or life-threatening): Anaphylaxis, decreased hematocrit, decreased hemoglobin, gastroesophageal reflux disease, hepatic insufficiency, hyperkalemia, increased uric acid, nausea, rhabdomyolysis, seizure, severe hypotension, Stevens-Johnson syndrome, tonic-clonic seizures, vomiting

Drug Interactions

Metabolism/Transport Effects Substrate of CYP3A4 (minor), P-glycoprotein; **Note:** Assignment of Major/Minor substrate status based on clinically relevant drug interaction potential

Avoid Concomitant Use

Avoid concomitant use of Aliskiren with any of the following: CycloSPORINE (Systemic); Itraconazole

Increased Effect/Toxicity

Aliskiren may increase the levels/effects of: ACE Inhibitors; Amifostine; Angiotensin II Receptor Blockers; Antipsychotic Agents (Second Generation [Atypical]); DULoxetine; Hypotension-Associated Agents; Levodopa

The levels/effects of Aliskiren may be increased by: Alfuzosin; AtorvaSTATin; Barbiturates; Brimonidine (Topical); Canagliflozin; CycloSPORINE (Systemic); Diazoxide; Drospirenone; Heparin; Heparin (Low Molecular Weight); Herbs (Hypotensive Properties); Itraconazole; Ketoconazole (Systemic); Lumacaftor; Molsidomine; Nicorandil; Nonsteroidal Anti-Inflammatory Agents; Obinutuzumab; Pentoxifylline; P-glycoprotein/ABCB1 Inhibitors; Phosphodiesterase 5 Inhibitors; Potassium Salts; Prostacyclin Analogues; Ranolazine; Verapamil

Decreased Effect

Aliskiren may decrease the levels/effects of: Furosemide

The levels/effects of Aliskiren may be decreased by: Amphetamines; Grapefruit Juice; Herbs (Hypertensive Properties); Lumacaftor; Methylphenidate; Nonsteroidal Anti-Inflammatory Agents; P-glycoprotein/ABCB1 Inducers; Yohimbine

Food Interactions High-fat meals decrease absorption. Grapefruit juice may decrease the serum concentration of aliskiren. Management: Administer at the same time each day; may take with or without a meal, but consistent administration with regards to meals is recommended. Avoid concomitant use of aliskiren and grapefruit juice.

Storage/Stability Store at 25°C (77°F); excursions permitted to 15°C to 30°C (59°F to 86°F). Protect from moisture.

Mechanism of Action Aliskiren is a direct renin inhibitor, resulting in blockade of the conversion of angiotensinogen to angiotensin I. Angiotensin I suppression decreases the formation of angiotensin II (Ang II), a potent blood pressure-elevating peptide (via direct vasoconstriction, aldosterone release, and sodium retention). Ang II also functions within the Renin-Angiotensin-Aldosterone System (RAAS) as a negative inhibitory feedback mediator within the renal parenchyma to suppress the further release of renin. Thus, reductions in Ang II levels suppress this feedback loop, leading to further increased plasma renin concentrations (PRC) and subsequent activity (PRA). This disinhibition effect can be potentially problematic for ACE inhibitor and ARB therapy, as increased PRA could partially overcome the pharmacologic inhibition of the RAAS. As aliskiren is a direct inhibitor of renin activity, blunting of PRA despite the increased PRC (from loss of the negative feedback) may be clinically advantageous. The effect of aliskiren on bradykinin levels is unknown.

Pharmacodynamics/Kinetics

Onset of action: Maximum antihypertensive effect: Within 2 weeks

Absorption: Poor; absorption decreased by high-fat meal. Aliskiren is a substrate of P-glycoprotein; concurrent use of P-glycoprotein inhibitors may increase absorption.

Metabolism: Extent of metabolism unknown; *in vitro* studies indicate metabolism via CYP3A4

Bioavailability: ~3%

Half-life elimination: ~24 hours (range: 16 to 32 hours)

Time to peak, plasma: 1 to 3 hours

Excretion: Urine (~25% of absorbed dose excreted unchanged in urine); feces (unchanged via biliary excretion)

Dosing

Adult Hypertension: Initial: 150 mg once daily; may increase to 300 mg once daily (maximum: 300 mg daily). Usual dosage range (ASH/ISH [Weber, 2014]): 150 to 300 mg once daily. **Note:** Prior to initiation, correct hypovolemia and/or closely monitor volume status in patients on concurrent diuretics during treatment initiation.

Geriatric Refer to adult dosing. No initial dosage adjustment required.

Renal Impairment

CrCl ≥30 mL/minute: No dosage adjustment necessary.

CrCl <30 mL/minute:

US labeling: There are no dosage adjustments provided in the manufacturer's labeling; however, no dosage adjustment necessary (Vaidyanathan, 2007). Risk of hyperkalemia and progressive renal dysfunction may occur; use with caution.

Canadian labeling: GFR <30 mL/minute/1.73 m²: Avoid use

ESRD (requiring hemodialysis): There are no dosage adjustments provided in the manufacturer's labeling; however, no dosage adjustment necessary (Khadzhynov, 2012). Risk of hyperkalemia is increased with chronic therapy; use with extreme caution. **Note:** Hemodialysis eliminates a minimal fraction; does not significantly alter overall aliskiren exposure.

Hepatic Impairment Initial: No dosage adjustment necessary.

Dietary Considerations May be taken with or without food; however, a high-fat meal reduces absorption. Consistent administration with regards to meals is recommended.

Administration Administer at the same time daily; may take with or without a meal, but consistent administration with regards to meals is recommended.

Monitoring Parameters Blood pressure; serum potassium, BUN, serum creatinine

Dosage Forms Excipient information presented when available (limited, particularly for generics); consult specific product labeling.

Tablet, Oral:

Tekturna: 150 mg, 300 mg

Aliskiren, Amlodipine, and Hydrochlorothiazide
(a lis KYE ren, am LOE di peen, & hye droe klor oh THYE a zide)

Brand Names: US Amturnide™

Index Terms Aliskiren, Hydrochlorothiazide, and Amlodipine; Amlodipine Besylate, Aliskiren Hemifumarate, and Hydrochlorothiazide; Amlodipine, Aliskiren, and Hydrochlorothiazide; Amlodipine, Hydrochlorothiazide, and Aliskiren; Hydrochlorothiazide, Aliskiren, and Amlodipine; Hydrochlorothiazide, Amlodipine, and Aliskiren

Pharmacologic Category Antianginal Agent; Antihypertensive; Calcium Channel Blocker; Calcium Channel Blocker, Dihydropyridine; Diuretic, Thiazide; Renin Inhibitor

Use Hypertension: Treatment of hypertension (not for initial therapy)

Dosing

Adult Note: Not for initial therapy. Dose is individualized; combination product may be substituted for individual components in patients currently maintained on all three agents separately, used to switch a patient on any dual combination of the components who is experiencing dose-limiting adverse reactions from an individual component (to a lower dose of that component), or used as add-on therapy in patients not adequately controlled with any two of the following: Aliskiren, dihydropyridine calcium channel blockers, and thiazide diuretics.

Hypertension: Oral: *Add-on/switch therapy/replacement therapy:* Aliskiren 150-300 mg and amlodipine 5-10 mg and hydrochlorothiazide 12.5-25 mg once daily; dose may be titrated after 2 weeks of therapy. Maximum recommended daily dose: Aliskiren 300 mg; amlodipine 10 mg; hydrochlorothiazide 25 mg

Geriatric Refer to adult dosing. Use of lower initial doses should be considered (use of individual components may be necessary).

Renal Impairment

CrCl ≥30 mL/minute: No dosage adjustment necessary.

CrCl <30 mL/minute: There are no dosage adjustments provided in the manufacturer's labeling (has not been studied); however, no dosage adjustment necessary for aliskiren or amlodipine (Doyle 1989; Vaidyanathan, 2007). Risk of hyperkalemia and progressive renal dysfunction may occur with aliskiren; use with caution. Hydrochlorothiazide is usually ineffective when CrCl <30 mL/minute and is contraindicated in patients who are anuric.

ESRD (requiring hemodialysis): There are no dosage adjustments provided in the manufacturer's labeling (has not been studied); however, no dosage adjustment necessary for aliskiren or amlodipine (Khadzhynov, 2012; Kungys 2003). Risk of hyperkalemia is increased with chronic aliskiren therapy; use with extreme caution. Hydrochlorothiazide is usually ineffective when CrCl <30 mL/minute and is contraindicated in patients who are anuric.

Hepatic Impairment Mild-to-severe: Use with caution and titrate slowly; amlodipine elimination prolonged; lower initial dose should be considered (possibly requiring use of the individual agents).

Additional Information Complete prescribing information should be consulted for additional detail.

Dosage Forms Excipient information presented when available (limited, particularly for generics); consult specific product labeling.

Tablet, oral:

Amturnide: Aliskiren 150 mg, amlodipine 5 mg, and hydrochlorothiazide 12.5 mg

Amturnide: Aliskiren 300 mg, amlodipine 5 mg, and hydrochlorothiazide 12.5 mg

Amturnide: Aliskiren 300 mg, amlodipine 5 mg, and hydrochlorothiazide 25 mg

Amturnide: Aliskiren 300 mg, amlodipine 10 mg, and hydrochlorothiazide 12.5 mg

Amturnide: Aliskiren 300 mg, amlodipine 10 mg, and hydrochlorothiazide 25 mg

Aliskiren and Hydrochlorothiazide
(a lis KYE ren & hye droe klor oh THYE a zide)

Brand Names: US Tekturna HCT

Brand Names: Canada Rasilez HCT

Index Terms Aliskiren Hemifumarate and Hydrochlorothiazide; Hydrochlorothiazide and Aliskiren

Pharmacologic Category Antihypertensive; Diuretic, Thiazide; Renin Inhibitor

Use Hypertension: Treatment of hypertension, including use as initial therapy in patients likely to need multiple antihypertensives for adequate control

Dosing

Adult Note: Dosage must be individualized. Combination product may be substituted for individual components in patients currently maintained on both agents separately or in patients not adequately controlled with monotherapy (using one of the agents or an agent within same antihypertensive class). The combination product is approved for use as initial therapy in the US labeling but is not approved for this indication in the Canadian labeling.

Hypertension: Oral:

Initial therapy: Aliskiren 150 mg and hydrochlorothiazide 12.5 mg once daily, dose may be titrated at 2- to 4-week intervals; maximum recommended daily doses: Aliskiren 300 mg; hydrochlorothiazide 25 mg

Add-on therapy: Initiate by adding the lowest available dose of the alternative component (aliskiren 150 mg or hydrochlorothiazide 12.5 mg); titrate to effect; maximum recommended daily doses: Aliskiren 300 mg; hydrochlorothiazide 25 mg

Replacement therapy: Substitute for the individually titrated components

Note: Prior to initiation, correct hypovolemia and/or closely monitor volume status in patients on concurrent diuretics during treatment initiation.

Geriatric Refer to adult dosing. No initial dosage adjustment required.

Renal Impairment

CrCl ≥30 mL/minute: No dosage adjustment necessary.

CrCl <30 mL/minute: There are no dosage adjustments provided in the manufacturer's labeling (has not been studied); however, no adjustment necessary for aliskiren (Vaidyanathan 2007). Risk of hyperkalemia and progressive renal dysfunction may occur with aliskiren (use with caution). Hydrochlorothiazide is usually ineffective when CrCl <30 mL/minute and is contraindicated in patients who are anuric. The Canadian labeling contraindicates use of aliskiren/hydrochlorothiazide if GFR <30 mL/minute/1.73 m².

ESRD (requiring hemodialysis): There are no dosage adjustments provided in the manufacturer's labeling (has not been studied); however, no dosage adjustment necessary for aliskiren (Khadzhynov 2012). Risk of hyperkalemia is increased with chronic aliskiren therapy; use with extreme caution. Hydrochlorothiazide is usually ineffective when CrCl <30 mL/minute and is contraindicated in patients who are anuric.

Hepatic Impairment

US labeling: Mild to severe impairment: No dosage adjustment necessary. Use with caution. See also Aliskiren and Hydrochlorothiazide individual monographs.

Canadian labeling:

Mild to moderate impairment: No dosage adjustment necessary. Use with caution.

Severe impairment: Use is not recommended.

Additional Information Complete prescribing information should be consulted for additional detail.

Dosage Forms Excipient information presented when available (limited, particularly for generics); consult specific product labeling.

Tablet, Oral:

Tekturna HCT:

150/12.5: Aliskiren 150 mg and hydrochlorothiazide 12.5 mg

150/25: Aliskiren 150 mg and hydrochlorothiazide 25 mg

300/12.5: Aliskiren 300 mg and hydrochlorothiazide 12.5 mg

300/25: Aliskiren 300 mg and hydrochlorothiazide 25 mg

Dosage Forms: Canada Excipient information presented when available (limited, particularly for generics); consult specific product labeling.

Tablet, Oral:

Rasilez HCT:

150/12.5: Aliskiren 150 mg and hydrochlorothiazide 12.5 mg

150/25: Aliskiren 150 mg and hydrochlorothiazide 25 mg

300/12.5: Aliskiren 300 mg and hydrochlorothiazide 12.5 mg

300/25: Aliskiren 300 mg and hydrochlorothiazide 25 mg

Allopurinol (al oh PURE i nole)

Brand Names: US Aloprim; Zyloprim

Brand Names: Canada Alloprin; Apo-Allopurinol; JAMP-Allopurinol; Mar-Allopurinol; Novo-Purol; Zyloprim

Index Terms Allopurinol Sodium

Pharmacologic Category Antigout Agent; Xanthine Oxidase Inhibitor

Use

Oral:

Calcium oxalate calculi: Management of recurrent calcium oxalate calculi (with uric acid excretion >800 mg/day in men and >750 mg/day in women)

Gout: Management of primary or secondary gout (acute attack, tophi, joint destruction, uric acid lithiasis, and/or nephropathy)

Lesch-Nyhan syndrome: *Canadian labeling: Additional use (not in U.S. labeling):* Management of hyperuricemia associated with Lesch-Nyhan syndrome

Malignancies: Management of hyperuricemia associated with cancer treatment for leukemia, lymphoma, or solid tumor malignancies

IV: **Malignancies:** Management of hyperuricemia associated with cancer treatment for leukemia, lymphoma, or solid tumor malignancies

Pregnancy Considerations Adverse events were observed in some animal reproduction studies. Allopurinol crosses the placenta (Torrance, 2009). An increased risk of adverse fetal events has not been observed (limited data) (Hoeltzenbein, 2013).

Breast-Feeding Considerations Allopurinol and its metabolite are excreted into breast milk; the metabolite was also detected in the serum of the nursing infant (Kamilli, 1993). The U.S. manufacturer recommends caution be used when administering allopurinol to nursing women. The Canadian labeling contraindicates use in nursing women except those with hyperuricemia secondary to malignancy.

Contraindications

Severe hypersensitivity reaction to allopurinol or any component of the formulation

Canadian labeling: Additional contraindications (not in U.S. labeling): Nursing mothers and children (except those with hyperuricemia secondary to malignancy or Lesch-Nyhan syndrome)

Warnings/Precautions Do not use to treat asymptomatic hyperuricemia. Has been associated with a number of hypersensitivity reactions, including severe reactions (vasculitis and Stevens-Johnson syndrome); discontinue at first sign of rash. Consider HLA-B*5801 testing in patients at a higher risk for allopurinol hypersensitivity syndrome (eg, Koreans with stage 3 or worse CKD and Han Chinese and Thai descent regardless of renal function) prior to initiation of therapy (ACR guidelines [Khanna, 2012]). Reversible hepatotoxicity has been reported; use with caution in patients with preexisting hepatic impairment. Bone marrow suppression has been reported; use caution with other drugs causing myelosuppression. Caution in renal impairment, dosage adjustments needed. Full effect on serum uric acid levels in chronic gout may take several weeks to become evident; gradual titration is recommended. Potentially significant drug-drug interactions may exist, requiring dose or frequency adjustment, additional monitoring, and/or selection of alternative therapy.

Adverse Reactions

Most commonly reported:

Dermatologic: Skin rash

Endocrine & metabolic: Gout (acute)

Gastrointestinal: Diarrhea, nausea

Hepatic: Increased liver enzymes, increased serum alkaline phosphatase

<1% (Limited to important or life-threatening): Ageusia, agranulocytosis, alopecia, angioedema, aplastic anemia, cataract, cholestatic jaundice, ecchymoses, eczematoid dermatitis, eosinophilia, exfoliative dermatitis, hepatic necrosis, hepatitis, hepatomegaly, hepatotoxicity (idiosyncratic) (Chalasani, 2014), hyperbilirubinemia, hypersensitivity reaction, leukocytosis, leukopenia, lichen planus, macular retinitis, myopathy, necrotizing angiitis, nephritis, neuritis, neuropathy, onycholysis, pancreatitis, purpura, renal failure, skin granuloma (annulare), Stevens-Johnson syndrome, thrombocytopenia, toxic epidermal necrolysis, toxic pustuloderma, uremia, vasculitis, vesicobullous dermatitis

Drug Interactions

Metabolism/Transport Effects None known.

Avoid Concomitant Use

Avoid concomitant use of Allopurinol with any of the following: Didanosine; Pegloticase; Tegafur

Increased Effect/Toxicity

Allopurinol may increase the levels/effects of: Amoxicillin; Ampicillin; AzaTHIOprine; Bendamustine; CarBAMazepine; ChlorproPAMIDE; Cyclophosphamide; Didanosine; Doxofylline; Mercaptopurine; Pegloticase; Theophylline Derivatives; Vitamin K Antagonists

The levels/effects of Allopurinol may be increased by: ACE Inhibitors; Loop Diuretics; Thiazide Diuretics

Decreased Effect

Allopurinol may decrease the levels/effects of: Tegafur

The levels/effects of Allopurinol may be decreased by: Antacids

Preparation for Administration Reconstitute powder for injection with SWFI. Further dilution with NS or D$_5$W (50 to 100 mL) to ≤6 mg/mL is recommended.

Storage/Stability

Powder for injection: Store at controlled room temperature of 20°C to 25°C (68°F to 77°F). Following preparation, intravenous solutions should be stored at 20°C to 25°C (68°F to 77°F). Do not refrigerate reconstituted and/or diluted product. Must be administered within 10 hours of solution preparation.

Tablet: Store at controlled room temperature of 20°C to 25°C (68°F to 77°F). Protect from moisture and light.

Mechanism of Action Allopurinol inhibits xanthine oxidase, the enzyme responsible for the conversion of hypoxanthine to xanthine to uric acid. Allopurinol is metabolized to oxypurinol which is also an inhibitor of xanthine oxidase; allopurinol acts on purine catabolism, reducing the production of uric acid without disrupting the biosynthesis of vital purines.

Pharmacodynamics/Kinetics

Onset of action: Gout: 2 to 3 days, peak effect: 1 to 2 weeks; Hyperuricemia associated with chemotherapy: Maximum effect: 27 hours (Coiffier, 2008)

Absorption: Oral: ~80% to 90% from GI tract; Rectal: Poor and erratic

Distribution: V_d: ~1.6 L/kg; V_{ss}: 0.84 to 0.87 L/kg; enters breast milk

Protein binding: <1%

Metabolism: ~75% to active metabolites, chiefly oxypurinol

Bioavailability: 49% to 53%

Half-life elimination:
Normal renal function: Parent drug: 1 to 3 hours; Oxypurinol: 18 to 30 hours
End-stage renal disease: Prolonged

Time to peak, plasma: Oral: Allopurinol: 1.54 hours; Oxipurinol: 4.5 hours

Excretion: Urine (76% as oxypurinol, 12% as unchanged drug); feces (20%)

Allopurinol and oxypurinol are dialyzable

Dosing

Adult & Geriatric Note: Oral doses >300 mg should be given in divided doses.

Gout (chronic): Oral:

Manufacturer's labeling: Initial: 100 mg once daily; increase at weekly intervals in increments of 100 mg/day as needed to achieve desired serum uric acid level. Usual dosage range: 200 to 300 mg/day in mild gout; 400 to 600 mg/day in moderate to severe tophaceous gout. Maximum daily dose: 800 mg/day.

Alternative dosing (off-label): Initial: 100 mg/day, increasing the dose gradually in increments of 100 mg/day every 2 to 5 weeks as needed to achieve desired serum uric acid level of ≤6 mg/dL (ACR guidelines [Khanna, 2012]; EULAR guidelines [Zhang, 2006]; McGill, 2010). Some patients may require therapy targeted at a serum uric acid level <5 mg/dL to control symptoms. Allopurinol may be initiated during an acute gout attack so long as antiinflammatory therapy has been initiated as well (ACR guidelines [Khanna, 2012]).

Management of hyperuricemia associated with chemotherapy and/or radiation therapy:
Oral:

U.S. labeling: 600 to 800 mg daily in divided doses

Canadian labeling: 600 to 800 mg daily in 2 to 3 divided doses for 2 to 3 days prior to chemotherapy/radiation therapy then adjust dose per serum uric acid level; for ongoing management, 300 to 400 mg daily is usually sufficient to control serum uric levels.

Alternative dosing (off-label; intermediate risk for tumor lysis syndrome): Intermediate risk for tumor lysis syndrome: 10 mg/kg daily divided every 8 hours (maximum dose: 800 mg daily) **or** 50 to 100 mg/m² every 8 hours (maximum dose: 300 mg/m² daily), begin 1 to 2 days before initiation of induction chemotherapy; may continue for 3 to 7 days after chemotherapy (Coiffier, 2008)

IV: **Note:** Intravenous daily dose can be given as a single infusion or in equally divided doses at 6-, 8-, or 12-hour intervals.

Manufacturer's labeling: 200 to 400 mg/m² daily (maximum: 600 mg daily) beginning 1 to 2 days before chemotherapy

Alternative dosing (off-label; intermediate risk for tumor lysis syndrome): 200 to 400 mg/m² daily (maximum dose: 600 mg daily) in 1 to 3 divided doses beginning 1 to 2 days before the start of induction chemotherapy; may continue for 3 to 7 days after chemotherapy (Coiffier, 2008)

Recurrent calcium oxalate stones: Oral: 200 to 300 mg daily in single or divided doses; may adjust dose as needed to control hyperuricosuria

Pediatric

Management of hyperuricemia associated with chemotherapy and/or radiation therapy:
Oral: **Note:** Oral doses >300 mg should be given in divided doses.

U.S. labeling:
Children <6 years: 150 mg daily
Children 6 to 10 years: 300 mg daily
Children >10 years: Refer to adult dosing.

Canadian labeling:
Children 6 to 10 years: 10 mg/kg daily (do not exceed adult dosing); adjust dose as necessary after 48 hours

Alternative dosing (off-label; intermediate risk for tumor lysis syndrome): Intermediate risk for tumor lysis syndrome: 10 mg/kg daily divided every 8 hours (maximum dose: 800 mg daily) **or** 50 to 100 mg/m² every 8 hours (maximum dose: 300 mg/m² daily), begin 12 to 24 hours (children) or 1 to 2 days (adults) before initiation of induction chemotherapy; may continue for 3 to 7 days after chemotherapy (Coiffier, 2008)

IV: **Note:** Intravenous daily dose can be given as a single infusion or in equally divided doses at 6-, 8-, or 12-hour intervals.

Manufacturer's labeling: Starting dose: 200 mg/m² daily beginning 1 to 2 days before chemotherapy

Alternative dosing (off-label; intermediate risk for tumor lysis syndrome) 200 to 400 mg/m² daily (maximum dose: 600 mg daily) in 1 to 3 divided doses beginning 1 to 2 days before the start of induction chemotherapy; may continue for 3 to 7 days after chemotherapy (Coiffier, 2008)

Management of hyperuricemia associated with Lesch-Nyhan syndrome: *Canadian labeling (not in U.S. labeling):* Children 6 to 10 years: Oral: 10 mg/kg daily in 1 to 3 divided doses; adjust dose as necessary after 48 hours

Renal Impairment

Manufacturer's labeling: Oral, IV: Lower doses are required in renal impairment due to potential for accumulation of allopurinol and metabolites.
CrCl 10 to 20 mL/minute: 200 mg daily
CrCl 3 to 10 mL/minute: ≤100 mg daily
CrCl <3 mL/minute: ≤100 mg/dose at extended intervals

Alternative dosing (off-label):
Management of hyperuricemia associated with chemotherapy: Dosage reduction of 50% is recommended in renal impairment (Coiffier, 2008)

Gout: Oral:
Initiate therapy with 50 to 100 mg daily, and gradually increase to a maintenance dose to achieve a serum uric acid level of ≤6 mg/dL (with close monitoring of serum uric acid levels and for hypersensitivity) (Dalbeth, 2007).

or

In patients with stage 4 CKD or worse, initiate therapy at 50 mg/day, increasing the dose every 2 to 5 weeks to achieve desired uric acid levels of ≤6 mg/dL; doses >300 mg/day are permitted so long as they are accompanied by appropriate patient education and monitoring for toxicity (eg, pruritus, rash, elevated hepatic transaminases). Some patients may require therapy targeted at a serum uric acid level <5 mg/dL to control symptoms (ACR guidelines; Khanna, 2012)

Hemodialysis: Initial: 100 mg alternate days given postdialysis, increase cautiously to 300 mg based on response. If dialysis is on a daily basis, an additional 50% of the dose may be required postdialysis (Dalbeth, 2007)

Hepatic Impairment There are no dosage adjustments provided in the U.S. manufacturer's labeling. The Canadian labeling suggests that a dose reduction is necessary but does not provide specific dosing recommendations.

Dietary Considerations Fluid intake should be administered to yield neutral or slightly alkaline urine and an output of ~2 L (in adults).

Administration

Oral: Administer after meals with plenty of fluid.

IV: The rate of infusion depends on the volume of the infusion; infuse maximum single daily doses (600 mg/day) over ≥30 minutes. Whenever possible, therapy should be initiated at 24 to 48 hours before the start of chemotherapy known to cause tumor lysis (including adrenocorticosteroids). IV daily dose can be administered as a single infusion or in equally divided doses at 6-, 8-, or 12-hour interval.

Monitoring Parameters CBC, serum uric acid levels every 2 to 5 weeks during dose titration until desired level is achieved; every 6 months thereafter (ACR guidelines [Khanna, 2012]), I & O, hepatic and renal function, especially at start of therapy; signs and symptoms of hypersensitivity

Reference Range Uric acid, serum: An increase occurs during childhood

Adults:

Males: 3.4 to 7 mg/dL or slightly more

Females: 2.4 to 6 mg/dL or slightly more

Target: ≤6 mg/dL

Values >7 mg/dL are sometimes arbitrarily regarded as hyperuricemia, but there is no sharp line between normals on the one hand, and the serum uric acid of those with clinical gout. Normal ranges cannot be adjusted for purine ingestion, but high purine diet increases uric acid. Uric acid may be increased with body size, exercise, and stress.

Dosage Forms Excipient information presented when available (limited, particularly for generics); consult specific product labeling. [DSC] = Discontinued product

Solution Reconstituted, Intravenous, as sodium [strength expressed as base, preservative free]:

Aloprim: 500 mg (1 ea)

Generic: 500 mg (1 ea [DSC])

Tablet, Oral:

Zyloprim: 100 mg, 300 mg [scored]

Generic: 100 mg, 300 mg

Dosage Forms: Canada Note: Refer also to Dosage Forms.

Excipient information presented when available (limited, particularly for generics); consult specific product labeling.

Tablet, Oral, as sodium:

Zyloprim: 200 mg [scored]

Extemporaneous Preparations A 20 mg/mL oral suspension may be made with tablets and either a 1:1 mixture of Ora-Sweet® and Ora-Plus® or a 1:1 mixture of Ora-Sweet® SF and Ora-Plus® or a 1:4 mixture of cherry syrup concentrate and simple syrup, NF. Crush eight 300 mg tablets in a mortar and reduce to a fine powder. Add small portions of chosen vehicle and mix to a uniform paste; mix while adding the vehicle in incremental proportions to **almost** 120 mL; transfer to a calibrated bottle, rinse mortar with vehicle, and add quantity of vehicle sufficient to make 120 mL. Label "shake well". Stable for 60 days refrigerated or at room temperature (Allen, 1996; Nahata, 2004).

Allen LV Jr and Erickson MA 3rd, "Stability of Acetazolamide, Allopurinol, Azathioprine, Clonazepam, and Flucytosine in Extemporaneously Compounded Oral Liquids," *Am J Health Syst Pharm*, 1996, 53(16):1944-9.

Nahata MC, Pai VB, and Hipple TF, *Pediatric Drug Formulations*, 5th ed, Cincinnati, OH: Harvey Whitney Books Co, 2004.

♦ **Allopurinol Sodium** see Allopurinol on page 73

♦ **All-trans Retinoic Acid** see Tretinoin (Systemic) on page 1838

♦ **All-trans Vitamin A Acid** see Tretinoin (Systemic) on page 1838

♦ **Almacone [OTC]** see Aluminum Hydroxide, Magnesium Hydroxide, and Simethicone on page 85

♦ **Almacone Double Strength [OTC]** see Aluminum Hydroxide, Magnesium Hydroxide, and Simethicone on page 85

Almotriptan (al moh TRIP tan)

Brand Names: US Axert

Brand Names: Canada Axert; Mylan-Almotriptan; Sandoz-Almotriptan

Index Terms Almotriptan Malate

Pharmacologic Category Antimigraine Agent; Serotonin 5-HT$_{1B, 1D}$ Receptor Agonist

Use Acute treatment of migraine with or without aura in adults (with a history of migraine) and adolescents (with a history of migraine lasting ≥4 hours when left untreated)

Pregnancy Considerations Adverse events were observed in animal reproduction studies. Information related to almotriptan use in pregnancy is limited (Källén, 2011; Nezvalová-Henriksen, 2010; Nezvalová-Henriksen, 2012). Until additional information is available, other agents are preferred for the initial treatment of migraine in pregnancy (Da Silva, 2012; MacGregor, 2012; Williams, 2012).

Breast-Feeding Considerations It is not known if almotriptan is excreted in breast milk. The manufacturer recommends that caution be exercised when administering almotriptan to nursing women.

Contraindications Hypersensitivity to almotriptan or any component of the formulation; hemiplegic or basilar migraine; known or suspected ischemic heart disease

(eg, angina pectoris, MI, documented silent ischemia, coronary artery vasospasm, Prinzmetal's variant angina); cerebrovascular syndromes (eg, stroke, transient ischemic attacks); peripheral vascular disease (eg, ischemic bowel disease); uncontrolled hypertension; use within 24 hours of another 5-HT$_1$ agonist; use within 24 hours of ergotamine derivatives and/or ergotamine-containing medications (eg, dihydroergotamine, ergotamine)

Warnings/Precautions Almotriptan is only indicated for the treatment of acute migraine headache; not indicated for migraine prophylaxis, or the treatment of cluster headaches, hemiplegic migraine, or basilar migraine. If a patient does not respond to the first dose, the diagnosis of acute migraine should be reconsidered.

Almotriptan should not be given to patients with documented ischemic or vasospastic CAD. Patients with risk factors for CAD (eg, hypertension, hypercholesterolemia, smoker, obesity, diabetes, strong family history of CAD, menopause, male >40 years of age) should undergo adequate cardiac evaluation prior to administration; if the cardiac evaluation is "satisfactory," the first dose of almotriptan should be given in the healthcare provider's office (consider ECG monitoring). All patients should undergo periodic evaluation of cardiovascular status during treatment. Cardiac events (coronary artery vasospasm, transient ischemia, myocardial infarction, ventricular tachycardia/fibrillation, cardiac arrest, and death), cerebral/subarachnoid hemorrhage, stroke, peripheral vascular ischemia, and colonic ischemia have been reported with 5-HT$_1$ agonist administration. Patients who experience sensations of chest pain/pressure/tightness or symptoms suggestive of angina following dosing should be evaluated for coronary artery disease or Prinzmetal's angina before receiving additional doses; if dosing is resumed and similar symptoms recur, monitor with ECG. Significant elevation in blood pressure, including hypertensive crisis, has also been reported on rare occasions following 5-HT$_1$ agonist administration in patients with and without a history of hypertension.

Acute migraine agents (eg, triptans, opioids, ergotamine, or a combination of the agents) used for 10 or more days per month may lead to worsening of headaches (medication overuse headache); withdrawal treatment may be necessary in the setting of overuse. Transient and permanent blindness and partial vision loss have been reported (rare) with 5-HT$_1$ agonist administration. Almotriptan contains a sulfonyl group which is structurally different from a sulfonamide. Cross-reactivity in patients with sulfonamide allergy has not been evaluated; however, the manufacturer recommends that caution be exercised in this patient population. Use with caution in liver or renal dysfunction. Symptoms of agitation, confusion, hallucinations, hyperreflexia, myoclonus, shivering, and tachycardia (serotonin syndrome) may occur with concomitant proserotonergic drugs (ie, SSRIs/SNRIs or triptans) or agents which reduce almotriptan's metabolism. Concurrent use of serotonin precursors (eg, tryptophan) is not recommended. If concomitant administration with SSRIs is warranted, monitor closely, especially at initiation and with dose increases.

Adverse Reactions

1% to 10%:

Central nervous system: Drowsiness (≤5%), dizziness (≤4%), headache (≤2%)

Gastrointestinal: Nausea (1% to 3%), vomiting (≤2%), xerostomia (1%)

Neuromuscular & skeletal: Paresthesia (≤1%)

<1% (Limited to important or life-threatening): Anaphylactic shock, anaphylaxis, angina pectoris, angioedema, colitis, coronary artery vasospasm, hemiplegia, hypersensitivity reaction, hypertension, ischemic heart disease, mastalgia, myocardial infarction, neuropathy, seizure, skin rash, syncope, tachycardia, ventricular fibrillation, ventricular tachycardia

Drug Interactions

Metabolism/Transport Effects Substrate of CYP2D6 (minor), CYP3A4 (minor); Note: Assignment of Major/Minor substrate status based on clinically relevant drug interaction potential

Avoid Concomitant Use

Avoid concomitant use of Almotriptan with any of the following: Dapoxetine; Ergot Derivatives; MAO Inhibitors

Increased Effect/Toxicity

Almotriptan may increase the levels/effects of: Antipsychotic Agents; Droxidopa; Ergot Derivatives; Metoclopramide; Serotonin Modulators

The levels/effects of Almotriptan may be increased by: Antiemetics (5HT3 Antagonists); Antipsychotic Agents; CYP3A4 Inhibitors (Strong); Dapoxetine; Ergot Derivatives; MAO Inhibitors; Metaxalone

Decreased Effect There are no known significant interactions involving a decrease in effect.

Storage/Stability Store at 25°C (77°F); excursions permitted to 15°C to 30°C (59°F to 86°F).

Mechanism of Action Selective agonist for serotonin (5-HT$_{1B}$ and 5-HT$_{1D}$ receptors) in cranial arteries; causes vasoconstriction and reduces sterile inflammation associated with antidromic neuronal transmission correlating with relief of migraine

Pharmacodynamics/Kinetics Note: Reported values are similar between adolescent and adult patients (Baldwin 2004).

Absorption: Well absorbed

Distribution: V$_d$: ~180 to 200 L

Protein binding: ~35%

Metabolism: Via MAO type A oxidative deamination (~27% of dose) and CYP3A4 and 2D6 (~12% of dose) to inactive metabolites

Bioavailability: ~70%

Half-life elimination: Mean: 3 to 5 hours (Baldwin 2004; McEnroe 2005)

Time to peak, plasma: 1 to 3 hours

Excretion: Urine (~75%; ~40% of total dose as unchanged drug); feces (~13% of total dose as unchanged drug and metabolites)

Dosing

Adult & Geriatric Migraine: Oral: Initial: 6.25-12.5 mg in a single dose; if the headache returns, repeat the dose after 2 hours; no more than 2 doses (maximum daily dose: 25 mg)

Note: The safety of treating more than 4 migraines/month has not been established.

Dosage adjustment with concomitant use of an enzyme inhibitor:

Patients receiving a potent CYP3A4 inhibitor: Initial: 6.25 mg in a single dose; maximum daily dose: 12.5 mg

Patients with renal impairment and concomitant use of a potent CYP3A4 inhibitor: Avoid use

Patients with hepatic impairment and concomitant use of a potent CYP3A4 inhibitor: Avoid use

Pediatric Migraine: Oral: Children ≥12 years: Refer to adult dosing.

Renal Impairment Severe renal impairment (CrCl ≤30 mL/minute): Initial: 6.25 mg in a single dose; maximum daily dose: 12.5 mg

Hepatic Impairment Initial: 6.25 mg in a single dose; maximum daily dose: 12.5 mg

Dietary Considerations May be taken without regard to meals.

Administration Administer without regard to meals.

Dosage Forms Excipient information presented when available (limited, particularly for generics); consult specific product labeling.

Tablet, Oral, as maleate:

Axert: 6.25 mg

Axert: 12.5 mg [contains fd&c blue #2 (indigotine)]

Generic: 6.25 mg, 12.5 mg

- ◆ Almotriptan Malate *see* Almotriptan *on page 75*
- ◆ Alocril *see* Nedocromil *on page 1265*
- ◆ Alocril® (Can) *see* Nedocromil *on page 1265*
- ◆ Alodox Convenience [DSC] *see* Doxycycline *on page 601*
- ◆ Aloe Vesta Antifungal [OTC] *see* Miconazole (Topical) *on page 1201*
- ◆ Alomide *see* Lodoxamide *on page 1094*
- ◆ Alomide® (Can) *see* Lodoxamide *on page 1094*
- ◆ Aloprim *see* Allopurinol *on page 73*
- ◆ Aloquin *see* Iodoquinol *on page 974*
- ◆ Alora *see* Estradiol (Systemic) *on page 681*
- ◆ Aloxi *see* Palonosetron *on page 1380*

Alpha-Galactosidase (AL fa ga lak TOE si days)

Brand Names: US beano® Meltaways [OTC]; beano® [OTC]

Index Terms Aspergillus niger

Pharmacologic Category Enzyme

Use Prevention of flatulence and bloating attributed to a variety of grains, cereals, nuts, and vegetables

Dosing

Adult & Geriatric Flatulence and bloating: Oral: Adjust dose according to the number of problem foods per meal:

Tablet, chewable (beano®): Usual dose: 2-3 tablets/meal

Tablet, orally disintegrating (beano® Meltaways): One tablet per meal

Pediatric Flatulence and bloating: Children ≥12 years: Refer to adult dosing.

Renal Impairment No dosage adjustment provided in the manufacturer's labeling.

Hepatic Impairment No dosage adjustment provided in the manufacturer's labeling.

Additional Information Complete prescribing information should be consulted for additional detail.

Dosage Forms Excipient information presented when available (limited, particularly for generics); consult specific product labeling.

Tablet, chewable, oral:

beano®: 150 Galactosidase units [scored]

Tablet, orally disintegrating, oral:

beano® Meltaways: 300 Galactosidase units [strawberry flavor]

- ◆ Alpha-Galactosidase-A (Recombinant) *see* Agalsidase Beta *on page 52*
- ◆ Alphagan *see* Brimonidine (Ophthalmic) *on page 254*
- ◆ Alphagan P *see* Brimonidine (Ophthalmic) *on page 254*
- ◆ 1α-Hydroxyergocalciferol *see* Doxercalciferol *on page 593*
- ◆ Alphanate *see* Antihemophilic Factor/von Willebrand Factor Complex (Human) *on page 133*
- ◆ AlphaNine SD *see* Factor IX (Human) *on page 737*
- ◆ Alphaquin HP *see* Hydroquinone *on page 893*
- ◆ AlphaTrex *see* Betamethasone (Topical) *on page 224*
- ◆ Alph-E [OTC] *see* Vitamin E *on page 1906*
- ◆ Alph-E-Mixed [OTC] *see* Vitamin E *on page 1906*
- ◆ Alph-E-Mixed 1000 [OTC] *see* Vitamin E *on page 1906*

ALPRAZolam (al PRAY zoe lam)

Brand Names: US ALPRAZolam Intensol; ALPRAZolam XR; Niravam; Xanax; Xanax XR

Brand Names: Canada Apo-Alpraz; Apo-Alpraz TS; Jamp-Alprazolam; Mylan-Alprazolam; Nat-Alprazolam; Riva-Alpraz; Teva-Alprazolam; Xanax; Xanax TS

Pharmacologic Category Benzodiazepine

Use Treatment of anxiety disorder (GAD); short-term relief of symptoms of anxiety; panic disorder, with or without agoraphobia; anxiety associated with depression

Pregnancy Considerations Benzodiazepines have the potential to cause harm to the fetus. Alprazolam and its metabolites cross the human placenta. Teratogenic effects have been observed with some benzodiazepines; however, additional studies are needed. The incidence of premature birth and low birth weights may be increased following maternal use of benzodiazepines; hypoglycemia and respiratory problems in the neonate may occur following exposure late in pregnancy. Neonatal withdrawal symptoms may occur within days to weeks after birth and "floppy infant syndrome" (which also includes withdrawal symptoms) has been reported with some benzodiazepines (Bergman, 1992; Iqbal, 2002; Wikner, 2007).

Breast-Feeding Considerations Benzodiazepines are excreted into breast milk. In a study of eight postpartum women, peak concentrations of alprazolam were found in breast milk ~1 hour after the maternal dose and the half-life was ~14 hours. Samples were obtained over 36 hours following a single oral dose of alprazolam 0.5 mg. Metabolites were not detected in the breast milk. In this study, the estimated exposure to the breast-feeding infant was ~3% of the weight-adjusted maternal dose (Oo, 1995). Drowsiness, lethargy, or weight loss in nursing infants have been observed in case reports following maternal use of some benzodiazepines (Iqbal, 2002). Breast-feeding is not recommended by the manufacturer.

Contraindications Hypersensitivity to alprazolam or any component of the formulation (cross-sensitivity with other benzodiazepines may exist); narrow-angle glaucoma; concurrent use with ketoconazole or itraconazole

Warnings/Precautions Rebound or withdrawal symptoms, including seizures, may occur following abrupt discontinuation or large decreases in dose (more common in adult patients receiving >4 mg/day or prolonged treatment); the risk of seizures appears to be greatest 24 to 72 hours following discontinuation of therapy. Breakthrough anxiety may occur at the end of dosing interval. Use with caution in patients receiving concurrent CYP3A4 inhibitors, moderate or strong CYP3A4 inducers, and major CYP3A4 substrates; consider alternative agents that avoid or lessen the potential for CYP-mediated interactions. Use with caution in renal impairment or predisposition to urate nephropathy; has weak uricosuric properties. Use with caution in or debilitated patients, patients with hepatic disease (including alcoholics) or respiratory

disease, or obese patients. Cigarette smoking may decrease alprazolam concentrations up to 50%.

Causes CNS depression (dose related) which may impair physical and mental capabilities. Patients must be cautioned about performing tasks that require mental alertness (eg, operating machinery or driving). Effects with other sedative drugs or ethanol may be potentiated. Benzodiazepines have been associated with falls and traumatic injury and should be used with extreme caution in patients who are at risk of these events.

Use caution in patients with depression, particularly if suicidal risk may be present. Episodes of mania or hypomania have occurred in depressed patients treated with alprazolam. May cause physical or psychological dependence. Acute withdrawal may be precipitated in patients after administration of flumazenil. Tolerance does not develop to the anxiolytic effects (Vinkers, 2012). Chronic use of this agent may increase the perioperative benzodiazepine dose needed to achieve desired effect.

Benzodiazepines have been associated with anterograde amnesia. Paradoxical reactions have been reported with benzodiazepines, particularly in adolescent/pediatric or psychiatric patients. Does not have analgesic, antidepressant, or antipsychotic properties.

Adverse Reactions

>10%:

Central nervous system: Ataxia, cognitive dysfunction, depression, dizziness, drowsiness, dysarthria, fatigue, irritability, memory impairment, sedation

Endocrine & metabolic: Decreased libido, weight gain, weight loss

Gastrointestinal: Change in appetite, constipation, xerostomia

Genitourinary: Difficulty in micturition

Respiratory: Nasal congestion

1% to 10%:

Cardiovascular: Chest pain, hypotension, palpitations, sinus tachycardia, syncope

Central nervous system: Abnormal dreams, agitation, akathisia, altered mental status, confusion, depersonalization, derealization, disinhibition, disorientation, disturbance in attention, dystonia, fear, hallucination, headache, hypersomnia, hypoesthesia, insomnia, lethargy, malaise, nervousness, nightmares, paresthesia, restlessness, seizure, talkativeness, vertigo

Dermatologic: Dermatitis, diaphoresis, skin rash

Endocrine & metabolic: Increased libido, menstrual disease

Gastrointestinal: Abdominal pain, anorexia, diarrhea, dyspepsia, nausea, sialorrhea, vomiting

Genitourinary: Dysmenorrhea, sexual disorder, urinary incontinence

Hepatic: Increased liver enzymes, increased serum bilirubin, jaundice

Neuromuscular & skeletal: Arthralgia, back pain, dyskinesia, muscle cramps, muscle twitching, myalgia, tremor, weakness

Ophthalmic: Blurred vision

Respiratory: Allergic rhinitis, dyspnea, hyperventilation, upper respiratory tract infection

<1% (Limited to important or life-threatening): Amnesia, angioedema, diplopia, falling, galactorrhea, gynecomastia, hepatic failure, hepatitis, homicidal ideation, hyperprolactinemia, hypomania, mania, peripheral edema, sleep apnea, Stevens-Johnson syndrome, suicidal ideation, tinnitus

Drug Interactions

Metabolism/Transport Effects Substrate of CYP3A4 (major); **Note:** Assignment of Major/Minor substrate status based on clinically relevant drug interaction potential; **Inhibits** CYP3A4 (weak)

Avoid Concomitant Use

Avoid concomitant use of ALPRAZolam with any of the following: Azelastine (Nasal); Conivaptan; Fusidic Acid (Systemic); Idelalisib; Indinavir; Itraconazole; Ketoconazole (Systemic); Methadone; OLANZapine; Orphenadrine; Paraldehyde; Pimozide; Sodium Oxybate; Thalidomide

Increased Effect/Toxicity

ALPRAZolam may increase the levels/effects of: Alcohol (Ethyl); ARIPiprazole; Azelastine (Nasal); Buprenorphine; CloZAPine; CNS Depressants; Dofetilide; Flibanserin; Hydrocodone; Lomitapide; Methadone; Methotrimeprazine; Metyrosine; Mirtazapine; NiMODipine; Orphenadrine; Paraldehyde; Pimozide; Pramipexole; ROPINIRole; Rotigotine; Selective Serotonin Reuptake Inhibitors; Sodium Oxybate; Suvorexant; Thalidomide; Zolpidem

The levels/effects of ALPRAZolam may be increased by: Aprepitant; Boceprevir; Brimonidine (Topical); Cannabis; Conivaptan; CYP3A4 Inhibitors (Moderate); CYP3A4 Inhibitors (Strong); Dasatinib; Doxylamine; Droperidol; FluvoxaMINE; Fosaprepitant; Fusidic Acid (Systemic); HydrOXYzine; Idelalisib; Indinavir; Itraconazole; Ivacaftor; Kava Kava; Ketoconazole (Systemic); Luliconazole; Macrolide Antibiotics; Magnesium Sulfate; Methotrimeprazine; Mifepristone; Minocycline; Nabilone; Netupitant; OLANZapine; Ombitasvir, Paritaprevir, and Ritonavir; Ombitasvir, Paritaprevir, Ritonavir, and Dasabuvir; Osimertinib; Palbociclib; Perampanel; Protease Inhibitors; Rufinamide; Simeprevir; Stiripentol; Tapentadol; Teduglutide; Telaprevir; Tetrahydrocannabinol

Decreased Effect

The levels/effects of ALPRAZolam may be decreased by: Bosentan; CYP3A4 Inducers (Moderate); CYP3A4 Inducers (Strong); Dabrafenib; Deferasirox; Enzalutamide; Mitotane; Osimertinib; Siltuximab; St Johns Wort; Theophylline Derivatives; Tocilizumab; Yohimbine

Food Interactions Alprazolam serum concentration is unlikely to be increased by grapefruit juice because of alprazolam's high oral bioavailability. The C_{max} of the extended release formulation is increased by 25% when a high-fat meal is given 2 hours before dosing. T_{max} is decreased 33% when food is given immediately prior to dose and increased by 33% when food is given ≥1 hour after dose. Management: Administer without regard to food.

Storage/Stability

Immediate release tablets: Store at 20°C to 25°C (68°F to 77°F).

Extended release tablets: Store at 25°C (77°F); excursions permitted to 15°C to 30°C (59°F to 86°F).

Orally-disintegrating tablet: Store at room temperature of 20°C to 25°C (68°F to 77°F). Protect from moisture. Seal bottle tightly and discard any cotton packaged inside bottle.

Mechanism of Action Binds to stereospecific benzodiazepine receptors on the postsynaptic GABA neuron at several sites within the central nervous system, including the limbic system, reticular formation. Enhancement of the inhibitory effect of GABA on neuronal excitability results by increased neuronal membrane permeability to chloride ions. This shift in chloride ions results in hyperpolarization (a less excitable state) and stabilization. Benzodiazepine receptors and effects appear to be linked to the GABA-A receptors. Benzodiazepines do not bind to GABA-B receptors.

Pharmacodynamics/Kinetics

Absorption: Readily absorbed; Extended release: Slower relative to immediate release formulation resulting in a concentration that is maintained 5 to 11 hours after dosing; rate increased following night time dosing (versus morning dosing)

Distribution: Immediate release: V_d: 0.84 to 1.42 L/kg (Greenblatt 1993)

Protein binding: 80%; primarily to albumin

Metabolism: Hepatic via CYP3A4; forms two active metabolites (4-hydroxyalprazolam and α-hydroxyalprazolam [about half as active as alprazolam]) and an inactive metabolite benzophenone metabolite, however, the active metabolites are unlikely to contribute to much of the pharmacologic effects because of their low concentrations and lesser potencies.

Bioavailability: Immediate release: 84% to 92% (Greenblatt 1993); Extended release: 90%

Half-life elimination:

Adults: 11.2 hours (Immediate release range: 6.3 to 26.9 hours; Extended release range: 10.7 to 15.8 hours); Orally-disintegrating tablet: Mean: 12.5 hours (range: 7.9 to 19.2 hours)

Alcoholic liver disease: 19.7 hours (range: 5.8 to 65.3 hours)

Obesity: 21.8 hours (range: 9.9 to 40.4 hours)

Elderly: 16.3 hours (range: 9 to 26.9 hours)

Time to peak, serum:

Immediate release: 1 to 2 hours

Extended release: Adolescents and Adults: ~9 hours, relatively steady from 4 to 12 hours (Glue 2006); decreased by 1 hour when administered at bedtime (as compared to morning administration); decreased by 33% when administered with a high-fat meal; increased by 33% when administered ≥1 hour after a high-fat meal

Orally-disintegrating tablet: 1.5 to 2 hours; occurs ~15 minutes earlier when administered with water; increased to ~4 hours when administered with a high-fat meal

Excretion: Urine (as unchanged drug and metabolites)

Dosing

Adult Note: Treatment >4 months should be re-evaluated to determine the patient's continued need for the drug

Anxiety: Oral: *Immediate release:* Initial: 0.25-0.5 mg 3 times/day; titrate dose upward every 3-4 days; usual maximum: 4 mg/day. Patients requiring doses >4 mg/day should be increased cautiously. Periodic reassessment and consideration of dosage reduction is recommended.

Panic disorder: Oral:
Immediate release: Initial: 0.5 mg 3 times/day; dose may be increased every 3-4 days in increments ≤1 mg/day. Mean effective dosage: 5-6 mg/day; some patients may require as much as 10 mg/day
Extended release: 0.5-1 mg once daily; may increase dose every 3-4 days in increments ≤1 mg/day (range: 3-6 mg/day)
Switching from immediate release to extended release: Patients may be switched to extended release tablets by taking the total daily dose of the immediate release tablets and giving it once daily using the extended release preparation.

Preoperative anxiety (off-label use): Oral: 0.5 mg 60-90 minutes before procedure (De Witte, 2002)

Dose reduction: Abrupt discontinuation should be avoided. Daily dose may be decreased by 0.5 mg every 3 days; however, some patients may require a slower reduction. If withdrawal symptoms occur, resume previous dose and discontinue on a less rapid schedule.

Geriatric Note: Titrate gradually, if needed and tolerated.
Immediate release: Initial 0.25 mg 2 to 3 times/day
Extended release: Initial: 0.5 mg once daily

Pediatric
Anxiety (off-label use): Oral: Immediate release: Initial: 0.005 mg/kg/dose or 0.125 mg/dose 3 times/day; increase in increments of 0.125-0.25 mg, up to a maximum of 0.02 mg/kg/dose or 0.06 mg/kg/day (range of doses reported in one study: 0.375-3 mg/day) (Pfefferbaum, 1987). See "Dose Reduction" comment in adult dosing.

Note: Treatment >4 months should be re-evaluated to determine the patient's continued need for the drug.

Renal Impairment No dosage adjustment provided in manufacturer's labeling; however, use caution.

Hepatic Impairment Advanced liver disease:
Immediate release: 0.25 mg 2-3 times/day; titrate gradually if needed and tolerated.
Extended release: 0.5 mg once daily; titrate gradually if needed and tolerate

Dietary Considerations Extended release tablet should be taken once daily in the morning.

Administration

Immediate release preparations: Can be administered sublingually if oral administration is not possible; absorption and onset of effect are comparable to oral administration (Scavone,1987; Scavone, 1992)

Extended release tablet: Should be taken once daily in the morning; do not crush, break, or chew.

Orally-disintegrating tablets: Using dry hands, place tablet on top of tongue and allow to disintegrate. If using one-half of tablet, immediately discard remaining half (may not remain stable). Administration with water is not necessary.

Monitoring Parameters Respiratory and cardiovascular status

Additional Information Not intended for management of anxieties and minor distresses associated with everyday life. Treatment longer than 4 months should be re-evaluated to determine the patient's need for the drug. Patients who become physically dependent on alprazolam tend to have a difficult time discontinuing it; withdrawal symptoms may be severe. To minimize withdrawal symptoms, taper dosage slowly; do not discontinue abruptly. Abrupt discontinuation after sustained use (generally >10 days) may cause withdrawal symptoms.

Dosage Forms Excipient information presented when available (limited, particularly for generics); consult specific product labeling. [DSC] = Discontinued product
Concentrate, Oral:
ALPRAZolam Intensol: 1 mg/mL (30 mL) [unflavored flavor]
Tablet, Oral:
Xanax: 0.25 mg [scored]
Xanax: 0.5 mg [scored; contains fd&c yellow #6 (sunset yellow)]
Xanax: 1 mg [scored; contains fd&c blue #2 (indigotine)]
Xanax: 2 mg [scored]
Generic: 0.25 mg, 0.5 mg, 1 mg, 2 mg
Tablet Dispersible, Oral:
Niravam: 0.25 mg, 0.5 mg [DSC], 1 mg [DSC], 2 mg [DSC] [scored; orange flavor]
Generic: 0.25 mg, 0.5 mg, 1 mg, 2 mg

Tablet Extended Release 24 Hour, Oral:
ALPRAZolam XR: 0.5 mg
ALPRAZolam XR: 1 mg [contains fd&c yellow #10 (quinoline yellow)]
ALPRAZolam XR: 2 mg [contains fd&c blue #2 (indigotine)]
ALPRAZolam XR: 3 mg [contains fd&c blue #2 (indigotine), fd&c yellow #10 (quinoline yellow)]
Xanax XR: 0.5 mg
Xanax XR: 1 mg [contains fd&c yellow #10 (quinoline yellow)]
Xanax XR: 2 mg [contains fd&c blue #2 (indigotine)]
Xanax XR: 3 mg [contains fd&c blue #2 (indigotine), fd&c yellow #10 (quinoline yellow)]
Generic: 0.5 mg, 1 mg, 2 mg, 3 mg

Controlled Substance C-IV

Extemporaneous Preparations Note: Commercial oral solution is available (Alprazolam Intensol™: 1 mg/mL [dye free, ethanol free, sugar free; contains propylene glycol])

A 1 mg/mL oral suspension may be made with tablets and one of three different vehicles (a 1:1 mixture of Ora-Sweet® and Ora-Plus®, a 1:1 mixture of Ora-Sweet® SF and Ora-Plus®, or a 1:4 mixture of cherry syrup with Simple Syrup, NF). Crush sixty 2 mg tablets in a mortar and reduce to a fine powder. Add 40 mL of vehicle and mix to a uniform paste; mix while adding the vehicle in incremental proportions to almost 120 mL; transfer to a calibrated bottle, rinse mortar with vehicle, and add a quantity of vehicle sufficient to make 120 mL. Label "shake well" and "refrigerate". Stable for 60 days.
Nahata MC, Pai VB, and Hipple TF, *Pediatric Drug Formulations*, 5th ed, Cincinnati, OH: Harvey Whitney Books Co, 2004.

◆ **ALPRAZolam Intensol** see ALPRAZolam *on page* 76
◆ **ALPRAZolam XR** see ALPRAZolam *on page* 76
◆ **Alprolix** see Factor IX (Recombinant) *on page* 738

Alprostadil (al PROS ta dill)

Brand Names: US Caverject; Caverject Impulse; Edex; Muse; Prostin VR
Brand Names: Canada Alprostadil Injection USP; Caverject; Muse Pellet; Prostin VR
Index Terms PGE₁; Prostaglandin E₁
Pharmacologic Category Prostaglandin; Vasodilator
Use

Prostin VR Pediatric: Temporary maintenance of patency of ductus arteriosus in neonates with ductal-dependent congenital heart disease until surgery can be performed. These defects include cyanotic (eg, pulmonary atresia, pulmonary stenosis, tricuspid atresia, Fallot's tetralogy, transposition of the great vessels) and acyanotic (eg, interruption of aortic arch, coarctation of aorta, hypoplastic left ventricle) heart disease.

Caverject, Caverject Impulse: Treatment of erectile dysfunction due to vasculogenic, psychogenic, neurogenic, or mixed etiology. May be a useful adjunct to other diagnostic tests in the diagnosis of erectile dysfunction

Edex, Muse: Treatment of erectile dysfunction due to vasculogenic, psychogenic, neurogenic, or mixed etiology

Pregnancy Considerations Adverse events were observed in animal reproduction studies. Alprostadil is not indicated for use in women. The manufacturer of Muse recommends a condom barrier when being used during sexual intercourse with a pregnant woman.

Breast-Feeding Considerations Alprostadil is not indicated for use in women.

Contraindications

Alprostadil (intracavernous):
Conditions predisposing patients to priapism (eg, sickle cell anemia or trait, multiple myeloma, leukemia); patients with anatomical deformation or fibrotic conditions of the penis (eg, angulation, cavernosal fibrosis, or Peyronie disease); penile implants.

Caverject, Caverject impulse: Hypersensitivity to alprostadil or any component of the formulation; use in men for whom sexual activity is inadvisable or contraindicated. Intracavernosal alprostadil is intended for use in adult men only and is not indicated for use in women, children, or newborns.

Alprostadil (transurethral): Hypersensitivity to alprostadil, use in patients with urethral stricture, balanitis (inflammation/infection of the glans penis), severe hypospadias and curvature, and in patients with acute or chronic urethritis; in patients who are prone to venous thrombosis or who have a hyperviscosity syndrome (eg, sickle cell anemia or trait, thrombocytopenia, polycythemia, multiple myeloma) and are therefore at increased risk of priapism (rigid erection lasting ≥6 hours). Should not be used in men for whom sexual activity is inadvisable or for sexual

intercourse with a pregnant woman unless the couple uses a condom barrier.

Alprostadil (intravenous): There are no contraindications listed in the manufacturer's labeling.

Warnings/Precautions

Prostin VR Pediatric: Use cautiously in neonates with bleeding tendencies. **[U.S. Boxed Warning]: Apnea may occur in 10% to 12% of neonates with congenital heart defects, especially in those weighing <2 kg at birth.** Apnea usually appears during the first hour of drug infusion. When used for patency of ductus arteriosus infuse for the shortest time at the lowest dose consistent with good patient care. Use for >120 hours has been associated with antral hyperplasia and gastric outlet obstruction.

Caverject, Caverject Impulse, Edex, Muse: When used in erectile dysfunction, priapism may occur; treat prolonged priapism (erection persisting for >4 hours) immediately to avoid penile tissue damage and permanent loss of potency; discontinue therapy if signs of penile fibrosis develop (penile angulation, cavernosal fibrosis, or Peyronie disease). Underlying causes of erectile dysfunction should be evaluated and treated prior to therapy. Treatment for erectile dysfunction should not be used in men whom sexual activity is inadvisable because of underlying cardiovascular status. When used in erectile dysfunction (Muse), syncope occurring within 1 hour of administration has been reported. The potential for drug-drug interactions may occur when Muse is prescribed concomitantly with antihypertensives. Instruct patients to avoid ethanol consumption; may have vasodilating effect.

Benzyl alcohol and derivatives: Some dosage forms may contain benzyl alcohol; large amounts of benzyl alcohol (≥99 mg/kg/day) have been associated with a potentially fatal toxicity ("gasping syndrome") in neonates; the "gasping syndrome" consists of metabolic acidosis, respiratory distress, gasping respirations, CNS dysfunction (including convulsions, intracranial hemorrhage), hypotension, and cardiovascular collapse (AAP ["Inactive" 1997]; CDC, 1982); some data suggests that benzoate displaces bilirubin from protein binding sites (Ahlfors 2001); avoid or use dosage forms containing benzyl alcohol with caution in neonates. See manufacturer's labeling.

Adverse Reactions

Intraurethral:

>10%: Genitourinary: Penile pain, urethral burning

2% to 10%:

Central nervous system: Dizziness, headache, pain

Genitourinary: Testicular pain, urethral bleeding (minor), vulvovaginal pruritus (female partner)

<2%: Tachycardia

Intracavernosal injection:

>10%: Genitourinary: Penile pain

1% to 10%:

Cardiovascular: Hypertension

Central nervous system: Dizziness, headache

Genitourinary: Prolonged erection (>4 hours, 4%), penile disease, penile rash, penile swelling, Peyronie's disease

Local: Bruising at injection site, hematoma at injection site

<1%: Balanitis, injection site hemorrhage, priapism (0.4%)

Intravenous:

>10%:

Cardiovascular: Flushing

Respiratory: Apnea

Miscellaneous: Fever

1% to 10%:

Cardiovascular: Bradycardia, cardiac arrest, edema, hypertension, hypotension, tachycardia

Central nervous system: Dizziness, headache, seizure

Endocrine & metabolic: Hypokalemia

Gastrointestinal: Diarrhea

Hematologic & oncologic: Disseminated intravascular coagulation

Infection: Sepsis

Local: Local pain (in structures other than the injection site)

Neuromuscular & skeletal: Back pain

Respiratory: Cough, flu-like symptoms, nasal congestion, sinusitis, upper respiratory tract infection

<1% (Limited to important or life-threatening): Anemia, anuria, bradypnea, cardiac failure, cerebral hemorrhage, gastroesophageal reflux disease, hematuria, hemorrhage, hyperbilirubinemia, hyperemia, hyperirritability, hyperkalemia, hypoglycemia, hypothermia, neck hyperextension, peritonitis, second degree atrioventricular block, shock, supraventricular tachycardia, thrombocytopenia, ventricular fibrillation

Drug Interactions

Metabolism/Transport Effects None known.

Avoid Concomitant Use

Avoid concomitant use of Alprostadil with any of the following: Phosphodiesterase 5 Inhibitors

Increased Effect/Toxicity

The levels/effects of Alprostadil may be increased by: Phosphodiesterase 5 Inhibitors

Decreased Effect There are no known significant interactions involving a decrease in effect.

Preparation for Administration

Caverject Impulse: Provided as a dual-chamber syringe with diluent in one chamber. To mix, hold syringe with needle pointing upward and turn plunger clockwise; turn upside down several times to mix. Device can be set to deliver specified dose, each device can be set at various increments.

Caverject powder: Use only the supplied diluent for reconstitution (ie, bacteriostatic/sterile water with benzyl alcohol 0.945%).

Edex: Reconstitute with NS; use immediately following reconstitution. Discard any remaining solution in cartridge.

Storage/Stability

Caverject Impulse: Store at or below 25°C (77°F); excursions are permitted between 15°C and 30°C (59°F and 86°F). Following reconstitution, use within 24 hours and discard any unused solution; for single use only.

Caverject powder: The 5 mcg, 10 mcg, and 20 mcg vials should be stored at or below 25°C (77°F). The 40 mcg vial should be stored at 2°C to 8°C (36°F to 46°F) until dispensed. After dispensing, stable for up to 3 months at or below 25°C (77°F). Following reconstitution, all strengths should be stored at or below 25°C (77°F); do not refrigerate or freeze; use within 24 hours.

Edex: Store at 25°C (77°F); excursions are permitted between 15°C and 30°C (59°F and 86°F).

Muse: Refrigerate at 2°C to 8°C (36°F to 46°F); may be stored at room temperature for up to 14 days.

Prostin VR Pediatric: Refrigerate at 2°C to 8°C (36°F to 46°F). The following stability information has also been reported: May be stored at 20°C for up to 34 days or 30°C for up to 26 days (Cohen 2007). Prior to infusion, dilute with D_5W, $D_{10}W$, or NS; use within 24 hours.

Mechanism of Action Causes vasodilation by means of direct effect on vascular and ductus arteriosus smooth muscle; relaxes trabecular smooth muscle by dilation of cavernosal arteries when injected along the penile shaft, allowing blood flow to and entrapment in the lacunar spaces of the penis (ie, corporeal veno-occlusive mechanism)

Pharmacodynamics/Kinetics

Onset of action: Erectile dysfunction: 5 to 20 minutes

Duration: Ductus arteriosus will begin to close within 1 to 2 hours after drug is stopped; Erectile dysfunction: Intended duration <1 hour

Distribution: Insignificant following penile injection

Protein binding, plasma: 81% to albumin

Metabolism: ~70% to 80% by oxidation during a single pass through the lungs; metabolite (13,14 dihydro-PGE1) is active and has been identified in neonates

Half-life elimination: 5 to 10 minutes

Time to Peak: Acyanotic congenital heart disease: Usual: 1.5 to 3 hours; range: 15 minutes to 11 hours; Cyanotic congenital heart disease: Usual: ~30 minutes

Excretion: Urine (90% as metabolites) within 24 hours

Dosing

Adult

Erectile dysfunction:

Intracavernous (Caverject, Caverject Impulse, Edex): Individualize dose by careful titration; doses >40 mcg (Edex) or >60 mcg (Caverject, Caverject Impulse) are not recommended: Initial dose must be titrated in physician's office. Patient must stay in the physician's office until complete detumescence occurs; if there is no response, then the next higher dose may be given within 1 hour; if there is still no response, a 1-day interval before giving the next dose is recommended; increasing the dose or concentration in the treatment of impotence results in increasing pain and discomfort. Initial dose titration:

Vasculogenic, psychogenic, or mixed etiology: Initiate dosage titration at 2.5 mcg.

If there is a partial response, increase dose by 2.5 mcg to a dose of 5 mcg and then, in increments of 5 to 10 mcg (depending on erectile response) until the dose that produces an erection suitable for intercourse and not exceeding a duration of 1 hour is reached.

If there is no response to the initial 2.5 mcg dose, the second dose may be increased to 7.5 mcg and administered within 1 hour, followed by increments of 5 to 10 mcg. According to the prescribing information for Caverject Impulse, no more than 2 doses during the initial titration should be given within a 24 hour period.

If there is a response, then there should be at least a 24 hour interval before the next dose is given.

Neurogenic etiology (eg, spinal cord injury): **Note:** Caverject powder must be used to prepare a 1.25 mcg dose: Initiate dosage titration at 1.25 mcg; may increase to a dose of 2.5 mcg within 1 hour and if necessary, to a dose of 5 mcg; may increase further in increments of 5 mcg until the dose is reached that produces an erection suitable for intercourse, not lasting >1 hour.

Maintenance: Once an appropriate dose has been determined, patient may self-administer injections at a frequency of no more than 3 times/week with at least 24 hours between doses

Intraurethral (Muse Pellet):
Initial: 125 to 250 mcg
Maintenance: Administer as needed to achieve an erection; duration of action is about 30-60 minutes; use only two systems per 24-hour period

Geriatric Elderly patients may have a greater frequency of renal dysfunction; lowest effective dose should be used. In clinical studies with Edex, higher minimally effective doses and a higher rate of lack of effect were noted.

Pediatric
Patent ductus arteriosus IV:
Prostin VR Pediatric: IV continuous infusion into a large vein, or alternatively through an umbilical artery catheter placed at the ductal opening: 0.05-0.1 mcg/kg/minute with therapeutic response, rate is reduced to lowest effective dosage. With unsatisfactory response, rate is increased gradually; maintenance: 0.01-0.4 mcg/kg/minute.

Note: Alprostadil is usually given at an infusion rate of 0.1 mcg/kg/minute, but it is often possible to reduce the dosage to 1/2 or even 1/10 without losing the therapeutic effect.

Note: Therapeutic response is indicated by increased pH in those with acidosis or by an increase in oxygenation (PO_2) usually evident within 30 minutes.

Renal Impairment There are no dosage adjustments provided in the manufacturer's labeling.

Hepatic Impairment There are no dosage adjustments provided in the manufacturer's labeling.

Usual Infusion Concentrations: Pediatric IV infusion: 10 mcg/mL **or** 20 mcg/mL

Administration
Patent ductus arteriosus (Prostin VR Pediatric): IV continuous infusion into a large vein or alternatively through an umbilical artery catheter placed at the ductal opening; manufacturer recommended maximum concentration for IV infusion: 20 mcg/mL

Erectile dysfunction: Intracavernous:
Caverject, Edex: Use a 1/2 inch, 27- to 30-gauge needle. Inject into the dorsolateral aspect of the proximal third of the penis, avoiding visible veins; alternate side of the penis for injections. Administer Edex over a 5- to 10-second interval.

Caverject Impulse consists of a disposable, single dose, dual chamber syringe system. After attaching the provided needle assembly, the dose to be given may be selected and after the site is cleansed with an alcohol swab, injected according to the prescribing information into the dorsolateral aspect of the proximal third of the penis, avoiding visible veins; alternate side of the penis for injections.

Monitoring Parameters Arterial pressure, respiratory rate, heart rate, temperature, degree of penile pain, duration of erection, adequate detumescence after dosing, signs of infection

Dosage Forms Excipient information presented when available (limited, particularly for generics); consult specific product labeling.

Kit, Intracavernosal:
Caverject Impulse: 10 mcg [contains benzyl alcohol]
Caverject Impulse: 20 mcg
Edex: 10 mcg, 20 mcg, 40 mcg
Pellet, Urethral:
Muse: 125 mcg (1 ea, 6 ea); 250 mcg (1 ea, 6 ea); 500 mcg (1 ea, 6 ea); 1000 mcg (1 ea, 6 ea)
Solution, Injection:
Prostin VR: 500 mcg/mL (1 mL) [contains benzyl alcohol]
Generic: 500 mcg/mL (1 mL)

Solution Reconstituted, Intracavernosal:
Caverject: 20 mcg (1 ea)
Caverject: 20 mcg (1 ea); 40 mcg (1 ea) [contains benzyl alcohol]

◆ **Alprostadil Injection USP (Can)** *see* Alprostadil *on page 78*
◆ **Alrex** *see* Loteprednol *on page 1110*
◆ **Alsuma** *see* SUMAtriptan *on page 1717*
◆ **Altabax** *see* Retapamulin *on page 1571*
◆ **Altacaine** *see* Tetracaine (Ophthalmic) *on page 1772*
◆ **Altace** *see* Ramipril *on page 1552*
◆ **Altachlore [OTC]** *see* Sodium Chloride *on page 1671*
◆ **Altamist Spray [OTC]** *see* Sodium Chloride *on page 1671*
◆ **Altarussin [OTC]** *see* GuaiFENesin *on page 860*
◆ **Altaryl [OTC]** *see* DiphenhydrAMINE (Systemic) *on page 561*
◆ **Altavera** *see* Ethinyl Estradiol and Levonorgestrel *on page 703*

Alteplase (AL te plase)

Brand Names: US Activase; Cathflo Activase
Brand Names: Canada Activase rt-PA; Cathflo Activase
Index Terms Alteplase, Recombinant; Alteplase, Tissue Plasminogen Activator, Recombinant; tPA
Pharmacologic Category Thrombolytic Agent
Use
Activase:
Acute ischemic stroke: Treatment of acute ischemic stroke (AIS)
Pulmonary embolism: Management of acute massive pulmonary embolism (PE)
ST-elevation myocardial infarction: Management of ST-elevation myocardial infarction (STEMI) for the lysis of thrombi in coronary arteries.
Limitations of use: The risk of stroke may outweigh the benefit produced by thrombolytic therapy in patients whose acute myocardial infarction (MI) puts them at low risk for death or heart failure.
Recommended criteria for treatment:
STEMI (ACCF/AHA [O'Gara 2013]): Ischemic symptoms within 12 hours of treatment or evidence of ongoing ischemia 12 to 24 hours after symptom onset with a large area of myocardium at risk or hemodynamic instability.
STEMI ECG definition: New ST-segment elevation at the J point in at least 2 contiguous leads of ≥2 mm (0.2 mV) in men or ≥1.5 mm (0.15 mV) in women in leads V_2-V_3 and/or of ≥1 mm (0.1 mV) in other contiguous precordial leads or limb leads. New or presumably new left bundle branch block (LBBB) may interfere with ST-elevation analysis and should not be considered diagnostic in isolation.
At non-PCI-capable hospitals, the ACCF/AHA recommends thrombolytic therapy administration when the anticipated first medical contact (FMC)-to-device time at a PCI-capable hospital is >120 minutes due to unavoidable delays.
AIS: Onset of stroke symptoms within 3 hours of treatment
Acute PE: Age ≤75 years: Documented massive PE (defined as acute PE with sustained hypotension [SBP <90 mm Hg for ≤15 minutes or requiring inotropic support], persistent profound bradycardia [HR <40 bpm with signs or symptoms of shock], or pulselessness); alteplase may be considered for submassive PE with clinical evidence of adverse prognosis (eg, new hemodynamic instability, worsening respiratory insufficiency, severe right ventricular (RV) dysfunction, or major myocardial necrosis) and low risk of bleeding complications. **Note:** Not recommended for patients with low-risk PE (eg, normotensive, no RV dysfunction, normal biomarkers) or submassive acute PE with minor RV dysfunction, minor myocardial necrosis, and no clinical worsening (AHA [Jaff 2011]).
Cathflo Activase: Restoration of function to central venous access device

Pregnancy Considerations Adverse events have been observed in animal reproduction studies. The risk of bleeding may be increased in pregnant women. Information related to alteplase use in pregnancy is limited (Leonhardt 2006; Li 2012) and most guidelines consider pregnancy to be a relative contraindication for its use (Jaff 2011; Jauch 2013; O'Gara 2013). Alteplase should not be withheld from pregnant women in life-threatening situations but should be avoided when safer alternatives are available (Bates 2012; Leonhardt 2006; Li 2012; Vanden Hoek 2010).

Breast-Feeding Considerations It is not known if alteplase is excreted in breast milk. The manufacturer recommends that caution be exercised when administering alteplase to nursing women.

Contraindications Hypersensitivity to alteplase or any component of the formulation

Treatment of STEMI or PE: Active internal bleeding; history of recent stroke; recent (within 3 months [ACCF/AHA: within 2 months]) intracranial or intraspinal surgery or serious head trauma; presence of intracranial conditions that may increase the risk of bleeding (eg, intracranial neoplasm, arteriovenous malformation, aneurysm); known bleeding diathesis; severe uncontrolled hypertension (ACCF/AHA: unresponsive to emergency therapy)

Additional contraindications according to the American Heart Association and American College of Cardiology Foundation (AHA [Jaff 2011]; ACCF/AHA [O'Gara 2013]): Active bleeding (excluding menses); any prior intracranial hemorrhage; suspected aortic dissection; ischemic stroke within 3 months **except** when within 4.5 hours; significant closed head or facial trauma within 3 months with radiographic evidence of bony fracture or brain injury

Treatment of AIS: Current intracranial hemorrhage; subarachnoid hemorrhage; active internal bleeding; recent (within 3 months) intracranial or intraspinal surgery or serious head trauma; presence of intracranial conditions that may increase the risk of bleeding (eg, intracranial neoplasm, arteriovenous malformation, aneurysm); known bleeding diathesis; severe uncontrolled hypertension

Additional contraindications according to the American Heart Association/American Stroke Association (AHA/ASA [Jauch 2013]): History of intracranial hemorrhage; suspicion of subarachnoid hemorrhage; stroke within 3 months; arterial puncture at a noncompressible site in previous 7 days; uncontrolled hypertension at time of treatment (eg, >185 mm Hg systolic or >110 mm Hg diastolic); multilobar cerebral infarction (hypodensity >$1/3$ cerebral hemisphere); known bleeding diathesis including but not limited to current use of oral anticoagulants with an INR >1.7 (or PT >15 seconds), current use of direct thrombin inhibitors or direct factor Xa inhibitors with elevated sensitive laboratory tests (eg, aPTT, INR, ECT, TT, or appropriate factor Xa activity assays) (see **"Note"**), administration of heparin within 48 hours preceding the onset of stroke with an elevated aPTT greater than the upper limit of normal, or platelet count <100,000/mm^3.

Note: The AHA/ASA guidelines do allow the use of alteplase in patients taking direct thrombin inhibitors (eg, dabigatran) or direct factor Xa inhibitors (eg, rivaroxaban) when sensitive laboratory tests (eg, aPTT, INR, ECT, TT, or appropriate direct factor Xa activity assays) are normal or the patient has not received a dose of these agents for >2 days (assuming normal renal function).

Additional exclusion criteria within clinical trials:

Presentation <3 hours after initial symptoms (NINDS, 1995): Time of symptom onset unknown, rapidly improving or minor symptoms, major surgery within 2 weeks, GI or urinary tract hemorrhage within 3 weeks, aggressive treatment required to lower blood pressure, glucose level <50 or >400 mg/dL, and lumbar puncture within 1 week.

Presentation 3 to 4.5 hours after initial symptoms (ECASS-III; Hacke 2008; AHA/ASA [Jauch 2013]): Age >80 years, time of symptom onset unknown, rapidly improving or minor symptoms, current use of oral anticoagulants regardless of INR, glucose level <50 or >400 mg/dL, aggressive intravenous treatment required to lower blood pressure, major surgery or severe trauma within 3 months, baseline National Institutes of Health Stroke Scale (NIHSS) score >25 [ie, severe stroke], and history of both stroke and diabetes.

Warnings/Precautions Internal bleeding (intracranial, retroperitoneal, gastrointestinal, genitourinary, respiratory) or external bleeding, especially at arterial and venous puncture, sites may occur (may be fatal). The total dose should not exceed 90 mg for acute ischemic stroke or 100 mg for acute myocardial infarction or pulmonary embolism. Doses ≥150 mg associated with significantly increased risk of intracranial hemorrhage compared to doses ≤100 mg. Bleeding risk is low. Monitor all potential bleeding sites; if serious bleeding occurs, the infusion of alteplase and any other concurrent anticoagulants (eg, heparin) should be stopped. Concurrent heparin anticoagulation may contribute to bleeding. In the treatment of acute ischemic stroke, concurrent use of anticoagulants was not permitted during the initial 24 hours of the <3 hour window trial (NINDS 1995). The AHA/ASA does not recommend initiation of anticoagulant therapy within 24 hours of treatment with alteplase (Jauch 2013). Initiation of SubQ heparin (≤10,000 units) or equivalent doses of low molecular weight heparin for prevention of DVT during the first 24 hours of the 3 to 4.5 hour window trial was permitted and did not increase the incidence of intracerebral hemorrhage (Hacke 2008). For acute PE, withhold heparin during the 2-hour infusion period. Intramuscular injections and nonessential handling of the patient should be avoided. Venipunctures should be performed carefully and only when necessary. Avoid internal jugular and subclavian venous punctures. If arterial puncture is necessary, use an upper extremity vessel that can be manually compressed. Avoid aspirin for 24 hours following administration of alteplase; administration within 24 hours increases the risk of hemorrhagic transformation.

For the following conditions, the risk of bleeding is higher with use of thrombolytics and should be weighed against the benefits of therapy: Recent major surgery or procedure (eg, CABG, obstetrical delivery, organ biopsy, previous puncture of noncompressible vessels), traumatic or prolonged (>10 minutes) CPR (ACCF/AHA [O'Gara 2013]), lumbar puncture within 10 days (ASRA [Horlocker 2012]), cerebrovascular disease, recent intracranial hemorrhage, recent gastrointestinal or genitourinary bleeding, recent trauma, hypertension (adults with systolic BP >175 mm Hg and/or diastolic BP >110 mm Hg), high likelihood of left heart thrombus (eg, mitral stenosis with atrial fibrillation), acute pericarditis, subacute bacterial endocarditis, hemostatic defects including ones caused by severe renal or hepatic dysfunction, significant hepatic dysfunction, advanced age, diabetic hemorrhagic retinopathy or other hemorrhagic ophthalmic conditions, septic thrombophlebitis or occluded AV cannula at seriously infected site and/or any other condition in which bleeding constitutes a significant hazard or would be particularly difficult to manage because of location. Use with caution in patients receiving oral anticoagulants. In the treatment of acute ischemic stroke (AIS) within 3 hours of symptom onset, the current use of oral anticoagulants is a contraindication per the manufacturer. According to the AHA/ASA, the current use of oral anticoagulants producing an INR >1.7, direct thrombin inhibitors, or direct factor Xa inhibitors with elevated sensitive laboratory tests are contraindications. However, alteplase may be administered to patients with AIS having received direct thrombin inhibitors (eg, dabigatran) or direct factor Xa inhibitors (eg, rivaroxaban) when sensitive laboratory tests (eg, aPTT, INR, platelet count, ECT, TT, or appropriate direct factor Xa activity assays) are normal or the patient has not received a dose of these agents for >2 days (assuming normal renal function). When treating AIS 3 to 4.5 hours after symptom onset, the use of alteplase should be avoided with current use of any oral anticoagulant regardless of INR (Jauch 2013). In the treatment of STEMI, adjunctive use of parenteral anticoagulants (eg, enoxaparin, heparin, or fondaparinux) is recommended to improve vessel patency and prevent reocclusion and may also contribute to bleeding; monitor for bleeding (ACCF/AHA; O'Gara 2013). Alteplase has not been shown to treat adequately underlying deep vein thrombosis in patients with PE. Consider the possible risk of re-embolization due to the lysis of underlying deep venous thrombi in this setting.

Coronary thrombolysis may result in reperfusion arrhythmias (eg, accelerated idioventricular rhythm) (Miller 1986). Patients who present **within 3 hours** of stroke symptom onset should be treated with alteplase unless contraindications exist. A longer time window (**3 to 4.5 hours** after symptom onset) has been shown to be safe and efficacious for select individuals (AHA/ASA [Jauch 2013]; Hacke 2008). Treatment of patients with minor neurological deficit or with rapidly improving symptoms is not recommended. Follow standard management for STEMI while infusing alteplase.

Cholesterol embolization has been reported rarely in patients treated with thrombolytic agents. Although typically mild and transient, orolingual angioedema has occurred during and up to 2 hours after alteplase infusion in patients treated for AIS and STEMI. The use of concomitant ACE inhibitors and strokes involving the insular and frontal cortex are associated with an increased risk (Foster-Goldman 2013). The manufacturer recommends monitoring patients during and for several hours after infusion for orolingual angioedema. If angioedema develops, discontinue the infusion and promptly institute appropriate therapy.

Cathflo Activase: When used to restore catheter function, use Cathflo cautiously in those patients with known or suspected catheter infections. Evaluate catheter for other causes of dysfunction before use. Avoid excessive pressure when instilling into catheter.

Some dosage forms may contain polysorbate 80 (also known as Tweens). Hypersensitivity reactions, usually a delayed reaction, have been reported following exposure to pharmaceutical products containing polysorbate 80 in certain individuals (Isaksson 2002; Lucente 2000; Shelley 1995). Thrombocytopenia, ascites, pulmonary deterioration, and renal and hepatic failure have been reported in premature neonates after receiving parenteral products containing polysorbate 80 (Alade 1986; CDC 1984). See manufacturer's labeling.

Adverse Reactions As with all drugs which may affect hemostasis, bleeding is the major adverse effect associated with alteplase. Hemorrhage may occur at virtually any site. Risk is dependent on multiple variables, including the dosage administered, concurrent use of multiple agents which alter hemostasis, and patient predisposition. Rapid lysis of coronary artery thrombi by thrombolytic agents may be associated with reperfusion-related atrial and/or ventricular arrhythmia. **Note:** Lowest rate of bleeding complications expected with dose used to restore catheter function.

1% to 10%:
Cardiovascular: Hypotension
Central nervous system: Fever
Dermatologic: Bruising (1%)
Gastrointestinal: GI hemorrhage (5%), nausea, vomiting
Genitourinary: GU hemorrhage (4%)
Hematologic: Bleeding (0.5% major, 7% minor: GUSTO trial)
Local: Bleeding at catheter puncture site (15.3%, accelerated administration)

<1% (Limited to important or life-threatening): Angioedema (orolingual), intracranial hemorrhage (0.4% to 0.87% when adult dose is ≤100 mg), retroperitoneal hemorrhage, pericardial hemorrhage, gingival hemorrhage, epistaxis, allergic reaction (anaphylaxis, anaphylactoid reactions, laryngeal edema, rash, and urticaria [<0.02%])
Additional cardiovascular events associated **with use in STEMI:** AV block, cardiogenic shock, heart failure, cardiac arrest, recurrent ischemia/infarction, myocardial rupture, electromechanical dissociation, pericardial effusion, pericarditis, mitral regurgitation, cardiac tamponade, thromboembolism, pulmonary edema, asystole, ventricular tachycardia, bradycardia, ruptured intracranial AV malformation, seizure, hemorrhagic bursitis, cholesterol crystal embolization
Additional events associated **with use in pulmonary embolism:** Pulmonary re-embolization, pulmonary edema, pleural effusion, thromboembolism
Additional events associated **with use in stroke:** Cerebral edema, cerebral herniation, seizure, new ischemic stroke

Drug Interactions
Metabolism/Transport Effects None known.
Avoid Concomitant Use There are no known interactions where it is recommended to avoid concomitant use.
Increased Effect/Toxicity
Alteplase may increase the levels/effects of: Anticoagulants; Dabigatran Etexilate; Prostacyclin Analogues

The levels/effects of Alteplase may be increased by: Agents with Antiplatelet Properties; Herbs (Anticoagulant/Antiplatelet Properties); Limaprost; Salicylates
Decreased Effect
The levels/effects of Alteplase may be decreased by: Aprotinin; Nitroglycerin
Preparation for Administration
Activase:
50 mg vial: Use accompanying diluent (50 mL vial of sterile water for injection); let stand undisturbed for several minutes to allow large bubbles to dissipate; mix by gentle swirling and/or slow inversion; do not shake. Vacuum is present in 50 mg vial. Final concentration: 1 mg/mL.
100 mg vial: Use transfer set with accompanying diluent (100 mL vial of sterile water for injection); let stand undisturbed for several minutes to allow large bubbles to dissipate; mix by gentle swirling; do not shake. No vacuum is present in 100 mg vial. Final concentration: 1 mg/mL.
Activase: ST-elevation MI: Accelerated infusion: Bolus dose may be prepared by one of three methods:
1) Removal of 15 mL reconstituted (1 mg/mL) solution from vial
2) Removal of 15 mL from a port on the infusion line after priming

3) Programming an infusion pump to deliver a 15 mL bolus at the initiation of infusion
Activase: Acute ischemic stroke: Bolus dose (10% of total dose) may be prepared by one of three methods:
1) Removal of the appropriate volume from reconstituted solution (1 mg/mL)
2) Removal of the appropriate volume from a port on the infusion line after priming
3) Programming an infusion pump to deliver the appropriate volume at the initiation of infusion
Cathflo Activase: Add 2.2 mL sterile water for injection to vial; let the vial stand undisturbed to allow large bubbles to dissipate. Mix by gently swirling until completely dissolved (complete dissolution should occur within 3 minutes); do not shake. Final concentration: 1 mg/mL.
Storage/Stability
Activase: Store intact vials at room temperature (not to exceed 30°C [86°F]), or under refrigeration at 2°C to 8°C (36°F to 46°F); protect from light. Store reconstituted solution at 2°C to 30°C (36°F to 86°F) and use within 8 hours. Discard any unused solution
Cathflo Activase: Store intact vials at 2°C to 8°C (36°F to 46°F); protect from light. Store reconstituted solution at 2°C to 30°C (36°F to 86°F) and use within 8 hours. Discard any unused solution.
Solutions of 0.5 mg/mL, 1 mg/mL, and 2 mg/mL in SWI retained ≥94% of fibrinolytic activity at 48 hours when stored at 2°C in plastic syringes; these solutions retained ≥90% of fibrinolytic activity when stored in plastic syringes at -25°C or -70°C for 7 or 14 days, thawed at room temperature and then stored at 2°C for 48 hours (Davis 2000). Solutions of 1 mg/mL in SWI were stable for 22 weeks in plastic syringes when stored at -30°C and for ~1 month in glass vials when stored at -20°C; bioactivity remained unchanged for 6 months in propylene containers when stored at -20°C and for 2 weeks in glass vials when stored at -70°C (Generali 2001).
Mechanism of Action Initiates local fibrinolysis by binding to fibrin in a thrombus (clot) and converts entrapped plasminogen to plasmin
Pharmacodynamics/Kinetics
Duration: >50% present in plasma cleared ~5 minutes after infusion terminated, ~80% cleared within 10 minutes; fibrinolytic activity persists for up to 1 hour after infusion terminated (Semba 2000)
Distribution: V_d (initial): Approximates plasma volume
Half-life elimination: Initial: 5 minutes
Excretion: Clearance (in patients with acute MI receiving accelerated regimen): Rapidly from circulating plasma (572 ± 132 mL/minute) (Tanswell 1992), primarily hepatic; >50% present in plasma is cleared within 5 minutes after the infusion is terminated, ~80% cleared within 10 minutes (Semba 2000)
Dosing
Adult & Geriatric
Acute ischemic stroke: Activase: IV: Within 3 hours of the onset of symptom onset (labeled use) **or** within 3 to 4.5 hours of symptom onset (off-label use; Hacke 2008; Jauch 2013): **Note:** Perform noncontrast-enhanced CT or MRI prior to administration. Initiation of anticoagulants (eg, heparin) or antiplatelet agents (eg, aspirin) within 24 hours after starting alteplase is not recommended; however, initiation of aspirin within 24 to 48 hours after stroke onset is recommended (Jauch 2013). Initiation of SubQ heparin (≤10,000 units) or equivalent doses of low molecular weight heparin for prevention of DVT during the first 24 hours of the 3 to 4.5 hour window trial did not increase incidence of intracerebral hemorrhage (Hacke 2008).
Recommended total dose: 0.9 mg/kg (maximum total dose: 90 mg)
Patients ≤100 kg: Load with 0.09 mg/kg (10% of 0.9 mg/kg dose) as an IV bolus over 1 minute, followed by 0.81 mg/kg (90% of 0.9 mg/kg dose) as a continuous infusion over 60 minutes.
Patients >100 kg: Load with 9 mg (10% of 90 mg) as an IV bolus over 1 minute, followed by 81 mg (90% of 90 mg) as a continuous infusion over 60 minutes.
Central venous catheter clearance: Cathflo Activase (1 mg/mL): Intracatheter:
Patients <30 kg: 110% of the internal lumen volume of the catheter, not to exceed 2 mg/2 mL; retain in catheter for 0.5 to 2 hours; may instill a second dose if catheter remains occluded
Patients ≥30 kg: 2 mg/2 mL; retain in catheter for 0.5 to 2 hours; may instill a second dose if catheter remains occluded
Pulmonary embolism (PE) (acute massive): Activase: IV: 100 mg over 2 hours; may be administered as a 10 mg bolus followed by 90 mg over 2 hours as was done in patients with submassive PE (Konstantinides 2002). Institute or resume parenteral anticoagulation

near the end of or immediately following the alteplase infusion when the partial thromboplastin time or thrombin time returns to twice normal or less. **Note:** Use in submassive PE is off-label.

ST-elevation myocardial infarction (STEMI): Activase: IV: **Note:** Manufacturer's labeling recommends 3-hour infusion regimen; however, accelerated regimen preferred by the ACCF/AHA (O'Gara 2013).

Accelerated regimen (weight-based):

Patients >67 kg: Total dose: 100 mg over 1.5 hours; administered as a 15 mg IV bolus over 1 to 2 minutes followed by infusions of 50 mg over 30 minutes, then 35 mg over 1 hour. Maximum total dose: 100 mg

Patients ≤67 kg: Infuse 15 mg IV bolus over 1 to 2 minutes followed by infusions of 0.75 mg/kg (not to exceed 50 mg) over 30 minutes then 0.5 mg/kg (not to exceed 35 mg) over 1 hour. Maximum total dose: 100 mg

Note: Thrombolytic should be administered within 30 minutes of hospital arrival. Generally, there is only a small trend for benefit of therapy after a delay of 12 to 24 hours from symptom onset, but thrombolysis may be considered for selected patients with ongoing ischemic pain and extensive ST elevation; however, primary PCI is preferred in these patients. Administer concurrent aspirin, clopidogrel, and anticoagulant therapy (ie, unfractionated heparin, enoxaparin, or fondaparinux) with alteplase (O'Gara 2013).

Acute peripheral arterial occlusion (off-label use): Intra-arterial:

Weight-based regimen: 0.001 to 0.02 mg/kg/hour (maximum dose: 2 mg/hour) (Semba 2000)

or

Fixed-dose regimen: 0.12 to 2 mg/hour (Semba 2000)

Note: The ACC/AHA guidelines state that thrombolysis is an effective and beneficial therapy for those with acute limb ischemia (Rutherford categories I and IIa) of <14 days duration (Hirsch 2006). The optimal dosage and concentration has not been established; a number of intra-arterial delivery techniques are employed with continuous infusion being the most common (Ouriel 2004). The Advisory Panel to the Society for Cardiovascular and Interventional Radiology on Thrombolytic Therapy recommends dosing of ≤2 mg/hour and concomitant administration of subtherapeutic heparin (aPTT 1.25 to 1.5 times baseline) (Semba 2000). Duration of alteplase infusion dependent upon size and location of the thrombus; typically between 6 to 48 hours (Disini 2008).

Frostbite (off-label use): Note: For use in patients with deep frostbite injury with potential significant morbidity (eg, extending proximally to the proximal interphalangeal joints of digits), without contraindications to the use of alteplase, who present within 24 hours of injury. Use of alteplase in the field is not recommended; administer treatment in a facility capable of intensive-care monitoring (WMS [McIntosh 2014]). Additional data may be necessary to further define the role of alteplase in the treatment of frostbite.

Intra-arterial: 2 to 4 mg bolus followed by a continuous intra-arterial infusion of 0.5 to 1 mg/hour (total dose if bilateral extremity involvement) via femoral or brachial artery; administer with continuous infusion heparin via an intra-arterial catheter. Discontinue alteplase if fibrinogen levels decrease to <150 mg/dL, if reperfusion is complete (as evidenced by angiography), or after a period of 48 hours whether or not reperfusion is achieved (Bruen 2007; Ibrahim 2015).

Parapneumonic effusions and empyema (off-label use): Intrapleural: 10 mg (diluted in 30 mL of normal saline) administered twice daily for a total of 3 days; each alteplase dose was followed >2 hours later by an intrapleural dornase alfa dose (with a 1-hour dwell time for each drug) (Rahman 2011). Some clinicians suggest consideration of fibrinolytic use in patients in whom treatment with at least 24 hours of chest tube drainage has failed and who are poor surgical candidates (Hamblin 2010). Dosing for this indication has not been established. Alteplase monotherapy dosing regimens have varied (range: 10 to 100 mg) and produced conflicting results in small trials and case series. These regimens have also included variations in chest tube sizes, number of doses, patient positions (still vs rotation), and clamping durations (Thommi 2007; Thommi 2012).

Prosthetic valve thrombosis, right-sided (any size thrombus) or left-sided (thrombus area <0.8 cm², recent onset [<14 days] of NYHA class I to II symptoms), or left-sided (thrombus area ≥0.8 cm²) when contraindications to surgery exist (off-label use) (ACCP [Guyatt 2012]; AHA/ACC [Nishimura 2014]; Alpert 2003; Roudaut 2003): IV:

High-dose regimen: Load with 10 mg, followed by 90 mg over 90 to 180 minutes (without heparin during infusion)

Low-dose regimen (preferred for very small adults): Load with 20 mg, followed by 10 mg/hour for 3 hours (without heparin during infusion)

Note: After successful administration of alteplase, heparin infusion should be introduced until warfarin achieves therapeutic INR (aortic: 3.0 to 4.0; mitral: 3.5 to 4.5) (Bonow 2008). The 2012 ACCP guidelines for antithrombotic therapy make no recommendation regarding INR range after prosthetic valve thrombosis.

Pulmonary embolism (PE) (submassive) (off-label use): Activase: IV: 100 mg over 2 hours; administered as a 10 mg bolus followed by 90 mg over 2 hours (Konstantinides 2002). Institute or resume parenteral anticoagulation near the end of or immediately following the alteplase infusion when the partial thromboplastin time or thrombin time returns to twice normal or less. **Note:** Not recommended for submassive PE with minor RV dysfunction, minor myocardial necrosis, and no clinical worsening or low-risk PE (ie, normotensive, no RV dysfunction, normal biomarkers) (AHA [Jaff 2011]).

Pediatric

Central venous catheter clearance: Intracatheter:

Patients <30 kg: 110% of the internal lumen volume of the catheter, not to exceed 2 mg/2 mL; retain in catheter for 0.5 to 2 hours; may instill a second dose if catheter remains occluded

Patients ≥30 kg: 2 mg/2 mL; retain in catheter for 0.5 to 2 hours; may instill a second dose if catheter remains occluded

Parapneumonic effusions and empyema (off-label use): Infants >3 months, Children, and Adolescents: Intrapleural: 4 mg (diluted in 40 mL of normal saline), with the first dose administered at time of chest tube placement (with a 1-hour dwell time); repeat every 24 hours for a total of 3 doses; or 0.1 mg/kg (maximum: 3 mg) (diluted in 10 to 30 mL of normal saline), with the first dose administered after pigtail catheter (chest tube) placement (45- to 60-minute dwell time) and repeat doses administered every 8 hours for 3 days (total of 9 doses) (Bradley 2011; Hawkins 2004; St Peter 2009). Dosing for this indication has not been established. Several intrapleural dosage regimens have been evaluated and have included variations in chest tube sizes, number of doses, patient positions (still vs rotation), and clamping durations.

Renal Impairment There are no dosage adjustments provided in the manufacturer's labeling. Plasma clearance is rapid and mediated primarily by the liver; therefore, degree of renal impairment is unlikely to influence elimination of alteplase. Hemostatic defects due to severe renal disease may increase the risk for bleeding.

Hepatic Impairment There are no dosage adjustments provided in the manufacturer's labeling. Plasma clearance is rapid and mediated primarily by the liver. Significant hepatic impairment and hemostatic defects due to severe hepatic disease may increase the risk for bleeding.

Usual Infusion Concentrations: Pediatric IV infusion: 0.5 mg/mL **or** 1 mg/mL

Usual Infusion Concentrations: Adult IV infusion: 1 mg/mL

Note: Concentrations for some indications (eg, peripheral arterial occlusion) may require further dilution (eg, 0.1 to 0.2 mg/mL [Chan 2001; Semba 2000]) and a usual concentration may not be established.

Administration

Activase: ST-elevation MI or acute ischemic stroke: Administer bolus dose (prepared by one of three methods) over 1 minute followed by infusion.

Infusion: Remaining dose for STEMI, AIS, or total dose for acute pulmonary embolism may be administered as follows: Any quantity of drug not to be administered to the patient must be removed from vial(s) prior to administration of remaining dose.

50 mg vial: Either PVC bag or glass vial and infusion set

100 mg vial: Insert spike end of the infusion set through the same puncture site created by transfer device and infuse from vial

If further dilution is desired, may be diluted in equal volume of 0.9% sodium chloride or D_5W to yield a final concentration of >0.5 mg/mL.

◀

Cathflo Activase: Intracatheter: Instill dose into occluded catheter. Do not force solution into catheter. After a 30-minute dwell time, assess catheter function by attempting to aspirate blood. If catheter is functional, aspirate 4 to 5 mL of blood in patients ≥10 kg or 3 mL in patients <10 kg to remove Cathflo Activase and residual clots. Gently irrigate the catheter with NS. If catheter remains nonfunctional, let Cathflo Activase dwell for another 90 minutes (total dwell time: 120 minutes) and reassess function. If catheter function is not restored, a second dose may be instilled.

Parapneumonic pleural effusions and empyemas (off-label use): Intrapleural: Instill dose into chest tube and clamp drain. Although the optimum dwell time has not been determined, clinical trials more often have used either a 45 minute (Hawkins 2004) or 1 hour (Rahman 2011; St. Peter 2009) dwell time; after dwell period, release clamp and connect chest tube to continuous suction.

Monitoring Parameters

Acute ischemic stroke (AIS): Baseline: Neurologic examination, head CT (without contrast), blood pressure, CBC, aPTT, PT/INR, glucose. During and after initiation: In addition to monitoring for bleeding complications, the 2013 AHA/ASA guidelines for the early management of AIS recommends the following:

Perform neurological assessments every 15 minutes during infusion and every 30 minutes thereafter for the next 6 hours, then hourly until 24 hours after treatment.

If severe headache, acute hypertension, nausea, or vomiting occurs, discontinue the infusion and obtain emergency CT scan.

Measure BP every 15 minutes for the first 2 hours of initiation then every 30 minutes for the next 6 hours, then hourly until 24 hours after initiation of alteplase. Increase frequency if a systolic BP is ≥180 mm Hg or if a diastolic BP is ≥105 mm Hg; administer antihypertensive medications to maintain BP at or below these levels.

Obtain a follow-up CT scan at 24 hours before starting anticoagulants or antiplatelet agents.

Central venous catheter clearance: Assess catheter function by attempting to aspirate blood.

Pulmonary embolism: Monitor BP and HR continually and for at least 24 hours after administration; assess invasive catheters hourly for bleeding (Smithburger 2013).

ST-elevation MI: Baseline: Blood pressure, serum cardiac biomarkers, CBC, PT/INR, aPTT. During and after initiation: Assess for evidence of cardiac reperfusion through resolution of chest pain, resolution of baseline ECG changes, preserved left ventricular function, cardiac enzyme washout phenomenon, and/or the appearance of reperfusion arrhythmias; assess for bleeding potential through clinical evidence of GI bleeding, hematuria, gingival bleeding, fibrinogen levels, fibrinogen degradation products, PT and aPTT.

Test Interactions Altered results of coagulation and fibrinolytic activity tests

Dosage Forms Excipient information presented when available (limited, particularly for generics); consult specific product labeling.

Solution Reconstituted, Injection:
Cathflo Activase: 2 mg (1 ea)
Solution Reconstituted, Intravenous:
Activase: 50 mg (1 ea); 100 mg (1 ea)

◆ Alteplase, Recombinant see Alteplase on page 80

◆ Alteplase, Tissue Plasminogen Activator, Recombinant see Alteplase on page 80

◆ Alti-Ipratropium (Can) see Ipratropium (Nasal) on page 978

◆ Alti-MPA (Can) see MedroxyPROGESTERone on page 1131

◆ Altoprev see Lovastatin on page 1110

Aluminum Hydroxide
(a LOO mi num hye DROKS ide)

Brand Names: US DermaMed [OTC]
Brand Names: Canada Amphojel; Basaljel
Pharmacologic Category Antacid; Antidote; Protectant, Topical
Use
Oral: Antacid: For the temporary relief of heartburn, acid indigestion, and sour stomach
Topical: Temporary protection and relief of chafed and abraded skin, minor burns and wounds, and skin irritations resulting from friction and rubbing.

Dosing
Adult & Geriatric
Antacid: 640 mg 5 to 6 times daily after meals and at bedtime (maximum: 3,840 mg in 24 hours)
Skin protectant: Topical: Apply to affected area as needed or as directed.
Hyperphosphatemia in chronic kidney disease (off-label use): Oral: Initial: 300 to 600 mg 3 times daily with meals. Note: The use of aluminum hydroxide should be reserved for serum phosphorus levels >7 mg/dL and limited to short-term use (4 weeks) given the toxicities associated with long-term use (NKF, 2003).
Pediatric
Skin protectant: Children and Adolescents: Topical: Refer to adult dosing.
Hyperphosphatemia in chronic kidney disease (off-label use): Adolescents: Oral: Initial: 300 to 600 mg 3 times daily with meals (Hudson, 2014). Note: The use of aluminum hydroxide should be reserved for serum phosphorus levels >7 mg/dL and limited to short-term use (4 to 6 weeks) given the toxicities associated with long-term use (NKF, 2005).
Renal Impairment Oral: Aluminum may accumulate in renal impairment.
Hepatic Impairment There are no dosage adjustments provided in the manufacturer's labeling.
Additional Information Complete prescribing information should be consulted for additional detail.
Dosage Forms Excipient information presented when available (limited, particularly for generics); consult specific product labeling. [DSC] = Discontinued product
Ointment, External:
DermaMed: (113 g)
Suspension, Oral:
Generic: 320 mg/5 mL (30 mL [DSC], 473 mL)

Aluminum Hydroxide and Magnesium Carbonate
(a LOO mi num hye DROKS ide & mag NEE zhum KAR bun nate)

Brand Names: US Acid Gone Extra Strength [OTC]; Acid Gone [OTC]; Gaviscon Extra Strength [OTC]; Gaviscon Liquid [OTC]
Index Terms Magnesium Carbonate and Aluminum Hydroxide
Pharmacologic Category Antacid
Use Antacid: Relief of heartburn, acid indigestion, sour stomach and GI upset associated with these symptoms
Dosing
Adult & Geriatric Antacid: Oral:
Chewable tablet: Acid Gone Extra Strength, Gaviscon Extra Strength (aluminum hydroxide 160 mg/magnesium carbonate 105 mg): Chew 2 to 4 tablets 4 times daily (maximum: 16 tablets per 24 hours)
Liquid:
Acid Gone, Gaviscon Regular Strength (aluminum hydroxide 31.7 mg/magnesium carbonate 119.3 mg per 5 mL): 15 to 30 mL 4 times daily (maximum: 120 mL per 24 hours)
Gaviscon Extra Strength (aluminum hydroxide 254 mg/magnesium carbonate 237.5 mg per 5 mL): 10 to 20 mL 4 times daily (maximum: 80 mL per 24 hours)
Pediatric Antacid: Oral: Children ≥12 years and Adolescents: Liquid: Acid Gone (aluminum hydroxide 31.7 mg/magnesium carbonate 119.3 mg per 5 mL): 15 to 30 mL 4 times daily (maximum: 120 mL per 24 hours)
Renal Impairment There are no dosage adjustments provided in the manufacturer's labeling; aluminum and/or magnesium may accumulate in renal impairment.
Hepatic Impairment
There are no dosage adjustments provided in the manufacturer's labeling.
Additional Information Complete prescribing information should be consulted for additional detail.
Dosage Forms Excipient information presented when available (limited, particularly for generics); consult specific product labeling.
Liquid:
Acid Gone: Aluminum hydroxide 31.7 mg and magnesium carbonate 119.3 mg per 5 mL (360 mL)
Gaviscon: Aluminum hydroxide 31.7 mg and magnesium carbonate 119.3 mg per 5 mL (355 mL) [contains sodium 0.57 mEq/5 mL and benzyl alcohol; cool mint flavor]
Gaviscon Extra Strength: Aluminum hydroxide 84.6 mg and magnesium carbonate 79.1 mg per 5 mL (355 mL) [contains sodium 0.9 mEq/5 mL and benzyl alcohol; cool mint flavor]

Tablet, chewable:

Acid Gone Extra Strength: Aluminum hydroxide 160 mg and magnesium carbonate 105 mg

Gaviscon Extra Strength: Aluminum hydroxide 160 mg and magnesium carbonate 105 mg [contains sodium 19 mg/tablet (1.3 mEq/tablet); cherry and original flavors]

Aluminum Hydroxide and Magnesium Hydroxide

(a LOO mi num hye DROKS ide & mag NEE zhum hye DROK side)

Brand Names: US Mag-Al [OTC]

Brand Names: Canada Diovol; Diovol Ex; Gelusil Extra Strength; Mylanta

Index Terms Magnesium Hydroxide and Aluminum Hydroxide

Pharmacologic Category Antacid

Use Antacid: Relief of heartburn, acid indigestion, sour stomach and GI upset associated with these symptoms

Dosing

Adult & Geriatric

Antacid: Oral: Liquid: Aluminum hydroxide 200 mg/magnesium hydroxide 200 mg per 5 mL: 10 to 20 mL 4 times daily (maximum: 80 mL per 24 hours)

Pediatric Antacid: Children ≥12 years and Adolescents: Refer to adult dosing.

Renal Impairment There are no dosage adjustments provided in the manufacturer's labeling; aluminum and/or magnesium may accumulate in renal impairment.

Hepatic Impairment There are no dosage adjustments provided in the manufacturer's labeling.

Additional Information Complete prescribing information should be consulted for additional detail.

Dosage Forms Excipient information presented when available (limited, particularly for generics); consult specific product labeling.

Liquid, oral:

Mag-Al: Aluminum hydroxide 200 mg and magnesium hydroxide 200 mg per 5 mL (30 mL) [dye free, ethanol free, sugar free; contains propylene glycol, sodium 4 mg/5 mL; peppermint flavor]

Aluminum Hydroxide and Magnesium Trisilicate

(a LOO mi num hye DROKS ide & mag NEE zhum trye SIL i kate)

Brand Names: US Gaviscon Tablet [OTC]

Index Terms Magnesium Trisilicate and Aluminum Hydroxide

Pharmacologic Category Antacid

Use Antacid: Temporary relief of heartburn and acid indigestion due to acid reflux

Dosing

Adult & Geriatric Antacid: Oral: Aluminum hydroxide 80 mg/magnesium trisilicate 14.2 mg: Chew 2 to 4 tablets 4 times daily (maximum: 16 tablets per 24 hours)

Renal Impairment There are no dosage adjustments provided in the manufacturer's labeling; aluminum and/or magnesium may accumulate in renal impairment.

Hepatic Impairment There are no dosage adjustments provided in the manufacturer's labeling

Additional Information Complete prescribing information should be consulted for additional detail.

Dosage Forms Excipient information presented when available (limited, particularly for generics); consult specific product labeling. [DSC] = Discontinued product

Tablet, chewable: Aluminum hydroxide 80 mg and magnesium trisilicate 20 mg

Gaviscon: Aluminum hydroxide 80 mg and magnesium trisilicate 20 mg [contains sodium 0.8 mEq/tablet; butterscotch flavor]

Aluminum Hydroxide, Magnesium Hydroxide, and Simethicone

(a LOO mi num hye DROKS ide, mag NEE zhum hye DROKS ide, & sye METH i kone)

Brand Names: US Alamag Plus [OTC]; Aldroxicon I [OTC]; Aldroxicon II [OTC]; Almacone Double Strength [OTC]; Almacone [OTC]; Gelusil [OTC]; Geri-Mox [OTC]; HyVee Advanced Antacid [OTC]; Maalox Advanced Maximum Strength [OTC]; Maalox Advanced Regular Strength [OTC]; Mi-Acid Maximum Strength [OTC] [DSC]; Mi-Acid [OTC]; Mintox Plus [OTC]; Mylanta Classic Maximum Strength Liquid [OTC]; Mylanta Classic Regular Strength Liquid [OTC]; Rulox [OTC]

Brand Names: Canada Diovol Plus; Gelusil; Mylanta Double Strength; Mylanta Extra Strength; Mylanta Regular Strength

Index Terms Magnesium Hydroxide, Aluminum Hydroxide, and Simethicone; Simethicone, Aluminum Hydroxide, and Magnesium Hydroxide

Pharmacologic Category Antacid; Antiflatulent

Use Antacid/antigas: Relief of acid indigestion, heartburn, sour stomach, or upset stomach and gas associated with these symptoms

Dosing

Adult & Geriatric

Antacid/antigas: Oral:

Products containing aluminum hydroxide 200 mg, magnesium hydroxide 200 mg, and simethicone 25 mg per tablet: 1 to 4 tablets 4 times daily; may also take as needed, up to 12 to 16 tablets in 24 hours

Products containing aluminum hydroxide 200 mg, magnesium hydroxide 200 mg, and simethicone 20 mg per 5 mL: 10 to 20 mL between meals, at bedtime, or as directed by health care provider; maximum: 80 to 120 mL in 24 hours

Products containing aluminum hydroxide 400 mg, magnesium hydroxide 400 mg, and simethicone 40 mg per 5 mL: 10 to 20 mL between meals, at bedtime, or as directed by health care provider; maximum: 40 to 60 mL in 24 hours

Pediatric Antacid/antigas: Children ≥12 years and Adolescents: Refer to adult dosing

Additional Information Complete prescribing information should be consulted for additional detail.

Dosage Forms Excipient information presented when available (limited, particularly for generics); consult specific product labeling. [DSC] = Discontinued product

Liquid, oral: Aluminum hydroxide 200 mg, magnesium hydroxide 200 mg, and simethicone 20 mg per 5 mL (360 mL); aluminum hydroxide 400 mg, magnesium hydroxide 400 mg, and simethicone 40 mg per 5 mL (360 mL)

Aldroxicon I: Aluminum hydroxide 200 mg, magnesium hydroxide 200 mg, and simethicone 20 mg per 5 mL (30 mL)

Aldroxicon II: Aluminum hydroxide 400 mg, magnesium hydroxide 400 mg, and simethicone 40 mg per 5 mL (30 mL)

Almacone: Aluminum hydroxide 200 mg, magnesium hydroxide 200 mg, and simethicone 20 mg per 5 mL (355 mL) [contains benzyl alcohol, ethanol <0.5%, magnesium 83 mg/5 mL]

Almacone Double Strength: Aluminum hydroxide 400 mg, magnesium hydroxide 400 mg, and simethicone 40 mg per 5 mL (360 mL)

Maalox Advanced Maximum Strength: Aluminum hydroxide 400 mg, magnesium hydroxide 400 mg, and simethicone 40 mg per 5 mL (355 mL, 769 mL [DSC]) [contains magnesium 167 mg/5 mL; cherry flavor]

Maalox Advanced Maximum Strength: Aluminum hydroxide 400 mg, magnesium hydroxide 400 mg, and simethicone 40 mg per 5 mL (355 mL, 769 mL) [contains magnesium 167 mg/5 mL; lemon flavor]

Maalox Advanced Maximum Strength: Aluminum hydroxide 400 mg, magnesium hydroxide 400 mg, and simethicone 40 mg per 5 mL (355 mL) [contains magnesium 167 mg/5 mL; mint flavor]

Maalox Advanced Maximum Strength: Aluminum hydroxide 400 mg, magnesium hydroxide 400 mg, and simethicone 40 mg per 5 mL (355 mL) [contains magnesium 167 mg/5 mL; vanilla crème flavor]

Maalox Advanced Regular Strength: Aluminum hydroxide 200 mg, magnesium hydroxide 200 mg, and simethicone 20 mg per 5 mL (360 mL, 780 mL) [contains magnesium 75 mg/5 mL, potassium 5 mg/5 mL, propylene glycol; mint flavor]

Mi-Acid: Aluminum hydroxide 200 mg, magnesium hydroxide 200 mg, and simethicone 20 mg per 5 mL (360 mL)

Mi-Acid Maximum Strength: Aluminum hydroxide 400 mg, magnesium hydroxide 400 mg, and simethicone 40 mg per 5 mL (360 mL)

Mylanta Classic Maximum Strength: Aluminum hydroxide 400 mg, magnesium hydroxide 400 mg, and simethicone 40 mg per 5 mL (360 mL, 720 mL) [original, cherry, orange creme, and mint flavors]

Mylanta Classic Regular Strength: Aluminum hydroxide 200 mg, magnesium hydroxide 200 mg, and simethicone 20 mg per 5 mL (360 mL) [original and mint flavors]

Suspension, oral: Aluminum hydroxide 225 mg, magnesium hydroxide 200 mg, and simethicone 25 mg per 5 mL (360 mL)

Geri-Mox: Aluminum hydroxide 200 mg, magnesium hydroxide 200 mg, and simethicone 25 mg per 5 mL (355 mL) [contains benzyl alcohol, magnesium 85 mg/5 mL; mint flavor]

HyVee Advanced Antacid: Aluminum hydroxide 400 mg, magnesium hydroxide 400 mg, and simethicone 40 mg per 5 mL (355 mL) [contains propylene glycol]

Rulox: Aluminum hydroxide 200 mg, magnesium hydroxide 200 mg, and simethicone 25 mg per 5 mL (355 mL) [contains magnesium 85 mg/5 mL; mint flavor]

Tablet, chewable: Aluminum hydroxide 200 mg, magnesium hydroxide 200 mg, and simethicone 25 mg

Alamag Plus: Aluminum hydroxide 200 mg, magnesium hydroxide 200 mg, and simethicone 25 mg [contains magnesium 83 mg/tablet, phenylalanine 2.6 mg/tablet; cherry flavor]

Almacone: Aluminum hydroxide 200 mg, magnesium hydroxide 200 mg, and simethicone 20 mg [dye free; contains magnesium 82 mg/tablet; peppermint flavor] [DSC]

Gelusil: Aluminum hydroxide 200 mg, magnesium hydroxide 200 mg, and simethicone 25 mg [peppermint flavor]

Mintox Plus: Aluminum hydroxide 200 mg, magnesium hydroxide 200 mg, and simethicone 25 mg [lemon crème flavor]

◆ Aluminum Sucrose Sulfate, Basic *see* Sucralfate *on page 1704*

◆ Alupent *see* Metaproterenol *on page 1156*

◆ Aluvea *see* Urea *on page 1853*

◆ Alvesco *see* Ciclesonide (Systemic) *on page 383*

Alvimopan (al VI moe pan)

Brand Names: US Entereg
Index Terms ADL-2698; LY246736
Pharmacologic Category Gastrointestinal Agent, Miscellaneous; Opioid Antagonist, Peripherally-Acting
Use Postoperative ileus: To accelerate the time to upper and lower GI recovery following surgeries including partial bowel resection with primary anastomosis
Pregnancy Considerations Adverse events have not been observed in animal reproduction studies.
Breast-Feeding Considerations It is not known if alvimopan is excreted in breast milk. The manufacturer recommends that caution be exercised when administering alvimopan to nursing women.
Prescribing and Access Restrictions As a requirement of the REMS program, access to this medication is restricted. Only hospitals enrolled in the ENTEREG Access Support and Education (E.A.S.E.™) Program may administer this medication. Hospital staff must be educated on the need to limit to short-term (no more than 15 doses) and inpatient use. Hospitals may contact the E.A.S.E.™ program at 1-800-278-0340.
Contraindications Patients who have taken therapeutic doses of opioids for more than 7 consecutive days immediately prior to alvimopan
Warnings/Precautions [U.S. Boxed Warning]: For short-term (≤15 doses) hospital use only. Only hospitals that have registered through the ENTEREG Access Support and Education (E.A.S.E.™) Program and met all requirements may use. It will not be dispensed to patients who have been discharged from the hospital. Use not recommended in patients with complete bowel obstruction or in patients having gastric or pancreatic anastomosis. Use with caution in patients with hepatic or renal impairment; use not recommended in patients with severe hepatic impairment or ESRD. Use with caution is patients recently exposed to opioids; may be more sensitive to gastrointestinal adverse effects (eg, abdominal pain, diarrhea, nausea and vomiting). Contraindicated in patients who have received therapeutic opioids for >7 consecutive days immediately prior to use. **[U.S. Boxed Warning]: A trend towards an increased incidence of MI was observed in alvimopan (low dose) treated patients compared to placebo in a 12-month study in patients treated with opioids for chronic pain. Other short-term studies have not observed this trend and a causal relationship has not been found.** MI was generally observed more frequently in the initial 1-4 months of treatment. Patients of Japanese descent should be monitored closely for gastrointestinal side effects (eg, abdominal pain, cramping, diarrhea) due to possibility of greater drug exposure; discontinue use if side effects occur.

Adverse Reactions Note: Incidence reported limited to bowel resection patients only.
1% to 10%:
Endocrine & metabolic: Hypokalemia (10%)
Gastrointestinal: Dyspepsia (2% to 7%)
Genitourinary: Urinary retention (3%)
Hematologic and oncologic: Anemia (5%)
Neuromuscular & skeletal: Back pain (3%)
Frequency not defined:
Cardiovascular: Myocardial infarction
Drug Interactions
Metabolism/Transport Effects None known.
Avoid Concomitant Use
Avoid concomitant use of Alvimopan with any of the following: Methylnaltrexone; Naloxegol
Increased Effect/Toxicity
Alvimopan may increase the levels/effects of: Naloxegol

The levels/effects of Alvimopan may be increased by: Analgesics (Opioid); Methylnaltrexone
Decreased Effect There are no known significant interactions involving a decrease in effect.
Food Interactions When administered with a high-fat meal, extent and rate of absorption may be reduced (C_{max} and AUC decreased by ~38% and 21%, respectively). Management: May administer with or without food.
Storage/Stability Store at 25°C (77°F); excursions permitted to 15°C to 30°C (59°F to 86°F).
Mechanism of Action An opioid receptor antagonist which blocks opioid binding at the mu receptor; alvimopan has restricted ability to cross the blood-brain barrier at therapeutic doses. It selectively and competitively binds to the GI tract mu opioid receptors and antagonizes the peripheral effects of opioids on gastrointestinal motility and secretion. Does not affect opioid analgesic effects or induce opioid withdrawal symptoms.
Pharmacodynamics/Kinetics
Distribution: V_d: 20-40 L
Protein binding: Parent drug: 80%; metabolite: 94% (both primarily to albumin)
Metabolism: Hydrolyzed to an amide hydrolysis compound (active metabolite) by gut microflora; further metabolism of active metabolite to glucuronide conjugates and other minor metabolites.
Bioavailability: ~6% (range: 1% to 19%)
Half-life elimination: 10-17 hours
Time to peak, plasma: Parent drug: ~2 hours; Metabolite: 36 hours
Excretion: Urine (~35% as unchanged drug and metabolites); feces (via biliary excretion)
Dosing
Adult & Geriatric Note: For hospital use only.
Management of postoperative ileus: Oral:
Initial: 12 mg administered 30 minutes to 5 hours prior to surgery
Maintenance: 12 mg twice daily beginning the day after surgery for a maximum of 7 days or until discharged from hospital (maximum total treatment: 15 doses)
Renal Impairment
Mild-to-severe impairment: No adjustment needed; use caution.
ESRD: Use not recommended.
Hepatic Impairment
Mild-to-moderate impairment (Child-Pugh class A or B): No adjustment needed; use caution.
Severe impairment (Child-Pugh class C): Use not recommended.
Dietary Considerations Take with or without food; high-fat meals may decrease the rate and extent of absorption
Administration Patient must be hospitalized. Initial dose should be administered 30 minutes to 5 hours prior to surgery. May be administered with or without food.
Dosage Forms Excipient information presented when available (limited, particularly for generics); consult specific product labeling.
Capsule, Oral:
Entereg: 12 mg

◆ ALX-0600 *see* Teduglutide *on page 1742*

◆ Alyacen 1/35 *see* Ethinyl Estradiol and Norethindrone *on page 708*

◆ Alyacen 7/7/7 *see* Ethinyl Estradiol and Norethindrone *on page 708*

◆ Alysena (Can) *see* Ethinyl Estradiol and Levonorgestrel *on page 703*

Amantadine (a MAN ta deen)

Brand Names: Canada Dom-Amantadine; Mylan-Amantadine; PHL-Amantadine; PMS-Amantadine

Index Terms Adamantanamine Hydrochloride; Amantadine Hydrochloride; Symmetrel

Pharmacologic Category Anti-Parkinson's Agent, Dopamine Agonist; Antiviral Agent; Antiviral Agent, Adamantane

Use

Drug-induced extrapyramidal reactions: Treatment of drug-induced extrapyramidal reactions.

Influenza A prophylaxis: Chemoprophylaxis against signs and symptoms of influenza A virus infection; also refer to current Advisory Committee on Immunization Practices (ACIP) guidelines for recommendations during current influenza season.

Influenza A treatment: Treatment of uncomplicated respiratory tract illness caused by influenza A virus strains; also refer to current ACIP guidelines for recommendations during current influenza season.

Parkinson disease: Treatment of idiopathic Parkinson disease (paralysis agitans), postencephalitic parkinsonism, parkinsonism in association with cerebral arteriosclerosis, and symptomatic parkinsonism, which may follow injury to the nervous system by carbon monoxide intoxication.

Pregnancy Considerations Adverse events have been observed in animal reproduction studies and teratogenic events have been observed in humans (case reports).

Untreated influenza infection is associated with an increased risk of adverse events to the fetus and an increased risk of complications or death to the mother. Other agents are currently recommended for the treatment or prophylaxis influenza in pregnant women and women up to 2 weeks postpartum. Appropriate antiviral agents are currently recommended as an adjunct to vaccination and should not be used as a substitute for vaccination in pregnant women (CDC 2011; CDC 2014).

Health care providers are encouraged to refer women exposed to influenza vaccine, or who have taken an antiviral medication during pregnancy to the Vaccines and Medications in Pregnancy Surveillance System (VAMPSS) by contacting The Organization of Teratology Information Specialists (OTIS) at (877) 311-8972

Breast-Feeding Considerations

Amantadine is excreted in breast milk. Breast-feeding is not recommended by the manufacturer.

Influenza may cause serious illness in postpartum women and prompt evaluation for febrile respiratory illnesses is recommended (Louie 2011).

Contraindications Hypersensitivity to amantadine or any component of the formulation

Warnings/Precautions May cause CNS depression, which may impair physical or mental abilities; patients must be cautioned about performing tasks that require mental alertness (eg, operating machinery or driving). There have been reports of suicidal ideation/attempt in patients with and without a history of psychiatric illness. Rarely, reversible elevations in transaminases have been reported. Use with caution in patients with hepatic impairment, a history of recurrent eczematoid dermatitis, uncontrolled psychosis or severe psychoneurosis, seizures, and in those receiving CNS stimulant drugs; reduce dose in renal impairment; when treating Parkinson disease, do not discontinue abruptly. In many patients, the therapeutic benefits of amantadine are limited to a few months. Abrupt discontinuation may cause agitation, anxiety, delirium, delusions, depression, hallucinations, paranoia, parkinsonian crisis, slurred speech, or stupor. Upon discontinuation of amantadine therapy, gradually taper dose. Elderly patients may be more susceptible to the CNS effects (using 2 divided daily doses may minimize this effect); may require dosage reductions. Use with caution in patients with heart failure, peripheral edema, or orthostatic hypotension; dosage reduction may be required. Avoid in untreated angle closure glaucoma. Potentially significant interactions may exist, requiring dose or frequency adjustment, additional monitoring, and/or selection of alternative therapy.

Dopamine agonists have been associated with compulsive behaviors and/or loss of impulse control, which has manifested as pathological gambling, libido increases (hypersexuality), and/or binge eating. Causality has not been established, and controversy exists as to whether this phenomenon is related to the underlying disease, prior behaviors/addictions, and/or drug therapy. Dose reduction or discontinuation of therapy has been reported to reverse these behaviors in some, but not all cases. Risk for melanoma development is increased in Parkinson disease patients; drug causation or factors contributing to risk have not been established. Patients should be monitored closely and periodic skin examinations should be performed.

Tolerance has also been reported with long-term use (Zubenko 1984).

Due to increased resistance, the ACIP has recommended that rimantadine and amantadine no longer be used for the treatment or prophylaxis of influenza A in the United States until susceptibility has been re-established; consult current guidelines (CDC 2011).

Some dosage forms may contain propylene glycol; large amounts are potentially toxic and have been associated hyperosmolality, lactic acidosis, seizures, and respiratory depression; use caution (AAP 1997; Zar 2007).

Adverse Reactions

1% to 10%:

Cardiovascular: Livedo reticularis, orthostatic hypotension, peripheral edema

Central nervous system: Abnormal dreams, agitation, anxiety, ataxia, confusion, delirium, depression, dizziness, drowsiness, fatigue, hallucination, headache, insomnia, irritability, nervousness

Gastrointestinal: Anorexia, constipation, diarrhea, nausea, xerostomia

Respiratory: Dry nose

<1% (Limited to important or life-threatening): Abnormal gait, acute respiratory tract failure, aggressive behavior, agranulocytosis, amnesia, anaphylaxis, cardiac arrest, cardiac arrhythmia, cardiac failure, coma, decreased libido, delusions, diaphoresis, dysphagia, dyspnea, eczema, EEG pattern changes, euphoria, fever, hyperkinesia, hypersensitivity reaction, hypertension, hypertonia, hypokinesia, hypotension, increased blood urea nitrogen, increased creatine phosphokinase, increased gamma-glutamyl transferase, increased lactate dehydrogenase, increased serum alkaline phosphatase, increased serum ALT, increased serum AST, increased serum bilirubin, increased serum creatinine, keratitis, leukocytosis, leukopenia, mania, muscle spasm, mydriasis, neuroleptic malignant syndrome (associated with dosage reduction or abrupt withdrawal of amantadine), neutropenia, oculogyric crisis, paranoia, paresthesia, pruritus, psychosis, pulmonary edema, seizure, skin photosensitivity, skin rash, slurred speech, stupor, suicidal ideation, suicide, suicide attempt, tachycardia, tachypnea, tremor, urinary retention, visual disturbance, vomiting, weakness

Drug Interactions

Metabolism/Transport Effects Substrate of OCT2

Avoid Concomitant Use

Avoid concomitant use of Amantadine with any of the following: Amisulpride

Increased Effect/Toxicity

Amantadine may increase the levels/effects of: BuPROPion; Glycopyrrolate; Glycopyrrolate (Systemic); Highest Risk QTc-Prolonging Agents; Memantine; Moderate Risk QTc-Prolonging Agents; Trimethoprim

The levels/effects of Amantadine may be increased by: Alcohol (Ethyl); BuPROPion; Methylphenidate; Mifepristone; Trimethoprim

Decreased Effect

Amantadine may decrease the levels/effects of: Amisulpride; Antipsychotic Agents (First Generation [Typical]); Influenza Virus Vaccine (Live/Attenuated)

The levels/effects of Amantadine may be decreased by: Amisulpride; Antipsychotic Agents (First Generation [Typical]); Antipsychotic Agents (Second Generation [Atypical]); Metoclopramide

Storage/Stability Store at 20°C to 25°C (68°F to 77°F); excursions permitted to 15°C to 30°C (59°F to 86°F). Protect capsules from moisture.

Mechanism of Action

Antiviral:

The mechanism of amantadine's antiviral activity has not been fully elucidated. It appears to primarily prevent the release of infectious viral nucleic acid into the host cell by interfering with the transmembrane domain of the viral M2 protein. Amantadine is also known to prevent viral assembly during replication. Amantadine inhibits the replication of influenza A virus isolates from each of the subtypes (ie, H1N1, H2N2 and H3N2), but has very little or no activity against influenza B virus isolates.

Parkinson disease:

The exact mechanism of amantadine in the treatment of Parkinson disease and drug-induced extrapyramidal reactions is not known. Data from early animal studies suggest that amantadine may have direct and indirect effects on dopamine neurons; however, recent studies have demonstrated that amantadine is a weak, noncompetitive NMDA receptor antagonist. Although amantadine has not been shown to possess direct anticholinergic activity, clinically, it exhibits

anticholinergic-like side effects (dry mouth, urinary retention, and constipation).

Pharmacodynamics/Kinetics

Onset of action: Antidyskinetic: Within 48 hours

Absorption: Well absorbed

Distribution: V_d: Normal: 3 to 8 L/kg; Renal failure: 5.1 ± 0.2 L/kg (Aoki 1988)

Protein binding: Normal renal function: ~67%; Hemodialysis: ~59% (Aoki 1988)

Metabolism: Not appreciable; small amounts of an acetyl metabolite identified

Bioavailability: 86% to 94% (Aoki 1988)

Half-life elimination: Normal renal function: 16 ± 6 hours (9 to 31 hours); Healthy, older (≥60 years) males: 29 hours (range: 20 to 41 hours) (Aoki 1988); End-stage renal disease: 8 days

Time to peak, plasma: 2 to 4 hours

Excretion: Urine (80% to 90% unchanged) by glomerular filtration and tubular secretion

Dosing

Adult

Influenza A treatment/prophylaxis: Note: Due to issues of resistance, amantadine is no longer recommended for the treatment or prophylaxis of influenza A (CDC 2011). Please refer to the current ACIP recommendations. The following is based on the manufacturer's labeling:

Influenza A treatment: Oral: 200 mg once daily **or** 100 mg twice daily (may be preferred to reduce CNS effects); **Note:** Initiate within 24 to 48 hours after onset of symptoms; continue for 24 to 48 hours after symptom resolution (duration of therapy is generally 5 days [CDC 2011]).

Influenza A prophylaxis: Oral: 200 mg once daily **or** 100 mg twice daily (may be preferred to reduce CNS effects). **Note:** Continue prophylaxis throughout the peak influenza activity in the community or throughout the entire influenza season in patients who cannot be vaccinated. Development of immunity following vaccination takes ~2 weeks; amantadine therapy should be considered for high-risk patients from the time of vaccination until immunity has developed.

Drug-induced extrapyramidal symptoms: Oral: 100 mg twice daily; may increase to 300 mg/day in divided doses, if needed

Parkinson's disease: Oral: Usual dose: 100 mg twice daily as monotherapy; may increase to 400 mg/day in divided doses, if needed, with close monitoring. **Note:** Patients with a serious concomitant illness or those receiving high doses of other anti-parkinson drugs should be started at 100 mg once daily; may increase to 100 mg twice daily, if needed, after one to several weeks.

Geriatric Patients ≥65 years: Adjust dose based on renal function; some patients tolerate the drug better when it is given in 2 divided daily doses (to avoid adverse neurologic reactions).

Influenza A treatment/prophylaxis: 100 mg once daily

Pediatric

Influenza A treatment/prophylaxis: Children and Adolescents: Oral: **Note:** Due to issues of resistance, amantadine is no longer recommended for the treatment or prophylaxis of influenza A (CDC 2011). Please refer to the current ACIP recommendations.

Influenza A treatment (CDC 2011):

1 to 9 years: 5 mg/kg/day in 2 divided doses (manufacturer's range: 4.4 to 8.8 mg/kg/day); maximum dose: 150 mg/day

≥10 years and <40 kg: 5 mg/kg/day in 2 divided doses

≥10 years and ≥40 kg: 100 mg twice daily

Note: Initiate within 24 to 48 hours after onset of symptoms; continue for 24 to 48 hours after symptom resolution (duration of therapy is generally 5 days)

Influenza A prophylaxis: Refer to "Influenza A treatment" dosing. **Note:** Continue prophylaxis throughout the peak influenza activity in the community or throughout the entire influenza season in patients who cannot be vaccinated. Development of immunity following vaccination takes ~2 weeks; amantadine therapy should be considered for high-risk patients from the time of vaccination until immunity has developed. For children <9 years receiving influenza vaccine for the first time, amantadine prophylaxis should continue for 6 weeks (4 weeks after the first dose and 2 weeks after the second dose).

Renal Impairment

CrCl 30 to 50 mL/minute: Administer 200 mg on day 1, then 100 mg/day

CrCl 15 to 29 mL/minute: Administer 200 mg on day 1, then 100 mg on alternate days

CrCl <15 mL/minute: Administer 200 mg every 7 days

Hemodialysis: Administer 200 mg every 7 days

Peritoneal dialysis: No supplemental dose is needed (Aronoff 2007)

Continuous renal replacement therapy: 100 mg once daily or every other day (Aronoff 2007)

Hepatic Impairment There are no dosage adjustments provided in the manufacturer's labeling; use with caution.

Monitoring Parameters Renal function, Parkinson's symptoms, mental status, influenza symptoms, blood pressure

Test Interactions May interfere with urine detection of amphetamines/methamphetamines (false-positive).

Dosage Forms Excipient information presented when available (limited, particularly for generics); consult specific product labeling.

Capsule, Oral, as hydrochloride:
Generic: 100 mg

Syrup, Oral, as hydrochloride:
Generic: 50 mg/5 mL (10 mL, 473 mL)

Tablet, Oral, as hydrochloride:
Generic: 100 mg

◆ Amantadine Hydrochloride *see* Amantadine *on page 86*

◆ Amaryl *see* Glimepiride *on page 842*

◆ Amatine (Can) *see* Midodrine *on page 1206*

◆ Ambi 10PEH/400GFN [OTC] *see* Guaifenesin and Phenylephrine *on page 862*

◆ AMBI 60PSE/400GFN/20DM *see* Guaifenesin, Pseudoephedrine, and Dextromethorphan *on page 864*

◆ Ambien *see* Zolpidem *on page 1940*

◆ Ambien CR *see* Zolpidem *on page 1940*

◆ Ambifed-G [OTC] *see* Guaifenesin and Pseudoephedrine *on page 863*

◆ AmBisome *see* Amphotericin B (Liposomal) *on page 119*

Ambrisentan (am bri SEN tan)

Brand Names: US Letairis

Brand Names: Canada Volibris

Index Terms BSF208075

Pharmacologic Category Endothelin Receptor Antagonist; Vasodilator

Use Pulmonary arterial hypertension: Treatment of pulmonary artery hypertension (PAH) (World Health Organization [WHO] Group I) to improve exercise ability and delay clinical worsening; in combination with tadalafil to reduce the risks of disease progression and hospitalization for worsening PAH, and to improve exercise ability. Studies establishing effectiveness included predominantly patients with WHO Functional Class II to III symptoms and etiologies of idiopathic or heritable PAH (60%) or PAH associated with connective tissue diseases (34%).

Note: According to treatment guidelines from the Fifth World Symposium on Pulmonary Hypertension (WSPH), only a small number of PAH patients with WHO-FC IV symptoms (ie, severely ill patients) were included in clinical trials, therefore, most experts consider ambrisentan second-line therapy in these patients (WSPH [Gailè 2013]).

Pregnancy Considerations [US Boxed Warning]: May cause birth defects; use in pregnancy is contraindicated. Exclude pregnancy prior to initiation of therapy and obtain pregnancy tests monthly during treatment and for 1 month after therapy is complete. Reliable contraception must be used during therapy and for 1 month after stopping treatment. Based on animal studies, ambrisentan is likely to produce major birth defects if used by pregnant women. Two reliable methods of contraception (eg, hormone method with a barrier method or 2 barrier methods) must be used throughout treatment and for 1 month after stopping treatment. Patients who have undergone a tubal ligation or the insertion of a contraceptive implant or intrauterine device (Copper T 380A or LNg 20) do not require additional contraceptive measures. A missed menses or suspected pregnancy should be reported to a healthcare provider and prompt immediate pregnancy testing. Sperm counts may be reduced in men during treatment (as observed with bosentan). In general, women with pulmonary hypertension should avoid pregnancy (Badesch, 2007; McLaughlin, 2009).

Breast-Feeding Considerations It is not known if ambrisentan is excreted in breast milk. Due to the potential for serious adverse reactions in the nursing infant, the US labeling recommends a decision be made whether to discontinue nursing or to discontinue the drug, taking into account the importance of treatment to the mother. The Canadian labeling contraindicates use in nursing women.

Prescribing and Access Restrictions As a requirement of the REMS program, access to this medication is restricted. Only prescribers and pharmacies registered with this program may prescribe and dispense ambrisentan. Further information may be obtained from the manufacturer, Gilead Sciences, Inc at www.letairisrems.com or 1-866-664-5327.

Medication Guide Available Yes

Contraindications

Pregnancy; idiopathic pulmonary fibrosis, including idiopathic pulmonary fibrosis with pulmonary hypertension (WHO Group 3)

Canadian labeling: Additional contraindications (not in US labeling): Hypersensitivity to ambrisentan or any component of the formulation; severe hepatic impairment (with or without cirrhosis); ALT or AST >3 times ULN at baseline; breast-feeding

Warnings/Precautions Hazardous agent - use appropriate precautions for handling and disposal (NIOSH 2014 [group 3]). **[US Boxed Warning]: May cause birth defects; use in pregnancy is contraindicated. Exclude pregnancy prior to initiation of therapy and obtain pregnancy tests monthly during treatment and for 1 month after therapy is complete. Reliable contraception must be used during therapy and for 1 month after stopping treatment.** Two reliable methods of contraception (eg, hormone method with a barrier method or 2 barrier methods) must be used throughout treatment and for 1 month after stopping treatment. Patients who have undergone a tubal ligation or the insertion of a contraceptive implant or intrauterine device (Copper T 380A or LNg 20) do not require additional contraceptive measures. A missed menses or suspected pregnancy should be reported to a healthcare provider and prompt immediate pregnancy testing. Women should also be educated on the appropriate use of emergency contraception if failure of contraceptive is known or suspected or in the event of unprotected sex.

[US Boxed Warning]: Because of the high likelihood of teratogenic effects, ambrisentan is only available through the Letairis REMS restricted distribution program. Female patients (regardless of reproductive potential), prescribers, and pharmacies must be registered with and meet conditions of the program. Call 1-866-664-5327 or visit www.letairisrems.com for more information.

Use caution in patients with low hemoglobin levels. May cause decreases in hemoglobin and hematocrit (monitoring of hemoglobin is recommended. Use not recommended in patients with clinically significant anemia. Development of peripheral edema due to treatment and/or disease state (pulmonary arterial hypertension) may occur; a higher incidence is seen in elderly patients. Sperm count may be reduced in men during treatment (as observed with bosentan). No changes in sperm function or hormone levels have been noted. Fertility issues may require discussion with patient. Increases in serum liver aminotransferases have been reported during postmarketing use; however, in the majority of the cases, alternative causes of hepatotoxicity could be identified. Perform liver enzyme testing when clinically indicated. Discontinue therapy if signs/symptoms of hepatic injury appear, if serum liver aminotransferases >5 times ULN (US labeling) or >3 times ULN (Canadian labeling) are observed, or if aminotransferases are increased in the presence of bilirubin >2 times ULN. Hepatotoxicity has been reported with other endothelin receptor antagonists (eg, bosentan); however, ambrisentan may be tried in patients that have experienced asymptomatic increases in liver enzymes caused by another endothelin receptor antagonist after the liver enzymes have returned to normal. Use caution in patients with mild hepatic impairment; US labeling does not recommend use in patients with moderate or severe impairment. The Canadian labeling recommends use with caution in moderate hepatic impairment and contraindicates use in severe hepatic impairment (with or without cirrhosis) and in patients with ALT or AST >3 times ULN at baseline. Development of peripheral edema due to treatment and/or disease state (pulmonary arterial hypertension) may occur; a higher incidence is seen with concomitant use of tadalafil and in elderly patients. There have also been postmarketing reports of fluid retention requiring treatment (eg, diuretics, fluid management, hospitalization). Further evaluation may be necessary to determine cause and appropriate treatment or discontinuation of therapy. Discontinue in any patient with pulmonary edema suggestive of pulmonary veno-occlusive disease (PVOD). Potentially significant drug-drug interactions may exist, requiring dose or frequency adjustment, additional monitoring, and/or selection of alternative therapy.

Adverse Reactions Frequency not always defined.

Cardiovascular: Peripheral edema (14% to 38%), flushing (4%)

Central nervous system: Headache (34%)

Gastrointestinal: Dyspepsia (3%)

Genitourinary: Oligospermia

Hematologic & oncologic: Decreased hemoglobin (7% to 10%; dose-dependent), anemia (7%), decreased hematocrit

Respiratory: Nasal congestion (6% to 16%), cough (13%), bronchitis (4%), sinusitis (3%)

<1% (Limited to important or life-threatening): Cardiac failure, dizziness, hypersensitivity, hypotension, increased liver enzymes, weakness

Drug Interactions

Metabolism/Transport Effects Substrate of CYP2C19 (minor), CYP3A4 (minor), P-glycoprotein, UGT1A3, UGT1A9, UGT2B7; **Note:** Assignment of Major/Minor substrate status based on clinically relevant drug interaction potential

Avoid Concomitant Use There are no known interactions where it is recommended to avoid concomitant use.

Increased Effect/Toxicity

The levels/effects of Ambrisentan may be increased by: CycloSPORINE (Systemic)

Decreased Effect There are no known significant interactions involving a decrease in effect.

Storage/Stability Store at 25°C (77°F); excursions are permitted between 15°C and 30°C (59°F and 86°F). Store in original packaging.

Mechanism of Action Blocks endothelin receptor subtypes ET_A and ET_B on vascular endothelium and smooth muscle. Stimulation of ET_A receptors, located primarily in pulmonary vascular smooth muscle cells is associated with vasoconstriction and cellular proliferation. Stimulation of ET_B receptors, located in both pulmonary vascular endothelial cells and smooth muscle cells is associated with vasodilation, antiproliferative effects, and endothelin clearance. Although ambrisentan blocks both ET_A and ET_B receptors, the affinity is greater for the ET_A receptor (>4,000-fold higher affinity).

Pharmacodynamics/Kinetics

Protein binding: 99%

Metabolism: Hepatic via CYP3A4, CYP2C19, and uridine 5'-diphosphate glucuronosyltransferases (UGTs) 1A9S, 2B7S, and 1A3S; *in vitro* studies also suggest it is a substrate of organic anion transporting polypeptides (OATP) 1B1 and 1B3 and P-glycoprotein (P-gp)

Half-life elimination: ~9 hours

Time to peak, plasma: ~2 hours

Excretion: Primarily nonrenal

Dosing

Adult & Geriatric

Pulmonary arterial hypertension: Oral: Initial: 5 mg once daily, with or without tadalafil; if tolerated, may increase at 4-week intervals to a maximum of 10 mg/day

Dosage adjustment for concomitant therapy: Coadministration with cyclosporine: Ambrisentan dose should not exceed 5 mg/day

Renal Impairment

US labeling:

Mild-to-moderate impairment: No dosage adjustment necessary.

Severe impairment: There are no dosage adjustments provided in the manufacturer's labeling (has not been studied).

Canadian labeling: No dosage adjustment necessary.

Hepatic Impairment

Preexisting impairment:

US labeling:

Mild impairment: There are no dosage adjustments provided in the manufacturer's labeling; exposure may be increased.

Moderate or severe impairment: Use not recommended.

Canadian labeling:

Mild or moderate impairment: There are no dosage adjustments provided in the manufacturer's labeling; use with caution and monitor closely.

Severe impairment: Use is contraindicated.

ALT or AST >3 times ULN at baseline: Use is contraindicated.

Impairment developing during therapy:

US labeling:

ALT or AST >5 times ULN: Discontinue therapy.

ALT or AST increased with signs/symptoms of hepatic injury or with bilirubin >2 times ULN: Discontinue therapy.

Canadian labeling:
ALT or AST >3 times ULN: Discontinue therapy.

ALT or AST increased with signs/symptoms of hepatic injury or with bilirubin >2 times ULN: Discontinue therapy.

May consider reinitiation after ALT or AST levels normalize and if there are no signs/symptoms of hepatic injury or jaundice.

Administration Oral: Swallow tablet whole. Do not split, crush, or chew tablets. Administer with or without food. Hazardous agent; use appropriate precautions for handling and disposal (NIOSH 2014 [group 3]).

Monitoring Parameters Monitor for significant peripheral edema and evaluate etiology if it occurs; hepatic enzyme testing when clinically appropriate. The Canadian labeling recommends hepatic function testing at baseline then as clinically indicated (all patients) and monthly during therapy (patients with moderate impairment or other risk factors [eg, significant right heart failure, preexisting hepatic disease or previously elevated transaminases, concurrent medications known to increase transaminases]).

A woman of childbearing potential must have a negative pregnancy test prior to the initiation of therapy, monthly during treatment, and 1 month after stopping treatment. Hemoglobin and hematocrit should be measured at baseline, at 1 month, and periodically thereafter (generally stabilizes after the first few weeks of treatment).

Dosage Forms Excipient information presented when available (limited, particularly for generics); consult specific product labeling.

Tablet, Oral:

Letairis: 5 mg, 10 mg [contains fd&c red #40 aluminum lake]

Dosage Forms: Canada

Excipient information presented when available (limited, particularly for generics); consult specific product labeling.

Tablet, Oral:

Volibris: 5 mg, 10 mg

◆ AMD3100 *see* Plerixafor *on page 1460*

◆ Amerge *see* Naratriptan *on page 1259*

◆ A-Methapred *see* MethylPREDNISolone *on page 1184*

◆ Amethia *see* Ethinyl Estradiol and Levonorgestrel *on page 703*

◆ Amethia Lo *see* Ethinyl Estradiol and Levonorgestrel *on page 703*

◆ Amethocaine Hydrochloride *see* Tetracaine (Ophthalmic) *on page 1772*

◆ Amethocaine Hydrochloride *see* Tetracaine (Systemic) *on page 1772*

◆ Amethocaine Hydrochloride *see* Tetracaine (Topical) *on page 1773*

◆ Amethopterin *see* Methotrexate *on page 1169*

◆ Amethyst *see* Ethinyl Estradiol and Levonorgestrel *on page 703*

◆ Ametop (Can) *see* Tetracaine (Topical) *on page 1773*

◆ Amfepramone *see* Diethylpropion *on page 546*

◆ AMG 073 *see* Cinacalcet *on page 387*

◆ AMG145 *see* Evolocumab *on page 725*

◆ AMG-162 *see* Denosumab *on page 515*

◆ AMG 531 *see* RomiPLOStim *on page 1615*

◆ Amicar *see* Aminocaproic Acid *on page 93*

◆ Amidate *see* Etomidate *on page 713*

Amifostine (am i FOS teen)

Brand Names: US Ethyol
Brand Names: Canada Ethyol
Index Terms Ethiofos; Gammaphos; WR-2721; YM-08310
Pharmacologic Category Antidote; Chemoprotective Agent
Use Reduce the incidence of moderate-to-severe xerostomia in patients undergoing postoperative radiation treatment for head and neck cancer, where the radiation port includes a substantial portion of the parotid glands; reduce the cumulative renal toxicity associated with repeated administration of cisplatin
Pregnancy Considerations Adverse events have been observed in animal reproduction studies.
Breast-Feeding Considerations It is not known if amifostine is excreted in breast milk. Due to the potential for adverse reactions in the nursing infant, the manufacturer recommends that breast-feeding should be discontinued during treatment.
Contraindications Hypersensitivity to aminothiol compounds or any component of the formulation

Warnings/Precautions Patients who are hypotensive or dehydrated should not receive amifostine. Interrupt antihypertensive therapy for 24 hours before treatment; patients who cannot safely stop their antihypertensives 24 hours before, should not receive amifostine. Adequately hydrated prior to treatment and keep in a supine position during infusion. Monitor blood pressure every 5 minutes during the infusion. If hypotension requiring interruption of therapy occurs, patients should be placed in the Trendelenburg position and given an infusion of normal saline using a separate IV line; subsequent infusions may require a dose reduction. Infusions >15 minutes are associated with a higher incidence of adverse effects. Use caution in patients with cardiovascular and cerebrovascular disease and any other patients in whom the adverse effects of hypotension may have serious adverse events.

Serious cutaneous reactions, including erythema multiforme, Stevens-Johnson syndrome, toxic epidermal necrolysis, toxoderma and exfoliative dermatitis have been reported with amifostine. May be delayed, developing up to weeks after treatment initiation. Cutaneous reactions have been reported more frequently when used as a radioprotectant. Discontinue treatment for severe/serious cutaneous reaction, or with fever. Withhold treatment and obtain dermatologic consultation for rash involving lips or mucosa (of unknown etiology outside of radiation port) and for bullous, edematous or erythematous lesions on hands, feet, or trunk; reinitiate only after careful evaluation.

Amifostine doses >300 mg/m^2 are associated with a moderate emetic potential (Dupuis, 2011). It is recommended that antiemetic medication, including dexamethasone 20 mg IV and a serotonin 5-HT$_3$ receptor antagonist be administered prior to and in conjunction with amifostine. Rare hypersensitivity reactions, including anaphylaxis and allergic reaction, have been reported; discontinue if allergic reaction occurs; do not rechallenge. Medications for the treatment of hypersensitivity reactions should be available.

Reports of clinically-relevant hypocalcemia are rare, but serum calcium levels should be monitored in patients at risk of hypocalcemia, such as those with nephrotic syndrome; may require calcium supplementation. Should not be used (in patients receiving chemotherapy for malignancies other than ovarian cancer) where chemotherapy is expected to provide significant survival benefit or in patients receiving definitive radiotherapy, unless within the context of a clinical trial.

Adverse Reactions

>10%:

Cardiovascular: Hypotension (15% to 61%; grades 3/4: 3% to 8%; dose dependent)

Gastrointestinal: Nausea/vomiting (53% to 96%; grades 3/4: 8% to 30%; dose dependent)

1% to 10%: Endocrine & metabolic: Hypocalcemia (clinically significant: 1%)

<1% (Limited to important or life-threatening): Apnea, anaphylactoid reactions, anaphylaxis, arrhythmia, atrial fibrillation, atrial flutter, back pain, bradycardia, cardiac arrest, chest pain, chest tightness, chills, cutaneous eruptions, dizziness, erythema multiforme, exfoliative dermatitis, extrasystoles, dyspnea, fever, flushing, hiccups, hypersensitivity reactions (fever, rash, hypoxia, dyspnea, laryngeal edema), hypertension (transient), hypoxia, malaise, MI, myocardial ischemia, pruritus, rash (mild), renal failure, respiratory arrest, rigors, seizure, sneezing, somnolence, Stevens-Johnson syndrome, supraventricular tachycardia, syncope, tachycardia, toxic epidermal necrolysis, toxoderma, urticaria

Drug Interactions

Metabolism/Transport Effects None known.

Avoid Concomitant Use There are no known interactions where it is recommended to avoid concomitant use.

Increased Effect/Toxicity

Amifostine may increase the levels/effects of: Antipsychotic Agents (Second Generation [Atypical]); DULOxetine

The levels/effects of Amifostine may be increased by: Alfuzosin; Barbiturates; Blood Pressure Lowering Agents; Brimonidine (Topical); Diazoxide; Herbs (Hypotensive Properties); Molsidomine; Nicorandil; Obinutuzumab; Pentoxifylline; Phosphodiesterase 5 Inhibitors; Prostacyclin Analogues

Decreased Effect There are no known significant interactions involving a decrease in effect.

Preparation for Administration For IV infusion, reconstitute intact vials with 9.7 mL 0.9% sodium chloride injection and dilute in 0.9% sodium chloride to a final concentration of 5-40 mg/mL. For SubQ administration, reconstitute with 2.5 mL NS or SWFI.

Storage/Stability Store intact vials of lyophilized powder at room temperature of 20°C to 25°C (68°F to 77°F). Reconstituted solutions (500 mg/10 mL) and solutions for infusion are chemically stable for up to 5 hours at room temperature (25°C) or up to 24 hours under refrigeration (2°C to 8°C).

Mechanism of Action Prodrug that is dephosphorylated by alkaline phosphatase in tissues to a pharmacologically-active free thiol metabolite. The free thiol is available to bind to, and detoxify, reactive metabolites of cisplatin; and can also act as a scavenger of free radicals that may be generated (by cisplatin or radiation therapy) in tissues.

Pharmacodynamics/Kinetics

Distribution: V_d: 3.5 L; unmetabolized prodrug is largely confined to the intravascular compartment; active metabolite is distributed into normal tissues with high concentrations in bone marrow, GI mucosa, skin, liver, and salivary glands

Protein binding: 4%

Metabolism: Hepatic dephosphorylation to two metabolites (active-free thiol and disulfide)

Half-life elimination: 9.3 minutes (Fouladi, 2001); Adults: ~8 to 9 minutes

Excretion: Urine (as metabolites)

Clearance, plasma: 2.17 L/minute

Dosing

Adult & Geriatric Note: Amifostine doses >300 mg/m² are associated with a moderate emetic potential. Antiemetic medication, including dexamethasone 20 mg IV and a serotonin 5-HT₃ receptor antagonist, is recommended prior to and in conjunction with amifostine.

Cisplatin-induced renal toxicity, reduction: IV: 910 mg/m² once daily over 15 minutes 30 minutes prior to cytotoxic therapy

For 910 mg/m² doses, the manufacturer suggests the following blood pressure-based adjustment schedule: *The infusion of amifostine should be interrupted if the systolic blood pressure decreases significantly from baseline, as defined below:*

Decrease of 20 mm Hg if baseline systolic blood pressure <100

Decrease of 25 mm Hg if baseline systolic blood pressure 100-119

Decrease of 30 mm Hg if baseline systolic blood pressure 120-139

Decrease of 40 mm Hg if baseline systolic blood pressure 140-179

Decrease of 50 mm Hg if baseline systolic blood pressure ≥180

If blood pressure returns to normal within 5 minutes (assisted by fluid administration and postural management) and the patient is asymptomatic, the infusion may be restarted so that the full dose of amifostine may be administered. If the full dose of amifostine cannot be administered, the dose of amifostine for subsequent cycles should be 740 mg/m².

Xerostomia from head and neck cancer, reduction:

IV: 200 mg/m² over 3 minutes once daily 15-30 minutes prior to radiation therapy **or**

SubQ (off-label route): 500 mg once daily prior to radiation therapy

Prevention of radiation proctitis in rectal cancer (off-label use): IV: 340 mg/m² once daily prior to radiation therapy (Keefe, 2007; Peterson, 2008)

Renal Impairment No dosage adjustment provided in manufacturer's labeling.

Hepatic Impairment No dosage adjustment provided in manufacturer's labeling.

Administration Amifostine doses >300 mg/m² are associated with a moderate emetic potential; antiemetics are recommended to prevent nausea/vomiting (Dupuis, 2011)

IV: Administer over 3 minutes (prior to radiation therapy) or 15 minutes (prior to cisplatin); administration as a longer infusion is associated with a higher incidence of side effects. Patients should be kept in supine position during infusion. **Note:** SubQ administration (off-label) has been used.

Monitoring Parameters Blood pressure should be monitored every 5 minutes during the infusion and after administration if clinically indicated; serum calcium levels (in patients at risk for hypocalcemia). Evaluate for cutaneous reactions prior to each dose.

Additional Information Oncology Comment: The American Society of Clinical Oncology (ASCO) guidelines for the use of protectants for chemotherapy and radiation (Hensley, 2008) recommend the use of amifostine for prevention of nephrotoxicity due to cisplatin-based chemotherapy and to decrease the incidence of acute and delayed radiation therapy-induced xerostomia. The ASCO guidelines do not recommend the use of amifostine to reduce the incidence of neutropenia or thrombocytopenia associated with chemotherapy or radiation therapy, neurotoxicity or ototoxicity associated with platinum-based chemotherapy, radiation therapy-induced mucositis associated with head and neck cancer, or esophagitis due to chemotherapy in patients with non-small cell lung cancer. Additionally, the guidelines do not support the use of amifostine in patients with head and neck cancer receiving concurrent platinum-based chemotherapy.

Dosage Forms Excipient information presented when available (limited, particularly for generics); consult specific product labeling.

Solution Reconstituted, Intravenous:

Ethyol: 500 mg (1 ea)

Generic: 500 mg (1 ea)

Solution Reconstituted, Intravenous [preservative free]:

Generic: 500 mg (1 ea)

Amikacin (am i KAY sin)

Brand Names: Canada Amikacin Sulfate Injection, USP; Amikin

Index Terms Amikacin Sulfate

Pharmacologic Category Antibiotic, Aminoglycoside

Use Treatment of serious infections (bone infections, respiratory tract infections, endocarditis, and septicemia) due to organisms resistant to gentamicin and tobramycin, including *Pseudomonas*, *Proteus*, *Serratia*, and other gram-negative bacilli; documented infection of mycobacterial organisms susceptible to amikacin

Pregnancy Considerations Adverse events were not observed in the initial animal reproduction studies. Amikacin crosses the placenta and produces detectable concentrations in the fetus. Aminoglycosides may cause fetal harm if administered to a pregnant woman. There are several reports of total irreversible bilateral congenital deafness in children whose mothers received another aminoglycoside (streptomycin) during pregnancy. Although serious side effects to the fetus/infant have not been reported following maternal use of all aminoglycosides, a potential for harm exists.

Due to pregnancy-induced physiologic changes, some pharmacokinetic parameters of amikacin may be altered (Bernard 1977).

Breast-Feeding Considerations Amikacin is excreted into breast milk (trace amounts) (Matsuda 1984). Due to the potential for serious adverse reactions in the nursing infant, the manufacturer recommends a decision be made whether to discontinue nursing or to discontinue the drug, taking into account the importance of treatment to the mother. As a class, aminoglycosides are expected to be poorly distributed into breast milk, limiting systemic exposure to a nursing infant. In general, modification of bowel flora may occur with any antibiotic exposure (Chung 2002).

Contraindications Hypersensitivity to amikacin sulfate or any component of the formulation; cross-sensitivity may exist with other aminoglycosides

Warnings/Precautions [US Boxed Warning]: Amikacin may cause neurotoxicity, nephrotoxicity, and/or neuromuscular blockade and respiratory paralysis; usual risk factors include preexisting renal impairment, concomitant neuro-/nephrotoxic medications, advanced age and dehydration. Dose and/or frequency of administration must be monitored and modified in patients with renal impairment. Drug should be discontinued if signs of ototoxicity, nephrotoxicity, or hypersensitivity occur. Ototoxicity is proportional to the amount of drug given and the duration of treatment. Tinnitus or vertigo may be indications of vestibular injury and impending bilateral irreversible damage. Renal damage is usually reversible. Use with caution in patients with neuromuscular disorders, hearing loss and hypocalcemia. Prolonged use may result in fungal or bacterial superinfection, including *C. difficile*-associated diarrhea (CDAD) and pseudomembranous colitis; CDAD has been observed >2 months postantibiotic treatment. Solution contains sodium metabisulfate; use caution in patients with sulfite allergy.

Adverse Reactions

1% to 10%:

Central nervous system: Neurotoxicity

Genitourinary: Nephrotoxicity

Otic: Auditory ototoxicity, vestibular ototoxicity

<1% (Limited to important or life-threatening): Dyspnea, eosinophilia, hypersensitivity reaction

Drug Interactions

Metabolism/Transport Effects None known.

Avoid Concomitant Use

Avoid concomitant use of Amikacin with any of the following: BCG (Intravesical); Foscarnet; Mannitol; Mannitol (Systemic); Mecamylamine

Increased Effect/Toxicity

Amikacin may increase the levels/effects of: AbobotulinumtoxinA; Bisphosphonate Derivatives; CARBOplatin; Colistimethate; CycloSPORINE (Systemic); Mecamylamine; Neuromuscular-Blocking Agents; OnabotulinumtoxinA; RimabotulinumtoxinB; Tenofovir Products

The levels/effects of Amikacin may be increased by: Amphotericin B; Capreomycin; Cefazedone; Cephalosporins (2nd Generation); Cephalosporins (3rd Generation); Cephalosporins (4th Generation); Cephradine; CISplatin; Foscarnet; Loop Diuretics; Mannitol; Mannitol (Systemic); Nonsteroidal Anti-Inflammatory Agents; Tenofovir Products; Vancomycin

Decreased Effect

Amikacin may decrease the levels/effects of: BCG (Intravesical); BCG Vaccine (Immunization); Sodium Picosulfate; Typhoid Vaccine

The levels/effects of Amikacin may be decreased by: Penicillins

Preparation for Administration Dilute in a compatible solution (eg, NS, D_5W) to a final concentration of 0.25-5 mg/mL.

Storage/Stability Store intact vials at 20°C to 25°C (68°F to 77°F). Following admixture at concentrations of 0.25-5 mg/mL, amikacin is stable for 24 hours at room temperature, 60 days at 4°C (39°F), or 30 days at -15°C (5°F). Previously refrigerated or thawed frozen solutions are stable for 24 hours when stored at 25°C (77°F).

Mechanism of Action Inhibits protein synthesis in susceptible bacteria by binding to 30S ribosomal subunits

Pharmacodynamics/Kinetics

Absorption:

IM: Rapid

Oral: Poorly absorbed

Distribution: V_d: 0.25 L/kg; primarily into extracellular fluid (highly hydrophilic); 12% of serum concentration penetrates into bronchial secretions; poor penetration into the blood-brain barrier even when meninges are inflamed; V_d is increased in neonates and patients with edema, ascites, fluid overload; Vd is decreased in patients with dehydration

Relative diffusion of antimicrobial agents from blood into CSF: Good only with inflammation (exceeds usual MICs)

CSF:blood level ratio: Normal meninges: 10% to 20%; Inflamed meninges: 15% to 24%

Protein-binding: 0% to 11%

Half-life elimination (renal function and age dependent):

Infants: Low birth weight (1 to 3 days): 7 to 9 hours; Full-term >7 days: 4 to 5 hours

Children: 1.6 to 2.5 hours

Adolescents: 1.5 ± 1 hour

Adults: Normal renal function: 1.4 to 2.3 hours; Anuria/end-stage renal disease: 28 to 86 hours

Time to peak, serum: IM: 45 to 120 minutes; IV: Within 30 minutes following a 30-minute infusion

Excretion: Urine (94% to 98%); excreted unchanged via glomerular filtration within 24 hours

Dosing

Adult & Geriatric Individualization is critical because of the low therapeutic index

In underweight and nonobese patients, use of total body weight (TBW) instead of ideal body weight for determining the initial mg/kg/dose is widely accepted (Nicolau, 1995). Ideal body weight (IBW) also may be used to determine doses for patients who are neither underweight nor obese (Gilbert 2009).

Initial and periodic peak and trough plasma drug levels should be determined, particularly in critically-ill patients with serious infections or in disease states known to significantly alter aminoglycoside pharmacokinetics (eg, cystic fibrosis, burns, or major surgery). Manufacturer recommends a maximum daily dose of 15 mg/kg/day (or 1.5 g/day in heavier patients). Higher doses may be warranted based on therapeutic drug monitoring or susceptibility information.

Usual dosage range:

IM, IV: 5-7.5 mg/kg/dose every 8 hours; **Note:** Some clinicians suggest a daily dose of 15-20 mg/kg for all patients with normal renal function. This dose is at least as efficacious with similar, if not less, toxicity than conventional dosing.

Intrathecal/intraventricular (off-label route): Meningitis (susceptible gram-negative organisms): 5-50 mg/day

Indication-specific dosing:

Endophthalmitis, bacterial (off-label use): Intravitreal: 0.4 mg/0.1 mL NS in combination with vancomycin

Hospital-acquired pneumonia (HAP): IV: 20 mg/kg/day with antipseudomonal beta-lactam or carbapenem (American Thoracic Society/ATS guidelines)

Meningitis (susceptible gram-negative organisms): IV: 5 mg/kg every 8 hours (administered with another bactericidal drug)

Intrathecal/intraventricular (off-label route): Usual dose: 30 mg/day (IDSA 2004); Range: 5-50 mg/day (with concurrent systemic antimicrobial therapy) (Gilbert, 1986; Guardado 2008; IDSA 2004; Kasiakou 2005)

***Mycobacterium avium* complex (MAC) (off-label use):** IV: Adjunct therapy (with macrolide, rifamycin, and ethambutol): 8-25 mg/kg 2-3 times weekly for first 2-3 months for severe disease (maximum single dose for age >50 years: 500 mg) (Griffith 2007)

***Mycobacterium fortuitum*, M. chelonae, or M. abscessus:** IV: 10-15 mg/kg daily for at least 2 weeks with high dose cefoxitin

Pediatric Usual dosage range: Infants and Children: IM, IV: 5-7.5 mg/kg/dose every 8 hours

Note: Individualization is critical because of the low therapeutic index

Use of ideal body weight (IBW) for determining the mg/kg/dose appears to be more accurate than dosing on the basis of total body weight (TBW)

Initial and periodic peak and trough plasma drug levels should be determined, particularly in critically-ill patients with serious infections or in disease states known to significantly alter aminoglycoside pharmacokinetics (eg, cystic fibrosis, burns, or major surgery). Manufacturer recommends a maximum daily dose of 15 mg/kg/day (or 1.5 g/day in heavier patients). Higher doses may be warranted based on therapeutic drug monitoring or susceptibility information.

Renal Impairment Some patients may require larger or more frequent doses if serum levels document the need (ie, cystic fibrosis or febrile granulocytopenic patients).

CrCl ≥60 mL/minute: Administer every 8 hours

CrCl 40-60 mL/minute: Administer every 12 hours

CrCl 20-40 mL/minute: Administer every 24 hours

CrCl <20 mL/minute: Loading dose, then monitor levels

Intermittent hemodialysis (IHD) (administer after hemodialysis on dialysis days): Dialyzable (20%; variable; dependent on filter, duration, and type of HD): 5-7.5 mg/kg every 48-72 hours. Follow levels. Redose when pre-HD concentration <10 mg/L; redose when post-HD concentration <6-8 mg/L (Heintz 2009). **Note:** Dosing dependent on the assumption of 3 times/week, complete IHD sessions.

Peritoneal dialysis (PD): Dose as CrCl <20 mL/minute: Follow levels.

Continuous renal replacement therapy (CRRT) (Heintz 2009; Trotman 2005): Drug clearance is highly dependent on the method of renal replacement, filter type, and flow rate. Appropriate dosing should consider monitoring of pharmacologic response, signs of adverse reactions due to drug accumulation, as well as drug concentrations in relation to target trough (if appropriate). The following are general recommendations only (based on dialysate flow/ultrafiltration rates of 1-2 L/hour and minimal residual renal function) and should not supersede clinical judgment:

CVVH/CVVHD/CVVHDF: Loading dose of 10 mg/kg followed by maintenance dose of 7.5 mg/kg every 24-48 hours

Note: For severe gram-negative rod infections, target peak concentration of 15-30 mg/L; redose when concentration <10 mg/L (Heintz 2009).

Hepatic Impairment No dosage adjustment provided in manufacturer's labeling.

Obesity In moderate obesity (TBW/IBW ≥1.25) or greater, (eg, morbid obesity [TBW/IBW >2]), initial dosage requirement may be estimated using a dosing weight of IBW + 0.4 (TBW - IBW) (Traynor, 1995).

Dietary Considerations Some products may contain sodium.

Administration

IM: Administer IM injection in large muscle mass.

IV: Infuse over 30-60 minutes (children and adults) or over 1-2 hours (infants).

Some penicillins (eg, carbenicillin, ticarcillin, and piperacillin) have been shown to inactivate *in vitro*. This has been observed to a greater extent with tobramycin and gentamicin, while amikacin has shown greater stability against inactivation. Concurrent use of these agents may pose a risk of reduced antibacterial efficacy *in vivo*, particularly in the setting of profound renal impairment. However,

definitive clinical evidence is lacking. If combination penicillin/aminoglycoside therapy is desired in a patient with renal dysfunction, separation of doses (if feasible), and routine monitoring of aminoglycoside levels, CBC, and clinical response should be considered.

Intrathecal/Intraventricular (off-label route): Reserved solely for meningitis due to susceptible gram-negative organisms.

Monitoring Parameters Urinalysis, BUN, serum creatinine, appropriately timed peak and trough concentrations, vital signs, temperature, weight, I & O, hearing parameters Initial and periodic peak and trough plasma drug levels should be determined, particularly in critically-ill patients with serious infections or in disease states known to significantly alter aminoglycoside pharmacokinetics (eg, cystic fibrosis, burns, or major surgery). Aminoglycoside levels measured from blood taken from Silastic® central catheters can sometimes give falsely high readings (draw levels from alternate lumen or peripheral stick, if possible).

Some penicillin derivatives may accelerate the degradation of aminoglycosides in vitro. This may be clinically-significant for certain penicillin (ticarcillin, piperacillin, carbenicillin) and aminoglycoside (gentamicin, tobramycin) combination therapy in patients with significant renal impairment. Close monitoring of aminoglycoside levels is warranted.

Reference Range

Therapeutic levels:

Peak:

Life-threatening infections: 25-40 mcg/mL

Serious infections: 20-25 mcg/mL

Urinary tract infections: 15-20 mcg/mL

Trough: <8 mcg/mL

The American Thoracic Society (ATS) recommends trough levels of <4-5 mcg/mL for patients with hospital-acquired pneumonia.

Toxic concentration: Peak: >40 mcg/mL; Trough: >10 mcg/mL

Timing of serum samples: Draw peak 30 minutes after completion of 30-minute infusion or at 1 hour following initiation of infusion or IM injection; draw trough within 30 minutes prior to next dose

Test Interactions Some penicillin derivatives may accelerate the degradation of aminoglycosides in vitro, leading to a potential underestimation of aminoglycoside serum concentration.

Dosage Forms Excipient information presented when available (limited, particularly for generics); consult specific product labeling.

Solution, Injection, as sulfate:

Generic: 500 mg/2 mL (2 mL); 1 g/4 mL (4 mL)

Solution, Injection, as sulfate [preservative free]:

Generic: 1 g/4 mL (4 mL)

◆ Amikacin Sulfate see Amikacin on page 91

◆ Amikacin Sulfate Injection, USP (Can) see Amikacin on page 91

◆ Amikin (Can) see Amikacin on page 91

AMILoride (a MIL oh ride)

Brand Names: US Midamor [DSC]
Brand Names: Canada Midamor
Index Terms Amiloride HCl; Amiloride Hydrochloride; Midamor
Pharmacologic Category Antihypertensive; Diuretic, Potassium-Sparing
Use

Heart failure or hypertension: Counteracts potassium loss induced by other diuretics in the treatment of hypertension or heart failure; usually used in conjunction with more potent diuretics such as thiazides or loop diuretics

According to the Eighth Joint National Committee (JNC 8) guidelines, potassium-sparing diuretics are not recommended for the initial treatment of hypertension (James, 2013). The American Society of Hypertension/International Society of Hypertension (ASH/ISH) suggests that amiloride in combination with other diuretics (eg, hydrochlorothiazide) may be used to prevent hypokalemia associated with diuretics used to manage hypertension (Weber, 2014).

Dosing

Adult

Hypertension, heart failure (to limit potassium loss): Oral: Initial: 5 mg once daily; may increase to 10 mg daily if necessary; doses >10 mg daily are usually not necessary; however, if patient is persistently hypokalemic, the dose may be increased in increments of 5 mg daily up to 20 mg daily with careful monitoring of electrolytes.

Ascites (off-label use): Initial: 10 mg twice daily. If no response, increase every 4 days in increments of 10 mg twice daily to a maximum dosage of 30 mg twice daily (Angeli 1994). American Association for the Study of Liver Diseases (AASLD) guidelines recommend a dosage range of 10 to 40 mg daily (AASLD [Runyon 2012]; EASL 2010).

Geriatric Oral: Geriatric patients also show decreased clearance of amiloride: use with caution. Refer to adult dosing.

Pediatric Hypertension (off-label use): Children and Adolescents 1 to 17 years: Oral: 0.4 to 0.625 mg/kg/day (maximum: 20 mg daily) (NHBPEP 2004)

Renal Impairment

Manufacturer's labeling: Use of amiloride in patients with diabetes mellitus, SCr >1.5 mg/dL, or BUN >30 mg/dL should be done with caution and careful monitoring; use is contraindicated in patients with anuria, acute or chronic renal insufficiency, or evidence of diabetic nephropathy.

Alternate recommendations:

CrCl 10 to 50 mL/minute: Administer at 50% of normal dose (Aronoff 2007). The Beers Criteria recommends avoiding use in older adults ≥65 years of age with a CrCl <30 mL/minute due to the risk of hyperkalemia and hyponatremia (Beers Criteria [AGS 2015]).

CrCl <10 mL/minute: Avoid use (Aronoff 2007).

Hepatic Impairment There are no dosage adjustments provided in the manufacturer's labeling; use with caution.

Additional Information Complete prescribing information should be consulted for additional detail.

Dosage Forms Excipient information presented when available (limited, particularly for generics); consult specific product labeling. [DSC] = Discontinued product

Tablet, Oral, as hydrochloride:

Midamor: 5 mg [DSC]

Generic: 5 mg

◆ Amiloride HCl see AMILoride on page 93

◆ Amiloride Hydrochloride see AMILoride on page 93

◆ 2-Amino-6-Mercaptopurine see Thioguanine on page 1783

◆ 2-Amino-6-Methoxypurine Arabinoside see Nelarabine on page 1265

◆ 2-Amino-6-Trifluoromethoxy-benzothiazole see Riluzole on page 1588

◆ Aminobenzylpenicillin see Ampicillin on page 122

Aminocaproic Acid (a mee noe ka PROE ik AS id)

Brand Names: US Amicar
Index Terms EACA; Epsilon Aminocaproic Acid
Pharmacologic Category Antifibrinolytic Agent; Antihemophilic Agent; Hemostatic Agent; Lysine Analog
Use To enhance hemostasis when fibrinolysis contributes to bleeding (causes may include cardiac surgery, hematologic disorders, neoplastic disorders, abruptio placentae, hepatic cirrhosis, and urinary fibrinolysis)
Dosing

Adult & Geriatric

Acute bleeding: Oral, IV: Loading dose: 4-5 g during the first hour, followed by 1 g/hour for 8 hours (or 1.25 g/hour using oral solution) or until bleeding controlled (maximum daily dose: 30 g)

Control of bleeding with severe thrombocytopenia (off-label use) (Bartholomew, 1989; Gardner, 1980): Initial: IV: 100 mg/kg (maximum dose: 5 g) over 30-60 minutes

Maintenance: Oral, IV: 1-4 g every 4-8 hours or 1 g/hour (maximum daily dose: 24 g)

Control of oral bleeding in congenital and acquired coagulation disorder (off-label use): Oral: 50-60 mg/kg every 4 hours (Mannucci, 1998)

Prevention of dental procedure bleeding in patients on oral anticoagulant therapy (off-label use): Oral rinse: Hold 4 g/10 mL in mouth for 2 minutes then spit out. Repeat every 6 hours for 2 days after procedure (Souto, 1996). Concentration and frequency may vary by institution and product availability.

Prevention of perioperative bleeding associated with cardiac surgery (off-label use): IV: Loading dose of 75-150 mg/kg (typically 5-10 g), followed by 10-15 mg/kg/hour (typically 1 g/hour); may add 2-2.5 g/L of cardiopulmonary bypass circuit priming solution (Gravlee, 2008)

or

Loading dose of 10 g followed by 2 g/hour during surgery; no medication added to the bypass circuit (Fergusson, 2008)

or

10 g over 20-30 minutes prior to skin incision, followed by 10 g after heparin administration then 10 g at discontinuation of cardiopulmonary bypass (Vander Salm, 1996)

Traumatic hyphema (off-label use): Oral: 50 mg/kg/dose every 4 hours (maximum daily dose: 30 g) for 5 days (Brandt, 2001; Crouch, 1999)

Pediatric

Prevention of perioperative bleeding associated with cardiac surgery (off-label use): IV: 100 mg/kg given over 20-30 minutes after induction and prior to incision, 100 mg/kg during cardiopulmonary bypass, and 100 mg/kg after heparin reversal over 3 hours (Chauhan, 2004)

Prevention of bleeding associated with extracorporeal membrane oxygenation (ECMO) (off-label use): IV: 100 mg/kg prior to or immediately after cannulation, followed by 25-30 mg/kg/hour for up to 72 hours (Downard, 2003; Horwitz, 1998; Wilson, 1993)

Prevention of perioperative bleeding associated with spinal surgery (eg, idiopathic scoliosis) (off-label use): Children and Adolescents: IV: 100 mg/kg given over 15-20 minutes after induction, followed by 10 mg/kg/hour for the remainder of the surgery; discontinue at time of wound closure (Florentino-Pineda, 2001; Florentino-Pineda, 2004)

Traumatic hyphema (off-label use): Oral: Refer to adult dosing.

Renal Impairment May accumulate in patients with decreased renal function. When used during cardiopulmonary bypass in anephric patients, a normal or slightly reduced loading dose and a continuous infusion rate of 5 mg/kg/hour has been recommended (Gravlee, 2008).

Hepatic Impairment No dosage adjustment provided in the manufacturer's labeling.

Additional Information Complete prescribing information should be consulted for additional detail.

Dosage Forms Excipient information presented when available (limited, particularly for generics); consult specific product labeling. [DSC] = Discontinued product

Solution, Intravenous:
Generic: 250 mg/mL (20 mL)

Solution, Oral:
Amicar: 25% (236.5 mL) [contains edetate disodium, methylparaben, propylparaben, saccharin sodium; raspberry flavor]

Syrup, Oral:
Amicar: 25% (473 mL) [raspberry flavor]
Generic: 25% (237 mL [DSC], 473 mL [DSC])

Tablet, Oral:
Amicar: 500 mg, 1000 mg [scored]
Generic: 500 mg [DSC], 1000 mg [DSC]

Aminolevulinic Acid (a MEE noh lev yoo lin ik AS id)

Brand Names: US Levulan Kerastick
Brand Names: Canada Levulan Kerastick
Index Terms 5-ALA; 5-Aminolevulinic Acid; ALA; Amino Levulinic Acid; Aminolevulinic Acid HCl; Aminolevulinic Acid Hydrochloride
Pharmacologic Category Photosensitizing Agent, Topical; Topical Skin Product
Use Actinic keratoses: Treatment of minimally to moderately thick actinic keratoses of the face or scalp; to be used in conjunction with blue light illumination
Dosing
Adult & Geriatric Note: Should only be applied by qualified medical personnel (not intended for application by patients).
Actinic keratoses: Topical: Apply to actinic keratoses (**not** perilesional skin) followed 14 to 18 hours later by blue light illumination. Application/treatment may be repeated at a treatment site (once) after 8 weeks.
Renal Impairment There are no dosage adjustments provided in the manufacturer's labeling.
Hepatic Impairment There are no dosage adjustments provided in the manufacturer's labeling.
Additional Information Complete prescribing information should be consulted for additional detail.

Dosage Forms Excipient information presented when available (limited, particularly for generics); consult specific product labeling.
Solution Reconstituted, External, as hydrochloride:
Levulan Kerastick: 20% (1 ea) [contains alcohol, usp, isopropyl alcohol, laureth, polyethylene glycol]

♦ Amino Levulinic Acid see Aminolevulinic Acid on page 94

♦ 5-Aminolevulinic Acid see Aminolevulinic Acid on page 94

♦ Aminolevulinic Acid HCl see Aminolevulinic Acid on page 94

♦ Aminolevulinic Acid Hydrochloride see Aminolevulinic Acid on page 94

♦ 4-aminopyridine see Dalfampridine on page 483

♦ 5-Aminosalicylic Acid see Mesalamine on page 1151

Amiodarone (a MEE oh da rone)

Brand Names: US Cordarone; Nexterone; Pacerone
Brand Names: Canada Amiodarone Hydrochloride For Injection; Apo-Amiodarone; Cordarone; Dom-Amiodarone; Mylan-Amiodarone; PHL-Amiodarone; PMS-Amiodarone; PRO-Amiodarone; Riva-Amiodarone; Sandoz-Amiodarone; Teva-Amiodarone
Index Terms Amiodarone Hydrochloride
Pharmacologic Category Antiarrhythmic Agent, Class III
Additional Appendix Information
Adult ACLS Algorithms on page 1993
Pediatric ALS (PALS) Algorithms on page 1990
Use Management of life-threatening recurrent ventricular fibrillation (VF) or recurrent hemodynamically-unstable ventricular tachycardia (VT) refractory to other antiarrhythmic agents or in patients intolerant of other agents used for these conditions
Pregnancy Considerations Adverse events have been observed in some animal reproduction studies. Amiodarone crosses the placenta (~10% to 50%) and may cause fetal harm when administered to a pregnant woman, leading to congenital goiter, hypo- or hyperthyroidism, neurodevelopmental, or neurological effects in the neonate. Growth retardation and premature birth have also been noted (ESG 2011). Amiodarone should be used in pregnant women only to treat arrhythmias that are life-threatening or refractory to other treatments (Blomström-Lundqvist 2003; ESG 2011).
Breast-Feeding Considerations Amiodarone and its active metabolite are excreted into human milk. Breast-feeding may lead to significant infant exposure and potential toxicity. Due to the long half-life, amiodarone may be present in breast milk for several days following discontinuation of maternal therapy (Hall 2003). The manufacturer recommends that breast-feeding be discontinued if treatment is needed.
Medication Guide Available Yes
Contraindications Hypersensitivity to amiodarone, iodine, or any component of the formulation; severe sinus-node dysfunction causing marked sinus bradycardia; second- and third-degree heart block (except in patients with a functioning artificial pacemaker); bradycardia causing syncope (except in patients with a functioning artificial pacemaker); cardiogenic shock
Warnings/Precautions Note: Although the US Boxed Warnings pertain to the tablet prescribing information, these effects may also be seen with intravenous administration depending on duration of use.

[US Boxed Warning (tablet)]: Only indicated for patients with life-threatening arrhythmias because of risk of substantial toxicity. Alternative therapies should be tried first before using amiodarone. Patients should be hospitalized when amiodarone is initiated. The 2015 ACLS guidelines recommend the consideration of IV amiodarone as the preferred antiarrhythmic for the treatment of pulseless VT/VF unresponsive to CPR, defibrillation, and vasopressor therapy (AHA [Link 2015]). In patients with non-life-threatening arrhythmias (eg, atrial fibrillation), amiodarone should be used only if the use of other antiarrhythmics has proven ineffective or are contraindicated.

[US Boxed Warning (tablet)]: Pulmonary toxicity (hypersensitivity pneumonitis or interstitial/alveolar pneumonitis and abnormal diffusion capacity without symptoms) may occur. Reports of acute-onset pulmonary injury (pulmonary infiltrates and/or mass on X-ray, pulmonary alveolar hemorrhage, pleural effusion, pulmonary fibrosis, bronchospasm, wheezing, fever, dyspnea, cough, hemoptysis, hypoxia) have occurred; some cases have progressed to respiratory failure and/or death.

Fatalities due to pulmonary toxicity occur in ~10% of cases; most fatalities due to sudden cardiac death occurred when amiodarone was discontinued; rule out other causes of respiratory impairment before discontinuing amiodarone in patients with life-threatening arrhythmias; use extreme caution if dose is decreased or discontinued. If hypersensitivity pneumonitis occurs, discontinue amiodarone and institute steroid therapy; if interstitial/alveolar pneumonitis occurs, institute steroid therapy and reduce amiodarone dose or preferably, discontinue. Some cases of interstitial/alveolar pneumonitis may resolve following dosage reduction and steroid therapy; rechallenge at a lower dose has not resulted in return of interstitial/alveolar pneumonitis in some patients; however, in some patients the pulmonary lesions have not been reversible. Educate patients about monitoring for symptoms (eg, nonproductive cough, dyspnea, pleuritic pain, hemoptysis, wheezing, weight loss, fever, malaise). Evaluate new respiratory symptoms; preexisting pulmonary disease does not increase risk of developing pulmonary toxicity, but if pulmonary toxicity develops then the prognosis is worse. Use of lower doses may be associated with a decreased incidence, but pulmonary toxicity has been reported in patients treated with low doses. The lowest effective dose should be used as appropriate for the acuity/severity of the arrhythmia being treated. **[US Boxed Warning (tablet)]: Liver toxicity is common, but usually mild with evidence of only increased liver enzymes; severe liver toxicity can occur and has been fatal in a few cases.** Hepatic enzyme levels are frequently elevated in patients exposed to amiodarone; most cases are asymptomatic. If increases >3x ULN (or ≥2x baseline in patients with preexisting elevations), consider dose reduction or discontinuation. Monitor hepatic enzymes regularly in patients on relatively high maintenance doses. Elevated bilirubin levels have been reported have been reported in patients administered IV amiodarone.

[US Boxed Warning (tablet)]: Amiodarone can exacerbate arrhythmias, by making them more difficult to tolerate or reverse; other types of arrhythmias have occurred, including significant heart block, sinus bradycardia, new ventricular fibrillation, incessant ventricular tachycardia, increased resistance to cardioversion, and polymorphic ventricular tachycardia associated with QTc prolongation (torsades de pointes [TdP]). Risk may be increased with concomitant use of other antiarrhythmic agents or drugs that prolong the QTc interval. Proarrhythmic effects may be prolonged. Amiodarone should not be used in patients with Wolff-Parkinson-White (WPW) syndrome and preexcited atrial fibrillation/flutter since ventricular fibrillation may result (AHA/ACC/HRS [January 2014]).

Monitor pacing or defibrillation thresholds in patients with implantable cardiac devices (eg, pacemakers, defibrillators). May cause hyper- or hypothyroidism; hyperthyroidism may result in thyrotoxicosis (including fatalities) and/or the possibility of arrhythmia breakthrough or aggravation. If any new signs of arrhythmia appear, consider the possibility of hyperthyroidism. Hypothyroidism (sometimes severe) may be primary or subsequent to resolution of preceding amiodarone-induced hyperthyroidism; myxedema (may be fatal) has been reported. If hyper- or hypothyroidism occurs, reduce dose or discontinue amiodarone. Thyroid nodules and/or thyroid cancer have also been reported. Use caution in patients with thyroid disease; thyroid function should be monitored prior to treatment and periodically thereafter, particularly in the elderly and in patients with underlying thyroid dysfunction. In acute myocardial infarction, beta-blocker therapy should still be initiated even though concomitant amiodarone therapy provides beta-blockade.

Regular ophthalmic examination (including slit lamp and fundoscopy) is recommended. May cause optic neuropathy and/or optic neuritis resulting in visual impairment (peripheral vision loss, changes in acuity) at any time during therapy; permanent blindness has occurred. If symptoms of optic neuropathy and/or optic neuritis occur, prompt ophthalmic evaluation is recommended. If diagnosis of optic neuropathy and/or optic neuritis is confirmed, reevaluate amiodarone therapy. Corneal microdeposits occur in a majority of adults and may cause visual disturbances in up to 10% of patients (blurred vision, halos); asymptomatic microdeposits may be reversible and are not generally considered a reason to discontinue treatment. Corneal refractive laser surgery is generally contraindicated in amiodarone users (from manufacturers of surgical devices).

Peripheral neuropathy has been reported rarely with chronic administration; may resolve when amiodarone is discontinued, but resolution may be slow and incomplete.

Amiodarone is a potent inhibitor of CYP enzymes and transport proteins (including p-glycoprotein), which may lead to increased serum concentrations/toxicity of a number of medications. Particular caution must be used when a drug with QTc-prolonging potential relies on metabolism via these enzymes, since the effect of elevated concentrations may be additive with the effect of amiodarone. Carefully assess risk:benefit of coadministration of other drugs which may prolong QTc interval. Additional potentially significant interactions may exist, requiring dose or frequency adjustment, additional monitoring, and/or selection of alternative therapy. Patients may still be at risk for amiodarone-related adverse reactions or drug interactions after the drug has been discontinued. The pharmacokinetics are complex (due to prolonged duration of action and half-life) and difficult to predict. Correct electrolyte disturbances, especially hypokalemia, hypomagnesemia, or hypocalcemia, prior to use and throughout therapy. Use caution when initiating amiodarone in patients on warfarin. Cases of increased INR with or without bleeding have occurred in patients treated with warfarin; monitor INR closely after initiating amiodarone in these patients.

May cause hypotension and bradycardia (infusion-rate related). May cause life-threatening or fatal cutaneous reactions, including Stevens-Johnson syndrome and toxic epidermal necrolysis (TEN). If symptoms or signs (eg, progressive skin rash often with blisters or mucosal lesions) occur, immediately discontinue. During long-term treatment, a blue-gray discoloration of exposed skin may occur; risk increased in patients with fair complexion or excessive sun exposure; may be related to cumulative dose and duration of therapy. There has been limited experience in patients receiving IV amiodarone for >3 weeks. Some dosage forms may contain polysorbate 80 (also known as Tweens). Hypersensitivity reactions, usually a delayed reaction, have been reported following exposure to pharmaceutical products containing polysorbate 80 in certain individuals (Isaksson, 2002; Lucente, 2000; Shelley, 1995). Thrombocytopenia, ascites, pulmonary deterioration, and renal and hepatic failure have been reported in premature neonates after receiving parenteral products containing polysorbate 80 (Alade, 1986; CDC, 1984). See manufacturer's labeling.

Use caution and close perioperative monitoring in surgical patients; may enhance myocardial depressant and conduction effects of halogenated inhalational anesthetics; adult respiratory distress syndrome (ARDS) has been reported postoperatively (fatal in rare cases). Hypotension upon discontinuation of cardiopulmonary bypass during open-heart surgery have been reported (rare); relationship to amiodarone is unknown. Commercially-prepared premixed infusion contains the excipient cyclodextrin (sulfobutyl ether beta-cyclodextrin), which may accumulate in patients with renal insufficiency, although the clinical significance of this finding is uncertain (Luke, 2010).

Adverse Reactions Frequency not always defined.

Cardiovascular: Hypotension (IV: 16%, refractory in rare cases), bradycardia (2% to 5%), atrioventricular block (<2% to 5%), cardiac arrest (3%), cardiac arrhythmia (1% to 3%), cardiac failure (1% to 3%), ventricular tachycardia (2%), asystole (≤2%; IV), atrial fibrillation (<2%), cardiogenic shock (<2%), torsades de pointes (<2%, rare), ventricular fibrillation (<2%), atrioventricular dissociation, cardiac conduction disturbance, edema, flushing, peripheral thrombophlebitis (IV, with concentrations >3 mg/mL), pulseless electrical activity (PEA)

Central nervous system: Abnormal gait (4% to 40%), ataxia (4% to 40%), dizziness (4% to 40%), fatigue (4% to 40%), involuntary body movements (4% to 40%), malaise (4% to 40%), peripheral neuropathy (4% to 40%), memory impairment (3% to 40%), paresthesia (4% to 9%), altered sense of smell (1% to 3%), headache (1% to 3%), insomnia (1% to 3%), sleep disorder (1% to 3%)

Dermatologic: Blue-gray skin pigmentation (oral: ≤15% with prolonged exposure to amiodarone), skin photosensitivity (4% to 10%)

Endocrine & metabolic: Hypothyroidism (1% to 10%), decreased libido (1% to 3%), hyperthyroidism (1% to 3%)

Gastrointestinal: Nausea (oral: 10% to 33%; IV: 4%), vomiting (10% to 33%), anorexia (≤25%), constipation (≤25%), altered salivation (1% to 3%), dysgeusia (1% to 3%), abdominal pain (1% to 3%), diarrhea (<2%)

Hematologic & oncologic: Blood coagulation disorder (1% to 3%)

Hepatic: Increased serum transaminases (IV: <2% to 54%; oral: 3% to 9%), abnormal hepatic function tests (4% to 9%), hepatic disease (1% to 3%)

Neuromuscular & skeletal: Tremor (≤40%)

Ophthalmic: Corneal deposits (>90%; causes visual disturbance in <10%), visual halos (≤10%), visual disturbance (2% to 9%), optic neuritis (1%), photophobia

Respiratory: Pulmonary toxicity (2% to 17%), pulmonary edema (IV: <2%), hypersensitivity pneumonitis, interstitial pneumonitis, pulmonary fibrosis

Miscellaneous: Fever

<1% (Limited to important or life-threatening): Acute pancreatitis, acute renal failure, agranulocytosis, alopecia, anaphylactic shock, anaphylactoid reaction, anaphylaxis, aplastic anemia, bronchiolitis obliterans organizing pneumonia, bullous dermatitis, cholestatic hepatitis, cholestasis, delirium, demyelinating polyneuropathy, disorientation, DRESS syndrome, drug-induced Parkinson disease, eosinophilic pneumonia, epididymitis (noninfectious), erythema multiforme, exfoliation of skin, granuloma, hallucination, hemolytic anemia, hemoptysis, hepatic cirrhosis, hepatic failure, hepatitis, hepatotoxicity (idiosyncratic) (Chalasani 2014), hypoesthesia, hypotension, hypoxia, impotence, increased intracranial pressure, increased lactate dehydrogenase, increased serum alkaline phosphatase, increased serum creatinine, jaundice, leukocytoclastic vasculitis, malignant neoplasm of skin, mass (pulmonary), myopathy, optic neuropathy, pancytopenia, pleural effusion, pleurisy, pseudotumor cerebri, pulmonary alveolar hemorrhage, pulmonary infiltrates, pulmonary phospholipidosis, prolonged Q-T interval on ECG (associated with worsening of arrhythmia), renal insufficiency, respiratory arrest, respiratory failure, rhabdomyolysis, SIADH, sinoatrial arrest, skin carcinoma, skin granuloma, skin sclerosis, spontaneous ecchymosis, Stevens-Johnson syndrome, superior vena cava syndrome, thrombocytopenia, thyroid cancer, thyroid nodule, thyrotoxicosis, tissue necrosis at injection site, toxic epidermal necrolysis, vasculitis, vortex keratopathy (Chan 2015)

Drug Interactions

Metabolism/Transport Effects Substrate of CYP1A2 (minor), CYP2C19 (minor), CYP2C8 (major), CYP2D6 (minor), CYP3A4 (major), P-glycoprotein; **Note:** Assignment of Major/Minor substrate status based on clinically relevant drug interaction potential; **Inhibits** CYP1A2 (weak), CYP2A6 (moderate), CYP2B6 (weak), CYP2C19 (weak), CYP2C9 (moderate), CYP2D6 (moderate), CYP3A4 (weak), OCT2, P-glycoprotein

Avoid Concomitant Use

Avoid concomitant use of Amiodarone with any of the following: Agalsidase Alfa; Agalsidase Beta; Antiarrhythmic Agents (Class Ia); Artesunate; Azithromycin (Systemic); Bosutinib; Ceritinib; Conivaptan; Daclatasvir; Fingolimod; Fusidic Acid (Systemic); Grapefruit Juice; Highest Risk QTc-Prolonging Agents; Idelalisib; Indinavir; Ivabradine; Lopinavir; Mifepristone; Moderate Risk QTc-Prolonging Agents; Nelfinavir; PAZOPanib; Pimozide; Propafenone; Ritonavir; Saquinavir; Silodosin; Sofosbuvir; Tegafur; Thioridazine; Tipranavir; Topotecan; VinCRIStine (Liposomal)

Increased Effect/Toxicity

Amiodarone may increase the levels/effects of: Afatinib; Amifostine; Antiarrhythmic Agents (Class Ia); Antipsychotic Agents (Second Generation [Atypical]); Artesunate; Beta-Blockers; Bosentan; Bosutinib; Bradycardia-Causing Agents; Brentuximab Vedotin; Brexpiprazole; Cannabis; Cardiac Glycosides; Carvedilol; Ceritinib; Colchicine; CycloSPORINE (Systemic); CYP2A6 Substrates; CYP2C9 Substrates; CYP2D6 Substrates; Dabigatran Etexilate; DOXOrubicin (Conventional); Dronabinol; DULoxetine; Edoxaban; Everolimus; Fesoterodine; Flecainide; Flibanserin; Fosphenytoin; Highest Risk QTc-Prolonging Agents; HMG-CoA Reductase Inhibitors; Hydrocodone; Hypotension-Associated Agents; Lacosamide; Ledipasvir; Levodopa; Lidocaine (Systemic); Lidocaine (Topical); Lomitapide; Loratadine; Metoprolol; Mipomersen; Naloxegol; Nebivolol; NiMODipine; PAZOPanib; P-glycoprotein/ABCB1 Substrates; Phenytoin; Pimozide; Porfimer; Propafenone; Prucalopride; Rifaximin; Silodosin; Tetrahydrocannabinol; Thioridazine; TiZANidine; Topotecan; Verteporfin; VinCRIStine (Liposomal); Vitamin K Antagonists

The levels/effects of Amiodarone may be increased by: Abiraterone Acetate; Aprepitant; Atazanavir; Azithromycin (Systemic); Barbiturates; Blood Pressure Lowering Agents; Boceprevir; Bretylium; Brimonidine (Topical); Calcium Channel Blockers (Nondihydropyridine); Cimetidine; Cobicistat; Conivaptan; Cyclophosphamide; CYP2C8 Inhibitors (Moderate); CYP2C8 Inhibitors (Strong); CYP3A4 Inhibitors (Moderate); CYP3A4 Inhibitors (Strong); Daclatasvir; Darunavir; Deferasirox; Diazoxide; Fingolimod; Fosamprenavir; Fosaprepitant; Fosphenytoin; Fusidic Acid (Systemic); Grapefruit Juice; Herbs (Hypotensive Properties); Idelalisib; Indinavir; Ivabradine; Ivacaftor; Lidocaine (Topical); Lopinavir;

Luliconazole; Mifepristone; Moderate Risk QTc-Prolonging Agents; Molsidomine; Nelfinavir; Netupitant; Nicorandil; Obinutuzumab; Ombitasvir, Paritaprevir, and Ritonavir; Ombitasvir, Paritaprevir, Ritonavir, and Dasabuvir; Palbociclib; Pentoxifylline; P-glycoprotein/ABCB1 Inhibitors; Phosphodiesterase 5 Inhibitors; Prostacyclin Analogues; QTc-Prolonging Agents (Indeterminate Risk and Risk Modifying); Ritonavir; Ruxolitinib; Saquinavir; Simeprevir; Sofosbuvir; Stiripentol; Telaprevir; Tipranavir; Tofacitinib

Decreased Effect

Amiodarone may decrease the levels/effects of: Agalsidase Alfa; Agalsidase Beta; Artesunate; Clopidogrel; Codeine; Sodium Iodide I131; Tamoxifen; Tegafur; TraMADol

The levels/effects of Amiodarone may be decreased by: Bile Acid Sequestrants; Bosentan; CYP2C8 Inducers (Strong); CYP3A4 Inducers (Moderate); CYP3A4 Inducers (Strong); Dabrafenib; Deferasirox; Enzalutamide; Etravirine; Fosphenytoin; Grapefruit Juice; Mitotane; Orlistat; P-glycoprotein/ABCB1 Inducers; Phenytoin; Rifampin; Siltuximab; St Johns Wort; Tocilizumab

Food Interactions Food increases the rate and extent of absorption of amiodarone. Grapefruit juice increases bioavailability of oral amiodarone by 50% and decreases the conversion of amiodarone to N-DEA (active metabolite); altered effects are possible. Management: Take consistently with regard to meals; grapefruit juice should be avoided during therapy.

Storage/Stability

Tablets: Store at 20°C to 25°C (68°F to 77°F); protect from light.

Injection: Store undiluted vials and premixed solutions (Nexterone) at 20°C to 25°C (68°F to 77°F); excursions are permitted between 15°C and 30°C (59°F and 86°F). Protect from light during storage; protect from excessive heat. There is no need to protect solutions from light during administration. When vial contents are admixed in D_5W to a final concentration of 1-6 mg/mL, amiodarone is stable for 24 hours in glass or polyolefin bottles and for 2 hours in polyvinyl chloride (PVC) bags; do not use evacuated glass containers as buffer may cause precipitation. Nexterone is available as premixed solutions. Although amiodarone adsorbs to PVC tubing, all clinical studies used PVC tubing and the recommended doses account for adsorption; in adults, PVC tubing is recommended. Discard any unused portions of premixed solutions.

Mechanism of Action Class III antiarrhythmic agent which inhibits adrenergic stimulation (alpha- and beta-blocking properties), affects sodium, potassium, and calcium channels, prolongs the action potential and refractory period in myocardial tissue; decreases AV conduction and sinus node function

Pharmacodynamics/Kinetics

Onset of action: Oral: 2 days to 3 weeks; IV: (electrophysiologic effects) within hours; Antiarrhythmic effects: 2 to 3 days to 1 to 3 weeks; mean onset of effect may be shorter in children vs adults and in patients receiving IV loading doses

Peak effect: 1 week to 5 months

Duration after discontinuing therapy: Variable, 2 weeks to months: Children: less than a few weeks; Adults: Several months

Note: Duration after discontinuation may be shorter in children than adults

Absorption: Oral: Slow and variable

Distribution:

IV: Rapid redistribution with a decrease to 10% of peak values within 30 to 45 minutes after completion of infusion

IV single dose: V_{dss}: Mean range: 40 to 84 L/kg

Oral: V_d: 66 L/kg (range: 18 to 148 L/kg)

Protein binding: >96%

Metabolism: Hepatic via CYP2C8 and 3A4 to active N-desethylamiodarone metabolite; possible enterohepatic recirculation

Bioavailability: Oral: ~50% (range: 35% to 65%)

Half-life elimination: **Note:** Half-life is shortened in children vs adults

Amiodarone:

Single dose: 58 days (range: 15 to 142 days)

Oral chronic therapy: Mean range: 40 to 55 days (range: 26 to 107 days)

IV single dose: Mean range: 9 to 36 days

N-desethylamiodarone (active metabolite):

Single dose: 36 days (range 14 to 75 days)

Oral chronic therapy: 61 days

IV single dose: Mean range: 9 to 30 days

Time to peak, serum: Oral: 3 to 7 hours

Excretion: Feces; urine (<1% as unchanged drug)

Dosing

Adult Note: Lower loading and maintenance doses are preferable in women and all patients with low body weight.

Ventricular arrhythmias:

Prevention of recurrent life-threatening ventricular arrhythmias (eg, VF or hemodynamically unstable VT): Oral: 800 to 1600 mg daily in 1 to 2 doses for 1 to 3 weeks, then when adequate arrhythmia control is achieved, decrease to 600 to 800 mg daily in 1 to 2 doses for 1 month; maintenance: 400 mg daily

Pulseless VT or VF (ACLS 2010; ACLS 2015): IV push, I.O.: Initial: 300 mg rapid bolus; if pulseless VT or VF continues after subsequent defibrillation attempt or recurs, administer supplemental dose of 150 mg. **Note:** In this setting, administering **undiluted** is preferred (Dager 2006; Skrifvars 2004). *The Handbook of Emergency Cardiovascular Care* (Hazinski 2015) and the ACLS guidelines do not make any specific recommendations regarding dilution of amiodarone in this setting. Experience limited with I.O. administration of amiodarone. Maximum recommended total daily dose is 2.2 g (ACLS 2010).

Upon return of spontaneous circulation, follow with an infusion of 1 mg/minute for 6 hours, then 0.5 mg/minute for 18 hours (mean daily doses >2.1 g daily have been associated with hypotension).

Stable VT: IV: 150 mg over 10 minutes, then 1 mg/minute for 6 hours, followed by 0.5 mg/minute; continue this rate for at least 18 hours (total infusion duration: 24 hours) **or** until complete transition to oral (see **Recommendations for conversion to oral amiodarone after IV administration**).

Breakthrough stable VT: 150 mg supplemental doses in 100 mL D_5W or NS over 10 minutes (mean daily doses >2.1 g/day have been associated with hypotension)

Supraventricular arrhythmias:

Atrial fibrillation:

Pharmacologic cardioversion (off-label use):

Oral: 600 to 800 mg daily in divided doses until 10 g total, then 200 mg daily as maintenance (AHA/ACC/HRS [January 2014]). Although not supported by clinical evidence, a maintenance dose of 100 mg daily is commonly used especially for the elderly or patients with low body mass (Zimetbaum 2007). **Note:** Other regimens have been described and may be used clinically:

800 mg daily for 14 days, followed by 600 mg daily for the next 14 days, then 300 mg daily for the remainder of the first year, then 200 mg daily thereafter (Singh 2005)

or

10 mg/kg/day for 14 days, followed by 300 mg daily for 4 weeks, followed by maintenance dosage of 200 mg daily (Roy 2000)

IV: 150 mg over 10 minutes, then 1 mg/minute for 6 hours, then 0.5 mg/minute for 18 hours or change to oral maintenance dosing (eg, 100 to 200 mg once daily) (AHA/ACC/HRS [January 2014]).

Maintenance of sinus rhythm (off-label use): Oral: 400 to 600 mg daily in divided doses for 2 to 4 weeks followed by a maintenance dose of 100 to 200 mg once daily (AHA/ACC/HRS [January 2014])

Prevention of postoperative atrial fibrillation and atrial flutter associated with cardiothoracic surgery (off-label use): **Note:** A variety of regimens have been used in clinical trials, including oral and intravenous regimens:

Oral: 200 mg 3 times daily for 7 days prior to surgery, followed by 200 mg daily until hospital discharge (Daoud, 1997).

IV:

Preoperative regimen: 150 mg loading dose, followed by 0.4 mg/**kg**/hour (~0.5 mg/minute for a 70 kg patient) for 3 days prior to surgery and for 5 days postoperative (Lee 2000).

Postoperative regimen: Starting at postop recovery, 1000 mg infused over 24 hours for 2 days (Guarnieri, 1999).

Rate control (off-label use): IV: 300 mg over 1 hour, then 10 to 50 mg/hour over 24 hours followed by an oral maintenance dose; usual maintenance dose: 100 to 200 mg once daily. **Note:** Amiodarone requires a longer time to achieve rate control as compared to nondihydropyridine calcium channel blockers (eg, diltiazem) (7 hours vs 3 hours, respectively) (AHA/ACC/HRS [January 2014]).

Supraventricular tachycardia (eg, AVNRT, AVRT): Note: Amiodarone is an effective therapeutic option with a variety of potential uses in the management of supraventricular tachycardia; however, safety risks

limit its therapeutic use. In many cases, amiodarone is reserved for use in patients who have failed other therapies or who have structural heart disease, including left ventricular dysfunction. In general, most patients do not require chronic long-term treatment with antiarrhythmic therapy.

Pharmacologic cardioversion (off-label use):

Oral: 600 to 800 mg daily in divided doses until 10 g total, then may administer 200 mg daily as maintenance (ACC/AHA/ESC [Blomström-Lundqvist 2003]; AHA/ACC/HRS [January 2014]).

IV: 150 mg over 10 minutes, then 1 mg/minute for 6 hours, then 0.5 mg/minute for 18 hours or may change to oral dosing (ACC/AHA/ESC [Blomström-Lundqvist 2003]; AHA/ACC/HRS [January 2014]).

Recommendations for conversion to oral amiodarone after IV administration: Use the following as a guide:

<1-week IV infusion: 800 to 1600 mg daily

1- to 3-week IV infusion: 600 to 800 mg daily

>3-week IV infusion: 400 mg

Note: Conversion from IV to oral therapy has not been formally evaluated. Some experts recommend a 1 to 2 day overlap when converting from IV to oral therapy especially when treating ventricular arrhythmias.

Recommendations for conversion to intravenous amiodarone after oral administration: During long-term amiodarone therapy (ie, ≥4 months), the mean plasma-elimination half-life of the active metabolite of amiodarone is 61 days. Replacement therapy may not be necessary in such patients if oral therapy is discontinued for a period <2 weeks, since any changes in serum amiodarone concentrations during this period may **not** be clinically significant.

Geriatric Refer to adult dosing. No specific guidelines available. Dose selection should be cautious, at low end of dosage range, and titration should be slower to evaluate response. Although not supported by clinical evidence, a maintenance dose of 100 mg daily is commonly used especially for the elderly or patients with low body mass (Zimetbaum 2007).

Pediatric

Pulseless VT or VF (PALS dosing): Infants, Children, and Adolescents: IV, I.O.: 5 mg/kg (maximum: 300 mg per dose) rapid bolus; may repeat twice up to a maximum total dose of 15 mg/kg during acute treatment (PALS 2010).

Perfusing tachycardias (PALS dosing): Infants, Children, and Adolescents: IV, I.O.: Loading dose: 5 mg/kg (maximum: 300 mg per dose) over 20 to 60 minutes; may repeat twice up to maximum total dose of 15 mg/kg during acute treatment (PALS 2010).

Renal Impairment No dosage adjustment necessary.

Hemodialysis: Not dialyzable (0% to 5%); supplemental dose is not necessary

Peritoneal dialysis: Not dialyzable (0% to 5%); supplemental dose is not necessary

Hepatic Impairment Dosage adjustment is probably necessary in substantial hepatic impairment. No specific guidelines available. If hepatic enzymes exceed 3 times normal or double in a patient with an elevated baseline, consider decreasing the dose or discontinuing amiodarone.

Dietary Considerations Take consistently with regard to meals. Amiodarone is a potential source of large amounts of inorganic iodine; ~3 mg of inorganic iodine per 100 mg of amiodarone is released into the systemic circulation. Recommended daily allowance for iodine in adults is 150 mcg.

Grapefruit juice is not recommended.

Usual Infusion Concentrations: Pediatric Note: Premixed solutions available.

IV infusion: 1.8 mg/mL

Usual Infusion Concentrations: Adult Note: Premixed solutions available.

IV infusion: 450 mg in 250 mL (concentration: 1.8 mg/mL) of D_5W or NS

Administration

Oral: Administer consistently with regard to meals. Take in divided doses with meals if GI upset occurs or if taking large daily dose. If GI intolerance occurs with single-dose therapy, use twice daily dosing.

IV: For infusions >1 hour, use concentrations ≤2 mg/mL unless a central venous catheter is used; commercially-prepared premixed solutions in concentrations of 1.5 mg/mL and 1.8 mg/mL are available. Use only volumetric infusion pump; use of drop counting may lead to underdosage. Administer through an IV line located as centrally as possible. For continuous infusions, an in-line

filter has been recommended during administration to reduce the incidence of phlebitis. During pulseless VT/VF, administering **undiluted** is preferred (Dager 2006; Skrifvars 2004). *The Handbook of Emergency Cardiovascular Care* (Hazinski 2015) and the ACLS guidelines do not make any specific recommendations regarding dilution of amiodarone in this setting.

Adjust administration rate to urgency (give more slowly when perfusing arrhythmia present). Slow the infusion rate if hypotension or bradycardia develops. Infusions >2 hours must be administered in a non-PVC container (eg, glass or polyolefin). PVC tubing is recommended for administration regardless of infusion duration. **Incompatible** with heparin; flush with saline prior to and following infusion. **Note:** IV administration at lower flow rates (potentially associated with use in pediatrics) and higher concentrations than recommended may result in leaching of plasticizers (DEHP) from intravenous tubing. DEHP may adversely affect male reproductive tract development. Alternative means of dosing and administration (1 mg/kg aliquots) may need to be considered.

Monitoring Parameters Blood pressure, heart rate (ECG) and rhythm throughout therapy; assess patient for signs of lethargy, edema of the hands or feet, weight loss, and pulmonary toxicity (baseline pulmonary function tests and chest X-ray; continue monitoring chest X-ray annually during therapy); liver function tests (semiannually); monitor serum electrolytes, especially potassium and magnesium. Assess thyroid function tests before initiation of treatment and then periodically thereafter (some experts suggest every 3-6 months). If signs or symptoms of thyroid disease or arrhythmia breakthrough/exacerbation occur then immediate re-evaluation is necessary. Amiodarone partially inhibits the peripheral conversion of thyroxine (T_4) to triiodothyronine (T_3); serum T_4 and reverse triiodothyronine (rT_3) concentrations may be increased and serum T_3 may be decreased; most patients remain clinically euthyroid, however, clinical hypothyroidism or hyperthyroidism may occur.

Perform regular ophthalmic exams.

Patients with implantable cardiac devices: Monitor pacing or defibrillation thresholds with initiation of amiodarone and during treatment.

Consult individual institutional policies and procedures.

Reference Range Therapeutic: 0.5-2.5 mg/L (SI: 1-4 micromole/L) (parent); desethyl metabolite is active and is present in equal concentration to parent drug

Dosage Forms Considerations Vials for injection contain benzyl alcohol which has been associated with "gasping syndrome" in neonates. Commercially-prepared premixed solutions do not contain benzyl alcohol.

Dosage Forms Excipient information presented when available (limited, particularly for generics); consult specific product labeling.

Solution, Intravenous, as hydrochloride:
Nexterone: 150 mg/100 mL (100 mL); 360 mg/200 mL (200 mL)
Generic: 150 mg/3 mL (3 mL); 450 mg/9 mL (9 mL); 900 mg/18 mL (18 mL)
Tablet, Oral, as hydrochloride:
Cordarone: 200 mg [scored]
Pacerone: 100 mg
Pacerone: 200 mg [scored; contains fd&c red #40, fd&c yellow #6 (sunset yellow)]
Pacerone: 400 mg [scored; contains fd&c yellow #10 aluminum lake]
Generic: 100 mg, 200 mg, 400 mg

Extemporaneous Preparations A 5 mg/mL oral suspension may be made with tablets and either a 1:1 mixture of Ora-Sweet® and Ora-Plus® or a 1:1 mixture of Ora-Sweet® SF and Ora-Plus® adjusted to a pH between 6-7 using a sodium bicarbonate solution (5 g/100 mL of distilled water). Crush five 200 mg tablets in a mortar and reduce to a fine powder. Add small portions of the chosen vehicle and mix to a uniform paste; mix while adding the vehicle in incremental proportions to **almost** 200 mL; transfer to a calibrated bottle, rinse mortar with vehicle, and add quantity of vehicle sufficient to make 200 mL. Label "shake well" and "protect from light". Stable for 42 days at room temperature or 91 days refrigerated (preferred) (Nahata, 2004).

Nahata MC, Pai VB, and Hipple TF, *Pediatric Drug Formulations*, 5th ed, Cincinnati, OH: Harvey Whitney Books Co, 2004.

◆ Amiodarone Hydrochloride see Amiodarone on page 94

◆ Amiodarone Hydrochloride For Injection (Can) see Amiodarone on page 94

◆ Amitiza see Lubiprostone on page 1113

Amitriptyline (a mee TRIP ti leen)

Brand Names: Canada Apo-Amitriptyline; Bio-Amitriptyline; Elavil; Levate; Novo-Triptyn; PMS-Amitriptyline
Index Terms Amitriptyline Hydrochloride; Elavil
Pharmacologic Category Antidepressant, Tricyclic (Tertiary Amine)
Use Depression: Treatment of depression
Pregnancy Considerations Adverse events have been observed in some animal reproduction studies. Amitriptyline crosses the human placenta; CNS effects, limb deformities, and developmental delay have been noted in case reports (causal relationship not established). Tricyclic antidepressants may be associated with irritability, jitteriness, and convulsions (rare) in the neonate (Yonkers, 2009).

The ACOG recommends that therapy for depression during pregnancy be individualized; treatment should incorporate the clinical expertise of the mental health clinician, obstetrician, primary healthcare provider, and pediatrician (ACOG, 2008). According to the American Psychiatric Association (APA), the risks of medication treatment should be weighed against other treatment options and untreated depression. For women who discontinue antidepressant medications during pregnancy and who may be at high risk for postpartum depression, the medications can be restarted following delivery (APA, 2010). Treatment algorithms have been developed by the ACOG and the APA for the management of depression in women prior to conception and during pregnancy (Yonkers, 2009). Although not a first-line agent, amitriptyline may be used for the treatment of post-traumatic stress disorder in pregnant women (Bandelow, 2008). Migraine prophylaxis should be avoided during pregnancy; if needed, amitriptyline may be used if other agents are ineffective or contraindicated (Pringsheim, 2012).

Breast-Feeding Considerations Amitriptyline is excreted into breast milk. Based on information from six mother/infant pairs, following maternal use of amitriptyline 75-175 mg/day, the estimated exposure to the breast-feeding infant would be 0.2% to 1.9% of the weight-adjusted maternal dose. Adverse events have not been reported in nursing infants (four cases). Infants should be monitored for signs of adverse events; routine monitoring of infant serum concentrations is not recommended (Fortinguerra, 2009). Migraine prophylaxis should be avoided in women who are nursing; if needed, amitriptyline may be used if other agents are ineffective or contraindicated (Pringsheim, 2012). Due to the potential for serious adverse reactions in the nursing infant, the manufacturer recommends a decision be made whether to discontinue nursing or to discontinue the drug, taking into account the importance of treatment to the mother.

Medication Guide Available Yes
Contraindications Hypersensitivity to amitriptyline or any component of the formulation; coadministration with or within 14 days of MAOIs; coadministration with cisapride; acute recovery phase following myocardial infarction

Documentation of allergenic cross-reactivity for tricyclic antidepressants is limited. However, because of similarities in chemical structure and/or pharmacologic actions, the possibility of cross-sensitivity cannot be ruled out with certainty.

Warnings/Precautions [US Boxed Warning]: Antidepressants increase the risk of suicidal thinking and behavior in children, adolescents, and young adults (18-24 years of age) with major depressive disorder (MDD) and other psychiatric disorders; consider risk prior to prescribing. Short-term studies did not show an increased risk in patients >24 years of age and showed a decreased risk in patients ≥65 years. Closely monitor for clinical worsening, suicidality, or unusual changes in behavior, particularly during the initial 1-2 months of therapy or during periods of dosage adjustments (increases or decreases); the patient's family or caregiver should be instructed to closely observe the patient and communicate condition with health care provider. A medication guide should be dispensed with each prescription. **Amitriptyline is not FDA-approved for use in children.**

The possibility of a suicide attempt is inherent in major depression and may persist until remission occurs. Worsening depression and severe abrupt suicidality that are not part of the presenting symptoms may require discontinuation or modification of drug therapy. The patient's family or caregiver should be alerted to monitor patients for the emergence of suicidality and associated behaviors (such as agitation, irritability, hostility, impulsivity, and hypomania) and notify healthcare provider.

May precipitate a shift to mania or hypomania in patients with bipolar disorder. Patients presenting with depressive symptoms should be screened for bipolar disorder. **Amitriptyline is not FDA approved for bipolar depression.**

The degree of sedation, anticholinergic effects, orthostasis, and conduction abnormalities are high relative to other antidepressants. Heart block may be precipitated in patients with preexisting conduction system disease and use is relatively contraindicated in patients with conduction abnormalities. May cause CNS depression, which may impair physical or mental abilities; patients must be cautioned about performing tasks that require mental alertness (eg, operating machinery or driving). Use with caution in patients with a history of cardiovascular disease (including previous MI, stroke, tachycardia, or conduction abnormalities). Use with caution in patients with urinary retention, benign prostatic hyperplasia, increased intraocular pressure (IOP), narrow-angle glaucoma, xerostomia, visual problems, constipation, or a history of bowel obstruction.

TCAs may rarely cause bone marrow suppression; monitor for any signs of infection and obtain CBC if symptoms (eg, fever, sore throat) evident. May alter glucose control - use with caution in patients with diabetes. Recommended by the manufacturer to discontinue prior to elective surgery; risks exist for drug interactions with anesthesia and for cardiac arrhythmias. However, definitive drug interactions have not been widely reported in the literature and continuation of tricyclic antidepressants is generally recommended as long as precautions are taken to reduce the significance of any adverse events that may occur (Pass, 2004). May lower seizure threshold - use caution in patients with a previous seizure disorder or condition predisposing to seizures such as brain damage, alcoholism, or concurrent therapy with other drugs which lower the seizure threshold. May increase the risks associated with electroconvulsive therapy. Bone fractures have been associated with antidepressant treatment. Consider the possibility of a fragility fracture if an antidepressant-treated patient presents with unexplained bone pain, point tenderness, swelling, or bruising (Rabenda, 2013; Rizzoli, 2012). Use with caution in patients with hepatic or renal dysfunction. May cause mild pupillary dilation which in susceptible individuals can lead to an episode of narrow-angle glaucoma. Consider evaluating patients who have not had an iridectomy for narrow-angle glaucoma risk factors. Therapy is relatively contraindicated in patients with symptomatic hypotension.

Abrupt discontinuation or interruption of antidepressant therapy has been associated with a discontinuation syndrome. Symptoms arising may vary with antidepressant however commonly include nausea, vomiting, diarrhea, headaches, light-headedness, dizziness, diminished appetite, sweating, chills, tremors, paresthesias, fatigue, somnolence, and sleep disturbances (eg, vivid dreams, insomnia). Greater risks for developing a discontinuation syndrome have been associated with antidepressants with shorter half-lives, longer durations of treatment, and abrupt discontinuation. For antidepressants of short or intermediate half-lives, symptoms may emerge within 2-5 days after treatment discontinuation and last 7-14 days (APA, 2010; Fava, 2006; Haddad, 2001; Shelton, 2001; Warner, 2006).

Adverse Reactions Anticholinergic effects may be pronounced; moderate to marked sedation can occur (tolerance to these effects usually occurs).

Frequency not defined.

Cardiovascular: Atrioventricular conduction disturbance, cardiac arrhythmia, cardiomyopathy (rare), cerebrovascular accident, ECG changes (nonspecific), edema, facial edema, heart block, hypertension, myocardial infarction, orthostatic hypotension, palpitations, syncope, tachycardia

Central nervous system: Anxiety, ataxia, cognitive dysfunction, coma, confusion, delusions, disorientation, dizziness, drowsiness, drug withdrawal (nausea, headache, malaise, irritability, restlessness, dream and sleep disturbance, mania [rare], and hypomania [rare]), dysarthria, EEG pattern changes, excitement, extrapyramidal reaction (including abnormal involuntary movements and tardive dyskinesia), fatigue, hallucination, headache, hyperpyrexia, insomnia, lack of concentration, nightmares, numbness, paresthesia, peripheral neuropathy, restlessness, sedation, seizure, tingling of extremities

Dermatologic: Allergic skin rash, alopecia, diaphoresis, skin photosensitivity, urticaria

Endocrine & metabolic: Altered serum glucose, decreased libido, galactorrhea, gynecomastia, increased libido, SIADH, weight gain, weight loss

Gastrointestinal: Ageusia, anorexia, constipation, diarrhea, melanoglossia, nausea, paralytic ileus, parotid gland enlargement, stomatitis, unpleasant taste, vomiting, xerostomia

Genitourinary: Breast hypertrophy, impotence, testicular swelling, urinary frequency, urinary retention, urinary tract dilation

Hematologic & oncologic: Bone marrow depression (including agranulocytosis, leukopenia, and thrombocytopenia), eosinophilia, purpura

Hepatic: Hepatic failure, hepatitis (rare; including altered liver function and jaundice)

Hypersensitivity: Tongue edema

Neuromuscular & skeletal: Lupus-like syndrome, tremor, weakness

Ophthalmic: Accommodation disturbance, blurred vision, increased intraocular pressure, mydriasis

Otic: Tinnitus

Limited to important or life-threatening: Angle-closure glaucoma, neuroleptic malignant syndrome (rare; Stevens, 2008), serotonin syndrome (rare)

Drug Interactions

Metabolism/Transport Effects Substrate of CYP1A2 (minor), CYP2B6 (minor), CYP2C19 (minor), CYP2C9 (minor), CYP2D6 (major), CYP3A4 (minor); **Note:** Assignment of Major/Minor substrate status based on clinically relevant drug interaction potential; **Inhibits** CYP1A2 (weak), CYP2C19 (weak), CYP2C9 (weak), CYP2D6 (weak), CYP2E1 (weak)

Avoid Concomitant Use

Avoid concomitant use of Amitriptyline with any of the following: Aclidinium; Azelastine (Nasal); Cimetropium; Cisapride; Dapoxetine; Dronedarone; Eluxadoline; Glucagon; Glycopyrrolate; Glycopyrrolate (Oral Inhalation); Iobenguane I 123; Ipratropium (Oral Inhalation); Levosulpiride; Linezolid; MAO Inhibitors; Methylene Blue; Moxonidine; Orphenadrine; Paraldehyde; Potassium Chloride; Thalidomide; Tiotropium; Umeclidinium

Increased Effect/Toxicity

Amitriptyline may increase the levels/effects of: AbobotulinumtoxinA; Alcohol (Ethyl); Alpha-/Beta-Agonists (Direct-Acting); Alpha1-Agonists; Amphetamines; Analgesics (Opioid); Anticholinergic Agents; Antipsychotic Agents; ARIPiprazole; Aspirin; Azelastine (Nasal); Beta2-Agonists; Buprenorphine; Cimetropium; Cisapride; Citalopram; CNS Depressants; Desmopressin; Dronedarone; Eluxadoline; Escitalopram; Fluconazole; Glucagon; Glycopyrrolate; Glycopyrrolate (Oral Inhalation); Highest Risk QTc-Prolonging Agents; Hydrocodone; Methotrimeprazine; Methylene Blue; Metyrosine; Mirabegron; Moderate Risk QTc-Prolonging Agents; Nicorandil; NSAID (COX-2 Inhibitor); NSAID (Nonselective); OnabotulinumtoxinA; Orphenadrine; Paraldehyde; Potassium Chloride; Pramipexole; QuiNIDine; Ramosetron; RimabotulinumtoxinB; ROPINIRole; Rotigotine; Serotonin Modulators; Sodium Phosphates; Sulfonylureas; Suvorexant; Thalidomide; Thiazide Diuretics; Tiotropium; TiZANidine; TraMADol; Vitamin K Antagonists; Yohimbine; Zolpidem

The levels/effects of Amitriptyline may be increased by: Abiraterone Acetate; Aclidinium; Altretamine; Antiemetics (5HT3 Antagonists); Antipsychotic Agents; Brimonidine (Topical); BuPROPion; Cannabis; Cimetidine; Cinacalcet; Citalopram; Cobicistat; CYP2D6 Inhibitors (Moderate); CYP2D6 Inhibitors (Strong); Dapoxetine; Darunavir; Dexmethylphenidate; Doxylamine; Dronabinol; Droperidol; DULoxetine; Escitalopram; Fluconazole; FLUoxetine; FluvoxaMINE; HydrOXYzine; Ipratropium (Oral Inhalation); Kava Kava; Linezolid; Lithium; Magnesium Sulfate; MAO Inhibitors; Metaxalone; Methotrimeprazine; Methylphenidate; Metoclopramide; Metyrosine; Mianserin; Mifepristone; Minocycline; Nabilone; Panobinostat; PARoxetine; Peginterferon Alfa-2b; Perampanel; Pramlintide; Protease Inhibitors; QuiNIDine; Rufinamide; Sertraline; Sodium Oxybate; Tapentadol; Tedizolid; Terbinafine (Systemic); Tetrahydrocannabinol; Thyroid Products; Topiramate; TraMADol; Umeclidinium; Valproate Products

Decreased Effect

Amitriptyline may decrease the levels/effects of: Acetylcholinesterase Inhibitors; Alpha1-Agonists; Alpha2-Agonists; Alpha2-Agonists (Ophthalmic); Gastrointestinal Agents (Prokinetic); Iobenguane I 123; Itopride; Levosulpiride; Moxonidine; Secretin

The levels/effects of Amitriptyline may be decreased by: Acetylcholinesterase Inhibitors; Barbiturates; CarBAMazepine; Peginterferon Alfa-2b; St Johns Wort

Storage/Stability Store at 20°C to 25°C (68°F to 77°F). Protect from light.

Mechanism of Action Increases the synaptic concentration of serotonin and/or norepinephrine in the central nervous system by inhibition of their reuptake by the presynaptic neuronal membrane pump.

Pharmacodynamics/Kinetics

Onset of action: Individual responses may vary; however, 4 to 8 weeks of treatment are needed before determining if a patient with depression is partially or non-responsive; similarly 8 to 12 weeks are required for an adequate migraine prophylaxis trial (APA, 2010; Prinsheim, 2012); desired therapeutic effect (for analgesia) may take as long as 1 to 3 weeks.

Absorption: Rapid, well absorbed

Distribution: V_d: ~18 to 22 L/kg (Schulz, 1985)

Protein binding: >90%

Metabolism: Rapid; hepatic N to demethylation to nortriptyline (active), hydroxy derivatives and conjugated derivatives

Bioavailability: ~43% to 46% (Schulz, 1985)

Half-life elimination: ~13 to 36 hours (Schulz, 1985)

Time to peak, serum: ~2 to 5 hours (Schulz, 1985)

Excretion: Urine (glucuronide or sulfate conjugate metabolites; 18% as unchanged drug); Feces (small amounts)

Special Populations: Elderly: May have increased plasma levels (Schulz, 1985)

Dosing

Adult

Depression: Oral: Initial: 25-50 mg daily single dose at bedtime or in divided doses; initial doses of 100 mg daily may be considered in hospitalized patients. Gradually increase dose to 100-300 mg daily (APA, 2010; Bauer 2013).

Chronic pain management (off-label use): Oral: Initial: 25-50 mg at bedtime; may increase as tolerated to 150 mg daily (McQuay, 1992; Pilowsky, 1982; Zitman, 1990).

Diabetic neuropathy (off-label use): Oral: 25-100 mg daily (Bril, 2011)

Interstitial cystitis (bladder pain syndrome) (off-label use): Oral: 10 to 25 mg daily titrated weekly over several weeks to a target dose of 75 to 100 mg as tolerated (AUA [Hanno, 2014]; Foster, 2010)

Migraine prophylaxis (off-label use): Oral: Initial: 10-25 mg at bedtime; increase at weekly increments of 10-25 mg daily based on response and tolerability up to 150 mg daily (Couch, 1976; Dodick, 2009; Evers, 2009; Keskinbora, 2008).

Post-traumatic stress disorder (PTSD) (off-label use): Oral: Initial: 50 mg daily; increase at 25 mg increments as tolerated to 100 mg within the first week; increase to 150 mg daily, then 200 mg daily before the end of 2 weeks; increase further if necessary and tolerated (Davidson, 1990).

Discontinuation of therapy: Upon discontinuation of antidepressant therapy, gradually taper the dose to minimize the incidence of withdrawal symptoms and allow for the detection of re-emerging symptoms. Evidence supporting ideal taper rates is limited. APA and NICE guidelines suggest tapering therapy over at least several weeks with consideration to the half-life of the antidepressant; antidepressants with a shorter half-life may need to be tapered more conservatively. In addition for long-term treated patients, WFSBP guidelines recommend tapering over 4-6 months. If intolerable withdrawal symptoms occur following a dose reduction, consider resuming the previously prescribed dose and/or decrease dose at a more gradual rate (APA, 2010; Bauer, 2002; Haddad, 2001; NCCMH, 2010; Schatzberg, 2006; Shelton, 2001; Warner, 2006).

MAO inhibitor recommendations:

Switching to or from an MAO inhibitor antidepressant:

Allow 14 days to elapse between discontinuing an MAO inhibitor intended to treat depression and initiation of amitriptyline.

Allow 14 days to elapse between discontinuing amitriptyline and initiation of an MAO inhibitor intended to treat depression.

Use with reversible MAO inhibitors (such as linezolid or IV methylene blue):

Do not initiate amitriptyline in patients receiving linezolid or IV methylene blue; consider other interventions for psychiatric condition.

If urgent treatment with linezolid or IV methylene blue is required in a patient already receiving amitriptyline and potential benefits outweigh potential risks, discontinue amitriptyline promptly and administer linezolid or IV methylene blue. Monitor for serotonin syndrome for 2 weeks or until 24 hours after the last dose of linezolid or IV methylene blue, whichever comes first. May resume amitriptyline 24 hours after the last dose of linezolid or IV methylene blue.

Geriatric

Depression: Oral: Usual dosage (recommended by the manufacturer): 10 mg 3 times daily and 20 mg at bedtime. In general, lower doses are recommended for elderly patients

Discontinuation of therapy: Refer to adult dosing.

MAO inhibitor recommendations: Refer to adult dosing.

Pediatric

Chronic pain management (off-label use): Oral: Initial: 0.1 mg/kg/day at bedtime, may advance as tolerated over 2-3 weeks to 0.5-2 mg/kg/day at bedtime (APS [Miaskowski, 2008]; Freidrichsdorf, 2007; Kliegman, 2011)

Depressive disorders: *Adolescents:* Usual dosage (recommended by the manufacturer): 10 mg three times daily and 20 mg at bedtime. In general, lower doses are recommended for adolescent patients. **Note:** Controlled clinical trials have not shown tricyclic antidepressants to be superior to placebo for the treatment of depression in children and adolescents; not recommended as first-line medication; may be beneficial for patient with comorbid conditions (Birmaher, 2007; Dopheide, 2006; Wagner, 2005).

Migraine prophylaxis (off-label use): Oral: Initial: 0.25 mg/kg/day, given at bedtime; increase dose by 0.25 mg/kg/day every 2 weeks to 1 mg/kg/day. Reported dosing range: 0.2-1.7 mg/kg/day (Hershey, 2000).

Discontinuation of therapy: Refer to adult dosing.

MAO inhibitor recommendations: Refer to adult dosing.

Renal Impairment There are no dosage adjustments provided in manufacturer's labeling; however, renally eliminated; use with caution.

Hepatic Impairment There are no dosage adjustments provided in manufacturer's labeling; however, hepatically metabolized; use with caution.

Administration Oral: Administer higher doses preferably at late afternoon or as bedtime doses to minimize daytime sedation.

Monitoring Parameters Evaluate mental status, suicide ideation (especially at the beginning of therapy or when doses are increased or decreased); anxiety, social functioning, mania, panic attacks or other unusual changes in behavior; heart rate, blood pressure and ECG in older adults and patients with preexisting cardiac disease; blood glucose; weight and BMI; blood levels are useful for therapeutic monitoring (APA, 2010).

Reference Range Therapeutic: Amitriptyline plus nortriptyline 80-250 ng/mL (SI: 288-900 nmol/L); amitriptyline plus nortriptyline levels >300 ng/mL are associated with increased side effects; plasma levels do not always correlate with clinical effectiveness (Am J Psychiatry, 1985; Boyer, 1984; Orsulak, 1979)

Dosage Forms Excipient information presented when available (limited, particularly for generics); consult specific product labeling.

Tablet, Oral, as hydrochloride:

Generic: 10 mg, 25 mg, 50 mg, 75 mg, 100 mg, 150 mg

Amitriptyline and Chlordiazepoxide
(a mee TRIP ti leen & klor dye az e POKS ide)

Index Terms Chlordiazepoxide and Amitriptyline Hydrochloride; Limbitrol

Pharmacologic Category Antidepressant, Tricyclic (Tertiary Amine); Benzodiazepine

Use Depression: Treatment of moderate-to-severe depression associated with moderate to severe anxiety

Medication Guide Available Yes

Dosing

Adult

Depression and anxiety: Oral: Amitriptyline 12.5 mg/chlordiazepoxide 5 mg or amitriptyline 25 mg/chlordiazepoxide 10 mg tablets:

Initial: 3 or 4 tablets daily in one or more divided doses; titrate to response; usual dose: 2 to 6 tablets daily in one or more divided doses.

Maximum daily dose: amitriptyline 150 mg/chlordiazepoxide 60 mg.

Discontinuation of therapy: Upon discontinuation of antidepressant therapy, gradually taper the dose to minimize the incidence of withdrawal symptoms and allow for the detection of re-emerging symptoms. Evidence supporting ideal taper rates is limited. APA and NICE guidelines suggest tapering therapy over at least several weeks with consideration to the half-life of the antidepressant; antidepressants with a shorter half-life may need to be tapered more conservatively. In addition for long-term treated patients, WFSBP guidelines

recommend tapering over 4 to 6 months. If intolerable withdrawal symptoms occur following a dose reduction, consider resuming the previously prescribed dose and/or decrease dose at a more gradual rate (APA, 2010; Bauer, 2002; Haddad, 2001; NCCMH, 2010; Schatzberg, 2006; Shelton, 2001; Warner 2006).

MAO inhibitor recommendations:
Switching to or from an MAO inhibitor intended to treat psychiatric disorders:
Allow 14 days to elapse between discontinuing an MAO inhibitor intended to treat psychiatric disorders and initiation of amitriptyline/chlordiazepoxide.
Allow 14 days to elapse between discontinuing amitriptyline/chlordiazepoxide and initiation of an MAO inhibitor intended to treat psychiatric disorders.
Use with reversible MAO inhibitors (such as linezolid or IV methylene blue):
Do not initiate amitriptyline/chlordiazepoxide in patients receiving linezolid or IV methylene blue; consider other interventions for psychiatric condition.
If urgent treatment with linezolid or IV methylene blue is required in a patient already receiving amitriptyline/chlordiazepoxide and potential benefits outweigh potential risks, discontinue amitriptyline/chlordiazepoxide promptly and administer linezolid or IV methylene blue. Monitor for serotonin syndrome for 2 weeks or until 24 hours after the last dose of linezolid or IV methylene blue, whichever comes first. May resume amitriptyline/chlordiazepoxide 24 hours after the last dose of linezolid or IV methylene blue.

Geriatric Refer to adult dosing. Lower initial doses should be considered; use with caution.

Renal Impairment There are no dosage adjustments provided in manufacturer's labeling; use with caution.

Hepatic Impairment There are no dosage adjustments provided in manufacturer's labeling; use with caution.

Additional Information Complete prescribing information should be consulted for additional detail.

Dosage Forms Excipient information presented when available (limited, particularly for generics); consult specific product labeling.
Tablet: 12.5/5: Amitriptyline hydrochloride 12.5 mg and chlordiazepoxide 5 mg; 25/10: Amitriptyline hydrochloride 25 mg and chlordiazepoxide 10 mg

Controlled Substance C-IV

Amitriptyline and Perphenazine
(a mee TRIP ti leen & per FEN a zeen)

Brand Names: Canada PMS-Levazine
Index Terms Perphenazine and Amitriptyline Hydrochloride
Pharmacologic Category Antidepressant, Tricyclic (Tertiary Amine); First Generation (Typical) Antipsychotic
Use Treatment of patients with moderate-to-severe anxiety and/or agitation and depression; schizophrenia with depressive symptoms
Medication Guide Available Yes
Dosing
Adult
Depression and anxiety: Oral:
Initial: One tablet (amitriptyline 25 mg/perphenazine 2 mg or amitriptyline 25 mg/perphenazine 4 mg) 3-4 times/day **or** 1 tablet (amitriptyline 50 mg/perphenazine 4 mg) 2 times/day; initial therapeutic response may be observed after several days or upwards of a few weeks or longer (maximum daily dose: amitriptyline 200 mg/perphenazine 16 mg)
Maintenance: Smallest dose necessary for symptom relief; usually 1 tablet (amitriptyline 25 mg/perphenazine 2 mg or amitriptyline 25 mg/perphenazine 4 mg) 2-4 times/day **or** 1 tablet (amitriptyline 50 mg/perphenazine 4 mg) 2 times/day

Schizophrenia and depression: Oral:
Initial: Two tablets (amitriptyline 25 mg/perphenazine 4 mg) 3 times/day; if necessary, a fourth dose may be given at bedtime; initial therapeutic response may be observed after several days or upwards of a few weeks or longer (maximum daily dose: amitriptyline 200 mg/perphenazine 16 mg) (maximum: 64 mg/day of perphenazine)
Maintenance: Smallest dose necessary for symptom relief; usually 1 tablet (amitriptyline 25 mg/perphenazine 2 mg or amitriptyline 25 mg/perphenazine 4 mg) 2-4 times/day **or** 1 tablet (amitriptyline 50 mg/perphenazine 4 mg) 2 times/day

Discontinuation of therapy: Upon discontinuation of antidepressant therapy, gradually taper the dose to minimize the incidence of withdrawal symptoms and allow for the detection of re-emerging symptoms. Evidence supporting ideal taper rates is limited. APA and

NICE guidelines suggest tapering therapy over at least several weeks with consideration to the half-life of the antidepressant; antidepressants with a shorter half-life may need to be tapered more conservatively. In addition for long-term treated patients, WFSBP guidelines recommend tapering over 4-6 months. If intolerable withdrawal symptoms occur following a dose reduction, consider resuming the previously prescribed dose and/or decrease dose at a more gradual rate (APA, 2010; Bauer, 2002; Haddad, 2001; NCCMH, 2010; Schatzberg, 2006; Shelton, 2001; Warner, 2006).

MAO inhibitor recommendations:
Switching to or from an MAO inhibitor intended to treat psychiatric disorders:
Allow 14 days to elapse between discontinuing an MAO inhibitor intended to treat psychiatric disorders and initiation of amitriptyline/perphenazine.
Allow 14 days to elapse between discontinuing amitriptyline/perphenazine and initiation of an MAO inhibitor intended to treat psychiatric disorders.
Use with reversible MAO inhibitors (such as linezolid or IV methylene blue):
Do not initiate amitriptyline/perphenazine in patients receiving linezolid or IV methylene blue; consider other interventions for psychiatric condition.
If urgent treatment with linezolid or IV methylene blue is required in a patient already receiving amitriptyline/perphenazine and potential benefits outweigh potential risks, discontinue amitriptyline/perphenazine promptly and administer linezolid or IV methylene blue. Monitor for serotonin syndrome for 2 weeks or until 24 hours after the last dose of linezolid or IV methylene blue, whichever comes first. May resume amitriptyline/perphenazine 24 hours after the last dose of linezolid or IV methylene blue.

Geriatric Oral: One tablet (amitriptyline 10 mg/perphenazine 4 mg) 3-4 times/day

Discontinuation of therapy: Refer to adult dosing.
MAO inhibitor recommendations: Refer to adult dosing.
Renal Impairment No dosage adjustment provided in manufacturer's labeling.
Hepatic Impairment Use caution; no dosage adjustment provided in manufacturer's labeling.
Additional Information Complete prescribing information should be consulted for additional detail.
Dosage Forms Excipient information presented when available (limited, particularly for generics); consult specific product labeling.
Tablet, Oral:
Amitriptyline hydrochloride 10 mg and perphenazine 2 mg
Amitriptyline hydrochloride 10 mg and perphenazine 4 mg
Amitriptyline hydrochloride 25 mg and perphenazine 2 mg
Amitriptyline hydrochloride 25 mg and perphenazine 4 mg
Amitriptyline hydrochloride 50 mg and perphenazine 4 mg

◆ Amitriptyline Hydrochloride *see* Amitriptyline on page 98
◆ AMJ 9701 *see* Palifermin on page 1374

AmLODIPine (am LOE di peen)

Brand Names: US Norvasc
Brand Names: Canada Accel-Amlodipine; ACT-Amlodipine; Amlodipine-Odan; Apo-Amlodipine; Auro-Amlodipine; Bio-Amlodipine; Dom-Amlodipine; GD-Amlodipine; JAMP-Amlodipine; Mar-Amlodipine; Mint-Amlodipine; Mylan-Amlodipine; Norvasc; PHL-Amlodipine; PMS-Amlodipine; Q-Amlodipine; RAN-Amlodipine; ratio-Amlodipine; Riva-Amlodipine; Sandoz Amlodipine; Septa-Amlodipine; Teva-Amlodipine
Index Terms Amlodipine Besylate
Pharmacologic Category Antianginal Agent; Antihypertensive; Calcium Channel Blocker; Calcium Channel Blocker, Dihydropyridine
Additional Appendix Information
Hypertension *on page 1996*
Use
Coronary artery disease (CAD):
Chronic stable angina: Treatment of symptomatic chronic stable angina. May be used alone or in combination with other antianginal agents.
Vasospastic angina (Prinzmetal or variant angina): Treatment of confirmed or suspected vasospastic angina.

May be used alone or in combination with other anti-anginal agents.

Angiographically documented CAD: Reduce the risk of hospitalization secondary to angina and to reduce the risk of a coronary revascularization procedure in patients with recently documented CAD by angiography (without heart failure or an ejection fraction of <40%).

The ACCF/AHA 2013 guidelines for management of heart failure state that, with the exception of amlodipine, calcium channel blockers should be avoided and withdrawn whenever possible in patients with heart failure with reduced ejection fraction (HFrEF). While amlodipine, like other calcium channel blockers, has no benefit on functioning or survival, it may be used for the treatment of hypertension or ischemic heart disease in patients with HFrEF (ACCF/AHA [Yancy 2013]).

Hypertension: Treatment of hypertension. May be used alone or in combination with other antihypertensive agents

The 2014 guideline for the management of high blood pressure in adults (JNC 8) recommends initiation of pharmacologic treatment to lower blood pressure for the following patients (JNC8 [James 2013]):

- Patients ≥60 years of age, with systolic blood pressure (SBP) ≥150 mm Hg or diastolic blood pressure (DBP) ≥90 mm Hg. Goal of therapy is SBP <150 mm Hg and DBP <90 mm Hg.
- Patients <60 years of age, with SBP ≥140 mm Hg or DBP ≥90 mm Hg. Goal of therapy is SBP <140 mm Hg and DBP <90 mm Hg.
- Patients ≥18 years of age with diabetes, with SBP ≥140 mm Hg or DBP ≥90 mm Hg. Goal of therapy is SBP <140 mm Hg and DBP <90 mm Hg.
- Patients ≥18 years of age with chronic kidney disease (CKD), with SBP ≥140 mm Hg or DBP ≥90 mm Hg. Goal of therapy is SBP <140 mm Hg and DBP <90 mm Hg.

In patients with chronic kidney disease (CKD), regardless of race or diabetes status, the use of an ACE inhibitor (ACEI) or angiotensin receptor blocker (ARB) as initial therapy is recommended to improve kidney outcomes. In the general nonblack population (without CKD) including those with diabetes, initial antihypertensive treatment should consist of a thiazide-type diuretic, calcium channel blocker, ACEI, or ARB. In the general black population (without CKD) including those with diabetes, initial antihypertensive treatment should consist of a thiazide-type diuretic or a calcium channel blocker **instead of** an ACEI or ARB.

Pregnancy Considerations Adverse events have been observed in some animal reproduction studies. Untreated chronic maternal hypertension is associated with adverse events in the fetus, infant, and mother. If treatment for hypertension during pregnancy is needed, other agents are preferred (ACOG 2013).

Breast-Feeding Considerations Amlodipine is excreted in breast milk. A study was conducted in 31 lactating women ~3 weeks postpartum. All women were administered amlodipine for pregnancy-induced hypertension (median daily dose 6.01 ± 2.31 mg). Sampling occurred ~10 days after dosing was initiated. The median predose amlodipine concentrations were 15.5 ng/mL (maternal serum) and 11.5 ng/mL (breast milk). The median estimated amlodipine exposure to the breast-feeding infant (relative infant dose) was 4.17 mcg/kg/day (median relative infant dose 4.18% based on the weight adjusted maternal dose). Variability was observed; the maximum relative infant dose calculated was 15.2% (Naito 2015). Breast-feeding is not recommended by the manufacturer.

Contraindications Hypersensitivity to amlodipine or any component of the formulation

Warnings/Precautions Increased angina and/or MI has occurred with initiation or dosage titration of calcium channel blockers. Symptomatic hypotension can occur; acute hypotension upon initiation is unlikely due to the gradual onset of action. Blood pressure must be lowered at a rate appropriate for the patient's clinical condition. Use caution in severe aortic stenosis and/or hypertrophic cardiomyopathy with outflow tract obstruction. Use caution in patients with hepatic impairment; may require lower starting dose; titrate slowly with severe hepatic impairment. The most common side effect is peripheral edema; occurs within 2 to 3 weeks of starting therapy. Reflex tachycardia may occur with use. Peak antihypertensive effect is delayed; dosage titration should occur after 7 to 14 days on a given dose. Initiate at a lower dose in the elderly.

Adverse Reactions

>10%:

Cardiovascular: Peripheral edema (2% to 11% dose related; female 15%; male 6%; HF patients 27% to 28% [Packer 1996; Packer 2013])

Respiratory: Pulmonary edema (HF patients 7% to 15% [Packer 1996; Packer 2013])

1% to 10%:

Cardiovascular: Palpitations (≤5%, dose related), flushing (≤3%, dose related, more frequent in females)

Central nervous system: Fatigue (5%), dizziness (1% to 3%, dose related), male sexual disorder (≤2%), drowsiness (1%)

Dermatologic: Pruritus (≤2%), skin rash (≤2%)

Gastrointestinal: Nausea (3%), abdominal pain (2%)

Neuromuscular & skeletal: Muscle cramps (≤2%), weakness (≤2%)

Respiratory: Dyspnea (≤2%)

<1% (Limited to important or life-threatening): Acute interstitial nephritis (Ejaz 2000), anorexia, atrial fibrillation, bradycardia, cholestasis, conjunctivitis, depression, diarrhea, difficulty in micturition, diplopia, dysphagia, epistaxis, erythema multiforme, exfoliative dermatitis, extrapyramidal reaction, eye pain, female sexual disorder, gingival hyperplasia, gynecomastia, hepatitis, hot flash, hyperglycemia, hypersensitivity angiitis, hypersensitivity reaction, hypoesthesia, increased serum transaminases, increased thirst, insomnia, leukopenia, maculopapular rash, myalgia, nocturia, orthostatic hypotension, osteoarthritis, pancreatitis, paresthesia, peripheral ischemia, peripheral neuropathy, phototoxicity, purpura, rigors, tachycardia, thrombocytopenia, tremor, vasculitis, ventricular tachycardia, weight gain

Drug Interactions

Metabolism/Transport Effects Substrate of CYP3A4 (major); **Note:** Assignment of Major/Minor substrate status based on clinically relevant drug interaction potential; **Inhibits** CYP1A2 (weak), CYP2A6 (weak), CYP2B6 (weak), CYP2C8 (weak), CYP2C9 (weak), CYP2D6 (weak), CYP3A4 (weak)

Avoid Concomitant Use

Avoid concomitant use of AmLODIPine with any of the following: Amodiaquine; Conivaptan; Fusidic Acid (Systemic); Idelalisib; Pimozide

Increased Effect/Toxicity

AmLODIPine may increase the levels/effects of: Amifostine; Amodiaquine; Antipsychotic Agents (Second Generation [Atypical]); ARIPiprazole; Atosiban; Calcium Channel Blockers (Nondihydropyridine); Dofetilide; DULoxetine; Flibanserin; Fosphenytoin; Hydrocodone; Hypotension-Associated Agents; Levodopa; Lomitapide; Magnesium Salts; Neuromuscular-Blocking Agents (Nondepolarizing); NiMODipine; Nitroprusside; Phenytoin; Pimozide; QuiNIDine; Simvastatin; Tacrolimus (Systemic); TiZANidine

The levels/effects of AmLODIPine may be increased by: Alfuzosin; Alpha1-Blockers; Antifungal Agents (Azole Derivatives, Systemic); Antihepaciviral Combination Products; Aprepitant; Barbiturates; Brimonidine (Topical); Calcium Channel Blockers (Nondihydropyridine); Conivaptan; CycloSPORINE (Systemic); CYP3A4 Inhibitors (Moderate); CYP3A4 Inhibitors (Strong); Dapoxetine; Dasatinib; Diazoxide; Fluconazole; Fosaprepitant; Fusidic Acid (Systemic); Grapefruit Juice; Herbs (Hypotensive Properties); Idelalisib; Ivacaftor; Luliconazole; Macrolide Antibiotics; Magnesium Salts; Mifepristone; Molsidomine; Netupitant; Nicorandil; Obinutuzumab; Osimertinib; Palbociclib; Pentoxifylline; Phosphodiesterase 5 Inhibitors; Prostacyclin Analogues; QuiNIDine; Simeprevir; Stiripentol

Decreased Effect

AmLODIPine may decrease the levels/effects of: Clopidogrel; QuiNIDine

The levels/effects of AmLODIPine may be decreased by: Amphetamines; Barbiturates; Bosentan; Calcium Salts; CarBAMazepine; CYP3A4 Inducers (Moderate); CYP3A4 Inducers (Strong); Dabrafenib; Deferasirox; Efavirenz; Enzalutamide; Herbs (Hypertensive Properties); Melatonin; Methylphenidate; Mitotane; Nafcillin; Osimertinib; Phenytoin; Rifamycin Derivatives; Siltuximab; St Johns Wort; Tocilizumab; Yohimbine

Food Interactions Grapefruit juice may modestly increase amlodipine levels. Management: Monitor closely with concurrent use.

Storage/Stability Store at 15°C to 30°C (59°F to 86°F).

Mechanism of Action Inhibits calcium ion from entering the "slow channels" or select voltage-sensitive areas of vascular smooth muscle and myocardium during depolarization, producing a relaxation of coronary vascular smooth muscle and coronary vasodilation; increases myocardial oxygen delivery in patients with vasospastic angina. Amlodipine directly acts on vascular smooth muscle to produce peripheral arterial vasodilation reducing peripheral vascular resistance and blood pressure.

Pharmacodynamics/Kinetics

Onset of action: Antihypertensive effect: Significant reductions in blood pressure at 24 to 48 hours after first dose; slight increase in heart rate within 10 hours of administration may reflect some vasodilating activity (Donnelly 1993)

Duration: Antihypertensive effect: At least 24 hours (Donnelly 1993); has been shown to extend to at least 72 hours when discontinued after 6 to 7 weeks of therapy (Biston 1999)

Absorption: Well absorbed (Meredith 1992)

Distribution: Mean V_d:

Children >6 years: Similar to adults on a mg per kg basis; **Note:** Weight-adjusted V_d in younger children (<6 years of age) may be greater than in older children (Flynn 2006)

Adults: 21 L/kg (Scholz 1997)

Protein binding: ~93%

Metabolism: Hepatic (~90%) to inactive metabolites

Bioavailability: 64% to 90%

Half-life elimination: Terminal (biphasic): 30 to 50 hours; increased with hepatic dysfunction

Time to peak, plasma: 6 to 12 hours

Excretion: Urine (10% of total dose as unchanged drug, 60% of total dose as metabolites)

Clearance: May be decreased in patients with hepatic insufficiency or moderate to severe heart failure; weight-adjusted clearance in children >6 years of age is similar to adults; **Note:** Weight-adjusted clearance in younger children (<6 years of age) may be greater than in older children (Flynn 2006)

Dosing

Adult

Coronary artery disease (CAD) (chronic stable angina, vasospastic angina, angiographically documented CAD [without heart failure or ejection fraction <40%]): Oral: 5 to 10 mg once daily

Hypertension: Oral: Initial: 5 mg once daily **or** 2.5 mg once daily in small or frail patients, or when adding amlodipine to other antihypertensive therapy; maximum dose: 10 mg once daily. In general, titrate every 7 to 14 days. Titrate more rapidly, however, if clinically warranted, provided the patient is assessed frequently. Usual dosage range (ASH/ISH [Weber 2014]): 5 to 10 mg once daily. Target dose (JNC8 [James 2013]): 10 mg once daily.

Geriatric Dosing should start at the lower end of dosing range and titrated to response due to possible increased incidence of hepatic, renal, or cardiac impairment. Elderly patients also show decreased clearance of amlodipine.

Coronary artery disease (CAD) (chronic stable angina, vasospastic angina, angiographically documented CAD without heart failure or ejection fraction <40%): Oral: Initial: 5 mg once daily

Hypertension: Oral: Initial: 2.5 mg once daily; maximum dose: 10 mg once daily. In general, titrate every 7 to 14 days. Titrate more rapidly, however, if clinically warranted, provided the patient is assessed frequently. Usual dosage range (ASH/ISH [Weber 2014]): 5 to 10 mg once daily. Target dose (JNC8 [James 2013]): 10 mg once daily.

Pediatric Hypertension: Children ≥6 years and Adolescents: Oral: 2.5 to 5 mg once daily

Renal Impairment

No dosage adjustment necessary (Doyle 1989; Kungys 2003).

End-stage renal disease (ESRD) on dialysis: Hemodialysis and peritoneal dialysis do not enhance elimination; supplemental dose is not necessary (Kungys 2003).

Hepatic Impairment

Coronary artery disease (CAD) (chronic stable angina, vasospastic angina, angiographically documented CAD without heart failure or ejection fraction <40%): Initial: 5 mg once daily; titrate slowly in patients with severe hepatic impairment.

Hypertension: Initial: 2.5 mg once daily; titrate slowly in patients with severe hepatic impairment.

Administration Oral: Administer without regard to meals.

Monitoring Parameters Heart rate, blood pressure

Dosage Forms Excipient information presented when available (limited, particularly for generics); consult specific product labeling.

Tablet, Oral:

Norvasc: 2.5 mg, 5 mg, 10 mg

Generic: 2.5 mg, 5 mg, 10 mg

Extemporaneous Preparations A 1 mg/mL oral suspension may be made with tablets and either a 1:1 mixture of simple syrup and 1% methylcellulose or a 1:1 mixture of Ora-Plus® and Ora-Sweet®. Crush fifty 5 mg tablets in a mortar and reduce to a fine powder. Add small portions of the chosen vehicle and mix to a uniform paste; mix while adding the vehicle in incremental proportions to almost 250 mL; transfer to a calibrated bottle, rinse mortar with vehicle, and add quantity of vehicle sufficient to make 250 mL. Label "shake well" and "refrigerate". Stable for 56 days at room temperature or 91 days refrigerated.

Nahata MC, Morosco RS, and Hipple TF, "Stability of Amlodipine Besylate in Two Liquid Dosage Forms," *J Am Pharm Assoc (Wash)* 1999, 39(3):375-7.

◆ Amlodipine, Aliskiren, and Hydrochlorothiazide *see* Aliskiren, Amlodipine, and Hydrochlorothiazide *on page 72*

Amlodipine and Atorvastatin
(am LOW di peen & a TORE va sta tin)

Brand Names: US Caduet®

Brand Names: Canada Caduet®

Index Terms Atorvastatin and Amlodipine; Atorvastatin Calcium and Amlodipine Besylate

Pharmacologic Category Antianginal Agent; Antihypertensive; Antilipemic Agent; HMG-CoA Reductase Inhibitor; Calcium Channel Blocker; Calcium Channel Blocker, Dihydropyridine

Use For use when treatment with both amlodipine and atorvastatin is appropriate:

Amlodipine: Treatment of hypertension; treatment of chronic stable angina, vasospastic (Prinzmetal's) angina (confirmed or suspected); prevention of hospitalization or to decrease coronary revascularization procedure due to angina with documented CAD (limited to patients without heart failure or ejection fraction <40%)

Atorvastatin: Treatment of dyslipidemias or primary prevention of cardiovascular disease (atherosclerotic) as detailed here:

Primary prevention of cardiovascular disease (high-risk for CVD): To reduce the risk of MI or stroke in patients without evidence of coronary heart disease who have multiple CVD risk factors or type 2 diabetes; also reduces the risk for angina or revascularization procedures in patients with multiple CVD risk factors without evidence of coronary heart disease

Secondary prevention of cardiovascular disease: To reduce the risk of MI, stroke, revascularization procedures, angina, and hospitalization for heart failure

Primary and secondary prevention of atherosclerotic cardiovascular disease (ASCVD) according to the American College of Cardiology/American Heart Association: To reduce the risk of ASCVD in patients with clinical ASCVD (eg, coronary heart disease, stroke/TIA, or peripheral arterial disease presumed to be of atherosclerotic origin); in patients without clinical ASCVD if LDL-C is 190 mg/dL or greater; in patients without clinical ASCVD who have type 1 or type 2 diabetes and are between 40 and 75 years of age; in patients with an estimated 10-year ASCVD risk 7.5% or greater and who are between 40 and 75 years of age (Stone, 2013). Specific recommendations from the Kidney Disease: Improving Global Outcomes (KDIGO) organization have also been released for patients with chronic kidney disease (KDIGO [Tonelli, 2013]).

Treatment of dyslipidemias: To reduce elevations in total cholesterol, LDL-C, apolipoprotein B, and triglycerides in patients with elevations of one or more components, and/or to increase low HDL-C as present in heterozygous familial/nonfamilial hypercholesterolemia and mixed dyslipidemia (Fredrickson type IIa and IIb hyperlipidemias); treatment of primary dysbetalipoproteinemia (Fredrickson type III), elevated serum TG levels (Fredrickson type IV), and homozygous familial hypercholesterolemia

Treatment of heterozygous familial hypercholesterolemia (HeFH) in adolescent patients (10 to 17 years of age, females >1 year postmenarche) having LDL-C ≥190 mg/dL or LDL-C ≥160 mg/dL with positive family history of premature cardiovascular disease (CVD) or with two or more CVD risk factors.

Dosing

Adult Note: Dose is individualized; combination product may be used as initial therapy or substituted for individual components in patients currently maintained on both agents separately or in patients not adequately controlled with monotherapy (using one of the agents or an agent within same pharmacologic class).

Hypertension, angina, and hyperlipidemia: Oral:

Initial therapy: Amlodipine 5 mg and atorvastatin 10-20 mg once daily; dose may be titrated after 1-2 weeks (amlodipine component) and after 2-4 weeks (atorvastatin component) to a maximum daily dose: Amlodipine 10 mg; atorvastatin 80 mg

Add-on therapy/replacement therapy: Amlodipine 5-10 mg and atorvastatin 10-80 mg once daily; dose may be titrated after 1-2 weeks (amlodipine component) and after 2-4 weeks (atorvastatin component) to a maximum daily dose: Amlodipine 10 mg; atorvastatin 80 mg

Dosage adjustment for atorvastatin with concomitant medications:
Boceprevir, nelfinavir: Use lowest effective atorvastatin dose (not to exceed 40 mg daily)
Clarithromycin, itraconazole, fosamprenavir, ritonavir (plus darunavir, fosamprenavir, or saquinavir): Use lowest effective atorvastatin dose (not to exceed 20 mg daily)

Geriatric Refer to adult dosing. Consider starting amlodipine at the lower end of dosing range due to increased incidence of hepatic, renal, or cardiac impairment. Elderly patients also show decreased clearance of amlodipine.

Pediatric Note: Dose is individualized; combination product may be used as initial therapy or substituted for individual components in patients currently maintained on both agents separately or in patients not adequately controlled with monotherapy (using one of the agents or an agent within same pharmacologic class).

Hypertension and hyperlipidemia: 10-17 years (females >1 year postmenarche): Oral:
Initial therapy: Amlodipine 2.5 mg and atorvastatin 10 mg once daily; dose may be titrated after 1-2 weeks (amlodipine component) and after 2-4 weeks (atorvastatin component) to a maximum daily dose: Amlodipine 5 mg; atorvastatin 20 mg
Add-on therapy/replacement therapy: Amlodipine 2.5-5 mg and atorvastatin 10-20 mg once daily; dose may be titrated after 1-2 weeks (amlodipine component) and after 2-4 weeks (atorvastatin component) to a maximum daily dose: Amlodipine 5 mg; atorvastatin 20 mg

Dosage adjustment for atorvastatin with concomitant medications: Refer to adult dosing.
Renal Impairment No dosage adjustment is necessary.
Hepatic Impairment Contraindicated in patients with active liver disease.
Additional Information Complete prescribing information should be consulted for additional detail.
Dosage Forms Excipient information presented when available (limited, particularly for generics); consult specific product labeling.
Tablet, oral: Amlodipine 2.5 mg and atorvastatin 10 mg; Amlodipine 2.5 mg and atorvastatin 20 mg; Amlodipine 2.5 mg and atorvastatin 40 mg; Amlodipine 5 mg and atorvastatin 10 mg; Amlodipine 5 mg and atorvastatin 20 mg; Amlodipine 5 mg and atorvastatin 40 mg; Amlodipine 5 mg and atorvastatin 80 mg; Amlodipine 10 mg and atorvastatin 10 mg; Amlodipine 10 mg and atorvastatin 20 mg; Amlodipine 10 mg and atorvastatin 40 mg; Amlodipine 10 mg and atorvastatin 80 mg
Caduet®:
2.5/10: Amlodipine 2.5 mg and atorvastatin 10 mg
2.5/20: Amlodipine 2.5 mg and atorvastatin 20 mg
2.5/40: Amlodipine 2.5 mg and atorvastatin 40 mg
5/10: Amlodipine 5 mg and atorvastatin 10 mg
5/20: Amlodipine 5 mg and atorvastatin 20 mg
5/40: Amlodipine 5 mg and atorvastatin 40 mg
5/80: Amlodipine 5 mg and atorvastatin 80 mg
10/10: Amlodipine 10 mg and atorvastatin 10 mg
10/20: Amlodipine 10 mg and atorvastatin 20 mg
10/40: Amlodipine 10 mg and atorvastatin 40 mg
10/80: Amlodipine 10 mg and atorvastatin 80 mg

Amlodipine and Benazepril
(am LOE di peen & ben AY ze pril)

Brand Names: US Lotrel
Index Terms Benazepril Hydrochloride and Amlodipine Besylate
Pharmacologic Category Angiotensin-Converting Enzyme (ACE) Inhibitor; Antianginal Agent; Antihypertensive; Calcium Channel Blocker; Calcium Channel Blocker, Dihydropyridine
Use Hypertension: Treatment of hypertension.
Dosing
Adult Note: Dose is individualized; combination product may be substituted for individual components in patients currently maintained on both agents separately or in patients not adequately controlled with monotherapy (using one of the agents or an agent within same antihypertensive class).

Hypertension: Oral: Initial: Amlodipine 2.5 mg/benazepril 10 mg once daily; based on clinical response, may titrate up to a maximum dose of amlodipine 10 mg/benazepril 40 mg once daily (based on dosage strength available).
Geriatric Initial dose: 2.5 mg (based on amlodipine component). Refer to adult dosing.
Renal Impairment
CrCl >30 mL/minute: No dosage adjustment necessary.
CrCl ≤30 mL/minute: Use is not recommended.
Hepatic Impairment Initial dose: 2.5 mg based on amlodipine component.
Additional Information Complete prescribing information should be consulted for additional detail.
Dosage Forms Excipient information presented when available (limited, particularly for generics); consult specific product labeling.
Capsule, oral:
2.5/10: Amlodipine 2.5 mg and benazepril hydrochloride 10 mg
5/10: Amlodipine 5 mg and benazepril hydrochloride 10 mg
5/20: Amlodipine 5 mg and benazepril hydrochloride 20 mg
5/40: Amlodipine 5 mg and benazepril hydrochloride 40 mg
10/20: Amlodipine 10 mg and benazepril hydrochloride 20 mg
10/40: Amlodipine 10 mg and benazepril hydrochloride 40 mg
Lotrel 2.5/10: Amlodipine 2.5 mg and benazepril hydrochloride 10 mg
Lotrel 5/10: Amlodipine 5 mg and benazepril hydrochloride 10 mg
Lotrel 5/20: Amlodipine 5 mg and benazepril hydrochloride 20 mg
Lotrel 5/40: Amlodipine 5 mg and benazepril hydrochloride 40 mg
Lotrel 10/20: Amlodipine 10 mg and benazepril hydrochloride 20 mg
Lotrel 10/40: Amlodipine 10 mg and benazepril hydrochloride 40 mg

Amlodipine and Olmesartan
(am LOE di peen & olme SAR tan)

Brand Names: US Azor
Index Terms Amlodipine Besylate and Olmesartan Medoxomil; Olmesartan and Amlodipine
Pharmacologic Category Angiotensin II Receptor Blocker; Antianginal Agent; Antihypertensive; Calcium Channel Blocker; Calcium Channel Blocker, Dihydropyridine
Use Hypertension: Treatment of hypertension
Dosing
Adult Dose is individualized; combination product may be substituted for individual components in patients currently maintained on both agents separately or in patients not adequately controlled with monotherapy (using one of the agents or an agent within the same antihypertensive class). May also be used as initial therapy in patients who are likely to need >1 antihypertensive to control blood pressure.
Hypertension: Oral:
Initial therapy (antihypertensive naive): Amlodipine 5 mg/olmesartan 20 mg once daily; dose may be increased after 1 to 2 weeks of therapy. Maximum dose: Amlodipine 10 mg/olmesartan 40 mg once daily.
Add-on/replacement therapy: Amlodipine 5 to 10 mg and olmesartan 20 to 40 mg once daily depending upon previous doses, current control, and goals of therapy; dose may be titrated after 2 weeks of therapy. Maximum dose: Amlodipine 10 mg/olmesartan 40 mg once daily.
Geriatric Initial therapy is not recommended in patients ≥75 years.
Renal Impairment Moderate to severe impairment (CrCl <40 mL/minute): No initial dosage adjustment necessary.
Hepatic Impairment Initial therapy is not recommended.
Additional Information Complete prescribing information should be consulted for additional detail.

Dosage Forms Excipient information presented when available (limited, particularly for generics); consult specific product labeling.
Tablet:
Azor 5/20: Amlodipine 5 mg and olmesartan medoxomil 20 mg
Azor 5/40: Amlodipine 5 mg and olmesartan medoxomil 40 mg
Azor 10/20: Amlodipine 10 mg and olmesartan medoxomil 20 mg
Azor 10/40: Amlodipine 10 mg and olmesartan medoxomil 40 mg

◆ Amlodipine and Telmisartan *see* Telmisartan and Amlodipine *on page 1748*

Amlodipine and Valsartan
(am LOE di peen & val SAR tan)

Brand Names: US Exforge®
Index Terms Amlodipine Besylate and Valsartan; Valsartan and Amlodipine
Pharmacologic Category Angiotensin II Receptor Blocker; Antianginal Agent; Antihypertensive; Calcium Channel Blocker; Calcium Channel Blocker, Dihydropyridine
Use Treatment of hypertension
Dosing
Adult Note: Dose is individualized; combination product may be used as initial therapy or substituted for individual components in patients currently maintained on both agents separately or in patients not adequately controlled with monotherapy (using one of the agents or an agent within same antihypertensive class).
Hypertension: Oral:
Initial therapy: Amlodipine 5 mg and valsartan 160 mg once daily, dose may be titrated after 1-2 weeks of therapy. Maximum recommended doses: Amlodipine 10 mg daily; valsartan 320 mg daily
Add-on/replacement therapy: Amlodipine 5-10 mg and valsartan 160-320 mg once daily; dose may be titrated after 3-4 weeks of therapy. Maximum recommended doses: Amlodipine 10 mg daily; valsartan 320 mg daily
Geriatric Refer to adult dosing. Use of lower initial doses should be considered.
Renal Impairment
CrCl ≥30 mL/minute: No dosage adjustment necessary.
CrCl <30 mL/minute: No dosage adjustment provided in manufacturer's labeling; safety and efficacy has not been established.
Hepatic Impairment
Mild-to-moderate impairment: Use with caution; amlodipine elimination prolonged and valsartan exposure doubled in patients with mild-to-moderate chronic disease compared to healthy volunteers. No dosage adjustment for valsartan is necessary; however, a lower initial amlodipine dose may be required (possibly requiring use of the individual agents).
Severe impairment: No dosage adjustment provided in manufacturer's labeling; however, similar to patients with mild to moderate impairment, a lower initial amlodipine dose may be required (possibly requiring use of the individual agents); titrate slowly.
Additional Information Complete prescribing information should be consulted for additional detail.
Dosage Forms Excipient information presented when available (limited, particularly for generics); consult specific product labeling.
Tablet, Oral:
Exforge:
5/160: Amlodipine 5 mg and valsartan 160 mg
5/320: Amlodipine 5 mg and valsartan 320 mg
10/160: Amlodipine 10 mg and valsartan 160 mg
10/320: Amlodipine 10 mg and valsartan 320 mg
Generic:
5/160: Amlodipine 5 mg and valsartan 160 mg
5/320: Amlodipine 5 mg and valsartan 320 mg
10/160: Amlodipine 10 mg and valsartan 160 mg
10/320: Amlodipine 10 mg and valsartan 320 mg

◆ Amlodipine Besylate *see* AmLODIPine *on page 101*
◆ Amlodipine Besylate, Aliskiren Hemifumarate, and Hydrochlorothiazide *see* Aliskiren, Amlodipine, and Hydrochlorothiazide *on page 72*
◆ Amlodipine Besylate and Olmesartan Medoxomil *see* Amlodipine and Olmesartan *on page 104*
◆ Amlodipine Besylate and Telmisartan *see* Telmisartan and Amlodipine *on page 1748*
◆ Amlodipine Besylate and Valsartan *see* Amlodipine and Valsartan *on page 105*

◆ Amlodipine Besylate, Olmesartan Medoxomil, and Hydrochlorothiazide *see* Olmesartan, Amlodipine, and Hydrochlorothiazide *on page 1321*
◆ Amlodipine Besylate, Valsartan, and Hydrochlorothiazide *see* Amlodipine, Valsartan, and Hydrochlorothiazide *on page 105*
◆ Amlodipine, Hydrochlorothiazide, and Aliskiren *see* Aliskiren, Amlodipine, and Hydrochlorothiazide *on page 72*
◆ Amlodipine, Hydrochlorothiazide, and Olmesartan *see* Olmesartan, Amlodipine, and Hydrochlorothiazide *on page 1321*
◆ Amlodipine, Hydrochlorothiazide, and Valsartan *see* Amlodipine, Valsartan, and Hydrochlorothiazide *on page 105*
◆ Amlodipine-Odan (Can) *see* AmLODIPine *on page 101*

Amlodipine, Valsartan, and Hydrochlorothiazide
(am LOE di peen, val SAR tan, & hye droe klor oh THYE a zide)

Brand Names: US Exforge HCT®
Index Terms Amlodipine Besylate, Valsartan, and Hydrochlorothiazide; Amlodipine, Hydrochlorothiazide, and Valsartan; Hydrochlorothiazide, Amlodipine, and Valsartan; Valsartan, Hydrochlorothiazide, and Amlodipine
Pharmacologic Category Angiotensin II Receptor Blocker; Antianginal Agent; Antihypertensive; Calcium Channel Blocker; Calcium Channel Blocker, Dihydropyridine; Diuretic, Thiazide
Use Treatment of hypertension (not for initial therapy)
Dosing
Adult Note: Not for initial therapy. Dose is individualized; combination product may be substituted for individual components in patients currently maintained on all three agents separately or in patients not adequately controlled with any two of the following antihypertensive classes: Calcium channel blockers, angiotensin II receptor blockers, and diuretics.

Hypertension: Oral: Add-on/switch/replacement therapy: Amlodipine 5-10 mg and valsartan 160-320 mg and hydrochlorothiazide 12.5-25 mg once daily; dose may be titrated after 2 weeks of therapy. Maximum recommended daily dose: Amlodipine 10 mg/valsartan 320 mg/hydrochlorothiazide 25 mg
Geriatric Refer to adult dosing. Use of lower initial doses should be considered.
Renal Impairment
CrCl ≥30 mL/minute: No dosage adjustment necessary.
CrCl <30 mL/minute: No dosage adjustment provided in manufacturer's labeling; safety and efficacy has not been established; hydrochlorothiazide is usually ineffective when CrCl <30 mL/minute and is contraindicated in patients who are anuric.
Hepatic Impairment
Mild-to-moderate impairment: Use with caution; amlodipine elimination prolonged and valsartan exposure doubled in patients with mild-to-moderate chronic disease compared to healthy volunteers. No dosage adjustment for valsartan is necessary; however, a lower initial amlodipine dose may be required (possibly requiring use of the individual agents).
Severe impairment: No dosage adjustment provided in manufacturer's labeling; however, similar to patients with mild to moderate impairment, a lower initial amlodipine dose may be required (possibly requiring use of the individual agents); titrate slowly.
Additional Information Complete prescribing information should be consulted for additional detail.
Dosage Forms Excipient information presented when available (limited, particularly for generics); consult specific product labeling.
Tablet, oral:
Exforge HCT:
Amlodipine 5 mg, valsartan 160 mg, and hydrochlorothiazide 12.5 mg
Amlodipine 5 mg, valsartan 160 mg, and hydrochlorothiazide 25 mg
Amlodipine 10 mg, valsartan 160 mg, and hydrochlorothiazide 12.5 mg
Amlodipine 10 mg, valsartan 160 mg, and hydrochlorothiazide 25 mg
Amlodipine 10 mg, valsartan 320 mg, and hydrochlorothiazide 25 mg

Generic:
Amlodipine 5 mg, valsartan 160 mg, and hydrochlorothiazide 12.5 mg
Amlodipine 5 mg, valsartan 160 mg, and hydrochlorothiazide 25 mg
Amlodipine 10 mg, valsartan 160 mg, and hydrochlorothiazide 12.5 mg
Amlodipine 10 mg, valsartan 160 mg, and hydrochlorothiazide 25 mg
Amlodipine 10 mg, valsartan 320 mg, and hydrochlorothiazide 25 mg

◆ Ammens® Original Medicated [OTC] *see* Zinc Oxide
on page 1929

◆ Ammens® Shower Fresh [OTC] *see* Zinc Oxide
on page 1929

◆ Ammonapse *see* Sodium Phenylbutyrate *on page 1677*

Ammonium Chloride (a MOE nee um KLOR ide)

Pharmacologic Category Electrolyte Supplement,
Parenteral
Use Treatment of hypochloremic states or metabolic alka-
losis
Dosing
Adult & Geriatric The following equations represent
different methods of correction utilizing either the body
chloride deficit or the body bicarbonate (HCO_3-) excess.
**These equations will yield different requirements of
ammonium chloride (NH_4Cl).**

**Dosing of mEq NH_4Cl via the chloride-deficit method
(hypochloremia) (Abouna 1974; Devlin 2014; Martin
1982):**
Dose of mEq NH_4Cl = [0.2 L/kg x body weight (kg)] x
[103 - observed serum chloride]; administer either
50% of the calculated dose over 12 to 24 hours **or**
the entire calculated dose over 12 to 24 hours, then re-
evaluate.
Note: 0.2 L/kg is the estimated chloride volume of
distribution and 103 is the average normal serum
chloride concentration (mEq/L)
**Dosing of mEq NH_4Cl via the bicarbonate-excess
method (refractory hypochloremic metabolic alkalosis) (Abouna 1974; Martin 1982):**
Dose of mEq NH_4Cl = [0.5 L/kg x body weight (kg)] x
(observed serum HCO_3^- - 24); administer 50% of dose
over 12 to 24 hours, then re-evaluate
Note: 0.5 L/kg is the estimated bicarbonate volume of
distribution and 24 is the average normal serum
bicarbonate concentration (mEq/L)
Pediatric Metabolic alkalosis: Refer to adult dosing.
Renal Impairment
Mild-to-moderate impairment: There are no dosage
adjustments provided in the manufacturer's labeling;
use with caution.
Severe impairment: Use is contraindicated.
Hepatic Impairment
Mild-to-moderate impairment: There are no dosage
adjustments provided in the manufacturer's labeling;
use with caution.
Severe impairment: Use is contraindicated.
Additional Information Complete prescribing information
should be consulted for additional detail.
Dosage Forms Excipient information presented when
available (limited, particularly for generics); consult specific
product labeling.
Injection, solution: Ammonium 5 mEq/mL and chloride 5
mEq/mL (20 mL) [equivalent to ammonium chloride
267.5 mg/mL]

◆ Ammonul *see* Sodium Phenylacetate and Sodium Benzoate *on page 1676*

◆ AMN107 *see* Nilotinib *on page 1282*

◆ Amnesteem *see* ISOtretinoin *on page 996*

Amobarbital (am oh BAR bi tal)

Brand Names: US Amytal Sodium
Index Terms Amobarbital Sodium; Amylobarbitone
Pharmacologic Category Barbiturate
Use Sedative/hypnotic: Use as a sedative, hypnotic, or
preanesthetic
Dosing
Adult
Hypnotic: IM, IV: 65 to 200 mg at bedtime (maximum
single dose: 1,000 mg)
Sedative: IM, IV: 30 to 50 mg 2 or 3 times daily (max-
imum single dose: 1,000 mg)

"Amytal interview" (off-label use): IV: 50 to 100 mg/mi-
nute for total dose of 200 to 1,000 mg or until patient
experiences drowsiness, impaired attention, slurred
speech, or nystagmus (Kavirajan 1999)
Wada test (off-label use): Intra-carotid: 60 to 200 mg
(usual dose: 125 mg) over 2 to 5 seconds via percutaneous transfemoral catheter; after 30 to 45 minutes has
elapsed since completion of first injection, may repeat
dose for evaluation of contralateral hemisphere
(Acharya 1997; Patel 2011). **Note:** Due to the adverse
effects associated with intra-carotid amobarbital and
questionable reliability and validity, other less invasive
tests (eg, functional MRI) may be recommended
(Sharan 2011).
Geriatric Avoid use due to risk of overdose with low
dosages, tolerance to sleep effects, and increased risk
of physical dependence (Beers Criteria).
Pediatric Sedative, hypnotic: Children ≥6 years and
Adolescents: IM (preferred), IV: 2 to 3 mg/kg/dose; maximum dose: 500 mg/dose (AHFS 2015; McEvoy 1993;
Nelson 1996). The manufacturer describes the ordinary
dose range in children 6 to 12 years as 65 to 500 mg and
specific dosing recommendations based on patient size
are not available; however, in several instances, this may
exceed expert weight-based recommendations; if using
manufacturer dosing, initiate therapy at the lower end of
the range and titrate the dose accordingly.
Renal Impairment There are no dosage adjustments
provided in the manufacturer's labeling; reduced doses
are recommended.
Hepatic Impairment There are no dosage adjustments
provided in the manufacturer's labeling; reduced doses
are recommended.
Additional Information Complete prescribing information
should be consulted for additional detail.
Dosage Forms Excipient information presented when
available (limited, particularly for generics); consult specific
product labeling.
Solution Reconstituted, Injection, as sodium:
Amytal Sodium: 500 mg (1 ea)
Controlled Substance C-II

◆ Amobarbital Sodium *see* Amobarbital *on page 106*

◆ Amoclan *see* Amoxicillin and Clavulanate *on page 111*

Amoxapine (a MOKS a peen)

Index Terms Asendin [DSC]
Pharmacologic Category Antidepressant, Tricyclic (Secondary Amine)
Use Depression: For the relief of symptoms of depression
in patients with neurotic or reactive depressive disorders
as well as endogenous and psychotic depressions; for
depression accompanied by anxiety or agitation.
Pregnancy Considerations Adverse events were
observed in some animal reproduction studies. Tricyclic
antidepressants may be associated with irritability, jitteriness, and convulsions (rare) in the neonate (Yonkers,
2009).

The ACOG recommends that therapy for depression during pregnancy be individualized; treatment should incorporate the clinical expertise of the mental health clinician,
obstetrician, primary healthcare provider, and pediatrician
(ACOG, 2008). According to the American Psychiatric
Association (APA), the risks of medication treatment
should be weighed against other treatment options and
untreated depression. For women who discontinue antidepressant medications during pregnancy and who may
be at high risk for postpartum depression, the medications
can be restarted following delivery (APA, 2010). Treatment
algorithms have been developed by the ACOG and the
APA for the management of depression in women prior to
conception and during pregnancy (Yonkers, 2009).
Breast-Feeding Considerations Amoxapine is excreted
into breast milk. A case report notes low concentrations of
amoxapine and its active metabolite in the milk of a non-
nursing woman who developed galactorrhea during therapy (Gelenberg, 1979). The manufacturer recommends
that caution be used if administered to a nursing woman.
Medication Guide Available Yes
Contraindications Hypersensitivity to amoxapine, any
component of the formulation, or dibenzoxazepine compounds; use with or within 14 days of MAO inhibitors;
acute recovery phase following myocardial infarction
**Warnings/Precautions [U.S. Boxed Warning]: Antide-
pressants increase the risk of suicidal thinking and
behavior in children, adolescents, and young adults
(18 to 24 years of age) with major depressive disorder
(MDD) and other psychiatric disorders;** consider risk
prior to prescribing. Short-term studies did not show an
increased risk in patients >24 years of age and showed a

decreased risk in patients ≥65 years. Closely monitor for clinical worsening, suicidality, or unusual changes in behavior, particularly during the initial 1 to 2 months of therapy or during periods of dosage adjustments (increases or decreases); the patient's family or caregiver should be instructed to closely observe the patient and communicate condition with healthcare provider. A medication guide should be dispensed with each prescription. **Amoxapine is not FDA approved for use in pediatric patients.**

The possibility of a suicide attempt is inherent in major depression and may persist until remission occurs. Use caution in high-risk patients. Worsening depression and severe abrupt suicidality that are not part of the presenting symptoms may require discontinuation or modification of drug therapy. The patient's family or caregiver should be alerted to monitor patients for the emergence of suicidality and associated behaviors (such as agitation, irritability, hostility, impulsivity, and hypomania) and notify the healthcare provider.

May precipitate a shift to mania or hypomania in patients with bipolar disorder. Patients presenting with depressive symptoms should be screened for bipolar disorder. Monotherapy in patients with bipolar disorder should be avoided. Patients presenting with depressive symptoms should be screened for bipolar disorder, including details regarding family history of suicide, bipolar disorder, and depression. **Amoxapine is not FDA approved for bipolar depression.** May cause extrapyramidal symptoms, including pseudoparkinsonism, acute dystonic reactions, akathisia, and tardive dyskinesia (risk of these reactions is low). Risk of dystonia (and possibly other EPS) may be greater with increased doses, use of conventional antipsychotics, males, and younger patients (APA, 2004). Risk of tardive dyskinesia (potentially irreversible) is often associated with total cumulative dose, therapy duration, and may also be increased in elderly patients (particularly elderly women); antipsychotics may also mask signs/symptoms of tardive dyskinesia. Therapy should be discontinued in any patient if signs/symptoms of tardive dyskinesia appear. May be associated with neuroleptic malignant syndrome.

May cause anticholinergic effects (constipation, xerostomia, blurred vision, urinary retention; use with caution in patients with decreased gastrointestinal motility, paralytic ileus, urinary retention, BPH, xerostomia, or visual problems. The degree of anticholinergic blockade produced by this agent is high relative to other antidepressants (Bauer, 2013). May cause CNS depression, which may impair physical or mental abilities; patients must be cautioned about performing tasks that require mental alertness (eg, operating machinery or driving). The degree of sedation is moderate relative to other antidepressants (Bauer, 2013). Use with caution in patients with a history of cardiovascular disease (including previous MI, stroke, tachycardia, or conduction abnormalities). May lower seizure threshold; use caution in patients with a previous seizure disorder or condition predisposing to seizures such as brain damage, alcoholism, or concurrent therapy with other drugs which lower the seizure threshold (APA, 2010). May increase the risks associated with electroconvulsive therapy. Bone fractures have been associated with antidepressant treatment. Consider the possibility of a fragility fracture if an antidepressant-treated patient presents with unexplained bone pain, point tenderness, swelling, or bruising (Rabenda, 2013; Rizzoli, 2012). Use with caution in patients with diabetes mellitus; may alter glucose regulation (APA, 2010).

May cause mild pupillary dilation which in susceptible individuals can lead to an episode of narrow-angle glaucoma. Consider evaluating patients who have not had an iridectomy for narrow-angle glaucoma risk factors. Use caution in elderly patients; may cause or exacerbate syndrome of inappropriate antidiuretic hormone secretion or hyponatremia; monitor sodium closely with initiation or dosage adjustments in older adults. May be inappropriate in older adults depending on comorbidities (eg, dementia, delirium, or in patients with a history of falls and fractures due to its potent anticholinergic effects (Beers Criteria). May also have increased risk of adverse events, including tardive dyskinesia (particularly older women) and sedation. Potentially significant interactions may exist, requiring dose or frequency adjustment, additional monitoring, and/ or selection of alternative therapy.

Abrupt discontinuation or interruption of antidepressant therapy has been associated with a discontinuation syndrome. Symptoms arising may vary with antidepressant however commonly include nausea, vomiting, diarrhea, headaches, lightheadedness, dizziness, diminished appetite, sweating, chills, tremors, paresthesias, fatigue, somnolence, and sleep disturbances (eg, vivid dreams,

insomnia). Greater risks for developing a discontinuation syndrome have been associated with antidepressants with shorter half-lives, longer durations of treatment, and abrupt discontinuation. For antidepressants of short or intermediate half-lives, symptoms may emerge within 2 to 5 days after treatment discontinuation and last 7 to 14 days (APA, 2010; Fava, 2006; Haddad, 2001; Shelton, 2001; Warner, 2006).

Adverse Reactions

>10%:
Central nervous system: Drowsiness (14%)
Gastrointestinal: Xerostomia (14%), constipation (12%)

1% to 10%:
Cardiovascular: Edema, palpitations
Central nervous system: Anxiety, ataxia, confusion, dizziness, EEG pattern changes, excitement, fatigue, headache, insomnia, nervousness, nightmares, restlessness
Dermatologic: Diaphoresis, skin rash
Endocrine & metabolic: Increased serum prolactin
Gastrointestinal: Increased appetite, nausea
Neuromuscular & skeletal: Tremor, weakness
Ophthalmic: Blurred vision (7%)

<1% (Limited to important or life-threatening): Accommodation disturbance, agranulocytosis, alopecia, altered serum glucose, anorexia, atrial arrhythmia, diarrhea, extrapyramidal reaction, galactorrhea, hallucination, heart block, hepatic insufficiency, hepatitis, hypersensitivity reaction, hypomania, impotence, increased intraocular pressure, lack of concentration, menstrual disease, mydriasis, myocardial infarction, neuroleptic malignant syndrome, numbness, painful ejaculation, pancreatitis, paralytic ileus, paresthesia, parotid swelling, petechia, purpura, SIADH, skin photosensitivity, syncope, tardive dyskinesia, testicular swelling, thrombocytopenia, tingling sensation, tinnitus, urinary retention, vasculitis, vomiting, weight gain

Drug Interactions

Metabolism/Transport Effects Substrate of CYP2D6 (major); **Note:** Assignment of Major/Minor substrate status based on clinically relevant drug interaction potential

Avoid Concomitant Use
Avoid concomitant use of Amoxapine with any of the following: Aclidinium; Azelastine (Nasal); Cimetropium; Dapoxetine; Dronedarone; Eluxadoline; Glucagon; Glycopyrrolate; Glycopyrrolate (Oral Inhalation); Iobenguane I 123; Ipratropium (Oral Inhalation); Levosulpiride; Linezolid; MAO Inhibitors; Methylene Blue; Moxonidine; Orphenadrine; Paraldehyde; Potassium Chloride; Thalidomide; Tiotropium; Umeclidinium

Increased Effect/Toxicity
Amoxapine may increase the levels/effects of: AbobotulinumtoxinA; Alcohol (Ethyl); Alpha-/Beta-Agonists (Direct-Acting); Alpha1-Agonists; Amphetamines; Analgesics (Opioid); Anticholinergic Agents; Antipsychotic Agents; Azelastine (Nasal); Beta2-Agonists; Buprenorphine; Cimetropium; Citalopram; CNS Depressants; Desmopressin; Dronedarone; Eluxadoline; Escitalopram; Glucagon; Glycopyrrolate; Glycopyrrolate (Oral Inhalation); Highest Risk QTc-Prolonging Agents; Hydrocodone; Methotrimeprazine; Methylene Blue; Metyrosine; Mirabegron; Moderate Risk QTc-Prolonging Agents; Nicorandil; OnabotulinumtoxinA; Orphenadrine; Paraldehyde; Potassium Chloride; Pramipexole; QuiNIDine; Ramosetron; RimabotulinumtoxinB; ROPINIRole; Rotigotine; Serotonin Modulators; Sodium Phosphates; Sulfonylureas; Suvorexant; Thalidomide; Thiazide Diuretics; Tiotropium; Topiramate; TraMADol; Vitamin K Antagonists; Yohimbine; Zolpidem

The levels/effects of Amoxapine may be increased by: Abiraterone Acetate; Aclidinium; Altretamine; Antiemetics (5HT3 Antagonists); Antipsychotic Agents; Brimonidine (Topical); Cannabis; Cimetidine; Cinacalcet; Citalopram; Cobicistat; CYP2D6 Inhibitors (Moderate); CYP2D6 Inhibitors (Strong); Dapoxetine; Darunavir; Dexmethylphenidate; Doxylamine; Dronabinol; Droperidol; DULoxetine; Escitalopram; FLUoxetine; FluvoxaMINE; HydrOXYzine; Ipratropium (Oral Inhalation); Kava Kava; Linezolid; Lithium; Magnesium Sulfate; MAO Inhibitors; Metaxalone; Methotrimeprazine; Methylphenidate; Metoclopramide; Metyrosine; Mianserin; Mifepristone; Minocycline; Nabilone; Panobinostat; PARoxetine; Peginterferon Alfa-2b; Perampanel; Pramlintide; Protease Inhibitors; QuiNIDine; Rufinamide; Sertraline; Sodium Oxybate; Tapentadol; Tedizolid; Tetrahydrocannabinol; Thyroid Products; TraMADol; Umeclidinium; Valproate Products

Decreased Effect
Amoxapine may decrease the levels/effects of: Acetylcholinesterase Inhibitors; Alpha1-Agonists; Alpha2-Agonists; Alpha2-Agonists (Ophthalmic); Gastrointestinal Agents (Prokinetic); Iobenguane I 123; Ioflupane I 123; Itopride; Levosulpiride; Moxonidine; Secretin

The levels/effects of Amoxapine may be decreased by: Acetylcholinesterase Inhibitors; Barbiturates; CarBAMazepine; Peginterferon Alfa-2b; St Johns Wort

Storage/Stability Store at 20°C to 25°C (68°F to 77°F).

Mechanism of Action Reduces the reuptake of serotonin and norepinephrine. The metabolite, 7-OH-amoxapine has significant dopamine receptor blocking activity similar to antipsychotic agents.

Pharmacodynamics/Kinetics

Onset of antidepressant effect: Usually occurs after 1 to 2 weeks, but may require 4 to 6 weeks

Absorption: Rapid and well absorbed

Distribution: V_d: 0.9 to 1.2 L/kg

Protein binding: ~90%

Metabolism: Extensively metabolized; hepatic hydroxylation produces two active metabolites, 7-hydroxyamoxapine (7-OH-amoxapine) and 8-hydroxyamoxapine (8-OH-amoxapine); metabolites undergo conjugation to form glucuronides

Half-life elimination: 8 hours; 8-hydroxyamoxapine metabolite: 30 hours

Time to peak, serum: ~90 minutes

Excretion: Urine

Dosing

Adult Depression: Oral: Initial: 50 mg once to 3 times daily. Doses may be increased to 100 mg 2 to 3 times daily by the end of the first week based on response and tolerability; if 300 mg daily has been reached and maintained for at least 2 weeks and no response is observed, may further increase to 400 mg daily. Hospitalized patients refractory to antidepressant therapy (and no history of seizures) may be cautiously titrated to 600 mg daily in divided doses. Usual dosage: 100 to 400 mg daily (Bauer, 2013). Once an effective dose is reached, doses ≤300 mg may be given once daily at bedtime and doses >300 mg daily should be divided. Maximum daily dose: 400 mg outpatient; 600 mg hospitalized patients.

Discontinuation of therapy: Upon discontinuation of antidepressant therapy, gradually taper the dose to minimize the incidence of withdrawal symptoms and allow for the detection of re-emerging symptoms. Evidence supporting ideal taper rates is limited. APA and NICE guidelines suggest tapering therapy over at least several weeks with consideration to the half-life of the antidepressant; antidepressants with a shorter half-life may need to be tapered more conservatively. In addition for long-term treated patients, WFSBP guidelines recommend tapering over 4 to 6 months. If intolerable withdrawal symptoms occur following a dose reduction, consider resuming the previously prescribed dose and/or decrease dose at a more gradual rate (APA, 2010; Bauer, 2002; Haddad, 2001; NCCMH, 2010; Schatzberg, 2006; Shelton, 2001; Warner 2006).

MAO inhibitor recommendations:

Switching to or from an MAO inhibitor intended to treat psychiatric disorders:

Allow 14 days to elapse between discontinuing an MAO inhibitor intended to treat psychiatric disorders and initiation of amoxapine.

Allow 14 days to elapse between discontinuing amoxapine and initiation of an MAO inhibitor intended to treat psychiatric disorders.

Use with reversible MAO inhibitors (such as linezolid or IV methylene blue):

Do not initiate amoxapine in patients receiving linezolid or IV methylene blue; consider other interventions for psychiatric condition.

If urgent treatment with linezolid or IV methylene blue is required in a patient already receiving amoxapine and potential benefits outweigh potential risks, discontinue amoxapine promptly and administer linezolid or IV methylene blue. Monitor for serotonin syndrome for 2 weeks or until 24 hours after the last dose of linezolid or IV methylene blue, whichever comes first. May resume amoxapine 24 hours after the last dose of linezolid or IV methylene blue.

Geriatric Depression: Oral: Initial: 25 mg 2 to 3 times daily. Dose may be increased to 50 mg 2 to 3 times daily by the end of the first week based on response and tolerability; if dose is ineffective, may further increase cautiously to 300 mg daily. Usual dosage: 100 to 150 mg daily. Once an effective dose is reached, doses ≤300 mg may be given once daily at bedtime. Maximum daily dose: 300 mg.

Discontinuation of therapy: Refer to adult dosing.

MAO inhibitor recommendations: Refer to adult dosing.

Renal Impairment There are no dosage adjustments provided in manufacturer's labeling. However, amoxapine is primarily eliminated renally, and renal failure may develop in overdoses; use with caution.

Hepatic Impairment There are no dosage adjustments provided in manufacturer's labeling.

Monitoring Parameters Evaluate mental status, suicide ideation (especially at the beginning of therapy or when doses are increased or decreased); anxiety, social functioning, mania, panic attacks, or other unusual changes in behavior; heart rate, blood pressure, and ECG in older adults and patients with preexisting cardiac disease; blood glucose; weight and BMI (APA, 2010).

Additional Information Extrapyramidal reactions and tardive dyskinesia may occur.

Dosage Forms Excipient information presented when available (limited, particularly for generics); consult specific product labeling.

Tablet, Oral:

Generic: 25 mg, 50 mg, 100 mg, 150 mg

Amoxicillin (a moks i SIL in)

Brand Names: US Moxatag

Brand Names: Canada Apo-Amoxi; Mylan-Amoxicillin; Novamoxin; NTP-Amoxicillin; Nu-Amoxi; PHL-Amoxicillin; PMS-Amoxicillin; Pro-Amox-250; Pro-Amox-500

Index Terms *p*-Hydroxyampicillin; Amoxicillin Trihydrate; Amoxil; Amoxycillin

Pharmacologic Category Antibiotic, Penicillin

Use

Ear, nose, and throat infection (pharyngitis/tonsillitis, otitis media, rhinosinusitis): Immediate-release: Treatment of infections due to beta-lactamase-negative *Streptococcus* spp (alpha- and beta-hemolytic isolates only), *Streptococcus pneumoniae*, *Staphylococcus* spp., or *Haemophilus influenzae*.

GU tract infections: Immediate-release: Treatment of infections of the GU tract due to beta-lactamase-negative *Escherichia coli*, *Proteus mirabilis*, or *Enterobacter faecalis*.

***Helicobacter pylori* infections (with active or 1 year history of duodenal ulcer disease):** Immediate-release: Eradication of *H. pylori* to reduce the risk of duodenal ulcer recurrence as a component of combination therapy (triple or dual therapy as clinically indicated).

Lower respiratory tract infections (including pneumonia): Immediate-release: Treatment of infections of the lower respiratory tract due to beta-lactamase-negative *Streptococcus* spp. (alpha- and beta-hemolytic strains only), *Streptococcus pneumoniae*, *Staphylococcus* spp., or *H. influenzae*.

Pharyngitis and tonsillitis: Extended-release tablets: Treatment of tonsillitis and/or pharyngitis due to *Streptococcus pyogenes* in adults and children 12 years of age and older.

Skin and skin structure infections: Immediate-release: Treatment of infections of the skin and skin structure due to beta-lactamase-negative *Streptococcus* spp. (alpha- and beta-hemolytic strains only), *Staphylococcus* spp., or *E. coli*.

Pregnancy Considerations Adverse events have not been observed in animal reproduction studies. Maternal use of amoxicillin has generally not resulted in an increased risk of adverse fetal effects; however, an increased risk of cleft lip with cleft palate has been observed in some studies. It is the drug of choice for the treatment of chlamydial infections in pregnancy and for anthrax prophylaxis when penicillin susceptibility is documented. Amoxicillin may be used in certain situations prior to vaginal delivery in women at high risk for endocarditis.

Due to pregnancy-induced physiologic changes, oral amoxicillin clearance is increased during pregnancy resulting in lower concentrations and smaller AUCs. Oral ampicillin-class antibiotics are poorly absorbed during labor.

Breast-Feeding Considerations Very small amounts of amoxicillin are excreted in breast milk. The manufacturer recommends that caution be exercised when administering amoxicillin to nursing women. Nondose-related effects could include modification of bowel flora and allergic sensitization of the infant.

Contraindications Serious hypersensitivity to amoxicillin (eg, anaphylaxis, Stevens-Johnson syndrome) or to other beta-lactams, or any component of the formulation

Warnings/Precautions In patients with renal impairment, doses and/or frequency of administration should be modified in response to the degree of renal impairment; in addition, use of certain dosage forms (eg, extended release 775 mg tablet and immediate release 875 mg tablet) should be avoided in patients with CrCl <30 mL/minute or patients requiring hemodialysis. A high

percentage of patients with infectious mononucleosis develop an erythematous rash during amoxicillin therapy; avoid use in these patients. Serious and occasionally severe or fatal hypersensitivity (anaphylactic) reactions have been reported in patients on penicillin therapy, including amoxicillin, especially with a history of beta-lactam hypersensitivity (including severe reactions with cephalosporins) and/or a history of sensitivity to multiple allergens. Prolonged use may result in fungal or bacterial superinfection, including *C. difficile*-associated diarrhea (CDAD) and pseudomembranous colitis; CDAD has been observed >2 months postantibiotic treatment. Potentially significant interactions may exist, requiring dose or frequency adjustment, additional monitoring, and/or selection of alternative therapy.

Chewable tablets may contain phenylalanine; see manufacturer's labeling.

Benzyl alcohol and derivatives: Some dosage forms may contain sodium benzoate/benzoic acid; benzoic acid (benzoate) is a metabolite of benzyl alcohol; large amounts of benzyl alcohol (≥99 mg/kg/day) have been associated with a potentially fatal toxicity ("gasping syndrome") in neonates; the "gasping syndrome" consists of metabolic acidosis, respiratory distress, gasping respirations, CNS dysfunction (including convulsions, intracranial hemorrhage), hypotension, and cardiovascular collapse (AAP ["Inactive" 1997]; CDC 1982); some data suggest that benzoate displaces bilirubin from protein binding sites (Ahlfors 2001); avoid or use dosage forms containing benzyl alcohol derivative with caution in neonates. See manufacturer's labeling.

Adverse Reactions Frequency not defined.
Cardiovascular: Hypersensitivity angiitis
Central nervous system: Agitation, anxiety, behavioral changes, confusion, dizziness, headache, hyperactivity (reversible), insomnia, seizure
Dermatologic: Acute generalized exanthematous pustulosis, erythematous maculopapular rash, erythema multiforme, exfoliative dermatitis, Stevens-Johnson syndrome, toxic epidermal necrolysis, urticaria
Gastrointestinal: Dental discoloration (brown, yellow, or gray; rare), diarrhea, hemorrhagic colitis, melanoglossia, mucocutaneous candidiasis, nausea, pseudomembranous colitis, vomiting
Genitourinary: Crystalluria
Hematologic & oncologic: Agranulocytosis, anemia, eosinophilia, hemolytic anemia, leukopenia, thrombocytopenia, thrombocytopenia purpura
Hepatic: Cholestatic hepatitis, cholestatic jaundice, hepatitis (acute cytolytic), increased serum ALT, increased serum AST
Hypersensitivity: Anaphylaxis
Immunologic: Serum sickness-like reaction

Drug Interactions
Metabolism/Transport Effects None known.
Avoid Concomitant Use
Avoid concomitant use of Amoxicillin with any of the following: BCG (Intravesical); Probenecid
Increased Effect/Toxicity
Amoxicillin may increase the levels/effects of: Methotrexate; Vitamin K Antagonists

The levels/effects of Amoxicillin may be increased by: Allopurinol; Probenecid
Decreased Effect
Amoxicillin may decrease the levels/effects of: BCG (Intravesical); BCG Vaccine (Immunization); Mycophenolate; Sodium Picosulfate; Typhoid Vaccine

The levels/effects of Amoxicillin may be decreased by: Tetracycline Derivatives
Storage/Stability
Amoxicillin 250 mg and 500 mg capsules, and 125 mg/5 mL and 250 mg/5 mL unreconstituted powder: Store at or below 20°C (68°F).
Amoxicillin 500 mg and 875 mg tablets, and 200 mg/5 mL and 400 mg/5mL unreconstituted powder: Store at or below 25°C (77°F).
Amoxil: Reconstituted oral suspension remains stable for 14 days at room temperature or if refrigerated (refrigeration preferred). Unit-dose antibiotic oral syringes are stable at room temperature for at least 72 hours (Tu 1988).
Moxatag: Store at 25°C (77°F); excursions permitted to 15°C to 30°C (59°F to 86°F).
Mechanism of Action Inhibits bacterial cell wall synthesis by binding to one or more of the penicillin-binding proteins (PBPs) which in turn inhibits the final transpeptidation step of peptidoglycan synthesis in bacterial cell walls, thus inhibiting cell wall biosynthesis. Bacteria eventually lyse due to ongoing activity of cell wall autolytic enzymes (autolysins and murein hydrolases) while cell wall assembly is arrested.

Pharmacodynamics/Kinetics
Absorption: Oral: Rapid and nearly complete (74% to 92% of a single dose is absorbed); food does not interfere
Extended-release tablet: Rate of absorption is slower compared to immediate-release formulations; food decreases the rate but not extent of absorption
Distribution: Readily into liver, lungs, prostate, muscle, middle ear effusions, maxillary sinus secretions, bone, gallbladder, bile, and into ascitic and synovial fluids; poor CSF penetration (except when meninges are inflamed)
CSF:blood level ratio: Normal meninges: <1%; Inflamed meninges: 8% to 90%
Protein binding: 17% to 20%, lower in neonates
Metabolism: Partially hepatic
Half-life elimination:
Neonates, full-term: 3.7 hours
Infants and Children: 1 to 2 hours
Adults: Normal renal function: 0.7 to 1.4 hours
CrCl <10 mL/minute: 7 to 21 hours
Time to peak: Capsule: 2 hours; Extended-release tablet: 3.1 hours; Suspension: Neonates: 3 to 4.5 hour, Children: 1 hour
Excretion: Urine (60% as unchanged drug); lower in neonates

Note: Extended-release tablets: In healthy volunteers, serum drug concentrations were below 0.25 mcg/mL and undetectable at 16 hours following dosing.
Dosing
Adult & Geriatric
Usual dosage range: Oral:
Mild or moderate infection: 250 every 8 hours or 500 mg every 12 hours
Mild or moderate infection (lower respiratory tract): 500 mg every 8 hours or 875 mg every 12 hours
Severe infection (as step-down therapy):
Immediate-release: 500 mg every 8 hours or 875 mg every 12 hours
Extended-release: 775 mg once daily

Indication-specific dosing:
Anthrax, inhalational prophylaxis (ACIP recommendations): Oral: 500 mg every 8 hours. **Note:** Use only if isolates of the specific *B. anthracis* are sensitive to amoxicillin (MIC ≤0.125 mcg/mL); may be administered to pregnant and breast-feeding women. Duration of antibiotic postexposure prophylaxis (PEP) is ≥60 days in a previously unvaccinated exposed person. Antimicrobial therapy should continue for 14 days after the third dose of PEP vaccine. Those who are partially or fully vaccinated should receive at least a 30-day course of antimicrobial PEP and continue with licensed vaccination regimen. Unvaccinated workers, even those wearing personal protective equipment with adequate respiratory protection, should receive antimicrobial PEP. Antimicrobial PEP is not required for fully vaccinated people (five-dose IM vaccination series with a yearly booster) who enter an anthrax area clothed in personal protective equipment. If respiratory protection is disrupted, a 30-day course of antimicrobial therapy is recommended (ACIP 2010).
Chlamydial infection during pregnancy (off-label use): Oral: 500 mg 3 times/day for 7 days (CDC 2010)
Ear, nose, throat, genitourinary tract, or skin/skin structure infections: Note: IDSA guidelines recommend amoxicillin-clavulanate as preferred first-line treatment of acute bacterial rhinosinusitis (ABRS)(IDSA [Chow 2012]); AAO-HNS guidelines for adult sinusitis recommend either amoxicillin or amoxicillin-clavulanate as initial first-line therapy of ABRS, with consideration given for amoxicillin-clavulanate instead of amoxicillin in certain patients (eg, moderate to severe ABRS symptoms, antibiotic use in past month, high prevalence of resistant bacteria in community, history of recurrent ABRS, presence of comorbidities) (AAO-HNS [Rosenfeld 2015]).
Mild-to-moderate: Oral: 500 mg every 12 hours **or** 250 mg every 8 hours
Severe: Oral: 875 mg every 12 hours **or** 500 mg every 8 hours
Tonsillitis and/or pharyngitis: Oral: Extended release tablet: 775 mg once daily
Endocarditis, prophylaxis (off-label use): Oral: 2 g 30 to 60 minutes before procedure. **Note:** American Heart Association (AHA) guidelines now recommend prophylaxis only in patients undergoing invasive procedures and in whom underlying cardiac conditions may predispose to a higher risk of adverse outcomes should infection occur. As of April 2007, routine prophylaxis for GI/GU procedures is no longer recommended by the AHA.

◄ **Erysipeloid (off-label use):** 500 mg 3 times daily for 7 to 10 days (IDSA [Stevens 2014])

***Helicobacter pylori* eradication (with active or 1 year history of duodenal ulcer disease):** 1,000 mg twice daily in combination therapy with clarithromycin and lansoprazole for 14 days; or 1,000 mg 3 times daily in combination with lansoprazole for 14 days (patients allergic/intolerant or suspected resistance to clarithromycin)

Lower respiratory tract infections: Oral: 875 mg every 12 hours **or** 500 mg every 8 hours

Lyme neuroborreliosis (off-label use): Oral: 500 mg every 6 to 8 hours (depending on size of patient) for 21 to 30 days

Periodontitis (aggressive) (in combination with metronidazole) associated with presence of *Actinobacillus actinomycetemcomitans* (AA): Oral: 500 mg every 8 hours for 10 days used in addition to scaling and root planing (Varela 2011)

Pharyngitis, group A streptococci (IDSA guidelines): 1,000 mg once daily or 500 mg twice daily (maximum daily dose: 1,000 mg) for 10 days (Shulman 2012)

Prophylaxis in total joint replacement patients undergoing dental procedures which produce bacteremia: Oral: 2 g 1 hour prior to procedure (ADA/AAOS 2003). **Note:** In general, patients with prosthetic joint implants do not require prophylactic antibiotics prior to dental procedures. In planning an invasive oral procedure, dental consultation with the patient's orthopedic surgeon may be advised to review the risks of infection (Sollecito 2015).

Prosthetic joint infection, chronic antimicrobial suppression of prosthetic joint infection associated with beta-hemolytic streptococci, penicillin-susceptible *Enterococcus* spp, or *Propionibacterium* spp (off-label use): Oral: 500 mg 3 times daily (Osmon 2013)

Pediatric

Usual dosage range:

Mild to moderate infection: Oral: Immediate-release: Infants ≤3 months:

Manufacturer's labeling: Up to 30 mg/kg/day divided every 12 hours (maximum dose: 30 mg/kg/day).

Alternate dosing (Red Book [AAP 2012]): 25 to 50 mg/kg/day divided every 8 hours.

Infants >3 months, Children, and Adolescents (<40 kg):

Manufacturer's labeling: 20 to 40 mg/kg/day in divided doses every 8 hours or 25 to 45 mg/kg/day in divided doses every 12 hours.

Alternate dosing (Red Book [AAP 2012]): 25 to 50 mg/kg/day in divided doses every 8 hours (maximum dose: 500 mg/dose).

Children and Adolescents (≥40 kg): Refer to adult dosing.

Severe infection (as step-down therapy):

Infants, Children, and Adolescents (Red Book [AAP 2012]): Oral: Immediate-release: 80 to 100 mg/kg/day in divided doses every 8 hours (maximum dose for most indications: 500 mg/dose).

Children ≥12 years and Adolescents: Oral: Extended-release: Refer to adult dosing.

Indication-specific dosing:

Infants, Children, and Adolescents: **Note:** In general, infants, children, and adolescents >3 months and ≥40 kg should be dosed according to the adult recommendations except where indicated.

Anthrax (off-label use): Oral: Immediate-release:

Cutaneous, community-acquired or bioterrorism-related (Stevens 2005):

Children <20 kg: 40 mg/kg/day in divided doses every 8 hours for 5 to 9 days.

Children ≥20 kg: 500 mg every 8 hours for 5 to 9 days.

Inhalational, postexposure prophylaxis (ACIP recommendations): **Note:** Use only if *B. anthracis* isolate is susceptible to amoxicillin (MIC ≤0.125 mcg/mL). Continue therapy for 30 to ≥60 days depending on vaccination status and for 14 days after the third vaccine dose (CDC 2010); see **"Note"** below.

Children <40 kg:

CDC recommendations: 45 mg/kg/day in divided doses every 8 hours (maximum dose: 500 mg/dose) (CDC 2010).

AAP recommendations: 80 mg/kg/day in divided doses every 8 hours (maximum dose: 500 mg/dose). The higher dose is recommended due to the lack of data on lower amoxicillin dosages for treating anthrax and the high mortality rate (Red Book [AAP 2012]).

Children ≥40 kg: 500 mg every 8 hours.

Note: Duration of antibiotic postexposure prophylaxis (PEP) is ≥60 days in a previously unvaccinated exposed person. Those who are partially or fully vaccinated should receive at least a 30-day course of antimicrobial PEP and continue with licensed vaccination regimen. Unvaccinated workers, even those wearing personal protective equipment with adequate respiratory protection, should receive antimicrobial PEP. Antimicrobial PEP is not required for fully vaccinated people (5-dose IM vaccination series with a yearly booster) who enter an anthrax area clothed in personal protective equipment. If respiratory protection is disrupted, a 30-day course of antimicrobial therapy is recommended (CDC 2010).

Endocarditis, prophylaxis (off-label use): Oral: Immediate-release: 50 mg/kg 1 hour before procedure (maximum dose: 2,000 mg/dose) (Wilson 2007). **Note:** American Heart Association (AHA) guidelines now recommend prophylaxis only in patients undergoing invasive procedures and in whom underlying cardiac conditions may predispose to a higher risk of adverse outcomes should infection occur. As of April 2007, routine prophylaxis for GI/GU procedures is no longer recommended by the AHA.

Lyme neuroborreliosis (off-label use): Infants, Children, and Adolescents: Oral: Immediate-release: 50 mg/kg/day divided every 8 hours (maximum dose: 500 mg/dose) (Halperin 2007, Wormser 2006).

Otitis media, acute: Infants ≥2 months and Children: Oral: Immediate-release: 80 to 90 mg/kg/day divided every 12 hours; variable duration of therapy, if <2 years of age or severe symptoms (any age): 10-day course; if 2 to 5 years of age with mild to moderate symptoms: 7-day course; ≥6 years of age with mild to moderate symptoms: 5- to 7-day course; some experts recommend initiating with 90 mg/kg/day (AAP [Lieberthal 2013]; Red Book [AAP 2012]); a maximum dose is not provided in the Guidelines for The Diagnosis and Management of Acute Otitis Media (AAP [Lieberthal 2013]); however, some experts suggest a maximum daily dose of 4,000 mg/day for high-dose amoxicillin therapy (Bradley 2015).

Peritonitis, prophylaxis (for patients receiving peritoneal dialysis who require dental procedures) (off-label use): Infants, Children, and Adolescents: Oral: Immediate-release: 50 mg/kg administered 30 to 60 minutes before dental procedure (maximum dose: 2000 mg/dose) (Warady 2012).

Pharyngitis (tonsillopharyngitis), group A streptococcal infection, treatment and primary prevention of rheumatic fever (off-label use): Oral:

Immediate release: Children and Adolescents 3 to 18 years: Oral: 50 mg/kg once daily **or** 25 mg/kg twice daily for 10 days (maximum daily dose: 1,000 mg/day) (Gerber 2009; Shulman 2012).

Extended release: Children ≥12 years and Adolescents: Oral: 775 mg once daily for 10 days.

Pneumococcal infection prophylaxis for anatomic or functional asplenia (eg, sickle cell disease ([SCD]) (off-label use) (Price 2007, Red Book [AAP 2012]): Oral: Immediate-release:

Infants (<2 months to 1 year, or as soon as SCD is diagnosed or asplenia occurs) and Children ≤5 years: 20 mg/kg/day in divided doses every 12 hours (maximum dose: 250 mg/dose).

Children ≥6 years and Adolescents: 250 mg every 12 hours. **Note:** The decision to discontinue penicillin prophylaxis after 5 years of age in children who have not experienced invasive pneumococcal infection and have received recommended pneumococcal immunizations is patient and clinician dependent.

Pneumonia, community-acquired (CAP) (Bradley 2011): Infants ≥3 months, Children, and Adolescents: Oral: Immediate-release: **Note:** In pediatric patients 5 to 15 years of age, a macrolide antibiotic may be a more reasonable first choice as *M. pneumoniae* is the chief cause of pneumonia in this age group.

Empiric treatment: 90 mg/kg/day in divided doses every 12 hours (maximum daily dose: 4,000 mg/day).

Group A *Streptococcus*: 50 to 75 mg/kg/day in divided doses every 12 hours (maximum daily dose: 4,000 mg/day).

H. influenzae: 75 to 100 mg/kg/day in divided doses every 8 hours (maximum daily dose: 4,000 mg/day).

S. pneumoniae (MICs to penicillin ≤2.0 mcg/mL), mild infection or step-down therapy: 90 mg/kg/day in divided doses every 12 hours or 45 mg/kg/day in divided doses every 8 hours (maximum daily dose: 4,000 mg/day).

Rhinosinusitis, acute bacterial; uncomplicated:
Note: AAP guidelines recommend amoxicillin as first-line empiric therapy for pediatric patients 1 to 18 years with uncomplicated cases and where resistance is not suspected; however, the IDSA guidelines consider amoxicillin/clavulanate as the preferred therapy (Chow 2012, Wald 2013):
Children and Adolescents: Oral: Immediate-release:
Low dose: 45 mg/kg/day in divided doses every 12 hours.
High dose (use reserved for select patients; see **"Note"**): 80 to 90 mg/kg/day in divided doses every 12 hours (maximum dose: 1,000 mg/dose). **Note:** Should only be used in the following: Mild to moderate infections in communities with a high prevalence of nonsusceptible *S. pneumoniae* resistance.

Renal Impairment Use of certain dosage forms (eg, extended-release 775 mg tablet and immediate-release 875 mg tablet) should be avoided in pediatric or adult patients with CrCl <30 mL/minute or patients requiring hemodialysis
Adults: Oral: Immediate-release:
CrCl ≥30 mL/minute: No dosage adjustment necessary.
CrCl 10 to 30 mL/minute: 250 to 500 mg every 12 hours.
CrCl <10 mL/minute: 250 to 500 mg every 24 hours.
ESRD on dialysis: Moderately dialyzable (20% to 50%); ~30% removed by 3-hour hemodialysis (Aronoff 2007): 250 to 500 mg every 24 hours; patients should receive an additional dose both during and after dialysis sessions.
Infants, Children, and Adolescents: Oral: Immediate-release:
Manufacturer's labeling: There are no dosage adjustments provided in the manufacturer's labeling.
Alternate dosing (Aronoff 2007):
Mild to moderate infection: Dosing based on 25 to 50 mg/kg/day divided every 8 hours in patients with normal renal function:
GFR ≥30 mL/minute/1.73 m^2: No dosage adjustment necessary.
GFR 10 to 29 mL/minute/1.73 m^2: 8 to 20 mg/kg/dose every 12 hours.
GFR <10 mL/minute/1.73 m^2: 8 to 20 mg/kg/dose every 24 hours.
End-stage renal disease (ESRD) on hemodialysis: Moderately dialyzable (20% to 50%); ~30% removed by 3-hour hemodialysis: 8 to 20 mg/kg/dose every 24 hours; give after dialysis.
Peritoneal dialysis: 8 to 20 mg/kg/dose every 24 hours.
Severe infection: Dosing based on 80 to 90 mg/kg/day divided every 12 hours in patients with normal renal function:
GFR ≥30 mL/minute/1.73 m^2: No dosage adjustment necessary.
GFR 10 to 29 mL/minute/1.73 m^2: 20 mg/kg/dose every 12 hours; do not use the 875 mg tablet.
GFR <10 mL/minute/1.73 m^2: 20 mg/kg/dose every 24 hours; do not use the 875 mg tablet.
ESRD on hemodialysis: Moderately dialyzable (20% to 50%); ~30% removed by 3-hour hemodialysis: 20 mg/kg/dose every 24 hours; give after dialysis.
Peritoneal dialysis: 20 mg/kg/dose every 24 hours.

Hepatic Impairment There are no dosage adjustments provided in the manufacturer's labeling.

Dietary Considerations May be taken with food. Some products may contain phenylalanine.
Moxatag: Take within 1 hour of finishing a meal.

Administration Administer around-the-clock to promote less variation in peak and trough serum levels. The appropriate amount of suspension may be mixed with formula, milk, fruit juice, water, ginger ale, or cold drinks; administer dose immediately after mixing.

Moxatag extended release tablet: Administer within 1 hour of finishing a meal.

Monitoring Parameters With prolonged therapy, monitor renal, hepatic, and hematologic function periodically; assess patient at beginning and throughout therapy for infection; monitor for signs of anaphylaxis during first dose

Test Interactions May interfere with urinary glucose tests using cupric sulfate (Benedict's solution, Clinitest)
Some penicillin derivatives may accelerate the degradation of aminoglycosides *in vitro*, leading to a potential underestimation of aminoglycoside serum concentration.

Dosage Forms Excipient information presented when available (limited, particularly for generics); consult specific product labeling.
Capsule, Oral:
Generic: 250 mg, 500 mg
Suspension Reconstituted, Oral:
Generic: 125 mg/5 mL (80 mL, 100 mL, 150 mL); 200 mg/5 mL (50 mL, 75 mL, 100 mL); 250 mg/5 mL (80 mL, 100 mL, 150 mL); 400 mg/5 mL (50 mL, 75 mL, 100 mL)
Tablet, Oral:
Generic: 500 mg, 875 mg
Tablet Chewable, Oral:
Generic: 125 mg, 250 mg
Tablet Extended Release 24 Hour, Oral:
Moxatag: 775 mg [contains cremophor el, fd&c blue #2 aluminum lake]
Generic: 775 mg

Amoxicillin and Clavulanate
(a moks i SIL in & klav yoo LAN ate)

Brand Names: US Amoclan; Augmentin; Augmentin ES-600; Augmentin XR
Brand Names: Canada Amoxi-Clav; Apo-Amoxi-Clav; Clavulin; Novo-Clavamoxin; ratio-Aclavulanate
Index Terms Amoxicillin and Clavulanate Potassium; Amoxicillin and Clavulanic Acid; Amoxicillin and Clavulanate Potassium; Amoxycillin and Clavulanic Acid; Clavulanic Acid and Amoxicillin; Clavulanic Acid and Amoxycillin; Co-Amoxiclav
Pharmacologic Category Antibiotic, Penicillin
Use
Pneumonia, community-acquired: Extended-release tablets only: Treatment of patients with community-acquired pneumonia (CAP) caused by confirmed or suspected beta-lactamase-producing pathogens (ie, *Haemophilus influenzae*, *Moraxella catarrhalis*, *Haemophilus parainfluenzae*, *Klebsiella pneumoniae*, methicillin-susceptible *Staphylococcus aureus*) and *Streptococcus pneumoniae* with reduced susceptibility to penicillin (penicillin minimum inhibitory concentration [MIC] = 2 mcg/mL).
Limitations of use: Augmentin XR is not indicated for the treatment of infections caused by *S. pneumoniae* with penicillin MIC of 4 mcg/mL or greater (limited data).
Otitis media, acute:
Immediate-release tablets, chewable tablets, oral suspension (400/57 mg per 5 mL, 250/62.5 mg per 5 mL, 200/28.5 mg per 5 mL, and 125/31.25 mg per 5 mL only): Treatment of otitis media caused by beta-lactamase-producing strains of *H. influenzae* and *M. catarrhalis*.
Oral suspension (600/42.9 mg per 5 mL concentration): Treatment of acute otitis media, recurrent or persistent, caused by *S. pneumoniae* (penicillin MIC = 2 mcg/mL or less), *H. influenzae* (including beta-lactamase-producing strains), and *M. catarrhalis* (including beta-lactamase-producing strains) in pediatric patients with a history of antibiotic exposure for acute otitis media in the preceding 3 months and who are either 2 years or younger or attend day care; treatment of otitis media caused by beta-lactamase-producing strains of *H. influenzae* and *M. catarrhalis*.
Respiratory tract infections, lower: Immediate-release tablets, chewable tablets, oral suspension (400/57 mg per 5 mL, 250/62.5 mg per 5 mL, 200/28.5 mg per 5 mL, and 125/31.25 mg per 5 mL only): Treatment of lower respiratory tract infection caused by beta-lactamase-producing strains of *H. influenzae* and *M. catarrhalis*.
Sinusitis, acute bacterial:
Extended-release tablets: Treatment of patients with acute bacterial sinusitis caused by confirmed or suspected beta-lactamase-producing pathogens (ie, *H. influenzae*, *M. catarrhalis*, *H. parainfluenzae*, *K. pneumoniae*, methicillin-susceptible *S. aureus*) and *S. pneumoniae* with reduced susceptibility to penicillin (penicillin MIC = 2 mcg/mL).

Limitations of use: Augmentin XR is not indicated for the treatment of infections caused by *S. pneumoniae* with penicillin MIC of 4 mcg/mL or greater (limited data). Immediate-release tablets, chewable tablets, oral suspension (400/57 mg per 5 mL, 250/62.5 mg per 5 mL, 200/28.5 mg per 5 mL, and 125/31.25 mg per 5 mL only): Treatment of sinusitis caused by beta-lactamase-producing strains of *H. influenzae* and *M. catarrhalis*.

Skin and skin structure infections: Immediate-release tablets, chewable tablets, oral suspension (400/57 mg per 5 mL, 250/62.5 mg per 5 mL, 200/28.5 mg per 5 mL, and 125/31.25 mg per 5 mL only): Treatment of skin and skin structure infections caused by beta-lactamase-producing strains of *S. aureus*, *Escherichia coli*, and *Klebsiella* spp.

Urinary tract infections: Immediate-release tablets, chewable tablets, oral suspension (400/57 mg per 5 mL, 250/62.5 mg per 5 mL, 200/28.5 mg per 5 mL, and 125/31.25 mg per 5 mL only): Treatment of urinary tract infections caused by beta-lactamase-producing strains of *E. coli*, *Klebsiella* spp, and *Enterobacter* spp.

Pregnancy Considerations Adverse events have not been observed in animal reproduction studies. Both amoxicillin and clavulanic acid cross the placenta. Maternal use of amoxicillin/clavulanate has generally not resulted in an increased risk of birth defects. A possible increased risk of necrotizing enterocolitis in neonates or bowel disorders in children exposed to amoxicillin/clavulanate *in utero* has been observed. In women with acute infections during pregnancy, amoxicillin/clavulanate may be given if an antibiotic is required and appropriate based on bacterial sensitivity; however, use is not recommended in the management of preterm premature rupture of membranes. Oral ampicillin-class antibiotics are poorly absorbed during labor.

Breast-Feeding Considerations Amoxicillin is found in breast milk. The manufacturer recommends that caution be used if administered to breast-feeding women. The use of amoxicillin/clavulanate may be safe while breast-feeding. However, the risk of adverse events in the infant may be increased when compared to the use of amoxicillin alone and the risk may be related to maternal dose.

Contraindications
Hypersensitivity to amoxicillin, clavulanic acid, other beta-lactam antibacterial drugs (eg, penicillins, cephalosporins), or any component of the formulation; history of cholestatic jaundice or hepatic dysfunction with amoxicillin/clavulanate potassium therapy

Augmentin XR: Additional contraindications: Severe renal impairment (creatinine clearance <30 mL/minute) and hemodialysis patients

Canadian labeling: Additional contraindications (not in US labeling): Suspected or confirmed mononucleosis

Warnings/Precautions Hypersensitivity reactions, including anaphylaxis (some fatal), have been reported. Prolonged use may result in fungal or bacterial superinfection, including *C. difficile*-associated diarrhea (CDAD) and pseudomembranous colitis; CDAD has been observed >2 months postantibiotic treatment. Although rarely fatal, hepatic dysfunction (eg, cholestatic jaundice, hepatitis) has been reported. Patients at highest risk include those with serious underlying disease or concomitant medications. Hepatic toxicity is usually reversible. Monitor liver function tests at regular intervals in patients with hepatic impairment. High percentage of patients with infectious mononucleosis have developed rash during therapy; ampicillin class antibiotics not recommended in these patients. Incidence of diarrhea is higher than with amoxicillin alone. Due to differing content of clavulanic acid, not all formulations are interchangeable; use of an inappropriate product for a specific dosage could result in either diarrhea (which may be severe) or subtherapeutic clavulanic acid concentrations leading to decreased clinical efficacy. Low incidence of cross-allergy with cephalosporins exists. Monitor renal, hepatic, and hematopoietic function if therapy extends beyond approved duration times. Some products contain phenylalanine. Potentially significant drug-drug interactions may exist, requiring dose or frequency adjustment, additional monitoring, and/or selection of alternative therapy.

Adverse Reactions
>10%: Gastrointestinal: Diarrhea (3% to 34%; incidence varies upon dose and regimen used)
1% to 10%:
  Dermatologic: Diaper rash, skin rash, urticaria
  Gastrointestinal: Abdominal distress, loose stools, nausea, vomiting

Genitourinary: Vaginitis
Infection: Candidiasis, vaginal mycosis
<1% (Limited to important or life-threatening): Cholestatic jaundice, flatulence, headache, hepatic insufficiency, hepatitis, hepatotoxicity (idiosyncratic) (Chalasani, 2014), increased liver enzymes, increased serum alkaline phosphatase, prolonged prothrombin time, thrombocythemia, vasculitis (hypersensitivity)

Additional adverse reactions seen with **ampicillin-class antibiotics:** Acute generalized exanthematous pustulosis, agitation, agranulocytosis, anaphylaxis, anemia, angioedema, anxiety, behavioral changes, confusion, convulsions, crystalluria, dental discoloration, dizziness, dyspepsia, enterocolitis, eosinophilia, erythema multiforme, exfoliative dermatitis, gastritis, glossitis, hematuria, hemolytic anemia, hemorrhagic colitis, hyperactivity, immune thrombocytopenia, increased serum bilirubin, increased serum transaminases, insomnia, interstitial nephritis, leukopenia, melanoglossia, mucocutaneous candidiasis, pruritus, pseudomembranous colitis, serum sickness-like reaction, Stevens-Johnson syndrome, stomatitis, thrombocytopenia, toxic epidermal necrolysis

Drug Interactions
Metabolism/Transport Effects None known.
Avoid Concomitant Use
  Avoid concomitant use of Amoxicillin and Clavulanate with any of the following: BCG (Intravesical); Probenecid
Increased Effect/Toxicity
  Amoxicillin and Clavulanate may increase the levels/effects of: Methotrexate; Vitamin K Antagonists

  The levels/effects of Amoxicillin and Clavulanate may be increased by: Allopurinol; Probenecid
Decreased Effect
  Amoxicillin and Clavulanate may decrease the levels/effects of: BCG (Intravesical); BCG Vaccine (Immunization); Mycophenolate; Sodium Picosulfate; Typhoid Vaccine

  The levels/effects of Amoxicillin and Clavulanate may be decreased by: Tetracycline Derivatives

Preparation for Administration Reconstitute powder for oral suspension with appropriate amount of water as specified in the manufacturer's labeling. Shake vigorously until suspended.

Storage/Stability
Powder for oral suspension: Store dry powder at or below 25°C (77°F). Reconstituted oral suspension should be kept in refrigerator. Discard unused suspension after 10 days (consult manufacturer's labeling for specific recommendations). Unit-dose antibiotic oral syringes are stable under refrigeration for 24 hours (Tu 1988).

Tablet: Store at or below 25°C (77°F). Dispense in original container.

Mechanism of Action Clavulanic acid binds and inhibits beta-lactamases that inactivate amoxicillin resulting in amoxicillin having an expanded spectrum of activity. Amoxicillin inhibits bacterial cell wall synthesis by binding to one or more of the penicillin-binding proteins (PBPs) which in turn inhibits the final transpeptidation step of peptidoglycan synthesis in bacterial cell walls, thus inhibiting cell wall biosynthesis. Bacteria eventually lyse due to ongoing activity of cell wall autolytic enzymes (autolysins and murein hydrolases) while cell wall assembly is arrested.

Pharmacodynamics/Kinetics Amoxicillin pharmacokinetics are not affected by clavulanic acid.
Amoxicillin: See individual Amoxicillin monograph.
Clavulanic acid:
  Protein binding: ~25%
  Half-life elimination: 1 hour
  Time to peak: 1.5 hours
  Excretion: Urine (25% to 40% as unchanged drug)

Dosing

Adult & Geriatric Note: Dose is based on the amoxicillin component; see "Augmentin Product-Specific Considerations" table.

Susceptible infections: Oral: 250 mg every 8 hours or 500 mg every 8 to 12 hours **or** 875 mg every 12 hours **or** 2,000 mg every 12 hours

Augmentin Product-Specific Considerations

Strength	Form	Consideration
125 mg	S	q8h dosing
	S	For adults having difficulty swallowing tablets, 125 mg/5 mL suspension may be substituted for 500 mg tablet.
200 mg	CT, S	q12h dosing
	CT	Contains phenylalanine
	S	For adults having difficulty swallowing tablets, 200 mg/5 mL suspension may be substituted for 875 mg tablet.
250 mg	S, T	q8h dosing
	T	Not for use in patients <40 kg; two 250 mg tablets are not equivalent to one 500 mg tablet
	S	For adults having difficulty swallowing tablets, 250 mg/5 mL suspension may be substituted for 500 mg tablet.
400 mg	CT, S	q12h dosing
	CT	Contains phenylalanine
	S	For adults having difficulty swallowing tablets, 400 mg/5 mL suspension may be substituted for 875 mg tablet.
500 mg	T	q8h or q12h dosing
600 mg	S	q12h dosing
		Not for use in adults, adolescents, or children ≥40 kg
		600 mg/5 mL suspension is not equivalent to or interchangeable with 200 mg/5 mL or 400 mg/5 mL due to differences in clavulanic acid.
875 mg	T	q12h dosing; not for use in CrCl <30 mL/minute
1,000 mg	XR	q12h dosing
		Not for use in children or adolescents <40 kg
		Not interchangeable with two 500 mg tablets
		Not for use if CrCl <30 mL/minute or hemodialysis

Legend: CT = chewable tablet, S = suspension, T = tablet, XR = extended release.

Bite wounds (animal/human) (off-label use): Oral: Immediate release: 875 mg every 12 hours (IDSA [Stevens 2014])

Chronic obstructive pulmonary disease (COPD) (off-label use): Oral: Immediate release: 500 mg every 8 hours (Llor 2012)

Impetigo (off-label use): Oral: Immediate release: 875 mg every 12 hours for 7 days, depending on response (IDSA [Stevens 2014])

Pneumonia, community-acquired (CAP) and respiratory tract infections, lower: *Manufacturer's labeling:* Oral:

Immediate release: 875 mg every 12 hours **or** 500 mg every 8 hours

Extended release: 2,000 mg every 12 hours for 7 to 10 days

Prosthetic joint infection, chronic antimicrobial suppression, oxacillin-susceptible *Staphylococci* (alternative to cephalexin or cefadroxil) (off-label use): Oral: Immediate release: 500 mg 3 times daily (IDSA [Osmon 2013])

Sinusitis, acute bacterial: Oral:

Manufacturer's labeling:

Immediate release: 500 mg every 8 hours or amoxicillin 875 mg every 12 hours

Extended release: Amoxicillin 2,000 mg every 12 hours for 10 days

Alternate dosing: IDSA recommendations:

Standard dose: Immediate release: 500 mg every 8 hours or 875 mg every 12 hours for 5 to 7 days

High dose: Extended release: 2,000 mg every 12 hours for 10 days. **Note:** Recommended for patients with any of the following: If initial therapy fails (as second-line therapy), in areas with high endemic rates of penicillin-nonsusceptible *S. pneumoniae*, those with severe infections, age >65 years, recent hospitalization, antibiotic use within the past month, or who are immunocompromised (AAO-HNS [Rosenfeld 2015]; IDSA [Chow 2012]).

Streptococci, group A, chronic carrier treatment (off-label use): Oral: Immediate release: Amoxicillin 40 mg/kg/day divided every 8 hours (maximum: amoxicillin 2,000 mg daily) for 10 days (IDSA [Shulman 2012])

Pediatric Note: Dose is based on the amoxicillin component; see "Augmentin Product-Specific Considerations" table.

Usual dosage range:

Infants <3 months: Oral: Amoxicillin 30 mg/kg/day divided every 12 hours using the 125 mg per 5 mL suspension **only**

Infants ≥3 months, Children, and Adolescents <40 kg: Oral: Immediate release:

Mild to moderate infections: Amoxicillin 25 mg/kg/day in divided doses twice daily (using the 200 mg per 5 mL or 400 mg per 5 mL suspension or 200 mg or 400 mg chewable tablets) **or** amoxicillin 20 mg/kg/day in divided doses 3 times daily (using the 125 mg per 5 mL or 250 mg per 5 mL suspension) (maximum single dose: 500 mg amoxicillin)

Severe infections: Amoxicillin 45 mg/kg/day in divided doses twice daily (using the 200 mg per 5 mL or 400 mg per 5 mL suspension or 200 mg or 400 mg **chewable** tablets) (maximum single dose: amoxicillin 875 mg) **or** amoxicillin 40 mg/kg/day in divided doses 3 times daily (using the 125 mg per 5 mL or 250 mg per 5 mL suspension) (maximum single dose: amoxicillin 500 mg)

Children and Adolescents ≥40 kg: Oral:

Mild to moderate infections: Immediate release: Amoxicillin 500 mg every 12 hours (using the 500 mg tablet; if difficulty swallowing the 125 mg per 5 mL or 250 mg per 5 mL suspension may be used) **or** 250 mg amoxicillin every 8 hours (using the 250 mg tablet)

Severe infections:

Immediate release: Amoxicillin 875 mg every 12 hours (using the 875 mg tablet; if difficulty swallowing, the 200 mg per 5 mL or 400 mg per 5 mL suspension may be used) **or** amoxicillin 500 mg every 8 hours (using the 500 mg tablet; if difficulty swallowing the 125 mg per 5 mL or 250 mg per 5 mL suspension may be used).

Extended release: Amoxicillin 2,000 mg every 12 hours

Indication-specific dosing:

Impetigo (off-label use): Infants ≥3 months, Children, and Adolescents: Oral: Immediate release: Amoxicillin 25 mg/kg/day in divided doses twice daily (using the 200 mg per 5 mL or 400 mg per 5 mL oral suspension or the 200 mg or 400 mg **chewable** tablets) (maximum single dose: 875 mg amoxicillin) (IDSA [Stevens 2014])

Otitis media, acute: Infants ≥6 months and Children: Oral: Immediate release: Amoxicillin 90 mg/kg/day divided every 12 hours (using the 600 mg per 5 mL suspension **only**) **Note:** Use for severe illness, those who have received amoxicillin in the past 30 days, who have treatment failure at 48 to 72 hours on first-line therapy, and when coverage for beta-lactamase positive *H. influenzae* and *M. catarrhalis* is needed. Variable duration of therapy; the manufacturer's labeling suggests 10-day course in all patients; however, new data suggest a shorter-course in some cases: If <2 years of age or severe symptoms (any age): 10-day course; if 2 to 5 years of age with mild to moderate symptoms: 7-day course; if ≥6 years of age with mild to moderate symptoms: 5- to 7-day course (AAP [Lieberthal 2013]). **Note:** Per the manufacturer, the 600 mg/5 mL formulation should only be used for patients weighing <40 kg.

Pneumonia, community-acquired (CAP) and respiratory tract infections, lower: Infants ≥3 months, Children, and Adolescents: Oral:

Manufacturer's labeling:

Patients weighing <40 kg: Immediate release: Amoxicillin 45 mg/kg/day in divided doses twice daily (using the 200 mg per 5 mL or 400 mg per 5 mL suspension or the 200 mg or 400 mg chewable tablets) (maximum single dose: amoxicillin 875 mg) **or** amoxicillin 40 mg/kg/day in divided doses 3 times daily (using the 125 mg per 5 mL or 250 mg per 5 mL suspension) (maximum single dose: amoxicillin 500 mg)

Patients weighing ≥40 kg:

Immediate release: Amoxicillin 875 mg every 12 hours using the 875 mg tablet or if difficulty swallowing, the 200 mg/5 mL or the 400 mg/5 mL oral suspension may be used **or** 500 mg amoxicillin every 8 hours using the 500 mg tablet or if difficulty swallowing, the 125 mg/5 mL or 250 mg/5 mL oral suspension may be used

Extended release: 2,000 mg amoxicillin every 12 hours

Alternate dosing (off-label dosing): Beta-lactamase positive *H. influenzae* strains (IDSA/PIDS [Bradley 2011]): Immediate release:

Standard dose: Amoxicillin 45 mg/kg/day in divided doses 3 times daily (using the 125 mg per 5 mL or 250 mg per 5 mL suspension) (maximum single dose: amoxicillin 500 mg)

High dose: Amoxicillin 90 mg/kg/day in divided doses 2 times daily (using the 600 mg per 5 mL suspension). **Note:** A wider dosing range of 80 to 100 mg/kg/day divided every 8 hours has also been used (Bradley 2002).

Sinusitis, acute bacterial: Oral:

IDSA recommendations:

Infants ≥3 months, Children, and Adolescents <40 kg: Immediate release:

Standard dose: Amoxicillin 45 mg/kg/day divided every 12 hours for 10 to 14 days (using the 200 mg per 5 mL or 400 mg per 5 mL suspension or 200 mg or 400 mg chewable tablets **only**) (IDSA [Chow 2012])

High dose (off-label dose): Amoxicillin 90 mg/kg/day divided every 12 hours for 10 to 14 days (using the 600 mg per 5 mL suspension **only**). **Note:** Use recommended in the following: If initial therapy fails (as second-line therapy), in areas with high endemic rates of penicillin-nonsusceptible *S. pneumoniae*, those with severe infections, daycare attendance, age <2 years, recent hospitalization, antibiotic use within the past month, or who are immunocompromised (IDSA [Chow 2012]).

Children and Adolescents ≥40 kg: Refer to adult dosing.

AAP recommendations: Children and Adolescents: Immediate release:

High dose (off-label dose): Amoxicillin 80 to 90 mg/kg/day divided every 12 hours (using the 600 mg per 5 mL oral suspension **only**); treatment duration variable: 10 to 28 days, some have suggested discontinuation of therapy 7 days after resolution of signs and symptoms of infection. **Note:** Recommended for patients with any of the following: moderate to severe infection, age <2 years, childcare attendance, or recent antibiotic treatment. (Wald 2013)

Streptococci, group A, chronic carrier treatment (off-label use): Infants ≥3 months, Children, and Adolescents: Oral: Immediate release: Amoxicillin 40 mg/kg/day divided every 8 hours for 10 days (using the 125 mg per 5 mL or 250 mg per 5 mL suspension) (IDSA [Shulman 2012])

Urinary tract infections: Infants and Children 2 to 24 months: Oral: Immediate release: Amoxicillin 20 to 40 mg/kg/day in divided doses 3 times daily (using the 125 mg per 5 mL or 250 mg per 5 mL suspension); (maximum single dose: amoxicillin 500 mg) (AAP 2011)

Renal Impairment

Adults: **Note:** Renally adjusted dose recommendations are based on the amoxicillin 250 mg/clavulanate 125 mg and amoxicillin 500 mg/clavulanate 125 mg tablets.

CrCl ≥30 mL/minute: No dosage adjustment necessary.

CrCl 10 to 30 mL/minute: 250 to 500 mg every 12 hours; do not use 875 mg tablet or extended-release tablets

CrCl <10 mL/minute: 250 to 500 mg every 24 hours; do not use 875 mg tablet or extended-release tablets

End-stage renal disease (ESRD) on hemodialysis: 250 to 500 mg amoxicillin every 24 hours; administer dose both during and after dialysis. Do not use 875 mg tablet or extended-release tablets.

Infants, Children, and Adolescents: There are no dosage adjustments provided in the manufacturer's labeling; however, the following adjustments have been recommended (Aronoff 2007):

Mild to moderate infection: Dosing based on amoxicillin 25 to 50 mg/kg/day divided every 8 hours:

GFR ≥30 mL/minute/1.73 m^2: No dosage adjustment necessary

GFR 10 to 29 mL/minute/1.73 m^2: Amoxicillin 8 to 20 mg/kg/dose every 12 hours

GFR <10 mL/minute/1.73 m^2: Amoxicillin 8 to 20 mg/kg/dose every 24 hours

End-stage renal disease (ESRD):

Hemodialysis: Amoxicillin 8 to 20 mg/kg/dose every 24 hours; give after dialysis

Peritoneal dialysis: Amoxicillin 8 to 20 mg/kg/dose every 24 hours

Severe infection (high dose): Dosing based on amoxicillin 80 to 90 mg/kg/day divided every 12 hours:

CrCl ≥30 mL/minute/1.73 m^2: No dosage adjustment necessary

CrCl 10 to 29 mL/minute/1.73 m^2: Amoxicillin 20 mg/kg/dose every 12 hours; do not use the 875 mg tablet

CrCl <10 mL/minute/1.73 m^2: Amoxicillin 20 mg/kg/dose every 24 hours; do not use the 875 mg tablet

End-stage renal disease (ESRD):

Hemodialysis: Amoxicillin 20 mg/kg/dose every 24 hours; give after dialysis; do not use the 875 mg tablet

Peritoneal dialysis: Amoxicillin 20 mg/kg/dose every 24 hours; do not use the 875 mg tablet

Hepatic Impairment There are no dosage adjustments provided in the manufacturer's labeling; use with caution. Use contraindicated in patients with a history of amoxicillin and clavulanate-associated hepatic dysfunction.

Dietary Considerations May be taken with meals or on an empty stomach; take with meals to increase absorption and decrease GI upset; may mix with milk, formula, or juice. Extended release tablets should be taken with food. Some products may contain sodium. Some products contain phenylalanine; if you have phenylketonuria or PKU, avoid use. All dosage forms contain potassium.

Administration Oral: Administer around-the-clock to promote less variation in peak and trough serum levels. Administer with food to increase absorption and decrease stomach upset; shake suspension well before use. Extended release tablets should be administered with food.

Monitoring Parameters Assess patient at beginning and throughout therapy for infection; with prolonged therapy, monitor renal, hepatic, and hematologic function periodically; monitor for signs of anaphylaxis during first dose

Test Interactions

May interfere with urinary glucose tests using cupric sulfate (Benedict's solution, Clinitest, Fehling's solution). Glucose tests based on enzymatic glucose oxidase reactions (eg, Clinistix) are recommended.

Ampicillin may transiently interfere with plasma concentrations of total conjugated estriol, estriol-glucuronide, conjugated estrone and estradiol in pregnant women.

Additional Information Two 250 mg tablets are not equivalent to a 500 mg tablet (both tablet sizes contain equivalent clavulanate). Two 500 mg tablets are not equivalent to a single 1000 mg extended release tablet.

Dosage Forms Excipient information presented when available (limited, particularly for generics); consult specific product labeling. [DSC] = Discontinued product

Powder for suspension, oral:

Generic: 200: Amoxicillin 200 mg and clavulanate potassium 28.5 mg per 5 mL (50 mL, 75 mL, 100 mL); 250: Amoxicillin 250 mg and clavulanate potassium 62.5 mg per 5 mL (75 mL, 100 mL, 150 mL); 400: Amoxicillin 400 mg and clavulanate potassium 57 mg per 5 mL (50 mL, 75 mL, 100 mL); 600: Amoxicillin 600 mg and clavulanate potassium 42.9 mg per 5 mL (75 mL, 125 mL, 200 mL)

Amoclan:

200: Amoxicillin 200 mg and clavulanate potassium 28.5 mg per 5 mL (50 mL, 75 mL, 100 mL) [contains phenylalanine 7 mg/5 mL and potassium 0.14 mEq/5 mL; fruit flavor]

400: Amoxicillin 400 mg and clavulanate potassium 57 mg per 5 mL (50 mL, 75 mL, 100 mL) [contains phenylalanine 7 mg/5 mL and potassium 0.29 mEq/5 mL; fruit flavor]

600: Amoxicillin 600 mg and clavulanate potassium 42.9 mg per 5 mL (75 mL, 125 mL, 200 mL) [contains phenylalanine 7 mg/5 mL, potassium 0.248 mEq/5 mL; orange flavor]

Augmentin:

125: Amoxicillin 125 mg and clavulanate potassium 31.25 mg per 5 mL (75 mL, 100 mL, 150 mL) [contains potassium 0.16 mEq/5 mL; banana flavor]

200: Amoxicillin 200 mg and clavulanate potassium 28.5 mg per 5 mL (50 mL, 75 mL, 100 mL) [contains phenylalanine 7 mg/5 mL and potassium 0.14 mEq/5 mL; orange flavor] [DSC]

250: Amoxicillin 250 mg and clavulanate potassium 62.5 mg per 5 mL (75 mL, 100 mL, 150 mL) [contains potassium 0.32 mEq/5 mL; orange flavor]

400: Amoxicillin 400 mg and clavulanate potassium 57 mg per 5 mL (50 mL, 75 mL, 100 mL) [contains phenylalanine 7 mg/5 mL and potassium 0.29 mEq/5 mL; orange flavor] [DSC]

Augmentin ES-600:

600: Amoxicillin 600 mg and clavulanate potassium 42.9 mg per 5 mL (75 mL, 125 mL, 200 mL) [contains phenylalanine 7 mg/5 mL, potassium 0.23 mEq/5 mL; strawberry cream flavor]

Tablet, oral:

Generic: 250: Amoxicillin 250 mg and clavulanate potassium 125 mg; 500: Amoxicillin 500 mg and clavulanate potassium 125 mg; 875: Amoxicillin 875 mg and clavulanate potassium 125 mg

Augmentin:

250: Amoxicillin 250 mg and clavulanate potassium 125 mg [contains potassium 0.63 mEq/tablet] [DSC]

500: Amoxicillin 500 mg and clavulanate potassium 125 mg [contains potassium 0.63 mEq/tablet]

875: Amoxicillin 875 mg and clavulanate potassium 125 mg [contains potassium 0.63 mEq/tablet]

Tablet, chewable, oral:

Generic: 200: Amoxicillin 200 mg and clavulanate potassium 28.5 mg [contains phenylalanine]; 400: Amoxicillin 400 mg and clavulanate potassium 57 mg [contains phenylalanine]

Tablet, extended release, oral:

Generic: Amoxicillin 1000 mg and clavulanate acid 62.5 mg

Augmentin XR: 1000: Amoxicillin 1000 mg and clavulanate acid 62.5 mg [contains potassium 12.6 mg (0.32 mEq) and sodium 29.3 mg (1.27 mEq) per tablet; packaged in either a 7-day or 10-day package]

Dosage Forms: Canada Note: Also refer to Dosage Forms. Excipient information presented when available (limited, particularly for generics); consult specific product labeling.

Powder for suspension, oral:

Clavulin:

125: Amoxicillin 125 mg and clavulanate potassium 31.25 mg per 5 mL (100 mL) [contains aspartame]

200: Amoxicillin 200 mg and clavulanate potassium 28.5 mg per 5 mL (70 mL) [contains aspartame]

250: Amoxicillin 250 mg and clavulanate potassium 62.5 mg per 5 mL (100 mL) [contains aspartame]

400: Amoxicillin 400 mg and clavulanate potassium 57 mg per 5 mL (70 mL) [contains aspartame]

Tablet, oral:

Clavulin:

500: Amoxicillin 500 mg and clavulanate potassium 125 mg

875: Amoxicillin 875 mg and clavulanate potassium 125 mg

◆ Amoxicillin and Clavulanate Potassium *see* Amoxicillin and Clavulanate *on page 111*

◆ Amoxicillin and Clavulanic Acid *see* Amoxicillin and Clavulanate *on page 111*

◆ Amoxicillin, Clarithromycin, and Lansoprazole *see* Lansoprazole, Amoxicillin, and Clarithromycin *on page 1035*

◆ Amoxicillin, Clarithromycin, and Omeprazole *see* Omeprazole, Clarithromycin, and Amoxicillin *on page 1333*

◆ Amoxicillin Trihydrate *see* Amoxicillin *on page 108*

◆ Amoxi-Clav (Can) *see* Amoxicillin and Clavulanate *on page 111*

◆ Amoxil *see* Amoxicillin *on page 108*

◆ Amoxycillin *see* Amoxicillin *on page 108*

◆ Amoxycillin and Clavulanate Potassium *see* Amoxicillin and Clavulanate *on page 111*

◆ Amoxycillin and Clavulanic Acid *see* Amoxicillin and Clavulanate *on page 111*

Amphetamine (am FET a meen)

Brand Names: US Evekeo

Index Terms Amphetamine Sulfate; Dyanavel XR; Racemic Amphetamine Sulfate

Pharmacologic Category Central Nervous System Stimulant

Use

Attention-deficit/hyperactivity disorder: Treatment of attention-deficit/hyperactivity disorder (ADHD)

Exogenous obesity (immediate release only): Short-term treatment of exogenous obesity as an adjunct to caloric restriction for patients refractory to alternative therapy (eg, repeated diets, group programs, and other drugs).

Narcolepsy (immediate release only): Treatment of narcolepsy.

Pregnancy Considerations Adverse effects have been observed in animal reproduction studies. The majority of human data are based on illicit amphetamine/methamphetamine exposure and not from therapeutic maternal use (Golub, 2005). Use of amphetamines during pregnancy may lead to an increased risk of premature birth and low birth weight; newborns may experience symptoms of withdrawal. Behavioral problems may also occur later in childhood (LaGasse, 2012).

Breast-Feeding Considerations Amphetamine is excreted in breast milk. The majority of human data are based on illicit amphetamine/methamphetamine exposure and not from therapeutic maternal use (Golub, 2005). Increased irritability, agitation, and crying have been reported in nursing infants (ACOG, 2011). Breast-feeding is not recommended by the manufacturer.

Contraindications

Immediate release: Hypersensitivity or idiosyncrasy to amphetamine or other sympathomimetic amines; advanced arteriosclerosis; symptomatic cardiovascular disease; moderate to severe hypertension; hyperthyroidism; agitated states; history of drug abuse; use during or within 14 days following MAO inhibitor.

Extended release: Hypersensitivity to amphetamine or any component of the formulation; use during or within 14 days following MAO inhibitor.

Documentation of allergenic cross-reactivity for amphetamines is limited. However, because of similarities in chemical structure and/or pharmacologic actions, the possibility of cross-sensitivity cannot be ruled out with certainty.

Warnings/Precautions [US Boxed Warning]: Potential for drug abuse and dependency exists; prolonged use may lead to drug dependency and must be avoided. Assess the risk for abuse prior to prescribing, and monitor for signs of abuse and dependence while on therapy. Consider the possibility of patients obtaining amphetamines for non-therapeutic use or distribution to others; prescribe sparingly. Use of immediate-release formulation is contraindicated in patients with history of drug abuse. Write prescriptions for the smallest quantity consistent with good patient care to minimize possibility of overdose.

[US Boxed Warning]: Misuse may cause serious cardiovascular events including sudden death. Adverse effects have been reported at usual doses in patients with preexisting structural cardiac abnormalities or other serious heart problems (sudden death in children and adolescents; sudden death, stroke, and MI in adults). These products should be avoided in the patients with known serious structural cardiac abnormalities, cardiomyopathy, serious heart rhythm abnormalities, coronary artery disease, or other serious cardiac problems that could increase the risk of sudden death that these conditions alone carry. Patients should be carefully evaluated for cardiac disease prior to initiation of therapy. Patients who develop symptoms such as exertional chest pain, unexplained syncope, or other symptoms suggestive of cardiac disease during treatment should undergo a prompt cardiac evaluation. Amphetamines may impair the ability to engage in potentially hazardous activities; patients must be cautioned about performing tasks that require mental alertness (eg, operating machinery or driving).

Stimulants are associated with peripheral vasculopathy, including Raynaud's phenomenon; signs/symptoms are usually mild and intermittent, and generally improve with dose reduction or discontinuation. Digital ulceration and/or soft tissue breakdown have been observed rarely; monitor for digital changes during therapy and seek further evaluation (eg, rheumatology) if necessary (Syed, 2008). Difficulty in accommodation and blurred vision has been reported with the use of stimulants. Use with caution in patients with hypertension and other cardiovascular conditions that might be exacerbated by increases in blood pressure or heart rate (eg, preexisting hypertension, heart failure, recent myocardial infarction, ventricular arrhythmia). Use of immediate-release formulation is contraindicated in patients with advanced arteriosclerosis, moderate to severe hypertension, or symptomatic cardiovascular disease. Use with caution in patients with preexisting psychosis or bipolar disorder; may exacerbate symptoms of behavior and thought disorder or induce mixed/manic episode, respectively. New-onset psychosis or mania may also occur with stimulant use. Screen patients with comorbid depressive symptoms prior to initiating treatment to determine if they are at risk for bipolar disorder, including a family history of suicide, bipolar disorder, and depression. May be associated with aggressive behavior or hostility (causal relationship not established); monitor for development or worsening of these behaviors. Limited information exists regarding amphetamine use in seizure disorder

(Cortese, 2013). Use with caution in patients with a history of seizure disorder; may lower seizure threshold leading to new onset or breakthrough seizure activity. Use with caution in patients with Tourette syndrome; stimulants may exacerbate tics (motor and phonic) and Tourette syndrome. Evaluate for tics and Tourette syndrome prior to therapy initiation (Pliszka, 2007). Potentially significant drug-drug interactions may exist, requiring dose or frequency adjustment, additional monitoring, and/or selection of alternative therapy.

Appetite suppression may occur in children; monitor weight during therapy. Use of stimulants has been associated with weight loss and slowing of growth rate; monitor growth rate and weight during treatment. Treatment interruption may be necessary in patients who are not increasing in height or gaining weight as expected.

Abrupt discontinuation following high doses or for prolonged periods may result in symptoms for withdrawal. Do not substitute extended-release formulation for other amphetamine products on a mg-per-mg basis since base composition and pharmacokinetic profiles are not similar.

Adverse Reactions Frequency not always defined.

Cardiovascular: Increased blood pressure, palpitations, tachycardia

Central nervous system: Dizziness, dysphoria, euphoria, exacerbation of Gilles de la Tourette's syndrome, exacerbation of tics, exacerbation of vocal tics, headache, insomnia, overstimulation, restlessness

Dermatologic: Urticaria

Endocrine & metabolic: Change in libido

Gastrointestinal: Upper abdominal pain (children: 4%), anorexia (when used for other than anorectic effect), constipation, diarrhea, dysgeusia, gastrointestinal distress, weight loss (when used for other than anorectic effect), xerostomia

Genitourinary: Impotence

Neuromuscular & skeletal: Dyskinesia, tremor

Respiratory: Allergic rhinitis (children: 4%), epistaxis (children: 4%)

<1% (Limited to important or life-threatening): Cardiomyopathy (with chronic use), peripheral vascular disease, psychosis (including delusions, hallucination, and mania in children and adolescents), Raynaud's phenomenon

Drug Interactions

Metabolism/Transport Effects None known.

Avoid Concomitant Use

Avoid concomitant use of Amphetamine with any of the following: Iobenguane I 123; MAO Inhibitors

Increased Effect/Toxicity

Amphetamine may increase the levels/effects of: Analgesics (Opioid); Doxofylline; Sympathomimetics

The levels/effects of Amphetamine may be increased by: Alkalinizing Agents; Antacids; AtoMOXetine; Cannabinoid-Containing Products; Carbonic Anhydrase Inhibitors; Linezolid; MAO Inhibitors; Proton Pump Inhibitors; Tedizolid; Tricyclic Antidepressants

Decreased Effect

Amphetamine may decrease the levels/effects of: Antihistamines; Antihypertensive Agents; Ethosuximide; Iobenguane I 123; Ioflupane I 123; PHENobarbital; Phenytoin

The levels/effects of Amphetamine may be decreased by: Ammonium Chloride; Antipsychotic Agents; Ascorbic Acid; Gastrointestinal Acidifying Agents; Lithium; Methenamine; Multivitamins/Fluoride (with ADE); Multivitamins/Minerals (with ADEK, Folate, Iron); Multivitamins/Minerals (with AE, No Iron); Urinary Acidifying Agents

Food Interactions Amphetamine serum levels may be reduced if taken with acidic food, juices, or vitamin C. Management: Monitor response when taken concurrently.

Storage/Stability Store at 20°C to 25°C (68°F to 77°F); excursions permitted from 15°C to 30°C (59°F to 86°F).

Mechanism of Action Amphetamines are noncatecholamine sympathomimetic amines that promote release of catecholamines (primarily dopamine and norepinephrine) from their storage sites in the presynaptic nerve terminals. A less significant mechanism may include their ability to block the reuptake of catecholamines by competitive inhibition. The anorexigenic effect is probably secondary to the CNS-stimulating effect; the site of action is probably the hypothalamic feeding center.

Pharmacodynamics/Kinetics

Absorption: Rapid (de la Torre 2004)

Distribution: V_d: 3 to 4 L/kg (de la Torre 2004)

Protein binding: 16% (de la Torre 2004)

Metabolism: Hepatic via oxidation, deamination, and CYP2D6

Bioavailability: Good (de la Torre 2004); Dyanavel XR: 106% of d-amphetamine and 111% for l-amphetamine

Half-life elimination: 12 hours (de la Torre 2004)

Dyanavel XR:
Children: d-amphetamine 10.43 ± 2.01 hours and l-amphetamine 12.14 ± 3.15 hours
Adults: d-amphetamine 12.36 ± 2.95 hours and l-amphetamine 15.12 ± 4.4 hours

Time to peak, serum: Within 4 hours (de la Torre 2004)

Dyanavel XR:
Children: Median time d-amphetamine 3.9 hours and l-amphetamine 4.5 hours
Adults: 4 (2 to 7) hours

Excretion: Urine (30% to 40%)

Dosing

Adult & Geriatric Note: Administer at the lowest effective dose.

Exogenous obesity (immediate release): Oral: Up to 30 mg daily in divided doses (5 to 10 mg per dose)

Narcolepsy (immediate release): Oral: Initial: 10 mg once daily; increase daily dose in 10 mg increments at weekly intervals until optimal response is obtained; usual dosage range: 5 to 60 mg daily in divided doses

Pediatric Note: Administer at the lowest effective dose.

Attention deficit/hyperactivity disorder:

Extended release: Children ≥6 years and Adolescents: Oral: Initial: 2.5 or 5 mg once daily; may increase in 2.5 to 10 mg/day increments every 4 to 7 days until optimal response is obtained (maximum: 20 mg/day)

Note: Do not substitute extended-release formulation for other amphetamine products on a mg-per-mg basis since base composition and pharmacokinetic profiles are not similar. If switching from other amphetamine products, discontinue that treatment, and titrate as per the recommended dosing schedule.

Immediate release: Oral:

Children 3 to 5 years: Initial: 2.5 mg once daily; increase daily dose in 2.5 mg increments at weekly intervals until optimal response is obtained. Only in rare cases will it be necessary to exceed 40 mg daily.

Children ≥6 years and Adolescents: Initial: 5 mg once or twice daily; increase daily dose in 5 mg increments at weekly intervals until optimal response is obtained. Only in rare cases will it be necessary to exceed 40 mg daily.

Exogenous obesity (immediate release): Oral: Children ≥12 years and Adolescents: Up to 30 mg daily in divided doses (5 to 10 mg per dose)

Narcolepsy (immediate release): Oral:

Children 6 to 12 years: Initial: 5 mg once daily; increase daily dose in 5 mg increments at weekly intervals until optimal response is obtained; usual dosage range: 5 to 60 mg daily in divided doses

Children ≥12 years and Adolescents: Initial: 10 mg once daily; increase daily dose in 10 mg increments at weekly intervals until optimal response is obtained; usual dosage range: 5 to 60 mg daily in divided doses

Renal Impairment There are no dosage adjustments provided in the manufacturer's labeling.

Hepatic Impairment There are no dosage adjustments provided in the manufacturer's labeling.

Administration Oral:

Extended release: Administer in the morning with or without food; use an oral dosing syringe or other suitable measuring device when dosing suspension. Shake bottle well prior to administration.

Immediate release: Administer with or without food; for short-term adjunct treatment of exogenous obesity, administer 30 to 60 minutes before meals. Administer the first dose on awakening; administer additional doses at intervals of 4 to 6 hours. Avoid late evening dosing.

Monitoring Parameters

CNS activity, blood pressure, pulse; height, weight, growth parameters; appetite; signs/symptoms of misuse, abuse, addiction, tolerance or dependence; behavioral changes; signs of peripheral vasculopathy (eg, digital changes)

When used for the treatment of ADHD, perform a targeted cardiac history (eg, patient history of previously detected cardiac disease, palpitations, syncope, or seizures; family history of sudden death in children or young adults; hypertrophic cardiomyopathy; long QT syndrome) and physician examination including cardiac examination. Monitor heart rate and blood pressure (baseline; follow-up within 1 to 3 months and routinely at 6 to 12 month intervals thereafter unless clinically indicated with dose titration and weaning of therapy) Consider obtaining ECG prior to initiation (Perrin, 2008; Vetter, 2008).

Test Interactions Amphetamines may elevate plasma corticosteroid levels; may interfere with urinary steroid determinations.

Product Availability Dyanavel XR extended-release oral suspension: FDA approved October 2015; availability anticipated in 2016. Dyanavel XR is indicated for the treatment of attention deficit hyperactivity disorder (ADHD) in children 6 years of age and older.

Dosage Forms Excipient information presented when available (limited, particularly for generics); consult specific product labeling.

Tablet, Oral, as sulfate:
Evekeo: 5 mg [scored]
Evekeo: 10 mg [scored; contains brilliant blue fcf (fd&c blue #1)]

Controlled Substance C-II

◆ Amphetamine and Dextroamphetamine *see* Dextroamphetamine and Amphetamine *on page 533*

◆ Amphetamine Sulfate *see* Amphetamine *on page 115*

◆ Amphojel (Can) *see* Aluminum Hydroxide *on page 84*

◆ Amphotec *see* Amphotericin B Cholesteryl Sulfate Complex *on page 117*

◆ Amphotec® (Can) *see* Amphotericin B Cholesteryl Sulfate Complex *on page 117*

Amphotericin B Cholesteryl Sulfate Complex
(am foe TER i sin bee kole LES te ril SUL fate KOM plecks)

Brand Names: US Amphotec
Brand Names: Canada Amphotec®
Index Terms ABCD; Amphotericin B Colloidal Dispersion
Pharmacologic Category Antifungal Agent, Parenteral
Use Treatment of invasive aspergillosis in patients who have failed amphotericin B deoxycholate treatment, or who have renal impairment or experience unacceptable toxicity which precludes treatment with amphotericin B deoxycholate in effective doses.

Dosing
Adult & Geriatric Note: Lipid-based amphotericin formulations (Amphotec) may be confused with conventional formulations (desoxycholate [Amphocin, Fungizone]). Lipid-based and conventional formulations are **not** interchangeable and have different dosing recommendations. Overdoses have occurred when conventional formulations were dispensed inadvertently for lipid-based products.

Aspergillosis (invasive), treatment: *Usual dosage range:* 3-4 mg/kg/day. **Note:** 6 mg/kg/day has been used for treatment of life-threatening invasive aspergillosis in immunocompromised patients (Bowden, 2002).
Premedication: For patients who experience chills, fever, hypotension, nausea, or other nonanaphylactic infusion-related immediate reactions, premedicate with the following drugs 30-60 minutes prior to drug administration: A nonsteroidal with or without diphenhydramine **or** acetaminophen with diphenhydramine **or** hydrocortisone 50-100 mg with or without a nonsteroidal and diphenhydramine (Paterson, 2008).
Test dose: For patients receiving their first dose in a new treatment course, a small amount (10 mL of the final preparation, containing between 1.6-8.3 mg) infused over 15-30 minutes is recommended. The patient should then be observed for an additional 30 minutes.

Pediatric Refer to adult dosing.

Renal Impairment
Mild to moderate impairment: No dosage adjustment provided in manufacturer's labeling. However, no pharmacokinetic changes were noted in patients with mild-to-moderate impairment.
Severe impairment: No dosage adjustment provided in manufacturer's labeling (has not been studied).

Hepatic Impairment No dosage adjustment provided in manufacturer's labeling (has not been studied).

Additional Information Complete prescribing information should be consulted for additional detail.

Dosage Forms Excipient information presented when available (limited, particularly for generics); consult specific product labeling.
Suspension Reconstituted, Intravenous:
Amphotec: 50 mg (1 ea); 100 mg (1 ea) [contains edetate disodium, hydrochloric acid, lactose, sodium cholesteryl sulfate, tromethamine]

◆ Amphotericin B Colloidal Dispersion *see* Amphotericin B Cholesteryl Sulfate Complex *on page 117*

Amphotericin B (Conventional)
(am foe TER i sin bee con VEN sha nal)

Brand Names: Canada Fungizone

Index Terms Amphotericin B Deoxycholate; Amphotericin B Desoxycholate; Conventional Amphotericin B
Pharmacologic Category Antifungal Agent, Parenteral
Use
Life-threatening fungal infections: Treatment of patients with progressive, potentially life-threatening fungal infections: Aspergillosis, cryptococcosis (torulosis), North American blastomycosis, systemic candidiasis, coccidioidomycosis, histoplasmosis, zygomycosis (including mucormycosis due to susceptible species of the genera *Absidia, Mucor,* and *Rhizopus*), and infections due to related susceptible species of *Conidiobolus, Basidiobolus,* and sporotrichosis.
Leishmaniasis: May be useful in the treatment of American mucocutaneous leishmaniasis, but it is not the drug of choice as primary therapy.

Dosing
Adult & Geriatric Note: Conventional amphotericin formulations (desoxycholate [Amphocin, Fungizone]) may be confused with lipid-based formulations (AmBisome, Abelcet, Amphotec). Lipid-based and conventional formulations are **not** interchangeable and have different dosage recommendations. Overdoses have occurred when conventional formulations were dispensed inadvertently for lipid-based products.
Note: Premedication: For patients who experience infusion-related immediate reactions, premedicate with the following drugs 30 to 60 minutes prior to drug administration: NSAID and/or diphenhydramine **or** acetaminophen with diphenhydramine **or** hydrocortisone. If the patient experiences rigors during the infusion, meperidine may be administered.
Test dose: IV: 1 mg infused over 20 to 30 minutes. Many clinicians believe a test dose is unnecessary.
Susceptible fungal infections: IV: Adults: 0.3 to 1.5 mg/kg/day; 1 to 1.5 mg/kg over 4 to 6 hours every other day may be given once therapy is established; aspergillosis, rhinocerebral mucormycosis, often require 1 to 1.5 mg/kg/day; do not exceed 1.5 mg/kg/day
Aspergillosis, disseminated: IV: 0.6 to 0.7 mg/kg/day for 3 to 6 months
Aspergillosis (invasive) in HIV-infected patients (off-label use): IV: 1 mg/kg once daily until infection resolution and CD4 count >200 cells/mm^3 (HHS [OI adult 2015])
Bone marrow transplantation (prophylaxis): IV: Low-dose amphotericin B 0.1 to 0.25 mg/kg/day has been administered after bone marrow transplantation to reduce the risk of invasive fungal disease.
Candidemia (neutropenic or non-neutropenic): IV: 0.5 to 1 mg/kg/day until 14 days after first negative blood culture and resolution of signs and symptoms (Pappas, 2009)
Candidiasis, chronic, disseminated: IV: 0.5 to 0.7 mg/kg/day for 3 to 6 months and resolution of radiologic lesions (Pappas, 2009)
Coccidioidomycosis in HIV-infected patients with severe, non-meningeal infection (ie, diffuse pulmonary or severely ill with extrathoracic disseminated disease) (off-label use): IV: 0.7 to 1 mg/kg/day until clinical improvement, then initiate triazole therapy (eg, fluconazole or itraconazole) (HHS [OI adult 2015])
Dematiaceous fungi: IV: 0.7 mg/kg/day in combination with an azole
Endocarditis: IV: 0.6 to 1 mg/kg/day (with or without flucytosine) for 6 weeks after valve replacement; **Note:** If isolates susceptible and/or clearance demonstrated, guidelines recommend step-down to fluconazole; also for long-term suppression therapy if valve replacement is not possible (Pappas, 2009)
Endophthalmitis, fungal (off-label use):
Intravitreal: 5 to 12.5 mcg (with or without concomitant systemic therapy) (Brod, 1990)
IV: 0.7 to 1 mg/kg/day (with flucytosine) for at least 4 to 6 weeks (Pappas, 2009)
Esophageal candidiasis: IV: 0.3 to 0.7 mg/kg/day for 14 to 21 days after clinical improvement (Pappas, 2009)
Histoplasmosis: Chronic, severe pulmonary or disseminated: IV: 0.5 to 1 mg/kg/day for 7 days, then 0.8 mg/kg every other day (or 3 times/week) until total dose of 10 to 15 mg/kg; may continue itraconazole as suppressive therapy (lifelong for immunocompromised patients)
Meningitis:
Candidal: IV: 0.7 to 1 mg/kg/day (with or without flucytosine) for at least 4 weeks; **Note:** Liposomal amphotericin favored by IDSA guidelines based on decreased risk of nephrotoxicity and potentially better CNS penetration (Pappas, 2009)

Cryptococcal or Coccidioides: Intrathecal: Initial: 0.01 to 0.05 mg as single daily dose; may increase daily in increments of 0.025 to 0.1 mg as tolerated (maximum: 1.5 mg/day; most patients will tolerate a maximum dose of ~0.5 mg/treatment). Once titration to a maximum tolerated dose is achieved, that dose is administered daily. Once CSF improvement noted, may decrease frequency on a weekly basis (eg, 5 times/week, then 3 times/week, then 2 times/week, then once weekly, then once every other week, then once every 2 weeks, etc) until administration occurs once every 6 weeks. Typically, concurrent oral azole therapy is maintained (Stevens, 2001). **Note:** IDSA notes that the use of intrathecal amphotericin for cryptococcal meningitis is generally discouraged and rarely necessary (Perfect, 2010).

Histoplasma: IV: 0.5 to 1 mg/kg/day for 7 days, then 0.8 mg/kg every other day (or 3 times/week) for 3 months total duration; follow with fluconazole suppressive therapy for up to 12 months

Meningoencephalitis, cryptococcal (Perfect, 2010): IV:

HIV positive: Induction: 0.7 to 1 mg/kg/day (plus flucytosine 100 mg/kg/day) for 2 weeks, then change to oral fluconazole for at least 8 weeks; alternatively, amphotericin (0.7 to 1 mg/kg/day) may be continued uninterrupted for 4 to 6 weeks; maintenance: amphotericin 1 mg/kg/week for ≥1 year may be considered, but inferior to use of azoles

HIV negative: Induction: 0.7 to 1 mg/kg/day (plus flucytosine 100 mg/kg/day) for 2 weeks (low-risk patients), ≥4 weeks (non-low-risk, but without neurologic complication, immunosuppression, underlying disease, and negative CSF culture at 2 weeks), >6 weeks (neurologic complication or patients intolerant of flucytosine) Follow with azole consolidation/maintenance treatment.

Oropharyngeal candidiasis: IV: 0.3 mg/kg/day for 7 to 14 days (Pappas, 2009)

Osteoarticular candidiasis: IV: 0.5 to 1 mg/kg/day for several weeks, followed by fluconazole for 6 to 12 months (osteomyelitis) or 6 weeks (septic arthritis) (Pappas, 2009)

Penicillium marneffei: IV: 0.6 mg/kg/day for 2 weeks

Pneumonia: Cryptococcal (mild to moderate): IV:

HIV positive: 0.5 to 1 mg/kg/day

HIV negative: 0.5 to 0.7 mg/kg/day (plus flucytosine) for 2 weeks

Sporotrichosis: Pulmonary, meningeal, osteoarticular or disseminated: IV: Total dose of 1 to 2 g, then change to oral itraconazole or fluconazole for suppressive therapy

Urinary tract candidiasis (IDSA [Pappas, 2009]):

Fungus balls: IV: 0.5 to 0.7 mg/kg/day with or without flucytosine 25 mg/kg 4 times daily

Pyelonephritis: IV: 0.5 to 0.7 mg/kg/day with or without flucytosine 25 mg/kg 4 times daily for 2 weeks

Symptomatic cystitis: IV: 0.3 to 0.6 mg/kg/day for 1 to 7 days

Bladder irrigation in patients with C. krusei or fluconazole-resistant C. glabrata: Irrigate with 50 mcg/mL solution instilled periodically or continuously for 5 to 7 days or until cultures are clear. **Note:** Recommended for use in conjunction with other treatment modalities (Fisher, 2011).

Pediatric Note: Conventional amphotericin formulations (desoxycholate [Amphocin, Fungizone]) may be confused with lipid-based formulations (AmBisome, Abelcet, Amphotec). Lipid-based and conventional formulations are **not** interchangeable and have different dosage recommendations. Overdoses have occurred when conventional formulations were dispensed inadvertently for lipid-based products.

Note: Premedication: For patients who experience infusion-related immediate reactions, premedicate with the following drugs 30 to 60 minutes prior to drug administration: NSAID and/or diphenhydramine **or** acetaminophen with diphenhydramine **or** hydrocortisone. If the patient experiences rigors during the infusion, meperidine may be administered.

Test dose: IV: Infants and Children: 0.1 mg/kg/dose to a maximum of 1 mg; infuse over 30 to 60 minutes. Many clinicians believe a test dose is unnecessary.

Susceptible fungal infections: IV: Infants and Children: Maintenance dose: 0.25 to 1 mg/kg/day given once daily; infuse over 2 to 6 hours. Once therapy has been established, amphotericin B can be administered on an every-other-day basis at 1 to 1.5 mg/kg/dose; cumulative dose: 1.5 to 2 g over 6 to 10 weeks

Note: Duration of therapy varies with nature of infection: Usual duration is 4 to 12 weeks or cumulative dose of 1 to 4 g.

Indication-specific dosing:

Infants and Children:

Aspergillosis (HIV-exposed/-positive): IV: 1 to 1.5 mg/kg/day once daily (CDC, 2009)

Candidiasis (HIV-exposed/-positive):

Invasive: IV: 0.5 to 1.5 mg/kg/day once daily (CDC, 2009)

Esophageal: IV: 0.3 to 0.5 mg/kg/day once daily (CDC, 2009)

Oropharyngeal, refractory: IV: 0.3 to 0.5 mg/kg/day (CDC, 2009)

Coccidioidomycosis (HIV-exposed/-positive): IV: 0.5 to 1 mg/kg/day (CDC, 2009)

***Cryptococcus,* CNS disease (HIV-exposed/-positive):** IV: 0.7 to 1 mg/kg/day plus flucytosine; **Note:** Minimum 2 week induction followed by consolidation and chronic suppressive therapy; may increase amphotericin dose to 1.5 mg/kg/day if flucytosine is not tolerated.

***Cryptococcus,* disseminated (non-CNS disease) or severe pulmonary disease (HIV-exposed/-positive):** IV: 0.7 to 1 mg/kg/day once daily with or without flucytosine

Histoplasma, CNS or severe disseminated: IV: 1 mg/kg/day once daily (CDC, 2009)

Adolescents:

Aspergillosis (invasive) in HIV-infected patients (off-label use): IV: Refer to adult dosing.

Coccidioidomycosis in HIV-infected patients with severe, non-meningeal infection (ie, diffuse pulmonary or severely ill with extrathoracic disseminated disease) (off-label use): IV: Refer to adult dosing.

Renal Impairment

If renal dysfunction is due to the drug, the daily total can be decreased by 50% or the dose can be given every other day. IV therapy may take several months.

Renal replacement therapy: Poorly dialyzed; no supplemental dose or dosage adjustment necessary, including patients on intermittent hemodialysis or CRRT.

Peritoneal dialysis (PD): Administration in dialysate: 1 to 2 mg/L of peritoneal dialysis fluid either with or without low-dose IV amphotericin B (a total dose of 2 to 10 mg/kg given over 7 to 14 days). Precipitate may form in ionic dialysate solutions.

Hepatic Impairment No dosage adjustment provided in manufacturer's labeling.

Additional Information Complete prescribing information should be consulted for additional detail.

Dosage Forms Excipient information presented when available (limited, particularly for generics); consult specific product labeling.

Solution Reconstituted, Injection, as desoxycholate:

Generic: 50 mg (1 ea)

◆ Amphotericin B Deoxycholate *see* Amphotericin B (Conventional) *on page 117*

◆ Amphotericin B Desoxycholate *see* Amphotericin B (Conventional) *on page 117*

Amphotericin B (Lipid Complex)
(am foe TER i sin bee LIP id KOM pleks)

Brand Names: US Abelcet

Brand Names: Canada Abelcet

Index Terms ABLC

Pharmacologic Category Antifungal Agent, Parenteral

Use Treatment of invasive fungal infection in patients who are refractory to or intolerant of conventional amphotericin B (amphotericin B deoxycholate) therapy

Dosing

Adult & Geriatric

Note: Lipid-based amphotericin formulations (Abelcet) may be confused with conventional formulations (desoxycholate [Amphocin, Fungizone]) or with other lipid-based amphotericin formulations (amphotericin B liposomal [AmBisome]; amphotericin B cholesteryl sulfate complex [Amphotec]). Lipid-based and conventional formulations are **not** interchangeable and have different dosing recommendations. Overdoses have occurred when conventional formulations were dispensed inadvertently for lipid-based products.

Note: Premedication: For patients who experience infusion-related immediate reactions, premedicate with the following drugs 30 to 60 minutes prior to drug administration: A nonsteroidal anti-inflammatory agent ± diphenhydramine **or** acetaminophen with diphenhydramine **or** hydrocortisone. If the patient experiences rigors during the infusion, meperidine may be administered.

Usual dose: IV: 5 mg/kg once daily
Manufacturer's labeling: Invasive fungal infections (when patients are intolerant or refractory to conventional amphotericin B): IV: 5 mg/kg/day

Indication-specific dosing:
Aspergillosis, invasive (alternative to preferred therapy): IV: 5 mg/kg/day; duration of treatment depends on site of infection, extent of disease and level of immunosuppression (Walsh 2008)
Aspergillosis (invasive) in HIV-infected patients (alternative to preferred therapy) (off-label use): 5 mg/kg/day; treat until infection appears to be resolved and CD4 count >200 cells/mm³ (HHS [OI adult 2015])
Blastomycosis, moderately severe to severe (off-label dose): IV: 3 to 5 mg/kg/day for 1 to 2 weeks or until improvement, followed by oral itraconazole (Chapman 2008)
Candidiasis (off-label dose): IV:
Chronic disseminated candidiasis, pericarditis or myocarditis due to Candida, suppurative thrombophlebitis: 3 to 5 mg/kg/day. **Note:** In chronic disseminated candidiasis, transition to fluconazole after several weeks in stable patients is preferred (Pappas 2009)
CNS candidiasis: 3 to 5 mg/kg/day (with or without flucytosine) for several weeks, followed by fluconazole (Pappas 2009)
Endocarditis due to Candida, infected pacemaker, ICD, or VAD: 3 to 5 mg/kg/day (with or without flucytosine); continue to treat for 4 to 6 weeks after device removal unless device cannot be removed then chronic suppression with fluconazole is recommended (Pappas 2009)
Coccidioidomycosis, progressive, disseminated (alternative to preferred therapy) (off-label dose): IV: 2 to 5 mg/kg/day (Galgiani 2005)
Coccidioidomycosis in HIV-infected patients with severe, nonmeningeal infection (ie, diffuse pulmonary or severely ill with extrathoracic disseminated disease) (off-label use): 4 to 6 mg/kg/day until clinical improvement, then switch to fluconazole or itraconazole (HHS [OI adult 2015])
Cryptococcosis: IV:
Cryptococcal meningitis in HIV-infected patients (alternative to preferred therapy) (off-label use): Induction therapy: 5 mg/kg/day with flucytosine for at least 2 weeks, followed by fluconazole for consolidation therapy (HHS [OI adult 2015]; Perfect 2010). **Note:** If flucytosine is not given due to intolerance, duration of amphotericin B lipid complex therapy should be 4 to 6 weeks (Perfect 2010).
Cryptococcal meningoencephalitis in HIV-negative patients and nontransplant patients (as an alternative to conventional amphotericin B): Induction therapy: 5 mg/kg/day (with flucytosine if possible) for ≥4 weeks followed by oral fluconazole. **Note:** If flucytosine is not given or treatment is interrupted, consider prolonging induction therapy for an additional 2 weeks (Perfect 2010).
Cryptococcal meningoencephalitis in transplant recipients: Induction therapy: 5 mg/kg/day (with flucytosine) for at least 2 weeks, followed by oral fluconazole **Note:** If flucytosine is not given, duration of amphotericin B lipid complex therapy should be 4 to 6 weeks (Perfect 2010).
Nonmeningeal cryptococcosis: Induction therapy: 5 mg/kg/day (with flucytosine if possible) for ≥4 weeks may be used for severe pulmonary cryptococcosis or for cryptococcemia with evidence of high fungal burden, followed by oral fluconazole. **Note:** If flucytosine is not given or treatment is interrupted, consider prolonging induction therapy for an additional 2 weeks (Perfect 2010).
Histoplasmosis: IV:
Acute pulmonary (moderately severe to severe): 5 mg/kg/day for 1 to 2 weeks, followed by oral itraconazole (Wheat 2007)
Moderate to severe disseminated disease in HIV-infected patients (alternative to preferred therapy) (off-label use): 3 mg/kg/day for at least 2 weeks, followed by itraconazole maintenance therapy (HHS [OI adult 2015])
Progressive disseminated (alternative to preferred therapy): 5 mg/kg/day for 1 to 2 weeks, followed by oral itraconazole (Wheat 2007)
Leishmaniasis (visceral) in HIV-infected patients (off-label use; HHS [OI adult 2015]):
Chronic maintenance therapy (for patients with a CD4 count <200 cells/mm³: 3 mg/kg every 21 days (HHS [OI adult 2015])
Sporotrichosis (off-label dose): IV:
Meningeal: 5 mg/kg/day for 4 to 6 weeks, followed by oral itraconazole (Kauffman 2007)

Pulmonary, osteoarticular, and disseminated: 3 to 5 mg/kg/day, followed by oral itraconazole after a favorable response is seen with amphotericin initial therapy (Kauffman 2007)
Pediatric
Note: Lipid-based amphotericin formulations (Abelcet) may be confused with conventional formulations (desoxycholate [Amphocin, Fungizone]) or with other lipid-based amphotericin formulations (amphotericin B liposomal [AmBisome]; amphotericin B cholesteryl sulfate complex [Amphotec]). Lipid-based and conventional formulations are **not** interchangeable and have different dosing recommendations. Overdoses have occurred when conventional formulations were dispensed inadvertently for lipid-based products.
Note: Premedication: For patients who experience infusion-related immediate reactions, premedicate with the following drugs 30 to 60 minutes prior to drug administration: A nonsteroidal anti-inflammatory agent ± diphenhydramine **or** acetaminophen with diphenhydramine **or** hydrocortisone. If the patient experiences rigors during the infusion, meperidine may be administered.

Usual dose: 5 mg/kg once daily
Manufacturer's labeling: Invasive fungal infections (when patients are intolerant or refractory to conventional amphotericin B): Children: IV: 5 mg/kg/day

Indication-specific dosing:
Aspergillosis (HIV-positive patients) (alternative to preferred therapy):
Infants and Children: IV: 5 mg/kg/day for ≥12 weeks (CDC [pediatric 2009])
Adolescents: Refer to adult dosing.
Candidiasis, invasive (HIV-positive patients) (alternative to preferred therapy): Infants and Children: IV: 5 mg/kg/day; treatment duration based on clinical response, treat until 2 to 3 weeks after last positive blood culture (CDC [pediatric 2009])
Coccidioidomycosis in HIV-infected patients with severe, nonmeningeal infection (ie, diffuse pulmonary or severely ill with extrathoracic disseminated disease) (off-label use): Adolescents: Refer to adult dosing.
Cryptococcosis:
Cryptococcus neoformans, disseminated disease (non-CNS disease) (HIV-positive patients): Infants and Children: IV: 5 mg/kg/day (with or without flucytosine); treatment duration of non-CNS disease varies by clinical response and site/severity of infection (CDC [pediatric 2009])
Cryptococcal meningitis in HIV-infected patients (as an alternative to preferred therapy) (off-label use): Adolescents: Refer to adult dosing.
Histoplasmosis in HIV-infected patients with moderate to severe disseminated disease (alternative to preferred therapy): Adolescents: Refer to adult dosing.
Leishmaniasis (visceral), chronic maintenance therapy in HIV-infected patients (off-label use): Adolescents: Refer to adult dosing.
Renal Impairment
Manufacturer's labeling: No dosage adjustment provided in manufacturer's labeling (has not been studied).
Alternate recommendations (Aronoff 2007):
Intermittent hemodialysis: Not hemodialyzable; no supplemental dosage necessary.
Peritoneal dialysis: No supplemental dosage necessary.
Continuous renal replacement therapy (CRRT): No supplemental dosage necessary.
Hepatic Impairment No dosage adjustment provided in manufacturer's labeling (has not been studied).
Additional Information Complete prescribing information should be consulted for additional detail.
Dosage Forms Excipient information presented when available (limited, particularly for generics); consult specific product labeling.
Suspension, Intravenous:
Abelcet: 5 mg/mL (20 mL)

Amphotericin B (Liposomal)
(am foe TER i sin bee lye po SO mal)

Brand Names: US AmBisome
Brand Names: Canada AmBisome
Index Terms Amphotericin B Liposome; L-AmB; Liposomal Amphotericin; Liposomal Amphotericin B
Pharmacologic Category Antifungal Agent, Parenteral

Use

Cryptococcal meningitis in HIV-infected patients: Treatment of cryptococcal meningitis in HIV-infected patients.

Fungal infections, empiric therapy: Empiric treatment in febrile neutropenic patients with presumed fungal infection.

Fungal infections, systemic therapy: Treatment of systemic infections caused by *Aspergillus* sp, *Candida* sp, and/or *Cryptococcus* sp in patients refractory to conventional amphotericin B deoxycholate therapy or when renal impairment or unacceptable toxicity precludes the use of the deoxycholate formulation.

Leishmaniasis (visceral): Treatment of visceral leishmaniasis.

Pregnancy Considerations Adverse events were not observed in animal reproduction studies. Amphotericin crosses the placenta and enters the fetal circulation. Amphotericin B is recommended for the treatment of serious systemic fungal diseases in pregnant women; refer to current guidelines (King 1998).

Breast-Feeding Considerations It is not known if amphotericin is excreted into breast milk. Due to its poor oral absorption, systemic exposure to the nursing infant is expected to be decreased; however, because of the potential for toxicity, breast-feeding is not recommended (Mactal-Haaf 2001).

Contraindications Hypersensitivity to amphotericin B deoxycholate or any component of the formulation

Warnings/Precautions Anaphylaxis has been reported with amphotericin B-containing drugs; facilities for cardiopulmonary resuscitation should be available during administration. Acute infusion reactions (including fever and chills) may occur 1 to 3 hours after starting infusions; reactions are more common with the first few doses and generally diminish with subsequent doses. Immediately discontinue infusion if a severe anaphylactic reaction occurs; the patient should not receive further infusions. Acute pulmonary toxicity has been reported in patients receiving simultaneous leukocyte transfusions and amphotericin B. Potentially significant interactions may exist, requiring dose or frequency adjustment, additional monitoring, and/or selection of alternative therapy.

Adverse Reactions Percentage of adverse reactions is dependent upon population studied and may vary with respect to premedications and underlying illness. Incidence of decreased renal function and infusion-related events are lower than rates observed with amphotericin B deoxycholate.

>10%:

Cardiovascular: Hypertension (8% to 20%), tachycardia (9% to 19%), peripheral edema (15%), edema (12% to 14%), hypotension (7% to 14%), chest pain (8% to 12%), localized phlebitis (9% to 11%)

Central nervous system: Chills (29% to 48%), insomnia (17% to 22%), headache (9% to 20%), pain (14%), anxiety (7% to 14%), confusion (9% to 13%)

Dermatologic: Skin rash (5% to 25%), pruritus (11%)

Endocrine & metabolic: Hypokalemia (31% to 51%), hypomagnesemia (15% to 50%), hyperglycemia (8% to 23%), hypocalcemia (5% to 18%), hyponatremia (9% to 12%), hypervolemia (8% to 12%)

Gastrointestinal: Nausea (16% to 40%), vomiting (11% to 32%), diarrhea (11% to 30%), abdominal pain (7% to 20%), constipation (15%), anorexia (10% to 14%)

Genitourinary: Nephrotoxicity (14% to 47%), hematuria (14%)

Hematologic & oncologic: Anemia (27% to 48%), leukopenia (15% to 17%), thrombocytopenia (6% to 13%)

Hepatic: Increased serum alkaline phosphatase (7% to 22%), hyperbilirubinemia (≤18%), increased serum ALT (15%), increased serum AST (13%), abnormal hepatic function tests (not specified) (4% to 13%)

Hypersensitivity: Transfusion reaction (9% to 18%)

Infection: Sepsis (7% to 14%), infection (11% to 13%)

Neuromuscular & skeletal: Weakness (6% to 13%), back pain (12%)

Renal: Increased serum creatinine (18% to 40%), increased blood urea nitrogen (7% to 21%)

Respiratory: Dyspnea (18% to 23%), pulmonary disease (14% to 18%), cough (2% to 18%), epistaxis (9% to 15%), pleural effusion (13%), rhinitis (11%)

Miscellaneous: Infusion related reactions (4% to 21%; fever [7% to 24%], chills [6% to 24%], vomiting [4% to 16%], nausea [8% to 14%], dyspnea [5% to 10%], tachycardia [2% to 10%], hypertension [2% to 9%], vasodilation [5%], hypotension [4%], hyperventilation [1%], hypoxia [≤1%])

2% to 10%:

Cardiovascular: Atrial fibrillation, bradycardia, cardiac arrest, cardiac arrhythmia, cardiomegaly, facial edema, flushing, heart valve disease, orthostatic hypotension, vascular disorder, vasodilatation

Central nervous system: Dizziness (7% to 9%), abnormality in thinking, agitation, coma, depression, drowsiness, dysesthesia, dystonia, hallucination, malaise, nervousness, paresthesia, rigors, seizure

Dermatologic: Diaphoresis (7%), alopecia, cellulitis, dermal ulcer, dermatological reaction, maculopapular rash, skin discoloration, urticaria, vesiculobullous dermatitis, xeroderma

Endocrine & metabolic: Hypernatremia (4%), acidosis, hyperchloremia, hyperkalemia, hypermagnesemia, hyperphosphatemia, hypophosphatemia, increased lactate dehydrogenase, increased nonprotein nitrogen

Gastrointestinal: Gastrointestinal hemorrhage (10%), aphthous stomatitis, dyspepsia, dysphagia, enlargement of abdomen, eructation, fecal incontinence, flatulence, gingival hemorrhage, hematemesis, hemorrhoids, hiccups, increased serum amylase, intestinal obstruction, mucositis, rectal disease, stomatitis, xerostomia

Genitourinary: Dysuria, toxic nephrosis, urinary incontence, vaginal hemorrhage

Hematologic & oncologic: Blood coagulation disorder, bruise, decreased prothrombin time, hemophthalmos, hemorrhage, hypoproteinemia, increased prothrombin time, oral hemorrhage, petechia, purpura

Hepatic: Hepatic injury, hepatic veno-occlusive disease, hepatomegaly

Hypersensitivity: Delayed hypersensitivity, hypersensitivity reaction

Immunologic: Graft versus host disease

Infection: Herpes simplex infection

Local: Inflammation at injection site

Neuromuscular & skeletal: Arthralgia, myalgia, neck pain, ostealgia, tremor

Ophthalmic: Conjunctivitis, dry eyes

Renal: Acute renal failure, renal failure, renal function abnormality

Respiratory: Hypoxia (6% to 8%), asthma, atelectasis, dry nose, flu-like symptoms, hemoptysis, hyperventilation, pharyngitis, pneumonia, pulmonary edema, respiratory alkalosis, respiratory failure, respiratory insufficiency, sinusitis

Miscellaneous: Procedural complication (8% to 10%)

Postmarketing and/or case reports: Agranulocytosis, angioedema, cyanosis, hemorrhagic cystitis, hypoventilation, rhabdomyolysis

Drug Interactions

Metabolism/Transport Effects None known.

Avoid Concomitant Use

Avoid concomitant use of Amphotericin B (Liposomal) with any of the following: Foscarnet; Saccharomyces boulardii

Increased Effect/Toxicity

Amphotericin B (Liposomal) may increase the levels/ effects of: Amifostine; Aminoglycosides; Antipsychotic Agents (Second Generation [Atypical]); Cardiac Glycosides; Colistimethate; CycloSPORINE (Systemic); DULoxetine; Flucytosine; Hypotension-Associated Agents; Levodopa

The levels/effects of Amphotericin B (Liposomal) may be increased by: Alfuzosin; Barbiturates; Blood Pressure Lowering Agents; Brimonidine (Topical); Corticosteroids (Orally Inhaled); Corticosteroids (Systemic); Diazoxide; Foscarnet; Herbs (Hypotensive Properties); Molsidomine; Nicorandil; Obinutuzumab; Pentoxifylline; Phosphodiesterase 5 Inhibitors; Prostacyclin Analogues

Decreased Effect

Amphotericin B (Liposomal) may decrease the levels/ effects of: Saccharomyces boulardii

The levels/effects of Amphotericin B (Liposomal) may be decreased by: Antifungal Agents (Azole Derivatives, Systemic)

Preparation for Administration Reconstitute with 12 mL SWFI to a concentration of 4 mg/mL. The use of any solution other than those recommended, or the presence of a bacteriostatic agent in the solution, may cause precipitation. **Shake the vial vigorously** for 30 seconds, until dispersed into a translucent yellow suspension.

Filtration and dilution: Withdraw appropriate amount of reconstituted solution into a syringe, attach a 5-micron filter, and inject contents of syringe through filter needle into an appropriate amount of D_5W. Dilute to a final concentration of 1-2 mg/mL (0.2-0.5 mg/mL for infants and small children).

Storage/Stability Store intact vials at ≤25°C (≤77°F). Reconstituted vials are stable at 2°C to 8°C (36°F to 46°F) for 24 hours. Do not freeze. Begin infusion within 6 hours of dilution with D$_5$W. Extended storage information may be available; contact product manufacturer to obtain current recommendations.

Mechanism of Action Binds to ergosterol altering cell membrane permeability in susceptible fungi and causing leakage of cell components with subsequent cell death. Proposed mechanism suggests that amphotericin causes an oxidation-dependent stimulation of macrophages (Lyman 1992).

Pharmacodynamics/Kinetics Note: Exhibits nonlinear kinetics (greater than proportional increase in serum concentration with an increase in dose)

Distribution: V$_d$: 0.1 to 0.16 L/kg

Half-life elimination: 7 to 10 hours (following a single 24-hour dosing interval); Terminal half to life: 100 to 153 hours (following multiple dosing up to 49 days)

Dosing

Adult & Geriatric Note: Lipid-based amphotericin formulations (AmBisome) may be confused with conventional formulations (desoxycholate [Amphocin, Fungizone]) or with other lipid-based amphotericin formulations (amphotericin B lipid complex [Abelcet], amphotericin B cholesteryl sulfate complex [Amphotec]). Lipid-based and conventional formulations are **not** interchangeable and have different dosing recommendations. Overdoses have occurred when conventional formulations were dispensed inadvertently for lipid-based products.

Usual dosage range: IV: 3 to 6 mg/kg/day; **Note:** Higher doses (7.5 to 15 mg/kg/day) have been used clinically in special cases (CDC 2013; Kauffman 2012; Walsh 2001)

Note: Premedication: For patients who experience non-anaphylactic immediate infusion-related reactions, premedicate with the following drugs 30 to 60 minutes prior to drug administration: A nonsteroidal anti-inflammatory agent ± diphenhydramine; **or** acetaminophen with diphenhydramine; **or** hydrocortisone. If the patient experiences rigors during the infusion, meperidine may be administered.

Indication-specific dosing: IV:

Aspergillus **(systemic infection):** 3 to 5 mg/kg/day

Aspergillosis (invasive) in HIV-infected patients (alternative to preferred therapy) (off-label use): 5 mg/kg/day until infection resolution and CD4 count >200 cells/mm^3 (HHS [OI adult 2015])

Candidiasis:

Empiric therapy: 3 to 5 mg/kg/day (Pappas 2009)

Endocarditis: 3 to 5 mg/kg/day (with or without flucytosine) for 6 weeks after valve replacement; Note: If isolates susceptible and/or clearance demonstrated, guidelines recommend step-down to fluconazole; also for long-term suppression therapy if valve replacement is not possible (Pappas 2009)

General invasive disease: 3 to 5 mg/kg/day with oral flucytosine (off-label combination; Pappas 2009)

Meningitis: 3 to 5 mg/kg/day with or without oral flucytosine (off-label combination; Pappas 2009)

Osteoarticular: 3 to 5 mg/kg/day for several weeks, followed by fluconazole for 6 to 12 months (osteomyelitis) or 6 weeks (septic arthritis) (Pappas 2009)

Systemic infection: Manufacturer's labeling: 3 to 5 mg/kg/day

Coccidioidomycosis in HIV-infected patients with severe, non-meningeal infection (ie, diffuse pulmonary or severely ill with extrathoracic, disseminated disease) (off-label use): 4 to 6 mg/kg/day until clinical improvement, then initiate triazole therapy (eg, fluconazole or itraconazole) (HHS [OI adult 2015])

Cryptococcus **(systemic infection):** 3 to 5 mg/kg/day

Cryptococcal meningitis in HIV-infected patients:

Manufacturer's labeling: 6 mg/kg/day

Alternate recommendations: 3 to 4 mg/kg/day in combination with oral flucytosine (HHS [OI adult 2015])

Fungal sinusitis: Limited data in immunocompromised patients have shown efficacy with 3 to 10 mg/kg/day (Barron 2005; Pagano 2004; Rokicka 2006). Note: An azole antifungal is recommended if causative organism is *Aspergillus* spp or *Pseudallescheria boydii* (*Scedosporium* sp).

Histoplasmosis in HIV-infected patients (off-label use; HHS [OI adult 2015]):

Moderately severe to severe disseminated disease: Induction therapy: 3 mg/kg/day for at least 2 weeks, followed by oral itraconazole for maintenance therapy

Histoplasma meningitis: Induction therapy: 5 mg/kg/day for 4 to 6 weeks, followed by oral itraconazole for maintenance therapy

Leishmaniasis (cutaneous) in HIV-infected patients (off-label use): 2 to 4 mg/kg/day for 10 days or an interrupted schedule (eg, 4 mg/kg on days 1 through 5, and then on days 10, 17, 24, 31, 38). Total dose administered should be 20 to 60 mg/kg (HHS [OI adult 2015])

Leishmaniasis (visceral):

Immunocompetent: 3 mg/kg/day on days 1 through 5, and 3 mg/kg/day on days 14 and 21; a repeat course may be given in patients who do not achieve parasitic clearance

Immunocompromised: 4 mg/kg/day on days 1 through 5, and 4 mg/kg/day on days 10, 17, 24, 31, and 38

Leishmaniasis (visceral) in HIV-infected patients (off-label use; HHS [OI adult 2015]):

Treatment: 2 to 4 mg/kg/day **or** an interrupted schedule (eg, 4 mg/kg on days 1 through 5, and then on days 10, 17, 24, 31, and 38). Total dose administered: 20 to 60 mg/kg

Chronic maintenance therapy (for patients with a CD4 count <200 cells/mm^3): 4 mg/kg every 2 to 4 weeks

Meningitis (secondary to contaminated [eg, Exserohilum rostratum] steroid products), severe or in patients not improving with voriconazole monotherapy (off-label use) (CDC 2013; Kauffman 2012): IV: 5 to 6 mg/kg/day in combination with voriconazole for ≥3 months; a higher dose (7.5 mg/kg/day) may be considered in patients who are not improving. **Note:** Consult an infectious disease specialist and current CDC guidelines for specific treatment recommendations.

Osteoarticular infection (secondary to contaminated [eg, *Exserohilum rostratum*] steroid products), severe or in patients with clinical instability (off-label use) (CDC 2013; Kauffman 2012): IV: 5 mg/kg/day in combination with voriconazole for ≥3 months. **Note:** Consult an infectious disease specialist and current CDC guidelines for specific treatment recommendations.

Penicillium marneffei **infection in HIV-infected patients (off-label use):** 3 to 5 mg/kg/day for 2 weeks, followed by oral itraconazole for 10 weeks, followed by chronic maintenance therapy (HHS [OI adult 2015])

Pediatric Note: Lipid-based amphotericin formulations (AmBisome) may be confused with conventional formulations (desoxycholate [Amphocin, Fungizone]) or with other lipid-based amphotericin formulations (amphotericin B lipid complex [Abelcet], amphotericin B cholesteryl sulfate complex [Amphotec]). Lipid-based and conventional formulations are **not** interchangeable and have different dosing recommendations. Overdoses have occurred when conventional formulations were dispensed inadvertently for lipid-based products.

Usual dosage range: Infants, Children, and Adolescents: IV: 3 to 6 mg/kg/day

Note: Premedication: For patients who experience nonanaphylactic immediate infusion-related reactions, premedicate with the following drugs 30 to 60 minutes prior to drug administration: A nonsteroidal anti-inflammatory agent ± diphenhydramine; **or** acetaminophen with diphenhydramine; **or** hydrocortisone. If the patient experiences rigors during the infusion, meperidine may be administered.

Indication-specific dosing:

Infants, Children, and Adolescents: IV:

Empiric therapy: 3 mg/kg/day

Cryptococcal meningitis in HIV-exposed/infected patients:

Infants and Children: 6 mg/kg/dose once daily; may coadminister with flucytosine (HHS [OI pediatric 2013]; off-label combination)

Adolescents: Refer to adult dosing.

Systemic fungal infections (*Aspergillus, Candida, Cryptococcus*); non-HIV-exposed/-infected: 3 to 5 mg/kg/day

Systemic fungal infections (HIV-exposed/-infected [HHS (OI pediatric 2013; OI adult 2015)]; off-label use):

Infants and Children:

Candidiasis, invasive: 5 mg/kg/dose once daily

Coccidioidomycosis (severe illness with respiratory compromise due to diffuse pulmonary or disseminated non-meningitic disease): 5 mg/kg/dose once daily until clinical improvement, then initiate triazole therapy (eg, fluconazole or itraconazole); dosage may be increased to 10 mg/kg/dose once daily for life-threatening infection.

Cryptococcus, disseminated (non-CNS): 3 to 5 mg/kg/dose once daily (may consider addition of oral flucytosine)

Histoplasmosis:
CNS infection: 5 mg/kg/dose once daily
Disseminated: 3 to 5 mg/kg/day once daily
Adolescents: Refer to adult dosing.
Leishmaniasis (cutaneous) in HIV-infected patients (off-label use): Adolescents: Refer to adult dosing.
Leishmaniasis (visceral):
Immunocompetent: 3 mg/kg/day on days 1 to 5, and 3 mg/kg/day on days 14 and 21; a repeat course may be given in patients who do not achieve parasitic clearance
Immunocompromised: 4 mg/kg/day on days 1 to 5, and 4 mg/kg/day on days 10, 17, 24, 31, and 38
Leishmaniasis (visceral) in HIV-infected patients (off-label use): Adolescents: Refer to adult dosing.
Penicillium marneffei **infection in HIV-infected patients (off-label use):** Adolescents: Refer to adult dosing.

Renal Impairment
There are no dosage adjustments provided in the manufacturer's labeling; has been successfully administered to patients with preexisting renal impairment.
End-stage renal disease (ESRD) on intermittent hemodialysis (IHD) (administer after hemodialysis on dialysis days): Poorly dialyzed; no dosage adjustment necessary (Heintz 2009)
CVVH/CVVHD/CVVHDF: No dosage adjustment necessary (Heintz 2009)

Hepatic Impairment There are no dosage adjustments provided in the manufacturer's labeling (has not been studied).

Dietary Considerations If on parenteral nutrition, may need to adjust the amount of lipid infused. The lipid portion of amphotericin B (liposomal) formulation contains 0.27 kcal per 5 mg (Sacks 1997).

Administration Administer via intravenous infusion, over a period of approximately 2 hours. Infusion time may be reduced to approximately 1 hour in patients in whom the treatment is well-tolerated. If the patient experiences discomfort during infusion, the duration of infusion may be increased. Existing intravenous line should be flushed with D₅W before and after infusion (if not feasible, administer through a separate line). An in-line membrane filter (not less than 1 micron) may be used.

For a patient who experiences chills, fever, hypotension, nausea, or other nonanaphylactic immediate infusion-related reactions, premedicate with the following drugs, 30 to 60 minutes prior to drug administration: A nonsteroidal (eg, ibuprofen, choline magnesium trisalicylate) ± diphenhydramine **or** acetaminophen with diphenhydramine **or** hydrocortisone. If the patient experiences rigors during the infusion, meperidine may be administered.

Monitoring Parameters Renal function (monitor frequently during therapy), electrolytes (especially potassium and magnesium), liver function tests, temperature, hematocrit, PT/PTT, CBC; monitor input and output; monitor for signs of hypokalemia (muscle weakness, cramping, drowsiness, ECG changes, etc); monitor cardiac function if used concurrently with corticosteroids

Test Interactions Falsely-elevated serum phosphate may occur when using the PHOSm assay.

Additional Information Amphotericin B (liposomal) is a true single bilayer liposomal drug delivery system. Liposomes are closed, spherical vesicles created by mixing specific proportions of amphiphilic substances such as phospholipids and cholesterol so that they arrange themselves into multiple concentric bilayer membranes when hydrated in aqueous solutions. Single bilayer liposomes are then formed by microemulsification of multilamellar vesicles using a homogenizer. Amphotericin B (liposomal) consists of these unilamellar bilayer liposomes with amphotericin B intercalated within the membrane. Due to the nature and quantity of amphophilic substances used, and the lipophilic moiety in the amphotericin B molecule, the drug is an integral part of the overall structure of the amphotericin B liposomal liposomes. Amphotericin B (liposomal) contains true liposomes that are <100 nm in diameter.

Dosage Forms Excipient information presented when available (limited, particularly for generics); consult specific product labeling.
Suspension Reconstituted, Intravenous:
AmBisome: 50 mg (1 ea) [contains cholesterol, distearoyl phosphatidylglycerol, hydrogenated soy phosphatidylcholine, sodium succinate hexahydrate, sucrose, tocopherol, dl-alpha]

◆ Amphotericin B Liposome *see* Amphotericin B (Liposomal) *on page 119*

Ampicillin (am pi SIL in)

Brand Names: Canada Ampicillin for Injection; Apo-Ampi; Novo-Ampicillin; Nu-Ampi
Index Terms Aminobenzylpenicillin; Ampicillin Sodium; Ampicillin Trihydrate; Principen
Pharmacologic Category Antibiotic, Penicillin
Use
Oral:
Genitourinary tract infections: Treatment of genitourinary tract infections caused by *Esherichia coli, Proteus mirabilis,* enterococci, *Shigella, Salmonella typhosa* and other *Salmonella,* and nonpenicillinase-producing *N. gonorrhoeae.* **Note:** Ampicillin is **not** recommended by the CDC as a first-line agent in the treatment of gonorrhea (CDC, 2010).
GI tract infections: Treatment of GI tract infections caused by *Shigella, S. typhosa* and other *Salmonella, E. coli, P. mirabilis,* and enterococci. **Note:** Ampicillin is not recommended as a first-line agent for Shigellosis, Salmonellosis (nontyphoid), or *Salmonella enterica* species (typhoid fever) due to development of resistance (CDC, 2014).
Respiratory tract infections: Treatment of respiratory tract infections caused by nonpenicillinase-producing *H. influenzae* and staphylococci, and streptococci, including *Streptococcus pneumoniae.*
Injection:
Bacterial meningitis: Treatment of bacterial meningitis caused by *E. coli,* group B streptococci, and other gram-negative bacteria (*Listeria monocytogenes, N. meningitidis*).
Gastrointestinal infections: Treatment of GI infections caused by *S. typhi* (typhoid fever), other *Salmonella* species and *Shigella* species (dysentery). **Note:** Ampicillin is **not** recommended as a first-line agent for Shigellosis, Salmonellosis (nontyphoid), or *S. enterica* species (typhoid fever) due to development of resistance (CDC, 2014).
Respiratory tract infections: Treatment of respiratory tract infections caused by *S. pneumoniae, Staphylococcus aureus* (penicillinase and nonpenicillinase producing), *H. influenzae,* and group A beta-hemolytic streptococci.
Septicemia and endocarditis: Treatment of septicemia and endocarditis caused by susceptible gram-positive organisms, including Streptococcus species, penicillin G-susceptible staphylococci, and enterococci; gram-negative sepsis caused by *E. coli, P. mirabilis,* and *Salmonella* species.
Urinary tract infections: Treatment of urinary tract infections caused by *E. coli* and *P. mirabilis.*

Pregnancy Considerations Adverse events have not been observed in animal reproduction studies. Ampicillin crosses the placenta, providing detectable concentrations in the cord serum and amniotic fluid (Bolognese, 1968; Fisher, 1967; MacAulay, 1966). Maternal use of ampicillin has generally not resulted in an increased risk of birth defects (Aselton, 1985; Czeizel, 2001b; Heinonen, 1977; Jick, 1981; Puhó, 2007). Ampicillin is recommended for use in pregnant women for the management of preterm premature rupture of membranes (PPROM) and for the prevention of early-onset group B streptococcal (GBS) disease in newborns. Ampicillin may also be used in certain situations prior to vaginal delivery in women at high risk for endocarditis (ACOG, 2013; ACOG No. 120, 2011; ACOG No. 485, 2011; CDC [RR-10], 2010).

The volume of distribution of ampicillin is increased during pregnancy and the half-life is decreased. As a result, serum concentrations in pregnant patients are approximately 50% of those in nonpregnant patients receiving the same dose. Higher doses may be needed during pregnancy. Although oral absorption is not altered during pregnancy, oral ampicillin is poorly absorbed during labor (Philipson, 1977; Philipson, 1978; Wasz-Höckert, 1970).

Breast-Feeding Considerations Ampicillin is excreted in breast milk. The manufacturer recommends that caution be exercised when administering ampicillin to nursing women. Due to the low concentrations in human milk, minimal toxicity would be expected in the nursing infant. Nondose-related effects could include modification of bowel flora and allergic sensitization.

Contraindications Hypersensitivity (eg, anaphylaxis) to ampicillin, any component of the formulation, or other penicillins; infections caused by penicillinase-producing organisms

Warnings/Precautions Dosage adjustment may be necessary in patients with renal impairment. Serious and occasionally severe or fatal hypersensitivity (anaphylactoid) reactions have been reported in patients on penicillin therapy, especially with a history of beta-lactam

hypersensitivity, history of sensitivity to multiple allergens, or previous IgE-mediated reactions (eg, anaphylaxis, angioedema, urticaria). Serious anaphylactoid reactions require emergency treatment and airway management. Appropriate treatments must be readily available. Use with caution in asthmatic patients. Appearance of any rash should be carefully evaluated to differentiate a nonallergic ampicillin rash from a hypersensitivity reaction. High percentage of patients with infectious mononucleosis have developed rash during therapy with ampicillin; ampicillin-class antibiotics not recommended in these patients This rash (generalized maculopapular and pruritic) usually appears 7 to 10 days after initiation and usually resolves within a week of discontinuation. It is not known whether these patients are truly allergic to ampicillin. Ampicillin rash occurs in 5% to 10% of children receiving ampicillin and is a generalized dull red, maculopapular rash, generally appearing 3 to 14 days after the start of therapy. It normally begins on the trunk and spreads over most of the body. It may be most intense at pressure areas, elbows, and knees. Prolonged use may result in fungal or bacterial superinfection, including *Clostridium difficile*-associated diarrhea (CDAD) and pseudomembranous colitis; CDAD has been observed >2 months postantibiotic treatment.

Adverse Reactions Frequency not defined.

Central nervous system: Brain disease (penicillin-induced), glossalgia, seizure, sore mouth

Dermatologic: Erythema multiforme, exfoliative dermatitis, skin rash, urticaria

Note: Appearance of a rash should be carefully evaluated to differentiate (if possible) nonallergic ampicillin rash from hypersensitivity reaction. Incidence is higher in patients with viral infection, *Salmonella* infection, lymphocytic leukemia, or patients that have hyperuricemia.

Gastrointestinal: Diarrhea, enterocolitis, glossitis, melanoglossia, nausea, oral candidiasis, pseudomembranous colitis, stomatitis, vomiting

Hematologic & oncologic: Agranulocytosis, anemia, eosinophilia, hemolytic anemia, immune thrombocytopenia, leukopenia

Hepatic: Increased serum AST

Hypersensitivity: Anaphylaxis

Immunologic: Serum sickness-like reaction

Renal: Interstitial nephritis (rare)

Respiratory: Stridor

Miscellaneous: Fever

Drug Interactions

Metabolism/Transport Effects None known.

Avoid Concomitant Use

Avoid concomitant use of Ampicillin with any of the following: BCG (Intravesical); Probenecid

Increased Effect/Toxicity

Ampicillin may increase the levels/effects of: Methotrexate; Vitamin K Antagonists

The levels/effects of Ampicillin may be increased by: Allopurinol; Probenecid

Decreased Effect

Ampicillin may decrease the levels/effects of: Atenolol; BCG (Intravesical); BCG Vaccine (Immunization); Mycophenolate; Sodium Picosulfate; Typhoid Vaccine

The levels/effects of Ampicillin may be decreased by: Chloroquine; Lanthanum; Tetracycline Derivatives

Food Interactions Food decreases ampicillin absorption rate; may decrease ampicillin serum concentration. Management: Take at equal intervals around-the-clock, preferably on an empty stomach (30 minutes before or 2 hours after meals). Maintain adequate hydration, unless instructed to restrict fluid intake.

Preparation for Administration

IM: Dissolve contents of vial in sterile water for injection or bacteriostatic water for injection; final concentration for IM injection is 125 mg/mL or 250 mg/mL. Solutions for IM injection should be freshly prepared and used within 1 hour.

IV:

Direct IV use: Dissolve contents of 125 mg, 250 mg, or 500 mg vial in 5 mL SWFI. Alternatively, dissolve contents of 1 g or 2 g vial in 7.4 or 14.8 mL SWFI, respectively.

Intermittent infusion: Minimum volume: Concentration should not exceed 30 mg/mL due to concentration-dependent stability restrictions. Standard diluent: 500 mg/50 mL NS; 1 g/50 mL NS; 2 g/100 mL NS.

Storage/Stability

Oral:

Capsules: Store at 20°C to 25°C (68°F to 77°F).

Oral suspension: Store dry powder at 20°C to 25°C (68°F to 77°F). Once reconstituted, oral suspension is stable for 14 days under refrigeration.

IV:

Store intact vials at 20°C to 25°C (68°F to 77°F). Solutions for IM or direct IV should be used within 1 hour. Stability of parenteral admixture in NS at 25°C (77°F) is 8 hours (concentrations up to 30 mg/mL) and at 4°C (39°F) is 24 hours (concentration of 30 mg/mL) or 48 hours (concentrations up to 20 mg/mL). Protect from freezing.

Mechanism of Action Inhibits bacterial cell wall synthesis by binding to one or more of the penicillin-binding proteins (PBPs) which in turn inhibits the final transpeptidation step of peptidoglycan synthesis in bacterial cell walls, thus inhibiting cell wall biosynthesis. Bacteria eventually lyse due to ongoing activity of cell wall autolytic enzymes (autolysins and murein hydrolases) while cell wall assembly is arrested.

Pharmacodynamics/Kinetics

Absorption: Oral: 50%

Distribution: Into bile; penetration into CSF occurs with inflamed meninges only

Protein binding: Neonates: 10%; Adults: 15% to 18%

Half-life elimination:

Neonates:

PNA 2 to 7 days: 4 hours

PNA 8 to 14 days: 2.8 hours

PNA 15 to 30 days: 1.7 hours

Children and Adults: 1 to 1.8 hours (Bergan 1979)

Anuric patients: 8 to 20 hours

Time to peak serum concentration: Oral: Within 1 to 2 hours

Excretion: Urine (~90%, unchanged within 24 hours); feces

Dosing

Adult & Geriatric

Usual dosage range:

Oral: 250 to 500 mg every 6 hours

IM, IV: 1 to 2 g every 4 to 6 hours or 50 to 250 mg/kg/day in divided doses (maximum: 12 g/day)

Endocarditis:

Treatment (off-label dose): IV: 2 g every 4 hours in combination with other antibiotics (Baddour, 2005)

Prophylaxis (off-label use): Dental, oral, or respiratory tract procedures: IM, IV: 2 g within 30 to 60 minutes prior to procedure in patients not allergic to penicillin and unable to take oral amoxicillin. IM injections should be avoided in patients who are receiving anticoagulant therapy. In these circumstances, orally administered regimens should be given whenever possible. Intravenously administered antibiotics should be used for patients who are unable to tolerate or absorb oral medications. **Note:** American Heart Association (AHA) guidelines now recommend prophylaxis only in patients undergoing invasive procedures and in whom underlying cardiac conditions may predispose to a higher risk of adverse outcomes should infection occur (Wilson, 2007).

Genitourinary and gastrointestinal tract procedures: IM, IV: **Note:** Routine prophylaxis for GI/GU procedures is no longer recommended by the AHA. Consider only in patients with the highest risk of adverse outcome from endocarditis (eg, prosthetic heart valve, previous endocarditis, some categories of congenital heart disease, cardiac valvulopathy in cardiac transplant patients) who have an established GI or GU enterococcal infection or for those already receiving antibiotic therapy to prevent a wound infection or sepsis associated with a GI or GU procedure in which enterococcal coverage is desired (Wilson, 2007).

High-risk patients: 2 g within 30 minutes prior to procedure, followed by ampicillin 1 g (or amoxicillin 1 g orally) 6 hours later; must be used in combination with gentamicin (Dajani, 1997).

Moderate-risk patients: 2 g within 30 minutes prior to procedure (Dajani, 1997).

Genitourinary or gastrointestinal infections: Oral, IM, IV: 500 mg every 6 hours

Group B streptococcus (maternal dose for neonatal prophylaxis) (off-label use): IV: 2 g initial dose, then 1 g every 4 hours until delivery (CDC, 2010)

***Listeria* infections (off-label dosing; Lorber, 1997):** IV:

Bacteremia: 200 mg/kg/day divided every 6 hours for ≥2 weeks

Brain abscess or rhombencephalitis: 200 mg/kg/day divided every 4 hours with concomitant aminoglycoside for ≥6 weeks

Endocarditis: 200 mg/kg/day divided every 6 hours with concomitant aminoglycoside for ≥4 to 6 weeks

Meningitis: 200 mg/kg/day divided every 4 hours with concomitant aminoglycoside for ≥3 weeks

Mild to moderate infections: Oral: 250 to 500 mg every 6 hours

Prosthetic joint infection, *Enterococcus* **spp (penicillin-susceptible) (off-label use):** IV: 12 g continuous infusion every 24 hours **or** 2 g every 4 hours for 4 to 6 weeks; consider addition of aminoglycoside (Osmon, 2013).

Prophylaxis in total joint replacement patients undergoing dental procedures which produce bacteremia (off-label use): Note: In general, patients with prosthetic joint implants do not require prophylactic antibiotics prior to dental procedures. In planning an invasive oral procedure, dental consultation with the patient's orthopedic surgeon may be advised to review the risks of infection (Sollecito, 2015).

IM, IV: 2 g 1 hour prior to procedure (ADA/AAOS, 2003).

Respiratory tract infections:
Oral: 250 mg 4 times daily
IM, IV: 250 to 500 mg every 6 hours

Sepsis/meningitis: IM, IV: **Note:** administer doses IV initially; IM may be used later in therapy course: 150 to 200 mg/kg/day divided every 3 to 4 hours (range: 6 to 12 g/day)

Surgical (perioperative) prophylaxis in liver transplantation (off-label use): IV: 2 g within 60 minutes prior to surgery in combination with cefotaxime. Doses may be repeated in 2 hours if procedure is lengthy or if there is excessive blood loss (Bratzler, 2013).

Urinary tract infections (ampicillin-susceptible *Enterococcus*; **off-label use):** IV: 1 to 2 g every 4 to 6 hours with or without an aminoglycoside (Heintz, 2010)

Pediatric
Usual dosage range: Infants, Children, and Adolescents:
Oral: 50 to 100 mg/kg/day divided every 6 hours (maximum: 2 to 4 g/day)
IM, IV: 25 to 200 mg/kg/day divided every 3 to 4 hours (maximum: 12 g/day)

Community-acquired pneumonia (CAP) (IDSA/PIDS, 2011): Infants >3 months, Children, and Adolescents: IV: **Note:** May consider addition of vancomycin or clindamycin to empiric therapy if community-acquired MRSA suspected. In children ≥5 years, a macrolide antibiotic should be added if atypical pneumonia cannot be ruled out. Maximum daily dose of ampicillin: 12 g/day (*Red Book* [AAP 2012]).
Empiric treatment or *S. pneumoniae* (moderate to severe; MICs to penicillin ≤2.0 mcg/mL) or *H. influenzae* (beta-lactamase negative) (preferred): 150 to 200 mg/kg/day divided every 6 hours
Group A *Streptococcus* (moderate to severe) (preferred): 200 mg/kg/day divided every 6 hours
S. pneumoniae (moderate to severe; MICs to penicillin ≥4.0 mcg/mL) (alternative to ceftriaxone): 300 to 400 mg/kg/day divided every 6 hours

Endocarditis prophylaxis (off-label use): Infants, Children, and Adolescents: IM, IV:
Dental, oral, or respiratory tract procedures: 50 mg/kg within 30 to 60 minutes prior to procedure in patients not allergic to penicillin and unable to take oral amoxicillin. Maximum single dose of ampicillin: 2 g. IM injections should be avoided in patients who are receiving anticoagulant therapy. In these circumstances, orally administered regimens should be given whenever possible. Intravenously administered antibiotics should be used for patients who are unable to tolerate or absorb oral medications (Wilson, 2007).
Note: American Heart Association (AHA) guidelines now recommend prophylaxis only in patients undergoing invasive procedures and in whom underlying cardiac conditions may predispose to a higher risk of adverse outcomes should infection occur.
Genitourinary and gastrointestinal tract procedures:
Note: Routine prophylaxis for GI/GU procedures is no longer recommended by the AHA. Consider only in patients with the highest risk of adverse outcome from endocarditis (eg, prosthetic heart valve, previous endocarditis, some categories of congenital heart disease, valvulopathy in cardiac transplant patients) who have an established GI or GU enterococcal infection or for those already receiving antibiotic therapy to prevent a wound infection or sepsis associated with a GI or GU procedure in which enterococcal coverage is desired (Wilson, 2007).
High-risk patients: 50 mg/kg (maximum: 2 g) within 30 minutes prior to procedure, followed by ampicillin 25 mg/kg (or amoxicillin 25 mg/kg orally) 6 hours later; must be used in combination with gentamicin. Maximum single dose of ampicillin: 2 g (Dajani, 1997). **Note:** Routine prophylaxis for GI/GU procedures is no longer recommended by the AHA (Wilson, 2007).

Moderate-risk patients: 50 mg/kg within 30 minutes prior to procedure Maximum single dose of ampicillin: 2 g (Dajani, 1997).

Endocarditis treatment (off-label dose): Infants, Children, and Adolescents: IV: 300 mg/kg/day in divided doses every 4 to 6 hours in combination with other antibiotics (maximum: 12 g/day) (Baddour, 2005)

Genitourinary or gastrointestinal infections:
Oral:
Infants and Children ≤20 kg: 100 mg/kg/day in divided doses 4 times daily
Children and Adolescents >20 kg: 500 mg 4 times daily
IM, IV:
Infants and Children <40 kg: 50 mg/kg/day in divided doses every 6 to 8 hours
Children and Adolescents ≥40 kg: 500 mg every 6 hours

Mild to moderate infections: Infants, Children, and Adolescents:
Oral: 50 to 100 mg/kg/day divided every 6 hours (maximum: 2 to 4 g/day) (*Red Book* [AAP 2012])
IM, IV: 100 to 150 mg/kg/day divided every 6 hours (maximum: 2 to 4 g/day) (*Red Book* [AAP 2012])

Respiratory tract infections:
Oral:
Infants and Children ≤20 kg: 50 mg/kg/day in divided doses 3 to 4 times daily
Children and Adolescents >20 kg: 250 mg 4 times daily
IM, IV:
Infants and Children <40 kg: 25 to 50 mg/kg/day in divided doses every 6 to 8 hours
Children and Adolescents ≥40 kg: 250 to 500 mg every 6 hours

Severe infections, meningitis, septicemia: Infants, Children, and Adolescents: IM, IV: **Note:** Treatment should be initiated with IV infusion therapy and may be continued with IM injections if preferred.
Manufacturer's labeling: 150 to 200 mg/kg/day in divided doses every 3 to 4 hours
Alternative recommendation: 200 to 400 mg/kg/day in divided doses every 6 hours (maximum: 6 to 12 g/day) (*Red Book* [AAP 2012])

Surgical (perioperative) prophylaxis in liver transplantation (off-label use): Children ≥1 year: IV: 50 mg/kg within 60 minutes prior to surgery (maximum: 2,000 mg/dose) in combination with cefotaxime. Doses may be repeated in 2 hours if procedure is lengthy or if there is excessive blood loss (Bratzler, 2013).

Renal Impairment There are no dosage adjustments provided in the manufacturer's labeling; however, the following adjustments have been recommended (Aronoff, 2007):
CrCl >50 mL/minute: Administer every 6 hours
CrCl 10 to 50 mL/minute: Administer every 6 to 12 hours
CrCl <10 mL/minute: Administer every 12 to 24 hours
End-stage renal disease (ESRD) on intermittent hemodialysis (IHD) (administer after hemodialysis on dialysis days): Dialyzable (20% to 50%): IV: 1 to 2 g every 12 to 24 hours (administer after hemodialysis on dialysis days) (Heintz, 2009). **Note:** Dosing dependent on the assumption of 3 times/week, complete IHD sessions.
Peritoneal dialysis (PD): IV: 250 mg every 12 hours (Aronoff, 2007)
Continuous renal replacement therapy (CRRT) (Heintz, 2009): Drug clearance is highly dependent on the method of renal replacement, filter type, and flow rate. Appropriate dosing requires close monitoring of pharmacologic response, signs of adverse reactions due to drug accumulation, as well as drug concentrations in relation to target trough (if appropriate). The following are general recommendations only (based on dialysate flow/ultrafiltration rates of 1 to 2 L/hour and minimal residual renal function) and should not supersede clinical judgment: IV:
CVVH: Loading dose of 2 g followed by 1 to 2 g every 8 to 12 hours
CVVHD: Loading dose of 2 g followed by 1 to 2 g every 8 hours
CVVHDF: Loading dose of 2 g followed by 1 to 2 g every 6 to 8 hours

Hepatic Impairment There are no dosage adjustments provided in the manufacturer's labeling.

Dietary Considerations Take on an empty stomach 30 minutes before or 2 hours after meals. Some products may contain sodium.

Administration Administer around-the-clock to promote less variation in peak and trough serum levels.

Oral: Administer on an empty stomach with a full glass (8 oz) of water (ie, 30 minutes prior to or 2 hours after meals) to increase total absorption.

IM.: Inject deep IM into a large muscle mass

IV: Direct IV bolus: Administer over 3 to 5 minutes (125 to 500 mg) or over 10 to 15 minutes (1 to 2 g). More rapid infusion may cause seizures.

Infusion: Rapid infusion may cause seizures. Adjust rate of infusion so that the total dose is administered before admixture stability expires.

Monitoring Parameters With prolonged therapy, monitor renal, hepatic, and hematologic function periodically; observe signs and symptoms of anaphylaxis during first dose

Test Interactions May interfere with urinary glucose tests using cupric sulfate (Benedict's solution, Clinitest®)

Some penicillin derivatives may accelerate the degradation of aminoglycosides *in vitro*, leading to a potential underestimation of aminoglycoside serum concentration.

Dosage Forms Excipient information presented when available (limited, particularly for generics); consult specific product labeling.

Capsule, Oral:
Generic: 250 mg, 500 mg

Solution Reconstituted, Injection, as sodium [strength expressed as base]:
Generic: 125 mg (1 ea); 250 mg (1 ea); 500 mg (1 ea); 1 g (1 ea); 2 g (1 ea); 10 g (1 ea)

Solution Reconstituted, Injection, as sodium [strength expressed as base, preservative free]:
Generic: 250 mg (1 ea); 500 mg (1 ea)

Solution Reconstituted, Intravenous, as sodium [strength expressed as base]:
Generic: 1 g (1 ea); 2 g (1 ea); 10 g (1 ea)

Solution Reconstituted, Intravenous, as sodium [strength expressed as base, preservative free]:
Generic: 10 g (1 ea)

Suspension Reconstituted, Oral:
Generic: 125 mg/5 mL (100 mL, 200 mL); 250 mg/5 mL (100 mL, 200 mL)

Ampicillin and Sulbactam
(am pi SIL in & SUL bak tam)

Brand Names: US Unasyn
Brand Names: Canada Unasyn
Index Terms Sulbactam and Ampicillin
Pharmacologic Category Antibiotic, Penicillin
Use Bacterial infections: Treatment of susceptible bacterial infections involved with skin and skin structure, intra-abdominal infections, gynecological infections; spectrum is that of ampicillin plus organisms producing beta-lactamases such as *S. aureus*, *H. influenzae*, *E. coli*, *Klebsiella*, *Acinetobacter*, *Enterobacter*, and anaerobes

Pregnancy Considerations Adverse events have not been observed in animal reproduction studies. Both ampicillin and sulbactam cross the placenta. Maternal use of penicillins has generally not resulted in an increased risk of birth defects. When used during pregnancy, pharmacokinetic changes have been observed with ampicillin alone (refer to the Ampicillin monograph for details). Ampicillin/sulbactam may be considered for prophylactic use prior to cesarean delivery (consult current guidelines).

Breast-Feeding Considerations Ampicillin and sulbactam are both excreted into breast milk in low concentrations. The manufacturer recommends that caution be used if administering to lactating women. Nondose-related effects could include modification of bowel flora and allergic sensitization of the infant. The maternal dose of sulbactam does not need altered in the postpartum period. Also refer to the Ampicillin monograph.

Contraindications Hypersensitivity (eg, anaphylaxis or Stevens-Johnson syndrome) to ampicillin, sulbactam, or to other beta-lactam antibacterial drugs (eg, penicillins, cephalosporins), or any component of the formulations; history of cholestatic jaundice or hepatic dysfunction associated with ampicillin/sulbactam

Warnings/Precautions Dosage adjustment may be necessary in patients with renal impairment. Serious and occasionally severe or fatal hypersensitivity (anaphylactic) reactions have been reported in patients on penicillin therapy, especially with a history of beta-lactam hypersensitivity, history of sensitivity to multiple allergens. Patients with a history of penicillin hypersensitivity have experienced severe reactions when treated with cephalosporins. Before initiating therapy, carefully investigate previous penicillin, cephalosporin, or other allergen hypersensitivity. If an allergic reaction occurs, discontinue and institute appropriate therapy. Hepatitis and cholestatic jaundice have been reported (including fatalities). Toxicity is usually reversible. Monitor hepatic function at regular intervals in patients with hepatic impairment. High percentage of patients with infectious mononucleosis have developed rash during therapy with ampicillin; ampicillin-class antibacterials are not recommended in these patients. Appearance of a rash should be carefully evaluated to differentiate a nonallergic ampicillin rash from a hypersensitivity reaction. Prolonged use may result in fungal or bacterial superinfection, including *C. difficile*-associated diarrhea (CDAD) and pseudomembranous colitis; CDAD has been observed >2 months postantibiotic treatment.

Adverse Reactions Also see Ampicillin.

>10%: Local: Pain at injection site (IM; 16%)

1% to 10%:
Cardiovascular: Thrombophlebitis (3%), phlebitis (1%)
Dermatologic: Skin rash (<2%)
Gastrointestinal: Diarrhea (3%)
Local: Pain at injection site (IV; 3%)

<1% (Limited to important or life-threatening): Acute generalized exanthematous pustulosis, agranulocytosis, anemia, basophilia, candidiasis, casts in urine (hyaline), chest pain, chills, cholestasis, cholestatic hepatitis, *clostridium difficile* associated diarrhea, convulsions, decreased neutrophils, decreased serum albumin, decreased serum total protein, dysuria, edema, eosinophilia, erythema, erythema multiforme, erythrocyturia, exfoliative dermatitis, gastritis, glossitis, hairy tongue, headache, hemolytic anemia, hepatic insufficiency, hepatitis, hyperbilirubinemia, hypersensitivity reaction, immune thrombocytopenia, increased blood urea nitrogen, increased lactate dehydrogenase, increased liver enzymes, increased monocytes, increased serum creatinine, injection site reaction, interstitial nephritis, lymphocytopenia, lymphocytosis (abnormal), nausea, positive direct Coombs test, pruritus, pseudomembranous colitis, Stevens-Johnson syndrome, stomatitis, thrombocythemia, thrombocytopenia, urinary retention, urticaria

Drug Interactions

Metabolism/Transport Effects None known.

Avoid Concomitant Use

Avoid concomitant use of Ampicillin and Sulbactam with any of the following: BCG (Intravesical); Probenecid

Increased Effect/Toxicity

Ampicillin and Sulbactam may increase the levels/effects of: Methotrexate; Vitamin K Antagonists

The levels/effects of Ampicillin and Sulbactam may be increased by: Allopurinol; Probenecid

Decreased Effect

Ampicillin and Sulbactam may decrease the levels/effects of: Atenolol; BCG (Intravesical); BCG Vaccine (Immunization); Mycophenolate; Sodium Picosulfate; Typhoid Vaccine

The levels/effects of Ampicillin and Sulbactam may be decreased by: Chloroquine; Lanthanum; Tetracycline Derivatives

Preparation for Administration

Direct IV administration and infusion: Reconstitute with sterile water for injection (SWFI). Sodium chloride 0.9% (NS) is the diluent of choice for IV infusion use.

IM administration: Reconstitute with SWFI or 0.5% or 2% lidocaine hydrochloride injection.

Storage/Stability

Prior to reconstitution, store at 20°C to 25°C (68°F to 77°F).

IM: Concentration of 375 mg/mL (250 mg ampicillin/125 mg sulbacatam) should be used within 1 hour after reconstitution.

Intermittent IV infusion: Solutions made in NS are stable up to 72 hours when refrigerated whereas dextrose solutions (same concentration) are stable for only 4 hours. For stability related to specific concentrations and temperatures, see prescribing information.

Mechanism of Action Inhibits bacterial cell wall synthesis by binding to one or more of the penicillin-binding proteins (PBPs) which in turn inhibits the final transpeptidation step of peptidoglycan synthesis in bacterial cell walls, thus inhibiting cell wall biosynthesis. Bacteria eventually lyse due to ongoing activity of cell wall autolytic enzymes (autolysins and murein hydrolases) while cell wall assembly is arrested. The addition of sulbactam, a beta-lactamase inhibitor, to ampicillin extends the spectrum of ampicillin to include some beta-lactamase-producing organisms.

Pharmacodynamics/Kinetics

Ampicillin: See Ampicillin monograph.

Sulbactam:

Distribution: Widely distributed to bile, blister, and tissue fluids; poor penetration into CSF with uninflamed meninges; higher concentrations attained with inflamed meninges; V_d (Nahata 1999):
Children 1 to 12 years: ~0.35 L/kg
Adults: 0.25 L/kg

Protein binding: 38%

Half-life elimination: Children 1 to 12 years (normal renal function): Mean range: ~0.7 to 0.9 hours (Nahata 1999); Adults (normal renal function): 1 to 1.3 hours; **Note:** Elimination kinetics of both ampicillin and sulbactam are similarly affected in patients with renal impairment, therefore, the blood concentration ratio is expected to remain constant regardless of renal function.

Excretion: Urine (~75% to 85% as unchanged drug) within 8 hours

Dosing

Adult & Geriatric Unasyn (ampicillin/sulbactam) is a combination product. **Note:** Dosage recommendations are expressed as grams of **ampicillin/sulbactam** combination.

Susceptible infections: IM, IV: 1.5 to 3 g every 6 hours (maximum: 12 g ampicillin/sulbactam daily)

Acute bacterial rhinosinusitis, severe infection requiring hospitalization (off-label use): IV: 1.5 to 3 g every 6 hours for 5 to 7 days (Chow 2012)

Amnionitis, cholangitis, diverticulitis, endomyometritis (with doxycycline), endophthalmitis, epididymitis/orchitis, liver abscess (with metronidazole), or peritonitis: IV: 3 g every 6 hours

Bite wounds (animal/human) (off-label use): IV: 1.5 to 3 g every 6 hours (human bites) or every 6 to 8 hours (animal bites) (IDSA [Stevens 2014])

Infective endocarditis (off-label use) (AHA/IDSA [Baddour 2005]):

Bartonella spp. (Native valve): IV: 3 g every 6 hours with concomitant gentamicin for 4 to 6 weeks.

Enterococcus organism (resistant to penicillin/susceptible to aminoglycoside and vancomycin): IV: 3 g every 6 hours with concomitant gentamicin for 6 weeks. **Note:** If enterococcus is gentamicin resistant, then >6 weeks of ampicillin-sulbactam therapy needed.

HACEK organism: IV: 3 g every 6 hours for 4 weeks

Intravascular catheter-associated bloodstream infection, *Acinetobacter* spp (off-label use) (IDSA 2009): IV: 3 g every 6 hours

Orbital cellulitis: IV: 3 g every 6 hours

Osteomyelitis (diabetic foot) (Lipsky 2004): IV: 3 g every 6 hours

Pelvic inflammatory disease (off-label use): IV: 3 g every 6 hours (for 24 hours after clinical improvement is noted) with doxycycline (continued for a total of 14 days) (CDC 2010)

Peritonitis associated with CAPD: Intraperitoneal:

Intermittent: 3 g added to one exchange every 12 hours; allow to dwell for at least 6 hours (Blackwell 1990; Li 2010)

Continuous: Loading dose: 1.5 g per liter of dialysate; maintenance dose: 150 mg per liter of dialysate (Li 2010)

Pneumonia (off-label use):

Aspiration or community-acquired: IV: 1.5 to 3 g every 6 hours for ≥5 days (Geckler 1994; Majcher-Peszynska 2014; Mandell 2007; Rossoff 1995). **Note:** In ICU patients, use in combination with azithromycin or a fluoroquinolone (Mandell 2007).

Hospital-acquired (empiric, early onset, no known risk for multidrug-resistant pathogens): IV: 3 g every 6 hours for ≥5 days (ATS 2005; Jauregui 1995).

Surgical (perioperative) prophylaxis (off-label use): IV: 3 g within 60 minutes prior to surgical incision. Doses may be repeated in 2 hours if procedure is lengthy or if there is excessive blood loss (Bratzler 2013).

Surgical site infections (intestinal or GI tract) (off-label use): IV: 3 g every 6 hours; in combination with gentamicin or tobramycin (IDSA [Stevens 2014])

Urinary tract infections, pyelonephritis: IV: 3 g every 6 hours for 14 days

Pediatric Unasyn (ampicillin/sulbactam) is a combination product. **Note:** Dosage recommendations are expressed as mg of the **ampicillin** component.

Susceptible infections: Children and Adolescents: IV: 100 to 200 mg **ampicillin**/kg/day divided every 6 hours (maximum: 8 g ampicillin daily or 12 g ampicillin/sulbactam daily).

Epiglottitis: Children and Adolescents: IV: 100 to 200 mg ampicillin/kg/day divided in 4 doses

Infective endocarditis (off-label use) (AHA/IDSA [Baddour 2005]): Infants, Children, and Adolescents:

Bartonella spp. (Native valve): IV: 200 mg ampicillin/kg/day in 4 or 6 divided doses with concomitant gentamicin for 4 to 6 weeks.

Enterococcus organism (resistant to penicillin/susceptible to aminoglycoside and vancomycin): IV: 200 mg ampicillin/kg/day in 4 divided doses with concomitant gentamicin for 6 weeks. **Note:** If enterococcus is

gentamicin resistant, then >6 weeks of ampicillin-sulbactam therapy needed.

HACEK organism: 200 mg ampicillin/kg/day in 4 or 6 divided doses for 4 weeks.

Intravascular catheter-associated bloodstream infection (off-label use) (IDSA 2009): Infants, Children, and Adolescents:

Infants: IV: 100 to 150 mg ampicillin/kg/day in 4 divided doses

Children and Adolescents: IV: 100 to 200 mg ampicillin/kg/day in 4 divided doses

Mild to moderate infections: Children and Adolescents: IV: 100 to 200 mg ampicillin/kg/day divided every 6 hours (maximum: 8 g ampicillin daily or 12 g ampicillin/sulbactam daily)

Peritonsillar and retropharyngeal abscess: Children and Adolescents: IV: 200 mg ampicillin/kg/day in 4 divided doses

Severe infections: Children and Adolescents: IV: 200 mg ampicillin/kg/day divided every 6 hours (maximum: 8 g ampicillin daily or 12 g ampicillin/sulbactam daily)

Surgical (perioperative) prophylaxis (off-label use): Children ≥1 year: IV: 50 mg ampicillin/kg within 60 minutes prior to surgical incision (maximum dose: 2000 mg ampicillin or 3 g ampicillin/sulbactam daily). Doses may be repeated in 2 hours if procedure is lengthy or if there is excessive blood loss (Bratzler 2013).

Renal Impairment Note: Estimation of renal function for the purpose of drug dosing should be done using the Cockcroft-Gault formula. Dosage recommendations are expressed as grams of **ampicillin/sulbactam** combination:

CrCl ≥30 mL/minute/1.73 m^2: No dosage adjustment necessary.

CrCl 15 to 29 mL/minute/1.73 m^2: 1.5 to 3 g every 12 hours

CrCl 5 to 14 mL/minute/1.73 m^2: 1.5 to 3 g every 24 hours

End stage renal disease (ESRD) on intermittent hemodialysis (IHD) (administer after hemodialysis on dialysis days): 1.5 to 3 g every 12 to 24 hours (Heintz 2009). **Note:** Dosing dependent on the assumption of 3 times weekly, complete IHD sessions.

Continuous renal replacement therapy (CRRT): Drug clearance is highly dependent on the method of renal replacement, filter type, and flow rate. Appropriate dosing requires close monitoring of pharmacologic response, signs of adverse reactions due to drug accumulation, as well as drug levels in relation to target trough (if appropriate). The following are general recommendations only (based on dialysate flow/ultrafiltration rates of 1 to 2 L/hour and minimal residual renal function) and should not supersede clinical judgment (Heintz 2009; Trotman 2005):

CVVH: Initial: 3 g; maintenance: 1.5 to 3 g every 8 to 12 hours

CVVHD: Initial: 3 g; maintenance: 1.5 to 3 g every 8 hours

CVVHDF: Initial: 3 g; maintenance: 1.5 to 3 g every 6 to 8 hours

Hepatic Impairment There is no dosage adjustment provided in the manufacturer's labeling.

Dietary Considerations Some products may contain sodium.

Administration Administer around-the-clock to promote less variation in peak and trough serum levels.

IV: Administer by slow injection over 10 to 15 minutes or as an IV infusion over 15 to 30 minutes. Ampicillin and gentamicin should not be mixed in the same IV tubing.

Some penicillins (eg, ampicillin, carbenicillin, ticarcillin, and piperacillin) have been shown to inactivate aminoglycosides *in vitro*. This has been observed to a greater extent with tobramycin and gentamicin, while amikacin has shown greater stability against inactivation. Concurrent Y-site administration should be avoided.

IM: Inject deep IM into large muscle mass; a concentration of 375 mg/mL ampicillin/sulbactam (250 mg ampicillin/125 mg sulbactam per mL) is recommended; may be diluted in sterile water or lidocaine 0.5% or lidocaine 2% for IM administration.

Monitoring Parameters With prolonged therapy, monitor hematologic, renal, and hepatic function; monitor for signs of anaphylaxis during first dose. In patients with preexisting hepatic impairment, monitor hepatic function at regular intervals.

Test Interactions May interfere with urinary glucose tests using cupric sulfate (Benedict's solution, Fehling's solution, or Clinitest®).

Some penicillin derivatives may accelerate the degradation of aminoglycosides *in vitro*, leading to a potential underestimation of aminoglycoside serum concentration.

Dosage Forms Excipient information presented when available (limited, particularly for generics); consult specific product labeling.

Injection, powder for reconstitution: 1.5 g: Ampicillin 1 g and sulbactam 0.5 g; 3 g: Ampicillin 2 g and sulbactam 1 g; 15 g: Ampicillin 10 g and sulbactam 5 g

Unasyn®:

1.5 g: Ampicillin 1 g and sulbactam 0.5 g [contains sodium 115 mg (5 mEq)/1.5 g)]

3 g: Ampicillin 2 g and sulbactam 1 g [contains sodium 115 mg (5 mEq)/1.5 g)]

15 g: Ampicillin 10 g and sulbactam 5 g [bulk package; contains sodium 115 mg (5 mEq)/1.5 g)]

Amyl Nitrite (AM il NYE trite)

Index Terms Isoamyl Nitrite
Pharmacologic Category Antianginal Agent; Antidote; Vasodilator
Use Coronary vasodilator in angina pectoris

Note: Given the widespread use of newer nitrate compounds, the use of amyl nitrite for patients experiencing angina pectoris has fallen out of favor.

Dosing

Adult & Geriatric

Angina: Inhalation: 2 to 6 nasal inhalations from 1 crushed ampul; may repeat in 3 to 5 minutes

Cyanide toxicity (off-label use): Inhalation: 0.3 mL ampul crushed into a gauze pad and placed in front of the patient's mouth (or endotracheal tube if patient is intubated) to inhale over 15 to 30 seconds; repeat every minute until sodium nitrite can be administered (Mokhlesi, 2003). **Note:** Must separate administrations by at least 30 seconds to allow for adequate oxygenation; each ampul will last for ~3 minutes. Amyl nitrite is a temporary intervention that should only be used until IV sodium nitrite infusion is ready for administration (ATSDR).

Pharmacologic provocation of latent left ventricular outflow tract (LVOT) gradient in hypertrophic cardiomyopathy (HCM) (off-label use): Nasal inhalation: 3 to 4 deep inhalations from 1 crushed ampul over a 10 to 15 second period (Gersh, 2011; Nagueh, 2011; Reagan, 2005). **Note:** The use of more physiologic testing (eg, treadmill testing with Doppler echocardiography) may be preferred over amyl nitrite inhalation (Maron, 2003; Nagueh, 2011).

Pediatric Cyanide toxicity (off-label use): Refer to adult dosing.

Additional Information Complete prescribing information should be consulted for additional detail.

Dosage Forms Excipient information presented when available (limited, particularly for generics); consult specific product labeling.

Liquid, for inhalation: USP: 85% to 103% (0.3 mL)

Anagrelide (an AG gre lide)

Brand Names: US Agrylin

Brand Names: Canada Agrylin; Dom-Anagrelide; Mylan-Anagrelide; PMS-Anagrelide; Sandoz-Anagrelide
Index Terms Anagrelide Hydrochloride; BL4162A
Pharmacologic Category Antiplatelet Agent; Phosphodiesterase-3 Enzyme Inhibitor
Use Thrombocythemia: Treatment of thrombocythemia associated with myeloproliferative disorders to reduce the risk of thrombosis and reduce associated symptoms (including thrombohemorrhagic events)

Dosing

Adult & Geriatric

Thrombocythemia: Oral: Initial: 0.5 mg 4 times daily or 1 mg twice daily (most patients will experience adequate response at dose ranges of 1.5 to 3 mg per day)

Note: Maintain initial dose for ≥1 week, then adjust to the lowest effective dose to reduce and maintain platelet count <600,000/mm^3 ideally to the normal range; the dose must not be increased by >0.5 mg per day in any 1 week; maximum single dose: 2.5 mg; maximum daily dose: 10 mg

Thrombocythemia, essential (off-label dosing): Oral: 0.5 mg twice daily for 1 week, then adjust dose to maintain platelet counts at normal (≤450,000/mm^3) or near normal (450,000/mm^3 to 600,000/mm^3) levels (Gisslinger, 2013).

Pediatric Thrombocythemia: Oral: Initial: 0.5 mg once daily (range: 0.5 mg 1 to 4 times daily)

Note: Maintain initial dose for ≥1 week, then adjust to the lowest effective dose to reduce and maintain platelet count <600,000/mm^3 ideally to the normal range; the dose must not be increased by >0.5 mg per day in any 1 week; maximum single dose: 2.5 mg; maximum daily dose: 10 mg

Renal Impairment No dosage adjustment necessary; monitor closely.

Hepatic Impairment

Moderate impairment (Child-Pugh score 7 to 9): Initial: 0.5 mg once daily; maintain for at least 1 week with careful monitoring of cardiovascular status; the dose must not be increased by >0.5 mg per day in any 1 week.

Severe impairment (Child-Pugh score ≥10): Avoid use.

Additional Information Complete prescribing information should be consulted for additional detail.

Dosage Forms Excipient information presented when available (limited, particularly for generics); consult specific product labeling.

Capsule, Oral:

Agrylin: 0.5 mg

Generic: 0.5 mg, 1 mg

Anakinra (an a KIN ra)

Brand Names: US Kineret
Brand Names: Canada Kineret
Index Terms IL-1Ra; Interleukin-1 Receptor Antagonist
Pharmacologic Category Antirheumatic, Disease Modifying; Interleukin-1 Receptor Antagonist
Use Treatment of moderately- to severely-active rheumatoid arthritis (RA) in adult patients who have failed one or more disease-modifying antirheumatic drugs (DMARDs; may be used alone or in combination with DMARDs [other than tumor necrosis factor-blocking agents]); treatment of neonatal-onset multisystem inflammatory disease (NOMID), which is a cryopyrin-associated periodic syndrome (CAPS)

Dosing

Adult & Geriatric

Neonatal-onset multisystem inflammatory disease (NOMID): SubQ: Initial: 1 to 2 mg/kg daily in 1 to 2 divided doses; adjust dose in 0.5 to 1 mg/kg increments as needed; usual maintenance dose: 3 to 4 mg/kg daily (maximum: 8 mg/kg daily). **Note:** Once-daily administration is preferred; however, the dose may also be divided and administered twice daily.

Rheumatoid arthritis (RA): SubQ: 100 mg once daily (administer at approximately the same time each day)

Pediatric

Neonatal-onset multisystem inflammatory disease (NOMID): Infants, Children, and Adolescents: SubQ: Refer to adult dosing.

Juvenile idiopathic arthritis, systemic (off-label use): Children and Adolescents: SubQ: Initial: 1 to 2 mg/kg once daily; maximum initial dose: 100 mg; if no response after 1 to 2 weeks, may titrate up to 4 mg/kg once daily (maximum daily dose: 200 mg) (Dewitt, 2012; Hedrich, 2012; Lequerré, 2008; Nigrovi, 2011; Quartier, 2011; Ringold, 2013).

Renal Impairment

CrCl ≥30 mL/minute: No dosage adjustment necessary.

CrCl <30 mL/minute:

RA: Adults: 100 mg every other day

NOMID: Infants, Children, Adolescents, and Adults: No dosage adjustment necessary; however, decrease frequency of administration to every other day.

ESRD (**Note:** <2.5% of the dose is removed by hemodialysis or CAPD):

RA: Adults: 100 mg every other day

NOMID: Infants, Children, Adolescents, and Adults: No dosage adjustment necessary; however, decrease frequency of administration to every other day.

Hepatic Impairment No dosage adjustments provided in the manufacturer's labeling (has not been studied).

Additional Information Complete prescribing information should be consulted for additional detail.

Dosage Forms Excipient information presented when available (limited, particularly for generics); consult specific product labeling.

Solution Prefilled Syringe, Subcutaneous [preservative free]:

Kineret: 100 mg/0.67 mL (0.67 mL) [contains disodium edta, polysorbate 80]

- ◆ Analpram E see Pramoxine and Hydrocortisone on page 1489
- ◆ Analpram HC see Pramoxine and Hydrocortisone on page 1489
- ◆ Anandron (Can) see Nilutamide on page 1283
- ◆ Anapen (Can) see EPINEPHrine (Systemic) on page 647
- ◆ Anapen Junior (Can) see EPINEPHrine (Systemic) on page 647
- ◆ Anaprox see Naproxen on page 1256
- ◆ Anaprox DS see Naproxen on page 1256
- ◆ Anascorp see Centruroides Immune F(ab')₂ (Equine) on page 358
- ◆ Anasept see Sodium Hypochlorite on page 1675
- ◆ Anaspaz see Hyoscyamine on page 899

Anastrozole (an AS troe zole)

Brand Names: US Arimidex

Brand Names: Canada ACH-Anastrozole; ACT-Anastrozole; Apo-Anastrozole; Arimidex; Auro-Anastrozole; Bio-Anastrozole; JAMP-Anastrozole; Mar-Anastrozole; Med-Anastrozole; Mint-Anastrozole; Mylan-Anastrozole; Nat-Anastrozole; PMS-Anastrozole; RAN-Anastrozole; Riva-Anastrozole; Sandoz-Anastrozole; Taro-Anastrozole; Teva-Anastrozole; Zinda-Anastrozole

Index Terms ICI-D1033; ZD1033

Pharmacologic Category Antineoplastic Agent, Aromatase Inhibitor

Use Breast cancer:

First-line treatment of locally-advanced or metastatic breast cancer (hormone receptor-positive or unknown) in postmenopausal women

Adjuvant treatment of early hormone receptor-positive breast cancer in postmenopausal women

Treatment of advanced breast cancer in postmenopausal women with disease progression following tamoxifen therapy

Pregnancy Considerations Adverse events were observed in animal reproduction studies. Anastrozole is contraindicated in women who are or may become pregnant (may cause fetal harm if administered during pregnancy). Use in premenopausal women with breast cancer does not provide any clinical benefit.

Breast-Feeding Considerations It is not known if anastrozole is excreted in breast milk. Due to the potential for serious adverse reactions in the nursing infant, a decision should be made whether to discontinue nursing or to discontinue the drug, taking into account the importance of treatment to the mother. The Canadian labeling contraindicates use in lactating women.

Contraindications Hypersensitivity to anastrozole or any component of the formulation; use in women who are or may become pregnant

Canadian labeling: Additional contraindications (not in U.S. labeling): Lactating women

Warnings/Precautions Hazardous agent - use appropriate precautions for handling and disposal (NIOSH 2014 [group 1]). Use is contraindicated in women who are or may become pregnant. Anastrozole offers no clinical benefit in premenopausal women with breast cancer. Patients with preexisting ischemic cardiac disease have an increased risk for ischemic cardiovascular events.

Due to decreased circulating estrogen levels, anastrozole is associated with a reduction in bone mineral density (BMD); decreases (from baseline) in total hip and lumbar spine BMD have been reported. Patients with preexisting osteopenia are at higher risk for developing osteoporosis (Eastell, 2008). When initiating anastrozole treatment, follow available guidelines for bone mineral density management in postmenopausal women with similar fracture risk; concurrent use of bisphosphonates may be useful in patients at risk for fractures.

Elevated total cholesterol levels (contributed to by LDL cholesterol increases) have been reported in patients receiving anastrozole; use with caution in patients with hyperlipidemias; cholesterol levels should be monitored/managed in accordance with current guidelines for patients with LDL elevations. Plasma concentrations in patients with stable hepatic cirrhosis were within the range of concentrations seen in normal subjects across all clinical trials; use has not been studied in patients with severe hepatic impairment.

Adverse Reactions

>10%:

Cardiovascular: Vasodilatation (25% to 36%), ischemic heart disease (4%; 17% in patients with preexisting ischemic heart disease), hypertension (2% to 13%), angina pectoris (2%; 12% in patients with preexisting ischemic heart disease), edema (7% to 11%)

Central nervous system: Fatigue (19%), mood disorder (19%), headache (9% to 18%), pain (11% to 17%), depression (2% to 13%)

Dermatologic: Skin rash (6% to 11%)

Endocrine & metabolic: Hot flash (12% to 36%)

Gastrointestinal: Gastrointestinal distress (29% to 34%), nausea (11% to 20%), vomiting (8% to 13%)

Neuromuscular & skeletal: Weakness (13% to 19%), arthritis (17%), arthralgia (2% to 15%), back pain (10% to 12%), ostealgia (6% to 12%), osteoporosis (11%)

Respiratory: Pharyngitis (6% to 14%), dyspnea (8% to 11%), increased cough (7% to 11%)

1% to 10%:

Cardiovascular: Peripheral edema (5% to 10%), chest pain (5% to 7%), venous thrombosis (2% to 4%; including pulmonary embolism, thrombophlebitis, retinal vein thrombosis), myocardial infarction (1%)

Central nervous system: Insomnia (2% to 10%), dizziness (5% to 8%), paresthesia (5% to 7%), anxiety (2% to 6%), confusion (2% to 5%), drowsiness (2% to 5%), malaise (2% to 5%), nervousness (2% to 5%), carpal tunnel syndrome (3%), hypertonia (3%), cerebrovascular insufficiency (2%), lethargy (1%)

Dermatologic: Alopecia (2% to 5%), pruritus (2% to 5%), diaphoresis (1% to 5%)

Endocrine & metabolic: Hypercholesterolemia (9%), increased serum cholesterol (9%), weight gain (2% to 9%), increased gamma-glutamyl transferase (2% to 5%), weight loss (2% to 5%)

Gastrointestinal: Constipation (7% to 9%), diarrhea (7% to 9%), abdominal pain (6% to 9%), anorexia (5% to 8%), dyspepsia (7%), gastrointestinal disease (7%), xerostomia (4% to 6%)

Genitourinary: Mastalgia (2% to 8%), urinary tract infection (2% to 8%), pelvic pain (5% to 7%), vulvovaginitis (6%), vaginal dryness (1% to 5%), vaginal hemorrhage (1% to 5%), vaginal discharge (4%), vaginitis (4%), leukorrhea (2% to 3%)

Hematologic & oncologic: Lymphedema (10%), breast neoplasm (5%), neoplasm (5%), anemia (2% to 5%), leukopenia (2% to 5%), tumor flare (3%)

Hepatic: Increased serum alkaline phosphatase (2% to 5%), increased serum ALT (2% to 5%), increased serum AST (2% to 5%)

Infection: Infection (2% to 9%)

Neuromuscular & skeletal: Bone fracture (1% to 10%), arthrosis (7%), myalgia (2% to 6%), neck pain (2% to 5%), pathological fracture (2% to 5%)

Ophthalmic: Cataract (6%)

Respiratory: Flu-like symptoms (2% to 7%), sinusitis (2% to 6%), bronchitis (2% to 5%), rhinitis (2% to 5%)

Miscellaneous: Accidental injury (2% to 10%), cyst (5%), fever (2% to 5%)

<1% (Limited to important or life-threatening): Anaphylaxis, angioedema, cerebral infarction, cerebral ischemia, dermal ulcer, endometrial carcinoma, erythema multiforme, hepatitis, hepatomegaly, hypercalcemia, hypersensitivity angiitis (including anaphylactoid purpura [IgA vasculitis]), jaundice, joint stiffness, pulmonary embolism, retinal thrombosis, skin blister, skin lesion, Stevens-Johnson syndrome, tenosynovitis (stenosing), urticaria

Drug Interactions

Metabolism/Transport Effects Inhibits CYP1A2 (weak), CYP2C8 (weak), CYP2C9 (weak)

Avoid Concomitant Use
Avoid concomitant use of Anastrozole with any of the following: Amodiaquine; Estrogen Derivatives

Increased Effect/Toxicity
Anastrozole may increase the levels/effects of: Amodiaquine; Methadone; TiZANidine

Decreased Effect
The levels/effects of Anastrozole may be decreased by: Estrogen Derivatives; Tamoxifen

Storage/Stability Store at 20°C to 25°C (68°F to 77°F).

Mechanism of Action Potent and selective nonsteroidal aromatase inhibitor. By inhibiting aromatase, the conversion of androstenedione to estrone, and testosterone to estradiol, is prevented, thereby decreasing tumor mass or delaying progression in patients with tumors responsive to hormones. Anastrozole causes an 85% decrease in estrone sulfate levels.

Pharmacodynamics/Kinetics
Onset of estradiol reduction: 70% reduction after 24 hours; 80% after 2 weeks of therapy

Duration of estradiol reduction: 6 days

Absorption: Well absorbed; extent of absorption not affected by food

Protein binding, plasma: 40%

Metabolism: Extensively hepatic (~85%) via N-dealkylation, hydroxylation, and glucuronidation; primary metabolite (triazole) inactive

Half-life elimination: ~50 hours

Time to peak, plasma: ~2 hours without food; 5 hours with food

Excretion: Feces; urine (urinary excretion accounts for ~10% of total elimination, mostly as metabolites)

Dosing
Adult & Geriatric
Breast cancer, advanced: Postmenopausal females: Oral: 1 mg once daily; continue until tumor progression

Breast cancer, early (adjuvant treatment): Postmenopausal females: Oral: 1 mg once daily. **Note:** The American Society of Clinical Oncology (ASCO) guidelines for Adjuvant Endocrine Therapy of Hormone-Receptor Positive Breast Cancer (Focused Update) recommend a maximum duration of 5 years of aromatase inhibitor (AI) therapy for postmenopausal women; AIs may be combined with tamoxifen for a total duration of up to 10 years of endocrine therapy. Refer to the guidelines for specific recommendations based on menopausal status and tolerability (Burstein, 2014).

Breast cancer, risk reduction (off-label use): Postmenopausal females ≥40 years: Oral: 1 mg once daily for 5 years (Cuzick, 2014)

Renal Impairment No dosage adjustment necessary.

Hepatic Impairment
Mild to moderate impairment or stable hepatic cirrhosis: No dosage adjustment necessary.

Severe hepatic impairment: There are no dosage adjustments provided in the manufacturer's labeling (has not been studied).

Administration May be administered with or without food. Hazardous agent; use appropriate precautions for handling and disposal (NIOSH 2014 [group 1]).

Monitoring Parameters
Bone mineral density; total cholesterol and LDL

Breast cancer risk reduction (off-label use): Bone mineral density at baseline, mammograms, and clinical breast exam at baseline and at least every 2 years (Cuzick, 2014)

Dosage Forms Excipient information presented when available (limited, particularly for generics); consult specific product labeling.

Tablet, Oral:
Arimidex: 1 mg
Generic: 1 mg

Anidulafungin (ay nid yoo la FUN jin)

Brand Names: US Eraxis
Brand Names: Canada Eraxis
Index Terms LY303366
Pharmacologic Category Antifungal Agent, Parenteral; Echinocandin
Use Treatment of candidemia and other forms of Candida infections (including those of intra-abdominal, peritoneal, and esophageal locus)

Dosing
Adult & Geriatric
Aspergillosis (invasive) in HIV-infected patients: IV: 200 mg on day 1, then 100 mg once daily until infection resolution and CD4 count >200 cells/mm³ (HHS [OI adult 2015])

Candidemia, intra-abdominal or peritoneal candidiasis: IV: Initial dose: 200 mg on day 1; subsequent dosing: 100 mg daily; treatment should continue until 14 days after last positive culture

Esophageal candidiasis: IV: Initial dose: 100 mg on day 1; subsequent dosing: 50 mg daily; treatment should continue for a minimum of 14 days and for at least 7 days after symptom resolution

Pediatric Aspergillosis (invasive) in HIV-infected patients (off-label use): Adolescents: IV: Refer to adult dosing.

Renal Impairment No dosage adjustment necessary, including dialysis patients.

Hepatic Impairment No dosage adjustment necessary.

Additional Information Complete prescribing information should be consulted for additional detail.

Dosage Forms Excipient information presented when available (limited, particularly for generics); consult specific product labeling.

Solution Reconstituted, Intravenous [preservative free]:
Eraxis: 50 mg (1 ea); 100 mg (1 ea) [contains polysorbate 80]

Anthralin (AN thra lin)

Brand Names: US Dritho-Creme HP; Dritho-Scalp [DSC]; Zithranol; Zithranol-RR
Brand Names: Canada Anthraforte; Anthranol; Anthrascalp; Micanol
Index Terms Dithranol
Pharmacologic Category Antipsoriatic Agent; Keratolytic Agent
Use Plaque psoriasis: Treatment of stable plaque psoriasis

Dosing
Adult & Geriatric Psoriasis: Topical:
Cream: Generally, apply once daily or as directed. The irritant potential of anthralin is directly related to the strength being used and each patient's individual tolerance. Always commence treatment using a short, daily contact time (5 to 10 minutes) for at least 1 week using the lowest strength possible. Contact time may be gradually increased (to 30 minutes) as tolerated.

Skin application: Apply sparingly only to psoriatic lesions and rub gently and carefully into the skin until absorbed. Avoid applying an excessive quantity which may cause unnecessary soiling and staining of the clothing or bed linen.

Scalp application: Comb hair to remove scalar debris, wet hair and, after suitably parting, rub cream well into the lesions, taking care to prevent the cream from spreading onto the forehead.

Note: Remove by washing or showering; optimal period of contact will vary according to the strength used and the patient's response to treatment. Continue treatment until the skin is entirely clear (ie, when there is nothing to feel with the fingers and the texture is normal).

Shampoo: Rub shampoo onto wet scalp, lather and leave on scalp for 3 to 5 minutes; rinse thoroughly; apply 3 to 4 times weekly

Pediatric Psoriasis: Children ≥12 years and Adolescents: Topical: Shampoo: Refer to adult dosing.

Renal Impairment There are no dosage adjustments provided in the manufacturer's labeling.

Hepatic Impairment There are no dosage adjustments provided in the manufacturer's labeling.

Additional Information Complete prescribing information should be consulted for additional detail.

Dosage Forms Excipient information presented when available (limited, particularly for generics); consult specific product labeling. [DSC] = Discontinued product

Cream, External:
Dritho-Creme HP: 1% (50 g) [contains methylparaben]
Dritho-Scalp: 0.5% (50 g) [DSC]
Zithranol-RR: 1.2% (45 g) [contains brilliant blue fcf (fd&c blue #1)]
Shampoo, External:
Zithranol: 1% (85 g) [contains brilliant blue fcf (fd&c blue #1)]

◆ Anthranol (Can) *see* Anthralin *on page 129*

◆ Anthrascalp (Can) *see* Anthralin *on page 129*

Anthrax Vaccine Adsorbed
(AN thraks vak SEEN ad SORBED)

Brand Names: US BioThrax
Index Terms AVA
Pharmacologic Category Vaccine; Vaccine, Inactivated (Bacterial)

Additional Appendix Information
Immunization Administration Recommendations *on page 1974*
Immunization Schedules *on page 1979*

Use
Anthrax immunization: Active immunization against *Bacillus anthracis* in persons 18 to 65 years of age.

Pre-exposure: For pre-exposure prophylaxis of disease in persons whose occupation or other activities place them at high risk of exposure.

Post-exposure: For post-exposure prophylaxis of disease following suspected or confirmed Bacillus anthracis exposure, when administered in conjunction with recommended antibacterial drugs.

The Advisory Committee on Immunization Practices (ACIP) recommends routine vaccination (preexposure vaccination) for the following (CDC [Wright 2010]):

• Persons who work directly with the organism in the laboratory

• Persons who handle animals or animal products only when
  - potentially infected in research settings;
  - in areas of high incidence of enzootic anthrax; or
  - where standards and restrictions are not sufficient to prevent exposure

• Military personnel deployed to areas with high risk of exposure as recommended by the Department of Defense (DoD)

• Persons engaged in environmental investigations or remediation efforts

Routine immunization for the general population is not recommended. Routine vaccination may be offered to emergency and other responders (police and fire departments, the National Guard, etc.) on a voluntary basis under the direction of a comprehensive occupational health and safety program (CDC [Wright 2010]).

The ACIP recommends postexposure prophylaxis after inhalation exposure to aerosolized *Bacillus anthracis* spores for the following (in the absence of completing a preexposure, routine vaccination schedule) (CDC [Wright 2010]):

• The general public, including pregnant and breast-feeding women
• Medical professionals
• Children ages 0 to 18 years as determined on an event-by-event basis
• Persons engaged in handling certain animals or animal products
• Persons who work directly with the organism in the laboratory (postexposure vaccination dependent upon pre-event vaccination status)
• Military personnel as recommended by the DoD
• Persons engaged in environmental investigations or remediation efforts (postexposure vaccination dependent upon pre-event vaccination status)
• Emergency and other responders (police and fire departments, the National Guard, etc.)
• Persons working in postal facilities

Prescribing and Access Restrictions Not commercially available in U.S.; presently, all anthrax vaccine lots are owned by the U.S. Department of Defense. The Center for Disease Control (CDC) does not currently recommend routine vaccination of the general public.

Medication Guide Available Yes

Dosing
Adult
Preexposure prophylaxis: Adults ≤65 years:
IM (preferred):
Primary immunization: Three injections of 0.5 mL each given at day 0, 1 month, and 6 months.
Booster injections: 0.5 mL each should be given 6 and 12 months after completion of the primary series and at 1-year intervals thereafter for persons who remain at risk
SubQ:
Primary immunization: Four injections of 0.5 mL each given at day 0, 2 weeks, 4 weeks, and 6 months.
Booster injections: 0.5 mL each should be given 6 and 12 months after completion of the primary series and at 1-year intervals thereafter for persons who remain at risk.
Note: SubQ administration is only to be used for primary immunization in persons who are at risk for hematoma formation following IM injection.

Postexposure prophylaxis (inhalation exposure):
SubQ: Three injections of 0.5 mL each given at day 0, 2 weeks, and 4 weeks post-exposure.
ACIP recommendations (CDC [Wright 2010]): Administer with a 60-day course of antibiotics. (Vaccination should begin within 10 days of exposure. Refer to guidelines provided as part of emergency use authorization [EUA] or investigational new drug [IND] application at the time of the event). **Note:** Additional considerations for postexposure prophylaxis following occupational exposures:

Fully vaccinated: Personnel who have completed the primary vaccination series and booster injections do not require postexposure prophylaxis if wearing protective equipment. If respiratory protection is disrupted, a 30-day course of antimicrobial therapy is recommended.

Previously unvaccinated: Workers should receive the vaccine as directed per postexposure prophylaxis along with the 60-day course of antimicrobial therapy (antimicrobial therapy should continue for 14 days after the third dose of PEP vaccine), then switch to the licensed regimen at the 6-month dose.

Partially vaccinated: Any person who started but did not complete the primary vaccination series should receive a 30-day course of antimicrobial therapy and continue with the primary vaccination schedule.

Geriatric Safety and efficacy have not been established in persons >65 years of age.

Pediatric Children <18 years: Safety and efficacy have not been established. **Note:** Use in children is recommended by the ACIP as determined on an event-by-event basis; refer to adult dosing for postexposure prophylaxis.

Additional Information Complete prescribing information should be consulted for additional detail.

Dosage Forms Excipient information presented when available (limited, particularly for generics); consult specific product labeling.
Injection, suspension:
BioThrax: *Bacillus anthracis* proteins (5 mL) [contains aluminum, natural rubber/natural latex in packaging]

◆ Anti-4 Alpha Integrin *see* Natalizumab *on page 1261*

◆ Anti-D Immunoglobulin *see* Rh₀(D) Immune Globulin
on page 1572

◆ Antibody-Drug Conjugate SGN-35 *see* Brentuximab
Vedotin *on page 250*

◆ Anti-CD20 Monoclonal Antibody *see* RiTUXimab
on page 1600

◆ Anti-CD30 ADC SGN-35 *see* Brentuximab Vedotin
on page 250

◆ Anti-CD30 Antibody-Drug Conjugate SGN-35 *see*
Brentuximab Vedotin *on page 250*

◆ Anti-CD52 Monoclonal Antibody *see* Alemtuzumab
on page 62

◆ anti-c-erB-2 *see* Trastuzumab *on page 1831*

◆ Anti-Dandruff [OTC] *see* Selenium Sulfide
on page 1647

◆ Anti-Diarrheal [OTC] *see* Loperamide *on page 1097*

◆ Antidigoxin Fab Fragments, Ovine *see* Digoxin Immune
Fab *on page 550*

◆ Antidiuretic Hormone *see* Vasopressin *on page 1879*

◆ Anti-EGFR Monoclonal Antibody IMC-11F8 *see* Necitumumab *on page 1263*

◆ anti-ERB-2 *see* Trastuzumab *on page 1831*

◆ Antifungal [OTC] *see* Miconazole (Topical)
on page 1201

◆ Anti-Fungal [OTC] *see* Tolnaftate *on page 1807*

Antihemophilic Factor (Human)
(an tee hee moe FIL ik FAK tor HYU man)

Brand Names: US Hemofil M; Koate-DVI; Monoclate-P
Brand Names: Canada Hemofil M
Index Terms AHF (Human); Factor VIII (Human); Kaote
DVI
Pharmacologic Category Antihemophilic Agent; Blood
Product Derivative
Use Hemophilia A: Prevention and treatment of hemor-
rhagic episodes in patients with hemophilia A (classic
hemophilia); perioperative management of hemophilia A.
Note: Can be of significant therapeutic value in patients
with acquired factor VIII inhibitors not exceeding 10
Bethesda units/mL
Limitations of use: Not effective in controlling bleeding in
patients with von Willebrand disease and therefore is not
indicated for this use.
Dosing
Adult & Geriatric Hemophilia: IV: Individualize dosage
based on coagulation studies performed prior to treatment and at regular intervals during treatment. In general,
administration of factor VIII 1 unit/kg will increase circulating factor VIII levels by ~2 units/dL. **Refer to product
information for specific manufacturer recommended
dosing.** Alternatively, the World Federation of Hemophilia (WFH) has recommended general dosing for factor
VIII products.

Dosage based on desired factor VIII increase (%):
To calculate dosage needed based on desired factor
VIII increase (%):
Body weight (kg) x 0.5 units/kg x desired factor VIII
increase (%) = units factor VIII required
For example:
50 kg x 0.5 units/kg x 30 (% increase) = 750 units
factor VIII
Dosage based on expected factor VIII increase (%):
It is also possible to calculate the **expected** % factor
VIII increase:
(# units administered x 2%/units/kg) divided by body
weight (kg) = expected % factor VIII increase
For example:
(1400 units x 2%/units/kg) divided by 70 kg = 40%

World Federation of Hemophilia (WFH) treatment
recommendations when no significant resource
constraint exists (WFH [Srivastava 2013]):

2013 World Federation of Hemophilia Treatment Recommendations (When No Significant Resource Constraint Exists)

Site of Hemorrhage/ Clinical Situation	Desired Factor VIII Level to Maintain	Duration
Joint	40 to 60 units/dL	1 to 2 days, may be longer if response is inadequate
Superficial muscle/no neurovascular compromise	40 to 60 units/dL	2 to 3 days, sometimes longer if response is inadequate
Iliopsoas and deep muscle with neurovascular injury, or substantial blood loss	*Initial:* 80 to 100 units/dL	*Initial:* 1 to 2 days
	Maintenance: 30 to 60 units/dL	*Maintenance:* 3 to 5 days, sometimes longer as secondary prophylaxis during physiotherapy
CNS/Head	*Initial:* 80 to 100 units/dL	*Initial:* 1 to 7 days
	Maintenance: 50 units/dL	*Maintenance:* 8 to 21 days
Throat and neck	*Initial:* 80 to 100 units/dL	*Initial:* 1 to 7 days
	Maintenance: 50 units/dL	*Maintenance:* 8 to 14 days
Gastrointestinal	*Initial:* 80 to 100 units/dL	*Initial:* 7 to 14 days
	Maintenance: 50 units/dL	*Maintenance:* Not specified
Renal	50 units/dL	3 to 5 days
Deep laceration	50 units/dL	5 to 7 days
Surgery (major)	*Preop:* 80 to 100 units/dL	
	Postop: 60 to 80 units/dL	*Postop:* 1 to 3 days
	Postop: 40 to 60 units/dL	*Postop:* 4 to 6 days
	Postop: 30 to 50 units/dL	*Postop:* 7 to 14 days
Surgery (minor)	*Preop:* 50 to 80 units/dL	
	Postop: 30 to 80 units/dL	*Postop:* 1 to 5 days depending on procedure type

Note: Factor VIII level may either be expressed as units/dL or as %. Dosing frequency most commonly corresponds to the half-life of factor VIII but should be determined based on an assessment of factor VIII levels before the next dose.

*Continuous infusion (for patients who require prolonged
periods of treatment [eg, intracranial hemorrhage or
surgery] to avoid peaks and troughs associated with
intermittent infusions) (Batorova 2002; Batorova 2012;
Poon 2012; Rickard 1995; WFH [Srivastava 2013]):*
Following initial bolus to achieve the desired factor VIII
level, initiate 2 to 4 units/kg/hour; adjust dose based on
frequent factor assays and calculation of factor VIII
clearance at steady-state using the following equations:
Factor VIII clearance (mL/kg/hour) = (current infusion
rate in units/kg/hour) divided by (plasma level in
units/mL)
New infusion rate (units/kg/hour) = (factor VIII clearance
in mL/kg/hour) x (desired plasma level in units/mL)
Pediatric Refer to adult dosing.
Renal Impairment There are no dosage adjustments
provided in the manufacturer's labeling.
Hepatic Impairment There are no dosage adjustments
provided in the manufacturer's labeling.
Additional Information Complete prescribing information
should be consulted for additional detail.
Dosage Forms Considerations
Strengths expressed with approximate values. Consult
individual vial labels for exact potency within each vial.
Hemofil M packaged contents may contain natural rubber
latex.
Dosage Forms Excipient information presented when
available (limited, particularly for generics); consult specific
product labeling. [DSC] = Discontinued product
Kit, Intravenous:
Monoclate-P: ~250 units, ~500 units, ~1000 units, ~1500
units [contains mouse protein (murine) (hamster)]
Solution Reconstituted, Intravenous:
Koate-DVI: ~500 units (1 ea) [contains albumin human,
polyethylene glycol, polysorbate 80]
Solution Reconstituted, Intravenous [preservative free]:
Hemofil M: ~250 units (1 ea) [contains albumin human,
mouse protein (murine) (hamster), polyethylene glycol]
Hemofil M: ~250 units (1 ea) [contains mouse protein
(murine) (hamster), polyethylene glycol]
Hemofil M: ~500 units (1 ea) [contains albumin human,
mouse protein (murine) (hamster), polyethylene glycol]
Hemofil M: ~500 units (1 ea) [contains mouse protein
(murine) (hamster), polyethylene glycol]
Hemofil M: ~1000 units (1 ea); ~1700 units (1 ea)
[contains albumin human, mouse protein (murine)
(hamster), polyethylene glycol]
Koate-DVI: ~250 units (1 ea); ~500 units (1 ea [DSC]);
~1000 units (1 ea) [contains albumin human, polyethylene glycol, polysorbate 80]

Antihemophilic Factor (Recombinant)
(an tee hee moe FIL ik FAK tor ree KOM be nant)

Brand Names: US Advate; Eloctate; Helixate FS; Kogenate FS; Kogenate FS Bio-Set; Novoeight; Nuwiq; Recombinate; Xyntha; Xyntha Solofuse

Brand Names: Canada Advate; Helixate FS; Kogenate FS; Xyntha; Xyntha Solofuse

Index Terms AHF (Recombinant); Efraloctocog Alfa; Factor VIII (Recombinant); Moroctocog Alfa; Octacog Alfa; rAHF

Pharmacologic Category Antihemophilic Agent

Use Hemophilia A:

Control and prevention of bleeding episodes: For the prevention and control of bleeding episodes in adults and children with hemophilia A.

Perioperative management: For surgical prophylaxis in adults and children with hemophilia A.

Routine prophylaxis to prevent or reduce the frequency of bleeding (Advate, Eloctate, Helixate FS, Kogenate FS, Novoeight, Nuwiq, Xyntha [Canadian labeling; not in US labeling]): For routine prophylactic treatment to prevent or reduce the frequency of bleeding episodes in adults and children with hemophilia A.

Routine prophylaxis to prevent bleeding episodes and joint damage (Helixate FS, Kogenate FS): For routine prophylactic treatment to reduce the frequency of bleeding episodes and the risk of joint damage in children without preexisting joint damage.

Dosing

Adult & Geriatric Hemophilia A: IV: Individualize dosage based on coagulation studies performed prior to treatment and at regular intervals during treatment. In general, administration of factor VIII 1 unit/kg will increase circulating factor VIII levels by ~2 units/dL. **Refer to product information for specific manufacturer recommended dosing.** Alternatively, the World Federation of Hemophilia (WFH) has recommended general dosing for factor VIII products.

Dosage based on desired factor VIII increase (%):
To calculate dosage needed based on desired factor VIII increase (%):
[Body weight (kg) x desired factor VIII increase (%)] divided by 2 (%/units/kg) = units factor VIII required
For example:
50 kg x 30 (% increase) divided by 2 = 750 units factor VIII

Dosage based on expected factor VIII increase (%):
It is also possible to calculate the **expected** % factor VIII increase:
[# units administered x 2 (%/units/kg)] divided by body weight (kg) = expected % factor VIII increase
For example:
[1,400 units x 2] divided by 70 kg = 40%

World Federation of Hemophilia (WFH) treatment recommendations when no significant resource constraint exists (WFH [Srivastava 2013]):

2013 World Federation of Hemophilia Treatment Recommendations (When No Significant Resource Constraint Exists)

Site of Hemorrhage/ Clinical Situation	Desired Factor VIII Level to Maintain	Duration
Joint	40 to 60 units/dL	1 to 2 days, may be longer if response is inadequate
Superficial muscle/no neurovascular compromise	40 to 60 units/dL	2 to 3 days, sometimes longer if response is inadequate
Iliopsoas and deep muscle with neurovascular injury, or substantial blood loss	Initial: 80 to 100 units/dL	Initial: 1 to 2 days
	Maintenance: 30 to 60 units/dL	Maintenance: 3 to 5 days, sometimes longer as secondary prophylaxis during physiotherapy
CNS/Head	Initial: 80 to 100 units/dL	Initial: 1 to 7 days
	Maintenance: 50 units/dL	Maintenance: 8 to 21 days
Throat and neck	Initial: 80 to 100 units/dL	Initial: 1 to 7 days
	Maintenance: 50 units/dL	Maintenance: 8 to 14 days
Gastrointestinal	Initial: 80 to 100 units/dL	Initial: 7 to 14 days
	Maintenance: 50 units/dL	Maintenance: Not specified
Renal	50 units/dL	3 to 5 days
Deep laceration	50 units/dL	5 to 7 days
Surgery (major)	Preop: 80 to 100 units/dL	
	Postop: 60 to 80 units/dL	Postop: 1 to 3 days
	Postop: 40 to 60 units/dL	Postop: 4 to 6 days
	Postop: 30 to 50 units/dL	Postop: 7 to 14 days
Surgery (minor)	Preop: 50 to 80 units/dL	
	Postop: 30 to 80 units/dL	Postop: 1 to 5 days depending on procedure type

Note: Factor VIII level may either be expressed as units/dL or as %. Dosing frequency most commonly corresponds to the half-life of factor VIII but should be determined based on an assessment of factor VIII levels before the next dose.

Continuous infusion *(for patients who require prolonged periods of treatment [eg, intracranial hemorrhage or surgery] to avoid peaks and troughs associated with intermittent infusions)* (Batorova 2002; Batorova 2012; Poon 2012; Rickard 1995; WFH [Srivastava 2013]): Following initial bolus to achieve the desired factor VIII level, initiate 2 to 4 units/kg/hour; adjust dose based on frequent factor assays and calculation of factor VIII clearance at steady-state using the following equations:
Factor VIII clearance (mL/kg/hour) = (current infusion rate in units/kg/hour) divided by (plasma level in units/mL)
New infusion rate (units/kg/hour) = (factor VIII clearance in mL/kg/hour) x (desired plasma level in units/mL)

Routine prophylaxis to prevent or reduce the frequency of bleeding episodes: IV:
Advate: 20 to 40 units/kg every other day (3 to 4 times weekly). Alternatively, an every-third-day dosing regimen may be used to target factor VIII trough levels of ≥1%.
Eloctate: 50 units/kg every 4 days; may adjust within the range of 25 to 65 units/kg at 3- to 5-day intervals based on patient response.
Helixate FS: 25 units/kg 3 times weekly
Kogenate FS: 25 units/kg 3 times weekly
Novoeight: 20 to 50 units/kg 3 times weekly **or** 20 to 40 units/kg every other day
Nuwiq: 30 to 40 units/kg every other day
Xyntha (Canadian labeling; not in US labeling): Treatment experienced patients: 25 to 35 units/kg 3 times weekly

Pediatric Hemophilia A: Children and Adolescents: IV: Refer to adult dosing. **Note:** Children <6 years may require higher doses and/or more frequent administration.
Routine prophylaxis to prevent bleeding episodes:
Advate: Refer to adult dosing.
Eloctate: 50 units/kg every 4 days; may adjust within the range of 25 to 65 units/kg at 3- to 5-day intervals based on patient response. More frequent or higher doses up to 80 units/kg may be required in children <6 years.
Helixate FS: Children: 25 units/kg every other day
Novoeight:
Children <12 years: 25 to 60 units per kg 3 times weekly **or** 25 to 50 units/kg every other day
Children ≥12 years and Adolescents: Refer to adult dosing.
Nuwiq:
Children 2 to 11 years: 30 to 50 units/kg every other day or 3 times weekly
Children ≥12 years and Adolescents: Refer to adult dosing.
Xyntha (Canadian labeling; not in US labeling): Adolescents (treatment experienced): Refer to adult dosing.
Routine prophylaxis to prevent bleeding episodes and joint damage (without preexisting joint damage) (Helixate FS, Kogenate FS): 25 units/kg every other day

Renal Impairment There are no dosage adjustments provided in the manufacturer's labeling.

Hepatic Impairment There are no dosage adjustments provided in the manufacturer's labeling.

Additional Information Complete prescribing information should be consulted for additional detail.

Dosage Forms Considerations
Strengths expressed with approximate values. Consult individual vial labels for exact potency within each vial.

Dosage Forms Excipient information presented when available (limited, particularly for generics); consult specific product labeling.
Kit, Intravenous:
Kogenate FS: 250 units, 500 units, 1000 units [contains mouse protein (murine) (hamster)]
Kit, Intravenous [preservative free]:
Helixate FS: 250 units, 500 units, 1000 units, 2000 units, 3000 units [contains polysorbate 80]
Kogenate FS: 2000 units, 3000 units [contains mouse protein (murine) (hamster)]
Kogenate FS Bio-Set: 250 units, 500 units, 1000 units, 2000 units, 3000 units
Nuwiq: 250 units, 500 units, 1000 units, 2000 units
Xyntha: 250 units, 500 units, 1000 units, 2000 units [albumin free; contains mouse protein (murine) (hamster), polysorbate 80]
Xyntha Solofuse: 250 units, 500 units, 1000 units, 2000 units, 3000 units [albumin free; contains mouse protein (murine) (hamster), polysorbate 80]

Solution Reconstituted, Intravenous [preservative free]:

Advate: 250 units (1 ea); 500 units (1 ea); 1000 units (1 ea); 1500 units (1 ea); 2000 units (1 ea); 3000 units (1 ea); 4000 units (1 ea) [albumin free; contains polysorbate 80]

Eloctate: 250 units (1 ea); 500 units (1 ea); 750 units (1 ea); 1000 units (1 ea); 1500 units (1 ea); 2000 units (1 ea); 3000 units (1 ea)

Novoeight: 250 units (1 ea); 500 units (1 ea); 1000 units (1 ea); 1500 units (1 ea); 2000 units (1 ea); 3000 units (1 ea) [contains mouse protein (murine) (hamster), polysorbate 80]

Nuwiq: 250 units (1 ea); 500 units (1 ea); 1000 units (1 ea); 2000 units (1 ea)

Recombinate: 220-400 units (1 ea); 401-800 units (1 ea); 801-1240 units (1 ea); 1241-1800 units (1 ea); 1801-2400 units (1 ea) [contains albumin human, polyethylene glycol, polysorbate 80]

Antihemophilic Factor (Recombinant [Porcine Sequence])

(an tee hee moe FIL ik FAK tor ree KOM be nant POR sine SEE kwens)

Brand Names: US Obizur

Index Terms AHF (Recombinant [Porcine Sequence]); Factor VIII (Recombinant [Porcine Sequence]); pFVIII; rAHF; rpFVIII

Pharmacologic Category Antihemophilic Agent

Use

Acquired hemophilia A: Treatment of bleeding episodes in adults with acquired hemophilia A

Limitations of use: Not indicated for the treatment of congenital hemophilia A or von Willebrand disease; safety and efficacy of has not been established in patients with baseline anti- porcine factor VIII inhibitor titer >20 BU.

Dosing

Adult & Geriatric

Acquired hemophilia A: IV: **Note:** Dose, dosing frequency, and duration based on location and severity of bleeding, target factor VIII levels, and clinical condition of the patient. Plasma levels of factor VIII should not exceed 200% of normal or 200 units/dL.

Minor to moderate hemorrhage: 200 units/kg initially to achieve factor VIII plasma level 50% to 100% of normal; titrate subsequent doses to maintain recommended factor VIII trough levels and individual clinical response; dose every 4 to 12 hours (frequency may be adjusted based on clinical response/factor VIII levels).

Major hemorrhage: 200 units/kg initially to achieve factor VIII plasma level 100% to 200% (for acute bleed) or 50% to 100% (after acute bleed is controlled, if required) of normal; titrate subsequent doses to maintain recommended factor VIII trough levels and individual clinical response; dose every 4 to 12 hours (frequency may be adjusted based on clinical response/factor VIII levels).

Renal Impairment There are no dosage adjustments provided in the manufacturer's labeling.

Hepatic Impairment There are no dosage adjustments provided in the manufacturer's labeling.

Additional Information Complete prescribing information should be consulted for additional detail.

Product Availability Obizur: Health Canada approved October 2015; anticipated availability is currently unknown.

Dosage Forms Excipient information presented when available (limited, particularly for generics); consult specific product labeling.

Solution Reconstituted, Intravenous:

Obizur: 500 units (1 ea) [contains mouse protein (murine) (hamster), polysorbate 80]

Antihemophilic Factor/von Willebrand Factor Complex (Human)

(an tee hee moe FIL ik FAK tor von WILL le brand FAK tor KOM plex HYU man)

Brand Names: US Alphanate; Humate-P; Wilate

Brand Names: Canada Humate-P

Index Terms AHF (Human); Factor VIII (Human)/von Willebrand Factor; Factor VIII Concentrate; FVIII/vWF; von Willebrand Factor/Factor VIII Complex; VWF/FVIII Concentrate; VWF:RCo; vWF:RCof

Pharmacologic Category Antihemophilic Agent; Blood Product Derivative

Use

Factor VIII deficiency: Alphanate, Humate-P: Prevention and treatment of hemorrhagic episodes in patients with hemophilia A (classical hemophilia); **Note:** Wilate is not approved for use in patients with hemophilia A or acquired factor VIII deficiency

von Willebrand disease (VWD):

Alphanate: Prophylaxis with surgical and/or invasive procedures in patients with VWD when desmopressin is either ineffective or contraindicated; **Note:** Not indicated for patients with severe VWD (type 3) undergoing major surgery

Humate-P: Treatment of spontaneous or trauma-induced bleeding, as well as prevention of excessive bleeding during and after surgery in patients with severe VWD, including mild or moderate disease where use of desmopressin is known or suspected to be inadequate; **Note:** Not indicated for the prophylaxis of spontaneous bleeding episodes

Wilate: Treatment of spontaneous and trauma-induced bleeding in patients with severe VWD, including mild or moderate disease where use of desmopressin is known or suspected to be inadequate or contraindicated; **Note:** Not indicated for prophylaxis of spontaneous bleeding or prevention of excessive bleeding during and after surgery

Dosing

Adult & Geriatric

Factor VIII deficiency: General guidelines (consult specific product labeling for Alphanate or Humate-P): IV:

Individualize dosage based on coagulation studies performed prior to treatment and at regular intervals during treatment; in general, administration of factor VIII 1 unit/kg will increase circulating factor VIII levels by ~2 units/dL.

Minor hemorrhage: Loading dose: FVIII:C 15 units/kg to achieve FVIII:C plasma level ~30% of normal. If second infusion is needed, half the loading dose may be given once or twice daily for 1 to 2 days.

Moderate hemorrhage: Loading dose: FVIII:C 25 units/kg to achieve FVIII:C plasma level ~50% of normal; Maintenance: FVIII:C 15 units/kg every 8 to 12 hours for 1 to 2 days in order to maintain FVIII:C plasma levels at 30% of normal. Repeat the same dose once or twice daily for up to 7 days or until adequate wound healing.

Life-threatening hemorrhage/major surgery: Loading dose: FVIII:C 40-50 units/kg; Maintenance: FVIII:C 20 to 25 units/kg every 8 to 12 hours to maintain FVIII:C plasma levels at 80% to 100% of normal for 7 days. Continue same dose once or twice daily for another 7 days in order to maintain FVIII:C levels at 30% to 50% of normal.

von Willebrand disease (VWD): Treatment:

Humate-P: IV: Individualize dosage based on coagulation studies performed prior to treatment and at regular intervals during treatment; in general, administration of factor VIII 1 unit/kg would be expected to raise circulating VWF:RCo ~5 units/dL

Type 1, mild VWD: Minor hemorrhage (if desmopressin is not appropriate) or major hemorrhage:

Loading dose: VWF:RCo 40 to 60 units/kg

Maintenance dose: VWF:RCo 40 to 50 units/kg every 8 to 12 hours for 3 days, keeping VWF:RCo nadir >50%; follow with 40 to 50 units/kg daily for up to 7 days

Type 1, moderate or severe VWD:

Minor hemorrhage: VWF:RCo 40 to 50 units/kg for 1 to 2 doses

Major hemorrhage:

Loading dose: VWF:RCo 50 to 75 units/kg

Maintenance dose: VWF:RCo 40 to 60 units/kg every 8 to 12 hours for 3 days to keep the VWF:RCo nadir >50%, then 40 to 60 units/kg daily for a total of up to 7 days

Types 2 and 3 VWD:

Minor hemorrhage: VWF:RCo 40 to 50 units/kg for 1 to 2 doses

Major hemorrhage:

Loading dose: VWF:RCo 60 to 80 units/kg

Maintenance dose: VWF:RCo 40 to 60 units/kg every 8 to 12 hours for 3 days, keeping the VWF:RCo nadir >50%; follow with 40 to 60 units/kg daily for a total of up to 7 days

Wilate: IV:

Minor hemorrhage:

Loading dose: VWF:RCo: 20 to 40 units/kg

Maintenance dose: 20 to 30 units/kg every 12 to 24 hours for ≤3 days, keeping the VWF:RCo nadir >30%

◀

Major hemorrhage:
Loading dose: VWF:RCo: 40 to 60 units/kg
Maintenance dose: 20 to 40 units/kg every 12 to 24 hours for 5 to 7 days, keeping the VWF:RCo nadir >50%

von Willebrand disease (VWD): Prophylaxis: IV:

Alphanate: Surgery/invasive procedure prophylaxis (except patients with type 3 undergoing major surgery):
Preoperative dose: VWF:RCo: 60 units/kg 1 hour prior to surgery
Maintenance dose: VWF:RCo: 40 to 60 units/kg every 8 to 12 hours as clinically needed. For minor procedures, maintain FVIII:C activity level of 40 to 50 units/dL during postoperative days 1 to 3; for major procedures maintain FVIII:C activity level of 100 units/dL for 3 to 7 days. Do not exceed FVIII:C activity level of 150 units/dL.

Humate-P: Surgery/procedure prevention of bleeding:
Emergency surgery: Administer VWF:RCo 50 to 60 units/kg; monitor trough coagulation factor levels for subsequent doses
Surgical management (nonemergency):
Loading dose calculation based on baseline target VWF:RCo: (Target peak VWF:RCo - Baseline VWF:RCo) x weight (in kg) / IVR = units VWF:RCo required. Administer loading dose 1 to 2 hours prior to surgery. **Note:** If *in vivo* recovery (IVR) not available, assume 2 units/dL per units/kg of VWF:RCo product administered.
Target concentrations for VWF:RCo following loading dose:
Major surgery: 100 units/dL
Minor surgery: 50 to 60 units/dL
Maintenance dose: Initial: One-half loading dose, followed by subsequent dosing determined by target trough concentrations, generally every 8 to 12 hours. Patients with shorter half-lives may require dosing every 6 hours.
Target maintenance trough VWF:RCo concentrations:
Major surgery: >50 units/dL for up to 3 days, followed by >30 units/dL for a minimum total treatment of 72 hours
Minor surgery: ≥30 units/dL for a minimum duration of 48 hours
Oral surgery: ≥30 units/dL for a minimum duration of 8 to 12 hours

Pediatric

Factor VIII deficiency: Refer to adult dosing.
von Willebrand disease (VWD): Treatment: Refer to adult dosing.
von Willebrand disease (VWD): Prophylaxis:
Surgery/invasive procedure prophylaxis (except patients with type 3 undergoing major surgery) (Alphanate): IV:
Preoperative dose: VWF:RCo: 75 units/kg 1 hour prior to surgery
Maintenance dose: VWF:RCo: 50 to 75 units/kg every 8 to 12 hours as clinically needed. For minor procedures, maintain FVIII:C activity level of 40 to 50 units/dL during postoperative days 1 to 3; for major procedures, maintain FVIII:C activity level of 100 units/dL for 3 to 7 days. Do not exceed FVIII:C activity level of 150 units/dL.
Surgery/procedure prevention of bleeding (Humate-P): Refer to adult dosing.

Renal Impairment There are no dosage adjustments provided in the manufacturer's labeling.

Hepatic Impairment There are no dosage adjustments provided in the manufacturer's labeling.

Additional Information Complete prescribing information should be consulted for additional detail.

Dosage Forms Considerations
Strengths expressed with approximate values. Consult individual vial labels for exact potency within each vial.

Dosage Forms Excipient information presented when available (limited, particularly for generics); consult specific product labeling. [DSC] = Discontinued product
Injection, powder for reconstitution [human derived]:
Alphanate:
250 units [Factor VIII and VWF:RCo ratio varies by lot; contains albumin and polysorbate 80; packaged with diluent]
500 units [Factor VIII and VWF:RCo ratio varies by lot; contains albumin and polysorbate 80; packaged with diluent]
1000 units [Factor VIII and VWF:RCo ratio varies by lot; contains albumin and polysorbate 80; packaged with diluent]

1500 units [Factor VIII and VWF:RCo ratio varies by lot; contains albumin and polysorbate 80; packaged with diluent]
2000 units [Factor VIII and VWF:RCo ratio varies by lot; contains albumin and polysorbate 80; packaged with diluent]
Humate-P:
FVIII 250 units and VWF:RCo 600 units [contains albumin; packaged with diluent]
FVIII 500 units and VWF:RCo 1200 units [contains albumin; packaged with diluent]
FVIII 1000 units and VWF:RCo 2400 units [contains albumin; packaged with diluent]
Wilate:
FVIII 450 units and VWF:RCo 450 units [contains polysorbate 80 (in diluent); packaged with diluent] [DSC]
FVIII 500 units and VWF:RCo 500 units [contains polysorbate 80 (in diluent); packaged with diluent]
FVIII 900 units and VWF:RCo 900 units [contains polysorbate 80 (in diluent); packaged with diluent] [DSC]
FVIII 1000 units and VWF:RCo 1000 units [contains polysorbate 80 (in diluent); packaged with diluent]

◆ Anti-Hist [OTC] [DSC] *see* DiphenhydrAMINE (Systemic) *on page 561*

◆ Anti-Hist Allergy [OTC] *see* DiphenhydrAMINE (Systemic) *on page 561*

Anti-inhibitor Coagulant Complex (Human)
(an TEE in HI bi tor coe AG yoo lant KOM pleks HYU man)

Brand Names: US FEIBA
Brand Names: Canada FEIBA NF
Index Terms Activated PCC; AICC; aPCC; Coagulant Complex Inhibitor; Factor Eight Inhibitor Bypassing Activity; Factor VIII Inhibitor Bypassing Activity; FEIBA NF; FEIBA VH
Pharmacologic Category Activated Prothrombin Complex Concentrate (aPCC); Antihemophilic Agent; Blood Product Derivative

Use

Hemorrhage in patients with hemophilia: For use in patients with hemophilia A and B with inhibitors for control and prevention of bleeding episodes.

Perioperative bleeding management in patients with hemophilia: For use in patients with hemophilia A and B with inhibitors for perioperative management.

Routine prophylaxis of bleeding events in patients with hemophilia: For use in patients with hemophilia A and B for routine prophylaxis to prevent or reduce the frequency of bleeding episodes.

Dosing

Adult & Geriatric Note: Anti-inhibitor coagulant complex (Human) contains mainly non-activated therapeutic levels of factors II, IX, and X and mainly activated factor VII

Control and prevention of bleeding episodes: IV:
Note: Considered a first-line treatment when factor VIII inhibitor titer is >5 Bethesda units (BU) (antihemophilic factor may be preferred when titer <5 BU)
General dosing guidelines: 50-100 units/kg per dose (maximum: 100 units/kg [single dose], 200 units/kg/day [total daily dose]). Dosage and duration of treatment depend on the location and extent of bleeding and clinical condition of the patient. If total single dose exceeds 100 units/kg or total daily dose exceeds 200 units/kg/day, monitor closely for DIC, coronary ischemia, and signs/symptoms of other thromboembolic events.
Joint hemorrhage: 50-100 units/kg every 12 hours until pain and acute disabilities are improved (maximum: 200 units/kg/day)
Mucous membrane bleeding: 50-100 units/kg every 6 hours for at least 1 day or until bleeding is resolved (maximum: 200 units/kg/day)
Soft tissue hemorrhage (eg, retroperitoneal bleed): 100 units/kg every 12 hours until resolution of bleed (maximum: 200 units/kg/day)
Other severe hemorrhage (eg, intracranial hemorrhage): 100 units/kg every 6-12 hours; continue until resolution of bleed (maximum: 200 units/kg/day).
Perioperative management:
Preoperative: 50-100 units/kg (single dose) administered immediately prior to surgery.
Postoperative: 50-100 units/kg every 6-12 hours until resolution of bleed and healing is achieved (maximum: 200 units/kg/day)
Routine prophylaxis: 85 units/kg every other day.

Hemorrhage (moderate-to-severe) due to acquired hemophilia (off-label use): IV: Optimal dosing has not been established: 50-100 units/kg every 8-12 hours until bleeding controlled has been suggested; may continue for 24-72 hours based on site, type, and severity of bleeding (maximum: 200 units/kg/day) (Huth-Kuhne, 2009; Sallah, 2004).

Life-threatening hemorrhage associated with dabigatran (off-label use): IV: Optimal dosing has not been established. Based on multiple case reports with various types of hemorrhage, a dosage range of 25 to 100 units/kg has been used (Dager, 2013; Faust, 2013; Kiraly, 2013; Neyens, 2014; Schulman, 2013). In one case study, after administration of 26 units/kg, an additional dose of 16 units/kg was administered for a concern of rebleeding (Dager, 2013). Others, including the European Heart Rhythm Association (EHRA), have recommended the use of 50 units/kg (EHRA [Heidbuchel, 2013];Weitz, 2012). Note: The use of anti-inhibitor coagulant complex (FEIBA, activated 4-factor PCC) may be associated with a higher risk of thrombosis compared to nonactivated PCCs especially with higher doses; monitor closely for arterial and venous thrombosis.

Pediatric Note: Anti-inhibitor coagulant complex (Human) contains mainly non-activated therapeutic levels of factors II, IX, and X and mainly *activated* factor VII

Control and prevention of bleeding episodes: Children and Adolescents: IV: **Note:** Considered a first-line treatment when factor VIII inhibitor titer is >5 Bethesda units (BU) (antihemophilic factor may be preferred when titer <5 BU)

General dosing guidelines: 50-100 units/kg per dose (maximum: 100 units/kg [single dose], 200 units/kg/day [total daily dose]). Dosage and duration of treatment depend on the location and extent of bleeding and clinical condition of the patient. If total single dose exceeds 100 units/kg or total daily dose exceeds 200 units/kg/day, monitor closely for DIC, coronary ischemia, and signs/symptoms of other thromboembolic events.

Joint hemorrhage: 50-100 units/kg every 12 hours until pain and acute disabilities are improved (maximum: 200 units/kg/day)

Mucous membrane bleeding: 50-100 units/kg every 6 hours for at least 1 day or until bleeding is resolved (maximum: 200 units/kg/day)

Soft tissue hemorrhage (eg, retroperitoneal bleed): 100 units/kg every 12 hours until resolution of bleed (maximum: 200 units/kg/day)

Other severe hemorrhage (eg, intracranial hemorrhage): 100 units/kg every 6-12 hours; continue until resolution of bleed (maximum: 200 units/kg/day).

Perioperative management:
Preoperative: 50-100 units/kg (single dose) administered immediately prior to surgery.
Postoperative: 50-100 units/kg every 6-12 hours until resolution of bleed and healing is achieved (maximum: 200 units/kg/day)

Routine prophylaxis: 85 units/kg every other day.

Renal Impairment No dosage adjustment provided in manufacturer's labeling.

Hepatic Impairment No dosage adjustment provided in manufacturer's labeling.

Additional Information Complete prescribing information should be consulted for additional detail.

Dosage Forms Considerations
FEIBA strengths expressed in terms of Factor VIII inhibitor bypassing activity with nominal strength values. Consult individual vial labels for exact potency within each vial.

Dosage Forms Excipient information presented when available (limited, particularly for generics); consult specific product labeling.
Solution Reconstituted, Intravenous [preservative free]:
FEIBA: 500 units (1 ea); 1000 units (1 ea); 2500 units (1 ea)

◆ Anti-Itch Maximum Strength [OTC] *see* Hydrocortisone (Topical) *on page 886*

◆ Anti-PD-1 Human Monoclonal Antibody MDX-1106 *see* Nivolumab *on page 1293*

◆ Anti-PD-1 Monoclonal Antibody MK-3475 *see* Pembrolizumab *on page 1414*

Antipyrine and Benzocaine
(an tee PYE reen & BEN zoe kane)

Brand Names: US Aurodex [DSC]
Brand Names: Canada Auralgan®
Index Terms Auralgan; Benzocaine and Antipyrine

Pharmacologic Category Otic Agent, Analgesic; Otic Agent, Cerumenolytic

Use Temporary relief of pain and reduction of swelling associated with acute congestive and serous otitis media; facilitates ear wax removal

Dosing
Adult & Geriatric
Pain and swelling associated with otitis media: Otic: Fill ear canal with solution; moisten cotton pledget with antipyrine and benzocaine solution, place in external ear, repeat every 1-2 hours until pain and congestion are relieved

Ear wax removal: Otic: Instill drops 3 times/day for 2-3 days; before and after ear wax removal, moisten cotton pledget with antipyrine and benzocaine solution and place in external ear after solution instillation.

Pediatric Refer to adult dosing.

Renal Impairment No dosage adjustment provided in manufacturer's labeling.

Hepatic Impairment No dosage adjustment provided in manufacturer's labeling.

Additional Information Complete prescribing information should be consulted for additional detail.

Dosage Forms Excipient information presented when available (limited, particularly for generics); consult specific product labeling. [DSC] = Discontinued product
Solution, otic [drops]:
Aurodex™: Antipyrine 5.4% and benzocaine 1.4% (10 mL [DSC])
Generic: Antipyrine 5.4% and benzocaine 1.4% (10 mL, 15 mL), Antipyrine 5.5% and benzocaine 1.4% (14 mL [DSC])

Antithrombin (an tee THROM bin)

Brand Names: US Thrombate III
Brand Names: Canada Antithrombin III NF; Thrombate III®
Index Terms Antithrombin Alfa; Antithrombin III; AT; AT-III; hpAT; rhAT; rhATIII
Pharmacologic Category Anticoagulant; Blood Product Derivative
Use
Treatment of antithrombin deficiency: Thrombate III: Antithrombin III (human) is indicated for the treatment of patients with hereditary antithrombin (AT) deficiency in connection with surgical or obstetrical procedures or when they suffer from thromboembolism.

Prevention of thromboembolic events: ATryn: Recombinant antithrombin is indicated for the prevention of perioperative and peripartum thromboembolic events in patients with hereditary antithrombin deficiency.

Limitations of use: ATryn is not indicated for treatment of thromboembolic events in patients with hereditary antithrombin deficiency.

Dosing
Adult & Geriatric Antithrombin deficiency: IV:
ATryn: Prophylaxis of thrombosis during perioperative and peripartum procedures:
Dosing is individualized based on pretherapy antithrombin (AT) activity levels. Therapy should begin before delivery or ~24 hours prior to surgery to obtain target AT activity levels. Dosing should be targeted to keep levels between 80% to 120% of normal. Loading dose should be given as a 15-minute infusion, followed by maintenance dose as a continuous infusion. Doses may be calculated based on the following formulas:
Surgical patients (nonpregnant):
Loading dose: [(100 - baseline AT activity level) **divided** by 2.3] x body weight (kg) = units of antithrombin required
Maintenance infusion: [(100 - baseline AT activity level) **divided** by 10.2] x body weight (kg) = units of antithrombin required/hour
Pregnant patients: Note: Pregnant women undergoing surgical procedures (other than a Cesarean section) should also be dosed according to the formula below.
Loading dose: [(100 - baseline AT activity level) **divided** by 1.3] x body weight (kg) = units of antithrombin required
Maintenance infusion: [(100 - baseline AT activity level) **divided** by 5.4] x body weight (kg) = units of antithrombin required/hour

Dosing adjustments: Adjustments should be made based on AT activity levels to maintain levels between 80% to 120% of normal. Surgery or delivery may rapidly decrease AT levels; check AT level just after surgery or delivery. The first AT level should be obtained 2 hours after initiation and adjusted as follows:

AT activity level <80%: Increase dose by 30%; recheck AT level 2 hours after adjustment. Alternatively, an additional bolus dose (using loading dose formula) may be needed to rapidly restore AT levels. Calculate the additional bolus/loading dose using the last available AT activity result. After additional loading/bolus dose given, resume maintenance infusion at the same rate prior to bolus administration.

AT activity level 80% to 120%: No dosage adjustment needed; recheck AT level in 6 hours

AT activity level >120%: Decrease dose by 30%; recheck AT level 2 hours after adjustment

Thrombate III: Prophylaxis of thrombosis during surgical or obstetrical procedures or treatment of thromboembolism:

Initial loading dose: Dosing is individualized based on pretherapy antithrombin (AT) levels. The initial dose should raise AT levels to 120% and may be calculated based on the following formula:

[(desired AT level % - baseline AT level %) x body weight (kg)] **divided** by 1.4 = units of antithrombin required

For example, if a 70 kg adult patient had a baseline AT level of 57%, the initial dose would be

[(120% - 57%) x 70] divided by 1.4 = 3150 units

Maintenance dose: In general, subsequent dosing should be targeted to keep levels between 80% to 120% which may be achieved by administering 60% of the initial loading dose every 24 hours. Adjustments may be made by adjusting dose or interval. Maintain level within normal range for 2-8 days depending on type of procedure/situation.

Renal Impairment There are no dosage adjustments provided in the manufacturer's labeling.

Hepatic Impairment There are no dosage adjustments provided in the manufacturer's labeling.

Additional Information Complete prescribing information should be consulted for additional detail.

Dosage Forms Excipient information presented when available (limited, particularly for generics); consult specific product labeling.

Solution Reconstituted, Intravenous:

Thrombate III: 500 units (1 ea); 1000 units (1 ea)

◆ Antithrombin III *see* Antithrombin *on page 135*

◆ Antithrombin III NF (Can) *see* Antithrombin *on page 135*

◆ Antithrombin Alfa *see* Antithrombin *on page 135*

Antithymocyte Globulin (Equine)
(an te THY moe site GLOB yu lin, E kwine)

Brand Names: US Atgam
Brand Names: Canada Atgam
Index Terms Anti-Thymocyte Globulin (Equine); Antithymocyte Immunoglobulin; ATG; Horse Antihuman Thymocyte Gamma Globulin; Lymphocyte Immune Globulin
Pharmacologic Category Immune Globulin; Immunosuppressant Agent; Polyclonal Antibody
Use

Aplastic anemia: Treatment of moderate-to-severe aplastic anemia in patients not considered suitable candidates for bone marrow transplantation

Limitations of use: The usefulness of antithymocyte globulin (equine) has not be demonstrated in patients with aplastic anemia who are suitable candidates for transplantation, or in aplastic anemia secondary to neoplastic disease, storage disease, myelofibrosis, Fanconi syndrome, or in patients with known prior treatment with myelotoxic agents or radiation therapy

Renal transplantation: Management of allograft rejection in renal transplantation (increases the frequency of resolution of acute rejection episode when administered with conventional therapy at the time of rejection)

Dosing

Adult Note: Test dose: A skin test is recommended prior to administration of the initial dose. Test initially with an epicutaneous prick of undiluted antithymocyte globulin (ATG); if no wheal in 10 minutes, then use 0.02 mL intradermally of a 1:1000 dilution of ATG in normal saline along with a separate saline control of 0.02 mL; observe in 10 minutes. A positive skin reaction consists of a wheal with the initial prick test (undiluted) or ≥3 mm in diameter

larger than the saline control with the diluted intradermal test. Alternatively, a 0.1 mL test dose (5 mg/mL concentration) may be administered intradermally along with a separate saline control; erythema larger than 5 mm in diameter (compared to the control) is considered a positive test (Molldrem, 2002). A positive skin test is suggestive of an increased risk for systemic allergic reactions with an infusion, although anaphylaxis may occur in patients who display negative skin tests. If ATG treatment is deemed appropriate following a positive skin test, the first infusion should be administered in a controlled environment with intensive life support immediately available. A systemic reaction precludes further administration.

Consider premedication with an antihistamine, corticosteroids, and/or an antipyretic. Concomitant immunosuppressants should also be administered.

Aplastic anemia: IV: 10 to 20 mg/kg once daily for 8 to 14 days, then if needed, may administer every other day for 7 more doses for a total of 21 doses in 28 days **or**

Off-label dosing: 40 mg/kg once daily for 4 days in combination with cyclosporine (Rosenfeld, 1995; Scheinberg, 2011)

Renal transplantation rejection (treatment): IV: 10 to 15 mg/kg once daily for 14 days, then if needed, may administer every other day for 7 more doses for a total of 21 doses in 28 days

Acute graft-versus-host disease (GVHD) treatment (off-label use): IV: 30 mg/kg every other day for 6 doses (MacMillan, 2007) **or** 15 mg/kg twice daily for 10 doses (MacMillan, 2002)

Myelodysplastic syndromes, refractory, lower-risk disease (off-label use): IV: 40 mg/kg once daily for 4 days; an intradermal test dose was administered prior to treatment (Molldrem, 2002)

Geriatric Refer to adult dosing. Begin at the lower end of dosing ranges.

Pediatric Note: See adult dosing for notes on intradermal skin testing and premedication.

Aplastic anemia: IV: 10 to 20 mg/kg once daily for 8 to 14 days; then if needed, may administer every other day for 7 more doses for a total of 21 doses in 28 days **or**

Off-label dosing (in combination with cyclosporine):
Children >10 kg and Adolescents: 40 mg/kg once daily for 4 days (Rosenfeld, 1995)
Children >2 years and Adolescents: 40 mg/kg once daily for 4 days (Scheinberg, 2011)

Renal transplantation rejection (treatment): IV: Rejection treatment: 10 to 15 mg/kg once daily for 14 days, then if needed, may administer every other day for 7 more doses for a total of 21 doses in 28 days

Acute graft-versus-host disease (GVHD) treatment (off-label use): IV: 30 mg/kg every other day for 6 doses (MacMillan, 2007) **or** 15 mg/kg twice daily for 10 doses (MacMillan, 2002)

Renal Impairment There are no dosage adjustments provided in the manufacturer's labeling.

Hepatic Impairment There are no dosage adjustments provided in the manufacturer's labeling.

Obesity *American Society for Blood and Marrow Transplantation (ASBMT) practice guideline committee position statement on chemotherapy dosing in obesity:* Utilize actual body weight (full weight) to calculate mg/kg dosing for hematopoietic stem cell transplant conditioning regimens (Bubalo, 2014).

Adjustment for Toxicity

Anaphylaxis: Discontinue infusion immediately; administer epinephrine. May require corticosteroids, respiration assistance, and/or other resuscitative measures. Do not resume infusion.

Hemolysis (severe and unremitting): May require discontinuation of treatment.

Leukopenia (severe and unremitting) in renal transplant patients: Discontinue treatment.

Thrombocytopenia (severe and unremitting) in renal transplant patients: Discontinue treatment.

Additional Information Complete prescribing information should be consulted for additional detail.

Dosage Forms Excipient information presented when available (limited, particularly for generics); consult specific product labeling.

Injectable, Intravenous:

Atgam: 50 mg/mL (5 mL) [thimerosal free]

◆ Anti-Thymocyte Globulin (Equine) *see* Antithymocyte Globulin (Equine) *on page 136*

Antithymocyte Globulin (Rabbit)
(an te THY moe site GLOB yu lin RAB bit)

Brand Names: US Thymoglobulin
Brand Names: Canada Thymoglobulin
Index Terms Antithymocyte Immunoglobulin; rATG
Pharmacologic Category Immune Globulin; Immunosuppressant Agent; Polyclonal Antibody
Use Renal transplant rejection: Treatment of acute renal transplant rejection (in conjunction with concomitant immunosuppression)

Dosing
Adult & Geriatric Note: Premedicate with corticosteroids, acetaminophen, and/or an antihistamine 1 hour prior to infusion to reduce the incidence and severity of infusion-related reactions. Antiviral prophylaxis is recommended.
   Renal transplant rejection, acute: IV: 1.5 mg/kg once daily for 7 to 14 days
Pediatric Refer to adult dosing.
Obesity *American Society for Blood and Marrow Transplantation (ASBMT) practice guideline committee position statement on chemotherapy dosing in obesity:* Utilize actual body weight (full weight) to calculate mg/kg dosing for hematopoietic stem cell transplant conditioning regimens (Bubalo 2014).
Adjustment for Toxicity
WBC count 2,000 to 3,000 cells/mm^3 or platelet count 50,000 to 75,000 cells/mm^3: Reduce dose by 50%.
WBC count <2,000 cells/mm^3 or platelet count <50,000 cells/mm^3: Consider discontinuing treatment.
Additional Information Complete prescribing information should be consulted for additional detail.
Dosage Forms Excipient information presented when available (limited, particularly for generics); consult specific product labeling.
Solution Reconstituted, Intravenous:
   Thymoglobulin: 25 mg (1 ea) [contains glycine, mannitol, sodium chloride]

- Antithymocyte Immunoglobulin *see* Antithymocyte Globulin (Equine) *on page 136*
- Antithymocyte Immunoglobulin *see* Antithymocyte Globulin (Rabbit) *on page 137*
- Antitumor Necrosis Factor Alpha (Human) *see* Adalimumab *on page 41*
- Anti-VEGF Monoclonal Antibody *see* Bevacizumab *on page 226*
- Anti-VEGF rhuMAb *see* Bevacizumab *on page 226*
- Antivenin *see* Crotalidae Immune F(ab')$_2$ (Equine) *on page 452*
- Antivenin (*Centruroides*) Immune F(ab')$_2$ (Equine) *see* Centruroides Immune F(ab')$_2$ (Equine) *on page 358*
- Antivenin (*Crotalidae*) Immune F(ab')2 (Equine) *see* Crotalidae Immune F(ab')$_2$ (Equine) *on page 452*
- Antivenin Scorpion *see* Centruroides Immune F(ab')$_2$ (Equine) *on page 358*
- Antivenom (*Centruroides*) Immune F(ab')$_2$ (Equine) *see* Centruroides Immune F(ab')$_2$ (Equine) *on page 358*
- Antivenom (*Crotalidae*) Immune F(ab')2 (Equine) *see* Crotalidae Immune F(ab')$_2$ (Equine) *on page 452*
- Antivenom Scorpion *see* Centruroides Immune F(ab')$_2$ (Equine) *on page 358*
- Antivert *see* Meclizine *on page 1131*
- Antivert [DSC] *see* Meclizine *on page 1131*
- Antizol *see* Fomepizole *on page 806*
- Anucort-HC *see* Hydrocortisone (Topical) *on page 886*
- Anusol-HC *see* Hydrocortisone (Topical) *on page 886*
- Anuzinc (Can) *see* Zinc Sulfate *on page 1929*
- Anzemet *see* Dolasetron *on page 581*
- 4-AP *see* Dalfampridine *on page 483*
- AP24534 *see* PONATinib *on page 1472*
- APAP (abbreviation is not recommended) *see* Acetaminophen *on page 25*
- APC8015 *see* Sipuleucel-T *on page 1662*
- aPCC *see* Anti-inhibitor Coagulant Complex (Human) *on page 134*
- ApexiCon *see* Diflorasone *on page 546*
- ApexiCon E *see* Diflorasone *on page 546*
- Apidra *see* Insulin Glulisine *on page 957*
- Apidra® (Can) *see* Insulin Glulisine *on page 957*
- Apidra SoloStar *see* Insulin Glulisine *on page 957*

Apixaban (a PIX a ban)

Brand Names: US Eliquis
Brand Names: Canada Eliquis
Pharmacologic Category Anticoagulant; Anticoagulant, Factor Xa Inhibitor
Additional Appendix Information
Oral Anticoagulant Comparison Chart *on page 1957*
Reversal of Oral Anticoagulants *on page 1959*
Use
Deep vein thrombosis: Treatment of deep vein thrombosis; to reduce the risk of recurrent deep vein thrombosis following initial therapy
Nonvalvular atrial fibrillation: To reduce the risk of stroke and systemic embolism in patients with nonvalvular atrial fibrillation (AF)
   Note: The 2014 American Heart Association/American College of Cardiology/Heart Rhythm Society guidelines for the management of AF recommend oral anticoagulation for patients with nonvalvular AF or atrial flutter with prior stroke, TIA, or a CHA$_2$DS$_2$-VASc score ≥2. As an alternative to warfarin, apixaban may also be used for 3 weeks prior and 4 weeks after cardioversion in patients with AF or atrial flutter of ≥48 hours duration or when the duration is unknown (January, 2014)
Postoperative venous thromboprophylaxis following hip or knee replacement surgery: Prophylaxis of deep vein thrombosis, which may lead to pulmonary embolism, in patients who have undergone hip or knee replacement surgery
Pulmonary embolism: Treatment of pulmonary embolism; to reduce the risk of recurrent pulmonary embolism following initial therapy
Pregnancy Considerations Adverse events were not observed in animal reproduction studies. Data are insufficient to evaluate the safety of oral factor Xa inhibitors during pregnancy; use during pregnancy should be avoided (Bates, 2012).
Breast-Feeding Considerations It is not known if apixaban is excreted in breast milk. Apixaban is not recommended for use in breast-feeding women; use of alternative anticoagulants is preferred (Bates, 2012)
Medication Guide Available Yes
Contraindications
U.S. labeling: Severe hypersensitivity reaction (ie, anaphylaxis) to apixaban or any component of the formulation; active pathological bleeding

Canadian labeling: Hypersensitivity to apixaban or any component of the formulation; clinically-significant active bleeding (including gastrointestinal bleeding); lesions or conditions at increased risk of clinically-significant bleeding (eg, cerebral infarct [ischemic or hemorrhagic], active peptic ulcer disease with recent bleeding; patients with spontaneous or acquired impairment of hemostasis); hepatic disease associated with coagulopathy and clinically-relevant bleeding risk; concomitant systemic treatment with agents that are strong inhibitors of both CYP3A4 and P-glycoprotein (P-gp); concomitant treatment with any other anticoagulant including unfractionated heparin (except at doses used to maintain patency of central venous or arterial catheter), low molecular weight heparins, heparin derivatives (eg, fondaparinux), and oral anticoagulants including warfarin, dabigatran, rivaroxaban except when transitioning to or from apixaban therapy
Warnings/Precautions [U.S. Boxed Warning]: Premature discontinuation of any oral anticoagulant, including apixaban, in the absence of adequate alternative anticoagulation increases the risk of thrombotic events. When used to prevent stroke in patients with nonvalvular atrial fibrillation, an increased risk of stroke was observed upon transition from apixaban to warfarin in clinical trials. If apixaban must be discontinued for reasons other than bleeding or completion of a course of therapy, consider the use of another anticoagulant to prevent stroke from occurring.

May increase the risk of bleeding; serious, potentially fatal bleeding may occur. Concomitant use of drugs that affect hemostasis increases the risk of bleeding. Monitor for signs and symptoms of bleeding. Discontinue therapy with active pathological hemorrhage and promptly evaluate for bleeding source. No specific antidote exists for apixaban reversal; hemodialysis does not appear to have a substantial impact on apixaban exposure. Although not evaluated in clinical trials, in the event of apixaban-related hemorrhage, the use of prothrombin complex concentrate (PCC), activated prothrombin complex concentrate, or recombinant factor VIIa may be considered. In vitro, PCC and aPCC seemed to be more efficient in restoring generation of thrombin, while rFVIIa was the quickest to produce a compact blood clot and most effective in studies

with blood circulating through a damaged blood vessel. These lab tests indicate that these agents may reverse the effects of apixaban, but more studies are needed to determine their clinical impact (Escolar, 2012). The use of activated oral charcoal may be considered if ingestion occurred within 2 to 6 hours of presentation.

[U.S. Boxed Warning]: Spinal or epidural hematomas resulting in long-term or permanent paralysis may occur with neuraxial anesthesia (epidural or spinal anesthesia) or spinal/epidural puncture; the risk is increased by the use of indwelling epidural catheters, with concomitant administration of other drugs that affect hemostasis (eg, NSAIDS, platelet inhibitors, other anticoagulants), in patients with a history of traumatic or repeated epidural or spinal punctures, a history of spinal deformity or surgery, or if optimal timing between the administration of apixaban and neuraxial procedures is not known. Consider the potential benefit versus risk prior to neuraxial intervention in patients who are anticoagulated or scheduled to be anticoagulated for thromboprophylaxis. In patients who receive both apixaban and neuraxial anesthesia, avoid removal of epidural or intrathecal catheter for at least 24 hours following last apixaban dose; avoid apixaban administration for at least 5 hours following catheter removal. If traumatic puncture occurs, delay administration of apixaban for at least 48 hours. **Monitor frequently for signs of neurologic impairment (eg, numbness/weakness of legs, bowel/bladder dysfunction). If neurologic impairment is noted, prompt treatment is necessary.**

In hemodynamically unstable patients with acute PE or patients with PE requiring thrombolysis or pulmonary embolectomy, the use of apixaban is not recommended as an alternative to unfractionated heparin for initial treatment. In a clinical trial of high-risk, post-acute coronary syndrome (ACS) patients (off-label use), use of apixaban in addition to standard antiplatelet therapy increased the incidence of major bleeding (including intracranial and fatal bleeding) without any significant clinical benefit (Alexander, 2011). In acutely ill patients (eg, heart failure, respiratory failure) at risk for venous thromboembolism (VTE) receiving apixaban for extended VTE prophylaxis, an increased incidence of major bleeding without greater efficacy was observed with extended apixaban therapy (eg, 30 days) versus low molecular weight heparin (enoxaparin) therapy for 1 to 2 weeks (Goldhaber, 2011). Canadian labeling: Use in patients undergoing hip fracture surgery has not been studied; avoid use in these patients.

Use with caution in moderate impairment (Child-Pugh class B) as there is limited clinical experience in these patients; dosing recommendations cannot be provided. Use in severe hepatic impairment (Child-Pugh class C) is not recommended. Systemic exposure increases with worsening renal function. Bleeding risk may be increased in severe renal impairment (CrCl <15 to 29 mL/minute); use with caution. Patients with significant renal impairment (eg, CrCl <30 mL/minute) were excluded from clinical trials. Patients with ESRD with or without hemodialysis have not been studied. Dosage reduction is recommended for patients with nonvalvular atrial fibrillation with a serum creatinine ≥1.5 mg/dL **and** are *either* ≥80 years of age or weigh ≤60 kg. Compared to warfarin, apixaban has been shown to be associated with less major bleeding among all ranges of estimated GFRs as determined by initial serum creatinine; however, patients with a serum creatinine >2.5 mg/dL or CrCl <25 mL/minute (as determined by Cockcroft-Gault equation) were excluded from the analysis (Hohnloser, 2012). Safety and efficacy have not been established in patients with prosthetic heart valves or significant rheumatic heart disease (eg, mitral stenosis); use is not recommended. Non-valvular atrial fibrillation is defined as atrial fibrillation that occurs in the absence of rheumatic mitral valve disease, mitral valve repair, or prosthetic heart valve (AHA/ACC/HRS [January, 2014]).

Potentially significant drug-drug interactions may exist, requiring dose or frequency adjustment, additional monitoring, and/or selection of alternative therapy. Systemic exposure is increased ~32% in patients >65 years of age and may be increased by 20% to 30% in patients <50 kg and decreased by 20% to 30% in patients >120 kg; dosage reduction is recommended for patients with nonvalvular atrial fibrillation with any 2 of the following: ≥80 years of age, weight ≤60 kg, or serum creatinine ≥1.5 mg/dL

Discontinue apixaban at least 24 to 48 hours prior to elective surgery or invasive procedures depending on risk or location of bleeding.

Adverse Reactions

>10%: Hematologic & oncologic: Hemorrhage (1% to 12%; major: ≤3%; clinically relevant nonmajor bleeding: 2% to 4%)

1% to 10%:
Endocrine & metabolic: Increased gamma-glutamyl transferase (≤1%)
Gastrointestinal: Nausea (3%), gingival hemorrhage (≤1%)
Genitourinary: Hematuria (≤2%), hypermenorrhea (1%)
Hematologic & oncologic: Anemia (3%), bruise (1% to 2%), hematoma (1% to 2%), postprocedural hemorrhage (≤1%), rectal hemorrhage (≤1%)
Hepatic: Increased serum transaminases (≤1%)
Respiratory: Epistaxis (≤4%), hemoptysis (1%)

<1%, postmarketing, and/or case reports: Abnormal uterine bleeding, acute posthemorrhagic anemia, anal hemorrhage, anaphylaxis, conjunctival hemorrhage, gastrointestinal hemorrhage, genital bleeding, hematoma at injection site, hemophthalmos, hemorrhoidal bleeding, hypersensitivity, hypotension, incision site hemorrhage, increased serum alkaline phosphatase, increased serum AST, increased serum bilirubin, intracranial hemorrhage, muscle hemorrhage, occult blood in urine, perioperative blood loss, periorbital hematoma, petechia, postoperative hematoma (incision site), postprocedural hemorrhage, puncture site bleeding, retinal hemorrhage, syncope, thrombocytopenia, traumatic hematoma, vaginal hemorrhage, wound hemorrhage, wound secretion

Drug Interactions

Metabolism/Transport Effects Substrate of BCRP, CYP1A2 (minor), CYP2C19 (minor), CYP2C8 (minor), CYP2C9 (minor), CYP3A4 (major), P-glycoprotein; **Note:** Assignment of Major/Minor substrate status based on clinically relevant drug interaction potential; **Inhibits** CYP2C19 (weak)

Avoid Concomitant Use
Avoid concomitant use of Apixaban with any of the following: Anticoagulants; CYP3A4 Inducers (Strong); Dabigatran Etexilate; Edoxaban; Hemin; Omacetaxine; Rivaroxaban; St Johns Wort; Urokinase; Vorapaxar

Increased Effect/Toxicity
Apixaban may increase the levels/effects of: Anticoagulants; Collagenase (Systemic); Deferasirox; Deoxycholic Acid; Ibritumomab; Nintedanib; Obinutuzumab; Omacetaxine; Rivaroxaban; Tositumomab and Iodine I 131 Tositumomab

The levels/effects of Apixaban may be increased by: Agents with Antiplatelet Properties; Antiplatelet Agents (P2Y12 Inhibitors); Aspirin; CYP3A4 Inhibitors (Moderate); CYP3A4 Inhibitors (Strong); Dabigatran Etexilate; Dasatinib; Edoxaban; Fusidic Acid (Systemic); Hemin; Herbs (Anticoagulant/Antiplatelet Properties); Ibrutinib; Inhibitors of CYP3A4 (Strong) and P-glycoprotein; Limaprost; Naproxen; Nonsteroidal Anti-Inflammatory Agents; NSAID (Nonselective); Omega-3 Fatty Acids; Osimertinib; Pentosan Polysulfate Sodium; Prostacyclin Analogues; Salicylates; Sugammadex; Thrombolytic Agents; Tibolone; Tipranavir; Urokinase; Vitamin E; Vitamin E (Oral); Vorapaxar

Decreased Effect
Apixaban may decrease the levels/effects of: Factor X (Human)

The levels/effects of Apixaban may be decreased by: Bosentan; CYP3A4 Inducers (Moderate); CYP3A4 Inducers (Strong); Dabrafenib; Deferasirox; Estrogen Derivatives; Osimertinib; Progestins; Siltuximab; St Johns Wort; Tocilizumab

Food Interactions Grapefruit juice may increase levels/effects of apixaban. Management: Advise patients who consume grapefruit juice during therapy to use caution; monitor for increased effects (eg, bleeding).

Storage/Stability Store at 20°C to 25°C (68°F to 77°F); excursions are permitted between 15°C and 30°C (59°F and 86°F).

Mechanism of Action Inhibits platelet activation and fibrin clot formation via direct, selective and reversible inhibition of free and clot-bound factor Xa (FXa). FXa, as part of the prothrombinase complex consisting also of factor Va, calcium ions, and phospholipid, catalyzes the conversion of prothrombin to thrombin. Thrombin both activates platelets and catalyzes the conversion of fibrinogen to fibrin.

Pharmacodynamics/Kinetics
Onset: 3 to 4 hours
Distribution: V_{ss}: ~21 L
Protein binding: ~87%
Metabolism: Hepatic predominantly via CYP3A4/5 and to a lesser extent via CYP1A2, 2C8, 2C9, 2C19, and 2J2 to inactive metabolites; substrate of P-glycoprotein (P-gp) and breast cancer resistant protein (BCRP)
Bioavailability: ~50%

Half-life elimination: ~12 hours

Time to peak: 3 to 4 hours

Excretion: Urine (~27% as parent drug); feces

Dosing

Adult

Deep venous thrombosis: Oral:

Treatment: 10 mg twice daily for 7 days followed by 5 mg twice daily

Reduction in the risk of recurrence: 2.5 mg twice daily after at least 6 months of treatment for DVT

Nonvalvular atrial fibrillation (to prevent stroke and systemic embolism): Oral: 5 mg twice daily **unless** patient has any 2 of the following: Age ≥80 years, body weight ≤60 kg, or serum creatinine ≥1.5 mg/dL, then reduce dose to 2.5 mg twice daily.

Postoperative venous thromboprophylaxis: Oral:

Hip replacement surgery: 2.5 mg twice daily beginning 12 to 24 hours postoperatively; duration: 35 days

Knee replacement surgery: 2.5 mg twice daily beginning 12 to 24 hours postoperatively; duration: 12 days

Pulmonary embolism (PE): Oral:

Treatment: 10 mg twice daily for 7 days followed by 5 mg twice daily

Reduction in the risk of recurrence: 2.5 mg twice daily after at least 6 months of treatment for PE

Conversion:

Conversion from warfarin to apixaban: Discontinue warfarin and initiate apixaban when INR is <2

Conversion from apixaban to warfarin: **Note:** Apixaban affects the INR; measuring the INR during coadministration with warfarin therapy may not be useful for determining an appropriate dose of warfarin

U.S. labeling: If continuous anticoagulation is necessary, discontinue apixaban and begin both a parenteral anticoagulant with warfarin when the next dose of apixaban is due; discontinue parenteral anticoagulant when INR reaches an acceptable range

Canadian labeling: Initiate warfarin or other vitamin K antagonist (VKA) at usual starting doses and continue apixaban until INR ≥2, then discontinue apixaban. During concomitant therapy, manufacturer recommends initiating INR testing on day 3 and just prior to each dose of apixaban.

Conversion from apixaban to other non-warfarin anticoagulants (oral or parenteral): Discontinue apixaban and begin taking the new non-warfarin anticoagulant at the usual time of the next scheduled dose of apixaban.

Conversion from other non-warfarin anticoagulants (oral or parenteral) to apixaban: Discontinue the other non-warfarin anticoagulant and begin taking apixaban at the usual time of the next scheduled dose of the other non-warfarin anticoagulant.

Dosage adjustment of apixaban with concomitant medications:

U.S. labeling: For patients receiving dual strong CYP3A4 and P-glycoprotein inhibitors (eg, clarithromycin, ketoconazole, itraconazole, ritonavir) and apixaban doses >2.5 mg twice daily, reduce apixaban dose by 50%. **Note:** Avoid concomitant use with dual strong CYP3A4 and P-glycoprotein inhibitors if patient is already taking apixaban 2.5 mg twice daily or patient meets 2 of the following criteria: Age ≥80 years, body weight ≤60 kg, or serum creatinine ≥1.5 mg/dL.

Canadian labeling: Dual CYP3A4 and P-glycoprotein inhibitors: No dosage adjustment necessary for moderate dual inhibitors. Use is contraindicated with strong dual inhibitors.

Geriatric Refer to adult dosing. Nonvalvular atrial fibrillation (to prevent stroke and systemic embolism): If patient is ≥80 years of age **and** *either* weighs ≤60 kg or has a serum creatinine ≥1.5 mg/dL, then reduce dose to 2.5 mg twice daily.

Renal Impairment

U.S. labeling:

Deep vein thrombosis (DVT), pulmonary embolism (PE), reduction in the risk of recurrent DVT and PE: No dosage adjustment is recommended by the manufacturer. However, it should be noted that patients with a serum creatinine >2.5 mg/dL or CrCl <25 mL/minute (as determined by Cockcroft-Gault equation) were excluded from the clinical trials (Agnelli, 2013a; Agnelli, 2013b).

Nonvalvular atrial fibrillation (to prevent stroke and systemic embolism):

Serum creatinine <1.5 mg/dL: No dosage adjustment necessary *unless* age ≥80 years **and** body weight ≤60 kg, then reduce dose to 2.5 mg twice daily (also refer to adult dosing).

Serum creatinine ≥1.5 mg/dL **and** *either* age ≥80 years **or** body weight ≤60 kg: 2.5 mg twice daily. **Note:** Patients with a serum creatinine >2.5 mg/dL or CrCl <25 mL/minute (as determined by Cockcroft-Gault equation) were excluded from clinical trials (Connolly, 2011; Granger, 2011). In patients with severe or end-stage chronic kidney disease, warfarin remains the anticoagulant of choice (AHA/ACC/HRS [January, 2014]).

ESRD requiring hemodialysis: 5 mg twice daily; reduce to 2.5 mg twice daily if age ≥80 years or body weight ≤60 kg. **Note:** This recommendation is made solely on a single dose pharmacokinetic and pharmacodynamic (anti-Xa activity) study. Clinical efficacy and long-term safety studies have not been done in this population; therefore, use with caution. In patients with severe or end-stage chronic kidney disease, warfarin remains the anticoagulant of choice (AHA/ACC/HRS [January, 2014]).

Postoperative (hip or knee replacement) venous thromboprophylaxis: No dosage adjustment is recommended by the manufacturer. However, it should be noted that patients with either clinically significant renal impairment (ADVANCE-1 [Lassen, 2009]), impaired renal function (ADVANCE-2 [Lassen, 2010b]), or CrCl <30 mL/minute (as determined by Cockcroft-Gault equation) (ADVANCE-3 [Lassen, 2010a]) were excluded from the respective clinical trials.

Canadian labeling: **Note:** Estimated creatinine clearance (eCrCl) may be calculated using Cockcroft-Gault equation.

Nonvalvular atrial fibrillation (to prevent stroke and systemic embolism):

eCrCl ≥25 mL/minute: No dosage adjustment necessary. Patients with serum creatinine ≥1.5 mg/dL (SI: ≥133 micromole/L) **and** *either* age ≥80 years **or** body weight ≤60 kg: 2.5 mg twice daily

eCrCl 15 to 24 mL/minute: There are no dosage adjustments provided in manufacturer's labeling (very limited data).

eCrCl <15 mL/minute: Use is not recommended.

Dialysis: Use is not recommended.

Postoperative (hip or knee replacement) venous thromboprophylaxis, deep vein thrombosis (DVT), pulmonary embolism (PE), reduction in the risk of recurrent DVT and PE:

eCrCl ≥30 mL/minute): No dosage adjustment required.

eCrCl 15 to 29 mL/minute: There are no dosage adjustments provided in manufacturer's labeling; use with caution as bleeding risk may be increased.

eCrCl <15 mL/minute: Use is not recommended.

Dialysis: Use is not recommended.

Hepatic Impairment

U.S. labeling:

Mild impairment (Child-Pugh class A): No dosage adjustment required.

Moderate impairment (Child-Pugh class B): There are no dosage adjustments provided in manufacturer's labeling; use with caution (limited clinical experience in these patients).

Severe impairment (Child-Pugh class C): Use is not recommended.

Canadian labeling:

Mild or moderate impairment (Child-Pugh class A or B): No dosage adjustment required; use with caution.

Severe impairment (Child-Pugh class C): Use is not recommended.

Note: Use is contraindicated in patients with hepatic disease associated with coagulopathy and clinically-relevant bleeding risk.

Administration Administer without regard to meals. After hip/knee replacement, initial dose should be administered 12 to 24 hours postoperatively. If patient unable to swallow whole tablets, may crush 5 mg or 2.5 mg tablets and suspend in 60 mL of D_5W followed by immediate delivery through a nasogastric tube. No information regarding administration of suspension by mouth is available.

Monitoring Parameters Renal function prior to initiation, when clinically indicated, and at least annually in all patients (AHA/ACC/HRS [January, 2014]), hepatic function; signs of bleeding. Routine monitoring of coagulation tests is not required. Although not recommended to assess effectiveness, the prothrombin time (PT), INR, and aPTT are prolonged with apixaban. Anti-FXa assay may be helpful (plasma concentrations and anti-FXa activity exhibit linear relationship) in guiding clinical decisions.

When converting from apixaban to a vitamin K antagonist (VKA), Canadian labeling recommends INR testing just prior to each dose of apixaban beginning on day 3 of concurrent therapy with the VKA.

Dosage Forms Excipient information presented when available (limited, particularly for generics); consult specific product labeling.
Tablet, Oral:
  Eliquis: 2.5 mg, 5 mg

Apraclonidine (a pra KLOE ni deen)

Brand Names: US Iopidine
Brand Names: Canada Iopidine
Index Terms Aplonidine; Apraclonidine Hydrochloride; p-Aminoclonidine
Pharmacologic Category Alpha$_2$ Agonist, Ophthalmic
Use
  0.5% solution: Short-term, adjunctive therapy in patients who require additional reduction of IOP
  1% solution: Prevention and treatment of postsurgical intraocular pressure (IOP) elevation following argon laser trabeculoplasty, argon laser iridotomy or Nd:YAG posterior capsulotomy
Dosing
Adult & Geriatric
  Intraocular pressure reduction: Ophthalmic:
    0.5%: Instill 1 to 2 drops in the affected eye(s) 3 times daily
    1%: Instill 1 drop in operative eye 1 hour prior to anterior segment laser surgery, second drop in same eye immediately upon completion of procedure
  Renal Impairment There are no dosage adjustments provided in the manufacturer's labeling; monitor cardiovascular parameters closely.
  Hepatic Impairment There are no dosage adjustments provided in the manufacturer's labeling; monitor cardiovascular parameters closely.
Additional Information Complete prescribing information should be consulted for additional detail.
Dosage Forms Excipient information presented when available (limited, particularly for generics); consult specific product labeling.
  Solution, Ophthalmic:
    Iopidine: 0.5% (5 mL, 10 mL); 1% (1 ea) [contains benzalkonium chloride]
    Generic: 0.5% (5 mL, 10 mL)

- Apraclonidine Hydrochloride *see* Apraclonidine on page 142

Apremilast (a PRE mi last)

Brand Names: US Otezla
Brand Names: Canada Otezla
Index Terms CC-10004
Pharmacologic Category Phosphodiesterase-4 Enzyme Inhibitor
Use
  Psoriasis: Treatment of patients with moderate to severe plaque psoriasis who are candidates for phototherapy or systemic therapy

Psoriatic arthritis: Treatment of adult patients with active psoriatic arthritis (PsA)

Pregnancy Considerations Adverse events were observed in some animal reproduction studies. A registry is available for women exposed to apremilast during pregnancy (877-311-8972). The Canadian labeling contraindicates use during pregnancy and recommends women attempting to conceive avoid use.

Breast-Feeding Considerations It is not known if apremilast is excreted into breast milk. The U.S. labeling recommends that caution be used if administered to a nursing woman. The Canadian labeling contraindicates use in nursing women.

Contraindications

Hypersensitivity to apremilast or any component of the formulation

Canadian labeling: Additional contraindications (not in US labeling): Pregnancy; breast-feeding

Warnings/Precautions Use caution in patients with latent infections such as tuberculosis, viral hepatitis, herpes viral infection and herpes zoster (limited experience). Use in patients with severe immunological diseases, severe acute infectious diseases, or psoriasis patients treated with immunosuppressive therapy has not been evaluated. May cause weight loss; monitor weight regularly. Discontinuation of therapy should be considered with unexplained or significant weight loss. Neuropsychiatric effects (eg, depression, suicidal ideation, mood changes) have been reported. Use with caution in patients with a history of depression and/or suicidal thoughts/behavior. Instruct patients/caregivers to report worsening psychiatric symptoms and consider risks/benefits of continuation of therapy in such patients. Use with caution in renal impairment. Systemic exposure is increased in patients with severe renal impairment (CrCl <30 mL/minute); dosage reduction is recommended. Potentially significant drug-drug interactions may exist, requiring dose or frequency adjustment, additional monitoring, and/or selection of alternative therapy.

Adverse Reactions

Frequency not always defined.

Central nervous system: Tension headache (7%), headache (6%), fatigue (3%), depression (2%), insomnia (2%), migraine (2%), paresthesia (<2%)

Dermatologic: Skin rash (<2%), folliculitis (1%)

Endocrine & metabolic: Weight loss (≥5% of body weight: 19%; ≥10% of body weight: 6%)

Gastrointestinal: Diarrhea (18%), nausea (17%), vomiting (4%), decreased appetite (3%), dyspepsia (3%), abdominal distress (2%), abdominal pain (2%), frequent bowel movements (2%), upper abdominal pain (2%), abdominal distention (<2%), gastroesophageal reflux disease (<2%)

Hypersensitivity: Hypersensitivity (<2%)

Infection: Influenza (<2%), tooth abscess (1%)

Neuromuscular & skeletal: Back pain (2%), arthralgia (<2%), muscle spasm (<2%), myalgia (<2%)

Respiratory: Upper respiratory tract infection (8%), nasopharyngitis (7%), sinusitis (2%), bronchitis (<2%), cough (<2%), pharyngitis (<2%), rhinitis (<2%), sinus headache (<2%)

<1% (Limited to important and life-threatening): Atrial fibrillation, exacerbation of psoriasis (rebound following discontinuation), tachyarrhythmia

Drug Interactions

Metabolism/Transport Effects Substrate of CYP3A4 (major), P-glycoprotein; **Note:** Assignment of Major/Minor substrate status based on clinically relevant drug interaction potential

Avoid Concomitant Use

Avoid concomitant use of Apremilast with any of the following: CYP3A4 Inducers (Strong)

Increased Effect/Toxicity

Apremilast may increase the levels/effects of: Riociguat

The levels/effects of Apremilast may be increased by: Osimertinib

Decreased Effect

The levels/effects of Apremilast may be decreased by: Bosentan; CYP3A4 Inducers (Moderate); CYP3A4 Inducers (Strong); Dabrafenib; Deferasirox; Osimertinib; Siltuximab; St Johns Wort; Tocilizumab

Storage/Stability Store below 30°C (86°F).

Mechanism of Action Apremilast inhibits phosphodiesterase 4 (PDE4) specific for cyclic adenosine monophosphate (cAMP) which results in increased intracellular cAMP levels and regulation of numerous inflammatory mediators (eg, decreased expression of nitric oxide synthase, TNF-α, and interleukin [IL]-23, as well as increased IL-10) (Schafer, 2012).

Pharmacodynamics/Kinetics

Absorption: Well absorbed

Distribution: V_d: 87 L

Protein binding: ~68%

Metabolism: Hepatic, primarily via CYP3A4; minor pathways include CYP1A2 and CYP2A6

Bioavailability: ~73%

Half-life elimination: ~6 to 9 hours

Time to peak: ~2.5 hours

Excretion: Urine (58%; 3% unchanged drug); feces (39%; 7% unchanged drug)

Dosing

Adult & Geriatric Active psoriatic arthritis or plaque psoriasis (moderate to severe): Oral: Initial: 10 mg in the morning. Titrate upward by additional 10 mg per day on days 2 to 5 as follows: Day 2: 10 mg twice daily; Day 3: 10 mg in the morning and 20 mg in the evening; Day 4: 20 mg twice daily; Day 5: 20 mg in the morning and 30 mg in the evening. Maintenance dose: 30 mg twice daily starting on day 6

Renal Impairment CrCl <30 mL/minute: Initial: 10 mg in the morning on days 1 to 3; titrate using morning doses only (skip evening doses) to 20 mg on days 4 and 5. Maintenance dose: 30 mg once daily in the morning starting on day 6.

Hepatic Impairment No dosage adjustment necessary.

Administration Oral: Administer without regard to food. Do not crush, chew, or split tablets.

Monitoring Parameters Monitor weight regularly during therapy; renal function; signs or symptoms of mood changes, depression, or suicidal thoughts

Dosage Forms Excipient information presented when available (limited, particularly for generics); consult specific product labeling.

Tablet, Oral:

Otezla: 30 mg

Tablet Therapy Pack, Oral:

Otezla: 10 & 20 & 30 MG (55 ea); 10 & 20 & 30 mg (27 ea)

Aprepitant (ap RE pi tant)

Brand Names: US Emend

Brand Names: Canada Emend

Index Terms L 754030; MK 869

Pharmacologic Category Antiemetic; Substance P/Neurokinin 1 Receptor Antagonist

Use

Chemotherapy-induced nausea and vomiting: Prevention of acute and delayed nausea and vomiting associated with moderately- and highly-emetogenic chemotherapy (in combination with other antiemetics) in patients ≥12 years and patients <12 years who weigh at least 30 kg.

Postoperative nausea and vomiting: Prevention of postoperative nausea and vomiting (PONV) in adults.

Limitations of use: Aprepitant has not been studied for the management of existing nausea and vomiting. Chronic, continuous administration is not recommended (chronic use may alter aprepitant's drug interaction profile).

Pregnancy Considerations Adverse events were not observed in animal reproduction studies. Efficacy of hormonal contraceptive may be reduced during and for 28 days following the last aprepitant dose; alternative or additional methods of contraception should be used both during treatment with fosaprepitant or aprepitant and for at least 1 month following the last fosaprepitant/aprepitant dose.

Breast-Feeding Considerations It is not known if aprepitant is excreted in breast milk. According to the manufacturer, the decision to breast-feed during therapy should take into account the risk of exposure to the infant and the benefits of treatment to the mother.

Contraindications Hypersensitivity to aprepitant or any component of the formulation; concurrent use with pimozide

Warnings/Precautions Potentially significant drug-drug interactions may exist, requiring dose or frequency adjustment, additional monitoring, and/or selection of alternative therapy. Use caution with severe hepatic impairment (Child-Pugh class C); has not been studied. Due to a risk of significantly increased pimozide plasma concentrations and potential for QT prolongation, concurrent use with pimozide is contraindicated. Other CYP3A4-mediated drug interactions may occur. In patients receiving concurrent warfarin, a clinically significant decrease in INR or prothrombin time (PT) may occur; monitor INR/PT for 2 weeks (particularly at 7 to 10 days) following aprepitant administration. Hypersensitivity reactions, including anaphylactic reactions have been reported. Pediatric patients should be at least 30 kg and be able to swallow capsules whole. Not approved for prevention of postoperative nausea and vomiting in children.

Adverse Reactions Adverse reactions may be reported in combination with other antiemetic agents. As reported for highly emetogenic cancer chemotherapy or moderately emetogenic cancer chemotherapy, unless otherwise noted as reported for postoperative nausea and vomiting (PONV).

>10%:

Central nervous system: Fatigue (adults: 13%; children & adolescents: 5%)

Hematologic & oncologic: Neutropenia (children & adolescents: 13%; adults: <3%)

0.5% to 10%:

Cardiovascular: Hypotension (PONV: 6%), bradycardia (PONV: <3%), flushing (<3%), palpitations (<3%), peripheral edema (<3%), syncope (PONV: <3%)

Central nervous system: Headache (children & adolescents: 9%), dizziness (<3% to 5%), anxiety (<3%), hypoesthesia (PONV: <3%), hypothermia (PONV: <3%), malaise (<3%), peripheral neuropathy (<3%)

Dermatologic: Alopecia (<3%), hyperhidrosis (<3%), skin rash (<3%), urticaria (<3%)

Endocrine & metabolic: Dehydration (≤3%), decreased serum albumin (PONV: <3%), decreased serum potassium (PONV: <3%), decreased serum sodium (<3%), hot flash (<3), hypokalemia (<3%), hypovolemia (PONV: <3%), increased serum glucose (PONV: <3%), weight loss (<3%)

Gastrointestinal: Constipation (PONV: 9%), diarrhea (6% to 9%), dyspepsia (≤7%), abdominal pain (≤6%), hiccups (4% to 5%), decreased appetite (<3% to 5%), dysgeusia (<3%), eructation (<3%), flatulence (<3%), gastritis (<3%), gastroesophageal reflux disease (<3%), nausea (<3%), vomiting (<3%), xerostomia (<3%)

Genitourinary: Proteinuria (<3%)

Hematologic & oncologic: Decreased hemoglobin (children & adolescents: 5%), decreased white blood cell count (≤4%), anemia (<3%), febrile neutropenia (<3%), hematoma (PONV: <3%), thrombocytopenia (<3%)

Hepatic: Increased serum ALT (3%), increased serum alkaline phosphatase (<3%), increased serum AST (<3%), increased serum bilirubin (PONV: <3%)

Infection: Candidiasis (<3%), postoperative infection (PONV: <3%)

Neuromuscular & skeletal: Weakness (≤7%), musculoskeletal pain (<3%)

Renal: Increased blood urea nitrogen (<3%)

Respiratory: Cough (<3% to 5%), dyspnea (<3%), hypoxia (PONV: <3%), oropharyngeal pain (<3%), pharyngitis (<3%), respiratory depression (PONV: <3%)

Miscellaneous: Wound dehiscence (PONV: <3%)

<0.5% (Limited to important or life-threatening): Anaphylaxis, angioedema, hypersensitivity reaction, pruritus, Stevens-Johnson syndrome, toxic epidermal necrolysis

Drug Interactions

Metabolism/Transport Effects Substrate of CYP1A2 (minor), CYP2C19 (minor), CYP3A4 (major); **Note:** Assignment of Major/Minor substrate status based on clinically relevant drug interaction potential; **Inhibits** CYP2C19 (weak), CYP2C9 (weak), CYP3A4 (moderate); **Induces** CYP2C9 (strong)

Avoid Concomitant Use

Avoid concomitant use of Aprepitant with any of the following: Bosutinib; Cisapride; Cobimetinib; Conivaptan; CYP3A4 Inducers (Strong); CYP3A4 Inhibitors (Moderate); CYP3A4 Inhibitors (Strong); Domperidone; Flibanserin; Fusidic Acid (Systemic); Ibrutinib; Idelalisib; Ivabradine; Lomitapide; Naloxegol; Olaparib; Pimozide; Simeprevir; Tolvaptan; Trabectedin; Ulipristal

Increased Effect/Toxicity

Aprepitant may increase the levels/effects of: Apixaban; ARIPiprazole; Avanafil; Bosentan; Bosutinib; Brexpiprazole; Bromocriptine; Budesonide (Systemic); Budesonide (Topical); Cannabis; Cilostazol; Cisapride; Cobimetinib; Colchicine; Corticosteroids (Systemic); CYP3A4 Substrates; Dapoxetine; Dofetilide; Domperidone; DOXOrubicin (Conventional); Dronabinol; Eletriptan; Eliglustat; Eplerenone; Everolimus; FentaNYL; Flibanserin; Halofantrine; Hydrocodone; Ibrutinib; Ifosfamide; Ivabradine; Ivacaftor; Lomitapide; Lurasidone; Naloxegol; NiMODipine; Olaparib; OxyCODONE; Pimecrolimus; Pimozide; Propafenone; Ranolazine; Salmeterol; Saxagliptin; Simeprevir; Sirolimus; Sonidegib; Suvorexant; Tetrahydrocannabinol; Tolvaptan; Trabectedin; Ulipristal; Vilazodone; Vindesine; Zopiclone; Zuclopenthixol

The levels/effects of Aprepitant may be increased by: Conivaptan; CYP3A4 Inhibitors (Moderate); CYP3A4 Inhibitors (Strong); Dasatinib; Fosaprepitant; Fusidic Acid (Systemic); Idelalisib; Luliconazole; Osimertinib; Palbociclib; Stiripentol

Decreased Effect

Aprepitant may decrease the levels/effects of: Contraceptives (Estrogens); Contraceptives (Progestins); CYP2C9 Substrates; Diclofenac (Systemic); PARoxetine; TOLBUTamide; Warfarin

The levels/effects of Aprepitant may be decreased by: Bosentan; CYP3A4 Inducers (Moderate); CYP3A4 Inducers (Strong); Dabrafenib; Deferasirox; Osimertinib; PARoxetine; Siltuximab; St Johns Wort; Tocilizumab

Food Interactions Aprepitant serum concentration may be increased when taken with grapefruit juice. Management: Avoid concurrent use.

Storage/Stability Store at room temperature of 20°C to 25°C (68°F to 77°F).

Mechanism of Action Prevents acute and delayed vomiting by inhibiting the substance P/neurokinin 1 (NK_1) receptor; augments the antiemetic activity of $5-HT_3$ receptor antagonists and corticosteroids to inhibit acute and delayed phases of chemotherapy-induced emesis.

Pharmacodynamics/Kinetics

Distribution: V_d: ~70 L; crosses the blood-brain barrier

Protein binding: >95%

Metabolism: Extensively hepatic via CYP3A4 (major); CYP1A2 and CYP2C19 (minor); forms 7 metabolites (weakly active)

Bioavailability: ~60% to 65%

Half-life elimination: Terminal: ~9 to 13 hours

Time to peak, plasma: Adult: ~3 hours; Pediatric: ~4 hours

Excretion: Primarily via metabolism

Dosing

Adult & Geriatric

Prevention of chemotherapy-induced nausea/vomiting:

Manufacturer's labeling:

Prevention of nausea/vomiting associated with highly-emetogenic chemotherapy: Oral: 125 mg 1 hour prior to chemotherapy on day 1, followed by 80 mg once daily on days 2 and 3 (in combination with a $5-HT_3$ antagonist antiemetic on day 1 and dexamethasone on days 1 to 4)

Prevention of nausea/vomiting associated with moderately-emetogenic chemotherapy: Oral: 125 mg 1 hour prior to chemotherapy on day 1, followed by 80 mg once daily on days 2 and 3 (in combination with a $5-HT_3$ antagonist antiemetic and dexamethasone on day 1)

Guideline recommendations:

Prevention of nausea/vomiting associated with highly-emetogenic chemotherapy (including anthracycline and cyclophosphamide [AC] regimens): Oral:

American Society of Clinical Oncology (ASCO; Basch, 2011): 125 mg prior to chemotherapy on day 1, followed by 80 mg once daily on days 2 and 3 (in combination with a $5-HT_3$ antagonist antiemetic on day 1 and dexamethasone on days 1 to 4 or days 1 to 3)

Multinational Association of Supportive Care in Cancer (MASCC) and European Society of Medical Oncology (ESMO) (Roila, 2010): 125 mg prior to chemotherapy on day 1, followed by 80 mg once daily on days 2 and 3 (in combination with a $5-HT_3$ antagonist antiemetic on day 1 and dexamethasone on days 1 to 4 or day 1 only [AC regimen])

Prevention of postoperative nausea/vomiting (PONV): Oral: 40 mg within 3 hours prior to anesthesia induction

Pediatric

Manufacturer's labeling:

Prevention of nausea/vomiting associated with highly-emetogenic chemotherapy: Children <12 years and ≥30 kg, Children ≥12 years, and Adolescents: Oral: 125 mg 1 hour prior to chemotherapy on day 1, followed by 80 mg once daily on days 2 and 3 (in combination with a $5-HT_3$ antagonist antiemetic on day 1 and dexamethasone on days 1 to 4 [reduce dexamethasone dose to 50% of recommended dose])

Prevention of nausea/vomiting associated with moderately-emetogenic chemotherapy: Children <12 years and ≥30 kg, Children ≥12 years, and Adolescents: Oral: 125 mg 1 hour prior to chemotherapy on day 1, followed by 80 mg once daily on days 2 and 3 (in combination with a $5-HT_3$ antagonist antiemetic and dexamethasone on day 1 [reduce dexamethasone dose to 50% of recommended dose])

Pediatric guideline recommendations: Prevention of nausea/vomiting associated with highly-emetogenic chemotherapy: Pediatric Oncology Group of Ontario (POGO): Children ≥12 years and Adolescents: Oral: 125 mg prior to chemotherapy on day 1, followed by 80 mg once daily on days 2 and 3 (Dupuis, 2013).

The antiemetic regimen also includes a 5-HT$_3$ antagonist and dexamethasone.

Renal Impairment
No dosage adjustment necessary.
ESRD undergoing dialysis: No dosage adjustment necessary.

Hepatic Impairment
Mild-to-moderate impairment (Child-Pugh class A or B): No dosage adjustment necessary.
Severe impairment (Child-Pugh class C): Use with caution; no data available; may require additional monitoring for adverse reactions.

Administration
Swallow capsule whole (according to the manufacturer).
Prevention of chemotherapy-induced nausea/vomiting: Administer with or without food. First dose should be given 1 hour prior to chemotherapy; subsequent doses should be given 1 hour prior to chemotherapy or in the morning (if no chemotherapy is administered).
Prevention of postoperative nausea/vomiting: Administer within 3 hours prior to induction; follow health care provider instructions about food/drink restrictions prior to surgery.

Monitoring Parameters In patients receiving concurrent warfarin, monitor INR/PT for 2 weeks (particularly at 7 to 10 days) following aprepitant administration; signs/symptoms of hypersensitivity reaction.

Product Availability Emend oral suspension: FDA approved December 2015; anticipated availability is currently unknown. Emend oral suspension is indicated for the prevention of chemotherapy induced nausea and vomiting in children ≥6 months of age. Information pertaining to this product within the monograph is pending revision.

Dosage Forms Excipient information presented when available (limited, particularly for generics); consult specific product labeling.
Capsule, Oral:
Emend: 40 mg, 80 mg, 125 mg, 80 mg & 125 mg

Extemporaneous Preparations A 20 mg/mL oral aprepitant suspension may be prepared with capsules and a 1:1 combination of Ora-Sweet and Ora-Plus (or Ora-Blend). Empty the contents of four 125 mg capsules into a mortar and reduce to a fine powder (process will take 10-15 minutes). Add small portions of vehicle and mix to a uniform paste. Add sufficient vehicle to form a liquid; transfer to a graduated cylinder, rinse mortar with vehicle, and add quantity of vehicle sufficient to make 25 mL. Label "shake well" and "refrigerate". Stable for 90 days refrigerated.
Dupuis LL, Lingertat-Walsh K, and Walker SE, "Stability of an Extemporaneous Oral Liquid Aprepitant Formulation," *Support Care Cancer*, 2009, 17(6):701-6.

Arformoterol (ar for MOE ter ol)

Brand Names: US Brovana
Index Terms (R,R)-Formoterol L-Tartrate; Arformoterol Tartrate
Pharmacologic Category Beta$_2$-Adrenergic Agonist; Beta$_2$-Adrenergic Agonist, Long-Acting
Use Chronic obstructive pulmonary disease: Long-term maintenance treatment of bronchoconstriction in patients with chronic obstructive pulmonary disease (COPD), including chronic bronchitis and emphysema
Medication Guide Available Yes
Dosing
Adult & Geriatric COPD: Nebulization: 15 mcg twice daily; maximum: 30 mcg daily
Renal Impairment No dosage adjustment necessary.
Hepatic Impairment No dosage adjustment necessary. Use with caution; systemic drug exposure prolonged.
Additional Information Complete prescribing information should be consulted for additional detail.
Dosage Forms Excipient information presented when available (limited, particularly for generics); consult specific product labeling.
Nebulization Solution, Inhalation:
Brovana: 15 mcg/2 mL (2 mL)

Argatroban (ar GA troh ban)

Pharmacologic Category Anticoagulant; Anticoagulant, Direct Thrombin Inhibitor
Additional Appendix Information
Reversal of Oral Anticoagulants *on page 1959*
Use
Heparin-induced thrombocytopenia: Prophylaxis or treatment of thrombosis in adult patients with heparin-induced thrombocytopenia (HIT)
Percutaneous coronary intervention: As an anticoagulant for percutaneous coronary intervention (PCI) in adult patients who have or are at risk of developing HIT
Pregnancy Considerations Adverse events have not been observed in animal reproduction studies. Information related to argatroban in pregnancy is limited. Use of parenteral direct thrombin inhibitors in pregnancy should be limited to those women who have severe allergic reactions to heparin, including heparin-induced thrombocytopenia, and who cannot receive danaparoid (Guyatt, 2012).
Breast-Feeding Considerations It is not known if argatroban is excreted in human milk. Due to the potential for serious adverse reactions in the nursing infant, the manufacturer recommends a decision be made whether to discontinue nursing or to discontinue the drug, taking into account the importance of treatment to the mother.
Contraindications Hypersensitivity to argatroban or any component of the formulation; major bleeding
Warnings/Precautions The most common complication is bleeding and can occur at any site in the body. Use with extreme caution in disease states and other circumstances in which there is an increased danger of bleeding (eg, hematologic conditions associated with increased bleeding tendencies such as congenital or acquired bleeding disorders and GI lesions such as ulcerations; recent puncture of large vessels or organ biopsy; spinal anesthesia or immediately following lumbar puncture; recent CVA, stroke, intracerebral surgery, or other neuraxial procedure; severe hypertension; renal impairment; recent major surgery; recent major bleeding (intracranial, GI, intraocular, or pulmonary). Monitor for signs and symptoms of bleeding. Airway, skin, and generalized hypersensitivity reactions have been reported. Use caution in critically-ill patients; reduced clearance may require dosage reduction. Use with caution in patients with hepatic impairment; may require >4 hours to achieve full reversal of argatroban's anticoagulant effect following treatment. Avoid use during PCI in patients with clinically significant hepatic disease or elevations of ALT/AST (≥3 times ULN) as use in these patients has not been evaluated. Limited pharmacokinetic and dosing information is available from use in critically-ill children with heparin-induced thrombocytopenia (HIT). Potentially significant interactions may exist, requiring

dose or frequency adjustment, additional monitoring, and/or selection of alternative therapy.

Adverse Reactions As with all anticoagulants, bleeding is the major adverse effect of argatroban. Hemorrhage may occur at virtually any site. Risk is dependent on multiple variables, including the intensity of anticoagulation and patient susceptibility.

>10%:

Cardiovascular: Chest pain (PCI related: <1% to 15%), hypotension (7% to 11%)

Genitourinary: Genitourinary tract hemorrhage (including hematuria; major: <1%; minor: 2% to 12%)

1% to 10%:

Cardiovascular: Vasodilation (1% to 10%), cardiac arrest (6%), bradycardia (5%), ventricular tachycardia (5%), myocardial infarction (PCI: 4%), angina pectoris (2%), coronary occlusion (2%), ischemic heart disease (2%), thrombosis (<1% to 2%)

Central nervous system: Headache (5%), pain (5%), intracranial hemorrhage (1% to 4%)

Dermatologic: Dermatological reaction (bullous eruption, rash; 1% to <10%)

Gastrointestinal: Nausea (5% to 7%), diarrhea (6%), vomiting (4% to 6%), abdominal pain (3% to 4%), gastrointestinal hemorrhage (major: <1% to 3%; minor: 3%)

Hematologic & oncologic: Decreased hematocrit (minor: ≤10%; major: <1%), decreased hemoglobin (minor: ≤10%; major: <1%; ≥2g/dL), groin bleeding (5%), brachial bleeding (2%), minor hemorrhage (CABG related: 2%)

Neuromuscular & skeletal: Back pain (PCI related: 8%)

Respiratory: Dyspnea (10%), cough (3% to 10%), hemoptysis (minor: ≤1% to 3%)

Miscellaneous: Fever (<1% to 7%)

<1% (Limited to important or life-threatening): Aortic valve stenosis, bleeding at injection site (or access site; minor), hypersensitivity reaction, local hemorrhage (limb and below-the-knee stump), pulmonary edema, retroperitoneal bleeding

Drug Interactions

Metabolism/Transport Effects None known.

Avoid Concomitant Use

Avoid concomitant use of Argatroban with any of the following: Apixaban; Dabigatran Etexilate; Edoxaban; Hemin; Omacetaxine; Rivaroxaban; Urokinase; Vorapaxar

Increased Effect/Toxicity

Argatroban may increase the levels/effects of: Anticoagulants; Collagenase (Systemic); Deferasirox; Deoxycholic Acid; Ibritumomab; Nintedanib; Obinutuzumab; Omacetaxine; Rivaroxaban; Tositumomab and Iodine I 131 Tositumomab

The levels/effects of Argatroban may be increased by: Agents with Antiplatelet Properties; Apixaban; Dabigatran Etexilate; Dasatinib; Edoxaban; Hemin; Herbs (Anticoagulant/Antiplatelet Properties); Ibrutinib; Limaprost; Nonsteroidal Anti-Inflammatory Agents; Omega-3 Fatty Acids; Pentosan Polysulfate Sodium; Prostacyclin Analogues; Salicylates; Sugammadex; Thrombolytic Agents; Tibolone; Tipranavir; Urokinase; Vitamin E; Vitamin E (Oral); Vorapaxar

Decreased Effect

The levels/effects of Argatroban may be decreased by: Estrogen Derivatives; Progestins

Preparation for Administration

Vials for injection, 2.5 mL (100 mg/mL) concentrate: Prior to administration, each vial must be diluted to a final concentration of 1 mg/mL. Solution may be mixed with sodium chloride 0.9% injection, dextrose 5% injection, or lactated Ringer's injection. Do not mix with other medications prior to dilution. To prepare solution for IV administration, dilute each 250 mg vial with 250 mL of diluent or dilute 500 mg per 500 mL of diluent. Mix by repeated inversion for 1 minute. A slight but brief haziness may occur upon mixing; use of diluent at room temperature is recommended.

Premixed vials (50 mL or 125 mL) and single-use bags for infusion (1 mg/mL): No further dilution is required.

Storage/Stability

Vials for injection, 2.5 mL (100 mg/mL) concentrate: Prior to use, store vial in original carton at 25°C (77°F); excursions permitted to 15°C to 30°C (59°F to 86°F). Do not freeze. Retain in the original carton to protect from light. The diluted, prepared solution is stable for 24 hours at 20°C to 25°C (68°F to 77°F) in ambient indoor light. Do not expose to direct sunlight. Prepared solutions that are protected from light and kept at 20°C to 25°C (68°F to 77°F) or under refrigeration at 2°C to 8°C (36°F to 46°F) are stable for up to 96 hours.

Premixed vials (50 mL or 125 mL) and single-use bags for infusion (1 mg/mL): Store at 20°C to 25°C (68°F to 77°F). Do not freeze. Protect from light.

Mechanism of Action A direct, highly-selective thrombin inhibitor. Reversibly binds to the active thrombin site of free and clot-associated thrombin. Inhibits fibrin formation; activation of coagulation factors V, VIII, and XIII; activation of protein C; and platelet aggregation.

Pharmacodynamics/Kinetics

Onset of action: Immediate

Distribution: 174 mL/kg

Protein binding: Albumin: 20%; alpha$_1$-acid glycoprotein: 35%

Metabolism: Hepatic via hydroxylation and aromatization (major route). Metabolism via CYP3A4/5 (minor route) to four known metabolites. Unchanged argatroban is the major plasma component. Plasma concentration of metabolite M1 is 0% to 20% of the parent drug and is three- to five-fold weaker.

Half-life elimination: 39-51 minutes; Hepatic impairment: ≤181 minutes

Time to peak: Steady-state: 1-3 hours

Excretion: Feces (65%; 14% unchanged); urine (22%; 16% unchanged); low quantities of metabolites M2-4 in urine

Clearance:

Pediatric patients (seriously ill): 0.16 L/kg/hour; 50% lower than healthy adults

Pediatric patients (seriously ill with elevated bilirubin due to hepatic impairment or cardiac complications; n=4): 0.03 L/kg/hour; 80% lower than pediatric patients with normal bilirubin

Adult: 0.31 L/kg/hour (5.1 mL/kg/minute); hepatic impairment: 1.9 mL/kg/minute

Dosing

Adult & Geriatric

Heparin-induced thrombocytopenia (HIT): IV:

Initial dose: 2 mcg/kg/minute

Obesity: Pharmacokinetics and pharmacodynamics have not been evaluated prospectively in obese patients; however, retrospective data suggest using actual body weight to dose and that adjustment of initial dose is unnecessary in obesity (BMI up to 51 kg/m^2) (Rice, 2007).

Maintenance dose: Patient may not be at steady-state but measure aPTT after 2 hours; adjust dose until the steady-state aPTT is 1.5 to 3 times the initial baseline value, not exceeding 100 seconds; dosage should not exceed 10 mcg/kg/minute

Note: Critically-ill patients with normal hepatic function have become excessively anticoagulated with FDA-approved or lower starting doses of argatroban. Doses between 0.15 to 1.3 mcg/kg/minute were required to maintain aPTTs in the target range (Reichert, 2003). In a prospective observational study of critically-ill patients with multiple organ dysfunction (MODS) and suspected or proven HIT, an initial infusion dose of 0.2 mcg/kg/minute was found to be sufficient and safe in this population (Beiderlinden, 2007). Consider reducing starting dose to 0.2 mcg/kg/minute in critically-ill patients with MODS defined as a minimum number of two organ failures. Another report of a cardiac patient with anasarca secondary to acute renal failure had a reduction in argatroban clearance similar to patients with hepatic dysfunction. Reduced clearance may have been due to reduced liver perfusion (de Denus, 2003). The American College of Chest Physicians has recommended an initial infusion rate of 0.5 to 1.2 mcg/kg/minute for patients with heart failure, MODS, severe anasarca, or postcardiac surgery (Linkins, 2012).

Conversion to oral anticoagulant: Because there may be a combined effect on the INR when argatroban is combined with warfarin, loading doses of warfarin should not be used. Warfarin therapy should be started at the expected daily dose.

Patients receiving ≤2 mcg/kg/minute of argatroban: Argatroban therapy can be stopped when the INR is >4 on combined warfarin and argatroban therapy; repeat INR measurement in 4 to 6 hours; if INR is below therapeutic level, argatroban therapy may be restarted. Repeat procedure daily until desired INR on warfarin alone is obtained.

Patients receiving >2 mcg/kg/minute of argatroban: In order to predict the INR on warfarin alone, reduce dose of argatroban to 2 mcg/kg/minute; measure INR for argatroban and warfarin 4 to 6 hours after dose reduction; argatroban therapy can be stopped when the INR on warfarin and argatroban combined therapy is >4. Repeat INR measurement in 4 to 6 hours; if INR is below therapeutic level, argatroban

therapy may be restarted. Repeat procedure daily until desired INR on warfarin alone is obtained.

Note: The American College of Chest Physicians suggests monitoring chromogenic factor X assay when transitioning from argatroban to warfarin (Garcia, 2012) or overlapping administration of warfarin for a minimum of 5 days until INR is within target range; recheck INR after anticoagulant effect of argatroban has dissipated (Guyatt, 2012). Factor X levels <45% have been associated with INR values >2 after the effects of argatroban have been eliminated (Arpino, 2005).

Prefilter administration for continuous renal replacement therapy (CRRT) in critically-ill patients with HIT (off-label use; Link, 2009): 0.1 to 1.5 mcg/kg/minute. **Note:** Loading dose of 100 mcg/kg was administered during clinical trial; however, this may be unnecessary.

Percutaneous coronary intervention (PCI): IV:
Initial: Begin infusion of 25 mcg/kg/minute and administer bolus dose of 350 mcg/kg (over 3 to 5 minutes). ACT should be checked 5 to 10 minutes after bolus infusion; proceed with procedure if ACT >300 seconds.
Obesity: Pharmacokinetics and pharmacodynamics have not been evaluated prospectively in obese patients; however, retrospective data suggest using actual body weight to dose and that adjustment of initial dose is unnecessary in obesity (BMI up to 51 kg/m^2) (Hursting, 2008).
Following initial bolus:
ACT <300 seconds: Give an additional 150 mcg/kg bolus, and increase infusion rate to 30 mcg/kg/minute (recheck ACT in 5 to 10 minutes)
ACT >450 seconds: Decrease infusion rate to 15 mcg/kg/minute (recheck ACT in 5 to 10 minutes)
Once a therapeutic ACT (300 to 450 seconds) is achieved, infusion should be continued at this dose for the duration of the procedure.
If dissection, impending abrupt closure, thrombus formation during PCI, or inability to achieve ACT >300 seconds: An additional bolus of 150 mcg/kg, followed by an increase in infusion rate to 40 mcg/kg/minute may be administered.
Note: Post-PCI anticoagulation, if required, may be achieved by continuing infusion at a reduced dose of 2 mcg/kg/minute, with close monitoring of aPTT; adjust infusion rate as needed.

Pediatric Heparin-induced thrombocytopenia (HIT) (dosing based on limited data from critically-ill patients): IV:
Initial dose: 0.75 mcg/kg/minute
Maintenance dose: Patient may not be at steady-state but measure aPTT after 2 hours; adjust dose until the steady-state aPTT is 1.5 to 3 times the initial baseline value, not exceeding 100 seconds; dosage may be adjusted in increments of 0.1 to 0.25 mcg/kg/minute. **Note:** Frequent dosage adjustments may be required to maintain desired anticoagulant activity.

Renal Impairment Dialyzable: 20%; removal during hemodialysis and continuous venovenous hemofiltration is clinically insignificant (Tang 2005). No dosage adjustment necessary.

Hepatic Impairment Decreased clearance and increased elimination half-life are seen with hepatic impairment; dose reduction and careful titration are required.
Adults: Per manufacturer labeling, the initial dose for moderate-to-severe hepatic impairment (Child-Pugh classes B and C) is 0.5 mcg/kg/minute; monitor aPTT closely and adjust dose as necessary. However, patients with severe hepatic impairment (Child-Pugh class C) may require further reduction of the initial dose. One case report describes a dose of 0.05 mcg/kg/minute required to maintain a stable, therapeutic aPTT in a patient with severe hepatic impairment (Yarbrough, 2012). **Note:** During PCI, avoid use in patients with elevations of ALT/AST (≥3 times ULN); the use of argatroban in these patients has not been evaluated.
Children: Initial dose: 0.2 mcg/kg/minute; adjust dose in increments of ≤0.05 mcg/kg/minute

Obesity Refer to indication-specific dosing for obesity-related information (may not be available for all indications).

Usual Infusion Concentrations: Pediatric Note: Premixed solutions available.
IV infusion: 1000 mcg/mL
Usual Infusion Concentrations: Adult Note: Premixed solutions available.
IV infusion: 250 mg in 250 mL (concentration: 1000 mcg/mL) in D$_5$W or NS

Administration The 2.5 mL (100 mg/mL) **concentrated** vial **must be diluted to 1 mg/mL** prior to administration. The premixed 50 mL or 125 mL vials and 250 mL bag (1 mg/mL) require no further dilution. The premixed 1 mg/mL vial may be inverted for use with an infusion set. Administer bolus dose over 3 to 5 minutes through a large bore intravenous line.

Monitoring Parameters Monitor hemoglobin, hematocrit, signs and symptoms of bleeding.

HIT: Obtain baseline aPTT prior to start of therapy. Patient may not be at steady-state but check aPTT 2 hours after start of therapy to adjust dose, keeping the steady-state aPTT 1.5 to 3 times the initial baseline value (not exceeding 100 seconds).

PCI: Monitor ACT before dosing, 5 to 10 minutes after bolus dosing, and after any change in infusion rate and at the end of the procedure. Additional ACT assessments should be made every 20 to 30 minutes during extended PCI procedures.

Test Interactions Argatroban may elevate PT/INR levels in the absence of warfarin. If warfarin is started, initial PT/INR goals while on argatroban may require modification. The American College of Chest Physicians suggests monitoring chromogenic factor X assay when transitioning from argatroban to warfarin (Garcia, 2012) or overlapping administration of warfarin for a minimum of 5 days until INR is within target range; recheck INR after anticoagulant effect of argatroban has dissipated (Guyatt, 2012). Factor Xa levels <45% have been associated with INR values >2 after the effects of argatroban have been eliminated (Arpino, 2005).

Additional Information Platelet counts recovered by day 3 in 53% of patients with heparin-induced thrombocytopenia and in 58% of patients with heparin-induced thrombocytopenia with thrombosis syndrome.

Dosage Forms Excipient information presented when available (limited, particularly for generics); consult specific product labeling.
Solution, Intravenous:
Generic: 125 mg/125 mL (125 mL); 250 mg/250 mL (250 mL); 250 mg/2.5 mL (2.5 mL)
Solution, Intravenous [preservative free]:
Generic: 50 mg/50 mL (50 mL); 250 mg/2.5 mL (2.5 mL)

Arginine (AR ji neen)

Brand Names: US R-Gene 10
Index Terms Arginine HCl; Arginine Hydrochloride; L-Arginine; L-Arginine Hydrochloride
Pharmacologic Category Diagnostic Agent
Use Diagnostic aid: As an intravenous (IV) stimulant to the pituitary for the release of human growth hormone (hGH) in patients in whom the measurement of pituitary reserve for hGH can be of diagnostic usefulness. Used as a diagnostic aid in such conditions as panhypopituitarism, pituitary dwarfism, chromophobe adenoma, postsurgical craniopharyngioma, hypophysectomy, pituitary trauma, acromegaly, gigantism, and problems of growth and stature.

Dosing
Adult & Geriatric
Diagnostic aid (pituitary function): Note: Dosing based on arginine hydrochloride product. IV: 30 g as a single dose
Pediatric
Diagnostic aid (pituitary function): Note: Dosing based on arginine hydrochloride product.
Infants, Children, and Adolescents <60 kg: IV: 0.5 g/kg as a single dose; (maximum dose: 30 g/dose)
Children and Adolescents ≥60 kg: Refer to adult dosing

Hyperammonemia, acute (urea cycle disorders) (off-label use): Limited data available: Infants, Children, and Adolescents: **Note:** Administered concomitantly with sodium benzoate and sodium phenylacetate. Dosage based on specific enzyme deficiency; therapy should continue until ammonia levels are in normal range. If patient already receiving arginine therapy, consider either a reduction in the loading dose or possible elimination (Batshaw 2001); if a loading dose is used, it should not be repeated (NORD 2012).
Dosing based on arginine hydrochloride product.
Weight-directed dosing:
Argininosuccinic acid lyase (ASL) or argininosuccinic acid synthetase (ASS, citrullinemia) deficiency: IV: Loading dose: 600 mg/kg followed by a continuous IV infusion of 600 mg/kg/day (Batshaw 2001; NORD 2012).

Carbamyl phosphate synthetase (CPS), ornithine transcarbamylase (OTC) or N-acetylglutamate synthetase (NAGS) deficiency: IV: Loading dose: 200 mg/kg followed by a continuous IV infusion of 200 mg/kg/day (Batshaw 2001; NORD 2012).

Unconfirmed/pending diagnosis: IV: Loading dose: 600 mg/kg followed by a continuous IV infusion of 600 mg/kg/day (NORD 2012). If ASS and ASL are excluded as diagnostic possibilities, reduce dose to 200 mg/kg/day.

BSA-directed dosing:

Argininosuccinic acid lyase (ASL) or argininosuccinic acid synthetase (ASS, citrullinemia) deficiency: IV: Loading dose: 12 g/m^2 followed by a continuous IV infusion of 12 g/m^2/day (Batshaw 2001; Brusilow 1996).

Carbamyl phosphate synthetase (CPS) or ornithine transcarbamylase (OTC) deficiency: IV: Loading dose: 4 g/m^2 followed by a continuous IV infusion of 4 g/m^2/day (Batshaw 2001; Brusilow 1996).

Urea cycle disorders, chronic therapy (off-label use): Limited data available: Infants, Children, and Adolescents: **Note:** Dose should be individualized based on patient response; doses may need to be increased by ~50% as part of a sick-day routine (Berry 2001). **Dosing based on arginine free base powder product:**
Weight-directed dosing:

Argininosuccinic acid lyase (ASL) or argininosuccinic acid synthetase (ASS, citrullinemia) deficiency: Oral: 400 to 700 mg/kg/day in 3 to 4 divided doses (Batshaw 2001; Berry 2001; Brusilow 1996; NORD 2012)

Carbamyl phosphate synthetase (CPS), ornithine transcarbamylase (OTC) or N-acetylglutamate synthetase (NAGS) deficiency: **Note:** Citrulline may be preferred for some patients: Oral: 170 mg/kg/day in 3 to 4 divided doses (Batshaw, 2001; Brusilow 1996; NORD 2012)

BSA-directed dosing:

Argininosuccinic acid lyase (ASL) or argininosuccinic acid synthetase (ASS, citrullinemia) deficiency: Oral: 8.8 to 15.4 g/m^2/day in 3 to 4 divided doses (Batshaw 2001; Berry 2001; Brusilow 1996; NORD 2012)

Carbamyl phosphate synthetase (CPS), ornithine transcarbamylase (OTC) or N-acetylglutamate synthetase (NAGS) deficiency: **Note:** Citrulline may be preferred for some patients: Oral: 3.8 g/m^2/day in 3 to 4 divided doses (Batshaw 2001; Brusilow 1996; NORD 2012)

Renal Impairment There are no dosage adjustments provided in the manufacturer's labeling; use with caution.

Hepatic Impairment There are no dosage adjustments provided in the manufacturer's labeling; use with caution.

Additional Information Complete prescribing information should be consulted for additional detail.

Dosage Forms Considerations
R-Gene 10 contains chloride 47.5 mEq per 100 mL

Dosage Forms Excipient information presented when available (limited, particularly for generics); consult specific product labeling.

Solution, Intravenous, as hydrochloride [preservative free]:
R-Gene 10: 10% (300 mL)

ARIPiprazole (ay ri PIP ray zole)

Brand Names: US Abilify; Abilify Discmelt [DSC]; Abilify Maintena

Brand Names: Canada Abilify; Abilify Maintena

Index Terms BMS 337039; OPC-14597

Pharmacologic Category Second Generation (Atypical) Antipsychotic

Use

Oral:

Bipolar I disorder: Acute treatment of manic and mixed episodes associated with bipolar I disorder.

Irritability associated with autistic disorder: Treatment of irritability associated with autistic disorder.

Major depressive disorder: Adjunctive treatment of major depressive disorder.

Schizophrenia: Treatment of schizophrenia.

Tourette disorder: Treatment of Tourette disorder.

Injection:

Agitation associated with schizophrenia or bipolar mania (immediate-release injection only): Treatment of agitation associated with schizophrenia or bipolar mania.

Schizophrenia (extended-release injection only): Treatment of schizophrenia.

Pregnancy Considerations Adverse events have been observed in animal reproduction studies. Aripiprazole crosses the placenta; aripiprazole and dehydro-aripiprazole can be detected in the cord blood at delivery (Nguyen, 2011; Watanabe, 2011). Antipsychotic use during the third trimester of pregnancy has a risk for abnormal muscle movements (extrapyramidal symptoms [EPS]) and/or withdrawal symptoms in newborns following delivery. Symptoms in the newborn may include agitation, feeding disorder, hypertonia, hypotonia, respiratory distress, somnolence, and tremor; these effects may be self-limiting or require hospitalization.

Treatment algorithms have been developed by the ACOG and the APA for the management of depression in women prior to conception and during pregnancy (Yonkers, 2009). The ACOG recommends that therapy during pregnancy be individualized; treatment with psychiatric medications during pregnancy should incorporate the clinical expertise of the mental health clinician, obstetrician, primary healthcare provider, and pediatrician. Safety data related to atypical antipsychotics during pregnancy is limited and routine use is not recommended. However, if a woman is inadvertently exposed to an atypical antipsychotic while pregnant, continuing therapy may be preferable to switching to a typical antipsychotic that the fetus has not yet been exposed to; consider risk:benefit (ACOG, 2008).

Healthcare providers are encouraged to enroll women exposed to aripiprazole during pregnancy in the National Pregnancy Registry for Atypical Antipsychotics (866-961-2388 or http://www.womensmentalhealth.org/clinical-and-research-programs/pregnancyregistry/).

Breast-Feeding Considerations Aripiprazole is excreted in breast milk (Schlotterbeck, 2007; Watanabe, 2011). In one case report, milk concentrations were ~20% of the maternal plasma concentration (maternal dose: 15 mg/day; ~6 months postpartum) (Schlotterbeck, 2007); however, aripiprazole was not detected in the breast milk in a second case (limit of detection 10 ng/mL; maternal dose: 15 mg/day; ~1 month postpartum) (Lutz, 2010). Aripiprazole was also detected in the neonatal blood 6 days after delivery in a breast-fed infant also exposed during pregnancy. In this case report, the authors suggest in utero exposure could have contributed to the findings due to the long elimination half-life of aripiprazole (Watanabe, 2011). In one report, lactation was not able to be established, possibly due to changes in maternal prolactin potentially caused by aripiprazole (Mendhekar, 2006). The manufacturer recommends a decision be made whether to discontinue nursing or to discontinue the drug, taking into account the importance of treatment to the mother. The manufacturer of the extended-release injection recommends the development and health benefits of breast-feeding be considered along with the mother's clinical need for therapy and any potential adverse effects on the breastfed infant from aripiprazole or from the underlying maternal condition.

Medication Guide Available Yes

Contraindications Hypersensitivity (eg, anaphylaxis, pruritus, urticaria) to aripiprazole or any component of the formulation.

Warnings/Precautions [US Boxed Warning]: Elderly patients with dementia-related psychosis treated with antipsychotics are at an increased risk of death compared to placebo. Most deaths appeared to be either cardiovascular (eg, heart failure, sudden death) or infectious (eg, pneumonia) in nature. In addition, an increased incidence of cerebrovascular effects (eg, transient ischemic attack, cerebrovascular accidents) has been reported in studies of placebo-controlled trials of aripiprazole in elderly patients with dementia-related psychosis. Use with caution in dementia with Lewy bodies; antipsychotics may worsen dementia symptoms and patients with dementia with Lewy bodies are more sensitive to the extrapyramidal side effects (APA, [Rabins, 2007]). **Aripiprazole is not approved for the treatment of dementia-related psychosis.**

[US Boxed Warning]: Antidepressants increase the risk of suicidal thinking and behavior in children, adolescents, and young adults (18 to 24 years of age) with major depressive disorder (MDD) and other psychiatric disorders; consider risk prior to prescribing. The possibility of a suicide attempt is inherent in major depression and may persist until remission occurs.

Patients treated with antidepressants should be observed for clinical worsening and suicidality, especially during the initial few months of a course of drug therapy, or at times of dose changes, either increases or decreases. Prescriptions should be written for the smallest quantity consistent with good patient care. The patient's family or caregiver should be alerted to monitor patients for the emergence of suicidality and associated behaviors; patients should be instructed to notify their healthcare provider if any of these symptoms or worsening depression or psychosis occur.

Leukopenia, neutropenia, and agranulocytosis (sometimes fatal) have been reported in clinical trials and postmarketing reports with antipsychotic use; presence of risk factors (eg, preexisting low WBC/ANC or history of drug-induced leuko-/neutropenia) should prompt periodic blood count assessment. Discontinue therapy at first signs of blood dyscrasias or if absolute neutrophil count <1,000/mm^3.

A medication guide concerning the use of antidepressants should be dispensed with each prescription. Aripiprazole is not FDA approved for adjunctive treatment of depression in children.

May cause extrapyramidal symptoms (EPS), including pseudoparkinsonism, acute dystonic reactions, akathisia, and tardive dyskinesia (risk of these reactions is very low relative to typical/conventional antipsychotics, frequencies reported are similar to placebo). Risk of dystonia (and probably other EPS) may be greater with increased doses, use of conventional antipsychotics, males, and younger patients. May be associated with neuroleptic malignant syndrome (NMS).

May cause CNS depression, which may impair physical or mental abilities; patients must be cautioned about performing tasks that require mental alertness (eg, operating machinery, driving). May cause orthostatic hypotension (although reported rates are similar to placebo); use caution in patients at risk of this effect or those who would not tolerate transient hypotensive episodes (cerebrovascular disease, cardiovascular disease, or other medications which may predispose). Case reports of new or worsening pathologic gambling have been reported in patients receiving aripiprazole (Gaboriau, 2014; Moore, 2014; Smith, 2011); patients with prior history of gambling disorders may be at increased risk.

Use caution in patients with Parkinson disease; antipsychotics may aggravate motor disturbances (APA [Lehman, 2004; Rabins, 2007]). Use with caution in patients with predisposition to seizures or severe cardiac disease. May alter cardiac conduction; life-threatening arrhythmias have occurred with therapeutic doses of antipsychotics. Esophageal dysmotility and aspiration have been associated with antipsychotic use; use caution in patients at risk for aspiration pneumonia (eg, Alzheimer dementia). May alter temperature regulation. Potentially significant interactions may exist, requiring dose or frequency adjustment, additional monitoring, and/or selection of alternative therapy.

Atypical antipsychotics have been associated with metabolic changes including loss of glucose control, lipid changes, and weight gain (>7% of baseline weight) (risk profile varies with product). Development of hyperglycemia in some cases, may be extreme and associated with ketoacidosis, hyperosmolar coma, or death. Reports of hyperglycemia with aripiprazole therapy have been few and specific risk associated with this agent is not known. Use caution in patients with diabetes or other disorders of glucose regulation; monitor for worsening of glucose control. Patients with risk factors for diabetes (eg, obesity or family history) should have a baseline fasting blood sugar (FBS) and periodic assessment of glucose regulation.

Tablets may contain lactose; avoid use in patients with galactose intolerance or glucose-galactose malabsorption.

Orally disintegrating tablets may contain phenylalanine.

There are two formulations available for intramuscular administration: Abilify is an immediate-release short-acting formulation and Abilify Maintena is an extended-release formulation. These products are **not** interchangeable.

Adverse Reactions Unless otherwise noted, frequency of adverse reactions is shown as reported for adult patients receiving aripiprazole monotherapy with oral administration. Spectrum and incidence of adverse effects similar in children; exceptions noted when incidence much higher in children.

>10%:

Central nervous system: Headache (adults 27%; children & adolescents 10% to 13%; injection 12%), extrapyramidal reaction (dose-related; children & adolescents 6% to 27%; adults 5% to 13%), drowsiness (children & adolescents 10% to 26%; adults 8% to 13%), akathisia (dose-related; adults 2% to 25%; children & adolescents 6% to 11%), fatigue (dose-related; children & adolescents 4% to 22%; adults 6%; injection 1% to 2%), sedation (dose-related; children & adolescents 9% to 21%; adults 5% to 7%), agitation (oral 19%; injection <1%), insomnia (18%; injection ≥1%), anxiety (oral 17%; injection ≥1%)

Endocrine & metabolic: Weight gain (children & adolescents 3% to 26%; injection 17% to 22%; adults 2% to 8%), increased serum cholesterol (injection 4% to 22%; oral 1% to 2%), increased serum triglycerides (adults 7% to 10%; children and adolescents 5%; injection 7% to 20%; oral 5% to 10%), increased serum glucose (adults 8% to 18%; children and adolescents 3% to 5%), decreased HDL cholesterol (injection 14%; children & adolescents 4%), increased LDL cholesterol (injection 10% to 14%)

Gastrointestinal: Nausea (8% to 15%), vomiting (oral 8% to 14%; injection: 3%), constipation (10% to 11%; children & adolescents 3%)

Neuromuscular & skeletal: Tremor (dose-related; oral 5% to 12%; injection 3%)

1% to 10%:

Cardiovascular: Tachycardia (injection ≤2%), hypertension (≥1%), peripheral edema (≥1%), orthostatic hypotension (including injection; ≤1%)

Central nervous system: Dizziness (3% to 10%), drooling (children & adolescents 3% to 9%), restlessness (oral 5% to 6%; injection ≥1%), lethargy (older adults 5%; children 3% to 5%; injection <1%), pain (3%), dystonia (2%), irritability (children & adolescents 2%; injection <1%), ataxia (≥1%), hypersomnia (≤1%)

Dermatologic: Skin rash (≤2%)

Endocrine & metabolic: Weight loss (injection 4%; oral ≥1%), increased thirst (children & adolescents 1%)

Gastrointestinal: Dyspepsia (oral 9%; injection <1%), sialorrhea (dose-related; 3% to 8%), decreased appetite (children & adolescents 5% to 7%; injection <1%), increased appetite (children & adolescents 7%), xerostomia (5%; injection: 4%; children & adolescents 1%), toothache (4%), diarrhea (3% to 4%), gastric distress (3%), upper abdominal pain (children & adolescents 3%; injection <1%), abdominal distress (2% to 3%), anorexia (≥1%)

Genitourinary: Urinary incontinence (older adults ≤5%; injection <1%), dysmenorrhea (children & adolescents 2%)

Hematologic & oncologic: Neutropenia (injection 6%)

Local: Pain at injection site (5%), injection site reaction (injection ≥1%; including erythema, induration, inflammation, hemorrhage, pruritus, swelling, rash)

Neuromuscular & skeletal: Arthralgia (injection 4%; children & adolescents 1%), back pain (injection 4%), limb pain (4%), myalgia (2% to 4%), stiffness (2% to 4%), musculoskeletal pain (injection 3%), muscle cramps (2%), muscle rigidity (children & adolescents 2%), muscle spasm (2%), weakness (1% to 2%), dyskinesia (children & adolescents 1%)

Ophthalmic: Blurred vision (oral 3% to 8%; injection <1%)

Respiratory: Nasopharyngitis (children & adolescents 6% to 9%; injection <1%), upper respiratory tract infection (4%), cough (3%), pharyngolaryngeal pain (3%), epistaxis (children & adolescents 2%), nasal congestion (injection: 2%; oral <1%), rhinorrhea (children & adolescents 2%), aspiration pneumonia (≥1%), dyspnea (≥1%)

Miscellaneous: Fever (children & adolescents 4% to 9%; injection <1%)

<1% (Limited to important or life-threatening): Abnormal bilirubin levels, abnormal gait, abnormal hepatic function tests, agranulocytosis, akinesia, alopecia, altered serum glucose, amenorrhea, angina pectoris, anorgasmia, atrial fibrillation, atrial flutter, atrioventricular block, bradycardia, bruxism, cardiopulmonary arrest, cardiorespiratory arrest, catatonia, cerebrovascular accident, chest discomfort, choreoathetosis, cogwheel rigidity, convulsions, decreased serum cholesterol, decreased serum triglycerides, delirium, depression, diabetes mellitus, diabetic ketoacidosis, diplopia, disruption of body temperature regulation, drug-induced Parkinson's disease, dry tongue, dysgeusia, dystonia (oromandibular), edema, erectile dysfunction, esophagitis, extrasystoles, eyelid edema, falling, gastroesophageal reflux disease, gynecomastia, hepatitis, hirsutism, homicidal ideation, hostility, hyperglycemia, hyperhidrosis, hyperinsulinism, hyperlipidemia, hypersensitivity, hypersexuality, hypertonia, hypoglycemia, hypokalemia, hypokinesia, hyponatremia, hypotension, hypotonia, impulse control disorder (including pathologic gambling and hypersexuality; Health Canada, Nov 2, 2015), increased blood urea nitrogen, increased creatinine clearance, increased creatine phosphokinase, increased gamma-glutamyl ▶

transferase, increased lactate dehydrogenase, increased serum prolactin, intentional injury, ischemic heart disease, jaundice, joint stiffness, leukopenia, mastalgia, memory impairment, mobility disorder, muscle twitching, myasthenia,myocardial infarction, myoclonus, neuroleptic malignant syndrome, obesity, oculogyric crisis, pancreatitis, panic attack, photopsia, pollakiuria presyncope, priapism, prolonged Q-T interval on ECG, psychosis, rhabdomyolysis, seizure (including injection), skin photosensitivity, sleep talking, somnambulism, suicidal ideation, suicidal tendencies, supraventricular tachycardia, syncope, tardive dyskinesia, thrombocytopenia, tics, tongue spasm, tonic-clonic seizures, transient ischemic attacks, urinary retention, ventricular tachycardia

Drug Interactions

Metabolism/Transport Effects Substrate of CYP2D6 (major), CYP3A4 (major); **Note:** Assignment of Major/Minor substrate status based on clinically relevant drug interaction potential

Avoid Concomitant Use

Avoid concomitant use of ARIPiprazole with any of the following: Amisulpride; Azelastine (Nasal); Conivaptan; Fusidic Acid (Systemic); Idelalisib; Metoclopramide; Orphenadrine; Paraldehyde; Sulpiride; Thalidomide

Increased Effect/Toxicity

ARIPiprazole may increase the levels/effects of: Alcohol (Ethyl); Amisulpride; Azelastine (Nasal); Buprenorphine; CNS Depressants; DULoxetine; FLUoxetine; Haloperidol; Highest Risk QTc-Prolonging Agents; Hydrocodone; Mequitazine; Methadone; Methotrimeprazine; Methylphenidate; Metyrosine; Mirtazapine; Moderate Risk QTc-Prolonging Agents; Orphenadrine; Paraldehyde; PARoxetine; Ritonavir; Selective Serotonin Reuptake Inhibitors; Serotonin Modulators; Sulpiride; Suvorexant; Thalidomide; Zolpidem

The levels/effects of ARIPiprazole may be increased by: Abiraterone Acetate; Acetylcholinesterase Inhibitors (Central); Aprepitant; Blood Pressure Lowering Agents; Brimonidine (Topical); Cannabis; Conivaptan; CYP2D6 Inhibitors (Moderate); CYP2D6 Inhibitors (Strong); CYP2D6 Inhibitors (Weak); CYP3A4 Inhibitors (Moderate); CYP3A4 Inhibitors (Strong); CYP3A4 Inhibitors (Weak); Dasatinib; Doxylamine; Dronabinol; Droperidol; DULoxetine; FLUoxetine; Fosaprepitant; Fusidic Acid (Systemic); Haloperidol; HydrOXYzine; Idelalisib; Ivacaftor; Kava Kava; Lithium; Luliconazole; Magnesium Sulfate; Methadone; Methotrimeprazine; Methylphenidate; Metoclopramide; Metyrosine; Mifepristone; Minocycline; Nabilone; Netupitant; Osimertinib; Palbociclib; Panobinostat; PARoxetine; Peginterferon Alfa-2b; Perampanel; Ritonavir; Serotonin Modulators; Sertraline; Simeprevir; Sodium Oxybate; Stiripentol; Tapentadol; Tetrahydrocannabinol

Decreased Effect

ARIPiprazole may decrease the levels/effects of: Amphetamines; Antidiabetic Agents; Anti-Parkinson's Agents (Dopamine Agonist); Haloperidol; Quinagolide

The levels/effects of ARIPiprazole may be decreased by: CYP3A4 Inducers; Dabrafenib; Deferasirox; Enzalutamide; Lithium; Mitotane; Osimertinib; Peginterferon Alfa-2b; Siltuximab; St Johns Wort; Tocilizumab

Food Interactions Ingestion with a high-fat meal delays time to peak plasma level. Management: Administer without regard to meals.

Preparation for Administration

Injection, powder (extended release):

Prefilled syringe: Reconstitute at room temperature. Rotate the syringe plunger rod to release diluent. Shake vigorously for 20 seconds or until the suspension is uniform; the resulting suspension will be milky white and opaque. (Refer to manufacturer's labeling for full preparation technique.) Inject full syringe contents immediately following reconstitution.

Vial for reconstitution: Reconstitute using 1.5 mL sterile water for injection (SWFI) (provided) for the 300 mg vial or 1.9 mL SWFI (provided) for the 400 mg vial to a final concentration of 200 mg/mL; residual SWFI should be discarded after reconstitution. Shake vigorously for 30 seconds or until the suspension is uniform; the resulting suspension will be milky white and opaque. If the suspension is not administered immediately after reconstitution, shake vigorously for 60 seconds prior to administration.

Storage/Stability

Injection, powder (extended release):

Prefilled syringe: Store below 30°C (86°F). Do not freeze. Protect from light and store in original package.

Vial for reconstitution: Store unused vials at 25°C (77°F); excursions permitted to 15°C to 30°C (59°F to 86°F). If the suspension is not administered immediately after reconstitution, store at room temperature in the vial (do not store in a syringe).

Injection, solution (immediate release): Store at 25°C (77°F); excursions permitted to 15°C to 30°C (59°F to 86°F). Protect from light. Retain in carton until time of use.

Oral solution and tablets: Store at 25°C (77°F); excursions permitted to 15°C to 30°C (59°F to 86°F). Use oral solution within 6 months after opening.

Mechanism of Action Aripiprazole is a quinolinone antipsychotic which exhibits high affinity for D_2, D_3, 5-HT$_{1A}$, and 5-HT$_{2A}$ receptors; moderate affinity for D_4, 5-HT$_{2C}$, 5-HT$_7$, alpha$_1$ adrenergic, and H$_1$ receptors. It also possesses moderate affinity for the serotonin reuptake transporter; has no affinity for muscarinic (cholinergic) receptors. Aripiprazole functions as a partial agonist at the D_2 and 5-HT$_{1A}$ receptors, and as an antagonist at the 5-HT$_{2A}$ receptor.

Pharmacodynamics/Kinetics Note: In pediatric patients 10 to 17 years of age, the pharmacokinetic parameters of aripiprazole and dehydro-aripiprazole have been shown to be similar to adult values when adjusted for weight.

Onset of action: Initial: 1 to 3 weeks

Absorption:

IM: Extended-release: Slow, prolonged

Oral: Well absorbed.

Distribution: V_d: 4.9 L/kg

Protein binding: ≥99%, primarily to albumin

Metabolism: Hepatic, via CYP2D6, CYP3A4 (dehydro-aripiprazole metabolite has affinity for D_2 receptors similar to the parent drug and represents 40% of the parent drug exposure in plasma)

Bioavailability: IM: 100%; Tablet: 87%; **Note:** Orally disintegrating tablets are bioequivalent to tablets; oral solution to tablet ratio of geometric mean for peak concentration is 122% and for AUC is 114%.

Half-life elimination: Aripiprazole: 75 hours; dehydro-aripiprazole: 94 hours; IM, extended release (terminal): ~30 to 47 days (dose-dependent)

CYP2D6 poor metabolizers: Aripiprazole: 146 hours

Time to peak, plasma:

IM:

Immediate release: 1 to 3 hours

Extended release (after multiple doses): 4 days (deltoid administration); 5 to 7 days (gluteal administration)

Tablet: 3 to 5 hours

With high-fat meal: Aripiprazole: Delayed by 3 hours; dehydro-aripiprazole: Delayed by 12 hours

Excretion: Feces (55%, ~18% of the total dose as unchanged drug); urine (25%, <1% of the total dose as unchanged drug)

Dosing

Adult & Geriatric Note: Oral solution may be substituted for the oral tablet on a mg-per-mg basis, up to 25 mg. Patients receiving 30 mg tablets should be given 25 mg oral solution. Orally disintegrating tablets (Abilify Discmelt) are bioequivalent to the immediate-release tablets (Abilify).

Acute agitation (schizophrenia/bipolar mania): IM, immediate release: 9.75 mg as a single dose (range: 5.25 to 15 mg; a lower dose of 5.25 mg IM may be considered when clinical factors warrant); repeated doses may be given at ≥2-hour intervals to a maximum of 30 mg/day. **Note:** If ongoing therapy with aripiprazole is necessary, transition to oral therapy as soon as possible.

Bipolar I disorder (acute manic or mixed episodes): Oral:

Monotherapy: Initial: 15 mg once daily. May increase to 30 mg once daily if clinically indicated (maximum 30 mg/day); safety of doses >30 mg/day has not been evaluated

Adjunct to lithium or valproic acid: Initial: 10 to 15 mg once daily. May increase to 30 mg once daily if clinically indicated (maximum 30 mg/day); safety of doses >30 mg/day has not been evaluated.

Depression (adjunctive with antidepressants): Oral: Initial: 2 to 5 mg/day (range: 2 to 15 mg/day); dose adjustments of up to 5 mg/day may be made in intervals of ≥1 week, up to a maximum of 15 mg/day. **Note:** Dosing based on patients already receiving antidepressant therapy.

Schizophrenia:

Oral: 10 or 15 mg once daily; may be increased to a maximum of 30 mg once daily (efficacy at dosages above 10 to 15 mg has not been shown to be increased). Dosage titration should not be more frequent than every 2 weeks.

IM, extended release: 400 mg once monthly (doses should be separated by ≥26 days); **Note:** Tolerability should be established using oral aripiprazole prior to initiation of parenteral therapy; due to the half-life of oral aripiprazole it may take up to 2 weeks to fully assess tolerability. Continue oral aripiprazole (or other oral antipsychotic) for 14 days during initiation of parenteral therapy.

Missed doses:

Second or third doses missed:
>4 weeks but <5 weeks since last dose: Administer next dose as soon as possible
>5 weeks since last dose: Administer oral aripiprazole for 14 days with next injection

Fourth or subsequent doses missed:
>4 weeks but <6 weeks since last dose: Administer next dose as soon as possible
>6 weeks since last dose: Administer oral aripiprazole for 14 days with next injection

Dosage adjustment for adverse effects: Consider reducing dose to 300 mg once monthly

Dosage adjustment with concurrent CYP450 inducer or inhibitor therapy:

Oral and IM, immediate release: **Note:** Dose reduction does not apply when adjunctive aripiprazole is administered to patients with major depressive disorder; follow usual dosing recommendations.

CYP3A4 inducers (eg, carbamazepine, rifampin): Aripiprazole dose should be doubled over 1 to 2 weeks; dose should be subsequently reduced to the original level over 1 to 2 weeks if concurrent inducer agent is discontinued.

Strong CYP3A4 inhibitors (eg, itraconazole, clarithromycin): Aripiprazole dose should be reduced to 50% of the usual dose, and proportionally increased upon discontinuation of the inhibitor agent.

Strong CYP2D6 inhibitors (eg, quinidine, fluoxetine, paroxetine): Aripiprazole dose should be reduced to 50% of the usual dose, and proportionally increased upon discontinuation of the inhibitor agent.

CYP3A4 and CYP2D6 inhibitors: Aripiprazole dose should be reduced to 25% of the usual dose. In patients receiving inhibitors of differing (eg, moderate 3A4/strong 2D6) or same (eg, moderate 3A4/moderate 2D6) potencies (excluding concurrent strong inhibitors), further dosage adjustments can be made to achieve the desired clinical response. In patients receiving strong CYP3A4 and 2D6 inhibitors, aripiprazole dose is proportionally increased upon discontinuation of one or both inhibitor agents.

IM, extended release: **Note:** Dosage adjustments are not recommended for concomitant use of CYP3A4 inhibitors, CYP2D6 inhibitors or CYP3A4 inducers for <14 days. In patients who had their aripiprazole dose adjusted for concomitant therapy, the aripiprazole dose may need to be increased if the CYP3A4 and/or CYP2D6 inhibitor is withdrawn.

CYP3A4 inducers: Avoid use; aripiprazole serum concentrations may fall below effective levels.

Strong CYP3A4 or CYP2D6 inhibitors:
Current aripiprazole dose of 300 mg once monthly: Reduce aripiprazole dose to 200 mg once monthly
Current aripiprazole dose of 400 mg once monthly: Reduce aripiprazole dose to 300 mg once monthly

Strong CYP3A4 inhibitors **and** CYPD2D6 inhibitors:
Current aripiprazole dose of 300 mg once monthly: Reduce aripiprazole dose to 160 mg once monthly
Current aripiprazole dose of 400 mg once monthly: Reduce aripiprazole dose to 200 mg once monthly

Dosage adjustment based on CYP2D6 metabolizer status:

Oral and IM, immediate release: Aripiprazole dose should be reduced to 50% of the usual dose in CYP2D6 poor metabolizers and to 25% of the usual dose in poor metabolizers receiving a concurrent strong CYP3A4 inhibitor (eg, itraconazole, clarithromycin); subsequently adjust dose for favorable clinical response.

IM, extended release: Reduce aripiprazole dose to 300 mg once monthly in CYP2D6 poor metabolizers; reduce dose to 200 mg once monthly in CYP2D6 poor metabolizers receiving a concurrent CYP3A4 inhibitor for >14 days.

Pediatric Note: Oral solution may be substituted for the oral tablet on a mg-per-mg basis, up to 25 mg. Patients receiving 30 mg tablets should be given 25 mg oral solution. Orally disintegrating tablets (Abilify Discmelt) are bioequivalent to the immediate-release tablets (Abilify).

Bipolar I disorder (acute manic or mixed episodes):

US labeling: Children ≥10 years and Adolescents: Oral: Initial: 2 mg once daily for 2 days, followed by 5 mg once daily for 2 days with a further increase to target dose of 10 mg once daily as monotherapy or as adjunct to lithium or valproic acid; subsequent dose increases may be made in 5 mg increments, up to a maximum of 30 mg/day.

Canadian labeling: Adolescents ≥13 years: Oral: Initial: 2 mg once daily for 2 days, followed by 5 mg once daily for 2 days with a further increase to target dose of 10 mg once daily as monotherapy; subsequent dose increases may be made in 5 mg increments, up to a maximum of 30 mg/day. **Note:** Not approved for maintenance or as adjunctive therapy.

Irritability associated with autistic disorder: Children ≥6 years and Adolescents: Oral: Initial: 2 mg once daily for 7 days, followed by an increase to 5 mg once daily; subsequent dose increases may be made in 5 mg increments at intervals of ≥1 week, up to a maximum of 15 mg/day. The need for ongoing treatment should be assessed periodically.

Schizophrenia: Adolescents ≥13 years (US labeling) or ≥15 years (Canadian labeling): Oral: Initial: 2 mg once daily for 2 days, followed by 5 mg once daily for 2 days with a further increase to target dose of 10 mg once daily; subsequent dose increases may be made in 5 mg increments up to a maximum of 30 mg/day (30 mg/day not shown to be more efficacious than 10 mg/day)

Tourette syndrome: Children ≥6 years and Adolescents: Oral:

<50 kg: Initial: 2 mg/day for 2 days then increase to a target dose of 5 mg/day; may increase dose up to a maximum of 10 mg/day based on response and tolerability; dosage adjustments should occur gradually at intervals of no less than 1 week. Assess the need for ongoing treatment periodically.

≥50 kg: Initial: 2 mg/day for 2 days, then increase to 5 mg/day for 5 days with a target dose of 10 mg/day on day 8; may increase dose up to a maximum of 20 mg/day, based on response and tolerability, in 5 mg/day increments at intervals no less than 1 week. Assess the need for ongoing treatment periodically.

Dosage adjustment with concurrent CYP450 inducer or inhibitor therapy, or adjustment based on CYP2D6 metabolizer status: Refer to adult dosing.

Renal Impairment No dosage adjustment necessary.

Hepatic Impairment No dosage adjustment necessary.

Dietary Considerations Some products may contain phenylalanine.

Administration

Injection: For IM use only; do not administer SubQ or IV; **Note:** Immediate-release and extended-release parenteral products are **not** interchangeable.

Immediate release: Inject slowly into deep muscle mass

Extended release: Inject slowly into deltoid or gluteal muscle using the appropriate provided needle; for non-obese patients, use the 1 inch (25 mm) needle with deltoid administration or the 1.5 inch (38 mm) needle with gluteal administration; for obese patients, use the 1.5 inch (38 mm) needle with deltoid administration or the 2 inch (50 mm) needle with gluteal administration. Do not massage muscle after administration. Rotate injection sites between the two deltoid or gluteal muscles. Administer monthly (doses should be separated by ≥26 days).

Oral: Administer with or without food. Tablet and oral solution may be interchanged on a mg-per-mg basis, up to 25 mg. Doses using 30 mg tablets should be exchanged for 25 mg oral solution. Orally disintegrating tablets (Abilify Discmelt) are bioequivalent to the immediate-release tablets (Abilify).

Orally disintegrating tablet: Remove from foil blister by peeling back (do not push tablet through the foil). Place tablet in mouth immediately upon removal. Tablet dissolves rapidly in saliva and may be swallowed without liquid. If needed, can be taken with liquid. Do not split tablet.

Monitoring Parameters Mental status; vital signs (as clinically indicated); blood pressure (baseline; repeat 3 months after antipsychotic initiation, then yearly); weight, height, BMI, waist circumference (baseline; repeat at 4, 8, and 12 weeks after initiating or changing therapy, then quarterly; consider switching to a different antipsychotic for a weight gain ≥5% of initial weight); CBC (as clinically indicated; monitor frequently during the first few months of therapy in patients with preexisting low WBC or history of drug-induced leukopenia/neutropenia); electrolytes and liver function (annually and as clinically indicated); personal and family history of obesity, diabetes, dyslipidemia, hypertension, or cardiovascular disease (baseline; repeat annually); fasting plasma glucose level/HbA$_{1c}$ (baseline;

repeat 3 months after starting antipsychotic, then yearly); fasting lipid panel (baseline; repeat 3 months after initiation of antipsychotic; if LDL level is normal repeat at 2- to 5-year intervals or more frequently if clinical indicated); changes in menstruation, libido, development of galactorrhea, erectile and ejaculatory function (yearly); abnormal involuntary movements or parkinsonian signs (baseline; repeat weekly until dose stabilized for at least 2 weeks after introduction and for 2 weeks after any significant dose increase); tardive dyskinesia (every 12 months; high-risk patients every 6 months); ocular examination (yearly in patients >40 years; every 2 years in younger patients) (ADA, 2004; Lehman, 2004; Marder, 2004).

Dosage Forms Considerations Oral solution contains fructose 200 mg and sucrose 400 mg per mL.

Dosage Forms Excipient information presented when available (limited, particularly for generics); consult specific product labeling. [DSC] = Discontinued product
Solution, Intramuscular:
Abilify: 9.75 mg/1.3 mL (1.3 mL [DSC])
Solution, Oral:
Abilify: 1 mg/mL (150 mL [DSC]) [contains methylparaben, propylene glycol, propylparaben; orange cream flavor]
Generic: 1 mg/mL (150 mL)
Suspension Reconstituted, Intramuscular:
Abilify Maintena: 300 mg (1 ea); 400 mg (1 ea)
Tablet, Oral:
Abilify: 2 mg
Abilify: 5 mg [contains fd&c blue #2 aluminum lake]
Abilify: 10 mg, 15 mg, 20 mg, 30 mg
Generic: 2 mg, 5 mg, 10 mg, 15 mg, 20 mg, 30 mg
Tablet Dispersible, Oral:
Abilify Discmelt: 10 mg [DSC], 15 mg [DSC] [contains aspartame, fd&c blue #2 aluminum lake]
Generic: 10 mg, 15 mg

Dosage Forms: Canada Note: Refer to Dosage Forms. Dispersible tablet and oral solution are not available in Canada.

ARIPiprazole Lauroxil (ay ri PIP ray zole lawr OX il)

Brand Names: US Aristada
Pharmacologic Category Second Generation (Atypical) Antipsychotic
Use Schizophrenia: Treatment of schizophrenia.
Medication Guide Available Yes>
Dosing
Adult
Schizophrenia: IM: Establish tolerability with oral aripiprazole prior to initiating treatment with aripiprazole lauroxil (may take up to 2 weeks). Base the initial aripiprazole lauroxil dose on the current oral aripiprazole dose and administer in conjunction with oral aripiprazole for 21 consecutive days. Adjust dose as needed; if a dose is required earlier than the recommended interval(s), do not administer <14 days after the previous injection.
Oral aripiprazole 10 mg/day: Initial intramuscular aripiprazole lauroxil dose: 441 mg per month
Oral aripiprazole 15 mg/day: Initial intramuscular aripiprazole lauroxil dose: 662 mg per month
Oral aripiprazole ≥20 mg/day: Initial intramuscular aripiprazole lauroxil dose: 882 mg every 4 or 6 weeks

Missed dose: Administer as soon as possible. Supplementation with oral aripiprazole may be required. In patients who require oral supplementation, administer the same dose of oral aripiprazole that the patient was receiving prior to initiation of aripiprazole lauroxil:
Current dose of aripiprazole lauroxil: 441 mg per month:
Last injection occurred ≤6 weeks ago: Administer aripiprazole lauroxil immediately; no oral aripiprazole supplementation required.
Last injection occurred >6 and ≤7 weeks ago: Administer aripiprazole lauroxil immediately in conjunction with oral aripiprazole supplementation for 7 days.
Last injection occurred >7 weeks ago: Administer aripiprazole lauroxil immediately in conjunction with oral aripiprazole supplementation for 21 days.
Current dose of aripiprazole lauroxil: 662 to 882 mg per month or 882 mg every 6 weeks:
Last injection occurred ≤8 weeks ago: Administer aripiprazole lauroxil immediately; no oral aripiprazole supplement.
Last injection occurred >8 and ≤12 weeks ago: Administer aripiprazole lauroxil immediately in conjunction with oral aripiprazole supplementation for 7 days.
Last injection occurred >12 weeks ago: Administer aripiprazole lauroxil immediately in conjunction with oral aripiprazole supplementation for 21 days.

Dosage adjustment for concomitant therapy (patients stabilized on aripiprazole lauroxil):
CYP450 modulators added for <2 weeks: No dosage adjustment necessary.
Initiation of a strong CYP3A4 inhibitor for ≥2 weeks: Reduce the dose of aripiprazole lauroxil to the next lower strength; in patients receiving 882 mg every 6 weeks, the next lower dose should be 441 mg every 4 weeks. If the patient is a known poor metabolizer of CYP2D6, reduce the aripiprazole lauroxil dose to 441 mg regardless of the current dose. In patients receiving aripiprazole lauroxil 441 mg, no dosage adjustment necessary, if tolerated.
Initiation of a strong CYP2D6 inhibitor for ≥2 weeks: Reduce the dose of aripiprazole lauroxil to the next lower strength; in patients receiving 882 mg every 6 weeks, the next lower dose should be 441 mg every 4 weeks. If the patient is a known poor metabolizer of CYP2D6 or if the patient is receiving aripiprazole lauroxil 441 mg, no dosage adjustment necessary, if tolerated.
Initiation of both a strong CYP3A4 and a strong CYP2D6 inhibitor for ≥2 weeks: Avoid use in patients receiving aripiprazole lauroxil 662 mg or 882 mg. In patients receiving aripiprazole lauroxil 441 mg, no dosage adjustment necessary, if tolerated.
Initiation of CYP3A4 inducer for ≥2 weeks: In patients receiving aripiprazole lauroxil 441 mg, increase the dose to 662 mg. In patients receiving aripiprazole lauroxil 662 mg or 882 mg, no dosage adjustment necessary.

Renal Impairment No dosage adjustment necessary.
Hepatic Impairment No dosage adjustment necessary.
Additional Information Complete prescribing information should be consulted for additional detail.
Dosage Forms Excipient information presented when available (limited, particularly for generics); consult specific product labeling.
Prefilled Syringe, Intramuscular:
Aristada: 441 mg/1.6 mL (1.6 mL); 662 mg/2.4 mL (2.4 mL); 882 mg/3.2 mL (3.2 mL)

◆ Aristada *see* ARIPiprazole Lauroxil *on page* 152

◆ Aristospan (Can) *see* Triamcinolone (Systemic) *on page* 1841

◆ Aristospan Intra-Articular *see* Triamcinolone (Systemic) *on page* 1841

◆ Aristospan Intralesional *see* Triamcinolone (Systemic) *on page* 1841

◆ Arixtra *see* Fondaparinux *on page* 807

Armodafinil (ar moe DAF i nil)

Brand Names: US Nuvigil
Index Terms R-modafinil
Pharmacologic Category Central Nervous System Stimulant
Use
Narcolepsy: To improve wakefulness in patients with excessive sleepiness associated with narcolepsy.
Obstructive sleep apnea: To improve wakefulness in patients with excessive sleepiness associated with obstructive sleep apnea (OSA).
Limitations of use: In OSA, armodafinil is indicated to treat excessive sleepiness and not as treatment for the underlying obstruction. If continuous positive airway pressure (CPAP) is the treatment of choice for a patient, a maximal effort to treat with CPAP for an adequate period of time should be made prior to initiating armodafinil for excessive sleepiness.
Shift-work disorder: To improve wakefulness in patients with excessive sleepiness associated with shift-work disorder.

Pregnancy Considerations Adverse events have been observed in animal reproduction studies. Efficacy of steroidal contraceptives may be decreased; alternate means of contraception should be considered during therapy and for 1 month after armodafinil is discontinued. A pregnancy registry has been established for patients exposed to armodafinil; healthcare providers are encouraged to register pregnant patients or pregnant women may register themselves by calling 1-866-404-4106.
Breast-Feeding Considerations It is not known if armodafinil is excreted into breast milk. The manufacturer recommends that caution be exercised when administering armodafinil to nursing women.
Medication Guide Available Yes
Contraindications Hypersensitivity to armodafinil, modafinil, or any component of the formulation.

Warnings/Precautions For use following complete evaluation of sleepiness and in conjunction with other standard treatments (eg, CPAP). The degree of sleepiness should be reassessed frequently; some patients may not return to a normal level of wakefulness. Patients with excessive sleepiness should be advised to avoid driving or any other potentially dangerous activity. Use >12 weeks has not been studied; patient should be reevaluated to determine effectiveness if use exceeds 12 weeks. Use is not recommended in patients with a history of angina or myocardial infarction, left ventricular hypertrophy, or patients with mitral valve prolapse who have developed mitral valve prolapse syndrome with previous CNS stimulant use. Patients with these conditions may also experience chest pain, palpitations, dyspnea, and transient ischemic T-wave changes on ECG. Increased blood pressure monitoring may be required in patients taking armodafinil. New or additional antihypertensive therapy may be needed.

Serious and life-threatening rashes including Stevens-Johnson syndrome, toxic epidermal necrolysis, and drug rash with eosinophilia and systemic symptoms (DRESS) have been reported. In modafinil clinical trials, rashes were more likely to occur in children; serious, postmarketing reactions have occurred with modafinil in adults and children as well as with armodafinil in adults. Most cases have been reported within the first 5 weeks of initiating therapy; however, rare cases have occurred after prolonged therapy. No risk factors have been identified to predict occurrence or severity of these reactions. Patients should be advised to discontinue use at first sign of rash (unless the rash is clearly not drug-related). Rare cases of multiorgan hypersensitivity reactions (with modafinil) and cases of angioedema and anaphylactoid reactions (armodafinil) have been reported. Signs and symptoms of multiorgan hypersensitivity reactions are diverse. Patients typically present with fever and rash associated with other organ system involvement. Patients should be advised to discontinue therapy and promptly report any signs or symptoms related to these adverse effects.

Caution should be exercised when modafinil is given to patients with a history of psychosis, depression, or mania; use may worsen symptoms (eg, mania, hallucinations, suicidal thoughts) of these disease; discontinue therapy if psychiatric symptoms develop. Use may impair the ability to engage in potentially hazardous activities; patients must be cautioned about performing tasks which require mental alertness (eg, operating machinery, driving). Use caution with hepatic impairment; consider use of a reduced dosage in patients with hepatic impairment or elderly patients. Use with caution in patients with a history of drug abuse; potential for drug dependency exists. Instruct patients to avoid concomitant ethanol consumption.

Adverse Reactions
>10%: Central nervous system: Headache (14% to 23%; dose related)
1% to 10%:
Cardiovascular: Palpitations (2%), increased heart rate (1%)
Central nervous system: Insomnia (4% to 6%; dose related), dizziness (5%), anxiety (4%), depression (1% to 3%; dose related), fatigue (2%), agitation (1%), depressed mood (1%), lack of concentration (1%), migraine (1%), nervousness (1%), pain (1%), paresthesia (1%)
Dermatologic: Skin rash (1% to 4%; dose related), contact dermatitis (1%), diaphoresis (1%)
Endocrine & metabolic: Increased gamma-glutamyl transferase (1%), increased thirst (1%)
Gastrointestinal: Nausea (6% to 9%; dose related), xerostomia (2% to 7%; dose related), diarrhea (4%), dyspepsia (2%), upper abdominal pain (2%), anorexia (1%), constipation (1%), decreased appetite (1%), loose stools (1%), vomiting (1%)
Hypersensitivity: Seasonal allergy (1%)
Neuromuscular & skeletal: Tremor (1%)
Renal: Polyuria (1%)
Respiratory: Dyspnea (1%), flu-like symptoms (1%)
Miscellaneous: Fever (1%)
<1% (Limited to important but life-threatening): Anaphylaxis, angioedema, DRESS syndrome, hypersensitivity, hypouricemia, increased liver enzymes, increased serum alkaline phosphatase, pancytopenia, Stevens-Johnson syndrome, suicidal ideation, systolic hypertension, toxic epidermal necrolysis

Drug Interactions
Metabolism/Transport Effects Substrate of CYP3A4 (major); **Note:** Assignment of Major/Minor substrate status based on clinically relevant drug interaction potential; **Inhibits** CYP2C19 (moderate); **Induces** CYP3A4 (weak)

Avoid Concomitant Use
Avoid concomitant use of Armodafinil with any of the following: Conivaptan; Fusidic Acid (Systemic); Idelalisib; Iobenguane I 123
Increased Effect/Toxicity
Armodafinil may increase the levels/effects of: Cilostazol; Citalopram; CYP2C19 Substrates; Doxofylline; Sympathomimetics

The levels/effects of Armodafinil may be increased by: Aprepitant; AtoMOXetine; Cannabinoid-Containing Products; Conivaptan; CYP3A4 Inhibitors (Moderate); CYP3A4 Inhibitors (Strong); Dasatinib; Fosaprepitant; Fusidic Acid (Systemic); Idelalisib; Ivacaftor; Linezolid; Luliconazole; Mifepristone; Netupitant; Osimertinib; Palbociclib; Simeprevir; Stiripentol; Tedizolid
Decreased Effect
Armodafinil may decrease the levels/effects of: ARIPiprazole; Clopidogrel; Contraceptives (Estrogens); CycloSPORINE (Systemic); Hydrocodone; Iobenguane I 123; NiMODipine; Saxagliptin

The levels/effects of Armodafinil may be decreased by: Bosentan; CYP3A4 Inducers (Moderate); CYP3A4 Inducers (Strong); Dabrafenib; Deferasirox; Enzalutamide; Mitotane; Osimertinib; Siltuximab; St Johns Wort; Tocilizumab

Food Interactions Food delays absorption, but minimal effects on bioavailability. Food may affect the onset and time course of armodafinil. Management: Administer without regard to meals.

Storage/Stability Store at 20°C to 25°C (68°F to 77°F).

Mechanism of Action The exact mechanism of action of armodafinil is unknown. It is the R-enantiomer of modafinil. Armodafinil binds to the dopamine transporter and inhibits dopamine reuptake, which may result in increased extracellular dopamine levels in the brain. However, it does not appear to be a dopamine receptor agonist and also does not appear to bind to or inhibit the most common receptors or enzymes that are relevant for sleep/wake regulation.

Pharmacodynamics/Kinetics
Absorption: Readily absorbed
Distribution: V_d: 42 L
Protein binding: ~60% (based on modafinil; primarily albumin)
Metabolism: Hepatic, multiple pathways, including amine hydrolysis and CYP3A4/5; metabolites include R-modafinil acid and modafinil sulfone
Half-life elimination: ~15 hours
Time to peak, plasma: 2 hours (fasted)
Excretion: Urine (based on modafinil: 80% predominantly as metabolites; <10% as unchanged drug)

Dosing
Adult
Narcolepsy: Oral: 150 to 250 mg once daily in the morning
Obstructive sleep apnea (OSA): Oral: 150 to 250 mg once daily in the morning; doses >150 mg have not been shown to have an increased benefit.
Shift-work disorder: Oral: 150 mg given once daily ~1 hour prior to work shift
Geriatric Refer to adult dosing. Consider lower initial dosage. Concentrations were almost doubled in clinical trials (based on modafinil).
Renal Impairment There are no dosage adjustments provided in the manufacturer's labeling.
Hepatic Impairment
Mild to moderate hepatic impairment: No dosage adjustment necessary.
Severe hepatic impairment: The manufacturer recommends a reduced dose; clearance of modafinil is decreased by ~60% and the steady-state concentration is doubled in this patient population.

Dietary Considerations Take with or without meals.
Administration May be administered without regard to food.
Monitoring Parameters Signs of hypersensitivity, rash, psychiatric symptoms, levels of sleepiness, blood pressure, and drug abuse
Dosage Forms Excipient information presented when available (limited, particularly for generics); consult specific product labeling.
Tablet, Oral:
Nuvigil: 50 mg, 150 mg, 200 mg, 250 mg
Controlled Substance C-IV

Arsenic Trioxide (AR se nik tri OKS id)

Brand Names: US Trisenox
Brand Names: Canada Trisenox
Index Terms Arsenic (III) Oxide; As_2O_3; ATO
Pharmacologic Category Antineoplastic Agent, Miscellaneous
Use Acute promyelocytic leukemia: Remission induction and consolidation in patients with acute promyelocytic leukemia (APL) who are refractory to, or have relapsed from, retinoid and anthracycline chemotherapy, and whose APL is characterized by the presence of the t(15;17) translocation or PML/RAR-alpha gene expression

Dosing

Adult Note: Arsenic trioxide is associated with a moderate emetic potential; antiemetics are recommended to prevent nausea and vomiting.

Acute promyelocytic leukemia (APL), relapsed or refractory: IV:
Induction: 0.15 mg/kg once daily until bone marrow remission; maximum: 60 doses for induction
Consolidation: 0.15 mg/kg once daily starting 3 to 6 weeks after completion of induction therapy; maximum: 25 doses over a period of up to 5 weeks for consolidation

APL, newly diagnosed (off-label use): IV:
Low/intermediate risk (Lo-Coco 2013):
Induction: 0.15 mg/kg/day; administer daily until bone marrow remission (in combination with tretinoin)
Consolidation: 0.15 mg/kg/day; administer 5 days/week for 4 weeks every 8 weeks for a total of 4 cycles (in combination with tretinoin)
High-risk:
Consolidation therapy after remission induction with tretinoin, daunorubicin and cytarabine (Powell 2010): Two consolidation courses (2 weeks apart): 0.15 mg/kg/day 5 days/week for 5 weeks
In combination with tretinoin in patients unable to tolerate anthracycline-based therapy (Estey 2006; Ravandi 2009):
Induction (beginning 10 days after initiation of tretinoin): 0.15 mg/kg/day until bone marrow remission; maximum: 75 doses for induction
Consolidation: 0.15 mg/kg/day Monday through Friday for 4 weeks every 8 weeks for 4 cycles (weeks 1 to 4, 9 to 12, 17 to 20, and 25 to 28)
APML 4 protocol (Iland 2012):
Induction: 0.15 mg/kg/day over 2 hours on days 9 to 36 (in combination with tretinoin and age-adjusted idarubicin)
Consolidation (2 cycles): 0.15 mg/kg/day on days 1 to 28 of consolidation cycle 1 (in combination with tretinoin); 0.15 mg/kg/day on days 1 to 5, 8 to 12, 15 to 19, 22 to 26, and 29 to 33 of consolidation cycle 2 (in combination with tretinoin)

Pediatric Note: Arsenic trioxide is associated with a moderate emetic potential; antiemetics are recommended to prevent nausea and vomiting (Dupuis 2011).

Acute promyelocytic leukemia (APL), relapsed or refractory: Children ≥4 years (US labeling) or ≥5 years (Canadian labeling): IV: Refer to adult dosing. **Note:** The Canadian labeling recommends dosing obese pediatric patients based on ideal body weight.

APL, newly diagnosed (off-label use): IV:
Induction, consolidation, and maintenance (Mathews 2006):
Induction: 0.15 mg/kg/day (maximum dose: 10 mg); administer daily until bone marrow remission; maximum: 60 doses for induction
Consolidation: 0.15 mg/kg/day (maximum dose: 10 mg) for 4 weeks, starting 4 weeks after completion of induction therapy
Maintenance: 0.15 mg/kg/dose (maximum dose: 10 mg) administered 10 days per month for 6 months, starting 4 weeks after completion of consolidation therapy
Children >1 year and Adolescents (APML 4 protocol; Iland 2012):
Induction: 0.15 mg/kg/day over 2 hours on days 9 to 36 (in combination with tretinoin and idarubicin)
Consolidation (2 cycles): 0.15 mg/kg/day on days 1 to 28 of consolidation cycle 1 (in combination with tretinoin); 0.15 mg/kg/day on days 1 to 5, 8 to 12, 15 to 19, 22 to 26, and 29 to 33 of consolidation cycle 2 (in combination with tretinoin)

Renal Impairment
Mild-to-moderate impairment (CrCl ≥30 mL/minute): There are no dosage adjustments provided in the manufacturer's labeling.

Severe renal impairment (CrCl <30 mL/minute): Use with caution (systemic exposure to metabolites may be higher); may require dosage reduction; monitor closely for toxicity.
Dialysis patients: There are no dosage adjustments provided in the manufacturer's labeling (has not been studied).

Hepatic Impairment There are no dosage adjustments provided in the manufacturer's labeling; use with caution. Patients with severe impairment (Child-Pugh class C) should be monitored closely for toxicity.

Adjustment for Toxicity Consider delaying infusion if a severe non-hematologic reaction occurs (eg, neurologic or dermatologic toxicity) until the toxicity has improved to ≤ grade 1.

Additional Information Complete prescribing information should be consulted for additional detail.

Dosage Forms Excipient information presented when available (limited, particularly for generics); consult specific product labeling.
Solution, Intravenous:
Trisenox: 10 mg/10 mL (10 mL)

♦ Artane *see* Trihexyphenidyl *on page 1846*
♦ Artemether and Benflumetol *see* Artemether and Lumefantrine *on page 154*

Artemether and Lumefantrine (ar TEM e ther & loo me FAN treen)

Brand Names: US Coartem
Index Terms Artemether and Benflumetol; Benflumetol and Artemether; Lumefantrine and Artemether
Pharmacologic Category Antimalarial Agent
Use Treatment of acute, uncomplicated malaria infections due to *Plasmodium falciparum*, including geographical regions where chloroquine resistance has been reported

Dosing

Adult Treatment of uncomplicated malaria: Three-day schedule: Oral:
Patients 25 to <35 kg: Three tablets at hour 0 and hour 8 on the first day, then 3 tablets twice daily on day 2 and day 3 (total of 18 tablets per treatment course)
Patients ≥35 kg: Four tablets at hour 0 and hour 8 on the first day, then 4 tablets twice daily on day 2 and day 3 (total of 24 tablets per treatment course)

Geriatric Refer to adult dosing:

Pediatric Treatment of uncomplicated malaria: Three-day schedule: Oral:
Children 2 months to ≤16 years:
5 to <15 kg: One tablet at hour 0 and hour 8 on the first day, then 1 tablet twice daily on day 2 and day 3 (total of 6 tablets per treatment course)
15 to <25 kg: Two tablets at hour 0 and hour 8 on the first day, then 2 tablets twice daily on day 2 and day 3 (total of 12 tablets per treatment course)
25 to <35 kg: Three tablets at hour 0 and hour 8 on the first day, then 3 tablets twice daily on day 2 and day 3 (total of 18 tablets per treatment course)
≥35 kg: Four tablets at hour 0 and hour 8 on the first day, then 4 tablets twice daily on day 2 and day 3 (total of 24 tablets per treatment course)
Children >16 years: Refer to adult dosing.

Renal Impairment Dosage adjustments are not recommended in mild or moderate impairment. Use caution in severe impairment (has not been studied).

Hepatic Impairment Dosage adjustments are not recommended in mild or moderate impairment. Use caution in severe impairment (has not been studied).

Additional Information Complete prescribing information should be consulted for additional detail.

Dosage Forms Excipient information presented when available (limited, particularly for generics); consult specific product labeling.
Tablet:
Coartem: Artemether 20 mg and lumefantrine 120 mg

♦ Artemisinin Derivative *see* Artesunate *on page 154*

Artesunate (ar TES oo nate)

Index Terms Artemisinin Derivative; Artesunic Acid; Dihydroartemisinin Hemisuccinate Sodium; Dihydroqinghaosu Hemisuccinate Sodium; Nuartez; P01BE03; Qinghao Derivative; Qinghaosu Derivative; Sodium Artesunate
Pharmacologic Category Antimalarial Agent; Artemisinin Derivative

Prescribing and Access Restrictions Investigational agent – not approved for use in the U.S.

Artesunate is available in the U.S. for IV use in patients with malaria through an Investigational New Drug (IND) protocol. To obtain artesunate via the IND protocol, clinicians must contact the Centers for Disease Control (CDC) Malaria Hotline at 770-488-7788 (business hours) or 770-488-7100 (nonbusiness hours) and request to speak with a CDC Malaria Branch clinician.

Eligibility criteria under the IND protocol include (Callender 2011; Hess 2010):
- **Patients must have malaria:** Confirmation by microscopy or undetermined but strong clinical suspicion of *Plasmodium falciparum* or other *Plasmodium* spp. infection
- **Patients must require parenteral therapy:** Unable to take oral medications, high-density parasitemia (eg, >5%), or diagnosis of severe malaria (eg, seizures, shock, hemoglobin <7 g/dL, disseminated intravascular coagulation, or acute respiratory distress syndrome [ARDS]).
- **IV artesunate must be the preferred treatment:** IV artesunate is at least as readily available as IV quinidine or the patient has experienced quinidine failure (eg, parasitemia >10% baseline after 48 hours of quinidine therapy), quinidine intolerance (eg, persistent hypotension, QRS prolongation >50% of baseline or QTc interval prolongation >25% of baseline), or contraindications to quinidine (eg, allergy, left bundle branch block, myasthenia gravis, digoxin toxicity).

For medical access to IV artesunate in Canada, please refer to special access information on the Public Health Agency of Canada website, http://www.phac-aspc.gc.ca/tmp-pmv/quinine/.

Dosing

Adult & Geriatric Treatment of severe malaria: IV: 2.4 mg/kg/dose initially, followed by 2.4 mg/kg/dose at 12 hours, 24 hours, and 48 hours after the initial dose for a total of 4 doses over a period of 3 days; longer treatment duration (eg, an additional 4 days [Hess 2010]) may be required in severely-ill patients or in patients unable to transition to oral therapy (Hess 2010; Rosenthal 2008). Transition to oral therapy at least 4 hours after the last dose of artesunate. Appropriate oral therapies include atovaquone-proguanil, doxycycline (in patients >8 years of age and nonpregnant adults), clindamycin, **or** mefloquine (CDC 2009; CDC 2014; Hess 2010; Rosenthal 2008).

Pediatric Refer to adult dosing.

Renal Impairment No dosage adjustment necessary (Rosenthal 2008), use with caution (WHO 2015).

Hepatic Impairment No dosage adjustment necessary (Rosenthal 2008), use with caution (WHO 2015).

Additional Information Complete prescribing information should be consulted for additional detail.

Dosage Forms Excipient information presented when available (limited, particularly for generics); consult specific product labeling.
Solution Reconstituted, Injection: 110 mg [phosphate buffer solution provided as diluent]

Ascorbic Acid (a SKOR bik AS id)

Brand Names: US Acerola C 500 [OTC]; Asco-Tabs-1000 [OTC]; Ascocid [OTC]; Ascocid-ISO-pH [OTC]; Ascor L 500 [OTC]; Ascor L NC [DSC]; BProtected Vitamin C [OTC]; C-500 [OTC]; C-Time [OTC]; Cemill SR [OTC]; Cemill [OTC]; Chew-C [OTC]; Fruit C 500 [OTC]; Fruit C [OTC]; Fruity C [OTC]; Mega-C/A Plus; Ortho-CS 250; Vita-C [OTC]

Brand Names: Canada Ascor L 500; Vitamin C

Index Terms Vitamin C

Pharmacologic Category Vitamin, Water Soluble

Use

Ascorbic acid deficiency: Treatment of symptoms of mild deficiency; use in conditions requiring an increased intake (eg, burns, wound healing)

Dietary supplement: As a dietary vitamin C supplement

Scurvy: Prevention and treatment of scurvy

Dosing

Adult & Geriatric

Recommended daily allowance (RDA) (IOM, 2000): Upper limit of intake should not exceed 2,000 mg daily
Males: 90 mg daily
Females: 75 mg daily
Pregnant females:
19 to 50 years: 85 mg daily; upper limit of intake should not exceed 2,000 mg daily
Lactating females:
19 to 50 years: 120 mg daily; upper limit of intake should not exceed 2,000 mg daily
Adult smoker: Add an additional 35 mg daily

Ascorbic acid deficiency: IM, IV, SubQ: 70 to 150 mg daily is an average protective dose; doses 3 to 5 times the RDA may be adequate for conditions with increased requirements.
Burns: IM, IV, SubQ: 1 to 2 g daily for severe burns; dose may be determined by extent of tissue injury
Wound healing: IM, IV, SubQ: 300 to 500 mg daily for 7 to 10 days pre- and post-operatively; larger doses have also been used

Scurvy:
IM, IV, SubQ: 300 to 1,000 mg daily; dose and duration of therapy should be individualized; doses up to 6 g per day have been administered (per manufacturer).
Oral: 100 to 300 mg daily until body stores are replenished; dose and duration of therapy should be individualized; doses as low as 10 mg may be effective (Hirschmann, 1999; Popovich, 2009; Weinstein, 2001).

Pediatric

Recommended adequate intake (AI) (IOM, 2000):
0 to 6 months: 40 mg daily
7 to 12 months: 50 mg daily

Recommended daily allowance (RDA) (IOM, 2000):
1 to 3 years: 15 mg daily; upper limit of intake should not exceed 400 mg daily
4 to 8 years: 25 mg daily; upper limit of intake should not exceed 650 mg daily
9 to 13 years: 45 mg daily; upper limit of intake should not exceed 1,200 mg daily
14 to 18 years: Upper limit of intake should not exceed 1,800 mg daily
Males: 75 mg daily
Females: 65 mg daily
Pregnant females: 80 mg daily; upper limit of intake should not exceed 1,800 mg daily
Lactating females: 115 mg daily; upper limit of intake should not exceed 1,800 mg daily

Scurvy: Oral: 100 to 300 mg daily until body stores are replenished; dose and duration of therapy should be individualized (Popovich, 2009; Weinstein, 2001)

Additional Information Complete prescribing information should be consulted for additional detail.

Dosage Forms Excipient information presented when available (limited, particularly for generics); consult specific product labeling. [DSC] = Discontinued product
Capsule Extended Release, Oral:
C-Time: 500 mg
Generic: 500 mg
Capsule Extended Release, Oral [preservative free]:
Generic: 500 mg
Crystals, Oral:
Vita-C: (120 g, 480 g) [animal products free, gelatin free, gluten free, lactose free, no artificial color(s), no artificial flavor(s), starch free, sugar free, yeast free]
Granules, Oral:
Generic: (1 g [DSC], 25 g [DSC], 100 g [DSC], 500 g [DSC], 1000 g [DSC], 5000 g [DSC], 12000 g [DSC])
Liquid, Oral:
BProtected Vitamin C: 500 mg/5 mL (236 mL) [contains propylene glycol, saccharin sodium, sodium benzoate; citrus flavor]
Generic: 500 mg/5 mL (473 mL)
Powder, Oral:
Ascocid: (227 g)
Generic: (113 g, 120 g, 480 g)

Powder Effervescent, Oral:
Ascocid-ISO-pH: (150 g) [corn free, rye free, wheat free]
Solution, Injection:
Generic: 500 mg/mL (50 mL)
Solution, Injection [preservative free]:
Ascor L 500: 500 mg/mL (50 mL)
Ascor L NC: 500 mg/mL (50 mL [DSC]) [corn free]
Mega-C/A Plus: 500 mg/mL (50 mL)
Solution, Injection, as sodium ascorbate [preservative free]:
Ortho-CS 250: 250 mg/mL (100 mL) [contains edetate disodium, water, sterile]
Generic: 250 mg/mL (30 mL)
Syrup, Oral:
Generic: 500 mg/5 mL (118 mL, 473 mL [DSC])
Tablet, Oral:
Asco-Tabs-1000: 1000 mg [color free, starch free, sugar free]
Generic: 100 mg, 250 mg, 500 mg, 1000 mg
Tablet, Oral [preservative free]:
Generic: 250 mg, 500 mg
Tablet Chewable, Oral:
Chew-C: 500 mg
Fruit C 500: 500 mg [animal products free, gelatin free, gluten free, kosher certified, lactose free, no artificial color(s), no artificial flavor(s), starch free, sugar free, yeast free]
Fruit C: 100 mg [animal products free, gelatin free, gluten free, lactose free, no artificial color(s), no artificial flavor(s), starch free, sugar free, yeast free]
Fruity C: 250 mg
Generic: 100 mg, 250 mg, 500 mg
Tablet Chewable, Oral [preservative free]:
C-500: 500 mg [animal products free, gluten free, soy free, starch free, yeast free]
Generic: 500 mg
Tablet Extended Release, Oral:
Cemill: 500 mg
Cemill SR: 1000 mg
Generic: 500 mg, 1000 mg, 1500 mg
Tablet Extended Release, Oral [preservative free]:
Generic: 1000 mg [DSC]
Wafer, Oral [preservative free]:
Acerola C 500: 500 mg (50 ea) [corn free, no artificial color(s), no artificial flavor(s), wheat free, yeast free; contains acerola (malpighia glabra)]

♦ Asco-Tabs-1000 [OTC] see Ascorbic Acid on page 155
♦ Ascriptin Maximum Strength [OTC] see Aspirin on page 157
♦ Ascriptin Regular Strength [OTC] see Aspirin on page 157

Asenapine (a SEN a peen)

Brand Names: US Saphris
Brand Names: Canada Saphris
Pharmacologic Category Antimanic Agent; Second Generation (Atypical) Antipsychotic
Use
Bipolar disorder: Treatment of acute manic or mixed episodes associated with bipolar I disorder (as monotherapy or adjunctive treatment with lithium or valproate)
Schizophrenia: Treatment of schizophrenia
Dosing
Adult & Geriatric Note: Safety of doses >20 mg/day has not been evaluated:
Schizophrenia: Sublingual: Initial: 5 mg twice daily; may increase to 10 mg twice daily after 1 week based on tolerability; maximum dose: 10 mg twice daily. Daily doses ≥20 mg/day in clinical trials did not appear to offer any additional benefit and had an increased risk of adverse effects.
Bipolar disorder: Sublingual:
Monotherapy: Initial: 10 mg twice daily; decrease to 5 mg twice daily if dose not tolerated; maximum dose: 10 mg twice daily.
Combination therapy (with lithium or valproate): Initial: 5 mg twice daily; may increase to 10 mg twice daily based on tolerability; maximum dose: 10 mg twice daily.
Pediatric Note: Safety of doses >20 mg/day has not been evaluated.
Bipolar disorder: Children ≥10 years and Adolescents ≤17 years: Sublingual: Monotherapy: Initial: 2.5 mg twice daily; may increase dose after 3 days to 5 mg twice daily, then after an additional 3 days to 10 mg twice daily based on tolerability (pediatric patients appear to be more sensitive to dystonia with initial dosing when the escalation schedule is not followed); maximum dose: 10 mg twice daily.
Renal Impairment No dosage adjustment necessary.

Hepatic Impairment
Mild-to-moderate hepatic impairment (Child-Pugh class A or B): No dosage adjustment necessary.
Severe hepatic impairment (Child-Pugh class C): Use is contraindicated.
Additional Information Complete prescribing information should be consulted for additional detail.
Dosage Forms Excipient information presented when available (limited, particularly for generics); consult specific product labeling.
Tablet Sublingual, Sublingual:
Saphris: 2.5 mg [black cherry flavor]
Saphris: 5 mg
Saphris: 5 mg [black cherry flavor]
Saphris: 10 mg
Saphris: 10 mg [black cherry flavor]

♦ Asendin [DSC] see Amoxapine on page 106
♦ Ashlyna see Ethinyl Estradiol and Levonorgestrel on page 703
♦ AsmalPred [DSC] see PrednisoLONE (Systemic) on page 1493
♦ AsmalPred Plus [DSC] see PrednisoLONE (Systemic) on page 1493
♦ Asmanex 7 Metered Doses see Mometasone (Oral Inhalation) on page 1225
♦ Asmanex 14 Metered Doses see Mometasone (Oral Inhalation) on page 1225
♦ Asmanex 30 Metered Doses see Mometasone (Oral Inhalation) on page 1225
♦ Asmanex 60 Metered Doses see Mometasone (Oral Inhalation) on page 1225
♦ Asmanex 120 Metered Doses see Mometasone (Oral Inhalation) on page 1225
♦ Asmanex HFA see Mometasone (Oral Inhalation) on page 1225
♦ Asmanex Twisthaler (Can) see Mometasone (Oral Inhalation) on page 1225

Asparaginase (Erwinia)
(a SPEAR a ji nase er WIN i ah)

Brand Names: US Erwinaze
Brand Names: Canada Erwinase
Index Terms Erwinia chrysanthemi; Asparaginase Erwinia chrysanthemi; L-asparaginase (Erwinia)
Pharmacologic Category Antineoplastic Agent, Enzyme; Antineoplastic Agent, Miscellaneous
Use Acute lymphoblastic leukemia: Treatment (in combination with other chemotherapy) of acute lymphoblastic leukemia (ALL) in patients with hypersensitivity to E. coli-derived asparaginase
Prescribing and Access Restrictions Erwinaze is distributed through Accredo Health Group, Inc. (1-877-900-9223).
Dosing
Adult Note: If administering IV, consider monitoring nadir serum asparaginase activity (NSAA) levels; if desired levels are not achieved, change to IM administration.
Acute lymphoblastic leukemia (ALL): IM, IV:
As a substitute for pegaspargase: 25,000 units/m² 3 times weekly (Mon, Wed, Fri) for 6 doses for each planned pegaspargase dose
As a substitute for asparaginase (E. coli): 25,000 units/m² for each scheduled asparaginase (E. coli) dose
ALL induction: Canadian labeling (not in the U.S. labeling): SubQ: 10,000 units/m² days 1, 3, and 5 of week 4 and day 1 of week 5 (in combination with prednisolone, vincristine, mercaptopurine, and methotrexate) **or** 10,000 units/m² 3 times weekly (starting week 4) for 4 weeks (in combination with prednisolone, vincristine, and daunorubicin)
Pediatric Note: If administering IV, consider monitoring nadir serum asparaginase activity (NSAA) levels; if desired levels are not achieved, change to IM administration.
Acute lymphoblastic leukemia (ALL): Children ≥1 year and Adolescents: IM, IV: Refer to adult dosing.
ALL induction: Canadian labeling (not in the U.S. labeling):
Children <14 years: IM: 6,000 units/m² 3 times weekly for 9 doses beginning day 4 of week 1 (in combination with vincristine, prednisone, methotrexate, and daunorubicin)
Children >14 years: SubQ: Refer to adult dosing.
Renal Impairment There are no dosage adjustments provided in the manufacturer's labeling.

Hepatic Impairment There are no dosage adjustments provided in the manufacturer's labeling; however, the following adjustments have been recommended for other asparaginase products for hepatotoxicity during treatment (Stock 2011):

ALT/AST >3 to 5 times ULN: Continue therapy

ALT/AST >5 to 20 times ULN: Delay next dose until transaminases <3 times ULN

ALT/AST >20 times ULN: Discontinue therapy if takes longer than 1 week for transaminases to return to <3 times ULN.

Direct bilirubin <3 mg/dL: Continue therapy

Direct bilirubin 3.1 to 5 mg/dL: Hold asparaginase and resume when direct bilirubin <2 mg/dL; consider switching to alternate asparaginase product.

Direct bilirubin >5 mg/dL: Discontinue asparaginase; do not substitute other asparaginase products; do not make up for missed doses.

Adjustment for Toxicity

Hemorrhagic or thrombotic event: Discontinue treatment; may resume treatment upon symptom resolution.

Pancreatitis:

Mild pancreatitis: Withhold treatment until signs and symptoms subside and amylase levels return to normal; may resume after resolution.

Severe or hemorrhagic pancreatitis (abdominal pain >72 hours and amylase ≥2 x ULN): Discontinue treatment; further use is contraindicated.

Serious hypersensitivity reaction: Discontinue treatment.

The following adjustments have also been recommended for asparaginase products (Stock 2011):

Hyperammonemia-related fatigue: Continue therapy for grade 2 toxicity. If grade 3 toxicity occurs, reduce dose by 25%; resume full dose when toxicity ≤ grade 2 (make up for missed doses). If grade 4 toxicity occurs, reduce dose by 50%; resume full dose when toxicity ≤ grade 2 (make up for missed doses).

Hyperglycemia: Continue therapy for uncomplicated hyperglycemia. If hyperglycemia requires insulin therapy, hold asparaginase (and any concomitant corticosteroids) until blood glucose controlled; resume dosing at prior dose level. For life-threatening hyperglycemia or toxicity requiring urgent intervention, hold asparaginase (and corticosteroids) until blood glucose is controlled with insulin; resume asparaginase and do not make up for missed doses.

Hypersensitivity reactions: May continue dosing for urticaria without bronchospasm, hypotension, edema, or need for parenteral intervention. If wheezing or other symptomatic bronchospasm with or without urticaria, angioedema, hypotension, and/or life-threatening hypersensitivity reactions occur, discontinue asparaginase.

Hypertriglyceridemia: If serum triglyceride level <1000 mg/dL, continue asparaginase but monitor closely for pancreatitis. If triglyceride level >1,000 mg/dL, hold asparaginase and monitor; resume therapy at prior dose level after triglyceride level returns to baseline.

Pancreatitis:

Asymptomatic amylase or lipase >3 times ULN (chemical pancreatitis) or radiologic abnormalities only: Continue asparaginase and monitor levels closely.

Symptomatic amylase or lipase >3 times ULN: Hold asparaginase until enzyme levels stabilize or are declining.

Symptomatic pancreatitis or clinical pancreatitis (abdominal pain with amylase or lipase >3 times ULN for >3 days and/or development of pancreatic pseudocyst): Permanently discontinue asparaginase.

Thrombosis and bleeding, CNS:

Thrombosis: Continue therapy for abnormal laboratory findings without a clinical correlate. If grade 3 toxicity occurs, discontinue therapy; if CNS signs/symptoms are fully resolved and further asparaginase doses are required, may resume therapy at a lower dose and/or longer intervals between doses. Discontinue therapy for grade 4 toxicity.

Hemorrhage: Discontinue therapy; do not withhold therapy for abnormal laboratory findings without a clinical correlate. If grade 3 toxicity occurs, discontinue therapy; if CNS signs/symptoms are fully resolved and further asparaginase doses are required, may resume therapy at a lower dose and/or longer intervals between doses. Discontinue therapy for grade 4 toxicity.

Thrombosis and bleeding, non-CNS:

Thrombosis: Continue therapy for abnormal laboratory findings without a clinical correlate. If grade 3 or 4 toxicity occurs, withhold therapy until acute toxicity and clinical signs resolve and anticoagulant therapy

is stable or completed. Do not withhold therapy for abnormal laboratory findings without clinical correlate.

Hemorrhage: If grade 2 bleeding in conjunction with hypofibrinogenemia occurs, withhold therapy until bleeding ≤ grade 1. Do not withhold therapy for abnormal laboratory findings without clinical correlate. For grade 3 or 4 bleeding, withhold therapy until bleeding ≤ grade 1 and until acute toxicity and clinical signs resolve and coagulant replacement therapy is stable or completed.

Additional Information Complete prescribing information should be consulted for additional detail.

Dosage Forms Excipient information presented when available (limited, particularly for generics); consult specific product labeling.

Solution Reconstituted, Intramuscular:

Erwinaze: 10,000 units (1 ea)

◆ Asparaginase *Erwinia chrysanthemi see* Asparaginase (*Erwinia*) *on page 156*

◆ Aspart Insulin *see* Insulin Aspart *on page 952*

◆ Aspercin [OTC] *see* Aspirin *on page 157*

◆ Aspergillus niger *see* Alpha-Galactosidase *on page 76*

Aspirin (AS pir in)

Brand Names: US Ascriptin Maximum Strength [OTC]; Ascriptin Regular Strength [OTC]; Aspercin [OTC]; Aspirlow [OTC]; Aspirtab [OTC]; Bayer Aspirin Extra Strength [OTC]; Bayer Aspirin Regimen Adult Low Strength [OTC]; Bayer Aspirin Regimen Children's [OTC]; Bayer Aspirin Regimen Regular Strength [OTC]; Bayer Genuine Aspirin [OTC]; Bayer Plus Extra Strength [OTC]; Bayer Women's Low Dose Aspirin [OTC]; Buffasal [OTC]; Bufferin Extra Strength [OTC]; Bufferin [OTC]; Buffinol [OTC]; Durlaza; Ecotrin Arthritis Strength [OTC]; Ecotrin Low Strength [OTC]; Ecotrin [OTC]; Halfprin [OTC]; St Joseph Adult Aspirin [OTC]; Tri-Buffered Aspirin [OTC]

Brand Names: Canada Asaphen; Asaphen E.C.; Entrophen; Novasen; Praxis ASA EC 81 Mg Daily Dose; Pro-AAS EC-80

Index Terms Acetylsalicylic Acid; ASA; Baby Aspirin

Pharmacologic Category Antiplatelet Agent; Salicylate

Additional Appendix Information

Oral Antiplatelet Comparison Chart *on page 1963*

Use

Immediate release:

Analgesic/Antipyretic: For the temporary relief of headache, pain, and fever caused by colds, muscle aches and pains, menstrual pain, toothache pain, and minor aches and pains of arthritis.

Revascularization procedures: In patients who have undergone revascularization procedures (ie, coronary artery bypass graft [CABG], percutaneous transluminal coronary angioplasty, or carotid endarterectomy).

Rheumatoid disease: For the relief of the signs and symptoms of rheumatoid arthritis (RA), juvenile idiopathic arthritis (formerly called juvenile RA), osteoarthritis, spondyloarthropathies, and arthritis and pleurisy associated with systemic lupus erythematosus.

Vascular indications (ischemic stroke, transient ischemic attack, acute myocardial infarction, prevention of recurrent myocardial infarction, unstable angina, and chronic stable angina): To reduce the combined risk of death and nonfatal stroke in patients who have had ischemic stroke or transient ischemia of the brain due to fibrin platelet emboli; to reduce the risk of vascular mortality in patients with a suspected acute myocardial infarction (MI); to reduce the combined risk of death and nonfatal MI in patients with a previous MI or unstable angina; to reduce the combined risk of MI and sudden death in patients with chronic stable angina.

Extended-release capsules:

Chronic coronary artery disease: To reduce the risk of death and MI in patients with chronic coronary artery disease (eg, history of MI, unstable angina, or chronic stable angina).

History of ischemic stroke or transient ischemic attack: To reduce the risk of death and recurrent stroke in patients who have had an ischemic stroke or transient ischemic attack (TIA).

Limitations of use: Do not use extended-release capsules in situations for which a rapid onset of action is required (such as acute treatment of MI or before percutaneous coronary intervention); use immediate-release formulations instead.

Pregnancy Considerations Salicylates have been noted to cross the placenta and enter fetal circulation. Adverse effects reported in the fetus include mortality, intrauterine growth retardation, salicylate intoxication, bleeding ▶

abnormalities, and neonatal acidosis. Use of aspirin close to delivery may cause premature closure of the ductus arteriosus. Adverse effects reported in the mother include anemia, hemorrhage, prolonged gestation, and prolonged labor (Østensen, 1998). Low-dose aspirin may be used to prevent preeclampsia in women with a history of early-onset preeclampsia and preterm delivery (<34 0/7 weeks), or preeclampsia in ≥1 prior pregnancy (ACOG, 2013). Low-dose aspirin is used to treat complications resulting from antiphospholipid syndrome in pregnancy (either primary or secondary to SLE) (ACCP [Guyatt, 2012]; Carp, 2004; Tincani, 2003). Low-dose aspirin to prevent thrombosis may also be used during the second and third trimesters in women with prosthetic valves (mechanical or bioprosthetic). The use of warfarin is recommended, along with low dose aspirin, in those with mechanical prosthetic valves (Nishimura, 2014). In general, low doses during pregnancy needed for the treatment of certain medical conditions have not been shown to cause fetal harm; however, discontinuing therapy prior to delivery is recommended (Østensen, 2006). Use of safer agents for routine management of pain or headache should be considered.

Breast-Feeding Considerations Low amounts of aspirin can be found in breast milk. Milk/plasma ratios ranging from 0.03 to 0.3 have been reported. Peak levels in breast milk are reported to be at ~9 hours after a dose. Metabolic acidosis was reported in one infant following an aspirin dose of 3.9 g/day in the mother. The WHO considers occasional doses of aspirin to be compatible with breast-feeding, but to avoid long-term therapy and consider monitoring the infant for adverse effects (WHO, 2002). Other sources suggest avoiding aspirin while breast-feeding due to the theoretical risk of Reye's syndrome (Bar-Oz, 2003; Spigset, 2000). When used for vascular indications, breast-feeding may be continued during low-dose aspirin therapy (ACCP [Guyatt, 2012]).

Contraindications

Hypersensitivity to NSAIDs; patients with asthma, rhinitis, and nasal polyps; use in children or teenagers for viral infections, with or without fever.

Documentation of allergenic cross-reactivity for salicylates is limited. However, because of similarities in chemical structure and/or pharmacologic actions, the possibility of cross-sensitivity cannot be ruled out with certainty.

Warnings/Precautions Use with caution in patients with platelet and bleeding disorders, renal dysfunction, dehydration, or erosive gastritis. Avoid use in patients with active peptic ulcer disease. Heavy ethanol use (>3 drinks/day) can increase bleeding risks. Avoid use in severe renal failure (GFR <10 mL/minute) or in severe hepatic failure. Low-dose aspirin for cardioprotective effects is associated with a two- to fourfold increase in UGI events (eg, symptomatic or complicated ulcers); risks of these events increase with increasing aspirin dose; during the chronic phase of aspirin dosing, doses >81 mg are not recommended unless indicated (Bhatt, 2008). Use of safer agents for routine management of pain or headache throughout pregnancy should be considered. If possible, avoid use during the third trimester of pregnancy.

Discontinue use if tinnitus or impaired hearing occurs. Caution in mild-to-moderate renal failure (only at high dosages). Patients with sensitivity to tartrazine dyes, nasal polyps, and asthma may have an increased risk of salicylate sensitivity. In the treatment of acute ischemic stroke, avoid aspirin for 24 hours following administration of alteplase; administration within 24 hours increases the risk of hemorrhagic transformation (Jauch, 2013). Concurrent use of aspirin and clopidogrel is not recommended for secondary prevention of ischemic stroke or TIA in patients unable to take oral anticoagulants due to hemorrhagic risk (Furie, 2011). Surgical patients should avoid ASA if possible, for 1 to 2 weeks prior to surgery, to reduce the risk of excessive bleeding (except in patients with cardiac stents that have not completed their full course of dual antiplatelet therapy [aspirin, clopidogrel]; patient-specific situations need to be discussed with cardiologist; AHA/ACC/SCAI/ACS/ADA Science Advisory provides recommendations). When used concomitantly with ≤325 mg of aspirin, NSAIDs (including selective COX-2 inhibitors) substantially increase the risk of gastrointestinal complications (eg, ulcer); concomitant gastroprotective therapy (eg, proton pump inhibitors) is recommended (Bhatt, 2008). Potentially significant drug-drug interactions may exist, requiring dose or frequency adjustment, additional monitoring, and/or selection of alternative therapy.

When used for self-medication (OTC labeling): Children and teenagers who have or are recovering from chickenpox or flu-like symptoms should not use this product. Changes in behavior (along with nausea and vomiting)

may be an early sign of Reye's syndrome; patients should be instructed to contact their healthcare provider if these occur.

Some dosage forms may contain polysorbate 80 (also known as Tweens). Hypersensitivity reactions, usually a delayed reaction, have been reported following exposure to pharmaceutical products containing polysorbate 80 in certain individuals (Isaksson, 2002; Lucente 2000; Shelley, 1995). Thrombocytopenia, ascites, pulmonary deterioration, and renal and hepatic failure have been reported in premature neonates after receiving parenteral products containing polysorbate 80 (Alade, 1986; CDC, 1984). See manufacturer's labeling.

Aspirin resistance is defined as measurable, persistent platelet activation that occurs in patients prescribed a therapeutic dose of aspirin. Clinical aspirin resistance, the recurrence of some vascular event despite a regular therapeutic dose of aspirin, is considered aspirin treatment failure. Estimates of biochemical aspirin resistance range from 5.5% to 60% depending on the population studied and the assays used (Gasparyan, 2008). Patients with aspirin resistance may have a higher risk of cardiovascular events compared to those who are aspirin sensitive (Gum, 2003).

Adverse Reactions As with all drugs which may affect hemostasis, bleeding is associated with aspirin. Hemorrhage may occur at virtually any site. Risk is dependent on multiple variables including dosage, concurrent use of multiple agents which alter hemostasis, and patient susceptibility. Many adverse effects of aspirin are dose related, and are extremely rare at low dosages. Other serious reactions are idiosyncratic, related to allergy or individual sensitivity. Accurate estimation of frequencies is not possible.

Cardiovascular: Cardiac arrhythmia, edema, hypotension, tachycardia

Central nervous system: Agitation, cerebral edema, coma, confusion, dizziness, fatigue, headache, hyperthermia, insomnia, lethargy, nervousness, Reye's syndrome

Dermatologic: Skin rash, urticaria

Endocrine & metabolic: Acidosis, dehydration, hyperglycemia, hyperkalemia, hypernatremia (buffered forms), hypoglycemia (children)

Gastrointestinal: Gastrointestinal ulcer (6% to 31%), duodenal ulcer, dyspepsia, epigastric distress, gastritis, gastrointestinal erosion, heartburn, nausea, stomach pain, vomiting

Genitourinary: Postpartum hemorrhage, prolonged gestation, prolonged labor, proteinuria, stillborn infant

Hematologic & oncologic: Anemia, blood coagulation disorder, disseminated intravascular coagulation, hemolytic anemia, hemorrhage, iron deficiency anemia, prolonged prothrombin time, thrombocytopenia

Hepatic: Hepatitis (reversible), hepatotoxicity, increased serum transaminases

Hypersensitivity: Anaphylaxis, angioedema

Neuromuscular & skeletal: Acetabular bone destruction, rhabdomyolysis, weakness

Otic: Hearing loss, tinnitus

Renal: Increased blood urea nitrogen, increased serum creatinine, interstitial nephritis, renal failure (including cases caused by rhabdomyolysis), renal insufficiency, renal papillary necrosis

Respiratory: Asthma, bronchospasm, dyspnea, hyperventilation, laryngeal edema, noncardiogenic pulmonary edema, respiratory alkalosis, tachypnea

Miscellaneous: Low birth weight

Postmarketing and/or case reports (Limited to important or life-threatening): Anorectal stenosis (suppository), atrial fibrillation (toxicity), cardiac conduction disturbance (toxicity), cerebral infarction (ischemic), cholestatic jaundice, colitis, colonic ulceration, coronary artery vasospasm, delirium, esophageal obstruction, esophagitis (with esophageal ulcer), hematoma (esophageal), macular degeneration (age-related) (Li 2014), periorbital edema, rhinosinusitis

Drug Interactions

Metabolism/Transport Effects Substrate of CYP2C9 (minor); **Note:** Assignment of Major/Minor substrate status based on clinically relevant drug interaction potential; **Induces** CYP2C19 (weak/moderate)

Avoid Concomitant Use

Avoid concomitant use of Aspirin with any of the following: Dexketoprofen; Floctafenine; Influenza Virus Vaccine (Live/Attenuated); Ketorolac (Nasal); Ketorolac (Systemic); Omacetaxine; Sulfinpyrazone; Urokinase

Increased Effect/Toxicity

Aspirin may increase the levels/effects of: ACE Inhibitors; Agents with Antiplatelet Properties; Alendronate; Anticoagulants; Apixaban; Blood Glucose Lowering Agents; Carbonic Anhydrase Inhibitors; Carisoprodol;

Collagenase (Systemic); Corticosteroids (Systemic); Dabigatran Etexilate; Deoxycholic Acid; Dexketoprofen; Edoxaban; Heparin; Ibritumomab; Methotrexate; Nicorandil; NSAID (COX-2 Inhibitor); Obinutuzumab; Omacetaxine; PRALAtrexate; Rivaroxaban; Salicylates; Talniflumate; Thrombolytic Agents; Ticagrelor; Tositumomab and Iodine I 131 Tositumomab; Urokinase; Valproate Products; Varicella Virus-Containing Vaccines; Vitamin K Antagonists

The levels/effects of Aspirin may be increased by: Agents with Antiplatelet Properties; Alcohol (Ethyl); Ammonium Chloride; Antidepressants (Tricyclic, Tertiary Amine); Calcium Channel Blockers (Nondihydropyridine); Dasatinib; Floctafenine; Ginkgo Biloba; Glucosamine; Herbs (Anticoagulant/Antiplatelet Properties); Ibrutinib; Influenza Virus Vaccine (Live/Attenuated); Ketorolac (Nasal); Ketorolac (Systemic); Limaprost; Loop Diuretics; Multivitamins/Fluoride (with ADE); Multivitamins/Minerals (with ADEK, Folate, Iron); Multivitamins/Minerals (with AE, No Iron); NSAID (Nonselective); Omega-3 Fatty Acids; Pentosan Polysulfate Sodium; Pentoxifylline; Potassium Acid Phosphate; Prostacyclin Analogues; Selective Serotonin Reuptake Inhibitors; Serotonin/Norepinephrine Reuptake Inhibitors; Tipranavir; Treprostinil; Vitamin E; Vitamin E (Oral)

Decreased Effect

Aspirin may decrease the levels/effects of: ACE Inhibitors; Benzbromarone; Carisoprodol; Dexketoprofen; Hyaluronidase; Lesinurad; Loop Diuretics; Multivitamins/Fluoride (with ADE); Multivitamins/Minerals (with ADEK, Folate, Iron); Multivitamins/Minerals (with AE, No Iron); NSAID (Nonselective); Probenecid; Sulfinpyrazone; Ticagrelor; Tiludronate

The levels/effects of Aspirin may be decreased by: Alcohol (Ethyl); Corticosteroids (Systemic); Dexketoprofen; Floctafenine; Ketorolac (Nasal); Ketorolac (Systemic); NSAID (Nonselective)

Food Interactions Food may decrease the rate but not the extent of oral absorption. Benedictine liqueur, prunes, raisins, tea, and gherkins have a potential to cause salicylate accumulation. Fresh fruits containing vitamin C may displace drug from binding sites, resulting in increased urinary excretion of aspirin. Curry powder, paprika, licorice; may cause salicylate accumulation. These foods contain 6 mg salicylate/100 g. An ordinary American diet contains 10-200 mg/day of salicylate. Management: Administer with food or large volume of water or milk to minimize GI upset. Limit curry powder, paprika, licorice.

Storage/Stability Store oral dosage forms (caplets, tablets, capsules) at room temperature; protect from moisture; see product-specific labeling for details. Keep suppositories in refrigerator; do not freeze. Hydrolysis of aspirin occurs upon exposure to water or moist air, resulting in salicylate and acetate, which possess a vinegar-like odor. Do not use if a strong odor is present.

Mechanism of Action Irreversibly inhibits cyclooxygenase-1 and 2 (COX-1 and 2) enzymes, via acetylation, which results in decreased formation of prostaglandin precursors; irreversibly inhibits formation of prostaglandin derivative, thromboxane A_2, via acetylation of platelet cyclooxygenase, thus inhibiting platelet aggregation; has antipyretic, analgesic, and anti-inflammatory properties

Pharmacodynamics/Kinetics

Onset: Immediate release: Platelet inhibition: Within 1 hour (nonenteric-coated). Onset of enteric-coated aspirin expected to be delayed (Eikelboom, 2012). **Note:** Chewing nonenteric-coated or enteric-coated tablets results in inhibition of platelet aggregation within 20 minutes; therefore, nonenteric-coated tablets should be chewed in settings where a more rapid onset is required (eg, acute MI) and enteric-coated tablets may be chewed when a rapid effect is required and immediate release nonenteric-coated tablets are not available (Eikelboom, 2012; Feldman, 1999; Sai, 2011).

Duration: Immediate release: 4 to 6 hours; however, platelet inhibitory effects last the lifetime of the platelet (~10 days) due to its irreversible inhibition of platelet COX-1 (Eikelboom, 2012).

Absorption: Immediate release: Rapidly absorbed in stomach and upper intestine (Eikelboom, 2012); Extended-release capsule: Rate of absorption is dependent upon food, alcohol, and gastric pH.

Distribution: V_d: 10 L; readily into most body fluids and tissues; hydrolyzed to salicylate (active) by esterases in the GI mucosa, red blood cells, synovial fluid and blood

Protein binding: Concentration dependent; as salicylate concentration increases, protein binding decreases: ~90% to 94% (to albumin) at concentrations ≤80 mcg/mL (Rosenberg 1981; Juurlink 2015); ~30% with concentrations seen in overdose (Juurlink, 2015).

Metabolism: Hydrolyzed to salicylate (active) by esterases in GI mucosa, red blood cells, synovial fluid, and blood; metabolism of salicylate occurs primarily by hepatic conjugation; metabolic pathways are saturable

Bioavailability: Immediate release: 50% to 75% reaches systemic circulation

Half-life elimination: Parent drug: Plasma concentration: 15 to 20 minutes; Salicylates (dose dependent): 3 hours at lower doses (300 to 600 mg), 5 to 6 hours (after 1 g), 10 hours with higher doses

Time to peak, serum: Immediate release: ~1 to 2 hours (nonenteric-coated), 3 to 4 hours (enteric-coated) (Eikelboom, 2012); Extended-release capsule: ~2 hours. **Note:** Chewing nonenteric-coated tablets results in a time to peak concentration of 20 minutes (Feldman, 1999). Chewing enteric-coated tablets results in a time to peak concentration of 2 hours (Sai, 2011).

Excretion: Urine (75% as salicyluric acid, 10% as salicylic acid)

Dosing

Adult & Geriatric Note: For most cardiovascular uses, typical maintenance dosing of aspirin is 81 mg once daily. Manufacturer recommended dosing for some indications have been superseded by more recent guideline recommended doses and therefore manufacturer recommended dosing may not be represented; terminologies may also differ from manufacturer's prescribing information.

Acute coronary syndrome (ST-elevation myocardial infarction [STEMI], unstable angina [UA]/non-ST-elevation myocardial infarction [NSTEMI]) (off-label dosing): Immediate release: Oral: Initial: 162 to 325 mg given on presentation (patient should chew nonenteric-coated aspirin especially if not taking before presentation); for patients unable to take oral, may use a rectal suppository dose of 600 mg (Maalouf, 2009). Maintenance (secondary prevention): 81 mg once daily preferred. When aspirin is used with ticagrelor, the recommended maintenance dose of aspirin is 81 mg/day (ACCF/AHA [Anderson 2013]; ACCF/AHA [O'Gara 2013]).

UA/NSTEMI: Concomitant antiplatelet therapy (ACCF/AHA [Anderson 2013]):

If invasive strategy chosen: Aspirin is recommended in combination with either clopidogrel, ticagrelor, (or prasugrel if at the time of PCI) or an IV GP IIb/IIIa inhibitor (if given before PCI, eptifibatide and tirofiban are preferred agents).

If noninvasive strategy chosen: Aspirin is recommended in combination with clopidogrel or ticagrelor and anticoagulant therapy.

Analgesic and antipyretic:

Oral: Immediate release: 325 to 650 mg as needed every 4 hours **or** 975 mg as needed every 6 hours **or** 500 to 1,000 mg as needed every 4 to 6 hours for no more than 10 days or as directed by health care provider; maximum daily dose: 4 g/day.

Rectal: 300 to 600 mg every 4 hours for no more than 10 days or as directed by health care provider

Anti-inflammatory (off-label dosing): Note: The use of non-aspirin NSAIDs has largely supplanted the use of aspirin for osteoarthritis, rheumatoid arthritis, and other inflammatory arthritides.

Immediate release: Oral: Usual maintenance dose: 2.1 to 7.3 g/day in divided doses (individualize dose); monitor serum salicylate concentrations especially when symptoms of salicylism (eg, tinnitus) appear; adjust dose accordingly (Csuka, 1989).

Aortic valve repair (off-label use): Immediate release: Oral: 50 to 100 mg once daily (ACCP [Guyatt 2012])

Atrial fibrillation (to prevent thromboembolism in patients not candidates for oral anticoagulation or at low risk of ischemic stroke [CHA$_2$DS$_2$-VASc score of 1]) (off-label use): Immediate release: Oral: 75 to 325 mg once daily (AHA/ACC/HRS [January 2014]; AHA/ASA [Furie 2011]). **Note:** Combination therapy with clopidogrel has been suggested over aspirin alone for those patients who are unsuitable for or choose not to take oral anticoagulant for reasons other than concerns for bleeding (ACCP [Guyatt 2012]).

As an alternative to adjusted-dose warfarin in patients with atrial fibrillation and mitral stenosis: 75 to 325 mg once daily with (preferred) or without clopidogrel (ACCP [Guyatt 2012])

Carotid artery stenosis (asymptomatic) (off-label use): Immediate release: Oral: 75 to 100 mg once daily (ACCP [Alonso-Coello, 2012]). **Note:** The addition of statin therapy has also been recommended for asymptomatic carotid stenosis (AHA/ASA [Meschia, 2014]). When symptomatic, the use of clopidogrel or aspirin/extended-release dipyridamole has been suggested over aspirin alone (ACCP [Alonso-Coello 2012]).

Carotid endarterectomy (off-label dosing): Immediate release: Oral: 75 to 100 mg once daily (ACCP [Alonso-Coello 2012]; AHA [Biller 1998]). The use of clopidogrel or aspirin/extended-release dipyridamole has been suggested over aspirin alone (ACCP [Alonso-Coello 2012]).

Colorectal cancer risk reduction (off-label use): Note: The optimal dose and duration of therapy for colorectal cancer risk reduction are unknown. Consider risk versus benefit ratio when initiating aspirin for this indication.

Primary/Secondary prevention: Immediate release: Oral: 75 to 325 mg once daily (Rothwell, 2010; Sandler, 2003; Ye, 2013)

Hereditary nonpolyposis colon cancer (HNPCC; Lynch Syndrome) carriers: Immediate release: Oral: 600 mg once daily for at least 2 years (ASCO [Stoffel 2014]; Burn, 2011)

Coronary artery disease (CAD), established or chronic:

Immediate release (off-label dosing): Oral: 75 to 100 mg once daily (ACCP [Guyatt 2012])

Extended-release capsule: Oral: 162.5 mg once daily

Percutaneous coronary intervention (PCI) (off-label dosing): Immediate release: Oral:

Non-emergent PCI: Preprocedure: 81 to 325 mg (325 mg [nonenteric coated] in aspirin-naive patients) starting at least 2 hours (preferably 24 hours) before procedure. Postprocedure: 81 mg once daily continued indefinitely (in combination with a P2Y$_{12}$ inhibitor [eg, clopidogrel, prasugrel, ticagrelor] up to 12 months) (ACCF/AHA/SCAI [Levine 2011])

Primary PCI: Preprocedure: 162 to 325 mg as early as possible prior to procedure; 325 mg preferred. Postprocedure: 81 mg once daily continued indefinitely (in combination with a P2Y12 inhibitor [eg, clopidogrel] for at least 14 days and up to 12 months) (ACCF/AHA [O'Gara 2013]).

Alternatively, in patients who have undergone elective PCI with either bare metal or drug-eluting stent placement: The American College of Chest Physicians recommends the use of 75 to 325 mg once daily (in combination with clopidogrel) for 1 month in patients receiving a bare metal stent or 3 to 6 months (dependent upon drug eluting stent type) followed by 75 to 100 mg once daily (in combination with clopidogrel) for up to 12 months. For patients who underwent PCI but did not have stent placement, 75 to 325 mg once daily (in combination with clopidogrel) for 1 month is recommended. In either case, single antiplatelet therapy (either aspirin or clopidogrel) is recommended indefinitely (ACCP [Guyatt 2012]).

Pericarditis (off-label use): Immediate release: Oral: Initial: 2.4 to 3.6 g daily in 3 to 4 divided doses; usual maintenance: 3.6 to 5.4 g daily in divided doses; gradually taper over 2- to 3-week period as appropriate (Imazio, 2004; Imazio, 2009).

Pericarditis in association with myocardial infarction (off-label use): Immediate release: Oral: Initial: 650 mg 4 times daily; may increase after 24 hours to 975 mg 4 times daily if necessary (ACCF/AHA [O'Gara 2013]; Berman, 1981).

Peripheral arterial disease (off-label use): Immediate release: Oral: 75 to 100 mg once daily (ACCP [Guyatt 2012]) **or** 75 to 325 mg once daily; may use in conjunction with clopidogrel in those who are not at an increased risk of bleeding but are of high cardiovascular risk. **Note:** These recommendations also pertain to those with intermittent claudication or critical limb ischemia, prior lower extremity revascularization, or prior amputation for lower extremity ischemia (Rooke, 2011).

Peripheral artery percutaneous transluminal angioplasty (with or without stenting) or peripheral artery bypass graft surgery, postprocedure (off-label use): Immediate release: Oral: 75 to 100 mg once daily (ACCP [Guyatt 2012]). **Note:** For below-knee bypass graft surgery with prosthetic grafts, combine with clopidogrel (ACCP [Guyatt 2012]).

Polycythemia vera (off-label use): Immediate release: Oral: 75 or 100 mg once daily. In pregnant women, administer 75 mg once daily throughout pregnancy and for 6 weeks after delivery (Barbui, 2006; McMullin, 2005).

Preeclampsia prevention (women at risk) (off-label use): Immediate release: Oral: 75 to 100 mg once daily starting in the second trimester (ACCP [Guyatt 2012]; USPSTF [LeFevre 2014]) **or** 60 to 80 mg once daily beginning late in the first trimester (ACOG, 2013).

Prevention (primary) of cardiovascular disease (off-label use): American College of Chest Physicians: Prevention of myocardial infarction and stroke: Select individuals ≥50 years of age (without symptomatic cardiovascular disease): Immediate release: Oral: 75 to 100 mg once daily (ACCP [Vandvik 2012])

Prevention (secondary) after coronary artery bypass graft (CABG) surgery (off-label dosing): Immediate release: Oral: 81 to 325 mg once daily administered preoperatively and within 6 hours postoperatively; continue indefinitely. Following off-pump CABG, administer aspirin 81 to 162 mg in combination with clopidogrel for 12 months (AHA [Kulik 2015]).

Prosthetic heart valve (thromboprophylaxis) (off-label use): Immediate release: Oral:

Bioprosthetic aortic valve (patient in normal sinus rhythm): 50 to 100 mg once daily (ACCP [Guyatt 2012]).

Bioprosthetic mitral valve: 50 to 100 mg once daily after 3 months of anticoagulation with warfarin (ACCP [Guyatt 2012]).

Mechanical aortic or mitral valve:

Low risk of bleeding: 50 to 100 mg once daily (in combination with warfarin) (ACCP [Guyatt 2012])

History of thromboembolism while receiving oral anticoagulants: 75 to 100 mg once daily (in combination with warfarin) (Furie, 2011)

Transcatheter aortic bioprosthetic valve: 50 to 100 mg once daily (in combination with clopidogrel) (ACCP [Guyatt 2012])

Pregnant women, mechanical or bioprosthetic: 75 to 100 mg once daily during the second and third trimesters (when used for mechanical prosthetic valve, combine with warfarin) (AHA/ACC [Nishimura 2014]).

Stroke/TIA: Oral:

Acute ischemic stroke/TIA:

Immediate release (off-label dosing): Initial: 160 to 325 mg within 48 hours of stroke/TIA onset, followed by 75 to 100 mg once daily (ACCP [Guyatt 2012]). The AHA/ASA recommends an initial dose of 325 mg within 24 to 48 hours after stroke; do not administer aspirin within 24 hours after administration of alteplase (Jauch, 2013).

Extended-release capsule: Maintenance (secondary prevention): 162.5 mg once daily. **Note:** Not for initial dosing during acute ischemic stroke or TIA (use immediate release)

Cardioembolic, secondary prevention (oral anticoagulation unsuitable) (off-label dosing: Immediate release: 75 to 100 mg once daily (in combination with clopidogrel) (ACCP [Guyatt 2012]; The ACTIVE Investigators [Connolly 2009])

Cryptogenic with patent foramen ovale (PFO) or atrial septal aneurysm (off-label use): Immediate release: 50 to 100 mg once daily (ACCP [Guyatt 2012])

Noncardioembolic, secondary prevention (off-label use): Immediate release: 75 to 325 mg once daily (Smith, 2011) **or** 75 to 100 mg once daily (ACCP [Guyatt 2012]). **Note:** Combination aspirin/extended release dipyridamole or clopidogrel is preferred over aspirin alone (ACCP [Guyatt 2012]).

Women at high risk for first stroke, primary prevention: Immediate release: 81 mg once daily **or** 100 mg every other day (AHA/ASA [Meschia 2014]).

Pediatric Note: Do not use aspirin in children <12 years (APS, 2008) and adolescents (per manufacturer) who have or who are recovering from chickenpox or flu symptoms due to the association with Reye's syndrome (APS, 2008).

Analgesic: Immediate release:

Infants, Children, and Adolescents weighing <50 kg (off-label use): Oral, rectal: 10 to 15 mg/kg/dose every 4 to 6 hours; maximum daily dose: The lesser value of either 90 mg/kg/day or 4 g/day (APS, 2008)

Children ≥12 years and Adolescents weighing ≥50 kg:

Oral: 325 to 650 mg as needed every 4 hours **or** 975 mg as needed every 6 hours **or** 500 to 1,000 mg as needed every 4 to 6 hours for no more than 10 days or as directed by health care provider; maximum daily dose: 4 g/day

Rectal: 300 to 600 mg every 4 hours for no more than 10 days or as directed by health care provider

Anti-inflammatory (off-label use): Immediate release: Oral: Initial: 60 to 90 mg/kg/day in divided doses; usual maintenance: 80 to 100 mg/kg/day divided every 6 to 8 hours; monitor serum concentrations

Antiplatelet effects (off-label use): Adequate pediatric studies have not been performed; pediatric dosage is derived from adult studies and clinical experience and is not well established. Doses are typically rounded to a convenient amount (eg, ½ of 81 mg tablet).

Acute ischemic stroke (AIS) (off-label use): Immediate release: Oral:

Noncardioembolic: 1 to 5 mg/kg/dose once daily for ≥2 years; patients with recurrent AIS or TIAs should be transitioned to clopidogrel, LMWH, or warfarin (ACCP [Monagle 2012])

Secondary to Moyamoya and non-Moyamoya vasculopathy: 1 to 5 mg/kg/dose once daily. **Note:** In non-Moyamoya vasculopathy, continue aspirin for 3 months, with subsequent use guided by repeat cerebrovascular imaging (ACCP [Monagle 2012]).

Norwood, Fontan surgery (postoperative) (primary prophylaxis) (off-label use): Immediate release: Oral: 1 to 5 mg/kg/dose once daily (ACCP [Monagle 2011]; AHA [Giglia 2013])

Prosthetic heart valve (off-label use): Immediate release: Oral:

Bioprosthetic aortic valve (in normal sinus rhythm): 1 to 5 mg/kg/dose once daily (ACCP [Guyatt 2012]; ACCP [Monagle 2012])

Mechanical aortic and/or mitral valve: Low-dose aspirin (eg, 1 to 5 mg/kg/day) combined with vitamin K antagonist (eg, warfarin) is recommended as first-line antithrombotic therapy (ACCP [Guyatt 2012]). Alternative regimens: 6 to 20 mg/kg/dose once daily in combination with dipyridamole (Bradley 1985; El Makhlouf 1987; LeBlanc 1993; Serra 1987; Solymar 1991)

Shunts: Blalock-Taussig or Glenn (primary prophylaxis) (off-label use): Immediate release: Oral: 1 to 5 mg/kg/dose once daily (AHA [Giglia 2013]; ACCP [Monagle 2012])

Transcatheter Atrial Septal Defect (ASD) or Ventricular Septal Defect (VSD) devices (postprocedure prophylaxis) (off-label use): Immediate release: Oral: 1 to 5 mg/kg/dose once daily starting one to several days prior to implantation and continued for at least 6 months. For older children and adolescents, after device closure of ASD, an additional anticoagulant may be given with aspirin for 3 to 6 months, but the aspirin should continue for at least 6 months (AHA [Giglia 2013]).

Ventricular assist device (VAD) placement (off-label use): Immediate release: Oral: 1 to 5 mg/kg/dose once daily initiated within 72 hours of VAD placement; should be used with heparin (initiated between 8 to 48 hours following implantation) (ACCP [Monagle 2012]).

Kawasaki disease (off-label use): Immediate release: Oral: 80 to 100 mg/kg/day divided every 6 hours for up to 14 days (until fever resolves for at least 48 hours); then decrease dose to 1 to 5 mg/kg/day once daily (AHA and AAP suggest 3 to 5 mg/kg/day). Combine initial high-dose treatment with IV immune globulin within first 10 days of symptom onset. In patients without coronary artery abnormalities, give lower dose for at least 6 to 8 weeks. In patients with coronary artery abnormalities, low-dose aspirin should be continued indefinitely (in combination with warfarin) (ACCP [Monagle 2012]; AHA [Giglia 2013]; Newburger, 2004; *Red Book* [AAP 2015]).

Rheumatic fever (off-label use): Limited data available: Infants, Children, and Adolescents: Oral: Initial: 100 mg/kg/day divided into 4 to 5 doses; if response inadequate, may increase dose to 125 mg/kg/day; continue for 2 weeks; then decrease dose to 60 to 70 mg/kg/day in divided doses for an additional 3 to 6 weeks (WHO Guidelines 2004)

Migratory polyarthritis, with carditis without cardiomegaly or congestive heart failure: Initial: 100 mg/kg/day in 4 divided doses for 3 to 5 days, followed by 75 mg/kg/day in 4 divided doses for 4 weeks (Kliegman 2011)

Carditis and cardiomegaly or congestive heart failure: At the beginning of the tapering of the prednisone dose, aspirin should be started at 75 mg/kg/day in 4 divided doses for 6 weeks (Kliegman 2011)

Renal Impairment

GFR <10 mL/minute: Avoid use.

Hemodialysis: Dialyzable (concentration dependent; higher salicylate concentrations are more readily dialyzable: 50% to 60%) (Rosenberg, 1981; Juurlink, 2015): Administer after hemodialysis on dialysis days (Aronoff, 2007).

Hepatic Impairment Avoid use in severe liver disease.

Administration

Oral:

Immediate-release tablets: Do not crush enteric-coated tablet. Administer with food or a full glass of water to minimize GI distress. In situations for which a rapid onset of action is required (eg, acute treatment of MI), have patient chew immediate-release tablet.

Extended-release capsules: Do not cut, crush, or chew. Administer with a full glass of water at the same time each day. Do not administer 2 hours before or 1 hour after alcohol consumption.

Rectal: Remove suppository from plastic packet and insert into rectum as far as possible.

Reference Range Timing of serum samples: Peak levels usually occur 2 hours after ingestion. Salicylate serum concentrations correlate with the pharmacological actions and adverse effects observed. The serum salicylate concentration (mcg/mL) and the corresponding clinical correlations are as follows: See table.

Serum Salicylate: Clinical Correlations

Serum Salicylate Concentration (mcg/mL)	Desired Effects	Adverse Effects / Intoxication
~100	Antiplatelet Antipyresis Analgesia	GI intolerance and bleeding, hypersensitivity, hemostatic defects
150-300	Anti-inflammatory	Mild salicylism
250-400	Treatment of rheumatic fever	Nausea/vomiting, hyperventilation, salicylism, flushing, sweating, thirst, headache, diarrhea, and tachycardia
>400-500		Respiratory alkalosis, hemorrhage, excitement, confusion, asterixis, pulmonary edema, convulsions, tetany, metabolic acidosis, fever, coma, cardiovascular collapse, renal and respiratory failure

Test Interactions False-negative results for glucose oxidase urinary glucose tests (Clinistix); false-positives using the cupric sulfate method (Clinitest); also, interferes with Gerhardt test, VMA determination; 5-HIAA, xylose tolerance test and T_3 and T_4

Dosage Forms Excipient information presented when available (limited, particularly for generics); consult specific product labeling.

Caplet, oral: 500 mg

Bayer Aspirin Extra Strength: 500 mg

Bayer Genuine Aspirin: 325 mg

Bayer Women's Low Dose Aspirin: 81 mg [contains elemental calcium 300 mg]

Caplet, oral [buffered]:

Ascriptin Maximum Strength: 500 mg [contains aluminum hydroxide, calcium carbonate, magnesium hydroxide]

Bayer Plus Extra Strength: 500 mg [contains calcium carbonate]

Caplet, enteric coated, oral:

Bayer Aspirin Regimen Regular Strength: 325 mg

Capsule Extended Release, oral:

Durlaza: 162.5 mg

Suppository, rectal: 300 mg (12s); 600 mg (12s)

Tablet, oral: 325 mg

Aspercin: 325 mg

Aspirtab: 325 mg

Bayer Genuine Aspirin: 325 mg

Tablet, oral [buffered]: 325 mg

Ascriptin Regular Strength: 325 mg [contains aluminum hydroxide, calcium carbonate, magnesium hydroxide]

Buffasal: 325 mg [contains magnesium oxide]

Bufferin: 325 mg [contains calcium carbonate, magnesium carbonate, magnesium oxide]

Bufferin Extra Strength: 500 mg [contains calcium carbonate, magnesium carbonate, magnesium oxide]

Buffinol: 324 mg [sugar free; contains magnesium oxide]

Tri-Buffered Aspirin: 325 mg [contains calcium carbonate, magnesium carbonate, magnesium oxide]

Tablet, chewable, oral: 81 mg

Bayer Aspirin Regimen Children's: 81 mg [cherry flavor]

Bayer Aspirin Regimen Children's: 81 mg [orange flavor]

St Joseph Adult Aspirin: 81 mg

Tablet, enteric coated, oral: 81 mg, 325 mg, 650 mg

Aspir-low: 81 mg

Bayer Aspirin Regimen Adult Low Strength: 81 mg

Ecotrin: 325 mg

Ecotrin Arthritis Strength: 500 mg

Ecotrin Low Strength: 81 mg

Halfprin: 81 mg

St Joseph Adult Aspirin: 81 mg

◆ Aspirin, Acetaminophen, and Caffeine *see* Acetaminophen, Aspirin, and Caffeine *on page 29*

◆ Aspirin and Carisoprodol *see* Carisoprodol and Aspirin *on page 320*

Aspirin and Diphenhydramine
(AS pir in & dye fen HYE dra meen)

Brand Names: US Bayer® PM [OTC]

Index Terms ASA and Diphenhydramine; Aspirin and Diphenhydramine Citrate; Diphenhydramine and ASA; Diphenhydramine and Aspirin; Diphenhydramine Citrate and Aspirin

Pharmacologic Category Analgesic, Miscellaneous

Use Aid in the relief of insomnia accompanied by minor pain or headache

Dosing

Adult & Geriatric Pain-associated insomnia: Oral: Two caplets (1000 mg aspirin/77 mg diphenhydramine citrate) at bedtime if needed or as directed by physician; do not exceed recommended dosage

Pediatric Children ≥12 years: Refer to adult dosing.

Additional Information Complete prescribing information should be consulted for additional detail.

Dosage Forms Excipient information presented when available (limited, particularly for generics); consult specific product labeling.

Caplet, oral:

Bayer® PM: Aspirin 500 mg and diphenhydramine citrate 38.3 mg

◆ **Aspirin and Diphenhydramine Citrate** *see* Aspirin and Diphenhydramine *on page 162*

Aspirin and Dipyridamole
(AS pir in & dye peer ID a mole)

Brand Names: US Aggrenox

Brand Names: Canada Aggrenox

Index Terms Aspirin and Extended-Release Dipyridamole; Dipyridamole and Aspirin

Pharmacologic Category Antiplatelet Agent

Use Stroke prevention: Reduction in the risk of stroke in patients who have had transient ischemia of the brain or complete ischemic stroke due to thrombosis.

Dosing

Adult

Stroke prevention: Oral: One capsule (dipyridamole extended release 200 mg/aspirin 25 mg) twice daily

Alternative regimen for patients with intolerable headache: Oral: One capsule (dipyridamole extended release 200 mg/aspirin 25 mg) at bedtime and low-dose aspirin in the morning. Return to usual dose (1 capsule twice daily) as soon as tolerance to headache develops (usually within a week).

Carotid artery stenosis, symptomatic (including recent carotid endarterectomy) (off-label use): Oral: One capsule (dipyridamole extended release 200 mg/ aspirin 25 mg) twice daily (Guyatt 2012)

Hemodialysis graft patency (off-label use): Oral: One capsule (dipyridamole extended release 200 mg/aspirin 25 mg) twice daily

Renal Impairment

GFR ≥10 mL/minute: There are no dosage adjustments provided in the manufacturer's labeling (has not been studied).

GFR <10 mL/minute: Avoid use.

Hepatic Impairment

Mild to moderate hepatic impairment: There are no dosage adjustments provided in the manufacturer's labeling (has not been studied).

Severe hepatic impairment: Avoid use.

Additional Information Complete prescribing information should be consulted for additional detail.

Dosage Forms Excipient information presented when available (limited, particularly for generics); consult specific product labeling.

Capsule Extended Release 12 Hour, Oral:

Aggrenox: Aspirin 25 mg [immediate release] and dipyridamole 200 mg [extended release]

Generic: Aspirin 25 mg [immediate release] and dipyridamole 200 mg [extended release] [dosage foc], Aspirin 25 mg [immediate release] and dipyridamole 200 mg [extended release]

◆ **Aspirin and Extended-Release Dipyridamole** *see* Aspirin and Dipyridamole *on page 162*

◆ **Aspirin and Oxycodone** *see* Oxycodone and Aspirin *on page 1362*

◆ **Aspirin, Caffeine and Acetaminophen** *see* Acetaminophen, Aspirin, and Caffeine *on page 29*

◆ **Aspirin, Caffeine, and Butalbital** *see* Butalbital, Aspirin, and Caffeine *on page 275*

◆ **Aspirin, Caffeine, and Orphenadrine** *see* Orphenadrine, Aspirin, and Caffeine *on page 1342*

◆ **Aspirin, Carisoprodol, and Codeine** *see* Carisoprodol, Aspirin, and Codeine *on page 320*

◆ **Aspirin, Dihydrocodeine, and Caffeine** *see* Dihydrocodeine, Aspirin, and Caffeine *on page 551*

◆ **Aspirin Free Anacin Extra Strength [OTC]** *see* Acetaminophen *on page 25*

◆ **Aspirin, Orphenadrine, and Caffeine** *see* Orphenadrine, Aspirin, and Caffeine *on page 1342*

◆ **Aspir-low [OTC]** *see* Aspirin *on page 157*

◆ **Aspirtab [OTC]** *see* Aspirin *on page 157*

◆ **Astagraf XL** *see* Tacrolimus (Systemic) *on page 1725*

◆ **Astelin [DSC]** *see* Azelastine (Nasal) *on page 187*

◆ **Astelin (Can)** *see* Azelastine (Nasal) *on page 187*

◆ **Astepro** *see* Azelastine (Nasal) *on page 187*

◆ **Asthmanefrin Refill [OTC]** *see* EPINEPHrine (Oral Inhalation) *on page 650*

◆ **Asthmanefrin Starter Kit [OTC]** *see* EPINEPHrine (Oral Inhalation) *on page 650*

◆ **Astramorph** *see* Morphine (Systemic) *on page 1230*

◆ **AT** *see* Antithrombin *on page 135*

◆ **AT-III** *see* Antithrombin *on page 135*

◆ **Atacand** *see* Candesartan *on page 294*

◆ **Atacand HCT** *see* Candesartan and Hydrochlorothiazide *on page 296*

◆ **Atacand Plus (Can)** *see* Candesartan and Hydrochlorothiazide *on page 296*

◆ **Atarax (Can)** *see* HydrOXYzine *on page 898*

◆ **Atasol (Can)** *see* Acetaminophen *on page 25*

Atazanavir (at a za NA veer)

Brand Names: US Reyataz

Brand Names: Canada Reyataz

Index Terms Atazanavir Sulfate; ATV; BMS-232632

Pharmacologic Category Antiretroviral, Protease Inhibitor (Anti-HIV)

Use

HIV-1 Infection:

US labeling: Treatment of HIV-1 infection in combination with other antiretroviral agents in patients ≥3 months weighing ≥5 kg

Limitations of use:

Not recommended for use in pediatric patients younger than 3 months due to the risk of kernicterus

Use in treatment-experienced patients should be guided by the number of baseline primary protease inhibitor resistance substitutions

Canadian labeling: Treatment of HIV-1 infection in combination with other antiretroviral agents in patients 6 years and older

Pregnancy Considerations Adverse events were not observed in animal reproduction studies. Atazanavir has a low level of transfer across the human placenta with cord blood concentrations reported as 13% to 21% of maternal serum concentrations at delivery. An increased risk of teratogenic effects has not been observed based on information collected by the antiretroviral pregnancy registry. A small increased risk of preterm birth has been associated with maternal use of protease inhibitor-based combination antiretroviral (ARV) therapy during pregnancy; however, the benefits of use generally outweigh this risk and protease inhibitors (PIs) should not be withheld if otherwise recommended. Hyperglycemia, new onset of diabetes mellitus, or diabetic ketoacidosis have been reported with PIs; it is not clear if pregnancy increases this risk. Hyperbilirubinemia or hypoglycemia may occur in neonates following *in utero* exposure to atazanavir, although data are conflicting.

The DHHS Perinatal HIV Guidelines recommend atazanavir as a preferred PI in antiretroviral-naive pregnant women when combined with low-dose ritonavir boosting. Pharmacokinetic studies suggest that standard dosing during pregnancy may provide decreased plasma concentrations and some experts recommend increased doses during the second and third trimesters. However, the manufacturer notes that dose adjustment is not required unless using concomitant H_2-receptor blockers or tenofovir or for ARV-naive pregnant women taking efavirenz. May give as once-daily dosing.

Regardless of CD4 count or HIV RNA copy number, all HIV-infected pregnant women should receive a combination antiretroviral (ARV) drug regimen. A combination of antepartum, intrapartum, and infant ARV prophylaxis is recommended. ARV therapy should be started as soon as possible in women with symptomatic infection. Although

earlier initiation may be more effective in reducing the perinatal transmission of HIV, initiation may be delayed until after 12 weeks gestation in women who do not require immediate treatment after careful consideration of maternal conditions (eg, nausea and vomiting) and the potential risks of first trimester fetal exposure for specific agents. A scheduled cesarean delivery at 38 weeks gestation is recommended for all women with HIV RNA >1000 copies/mL or unknown concentrations near delivery in order to decrease transmission. If ARV therapy must be interrupted for <24 hours during the peripartum period, stop then restart all medications simultaneously in order to decrease the chance of developing resistance. Long-term follow-up is recommended for all infants exposed to ARV medications. In couples who want to conceive, the HIV-infected partner should attain maximum viral suppression prior to conception.

Healthcare providers are encouraged to enroll pregnant women exposed to antiretroviral medications in the Antiretroviral Pregnancy Registry (1-800-258-4263 or www.-APRegistry.com). Healthcare providers caring for HIV-infected women and their infants may contact the National Perinatal HIV Hotline (888-448-8765) for clinical consultation (DHHS [perinatal], 2014).

Breast-Feeding Considerations Atazanavir is excreted into breast milk. Maternal or infant antiretroviral therapy does not completely eliminate the risk of postnatal HIV transmission. In addition, multiclass-resistant virus has been detected in breast-feeding infants despite maternal therapy. Therefore, in the United States, where formula is accessible, affordable, safe, and sustainable, and the risk of infant mortality due to diarrhea and respiratory infections is low, complete avoidance of breast-feeding by HIV-infected women is recommended to decrease potential transmission of HIV (DHHS [perinatal], 2014).

Contraindications

Hypersensitivity (eg, Stevens-Johnson syndrome, erythema multiforme, or toxic skin eruptions) to atazanavir or any component of the formulation; concurrent therapy with alfuzosin, cisapride, ergot derivatives (dihydroergotamine, ergonovine, ergotamine, methylergonovine), indinavir, irinotecan, lovastatin, midazolam (oral), nevirapine, pimozide, rifampin, sildenafil (when used for pulmonary artery hypertension [eg, Revatio]), simvastatin, St. John's wort, or triazolam

Canadian labeling: Additional contraindications (not in US labeling): Concomitant use of quinidine or bepridil (currently not marketed in Canada)

Warnings/Precautions Atazanavir may prolong PR interval; ECG monitoring should be considered in patients with preexisting conduction abnormalities or with medications which prolong AV conduction (dosage adjustment required with some agents); rare cases of second-degree AV block have been reported. May cause or exacerbate preexisting hepatic dysfunction; use caution in patients with transaminase elevations prior to therapy or underlying hepatic disease, such as hepatitis B or C or cirrhosis; monitor closely at baseline and during treatment. Not recommended in patients with severe hepatic impairment. In combination with ritonavir, is not recommended in patients with any degree of hepatic impairment.

Asymptomatic elevations in bilirubin (unconjugated) occur commonly during therapy with atazanavir; consider alternative therapy if bilirubin is >5 times ULN. Evaluate alternative etiologies if transaminase elevations also occur.

Cases of nephrolithiasis have been reported in postmarketing surveillance; temporary or permanent discontinuation of therapy should be considered if symptoms develop. Not recommended for use in treatment-experienced patients with end stage renal disease (ESRD) on hemodialysis.

Protease inhibitors have been associated with a variety of hypersensitivity events (some severe), including rash, anaphylaxis (rare), angioedema, bronchospasm, erythema multiforme, Stevens-Johnson syndrome (rare) and/or toxic skin eruptions (including DRESS [drug rash, eosinophilia and systemic symptoms] syndrome). It is generally recommended to discontinue treatment if severe rash or moderate symptoms accompanied by other systemic symptoms occur.

Use with caution in patients with hemophilia A or B; increased bleeding during protease inhibitor therapy has been reported. Changes in glucose tolerance, hyperglycemia, exacerbation of diabetes, DKA, and new-onset diabetes mellitus have been reported in patients receiving protease inhibitors. May be associated with fat redistribution (buffalo hump, increased abdominal girth, breast engorgement, facial atrophy). Immune reconstitution syndrome may develop resulting in the occurrence of an inflammatory response to an indolent or residual opportunistic infection during initial HIV treatment or activation of autoimmune disorders (eg, Graves' disease, polymyositis, Guillain-Barré syndrome) later in therapy; further evaluation and treatment may be required. Oral powder contains phenylalanine; avoid or use with caution in patients with phenylketonuria. Oral powder is not recommended for use in children <5 kg. Do not use in children <3 months of age due to potential for kernicterus. Potentially significant drug-drug interactions may exist, requiring dose or frequency adjustment, additional monitoring, and/or selection of alternative therapy. Do not use atazanavir/ritonavir plus abacavir/lamivudine in adolescent and adult HIV-1 patients with a pre-ART HIV RNA >100,000 copies/mL (HHS [adult] 2015).

Adverse Reactions Includes data from both treatment-naive and treatment-experienced patients. Unless otherwise noted, frequency of adverse events is as reported in adults receiving combination antiretroviral therapy.

>10%:

Dermatologic: Skin rash (adults 3% to 21%; median onset: 7 weeks; children 14%)

Endocrine & metabolic: Increased serum cholesterol (≥240 mg/dL: 6% to 25%), increased amylase (adults: >2 x ULN: ≤14%)

Gastrointestinal: Nausea (3% to 14%)

Hepatic: Increased serum bilirubin (≥2.6 x ULN: adults 35% to 49%; children 16%), jaundice (children 13% to 15%; adults 5% to 9%)

Neuromuscular & skeletal: Increased creatine phosphokinase (>5 times ULN: 6% to 11%)

Respiratory: Cough (children 21%)

Miscellaneous: Fever (children 18% to 19%; adults 2%)

1% to 10%:

Cardiovascular: Peripheral edema (children 7%), first degree atrioventricular block (6%), second degree atrioventricular block (children ≤2%; adults [rare])

Central nervous system: Headache (adults 1% to 6%; children 7% to 8%), peripheral neuropathy (<1% to 4%), insomnia (<1% to 3%), depression (2%), dizziness (<1% to 2%)

Endocrine & metabolic: Increased serum triglycerides (≥751 mg/dL: <1% to 8%), hyperglycemia (≥251 mg/dL: 5%), hypoglycemia (children: grades 3/4: 4%)

Gastrointestinal: Vomiting (children 8% to 12%; adults 3% to 4%), diarrhea (children 8% to 9%; adults 1% to 3%), increased serum lipase (adults: >2 x ULN: ≤5%), abdominal pain (4%)

Hematologic & oncologic: Decreased neutrophils (<750 cells/mm³: 3% to 7%), decreased hemoglobin (<8.0 g/dL: <1% to 5%), decreased platelet count (<50,000 cells/mm³: 2%)

Hepatic: Increased serum ALT (adults and children: >5 x ULN: 3% to 9%; 10% to 25% in adult patients co-infected with hepatitis B and/or C), increased serum AST (>5 times ULN: 2% to 7%; 9% to 10% in patients co-infected with hepatitis B and/or C)

Neuromuscular & skeletal: Myalgia (4%), limb pain (children 6%)

Respiratory: Nasal congestion (children 6%), oropharyngeal pain (children 6%), rhinorrhea (children 6%), wheezing (children 6%)

Postmarketing and/or case reports (Limited to important or life-threatening): Cholecystitis, cholelithiasis, cholestasis, complete atrioventricular block (rare), diabetes mellitus, DRESS syndrome, edema, erythema multiforme, immune reconstitution syndrome, interstitial nephritis, left bundle branch block, maculopapular rash, nephrolithiasis, pancreatitis, prolongation P-R interval on ECG, prolonged Q-T interval on ECG, Stevens-Johnson syndrome, torsades de pointes

Drug Interactions

Metabolism/Transport Effects Substrate of CYP3A4 (major); **Note:** Assignment of Major/Minor substrate status based on clinically relevant drug interaction potential; **Inhibits** CYP1A2 (weak), CYP2C8 (weak), CYP2C9 (weak), CYP3A4 (strong), SLCO1B1, UGT1A1

Avoid Concomitant Use

Avoid concomitant use of Atazanavir with any of the following: Ado-Trastuzumab Emtansine; Alfuzosin; Amodiaquine; Aprepitant; Astemizole; Avanafil; Axitinib; Barnidipine; Belinostat; Bosutinib; Bromocriptine; Buprenorphine; Cabozantinib; Ceritinib; Cisapride; Cobimetinib; Conivaptan; Crizotinib; Dabrafenib; Dapoxetine; Domperidone; Dronedarone; Eletriptan; Eplerenone; Ergot Derivatives; Everolimus; Flibanserin; Fusidic Acid (Systemic); Halofantrine; Ibrutinib; Idelalisib; Indinavir; Irinotecan Products; Isavuconazonium Sulfate; Ivabradine; Lapatinib; Lercanidipine; Lomitapide; Lovastatin; Lurasidone; Macitentan; Midazolam; Naloxegol; Nevirapine; Nilotinib; NiMODipine; Nisoldipine; Olaparib; Ombitasvir, Paritaprevir, and Ritonavir; Osimertinib;

PACLitaxel (Conventional); Palbociclib; Pimozide; Ranolazine; Red Yeast Rice; Regorafenib; Repaglinide; Rifampin; Salmeterol; Silodosin; Simeprevir; Simvastatin; Sonidegib; St Johns Wort; Suvorexant; Tamsulosin; Terfenadine; Ticagrelor; Tipranavir; Tolvaptan; Toremifene; Trabectedin; Triazolam; Ulipristal; Vemurafenib; VinCRIStine (Liposomal); Vorapaxar; Voriconazole

Increased Effect/Toxicity

Atazanavir may increase the levels/effects of: Ado-Trastuzumab Emtansine; Alfuzosin; Alitretinoin (Systemic); Almotriptan; Alosetron; ALPRAZolam; Amiodarone; Amodiaquine; Apixaban; Aprepitant; ARIPiprazole; ARIPiprazole Lauroxil; Astemizole; AtorvaSTATin; Avanafil; Axitinib; Barnidipine; Bedaquiline; Belinostat; Bortezomib; Bosentan; Bosutinib; Brentuximab Vedotin; Brexpiprazole; Brinzolamide; Bromocriptine; Budesonide (Nasal); Budesonide (Oral Inhalation); Budesonide (Systemic); Budesonide (Topical); Buprenorphine; Cabazitaxel; Cabozantinib; Calcium Channel Blockers (Nondihydropyridine); Cannabis; CarBAMazepine; Cariprazine; Ceritinib; Cilostazol; Cisapride; Clarithromycin; Cobimetinib; Colchicine; Conivaptan; Contraceptives (Progestins); Corticosteroids (Orally Inhaled); Corticosteroids (Systemic); Crizotinib; Cyclophosphamide; CycloSPORINE (Systemic); CYP3A4 Substrates; Dabrafenib; Daclatasvir; Dapoxetine; Dasatinib; Digoxin; Domperidone; DOXOrubicin (Conventional); Dronabinol; Dronedarone; Dutasteride; Eletriptan; Eliglustat; Eluxadoline; Elvitegravir; Enfuvirtide; Eplerenone; Ergot Derivatives; Erlotinib; Estazolam; Etizolam; Etravirine; Everolimus; FentaNYL; Fesoterodine; Flibanserin; Fluticasone (Nasal); Fluticasone (Oral Inhalation); Fluvastatin; Gefitinib; GuanFACINE; Halofantrine; Highest Risk QTc-Prolonging Agents; Hydrocodone; Ibrutinib; Iloperidone; Imatinib; Imidafenacin; Indinavir; Irinotecan Products; Isavuconazonium Sulfate; Ivabradine; Ivacaftor; Ixabepilone; Lacosamide; Lapatinib; Lercanidipine; Levobupivacaine; Levomilnacipran; Lomitapide; Lovastatin; Lurasidone; Macitentan; Maraviroc; Meperidine; Methyl-PREDNISolone; Midazolam; Mifepristone; Minoxidil (Systemic); Moderate Risk QTc-Prolonging Agents; Naloxegol; Nefazodone; Nevirapine; Nilotinib; NiMODipine; Nisoldipine; Olaparib; Ombitasvir, Paritaprevir, and Ritonavir; Ombitasvir, Paritaprevir, Ritonavir, and Dasabuvir; Osimertinib; Ospemifene; Oxybutynin; OxyCODONE; PACLitaxel (Conventional); Palbociclib; Panobinostat; Parecoxib; Paricalcitol; PAZOPanib; Pimecrolimus; Pimozide; Pitavastatin; PONATinib; Pranlukast; PrednisoLONE (Systemic); PredniSONE; Propafenone; Protease Inhibitors; QUEtiapine; QuiNIDine; Ramelteon; Ranolazine; Red Yeast Rice; Regorafenib; Repaglinide; Retapamulin; Rifabutin; Rilpivirine; Riociguat; RomiDEPsin; Rosiglitazone; Rosuvastatin; Ruxolitinib; Salmeterol; Saxagliptin; Sildenafil; Silodosin; Simeprevir; Simvastatin; Sonidegib; SORAfenib; Suvorexant; Tacrolimus (Systemic); Tacrolimus (Topical); Tadalafil; Tamsulosin; Tasimelteon; Temsirolimus; Tenofovir Disoproxil Fumarate; Terfenadine; Tetrahydrocannabinol; Ticagrelor; TiZANidine; Tofacitinib; Tolterodine; Tolvaptan; Toremifene; Trabectedin; TraMADol; TraZODone; Triazolam; Tricyclic Antidepressants; Ulipristal; Vardenafil; Vemurafenib; Vilazodone; VinCRIStine (Liposomal); Vindesine; Vinorelbine; Vorapaxar; Voriconazole; Warfarin; Zopiclone; Zuclopenthixol

The levels/effects of Atazanavir may be increased by: Clarithromycin; Conivaptan; CycloSPORINE (Systemic); CYP3A4 Inhibitors (Moderate); CYP3A4 Inhibitors (Strong); Dapsone (Systemic); Delavirdine; Enfuvirtide; Fusidic Acid (Systemic); Idelalisib; Indinavir; Luliconazole; Mifepristone; Netupitant; Posaconazole; Simeprevir; Stiripentol; Telaprevir

Decreased Effect

Atazanavir may decrease the levels/effects of: Abacavir; Antidiabetic Agents; Boceprevir; Clarithromycin; Contraceptives (Estrogens); Delavirdine; Didanosine; Disulfiram; Ifosfamide; LamoTRIgine; Meperidine; Prasugrel; Telaprevir; Ticagrelor; Valproate Products; Voriconazole; Zidovudine

The levels/effects of Atazanavir may be decreased by: Antacids; Boceprevir; Bosentan; Buprenorphine; CarBAMazepine; CYP3A4 Inducers (Moderate); CYP3A4 Inducers (Strong); Deferasirox; Didanosine; Efavirenz; Enzalutamide; Etravirine; Garlic; H2-Antagonists; Minocycline; Mitotane; Nevirapine; Proton Pump Inhibitors; Rifampin; Siltuximab; St Johns Wort; Tenofovir Disoproxil Fumarate; Tipranavir; Tocilizumab; Voriconazole

Food Interactions Bioavailability of atazanavir increased when taken with food. Management: Administer with food.

Preparation for Administration

Oral powder: It is preferable to mix oral powder with food such as applesauce or yogurt. Mixing oral powder with a beverage (eg, milk, infant formula, water) may be used for patients who can drink from a cup. For young infants (less than 6 months) who cannot eat solid food or drink from a cup, oral powder should be mixed with infant formula and given using an oral dosing syringe. Administration of atazanavir and infant formula using an infant bottle is not recommended because full dose may not be delivered.

Determine the number of packets (4 or 5 packets) needed. Mix with a small amount (one tablespoon) of soft food (preferred [eg, applesauce, yogurt]) or beverage (milk, formula, water). After administration, add an additional small amount of soft food or beverage to the container, mix, and feed the residual amount to insure that the entire dose has been consumed.

Storage/Stability

Store capsules at 25°C (77°F); excursions are permitted between 15°C and 30°C (59°F and 86°F).

Store oral powder below 30°C (86°F). Store oral powder in the original packet and do not open until ready to use. Once the oral powder is mixed with food or beverage, it may be kept at 20°C to 30°C (68°F to 86°F) for up to 1 hour prior to administration.

Mechanism of Action Binds to the site of HIV-1 protease activity and inhibits cleavage of viral Gag-Pol polyprotein precursors into individual functional proteins required for infectious HIV. This results in the formation of immature, noninfectious viral particles.

Pharmacodynamics/Kinetics

Absorption: Rapid; enhanced with food

Distribution: CSF: Plasma concentration ratio (range): 0.0021 to 0.0226

Protein binding: 86%; binds to both alpha$_1$-acid glycoprotein and albumin (similar affinity)

Metabolism: Hepatic, primarily by cytochrome P450 isoenzyme CYP3A; also undergoes biliary elimination; major biotransformation pathways include mono-oxygenation and deoxygenation; minor pathways for parent drug or metabolites include glucuronidation, N-dealkylation, hydrolysis and oxygenation with dehydrogenation; 2 minor inactive metabolites have been identified

Half-life elimination: Unboosted therapy: 7 to 8 hours; Boosted therapy (with ritonavir): 9 to 18 hours; 12 hours in patients with hepatic impairment

Time to peak, plasma: 2 to 3 hours

Excretion: Feces (79%, 20% of total dose as unchanged drug); urine (13%, 7% of total dose as unchanged drug)

Dosing

Adult & Geriatric

Treatment of HIV-1 infection: Oral:

Antiretroviral-naive patients: Atazanavir 300 mg once daily **plus** ritonavir 100 mg **or** cobicistat 150 mg once daily **or** atazanavir 400 mg once daily in patients unable to tolerate ritonavir.

Antiretroviral-experienced patients: Atazanavir 300 mg once daily **plus** ritonavir 100 mg **or** cobicistat 150 mg once daily. **Note:** Atazanavir without ritonavir is not recommended in antiretroviral-experienced patients with prior virologic failure.

Pregnant patients, antiretroviral naive or experienced: Atazanavir 300 mg once daily **plus** ritonavir 100 mg once daily. **Note:** Preferred regimen for pregnant patients who are antiretroviral-naive (DHHS [perinatal], 2014). Postpartum dosage adjustment not needed. Observe patient for adverse events, especially within 2 months after delivery. Dose adjustments required for treatment-experienced patients during their second and third trimester if concomitant tenofovir *or* H$_2$ antagonist use (insufficient information for dose adjustment if *both* tenofovir and an H$_2$ antagonist are used). Some experts recommend atazanavir 400 mg plus ritonavir 100 mg in all pregnant women during the second and third trimesters due to decreased plasma concentrations (DHHS [perinatal], 2014).

Dosage adjustments for concomitant therapy:
Coadministration with efavirenz:

Antiretroviral-naive patients: Atazanavir 400 mg plus ritonavir 100 mg given with efavirenz 600 mg (all once daily but administered at different times; atazanavir and ritonavir with food and efavirenz on an empty stomach).

Antiretroviral-experienced patients: Concurrent use not recommended due to decreased atazanavir exposure.

Coadministration with didanosine buffered or enteric-coated formulations: Administer atazanavir 2 hours before or 1 hour after didanosine buffered or enteric coated formulations

Coadministration with H$_2$ antagonists:

Antiretroviral-naive patients: Atazanavir 300 mg plus ritonavir 100 mg given simultaneously with, or at least 10 hours after an H$_2$ antagonist equivalent dose of ≤80 mg famotidine/day

Patients unable to tolerate ritonavir: Atazanavir 400 mg once daily given at least 2 hours before or at least 10 hours after an H$_2$ antagonist equivalent daily dose of ≤40 mg famotidine (single dose ≤20 mg)

Antiretroviral-experienced patients: Atazanavir 300 mg plus ritonavir 100 mg given simultaneously with, or at least 10 hours after an H$_2$ antagonist equivalent dose of ≤40 mg famotidine/day

Antiretroviral-experienced pregnant patients in the second or third trimester: Atazanavir 400 mg plus ritonavir 100 mg simultaneously with, or at least 10 hours after an H$_2$ antagonist. **Note:** Insufficient information for dose adjustment if tenofovir **and** an H$_2$ antagonist are used.

Coadministration with proton pump inhibitors:

U.S. labeling:

Antiretroviral-naive patients: Atazanavir 300 mg plus ritonavir 100 mg given 12 hours after a proton pump inhibitor equivalent dose of ≤20 mg omeprazole/day

Antiretroviral-experienced patients: Concurrent use not recommended. (**Note:** One study noted adequate serum concentrations when atazanavir 400 mg plus ritonavir 100 mg was given at the same time or 12 hours after omeprazole 20 mg.)

Canadian labeling: Concurrent use is not recommended; however, if unavoidable, administer atazanavir 400 mg plus ritonavir 100 mg once daily with proton pump inhibitor equivalent dose of ≤20 mg omeprazole/day. **Note:** Manufacturer's labeling does not specify patient population (antiretroviral-naive and/or experienced) to which dosing recommendation applies.

Coadministration with tenofovir:

Antiretroviral-naive patients: Atazanavir 300 mg plus ritonavir 100 mg given with tenofovir 300 mg (all as a single daily dose)

Antiretroviral-experienced patients: Atazanavir 300 mg plus ritonavir 100 mg given with tenofovir 300 mg (all as a single daily dose); if H$_2$ antagonist coadministered (not to exceed equivalent daily dose of ≤40 mg famotidine), increase atazanavir to 400 mg (plus ritonavir 100 mg) once daily

Antiretroviral-experienced pregnant patients in the second or third trimester: Atazanavir 400 mg plus ritonavir 100 mg. **Note:** Insufficient information for dose adjustment if tenofovir **and** an H$_2$ antagonist are used

Pediatric

Treatment of HIV-1 infection: Infants ≥3 months, Children and Adolescents <18 years: Oral: **Note:** Ritonavir-boosted atazanavir dosing regimen is preferred. Atazanavir is not approved for use in pediatric patients <6 years in the Canadian labeling.

Ritonavir-unboosted regimen:

Antiretroviral-naive patients:

Children 6 years to <13 years: Dose not established; use not recommended

Adolescents <40 kg **who are not able to tolerate ritonavir:** No dosage recommendations provided in the manufacturer's labeling.

Adolescents ≥40 kg **who are not able to tolerate ritonavir:** Atazanavir 400 mg once daily (without ritonavir). **Note:** Ritonavir boosted atazanavir dosing regimen is preferred; data indicate that higher atazanavir dosing (ie, higher on a mg/kg or mg/m^2 basis than predicted by adult dosing guidelines) may be needed when atazanavir is used without ritonavir boosting in children and adolescents (DHHS [pediatric], 2014).

Ritonavir-boosted regimen: **Note:** An increase to atazanavir 300 mg for patients ≥35 kg, especially when given with tenofovir, may be considered (DHHS [pediatric], 2014)

Antiretroviral-naive patients: Oral powder: Infants ≥3 months and Children weighing 5 to <10 kg: Atazanavir 200 mg (4 packets) **plus** ritonavir 80 mg once daily **or**, if not tolerated, atazanavir 150 mg (3 packets) **plus** ritonavir 80 mg once daily with close HIV viral load monitoring

Antiretroviral-naive and experienced patients:

Oral powder: Infants ≥3 months and Children and Adolescents weighing ≥5 kg:

5 to <15 kg: Atazanavir 200 mg (4 packets) **plus** ritonavir 80 mg once daily. In antiretroviral-naïve patients weighing 5 to <10 kg unable to tolerate this dose, may use atazanavir 150 mg (3 packets) **plus** ritonavir 80 mg once daily with close HIV viral load monitoring.

15 to <25 kg: Atazanavir 250 mg (5 packets) **plus** ritonavir 80 mg once daily

≥25 kg, patient cannot swallow capsules: Atazanavir 300 mg (6 packets) **plus** ritonavir 100 mg once daily

Oral capsules: Children ≥6 years and Adolescents <18 years:

15 to <20 kg: Atazanavir 150 mg once daily **plus** ritonavir 100 mg once daily

20 to <40 kg: Atazanavir 200 mg once daily **plus** ritonavir 100 mg once daily

≥40 kg: Atazanavir 300 mg once daily **plus** ritonavir 100 mg once daily

Dosage adjustment for concomitant therapy: Antiretroviral-experienced or antiretroviral-naive patients: Coadministration with H$_2$ antagonists, proton pump inhibitors, or other antiretroviral agents (eg, efavirenz, tenofovir, didanosine):

Infants ≥3 months, Children and Adolescents: Refer to adult dosing for recommendations regarding the timing and maximum doses of concomitant proton pump inhibitors, H$_2$ antagonists, and other antiretroviral agents.

Renal Impairment

Mild to severe impairment: No dosage adjustment necessary.

ESRD receiving IHD:

Antiretroviral-naive patients: Use boosted therapy of atazanavir 300 mg with ritonavir 100 mg once daily

Antiretroviral-experienced patients: Not recommended.

Hepatic Impairment

Atazanavir: *Antiretroviral-naive patients:*

Mild impairment (Child-Pugh class A): Atazanavir 400 mg once daily

Moderate impairment (Child-Pugh class B): Atazanavir 300 mg once daily

Severe impairment (Child-Pugh class C): Use is not recommended.

Note: Patients with underlying hepatitis B or C may be at increased risk of hepatic decompensation.

Atazanavir/ritonavir: Mild to severe impairment: Use is not recommended (has not been studied).

Dietary Considerations Must be taken with food; enhances absorption.

Administration Administer with food. Administer atazanavir 2 hours before or 1 hour after didanosine buffered formulations, didanosine enteric-coated capsules, other buffered medications, or antacids. Administer atazanavir (with ritonavir) simultaneously with, or at least 10 hours after, H$_2$-receptor antagonists; administer atazanavir (without ritonavir) at least 2 hours before or at least 10 hours after H$_2$-receptor antagonist. Administer atazanavir (with ritonavir) 12 hours after proton pump inhibitor.

Additional formulation specific information:

Oral capsules: Swallow capsules whole, do not open.

Oral powder: Mixing with food: Using a spoon, mix the recommended number of oral powder packets with a minimum of one tablespoon of food (such as applesauce or yogurt) in a small container. Feed the mixture to the patient. Add an additional one tablespoon of food to the container, mix, and feed the patient the residual mixture.

Mixing with a beverage such as milk or water in a small drinking cup: Using a spoon, mix the recommended number of oral powder packets with a minimum of 30 mL of the beverage in a drinking cup. Have the patient drink the mixture. Add an additional 15 mL more of beverage to the cup, mix, and have the patient drink the residual mixture. If water is used, food should also be taken at the same time.

Mixing with liquid infant formula using an oral dosing syringe and a small medicine cup: Using a spoon, mix the recommended number of oral powder packets with 10 mL of prepared liquid infant formula in the medicine cup. Draw up the full amount of the mixture into an oral syringe and administer into either right or left inner cheek of infant. Pour another 10 mL of formula into the medicine cup to rinse off remaining oral powder in cup. Draw up residual mixture into the syringe and administer into either right or left inner cheek of infant.

Administer the entire dosage of oral powder (mixed in the food or beverage) within one hour of preparation (may leave the mixture at room temperature during this one hour period). Ensure that the patient eats or drinks all

the food or beverage that contains the powder. Additional food may be given after consumption of the entire mixture. Administer ritonavir immediately following oral powder administration.

Monitoring Parameters Viral load, CD4, serum glucose; liver function tests, bilirubin, drug levels (with certain concomitant medications), ECG monitoring in patients with preexisting prolonged PR interval or with concurrent AV nodal blocking drugs

Additional Information A listing of medications that should not be used concurrently is available with each bottle and patients should be provided with this information.

Dosage Forms Excipient information presented when available (limited, particularly for generics); consult specific product labeling.

Capsule, Oral, as sulfate:
Reyataz: 150 mg, 200 mg, 300 mg [contains fd&c blue #2 (indigotine)]
Packet, Oral, as sulfate:
Reyataz: 50 mg (30 ea) [contains aspartame; orange-vanilla flavor]

◆ Atazanavir Sulfate see Atazanavir on page 162
◆ Atelvia see Risedronate on page 1591

Atenolol (a TEN oh lole)

Brand Names: US Tenormin
Brand Names: Canada Apo-Atenol; Ava-Atenolol; CO Atenolol; Dom-Atenolol; JAMP-Atenolol; Mint-Atenolol; Mylan-Atenolol; Nu-Atenol; PMS-Atenolol; RAN-Atenolol; ratio-Atenolol; Riva-Atenolol; Sandoz-Atenolol; Septa-Atenolol; Tenormin; Teva-Atenolol
Pharmacologic Category Antianginal Agent; Antihypertensive; Beta-Blocker, Beta-1 Selective

Use
Hypertension: Treatment of hypertension, alone or in combination with other agents; management of angina pectoris; secondary prevention postmyocardial infarction

Guideline recommendations:
Hypertension: The 2014 guideline for the management of high blood pressure in adults (Eighth Joint National Committee [JNC 8]) recommends initiation of pharmacologic treatment to lower blood pressure for the following patients (JNC8 [James, 2013]):
• Patients ≥60 years of age with systolic blood pressure (SBP) ≥150 mm Hg or diastolic blood pressure (DBP) ≥90 mm Hg. Goal of therapy is SBP <150 mm Hg and DBP <90 mm Hg.
• Patients <60 years of age with SBP ≥140 mm Hg or DBP is ≥90 mm Hg. Goal of therapy is SBP <140 mm Hg and DBP <90 mm Hg.
• Patients ≥18 years of age with diabetes and SBP ≥140 mm Hg or DBP ≥90 mm Hg. Goal of therapy is SBP <140 mm Hg and DBP <90 mm Hg.
• Patients ≥18 years of age with chronic kidney disease (CKD) and SBP ≥140 mm Hg or DBP ≥90 mm Hg. Goal of therapy is SBP <140 mm Hg and DBP <90 mm Hg.
Chronic kidney disease (CKD) and hypertension: Regardless of race or diabetes status, the use of an ACE inhibitor (ACEI) or angiotensin receptor blocker (ARB) as initial therapy is recommended to improve kidney outcomes. In the general nonblack population (without CKD) including those with diabetes, initial antihypertensive treatment should consist of a thiazide-type diuretic, calcium channel blocker, ACEI, or ARB. In the general black population (without CKD) including those with diabetes, initial antihypertensive treatment should consist of a thiazide-type diuretic or a calcium channel blocker **instead of** an ACEI or ARB.
Coronary artery disease (CAD) and hypertension: The American Heart Association, American College of Cardiology and American Society of Hypertension (AHA/ACC/ASH) 2015 scientific statement for the treatment of hypertension in patients with coronary artery disease (CAD) recommends the use of a beta blocker as part of a regimen in patients with hypertension and chronic stable angina with a history of prior MI. A BP target of <140/90 mm Hg is reasonable for the secondary prevention of cardiovascular events. A lower target BP (<130/80 mm Hg) may be appropriate in some individuals with CAD, previous MI, stroke or transient ischemic attack, or CAD risk equivalents (AHA/ACC/ASH [Rosendorff 2015]).

Pregnancy Considerations Studies in pregnant women have demonstrated a risk to the fetus; therefore, the manufacturer classifies atenolol as pregnancy category D. Atenolol crosses the placenta and is found in cord blood. In a cohort study, an increased risk of cardiovascular defects was observed following maternal use of beta-blockers during pregnancy. Intrauterine growth restriction (IUGR), small placentas, as well as fetal/neonatal bradycardia, hypoglycemia, and/or respiratory depression have been observed following in utero exposure to beta-blockers as a class. Adequate facilities for monitoring infants at birth should be available. Untreated chronic maternal hypertension and pre-eclampsia are also associated with adverse events in the fetus, infant, and mother. The maternal pharmacokinetic parameters of atenolol during the second and third trimesters are within the ranges reported in nonpregnant patients. Although atenolol has shown efficacy in the treatment of hypertension in pregnancy, it is not the drug of choice due to potential IUGR in the infant.

Breast-Feeding Considerations Atenolol is excreted in breast milk and has been detected in the serum and urine of nursing infants. Peak concentrations in breast milk have been reported to occur between 2 to 8 hours after the maternal dose and in some cases are higher than the peak maternal serum concentration. Although most studies have not reported adverse events in nursing infants, avoiding maternal use while nursing infants with renal dysfunction or infants <44 weeks postconceptual age has been suggested. Beta-blockers with less distribution into breast milk may be preferred. The manufacturer recommends that caution be exercised when administering atenolol to nursing women.

Contraindications Hypersensitivity to atenolol or any component of the formulation; sinus bradycardia; sinus node dysfunction; heart block greater than first-degree (except in patients with a functioning artificial pacemaker); cardiogenic shock; uncompensated cardiac failure; pulmonary edema; pregnancy

Warnings/Precautions Consider preexisting conditions such as sick sinus syndrome before initiating. Administer cautiously in compensated heart failure and monitor for a worsening of the condition (efficacy of atenolol in heart failure has not been established). **[US Boxed Warning]: Beta-blocker therapy should not be withdrawn abruptly (particularly in patients with CAD), but gradually tapered to avoid acute tachycardia, hypertension, and/or ischemia.** Beta-blockers without alpha1-adrenergic receptor blocking activity should be avoided in patients with Prinzmetal variant angina (Mayer, 1998). Chronic beta-blocker therapy should not be routinely withdrawn prior to major surgery. Beta-blockers should be avoided in patients with bronchospastic disease (asthma). Atenolol, with B$_1$ selectivity, has been used cautiously in bronchospastic disease with close monitoring. May precipitate or aggravate symptoms of arterial insufficiency in patients with PVD and Raynaud's disease; use with caution and monitor for progression of arterial obstruction. Use cautiously in patients with diabetes - may mask hypoglycemic symptoms. May mask signs of hyperthyroidism (eg, tachycardia); use caution if hyperthyroidism is suspected, abrupt withdrawal may precipitate thyroid storm. Alterations in thyroid function tests may be observed. Use cautiously in the renally impaired (dosage adjustment required). Caution in myasthenia gravis or psychiatric disease (may cause CNS depression). Bradycardia may be observed more frequently in elderly patients (>65 years of age); dosage reductions may be necessary. Adequate alpha-blockade is required prior to use of any beta-blocker for patients with untreated pheochromocytoma. May induce or exacerbate psoriasis. Use caution with history of severe anaphylaxis to allergens; patients taking beta-blockers may become more sensitive to repeated challenges. Treatment of anaphylaxis (eg, epinephrine) in patients taking beta-blockers may be ineffective or promote undesirable effects. Use with caution in patients on concurrent digoxin, verapamil, or diltiazem; bradycardia or heart block can occur. Use with caution in patients receiving inhaled anesthetic agents known to depress myocardial contractility.

Adverse Reactions
1% to 10%:
Cardiovascular: Bradycardia (persistent), cardiac failure, chest pain, cold extremities, complete atrioventricular block, edema, hypotension, Raynaud's phenomenon, second degree atrioventricular block
Central nervous system: Confusion, decreased mental acuity, depression, dizziness, fatigue, headache, insomnia, lethargy, nightmares
Gastrointestinal: Constipation, diarrhea, nausea
Genitourinary: Impotence
<1% (Limited to important or life-threatening): Alopecia, dyspnea (especially with large doses), hallucination, increased liver enzymes, lupus-like syndrome, Peyronie's disease, positive ANA titer, psoriasiform eruption, psychosis, thrombocytopenia, wheezing

Drug Interactions

Metabolism/Transport Effects None known.

Avoid Concomitant Use

Avoid concomitant use of Atenolol with any of the following: Ceritinib; Floctafenine; Methacholine; Rivastigmine

Increased Effect/Toxicity

Atenolol may increase the levels/effects of: Alpha-/Beta-Agonists (Direct-Acting); Alpha1-Blockers; Alpha2-Agonists; Amifostine; Antipsychotic Agents (Second Generation [Atypical]); Bradycardia-Causing Agents; Bupivacaine; Cardiac Glycosides; Ceritinib; Cholinergic Agonists; Disopyramide; DULoxetine; Ergot Derivatives; Fingolimod; Grass Pollen Allergen Extract (5 Grass Extract); Hypotension-Associated Agents; Insulin; Ivabradine; Lacosamide; Levodopa; Lidocaine (Systemic); Lidocaine (Topical); Mepivacaine; Methacholine; Midodrine; Sulfonylureas

The levels/effects of Atenolol may be increased by: Acetylcholinesterase Inhibitors; Alpha2-Agonists; Amiodarone; Anilidopiperidine Opioids; Barbiturates; Bretylium; Brimonidine (Topical); Calcium Channel Blockers (Nondihydropyridine); Diazoxide; Dipyridamole; Disopyramide; Dronedarone; Floctafenine; Glycopyrrolate; Glycopyrrolate (Systemic); Herbs (Hypotensive Properties); Molsidomine; Nicorandil; NIFEdipine; Obinutuzumab; Pentoxifylline; Phosphodiesterase 5 Inhibitors; Prostacyclin Analogues; Regorafenib; Reserpine; Rivastigmine; Ruxolitinib; Tofacitinib

Decreased Effect

Atenolol may decrease the levels/effects of: Beta2-Agonists; Theophylline Derivatives

The levels/effects of Atenolol may be decreased by: Amphetamines; Ampicillin; Herbs (Hypertensive Properties); Methylphenidate; Nonsteroidal Anti-Inflammatory Agents; Yohimbine

Food Interactions Atenolol serum concentrations may be decreased if taken with food. Management: Administer without regard to meals.

Storage/Stability Store at 20°C to 25°C (68°F to 77°F).

Mechanism of Action Competitively blocks response to beta-adrenergic stimulation, selectively blocks beta$_1$-receptors with little or no effect on beta$_2$-receptors except at high doses

Pharmacodynamics/Kinetics

Onset of action: Beta-blocking effect: Onset: Oral: ≤1 hour; Peak effect: Oral: 2 to 4 hours

Duration: Normal renal function: Beta-blocking effect: 12 to 24 hours; Antihypertensive effect: Oral: 24 hours

Absorption: Oral: Rapid, incomplete (~50%)

Distribution: Low lipophilicity; does not cross blood-brain barrier

Protein binding: 6% to 16%

Metabolism: Limited hepatic

Half-life elimination: Beta:

Newborns (<24 hours of age) born to mothers receiving atenolol: Mean: 16 hours; up to 35 hours (Rubin 1983)

Children and Adolescents 5 to 16 years of age: Mean: 4.6 hours; range: 3.5 to 7 hours; Patients >10 years of age may have longer half-life (>5 hours) compared to children 5 to 10 years of age (<5 hours) (Buck 1989)

Adults: Normal renal function: 6 to 7 hours, prolonged with renal impairment; End-stage renal disease (ESRD): 15 to 35 hours

Time to peak, plasma: Oral: 2 to 4 hours

Excretion: Feces (50%); urine (40% as unchanged drug)

Dosing

Adult

Hypertension: Oral: Initial: 25 to 50 mg once daily, after 1 to 2 weeks, may increase to 100 mg once daily; usual dose (ASH/ISH [Weber, 2014]): 100 mg once daily; target dose (JNC 8 [James, 2013]): 100 mg once daily. Doses >100 mg are unlikely to produce any further benefit.

Angina pectoris: Oral: 50 mg once daily; may increase to 100 mg daily. Some patients may require 200 mg daily.

Postmyocardial infarction: Oral: 100 mg/day or 50 mg twice daily for 6 to 9 days postmyocardial infarction

Atrial fibrillation (rate control) (off-label use): Usual maintenance dose: 25 to 100 mg once daily (AHA/ACC/HRS [January, 2014])

Thyrotoxicosis (off-label use): Oral: 25 to 100 mg once or twice daily (Bahn, 2011)

Geriatric Refer to adult dosing. In the management of hypertension, consider lower initial doses and titrate to response (Aronow, 2011).

Pediatric Hypertension: Oral: Children: 0.5 to 1 mg/kg dose given daily; range of 0.5 to 1.5 mg/kg/day; maximum dose: 2 mg/kg/day up to 100 mg/day

Renal Impairment

CrCl >35 mL/minute/1.73 m^2: No dosage adjustment necessary.

CrCl 15 to 35 mL/minute/1.73 m^2: Maximum dose: 50 mg daily

CrCl <15 mL/minute/1.73 m^2: Maximum dose: 25 mg daily

Hemodialysis: Moderately dialyzable (20% to 50%) via hemodialysis; administer dose postdialysis or administer 25 to 50 mg supplemental dose.

Peritoneal dialysis: Elimination is not enhanced; supplemental dose is not necessary.

Hepatic Impairment There are no dosage adjustments provided in the manufacturer's labeling; however, atenolol undergoes minimal hepatic metabolism.

Dietary Considerations May be taken without regard to meals.

Administration When administered acutely for cardiac treatment, monitor ECG and blood pressure. May be administered without regard to meals.

Monitoring Parameters Acute cardiac treatment: Monitor ECG and blood pressure

Test Interactions Increased glucose; decreased HDL

Dosage Forms Excipient information presented when available (limited, particularly for generics); consult specific product labeling. [DSC] = Discontinued product

Tablet, Oral:

Tenormin: 25 mg, 50 mg

Tenormin: 50 mg [DSC] [scored]

Tenormin: 100 mg

Generic: 25 mg, 50 mg, 100 mg

Extemporaneous Preparations A 2 mg/mL oral suspension may be made with tablets. Crush four 50 mg tablets in a mortar and reduce to a fine powder. Add a small amount of glycerin and mix to a uniform paste. Mix while adding Ora-Sweet® SF vehicle in incremental proportions to **almost** 100 mL; transfer to a calibrated bottle, rinse mortar with vehicle, and add quantity of vehicle sufficient to make 100 mL. Label "shake well" and "refrigerate". Stable for 90 days.

Nahata MC, Pai VB, and Hipple TF, *Pediatric Drug Formulations*, 5th ed, Cincinnati, OH: Harvey Whitney Books Co, 2004.

♦ **ATG** see Antithymocyte Globulin (Equine) on page 136

♦ **Atgam** see Antithymocyte Globulin (Equine) on page 136

♦ **Athletes Foot Spray [OTC]** see Tolnaftate on page 1807

♦ **Ativan** see LORazepam on page 1103

♦ **Atlizumab** see Tocilizumab on page 1802

♦ **ATNAA** see Atropine and Pralidoxime on page 179

♦ **ATO** see Arsenic Trioxide on page 154

AtoMOXetine (AT oh mox e teen)

Brand Names: US Strattera

Brand Names: Canada Apo-Atomoxetine; DOM-Atomoxetine; Mylan-Atomoxetine; PMS-Atomoxetine; RIVA-Atomoxetine; Sandoz-Atomoxetine; Strattera; Teva-Atomoxetine

Index Terms Atomoxetine Hydrochloride; LY139603; Methylphenoxy-Benzene Propanamine; Tomoxetine

Pharmacologic Category Norepinephrine Reuptake Inhibitor, Selective

Use Attention-deficit/hyperactivity disorder: Treatment of attention-deficit/hyperactivity disorder (ADHD)

Pregnancy Considerations Adverse events have been observed in animal reproduction studies. Information related to atomoxetine use in pregnancy is limited; appropriate contraception is recommended for sexually active women of childbearing potential (Heiligenstein, 2003).

Breast-Feeding Considerations It is not known if atomoxetine is excreted in breast milk. The manufacturer recommends that caution be exercised when administering atomoxetine to nursing women.

Medication Guide Available Yes

Contraindications Hypersensitivity to atomoxetine or any component of the formulation; use with or within 14 days of MAO inhibitors; narrow-angle glaucoma; current or past history of pheochromocytoma; severe cardiac or vascular disorders in which the condition would be expected to deteriorate with clinically important increases in blood pressure (eg, 15 to 20 mm Hg) or heart rate (eg, 20 beats/minute).

Canadian labeling: Additional contraindications (not in U.S. labeling): Symptomatic cardiovascular diseases, moderate-to-severe hypertension; advanced arteriosclerosis; uncontrolled hyperthyroidism

Warnings/Precautions [US Boxed Warning]: Use caution in pediatric patients; may be an increased risk of suicidal ideation. Closely monitor for clinical worsening, suicidality, or unusual changes in behavior; especially

during the initial few months of a course of drug therapy, or at times of dose changes, either increases or decreases. The family or caregiver should be instructed to closely observe the patient and communicate condition with healthcare provider. New or worsening symptoms of hostility or aggressive behaviors have been associated with atomoxetine, particularly with the initiation of therapy. Treatment-emergent psychotic or manic symptoms (eg, hallucinations, delusional thinking, mania) may occur in children and adolescents without a prior history of psychotic illness or mania; consider discontinuation of treatment if symptoms occur. Use caution in patients with comorbid bipolar disorder; therapy may induce mixed/manic episode. Atomoxetine is not approved for major depressive disorder. Patients presenting with depressive symptoms should be screened for bipolar disorder. Recommended to be used as part of a comprehensive treatment program for attention deficit disorders. Atomoxetine does not worsen anxiety in patients with existing anxiety disorders or tics related to Tourette's disorder.

Use caution with hepatic disease (dosage adjustments necessary in moderate and severe hepatic impairment). Use may be associated with rare but severe hepatotoxicity, including hepatic failure; discontinue and do not restart if signs or symptoms of hepatotoxic reaction (eg, jaundice, pruritus, flu-like symptoms, dark urine, right upper quadrant tenderness) or laboratory evidence of liver disease are noted. Use caution in patients who are poor metabolizers of CYP2D6 metabolized drugs ("poor metabolizers"), bioavailability increases; dosage adjustments are recommended in patients known to be CYP2D6 poor metabolizers. In clinical trials, at therapeutic doses, atomoxetine consistently did not prolong the QT/QTc interval; however, one placebo-controlled study in healthy CYP2D6 poor metabolizers demonstrated a statistically significant increase in QTc with increasing atomoxetine concentrations (Loghin 2012; Martinez-Raga 2013). Case reports suggest that atomoxetine overdose may increase the QT interval; however, this occurred when atomoxetine was combined with other agents known to have QT prolongation potential or inhibit CYP2D6 (Barker 2004; Sawant 2004). Atomoxetine, at high concentrations ex vivo, has demonstrated hERG channel block (Scherer 2009).

Orthostasis can occur; use caution in patients predisposed to hypotension or those with abrupt changes in heart rate or blood pressure. Atomoxetine has been associated with serious cardiovascular events including sudden death in patients with preexisting structural cardiac abnormalities or other serious heart problems (sudden death in children and adolescents; sudden death, stroke, and MI in adults). Atomoxetine should be avoided in patients with known serious structural cardiac abnormalities, cardiomyopathy, serious heart rhythm abnormalities, or other serious cardiac problems that could increase the risk of sudden death that these conditions alone carry. Patients should be carefully evaluated for cardiac disease prior to initiation of therapy. Perform a prompt cardiac evaluation in patients who develop symptoms of exertional chest pain, unexplained syncope, or other symptoms suggestive of cardiac disease during treatment. May cause increased heart rate or blood pressure; use caution with hypertension or other cardiovascular or cerebrovascular disease; CYP2D6 poor metabolizers may experience greater increases in blood pressure and heart rate effects. Use caution in patients with a history of urinary retention or bladder outlet obstruction; may cause urinary retention/hesitancy; use caution in patients with history of urinary retention or bladder outlet obstruction. Prolonged and painful erections (priapism), sometimes requiring surgical intervention, have been reported with stimulant and atomoxetine use in pediatric and adult patients. Priapism has been reported to develop after some time on the drug, often subsequent to an increase in dose and also during a period of drug withdrawal (drug holidays or discontinuation). Patients with certain hematological dyscrasias (eg, sickle cell disease), malignancies, perineal trauma, or concomitant use of alcohol, illicit drugs, or other medications associated with priapism may be at increased risk. Patients who develop abnormally sustained or frequent and painful erections should discontinue therapy and seek immediate medical attention. An emergent urological consultation should be obtained in severe cases. Use has been associated with different dosage forms and products; it is not known if rechallenge with a different formulation will risk recurrence. Avoidance of stimulants and atomoxetine may be preferred in patients with severe cases that were slow to resolve and/or required detumescence (Eiland, 2014). Allergic reactions (including anaphylactic reactions, angioneurotic edema, urticaria, and rash) may occur (rare).

Growth in pediatric patients should be monitored during treatment. Height and weight gain may be reduced during the first 9 to 12 months of treatment, but should recover by 3 years of therapy.

Adverse Reactions Percentages as reported in children and adults; some adverse reactions may be increased in "poor metabolizers" (CYP2D6). Frequency not always defined.

>10%:
Central nervous system: Headache (19%; children and adolescents), insomnia (1% to 19%), drowsiness (8% to 11%)
Dermatologic: Hyperhidrosis (4% to 15%)
Gastrointestinal: Xerostomia (17% to 35%), nausea (7% to 26%), decreased appetite (15% to 23%), abdominal pain (7% to 18%), vomiting (4% to 11%), constipation (1% to 11%)
Genitourinary: Erectile dysfunction (8% to 21%)
1% to 10%:
Cardiovascular: Increased diastolic blood pressure (5% to 9%; ≥15 mm Hg), systolic hypertension (4% to 5%), palpitations (3%), cold extremities (1% to 3%), syncope (≤3%), flushing (≥2%), orthostatic hypotension (≤2%), tachycardia (≤2%), prolonged Q-T interval on ECG
Central nervous system: Fatigue (6% to 10%), dizziness (5% to 8%), depression (4% to 7%), disturbed sleep (3% to 7%), irritability (5% to 6%), jitteriness (2% to 5%), abnormal dreams (4%), chills (3%), paresthesia (adults 3%; postmarketing observation in children), anxiety (≥2%), hostility (children and adolescents 2%), emotional lability (1% to 2%), agitation, restlessness, sensation of cold
Dermatologic: Excoriation (2% to 4%), skin rash (2%), pruritus, urticaria
Endocrine & metabolic: Weight loss (2% to 7%), decreased libido (3%), hot flash (3%), increased thirst (2%), menstrual disease
Gastrointestinal: Dyspepsia (4%), anorexia (3%), dysgeusia, flatulence
Genitourinary: Ejaculatory disorder (2% to 6%), urinary retention (1% to 6%), dysmenorrhea (3%), dysuria (2%), orgasm abnormal, pollakiuria, prostatitis, testicular pain, urinary frequency
Neuromuscular & skeletal: Tremor (1% to 5%), muscle spasm, weakness
Ophthalmic: Blurred vision (1% to 4%), conjunctivitis (1% to 3%), mydriasis
Respiratory: Pharyngolaryngeal pain
Miscellaneous: Therapeutic response unexpected (2%)
<1% (Limited to important or life-threatening): Cerebrovascular accident, delusions, growth suppression (children), hallucination, hepatotoxicity, hypersensitivity reaction, hypomania, impulsivity, mania, myocardial infarction, panic attack, pelvic pain, priapism, Raynaud's phenomenon, rhabdomyolysis, seizure (including patients with no prior history or known risk factors for seizure), severe hepatic disease, suicidal ideation, tics

Drug Interactions
Metabolism/Transport Effects Substrate of CYP2C19 (minor), CYP2D6 (major); **Note:** Assignment of Major/Minor substrate status based on clinically relevant drug interaction potential; **Inhibits** CYP2D6 (weak)
Avoid Concomitant Use
Avoid concomitant use of AtoMOXetine with any of the following: Iobenguane I 123; MAO Inhibitors
Increased Effect/Toxicity
AtoMOXetine may increase the levels/effects of: ARIPiprazole; Beta2-Agonists; Highest Risk QTc-Prolonging Agents; Moderate Risk QTc-Prolonging Agents; Sympathomimetics

The levels/effects of AtoMOXetine may be increased by: Abiraterone Acetate; Cobicistat; CYP2D6 Inhibitors (Moderate); CYP2D6 Inhibitors (Strong); Darunavir; MAO Inhibitors; Mifepristone; Panobinostat; Peginterferon Alfa-2b
Decreased Effect
AtoMOXetine may decrease the levels/effects of: Iobenguane I 123

The levels/effects of AtoMOXetine may be decreased by: Peginterferon Alfa-2b
Storage/Stability Store at 25°C (77°F); excursions are permitted between 15°C and 30°C (59°F and 86°F).
Mechanism of Action Selectively inhibits the reuptake of norepinephrine (Ki 4.5 nM) with little to no activity at the other neuronal reuptake pumps or receptor sites.
Pharmacodynamics/Kinetics
Note: The pharmacokinetics in pediatric patients ≥6 years of age have been shown to be similar to those of adult patients.
Absorption: Rapid

Distribution: V_d: IV: 0.85 L/kg

Protein binding: 98%, primarily albumin

Metabolism: Hepatic, via CYP2D6 and CYP2C19; forms metabolites (4-hydroxyatomoxetine, active, equipotent to atomoxetine; N-desmethylatomoxetine, limited activity); **Note:** CYP2D6 poor metabolizers have atomoxetine AUCs that are ~10-fold higher and peak concentrations that are ~fivefold greater than extensive metabolizers; 4-hyroxyatomoxetine plasma concentrations are very low (extensive metabolizers: 1% of atomoxetine concentrations; poor metabolizers: 0.1% of atomoxetine concentrations

Bioavailability: 63% in extensive metabolizers; 94% in poor metabolizers

Half-life elimination: Atomoxetine: 5 hours (up to 24 hours in poor metabolizers); Active metabolites: 4-hydroxyatomoxetine: 6-8 hours; N-desmethylatomoxetine: 6-8 hours (34-40 hours in poor metabolizers)

Time to peak, plasma: 1-2 hours; delayed 3 hours by high-fat meal

Excretion: Urine (80%, as conjugated 4-hydroxy metabolite; <3% is excreted unchanged); feces (17%)

Dosing

Adult Attention deficit hyperactivity disorder (ADHD) treatment: Oral: **Note:** Atomoxetine may be discontinued without the need for tapering dose.

U.S. labeling:

Initial: 40 mg/day, increased after minimum of 3 days to ~80 mg/day; may administer as either a single daily dose or 2 evenly divided doses in morning and late afternoon/early evening. May increase to 100 mg/day in 2-4 additional weeks to achieve optimal response. Maximum daily dose: 100 mg/day.

Dosage adjustment in patients receiving strong CYP2D6 inhibitors (eg, paroxetine, fluoxetine, quinidine) or patients known to be CYP2D6 poor metabolizers: Initial: 40 mg/day; if tolerating therapy but inadequate response, may increase after minimum of 4 weeks to 80 mg/day.

Canadian labeling:

Initial: 40 mg/day for 7-14 days (Step 1); if tolerated, may increase dose at 7-14 day intervals to 60 mg/day (Step 2) then to 80 mg/day (Step 3). If optimal response is not obtained after 2-4 additional weeks, may increase to a maximum dose of 100 mg/day.

Dosage adjustment in patients receiving strong CYP2D6 inhibitors: Initial: 40 mg/day; may increase to next dosage level after 14 days if previous dose is well tolerated but response is inadequate. **Note:** Canadian labeling does not include specific dosing recommendations in regards to patients who are poor CYP2D6 metabolizers although similar dose reductions would appear necessary.

Geriatric Use has not been evaluated in the elderly.

Pediatric ADHD treatment: Oral: **Note:** Atomoxetine may be discontinued without the need for tapering dose.

Children ≥6 years and ≤70 kg:

U.S. labeling:

Initial: 0.5 mg/kg/day, increase after minimum of 3 days to ~1.2 mg/kg/day; may administer as either a single daily dose or 2 evenly divided doses in morning and late afternoon/early evening. Maximum daily dose: 1.4 mg/kg or 100 mg, whichever is less.

Dosage adjustment in patients receiving strong CYP2D6 inhibitors (eg, paroxetine, fluoxetine, quinidine) or patients known to be CYP2D6 poor metabolizers: Initial: 0.5 mg/kg/day; if tolerating therapy but inadequate response, may increase after minimum of 4 weeks to 1.2 mg/kg/day.

Canadian labeling:

Initial: ~0.5 mg/kg/day for 7-14 days (Step 1); if tolerated, may increase to ~0.8 mg/kg/day for 7-14 days (Step 2), then to ~1.2 mg/kg/day (Step 3); re-evaluate after ≥30 days and adjust for response if necessary. Maximum daily dose: 1.4 mg/kg or 100 mg, whichever is less. **Note:** Children should weigh at least 20 kg at the time of initiation as 10 mg is the lowest available capsule strength and capsules are to be swallowed whole.

Dosing recommendations according to weight:

Initial (Step 1):
20-29 kg: 10 mg/day
30-44 kg: 18 mg/day
45-64 kg: 25 mg/day
65-70 kg: 40 mg/day

First titration (Step 2):
20-29 kg: 18 mg/day
30-44 kg: 25 mg/day
45-64 kg: 40 mg/day
65-70 kg: 60 mg/day

Second titration (Step 3):
20-29 kg: 25 mg/day
30-44 kg: 40 mg/day
45-64 kg: 60 mg/day
65-70 kg: 80 mg/day

Dosage adjustment in patients receiving strong CYP2D6 inhibitors: Initial: 0.5 mg/kg/day; may increase to next dosage level after 14 days if previous dose is well tolerated but response is inadequate. **Note:** Canadian labeling does not include specific dosing recommendations in regards to patients who are poor CYP2D6 metabolizers although similar dose reductions would appear necessary.

Children ≥6 years and >70 kg: Refer to adult dosing.

Renal Impairment No dosage adjustment necessary.

Hepatic Impairment

Mild impairment (Child-Pugh class A): No dosage adjustment provided in manufacturer's labeling.

Moderate impairment (Child-Pugh class B): All doses should be reduced to 50% of normal.

Severe impairment (Child-Pugh class C): All doses should be reduced to 25% of normal.

Administration Administer with or without food as a single daily dose in the morning or as two evenly divided doses in morning and late afternoon/early evening. Swallow capsules whole; do not open capsules. If opened accidentally, do not touch eyes; wash hands immediately (product is an ocular irritant).

Monitoring Parameters Patient growth (weight/height gain in children); attention, hyperactivity, anxiety, worsening of aggressive behavior or hostility; blood pressure and pulse (baseline and following dose increases and periodically during treatment)

Family members and caregivers need to monitor patient daily for emergence of irritability, agitation, unusual changes in behavior, and suicide ideation. Pediatric patients should be monitored closely for suicidality, clinical worsening, or unusual changes in behavior, especially during the initial for months of therapy or at times of dose changes. Appearance of symptoms needs to be immediately reported to healthcare provider.

Thoroughly evaluate for cardiovascular risk. Monitor heart rate, blood pressure, and consider obtaining ECG prior to initiation (Martinez-Raga, 2013; Vetter, 2008). Periodically reevaluate the long-term usefulness of the drug for the individual patient.

Dosage Forms Excipient information presented when available (limited, particularly for generics); consult specific product labeling.

Capsule, Oral:

Strattera: 10 mg, 18 mg, 25 mg, 40 mg, 60 mg

Strattera: 80 mg, 100 mg [contains fd&c blue #2 (indigotine)]

◆ Atomoxetine Hydrochloride *see* AtoMOXetine *on page 167*

AtorvaSTATin (a TORE va sta tin)

Brand Names: US Lipitor

Brand Names: Canada ACT Atorvastatin; Apo-Atorvastatin; Auro-Atorvastatin; Ava-Atorvastatin; Dom-Atorvastatin; GD-Atorvastatin; JAMP-Atorvastatin; Lipitor; Mylan-Atorvastatin; Novo-Atorvastatin; PMS-Atorvastatin; RAN-Atorvastatin; ratio-Atorvastatin; Reedy-Atorvastatin; Riva-Atorvastatin; Sandoz-Atorvastatin

Index Terms Atorvastatin Calcium

Pharmacologic Category Antilipemic Agent, HMG-CoA Reductase Inhibitor

Use

Dyslipidemias:

Dysbetalipoproteinemia: Treatment of primary dysbetalipoproteinemia (Fredrickson type III).

Heterozygous familial and nonfamilial hypercholesterolemia and mixed dyslipidemia: To reduce elevated total cholesterol (total-C), low-density lipoprotein cholesterol (LDL-C), apolipoprotein B (apo B), and triglyceride levels, and to increase HDL-C in patients with primary hypercholesterolemia (heterozygous familial and nonfamilial) and mixed dyslipidemia (Fredrickson type IIa and IIb).

Heterozygous familial hypercholesterolemia: To reduce total-C, LDL-C, and apo B levels in boys and postmenarche girls 10 to 17 years of age with heterozygous familial hypercholesterolemia with LDL-C ≥190 mg/dL, LDL-C ≥160 mg/dL with positive family history of premature cardiovascular disease (CVD), or LDL-C ≥160 mg/dL with two or more other CVD risk factors.

Homozygous familial hypercholesterolemia: To reduce total-C and LDL-C in patients with homozygous familial hypercholesterolemia as an adjunct to other lipid-lowering treatments (eg, LDL apheresis) or if such treatments are unavailable.

Hypertriglyceridemia: Treatment of elevated serum triglyceride levels (Fredrickson type IV).

Limitations of use: Has not been studied in conditions where the major lipid abnormality is elevation of chylomicrons (Fredrickson types I and V).

Prevention of cardiovascular disease (CVD):

Primary prevention of cardiovascular disease (high-risk for CVD): To reduce the risk of MI, stroke, and revascularization procedures and angina in adult patients without clinically evident coronary heart disease (CHD) who have multiple CHD risk factors (eg, age, smoking, hypertension, low high-density lipoprotein cholesterol [HDL-C], family history of early CHD); to reduce the risk of MI and stroke in patients with type 2 diabetes and without clinically evident CHD but with multiple risk factors for CHD (eg, retinopathy, albuminuria, smoking, hypertension).

Secondary prevention of cardiovascular disease: To reduce the risk of nonfatal MI, fatal and nonfatal stroke, revascularization procedures, hospitalization for decompensated heart failure, and angina in patients with clinically evident CHD.

Primary and secondary prevention of atherosclerotic cardiovascular disease (ASCVD) according to the American College of Cardiology/American Heart Association: To reduce the risk of ASCVD in patients with clinical ASCVD (eg, coronary heart disease, stroke/TIA, or peripheral arterial disease presumed to be of atherosclerotic origin); in patients without clinical ASCVD if LDL-C is 190 mg/dL or greater; in patients without clinical ASCVD who have type 1 or type 2 diabetes and are between 40 and 75 years of age; in patients with an estimated 10-year ASCVD risk 7.5% or greater and who are between 40 and 75 years of age (Stone 2013). Specific recommendations from the Kidney Disease: Improving Global Outcomes (KDIGO) organization have also been released for patients with chronic kidney disease (KDIGO [Tonelli 2013]).

Pregnancy Considerations Studies in animals and pregnant women have shown evidence of fetal abnormalities and use is contraindicated in women who are or may become pregnant. There are reports of congenital anomalies following maternal use of HMG-CoA reductase inhibitors in pregnancy; however, maternal disease, differences in specific agents used, and the low rates of exposure limit the interpretation of the available data (Godfrey 2012; Lecarpentier 2012). Cholesterol biosynthesis may be important in fetal development; serum cholesterol and triglycerides increase normally during pregnancy. The discontinuation of lipid lowering medications temporarily during pregnancy is not expected to have significant impact on the long term outcomes of primary hypercholesterolemia treatment.

HMG-CoA reductase inhibitors should be discontinued prior to pregnancy (ADA 2013). If treatment of dyslipidemias is needed in pregnant women or in women of reproductive age, other agents are preferred (Berglund 2012; Stone 2013). The manufacturer recommends administration to women of childbearing potential only when conception is highly unlikely and patients have been informed of potential hazards.

Breast-Feeding Considerations It is not known if atorvastatin is excreted in breast milk. Due to the potential for serious adverse reactions in a nursing infant, use while breast-feeding is contraindicated by the manufacturer.

Contraindications
Hypersensitivity to atorvastatin or any component of the formulation; active liver disease; unexplained persistent elevations of serum transaminases; pregnancy or women who may become pregnant; breast-feeding
Canadian labeling: Additional contraindications (not in US labeling): Telaprevir Canadian product monograph contraindicates use with atorvastatin.

Warnings/Precautions Secondary causes of hyperlipidemia should be ruled out prior to therapy. Drug therapy should be only one component of multiple risk factor intervention in patients at significantly increased risk for atherosclerotic vascular disease due to hypercholesterolemia. In patients with CHD or multiple risk factors for CHD, initiate therapy simultaneously with diet. Rhabdomyolysis with acute renal failure secondary to myoglobinuria and/or myopathy has been reported; patients should be monitored closely. This risk is dose-related and is increased with concurrent use of strong CYP3A4 inhibitors (eg, clarithromycin, itraconazole, protease inhibitors), cyclosporine, fibric acid derivatives (eg, gemfibrozil), or niacin

(doses ≥1 g/day); if concurrent use is warranted, consider lower starting and maintenance doses of atorvastatin. Use caution in patients with inadequately treated hypothyroidism, and those taking other drugs associated with myopathy (eg, colchicine); these patients are predisposed to myopathy. Uncomplicated myalgia immune-mediated necrotizing myopathy (IMNM) associated with HMG-CoA reductase inhibitors use has also been reported. Patients should be instructed to report unexplained muscle pain, tenderness, weakness, or brown urine, particularly if accompanied by malaise or fever. Discontinue therapy if markedly elevated CPK levels occur or myopathy is diagnosed/suspected.

Persistent elevations in serum transaminases have been reported; upon dose reduction, drug interruption, or discontinuation, transaminase levels returned to or near pretreatment levels. Postmarketing reports of fatal and nonfatal hepatic failure have been reported and are rare. If serious hepatotoxicity with clinical symptoms and/or hyperbilirubinemia or jaundice occurs during treatment, interrupt therapy promptly. If an alternate etiology is not identified, do not restart atorvastatin. Liver enzyme tests should be obtained at baseline and as clinically indicated and if signs/symptoms of liver injury occur. Ethanol may enhance the potential of adverse hepatic effects; instruct patients to avoid excessive ethanol consumption. Increases in HbA_{1c} and fasting blood glucose have been reported. Use with caution in patients who consume large amounts of ethanol or have a history of liver disease; use is contraindicated in patients with active liver disease or unexplained persistent elevations of serum transaminases. Use with caution in patients with renal impairment and the elderly; these patients are predisposed to myopathy.

Patients with recent stroke or TIA receiving long-term therapy with high-dose (ie, 80 mg/day) atorvastatin may be at increased risk for hemorrhagic stroke (SPARCL Investigators 2006). A subsequent post-hoc analysis demonstrated that patients with lacunar or hemorrhagic stroke may be at higher risk of hemorrhagic stroke; however, this finding was determined to be hypothesis generating. The overall benefit of treatment with atorvastatin (ie, reduced risk of stroke and cardiovascular events) in this population seems to outweigh the increased risk of hemorrhagic stroke if one truly exists (Goldstein 2008). The manufacturer recommends temporary discontinuation for elective major surgery, acute medical or surgical conditions, or in any patient experiencing an acute, serious condition suggestive of a myopathy or having a risk factor predisposing to the development of renal failure secondary to rhabdomyolysis (eg, sepsis, hypotension, trauma, uncontrolled seizures, severe metabolic, endocrine, or electrolyte disorders). Based on current research and clinical guidelines, HMG-CoA reductase inhibitors should be continued in the perioperative period (ACC/AHA [Fleisher 2014]. Postoperative discontinuation of statin therapy is associated with an increased risk of cardiac morbidity and mortality. Potentially significant interactions may exist, requiring dose or frequency adjustment, additional monitoring, and/or selection of alternative therapy. Consult drug interactions database for more detailed information.

Some dosage forms may contain polysorbate 80 (also known as Tweens). Hypersensitivity reactions, usually a delayed reaction, have been reported following exposure to pharmaceutical products containing polysorbate 80 in certain individuals (Isaksson 2002; Lucente 2000; Shelley 1995).

Adverse Reactions
>10%:
Gastrointestinal: Diarrhea (7% to 14%)
Neuromuscular & skeletal: Arthralgia (9% to 12%)
Respiratory: Nasopharyngitis (13%)
2% to 10%:
Cardiovascular: Hemorrhagic stroke (2%)
Central nervous system: Insomnia (5%)
Endocrine & metabolic: Diabetes mellitus (6%)
Gastrointestinal: Nausea (7%), dyspepsia (6%)
Genitourinary: Urinary tract infection (7% to 8%), cystitis (interstitial; Huang 2015)
Hepatic: Increased serum transaminases (≤2%)
Neuromuscular & skeletal: Limb pain (9%), myalgia (4% to 8%), musculoskeletal pain (5%), muscle spasm (4% to 5%)
Respiratory: Pharyngolaryngeal pain (3% to 4%)
<2% (Limited to important or life-threatening): Abdominal pain, abnormal hepatic function tests, alopecia, anaphylaxis, anemia, angioedema, anorexia, cholestasis, cholestatic jaundice, cognitive dysfunction (reversible), confusion (reversible), depression, elevated glycosylated hemoglobin (HbA_{1c}), epistaxis, eructation, erythema multiforme, gynecomastia, hematuria, hepatic failure,

hepatitis, hyperglycemia, hypoesthesia, increased creatinine phosphokinase, increased serum alkaline phosphatase, increased serum glucose, jaundice, joint swelling, muscle fatigue, myasthenia, myopathy, myositis, neck stiffness, nightmares, pancreatitis, paresthesia, peripheral edema, peripheral neuropathy, rhabdomyolysis, rupture of tendon, Stevens-Johnson syndrome, thrombocytopenia, toxic epidermal necrolysis

Drug Interactions

Metabolism/Transport Effects Substrate of CYP3A4 (major), P-glycoprotein, SLCO1B1; **Note:** Assignment of Major/Minor substrate status based on clinically relevant drug interaction potential; **Inhibits** CYP3A4 (weak), P-glycoprotein

Avoid Concomitant Use

Avoid concomitant use of AtorvaSTATin with any of the following: Bosutinib; Conivaptan; CycloSPORINE (Systemic); Fusidic Acid (Systemic); Gemfibrozil; Idelalisib; PAZOPanib; Pimozide; Posaconazole; Red Yeast Rice; Silodosin; Telaprevir; Tipranavir; Topotecan; VinCRIStine (Liposomal)

Increased Effect/Toxicity

AtorvaSTATin may increase the levels/effects of: Afatinib; Aliskiren; ARIPiprazole; Bosutinib; Brentuximab Vedotin; Cimetidine; Colchicine; DAPTOmycin; Digoxin; Diltiazem; Dofetilide; DOXOrubicin (Conventional); Edoxaban; Everolimus; Flibanserin; Hydrocodone; Ketoconazole (Systemic); Ledipasvir; Lomitapide; Midazolam; Naloxegol; NiMODipine; PAZOPanib; P-glycoprotein/ABCB1 Substrates; Pimozide; Prucalopride; Rifaximin; Silodosin; Spironolactone; Topotecan; Trabectedin; Verapamil; VinCRIStine (Liposomal)

The levels/effects of AtorvaSTATin may be increased by: Acipimox; Amiodarone; Aprepitant; Azithromycin (Systemic); Bezafibrate; Boceprevir; Ciprofibrate; Clarithromycin; Cobicistat; Colchicine; Conivaptan; CycloSPORINE (Systemic); CYP3A4 Inhibitors (Moderate); CYP3A4 Inhibitors (Strong); Cyproterone; Daclatasvir; Danazol; Dasatinib; Diltiazem; Dronedarone; Eltrombopag; Erythromycin (Systemic); Fenofibrate and Derivatives; Fluconazole; Fosaprepitant; Fusidic Acid (Systemic); Gemfibrozil; Grapefruit Juice; Idelalisib; Itraconazole; Ivacaftor; Ketoconazole (Systemic); Luliconazole; Mifepristone; Netupitant; Niacin; Niacinamide; Ombitasvir, Paritaprevir, Ritonavir, and Dasabuvir; Osimertinib; Palbociclib; P-glycoprotein/ABCB1 Inhibitors; Posaconazole; Protease Inhibitors; QuiNINE; Raltegravir; Ranolazine; Red Yeast Rice; Sacubitril; Simeprevir; Stiripentol; Telaprevir; Telithromycin; Teriflunomide; Ticagrelor; Tipranavir; Verapamil; Voriconazole

Decreased Effect

AtorvaSTATin may decrease the levels/effects of: Dabigatran Etexilate; Lanthanum

The levels/effects of AtorvaSTATin may be decreased by: Antacids; Bexarotene (Systemic); Bile Acid Sequestrants; Bosentan; CYP3A4 Inducers (Moderate); CYP3A4 Inducers (Strong); Dabrafenib; Deferasirox; Efavirenz; Enzalutamide; Etravirine; Fosphenytoin; Mitotane; Osimertinib; P-glycoprotein/ABCB1 Inducers; Phenytoin; Rifamycin Derivatives; Siltuximab; St Johns Wort; Tocilizumab

Food Interactions Atorvastatin serum concentrations may be increased by grapefruit juice. Management: Avoid concurrent intake of large quantities of grapefruit juice (>1 quart/day).

Storage/Stability Store at 20°C to 25°C (68°F to 77°F).

Mechanism of Action Inhibitor of 3-hydroxy-3-methylglutaryl coenzyme A (HMG-CoA) reductase, the rate-limiting enzyme in cholesterol synthesis (reduces the production of mevalonic acid from HMG-CoA); this then results in a compensatory increase in the expression of LDL receptors on hepatocyte membranes and a stimulation of LDL catabolism. In addition to the ability of HMG-CoA reductase inhibitors to decrease levels of high-sensitivity C-reactive protein (hsCRP), they also possess pleiotropic properties including improved endothelial function, reduced inflammation at the site of the coronary plaque, inhibition of platelet aggregation, and anticoagulant effects (de Denus 2002; Ray 2005).

Pharmacodynamics/Kinetics

Onset of action: Initial changes: 3 to 5 days; Maximal reduction in plasma cholesterol and triglycerides: 2 to 4 weeks; LDL reduction: 10 mg/day: 39% (for each doubling of this dose, LDL is lowered approximately 6%)

Absorption: Oral: Rapidly absorbed; extensive first-pass metabolism in GI mucosa and liver

Distribution: V_d: ~381 L

Protein binding: ≥98%

Metabolism: Hepatic via CYP3A4; forms active ortho- and parahydroxylated derivatives and an inactive beta-oxidation product; plasma concentrations are elevated in patients with chronic alcoholic liver disease and Childs-Pugh class A and B liver disease

Bioavailability: ~14% (parent drug); ~30% (parent drug and equipotent metabolites)

Half-life elimination: Parent drug: ~14 hours; Equipotent metabolites: 20 to 30 hours

Time to peak, serum: 1 to 2 hours

Excretion: Bile (following hepatic and/or extra-hepatic metabolism; does not appear to undergo enterohepatic recirculation); urine (<2% as unchanged drug)

Dosing

Adult & Geriatric

Primary prevention: Note: Doses should be individualized according to the baseline LDL-cholesterol concentrations and patient response; adjustments should be made at intervals of 2 to 4 weeks

Hypercholesterolemia (heterozygous familial and nonfamilial) and mixed hyperlipidemia (Fredrickson types IIa and IIb): Oral: Initial: 10 or 20 mg once daily; patients requiring >45% reduction in LDL-C may be started at 40 mg once daily; range: 10 to 80 mg once daily

Homozygous familial hypercholesterolemia: Oral: 10 to 80 mg once daily

Prevention of cardiovascular disease: ACC/AHA Blood Cholesterol Guideline recommendations to reduce the risk of atherosclerotic cardiovascular disease (ASCVD) (Stone 2013): Adults ≥21 years:

Primary Prevention:

LDL-C ≥190 mg/dL: High-intensity therapy: 80 mg once daily; if unable to tolerate, may reduce dose to 40 mg once daily

Type 1 or 2 diabetes and age 40 to 75 years: Moderate-intensity therapy: 10 to 20 mg once daily

Type 1 or 2 diabetes, age 40 to 75 years, and an estimated 10-year ASCVD risk ≥7.5%: High-intensity therapy: 80 mg once daily; if unable to tolerate, may reduce dose to 40 mg once daily

Age 40 to 75 years and an estimated 10-year ASCVD risk ≥7.5%: Moderate- to high-intensity therapy: 10 to 80 mg once daily

Secondary prevention:

Patient has clinical ASCVD (eg, coronary heart disease, stroke/TIA, or peripheral arterial disease presumed to be of atherosclerotic origin) or is post-CABG (AHA [Kulik 2015]) **and:**

Age ≤75 years: High-intensity therapy: 80 mg once daily; if unable to tolerate, may reduce dose to 40 mg once daily

Age >75 years or not a candidate for high intensity therapy: Moderate-intensity therapy: 10 to 20 mg once daily

Intensive lipid-lowering after an ACS event regardless of baseline LDL (off-label use): Oral: Initial: 80 mg once daily; adjust based on patient tolerability (Cannon 2004; Pederson 2005; Schwartz 2001). **Note:** Currently, the ACC/AHA guidelines for UA/NSTEMI do not specify which statin to use (ACCF/AHA [Anderson 2013]). Also consider the ACC/AHA Blood Cholesterol Guideline recommendations (Stone 2013).

Noncardioembolic stroke/TIA (off-label use): Oral: Initial: 80 mg once daily; adjust based on patient tolerability (Adams 2008; Amarenco 2006). Also consider the ACC/AHA Blood Cholesterol Guideline recommendations (Stone 2013).

Dosage adjustment for atorvastatin with concomitant medications:

Boceprevir, nelfinavir: Use lowest effective atorvastatin dose (not to exceed 40 mg daily)

Clarithromycin, itraconazole, fosamprenavir, ritonavir (plus darunavir, fosamprenavir, or saquinavir): Use lowest effective atorvastatin dose (not to exceed 20 mg daily)

Lomitapide: Consider atorvastatin dose reduction (per lomitapide manufacturer)

Pediatric Note: Doses should be individualized according to the baseline LDL-cholesterol concentrations and patient response; adjustments should be made at intervals of 4 weeks

Heterozygous familial hypercholesterolemia: Children ≥10 years and Adolescents (females postmenarche): Oral: 10 mg once daily (maximum: 20 mg/day)

Dosage adjustment for atorvastatin with concomitant medications: Refer to adult dosing.

Renal Impairment No dosage adjustment necessary. Dialysis: Due to the high protein binding, atorvastatin is not expected to be cleared by dialysis (not studied)

Hepatic Impairment Contraindicated in active liver disease or in patients with unexplained persistent elevations of serum transaminases.

Adjustment for Toxicity

Severe muscle symptoms or fatigue: Promptly discontinue use; evaluate CPK, creatinine, and urinalysis for myoglobinuria (Stone 2013).

Mild to moderate muscle symptoms: Discontinue use until symptoms can be evaluated; evaluate patient for conditions that may increase the risk for muscle symptoms (eg, hypothyroidism, reduced renal or hepatic function, rheumatologic disorders such as polymyalgia rheumatica, steroid myopathy, vitamin D deficiency, or primary muscle diseases). Upon resolution, resume the original or lower dose of atorvastatin. If muscle symptoms recur, discontinue atorvastatin use. After muscle symptom resolution, may then use a low dose of a different statin; gradually increase if tolerated. In the absence of continued statin use, if muscle symptoms or elevated CPK continues after 2 months, consider other causes of muscle symptoms. If determined to be due to another condition aside from statin use, may resume statin therapy at the original dose (Stone 2013).

Dietary Considerations Before initiation of therapy, patients should be placed on a standard cholesterol-lowering diet for 3 to 6 months and the diet should be continued during drug therapy. Atorvastatin serum concentration may be increased when taken with grapefruit juice; avoid concurrent intake of large quantities (>1 quart/day).

Red yeast rice contains variable amounts of several compounds that are structurally similar to HMG-CoA reductase inhibitors, primarily monacolin K (or mevinolin) which is structurally identical to lovastatin; concurrent use of red yeast rice with HMG-CoA reductase inhibitors may increase the incidence of adverse and toxic effects (Lapi 2008; Smith 2003).

Administration Administer with or without food; may take without regard to time of day. The manufacturer's labeling states tablets should not be broken; however, available data do not indicate any safety or efficacy concerns with this practice.

Monitoring Parameters

2013 ACC/AHA Blood Cholesterol Guideline recommendations (Stone 2013):

Lipid panel (total cholesterol, HDL, LDL, triglycerides): Baseline lipid panel; fasting lipid profile within 4-12 weeks after initiation or dose adjustment and every 3-12 months (as clinically indicated) thereafter. If 2 consecutive LDL levels are <40 mg/dL, consider decreasing the dose.

Hepatic transaminase levels: Baseline measurement of hepatic transaminase levels (ie, ALT); measure hepatic function if symptoms suggest hepatotoxicity (eg, unusual fatigue or weakness, loss of appetite, abdominal pain, dark-colored urine or yellowing of skin or sclera) during therapy.

CPK: CPK should not be routinely measured. Baseline CPK measurement is reasonable for some individuals (eg, family history of statin intolerance or muscle disease, clinical presentation, concomitant drug therapy that may increase risk of myopathy). May measure CPK in any patient with symptoms suggestive of myopathy (pain, tenderness, stiffness, cramping, weakness, or generalized fatigue).

Evaluate for new-onset diabetes mellitus during therapy; if diabetes develops, continue statin therapy and encourage adherence to a heart-healthy diet, physical activity, a healthy body weight, and tobacco cessation.

If patient develops a confusional state or memory impairment, may evaluate patient for nonstatin causes (ie, exposure to other drugs), systemic and neuropsychiatric causes, and the possibility of adverse effects associated with statin therapy.

Manufacturer's labeling: Liver enzyme tests at baseline and repeated when clinically indicated. Measure CPK when myopathy is being considered or may measure CPK periodically in high risk patients (eg, drug-drug interaction). Upon initiation or titration, lipid panel should be analyzed within 2-4 weeks.

Dosage Forms Excipient information presented when available (limited, particularly for generics); consult specific product labeling.

Tablet, Oral:

Lipitor: 10 mg, 20 mg, 40 mg, 80 mg

Generic: 10 mg, 20 mg, 40 mg, 80 mg

◆ Atorvastatin and Amlodipine *see* Amlodipine and Atorvastatin *on page 103*

◆ Atorvastatin and Ezetimibe *see* Ezetimibe and Atorvastatin *on page 730*

◆ Atorvastatin Calcium *see* AtorvaSTATin *on page 169*

◆ Atorvastatin Calcium and Amlodipine Besylate *see* Amlodipine and Atorvastatin *on page 103*

Atovaquone (a TOE va kwone)

Brand Names: US Mepron

Brand Names: Canada Mepron

Pharmacologic Category Antiprotozoal

Use

Pneumocystis jirovecii pneumonia (PCP), prophylaxis: Prevention of PCP in adults and adolescents 13 years and older who are intolerant to trimethoprim-sulfamethoxazole (TMP-SMZ)

Pneumocystis jirovecii pneumonia (PCP), treatment: Acute oral treatment of mild-to-moderate PCP in adults and adolescents 13 years and older who are intolerant to TMP-SMZ

Pregnancy Considerations Adverse events were observed in animal reproduction studies. Diagnosis and treatment of *Pneumocystis jirovecii* pneumonia (PCP) in pregnant women is the same as in nonpregnant women; however, information specific to the use of atovaquone in pregnancy is limited (HHS [OI adult 2015]).

Breast-Feeding Considerations It is not known if atovaquone is excreted in breast milk. The manufacturer recommends that caution be exercised when administering atovaquone to nursing women.

Contraindications Hypersensitivity to atovaquone or any component of the formulation

Warnings/Precautions Hypersensitivity reactions (eg, angioedema, bronchospasm, throat tightness, urticaria) have occurred. When used for *Pneumocystis jirovecii* pneumonia (PCP) treatment, has only been indicated in mild-to-moderate PCP; not studied for use in severe PCP; atovaquone has less adverse effects than trimethoprim-sulfamethoxazole ([TMP-SMZ], the treatment of choice for mild-to-moderate PCP), although atovaquone is less effective than TMP-SMZ (HHS [OI adult 2015]). Use with caution in elderly patients. Absorption may be decreased in patients who have diarrhea or vomiting; monitor closely and consider use of an antiemetic; if severe, consider use of an alternative antiprotozoal. Consider parenteral therapy with alternative agents in patients who have difficulty taking atovaquone with food; gastrointestinal disorders may limit absorption of oral medications; may not achieve adequate plasma levels. Use with caution in patients with severe hepatic impairment; monitor closely; rare cases of cholestatic hepatitis, elevated liver function tests, and fatal liver failure have been reported. Potentially significant drug-drug interactions may exist, requiring dose or frequency adjustment, additional monitoring, and/or selection of alternative therapy.

Benzyl alcohol and derivatives: Some dosage forms may contain benzyl alcohol; large amounts of benzyl alcohol (≥99 mg/kg/day) have been associated with a potentially fatal toxicity ("gasping syndrome") in neonates; the "gasping syndrome" consists of metabolic acidosis, respiratory distress, gasping respirations, CNS dysfunction (including convulsions, intracranial hemorrhage), hypotension and cardiovascular collapse (AAP ["Inactive" 1997]; CDC 1982); some data suggests that benzoate displaces bilirubin from protein binding sites (Ahlfors 2001); avoid or use dosage forms containing benzyl alcohol with caution in neonates. See manufacturer's labeling.

Adverse Reactions Note: Adverse reaction statistics have been compiled from studies including patients with advanced HIV disease. Consequently, it is difficult to distinguish reactions attributed to atovaquone from those caused by the underlying disease or a combination thereof.

>10%:

Central nervous system: Headache (16% to 31%), insomnia (10% to 19%), depression, pain

Dermatologic: Skin rash (22% to 46%), pruritus (5% to ≥10%), diaphoresis

Gastrointestinal: Diarrhea (19% to 42%), nausea (21% to 32%), vomiting (14% to 22%), abdominal pain (4% to 21%)

Infection: Infection (18% to 22%)

Neuromuscular & skeletal: Weakness (8% to 31%), myalgia

Respiratory: Cough (14% to 25%), rhinitis (5% to 24%), dyspnea (15% to 21%), sinusitis (7% to ≥10%), flu-like symptoms

Miscellaneous: Fever (14% to 40%)

1% to 10%:

Cardiovascular: Hypotension (≤1%)

Central nervous system: Dizziness (3% to 8%), anxiety (≤7%)

Endocrine & metabolic: Hyponatremia (7% to 10%), hyperglycemia (≤9%), increased amylase (7% to 8%), hypoglycemia (≤1%)

Gastrointestinal: Oral candidiasis (5% to 10%), anorexia (≤7%), dyspepsia (≤5%), constipation (≤3%), dysgeusia (≤3%)

Hematologic & oncologic: Anemia (4% to 6%), neutropenia (3% to 5%)

Hepatic: Increased liver enzymes (4% to 8%)

Renal: Increased blood urea nitrogen (≤1%), increased serum creatinine (≤1%)

Respiratory: Bronchospasm (2% to 4%)

Postmarketing and/or case reports (Limited to important or life-threatening): Acute renal failure, angioedema, constriction of the pharynx, corneal disease (vortex keratopathy), desquamation, erythema multiforme, hepatic failure (rare), hepatitis (rare), hypersensitivity reaction, methemoglobinemia, pancreatitis, Stevens-Johnson syndrome, thrombocytopenia, urticaria

Drug Interactions

Metabolism/Transport Effects None known.

Avoid Concomitant Use

Avoid concomitant use of Atovaquone with any of the following: Rifamycin Derivatives; Ritonavir

Increased Effect/Toxicity

Atovaquone may increase the levels/effects of: Etoposide

Decreased Effect

Atovaquone may decrease the levels/effects of: Indinavir

The levels/effects of Atovaquone may be decreased by: Efavirenz; Metoclopramide; Rifamycin Derivatives; Ritonavir; Tetracycline

Food Interactions Ingestion with a fatty meal increases absorption. Management: Administer with food, preferably high-fat meals (peanuts or ice cream).

Storage/Stability Store at 15°C to 25°C (59°F to 77°F). Do not freeze.

Mechanism of Action Inhibits electron transport in mitochondria resulting in the inhibition of key metabolic enzymes responsible for the synthesis of nucleic acids and ATP

Pharmacodynamics/Kinetics

Absorption:

Infants and Children <2 years of age: Decreased absorption

Adults: Oral suspension: Absorption is enhanced 1.4-fold with food; decreased absorption with single doses exceeding 750 mg

Distribution: V_{dss}: 0.6 ± 0.17 L/kg; CSF concentration is <1% of the plasma concentration

Protein binding: >99%

Metabolism: Undergoes enterohepatic recirculation

Bioavailability: Suspension (administered with food): 47% ± 15%

Half-life elimination:

Children (4 months to 12 years): 60 hours (range: 31 to 163 hours)

Adults: 2.9 days

Adults with AIDS: 2.2 days

Time to peak, serum: Dual peak serum concentrations at 1 to 8 hours and at 24 to 96 hours after dose due to enterohepatic cycling

Excretion: Feces (>94% as unchanged drug); urine (<1%)

Dosing

Adult & Geriatric

Pneumocystis jirovecii pneumonia (PCP), prevention: Oral: 1,500 mg once daily with food

PCP, mild-to-moderate, treatment: Oral: 750 mg twice daily with food for 21 days

Babesiosis (off-label use): Oral: 750 mg twice daily with azithromycin for 7 to 10 days; **Note:** Relapsing infection may require at least 6 weeks of therapy (Krauss 2000; Vannier 2012).

Toxoplasma gondii encephalitis in HIV-infected patients (off-label use) (HHS [OI adult 2015]): Oral:

Prophylaxis: 1,500 mg once daily with food (either as monotherapy or with pyrimethamine plus leucovorin)

Treatment: 1,500 mg twice daily with food (either with pyrimethamine plus leucovorin, or with sulfadiazine, or as monotherapy) for at least 6 weeks (longer if extensive disease or incomplete response)

Chronic maintenance: 750 to 1,500 mg twice daily with food (either with pyrimethamine plus leucovorin, or with sulfadiazine, or as monotherapy); may discontinue when asymptomatic and CD4 count >200 cells/mm³ for 6 months

Pediatric

Pneumocystis jirovecii pneumonia (PCP), prevention:

Infants and Children <13 years (off-label use) (CDC 2009): Oral:

1 to 3 months: 30 mg/kg once daily with food

4 to 24 months: 45 mg/kg once daily with food

>24 months: 30 mg/kg once daily with food

Adolescents ≥13 years: Refer to adult dosing.

PCP, mild-to-moderate, treatment:

Infants and Children <13 years (off-label use) (CDC 2009): Oral:

Birth to 3 months: 30 to 40 mg/kg/day in 2 divided doses with food (maximum: 1,500 mg daily)

3 to 24 months: 45 mg/kg/day in 2 divided doses with food (maximum: 1,500 mg daily)

≥24 months: 30 to 40 mg/kg/day in 2 divided doses with food (maximum: 1,500 mg daily)

Adolescents ≥13 years: Refer to adult dosing

Toxoplasma gondii encephalitis in HIV-exposed/infected patients (off-label use):

Infants and Children <13 years: Prophylaxis (either as monotherapy or with pyrimethamine plus leucovorin) (CDC 2009): Oral:

1 to 3 months: 30 mg/kg once daily with food

4 to 24 months: 45 mg/kg once daily with food

>24 months: 30 mg/kg once daily with food

Adolescents: Prophylaxis, treatment, and chronic maintenance (HHS [OI adult 2015]): Refer to adult dosing.

Babesiosis (off-label use): Children: Oral: 40 mg/kg/day in 2 divided doses with azithromycin for 7 to 10 days (maximum: 1,500 mg daily). **Note:** Relapsing infection may require at least 6 weeks of therapy (Vannier 2012).

Renal Impairment There are no dosage adjustments provided in the manufacturer's labeling (has not been studied). However, atovaquone is not appreciably renally excreted.

Hepatic Impairment There are no dosage adjustments provided in the manufacturer's labeling (has not been studied). Atovaquone undergoes enterohepatic cycling and primarily hepatic excretion. Use caution in patients with severe impairment; monitor closely.

Dietary Considerations Must be taken with food.

Administration Oral: Must administer with food. Shake suspension gently before use. Once opened, a foil pouch can be emptied on a dosing spoon, in a cup, or directly into the mouth.

Monitoring Parameters Hepatic function at baseline (monitor closely during treatment in patients with severe hepatic impairment), hypersensitivity reactions, CD4 count (for chronic maintenance treatment in toxoplasmosis), patient's food tolerance/ability to take atovaquone, post-dose vomiting, diarrhea

Dosage Forms Excipient information presented when available (limited, particularly for generics); consult specific product labeling.

Suspension, Oral:

Mepron: 750 mg/5 mL (5 mL, 210 mL) [contains benzyl alcohol; citrus flavor]

Generic: 750 mg/5 mL (210 mL)

Atovaquone and Proguanil
(a TOE va kwone & pro GWA nil)

Brand Names: US Malarone®

Brand Names: Canada Malarone®; Malarone® Pediatric

Index Terms Atovaquone and Proguanil Hydrochloride; Proguanil and Atovaquone; Proguanil Hydrochloride and Atovaquone

Pharmacologic Category Antimalarial Agent

Use

Malaria prevention: Prophylaxis of *Plasmodium falciparum* malaria, including areas where chloroquine resistance has been reported

Malaria treatment: Treatment of acute, uncomplicated *P. falciparum* malaria

Dosing

Adult & Geriatric

Prevention of malaria: Oral: Atovaquone/proguanil 250 mg/100 mg once daily; start 1-2 days prior to entering a malaria-endemic area, continue throughout the stay and for 7 days after returning.

Treatment of acute malaria: Oral: Atovaquone/proguanil 1000 mg/400 mg as a single dose, once daily for 3 consecutive days

Pediatric

Prevention of malaria: Oral: Start 1-2 days prior to entering a malaria-endemic area, continue throughout the stay and for 7 days after returning. Take as a single dose, once daily.

5-8 kg (off-label dosing): Atovaquone/proguanil 31.25 mg/12.5 mg (Boggild, 2007)

9-10 kg (off-label dosing): Atovaquone/proguanil 46.8 mg/18.75 mg (Boggild, 2007)

11-20 kg: Atovaquone/proguanil 62.5 mg/25 mg

21-30 kg: Atovaquone/proguanil 125 mg/50 mg

31-40 kg: Atovaquone/proguanil 187.5 mg/75 mg

>40 kg: Atovaquone/proguanil 250 mg/100 mg

Treatment of acute malaria: Oral: Take as a single dose, once daily for 3 consecutive days.

5-8 kg: Atovaquone/proguanil 125 mg/50 mg

9-10 kg: Atovaquone/proguanil 187.5 mg/75 mg

11-20 kg: Atovaquone/proguanil 250 mg/100 mg

21-30 kg: Atovaquone/proguanil 500 mg/200 mg

31-40 kg: Atovaquone/proguanil 750 mg/300 mg

>40 kg: Atovaquone/proguanil 1000 mg/400 mg

Renal Impairment

CrCl ≥30 mL/minute: No dosage adjustment necessary.

CrCl <30 mL/minute:

Prophylaxis: Use is contraindicated.

Treatment: No dosage adjustment necessary; however, use with extreme caution and only if the benefits outweigh the risks.

Hepatic Impairment

Mild-to-moderate impairment: No dosage adjustment necessary.

Severe impairment; No dosage adjustment provided in manufacturer's labeling (has not been studied).

Additional Information Complete prescribing information should be consulted for additional detail.

Dosage Forms Excipient information presented when available (limited, particularly for generics); consult specific product labeling.

Tablet, oral: Atovaquone 250 mg and proguanil hydrochloride 100 mg

Malarone®: Atovaquone 250 mg and proguanil hydrochloride 100 mg

Tablet, oral [pediatric]:

Malarone®: Atovaquone 62.5 mg and proguanil hydrochloride 25 mg

♦ Atovaquone and Proguanil Hydrochloride *see* Atovaquone and Proguanil *on page 173*

♦ ATRA *see* Tretinoin (Systemic) *on page 1838*

♦ Atrac-Tain [OTC] *see* Urea *on page 1853*

Atracurium (a tra KYOO ree um)

Brand Names: Canada Atracurium Besylate Injection

Index Terms Atracurium Besylate

Pharmacologic Category Neuromuscular Blocker Agent, Nondepolarizing

Use

Neuromuscular blockade: As an adjunct to general anesthesia, to facilitate endotracheal intubation and to provide skeletal muscle relaxation during surgery or mechanical ventilation.

Note: Atracurium does not relieve pain or produce sedation.

Pregnancy Considerations Adverse events were observed in animal reproduction studies. Small amounts of atracurium have been shown to cross the placenta when given to women during cesarean section.

Breast-Feeding Considerations It is not known if atracurium is excreted in breast milk. The manufacturer recommends that caution be exercised when administering atracurium to nursing women.

Contraindications

Hypersensitivity to atracurium besylate or any component of the formulation. Multiple-dose vials contain benzyl alcohol as a preservative; use is contraindicated in patients with a known hypersensitivity to benzyl alcohol.

Documentation of allergenic cross-reactivity for neuromuscular blockers is limited. However, because of similarities in chemical structure and/or pharmacologic actions, the possibility of cross-sensitivity cannot be ruled out with certainty.

Warnings/Precautions Severe anaphylactic reactions have been reported with atracurium use; some life-threatening and fatal. Appropriate emergency treatment (including epinephrine 1:1000) should be immediately available during use. Reduce initial dosage and inject slowly (over 1 to 2 minutes) in patients in whom substantial histamine release would be potentially hazardous (eg, patients with clinically-important cardiovascular disease). Cross-sensitivity with other neuromuscular-blocking agents may occur; use extreme caution in patients with previous anaphylactic reactions. Maintenance of an adequate airway and respiratory support is critical. Certain clinical conditions may result in potentiation or antagonism of neuromuscular blockade:

Antagonism: Respiratory alkalosis, hypercalcemia, demyelinating lesions, peripheral neuropathies, denervation, and muscle trauma

Potentiation: Electrolyte abnormalities (eg, severe hypocalcemia, severe hypokalemia, hypermagnesemia), neuromuscular diseases, metabolic acidosis, metabolic alkalosis, respiratory acidosis, Eaton-Lambert syndrome and myasthenia gravis

Resistance may occur in burn patients (≥20% of total body surface area), usually several days after the injury, and may persist for several months after wound healing. Resistance may occur in patients who are immobilized. Use caution in the elderly. Bradycardia may be more common with atracurium than with other neuromuscular-blocking agents since it has no clinically-significant effects on heart rate to counteract the bradycardia produced by anesthetics. Should be administered by adequately trained individuals familiar with its use. Potentially significant drug-drug interactions may exist, requiring dose or frequency adjustment, additional monitoring, and/or selection of alternative therapy.

Benzyl alcohol and derivatives: Some dosage forms may contain benzyl alcohol; large amounts of benzyl alcohol (≥99 mg/kg/day) have been associated with a potentially fatal toxicity ("gasping syndrome") in neonates; the "gasping syndrome" consists of metabolic acidosis, respiratory distress, gasping respirations, CNS dysfunction (including convulsions, intracranial hemorrhage), hypotension and cardiovascular collapse (AAP ["Inactive" 1997]; CDC 1982); some data suggests that benzoate displaces bilirubin from protein binding sites (Ahlfors 2001); avoid or use dosage forms containing benzyl alcohol with caution in neonates. See manufacturer's labeling.

Adverse Reactions Mild, rare, and generally suggestive of histamine release

1% to 10%: Cardiovascular: Flushing

<1%: Bronchial secretions, erythema, hives, itching, wheezing

Postmarketing and/or case reports: Allergic reaction, bradycardia, bronchospasm, dyspnea, hypotension, injection site reaction, seizure, acute quadriplegic myopathy syndrome (prolonged use), laryngospasm, myositis ossificans (prolonged use), tachycardia, urticaria

Causes of prolonged neuromuscular blockade: Excessive drug administration; cumulative drug effect, metabolism/excretion decreased (hepatic and/or renal impairment); accumulation of active metabolites; electrolyte imbalance (hypokalemia, hypocalcemia, hypermagnesemia, hypernatremia); hypothermia

Drug Interactions

Metabolism/Transport Effects None known.

Avoid Concomitant Use

Avoid concomitant use of Atracurium with any of the following: QuiNINE

Increased Effect/Toxicity

Atracurium may increase the levels/effects of: Cardiac Glycosides; Corticosteroids (Systemic); OnabotulinumtoxinA; RimabotulinumtoxinB

The levels/effects of Atracurium may be increased by: AbobotulinumtoxinA; Aminoglycosides; Calcium Channel Blockers; Capreomycin; Clindamycin (Topical); Colistimethate; CycloSPORINE (Systemic); Fosphenytoin-Phenytoin; Inhalational Anesthetics; Ketorolac (Nasal); Ketorolac (Systemic); Lincosamide Antibiotics; Lithium; Loop Diuretics; Magnesium Salts; Minocycline; Polymyxin B; Procainamide; QuiNIDine; QuiNINE; Spironolactone; Tetracycline Derivatives; Vancomycin

Decreased Effect

The levels/effects of Atracurium may be decreased by: Acetylcholinesterase Inhibitors; Fosphenytoin-Phenytoin; Loop Diuretics

Preparation for Administration May prepare an infusion solution (final concentrations: 0.2 mg/mL or 0.5 mg/mL) by admixing with an appropriate diluent (eg, NS, D_5W, D_5NS). Do not mix with alkaline solutions.

Storage/Stability Store intact vials at 2°C to 8°C (36°F to 46°F). Do not freeze. Upon removal from refrigeration to room temperature storage conditions (25°C/77°F), use within 14 days even if re-refrigerated. Dilutions of 0.2 mg/mL or 0.5 mg/mL in 0.9% sodium chloride, dextrose 5% in water, or 5% dextrose in sodium chloride 0.9% are stable for up to 24 hours at room temperature or under refrigeration.

Mechanism of Action Blocks neural transmission at the myoneural junction by binding with cholinergic receptor sites

Pharmacodynamics/Kinetics
Onset of action (dose dependent): 2 to 3 minutes; Peak effect: 3 to 5 minutes
Duration: Recovery begins in 20 to 35 minutes following initial dose of 0.4 to 0.5 mg/kg under balanced anesthesia; recovery to 95% of control takes 60 to 70 minutes
Distribution: V_d:
Infants: 0.21 L/kg
Children: 0.13 L/kg
Adults: 0.1 L/kg
Metabolism: Undergoes ester hydrolysis and Hofmann elimination (nonbiologic process independent of renal, hepatic, or enzymatic function); metabolites have no neuromuscular blocking properties; laudanosine, a product of Hofmann elimination, is a CNS stimulant and can accumulate with prolonged use. Laudanosine is hepatically metabolized.
Half-life elimination:
Infants: 20 minutes
Children: 17 minutes
Adults: Biphasic: Initial (distribution): 2 minutes; Terminal: 20 minutes
Excretion: Urine (<5%)
Clearance:
Infants: 7.9 mL/kg/minute
Children: 6.8 mL/kg/minute
Adults: 5.3 mL/kg/minute

Dosing
Adult & Geriatric For IV administration only (not to be used IM): Dose to effect; doses must be individualized due to interpatient variability

Adjunct to surgical anesthesia (neuromuscular blockade):
IV (bolus): 0.4 to 0.5 mg/kg, then 0.08 to 0.1 mg/kg administered 20 to 45 minutes after initial dose to maintain neuromuscular block; repeat dose at 15- to 25-minute intervals as needed. **Note:** Initial dose may be reduced to 0.3 to 0.4 mg/kg in patients with significant cardiovascular disease or history of elevated risk of histamine release (eg, severe anaphylactoid reactions or asthma).
Initial dose after succinylcholine for intubation (balanced anesthesia): 0.3 to 0.4 mg/kg
Pretreatment/priming: 10% of intubating dose (eg, 0.04 to 0.05 mg/kg) given 2 to 4 minutes before the larger second dose (Mehta 1985; Miller 2010). **Note:** Although priming has been advocated by some, priming may either be uncomfortable for the patient, increase the risk of aspiration and difficulty swallowing, or intubating conditions after priming may not be as good as that seen with succinylcholine (Miller 2010).
Maintenance infusion for continued surgical relaxation during extended surgical procedures: At initial signs of recovery from bolus dose, a continuous infusion may be initiated at a rate of 9 to 10 mcg/kg/**minute** (0.54 to 0.6 mg/kg/**hour**); block usually maintained by a rate of 5 to 9 mcg/kg/**minute** (0.3 to 0.54 mg/kg/**hour**) under balanced anesthesia; range: 2 to 15 mcg/kg/**minute** (0.12 to 0.9 mg/kg/**hour**)
ICU paralysis (eg, facilitate mechanical ventilation) in selected adequately sedated patients (off-label dosing): IV: Initial bolus of 0.4 to 0.5 mg/kg, followed by 4 to 20 mcg/kg/**minute** (0.24 to 1.2 mg/kg/**hour**) (ACCM/SCCM/ASHP [Murray 2002]; Greenberg 2013)
Pediatric Adjunct to surgical anesthesia: IV (not to be used IM): Dose to effect; doses must be individualized due to interpatient variability; use ideal body weight for obese patients
Infants and Children 1 month to 2 years: Initial: 0.3 to 0.4 mg/kg followed by maintenance doses as needed to maintain neuromuscular blockade. **Note:** Maintenance doses may be required with slightly greater frequency in infants and children compared to adults.
Children >2 years and Adolescents: 0.4 to 0.5 mg/kg, then 0.08 to 0.1 mg/kg administered 20 to 45 minutes after initial dose to maintain neuromuscular block; repeat dose at 15- to 25-minute intervals as needed. **Note:** Initial dose may be reduced to 0.3 to 0.4 mg/kg in patients with significant cardiovascular disease or

history of elevated risk of histamine release (eg, severe anaphylactoid reactions or asthma).
Pretreatment/priming: 10% of intubating dose (eg, 0.04 to 0.05 mg/kg) given 2 to 4 minutes before the larger second dose (Mehta 1985; Miller 2010). **Note:** Although priming has been advocated by some, priming may either be uncomfortable for the patient, increase the risk of aspiration and difficulty swallowing, or intubating conditions after priming may not be as good as that seen with succinylcholine (Miller 2010).
Maintenance infusion for continued surgical relaxation during extended surgical procedures: At initial signs of recovery from bolus dose, a continuous infusion may be initiated at a rate of 9 to 10 mcg/kg/**minute** (0.54 to 0.6 mg/kg/**hour**); block usually maintained by a rate of 5 to 9 mcg/kg/**minute** (0.3 to 0.54 mg/kg/**hour**) under balanced anesthesia; range: 2 to 15 mcg/kg/**minute** (0.12 to 0.9 mg/kg/**hour**)

Renal Impairment No dosage adjustment necessary.
Hepatic Impairment No dosage adjustment necessary.
Obesity Morbidly-obese patients should be dosed using ideal body weight or an adjusted body weight (ie, between IBW and total body weight [TBW]) (Erstad 2004). In a bariatric surgical population of morbidly-obese patients who were administered an induction dose of atracurium based on TBW as compared to IBW, time to recovery of twitch response was prolonged (Kralingen 2011).

Usual Infusion Concentrations: Adult IV infusion: 20 mg in 100 mL (concentration: 0.2 mg/mL) **or** 50 mg in 100 mL (concentration: 0.5 mg/mL) of D_5W, D_5NS, or NS.

Administration May be given undiluted as a bolus injection; do **not** administer IM (excessive tissue irritation). May also administer via continuous infusion; requires the use of an infusion pump. Use infusion solutions within 24 hours of preparation.

Monitoring Parameters Vital signs (heart rate, blood pressure, respiratory rate); degree of muscle relaxation (via peripheral nerve stimulator and presence of spontaneous movement)
In the ICU setting, prolonged paralysis and generalized myopathy, following discontinuation of agent, may be minimized by appropriately monitoring degree of blockade.

Additional Information Atracurium is classified as an intermediate-duration neuromuscular-blocking agent. It does not appear to have a cumulative effect on the duration of blockade.

Dosage Forms Excipient information presented when available (limited, particularly for generics); consult specific product labeling.
Solution, Intravenous, as besylate:
Generic: 50 mg/5 mL (5 mL); 100 mg/10 mL (10 mL)
Solution, Intravenous, as besylate [preservative free]:
Generic: 50 mg/5 mL (5 mL)

◆ Atracurium Besylate see Atracurium on page 174

◆ Atracurium Besylate Injection (Can) see Atracurium on page 174

◆ Atralin see Tretinoin (Topical) on page 1841

◆ Atrapro Dermal Spray see Sodium Chloride on page 1671

◆ Atriance (Can) see Nelarabine on page 1265

◆ Atripla see Efavirenz, Emtricitabine, and Tenofovir Disoproxil Fumarate on page 621

◆ AtroPen see Atropine (Systemic) on page 175

Atropine (Systemic) (A troe peen)

Brand Names: US AtroPen
Index Terms Atropine Sulfate
Pharmacologic Category Anticholinergic Agent; Antidote; Antispasmodic Agent, Gastrointestinal
Additional Appendix Information
Adult ACLS Algorithms on page 1993
Pediatric ALS (PALS) Algorithms on page 1990
Use
Preoperative medication to inhibit salivation and secretions; treatment of symptomatic sinus bradycardia, AV block (nodal level); antidote for anticholinesterase poisoning (carbamate insecticides, nerve agents, organophosphate insecticides); adjuvant use with anticholinesterases (eg, edrophonium, neostigmine) to decrease their side effects during reversal of neuromuscular blockade
Note: Use is no longer recommended in the management of asystole or pulseless electrical activity (PEA) (ACLS 2010).

Pregnancy Considerations Adverse events were not observed in animal reproduction studies (studies not conducted by all manufacturers). Atropine has been found to cross the human placenta (Kanto 1981).

Breast-Feeding Considerations Trace amounts of atropine are excreted into breast milk. Atropine may suppress lactation or cause adverse events in the nursing infant (data is conflicting). The manufacturer recommends that caution be exercised when administering atropine to nursing women.

Prescribing and Access Restrictions The AtroPen formulation is available for use primarily by the Department of Defense.

Contraindications

Hypersensitivity to atropine or any component of the formulation

Note: No contraindications exist in the treatment of life-threatening organophosphate or carbamate insecticide or nerve agent poisoning.

Warnings/Precautions Heat prostration may occur in the presence of high environmental temperatures. Psychosis may occur in sensitive individuals or following use of excessive doses. Avoid use if possible in patients with obstructive uropathy or in other conditions resulting in urinary retention; use is contraindicated in patients with prostatic hypertrophy. Avoid use in patients with paralytic ileus, intestinal atony of the elderly or debilitated patient, severe ulcerative colitis, and toxic megacolon complicating ulcerative colitis. Use with caution in patients with autonomic neuropathy, hyperthyroidism, renal or hepatic impairment, myocardial ischemia, HF, tachyarrhythmias (including sinus tachycardia), hypertension, and hiatal hernia associated with reflux esophagitis. Treatment-related blood pressure increases and tachycardia may lead to ischemia, precipitate an MI, or increase arrhythmogenic potential. In heart transplant recipients, atropine will likely be ineffective in treatment of bradycardia due to lack of vagal innervation of the transplanted heart; cholinergic reinnervation may occur over time (years), so atropine may be used cautiously; however, some may experience paradoxical slowing of the heart rate and high-degree AV block upon administration (ACLS, 2010; Bernheim, 2004).

Avoid relying on atropine for effective treatment of type II second-degree or third-degree AV block (with or without a new wide QRS complex). Asystole or bradycardic pulseless electrical activity (PEA): Although no evidence exists for significant detrimental effects, routine use is unlikely to have a therapeutic benefit and is no longer recommended (ACLS, 2010).

AtroPen®: There are no absolute contraindications for the use of atropine in severe organophosphate or carbamate insecticide or nerve agent poisonings; however in mild poisonings, use caution in those patients where the use of atropine would be otherwise contraindicated. Formulation for use by trained personnel only. Clinical symptoms consistent with highly-suspected organophosphate or carbamate insecticides or nerve agent poisoning should be treated with antidote immediately; administration should not be delayed for confirmatory laboratory tests. Signs of atropinization include flushing, mydriasis, tachycardia, and dryness of the mouth or nose. Monitor effects closely when administering subsequent injections as necessary. The presence of these effects is not indicative of the success of therapy; inappropriate use of mydriasis as an indicator of successful treatment has resulted in atropine toxicity. Reversal of bronchial secretions is the preferred indicator of success. Adjunct treatment with a cholinesterase reactivator (eg, pralidoxime) may be required in patients with toxicity secondary to organophosphorus insecticides or nerve agents. Treatment should always include proper evacuation and decontamination procedures; medical personnel should protect themselves from inadvertent contamination. Antidotal administration is intended only for initial management; definitive and more extensive medical care is required following administration. Individuals should not rely solely on antidote for treatment, as other supportive measures (eg, artificial respiration) may still be required. Atropine reverses the muscarinic but not the nicotinic effects associated with anticholinesterase toxicity.

Children may be more sensitive to the anticholinergic effects of atropine; use with caution in children with spastic paralysis.

Adverse Reactions Frequency not always defined. Severity and frequency of adverse reactions are dose related.

Cardiovascular: Asystole, atrial arrhythmia, atrial fibrillation, atrioventricular dissociation (transient), bigeminy, bradycardia, cardiac dilatation, chest pain, decreased blood pressure, ECG changes (prolonged P wave, shortened PR segment, R on T phenomenon, shortened RT duration, prolonged QT interval, widening of QRS complex, flattened T wave, repolarization abnormalities, ST segment elevation, retrograde conduction), ectopic beats (atrial), extrasystoles (nodal, ventricular, supraventricular), flushing, increased blood pressure, left heart failure, myocardial infarction, nodal arrhythmia (no P wave on ECG), palpitations, sinus tachycardia, supraventricular tachycardia (including junctional tachycardia), tachycardia, trigeminy, ventricular arrhythmia, ventricular fibrillation, ventricular flutter, ventricular premature contractions, ventricular tachycardia, weak pulse (or impalpable peripheral pulses)

Central nervous system: Abnormal electroencephalogram (runs of alpha waves, increase in photic stimulation, and signs of drowsiness), agitation (children), amnesia, anxiety, ataxia, behavioral changes, coma, confusion, decreased deep tendon reflex, delirium, dizziness, drowsiness, dysarthria, dysmetria, excitement, feeling hot, hallucination (visual or aural), headache, hyperpyrexia, hyperreflexia, hypertonia, insomnia, intoxicated feeling, irritability (children), lack of concentration, lethargy (children), mania, mental disorders, myoclonus, neurologic abnormality, nocturnal enuresis, opisthotonus, paranoia, positive Babinski sign, restlessness, seizure (generally tonic-clonic), stupor, unsociability, vertigo

Dermatologic: Anhidrosis, cold skin, dermatitis, dry and hot skin, erythematous rash, hyperhidrosis, macular eruption, maculopapular rash, papular rash, scarlatiniform rash, skin rash

Endocrine & metabolic: Dehydration, hyperglycemia, hypoglycemia, hypokalemia, hyponatremia, increased thirst, loss of libido

Gastrointestinal: Abdominal and bladder distension, abdominal pain, constipation, delayed gastric emptying, diminished bowel sounds, dry mucous membranes, dysphagia, malabsorption, nausea, oral lesion, paralytic ileus, salivation, vomiting, xerostomia

Genitourinary: Difficulty in micturition, impotence, urinary hesitancy, urinary retention, urinary urgency

Hematologic & oncologic: Decreased hemoglobin, increased hemoglobin, increased red blood cell count, leukocytosis, petechia

Hypersensitivity: Hypersensitivity reaction

Local: Injection site reaction

Neuromuscular & skeletal: Laryngospasm, muscle twitching, weakness

Ophthalmic: Abnormal eye movements (cyclophoria and heterophoria), angle-closure glaucoma (acute), blepharitis, blindness, blurred vision, conjunctivitis, crusted of eyelid, cycloplegia, decreased accommodation, decreased visual acuity, dry eye syndrome, eye irritation, keratoconjunctivitis sicca, lacrimation, mydriasis, photophobia, strabismus

Renal: Increased blood urea nitrogen

Respiratory: Bradypnea, changes in respiration (labored respiration), cyanosis, dyspnea, laryngitis, pulmonary edema, respiratory failure, stridor (inspiratory), tachypnea

Miscellaneous: Failure to thrive, fever (secondary to decreased sweat gland activity), swelling (children), tongue biting

Drug Interactions

Metabolism/Transport Effects None known.

Avoid Concomitant Use

Avoid concomitant use of Atropine (Systemic) with any of the following: Aclidinium; Cimetropium; Eluxadoline; Glucagon; Glycopyrrolate; Glycopyrrolate (Oral Inhalation); Ipratropium (Oral Inhalation); Levosulpiride; Potassium Chloride; Tiotropium; Umeclidinium

Increased Effect/Toxicity

Atropine (Systemic) may increase the levels/effects of: AbobotulinumtoxinA; Analgesics (Opioid); Anticholinergic Agents; Cannabinoid-Containing Products; Cimetropium; Eluxadoline; Glucagon; Glycopyrrolate; Glycopyrrolate (Oral Inhalation); Mirabegron; OnabotulinumtoxinA; Potassium Chloride; Ramosetron; RimabotulinumtoxinB; Thiazide Diuretics; Tiotropium; Topiramate

The levels/effects of Atropine (Systemic) may be increased by: Aclidinium; Ipratropium (Oral Inhalation); Mianserin; Pramlintide; Umeclidinium

Decreased Effect

Atropine (Systemic) may decrease the levels/effects of: Acetylcholinesterase Inhibitors; Gastrointestinal Agents (Prokinetic); Itopride; Levosulpiride; Secretin

The levels/effects of Atropine (Systemic) may be decreased by: Acetylcholinesterase Inhibitors

Preparation for Administration Preparation of bulk atropine solution for mass chemical terrorism: Add atropine sulfate powder to 100 mL NS in polyvinyl chloride bags to yield a final concentration of 1 mg/mL (Dix 2003).

Storage/Stability Store injection at controlled room temperature of 15°C to 30°C (59°F to 86°F); avoid freezing. In addition, AtroPen should be protected from light. Preparation of bulk atropine solution for mass chemical terrorism at a concentration of 1 mg/mL is stable for 72 hours at 4°C to 8°C (39°F to 46°F); 20°C to 25°C (68°F to 77°F); 32°C to 36°C (90°F to 97°F) (Dix 2003).

Mechanism of Action Blocks the action of acetylcholine at parasympathetic sites in smooth muscle, secretory glands, and the CNS; increases cardiac output, dries secretions. Atropine reverses the muscarinic effects of cholinergic poisoning due to agents with acetylcholinesterase inhibitor activity by acting as a competitive antagonist of acetylcholine at muscarinic receptors. The primary goal in cholinergic poisonings is reversal of bronchorrhea and bronchoconstriction. Atropine has no effect on the nicotinic receptors responsible for muscle weakness, fasciculations, and paralysis.

Pharmacodynamics/Kinetics

Onset of action:

Inhibition of salivation: IM: 30 minutes; maximum effect: 1 to 1.6 hours

Increased heart rate: IM: 5 to 40 minutes; maximum effect: IM: 20 minutes to 1 hour; IV: 2 to 4 minutes

Duration: Inhibition of salivation: IM: Up to 4 hours

Absorption: Rapid and well absorbed from all dosage forms

Distribution: Widely throughout the body; crosses blood-brain barrier

Protein binding: 14% to 22%

Metabolism: Hepatic via enzymatic hydrolysis

Half-life elimination: Children <2 years: 6.9 ± 3 hours; Children >2 years: 2.5 ± 1.2 hours; Adults: 3 ± 0.9 hours; Elderly 65 to 75 years of age: 10 hours

Time to peak: IM: Auto-injector: 3 minutes

Excretion: Urine (30% to 50% as unchanged drug and metabolites)

Dosing

Adult & Geriatric Doses <0.5 mg have been associated with paradoxical bradycardia.

Inhibit salivation and secretions (preanesthesia): IM, IV, SubQ: 0.4 to 0.6 mg 30 to 60 minutes preop and repeat every 4 to 6 hours as needed.

Bradycardia (Note: Atropine may be ineffective in heart transplant recipients): IV: 0.5 mg every 3 to 5 minutes, not to exceed a total of 3 mg or 0.04 mg/kg (ACLS 2010)

Neuromuscular blockade reversal: IV: Neuromuscular blockade reversal: IV: 15 to 30 mcg/kg administered with neostigmine or 7 to 10 mcg/kg administered with edrophonium (Cronnelly 1982; Miller 2010; Mirakhur 1981; Naguib 1989)

Organophosphate or carbamate insecticide or nerve agent poisoning: Note: The dose of atropine required varies considerably with the severity of poisoning. The total amount of atropine used for carbamate poisoning is usually less than with organophosphate insecticide or nerve agent poisoning. Severely poisoned patients may exhibit significant tolerance to atropine; ≥2 times the suggested doses may be needed. Titrate to pulmonary status (decreased bronchial secretions); consider administration of atropine via continuous IV infusion in patients requiring large doses of atropine. Once patient is stable for a period of time, the dose/dosing frequency may be decreased. Pralidoxime is a component of the management of organophosphate insecticide and nerve agent toxicity; refer to Pralidoxime monograph for the specific route and dose.

IV, IM (off-label dose): Initial: 1 to 6 mg (ATSDR 2011; Roberts 2007); repeat every 3 to 5 minutes as needed, doubling the dose if previous dose did not induce atropinization (Eddleston 2004b; Roberts 2007). Maintain atropinization by administering repeat doses as needed for ≥2 to 12 hours based on recurrence of symptoms (Reigart, 1999).

IV Infusion (off-label dose): Following atropinization, administer 10% to 20% of the total loading dose required to induce atropinization as a continuous IV infusion per hour; adjust as needed to maintain adequate atropinization without atropine toxicity (Eddleston 2004b; Roberts 2007)

IM (AtroPen):

Mild symptoms (≥2 mild symptoms): Administer 2 mg as soon as an exposure is known or strongly suspected. If severe symptoms develop after the first dose, 2 additional doses should be repeated in rapid succession 10 minutes after the first dose; do not administer more than 3 doses. If profound anticholinergic effects occur in the absence of excessive bronchial secretions, further doses of atropine should be withheld.

Severe symptoms (≥1 severe symptoms): Immediately administer **three** 2 mg doses in rapid succession.

Symptoms of insecticide or nerve agent poisoning, as provided by manufacturer in the AtroPen product labeling, to guide therapy:

Mild symptoms: Blurred vision, bradycardia, breathing difficulties, chest tightness, coughing, drooling, miosis, muscular twitching, nausea, runny nose, salivation increased, stomach cramps, tachycardia, teary eyes, tremor, vomiting, or wheezing

Severe symptoms: Breathing difficulties (severe), confused/strange behavior, defecation (involuntary), muscular twitching/generalized weakness (severe), respiratory secretions (severe), seizure, unconsciousness, urination (involuntary)

Stress echocardiography (adjunct chronotropic agent) (off-label use): IV: 0.25 to 0.5 mg up to a total dose of 1 to 2 mg until 85% of target heart rate is achieved (ASNC [Henzlova 2009])

Pediatric Note: Doses <0.1 mg have been associated with paradoxical bradycardia.

Inhibit salivation and secretions (preanesthesia) (Nelson, 1996): Infants, Children, and Adolescents: IM, IV, SubQ: Administer dose 30 to 60 minutes preoperatively then every 4 to 6 hours as needed:

Infants <5 kg: 0.02 mg/kg/dose; use of a minimum dosage of 0.1 mg will result in dosages >0.02 mg/kg; there is no documented minimum dosage in this age group.

Infants and Children ≥5 kg: 0.01 to 0.02 mg/kg/dose; maximum single dose: 0.4 mg; minimum dose: 0.1 mg

Alternate dosing:

3 to 7 kg (7 to 16 lb): 0.1 mg

8 to 11 kg (17 to 24 lb): 0.15 mg

11 to 18 kg (24 to 40 lb): 0.2 mg

18 to 29 kg (40 to 65 lb): 0.3 mg

>30 kg (>65 lb): 0.4 mg

Bradycardia:

IV, I.O.: Infants, Children, and Adolescents: 0.02 mg/kg, minimum dose recommended by PALS: 0.1 mg; however, use of a minimum dosage of 0.1 mg in patients <5 kg will result in dosages >0.02 mg/kg and is not recommended (Barrington 2011); there is no documented minimum dosage in this age group; maximum single dose: 0.5 mg; may repeat once in 3 to 5 minutes; maximum total dose: 1 mg (PALS 2010).

Endotracheal: Infants, Children, and Adolescents: 0.04 to 0.06 mg/kg; may repeat once if needed (PALS 2010)

Organophosphate or carbamate insecticide or nerve agent poisoning: Infants, Children, and Adolescents: **Note:** The dose of atropine required varies considerably with the severity of poisoning. The total amount of atropine used for carbamate poisoning is usually less than with organophosphate insecticide or nerve agent poisoning. Severely poisoned patients may exhibit significant tolerance to atropine; ≥2 times the suggested doses may be needed. Titrate to pulmonary status (decreased bronchial secretions); consider administration of atropine via continuous IV infusion in patients requiring large doses of atropine. Once patient is stable for a period of time, the dose/dosing frequency may be decreased. Pralidoxime is a component of the management of organophosphate insecticide and nerve agent toxicity; refer to Pralidoxime monograph for the specific route and dose.

IV, IM (off-label dose): Initial: 0.05 to 0.1 mg/kg; repeat every 5 to 10 minutes as needed, doubling the dose if previous dose does not induce atropinization (Hegenbarth 2008; Rotenberg 2003). Maintain atropinization by administering repeat doses as needed for ≥2 to 12 hours based on recurrence of symptoms (Reigart, 1999).

IV infusion (off-label dose): Following atropinization, administer 10% to 20% of the total loading dose required to induce atropinization as a continuous IV infusion per hour; adjust as needed to maintain adequate atropinization without atropine toxicity (Eddleston 2004b; Roberts 2007).

IM (AtroPen):

Mild symptoms (≥2 mild symptoms): Administer the weight-based dose listed below as soon as an exposure is known or strongly suspected. If severe symptoms develop after the first dose, 2 additional doses should be repeated in rapid succession 10 minutes after the first dose; do not administer more than 3 doses. If profound anticholinergic effects occur in the absence of excessive bronchial secretions, further doses of atropine should be withheld.

◀

Severe symptoms (≥1 severe symptoms): Immediately administer **three** weight-based doses in rapid succession.

Weight-based dosing:

<6.8 kg (15 lb): 0.25 mg/dose

6.8 to 18 kg (15 to 40 lb): 0.5 mg/dose

18 to 41 kg (40 to 90 lb): 1 mg/dose

>41 kg (>90 lb): 2 mg/dose

Symptoms of insecticide or nerve agent poisoning, as provided by manufacturer in the AtroPen product labeling, to guide therapy:

Mild symptoms: Blurred vision, bradycardia, breathing difficulties, chest tightness, coughing, drooling, miosis, muscular twitching, nausea, runny nose, salivation increased, stomach cramps, tachycardia, teary eyes, tremor, vomiting, or wheezing

Severe symptoms: Breathing difficulties (severe), confused/strange behavior, defecation (involuntary), muscular twitching/generalized weakness (severe), respiratory secretions (severe), seizure, unconsciousness, urination (involuntary); **Note:** Infants may become drowsy or unconscious with muscle floppiness as opposed to muscle twitching.

Endotracheal (off-label route): Increase the dose by 2-3 times the usual IV dose. Mix with 3 to 5 mL of normal saline and administer. Flush with 3 to 5 mL of NS and follow with 5 assisted manual ventilations (Rotenberg 2003).

Renal Impairment No dosage adjustment provided in manufacturer's labeling.

Hepatic Impairment No dosage adjustment provided in manufacturer's labeling.

Administration

IM: AtroPen: Administer to the outer thigh. Firmly grasp the autoinjector with the green tip (0.5 mg, 1 mg, and 2 mg autoinjector) or black tip (0.25 mg autoinjector) pointed down; remove the yellow safety release (0.5 mg, 1 mg, and 2 mg autoinjector) or gray safety release (0.25 mg autoinjector). Jab the green tip at a 90° angle against the outer thigh; may be administered through clothing as long as pockets at the injection site are empty. In thin patients or patients <6.8 kg (15 lb), bunch up the thigh prior to injection. Hold the autoinjector in place for 10 seconds following the injection; remove the autoinjector and massage the injection site. After administration, the needle will be visible; if the needle is not visible, repeat the above steps. After use, bend the needle against a hard surface (needle does not retract) to avoid accidental injury.

IV: Administer undiluted by rapid IV injection; slow injection may result in paradoxical bradycardia. In bradycardia, atropine administration should not delay treatment with external pacing.

Endotracheal: Dilute in NS or sterile water. Absorption may be greater with sterile water. Stop compressions (if using for cardiac arrest), spray the drug quickly down the tube. Follow immediately with several quick insufflations and continue chest compressions.

Monitoring Parameters Heart rate, blood pressure, pulse, mental status; intravenous administration requires a cardiac monitor

Organophosphate or carbamate insecticide or nerve agent poisoning: Heart rate, blood pressure, respiratory status, oxygenation secretions. Maintain atropinization with repeated dosing as indicated by clinical status. Crackles in lung bases, or continuation of cholinergic signs, may be signs of inadequate dosing. Pulmonary improvement may not parallel other signs of atropinization. Monitor for signs and symptoms of atropine toxicity (eg, fever, muscle fasciculations, delirium); if toxicity occurs, discontinue atropine and monitor closely.

Consult individual institutional policies and procedures.

Dosage Forms Excipient information presented when available (limited, particularly for generics); consult specific product labeling.

Device, Intramuscular, as sulfate:

AtroPen: 0.25 mg/0.3 mL (0.3 mL) [pyrogen free]

AtroPen: 0.5 mg/0.7 mL (0.7 mL); 1 mg/0.7 mL (0.7 mL); 2 mg/0.7 mL (0.7 mL) [pyrogen free; contains phenol]

Solution, Injection, as sulfate:

Generic: 0.05 mg/mL (5 mL); 0.1 mg/mL (5 mL, 10 mL); 0.4 mg/mL (1 mL, 20 mL); 1 mg/mL (1 mL)

Solution, Injection, as sulfate [preservative free]:

Generic: 0.4 mg/mL (1 mL); 0.8 mg/mL (0.5 mL); 1 mg/mL (1 mL)

Atropine (Ophthalmic) (A troe peen)

Brand Names: US Atropine-Care [DSC]; Isopto Atropine [DSC]

Brand Names: Canada Dioptic's Atropine Solution; Isopto Atropine

Index Terms Atropine Sulfate

Pharmacologic Category Anticholinergic Agent, Ophthalmic; Ophthalmic Agent, Mydriatic

Use Produce mydriasis and cycloplegia for examination of the retina and optic disc and accurate measurement of refractive errors; produce papillary dilation in inflammatory conditions of the iris and uveal tract (eg, uveitis); penalization of the healthy eye in the treatment of amblyopia

Pregnancy Considerations Animal reproduction studies have not been conducted. Atropine is absorbed systemically following ophthalmic administration (variable concentrations). Atropine has been found to cross the human placenta.

Breast-Feeding Considerations Trace amounts of atropine are excreted into breast milk. Atropine may suppress lactation or cause adverse events in the nursing infant (data is conflicting). The manufacturer recommends that caution be exercised when administering atropine to nursing women.

Contraindications Hypersensitivity to atropine or any component of the formulation

Warnings/Precautions Photophobia or blurred vision may last up to 2 weeks due to pupil unresponsiveness and cycloplegia. Elevated blood pressure may occur due to systemic absorption following conjunctival instillation.

Adverse Reactions Frequency not defined. Severity and frequency of adverse reactions are dose related.

Cardiovascular: Delirium, flushing, hypotension, increased blood pressure

Central nervous system: Irritability, restlessness

Dermatologic: Contact dermatitis, xeroderma

Gastrointestinal: Xerostomia

Ophthalmic: Blurred vision, decreased lacrimation, eye irritation, eyelid edema, eye pain, papillary conjunctivitis, photophobia, stinging of eyes, superficial keratitis

Respiratory: Dry throat, respiratory depression

Drug Interactions

Metabolism/Transport Effects None known.

Avoid Concomitant Use

Avoid concomitant use of Atropine (Ophthalmic) with any of the following: Aclidinium; Cimetropium; Eluxadoline; Glucagon; Glycopyrrolate; Glycopyrrolate (Oral Inhalation); Ipratropium (Oral Inhalation); Levosulpiride; MAO Inhibitors; Potassium Chloride; Tiotropium; Umeclidinium

Increased Effect/Toxicity

Atropine (Ophthalmic) may increase the levels/effects of: AbobotulinumtoxinA; Analgesics (Opioid); Anticholinergic Agents; Cannabinoid-Containing Products; Cimetropium; Eluxadoline; Glucagon; Glycopyrrolate; Glycopyrrolate (Oral Inhalation); Mirabegron; OnabotulinumtoxinA; Potassium Chloride; Ramosetron; RimabotulinumtoxinB; Thiazide Diuretics; Tiotropium; Topiramate

The levels/effects of Atropine (Ophthalmic) may be increased by: Aclidinium; Ipratropium (Oral Inhalation); MAO Inhibitors; Mianserin; Pramlintide; Umeclidinium

Decreased Effect

Atropine (Ophthalmic) may decrease the levels/effects of: Acetylcholinesterase Inhibitors; Gastrointestinal Agents (Prokinetic); Itopride; Levosulpiride; Secretin

The levels/effects of Atropine (Ophthalmic) may be decreased by: Acetylcholinesterase Inhibitors

Storage/Stability Ophthalmic products: Store at 20°C to 25°C (68°F to 77°F); keep tightly closed.

Mechanism of Action Blocks the action of acetylcholine at parasympathetic sites in smooth muscle, secretory glands, and the CNS

Pharmacodynamics/Kinetics

Onset of action: Ophthalmic solution: Within 40 minutes; maximum effect: 2 hours

Duration: Up to 2 weeks in a normal eye

Absorption: Well absorbed from all dosage forms

Metabolism: Hepatic via enzymatic hydrolysis

Bioavailability: Ophthalmic solution: 63.5 ± 29% (range: 19% to 95%)

Half-life elimination: 2.5 ± 0.8 hours

Time to peak: 28 ± 27 minutes

Excretion: Urine (13% to 50% as unchanged drug and metabolites)

Dosing

Adult

Mydriasis, cycloplegia (preprocedure): Ophthalmic: Solution (1%): Instill 1 to 2 drops 1 hour before procedure.

Uveitis: Ophthalmic:
Ointment: Apply a small amount in the conjunctival sac 1 to 2 times/day; compress the lacrimal sac by digital pressure for 1 to 3 minutes after instillation
Solution (1%): Instill 1 to 2 drops up to 4 times/day
Terminal respiratory sections (off-label use): Sublingual (using 1% ophthalmic solution): Initial: 1 to 2 drops every 2 to 4 hours; usual dose range: 2 to 4 drops every 2 to 4 hours (Protus 2013)

Pediatric
Amblyopia, healthy eye penalization: Children ≥3 years and Adolescents: Ophthalmic: Solution (1%): Instill 1 drop once daily to healthy eye; dose may be repeated up to twice daily if needed (Repka 2014; Scheiman 2008)
Mydriasis, cycloplegia (preprocedure):
Infants ≥3 months and Children <3 years: Ophthalmic: Solution (1%): Instill 1 drop 40 minutes prior to intended maximal dilation time. Maximum dose: 1 drop per eye per day.
Children ≥3 years and Adolescents: Ophthalmic: Solution (1%): Instill 1 to 2 drops 40 minutes prior to intended maximal dilation time (Nelson 1996)

Renal Impairment There are no dosage adjustments provided in the manufacturer's labeling.
Hepatic Impairment There are no dosage adjustments provided in the manufacturer's labeling.
Administration Solution: Instill solution into conjunctival sac of affected eye(s); compress lacrimal sac with digital pressure for 2 to 3 minutes after instillation; avoid contact of bottle tip with eye or skin
Dosage Forms Excipient information presented when available (limited, particularly for generics); consult specific product labeling. [DSC] = Discontinued product
Ointment, Ophthalmic, as sulfate:
Generic: 1% (3.5 g)
Solution, Ophthalmic, as sulfate:
Atropine-Care: 1% (2 mL [DSC], 5 mL [DSC], 15 mL [DSC]) [contains benzalkonium chloride, edetate disodium]
Isopto Atropine: 1% (5 mL [DSC], 15 mL [DSC])
Generic: 1% (2 mL, 5 mL, 15 mL)

◆ Atropine and Diphenoxylate see Diphenoxylate and Atropine on page 564

Atropine and Pralidoxime
(A troe peen & pra li DOKS eem)

Brand Names: US ATNAA; Duodote
Index Terms Atropine and Pralidoxime Chloride; Mark 1; NAAK; Nerve Agent Antidote Kit; Pralidoxime and Atropine
Pharmacologic Category Anticholinergic Agent; Antidote
Use
ATNAA: Treatment of poisoning in patients who have been exposed to organophosphate nerve agents (eg, tabun, sarin, soman) that have acetylcholinesterase-inhibiting activity for self- or buddy-administration by military personnel
Duodote™: Treatment of poisoning by organophosphate nerve agents (eg, tabun, sarin, soman) or organophosphate insecticides for use by trained emergency medical services personnel
Prescribing and Access Restrictions
ATNAA (**A**ntidote **T**reatment-**N**erve **A**gent **A**uto-Injector) is only available for use by U.S. Armed Forces military personnel. Information on distribution is available at Defense Services Supply Center-Philadelphia at 215-737-2341.
Duodote is only available for use by trained emergency medical services personnel to treat civilians. Distribution is limited to directly from manufacturer (Meridian Medical Technologies, Inc) to emergency medical service organizations or their suppliers.
Dosing
Adult Organophosphate insecticide or nerve agent:
IM: **Note:** If exposure is suspected, antidotal therapy should be given immediately as soon as symptoms appear (critical to administer immediately in case of soman exposure). Definitive medical care should be sought after any injection given. One injection only may be given as self-aid. If repeat injections needed, administration must be done by another trained individual. Emergency medical personnel who have self-administered a dose must determine capacity to continue to provide care.

ATNAA:
Mild symptoms (some or all mild symptoms): Self-Aid or Buddy-Aid: 1 injection (wait 10-15 minutes for effect); if the patient is able to ambulate, and knows who and where they are, then no further injections are needed.

If symptoms still present: Buddy-Aid: May repeat 1-2 more injections
Severe symptoms (if most or all): Buddy-Aid: If no self-aid given, 3 injections in rapid succession; if 1 self-aid injection given, 2 injections in rapid succession
Maximum cumulative dose: 3 injections
Symptoms of organophosphate insecticide or nerve agent poisoning, as provided by manufacturer in the ATNAA product labeling to guide therapy:
Mild symptoms: Breathing difficulties, chest tightness, coughing, difficulty in seeing, drooling, headache, localized sweating and muscular twitching, miosis, nausea (with or without vomiting), runny nose, stomach cramps, tachycardia (followed by bradycardia), wheezing
Severe symptoms: Bradycardia, confused/strange behavior, convulsions, increased wheezing and breathing difficulties, involuntary urination/defecation, miosis (severe), muscular twitching/generalized weakness (severe), red/teary eyes, respiratory failure, unconsciousness, vomiting

Duodote™:
Mild symptoms (≥2 mild symptoms): 1 injection (wait 10-15 minutes for effect); if after 10-15 minutes no severe symptoms emerge, no further injections are indicated; if any severe symptoms emerge at any point following initial injection, repeat dose by giving 2 additional injections in rapid succession. Transport to medical care facility.
Severe symptoms (≥1 severe symptom): 3 injections in rapid succession. Transport to medical care facility.
Maximum cumulative dose: 3 injections unless medical care support (eg, hospital, respiratory support) is available
Symptoms of organophosphate insecticide or nerve agent poisoning, as provided by manufacturer in the Duodote™ product labeling to guide therapy:
Mild symptoms: Airway secretions increased, blurred vision, bradycardia, breathing difficulties, chest tightness, drooling miosis, nausea, vomiting, runny nose, salivation, stomach cramps (acute onset), tachycardia, teary eyes, tremors/muscular twitching, wheezing/coughing
Severe symptoms: Breathing difficulties (severe), confused/strange behavior, convulsions, copious secretions from lung or airway, involuntary urination/defecation, muscular twitching/generalized weakness (severe)

Geriatric Refer to adult dosing. No dosing adjustment recommended.
Renal Impairment Use caution in renal impairment; pralidoxime is renally eliminated.
Hepatic Impairment No dosage adjustment provided in manufacturer's labeling.
Additional Information Complete prescribing information should be consulted for additional detail.
Dosage Forms Excipient information presented when available (limited, particularly for generics); consult specific product labeling.
Injection, solution:
ATNAA, Duodote™: Atropine 2.1 mg/0.7 mL and pralidoxime chloride 600 mg/2 mL [contains benzyl alcohol; prefilled autoinjector]

◆ Atropine and Pralidoxime Chloride see Atropine and Pralidoxime on page 179
◆ Atropine-Care [DSC] see Atropine (Ophthalmic) on page 178
◆ Atropine, Hyoscyamine, Phenobarbital, and Scopolamine see Hyoscyamine, Atropine, Scopolamine, and Phenobarbital on page 900
◆ Atropine Sulfate see Atropine (Ophthalmic) on page 178
◆ Atropine Sulfate see Atropine (Systemic) on page 175
◆ Atrovent see Ipratropium (Nasal) on page 978
◆ Atrovent® (Can) see Ipratropium (Nasal) on page 978
◆ Atrovent HFA see Ipratropium (Systemic) on page 977
◆ ATV see Atazanavir on page 162
◆ ATX-101 see Deoxycholic Acid on page 518
◆ Aubagio see Teriflunomide on page 1763
◆ Aubra see Ethinyl Estradiol and Levonorgestrel on page 703
◆ Augmentin see Amoxicillin and Clavulanate on page 111
◆ Augmentin ES-600 see Amoxicillin and Clavulanate on page 111
◆ Augmentin XR see Amoxicillin and Clavulanate on page 111
◆ Auralgan see Antipyrine and Benzocaine on page 135

◆ Auralgan® (Can) *see* Antipyrine and Benzocaine *on page 135*

Auranofin (au RANE oh fin)

Brand Names: US Ridaura
Brand Names: Canada Ridaura®
Pharmacologic Category Gold Compound
Use Management of active stage classic or definite rheumatoid arthritis in patients who do not respond to or tolerate other agents
Dosing
Adult & Geriatric Rheumatoid arthritis: Oral: Initial: 6 mg/day in 1-2 divided doses; after 6 months may be increased to 9 mg/day in 3 divided doses; discontinue therapy if no response after 3 months at 9 mg/day
Note: Signs of clinical improvement may not be evident until after 3 months of therapy.
Renal Impairment There are no dosage adjustments provided in the manufacturer's labeling. The following guidelines have been used by some clinicians (Aronoff 2007):
CrCl 50 to 80 mL/minute: Administer 50% of dose.
CrCl <50 mL/minute: Avoid use.
Hepatic Impairment No dosage adjustment provided in manufacturer's labeling.
Additional Information Complete prescribing information should be consulted for additional detail.
Dosage Forms Excipient information presented when available (limited, particularly for generics); consult specific product labeling.
Capsule, Oral:
Ridaura: 3 mg [contains benzyl alcohol]

◆ Auraphene-B [OTC] *see* Carbamide Peroxide *on page 307*
◆ Auro-Alendronate (Can) *see* Alendronate *on page 66*
◆ Auro-Amlodipine (Can) *see* AmLODIPine *on page 101*
◆ Auro-Anastrozole (Can) *see* Anastrozole *on page 128*
◆ Auro-Atorvastatin (Can) *see* AtorvaSTATin *on page 169*
◆ Auro-Carvedilol (Can) *see* Carvedilol *on page 323*
◆ Auro-Cefixime (Can) *see* Cefixime *on page 335*
◆ Auro-Cefprozil (Can) *see* Cefprozil *on page 343*
◆ Auro-Cefuroxime (Can) *see* Cefuroxime *on page 353*
◆ Auro-Ciprofloxacin (Can) *see* Ciprofloxacin (Systemic) *on page 388*
◆ Auro-Citalopram (Can) *see* Citalopram *on page 398*
◆ Auro-Clindamycin (Can) *see* Clindamycin (Systemic) *on page 405*
◆ Auro-Clopidogrel (Can) *see* Clopidogrel *on page 424*
◆ Auro-Cyclobenzaprine (Can) *see* Cyclobenzaprine *on page 454*
◆ Aurodex [DSC] *see* Antipyrine and Benzocaine *on page 135*
◆ Auro-Donepezil (Can) *see* Donepezil *on page 583*
◆ Auro-Finasteride (Can) *see* Finasteride *on page 769*
◆ Auro-Gabapentin (Can) *see* Gabapentin *on page 823*
◆ Auro-Galantamine ER (Can) *see* Galantamine *on page 826*
◆ Auro-Irbesartan (Can) *see* Irbesartan *on page 979*
◆ Auro-Lamotrigine (Can) *see* LamoTRIgine *on page 1027*
◆ Auro-Letrozole (Can) *see* Letrozole *on page 1048*
◆ Auro-Levetiracetam (Can) *see* LevETIRAcetam *on page 1056*
◆ Auro-Lisinopril (Can) *see* Lisinopril *on page 1088*
◆ Auro-Losartan (Can) *see* Losartan *on page 1107*
◆ Auro-Losartan HCT (Can) *see* Losartan and Hydrochlorothiazide *on page 1109*
◆ Auro-Meloxicam (Can) *see* Meloxicam *on page 1137*
◆ Auro-Metformin (Can) *see* MetFORMIN *on page 1156*
◆ Auro-Mirtazapine (Can) *see* Mirtazapine *on page 1216*
◆ Auro-Mirtazapine OD (Can) *see* Mirtazapine *on page 1216*
◆ Auro-Modafinil (Can) *see* Modafinil *on page 1222*
◆ Auro-Montelukast (Can) *see* Montelukast *on page 1229*
◆ Auro-Montelukast Chewable Tablets (Can) *see* Montelukast *on page 1229*
◆ Auro-Nevirapine (Can) *see* Nevirapine *on page 1270*
◆ Auro-Omeprazole (Can) *see* Omeprazole *on page 1330*
◆ Auro-Paroxetine (Can) *see* PARoxetine *on page 1399*
◆ Auro-Pioglitazone (Can) *see* Pioglitazone *on page 1454*

◆ Auro-Pramipexole (Can) *see* Pramipexole *on page 1486*
◆ Auro-Pregabalin (Can) *see* Pregabalin *on page 1500*
◆ Auro-Quetiapine (Can) *see* QUEtiapine *on page 1536*
◆ Auro-Ramipri (Can) *see* Ramipril *on page 1552*
◆ Auro-Repaglinide (Can) *see* Repaglinide *on page 1569*
◆ Auro-Risedronate (Can) *see* Risedronate *on page 1591*
◆ Auro-Sertraline (Can) *see* Sertraline *on page 1649*
◆ Auro-Simvastatin (Can) *see* Simvastatin *on page 1659*
◆ Auro-Terbinafine (Can) *see* Terbinafine (Systemic) *on page 1759*
◆ AURO-Topiramate (Can) *see* Topiramate *on page 1810*
◆ Auro-Valsartan (Can) *see* Valsartan *on page 1865*
◆ Auryxia *see* Ferric Citrate *on page 760*
◆ Auvi-Q [DSC] *see* EPINEPHrine (Systemic) *on page 647*
◆ AVA *see* Anthrax Vaccine Adsorbed *on page 130*
◆ Ava-Acebutolol (Can) *see* Acebutolol *on page 24*
◆ Ava-Atenolol (Can) *see* Atenolol *on page 166*
◆ Ava-Atorvastatin (Can) *see* AtorvaSTATin *on page 169*
◆ Ava-Bisoprolol (Can) *see* Bisoprolol *on page 233*
◆ Ava-Cefprozil (Can) *see* Cefprozil *on page 343*
◆ Ava-Clindamycin (Can) *see* Clindamycin (Systemic) *on page 405*
◆ Ava-Cyclobenzaprine (Can) *see* Cyclobenzaprine *on page 454*
◆ Ava-Famciclovir (Can) *see* Famciclovir *on page 739*
◆ Ava-Fenofibrate Micro (Can) *see* Fenofibrate and Derivatives *on page 746*
◆ Ava-Fluoxetine (Can) *see* FLUoxetine *on page 786*
◆ Ava-Fluvoxamine (Can) *see* FluvoxaMINE *on page 801*
◆ Ava-Fosinopril (Can) *see* Fosinopril *on page 814*
◆ AVA-Furosemide (Can) *see* Furosemide *on page 821*
◆ Avage *see* Tazarotene *on page 1740*
◆ Ava-Glyburide (Can) *see* GlyBURIDE *on page 847*
◆ Ava-Hydrochlorothiazide (Can) *see* Hydrochlorothiazide *on page 881*
◆ Ava-Irbesartan (Can) *see* Irbesartan *on page 979*
◆ Avakine *see* InFLIXimab *on page 941*
◆ Avalide *see* Irbesartan and Hydrochlorothiazide *on page 980*
◆ Ava-Metoprolol (Can) *see* Metoprolol *on page 1193*
◆ Ava-Metoprolol (Type L) (Can) *see* Metoprolol *on page 1193*
◆ Ava-Mirtazapine (Can) *see* Mirtazapine *on page 1216*
◆ Avamys (Can) *see* Fluticasone (Nasal) *on page 795*

Avanafil (a VAN a fil)

Brand Names: US Stendra
Index Terms Stendra
Pharmacologic Category Phosphodiesterase-5 Enzyme Inhibitor
Use Erectile dysfunction: Treatment of erectile dysfunction
Pregnancy Considerations Based on data from animal reproduction studies, avanafil is predicted to have a low risk for major developmental abnormalities in humans. This product is not indicated for use in women.
Breast-Feeding Considerations This product is not indicated for use in women.
Contraindications Hypersensitivity to avanafil or any component of the formulation; coadministration with any form of organic nitrates (either regularly or intermittently) or guanylate cyclase stimulators (eg, riociguat)
Warnings/Precautions There is a degree of cardiac risk associated with sexual activity; therefore, physicians may wish to consider the patient's cardiovascular status prior to initiating any treatment for erectile dysfunction. Use caution in patients with anatomical deformation of the penis (angulation, cavernosal fibrosis, or Peyronie's disease) and in patients who have conditions which may predispose them to priapism (sickle cell anemia, multiple myeloma, leukemia). Priapism, painful erection >6 hours in duration has been reported (rarely). Instruct patients to seek immediate medical attention if erection persists >4 hours.

Use is not recommended in patients with hypotension (<90/50 mm Hg); uncontrolled hypertension (>170/100 mm Hg); unstable angina or angina during intercourse; life-threatening arrhythmias, stroke, or MI within the last 6 months; cardiac failure or coronary artery disease causing unstable angina. Safety and efficacy have not been

studied in these patients. Use caution in patients with left ventricular outflow obstruction (eg, aortic stenosis, hypertrophic cardiomyopathy with outflow tract obstruction). Use caution with alpha-blockers; dosage adjustment is needed. Patients should avoid or limit concurrent substantial alcohol consumption as this may increase the risk of symptomatic hypotension.

Rare cases of nonarteritic ischemic optic neuropathy (NAION) have been reported; patients who have already experienced NAION are at an increased risk of recurrence. Other risk factors for NAION include heart disease, diabetes, hypertension, smoking, age >50 years, or history of certain eye problems. Use with caution in these patients only when the benefits outweigh the risks. Sudden decrease or loss of hearing has been reported rarely; hearing changes may be accompanied by tinnitus and dizziness.

Safety and efficacy have not been studied in patients with the following conditions, therefore, use in these patients is not recommended at this time: Severe hepatic impairment (Child-Pugh class C); severe renal impairment; end-stage renal disease requiring dialysis; retinitis pigmentosa or other degenerative retinal disorders. Potentially significant drug-drug interactions may exist, requiring dose or frequency adjustment, additional monitoring, and/or selection of alternative therapy. Use of avanafil is contraindicated in patients currently taking nitrate preparations. According to the manufacturer, when nitrate administration is deemed medically necessary in a life-threatening situation, may administer nitrates only if 12 hours has elapsed after avanafil use. Of note, the elimination half-life of avanafil is similar to that of sildenafil and vardenafil which both require 24 hours to elapse prior to administration of nitrates (ACCF/AHA [Anderson, 2013]; ACCF/AHA [O'Gara, 2013]). Potential underlying causes of erectile dysfunction should be evaluated prior to treatment.

Adverse Reactions

>10%: Central nervous system: Headache (1% to 12%)

2% to 10%:
Cardiovascular: Flushing (3% to 10%), ECG abnormality (1% to 3%)
Central nervous system: Dizziness (1% to 2%)
Gastrointestinal: Viral gastroenteritis (≤2%)
Neuromuscular & skeletal: Back pain (1% to 3%)
Respiratory: Nasopharyngitis (1% to 5%), nasal congestion (1% to 3%), upper respiratory tract infection (1% to 3%)

<2% (Limited to important or life-threatening): Angina pectoris, anterior ischemic optic neuropathy (nonarteritic), balanitis, deep vein thrombosis, depression, gastritis, gastroesophageal reflux disease, hearing loss, hematuria, hyperglycemia, hypertension, hypoglycemia, hypotension, increased serum ALT, myalgia, nausea, nephrolithiasis, palpitations, peripheral edema, pollakiuria, priapism, skin rash, urinary tract infection, vision color changes, vision loss (temporary or permanent), wheezing

Drug Interactions

Metabolism/Transport Effects Substrate of CYP3A4 (major); **Note:** Assignment of Major/Minor substrate status based on clinically relevant drug interaction potential

Avoid Concomitant Use
Avoid concomitant use of Avanafil with any of the following: Alprostadil; Amyl Nitrite; Conivaptan; CYP3A4 Inhibitors (Strong); Dapoxetine; Fusidic Acid (Systemic); Idelalisib; Itraconazole; Ketoconazole (Systemic); Molsidomine; Phosphodiesterase 5 Inhibitors; Posaconazole; Riociguat; Vasodilators (Organic Nitrates); Voriconazole

Increased Effect/Toxicity
Avanafil may increase the levels/effects of: Alpha1-Blockers; Alprostadil; Amyl Nitrite; Blood Pressure Lowering Agents; Bosentan; Phosphodiesterase 5 Inhibitors; Riociguat; Vasodilators (Organic Nitrates)

The levels/effects of Avanafil may be increased by: Alcohol (Ethyl); Conivaptan; CYP3A4 Inhibitors (Moderate); CYP3A4 Inhibitors (Strong); Dapoxetine; Dasatinib; Fluconazole; Fosaprepitant; Fusidic Acid (Systemic); Idelalisib; Itraconazole; Ivacaftor; Ketoconazole (Systemic); Lorcaserin; Luliconazole; Mifepristone; Molsidomine; Osimertinib; Palbociclib; Posaconazole; Sapropterin; Simeprevir; Stiripentol; Voriconazole

Decreased Effect
The levels/effects of Avanafil may be decreased by: Bosentan; CYP3A4 Inducers (Moderate); CYP3A4 Inducers (Strong); Dabrafenib; Deferasirox; Enzalutamide; Etravirine; Mitotane; Osimertinib; Siltuximab; St Johns Wort; Tocilizumab

Food Interactions Grapefruit juice may increase serum levels/toxicity of avanafil. Management: Avoid grapefruit juice.

Storage/Stability Store at 20°C to 25°C (68°F to 77°F); excursions are permitted to 30°C (86°F). Protect from light.

Mechanism of Action Does not directly cause penile erections, but affects the response to sexual stimulation. The physiologic mechanism of erection of the penis involves release of nitric oxide (NO) in the corpus cavernosum during sexual stimulation. NO then activates the enzyme guanylate cyclase, which results in increased levels of cyclic guanosine monophosphate (cGMP), producing smooth muscle relaxation and inflow of blood to the corpus cavernosum. Avanafil enhances the effect of NO by inhibiting phosphodiesterase type 5 (PDE-5), which is responsible for degradation of cGMP in the corpus cavernosum; when sexual stimulation causes local release of NO, inhibition of PDE-5 by avanafil causes increased levels of cGMP in the corpus cavernosum, resulting in smooth muscle relaxation and inflow of blood to the corpus cavernosum; at recommended doses, it has no effect in the absence of sexual stimulation.

Pharmacodynamics/Kinetics

Absorption: Rapid
Protein binding: ~99%
Metabolism: Hepatic via CYP3A4 (major), CYP2C (minor); forms metabolites (active and inactive)
Half-life elimination: Terminal: ~5 hours
Time to peak, plasma: 30 to 45 minutes (fasting); 1.12 to 1.25 hours (high-fat meal)
Excretion: Feces (~62%); urine (~21%)

Dosing

Adult Erectile dysfunction: Oral: Initial: 100 mg taken ~15 minutes prior to sexual activity; taken as one single dose and not more than once daily; dose may be increased to 200 mg ~15 minutes prior to sexual activity or decreased to 50 mg ~30 minutes prior to sexual activity using the lowest dose that provides benefit; maximum 200 mg daily

Dosing adjustment with concomitant medications:
Alpha-blocker (dose should be stable at time of avanafil initiation): Initial avanafil dose: 50 mg taken as one single dose and not more than once daily.
Moderate CYP34A inhibitors (including amprenavir, aprepitant, diltiazem, erythromycin, fluconazole, fosamprenavir, verapamil): Maximum avanafil dose: 50 mg taken as one single dose and not more than once daily.
Strong CYP3A4 inhibitors (including atazanavir, clarithromycin, indinavir, itraconazole, ketoconazole, nefazodone, nelfinavir, saquinavir, ritonavir, telithromycin): Avoid concomitant use of avanafil.

Geriatric Elderly ≥65 years: Refer to adult dosing.

Renal Impairment
CrCl ≥30 mL/minute: No dosage adjustment necessary.
CrCl <30 mL/minute: Has not been studied; use is not recommended by the manufacturer.
ESRD requiring hemodialysis: Has not been studied; use is not recommended by the manufacturer.

Hepatic Impairment
Mild-to-moderate hepatic impairment (Child-Pugh class A or B): No dosage adjustment necessary.
Severe hepatic impairment (Child-Pugh class C): Has not been studied; use is not recommended by the manufacturer.

Dietary Considerations Avoid grapefruit juice.

Administration May be administered with or without food, ~15 to 30 minutes prior to sexual activity.

Monitoring Parameters Monitor for response, adverse reactions, blood pressure, and heart rate.

Dosage Forms Excipient information presented when available (limited, particularly for generics); consult specific product labeling.
Tablet, Oral:
Stendra: 50 mg, 100 mg, 200 mg

Axitinib (ax I ti nib)

Brand Names: US Inlyta
Brand Names: Canada Inlyta
Index Terms AG-013736
Pharmacologic Category Antineoplastic Agent, Tyrosine Kinase Inhibitor; Antineoplastic Agent, Vascular Endothelial Growth Factor (VEGF) Inhibitor
Use Renal cell carcinoma, advanced: Treatment of advanced renal cell carcinoma after failure of one prior systemic therapy.
Pregnancy Considerations Teratogenic, embryotoxic, and fetotoxic events were observed in animal reproduction studies when administered in doses less than the normal human dose. Based on its mechanism of action and because axitinib inhibits angiogenesis (a critical component of fetal development), adverse effects on pregnancy would be expected. Women of childbearing potential should be advised to avoid pregnancy during therapy.
Breast-Feeding Considerations It is not known if axitinib is excreted in breast milk. Due to the potential for serious adverse reactions in the nursing infant, the manufacturer recommends a decision be made whether to discontinue nursing or to discontinue the drug, taking into account the importance of treatment to the mother.
Prescribing and Access Restrictions Available from select specialty pharmacies. Further information may be obtained at 877-744-5675 or www.inlytahcp.com.
Contraindications There are no contraindications listed within the manufacturer's labeling.
Warnings/Precautions Hazardous agent - use appropriate precautions for handling and disposal (meets NIOSH 2014 criteria). May cause hypertension; the median onset is within the first month, and has been observed as early as 4 days after treatment initiation. Hypertensive crisis has been reported. Blood pressure should be well-controlled prior to treatment initiation. Monitor blood pressure and treat with standard antihypertensive therapy. Persistent hypertension (despite antihypertensive therapy) may require dose reduction; discontinue if severe and persistent despite concomitant antihypertensives (or dose reduction), or with evidence of hypertensive crisis. Monitor for hypotension if on antihypertensive therapy and axitinib is withheld or discontinued. Cardiac failure, including fatal events, has been observed rarely. Monitor for signs/symptoms of cardiac failure throughout therapy; management may require permanent therapy discontinuation.

Gastrointestinal perforation and fistulas (including a fatality) have been reported. Monitor for signs/symptoms throughout treatment. Has not been studied in patients with recent active gastrointestinal bleeding; use is not recommended.

Arterial thrombotic events (cerebrovascular accident, MI, retinal artery occlusion, and transient ischemic attack), with fatalities, have been reported. Venous thrombotic events, including pulmonary embolism, deep vein thrombosis, retinal vein occlusion and retinal vein thrombosis, have been observed (with some fatalities). Use with caution in patients with a history of or risks for arterial or venous thrombotic events; has not been studied in patients within 12 months of an arterial thrombotic event or within 6 months of a venous thrombotic event. Hemorrhagic events (cerebral hemorrhage, gastrointestinal hemorrhage, hematuria, hemoptysis, and melena) have been reported (with some fatalities). Temporarily interrupt treatment with any hemorrhage requiring medical intervention.

Cases of reversible posterior leukoencephalopathy syndrome (RPLS) have been reported. Symptoms of RPLS include confusion, headache, hypertension (mild-to-severe), lethargy, seizure, blindness and/or other vision, or neurologic disturbances; interrupt treatment and manage hypertension. MRI is recommended to confirm RPLS diagnosis. Discontinue axitinib if RPLS is confirmed. The safety of reinitiating axitinib in patients previously experiencing RPLS is unknown.

Hypothyroidism occurs commonly with tyrosine kinase inhibitors, including axitinib. Hyperthyroidism has also been reported. Monitor thyroid function at baseline and periodically throughout therapy. Thyroid disorders should be treated according to standard practice to achieve/maintain euthyroid state. Proteinuria is associated with use. Monitor for proteinuria at baseline and periodically throughout therapy. If moderate or severe proteinuria occurs, reduce dose or temporarily withhold treatment. Although the effect on wound healing has not been studied with axitinib, vascular endothelial growth factor (VEGF) receptor inhibitors are associated with impaired wound healing. Discontinue treatment at least 24 hours prior to scheduled surgery; treatment reinitiation should be guided by clinical judgment and wound assessment. Has not been studied in patients with evidence of untreated brain metastases; use is not recommended. Systemic exposure to axitinib is increased in patients with moderate hepatic impairment; dose reductions are recommended. Has not been studied in patients with severe hepatic impairment. Increases in ALT have been observed during treatment; monitor liver function tests. Potentially significant drug-drug interactions may exist, requiring dose or frequency adjustment, additional monitoring, and/or selection of alternative therapy.

Adverse Reactions
>10%:
Cardiovascular: Hypertension (40%; grades 3/4: 16%)
Central nervous system: Fatigue (39%), dysphonia (31%), headache (14%)
Dermatologic: Palmar-plantar erythrodysesthesia syndrome (27%; grades 3/4: 5%), rash (13%; grades 3/4: <1%)
Endocrine & metabolic: Bicarbonate decreased (44%), hypocalcemia (39%), hyperglycemia (28%), hypothyroidism (19%; grades 3/4: <1%), hypernatremia (17%), hyperkalemia (15%), hypoalbuminemia (15%), hyponatremia (13%), hypophosphatemia (13%), hypoglycemia (11%)
Gastrointestinal: Diarrhea (55%; grades 3/4: 11%), appetite decreased (34%), nausea (32%; grades 3/4: 3%), lipase increased (3% to 27%), amylase increased (25%), weight loss (25%), vomiting (24%; grades 3/4: 3%), constipation (20%), mucosal inflammation (15%), stomatitis (15%), abdominal pain (8% to 14%), taste alteration (11%)
Hematologic: Anemia (4% to 35%; grades 3/4: <1%), lymphopenia (33%; grades 3/4: 3%), hemorrhage (16%; grades 3/4 1%), thrombocytopenia (15%; grades 3/4: <1%), leukopenia (11%)
Hepatic: Alkaline phosphatase increased (30%), ALT increased (22%; grades 3/4: <1%), AST increased (20%; grades 3/4: <1%)

Neuromuscular & skeletal: Weakness (21%), arthralgia (15%), limb pain (13%)

Renal: Creatinine increased (55%), proteinuria (11%; grade 3: 3%)

Respiratory: Cough (15%), dyspnea (15%)

1% to 10%:

Cardiovascular: Venous thrombotic events (grades 3/4: 3%), arterial thrombotic events (2%; grade 3/4: 1%), deep vein thrombosis (1%), transient ischemic attack (1%)

Central nervous system: Dizziness (9%)

Dermatologic: Dry skin (10%), pruritus (7%), alopecia (4%), erythema (2%)

Endocrine & metabolic: Dehydration (6%), hyperthyroidism (1%)

Gastrointestinal: Dyspepsia (10%), hemorrhoids (4%), rectal hemorrhage (2%), fistula (1%), gastrointestinal perforation (≤1%)

Hematologic: Hemoglobin increased (9%), polycythemia (1%)

Neuromuscular & skeletal: Myalgia (7%)

Ocular: Retinal vein occlusion/thrombosis (1%)

Otic: Tinnitus (3%)

Renal: Hematuria (3%)

Respiratory: Epistaxis (6%), hemoptysis (2%), pulmonary embolism (2%)

<1% (Limited to important or life-threatening): Cerebral bleeding, cerebrovascular accident, fever, hypertensive crisis, heart failure, neutropenia, reversible posterior leukoencephalopathy syndrome (RPLS)

Drug Interactions

Metabolism/Transport Effects Substrate of CYP1A2 (minor), CYP2C19 (minor), CYP3A4 (major), UGT1A1; **Note:** Assignment of Major/Minor substrate status based on clinically relevant drug interaction potential

Avoid Concomitant Use

Avoid concomitant use of Axitinib with any of the following: Conivaptan; CYP3A4 Inducers (Moderate); CYP3A4 Inducers (Strong); CYP3A4 Inhibitors (Strong); Fusidic Acid (Systemic); Grapefruit Juice; Idelalisib; St Johns Wort

Increased Effect/Toxicity

Axitinib may increase the levels/effects of: Bisphosphonate Derivatives

The levels/effects of Axitinib may be increased by: Aprepitant; Conivaptan; CYP3A4 Inhibitors (Moderate); CYP3A4 Inhibitors (Strong); Dasatinib; Fosaprepitant; Fusidic Acid (Systemic); Grapefruit Juice; Idelalisib; Ivacaftor; Luliconazole; Mifepristone; Netupitant; Osimertinib; Palbociclib; Simeprevir; Stiripentol

Decreased Effect

The levels/effects of Axitinib may be decreased by: CYP3A4 Inducers (Moderate); CYP3A4 Inducers (Strong); Deferasirox; Osimertinib; Siltuximab; St Johns Wort; Tocilizumab

Food Interactions Axitinib serum concentrations may be increased when taken with grapefruit or grapefruit juice. Management: Avoid concurrent use.

Storage/Stability Store at 20°C to 25°C (68°F to 77°F); excursions permitted to 15°C to 30°C (59°F to 86°F).

Mechanism of Action Axitinib is a selective second generation tyrosine kinase inhibitor which blocks angiogenesis and tumor growth by inhibiting vascular endothelial growth factor receptors (VEGFR-1, VEGFR-2, and VEGFR-3).

Pharmacodynamics/Kinetics

Absorption: Rapid (Rugo, 2005)

Distribution: V_d: 160 L

Protein binding: >99%; to albumin (primarily) and to alpha$_1$ acid glycoprotein (AAG)

Metabolism: Hepatic; primarily via CYP3A4/5 and to a lesser extend via CYP1A2, CYP2C19 and UGT1A1

Bioavailability: 58%

Half-life elimination: 2.5 to 6 hours

Time to peak: 2.5 to 4 hours

Excretion: Feces (~41%; 12% as unchanged drug); urine (~23%; as metabolites)

Dosing

Adult Renal cell cancer, advanced: Oral: Initial: 5 mg twice daily (approximately every 12 hours)

Dose increases: If dose is tolerated (no adverse events above grade 2, blood pressure is normal and no antihypertensive use) for at least 2 consecutive weeks, may increase the dose to 7 mg twice daily, and then further increase (using the same tolerance criteria) to 10 mg twice daily.

Dose decreases: For adverse events, reduce dose from 5 mg twice daily to 3 mg twice daily; further reduce to 2 mg twice daily if adverse events persist.

Dosage adjustment for strong CYP3A4 inhibitors: Avoid concomitant administration with strong CYP3A4 inhibitors (eg, clarithromycin, itraconazole, ketoconazole, nefazodone, protease inhibitors, telithromycin, voriconazole, grapefruit juice); if concomitant administration with a strong CYP3A4 inhibitor cannot be avoided, ~50% dosage reduction is recommended; adjust dose based on individual tolerance and safety. When the strong CYP3A4 inhibitor is discontinued, resume previous axitinib dose after 3-5 half-lives of the inhibitor have passed.

Geriatric Refer to adult dosing. No adjustment necessary.

Renal Impairment

Mild to severe renal impairment (CrCl 15 to <89 mL/minute): No initial dosage adjustment necessary.

End-stage renal disease (ESRD) There are no dosage adjustments provided in the manufacturer's labeling; use with caution.

Hepatic Impairment

Mild impairment (Child-Pugh class A): No starting dosage adjustment necessary.

Moderate impairment (Child-Pugh class B): Reduce starting dose by ~50%; increase or decrease based on individual tolerance.

Severe impairment (Child-Pugh class C): There are no dosage adjustments provided in the manufacturer's labeling (has not been studied).

Adjustment for Toxicity

Adverse events: May require temporary interruption, dose decreases (reduce dose from 5 mg twice daily to 3 mg twice daily; further reduce to 2 mg twice daily) or discontinuation

Cardiac failure: May require permanent discontinuation

Hypertension: Treat with standard antihypertensive therapy.

Persistent hypertension: May require dose reduction

Severe, persistent (despite antihypertensives and dose reduction), or evidence of hypertensive crisis: Discontinue treatment

Hemorrhage: Any bleeding requiring medical intervention: Temporarily interrupt treatment.

Proteinuria (moderate-to-severe): Reduce dose or temporarily interrupt treatment.

Dietary Considerations May be taken without regard to food. Avoid grapefruit and grapefruit juice.

Administration Oral: Swallow tablet whole with a glass of water. May be taken with or without food. If a dose is missed or vomited, do not make up; resume dosing with the next scheduled dose. A suspension may be prepared for nasogastric administration (refer to Extemporaneous Preparations information).

Hazardous agent; use appropriate precautions for handling and disposal (meets NIOSH 2014 criteria).

Monitoring Parameters Hepatic function (ALT, AST, and bilirubin; baseline and periodic), thyroid function (baseline and periodic), urinalysis (for proteinuria; baseline and periodically); blood pressure, signs/symptoms of RPLS, gastrointestinal bleeding/perforation/fistula, signs/symptoms cardiac failure

Thyroid function testing recommendations (Hamnvik, 2011):

Preexisting levothyroxine therapy: Obtain baseline TSH levels, then monitor every 4 weeks until levels and levothyroxine dose are stable, then monitor every 2 months

Without preexisting thyroid hormone replacement: TSH at baseline, then monthly for 4 months, then every 2-3 months

Dosage Forms Excipient information presented when available (limited, particularly for generics); consult specific product labeling.

Tablet, Oral:

Inlyta: 1 mg, 5 mg

Extemporaneous Preparations Hazardous agent – use appropriate precautions for handling and disposal (meets NIOSH 2014 criteria). For patients unable to swallow tablets whole, a suspension may be prepared for nasogastric tube administration (for doses of 2 to 10 mg). Place a 20 mL tightly capped amber syringe in a small drinking glass, with the open end of the syringe pointing up. Place the appropriate axitinib dose in the open syringe barrel; add 15 mL of USP grade water (do not use tap water or bottled water) to the syringe. Allow at least 10 minutes to dissolve the tablets; avoid direct light. Place the plunger of the syringe into the barrel, invert the syringe so the tip is pointing upward and remove the cap. Expel excess air; replace the cap until ready for use (keep syringe tip facing up). Prior to administration, gently invert the syringe several times to ensure a uniform suspension. Flush the nasogastric feeding tube with 15 mL of USP grade water before administration. After administering the dose, draw

up 10 mL of USP grade water (into the same syringe which contained the dose) and flush the feeding tube; repeat this step 5 additional times to ensure the entire dose has been administered. Lastly, flush the feeding tube with a separate syringe containing 15 mL of USP grade water. Administer within 15 minutes of preparation.

Borst DL, Arruda LS, MacLean E, Pithavala YK, Morgado JE. Common questions regarding clinical use of axitinib in advanced renal cell carcinoma. *Am J Health Syst Pharm.* 2014;71(13):1092-1096.

AzaCITIDine (ay za SYE ti deen)

Brand Names: US Vidaza
Brand Names: Canada Vidaza
Index Terms 5-Azacytidine; 5-AZC; AZA-CR; Azacytidine; Ladakamycin
Pharmacologic Category Antineoplastic Agent, Antimetabolite; Antineoplastic Agent, DNA Methylation Inhibitor

Use

US labeling:

Myelodysplastic syndromes: Treatment of myelodysplastic syndromes (MDS) in patients with the following French-American-British (FAB) classification subtypes: Refractory anemia or refractory anemia with ringed sideroblasts (if accompanied by neutropenia or thrombocytopenia or requiring transfusions), refractory anemia with excess blasts, refractory anemia with excess blasts in transformation, and chronic myelomonocytic leukemia.

Canadian labeling:

Acute myeloid leukemia: Treatment of acute myeloid leukemia (AML) with 20% to 30% blasts and myelodysplasia-related features (previously referred to as multilineage dysplasia), according to World Health Organization (WHO) classification.

Myelodysplastic syndromes: Treatment of Intermediate-2 and high-risk myelodysplastic syndromes (MDS) (according to International Prognostic Scoring System) in adults who are not eligible for hematopoietic stem cell transplantation.

Dosing

Adult Note: Azacitidine is associated with a moderate emetic potential (Basch 2011; Roila 2010); antiemetics are recommended to prevent nausea and vomiting.

Myelodysplastic syndromes (MDS):

US labeling: IV, SubQ: Initial cycle: 75 mg/m²/day for 7 days. Subsequent cycles: 75 mg/m²/day for 7 days every 4 weeks; dose may be increased to 100 mg/m²/day if no benefit is observed after 2 cycles and no toxicity other than nausea and vomiting have occurred. Patients should be treated for a minimum of 4 to 6 cycles; treatment may be continued as long as patient continues to benefit.

Canadian labeling: SubQ: Initial cycle: 75 mg/m²/day for 7 days. Subsequent cycles: If no toxicity observed with initial treatment continue 75 mg/m²/day for 7 days every 4 weeks; dose reductions and/or therapy interruption may be required for hematologic or renal toxicity. Patients should be treated for a minimum of 6 cycles and then as long as patient continues to benefit or until disease progression.

Note: Alternate (off-label) schedules (which have produced hematologic response) have been used for convenience in community oncology centers (Lyons 2009): SubQ:

75 mg/m²/day for 5 days (Mon-Fri), 2 days rest (Sat, Sun), then 75 mg/m²/day for 2 days (Mon, Tues); repeat cycle every 28 days **or**

50 mg/m²/day for 5 days (Mon-Fri), 2 days rest (Sat, Sun), then 50 mg/m²/day for 5 days (Mon-Fri); repeat cycle every 28 days **or**

75 mg/m²/day for 5 days (Mon-Fri), repeat cycle every 28 days

Acute myeloid leukemia (AML): Canadian labeling (off-label use in US): SubQ: 75 mg/m²/day for 7 days every 4 weeks for at least 6 cycles; treatment may be continued as long as patient continues to benefit or until disease progression or unacceptable toxicity (Fenaux 2010). Dose reductions and/or therapy interruption may be required for hematologic or renal toxicity.

Dosage adjustment based on serum electrolytes: If serum bicarbonate falls to <20 mEq/L (unexplained decrease): Reduce dose by 50% for next treatment course.

Geriatric Refer to adult dosing. Due to the potential for decreased renal function in the elderly, select dose carefully and closely monitor renal function.

Renal Impairment

Renal impairment at *baseline:*

Mild to moderate impairment (CrCl ≥30 mL/minute): No dosage adjustment necessary (Douvali 2012).

Severe impairment (CrCl <30 mL/minute): No dosage adjustment necessary for cycle 1; due to renal excretion of azacitidine and metabolites, monitor closely for toxicity.

Renal toxicity *during* treatment:

US labeling: Unexplained increases in BUN or serum creatinine: Delay next cycle until values reach baseline or normal, then reduce dose by 50% for next treatment course.

Canadian labeling: Unexplained increases in serum creatinine or BUN 2 fold above baseline and above the upper limit of normal (ULN): Delay next cycle until values reach baseline or normal, then reduce dose by 50% for next treatment course.

Hepatic Impairment No dosage adjustment provided in the manufacturer's labeling (has not been studied). Use is contraindicated in patients with advanced malignant hepatic tumors.

Adjustment for Toxicity

US labeling: Hematologic toxicity: MDS:

For baseline WBC ≥3 x 10⁹/L, ANC ≥1.5 x 10⁹/L, and platelets ≥75 x 10⁹/L:

Nadir count: ANC <0.5 x 10⁹/L or platelets <25 x 10⁹/L: Administer 50% of dose during next treatment course

Nadir count: ANC 0.5 to 1.5 x 10⁹/L or platelets 25-50 x 10⁹/L: Administer 67% of dose during next treatment course

Nadir count: ANC >1.5 x 10⁹/L or platelets >50 x 10⁹/L: Administer 100% of dose during next treatment course

For baseline WBC <3 x 10⁹/L, ANC <1.5 x 10⁹/L, or platelets <75 x 10⁹/L: Adjust dose as follows based on nadir counts and bone marrow biopsy cellularity at the time of nadir, unless clear improvement in differentiation at the time of the next cycle:

WBC or platelet nadir decreased 50% to 75% from baseline and bone marrow biopsy cellularity at time of nadir 30% to 60%: Administer 100% of dose during next treatment course

WBC or platelet nadir decreased 50% to 75% from baseline and bone marrow biopsy cellularity at time of nadir 15% to 30%: Administer 50% of dose during next treatment course

WBC or platelet nadir decreased 50% to 75% from baseline and bone marrow biopsy cellularity at time of nadir <15%: Administer 33% of dose during next treatment course

WBC or platelet nadir decreased >75% from baseline and bone marrow biopsy cellularity at time of nadir 30% to 60%: Administer 75% of dose during next treatment course

WBC or platelet nadir decreased >75% from baseline and bone marrow biopsy cellularity at time of nadir 15% to 30%: Administer 50% of dose during next treatment course

WBC or platelet nadir decreased >75% from baseline and bone marrow biopsy cellularity at time of nadir <15%: Administer 33% of dose during next treatment course

Note: If a nadir defined above occurs, administer the next treatment course 28 days after the start of the preceding course as long as WBC and platelet counts are >25% above the nadir and rising. If a >25% increase above the nadir is not seen by day 28, reassess counts every 7 days. If a 25% increase is not seen by day 42, administer 50% of the scheduled dose.

Canadian labeling: **AML, MDS:**

For baseline WBC ≥3 x 10^9/L, ANC ≥1.5 x 10^9/L, and platelets ≥75 x 10^9/L prior to first treatment:

Nadir count: ANC ≤1 x 10^9/L or platelets ≤50 x 10^9/L: If hematologic toxicity is observed, delay treatment

Nadir count: ANC ≤1 x 10^9/L or platelets ≤50 x 10^9/L: Delay treatment until ANC and platelets have recovered (to at least the nadir plus half the difference between nadir and baseline); if recovery achieved within 14 days, no dosage adjustment is necessary; if recovery not achieved within 14 days administer 50% of dose during next treatment course

Nadir count: ANC >1 x 10^9/L or platelets >50 x 10^9/L: If recovery not achieved within 14 days administer 100% of dose during next treatment course

For baseline WBC <3 x 10^9/L, ANC <1.5 x 10^9/L, or platelets <75 x 10^9/L prior to first treatment:

WBC or ANC or platelets decreased <50%, or decreased >50% but with improvement in any cell line differentiation: No delay or dose adjustment is necessary during next treatment course.

WBC or ANC or platelets decreased >50% with no improvement in cell line differentiation: Delay treatment until platelet count and ANC recovery. If recovery occurs within 14 days no dosage adjustment is necessary in the next treatment course. If recovery is not achieved within 14 days determine bone marrow cellularity. If bone marrow cellularity is >50% no dosage adjustment is necessary during next treatment course. If bone marrow cellularity is ≤50% delay treatment until recovery and reduce dose during next treatment course as follows:

Bone marrow cellularity 15 to 50%: Administer 50% of dose if recovery achieved >21 days or administer 100% of dose if recovery achieved >14 to ≤21 days

Bone marrow cellularity <15%: Administer 33% of dose if recovery achieved >21 days or administer 100% of dose if recovery achieved >14 to ≤21 days

Note: Resume 28 day treatment cycles following dose modifications.

Missed doses: Missed doses should be added to the end of the current dosing cycle; do not administer at time of next dose (ie, double dose).

Additional Information Complete prescribing information should be consulted for additional detail.

Dosage Forms Excipient information presented when available (limited, particularly for generics); consult specific product labeling.

Suspension Reconstituted, Injection:

Generic: 100 mg (1 ea)

Suspension Reconstituted, Injection [preservative free]:

Vidaza: 100 mg (1 ea)

Generic: 100 mg (1 ea)

◆ AZA-CR *see* AzaCITIDine *on page 184*
◆ Azactam *see* Aztreonam (Systemic) *on page 193*
◆ Azactam in Dextrose *see* Aztreonam (Systemic) *on page 193*
◆ Azacytidine *see* AzaCITIDine *on page 184*
◆ 5-Azacytidine *see* AzaCITIDine *on page 184*
◆ 5-Aza-dCyd *see* Decitabine *on page 508*
◆ Azaepothilone B *see* Ixabepilone *on page 1006*
◆ Azasan *see* AzaTHIOprine *on page 185*
◆ AzaSite *see* Azithromycin (Ophthalmic) *on page 193*

AzaTHIOprine (ay za THYE oh preen)

Brand Names: US Azasan; Imuran
Brand Names: Canada Apo-Azathioprine; Imuran; Mylan-Azathioprine; Teva-Azathioprine
Index Terms Azathioprine Sodium
Pharmacologic Category Immunosuppressant Agent
Use

Renal transplantation: Adjunctive therapy in prevention of rejection of kidney transplants

Rheumatoid arthritis: Treatment of active rheumatoid arthritis (RA), to reduce signs and symptoms

Pregnancy Considerations Adverse events have been observed in animal reproduction studies. Azathioprine crosses the placenta in humans; congenital anomalies, immunosuppression, hematologic toxicities (lymphopenia, pancytopenia), and intrauterine growth retardation have

been reported. Azathioprine should not be used to treat rheumatoid arthritis during pregnancy. Women of childbearing potential should avoid becoming pregnant during treatment.

The National Transplantation Pregnancy Registry (NTPR, Temple University) is a registry for pregnant women taking immunosuppressants following any solid organ transplant. The NTPR encourages reporting of all immunosuppressant exposures during pregnancy in transplant recipients at 877-955-6877.

Breast-Feeding Considerations Azathioprine is excreted in breast milk. Due to potential for serious adverse reactions in the nursing infant, breast-feeding is not recommended by the manufacturer.

Contraindications Hypersensitivity to azathioprine or any component of the formulation; pregnancy (in patients with rheumatoid arthritis); patients with rheumatoid arthritis and a history of treatment with alkylating agents (eg, cyclophosphamide, chlorambucil, melphalan) may have a prohibitive risk of malignancy with azathioprine treatment

Warnings/Precautions Hazardous agent - use appropriate precautions for handling and disposal (NIOSH 2014 [group 2]).

[US Boxed Warning]: Chronic immunosuppression with azathioprine (a purine antimetabolite), increases the risk of malignancy. Malignancies reported have included post-transplant lymphoma and hepatosplenic T-cell lymphoma (HSTCL) in patients with inflammatory bowel disease. Health care providers using this drug should be very familiar with this risk, as well as with the mutagenic potential to both men and women, and with possible hematologic toxicities. Patients should be informed of the risk for malignancy development. HSTCL is a rare white blood cell cancer that is usually fatal and has predominantly occurred in adolescents and young adults treated for Crohn disease or ulcerative colitis and receiving TNF blockers (eg, adalimumab, certolizumab pegol, etanercept, golimumab), azathioprine, and/or mercaptopurine. Most cases of HSTCL have occurred in patients treated with a combination of immunosuppressant agents, although there have been reports of HSTCL in patients receiving azathioprine or mercaptopurine monotherapy. Renal transplant patients are also at increased risk for malignancy (eg, skin cancer, lymphoma); limit sun and ultraviolet light exposure and use appropriate sun protection.

Dose-related hematologic toxicities (leukopenia, thrombocytopenia, and anemias, including macrocytic anemia, or pancytopenia) may occur; may be severe and/or delayed. Thiopurine methyltransferase (TPMT) genotyping or phenotyping may help to identify patients who are at an increased risk for developing azathioprine toxicity. Patients with intermediate TPMT activity may be at increased risk for hematologic toxicity at conventional azathioprine doses; patients with low or absent TPMT activity are at risk for severe, life-threatening myelotoxicity. Myelosuppression may be more severe with renal transplants undergoing rejection. Monitor CBC with differential and platelets weekly during the first month, then twice a month for 2 months, then monthly (or more frequently if clinically indicated). May require treatment interruption or dose reduction. Leukopenia does not correlate with therapeutic effect and the dose should not be increased intentionally to lower the white blood cell count.

Chronic immunosuppression increases the risk of serious, sometimes fatal, infections (bacterial, viral, fungal, protozoal, and opportunistic) including reactivation of latent infections. Cases of JC virus-associated infection resulting in progressive multifocal leukoencephalopathy (PML), have been reported in patients treated with immunosuppressants, including azathioprine (some cases have been fatal). Risk factors for PML include treatment with immunosuppressants and immune system impairment. Consider a diagnosis of PML in any patient presenting with new-onset neurological manifestations; consultation with a neurologist as clinically indicated may be warranted. Consider decreasing the degree of immunosuppression with respect to the risk of organ rejection in transplant patients.

Use with caution in patients with liver disease or renal impairment; monitor hematologic function closely. Azathioprine is metabolized to mercaptopurine; concomitant use may result in profound myelosuppression and should be avoided. Patients with genetic deficiency of TPMT or concurrent therapy with drugs which may inhibit TPMT are more sensitive to myelosuppressive effects. Patients with intermediate TPMT activity may be at risk for increased myelosuppression; those with low or absent TPMT activity are at risk for developing severe myelotoxicity. TPMT genotyping or phenotyping may assist in

identifying patients at risk for developing toxicity. Consider TPMT testing in patients with abnormally low CBC unresponsive to dose reduction. TPMT testing does not substitute for CBC monitoring. Potentially significant drug-drug interactions may exist, requiring dose or frequency adjustment, additional monitoring, and/or selection of alternative therapy. Xanthine oxidase inhibitors may increase risk for hematologic toxicity; reduce azathioprine dose when used concurrently with allopurinol; patients with low or absent TPMT activity may require further dose reductions or discontinuation.

Hepatotoxicity (transaminase, bilirubin, and alkaline phosphatase elevations) may occur, usually in renal transplant patients and generally within 6 months of transplant; normally reversible with discontinuation; monitor liver function periodically. Rarely, hepatic sinusoidal obstruction syndrome (SOS; formerly called veno-occlusive disease) has been reported; discontinue if hepatic SOS is suspected. Severe nausea, vomiting, diarrhea, rash, fever, malaise, myalgia, hypotension, and liver enzyme abnormalities may occur within the first several weeks of treatment and are generally reversible upon discontinuation. **[U.S. Boxed Warning]: Should be prescribed by physicians familiar with the risks, including hematologic toxicities and mutagenic potential.** Immune response to vaccines may be diminished.

Adverse Reactions Frequency not always defined; dependent upon dose, duration, indication, and concomitant therapy.

Central nervous system: Malaise

Gastrointestinal: Nausea and vomiting (rheumatoid arthritis: 12%), diarrhea

Hematologic & oncologic: Leukopenia (renal transplant: >50%; rheumatoid arthritis: 28%), neoplasia (renal transplant 3% [other than lymphoma], 0.5% [lymphoma]), thrombocytopenia

Hepatic: Hepatotoxicity, increased serum alkaline phosphatase, increased serum bilirubin, increased serum transaminases

Infection: Increased susceptibility to infection (renal transplant 20%; rheumatoid arthritis <1%; includes bacterial, fungal, protozoal, viral, opportunistic, and reactivation of latent infections)

Neuromuscular & skeletal: Myalgia

Miscellaneous: Fever

<1% (Limited to important or life-threatening): Abdominal pain, acute myelocytic leukemia, alopecia, anemia, arthralgia, bone marrow depression, hemorrhage, hepatic veno-occlusive disease, hepatosplenic T-cell lymphomas, hepatotoxicity (idiosyncratic) (Chalasani, 2014), hypersensitivity, hypotension, interstitial pneumonitis (reversible), JC virus infection, macrocytic anemia, malignant lymphoma, malignant neoplasm of skin, negative nitrogen balance, pancreatitis, pancytopenia, progressive multifocal leukoencephalopathy, skin rash, steatorrhea, Sweet's syndrome (acute febrile neutrophilic dermatosis)

Drug Interactions

Metabolism/Transport Effects None known.

Avoid Concomitant Use

Avoid concomitant use of AzaTHIOprine with any of the following: BCG (Intravesical); Febuxostat; Mercaptopurine; Natalizumab; Pimecrolimus; Tacrolimus (Topical); Tofacitinib

Increased Effect/Toxicity

AzaTHIOprine may increase the levels/effects of: Cyclophosphamide; Fingolimod; Leflunomide; Mercaptopurine; Natalizumab; Tofacitinib; Vaccines (Live)

The levels/effects of AzaTHIOprine may be increased by: 5-ASA Derivatives; ACE Inhibitors; Allopurinol; Denosumab; Febuxostat; Pimecrolimus; Ribavirin (Oral Inhalation); Ribavirin (Systemic); Roflumilast; Sulfamethoxazole; Tacrolimus (Topical); Trastuzumab; Trimethoprim

Decreased Effect

AzaTHIOprine may decrease the levels/effects of: BCG (Intravesical); Coccidioides immitis Skin Test; Sipuleucel-T; Vaccines (Inactivated); Vaccines (Live); Vitamin K Antagonists

The levels/effects of AzaTHIOprine may be decreased by: Echinacea

Preparation for Administration Hazardous agent; use appropriate precautions for handling and disposal (NIOSH 2014 [group 2]).

Powder for injection [Canadian product]: Reconstitute each vial with 5 to 10 mL sterile water for injection (adding 5 mL will result in a 10 mg/mL solution); gently swirl to dissolve. May further dilute in NS for infusion.

Storage/Stability

Tablet: Store at 15°C to 25°C (59°F to 77°F). Protect from light and moisture.

Powder for injection [Canadian product]: Store intact vials at 15°C to 25°C (59°F to 77°F). Protect from light. Use immediately after preparation; discard unused portion.

Mechanism of Action Azathioprine is an imidazolyl derivative of mercaptopurine; metabolites are incorporated into replicating DNA and halt replication; also block the pathway for purine synthesis (Taylor, 2005). The 6-thioguanine nucleotide metabolites appear to mediate the majority of azathioprine's immunosuppressive and toxic effects.

Pharmacodynamics/Kinetics

Absorption: Oral: Well absorbed

Protein binding: ~30%

Metabolism: Hepatic; metabolized to 6-mercaptopurine via glutathione S-transferase (GST) reduction. Further metabolized (in the liver and GI tract) via three major pathways: Hypoxanthine guanine phosphoribosyltransferase (to active metabolites: 6-thioguanine-nucleotides, or 6-TGNs), xanthine oxidase (to inactive metabolite: 6-thiouric acid), and thiopurine methyltransferase (TPMT) (to inactive metabolite: 6-methylmercaptopurine)

Half-life elimination: Azathioprine and mercaptopurine: Variable: ~2 hours (Taylor, 2005)

Time to peak: Oral: 1 to 2 hours (including metabolites)

Excretion: Urine (primarily as metabolites)

Dosing

Adult & Geriatric Note: Patients with intermediate TPMT activity may be at risk for increased myelosuppression; those with low or absent TPMT activity receiving conventional azathioprine doses are at risk for developing severe, life-threatening myelotoxicity. Dosage reductions are recommended for patients with reduced TPMT activity; consider discontinuing in patients with abnormal blood counts that do not respond to dose reduction.

Renal transplantation (treatment usually started the day of transplant, however, has been initiated [rarely] 1 to 3 days prior to transplant):

Oral: Initial: 3 to 5 mg/kg once daily (usually given as a single daily dose), then 1 to 3 mg/kg once daily maintenance

IV: [Canadian product]: Initial: 3 to 5 mg/kg daily; Maintenance: dose reduction to 1 to 3 mg/kg daily is usually possible. **Note:** IV is indicated only in patients unable to tolerate oral medications (dosing should be transitioned from IV to oral as soon as tolerated).

Rheumatoid arthritis:

Oral:

Initial: 1 mg/kg/day (50 to 100 mg) given once daily or divided twice daily for 6 to 8 weeks; may increase by 0.5 mg/kg every 4 weeks until response or up to 2.5 mg/kg/day; an adequate trial should be a minimum of 12 weeks

Maintenance dose: Reduce dose by 0.5 mg/kg (~25 mg daily) every 4 weeks until lowest effective dose is reached; optimum duration of therapy not specified; may be discontinued abruptly (monitor for delayed toxicities)

IV [Canadian product]: **Note:** IV is indicated only in patients unable to tolerate oral medications (dosing should be transitioned from IV to oral as soon as tolerated):

Initial: ~1 mg/kg/day (50 to 100 mg) given once daily or divided twice daily for 6 to 8 weeks; may increase by 0.5 mg/kg every 4 weeks until response or up to 2.5 mg/kg/day; an adequate trial should be a minimum of 12 weeks

Maintenance dose: Reduce dose by 0.5 mg/kg (~25 mg daily) every 4 weeks until lowest effective dose is reached; optimum duration of therapy not specified; may be discontinued abruptly (monitor for delayed toxicities)

Crohn disease, remission maintenance or reduction of steroid use (off-label use): Oral: 2 to 3 mg/kg/day (Lichtenstein, 2009)

Dermatomyositis/polymyositis, adjunctive management (off-label use): Oral: 50 mg/day in conjunction with prednisone; increase by 50 mg/week to total dose of 2 to 3 mg/kg/day (Briemberg, 2003); **Note:** Onset of beneficial effects may take 3 to 6 months; however, may be preferred over methotrexate in patients with pulmonary or hepatic toxicity.

Immune thrombocytopenia (ITP), chronic refractory (off-label use): Oral: Maintenance: 100 to 200 mg/day (Boruchov, 2007)

Lupus nephritis, maintenance (off-label use): Oral: Initial: 2 mg/kg/day; may reduce to 1.5 mg/kg/day after 1 month (if proteinuria <1 g/day and serum creatinine stable) (Moroni, 2006) **or** target dose: 2 mg/kg/day (Hahn, 2012; Houssiau, 2010)

Ulcerative colitis, remission maintenance or reduction of steroid use (off-label use): Oral: 1.5 to 2.5 mg/kg/day (Kornbluth, 2010)

Dosage adjustment for concomitant use with allopurinol: Reduce azathioprine dose to one-third or one-fourth the usual dose when used concurrently with allopurinol. Patients with low or absent TPMT activity may require further dose reductions or discontinuation.

Renal Impairment There are no specific dosage adjustments provided in the manufacturer's labeling; however, oliguric patients, particularly those with tubular necrosis in the immediate post-transplant period (cadaveric transplant) may have delayed clearance and typically receive lower doses. The following adjustments have been recommended (Aronoff, 2007):

CrCl >50 mL/minute: No adjustment recommended.
CrCl 10-50 mL/minute: Administer 75% of normal dose.
CrCl <10 mL/minute: Administer 50% of normal dose.
Hemodialysis (dialyzable; ~45% removed in 8 hours): Administer 50% of normal dose; supplement: 0.25 mg/kg
CRRT: Administer 75% of normal dose

Hepatic Impairment There are no dosage adjustments provided in the manufacturer's labeling.

Adjustment for Toxicity

Rapid WBC count decrease, persistently low WBC count, or serious infection: Reduce dose or temporarily withhold treatment.

Severe toxicity (hematologic or other) in renal transplantation: May require discontinuation.

Hepatic sinusoidal obstruction syndrome (SOS; veno-occlusive disease): Permanently discontinue.

Administration

Oral: Administering tablets after meals or in divided doses may decrease adverse GI events.

IV [Canadian product]: Infusion is usually administered over 30 to 60 minutes, although may be infused over 5 minutes up to over 8 hours.

Hazardous agent; use appropriate precautions for handling and disposal (NIOSH 2014 [group 2]). NIOSH recommends single gloving for administration of intact tablets (NIOSH 2014).

Monitoring Parameters CBC with differential and platelets (weekly during first month, twice monthly for months 2 and 3, then monthly; monitor more frequently with dosage modifications), total bilirubin, liver function tests, creatinine clearance, TPMT genotyping or phenotyping (consider TPMT testing in patients with abnormally low CBC unresponsive to dose reduction); monitor for symptoms of infection

For use as immunomodulatory therapy in CD or UC, monitor CBC with differential weekly for 1 month, then biweekly for 1 month, followed by monitoring every 1 to 2 months throughout the course of therapy; monitor more frequently if symptomatic. LFTs should be assessed every 3 months. Monitor for signs/symptoms of malignancy (eg, splenomegaly, hepatomegaly, abdominal pain, persistent fever, night sweats, weight loss).

Test Interactions TPMT phenotyping results will not be accurate following recent blood transfusions.

Dosage Forms Excipient information presented when available (limited, particularly for generics); consult specific product labeling. [DSC] = Discontinued product

Solution Reconstituted, Injection:
Generic: 100 mg (1 ea [DSC])
Tablet, Oral:
Azasan: 75 mg, 100 mg [scored]
Imuran: 50 mg [scored]
Generic: 50 mg

Dosage Forms: Canada Note: Refer also to Dosage Forms.

Injection, powder for reconstitution [preservative free]:
Imuran: 50 mg

Extemporaneous Preparations Hazardous agent: Use appropriate precautions for handling and disposal (NIOSH 2014 [group 2]). When compounding an oral liquid or suspension, NIOSH recommends double gloving, a protective gown, and preparation in a controlled device; if not prepared in a controlled device, respiratory and eye protection as well as ventilated engineering controls are recommended (NIOSH 2014).

A 50 mg/mL oral suspension may be prepared with tablets. Crush one-hundred-twenty 50 mg tablets in a mortar and reduce to a fine powder. Add 40 mL of either cherry syrup (diluted 1:4 with Simple Syrup, USP); a 1:1 mixture of Ora-Sweet® and Ora-Plus; or a 1:1 mixture of Ora-Sweet SF and Ora-Plus®, and mix to a uniform paste. Mix while adding the vehicle in incremental proportions to **almost** 120 mL; transfer to a calibrated bottle, rinse mortar with vehicle, and add quantity of vehicle sufficient to make 120 mL. Label "shake well", "refrigerate", and "protect from light". Stable for 60 days refrigerated.

Allen LV Jr and Erickson MA 3rd, "Stability of Acetazolamide, Allopurinol, Azathioprine, Clonazepam, and Flucytosine in Extemporaneously Compounded Oral Liquids," *Am J Health Syst Pharm*, 1996, 53(16):1944-9.

◆ Azathioprine Sodium *see* AzaTHIOprine *on page* 185
◆ 5-AZC *see* AzaCITIDine *on page* 184
◆ AZD2281 *see* Olaparib *on page* 1318
◆ AZD6140 *see* Ticagrelor *on page* 1786
◆ AZD6474 *see* Vandetanib *on page* 1873
◆ AZD9291 *see* Osimertinib *on page* 1346

Azelaic Acid (a zeh LAY ik AS id)

Brand Names: US Azelex; Finacea
Brand Names: Canada Finacea
Index Terms Anchoic Acid; Lepargylic Acid
Pharmacologic Category Topical Skin Product, Acne
Use

Acne vulgaris (cream): Treatment of mild to moderate inflammatory acne vulgaris.

Rosacea (foam, gel): Treatment of inflammatory papules and pustules of mild to moderate rosacea.

Limitations of use: Efficacy for treatment of erythema in rosacea in the absence of papules and pustules has not been evaluated.

Dosing

Adult & Geriatric

Acne vulgaris: Topical: Cream 20%: Apply a thin film to the affected area(s) twice daily, in the morning and evening; may reduce to once daily if persistent skin irritation occurs. Improvement in condition is usually seen within 4 weeks.

Rosacea: Topical: Gel 15% and foam 15%: Apply a thin layer to the affected area(s) of the face twice daily, in the morning and evening; reassess if no improvement after 12 weeks of therapy.

Pediatric Acne vulgaris: Children ≥12 years and Adolescents: Refer to adult dosing.

Renal Impairment There are no dosage adjustments provided in the manufacturer's labeling. However, dosage adjustment unlikely due to low systemic absorption.

Hepatic Impairment There are no dosage adjustments provided in the manufacturer's labeling. However, dosage adjustment unlikely due to low systemic absorption.

Additional Information Complete prescribing information should be consulted for additional detail.

Dosage Forms Excipient information presented when available (limited, particularly for generics); consult specific product labeling.

Cream, External:
Azelex: 20% (30 g, 50 g)
Foam, External:
Finacea: 15% (50 g) [contains benzoic acid, cetostearyl alcohol, polysorbate 80, propylene glycol]
Gel, External:
Finacea: 15% (50 g) [contains benzoic acid, disodium edta, polysorbate 80, propylene glycol]

Azelastine (Nasal) (a ZEL as teen)

Brand Names: US Astelin [DSC]; Astepro
Brand Names: Canada Astelin
Index Terms Azelastine Hydrochloride
Pharmacologic Category Histamine H_1 Antagonist; Histamine H_1 Antagonist, Second Generation
Use

Perennial allergic rhinitis: Relief of symptoms of perennial allergic rhinitis in patients ≥6 months.

Seasonal allergic rhinitis: Relief of symptoms of seasonal allergic rhinitis in patients ≥2 years.

Dosing

Adult & Geriatric

Perennial allergic rhinitis: Intranasal: 0.15% solution: Two sprays in each nostril twice daily.

Seasonal allergic rhinitis: Intranasal: 0.1% or 0.15% solution: 1 to 2 sprays in each nostril twice daily **or** 2 sprays of 0.15% solution in each nostril once daily

Pediatric

Perennial allergic rhinitis: Intranasal:

Infants ≥6 months and Children ≤5 years: 0.1% solution: One spray in each nostril twice daily.

Children 6 to <12 years: 0.1% or 0.15% solution: One spray in each nostril twice daily.

Children ≥12 years and Adolescents: Refer to adult dosing.

Seasonal allergic rhinitis: Intranasal:

Children 2 to 5 years: 0.1% solution: One spray in each nostril twice daily.

Children 6 to <12 years: 0.1% or 0.15% solution: One spray in each nostril twice daily.

Children ≥12 years and Adolescents: Refer to adult dosing.

Renal Impairment There are no dosage adjustments provided in the manufacturer's labeling.

Hepatic Impairment There are no dosage adjustments provided in the manufacturer's labeling.

Additional Information Complete prescribing information should be consulted for additional detail.

Dosage Forms Considerations

Astelin and Astepro 30 mL bottles contain 200 sprays each.

Dosage Forms Excipient information presented when available (limited, particularly for generics); consult specific product labeling. [DSC] = Discontinued product

Solution, Nasal, as hydrochloride:

Astelin: 137 mcg/spray (30 mL [DSC]) [contains benzalkonium chloride, edetate disodium]

Astepro: 0.15% (30 mL) [contains benzalkonium chloride, edetate disodium]

Generic: 0.1% (30 mL); 0.15% (30 mL)

Azelastine (Ophthalmic) (a ZEL as teen)

Brand Names: US Optivar [DSC]

Index Terms Azelastine Hydrochloride; Optivar

Pharmacologic Category Histamine H₁ Antagonist; Histamine H₁ Antagonist, Second Generation

Use Treatment of itching of the eye associated with seasonal allergic conjunctivitis

Dosing

Adult & Geriatric Seasonal allergic conjunctivitis: Ophthalmic: Instill 1 drop into affected eye(s) twice daily.

Pediatric Seasonal allergic conjunctivitis: Ophthalmic: Children ≥3 years: Refer to adult dosing.

Renal Impairment No dosage adjustment provided in the manufacturer's labeling.

Hepatic Impairment No dosage adjustment provided in manufacturer's labeling.

Additional Information Complete prescribing information should be consulted for additional detail.

Dosage Forms Excipient information presented when available (limited, particularly for generics); consult specific product labeling. [DSC] = Discontinued product

Solution, Ophthalmic, as hydrochloride:

Optivar: 0.05% (6 mL [DSC]) [contains benzalkonium chloride]

Generic: 0.05% (6 mL)

Azelastine and Fluticasone
(a ZEL as teen & floo TIK a sone)

Brand Names: US Dymista

Brand Names: Canada Dymista

Index Terms Fluticasone Propionate and Azelastine Hydrochloride

Pharmacologic Category Corticosteroid, Nasal; Histamine H₁ Antagonist, Second Generation

Use Seasonal allergic rhinitis:

US labeling: Relief of symptoms of seasonal allergic rhinitis in patients 6 years and older

Canadian labeling: Symptomatic treatment of moderate to severe seasonal allergic rhinitis and associated ocular symptoms in patients 12 years and older who have an inadequate response to monotherapy with antihistamines or intranasal corticosteroids

Dosing

Adult & Geriatric Seasonal allergic rhinitis: Intranasal: One spray (137 mcg azelastine/50 mcg fluticasone) per nostril twice daily

Pediatric Seasonal allergic rhinitis:

US labeling: Children ≥6 years and Adolescents: Refer to adult dosing.

Canadian labeling: Children ≥12 years and Adolescents: Refer to adult dosing.

Renal Impairment There are no dosage adjustments provided in the manufacturer's labeling.

Hepatic Impairment There are no dosage adjustments provided in the manufacturer's labeling.

Additional Information Complete prescribing information should be consulted for additional detail.

Dosage Forms Excipient information presented when available (limited, particularly for generics); consult specific product labeling.

Suspension, intranasal [spray]:

Dymista: Azelastine hydrochloride 0.1% [137 mcg/spray] and fluticasone propionate 0.037% [50 mcg/spray] (23 g) [contains benzalkonium chloride; 120 metered sprays]

◆ Azelastine Hydrochloride *see* Azelastine (Nasal) *on page 187*

◆ Azelastine Hydrochloride *see* Azelastine (Ophthalmic) *on page 188*

◆ Azelex *see* Azelaic Acid *on page 187*

◆ Azidothymidine *see* Zidovudine *on page 1926*

◆ Azidothymidine, Abacavir, and Lamivudine *see* Abacavir, Lamivudine, and Zidovudine *on page 18*

◆ Azilect *see* Rasagiline *on page 1560*

Azilsartan (ay zil SAR tan)

Brand Names: US Edarbi

Brand Names: Canada Edarbi

Index Terms Azilsartan Medoxomil; AZL-M

Pharmacologic Category Angiotensin II Receptor Blocker; Antihypertensive

Use

Hypertension: Treatment of hypertension; may be used alone or in combination with other antihypertensives

Guideline recommendations:

Hypertension: The 2014 guideline for the management of high blood pressure in adults (Eighth Joint National Committee [JNC 8]) recommends initiation of pharmacologic treatment to lower blood pressure for the following patients:

• Patients ≥60 years of age with systolic blood pressure (SBP) ≥150 mm Hg or diastolic blood pressure (DBP) ≥90 mm Hg. Goal of therapy is SBP <150 mm Hg and DBP <90 mm Hg.

• Patients <60 years of age with SBP ≥140 mm Hg or DBP ≥90 mm Hg. Goal of therapy is SBP <140 mm Hg and DBP <90 mm Hg.

• Patients ≥18 years of age with diabetes and SBP ≥140 mm Hg or DBP ≥90 mm Hg. Goal of therapy is SBP <140 mm Hg and DBP <90 mm Hg.

• Patients ≥18 years of age with chronic kidney disease (CKD) and SBP ≥140 mm Hg or DBP ≥90 mm Hg. Goal of therapy is SBP <140 mm Hg and DBP <90 mm Hg.

Chronic kidney disease (CKD) and hypertension: Regardless of race or diabetes status, the use of an ACE inhibitor (ACEI) or angiotensin receptor blocker (ARB) as initial therapy is recommended to improve kidney outcomes. In the general nonblack population (without CKD) including those with diabetes, initial antihypertensive treatment should consist of a thiazide-type diuretic, calcium channel blocker, ACEI, or ARB. In the general black population (without CKD) including those with diabetes, initial antihypertensive treatment should consist of a thiazide-type diuretic or a calcium channel blocker instead of an ACEI or ARB.

Coronary artery disease and hypertension: The American Heart Association, American College of Cardiology and American Society of Hypertension (AHA/ACC/ASH) 2015 scientific statement for the treatment of hypertension in patients with coronary artery disease (CAD) recommends the use of an ARB (or ACE inhibitor) as part of a regimen in patients with hypertension and chronic stable angina if there is prior MI, LV systolic dysfunction, diabetes mellitus, or CKD. A BP target of <140/90 mm Hg is reasonable for the secondary prevention of cardiovascular events. A lower target BP (<130/80 mm Hg) may be appropriate in some individuals with CAD, previous MI, stroke or transient ischemic attack, or CAD risk equivalents (AHA/ACC/ASH [Rosendorff 2015]).

Pregnancy Considerations [US Boxed Warning]: Drugs that act on the renin-angiotensin system can cause injury and death to the developing fetus. Discontinue as soon as possible once pregnancy is detected. The use of drugs which act on the renin-angiotensin system are associated with oligohydramnios. Oligohydramnios, due to decreased fetal renal function, may lead to fetal lung hypoplasia and skeletal malformations. Use is also associated with anuria, hypotension, renal failure, skull hypoplasia, and death in the fetus/neonate. The exposed fetus should be monitored for fetal growth, amniotic fluid volume, and organ formation. Infants

exposed *in utero* should be monitored for hyperkalemia, hypotension, and oliguria (exchange transfusions or dialysis may be needed). These adverse events are generally associated with maternal use in the second and third trimesters.

Untreated chronic maternal hypertension is also associated with adverse events in the fetus, infant, and mother. The use of angiotensin II receptor blockers is not recommended to treat chronic uncomplicated hypertension in pregnant women and should generally be avoided in women of reproductive potential (ACOG, 2013). The Canadian labeling contraindicates use in pregnant women.

Breast-Feeding Considerations It is not known if azilsartan is excreted into breast milk. Due to the potential for serious adverse reactions in the nursing infant, the US labeling recommends a decision be made whether to discontinue nursing or to discontinue the drug, taking into account the importance of treatment to the mother. The Canadian labeling contraindicates use in nursing women.

Contraindications

US labeling: Concomitant use with aliskiren in patients with diabetes mellitus

Canadian labeling: Hypersensitivity to azilsartan medoxomil or any component of the formulation; concomitant use with aliskiren-containing drugs in patients with diabetes or moderate-to-severe renal impairment (GFR <60 mL/minute/1.73 m^2); pregnancy; breast-feeding

Warnings/Precautions [US Boxed Warning]: Drugs that act on the renin-angiotensin system can cause injury and death to the developing fetus. Discontinue as soon as possible once pregnancy is detected. Angiotensin II receptor blockers may cause hyperkalemia; avoid potassium supplementation unless specifically required by healthcare provider. Avoid use or use a smaller dose in patients who are volume depleted; correct depletion first. May be associated with deterioration of renal function and/or increases in serum creatinine, particularly in patients with low renal blood flow (eg, renal artery stenosis, heart failure, volume depletion) whose glomerular filtration rate (GFR) is dependent on efferent arteriolar vasoconstriction by angiotensin II. Use with caution in unstented unilateral/bilateral renal artery stenosis. When unstented bilateral renal artery stenosis is present, use is generally avoided due to the elevated risk of deterioration in renal function unless possible benefits outweigh risks. Use with caution in preexisting renal insufficiency; significant aortic/mitral stenosis. Potentially significant drug-drug interactions may exist, requiring dose or frequency adjustment, additional monitoring, and/or selection of alternative therapy. In surgical patients on chronic angiotensin receptor blocker (ARB) therapy, intraoperative hypotension may occur with induction and maintenance of general anesthesia; however, discontinuation of therapy prior to surgery is controversial. If continued preoperatively, avoidance of hypotensive agents during surgery is prudent (Hillis, 2011).

Angioedema has been reported rarely with some angiotensin II receptor antagonists (ARBs) and may occur at any time during treatment (especially following first dose). It may involve the head and neck (potentially compromising airway) or the intestine (presenting with abdominal pain). Patients with idiopathic or hereditary angioedema or previous angioedema associated with ACE-inhibitor therapy may be at an increased risk. Prolonged frequent monitoring may be required, especially if tongue, glottis, or larynx are involved, as they are associated with airway obstruction. Patients with a history of airway surgery may have a higher risk of airway obstruction. Discontinue therapy immediately if angioedema occurs. Aggressive early management is critical. Intramuscular (IM) administration of epinephrine may be necessary. Do not readminister to patients who have had angioedema with ARBs.

Adverse Reactions Frequency not always defined.

Cardiovascular: Hypotension, orthostatic hypotension

Central nervous system: Dizziness, fatigue

Gastrointestinal: Diarrhea (2%), nausea

Hematologic & oncologic: Decreased hemoglobin, decreased hematocrit, decreased red blood cells, leukopenia (rare), thrombocytopenia (rare)

Neuromuscular & skeletal: Muscle spasm, weakness

Renal: Increased serum creatinine

Respiratory: Cough

<1% (Limited to important or life-threatening): Angioedema, pruritus, skin rash

Drug Interactions

Metabolism/Transport Effects Substrate of CYP2C9 (minor); **Note:** Assignment of Major/Minor substrate status based on clinically relevant drug interaction potential

Avoid Concomitant Use There are no known interactions where it is recommended to avoid concomitant use.

Increased Effect/Toxicity

Azilsartan may increase the levels/effects of: ACE Inhibitors; Amifostine; Antipsychotic Agents (Second Generation [Atypical]); Ciprofloxacin (Systemic); CycloSPORINE (Systemic); Drospirenone; DULoxetine; Hypotension-Associated Agents; Levodopa; Lithium; Nonsteroidal Anti-Inflammatory Agents; Potassium-Sparing Diuretics; Sodium Phosphates

The levels/effects of Azilsartan may be increased by: Alfuzosin; Aliskiren; Barbiturates; Brimonidine (Topical); Canagliflozin; Dapoxetine; Diazoxide; Eplerenone; Heparin; Heparin (Low Molecular Weight); Herbs (Hypotensive Properties); Molsidomine; Nicorandil; Obinutuzumab; Pentoxifylline; Phosphodiesterase 5 Inhibitors; Potassium Salts; Prostacyclin Analogues; Tolvaptan; Trimethoprim

Decreased Effect

The levels/effects of Azilsartan may be decreased by: Amphetamines; Herbs (Hypertensive Properties); Methylphenidate; Nonsteroidal Anti-Inflammatory Agents; Yohimbine

Storage/Stability Store at 25°C (77°F); excursions permitted to 15°C to 30°C (59°F to 86°F). Protect from moisture and light. Dispense and store in original container.

Mechanism of Action Angiotensin II (which is formed by enzymatic conversion from angiotensin I) is the primary pressor agent of the renin-angiotensin system. Effects of angiotensin II include vasoconstriction, stimulation of aldosterone synthesis/release, cardiac stimulation, and renal sodium reabsorption. Azilsartan inhibits angiotensin II's vasoconstrictor and aldosterone-secreting effects by selectively blocking the binding of angiotensin II to the AT$_1$ receptor in vascular smooth muscle and adrenal gland tissues (azilsartan has a stronger affinity for the AT$_1$ receptor than the AT$_2$ receptor). The action is independent of the angiotensin II synthesis pathways. Azilsartan does not inhibit ACE (kininase II), therefore it does not affect the response to bradykinin (the clinical relevance of this is unknown) and does not bind to or inhibit other receptors or ion channels of importance in cardiovascular regulation.

Pharmacodynamics/Kinetics

Distribution: V$_d$: ~16 L

Protein binding: >99%; primarily to serum albumin

Metabolism: Gut: prodrug hydrolyzed to active metabolite; Hepatic: primarily via CYP2C9 to inactive metabolites

Bioavailability: ~60%

Half-life elimination: ~11 hours

Time to peak, serum: 1.5-3 hours

Excretion: Feces (~55%); urine (~42%, 15% as unchanged drug)

Clearance: 2.3 mL/minute

Dosing

Adult & Geriatric Hypertension: Oral:

US labeling: 80 mg once daily; consider initial dose of 40 mg once daily in patients with volume depletion (eg, patients receiving high-dose diuretics); usual dosage (ASH/ISH [Weber, 2014]): 80 mg daily

Canadian labeling: Initial: 40 mg once daily; may increase to 80 mg once daily if necessary

Renal Impairment

US labeling: No dosage adjustment necessary; however, carefully monitor the patient.

Canadian labeling:

Mild-to-moderate impairment: No dosage adjustment is necessary; however, carefully monitor the patient.

Severe impairment or end stage renal disease (ESRD): No dosage adjustment provided in manufacturer's labeling (has not been studied). Use with caution.

Hepatic Impairment

US labeling:

Mild-to-moderate impairment: No dosage adjustment necessary; however, carefully monitor the patient.

Severe impairment: No dosage adjustment provided in manufacturer's labeling (has not been studied).

Canadian labeling:

Mild-to-moderate impairment: There is no specific dosage adjustment provided in manufacturer's labeling; however, a reduced initial dose is recommended. Do not exceed daily dose of 80 mg.

Severe impairment: Use is not recommended.

Dietary Considerations May be taken with or without food.

Administration Administer without regard to food.

Monitoring Parameters Electrolytes, serum creatinine, BUN; blood pressure

Dosage Forms Excipient information presented when available (limited, particularly for generics); consult specific product labeling.

Tablet, Oral, as medoxomil:

Edarbi: 40 mg, 80 mg

Azilsartan and Chlorthalidone
(ay zil SAR tan & klor THAL i done)

Brand Names: US Edarbyclor
Brand Names: Canada Edarbyclor
Index Terms Azilsartan Medoxomil and Chlorthalidone; Chlorthalidone and Azilsartan
Pharmacologic Category Angiotensin II Receptor Blocker; Antihypertensive; Diuretic, Thiazide-Related
Use Hypertension: Treatment of hypertension (when blood pressure control is inadequate with monotherapy or as initial therapy when multiple agents are required to achieve satisfactory blood pressure control)

Dosing
Adult & Geriatric Dose is individualized; combination product may be substituted for individual components in patients currently maintained on both agents separately or in patients not adequately controlled with monotherapy (using one of the agents or an agent within the same antihypertensive class). May also be used as initial therapy in patients who are likely to need >1 antihypertensive to control blood pressure.

Hypertension: Oral: *Initial therapy:* Azilsartan 40 mg/chlorthalidone 12.5 mg once daily; dose may be increased after 2-4 weeks of therapy to azilsartan 40 mg/chlorthalidone 25 mg once daily. Maximum recommended dose: Azilsartan 40 mg/day; chlorthalidone 25 mg/day

Renal Impairment
Mild-to-moderate renal impairment (eGFR 30-90 mL/minute/1.73 m^2): No dosage adjustment necessary.
Severe renal impairment (eGFR <30 mL/minute/1.73 m^2): No dosage adjustment provided in manufacturer's labeling (has not been studied); use with caution.

Hepatic Impairment
US labeling:
Mild-to-moderate hepatic impairment: No initial dosage adjustment necessary; monitor patient carefully.
Severe hepatic impairment: No dosage adjustment provided in manufacturer's labeling (has not been studied); use with caution.
Canadian labeling:
Mild-to-moderate hepatic impairment: Initial dosage reduction is recommended although specific adjustments are not provided in the manufacturer's labeling; monitor patient carefully.
Severe hepatic impairment: Use is not recommended (has not been studied).

Additional Information Complete prescribing information should be consulted for additional detail.

Dosage Forms Excipient information presented when available (limited, particularly for generics); consult specific product labeling.
Tablet, Oral:
Edarbyclor: 40/25: Azilsartan medoxomil 40 mg and chlorthalidone 25 mg, 40/12.5: Azilsartan medoxomil 40 mg and chlorthalidone 12.5 mg

◆ Azilsartan Medoxomil *see* Azilsartan *on page 188*
◆ Azilsartan Medoxomil and Chlorthalidone *see* Azilsartan and Chlorthalidone *on page 190*

Azithromycin (Systemic) (az ith roe MYE sin)

Brand Names: US Zithromax; Zithromax Tri-Pak; Zithromax Z-Pak; Zmax
Brand Names: Canada ACT-Azithromycin; Apo-Azithromycin; Apo-Azithromycin Z; Azithromycin for Injection; Azithromycin for Injection, USP; Dom-Azithromycin; GD-Azithromycin; Mylan-Azithromycin; Novo-Azithromycin; PHL-Azithromycin; PMS-Azithromycin; PRO-Azithromycine; Riva-Azithromycin; Sandoz-Azithromycin; Zithromax; Zithromax For Intravenous Injection; Zmax SR
Index Terms Azithromycin Dihydrate; Azithromycin Monohydrate; Z-Pak; Zithromax TRI-PAK; Zithromax Z-PAK
Pharmacologic Category Antibiotic, Macrolide
Use Oral, IV: Treatment of acute otitis media due to *H. influenzae*, *M. catarrhalis*, or *S. pneumoniae*; pharyngitis/tonsillitis due to *S. pyogenes*, community-acquired pneumonia due to *Chlamydia* (also known as *Chlamydophila*) *pneumoniae*, *H. influenzae*, *M. pneumoniae*, or *S. pneumoniae*; pelvic inflammatory disease (PID) due to *C. trachomatis*, *N. gonorrhoeae*, or *M. hominis*; genital ulcer disease (in men) due to *H. ducreyi* (chancroid); acute bacterial exacerbations of chronic obstructive pulmonary disease (COPD) due to *H. influenzae*, *M. catarrhalis*, or *S. pneumoniae*; acute bacterial sinusitis due to *H. influenzae*, *M. catarrhalis*, or *S. pneumoniae*; prevention of *Mycobacterium avium* complex (MAC) (alone or in combination with rifabutin) in patients with advanced HIV infection; treatment of disseminated MAC (in combination with ethambutol) in patients with advanced HIV infection; skin and skin structure infections (uncomplicated) due to *S. aureus*, *S. pyogenes*, or *S. agalactiae*; urethritis and cervicitis due to *C. trachomatis* or *N. gonorrhoeae*

Pregnancy Considerations Adverse events were not observed in animal reproduction studies. Azithromycin crosses the placenta (Ramsey 2003). The maternal serum half-life of azithromycin is unchanged in early pregnancy and decreased at term; however, high concentrations of azithromycin are sustained in the myometrium and adipose tissue (Fischer 2012; Ramsey 2003). Azithromycin is recommended for the treatment of several infections, including chlamydia, gonococcal infections, granuloma inguinale (donovanosis) and *Mycobacterium avium* complex (MAC) in pregnant patients (consult current guidelines) (CDC [Workowski 2015]; DHHS 2013).

Breast-Feeding Considerations Azithromycin is excreted in low amounts into breast milk (Kelsey 1994). Decreased appetite, diarrhea, rash, and somnolence have been reported in nursing infants exposed to macrolide antibiotics (Goldstein 2009). The manufacturer recommends that caution be exercised when administering azithromycin to breast-feeding women.

Contraindications Hypersensitivity to azithromycin, other macrolide (eg, azalide or ketolide) antibiotics, or any component of the formulation; history of cholestatic jaundice/hepatic dysfunction associated with prior azithromycin use

Note: The manufacturer does not list concurrent use of pimozide as a contraindication; however, azithromycin is listed as a contraindication in the manufacturer's labeling for pimozide.

Warnings/Precautions Use with caution in patients with preexisting liver disease; hepatocellular and/or cholestatic hepatitis, with or without jaundice, hepatic necrosis, failure and death have occurred. Discontinue immediately if symptoms of hepatitis occur (malaise, nausea, vomiting, abdominal colic, fever). Allergic reactions have been reported (rare); reappearance of allergic reaction may occur shortly after discontinuation without further azithromycin exposure. May mask or delay symptoms of incubating gonorrhea or syphilis, so appropriate culture and susceptibility tests should be performed prior to initiating a treatment regimen. Prolonged use may result in fungal or bacterial superinfection, including *C. difficile*-associated diarrhea (CDAD); CDAD has been observed >2 months postantibiotic treatment. Use caution with renal dysfunction. Macrolides (especially erythromycin) have been associated with rare QTc prolongation and ventricular arrhythmias, including torsade de pointes; consider avoiding use in patients with prolonged QT interval, congenital long QT syndrome, history of torsade de pointes, bradyarrhythmias, uncorrected hypokalemia or hypomagnesemia, clinically significant bradycardia, uncompensated heart failure, or concurrent use of Class IA (eg, quinidine, procainamide) or Class III (eg, amiodarone, dofetilide, sotalol) antiarrhythmic agents or other drugs known to prolong the QT interval. Use with caution in patients with myasthenia gravis.

Oral suspensions (immediate release and extended release) are not interchangeable.

Adverse Reactions
>10%: Gastrointestinal: Loose stools (≤14%; single-dose regimens tend to be associated with increased incidence), vomiting (children, single-dose regimens tend to be associated with increased incidence: 1% to 14%; adults: ≤2%; adults, single 2 g dose: 1% to 7%), diarrhea (2% to 9%; single-dose regimens 4% to 14%), nausea (≤7%; high single-dose regimens 4% to 18%)
2% to 10%:
Cardiovascular: Chest pain (≤1%), palpitations (≤1%)
Central nervous system: Dizziness (≤1%), drowsiness (≤1%), fatigue (≤1%), headache (≤1%), vertigo (≤1%)
Dermatologic: Skin rash (≤5%; single-dose regimens tend to be associated with increased incidence), dermatitis (children: ≤2%), pruritus (≤2%), skin photosensitivity (≤1%)
Endocrine & metabolic: Increased lactate dehydrogenase (1% to 3%), increased gamma-glutamyl transferase (1% to 2%), increased serum potassium (1% to 2%), decreased serum bicarbonate (adults: ≥1%), decreased serum glucose (adults: >1%)
Gastrointestinal: Abdominal pain (1% to 7%; single-dose regimens tend to be associated with increased incidence), anorexia (≤2%), dysgeusia (≤1%), dyspepsia (≤1%), flatulence (≤1%), gastritis (≤1%), melena (adults, multiple-dose regimens: ≤1%), mucositis (≤1%), oral candidiasis (≤1%)
Genitourinary: Vaginitis (≤3%), genital candidiasis (adults, multiple-dose regimens: ≤1%)

Hematologic & oncologic: Decrease in absolute neutrophil count (children: 15% to 16%; 500 to 1500 cells/mm^3), decreased hematocrit (adults: >1%), decreased hemoglobin (adults: >1%), increased neutrophils (adults: >1%), thrombocythemia (adults: >1%), change in neutrophil count (children: ≥1%), eosinophilia (≥1%), lymphocytopenia (≥1%)

Hepatic: Increased serum ALT (≤6%), increased serum AST (≤6%), increased serum bilirubin (≤3%), cholestatic jaundice (≤1%)

Local (adults with IV administration): Pain at injection site (7%), local inflammation (3%)

Neuromuscular & skeletal: Increased creatine phosphokinase (1% to 2%)

Renal: Increased serum creatinine (≤6%), increased blood urea nitrogen (≤1%), nephritis (adults, multiple-dose regimens: ≤1%)

Respiratory: Bronchospasm (≤1%)

Miscellaneous: Fever (children: (≤2%)

≤1% (Limited to important or life-threatening): Abnormal stools, acute renal failure, ageusia, agitation, aggressive behavior, alteration in sodium, altered sense of smell, altered serum glucose, anaphylaxis, anemia, angioedema, anosmia, anxiety, arthralgia, asthma, basophilia, bronchitis, cardiac arrhythmia, change in serum potassium, conjunctivitis (children), constipation, cough, deafness, decreased serum potassium, decreased serum sodium, diaphoresis, DRESS syndrome, dyspnea, dysuria, eczema, edema, emotional lability, enteritis, erythema multiforme, facial edema, flu-like symptoms (children), fungal dermatitis (children), fungal infection (children), gastrointestinal disease, hearing loss, hepatic failure, hepatic insufficiency, hepatic necrosis, hepatitis, hepatotoxicity (idiosyncratic) (Chalasani 2014), hostility, hyperactivity, hyperkinesia, hypersensitivity reaction, hypotension, increased monocytes, increased serum alkaline phosphatase, increased serum bicarbonate, increased serum phosphate, interstitial nephritis, insomnia, irritability, jaundice, leukopenia, maculopapular rash, malaise, nervousness, neutropenia, otitis media, pain, pancreatitis, paresthesia, pharyngitis, pleural effusion, prolonged Q-T interval on ECG, pseudomembranous colitis, pyloric stenosis, rhinitis, seizure, Stevens-Johnson syndrome, syncope, thrombocytopenia, tinnitus, tongue discoloration, toxic epidermal necrolysis, urticaria, ventricular tachycardia, vesiculobullous dermatitis, weakness

Drug Interactions

Metabolism/Transport Effects Substrate of CYP3A4 (minor); **Note:** Assignment of Major/Minor substrate status based on clinically relevant drug interaction potential; **Inhibits** CYP1A2 (weak), P-glycoprotein

Avoid Concomitant Use

Avoid concomitant use of Azithromycin (Systemic) with any of the following: Amiodarone; BCG (Intravesical); Bosutinib; Highest Risk QTc-Prolonging Agents; Ivabradine; Mifepristone; PAZOPanib; Pimozide; QuiNINE; Silodosin; Terfenadine; Topotecan; VinCRIStine (Liposomal)

Increased Effect/Toxicity

Azithromycin (Systemic) may increase the levels/effects of: Afatinib; Amiodarone; AtorvaSTATin; Bosutinib; Brentuximab Vedotin; Cardiac Glycosides; Colchicine; CycloSPORINE (Systemic); Dabigatran Etexilate; DOXOrubicin (Conventional); Edoxaban; Everolimus; Highest Risk QTc-Prolonging Agents; Ivermectin (Systemic); Ledipasvir; Lovastatin; Moderate Risk QTc-Prolonging Agents; Naloxegol; PAZOPanib; P-glycoprotein/ABCB1 Substrates; Pimozide; Prucalopride; QuiNINE; Ranolazine; Rifaximin; Rilpivirine; Silodosin; Simvastatin; Tacrolimus (Systemic); Tacrolimus (Topical); Terfenadine; TiZANidine; Topotecan; VinCRIStine (Liposomal); Vitamin K Antagonists

The levels/effects of Azithromycin (Systemic) may be increased by: Ivabradine; Mifepristone; Nelfinavir; QTc-Prolonging Agents (Indeterminate Risk and Risk Modifying)

Decreased Effect

Azithromycin (Systemic) may decrease the levels/effects of: BCG (Intravesical); BCG Vaccine (Immunization); Sodium Picosulfate; Typhoid Vaccine

Food Interactions Rate and extent of GI absorption may be altered depending upon the formulation. Azithromycin suspension, not tablet form, has significantly increased absorption (46%) with food. Management: Immediate release suspension and tablet may be taken without regard to food; extended release suspension should be taken on an empty stomach (at least 1 hour before or 2 hours following a meal).

Preparation for Administration Injection (Zithromax®): Prepare initiation solution by adding 4.8 mL of sterile water for injection to the 500 mg vial (resulting concentration: 100 mg/mL). Use of a standard syringe is recommended due to the vacuum in the vial (which may draw additional solution through an automated syringe).

The initial solution should be further diluted to a concentration of 1 mg/mL (500 mL) to 2 mg/mL (250 mL) in 0.9% sodium chloride, 5% dextrose in water, or lactated Ringer's.

Storage/Stability

Injection (Zithromax): Store intact vials of injection at room temperature. Reconstituted solution is stable for 24 hours when stored below 30°C (86°F). The diluted solution is stable for 24 hours at or below room temperature (30°C [86°F]) and for 7 days if stored under refrigeration (5°C [41°F]).

Suspension, immediate release (Zithromax): Store dry powder below 30°C (86°F). Store reconstituted suspension at 5°C to 30°C (41°F to 86°F) and use within 10 days.

Suspension, extended release (Zmax): Store dry powder ≤30°C (86°F). Following reconstitution, store at 25°C (77°F); excursions permitted to 15°C to 30°C (59°F to 86°F); do not refrigerate or freeze. Should be consumed within 12 hours following reconstitution.

Tablet (Zithromax): Store between 15°C to 30°C (59°F to 86°F).

Mechanism of Action Inhibits RNA-dependent protein synthesis at the chain elongation step; binds to the 50S ribosomal subunit resulting in blockage of transpeptidation

Pharmacodynamics/Kinetics

Absorption: Oral: Rapid from the GI tract

Distribution: Extensive tissue; distributes well into skin, lungs, sputum, tonsils, and cervix; penetration into CSF is poor; V$_d$: 31 to 33 L/kg

Protein binding (concentration dependent and dependent on alpha1-acid glycoprotein concentrations): Oral, IV: 7% to 51%

Metabolism: Hepatic to inactive metabolites

Bioavailability: Oral: Tablet, immediate release oral suspension: 34% to 52%; extended release oral suspension: 28% to 43%; variable effect with food (increased with immediate or delayed release oral suspension, unchanged with tablet)

Half-life elimination: Terminal: Oral, IV:
  Infants and Children 4 months to 15 years: 54.5 hours
  Adults: Immediate release: 68-72 hours; Extended release: 59 hours

Time to peak, serum: Oral: Immediate release: 2-3 hours; Extended release: 3-5 hours

Excretion: Oral, IV: Biliary (major route 50%, unchanged); urine (6% to 14% unchanged)

Dosing

Adult & Geriatric Note: Extended release suspension (Zmax) is not interchangeable with immediate release formulations. Use should be limited to approved indications. All doses are expressed as immediate release azithromycin unless otherwise specified.

Babesiosis (off-label use): Oral: 500 to 1,000 mg on day 1, followed by 250 mg once daily for 7 to 10 days with atovaquone; higher doses may be required in immunocompromised patients (600 to 1,000 mg daily). **Note:** Relapsing infection may require at least 6 weeks of therapy (Krause 2000; Vannier 2012; IDSA [Wormser 2006]).

Bacterial sinusitis: Oral: 500 mg daily for a total of 3 days
  Extended release suspension (Zmax): 2 g as a single dose

Bronchiolitis obliterans syndrome (off-label use): Oral: 250 mg daily for 5 days, followed by 250 mg 3 times per week for a minimum of 3 months (Meyer 2014). **Note:** It is unclear whether azithromycin should be continued long-term if a benefit is observed or if it should be discontinued if lung function does not improve (Meyer 2014).

Cat scratch disease (off-label use): Oral: ≥45.5 kg: 500 mg as a single dose, then 250 mg once daily for 4 additional days (Bass 1998; Stevens 2014)

Chancroid due to *H. ducreyi*: Oral: 1 g as a single dose. **Note:** Data are limited concerning the efficacy in HIV infected patients (CDC [Workowski 2015]).

***Chlamydia trachomatis* infection:** Oral: 1 g as a single dose (CDC [Workowski 2015])

Community-acquired pneumonia:
  Oral: 500 mg on day 1 followed by 250 mg once daily on days 2-5
  Extended release suspension (Zmax): 2 g as a single dose

IV: 500 mg as a single dose for at least 2 days, follow IV therapy by the oral route with a single daily dose of 500 mg to complete a 7- to 10-day course of therapy.

Disseminated *M. avium* complex disease in patients with advanced HIV infection: Oral:

Treatment: 600 mg daily in combination with ethambutol

Primary prophylaxis: 1,200 mg once weekly (preferred), with or without rifabutin **or** alternatively, 600 mg twice weekly (DHHS 2013)

Secondary prophylaxis: 500 to 600 mg daily in combination with ethambutol (DHHS 2013)

Gonococcal infection, conjunctivitis (off-label use): Oral: 1 g as a single dose in combination with ceftriaxone (CDC [Workowski 2015])

Gonococcal infection, disseminated (arthritis, arthritis-dermatitis, meningitis, endocarditis) (off-label use): Oral: 1 g as a single dose in combination with ceftriaxone (CDC [Workowski 2015])

Gonococcal infection, expedited partner therapy (off-label use): Oral: 1 g as a single dose in combination with cefixime (CDC [Workowski 2015]). **Note:** To be used only for heterosexual partners with gonorrhea if health department partner-management strategies are impractical/unavailable and there is concern by the provider for the prompt evaluation and treatment of the partner; medication may be delivered to partner by patient, collaborating pharmacy, or disease investigation specialist as permitted by law; written materials to educate partners about their exposure to gonorrhea, importance of therapy, and when to seek clinical evaluation for adverse reactions/complications must also be provided with the medication (CDC [Workowski 2015]).

Gonococcal infection, uncomplicated (cervix, rectum [off-label use], urethra) (off-label regimen): Oral: 1 g as a single dose in combination with ceftriaxone (preferred) or cefixime (only if ceftriaxone unavailable) (CDC [Workowski 2015]).

Patients with severe cephalosporin allergy (off-label regimen): 2 g as a single dose in combination with gemifloxacin or gentamicin IM (CDC [Workowski 2015])

Gonococcal infection, uncomplicated (pharynx) (off-label use): Oral: 1 g as a single dose in combination with ceftriaxone (CDC [Workowski 2015])

Granuloma inguinale (donovanosis) (off-label use): Oral: 1 g once weekly **or** 500 mg once daily for at least 3 weeks and until lesions have healed. **Note:** If symptoms do not improve within the first few days of therapy, the addition of gentamicin may be considered (CDC [Workowski 2015])

Mild to moderate respiratory tract, skin, and soft tissue infections: Oral: 500 mg in a single loading dose on day 1 followed by 250 mg daily as a single dose on days 2-5

Alternative regimen: Bacterial exacerbation of COPD: 500 mg daily for a total of 3 days

Pelvic inflammatory disease (PID): IV: 500 mg as a single dose for 1 to 2 days, follow IV therapy by the oral route with a single daily dose of 250 mg to complete a 7-day course of therapy.

Pertussis (off-label use) (CDC 2005): Oral: 500 mg on day 1 followed by 250 mg daily on days 2 to 5 (maximum: 500 mg daily)

Pharyngitis (including susceptible group A streptococci, tonsillitis (as an alternative agent in penicillin-allergic patients): Oral: 12 mg/kg (maximum: 500 mg) on day 1 followed by 6 mg/kg (maximum: 250 mg) once daily on days 2 through 5. **Note:** Regimen is also recommended by the Infectious Disease Society of America (IDSA) (Shulman 2012).

Prevention of pulmonary exacerbations in patients with noncystic fibrosis bronchiectasis (off-label use): Oral: 500 mg 3 days per week. **Note:** Duration of treatment in clinical trial was 6 months; durations >6 months have not been evaluated. Trial patients had ≥1 exacerbation in the past year, no macrolide treatment for >3 months in the past 6 months, and were screened for nontuberculous mycobacterial infection prior to treatment (Wong 2012). A more selective approach for patients with functionally mild disease has been suggested (Wilson 2012).

Prophylaxis against infective endocarditis (off-label use): Oral: 500 mg 30 to 60 minutes prior to the procedure. **Note:** American Heart Association (AHA) guidelines now recommend prophylaxis only in patients undergoing invasive procedures and in whom underlying cardiac conditions may predispose to a higher risk of adverse outcomes should infection occur. As of April 2007, routine prophylaxis for GI/GU procedures is no longer recommended by the AHA.

Prophylaxis against sexually transmitted diseases following sexual assault (off-label use): Oral: 1 g as a single dose in combination with ceftriaxone (plus metronidazole or tinidazole) (CDC [Workowski 2015])

Shigella dysentery type 1 (off-label use): Oral: 1,000 to 1,500 mg once daily for 1 to 5 days (WHO 2005)

Traveler's diarrhea (off-label use): Oral: 1,000 mg as a single dose **or** 500 mg once daily for 1 to 3 days with or without concomitant loperamide (CDC 2015; Ericsson 2007; Tribble 2007). **Note:** Increased nausea may occur with the 1,000 mg single dose regimen (Tribble 2007).

Urethritis/cervicitis (nongonococcal): Oral: 1 g as a single dose

Urethritis/cervicitis due to or likely due to *M. genitalium* infections (off-label use): Oral: 1 g as a single dose **or** 500 mg on day 1, followed by 250 mg daily on days 2 through 5 (CDC [Workowski 2015]; Manhart 2011)

Pediatric Note: Extended release suspension (Zmax) is not interchangeable with immediate release formulations. Use should be limited to approved indications. All doses are expressed as immediate release azithromycin unless otherwise specified.

Note: Adolescents ≥16 years: Refer to adult dosing.

Bacterial sinusitis: Children ≥6 months: Oral: 10 mg/kg once daily for 3 days (maximum: 500 mg daily)

Cat scratch disease (off-label use) (Bass 1998; Stevens 2014): Oral:

<45.5 kg: 10 mg/kg as a single dose, then 5 mg/kg once daily for 4 additional days

≥45.5 kg: Refer to adult dosing.

***Chlamydia trachomatis* infection (off-label use):** Oral: Children ≥45 kg: 1 g as a single dose (CDC [Workowski 2015])

Community-acquired pneumonia (CAP) (IDSA/PIDS 2011): Infants >3 months and Children: **Note:** A beta-lactam antibiotic should be added if typical bacterial pneumonia cannot be ruled out

Presumed mild infection or step-down therapy, atypical *(M. pneumoniae, Chlamydophila* [also known as *Chlamydia*] *pneumoniae, C. trachomatis)* (preferred): Oral: 10 mg/kg (maximum dose: 500 mg) as a single dose on the first day, followed by 5 mg/kg/day (maximum dose: 250 mg) on days 2 through 5.

Presumed moderate to severe infection, atypical *(M. pneumoniae, Chlamydophila* [also known as *Chlamydia*] *pneumoniae, C. trachomatis):* IV: 10 mg/kg/day on days 1 and 2, then switch to oral azithromycin therapy if possible to finish the 5-day course

Alternative regimens for community-acquired pneumonia: Oral: 10 mg/kg (maximum dose: 500 mg) once daily for 3 days (Kogan 2003)

Extended release suspension (Zmax):

<75 lbs (34 kg): 60 mg/kg as a single dose

≥75 lbs (34 kg): Refer to adult dosing

Disseminated *M. avium* complex disease in patients with advanced HIV infection (off-label use) (DHHS 2013): Oral:

Treatment: 10 to 12 mg/kg/day (maximum: 500 mg) in combination with ethambutol; patients with severe disease should also receive rifabutin

Primary prophylaxis: 20 mg/kg (maximum: 1,200 mg) once weekly (preferred) or alternatively, 5 mg/kg/day once daily (maximum: 250 mg daily)

Secondary prophylaxis: 5 mg/kg/day once daily (maximum: 250 mg daily) in combination with ethambutol, with or without rifabutin

Gonococcal infection, conjunctivitis (off-label use): Adolescents: Refer to adult dosing.

Gonococcal infection, disseminated (arthritis, arthritis-dermatitis, meningitis, endocarditis) (off-label use): Adolescents: Refer to adult dosing.

Gonococcal infection, uncomplicated (cervix, rectum [off-label use], urethra) (off-label regimen): Adolescents: Refer to adult dosing.

Gonococcal infection, uncomplicated (pharynx) (off-label use): Adolescents: Refer to adult dosing.

Otitis media: Children ≥6 months: Oral:

1-day regimen: 30 mg/kg as a single dose (maximum dose: 1,500 mg)

3-day regimen: 10 mg/kg once daily for 3 days (maximum: 500 mg daily)

5-day regimen: 10 mg/kg on day 1 (maximum: 500 mg daily) followed by 5 mg/kg/day once daily on days 2 to 5 (maximum: 250 mg daily)

Pertussis (off-label use) (CDC 2005): Oral:

Children <6 months: 10 mg/kg/day for 5 days

Children ≥6 months: 10 mg/kg on day 1 (maximum: 500 mg daily) followed by 5 mg/kg/day once daily on days 2 to 5 (maximum: 250 mg daily)

Pharyngitis (including susceptible group A strepto-cocci), tonsillitis (as an alternative agent in penicillin allergic patients):
Manufacturer's labeling and AHA/AAP recommendations: Children ≥2 years and Adolescents: Oral: 12 mg/kg/dose once daily for 5 days (maximum: 500 mg daily) (AHA guidelines [Gerber 2009]; *Red Book* [AAP 2012])
Alternative recommendations: Children and Adolescents: Oral: 12 mg/kg (maximum: 500 mg) on day 1 followed by 6 mg/kg/dose (maximum: 250 mg) once daily on days 2 through 5 (IDSA guidelines [Shulman 2012])

Prophylaxis against infective endocarditis (off-label use): Oral: 15 mg/kg 30 to 60 minutes before procedure. **Note:** American Heart Association (AHA) guidelines now recommend prophylaxis only in patients undergoing invasive procedures and in whom underlying cardiac conditions may predispose to a higher risk of adverse outcomes should infection occur. As of April 2007, routine prophylaxis for GI/GU procedures is no longer recommended by the AHA.

Prophylaxis against sexually transmitted diseases following sexual assault (off-label use): Adolescents: Refer to adult dosing.

Shigella dysentery type 1 (off-label use): Oral: 6 to 20 mg/kg/day for 1 to 5 days (WHO 2005)

Renal Impairment
Use with caution in patients with GFR <10 mL/minute (AUC increased by 35% compared to patients with normal renal function); however, no dosage adjustment is provided in the manufacturer's labeling.
No supplemental dose or dosage adjustment necessary, including patients on intermittent hemodialysis, peritoneal dialysis, or continuous renal replacement therapy (eg, CVVHD) (Aronoff 2007; Heintz 2009).

Hepatic Impairment Azithromycin is predominantly hepatically eliminated; however, there is no dosage adjustment provided in the manufacturer's labeling, Use with caution due to potential for hepatotoxicity (rare); discontinue immediately for signs or symptoms of hepatitis.

Dietary Considerations
Some products may contain sodium and/or sucrose.
Oral suspension, immediate release, may be administered with or without food.
Oral suspension, extended release, should be taken on an empty stomach (at least 1 hour before or 2 hours following a meal).
Tablet may be administered with food to decrease GI effects.

Administration
IV: Infuse over 1 hour (2 mg/mL infusion) or over 3 hours (1 mg/mL infusion). Not for IM or IV bolus administration.
Oral: Immediate release suspension and tablet may be taken without regard to food; extended release suspension should be taken on an empty stomach (at least 1 hour before or 2 hours following a meal), within 12 hours of reconstitution.

Monitoring Parameters Liver function tests, CBC with differential

Additional Information Zithromax® tablets and immediate release suspension may be interchanged (eg, two Zithromax® 250 mg tablets may be substituted for one Zithromax® 500 mg tablet or the tablets may be substituted with the immediate release suspension); however, the extended release suspension (Zmax®) is not bioequivalent with Zithromax® and therefore should not be interchanged.

Azithromycin is not recommended for treatment of early syphilis (ie, primary or secondary syphilis); the 23S rRNA mutation, which has been associated with macrolide resistance, has been documented in multiple geographic areas and in the MSM population. If a penicillin allergic patient cannot take doxycycline (preferred alternative to penicillin), azithromycin (single 2 g dose orally) may be considered but close clinical follow-up is needed (Ghanem 2011; CDC [Workowski 2015]).

Dosage Forms Excipient information presented when available (limited, particularly for generics); consult specific product labeling.
Packet, Oral:
Zithromax: 1 g (3 ea, 10 ea) [cherry-banana flavor]
Generic: 1 g (3 ea, 10 ea)
Solution Reconstituted, Intravenous:
Zithromax: 500 mg (1 ea)
Generic: 500 mg (1 ea); 2.5 g (1 ea)
Solution Reconstituted, Intravenous [preservative free]:
Generic: 500 mg (1 ea)

Suspension Reconstituted, Oral:
Zithromax: 100 mg/5 mL (15 mL) [cherry-vanilla-banana flavor]
Zithromax: 200 mg/5 mL (15 mL, 22.5 mL, 30 mL) [cherry flavor]
Zmax: 2 g (1 ea) [cherry-banana flavor]
Generic: 100 mg/5 mL (15 mL); 200 mg/5 mL (15 mL, 22.5 mL, 30 mL)
Tablet, Oral:
Zithromax: 250 mg, 500 mg, 600 mg
Zithromax Tri-Pak: 500 mg
Zithromax Z-Pak: 250 mg
Generic: 250 mg, 500 mg, 600 mg

Azithromycin (Ophthalmic) (az ith roe MYE sin)

Brand Names: US AzaSite
Pharmacologic Category Antibiotic, Macrolide; Antibiotic, Ophthalmic
Use Treatment of bacterial conjunctivitis caused by susceptible microorganisms
Dosing
Adult & Geriatric Bacterial conjunctivitis: Ophthalmic: Instill 1 drop into affected eye(s) twice daily (8-12 hours apart) for 2 days, then 1 drop into affected eye(s) once daily for 5 days
Pediatric Bacterial conjunctivitis: Children ≥1 year: Refer to adult dosing.
Additional Information Complete prescribing information should be consulted for additional detail.
Dosage Forms Excipient information presented when available (limited, particularly for generics); consult specific product labeling.
Solution, Ophthalmic:
AzaSite: 1% (2.5 mL) [contains benzalkonium chloride, disodium edta]

♦ Azithromycin Dihydrate *see* Azithromycin (Systemic) *on page 190*

♦ Azithromycin for Injection (Can) *see* Azithromycin (Systemic) *on page 190*

♦ Azithromycin for Injection, USP (Can) *see* Azithromycin (Systemic) *on page 190*

♦ Azithromycin Monohydrate *see* Azithromycin (Systemic) *on page 190*

♦ AZL-M *see* Azilsartan *on page 188*

♦ Azo-Gesic [OTC] *see* Phenazopyridine *on page 1435*

♦ Azolen Tincture [OTC] *see* Miconazole (Topical) *on page 1201*

♦ Azopt *see* Brinzolamide *on page 254*

♦ Azopt® (Can) *see* Brinzolamide *on page 254*

♦ Azor *see* Amlodipine and Olmesartan *on page 104*

♦ AZT (Can) *see* Zidovudine *on page 1926*

♦ AZT + 3TC (error-prone abbreviation) *see* Lamivudine and Zidovudine *on page 1026*

♦ AZT, Abacavir, and Lamivudine *see* Abacavir, Lamivudine, and Zidovudine *on page 18*

♦ AZT (error-prone abbreviation) *see* Zidovudine *on page 1926*

♦ Azthreonam *see* Aztreonam (Oral Inhalation) *on page 195*

♦ Azthreonam *see* Aztreonam (Systemic) *on page 193*

Aztreonam (Systemic) (AZ tree oh nam)

Brand Names: US Azactam; Azactam in Dextrose
Index Terms Azthreonam
Pharmacologic Category Antibiotic, Miscellaneous
Use Treatment of patients with urinary tract infections, lower respiratory tract infections, septicemia, skin/skin structure infections, intra-abdominal infections, and gynecological infections caused by susceptible gram-negative bacilli
Pregnancy Considerations Adverse events have not been observed in animal reproduction studies. Aztreonam crosses the placenta and can be detected in the fetus.
Breast-Feeding Considerations Aztreonam is excreted into breast milk in concentrations <1% of the corresponding maternal serum concentration. The manufacturer suggests consideration be given to temporarily discontinuing nursing during therapy.
Contraindications Hypersensitivity to aztreonam or any component of the formulation

Warnings/Precautions Rare cross-allergenicity to penicillins, cephalosporins, or carbapenems may occur; use with caution in patients with a history of hypersensitivity to beta-lactams. Use caution in renal impairment; dosing adjustment required for the injectable formulation. Prolonged use may result in fungal or bacterial superinfection, including *C. difficile*-associated diarrhea (CDAD) and pseudomembranous colitis; CDAD has been observed >2 months postantibiotic treatment. Use with caution in bone marrow transplant patients with multiple risk factors for toxic epidermal necrolysis (TEN) (eg, sepsis, radiation therapy, drugs known to cause TEN); rare cases of TEN in this population have been reported. Patients colonized with *Burkholderia cepacia* have not been studied. Potentially significant interactions may exist, requiring dose or frequency adjustment, additional monitoring, and/or selection of alternative therapy.

Adverse Reactions

>10%:

Hematologic & oncologic: Neutropenia (children 3% to 11%; adults <1%)

Hepatic: Increased serum transaminases (children, high dose: >3 times ULN: 15% to 20%; children, standard dose: increased serum AST 4%, increased serum ALT 7%)

Local: Pain at injection site (children 12%, adults 2%)

1% to 10%:

Cardiovascular: Phlebitis (intravenous: ≤2%), thrombophlebitis (intravenous: ≤2%)

Dermatologic: Skin rash (children 4%, adults ≤1%)

Gastrointestinal: Diarrhea (≤1%), nausea (≤1%), vomiting (≤1%)

Hematologic & oncologic: Eosinophilia (children 6%, adults <1%), thrombocythemia (children 4%, adults <1%)

Local: Erythema at injection site (intravenous: Children 3%, adults <1%), discomfort at injection site (intramuscular: ≤2%), swelling at injection site (intramuscular: ≤2%)

Renal: Increased serum creatinine (children 6%)

Miscellaneous: Fever (≤1%)

<1% (Limited to important or life-threatening): Abdominal cramps, anaphylaxis, anemia, angioedema, breast tenderness, bronchospasm, chest pain, *Clostridium difficile* associated diarrhea, confusion, diaphoresis, diplopia, dizziness, dysgeusia, dyspnea, erythema multiforme, exfoliative dermatitis, flushing, gastrointestinal hemorrhage, hepatitis, hepatobiliary disease, hypotension, increased serum alkaline phosphatase, increased serum ALT (adults), increased serum AST (adults), induration at injection site, insomnia, jaundice, leukocytosis, malaise, myalgia, numbness of tongue, oral mucosa ulcer, pancytopenia, paresthesia, petechia, positive direct Coombs test, prolonged partial thromboplastin time, prolonged prothrombin time, pruritus, pseudomembranous colitis, purpura, seizure, thrombocytopenia, tinnitus, toxic epidermal necrolysis, urticaria, vaginitis, ventricular bigeminy (transient), ventricular premature contractions (transient), vertigo, vulvovaginal candidiasis, weakness, wheezing

Drug Interactions

Metabolism/Transport Effects None known.

Avoid Concomitant Use

Avoid concomitant use of Aztreonam (Systemic) with any of the following: BCG (Intravesical)

Increased Effect/Toxicity There are no known significant interactions involving an increase in effect.

Decreased Effect

Aztreonam (Systemic) may decrease the levels/effects of: BCG (Intravesical); BCG Vaccine (Immunization); Sodium Picosulfate; Typhoid Vaccine

Preparation for Administration

IM: Reconstitute vial with at least 3 mL SWFI, sterile bacteriostatic water for injection, NS, or bacteriostatic sodium chloride per gram of aztreonam; immediately shake vigorously.

IV:

Bolus injection: Reconstitute vial with 6-10 mL SWFI; immediately shake vigorously.

Infusion: Reconstitute vial with at least 3 mL SWFI per gram of aztreonam; immediately shake vigorously. Reconstituted solutions are colorless to light yellow straw and may turn pink upon standing without affecting potency. Further dilute in an appropriate solution for infusion to a final concentration ≤2% (ie, final concentration should not exceed 20 mg/mL).

Storage/Stability

Vials: Prior to reconstitution, store at room temperature; avoid excessive heat. After reconstitution, solutions for infusion with a final concentration of ≤20 mg/mL should be used within 48 hours if stored at room temperature or within 7 days if refrigerated. Solutions for infusion with a final concentration of >20 mg/mL (if prepared with SWFI or NS **only**) should also be used within 48 hours if stored at room temperature or within 7 days if refrigerated; all other solutions for infusion with a final concentration >20 mg/mL must be used immediately after preparation (unless prepared with SWFI or NS).

Premixed frozen containers: Store unused container frozen at ≤-20°C (-4°F). Frozen container can be thawed at room temperature of 25°C (77°F) or in a refrigerator, 2°C to 8°C (36°F to 46°F). Thawed solution should be used within 48 hours if stored at room temperature or within 14 days if stored under refrigeration. **Do not freeze.**

Mechanism of Action Inhibits bacterial cell wall synthesis by binding to one or more of the penicillin-binding proteins (PBPs) which in turn inhibits the final transpeptidation step of peptidoglycan synthesis in bacterial cell walls, thus inhibiting cell wall biosynthesis. Bacteria eventually lyse due to ongoing activity of cell wall autolytic enzymes (autolysins and murein hydrolases) while cell wall assembly is arrested. Monobactam structure makes cross-allergenicity with beta-lactams unlikely.

Pharmacodynamics/Kinetics

Absorption: IM: Well absorbed; IM and IV doses produce comparable serum concentrations

Distribution: Injection: Widely into body tissues, cerebrospinal fluid, bronchial secretions, peritoneal fluid, bile, and bone

V_d: Neonates: 0.26 to 0.36 L/kg; Children: 0.2 to 0.29 L/kg; Adults: 0.2 L/kg

Relative diffusion of antimicrobial agents from blood into CSF: Good only with inflammation (exceeds usual MICs)

CSF:blood level ratio: Meninges: Inflamed: 8% to 40%; Normal: ~1%

Protein binding: 56%

Metabolism: Injection: Hepatic (minor %)

Half-life elimination: Injection:

Neonates: <7 days, ≤2.5 kg: 5.5 to 9.9 hours; <7 days, >2.5 kg: 2.6 hours; 1 week to 1 month: 2.4 hours

Children 2 months to 12 years: 1.7 hours

Children with cystic fibrosis: 1.3 hours

Adults: Normal renal function: 1.7 to 2.9 hours

End-stage renal disease (ESRD): 6 to 8 hours

Time to peak: IM, IV push: Within 60 minutes; IV infusion: 1.5 hours

Excretion: Injection: Urine (60% to 70% as unchanged drug); feces (~13% to 15%)

Dosing

Adult & Geriatric

Urinary tract infection: IM, IV: 500 mg to 1 g every 8 to 12 hours

Moderately severe systemic infections: 1 g IV or IM or 2 g IV every 8 to 12 hours. **Note:** IV route preferred for septicemia, intra-abdominal abscess, or peritonitis; higher doses (8 to 12 g daily) may be needed for patients with cystic fibrosis (Zobell, 2013) or other infections (Solomkin, 2010).

Severe systemic or life-threatening infections (eg, *Pseudomonas aeruginosa*): IV: 2 g every 6 to 8 hours; maximum: 8 g daily. **Note:** Higher doses (8 to 12 g daily) may be needed for patients with cystic fibrosis (Zobell, 2013) or other infections (Solomkin, 2010).

Surgical (perioperative) prophylaxis (off-label use): IV: 2 g within 60 minutes prior to surgery. Doses may be repeated in 4 hours if procedure is lengthy or if there is excessive blood loss (Bratzler, 2013).

Pediatric

Mild-to-moderate infections: Infants ≥9 months, Children, and Adolescents: IV: 30 mg/kg/dose every 8 hours; maximum: 120 mg/kg/day (8 g daily)

Moderate-to-severe infections: Infants ≥9 months, Children, and Adolescents: IV: 30 mg/kg/dose every 6 to 8 hours; maximum: 120 mg/kg/day (8 g daily)

Cystic fibrosis: Infants ≥9 months, Children, and Adolescents: IV: 50 mg/kg/dose every 6 to 8 hours (ie, up to 200 mg/kg/day); maximum: 8 g daily. **Note:** Higher doses (8 to 12 g daily) may be needed for patients with cystic fibrosis (Zobell, 2013).

Surgical (perioperative) prophylaxis (off-label use): Children ≥1 year and Adolescents: IV: 30 mg/kg within 60 minutes prior to surgery (maximum: 2,000 mg per dose). Doses may be repeated in 4 hours if procedure is lengthy or if there is excessive blood loss (Bratzler, 2013).

Renal Impairment

IM, IV: Adults: Following initial dose, maintenance doses should be given as follows:

CrCl 10 to 30 mL/minute: 50% of usual dose at the usual interval

CrCl <10 mL/minute: 25% of usual dosage at the usual interval

Intermittent hemodialysis (IHD): Dialyzable (20% to 50%): Loading dose of 500 mg, 1 g, or 2 g, followed by 25% of initial dose at usual interval; for serious/life-threatening infections, administer 12.5% of initial dose after each hemodialysis session (given in addition to the maintenance doses). Alternatively, may administer 500 mg every 12 hours (Heintz, 2009). **Note:** Dosing dependent on the assumption of 3 times/week, complete IHD sessions.

Peritoneal dialysis (PD): Administer as for CrCl <10 mL/minute (Aronoff, 2007)

Continuous renal replacement therapy (CRRT) (Heintz, 2009; Trotman, 2005): Drug clearance is highly dependent on the method of renal replacement, filter type, and flow rate. Appropriate dosing requires close monitoring of pharmacologic response, signs of adverse reactions due to drug accumulation, as well as drug concentrations in relation to target trough (if appropriate). The following are general recommendations only (based on dialysate flow/ultrafiltration rates of 1 to 2 L/hour and minimal residual renal function) and should not supersede clinical judgment:

CVVH: Loading dose of 2 g followed by 1 to 2 g every 12 hours

CVVHD/CVVHDF: Loading dose of 2 g followed by either 1 g every 8 hours **or** 2 g every 12 hours (Heintz, 2009)

Hepatic Impairment No dosage adjustment provided in manufacturer's labeling. Use with caution (minor hepatic elimination occurs).

Administration

Injection: Doses >1 g should be administered IV

IM: Administer by deep injection into large muscle mass, such as upper outer quadrant of gluteus maximus or the lateral part of the thigh

IV: Administer by slow IV push over 3 to 5 minutes or by intermittent infusion over 20 to 60 minutes.

Monitoring Parameters Injection: Periodic liver function test; monitor for signs of anaphylaxis during first dose

Test Interactions May interfere with urine glucose tests containing cupric sulfate (Benedict's solution, Clinitest); positive Coombs' test

Additional Information Although marketed as an agent similar to aminoglycosides, aztreonam is a monobactam antimicrobial with almost pure gram-negative aerobic activity. It cannot be used for gram-positive infections.

Dosage Forms Excipient information presented when available (limited, particularly for generics); consult specific product labeling.

Solution, Intravenous:

Azactam in Dextrose: 1 g (50 mL); 2 g (50 mL) [sodium free]

Solution Reconstituted, Injection:

Azactam: 1 g (1 ea); 2 g (1 ea) [sodium free]

Generic: 1 g (1 ea); 2 g (1 ea)

Aztreonam (Oral Inhalation) (AZ tree oh nam)

Brand Names: US Cayston

Brand Names: Canada Cayston

Index Terms Azthreonam

Pharmacologic Category Antibiotic, Miscellaneous

Use Cystic fibrosis: Improve respiratory symptoms in cystic fibrosis (CF) patients with pulmonary *Pseudomonas aeruginosa* infections

Pregnancy Considerations Animal reproduction studies have not been conducted with aztreonam solution for inhalation; however, adverse events were not observed in animal reproduction studies conducted with the injection. Aztreonam crosses the placenta and reaches the fetal circulation following IV administration; however, peak plasma concentrations following inhalation of aztreonam are significantly less than those observed following aztreonam IV.

Breast-Feeding Considerations Aztreonam is excreted into breast milk following intravenous administration. The peak plasma concentration of aztreonam following inhalation is <1% of the peak concentration seen following IV administration. Maternal use of inhaled aztreonam is not likely to pose a risk to breast-feeding infants.

Prescribing and Access Restrictions Cayston (aztreonam inhalation solution) is only available through a select group of specialty pharmacies and cannot be obtained through a retail pharmacy. Because Cayston may only be used with the Altera Nebulizer System, it can only be obtained from the following specialty pharmacies: IV Solutions/Maxor; Foundation Care; Pharmaceutical Specialties Inc; TLCRx/ ModernHEALTH; and Walgreens Specialty Pharmacy. This network of specialty pharmacies ensures proper access to both the drug and device. To obtain the medication and proper nebulizer, contact the Cayston Access Program at 1-877-7CAYSTON (1-877-722-9786) or at www.cayston.com. In Canada, Cayston is distributed by Innomar Solutions specialty pharmacy; Canadian healthcare providers and patients may obtain additional information at http://cayston.ca/

Contraindications Hypersensitivity to aztreonam or any component of the formulation

Warnings/Precautions Rare cross-allergenicity to penicillins, cephalosporins, or carbapenems may occur; use with caution in patients with a history of hypersensitivity to beta-lactams. Patients colonized with *Burkholderia cepacia* have not been studied. Safety and efficacy has not been established in patients with FEV_1 <25% or >75% predicted. Compare patient's baseline FEV_1 prior to therapy and the presence of other symptoms when deciding if post-treatment FEV_1 changes (eg, decline) are caused by a pulmonary exacerbation. Reserve use for CF patients with known *Pseudomonas aeruginosa*. Bronchospasm may occur following nebulization; administer a bronchodilator prior to treatment.

Adverse Reactions

>10%:

Gastrointestinal: Pharyngolaryngeal pain (12%)

Respiratory: Cough (54%), nasal congestion (16%), wheezing (16%)

Miscellaneous: Fever (13%; more common in children)

1% to 10%:

Cardiovascular: Chest discomfort (8%)

Dermatologic: Skin rash (2%)

Gastrointestinal: Abdominal pain (7%), vomiting (6%)

Respiratory: Bronchospasm (3%; patients experienced ≥15% reduction in FEV_1)

<1% (Limited to important or life-threatening): Arthralgia, facial rash, facial swelling, hypersensitivity reaction, joint swelling, pharyngeal edema

Drug Interactions

Metabolism/Transport Effects None known.

Avoid Concomitant Use There are no known interactions where it is recommended to avoid concomitant use.

Increased Effect/Toxicity There are no known significant interactions involving an increase in effect.

Decreased Effect There are no known significant interactions involving a decrease in effect.

Preparation for Administration Reconstitute with 1 mL of sterile diluent (saline) immediately prior to use. Squeeze diluent into opened glass vial. Replace rubber stopper and gently swirl vial until contents have completely dissolved.

Storage/Stability Prior to reconstitution, store at 2°C to 8°C (36°F to 46°F). Once removed from refrigeration, aztreonam and the diluent may be stored at room temperature (up to 25°C [77°F]) for ≤28 days. Protect from light. Use immediately after reconstitution.

Mechanism of Action Inhibits bacterial cell wall synthesis by binding to one or more of the penicillin-binding proteins (PBPs), which in turn inhibits the final transpeptidation step of peptidoglycan synthesis in bacterial cell walls, thus inhibiting cell wall biosynthesis. Bacteria eventually lyse due to ongoing activity of cell wall autolytic enzymes (autolysins and murein hydrolases), while cell wall assembly is arrested. Monobactam structure makes cross-allergenicity with beta-lactams unlikely.

Pharmacodynamics/Kinetics

Absorption: Low systemic absorption

Protein binding: 56%

Half-life elimination: Adults: 2.1 hours

Excretion: Urine (10% [compared with 60% to 70% for injection] as unchanged drug)

Dosing

Adult Cystic fibrosis: Inhalation (nebulizer): 75 mg 3 times daily (at least 4 hours apart) for 28 days; do not repeat for 28 days after completion. **Note:** Pretreatment with a bronchodilator is recommended

Pediatric Cystic fibrosis: Note: Pretreatment with a bronchodilator is recommended.

US labeling: Children ≥7 years and Adolescents: Inhalation (nebulizer): Refer to adult dosing.

Canadian labeling: Children ≥6 years and Adolescents: Inhalation (nebulizer): Refer to adult dosing.

Renal Impairment No dosage adjustment necessary.

Hepatic Impairment

US labeling: There are no dosage adjustments provided in the manufacturer's labeling.

Canadian labeling: No dosage adjustment is necessary; minimal systemic absorption following inhalation.

Administration Administer using only an Altera nebulizer system; **administer alone; do not mix with other nebulizer medications.** Administer a bronchodilator before administration of aztreonam (short-acting: 15 minutes to 4 hours before; long-acting: 30 minutes to 12 hours before). For patients on multiple inhaled therapies, administer bronchodilator first, then mucolytic, and lastly, aztreonam.

To administer Cayston, pour reconstituted solution into the handset of the nebulizer system, turn unit on. Place the mouthpiece in the patient's mouth and encourage to breathe normally through the mouth. Administration time is usually 2 to 3 minutes. Administer doses ≥4 hours apart.

Monitoring Parameters Consider measuring FEV_1 prior to initiation of therapy

Dosage Forms Excipient information presented when available (limited, particularly for generics); consult specific product labeling.

Solution Reconstituted, Inhalation [preservative free]:
Cayston: 75 mg (84 mL) [arginine free]

◆ **Azulfidine** see SulfaSALAzine on page 1714

◆ **Azulfidine EN-tabs** see SulfaSALAzine on page 1714

◆ **Azuphen MB** see Methenamine, Sodium Phosphate Monobasic, Phenyl Salicylate, Methylene Blue, and Hyoscyamine on page 1166

◆ **Azurette** see Ethinyl Estradiol and Desogestrel on page 701

◆ **B-2-400 [OTC]** see Riboflavin on page 1579

◆ **B6** see Pyridoxine on page 1533

◆ **B-12 Compliance Injection** see Cyanocobalamin on page 453

◆ **B1939** see Eribulin on page 664

◆ **B2036-PEG** see Pegvisomant on page 1414

◆ **Baby Anbesol [OTC]** see Benzocaine on page 217

◆ **Baby Aspirin** see Aspirin on page 157

◆ **Baby Ayr Saline [OTC]** see Sodium Chloride on page 1671

◆ **BabyBIG®** see Botulism Immune Globulin (Intravenous-Human) on page 249

◆ **BACiiM** see Bacitracin (Systemic) on page 196

◆ **BaciJect (Can)** see Bacitracin (Systemic) on page 196

◆ **Bacillus Calmette-Guérin (BCG) Live** see BCG (Intravesical) on page 203

◆ **Bacillus Calmette-Guérin (BCG) Live** see BCG Vaccine (Immunization) on page 203

◆ **Bacitin (Can)** see Bacitracin (Topical) on page 196

Bacitracin (Systemic) (bas i TRAY sin)

Brand Names: US BACiiM
Brand Names: Canada BaciJect
Pharmacologic Category Antibiotic, Miscellaneous
Use Pneumonia and empyema: Treatment of pneumonia and empyema in infants caused by susceptible staphylococci; due to toxicity risks, systemic uses of bacitracin should be limited to situations where less toxic alternatives would not be effective

Dosing
Pediatric Do not administer IV
Treatment of pneumonia and empyema: Infants: IM:
≤2.5 kg: 900 units/kg/day in 2 to 3 divided doses
>2.5 kg: 1000 units/kg/day in 2 to 3 divided doses
Additional Information Complete prescribing information should be consulted for additional detail.
Dosage Forms Excipient information presented when available (limited, particularly for generics); consult specific product labeling.
Solution Reconstituted, Intramuscular:
BACiiM: 50,000 units (1 ea)
Generic: 50,000 units (1 ea)
Solution Reconstituted, Intramuscular [preservative free]:
Generic: 50,000 units (1 ea)

Bacitracin (Ophthalmic) (bas i TRAY sin)

Pharmacologic Category Antibiotic, Ophthalmic
Use Superficial ocular infections: Treatment of superficial ocular infections involving the conjunctiva or cornea due to susceptible organisms

Dosing
Adult & Geriatric Ophthalmic infection: Ophthalmic: Apply 1 to 3 times daily
Pediatric Ophthalmic infection: Children and Adolescents: Ophthalmic: Refer to adult dosing.
Additional Information Complete prescribing information should be consulted for additional detail.
Dosage Forms Excipient information presented when available (limited, particularly for generics); consult specific product labeling.
Ointment, Ophthalmic:
Generic: 500 units/g (1 g, 3.5 g)

Bacitracin (Topical) (bas i TRAY sin)

Brand Names: Canada Bacitin
Pharmacologic Category Antibiotic, Topical
Use Topical infection prevention: Prevention of infection in minor cuts, scrapes, or burns
Dosing
Adult & Geriatric Prevention of infection: Topical: Apply 1 to 3 times daily.
Pediatric Prevention of infection: Children and Adolescents: Topical: Refer to adult dosing.
Additional Information Complete prescribing information should be consulted for additional detail.
Dosage Forms Excipient information presented when available (limited, particularly for generics); consult specific product labeling.
Ointment, External, as zinc [strength expressed as base]:
Generic: 500 units/g (1 ea, 1 g, 14 g, 14.2 g, 15 g, 28 g, 28.35 g, 28.4 g, 30 g, 120 g, 453.9 g, 454 g)

Bacitracin and Polymyxin B (Ophthalmic) (bas i TRAY sin & pol i MIKS in bee)

Brand Names: US AK-Poly-Bac; Polycin; Polycin B [DSC]
Brand Names: Canada LID-Pack; Optimyxin
Index Terms Polymyxin B and Bacitracin
Pharmacologic Category Antibiotic, Ophthalmic
Use Superficial ocular infections: Treatment of superficial infections caused by susceptible organisms
Dosing
Adult & Geriatric Superficial ocular infections: Ophthalmic: Apply to affected eye(s) every 3 to 4 hours for 7 to 10 days
Pediatric Conjunctivitis: Infants, Children, and Adolescents: Ophthalmic: Apply to affected eye(s) 4 times daily (Giggliotti 1984; Ward 1997)
Renal Impairment There are no dosage adjustments provided in the manufacturer's labeling.
Hepatic Impairment There are no dosage adjustments provided in the manufacturer's labeling.
Additional Information Complete prescribing information should be consulted for additional detail.
Dosage Forms Excipient information presented when available (limited, particularly for generics); consult specific product labeling. [DSC] = Discontinued product
Ointment, Ophthalmic:
Polycin: Bacitracin 500 units and polymyxin B 10,000 units per g (3.5 g)
Polycin B: Bacitracin 500 units and polymyxin B 10,000 units per g (3.5 g [DSC])
Generic: Bacitracin 500 units and polymyxin B 10,000 units per g (3.5 g)
Ointment, Ophthalmic [preservative free]:
AK-Poly-Bac: Bacitracin 500 units and polymyxin B 10,000 units per g (3.5 g)

Bacitracin and Polymyxin B (Topical) (bas i TRAY sin & pol i MIKS in bee)

Brand Names: US Double Antibiotic [OTC]; Polysporin [OTC]
Index Terms Polymyxin B and Bacitracin
Pharmacologic Category Antibiotic, Topical
Use Topical infection prevention: Prevention of infection in minor cuts, scrapes, or burns
Dosing
Adult & Geriatric Topical infection prevention: Topical: Apply to affected area 1 to 3 times/day; may cover with sterile bandage if needed.
Pediatric Topical infection prevention: Children and Adolescents: Refer to adult dosing.
Additional Information Complete prescribing information should be consulted for additional detail.
Dosage Forms Excipient information presented when available (limited, particularly for generics); consult specific product labeling.
Ointment, External:
Double Antibiotic: 500-10,000 units/g (1 ea, 14.17 g, 28.35 g)
Polysporin: 500-10,000 units/g (1 ea, 14.2 g, 28.3 g)

Bacitracin, Neomycin, and Polymyxin B (Ophthalmic) (bas i TRAY sin, nee oh MYE sin, & pol i MIKS in bee)

Brand Names: US Neo-Polycin
Index Terms Neomycin, Bacitracin, and Polymyxin B; Polymyxin B, Bacitracin, and Neomycin
Pharmacologic Category Antibiotic, Ophthalmic

Use Superficial ocular infections: Short-term treatment of superficial external ocular infections caused by susceptible organisms

Dosing

Adult & Geriatric Superficial ocular infections: Ophthalmic: Apply every 3 to 4 hours for 7 to 10 days for acute infections.

Pediatric Conjunctivitis: Limited data available: Children and Adolescents: Ophthalmic: Ointment: Apply 0.5 inch ribbon every 3 to 4 hours for acute infections, or 2 to 3 times per day for mild to moderate infections, for 7 to 10 days (Pichichero 2011).

Renal Impairment There are no dosage adjustments provided in the manufacturer's labeling.

Hepatic Impairment There are no dosage adjustments provided in the manufacturer's labeling.

Additional Information Complete prescribing information should be consulted for additional detail.

Dosage Forms Excipient information presented when available (limited, particularly for generics); consult specific product labeling.

Ointment, Ophthalmic:

Neo-Polycin: Bacitracin 400 units, neomycin 3.5 mg, and polymyxin B 10,000 units per g (3.5 g)

Generic: 5-400-10000 (3.5 g); Bacitracin 400 units, neomycin 3.5 mg, and polymyxin B 10,000 units per g (3.5 g)

Bacitracin, Neomycin, and Polymyxin B (Topical) (bas i TRAY sin, nee oh MYE sin, & pol i MIKS in bee)

Brand Names: US Medi-First Triple Antibiotic [OTC]; Neosporin Original [OTC]; Triple Antibiotic [OTC]

Index Terms Neomycin, Bacitracin, and Polymyxin B; Polymyxin B, Bacitracin, and Neomycin; Triple Antibiotic

Pharmacologic Category Antibiotic, Topical

Use Topical infection prevention: Prevention of infection in minor cuts

Dosing

Adult & Geriatric Topical infection prevention: Topical: Apply 1 to 3 times/day to infected area; may cover with sterile bandage if necessary.

Pediatric Topical infection prevention: Children and Adolescents: Refer to adult dosing.

Renal Impairment There are no dosage adjustments provided in the manufacturer's labeling. However, dosage adjustment unlikely due to low systemic absorption.

Hepatic Impairment There are no dosage adjustments provided in the manufacturer's labeling. However, dosage adjustment unlikely due to low systemic absorption.

Additional Information Complete prescribing information should be consulted for additional detail.

Dosage Forms Excipient information presented when available (limited, particularly for generics); consult specific product labeling.

Ointment, External:

Medi-First Triple Antibiotic: Bacitracin 400 units, neomycin 3.5 mg, and polymyxin B 5000 units per g (1 ea)

Neosporin Original: Bacitracin 400 units, neomycin 3.5 mg, and polymyxin B 5000 units per g (1 ea, 14.2 g, 15 g, 28.3 g)

Triple Antibiotic: Bacitracin 400 units, neomycin 3.5 mg, and polymyxin B 5000 units per g (1 ea, 1 g, 9.4 g, 14 g, 14.2 g, 15 g, 28 g, 28.4 g, 30 g, 453.9 g)

Generic: Bacitracin 400 units, neomycin 3.5 mg, and polymyxin B 5000 units per g (1 ea, 15 g, 28.35 g)

Bacitracin, Neomycin, Polymyxin B, and Hydrocortisone (Ophthalmic)

(bas i TRAY sin, nee oh MYE sin, pol i MIKS in bee, & hye droe KOR ti sone)

Brand Names: US Neo-Polycin HC

Index Terms Hydrocortisone, Bacitracin, Neomycin, and Polymyxin B; Neomycin, Bacitracin, Polymyxin B, and Hydrocortisone; Polymyxin B, Bacitracin, Neomycin, and Hydrocortisone

Pharmacologic Category Antibiotic, Ophthalmic; Corticosteroid, Ophthalmic

Use Inflammatory ocular conditions: Corticosteroid-responsive inflammatory ocular conditions where bacterial infection or risk of bacterial infection exists

Dosing

Adult & Geriatric Inflammatory ocular conditions: Ophthalmic: Apply to inside of lower lid of affected eye(s) every 3 or 4 hours (depending on severity of condition)

Renal Impairment There are no dosage adjustments provided in the manufacturer's labeling. Dosage adjustment unlikely due to low systemic absorption.

Hepatic Impairment There are no dosage adjustments provided in the manufacturer's labeling. Dosage adjustment unlikely due to low systemic absorption.

Additional Information Complete prescribing information should be consulted for additional detail.

Dosage Forms Excipient information presented when available (limited, particularly for generics); consult specific product labeling.

Ointment, ophthalmic:

Generic: Bacitracin 400 units, neomycin 3.5 mg, polymyxin B 10,000 units, and hydrocortisone 10 mg per g (3.5 g)

Neo-Polycin HC: Bacitracin 400 units, neomycin 3.5 mg, polymyxin B 10,000 units, and hydrocortisone 10 mg per g (3.5 g)

Bacitracin, Neomycin, Polymyxin B, and Hydrocortisone (Topical)

(bas i TRAY sin, nee oh MYE sin, pol i MIKS in bee, & hye droe KOR ti sone)

Brand Names: US Cortisporin Ointment

Brand Names: Canada Cortisporin Topical Ointment

Index Terms Hydrocortisone, Bacitracin, Neomycin, and Polymyxin B; Neomycin, Bacitracin, Polymyxin B, and Hydrocortisone; Polymyxin B, Bacitracin, Neomycin, and Hydrocortisone

Pharmacologic Category Antibiotic, Topical; Corticosteroid, Topical

Use Superficial dermal infection: Treatment of corticosteroid-responsive dermatoses with secondary infection

Dosing

Adult & Geriatric Superficial dermal infection: Topical: Apply sparingly to affected area 2 to 4 times daily for up to 7 days

Renal Impairment There are no dosage adjustments provided in the manufacturer's labeling.

Hepatic Impairment There are no dosage adjustments provided in the manufacturer's labeling.

Additional Information Complete prescribing information should be consulted for additional detail.

Dosage Forms Excipient information presented when available (limited, particularly for generics); consult specific product labeling.

Ointment, topical:

Cortisporin: Bacitracin 400 units, neomycin 3.5 mg, polymyxin B 5000 units, and hydrocortisone 10 mg per g (15 g)

Baclofen (BAK loe fen)

Brand Names: US Ed Baclofen [DSC]; EnovaRX-Baclofen; Equipto-Baclofen; Gablofen; Lioresal

Brand Names: Canada Apo-Baclofen; Dom-Baclofen; Lioresal; Lioresal D.S.; Lioresal Intrathecal; Mylan-Baclofen; Novo-Baclofen; PHL-Baclofen; PMS-Baclofen; ratio-Baclofen; Riva-Baclofen; VPI-Baclofen Intrathecal

Pharmacologic Category Skeletal Muscle Relaxant

Use

Spasticity:

Oral: Management of reversible spasticity associated with multiple sclerosis or spinal cord lesions

Intrathecal: Management of severe spasticity of spinal cord origin (eg, spinal cord injury, multiple sclerosis) or cerebral origin (eg, cerebral palsy, traumatic brain injury) in patients ≥4 years; may be considered as an alternative to destructive neurosurgical procedures.

Limitations of use: Patients should first respond to a screening dose of intrathecal baclofen prior to consideration for long term infusion via an implantable pump. For spasticity of spinal cord origin, chronic infusion via an implantable pump should be reserved for patients unresponsive to oral baclofen therapy, or those who experience intolerable CNS side effects at effective doses. Patients with spasticity due to traumatic brain injury should wait at least one year after the injury before consideration of long term intrathecal baclofen therapy.

Pregnancy Considerations Adverse events were observed in animal reproduction studies. Withdrawal symptoms in the neonate were noted in a case report following the maternal use of oral baclofen 20 mg 4 times/day throughout pregnancy (Ratnayaka, 2001). Plasma concentrations following administration of intrathecal baclofen are significantly less than those with oral doses; exposure to the fetus is expected to be limited (Morton, 2009).

◄ **Breast-Feeding Considerations** Baclofen is excreted into breast milk. Very small amounts were found in the breast milk of a woman 14 days postpartum after oral use. Following a single oral dose of baclofen 20 mg, the total amount of baclofen excreted in breast milk within 26 hours was 22 mcg (Eriksson, 1981). Adverse events were not observed in a nursing infant following maternal use of intrathecal baclofen 200 mcg/day throughout pregnancy and while nursing (Morton, 2009). Due to the potential for adverse events in the nursing infant, breast-feeding is not recommended by the manufacturer.

Contraindications

Hypersensitivity to baclofen or any component of the formulation

Intrathecal: IV, IM, SubQ, or epidural administration

Warnings/Precautions [US Boxed Warning]: **Abrupt withdrawal of intrathecal baclofen has resulted in severe sequelae (hyperpyrexia, obtundation, rebound/exaggerated spasticity, muscle rigidity, and rhabdomyolysis), leading to organ failure and some fatalities. Prevention of abrupt discontinuation requires careful attention to programming and monitoring of infusion system, refill scheduling and procedures, and pump alarms. Risk may be higher in patients with injuries at T-6 or above, history of baclofen withdrawal, or limited ability to communicate.** Abrupt withdrawal of oral therapy has been associated with hallucinations and seizures; gradual dose reductions (over ~1 to 2 weeks) are recommended in the absence of severe adverse reactions.

Patients receiving intrathecal baclofen should be infection-free prior to the test dose and pump implantation. Clinicians should be experienced with chronic intrathecal infusion therapy. Pump should only be implanted if patients' response to bolus intrathecal baclofen was adequately evaluated and found to be safe and effective. Resuscitative equipment should be readily available. Monitor closely during the initial phase of pump use and when adjusting the dosing rate and/or the concentration in the reservoir. Educate patients and caregivers on proper home care of the pump and insertion site; early symptoms of baclofen withdrawal (eg, return of baseline spasticity, hypotension, paresthesia, pruritus); signs/symptoms of overdose (eg, dizziness, somnolence, respiratory depression, seizures); and appropriate actions in the event of an overdose. Cases (most from pharmacy compounded preparations) of intrathecal mass formation at the implanted catheter tip have been reported; may lead to loss of clinical response, pain or new/worsening neurological effects. Neurosurgical evaluation and/or an appropriate imaging study should be considered if a mass is suspected. Use caution with history of autonomic dysreflexia; presence of nociceptive stimuli or abrupt baclofen withdrawal may cause an autonomic dysreflexia episode.

May cause CNS depression, which may impair physical or mental abilities; patients must be cautioned about performing tasks which require mental alertness (eg, operating machinery or driving). Elderly patients are more sensitive to the effects of baclofen and are more likely to experience adverse CNS effects at higher doses. Use with caution in patients with seizure disorder, respiratory disease, psychiatric disease, peptic ulcer disease, decreased GI motility, and/or gastrointestinal obstructive disorders.

Use with caution in patients with renal impairment; baclofen is eliminated primarily unchanged via the kidneys. Multiple cases describing neurotoxicity due to oral baclofen accumulation in adult patients with varying levels of renal impairment have been reported in the literature. In patients with renal impairment, initiation of oral baclofen at lower doses and/or extended intervals has been suggested (Aisen 1994; Chen 1997; Chou 2006; El-Husseini 2011; Peces 1998; Su 2009; Vlavonu 2014).

Efficacy of oral baclofen has not been established in patients with stroke, Parkinson disease, or cerebral palsy; therefore, use is not recommended. Not indicated for spasticity associated with rheumatic disorders. Use with caution when spasticity is utilized to sustain upright posture and balance in locomotion, or when spasticity is necessary to obtain increased function. Adverse effects are more likely in patients with spastic states of cerebral origin; cautious dosing and careful monitoring are necessary.

Animal studies have shown an increased incidence in ovarian cysts; however, incidence observed in multiple sclerosis patients treated with baclofen for up to one year was similar to the estimated incidence in healthy females. Spontaneous resolution occurred in most of these MS patients while continuing treatment. May cause acute urinary retention (may be related to underlying disease);

use with caution in patients with urinary obstruction. Potentially significant drug-drug interactions may exist, requiring dose or frequency adjustment, additional monitoring, and/or selection of alternative therapy.

Adverse Reactions

>10%:

Central nervous system: Hypotonia (2% to 35%), drowsiness (6% to 21%), confusion (1% to 11%), headache (2% to 11%)

Gastrointestinal: Nausea (1% to 12%), vomiting (2% to 11%)

1% to 10%:

Cardiovascular: Hypotension (≤9%), peripheral edema (≤3%)

Central nervous system: Convulsions (≤10%), dizziness (2% to 8%), insomnia (≤7%), paresthesia (≤7%), hypertonia (≤6%), pain (≤4%), speech disturbance (≤4%), depression (2%), coma (≤2%), abnormality in thinking (≤1%), agitation (≤1%), chills (≤1%)

Dermatologic: Pruritus (4%), urticaria (≤1%)

Gastrointestinal: Constipation (≤6%), sialorrhea (3%), xerostomia (≤3%), diarrhea (≤2%)

Genitourinary: Urinary retention (≤8%), urinary frequency (≤6%), difficulty in micturition (2%), impotence (≤2%), urinary incontinence (≤2%)

Neuromuscular & skeletal: Back pain (≤2%), weakness (≤2%), tremor (≤1%)

Ophthalmic: Amblyopia (≤2%)

Respiratory: Hypoventilation (≤4%), pneumonia (≤2%), dyspnea (≤1%)

Miscellaneous: Accidental injury (≤4%)

<1% (Limited to important or life-threatening): Accommodation disturbance, akathisia, albuminuria, alopecia, amnesia, apnea, ataxia, blurred vision, bradycardia, bradypnea, carcinoma, chest pain, decreased appetite, deep vein thrombosis, dehydration, diaphoresis, diplopia, disorientation, dysarthria, dysautonomia, dysgeusia, dysphagia, dysphoria, dystonia, dysuria, epilepsy, facial edema, fecal incontinence, gastrointestinal hemorrhage, hyperglycemia, hyperhidrosis, hypertension, hyperventilation, hypothermia, hysteria, inhibited ejaculation, intestinal obstruction, lethargy, leukocytosis, loss of postural reflex, lower extremity weakness, malaise, miosis, muscle rigidity, myalgia, mydriasis, nephrolithiasis, nocturia, nystagmus, occult blood in stools, oliguria, opisthotonus, pallor, palpitations, petechial rash, pulmonary embolism, respiratory depression, sedation, slurred speech, strabismus, suicidal ideation, syncope, vasodilatation

Withdrawal reactions have occurred with abrupt discontinuation (particularly severe with intrathecal use).

Drug Interactions

Metabolism/Transport Effects None known.

Avoid Concomitant Use

Avoid concomitant use of Baclofen with any of the following: Azelastine (Nasal); Orphenadrine; Paraldehyde; Thalidomide

Increased Effect/Toxicity

Baclofen may increase the levels/effects of: Alcohol (Ethyl); Azelastine (Nasal); Buprenorphine; CNS Depressants; Hydrocodone; Lacidipine; Methotrimeprazine; Metyrosine; Mirtazapine; Orphenadrine; Paraldehyde; Pramipexole; ROPINIRole; Rotigotine; Selective Serotonin Reuptake Inhibitors; Suvorexant; Thalidomide; Zolpidem

The levels/effects of Baclofen may be increased by: Brimonidine (Topical); Cannabis; Doxylamine; Dronabinol; Droperidol; HydrOXYzine; Kava Kava; Magnesium Sulfate; Methotrimeprazine; Minocycline; Nabilone; Perampanel; Rufinamide; Sodium Oxybate; Tapentadol; Tetrahydrocannabinol

Decreased Effect There are no known significant interactions involving a decrease in effect.

Preparation for Administration Intrathecal: Screening doses are a 50 mcg/mL concentration and only the 1 mL screening ampul or screening syringe (50 mcg/mL) is used; do not further dilute. Maintenance infusions for patients who require concentrations other than 500 mcg/mL, 1,000 mcg/mL, or 2,000 mcg/mL must be diluted with preservative-free sodium chloride. Discard any unused solution.

Storage/Stability

Injection: Do not store above 30°C (86°F). Does not require refrigeration. Do not freeze or heat sterilize.

Tablets: Store at 20°C to 25°C (68°F to 77°F).

Mechanism of Action Inhibits the transmission of both monosynaptic and polysynaptic reflexes at the spinal cord level, possibly by hyperpolarization of primary afferent fiber terminals, with resultant relief of muscle spasticity

Pharmacodynamics/Kinetics

Onset of action: Intrathecal bolus: 30 minutes to 1 hour; Continuous infusion: 6 to 8 hours after infusion initiation

Peak effect: Intrathecal bolus: 4 hours (effects may last 4 to 8 hours); Continuous infusion: 24 to 48 hours

Absorption (dose dependent): Oral: Rapid; absorption from the GI tract is thought to be dose dependent; in pediatric patients (age range: 2 to 17 years) with cerebral palsy, absorption from GI tract highly variable and delayed (reported time lag: 0.59 ± 0.28 hours) (He 2014)

Protein binding: 30%

Volume of distribution: Pediatric patients (age range: 2 to 17 years): Oral: Highly variable: 1.16 L/kg with 43.5% interindividual variability (He 2014)

Metabolism: Hepatic (15% of dose) (He 2014)

Half-life elimination: Oral:

Pediatric patients with cerebral palsy (age range: 2 to 17 years): Oral: 4.5 hours (He 2014)

Adults: 3.75 ± 0.96 hours (Brunton 2011); Intrathecal: CSF elimination half-life: 1.5 hours over the first 4 hours

Time to peak, serum: Oral: 1 hour (0.5 to 4 hours) (Brunton 2011)

Excretion: Urine (>70% as unchanged drug) and feces (Brunton 2011)

Dosing

Adult

Spasticity:

Oral: Initial: 5 mg 3 times daily; may increase by 5 mg per dose every 3 days (ie, 5 mg 3 times daily for 3 days, then 10 mg 3 times daily for 3 days, etc.) until optimal response is reached. Usual dosage range: 40 to 80 mg daily. Do not exceed 80 mg daily (20 mg 4 times daily).

Intrathecal:

Screening dose:

U.S. labeling: Initial: 50 mcg (1 mL) for 1 dose; following initial administration, observe patient for 4 to 8 hours. A positive response consists of a significant decrease in muscle tone and/or frequency and/or severity of spasms. If response is inadequate, may give 75 mcg as a second screening dose 24 hours after the first screening dose; observe patient for 4 to 8 hours. If response is still inadequate, may repeat a final screening dose of 100 mcg given 24 hours after the second screening dose. Patients not responding to screening dose of 100 mcg should not be considered for chronic infusion/implanted pump.

Canadian labeling: Initial: 25 to 50 mcg for 1 dose; titrate up in 25 mcg increments at least 24 hours apart until an approximately 4 to 8 hour response is observed. Patients not responding to screening dose of 100 mcg should not be given further increases in dose or be considered for chronic infusion/implanted pump; however, some patients, particularly those with spasticity of cerebral origin, have in rare instances received higher test bolus doses. **Note:** A 10 mcg dose may be administered if adverse reactions occur with a 25 mcg dose.

Dose titration following pump implant: After positive response to screening dose, a maintenance intrathecal infusion can be administered via an implanted intrathecal pump.

Initial total daily dose via pump: Double the screening dose that gave a positive response and administer over 24 hours, unless efficacy of the bolus dose was maintained for >8 hours (US labeling) or >12 hours (Canadian labeling), then infuse a dose equivalent to the screening dose over 24hours. Do not increase dose in first 24 hours (to allow steady state to be achieved); thereafter, dosage adjustments may be made as follows:

US labeling: Increase daily dose slowly by 10% to 30% (spasticity of spinal cord origin) or 5% to 15% (spasticity of cerebral origin) once every 24 hours until satisfactory response

Canadian labeling: Increase daily dose slowly by 10% to 30% once every 24 hours (if using a programmable pump) or once every 48 hours (if using a nonprogrammable pump)

Maintenance:

US labeling: Daily dose may be increased 5% to 20% (maximum increase: 20%) (spasticity of cerebral origin) or by 10% to 40% (maximum increase: 40%) (spasticity of spinal cord origin). Dose may also be decreased 10% to 20% for adverse effects. Most patients have been adequately maintained on 90 mcg to 703 mcg daily (spasticity of cerebral origin) or 300 mcg to 800 mcg daily (spasticity of spinal cord origin). Experience with doses >1,000 mcg daily is limited.

Canadian labeling: Daily dose may be increased 10% to 30%. Dose may also be decreased 10% to 20% for adverse effects. Most patients have been adequately maintained on 300 mcg to 800 mcg daily.

Note: Dosage adjustments may be required often during the first few months of therapy to adjust for life style changes due to alleviation of spasticity. Maintain lowest dose that produces adequate response. Most patients require gradual increases over time to maintain optimal response. Sudden large requirements for a dose increase may indicate a catheter complication (eg, kink, dislodgement). Titrate dose to allow sufficient muscle tone and occasional spasms to optimize activities of daily living, support circulation, and possibly prevent DVT formation. Use extreme caution when filling the pump; follow manufacturer instructions carefully. 5% to 10% of patients receiving chronic therapy become refractory to dose adjustments; may consider a drug holiday (hospitalized patients only) with a gradual withdrawal over 2 to 4 weeks and use of alternative spasticity management methods. Following the drug holiday intrathecal baclofen may be resumed at the initial continuous infusion dose.

Hiccups (off-label use): Oral: 5 to 10 mg 3 times daily (maximum: 75 mg daily in divided doses) (Guelaud 1995; Zhang 2014)

Geriatric Oral: Refer to adult dosing; use with caution. If benefits are not observed, withdraw the drug slowly.

Pediatric

Oral: **Note:** Use the lowest effective dose; patients who fail to respond within a reasonable amount of time should be slowly withdrawn from therapy (avoid abrupt withdrawal of drug).

Spasticity:

Oral:

Children ≥12 years and Adolescents: Refer to adult dosing.

Infants, Children, and Adolescents (off-label): **Note:** Dose-related side effects (eg, sedation) may be minimized by slow titration; lower initial doses than described below (2.5 to 10 mg **daily**) may be used with subsequent titration to 8 hourly doses. There is limited published data in infants and children; the following is a compilation of small prospective studies (Milla 1977; Scheinberg 2006) and one large retrospective analysis of baclofen use in children (Lubsch 2006). Efficacy results variable (AAN [Delgado] 2010)

Infants ≥4 months and Children <2 years: Limited data available: 10 to 20 mg **daily** divided every 8 hours; begin at low end of range and titrate dose to patient response, titration intervals of every 3 days to weekly have been used in pediatric patients ≥2 years (Millia 1997; Scheinberg 2006). Maximum daily dose: 40 mg/**day** (Lubsch 2006). **Note:** To minimize dose-related side effects (eg, sedation), lower initial doses (eg, 2.5 mg once daily) and slower titration may be considered (eg, weekly) and has been reported in pediatric patients >2 years (Scheinberg 2006).

2 to 7 years: Limited data available: 20 to 40 mg **daily** divided every 8 hours; begin at low end of range (or even lower [2.5 to 10 mg **daily**] and titrate dose to patient response; titration intervals of every 3 days to weekly have been used in pediatric patients. Maximum daily dose: 60 mg/day (Lubsch 2006; Millia 1997; Scheinberg 2006).

≥8 years and Adolescents: Limited data available in children <12 years: 30 to 40 mg **daily** divided every 8 hours; begin at low end of range (or even lower [10 mg to 15 mg **daily** in 3 divided doses]) and titrate dose to patient response, titration intervals of every 3 days to weekly have been used (Millia 1997; Scheinberg 2006); some patients ≥12 years may require every 6 hour dosing; usual maximum daily dose range: 60 to 80 mg/**day** (Lubsch 2006; Millia 1977). **Note:** Higher maximum daily doses (up to 200 mg/day) have been described in some patients in a retrospective review, usually the higher doses were needed over time (Lubsch 2006).

Intrathecal: Children ≥4 years and Adolescents (US labeling):

Screening dose: Initial: 50 mcg (1 mL) for 1 dose; following initial administration, observe patient for 4 to 8 hours. A positive response consists of a significant decrease in muscle tone and/or frequency and/or severity of spasms. If response is inadequate, may give 75 mcg as a second screening dose 24 hours after the first screening dose; observe patient for 4 to 8 hours. If response is still inadequate, may

repeat a final screening dose of 100 mcg given 24 hours after the second screening dose. Patients not responding to screening dose of 100 mcg should not be considered for chronic infusion/implanted pump. **Note:** A 25 mcg initial screening dose may be considered in very small pediatric patients.

Dose titration following pump implant: After positive response to screening dose, a maintenance intrathecal infusion can be administered via an implanted intrathecal pump.

Initial total daily dose via pump: Double the screening dose that gave a positive response and administer over 24 hours, unless efficacy of the bolus dose was maintained for >8 hours, then infuse a dose equivalent to the screening dose over 24 hours. Do not increase dose in first 24 hours (to allow steady state to be achieved); thereafter, increase daily dose slowly by 5% to 15% once every 24 hours until satisfactory response.

Maintenance: Daily dose may be increased 5% to 20% (maximum increase: 20%). Dose may also be decreased 10% to 20% for adverse effects. Patients <12 years required lower daily doses in clinical trials (average dose: 274 mcg daily; dosage range: 24 mcg to 1,199 mcg/day); dose requirements of patients >12 years were similar to that of adults.

Note: Dosage adjustments may be required often during the first few months of therapy to adjust for life style changes due to alleviation of spasticity. Maintain lowest dose that produces adequate response. Most patients require gradual increases over time to maintain optimal response. Sudden large requirements for a dose increase may indicate a catheter complication (eg, kink, dislodgement). Titrate dose to allow sufficient muscle tone and occasional spasms to optimize activities of daily living, support circulation, and possibly prevent DVT formation. **Use extreme caution when filling the pump; follow manufacturer instructions carefully.** 5% to 10% of patients receiving chronic therapy become refractory to dose adjustments; may consider a drug holiday (hospitalized patients only) with a gradual withdrawal over 2 to 4 weeks and use of alternative spasticity management methods. Following the drug holiday intrathecal baclofen may be resumed at the initial continuous infusion dose.

Renal Impairment

Oral: There are no dosage adjustments provided in the manufacturer's labeling. However, baclofen is primarily renally eliminated; use with caution; dosage reduction may be necessary.

Hemodialysis:
US labeling: There are no dosage adjustments provided in the manufacturer's labeling.
Canadian labeling: 5 mg once daily

Hepatic Impairment

Oral:
US labeling: There are no dosage adjustments provided in the manufacturer's labeling.
Canadian labeling: No dosage adjustment necessary; use with caution in severe impairment.

Administration

Intrathecal: For screening dosages, administer as a bolus injection (50 mcg/mL concentration) by barbotage into the subarachnoid space over at least 1 minute, followed by maintenance continuous infusion.

Oral: The Canadian labeling recommends administering with food or milk in patients with persistent nausea despite dose reductions.

Monitoring Parameters Regular electroencephalogram (EEG) in patients with epilepsy (loss of seizure control has been reported).

Dosage Forms Considerations EnovaRX-Baclofen and Equipto-Baclofen creams are compounded from kits. Refer to manufacturer's labeling for compounding instructions.

Dosage Forms Excipient information presented when available (limited, particularly for generics); consult specific product labeling. [DSC] = Discontinued product

Cream, External:
EnovaRX-Baclofen: 1% (60 g, 120 g) [contains cetyl alcohol]
Equipto-Baclofen: 2% (120 g)
Generic: 2% (60 g)

Solution, Intrathecal [preservative free]:
Gablofen: 50 mcg/mL (1 mL); 10,000 mcg/20 mL (20 mL); 20,000 mcg/20 mL (20 mL); 40,000 mcg/20 mL (20 mL) [antioxidant free]
Lioresal: 0.05 mg/mL (1 mL); 10 mg/20 mL (20 mL); 10 mg/5 mL (5 mL); 40 mg/20 mL (20 mL) [antioxidant free]

Tablet, Oral:
Ed Baclofen: 10 mg [DSC]
Generic: 10 mg, 20 mg

Extemporaneous Preparations A 5 mg/mL oral suspension may be made with tablets. Crush thirty 20 mg tablets in a mortar and reduce to a fine powder. Add a small amount of glycerin and mix to a uniform paste. Mix while adding Simple Syrup, NF in incremental proportions to **almost** 120 mL; transfer to a calibrated bottle, rinse mortar with vehicle, and add a sufficient quantity of vehicle to make 120 mL. Label "shake well" and "refrigerate". Stable for 35 days (Johnson, 1993).

A 10 mg/mL oral suspension may be made with tablets. Crush one-hundred-twenty 10 mg tablets in a mortar and reduce to a fine powder. Add small portions (60 mL) of a 1:1 mixture of Ora-Sweet® and Ora-Plus® and mix to a uniform paste; mix while adding the vehicle in incremental proportions to **almost** 120 mL; transfer to a calibrated bottle, rinse mortar with vehicle, and add quantity of vehicle sufficient to make 120 mL. Label "shake well" and "refrigerate". Stable for 60 days (Allen, 1996).

Allen LV Jr and Erickson MA 3rd, "Stability of Baclofen, Captopril, Diltiazem Hydrochloride, Dipyridamole, and Flecainide Acetate in Extemporaneously Compounded Oral Liquids," *Am J Health Syst Pharm*, 1996, 53(18):2179-84.

Johnson CE and Hart SM, "Stability of an Extemporaneously Compounded Baclofen Oral Liquid," *Am J Hosp Pharm*, 1993, 50 (11):2353-5.

◆ **Bactocill in Dextrose** *see* Oxacillin *on page 1348*

◆ **Bactrim** *see* Sulfamethoxazole and Trimethoprim *on page 1710*

◆ **Bactrim DS** *see* Sulfamethoxazole and Trimethoprim *on page 1710*

◆ **Bactroban** *see* Mupirocin *on page 1239*

◆ **Bactroban Nasal** *see* Mupirocin *on page 1239*

◆ **Baking Soda** *see* Sodium Bicarbonate *on page 1669*

◆ **BAL** *see* Dimercaprol *on page 557*

◆ **BAL8557** *see* Isavuconazonium Sulfate *on page 988*

◆ **Bal in Oil** *see* Dimercaprol *on page 557*

◆ **Balmex® [OTC]** *see* Zinc Oxide *on page 1929*

◆ **Balminil Codeine + Decongestant + Expectorant (Can)** *see* Guaifenesin, Pseudoephedrine, and Codeine *on page 863*

◆ **Balminil Decongestant (Can)** *see* Pseudoephedrine *on page 1527*

◆ **Balminil DM D (Can)** *see* Pseudoephedrine and Dextromethorphan *on page 1528*

◆ **Balminil DM + Decongestant + Expectorant (Can)** *see* Guaifenesin, Pseudoephedrine, and Dextromethorphan *on page 864*

◆ **Balminil DM + Decongestant + Expectorant Extra Strength (Can)** *see* Guaifenesin, Pseudoephedrine, and Dextromethorphan *on page 864*

◆ **Balminil DM E (Can)** *see* Guaifenesin and Dextromethorphan *on page 861*

◆ **Balminil Expectorant (Can)** *see* GuaiFENesin *on page 860*

Balsalazide (bal SAL a zide)

Brand Names: US Colazal; Giazo

Index Terms Balsalazide Disodium

Pharmacologic Category 5-Aminosalicylic Acid Derivative; Anti-inflammatory Agent

Use Treatment of mildly- to moderately-active ulcerative colitis

Giazo™: Only approved in males ≥18 years; effectiveness in females was not demonstrated

Pregnancy Considerations Adverse events have not been observed in animal reproduction studies. Mesalamine (5-aminosalicylic acid) is the active metabolite of balsalazide; mesalamine is known to cross the placenta. Refer to the Mesalamine monograph for additional information.

Breast-Feeding Considerations It is not known if balsalazide is excreted in breast milk. The manufacturer recommends that caution be exercised when administering balsalazide to nursing women. Mesalamine, 5-aminosalicylic acid, is the active metabolite of balsalazide. Low levels of mesalamine enter breast milk; refer to the Mesalamine monograph for additional information.

Contraindications Hypersensitivity to balsalazide or its metabolites, salicylates, or any component of the formulation

Warnings/Precautions Pyloric stenosis may prolong gastric retention of balsalazide. Renal toxicity and hepatic failure have been observed with other mesalamine (5-aminosalicylic acid) products; use with caution in patients with known renal or hepatic disease. Symptomatic worsening of ulcerative colitis may occur following initiation of treatment. May cause an acute intolerance syndrome (cramping, acute abdominal pain, bloody diarrhea; sometimes fever, headache, rash); discontinue if this occurs. May cause staining of teeth or tongue if capsule is opened and sprinkled on food.

Adverse Reactions

>10%:

Central nervous system: Headache (children 15%; adults 8%)

Gastrointestinal: Abdominal pain (children 12% to 13%; adults ≤6%)

1% to 10%:

Central nervous system: Insomnia (adults 2%), fatigue (children 4%; adults ≤2%), fever (children 6%; adults 2%)

Endocrine & metabolic: Dysmenorrhea (children 3%)

Gastrointestinal: Vomiting (children 10%; adults ≤4%), diarrhea (children 9%; adults ≤5%), ulcerative colitis exacerbation (children 6%; adults 1%), nausea (children 4%; adults 5%), hematochezia (children 4%), stomatitis (children 3%), anorexia (adults 2%), dyspepsia (adults 2%), flatulence (adults ≤2%), cramps (adults 1%), constipation (adults ≤1%), xerostomia (adults ≤1%)

Genitourinary: Urinary tract infection (adults 1% to 4%)

Hematologic: Anemia (4%)

Neuromuscular & skeletal: Arthralgia (adults ≤4%), musculoskeletal pain (adults 2%), myalgia (adults ≤1%)

Respiratory: Respiratory infection (adults ≤4%), cough (children 3%; adults 2%), pharyngitis (children 6%; adults 2%), pharyngolaryngeal pain (children 3%; adults 4%), rhinitis (adults 2%)

Miscellaneous: Flu-like syndrome (children 4%; adults 1%)

<1% (Limited to important or life-threatening): Alopecia, alveolitis, AST increased, back pain, blood pressure increased, cholestatic jaundice, cirrhosis, defecation urgency, dizziness, dyspnea, edema, erythema nodosum, facial edema, fever, gastroenteritis, gastroesophageal reflux, hard stool, heart rate increased, hepatocellular damage, hepatotoxicity, hyperbilirubinemia, hypersensitivity, interstitial nephritis, jaundice, Kawasaki-like syndrome, lethargy, liver failure, liver necrosis, liver function tests increased, malaise, myocarditis, pain, pancreatitis, pericarditis, pleural effusion, pneumonia (with and without eosinophilia), pruritus, rash, renal failure, vasculitis

Drug Interactions

Metabolism/Transport Effects None known.

Avoid Concomitant Use There are no known interactions where it is recommended to avoid concomitant use.

Increased Effect/Toxicity

Balsalazide may increase the levels/effects of: Heparin; Heparin (Low Molecular Weight); Thiopurine Analogs; Varicella Virus-Containing Vaccines

The levels/effects of Balsalazide may be increased by: Nonsteroidal Anti-Inflammatory Agents

Decreased Effect

Balsalazide may decrease the levels/effects of: Cardiac Glycosides

Storage/Stability Store at controlled room temperature of 20°C to 25°C (68°F to 77°F); excursions permitted to 15°C to 30°C (59°F to 86°F).

Mechanism of Action Balsalazide is a prodrug, converted by bacterial azoreduction to 5-aminosalicylic acid (mesalamine, active), 4-aminobenzoyl-β-alanine (inert), and their metabolites. 5-aminosalicylic acid may decrease inflammation by blocking the production of arachidonic acid metabolites topically in the colon mucosa.

Pharmacodynamics/Kinetics

Onset of action: Delayed; may require several days to weeks (2 weeks); similar in adults and children

Absorption: Very low and variable; in children, reported systemic absorption of 5-ASA (active) lower than adults (C_{max}: 67% lower, AUC: 64% lower)

Protein binding: Balsalazide: ≥99%

Metabolism: Azoreduced in the colon to 5-aminosalicylic acid (active), 4-aminobenzoyl-β-alanine (inert), and N-acetylated metabolites

Half-life elimination: Primary effect is topical (colonic mucosa); therapeutic effect appears not to be influenced by the systemic half-life of balsalazide (1.9 hours) or its metabolites (5-ASA [9.5 hours], N-Ac-5-ASA [10.4 hours])

Time to peak: Balsalazide: Capsule: 1 to 2 hours; Tablet: 0.5 hours

Excretion: Feces (65% as 5-aminosalicylic acid, 4-aminobenzoyl-β-alanine, and N-acetylated metabolites); urine (<16% as N-acetylated metabolites); Parent drug: Urine or feces (<1%)

Dosing

Adult & Geriatric Ulcerative colitis: Oral:

Capsule: 2.25 g (three 750 mg capsules) 3 times daily for up to 8-12 weeks

Tablet (Giazo™): Males: 3.3 g (three 1.1 g tablets) twice daily for up to 8 weeks

Pediatric Ulcerative colitis: Oral: Capsule: Children 5-17 years: 750 mg 3 times daily for up to 8 weeks **or** 2.25 g (three 750 mg capsules) 3 times daily for up to 8 weeks

Renal Impairment No dosage adjustment provided in manufacturer's labeling. Renal toxicity has been observed with other 5-aminosalicylic acid products; use with caution.

Hepatic Impairment No dosage adjustment provided in manufacturer's labeling.

Dietary Considerations Some products may contain sodium. Take tablets with or without food.

Administration

Capsule: Should be swallowed whole or may be opened and sprinkled on applesauce. Applesauce mixture may be chewed; swallow immediately, do not store mixture for later use. When sprinkled on food, may cause staining of teeth or tongue.

Tablet: Administer with or without food.

Monitoring Parameters Improvement or worsening of symptoms; renal function (prior to initiation, then periodically); liver function tests

Additional Information Balsalazide 750 mg is equivalent to mesalamine 267 mg

Dosage Forms Excipient information presented when available (limited, particularly for generics); consult specific product labeling.

Capsule, Oral, as disodium:
Colazal: 750 mg
Generic: 750 mg

Tablet, Oral, as disodium:
Giazo: 1.1 g

Basiliximab (ba si LIK si mab)

Brand Names: US Simulect

Brand Names: Canada Simulect

Pharmacologic Category Immunosuppressant Agent; Monoclonal Antibody

Use Renal transplant rejection: Prophylaxis of acute organ rejection in renal transplantation in combination with cyclosporine (modified) and corticosteroids

Pregnancy Considerations Adverse effects were not observed in animal reproduction studies. IL-2 receptors play an important role in the development of the immune system. Women of childbearing potential should use effective contraceptive measures before beginning treatment, during, and for 4 months after completion of basiliximab treatment. The National Transplantation Pregnancy Registry (NTPR, Temple University) is a registry for pregnant women taking immunosuppressants following any solid organ transplant. The NTPR encourages reporting of all immunosuppressant exposures during pregnancy in transplant recipients at 877-955-6877.

Breast-Feeding Considerations It is not known if basiliximab is excreted in human milk. Because many immunoglobulins are secreted in milk and the potential for serious adverse reactions exists, a decision should be made to discontinue nursing or discontinue the drug, taking into account the importance of the drug to the mother. The Canadian labeling recommends women avoid nursing for 4 months following the last dose.

Contraindications Known hypersensitivity to basiliximab or any component of the formulation

◄ **Warnings/Precautions** To be used as a component of an immunosuppressive regimen which includes cyclosporine and corticosteroids. The incidence of lymphoproliferative disorders and/or opportunistic infections may be increased by immunosuppressive therapy. Severe hypersensitivity reactions, occurring within 24 hours, have been reported. Reactions, including anaphylaxis, have occurred both with the initial exposure and/or following re-exposure after several months. Use caution during re-exposure to a subsequent course of therapy in a patient who has previously received basiliximab; patients in whom concomitant immunosuppression was prematurely discontinued due to abandoned transplantation or early graft loss are at increased risk for developing a severe hypersensitivity reaction upon re-exposure. Discontinue permanently if a severe reaction occurs. Medications for the treatment of hypersensitivity reactions should be available for immediate use. Treatment may result in the development of human antimurine antibodies (HAMA); however, limited evidence suggesting the use of muromonab-CD3 or other murine products is not precluded. **[U.S. Boxed Warning]: Should be administered under the supervision of a physician experienced in immunosuppression therapy and organ transplant management.** In renal transplant patients receiving basiliximab plus prednisone, cyclosporine, and mycophenolate, new-onset diabetes, glucose intolerance, and impaired fasting glucose were observed at rates significantly higher than observed in patients receiving prednisone, cyclosporine, and mycophenolate without basiliximab (Aasebo, 2010). Potentially significant drug-drug interactions may exist, requiring dose or frequency adjustment, additional monitoring, and/or selection of alternative therapy.

Adverse Reactions Administration of basiliximab did not appear to increase the incidence or severity of adverse effects in clinical trials. Adverse events were reported in 96% of both the placebo and basiliximab groups.

>10%:
Cardiovascular: Hypertension, peripheral edema
Central nervous system: Fever, headache, insomnia, pain
Dermatologic: Acne, wound complications
Endocrine & metabolic: Hypercholesterolemia, hyperglycemia, hyper-/hypokalemia, hyperuricemia, hypophosphatemia
Gastrointestinal: Abdominal pain, constipation, diarrhea, dyspepsia, nausea, vomiting
Genitourinary: Urinary tract infection
Hematologic: Anemia
Neuromuscular & skeletal: Tremor
Respiratory: Dyspnea, infection (upper respiratory)
Miscellaneous: Viral infection
3% to 10%:
Cardiovascular: Abnormal heart sounds, angina, arrhythmia, atrial fibrillation, chest pain, generalized edema, heart failure, hypotension, tachycardia
Central nervous system: Agitation, anxiety, depression, dizziness, fatigue, hypoesthesia, malaise
Dermatologic: Cyst, hypertrichosis, pruritus, rash, skin disorder, skin ulceration
Endocrine & metabolic: Acidosis, dehydration, diabetes mellitus, fluid overload, glucocorticoids increased, hyper-/hypocalcemia, hyperlipemia, hypertriglyceridemia, hypoglycemia, hypomagnesemia, hyponatremia, hypoproteinemia
Gastrointestinal: Abdomen enlarged, esophagitis, flatulence, gastroenteritis, GI hemorrhage, gingival hyperplasia, melena, moniliasis, stomatitis (including ulcerative), weight gain
Genitourinary: Bladder disorder, dysuria, genital edema (male), impotence, ureteral disorder, urinary frequency, urinary retention
Hematologic: Hematoma, hemorrhage, leukopenia, polycythemia, purpura, thrombocytopenia, thrombosis
Neuromuscular & skeletal: Arthralgia, arthropathy, back pain, cramps, fracture, hernia, leg pain, myalgia, neuropathy, paresthesia, rigors, weakness
Ocular: Abnormal vision, cataract, conjunctivitis
Renal: Albuminuria, hematuria, nonprotein nitrogen increased, oliguria, renal function abnormal, renal tubular necrosis
Respiratory: Bronchitis, bronchospasm, cough, pharyngitis, pneumonia, pulmonary edema, rhinitis, sinusitis
Miscellaneous: Accidental trauma, cytomegalovirus (CMV) infection, herpes infection (simplex and zoster), infection, sepsis
Postmarketing and/or case reports: Anaphylaxis, capillary leak syndrome, cytokine release syndrome, diabetes (new onset), fasting glucose impaired, glucose intolerance, hypersensitivity reaction (including heart failure, hypotension, tachycardia, bronchospasm, dyspnea,

pulmonary edema, respiratory failure, sneezing, pruritus, rash, urticaria), lymphoproliferative disease

Drug Interactions
Metabolism/Transport Effects None known.
Avoid Concomitant Use
Avoid concomitant use of Basiliximab with any of the following: BCG (Intravesical); Belimumab; Natalizumab; Pimecrolimus; Tacrolimus (Topical); Tofacitinib; Vaccines (Live)
Increased Effect/Toxicity
Basiliximab may increase the levels/effects of: Belimumab; Fingolimod; Leflunomide; Natalizumab; Tofacitinib; Vaccines (Live)

The levels/effects of Basiliximab may be increased by: Denosumab; Pimecrolimus; Roflumilast; Tacrolimus (Topical); Trastuzumab
Decreased Effect
Basiliximab may decrease the levels/effects of: BCG (Intravesical); Coccidioides immitis Skin Test; Sipuleucel-T; Vaccines (Inactivated); Vaccines (Live)

The levels/effects of Basiliximab may be decreased by: Echinacea

Preparation for Administration Reconstitute with preservative-free sterile water for injection (reconstitute 10 mg vial with 2.5 mL, 20 mg vial with 5 mL). Shake gently to dissolve. May further dilute reconstituted solution with 25 mL (10 mg) or 50 mL (20 mg) 0.9% sodium chloride or dextrose 5% in water. When mixing the solution, gently invert the bag to avoid foaming. Do not shake solutions diluted for infusion.

Storage/Stability Store intact vials refrigerated at 2°C to 8°C (36°F to 46°F). Should be used immediately after reconstitution; however, if not used immediately, reconstituted solution may be stored at 2°C to 8°C for up to 24 hours or at room temperature for up to 4 hours. Discard the reconstituted solution if not used within 24 hours.

Mechanism of Action Chimeric (murine/human) immunosuppressant monoclonal antibody which blocks the alpha-chain of the interleukin-2 (IL-2) receptor complex; this receptor is expressed on activated T lymphocytes and is a critical pathway for activating cell-mediated allograft rejection

Pharmacodynamics/Kinetics
Duration: Mean: 36 days ± 14 days (determined by IL-2R alpha saturation in patients also on cyclosporine and corticosteroids)
Distribution: Mean: V_d: Children 1 to 11 years: 4.8 ± 2.1 L; Adolescents 12 to 16 years: 7.8 ± 5.1 L; Adults: 8.6 ± 4.1 L
Half-life elimination: Children 1 to 11 years: 9.5 ± 4.5 days; Adolescents 12 to 16 years: 9.1 ± 3.9 days; Adults: Mean: 7.2 ± 3.2 days
Excretion: Clearance:
Children 1 to 11 years: 17 ± 6 mL/hour; in pediatric liver transplant patients, significant basiliximab loss through ascites fluid can increase total body clearance and reduce IL-2R (CD25) saturation duration; dosage adjustments may be necessary (Cintorino 2006; Kovarik 2002; Spada 2006)
Adolescents 12 to 16 years: 31 ±19 mL/hour
Adults: 41 ± 19 mL/hour

Dosing
Adult & Geriatric Note: Patients previously administered basiliximab should only be re-exposed to a subsequent course of therapy with extreme caution.
Acute renal transplant rejection prophylaxis: IV: 20 mg within 2 hours prior to transplant surgery, followed by a second 20 mg dose 4 days after transplantation. The second dose should be withheld if complications occur (including severe hypersensitivity reactions or graft loss).
Acute cardiac transplant rejection prophylaxis (off-label use): IV: 20 mg on the day of transplant, followed by a second dose 4 days after transplantation (Mehra, 2005); usually given within the first hour postoperatively
Acute liver transplant rejection prophylaxis (off-label use): IV: 20 mg within 6 hours of organ reperfusion, followed by a second 20 mg dose 4 days after transplantation (Neuhaus, 2002)
Treatment of refractory acute GVHD (off-label use): IV: 20 mg on days 1 and 4; may repeat for recurrent acute GVHD (Schmidt-Hieber, 2005). Additional data may be necessary to further define the role of basiliximab in this condition.
Pediatric Note: Patients previously administered basiliximab should only be re-exposed to a subsequent course of therapy with extreme caution.
Acute renal transplant rejection prophylaxis: IV:
Note: Use in pediatric patients is not approved in the Canadian labeling (limited pharmacokinetic data available).

Children <35 kg: 10 mg within 2 hours prior to transplant surgery, followed by a second 10 mg dose 4 days after transplantation; the second dose should be withheld if complications occur (including severe hypersensitivity reactions or graft loss)

Children ≥35 kg: Refer to adult dosing

Renal Impairment There are no dosage adjustments provided in the manufacturer's labeling.

Hepatic Impairment There are no dosage adjustments provided in the manufacturer's labeling.

Administration For intravenous administration only. Infuse as a bolus or IV infusion over 20-30 minutes. (Bolus dosing is associated with nausea, vomiting, and local pain at the injection site.) Administer only after assurance that patient will receive renal graft and immunosuppression. For the treatment of acute GVHD (off-label use), the dose was diluted in 250 mL NS and administered over 30 minutes (Schmidt-Hieber, 2005).

Monitoring Parameters Signs and symptoms of acute rejection; hypersensitivity, infection

Dosage Forms Excipient information presented when available (limited, particularly for generics); consult specific product labeling.

Solution Reconstituted, Intravenous [preservative free]:
Simulect: 10 mg (1 ea); 20 mg (1 ea)

◆ BAY 43-9006 *see* SORAfenib *on page 1691*
◆ BAY 59-7939 *see* Rivaroxaban *on page 1604*
◆ BAY 63-2521 *see* Riociguat *on page 1589*
◆ BAY 73-4506 *see* Regorafenib *on page 1565*
◆ Baycadron [DSC] *see* Dexamethasone (Systemic) *on page 525*
◆ Bayer Aspirin Extra Strength [OTC] *see* Aspirin *on page 157*
◆ Bayer Aspirin Regimen Adult Low Strength [OTC] *see* Aspirin *on page 157*
◆ Bayer Aspirin Regimen Children's [OTC] *see* Aspirin *on page 157*
◆ Bayer Aspirin Regimen Regular Strength [OTC] *see* Aspirin *on page 157*
◆ Bayer Genuine Aspirin [OTC] *see* Aspirin *on page 157*
◆ Bayer Plus Extra Strength [OTC] *see* Aspirin *on page 157*
◆ Bayer® PM [OTC] *see* Aspirin and Diphenhydramine *on page 162*
◆ Bayer Women's Low Dose Aspirin [OTC] *see* Aspirin *on page 157*
◆ Baza Antifungal [OTC] *see* Miconazole (Topical) *on page 1201*
◆ Baza® Clear [OTC] *see* Vitamin A and Vitamin D (Topical) *on page 1906*
◆ Bazedoxifene and Estrogens (Conjugated/Equine) *see* Estrogens (Conjugated/Equine) and Bazedoxifene *on page 693*
◆ B-Caro-T [OTC] *see* Beta-Carotene *on page 221*

BCG (Intravesical) (bee see jee)

Brand Names: US TheraCys; Tice BCG
Brand Names: Canada ImmuCyst; Oncotice
Index Terms Bacillus Calmette-Guérin (BCG) Live; BCG, Live
Pharmacologic Category Antineoplastic Agent, Biological Response Modulator
Use
Bladder cancer: Treatment and prophylaxis of carcinoma in situ of the urinary bladder; prophylaxis of primary or recurrent superficial or minimally invasive (stage Ta and/or T1) papillary tumors following transurethral resection
Limitations of use: BCG (intravesical) is not recommended for stage Ta low-grade papillary tumors unless judged to be at high risk for recurrence. BCG (intravesical) is not recommended for immunization against tuberculosis.
Dosing
Adult & Geriatric
Bladder cancer: Intravesicular:
TheraCys: Induction: One dose (81 mg or one vial) instilled into bladder (retain for up to 2 hours) once weekly for 6 weeks beginning at least 14 days after biopsy or transurethral resection, followed by maintenance therapy of 81 mg (one vial) at 3, 6, 12, 18, and 24 months after initial dose.
TICE BCG: Induction: One dose (~50 mg or one vial) instilled into the bladder (retain for 2 hours) once weekly for 6 weeks beginning 7 to 14 days after biopsy (may repeat cycle 1 time if tumor remission not achieved), followed by maintenance therapy of

~50 mg (one vial) approximately once a month for at least 6 to 12 months.

Renal Impairment There are no dosage adjustments provided in the manufacturer's labeling.

Hepatic Impairment There are no dosage adjustments provided in the manufacturer's labeling.

Adjustment for Toxicity
Bacterial urinary tract infection: Withhold treatment until complete resolution.
Persistent fever or acute febrile illness consistent with BCG infection: Discontinue treatment.

Additional Information Complete prescribing information should be consulted for additional detail.

Dosage Forms Excipient information presented when available (limited, particularly for generics); consult specific product labeling.
Suspension Reconstituted, Intravesical:
Tice BCG: 50 mg (1 ea)
Suspension Reconstituted, Intravesical [preservative free]:
TheraCys: 81 mg (1 ea) [contains monosodium glutamate (sodium glutamate)]

◆ BCG, Live *see* BCG (Intravesical) *on page 203*
◆ BCG, Live *see* BCG Vaccine (Immunization) *on page 203*
◆ BCG Vaccine (Can) *see* BCG Vaccine (Immunization) *on page 203*

BCG Vaccine (Immunization) (bee see jee vak SEEN)

Brand Names: Canada BCG Vaccine
Index Terms Bacillus Calmette-Guérin (BCG) Live; BCG Vaccine U.S.P. *(percutaneous use product)*; BCG, Live
Pharmacologic Category Vaccine; Vaccine, Live (Bacterial)
Additional Appendix Information
Immunization Administration Recommendations *on page 1974*
Immunization Schedules *on page 1979*
Use *Mycobacterium tuberculosis* **disease prevention:** Active immunization against *Mycobacterium tuberculosis* in persons not previously infected and who are at high risk for exposure
BCG vaccine is not routinely administered for the prevention of *M. tuberculosis* in the United States. The Advisory Committee on Immunization Practices (ACIP) recommends vaccination be considered for the following (CDC/ACIP [Villarino 1996]):
- Infants and children with a negative tuberculin skin test who are continually exposed to (and cannot be separated from) patients who are untreated or ineffectively treated for infectious pulmonary TB disease when the child cannot be given long-term treatment for infection **or** if the patient has infectious pulmonary TB caused by strains resistant to isoniazid and rifampin.
- Health care workers with a high percentage of patients with *M. tuberculosis* strains resistant to both isoniazid and rifampin, if there is ongoing transmission of the resistant strains and subsequent infection is likely, or if comprehensive infection-control precautions have not been successful. In addition, health care workers should be counseled on the risks and benefits of vaccination and treatment of latent TB infection
Dosing
Adult & Geriatric Immunization against tuberculosis:
US labeling: Percutaneous: 0.2 to 0.3 mL (full strength dilution); conduct postvaccinal tuberculin test (5 TU of PPD) in 2 to 3 months; if test is negative, repeat vaccination. **Note:** Initial lesions usually appear after 10 to 14 days and consist of small, red papules at injection site, which reach maximum diameter of 3 mm in 4 to 6 weeks.
Canadian labeling: Intradermal: 0.1 mL (0.1 mg) as a single dose.
Pediatric Immunization against tuberculosis:
US labeling:
Neonates <1 month: Percutaneous: 0.2 to 0.3 mL (half-strength dilution). Administer tuberculin test (5 TU) after 2 to 3 months; repeat vaccination after 1 year of age for negative tuberculin test if indications persist. **Note:** Initial lesions usually appear after 10 to 14 days and consist of small, red papules at injection site, which reach maximum diameter of 3 mm in 4 to 6 weeks.
Infants, Children, and Adolescents: Refer to adult dosing.

Canadian labeling:
Neonates and Infants ≤12 months: Intradermal: 0.05 mL (0.05 mg) as a single dose.
Children >1 year and Adolescents: Intradermal: Refer to adult dosing.

Renal Impairment There are no dosage adjustments provided in the manufacturer's labeling.

Hepatic Impairment There are no dosage adjustments provided in the manufacturer's labeling.

Additional Information Complete prescribing information should be consulted for additional detail.

Dosage Forms Excipient information presented when available (limited, particularly for generics); consult specific product labeling.
Injectable, Injection:
Generic: 50 mg (1 ea)

Dosage Forms: Canada Excipient information presented when available (limited, particularly for generics); consult specific product labeling.
Injection, powder for reconstitution, Intradermal:
BCG Vaccine: 1.5 mg (1 ea) [contains monosodium glutamate (sodium glutamate), vial stopper contain natural rubber/natural latex, polysorbate 80 (in diluent)]

◆ BCG Vaccine U.S.P. *(percutaneous use product) see* BCG Vaccine (Immunization) *on page 203*

◆ BCNU *see* Carmustine *on page 320*

◆ BCX-1812 *see* Peramivir *on page 1428*

◆ B-Donna *see* Hyoscyamine, Atropine, Scopolamine, and Phenobarbital *on page 900*

◆ beano® [OTC] *see* Alpha-Galactosidase *on page 76*

◆ beano® Meltaways [OTC] *see* Alpha-Galactosidase *on page 76*

◆ Bebulin *see* Factor IX Complex (Human) [(Factors II, IX, X)] *on page 734*

◆ Bebulin VH *see* Factor IX Complex (Human) [(Factors II, IX, X)] *on page 734*

Becaplermin (be KAP ler min)

Brand Names: US Regranex

Index Terms Recombinant Human Platelet-Derived Growth Factor B; rPDGF-BB

Pharmacologic Category Growth Factor, Platelet-Derived; Topical Skin Product

Use Diabetic ulcers: Adjunctive treatment of lower extremity diabetic neuropathic ulcers that extend into the subcutaneous tissue or beyond and have an adequate blood supply.

Limitations of use: Efficacy has not been established for pressure and venous stasis ulcers; has not been evaluated for diabetic neuropathic ulcers that do not extend through the dermis into subcutaneous tissue (stage I or II, International Association of Enterostomal Therapy [IAET] staging classification) or ischemic diabetic ulcers.

Dosing

Adult & Geriatric Diabetic ulcers (lower extremity): Topical: Apply appropriate amount of gel once daily with a cotton swab, tongue depressor, or similar tool, as a coating over the ulcer. The amount of becaplermin to be applied will vary depending on the size of the ulcer area.

Note: If the ulcer does not decrease in size by ~30% after 10 weeks of treatment or complete healing has not occurred in 20 weeks, continued treatment with becaplermin should be reassessed.

Estimation of gel requirement: To calculate the length of gel applied to the ulcer, measure the greatest length of the ulcer by the greatest width of the ulcer. Tube size and unit of measure will determine the formula used in the calculation. Recalculate amount of gel needed every 1 to 2 weeks, depending on the rate of change in ulcer area.

Centimeters:
15 g tube: [ulcer length (cm) x width (cm)] divided by 4 = length of gel (cm)
2 g tube: [ulcer length (cm) x width (cm)] divided by 2 = length of gel (cm)

Inches:
15 g tube: [length (in) x width (in)] x 0.6 = length of gel (in)
2 g tube: [length (in) x width (in)] x 1.3 = length of gel (in)

Pediatric Diabetic ulcers (lower extremity): Adolescents ≥16 years: Refer to adult dosing

Renal Impairment There are no dosage adjustments provided in the manufacturer's labeling. However, dosage adjustment unlikely due to low systemic absorption.

Hepatic Impairment There are no dosage adjustments provided in the manufacturer's labeling. However, dosage adjustment unlikely due to low systemic absorption.

Additional Information Complete prescribing information should be consulted for additional detail.

Dosage Forms Excipient information presented when available (limited, particularly for generics); consult specific product labeling.
Gel, External:
Regranex: 0.01% (15 g) [contains metacresol, methylparaben, propylparaben]

◆ Becenum *see* Carmustine *on page 320*

Beclomethasone (Systemic)
(be kloe METH a sone)

Brand Names: US Qvar

Brand Names: Canada QVAR

Index Terms Vanceril

Pharmacologic Category Corticosteroid, Inhalant (Oral)

Additional Appendix Information
Inhaled Corticosteroids *on page 1951*

Use

Asthma: Maintenance and prophylactic treatment of asthma in patients ≥5 years (including those who require corticosteroids and those who may benefit from a dose reduction/elimination of systemically administered corticosteroids).

Limitations of use: Not for relief of acute bronchospasm.

Guideline recommendations: A low-dose inhaled corticosteroid (in addition to an as-needed short acting beta$_2$-agonist) is the initial preferred long-term control medication for children, adolescents, and adult patients with persistent asthma who are candidates for treatment according to a step-wise treatment approach (NAEPP 2007; GINA 2015).

Pregnancy Considerations Adverse events have been observed in animal reproduction studies. Hypoadrenalism may occur in newborns following maternal use of corticosteroids in pregnancy. Based on available data, an overall increased risk of congenital malformations or a decrease in fetal growth has not been associated with maternal use of inhaled corticosteroids during pregnancy (Bakhireva, 2005; NAEPP, 2005; Namazy, 2004). Uncontrolled asthma is associated with adverse events in pregnancy (increased risk of perinatal mortality, pre-eclampsia, preterm birth, low birth weight infants). Inhaled corticosteroids are recommended for the treatment of asthma during pregnancy (most information available using budesonide) (ACOG, 2008; NAEPP, 2005).

Breast-Feeding Considerations Other corticosteroids have been found in breast milk; however, information for beclomethasone is not available. Due to the potential for serious adverse reactions in the nursing infant, the manufacturer recommends a decision be made whether to discontinue nursing or to discontinue the drug, taking into account the importance of treatment to the mother. Use of inhaled corticosteroids is not a contraindication to breast-feeding (NAEPP, 2005).

Contraindications

Hypersensitivity to beclomethasone or any component of the formulation; status asthmaticus, or other acute asthma episodes requiring intensive measures

Documentation of allergenic cross-reactivity for corticosteroids is limited. However, because of similarities in chemical structure and/or pharmacologic actions, the possibility of cross-sensitivity cannot be ruled out with certainty.

Canadian labeling: Additional contraindications (not in US labeling): Moderate to severe bronchiectasis requiring intensive measures; untreated fungal, bacterial, or tubercular infections of the respiratory tract

Warnings/Precautions May cause hypercorticism or suppression of hypothalamic-pituitary-adrenal (HPA) axis, particularly in younger children or in patients receiving high doses for prolonged periods. HPA axis suppression may lead to adrenal crisis. Withdrawal and discontinuation of a corticosteroid should be done slowly and carefully. Particular care is required when patients are transferred from systemic corticosteroids to inhaled products due to possible adrenal insufficiency or withdrawal from steroids, including an increase in allergic symptoms. Patients receiving >20 mg per day of prednisone (or equivalent) may be most susceptible. Fatalities have occurred due to adrenal insufficiency in asthmatic patients during and after transfer from systemic corticosteroids to aerosol steroids; aerosol steroids do **not** provide the systemic steroid

needed to treat patients having trauma, surgery, or infections (particularly gastroenteritis), or other conditions with severe electrolyte loss. Select surgical patients on long-term, high-dose, inhaled corticosteroid (ICS), should be given stress doses of hydrocortisone intravenously during the surgical period and the dose reduced rapidly within 24 hours after surgery (Expert Panel Report 3, 2007).

Bronchospasm may occur with wheezing after inhalation (possibly life-threatening); if bronchospasm occurs, discontinue steroid and treat with a fast-acting bronchodilator. Supplemental steroids (oral or parenteral) may be needed during stress or severe asthma attacks. Not to be used in status asthmaticus or for the relief of acute bronchospasm. Immediate hypersensitivity reactions may occur, including angioedema, bronchospasm, rash, and urticaria; discontinue use if reaction occurs. Corticosteroid use may cause psychiatric disturbances, including depression, euphoria, insomnia, mood swings, and personality changes. Preexisting psychiatric conditions may be exacerbated by corticosteroid use. Prolonged use of corticosteroids may also increase the incidence of secondary infection, mask acute infection (including fungal infections), prolong or exacerbate viral infections, or limit response to vaccines. Avoid use, if possible, in patients with ocular herpes, active or quiescent respiratory or untreated viral, fungal, parasitic or bacterial systemic infections (Canadian labeling contraindicates use with untreated respiratory infections). Exposure to chickenpox or measles should be avoided. Close observation is required in patients with latent tuberculosis and/or TB reactivity; restrict use in active TB. Prolonged treatment with corticosteroids has been associated with the development of Kaposi sarcoma (case reports); if noted, discontinuation of therapy should be considered. *Candida albicans* infections may occur in the mouth and pharynx; rinsing (and spitting) with water after inhaler use may decrease risk. Rare cases of vasculitis (Churg-Strauss syndrome) or other systemic eosinophilic conditions can occur; often associated with decrease and/or withdrawal of oral corticosteroid therapy following initiation of inhaled corticosteroid.

Use with caution in patients with major risk factors for decreased bone mineral count. Use with caution in patients with thyroid disease, hepatic impairment, renal impairment, cardiovascular disease, diabetes, glaucoma, cataracts, myasthenia gravis, patients at risk for seizures, or GI diseases (diverticulitis, peptic ulcer, ulcerative colitis). Use caution following acute MI (corticosteroids have been associated with myocardial rupture). Because of the risk of adverse effects, systemic corticosteroids should be used cautiously in elderly patients in the smallest possible effective dose for the shortest duration.

Orally inhaled corticosteroids may cause a reduction in growth velocity in pediatric patients (~1 centimeter per year [range: 0.3 to 1.8 cm per year] and related to dose and duration of exposure). To minimize the systemic effects of orally inhaled corticosteroids, each patient should be titrated to the lowest effective dose. Growth should be routinely monitored in pediatric patients. A gradual tapering of dose may be required prior to discontinuing therapy; there have been reports of systemic corticosteroid withdrawal symptoms (eg, joint/muscle pain, lassitude, depression) when withdrawing oral inhalation therapy. When transferring from oral inhalation therapy from systemic corticosteroid therapy; previously suppressed allergic conditions (rhinitis, conjunctivitis, eczema, arthritis, and eosinophilic conditions) may be unmasked; during transition monitor pulmonary function tests (FEV$_1$ or PEF), beta-agonist use, and asthma symptoms and observe for signs and symptoms of adrenal insufficiency.

Adverse Reactions

>10%: Central nervous system: Headache (12%)
1% to 10%:
Central nervous system: Voice disorder (1% to 3%), pain (2%)
Gastrointestinal: Nausea (1%)
Genitourinary: Dysmenorrhea (1% to 3%)
Neuromuscular & skeletal: Back pain (1%)
Respiratory: Upper respiratory tract infection (9%), pharyngitis (8%), rhinitis (6%), sinusitis (3%), cough (1% to 3%)
<1%, postmarketing, and/or case reports: Anaphylactoid reaction, anaphylaxis, behavioral changes (such as aggressiveness, depression, sleep disturbances, psychomotor hyperactivity, suicidal ideation; more common in children), decreased linear skeletal growth rate (in children/adolescents), hypersensitivity reaction (immediate and delayed; including angioedema, bronchospasm, rash, urticaria), HPA-axis suppression; rarely glaucoma, increased intraocular pressure, and cataracts have been reported with inhaled corticosteroids

Drug Interactions

Metabolism/Transport Effects None known.

Avoid Concomitant Use

Avoid concomitant use of Beclomethasone (Oral Inhalation) with any of the following: Aldesleukin; BCG (Intravesical); Loxapine; Natalizumab; Pimecrolimus; Tacrolimus (Topical); Tofacitinib

Increased Effect/Toxicity

Beclomethasone (Oral Inhalation) may increase the levels/effects of: Amphotericin B; Ceritinib; Deferasirox; Fingolimod; Leflunomide; Loop Diuretics; Loxapine; Natalizumab; Thiazide Diuretics; Tofacitinib

The levels/effects of Beclomethasone (Oral Inhalation) may be increased by: Denosumab; Pimecrolimus; Tacrolimus (Topical); Trastuzumab

Decreased Effect

Beclomethasone (Oral Inhalation) may decrease the levels/effects of: Aldesleukin; BCG (Intravesical); Coccidioides immitis Skin Test; Corticorelin; Hyaluronidase; Sipuleucel-T; Vaccines (Inactivated)

The levels/effects of Beclomethasone (Oral Inhalation) may be decreased by: Echinacea

Storage/Stability Store at 25°C (77°F); excursions are permitted between 15°C and 30°C (59°F and 86°F). Do not use or store near heat or open flame. Do not puncture canisters. Store on concave end of canister with actuator on top.

Mechanism of Action Controls the rate of protein synthesis; depresses the migration of polymorphonuclear leukocytes, fibroblasts; reverses capillary permeability and lysosomal stabilization at the cellular level to prevent or control inflammation

Pharmacodynamics/Kinetics

Onset of action: Within 1 to 2 days in some patients; usually within 1 to 2 weeks; Maximum effect: 3 to 4 weeks

Absorption: Readily; quickly hydrolyzed by pulmonary esterases to active metabolite (beclomethasone-17-monoproprionate [17-BMP]) during absorption

Distribution: V$_d$: Beclomethasone dipropionate (BDP): 20 L; 17-BMP: 424 L

Protein binding: BDP 87%; 17-BMP: 94% to 96%

Metabolism: BDP is a pro-drug (inactive); undergoes rapid conversion to 17-BMP during absorption; followed by additional metabolism via CYP3A4 to other, less active metabolites (beclomethasone-21-monopropionate [21-BMP] and beclomethasone [BOH])

Half-life elimination: BDP: 0.5 hours; 17-BMP: 2.7 hours

Time to peak, plasma: Oral inhalation: BDP: 0.5 hours; 17-BMP: 0.7 hours

Excretion: Primary route of excretion is via feces (~60%); <10% to 12% of oral dose excreted in urine as metabolites

Dosing

Adult & Geriatric

Asthma: Inhalation, oral (doses should be titrated to the lowest effective dose once asthma is controlled):

US labeling:

Patients previously on bronchodilators only: Initial dose 40 to 80 mcg twice daily; maximum dose: 320 mcg twice daily

Patients previously on inhaled corticosteroids: Initial dose 40 to 160 mcg twice daily; maximum dose: 320 mcg twice daily

Canadian labeling:

Mild asthma: 50 to 100 mcg twice daily; maximum dose: 100 mcg twice daily

Moderate asthma: 100 to 250 mcg twice daily; maximum dose: 250 mcg twice daily

Severe asthma: 300 to 400 mcg twice daily; maximum dose: 400 mcg twice daily

Asthma Guidelines:

National Asthma Education and Prevention Program guidelines (NAEPP, 2007): HFA inhaler (refers to Qvar 40 mcg and 80 mcg strengths available in US):

"Low" dose: 80 to 240 mcg daily

"Medium" dose: >240 to 480 mcg daily

"High" dose: >480 mcg daily

Global Initiative for Asthma guidelines (GINA 2015): HFA inhaler (refers to Qvar 50 mcg and 100 mcg strengths available in Canada):

"Low" dose: 100 to 200 mcg daily

"Medium" dose: >200 to 400 mcg daily

"High" dose: >400 mcg daily

Conversion: Conversion from oral systemic corticosteroid to orally inhaled corticosteroid: Initiation of oral inhalation therapy should begin in patients whose asthma is reasonably stabilized on oral corticosteroids (OCS). A gradual dose reduction of OCS should begin ~7 days after starting inhaled therapy. US labeling recommends reducing prednisone dose no more ▶

rapidly than ≤2.5 mg/day (or equivalent of other OCS) every 1 to 2 weeks. The Canadian labeling recommends decreasing the daily dose of prednisone by 1 mg (or equivalent of other OCS) every 7 days or more in closely monitored patients. If adrenal insufficiency occurs, temporarily increase the OCS dose and follow with a more gradual withdrawal. **Note:** When transitioning from systemic to inhaled corticosteroids, supplemental systemic corticosteroid therapy may be necessary during periods of stress or during severe asthma attacks.

Chronic obstructive pulmonary disease (stable) (off-label use): Inhalation, oral: 50 to 400 mcg daily in combination with a long-acting bronchodilator (GOLD, 2014).

Pediatric

Asthma: Inhalation, oral (doses should be titrated to the lowest effective dose once asthma is controlled):

US labeling:

Children 5 to 11 years: Initial: 40 mcg twice daily; maximum dose: 80 mcg twice daily

Children ≥12 years and Adolescents: Refer to adult dosing

Canadian labeling:

Children 5 to 11 years: Initial: 50 mcg twice daily; maximum dose: 100 mcg twice daily

Children ≥12 years and Adolescents: Refer to adult dosing.

Asthma Guidelines:

National Asthma Education and Prevention Program guidelines (NAEPP, 2007): HFA inhaler (refers to Qvar 40 mcg and 80 mcg strengths available in US):

Children 5 to 11 years:

"Low" dose: 80 to 160 mcg daily

"Medium" dose: >160 to 320 mcg daily

"High" dose: >320 mcg daily

Children ≥12 years and Adolescents: Refer to adult dosing.

Global Initiative for Asthma guidelines (GINA, 2015): HFA inhaler (refers to Qvar 50 mcg and 100 mcg strengths available in Canada):

Children ≤5 years: "Low" dose: 100 mcg daily

Children 6 to 11 years:

"Low" dose: 50 to 100 mcg daily

"Medium" dose: >100 to 200 mcg daily

"High" dose: >200 mcg daily

Children ≥12 years and Adolescents: Refer to adult dosing.

Conversion: *Conversion from oral systemic corticosteroid to orally inhaled corticosteroid:* Initiation of oral inhalation therapy should begin in patients whose asthma is reasonably stabilized on oral corticosteroids (OCS). A gradual dose reduction of OCS should begin ~7 days after starting inhaled therapy. US labeling recommends reducing prednisone dose no more rapidly than ≤2.5 mg/day (or equivalent of other OCS) every 1 to 2 weeks. The Canadian labeling recommends decreasing the daily dose of prednisone by 1 mg (or equivalent of other OCS) every 7 days or more in closely monitored patients. If adrenal insufficiency occurs, temporarily increase the OCS dose and follow with a more gradual withdrawal. **Note:** When transitioning from systemic to inhaled corticosteroids, supplemental systemic corticosteroid therapy may be necessary during periods of stress or during severe asthma attacks.

Renal Impairment There are no dosage adjustments provided in the manufacturer's labeling

Hepatic Impairment There are no dosage adjustments provided in the manufacturer's labeling

Administration Canister does not need shaken prior to use. Prime canister by spraying twice into the air prior to initial use or if not in use for >10 days. Avoid spraying in face or eyes. Exhale fully prior to bringing inhaler to mouth. Place inhaler in mouth, close lips around mouthpiece, and inhale slowly and deeply. Remove inhaler and hold breath for approximately 5 to 10 seconds. Rinse mouth and throat with water (and spit) after use to prevent *Candida* infection. Do not wash or put inhaler in water; mouth piece may be cleaned with a dry tissue or cloth. Discard the inhaler when the dose counter displays "0". Patients using a spacer should inhale immediately due to decreased amount of medication that is delivered with a delayed inspiration.

Monitoring Parameters Growth (adolescents) and signs/symptoms of HPA axis suppression/adrenal insufficiency; signs/symptoms of oral candidiasis; ocular effects (eg, cataracts, increased intraocular pressure, glaucoma)

Additional Information Effects of inhaled steroids on growth have been observed in the absence of laboratory evidence of HPA axis suppression, suggesting that growth velocity is a more sensitive indicator of systemic corticosteroid exposure in pediatric patients than some commonly used tests of HPA axis function. The long-term effects of this reduction in growth velocity associated with orally-inhaled corticosteroids, including the impact on final adult height, are unknown. The potential for "catch up" growth following discontinuation of treatment with inhaled corticosteroids has not been adequately studied.

Dosage Forms Considerations QVAR 8.7 g canisters contain 120 inhalations.

Dosage Forms Excipient information presented when available (limited, particularly for generics); consult specific product labeling.

Aerosol Solution, Inhalation, as dipropionate:

Qvar: 40 mcg/actuation (8.7 g); 80 mcg/actuation (8.7 g)

Dosage Forms: Canada Excipient information presented when available (limited, particularly for generics); consult specific product labeling.

Aerosol, for oral inhalation, as dipropionate:

QVAR: 50 mcg/inhalation (6.5 g) [chlorofluorocarbon free; contains ethanol; 100 metered actuations]

QVAR: 50 mcg/inhalation (12.4 g) [chlorofluorocarbon free; contains ethanol; 200 metered actuations]

QVAR: 100 mcg/inhalation (6.5 g) [chlorofluorocarbon free; contains ethanol; 100 metered actuations]

QVAR: 100 mcg/inhalation (12.4 g) [chlorofluorocarbon free; contains ethanol; 200 metered actuations]

Beclomethasone (Nasal) (be kloe METH a sone)

Brand Names: US Beconase AQ; Qnasl; Qnasl Childrens

Brand Names: Canada Apo-Beclomethasone; Mylan-Beclo AQ; Rivanase AQ

Index Terms Beclomethasone Dipropionate; Vancenase AQ

Pharmacologic Category Corticosteroid, Nasal

Additional Appendix Information

Inhaled Corticosteroids *on page 1951*

Use

Nasal polyps Beconase AQ only: Prevention of recurrence of nasal polyps following surgical removal

Rhinitis:

Beconase AQ: Relief of symptoms of seasonal or perennial allergic rhinitis and nonallergic (vasomotor) rhinitis

Qnasl: Treatment of the nasal symptoms associated with seasonal or perennial allergic rhinitis in patients 4 years and older.

Dosing

Adult & Geriatric

Beconase AQ: Rhinitis, nasal polyps (postsurgical prophylaxis): Inhalation, nasal: One or two inhalations (42 or 84 mcg) in each nostril twice daily; total dose: 168 to 336 mcg daily; maximum dose: 336 mcg daily

Qnasl: Allergic rhinitis: Inhalation, nasal: Qnasl 80 mcg: Two inhalations (160 mcg) in each nostril once daily (maximum: 320 mcg daily)

Pediatric

Beconase AQ: Rhinitis, nasal polyps (postsurgical prophylaxis): Inhalation, nasal:

Children 6 to 11 years: Initial: One inhalation (42 mcg) in each nostril twice daily (total dose: 168 mcg daily); if response inadequate, may increase to 2 inhalations (84 mcg) in each nostril twice daily (total dose: 336 mcg daily); once adequate control is achieved, decreased to 1 inhalation (42 mcg) in each nostril twice daily (total dose: 168 mcg daily)

Children ≥12 years and Adolescents: Refer to adult dosing.

Qnasl: Allergic rhinitis: Inhalation, nasal:

Children 4 to 11 years: Qnasl 40 mcg: One inhalation (40 mcg) in each nostril once daily (maximum: 80 mcg daily)

Children ≥12 years and Adolescents: Qnasl 80 mcg: Refer to adult dosing.

Renal Impairment There are no dosage adjustments provided in the manufacturer's labeling.

Hepatic Impairment There are no dosage adjustments provided in the manufacturer's labeling.

Additional Information Complete prescribing information should be consulted for additional detail.

Dosage Forms Considerations

Beconase AQ 25 g bottles contain 180 sprays.

Qnasl 8.7 g bottles contain 120 actuations.

Dosage Forms Excipient information presented when available (limited, particularly for generics); consult specific product labeling.

Aerosol Solution, Nasal, as dipropionate:

Qnasl: 80 mcg/actuation (8.7 g)

Qnasl Childrens: 40 mcg/actuation (4.9 g)

Suspension, Nasal, as dipropionate:
Beconase AQ: 42 mcg/spray (25 g) [contains benzalkonium chloride]

♦ **Beclomethasone Dipropionate** *see* Beclomethasone (Nasal) *on page 206*

♦ **Beconase AQ** *see* Beclomethasone (Nasal) *on page 206*

Bedaquiline (bed AK wi leen)

Brand Names: US Sirturo
Index Terms AIDS222089; R207910; TMC207
Pharmacologic Category Antitubercular Agent
Use
Multidrug-resistant pulmonary tuberculosis: Treatment of pulmonary multidrug-resistant tuberculosis (MDR-TB) in adults (≥18 years of age) when other alternatives are not available.
Limitations of use: Not for use in extrapulmonary TB, latent infection due to TB, drug-sensitive TB, or treatment of other mycobacteria. Clinical data in HIV-1 infected patients coinfected with MDR-TB are limited (safety and efficacy has not been established).
Medication Guide Available Yes
Dosing
Adult & Geriatric Note: Use with ≥3 drugs also active against the patient's *M. tuberculosis* isolate.
Tuberculosis (multidrug-resistant), pulmonary: Oral: Directly observed therapy (DOT):
Weeks 1-2: 400 mg once daily. **Note:** If a dose is missed during weeks 1-2, do not make up the missed dose, and continue the usual dosing schedule.
Weeks 3-24: 200 mg 3 times weekly (total weekly dose: 600 mg). **Note:** Space doses at least 48 hours apart. If a dose is missed during weeks 3-24, administer the missed dose as soon as possible, and resume the 3-times-weekly schedule.
Renal Impairment
Mild-to-moderate renal impairment: No dosage adjustment necessary.
Severe renal impairment: No dosage adjustment provided in manufacturer's labeling; use with caution. Manufacturer's labeling recommends monitoring for adverse reactions in this population.
Intermittent hemodialysis (IHD) or peritoneal dialysis (PD): No dosage adjustment provided in manufacturer's labeling. Use with caution (CDC 2013); bedaquiline is highly protein bound and not likely to be removed by dialysis. Manufacturer's labeling recommends monitoring for adverse reactions in this population.
Hepatic Impairment
Mild or moderate impairment (Child-Pugh class A or B): No dosage adjustment necessary.
Severe impairment (Child-Pugh class C): No dosage adjustment provided in manufacturer's labeling; use with caution (has not been studied). Manufacturer's labeling recommends monitoring for adverse reactions in this population.
Additional Information Complete prescribing information should be consulted for additional detail.
Dosage Forms Excipient information presented when available (limited, particularly for generics); consult specific product labeling.
Tablet, Oral:
Sirturo: 100 mg

♦ **Behenyl Alcohol** *see* Docosanol *on page 578*

♦ **Bekyree** *see* Ethinyl Estradiol and Desogestrel *on page 701*

Belatacept (bel AT a sept)

Brand Names: US Nulojix
Index Terms BMS-224818; LEA29Y
Pharmacologic Category Selective T-Cell Costimulation Blocker
Use
Kidney transplant: Prophylaxis of organ rejection concomitantly with basiliximab induction, mycophenolate, and corticosteroids in adult Epstein-Barr virus (EBV) seropositive kidney transplant recipients
Limitations of use: Use only in EBV seropositive patients; use for prophylaxis of organ rejection in transplanted organs other than the kidney has not been established.
Pregnancy Considerations Adverse events have been observed in animal reproduction studies. According to the manufacturer, do not use belatacept in pregnancy unless the potential benefit to the mother outweighs the potential risk to the fetus. A pregnancy registry has been established to monitor outcomes of women exposed to belatacept during pregnancy (1-877-955-6877).

Breast-Feeding Considerations It is not known if belatacept is excreted in breast milk. Due to the potential for serious adverse reactions in the nursing infant, the manufacturer recommends a decision be made whether to discontinue nursing or to discontinue the drug, taking into account the importance of treatment to the mother.
Prescribing and Access Restrictions The ENLiST registry has been created to further determine the safety of belatacept, particularly the incidence of post-transplant lymphoproliferative disorder (PTLD), CNS PTLD, and progressive multifocal leukoencephalopathy (PML), in U.S. adult EBV-seropositive kidney transplant patients. Transplant centers are encouraged to participate (1-800-321-1335).
Medication Guide Available Yes
Contraindications Transplant patients who are Epstein-Barr virus (EBV) seronegative or with unknown EBV serostatus
Warnings/Precautions [U.S. Boxed Warning]: Risk of post-transplant lymphoproliferative disorder (PTLD) is increased, primarily involving the CNS, in patients receiving belatacept compared to patients receiving cyclosporine-based regimens. Degree of immunosuppression is a risk factor for PTLD developing; do not exceed recommended dosing. Patients who are Epstein-Barr virus seronegative (EBV) are at an even higher risk; use is contraindicated in patients without evidence of immunity to EBV. Therapy is only appropriate in patients who are EBV seropositive via evidence of acquired immunity, such as presence of IgG antibodies to viral capsid antigen [VCA] and EBV nuclear antigen [EBNA]. Cytomegalovirus (CMV) infection and T-cell depleting therapy also increases the risk for PTLD; T-cell depleting therapies to treat acute rejection should be used with caution. Although CMV disease is a risk for PTLD and CMV seronegative patients are at an increased risk for CMV disease, the clinical role, if any, of determining CMV serology to determine risk of PTLD development has not been determined.

[U.S. Boxed Warning]: Risk for infection is increased. Immunosuppressive therapy may lead to bacterial, viral (CMV and herpes), fungal, and protozoal infections, including opportunistic infections (may be fatal). Tuberculosis (TB) is increased; test patients for latent TB prior to initiation, and treat latent TB infection prior to use. Prophylaxis for CMV is recommended for at least 3 months after transplantation; prophylaxis for *Pneumocystis jiroveci* is recommended after transplantation. Patients receiving immunosuppressive therapy are at an increased risk of activation of latent viral infections, including John Cunningham virus (JCV) and BK virus infection. Activation of JCV may result in progressive multifocal leukoencephalopathy (PML), a rare and potentially fatal condition affecting the CNS. Symptoms of PML include apathy, ataxia, cognitive deficiencies, confusion, and hemiparesis. Polyoma virus-associated nephropathy (PVAN), primarily from activation of BK virus, may also occur and lead to the deterioration of renal function and/or renal graft loss. Risk factors for the development of PML and PVAN include immunosuppression and treatment with immunosuppressant therapy. The onset of PML or PVAN may warrant a reduction in immunosuppressive therapy; however, in transplant recipients, the risk of reduced immunosuppression and graft rejection should be considered.

[U.S. Boxed Warning]: Risk for malignancy is increased. Malignancy, including skin malignancy and PTLD, is associated with the use of belatacept; higher than recommended doses or more frequent dosing is not recommended; patients should be advised to limit their exposure to sunlight/UV light.

[U.S. Boxed Warning]: Therapy is not recommended in liver transplant patients due to increased risk of graft loss and death. [U.S. Boxed Warning]: Should be administered under the supervision of a physician experienced in immunosuppressive therapy. Increased rate and grade of acute rejection, particularly grade 3 rejection, and graft loss has been observed with belatacept when corticosteroids were minimized to 5 mg daily between day 3 and week 6 post-transplant; corticosteroid dosing should be consistent with clinical trial experience (ie, tapered to ~15 mg [10 to 20 mg] daily by the first 6 weeks post-transplant and remain at ~10 mg [5 to 10 mg] daily for the first 6 months post-transplant). Immunization with live vaccines should be avoided during treatment. Potentially significant drug-drug interactions may exist, requiring dose or frequency adjustment, additional monitoring, and/or selection of alternative therapy.

◄ **Adverse Reactions** Incidences reported occurred during clinical trials using belatacept compared to a cyclosporine control regimen. All patients also received basiliximab induction, mycophenolate mofetil, and corticosteroids, and were followed up to 3 years.

>10%:

Cardiovascular: Peripheral edema (34%), hypertension (32%), hypotension (18%)

Central nervous system: Fever (28%), headache (21%), insomnia (15%)

Endocrine & metabolic: Hypokalemia (21%), hyperkalemia (20%), hypophosphatemia (19%), lipid metabolism disorder (19%), hyperglycemia (16%), hypocalcemia (13%), hypercholesterolemia (11%)

Gastrointestinal: Diarrhea (39%), constipation (33%), nausea (24%), vomiting (22%), abdominal pain (19%)

Genitourinary: Urinary tract infection (37%), dysuria (11%)

Hematologic & oncologic: Anemia (45%), leukopenia (20%)

Infection: Increased susceptibility to infection (72% to 82%, serious infection 24% to 36%), herpes (7% to 14%), cytomegalovirus disease (11% to 13%), influenza (11%)

Neuromuscular & skeletal: Arthralgia (17%), back pain (13%)

Renal: Proteinuria (16%; up to 33% 2+ proteinuria at 1 month post-transplant), renal graft dysfunction (25%), hematuria (16%), increased serum creatinine (15%)

Respiratory: Cough (24%), upper respiratory tract infection (15%), nasopharyngitis (13%), dyspnea (12%)

1% to 10%:

Cardiovascular: Arteriovenous fistula site complication (thrombosis, <10%), atrial fibrillation (<10%)

Central nervous system: Anxiety (10%), Guillain-Barré syndrome (<10%), dizziness (9%)

Dermatologic: Alopecia (<10%), hyperhidrosis (<10%), acne vulgaris (8%)

Endocrine & metabolic: Diabetes mellitus (new onset, 5% to 8%), hypomagnesemia (7%), hyperuricemia (5%)

Gastrointestinal: Stomatitis (<10%), upper abdominal pain (9%)

Genitourinary: Urinary incontinence (<10%)

Hematologic & oncologic: Hematoma (<10%), lymphocele (<10%), neutropenia (<10%), malignant neoplasm (4%), malignant neoplasm of skin (nonmelanoma, 2%)

Immunologic: Antibody development (2%)

Infection: Polyoma virus (3% to 4%)

Neuromuscular & skeletal: Musculoskeletal pain (<10%), tremor (8%)

Renal: Acute renal failure (<10%), chronic allograft nephropathy (<10%), hydronephrosis (<10%), renal insufficiency (<10%), renal artery stenosis (<10%), renal tubular necrosis (9%), renal disease (BK virus-associated, 1%)

Respiratory: Bronchitis (10%), tuberculosis (1% to 2%)

Miscellaneous: Infusion related reaction (5%)

<1%, postmarketing, and/or case reports (Limited to important or life-threatening): Aspergillosis (cerebral; higher dosing regimen), encephalitis (Chagas, West Nile; higher dosing regimen), lymphoproliferative disorder (post-transplant; incidence is 9-fold higher in non-EBV seropositive patients), meningitis (cryptococcal), progressive multifocal leukoencephalopathy (higher dosing regimen), renal graft rejection

Drug Interactions

Metabolism/Transport Effects None known.

Avoid Concomitant Use

Avoid concomitant use of Belatacept with any of the following: BCG (Intravesical); Belimumab; Natalizumab; Pimecrolimus; Tacrolimus (Topical); Tofacitinib; Vaccines (Live)

Increased Effect/Toxicity

Belatacept may increase the levels/effects of: Belimumab; Fingolimod; Leflunomide; Natalizumab; Tofacitinib; Vaccines (Live)

The levels/effects of Belatacept may be increased by: Denosumab; Pimecrolimus; Roflumilast; Tacrolimus (Topical); Trastuzumab

Decreased Effect

Belatacept may decrease the levels/effects of: BCG (Intravesical); Coccidioides immitis Skin Test; Sipuleucel-T; Vaccines (Inactivated); Vaccines (Live)

The levels/effects of Belatacept may be decreased by: Echinacea

Preparation for Administration Reconstitute each vial with 10.5 mL of diluent (SWFI, NS, or D₅W only) using the provided silicone-free disposable syringe, and an 18- to 21-gauge needle. Reconstitute using **only** the silicone-free syringe provided; if the provided silicone-free syringe is dropped or becomes contaminated, use a new silicone-free disposable syringe from inventory (contact the manufacturer on obtaining additional silicone-free disposable syringes). If powder is inadvertently mixed using a siliconized syringe, discard solution; translucent particles may develop. Inject the diluent down the side of the vial to avoid foaming. Rotate the vial and invert with gentle swirling until completely dissolved; do **not** shake vial. Immediately transfer the reconstituted solution using the same silicone-free syringe to an infusion bag or bottle with NS or D₅W (if NS or D₅W were used to reconstitute, the same fluid should be used to further dilute). Gently rotate the infusion bag or bottle; do not shake. The final concentration should range from 2 mg/mL and 10 mg/mL (typical infusion volume is 100 mL; volumes ranging from 50 mL to 250 mL may be used). Prior to adding belatacept to the infusion solution, the manufacturer recommends withdrawing a volume equal to the amount of belatacept to be added.

Storage/Stability Prior to use, store refrigerated at 2°C to 8°C (36°F to 46°F). Protect from light. After dilution, the reconstituted solution should be transferred from the vial to infusion bag or bottle immediately; infusion solution may be stored refrigerated for up to 24 hours, with a maximum of 4 hours of the 24 hours at room temperature, 20°C to 25°C (68°F to 77°F), and room light. Infusion must be completed within 24 hours of reconstitution. Discard unused solution in vials.

Mechanism of Action Fusion protein which acts as a selective T-cell (lymphocyte) costimulation blocker by binding to CD80 and CD86 receptors on antigen presenting cells (APC), blocking the required CD28 mediated interaction between APCs and T cells needed to activate T lymphocytes. T-cell stimulation results in cytokine production and proliferation, mediators in immunologic rejection associated with kidney transplantation.

Pharmacodynamics/Kinetics

Distribution: V_{ss}: 0.11 L/kg (transplant patients)

Half-life elimination: ~10 days (healthy patients and kidney transplant patients)

Dosing

Adult Note: Dosing is based on actual body weight at the time of transplantation; do not modify weight-based dosing during course of therapy unless the change in body weight is >10%. The prescribed dose must be evenly divisible by 12.5 mg to allow accurate preparation of the reconstituted solution using the provided required disposable syringe for preparation. For example, the calculated dose for a 64 kg patient: 64 kg x 10 mg per kg = 640 mg. The nearest doses to 640 mg that are evenly divisible by 12.5 mg would be 637.5 mg or 650 mg; the closest dose to the calculated dose is 637.5 mg, therefore, 637.5 should be the actual prescribed dose for the patient.

Kidney transplant, prophylaxis of organ rejection: IV:

Note: Use in combination with basiliximab induction, mycophenolate mofetil, and corticosteroids.

Initial phase: 10 mg/kg on Day 1 (day of transplant, prior to implantation) and on Day 5 (~96 hours after Day 1 dose), followed by 10 mg/kg at the end of Week 2, Week 4, Week 8, and Week 12 following transplantation

Maintenance phase: 5 mg/kg every 4 weeks (plus or minus 3 days) beginning at the end of Week 16 following transplantation

Geriatric Refer to adult dosing

Renal Impairment There are no dosage adjustments provided in the manufacturer's labeling; however, renal function did not affect clearance in pharmacokinetic studies of kidney transplant patients.

Hepatic Impairment There are no dosage adjustments provided in the manufacturer's labeling; however, hepatic function did not affect clearance in pharmacokinetic studies of kidney transplant patients.

Administration Administer as an IV infusion over 30 minutes using an infusion set with a 0.2 to 1.2 micron low protein-binding filter. The infusion must be completed within 24 hours of reconstitution of the lyophilized powder. Infuse in a separate line from other infused agents.

Monitoring Parameters New-onset or worsening neurological, cognitive, or behavioral signs/symptoms; signs/symptoms of infection or malignancy; TB screening prior to therapy initiation; EBV seropositive verification prior to therapy initiation

Additional Information If additional silicone-free disposable syringes are needed, contact Bristol-Myers Squibb at 1-888-NULOJIX.

Dosage Forms Excipient information presented when available (limited, particularly for generics); consult specific product labeling.
Solution Reconstituted, Intravenous:
Nulojix: 250 mg (1 ea)

◆ Belbuca see Buprenorphine on page 263
◆ Beleodaq see Belinostat on page 210

Belimumab (be LIM yoo mab)

Brand Names: US Benlysta
Brand Names: Canada Benlysta
Pharmacologic Category Monoclonal Antibody
Use
Systemic lupus erythematosus: Treatment of adult patients with active, autoantibody-positive systemic lupus erythematosus (SLE) who are receiving standard therapy.
Limitations of use: Use is not recommended in patients with severe active lupus nephritis, severe active CNS lupus, or in combination with other biologics, including B-cell targeted therapies or intravenous (IV) cyclophosphamide.
Pregnancy Considerations Adverse events were observed in some animal reproduction studies. IgG molecules are known to cross the placenta (belimumab is an engineered IgG molecule). Effective contraception should be used during and for at least 4 months following treatment in women of childbearing potential. Healthcare providers are encouraged to enroll women exposed to belimumab during pregnancy in a pregnancy registry (877-681-6296); patients may also enroll themselves.
Breast-Feeding Considerations It is not known if belimumab is excreted in breast milk. Because IgG molecules are excreted in breast milk, a decision should be made whether to discontinue nursing or to discontinue the drug, taking into account the importance of treatment to the mother.
Medication Guide Available Yes
Contraindications Hypersensitivity (anaphylaxis) to belimumab or any component of the formulation
Warnings/Precautions Deaths due to infection, cardiovascular disease, and suicide were higher in belimumab patients compared to placebo during clinical trials. Serious and potentially fatal infections may occur during treatment. Use with caution in patients with chronic infections; treatment should not be undertaken if receiving therapy for chronic infection. Consider interrupting belimumab in patients who develop new infections and initiate appropriate anti-infective treatment; monitor closely. Cases of progressive multifocal leukoencephalopathy (PML) associated with JC virus (some fatal) have been reported in patients with SLE receiving immunosuppressants, including belimumab. Risk factors for PML include immunosuppressant therapies and impaired immune function. Consider diagnosis of PML in any patient presenting with new-onset or deteriorating neurologic signs/symptoms; consult a neurologist (or other appropriate specialist). If PML is confirmed, consider discontinuing immunosuppressant treatment, including belimumab.

Acute hypersensitivity reactions including anaphylaxis (with fatalities) and infusion-related reactions (eg, bradycardia, hypotension, myalgia, headache, rash, and urticaria) have been reported, including patients who had previously tolerated infusions of belimumab; onset may occur within hours of the infusion or may be delayed. Monitor for an appropriate time following administration. Discontinue for severe reactions (anaphylaxis, angioedema); infusion may be slowed or temporarily interrupted for other infusion-related reactions. Risk for hypersensitivity reactions may be increased with history of multiple drug allergies or significant hypersensitivity. Immunosuppressants may increase risk of malignancy. May cause psychiatric adverse effects, including anxiety, insomnia, or new/worsening depression. Potentially significant drug-drug interactions may exist, requiring dose or frequency adjustment, additional monitoring, and/or selection of alternative therapy. Live vaccines should not be given within 30 days before or concurrently with belimumab. Black/African-American patients may have a lower response rate; use with caution.
Adverse Reactions
>10%:
Gastrointestinal: Nausea (15%), diarrhea (12%)
Hypersensitivity: Hypersensitivity (13%)
Miscellaneous: Infusion related reaction (17%)
≥3% to 10%:
Central nervous system: Insomnia (6% to 7%), depression (5% to 6%), migraine (5%), anxiety (4%), headache (≥3%)

Dermatologic: Dermatological reaction (≥3%)
Gastrointestinal: Viral gastroenteritis (3%)
Genitourinary: Urinary tract infection (site not specified >5%), cystitis (4%)
Hematologic & oncologic: Leukopenia (4%)
Infection: Influenza (>5%)
Neuromuscular & skeletal: Limb pain (6%)
Respiratory: Bronchitis (9%), nasopharyngitis (9%), sinusitis (>5%), upper respiratory tract infection (>5%), pharyngitis (5%)
Miscellaneous: Fever (10%)
<3% (Limited to important or life-threatening): Anaphylaxis (including fatalities), antibody development, bradycardia, cellulitis, myalgia, pneumonia, progressive multifocal leukoencephalopathy (immune compromised), suicidal tendencies
Drug Interactions
Metabolism/Transport Effects None known.
Avoid Concomitant Use
Avoid concomitant use of Belimumab with any of the following: Abatacept; BCG (Intravesical); Belatacept; Cyclophosphamide; Etanercept; Monoclonal Antibodies; Natalizumab; Pimecrolimus; Tacrolimus (Topical); Tofacitinib; Vaccines (Live)
Increased Effect/Toxicity
Belimumab may increase the levels/effects of: Cyclophosphamide; Fingolimod; Leflunomide; Natalizumab; Tofacitinib; Vaccines (Live)

The levels/effects of Belimumab may be increased by: Abatacept; Belatacept; Etanercept; Monoclonal Antibodies; Pimecrolimus; Roflumilast; Tacrolimus (Topical)
Decreased Effect
Belimumab may decrease the levels/effects of: BCG (Intravesical); Coccidioides immitis Skin Test; Sipuleucel-T; Vaccines (Inactivated)

The levels/effects of Belimumab may be decreased by: Echinacea
Preparation for Administration To reconstitute, remove vial from the refrigerator and allow to stand 10 to 15 minutes to reach room temperature. Reconstitute 120 mg vial with 1.5 mL of sterile water for injection (SWFI). Reconstitute 400 mg vial with 4.8 mL of SWFI. To minimize foaming, direct SWFI toward the side of the vial. Gently swirl for 60 seconds every 5 minutes until powder has dissolved (usual reconstitution time is 10-15 minutes, but may take up to 30 minutes); do not shake. If utilizing a mechanical reconstitution device, do not exceed 500 rpm or 30 minutes. Further dilute reconstituted solution in 250 mL of 0.9% sodium chloride (dilute only in 0.9% sodium chloride) by first removing and discarding the volume equivalent to the volume of the reconstituted solution to be added to prepare the appropriate dose; add the appropriate volume of the reconstituted solution to the infusion container and gently invert to mix solution. Protect from light. Solution may be stored refrigerated or at room temperature.
Storage/Stability Prior to reconstitution, store unused vials between 2°C and 8°C (36°F and 46°F); do not freeze. Protect from light. Avoid exposure to heat. Prior to further dilution, the reconstituted solution must be stored under refrigeration. The diluted solution may be stored refrigerated or at room temperature. Infusion must be completed within 8 hours of reconstitution.
Mechanism of Action Belimumab is an IgG1-lambda monoclonal antibody that prevents the survival of B lymphocytes by blocking the binding of soluble human B lymphocyte stimulator protein (BLyS) to receptors on B lymphocytes. This reduces the activity of B-cell mediated immunity and the autoimmune response.
Pharmacodynamics/Kinetics
Onset of action: B cells: 8 weeks; Clinical improvement (SLE Responder Index and flare reduction): 16 weeks (Navarra, 2011)
Distribution: V_d: 5.29 L
Half-life elimination: 19.4 days
Dosing
Adult & Geriatric Systemic lupus erythematosus (SLE): IV: Initial: 10 mg/kg every 2 weeks for 3 doses; Maintenance: 10 mg/kg every 4 weeks
Renal Impairment
CrCl ≥15 mL/minute: No dosage adjustment necessary.
CrCl <15 mL/minute: There are no dosage adjustments provided in the manufacturer's labeling (has not been studied).
Hepatic Impairment There are no dosage adjustments provided in the manufacturer's labeling (has not been studied).
Administration Administer intravenously over 1 hour through a dedicated IV line. Do **NOT** administer as an IV push or bolus. Discontinue infusion for severe hypersensitivity reaction (eg, anaphylaxis, angioedema). The infusion

may be slowed or temporarily interrupted for minor reactions. Consider premedicating with an antihistamine and antipyretic for prophylaxis against hypersensitivity or infusion reactions.

Monitoring Parameters Monitor for hypersensitivity and/or infusion reactions; infections; worsening of depression, mood changes, or suicidal thoughts

Dosage Forms Excipient information presented when available (limited, particularly for generics); consult specific product labeling.

Solution Reconstituted, Intravenous [preservative free]:

Benlysta: 120 mg (1 ea); 400 mg (1 ea) [contains polysorbate 80]

Belinostat (be LIN oh stat)

Brand Names: US Beleodaq

Index Terms PXD101

Pharmacologic Category Antineoplastic Agent, Histone Deacetylase (HDAC) Inhibitor

Use Peripheral T-cell lymphoma: Treatment of relapsed or refractory peripheral T-cell lymphoma (PTCL)

Pregnancy Considerations Animal reproduction studies have not been conducted. Belinostat is a genotoxic drug that targets dividing cells; embryofetal toxicity is expected if exposure occurs during pregnancy. Based on animal data, belinostat may also impair male fertility. Women of reproductive potential should avoid pregnancy during treatment with belinostat.

Breast-Feeding Considerations It is not known if belinostat is excreted in breast milk. Due to the potential for serious adverse reactions in the nursing infant, the manufacturer recommends that a decision be made whether to discontinue nursing or to discontinue the drug, taking into account the importance of treatment to the mother.

Contraindications There are no contraindications listed in the manufacturer's labeling.

Warnings/Precautions Hazardous agent – Use appropriate precautions for handling and disposal (meets NIOSH 2014 criteria).

May cause thrombocytopenia, leukopenia (neutropenia and lymphopenia), and/or anemia. Monitor blood counts at baseline and weekly during treatment. May require dosage reduction, treatment delay, or discontinuation. Serious infections (occasionally fatal), including pneumonia and sepsis, have occurred with treatment. Do not administer in patients with an active infection. Heavily pretreated patients (history of extensive or intensive prior chemotherapy) may be at higher risk for life-threatening infections.

May cause liver function test abnormalities and fatal hepatotoxicity. Monitor liver function tests at baseline and prior to each cycle. May require dosage reduction, treatment delay, or permanent discontinuation (based on the severity of the hepatotoxicity). Belinostat is metabolized hepatically and increased exposure is expected to occur in patients with hepatic impairment. Patients with moderate to severe hepatic impairment (total bilirubin >1.5 times ULN) were excluded from clinical studies. Tumor lysis syndrome (TLS) has been observed; closely monitor patients with advanced disease and/or high tumor burden. If TLS occurs, initiate appropriate treatment. Nausea, vomiting, and diarrhea occur with belinostat; may require management with antiemetic and antidiarrheal medications. In a phase 1 study, nausea/vomiting generally occurred at the end of the infusion each day (rarely persisting beyond day 5 each cycle) and was managed with standard antiemetics (Steele, 2011).

Belinostat is primarily metabolized by UGT1A1; the initial dose should be reduced in patients known to be homozygous for UGT1A1*28 allele. Potentially significant drug-drug interactions may exist, requiring dose or frequency adjustment, additional monitoring, and/or selection of alternative therapy.

Adverse Reactions

>10%:

Cardiovascular: Peripheral edema (20%), prolonged Q-T interval on ECG (11%; grades 3/4: 4%)

Central nervous system: Fatigue (37%; grades 3/4: 5%), chills (16%; grades 3/4: 1%), headache (15%)

Dermatologic: Skin rash (20%; grades 3/4: 1%), pruritus (16%; grades 3/4: 3%)

Endocrine & metabolic: Increased lactate dehydrogenase (16%; grades 3/4: 2%), hypokalemia (12%; grades 3/4: 4%)

Gastrointestinal: Nausea (42%; grades 3/4: 1%), vomiting (29%; grades 3/4: 1%), constipation (23%; grades 3/4: 1%), diarrhea (23%; grades 3/4: 2%), decreased appetite (15%; grades 3/4: 2%), abdominal pain (11%; grades 3/4: 1%)

Hematologic & oncologic: Anemia (32%; grades 3/4: 11%), thrombocytopenia (16%; grades 3/4: 7%)

Local: Pain at injection site (14%)

Respiratory: Dyspnea (22%; grades 3/4: 6%), cough (19%)

Miscellaneous: Fever (35%; grades 3/4: 2%)

1% to 10%:

Cardiovascular: Hypotension (10%; grades 3/4: 3%), phlebitis (10%; grades 3/4: 1%)

Central nervous system: Dizziness (10%)

Infection: Infection (>2%)

Renal: Increased serum creatinine (>2%)

Respiratory: Pneumonia (>2%)

Miscellaneous: Multi-organ failure (>2%)

<1% (Limited to important or life-threatening): Hepatic failure, leukopenia, sepsis, tumor lysis syndrome, ventricular fibrillation

Drug Interactions

Metabolism/Transport Effects Substrate of CYP2A6 (minor), CYP2C9 (minor), CYP3A4 (minor), P-glycoprotein, UGT1A1; **Note:** Assignment of Major/Minor substrate status based on clinically relevant drug interaction potential; **Inhibits** CYP2C8 (weak), CYP2C9 (weak)

Avoid Concomitant Use

Avoid concomitant use of Belinostat with any of the following: Amodiaquine; Atazanavir; BCG (Intravesical); Deferiprone; Dipyrone

Increased Effect/Toxicity

Belinostat may increase the levels/effects of: Amodiaquine; CloZAPine; Deferiprone

The levels/effects of Belinostat may be increased by: Atazanavir; Dipyrone

Decreased Effect

Belinostat may decrease the levels/effects of: BCG (Intravesical)

Preparation for Administration Hazardous agent; use appropriate precautions for handling and disposal (meets NIOSH 2014 criteria). Reconstitute each 500 mg vial with SWFI 9 mL to a concentration of 50 mg/mL. Swirl contents until there are no visible particles in the reconstituted solution. Further dilute the appropriate dose in NS 250 mL; do not use if cloudy or precipitate is present.

Storage/Stability Store intact vials at 20°C to 25°C (68°F to 77°F); excursions are permitted between 15°C and 30°C (59°F and 86°F). Retain in original package until use. The reconstituted solution may be stored for 12 hours at 15°C to 25°C (59°F to 77°F). Solutions diluted for infusion may be stored for up to 36 hours (including infusion time) at 15°C to 25°C (59°F to 77°F).

Mechanism of Action Histone deacetylase (HDAC) inhibitor which catalyzes acetyl group removal from protein lysine residues (of histone and some nonhistone proteins). Inhibition of histone deacetylase results in accumulation of acetyl groups, leading to cell cycle arrest and apoptosis. Belinostat has preferential cytotoxicity toward tumor cells versus normal cells.

Pharmacodynamics/Kinetics

Distribution: ~114 L/m^2 (Steele, 2011); mean volume of distribution approaches total body water

Protein binding: 93% to 96%

Metabolism: Hepatic; predominantly via UGT1A1, also by CYP2A6, CYP2C9, and CYP3A4 to the amide and acid metabolites

Half-life elimination: 1.1 hours

Time to peak: At end of infusion (Steele, 2011)

Excretion: Urine (~40%, predominantly as metabolites; <2% as unchanged drug)

Dosing

Adult & Geriatric Note: ANC should be ≥1000/mm^3 and platelets should be ≥50,000/mm^3 prior to each cycle

Peripheral T-cell lymphoma, relapsed or refractory: IV: 1000 mg/m^2 daily on days 1 to 5 every 21 days until disease progression or unacceptable toxicity (O'Connor, 2013)

Dosage adjustment for patients with reduced UGT1A1 activity: Reduce initial dose to 750 mg/m^2 for patients known to be homozygous for UGT1A1*28 allele.

Renal Impairment

CrCl >39 mL/minute: Exposure is not altered (dosage adjustment is not likely necessary).

CrCl ≤39 mL/minute: There are no dosage adjustments provided in the manufacturer's labeling (data is insufficient to recommend a dose).

Hepatic Impairment

Mild hepatic impairment: There are no dosage adjustments provided in the manufacturer's labeling (exposure is expected to be increased in hepatic impairment).

Moderate to severe hepatic impairment (total bilirubin >1.5 times ULN): There are no dosage adjustments provided in the manufacturer's labeling (data is insufficient to recommend a dose).

Obesity *ASCO Guidelines for appropriate chemotherapy dosing in obese adults with cancer:* Utilize patient's actual body weight (full weight) for calculation of body surface area- or weight-based dosing, particularly when the intent of therapy is curative; manage regimen-related toxicities in the same manner as for nonobese patients; if a dose reduction is utilized due to toxicity, consider resumption of full weight-based dosing with subsequent cycles, especially if cause of toxicity (eg, hepatic or renal impairment) is resolved (Griggs, 2012).

Adjustment for Toxicity

Hematologic toxicity: ANC should be ≥1000/mm^3 and platelets should be ≥50,000/mm^3 prior to each cycle and prior to resuming treatment following a delay due to toxicity. Resume subsequent treatment according to the following parameters:

Platelets ≥25,000/mm^3 and nadir ANC ≥500/mm^3: No dosage adjustment necessary (continue treatment without modification).

Nadir ANC <500/mm^3 and any platelet count: Reduce dose by 25% (to 750 mg/m^2).

Platelets <25,000/mm^3 and any nadir ANC: Reduce dose by 25% (to 750 mg/m^2).

Recurrent nadir ANC <500/mm^3 and/or recurrent nadir platelets <25,000/mm^3 following 2 dosage reductions: Discontinue treatment.

Nonhematologic toxicity: Nonhematologic toxicities should be grade 2 or lower prior to retreatment. Resume subsequent treatment according to the following parameters:

Any grade 3 or 4 toxicity (except nausea, vomiting, or diarrhea): Reduce dose by 25% (to 750 mg/m^2).

Recurrent grade 3 or 4 toxicity following 2 dosage reductions: Discontinue treatment.

Grade 3 or 4 nausea, vomiting, or diarrhea: Manage with supportive care; reduce the dose only if duration is >7 days with supportive management.

Administration IV: Infuse over 30 minutes using a 0.22-micron inline filter; if infusion site pain or other symptoms associated with infusion occur, may increase infusion time to 45 minutes.

Hazardous agent; use appropriate precautions for handling and disposal (meets NIOSH 2014 criteria).

Monitoring Parameters Monitor CBC with platelets and differential at baseline and weekly; serum chemistries (including renal and hepatic functions tests) at baseline and before each cycle; monitor for signs/symptoms of gastrointestinal toxicity (eg, nausea, vomiting, diarrhea), tumor lysis syndrome, and infection.

Dosage Forms Excipient information presented when available (limited, particularly for generics); consult specific product labeling.

Solution Reconstituted, Intravenous:

Beleodaq: 500 mg (1 ea)

◆ Belladonna Alkaloids With Phenobarbital *see* Hyoscyamine, Atropine, Scopolamine, and Phenobarbital *on page 900*

Belladonna and Opium (bel a DON a & OH pee um)

Index Terms B&O; Opium and Belladonna

Pharmacologic Category Analgesic Combination (Opioid); Analgesic, Opioid; Antispasmodic Agent, Urinary

Use Relief of moderate-to-severe pain associated with ureteral spasms not responsive to nonopioid analgesics and to space intervals between injections of opioids

Dosing

Adult & Geriatric Pain: Rectal: One suppository 1 to 2 times daily; maximum: 4 doses/day

Pediatric Pain: Adolescents: Refer to adult dosing.

Additional Information Complete prescribing information should be consulted for additional detail.

Dosage Forms Excipient information presented when available (limited, particularly for generics); consult specific product labeling.

Suppository: Belladonna extract 16.2 mg and opium 30 mg; belladonna extract 16.2 mg and opium 60 mg

Controlled Substance C-II

◆ Belsomra *see* Suvorexant *on page 1723*

◆ Belviq *see* Lorcaserin *on page 1105*

◆ Benadryl *see* DiphenhydrAMINE (Systemic) *on page 561*

◆ Benadryl [OTC] *see* DiphenhydrAMINE (Systemic) *on page 561*

◆ Benadryl-D® Allergy & Sinus [OTC] *see* Diphenhydramine and Phenylephrine *on page 564*

◆ Benadryl-D® Children's Allergy & Sinus [OTC] *see* Diphenhydramine and Phenylephrine *on page 564*

◆ Benadryl Allergy [OTC] *see* DiphenhydrAMINE (Systemic) *on page 561*

◆ Benadryl Allergy Childrens [OTC] *see* DiphenhydrAMINE (Systemic) *on page 561*

◆ Benadryl Dye-Free Allergy [OTC] *see* DiphenhydrAMINE (Systemic) *on page 561*

Benazepril (ben AY ze pril)

Brand Names: US Lotensin

Brand Names: Canada Lotensin

Index Terms Benazepril Hydrochloride

Pharmacologic Category Angiotensin-Converting Enzyme (ACE) Inhibitor; Antihypertensive

Use

Hypertension: Treatment of hypertension, either alone or in combination with other antihypertensive agents

Guideline recommendations:

Hypertension: The 2014 guideline for the management of high blood pressure in adults (Eighth Joint National Committee [JNC 8]) recommends initiation of pharmacologic treatment to lower blood pressure for the following patients:

• Patients ≥60 years of age with systolic blood pressure (SBP) ≥150 mm Hg or diastolic blood pressure (DBP) ≥90 mm Hg. Goal of therapy is SBP <150 mm Hg and DBP <90 mm Hg.

• Patients <60 years of age with SBP ≥140 mm Hg or DBP is ≥90 mm Hg. Goal of therapy is SBP <140 mm Hg and DBP <90 mm Hg.

• Patients ≥18 years of age with diabetes and SBP ≥140 mm Hg or DBP ≥90 mm Hg. Goal of therapy is SBP <140 mm Hg and DBP <90 mm Hg.

• Patients ≥18 years of age with chronic kidney disease (CKD) and SBP ≥140 mm Hg or DBP ≥90 mm Hg. Goal of therapy is SBP <140 mm Hg and DBP <90 mm Hg.

Chronic kidney disease (CKD) and hypertension: Regardless of race or diabetes status, the use of an ACE inhibitor (ACEI) or angiotensin receptor blocker (ARB) as initial therapy is recommended to improve kidney outcomes. In the general nonblack population (without CKD) including those with diabetes, initial antihypertensive treatment should consist of a thiazide-type diuretic, calcium channel blocker, ACEI, or ARB. In the general black population (without CKD) including those with diabetes, initial antihypertensive treatment should consist of a thiazide-type diuretic or a calcium channel blocker **instead of** an ACEI or ARB.

Coronary artery disease (CAD) and hypertension: The American Heart Association, American College of Cardiology and American Society of Hypertension (AHA/ACC/ASH) 2015 scientific statement for the treatment of hypertension in patients with CAD recommends the use of an ACE inhibitor (or an ARB) as part of a regimen in patients with hypertension and chronic stable angina if there is prior MI, LV systolic dysfunction, diabetes mellitus, or CKD. A BP target of <140/90 mm Hg is reasonable for the secondary prevention of cardiovascular events. A lower target BP (<130/80 mm Hg) may be appropriate in some individuals with CAD, previous MI, stroke or transient ischemic attack, or CAD risk equivalents(AHA/ACC/ASH [Rosendorff 2015]).

Pregnancy Considerations [U.S. Boxed Warning]: Drugs that act on the renin-angiotensin system can cause injury and death to the developing fetus. Discontinue as soon as possible once pregnancy is detected. Benazepril crosses the placenta. Drugs that act on the renin-angiotensin system are associated with oligohydramnios. Oligohydramnios, due to decreased fetal renal function, may lead to fetal lung hypoplasia and skeletal malformations. Their use in pregnancy is also associated with anuria, hypotension, renal failure, skull hypoplasia, and death in the fetus/neonate. Teratogenic effects may occur following maternal use of an ACE inhibitor during the first trimester, although this finding may be confounded by maternal disease. Because adverse fetal events are well documented with exposure later in pregnancy, ACE inhibitor use in pregnant women is not recommended (Seely 2014; Weber 2014). Infants exposed to an ACE inhibitor in utero should be monitored for hyperkalemia, hypotension, and oliguria. Oligohydramnios may not appear until after irreversible fetal injury has occurred. Exchange transfusions or dialysis may be required to reverse hypotension or improve renal function,

although data related to the effectiveness in neonates is limited.

Chronic maternal hypertension itself is also associated with adverse events in the fetus/infant and mother. ACE inhibitors are not recommended for the treatment of uncomplicated hypertension in pregnancy (ACOG 2013) and they are specifically contraindicated for the treatment of hypertension and chronic heart failure during pregnancy by some guidelines (Regitz-Zagrosek 2011). In addition, ACE inhibitors should generally be avoided in women of reproductive age (ACOG 2013). If treatment for hypertension or chronic heart failure in pregnancy is needed, other agents should be used (ACOG 2013; Regitz-Zagrosek 2011).

Breast-Feeding Considerations Small amounts of benazepril and benazeprilat are found in breast milk. Some guidelines consider benazepril to be acceptable for use in breast-feeding women. Monitoring of the nursing child's weight for the first 4 weeks is recommended (Regitz-Zagrosek 2011).

Contraindications Hypersensitivity to benazepril or any component of the formulation; patients with a history of angioedema (with or without prior ACE inhibitor therapy); concomitant use with aliskiren in patients with diabetes mellitus

Canadian labeling: Additional contraindications (not in U.S. labeling): Concomitant use with aliskiren in patients with moderate to severe renal impairment (GFR <60 mL/minute/1.73 m^2); pregnancy; breast-feeding; rare hereditary problems of galactose intolerance (eg, galactosemia, Lapp Lactase deficiency or glucose-galactose malabsorption)

Warnings/Precautions Anaphylactic reactions may occur rarely with ACE inhibitors. At any time during treatment (especially following first dose) angioedema may occur rarely with ACE inhibitors. It may involve the head and neck (potentially compromising airway) or the intestine (presenting with abdominal pain). African-Americans and patients with idiopathic or hereditary angioedema may be at an increased risk. Risk may also be increased with concomitant use of mTOR inhibitor (eg, everolimus) therapy. Prolonged frequent monitoring may be required especially if tongue, glottis, or larynx are involved as they are associated with airway obstruction. Patients with a history of airway surgery may have a higher risk of airway obstruction. Aggressive early and appropriate management is critical. Contraindicated in patients with history of angioedema with or without prior ACE inhibitor therapy. Hypersensitivity reactions may be seen during hemodialysis (eg, CVVHD) with high-flux dialysis membranes (eg, AN69), and rarely, during low density lipoprotein apheresis with dextran sulfate cellulose. Rare cases of anaphylactoid reactions have been reported in patients undergoing sensitization treatment with hymenoptera (bee, wasp) venom while receiving ACE inhibitors.

Symptomatic hypotension with or without syncope can occur with ACE inhibitors (usually with the first several doses); effects are most often observed in volume depleted patients; close monitoring of patient is required especially with initial dosing and dosing increases; blood pressure must be lowered at a rate appropriate for the patient's clinical condition. Initiation of therapy in patients with ischemic heart disease or cerebrovascular disease warrants close observation due to the potential consequences posed by falling blood pressure (eg, MI, stroke). Use with caution in hypertrophic cardiomyopathy with outflow tract obstruction and severe aortic stenosis. In patients on chronic ACE inhibitor therapy, intraoperative hypotension may occur with induction and maintenance of general anesthesia; use with caution before, during, or immediately after major surgery. Cardiopulmonary bypass, intraoperative blood loss, or vasodilating anesthesia increases endogenous renin release. Use of ACE inhibitors perioperatively will blunt angiotensin II formation and may result in hypotension. However, discontinuation of therapy prior to surgery is controversial. If continued preoperatively, avoidance of hypotensive agents during surgery is prudent (Hillis, 2011). **[US Boxed Warning]: Drugs that act on the renin-angiotensin system can cause injury and death to the developing fetus. Discontinue as soon as possible once pregnancy is detected.**

Hyperkalemia may occur with ACE inhibitors; risk factors include renal dysfunction, diabetes mellitus, concomitant use of potassium-sparing diuretics, potassium supplements and/or potassium-containing salts. Use cautiously, if at all, with these agents and monitor potassium periodically. Cough may occur with ACE inhibitors. Other causes of cough should be considered (eg, pulmonary congestion in patients with heart failure) and excluded prior to discontinuation. Use with caution in patients with diabetes

receiving insulin or oral antidiabetic agents; may be at increased risk for episodes of hypoglycemia.

May be associated with deterioration of renal function and/or increases in serum creatinine, particularly in patients with low renal blood flow (eg, renal artery stenosis, heart failure) whose glomerular filtration rate (GFR) is dependent on efferent arteriolar vasoconstriction by angiotensin II; deterioration may result in oliguria, acute renal failure, and progressive azotemia. Small increases in serum creatinine may occur following initiation; consider discontinuation only in patients with progressive and/or significant deterioration in renal function. Use with caution in patients with unstented unilateral/bilateral renal artery stenosis. When unstented bilateral renal artery stenosis is present, use is generally avoided due to the elevated risk of deterioration in renal function unless possible benefits outweigh risks. Potentially significant drug-drug interactions may exist, requiring dose or frequency adjustment, additional monitoring, and/or selection of alternative therapy.

Rare toxicities associated with ACE inhibitors include cholestatic jaundice (which may progress to fulminant hepatic necrosis), agranulocytosis, neutropenia, or leukopenia with myeloid hypoplasia. Patients with collagen vascular diseases (especially with concomitant renal impairment) or renal impairment alone may be at increased risk for hematologic toxicity; periodically monitor CBC with differential in these patients.

Adverse Reactions

1% to 10%:

Central nervous system: Headache (6%), dizziness (4%), drowsiness (2%), orthostatic dizziness (2%)

Renal: Increased serum creatinine (2%), renal insufficiency (may occur in patients with bilateral renal artery stenosis or hypovolemia)

Respiratory: Cough (1% to 10%)

<1%, postmarketing, and/or case reports (Limited to important or life-threatening): Agranulocytosis, alopecia, anaphylactoid reaction, angina pectoris, angioedema (includes head, neck, and intestinal angioedema), arthralgia, arthritis, asthma, dermatitis, dyspnea, ECG changes, eosinophilia, flushing, gastritis, hemolytic anemia, hyperbilirubinemia, hyperglycemia, hyperkalemia, hypersensitivity, hypertonia, hyponatremia, hypotension, impotence, increased blood urea nitrogen (transient), increased serum transaminases, increased uric acid, insomnia, leukopenia, myalgia, neutropenia, orthostatic hypotension, palpitations, pancreatitis, paresthesia, pemphigus, peripheral edema, proteinuria, pruritus, shock, skin photosensitivity, skin rash, Stevens-Johnson syndrome, syncope, thrombocytopenia, vomiting

Eosinophilic pneumonitis, anaphylaxis, neutropenia, agranulocytosis, renal insufficiency, and renal failure have been reported with other ACE inhibitors. In addition, a syndrome including fever, myalgia, arthralgia, interstitial nephritis, vasculitis, rash, eosinophilia, and elevated ESR has been reported to be associated with ACE inhibitors.

Drug Interactions

Metabolism/Transport Effects None known.

Avoid Concomitant Use

Avoid concomitant use of Benazepril with any of the following: Sacubitril

Increased Effect/Toxicity

Benazepril may increase the levels/effects of: Allopurinol; Amifostine; Antipsychotic Agents (Second Generation [Atypical]); AzaTHIOprine; Ciprofloxacin (Systemic); Drospirenone; DULoxetine; Ferric Gluconate; Gold Sodium Thiomalate; Grass Pollen Allergen Extract (5 Grass Extract); Hypotension-Associated Agents; Iron Dextran Complex; Levodopa; Lithium; Nonsteroidal Anti-Inflammatory Agents; Pregabalin; Sacubitril; Sodium Phosphates

The levels/effects of Benazepril may be increased by: Alfuzosin; Aliskiren; Angiotensin II Receptor Blockers; Barbiturates; Brimonidine (Topical); Canagliflozin; Dapoxetine; Diazoxide; DPP-IV Inhibitors; Eplerenone; Everolimus; Heparin; Heparin (Low Molecular Weight); Herbs (Hypotensive Properties); Hydrochlorothiazide; Loop Diuretics; Molsidomine; Nicorandil; Obinutuzumab; Pentoxifylline; Phosphodiesterase 5 Inhibitors; Potassium Salts; Potassium-Sparing Diuretics; Prostacyclin Analogues; Salicylates; Sirolimus; Temsirolimus; Thiazide Diuretics; TiZANidine; Tolvaptan; Trimethoprim

Decreased Effect

Benazepril may decrease the levels/effects of: Hydrochlorothiazide

The levels/effects of Benazepril may be decreased by: Amphetamines; Aprotinin; Herbs (Hypertensive Properties); Icatibant; Lanthanum; Methylphenidate; Nonsteroidal Anti-Inflammatory Agents; Salicylates; Yohimbine

Storage/Stability Store at ≤30°C (86°F). Protect from moisture.

Mechanism of Action Competitive inhibition of angiotensin I being converted to angiotensin II, a potent vasoconstrictor, through the angiotensin I-converting enzyme (ACE) activity, with resultant lower levels of angiotensin II which causes an increase in plasma renin activity and a reduction in aldosterone secretion

Pharmacodynamics/Kinetics

Reduction in plasma angiotensin-converting enzyme (ACE) activity:
Onset of action: Peak effect: 1 to 2 hours after 2 to 20 mg dose (Nussberger 1987; Nussberger 1989)
Duration: >90% inhibition for 24 hours after 5 to 20 mg dose (Balfour 1991)
Reduction in blood pressure:
Peak effect: Single dose: 2 to 4 hours; Continuous therapy: 2 weeks (Fogari 1990)
Absorption: Rapid (37%); food does not alter significantly; metabolite (benazeprilat) itself unsuitable for oral administration due to poor absorption
Distribution: V_d: ~8.7 L (Balfour 1991)
Protein binding:
Benazepril: ~97%
Benazeprilat: ~95%
Metabolism: Rapidly and extensively hepatic to its active metabolite, benazeprilat, via enzymatic hydrolysis; extensive first-pass effect
Half-life elimination: Benazeprilat: Effective: 10 to 11 hours; Terminal: Children: 5 hours, Adults: 22 hours
Time to peak: Parent drug: 0.5 to 1 hour
Excretion:
Urine (trace amounts as benazepril; 20% as benazeprilat; 12% as other metabolites)
Clearance: Nonrenal clearance (ie, biliary, metabolic) appears to contribute to the elimination of benazeprilat (11% to 12%), particularly patients with severe renal impairment; hepatic clearance is the main elimination route of unchanged benazepril
Dialysis: ~6% of metabolite removed within 4 hours of dialysis following 10 mg of benazepril administered 2 hours prior to procedure; parent compound not found in dialysate

Dosing

Adult Hypertension: Oral: Initial: 10 mg/day in patients not receiving a diuretic; 20 to 80 mg daily as a single dose or 2 divided doses; the need for twice-daily dosing should be assessed by monitoring peak (2 to 6 hours after dosing) and trough responses. Usual dosage (ASH/ISH [Weber, 2014]): 10 to 40 mg daily.
Note: Patients taking diuretics should have them discontinued 2 to 3 days prior to starting benazepril. If they cannot be discontinued, then initial dose should be 5 mg; restart after blood pressure is stabilized if needed.

Nephropathy (Nondiabetic) (off-label use): Oral: Initial: 10 mg once daily. If tolerated well after 2 to 4 weeks of therapy, may increase to 10 mg twice daily (Hou, 2006; Maschio, 1996).

Geriatric Oral: Consider lower initial doses (MacDonald, 1993; Reid, 1989). Also see **"Note"** in adult dosing.

Pediatric Hypertension: Children ≥6 years and Adolescents: Oral: Initial: 0.2 mg/kg/day (up to 10 mg daily) as monotherapy; dosing range: 0.1 to 0.6 mg/kg/day (maximum dose: 40 mg daily)

Renal Impairment

CrCl ≥30 mL/minute/1.73m²: No dosage adjustment necessary.
CrCl <30 mL/minute/1.73m²:
Adults: Initial: 5 mg once daily; maximum daily dose: 40 mg.
Children: Use is not recommended (insufficient data exists; dose not established).
Hemodialysis: 25% to 50% of usual dose; supplemental dose is not necessary (Aronoff, 2007).
Peritoneal dialysis: 25% to 50% of usual dose; supplemental dose is not necessary (Aronoff, 2007).

Hepatic Impairment There are no dosage adjustments provided in the manufacturer's labeling.

Monitoring Parameters Blood pressure; serum creatinine and potassium; if patient has collagen vascular disease and/or renal impairment, periodically monitor CBC with differential

Dosage Forms Excipient information presented when available (limited, particularly for generics); consult specific product labeling.
Tablet, Oral, as hydrochloride:
Lotensin: 10 mg, 20 mg, 40 mg
Generic: 5 mg, 10 mg, 20 mg, 40 mg

Extemporaneous Preparations A 2 mg/mL oral suspension may be made with tablets. Mix fifteen benazepril 20 mg tablets in an amber polyethylene terephthalate

bottle with Ora-Plus® 75 mL. Shake for 2 minutes, allow suspension to stand for ≥1 hour, then shake again for at least 1 additional minute. Add Ora-Sweet® 75 mL to suspension and shake to disperse. Will make 150 mL of a 2 mg/mL suspension. Label "shake well" and "refrigerate". Stable for 30 days.
Lotensin® prescribing information, Novartis Pharmaceuticals Corporation, Suffern, NY, 2015.

Benazepril and Hydrochlorothiazide
(ben AY ze pril & hye droe klor oh THYE a zide)

Brand Names: US Lotensin HCT®
Index Terms Benazepril Hydrochloride and Hydrochlorothiazide; Hydrochlorothiazide and Benazepril
Pharmacologic Category Angiotensin-Converting Enzyme (ACE) Inhibitor; Antihypertensive; Diuretic, Thiazide
Use Treatment of hypertension

Dosing

Adult & Geriatric Note: Not for initial therapy; dose should be individualized.
Hypertension: Oral: Range: Benazepril: 5 to 20 mg; Hydrochlorothiazide: 6.25 to 25 mg/day
Add-on therapy:
Patients not adequately controlled on benazepril or hydrochlorothiazide monotherapy: Initiate benazepril 10 mg/hydrochlorothiazide 12.5 mg; titrate to effect at 2- to 3-week intervals (maximum daily dose: benazepril 20 mg/hydrochlorothiazide 25 mg).
Replacement therapy: Substitute for the individually titrated components

Renal Impairment

CrCl >30 mL/minute: No dosage adjustment necessary.
CrCl ≤30 mL/minute: Use not recommended. Hydrochlorothiazide is usually ineffective with a GFR <30 mL/minute; use contraindicated in patients with anuria.

Hepatic Impairment

Mild to moderate impairment: Initial: No dosage adjustment necessary.
Severe impairment: There are no dosage adjustments provided in the manufacturer's labeling. Use with caution; hydrochlorothiazide may precipitate hepatic coma.

Additional Information Complete prescribing information should be consulted for additional detail.

Dosage Forms Excipient information presented when available (limited, particularly for generics); consult specific product labeling.
Tablet: 5/6.25: Benazepril hydrochloride 5 mg and hydrochlorothiazide 6.25 mg; 10/12.5: Benazepril hydrochloride 10 mg and hydrochlorothiazide 12.5 mg; 20/12.5: Benazepril hydrochloride 20 mg and hydrochlorothiazide 12.5 mg; 20/25: Benazepril hydrochloride 20 mg and hydrochlorothiazide 25 mg
Lotensin HCT® 10/12.5: Benazepril hydrochloride 10 mg and hydrochlorothiazide 12.5 mg
Lotensin HCT® 20/12.5: Benazepril hydrochloride 20 mg and hydrochlorothiazide 12.5 mg
Lotensin HCT® 20/25: Benazepril hydrochloride 20 mg and hydrochlorothiazide 25 mg

◆ Benazepril Hydrochloride see Benazepril on page 211

◆ Benazepril Hydrochloride and Amlodipine Besylate see Amlodipine and Benazepril on page 104

◆ Benazepril Hydrochloride and Hydrochlorothiazide see Benazepril and Hydrochlorothiazide on page 213

Bendamustine (ben da MUS teen)

Brand Names: US Bendeka; Treanda
Brand Names: Canada Treanda
Index Terms Bendamustine Hydrochloride; Bendeka; Cytostasan; SDX-105
Pharmacologic Category Antineoplastic Agent, Alkylating Agent; Antineoplastic Agent, Alkylating Agent (Nitrogen Mustard)

Use

Chronic lymphocytic leukemia: Treatment of chronic lymphocytic leukemia (CLL)
Non-Hodgkin lymphoma: Treatment of indolent B-cell non-Hodgkin lymphoma (NHL) which has progressed during or within 6 months of rituximab treatment or a rituximab-containing regimen

Pregnancy Considerations Adverse events were observed in animal reproduction studies. May cause fetal harm if administered during pregnancy. For women and men of reproductive potential, the US labels recommend effective contraception during and for 3 months after treatment. The Canadian labeling recommends effective contraception beginning 2 weeks prior to treatment and for ≥1 month after treatment.

Breast-Feeding Considerations It is not known if bendamustine is excreted in breast milk. Due to the potential for serious adverse reactions in the nursing infant, a decision should be made to discontinue bendamustine or discontinue breast-feeding, taking into account the benefits of treatment to the mother.

Contraindications Hypersensitivity (eg, anaphylactic or anaphylactoid reactions) to bendamustine or any component of the formulation. Bendeka is also contraindicated in patients with hypersensitivity to polyethylene glycol 400, propylene glycol, or monothioglycerol.

Warnings/Precautions Hazardous agent - use appropriate precautions for handling and disposal (NIOSH 2014 [group 1]). Myelosuppression (neutropenia, thrombocytopenia, and anemia) is a common toxicity; may require therapy delay and/or dose reduction; monitor blood counts frequently (nadirs typically occurred in the third week of treatment). Complications due to febrile neutropenia and severe thrombocytopenia have been reported (some fatal). ANC should recover to ≥1000/mm^3 and platelets to ≥75,000/mm^3 prior to cycle initiation. Pneumonia, hepatitis, sepsis, and septic shock have been reported; fatalities due to infection have occurred; patients with myelosuppression are more susceptible to infection; monitor closely. Reactivation of hepatitis B, cytomegalovirus, Mycobacterium tuberculosis, and herpes zoster infection may occur in patients receiving bendamustine. Monitor; may require infection prophylaxis and/or treatment prior to bendamustine administration.

Infusion reactions, including chills, fever, pruritus, and rash are common; rarely, anaphylactic and anaphylactoid reactions have occurred, particularly with the second or subsequent cycle(s). Patients who experienced grade 3 or higher allergic reactions should not be rechallenged. Consider premedication with antihistamines, antipyretics, and corticosteroids for patients with a history of grade 1 or 2 infusion reaction. Discontinue for severe allergic reaction or grade 4 infusion reaction; consider discontinuation with grade 3 infusion reaction. Rash, toxic skin reactions and bullous exanthema have been reported with monotherapy and in combination with other antineoplastics; may be progressive or worsen with continued treatment; discontinue bendamustine treatment for severe or progressive skin reaction; monitor closely; withhold or discontinue bendamustine treatment for severe or progressive skin reaction. The risk for severe skin toxicity is increased with concurrent use of allopurinol and other medications known to cause skin toxicity; Stevens-Johnson syndrome (SJS) and toxic epidermal necrolysis (TEN) have been reported. TEN has also been reported when used in combination with rituximab. Bendamustine is an irritant with vesicant-like properties; ensure proper needle or catheter placement prior to and during infusion; avoid extravasation; erythema, marked swelling, and pain have been reported with extravasation. Bendamustine is associated with a moderate emetic potential (Basch 2011; Dupuis 2011; Roila 2010); antiemetics are recommended to prevent nausea and vomiting.

Tumor lysis syndrome (usually occurring in the first treatment cycle) may occur as a consequence of antineoplastic treatment, including treatment with bendamustine. May lead to life-threatening acute renal failure; vigorous hydration and prophylactic measures (eg, antihyperuricemic therapy) should be instituted prior to treatment in high-risk patients; monitor closely. **Note:** Allopurinol may increase the risk for bendamustine skin toxicity. May cause hypokalemia; monitor potassium closely during therapy, particularly in patients with cardiac disease.

Per manufacturer's labeling, use with caution in patients with mild hepatic impairment. However, a pharmacokinetic study showed only slight differences in bendamustine AUC and C_{max} in patients with mild hepatic impairment (defined in the study as total bilirubin 1 to 1.5 times ULN or AST greater than ULN, as compared to patients with normal hepatic function (Owen 2010). Use is not recommended in patients with moderate (AST or ALT 2.5 to 10 times ULN and total bilirubin 1.5 to 3 times ULN) or severe (total bilirubin >3 times ULN) hepatic impairment.

Use with caution in patients with mild-to-moderate renal impairment. The US and Canadian product labels do not recommend use in patients with CrCl <40 mL/minute. A pharmacokinetic study illustrated only slight differences in bendamustine AUC and C_{max} in patients with mild (CrCl >50 to ≤80 mL/minute) and moderate (CrCl >30 to ≤50 mL/minute) renal dysfunction, compared to patients with normal renal function (Owen 2010). A retrospective safety study found no significant difference in lab toxicities between CLL patients with renal impairment (CrCl <40 mL/minute) compared to those without renal impairment, although an increase in grades 3/4 thrombocytopenia and

grades 3/4 BUN increases were detected in patients with renal impairment (Nordstrom 2012); monitor blood counts and renal function. **Note:** UK labeling (Levact prescribing information, October 2010) recommends no dosage adjustment for patients with CrCl >10 mL/minute. Secondary malignancies (including myelodysplastic syndrome, myeloproliferative disorders, acute myeloid leukemia and bronchial cancer) and premalignant diseases have been reported in patients who have received bendamustine. Potentially significant drug-drug interactions may exist, requiring dose or frequency adjustment, additional monitoring, and/or selection of alternative therapy.

Several formulations of bendamustine are available: a liquid solution formulation (45 mg/0.5 mL and 180 mg/2 mL [Treanda] and 100 mg/4 mL [Bendeka]) and a powder for reconstitution (5 mg/mL after reconstitution [Treanda]). Concentrations, storage, and compatibility differ between formulations. Use caution when selecting bendamustine formulation for preparation and administration. Do not mix or combine the formulations. Bendamustine solution (Treanda: 45 mg/0.5 mL and 180 mg/2 mL) contains N, N-dimethylacetamide, which is incompatible with closed-system transfer devices (CSTDs), adapters, and syringes containing polycarbonate or acrylonitrile-butadiene-styrene (ABS). When used to prepare or transfer the concentrated bendamustine solution into the infusion bag, the plastic components of these devices may dissolve, resulting in subsequent leakage and potential infusion of dissolved plastic into the patient (ISMP [Smetzer 2015]). Do not use the liquid solution formulation if CSTDs, adapters, and syringes containing polycarbonate or ABS are used **prior** to dilution in the infusion bag; according to the Treanda manufacturer, after dilution into the infusion bag, devices containing polycarbonate or ABS (including infusion sets) may be used. Some dosage forms may contain propylene glycol; large amounts are potentially toxic and have been associated with hyperosmolality, lactic acidosis, seizures and respiratory depression; use caution (AAP 1997; Zar 2007). See manufacturer's labeling.

Adverse Reactions

>10%:

Cardiovascular: Peripheral edema (NHL 13%; grades 3/4: <1%)

Central nervous system: Fatigue (NHL 57% [grades 3/4: 11%]; CLL 9%), headache (21%), dizziness (14%), chills (6% to 14%), insomnia (13%)

Dermatologic: Skin rash (8% to 16%; grades 3/4: ≤3%)

Endocrine & metabolic: Weight loss (NHL 18% [grades 3/4: 2%]; CLL 7%), dehydration (14%)

Gastrointestinal: Nausea (NHL 75% [grades 3/4: 4%]; CLL 20% [grades 3/4: <1%]), vomiting (NHL 40% [grades 3/4: 3%]; CLL 16% [grades 3/4: <1%]), diarrhea (NHL 37% [grades 3/4: 3%]; CLL 9% [grades 3/4: 1%]), constipation (NHL 29%; grades 3/4: <1%), anorexia (NHL 23%; grades 3/4: 2%), stomatitis (NHL 15%; grades 3/4: <1%), decreased appetite (NHL 13%; grades 3/4: <1%), abdominal pain (NHL 5% to 13%; grades 3/4: 1%), dyspepsia (11%)

Hematologic & oncologic: Lymphocytopenia (NHL 99% [grades 3/4: 94%]; CLL 68% [grades 3/4: 47%]), bone marrow depression (grades 3/4: 98%; nadir: In week 3), leukopenia (NHL 94% [grades 3/4: 56%]; CLL 61% [grades 3/4: 28%]), decreased hemoglobin (88% to 89%; grades 3/4: 11% to 13%), decreased neutrophils (NHL 86% [grades 3/4: 60%]; CLL 75% [grades 3/4: 43%]), thrombocytopenia (77% to 86%; grades 3/4: NHL 25%; CLL 11%)

Hepatic: Increased serum bilirubin (34%; grades 3/4: 3%)

Neuromuscular & skeletal: Back pain (14%), weakness (8% to 11%)

Respiratory: Cough (NHL 22%; CLL 4%), dyspnea (16%)

Miscellaneous: Fever (NHL 34%; CLL 24%)

1% to 10%:

Cardiovascular: Tachycardia (7%), chest pain (6%), hypotension (6%), exacerbation of hypertension (≤3%)

Central nervous system: Anxiety (8%), depression (6%), pain (6%)

Dermatologic: Pruritus (5% to 6%), hyperhidrosis (5%), night sweats (5%), xeroderma (5%)

Endocrine & metabolic: Hypokalemia (9%), hyperuricemia (7%; grades 3/4: 2%), hyperglycemia (grades 3/4: 3%), hypocalcemia (grades 3/4: 2%), hyponatremia (grades 3/4: 2%)

Gastrointestinal: Gastroesophageal reflux disease (10%), xerostomia (9%), dysgeusia (7%), oral candidiasis (6%), abdominal distention (5%)

Genitourinary: Urinary tract infection (10%)

Hematologic & oncologic: Febrile neutropenia (6%)

Hepatic: Increased serum ALT (grades 3/4: 3%), increased serum AST (grades 3/4: 1%)

Hypersensitivity: Hypersensitivity (5%; grades 3/4: 1%)

Infection: Herpes zoster (10%), infection (6%; grades 3/4: 2%), herpes simplex infection (3%)

Local: Infusion site reaction (6%), catheter pain (5%)

Neuromuscular & skeletal: Arthralgia (6%), limb pain (5%), ostealgia (5%)

Renal: Increased serum creatinine (grades 3/4: 2%)

Respiratory: Upper respiratory tract infection (10%), sinusitis (9%), pharyngolaryngeal pain (8%), pneumonia (8%), nasopharyngitis (6% to 7%), nasal congestion (5%), wheezing (5%)

<1% (Limited to important or life-threatening): Acute renal failure, alopecia, anaphylaxis, bronchogenic carcinoma, bullous rash, cardiac failure, dermatitis, dermatological reaction (toxic), drowsiness, erythema, exacerbation of hepatitis B, hemolysis, infusion related reaction, mucositis, myelodysplastic syndrome, myeloid leukemia (acute), myeloproliferative disease, pneumonitis, pulmonary fibrosis, sepsis, septic shock, skin necrosis, Stevens-Johnson syndrome, toxic epidermal necrolysis, tumor lysis syndrome

Drug Interactions

Metabolism/Transport Effects Substrate of BCRP, CYP1A2 (minor), P-glycoprotein; **Note:** Assignment of Major/Minor substrate status based on clinically relevant drug interaction potential

Avoid Concomitant Use

Avoid concomitant use of Bendamustine with any of the following: BCG (Intravesical); Deferiprone; Dipyrone

Increased Effect/Toxicity

Bendamustine may increase the levels/effects of: CloZAPine; Deferiprone

The levels/effects of Bendamustine may be increased by: Allopurinol; CYP1A2 Inhibitors (Strong); Dipyrone

Decreased Effect

Bendamustine may decrease the levels/effects of: BCG (Intravesical)

The levels/effects of Bendamustine may be decreased by: CYP1A2 Inducers (Strong)

Preparation for Administration Hazardous agent; use appropriate precautions for handling and disposal (NIOSH 2014 [group 1]).

Several formulations of bendamustine are available: a liquid solution formulation (45 mg/0.5 mL and 180 mg/2 mL [Treanda] and 100 mg/4 mL [Bendeka]) and the powder for reconstitution (5 mg/mL after reconstitution [Treanda]). Concentrations, storage, and compatibility differ between formulations. Use caution when selecting bendamustine formulation for preparation and administration. Do not mix or combine the formulations.

Bendeka: Prior to administration, allow vial(s) to reach room temperature. Dilute appropriate dose in 50 mL of NS, D2.5¹/₂NS, or D5W to a final concentration of 1.85 to 5.6 mg/mL; thoroughly mix. The resulting solution should be clear and colorless to yellow.

Treanda:

Powder for solution (for reconstitution): Reconstitute 25 mg vial with 5 mL and 100 mg vial with 20 mL of sterile water for injection to a concentration of 5 mg/mL; powder usually dissolves within 5 minutes (do not use if particulates are visible). Within 30 minutes of reconstitution, dilute appropriate dose for infusion in 500 mL NS (or D₂.₅¹/₂NS) to a final concentration of 0.2 to 0.6 mg/mL; mix thoroughly. Closed-system transfer devices (CSTDs) or adaptors containing polycarbonate or acrylonitrile-butadiene-styrene (ABS) are safe to use with the lyophilized powder formulation.

Solution: Prior to administration, dilute appropriate dose (using polypropylene syringes with a metal needle and polypropylene hub) in 500 mL NS (or D₂.₅¹/₂NS) to a final concentration of 0.2 to 0.7 mg/mL; resulting solution should be colorless to yellow. Bendamustine contains N,N-dimethylacetamide, which is incompatible with CSTDs, adapters, and syringes containing polycarbonate or ABS. When used to prepare or transfer the concentrated bendamustine solution into the infusion bag, the plastic components of these devices may dissolve, resulting in subsequent leakage and potential infusion of dissolved plastic into the patient (ISMP [Smetzer 2015]). If using a syringe to withdraw and transfer the bendamustine solution from the vial into the infusion bag, only use polypropylene syringes (translucent in appearance) with a metal needle and polypropylene hub. **After** dilution into the infusion bag, devices containing polycarbonate or ABS (including infusion sets) may be used.

Storage/Stability

Bendeka:

Solution: Store intact vials between 2°C to 8°C (36°F to 46°F); protect from light. Solutions for infusion should be prepared as close as possible to administration. Solutions diluted with NS or D₂.₅¹/₂NS are stable for

up to 24 hours when stored at 2°C to 8°C (36°F to 46°F) or for up to 6 hours when stored at 15°C to 30°C (59°F to 86°F) and room light. Solutions diluted with D5W are stable for up to 24 hours when stored at 2°C to 8°C (36°F to 46°F) or for up to 3 hours when stored at 15°C to 30°C (59°F to 86°F) and room light. Infusion must be completed within these time frames. Bendeka is a multiple-dose vial; after the first use, partially used vials are stable for up to 28 days when stored in the original carton at 2°C to 8°C (36°F to 46°F). Do not withdraw more than 6 doses from each vial.

Treanda:

Powder for solution: Prior to reconstitution, store intact vials up to 25°C (77°F); excursions are permitted up to 30°C (86°F). Protect from light. The solution in the vial (reconstituted with SWFI) is stable for 30 minutes (transfer to 500 mL infusion bag within that 30 minutes). The solution diluted in 500 mL for infusion is stable for 24 hours refrigerated (2°C to 8°C ([36°F to 46°F]) or 3 hours at room temperature (15°C to 30°C [59°F to 86°F]) and room light. Infusion must be completed within these time frames.

Solution: Store intact vials between 2°C to 8°C (36°F to 46°F); protect from light. Solutions diluted for infusion are stable for up to 24 hours when stored at 2°C to 8°C (36°F to 46°F) or for up to 2 hours when stored at 15°C to 30°C (59°F to 86°F) and room light. Infusion must be completed within these time frames.

Mechanism of Action Bendamustine is an alkylating agent (nitrogen mustard derivative) with a benzimidazole ring (purine analog) which demonstrates only partial cross-resistance (*in vitro*) with other alkylating agents. It leads to cell death via single and double strand DNA cross-linking. Bendamustine is active against quiescent and dividing cells. The primary cytotoxic activity is due to bendamustine (as compared to metabolites).

Pharmacodynamics/Kinetics

Distribution: V_{ss}: ~20 to 25 L

Protein binding: 94% to 96%

Metabolism: Hepatic (extensive), via CYP1A2 to active (minor) metabolites gamma-hydroxy bendamustine (M3) and N-desmethyl-bendamustine (M4); also via hydrolysis to low cytotoxic metabolites, monohydroxy bendamustine (HP1) and dihydroxy bendamustine (HP2)

Half-life elimination: Bendamustine: ~40 minutes; M3: ~3 hours; M4: ~30 minutes

Time to peak, serum: At end of infusion

Excretion: Feces (~25%); urine (~50%; ~3% as active parent drug)

Pharmacokinetic note: In a pharmacokinetic study, a 10 minute infusion of Bendeka (120 mg/m²) resulted in higher maximum plasma concentrations and equivalent systemic exposure as the same dose of Treanda infused over 60 minutes.

Dosing

Adult & Geriatric Note: Bendamustine is associated with a moderate emetic potential (Basch 2011; Roila 2010); antiemetics are recommended to prevent nausea and vomiting.

Chronic lymphocytic leukemia (CLL): IV: 100 mg/m² on days 1 and 2 of a 28-day treatment cycle (as a single agent) for up to 6 cycles (Knauf 2009; Knauf 2012)

CLL, first-line treatment (off-label dosing): IV: 90 mg/m² on days 1 and 2 of a 28-day treatment cycle (in combination with rituximab) for up to 6 cycles (Fischer 2012)

CLL, relapsed/refractory (off-label dosing): IV: 70 mg/m² on days 1 and 2 of a 28-day treatment cycle (in combination with rituximab) for up to 6 cycles (Fischer 2011)

Non-Hodgkin lymphomas: IV:

Lymphoma, indolent B-cell, refractory: 120 mg/m² on days 1 and 2 of a 21-day treatment cycle (as a single agent) for up to 8 cycles (Kahl 2010)

Lymphoma, indolent B-cell, follicular, or mantle cell, first-line (off-label use): 90 mg/m² over 30 to 60 minutes on days 1 and 2 of a 28-day treatment cycle (in combination with rituximab) for up to 6 cycles (Rummel, 2013) **or** 90 mg/m² over 30 minutes on days 1 and 2 of a 28-day treatment cycle (in combination with rituximab) for 6 to 8 cycles (Flinn, 2014)

Lymphoma, follicular, relapsed or refractory (off-label use): 90 mg/m² over 60 minutes on days 1 and 2 of a 35-day treatment cycle (in combination with bortezomib and rituximab) for 5 cycles (Fowler 2011)

Lymphoma, mantle cell, relapsed or refractory (off-label use): 90 mg/m² over 30 minutes on days 2 and 3 of a 28-day treatment cycle (in combination with rituximab) for up to 4 cycles (Rummel 2005)

Hodgkin lymphoma, relapsed or refractory (off-label use): IV: 120 mg/m^2 over 30 minutes on days 1 and 2 of a 28-day treatment cycle for up to 6 cycles (Moskowitz 2013)

Multiple myeloma, salvage therapy (off-label use): IV: 90 to 100 mg/m^2 on days 1 and 2 of a 28-day treatment cycle for at least 2 cycles (Knop, 2005) **or** 75 mg/m^2 on days 1 and 2 of a 28-day treatment cycle (in combination with lenalidomide and dexamethasone) for up to 8 cycles (Lentzsch, 2012)

Waldenström macroglobulinemia, refractory (off-label use): IV: 90 mg/m^2 on days 1 and 2 of a 28-day treatment cycle (in combination with rituximab) for 6 cycles (Treon 2011) **or** 90 mg/m^2 over 30 minutes on days 2 and 3 of a 28-day treatment cycle (in combination with rituximab) for 4 cycles (Rummel 2005)

Renal Impairment

CrCl <40 mL/minute: Use is not recommended in the US and Canadian manufacturers' labeling.

Study data suggest minor changes in systemic exposure may occur with mild-to-moderate renal impairment. Based on a pharmacokinetic study (patients receiving 120 mg/m^2 for 2 days every 21 days), only slight differences in bendamustine AUC and C$_{max}$ were demonstrated in patients with mild (CrCl >50 to ≤80 mL/minute) and moderate (CrCl >30 to ≤50 mL/minute) renal dysfunction, compared to patients with normal renal function (Owen 2010). A retrospective study of bendamustine in CLL and NHL patients with renal impairment (CrCl <40 mL/minute) compared to those without (CrCl ≥60 mL/minute) found no significant difference in lab toxicities in CLL patients with renal impairment compared to those without renal impairment, although an increase in grades 3/4 thrombocytopenia was noted in NHL patients and grades 3/4 BUN increases were higher when combining data for CLL and NHL (Nordstrom 2012).

Note: UK manufacturer's labeling (Levact [prescribing information], October 2010) recommends no dosage adjustment for patients with CrCl >10 mL/minute.

Hepatic Impairment

Mild impairment: Per US and Canadian manufacturers' labeling, use with caution. However, a pharmacokinetic study showed only slight differences in bendamustine AUC and C$_{max}$ in patients with mild hepatic impairment (defined in the study as total bilirubin 1 to 1.5 times ULN or AST greater than ULN), compared to patients with normal hepatic function (Owen 2010).

Moderate impairment (AST or ALT 2.5 to 10 times ULN and total bilirubin 1.5 to 3 times ULN): Use is not recommended.

Severe impairment (total bilirubin >3 times ULN): Use is not recommended.

Obesity *American Society of Clinical Oncology (ASCO) Guidelines for appropriate chemotherapy dosing in obese adults with cancer:* Utilize patient's actual body weight (full weight) for calculation of body surface area- or weight-based dosing, particularly when the intent of therapy is curative; manage regimen-related toxicities in the same manner as for nonobese patients; if a dose reduction is utilized due to toxicity, consider resumption of full weight-based dosing with subsequent cycles, especially if cause of toxicity (eg, hepatic or renal impairment) is resolved (Griggs 2012).

Adjustment for Toxicity

Infusion reactions:

Grade 1 or 2: Consider premedication with antihistamines, antipyretics, and corticosteroids in subsequent cycles

Grade 3: Consider discontinuing treatment

Grade 4: Discontinue treatment

Skin reaction, severe or progressive: Withhold or discontinue treatment

Treatment delay:

Hematologic toxicity ≥ grade 4: Delay treatment until resolves (ANC ≥1000/mm^3, platelets ≥75,000/mm^3)

Nonhematologic toxicity ≥ grade 2 (clinically significant): Delay treatment until resolves to ≤ grade 1

Dose modification CLL:

Hematologic toxicity ≥ grade 3: Reduce dose to 50 mg/m^2 on days 1 and 2 of each treatment cycle. For recurrent hematologic toxicity (≥grade 3), further reduce dose to 25 mg/m^2 on days 1 and 2 of the treatment cycle. May cautiously re-escalate dose in subsequent cycles.

Nonhematologic toxicity ≥ grade 3 (clinically significant): Reduce dose to 50 mg/m^2 on days 1 and 2 of the treatment cycle with discretion. May cautiously re-escalate dose in subsequent cycles.

Dose modification in NHL:

Hematologic toxicity grade 4: Reduce dose to 90 mg/m^2 on days 1 and 2 of each treatment cycle. For recurrent hematologic toxicity (grade 4), further reduce dose to 60 mg/m^2 on days 1 and 2 of each treatment cycle.

Nonhematologic toxicity ≥ grade 3: Reduce dose to 90 mg/m^2 on days 1 and 2 of the treatment cycle with discretion. For recurrent toxicity ≥ grade 3, further reduce dose to 60 mg/m^2 on days 1 and 2 of each treatment cycle.

Administration For chronic lymphocytic leukemia, infuse over 30 minutes (Treanda) or 10 minutes (Bendeka). For non-Hodgkin lymphoma, infuse over 60 minutes (Treanda) or 10 minutes (Bendeka). Administration times for off-label uses/doses vary by protocol.

Bendamustine solution (45 mg/0.5 mL and 180 mg/2 mL [Treanda]) contains N, N-dimethylacetamide, which is incompatible with closed-system transfer devices (CSTDs), adapters, and syringes containing polycarbonate or acrylonitrile-butadiene-styrene (ABS). After dilution of bendamustine solution (Treanda) into the infusion bag, devices containing polycarbonate or ABS (including infusion sets) may be used.

Consider premedication with antihistamines, antipyretics, and corticosteroids for patients with a previous grade 1 or 2 infusion reaction to bendamustine. Bendamustine is associated with a moderate emetic potential (Basch 2011; Dupuis 2011; Roila 2010); antiemetics are recommended to prevent nausea and vomiting.

Irritant with vesicant-like properties; ensure proper needle or catheter placement prior to and during infusion. Avoid extravasation; monitor IV site for redness, swelling, or pain.

Extravasation management: If extravasation occurs, stop infusion immediately and disconnect (leave cannula/needle in place); gently aspirate extravasated solution (do **NOT** flush the line); remove needle/cannula; elevate extremity. Apply dry cold compresses for 20 minutes 4 times daily (Perez Fildago 2012). May be managed by sodium thiosulfate in the same manner as mechlorethamine extravasation (Schulmeister 2011).

Sodium thiosulfate 1/6 M solution (instructions for mechlorethamine): Inject subcutaneously into extravasation area using 2 mL for each mg of drug suspected to have extravasated (Perez Fidalgo 2012; Polovich 2009).

Hazardous agent; use appropriate precautions for handling and disposal (NIOSH 2014 [group 1]).

Monitoring Parameters CBC with differential and platelets (monitored weekly [initially] in clinical trials); serum creatinine; ALT, AST, and total bilirubin; monitor potassium and uric acid levels in patients at risk for tumor lysis syndrome; monitor for infusion reactions anaphylaxis, infection (including reactivations), and dermatologic toxicity; monitor IV site during and after infusion.

Canadian labeling also recommends periodic monitoring of blood pressure, serum glucose, and ECG (in patients with cardiac disease particularly if concomitant electrolyte disturbances).

Product Availability Bendeka: FDA approved December 2015; availability anticipated in the first quarter of 2016. Bendeka is a liquid, low-volume (50 mL) and short-time (10-minute) infusion formulation of bendamustine. Information pertaining to this product within the monograph is pending revision.

Dosage Forms Excipient information presented when available (limited, particularly for generics); consult specific product labeling.

Solution, Intravenous, as hydrochloride:

Bendeka: 100 mg/4 mL (4 mL) [contains polyethylene glycol, propylene glycol]

Treanda: 45 mg/0.5 mL (0.5 mL); 180 mg/2 mL (2 mL) [contains propylene glycol]

Solution Reconstituted, Intravenous, as hydrochloride:

Treanda: 25 mg (1 ea); 100 mg (1 ea)

Bentoquatam (BEN toe kwa tam)

Brand Names: US Ivy Block [OTC]
Index Terms Quaternium-18 Bentonite
Pharmacologic Category Topical Skin Product
Use Skin protectant for the prevention of poison ivy, poison oak, and poison sumac
Dosing
  Adult & Geriatric Skin protectant: Topical: Apply to skin 15 minutes prior to potential exposure to poison ivy, poison oak, or poison sumac; may reapply every 4 hours
  Pediatric Children ≥6 years: Refer to adult dosing.
Additional Information Complete prescribing information should be consulted for additional detail.
Dosage Forms Excipient information presented when available (limited, particularly for generics); consult specific product labeling.
  Lotion, topical:
    Ivy Block: 5% (30 mL, 120 mL) [contains benzyl alcohol, ethanol 25%]

Benzocaine (BEN zoe kane)

Brand Names: US Anacaine; Anbesol Cold Sore Therapy [OTC]; Anbesol JR [OTC]; Anbesol Maximum Strength [OTC]; Anbesol [OTC]; Baby Anbesol [OTC]; Benz-O-Sthetic [OTC]; Benzocaine Oral Anesthetic [OTC]; Bi-Zets/Benzotroches [OTC]; Blistex Medicated [OTC]; Cepacol Dual Relief [OTC]; Cepacol Sensations Hydra [OTC]; Cepacol Sensations Warming [OTC]; Chiggerex [OTC]; Chiggertox [OTC]; Dent-O-Kain/20 [OTC]; Dentapaine [OTC]; Dermoplast [OTC]; Foille [OTC]; HurriCaine One [OTC]; Hurricaine [OTC]; Ivy-Rid [OTC]; Kank-A Mouth Pain [OTC]; Ora-film [OTC]; Oral Pain Relief Max St [OTC] [DSC]; Pinnacaine Otic [DSC]; Sore Throat Relief [OTC]; Topex Topical Anesthetic; Trocaine Throat [OTC]; Zilactin Baby [OTC]
Brand Names: Canada Anbesol® Baby; Zilactin Baby®; Zilactin-B®

Index Terms Ethyl Aminobenzoate
Pharmacologic Category Antihemorrhoidal Agent; Local Anesthetic
Use Temporary relief of pain associated with pruritic dermatosis, pruritus, minor burns, acute congestive, bee stings, and insect bites; mouth and gum irritations (toothache, minor sore throat pain, canker sores, dentures, orthodontia, teething, mucositis, stomatitis); sunburn; hemorrhoids; anesthetic lubricant for passage of catheters and endoscopic tubes
Dosing
  Adult & Geriatric Note: These are general dosing guidelines; Refer to specific product labeling for dosing instructions.

  Bee stings, insect bites, minor burns, sunburn: Topical 5% to 20%: Apply to affected area 3-4 times a day as needed. In cases of bee stings, remove stinger before treatment.

  Boils: Topical 20%: Apply to affected area up to 2 times daily (maximum: 2 times/day)
  Lubricant for passage of catheters and instruments: Topical 20%: Apply evenly to exterior of instrument prior to use.
  Mouth and gum irritation: Topical (oral) 10% to 20%: Apply thin layer to affected area up to 4 times daily
  Sore throat:
    Oral: Allow 1 lozenge (10-15 mg) to dissolve slowly in mouth; may repeat every 2 hours as needed
  Hemorrhoids: Rectal 5% to 20%: Apply externally to affected area up to 6 times daily
  Pediatric Note: These are general dosing guidelines; refer to specific product labeling for dosing instructions.

  Teething pain: Children ≥4 months: Topical (oral): 7.5% to 10%: Apply to affected gum area up to 4 times daily
  Bee stings, boils, insect bites, minor burns, sunburn: Topical: Children ≥2 years: Refer to adult dosing.
  Lubricant for passage of catheters and instruments: Topical: Children ≥2 years: Refer to adult dosing.
  Mouth and gum irritation: Topical (oral) 10% to 20%: Children ≥2 years: Refer to adult dosing.
  Sore throat:
    Oral: Children ≥5 years: Refer to adult dosing.
  Hemorrhoids: Rectal 5% to 20%: Children ≥12 years: Refer to adult dosing.
Additional Information Complete prescribing information should be consulted for additional detail.
Dosage Forms Excipient information presented when available (limited, particularly for generics); consult specific product labeling. [DSC] = Discontinued product
  Aerosol, External:
    Dermoplast: Benzocaine 20% and menthol 0.5% (56 g) [contains methylparaben]
    Ivy-Rid: 2% (82.5 mL)
  Gel, Mouth/Throat:
    Anbesol: 10% (9 g) [contains benzyl alcohol, brilliant blue fcf (fd&c blue #1), fd&c yellow #10 (quinoline yellow), fd&c yellow #6 (sunset yellow), methylparaben, propylene glycol, saccharin; cool mint flavor]
    Anbesol JR: 10% (9 g) [contains methylparaben]
    Anbesol Maximum Strength: 20% (9 g) [contains brilliant blue fcf (fd&c blue #1), fd&c red #40, fd&c yellow #10 (quinoline yellow), methylparaben, saccharin]
    Baby Anbesol: 7.5% (9 g)
    Benz-O-Sthetic: 20% (15 g) [contains benzyl alcohol, saccharin sodium]
    Benz-O-Sthetic: 20% (29 g) [contains benzyl alcohol, saccharin sodium; bubble-gum flavor]
    Benz-O-Sthetic: 20% (29 g) [contains benzyl alcohol, saccharin sodium; cherry flavor]
    Dentapaine: 20% (11 g)
    Hurricaine: 20% (5.25 g) [contains polyethylene glycol, saccharin sodium]
    Hurricaine: 20% (28.4 g) [contains polyethylene glycol, saccharin sodium; mint flavor]
    Hurricaine: 20% (30 g) [contains polyethylene glycol, saccharin sodium; pina colada flavor]
    Hurricaine: 20% (30 g) [contains polyethylene glycol, saccharin sodium; watermelon flavor]
    Hurricaine: 20% (5.25 g, 30 g) [contains polyethylene glycol, saccharin sodium; wild cherry flavor]
    Oral Pain Relief Max St: 20% (14.2 g [DSC]) [contains saccharin sodium]
    Zilactin Baby: 10% (9.4 g) [alcohol free, dye free, saccharin free]
  Liquid, External:
    Chiggertox: 2.1% (30 mL)

Liquid, Mouth/Throat:
Anbesol: 10% (12 mL) [contains brilliant blue fcf (fd&c blue #1), fd&c yellow #10 (quinoline yellow), fd&c yellow #6 (sunset yellow), methylparaben, saccharin; cool mint flavor]
Anbesol Maximum Strength: 20% (12 mL) [contains benzyl alcohol, brilliant blue fcf (fd&c blue #1), fd&c red #40, fd&c yellow #10 (quinoline yellow), methylparaben, polyethylene glycol, propylene glycol, saccharin]
Benz-O-Sthetic: 20% (56 g) [contains benzyl alcohol, brilliant blue fcf (fd&c blue #1), fd&c red #40, fd&c yellow #10 (quinoline yellow), polyethylene glycol, propylene glycol, saccharin]
Cepacol Dual Relief: 5% (22.2 mL) [sugar free; cherry flavor]
Dent-O-Kain/20: 20% (9 mL) [contains benzyl alcohol, brilliant blue fcf (fd&c blue #1), d&c yellow #11 (quinoline yellow ss), fd&c red #40, propylene glycol, saccharin]
Oral Pain Relief Max St: 20% (15 mL [DSC]) [contains benzyl alcohol, brilliant blue fcf (fd&c blue #1), fd&c red #40, fd&c yellow #10 (quinoline yellow), methylparaben, polyethylene glycol, propylene glycol, saccharin]
Lozenge, Mouth/Throat:
Bi-Zets/Benzotroches: 15 mg (10 ea) [orange flavor]
Cepacol Sensations Hydra: 3 mg (20 ea) [contains brilliant blue fcf (fd&c blue #1), fd&c yellow #10 (quinoline yellow)]
Cepacol Sensations Warming: 4 mg (20 ea) [contains fd&c red #40, fd&c yellow #10 (quinoline yellow)]
Sore Throat Relief: 10 mg (2 ea) [wild cherry flavor]
Trocaine Throat: 10 mg (1 ea)
Ointment, External:
Anacaine: 10% (30 g)
Anbesol Cold Sore Therapy: 20% (9 g) [contains aloe, vitamin e]
Blistex Medicated: (6.3 g) [contains cetyl alcohol, edetate calcium disodium, saccharin sodium, sd alcohol]
Chiggerex: 2% (52.5 g)
Foille: 5% (28 g)
Solution, Mouth/Throat:
Benz-O-Sthetic: 20% (30 mL) [contains polyethylene glycol, saccharin]
Benzocaine Oral Anesthetic: 20% (59.7 g) [contains alcohol, usp, polyethylene glycol, saccharin sodium]
Hurricaine: 20% (57 g) [contains polyethylene glycol, saccharin sodium]
Hurricaine: 20% (30 mL) [contains polyethylene glycol, saccharin sodium; pina colada flavor]
Hurricaine: 20% (57 g, 30 mL) [contains polyethylene glycol, saccharin sodium; wild cherry flavor]
HurriCaine One: 20% (2 ea, 25 ea) [contains polyethylene glycol, saccharin sodium]
Kank-A Mouth Pain: 20% (9.75 mL) [contains benzyl alcohol, propylene glycol, saccharin sodium]
Topex Topical Anesthetic: 20% (57 g) [cherry flavor]
Solution, Otic:
Pinnacaine Otic: 20% (15 mL [DSC])
Strip, Mouth/Throat:
Ora-film: 6% (12 ea) [contains brilliant blue fcf (fd&c blue #1), menthol, methylparaben, propylparaben, tartrazine (fd&c yellow #5)]
Swab, Mouth/Throat:
Benz-O-Sthetic: 20% (2 ea [DSC]) [contains benzyl alcohol, polyethylene glycol, saccharin sodium]
Benz-O-Sthetic: 20% (2 ea) [contains benzyl alcohol, polyethylene glycol, saccharin sodium; cherry flavor]
Hurricaine: 20% (72 ea) [contains polyethylene glycol, saccharin sodium; wild cherry flavor]

◆ Benzocaine and Antipyrine see Antipyrine and Benzocaine on page 135

Benzocaine, Butamben, and Tetracaine
(BEN zoe kane, byoo TAM ben, & TET ra kane)

Brand Names: US Cetacaine
Index Terms Benzocaine, Butamben, and Tetracaine Hydrochloride; Benzocaine, Butyl Aminobenzoate, and Tetracaine; Butamben, Tetracaine, and Benzocaine; Exactacain; Tetracaine, Benzocaine, and Butamben
Pharmacologic Category Local Anesthetic
Use Topical anesthetic to control pain in surgical or endoscopic procedures, or other procedures in the ear, nose, mouth, pharynx, larynx, trachea, bronchi, and esophagus (may also be used for vaginal or rectal procedure, when feasible); anesthetic for accessible mucous membranes except for the eyes; to control pain or gagging (spray only)

Dosing
Adult Anesthesia: Topical: Cetacaine:
Spray: Apply for ≤1 second; use of sprays >2 seconds is contraindicated. **Note:** Spray provides ~200 mg/second
Gel: Apply 200 mg (~¼ to ½ inch); application of >400 mg (>1 inch) is contraindicated
Liquid: Apply 200 mg (~0.2 mL); application of >400 mg (~0.4 mL) is contraindicated
Geriatric Dose reduction is suggested; refer to adult dosing.
Pediatric Dose has not been established; dose reduction is suggested
Renal Impairment No dosage adjustment provided in manufacturer's labeling.
Hepatic Impairment No dosage adjustment provided in manufacturer's labeling.
Additional Information Complete prescribing information should be consulted for additional detail.
Dosage Forms Excipient information presented when available (limited, particularly for generics); consult specific product labeling.
Aerosol, spray, topical [kit]:
Cetacaine: Benzocaine 14%, butamben 2%, and tetracaine hydrochloride 2% (56 g) [delivers benzocaine 28 mg, butamben 4 mg, and tetracaine hydrochloride 4 mg per second; contains benzalkonium chloride, chlorofluorocarbon; packaged with cannula assortment]
Aerosol, spray, topical:
Cetacaine: Benzocaine 14%, butamben 2%, and tetracaine hydrochloride 2% (20 g, 56 g) [delivers benzocaine 28 mg, butamben 4 mg, and tetracaine hydrochloride 4 mg per second; contains benzalkonium chloride, chlorofluorocarbon; packaged with cannula]
Gel, topical:
Cetacaine: Benzocaine 14%, butamben 2%, and tetracaine hydrochloride 2% (32 g) [delivers benzocaine 28 mg, butamben 4 mg and tetracaine hydrochloride 4 mg per pump actuation ~0.25 inch (6.5 mm) x 0.5 inch (13 mm) long application; contains benzalkonium chloride]
Liquid, topical [kit]:
Cetacaine: Benzocaine 14%, butamben 2%, and tetracaine hydrochloride 2% (14 g, 30 g) [provides benzocaine 28 mg, butamben 4 mg, and tetracaine hydrochloride 4 mg per 6-7 drops (0.2 mL); contains benzalkonium chloride; packaged with syringes and applicator tips]
Liquid, topical:
Cetacaine: Benzocaine 14%, butamben 2%, and tetracaine hydrochloride 2% (14 g, 30 g) [provides benzocaine 28 mg, butamben 4 mg, and tetracaine hydrochloride 4 mg per 6-7 drops (0.2 mL); contains benzalkonium chloride]

◆ Benzocaine, Butamben, and Tetracaine Hydrochloride see Benzocaine, Butamben, and Tetracaine on page 218
◆ Benzocaine, Butyl Aminobenzoate, and Tetracaine see Benzocaine, Butamben, and Tetracaine on page 218
◆ Benzocaine Oral Anesthetic [OTC] see Benzocaine on page 217
◆ Benzoic Acid, Hyoscyamine, Methenamine, Methylene Blue, and Phenyl Salicylate see Methenamine, Phenyl Salicylate, Methylene Blue, Benzoic Acid, and Hyoscyamine on page 1166
◆ Benzoic Acid, Methenamine, Methylene Blue, Phenyl Salicylate, and Hyoscyamine see Methenamine, Phenyl Salicylate, Methylene Blue, Benzoic Acid, and Hyoscyamine on page 1166

Benzonatate (ben ZOE na tate)

Brand Names: US Tessalon Perles; Tessalon [DSC]; Zonatuss
Index Terms Tessalon Perles
Pharmacologic Category Antitussive
Use Symptomatic relief of nonproductive cough
Dosing
Adult & Geriatric Cough: Oral: 100-200 mg 3 times/day as needed; maximum dose: 600 mg/day
Pediatric Children >10 years: Refer to adult dosing.
Renal Impairment No dosage adjustment provided in manufacturer's labeling.
Hepatic Impairment No dosage adjustment provided in manufacturer's labeling.
Additional Information Complete prescribing information should be consulted for additional detail.
Dosage Forms Excipient information presented when available (limited, particularly for generics); consult specific product labeling. [DSC] = Discontinued product

Capsule, Oral:
Tessalon: 200 mg [DSC] [contains fd&c yellow #10 (quinoline yellow), methylparaben, propylparaben]
Tessalon Perles: 100 mg
Zonatuss: 150 mg [contains brilliant blue fcf (fd&c blue #1)]
Generic: 100 mg, 150 mg, 200 mg

◆ Benz-O-Sthetic [OTC] see Benzocaine on page 217
◆ Benzoyl Peroxide and Adapalene see Adapalene and Benzoyl Peroxide on page 44
◆ Benzoyl Peroxide and Erythromycin see Erythromycin and Benzoyl Peroxide on page 673

Benzoyl Peroxide and Hydrocortisone
(BEN zoe il peer OKS ide & hye droe KOR ti sone)

Brand Names: US Vanoxide-HC®
Brand Names: Canada Vanoxide-HC®
Index Terms Hydrocortisone and Benzoyl Peroxide
Pharmacologic Category Acne Products; Topical Skin Product; Topical Skin Product, Acne
Use Treatment of acne vulgaris and oily skin
Dosing
Adult & Geriatric Acne vulgaris: Topical: Apply thin film 1-3 times/day
Pediatric Adolescents ≥12 years: Refer to adult dosing.
Additional Information Complete prescribing information should be consulted for additional detail.
Dosage Forms Excipient information presented when available (limited, particularly for generics); consult specific product labeling.
Lotion, topical:
Vanoxide-HC®: Benzoyl peroxide 5% and hydrocortisone 0.5% (25 g)

Benztropine (BENZ troe peen)

Brand Names: US Cogentin
Brand Names: Canada Benztropine Omega; Kynesia; PMS-Benztropine
Index Terms Benzatropine; Benztropine Mesylate; Cogentin
Pharmacologic Category Anti-Parkinson's Agent, Anticholinergic; Anticholinergic Agent
Use
Extrapyramidal disorders: Aid in the control of extrapyramidal disorders (except tardive dyskinesia) due to neuroleptic drugs (eg, phenothiazines).
Parkinsonism: Adjunctive therapy of all forms of parkinsonism.
Pregnancy Considerations Animal reproduction studies have not been conducted. Paralytic ileus (which resolved rapidly) was reported in two newborns exposed to a combination of benztropine and chlorpromazine during the second and third trimesters and the last 6 weeks of pregnancy, respectively (Falterman, 1980).
Breast-Feeding Considerations It is not known if benztropine is excreted in breast milk. Anticholinergic agents may suppress lactation.
Contraindications Hypersensitivity to benztropine or any component of the formulation; children <3 years of age (due to atropine-like adverse effects)
Warnings/Precautions May cause anticholinergic effects (constipation, xerostomia, blurred vision, urinary retention). Use with caution in children >3 years of age due to its anticholinergic effects (dose has not been established). Use is contraindicated in children <3 years of age. Use with caution in hot weather or during exercise. May cause anhidrosis and hyperthermia, which may be severe. The risk is increased in hot environments, particularly in the elderly, alcoholics, patients with CNS disease, and those with prolonged outdoor exposure. If there is evidence of anhidrosis, consider decreasing dose so the ability to maintain body heat equilibrium by perspiration is not impaired.

Use with caution in patients >65 years of age; response in elderly may be altered. Initiate at low doses in the elderly and increase as needed while monitoring for adverse events.

Use with caution in patients with tachycardia, glaucoma, prostatic hyperplasia (especially in the elderly), any tendency toward urinary retention, and obstructive disease of the GI or GU tracts. Avoid use in angle-closure glaucoma. When given in large doses or to susceptible patients, may cause weakness and inability to move particular muscle groups.

May be associated with confusion, visual hallucinations, or excitement (generally at higher dosages). Intensification of symptoms or toxic psychosis may occur in patients with mental disorders. May cause CNS depression, which may impair physical or mental abilities; patients must be cautioned about performing tasks which require mental alertness (eg, operating machinery or driving). Benztropine does not relieve symptoms of tardive dyskinesia and may potentially exacerbate symptoms.

Potentially significant drug-drug interactions may exist, requiring dose or frequency adjustment, additional monitoring, and/or selection of alternative therapy.
Adverse Reactions Frequency not defined.
Cardiovascular: Tachycardia
Central nervous system: Confusion, depression, disorientation, heatstroke, hyperthermia, lethargy, memory impairment, nervousness, numbness of fingers, psychotic symptoms (exacerbation of preexisting symptoms), toxic psychosis, visual hallucination
Dermatologic: Skin rash
Gastrointestinal: Constipation, nausea, paralytic ileus, vomiting, xerostomia
Genitourinary: Dysuria, urinary retention
Ophthalmic: Blurred vision, mydriasis
Drug Interactions
Metabolism/Transport Effects Substrate of CYP2D6 (minor); **Note:** Assignment of Major/Minor substrate status based on clinically relevant drug interaction potential
Avoid Concomitant Use
Avoid concomitant use of Benztropine with any of the following: Aclidinium; Cimetropium; Eluxadoline; Glucagon; Glycopyrrolate; Glycopyrrolate (Oral Inhalation); Ipratropium (Oral Inhalation); Levosulpiride; Potassium Chloride; Tiotropium; Umeclidinium
Increased Effect/Toxicity
Benztropine may increase the levels/effects of: AbobotulinumtoxinA; Analgesics (Opioid); Anticholinergic Agents; Cannabinoid-Containing Products; Cimetropium; Eluxadoline; Glucagon; Glycopyrrolate; Glycopyrrolate (Oral Inhalation); Mirabegron; OnabotulinumtoxinA; Potassium Chloride; Ramosetron; RimabotulinumtoxinB; Thiazide Diuretics; Tiotropium; Topiramate

The levels/effects of Benztropine may be increased by: Aclidinium; Ipratropium (Oral Inhalation); Mianserin; Pramlintide; Umeclidinium
Decreased Effect
Benztropine may decrease the levels/effects of: Acetylcholinesterase Inhibitors; Gastrointestinal Agents (Prokinetic); Ioflupane I 123; Itopride; Levosulpiride; Secretin

The levels/effects of Benztropine may be decreased by: Acetylcholinesterase Inhibitors
Storage/Stability Store at 20°C to 25°C (68°F to 77°F).
Mechanism of Action Possesses both anticholinergic and antihistaminic effects. *In vitro* anticholinergic activity approximates that of atropine; *in vivo* it is only about half as active as atropine. Animal data suggest its antihistaminic activity and duration of action approach that of pyrilamine maleate.
Pharmacodynamics/Kinetics
Onset of action:
IM, IV: Within a few minutes; there is no significant difference between onset of effect after intravenous or intramuscular injection
Oral: Within 1 hour
Metabolism: Hepatic (N-oxidation, N-dealkylation, and ring hydroxylation) (from animal studies only) (Brocks 1999)
Time to peak, plasma: Oral: 7 hours (Brocks 1999)
Dosing
Adult
Drug-induced extrapyramidal symptoms: Oral, IM, IV: Initial: 1 to 2 mg 2 to 3 times daily for reactions developing soon after initiation of antipsychotic medication. Usually provides relief within 1 to 2 days. Titrate gradually at 0.5 mg increments at 5- to 6-day intervals based on response and tolerability. Usual dosage is 1 to 4 mg once or twice daily up to a maximum daily dose of 6 mg. Treatment may be continued for 1 to 2 weeks, after which treatment should be withdrawn to reassess continued need for therapy. May reinitiate benztropine if symptoms recur (Holloman, 1997; Tonda, 1994). **Note:** Certain drug-induced extrapyramidal disorders that develop slowly may not respond to benztropine.
Acute dystonic reactions: 1 to 2 mg to treat acute reactions followed by 1 to 2 mg (orally) 1 to 2 times daily for up to 7 to 28 days to prevent recurrence. **Note:** IM/IV administration is preferred over oral administration for severe acute reactions due to the faster onset of action (Holloman, 1997; Tonda, 1994).

Parkinsonism: Oral, IM, IV:

Idiopathic parkinsonism: Initial: 0.5 to 1 mg daily at bedtime or in 2 to 4 divided doses. Titrate in 0.5 mg increments every 5 to 6 days based on response and tolerability. Usual dose: 1 to 2 mg daily (range: 0.5 to 6 mg daily) although some patients may need 4 to 6 mg daily; maximum: 6 mg daily

Postencephalitic parkinsonism: Initial: 2 mg daily as a single dose at bedtime or in 2 to 4 divided doses; a lower initial dose of 0.5 mg at bedtime may be considered in highly sensitive patients. Titrate in 0.5 mg increments every 5 to 6 days based on response and tolerability. Usual dose: 1 to 2 mg daily (range: 0.5 to 6 mg daily); maximum: 6 mg daily.

Note: Lower initial doses may be appropriate for older and thinner patients.

Geriatric Refer to adult dosing. Start at low end of dosing range and increase only as needed and as tolerated.

Pediatric

Drug-induced extrapyramidal symptoms: Oral, IM, IV: Children ≥3 years (off-label dose): 0.02 to 0.05 mg/kg/dose 1 to 2 times daily (Bellman, 1974; Habre, 1999; Joseph, 1995; Teoh, 2002)

Adolescents (off-label dose): 1 to 4 mg every 12 to 24 hours (Nelson, 1996)

Renal Impairment There are no dosage adjustments provided in the manufacturer's labeling.

Hepatic Impairment There are no dosage adjustments provided in the manufacturer's labeling.

Dietary Considerations Tablet may be taken with or without food.

Administration

Oral: Administer with or without food.

Injectable: Administer IM or IV if oral route is unacceptable. Manufacturer's labeling states there is no difference in onset of effect after IV or IM injection and therefore there is usually no need to use the IV route. No specific instructions on administering benztropine IV are provided in the labeling. The IV route has been reported in the literature (slow IV push when reported), although specific instructions are lacking (Duncan, 2001; Lydon, 1998; Sachdev, 1993; Schramm, 2002).

Monitoring Parameters Pulse, anticholinergic effects

Dosage Forms Excipient information presented when available (limited, particularly for generics); consult specific product labeling.

Solution, Injection, as mesylate:
Cogentin: 1 mg/mL (2 mL)
Generic: 1 mg/mL (2 mL)
Tablet, Oral, as mesylate:
Generic: 0.5 mg, 1 mg, 2 mg

- ◆ Benztropine Mesylate *see* Benztropine *on page 219*
- ◆ Benztropine Omega (Can) *see* Benztropine *on page 219*

Benzyl Alcohol (BEN zill AL koe hol)

Brand Names: US Ulesfia; Zilactin [OTC]

Pharmacologic Category Analgesic, Topical; Antiparasitic Agent, Topical; Pediculocide; Topical Skin Product

Use

Oral pain (gel only): Temporary relief of pain from cold sores/fever blisters, canker sores, mouth sores, and/or gum irritations

Head lice (lotion only): Treatment of head lice infestation in patients 6 months and older

Dosing

Adult & Geriatric

Oral pain: Topical: Gel: Apply to affected area up to 4 times daily

Head lice: Topical: Lotion: Apply appropriate volume for hair length to dry hair and completely saturate the scalp; leave on for 10 minutes; rinse thoroughly with water; repeat in 7 days

Hair length 0 to 2 inches: 4 to 6 ounces
Hair length 2 to 4 inches: 6 to 8 ounces
Hair length 4 to 8 inches: 8 to 12 ounces
Hair length 8 to 16 inches: 12 to 24 ounces
Hair length 16 to 22 inches: 24 to 32 ounces
Hair length >22 inches: 32 to 48 ounces

Pediatric

Oral pain: Topical: Gel: Children ≥2 years and Adolescents: Refer to adult dosing.

Head lice: Topical: Lotion: Infants ≥6 months, Children, and Adolescents: Refer to adult dosing.

Renal Impairment There are no dosage adjustments provided in the manufacturer's labeling.

Hepatic Impairment There are no dosage adjustments provided in the manufacturer's labeling.

Additional Information Complete prescribing information should be consulted for additional detail.

Dosage Forms Excipient information presented when available (limited, particularly for generics); consult specific product labeling.

Gel, Mouth/Throat:
Zilactin: 10% (7.1 g) [contains propylene glycol, sd alcohol]
Lotion, External:
Ulesfia: 5% (227 g) [contains polysorbate 80, trolamine (triethanolamine)]

- ◆ Benzylpenicillin Benzathine *see* Penicillin G Benzathine *on page 1419*
- ◆ Benzylpenicillin Potassium *see* Penicillin G (Parenteral/Aqueous) *on page 1420*
- ◆ Benzylpenicillin Sodium *see* Penicillin G (Parenteral/Aqueous) *on page 1420*

Bepotastine (be poe TAS teen)

Brand Names: US Bepreve

Index Terms Bepotastine Besilate

Pharmacologic Category Histamine H$_1$ Antagonist; Histamine H$_1$ Antagonist, Second Generation; Mast Cell Stabilizer

Use Treatment of itching associated with allergic conjunctivitis

Dosing

Adult & Geriatric Allergic conjunctivitis: Ophthalmic: Instill 1 drop into the affected eye(s) twice daily

Pediatric Allergic conjunctivitis: Ophthalmic: Children ≥2 years: Refer to adult dosing.

Additional Information Complete prescribing information should be consulted for additional detail.

Dosage Forms Excipient information presented when available (limited, particularly for generics); consult specific product labeling.

Solution, Ophthalmic, as besilate:
Bepreve: 1.5% (5 mL, 10 mL) [contains benzalkonium chloride]

- ◆ Bepotastine Besilate *see* Bepotastine *on page 220*
- ◆ Bepreve *see* Bepotastine *on page 220*

Beractant (ber AKT ant)

Brand Names: US Survanta

Brand Names: Canada Survanta®

Index Terms Bovine Lung Surfactant; Natural Lung Surfactant

Pharmacologic Category Lung Surfactant

Use Prevention and treatment of respiratory distress syndrome (RDS) in premature infants

Prophylactic therapy: Body weight <1250 g in infants at risk for developing, or with evidence of, surfactant deficiency (administer within 15 minutes of birth)

Rescue therapy: Treatment of infants with RDS confirmed by x-ray and requiring mechanical ventilation (administer as soon as possible - within 8 hours of age)

Pregnancy Considerations Beractant is only indicated for use in premature infants.

Contraindications There are no contraindications listed within the FDA-approved labeling

Warnings/Precautions For endotracheal administration only. Rapidly affects oxygenation and lung compliance; restrict use to a highly-supervised clinical setting with immediate availability of clinicians experienced in intubation and ventilatory management of premature infants. Transient episodes of bradycardia and decreased oxygen saturation occur. Discontinue dosing procedure and initiate measures to alleviate the condition; may reinstitute after the patient is stable. Produces rapid improvements in lung oxygenation and compliance that may require frequent adjustments to oxygen delivery and ventilator settings.

Adverse Reactions During the dosing procedure:
>10%: Cardiovascular: Transient bradycardia
1% to 10%: Respiratory: Oxygen desaturation
<1% (Limited to important or life-threatening): Apnea, endotracheal tube blockage, hypercarbia, hyper-/hypotension, post-treatment nosocomial sepsis probability increased, pulmonary air leaks, pulmonary interstitial emphysema, vasoconstriction

Drug Interactions

Metabolism/Transport Effects None known.

Avoid Concomitant Use

Avoid concomitant use of Beractant with any of the following: Ceritinib

Increased Effect/Toxicity

Beractant may increase the levels/effects of: Bradycardia-Causing Agents; Ceritinib; Ivabradine; Lacosamide

The levels/effects of Beractant may be increased by: Bretylium; Ruxolitinib; Tofacitinib

Decreased Effect There are no known significant interactions involving a decrease in effect.

Storage/Stability Refrigerate; protect from light. Prior to administration, warm by standing at room temperature for 20 minutes or held in hand for 8 minutes. **Artificial warming methods should not be used.** Unused, unopened vials warmed to room temperature may be returned to the refrigerator within 24 hours of warming only once.

Mechanism of Action Replaces deficient or ineffective endogenous lung surfactant in neonates with respiratory distress syndrome (RDS) or in neonates at risk of developing RDS. Surfactant prevents the alveoli from collapsing during expiration by lowering surface tension between air and alveolar surfaces.

Pharmacodynamics/Kinetics Excretion: Clearance: Alveolar clearance is rapid

Dosing

Pediatric

Respiratory distress treatment: Premature infants:
Prophylactic treatment: Endotracheal: Administer 4 mL/kg (100 mg phospholipids/kg) as soon as possible; as many as 4 doses may be administered during the first 48 hours of life, no more frequently than 6 hours apart. The need for additional doses is determined by evidence of continuing respiratory distress; if the infant is still intubated and requiring at least 30% inspired oxygen to maintain a PaO$_2$ ≤80 torr.
Rescue treatment: Endotracheal: Administer 4 mL/kg (100 mg phospholipids/kg) as soon as the diagnosis of RDS is made; may repeat if needed, no more frequently than every 6 hours to a maximum of 4 doses

Renal Impairment No dosage adjustment provided in manufacturer's labeling.

Hepatic Impairment No dosage adjustment provided in manufacturer's labeling.

Administration

For endotracheal administration only

Suction infant prior to administration. Inspect solution to verify complete mixing of the suspension (may swirl gently, but DO NOT SHAKE). Do not filter dose and avoid shaking.

Administer endotracheally by instillation through a 5-French end-hole catheter inserted into the infant's endotracheal tube.

Administer the dose in four 1 mL/kg aliquots. Each quarter-dose is instilled over 2-3 seconds followed by at least 30 seconds of manual ventilation or until stable; each quarter-dose is administered with the infant in a different position. Slightly downward inclination with head turned to the right, then repeat with head turned to the left; then slightly upward inclination with head turned to the right, then repeat with head turned to the left. Following administration of one full dose, withhold suctioning for 1 hour unless signs of significant airway obstruction.

Monitoring Parameters Continuous ECG and transcutaneous O$_2$ saturation should be monitored during administration; frequent arterial blood gases are necessary to prevent postdosing hyperoxia and hypocarbia

Additional Information Each mL contains 25 mg phospholipids suspended in 0.9% sodium chloride solution. Contents of 1 mL: 0.5-1.75 mg triglycerides, 1.4-3.5 mg free fatty acids, and <1 mg protein.

Dosage Forms Excipient information presented when available (limited, particularly for generics); consult specific product labeling.
Suspension, Inhalation:
Survanta: Phospholipids 25 mg/mL (4 mL, 8 mL)

◆ Berinert *see* C1 Inhibitor (Human) *on page 276*

◆ Beriplex P/N *see* Prothrombin Complex Concentrate (Human) [(Factors II, VII, IX, X), Protein C, and Protein S] *on page 1525*

Besifloxacin (be si FLOX a sin)

Brand Names: US Besivance
Brand Names: Canada Besivance
Index Terms Besifloxacin Hydrochloride; BOL-303224-A; SS734
Pharmacologic Category Antibiotic, Fluoroquinolone; Antibiotic, Ophthalmic
Use Bacterial conjunctivitis: Treatment of bacterial conjunctivitis caused by susceptible isolates of the following bacteria: *Aerococcus viridans*, CDC coryneform group G, *Haemophilus influenzae*, *Staphylococcus aureus*,

Staphylococcus epidermidis, Streptococcus mitis group, *Streptococcus oralis, Streptococcus pneumoniae, Corynebacterium pseudodiphtheriticum, Corynebacterium striatum, Moraxella lacunata, Moraxella catarrhalis, Pseudomonas aeruginosa, Staphylococcus hominis, Staphylococcus lugdunensis, Staphylococcus warneri, Streptococcus salivarius.*

Dosing

Adult & Geriatric Bacterial conjunctivitis: Ophthalmic: Instill 1 drop into affected eye(s) 3 times daily (4 to 12 hours apart) for 7 days

Pediatric Bacterial conjunctivitis: Children ≥1 year and Adolescents: Ophthalmic: Refer to adult dosing.

Renal Impairment There are no dosage adjustments provided in the manufacturer's labeling. However, dosage adjustment unlikely due to low systemic absorption.

Hepatic Impairment There are no dosage adjustments provided in the manufacturer's labeling. However, dosage adjustment unlikely due to low systemic absorption.

Additional Information Complete prescribing information should be consulted for additional detail.

Dosage Forms Excipient information presented when available (limited, particularly for generics); consult specific product labeling.
Suspension, Ophthalmic:
Besivance: 0.6% (5 mL) [contains benzalkonium chloride, edetate disodium dihydrate]

◆ Besifloxacin Hydrochloride *see* Besifloxacin *on page 221*

◆ Besivance *see* Besifloxacin *on page 221*

◆ β,β-Dimethylcysteine *see* PenicillAMINE *on page 1418*

◆ 9-Beta-D-Ribofuranosyladenine *see* Adenosine *on page 46*

◆ Betacaine (Can) *see* Lidocaine (Topical) *on page 1074*

◆ Beta Care Betamide [OTC] *see* Urea *on page 1853*

◆ β Carotene *see* Beta-Carotene *on page 221*

Beta-Carotene (BAY ta KARE oh teen)

Brand Names: US A-Caro-25 [OTC]; B-Caro-T [OTC]; Caroguard [OTC]
Index Terms β Carotene; β-Carotene
Pharmacologic Category Vitamin, Fat Soluble
Use Prophylaxis against photosensitivity reactions in erythropoietic protoporphyria (EPP)
Dosing

Adult & Geriatric Erythropoietic protoporphyria (EPP) (Lumitene™): Oral: 30-300 mg/day

Pediatric Erythropoietic protoporphyria (EPP) (Lumitene™): Oral: Children <14 years: 30-150 mg/day

Renal Impairment No dosage adjustment provided in manufacturer's labeling (has not been studied); use with caution.

Hepatic Impairment No dosage adjustment provided in manufacturer's labeling (has not been studied); use with caution.

Additional Information Complete prescribing information should be consulted for additional detail.

Dosage Forms Excipient information presented when available (limited, particularly for generics); consult specific product labeling.
Capsule, Oral:
A-Caro-25: 25,000 units [contains soybean lecithin, soybean oil]
Generic: 25,000 units
Capsule, Oral [preservative free]:
B-Caro-T: 15 mg [dye free]
Caroguard: 15 mg [dye free]
Generic: 25,000 units

◆ Betaderm (Can) *see* Betamethasone (Topical) *on page 224*

◆ Betagan *see* Levobunolol *on page 1059*

◆ Betagan® (Can) *see* Levobunolol *on page 1059*

◆ Beta HC [OTC] *see* Hydrocortisone (Topical) *on page 886*

Betaine (BAY ta een)

Brand Names: US Cystadane
Brand Names: Canada Cystadane
Index Terms Betaine Anhydrous
Pharmacologic Category Homocystinuria, Treatment Agent
Use Homocystinuria: Treatment of homocystinuria including deficiencies or defects in cystathionine beta-synthase (CBS), 5,10-methylene tetrahydrofolate reductase (MTHFR), and cobalamin cofactor metabolism (CBL).

Prescribing and Access Restrictions Cystadane may be obtained by contacting AnovoRx at wholesale@anovorx.com.

Dosing

Adult & Geriatric

Homocystinuria: Oral: 3 g twice daily. Dosages of up to 20 g/day have been necessary to control homocysteine levels in some patients.

Note: Dosage in all patients can be gradually increased until plasma total homocysteine is undetectable or present only in small amounts. One in vitro study indicated minimal benefit from exceeding a twice daily dosing schedule and a 150 mg/kg/day dosage.

Pediatric

Homocystinuria: Oral:

Infants and Children <3 years: Initial dose: 100 mg/kg/day in 2 divided doses; increase weekly by 50 mg/kg increments, as needed

Children ≥3 years and Adolescents: Refer to adult dosing.

Note: Dosage in all patients can be gradually increased until plasma total homocysteine is undetectable or present only in small amounts. One in vitro study indicated minimal benefit from exceeding a twice daily dosing schedule and a 150 mg/kg/day dosage.

Renal Impairment There are no dosage adjustments provided in the manufacturer's labeling.

Hepatic Impairment There are no dosage adjustments provided in the manufacturer's labeling.

Additional Information Complete prescribing information should be consulted for additional detail.

Dosage Forms Excipient information presented when available (limited, particularly for generics); consult specific product labeling.

Powder, Oral, as anhydrous:
Cystadane: 1 g/scoop (180 g)
Tablet, Oral, as anhydrous:
Generic: 300 mg

◆ Betaine Anhydrous *see* Betaine *on page 221*

◆ Betaject (Can) *see* Betamethasone (Systemic) *on page 222*

◆ Betaloc (Can) *see* Metoprolol *on page 1193*

Betamethasone (Systemic) (bay ta METH a sone)

Brand Names: US Celestone Soluspan; Celestone [DSC]
Brand Names: Canada Betaject; Celestone Soluspan
Index Terms Betamethasone Acetate; Betamethasone Sodium Phosphate; Flubenisolone
Pharmacologic Category Corticosteroid, Systemic
Additional Appendix Information
Corticosteroids Systemic Equivalencies *on page 1950*
Use

Intramuscular:

Allergic states: Control of severe or incapacitating allergic conditions intractable to adequate trials of conventional treatment in asthma, atopic dermatitis, contact dermatitis, drug hypersensitivity reactions, perennial or seasonal allergic rhinitis, serum sickness, transfusion reactions

Dermatologic diseases: Bullous dermatitis herpetiformis, exfoliative erythroderma, mycosis fungoides, pemphigus, severe erythema multiforme (Stevens-Johnson syndrome)

Endocrine disorders: Congenital adrenal hyperplasia, hypercalcemia associated with cancer, nonsuppurative thyroiditis. Hydrocortisone or cortisone is the drug of choice in primary or secondary adrenocortical insufficiency. Synthetic analogs may be used in conjunction with mineralocorticoids where applicable; in infancy mineralocorticoid supplementation is of particular importance

Gastrointestinal diseases: To tide the patient over a critical period of the disease in regional enteritis and ulcerative colitis

Hematologic disorders: Acquired (autoimmune) hemolytic anemia, Diamond-Blackfan anemia, pure red cell aplasia, selected cases of secondary thrombocytopenia

Neoplastic diseases: Palliative management of leukemias and lymphomas

Nervous system: Acute exacerbations of multiple sclerosis; cerebral edema associated with primary or metastatic brain tumor or craniotomy

Ophthalmic diseases: Sympathetic ophthalmia, temporal arteritis, uveitis and ocular inflammatory conditions unresponsive to topical corticosteroids

Renal diseases: To induce diuresis or remission of proteinuria in idiopathic nephrotic syndrome or that due to lupus erythematosus

Respiratory diseases: Berylliosis, fulminating or disseminated pulmonary tuberculosis when used concurrently with appropriate antituberculous chemotherapy, idiopathic eosinophilic pneumonias, symptomatic sarcoidosis

Rheumatic disorders: Adjunctive therapy for short-term administration (to tide the patient over an acute episode or exacerbation) in acute gouty arthritis; acute rheumatic carditis; ankylosing spondylitis; psoriatic arthritis; rheumatoid arthritis, including juvenile rheumatoid arthritis (selected cases may require low-dose maintenance therapy); treatment of dermatomyositis, polymyositis, and systemic lupus erythematosus.

Miscellaneous: Trichinosis with neurologic or myocardial involvement, tuberculous meningitis with subarachnoid block or impending block when used with appropriate antituberculous chemotherapy

Intra-articular or soft tissue administration:

Adjunctive therapy for short-term administration (to tide the patient over an acute episode or exacerbation) in acute gouty arthritis, acute and subacute bursitis, acute nonspecific tenosynovitis, epicondylitis, rheumatoid arthritis, synovitis of osteoarthritis

Intralesional:

Treatment of alopecia areata; discoid lupus erythematosus; keloids; localized hypertrophic, infiltrated, inflammatory lesions of granuloma annulare, lichen planus, lichen simplex chronicus (neurodermatitis), and psoriatic plaques; necrobiosis lipoidica diabeticorum

Pregnancy Considerations Adverse events have been observed with corticosteroids in animal reproduction studies. Betamethasone crosses the placenta (Brownfoot, 2013); and is partially metabolized by placental enzymes to an inactive metabolite (Murphy, 2007). Some studies have shown an association between first trimester systemic corticosteroid use and oral clefts (Park-Wyllie, 2000; Pradat, 2003). Systemic corticosteroids may have an effect on fetal growth (decreased birth weight); however, information is conflicting (Lunghi, 2010). Hypoadrenalism may occur in newborns following maternal use of corticosteroids during pregnancy; monitor.

Because antenatal corticosteroid administration may reduce the incidence of intraventricular hemorrhage, necrotizing enterocolitis, neonatal mortality, and respiratory distress syndrome, the injection is often used in patients with preterm premature rupture of membranes (membrane rupture between 24 0/7 weeks and 34 0/7 weeks of gestation) who are at risk of preterm delivery (ACOG, 2013). When systemic corticosteroids are needed in pregnancy, it is generally recommended to use the lowest effective dose for the shortest duration of time, avoiding high doses during the first trimester (Leachman, 2006; Lunghi, 2010; Makol, 2011; Østensen, 2009).

Women exposed to betamethasone during pregnancy for the treatment of an autoimmune disease may contact the OTIS Autoimmune Diseases Study at 877-311-8972.

Breast-Feeding Considerations Corticosteroids are excreted in human milk. The onset of milk secretion after birth may be delayed and the volume of milk produced may be decreased by antenatal betamethasone therapy; this affect was seen when delivery occurred 3-9 days after the betamethasone dose in women between 28 and 34 weeks gestation. Antenatal betamethasone therapy did not affect milk production when birth occurred <3 days or >10 days of treatment (Henderson, 2008).

The manufacturer notes that when used systemically, maternal use of corticosteroids have the potential to cause adverse events in a nursing infant (eg, growth suppression, interfere with endogenous corticosteroid production) and therefore recommends that caution be exercised when administering betamethasone to nursing women. If there is concern about exposure to the infant, some guidelines recommend waiting 4 hours after the maternal dose of an oral systemic corticosteroid before breast-feeding in order to decrease potential exposure to the infant (based on a study using prednisolone) (Bae, 2011; Leachman, 2006; Makol, 2011; Ost, 1985).

Contraindications

Hypersensitivity to any component of the formulation; IM administration contraindicated in idiopathic thrombocytopenic purpura.

Documentation of allergenic cross-reactivity for glucocorticoids is limited. However, because of similarities in chemical structure and/or pharmacologic actions, the possibility of cross-sensitivity cannot be ruled out with certainty.

Warnings/Precautions Avoid concurrent use of other corticosteroids.

May cause hypercorticism or suppression of hypothalamic-pituitary-adrenal (HPA) axis, particularly in younger children or in patients receiving high doses for prolonged periods. HPA axis suppression may lead to adrenal crisis. Withdrawal and discontinuation of a corticosteroid should be done slowly and carefully. Particular care is required when patients are transferred from systemic corticosteroids to inhaled products due to possible adrenal insufficiency or withdrawal from steroids, including an increase in allergic symptoms. Patients receiving >20 mg per day of prednisone (or equivalent) may be most susceptible. Fatalities have occurred due to adrenal insufficiency in asthmatic patients during and after transfer from systemic corticosteroids to aerosol steroids; aerosol steroids do not provide the systemic steroid needed to treat patients having trauma, surgery, or infections. In stressful situations, HPA axis-suppressed patients should receive adequate supplementation with natural glucocorticoids (hydrocortisone or cortisone) rather than betamethasone (due to lack of mineralocorticoid activity).

Acute myopathy has been reported with high-dose corticosteroids, usually in patients with neuromuscular transmission disorders; may involve ocular and/or respiratory muscles; monitor creatine kinase; recovery may be delayed. Corticosteroid use may cause psychiatric disturbances, including depression, euphoria, insomnia, mood swings, and personality changes. Preexisting psychiatric conditions may be exacerbated by corticosteroid use. Prolonged use of corticosteroids may also increase the incidence of secondary infection, mask acute infection (including fungal infections), prolong or exacerbate viral infections, or limit response to killed or inactivated vaccines. Special pathogens (Amoeba, Candida, Cryptococcus, Mycobacterium, Nocardia, Pneumocystis, Strongyloides, or Toxoplasma) may be activated or an infection exacerbation may occur (may be fatal). Amebiasis or Strongyloides infections should be particularly ruled out. Exposure to varicella zoster (chickenpox) should be avoided; corticosteroids should not be used to treat ocular herpes simplex. Corticosteroids should not be used for cerebral malaria or viral hepatitis. Close observation is required in patients with latent tuberculosis and/or TB reactivity; restrict use in active TB (only in conjunction with antituberculosis treatment). Prolonged treatment with corticosteroids has been associated with the development of Kaposi sarcoma (case reports); if noted, discontinuation of therapy should be considered. High-dose corticosteroids should not be used to manage acute head injury. Rare cases of anaphylactoid reactions have been observed in patients receiving corticosteroids.

Use with caution in patients with thyroid disease, hepatic impairment, renal impairment, cardiovascular disease, diabetes, glaucoma, cataracts, myasthenia gravis, patients at risk for osteoporosis, patients at risk for seizures, or GI diseases (diverticulitis, fresh intestinal anastomoses, peptic ulcer, ulcerative colitis) due to perforation risk. Use caution following acute MI (corticosteroids have been associated with myocardial rupture). Use with caution in patients with HF and/or hypertension; long-term use has been associated with fluid retention and electrolyte disturbances. Dietary modifications may be necessary. Use with caution in patients with a recent history of myocardial infarction (MI); left ventricular free wall rupture has been reported after the use of corticosteroids. Use with caution in patients with renal impairment; fluid and sodium retention and increased potassium and calcium excretion may occur. Dietary modifications may be necessary. Not recommended for the treatment of optic neuritis; may increase frequency of new episodes. Intra-articular injection may result in joint tissue damage. Injection into an infected site should be avoided. Injection into a previously infected join is usually not recommended. If infection is suspected, joint fluid examination is recommended. If septic arthritis occurs after injection, institute appropriate antimicrobial therapy. Suspension for injection is for intramuscular, intra-articular or intralesional use only, do not administer intravenously. Corticosteroids are not approved for epidural injection. Serious neurologic events (eg, spinal cord infarction, paraplegia, quadriplegia, cortical blindness, stroke), some resulting in death, have been reported with epidural injection of corticosteroids, with and without use of fluoroscopy. Intra-articular injected corticosteroids may be systemically absorbed. May produce systemic as well as local effects. Appropriate examination of any joint fluid present is necessary to exclude a septic process. Avoid injection into an infected site. Do not inject into unstable joints. Intra-articular injection may result in damage to joint tissues. Potentially significant drug-drug interactions may exist, requiring dose or frequency adjustment, additional monitoring, and/or selection of alternative therapy. Because of the risk of adverse effects, systemic corticosteroids should be used cautiously in the elderly in the smallest possible effective dose for the shortest duration. Withdraw therapy with gradual tapering of dose.

Prolonged use in children may affect growth velocity; growth should be routinely monitored in pediatric patients.

Adverse Reactions

Cardiovascular: Congestive heart failure, edema, hyper-/hypotension

Central nervous system: Dizziness, headache, insomnia, intracranial pressure increased, lightheadedness, nervousness, pseudotumor cerebri, seizure, vertigo

Dermatologic: Ecchymoses, facial erythema, fragile skin, hirsutism, hyper-/hypopigmentation, perioral dermatitis (oral), petechiae, striae, wound healing impaired

Endocrine & metabolic: Amenorrhea, Cushing's syndrome, diabetes mellitus, growth suppression, hyperglycemia, hypokalemia, menstrual irregularities, pituitary-adrenal axis suppression, protein catabolism, sodium retention, water retention

Gastrointestinal: Abdominal distention, appetite increased, hiccups, indigestion, peptic ulcer, pancreatitis, ulcerative esophagitis

Local: Injection site reactions (intra-articular use), sterile abscess

Neuromuscular & skeletal: Arthralgia, muscle atrophy, fractures, muscle weakness, myopathy, osteoporosis, necrosis (femoral and humeral heads)

Ocular: Cataracts, glaucoma, intraocular pressure increased

Miscellaneous: Anaphylactoid reaction, diaphoresis, hypersensitivity, secondary infection

Drug Interactions

Metabolism/Transport Effects None known.

Avoid Concomitant Use

Avoid concomitant use of Betamethasone (Systemic) with any of the following: Aldesleukin; BCG (Intravesical); Indium 111 Capromab Pendetide; Mifepristone; Natalizumab; Pimecrolimus; Tacrolimus (Topical); Tofacitinib

Increased Effect/Toxicity

Betamethasone (Systemic) may increase the levels/effects of: Acetylcholinesterase Inhibitors; Amphotericin B; Androgens; Ceritinib; Deferasirox; Fingolimod; Leflunomide; Loop Diuretics; Natalizumab; Nicorandil; NSAID (COX-2 Inhibitor); NSAID (Nonselective); Quinolone Antibiotics; Thiazide Diuretics; Tofacitinib; Vaccines (Live); Warfarin

The levels/effects of Betamethasone (Systemic) may be increased by: Aprepitant; CYP3A4 Inhibitors (Strong); Denosumab; Estrogen Derivatives; Fosaprepitant; Indacaterol; Mifepristone; Neuromuscular-Blocking Agents (Nondepolarizing); Pimecrolimus; Roflumilast; Salicylates; Tacrolimus (Topical); Telaprevir; Trastuzumab

Decreased Effect

Betamethasone (Systemic) may decrease the levels/effects of: Aldesleukin; Antidiabetic Agents; BCG (Intravesical); Calcitriol (Systemic); Coccidioides immitis Skin Test; Corticorelin; Hyaluronidase; Indium 111 Capromab Pendetide; Isoniazid; Salicylates; Sipuleucel-T; Telaprevir; Urea Cycle Disorder Agents; Vaccines (Inactivated); Vaccines (Live)

The levels/effects of Betamethasone (Systemic) may be decreased by: CYP3A4 Inducers (Strong); Echinacea; Mifepristone; Mitotane

Storage/Stability Store at 25°C (77°F); excursions are permitted between 15°C and 30°C (59°F and 86°F). Protect from light.

Mechanism of Action Controls the rate of protein synthesis; depresses the migration of polymorphonuclear leukocytes, fibroblasts; reverses capillary permeability and lysosomal stabilization at the cellular level to prevent or control inflammation

Dosing

Adult Note: Dosages expressed as combined amount of betamethasone sodium phosphate and betamethasone acetate; 1 mg is equivalent to betamethasone sodium phosphate 0.5 mg and betamethasone acetate 0.5 mg. Base dosage on severity of disease and patient response.

Usual dosage range: IM: Initial: 0.25 to 9 mg daily

Indication-specific dosing:

Antenatal fetal maturation (off-label use): IM: In women with preterm premature rupture of membranes (membrane rupture between 24 0/7 weeks and 34 0/7 weeks of gestation), a single course of corticosteroids is recommended if there is a risk of preterm delivery (ACOG, 2013). Although the optimal corticosteroid and dose have not been determined, betamethasone ▶

12 mg every 24 hours for a total of 2 doses has been used in most studies (Brownfoot, 2013).

Bursitis (other than of foot), tenosynovitis, peritendinitis: Intrabursal: 3 to 6 mg (0.5 to 1 mL) for one dose; several injections may be required for acute exacerbations or chronic conditions; reduced doses may be warranted for repeat injections.

Dermatologic: Intralesional: 1.2 mg/cm^2 (0.2 mL/cm^2) for one dose (maximum: 6 mg [1 mL] weekly).

Foot disorders: Intra-articular: 1.5 mg to 6 mg (0.25 to 1 mL) per dose at 3 to 7 day intervals. Dose is based upon condition:
Bursitis: 1.5 mg to 3 mg (0.25 to 0.5 mL)
Tenosynovitis: 3 mg (0.5 mL)
Acute gouty arthritis: 3 mg to 6 mg (0.5 to 1 mL)

Multiple sclerosis: IM: 30 mg daily for 1 week, followed by 12 mg every other day for 4 weeks.

Rheumatoid and osteoarthritis: Intra-articular: 3 mg to 12 mg (0.5 to 2 mL) for one dose. Dose is based upon the joint size:
Very large (eg, hip): 6 to 12 mg (1 to 2 mL)
Large (eg, knee, ankle, shoulder): 6 mg (1 mL)
Medium (eg, elbow, wrist): 3 mg to 6 mg (0.5 to 1 mL)
Small (eg, inter- or metacarpophalangeal, sternoclavicular): 1.5 mg to 3 mg (0.25 to 0.5 mL)

Geriatric Refer to adult dosing. Use the lowest effective dose.

Pediatric Note: Dosages expressed as combined amount of betamethasone sodium phosphate and betamethasone acetate; 1 mg is equivalent to betamethasone sodium phosphate 0.5 mg and betamethasone acetate 0.5 mg. Base dosage on severity of disease and patient response.

Inflammatory conditions: Children and Adolescents: IM: 0.02 to 0.3 mg/kg/day (0.6 to 9 mg/m^2/day) in 3 or 4 divided doses

Renal Impairment There are no dosage adjustments provided in the manufacturer's labeling.

Hepatic Impairment There are no dosage adjustments provided in the manufacturer's labeling.

Administration If suspension is coadministered with a local anesthetic, it may be mixed in syringe with 1% or 2% lidocaine HCl (without parabens) or similar parabens-free local anesthetic. Withdraw the dose of betamethasone suspension from the vial into the syringe, then draw up the local anesthetic into the syringe and shake the syringe briefly. Do not inject the local anesthetic directly into the suspension vial.

IM: Do **not** give injectable sodium phosphate/acetate suspension IV or epidurally

Intrabursal: Tendinitis, tenosynovitis: Inject into affected tendon sheaths (not directly into tendons).

Intradermal: Using a 25-gauge 1 mL (eg, tuberculin) syringe with 1/2-inch needle inject a uniform depot. Do **not** inject subcutaneously

Monitoring Parameters Growth in children

Test Interactions May suppress the wheal and flare reactions to skin test antigens

Dosage Forms Excipient information presented when available (limited, particularly for generics); consult specific product labeling. [DSC] = Discontinued product
Solution, Oral, as base:
Celestone: 0.6 mg/5 mL (118 mL [DSC]) [cherry-orange flavor]
Suspension, Injection:
Celestone Soluspan: Betamethasone sodium phosphate 3 mg and betamethasone acetate 3 mg per 1 mL (5 mL) [contains benzalkonium chloride, edetate disodium]
Generic: Betamethasone sodium phosphate 3 mg and betamethasone acetate 3 mg per 1 mL (5 mL)

Betamethasone (Topical) (bay ta METH a sone)

Brand Names: US AlphaTrex; Diprolene; Diprolene AF; Luxiq

Brand Names: Canada Betaderm; Betnesol; Celestoderm V; Celestoderm V/2; Diprolene; Diprosone; Luxiq; Prevex B; ratio-Ectosone; Ratio-Topilene; Ratio-Topisone; Rivasone; Rolene; Rosone; Taro-Sone; Valisone Scalp Lotion

Index Terms Betamethasone Dipropionate; Betamethasone Dipropionate, Augmented; Betamethasone Valerate

Pharmacologic Category Corticosteroid, Topical

Additional Appendix Information
Corticosteroids Systemic Equivalencies *on page 1950*
Topical Corticosteroids *on page 1952*

Use
Dermatoses: Relief of inflammatory and pruritic manifestations of corticosteroid-responsive dermatoses.

Dermatoses of the scalp (foam only): Relief of inflammatory and pruritic manifestations of corticosteroid-responsive dermatoses of the scalp.

Dosing
Adult Note: Base dosage on severity of disease and patient response.

Corticosteroid-responsive dermatoses: Topical: **Note:** Therapy should be discontinued when control is achieved.

Cream, augmented formulation: Betamethasone dipropionate 0.05%: Apply once or twice daily (maximum: 50 g weekly).

Cream, unaugmented formulation:
Betamethasone dipropionate 0.05%: Apply once daily; may increase to twice daily if needed
Betamethasone valerate 0.1%: Apply 1 to 3 times daily. **Note:** Once- or twice-daily applications are usually effective.

Foam: Apply to the scalp twice daily, once in the morning and once at night. **Note:** Reassess if no improvement after 2 weeks of treatment.

Gel, augmented formulation: Apply once or twice daily; rub in gently (maximum: 50 g weekly). **Note:** Reassess if no improvement after 2 weeks of treatment.

Lotion, augmented formulation: Betamethasone dipropionate 0.05%: Apply a few drops once or twice daily (maximum: 50 mL weekly). **Note:** Reassess if no improvement after 2 weeks of treatment.

Lotion, unaugmented formulation:
Betamethasone dipropionate 0.05%: Apply a few drops twice daily
Betamethasone valerate 0.1%: Apply a few drops twice daily; may consider increasing dose for resistant cases. Following improvement, may apply once daily.

Ointment, augmented formulation: Betamethasone dipropionate 0.05%: Apply once or twice daily (maximum: 50 g weekly). **Note:** Reassess if no improvement after 2 weeks of treatment.

Ointment, unaugmented formulation:
Betamethasone dipropionate 0.05%: Apply once daily; may increase to twice daily if needed
Betamethasone valerate 0.1%: Apply 1 to 3 times daily. **Note:** Once- or twice-daily applications are usually effective.

Geriatric Refer to adult dosing. Use the lowest effective dose.

Pediatric
Corticosteroid-responsive dermatoses: Topical:
Children: Cream, lotion or ointment: Unaugmented formulation: Refer to adult dosing.
Adolescents: Cream, gel, lotion, or ointment: Augmented formulation: Refer to adult dosing.

Renal Impairment There are no dosage adjustments provided in the manufacturer's labeling.

Hepatic Impairment There are no dosage adjustments provided in the manufacturer's labeling.

Additional Information Complete prescribing information should be consulted for additional detail.

Dosage Forms Excipient information presented when available (limited, particularly for generics); consult specific product labeling.
Cream, External, as dipropionate [strength expressed as base]:
Generic: 0.05% (15 g, 45 g)
Cream, External, as dipropionate augmented [strength expressed as base]:
Diprolene AF: 0.05% (15 g, 50 g)
Generic: 0.05% (15 g, 50 g)
Cream, External, as valerate [strength expressed as base]:
Generic: 0.1% (15 g, 45 g)
Foam, External, as valerate:
Luxiq: 0.12% (50 g, 100 g) [contains alcohol, usp, cetyl alcohol, propylene glycol]
Generic: 0.12% (50 g, 100 g)
Gel, External, as dipropionate augmented [strength expressed as base]:
AlphaTrex: 0.05% (15 g, 50 g)
Generic: 0.05% (15 g, 50 g)
Lotion, External, as dipropionate [strength expressed as base]:
Generic: 0.05% (60 mL)
Lotion, External, as dipropionate augmented [strength expressed as base]:
Diprolene: 0.05% (30 mL, 60 mL) [contains isopropyl alcohol, propylene glycol]
Generic: 0.05% (30 mL, 60 mL)
Lotion, External, as valerate [strength expressed as base]:
Generic: 0.1% (60 mL)
Ointment, External, as dipropionate [strength expressed as base]:
Generic: 0.05% (15 g, 45 g)

Ointment, External, as dipropionate augmented [strength expressed as base]:
Diprolene: 0.05% (15 g, 50 g)
Generic: 0.05% (15 g, 45 g, 50 g)
Ointment, External, as valerate [strength expressed as base]:
Generic: 0.1% (15 g, 45 g)

◆ Betamethasone Acetate see Betamethasone (Systemic) on page 222

Betamethasone and Clotrimazole
(bay ta METH a sone & kloe TRIM a zole)

Brand Names: US Lotrisone
Brand Names: Canada Lotriderm
Index Terms Clotrimazole and Betamethasone
Pharmacologic Category Antifungal Agent, Topical; Corticosteroid, Topical
Use
Fungal infections: Topical treatment of symptomatic inflammatory tinea pedis, tinea cruris, and tinea corporis caused by *Trichophyton rubrum*, *T. mentagrophytes*, and *Epidermophyton floccosum* in patients ≥17 years
Limitations of use: Efficacy of betamethasone/clotrimazole lotion in the treatment of zoophilic dermatophytes (eg, Microsporum canis) has not been established.
Dosing
Adult
Tinea corporis, tinea cruris: Topical:
Cream: Massage into affected area twice daily, morning and evening for 1 week; re-evaluate after 1 week if no clinical improvement; do not exceed 45 g cream per week; maximum duration: 2 weeks.
Lotion: Massage into affected area twice daily, morning and evening; re-evaluate after 1 week if no clinical improvement; do not exceed 45 mL lotion per week; maximum duration: 2 weeks.
Tinea pedis: Topical:
Cream: Massage into affected area twice daily, morning and evening for 2 weeks; re-evaluate after 2 weeks if no clinical improvement; do not exceed 45 g cream per week; maximum duration: 4 weeks.
Lotion: Massage into affected area twice daily, morning and evening; re-evaluate after 2 weeks if no clinical improvement; do not exceed 45 mL lotion per week; maximum duration: 4 weeks.
Geriatric Refer to adult dosing. Use with caution. Skin atrophy and skin ulceration (rare) have been reported in patients with thinning skin. Do not use for diaper dermatitis or under occlusive dressings.
Pediatric
Infants, Children, and Adolescents <17 years: Do not use.
Adolescents ≥17 years: Refer to adult dosing.
Renal Impairment There are no dosage adjustments provided in the manufacturer's labeling.
Hepatic Impairment There are no dosage adjustments provided in the manufacturer's labeling.
Additional Information Complete prescribing information should be consulted for additional detail.
Dosage Forms Excipient information presented when available (limited, particularly for generics); consult specific product labeling.
Cream: Betamethasone dipropionate 0.05% (base) and clotrimazole 1% (15 g, 45 g)
Lotrisone: Betamethasone dipropionate 0.05% (base) and clotrimazole 1% (15 g, 45 g) [contains benzyl alcohol]
Lotion: Betamethasone dipropionate 0.05% (base) and clotrimazole 1% (30 mL)
Lotrisone: Betamethasone dipropionate 0.05% (base) and clotrimazole 1% (30 mL) [contains benzyl alcohol]

◆ Betamethasone Dipropionate see Betamethasone (Topical) on page 224

◆ Betamethasone Dipropionate and Calcipotriene Hydrate see Calcipotriene and Betamethasone on page 282

◆ Betamethasone Dipropionate, Augmented see Betamethasone (Topical) on page 224

◆ Betamethasone Sodium Phosphate see Betamethasone (Systemic) on page 222

◆ Betamethasone Valerate see Betamethasone (Topical) on page 224

◆ Betapace see Sotalol on page 1694

◆ Betapace AF see Sotalol on page 1694

◆ Betasept Surgical Scrub [OTC] see Chlorhexidine Gluconate on page 373

◆ Betaseron see Interferon Beta-1b on page 972

◆ Betaxin (Can) see Thiamine on page 1782

Betaxolol (Systemic) (be TAKS oh lol)

Brand Names: US Kerlone
Index Terms Betaxolol Hydrochloride
Pharmacologic Category Antihypertensive; Beta-Blocker, Beta-1 Selective
Use
Hypertension: Management of hypertension

Guideline recommendations:
Hypertension: The 2014 guideline for the management of high blood pressure in adults (Eighth Joint National Committee [JNC 8]) recommends initiation of pharmacologic treatment to lower blood pressure for the following patients (JNC8 [James, 2013]):
• Patients ≥60 years of age, with systolic blood pressure (SBP) ≥150 mm Hg or diastolic blood pressure (DBP) ≥90 mm Hg. Goal of therapy is SBP <150 mm Hg and DBP <90 mm Hg.
• Patients <60 years of age, with SBP ≥140 mm Hg or DBP ≥90 mm Hg. Goal of therapy is SBP <140 mm Hg and DBP <90 mm Hg.
• Patients ≥18 years of age with diabetes, with SBP ≥140 mm Hg or DBP ≥90 mm Hg. Goal of therapy is SBP <140 mm Hg and DBP <90 mm Hg.
• Patients ≥18 years of age with chronic kidney disease (CKD), with SBP ≥140 mm Hg or DBP ≥90 mm Hg. Goal of therapy is SBP <140 mm Hg and DBP <90 mm Hg.
Chronic kidney disease (CKD) and hypertension: Regardless of race or diabetes status, the use of an ACE inhibitor (ACEI) or angiotensin receptor blocker (ARB) as initial therapy is recommended to improve kidney outcomes. In the general nonblack population (without CKD) including those with diabetes, initial antihypertensive treatment should consist of a thiazide-type diuretic, calcium channel blocker, ACEI, or ARB. In the general black population (without CKD) including those with diabetes, initial antihypertensive treatment should consist of a thiazide-type diuretic or a calcium channel blocker **instead of** an ACEI or ARB.
Coronary artery disease (CAD) and hypertension: The American Heart Association, American College of Cardiology and American Society of Hypertension (AHA/ACC/ASH) 2015 scientific statement for the treatment of hypertension in patients with coronary artery disease (CAD) recommends the use of a beta blocker as part of a regimen in patients with hypertension and chronic stable angina with a history of prior MI. A BP target of <140/90 mm Hg is reasonable for the secondary prevention of cardiovascular events. A lower target BP (<130/80 mm Hg) may be appropriate in some individuals with CAD, previous MI, stroke or transient ischemic attack, or CAD risk equivalents (AHA/ACC/ASH [Rosendorff 2015]).
Dosing
Adult
Hypertension: Oral: Initial: 10 mg once daily; may increase dose to 20 mg daily after 7 to 14 days if desired response is not achieved. Increasing the dose beyond 20 mg daily has not been shown to produce further antihypertensive effect.
Atrial fibrillation (rate control) (off-label use): 20 mg once daily; may use in combination with digoxin (Koh 1995)
Chronic stable angina (off-label use): 20 mg once daily (Glasser 1994)
Postoperative atrial fibrillation associated with cardiac surgery (prevention) (off-label use): 20 mg once daily (Iliuta 2009)
Geriatric Hypertension: Oral: Refer to adult dosing. Initial: 5 mg daily
Renal Impairment
Severe impairment: Initial dose: 5 mg once daily; may increase every 2 weeks up to a maximum of 20 mg once daily
Hemodialysis: Initial dose: 5 mg once daily; may increase every 2 weeks up to a maximum of 20 mg once daily. Supplemental dose not required.
Hepatic Impairment Dosage adjustments are not routinely required.
Additional Information Complete prescribing information should be consulted for additional detail.
Dosage Forms Excipient information presented when available (limited, particularly for generics); consult specific product labeling.
Tablet, Oral, as hydrochloride:
Kerlone: 10 mg [scored]
Kerlone: 20 mg
Generic: 10 mg, 20 mg

Betaxolol (Ophthalmic) (be TAKS oh lol)

Brand Names: US Betoptic-S
Brand Names: Canada Betoptic S; Sandoz-Betaxolol
Index Terms Betaxolol Hydrochloride
Pharmacologic Category Ophthalmic Agent, Antiglaucoma
Use Treatment of chronic open-angle glaucoma or ocular hypertension
Dosing
Adult & Geriatric
Glaucoma: Ophthalmic:
Solution: Instill 1-2 drops into affected eye(s) twice daily.
Suspension (Betoptic® S): Instill 1 drop into affected eye(s) twice daily.
Pediatric Elevated intraocular pressure: Ophthalmic suspension (Betoptic® S): Instill 1 drop into affected eye(s) twice daily.
Additional Information Complete prescribing information should be consulted for additional detail.
Dosage Forms Excipient information presented when available (limited, particularly for generics); consult specific product labeling.
Solution, Ophthalmic:
Generic: 0.5% (5 mL, 10 mL, 15 mL)
Suspension, Ophthalmic:
Betoptic-S: 0.25% (10 mL, 15 mL)

- ◆ Betaxolol Hydrochloride *see* Betaxolol (Ophthalmic) *on page 226*
- ◆ Betaxolol Hydrochloride *see* Betaxolol (Systemic) *on page 225*

Bethanechol (be THAN e kole)

Brand Names: US Urecholine
Brand Names: Canada Duvoid; PHL-Bethanechol; PMS-Bethanechol
Index Terms Bethanechol Chloride
Pharmacologic Category Cholinergic Agonist
Use
Neurogenic bladder: Treatment of neurogenic atony of the urinary bladder with retention
Urinary retention: Treatment of acute postoperative and postpartum nonobstructive (functional) urinary retention
Dosing
Adult & Geriatric
Urinary retention, neurogenic bladder: Oral: Initial (to determine minimal effective dose): 5 to 10 mg; repeat the same dose hourly until effective response or cumulative dose of 50 mg is reached; usual dose: 10 to 50 mg 3 to 4 times daily. Cholinergic effects at higher oral dosages may be cumulative.
Renal Impairment There are no dosage adjustments provided in the manufacturer's labeling.
Hepatic Impairment There are no dosage adjustments provided in the manufacturer's labeling.
Additional Information Complete prescribing information should be consulted for additional detail.
Dosage Forms Excipient information presented when available (limited, particularly for generics); consult specific product labeling.
Tablet, Oral, as chloride:
Urecholine: 5 mg, 10 mg [scored]
Urecholine: 25 mg, 50 mg [scored; contains fd&c yellow #10 (quinoline yellow), fd&c yellow #6 (sunset yellow)]
Generic: 5 mg, 10 mg, 25 mg, 50 mg
Dosage Forms: Canada Excipient information presented when available (limited, particularly for generics); consult specific product labeling.
Tablet, as chloride:
Duvoid: 10 mg, 25 mg, 50 mg

- ◆ Bethanechol Chloride *see* Bethanechol *on page 226*
- ◆ Bethkis *see* Tobramycin (Oral Inhalation) *on page 1802*
- ◆ Betimol *see* Timolol (Ophthalmic) *on page 1790*
- ◆ Betnesol (Can) *see* Betamethasone (Topical) *on page 224*
- ◆ Betoptic-S *see* Betaxolol (Ophthalmic) *on page 226*
- ◆ Betoptic S (Can) *see* Betaxolol (Ophthalmic) *on page 226*

Bevacizumab (be vuh SIZ uh mab)

Brand Names: US Avastin
Brand Names: Canada Avastin
Index Terms Anti-VEGF Monoclonal Antibody; rhuMAb; rhuMAb-VEGF

Pharmacologic Category Antineoplastic Agent, Monoclonal Antibody; Antineoplastic Agent, Vascular Endothelial Growth Factor (VEGF) Inhibitor; Vascular Endothelial Growth Factor (VEGF) Inhibitor
Use
Cervical cancer, persistent/recurrent/metastatic: Treatment of persistent, recurrent, or metastatic cervical cancer (in combination with paclitaxel and either cisplatin or topotecan). **Note:** Not an approved use in Canada.
Colorectal cancer, metastatic: First- or second-line treatment of metastatic colorectal cancer (CRC) (in combination with fluorouracil-based chemotherapy); second-line treatment of metastatic CRC (in combination with fluoropyrimidine-irinotecan- or fluoropyrimidine-oxaliplatin-based chemotherapy) after progression on a first-line treatment containing bevacizumab.
Limitations of use: Not indicated for the adjuvant treatment of colon cancer.
Glioblastoma: Treatment of progressive glioblastoma (as a single agent).
Limitations of use: Effectiveness is based on improvement in objective response rate.
Non-small cell lung cancer, nonsquamous: First-line treatment of unresectable, locally advanced, recurrent or metastatic nonsquamous non-small cell lung cancer (NSCLC) (in combination with carboplatin and paclitaxel).
Ovarian (epithelial), fallopian tube, or primary peritoneal cancer (platinum-resistant recurrent): Treatment of platinum-resistant recurrent epithelial ovarian, fallopian tube, or primary peritoneal cancer (in combination with paclitaxel, doxorubicin [liposomal], or topotecan) in patients who received no more than 2 prior chemotherapy regimens. According to the Canadian labeling, patients should not have received prior VEGF-targeted therapy (including bevacizumab).
Ovarian (epithelial), fallopian tube, or primary peritoneal cancer (platinum-sensitive recurrent): Canadian labeling: Treatment of first recurrence platinum-sensitive epithelial ovarian, fallopian tube, or primary peritoneal cancer (in combination with carboplatin and gemcitabine). Patients should not have received prior VEGF-targeted therapy (including bevacizumab).
Renal cell carcinoma, metastatic: Treatment of metastatic renal cell carcinoma (RCC) (in combination with interferon alfa). **Note:** Not an approved use in Canada.
Pregnancy Considerations Based on its mechanism of action, bevacizumab would be expected to cause fetal harm if administered to a pregnant woman. Information from postmarketing reports following exposure in pregnancy is limited. Adequate contraception during therapy and for ≥6 months following the last dose is recommended due to the long half-life of bevacizumab. Bevacizumab treatment may also increase the risk of ovarian failure and impair fertility; long term effects on fertility are not known.
Breast-Feeding Considerations It is not known if bevacizumab is excreted in breast milk. Immunoglobulins are excreted in breast milk, and it is assumed that bevacizumab may appear in breast milk. Because of the potential for serious adverse reactions in the nursing infant, breast-feeding is not recommended. The half-life of bevacizumab is up to 50 days (average 20 days), and this should be considered when decisions are made concerning breast-feeding resumption.

Note: Canadian labeling recommends to discontinue breast-feeding during treatment and to avoid breast-feeding a minimum of 6 months following discontinuation of treatment.
Contraindications
There are no contraindications listed in the manufacturer's labeling.
Canadian labeling: Hypersensitivity to bevacizumab, any component of the formulation, Chinese hamster ovary cell products or other recombinant human or humanized antibodies; untreated CNS metastases
Warnings/Precautions [US Boxed Warning]: Gastrointestinal (GI) perforation (sometimes fatal) has occurred in 0.3 to 3.2% of clinical study patients receiving bevacizumab; discontinue (permanently) if GI perforation occurs. All cervical cancer patients with GI perforation had a history of prior pelvic radiation. GI perforation was observed in patients with platinum-resistant ovarian cancer, although patients with evidence of recto-sigmoid involvement (by pelvic exam), bowel involvement (on CT scan), or clinical symptoms of bowel obstruction were excluded from the study; avoid bevacizumab use in these ovarian cancer patient populations. Most cases occur within 50 days of treatment initiation; monitor patients for signs/symptoms (eg, fever, abdominal pain with constipation and/or nausea/vomiting). GI fistula (including enterocutaneous, esophageal, duodenal, and rectal fistulas), and intra-abdominal abscess have been

reported in patients receiving bevacizumab for colorectal cancer, ovarian cancer, and other cancers (not related to treatment duration). Non-GI fistula formation (including tracheoesophageal, bronchopleural, biliary, vaginal, vesical, renal, bladder, and female tract fistulas) has been observed (rarely fatal), most commonly within the first 6 months of treatment. Gastrointestinal-vaginal fistulas have been reported in cervical cancer patients, all of whom had received prior pelvic radiation; patients may also have bowel obstructions requiring surgical intervention and diverting ostomies. Permanently discontinue in patients who develop internal organ fistulas, tracheoesophageal (TE) fistula, or any grade 4 fistula. **[US Boxed Warning]: The incidence of wound healing and surgical complications, including serious and fatal events, is increased in patients who have received bevacizumab; discontinue with wound dehiscence. Although the appropriate interval between withholding bevacizumab and elective surgery has not been defined, bevacizumab should be discontinued at least 28 days prior to surgery and should not be reinitiated for at least 28 days after surgery and until wound is fully healed.** In a retrospective review of central venous access device placements, a greater risk of wound dehiscence was observed when port placement and bevacizumab administration were separated by <14 days (Erinjeri 2011).

[US Boxed Warning]: Severe or fatal hemorrhage, including hemoptysis, gastrointestinal bleeding, central nervous system hemorrhage, epistaxis, and vaginal bleeding have been reported (up to 5 times more frequently if receiving bevacizumab). Avoid use in patients with serious hemorrhage or recent hemoptysis (≥2.5 mL blood). Serious or fatal pulmonary hemorrhage has been reported in patients receiving bevacizumab (primarily in patients with non–small cell lung cancer with squamous cell histology [not an FDA-approved indication]). Intracranial hemorrhage, including cases of grade 3 or 4 hemorrhage, has occurred in patients with previously treated glioblastoma. Treatment discontinuation is recommended in all patients with intracranial or other serious hemorrhage. Use with caution in patients with CNS metastases; once case of CNS hemorrhage was observed in an ongoing study of NSCLC patients with CNS metastases. Use in patients with untreated CNS metastases is contraindicated in the Canadian labeling. Use with caution in patients at risk for thrombocytopenia.

Bevacizumab is associated with an increased risk for arterial thromboembolic events (ATE), including cerebral infarction, stroke, MI, TIA, angina, and other ATEs, when used in combination with chemotherapy. History of ATE, diabetes, or ≥65 years of age may present an even greater risk. Although patients with cancer are already at risk for venous thromboembolism (VTE), a meta-analysis of 15 controlled trials has demonstrated an increased risk for VTE in patients who received bevacizumab (Nalluri 2008). Cervical cancer patients receiving bevacizumab plus chemotherapy may be at increased risk of grade 3 or higher VTE compared to those patients who received chemotherapy alone. Permanently discontinue therapy in patients with severe ATE or life-threatening (grade 4) VTE, including pulmonary embolism; the safety of treatment reinitiation after ATE has not been studied.

Use with caution in patients with cardiovascular disease. Among approved and nonapproved uses evaluated thus far, the incidence of heart failure (HF) and/or left ventricular dysfunction (including LVEF decline), is higher in patients receiving bevacizumab plus chemotherapy when compared to chemotherapy alone. Bevacizumab may potentiate the cardiotoxic effects of anthracyclines. HF is more common with prior anthracycline exposure and/or left chest wall irradiation. The safety of therapy resumption or continuation in patients with cardiac dysfunction has not been studied. In studies of patients with metastatic breast cancer (an off-label use), the incidence of grades 3 or 4 HF was increased in patients receiving bevacizumab plus paclitaxel, compared to the control arm. Patients with metastatic breast cancer who had received prior anthracycline therapy had a higher rate of HF compared to those receiving paclitaxel alone (3.8% vs 0.6% respectively). A meta-analysis of 5 studies which enrolled patients with metastatic breast cancer who received bevacizumab suggested an association with an increased risk of heart failure; all trials included in the analysis enrolled patients who either received prior or were receiving concurrent anthracycline therapy (Choueiri 2011).

Bevacizumab may cause and/or worsen hypertension; the incidence of severe hypertension in increased with bevacizumab. Use caution in patients with preexisting hypertension and monitor BP closely (every 2 to 3 weeks during treatment; regularly after discontinuation if bevacizumab-induced hypertension occurs or worsens). Permanent discontinuation is recommended in patients who experience a hypertensive crisis or hypertensive encephalopathy. Temporarily discontinue in patients who develop uncontrolled hypertension. An increase in diastolic and systolic blood pressures were noted in a retrospective review of patients with renal insufficiency (CrCl ≤60 mL/minute) who received bevacizumab for renal cell cancer (Gupta 2011). Cases of posterior reversible encephalopathy syndrome (PRES) have been reported. Symptoms (which include headache, seizure, confusion, lethargy, blindness and/or other vision, or neurologic disturbances) may occur from 16 hours to 1 year after treatment initiation. Resolution of symptoms usually occurs within days after discontinuation; however, neurologic sequelae may remain. PRES may be associated with hypertension; discontinue bevacizumab and begin management of hypertension, if present. The safety of treatment reinitiation after PRES is not known.

Infusion reactions (eg, hypertension, hypertensive crisis, wheezing, oxygen desaturation, hypersensitivity [including anaphylactic/anaphylactoid reactions], chest pain, rigors, headache, diaphoresis) may occur with the first infusion (uncommon); interrupt therapy in patients experiencing severe infusion reactions and administer appropriate therapy; there are no data to address routine premedication use or reinstitution of therapy in patients who experience severe infusion reactions. Cases of necrotizing fasciitis, including fatalities, have been reported (rarely); usually secondary to wound healing complications, GI perforation or fistula formation. Discontinue in patients who develop necrotizing fasciitis. Proteinuria and/or nephrotic syndrome have been associated with bevacizumab; risk may be increased in patients with a history of hypertension; thrombotic microangiopathy has been associated with bevacizumab-induced proteinuria. Withhold treatment for ≥2 g proteinuria/24 hours and resume when proteinuria is <2 g/24 hours; discontinue in patients with nephrotic syndrome. Elderly patients (≥65 years of age) are at higher risk for adverse events, including thromboembolic events and proteinuria; serious adverse events occurring more frequently in the elderly also include weakness, deep thrombophlebitis, sepsis, hyper-/hypotension, MI, CHF, diarrhea, constipation, anorexia, leukopenia, anemia, dehydration, hypokalemia, and hyponatremia. Potentially significant drug-drug interactions may exist, requiring dose or frequency adjustment, additional monitoring, and/or selection of alternative therapy. Microangiopathic hemolytic anemia (MAHA) has been reported when bevacizumab has been used in combination with sunitinib. Concurrent therapy with sunitinib and bevacizumab is also associated with dose-limiting hypertension in patients with metastatic renal cell cancer. The incidence of hand-foot syndrome is increased in patients treated with bevacizumab plus sorafenib in comparison to those treated with sorafenib monotherapy. When used in combination with myelosuppressive chemotherapy, increased rates of severe or febrile neutropenia and neutropenic infection were reported. Bevacizumab, in combination with chemotherapy (or biologic therapy), is associated with an increased risk of treatment-related mortality; a higher risk of fatal adverse events was identified in a meta-analysis of 16 trials in which bevacizumab was used for the treatment of various cancers (breast cancer, colorectal cancer, non-small cell lung cancer, pancreatic cancer, prostate cancer, and renal cell cancer) and compared to chemotherapy alone (Ranpura 2011). When bevacizumab is used in combination with myelosuppressive chemotherapy, increased rates of severe or febrile neutropenia and neutropenic infection have been reported. In premenopausal women receiving bevacizumab in combination with mFOLFOX (fluorouracil/oxaliplatin based chemotherapy) the incidence of ovarian failure (amenorrhea ≥3 months) was higher (34%) compared to women who received mFOLFOX alone (2%); ovarian function recovered in some patients after treatment was discontinued; premenopausal women should be informed of the potential risk of ovarian failure. Serious eye infections and vision loss due to endophthalmitis have been reported from intravitreal administration (off-label use/route).

Adverse Reactions Percentages reported as monotherapy and as part of combination chemotherapy regimens. Some studies only reported hematologic toxicities grades ≥4 and nonhematologic toxicities grades ≥3.
>10%:
  Cardiovascular: Hypertension (12% to 34%; grades 3/4: 5% to 18%), venous thromboembolism (secondary: 21%; with oral anticoagulants), peripheral edema (15%), hypotension (7% to 15%), venous thromboembolism (8% to 14%; grades 3/4: 5% to 15%), arterial thrombosis (6%; grades 3/4: 3%)

227

◀

Central nervous system: Fatigue (33% to 80%; grades 3/4: 4% to 19%), pain (8% to 62%; grades 3/4: 8%), headache (22% to 37%; grades 3/4: 3% to 4%), dizziness (19% to 26%), taste disorder (14% to 21%), peripheral sensory neuropathy (17% to 18%), anxiety (17%)

Dermatologic: Alopecia (6% to 32%), palmar-plantar erythrodysesthesia (11%), exfoliative dermatitis (>10%), xeroderma (>10%)

Endocrine & metabolic: Ovarian failure (34%), hyperglycemia (26%), hypomagnesemia (24%), weight loss (15% to 21%), hyponatremia (19%; grades 3/4: 4%), hypoalbuminemia (16%)

Gastrointestinal: Abdominal pain (50% to 61%; grades 3/4: 8%), vomiting (47% to 52%; grades 3/4: 11%), anorexia (35% to 43%), constipation (40%; grades 3/4: 4%), decreased appetite (34%), diarrhea (21%; grades 3/4: 1% to 34%), stomatitis (15% to 32%), gastrointestinal hemorrhage (19% to 24%), dyspepsia (17% to 24%), nausea (grades 3/4: 12%)

Genitourinary: Proteinuria (4% to 36%; grades >2%: grades 3/4: ≤7%; median onset: 5.6 months; median time to resolution: 6.1 months), urinary tract infection (22%; grades 3/4: -8%), pelvic pain (14%; grades 3/4: 6%)

Hematologic & oncologic: Hemorrhage (40%; grades 3/4: ≤7%), leukopenia (grades 3/4: 37%), pulmonary hemorrhage (4% to 31%), neutropenia (12%; grades ≥3: 8% to 27%, grade 4: 27%), lymphocytopenia (12%; grades 3/4: 6%)

Infection: Infection (55%; serious: 7% to 14%; pneumonia, catheter infection, or wound infection)

Neuromuscular & skeletal: Myalgia (19%), back pain (12%; grades 3/4: 6%)

Renal: Increased serum creatinine (16%)

Respiratory: Upper respiratory tract infection (40% to 47%), epistaxis (17% to 35%), dyspnea (25% to 26%), rhinitis (3% to >10%)

Miscellaneous: Postoperative wound complication (including dehiscence, 1% to 15%)

1% to 10%:

Cardiovascular: Thrombosis (8% to 10%), deep vein thrombosis (6% to 9%; grades 3/4: 9%), syncope (grades 3/4: 3%), intra-abdominal thrombosis (venous, grades 3/4: 3%), left ventricular dysfunction (grades 3/4: 1%), pulmonary embolism (1%)

Central nervous system: Voice disorder (5% to 9%)

Dermatologic: Dermal ulcer (6%), cellulitis (grades 3/4: 3%), acne vulgaris (1%)

Endocrine & metabolic: Dehydration (grades 3/4: 4% to 10%), hypokalemia (grades 3/4: 7%)

Gastrointestinal: Xerostomia (4% to 7%), rectal pain (6%), colitis (1% to 6%), intestinal obstruction (grades 3/4: 4%), gingival hemorrhage (minor, 2% to 4%), gastrointestinal perforation (≤3%), gastroesophageal reflux disease (2%), gastrointestinal fistula (≤2%), gingivitis (2%), oral mucosa ulcer (2%), gastritis (1%), gingival pain (1%)

Genitourinary: Vaginal hemorrhage (4%)

Hematologic & oncologic: Febrile neutropenia (5%), neutropenic infection (grades 3/4: 5%), thrombocytopenia (5%), hemorrhage (CNS; 5%; grades 3/4: 1%)

Infection: Abscess (tooth, 2%)

Neuromuscular & skeletal: Weakness (grades 3/4: 10%), dysarthria (8%)

Ophthalmic: Blurred vision (2%)

Otic: Tinnitus (2%), deafness (1%)

Respiratory: Pneumonitis (grades 3/4: 5%),

Miscellaneous: Fistula (gastrointestinal-vaginal; 8%), fistula (anal; 6%; grades 3/4: 4%), infusion related reaction (<3%), fistula (≤2%)

Miscellaneous: Fistula (gastrointestinal-vaginal; 8%), fistula (anal; 6%; grades 3/4: 4%), infusion related reaction (<3%), fistula (≤2%)

<1% (Limited to important or life-threatening): Angina pectoris, antibody development (anti-bevacizumab and neutralizing), bladder fistula, bronchopleural fistula, cerebral infarction, conjunctival hemorrhage, endophthalmitis (infectious and sterile), fistula of bile duct, fulminant necrotizing fasciitis, gallbladder perforation, gastrointestinal ulcer, hemolytic anemia (microangiopathic; when used in combination with sunitinib), hemoptysis, hemorrhagic stroke, hypersensitivity, hypertensive crisis, hypertensive encephalopathy, increased intraocular pressure, intestinal necrosis, intraocular inflammation (iritis, vitritis), mesenteric thrombosis, myocardial infarction, nasal septum perforation, ocular hyperemia, osteonecrosis of the jaw, ovarian failure, pancytopenia, polyserositis, pulmonary hypertension, rectal fistula, renal failure, renal fistula, renal thrombotic microangiopathy, retinal detachment, retinal hemorrhage, reversible posterior leukoencephalopathy syndrome, sepsis, tracheoesophageal fistula, vaginal fistula, vitreous hemorrhage, vitreous opacity

Drug Interactions

Metabolism/Transport Effects None known.

Avoid Concomitant Use

Avoid concomitant use of Bevacizumab with any of the following: BCG (Intravesical); Belimumab; Deferiprone; Dipyrone; SUNItinib

Increased Effect/Toxicity

Bevacizumab may increase the levels/effects of: Antineoplastic Agents (Anthracycline, Systemic); Belimumab; Bisphosphonate Derivatives; CloZAPine; Deferiprone; SORAfenib; SUNItinib

The levels/effects of Bevacizumab may be increased by: Dipyrone; SUNItinib

Decreased Effect

Bevacizumab may decrease the levels/effects of: BCG (Intravesical)

Preparation for Administration Dilute in 100 mL NS prior to infusion (the manufacturer recommends a total volume of 100 mL). Do not mix with dextrose-containing solutions.

Storage/Stability Store intact vials at 2°C to 8°C (36°F to 46°F) in original carton; do not freeze. Protect from light; do not shake. Diluted solutions are stable for up to 8 hours under refrigeration. Discard unused portion of vial.

Mechanism of Action Bevacizumab is a recombinant, humanized monoclonal antibody which binds to, and neutralizes, vascular endothelial growth factor (VEGF), preventing its association with endothelial receptors, Flt-1 and KDR. VEGF binding initiates angiogenesis (endothelial proliferation and the formation of new blood vessels). The inhibition of microvascular growth is believed to retard the growth of all tissues (including metastatic tissue).

Pharmacodynamics/Kinetics

Distribution: V_d: 46 mL/kg

Half-life elimination:

IV:

Pediatric patients (age: 1 to 21 years): Median: 11.8 days (range: 4.4 to 14.6 days) (Glade Bender 2008)

Adults: ~20 days (range: 11 to 50 days)

Intravitreal: ~5 to 10 days (Bakri 2007; Krohne 2008)

Dosing

Adult & Geriatric

Cervical cancer, persistent/recurrent/metastatic: IV: 15 mg/kg every 3 weeks (in combination with paclitaxel and either cisplatin or topotecan) until disease progression or unacceptable toxicity (Tewari 2014)

Colorectal cancer, metastatic, in combination with fluorouracil-based chemotherapy: IV: 5 mg/kg every 2 weeks (in combination with bolus-IFL) **or** 10 mg/kg every 2 weeks (in combination with FOLFOX4)

Canadian labeling: 5 mg/kg every 2 weeks (in combination with fluorouracil-based chemotherapy)

Colorectal cancer, metastatic, following first-line therapy containing bevacizumab: IV: 5 mg/kg every 2 weeks **or** 7.5 mg/kg every 3 weeks (in combination with fluoropyrimidine-irinotecan or fluoropyrimidine-oxaliplatin based regimen)

Glioblastoma: IV: 10 mg/kg every 2 weeks as monotherapy **or** (off-label dosing) 10 mg/kg every 2 weeks (in combination with irinotecan) (Vredenburgh 2007)

Non-small cell lung cancer (nonsquamous cell histology): IV: 15 mg/kg every 3 weeks (in combination with carboplatin and paclitaxel) for 6 cycles followed by maintenance treatment (off-label use) of bevacizumab 15 mg/kg every 3 weeks as monotherapy until disease progression or unacceptable toxicity

Ovarian (epithelial), fallopian tube, or primary peritoneal cancer (platinum-resistant recurrent): IV: 10 mg/kg every 2 week (in combination with weekly paclitaxel, every 4 week doxorubicin [liposomal], or days 1, 8, and 15 topotecan) **or** 15 mg/kg every 3 weeks (in combination with every 3 week topotecan) (Pujade-Lauraine 2014)

Ovarian (epithelial), fallopian tube, or primary peritoneal cancer (platinum-sensitive recurrent): Canadian labeling: IV: 15 mg/kg every 3 weeks (in combination with carboplatin and gemcitabine) for 6 to 10 cycles then continue with bevacizumab (monotherapy) until disease progression or unacceptable toxicity (Aghajanian 2012).

Renal cell cancer, metastatic: IV: 10 mg/kg every 2 weeks (in combination with interferon alfa) **or** (off-label dosing) 10 mg/kg every 2 weeks as monotherapy (Yang 2003)

Age-related macular degeneration (off-label use/route): Intravitreal: 1.25 mg (0.05 mL) monthly for 3 months, then may be given scheduled (monthly) or as needed based on monthly ophthalmologic assessment (Chakravarthy 2013; Martin 2012)

Breast cancer, metastatic (off-label use): IV: 10 mg/kg every 2 weeks (in combination with paclitaxel) (Miller 2007)

Endometrial cancer, recurrent or persistent (off-label use): IV: 15 mg/kg every 3 weeks (as monotherapy) until disease progression or unacceptable toxicity (Aghajanian 2011)

Soft tissue sarcoma, angiosarcoma, metastatic or locally advanced (off-label use): IV: 15 mg/kg every 3 weeks until disease progression or unacceptable toxicity (Agulnik 2013). Additional data may be necessary to further define the role of bevacizumab in this condition.

Renal Impairment There are no dosage adjustments provided in the manufacturer's labeling.

Hepatic Impairment There are no dosage adjustments provided in the manufacturer's labeling.

Adjustment for Toxicity IV administration (systemic): There are no recommended dosage reductions. Temporary suspension is recommended for severe infusion reactions, at least 4 weeks prior to (and after) elective surgery, in moderate-to-severe proteinuria (in most studies, treatment was withheld for ≥2 g proteinuria/24 hours), or in patients with severe hypertension which is not controlled with medical management. Permanent discontinuation is recommended (by the manufacturer) in patients who develop wound dehiscence and wound healing complications requiring intervention, necrotizing fasciitis, fistula (gastrointestinal and nongastrointestinal), gastrointestinal perforation, intra-abdominal abscess, hypertensive crisis, hypertensive encephalopathy, serious bleeding/hemorrhage, severe arterial thromboembolic event, life-threatening (grade 4) venous thromboembolic events (including pulmonary embolism), nephrotic syndrome, or PRES.

Administration

IV: Infuse the initial dose over 90 minutes. The second infusion may be shortened to 60 minutes if the initial infusion is well tolerated. The third and subsequent infusions may be shortened to 30 minutes if the 60-minute infusion is well tolerated. Monitor closely during the infusion for signs/symptoms of an infusion reaction. After tolerance at the 90-, 60-, and 30-minute infusion rates has been established, some institutions use an off-label 10-minute infusion rate (0.5 mg/kg/minute) for bevacizumab dosed at 5 mg/kg (Reidy 2007). In a study evaluating the safety of the 0.5 mg/kg/minute infusion rate, proteinuria and hypertension incidences were not increased with the shorter infusion time (Shah 2013). Do not administer IV push. Do not administer with dextrose solutions. Temporarily withhold bevacizumab for 4 weeks prior to elective surgery and for at least 4 weeks (and until the surgical incision is fully healed) after surgery.

Intravitreal injection (off-label use/route): Adequate local anesthesia and a topical broad-spectrum antimicrobial agent should be administered prior to the procedure.

Monitoring Parameters Monitor closely during the infusion for signs/symptoms of an infusion reaction. Monitor CBC with differential; signs/symptoms of gastrointestinal perforation, fistula, or abscess (including abdominal pain, constipation, vomiting, and fever); signs/symptoms of bleeding, including hemoptysis, gastrointestinal, and/or CNS bleeding, and/or epistaxis. Monitor blood pressure every 2 to 3 weeks; more frequently if hypertension develops during therapy. Continue to monitor blood pressure after discontinuing due to bevacizumab-induced hypertension. Monitor for proteinuria/nephrotic syndrome with urine dipstick; collect 24-hour urine in patients with ≥2+ reading. Monitor for signs/symptoms of thromboembolism (arterial and venous).

AMD (off-label use): Monitor intraocular pressure and retinal artery perfusion

Dosage Forms Excipient information presented when available (limited, particularly for generics); consult specific product labeling.
Solution, Intravenous [preservative free]:
Avastin: 100 mg/4 mL (4 mL); 400 mg/16 mL (16 mL)

Bexarotene (Systemic) (beks AIR oh teen)

Brand Names: US Targretin
Index Terms 3-methyl TTNEB
Pharmacologic Category Antineoplastic Agent, Retinoic Acid Derivative
Additional Appendix Information
Oral Dosages That Should Not Be Crushed *on page 2003*
Use Cutaneous T-cell lymphoma, refractory: Treatment of cutaneous manifestations of cutaneous T-cell lymphoma in patients who are refractory to at least one prior systemic therapy

Dosing
Adult & Geriatric

Cutaneous T-cell lymphoma, refractory: Oral: Initial: 300 mg/m^2 once daily taken as a single daily dose; if well tolerated, but no tumor response after 8 weeks, may increase to 400 mg/m^2 once daily; continue as long as clinical benefit is demonstrated (bexarotene was administered in studies for up to 97 weeks).

Mycosis fungoides/Sezary syndrome, refractory/resistant (off-label dose): Oral: 75 to 150 mg daily in combination with PUVA; maximum dose: 300 mg daily (Rupoli, 2010; Singh, 2004)

Renal Impairment There are no dosage adjustments provided in the manufacturer's labeling (has not been studied); however, although renal elimination is a minor excretion pathway, renal insufficiency may result in significant protein binding changes and alter pharmacokinetics of bexarotene.

Hepatic Impairment There are no dosage adjustments provided in the manufacturer's labeling (has not been studied); however, hepatic impairment would be expected to result in decreased clearance of bexarotene due to the extensive hepatic contribution to elimination.

Obesity *ASCO Guidelines for appropriate chemotherapy dosing in obese adults with cancer:* Utilize patient's actual body weight (full weight) for calculation of body surface area- or weight-based dosing, particularly when the intent of therapy is curative; manage regimen-related toxicities in the same manner as for nonobese patients; if a dose reduction is utilized due to toxicity, consider resumption of full weight-based dosing with subsequent cycles, especially if cause of toxicity (eg, hepatic or renal impairment) is resolved (Griggs, 2012).

Adjustment for Toxicity If necessitated by toxicity, may decrease dose from 300 mg/m^2/day to 200 mg/m^2/day, then to 100 mg/m^2/day, or temporarily hold. Upon recovery, may titrate dose upward with careful monitoring.
Hepatotoxicity: If AST, ALT, or bilirubin >3 times ULN, consider withholding or discontinuing therapy.
Hypertriglyceridemia: Consider dose reduction, treatment interruption, or and antilipemic therapy.
Leukopenia and neutropenia: Leukopenia and neutropenia resolved after dose reduction or discontinuation.

Additional Information Complete prescribing information should be consulted for additional detail.

Dosage Forms Excipient information presented when available (limited, particularly for generics); consult specific product labeling.
Capsule, Oral:
Targretin: 75 mg
Generic: 75 mg

Bexarotene (Topical) (beks AIR oh teen)

Brand Names: US Targretin
Pharmacologic Category Antineoplastic Agent, Retinoic Acid Derivative
Use Cutaneous T-cell lymphoma: Topical treatment of cutaneous lesions in patients with refractory or persistent cutaneous T-cell lymphoma (stage 1A and 1B) or who have not tolerated other therapies

Dosing
Adult & Geriatric

Cutaneous T-cell lymphoma: Topical: Apply to lesions once every other day for first week, then increase on a weekly basis to once daily, 2 times daily, 3 times daily, and finally 4 times daily, according to individual lesion tolerance. Continue as long as deriving benefit. Response is usually observed with application at 2 to 4 times daily. May decrease frequency if local toxicity occurs; for severe irritation, temporarily withhold for a few days until symptoms subside.

Renal Impairment There are no dosage adjustments provided in the manufacturer's labeling (has not been studied); however, although renal elimination is a minor excretion pathway, renal insufficiency may result in significant protein binding changes and altered pharmacokinetics of bexarotene.

Hepatic Impairment There are no dosage adjustments provided in the manufacturer's labeling (has not been studied); however, hepatic impairment would be expected to result in decreased clearance of bexarotene due to the extensive hepatic contribution to elimination.

Additional Information Complete prescribing information should be consulted for additional detail.

Dosage Forms Excipient information presented when available (limited, particularly for generics); consult specific product labeling.
Gel, External:
Targretin: 1% (60 g) [contains alcohol, usp]

◆ Beyaz see Ethinyl Estradiol, Drospirenone, and Levomefolate on page 712

◆ BG-12 see Dimethyl Fumarate on page 557

◆ BI 397 see Dalbavancin on page 482

◆ BI-1356 see Linagliptin on page 1078

◆ BI10773 see Empagliflozin on page 632

◆ Biaxin see Clarithromycin on page 401

◆ Biaxin XL see Clarithromycin on page 401

◆ Biaxin XL Pac see Clarithromycin on page 401

◆ Biaxin BID (Can) see Clarithromycin on page 401

◆ BIBF1120 see Nintedanib on page 1284

◆ BIBW 2992 see Afatinib on page 50

Bicalutamide (bye ka LOO ta mide)

Brand Names: US Casodex

Brand Names: Canada ACH-Bicalutamide; ACT Bicalutamide; Apo-Bicalutamide; Casodex; Dom-Bicalutamide; JAMP-Bicalutamide; Mylan-Bicalutamide; PHL-Bicalutamide; PMS-Bicalutamide; PRO-Bicalutamide; RAN-Bicalutamide; Sandoz-Bicalutamide; Teva-Bicalutamide

Index Terms CDX; ICI-176334

Pharmacologic Category Antineoplastic Agent, Antiandrogen

Use

Prostate cancer, metastatic: Treatment of stage D_2 metastatic prostate cancer (in combination with an LHRH agonist)

Limitation of use: Bicalutamide 150 mg daily is not approved for use alone or with other treatments

Pregnancy Considerations Adverse events were observed in animal reproduction studies. Bicalutamide use is contraindicated in women. Androgen receptor inhibition during pregnancy may affect fetal development.

Breast-Feeding Considerations Bicalutamide is not indicated for use in women.

Contraindications

Hypersensitivity to bicalutamide or any component of the formulation; use in women, especially women who are or may become pregnant

Canadian labeling: Additional contraindications (not in U.S. labeling): Patients with localized prostate cancer undergoing watchful waiting; children

Warnings/Precautions Hazardous agent - use appropriate precautions for handling and disposal (NIOSH 2014 [group 1]). Rare cases of death or hospitalization due to hepatitis have been reported postmarketing. Use with caution in moderate-to-severe hepatic dysfunction. Hepatotoxicity generally occurs within the first 3 to 4 months of use; patients should be monitored for signs and symptoms of liver dysfunction. Bicalutamide should be discontinued if patients have jaundice or ALT is >2 times the upper limit of normal. Androgen-deprivation therapy may increase the risk for cardiovascular disease (Levine, 2010). Androgen deprivation therapy may cause prolongation of the QT/QTc interval (Garnick, 2004); evaluate risk versus benefit in patients with congenital long QT syndrome, heart failure, frequent electrolyte abnormalities, and in patients taking medication known to prolong the QT interval. Correct electrolytes prior to initiation and consider periodic electrolyte and ECG monitoring.

Anemia may occur with testosterone suppression; monitor CBC periodically as indicated. Interstitial lung disease has been reported rarely (including fatalities) although mostly at dosages greater than what is recommended; promptly evaluate any worsening of respiratory symptoms (eg, dyspnea, cough and fever). Prolonged use of antiandrogen therapy is associated with decreased bone mineral density and an increased risk of osteoporosis and fracture (Smith, 2003); alcohol abuse, familial history of osteoporosis, and/or chronic use of drugs capable of decreasing bone mass (eg, corticosteroids) may increase risk. Evaluate risk carefully before initiating therapy.

May cause gynecomastia, breast pain, or lead to spermatogenesis inhibition. When used in combination with LHRH agonists, a loss of glycemic control and decrease in glucose tolerance has been reported in patients with diabetes; monitor. May cause gynecomastia or breast pain (at higher, off-label doses), or lead to spermatogenesis inhibition. Potentially significant drug-drug interactions may exist, requiring dose or frequency adjustment, additional monitoring, and/or selection of alternative therapy. Discontinue use immediately if disease worsens; decreased prostate specific antigen (PSA) levels and/or clinical improvement may be observed in some patients when antiandrogen therapy is held due to worsening of disease. The Canadian labeling recommends monitoring

patients for 6 to 8 weeks after interrupting therapy to observe for withdrawal response.

Adverse Reactions Adverse reaction percentages reported as part of combination regimen with an LHRH analogue unless otherwise noted.

>10%:

Cardiovascular: Peripheral edema (13%)

Central nervous system: Pain (35%)

Endocrine & metabolic: Hot flash (53%), gynecomastia (9%; monotherapy [150 mg]: 38% to 73% [McLeod 2006])

Gastrointestinal: Constipation (22%), nausea (15%), diarrhea (12%), abdominal pain (11%)

Genitourinary: Mastalgia (6%; monotherapy [150 mg]: 39% to 85% [McLeod 2006]), pelvic pain (21%), hematuria (12%), nocturia (12%)

Hematologic & oncologic: Anemia (11%)

Infection: Infection (18%)

Neuromuscular & skeletal: Back pain (25%), weakness (22%)

Respiratory: Dyspnea (13%)

≥2% to 10%:

Cardiovascular: Chest pain (8%), hypertension (8%), angina pectoris (2% to <5%), cardiac arrest (2% to <5%), cardiac failure (2% to <5%), coronary artery disease (2% to <5%), edema (2% to <5%), myocardial infarction (2% to <5%), syncope (2% to <5%)

Central nervous system: Dizziness (10%), paresthesia (8%), headache (7%), insomnia (7%), myasthenia (7%), anxiety (5%), chills (2% to <5%), confusion (2% to <5%), drowsiness (2% to <5%), hypertonia (2% to <5%), nervousness (2% to <5%), neuropathy (2% to <5%), depression (4%)

Dermatologic: Skin rash (9%), diaphoresis (6%), alopecia (2% to <5%), pruritus (2% to <5%), xeroderma (2% to <5%)

Endocrine & metabolic: Weight loss (7%), hyperglycemia (6%), weight gain (5%), decreased libido (2% to <5%), dehydration (2% to <5%), gout (2% to <5%), hypercholesterolemia (2% to <5%)

Gastrointestinal: Dyspepsia (7%), anorexia (6%), flatulence (6%), vomiting (6%), dysphagia (2% to <5%), hernia (2% to <5%), melena (2% to <5%), periodontal abscess (2% to <5%), xerostomia (2% to <5%)

Genitourinary: Urinary tract infection (9%), impotence (7%), difficulty in micturition (5%), urinary retention (5%), dysuria (2% to <5%), urinary urgency (2% to <5%), urinary incontinence (4%)

Hematologic & oncologic: Gastrointestinal carcinoma (2% to <5%), rectal hemorrhage (2% to <5%), skin carcinoma (2% to <5%)

Hepatic: Increased liver enzymes (7%), increased serum alkaline phosphatase (5%)

Infection: Herpes zoster (2% to <5%), sepsis (2% to <5%)

Neuromuscular & skeletal: Ostealgia (9%), arthritis (5%), leg cramps (2% to <5%), myalgia (2% to <5%), neck pain (2% to <5%), pathological fracture (4%)

Ophthalmic: Cataract (2% to <5%)

Renal: Polyuria (6%), hydronephrosis (2% to <5%), increased blood urea nitrogen (2% to <5%), increased serum creatinine (2% to <5%)

Respiratory: Cough (8%), pharyngitis (8%), flu-like symptoms (7%), bronchitis (6%), asthma (2% to <5%), epistaxis (2% to <5%), sinusitis (2% to <5%), pneumonia (4%), rhinitis (4%)

Miscellaneous: Cyst (2% to <5%), fever (2% to <5%)

<1% (Limited to important or life-threatening): Decreased glucose tolerance, decreased hemoglobin, decreased white blood cell count, hepatic failure, hepatitis, hepatotoxicity, hypersensitivity (including angioedema and urticaria), increased serum bilirubin, interstitial pneumonitis, interstitial pulmonary disease, pulmonary fibrosis

Drug Interactions

Metabolism/Transport Effects Inhibits CYP3A4 (weak)

Avoid Concomitant Use

Avoid concomitant use of Bicalutamide with any of the following: Astemizole; Cisapride; Indium 111 Capromab Pendetide; Pimozide; Terfenadine

Increased Effect/Toxicity

Bicalutamide may increase the levels/effects of: ARIPiprazole; Astemizole; Cisapride; Dofetilide; Flibanserin; Hydrocodone; Lomitapide; NiMODipine; Pimozide; Porfimer; Terfenadine; Verteporfin; Vitamin K Antagonists

Decreased Effect

Bicalutamide may decrease the levels/effects of: Choline C 11; Indium 111 Capromab Pendetide

Storage/Stability Store at room temperature of 20°C to 25°C (68°F to 77°F).

Mechanism of Action Androgen receptor inhibitor; pure nonsteroidal antiandrogen that binds to androgen receptors; specifically a competitive inhibitor for the binding of dihydrotestosterone and testosterone; prevents testosterone stimulation of cell growth in prostate cancer

Pharmacodynamics/Kinetics

Absorption: Well absorbed; unaffected by food

Protein binding: 96%

Metabolism: Extensively hepatic; glucuronidation and oxidation of the R (active) enantiomer to inactive metabolites; the S enantiomer is inactive

Half-life elimination:

Active enantiomer: ~6 days

Active enantiomer (in patients with severe liver disease): ~10 days

R-isomer (in patients with severe liver disease): Increased ~76%

Time to peak, plasma: Active enantiomer: ~31 hours

Excretion: Urine and feces

Dosing

Adult & Geriatric

Prostate cancer, metastatic: Oral: 50 mg once daily (in combination with an LHRH analogue)

Prostate cancer, locally-advanced, high recurrence risk (off-label use): Oral: 150 mg once daily (as monotherapy) (McLeod, 2006). Additional trials may be necessary to further define the role of bicalutamide in this condition.

Renal Impairment No dosage adjustment necessary.

Hepatic Impairment

Hepatic impairment at treatment initiation: Mild, moderate, or severe impairment: No dosage adjustment is necessary. Use with caution in patients with moderate-to-severe impairment; clearance may be delayed in severe impairment (based on a limited number of patients).

Hepatic impairment during treatment: ALT >2 times ULN or jaundice develops: Discontinue immediately.

Administration Dose should be taken at the same time each day, either in the morning or in the evening. May be administered with or without food. Treatment for metastatic cancer should be started concomitantly with an LHRH analogue.

Hazardous agent; use appropriate precautions for handling and disposal (NIOSH 2014 [group 1]).

Monitoring Parameters Periodically monitor CBC, ECG, echocardiograms, serum testosterone, luteinizing hormone, and prostate specific antigen (PSA). Liver function tests should be obtained at baseline and repeated regularly during the first 4 months of treatment, and periodically thereafter; monitor for signs and symptoms of liver dysfunction (discontinue if jaundice is noted or ALT is >2 times the upper limit of normal). Monitor blood glucose in patients with diabetes. If initiating bicalutamide in patients who are on warfarin, closely monitor prothrombin time.

Dosage Forms Excipient information presented when available (limited, particularly for generics); consult specific product labeling.

Tablet, Oral:

Casodex: 50 mg

Generic: 50 mg

♦ Bicillin L-A *see* Penicillin G Benzathine *on page 1419*

♦ Bicillin® C-R *see* Penicillin G Benzathine and Penicillin G Procaine *on page 1420*

♦ Bicillin® C-R 900/300 *see* Penicillin G Benzathine and Penicillin G Procaine *on page 1420*

♦ Bicitra *see* Sodium Citrate and Citric Acid *on page 1673*

♦ BiCNU *see* Carmustine *on page 320*

♦ Bidex [OTC] *see* GuaiFENesin *on page 860*

♦ BiDil *see* Isosorbide Dinitrate and Hydralazine *on page 994*

♦ BIG-IV *see* Botulism Immune Globulin (Intravenous-Human) *on page 249*

♦ Biltricide *see* Praziquantel *on page 1492*

Bimatoprost (bi MAT oh prost)

Brand Names: US Latisse; Lumigan

Brand Names: Canada Latisse; Lumigan; Lumigan RC

Pharmacologic Category Ophthalmic Agent, Antiglaucoma; Prostaglandin, Ophthalmic

Use

Elevated intraocular pressure (Lumigan only): Reduction of elevated intraocular pressure (IOP) in patients with open-angle glaucoma or ocular hypertension

Hypotrichosis of the eyelashes (Latisse only): Treatment of hypotrichosis of the eyelashes

Dosing

Adult & Geriatric

Elevated intraocular pressure (Lumigan): Ophthalmic: Instill 1 drop into affected eye(s) once daily in the evening; do not exceed once-daily dosing (may decrease IOP-lowering effect). If used with other topical ophthalmic agents, separate administration by at least 5 minutes.

Hypotrichosis of the eyelashes (Latisse): Ophthalmic, topical: Place one drop on applicator and apply evenly along the skin of the upper eyelid at base of eyelashes once daily at bedtime; repeat procedure for second eye (use a clean applicator).

Pediatric

Elevated intraocular pressure (Lumigan): Adolescents ≥16 years: Refer to adult dosing.

Hypotrichosis of the eyelashes (Latisse): Children ≥5 years and Adolescents: Refer to adult dosing.

Renal Impairment There are no dosage adjustments provided in the manufacturer's labeling.

Hepatic Impairment There are no dosage adjustments provided in the manufacturer's labeling.

Additional Information Complete prescribing information should be consulted for additional detail.

Dosage Forms Excipient information presented when available (limited, particularly for generics); consult specific product labeling. [DSC] = Discontinued product

Solution, External:

Latisse: 0.03% (3 mL, 5 mL) [contains benzalkonium chloride]

Solution, Ophthalmic:

Lumigan: 0.01% (2.5 mL, 5 mL, 7.5 mL); 0.03% (2.5 mL [DSC], 5 mL [DSC], 7.5 mL [DSC]) [contains benzalkonium chloride]

Generic: 0.03% (2.5 mL, 5 mL, 7.5 mL)

♦ Binosto *see* Alendronate *on page 66*

♦ Bio-Amitriptyline (Can) *see* Amitriptyline *on page 98*

♦ Bio-Amlodipine (Can) *see* AmLODIPine *on page 101*

♦ Bio-Anastrozole (Can) *see* Anastrozole *on page 128*

♦ Bio-Celecoxib (Can) *see* Celecoxib *on page 355*

♦ Bio-Diazepam (Can) *see* Diazepam *on page 537*

♦ Bio-Donepezil (Can) *see* Donepezil *on page 583*

♦ Bio-Ezetimibe (Can) *see* Ezetimibe *on page 729*

♦ Bio-Flurazepam (Can) *see* Flurazepam *on page 791*

♦ Bio-Furosemide (Can) *see* Furosemide *on page 821*

♦ Bio Glo *see* Fluorescein *on page 782*

♦ Bio-Hydrochlorothiazide (Can) *see* Hydrochlorothiazide *on page 881*

♦ Bio-Letrozole (Can) *see* Letrozole *on page 1048*

♦ Bio-Modafinil (Can) *see* Modafinil *on page 1222*

♦ Bionect *see* Hyaluronate and Derivatives *on page 879*

♦ Bioniche Promethazine (Can) *see* Promethazine *on page 1510*

♦ Bio-Oxazepam (Can) *see* Oxazepam *on page 1352*

♦ BioQuin Durules (Can) *see* QuiNIDine *on page 1542*

♦ Bio-Statin *see* Nystatin (Oral) *on page 1304*

♦ BioThrax *see* Anthrax Vaccine Adsorbed *on page 130*

♦ Biphentin (Can) *see* Methylphenidate *on page 1180*

♦ Bird Flu Vaccine *see* Influenza A Virus Vaccine (H5N1) *on page 944*

♦ Bisac-Evac [OTC] *see* Bisacodyl *on page 231*

Bisacodyl (bis a KOE dil)

Brand Names: US Bisac-Evac [OTC]; Bisacodyl EC [OTC]; Bisacodyl Laxative [OTC]; Biscolax [OTC]; Correct [OTC]; Ducodyl [OTC]; Dulcolax [OTC]; Ex-Lax Ultra [OTC]; Fematrol [OTC] [DSC]; Fleet Bisacodyl [OTC]; Fleet Laxative [OTC]; Gentle Laxative [OTC]; Laxative [OTC]; Stimulant Laxative [OTC]; The Magic Bullet [OTC]; Womens Laxative [OTC]

Brand Names: Canada Apo-Bisacodyl [OTC]; Bisacodyl-Odan [OTC]; Bisacolax [OTC]; Carter's Little Pills [OTC]; Codulax [OTC]; Dulcolax For Women [OTC]; Dulcolax [OTC]; PMS-Bisacodyl [OTC]; ratio-Bisacodyl [OTC]; Silver Bullet Suppository [OTC]; Soflax EX [OTC]; The Magic Bullet [OTC]; Woman's Laxative [OTC]

Index Terms Doxidan

Pharmacologic Category Laxative, Stimulant

Use Treatment of constipation; colonic evacuation prior to procedures or examination ▶

Dosing

Adult & Geriatric

Relief of constipation:

Oral: 5-15 mg as single dose (up to 30 mg when complete evacuation of bowel is required)

Rectal: Suppository: 10 mg as single dose

Pediatric

Relief of constipation:

Oral: Children >6 years: 5-10 mg (0.3 mg/kg) at bedtime or before breakfast

Rectal (suppository): Children:

<2 years: 5 mg as a single dose

>2 years: 10 mg

Renal Impairment No dosage adjustment provided in manufacturer's labeling. Use with caution in patients with impaired renal function.

Hepatic Impairment No dosage adjustment provided in manufacturer's labeling.

Additional Information Complete prescribing information should be consulted for additional detail.

Dosage Forms Excipient information presented when available (limited, particularly for generics); consult specific product labeling. [DSC] = Discontinued product

Enema, Rectal:

Fleet Bisacodyl: 10 mg/30 mL (37 mL)

Suppository, Rectal:

Bisac-Evac: 10 mg (1 ea, 8 ea, 12 ea, 50 ea, 100 ea, 500 ea, 1000 ea)

Bisacodyl Laxative: 10 mg (12 ea)

Biscolax: 10 mg (12 ea, 100 ea)

Dulcolax: 10 mg (4 ea, 8 ea, 16 ea, 28 ea, 50 ea)

Gentle Laxative: 10 mg (4 ea, 8 ea, 12 ea)

Laxative: 10 mg (12 ea, 100 ea)

The Magic Bullet: 10 mg (10 ea, 12 ea [DSC], 100 ea)

Generic: 10 mg (12 ea, 50 ea, 100 ea)

Tablet Delayed Release, Oral:

Bisac-Evac: 5 mg [DSC] [contains fd&c yellow #10 aluminum lake, fd&c yellow #6 aluminum lake]

Bisacodyl EC: 5 mg

Bisacodyl EC: 5 mg [contains fd&c yellow #10 (quinoline yellow), fd&c yellow #6 (sunset yellow)]

Bisacodyl EC: 5 mg [contains fd&c yellow #10 aluminum lake, fd&c yellow #6 aluminum lake]

Bisacodyl EC: 5 mg [contains fd&c yellow #10 aluminum lake, fd&c yellow #6 aluminum lake, methylparaben, propylparaben, sodium benzoate]

Correct: 5 mg

Ducodyl: 5 mg

Dulcolax: 5 mg [contains fd&c yellow #10 (quinoline yellow), methylparaben, propylparaben, sodium benzoate]

Ex-Lax Ultra: 5 mg [contains fd&c yellow #6 (sunset yellow), methylparaben]

Fematrol: 5 mg [DSC]

Fleet Laxative: 5 mg

Gentle Laxative: 5 mg

Stimulant Laxative: 5 mg

Stimulant Laxative: 5 mg [contains fd&c yellow #10 aluminum lake, fd&c yellow #6 aluminum lake]

Womens Laxative: 5 mg

Womens Laxative: 5 mg [contains fd&c blue #1 aluminum lake, sodium benzoate, tartrazine (fd&c yellow #5)]

- ◆ Bisacodyl EC [OTC] *see* Bisacodyl *on page 231*
- ◆ Bisacodyl Laxative [OTC] *see* Bisacodyl *on page 231*
- ◆ Bisacodyl-Odan [OTC] (Can) *see* Bisacodyl *on page 231*
- ◆ Biscolax [OTC] (Can) *see* Bisacodyl *on page 231*
- ◆ bis(chloroethyl) nitrosourea *see* Carmustine *on page 320*
- ◆ bis-chloronitrosourea *see* Carmustine *on page 320*
- ◆ Biscolax [OTC] *see* Bisacodyl *on page 231*
- ◆ Bismatrol *see* Bismuth Subsalicylate *on page 232*
- ◆ Bismatrol [OTC] *see* Bismuth Subsalicylate *on page 232*
- ◆ Bismatrol Maximum Strength [OTC] *see* Bismuth Subsalicylate *on page 232*

Bismuth Subsalicylate (BIZ muth sub sa LIS i late)

Brand Names: US Bismatrol Maximum Strength [OTC]; Bismatrol [OTC]; Diotame [OTC]; Geri-Pectate [OTC]; Kao-Tin [OTC]; Peptic Relief [OTC]; Pepto-Bismol To-Go [OTC]; Pepto-Bismol [OTC]; Pink Bismuth [OTC]; Stomach Relief Max St [OTC]; Stomach Relief Plus [OTC]; Stomach Relief [OTC]

Index Terms Bismatrol; BSS; Pink Bismuth

Pharmacologic Category Antidiarrheal

Use

Diarrhea: To control diarrhea, reduce number of bowel movements, and firm stool.

Dyspepsia: Relief of gas, upset stomach, indigestion, heartburn, and nausea.

Pregnancy Considerations Following oral administration, bismuth and salicylates cross the placenta. The use of salicylates in pregnancy may adversely affect the newborn (Lione, 1988). Use during pregnancy is not recommended (Mahadevan 2007).

Breast-Feeding Considerations Low amounts of salicylates enter breast milk; refer to the aspirin monograph for additional information (Bar-Oz, 2004). A case report describes bowel obstruction in a breast-fed infant whose mother applied a bismuth-containing ointment to her nipples prior to breast-feeding (Anonymous 1974).

Contraindications OTC labeling: When used for self-medication, do not use if you are allergic to salicylates or are taking other salicylates; have an ulcer, bleeding problem or bloody/black stool

Warnings/Precautions Bismuth subsalicylate should be used with caution if patient is taking aspirin. Bismuth products may be neurotoxic with very large doses. Some dosage forms may contain sodium benzoate/benzoic acid; benzoic acid (benzoate) is a metabolite of benzyl alcohol; large amounts of benzyl alcohol (≥99 mg/kg/day) have been associated with a potentially fatal toxicity ("gasping syndrome") in neonates; the "gasping syndrome" consists of metabolic acidosis, respiratory distress, gasping respirations, CNS dysfunction (including convulsions, intracranial hemorrhage), hypotension and cardiovascular collapse (AAP ["Inactive" 1997]; CDC 1982); some data suggests that benzoate displaces bilirubin from protein binding sites (Ahlfors 2001); avoid or use dosage forms containing benzyl alcohol derivative with caution in neonates. Potentially significant drug-drug interactions may exist, requiring dose or frequency adjustment, additional monitoring, and/or selection of alternative therapy.

When used for self-medication (OTC labeling): Children and teenagers who have or are recovering from chickenpox or flu-like symptoms should not use subsalicylate. Changes in behavior (along with nausea and vomiting) may be an early sign of Reye syndrome; patients should be instructed to contact their health care provider if these occur. A temporary harmless darkening of the stool and/or tongue may occur with use. Contact a health care provider before use if fever or mucus in the stool occurs. Discontinue use and contact health care provider if any of the following occur: diarrhea lasts >2 days or other symptoms lasts >14 days, diarrhea with a fever, symptoms get worse, hearing loss, or ringing in the ears.

Adverse Reactions Frequency not defined; subsalicylate formulation:

Central nervous system: Anxiety, confusion, depression, headache, slurred speech

Gastrointestinal: Fecal discoloration (grayish black; impaction may occur in infants and debilitated patients), tongue discoloration (darkening)

Neuromuscular & skeletal: Muscle spasm, weakness

Otic: Hearing loss, tinnitus

Drug Interactions

Metabolism/Transport Effects None known.

Avoid Concomitant Use

Avoid concomitant use of Bismuth Subsalicylate with any of the following: Bismuth Subcitrate; Dexketoprofen; Influenza Virus Vaccine (Live/Attenuated); Sulfinpyrazone

Increased Effect/Toxicity

Bismuth Subsalicylate may increase the levels/effects of: ACE Inhibitors; Anticoagulants; Bismuth Subcitrate; Blood Glucose Lowering Agents; Carbonic Anhydrase Inhibitors; Corticosteroids (Systemic); Dexketoprofen; Methotrexate; PRALAtrexate; Salicylates; Thrombolytic Agents; Valproate Products; Varicella Virus-Containing Vaccines; Vitamin K Antagonists

The levels/effects of Bismuth Subsalicylate may be increased by: Agents with Antiplatelet Properties; Ammonium Chloride; Calcium Channel Blockers (Nondihydropyridine); Ginkgo Biloba; Herbs (Anticoagulant/Antiplatelet Properties); Influenza Virus Vaccine (Live/Attenuated); Loop Diuretics; NSAID (Nonselective); Potassium Acid Phosphate; Treprostinil

Decreased Effect

Bismuth Subsalicylate may decrease the levels/effects of: ACE Inhibitors; Benzbromarone; Dexketoprofen; Hyaluronidase; Loop Diuretics; NSAID (Nonselective); Probenecid; Sulfinpyrazone; Tetracycline Derivatives

The levels/effects of Bismuth Subsalicylate may be decreased by: Corticosteroids (Systemic); Dexketoprofen; NSAID (Nonselective)

Storage/Stability Store at room temperature. Avoid excessive heat. Protect from freezing.

Mechanism of Action Bismuth subsalicylate exhibits both antisecretory and antimicrobial action. This agent may provide some anti-inflammatory action as well. The salicylate moiety provides antisecretory effect and the bismuth exhibits antimicrobial directly against bacterial and viral gastrointestinal pathogens.

Pharmacodynamics/Kinetics

Absorption: Bismuth: <1%; Subsalicylate: >80%

Distribution: Salicylate: V_d: 170 mL/kg

Protein binding, plasma: Bismuth and salicylate: >90%

Metabolism: Bismuth subsalicylate is converted to bismuth and salicylic acid in the GI tract.

Half-life elimination: Terminal: Bismuth: 21 to 72 days; Salicylate: 2 to 5 hours

Excretion: Bismuth: Urine and biliary; Salicylate: Urine (10% excreted unchanged)

Dosing

Adult & Geriatric

Diarrhea/dyspepsia: Oral: ~525 mg every 30 to 60 minutes or 1,050 mg every 60 minutes as needed for up to 2 days (maximum: ~4,200 mg [8 doses (regular strength); 4 doses (maximum strength)]/24 hours)

Traveler's diarrhea (off-label use): Oral: 524 mg every 30 minutes as needed up to 8 doses/24 hours (Castelli 2006; Hill 2006; "What to do" 2002)

Helicobacter pylori **eradication (off-label use):** Oral: 525 mg 4 times daily (in combination with metronidazole, tetracycline, and a PPI or H_2-antagonist) for 10 to 14 days (ACG [Chey 2007])

Pediatric Diarrhea/dyspepsia: Children ≥12 years and Adolescents: Refer to adult dosing.

Renal Impairment There are no dosage adjustments provided in the manufacturer's labeling; use with caution.

Hepatic Impairment There are no dosage adjustments provided in the manufacturer's labeling.

Dietary Considerations Drink plenty of fluids to help prevent dehydration caused by diarrhea. Some products may contain phenylalanine, potassium, and/or sodium.

Administration Oral: Shake liquids well prior to use. Chew tablets thoroughly or allow to dissolve in the mouth before swallowing. Nonchewable tablets should be swallowed whole with a full glass of water.

Test Interactions Increased uric acid, increased AST; bismuth absorbs x-rays and may interfere with diagnostic procedures of GI tract

Additional Information Bismuth subcitrate potassium is bismuth salt that is only available in the combination product Pylera, approved for use as part of a multidrug regimen for *H. pylori* eradication. It is not available as a single-agent product.

Dosage Forms Excipient information presented when available (limited, particularly for generics); consult specific product labeling. [DSC] = Discontinued product

Suspension, Oral, as subsalicylate:

Bismatrol: 262 mg/15 mL (236 mL) [contains benzoic acid, d&c red #22 (eosine), saccharin sodium; wintergreen flavor]

Bismatrol Maximum Strength: 525 mg/15 mL (236 mL) [contains benzoic acid, d&c red #22 (eosine), saccharin sodium; wintergreen flavor]

Geri-Pectate: 262 mg/15 mL (355 mL)

Kao-Tin: 262 mg/15 mL (236 mL, 473 mL) [contains fd&c red #40, saccharin sodium, sodium benzoate]

Peptic Relief: 262 mg/15 mL (237 mL) [sugar free; contains benzoic acid, d&c red #22 (eosine), saccharin sodium; mint flavor]

Pepto-Bismol: 262 mg/15 mL (473 mL) [contains benzoic acid, d&c red #22 (eosine), saccharin sodium]

Pepto-Bismol: 524 mg/30 mL (118 mL)

Pink Bismuth: 262 mg/15 mL (236 mL)

Pink Bismuth: 262 mg/15 mL (473 mL) [contains benzoic acid, d&c red #22 (eosine), saccharin sodium]

Stomach Relief: 262 mg/15 mL (237 mL, 355 mL) [contains d&c red #22 (eosine), saccharin sodium]

Stomach Relief: 527 mg/30 mL (240 mL, 480 mL)

Stomach Relief Max St: 525 mg/15 mL (237 mL) [contains d&c red #22 (eosine), saccharin sodium]

Stomach Relief Plus: 525 mg/15 mL (240 mL, 480 mL)

Tablet Chewable, Oral:

Stomach Relief: 262 mg [contains aspartame]

Tablet Chewable, Oral, as subsalicylate:

Bismatrol: 262 mg [contains aspartame]

Diotame: 262 mg

Peptic Relief: 262 mg [DSC]

Peptic Relief: 262 mg [contains saccharin sodium]

Pepto-Bismol To-Go: 262 mg [sugar free; contains fd&c red #40 aluminum lake, cherry flavor]

Pink Bismuth: 262 mg

Pink Bismuth: 262 mg [contains saccharin sodium]

Generic: 262 mg

Bisoprolol (bis OH proe lol)

Brand Names: US Zebeta

Brand Names: Canada Apo-Bisoprolol; Ava-Bisoprolol; Mylan-Bisoprolol; Novo-Bisoprolol; PHL-Bisoprolol; PMS-Bisoprolol; PRO-Bisoprolol; Sandoz-Bisoprolol; Teva-Bisoprolol

Index Terms Bisoprolol Fumarate

Pharmacologic Category Antihypertensive; Beta-Blocker, Beta-1 Selective

Use

Hypertension: Treatment of hypertension, alone or in combination with other agents

Guideline recommendations:

Hypertension: The 2014 guideline for the management of high blood pressure in adults (Eighth Joint National Committee [JNC 8]) recommends initiation of pharmacologic treatment to lower blood pressure for the following patients (JNC8 [James, 2013]):

• Patients ≥60 years of age, with systolic blood pressure (SBP) ≥150 mm Hg or diastolic blood pressure (DBP) ≥90 mm Hg. Goal of therapy is SBP <150 mm Hg and DBP <90 mm Hg.

• Patients <60 years of age, with SBP ≥140 mm Hg or DBP ≥90 mm Hg. Goal of therapy is SBP <140 mm Hg and DBP <90 mm Hg.

• Patients ≥18 years of age with diabetes, with SBP ≥140 mm Hg or DBP ≥90 mm Hg. Goal of therapy is SBP <140 mm Hg and DBP <90 mm Hg.

• Patients ≥18 years of age with chronic kidney disease (CKD), with SBP ≥140 mm Hg or DBP ≥90 mm Hg. Goal of therapy is SBP <140 mm Hg and DBP <90 mm Hg.

Chronic kidney disease (CKD) and hypertension: Regardless of race or diabetes status, the use of an ACE inhibitor (ACEI) or angiotensin receptor blocker (ARB) as initial therapy is recommended to improve kidney outcomes. In the general nonblack population (without CKD) including those with diabetes, initial antihypertensive treatment should consist of a thiazide-type diuretic, calcium channel blocker, ACEI, or ARB. In the general black population (without CKD) including those with diabetes, initial antihypertensive treatment should consist of a thiazide-type diuretic or a calcium channel blocker **instead of** an ACEI or ARB.

Coronary artery disease (CAD) and hypertension: The American Heart Association, American College of Cardiology and American Society of Hypertension (AHA/ACC/ASH) 2015 scientific statement for the treatment of hypertension in patients with coronary artery disease (CAD) recommends the use of a beta blocker as part of a regimen in patients with hypertension and chronic stable angina with a history of prior MI. A BP target of <140/90 mm Hg is reasonable for the secondary prevention of cardiovascular events. A lower target BP (<130/80 mm Hg) may be appropriate in some individuals with CAD, previous MI, stroke or transient ischemic attack, or CAD risk equivalents (AHA/ACC/ASH [Rosendorff 2015]).

Pregnancy Considerations Adverse events were observed in animal reproduction studies; therefore, the manufacturer classifies bisoprolol as pregnancy category C. In a cohort study, an increased risk of cardiovascular defects was observed following maternal use of beta-blockers during pregnancy. Intrauterine growth restriction (IUGR), small placentas, as well as fetal/neonatal bradycardia, hypoglycemia, and/or respiratory depression have been observed following *in utero* exposure to beta-blockers as a class. Adequate facilities for monitoring infants at birth should be available. Untreated chronic maternal hypertension and pre-eclampsia are also associated with adverse events in the fetus, infant, and mother. Limited information is available related to the use of bisoprolol for the treatment of hypertension in pregnancy; other agents may be more appropriate for use.

Breast-Feeding Considerations It is not known if bisoprolol is excreted into breast milk. The manufacturer recommends that caution be exercised when administering bisoprolol to nursing women.

Contraindications Cardiogenic shock; overt cardiac failure; marked sinus bradycardia or heart block greater than first-degree (except in patients with a functioning artificial pacemaker)

Warnings/Precautions Consider preexisting conditions such as sick sinus syndrome before initiating. Use caution in patients with heart failure; use gradual and careful titration; monitor for symptoms of congestive heart failure. Beta-blockers without alpha1-adrenergic receptor blocking activity should be avoided in patients with Prinzmetal variant angina (Mayer, 1998). Use with caution in patients with myasthenia gravis, psychiatric disease (may cause

CNS depression), bronchospastic disease, undergoing anesthesia; and in those with impaired hepatic function. Bradycardia may be observed more frequently in elderly patients (>65 years of age); dosage reductions may be necessary. Beta-blocker therapy should not be withdrawn abruptly (particularly in patients with CAD), but gradually tapered to avoid acute tachycardia, hypertension, and/or ischemia. Chronic beta-blocker therapy should not be routinely withdrawn prior to major surgery. Can precipitate or aggravate symptoms of arterial insufficiency in patients with PVD and Raynaud's disease; use with caution and monitor for progression of arterial obstruction. Use caution with concurrent use of digoxin, verapamil, or diltiazem; bradycardia or heart block may occur. Use with caution in patients receiving inhaled anesthetic agents known to depress myocardial contractility. Bisoprolol, with beta$_1$-selectivity, may be used cautiously in bronchospastic disease with close monitoring. Use cautiously in patients with diabetes because it can mask prominent hypoglycemic symptoms. May mask signs of hyperthyroidism (eg, tachycardia); use caution if hyperthyroidism is suspected, abrupt withdrawal may precipitate thyroid storm. Dosage adjustment is required in patients with significant hepatic or renal dysfunction. Adequate alpha-blockade is required prior to use of any beta-blocker for patients with untreated pheochromocytoma. May induce or exacerbate psoriasis. Use caution with history of severe anaphylaxis to allergens; patients taking beta-blockers may become more sensitive to repeated challenges. Treatment of anaphylaxis (eg, epinephrine) in patients taking beta-blockers may be ineffective or promote undesirable effects.

Adverse Reactions

1% to 10%:
Cardiovascular: Chest pain (1% to 2%)
Central nervous system: Fatigue (dose related; 6% to 8%), insomnia (2% to 3%), hypoesthesia (1% to 2%)
Gastrointestinal: Diarrhea (dose related; 3% to 4%), nausea (2%), vomiting (1% to 2%)
Neuromuscular & skeletal: Arthralgia (2% to 3%), weakness (dose related; ≤2%)
Respiratory: Upper respiratory infection (5%), rhinitis (3% to 4%), sinusitis (2%), dyspnea (1% to 2%)
<1% (Limited to important or life-threatening): Abdominal pain, abnormal lacrimation, acne vulgaris, alopecia, amnesia, angioedema, anxiety, asthma, back pain, bradycardia (dose related), bronchitis, bronchospasm, cardiac arrhythmia, claudication, cold extremities, confusion (especially in the elderly), congestive heart failure, constipation, cough, cystitis, decreased libido, depression, dermatitis, dizziness, drowsiness, dysgeusia, dyspepsia, dyspnea on exertion, eczema, edema, exfoliative dermatitis, eye pain, flushing, gastritis, gout, hallucination, headache, hearing loss, hyperesthesia, hyperglycemia, hyperkalemia, hyperphosphatemia, hypersensitivity angiitis, hypertriglyceridemia, hypotension, impotence, increased blood urea nitrogen, increased serum creatinine, increased serum transaminases, increased uric acid, insomnia, leukopenia, malaise, muscle cramps, myalgia, neck pain, nervousness, orthostatic hypotension, palpitations, paresthesia, peptic ulcer, Peyronie's disease, pharyngitis, polyuria, positive ANA titer, pruritus, psoriasiform eruption, psoriasis, purpura, renal colic, restlessness, sensation of eye pressure, skin rash, syncope, thrombocytopenia, tinnitus, tremor, twitching, vasculitis, vertigo, visual disturbance, weight gain, xerostomia

Drug Interactions

Metabolism/Transport Effects Substrate of CYP2D6 (minor), CYP3A4 (major); **Note:** Assignment of Major/Minor substrate status based on clinically relevant drug interaction potential

Avoid Concomitant Use

Avoid concomitant use of Bisoprolol with any of the following: Ceritinib; Conivaptan; Floctafenine; Fusidic Acid (Systemic); Idelalisib; Methacholine; Rivastigmine

Increased Effect/Toxicity

Bisoprolol may increase the levels/effects of: Alpha-/Beta-Agonists (Direct-Acting); Alpha1-Blockers; Alpha2-Agonists; Amifostine; Antipsychotic Agents (Phenothiazines); Antipsychotic Agents (Second Generation [Atypical]); Bradycardia-Causing Agents; Bupivacaine; Cardiac Glycosides; Ceritinib; Cholinergic Agonists; Disopyramide; DULoxetine; Ergot Derivatives; Fingolimod; Grass Pollen Allergen Extract (5 Grass Extract); Hypotension-Associated Agents; Insulin; Ivabradine; Lacosamide; Levodopa; Lidocaine (Systemic); Lidocaine (Topical); Mepivacaine; Methacholine; Midodrine; Sulfonylureas

The levels/effects of Bisoprolol may be increased by: Acetylcholinesterase Inhibitors; Alpha2-Agonists; Aminoquinolines (Antimalarial); Amiodarone; Anilidopiperidine Opioids; Antipsychotic Agents (Phenothiazines); Aprepitant; Barbiturates; Bretylium; Brimonidine (Topical);

Calcium Channel Blockers (Nondihydropyridine); Conivaptan; CYP3A4 Inhibitors (Moderate); CYP3A4 Inhibitors (Strong); Dasatinib; Diazoxide; Dipyridamole; Disopyramide; Dronedarone; Floctafenine; Fosaprepitant; Fusidic Acid (Systemic); Herbs (Hypotensive Properties); Idelalisib; Ivacaftor; Luliconazole; Mifepristone; Molsidomine; Netupitant; Nicorandil; NIFEdipine; Obinutuzumab; Osimertinib; Palbociclib; Pentoxifylline; Phosphodiesterase 5 Inhibitors; Propafenone; Prostacyclin Analogues; Regorafenib; Reserpine; Rivastigmine; Ruxolitinib; Simeprevir; Stiripentol; Tofacitinib

Decreased Effect

Bisoprolol may decrease the levels/effects of: Beta2-Agonists; Theophylline Derivatives

The levels/effects of Bisoprolol may be decreased by: Amphetamines; Barbiturates; Bosentan; CYP3A4 Inducers (Moderate); CYP3A4 Inducers (Strong); Dabrafenib; Deferasirox; Enzalutamide; Herbs (Hypertensive Properties); Methylphenidate; Mitotane; Nonsteroidal Anti-Inflammatory Agents; Osimertinib; Siltuximab; St Johns Wort; Tocilizumab; Yohimbine

Storage/Stability Store at controlled room temperature 20°C to 25°C (68°F to 77°F). Protect from moisture.

Mechanism of Action Selective inhibitor of beta$_1$-adrenergic receptors; competitively blocks beta$_1$-receptors, with little or no effect on beta$_2$-receptors at doses ≤20 mg

Pharmacodynamics/Kinetics

Onset of action: 1 to 2 hours
Absorption: Rapid and almost complete
Distribution: Widely; highest concentrations in heart, liver, lungs, and saliva; crosses blood-brain barrier
Protein binding: ~30%
Metabolism: Extensively hepatic; significant first-pass effect (~20%)
Bioavailability: ~80%
Half-life elimination: Normal renal function: 9 to 12 hours; CrCl <40 mL/minute: 27 to 36 hours; Hepatic cirrhosis: 8 to 22 hours
Time to peak: 2 to 4 hours
Excretion: Urine (50% as unchanged drug, remainder as inactive metabolites); feces (<2%)

Dosing

Adult & Geriatric

Hypertension: Oral: Initial: 2.5 to 5 mg once daily; may be increased to 10 mg and then up to 20 mg once daily, if necessary; usual dose range (ASH/ISH [Weber, 2014]): 5 to 10 mg once daily

Atrial fibrillation (rate control) (off-label use): Usual maintenance dose: 2.5 to 10 mg once daily (AHA/ACC/HRS [January, 2014])

Heart failure (off-label use): Oral: Initial: 1.25 mg once daily; maximum dose: 10 mg once daily. **Note:** Initiate only in stable patients or hospitalized patients after volume status has been optimized and IV diuretics, vasodilators, and inotropic agents have all been successfully discontinued. Caution should be used when initiating in patients who required inotropes during their hospital course. Increase dose gradually and monitor for congestive signs and symptoms of HF making every effort to achieve target dose shown to be effective (ACCF/AHA [Yancy, 2013]; CIBIS-II Investigators and Committees, 1999; HFSA [Lindenfeld, 2010]).

Renal Impairment

Hypertension: CrCl <40 mL/minute: Initial: 2.5 mg daily; increase cautiously.

Heart failure (off-label use): In clinical trials, the initial recommended dosage (ie, 1.25 mg once daily) was not reduced further based on CrCl; however, patients with serum creatinine ≥3.4 mg/dL were excluded in one trial (CIBIS-II Investigators and Committees, 1999) and those with a serum creatinine ≥2.5 mg/dL were excluded in another trial (Willenheimer, 2005).

Hemodialysis: Not dialyzable

Hepatic Impairment Hepatitis or cirrhosis: Initial: 2.5 mg daily; increase cautiously.

Dietary Considerations May be taken without regard to meals.

Administration May be administered without regard to meals.

Monitoring Parameters Blood pressure, heart rate, ECG; serum glucose regularly (in patients with diabetes)

Dosage Forms Excipient information presented when available (limited, particularly for generics); consult specific product labeling.

Tablet, Oral, as fumarate:
Zebeta: 5 mg [scored]
Zebeta: 10 mg
Generic: 5 mg, 10 mg

Bisoprolol and Hydrochlorothiazide
(bis OH proe lol & hye droe klor oh THYE a zide)

Brand Names: US Ziac®
Brand Names: Canada Ziac®
Index Terms Bisoprolol Fumarate and Hydrochlorothiazide; Hydrochlorothiazide and Bisoprolol
Pharmacologic Category Antihypertensive; Beta-Blocker, Beta-1 Selective; Diuretic, Thiazide
Use Hypertension: Management of hypertension.
Dosing
Adult & Geriatric
Hypertension: Oral: Initial: Bisoprolol 2.5 mg /hydrochlorothiazide 6.25 mg once daily; dose may be titrated at ≥2-week intervals. Maximum dose: Bisoprolol 20 mg/ hydrochlorothiazide 12.5 mg once daily.
Add-on/replacement therapy: Bisoprolol 2.5 to 20 mg/ hydrochlorothiazide 6.25 to 12.5 mg once daily.
Pediatric Hypertension (off-label use): Oral: Initial: Bisoprolol 2.5 mg/hydrochlorothiazide 6.25 mg once daily; may increase up to bisoprolol 10 mg/hydrochlorothiazide 6.25 mg once daily (Sorof 2002).
Renal Impairment There are no dosage adjustments provided in the manufacturer's labeling; use with caution when dosing/titrating patients with renal impairment. Discontinue use with progressive renal impairment; use is contraindicated in patients with anuria.
Hepatic Impairment There are no dosage adjustments provided in the manufacturer's labeling; use with caution should be used when dosing/titrating patients with hepatic impairment.
Additional Information Complete prescribing information should be consulted for additional detail.
Dosage Forms Excipient information presented when available (limited, particularly for generics); consult specific product labeling.
Tablet, oral: 2.5/6.25: Bisoprolol fumarate 2.5 mg and hydrochlorothiazide 6.25 mg; 5/6.25: Bisoprolol fumarate 5 mg and hydrochlorothiazide 6.25 mg; 10/6.25: Bisoprolol fumarate 10 mg and hydrochlorothiazide 6.25 mg
Ziac: 2.5/6.25: Bisoprolol fumarate 2.5 mg and hydrochlorothiazide 6.25 mg
Ziac: 5/6.25: Bisoprolol fumarate 5 mg and hydrochlorothiazide 6.25 mg
Ziac: 10/6.25: Bisoprolol fumarate 10 mg and hydrochlorothiazide 6.25 mg

♦ Bisoprolol Fumarate *see* Bisoprolol *on page 233*
♦ Bisoprolol Fumarate and Hydrochlorothiazide *see* Bisoprolol and Hydrochlorothiazide *on page 235*
♦ Bis-POM PMEA *see* Adefovir *on page 45*
♦ Bistropamide *see* Tropicamide *on page 1848*
♦ Bivalent Human Papillomavirus Vaccine *see* Papillomavirus (Types 16, 18) Vaccine (Human, Recombinant) *on page 1394*

Bivalirudin (bye VAL i roo din)

Brand Names: US Angiomax
Brand Names: Canada Angiomax
Index Terms Hirulog
Pharmacologic Category Anticoagulant; Anticoagulant, Direct Thrombin Inhibitor
Use Anticoagulant used in conjunction with aspirin for patients with unstable angina undergoing percutaneous transluminal coronary angioplasty (PTCA) or percutaneous coronary intervention (PCI) with provisional glycoprotein IIb/IIIa inhibitor; anticoagulant used in conjunction with aspirin for patients undergoing PCI with (or at risk of) heparin-induced thrombocytopenia (HIT) / thrombosis syndrome (HITTS)

Canadian labeling: Additional uses (not in U.S. labeling): In conjunction with aspirin for treatment of patients with ST-elevation myocardial infarction (STEMI) undergoing primary PCI; anticoagulant with or without glycoprotein IIb/IIIa inhibitor; anticoagulant used in conjunction with aspirin for patients undergoing cardiac surgery with (or at risk of) heparin-induced thrombocytopenia (HIT) / thrombosis syndrome (HITTS)
Pregnancy Considerations Adverse events have not been observed in animal reproduction studies. Bivalirudin is used in conjunction with aspirin, which may lead to maternal or fetal adverse effects, especially during the third trimester. Use of parenteral direct thrombin inhibitors in pregnancy should be limited to those women who have severe allergic reactions to heparin, including heparin-induced thrombocytopenia, and who cannot receive danaparoid (Guyatt, 2012).

Breast-Feeding Considerations It is not known if bivalirudin is excreted in breast milk. The manufacturer recommends that caution be exercised when administering bivalirudin to nursing women.
Contraindications Hypersensitivity to bivalirudin or any component of the formulation; active major bleeding

Canadian labeling: Additional contraindications (not in U.S. labeling): Major blood clotting disorders; acute gastric or duodenal ulcer; cerebral hemorrhage; severe cerebro-spinal trauma; bacterial endocarditis; severe uncontrolled hypertension; diabetic or hemorrhagic retinopathy; proximal use of spinal/epidural anesthesia
Warnings/Precautions Not for intramuscular use. Safety and efficacy have not been established in patients with unstable angina or acute coronary syndromes who are not undergoing PTCA or PCI. Increased risk of thrombus formation (some fatal) has been reported with bivalirudin use in gamma brachytherapy. As with all anticoagulants, bleeding may occur at any site and should be considered following an unexplained fall in blood pressure or hematocrit, or any unexplained symptom. Use with caution in patients with disease states associated with increased risk of bleeding. Use with caution in patients with renal impairment; dosage reduction required.
Adverse Reactions As with all anticoagulants, bleeding is the major adverse effect of bivalirudin. Hemorrhage may occur at virtually any site. Risk is dependent on multiple variables, including the intensity of anticoagulation, concurrent use of a glycoprotein IIb/IIIa inhibitor, and patient susceptibility. Additional adverse effects are often related to idiosyncratic reactions, and the frequency is difficult to estimate. Adverse reactions reported were generally less than those seen with heparin.

>10%:
Cardiovascular: Hypotension (≤12%)
Central nervous system: Pain (≤15%), headache (≤12%)
Gastrointestinal: Nausea (≤15%)
Hematologic & oncologic: Minor hemorrhage (Protocol defined: 14%; heparin 26%; TIMI defined: 1%; heparin 3% [Lincoff, 2003])
Neuromuscular & skeletal: Back pain (9% to 42%)
1% to 10%:
Cardiovascular: Hypertension (6%), bradycardia (5%), angina pectoris (≤5%)
Central nervous system: Insomnia (7%), anxiety (6%), nervousness (5%)
Gastrointestinal: Vomiting (≤6%), abdominal pain (5%), dyspepsia (5%)
Genitourinary: Pelvic pain (6%), urinary retention (4%)
Hematologic & oncologic: Major hemorrhage (Protocol defined: 2% to 4%; heparin 4% to 9%; TIMI defined: 0.6%; heparin 0.9%; transfusion required: 1% to 2%; heparin 2% to 6% [Lincoff, 2003])
Local: Pain at injection site (≤8%)
Miscellaneous: Fever (5%)
<1% (Limited to important or life-threatening): Cerebral ischemia, confusion, facial paralysis, hemorrhage (fatal), hypersensitivity reaction (including anaphylaxis), increased susceptibility to infection, intracranial hemorrhage, oliguria, pulmonary edema, renal failure, retroperitoneal hemorrhage, sepsis, syncope, thrombocytopenia, vascular disease, venous thrombosis (during PCI, including intracoronary brachytherapy), ventricular fibrillation
Drug Interactions
Metabolism/Transport Effects None known.
Avoid Concomitant Use
Avoid concomitant use of Bivalirudin with any of the following: Apixaban; Dabigatran Etexilate; Edoxaban; Hemin; Omacetaxine; Rivaroxaban; Urokinase; Vorapaxar
Increased Effect/Toxicity
Bivalirudin may increase the levels/effects of: Anticoagulants; Collagenase (Systemic); Deferasirox; Deoxycholic Acid; Ibritumomab; Nintedanib; Obinutuzumab; Omacetaxine; Rivaroxaban; Tositumomab and Iodine I 131 Tositumomab

The levels/effects of Bivalirudin may be increased by: Agents with Antiplatelet Properties; Apixaban; Dabigatran Etexilate; Dasatinib; Edoxaban; Hemin; Herbs (Anticoagulant/Antiplatelet Properties); Ibrutinib; Limaprost; Nonsteroidal Anti-Inflammatory Agents; Omega-3 Fatty Acids; Pentosan Polysulfate Sodium; Prostacyclin Analogues; Salicylates; Sugammadex; Thrombolytic Agents; Tibolone; Tipranavir; Urokinase; Vitamin E; Vitamin E (Oral); Vorapaxar
Decreased Effect
The levels/effects of Bivalirudin may be decreased by: Estrogen Derivatives; Progestins

Preparation for Administration Reconstitute each 250 mg with 5 mL SWFI. Gently swirl to dissolve. Further dilution in D_5W or NS (50 mL to make 5 mg/mL solution **or** 500 mL to make 0.5 mg/mL solution) is required prior to infusion.

Storage/Stability Store unopened vials at 20°C to 25°C (68°F to 77°F); excursions permitted between 15°C to 30°C. Following reconstitution, vials should be stored at 2°C to 8°C for up to 24 hours. Do not freeze. Final dilutions of 0.5 mg/mL or 5 mg/mL are stable at room temperature for up to 24 hours.

Mechanism of Action Bivalirudin acts as a specific and reversible direct thrombin inhibitor; it binds to the catalytic and anionic exosite of both circulating and clot-bound thrombin. Catalytic binding site occupation functionally inhibits coagulant effects by preventing thrombin-mediated cleavage of fibrinogen to fibrin monomers, and activation of factors V, VIII, and XIII. Shows linear dose- and concentration-dependent prolongation of ACT, aPTT, PT, and TT.

Pharmacodynamics/Kinetics

Onset of action: Immediate

Duration: Coagulation times return to baseline ~1 hour following discontinuation of infusion

Distribution: 0.2 L/kg

Protein binding, plasma: Does not bind other than thrombin

Metabolism: Blood proteases

Half-life elimination:

Normal renal function (CrCl ≥90 mL/minute): 25 minutes

Severe renal impairment (CrCl 10 to 29 mL/minute): 57 minutes

Dialysis-dependent patients (off dialysis): 3.5 hours

Excretion: Urine (20%), proteolytic cleavage

Dosing

Adult Note: If clinically indicated, provisional glycoprotein (GP) IIb/IIIa inhibition (eg, abciximab, eptifibatide, tirofiban) may be concomitantly administered during percutaneous coronary intervention (PCI). In addition to aspirin, concomitant administration of clopidogrel, prasugrel, or ticagrelor is also recommended for patients undergoing PCI (ACCF/AHA/SCAI [Levine, 2011]).

PTCA/PCI with or without HIT/HITTS: IV: Initial: 0.75 mg/kg bolus immediately prior to procedure, followed by 1.75 mg/kg/hour for the duration of procedure and up to 4 hours postprocedure if needed (according to the manufacturer); may determine ACT 5 minutes after bolus dose; may administer additional bolus of 0.3 mg/kg if necessary. If continued anticoagulation is needed after the initial 4-hour postprocedure infusion, the infusion may be continued at 0.2 mg/kg/hour for up to an additional 20 hours (U.S. labeling) or 0.25 mg/kg/hour for 4 to 12 hours post procedure (Canadian labeling).

Unstable angina/non-ST-elevation myocardial infarction (UA/NSTEMI) (moderate-high risk) undergoing early invasive strategy: IV:

During PCI: 0.75 mg/kg bolus prior to procedure, followed by 1.75 mg/kg/hour (ACCF/AHA [Anderson, 2013]).

Prior to PCI (U.S. off-label dose): Alternatively, may administer an initial 0.1 mg/kg bolus prior to diagnostic angiography, followed by 0.25 mg/kg/hour. Once PCI is determined to be necessary, give an additional bolus of 0.5 mg/kg and increase infusion rate to 1.75 mg/kg/hour; may discontinue at end of procedure or continue for up to 4 hours postprocedure if necessary (Stone, 2006). If after angiography, cardiac surgery is deemed necessary, discontinue bivalirudin 3 hours prior to surgery and dose with unfractionated heparin per institutional practice. If medical management is the decided treatment approach, may either discontinue bivalirudin or continue at 0.25 mg/kg/hour for up to 72 hours (ACCF/AHA [Anderson, 2013]).

Canadian labeling: Initial: 0.1 mg/kg bolus, followed by 0.25 mg/kg/hour for up to 72 hours if patient is medically managed. If PCI is determined to be necessary, give an additional bolus of 0.5 mg/kg and increase infusion rate to 1.75 mg/kg/hour; may resume infusion at 0.25 mg/kg/hour for 4-12 hours following PCI if necessary. If coronary artery bypass graft (CABG) surgery is deemed necessary, discontinue bivalirudin infusion 1 hour prior to CABG (on-pump) surgery and dose with unfractionated heparin or continue infusion until time of CABG (off-pump) surgery then give 0.5 mg/kg bolus and increase infusion rate to 1.75 mg/kg/hour until end of surgery.

STEMI undergoing primary PCI *(U.S. off-label use):* IV: Initial: 0.75 mg/kg bolus, followed by 1.75 mg/kg/hour for the duration of procedure; may continue postprocedure at a reduced dose if clinically indicated (ACCF/AHA [O'Gara, 2013]; Stone, 2008). In STEMI patients who are at a high risk of bleeding, it is reasonable to use bivalirudin monotherapy in preference to the combination of unfractionated heparin and a GP IIb/IIIa receptor antagonist (ACCF/AHA [O'Gara 2013]). Of note, a single-center, open-label, randomized controlled trial comparing heparin to bivalirudin in patients with STEMI undergoing primary PCI (mostly with a radial approach) demonstrated that heparin reduces the incidence of major adverse cardiovascular events with no increase in bleeding as compared to bivalirudin (Shahzad, 2014).

If patient received unfractionated heparin (UFH) prior to procedure and bivalirudin is the desired anticoagulant: Discontinue heparin if infusing; without measurement of ACT, may initiate bivalirudin ≥30 minutes after the last UFH bolus but before PCI occurs (Stone, 2008). Switching patients from UFH to bivalirudin has been shown to be safe compared to continuing with UFH and as needed glycoprotein IIb/IIIa inhibition; median time from prerandomization UFH bolus to bivalirudin administration within the HORIZONS-AMI trial was 64 ± 61 minutes (Dangas, 2011).

Canadian labeling: Initial: 0.1 mg/kg bolus, followed by 0.25 mg/kg/hour for up to 72 hours if patient is medically managed. If PCI is determined to be necessary, give an additional bolus of 0.5 mg/kg and increase infusion rate to 1.75 mg/kg/hour; may resume infusion at 0.25 mg/kg/hour for 4-12 hours following PCI if necessary. If coronary artery bypass graft (CABG) surgery is deemed necessary, discontinue bivalirudin infusion 1 hour prior to CABG (on-pump) surgery and dose with unfractionated heparin or continue infusion until time of CABG (off-pump) surgery then give 0.5 mg/kg bolus and increase infusion rate to 1.75 mg/kg/hour until end of surgery.

Cardiac surgery in patients with acute or subacute heparin-induced thrombocytopenia, urgent surgery required: *U.S. off-label use* (Linkins, 2012): IV: Intraoperative:

Off-pump: Initial bolus: 0.75 mg/kg, followed by continuous infusion 1.75 mg/kg/hour to maintain ACT >300 seconds (Dyke, 2007). If patient needs to go on-pump, Canadian labeling recommends an additional 0.25 mg/kg bolus and increasing the infusion rate to 2.5 mg/kg/hour.

On-pump: Initial bolus: 1 mg/kg, followed by continuous infusion 2.5 mg/kg/hour; 50 mg bolus added to priming solution of cardiopulmonary bypass (CPB) circuit. Additional boluses of 0.1-0.5 mg/kg may be given to maintain ACT >2.5 times baseline ACT. **Note:** Special maneuvers needed to prevent stasis and consequent clotting within CPB circuit during or after surgery (Koster, 2007). Per Canadian labeling, after completion of CPB, provision to allow recirculation of the circuit may be done by administering 50 mg **into the circuit** followed by a continuous infusion of 50 mg/hour **into the circuit.**

Canadian labeling: Pre -and post-cardiac surgery administration: Initial bolus: 0.1 mg/kg, followed by continuous infusion 0.2 mg/kg/hour for up to 48 hours prior to surgery or for up to 14 days after surgery; maintain aPTT 1.5-2.5 times baseline aPTT.

Heparin-induced thrombocytopenia (HIT) (off-label use): IV: Initial dose: 0.15-0.2 mg/kg/hour; adjust to aPTT 1.5-2.5 times baseline value (Linkins, 2012). **Note:** Although the use of bivalirudin is not a currently recommended treatment for HIT due to insufficient evidence, the American College of Chest Physicians recommends overlapping administration of warfarin for a minimum of 5 days until INR is within target range; recheck INR after the non-heparin anticoagulant effect has dissipated (Linkins, 2012).

Geriatric Refer to adult dosing. No dosage adjustment is needed in elderly patients with normal renal function. Puncture site hemorrhage and catheterization site hemorrhage were seen in more patients ≥65 years of age than in patients <65 years of age.

Renal Impairment Infusion dose should be reduced based on degree of renal impairment. Initial bolus dose remains unchanged. Monitor activated coagulation time (ACT) or aPTT depending on indication.

For use in PCI:

U.S. labeling:

CrCl ≥30 mL/minute: No adjustment required.

CrCl 10-29 mL/minute: Decrease infusion rate to 1 mg/kg/hour

Dialysis-dependent patients (off dialysis during administration): Decrease infusion rate to 0.25 mg/kg/hour

Hemodialysis: Approximately 25% removed during hemodialysis

Canadian labeling: **Note:** Check ACT following dose alterations at 5 and 45 minutes in renally impaired patients. If ACT ≤250 seconds give additional bolus 0.3 mg/kg and double infusion rate to maintain ACT ~350 seconds; if ACT 250-300 seconds give additional bolus 0.3 mg/kg to maintain ACT ~350 seconds. CrCl ≥30 mL/minute: No adjustment required.
CrCl 10-29 mL/minute: Decrease infusion rate to 1 mg/kg/hour
Dialysis-dependent patients (off dialysis during administration): Decrease infusion rate to 0.25 mg/kg/hour

For use in cardiac surgery:
Canadian labeling:
CrCl ≥30 mL/minute: No adjustment required; monitor ACT.
CrCl <30 mL/minute: There are no dosage adjustments provided in the manufacturer's labeling; has not been studied; monitor ACT.

For use in HIT: There are no dosage adjustments provided in the manufacturer's labeling for this population; however, the following dose ranges have been observed in small retrospective observational studies (Kiser 2006; Kiser, 2008; Tsu, 2011). Of note, critically-ill patients comprised a significant proportion of patients in these observational studies. The following dose recommendations are based on the mean dose achieving aPTT goal within these studies; overlaps may exist; **Note:** The Cockcroft-Gault equation was used in all studies to define creatinine clearance:
CrCl >60 mL/minute: 0.13 mg/kg/hour
CrCl 30-60 mL/minute: 0.08-0.1 mg/kg/hour
CrCl <30 mL/minute: 0.04-0.05 mg/kg/hour
Intermittent hemodialysis (IHD): 0.07 mg/kg/hour (Tsu, 2011)
CRRT (eg, CVVH or CVVHDF): 0.03-0.07 mg/kg/hour (Kiser, 2006; Tsu, 2011)
Sustained low-efficiency daily diafiltration (SLEDD): 0.09 mg/kg/hour (Tsu, 2011)

Hepatic Impairment No dosage adjustment necessary.

Usual Infusion Concentrations: Adult IV infusion: 250 mg in 500 mL (concentration: 0.5 mg/mL) **or** 250 mg in 50 mL (concentration: 5 mg/mL) of D_5W or NS

Administration For IV administration only.

Monitoring Parameters Depends upon indication for use of bivalirudin: ACT or aPTT

Test Interactions PT/INR levels may become elevated in the absence of warfarin. If warfarin is initiated, initial PT/INR goals while on bivalirudin may require modification.

Dosage Forms Excipient information presented when available (limited, particularly for generics); consult specific product labeling.
Solution Reconstituted, Intravenous:
Angiomax: 250 mg (1 ea)
Generic: 250 mg (1 ea)

◆ Bivigam *see* Immune Globulin *on page 927*
◆ Bi-Zets/Benzotroches [OTC] *see* Benzocaine *on page 217*
◆ BL4162A *see* Anagrelide *on page 127*
◆ Blanche *see* Hydroquinone *on page 893*
◆ Blenoxane *see* Bleomycin *on page 237*
◆ Bleo *see* Bleomycin *on page 237*

Bleomycin (blee oh MYE sin)

Brand Names: Canada Blenoxane; Bleomycin Injection, USP

Index Terms Blenoxane; Bleo; Bleomycin Sulfate; BLM

Pharmacologic Category Antineoplastic Agent, Antibiotic

Use
Head and neck cancers: Treatment of squamous cell carcinomas of the head and neck
Hodgkin lymphoma: Treatment of Hodgkin lymphoma
Malignant pleural effusion: Sclerosing agent for malignant pleural effusion
Testicular cancer: Treatment of testicular cancer

Dosing
Adult Note: The risk for pulmonary toxicity increases with age >70 years and cumulative lifetime dose of >400 units. **International considerations:** Dosages below expressed as USP units; 1 USP unit = 1 mg (by potency) = 1,000 international units (Stefanou, 2001).

Test dose for lymphoma patients: IM, IV, SubQ: Because of the possibility of an anaphylactoid reaction, the manufacturer recommends administering 1 to 2 units of bleomycin before the first 1 to 2 doses; monitor vital signs every 15 minutes; wait a minimum of 1 hour before administering remainder of dose; if no acute reaction occurs, then the regular dosage schedule

may be followed. **Note:** Test doses may not be predictive of a reaction (Lam, 2005) and/or may produce false-negative results.

Hodgkin lymphoma (off-label dosing): IV:
ABVD: 10 units/m² days 1 and 15 of a 28-day treatment cycle (in combination with doxorubicin, vinblastine, and dacarbazine) (Straus, 2004)
BEACOPP: 10 units/m² day 8 of a 21-day treatment cycle (in combination with etoposide, doxorubicin, cyclophosphamide, vincristine, procarbazine, and prednisone) (Dann, 2007; Diehl, 2003)
Stanford V: 5 units/m²/dose in weeks 2, 4, 6, 8, 10 and 12 (in combination with mechlorethamine, vinblastine, vincristine, doxorubicin, etoposide, and prednisone) (Horning, 2002; Horning, 2000)

Testicular cancer (off-label dosing): IV: BEP: 30 units/dose days 1, 8, and 15 of a 21-day treatment cycle for 4 cycles (in combination with etoposide and cisplatin) (Culine, 2008; Nichols, 1998)

Ovarian germ cell cancer (off-label use): IV: 30 units/dose days 1, 8, and 15 of a 21-day treatment cycle for 3 cycles (Williams, 1994) **or** 15 units/m² day 1 of a 21-day treatment cycle for 4 cycles (Cushing, 2004); in combination with etoposide and cisplatin

Malignant pleural effusion: Intrapleural: 60 units as a single instillation; mix in 50 to 100 mL of NS

Geriatric Refer to adult dosing. The incidence of pulmonary toxicity is higher in patients >70 years of age.

Pediatric Note: The risk for pulmonary toxicity increases with age >70 years and cumulative lifetime dose of >400 units. **International considerations:** Dosages below expressed as USP units; 1 USP unit = 1 mg (by potency) = 1,000 international units (Stefanou, 2001).

Test dose for lymphoma patients: IM, IV, SubQ: Because of the possibility of an anaphylactoid reaction, the manufacturer recommends administering 1 to 2 units of bleomycin before the first 1 to 2 doses; monitor vital signs every 15 minutes; wait a minimum of 1 hour before administering remainder of dose; if no acute reaction occurs, then the regular dosage schedule may be followed. **Note:** Test doses may not be predictive of a reaction (Lam, 2005) and/or may produce false-negative results.

Hodgkin lymphoma (off-label dosing): IV: ABVD: IV: 10 units/m² days 1 and 15 of a 28-day treatment cycle (in combination with doxorubicin, vinblastine, and dacarbazine) (Hutchinson, 1998)

Renal Impairment
The U.S. labeling recommends the following adjustments (creatinine clearance should be estimated using the Cockcroft-Gault formula):
CrCl >50 mL/minute: No dosage adjustment necessary.
CrCl 40-50 mL/minute: Administer 70% of normal dose
CrCl 30-40 mL/minute: Administer 60% of normal dose
CrCl 20-30 mL/minute: Administer 55% of normal dose
CrCl 10-20 mL/minute: Administer 45% of normal dose
CrCl 5-10 mL/minute: Administer 40% of normal dose
The Canadian labeling recommends the following adjustment: CrCl ≤40 mL/minute: Reduce dose by 40% to 75%.
The following adjustments have also been recommended:
Aronoff, 2007: Adults: Continuous renal replacement therapy (CRRT): Administer 75% of dose
Kintzel, 1995: Adults:
CrCl 46-60 mL/minute: Administer 70% of dose
CrCl 31-45 mL/minute: Administer 60% of dose
CrCl <30 mL/minute: Consider use of alternative drug

Hepatic Impairment There are no dosage adjustments provided in the manufacturer's labeling (has not been studied); however, adjustment for hepatic impairment is not necessary (King, 2001).

Obesity *ASCO Guidelines for appropriate chemotherapy dosing in obese adults with cancer:* Fixed doses (dosing which is independent of body weight or BSA), are used in some protocols (eg, testicular cancer); due to toxicity concerns, the same fixed dose should also be considered for obese patients (Griggs, 2012).

Adjustment for Toxicity
Pulmonary changes: Discontinue until determined not to be drug-related.
Pulmonary diffusion capacity for carbon monoxide (DL_{CO}) <30% to 35% of baseline: Discontinue treatment.

Additional Information Complete prescribing information should be consulted for additional detail.

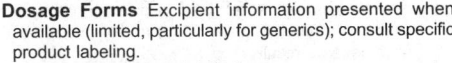

Dosage Forms Excipient information presented when available (limited, particularly for generics); consult specific product labeling.
Solution Reconstituted, Injection:
Generic: 15 units (1 ea); 30 units (1 ea)
Solution Reconstituted, Injection [preservative free]:
Generic: 15 units (1 ea); 30 units (1 ea)

◆ Bleomycin Injection, USP (Can) see Bleomycin on page 237

◆ Bleomycin Sulfate see Bleomycin on page 237

◆ Bleph-10 see Sulfacetamide (Ophthalmic) on page 1707

◆ Bleph 10 DPS (Can) see Sulfacetamide (Ophthalmic) on page 1707

◆ Blephamide see Sulfacetamide and Prednisolone on page 1708

Blinatumomab (blin a TOOM oh mab)

Brand Names: US Blincyto
Index Terms MT103
Pharmacologic Category Antineoplastic Agent, Anti-CD19/CD3; Antineoplastic Agent, Monoclonal Antibody
Use Acute lymphoblastic leukemia: Treatment of Philadelphia chromosome-negative (Ph-) relapsed or refractory B-cell precursor acute lymphoblastic leukemia (ALL)
Pregnancy Considerations Animal reproductions studies have not been conducted.
Breast-Feeding Considerations It is not known if blinatumomab is excreted in breast milk. Due to the potential for serious adverse reactions in the nursing infant, the manufacturer recommends a decision to discontinue nursing or to discontinue the drug, taking into account the importance of treatment to the mother.
Medication Guide Available Yes
Contraindications Known hypersensitivity to blinatumomab or any component of the formulation
Warnings/Precautions [U.S. Boxed Warning]: Cytokine release syndrome (CRS), which may be life-threatening or fatal, has occurred. Interrupt or discontinue therapy as recommended. Infusion reactions have also occurred, and may be difficult to distinguish from CRS. CRS symptoms may include pyrexia, headache, nausea, weakness, hypotension, increased transaminases, and elevated total bilirubin. In some patients, disseminated intravascular coagulation (DIC), capillary leak syndrome (CLS), and hemophagocytic lymphohistiocytosis/macrophage activation syndrome (HLH/MAS) have been reported in the setting of CRS. Monitor closely for signs/symptoms of these conditions; may require therapy interruption or discontinuation. CRS which was life-threatening or fatal occurred rarely. **[U.S. Boxed Warning]: Neurological toxicities, which may be severe, life-threatening, or fatal, have occurred. Interrupt or discontinue therapy as recommended.** Neurotoxicity has occurred in approximately half of patients in clinical trials. The median time to onset was 7 days. Grade 3 or higher neurotoxicity (eg, encephalopathy, convulsions, speech disorders, disturbances in consciousness, confusion and disorientation, and coordination and balance disorders) has also been observed. Patients are at risk for loss of consciousness due to neurologic events while taking blinatumomab; advise patients to avoid driving, participating in hazardous occupations, or operating heavy or dangerous machinery during treatment. Monitor patients for signs/symptoms of neurotoxicity; may require therapy interruption or discontinuation. The majority of symptoms resolved after interrupting therapy. Leukoencephalopathy (as seen on MRI) has been reported, particularly in those patients who received prior treatment with cranial irradiation and antileukemia chemotherapy (eg, high dose methotrexate or intrathecal cytarabine).

Neutropenia and neutropenic fever, including life-threatening episodes, have been reported. Monitor blood counts throughout therapy; may require therapy interruption if prolonged neutropenia occurs. Anemia and thrombocytopenia may also occur. Serious infections such as sepsis, pneumonia, bacteremia, opportunistic infections, and catheter-related infections have been reported in approximately one-fourth of patients in clinical trials (may be life-threatening or fatal). Consider prophylactic antibiotics if appropriate, and monitor closely for signs/symptoms of infection. Treat promptly if infection occurs. Transient increases in liver enzymes (associated both with and without CRS) may occur during therapy. The median time to enzyme elevation was 15 days; grade 3 or higher elevations were observed in a small percentage of patients. Monitor ALT, AST, GGT, and total bilirubin at baseline and during treatment. Interrupt therapy if transaminases

are >5 times ULN or if bilirubin is >3 times ULN. Life-threatening or fatal tumor lysis syndrome (TLS) has been observed. Administer measures to prevent TLS (eg, pretreatment nontoxic cytoreduction, and hydration during treatment). Monitor for signs/symptoms of TLS (eg, acute renal failure, hyperkalemia, hypocalcemia, hyperuricemia, and/or hyperphosphatemia); may require treatment interruption or discontinuation. Elderly patients experienced an increased rate of neurotoxicity (including cognitive disorder), encephalopathy, confusion, and serious infections as compared to patients less than 65 years. Preparation and administration errors have occurred. Preparation and administration errors have occurred. Do not flush infusion line, particularly when changing infusion bags or at completion of infusion; may result in overdose and complications. IV bag volume will be more than the volume administered to the patient (240 mL) to account for IV line priming and to ensure that the full dose is administered. Follow preparation and administration instructions carefully. Refer to manufacturer labeling for further information.
Adverse Reactions
>10%:
Cardiovascular: Peripheral edema (25%; ≥ grade 3: <1%), chest pain (11%; ≥ grade 3: 1%), hypotension (11%; ≥ grade 3: 2%)
Central nervous system: Neurotoxicity (50%; ≥ grade 3: 15%; incidence increased in older adults), headache (36%; ≥ grade 3: 3%), fatigue (17%; ≥ grade 3: 1%), chills (15%), insomnia (15%), dizziness (14%; ≥ grade 3: <1%)
Dermatologic: Skin rash (21%; ≥ grade 3: 2%)
Endocrine & metabolic: Hypokalemia (23%; ≥ grade 3: 6%), hypomagnesemia (12%), hyperglycemia (11%; ≥ grade 3: 7%), weight gain (11%)
Gastrointestinal: Nausea (25%), constipation (20%; ≥ grade 3: <1%), diarrhea (20%; ≥ grade 3: 1%), abdominal pain (15%; ≥ grade 3: 2%), vomiting (13%)
Hematologic & oncologic: Febrile neutropenia (25%; ≥ grade 3: 23%), anemia (18%; ≥ grade 3: 13%), neutropenia (16%; ≥ grade 3: 15%), thrombocytopenia (11%; ≥ grade 3: 8%)
Hepatic: Increased serum ALT (12%; ≥ grade 3: 6%), increased serum AST (11%; ≥ grade 3: 4%)
Hypersensitivity: Cytokine release syndrome (including cytokine storms) (11%; ≥ grade 3: 1%)
Infection: Infection (44%; ≥ grade 3: 25%), bacterial infection (19%; ≥ grade 3: 12%), fungal infection (15%; ≥ grade 3: 7%), viral infection (13%; ≥ grade 3: 4%)
Neuromuscular & skeletal: Tremor (20%; ≥ grade 3: 1%), back pain (14%; ≥ grade 3: 2%), limb pain (12%; ≥ grade 3: 1%), ostealgia (11%; ≥ grade 3: 3%)
Respiratory: Cough (19%), dyspnea (15%; ≥ grade 3: 5%)
Miscellaneous: Fever (62%; ≥ grade 3: 7%)
1% to 10%:
Cardiovascular: Hypertension (8%; ≥ grade 3: 5%), tachycardia (8%), edema (5%)
Central nervous system: Confusion (7%), brain disease (5%), paresthesia (5%), aphasia (4%), disorientation (3%), convulsions (2%), memory impairment (2%), cognitive dysfunction (1%), loss of consciousness
Endocrine & metabolic: Hypophosphatemia (6%; ≥ grade 3: 5%), increased gamma-glutamyl transferase (6%), hypoalbuminemia (4%)
Gastrointestinal: Decreased appetite (10%; ≥ grade 3: 3%)
Hematologic & oncologic: Decreased serum immunoglobulins (9%), leukopenia (9%; ≥ grade 3: 8%), tumor lysis syndrome (4%), leukocytosis (2%), lymphocytopenia (1%)
Hepatic: Increased serum bilirubin (8%), increased liver enzymes (1%)
Hypersensitivity: Cytokine storm (1%), hypersensitivity (1%)
Infection: Sepsis (7%; ≥ grade 3: 6%)
Neuromuscular & skeletal: Arthralgia (10%; ≥ grade 3: 2%)
Respiratory: Pneumonia (9%; ≥ grade 3: 8%)
<1% (Limited to important or life-threatening): Bronchospasm, capillary leak syndrome, leukoencephalopathy, speech disturbance
Drug Interactions
Metabolism/Transport Effects None known.
Avoid Concomitant Use
Avoid concomitant use of Blinatumomab with any of the following: BCG (Intravesical); Deferiprone; Dipyrone; Natalizumab; Pimecrolimus; Tacrolimus (Topical); Tofacitinib; Vaccines (Live)
Increased Effect/Toxicity
Blinatumomab may increase the levels/effects of: CloZA-Pine; Deferiprone; Fingolimod; Leflunomide; Natalizumab; Tofacitinib; Vaccines (Live)

The levels/effects of Blinatumomab may be increased by: Denosumab; Dipyrone; Pimecrolimus; Roflumilast; Tacrolimus (Topical); Trastuzumab

Decreased Effect

Blinatumomab may decrease the levels/effects of: BCG (Intravesical); Coccidioides immitis Skin Test; Sipuleucel-T; Vaccines (Inactivated); Vaccines (Live)

The levels/effects of Blinatumomab may be decreased by: Echinacea

Preparation for Administration All doses should be prepared in a prefilled 250 mL NS bag. Prefilled 250 mL NS bags typically contain overfill to a volume of 265 to 275 mL and dose calculations are based on a starting volume of 265 to 275 mL (if necessary, adjust the bag volume to achieve a starting volume between 265 and 275 mL). Final bag volume will be more than the volume administered to the patient (240 mL) to account for IV line priming and to ensure that the full dose is administered. Use only poly-olefin, PVC non-di-ethylhexylphthalate (non-DEHP), or ethyl vinyl acetate (EVA) infusion bags or pump cassettes. IV solution stabilizer provided is used to coat the prefilled NS bag prior to addition of reconstituted blinatumomab. Therefore, the IV solution stabilizer is added to the NS bag; do NOT use IV solution stabilizer for reconstitution of blinatumomab. Preparation and administration errors have occurred; follow preparation instructions carefully. Refer to manufacturer labeling for further information.

9 mcg daily dose infused over 24 hours at a rate of 10 mL/hour: Transfer **5.5 mL** of IV solution stabilizer to the prefilled 250 mL NS bag using a 10 mL syringe; gently mix to avoid foaming. Reconstitute **one** vial of lyophilized powder with 3 mL of preservative-free SWFI; direct stream toward the side of the vial and gently swirl to avoid excess foaming. Do not shake; final reconstituted concentration is 12.5 **mcg**/mL. Reconstituted solution should be clear to slightly opalescent, colorless to slightly yellow; do not use if cloudy or if precipitation occurs. Transfer **0.83 mL** of reconstituted solution into the pre-filled NS bag; gently mix. Remove air from the IV bag; prime IV line with the prepared infusion solution only (do not prime with NS). If not used immediately, store at 2°C to 8°C (36°F to 46°F) for up to 8 days (infusion must be completed within this time frame).

9 mcg daily dose infused over 48 hours at a rate of 5 mL/hour: Transfer **5.5 mL** of IV solution stabilizer to the prefilled 250 mL NS bag using a 10 mL syringe; gently mix to avoid foaming. Reconstitute **one** vial of lyophilized powder with 3 mL of preservative-free SWFI; direct stream toward the side of the vial and gently swirl to avoid excess foaming. Do not shake; final reconstituted concentration is 12.5 **mcg**/mL. Reconstituted solution should be clear to slightly opalescent, colorless to slightly yellow; do not use if cloudy or if precipitation occurs. Transfer **1.7 mL** of reconstituted solution into the prefilled NS bag; gently mix. Remove air from the IV bag; prime IV line with the prepared infusion solution only (do not prime with NS). If not used immediately, store at 2°C to 8°C (36°F to 46°F) for up to 8 days (infusion must be completed within this time frame).

28 mcg daily dose infused over 24 hours at a rate of 10 mL/hour: Transfer **5.6 mL** of IV solution stabilizer to the prefilled 250 mL NS bag using a 10 mL syringe; gently mix to avoid foaming. Reconstitute **one** vial of lyophilized powder with 3 mL of preservative-free SWFI; direct stream toward the side of the vial and gently swirl to avoid excess foaming. Do not shake; final reconstituted concentration is 12.5 **mcg**/mL. Reconstituted solution should be clear to slightly opalescent, colorless to slightly yellow; do not use if cloudy or if precipitation occurs. Transfer **2.6 mL** of reconstituted solution into the prefilled NS bag; gently mix. Remove air from the IV bag; prime IV line with the prepared infusion solution only (do not prime with NS). If not used immediately, store at 2°C to 8°C (36°F to 46°F) for up to 8 days (infusion must be completed within this time frame).

28 mcg daily dose infused over 48 hours at a rate of 5 mL/hour: Transfer **5.6 mL** of IV solution stabilizer to the prefilled 250 mL NS bag using a 10 mL syringe; gently mix to avoid foaming. Use 2 vials of lyophilized powder; reconstitute each vial with 3 mL of preservative-free SWFI; direct stream toward the side of the vial and gently swirl to avoid excess foaming. Do not shake; final reconstituted concentration in each vial is 12.5 mcg/mL. Reconstituted solution should be clear to slightly opalescent, colorless to slightly yellow; do not use if cloudy or if precipitation occurs. Transfer **5.2 mL** (2.7 mL from one vial and the remaining 2.5 mL from the second vial) of reconstituted solution into the prefilled NS bag; gently mix. Remove air from the IV bag; prime IV line with the prepared infusion solution only (do not prime with NS). If

not used immediately, store at 2°C to 8°C (36°F to 46°F) for up to 8 days (infusion must be completed within this time frame).

Storage/Stability Store intact vials (drug and solution stabilizer) in the original package at 2°C to 8°C (36°F to 46°F); protect from light. Do not freeze. Intact vials of both drug and stabilizer may be stored for up to 8 hours at room temperature. Reconstituted solution is stable for up to 4 hours at 23°C to 27°C (73°F to 81°F) or up to 24 hours at 2°C to 8°C (36°F to 46°F). Solutions diluted for infusion are stable for up to 48 hours at 23°C to 27°C (73°F to 81°F) or up to 8 days at 2°C to 8°C (36°F to 46°F). Infusion should be completed within these time frames; if IV bag of solution for infusion is not administered within the time frames and temperatures indicated, discard; do not refrigerate again.

Mechanism of Action Blinatumomab is a bispecific CD19-directed CD3 T-cell engager which binds to CD19 expressed on B-cells and CD3 expressed on T-cells. It activates endogenous T cells by connecting CD3 in the T-cell receptor complex with CD19 on B-cells (malignant and benign), thus forming a cytolytic synapse between a cytotoxic T-cell and the cancer target B-cell (Topp, 2014). Blinatumomab mediates the production of cytolytic pro-teins, release of inflammatory cytokines, and proliferation of T cells, which result in lysis of CD19-positive cells.

Pharmacodynamics/Kinetics

Distribution: 4.52 L

Half-life elimination: 2.11 hours

Excretion: Urine (negligible amounts)

Dosing

Adult & Geriatric Note: Hospitalization is recommended for the first 9 days of cycle 1, and the first 2 days of cycle 2. Consider hospitalization or close observation by a healthcare professional (or hospitalization) is recom-mended for initiation of all subsequent cycles or for therapy reinitiation (eg, treatment is interrupted for 4 or more hours). Do **not** flush infusion line, particularly when changing infusion bags or at completion of infusion; may result in overdose and complications. Premedicate with dexamethasone 20 mg IV one hour prior to the first dose of each cycle, prior to a step dose (eg, Cycle 1 day 8), or when restarting therapy after an interruption of ≥4 hours.

Acute lymphoblastic leukemia (B-cell precursor), Philadelphia chromosome-negative, relapsed/refractory: Adults ≥45 kg: IV: Each treatment cycle consists of 4 weeks of continuous infusion followed by a 2-week treatment-free interval (allow at least 2 weeks treatment-free between cycles). Therapy involves 2 induction cycles followed by 3 additional cycles for consolidation (total of up to 5 cycles).

Cycle 1: 9 **mcg** daily administered as a continuous infusion on days 1 to 7, followed by 28 **mcg** daily as a continuous infusion on days 8 to 28 of a 6-week treatment cycle

Cycles 2 through 5: 28 **mcg** daily administered as a continuous infusion on days 1 to 28 of a 6-week treatment cycle

Renal Impairment

CrCl ≥30 mL/minute: No dosage adjustment necessary.

CrCl <30 mL/minute: There are no dosage adjustments provided in the manufacturer's labeling (has not been studied).

Hemodialysis: There are no dosage adjustments pro-vided in the manufacturer's labeling (has not been studied).

Hepatic Impairment

There are no dosage adjustments provided in the man-ufacturer's labeling (has not been studied).

Hepatotoxicity during treatment: Interrupt therapy if trans-aminases are >5 times ULN or if bilirubin is >3 times ULN.

Adjustment for Toxicity If the interruption after an adverse event is no longer than 7 days, continue the same cycle to a total of 28 days of infusion inclusive of days before and after the interruption in that cycle. If an interruption due to an adverse event is longer than 7 days, start a new cycle.

Cytokine release syndrome (CRS):

Grade 3: Interrupt therapy until resolved, then resume dosing at 9 **mcg** daily. Increase dose to 28 **mcg** daily after 7 days if toxicity does not recur.

Grade 4: Discontinue permanently

Neurologic toxicity:

Grade 3: Interrupt therapy for at least 3 days and until toxicity is ≤ grade 1 (mild), then resume dosing at 9 **mcg** daily. Increase dose to 28 **mcg** daily after 7 days if toxicity does not recur. If toxicity occurred at the 9 **mcg** daily dose, or if it takes more than 7 days to resolve, discontinue permanently.

Grade 4: Discontinue permanently

Seizure: Discontinue permanently if more than 1 seiz-ure occurs.

Other clinically relevant toxicity:

Grade 3: Interrupt therapy until toxicity is ≤ grade 1 (mild), then resume dosing at 9 mcg daily. Increase dose to 28 mcg daily after 7 days if toxicity does not recur. If toxicity takes more than 14 days to resolve, discontinue permanently.

Grade 4: Discontinue permanently

Administration IV: Administer 240 mL as a continuous IV infusion at a constant flow rate of 10 mL/hour for 24 hours or 5 mL/hour for 48 hours (depending on dose, duration, and/or concentration) through a dedicated lumen. Use a programmable, lockable, non-elastomeric infusion pump with an alarm; IV tubing should include a sterile, non-pyrogenic, low protein-binding, 0.2 micron in-line filter. Only use polyolefin, PVC non-di-ethylhexylphthalate (non-DEHP), or ethyl vinyl acetate (EVA) infusion bags, pump cassettes and IV tubing. IV tubing should be primed with prepared infusion solution, not NS. Premedicate with dexamethasone 20 mg IV one hour prior to the first dose of each cycle, prior to a step dose (such as cycle 1 day 8), or when restarting therapy after an interruption of ≥4 hours.

Do not flush infusion line, particularly when changing infusion bags or at completion of infusion; may result in excess dosage and complications. Do not infuse other medications through the same line.

Monitoring Parameters CBC with differential, liver function tests (ALT, AST, GGT, and total bilirubin) at baseline and throughout therapy; signs/symptoms of cytokine release syndrome, neurotoxicity, infection, and tumor lysis syndrome

Dosage Forms Excipient information presented when available (limited, particularly for generics); consult specific product labeling.

Solution Reconstituted, Intravenous [preservative free]:

Blincyto: 35 mcg (1 ea) [contains polysorbate 80]

♦ Blincyto *see* Blinatumomab *on page 238*

♦ Blisovi 24 Fe *see* Ethinyl Estradiol and Norethindrone *on page 708*

♦ Blisovi Fe 1/20 *see* Ethinyl Estradiol and Norethindrone *on page 708*

♦ Blistex Medicated [OTC] *see* Benzocaine *on page 217*

♦ BLM *see* Bleomycin *on page 237*

♦ Bloxiverz *see* Neostigmine *on page 1268*

♦ BMS-188667 *see* Abatacept *on page 18*

♦ BMS 201038 *see* Lomitapide *on page 1094*

♦ BMS-224818 *see* Belatacept *on page 207*

♦ BMS-232632 *see* Atazanavir *on page 162*

♦ BMS-247550 *see* Ixabepilone *on page 1006*

♦ BMS 337039 *see* ARIPiprazole *on page 148*

♦ BMS-354825 *see* Dasatinib *on page 501*

♦ BMS-477118 *see* Saxagliptin *on page 1638*

♦ BMS-901608 *see* Elotuzumab *on page 625*

♦ BMS-936558 *see* Nivolumab *on page 1293*

♦ B&O *see* Belladonna and Opium *on page 211*

Boceprevir (boe SE pre vir)

Brand Names: US Victrelis
Brand Names: Canada Victrelis
Index Terms SCH503034
Pharmacologic Category Antihepaciviral, Protease Inhibitor (Anti-HCV)

Use Chronic hepatitis C: Treatment of chronic hepatitis C (CHC) genotype 1 (in combination with peginterferon alfa and ribavirin) in adult patients with compensated liver disease (including cirrhosis) who were previously untreated or have failed prior therapy with peginterferon alfa and ribavirin therapy including prior null responders, partial responders, and relapsers

Pregnancy Considerations Adverse events were not observed with boceprevir in animal reproduction studies; however, boceprevir must not be used as monotherapy (must be used in combination with peginterferon alfa and ribavirin). Adverse events have been observed with ribavirin and interferons (specific studies with peginterferon alfa-2a have not been conducted) in animal reproduction studies. Use of ribavirin in combination with peginterferon alfa-2a is contraindicated in pregnant women and males whose female partners are pregnant. A negative pregnancy test is required before initiation of therapy and pregnancy testing should be conducted monthly during treatment and for 6 months after therapy has ended. Women of childbearing potential and males must use at least 2 effective forms of contraception during treatment and continue contraceptive measures for at least 6 months after completion of therapy. One of the two forms of effective contraception may be a combined oral contraceptive product with at least 1 mg of norethindrone; oral contraceptives with <1 mg of norethindrone and other forms of hormonal contraception are contraindicated because they have not been studied. If patient or female partner becomes pregnant during treatment, she should be counseled about potential risks of exposure. Health care providers and patients are encouraged to enroll women exposed to ribavirin during pregnancy or within 6 months after treatment in the Ribavirin Pregnancy Registry (800-593-2214).

Breast-Feeding Considerations It is not known if boceprevir is excreted into breast milk. According to the manufacturer, due to the potential for serious adverse reactions in the nursing infant, a decision should be made whether to discontinue nursing or to discontinue the drug, taking into account the importance of treatment to the mother.

Breast-feeding is not linked to the spread of hepatitis C virus; however, if nipples are cracked or bleeding, breast-feeding is not recommended (CDC, 2010).

Medication Guide Available Yes

Contraindications

Hypersensitivity to boceprevir or any component of the formulation; pregnancy; male partners of pregnant women

Coadministration with CYP3A4/5 highly-dependent substrates (alfuzosin, cisapride, doxazosin, drospirenone, ergot derivatives [dihydroergotamine, ergonovine, ergotamine, methylergonovine], lovastatin, midazolam [oral], pimozide, sildenafil/tadalafil [when used for treatment of pulmonary arterial hypertension], silodosin, simvastatin, tamsulosin, triazolam) or strong CYP3A4/5 inducers (carbamazepine, phenobarbital, phenytoin, rifampin, St John's wort)

Refer to Peginterferon Alfa and Ribavirin monographs for individual product contraindications.

Canadian labeling: Additional contraindications (not in U.S. labeling): Autoimmune hepatitis, hepatic decompensation (Child-Pugh class B or C); coadministration with amiodarone, astemizole, propafenone, quinidine, terfenadine

Warnings/Precautions Combination therapy with ribavirin and interferons may cause birth defects; avoid pregnancy in females and female partners of male patients during therapy and for 6 months following treatment; two forms of effective contraception should be used. Combination therapy with ribavirin and peginterferon alfa-2a is contraindicated in pregnancy. Serious acute hypersensitivity reactions, angioedema and urticaria have been reported with boceprevir, peginterferon alfa, and ribavirin combination therapy. Discontinuation of combination therapy and institution of supportive measures may be necessary. Safety and efficacy have not been established in patients who have uncompensated cirrhosis or have received organ transplants. Monotherapy is not effective for chronic hepatitis C infection. Patients who have less than 0.5-$\log_{10}$ HCV-RNA decline at treatment week 4 with peginterferon alfa and ribavirin when **initiating** boceprevir therapy are predicted to have less than a 2-$\log_{10}$ HCV-RNA decline by treatment week 12. Those poor responders treated with boceprevir will likely not have a sustained virologic response (SVR) and have a predisposition to viral resistance at treatment failure.

Anemia has been reported with peginterferon alfa and ribavirin; addition of boceprevir is associated with further hemoglobin decreases. With anemia management, average hemoglobin decrease in clinical trials was ~1 g/dL. Dose reduction of ribavirin therapy is recommended for the initial management of anemia if hemoglobin <10 g/dL; permanent discontinuation of ribavirin treatment is recommended if hemoglobin <8.5 g/dL. The addition of boceprevir to peginterferon alfa and ribavirin therapy is also associated with a higher incidence of neutropenia. May be severe or life-threatening (rare); discontinuation of therapy may be necessary. Dose reductions of peginterferon alfa and ribavirin were needed more often in patients also taking boceprevir. Serious cases of pancytopenia have been reported in patients receiving boceprevir in combination with peginterferon alfa and ribavirin. Complete blood counts with differential should be obtained pretreatment and at weeks 2, 4, 8, and 12, as well as other times during treatment. If ribavirin is permanently discontinued, boceprevir and peginterferon alfa must also be discontinued.

Adverse Reactions

>10%:

Central nervous system: Fatigue (55% to 58%), chills (33% to 34%), insomnia (30% to 34%), irritability (21% to 22%), dizziness (16% to 19%), headache

Dermatologic: Alopecia (22% to 27%), dry skin (18% to 22%), rash (16% to 17%)

Gastrointestinal: Nausea (43% to 46%), abnormal taste (35% to 44%), appetite decreased (25% to 26%), diarrhea (24% to 25%), vomiting (15% to 20%), xerostomia (11% to 15%)

Hematologic: Anemia (45% to 50%), neutropenia (14% to 31%)

Neuromuscular & skeletal: Arthralgia (19% to 23%), weakness (15% to 21%)

Respiratory: Dyspnea (8% to 11%)

1% to 10%: Hematologic: Thrombocytopenia

<1% (Limited to important or life-threatening): Agranulocytosis, angioedema, drug rash with eosinophilia and systemic symptoms (DRESS) syndrome, exfoliative dermatitis, exfoliative rash, mouth ulceration, pancytopenia, pneumonia, sepsis, Stevens-Johnson syndrome, stomatitis, thromboembolic events, toxic skin eruption, toxicoderma, urticaria

Drug Interactions

Metabolism/Transport Effects Substrate of BCRP, CYP3A4 (major), P-glycoprotein; **Note:** Assignment of Major/Minor substrate status based on clinically relevant drug interaction potential; **Inhibits** CYP3A4 (strong), P-glycoprotein

Avoid Concomitant Use

Avoid concomitant use of Boceprevir with any of the following: Ado-Trastuzumab Emtansine; Alfuzosin; Aprepitant; Astemizole; Avanafil; Axitinib; Barnidipine; Bosutinib; Bromocriptine; Cabozantinib; CarBAMazepine; Ceritinib; Cisapride; Cobicistat; Cobimetinib; Conivaptan; Crizotinib; CYP3A4 Inducers (Strong); Dabrafenib; Dapoxetine; Dihydroergotamine; Domperidone; Doxazosin; Dronedarone; Drospirenone; Efavirenz; Eletriptan; Eplerenone; Ergoloid Mesylates; Ergonovine; Ergotamine; Etravirine; Everolimus; Flibanserin; Fosphenytoin; Halofantrine; Ibrutinib; Irinotecan Products; Isavuconazonium Sulfate; Ivabradine; Lapatinib; Lercanidipine; Lomitapide; Lovastatin; Lurasidone; Macitentan; Methylergonovine; Midazolam; Naloxegol; Nilotinib; NiMODipine; Nisoldipine; Olaparib; Osimertinib; Palbociclib; PHENobarbital; Phenytoin; Pimozide; Primidone; Ranolazine; Red Yeast Rice; Regorafenib; Rifabutin; Rifampin; Salmeterol; Sildenafil; Silodosin; Simeprevir; Simvastatin; Sonidegib; St Johns Wort; Suvorexant; Tamsulosin; Terfenadine; Ticagrelor; Tipranavir; Tolvaptan; Toremifene; Trabectedin; Triazolam; Ulipristal; Vemurafenib; VinCRIStine (Liposomal); Vorapaxar

Increased Effect/Toxicity

Boceprevir may increase the levels/effects of: Ado-Trastuzumab Emtansine; Alfuzosin; Alitretinoin (Systemic); Almotriptan; Alosetron; ALPRAZolam; Amiodarone; Apixaban; Aprepitant; ARIPiprazole; ARIPiprazole Lauroxil; Astemizole; AtorvaSTATin; Avanafil; Axitinib; Barnidipine; Bedaquiline; Bepridil; Bortezomib; Bosentan; Bosutinib; Brentuximab Vedotin; Brexpiprazole; Brinzolamide; Bromocriptine; Budesonide (Nasal); Budesonide (Oral Inhalation); Budesonide (Systemic); Budesonide (Topical); Buprenorphine; Cabazitaxel; Cabozantinib; Cannabis; Cariprazine; Ceritinib; Cilostazol; Cisapride; Clarithromycin; Cobimetinib; Colchicine; Conivaptan; Contraceptives (Progestins); Corticosteroids (Orally Inhaled); Corticosteroids (Systemic); Crizotinib; CycloSPORINE (Systemic); CYP3A4 Substrates; Dabrafenib; Daclatasvir; Dapoxetine; Dasatinib; Desipramine; Digoxin; Dihydroergotamine; Dofetilide; Domperidone; Doxazosin; DOXOrubicin (Conventional); Dronabinol; Dronedarone; Drospirenone; Dutasteride; Efavirenz; Eletriptan; Eliglustat; Eplerenone; Ergoloid Mesylates; Ergonovine; Ergotamine; Erlotinib; Estazolam; Etizolam; Everolimus; FentaNYL; Fesoterodine; Flecainide; Flibanserin; Fluticasone (Nasal); Fluticasone (Oral Inhalation); Fluvastatin; Gefitinib; GuanFACINE; Halofantrine; Hydrocodone; Ibrutinib; Idelalisib; Iloperidone; Imatinib; Imidafenacin; Irinotecan Products; Isavuconazonium Sulfate; Itraconazole; Ivabradine; Ivacaftor; Ixabepilone; Ketoconazole (Systemic); Lacosamide; Lapatinib; Lercanidipine; Levobupivacaine; Levomilnacipran; Lomitapide; Lovastatin; Lumefantrine; Lurasidone; Macitentan; Maraviroc; Methadone; Methylergonovine; MethylPREDNISolone; Midazolam; Mifepristone; Naloxegol; Nilotinib; NiMODipine; Nisoldipine; Olaparib; Osimertinib; Ospemifene; Oxybutynin; OxyCODONE; Palbociclib; Panobinostat; Parecoxib; Paricalcitol; PAZOPanib; Pimecrolimus; Pimozide; Pitavastatin; PONATinib; Posaconazole; Pranlukast; Pravastatin; PrednisoLONE (Systemic); PredniSONE; Propafenone; QUEtiapine; QuiNIDine; Ramelteon; Ranolazine; Red Yeast Rice; Regorafenib; Repaglinide; Retapamulin; Rifabutin; Rilpivirine; RomiDEPsin; Rosuvastatin; Ruxolitinib; Salmeterol; Saxagliptin; Sildenafil; Silodosin; Simeprevir; Simvastatin; Sirolimus; Sonidegib; SORAfenib; Suvorexant; Tacrolimus (Systemic); Tadalafil; Tamsulosin; Tasimelteon; Terfenadine; Tetrahydrocannabinol; Ticagrelor; Tofacitinib;

Tolterodine; Tolvaptan; Toremifene; Trabectedin; TraMADol; TraZODone; Triazolam; Ulipristal; Vardenafil; Vemurafenib; Vilazodone; VinCRIStine (Liposomal); Vindesine; Vinorelbine; Vorapaxar; Voriconazole; Warfarin; Zopiclone; Zuclopenthixol

The levels/effects of Boceprevir may be increased by: Clarithromycin; Cobicistat; CycloSPORINE (Systemic); Itraconazole; Ketoconazole (Systemic); Posaconazole; Voriconazole

Decreased Effect

Boceprevir may decrease the levels/effects of: Buprenorphine; Contraceptives (Estrogens); Escitalopram; Etravirine; Ifosfamide; Methadone; Prasugrel; Protease Inhibitors; Ritonavir; Ticagrelor; Tipranavir; Warfarin

The levels/effects of Boceprevir may be decreased by: Bosentan; CarBAMazepine; CYP3A4 Inducers (Moderate); CYP3A4 Inducers (Strong); Deferasirox; Efavirenz; Fosphenytoin; PHENobarbital; Phenytoin; Primidone; Protease Inhibitors; Rifabutin; Rifampin; Ritonavir; Siltuximab; St Johns Wort; Tipranavir; Tocilizumab

Storage/Stability Store refrigerated at 2°C to 8°C (36°F to 46°F). After dispensing, may be stored at room temperature of up to 25°C (77°F) for 3 months; keep container closed tightly; avoid excessive heat.

Mechanism of Action Binds reversibly to nonstructural protein 3 (NS 3) serine protease and inhibits replication of the hepatitis C virus. Considered a direct-acting antiviral treatment for HCV, also called a specifically targeted antiviral therapy for HCV (STAT-C).

Pharmacodynamics/Kinetics

Absorption: Food (type or timing is not important) enhances absorption by up to 65%

Distribution: V_d: ~772 L

Protein binding: ~75%

Metabolism: Primarily hepatic via aldo-ketoreductase pathway to inactive metabolites. Also some oxidative CYP 3A4/5 metabolism.

Half-life elimination: Plasma: Adults: ~3.4 hours

Time to peak, serum: 2 hours

Excretion: Feces (79%); urine (9%)

Dosing

Adult & Geriatric Note: Victrelis is no longer available in the US.

Treatment of chronic hepatitis C (CHC): Oral: 800 mg 3 times daily (in combination with peginterferon alfa and ribavirin). Missed doses: If a dose is missed, skip dose if it is <2 hours before the next dose; if ≥2 hours before next dose is due, take dose with food and resume normal dosing schedule. **Note:** Boceprevir-containing regimens are **not** recommended for treatment-naive patients or for prior relapse patients nonresponsive to peginterferon/ribavirin regimens with or without an HCV protease inhibitor (AASLD/IDSA, 2014)

Treatment-naive patients without cirrhosis (interferon-responsive [≥1-log₁₀ HCV-RNA decline in viral load] at week 4):

Weeks 1 to 4: Peginterferon alfa with concomitant ribavirin only

Weeks 5 to 8: Boceprevir 800 mg 3 times daily with continued peginterferon alfa and ribavirin

Weeks 9 to 24 (based on HCV-RNA results at week 8):

HCV-RNA **undetectable** or **detectable** at a level of <100 units/mL: Boceprevir 800 mg 3 times daily with continued peginterferon alfa and ribavirin

HCV-RNA ≥100 units/mL but <1,000 units/mL: Boceprevir 800 mg 3 times daily with continued peginterferon alfa and ribavirin. Recheck HCV-RNA at week 12. If HCV-RNA ≥100 units/mL at week 12, discontinue treatment (boceprevir, peginterferon alfa, and ribavirin).

HCV-RNA ≥1,000 units/mL: Discontinue treatment (boceprevir, peginterferon alfa, and ribavirin)

Weeks ≥24:

HCV-RNA **undetectable** at week 8 and week 24: Boceprevir 800 mg 3 times daily with continued peginterferon alfa and ribavirin for 4 additional weeks (through week 28)

HCV-RNA **detectable** (≥100 units/mL but <1,000 units/mL) at week 8 and **undetectable** at week 24:

U.S. labeling: Boceprevir 800 mg 3 times daily with continued peginterferon alfa and ribavirin for 12 additional weeks (through week 36), followed by peginterferon alfa and ribavirin for additional 12 weeks (through week 48)

Canadian labeling: Boceprevir 800 mg 3 times daily with continued peginterferon alfa and ribavirin for 4 additional weeks (through week 28), followed by peginterferon alfa and ribavirin for additional 20 weeks (through week 48)

HCV-RNA **detectable** at week 24: Discontinue treatment (boceprevir, peginterferon alfa, and ribavirin)

Treatment-naive patients (interferon nonresponsive [<0.5-log₁₀ HCV-RNA decline in viral load] at week 4):

Treatment-naive patients (interferon nonresponsive [<0.5-log_{10} HCV-RNA decline in viral load] at week 4):
Note: Manufacturer also recommends consideration of treatment of poor responders [<1-log_{10} HCV-RNA decline in viral load at week 4] in order to maximize rate of sustained virologic response (SVR):
Weeks 1 to 4: Peginterferon alfa with concomitant ribavirin only
Weeks 5 to 48: Boceprevir 800 mg 3 times daily with continued peginterferon alfa and ribavirin

Previously-treated patients without cirrhosis (partial response or relapser): **Note:** Previously treated does not include prior treatment with boceprevir. "Partial response" includes patients with a $≥2$-log_{10} HCV-RNA decrease by week 12, but a nonsustained virologic response thereafter. "Relapser" includes patients with an undetectable HCV-RNA upon completion of previous treatment, but with detectable HCV-RNA during the follow-up period.
Weeks 1 to 4: Peginterferon alfa with concomitant ribavirin only
Weeks 5 to 8: Boceprevir 800 mg 3 times daily with continued peginterferon alfa and ribavirin
Weeks 9 to 24 (based on HCV-RNA results at week 8):
HCV-RNA **undetectable** or <100 units/mL: Boceprevir 800 mg 3 times daily with continued peginterferon alfa and ribavirin
HCV-RNA $≥100$ units/mL but <1,000 units/mL: Boceprevir 800 mg 3 times daily with continued peginterferon alfa and ribavirin. Recheck HCV-RNA at week 12. If HCV-RNA $≥100$ units/mL at week 12, discontinue treatment (boceprevir, peginterferon alfa, and ribavirin).
HCV-RNA $≥1,000$ units/mL: Discontinue treatment (boceprevir, peginterferon alfa, and ribavirin)
Weeks $≥24$:
HCV-RNA **undetectable** at week 8 and week 24: Boceprevir 800 mg 3 times daily with continued peginterferon alfa and ribavirin for 12 additional weeks (through week 36)
HCV-RNA **detectable** ($≥100$ units/mL but <1,000 units/mL) at week 8 and **undetectable** at week 24: Boceprevir 800 mg 3 times daily with continued peginterferon alfa and ribavirin for 12 additional weeks (through week 36), followed by peginterferon alfa and ribavirin for additional 12 weeks (through week 48)
HCV-RNA **detectable** at week 24: Discontinue treatment (boceprevir, peginterferon alfa, and ribavirin)

Previously treated patients with <2-log_{10} HCV-RNA decline by week 12 (prior null responders):
Weeks 1 to 4: Peginterferon alfa with concomitant ribavirin only
Weeks 5 to 8: Boceprevir 800 mg 3 times daily with continued peginterferon alfa and ribavirin
Weeks 9 to 24 (based on HCV-RNA results at week 8):
HCV-RNA **undetectable** or <100 units/mL: Boceprevir 800 mg 3 times daily with continued peginterferon alfa and ribavirin
HCV-RNA $≥100$ units/mL but <1,000 units/mL: Boceprevir 800 mg 3 times daily with continued peginterferon alfa and ribavirin. Recheck HCV-RNA at week 12. If HCV-RNA $≥100$ units/mL at week 12, discontinue treatment (boceprevir, peginterferon alfa, and ribavirin).
HCV-RNA $≥1,000$ units/mL: Discontinue treatment (boceprevir, peginterferon alfa, and ribavirin)
Weeks $≥24$:
HCV-RNA **undetectable** at week 24: Boceprevir 800 mg 3 times daily with continued peginterferon alfa and ribavirin for 24 additional weeks (through week 48)
HCV-RNA **detectable** at week 24: Discontinue treatment (boceprevir, peginterferon alfa, and ribavirin)

Cirrhosis, compensated:
Weeks 1 to 4: Peginterferon alfa with concomitant ribavirin only
Weeks 5 to 8: Boceprevir 800 mg 3 times daily with continued peginterferon alfa and ribavirin
Weeks 9 to 24 (based on HCV-RNA results at week 8):
HCV-RNA **undetectable** or <100 units/mL: Boceprevir 800 mg 3 times daily with continued peginterferon alfa and ribavirin
HCV-RNA $≥100$ units/mL but <1,000 units/mL: Boceprevir 800 mg 3 times daily with continued peginterferon alfa and ribavirin. Recheck HCV-RNA at week 12. If HCV-RNA $≥100$ units/mL at week 12, discontinue treatment (boceprevir, peginterferon alfa, and ribavirin).
HCV-RNA $≥1,000$ units/mL: Discontinue treatment (boceprevir, peginterferon alfa, and ribavirin)

Weeks $≥24$:
HCV-RNA **undetectable** at week 24: Boceprevir 800 mg 3 times daily with continued peginterferon alfa and ribavirin for 24 additional weeks (through week 48)
HCV-RNA **detectable** at week 24: Discontinue treatment (boceprevir, peginterferon alfa, and ribavirin)

Renal Impairment
Mild-to-severe impairment: No dosage adjustment necessary.
ESRD requiring hemodialysis: No dosage adjustment necessary. Not removed by hemodialysis.

Hepatic Impairment
Mild, moderate, or severe impairment: No dosage adjustment necessary.
Compensated cirrhosis: Consider risks and benefits before initiating therapy in patients with compensated cirrhosis who have platelet count less than 100,000/mm³ and serum albumin less than 3.5 g/dL at baseline. Monitor closely for signs of infection and worsening of liver function. Also refer to Peginterferon Alfa and Ribavirin individual monographs.
Decompensated cirrhosis: There are no dosage adjustments provided in manufacturer's labeling (has not been studied); not approved for use in decompensated cirrhosis (safety/efficacy not established). Also refer to Peginterferon Alfa and Ribavirin individual monographs.

Dietary Considerations Take with food. The type or timing of a meal is not important as long as dose is taken with food.

Administration Administer with food (a meal or light snack). Doses should be taken approximately every 7-9 hours. Administer concurrently with peginterferon alfa and ribavirin.

Monitoring Parameters
CBC with differential and platelet count at baseline and at weeks 2, 4, 8 and 12, then periodically (and when clinically indicated)
Baseline serum albumin (patients with compensated cirrhosis)
Serum HCV RNA at baseline, weeks 4, 8, 12 and 24, end of treatment, during treatment follow up, and when clinically indicated
Pretreatment and monthly pregnancy test up to 6 months following discontinuation of therapy for women of childbearing age
Signs of infection and worsening of liver function (especially in compensated cirrhosis)

Reference Range
Treatment futility: HCV-RNA $≥1000$ units/mL at treatment week 8, $≥100$ units/mL at treatment week 12, or confirmed, detectable HCV-RNA at treatment week 24
Rapid virological response (RVR): Absence of detectable HCV RNA after 4 weeks of treatment
Early viral response (EVR): $≥2$-log decrease in HCV RNA after 8-12 weeks of treatment
End of treatment response (ETR): Absence of detectable HCV RNA at end of the recommended treatment period
Sustained treatment response (STR): Absence of HCV RNA in the serum 6 months following completion of full treatment course
Sustained virologic response (SVR): Plasma HCV RNA <25 units/mL at follow up week 24

Additional Information In clinical studies of treatment-naive patients, a sustained virologic response (SVR) with peginterferon alfa, ribavirin, and boceprevir was achieved in ~68% of non-African-American patients versus 40% of controls (peginterferon alfa and ribavirin only). African-American patients had a lower rate of SVR compared to controls (42% to 53% dependent upon treatment duration versus 23% of controls). Rapid virologic response (RVR) at week 4 of lead-in treatment with peginterferon alfa and ribavirin can predict patient success after the addition of boceprevir and guide treatment duration. Patients who have marginal response during the lead-in treatment phase have a lower SVR after the addition of boceprevir; these patients may need close monitoring for regimen adherence and resistance development.

Product Availability Note: Victrelis is no longer available in the US.

Dosage Forms Excipient information presented when available (limited, particularly for generics); consult specific product labeling.
Capsule, Oral:
Victrelis: 200 mg [contains brilliant blue fcf (fd&c blue #1), fd&c red #40, fd&c yellow #10 (quinoline yellow), fd&c yellow #6 (sunset yellow)]

◆ BOL-303224-A see Besifloxacin on page 221
◆ Boniva see Ibandronate on page 901
◆ Boostrix see Diphtheria and Tetanus Toxoids, and Acellular Pertussis Vaccine on page 567

◆ Boostrix-Polio (Can) *see* Diphtheria and Tetanus Toxoids, Acellular Pertussis, and Poliovirus Vaccine *on page 566*

Bortezomib (bore TEZ oh mib)

Brand Names: US Velcade
Brand Names: Canada Bortezomib For Injection; Velcade
Index Terms LDP-341; MLN341; PS-341
Pharmacologic Category Antineoplastic Agent, Proteasome Inhibitor
Use
Mantle cell lymphoma: Treatment of mantle cell lymphoma
Multiple myeloma: Treatment of multiple myeloma
Pregnancy Considerations Adverse effects (fetal loss and decreased fetal weight) were observed in animal reproduction studies at doses less than the equivalent human dose (based on BSA). Women of reproductive potential should avoid becoming pregnant and should use effective contraception during treatment. The Canadian labeling recommends that females and males of reproductive potential use effective contraception during treatment and for 3 months following treatment.
Breast-Feeding Considerations It is not known if bortezomib is excreted in breast milk. Due to the potential for serious adverse reactions in the nursing infant, the decision to discontinue bortezomib or to discontinue breast-feeding should take into account the benefits of treatment to the mother.
Contraindications Hypersensitivity (excluding local reactions) to bortezomib, boron, mannitol, or any component of the formulation; administration via the intrathecal route
Warnings/Precautions Hazardous agent - use appropriate precautions for handling and disposal (NIOSH 2014 [group 1]). May cause or worsen peripheral neuropathy (usually sensory but may be mixed sensorimotor); risk may be increased with previous use of neurotoxic agents or preexisting peripheral neuropathy (patients with preexisting neuropathy should use only after risk versus benefit assessment); monitor for signs and symptoms; adjustment of dose and/or schedule may be required. The incidence of grades 2 and 3 peripheral neuropathy may be lower with SubQ route (compared to IV); consider subQ administration in patients with preexisting or at high risk for peripheral neuropathy; the majority of patients with ≥ grade 2 peripheral neuropathy have improvement in or resolution of symptoms with dose adjustments or discontinuation; in a study of elderly patients receiving a weekly bortezomib schedule with combination chemotherapy, the incidence of peripheral neuropathy was significantly reduced without an effect on outcome (Boccadoro, 2010; Palumbo, 2009). May cause hypotension (including postural and orthostatic); use caution with dehydration, history of syncope, or medications associated with hypotension (may require adjustment of antihypertensive medication, hydration, and mineralocorticoids and/or sympathomimetics). Has been associated with the development or exacerbation of heart failure (HF) and decreased left ventricular ejection fraction (LVEF); monitor closely in patients with risk factors for HF or existing heart disease, although HF and decreased LVEF have been observed in patients without risk factors. Has also been associated with isolated reports of QTc prolongation.

Pulmonary disorders (some fatal) including pneumonitis, interstitial pneumonia, lung infiltrates, and acute respiratory distress syndrome (ARDS) have been reported. Pulmonary hypertension (without left heart failure or significant pulmonary disease has been reported rarely). Promptly evaluate with new or worsening cardiopulmonary symptoms; therapy interruption may be required. Tumor lysis syndrome has been reported; risk is increased in patients with high tumor burden prior to treatment. Posterior reversible leukoencephalopathy syndrome (PRES, formerly RPLS) has been reported (rarely). Symptoms of PRES include confusion, headache, hypertension, lethargy, seizure, blindness and/or other vision, or neurologic disturbances; discontinue bortezomib if PRES occurs. MRI is recommended to confirm PRES diagnosis. The safety of reinitiating bortezomib in patients previously experiencing PRES is unknown. Progressive multifocal leukoencephalopathy (PML) has been rarely observed; monitor closely and evaluate promptly. Herpes (zoster and simplex) reactivation has been reported with bortezomib; consider antiviral prophylaxis during therapy. Hematologic toxicity, including grade 3 and 4 neutropenia and severe thrombocytopenia, may occur (nadirs generally occur following the last dose of a cycle and recover prior to the next cycle); risk is increased in patients with pretreatment platelet counts <75,000/µL; frequent monitoring is required throughout treatment; may require dosage or schedule adjustments; withhold treatment for platelets <30,000/µL. Management with platelet transfusions and supportive care may be necessary. Hemorrhage (gastrointestinal and intracerebral) due to low platelet count has been observed. Acute liver failure has been reported (rarely) in patients receiving multiple concomitant medications and with serious underlying conditions. Hepatitis, transaminase increases, and hyperbilirubinemia have also been reported; interrupt therapy to assess reversibility. Use caution in patients with hepatic dysfunction; reduced initial doses are recommended for moderate and severe hepatic impairment (exposure is increased); closely monitor for toxicities. Hyper- and hypoglycemia may occur in diabetic patients receiving oral hypoglycemics; may require adjustment of diabetes medications. Nausea, vomiting, diarrhea or constipation may occur; may require antiemetics or antidiarrheals; ileus may occur; administer fluid and electrolytes to prevent dehydration (monitor closely); interrupt therapy for severe symptoms.

Potentially significant drug-drug/drug-food interactions may exist, requiring dose or frequency adjustment, additional monitoring, and/or selection of alternative therapy. Coadministration of strong CYP3A4 inhibitors may increase bortezomib exposure; monitor for toxicity and consider dose reduction if concurrent therapy cannot be avoided. Efficacy may be reduced when administered with strong CYP3A4 inducers; concomitant use is not recommended.

For IV or SubQ administration only. Intrathecal administration is contraindicated; inadvertent intrathecal administration has resulted in death. Bortezomib should **NOT** be prepared during the preparation of any intrathecal medications. After preparation, keep bortezomib in a location **away** from the separate storage location recommended for intrathecal medications. Bortezomib should **NOT** be delivered to the patient at the same time with any medications intended for central nervous system administration. The reconstituted concentrations for IV and SubQ administration are different; use caution when calculating the volume for each route and dose. The manufacturer provides stickers to facilitate identification of the route for reconstituted vials.

Adverse Reactions Incidences reported are associated with monotherapy. Additional adverse reactions reported with mono- or combination therapy; frequency not defined.
Cardiovascular: Hypotension (8% to 9%; grades 3/4: ≤2%), cardiac disease (treatment emergent; 8%), acute pulmonary edema (≤1%), cardiac failure (≤1%), cardiogenic shock (≤1%), pulmonary edema (≤1%), aggravated atrial fibrillation, angina pectoris, atrial flutter, atrioventricular block, bradycardia, cerebrovascular accident, deep vein thrombosis, edema, embolism (peripheral), facial edema, hemorrhagic stroke, hypertension, ischemic heart disease, myocardial infarction, pericardial effusion, pericarditis, peripheral edema, phlebitis, portal vein thrombosis, pulmonary embolism, septic shock, sinoatrial arrest, subdural hematoma, torsades de pointes, transient ischemic attacks, ventricular tachycardia
Central nervous system: Peripheral neuropathy (IV 35% to 54%; SubQ 37%; grade ≥2: 24% to 39%; grade ≥3: SubQ 5% to 6%; IV 7% to 15%; grade 4: <1%), fatigue (7% to 52%), neuralgia (23%), headache (10% to 19%), paresthesia (7% to 19%), dizziness (10% to 18%; excludes vertigo), agitation, anxiety, ataxia, brain disease, cerebral hemorrhage, chills, coma, confusion, cranial nerve palsy, dysarthria, dysautonomia, dysesthesia, insomnia, malaise, mental status changes, motor dysfunction, paralysis, psychosis, seizure, spinal cord compression, suicidal ideation, vertigo
Dermatologic: Skin rash (12% to 23%), pruritus, urticaria
Endocrine & metabolic: Dehydration (2%), amyloid heart disease, hyperglycemia (diabetic patients), hyperkalemia, hypernatremia, hyperuricemia, hypocalcemia, hypoglycemia (diabetic patients), hypokalemia, hyponatremia, weight loss
Gastrointestinal: Diarrhea (19% to 52%), nausea (14% to 52%), constipation (24% to 34%), vomiting (9% to 29%), anorexia (14% to 21%), abdominal pain (11%), decreased appetite (11%), cholestasis, duodenitis (hemorrhagic), dysphagia, fecal impaction, gastritis (hemorrhagic), gastroenteritis, gastroesophageal reflux disease, hematemesis, intestinal obstruction, intestinal perforation, melena, oral candidiasis, pancreatitis, paralytic ileus, peritonitis, stomatitis
Genitourinary: Bladder spasm, hematuria, hemorrhagic cystitis, urinary incontinence, urinary retention, urinary tract infection

Hematologic & oncologic: Thrombocytopenia (16% to 52%; grade 3: 5% to 24%; grade 4: 3% to 7%; nadir: Day 11; recovery: By day 21), neutropenia (5% to 27%; grade 3: 8% to 18%; grade 4: 2% to 4%; nadir: Day 11; recovery: By day 21), anemia (12% to 23%; grade 3: 4% to 6%; grade 4: <1%). leukopenia (18% to 20%; grade 3: 5%; grade 4: ≤1%), hemorrhage (≥ grade 3: 2%), disseminated intravascular coagulation, febrile neutropenia, lymphocytopenia, oral mucosal petechiae

Hepatic: Ascites, hepatic failure, hepatic hemorrhage, hepatitis, hyperbilirubinemia

Hypersensitivity: Anaphylaxis, angioedema, hypersensitivity, hypersensitivity angiitis

Infection: Herpes zoster (reactivation; 6% to 11%), herpes simplex infection (1% to 3%), herpes zoster (1% to 2%), aspergillosis, bacteremia, listeriosis, toxoplasmosis

Local: Injection site reaction (mostly redness; SubQ 6%), irritation at injection site (IV 5%), catheter infection

Neuromuscular & skeletal: Weakness (7% to 16%), arthralgia, back pain, bone fracture, limb pain, myalgia, ostealgia

Ophthalmic: Blurred vision, conjunctival infection, conjunctival irritation, diplopia

Otic: Auditory impairment

Renal: Bilateral hydronephrosis, nephrolithiasis, proliferative glomerulonephritis, renal failure

Respiratory: Dyspnea (11%), pneumonia (1% to 3%), adult respiratory distress syndrome, aspiration pneumonia, atelectasis, bronchitis, chronic obstructive pulmonary disease (exacerbation), cough, epistaxis, hemoptysis, hypoxia, laryngeal edema, nasopharyngitis, pleural effusion, pneumonitis, pulmonary hypertension, pulmonary infiltrates (including diffuse), respiratory tract infection, sinusitis

Miscellaneous: Fever (8% to 23%)

<1% (Limited to important or life-threatening): Acute ischemic stroke, amyloidosis, blindness, cardiac arrest, cardiac tamponade, deafness (bilateral), decreased left ventricular ejection fraction, dysgeusia, dyspepsia, herpes meningoencephalitis, increased gamma-glutamyl transferase, increased serum alkaline phosphatase, increased serum transaminases, interstitial pneumonitis, ischemic colitis, ocular herpes simplex, optic neuritis, progressive multifocal leukoencephalopathy, prolonged QT interval on ECG, respiratory failure, reversible posterior leukoencephalopathy syndrome, sepsis, SIADH, Stevens-Johnson syndrome, subarachnoid hemorrhage, Sweet syndrome, syncope, tachycardia, toxic epidermal necrolysis, tumor lysis syndrome

Drug Interactions

Metabolism/Transport Effects Substrate of CYP1A2 (minor), CYP2C19 (major), CYP2C9 (minor), CYP2D6 (minor), CYP3A4 (major); **Note:** Assignment of Major/Minor substrate status based on clinically relevant drug interaction potential; **Inhibits** CYP1A2 (weak), CYP2C19 (moderate), CYP2C9 (weak), CYP2D6 (weak)

Avoid Concomitant Use

Avoid concomitant use of Bortezomib with any of the following: BCG (Intravesical); CYP3A4 Inducers (Strong); Deferiprone; Dipyrone; Green Tea; St Johns Wort

Increased Effect/Toxicity

Bortezomib may increase the levels/effects of: Amifostine; Antipsychotic Agents (Second Generation [Atypical]); ARIPiprazole; Cilostazol; Citalopram; CloZAPine; CYP2C19 Substrates; Deferiprone; DULoxetine; Highest Risk QTc-Prolonging Agents; Hypotension-Associated Agents; Levodopa; Moderate Risk QTc-Prolonging Agents; TiZANidine

The levels/effects of Bortezomib may be increased by: Alfuzosin; Barbiturates; Blood Pressure Lowering Agents; Brimonidine (Topical); CYP3A4 Inhibitors (Strong); Diazoxide; Dipyrone; Herbs (Hypotensive Properties); Mifepristone; Molsidomine; Nicorandil; Obinutuzumab; Osimertinib; Pentoxifylline; Phosphodiesterase 5 Inhibitors; Prostacyclin Analogues

Decreased Effect

Bortezomib may decrease the levels/effects of: BCG (Intravesical); Clopidogrel

The levels/effects of Bortezomib may be decreased by: Ascorbic Acid; Bosentan; CYP2C19 Inducers (Strong); CYP3A4 Inducers (Moderate); CYP3A4 Inducers (Strong); Dabrafenib; Deferasirox; Green Tea; Multivitamins/Fluoride (with ADE); Multivitamins/Minerals (with ADEK, Folate, Iron); Multivitamins/Minerals (with AE, No Iron); Osimertinib; Siltuximab; St Johns Wort; Tocilizumab

Preparation for Administration Note: The reconstituted concentrations for IV and SubQ administration are different; the manufacturer provides stickers to facilitate identification of the route for reconstituted vials. The amount contained in each vial may exceed the prescribed dose; use care with dosage and volume calculations.

Hazardous agent; use appropriate precautions for handling and disposal (NIOSH 2014 [group 1]). Reconstitute only with normal saline (NS). Reconstituted solutions should be clear and colorless.

IV: Reconstitute each 3.5 mg vial with 3.5 mL NS to a concentration of 1 mg/mL.

SubQ: Reconstitute each 3.5 mg vial with 1.4 mL NS to a concentration of 2.5 mg/mL (Moreau, 2011). If injection site reaction occurs, the more dilute 1 mg/mL concentration may be used SubQ.

Storage/Stability Prior to reconstitution, store intact vials at 25°C (77°F); excursions are permitted between 15°C and 30°C (59°F and 86°F). Once reconstituted, the manufacturer recommends use within 8 hours of reconstitution. However, stability studies have demonstrated solutions of 1 mg/mL (vial or syringe) may be stored at room temperature for up to 3 days, or under refrigeration for up to 5 days (Andre, 2005); or refrigerated in the original vial for up to 15 days (Vanderloo, 2010). Protect from light. After preparation, keep bortezomib in a location away from the separate storage location recommended for intrathecal medications.

Mechanism of Action Bortezomib inhibits proteasomes, enzyme complexes which regulate protein homeostasis within the cell. Specifically, it reversibly inhibits chymotrypsin-like activity at the 26S proteasome, leading to activation of signaling cascades, cell-cycle arrest, and apoptosis.

Pharmacodynamics/Kinetics

Distribution: 498 to 1884 L/m^2; distributes widely to peripheral tissues

Protein binding: ~83%

Metabolism: Hepatic primarily via CYP2C19 and 3A4 and to a lesser extent CYP1A2; forms metabolites (inactive) via deboronization followed by hydroxylation

Half-life elimination: Single dose: IV: 9 to 15 hours; Multiple dosing: 1 mg/m^2: 40 to 193 hours; 1.3 mg/m^2: 76 to 108 hours

Dosing

Adult & Geriatric Note: Consecutive doses should be separated by at least 72 hours.

Multiple myeloma (first-line therapy; in combination with melphalan and prednisone): IV, SubQ: 1.3 mg/m^2 days 1, 4, 8, 11, 22, 25, 29, and 32 of a 42-day treatment cycle for 4 cycles, followed by 1.3 mg/m^2 days 1, 8, 22, and 29 of a 42-day treatment cycle for 5 cycles.

Retreatment may be considered for multiple myeloma patients who had previously responded to bortezomib (either as monotherapy or in combination) and who have relapsed at least 6 months after completing prior bortezomib therapy; initiate at the last tolerated dose.

Transplant-eligible patients (first-line therapy; in combination with other chemotherapy agents) (Canadian labeling): IV: 1.3 mg/m^2 days 1, 4, 8, and 11 followed by a rest period of up to 20 days (equals one treatment cycle); administer 3 to 6 cycles.

Alternative first-line therapy (off-label dosing):

CyBorD regimen: IV: 1.5 mg/m^2 days 1, 8, 15, and 22 of a 28-day treatment cycle for 4 cycles (may continue beyond 4 cycles) in combination with cyclophosphamide and dexamethasone (Khan, 2012)

PAD regimen: IV: Induction: 1.3 mg/m^2 days 1, 4, 8, and 11 of a 28-day treatment cycle for 3 cycles (in combination with doxorubicin and dexamethasone), followed by conditioning/stem cell transplantation, and then maintenance bortezomib 1.3 mg/m^2 once every 2 weeks for 2 years (Sonneveld, 2012)

VRd regimen: IV: 1.3 mg/m^2 days 1, 4, 8, and 11 of a 21-day treatment cycle for 8 cycles (in combination with lenalidomide and dexamethasone) (Kumar, 2012; Richardson, 2010)

Patients ≥65 years: IV: 1.3 mg/m^2 days 1, 8, 15, and 22 of a 35-day treatment cycle, in combination with **either** melphalan and prednisone or melphalan, prednisone, and thalidomide (Boccadoro, 2010; Bringhen, 2010; Palumbo, 2009)

Multiple myeloma (relapsed): IV, SubQ: 1.3 mg/m^2 twice weekly for 2 weeks on days 1, 4, 8, and 11 of a 21-day treatment cycle. Therapy extending beyond 8 cycles may be administered by the standard schedule or may be given once weekly for 4 weeks (days 1, 8, 15, and 22), followed by a 13-day rest (days 23 through 35).

Retreatment may be considered for multiple myeloma patients who had previously responded to bortezomib (either as monotherapy or in combination) and who have relapsed at least 6 months after completing prior

bortezomib therapy; initiate at the last tolerated dose. Administer twice weekly for 2 weeks on days 1, 4, 8, and 11 of a 21-day treatment cycle (either as a single-agent or in combination with dexamethasone) for a maximum of 8 cycles.

Alternative relapsed therapy (off-label dosing): IV: 1.3 mg/m^2 days 1, 4, 8, and 11 of a 21-day treatment cycle for at least 8 cycles or until disease progression or unacceptable toxicity (in combination with liposomal doxorubicin) (Orlowski, 2007)

Mantle cell lymphoma (first-line therapy; in combination with rituximab, cyclophosphamide, doxorubicin, and prednisone [VcR-CAP]): IV: 1.3 mg/m^2 days 1, 4, 8, 11 of a 21-day treatment cycle for 6 cycles. If response first documented at cycle 6, treatment for an additional 2 cycles is recommended.

Mantle cell lymphoma (relapsed): IV, SubQ: 1.3 mg/m^2 twice weekly for 2 weeks on days 1, 4, 8, and 11 of a 21-day treatment cycle. Therapy extending beyond 8 cycles may be administered by the standard schedule or may be given once weekly for 4 weeks (days 1, 8, 15, and 22), followed by a 13-day rest (days 23 through 35).

Cutaneous or peripheral T-cell lymphoma, relapsed/refractory (off-label use): IV: 1.3 mg/m^2 twice weekly for 2 weeks on days 1, 4, 8, and 11 of a 21-day treatment cycle (Zinzani, 2007); additional data may be necessary to further define the role of bortezomib in this condition.

Follicular lymphoma, relapsed/refractory (off-label use): IV: 1.3 mg/m^2 days 1, 4, 8, and 11 of a 28-day treatment cycle, in combination with bendamustine and rituximab for 6 cycles (Friedberg, 2011) **or** 1.6 mg/m^2 days 1, 8, 15, and 22 of a 35-day treatment cycle, in combination with bendamustine and rituximab for 5 cycles (Fowler, 2011)

Systemic light-chain amyloidosis (off-label use): IV: 1.3 mg/m^2 days 1, 4, 8, and 11 of a 21-day treatment cycle (with or without dexamethasone) (Kastritis, 2010)

Waldenström's macroglobulinemia, relapsed/refractory (off-label use): IV: 1.3 mg/m^2 days 1, 4, 8, and 11 of a 21-day treatment cycle (Chen, 2007) **or** 1.3 mg/m^2 days 1, 4, 8, and 11 of a 21-day treatment cycle (in combination with dexamethasone and rituximab) (Treon, 2009) **or** 1.6 mg/m^2 days 1, 8, and 15 of a 28-day treatment cycle (in combination with rituximab) (Ghobrial, 2010)

Renal Impairment No dosage adjustment is necessary. Dialysis may reduce bortezomib concentrations; administer postdialysis (Leal, 2011).

Hepatic Impairment

Mild impairment (bilirubin ≤1 times ULN and AST >ULN or bilirubin >1 to 1.5 times ULN): No initial dose adjustment is necessary (LoRusso, 2012).

Moderate (bilirubin >1.5 to 3 times ULN) and severe impairment (bilirubin >3 times ULN): Reduce initial dose to 0.7 mg/m^2 in the first cycle; based on patient tolerance, may consider dose escalation to 1 mg/m^2 (LoRusso, 2012) or further dose reduction to 0.5 mg/m^2 in subsequent cycles

Obesity *ASCO Guidelines for appropriate chemotherapy dosing in obese adults with cancer:* Utilize patient's actual body weight (full weight) for calculation of body surface area- or weight-based dosing, particularly when the intent of therapy is curative; manage regimen-related toxicities in the same manner as for nonobese patients; if a dose reduction is utilized due to toxicity, consider resumption of full weight-based dosing with subsequent cycles, especially if cause of toxicity (eg, hepatic or renal impairment) is resolved (Griggs, 2012).

Adjustment for Toxicity

Myeloma (first-line therapy):

Platelets should be ≥70,000/mm^3, ANC should be ≥1000/mm^3, and nonhematologic toxicities should resolve to grade 1 or baseline prior to therapy initiation.

Platelets ≤30,000/mm^3 or ANC ≤750/mm^3 on bortezomib day(s) (except day 1): Withhold bortezomib; if several bortezomib doses in consecutive cycles are withheld, reduce dose 1 level (1.3 mg/m^2/dose reduced to 1 mg/m^2/dose; 1 mg/m^2/dose reduced to 0.7 mg/m^2/dose)

Grade ≥3 nonhematological toxicity (other than neuropathy): Withhold bortezomib until toxicity resolves to grade 1 or baseline. May reinitiate bortezomib at 1 dose level reduction (1.3 mg/m^2/dose reduced to 1 mg/m^2/dose; 1 mg/m^2/dose reduced to 0.7 mg/m^2/dose).

Neuropathic pain and/or peripheral sensory or motor neuropathy: See "Neuropathic pain and/or peripheral sensory or motor neuropathy" toxicity adjustment guidelines below.

Mantle cell lymphoma (first-line therapy):

Platelets should be ≥100,000/mm^3, ANC should be ≥1,500/mm^3, hemoglobin should be ≥8 g/dL, and nonhematologic toxicities should resolve to grade 1 or baseline prior to each cycle (cycle 2 and beyond).

Platelets <25,000/mm^3 or ≥ grade 3 neutropenia on bortezomib day(s) (except day 1): Withhold bortezomib for up to 2 weeks until platelets are ≥25,000/mm^3 and/or ANC ≥750/mm^3, then reduce dose 1 level (1.3 mg/m^2/dose reduced to 1 mg/m^2/dose; 1 mg/m^2/dose reduced to 0.7 mg/m^2/dose). If hematologic toxicity does not resolve after withholding therapy, discontinue bortezomib.

Grade ≥3 nonhematological toxicity (other than neuropathy): Withhold bortezomib until toxicity resolves to ≤ grade 2. May reinitiate bortezomib at 1 dose level reduction (1.3 mg/m^2/dose reduced to 1 mg/m^2/dose; 1 mg/m^2/dose reduced to 0.7 mg/m^2/dose).

Neuropathic pain and/or peripheral sensory or motor neuropathy: See "Neuropathic pain and/or peripheral sensory or motor neuropathy" toxicity adjustment guidelines below.

Relapsed multiple myeloma and mantle cell lymphoma:

Grade 3 nonhematological (excluding neuropathy) or grade 4 hematological toxicity: Withhold until toxicity resolved; may reinitiate with a 25% dose reduction (1.3 mg/m^2/dose reduced to 1 mg/m^2/dose; 1 mg/m^2/dose reduced to 0.7 mg/m^2/dose)

Neuropathic pain and/or peripheral sensory, motor, or autonomic neuropathy:

Note: Consider subQ administration in patients with preexisting or at high risk for peripheral neuropathy.

Grade 1 (asymptomatic; deep tendon reflex loss or paresthesia) without pain or loss of function: No action needed

Grade 1 with pain or grade 2 (moderate symptoms; limiting instrumental activities of daily living): Reduce dose to 1 mg/m^2

Grade 2 with pain or grade 3 (severe symptoms; limiting self-care activities of daily living): Withhold until toxicity resolved, may reinitiate at 0.7 mg/m^2 once weekly

Grade 4 (life-threatening consequences with urgent intervention indicated) and/or severe autonomic neuropathy: Discontinue therapy.

Dietary Considerations Green tea and green tea extracts may diminish the therapeutic effect of bortezomib and should be avoided (Golden, 2009). Avoid grapefruit juice. Avoid additional, nondietary sources of ascorbic acid supplements, including multivitamins containing ascorbic acid (may diminish bortezomib activity) during treatment, especially 12 hours before and after bortezomib treatment (Perrone, 2009).

Administration Note: The reconstituted concentrations for IV and SubQ administration are different; use caution when calculating the volume for each route and dose. Consider SubQ administration in patients with preexisting or at high risk for peripheral neuropathy.

IV: Administer via rapid IV push (3-5 seconds). When administering in combination with rituximab for first-line therapy of mantle cell lymphoma, administer bortezomib prior to rituximab.

SubQ: Subcutaneous administration of bortezomib 1.3 mg/m^2 days 1, 4, 8, and 11 of a 21-day treatment cycle has been studied in a limited number of patients with relapsed multiple myeloma; doses were administered subcutaneously (concentration of 2.5 mg/mL) into the thigh or abdomen, rotating the injection site with each dose; injections at the same site within a single cycle were avoided (Moreau, 2010; Moreau, 2011). Response rates were similar to IV administration; decreased incidence of grade 3 or higher adverse events were observed with SubQ administration. Administer at least 1 inch from an old site and never administer to tender, bruised, erythematous, or indurated sites. If injection site reaction occurs, the more dilute 1 mg/mL concentration may be used SubQ (or IV administration of 1 mg/mL concentration may be considered).

For IV or SubQ administration only; fatalities have been reported with inadvertent intrathecal administration. Bortezomib should **NOT** be delivered to the patient at the same time with any medications intended for central nervous system administration.

Hazardous agent; use appropriate precautions for handling and disposal (NIOSH 2014 [group 1]).

Monitoring Parameters CBC with differential and platelets (monitor frequently throughout therapy); liver function tests (in patients with existing hepatic impairment); signs/symptoms of peripheral neuropathy, dehydration, hypotension, PRES, or PML; renal function, baseline chest x-ray

and then periodic pulmonary function testing (with new or worsening pulmonary symptoms)

Dosage Forms Excipient information presented when available (limited, particularly for generics); consult specific product labeling.

Solution Reconstituted, Injection:
Velcade: 3.5 mg (1 ea)

◆ Bortezomib For Injection (Can) *see* Bortezomib on page 243

Bosentan (boe SEN tan)

Brand Names: US Tracleer

Brand Names: Canada ACT Bosentan; Mylan-Bosentan; PMS-Bosentan; Sandoz-Bosentan; Teva-Bosentan; Tracleer

Pharmacologic Category Endothelin Receptor Antagonist; Vasodilator

Use Treatment of pulmonary artery hypertension (PAH) (WHO Group I) in patients with WHO/NYHA Class II, III, or IV symptoms to improve exercise capacity and decrease the rate of clinical deterioration. **Note:** According to treatment guidelines from the Fifth World Symposium on Pulmonary Hypertension (WSPH), only a small number of PAH patients with WHO-FC IV symptoms (ie, severely ill patients) were included in clinical trials, therefore, most experts consider bosentan second-line therapy in these patients (WSPH [Gailè 2013]).

Pregnancy Considerations [U.S. Boxed Warning]: May cause birth defects; use in pregnancy is contraindicated. Exclude pregnancy prior to initiation of therapy and obtain pregnancy tests monthly during treatment. Reliable contraception must be used during therapy and for 1 month after stopping treatment. Hormonal contraceptives (oral, injectable, transdermal, or implantable) may not be effective and a second method of contraception (nonhormonal) is required. Patients with tubal ligation or an implanted IUD (Copper T 380A or LNg 20) do not need additional contraceptive measures. When a hormonal or barrier contraceptive is used, one additional method of contraception is still needed if a male partner has had a vasectomy. When initiating treatment for women of reproductive potential, a negative pregnancy test should be documented within the first 5 days of a normal menstrual period and ≥11 days after the last unprotected intercourse. A missed menses or suspected pregnancy should be reported to a healthcare provider and prompt immediate pregnancy testing. Sperm counts may be reduced in men during treatment. Women of childbearing potential should avoid splitting, crushing, or handling broken tablets and exposure to the generated dust (tablet splitting is currently outside of product labeling).

Breast-Feeding Considerations It is not known if bosentan is excreted in breast milk. Due to the potential for serious adverse reactions in the nursing infant, the manufacturer recommends a decision be made whether to discontinue nursing or to discontinue the drug, taking into account the importance of treatment to the mother.

Prescribing and Access Restrictions As a requirement of the REMS program, access to this medication is restricted. Bosentan (Tracleer) is only available through Tracleer REMS Program. Only prescribers and pharmacies registered with Tracleer REMS Program may prescribe and dispense bosentan. Further information may be obtained from the manufacturer, Actelion Pharmaceuticals (1-866-228-3546 or http://www.tracleer.com/hcp/prescribing-tracleer.asp).

Medication Guide Available Yes

Contraindications Hypersensitivity to bosentan or any component of the formulation; concurrent use of cyclosporine or glyburide; pregnancy

Canadian labeling: Additional contraindications (not in U.S. labeling): Moderate-to-severe hepatic impairment and/or baseline ALT or AST >3 times the upper limit of normal (ULN), particularly when total bilirubin >2 times ULN

Warnings/Precautions Hazardous agent - use appropriate precautions for handling and disposal (NIOSH 2014 [group 3]). **[U.S. Boxed Warning]: May cause hepatotoxicity; has been associated with a high incidence (~11%) of significant transaminase elevations (ALT or AST ≥3 times ULN) with or without elevations in bilirubin and rare cases of unexplained hepatic cirrhosis (after >12 months of therapy) or hepatic failure. Monitor transaminases at baseline then monthly thereafter. Adjust dosage if elevations in liver enzymes occur without symptoms of hepatic injury or elevated bilirubin. Treatment should be stopped in patients who develop elevated transaminases either in combination with symptoms of hepatic injury (unusual fatigue, jaundice, nausea, vomiting, abdominal pain, and/or fever) or elevated bilirubin (≥2 times ULN); safety of reintroduction is unknown. Avoid use in patients with baseline serum transaminases >3 times ULN or moderate-to-severe hepatic impairment.** Transaminase elevations are dose dependent, generally asymptomatic, occur both early and late in therapy, progress slowly, and are usually reversible after treatment interruption or discontinuation. Consider the benefits of treatment versus the risk of hepatotoxicity when initiating therapy in patients with WHO Class II symptoms.

[U.S. Boxed Warning]: May cause birth defects; use in pregnancy is contraindicated. Exclude pregnancy prior to initiation of therapy and obtain pregnancy tests monthly during treatment. Reliable contraception must be used during therapy and for 1 month after stopping treatment. Hormonal contraceptives (oral, injectable, transdermal, or implantable) may not be effective and a second method of contraception (nonhormonal) is required. Patients with tubal ligation or an implanted IUD (Copper T 380A or LNg 20) do not need additional contraceptive measures. (See Pregnancy Considerations.)

[U.S. Boxed Warning]: Because of the risks of hepatic impairment and the high likelihood of teratogenic effects, bosentan is only available through the T.A.P. restricted distribution program. Patients, prescribers, and pharmacies must be registered with and meet conditions of T.A.P. Call 1-866-228-3546 or visit http://www.tracleer.com/hcp/prescribing-tracleer.asp for more information.

A reduction in hematocrit/hemoglobin may be observed within the first few weeks of therapy with subsequent stabilization of levels. Hemoglobin reductions >15% have been observed in some patients. Measure hemoglobin prior to initiating therapy, at 1 and 3 months, and every 3 months thereafter. Significant decreases in hemoglobin in the absence of other causes may warrant the discontinuation of therapy.

Development of peripheral edema due to treatment and/or disease state (pulmonary arterial hypertension) may occur. There have also been postmarketing reports of fluid retention requiring treatment (eg, diuretics, fluid management, hospitalization). Further evaluation may be necessary to determine cause and appropriate treatment or discontinuation of therapy. Bosentan should be discontinued in any patient with pulmonary edema suggestive of pulmonary veno-occlusive disease (PVOD). Bosentan may interact with many medications, resulting in potentially serious and/or life-threatening adverse events (see Drug Interactions).

Adverse Reactions

>10%:
Cardiovascular: Edema (11%)
Central nervous system: Headache (15%)
Genitourinary: Inhibition of spermatogenesis (25%)
Hematologic & oncologic: Decreased hemoglobin (typically in first 6 weeks of therapy; ≥1 g/dL: ≤57%; <11 g/dL: 3% to 6%)
Hepatic: Increased serum transaminases (≥3 times ULN: ≤12%; dose-related)
Respiratory: Respiratory tract infection (22%)

1% to 10%:
Cardiovascular: Chest pain (5%), syncope (5%), flushing (4%), hypotension (4%), palpitations (4%)
Dermatologic: Pruritus (2%)
Hematologic & oncologic: Anemia (3%)
Hepatic: Hepatic insufficiency (4%)
Neuromuscular & skeletal: Arthralgia (4%)
Respiratory: Sinusitis (4%)

<1% (Limited to important or life-threatening): Anaphylaxis, angioedema, hepatic cirrhosis (prolonged therapy), hepatic failure (rare), hyperbilirubinemia, hypersensitivity, hypersensitivity angiitis, jaundice, leukopenia, neutropenia, peripheral edema, skin rash, thrombocytopenia, weight gain, worsening of heart failure

Drug Interactions

Metabolism/Transport Effects Substrate of CYP2C9 (minor), CYP3A4 (minor), SLCO1B1; **Note:** Assignment of Major/Minor substrate status based on clinically relevant drug interaction potential; **Induces** CYP2C9 (weak/moderate), CYP3A4 (moderate)

Avoid Concomitant Use

Avoid concomitant use of Bosentan with any of the following: Antihepaciviral Combination Products; Axitinib; Bedaquiline; Bosutinib; Cobimetinib; CycloSPORINE (Systemic); Flibanserin; GlyBURIDE; Nisoldipine; Olaparib; Palbociclib; Ranolazine; Simeprevir; Sonidegib; Ulipristal

Increased Effect/Toxicity

Bosentan may increase the levels/effects of: Clarithromycin; Ifosfamide

The levels/effects of Bosentan may be increased by: Atazanavir; Boceprevir; Clarithromycin; Cobicistat; CycloSPORINE (Systemic); CYP2C9 Inhibitors (Moderate); CYP2C9 Inhibitors (Strong); CYP3A4 Inhibitors (Moderate); CYP3A4 Inhibitors (Strong); Darunavir; Eltrombopag; Fosamprenavir; GlyBURIDE; Indinavir; Lopinavir; Nelfinavir; Phosphodiesterase 5 Inhibitors; Rifampin; Ritonavir; Saquinavir; Telaprevir; Teriflunomide; Tipranavir

Decreased Effect

Bosentan may decrease the levels/effects of: Antihepaciviral Combination Products; ARIPiprazole; Atazanavir; Axitinib; Bedaquiline; Boceprevir; Bosutinib; Clarithromycin; Cobimetinib; Contraceptives (Estrogens); Contraceptives (Progestins); CycloSPORINE (Systemic); CYP3A4 Substrates; Daclatasvir; Darunavir; FentaNYL; Flibanserin; Fosamprenavir; GlyBURIDE; Hydrocodone; Ibrutinib; Ifosfamide; Indinavir; Lopinavir; Nelfinavir; NiMODipine; Nisoldipine; Olaparib; Palbociclib; Phosphodiesterase 5 Inhibitors; Ranolazine; Rolapitant; Saquinavir; Saxagliptin; Simeprevir; Simvastatin; Sonidegib; Telaprevir; Tipranavir; Ulipristal; Vitamin K Antagonists

The levels/effects of Bosentan may be decreased by: GlyBURIDE; Rifampin

Food Interactions Bioavailability of bosentan is not affected by food. Bosentan serum concentrations may be increased by grapefruit juice. Management: Avoid grapefruit/grapefruit juice.

Storage/Stability Store at 20°C to 25°C (68°F to 77°F); excursions permitted to 15°C to 30°C (59°F to 86°F).

Mechanism of Action Blocks endothelin receptors on vascular endothelium and smooth muscle. Stimulation of these receptors is associated with vasoconstriction. Although bosentan blocks both ET_A and ET_B receptors, the affinity is higher for the A subtype.

Pharmacodynamics/Kinetics

Distribution: V_d: ~18 L (does not distribute into RBCs)

Protein binding, plasma: >98% primarily to albumin

Metabolism: Hepatic via CYP2C9 and 3A4 to three primary metabolites (one contributing ~10% to 20% pharmacologic activity); steady-state plasma concentrations are 50% to 65% of those attained after single dose (most likely due to autoinduction of liver enzymes); steady-state is attained within 3 to 5 days

Bioavailability: ~50%

Half-life elimination: 5 hours; prolonged with heart failure, possibly in PAH

Time to peak, plasma: 3 to 5 hours

Excretion: Feces (as metabolites); urine (<3% as unchanged drug)

Dosing

Adult & Geriatric

Pulmonary artery hypertension: Oral:

<40 kg: Initial and maintenance: 62.5 mg twice daily

≥40 kg: Initial: 62.5 mg twice daily for 4 weeks; increase to maintenance dose of 125 mg twice daily. Doses >125 mg twice daily do not appear to confer additional clinical benefit but may increase risk of liver toxicity.

Note: When discontinuing treatment, consider a reduction in dosage to 62.5 mg twice daily for 3-7 days (to avoid clinical deterioration).

Coadministration with protease inhibitor regimen: Oral:

Dosage adjustment for concurrent use with atazanavir/ritonavir, darunavir/ritonavir, fosamprenavir, lopinavir/ritonavir, ritonavir, saquinavir/ritonavir, tipranavir/ritonavir:

Coadministration of bosentan in patients currently receiving one of these protease inhibitor regimens for at least 10 days: Begin with bosentan 62.5 mg once daily or every other day based on tolerability

Coadministration of one of these protease inhibitor regimens in patients currently receiving bosentan: Discontinue bosentan 36 hours prior to the initiation of an above regimen. After at least 10 days of the protease inhibitor regimen, resume bosentan 62.5 mg once daily or every other day based on tolerability.

Dosage adjustment for concurrent use with indinavir or nelfinavir:

Coadministration of bosentan in patients currently receiving indinavir or nelfinavir: Begin with bosentan 62.5 mg once daily or every other day based on tolerability

Coadministration of indinavir or nelfinavir in patients currently receiving bosentan: Adjust bosentan to 62.5 mg once daily or every other day based on tolerability

Pediatric Pulmonary artery hypertension: Adolescents >12 years: Refer to adult dosing.

Canadian labeling (not in U.S. labeling): Children 3-18 years: Oral:

10-20 kg: Initial: 31.25 mg once daily for 4 weeks; increase to maintenance dose of 31.25 mg twice daily

>20-40 kg: Initial: 31.25 mg twice daily for 4 weeks; increase to maintenance dose of 62.5 mg twice daily

>40 kg: Initial: 62.5 mg twice daily for 4 weeks; increase to maintenance dose of 125 mg twice daily

Renal Impairment No dosage adjustment necessary.

Hepatic Impairment

Mild impairment (Child-Pugh class A): No dosage adjustment necessary.

Moderate-to-severe impairment (Child-Pugh class B and C) and/or baseline transaminase >3 times ULN: Use not recommended; systemic exposure significantly increased in patients with moderate impairment (not studied in patients with severe impairment).

Modification based on transaminase elevation:

If any elevation, regardless of degree, is accompanied by clinical symptoms of hepatic injury (unusual fatigue, nausea, vomiting, abdominal pain, fever, or jaundice) or a serum bilirubin ≥2 times ULN, treatment should be stopped.

AST/ALT >3 times but ≤5 times ULN: Confirm with additional test; if confirmed, reduce dose to 62.5 mg twice daily or interrupt treatment and monitor every 2 weeks. If transaminase levels return to pretreatment values, may continue or reintroduce treatment at the starting dose, as appropriate. When reintroducing treatment, recheck transaminases within 3 days and at least every 2 weeks thereafter.

AST/ALT >5 times but ≤8 times ULN: Confirm with additional test; if confirmed, stop treatment. Monitor transaminase levels at least every 2 weeks. May reintroduce treatment, as appropriate, at starting dose, following return to pretreatment values. Recheck within 3 days and at least every 2 weeks thereafter following reinitiation.

AST/ALT >8 times ULN: Stop treatment and do not reintroduce.

Dietary Considerations May be taken with or without food. Avoid grapefruit and grapefruit juice.

Administration May be administered with or without food, once in the morning and once in the evening. Women of childbearing potential should avoid excessive handling of broken tablets.

Hazardous agent; use appropriate precautions for handling and disposal (NIOSH 2014 [group 3]).

Monitoring Parameters Serum transaminase (AST and ALT) and bilirubin should be determined prior to the initiation of therapy and at monthly intervals thereafter. Monitor for clinical signs and symptoms of liver injury (eg, abdominal pain, fatigue, fever, jaundice, nausea, vomiting). Hemoglobin and hematocrit should be measured at baseline, at 1 month and 3 months of treatment, and every 3 months thereafter (generally stabilizes after 4-12 weeks of treatment).

A woman of childbearing potential must have a negative pregnancy test prior to the initiation of therapy and monthly thereafter (prior to shipment of monthly refill).

Dosage Forms Excipient information presented when available (limited, particularly for generics); consult specific product labeling.

Tablet, Oral:

Tracleer: 62.5 mg, 125 mg

Extemporaneous Preparations Hazardous agent; use appropriate precautions for handling and disposal (NIOSH 2014 [group 3]).

Note: Tablets are not scored; a commercial pill cutter should be used to prepare a 31.25 mg dose from the 62.5 mg tablet; the half-cut 62.5 mg tablets are stable for up to 4 weeks when stored at room temperature in the high-density polyethylene plastic bottle provided by the manufacturer. Since bosentan is classified as a teratogen (Pregnancy Risk Factor X), individuals should avoid exposure to bosentan powder (dust) by taking appropriate measures (eg, using gloves and mask); women of childbearing potential should avoid exposure to dust generated from broken or split tablets.

Crushing of the tablets is not recommended; bosentan tablets will disintegrate rapidly (within 5 minutes) in 5-25 mL of water to create a suspension. An appropriate aliquot of the suspension can be used to deliver the prescribed

dose. Any remaining suspension should be discarded. Bosentan should not be mixed or dissolved in liquids with a low (acidic) pH (eg, fruit juices) due to poor solubility; the drug is most soluble in solutions with a pH >8.5.

◆ **Bosulif** see Bosutinib on page 248

Bosutinib (boe SUE ti nib)

Brand Names: US Bosulif
Brand Names: Canada Bosulif
Index Terms Bosutinib Monohydrate; SKI-606
Pharmacologic Category Antineoplastic Agent, BCR-ABL Tyrosine Kinase Inhibitor; Antineoplastic Agent, Tyrosine Kinase Inhibitor
Use Chronic myelogenous leukemia (CML):
  US labeling: Treatment of chronic, accelerated, or blast phase Philadelphia chromosome-positive (Ph+) CML in patients resistant or intolerant to prior therapy
  Canadian labeling: Treatment of chronic, accelerated or blast phase Philadelphia chromosome-positive (Ph+) CML in patients resistant or intolerant to prior therapy and for whom subsequent treatment with imatinib, nilotinib, and dasatinib is not appropriate
Pregnancy Considerations Adverse events were observed in animal reproduction studies. Based on the mechanism of action, bosutinib may cause fetal harm if administered in pregnancy. Females of reproductive potential should use effective contraception during bosutinib treatment and for at least 30 days after completion of treatment. The Canadian labeling suggests that semen from male patients (including those who have undergone successful vasectomy) receiving bosutinib may pose a risk to a developing fetus and recommends that male patients use effective contraception while receiving treatment, during any treatment interruptions, and for at least 4 weeks after discontinuation of treatment.
Breast-Feeding Considerations It is not known if bosutinib is excreted in breast milk. Due to the potential for serious adverse reactions in the nursing infant, the decision to discontinue bosutinib or discontinue breast-feeding should take into account the benefits of treatment to the mother.
Contraindications
  Hypersensitivity to bosutinib or any component of the formulation
  Canadian labeling: Additional contraindications (not in US labeling): History of long QT syndrome or with persistent QT interval >480 milliseconds; uncorrected hypokalemia or hypomagnesemia; hepatic impairment
Warnings/Precautions Hazardous agent - use appropriate precautions for handling and disposal (meets NIOSH 2014 criteria).

Diarrhea, nausea, vomiting, and abdominal pain may occur. Monitor; may require treatment interruption, dose reduction, or discontinuation. For patients experiencing diarrhea (all grades), the median time to onset was 2 days; median duration (per event) was 1 day; manage diarrhea with antidiarrheals and/or fluid replacement. Nausea and vomiting may be managed with antiemetics and fluid replacement. Acute pancreatitis has been reported; use caution in patients with a prior history of pancreatitis. The Canadian labeling recommends interruption of therapy in patients with elevated amylase/lipase accompanied by abdominal symptoms and evaluation to rule out pancreatitis.

Bleeding events (eg, GI, ophthalmic, pericardial, cerebral, vaginal) have been reported. Anemia, neutropenia, and thrombocytopenia may also occur. May require treatment interruption, dose reduction, or discontinuation. Monitor blood counts weekly during first month, then monthly thereafter (or as clinically indicated). Fluid retention, manifesting as pericardial effusion, pleural effusion, pulmonary edema and/or peripheral edema may occur; may be severe. Monitor for fluid retention (eg, weight gain) and manage appropriately; may require treatment interruption, dose reduction, or discontinuation. QTcF >500 milliseconds was observed rarely (≤0.8%) in clinical trials (Abbas 2012; Cortes 2012); patients with significant or uncontrolled cardiovascular disease (including prolonged QT interval at baseline) were not studied. The Canadian labeling recommends obtaining an ECG (baseline and as clinically indicated thereafter), correction of preexisting hypokalemia and/or hypomagnesemia and periodic monitoring of serum potassium and magnesium.

Bosutinib exposure is increased in patients with hepatic impairment; dose reduction is recommended (Canadian labeling contraindicates use in patients with hepatic impairment at baseline). Hepatotoxicity has been reported during treatment; dose reductions may be necessary. Monitor

liver function. ALT and AST elevations may occur, usually with an onset in the first 3 months of treatment (median onset was ~30 to 33 days; median duration was 21 days). One case of drug-induced liver injury has been reported; full recovery occurred after discontinuation. Bosutinib exposure is increased in patients with moderate or severe renal impairment. Declines in glomerular filtration rates throughout bosutinib treatment have been observed in clinical studies; monitor renal function at baseline and during therapy, particularly in patients with preexisting impairment or other risk factors for renal dysfunction. Consider dosage adjustment in patients with renal dysfunction at baseline or with treatment emergent impairment. Bone fracture and mineral abnormalities (eg, hypophosphatemia) has been reported (Bosulif Canadian product monograph 2014); monitor patients with severe osteoporosis or endocrine disease (eg, hyperparathyroidism) for mineral abnormalities and/or changes in bone density.

Potentially significant drug-drug interactions may exist, requiring dose or frequency adjustment, additional monitoring, and/or selection of alternative therapy. Proton pump inhibitors (PPIs) may decrease bosutinib effects; consider using short acting antacids or H$_2$ antagonists instead of PPIs; separate administration of antacids or H$_2$ antagonists from bosutinib by at least 2 hours.
Adverse Reactions
  >10%:
    Cardiovascular: Edema (14%; grades 3/4: <1%)
    Cardiovascular: Edema (14%; grades 3/4: <1%)
    Central nervous system: Fatigue (20% to 26%), headache (18% to 20%), dizziness (10% to 13%)
    Dermatologic: Skin rash (34% to 35%), pruritus (8% to 11%)
    Endocrine & metabolic: Hypophosphatemia (50% [Gambacorti–Passerini 2014]; grades 3/4: 7%), hypokalemia (18%; grades 3/4: 2% [Gambacorti-Passerini 2014])
    Gastrointestinal: Diarrhea (76% to 84%; grades 3/4: 5% to 9%), nausea (46% to 47%; grades 3/4: 1% to 2%), vomiting (37% to 42%; grades 3/4: 3% to 4%), abdominal pain (29% to 40%; grades 3/4: 1% to 5%), increase serum lipase (15% to 38%; grades 3/4: 3% to 9% [Cortes 2012, Gambacorti–Passerini 2014]), decreased appetite (13% to 14%)
    Hematologic & oncologic: Thrombocytopenia (40% to 42%; grades 3/4: 26% to 37%), anemia (23% to 37%; grades 3/4: 9% to 26%), neutropenia (16% to 19%; grades 3/4: 11% to 18%)
    Hepatic: Increased serum ALT (10% to 20%; grades 3/4: 5% to 7%), increased serum AST (11% to 16%; grades 3/4: 3% to 4%)
    Neuromuscular & skeletal: Arthralgia (13% to 14%), back pain (7% to 12%), weakness (10% to 11%)
    Respiratory: Cough (20% to 21%), dyspnea (10% to 19%), respiratory tract infection (10% to 12%), nasopharyngitis (5% to 12%)
    Miscellaneous: Fever (22% to 36%)
  1% to 10%:
    Cardiovascular: Pericardial effusion (grades 3/4: <1%), chest pain, prolonged Q-T interval on ECG
    Central nervous system: Pain
    Dermatologic: Acne vulgaris, urticaria
    Endocrine & metabolic: Dehydration, hyperkalemia
    Gastrointestinal: Dysgeusia, gastritis
    Hematologic & oncologic: Febrile neutropenia
    Hepatic: Hepatic insufficiency, hepatotoxicity, increased serum bilirubin
    Hypersensitivity: Hypersensitivity reaction
    Infection: Influenza
    Neuromuscular & skeletal: Increased creatine phosphokinase, myalgia
    Otic: Tinnitus
    Renal: Increased serum creatinine, renal failure
    Respiratory: Bronchitis, pleural effusion, pneumonia
  <1% (Limited to important or life-threatening): Anaphylactic shock, erythema multiforme, exfoliative dermatitis, gastrointestinal hemorrhage, pancreatitis, pericarditis, pulmonary edema, pulmonary hypertension, respiratory failure
Drug Interactions
  Metabolism/Transport Effects Substrate of CYP3A4 (major); **Note:** Assignment of Major/Minor substrate status based on clinically relevant drug interaction potential; **Inhibits** P-glycoprotein
Avoid Concomitant Use
  Avoid concomitant use of Bosutinib with any of the following: BCG (Intravesical); Bitter Orange; Conivaptan; CYP3A4 Inducers (Moderate); CYP3A4 Inducers (Strong); CYP3A4 Inhibitors (Moderate); CYP3A4 Inhibitors (Strong); Deferiprone; Dipyrone; Fusidic Acid (Systemic); Idelalisib; P-glycoprotein/ABCB1 Inhibitors; Pomegranate; St Johns Wort; Star Fruit

Increased Effect/Toxicity

Bosutinib may increase the levels/effects of: CloZAPine; Deferiprone; Highest Risk QTc-Prolonging Agents; Moderate Risk QTc-Prolonging Agents

The levels/effects of Bosutinib may be increased by: Bitter Orange; Conivaptan; CYP3A4 Inhibitors (Moderate); CYP3A4 Inhibitors (Strong); Dasatinib; Dipyrone; Fosaprepitant; Fusidic Acid (Systemic); Idelalisib; Luliconazole; Osimertinib; Palbociclib; P-glycoprotein/ABCB1 Inhibitors; Pomegranate; Star Fruit; Stiripentol

Decreased Effect

Bosutinib may decrease the levels/effects of: BCG (Intravesical)

The levels/effects of Bosutinib may be decreased by: Antacids; CYP3A4 Inducers (Moderate); CYP3A4 Inducers (Strong); Deferasirox; H2-Antagonists; Osimertinib; Proton Pump Inhibitors; Siltuximab; St Johns Wort; Tocilizumab

Food Interactions Grapefruit juice may increase bosutinib plasma concentration. Management: Avoid grapefruit juice during bosutinib therapy. Additionally the Canadian labeling recommends avoiding products containing Seville oranges, pomegranate and star fruit during therapy; may increase bosutinib plasma concentrations.

Storage/Stability Store at 20°C to 25°C (68°F to 77°F); excursions permitted to 15°C to 30°C (59°F to 86°F).

Mechanism of Action BCR-ABL tyrosine kinase inhibitor (TKI); inhibits BCR-ABL kinase that promotes CML. Also inhibits SRC family (including SRC, LYN, and HCK). Bosutinib has minimal activity against c-KIT and platelet-derived growth factor receptor (PDGFR), which are non-specific targets associated with toxicity in other TKIs (Cortes 2012). Bosutinib has activity in 16 of 18 imatinib-resistant BCR-ABL mutations, with the exceptions of the T315I and V299L mutants (Cortes 2011).

Pharmacodynamics/Kinetics

Onset:
Median time to complete hematologic response (in responders): 2 weeks (Cortes 2011)
Median time to major cytogenetic response (in responders): 12.3 weeks (Cortes 2011)
Median time to first complete cytogenic response: 12.9 weeks (Cortes 2012)

Absorption: Slow (Abbas 2012)
Distribution: V_d: 6,080 ± 1,230 L
Protein binding: 94% to plasma proteins
Metabolism: Hepatic via CYP3A4, primarily to inactive metabolites oxydechlorinated (M2) bosutinib and *N*-desmethylated (M5) bosutinib, also to bosutinib *N*-oxide (M6)
Half-life elimination: 22 to 27 hours (Cortes 2011)
Time to peak: 4 to 6 hours
Excretion: Feces (~91%); urine (3%)

Dosing

Adult & Geriatric Philadelphia chromosome-positive chronic myelogenous leukemia (Ph+CML): Oral: 500 mg once daily; continue until disease progression or unacceptable toxicity. **Note:** If complete hematologic response is not achieved by week 8 or complete cytogenetic response is not achieved by week 12, in the absence of grade 3 or higher adverse reactions, consider increasing the dose from 500 mg once daily to 600 mg once daily.

Missed doses: If a dose is missed beyond 12 hours, skip the dose and resume the usual dose the following day

Renal Impairment

Preexisting impairment:
Mild impairment (CrCl >50 to 80 mL/minute): There are no dosage adjustments provided in manufacturer's labeling, however, based on the pharmacokinetics, the need for dosage adjustment is not likely.
Moderate impairment (CrCl 30 to 50 mL/minute): Initial: 400 mg once daily.
Severe impairment (CrCl <30 mL/minute): Reduce dose to 300 mg once daily (this dose is predicted to result in an AUC similar to that of patients with normal renal function, however, there is no efficacy data for this dose in CML patients with renal impairment).

Renal toxicity during treatment: If unable to tolerate initial dose, reduce dose per adjustment recommendations for toxicity (withhold treatment until resolved, then consider resuming at 400 mg once daily; if clinically appropriate, may re-escalate dose to 500 mg once daily).

Hemodialysis: There are no dosage adjustments provided in the manufacturer's labeling (has not been studied).

Hepatic Impairment

Preexisting impairment (mild, moderate, or severe):
US labeling: Child-Pugh class A, B, or C: Reduce initial dose to 200 mg once daily (this dose is predicted to result in an AUC similar to that of patients with normal hepatic function, however, there is no efficacy data for this dose in CML patients with hepatic impairment).
Canadian labeling: Use is contraindicated in hepatic impairment.

Hepatotoxicity during treatment:
ALT or AST >5 times ULN: Withhold treatment until recovery to ≤2.5 times ULN and resume at 400 mg once daily thereafter. If recovery to ≤2.5 times ULN takes >4 weeks: Discontinue bosutinib.
ALT or AST ≥3 times ULN in conjunction with bilirubin elevation >2 times ULN and alkaline phosphatase <2 times ULN: Discontinue bosutinib.

Adjustment for Toxicity

Hematologic toxicity: ANC <1000/mm^3 or platelets <50,000/mm^3: Withhold treatment until ANC ≥1000/mm^3 **and** platelets ≥50,000/mm^3; if recovery occurs within 2 weeks, resume treatment at the same dose. If ANC and platelets remain low for >2 weeks, upon recovery, resume treatment with the dose reduced by 100 mg. If cytopenia recurs, withhold until recovery and resume treatment with the dose reduced by an additional 100 mg. Doses <300 mg daily have not been evaluated.

Nonhematologic toxicity:
Diarrhea: Grade 3 or 4 (≥7 stools/day increase over baseline): Withhold treatment until recovery to ≤ grade 1; may resume at 400 mg once daily.
Other clinically significant nonhematologic toxicity, moderate or severe: Withhold treatment until resolved, then consider resuming at 400 mg once daily; may re-escalate dose to 500 mg once daily if clinically appropriate.

Dietary Considerations Take with food.

Administration Oral: Administer with food. Swallow tablet whole; do not crush or break. Hazardous agent; use appropriate precautions for handling and disposal (meets NIOSH 2014 criteria).

Monitoring Parameters CBC with differential and platelets (weekly during first month, then monthly thereafter, or as clinically indicated); hepatic enzymes (monthly for first 3 months or as clinically indicated; monitor more frequently with transaminase elevations); renal function (at baseline and throughout therapy); diarrhea episodes; fluid/edema status (eg, weight gain)

Canadian labeling: Additional recommendations (not in US labeling): ECG (baseline then as clinically indicated); serum electrolytes and lipase/amylase (baseline, frequently during treatment, and as clinically indicated); bone density (patients with severe osteoporosis or endocrine disease)

Dosage Forms Excipient information presented when available (limited, particularly for generics); consult specific product labeling.
Tablet, Oral:
Bosulif: 100 mg, 500 mg

Botulism Immune Globulin (Intravenous-Human)

(BOT yoo lism i MYUN GLOB you lin, in tra VEE nus, YU man)

Brand Names: US BabyBIG®
Index Terms BIG-IV
Pharmacologic Category Blood Product Derivative; Immune Globulin

Use Treatment of infant botulism caused by toxin type A or B

Prescribing and Access Restrictions Access to botulism immune globulin is restricted through the Infant Botulism Treatment and Prevention Program (IBTPP). Healthcare providers must contact the IBTPP on-call physician at (510) 231-7600 to review treatment indications and to obtain the medication. For more information,

refer to http://www.infantbotulism.org or contact
IBTPP@infantbotulism.org.

Dosing

Pediatric Infant botulism: Infants <1 year: IV: 50 mg/kg as
a single dose as soon as diagnosis of infant botulism is
made. **Note:** The recommended dose may vary with
each manufactured sublot; verify dose with the prescribing information and guidance provided with each product
shipment.

Renal Impairment Use with caution; the rate of infusion
and concentration of solution should be minimized in
patients with renal impairment or those at risk for renal
dysfunction.

Hepatic Impairment No dosage adjustment provided in
manufacturer's labeling.

Adjustment for Toxicity Infusion reactions: Slow the
infusion rate or temporarily interrupt infusion for minor
reaction (ie, flushing). Discontinue infusion and administer epinephrine for anaphylactic reaction or significant
hypotension.

Additional Information Complete prescribing information
should be consulted for additional detail.

Dosage Forms Excipient information presented when
available (limited, particularly for generics); consult specific
product labeling.

Injection, powder for reconstitution [preservative free]:
BabyBIG®: ~100 mg [contains albumin (human),
sucrose; supplied with diluent]

Brentuximab Vedotin (bren TUX i mab ve DOE tin)

Brand Names: US Adcetris
Brand Names: Canada Adcetris
Index Terms Anti-CD30 ADC SGN-35; Anti-CD30 Anti-
body-Drug Conjugate SGN-35; Antibody-Drug Conjugate
SGN-35; Brentuximab; SGN-35
Pharmacologic Category Antineoplastic Agent, Anti-
CD30; Antineoplastic Agent, Antibody Drug Conjugate;
Antineoplastic Agent, Monoclonal Antibody

Use

Anaplastic large cell lymphoma (systemic): Treatment
of systemic anaplastic large cell lymphoma after failure of
at least 1 prior multiagent chemotherapy regimen

Hodgkin lymphoma: Treatment of classical Hodgkin lymphoma after failure of at least 2 prior multiagent chemotherapy regimens (in patients who are not autologous
hematopoietic stem cell transplant candidates) or after
failure of autologous hematopoietic stem cell transplant

**Hodgkin lymphoma (post-autologous hematopoietic
stem cell transplantation):** Treatment (maintenance
therapy) of classical Hodgkin lymphoma in patients at
high risk of relapse or progression as post–autologous
hematopoietic stem cell transplant consolidation

Pregnancy Considerations Adverse events were
observed in animal reproduction studies. Based on the
mechanism of action, may cause fetal harm if administered
to a pregnant woman.

Breast-Feeding Considerations It is not known if brentuximab vedotin is excreted in breast milk. Due to the
potential for serious adverse reactions in the nursing
infant, the manufacturer recommends a decision be made
to discontinue nursing or to discontinue the drug, taking
into account the importance of treatment to the mother.

Contraindications

US labeling: Concurrent use with bleomycin
Canadian labeling: Hypersensitivity to brentuximab or any
component of the formulation; concurrent use with bleomycin; patients who have or have history of progressive
multifocal leukoencephalopathy

Warnings/Precautions Hazardous agent - use appropriate precautions for handling and disposal (NIOSH 2014
[group 1]).

**[US Boxed Warning]: Cases of progressive multifocal
leukoencephalopathy (PML) and death due to JC virus
infection have been reported.** Immunosuppression due
to prior chemotherapy treatments or underlying disease
may also contribute to PML development. New-onset
signs/symptoms of central nervous system abnormalities
(eg, changes in mood, memory, cognition, motor incoordination and/or weakness, speech and/or visual disturbances) should receive prompt evaluation with neurology
consultation, brain MRI, and lumbar puncture or brain
biopsy. The time to initial symptom onset varies from
treatment initiation, with some cases occurring within 3
months of initial drug treatment. Withhold treatment with
new-onset symptoms suggestive of PML; discontinue if
diagnosis of PML is confirmed.

Peripheral neuropathy is common and is generally cumulative; usually sensory neuropathy, although motor neuropathy has also been observed; neuropathy completely
resolved in nearly half of patients; almost one-third had
partial improvement. Monitor for symptoms of neuropathy
(hypoesthesia, hyperesthesia, paresthesia, discomfort,
burning sensation, neuropathic pain, or weakness); dose
interruption, reduction or discontinuation may be recommended for new or worsening neuropathy.

Grade 3 or 4 neutropenia, thrombocytopenia, and anemia
may occur; neutropenia may be severe and/or prolonged
(≥1 week); neutropenic fever also has been reported;
monitor blood counts prior to each dose and consider more
frequent monitoring for patients with Grade 3 or 4 neutropenia; may require growth factor support, dose interruption, reduction or discontinuation. Serious infections,
including opportunistic infections (eg, pneumonia, bacteremia, sepsis/septic shock) have been reported (some
fatal); monitor for signs or symptoms of bacterial, fungal,
or viral infections. Infusion reactions, including anaphylaxis
have been reported; monitor during infusion. For anaphylaxis, immediately and permanently discontinue and
administer appropriate medical intervention. For infusion-
related reaction, interrupt infusion and administer appropriate medical intervention; premedicate for subsequent
infusions (with acetaminophen, an antihistamine, and/or
a corticosteroid).

Noninfectious pulmonary toxicity (eg, pneumonitis, interstitial lung disease, acute respiratory distress syndrome),
some fatal, has been reported in patients receiving brentuximab vedotin. Monitor for signs/symptoms of pulmonary
toxicity (eg, cough, dyspnea). Withhold treatment and
perform prompt diagnostic evaluation and management
for new or worsening pulmonary symptoms. Due to the
risk for pulmonary injury, concurrent use with bleomycin is
contraindicated. In a study comparing brentuximab combined with ABVD (doxorubicin, bleomycin, vinblastine, and
dacarbazine) to brentuximab combined with AVD (doxorubicin, vinblastine, and dacarbazine), the occurrence of
pulmonary toxicity was higher in the brentuximab/ABVD
group. Pulmonary symptoms/toxicities reported with brentuximab in combination with ABVD consisted of cough,
dyspnea, and interstitial infiltration/inflammation; most
patients responded to corticosteroids. Potentially significant drug-drug interactions may exist, requiring dose or
frequency adjustment, additional monitoring, and/or selection of alternative therapy.

Serious hepatotoxicity, including fatalities, has occurred;
cases were consistent with hepatocellular injury, with elevations of transaminases and/or bilirubin. Some have
occurred after the initial dose or after rechallenge. The risk
for hepatotoxicity may be increased with preexisting liver
disease, elevated baseline liver enzymes, and concurrent
medications. Monitor liver enzymes and bilirubin. Treatment delay, dose reduction or discontinuation may be
required for new, worsening, or recurrent hepatotoxicity.
Avoid use in patients with moderate to severe hepatic
impairment (Child-Pugh classes B and C). The frequency
of grade 3/4 toxicities (and deaths) was increased in
patients with moderate or severe impairment (compared
to patients with normal hepatic function). A component of
brentuximab vedotin, the microtubule-disrupting agent
monomethylauristatin E (MMAE) is excreted hepatically.
MMAE exposure is increased ~2.2-fold in patients with
hepatic impairment.

Avoid use in patients with severe renal impairment (CrCl
<30 mL/minute). The frequency of grade 3/4 toxicities (and
deaths) was increased in patients with severe impairment
(compared to patients with normal renal function). A component of brentuximab vedotin, the microtubule-disrupting
agent MMAE is excreted renally; MMAE exposure is

increased in patients with severe impairment. Stevens-Johnson syndrome (SJS) and toxic epidermal necrolysis (TEN) have been reported (some fatal). Discontinue (and begin appropriate management) if SJS or TEN occur. Tumor lysis syndrome (TLS) may occur; risk of TLS is higher in patients with a high tumor burden or with rapid tumor proliferation; monitor closely.

Adverse Reactions

>10%:

Cardiovascular: Peripheral edema (4% to 16%)

Central nervous system: Peripheral sensory neuropathy (2% to 56%; grade 3: 8% to 10%), fatigue (24% to 49%), pain (7% to 28%), headache (11% to 19%), insomnia (14% to 16%), dizziness (11% to 16%), peripheral motor neuropathy (4% to 23%; grade 3: 3% to 6%), chills (10% to 13%), anxiety (7% to 11%)

Dermatologic: Skin rash (27% to 31%), pruritus (12% to 19%), alopecia (13% to 14%), night sweats (9% to 12%)

Endocrine & metabolic: Weight loss (6% to 19%)

Gastrointestinal: Nausea (2% to 42%), diarrhea (20% to 36%), abdominal pain (3% to 25%), vomiting (3% to 22%), constipation (13% to 19%), decreased appetite (11% to 16%)

Hematologic & oncologic: Neutropenia (54% to 78%; grade 3: 12% to 30%; grade 4: 6% to 9%), anemia (27% to 52%; grade 3: 2% to 8%; grade 4: 4%), thrombocytopenia (16% to 41%; grade 3: 5% to 7%; grade 4: 2% to 5%), lymphadenopathy (10% to 11%)

Immunologic: Antibody development (antibrentuximab; transient: 30%; persistent: 7%)

Neuromuscular & skeletal: Arthralgia (9% to 19%), myalgia (11% to 17%), back pain (10% to 14%), muscle spasm (9% to 11%)

Respiratory: Upper respiratory tract infection (12% to 47%), cough (17% to 25%), dyspnea (13% to 19%), oropharyngeal pain (9% to 11%)

Miscellaneous: Fever (2% to 38%), infusion related reaction (12% to 15%)

1% to 10%:

Cardiovascular: Septic shock (3%), supraventricular cardiac arrhythmia (3%), pulmonary embolism (2%)

Dermatologic: Xeroderma (4% to 10%)

Genitourinary: Urinary tract infection (3%)

Hepatic: Hepatotoxicity (2%)

Neuromuscular & skeletal: Limb pain (3% to 10%)

Renal: Pyelonephritis (2%)

Respiratory: Pulmonary toxicity (5%, noninfectious), pneumonia (4%), pneumonitis (2%), pneumothorax (2%)

<1% (Limited to important or life-threatening): Anaphylaxis, febrile neutropenia, hyperglycemia, pancreatitis, progressive multifocal leukoencephalopathy, opportunistic infection, serious infection, Stevens-Johnson syndrome, tumor lysis syndrome

Drug Interactions

Metabolism/Transport Effects Substrate of CYP3A4 (minor), P-glycoprotein; **Note:** Assignment of Major/Minor substrate status based on clinically relevant drug interaction potential

Avoid Concomitant Use

Avoid concomitant use of Brentuximab Vedotin with any of the following: BCG (Intravesical); Belimumab; Bleomycin; Natalizumab; Pimecrolimus; Tacrolimus (Topical); Tofacitinib; Vaccines (Live)

Increased Effect/Toxicity

Brentuximab Vedotin may increase the levels/effects of: Belimumab; Bleomycin; Fingolimod; Leflunomide; Natalizumab; Tofacitinib; Vaccines (Live)

The levels/effects of Brentuximab Vedotin may be increased by: CYP3A4 Inhibitors (Strong); Denosumab; Lumacaftor; P-glycoprotein/ABCB1 Inhibitors; Pimecrolimus; Ranolazine; Roflumilast; Tacrolimus (Topical); Trastuzumab

Decreased Effect

Brentuximab Vedotin may decrease the levels/effects of: BCG (Intravesical); Coccidioides immitis Skin Test; Sipuleucel-T; Vaccines (Inactivated); Vaccines (Live)

The levels/effects of Brentuximab Vedotin may be decreased by: CYP3A4 Inducers (Strong); Echinacea; Lumacaftor; P-glycoprotein/ABCB1 Inducers

Preparation for Administration Hazardous agent: Use appropriate precautions for handling and disposal (NIOSH 2014 [group 1]). Reconstitute each 50 mg vial with 10.5 mL sterile water for injection (SWFI), resulting in a concentration of 5 mg/mL. Direct SWFI toward the vial wall; do not direct toward the cake or powder. Swirl gently to dissolve, do not shake. Reconstituted solution should be clear to slightly opalescent without visible particles. Further dilute in at least 100 mL of either NS, D₅W, or lactated Ringer's to a final concentration of 0.4 to 1.8 mg/mL; gently invert

bag to mix. Do not mix with other medications. Use within 24 hours of initial reconstitution.

Storage/Stability Store intact vials refrigerated at 2°C to 8°C (36°F to 46°F) in the original carton. Protect from light. Reconstituted solution should be diluted immediately; however, may be stored refrigerated for up to 24 hours; do not freeze. Solutions diluted for infusion should be used immediately after preparation; however, may be stored for 24 hours refrigerated (do not freeze); use within 24 hours of initial reconstitution.

Mechanism of Action Brentuximab vedotin is an antibody drug conjugate (ADC) directed at CD30 consisting of 3 components: 1) a CD30-specific chimeric IgG1 antibody cAC10; 2) a microtubule-disrupting agent, monomethylauristatin E (MMAE); and 3) a protease cleavable dipeptide linker (which covalently conjugates MMAE to cAC10). The conjugate binds to cells which express CD30, and forms a complex which is internalized within the cell and releases MMAE. MMAE binds to the tubules and disrupts the cellular microtubule network, inducing cell cycle arrest (G2/M phase) and apoptosis.

Pharmacodynamics/Kinetics

Distribution: V_{dss}: ADC: 6 to 10 L

Metabolism: MMAE: Minimal, primarily via oxidation by CYP3A4/5

Half-life elimination: Terminal: ADC: ~4 to 6 days

Time to peak: ADC: At end of infusion; MMAE: ~1 to 3 days

Excretion: MMAE: Feces (~72%, primarily unchanged); urine

Dosing

Adult & Geriatric

Hodgkin lymphoma, refractory: IV: 1.8 mg/kg (maximum dose: 180 mg) every 3 weeks, continue until disease progression or unacceptable toxicities

Hodgkin lymphoma, maintenance therapy after autologous hematopoietic stem cell transplantation (HSCT): IV: 1.8 mg/kg (maximum dose: 180 mg) every 3 weeks, continue until a maximum of 16 cycles, disease progression, or unacceptable toxicity. Begin therapy within 4 to 6 weeks post HSCT or upon recovery from HSCT.

Systemic anaplastic large cell lymphoma (sALCL), refractory: IV: 1.8 mg/kg (maximum dose: 180 mg) every 3 weeks, continue until disease progression or unacceptable toxicities

Renal Impairment

CrCl ≥30 mL/minute: Initial: No dosage adjustment necessary.

CrCl <30 mL/minute: Initial: Avoid use.

Hepatic Impairment

Mild impairment (Child-Pugh class A): Initial: 1.2 mg/kg (maximum dose: 120 mg) every 3 weeks.

Moderate to severe impairment (Child-Pugh class B or C): Avoid use.

Adjustment for Toxicity

Hematologic toxicity:

Grade 3 or 4 neutropenia: Withhold treatment until resolves to baseline or ≤ grade 2, consider growth factor support in subsequent cycles.

Recurrent grade 4 neutropenia (despite the use of growth factor support): Consider reducing the dose to 1.2 mg/kg or discontinuing treatment

Grade 3 or 4 thrombocytopenia (Canadian labeling): Monitor closely; dose delays or platelet transfusions may be considered.

Nonhematologic toxicities:

Anaphylaxis: Discontinue immediately and permanently

Infusion reaction: Interrupt infusion and administer appropriate medical intervention. Premedicate subsequent infusions with acetaminophen, an antihistamine, and/or a corticosteroid.

Peripheral neuropathy, new or worsening grade 2 or 3: Withhold treatment until improves or returns to grade 1 or baseline; then resume with dose reduced to 1.2 mg/kg

Peripheral neuropathy, grade 4: Discontinue treatment

Progressive multifocal leukoencephalopathy (PML): Withhold treatment with new-onset symptoms suggestive of PML; discontinue if PML diagnosis confirmed

Pulmonary toxicity: Withhold treatment with new-onset or worsening pulmonary symptoms during evaluation and until symptomatic improvement

Stevens-Johnson syndrome or toxic epidermal necrolysis: Discontinue and administer appropriate medical intervention

Administration Infuse over 30 minutes. Do not administer as IV push or bolus; do not mix or infuse with other medications. Hazardous agent; use appropriate precautions for handling and disposal (NIOSH 2014 [group 1]).

Monitoring Parameters CBC with differential prior to each dose (more frequently if clinically indicated); liver and renal function tests. Monitor for infusion reaction, tumor lysis syndrome, signs/symptoms of progressive multifocal leukoencephalopathy (PML), and for signs of neuropathy (hypoesthesia, hyperesthesia, paresthesia, discomfort, burning sensation, or neuropathic pain or weakness), dermatologic toxicity, pulmonary toxicity, or infection.

Dosage Forms Excipient information presented when available (limited, particularly for generics); consult specific product labeling.
Solution Reconstituted, Intravenous [preservative free]:
Adcetris: 50 mg (1 ea) [contains polysorbate 80]

Brexpiprazole (breks PIP ray zole)

Brand Names: US Rexulti
Index Terms OPC-34712
Pharmacologic Category Second Generation (Atypical) Antipsychotic
Use
Major depressive disorder: Adjunctive treatment of major depressive disorder (MDD)
Schizophrenia: Treatment of schizophrenia
Pregnancy Considerations Adverse events were observed in some animal reproduction studies. Antipsychotic use during the third trimester of pregnancy has a risk for abnormal muscle movements (extrapyramidal symptoms [EPS]) and/or withdrawal symptoms in newborns following delivery. Symptoms in the newborn may include agitation, feeding disorder, hypertonia, hypotonia, respiratory distress, somnolence, and tremor; these effects may be self-limiting or require hospitalization.

Treatment algorithms have been developed by the ACOG and the APA for the management of depression in women prior to conception and during pregnancy (Yonkers 2009). The ACOG recommends that therapy during pregnancy be individualized; treatment with psychiatric medications during pregnancy should incorporate the clinical expertise of the mental health clinician, obstetrician, primary health care provider, and pediatrician. Safety data related to atypical antipsychotics during pregnancy is limited and routine use is not recommended. However, if a woman is inadvertently exposed to an atypical antipsychotic while pregnant, continuing therapy may be preferable to switching to a typical antipsychotic that the fetus has not yet been exposed to; consider risk:benefit (ACOG 2008).

Health care providers are encouraged to enroll women exposed to brexpiprazole during pregnancy in the National Pregnancy Registry for Atypical Antipsychotics (866-961-2388 or http://www.womensmentalhealth.org/clinical-and-research-programs/pregnancyregistry/).
Breast-Feeding Considerations It is not known if brexpiprazole is excreted in breast milk. According to the manufacturer, the decision to continue or discontinue breast-feeding during therapy should take into account the risk of exposure to the infant and the benefits of treatment to the mother.
Contraindications Hypersensitivity (eg, anaphylaxis, facial swelling, rash, urticaria) to brexpiprazole or any component of the formulation
Warnings/Precautions [US Boxed Warning]: Elderly patients with dementia-related psychosis treated with antipsychotics are at an increased risk of death compared to placebo. Most deaths appeared to be either cardiovascular (eg, heart failure, sudden death) or infectious (eg, pneumonia) in nature. Use with caution in dementia with Lewy bodies; antipsychotics may worsen dementia symptoms and patients with dementia with Lewy bodies are more sensitive to the extrapyramidal side effects (APA [Rabins 2007]). Brexpiprazole is not approved for the treatment of dementia-related psychosis.

[US Boxed Warning]: Antidepressants increase the risk of suicidal thinking and behavior in children, adolescents, and young adults (≤24 years of age). Short-term studies did not show an increased risk in patients >24 years of age and showed a decreased risk in patients ≥65 years. **Closely monitor patients for clinical worsening and suicidality** particularly during the initial 1 to 2 months of therapy or during periods of dosage adjustments (increases or decreases); the patient's family or caregiver should be instructed to closely observe the patient and communicate condition with healthcare provider. **Safety and efficacy have not been established in pediatric patients.**

Leukopenia, neutropenia, and agranulocytosis (sometimes fatal) have been reported in clinical trials and postmarketing reports with antipsychotic use; presence of risk factors (eg, preexisting low WBC/ANC or history of drug-induced leuko-/neutropenia) should prompt periodic blood count assessment. Discontinue therapy at first signs of blood dyscrasias or if absolute neutrophil count <1,000/mm³.

May cause extrapyramidal symptoms, including pseudoparkinsonism, acute dystonic reactions, akathisia, and tardive dyskinesia (risk of these reactions is generally much lower relative to typical/conventional antipsychotics). Risk of dystonia (and probably other EPS) may be greater with increased doses, use of conventional antipsychotics, males, and younger patients. Factors associated with greater vulnerability to tardive dyskinesia include older in age, female gender combined with postmenopausal status, Parkinson disease, pseudoparkinsonism symptoms, affective disorders (particularly major depressive disorder), concurrent medical diseases such as diabetes, previous brain damage, alcoholism, poor treatment response, and use of high doses of antipsychotics (APA [Lehman 2004]; Soares-Weiser 2007). Consider therapy discontinuation with signs/symptoms of tardive dyskinesia. Use may be associated with neuroleptic malignant syndrome (NMS); monitor for mental status changes, fever, muscle rigidity, and/or autonomic instability.

May cause CNS depression, which may impair physical or mental abilities; patients must be cautioned about performing tasks that require mental alertness (eg, operating machinery, driving). May cause orthostatic hypotension; increased risk at initiation of therapy or during dose escalation. Use with caution in patients at risk of this effect or in those who would not tolerate transient hypotensive episodes (patients who are antipsychotic-naive or have cerebrovascular disease, cardiovascular disease, hypovolemia, dehydration, or are taking concurrent medication use which may predispose to hypotension/bradycardia). Consider using lower starting dosages and slower titrations in these patients.

Use with caution in patients with Parkinson disease; antipsychotics may aggravate motor disturbances (APA [Lehman 2004; Rabins 2007]). Use with caution in patients at risk of seizures or with conditions that potentially lower the seizure threshold. Elderly patients may be at increased risk of seizures due to an increased prevalence of predisposing factors. An increased incidence of cerebrovascular effects (eg, transient ischemic attack, stroke), including fatalities, has been reported in placebo-controlled trials of antipsychotics for the unapproved use in elderly patients with dementia-related psychosis. Antipsychotic use has been associated with esophageal dysmotility and aspiration; use with caution in patients at risk for aspiration pneumonia (eg, Alzheimer dementia) (Maddalena 2004).

Dyslipidemia has been reported with atypical antipsychotics; risk profile may differ between agents. In clinical trials, the incidence of hypertriglyceridemia observed with brexpiprazole was greater than observed with placebo, while changes in fasting total cholesterol, LDL, and HDL were similar. Atypical antipsychotics have been associated with development of hyperglycemia; in some cases, may be extreme and associated with ketoacidosis, hyperosmolar coma, or death. All patients should be monitored for symptoms of hyperglycemia (eg, polydipsia, polyuria, polyphagia, weakness). Use with caution in patients with diabetes or other disorders of glucose regulation; monitor for worsening of glucose control. Patients with risk factors for diabetes (eg, obesity or family history) should have a baseline fasting blood sugar (FBS) and periodic assessment of glucose regulation. Hyperglycemia may resolve with discontinuation of antipsychotic; some patients may require treatment of diabetes after discontinuation of therapy.

Antipsychotic use has been associated with impaired core body temperature regulation; caution with strenuous exercise, heat exposure, dehydration, and concomitant medication possessing anticholinergic effects. Significant

weight gain has been observed with antipsychotic therapy; incidence varies with product. Monitoring of weight is recommended.

Use in elderly patients with dementia-related psychosis is associated with an increased risk of mortality and cerebrovascular accidents. Brexpiprazole is not approved for the treatment of dementia-related psychosis; avoid antipsychotic use for behavioral problems associated with dementia unless alternative nonpharmacologic therapies have failed and patient may harm self or others. In addition, antipsychotic use may cause or exacerbate syndrome of inappropriate antidiuretic hormone secretion or hyponatremia; monitor sodium closely with initiation or dosage adjustments in older adults (Beers Criteria).

Potentially significant interactions may exist, requiring dose or frequency adjustment, additional monitoring, and/or selection of alternative therapy. Tablets may contain lactose; avoid use in patients with galactose intolerance or glucose-galactose malabsorption.

Adverse Reactions

>10%:
Central nervous system: Akathisia (4% to 14%; dose-related)
Endocrine & metabolic: Increased serum triglycerides (<500 mg/dL: 8% to 13%; ≥500 mg/dL: <1%), weight gain (3% to 11%)

1% to 10%:
Central nervous system: Headache (major depressive disorder: 9%), drug-induced extrapyramidal reaction (5% to 6%), drowsiness (4% to 6%), fatigue (major depressive disorder: 3% to 5%), dizziness (major depressive disorder: 2% to 5%), anxiety (major depressive disorder: 2% to 4%), restlessness (major depressive disorder: 2% to 4%; dose-related), sedation (2% to 3%), abnormal dreams (≥1%), insomnia (≥1%)
Dermatologic: Hyperhidrosis (≥1%)
Endocrine & metabolic: Decreased cortisol (major depressive disorder: 3% to 4%), increased serum prolactin (≥1%)
Gastrointestinal: Dyspepsia (schizophrenia: 3% to 6%), increased appetite (major depressive disorder: 3%), constipation (major depressive disorder: 2% to 3%), diarrhea (schizophrenia: 2%), abdominal pain (≥1%), flatulence (≥1%), nausea (≥1%), sialorrhea (≥1%), xerostomia (≥1%)
Genitourinary: Urinary tract infection (≥1%)
Neuromuscular & skeletal: Tremor (2% to 5%), increased creatine phosphokinase (schizophrenia: 2% to 4%), myalgia (≥1%)
Ophthalmic: Blurred vision (≥1%)
Respiratory: Nasopharyngitis (major depressive disorder: 3% to 7%)
<1% (Limited to important or life-threatening): Dystonia (excluding akathisia), orthostatic hypotension, syncope

Drug Interactions

Metabolism/Transport Effects Substrate of CYP2D6 (major), CYP3A4 (major); **Note:** Assignment of Major/Minor substrate status based on clinically relevant drug interaction potential

Avoid Concomitant Use
Avoid concomitant use of Brexpiprazole with any of the following: Amisulpride; Azelastine (Nasal); Conivaptan; Fusidic Acid (Systemic); Idelalisib; Metoclopramide; Orphenadrine; Paraldehyde; Sulpiride; Thalidomide

Increased Effect/Toxicity
Brexpiprazole may increase the levels/effects of: Alcohol (Ethyl); Amisulpride; Azelastine (Nasal); Buprenorphine; CNS Depressants; Hydrocodone; Mequitazine; Methotrimeprazine; Methylphenidate; Metyrosine; Mirtazapine; Orphenadrine; Paraldehyde; Selective Serotonin Reuptake Inhibitors; Serotonin Modulators; Sulpiride; Suvorexant; Thalidomide; Zolpidem

The levels/effects of Brexpiprazole may be increased by: Abiraterone Acetate; Acetylcholinesterase Inhibitors (Central); Aprepitant; Blood Pressure Lowering Agents; Brimonidine (Topical); Cannabis; Conivaptan; CYP2D6 Inhibitors (Moderate); CYP2D6 Inhibitors (Strong); CYP3A4 Inhibitors (Moderate); CYP3A4 Inhibitors (Strong); Dasatinib; Doxylamine; Dronabinol; Droperidol; Fosaprepitant; Fusidic Acid (Systemic); HydrOXYzine; Idelalisib; Ivacaftor; Kava Kava; Lithium; Luliconazole; Magnesium Sulfate; Methotrimeprazine; Methylphenidate; Metoclopramide; Metyrosine; Mifepristone; Minocycline; Nabilone; Netupitant; Osimertinib; Palbociclib; Panobinostat; Peginterferon Alfa-2b; Perampanel; Rufinamide; Serotonin Modulators; Simeprevir; Sodium Oxybate; Stiripentol; Tapentadol; Tetrabenazine; Tetrahydrocannabinol

Decreased Effect
Brexpiprazole may decrease the levels/effects of: Amphetamines; Antidiabetic Agents; Anti-Parkinson's Agents (Dopamine Agonist); Quinagolide

The levels/effects of Brexpiprazole may be decreased by: Bosentan; CYP3A4 Inducers (Moderate); CYP3A4 Inducers (Strong); Dabrafenib; Deferasirox; Enzalutamide; Lithium; Mitotane; Osimertinib; Peginterferon Alfa-2b; Siltuximab; St Johns Wort; Tocilizumab

Storage/Stability Store at 20°C to 25°C (68°F to 77°F); excursions permitted to 15°C to 30°C (59°F to 86°F).

Mechanism of Action Brexpiprazole exhibits partial agonist activity for 5-HT$_{1A}$ and D$_2$ receptors and antagonist activity for 5-HT$_{2A}$ receptors.

Pharmacodynamics/Kinetics
Distribution: V$_d$: IV: 1.56 L/kg
Protein binding: >99%, primarily to serum albumin and alpha$_1$-acid glycoprotein
Metabolism: Hepatic, primarily by CYP3A4 and CYP2D6; major metabolite, DM-3411 (inactive)
Bioavailability: 95%
Half-life elimination: Terminal: Brexpiprazole: 91 hours; DM-3411: 86 hours
Time to peak, plasma: Within 4 hours
Excretion: Feces (46%, ~14% of the total dose as unchanged drug); urine (25%, <1% of the total dose as unchanged drug)

Dosing
Adult
Major Depressive disorder (adjunct to antidepressants): Oral: Initial: 0.5 mg or 1 mg once daily; titrate at weekly intervals based on response and tolerability to 1 mg once daily (if initial dose is 0.5 mg), followed by 2 mg once daily; maximum daily dose: 3 mg
Schizophrenia: Oral: Initial: 1 mg once daily for 4 days, titrate based on response and tolerability to 2 mg once daily for 3 days, followed by 4 mg on day 8; maximum daily dose: 4 mg

Dosage adjustment for CYP2D6 poor metabolizers:
CYP2D6 poor metabolizers: Administer 1/2 of the usual dose
Known CYP2D6 poor metabolizers taking moderate/strong CYP3A4 inhibitors: Administer 1/4 of the usual dose

Dosage adjustment with concomitant therapy: Note: If the coadministered drug is discontinued, adjust brexpiprazole to original dose; if the coadministered CYP3A4 inducer is discontinued, reduce brexpiprazole to original dose over 1 to 2 weeks.
Strong CYP2D6 inhibitors:
Major depressive disorder: Dosage adjustment not necessary.
Schizophrenia: Administer 1/2 of the usual dose
Strong CYP3A4 inhibitors: Administer 1/2 of the usual dose
Moderate/strong CYP2D6 inhibitors in combination with moderate/strong CYP3A4 inhibitors: Administer 1/4 of the usual dose
Strong CYP3A4 inducers: Double the usual dose over 1 to 2 weeks

Geriatric Refer to adult dosing

Renal Impairment
CrCl ≥60 mL/minute: No dosage adjustment necessary.
CrCl <60 mL/minute: Maximum dose:
Major depressive disorder: 2 mg once daily
Schizophrenia: 3 mg once daily
Hemodialysis: There are no dosage adjustments provided in the manufacturer's labeling (has not been studied); however, removal by dialysis unlikely since brexpiprazole is highly protein bound.

Hepatic Impairment
Mild impairment (Child-Pugh class A): There are no dosage adjustments provided in the manufacturer's labeling.
Moderate to severe impairment (Child-Pugh class B or C): Maximum dose:
Major depressive disorder: 2 mg once daily
Schizophrenia: 3 mg once daily

Administration Oral: Administer with or without food.

Monitoring Parameters Mental status; vital signs (as clinically indicated); blood pressure (baseline; repeat 3 months after antipsychotic initiation, then yearly); weight, height, BMI, waist circumference (baseline; repeat at 4, 8, and 12 weeks after initiating or changing therapy, then quarterly; consider switching to a different antipsychotic for a weight gain ≥5% of initial weight); CBC (as clinically indicated; monitor frequently during the first few months of therapy in patients with preexisting low WBC or history of drug-induced leukopenia/neutropenia); electrolytes and liver function (annually and as clinically indicated);

personal and family history of obesity, diabetes, dyslipide-mia, hypertension, or cardiovascular disease (baseline; repeat annually); fasting plasma glucose level/HbA$_{1c}$ (baseline; repeat 3 months after starting antipsychotic, then yearly); fasting lipid panel (baseline; repeat 3 months after initiation of antipsychotic; if LDL level is normal repeat at 2- to 5-year intervals or more frequently if clinical indicated); changes in menstruation, libido, development of galactorrhea, erectile and ejaculatory function (yearly); abnormal involuntary movements or parkinsonian signs (baseline; repeat weekly until dose stabilized for at least 2 weeks after introduction and for 2 weeks after any significant dose increase); tardive dyskinesia (every 12 months; high-risk patients every 6 months); ocular exami-nation (yearly in patients >40 years; every 2 years in younger patients) (ADA 2004; Lehman 2004; Marder 2004).

Dosage Forms Excipient information presented when available (limited, particularly for generics); consult specific product labeling.
Tablet, Oral:
Rexulti: 0.25 mg, 0.5 mg, 1 mg, 2 mg, 3 mg, 4 mg

- ◆ Bricanyl see Terbutaline on page 1761
- ◆ Bricanyl Turbuhaler (Can) see Terbutaline on page 1761
- ◆ Bridion see Sugammadex on page 1706
- ◆ Briellyn see Ethinyl Estradiol and Norethindrone on page 708
- ◆ Brilinta see Ticagrelor on page 1786

Brimonidine (Ophthalmic) (bri MOE ni deen)

Brand Names: US Alphagan P
Brand Names: Canada Alphagan; Alphagan P; Apo-Brimonidine; Brimonidine P; PMS-Brimonidine; ratio-Bri-monidine; Sandoz-Brimonidine
Index Terms Alphagan; Brimonidine Tartrate
Pharmacologic Category Alpha$_2$ Agonist, Ophthalmic; Ophthalmic Agent, Antiglaucoma
Use Elevated intraocular pressure: Reduction of elevated intraocular pressure (IOP) in patients with open-angle glaucoma or ocular hypertension
Dosing
Adult & Geriatric
Elevated intraocular pressure:
US labeling: Ophthalmic: Instill 1 drop in affected eye(s) 3 times/day (approximately every 8 hours)
Canadian labeling: Ophthalmic:
Solution 0.15%: Instill 1 drop in affected eye(s) 3 times/day (approximately every 8 hours)
Solution 0.2%: Instill 1 drop in affected eye(s) 2 times/day (approximately every 12 hours)
Pediatric
US labeling: Children ≥2 years and Adolescents: Refer to adult dosing.
Canadian labeling: Children ≥2 years and Adolescents: Use is not recommended.
Renal Impairment There are no dosage adjustments provided in the manufacturer's labeling (has not been studied).
Additional Information Complete prescribing information should be consulted for additional detail.
Dosage Forms Excipient information presented when available (limited, particularly for generics); consult specific product labeling.
Solution, Ophthalmic, as tartrate:
Alphagan P: 0.1% (5 mL, 10 mL, 15 mL); 0.15% (5 mL, 10 mL, 15 mL) [contains carboxymethylcellulose sodium]
Generic: 0.15% (5 mL, 10 mL, 15 mL); 0.2% (5 mL, 10 mL, 15 mL)
Dosage Forms: Canada Excipient information presented when available (limited, particularly for generics); consult specific product labeling.
Solution, Ophthalmic, as tartrate:
Alphagan: 0.2% (5 mL, 10 mL) [contains benzalkonium chloride]
Alphagan P: 0.15% (5 mL, 10 mL) [contains carboxyme-thylcellulose sodium]

Brimonidine (Topical) (bri MOE ni deen)

Brand Names: US Mirvaso
Index Terms Brimonidine Tartrate
Pharmacologic Category Alpha$_2$-Adrenergic Agonist
Use Rosacea: Topical treatment of persistent (nontran-sient) facial erythema of rosacea in adults

Dosing
Adult & Geriatric Rosacea: Topical: Apply a pea-size amount once daily as a thin layer across the entire face covering the central forehead, each cheek, nose, and chin. Do not apply to eyes or lips.
Additional Information Complete prescribing information should be consulted for additional detail.
Dosage Forms Excipient information presented when available (limited, particularly for generics); consult specific product labeling.
Gel, External:
Mirvaso: 0.33% (30 g) [contains methylparaben, propy-lene glycol]

Brimonidine and Timolol
(bri MOE ni deen & TIM oh lol)

Brand Names: US Combigan
Brand Names: Canada Combigan
Index Terms Brimonidine Tartrate and Timolol Maleate; Timolol and Brimonidine
Pharmacologic Category Alpha$_2$ Agonist, Ophthalmic; Beta-Blocker, Nonselective; Ophthalmic Agent, Antiglau-coma
Use Reduction of intraocular pressure (IOP) in patients with glaucoma or ocular hypertension
Dosing
Adult & Geriatric Glaucoma, ocular hypertension: Oph-thalmic: Instill 1 drop into affected eye(s) twice daily
Pediatric Glaucoma, ocular hypertension: Children ≥2 years: Ophthalmic: Instill 1 drop into affected eye(s) twice daily
Note: In the Canadian labeling, use in children (at any age) is not recommended
Additional Information Complete prescribing information should be consulted for additional detail.
Dosage Forms Excipient information presented when available (limited, particularly for generics); consult specific product labeling.
Solution, ophthalmic [drops]:
Combigan: Brimonidine tartrate 0.2% and timolol 0.5% (5 mL,10 mL) [contains benzalkonium chloride]
Dosage Forms: Canada Excipient information presented when available (limited, particularly for generics); consult specific product labeling.
Solution, ophthalmic [drops]:
Combigan: Brimonidine tartrate 0.2% and timolol maleate 0.5% (2.5 mL, 5 mL,10 mL) [contains benzalkonium chloride]

- ◆ Brimonidine P (Can) see Brimonidine (Ophthalmic) on page 254
- ◆ Brimonidine Tartrate see Brimonidine (Ophthalmic) on page 254
- ◆ Brimonidine Tartrate see Brimonidine (Topical) on page 254
- ◆ Brimonidine Tartrate and Timolol Maleate see Brimo-nidine and Timolol on page 254
- ◆ Brintellix see Vortioxetine on page 1914

Brinzolamide (brin ZOH la mide)

Brand Names: US Azopt
Brand Names: Canada Azopt®
Pharmacologic Category Carbonic Anhydrase Inhibitor (Ophthalmic); Ophthalmic Agent, Antiglaucoma
Use Treatment of elevated intraocular pressure in patients with ocular hypertension or open-angle glaucoma
Dosing
Adult & Geriatric Ocular hypertension or open-angle glaucoma: Ophthalmic: Instill 1 drop in affected eye(s) 3 times/day
Renal Impairment Severe renal impairment (CrCl <30 mL/minute): Use is not recommended (has not been studied; brinzolamide and metabolite are excreted pre-dominately by the kidney).
Hepatic Impairment No dosage adjustment provided in manufacturer's labeling.
Additional Information Complete prescribing information should be consulted for additional detail.
Dosage Forms Excipient information presented when available (limited, particularly for generics); consult specific product labeling.
Suspension, Ophthalmic:
Azopt: 1% (10 mL, 15 mL)

- ◆ Brisdelle see PARoxetine on page 1399
- ◆ British Anti-Lewisite see Dimercaprol on page 557
- ◆ BRL 43694 see Granisetron on page 857
- ◆ Bromday [DSC] see Bromfenac on page 255

Bromfenac (BROME fen ak)

Brand Names: US Bromday [DSC]; Prolensa
Index Terms Bromfenac Sodium
Pharmacologic Category Nonsteroidal Anti-inflammatory Drug (NSAID), Ophthalmic
Use Treatment of postoperative inflammation and reduction in ocular pain following cataract removal
Dosing
Adult & Geriatric Pain, inflammation associated with cataract surgery: Ophthalmic (0.07%, 0.09%): Instill 1 drop into affected eye(s) once daily beginning 1 day prior to surgery and continuing on the day of surgery and for 2 weeks postoperatively
Renal Impairment There are no dosage adjustments provided in the manufacturer's labeling. However, dosage adjustment unlikely due to low systemic absorption.
Hepatic Impairment There are no dosage adjustments provided in the manufacturer's labeling. However, dosage adjustment unlikely due to low systemic absorption.
Additional Information Complete prescribing information should be consulted for additional detail.
Dosage Forms Excipient information presented when available (limited, particularly for generics); consult specific product labeling. [DSC] = Discontinued product
Solution, Ophthalmic:
Bromday: 0.09% (1.7 mL [DSC]) [contains benzalkonium chloride, edetate disodium, polysorbate 80, sodium sulfite]
Prolensa: 0.07% (1.6 mL [DSC], 3 mL) [contains benzalkonium chloride, edetate disodium, sodium sulfite]
Generic: 0.09% (1.7 mL, 2.5 mL, 5 mL [DSC])

◆ *Bromfenac Sodium see Bromfenac on page 255*

Bromocriptine (broe moe KRIP teen)

Brand Names: US Cycloset; Parlodel
Brand Names: Canada Dom-Bromocriptine; PMS-Bromocriptine
Index Terms Bromocriptine Mesylate; Cycloset
Pharmacologic Category Anti-Parkinson's Agent, Dopamine Agonist; Antidiabetic Agent, Dopamine Agonist; Ergot Derivative
Use
Acromegaly (excluding Cycloset): Treatment of acromegaly
Hyperprolactinemia (excluding Cycloset): Treatment of prolactin-secreting pituitary adenoma or disorders associated with hyperprolactinemia including amenorrhea with or without galactorrhea, hypogonadism, or infertility
Parkinson disease (excluding Cycloset): Treatment of the signs and symptoms of idiopathic or postencephalitic Parkinson disease; as adjunctive treatment to levodopa (alone or with a peripheral decarboxylase inhibitor)
Type 2 diabetes mellitus (Cycloset only): To improve glycemic control in adults with type 2 diabetes mellitus (noninsulin dependent, NIDDM) as an adjunct to diet and exercise
Dosing
Adult & Geriatric
Acromegaly: Oral: Initial: 1.25 to 2.5 mg daily increasing by 1.25 to 2.5 mg daily as necessary every 3 to 7 days; usual dose: 20 to 30 mg daily (maximum: 100 mg/day)
Hyperprolactinemia: Oral: Initial: 1.25 to 2.5 mg daily; may be increased by 2.5 mg daily as tolerated every 2 to 7 days until optimal response (range: 2.5 to 15 mg/day)
Parkinsonism: Oral: 1.25 mg twice daily, increased by 2.5 mg daily in 2- to 4-week intervals as needed (maximum: 100 mg/day)
Type 2 diabetes (Cycloset only): Oral: Initial: 0.8 mg once daily; may increase at weekly intervals in 0.8 mg increments as tolerated; usual dose: 1.6 to 4.8 mg once daily (maximum: 4.8 mg/day)
Cycloset dosing adjustment for concomitant therapy:
Moderate CYP3A4 inhibitor (eg, erythromycin): Maximum 1.6 mg/day
Strong CYP3A4 inhibitors (eg, azole antimycotics, HIV protease inhibitors): Avoid concomitant use and unsure adequate washout of the strong CYP3A4 inhibitor prior to bromocriptine initiation.
Neuroleptic malignant syndrome (off-label use): Oral: 2.5 mg (orally or via gastric tube) every 8 to 12 hours, increased to a maximum of 45 mg daily, if needed; continue therapy until NMS is controlled, then taper slowly (Gortney 2009; Strawn 2007)
Pediatric
Hyperprolactinemia: Oral:
Children and Adolescents 11 to 15 years (based on limited information): Initial: 1.25 to 2.5 mg daily.

Dosage may be increased as tolerated to achieve a therapeutic response (range: 2.5 to 10 mg/day). Children ≥16 years: Refer to adult dosing.
Renal Impairment There are no dosage adjustments provided in the manufacturer's labeling (has not been studied).
Hepatic Impairment There are no dosage adjustments provided in the manufacturer's labeling. However, adjustment may be necessary due to extensive hepatic metabolism; use with caution.
Additional Information Complete prescribing information should be consulted for additional detail.
Dosage Forms Excipient information presented when available (limited, particularly for generics); consult specific product labeling. [DSC] = Discontinued product
Capsule, Oral:
Parlodel: 5 mg
Generic: 5 mg
Tablet, Oral:
Cycloset: 0.8 mg
Parlodel: 2.5 mg [DSC] [scored]
Generic: 2.5 mg

◆ *Bromocriptine Mesylate see Bromocriptine on page 255*

Brompheniramine (brome fen IR a meen)

Brand Names: US J-Tan PD [OTC]; Respa-BR
Index Terms Brompheniramine Maleate; Brompheniramine Tannate
Pharmacologic Category Alkylamine Derivative; Histamine H₁ Antagonist; Histamine H₁ Antagonist, First Generation
Use Upper respiratory allergies: Temporary relief of sneezing; itchy, watery eyes; itchy nose or throat; and runny nose caused by hay fever (allergic rhinitis) or other upper respiratory allergies.
Dosing
Pediatric
Upper respiratory allergies: Oral:
Children 2 to <6 years: 1 mg (1 mL) every 4 to 6 hours (maximum: 6 mg [6 mL] per 24 hours)
Children 6 to <12 years: 2 mg (2 mL) every 4-6 hours (maximum: 12 mg [12 mL] per 24 hours)
Additional Information Complete prescribing information should be consulted for additional detail.
Dosage Forms Excipient information presented when available (limited, particularly for generics); consult specific product labeling.
Liquid, Oral, as maleate:
J-Tan PD: 1 mg/mL (30 mL) [alcohol free, dye free, sugar free; contains propylene glycol, saccharin sodium; strawberry-banana flavor]
Tablet Extended Release 12 Hour, Oral, as maleate:
Respa-BR: 11 mg [dye free]

◆ *Brompheniramine Maleate see Brompheniramine on page 255*

◆ *Brompheniramine Tannate see Brompheniramine on page 255*

◆ *Broncho Saline [OTC] see Sodium Chloride on page 1671*

◆ *Brovana see Arformoterol on page 145*

◆ *BSF208075 see Ambrisentan on page 88*

◆ *BSS see Bismuth Subsalicylate on page 232*

◆ *BTK inhibitor PCI-32765 see Ibrutinib on page 902*

◆ *BTX-A see OnabotulinumtoxinA on page 1333*

◆ *B-type Natriuretic Peptide (Human) see Nesiritide on page 1269*

◆ *Buckleys Chest Congestion [OTC] see GuaiFENesin on page 860*

◆ *Budeprion XL [DSC] see BuPROPion on page 269*

◆ *Budeprion SR see BuPROPion on page 269*

◆ *Budeprion SR [DSC] see BuPROPion on page 269*

Budesonide (Systemic) (byoo DES oh nide)

Brand Names: US Entocort EC; Uceris
Brand Names: Canada Entocort
Pharmacologic Category Corticosteroid, Systemic
Additional Appendix Information
Oral Dosages That Should Not Be Crushed on page 2003 ▶

Use

Oral capsule: Treatment of active Crohn disease (mild-to-moderate) involving the ileum and/or ascending colon; maintenance of remission (for up to 3 months) of Crohn disease (mild-to-moderate) involving the ileum and/or ascending colon

Oral tablet: Induction of remission in patients with active ulcerative colitis (mild-to-moderate)

Pregnancy Considerations Adverse events have been observed with corticosteroids in animal reproduction studies. Some studies have shown an association between first trimester systemic corticosteroid use and oral clefts (Park-Wyllie 2000; Pradat 2003). Systemic corticosteroids may also influence fetal growth (decreased birth weight); however, information is conflicting (Lunghi 2010). Hypoadrenalism may occur in newborns following maternal use of corticosteroids in pregnancy; monitor. When systemic corticosteroids are needed in pregnancy, it is generally recommended to use the lowest effective dose for the shortest duration of time, avoiding high doses during the first trimester (Leachman 2006; Lunghi 2010). Budesonide may be used for the induction of remission in pregnant women with inflammatory bowel disease (Habal 2012).

Based on available data, an overall increased risk of congenital malformations or a decrease in fetal growth has not been associated with maternal use of inhaled corticosteroids during pregnancy (Bakhireva 2005; NAEPP 2005; Namazy 2004). In addition, studies of pregnant women specifically using inhaled budesonide have not demonstrated an increased risk of congenital abnormalities. Uncontrolled asthma is associated with adverse events on pregnancy (increased risk of perinatal mortality, pre-eclampsia, preterm birth, low birth weight infants). Inhaled corticosteroids are recommended for the treatment of asthma during pregnancy; budesonide is preferred (ACOG 2008; NAEPP 2005).

Breast-Feeding Considerations Due to the potential for serious adverse reactions in the nursing infant, the manufacturers of the oral tablets and capsules recommend a decision be made whether to discontinue nursing or to discontinue the drug, taking into account the importance of treatment to the mother. If there is concern about exposure to the infant, some guidelines recommend waiting 4 hours after the maternal dose of an oral systemic corticosteroid before breast-feeding in order to decrease potential exposure to the nursing infant (based on a study using prednisolone) (Habal 2012; Ost 1985).

According to the manufacturer of the product for inhalation, the decision to continue or discontinue breast-feeding during therapy should take into account the risk of minimal exposure to the infant and the benefits of breast-feeding to the mother. The use of inhaled corticosteroids is not considered a contraindication to breast-feeding (NAEPP 2005).

Contraindications Hypersensitivity to budesonide or any component of the formulation; primary treatment of status asthmaticus, acute episodes of asthma; not for relief of acute bronchospasm

Warnings/Precautions May cause hypercorticism or suppression of hypothalamic-pituitary-adrenal (HPA) axis, particularly in younger children, in patients receiving high doses for prolonged periods, or with concomitant CYP3A4 inhibitor use. HPA axis suppression may lead to adrenal crisis. Withdrawal and discontinuation of a corticosteroid should be done slowly and carefully. Particular care is required when patients are transferred from systemic corticosteroids to inhaled products or corticosteroids with lower systemic effect due to possible adrenal insufficiency or withdrawal from steroids, including an increase in allergic symptoms. Adult patients receiving >20 mg per day of prednisone (or equivalent) may be most susceptible. Fatalities have occurred due to adrenal insufficiency in asthmatic patients during and after transfer from systemic corticosteroids to aerosol steroids; aerosol steroids do not provide the systemic steroid needed to treat patients having trauma, surgery, or infections. Do not use this product to transfer patients directly from oral corticosteroid therapy. Select surgical patients on long-term, high-dose, inhaled corticosteroid (ICS), should be given stress doses of hydrocortisone intravenously during the surgical period and the dose reduced rapidly within 24 hours after surgery (NAEPP 2007).

Acute myopathy has been reported with high-dose corticosteroids, usually in patients with neuromuscular transmission disorders; may involve ocular and/or respiratory muscles; monitor creatine kinase; recovery may be delayed. Corticosteroid use may cause psychiatric disturbances, including depression, euphoria, insomnia, mood swings, and personality changes. Preexisting psychiatric conditions may be exacerbated by corticosteroid use.

Prolonged use of corticosteroids may also increase the incidence of secondary infection, mask acute infection (including fungal infections), prolong or exacerbate viral infections, or limit response to vaccines. Exposure to chickenpox should be avoided; corticosteroids should not be used to treat ocular herpes simplex. Corticosteroids should not be used for viral hepatitis. Close observation is required in patients with latent tuberculosis and/or TB reactivity; restrict use in active TB (only in conjunction with antituberculosis treatment). Prolonged treatment with corticosteroids has been associated with the development of Kaposi sarcoma (case reports); if noted, discontinuation of therapy should be considered.

Use with caution in patients with thyroid disease, hepatic impairment, renal impairment, cardiovascular disease, diabetes, glaucoma, cataracts, myasthenia gravis, patients at risk for osteoporosis, patients at risk for seizures, or GI diseases (diverticulitis, peptic ulcer, ulcerative colitis) due to perforation risk. Use caution following acute MI (corticosteroids have been associated with myocardial rupture).

Potentially significant interactions may exist, requiring dose or frequency adjustment, additional monitoring, and/or selection of alternative therapy.

Some dosage forms may contain polysorbate 80 (also known as Tweens). Hypersensitivity reactions, usually a delayed reaction, have been reported following exposure to pharmaceutical products containing polysorbate 80 in certain individuals (Isaksson 2002; Lucente 2000; Shelley 1995). Thrombocytopenia, ascites, pulmonary deterioration, and renal and hepatic failure have been reported in premature neonates after receiving parenteral products containing polysorbate 80 (Alade 1986; CDC 1984). See manufacturer's labeling.

Adverse Reactions

>10%:

Central nervous system: Headache (15% to 21%)

Dermatologic: Acne vulgaris (≤5%)

Endocrine & metabolic: Redistribution of body fat (1%)

Gastrointestinal: Nausea (5% to 11%)

Respiratory: Respiratory tract infection (11%)

1% to 10%:

Cardiovascular: Edema (<5%), chest pain (<5%), facial edema (<5%), flushing (<5%), hypertension (<5%), palpitations (<5%), tachycardia (<5%)

Central nervous system: Dizziness (<5% to 7%), fatigue (3% to 5%), agitation (<5%), amnesia (<5%), confusion (<5%), drowsiness (<5%), insomnia (<5%), malaise (<5%), nervousness (<5%), paresthesia (<5%), sleep disorder (<5%), vertigo (<5%)

Dermatologic: Alopecia (<5%), dermatitis (<5%), dermatological disease (<5%), diaphoresis (<5%), eczema (<5%)

Endocrine & metabolic: Hirsutism (<1% to 5%), hypokalemia (1% to <5%), intermenstrual bleeding (<5%), menstrual disease (<5%), weight gain (<5%), decreased cortisol (2% to 4%), adrenocortical insufficiency (>1%)

Gastrointestinal: Diarrhea (10%), dyspepsia (6%), anal disease (<5%), enteritis (<5%), epigastric pain (<5%), exacerbation of Crohn's disease (<5%), gastrointestinal fistula (<5%), glossitis (<5%), hemorrhoids (<5%), increased appetite (<5%), intestinal obstruction (<5%), oral candidiasis (<5%), upper abdominal pain (3% to 4%), flatulence (3%), abdominal distention (2%), constipation (2%)

Genitourinary: Dysuria (<5%), nocturia (<5%), urinary frequency (<5%), urinary tract infection (2% to <5%), hematuria (≥1%), pyuria (≥1%)

Hematologic & oncologic: C-reactive protein increased (1% to <5%), leukocytosis (1% to <5%), purpura (<5%), abnormal neutrophils (≥1%), anemia (≥1%), increased erythrocyte sedimentation rate (≥1%)

Hepatic: Increased serum alkaline phosphatase (≥1%)

Hypersensitivity: Tongue edema (<5%)

Infection: Viral infection (6%), abscess (<5%)

Neuromuscular & skeletal: Arthralgia (5%), arthritis (≤5%), hyperkinesia (<5%), muscle cramps (<5%), myalgia (<5%), tremor (<5%), weakness (<5%)

Ophthalmic: Eye disease (<5%), visual disturbance (<5%)

Otic: Otic infection (<5%)

Respiratory: Sinusitis (8%), bronchitis (<5%), dyspnea (<5%), flu-like symptoms (<5%), pharyngeal disease (<5%), rhinitis (<5%)

Miscellaneous: Fever (<5%)

<1% (Limited to important or life-threatening): Anaphylaxis, intracranial hypertension (benign), peripheral edema, rectal bleeding

Drug Interactions

Metabolism/Transport Effects Substrate of CYP3A4 (major); **Note:** Assignment of Major/Minor substrate status based on clinically relevant drug interaction potential

Avoid Concomitant Use

Avoid concomitant use of Budesonide (Systemic) with any of the following: Aldesleukin; BCG (Intravesical); Conivaptan; Fusidic Acid (Systemic); Grapefruit Juice; Idelalisib; Natalizumab; Pimecrolimus; Tacrolimus (Topical); Tofacitinib

Increased Effect/Toxicity

Budesonide (Systemic) may increase the levels/effects of: Deferasirox; Fingolimod; Leflunomide; Natalizumab; Tofacitinib

The levels/effects of Budesonide (Systemic) may be increased by: Conivaptan; CYP3A4 Inhibitors (Moderate); CYP3A4 Inhibitors (Strong); Dasatinib; Denosumab; Fosaprepitant; Fusidic Acid (Systemic); Grapefruit Juice; Idelalisib; Ivacaftor; Luliconazole; Mifepristone; Osimertinib; Palbociclib; Pimecrolimus; Roflumilast; Simeprevir; Stiripentol; Tacrolimus (Topical); Trastuzumab

Decreased Effect

Budesonide (Systemic) may decrease the levels/effects of: Aldesleukin; BCG (Intravesical); Coccidioides immitis Skin Test; Corticorelin; Hyaluronidase; Sipuleucel-T; Vaccines (Inactivated)

The levels/effects of Budesonide (Systemic) may be decreased by: Antacids; Bile Acid Sequestrants; Echinacea; Osimertinib

Food Interactions Grapefruit juice may double systemic exposure of orally administered budesonide. Administration of capsules with a high-fat meal delays peak concentration, but does not alter the extent of absorption; administration of tablets with a high-fat meal decreases peak concentration (~27%). Management: Avoid grapefruit juice when using oral capsules or tablets.

Storage/Stability Oral capsules and tablets: Store at 25°C (77°F); excursions permitted to 15°C to 30°C (59°F to 86°F); keep container tightly closed.

Mechanism of Action Controls the rate of protein synthesis; depresses the migration of polymorphonuclear leukocytes, fibroblasts; reverses capillary permeability and lysosomal stabilization at the cellular level to prevent or control inflammation. Has potent glucocorticoid activity and weak mineralocorticoid activity.

Pharmacodynamics/Kinetics

Distribution:
Children 4 to 6 years: 3 L/kg
Adults: 2.2 to 3.9 L/kg
Protein binding: 85% to 90%
Metabolism: Hepatic via CYP3A4 to two metabolites: 16 alpha-hydroxyprednisolone and 6 beta-hydroxybudesonide; both are <1% as active as parent
Bioavailability: Limited by high first-pass effect; Capsule: 9% in healthy volunteers and 21% in patients with Crohn's disease
Half-life elimination: IV:
Children 10 to 14 years: 1.5 hours
Adults: 2 to 3.6 hours
Time to peak: Capsule: 0.5 to 10 hours (variable in Crohn disease); Tablet (extended release): ~13 hours
Excretion: Urine (60%) and feces as metabolites

Dosing

Adult & Geriatric

Crohn disease (active): Oral: Capsule: 9 mg once daily in the morning for up to 8 weeks; recurring episodes may be treated with a repeat 8-week course of treatment.

Maintenance of remission: Following treatment of active disease (control of symptoms with CDAI <150), treatment may be continued at a dosage of 6 mg once daily for up to 3 months. If symptom control is maintained for 3 months, tapering of the dosage to complete cessation is recommended. Continued dosing beyond 3 months has not been demonstrated to result in substantial benefit.

Ulcerative colitis (active): Oral: Tablet: 9 mg once daily in the morning for up to 8 weeks

Renal Impairment There are no dosage adjustments provided in the manufacturer's labeling (has not been studied).

Hepatic Impairment There are no specific dosage adjustments provided in the manufacturer's labeling (has not been studied). Manufacturer labeling for oral budesonide suggests a dosage reduction may be necessary with moderate to severe impairment. Budesonide undergoes hepatic metabolism; bioavailability increased in cirrhosis; monitor closely for signs and symptoms of hypercorticism.

Dietary Considerations Oral capsules, tablets: Avoid grapefruit juice.

Administration Oral capsule, tablet: May be administered without regard to meals. Swallow whole; do not crush, chew, or break.

Monitoring Parameters Monitor growth in pediatric patients; blood pressure, serum glucose, weight with high-dose or long-term oral use; signs and symptoms of hypercorticism or adrenal suppression

Dosage Forms Excipient information presented when available (limited, particularly for generics); consult specific product labeling.

Capsule Extended Release 24 Hour, Oral:
Entocort EC: 3 mg
Generic: 3 mg
Tablet Extended Release 24 Hour, Oral:
Uceris: 9 mg

Budesonide (Nasal) (byoo DES oh nide)

Brand Names: US Rhinocort Aqua
Brand Names: Canada Mylan-Budesonide AQ; Rhinocort Aqua; Rhinocort Turbuhaler
Index Terms Rhinocort Allergy OTC
Pharmacologic Category Corticosteroid, Nasal
Additional Appendix Information
Inhaled Corticosteroids *on page 1951*
Use Management of symptoms of seasonal or perennial rhinitis
Canadian labeling: Additional use (not in U.S. labeling): Prevention and treatment of nasal polyps

Dosing

Adult & Geriatric

Nasal polyps: *Nasal inhalation:*
Canadian labeling:
Rhinocort Aqua: 256 mcg/day administered as a single 64 mcg spray in each nostril twice daily; maximum dose: 256 mcg/day
Rhinocort Turbuhaler: 100 mcg into each nostril twice daily; maximum: 400 mcg/day

Rhinitis: *Nasal inhalation:*
U.S. labeling (Rhinocort Aqua): 64 mcg/day as a single 32 mcg spray in each nostril. Some patients who do not achieve adequate control may benefit from increased dosage. A reduced dosage may be effective after initial control is achieved
Maximum dose: Children <12 years: 128 mcg/day; Adults: 256 mcg/day
Canadian labeling:
Rhinocort Aqua: Initial: 256 mcg/day administered as two 64 mcg sprays in each nostril once daily or a single 64 mcg spray in each nostril twice daily; Maintenance: Individualize, lowest effective dose (maximum dose: 256 mcg/day)
Rhinocort Turbuhaler: Initial: 200 mcg into each nostril once daily; Maintenance: Individualize, lowest effective dose (maximum: 400 mcg/day)

Pediatric

Nasal polyps: *Nasal inhalation:*
Canadian labeling: Children ≥6 years: Refer to adult dosing.

Rhinitis: *Nasal inhalation:*
U.S. labeling (Rhinocort Aqua): Children ≥6 years: Refer to adult dosing.
Canadian labeling (Rhinocort Aqua, Rhinocort Turbuhaler): Children ≥6 years: Refer to adult dosing.

Renal Impairment No dosage adjustment provided in manufacturer's labeling (has not been studied).

Hepatic Impairment No dosage adjustment provided in manufacturer's labeling. Systemic availability of budesonide may be increased in patients with cirrhosis; monitor closely for signs and symptoms of hypercorticism; dosage reduction may be required.

Additional Information Complete prescribing information should be consulted for additional detail.

Product Availability Rhinocort Allergy OTC: FDA approved March 2015; anticipated availability is currently unknown.

Dosage Forms Considerations Rhinocort Aqua 8.6 g bottles contain 120 sprays.

Dosage Forms Excipient information presented when available (limited, particularly for generics); consult specific product labeling.

Suspension, Nasal:
Rhinocort Aqua: 32 mcg/actuation (8.6 g) [contains disodium edta, polysorbate 80]
Generic: 32 mcg/actuation (8.6 g)

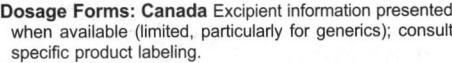

Dosage Forms: Canada Excipient information presented when available (limited, particularly for generics); consult specific product labeling.

Powder for nasal inhalation:

Rhinocort Turbuhaler: 100 mcg/inhalation [delivers 200 metered actuations]

Suspension, intranasal [spray]:

Rhinocort Aqua: 64 mcg/inhalation [120 metered actuations]

Budesonide (Oral Inhalation)
(byoo DES oh nide)

Brand Names: US Pulmicort; Pulmicort Flexhaler
Brand Names: Canada Pulmicort Turbuhaler
Pharmacologic Category Corticosteroid, Inhalant (Oral)
Additional Appendix Information

Inhaled Corticosteroids *on page 1951*

Use

Nebulization: Maintenance and prophylactic treatment of asthma

Oral inhalation: Maintenance and prophylactic treatment of asthma; includes patients who require oral corticosteroids and those who may benefit from systemic dose reduction/elimination

Guideline recommendations: Asthma: A low-dose inhaled corticosteroid (*in addition to an as-needed short acting beta2-agonist*) is the initial preferred long term control medication for children, adolescents, and adult patients with persistent asthma who are candidates for treatment according to a step-wise treatment approach (GINA 2015; NAEPP 2007).

Pregnancy Considerations Adverse events have been observed with corticosteroids in animal reproduction studies. Some studies have shown an association between first trimester systemic corticosteroid use and oral clefts (Park-Wyllie 2000; Pradat 2003). Systemic corticosteroids may also influence fetal growth (decreased birth weight); however, information is conflicting (Lunghi 2010). Hypoadrenalism may occur in newborns following maternal use of corticosteroids in pregnancy; monitor. When systemic corticosteroids are needed in pregnancy, it is generally recommended to use the lowest effective dose for the shortest duration of time, avoiding high doses during the first trimester (Leachman 2006; Lunghi 2010). Budesonide may be used for the induction of remission in pregnant women with inflammatory bowel disease (Habal 2012).

Based on available data, an overall increased risk of congenital malformations or a decrease in fetal growth has not been associated with maternal use of inhaled corticosteroids during pregnancy (Bakhireva 2005; NAEPP 2005; Namazy 2004). In addition, studies of pregnant women specifically using inhaled budesonide have not demonstrated an increased risk of congenital abnormalities. Uncontrolled asthma is associated with adverse events on pregnancy (increased risk of perinatal mortality, pre-eclampsia, preterm birth, low birth weight infants). Inhaled corticosteroids are recommended for the treatment of asthma during pregnancy; budesonide is preferred (ACOG 2008; NAEPP 2005).

Breast-Feeding Considerations Following use of the powder for oral inhalation, ~0.3% to 1% of the maternal dose was found in breast milk. The maximum concentration appeared within 45 minutes of dosing. Plasma budesonide levels obtained from infants ~90 minutes after breast-feeding (~140 minutes after maternal dose) were below the limit of quantification. Concentrations of budesonide in breast milk are expected to be higher following administration of oral capsules/tablets than after an inhaled dose.

According to the manufacturer of the product for inhalation, the decision to continue or discontinue breast-feeding during therapy should take into account the risk of minimal exposure to the infant and the benefits of breast-feeding to the mother. The use of inhaled corticosteroids is not considered a contraindication to breast-feeding (NAEPP 2005).

Contraindications

Hypersensitivity to budesonide or any component of the formulation; primary treatment of status asthmaticus, acute episodes of asthma; not for relief of acute bronchospasm

Canadian labeling: Additional contraindications (not in US labeling): Moderate-to-severe bronchiectasis, pulmonary tuberculosis (active or quiescent), untreated respiratory infection (bacterial, fungal, or viral)

Warnings/Precautions May cause hypercorticism or suppression of hypothalamic-pituitary-adrenal (HPA) axis, particularly in younger children, in patients receiving high doses for prolonged periods, or with concomitant CYP3A4 inhibitor use. HPA axis suppression may lead to adrenal

crisis. Withdrawal and discontinuation of a corticosteroid should be done slowly and carefully. Particular care is required when patients are transferred from systemic corticosteroids to inhaled products or corticosteroids with lower systemic effect due to possible adrenal insufficiency or withdrawal from steroids, including an increase in allergic symptoms. Adult patients receiving >20 mg per day of prednisone (or equivalent) may be most susceptible. Fatalities have occurred due to adrenal insufficiency in asthmatic patients during and after transfer from systemic corticosteroids to aerosol steroids; aerosol steroids do not provide the systemic steroid needed to treat patients having trauma, surgery, or infections. Do not use this product to transfer patients directly from oral corticosteroid therapy. Select surgical patients on long-term, high-dose, inhaled corticosteroid (ICS), should be given stress doses of hydrocortisone intravenously during the surgical period and the dose reduced rapidly within 24 hours after surgery (NAEPP 2007). Rare cases of vasculitis (Churg-Strauss syndrome) or other systemic eosinophilic conditions can occur; often associated with decrease and/or withdrawal of oral corticosteroid therapy following initiation of inhaled corticosteroid.

Bronchospasm may occur with wheezing after inhalation; if this occurs stop steroid and treat with a fast-acting bronchodilator (eg, albuterol). Supplemental steroids (oral or parenteral) may be needed during stress or severe asthma attacks. Not to be used in status asthmaticus or for the relief of acute bronchospasm. Acute myopathy has been reported with high-dose corticosteroids, usually in patients with neuromuscular transmission disorders; may involve ocular and/or respiratory muscles; monitor creatine kinase; recovery may be delayed. Corticosteroid use may cause psychiatric disturbances, including depression, euphoria, insomnia, mood swings, and personality changes. Preexisting psychiatric conditions may be exacerbated by corticosteroid use. Prolonged use of corticosteroids may also increase the incidence of secondary infection, mask acute infection (including fungal infections), prolong or exacerbate viral infections, or limit response to vaccines. Exposure to chickenpox should be avoided; corticosteroids should not be used to treat ocular herpes simplex. Corticosteroids should not be used for viral hepatitis. Close observation is required in patients with latent tuberculosis and/or TB reactivity; restrict use in active TB (only in conjunction with antituberculosis treatment). *Candida albicans* infections may occur in the mouth and pharynx; rinsing (and spitting) with water after inhaler use may decrease risk. Prolonged treatment with corticosteroids has been associated with the development of Kaposi sarcoma (case reports); if noted, discontinuation of therapy should be considered.

Use with caution in patients with thyroid disease, hepatic impairment, cardiovascular disease, diabetes, glaucoma, cataracts, myasthenia gravis, patients at risk for osteoporosis, patients at risk for seizures, or GI diseases (diverticulitis, peptic ulcer, ulcerative colitis) due to perforation risk. Use caution following acute MI (corticosteroids have been associated with myocardial rupture).

Potentially significant interactions may exist, requiring dose or frequency adjustment, additional monitoring, and/or selection of alternative therapy.

Orally-inhaled corticosteroids may cause a reduction in growth velocity in pediatric patients (~1 centimeter per year [range: 0.3 to 1.8 cm per year]) and related to dose and duration of exposure). To minimize the systemic effects of orally-inhaled corticosteroids, each patient should be titrated to the lowest effective dose. Growth should be routinely monitored in pediatric patients. Withdraw systemic therapy with gradual tapering of dose. There have been reports of systemic corticosteroid withdrawal symptoms (eg, joint/muscle pain, lassitude, depression) when withdrawing oral inhalation therapy. Pulmicort Flexhaler contains lactose; very rare anaphylactic reactions have been reported in patients with severe milk protein allergy. Some dosage forms may contain polysorbate 80 (also known as Tweens). Hypersensitivity reactions, usually a delayed reaction, have been reported following exposure to pharmaceutical products containing polysorbate 80 in certain individuals (Isaksson 2002; Lucente 2000; Shelley 1995). Thrombocytopenia, ascites, pulmonary deterioration, and renal and hepatic failure have been reported in premature neonates after receiving parenteral products containing polysorbate 80 (Alade 1986; CDC 1984). See manufacturer's labeling.

Adverse Reactions
Oral inhaler (Pulmicort Flexhaler):
1% to 10%:

Cardiovascular: Syncope (1% to 3%)

Central nervous system: Headache (≥3%), pain (≥3%), hypertonia (1% to 3%), insomnia (1% to 3%), voice disorder (1% to 3%)

Endocrine & metabolic: Weight gain (1% to 3%)

Gastrointestinal: Dyspepsia (≥5%), nausea (2% to ≥5%), abdominal pain (1% to 3%), dysgeusia (1% to 3%), vomiting (1% to 3%), xerostomia (1% to 3%), viral gastroenteritis (2%), oral candidiasis (1%)

Hematologic & oncologic: Bruise (1% to 3%)

Infection: Infection (1% to 3%)

Neuromuscular & skeletal: Arthralgia (≥5%), weakness (≥5%), back pain (≥3%), bone fracture (1% to 3%), myalgia (1% to 3%), neck pain (1% to 3%)

Otic: Otitis media (1%)

Respiratory: Nasopharyngitis (9%), cough (≥5%), rhinitis (≥5%), respiratory tract infection (≥3%), sinusitis (≥3%), nasal congestion (3%), pharyngitis (3%), allergic rhinitis (2%), viral upper respiratory tract infection (2%)

Miscellaneous: Fever (≥3%)

Postmarketing and/or case reports (Limited to important or life-threatening): Adrenocortical insufficiency, aggressive behavior, cataract, depression, glaucoma, hypercorticoidism, hypersensitivity (immediate and delayed [includes rash, contact dermatitis, angioedema, bronchospasm, urticaria]), increased intraocular pressure, psychosis, wheezing (patients with severe milk allergy)

Suspension for nebulization:
>10%:

Otic: Otitis media (12%)

Respiratory: Respiratory infection (38%), rhinitis (11% to 12%)

1% to 10%:

Cardiovascular: Chest pain (1% to <3%)

Central nervous system: Emotional lability (1% to <3%), fatigue (1% to <3%), voice disorder (1% to <3%)

Dermatologic: Skin rash (4%), contact dermatitis (1% to <3%), eczema (1% to <3%), pruritus (1% to <3%), pustular rash (1% to <3%)

Gastrointestinal: Gastroenteritis (5%), diarrhea (4%), vomiting (4%), abdominal pain (3%), anorexia (1% to <3%)

Hematologic & oncologic: Cervical lymphadenopathy (1% to <3%), purpura (1% to <3%)

Hypersensitivity: Hypersensitivity reaction (1% to <3%)

Infection: Candidiasis (4% to 5%), viral infection (4% to 5%), herpes simplex infection (1% to <3%), infection (1% to <3%)

Neuromuscular & skeletal: Bone fracture (1% to <3%), hyperkinesia (1% to <3%), myalgia (1% to <3%)

Ophthalmic: Conjunctivitis (4%), eye infection (1% to <3%)

Otic: Otic infection (5%), otalgia (1% to <3%), otitis externa (1% to <3%)

Respiratory: Cough (8% to 9%), epistaxis (2% to 4%), flu-like symptoms (1% to <3%), stridor (1% to <3%)

Postmarketing and/or case reports (Limited to important or life-threatening): Adrenocortical insufficiency, aggressive behavior, avascular necrosis of femoral head, bronchitis, cataract, depression, glaucoma, growth suppression, hypercorticoidism, hypersensitivity (immediate and delayed [includes angioedema, bronchospasm, urticaria]), increased intraocular pressure, osteoporosis, psychosis

Drug Interactions
Metabolism/Transport Effects None known.

Avoid Concomitant Use

Avoid concomitant use of Budesonide (Oral Inhalation) with any of the following: Aldesleukin; Loxapine

Increased Effect/Toxicity

Budesonide (Oral Inhalation) may increase the levels/effects of: Amphotericin B; Ceritinib; Deferasirox; Loop Diuretics; Loxapine; Thiazide Diuretics

The levels/effects of Budesonide (Oral Inhalation) may be increased by: CYP3A4 Inhibitors (Strong); Telaprevir

Decreased Effect

Budesonide (Oral Inhalation) may decrease the levels/effects of: Aldesleukin; Corticorelin; Hyaluronidase

Storage/Stability
Oral inhaler (Pulmicort Flexhaler): Store at controlled room temperature of 20°C to 25°C (68°F to 77°F). Protect from moisture.

Suspension for nebulization: Store upright at 20°C to 25°C (68°F to 77°F). Protect from light. Do not refrigerate or freeze. Once aluminum package is opened, solution should be used within 2 weeks. Continue to protect from light.

Mechanism of Action
Controls the rate of protein synthesis; depresses the migration of polymorphonuclear leukocytes, fibroblasts; reverses capillary permeability and lysosomal stabilization at the cellular level to prevent or control inflammation. Has potent glucocorticoid activity and weak mineralocorticoid activity.

Pharmacodynamics/Kinetics
Onset of action: Nebulization: 2 to 8 days; Inhalation: 24 hours

Peak effect: Nebulization: 4 to 6 weeks; Inhalation: 1 to 2 weeks

Distribution:

Children 4 to 6 years: 3 L/kg

Adults: 2.2 to 3.9 L/kg

Protein binding: 85% to 90%

Metabolism: Hepatic via CYP3A4 to two metabolites: 16 alpha-hydroxyprednisolone and 6 beta-hydroxybudesonide; both are <1% as active as parent

Bioavailability:

Nebulization: Children 4 to 6 years: 6%

Oral inhalation: 39% of an inhaled metered dose is available systemically

Half-life elimination:

Children 4 to 6 years: 2.3 hours (after nebulization)

Children and Adolescents 10 to 14 years: 1.5 hours

Adults: 2 to 3.6 hours

Time to peak:

Nebulization: Pulmicort Respules: Children: 20 minutes

Oral inhalation: Pulmicort Flexhaler:

Children and Adolescents: 15 to 30 minutes

Adults: 10 minutes

Excretion: Urine (60%) and feces as metabolites

Clearance:

Children 4 to 6 years: 0.5 L/minute (~50% greater than healthy adults after weight adjustment)

Adults: 0.9 to 1.8 L/minute

Dosing
Adult & Geriatric
Asthma: Oral inhalation: Titrate to lowest effective dose once patient is stable.

US labeling: Pulmicort Flexhaler: Initial: 360 mcg twice daily (selected patients may be initiated at 180 mcg twice daily); maximum: 720 mcg twice daily; **Note:** May increase dose after 1 to 2 weeks of therapy in patients who are not adequately controlled

Canadian labeling: Pulmicort Turbuhaler:

Initial (or during periods of severe asthma or when switching from oral corticosteroid therapy): 400 to 2400 mcg daily in 2 to 4 divided doses

Maintenance: 200 to 400 mcg twice daily (higher doses may be needed for some patients). Patients taking 400 mcg/day may take as a single daily dose.

Asthma guidelines:

National Asthma Education and Prevention Program guidelines (NAEPP 2007): Dry powder inhaler (refers to the Pulmicort Flexhaler available in US). **Note:** Administer in divided doses twice daily.

"Low" dose: 180 to 600 mcg/day

"Medium" dose: >600 to 1,200 mcg/day

"High" dose: >1,200 mcg/day

Global Initiative for Asthma guidelines (GINA 2015): Dry powder inhaler (refers to the Pulmicort Turbuhaler available in Canada):

"Low" dose: 200 to 400 mcg daily

"Medium" dose: >400 to 800 mcg daily

"High" dose: >800 mcg daily

Conversion: Conversion from oral systemic corticosteroid to orally inhaled corticosteroid: Initiation of oral inhalation therapy should begin in patients whose asthma is reasonably stabilized on oral corticosteroids (OCS). A gradual dose reduction of OCS should begin ~7 to 10 days after starting inhaled therapy. US labeling recommends reducing prednisone dose by 2.5 mg/day (or equivalent of other OCS) on a weekly basis (patients using oral inhaler) or by ≤25% every 1 to 2 weeks (patients using respules). Canadian labeling recommends reducing prednisone dose by 2.5 mg/day (or equivalent of other OCS) every 4 days in closely monitored patients or every 10 days if not closely monitored. If adrenal insufficiency occurs, temporarily increase the OCS dose and follow with a more gradual withdrawal. **Note:** When transitioning from systemic to inhaled corticosteroids, supplemental systemic corticosteroid therapy may be necessary during periods of stress or during severe asthma attacks.

Chronic obstructive pulmonary disease (acute exacerbation) (off-label use): Nebulization: 2 mg every 6 hours (Maltais 2002)

Chronic obstructive pulmonary disease (stable) (off-label use): Oral inhalation: 100 to 400 mcg daily in combination with a long-acting bronchodilator (GOLD 2014)

Pediatric

Asthma: Titrate to lowest effective dose once patient is stable.

Oral inhalation:

US labeling: Pulmicort Flexhaler: Children ≥6 years: Initial: 180 mcg twice daily (some patients may be initiated at 360 mcg twice daily); maximum: 360 mcg twice daily; **Note:** May increase dose after 1 to 2 weeks of therapy in patients who are not adequately controlled.

Canadian labeling: Pulmicort Turbuhaler:

Children 6 to 11 years:

Initial (or during periods of severe asthma or when switching from oral corticosteroid therapy): 200 to 400 mcg daily in 2 divided doses

Maintenance: Individualized, lowest effective dose in 2 divided doses

Children ≥12 years: Refer to adult dosing.

Asthma guidelines:

National Asthma Education and Prevention Program guidelines (NAEPP 2007): Dry powder inhaler (refers to the Pulmicort Flexhaler available in US). **Note:** Administer in divided doses twice daily.

Children 5 to 11 years:

"Low" dose: 180 to 400 mcg/day

"Medium" dose: >400 to 800 mcg/day

"High" dose: >800 mcg/day

Children ≥12 years and Adolescents: Refer to adult dosing.

Global Initiative for Asthma guidelines (GINA 2015): Dry powder inhaler (refers to the Pulmicort Turbuhaler available in Canada):

Children 6 to 11 years:

"Low" dose: 100 to 200 mcg daily

"Medium" dose: >200 to 400 mcg daily

"High" dose: >400 mcg daily

Children ≥12 years and Adolescents: Refer to adult dosing.

Conversion: *Conversion from oral systemic corticosteroid to orally inhaled corticosteroid:* Initiation of oral inhalation therapy should begin in patients whose asthma is reasonably stabilized on oral corticosteroids (OCS). A gradual dose reduction of OCS should begin ~7 to 10 days after starting inhaled therapy. US labeling recommends reducing prednisone dose by 2.5 mg/day (or equivalent of other OCS) on a weekly basis (patients using oral inhaler) or by ≤25% every 1 to 2 weeks (patients using respules). Canadian labeling recommends reducing prednisone dose by 2.5 mg/day (or equivalent of other OCS) every 4 days in closely monitored patients or every 10 days if not closely monitored. If adrenal insufficiency occurs, temporarily increase the OCS dose and follow with a more gradual withdrawal. **Note:** When transitioning from systemic to inhaled corticosteroids, supplemental systemic corticosteroid therapy may be necessary during periods of stress or during severe asthma attacks.

Nebulization: Pulmicort Respules: Children 12 months to 8 years: Titrate to lowest effective dose once patient is stable; start at 0.25 mg/day or use as follows:

Previous therapy of bronchodilators alone: 0.5 mg/day administered as a single dose or divided twice daily (maximum daily dose: 0.5 mg)

Previous therapy of inhaled corticosteroids: 0.5 mg/day administered as a single dose or divided twice daily (maximum daily dose: 1 mg)

Previous therapy of oral corticosteroids: 1 mg/day administered as a single dose or divided twice daily (maximum daily dose: 1 mg)

Asthma guidelines:

National Asthma Education and Prevention Program guidelines (NAEPP 2007):

Children 0 to 4 years:

"Low" dose: 0.25 to 0.5 mg/day

"Medium" dose: >0.5 to 1 mg/day

"High" dose: >1 mg/day

Children 5 to 11 years:

"Low" dose: 0.5 mg/day

"Medium" dose: 1 mg/day

"High" dose: 2 mg/day

Global Initiative for Asthma guidelines (GINA 2015):

Children ≤5 years: "Low" dose: 0.5 mg daily

Children 6 to 11 years:

"Low" dose: 0.25 to 0.5 mg daily

"Medium" dose: >0.5 to 1 mg daily

"High" dose: >1 mg daily

Renal Impairment There are no dosage adjustments provided in the manufacturer's labeling (has not been studied).

Hepatic Impairment There are no dosage adjustments provided in the manufacturer's labeling (has not been studied). However, budesonide undergoes hepatic metabolism; drug may accumulate with hepatic impairment; use with caution; monitor closely for signs and symptoms of hypercorticism.

Administration

Powder for inhalation:

Pulmicort Flexhaler: Hold inhaler in upright position (mouthpiece up) to load dose. Do not shake prior to use. Unit should be primed prior to first use only. It will not need primed again, even if not used for a long time. Place mouthpiece between lips and inhale forcefully and deeply. Do not exhale through inhaler; do not use a spacer. Dose indicator does not move with every dose, usually only after 5 doses. Discard when dose indicator reads "0". Rinse mouth with water after each use to reduce incidence of candidiasis.

Pulmicort Turbuhaler [CAN, not available in the US]: Hold inhaler in upright position (mouthpiece up) to load dose. Do not shake inhaler after dose is loaded. Unit should be primed prior to first use. Place mouthpiece between lips and inhale forcefully and deeply; mouthpiece should face up. Do not exhale through inhaler; do not use a spacer. When a red mark appears in the dose indicator window, 20 doses are left. When the red mark reaches the bottom of the window, the inhaler should be discarded. Rinse mouth with water after use to reduce incidence of candidiasis.

Suspension for nebulization: Shake well before using. Use Pulmicort Respules with jet nebulizer connected to an air compressor; administer with mouthpiece or facemask. Do not use ultrasonic nebulizer. Do not mix with other medications in nebulizer. Rinse mouth following treatments to decrease risk of oral candidiasis (wash face if using face mask).

Monitoring Parameters

Monitor growth in pediatric patients; blood pressure, serum glucose, weight with high-dose or long-term oral use; signs and symptoms of hypercorticism or adrenal suppression

Asthma: FEV_1, peak flow, and/or other pulmonary function tests

Additional Information Effects of inhaled steroids on growth have been observed in the absence of laboratory evidence of HPA axis suppression, suggesting that growth velocity is a more sensitive indicator of systemic corticosteroid exposure in pediatric patients than some commonly used tests of HPA axis function. The long-term effects of this reduction in growth velocity associated with orally-inhaled corticosteroids, including the impact on final adult height, are unknown. The potential for "catch up" growth following discontinuation of treatment with inhaled corticosteroids has not been adequately studied.

Dosage Forms Considerations Pulmicort Flexhaler 180 mcg/actuation canisters contain 120 actuations and the 90 mcg/actuation canisters contain 60 inhalations.

Dosage Forms Excipient information presented when available (limited, particularly for generics); consult specific product labeling.

Aerosol Powder Breath Activated, Inhalation:

Pulmicort Flexhaler: 90 mcg/actuation (1 ea); 180 mcg/actuation (1 ea) [contains milk protein]

Suspension, Inhalation:

Pulmicort: 0.25 mg/2 mL (2 mL); 0.5 mg/2 mL (2 mL); 1 mg/2 mL (2 mL) [contains disodium edta, polysorbate 80]

Generic: 0.25 mg/2 mL (2 mL); 0.5 mg/2 mL (2 mL)

Dosage Forms: Canada Excipient information presented when available (limited, particularly for generics); consult specific product labeling.

Powder for oral inhalation:

Pulmicort Turbuhaler: 100 mcg/inhalation [delivers 200 metered actuations]; 200 mcg/inhalation [delivers 200 metered actuations]; 400 mcg/inhalation [delivers 200 metered actuations]

◆ Budesonide and Eformoterol *see* Budesonide and Formoterol *on page 260*

Budesonide and Formoterol

(byoo DES oh nide & for MOH te rol)

Brand Names: US Symbicort
Brand Names: Canada Symbicort
Index Terms Budesonide and Eformoterol; Eformoterol and Budesonide; Formoterol and Budesonide; Formoterol Fumarate Dihydrate and Budesonide

Pharmacologic Category Beta₂ Agonist; Beta₂-Adrenergic Agonist, Long-Acting; Corticosteroid, Inhalant (Oral)

Use Treatment of asthma in patients ≥12 years of age where combination therapy is indicated; maintenance treatment of airflow obstruction associated with chronic obstructive pulmonary disease (COPD; including chronic bronchitis and emphysema)

Medication Guide Available Yes

Dosing

Adult & Geriatric

Asthma: Oral inhalation:

U.S. labeling: Symbicort 80/4.5, Symbicort 160/4.5: Two inhalations twice daily (maximum: 4 inhalations/day). Recommended starting dose combination is determined according to asthma severity. In patients not adequately controlled on the lower combination dose following 1 to 2 weeks of therapy, consider the higher dose combination.

Canadian labeling:

Symbicort 100 Turbuhaler [CAN; not available in U.S.], Symbicort 200 Turbuhaler [CAN; not available in U.S.]:

Initial: 1 to 2 inhalations twice daily until symptom control, then titrate to lowest effective dosage to maintain control

Maintenance: 1 to 2 inhalations once or twice daily (maximum: 8 inhalations/day as temporary treatment in periods of worsening asthma)

Symbicort Maintenance and Reliever Therapy (Symbicort SMART): **Note:** Not approved in the U.S.:

Maintenance: Symbicort 100 Turbuhaler [CAN] **or** Symbicort 200 Turbuhaler [CAN]: 1 to 2 inhalations twice daily **or** 2 inhalations once daily

Reliever therapy: Symbicort 100 Turbuhaler [CAN] **or** Symbicort 200 Turbuhaler [CAN]: 1 additional inhalation as needed, may repeat if no relief for up to 6 inhalations total (maximum: 8 inhalations/day)

COPD: Oral inhalation:

U.S. labeling: Symbicort 160/4.5: Two inhalations twice daily (maximum: 4 inhalations/day)

Canadian labeling: Symbicort 200 Turbuhaler [CAN; not available in U.S.]: Two inhalations twice daily (maximum: 4 inhalations/day)

Pediatric Asthma: Oral inhalation:

Children 5 to 11 years (off-label): Symbicort 80/4.5: Two inhalations twice daily. Do not exceed 4 inhalations per day (Morice, 2008; NAEPP, 2007).

Children ≥12 years: Refer to adult dosing.

Renal Impairment No dosage adjustment provided in the manufacturer's labeling (has not been studied).

Hepatic Impairment No dosage adjustment provided in manufacturer's labeling (has not been studied). However, close monitoring of patients with hepatic disease may be warranted due to hepatic metabolism of both agents.

Additional Information Complete prescribing information should be consulted for additional detail.

Dosage Forms Excipient information presented when available (limited, particularly for generics); consult specific product labeling.

Aerosol for oral inhalation:

Symbicort 80/4.5: Budesonide 80 mcg and formoterol fumarate dihydrate 4.5 mcg per actuation (6.9 g) [60 metered inhalations]; budesonide 80 mcg and formoterol fumarate dihydrate 4.5 mcg per actuation (10.2 g) [120 metered inhalations]

Symbicort 160/4.5: Budesonide 160 mcg and formoterol fumarate dihydrate 4.5 mcg per actuation (6 g) [60 metered inhalations]; budesonide 160 mcg and formoterol fumarate dihydrate 4.5 mcg per actuation (10.2 g) [120 metered inhalations]

Dosage Forms: Canada Excipient information presented when available (limited, particularly for generics); consult specific product labeling.

Powder for oral inhalation:

Symbicort 100 Turbuhaler: Budesonide 100 mcg and formoterol dihydrate 6 mcg per inhalation (available in 60 or 120 metered doses) [delivers ~80 mcg budesonide and 4.5 mcg formoterol per inhalation; contains lactose]

Symbicort 200 Turbuhaler: Budesonide 200 mcg and formoterol dihydrate 6 mcg per inhalation (available in 60 or 120 metered doses) [delivers ~160 mcg budesonide and 4.5 mcg formoterol per inhalation; contains lactose]

◆ Buffasal [OTC] *see* Aspirin *on page 157*

◆ Bufferin [OTC] *see* Aspirin *on page 157*

◆ Bufferin Extra Strength [OTC] *see* Aspirin *on page 157*

◆ Buffinol [OTC] *see* Aspirin *on page 157*

Bumetanide (byoo MET a nide)

Brand Names: US Bumex

Brand Names: Canada Burinex

Index Terms Bumex

Pharmacologic Category Antihypertensive; Diuretic, Loop

Use Management of edema secondary to heart failure or hepatic or renal disease (including nephrotic syndrome)

Pregnancy Considerations Adverse events have been observed in some animal reproduction studies.

Breast-Feeding Considerations It is not known if bumetanide is excreted in breast milk. Breast-feeding is not recommended by the manufacturer. Diuretics have the potential to decrease milk volume and suppress lactation.

Contraindications Hypersensitivity to bumetanide or any component of the formulation; anuria; patients with hepatic coma or in states of severe electrolyte depletion until the condition improves or is corrected

Warnings/Precautions [U.S. Boxed Warning]: Excessive amounts can lead to profound diuresis with fluid and electrolyte loss; close medical supervision and dose evaluation are required. Potassium supplementation and/or use of potassium-sparing diuretics may be necessary to prevent hypokalemia. In contrast to thiazide diuretics, a loop diuretic can also lower serum calcium concentrations. Electrolyte disturbances can predispose a patient to serious cardiac arrhythmias. In cirrhosis, initiate bumetanide therapy with conservative dosing and close monitoring of electrolytes; avoid sudden changes in fluid and electrolyte balance and acid/base status which may lead to hepatic encephalopathy. *In vitro* studies using pooled sera from critically-ill neonates have shown bumetanide to be a potent displacer of bilirubin; avoid use in neonates at risk for kernicterus. Coadministration of antihypertensives may increase the risk of hypotension.

Monitor fluid status and renal function in an attempt to prevent oliguria, azotemia, and reversible increases in BUN and creatinine; close medical supervision of aggressive diuresis required. Larger doses may be necessary in patients with impaired renal function to obtain the same therapeutic response (Brater, 1998). Diuretic resistance may occur in some patients, despite higher doses of loop diuretic treatment, and can usually be overcome by intravenous administration, the use of two diuretics together (eg, furosemide and chlorothiazide), or the use of a diuretic with a positive inotropic agent. When such combinations are used, serum electrolytes need to be monitored even more closely (ACC/AHA [Yancy 2013]; Cody 1994; HFSA 2010). Bumetanide-induced ototoxicity (usually transient) may occur with rapid IV administration, renal impairment, excessive doses, and concurrent use of other ototoxins (eg, aminoglycosides). Asymptomatic hyperuricemia has been reported with use. If given the morning of surgery, bumetanide may render the patient volume depleted and blood pressure may be labile during general anesthesia.

Benzyl alcohol and derivatives: Some dosage forms may contain benzyl alcohol; large amounts of benzyl alcohol (≥99 mg/kg/day) have been associated with a potentially fatal toxicity ("gasping syndrome") in neonates; the "gasping syndrome" consists of metabolic acidosis, respiratory distress, gasping respirations, CNS dysfunction (including convulsions, intracranial hemorrhage), hypotension and cardiovascular collapse (AAP ["Inactive" 1997]; CDC 1982); some data suggests that benzoate displaces bilirubin from protein binding sites (Ahlfors, 2001); avoid or use dosage forms containing benzyl alcohol with caution in neonates. See manufacturer's labeling.

Sulfonamide ("sulfa") allergy: The FDA-approved product labeling for many medications containing a sulfonamide chemical group includes a broad contraindication in patients with a prior allergic reaction to sulfonamides. There is a potential for cross-reactivity between members of a specific class (eg, two antibiotic sulfonamides). However, concerns for cross-reactivity have previously extended to all compounds containing the sulfonamide structure (SO_2NH_2). An expanded understanding of allergic mechanisms indicates cross-reactivity between antibiotic sulfonamides and nonantibiotic sulfonamides may not occur or at the very least this potential is extremely low (Brackett 2004; Johnson 2005; Slatore 2004; Tornero 2004). In particular, mechanisms of cross-reaction due to antibody production (anaphylaxis) are unlikely to occur with nonantibiotic sulfonamides. T-cell-mediated (type IV) reactions (eg, maculopapular rash) are less well understood and it is not possible to completely exclude this potential based on current insights. In cases where prior reactions were severe (Stevens-Johnson syndrome/TEN), some clinicians choose to avoid exposure to these classes.

Adverse Reactions

>10%:

Endocrine & metabolic: Hyperuricemia (18%), hypochloremia (15%), hypokalemia (15%)

Genitourinary: Azotemia (11%)

1% to 10%:

Central nervous system: Dizziness (1%)

Endocrine & metabolic: Hyponatremia (9%), hyperglycemia (7%), phosphorus change (5%), variations in bicarbonate (3%), abnormal serum calcium (2%), abnormal lactate dehydrogenase (1%)

Neuromuscular & skeletal: Muscle cramps (1%)

Renal: Increased serum creatinine (7%)

Respiratory: Variations in CO_2 content (4%)

<1% (Limited to important or life-threatening): Abdominal pain, abnormal alkaline phosphatase, abnormal bilirubin levels, abnormal hematocrit, abnormal hemoglobin level, abnormal transaminase, arthritic pain, asterixis, auditory impairment, blood cholesterol abnormal, brain disease (in patients with preexisting liver disease), change in creatinine clearance, change in prothrombin time, change in WBC count, chest pain, dehydration, diaphoresis, diarrhea, dyspepsia, ECG changes, erectile dysfunction, fatigue, glycosuria, headache, hyperventilation, hypotension, musculoskeletal pain, nausea, nipple tenderness, orthostatic hypotension, otalgia, ototoxicity, premature ejaculation, proteinuria, pruritus, renal failure, skin rash, Stevens-Johnson syndrome, thrombocytopenia, toxic epidermal necrolysis, urticaria, vertigo, vomiting, weakness, xerostomia

Drug Interactions

Metabolism/Transport Effects None known.

Avoid Concomitant Use

Avoid concomitant use of Bumetanide with any of the following: Levosulpiride; Mecamylamine

Increased Effect/Toxicity

Bumetanide may increase the levels/effects of: ACE Inhibitors; Allopurinol; Amifostine; Aminoglycosides; Antipsychotic Agents (Second Generation [Atypical]); Cardiac Glycosides; Cefotiam; Ceftizoxime; CISplatin; Dofetilide; DULoxetine; Foscarnet; Hypotension-Associated Agents; Ivabradine; Levodopa; Levosulpiride; Lithium; Mecamylamine; Methotrexate; Neuromuscular-Blocking Agents; Nonsteroidal Anti-Inflammatory Agents; RisperiDONE; Salicylates; Sodium Phosphates; Tobramycin (Oral Inhalation); Topiramate

The levels/effects of Bumetanide may be increased by: Alfuzosin; Analgesics (Opioid); Barbiturates; Beta2-Agonists; Brimonidine (Topical); Canagliflozin; Cefazedone; Cephradine; Corticosteroids (Orally Inhaled); Corticosteroids (Systemic); CycloSPORINE (Systemic); Diazoxide; Empagliflozin; Herbs (Hypotensive Properties); Licorice; Methotrexate; Molsidomine; Nicorandil; Obinutuzumab; Pentoxifylline; Phosphodiesterase 5 Inhibitors; Probenecid; Prostacyclin Analogues

Decreased Effect

Bumetanide may decrease the levels/effects of: Antidiabetic Agents; Lithium; Neuromuscular-Blocking Agents

The levels/effects of Bumetanide may be decreased by: Amphetamines; Bile Acid Sequestrants; Fosphenytoin; Herbs (Hypertensive Properties); Methotrexate; Methylphenidate; Nonsteroidal Anti-Inflammatory Agents; Phenytoin; Probenecid; Salicylates; Yohimbine

Food Interactions Bumetanide serum levels may be decreased if taken with food. Management: It has been recommended that bumetanide be administered without food (Bard, 2004).

Storage/Stability

IV: Store vials at 15°C to 30°C (59°F to 86°F). Infusion solutions should be used within 24 hours after preparation. Light sensitive; discoloration may occur when exposed to light.

Tablet: Store at 15°C to 30°C (59°F to 86°F); protect from light.

Mechanism of Action Inhibits reabsorption of sodium and chloride in the ascending loop of Henle and proximal renal tubule, interfering with the chloride-binding cotransport system, thus causing increased excretion of water, sodium, chloride, magnesium, phosphate, and calcium; it does not appear to act on the distal tubule

Pharmacodynamics/Kinetics

Onset of action: Oral, IM: 0.5 to 1 hour; IV: 2 to 3 minutes

Peak effect: Oral: 1 to 2 hours; IV: 15 to 30 minutes

Duration: Oral: 4 to 6 hours; IV: 2 to 3 hours

Distribution: V_d: Neonates and Infants: 0.26 to 0.39 L/kg; Adults: 9 to 25 L

Protein binding: 94% to 96%; Neonates: 97%

Metabolism: Partially hepatic

Bioavailability: 59% to 89% (median: 80%)

Half-life elimination:

Premature and full term neonates: 6 hours (range up to 15 hours)

Infants <2 months: 2.5 hours

Infants 2 to 6 months: 1.5 hours

Adults: 1 to 1.5 hours

Excretion: Urine (81% of total dose; 45% of which is unchanged drug); feces (2% of total dose)

Clearance:

Preterm and full term neonates: 0.2 to 1.1 mL/minute/kg

Infants <2 months: 2.17 mL/minute/kg

Infants 2 to 6 months: 3.8 mL/minute/kg

Adults: 2.9 ± 0.2 mL/minute/kg

Dosing

Adult & Geriatric Note: Dose equivalency for patients with normal renal function (approximate): Bumetanide 1 mg = furosemide 40 mg = torsemide 20 mg = ethacrynic acid 50 mg

Edema, heart failure:

Oral: 0.5-2 mg/dose 1-2 times daily; if diuretic response to initial dose is not adequate, may repeat in 4-5 hours for up to 2 doses (maximum dose: 10 mg daily). ACCF/AHA 2013 heart failure guidelines recommend initial dosing of 0.5-1 mg once or twice daily and a maximum total daily dose of 10 mg (Yancy, 2013).

IM, IV: 0.5-1 mg/dose; if diuretic response to initial dose is not adequate, may repeat in 2-3 hours for up to 2 doses (maximum dose: 10 mg daily)

Continuous IV infusion (off-label dose): Initial: 1 mg IV load then 0.5-2 mg/hour; repeat loading dose before increasing infusion rate (ACCF/AHA [Yancy, 2013]; Brater, 1998). **Note:** With lower baseline CrCl (eg, CrCl <25 mL/minute), the upper end of the initial infusion dosage range should be considered.

Pediatric Edema: Oral, IM, IV: Infants and Children: 0.015-0.1 mg/kg/dose every 6-24 hours (maximum dose: 10 mg/day)

Renal Impairment Use is contraindicated in anuria. Use with caution in renal insufficiency due to increased risk of adverse effects.

Hepatic Impairment Use is contraindicated in hepatic coma. Use with caution in cirrhosis and ascites due to increased risk of precipitating hepatic coma; initiate with conservative doses and monitoring.

Dietary Considerations Administration with food slows the rate and reduces the extent of absorption and may reduce diuretic efficacy (Bard, 2004). May require increased intake of potassium-rich foods.

Administration

IV: Administer slowly, over 1-2 minutes.

Oral: An alternate-day schedule or a 3-4 daily dosing regimen with rest periods of 1-2 days in between may be the most tolerable and effective regimen for the continued control of edema.

Monitoring Parameters Blood pressure; serum electrolytes, renal function; fluid status (weight and I & O), blood pressure

Dosage Forms Excipient information presented when available (limited, particularly for generics); consult specific product labeling.

Solution, Injection:

Generic: 0.25 mg/mL (2 mL, 4 mL, 10 mL)

Tablet, Oral:

Bumex: 0.5 mg [contains fd&c blue #1 aluminum lake, fd&c yellow #10 aluminum lake]

Bumex: 1 mg [contains fd&c yellow #10 (quinoline yellow)]

Bumex: 2 mg

Generic: 0.5 mg, 1 mg, 2 mg

Dosage Forms: Canada Note: Solution for injection is not available in Canada. Excipient information presented when available (limited, particularly for generics); consult specific product labeling.

Tablet, Oral:

Burinex: 1 mg, 5 mg

◆ Bumex see Bumetanide on page 261

◆ Buminate see Albumin on page 55

◆ Buminate-5% (Can) see Albumin on page 55

◆ Buminate-25% (Can) see Albumin on page 55

◆ Bunavail see Buprenorphine and Naloxone on page 267

◆ Bupap see Butalbital and Acetaminophen on page 275

◆ Buphenyl see Sodium Phenylbutyrate on page 1677

Bupivacaine (byoo PIV a kane)

Brand Names: US Bupivacaine Spinal; Marcaine; Marcaine Preservative Free; Marcaine Spinal; Sensorcaine; Sensorcaine-MPF; Sensorcaine-MPF Spinal

Brand Names: Canada Marcaine®; Sensorcaine®

Index Terms Bupivacaine Hydrochloride
Pharmacologic Category Local Anesthetic
Use Local or regional anesthesia; spinal anesthesia (0.75% in dextrose 8.25% injection); diagnostic and therapeutic procedures; obstetrical procedures (only 0.25% and 0.5% concentrations)

  0.25%: Local infiltration, peripheral nerve block, sympathetic block, caudal or epidural block

  0.5%: Peripheral nerve block, caudal and epidural block

  0.75% **(not for obstetrical anesthesia)**: Retrobulbar block, epidural block. **Note:** Reserve for surgical procedures where a high degree of muscle relaxation and prolonged effect are necessary

Dosing
Adult & Geriatric Note: Dose varies with procedure, depth of anesthesia, vascularity of tissues, duration of anesthesia, and condition of patient. Do not use solutions containing preservatives for caudal or epidural block.

Local anesthesia: Infiltration: 0.25% infiltrated locally; maximum: 175 mg. **Note:** Aspiration should be performed prior to each injection; however, absence of blood in the syringe does not guarantee that intravascular injection has been avoided (Mulroy 2010).

Caudal block (preservative free): 15 to 30 **mL** of 0.25% or 0.5%

Epidural block (other than caudal block; preservative free): Administer in 3 to 5 **mL** increments, allowing sufficient time to detect toxic manifestations of inadvertent IV or intrathecal administration: 10 to 20 **mL** of 0.25% or 0.5%

  Surgical procedures requiring a high degree of muscle relaxation and prolonged effects **only**: 10 to 20 **mL** of 0.75% **(Note:** Not to be used in obstetrical cases)

Peripheral nerve block: 5 **mL** of 0.25% or 0.5%; maximum: 400 mg/day

Sympathetic nerve block: 20 to 50 **mL** of 0.25%

Retrobulbar anesthesia: 2 to 4 **mL** of 0.75%

Spinal anesthesia: Preservative free solution of 0.75% bupivacaine in 8.25% dextrose:

  Lower extremity and perineal procedures: 1 **mL**

  Lower abdominal procedures: 1.6 **mL**

  Normal vaginal delivery: 0.8 **mL** (higher doses may be required in some patients)

  Cesarean delivery: 1 to 1.4 **mL**

Combined spinal-epidural (CSE) technique for labor analgesia (off-label dosing [spinal component]): 1.75 to 2.5 mg combined with fentanyl 15 mcg (Eltzschig 2003; Ngan Kee 2014; Whitty 2007).

Combined spinal-epidural (CSE) technique for anesthesia for Cesarean delivery (off-label dosing [spinal component]): 9 to 12 mg combined with fentanyl 15 mcg; in addition to fentanyl, may also include a longer-acting opioid (ie, morphine 100 to 150 **mcg**) for postoperative analgesia (Santos 2015).

Pediatric Note: Dose varies with procedure, depth of anesthesia, vascularity of tissues, duration of anesthesia, and condition of patient. Do not use solutions containing preservatives for caudal or epidural block.

Caudal block, epidural block, local anesthesia: Adolescents: Refer to adult dosing.

Peripheral or sympathetic nerve block: Adolescents: Refer to adult dosing.

Retrobulbar anesthesia: Adolescents: Refer to adult dosing.

Renal Impairment There are no dosage adjustments provided in the manufacturer's labeling; use with caution.

Hepatic Impairment There are no dosage adjustments provided in the manufacturer's labeling; use with caution.

Additional Information Complete prescribing information should be consulted for additional detail.

Dosage Forms Excipient information presented when available (limited, particularly for generics); consult specific product labeling.

Solution, Injection, as hydrochloride:

  Marcaine: 0.25% (50 mL); 0.5% (50 mL) [contains methylparaben]

  Sensorcaine: 0.25% (50 mL); 0.5% (50 mL) [contains methylparaben]

  Sensorcaine-MPF: 0.25% (10 mL, 30 mL); 0.5% (10 mL, 30 mL); 0.75% (10 mL, 30 mL) [methylparaben free]

  Generic: 0.25% (10 mL, 30 mL, 50 mL); 0.5% (10 mL, 30 mL, 50 mL); 0.75% (10 mL, 30 mL)

Solution, Injection, as hydrochloride [preservative free]:

  Marcaine: 0.75% (10 mL, 30 mL)

  Marcaine Preservative Free: 0.25% (10 mL, 30 mL); 0.5% (10 mL, 30 mL)

  Generic: 0.25% (10 mL, 20 mL, 30 mL); 0.5% (10 mL, 20 mL, 30 mL); 0.75% (10 mL, 20 mL, 30 mL)

Solution, Intrathecal, as hydrochloride [preservative free]:

  Bupivacaine Spinal: 0.75% [7.5 mg/mL] (2 mL)

  Marcaine Spinal: 0.75% [7.5 mg/mL] (2 mL)

  Sensorcaine-MPF Spinal: 0.75% [7.5 mg/mL] (2 mL)

♦ **Bupivacaine Hydrochloride** *see* Bupivacaine *on page 262*

Bupivacaine (Liposomal) (byoo PIV a kane lye po SO mal)

Brand Names: US Exparel
Index Terms Bupivacaine Liposome; DepoFoam Bupivacaine; Exparel; Liposomal Bupivacaine
Pharmacologic Category Analgesic, Nonopioid
Use Injected into the surgical site (eg, bunionectomy, hemorrhoidectomy) to provide postoperative analgesia
Dosing
Adult Postoperative analgesia: Infiltration (local): Dose is based on surgical site and volume required to cover the area (in general, the maximum total dose is 266 mg).

  Bunionectomy: 7 mL into the tissues surrounding the osteotomy and 1 mL into the subcutaneous tissue of the surgical site (total dose = 8 mL [106 mg])

  Hemorrhoidectomy: 30 mL (20 mL vial diluted with 10 mL NS or LR) divided and administered as 6 injections of 5 mL each (total dose = 30 mL [266 mg])

Renal Impairment There are no dosage adjustments provided in manufacturer's labeling; however, renal impairment may reduce bupivacaine elimination increasing systemic exposure and the risk of adverse effects or toxicities; use with caution.

Hepatic Impairment There are no dosage adjustments provided in manufacturer's labeling; however, moderate-to-severe impairment may reduce bupivacaine metabolism increasing systemic exposure and the risk of adverse effects or toxicities; use with caution.

Additional Information Complete prescribing information should be consulted for additional detail.

Dosage Forms Excipient information presented when available (limited, particularly for generics); consult specific product labeling.

Suspension, Injection:

  Exparel: 1.3% (20 mL)

♦ **Bupivacaine Liposome** *see* Bupivacaine (Liposomal) *on page 263*

♦ **Bupivacaine Spinal** *see* Bupivacaine *on page 262*

♦ **Buprenex** *see* Buprenorphine *on page 263*

Buprenorphine (byoo pre NOR feen)

Brand Names: US Belbuca; Buprenex; Butrans; Subutex [DSC]
Brand Names: Canada Butrans
Index Terms Buprenorphine Hydrochloride; Subutex
Pharmacologic Category Analgesic, Opioid; Analgesic, Opioid Partial Agonist
Additional Appendix Information
  Opioid Conversion Table and Morphine Equivalent Dose Table *on page 1955*
Use
  Buccal film, transdermal patch: Management of pain severe enough to require around-the-clock, long-term, opioid treatment and for which alternative treatment options (eg, nonopioid analgesics or immediate-release opioids) are inadequate.

  Limitations of use: Not indicated as an as-needed analgesic.

  Injection: Management of moderate to severe pain

  Sublingual tablet: Treatment of opioid dependence

Pregnancy Considerations Adverse effects have been observed in some animal reproduction studies. Buprenorphine crosses the placenta; buprenorphine and norbuprenorphine can be detected in newborn serum, urine, and meconium following in utero exposure (CSAT 2004). **[US Boxed Warning]: Prolonged use can result in neonatal opioid withdrawal syndrome. If not recognized and treated, this may be life-threatening and require management according to protocols developed by neonatology experts.** Following chronic opioid therapy in pregnancy, adverse events in the newborn (including withdrawal) may occur; monitoring of the neonate is recommended. The minimum effective dose should be used if opioids are needed (Chou 2009). The onset of withdrawal in infants of women receiving buprenorphine during pregnancy ranged from day 1 to day 8 of life, most occurring on day 1. Symptoms of withdrawal may include agitation, apnea, bradycardia, convulsions, hypertonia, myoclonus, respiratory depression, and tremor.

Buprenorphine is currently considered an alternate treatment for pregnant women who need therapy for opioid addiction (CSAT 2004; Dow 2012); however, use in pregnancy for this purpose is increasing (ACOG 2012; Soyka 2013). Buprenorphine should not be used to treat pain

during labor. Women receiving buprenorphine for the treatment of addiction should be maintained on their daily dose of buprenorphine in addition to receiving the same pain management options during labor and delivery as opioid-naive women; maintenance doses of buprenorphine will not provide adequate pain relief. Narcotic agonist-antagonists should be avoided for the treatment of labor pain in women maintained on buprenorphine due to the risk of precipitating acute withdrawal. In addition, buprenorphine should not be given to women in labor taking methadone (ACOG 2012).

Amenorrhea may develop secondary to substance abuse; pregnancy may occur following the initiation of buprenorphine maintenance treatment. Contraception counseling is recommended to prevent unplanned pregnancies (Dow 2012). Long-term opioid use may cause secondary hypogonadism, which may lead to sexual dysfunction or infertility (Brennan 2013).

Breast-Feeding Considerations Buprenorphine is excreted in breast milk. Breast-feeding is not recommended by the manufacturer. Nursing infants exposed to large doses of opioids should be monitored for apnea and sedation (Montgomery 2012).

When buprenorphine is used to treat opioid addiction in nursing women, most guidelines do not contraindicate breast-feeding as long as the infant is tolerant to the dose and other contraindications do not exist; caution should be used when nursing infants not previously exposed (ACOG 2012; CSAT 2004; Montgomery 2012). If additional illicit substances are being abused, women treated with buprenorphine should pump and discard breast milk until sobriety is established (ACOG 2012; Dow 2012).

Prescribing and Access Restrictions Prescribing of tablets for opioid dependence is limited to physicians who have met the qualification criteria and have received a DEA number specific to prescribing this product. Tablets will be available through pharmacies and wholesalers which normally provide controlled substances.

Medication Guide Available Yes

Contraindications

Hypersensitivity to buprenorphine or any component of the formulation

Buccal film, transdermal patch: Additional contraindications: Significant respiratory depression; acute or severe asthma; known or suspected GI obstruction, including paralytic ileus

Documentation of allergenic cross-reactivity for morphine and related drugs in this class is limited. However, because of similarities in chemical structure and/or pharmacologic actions, the possibility of cross-sensitivity cannot be ruled out with certainty.

Warnings/Precautions An opioid-containing analgesic regimen should be tailored to each patient's needs and based upon the type of pain being treated (acute versus chronic), the route of administration, degree of tolerance for opioids (naive versus chronic user), age, weight, and medical condition. The optimal analgesic dose varies widely among patients. Doses should be titrated to pain relief/prevention.

May cause CNS depression, which may impair physical or mental abilities; patients must be cautioned about performing tasks which require mental alertness (eg, operating machinery or driving). May cause respiratory depression; use with extreme caution in patients with preexisting respiratory compromise (hypoxia and/or hypercapnia), COPD or other obstructive pulmonary disease, and kyphoscoliosis or other skeletal disorder which may alter respiratory function; critical respiratory depression may occur, even at therapeutic dosages. Use with caution in the elderly; may be more sensitive to adverse effects (eg, life-threatening respiratory depression). Also use with caution in debilitated or cachectic patients; there is a greater potential for life-threatening respiratory depression, even at therapeutic dosages. Hypersensitivity reactions, including bronchospasm, angioneurotic edema, and anaphylactic shock, have been reported. Potential for drug dependency exists, abrupt cessation may precipitate withdrawal.

Hepatitis has been reported with buprenorphine use; hepatic events ranged from transient, asymptomatic transaminase elevations to hepatic failure; in many cases, patients had preexisting hepatic dysfunction. Monitor liver function tests in patients at increased risk for hepatotoxicity (eg, history of alcohol abuse, preexisting hepatic dysfunction, IV drug abusers) prior to and during therapy. Use with caution in patients with moderate hepatic impairment; dosage adjustment recommended in severe hepatic impairment.

Avoid use in patients with CNS depression or coma as these patients are susceptible to intracranial effects of CO_2 retention. Use with extreme caution in patients with head injury, intracranial lesions, or elevated intracranial pressure; exaggerated elevation of ICP may occur. May cause severe hypotension, including orthostatic hypotension and syncope; use with caution in patients with hypovolemia, cardiovascular disease (including acute MI, or drugs which may exaggerate hypotensive effects (including phenothiazines or general anesthetics). Avoid use in patients with circulatory shock; may cause vasodilation that can further reduce cardiac output and blood pressure. May obscure diagnosis or clinical course of patients with acute abdominal conditions. Use with caution in patients with a history of ileus or bowel obstruction; use of buccal film is contraindicated in patients with known or suspected gastrointestinal obstruction, including paralytic ileus, and transdermal patch is contraindicated in patients with known or suspected paralytic ileus. Use with caution in patients with biliary tract dysfunction, including acute pancreatitis; may cause constriction of sphincter of Oddi. Opioid therapy may lower seizure threshold; use caution in patients with a history of seizure disorders. Use with caution in patients with adrenal insufficiency, including Addison's disease. Chronic opioid use may cause secondary hypogonadism, although this may not occur with buprenorphine (Aurilio 2001; Bliesener 2005; Brennan 2013). Use with caution in patients with renal impairment, morbid obesity, toxic psychosis, thyroid dysfunction, or prostatic hyperplasia and/or urinary stricture. Potentially significant drug-drug interactions may exist, requiring dose or frequency adjustment, additional monitoring, and/or selection of alternative therapy.

Buccal film, transdermal patch: Indicated for the management of pain severe enough to require daily, around the clock, long-term opioid treatment; should not be used for as-needed pain relief. **[US Boxed Warning]: May cause potentially life-threatening respiratory depression; monitor for respiratory depression, especially during initiation or dose escalation. Misuse or abuse by chewing, swallowing, snorting, or injecting buprenorphine extracted from the transdermal system will result in the uncontrolled delivery of buprenorphine and pose a significant risk of overdose and death. Accidental exposure to even one dose, especially in children, can result in a fatal overdose.** Do not exceed a dose of 900 mcg every 12 hours buccal film or one 20 mcg/hour transdermal patch due to the risk of QTc-interval prolongation. Avoid using in patients with a personal or family history of long QT syndrome or in patients taking concurrent class IA or III antiarrhythmics or other medications that prolong the QT interval. Use with caution in patients with hypokalemia, hypomagnesemia, or clinically unstable cardiac disease, including unstable heart failure, unstable atrial fibrillation, symptomatic bradycardia, or active MI. **[US Boxed Warning]: Abuse, misuse, and addiction, which can lead to overdose and death, may occur.** Risk of opioid abuse is increased in patients with a history or family history of alcohol or drug abuse or mental illness (eg, major depression). Assess each patient's risk before prescribing, and monitor all patients for the development of these behaviors or conditions. The misuse of buccal film by swallowing or transdermal patch by placing it in the mouth, chewing it, swallowing it, or using it in ways other than indicated may cause choking, overdose, and death. To properly dispose of Butrans patch, fold it over on itself and flush down the toilet; alternatively, seal the used patch in the provided Patch-Disposal Unit and dispose of in the trash. Avoid exposure of application site and surrounding area to direct external heat sources (eg, heating pads, electric blankets, heating lamps, saunas, hot water, or direct sunlight). Buprenorphine release from the patch is temperature-dependent and may result in overdose. Patients who experience fever or increase in core temperature should be monitored closely and adjust dose if signs or respiratory depression or central nervous system depression occur. Application site reactions, including rare cases of severe reactions (eg, vesicles, discharge, "burns"), have been observed with use; onset varies from days to months after initiation; patients should be instructed to report severe reactions promptly and discontinue therapy. Oral mucositis may result in more rapid absorption and higher buprenorphine plasma levels in patients using buccal film; reduce dose in patients with oral mucositis and monitor closely for signs and symptoms of toxicity or overdose. Therapy with the buccal film or transdermal patch is not appropriate for use in the management of addictions. **[US Boxed Warning]: Prolonged use during pregnancy may result in neonatal abstinence syndrome (NAS) in neonates and infants. If not recognized and treated, this may be life-threatening and require management according**

to protocols developed by neonatology experts. Monitor neonate closely. Signs and symptoms include irritability, hyperactivity and abnormal sleep pattern, high pitched cry, tremor, vomiting, diarrhea and failure to gain weight. Onset, duration and severity depend on the drug used, duration of use, maternal dose, and rate of drug elimination by the newborn.

Reversal of partial opioid agonists or mixed opioid agonist/antagonists (eg, buprenorphine, pentazocine) may be incomplete and large doses of naloxone may be required. Concurrent use of agonist/antagonist analgesics may precipitate withdrawal symptoms and/or reduced analgesic efficacy in patients following prolonged therapy with mu opioid agonists. Abrupt discontinuation following prolonged use may also lead to withdrawal symptoms and is not recommended; taper dose gradually when discontinuing.

Sublingual tablets, which are used for induction treatment of opioid dependence, should not be started until effects of withdrawal are evident.

Adverse Reactions

Injection:

>10%: Central nervous system: Sedation (≤66%)

1% to 10%:

Cardiovascular: Hypotension (1% to 5%)

Central nervous system: Dizziness (5% to 10%), headache (1% to 5%)

Dermatologic: Diaphoresis (1% to 5%)

Gastrointestinal: Nausea (5% to 10%), vomiting (1% to 5%)

Ophthalmic: Miosis (1% to 5%)

Respiratory: Respiratory depression (1% to 5%)

<1%: (Limited to important or life-threatening): Amblyopia, anaphylactic shock, apnea, bradycardia, conjunctivitis, coma, cyanosis, depersonalization, depression, diplopia, euphoria, hallucination, hypersensitivity, hypertension, hypogonadism (Brennan, 2013; Debono, 2011), injection site reaction, psychosis, seizure, slurred speech, tachycardia, urinary retention, Wenckebach period on ECG

Tablet:

>10%:

Central nervous system: Headache (30%), insomnia (21% to 25%), pain (24%), withdrawal syndrome (18% to 22%; placebo 37%), anxiety (12%), depression (11%)

Dermatologic: Diaphoresis (12% to 13%)

Gastrointestinal: Nausea (10% to 14%), abdominal pain (12%), constipation (8% to 11%)

Infection: Infection (12% to 20%)

Neuromuscular & skeletal: Back pain (14%), weakness (14%)

Respiratory: Rhinitis (11%)

1% to 10%:

Central nervous system: Chills (6%), nervousness (6%), drowsiness (5%), dizziness (4%)

Gastrointestinal: Vomiting (5% to 8%), diarrhea (5%), dyspepsia (3%)

Infection: Abscess (2%)

Ophthalmic: Lacrimation (5%)

Respiratory: Flu-like symptoms (6%), cough (4%), pharyngitis (4%)

Miscellaneous: Fever (3%)

<1% (Limited to important or life-threatening): Anaphylactic shock, angioedema, hepatic encephalopathy, hepatic failure, hepatic necrosis, hepatitis (including cytolytic), hepatorenal syndrome, hypersensitivity, hypogonadism (Brennan, 2013; Debono, 2011), increased serum transaminases

Transdermal patch:

>10%:

Central nervous system: Headache (3% to 14%), dizziness (2% to 15%), drowsiness (2% to 13%)

Gastrointestinal: Nausea (6% to 23%), constipation (3% to 13%)

Local: Local pruritus (4% to 15%)

1% to 10%:

Cardiovascular: Chest pain (1% to <5%), hypertension (1% to <5%), peripheral edema (1% to <5%)

Central nervous system: Anxiety (1% to <5%), depression (1% to <5%), fatigue (1% to <5%), hypoesthesia (1% to <5%), insomnia (1% to <5%), migraine (1% to <5%), pain (1% to <5%), paresthesia (1% to <5%)

Dermatologic: Diaphoresis (1% to <5%), pruritus (1% to <5%), skin rash (1% to <5%)

Gastrointestinal: Vomiting (4% to 9%), xerostomia (6%), anorexia (1% to <5%), diarrhea (1% to <5%), dyspepsia (1% to <5%), upper abdominal pain (1% to <5%), abdominal distress (2%)

Genitourinary: Urinary tract infection (1% to <5%)

Local: Application site erythema (3% to 10%), application site rash (3% to 8%), application site irritation (1% to 6%)

Neuromuscular & skeletal: Arthralgia (1% to <5%), back pain (1% to <5%), joint swelling (1% to <5%), limb pain (1% to <5%), muscle spasm (1% to <5%), musculoskeletal pain (1% to <5%), myalgia (1% to <5%), neck pain (1% to <5%), tremor (1% to <5%), weakness (1% to <5%)

Respiratory: Bronchitis (1% to <5%), cough (1% to <5%), dyspnea (1% to <5%), flu-like symptoms (1% to <5%), nasopharyngitis (1% to <5%), pharyngolaryngeal pain (1% to <5%), sinusitis (1% to <5%), upper respiratory tract infection (1% to <5%)

Miscellaneous: Fever (1% to <5%)

<1% (Limited to important or life-threatening): Angina pectoris, angioedema, application site dermatitis, bradycardia, contact dermatitis, diverticulitis, exacerbation of asthma, hallucination, hyperventilation, hypersensitivity reaction, hypogonadism (Brennan, 2013; Debono, 2011), hypotension, hypoventilation, increased serum ALT, intestinal obstruction, loss of consciousness, memory impairment, mental deficiency, mental status changes, miosis (dose-related), orthostatic hypotension, psychosis, respiratory depression, respiratory distress, respiratory failure, syncope, tachycardia, urinary incontinence, urinary retention, vasodilatation, visual disturbance, withdrawal syndrome

Drug Interactions

Metabolism/Transport Effects Substrate of CYP3A4 (major); **Note:** Assignment of Major/Minor substrate status based on clinically relevant drug interaction potential; **Inhibits** CYP1A2 (weak), CYP2A6 (weak), CYP2C19 (weak), CYP2D6 (weak)

Avoid Concomitant Use

Avoid concomitant use of Buprenorphine with any of the following: Analgesics (Opioid); Atazanavir; Azelastine (Nasal); Conivaptan; Eluxadoline; Fusidic Acid (Systemic); Highest Risk QTc-Prolonging Agents; Idelalisib; Ivabradine; MAO Inhibitors; Mifepristone; Mixed Agonist / Antagonist Opioids; Moderate Risk QTc-Prolonging Agents; Orphenadrine; Paraldehyde; Thalidomide

Increased Effect/Toxicity

Buprenorphine may increase the levels/effects of: Alvimopan; Azelastine (Nasal); Desmopressin; Diuretics; Eluxadoline; Highest Risk QTc-Prolonging Agents; MAO Inhibitors; Methotrimeprazine; Metyrosine; Orphenadrine; Paraldehyde; Pramipexole; Ramosetron; ROPINIRole; Rotigotine; Selective Serotonin Reuptake Inhibitors; Suvorexant; Thalidomide; TiZANidine; Zolpidem

The levels/effects of Buprenorphine may be increased by: Alcohol (Ethyl); Amphetamines; Anticholinergic Agents; Aprepitant; Atazanavir; Boceprevir; Brimonidine (Topical); Cannabis; CNS Depressants; Cobicistat; Conivaptan; CYP3A4 Inhibitors (Moderate); CYP3A4 Inhibitors (Strong); Dronabinol; Fosaprepitant; Fusidic Acid (Systemic); Idelalisib; Ivabradine; Ivacaftor; Kava Kava; Luliconazole; Magnesium Sulfate; Methotrimeprazine; Mifepristone; Minocycline; Moderate Risk QTc-Prolonging Agents; Nabilone; Netupitant; Ombitasvir, Paritaprevir, and Ritonavir; Ombitasvir, Paritaprevir, Ritonavir, and Dasabuvir; Palbociclib; Perampanel; QTc-Prolonging Agents (Indeterminate Risk and Risk Modifying); Rufinamide; Simeprevir; Sodium Oxybate; Stiripentol; Succinylcholine; Tetrahydrocannabinol

Decreased Effect

Buprenorphine may decrease the levels/effects of: Analgesics (Opioid); Atazanavir; Pegvisomant

The levels/effects of Buprenorphine may be decreased by: Ammonium Chloride; Boceprevir; Bosentan; CYP3A4 Inducers (Moderate); CYP3A4 Inducers (Strong); Dabrafenib; Deferasirox; Efavirenz; Enzalutamide; Etravirine; Mitotane; Mixed Agonist / Antagonist Opioids; Naltrexone; Siltuximab; St Johns Wort; Tocilizumab

Storage/Stability

Injection: Protect from excessive heat >40°C (>104°F). Protect from light.

Film, patch, tablet: Store at 25°C (77°F); excursions permitted between 15°C to 30°C (59°F to 86°F).

Mechanism of Action Buprenorphine exerts its analgesic effect via high affinity binding to μ opiate receptors in the CNS; displays partial mu agonist and weak kappa antagonist activity. Due to it being a partial mu agonist, its analgesic effects plateau at higher doses and it then behaves like an antagonist.

Pharmacodynamics/Kinetics

Onset of action: Analgesic: IM: Within 15 minutes

Peak effect: IM: ~1 hour; Transdermal patch: Steady state achieved by day 3

Duration: IM: ≥6 hours

Absorption: IM, SubQ: 30% to 40%. Application of a heating pad onto the transdermal system may increase blood concentrations of buprenorphine 26% to 55%. Ingestion of liquids decreases systemic exposure to buprenorphine from buccal film by 23% to 37%.

Distribution: CSF concentrations are ~15% to 25% of plasma concentrations

V_d:

Premature neonates (GA: 27 to 32 weeks): 6.2 ± 2.1 L/kg (Barrett 1993)

Children 4 to 7 years: 3.2 ± 2 L/kg (Olkkola 1989)

Adults: 97 to 187 L/kg

Protein binding: High (~96%, primarily to alpha- and beta globulin)

Metabolism: Primarily hepatic via N-dealkylation by CYP3A4 to norbuprenorphine (active metabolite), and to a lesser extent via glucuronidation by UGT1A1 and 2B7 to buprenorphine 3-O-glucuronide; the major metabolite, norbuprenorphine, also undergoes glucuronidation via UGT1A3; extensive first-pass effect

Bioavailability (relative to IV administration): Buccal film: 46% to 65%; IM: 70%; Sublingual tablet: 29%; Transdermal patch: ~15%

Half-life elimination:

Premature neonates (GA: 27 to 32 weeks): IV: 20 ± 8 hours (Barrett 1993)

Children 4 to 7 years: IV: ~1 hour (Olkkola 1989)

Adults: IV: 2.2 to 3 hours; Buccal film: 27.6 ± 11.2 hours; Apparent terminal half-life: Sublingual tablet: ~37 hours; Transdermal patch: ~26 hours. **Note:** Extended elimination half-life for sublingual administration may be due to depot effect (Kuhlman 1996).

Time to peak, plasma: Buccal film: 2.5 to 3 hours; Sublingual: 30 minutes to 1 hour (Kuhlman 1996); Transdermal patch: Steady state achieved by day 3

Excretion: Feces (~70%; 33% as unchanged drug; 5% as conjugated drug; 21% as norbuprenorphine; and 2% as conjugated norbuprenorphine); urine (27% to 30%; 1% as unchanged drug; 9.4% as conjugated drug; 2.7% as norbuprenorphine; and 11% as conjugated norbuprenorphine)

Clearance: Related to hepatic blood flow

Premature neonates (GA: 27 to 32 weeks): 0.23 ± 0.07 L/hour/kg (Barrett 1993)

Children 4 to 7 years: 3.6 ± 1.1 L/hour/kg (Olkkola 1989)

Adults: 0.78 to 1.32 L/hour/kg

Dosing

Adult

Acute pain (moderate to severe): Note: Long-term use is not recommended. The following recommendations are guidelines and do not represent the maximum doses that may be required in all patients. Doses should be titrated to pain relief/prevention. In high-risk patients (eg, elderly, debilitated, presence of respiratory disease) and/or concurrent CNS depressant use, reduce dose by one-half. Buprenorphine has an analgesic ceiling.

IM: Initial: Opioid-naive: 0.3 mg every 6 to 8 hours as needed; initial dose (up to 0.3 mg) may be repeated once in 30 to 60 minutes after the initial dose if needed; usual dosage range: 0.15 to 0.6 mg every 4 to 8 hours as needed

Slow IV: Initial: Opioid-naive: 0.3 mg every 6 to 8 hours as needed; initial dose (up to 0.3 mg) may be repeated once in 30 to 60 minutes after the initial dose if needed

Chronic pain (moderate to severe):

Buccal film:

Note: Buprenorphine buccal film doses of 600, 750, and 900 mcg are only for use following titration from lower doses (maximum dose: 900 mcg every 12 hours).

Opioid-naive patients: Initial: 75 mcg once daily or, if tolerated, every 12 hours for at least 4 days, then increase to 150 mcg every 12 hours.

Opioid-experienced patients (conversion from other opioids to buprenorphine): Taper patient's current opioid to no more than 30 mg oral morphine sulfate equivalents daily before initiating buprenorphine. Following analgesic taper, base the initial buprenorphine dose on the patient's daily opioid dose prior to taper. Patients may require additional short-acting analgesics during the taper period.

Patients who were receiving daily dose of <30 mg of oral morphine equivalents: Initial: 75 mcg once daily or every 12 hours

Patients who were receiving daily dose of 30 to 89 mg of oral morphine equivalents: Initial: 150 mcg every 12 hours

Patients who were receiving daily dose of 90 to 160 mg of oral morphine equivalents: Initial: 300 mcg every 12 hours

Patients who were receiving daily dose of >160 mg of oral morphine equivalents: Buprenorphine buccal film may not provide adequate analgesia; **consider the use of an alternate analgesic.**

Conversion from methadone: Close monitoring is required when converting methadone to another opioid. Ratio between methadone and other opioid agonists varies widely according to previous dose exposure. Methadone has a long half-life and can accumulate in the plasma.

Dose titration (opioid-naive or opioid-experienced patients): Individually titrate in increments of 150 mcg every 12 hours, no more frequently than every 4 days, to a dose that provides adequate analgesia and minimizes adverse reactions (maximum dose: 900 mcg every 12 hours; doses up to 450 mcg every 12 hours were studied in opioid naïve patients). Patients may require additional short-acting analgesics during titration.

Discontinuation of therapy: Use a gradual downward titration of the dose to prevent withdrawal; do not abruptly discontinue.

Patients with oral mucositis: Reduce the starting dose and titration incremental dose by 50%.

Transdermal patch:

Opioid-naive patients: Initial: 5 **mcg**/hour applied once every 7 days

Opioid-experienced patients (conversion from other opioids to buprenorphine): Discontinue all other around-the-clock opioid drugs when buprenorphine therapy is initiated. Short-acting analgesics as needed may be continued until analgesia with transdermal buprenorphine is attained. There is a potential for buprenorphine to precipitate withdrawal in patients already receiving opioids.

Patients who were receiving daily dose of <30 mg of oral morphine equivalents: Initial: 5 **mcg**/hour applied once every 7 days

Patients who were receiving daily dose of 30 to 80 mg of oral morphine equivalents: Taper the current around-the-clock opioid for up to 7 days to ≤30 mg/day of oral morphine or equivalent before initiating therapy. Initial: 10 **mcg**/hour applied once every 7 days

Patient who were receiving daily dose of >80 mg of oral morphine equivalents: Buprenorphine transdermal patch, even at the maximum dose of 20 **mcg**/hour applied once every 7 days, may not provide adequate analgesia; **consider the use of an alternate analgesic.**

Dose titration (opioid-naive or opioid-experienced patients): May increase dose in 5 mcg/hour, 7.5 mcg/hour, or 10 mcg/hour increments (using no more than two patches), based on patient's supplemental short-acting analgesic requirements, with a minimum titration interval of 72 hours (maximum dose: 20 **mcg**/hour applied once every 7 days; risk for QTc prolongation increases with doses >20 **mcg**/hour patch).

Discontinuation of therapy: Taper dose gradually over 7 days to prevent withdrawal in the physically dependent patient; consider initiating immediate-release opioids, if needed.

Opioid withdrawal in heroin-dependent hospitalized patients (off-label use): IV infusion: 0.3 to 0.9 mg (diluted in 50 to 100 mL of NS) over 20 to 30 minutes every 6 to 12 hours (Welsh 2002)

Opioid dependence: Sublingual tablet: **Note:** The combination product, buprenorphine and naloxone, is preferred therapy over buprenorphine monotherapy for induction treatment (and stabilization/maintenance treatment) for short-acting opioid dependence (US Department of Health and Human Services 2005).

Manufacturer's labeling:

Induction: Day 1: 8 mg; Day 2 and subsequent induction days: 16 mg; usual induction dosage range: 12 to 16 mg/day (induction usually accomplished over 3 to 4 days). Treatment should begin at least 4 hours after last use of heroin or other short-acting opioids, preferably when first signs of withdrawal appear. Titrating dose to clinical effectiveness should be done as rapidly as possible to prevent undue withdrawal symptoms and patient drop-out during the induction period. There is little controlled experience with induction in patients on methadone or other long-acting opioids; consult expert physician experienced with this procedure.

Maintenance: Target dose: 16 mg/day; in some patients 12 mg/day may be effective; patients should be switched to the buprenorphine/naloxone combination product for maintenance and unsupervised therapy

Geriatric

Acute pain (moderate to severe): IM, slow IV: 0.15 mg every 6 hours; elderly patients are more likely to suffer from confusion and drowsiness compared to younger patients. **Long-term use is not recommended.**

Chronic pain (moderate to severe): Buccal film, transdermal patch: No specific dosage adjustments required; use caution due to potential for increased risk of adverse events.

Pediatric

Acute pain (moderate-to-severe):

Children 2 to 12 years: IM, slow IV: 2 to 6 **mcg**/kg every 4 to 6 hours

Children ≥13 years: Refer to adult dosing.

Opioid dependence: Children ≥16 years: Refer to adult dosing.

Renal Impairment Buccal film, injection, sublingual, transdermal: There are no dosage adjustments provided in the manufacturer's labeling (has not been adequately studied); use with caution.

Hepatic Impairment

Buccal film:

Mild impairment (Child-Pugh class A): No dosage adjustment necessary.

Moderate impairment (Child-Pugh class B): No dosage adjustment necessary; use caution and monitor for signs and symptoms of toxicity or overdose.

Severe impairment (Child-Pugh class C): Reduce starting dose and reduce titration dose by 50% (ie, from 150 mcg to 75 mcg).

Injection: There are no dosage adjustments provided in the manufacturer's labeling; undergoes extensive hepatic metabolism; use with caution, especially in severe impairment.

Sublingual:

Mild impairment: No dosage adjustment necessary.

Moderate impairment: No dosage adjustment necessary; use caution and monitor for signs and symptoms of toxicity or overdose.

Severe impairment: Consider reducing initial and titration incremental dose by 50%; monitor for signs and symptoms of toxicity or overdose.

Transdermal patch: Severe impairment: There are no dosage adjustments provided in the manufacturer's labeling (has not been studied); consider alternative therapy with more flexibility for dosing adjustments.

Administration

IM: Administer via deep IM injection

IV: Administer slowly, over at least 2 minutes. Administration over 20 to 30 minutes preferred when managing opioid withdrawal in heroin-dependent hospitalized patients (Welsh 2002).

Oral:

Buccal film: Prior to placing the film, moisten inside of cheek with tongue or water. Apply film with a dry finger immediately after removing it from packaging. Place yellow side of film against the inside of the moistened cheek; press and hold the film in place for 5 seconds with finger (film should stay in place after this period). Keep film in place until it dissolves completely (usually within 30 minutes of application). Do not chew, swallow, touch, or move film after placement. Liquids and food can be consumed after film dissolves. Do not cut or tear the film. Avoid application to areas of the mouth with any open sores or lesions. To dispose of film; remove foil overwrap from any unused, unneeded films and dispose by flushing down the toilet.

Sublingual tablet: Tablet should be placed under the tongue until dissolved; should not be swallowed. If two or more tablets are needed per dose, all may be placed under the tongue at once, or two at a time. To ensure consistent bioavailability, subsequent doses should always be taken the same way.

Transdermal patch: Apply patch to intact, nonirritated skin only. Apply to a hairless or nearly hairless skin site. If hairless site is not available, do not shave skin; hair at application site should be clipped. Prior to application, if the site must be cleaned, clean with clear water and allow to dry completely; do not use soaps, alcohol, oils, lotions, or abrasives due to potential for increased skin absorption. Do not use any patch that has been damaged, cut or manipulated in any way. Remove patch from protective pouch immediately before application. Remove the protective backing, and apply the sticky side of the patch to one of eight possible application sites (upper outer arm, upper chest, upper back or the side of the chest [each site on either side of the body]). Up to 2 patches may be applied at the same time adjacent to one another at the same application site. Firmly press patch in place and hold for ~15 seconds. Change patch every 7 days. Rotate patch application sites; wait ≥21 days before reapplying another patch to the same skin site. Avoid exposing application site to external heat sources (eg, heating pad, electric blanket, heat lamp, hot tub). Incidental exposure to water while bathing or showering is acceptable based on experience during clinical studies. If there is difficulty with patch adhesion, the edges of the system may be taped in place with first-aid tape. If ineffective, the system may be covered with waterproof or semipermeable adhesive dressings suitable for 7 days of wear. If the patch falls off during the 7-day dosing interval, dispose of the patch and apply a new patch to a different skin site. Dispose of patches using the Patch-Disposal Unit or by folding the adhesive sides of the patch together and then flushing down the toilet.

Monitoring Parameters Pain relief, respiratory and mental status, CNS depression (especially in elderly, debilitated or cachectic patients particularly during treatment initiation or titration, or when using concomitant CNS depressants), blood pressure (monitor for hypotension during initiation and titration); LFTs (prior to initiation and during therapy); signs of addiction, abuse, or misuse; symptoms of withdrawal; patients with biliary tract disease for worsening symptoms; application site reactions (transdermal patch); signs or symptoms of hypogonadism or hypoadrenalism (Brennan 2013); signs and symptoms of toxicity or overdose (especially in patients with hepatic impairment).

Product Availability Belbuca (buprenorphine buccal film): FDA approved October 2015; availability anticipated in the first quarter of 2016. Belbuca is indicated for the management of severe pain requiring daily, around-the-clock, long-term opioid treatment and for which alternative treatment options are inadequate. Consult prescribing information for additional information.

Dosage Forms Excipient information presented when available (limited, particularly for generics); consult specific product labeling. [DSC] = Discontinued product

Film, Buccal:

Belbuca: 75 mcg (60 ea); 150 mcg (60 ea); 300 mcg (60 ea); 450 mcg (60 ea); 600 mcg (60 ea); 750 mcg (60 ea); 900 mcg (60 ea) [contains methylparaben, propylparaben, saccharin sodium, sodium benzoate; peppermint flavor]

Patch Weekly, Transdermal:

Butrans: 5 mcg/hr (4 ea); 7.5 mcg/hr (4 ea); 10 mcg/hr (4 ea); 15 mcg/hr (4 ea); 20 mcg/hr (4 ea)

Solution, Injection:

Buprenex: 0.3 mg/mL (1 mL)

Generic: 0.3 mg/mL (1 mL)

Tablet Sublingual, Sublingual:

Subutex: 2 mg [DSC], 8 mg [DSC]

Generic: 2 mg, 8 mg

Controlled Substance C-III

Extemporaneous Preparations A 0.075 mg/mL solution can be made using the 0.3 mg/mL injection, 95% ethanol, and simple syrup. Add 1.26 mL of 95% ethanol to 0.3 mg buprenorphine obtained from an 0.3 mg/1 mL ampule, mix well, and add quantity of simple syrup sufficient to obtain 4 mL (final volume). Solution is stable under refrigeration and at room temperature for 30 days when stored in amber glass bottles and for 7 days when stored in oral syringes (Anagnostis, 2011; Anagnostis, 2013).

Anagnostis EA, Sadaka RE, Sailor LA, et al, "Formulation of Buprenorphine for Sublingual Use in Neonates," J Pediatr Pharmacol Ther, 2011, 16(4):281-4.

Anagnostis EA, personal communication, March 2013.

Buprenorphine and Naloxone

(byoo pre NOR feen & nal OKS one)

Brand Names: US Bunavail; Suboxone; Zubsolv

Brand Names: Canada Mylan-Buprenorphine/Naloxone; Suboxone; Teva-Buprenorphine/Naloxone

Index Terms Buprenorphine Hydrochloride and Naloxone Hydrochloride Dihydrate; Naloxone and Buprenorphine; Naloxone Hydrochloride Dihydrate and Buprenorphine Hydrochloride

Pharmacologic Category Analgesic, Opioid; Analgesic, Opioid Partial Agonist

Use

Opioid dependence: Treatment of opioid dependence. *General information:* Buprenorphine/naloxone should be used as part of a complete treatment plan to include counseling and psychosocial support

Prescribing and Access Restrictions In the US prescribing of tablets for opioid dependence is limited to physicians who have met the qualification criteria and have received a DEA number specific to prescribing this product. Tablets will be available through pharmacies and wholesalers which normally provide controlled substances.

In Canada, buprenorphine/naloxone sublingual tablets may be prescribed only by physicians experienced in substitution treatment in opioid dependence and who have completed a recognized buprenorphine/naloxone education program. Components of the program include: Training of physicians in the use of buprenorphine/naloxone; maintenance of a list of physicians who have completed training; daily dosing supervision by a health care professional until the patient is clinically stable and able to safely store buprenorphine/naloxone. Take-home doses should be assessed and reviewed regularly. Further information about the program may be obtained by contacting the manufacturer.

Medication Guide Available Yes

Dosing

Adult & Geriatric

Opioid dependence: Sublingual:

US labeling:

Induction: Heroin or other short-acting opioid dependency:

Notes:

Buprenorphine/naloxone is not recommended for use during the induction period for long-acting opioids or methadone; initial treatment should begin using buprenorphine monotherapy under supervision. Patients should be switched to the combination product for maintenance and unsupervised therapy.

Buprenorphine/naloxone sublingual film and tablets (Zubsolv) may be used during the induction period for short-acting opioids or heroin; initial treatment may begin using buprenorphine/naloxone sublingual film or tablets or using buprenorphine sublingual monotherapy when signs of moderate opioid withdrawal appear and not less than 6 hours after last opioid use. Titrate to adequate maintenance dose as rapidly as possible based on control of acute withdrawal symptoms.

Sublingual film:

Day 1 induction dose: Initial: Buprenorphine 2 mg/naloxone 0.5 mg or buprenorphine 4 mg/naloxone 1 mg; may titrate dose, based on control of acute withdrawal symptoms, in buprenorphine 2 to 4 mg/naloxone 0.5 to 1 mg increments approximately every 2 hours up to a total dose of buprenorphine 8 mg/naloxone 2 mg.

Day 2 induction dose: Up to buprenorphine 16 mg/naloxone 4 mg once daily

Sublingual tablet (Zubsolv; Buprenorphine 1.4 mg/naloxone 0.36 mg, buprenorphine 2.9 mg/naloxone 0.71 mg, buprenorphine 5.7 mg/naloxone 1.4 mg, buprenorphine 8.6 mg/naloxone 2.1 mg, or buprenorphine 11.4 mg/naloxone 2.9 mg):

Day 1 induction dose: Initial: Buprenorphine 1.4 mg/naloxone 0.36 mg; may titrate dose, based on control of acute withdrawal symptoms in increments of buprenorphine 1.4 mg or 2.8 mg/naloxone 0.36 or 0.72 mg every 1.5 to 2 hours to a total day 1 dose up to buprenorphine 5.7 mg/naloxone 1.4 mg. Some patients (eg, those with recent exposure to buprenorphine) may tolerate up to buprenorphine 4.2 mg/naloxone 1.08 mg as a single, second dose.

Day 2 induction dose: Up to buprenorphine 11.4 mg/naloxone 2.9 mg once daily

Maintenance:

Buccal film (Bunavail: Buprenorphine 2.1 mg/naloxone 0.3 mg, buprenorphine 4.2 mg/naloxone 0.7 mg, buprenorphine 6.3 mg/naloxone 1 mg): Target dose: Buprenorphine 8.4 mg/naloxone 1.4 mg once daily; dosage should be adjusted in increments/decrements of buprenorphine 2.1 mg/naloxone 0.3 mg to a level that maintains treatment and suppresses opioid withdrawal symptoms; usual range: Buprenorphine 2.1 to 12.6 mg/naloxone 0.3 to 2.1 mg once daily

Sublingual film and sublingual tablet (buprenorphine 2 mg/naloxone 0.5 mg or buprenorphine 8 mg/naloxone 2 mg): Target dose: Buprenorphine 16 mg/naloxone 4 mg once daily; dosage should be adjusted in increments of buprenorphine 2 mg or 4 mg/naloxone 0.5 mg or buprenorphine 4 mg/naloxone 1 mg to a level that maintains treatment and suppresses opioid withdrawal symptoms; usual range: Buprenorphine 4 to 24 mg/naloxone 1 to 6 mg once daily

Sublingual tablet (Zubsolv: Buprenorphine 1.4 mg/naloxone 0.36 mg, buprenorphine 2.9 mg/naloxone 0.71 mg, buprenorphine 5.7 mg/naloxone 1.4 mg, buprenorphine 8.6 mg/naloxone 2.1 mg, or buprenorphine 11.4 mg/naloxone 2.9 mg): Target dose: Buprenorphine 11.4 mg/naloxone 2.9 mg once daily; dosage should be adjusted in increments/decrements of buprenorphine 1.4 mg or 2.9 mg/naloxone 0.36 or 0.71 mg to a level that maintains treatment and suppresses opioid withdrawal symptoms; usual range: Buprenorphine 2.9 to 17.2 mg/naloxone 0.71 to 4.2 mg once daily.

Off-label dosing recommendations (U.S. Department of Health and Human Services, 2004): Doses provided based on buprenorphine content.

Induction (only administer combination product for induction in patients who are dependent on **short-acting** opioids and whose last dose of opioids was >12 to 24 hours prior to induction):

Day 1 induction dose: Initial: 4 mg; may repeat dose after >2 hours if withdrawal symptoms not relieved; maximum daily dose on day 1: 8 mg daily

Day 2 induction dose: Previous dose from day 1 if no withdrawal symptoms present; if symptoms of withdrawal present, increase day 1 dose by 4 mg. If withdrawal symptoms not relieved after >2 hours, may administer 4 mg; maximum daily dose on day 2: 16 mg daily

Subsequent induction days: If withdrawal symptoms are not present, daily dose is established. If withdrawal symptoms are present, increase dose in increments of 2 mg or 4 mg each day as needed for symptom relief. Target daily dose by the end of the first week: 12 mg or 16 mg daily; maximum daily dose: 32 mg daily

Stabilization: Usual dose: 16 to 24 mg daily; maximum dose: 32 mg daily

Switching between sublingual tablets and sublingual film: Same dosage should be used as the previous administered product. **Note:** Potential for greater bioavailability with certain sublingual film strengths compared to the same strength of the sublingual tablet; monitor closely for either over- or underdosing when switching patients from one formulation to another.

Switching between buccal film and sublingual tablets or films: Due to differences in the bioavailability of Bunavail buccal films compared to other buprenorphine/naloxone sublingual tablets, different strengths must be given to achieve equivalent doses. When switching between Bunavail and other sublingual tablets, corresponding dosage strengths are as follows:

Bunavail buprenorphine 2.1 mg/naloxone 0.3 mg = buprenorphine 4 mg/naloxone 1 mg sublingual tablets or films

Bunavail buprenorphine 4.2 mg/naloxone 0.7 mg = buprenorphine 8 mg/naloxone 2 mg sublingual tablets or films

Bunavail buprenorphine 6.3 mg/naloxone 1 mg = buprenorphine 12 mg/naloxone 3 mg sublingual tablets or films

Switching between sublingual film strengths: Systemic exposure may be different with various combinations of sublingual film strengths; pharmacists should not substitute one or more film strengths for another (eg, switching from three buprenorphine 4 mg/naloxone 1 mg films to a single buprenorphine 12 mg/naloxone 3 mg film, or vice-versa) without health care provider approval, and patients should be monitored closely for either over- or underdosing when switching between film strengths.

Switching between sublingual and buccal sites of administration (Suboxone): Systemic exposure between buccal and sublingual administration of buprenorphine/naloxone sublingual film is similar. Once induction is complete, patients can switch between buccal and sublingual administration without significant risk of under or overdosing.

Switching between sublingual tablet products: Due to differences in the bioavailability of Zubsolv sublingual tablets compared to other buprenorphine/naloxone sublingual tablets, different strengths must be given to achieve equivalent doses. When switching between Zubsolv and other sublingual tablets, corresponding dosage strengths are as follows:

Zubsolv buprenorphine 1.4 mg/naloxone 0.36 mg sublingual tablets = buprenorphine 2 mg/naloxone 0.5 mg sublingual tablets

Zubsolv buprenorphine 2.9 mg/naloxone 0.71 mg sublingual tablets = buprenorphine 4 mg/naloxone 1 mg (as two buprenorphine 2 mg/naloxone 0.5 mg sublingual tablets)

Zubsolv buprenorphine 5.7 mg/naloxone 1.4 mg sublingual tablets = buprenorphine 8 mg/naloxone 2 mg sublingual tablets

Zubsolv buprenorphine 8.6 mg/naloxone 2.1 mg sublingual tablet = buprenorphine 12 mg/naloxone 3 mg sublingual tablets (as one buprenorphine 8 mg/naloxone 2 mg sublingual tablets and two buprenorphine 2 mg/naloxone 0.5 mg sublingual tablets)

Zubsolv buprenorphine 11.4 mg/naloxone 2.9 mg sublingual tablet = buprenorphine 16 mg/naloxone 4 mg sublingual tablets (as two buprenorphine 8 mg/naloxone 2 mg sublingual tablets)

Canadian labeling: Sublingual tablet: **Note:** Dose based on buprenorphine content. Prior to induction, consider patient's type of dependence (ie, long- or short-acting opiate), time since last use of opiate and extent of dependence. Initiate buprenorphine/naloxone when early signs of opiate withdrawal appear but no sooner than 6 hours after the last use of heroin or other short-acting opiates. Patients on methadone should have their methadone maintenance dose reduced to the minimum tolerable dose; initiate buprenorphine/naloxone only when early signs of withdrawal appear but no sooner than 24 hours after the last methadone dose.

Induction: Day 1: Initial: 4 mg as single dose; may repeat dose if necessary depending on patient's requirement; target dose: 8 to 12 mg.

Maintenance: Day 2 and beyond: Titrate per response in increments or decrements of 2 to 8 mg; usual maintenance dose: 12 to 16 mg once daily (maximum: 24 mg/day). Upon stabilization, may consider less frequent administration of corresponding equivalent dose (eg, 16 mg every other day instead of 8 mg/day or 3 times/week dosing [eg, Monday-Wednesday-Friday] with twice the maintenance dose on Monday and Wednesday and three times the maintenance dose on Friday); continue to limit maximum dose to 24 mg/day on any single day. **Note:** When switching dosing to less than once daily, monitor all patients for at least 90 minutes following the initial dose of the new regimen. The less frequent dosing regimen is not recommended in patients dependent on concurrent CNS-active drugs, including ethanol.

Missed doses: Reassess patients who have missed multiple doses; initial induction doses may be required when resuming therapy.

Pediatric Opioid dependence: Adolescents ≥16 years: Refer to adult dosing. Canadian labeling does not approve of use in patients <18 years.

Renal Impairment

US labeling: There are no dosage adjustments provided in the manufacturer's labeling (has not been adequately studied); use with caution.

Canadian labeling:

CrCl ≥30 mL/minute: No dosage adjustment necessary.

CrCl <30 mL/minute: Use with caution in severe impairment; dosage adjustment may be required.

Hepatic Impairment

US labeling:

Mild hepatic impairment: No dosage adjustment necessary.

Moderate hepatic impairment: Use with caution during maintenance treatment (due to extensive metabolism of buprenorphine and naloxone, use may not be appropriate). Suboxone use is not recommended during induction therapy.

Severe hepatic impairment: Use is not recommended.

Canadian labeling:

Mild to moderate impairment: There are no specific dosage adjustments provided in the manufacturer's labeling; however, a dosage adjustment may be considered. Because of extensive metabolism of buprenorphine and naloxone, use may not be appropriate in moderate impairment; use with caution and monitor closely.

Severe impairment: Use is contraindicated.

Additional Information Complete prescribing information should be consulted for additional detail.

Dosage Forms Excipient information presented when available (limited, particularly for generics); consult specific product labeling.

Film, buccal:

Bunavail: Buprenorphine 2.1 mg and naloxone 0.3 mg (30s); buprenorphine 4.2 mg and naloxone 0.7 mg (30s); buprenorphine 6.3 mg and naloxone 1 mg (30s) [citrus flavor]

Film, sublingual:

Suboxone: Buprenorphine 2 mg and naloxone 0.5 mg (30s); buprenorphine 4 mg and naloxone 1 mg (30s); buprenorphine 8 mg and naloxone 2 mg (30s); buprenorphine 12 mg and naloxone 3 mg (30s) [lime flavor]

Tablet, sublingual: Buprenorphine 2 mg and naloxone 0.5 mg; buprenorphine 8 mg and naloxone 2 mg

Zubsolv: Buprenorphine 1.4 mg and naloxone 0.36 mg; buprenorphine 2.9 mg and naloxone 0.71 mg; buprenorphine 5.7 mg and naloxone 1.4 mg; buprenorphine 8.6 mg and naloxone 2.1 mg; buprenorphine 11.4 mg and naloxone 2.9 mg [menthol flavor]

Dosage Forms: Canada Excipient information presented when available (limited, particularly for generics); consult specific product labeling.

Tablet, Sublingual:

Suboxone: Buprenorphine 2 mg and naloxone 0.5 mg; buprenorphine 8 mg and naloxone 2 mg

Controlled Substance C-III

◆ **Buprenorphine Hydrochloride** *see* Buprenorphine *on page 263*

◆ **Buprenorphine Hydrochloride and Naloxone Hydrochloride Dihydrate** *see* Buprenorphine and Naloxone *on page 267*

◆ **Buproban** *see* BuPROPion *on page 269*

BuPROPion (byoo PROE pee on)

Brand Names: US Aplenzin; Budeprion SR [DSC]; Budeprion XL [DSC]; Buproban; Forfivo XL; Wellbutrin; Wellbutrin SR; Wellbutrin XL; Zyban

Brand Names: Canada Bupropion SR; Mylan-Bupropion XL; Novo-Bupropion SR; PMS-Bupropion SR; ratio-Bupropion SR; Sandoz-Bupropion SR; Wellbutrin SR; Wellbutrin XL; Zyban

Index Terms Budeprion SR; Bupropion Hydrobromide; Bupropion Hydrochloride

Pharmacologic Category Antidepressant, Dopamine/Norepinephrine-Reuptake Inhibitor; Smoking Cessation Aid

Use

Major depressive disorder (Aplenzin, Forfivo XL, Wellbutrin, Wellbutrin SR, Wellbutrin XL): Treatment of major depressive disorder (MDD).

Seasonal affective disorder (Aplenzin, Wellbutrin XL): Prevention of seasonal major depressive episodes in patients with a diagnosis of seasonal affective disorder (SAD).

Smoking cessation (Buproban and Zyban): As an aid to smoking cessation treatment.

Pregnancy Considerations Adverse events have been observed in some animal reproduction studies. Bupropion and its metabolites were found to cross the placenta in *in vitro* studies (Earhart 2012). An increased risk of congenital malformations has not been observed following maternal use of bupropion during pregnancy; however, data specific to cardiovascular malformations is inconsistent. The long-term effects on development and behavior have not been studied. The ACOG recommends that antidepressant therapy during pregnancy be individualized; treatment of depression during pregnancy should incorporate the clinical expertise of the mental health clinician, obstetrician, primary healthcare provider, and pediatrician. According to the American Psychiatric Association (APA), the risks of medication treatment should be weighed against other treatment options and untreated depression. For women who discontinue antidepressant medications during pregnancy and who may be at high risk for postpartum depression, the medications can be restarted following delivery. Treatment algorithms have been developed by the ACOG and the APA for the management of depression in women prior to conception and during pregnancy (ACOG 2008; APA 2010; Yonkers 2009). There is insufficient information related to the use of bupropion to recommend use in pregnancy (ACOG 2010).

Breast-Feeding Considerations Bupropion and its metabolites are excreted into breast milk. The estimated dose to a nursing infant varies by study and has been reported as ~2% of the weight-adjusted maternal dose (range: 1.4% to 10.6%) (Davis 2009; Haas 2004). Adverse events have been reported with some antidepressants and a seizure was noted in one 6-month old nursing infant exposed to bupropion (a causal effect could not be confirmed) (Chaudron 2004; Hale 2010). Recommendations for use in nursing women vary by manufacturer labeling.

Medication Guide Available Yes

Contraindications Hypersensitivity to bupropion or any component of the formulation; seizure disorder; history of anorexia/bulimia; patients undergoing abrupt discontinuation of ethanol or sedatives, including benzodiazepines, barbiturates, or antiepileptic drugs; use of MAO inhibitors or MAO inhibitors intended to treat psychiatric disorders (concurrently or within 14 days of discontinuing either bupropion or the MAO inhibitor); initiation of bupropion in

◄ a patient receiving linezolid or intravenous methylene blue; patients receiving other dosage forms of bupropion

Aplenzin, Wellbutrin XL: Additional contraindications: Other conditions that increase seizure risk, including arteriovenous malformation, severe head injury, severe stroke, CNS tumor, CNS infection

Warnings/Precautions [US Boxed Warning]: Use in treating psychiatric disorders: Antidepressants increase the risk of suicidal thinking and behavior in children, adolescents, and young adults (18 to 24 years of age) with major depressive disorder (MDD) and other psychiatric disorders; consider risk prior to prescribing. Short-term studies did not show an increased risk in patients >24 years of age and showed a decreased risk in patients ≥65 years. All patients must be closely monitored for clinical worsening, suicidality, or unusual changes in behavior, especially during the initiation of therapy (generally first 1 to 2 months) or following an increase or decrease in dosage. The patient's family or caregiver should be instructed to closely observe the patient and communicate condition with healthcare provider. A medication guide should be dispensed with each prescription.

[US Boxed Warning]: Use in smoking cessation: Serious neuropsychiatric events have occurred in patients taking bupropion for smoking cessation, including changes in mood (eg, depression, mania), psychosis, hallucinations, paranoia, delusions, homicidal ideation, hostility, agitation, aggression, anxiety, panic, suicidal ideation, suicide attempt and completed suicide. **The majority occurred during bupropion treatment; some occurred during treatment discontinuation. A causal relationship is uncertain as depressed mood may be a symptom of nicotine withdrawal. Some cases also occurred in patients taking bupropion who continued to smoke. Observe all patients taking bupropion for neuropsychiatric reactions. Instruct patients to contact a health care provider if neuropsychiatric reactions occur.**

The possibility of a suicide attempt is inherent in major depression and may persist until remission occurs. Worsening depression and severe abrupt suicidality that are not part of the presenting symptoms may require discontinuation or modification of drug therapy. Use caution in high-risk patients during initiation of therapy. Prescriptions should be written for the smallest quantity consistent with good patient care. The patient's family or caregiver should be alerted to monitor patients for the emergence of suicidality and associated behaviors such as anxiety, agitation, panic attacks, insomnia, irritability, hostility, impulsivity, akathisia, hypomania, and mania; patients should be instructed to notify their healthcare provider if any of these symptoms or worsening depression or psychosis occur.

May cause delusions, hallucinations, psychosis, concentration disturbance, paranoia, and confusion; most common in depressed patients and patients with a diagnosis of bipolar disorder. Symptoms may abate with dose reduction and/or withdrawal of treatment. May precipitate a manic, mixed, or hypomanic episode; risk is increased in patients with bipolar disorder or who have risk factors for bipolar disorder. Screen patients for a history of bipolar disorder and the presence of risk factors including a family history of bipolar disorder, suicide, or depression. **Bupropion is not FDA approved for bipolar depression.**

May cause a dose-related risk of seizures. Use is contraindicated in patients with a history of seizures or certain conditions with high seizure risk (eg, arteriovenous malformation, severe head injury, severe stroke, CNS tumor, or CNS infection, history of anorexia/bulimia, or patients undergoing abrupt discontinuation of ethanol, benzodiazepines, barbiturates, or antiepileptic drugs). Use caution with concurrent use of antipsychotics, antidepressants, theophylline, systemic corticosteroids, stimulants (including cocaine), anorectants, or hypoglycemic agents, or with excessive use of ethanol, benzodiazepines, sedative/hypnotics, or opioids. Use with caution in seizure-potentiating metabolic disorders (hypoglycemia, hyponatremia, severe hepatic impairment, and hypoxia). The dose-dependent risk of seizures may be reduced by gradual dose increases and by not exceeding the maximum daily dose. Use of multiple bupropion formulations is contraindicated. Permanently discontinue if seizure occurs during therapy. Chewing, crushing, or dividing long-acting products may increase seizure risk.

May cause CNS stimulation (restlessness, anxiety, insomnia) or anorexia. May increase the risks associated with electroconvulsive therapy (ECT). Consider discontinuing, when possible, prior to ECT. May cause weight loss; use caution in patients where weight loss is not desirable. The incidence of sexual dysfunction with bupropion is generally lower than with SSRIs.

May elevate blood pressure and cause hypertension. Events have been observed in patients with or without evidence of preexisting hypertension. The risk is increased when used concomitantly with monoamine oxidase inhibitors, nicotine replacement, or other drugs that increase dopaminergic or noradrenergic activity. Assess blood pressure before treatment and monitor periodically. Use caution in patients with cardiovascular disease. All children diagnosed with ADHD who may be candidates for stimulant medications should have a thorough cardiovascular assessment to identify risk factors for sudden cardiac death prior to initiation of drug therapy. Use with caution in patients with hepatic or renal dysfunction and in elderly patients; reduced dose and/or frequency may be recommended; Forfivo XL is not recommended in patients with hepatic or renal impairment. Elderly patients may be at greater risk of accumulation during chronic dosing. May cause motor or cognitive impairment in some patients; use with caution if tasks requiring alertness such as operating machinery or driving are undertaken. May cause mild pupillary dilation, which in susceptible individuals can lead to an episode of narrow-angle glaucoma. Consider evaluating patients who have not had an iridectomy for narrow-angle glaucoma risk factors. Anaphylactoid/anaphylactic reactions have occurred, with symptoms of pruritus, urticaria, angioedema, and dyspnea. Serious reactions have been (rarely) reported, including erythema multiforme, Stevens-Johnson syndrome and anaphylactic shock. Arthralgia, myalgia, and fever with rash and other symptoms suggestive of delayed hypersensitivity resembling serum sickness have been reported. Potentially significant drug-drug interactions may exist, requiring dose or frequency adjustment, additional monitoring, and/or selection of alternative therapy.

Extended release tablet: Insoluble tablet shell may remain intact and be visible in the stool.

Adverse Reactions
>10%:
Cardiovascular: Tachycardia (11%)
Central nervous system: Headache (25% to 34%), agitation (2% to 32%), dizziness (6% to 22%), insomnia (11% to 20%)
Dermatologic: Diaphoresis (5% to 22%)
Endocrine & metabolic: Weight loss (14% to 23%)
Gastrointestinal: Xerostomia (17% to 28%), nausea (1% to 18%)
Ophthalmic: Blurred vision (2% to 15%)
Respiratory: Pharyngitis (3% to 13%)
1% to 10%:
Cardiovascular: Palpitations (2% to 6%), cardiac arrhythmia (5%), chest pain (3% to 4%), hypertension (2% to 4%; may be severe), flushing (1% to 4%), hypotension (3%)
Central nervous system: Confusion (8%), anxiety (3% to 7%), hostility (6%), nervousness (3% to 5%), sensory disturbance (4%), sleep disorder (4%), migraine (1% to 4%), abnormal dreams (3%), memory impairment (≤3%), drowsiness (2% to 3%), irritability (2% to 3%), pain (2% to 3%), akathisia (≤2%), central nervous system stimulation (1% to 2%), paresthesia (1% to 2%), twitching (1% to 2%), depression
Dermatologic: Skin rash (1% to 8%), pruritus (2% to 4%), urticaria (1% to 2%)
Endocrine & metabolic: Weight gain (9%), menstrual disease (2% to 5%), decreased libido (3%), hot flash (1% to 3%)
Gastrointestinal: Constipation (5% to 10%), abdominal pain (2% to 9%), diarrhea (5% to 7%), flatulence (6%), anorexia (3% to 5%), increased appetite (4%), dysgeusia (2% to 4%), vomiting (2% to 4%), dyspepsia (3%), dysphagia (≤2%)
Genitourinary: Urinary urgency (≤2%), vaginal hemorrhage (≤2%), urinary tract infection (≤1%)
Hypersensitivity: Hypersensitivity reaction (including anaphylaxis, pruritus, urticaria)
Infection: Infection (8% to 9%)
Neuromuscular & skeletal: Tremor (3% to 6%), myalgia (2% to 6%), weakness (2% to 4%), arthralgia (1% to 4%), arthritis (≤2%), neck pain
Otic: Tinnitus (3% to 6%), auditory disturbance (5%)
Renal: Polyuria (2% to 5%)
Respiratory: Upper respiratory infection (9%), cough (1% to 4%), sinusitis (1% to 5%)
Miscellaneous: Fever (1% to 2%)
<1% (Limited to important or life-threatening): Abnormal accommodation, akinesia, alopecia, amnesia, anaphylactic shock, anaphylactoid reaction, anemia, angioedema, angle-closure glaucoma, aphasia, ataxia, atrioventricular block, cerebrovascular accident, colitis,

coma, cystitis, deafness, delayed hypersensitivity, delirium, delusions, depersonalization, derealization, diplopia, dysarthria, dyskinesia, dyspareunia, dysphoria, dystonia, dysuria, edema, EEG pattern changes, erythema multiforme, esophagitis, euphoria, exfoliative dermatitis, extrapyramidal reaction, extrasystoles, facial edema, gastric ulcer, gastroesophageal reflux disease, gastrointestinal hemorrhage, gingival hemorrhage, glossitis, glycosuria, gynecomastia, hallucination, hepatic injury, hepatic insufficiency, hepatitis, hirsutism, hyperglycemia, hyperkinesia, hypertonia, hypoglycemia, hypokinesia, hypomania, impotence, increased intraocular pressure, increased libido, intestinal perforation, jaundice, leukocytosis, leukopenia, lymphadenopathy, manic behavior, myasthenia, mydriasis, myocardial infarction, myoclonus, neuralgia, neuropathy, orthostatic hypotension, painful erection, pancreatitis, pancytopenia, paranoia, pneumonia, psychiatric signs and symptoms, pulmonary embolism, rhabdomyolysis, salpingitis, sciatica, seizure (dose-related), SIADH, skin photosensitivity, Stevens-Johnson syndrome, stomatitis, suicidal ideation, syncope, tardive dyskinesia, thrombocytopenia, tongue edema, urinary incontinence, urinary retention, vasodilatation

Drug Interactions

Metabolism/Transport Effects Substrate of CYP1A2 (minor), CYP2A6 (minor), CYP2B6 (major), CYP2C9 (minor), CYP2D6 (minor), CYP2E1 (minor), CYP3A4 (minor); **Note:** Assignment of Major/Minor substrate status based on clinically relevant drug interaction potential; **Inhibits** CYP2D6 (strong), OCT2

Avoid Concomitant Use

Avoid concomitant use of BuPROPion with any of the following: MAO Inhibitors; Mequitazine; Pimozide; Tamoxifen; Thioridazine

Increased Effect/Toxicity

BuPROPion may increase the levels/effects of: Alcohol (Ethyl); ARIPiprazole; ARIPiprazole Lauroxil; AtoMOXetine; Brexpiprazole; Citalopram; CYP2D6 Substrates; Dapoxetine; DOXOrubicin (Conventional); DULoxetine; Eliglustat; Fesoterodine; FLUoxetine; FluvoxaMINE; Iloperidone; Lorcaserin; Mequitazine; Metoprolol; Nebivolol; OCT2 Substrates; PARoxetine; Pimozide; Propafenone; Tamsulosin; Tetrabenazine; Thioridazine; TraMADol; Tricyclic Antidepressants; Vortioxetine

The levels/effects of BuPROPion may be increased by: Alcohol (Ethyl); Anti-Parkinson's Agents (Dopamine Agonist); CYP2B6 Inhibitors (Moderate); MAO Inhibitors; Mifepristone; Quazepam

Decreased Effect

BuPROPion may decrease the levels/effects of: Codeine; Hydrocodone; Iloperidone; Ioflupane I 123; Tamoxifen; TraMADol

The levels/effects of BuPROPion may be decreased by: Antihepaciviral Combination Products; CYP2B6 Inducers (Strong); Dabrafenib; Efavirenz; Isavuconazonium Sulfate; Lopinavir; Lumacaftor; Ritonavir

Storage/Stability

Store at 15°C to 30°C (59°F to 86°F).

Wellbutrin, Wellbutrin XL, Zyban: Protect from light and moisture.

Mechanism of Action Aminoketone antidepressant structurally different from all other marketed antidepressants; like other antidepressants the mechanism of bupropion's activity is not fully understood. Bupropion is a relatively weak inhibitor of the neuronal uptake of norepinephrine and dopamine, and does not inhibit monoamine oxidase or the reuptake of serotonin. Metabolite inhibits the reuptake of norepinephrine. The primary mechanism of action is thought to be dopaminergic and/or noradrenergic.

Pharmacodynamics/Kinetics

Onset of action: 1 to 2 weeks

Duration of action: 1 to 2 days

Absorption: Rapid

Distribution: V_d: ~20 to 47 L/kg (Laizure 1985)

Protein binding: 84%

Metabolism: Extensively hepatic via CYP2B6 to hydroxybupropion; non-CYP-mediated metabolism to erythrohydrobupropion and threohydrobupropion. Metabolite activity ranges from 20% to 50% potency of bupropion. Bupropion also undergoes oxidation to form the glycine conjugate of meta-chlorobenzoic acid, the major urinary metabolite.

Half-life:

Distribution: 3 to 4 hours

Elimination: ~21 hours after chronic dosing (range: 12 to 30 hours); Metabolites (after a single dose): Hydroxybupropion: 20 ± 5 hours; Erythrohydrobupropion: 33 ± 10 hours; Threohydrobupropion: 37 ± 13 hours

Extended release (Aplenzin): 21 ± 7 hours; Metabolites: Hydroxybupropion: 24 ± 5 hours; Erythrohydrobupropion: 31 ± 8 hours; Threohydrobupropion: 51 ± 9 hours

Time to peak, serum:

Bupropion: Immediate release: Within 2 hours; Sustained release: Within 3 hours; Extended release: ~5 hours (Forfivo XL: 5 hours [fasting]; 12 hours [fed])

Metabolite: Hydroxybupropion: Immediate release: ~3 hours; Extended release, sustained release: ~6 to 7 hours

Excretion: Urine (87%, primarily as metabolites); feces (10%, primarily as metabolites)

Dosing

Adult

Depression: Oral: **Note:** Treatment should be periodically evaluated at appropriate intervals to ensure lowest effective dose is used.

Immediate release hydrochloride salt: Initial: 100 mg twice daily; after 3 days may increase to the usual dose of 100 mg 3 times a day; if no clinical improvement after several weeks, may increase to a maximum dose of 450 mg daily in 3 or 4 divided doses; do not exceed 150 mg in a single dose

Sustained release hydrochloride salt: Initial: 150 mg daily in the morning; if tolerated, after 3 days, may increase to a target dose of 150 mg twice daily; if no clinical improvement after several weeks, may increase to a maximum dose of 200 mg twice daily

Extended release:

Hydrochloride salt (Wellbutrin XL): Initial: 150 mg once daily in the morning; if tolerated, as early as day 4, may increase to 300 mg once daily (maximum dose: 300 mg/day; however, guidelines suggest up to 450 mg/day may be used [APA 2010]). **Note:** Forfivo XL may only be used after initial dose titration with other bupropion products.

Hydrochloride salt (Forfivo XL): *Switching from Wellbutrin immediate release, SR, or XL to Forfivo XL:* Patients receiving 300 mg daily of bupropion hydrochloride for at least 2 weeks and requiring a dose increase or patients already taking 450 mg daily of bupropion hydrochloride may switch to Forfivo XL 450 mg once daily.

Hydrobromide salt (Aplenzin): Initial: 174 mg once daily in the morning; may increase as early as day 4 of dosing to 348 mg once daily (target dose); maximum dose: 522 mg daily.

Switching from hydrochloride salt formulation (eg, Wellbutrin immediate release, SR, XL, or Forfivo XL) to hydrobromide salt formulation (Aplenzin):

Bupropion hydrochloride 150 mg daily is equivalent to bupropion hydrobromide 174 mg once daily

Bupropion hydrochloride 300 mg daily is equivalent to bupropion hydrobromide 348 mg once daily

Bupropion hydrochloride 450 mg daily is equivalent to bupropion hydrobromide 522 mg once daily

Seasonal affective disorder (SAD): Initial: 150 mg once daily (Wellbutrin XL) or 174 mg once daily (Aplenzin) in the morning; if tolerated, may increase after 1 week to 300 mg once daily (Wellbutrin XL) or 348 mg once daily (Aplenzin) in the morning.

Note: Prophylactic treatment should be reserved for those patients with frequent depressive episodes and/or significant impairment. Initiate treatment in the Autumn prior to symptom onset, and discontinue in early Spring with dose tapering. Doses >300 mg daily (Wellbutrin XL) or >348 mg daily (Aplenzin) have not been studied in SAD (maximum: Wellbutrin XL 300 mg daily; Aplenzin 522 mg daily).

Smoking cessation (Zyban, Buproban): Initial: 150 mg once daily for 3 days; increase to 150 mg twice daily; treatment should continue for 7 to 12 weeks (maximum dose: 300 mg daily).

Note: Therapy should begin at least 1 week before target quit date. Target quit dates are generally in the second week of treatment. If patient successfully quits smoking after 7 to 12 weeks, may consider ongoing maintenance therapy based on individual patient risk:benefit. Efficacy of maintenance therapy (300 mg daily) has been demonstrated for up to 6 months. Conversely, if significant progress has not been made by the seventh week of therapy, success is unlikely and treatment discontinuation should be considered.

Dosing conversion between hydrochloride salt immediate (Wellbutrin), sustained (Wellbutrin SR), and extended release (Wellbutrin XL, Forfivo XL) products: Convert using same total daily dose (up to the maximum recommended dose for a given dosage form), but adjust frequency as indicated for sustained (twice daily) or extended (once daily) release products.

Discontinuation of therapy: Upon discontinuation of antidepressant therapy, gradually taper the dose to allow for the detection of re-emerging symptoms.

Withdrawal symptoms resulting from abrupt discontinuation are unlikely because bupropion has minimal serotonergic activity (APA 2010).

Manufacturer's labeling:

Aplenzin: In patients receiving 348 mg once daily, taper dose down to 174 mg once daily for 2 weeks prior to discontinuing.

Wellbutrin XL: In patients receiving 300 mg once daily, taper dose down to 150 mg once daily for 2 weeks prior to discontinuing.

MAO inhibitor recommendations:

Switching to or from an MAO inhibitor antidepressant:

Allow 14 days to elapse between discontinuing an MAO inhibitor intended to treat depression and initiation of bupropion.

Allow 14 days to elapse between discontinuing bupropion and initiation of an MAO inhibitor intended to treat depression.

Use with reversible MAO inhibitors (such as linezolid or IV methylene blue):

Do not initiate bupropion in patients receiving linezolid or IV methylene blue; consider other interventions for psychiatric condition.

If urgent treatment with linezolid or IV methylene blue is required in a patient already receiving bupropion and potential benefits outweigh potential risks, discontinue bupropion promptly and administer linezolid or IV methylene blue. Monitor for increased risk of hypertensive reactions for 2 weeks or until 24 hours after the last dose of linezolid or IV methylene blue, whichever comes first. May resume bupropion 24 hours after the last dose of linezolid or IV methylene blue.

Geriatric

Depression: Oral (hydrochloride salt): Initial: 37.5 mg of immediate release tablets twice daily or 100 mg daily of sustained release tablets; increase by 37.5 to 100 mg every 3 to 4 days as tolerated to a maximum dose of 300 mg daily (in divided doses). There is evidence that the elderly respond at 150 mg daily in divided doses, but some may require a higher dose. **Note:** Patients with Alzheimer's dementia-related depression may require a lower starting dosage of 37.5 mg once or twice daily (100 mg daily sustained release), increased as needed up to 300 mg daily in divided doses (300 mg daily for sustained release) (Rabins 2007).

Smoking cessation: Refer to adult dosing.

Discontinuation of therapy: Refer to adult dosing.

MAO inhibitor recommendations: Refer to adult dosing.

Pediatric

ADHD (off-label use): Oral (hydrochloride salt): Children and Adolescents: 1.4 to 6 mg/kg/day (Barrickman 1995; Conners 1996)

MAO inhibitor recommendations: Refer to adult dosing.

Renal Impairment

Use with caution; manufacturer's labeling suggests a reduction in dose and/or frequency be considered but does not provide specific dosing recommendations. Aplenzin, Wellbutrin, Wellbutrin SR, Wellbutrin XL, and Zyban product labeling defines renal impairment as GFR <90 mL/minute.

Forfivo XL: Use is not recommended.

Hepatic Impairment

Mild impairment (Child-Pugh score 5 to 6): Use with caution; manufacturer's labeling suggests a reduction in dose and/or frequency be considered but does not provide specific dosing recommendations.

Forfivo XL: Use is not recommended.

Moderate to severe impairment, including severe hepatic cirrhosis (Child-Pugh score 7 to 15): Use with extreme caution; maximum dose:

Aplenzin: 174 mg every other day

Buproban: Severe hepatic cirrhosis: 150 mg every other day

Forfivo XL: Use is not recommended.

Wellbutrin: 75 mg once daily

Wellbutrin SR: 100 mg once daily or 150 mg every other day

Wellbutrin XL, Zyban: 150 mg every other day

Administration

May be taken without regard to meals. The manufacturer states that tablets should be swallowed whole; do not crush, chew, or divide.

Extended release: Administer once daily with at least 24 hours between successive doses.

Immediate release: Administer 3 to 4 times daily with at least 6 hours between successive doses; do not exceed 150 mg in a single dose.

Sustained release: Administer 2 times daily with at least 8 hours between successive doses.

Monitoring Parameters Body weight; mental status for depression, suicidal ideation (especially at the beginning of therapy or when doses are increased or decreased), anxiety, social functioning, mania, panic attacks; blood pressure (baseline and periodically especially when used in conjunction with nicotine transdermal replacement); renal and hepatic function

When used for the treatment of ADHD, thoroughly evaluate for cardiovascular risk. Monitor heart rate, blood pressure, and consider obtaining ECG prior to initiation (Vetter 2008).

Reference Range Therapeutic levels (trough, 12 hours after last dose): 50 to 100 ng/mL

Test Interactions May interfere with urine detection of amphetamine/methamphetamine (false-positive). Decreased prolactin levels.

Additional Information Risk of seizures: When using bupropion hydrochloride immediate release tablets, seizure risk is increased at total daily dosage >450 mg, individual dosages >150 mg, or by sudden, large increments in dose. Data for the immediate-release formulation of bupropion revealed a seizure incidence of 0.4% in patients treated at doses in the 300-450 mg/day range. The estimated seizure incidence increases almost 10-fold between 450 mg and 600 mg per day. Data for the sustained release dosage form revealed a seizure incidence of 0.1% in patients treated at a dosage range of 100-300 mg/day, and increases to ~0.4% at the maximum recommended dose of 400 mg/day.

Dosage Forms Excipient information presented when available (limited, particularly for generics); consult specific product labeling. [DSC] = Discontinued product

Tablet, Oral, as hydrochloride:

Wellbutrin: 75 mg, 100 mg

Generic: 75 mg, 100 mg

Tablet Extended Release 12 Hour, Oral:

Generic: 100 mg, 150 mg

Tablet Extended Release 12 Hour, Oral, as hydrochloride:

Budeprion SR: 100 mg [DSC] [contains tartrazine (fd&c yellow #5)]

Budeprion SR: 150 mg [DSC]

Buproban: 150 mg

Wellbutrin SR: 100 mg, 150 mg, 200 mg

Zyban: 150 mg

Generic: 100 mg, 150 mg, 200 mg

Tablet Extended Release 24 Hour, Oral, as hydrobromide:

Aplenzin: 174 mg, 348 mg, 522 mg

Tablet Extended Release 24 Hour, Oral, as hydrochloride:

Budeprion XL: 150 mg [DSC]

Budeprion XL: 300 mg [DSC] [contains fd&c red #40, tartrazine (fd&c yellow #5)]

Forfivo XL: 450 mg

Wellbutrin XL: 150 mg, 300 mg

Generic: 150 mg, 300 mg

Dosage Forms: Canada Refer to Dosage Forms. **Note:** Aplenzin, Buproban, and Forfivo XL are not available in Canada.

◆ **Bupropion and Naltrexone** *see* Naltrexone and Bupropion *on page 1254*

◆ **Bupropion Hydrobromide** *see* BuPROPion *on page 269*

◆ **Bupropion Hydrochloride** *see* BuPROPion *on page 269*

◆ **Bupropion Hydrochloride and Naltrexone Hydrochloride** *see* Naltrexone and Bupropion *on page 1254*

◆ **Bupropion SR (Can)** *see* BuPROPion *on page 269*

◆ **Burinex (Can)** *see* Bumetanide *on page 261*

◆ **Buscopan (Can)** *see* Scopolamine (Systemic) *on page 1640*

◆ **BuSpar** *see* BusPIRone *on page 272*

BusPIRone (byoo SPYE rone)

Brand Names: Canada Apo-Buspirone; Dom-Buspirone; PMS-Buspirone; Riva-Buspirone; Teva-Buspirone

Index Terms BuSpar; Buspirone Hydrochloride

Pharmacologic Category Antianxiety Agent, Miscellaneous

Use Management of generalized anxiety disorder (GAD)

Pregnancy Considerations Adverse events have not been observed in animal reproduction studies.

Breast-Feeding Considerations It is not known if buspirone is excreted in breast milk. Breast-feeding is not recommended by the manufacturer.

Contraindications Hypersensitivity to buspirone or any component of the formulation

Warnings/Precautions Use in severe hepatic or renal impairment is not recommended. Low potential for cognitive or motor impairment; until effects on patient known, patients should be warned to use caution when performing tasks which require mental alertness (eg, operating machinery or driving). Effects may be potentiated when used with other sedative drugs or ethanol. Use with MAO inhibitors may result in hypertensive reactions; concurrent use is not recommended. Restlessness syndrome has been reported in small number of patients; may be attributable to buspirone's antagonism of central dopamine receptors. Monitor for signs of any dopamine-related movement disorders (eg, dystonia, akathisia, pseudo-parkinsonism). Buspirone does not exhibit cross-tolerance with benzodiazepines or other sedative/hypnotic agents. If substituting buspirone for any of these agents, gradually withdraw the drug(s) prior to initiating buspirone.

Adverse Reactions
>10%: Central nervous system: Dizziness (3% to 12%)
1% to 10%:
Cardiovascular: Chest pain (≥1%)
Central nervous system: Drowsiness (10%), headache (6%), nervousness (5%), confusion (2%), excitement (2%), numbness (2%), outbursts of anger (2%), abnormal dreams (≥1%), ataxia (1%) paresthesia (1%)
Dermatologic: Diaphoresis (1%), skin rash (1%)
Gastrointestinal: Nausea (8%), diarrhea (2%), sore throat (≥1%)
Neuromuscular & skeletal: Weakness (2%), musculoskeletal pain (1%), tremor (1%)
Ophthalmic: Blurred vision (2%)
Otic: Tinnitus (≥1%)
Respiratory: Nasal congestion (≥1%)
<1% (Limited to important or life-threatening): Alcohol abuse, alopecia, amenorrhea, angioedema, anorexia, bradycardia, bruise, cardiac failure, cardiomyopathy, cerebrovascular accident, claustrophobia, cogwheel rigidity, conjunctivitis, dyskinesia, dystonia, edema, eosinophilia, epistaxis, extrapyramidal reaction, galactorrhea, hallucination, hemorrhagic diathesis, hypersensitivity reaction, hypertension, hyperventilation, hypotension, increased intraocular pressure, increased serum ALT, increased serum AST, increased serum transaminases, irritable bowel syndrome, leukopenia, memory impairment, menstrual disease, myocardial infarction, parkinsonian-like syndrome, pelvic inflammatory disease, personality disorder, photophobia, psychosis, rectal hemorrhage, restless leg syndrome, seizure, serotonin syndrome, slowed reaction time, slurred speech, suicidal ideation, syncope, thrombocytopenia, thyroid disease, urinary incontinence, visual disturbance (tunnel vision)

Drug Interactions
Metabolism/Transport Effects Substrate of CYP2D6 (minor), CYP3A4 (major); **Note:** Assignment of Major/Minor substrate status based on clinically relevant drug interaction potential

Avoid Concomitant Use
Avoid concomitant use of BusPIRone with any of the following: Azelastine (Nasal); Conivaptan; Dapoxetine; Fusidic Acid (Systemic); Idelalisib; MAO Inhibitors; Methylene Blue; Orphenadrine; Paraldehyde; Thalidomide

Increased Effect/Toxicity
BusPIRone may increase the levels/effects of: Alcohol (Ethyl); Antidepressants (Serotonin Reuptake Inhibitor/Antagonist); Antipsychotic Agents; Azelastine (Nasal); Buprenorphine; CNS Depressants; Hydrocodone; MAO Inhibitors; Methotrimeprazine; Methylene Blue; Metoclopramide; Metyrosine; Orphenadrine; Paraldehyde; Pramipexole; ROPINIRole; Rotigotine; Selective Serotonin Reuptake Inhibitors; Serotonin Modulators; Suvorexant; Thalidomide; Zolpidem

The levels/effects of BusPIRone may be increased by: Antiemetics (5HT3 Antagonists); Antifungal Agents (Azole Derivatives, Systemic); Antipsychotic Agents; Aprepitant; Brimonidine (Topical); Calcium Channel Blockers (Nondihydropyridine); Cannabis; Conivaptan; CYP3A4 Inhibitors (Moderate); CYP3A4 Inhibitors (Strong); Dapoxetine; Dasatinib; Doxylamine; Dronabinol; Droperidol; Fosaprepitant; Fusidic Acid (Systemic); Grapefruit Juice; HydrOXYzine; Idelalisib; Ivacaftor; Kava Kava; Luliconazole; Macrolide Antibiotics; Magnesium Sulfate; Metaxalone; Methotrimeprazine; Mifepristone; Minocycline; Nabilone; Netupitant; Osimertinib; Palbociclib; Perampanel; Resveratrol; Rufinamide; Selective Serotonin Reuptake Inhibitors; Simeprevir; Sodium Oxybate; Stiripentol; Tapentadol; Tetrahydrocannabinol

Decreased Effect
BusPIRone may decrease the levels/effects of: Ioflupane I 123

The levels/effects of BusPIRone may be decreased by: Bosentan; CYP3A4 Inducers (Moderate); CYP3A4 Inducers (Strong); Dabrafenib; Deferasirox; Enzalutamide; Mitotane; Osimertinib; Rifamycin Derivatives; Siltuximab; St Johns Wort; Tocilizumab; Yohimbine

Food Interactions Food may decrease the absorption of buspirone, but it may also decrease the first-pass metabolism, thereby increasing the bioavailability of buspirone. Grapefruit juice may cause increased buspirone concentrations. Management: Administer with or without food, but must be consistent. Avoid intake of large quantities of grapefruit juice.

Storage/Stability Store at 25°C (77°F); excursions permitted between 15°C to 30°C (59°F to 86°F). Protect from light.

Mechanism of Action The mechanism of action of buspirone is unknown. Buspirone has a high affinity for serotonin 5-HT$_{1A}$ and 5-HT$_2$ receptors, without affecting benzodiazepine-GABA receptors. Buspirone has moderate affinity for dopamine D$_2$ receptors.

Pharmacodynamics/Kinetics
Onset of action: Within 2 weeks
Absorption: Rapid and complete; bioavailability is limited by extensive first-pass effect; only 1.5% to 13% (mean 4%) of the oral dose reaches the systemic circulation unchanged
Distribution: V$_d$: 5.3 L/kg
Protein binding: 86%
Metabolism: Hepatic oxidation, primarily via CYP3A4 to several metabolites including an active metabolite, 1-pyrimidinylpiperazine (1-PP; exhibits about 25% of the activity of buspirone); extensive first-pass effect
Half-life elimination: 2 to 3 hours; increased with renal or hepatic impairment
Time to peak, serum: 40 to 90 minutes
Excretion: Urine: 29% to 63% (primarily as metabolites); feces: 18% to 38%

Dosing
Adult & Geriatric
Generalized anxiety disorder (GAD): Oral: Initial: 7.5 mg twice daily; may increase every 2-3 days in increments of 2.5 mg twice daily to a maximum of 30 mg twice daily; a dose of 10-15 mg twice daily was most often used in clinical trials that allowed for dose titration
Augmentation agent for antidepressants (off-label use): Oral: Initial: 7.5 mg twice daily; may increase weekly in increments of 7.5 mg twice daily to a maximum of 30 mg twice daily (Trivedi, 2006).

Renal Impairment Patients with impaired renal function demonstrated increased plasma levels and a prolonged half-life of buspirone. Use in patients with severe renal impairment not recommended.

Hepatic Impairment Patients with impaired hepatic function demonstrated increased plasma levels and a prolonged half-life of buspirone. Use in patients with severe hepatic impairment not recommended.

Dietary Considerations May be taken with or without food, but must be consistent. Avoid large quantities of grapefruit juice.

Administration May be administered with or without food, but must be consistent.

Monitoring Parameters Mental status, symptoms of anxiety

Test Interactions The presence of buspirone may result in a false positive on a urinary assay for metanephrine/catecholamine; discontinue buspirone ≥48 hours prior to collection of urine sample for catecholamines

Additional Information Has shown little potential for abuse; needs continuous use. Because of slow onset, not appropriate for "as needed" (prn) use or for brief, situational anxiety. Ineffective for treatment of benzodiazepine or ethanol withdrawal.

Dosage Forms Excipient information presented when available (limited, particularly for generics); consult specific product labeling.
Tablet, Oral, as hydrochloride:
Generic: 5 mg, 7.5 mg, 10 mg, 15 mg, 30 mg

◆ Buspirone Hydrochloride see BusPIRone on page 272
◆ Bussulfam see Busulfan on page 273

Busulfan (byoo SUL fan)

Brand Names: US Busulfex; Myleran
Brand Names: Canada Busulfex; Myleran
Index Terms Bussulfam; Busulfanum; Busulphan
Pharmacologic Category Antineoplastic Agent, Alkylating Agent

Use

Chronic myeloid leukemia (CML):

Injection: Conditioning regimen prior to allogeneic hematopoietic progenitor cell transplantation for CML (in combination with cyclophosphamide)

Tablets: Palliative treatment of CML

Dosing

Adult Note: Premedicate with prophylactic anticonvulsant therapy (eg, phenytoin, levetiracetam, benzodiazepines, or valproic acid) beginning 12 hours prior to high-dose busulfan treatment and continuing for 24 hours after the last busulfan dose. Busulfan is associated with a moderate emetic potential (depending on dose and/or administration route); antiemetics may be recommended to prevent nausea and vomiting (Dupuis 2011). Antiemetics are recommended when used for transplantation.

Chronic myelogenous leukemia (CML), palliation (manufacturer's labeling): *Oral:*

Remission induction: 60 mcg/kg/day or 1.8 mg/m²/day; usual range: 4 to 8 mg/day; titrate dose (or withhold) to maintain leukocyte counts ≥15,000/mm³ (doses >4 mg/day should be reserved for patients with the most compelling symptoms)

Maintenance: When leukocyte count ≥50,000/mm³: Resume induction dose **or** (if remission <3 months) 1 to 3 mg/day (to control hematologic status and prevent relapse)

Hematopoietic stem cell (HSCT) conditioning regimen:

IV: 0.8 mg/kg/dose (ideal or actual body weight, whichever is lower) every 6 hours for 4 days (a total of 16 doses) beginning 7 days prior to transplant (followed by cyclophosphamide).

Obesity: For severely or severely-obese patients, use of an adjusted body weight [IBW + 0.25 x (actual – IBW)] is recommended (by the manufacturer).

Reduced intensity conditioning regimen (off-label dosing): 0.8 mg/kg/day for 4 days starting 5 days prior to transplant (in combinations with fludarabine) (Ho 2009)

Oral (off-label use): 1 mg/kg/dose every 6 hours for 16 doses (in combination with cyclophosphamide) (Socié 2001) **or** 1 mg/kg/dose every 6 hours for 16 doses beginning 9 days prior to transplant (in combination with cyclophosphamide) (Cassileth 1993) **or** 0.44 mg/kg/dose every 6 hours for 16 doses (in combination with cyclophosphamide) (Anderson 1996) **or** 1 mg/kg/dose every 6 hours for 16 doses beginning 6 days prior to transplant (in combination with melphalan) (Fermand 2005)

Essential thrombocythemia (off-label use): Oral: 2 to 4 mg daily (Fabris 2009; Tefferi 2011)

Polycythemia vera, refractory (off-label use): Oral: 2 to 4 mg daily (Tefferi 2011)

Geriatric Oral (refer to individual protocols): Start with lowest recommended doses for adults.

Pediatric Note: Premedicate with prophylactic anticonvulsant therapy (eg, phenytoin, levetiracetam, benzodiazepines, or valproic acid) beginning 12 hours prior to high-dose busulfan treatment and continuing for 24 hours after the last busulfan dose. Busulfan is associated with a moderate emetic potential (depending on dose and/or administration route); antiemetics may be recommended to prevent nausea and vomiting (Dupuis 2011). Antiemetics are recommended when used for transplantation.

Chronic myelogenous leukemia (CML), palliation (manufacturer's labeling): *Oral:*

Remission induction: 60 mcg/kg/day or 1.8 mg/m²/day; titrate dose (or withhold) to maintain leukocyte counts ≥15,000/mm³ (doses >4 mg/day should be reserved for patients with the most compelling symptoms)

Maintenance: When leukocyte count ≥50,000/mm³: Resume induction dose **or** (if remission <3 months) 1 to 3 mg/day (to control hematologic status and prevent relapse)

Hematopoietic stem cell transplant (HSCT) conditioning regimens:

IV:

≤12 kg: 1.1 mg/kg/dose (actual body weight) every 6 hours for 16 doses (over 4 days) (followed by cyclophosphamide)

>12 kg: 0.8 mg/kg/dose (actual body weight) every 6 hours for 16 doses (over 4 days) (followed by cyclophosphamide)

Adjust dose to desired AUC (900 to 1,350 micromolar•minute) at the completion of dose 1 using the following formula:

Adjusted dose (mg) = Actual dose (mg) x [target AUC (micromolar•minute) / actual AUC (micromolar•minute)]

Reduced intensity conditioning regimen (off-label dosing): 0.8 mg/kg/dose for 1 dose 7 to 10 days prior to transplant, followed by ~0.8 mg/kg/dose (busulfan kinetics calculated after initial dose) every 6 hours for 7 doses beginning 3 to 6 days prior to transplant (in combination with fludarabine and antithymocyte globulin) (Pulsipher 2009)

Oral (off-label use): 1 mg/kg/dose every 6 hours for 16 doses beginning 9 days prior to transplant (in combination with cyclophosphamide) (Cassileth 1998)

Renal Impairment

IV: There are no dosage adjustments provided in the manufacturer's labeling (has not been studied).

Oral: There are no dosage adjustments provided in the manufacturer's labeling (elimination appears to be independent of renal function); however, it has been suggested that adjustment is not necessary (Aronoff 2007).

Hepatic Impairment

IV: There are no dosage adjustments provided in the manufacturer's labeling (has not been studied).

Oral: There are no dosage adjustments provided in the manufacturer's labeling.

Obesity *American Society for Blood and Marrow Transplantation (ASBMT) practice guideline committee position statement on chemotherapy dosing in obesity (Bubalo 2014):*

Busulfan (oral): **Note:** For doses over 12 mg/kg, utilize pharmacokinetically targeted dosage (as appropriate for disease state). When busulfan and cyclophosphamide are used in combination for HSCT conditioning, the maximum tolerated busulfan dose is 4 mg/kg/day for 4 days. The maximum tolerated busulfan dose has not been determined when used in combination with other agents.

Body surface area (BSA) dosing: Adults and pediatrics: Utilize actual body weight (ABW) to calculate BSA

Weight based dosing (mg/kg): Adults: Utilize ABW25 for obese and nonobese patients; Pediatric: Utilize actual body weight (ABW)

ABW25: Adjusted wt (kg) = Ideal body weight (kg) + 0.25 [actual wt (kg) - ideal body weight (kg)]

Additional Information Complete prescribing information should be consulted for additional detail.

Dosage Forms Excipient information presented when available (limited, particularly for generics); consult specific product labeling.

Solution, Intravenous:

Busulfex: 6 mg/mL (10 mL)

Tablet, Oral:

Myleran: 2 mg

◆ Busulfanum *see* Busulfan *on page 273*

◆ Busulfex *see* Busulfan *on page 273*

◆ Busulphan *see* Busulfan *on page 273*

Butabarbital (byoo ta BAR bi tal)

Brand Names: US Butisol Sodium

Pharmacologic Category Barbiturate

Use Sedative/Hypnotic: Use as a sedative or hypnotic.

Dosing

Adult Note: Butisol sodium elixir has been discontinued in the US for more than 1 year.

Daytime sedation: Oral: 15 to 30 mg 3 to 4 times daily

Hypnotic: Oral: 50 to 100 mg at bedtime. When used for insomnia, treatment should be limited since barbiturates lose effectiveness for sleep induction and maintenance after 2 weeks.

Preoperative sedation: Oral: 50 to 100 mg 60 to 90 minutes before surgery

Geriatric Avoid use due to risk of overdose with low dosages, tolerance to sleep effects, and increased risk of physical dependence (Beers Criteria).

Pediatric Note: Butisol sodium elixir has been discontinued in the US for more than 1 year.

Preoperative sedation: Children and Adolescents: Oral: 2 to 6 mg/kg 60 to 90 minutes before surgery; maximum: 100 mg

Renal Impairment There are no dosage adjustments provided in the manufacturer's labeling; reduced doses are recommended.

Hepatic Impairment There are no dosage adjustments provided in the manufacturer's labeling; reduced doses are recommended.

Additional Information Complete prescribing information should be consulted for additional detail.

Product Availability Butisol sodium elixir has been discontinued in the US for more than 1 year.

Dosage Forms Excipient information presented when available (limited, particularly for generics); consult specific product labeling. [DSC] = Discontinued product

Elixir, Oral, as sodium:
  Butisol Sodium: 30 mg/5 mL (473 mL [DSC]) [contains alcohol, usp, tartrazine (fd&c yellow #5); mint flavor]
Tablet, Oral, as sodium:
  Butisol Sodium: 30 mg, 50 mg [scored; contains tartrazine (fd&c yellow #5)]
Controlled Substance C-III

Butalbital, Acetaminophen, and Caffeine
(byoo TAL bi tal, a seet a MIN oh fen, & KAF een)

Brand Names: US Alagesic LQ; Dolgic Plus [DSC]; Esgic; Esgic-Plus; Fioricet; Margesic; Zebutal
Index Terms Acetaminophen, Butalbital, and Caffeine; Esgic-Plus
Pharmacologic Category Barbiturate
Use Tension or muscle contraction headache: Relief of symptom complex of tension or muscle contraction headache
Dosing
  Adult & Geriatric Tension or muscle contraction headache: Oral: 1-2 tablets or capsules (or 15-30 mL solution) every 4 hours; not to exceed 6 tablets or capsules (or 90 mL solution) daily
  Renal Impairment No dosage adjustment provided in the manufacturer's labeling; use with caution, especially with severe impairment.
  Hepatic Impairment No dosage adjustment provided in the manufacturer's labeling; use with caution, especially with severe impairment.
Additional Information Complete prescribing information should be consulted for additional detail.
Dosage Forms Excipient information presented when available (limited, particularly for generics); consult specific product labeling. [DSC] = Discontinued product
Capsule, oral:
  Esgic: Butalbital 50 mg, acetaminophen 325 mg, and caffeine 40 mg
  Fioricet: Butalbital 50 mg, acetaminophen 300 mg, and caffeine 40 mg
  Margesic: Butalbital 50 mg, acetaminophen 325 mg, and caffeine 40 mg
  Zebutal: Butalbital 50 mg, acetaminophen 325 mg, and caffeine 40 mg; Butalbital 50 mg, acetaminophen 500 mg, and caffeine 40 mg [DSC]
  Generic: Butalbital 50 mg, acetaminophen 300 mg, and caffeine 40 mg; Butalbital 50 mg, acetaminophen 325 mg, and caffeine 40 mg
Liquid, oral:
  Alagesic LQ: Butalbital 50 mg, acetaminophen 325 mg, and caffeine 40 mg per 15 mL (480 mL) [contains ethanol 7%; propylene glycol]
Tablet, oral:
  Dolgic Plus: Butalbital 50 mg, acetaminophen 750 mg, and caffeine 40 mg [DSC]
  Esgic, Fioricet [DSC]: Butalbital 50 mg, acetaminophen 325 mg, and caffeine 40 mg
  Esgic-Plus: Butalbital 50 mg, acetaminophen 500 mg, and caffeine 40 mg [DSC]
  Generic: Butalbital 50 mg, acetaminophen 325 mg, and caffeine 40 mg

Butalbital and Acetaminophen
(byoo TAL bi tal & a seet a MIN oh fen)

Brand Names: US Bupap; Orviban CF; Phrenilin Forte; Promacet
Index Terms Acetaminophen and Butalbital
Pharmacologic Category Analgesic, Miscellaneous; Barbiturate
Use Relief of the symptomatic complex of tension or muscle contraction headache
Dosing
  Adult & Geriatric Tension or muscle contraction headache: Oral:
  Butalbital 50 mg and acetaminophen 300-325 mg: 1-2 tablets every 4 hours as needed (maximum: 6 tablets/24 hours)
  Butalbital 50 mg and acetaminophen 650 mg: One tablet/capsule every 4 hours as needed (maximum: 6 doses/24 hours)
  Pediatric Tension or muscle contraction headache: Children ≥12 years: Oral: Refer to adult dosing.
  Renal Impairment No dosage adjustment provided in the manufacturer's labeling; however, use with caution; dose reduction or alternate therapy should be considered, especially with severe impairment.

Hepatic Impairment No dosage adjustment provided in the manufacturer's labeling; however, use with caution; dose reduction or alternate therapy should be considered, especially with severe impairment.
Additional Information Complete prescribing information should be consulted for additional detail.
Dosage Forms Excipient information presented when available (limited, particularly for generics); consult specific product labeling. [DSC] = Discontinued product
  Tablet, oral: Butalbital 50 mg and acetaminophen 325 mg
  Bupap [DSC], Promacet: Butalbital 50 mg and acetaminophen 650 mg
  Bupap, Orbivan CF: Butalbital 50 mg and acetaminophen 300 mg
Capsule, oral:
  PhrenilinForte: Butalbital 50 mg and acetaminophen 650 mg [may contain benzyl alcohol]

Butalbital, Aspirin, and Caffeine
(byoo TAL bi tal, AS pir in, & KAF een)

Brand Names: US Fiorinal
Brand Names: Canada Fiorinal
Index Terms Aspirin, Caffeine, and Butalbital; Butalbital Compound
Pharmacologic Category Barbiturate
Use Tension or muscle contraction headache: Relief of the symptomatic complex of tension (or muscle contraction) headache
Dosing
  Adult Tension or muscle contraction headache: Oral: 1 to 2 capsules every 4 hours as needed (Canadian labeling: 2 capsules at once, followed by 1 capsule every 3 to 4 hours as needed); maximum: 6 capsules per day.
  Geriatric Not recommended for use in the elderly (American Geriatrics Society, 2012).
  Renal Impairment There are no dosage adjustments provided in the manufacturer's labeling; use with caution in severe renal impairment.
  Hepatic Impairment There are no dosage adjustments provided in the manufacturer's labeling; use with caution with severe hepatic impairment.
Additional Information Complete prescribing information should be consulted for additional detail.
Dosage Forms Excipient information presented when available (limited, particularly for generics); consult specific product labeling.
  Capsule: Butalbital 50 mg, aspirin 325 mg, and caffeine 40 mg
  Fiorinal: Butalbital 50 mg, aspirin 325 mg, and caffeine 40 mg
  Tablet: Butalbital 50 mg, aspirin 325 mg, and caffeine 40 mg [DSC]
Controlled Substance C-III

◆ Butalbital Compound see Butalbital, Aspirin, and Caffeine on page 275

◆ Butamben, Tetracaine, and Benzocaine see Benzocaine, Butamben, and Tetracaine on page 218

Butenafine (byoo TEN a feen)

Brand Names: US Lotrimin Ultra [OTC]; Mentax
Index Terms Butenafine Hydrochloride
Pharmacologic Category Antifungal Agent, Topical
Use
  Topical infections: Topical treatment of tinea (pityriasis) versicolor due to *Malassezia furfur*
  OTC labeling: Topical treatment of tinea pedis (athlete's foot), tinea cruris (jock itch), and tinea corporis (ringworm)
Dosing
  Adult & Geriatric
    Tinea corporis, tinea cruris: Topical: Apply once daily for 2 weeks to affected area
    Tinea versicolor: Topical: Apply once daily for 2 weeks to affected area and surrounding skin
    Tinea pedis: Topical: Apply twice daily for 1 week or once daily for 4 weeks to affected skin between and around the toes
  Pediatric Children ≥12 years and Adolescents: Refer to adult dosing.
  Renal Impairment There are no dosage adjustments provided in the manufacturer's labeling. However, dosage adjustment unlikely due to low systemic absorption.
  Hepatic Impairment There are no dosage adjustments provided in the manufacturer's labeling. However, dosage adjustment unlikely due to low systemic absorption.
Additional Information Complete prescribing information should be consulted for additional detail.

Dosage Forms Excipient information presented when available (limited, particularly for generics); consult specific product labeling.

Cream, External, as hydrochloride:

Lotrimin Ultra: 1% (30 g) [contains benzyl alcohol, cetyl alcohol, propylene glycol, sodium benzoate]

Mentax: 1% (15 g, 30 g) [contains benzyl alcohol, sodium benzoate]

◆ Butenafine Hydrochloride see Butenafine on page 275

◆ Butisol Sodium see Butabarbital on page 274

Butoconazole (byoo toe KOE na zole)

Brand Names: US Gynazole-1

Index Terms Butoconazole Nitrate

Pharmacologic Category Antifungal Agent, Imidazole Derivative; Antifungal Agent, Vaginal

Use Vulvovaginal candidiasis: Local treatment of vulvo-vaginal candidiasis due to *Candida albicans*

Dosing

Adult & Geriatric Vulvovaginal candidiasis: Intravaginal: Insert 1 applicatorful (~5 g) intravaginally as a single dose

Renal Impairment There are no dosage adjustments provided in the manufacturer's labeling.

Hepatic Impairment There are no dosage adjustments provided in the manufacturer's labeling.

Additional Information Complete prescribing information should be consulted for additional detail.

Dosage Forms Excipient information presented when available (limited, particularly for generics); consult specific product labeling. [DSC] = Discontinued product

Cream, Vaginal, as nitrate:

Gynazole-1: 2% (5 g, 5.8 g [DSC]) [contains edetate disodium, methylparaben, propylene glycol, propylparaben]

◆ Butoconazole Nitrate see Butoconazole on page 276

Butorphanol (byoo TOR fa nole)

Brand Names: Canada Butorphanol (Nasal Spray); PMS-Butorphanol

Index Terms Butorphanol Tartrate; Stadol

Pharmacologic Category Analgesic, Opioid; Analgesic, Opioid Partial Agonist

Additional Appendix Information

Opioid Conversion Table and Morphine Equivalent Dose Table on page 1955

Use

Parenteral: Management of pain when the use of an opioid analgesic is appropriate; preoperative or preanesthetic medication; supplement to balanced anesthesia; management of pain during labor.

Nasal spray: Management of pain when the use of an opioid analgesic is appropriate.

Dosing

Adult Note: These are guidelines and do not represent the maximum doses that may be required in all patients. Doses should be titrated to pain relief/prevention. Butorphanol has an analgesic ceiling.

Pain:

IM: Initial: 2 mg, may repeat every 3-4 hours as needed; usual range: 1-4 mg every 3-4 hours as needed

IV: Initial: 1 mg, may repeat every 3-4 hours as needed; usual range: 0.5-2 mg every 3-4 hours as needed

Intranasal (spray): Initial: 1 spray (~1 mg per spray) in 1 nostril; if adequate pain relief is not achieved within 60-90 minutes, an additional 1 spray in 1 nostril may be given; may repeat initial dose sequence in 3-4 hours after the last dose as needed

Alternatively, an initial dose of 2 mg (1 spray in each nostril) may be used in patients who will be able to remain recumbent (in the event drowsiness or dizziness occurs); additional 2 mg doses should not be given for 3-4 hours

Preoperative medication: *IM:* 2 mg 60-90 minutes before surgery

Supplement to balanced anesthesia: *IV:* 2 mg shortly before induction and/or an incremental dose of 0.5-1 mg (up to 0.06 mg/kg), depending on previously administered sedative, analgesic, and hypnotic medications

Pain during labor (fetus >37 weeks gestation and no signs of fetal distress):

IM, IV: 1-2 mg; may repeat in 4 hours

Note: Alternative analgesia should be used for pain associated with delivery or if delivery is anticipated within 4 hours

Geriatric

IM, IV: Initial dosage should generally be $1/2$ of the recommended dose; repeated dosing must be based on initial response rather than fixed intervals, but generally should be at least 6 hours apart

Nasal spray: Initial dose should not exceed 1 mg; a second dose may be given after 90-120 minutes if needed. In Canadian labeling, repeated dosing must be based on initial response rather than fixed intervals, but generally should be at least 6 hours apart.

Renal Impairment

IM, IV: Initial dosage should generally be $1/2$ of the recommended dose; repeated dosing must be based on initial response rather than fixed intervals, but generally should be at least 6 hours apart

Nasal spray: Initial dose should not exceed 1 mg; a second dose may be given after 90-120 minutes if needed. Repeated dosing must be based on initial response rather than fixed intervals, but generally should be at least 6 hours apart.

Canadian labeling: CrCl <30 mL/minute: Increase initial dosing interval to 6-8 hours.

Hepatic Impairment

IM, IV: Initial dosage should generally be $1/2$ of the recommended dose; repeated dosing must be based on initial response rather than fixed intervals, but generally should be at least 6 hours apart

Nasal spray: Initial dose should not exceed 1 mg; a second dose may be given after 90-120 minutes if needed. Repeated dosing must be based on initial response rather than fixed intervals, but generally should be at least 6 hours apart.

Canadian labeling: Increase interval of repeat dosing to 6-12 hours.

Additional Information Complete prescribing information should be consulted for additional detail.

Dosage Forms Excipient information presented when available (limited, particularly for generics); consult specific product labeling.

Solution, Injection, as tartrate:

Generic: 1 mg/mL (1 mL); 2 mg/mL (1 mL, 2 mL, 10 mL)

Solution, Injection, as tartrate [preservative free]:

Generic: 1 mg/mL (1 mL); 2 mg/mL (1 mL)

Solution, Nasal, as tartrate:

Generic: 10 mg/mL (2.5 mL)

Controlled Substance C-IV

◆ Butorphanol (Nasal Spray) (Can) see Butorphanol on page 276

◆ Butorphanol Tartrate see Butorphanol on page 276

◆ Butrans see Buprenorphine on page 263

◆ BW-430C see LamoTRIgine on page 1027

◆ BW524W91 see Emtricitabine on page 634

◆ Bydureon see Exenatide on page 727

◆ Byetta (Can) see Exenatide on page 727

◆ Byetta 5 MCG Pen see Exenatide on page 727

◆ Byetta 10 MCG Pen see Exenatide on page 727

◆ Bystolic see Nebivolol on page 1263

◆ C1 Esterase Inhibitor see C1 Inhibitor (Human) on page 276

◆ C1 Esterase Inhibitor see C1 Inhibitor (Recombinant) on page 277

◆ C1-INH see C1 Inhibitor (Human) on page 276

◆ C1-INH see C1 Inhibitor (Recombinant) on page 277

◆ C1-Inhibitor see C1 Inhibitor (Human) on page 276

◆ C1-Inhibitor see C1 Inhibitor (Recombinant) on page 277

◆ C1INHRP see C1 Inhibitor (Human) on page 276

◆ C2B8 Monoclonal Antibody see RiTUXimab on page 1600

◆ 2C4 Antibody see Pertuzumab on page 1433

◆ C7E3 see Abciximab on page 20

◆ 311C90 see ZOLMitriptan on page 1938

◆ C225 see Cetuximab on page 366

◆ C-500 [OTC] see Ascorbic Acid on page 155

C1 Inhibitor (Human) (cee won in HIB i ter HYU man)

Brand Names: US Berinert; Cinryze

Brand Names: Canada Berinert

Index Terms C1 Esterase Inhibitor; C1-INH; C1-Inhibitor; C1INHRP; Human C1 Inhibitor

Pharmacologic Category Blood Product Derivative; C1 Esterase Inhibitor

Use

Hereditary angioedema:

Berinert: Treatment of acute abdominal, facial, or laryngeal attacks of hereditary angioedema (HAE) in adult and adolescent patients

Cinryze: Routine prophylaxis against angioedema attacks in adult and adolescent patients with HAE

Prescribing and Access Restrictions Assistance with procurement and reimbursement of Cinryze is available for healthcare providers and patients through the CINRYZE-Solutions program (telephone: 1-877-945-1000) or at http://www.cinryze.com/Cinryze_Solutions/Default.aspx

Dosing

Adult & Geriatric

Routine prophylaxis against hereditary angioedema (HAE) attacks (Cinryze): IV: 1,000 units every 3 to 4 days

Treatment of abdominal, facial, or laryngeal HAE attacks (Berinert): IV: 20 units/kg

Pediatric

Children: Dosage not established.

Adolescents: Refer to adult dosing.

Renal Impairment There are no dosage adjustments provided in the manufacturer's labeling (has not been studied).

Hepatic Impairment There are no dosage adjustments provided in the manufacturer's labeling (has not been studied).

Additional Information Complete prescribing information should be consulted for additional detail.

Dosage Forms Excipient information presented when available (limited, particularly for generics); consult specific product labeling.

Kit, Intravenous:

Berinert: 500 units

Solution Reconstituted, Intravenous [preservative free]:

Cinryze: 500 units (1 ea)

Dosage Forms: Canada Excipient information presented when available (limited, particularly for generics); consult specific product labeling.

Kit, Intravenous:

Berinert: 1,500 units

C1 Inhibitor (Recombinant)
(cee won in HIB i ter ree KOM be nant)

Brand Names: US Ruconest

Index Terms C1 Esterase Inhibitor; C1-INH; C1-Inhibitor; Conestat Alfa; Recombinant C1 Inhibitor

Pharmacologic Category C1 Esterase Inhibitor

Use

Hereditary angioedema: Treatment of acute attacks of hereditary angioedema (HAE) in adult and adolescent patients

Limitations of use: Effectiveness not established in HAE patients with laryngeal attacks.

Pregnancy Considerations Adverse events were not observed in animal reproduction studies. Human C1 inhibitor concentrate is the preferred treatment for HAE during pregnancy; recombinant C1 inhibitor should be avoided until more data is available. Current guidelines recommend discontinuing the recombinant product 1 week prior to conception. Women with HAE should be monitored closely during pregnancy and for at least 72 hours after delivery (Caballero, 2012).

Breast-Feeding Considerations It is not known if C1 Inhibitor (recombinant) is excreted into breast milk. The manufacturer recommends that caution be used if administered to a nursing woman. Until more data is available, current guidelines recommend plasma-derived human C1 inhibitor concentrate as the preferred treatment for HAE during lactation (Caballero, 2012).

Contraindications Life-threatening immediate hypersensitivity reactions, including anaphylaxis, to C1 esterase inhibitor preparations or any component of the formulation; allergy to rabbits or rabbit-derived products

Warnings/Precautions Severe hypersensitivity reactions (eg, urticaria, hives, tightness of the chest, wheezing, hypotension, anaphylaxis) may occur during or after administration. Signs/symptoms of hypersensitivity reactions may be similar to the attacks associated with hereditary angioedema, therefore, consideration should be given to treatment methods. In the event of acute hypersensitivity reactions C1 inhibitor therapy should be discontinued and appropriate treatment should be instituted. Serious arterial and venous thromboembolic events have been reported at recommended doses in patients with risk factors (eg, presence of an indwelling venous catheter/access device, prior history of thrombosis, underlying atherosclerosis, use of oral contraceptives or certain androgens, morbid obesity, immobility). Closely monitor patients with preexisting risks for thrombotic events during and after administration.

Adverse Reactions

>10%:

Central nervous system: Headache (more common in adolescents than in adults)

Gastrointestinal: Abdominal pain (adolescents: ≥12%)

Respiratory: Oropharyngeal pain (adolescents: ≥12%)

1% to 10%:

Central nervous system: Vertigo (3%)

Dermatologic: Burning sensation of skin (2%), erythema (2%; marginatum)

Gastrointestinal: Diarrhea (≥2%), nausea (≥2%)

Hematologic & oncologic: C-reactive protein increased (2%), increased fibrin (2%), lipoma (2%)

Hypersensitivity: Angioedema (3%)

Immunologic: Antibody development (after repeat therapy exposure, non-neutralizing)

Neuromuscular & skeletal: Back pain (3%)

Respiratory: Sneezing (2%)

Limited to important or life-threatening: Abdominal pain, arterial thromboembolism, hypersensitivity reaction, venous thromboembolism

Drug Interactions

Metabolism/Transport Effects None known.

Avoid Concomitant Use There are no known interactions where it is recommended to avoid concomitant use.

Increased Effect/Toxicity

The levels/effects of C1 Inhibitor (Recombinant) may be increased by: Androgens; Estrogen Derivatives; Progestins

Decreased Effect There are no known significant interactions involving a decrease in effect.

Preparation for Administration Allow diluent and C1 inhibitor to warm to room temperature. Reconstitute with 14 mL SWFI. Slowly add SWFI and swirl slowly to mix; avoid foaming. Resulting concentration is 150 units/mL. If patient requires contents of ≥1 vial, contents of multiple vials may be pooled into a single syringe.

Storage/Stability Store intact vials at 2°C to 25°C (36°F to 77°F) for up to 48 months; do not freeze. Protect from light. Reconstituted solution may be stored at 2°C to 8°C (36°F to 46°F) for ≤8 hours; do not freeze. Discard unused portion.

Mechanism of Action C1 inhibitor, a serine protease inhibitor (serpin), regulates the activation of the complement and contact system pathways by irreversibly binding target proteases. Suppression of contact system activation by C1 inhibitor through the inactivation of plasma kallikrein and factor XIIa is thought to modulate vascular permeability that leads to clinical manifestations of hereditary angioedema (HAE) attacks by preventing the generation of bradykinin.

Pharmacodynamics/Kinetics

Onset of action: Onset of symptom relief: Median: 90 minutes

Distribution: V_{ss}: ~3 L

Half-life elimination: ~2.5 hours

Time to peak: ~0.3 hours

Dosing

Adult & Geriatric

Hereditary angioedema (HAE): IV: 50 units/kg as a single dose for patients weighing <84 kg; 4,200 units as a single dose for patients weighing ≥84 kg. Maximum dose: 4,200 units. If attack symptoms persist, one additional dose may be administered; no more than 2 doses may be administered per 24 hours.

Pediatric

Hereditary angioedema (HAE): Adolescents: IV: Refer to adult dosing.

Renal Impairment There are no dosage adjustments provided in the manufacturer's labeling (has not been studied).

Hepatic Impairment There are no dosage adjustments provided in the manufacturer's labeling (has not been studied).

Administration Administer by a separate infusion line as a slow IV injection over ~5 minutes. Appropriately trained patients may self-administer upon recognition of an HAE attack.

Monitoring Parameters Monitor for signs/symptoms of hypersensitivity reactions and thrombotic events.

Dosage Forms Excipient information presented when available (limited, particularly for generics); consult specific product labeling.

Solution Reconstituted, Intravenous [preservative free]:

Ruconest: 2100 units (1 ea) [contains rabbit protein]

Cabazitaxel (ca baz i TAKS el)

Brand Names: US Jevtana

◀ **Brand Names: Canada** Jevtana

Index Terms RPR-116258A; XRP6258

Pharmacologic Category Antineoplastic Agent, Antimicrotubular; Antineoplastic Agent, Taxane Derivative

Use Prostate cancer, metastatic: Treatment of hormone-refractory metastatic prostate cancer (in combination with prednisone) in patients previously treated with a docetaxel-containing regimen

Pregnancy Considerations Adverse events have been observed in animal reproduction studies. Cabazitaxel is not indicated for use in women. May cause fetal harm if administered during pregnancy. Pregnant women should avoid exposure to cabazitaxel.

Breast-Feeding Considerations It is not known if cabazitaxel is excreted in breast milk. Cabazitaxel is not indicated for use in women. Due to the potential for serious adverse reactions in the nursing infant, the manufacturer recommends a decision be made to discontinue nursing or to discontinue the drug, taking into account the importance of treatment to the mother.

Contraindications Severe hypersensitivity to cabazitaxel or any component of the formulation, or to other medications formulated with polysorbate 80; neutrophil count ≤1,500/mm³; severe hepatic impairment (total bilirubin >3 times ULN)

Canadian labeling: Additional contraindications (not in US labeling): Hepatic impairment (bilirubin ≥ULN or AST and/or ALT ≥1.5 times ULN); concomitant vaccination with yellow fever vaccine

Warnings/Precautions Hazardous agent - use appropriate precautions for handling and disposal (NIOSH 2014 [group 1]). **[US Boxed Warning]: Severe hypersensitivity reactions, including generalized rash, erythema, hypotension, and bronchospasm may occur; immediate discontinuation is required if hypersensitivity is severe; administer appropriate supportive medications. Premedicate with an IV antihistamine, corticosteroid and H₂ antagonist prior to infusion. Use in patients with history of severe hypersensitivity to cabazitaxel or other medications formulated with polysorbate 80 is contraindicated.** Observe closely during infusion, especially during the first and second infusions; reaction may occur within minutes. Do not rechallenge after severe hypersensitivity reactions.

[US Boxed Warning]: Deaths due to neutropenia have been reported. Cabazitaxel is contraindicated in patients with neutrophil count ≤1,500/mm³; monitor blood counts frequently. Neutropenia, anemia, thrombocytopenia, and/or pancytopenia may occur with use; grade 3 and 4 neutropenia was observed in over 80% of patients treated with cabazitaxel in a clinical trial. Dose reductions are recommended following neutropenic fever or prolonged neutropenia. Administration of WBC growth factors may reduce the risk of complications due to neutropenia; consider primary WBC growth factor prophylaxis in high-risk patients (eg, >65 years of age, poor performance status, history of neutropenic fever, extensive prior radiation, poor nutrition status, or other serious comorbidities); secondary prophylaxis and therapeutic WBC growth factors should be considered in all patients with increased risk for neutropenic complications. Use cautiously in patients with hemoglobin <10 g/dL. Monitor complete blood counts weekly during cycle 1 and prior to subsequent treatment cycles, or as clinically indicated. Patients ≥65 years of age are more likely to experience certain adverse reactions, including grade 3 and 4 neutropenia and neutropenic fever. Fatigue, asthenia, pyrexia, dizziness, urinary tract infection, and dehydration also occurred more frequently in elderly patients compared to younger patients. Death due to causes other than disease progression (within 30 days of the last cabazitaxel dose) was higher in elderly patients versus younger patients.

Use is contraindicated in patients with severe hepatic impairment (total bilirubin >3 times ULN). Dose reduction is necessary in patients with mild impairment (total bilirubin >1 to ≤1.5 times ULN or AST >1.5 times ULN) and moderate impairment (total bilirubin >1.5 to ≤3 times ULN); use with caution and monitor closely. Due to extensive hepatic metabolism, cabazitaxel exposure is increased in patients with hepatic impairment. Renal failure (including rare fatalities) has been reported from clinical trials; generally associated with dehydration, sepsis, or obstructive uropathy; use with caution in patients with severe renal impairment (CrCl <30 mL/minute) and end-stage renal disease. Nausea, vomiting, and diarrhea may occur. Diarrhea may be severe and may result in dehydration and electrolyte imbalance; fatalities have been reported. Per the manufacturer, antiemetic prophylaxis is recommended. Antidiarrheal medication and fluid and electrolyte replacement may be necessary. Diarrhea ≥ grade 3 may require treatment delay and or dosage reduction. Gastrointestinal hemorrhage and perforation, enterocolitis, neutropenic enterocolitis, and ileus (some fatal) have also been observed. Use with caution in patients at risk of developing gastrointestinal complications (eg, elderly patients, those with neutropenia or a prior history of pelvic radiation, adhesions, GI ulceration or bleeding, concomitant use of steroids, NSAIDs, antiplatelet or anticoagulant medications). Evaluate promptly if symptoms such as abdominal pain and tenderness, fever, persistent constipation, and diarrhea (with or without neutropenia) occur. May require treatment interruption and/or therapy discontinuation.

Failure to properly reconstitute the concentrated vial of cabazitaxel with the correct amount of diluent may lead to higher dosage being administered and increased risk of toxicity. Follow manufacturer instructions carefully. Potentially significant drug-drug interactions may exist, requiring dose or frequency adjustment, additional monitoring, and/ or selection of alternative therapy.

Some dosage forms may contain polysorbate 80 (also known as Tweens). Hypersensitivity reactions, usually a delayed reaction, have been reported following exposure to pharmaceutical products containing polysorbate 80 in certain individuals (Isaksson 2002; Lucente 2000; Shelley 1995). Thrombocytopenia, ascites, pulmonary deterioration, and renal and hepatic failure have been reported in premature neonates after receiving parenteral products containing polysorbate 80 (Alade 1986; CDC 1984). See manufacturer's labeling.

Adverse Reactions Note: Adverse reactions reported for combination therapy with prednisone.

>10%:

Central nervous system: Fatigue (37%), fever (12%)

Gastrointestinal: Diarrhea (47%; grades 3/4: 6%), nausea (34%), vomiting (22%), constipation (20%), abdominal pain (17%), anorexia (16%), taste alteration (11%)

Hematologic: Anemia (98%; grades 3/4: 11%), leukopenia (96%; grades 3/4: 69%), neutropenia (94%; grades 3/4: 82%; nadir: 12 days [range: 4-17 days]), thrombocytopenia (48%; grades 3/4: 4%)

Neuromuscular & skeletal: Weakness (20%), back pain (16%), peripheral neuropathy (13%; grades 3/4: <1%), arthralgia (11%)

Renal: Hematuria (17%)

Respiratory: Dyspnea (12%), cough (11%)

1% to 10%:

Cardiovascular: Peripheral edema (9%), arrhythmia (5%), hypotension (5%)

Central nervous system: Dizziness (8%), headache (8%), pain (5%)

Dermatologic: Alopecia (10%)

Endocrine & metabolic: Dehydration (5%)

Gastrointestinal: Dyspepsia (10%), weight loss (9%), mucosal inflammation (6%)

Genitourinary: Urinary tract infection (8%), dysuria (7%)

Hematologic: Neutropenic fever (grades 3/4: 7%)

Hepatic: ALT increased (grades 3/4: ≤1%), AST increased (grades 3/4: ≤1%), bilirubin increased (grades 3/4: ≤1%)

Neuromuscular & skeletal: Muscle spasm (7%)

<1% (Limited to important or life-threatening): Colitis, electrolyte imbalance, enterocolitis, gastritis, gastrointestinal hemorrhage, gastrointestinal perforation, hypersensitivity (eg, rash, erythema, hypotension, bronchospasm), intestinal obstruction, neutropenic enterocolitis, renal failure, sepsis, septic shock

Drug Interactions

Metabolism/Transport Effects Substrate of CYP2C8 (minor), CYP3A4 (major); **Note:** Assignment of Major/Minor substrate status based on clinically relevant drug interaction potential

Avoid Concomitant Use

Avoid concomitant use of Cabazitaxel with any of the following: BCG (Intravesical); Conivaptan; Deferiprone; Dipyrone; Fusidic Acid (Systemic); Idelalisib; Natalizumab; Pimecrolimus; Tacrolimus (Topical); Tofacitinib; Vaccines (Live)

Increased Effect/Toxicity

Cabazitaxel may increase the levels/effects of: Antineoplastic Agents (Anthracycline, Systemic); CloZAPine; Deferiprone; DOXOrubicin (Conventional); Fingolimod; Leflunomide; Natalizumab; Tofacitinib; Vaccines (Live)

The levels/effects of Cabazitaxel may be increased by: Aprepitant; Conivaptan; CYP3A4 Inhibitors (Moderate); CYP3A4 Inhibitors (Strong); Dasatinib; Denosumab; Dipyrone; Fosaprepitant; Fusidic Acid (Systemic); Idelalisib; Ivacaftor; Luliconazole; Mifepristone; Netupitant; Osimertinib; Palbociclib; Pimecrolimus; Platinum

Derivatives; Roflumilast; Simeprevir; Stiripentol; Tacrolimus (Topical); Trastuzumab

Decreased Effect

Cabazitaxel may decrease the levels/effects of: BCG (Intravesical); Coccidioides immitis Skin Test; Sipuleucel-T; Vaccines (Inactivated); Vaccines (Live)

The levels/effects of Cabazitaxel may be decreased by: Bosentan; CYP3A4 Inducers (Moderate); CYP3A4 Inducers (Strong); Dabrafenib; Deferasirox; Echinacea; Enzalutamide; Mitotane; Osimertinib; Siltuximab; St Johns Wort; Tocilizumab

Food Interactions Grapefruit juice may increase the levels/effects of cabazitaxel. Management: Avoid grapefruit juice.

Preparation for Administration Hazardous agent; use appropriate precautions for handling and disposal (NIOSH 2014 [group 1]). Do not prepare or administer in PVC-containing infusion containers or polyurethane infusion sets. Cabazitaxel and diluent vials contain overfill. **Preparation requires 2 steps.** Slowly inject the **entire contents** of the provided diluent vial into the cabazitaxel 60 mg/1.5 mL vial, directing the diluent down the vial wall. Mix gently by inverting the vial for at least 45 seconds; do not shake. Allow vial to sit so that foam dissipates and solution appears homogeneous. This results in an intermediate reconstituted concentration of 10 mg/mL. The US labeling recommends to further dilute within 30 minutes into a 250 mL D_5W or NS non-PVC infusion container to final concentration of 0.1 to 0.26 mg/mL (total doses >65 mg will require a larger infusion volume; final concentration should not exceed 0.26 mg/mL). The Canadian labeling recommends further dilution of the reconstituted vial occur within 60 minutes. Gently invert container to mix. Do not use infusion solutions if crystals or precipitate appear; discard if this occurs. Infusion should be completed within 8 hours if stored at room temperature. For infusion solutions stored under refrigeration, the US labeling recommends that the infusion be completed within 24 hours. The Canadian labeling recommends that the infusion be completed within 48 hours.

Storage/Stability Store intact vials at 25°C (77°F); excursions permitted between 15°C and 30°C (59°F and 86°F). Do not refrigerate. Do not prepare or administer in PVC-containing infusion containers or polyurethane infusion sets. The US labeling indicates the initial reconstituted solution (at 10 mg/mL) is stable for 30 minutes in the vial and that solutions for infusion are stable for up to 8 hours at room temperature (includes the 1 hour infusion) or 24 hours refrigerated (includes the 1 hour infusion). The Canadian labeling indicates the initial reconstituted solution (at 10 mg/mL) is stable for 1 hour in the vial and that solutions for infusion are stable for up to 8 hours at room temperature (includes the 1 hour infusion) or 48 hours refrigerated (includes the 1 hour infusion).

Mechanism of Action Cabazitaxel is a taxane derivative which is a microtubule inhibitor; it binds to tubulin promoting assembly into microtubules and inhibiting disassembly which stabilizes microtubules. This inhibits microtubule depolymerization and cell division, arresting the cell cycle and inhibiting tumor proliferation. Unlike other taxanes, cabazitaxel has a poor affinity for multidrug resistance (MDR) proteins, therefore conferring activity in resistant tumors.

Pharmacodynamics/Kinetics

Distribution: V_{dss}: 4,864 L; has greater CNS penetration than other taxanes

Protein binding: 89% to 92%; primarily to serum albumin and lipoproteins

Metabolism: Extensively hepatic; primarily via CYP3A4 and 3A5; also via CYP2C8 (minor)

Half-life elimination: Terminal: 95 hours

Excretion: Feces (76% as metabolites); Urine (~4%)

Dosing

Adult Note: Premedicate at least 30 minutes prior to each dose of cabazitaxel with an antihistamine (eg, diphenhydramine IV 25 mg or equivalent), a corticosteroid (eg, dexamethasone 8 mg IV or equivalent), and an H_2 antagonist (eg, ranitidine 50 mg IV or equivalent). Per the manufacturer, antiemetic prophylaxis (oral or IV) is also recommended.

Prostate cancer, metastatic: IV: 25 mg/m² once every 3 weeks (in combination with prednisone)

Dosage adjustment for concomitant use with strong CYP3A inhibitors: Concomitant use with strong CYP3A inhibitors (eg, ketoconazole, itraconazole, clarithromycin, protease inhibitors, nefazodone, telithromycin, voriconazole) may increase cabazitaxel plasma concentrations; avoid concurrent use. If concomitant use cannot be avoided, consider reducing cabazitaxel dose by 25%.

Renal Impairment

Mild to moderate renal impairment (CrCl ≥30 mL/minute): No dosage adjustment necessary.

Severe renal impairment (CrCl <30 mL/minute) or end-stage renal disease: Use with caution; monitor closely.

Hepatic Impairment

US labeling:

Mild impairment (total bilirubin >1 to ≤1.5 times ULN or AST ≥1.5 times ULN): Reduce dose to 20 mg/m².

Moderate impairment (total bilirubin >1.5 to ≤3 times ULN with any AST): Reduce dose to 15 mg/m² (based on tolerability; efficacy of this dose is not known).

Severe impairment (total bilirubin >3 times ULN): Use is contraindicated.

Canadian labeling: Hepatic impairment (bilirubin ≥1 times ULN or AST and/or ALT ≥1.5 times ULN): Use is contraindicated.

Obesity ASCO Guidelines for appropriate chemotherapy dosing in obese adults with cancer: Utilize patient's actual body weight (full weight) for calculation of body surface area- or weight-based dosing, particularly when the intent of therapy is curative; manage regimen-related toxicities in the same manner as for nonobese patients; if a dose reduction is utilized due to toxicity, consider resumption of full weight-based dosing with subsequent cycles, especially if cause of toxicity (eg, hepatic or renal impairment) is resolved (Griggs 2012).

Adjustment for Toxicity

Hematologic toxicity:

Neutropenia ≥ grade 3 for >1 week despite WBC growth factors: Delay treatment until ANC >1,500/mm³ and then reduce dose to 20 mg/m² with continued WBC growth factor secondary prophylaxis.

Neutropenic fever or neutropenic infection: Delay treatment until improvement/resolution and ANC >1,500/mm³ and then reduce dose to 20 mg/m² with continued WBC growth factor secondary prophylaxis.

Persistent hematologic toxicity (despite dosage reduction): Discontinue treatment.

Nonhematologic toxicity:

Severe hypersensitivity: Discontinue immediately.

Diarrhea ≥ grade 3 or persistent despite appropriate medication, fluids, and electrolyte replacement: Delay treatment until improves or resolves and then reduce dose to 20 mg/m².

Persistent diarrhea (despite dosage reduction): Discontinue treatment.

Peripheral neuropathy (grade 2): Delay treatment until improves or resolves and then reduce dose to 20 mg/m²

Persistent peripheral neuropathy (despite dosage reduction) or ≥ grade 3 peripheral neuropathy: Discontinue treatment

Dietary Considerations Avoid grapefruit juice.

Administration IV: Infuse over 1 hour using a 0.22-micron inline filter. Do not use polyurethane-containing infusion sets for administration. Allow to reach room temperature prior to infusion. Premedicate with an antihistamine, a corticosteroid, and an H_2 antagonist at least 30 minutes prior to infusion. Observe closely during infusion (for hypersensitivity). Per the manufacturer, antiemetic prophylaxis (oral or IV) is also recommended.

Hazardous agent; use appropriate precautions for handling and disposal (NIOSH 2014 [group 1]).

Monitoring Parameters CBC with differential and platelets (weekly during first cycle, then prior to each treatment cycle and as clinically indicated); hepatic/renal function. Monitor for hypersensitivity reactions (especially during the first and second infusions). Monitor for signs/symptoms of gastrointestinal disorders (eg, nausea, vomiting, diarrhea, gastrointestinal hemorrhage and perforation, ileus, colitis, abdominal pain/tenderness)

Dosage Forms Excipient information presented when available (limited, particularly for generics); consult specific product labeling.

Solution, Intravenous:

Jevtana: 60 mg/1.5 mL (1.5 mL) [contains alcohol, usp, polysorbate 80]

Cabergoline (ca BER goe leen)

Brand Names: Canada ACT Cabergoline; Dostinex

Index Terms Dostinex

Pharmacologic Category Ergot Derivative

Use

Hyperprolactinemic disorders: Treatment of hyperprolactinemic disorders, either idiopathic or caused by pituitary adenomas.

Limitations of use: Not indicated for inhibition or suppression of physiologic lactation.

Canadian labeling: Additional use (not in U.S. labeling): Prevention of the onset of physiological lactation in the puerperium when clinically indicated (eg, still born baby or neonatal death, conditions that interfere with suckling, severe acute or chronic mental illness, maternal disease which may be transmitted to the baby that require medications which are excreted in the milk).

Limitations of use: Not indicated for suppression of already established postpartum lactation.

Dosing

Adult

Hyperprolactinemia: Oral:

U.S. labeling: Initial dose: 0.25 mg twice weekly; the dose may be increased by 0.25 mg twice weekly up to a maximum of 1 mg twice weekly according to the patient's serum prolactin level. Dosage increases should not occur more rapidly than every 4 weeks. Once a normal serum prolactin level is maintained for 6 months, discontinue cabergoline and monitor prolactin levels to determine if cabergoline should be reinstituted. The durability of efficacy beyond 24 months of therapy has not been established.

Canadian labeling: Initial dose: 0.5 mg once weekly or 0.25 mg twice weekly; weekly dose may be increased by 0.5 mg per week at 4 week intervals until optimal therapeutic response. Therapeutic dose: Usual: 1 mg/week (range: 0.25 to 2 mg/week). Once a normal serum prolactin level is maintained for 6 months, discontinue cabergoline and monitor prolactin levels to determine if cabergoline should be reinstituted. **Note:** May divide weekly dose into 2 or more divided doses per week (recommended for doses >1 mg/week) based on tolerability.

Lactation inhibition *(Canadian labeling; not in U.S. labeling):* Oral: 1 mg single dose on first day postpartum

Geriatric Refer to adult dosing. Start at the low end of the dosage range.

Renal Impairment There are no dosage adjustments provided in the manufacturer's labeling; however, cabergoline pharmacokinetics are not altered in patients with moderate to severe renal impairment.

Hepatic Impairment There are no dosage adjustments provided in the manufacturer's labeling; however, use caution in patients with severe hepatic impairment (Child-Pugh class C) (cabergoline bioavailability is increased).

Additional Information Complete prescribing information should be consulted for additional detail.

Dosage Forms Excipient information presented when available (limited, particularly for generics); consult specific product labeling.

Tablet, Oral:

Generic: 0.5 mg

◆ Caduet® *see* Amlodipine and Atorvastatin *on page* 103

◆ CaEDTA *see* Edetate CALCIUM Disodium *on page* 616

◆ Caelyx (Can) *see* DOXOrubicin (Liposomal) *on page* 597

◆ Cafcit *see* Caffeine *on page* 280

◆ CAFdA *see* Clofarabine *on page* 413

Caffeine (KAF een)

Brand Names: US Cafcit; Keep Alert [OTC]; No Doz Maximum Strength [OTC]; Stay Awake Maximum Strength [OTC]; Stay Awake [OTC]; Vivarin [OTC]

Index Terms Caffeine and Sodium Benzoate; Caffeine Citrate; Caffeine Sodium Benzoate; Sodium Benzoate and Caffeine

Pharmacologic Category Central Nervous System Stimulant; Phosphodiesterase Enzyme Inhibitor, Nonselective

Use

Caffeine citrate: Treatment of idiopathic apnea of prematurity

Caffeine and sodium benzoate: Treatment of acute respiratory depression (not a preferred agent)

Caffeine [OTC labeling]: Restore mental alertness or wakefulness when experiencing fatigue

Pregnancy Considerations Adverse events were observed in animal reproduction studies. Caffeine crosses the placenta; serum concentrations in the fetus are similar to those in the mother (Grosso, 2005). Based on current studies, usual dietary exposure to caffeine is unlikely to cause congenital malformations (Brent, 2011). However, available data shows conflicting results related to maternal caffeine use and the risk of other adverse events, such as spontaneous abortion or growth retardation (Brent, 2011; Jahanfar, 2013). The half-life of caffeine is prolonged during the second and third trimesters of pregnancy and maternal and fetal exposure is also influenced by maternal smoking or drinking (Brent, 2011; Koren, 2000). Current guidelines recommend limiting caffeine intake from all sources to ≤200 mg/day (ACOG, 2010).

Breast-Feeding Considerations Caffeine is detected in breast milk (Berlin, 1981; Hildebrant, 1983; Ryu, 1985a); concentrations may be dependent upon maternal consumption and her ability to metabolize (eg, smoker versus nonsmoker) (Brent, 2011). The ability of the breast-feeding child to metabolize caffeine is age-dependent (Hildebrant, 1983). Irritability and jitteriness have been reported in the nursing infant exposed to high concentrations of caffeine in breast milk (Martin, 2007). Infant heart rates and sleep patterns were not found to be affected in normal, full-term infants exposed to lesser amounts of caffeine (Ryu, 1985b).

Contraindications Hypersensitivity to caffeine or any component of the formulation; sodium benzoate is not for use in neonates

Warnings/Precautions Use with caution in patients with a history of peptic ulcer, gastroesophageal reflux, impaired renal or hepatic function, seizure disorders, or cardiovascular disease. Avoid use in patients with symptomatic cardiac arrhythmias, agitation, anxiety, or tremor. Over-the-counter [OTC] products contain an amount of caffeine similar to one cup of coffee; limit the use of other caffeine-containing beverages or foods.

Caffeine citrate should not be interchanged with caffeine and sodium benzoate. Avoid use of products containing sodium benzoate in neonates; has been associated with a potentially fatal toxicity ("gasping syndrome"). Neonates receiving caffeine citrate should be closely monitored for the development of necrotizing enterocolitis. Caffeine serum levels should be closely monitored to optimize therapy and prevent serious toxicity. Concomitant use with transcutaneous electrical nerve stimulation may lessen analgesia (Marchand, 1995).

Adverse Reactions Frequency not specified; primarily serum-concentration related.

Cardiovascular: Angina pectoris, chest pain, flushing, palpitations, sinus tachycardia, supraventricular tachycardia, vasodilatation, ventricular arrhythmia

Central nervous system: Agitation, delirium, dizziness, hallucination, headache, insomnia, irritability, psychosis, restlessness

Dermatologic: Urticaria

Gastrointestinal: Esophageal motility disorder (sphincter tone decreased), gastritis

Genitourinary: Diuresis

Neuromuscular & skeletal: Fasciculations

Ophthalmic: Increased intraocular pressure (>180 mg caffeine), miosis

Drug Interactions

Metabolism/Transport Effects Substrate of CYP1A2 (major), CYP2C9 (minor), CYP2D6 (minor), CYP2E1 (minor), CYP3A4 (minor); **Note:** Assignment of Major/Minor substrate status based on clinically relevant drug interaction potential; **Inhibits** CYP1A2 (weak)

Avoid Concomitant Use

Avoid concomitant use of Caffeine with any of the following: Doxofylline; Iobenguane I 123; Stiripentol

Increased Effect/Toxicity

Caffeine may increase the levels/effects of: Doxofylline; Formoterol; Indacaterol; Olodaterol; Sympathomimetics; TiZANidine

The levels/effects of Caffeine may be increased by: Abiraterone Acetate; AtoMOXetine; Cannabinoid-Containing Products; Ciprofloxacin (Systemic); CYP1A2 Inhibitors (Moderate); CYP1A2 Inhibitors (Strong); Deferasirox; Linezolid; Norfloxacin; Peginterferon Alfa-2b; Stiripentol; Tedizolid; Vemurafenib

Decreased Effect

Caffeine may decrease the levels/effects of: Adenosine; Iobenguane I 123; Lithium; Regadenoson

The levels/effects of Caffeine may be decreased by: Teriflunomide

Preparation for Administration Parenteral:

Caffeine citrate: May administer without dilution or diluted with D₅W to 10 mg caffeine citrate/mL.

Caffeine and sodium benzoate: For spinal headaches, dilute in 1000 mL NS.

Storage/Stability Store at 20°C to 25°C (68°F to 77°F).

Caffeine citrate: Injection and oral solution contain no preservatives; injection is chemically stable for at least 24 hours at room temperature when diluted to 10 mg/mL (as caffeine citrate) with D₅W, D₅₀W, Intralipid® 20%, and Aminosyn® 8.5%; also compatible with dopamine (600 mcg/mL), calcium gluconate 10%, heparin (1 unit/mL), and fentanyl (10 mcg/mL) at room temperature for 24 hours.

Mechanism of Action Increases levels of 3'5' cyclic AMP by inhibiting phosphodiesterase; CNS stimulant which increases medullary respiratory center sensitivity to carbon dioxide, stimulates central inspiratory drive, and improves skeletal muscle contraction (diaphragmatic contractility); prevention of apnea may occur by competitive inhibition of adenosine

Pharmacodynamics/Kinetics

Distribution: V_d:

Neonates: 0.8-0.9 L/kg

Children >9 months to Adults: 0.6 L/kg

Protein binding: 17% (children) to 36% (adults)

Metabolism: Hepatic, via demethylation by CYP1A2. **Note:** In neonates, interconversion between caffeine and theophylline has been reported (caffeine levels are ~25% of measured theophylline after theophylline administration and ~3% to 8% of caffeine would be expected to be converted to theophylline)

Half-life elimination:

Neonates: 72-96 hours (range: 40-230 hours)

Children >9 months and Adults: 5 hours

Time to peak, serum: Oral: Within 30 minutes to 2 hours

Excretion:

Neonates ≤1 month: 86% excreted unchanged in urine

Infants >1 month and Adults: In urine, as metabolites

Clearance:

Neonates: 8.9 mL/hour/kg (range: 2.5-17)

Adults: 94 mL/hour/kg

Dosing

Adult & Geriatric Note: Caffeine citrate should not be interchanged with the caffeine sodium benzoate formulation.

Caffeine and sodium benzoate:

Electroconvulsive therapy: IV: 300-2000 mg

Respiratory depression: IM, IV: 250 mg as a single dose; may repeat as needed. Maximum single dose should be limited to 500 mg; maximum amount in any 24-hour period should generally be limited to 2500 mg.

Spinal puncture headache (off-label use):

IV: 500 mg in 1000 mL NS infused over 1 hour, followed by 1000 mL NS infused over 1 hour; a second course of caffeine can be given for unrelieved headache pain in 4 hours.

Oral: 300 mg as a single dose

Stimulant/diuretic (off-label use): IM, IV: 500 mg, maximum single dose: 1 g

OTC labeling (stimulant): Oral: 100-200 mg every 3-4 hours as needed

Pediatric Note: Caffeine citrate should not be interchanged with the caffeine sodium benzoate formulation.

Caffeine citrate: Apnea of prematurity: Neonates: Oral, IV:

Loading dose: 10-20 mg/kg as caffeine citrate (5-10 mg/kg as caffeine base). If theophylline has been administered to the patient within the previous 3 days, a full or modified loading dose (50% to 75% of a loading dose) may be given.

Maintenance dose: 5 mg/kg/day as caffeine citrate (2.5 mg/kg/day as caffeine base) once daily starting 24 hours after the loading dose. Maintenance dose is adjusted based on patient's response and serum caffeine concentrations.

Caffeine and sodium benzoate: Stimulant:

IM, IV, SubQ: 8 mg/kg every 4 hours as needed

Oral: OTC labeling: Children ≥12 years: Refer to adult dosing.

Renal Impairment No dosage adjustment required.

Dietary Considerations Oral formulations may be taken without regard to feedings or meals.

Administration

Oral: May be administered without regard to feedings or meals. May administer injectable formulation (caffeine citrate) orally.

Parenteral:

Caffeine citrate: Infuse loading dose over at least 30 minutes; maintenance dose may be infused over at least 10 minutes. May administer without dilution.

Caffeine and sodium benzoate: IV as slow direct injection. For spinal headaches, infuse diluted solution over 1 hour. Follow with 1000 mL NS; infuse over 1 hour. May administer IM undiluted.

Reference Range

Therapeutic: Apnea of prematurity: 8-20 mcg/mL

Potentially toxic: >20 mcg/mL

Toxic: >50 mcg/mL

Dosage Forms Excipient information presented when available (limited, particularly for generics); consult specific product labeling. [DSC] = Discontinued product

Injection, solution, as citrate [preservative free]:

Cafcit: 60 mg/3 mL (3 mL) [equivalent to 10 mg/mL caffeine base]

Generic: 60 mg/3 mL (3 mL) [equivalent to 10 mg/mL caffeine base]

Injection, solution [with sodium benzoate]:

Generic: Caffeine 125 mg/mL and sodium benzoate 125 mg/mL (2 mL)

Solution, oral, as citrate [preservative free]:

Cafcit: 60 mg/3 mL (3 mL) [equivalent to 10 mg/mL caffeine base] [DSC]

Generic: 60 mg/3 mL (3 mL) [equivalent to 10 mg/mL caffeine base]

Tablet, oral:

Keep Alert: 200 mg

NoDoz Maximum Strength: 200 mg

Stay Awake: 200 mg

Stay Awake Maximum Strength: 200 mg

Vivarin: 200 mg

Generic: 200 mg

Extemporaneous Preparations A 10 mg/mL oral solution of caffeine (as citrate) may be prepared from 10 g citrated caffeine powder combined with 10 g citric acid USP and dissolved in 1000 mL sterile water. Label "shake well". Stable for 3 months at room temperature (Nahata, 2004).

A 20 mg/mL oral solution of caffeine (as citrate) may be made from 10 g citrated caffeine powder and dissolved in 250 mL sterile water for irrigation. Stir solution until completely clear, then add a 2:1 mixture of simple syrup and cherry syrup in sufficient quantity to make 500 mL. Label "shake well" and "refrigerate". Stable for 90 days (Eisenberg, 1984).

Eisenberg MG and Kang N, "Stability of Citrated Caffeine Solutions for Injectable and Enteral Use," *Am J Hosp Pharm*, 1984, 41(11):2405-6.

Nahata MC, Pai VB, and Hipple TF, *Pediatric Drug Formulations*, 5th ed, Cincinnati, OH: Harvey Whitney Books Co, 2004.

Calamine (KAL a meen)

Index Terms Calamine Lotion

Pharmacologic Category Topical Skin Product

Use Employed primarily as an astringent, protectant, and soothing agent for conditions such as poison ivy, poison oak, poison sumac, sunburn, insect bites, or minor skin irritations

Dosing

Adult Skin protectant: Topical: Apply to affected area as often as needed

Pediatric Refer to adult dosing.

Additional Information Complete prescribing information should be consulted for additional detail.

Dosage Forms Excipient information presented when available (limited, particularly for generics); consult specific product labeling.

Lotion, External:

Generic: 8% (120 mL, 180 mL, 240 mL)

◆ Calcio del Mar [OTC] [DSC] *see* Calcium Carbonate *on page 287*

◆ Calcionate [OTC] *see* Calcium Glubionate *on page 290*

Calcipotriene (kal si POE try een)

Brand Names: US Calcitrene; Dovonex; Sorilux
Brand Names: Canada Dovonex
Index Terms Calcipotriol
Pharmacologic Category Topical Skin Product; Vitamin D Analog
Use Plaque psoriasis: Treatment of plaque psoriasis of the body (cream, foam, ointment) or of the scalp (foam, solution)

Dosing
Adult & Geriatric
  Plaque psoriasis: Topical:
    US labeling:
    Cream: Apply a thin film to the affected skin twice daily
    Foam: Apply a thin film to the affected skin or scalp twice daily
    Ointment: Apply a thin film to the affected skin once or twice daily
    Solution: Apply to the affected scalp twice daily
    Canadian labeling: Cream, ointment, solution: Apply a thin film to the affected skin twice daily; decrease application to once daily for maintenance treatment when appropriate. If used in combination with a moderately potent to very potent topical corticosteroid apply calcipotriene and the steroid once daily at alternate times (ie, morning versus evening application). Maximum weekly dose:
    Cream: 100 g per week
    Ointment: 100 g per week
    Solution: 60 mL per week

Pediatric
  Plaque psoriasis: Children and Adolescents: *Canadian labeling:* Topical: Cream, ointment: Apply a thin film to the affected skin twice daily; decrease application to once daily for maintenance treatment when appropriate. Maximum weekly dose:
    2 to 5 years: 25 g per week
    6 to 10 years: 50 g per week
    11 to 14 years: 75 g per week
    >14 years: 100 g per week

Renal Impairment There are no dosage adjustments provided in the manufacturer's labeling.
Hepatic Impairment There are no dosage adjustments provided in the manufacturer's labeling.
Additional Information Complete prescribing information should be consulted for additional detail.
Dosage Forms Excipient information presented when available (limited, particularly for generics); consult specific product labeling. [DSC] = Discontinued product
Cream, External:
  Dovonex: 0.005% (60 g, 120 g) [contains cetearyl alcohol, disodium edta]
  Generic: 0.005% (60 g, 120 g)
Foam, External:
  Sorilux: 0.005% (60 g, 120 g) [contains cetyl alcohol, edetate disodium, propylene glycol]
Ointment, External:
  Calcitrene: 0.005% (60 g, 120 g) [contains disodium edta, propylene glycol]
  Generic: 0.005% (60 g, 120 g)
Solution, External:
  Dovonex: 0.005% (60 mL [DSC]) [contains menthol, propylene glycol]
  Generic: 0.005% (60 mL)

Calcipotriene and Betamethasone
(kal si POE try een & bay ta METH a sone)

Brand Names: US Enstilar; Taclonex
Brand Names: Canada Dovobet
Index Terms Betamethasone Dipropionate and Calcipotriene Hydrate; Calcipotriol and Betamethasone Dipropionate; Enstilar
Pharmacologic Category Corticosteroid, Topical; Vitamin D Analog
Use Plaque psoriasis:
  Foam: Treatment of plaque psoriasis in patients 18 years and older.
  Ointment: Treatment of plaque psoriasis in patients 12 years and older.
  Suspension: Treatment of plaque psoriasis of the scalp (patients 12 years and older) and body (adults).

Dosing
Adult & Geriatric
  Plaque psoriasis: Topical:
    Foam: Apply to affected area of skin once daily for up to 4 weeks (maximum dose: 60 g every 4 days).
    Ointment: Apply to affected area of skin once daily for up to 4 weeks (maximum dose: 100 g weekly). Application to >30% of body surface area is not recommended.
    Suspension: Apply to affected area of skin or scalp once daily for up to 8 weeks (maximum dose: 100 g weekly)
Pediatric
  Plaque psoriasis: Children ≥12 years and Adolescents: Topical:
    Ointment: Apply to affected area of skin once daily for up to 4 weeks (maximum dose: 60 g weekly). Application to >30% of body surface area is not recommended.
    Suspension: Apply to affected area of the scalp once daily for up to 8 weeks (maximum dose: 60 g weekly).
Renal Impairment There are no dosage adjustments provided in the manufacturer's labeling.
Hepatic Impairment There are no dosage adjustments provided in the manufacturer's labeling.
Additional Information Complete prescribing information should be consulted for additional detail.
Product Availability Enstilar foam: FDA approved October 2015; anticipated availability is currently unknown. Enstilar is indicated for the treatment of plaque psoriasis.
Dosage Forms Excipient information presented when available (limited, particularly for generics); consult specific product labeling.
Foam, topical:
  Enstilar: Calcipotriene 0.005% and betamethasone dipropionate 0.064% (60 g)
Ointment, topical:
  Taclonex: Calcipotriene 0.005% and betamethasone dipropionate 0.064% (60 g, 100 g)
  Generic: Calcipotriene 0.005% and betamethasone dipropionate 0.064% (60 g, 100 g)
Suspension, topical:
  Taclonex: Calcipotriene 0.005% and betamethasone dipropionate 0.064% (60 g, 120 g) [contains castor oil]
Dosage Forms: Canada Excipient information presented when available (limited, particularly for generics); consult specific product labeling.
Ointment, topical:
  Dovobet: Calcipotriol 50 mcg/g and betamethasone 0.5 mg/g (30 g, 60 g, 120 g)

◆ Calcipotriol *see* Calcipotriene *on page 282*
◆ Calcipotriol and Betamethasone Dipropionate *see* Calcipotriene and Betamethasone *on page 282*
◆ Calcite-500 (Can) *see* Calcium Carbonate *on page 287*

Calcitonin (kal si TOE nin)

Brand Names: US Fortical; Miacalcin
Brand Names: Canada Calcimar
Index Terms Calcitonin (Salmon); Salcatonin
Pharmacologic Category Antidote; Hormone
Use
Injection:
  Hypercalcemia: Adjunctive therapy for hypercalcemia
  Paget disease: Treatment of symptomatic Paget disease of bone (osteitis deformans) in patients who are nonresponsive or intolerant to alternative therapy
  Postmenopausal osteoporosis: Treatment of osteoporosis in women more than 5 years postmenopause
Intranasal:
  Postmenopausal osteoporosis: Treatment of postmenopausal osteoporosis in women more than 5 years postmenopause
Pregnancy Considerations Adverse events have been observed in animal reproduction studies. Calcitonin does not cross the placenta.
Breast-Feeding Considerations It is not known if calcitonin is excreted in human breast milk. Calcitonin has been shown to decrease milk production in animals. The manufacturer recommends that caution be exercised when administering calcitonin to nursing women.
Contraindications Hypersensitivity to calcitonin salmon or any component of the formulation
Warnings/Precautions A skin test should be performed prior to initiating therapy of calcitonin salmon in patients with suspected sensitivity; anaphylactic shock, anaphylaxis, bronchospasm, and swelling of the tongue or throat have been reported; have epinephrine immediately available for a possible hypersensitivity reaction. A detailed skin testing protocol is available from the manufacturers.

Rhinitis and epistaxis have been reported; mucosal alterations may occur. Perform nasal examinations with visualization of the nasal mucosa, turbinates, septum and mucosal blood vessels prior to initiation of therapy, periodically during therapy, and at any time nasal symptoms occur. Temporarily withdraw use if ulceration of nasal mucosa occurs. Discontinue for severe ulcerations >1.5 mm, those that penetrate below the mucosa, or those associated with heavy bleeding. Patients >65 years of age may experience a higher incidence of nasal adverse events with calcitonin nasal spray.

Hypocalcemia with tetany and seizure activity has been reported. Hypocalcemia and other disorders affecting mineral metabolism (eg, vitamin D deficiency) should be corrected before initiating therapy; monitor serum calcium and symptoms of hypocalcemia during therapy. Administer in conjunction with calcium and vitamin D. Fracture reduction efficacy has not been demonstrated; use has not been shown to increase spinal bone mineral density in early postmenopausal women. Use should be reserved for patients for whom alternative treatments are not suitable (eg, patients for whom other therapies are contraindicated or for patients who are intolerant or unwilling to use other therapies). Analyses of randomized controlled trials (in osteoporosis and osteoarthritis) using the nasal spray and oral formulations have demonstrated a statistically significant increase in the risk of the development of cancer in calcitonin-treated patients (compared to placebo). The risk for malignancies is associated with long-term use of calcitonin (trials ranged from 6 months to 5 years in duration). Periodically reassess continued use of calcitonin therapy, carefully considering the risks versus benefits. Similar risk for other routes (subcutaneous, IM, IV) cannot be ruled out. Definitive efficacy of calcitonin-salmon in decreasing fractures is lacking compared to other agents approved for osteoporosis treatment; consider potential benefits of therapy against risks in osteoporosis treatment, including the potential risk for malignancy with long-term use.

Adverse Reactions Unless otherwise noted, frequencies reported are with nasal spray.

>10%: Respiratory: Rhinitis (<12%, including ulcerative)
1% to 10%:
Cardiovascular: Flushing (injection: 2% to 5%, hands or face; nasal spray: <1%)
Central nervous system: Depression (1% to 3%), dizziness (1% to 3%), paresthesia (1% to 3%)
Dermatologic: Erythematous rash (1% to 3%)
Gastrointestinal: Nausea (injection: 10%; nasal spray: 1% to 3%), abdominal pain (1% to 3%)
Hematologic & oncologic: Malignant neoplasm (5%), lymphadenopathy (1% to 3%)
Infection: Infection (1% to 3%)
Local: Injection site reaction (injection: 10%)
Neuromuscular & skeletal: Back pain (5%), myalgia (1% to 3%), osteoarthritis (1% to 3%)
Ophthalmic: Abnormal lacrimation (1% to 3%), conjunctivitis (1% to 3%)
Respiratory: Bronchospasm (1% to 3%), flu-like symptoms (1% to 3%), sinusitis (1% to 3%), upper respiratory tract infection (1% to 3%)
<1% (Limited to important or life-threatening; all routes): Alopecia, altered sense of smell, anorexia, antibody development (drug efficacy can be affected), edema, excoriation (nasal mucosa), hearing loss, hypersensitivity reaction, nocturia, polyuria, tachycardia

Drug Interactions
Metabolism/Transport Effects None known.
Avoid Concomitant Use There are no known interactions where it is recommended to avoid concomitant use.
Increased Effect/Toxicity
Calcitonin may increase the levels/effects of: Zoledronic Acid
Decreased Effect
Calcitonin may decrease the levels/effects of: Lithium
Preparation for Administration Injection: NS has been recommended for the dilution to prepare a skin test in patients with suspected sensitivity.
Storage/Stability
Injection: Store under refrigeration at 2°C to 8°C (36°F to 46°F); protect from freezing. The following stability information has also been reported: May be stored at room temperature for up to 14 days (Cohen, 2007).
Nasal: Store unopened bottle under refrigeration at 2°C to 8°C (36°F to 46°F); do not freeze.
Fortical: After opening, store for up to 30 days at 20°C to 25°C (68°F to 77°F); excursions permitted to 15°C to 30°C (59°F to 86°F). Store in upright position.
Miacalcin: After opening, store for up to 35 days at room temperature of 15°C to 30°C (59°F to 86°F). Store in upright position.

Mechanism of Action Peptide sequence similar to human calcitonin; functionally antagonizes the effects of parathyroid hormone. Directly inhibits osteoclastic bone resorption; promotes the renal excretion of calcium, phosphate, sodium, magnesium, and potassium by decreasing tubular reabsorption; increases the jejunal secretion of water, sodium, potassium, and chloride
Pharmacodynamics/Kinetics
Onset of action:
Hypercalcemia: IM, SubQ: ~2 hours
Paget's disease: Within a few months; may take up to 1 year for neurologic symptom improvement
Duration: Hypercalcemia: IM, SubQ: 6 to 8 hours
Absorption: Intranasal: Rapidly but highly variable and lower than IM administration
Distribution: V_d: 0.15 to 0.3 L/kg
Metabolism: Metabolized in kidneys, blood and peripheral tissue
Bioavailability: IM: 66%; SubQ: 71%; Nasal: ~3% to 5% (relative to IM)
Half-life elimination (terminal): IM 58 minutes; SubQ 59 to 64 minutes; Nasal: ~18 to 23 minutes
Time to peak, plasma: SubQ ~23 minutes; Nasal: ~10 to 13 minutes
Excretion: Urine (as inactive metabolites)
Clearance: Salmon calcitonin: 3.1 mL/kg/minute
Dosing
Adult & Geriatric
Paget's disease, symptomatic *(Miacalcin)*: IM, SubQ: 100 units daily. **Note:** Due to the risk of malignancy associated with prolonged calcitonin use, the Canadian labeling recommends limiting therapy in most patients to ≤3 months; under exceptional circumstances (eg, impending pathologic fracture), therapy may be extended to ≤6 months
Hypercalcemia *(Miacalcin)*: Initial: IM, SubQ: 4 units/kg every 12 hours; after 1 to 2 days, may increase up to 8 units/kg every 12 hours; if the response remains unsatisfactory after 2 more days, may further increase up to a maximum of 8 units/kg every 6 hours
Postmenopausal osteoporosis:
Miacalcin: IM, SubQ: 100 units daily
Fortical, Miacalcin: Intranasal: 200 units (1 spray) in one nostril once daily
Renal Impairment There are no dosage adjustments provided in the manufacturer's labeling.
Hepatic Impairment There are no dosage adjustments provided in the manufacturer's labeling.
Dietary Considerations Patients with Paget's disease and hypercalcemia should follow a low calcium diet as prescribed. Recommended amounts of vitamin D and calcium intake is essential for preventing/treating osteoporosis. If dietary intake is inadequate, dietary supplementation is recommended. Women and men should consume:
Calcium: 1,000 mg/day (men: 50 to 70 years) **or** 1,200 mg/day (women ≥51 years and men ≥71 years) (IOM, 2011; NOF [Cosman 2014])
Vitamin D: 800 to 1,000 units/day (men and women ≥50 years) (NOF [Cosman, 2014]). Recommended Dietary Allowance (RDA): 600 units/day (men and women ≤70 years) **or** 800 units/day (men and women ≥71 years) (IOM, 2011).
Administration
Injection: May be administered IM or SubQ. IM route is preferred if the injection volume is >2 mL (use multiple injection sites if dose volume is >2 mL). SubQ route is preferred for outpatient self-administration unless the injection volume is >2 mL.
Nasal spray: Before first use, allow bottle to reach room temperature, then prime pump by releasing at least 5 sprays until full spray is produced. To administer, place nozzle into nostril with head in upright position. Alternate nostrils daily. Do not prime pump before each daily use. Discard after 30 doses.
Monitoring Parameters
Osteoporosis: Bone mineral density (BMD) should be evaluated 1 to 2 years after initiating therapy and every 2 years thereafter (NOF [Cosman, 2014]); annual measurements of height and weight, assessment of chronic back pain; serum calcium and 25(OH)D; consider measuring biochemical markers of bone turnover
Paget disease: Alkaline phosphatase; pain; serum calcium and 25(OH)D
Nasal formulation: Visualization of nasal mucosa, turbinate, septum, and mucosal blood vessels (at baseline and with nasal complaints)
Consider periodic examinations of urine sediment
Reference Range
Calcium (total): Adults: 9.0 to 11.0 mg/dL (2.05 to 2.54 mmol/L), may slightly decrease with aging
Phosphorus: 2.5 to 4.5 mg/dL (0.81 to 1.45 mmol/L)

Vitamin D: There is no clear consensus on a reference range for total serum 25(OH)D concentrations or the validity of this level as it relates clinically to bone health. In addition, there is significant variability in the reporting of serum 25(OH)D levels as a result of different assay types in use; however, the following ranges have been suggested:

Adults (IOM, 2011): Sufficient levels in practically all persons: ≥20 ng/mL (50 nmol/L); concern for risk of toxicity: >50 ng/mL (125 nmol/L)

Osteoporosis patients (NOF [Cosman 2014]): Recommended level to reach and maintain: ~30 ng/mL (75 nmol/L)

Dosage Forms Excipient information presented when available (limited, particularly for generics); consult specific product labeling.

Solution, Injection:
Miacalcin: 200 units/mL (2 mL) [contains phenol]

Solution, Nasal:
Fortical: 200 units/actuation (3.7 mL)
Miacalcin: 200 units/actuation (3.7 mL)
Generic: 200 units/actuation (3.7 mL)

Dosage Forms: Canada Refer to Dosage Forms. Intranasal solution is not available in Canada.

◆ Calcitonin (Salmon) see Calcitonin on page 282

◆ Calcitrate [OTC] see Calcium and Vitamin D on page 286

◆ Cal-Citrate [OTC] see Calcium Citrate on page 290

◆ Calcitrene see Calcipotriene on page 282

Calcitriol (kal si TRYE ole)

Brand Names: US Calcijex [DSC]; Rocaltrol; Vectical
Brand Names: Canada Calcijex; Calcitriol Injection; Calcitriol-Odan; Rocaltrol; Silkis
Index Terms 1,25 Dihydroxycholecalciferol
Pharmacologic Category Vitamin D Analog
Use

Management of hypocalcemia in patients on chronic renal dialysis (oral, injection); management of secondary hyperparathyroidism in patients with chronic kidney disease (CKD) not yet on dialysis (predialysis patients) (oral); management of hypocalcemia in patients with hypoparathyroidism and pseudohypoparathyroidism (oral); management of mild-to-moderate plaque psoriasis (topical)

Canadian labeling: Additional uses (not in U.S. labeling): Vitamin D-resistant rickets (oral)

Pregnancy Considerations Teratogenic effects have been observed in some animal reproduction studies. Mild hypercalcemia has been reported in a newborn following maternal use of calcitriol during pregnancy. Adverse effects on fetal development were not observed with use of calcitriol during pregnancy in women (N=9) with pseudovitamin D-dependent rickets. Doses were adjusted every 4 weeks to keep calcium concentrations within normal limits (Edouard, 2011). If calcitriol is used for the management of hypoparathyroidism in pregnancy, dose adjustments may be needed as pregnancy progresses and again following delivery. Vitamin D and calcium levels should be monitored closely and kept in the lower normal range.

Breast-Feeding Considerations Low levels are found in breast milk (~2 pg/mL)

Contraindications

U.S. labeling:

Oral, injection: Hypersensitivity to calcitriol or any component of the formulation; hypercalcemia, vitamin D toxicity

Topical: There are no contraindications listed in the manufacturer's labeling.

Canadian labeling:

Oral, injection: Hypersensitivity to calcitriol, vitamin D or its analogues or derivatives, or any component of the formulation or container; hypercalcemia, vitamin D toxicity

Topical: Ophthalmic or internal use; hypercalcemia or a history of abnormal calcium metabolism; concurrent systemic treatment of calcium homeostasis; severe renal impairment or end-stage renal disease (ESRD)

Warnings/Precautions Oral, injection: Adequate dietary (supplemental) calcium is necessary for clinical response to vitamin D. Excessive vitamin D may cause severe hypercalcemia, hypercalciuria, and hyperphosphatemia. Discontinue use immediately in adult patients with a calcium-phosphate product (serum calcium times phosphorus) >70 mg^2/dL^2, may resume therapy at decreased doses when levels are appropriate. Other forms of vitamin D should be withheld during therapy to avoid the potential for hypercalcemia to develop. In addition, several months

may be required for ergocalciferol levels to return to baseline in patients switching from ergocalciferol therapy to calcitriol. Monitor calcium levels closely with initiation of therapy and with dose adjustments; discontinue use promptly in patients who develop hypercalcemia. Avoid abrupt dietary modifications (eg, increased intake of dairy products) which may lead to hypercalcemia; adjust calcium intake if indicated and maintain adequate hydration. Chronic hypercalcemia can result in generalized vascular and soft tissue calcification. Immobilized patients may be at a higher risk for hypercalcemia.

Use oral calcitriol with caution in patients with malabsorption syndromes (efficacy may be limited and/or response may be unpredictable). Use of calcitriol for the treatment of secondary hyperparathyroidism associated with CKD is not recommended in patients with rapidly worsening kidney function or in noncompliant patients. Increased serum phosphate levels in patients with renal failure may lead to calcification; the use of an aluminum-containing phosphate binder is recommended along with a low phosphate diet in these patients. Use with caution in patients taking cardiac glycosides; digitalis toxicity is potentiated by hypocalcemia. Concomitant use with magnesium-containing products such as antacids may lead to hypermagnesemia in patients receiving chronic renal dialysis.

Aluminum: The parenteral product may contain aluminum; toxic aluminum concentrations may be seen with high doses, prolonged use, or renal dysfunction. Premature neonates are at higher risk due to immature renal function and aluminum intake from other parenteral sources. Parenteral aluminum exposure of >4 to 5 mcg/kg/day is associated with CNS and bone toxicity; tissue loading may occur at lower doses (Federal Register, 2002). See manufacturer's labeling. Products may contain coconut (capsule) or palm seed oil (oral solution). Some products may contain tartrazine.

Topical: May cause hypercalcemia; if alterations in calcium occur, discontinue treatment until levels return to normal. For external use only; not for ophthalmic, oral, or intravaginal use. Do not apply to facial skin, eyes, or lips. Absorption may be increased with occlusive dressings. Avoid or limit excessive exposure to natural or artificial sunlight, or phototherapy. The safety and effectiveness has not been evaluated in patients with erythrodermic, exfoliative, or pustular psoriasis. Canadian labeling does not recommend use in patients with hepatic or renal impairment.

Adverse Reactions

Oral, IV: Frequency not defined.

Cardiovascular: Cardiac arrhythmia, hypertension

Central nervous system: Apathy, drowsiness, headache, hyperthermia, metallic taste, psychosis, sensory disturbance

Dermatologic: Erythema, erythema multiforme, pruritus, skin rash, urticaria

Endocrine & metabolic: Albuminuria, calcinosis, decreased libido, dehydration, growth suppression, hypercalcemia, hypercholesterolemia, polydipsia, weight loss

Gastrointestinal: Abdominal pain, anorexia, constipation, nausea, pancreatitis, stomach pain, vomiting, xerostomia

Genitourinary: Hypercalciuria, nocturia, urinary tract infection

Hepatic: Increased serum ALT, increased serum AST

Hypersensitivity: Hypersensitivity reaction

Local: Pain at injection site (mild)

Neuromuscular & skeletal: Dystrophy, myalgia, ostealgia, weakness

Ophthalmic: Conjunctivitis, photophobia

Renal: Calcium nephrolithiasis, increased blood urea nitrogen, increased serum creatinine, polyuria

Respiratory: Rhinorrhea

Postmarketing and/or case reports: Anaphylaxis

Topical:

>10%: Endocrine: Hypercalcemia (24%)

1% to 10%:

Dermatologic: Psoriasis (4%), skin discomfort (3%), pruritus (1% to 3%)

Genitourinary: Urine abnormality (4%), hypercalciuria (3%)

<1%, postmarketing, and/or case reports: Nephrolithiasis

Drug Interactions

Metabolism/Transport Effects Substrate of CYP3A4 (major); **Note:** Assignment of Major/Minor substrate status based on clinically relevant drug interaction potential; **Induces** CYP3A4 (weak)

Avoid Concomitant Use

Avoid concomitant use of Calcitriol with any of the following: Aluminum Hydroxide; Conivaptan; Fusidic Acid

(Systemic); Idelalisib; Multivitamins/Fluoride (with ADE); Multivitamins/Minerals (with ADEK, Folate, Iron); Sucralfate; Vitamin D Analogs

Increased Effect/Toxicity

Calcitriol may increase the levels/effects of: Aluminum Hydroxide; Cardiac Glycosides; Magnesium Salts; Sucralfate; Vitamin D Analogs

The levels/effects of Calcitriol may be increased by: Aprepitant; Calcium Salts; Ceritinib; Conivaptan; CYP3A4 Inhibitors (Moderate); CYP3A4 Inhibitors (Strong); Danazol; Dasatinib; Fosaprepitant; Fusidic Acid (Systemic); Idelalisib; Ivacaftor; Luliconazole; Mifepristone; Multivitamins/Fluoride (with ADE); Multivitamins/Minerals (with ADEK, Folate, Iron); Netupitant; Palbociclib; Simeprevir; Stiripentol; Thiazide Diuretics

Decreased Effect

Calcitriol may decrease the levels/effects of: ARIPiprazole; Hydrocodone; Saxagliptin

The levels/effects of Calcitriol may be decreased by: Bile Acid Sequestrants; Bosentan; Corticosteroids (Systemic); CYP3A4 Inducers (Moderate); CYP3A4 Inducers (Strong); Dabrafenib; Deferasirox; Mineral Oil; Mitotane; Orlistat; Sevelamer; Siltuximab; St Johns Wort; Tocilizumab

Storage/Stability

Oral capsule, injection, solution: Store at room temperature of 15°C to 30°C (59°F to 86°F). Protect from light.

Topical: Store at room temperature of 25°C (77°F); excursions permitted to 15°C to 30°C (59°F to 86°F); do not refrigerate; do not freeze.

Mechanism of Action

Calcitriol, the active form of vitamin D (1,25 hydroxyvitamin D_3), binds to and activates the vitamin D receptor in kidney, parathyroid gland, intestine, and bone, stimulating intestinal calcium transport and absorption. It reduces PTH levels and improves calcium and phosphate homeostasis by stimulating bone resorption of calcium and increasing renal tubular reabsorption of calcium. Decreased renal conversion of vitamin D to its primary active metabolite (1,25 hydroxyvitamin D) in chronic renal failure leads to reduced activation of vitamin D receptor, which subsequently removes inhibitory suppression of parathyroid hormone (PTH) release; increased serum PTH (secondary hyperparathyroidism) reduces calcium excretion and enhances bone resorption.

The mechanism by which calcitriol is beneficial in the treatment of psoriasis has not been established.

Pharmacodynamics/Kinetics

Onset of action: Oral: 2 hours; maximum effect: 10 hours

Duration: Oral, IV: 3 to 5 days

Absorption: Oral: Rapid

Protein binding: 99.9%

Metabolism: Primarily to calcitroic acid and a lactone metabolite

Half-life elimination: Children 1.8-16 years undergoing peritoneal dialysis: 27.4 hours; Healthy adults: 5 to 8 hours; Hemodialysis: 16 to 22 hours

Time to peak, serum: Oral: 3 to 6 hours; Hemodialysis: 8 to 12 hours

Excretion: Feces (27%); urine (7%, unchanged in 24 hours)

Clearance: Children 1.8 to 16 years undergoing peritoneal dialysis: 15.3 mL/hour/kg

Dosing

Adult

Hypocalcemia in patients on chronic renal dialysis:

Oral: Initial: 0.25 mcg daily; may increase dose by 0.25 mcg daily at 4- to 8-week intervals, up to 0.5-1 mcg daily; patients with normal or mildly decreased serum calcium levels may respond to 0.25 mcg every other day

IV:

U.S. labeling: Initial: 1-2 mcg 3 times weekly approximately every other day. Adjust dose by 0.5-1 mcg at 2- to 4-week intervals; dosing range: 0.5-4 mcg 3 times weekly. Gradual dose reduction and discontinuation of therapy may be necessary as PTH levels decrease below target of (1.5-3 x ULN) in response to therapy.

Canadian labeling: Initial: 0.5 mcg 3 times weekly, approximately every other day. Adjust dose by 0.25-0.5 mcg at 2- to 4-week intervals; dosing range: 0.5-3 mcg 3 times weekly

Hypocalcemia in hypoparathyroidism/pseudohypoparathyroidism: Oral:

U.S. labeling: Initial: 0.25 mcg daily (may adjust dose at 2- to 4-week intervals); range: 0.5-2 mcg once daily

Canadian labeling: Initial: 0.25 mcg daily; may increase dose by 0.25 mcg daily at 2- to 4-week intervals. Discontinue use immediately for hypercalcemia; may resume therapy after calcium levels normalize.

Psoriasis: Topical: Apply twice daily to affected areas (maximum: 200 g weekly); Canadian labeling recommends maximum of 30 g daily

Secondary hyperparathyroidism associated with moderate-to-severe CKD in patients not yet on dialysis: Oral: 0.25 mcg daily; may increase to 0.5 mcg daily

Note: KDIGO guidelines do not recommend routine vitamin D therapy (with vitamin D supplements or a vitamin D analog [eg, calcitriol]) for progressive or persistently elevated PTH concentrations in CKD patients (stages 3-5) not on dialysis in the absence of suspected/documented Vitamin D deficiency. Caution is advised to avoid hypercalcemia or elevated phosphate levels (KDIGO, 2009; KDIGO, 2012; Uhlig, 2010).

Vitamin D-dependent rickets type 1/pseudovitamin D deficiency rickets (PDDR): *U.S. off-label use:* Oral: Initial: 0.5 mcg twice daily; subsequent dosing adjusted to maintain normal serum calcium and PTH levels; median dose after 2 years: 0.25 mcg daily (range: 0.1-0.5 mcg daily) (Edouard, 2011)

Vitamin D-resistant rickets: *Canadian labeling (not in U.S. labeling):* Oral: Initial: 0.25 mcg daily; may increase dose by 0.25 mcg daily at 2- to 4-week intervals if response is inadequate; discontinue use immediately for hypercalcemia and do not resume until calcium levels normalize.

Geriatric Refer to adult dosing. Start at the lower end of the dosage range.

Pediatric

Hypocalcemia in hypoparathyroidism/pseudohypoparathyroidism:

U.S. labeling: Oral:

Children 1-5 years: Usual dosage range: 0.25-0.75 mcg once daily (may adjust dose at 2- to 4-week intervals)

Children ≥6 years: Refer to adult dosing.

Canadian labeling: Oral: Children: Initial: 0.03-0.05 mcg/kg/day; evaluate response after 2 weeks and increase dose by 25% if response is inadequate. Dose may be increased or decreased by 25% every 2 weeks thereafter until therapeutic response is achieved. **Note:** May consider initial dose of 0.05 mcg/kg/day for severe hypocalcemia/ symptoms (hospitalization recommended with close monitoring and dose reduction as soon as clinically possible). Maintenance dose: 0.014-0.04 mcg/kg/day

Secondary hyperparathyroidism associated with moderate-to-severe CKD in patients not yet on dialysis: Oral:

U.S. labeling:

Children <3 years: Initial dose: 0.01-0.015 mcg/kg/day

Children ≥3 years and Adolescents: Refer to adult dosing.

Vitamin D-dependent rickets type 1/pseudovitamin D deficiency rickets (PDDR): Oral:

U.S. off-label use: Children: Refer to adult dosing.

Canadian labeling: Children: Initial: 0.01-0.025 mcg/kg/day; evaluate response after two weeks and increase dose by 25% if response is inadequate. Dose may be increased or decreased by 25% every 2 weeks thereafter until therapeutic response is achieved. **Note:** May consider initial dose of 0.05 mcg/kg/day for severe hypocalcemia/ symptoms (hospitalization recommended with close monitoring and dose reduction as soon as clinically possible). Maintenance dose: 0.0046-0.015 mcg/kg/day.

X-linked hypophosphatemic rickets: *Canadian labeling (not in U.S. labeling):* Children: Oral: Initial: 0.01-0.02 mcg/kg/day; evaluate response after 2 weeks and increase dose by 25% if response is inadequate. Dose may be increased or decreased by 25% every two weeks thereafter until therapeutic response is achieved. **Note:** May consider initial dose of 0.05 mcg/kg/day for severe hypocalcemia/ symptoms (hospitalization recommended with close monitoring and dose reduction as soon as clinically possible). Maintenance dose: 0.01-0.05 mcg/kg/day.

Renal Impairment No dosage adjustment necessary.

Hepatic Impairment There are no dosage adjustments provided in the manufacturer's labeling.

Dietary Considerations May be taken without regard to food. Give with meals to reduce GI problems. Adequate calcium intake should be maintained during therapy; dietary phosphorous may need to be restricted.

Administration

IV: May be administered as a bolus dose IV through the catheter at the end of hemodialysis.

Oral: May be administered without regard to food. Administer with meals to reduce GI problems.

Topical: Apply externally; not for ophthalmic, oral, or intravaginal use. Do not apply to eyes, lips, or facial skins. Rub in gently so that no medication remains visible. Limit application to only the areas of skin affected by psoriasis.

Monitoring Parameters

Manufacturer's labeling:

Oral therapy:

Dialysis patients: Serum calcium, phosphorus, magnesium, and alkaline phosphate monitored periodically

Hypoparathyroid patients: Serum calcium, phosphorus, 24 hour urinary calcium monitored periodically

Predialysis patients: Serum calcium, phosphorus, alkaline phosphatase, creatinine, and intact PTH, initially; then serum calcium, phosphorus, alkaline phosphatase, and creatinine monthly x 6 months, then periodically. Intact PTH should be monitored every 3-4 months. During titration periods (all patients), monitor serum calcium levels at least twice weekly.

IV therapy: Serum calcium and phosphorus twice weekly (following initiation and during dosage adjustments) and periodically during therapy; periodic magnesium, alkaline phosphatase, 24 hour urinary calcium and phosphorous

KDIGO guidelines (2009):

Serum calcium, phosphorus, and PTH: CKD stages 3-5D: Frequency of monitoring should be based on the presence and magnitude of abnormalities, as well as the rate of CKD progression. Reasonable intervals are:

CKD stage 3: Serum calcium and phosphorus, every 6 to 12 months; PTH: monitor based on baseline level and CKD progression

CKD stage 4: Serum calcium and phosphorus every 3 to 6 months; PTH every 6 to 12 months

CKD stage 5 (includes 5D): Serum calcium and phosphorus every 1 to 3 months; PTH every 3 to 6 months

Alkaline phosphatase: CKD stages 4-5D: Monitor every 12 months or more frequently in the presence of increased PTH levels

Reference Range

Corrected total serum calcium: KDIGO guidelines recommend maintaining normal ranges for all stages of CKD (3-5D) (KDIGO, 2009)

Phosphorus: KDIGO guidelines recommend maintaining normal ranges for CKD stages 3-5 and lowering elevated phosphorus levels toward the normal range for CKD stage 5D (KDIGO, 2009)

PTH: Whole molecule, immunochemiluminometric assay (ICMA): 1 to 5.2 pmol/L; whole molecule, radioimmunoassay (RIA): 10 to 65 pg/mL; whole molecule, immunoradiometric, double antibody (IRMA): 1 to 6 pmol/L

Target ranges by stage of chronic kidney disease (KDIGO, 2009): CKD stage 3-5: Optimal iPTH is unknown; maintain normal range (assay-dependent); CKD stage 5D: Maintain iPTH within 2-9 times the upper limit of normal for the assay used

Dosage Forms Excipient information presented when available (limited, particularly for generics); consult specific product labeling. [DSC] = Discontinued product

Capsule, Oral:

Rocaltrol: 0.25 mcg, 0.5 mcg [contains fd&c yellow #6 (sunset yellow), methylparaben, propylparaben]

Generic: 0.25 mcg, 0.5 mcg

Ointment, External:

Vectical: 3 mcg/g (100 g)

Generic: 3 mcg/g (100 g)

Solution, Intravenous:

Calcijex: 1 mcg/mL (1 mL [DSC])

Generic: 1 mcg/mL (1 mL)

Solution, Oral:

Rocaltrol: 1 mcg/mL (15 mL)

Generic: 1 mcg/mL (15 mL)

Dosage Forms: Canada Excipient information presented when available (limited, particularly for generics); consult specific product labeling.

Ointment, topical:

Silkis™: 3 mcg/g (5 g, 30 g, 100 g)

◆ Calcitriol Injection (Can) see Calcitriol *on page 284*

◆ Calcitriol-Odan (Can) see Calcitriol *on page 284*

◆ Calcium 600 [OTC] see Calcium Carbonate *on page 287*

Calcium Acetate (KAL see um AS e tate)

Brand Names: US Calphron [OTC]; Eliphos; PhosLo; Phoslyra

Brand Names: Canada PhosLo®

Pharmacologic Category Antidote; Calcium Salt; Phosphate Binder

Use Control of hyperphosphatemia in end-stage renal failure; does not promote aluminum absorption

Dosing

Adult & Geriatric Control of hyperphosphatemia (ESRD, on dialysis): Oral: Initial: 1334 mg with each meal, can be increased gradually (ie, every 2-3 weeks) to bring the serum phosphate value <6 mg/dL as long as hypercalcemia does not develop (usual dose: 2001-2668 mg calcium acetate with each meal); do not give additional calcium supplements

Renal Impairment No dosage adjustment necessary.

Hepatic Impairment No dosage adjustment provided in manufacturer's labeling.

Additional Information Complete prescribing information should be consulted for additional detail.

Dosage Forms Considerations

Calcium acetate is approximately 25% elemental calcium

Calcium acetate 667 mg = elemental calcium 169 mg = calcium 8.45 mEq = calcium 4.23 mmol

Dosage Forms Excipient information presented when available (limited, particularly for generics); consult specific product labeling.

Capsule, Oral:

PhosLo: 667 mg

Generic: 667 mg

Solution, Oral:

Phoslyra: 667 mg/5 mL (473 mL) [contains methylparaben, propylene glycol]

Tablet, Oral:

Calphron: 667 mg

Eliphos: 667 mg

Generic: 667 mg, 668 mg

◆ Calcium Acetylhomotaurinate see Acamprosate *on page 24*

Calcium and Vitamin D (KAL see um & VYE ta min dee)

Brand Names: US Cal-CYUM [OTC] [DSC]; Calcet Petites [OTC]; Calcitrate [OTC]; Caltrate 600+D [OTC]; Caltrate 600+Soy [OTC]; Caltrate ColonHealth [OTC]; Caltrate Gummy Bites [OTC]; Citracal Maximum [OTC]; Citracal Petites [OTC]; Citracal Regular [OTC]; Os-Cal Calcium + D3 [OTC]; Os-Cal Extra D3 [OTC]; Os-Cal [OTC]; Oysco 500+D [OTC]; Oysco D [OTC]

Index Terms Calcium Citrate and Vitamin D; Vitamin D and Calcium Carbonate

Pharmacologic Category Calcium Salt; Electrolyte Supplement, Oral; Vitamin, Fat Soluble

Use Dietary supplement, antacid

Dosing

Adult & Geriatric Calcium supplement, hyperphosphatemia: Oral: Refer to individual monographs for dietary reference intake.

Renal Impairment Use caution in severe renal impairment.

Additional Information Complete prescribing information should be consulted for additional detail.

Dosage Forms Excipient information presented when available (limited, particularly for generics); consult specific product labeling. [DSC] = Discontinued product

Caplet, oral:

Citracal Maximum: Calcium 315 mg and vitamin D 250 units [gluten free]

Os-Cal Calcium + D3: Calcium 500 mg and vitamin D 200 units

Os-Cal Extra D3: Calcium 500 mg and vitamin D 600 units

Capsule, oral:

Generic: Calcium 600 mg and vitamin D 100 units, calcium 600 mg and vitamin D 400 units, calcium 600 mg and vitamin D 500 units, calcium 600 mg and vitamin D 1000 units

Tablet, oral:

Calcet Petites: Calcium 200 mg and vitamin D 250 units [gluten free; contains tartrazine]

Calcitrate: Calcium 315 mg and vitamin D 250 units

Caltrate 600+D: Calcium 600 mg and vitamin D 200 units [contains soybean oil]

Caltrate 600+Soy: Calcium 600 mg and vitamin D 200 units [contains soy isoflavones 25 mg]

Caltrate ColonHealth: Calcium 600 mg and vitamin D 200 units [contains soybean oil]

Citracal Petites: Calcium 200 mg and vitamin D 250 units [gluten free]

Citracal Regular: Calcium 250 mg and vitamin D 200 units [gluten free]

Oysco D: Calcium 250 mg and vitamin D 125 units [contains brilliant blue fcf (fd&c blue #1), fd&c yellow #10 (quinoline yellow)]

Oysco 500+D: Calcium 500 mg and vitamin D 200 units [contains tartrazine]

Generic: Calcium 250 mg and vitamin D 125 units; calcium 315 mg and vitamin D 200 units; calcium 500 mg and vitamin D 125 units; calcium 500 mg and vitamin D 200 units; calcium 500 mg and vitamin D 400 units; calcium 500 mg and vitamin D 600 units; calcium 600 mg and vitamin D 125 units; calcium 600 mg and vitamin D 200 units; calcium 600 mg and vitamin D 400 units; calcium 600 mg and vitamin D 800 units

Tablet, chewable:

Caltrate Gummy Bites: Calcium 250 mg and vitamin D 400 units

Os-Cal: Calcium 500 mg and vitamin D 600 units [sugar free; contains phenylalanine; lemon chiffon flavor]

Generic: Calcium 500 mg and vitamin D 100 units; calcium 500 mg and vitamin D 200 units; calcium 500 mg and vitamin D 600 units; calcium 600 mg and vitamin D 400 units

Wafer, chewable:

Cal-CYUM: Calcium 519 mg and vitamin D 150 units (50s) [dye free; vanilla flavor] [DSC]

◆ Calcium Antacid [OTC] *see* Calcium Carbonate *on page 287*

◆ Calcium Antacid Extra Strength [OTC] *see* Calcium Carbonate *on page 287*

◆ Calcium Antacid Ultra Max St [OTC] *see* Calcium Carbonate *on page 287*

Calcium Carbonate (KAL see um KAR bun ate)

Brand Names: US Alcalak [OTC]; Antacid Calcium Extra Strength [OTC]; Antacid Calcium [OTC]; Antacid Extra Strength [OTC]; Antacid [OTC]; Cal-Carb Forte [OTC]; Cal-CO3S [OTC] [DSC]; Cal-Gest Antacid [OTC]; Cal-Mint [OTC]; Calcarb 600 [OTC]; Calci-Chew [OTC]; Calci-Mix [OTC] [DSC]; Calcio del Mar [OTC] [DSC]; Calcium 600 [OTC]; Calcium Antacid Extra Strength [OTC]; Calcium Antacid Ultra Max St [OTC]; Calcium Antacid [OTC]; Calcium High Potency [OTC]; Caltrate 600 [OTC]; Florical [OTC]; Maalox Childrens [OTC]; Maalox [OTC]; Os-Cal [OTC] [DSC]; Oysco 500 [OTC]; Oyst-Cal [OTC] [DSC]; Rolaids Extra Strength [OTC] [DSC]; Titralac [OTC]; Tums Chewy Delights [OTC]; Tums E-X 750 [OTC]; Tums Freshers [OTC]; Tums Kids [OTC]; Tums Lasting Effects [OTC]; Tums Smoothies [OTC]; Tums Ultra 1000 [OTC]; Tums [OTC]

Brand Names: Canada Apo-Cal; Calcite-500; Caltrate; Caltrate Select; Os-Cal; Tums Chews Extra Strength; Tums Extra Strength; Tums Regular Strength; Tums Smoothies; Tums Ultra Strength

Index Terms Oscal

Pharmacologic Category Antacid; Antidote; Calcium Salt; Electrolyte Supplement, Oral; Phosphate Binder

Use

Antacid: For the relief of acid indigestion, heartburn, sour stomach, and GI upset associated with these symptoms

Calcium supplementation: For use as a dietary supplement when calcium intake may be inadequate (eg, osteoporosis, osteomalacia, hypocalcemic rickets) (IOM, 2011)

Dosing

Adult Dosage is in terms of calcium **carbonate** except where noted; calcium carbonate generally provides approximately 40% elemental calcium:

Dietary Reference Intake for Calcium: Oral:

Adults, Females/Males: RDA:

19 to 50 years: 1,000 mg **elemental calcium** daily

≥51 years, females: 1,200 mg **elemental calcium** daily

51 to 70 years, males: 1,000 mg **elemental calcium** daily

Female: Pregnancy/Lactating: RDA: Requirements are the same as in nonpregnant or nonlactating females (IOM 2011)

Calcium supplementation: Oral: 500 mg to 4 g daily in 1 to 3 divided doses

Antacid: Oral: Generally, 1 to 4 tablets as symptoms occur; maximum: 8,000 mg daily for up to 2 weeks; OTC dosing recommendations may vary by product and/or manufacturer; specific product labeling should be consulted

Hyperphosphatemia in chronic kidney disease (off-label use): Total dose of elemental calcium (including dietary sources and calcium-based phosphate binders) should not exceed 2000 mg daily (Eknoyan 2003).

Geriatric

Dietary Reference Intake for Calcium:

Females: Refer to adult dosing.

Males ≤70 years: Refer to adult dosing.

Males >70 years: 1200 mg **elemental calcium** daily (IOM 2011)

All other indications: Refer to adult dosing.

Pediatric Dosage is in terms of calcium **carbonate**, except where noted; calcium carbonate generally provides approximately 40% elemental calcium:

Dietary Reference Intake for Calcium: Oral:

0 to <6 months: Adequate intake: 200 mg **elemental calcium** daily

6 to 12 months: Adequate intake: 260 mg **elemental calcium** daily

1 to 3 years: RDA: 700 mg **elemental calcium** daily

4 to 8 years: RDA: 1,000 mg **elemental calcium** daily

9 to 18 years: RDA: 1,300 mg **elemental calcium** daily

Females: Pregnancy/Lactating: RDA: Requirements are the same as in nonpregnant or nonlactating females (IOM 2011).

Antacid: Oral:

Children 2 to 5 years (10.9 to 21.3 kg): 375 to 400 mg as symptoms occur; maximum: 1,500 mg daily for up to 2 weeks; OTC dosing recommendations may vary by product and/or manufacturer; specific product labeling should be consulted.

Children 6 to11 years (≥21.8 kg): 750 to 800 mg as symptoms occur; maximum: 3,000 mg daily for up to 2 weeks; OTC dosing recommendations may vary by product and/or manufacturer; specific product labeling should be consulted.

Children ≥12 years and Adolescents: 500 to 3,000 mg as symptoms occur for up to 2 weeks; maximum daily dose: 7,500 mg/day; OTC dosing recommendations may vary by product and/or manufacturer; specific product labeling should be consulted.

Calcium supplementation: Oral:

Children 2 to 4 years: 750 mg twice daily

Children ≥4 years and Adolescents: 750 mg 3 times daily

Renal Impairment CrCl <25 mL/minute: Dosage adjustments may be necessary depending on the serum calcium levels.

Hepatic Impairment There are no dosage adjustments provided in the manufacturer's labeling (has not been studied).

Additional Information Complete prescribing information should be consulted for additional detail.

Dosage Forms Considerations 1 g calcium carbonate = elemental calcium 400 mg = calcium 20 mEq = calcium 10 mmol

Dosage Forms Excipient information presented when available (limited, particularly for generics); consult specific product labeling. [DSC] = Discontinued product

Capsule, Oral:

Calci-Mix: 1250 mg (elemental calcium 500 mg) [DSC]

Florical: 364 mg

Capsule, Oral [preservative free]:

Cal-CO3S: 200 mg [DSC] [dye free]

Powder, Oral:

Generic: 800 mg/2 g (480 g)

Suspension, Oral:

Generic: 1250 (500 Ca) mg/5 mL (5 mL, 473 mL); 1250 mg (elemental calcium 500 mg) per 5 mL (500 mL)

Tablet, Oral:

Cal-Carb Forte: 1250 (500 Ca) mg

Calcarb 600: 1500 (600 Ca) mg [scored]

Calcio del Mar: 1250 (500 Ca) mg [DSC]

Calcium 600: 600 mg [scored]

Calcium 600: 600 mg [contains fd&c yellow #6 aluminum lake, soy polysaccarides]

Calcium High Potency: 600 mg

Caltrate 600: 1500 mg (elemental calcium 600 mg) [scored]

Florical: 364 mg

Oysco 500: 500 mg [contains brilliant blue fcf (fd&c blue #1), tartrazine (fd&c yellow #5)]

Oyst-Cal: 500 mg [DSC]

Generic: 500 mg, 600 mg, 648 mg, 1250 (500 Ca) mg, 1250 mg (elemental calcium 500 mg), 1500 (600 Ca) mg [DSC]

Tablet, Oral [preservative free]:

Calcium 600: 600 mg [lactose free, salt free, sugar free]

Generic: 500 mg, 600 mg, 1250 (500 Ca) mg

Tablet Chewable, Oral:

Alcalak: 420 mg [mint flavor]

Antacid: 420 mg [mint flavor]

Antacid: 500 mg

Antacid: 500 mg [assorted fruit flavor]

Antacid: 500 mg [peppermint flavor]

Antacid: 500 mg [contains brilliant blue fcf (fd&c blue #1), fd&c yellow #10 (quinoline yellow), fd&c yellow #6 (sunset yellow)]

Antacid: 500 mg [contains fd&c blue #1 aluminum lake, fd&c red #40 aluminum lake, fd&c yellow #5 aluminum lake, fd&c yellow #6 aluminum lake]

Antacid Calcium: 500 mg [peppermint flavor]

Antacid Calcium: 500 mg [gluten free; peppermint flavor]

Antacid Calcium Extra Strength: 750 mg [contains fd&c blue #1 aluminum lake, fd&c red #40 aluminum lake; assorted flavor]

Antacid Calcium Extra Strength: 750 mg [gluten free; contains fd&c blue #1 aluminum lake, fd&c red #40 aluminum lake; assorted fruit flavor]

Antacid Extra Strength: 750 mg [contains brilliant blue fcf (fd&c blue #1), fd&c red #40]

Antacid Extra Strength: 750 mg [contains fd&c red #40, fd&c yellow #6 (sunset yellow), tartrazine (fd&c yellow #5)]

Cal-Gest Antacid: 500 mg [DSC] [contains fd&c blue #1 aluminum lake, fd&c yellow #10 aluminum lake, fd&c yellow #6 aluminum lake]

Cal-Gest Antacid: 500 mg [contains fd&c blue #1 aluminum lake, fd&c yellow #10 aluminum lake, fd&c yellow #6 aluminum lake; assorted fruit flavor]

Cal-Mint: 260 mg [animal products free, gelatin free, gluten free, lactose free, no artificial color(s), no artificial flavor(s), starch free, sugar free, yeast free]

Calci-Chew: 1250 (500 Ca) mg [cherry flavor]

Calcium Antacid: 500 mg [DSC]

Calcium Antacid: 500 mg [DSC] [assorted fruit flavor]

Calcium Antacid: 500 mg [DSC] [peppermint flavor]

Calcium Antacid: 500 mg [contains brilliant blue fcf (fd&c blue #1), fd&c red #40, fd&c yellow #6 (sunset yellow), soybeans (glycine max), tartrazine (fd&c yellow #5); assorted flavor]

Calcium Antacid: 500 mg [contains fd&c blue #1 aluminum lake]

Calcium Antacid: 500 mg [contains fd&c blue #1 aluminum lake, fd&c yellow #10 aluminum lake, fd&c yellow #6 aluminum lake; assorted fruit flavor]

Calcium Antacid Extra Strength: 750 mg [DSC] [assorted fruit flavor]

Calcium Antacid Extra Strength: 750 mg [contains brilliant blue fcf (fd&c blue #1), fd&c red #40, fd&c yellow #6 (sunset yellow), tartrazine (fd&c yellow #5); assorted flavor]

Calcium Antacid Extra Strength: 750 mg [contains fd&c blue #1 aluminum lake, fd&c red #40 aluminum lake]

Calcium Antacid Extra Strength: 750 mg [gluten free; contains brilliant blue fcf (fd&c blue #1), fd&c yellow #10 (quinoline yellow), fd&c yellow #6 (sunset yellow)]

Calcium Antacid Ultra Max St: 1000 mg [contains brilliant blue fcf (fd&c blue #1), fd&c red #40, fd&c yellow #6 (sunset yellow), soybeans (glycine max), tartrazine (fd&c yellow #5)]

Maalox: 600 mg [contains aspartame; wild berry flavor]

Maalox Childrens: 400 mg [contains aspartame; wild berry flavor]

Os-Cal: 1250 mg (elemental calcium 500 mg) [DSC]

Rolaids Extra Strength: 1177 mg [DSC] [contains fd&c red #40 aluminum lake, soybean lecithin]

Titralac: 420 mg [low sodium, sugar free; contains saccharin]

Tums: 500 mg [gluten free]

Tums: 500 mg [gluten free; contains fd&c blue #1 aluminum lake, fd&c red #40 aluminum lake, fd&c yellow #6 aluminum lake, tartrazine (fd&c yellow #5)]

Tums Chewy Delights: 1177 mg [contains fd&c red #40 aluminum lake, soybean lecithin; cherry flavor]

Tums E-X 750: 750 mg

Tums E-X 750: 750 mg [assorted flavor]

Tums E-X 750: 750 mg [gluten free; contains fd&c blue #1 aluminum lake, fd&c red #40 aluminum lake; assorted berries flavor]

Tums E-X 750: 750 mg [gluten free; contains fd&c blue #1 aluminum lake, fd&c red #40 aluminum lake, fd&c yellow #5 aluminum lake, fd&c yellow #6 aluminum lake; assorted fruit flavor]

Tums E-X 750: 750 mg [sugar free]

Tums Freshers: 500 mg [gluten free; contains brilliant blue fcf (fd&c blue #1); mint flavor]

Tums Freshers: 500 mg [kosher certified; contains brilliant blue fcf (fd&c blue #1), tartrazine (fd&c yellow #5); spearmint flavor]

Tums Kids: 750 mg [scored; contains fd&c blue #1 aluminum lake, fd&c red #40 aluminum lake; cherry flavor]

Tums Lasting Effects: 500 mg [contains fd&c red #40 aluminum lake, fd&c yellow #6 aluminum lake, tartrazine (fd&c yellow #5)]

Tums Smoothies: 750 mg [DSC]

Tums Smoothies: 750 mg [peppermint flavor]

Tums Smoothies: 750 mg [contains fd&c blue #1 aluminum lake, fd&c red #40 aluminum lake, fd&c yellow #6 aluminum lake, soybeans (glycine max); assorted tropical fruit flavor]

Tums Smoothies: 750 mg [contains fd&c blue #1 aluminum lake, fd&c red #40 aluminum lake, soybeans (glycine max); berry flavor]

Tums Smoothies: 750 mg [gluten free; contains fd&c blue #1 aluminum lake, fd&c red #40 aluminum lake, fd&c yellow #5 aluminum lake, fd&c yellow #6 aluminum lake, milk (cow)]

Tums Ultra 1000: 1000 mg [peppermint flavor]

Tums Ultra 1000: 1000 mg [contains fd&c blue #1 aluminum lake, fd&c red #40 aluminum lake, fd&c yellow #5 aluminum lake, fd&c yellow #6 aluminum lake; assorted berries flavor]

Tums Ultra 1000: 1000 mg [DSC] [contains fd&c red #40 aluminum lake, fd&c yellow #6 aluminum lake, tartrazine (fd&c yellow #5)]

Tums Ultra 1000: 1000 mg [contains fd&c red #40 aluminum lake, fd&c yellow #6 aluminum lake, tartrazine (fd&c yellow #5); assorted tropical fruit flavor]

Tums Ultra 1000: 1000 mg [DSC] [gluten free]

Tums Ultra 1000: 1000 mg [gluten free; contains fd&c blue #1 aluminum lake, fd&c red #40 aluminum lake, fd&c yellow #6 aluminum lake, tartrazine (fd&c yellow #5)]

Generic: 260 mg, 500 mg, 750 mg

Calcium Carbonate and Magnesium Hydroxide
(KAL see um KAR bun ate & mag NEE zhum hye DROKS ide)

Brand Names: US Geri-Lanta Supreme [OTC]; Mi-Acid Double Strength [OTC]; Mylanta Supreme [OTC]; Mylanta Ultra [OTC] [DSC]

Index Terms Magnesium Hydroxide and Calcium Carbonate; Rolaids

Pharmacologic Category Antacid

Use Antacid: Relief of heartburn, acid indigestion, sour stomach and GI upset associated with these symptoms

Dosing

Adult & Geriatric Antacid: Oral:

Chewable tablet: Calcium carbonate 700 mg/magnesium hydroxide 300 mg: Chew 2 to 4 tablets 4 times daily (maximum: 8 tablets per 24 hours)

Liquid: Calcium carbonate 400 mg/magnesium hydroxide 135 mg per 5 mL: 10 to 20 mL 4 times daily (maximum: 90 mL per 24 hours)

Renal Impairment There are no dosage adjustments provided in the manufacturer's labeling; magnesium may accumulate in renal impairment.

Hepatic Impairment

There are no dosage adjustments provided in the manufacturer's labeling.

Additional Information Complete prescribing information should be consulted for additional detail.

Dosage Forms Excipient information presented when available (limited, particularly for generics); consult specific product labeling. [DSC] = Discontinued product.

Liquid, Oral:

Geri-Lanta Supreme: Calcium carbonate 400 mg and magnesium hydroxide 135 mg per 5 mL (355 mL) [cherry flavor]

Mylanta Supreme: Calcium carbonate 400 mg and magnesium hydroxide 135 mg per 5 mL (360 mL, 720 mL) [cherry flavor]

Tablet, chewable, Oral:

Mi-Acid Double Strength: Calcium carbonate 700 mg and magnesium hydroxide 300 mg

Mylanta Ultra: Calcium carbonate 700 mg and magnesium hydroxide 300 mg [cherry créme and cool mint flavors] [DSC]

Calcium Chloride (KAL see um KLOR ide)

Pharmacologic Category Calcium Salt; Electrolyte Supplement, Parenteral

Use Treatment of hypocalcemia and conditions secondary to hypocalcemia (eg, tetany, seizures, arrhythmias); emergent treatment of severe hypermagnesemia

Pregnancy Considerations Animal reproduction studies have not been conducted. Calcium crosses the placenta. The amount of calcium reaching the fetus is determined by maternal physiological changes. Calcium requirements are the same in pregnant and nonpregnant females (IOM, 2011). Information related to use as an antidote in pregnancy is limited. In general, medications used as antidotes should take into consideration the health and prognosis of the mother; antidotes should be administered to pregnant women if there is a clear indication for use and should not

be withheld because of fears of teratogenicity (Bailey, 2003).

Breast-Feeding Considerations Calcium is excreted in breast milk. The amount of calcium in breast milk is homeostatically regulated and not altered by maternal calcium intake. Calcium requirements are the same in lactating and nonlactating females (IOM, 2011).

Contraindications Known or suspected digoxin toxicity; not recommended as routine treatment in cardiac arrest (includes asystole, ventricular fibrillation, pulseless ventricular tachycardia, or pulseless electrical activity)

Warnings/Precautions For IV use only; do not inject SubQ or IM; avoid rapid IV administration (do not exceed 100 mg/minute except in emergency situations). Vesicant; ensure proper catheter or needle position prior to and during infusion; avoid extravasation; extravasation may result in severe necrosis and sloughing. Monitor the IV site closely. Use with caution in patients with hyperphosphatemia, respiratory acidosis, renal impairment, or respiratory failure; acidifying effect of calcium chloride may potentiate acidosis. Use with caution in patients with chronic renal failure to avoid hypercalcemia; frequent monitoring of serum calcium and phosphorus is necessary. Use with caution in hypokalemic or digitalized patients since acute rises in serum calcium levels may precipitate cardiac arrhythmias; use is contraindicated with known or suspected digoxin toxicity. Hypomagnesemia is a common cause of hypocalcemia; therefore, correction of hypocalcemia may be difficult in patients with concomitant hypomagnesemia. Evaluate serum magnesium and correct hypomagnesemia (if necessary), particularly if initial treatment of hypocalcemia is refractory. The parenteral product may contain aluminum; toxic aluminum concentrations may be seen with high doses, prolonged use, or renal dysfunction. Premature neonates are at higher risk due to immature renal function and aluminum intake from other parenteral sources. Parenteral aluminum exposure of >4 to 5 mcg/kg/day is associated with CNS and bone toxicity; tissue loading may occur at lower doses (Federal Register, 2002). See manufacturer's labeling. Avoid metabolic acidosis (ie, administer only up to 2 to 3 days then change to another calcium salt).

Ceftriaxone may complex with calcium causing precipitation. Fatal lung and kidney damage associated with calcium-ceftriaxone precipitates has been observed in premature and term neonates. Due to reports of precipitation reaction in neonates, do not coadminister ceftriaxone with calcium-containing solutions, even via separate infusion lines/sites or at different times in any neonate. Ceftriaxone should not be administered simultaneously with any calcium-containing solution via a Y-site in any patient. However, ceftriaxone and calcium-containing solutions may be administered sequentially of one another for use in patients **other than neonates** if infusion lines are thoroughly flushed (with a compatible fluid) between infusions. Multiple salt forms of calcium exist; close attention must be paid to the salt form when ordering and administering calcium; incorrect selection or substitution of one salt for another without proper dosage adjustment may result in serious over or under dosing.

Adverse Reactions Frequency not defined. IV:

Cardiovascular (following rapid IV injection): Bradycardia, cardiac arrest, cardiac arrhythmia, hypotension, syncope, vasodilatation

Central nervous system: Feeling abnormal (sense of oppression; with rapid IV injection), tingling sensation (with rapid IV injection)

Endocrine & metabolic: Hot flash (with rapid IV injection), hypercalcemia

Gastrointestinal: Dysgeusia (chalky taste), gastrointestinal irritation, increased serum amylase

Local: Local tissue necrosis (following extravasation)

Renal: Nephrolithiasis

Postmarketing and/or case reports (Limited to important or life-threatening): Cutaneous calcification

Drug Interactions

Metabolism/Transport Effects None known.

Avoid Concomitant Use

Avoid concomitant use of Calcium Chloride with any of the following: Calcium Acetate

Increased Effect/Toxicity

Calcium Chloride may increase the levels/effects of: Calcium Acetate; Cardiac Glycosides; CefTRIAXone; Vitamin D Analogs

The levels/effects of Calcium Chloride may be increased by: Multivitamins/Fluoride (with ADE); Multivitamins/Minerals (with ADEK, Folate, Iron); Thiazide Diuretics

Decreased Effect

Calcium Chloride may decrease the levels/effects of: Bisphosphonate Derivatives; Calcium Channel Blockers; Deferiprone; DOBUTamine; Dolutegravir; Eltrombopag;

Multivitamins/Fluoride (with ADE); Phosphate Supplements; Tetracycline Derivatives; Thyroid Products; Trientine

The levels/effects of Calcium Chloride may be decreased by: Trientine

Preparation for Administration IV: For intermittent IV infusion, dilute to a maximum concentration of 20 mg/mL.

Storage/Stability Store intact vials at 20°C to 25°C (68°F to 77°F); excursions permitted to 15°C to 30°C (59°F to 86°F). Do not refrigerate solutions; IV infusion solutions are stable for 24 hours at room temperature.

Although calcium chloride is not routinely used in the preparation of parenteral nutrition, it is important to note that phosphate salts may precipitate when mixed with calcium salts. Solubility is improved in amino acid parenteral nutrition solutions. Check with a pharmacist to determine compatibility.

Mechanism of Action Moderates nerve and muscle performance via action potential excitation threshold regulation

Pharmacodynamics/Kinetics

Protein binding: ~40%, primarily to albumin (Wills, 1971)

Excretion: Primarily feces (80% as insoluble calcium salts); urine (20%)

Dosing

Adult & Geriatric Note: One gram of calcium chloride salt is equal to 270 mg of elemental calcium.

Dosages are expressed in terms of the calcium chloride salt based on a solution concentration of 100 mg/mL (10%) containing 1.4 mEq (27 mg)/mL elemental calcium.

Hypocalcemia: IV:

Acute, symptomatic: Manufacturer's labeling: 200 to 1,000 mg every 1 to 3 days

Severe, symptomatic (eg, seizure, tetany): 1,000 mg over 10 minutes; repeat every 60 minutes until symptoms resolve (French, 2012)

Note: In general, IV calcium gluconate is preferred over IV calcium chloride in nonemergency settings due to the potential for extravasation with calcium chloride.

Cardiac arrest or cardiotoxicity in the presence of hyperkalemia, hypocalcemia, or hypermagnesemia: IV: 500 to 1,000 mg over 2 to 5 minutes; may repeat as necessary (AHA [Vanden Hoek, 2010])

Note: Routine use in cardiac arrest is not recommended due to the lack of improved survival (AHA [Neumar, 2010]).

Beta-blocker overdose, refractory to glucagon and high-dose vasopressors (off-label use): Note: Optimal dose has not been established (DeWitt, 2004): IV: 20 mg/kg over 5 to 10 minutes followed by an infusion of 20 mg/kg/hour titrated to adequate hemodynamic response (AHA [Vanden Hoek, 2010])

Calcium channel blocker overdose (off-label use): Note: Optimal dose has not been established DeWitt, 2004.

IV: Initial: 1,000 to 2,000 mg over 5 minutes; may repeat every 10 to 20 minutes with 3 to 4 additional doses **or** 1,000 mg every 2 to 3 minutes until clinical effect is achieved (DeWitt, 2004); if favorable response obtained, consider IV infusion

IV infusion: 20 to 40 mg/kg/hour (DeWitt, 2004; Salhanick, 2003)

Pediatric Note: One gram of calcium chloride salt is equal to 270 mg of elemental calcium.

Dosages are expressed in terms of the calcium chloride salt based on a solution concentration of 100 mg/mL (10%) containing 1.4 mEq (27 mg)/mL elemental calcium.

Hypocalcemia: *Acute, symptomatic: Manufacturer's recommendations:* Children: IV: 2.7 to 5 mg/kg/dose every 4 to 6 hours

Note: In general, IV calcium gluconate is preferred over IV calcium chloride in nonemergency settings due to the potential for extravasation with calcium chloride.

Cardiac arrest or cardiotoxicity in the presence of hyperkalemia, hypocalcemia, or hypermagnesemia: Infants and Children: IV, I.O.: 20 mg/kg (maximum: 2,000 mg/dose); may repeat as necessary (AHA [Kleinman, 2010]; Hegenbarth, 2008)

Note: Routine use in cardiac arrest is not recommended due to the lack of improved survival (AHA [Kleinman, 2010]).

◀

Calcium channel blocker overdose (off-label use):
Note: Optimal dose has not been established (DeWitt, 2004): Infants and Children:

IV, I.O.: Initial: 10 to 20 mg/kg (maximum: 2,000 mg/dose) over 10 to 15 minutes; may repeat every 10 to 15 minutes (AHA [Kleinman, 2010]; Arroyo, 2009); if favorable response obtained, consider IV infusion
IV infusion: 20 to 50 mg/kg/hour (Arroyo, 2009)

Renal Impairment No initial dosage adjustment necessary; however, accumulation may occur with renal impairment and subsequent doses may require adjustment based on serum calcium concentrations.

Hepatic Impairment No initial dosage adjustment necessary; subsequent doses should be guided by serum calcium concentrations.

Administration For IV administration only. Not for IM or SubQ administration (severe necrosis and sloughing may occur). Avoid rapid administration (do not exceed 100 mg/minute except in emergency situations). For intermittent IV infusion, infuse diluted solution over 1 hour or no greater than 45-90 mg/kg/hour (0.6-1.2 mEq/kg/hour); administration via a central or deep vein is preferred; do not use scalp, small hand or foot veins for IV administration (severe necrosis and sloughing may occur). Monitor ECG if calcium is infused faster than 2.5 mEq/minute; **stop the infusion if the patient complains of pain or discomfort.** Warm solution to body temperature prior to administration. **Do not infuse calcium chloride in the same IV line as phosphate-containing solutions.**

Vesicant; ensure proper needle or catheter placement prior to and during IV infusion. Avoid extravasation.

Extravasation management: If extravasation occurs, stop infusion immediately and disconnect (leave needle/cannula in place); gently aspirate extravasated solution (do **NOT** flush the line); initiate hyaluronidase antidote; remove needle/cannula; apply dry cold compresses (Hurst, 2004); elevate extremity.

Hyaluronidase: Intradermal or SubQ: Inject a total of 1 mL (15 units/mL) as five separate 0.2 mL injections (using a 25-gauge needle) into area of extravasation at the leading edge in a clockwise manner (MacCara, 1983; Zenk, 1981).

Monitoring Parameters Monitor infusion site, ECG when appropriate; serum calcium and ionized calcium (normal: 8.5-10.2 mg/dL [total]; 4.5-5.0 mg/dL [ionized]), albumin, serum phosphate; magnesium (to facilitate calcium repletion)

Calcium channel blocker overdose, beta-blocker overdose: Hemodynamic response, serum ionized calcium concentration

Reference Range
Serum total calcium: 8.4-10.2 mg/dL (2.1-2.55 mmol/L).
Note: Due to a poor correlation between the serum ionized calcium (free) and total serum calcium, particularly in states of low albumin or acid/base imbalances, direct measurement of ionized calcium is recommended.
In low albumin states, the corrected **total** serum calcium may be estimated by the following equation (assuming a normal albumin of 4 g/dL [40 g/L]).

Corrected total calcium (mg/dL) = measured total calcium (mg/mL) + 0.8 [4 - measured serum albumin(g/dL)]
or
Corrected total calcium (mmol/L) = measured total calcium (mmol/L) + 0.02 [40-measured serum albumin (g/L)]

Additional Information 14 mEq calcium/g (10 mL); 270 mg elemental calcium/g calcium chloride (27% elemental calcium)

Dosage Forms Considerations 1 g calcium chloride = elemental calcium 273 mg = calcium 13.6 mEq = calcium 6.8 mmol

Dosage Forms Excipient information presented when available (limited, particularly for generics); consult specific product labeling.
Solution, Intravenous:
Generic: 10% (10 mL)
Solution, Intravenous [preservative free]:
Generic: 10% (10 mL)

Calcium Citrate (KAL see um SIT rate)

Brand Names: US Cal-Citrate [OTC]; Calcitrate [OTC]
Brand Names: Canada Osteocit®
Pharmacologic Category Calcium Salt
Use Dietary supplement

Dosing
Adult Oral: Dosage is in terms of **elemental** calcium
Dietary Reference Intake for Calcium:
Adults, Females/Males: RDA:
19-50 years: 1000 mg/day
≥51 years, females: 1200 mg/day
51-70 years, males: 1000 mg/day
Females: Pregnancy/Lactating: RDA: Requirements are the same as in nonpregnant or nonlactating females
Geriatric Dietary Reference Intake for Calcium: RDA:
Females: Refer to adult dosing.
Males ≤70 years: Refer to adult dosing.
Males >70 years: 1200 mg/day
Pediatric Oral: Dosage is in terms of **elemental** calcium
Dietary Reference Intake for Calcium:
1-6 months: Adequate intake: 200 mg/day
7-12 months: Adequate intake: 260 mg/day
1-3 years: RDA: 700 mg/day
4-8 years: RDA: 1000 mg/day
9-18 years: RDA: 1300 mg/day
Females: Pregnancy/Lactating: RDA: Requirements are the same as in nonpregnant or nonlactating females
Additional Information Complete prescribing information should be consulted for additional detail.
Dosage Forms Considerations 1 g calcium citrate = elemental calcium 211 mg = calcium 10.5 mEq = calcium 5.25 mmol
Dosage Forms Excipient information presented when available (limited, particularly for generics); consult specific product labeling.
Capsule, Oral [preservative free]:
Cal-Citrate: 150 mg [dye free]
Granules, Oral:
Generic: 760 mg/3.5 g (480 g)
Tablet, Oral:
Generic: 250 mg, 950 mg, 1040 mg
Tablet, Oral [preservative free]:
Calcitrate: 950 mg [lactose free, milk derivatives/products, no artificial color(s), no artificial flavor(s), sodium free, soy free, sugar free, wheat free, yeast free]

◆ **Calcium Citrate and Vitamin D** *see* Calcium and Vitamin D *on page 286*

◆ **Calcium Disodium Edetate** *see* Edetate CALCIUM Disodium *on page 616*

◆ **Calcium Disodiumethylenediaminetetraacetic Acid** *see* Edetate CALCIUM Disodium *on page 616*

◆ **Calcium Folinate** *see* Leucovorin Calcium *on page 1049*

Calcium Glubionate (KAL see um gloo BYE oh nate)

Brand Names: US Calcionate [OTC]
Pharmacologic Category Calcium Salt
Use Dietary supplement
Dosing
Adult Dosage is in terms of **elemental** calcium
Dietary Reference Intake for Calcium: Oral:
Adults, Females/Males: RDA:
19 to 50 years: 1000 mg daily
≥51 years, females: 1200 mg daily
51 to 70 years, males: 1000 mg daily
Females: Pregnancy/Lactating: RDA: Requirements are the same as in nonpregnant or nonlactating females
Dietary supplement: Oral: **Note:** Each 5 mL contains elemental calcium 115 mg: 15 mL 3 times daily or 15 mL 4 times daily (pregnancy/lactating)
Geriatric
Dietary Reference Intake for Calcium: RDA: Oral:
Females: Refer to adult dosing.
Males ≤70 years: Refer to adult dosing.
Males >70 years: 1200 mg/day
Dietary supplement: Refer to adult dosing.
Pediatric Dosage is in terms of **elemental** calcium
Dietary Reference Intake for Calcium: Oral:
1 to 6 months: Adequate intake: 200 mg daily
7 to 12 months: Adequate intake: 260 mg daily
1 to 3 years: RDA: 700 mg daily
4 to 8 years: RDA: 1000 mg daily
9 to 18 years: RDA: 1300 mg daily
Females: Pregnancy/Lactating: RDA: Requirements are the same as in nonpregnant or nonlactating females
Dietary supplement: Oral: **Note:** Each 5 mL contains elemental calcium 115 mg
Infants <12 months: 5 mL 5 times daily; may mix with juice or formula
Children <4 years: 10 mL 3 times daily
Children ≥4 years and Adolescents: Refer to adult dosing.
Additional Information Complete prescribing information should be consulted for additional detail.

Dosage Forms Considerations 1 g calcium glubionate = elemental calcium 63.8 mg = calcium 3.2 mEq = calcium 1.6 mmol

Dosage Forms Excipient information presented when available (limited, particularly for generics); consult specific product labeling.

Syrup, Oral:

Calcionate: 1.8 g/5 mL (473 mL) [fruit flavor]

Calcium Gluconate (KAL see um GLOO koe nate)

Brand Names: US Cal-Glu [OTC]

Pharmacologic Category Calcium Salt; Electrolyte Supplement, Oral; Electrolyte Supplement, Parenteral

Use

IV: Treatment of hypocalcemia and conditions secondary to hypocalcemia (eg, tetany, seizures, arrhythmias); treatment of cardiac disturbances secondary to hyperkalemia; adjunctive treatment of rickets, osteomalacia, and magnesium sulfate overdose; decrease capillary permeability in allergic conditions, nonthrombocytopenic purpura, and exudative dermatoses (eg, dermatitis herpetiformis, pruritus secondary to certain drugs); treatment of black widow spider bites to relieve muscle cramping

Oral: Dietary calcium supplementation

Pregnancy Considerations Animal reproduction studies have not been conducted. Calcium crosses the placenta. The amount of calcium reaching the fetus is determined by maternal physiological changes. Calcium requirements are the same in pregnant and nonpregnant females (IOM, 2011). Information related to use as an antidote in pregnancy is limited. In general, medications used as antidotes should take into consideration the health and prognosis of the mother; antidotes should be administered to pregnant women if there is a clear indication for use and should not be withheld because of fears of teratogenicity (Bailey, 2003).

Breast-Feeding Considerations Calcium is excreted in breast milk. The amount of calcium in breast milk is homeostatically regulated and not altered by maternal calcium intake. Calcium requirements are the same in lactating and nonlactating females (IOM, 2011).

Contraindications Ventricular fibrillation; hypercalcemia; concomitant use of IV calcium gluconate and ceftriaxone in neonates

Warnings/Precautions Multiple salt forms of calcium exist; close attention must be paid to the salt form when ordering and administering calcium; incorrect selection or substitution of one salt for another without proper dosage adjustment may result in serious over or under dosing. Avoid too rapid IV administration (do not exceed 200 mg/minute except in emergency situations);may result in vasodilation, hypotension, bradycardia, arrhythmias, and cardiac arrest. Parenteral calcium is a vesicant; ensure proper catheter or needle position prior to and during infusion. Avoid extravasation; may result in necrosis. Monitor the IV site closely. Use with caution in severe hyperphosphatemia or severe hypokalemia. Hypercalcemia may occur in patients with renal failure; frequent determination of serum calcium is necessary. Use caution with chronic renal disease. Use caution when administering calcium supplements to patients with a history of kidney stones. Hypomagnesemia is a common cause of hypocalcemia; therefore, correction of hypocalcemia may be difficult in patients with concomitant hypomagnesemia. Evaluate serum magnesium and correct hypomagnesemia (if necessary), particularly if initial treatment of hypocalcemia is refractory.

The parenteral product may contain aluminum; toxic aluminum concentrations may be seen with high doses, prolonged use, or renal dysfunction. Premature neonates are at higher risk due to immature renal function and aluminum intake from other parenteral sources. Parenteral aluminum exposure of >4 to 5 mcg/kg/day is associated with CNS and bone toxicity; tissue loading may occur at lower doses (Federal Register, 2002). See manufacturer's labeling.

Constipation, bloating, and gas are common with oral calcium supplements (especially carbonate salt). Administering oral calcium with food and vitamin D will optimize calcium absorption. Some products may contain tartrazine, which may cause allergic reactions in susceptible individuals.

Potentially significant drug-drug interactions may exist, requiring dose or frequency adjustment, additional monitoring, and/or selection of alternative therapy.

Adverse Reactions Frequency not defined.

IV:

Cardiovascular (with rapid IV injection): Arrhythmia, bradycardia, cardiac arrest, hypotension, syncope, vasodilation

Central nervous system: Sense of oppression (with rapid IV injection)

Endocrine & metabolic: Hypercalcemia

Gastrointestinal: Chalky taste

Neuromuscular & skeletal: Tingling sensation (with rapid IV injection)

Miscellaneous: Heat waves (with rapid IV injection)

Postmarketing and/or case reports: Calcinosis cutis

Oral: Gastrointestinal: Constipation

Drug Interactions

Metabolism/Transport Effects None known.

Avoid Concomitant Use

Avoid concomitant use of Calcium Gluconate with any of the following: Calcium Acetate

Increased Effect/Toxicity

Calcium Gluconate may increase the levels/effects of: Calcium Acetate; Cardiac Glycosides; CefTRIAXone; Vitamin D Analogs

The levels/effects of Calcium Gluconate may be increased by: Multivitamins/Fluoride (with ADE); Multivitamins/Minerals (with ADEK, Folate, Iron); Thiazide Diuretics

Decreased Effect

Calcium Gluconate may decrease the levels/effects of: Alpha-Lipoic Acid; Bisphosphonate Derivatives; Calcium Channel Blockers; Deferiprone; DOBUTamine; Dolutegravir; Eltrombopag; Estramustine; Multivitamins/Fluoride (with ADE); Phosphate Supplements; Quinolone Antibiotics; Strontium Ranelate; Tetracycline Derivatives; Thyroid Products; Trientine

The levels/effects of Calcium Gluconate may be decreased by: Alpha-Lipoic Acid; Trientine

Preparation for Administration

IV: Observe the vial for the presence of particulates. If particulates are observed, place vial in a 60°C to 80°C water bath for 15 to 30 minutes (or until solution is clear); occasionally shake to dissolve; cool to body/room temperature before use. Do not use vial if particulates do not dissolve. **Note:** Due to the potential presence of particulates, American Regent, Inc recommends the use of a 5 micron filter when preparing calcium gluconate-containing IV solutions (Important Drug Administration Information, American Regent, 2013); a similar recommendation has not been noted by other manufacturers. Usual concentrations: 1 g/100 mL D₅W or NS; 2 g/100 mL D₅W or NS. Maximum concentration in parenteral nutrition solutions is variable depending upon concentration and solubility (consult detailed reference).

Inhalation: Treatment of hydrofluoric acid burns (off-label use): Mix 1 mL of 10% calcium gluconate solution with 4 mL NS to make a 2.5% solution.

Storage/Stability

IV: Store intact vials at 20°C to 25°C (68°F to 77°F); excursions are permitted between 15°C and 30°C (59°F and 86°F). Do not freeze. Calcium-phosphate stability in parenteral nutrition solutions is dependent upon the pH of the solution, temperature, and relative concentration of each ion. The pH of the solution is primarily dependent upon the amino acid concentration. The higher the percentage amino acids the lower the pH, the more soluble the calcium and phosphate. Individual commercially available amino acid solutions vary significantly with respect to pH lowering potential and consequent calcium phosphate compatibility.

Oral: Store at room temperature; consult product labeling for specific requirements.

Mechanism of Action Moderates nerve and muscle performance via action potential threshold regulation.

In hydrogen fluoride exposures, calcium gluconate provides a source of calcium ions to complex free fluoride ions and prevent or reduce toxicity; administration also helps to correct fluoride-induced hypocalcemia.

Pharmacodynamics/Kinetics

Absorption: Oral: Minimal unless chronic, high doses are given; predominantly in the duodenum and dependent on calcitriol and vitamin D; mean absorption of calcium intake varies with age (infants 60%, prepubertal children 28%, pubertal children 34%, adults 25%); during pregnancy, calcium absorption doubles; calcium is absorbed in soluble, ionized form; solubility of calcium is increased in an acidic environment (IOM 2011); decreased absorption occurs in patients with achlorhydria, renal osteodystrophy, steatorrhea, or uremia

Distribution: Primarily in bones, teeth (IOM 2011)
Protein binding: ~40%, primarily to albumin (Wills 1971)
Excretion: Primarily feces (75%; as unabsorbed calcium salts); urine (20%) (IOM 2011)

Dosing

Adult Note: One gram of calcium gluconate salt is equal to 93 mg of elemental calcium.

Dosages are expressed in terms of the calcium gluconate salt (unless otherwise specified as elemental calcium). Dosages expressed in terms of the calcium gluconate salt are based on a solution concentration of 100 mg/mL (10%) containing 0.465 mEq (9.3 mg)/mL elemental calcium, except where noted.

Dietary Reference Intake for Calcium (IOM, 2011):
Oral: **Note:** Dose expressed as elemental calcium:
Adults, Females/Males: RDA:
19 to 50 years: 1000 mg **elemental calcium** daily
≥51 years, females: 1200 mg **elemental calcium** daily
51 to 70 years, males: 1000 mg **elemental calcium** daily
Females: Pregnancy/Lactating: RDA: Requirements are the same as in nonpregnant or nonlactating females

Hypocalcemia: IV:
Mild (ionized calcium: 4 to 5 mg/dL [1 to 1.2 mmol/L]): 1000 to 2000 mg over 2 hours; asymptomatic patients may be given oral calcium (Ariyan, 2004; French, 2012)
Moderate-to-severe (without seizure or tetany; ionized calcium: <4 mg/dL [<1 mmol/L]): 4000 mg over 4 hours (French, 2012)
Severe symptomatic (eg, seizure, tetany): 1000 to 2000 mg over 10 minutes; repeat every 60 minutes until symptoms resolve (French, 2012)
Note: Repeat ionized calcium measurement 6 to 10 hours after completion of administration. Check for hypomagnesemia and correct if present. Consider continuous infusion if hypocalcemia is likely to recur due to ongoing losses (French, 2012).
Continuous infusion: 5 to 20 mg/kg/hour (Pai, 2011)

Cardiac arrest or cardiotoxicity in the presence of hyperkalemia, hypocalcemia, or hypermagnesemia: IV: 1500 to 3000 mg over 2 to 5 minutes (Vanden Hoek, 2010)
Note: Routine use in cardiac arrest is not recommended due to the lack of improved survival (Neumar, 2010):

Parenteral nutrition, maintenance requirement: IV (Mirtallo, 2004): **Note:** Expressed in terms of **elemental calcium:** 10 to 20 **mEq elemental calcium** daily

Calcium channel blocker overdose (off-label use):
Hypotension/conduction disturbances: IV: 60 to 120 mg/kg/**hour** (Salhanick, 2003) **or** 60 mg/kg/dose over 5 minutes (maximum: 3000 to 6000 mg/dose) every 10 to 20 minutes; may repeat for 3 to 4 additional doses (Vanden Hoek, 2010; DeWitt, 2004). In life-threatening situations, 1000 mg has been administered every 2 to 3 minutes until clinical effect is achieved (Buckley, 1994). In one report, 18 **g** was administered over a 3-hour period (Luscher, 1994).

Hydrofluoric acid burns, treatment (off-label route/use):
SubQ (off-label route/use): 5% to 10% solution: 0.5 **mL**/cm² of burned tissue (Dibbell, 1970; Hatzifotis, 2004; Kirkpatrick, 1995; Krenzelok, 1999). Infiltration should be carried 0.5 cm away from the margin of the injured tissue into the surrounding uninjured areas. Repeat if pain recurs. Local anesthesia may be required to perform procedure; pain resolution is the therapeutic endpoint and if a local anesthetic is utilized, it may be difficult to determine the success of therapy (**Note: Never use calcium chloride for subcutaneous injection**).
Intra-arterial (off-label route/use): Add 10 **mL** of a 10% solution to 50 mL of D₅W. Infuse over 4 hours into the artery that provides the vascular supply to the affected area (Hatzifotis, 2004; Kirkpatrick, 1995). Pain usually resolves by the end of the infusion; repeat if pain recurs. **This intervention should be used only by those accustomed to this technique. Extreme care should be taken to avoid the extravasation.** A poison information center or clinical toxicologist should be consulted prior to implementation.
Inhalation (off-label route/use): 2.5% nebulization solution: Mix 1 **mL** of 10% calcium gluconate solution with 4 mL NS to make a 2.5% solution and administer via nebulization (Hatzifotis, 2004).

Geriatric Note: One gram of calcium gluconate salt is equal to 93 mg of elemental calcium.

Dosages are expressed in terms of the calcium gluconate salt (unless otherwise specified as elemental calcium). Dosages expressed in terms of the calcium gluconate salt are based on a solution concentration of 100 mg/mL (10%) containing 0.465 mEq (9.3 mg)/mL elemental calcium, except where noted.

Dietary Reference Intake for Calcium (IOM, 2011):
Oral: **Note:** Dose expressed as elemental calcium: RDA:
Females: Refer to adult dosing.
Males ≤70 years: Refer to adult dosing.
Males >70 years: 1200 mg **elemental calcium** daily
All other indications: Refer to adult dosing.

Pediatric Note: One gram of calcium gluconate salt is equal to 93 mg of elemental calcium.

Dosages are expressed in terms of the calcium gluconate salt (unless otherwise specified as elemental calcium). Dosages expressed in terms of the calcium gluconate salt are based on a solution concentration of 100 mg/mL (10%) containing 0.465 mEq (9.3 mg)/mL elemental calcium, except where noted.

Dietary Reference Intake for Calcium (IOM, 2011):
Oral: **Note:** Dose expressed as elemental calcium:
1 to 6 months: Adequate intake: 200 mg **elemental calcium** daily
7 to 12 months: Adequate intake: 260 mg **elemental calcium** daily
1 to 3 years: RDA: 700 mg **elemental calcium** daily
4 to 8 years: RDA: 1000 mg **elemental calcium** daily
9 to 18 years: RDA: 1300 mg **elemental calcium** daily
Females: Pregnancy/Lactating: RDA: Requirements are the same as in nonpregnant or nonlactating females

Hypocalcemia:
General dosing: Infants, Children, and Adolescents: IV: 200 to 500 mg/kg/day as a continuous infusion or in 4 divided doses (maximum dose: 1000 mg/dose [Infants, Children]; 2000 to 3000 mg/dose [Adolescents]) (Edmondson, 1990; Zhou, 2009)
Symptomatic (ie, seizures, tetany): Infants, Children, and Adolescents: IV: 100 to 200 mg/kg/dose over 5 to 10 minutes; usual adult dose: 1000 to 2000 mg/dose; may repeat after 6 hours or follow with a continuous infusion of 200 to 800 mg/kg/day (Edmondson, 1990; Kelly, 2013; Misra, 2008; Nelson, 1996; Zhou, 2009)

Cardiac arrest or cardiotoxicity in the presence of hyperkalemia, hypocalcemia, or hypermagnesemia:
Infants, Children, and Adolescents: IV, intraosseous: 60 to 100 mg/kg/dose (maximum: 3000 mg/dose); may repeat in 10 minutes if necessary; if effective, consider IV infusion (Hegenbarth, 2008)
Note: Routine use in cardiac arrest is not recommended due to the lack of improved survival (Kleinman, 2010; Neumar, 2010)

Parenteral nutrition, maintenance requirement: IV:
Infants and Children (≤50 kg) (Mirtallo, 2004): **Note:** Dose expressed as **elemental calcium:** 0.5 to 4 **mEq elemental calcium**/kg/day
Children (>50 kg) and Adolescents: Refer to adult dosing.

Calcium channel blocker overdose (off-label use):
Hypotension/conduction disturbances: Infants, Children, and Adolescents: IV, intraosseous: 60 mg/kg/dose administered over 30 to 60 minutes (Hegenbarth, 2008). **Note:** Calcium chloride may provide a more rapid increase of ionized calcium in critically-ill children. Calcium gluconate may be substituted if calcium chloride is not available.

Hydrofluoric acid burns, treatment (off-label route/use): Children and Adolescents: Refer to adult dosing.

Renal Impairment No initial dosage adjustment necessary; however, accumulation may occur with renal impairment and subsequent doses may require adjustment based on serum calcium concentrations.

Hepatic Impairment No initial dosage adjustment necessary; subsequent doses should be guided by serum calcium concentrations. In patients in the anhepatic stage of liver transplantation, equal rapid increases in ionized concentrations occur suggesting that calcium gluconate does not require hepatic metabolism for release of ionized calcium (Martin, 1990).

Administration

Oral: Administer with plenty of fluids with or following meals. The 10% calcium gluconate injection may be administered orally in young pediatric patients (Mimouni, 1994).

IV: Administer slowly (~1.5 mL calcium gluconate 10% per minute; not to exceed 200 mg/minute except in emergency situations) through a small needle into a large vein in order to avoid too rapid increases in the serum calcium and extravasation. **Note:** Due to the potential presence of particulates, American Regent, Inc recommends the use of a 0.22 micron inline filter for IV administration (1.2 micron filter if admixture contains lipids) (Important Drug Administration Information, American Regent, 2013); a similar recommendation has not been noted by other manufacturers. Not for IM administration. In acute situations of symptomatic hypocalcemia, infusions over 5 to 10 minutes have been described in pediatric patients (Kelly, 2013; Misra, 2008).

Vesicant; ensure proper needle or catheter placement prior to and during IV infusion. Avoid extravasation.

Extravasation management: If extravasation occurs, stop infusion immediately and disconnect (leave needle/cannula in place); gently aspirate extravasated solution (do **NOT** flush the line); initiate hyaluronidase antidote; remove needle/cannula; apply dry cold compresses (Hurst, 2004); elevate extremity.

Hyaluronidase: Intradermal or SubQ: Inject a total of 1 mL (15 units/mL) as five separate 0.2 mL injections (using a 25-gauge needle) into area of extravasation at the leading edge in a clockwise manner (MacCara, 1983; Zenk, 1981).

Treatment of hydrofluoric acid burns (off-label use):

SubQ infiltration (off-label route): Using a 27- or 30-gauge needle, approach the wound from the distal point of injury and infiltrate directly into the affected dermis and subcutaneous tissue. The infiltration should be carried 0.5 cm away from the margin of the injured tissue into the surrounding uninjured areas (Dibbell, 1970). Avoid excessive administration as it can cause compartment syndrome and further exacerbate tissue damage. Following subungual exposure, administer to the affected area via the lateral or volar route through the fat pad (under digital nerve block); administration may also require removal of the nailbed, splitting the distal nail from the nailbed, or trimming the nail to the nailbed to reach the affected area (Kirkpatrick, 1995; Roberts, 1989).

Intra-arterial (off-label route): Requires radiology to place an arterial catheter in an artery supplying blood to the area of exposure; infuse over four hours (Vance, 1986). **This intervention should be used only by those accustomed to this technique. Care should be taken to avoid the extravasation.** A poison information center or clinical toxicologist should be consulted prior to implementation.

Inhalation: Dilute 10% calcium gluconate solution to a 2.5% solution and administer via nebulization.

Reference Range

Serum total calcium: 8.4 to 10.2 mg/dL (2.1 to 2.55 mmol/L). **Note:** Due to a poor correlation between the serum ionized calcium (free) and total serum calcium, particularly in states of low albumin or acid/base imbalances, direct measurement of ionized calcium is recommended. In low albumin states, the corrected **total** serum calcium may be estimated by the following equation (assuming a normal albumin of 4 g/dL [40 g/L]).

Corrected total calcium (mg/dL) = measured total calcium (mg/mL) + 0.8 [4 - measured serum albumin(g/dL)]

or

Corrected total calcium (mmol/L) = measured total calcium (mmol/L) + 0.02 [40-measured serum albumin (g/L)]

Test Interactions IV administration may produce falsely decreased serum and urine magnesium concentrations

Dosage Forms Considerations 1 g calcium gluconate = elemental calcium 93 mg = calcium 4.65 mEq = calcium 2.33 mmol

Dosage Forms Excipient information presented when available (limited, particularly for generics); consult specific product labeling. [DSC] = Discontinued product
Capsule, Oral [preservative free]:
  Cal-Glu: 500 mg [dye free]
Solution, Intravenous:
  Generic: 10% (10 mL, 50 mL, 100 mL, 200 mL [DSC])
Solution, Intravenous [preservative free]:
  Generic: 10% (100 mL)
Tablet, Oral:
  Generic: 50 mg, 500 mg, 648 mg [DSC]

◆ Calcium High Potency [OTC] see Calcium Carbonate on page 287

◆ Calcium Leucovorin see Leucovorin Calcium on page 1049

◆ Calcium Levoleucovorin see LEVOleucovorin on page 1063

◆ Cal-CO3S [OTC] [DSC] see Calcium Carbonate on page 287

◆ Cal-CYUM [OTC] [DSC] see Calcium and Vitamin D on page 286

◆ Caldolor see Ibuprofen on page 905

Calfactant (kaf AKT ant)

Brand Names: US Infasurf
Index Terms Bovine Lung Surfactant
Pharmacologic Category Lung Surfactant
Use Prevention of respiratory distress syndrome (RDS) in premature infants at high risk for RDS and for the treatment ("rescue") of premature infants who develop RDS

Prophylaxis: Therapy at birth with calfactant is indicated for premature infants <29 weeks of gestational age at significant risk for RDS. Should be administered as soon as possible, preferably within 30 minutes after birth.

Treatment: For infants ≤72 hours of age with RDS (confirmed by clinical and radiologic findings) and requiring endotracheal intubation.

Dosing

Pediatric Prevention or treatment of RDS in premature infants: Intratracheal administration **only:** Each dose is 3 mL/kg body weight at birth; should be administered every 12 hours for a total of up to 3 doses

Renal Impairment No dosage adjustment provided in manufacturer's labeling.

Hepatic Impairment No dosage adjustment provided in manufacturer's labeling.

Additional Information Complete prescribing information should be consulted for additional detail.

Dosage Forms Excipient information presented when available (limited, particularly for generics); consult specific product labeling.
Suspension, Inhalation:
  Infasurf: 35 mg phospholipids and 0.7 mg protein per mL (3 mL, 6 mL)

◆ Cal-Gest Antacid [OTC] see Calcium Carbonate on page 287

◆ Cal-Glu [OTC] see Calcium Gluconate on page 291

◆ Cal-Mint [OTC] see Calcium Carbonate on page 287

◆ Calmylin PSE with Codeine (Can) see Guaifenesin, Pseudoephedrine, and Codeine on page 863

◆ CaloMist see Cyanocobalamin on page 453

◆ Calphron [OTC] see Calcium Acetate on page 286

◆ Caltrate (Can) see Calcium Carbonate on page 287

◆ Caltrate 600 [OTC] see Calcium Carbonate on page 287

◆ Caltrate 600+D [OTC] see Calcium and Vitamin D on page 286

◆ Caltrate 600+Soy [OTC] see Calcium and Vitamin D on page 286

◆ Caltrate ColonHealth [OTC] see Calcium and Vitamin D on page 286

◆ Caltrate Gummy Bites [OTC] see Calcium and Vitamin D on page 286

◆ Caltrate Select (Can) see Calcium Carbonate on page 287

◆ Cambia see Diclofenac (Systemic) on page 540

◆ Camila see Norethindrone on page 1298

◆ Campath see Alemtuzumab on page 62

◆ Campath-1H see Alemtuzumab on page 62

◆ Camphorated Tincture of Opium (error-prone synonym) see Paregoric on page 1396

◆ Campral see Acamprosate on page 24

◆ Campral [DSC] see Acamprosate on page 24

◆ Campral® (Can) see Acamprosate on page 24

◆ Camptosar see Irinotecan (Conventional) on page 980

◆ Camptothecin-11 see Irinotecan (Conventional) on page 980

◆ camrese see Ethinyl Estradiol and Levonorgestrel on page 703

◆ camrese lo see Ethinyl Estradiol and Levonorgestrel on page 703

Canakinumab (can a KIN ue mab)

Brand Names: US Ilaris

Brand Names: Canada Ilaris
Index Terms ACZ885
Pharmacologic Category Interleukin-1 Beta Inhibitor; Interleukin-1 Inhibitor; Monoclonal Antibody
Use

Cryopyrin-associated periodic syndromes:

U.S. labeling: Treatment of cryopyrin-associated periodic syndromes (CAPS) in adults and children 4 years and older, including familial cold autoinflammatory syndrome (FCAS) and Muckle-Wells syndrome (MWS).

Canadian labeling: Treatment of cryopyrin-associated periodic syndromes (CAPS) in adults and children 2 years and older, including familial cold autoinflammatory syndrome (FCAS) and Muckle-Wells syndrome (MWS). May also be used in Neonatal-Onset Multisystem Inflammatory Disease (NOMID) although clinical data has not confirmed improvement of CNS symptoms in this patient population.

Systemic juvenile idiopathic arthritis: Treatment of active systemic juvenile idiopathic arthritis (SJIA) in patients 2 years and older.

Medication Guide Available Yes
Dosing

Adult & Geriatric

Cryopyrin-associated periodic syndromes (CAPS):
Adults >40 kg: SubQ:

U.S. labeling: 150 mg every 8 weeks

Canadian labeling: 150 mg every 8 weeks; if inadequate response after 7 days may consider further titration by 150 mg every 7 days up to a maximum dose of 600 mg. The dose at which a satisfactory response is achieved should be maintained and administered every 8 weeks.

Pediatric

Cryopyrin-associated periodic syndromes (CAPS):
SubQ:

U.S. labeling:

Children ≥4 years and Adolescents:
15 to 40 kg: 2 mg/kg every 8 weeks; may increase to 3 mg/kg if response inadequate
>40 kg: 150 mg every 8 weeks

Canadian labeling:

Children ≥2 years and Adolescents:
15 to 40 kg: Initial: 2 mg/kg every 8 weeks; if inadequate response after 7 days may consider further titration by 2 mg/kg every 7 days up to a maximum dose of 8 mg/kg (do not exceed 600 mg). The dose at which a satisfactory response is achieved should be maintained and administered every 8 weeks.
>40 kg: 150 mg every 8 weeks; if inadequate response after 7 days may consider further titration by 150 mg every 7 days up to a maximum dose of 600 mg. The dose at which a satisfactory response is achieved should be maintained and administered every 8 weeks.

Systemic juvenile idiopathic arthritis (SJIA): SubQ: Children ≥2 years and ≥7.5 kg (U.S. labeling) or >9 kg (Canadian labeling) and Adolescents: 4 mg/kg every 4 weeks (maximum: 300 mg per dose)

Renal Impairment

U.S. labeling: There are no dosage adjustments provided in the manufacturer's labeling.

Canadian labeling: No dosage adjustment necessary; limited data in this population.

Hepatic Impairment There are no dosage adjustments provided in the manufacturer's labeling (has not been studied).

Additional Information Complete prescribing information should be consulted for additional detail.

Dosage Forms Excipient information presented when available (limited, particularly for generics); consult specific product labeling.
Solution Reconstituted, Subcutaneous [preservative free]:
Ilaris: 180 mg (1 ea) [contains polysorbate 80]

Dosage Forms: Canada Excipient information presented when available (limited, particularly for generics); consult specific product labeling.
Injection, powder for reconstitution:
Ilaris: 150 mg [contains polysorbate 80, sucrose]

◆ Canasa see Mesalamine on page 1151
◆ Cancidas see Caspofungin on page 325

Candesartan (kan de SAR tan)

Brand Names: US Atacand
Brand Names: Canada ACH Candesartan; Apo-Candesartan; Atacand; CO Candesartan; DOM-Candesartan; JAMP-Candesartan; Mylan-Candesartan; PMS-Candesartan; Ran-Candesartan; Sandoz-Candesartan; Teva-Candesartan

Index Terms Candesartan Cilexetil
Pharmacologic Category Angiotensin II Receptor Blocker; Antihypertensive
Use

Heart failure: Treatment of heart failure (NYHA class II-IV)
Hypertension: Alone or in combination with other antihypertensive agents in treating hypertension

Guideline recommendations:

Heart failure: The ACCF/AHA 2013 heart failure guidelines recommend the use of ARBs (ie, candesartan, losartan, and valsartan) in patients with HF with reduced ejection fraction who cannot tolerate ACE inhibitors (due to cough) to reduce morbidity and mortality. They also suggest that ARBs are reasonable first-line alternatives to ACE inhibitors in patients already maintained on an ARB for other indications (ACCF/AHA [Yancy, 2013]).

Hypertension: The 2014 guideline for the management of high blood pressure in adults (Eighth Joint National Committee [JNC 8; James, 2013]) recommends initiation of pharmacologic treatment to lower blood pressure for the following patients:
• Patients ≥60 years of age with systolic blood pressure (SBP) ≥150 mm Hg or diastolic blood pressure (DBP) ≥90 mm Hg. Goal of therapy is SBP <150 mm Hg and DBP <90 mm Hg.
• Patients <60 years of age with SBP ≥140 mm Hg or DBP ≥90 mm Hg. Goal of therapy is SBP <140 mm Hg and DBP <90 mm Hg.
• Patients ≥18 years of age with diabetes and SBP ≥140 mm Hg or DBP ≥90 mm Hg. Goal of therapy is SBP <140 mm Hg and DBP <90 mm Hg.
• Patients ≥18 years of age with chronic kidney disease (CKD) and SBP ≥140 mm Hg or DBP ≥90 mm Hg. Goal of therapy is SBP <140 mm Hg and DBP <90 mm Hg.

Chronic kidney disease (CKD) and hypertension: Regardless of race or diabetes status, the use of an ACE inhibitor (ACEI) or angiotensin receptor blocker (ARB) as initial therapy is recommended to improve kidney outcomes. In the general nonblack population (without CKD), including those with diabetes, initial antihypertensive treatment should consist of a thiazide-type diuretic, calcium channel blocker, ACEI, or ARB. In the general black population (without CKD), including those with diabetes, initial antihypertensive treatment should consist of a thiazide-type diuretic or a calcium channel blocker instead of an ACEI or ARB.

Coronary artery disease and hypertension: The American Heart Association, American College of Cardiology and American Society of Hypertension (AHA/ACC/ASH) 2015 scientific statement for the treatment of hypertension in patients with coronary artery disease (CAD) recommends the use of an ARB (or ACE inhibitor) as part of a regimen in patients with hypertension and chronic stable angina if there is prior MI, LV systolic dysfunction, diabetes mellitus, or CKD. A BP target of <140/90 mm Hg is reasonable for the secondary prevention of cardiovascular events. A lower target BP (<130/80 mm Hg) may be appropriate in some individuals with CAD, previous MI, stroke or transient ischemic attack, or CAD risk equivalents (AHA/ACC/ASH [Rosendorff 2015]).

Pregnancy Considerations [U.S. Boxed Warning]: Drugs that act on the renin-angiotensin system can cause injury and death to the developing fetus. Discontinue as soon as possible once pregnancy is detected. The use of drugs which act on the renin-angiotensin system are associated with oligohydramnios. Oligohydramnios, due to decreased fetal renal function, may lead to fetal lung hypoplasia and skeletal malformations. Use is also associated with anuria, hypotension, renal failure, skull hypoplasia, and death in the fetus/neonate. The exposed fetus should be monitored for fetal growth, amniotic fluid volume, and organ formation. Infants exposed *in utero* should be monitored for hyperkalemia, hypotension, and oliguria (exchange transfusions or dialysis may be needed). These adverse events are generally associated with maternal use in the second and third trimesters.

Untreated chronic maternal hypertension is also associated with adverse events in the fetus, infant, and mother. The use of angiotensin II receptor blockers is not recommended to treat chronic uncomplicated hypertension in pregnant women and should generally be avoided in women of reproductive potential (ACOG, 2013).

Breast-Feeding Considerations It is not known if candesartan is excreted into breast milk. Due to the potential for serious adverse reactions in the nursing infant, the manufacturer recommends a decision be made whether

to discontinue nursing or to discontinue the drug, taking into account the importance of treatment to the mother. The Canadian labeling contraindicates use in breast-feeding women.

Contraindications

Hypersensitivity to candesartan or any component of the formulation; concomitant use with aliskiren in patients with diabetes mellitus

Canadian labeling: Additional contraindications (not in U.S. labeling): Concomitant use with aliskiren in patients with moderate-to-severe renal impairment (GFR <60 mL/minute/1.73 m^2); pregnancy; breast-feeding; children <1 year of age; rare hereditary problems of galactose intolerance, Lapp lactase deficiency or glucose-galactose malabsorption

Warnings/Precautions [U.S. Boxed Warning]: Drugs that act on the renin-angiotensin system can cause injury and death to the developing fetus. Discontinue as soon as possible once pregnancy is detected. May

cause hyperkalemia; avoid potassium supplementation unless specifically required by healthcare provider. Avoid use or use a smaller dose in patients who are volume depleted; correct depletion first. May be associated with deterioration of renal function and/or increases in serum creatinine, particularly in patients with low renal blood flow (eg, renal artery stenosis, heart failure) whose glomerular filtration rate (GFR) is dependent on efferent arteriolar vasoconstriction by angiotensin II; deterioration may result in oliguria, acute renal failure, and progressive azotemia. Small increases in serum creatinine may occur following initiation; consider discontinuation only in patients with progressive and/or significant deterioration in renal function. Use with caution in unstented unilateral/bilateral renal artery stenosis, preexisting renal insufficiency, or significant aortic/mitral stenosis. Systemic exposure increases in hepatic impairment. U.S. manufacturer labeling recommends a dosage adjustment in patients with moderate hepatic impairment; pharmacokinetics have not been studied in severe hepatic impairment. Use caution when initiating in heart failure; may need to adjust dose, and/or concurrent diuretic therapy, because of candesartan-induced hypotension. In surgical patients on chronic angiotensin receptor blocker (ARB) therapy, intraoperative hypotension may occur with induction and maintenance of general anesthesia Potentially significant drug-drug interactions may exist, requiring dose or frequency adjustment, additional monitoring, and/or selection of alternative therapy. Pediatric patients with a GFR <30 mL/minute/1.73 m^2 should not receive candesartan; has not been evaluated. Avoid use in infants <1 year of age due to potential effects on the development of immature kidneys.

Angioedema has been reported rarely with some angiotensin II receptor antagonists (ARBs) and may occur at any time during treatment (especially following first dose). It may involve the head and neck (potentially compromising airway) or the intestine (presenting with abdominal pain). Patients with idiopathic or hereditary angioedema or previous angioedema associated with ACE-inhibitor therapy may be at an increased risk. Prolonged frequent monitoring may be required, especially if tongue, glottis, or larynx are involved, as they are associated with airway obstruction. Patients with a history of airway surgery may have a higher risk of airway obstruction. Discontinue therapy immediately if angioedema occurs. Aggressive early management is critical. Intramuscular (IM) administration of epinephrine may be necessary. Do not readminister to patients who have had angioedema with ARBs.

Adverse Reactions Frequency not always defined.

Cardiovascular: Hypotension (heart failure 19%), angina pectoris, myocardial infarction, palpitations, tachycardia

Central nervous system: Anxiety, depression, dizziness, drowsiness, headache, paresthesia, vertigo

Dermatologic: Diaphoresis, skin rash

Endocrine & metabolic: Hyperkalemia (heart failure <1% to 6%), hyperglycemia, hypertriglyceridemia, hyperuricemia

Gastrointestinal: Dyspepsia, gastroenteritis

Genitourinary: Hematuria

Neuromuscular & skeletal: Back pain, increased creatine phosphokinase, myalgia, weakness

Renal: Increased serum creatinine (≤13% in patients with heart failure with drug discontinuation required in 6%)

Respiratory: Dyspnea, epistaxis, pharyngitis, rhinitis, upper respiratory tract infection

Miscellaneous: Fever

<1% (Limited to important or life-threatening): Atrial fibrillation, bradycardia, cardiac failure, cerebrovascular accident, confusion, hepatic insufficiency, hepatitis, hypersensitivity, leukopenia, loss of consciousness, pancreatitis, pneumonia, presyncope, pulmonary edema, renal failure, rhabdomyolysis, thrombocytopenia

Drug Interactions

Metabolism/Transport Effects Substrate of CYP2C9 (minor); **Note:** Assignment of Major/Minor substrate status based on clinically relevant drug interaction potential; **Inhibits** CYP2C8 (weak), CYP2C9 (weak)

Avoid Concomitant Use

Avoid concomitant use of Candesartan with any of the following: Amodiaquine

Increased Effect/Toxicity

Candesartan may increase the levels/effects of: ACE Inhibitors; Amifostine; Amodiaquine; Antipsychotic Agents (Second Generation [Atypical]); Ciprofloxacin (Systemic); CycloSPORINE (Systemic); Drospirenone; DULoxetine; Hypotension-Associated Agents; Levodopa; Lithium; Nonsteroidal Anti-Inflammatory Agents; Potassium-Sparing Diuretics; Sodium Phosphates

The levels/effects of Candesartan may be increased by: Alfuzosin; Aliskiren; Barbiturates; Brimonidine (Topical); Canagliflozin; Dapoxetine; Diazoxide; Eplerenone; Heparin; Heparin (Low Molecular Weight); Herbs (Hypotensive Properties); Molsidomine; Nicorandil; Obinutuzumab; Pentoxifylline; Phosphodiesterase 5 Inhibitors; Potassium Salts; Prostacyclin Analogues; Tolvaptan; Trimethoprim

Decreased Effect

The levels/effects of Candesartan may be decreased by: Amphetamines; Herbs (Hypertensive Properties); Methylphenidate; Nonsteroidal Anti-Inflammatory Agents; Yohimbine

Storage/Stability Store at 25°C (77°F); excursions permitted to 15°C to 30°C (59°F to 86°F).

Mechanism of Action Candesartan is an angiotensin receptor antagonist. Angiotensin II acts as a vasoconstrictor. In addition to causing direct vasoconstriction, angiotensin II also stimulates the release of aldosterone. Once aldosterone is released, sodium as well as water are reabsorbed. The end result is an elevation in blood pressure. Candesartan binds to the AT1 angiotensin II receptor. This binding prevents angiotensin II from binding to the receptor thereby blocking the vasoconstriction and the aldosterone secreting effects of angiotensin II.

Pharmacodynamics/Kinetics

Onset of action: 2 to 3 hours; antihypertensive effect: Within 2 weeks

Peak effect: 6 to 8 hours; maximum antihypertensive effect: 4 to 6 weeks

Duration: >24 hours

Absorption: Candesartan: Rapid and complete following conversion from candesartan cilexetil by GI esterases

Distribution: V_d: 0.13 L/kg

Protein binding: >99%

Metabolism: Converted to active candesartan, via ester hydrolysis during absorption from GI tract; hepatic (minor) via O-deethylation to inactive metabolite

Bioavailability, absolute: Candesartan: 15%

Half-life elimination (dose dependent): 5 to 9 hours

Time to peak: Children (1 to 17 years); Adults: 3 to 4 hours

Excretion: Feces (67%); urine (33%; 26% as unchanged drug)

Clearance: Total body: 0.37 mL/minute/kg; Renal: 0.19 mL/minute/kg; decreased with severe renal impairment

Dosing

Adult

Hypertension: Oral: **Note:** Antihypertensive effect usually observed within 2 weeks; maximum antihypertensive effect seen within 4 to 6 weeks. Dosage must be individualized. Consider lower initial dosages in volume depleted patients; if possible, correct volume depletion prior to administration. Initial: 16 mg once daily; titrate to response; usual range: 8 to 32 mg daily in 1 to 2 divided doses; target dose (JNC 8 [James, 2013]): 12 to 32 mg daily; maximum daily dose: 32 mg daily.

Heart failure: Oral: Initial: 4 mg once daily (U.S. labeling) or alternatively 4 to 8 mg once daily (ACCF/AHA [Yancy, 2013]; double the dose at 2-week intervals, as tolerated; target dose: 32 mg once daily (ACCF/AHA [Yancy, 2013]).

Note: Concurrent therapy with an ACE inhibitor may provide additional benefit in patients with HF with reduced EF who remain symptomatic on standard therapy and are unable to receive an aldosterone antagonist (ACCF/AHA [Yancy, 2013]).

Canadian labeling: Initial: 4 mg once daily; double the dose at 2-week intervals as tolerated; target dose: 32 mg once daily

Geriatric: Refer to adult dosing. No initial dosage adjustment is necessary for elderly patients (although higher concentrations (C_{max}) and AUC were observed in this population).

◄

Pediatric Hypertension: Oral: **Note:** Antihypertensive effect usually observed within 2 weeks; maximum antihypertensive effect seen within 4 to 6 weeks. Consider lower initial dosages in volume depleted patients; if possible, correct volume depletion prior to administration. Use in children <6 years is not approved in the Canadian labeling.

Children 1 to <6 years: Initial: 0.2 mg/kg/day in 1 to 2 divided doses; titrate to response; usual range: 0.05 to 0.4 mg/kg/day; maximum daily dose: 0.4 mg/kg/day

Children ≥6 years and Adolescents <17 years: *U.S. labeling:*

<50 kg: Initial: 4 to 8 mg daily in 1 to 2 divided doses; titrate to response; usual range: 2 to 16 mg daily; maximum daily dose: 32 mg daily

≥50 kg: Initial: 8 to 16 mg daily in 1 to 2 divided doses; titrate to response; usual range: 4 to 32 mg daily; maximum daily dose: 32 mg daily

Children ≥6 years and Adolescents ≤17 years: *Canadian labeling:*

<50 kg: Initial: 4 mg once daily; titrate to response; maximum dose: 8 mg daily

≥50 kg: Initial: 8 mg once daily; titrate to response; maximum dose: 8 mg daily

Renal Impairment

U.S. labeling:

Adults: No initial dosage adjustment necessary; however, in patients with severe renal impairment (CrCl <30 mL/minute/1.73 m^2) AUC and C_{max} were approximately doubled after repeated dosing.

Children ≥1 and Adolescents <17 years: There are no dosage adjustments provided in the manufacturer's labeling (has not been studied). Children with GFR <30 mL/minute/1.73 m^2 should not receive candesartan.

Canadian labeling:

Adults:

Mild impairment: No dosage adjustment necessary.

Moderate or severe impairment: Consider initial dose of 4 mg once daily in patients with hypertension.

Dialysis: Consider initial dose of 4 mg once daily in patients with hypertension.

Children ≥6 and Adolescents ≤17 years: There are no dosage adjustments provided in the manufacturer's labeling (has not been studied).

Hepatic Impairment

U.S. labeling:

Mild impairment (Child-Pugh class A): No initial dosage adjustment necessary.

Moderate impairment (Child-Pugh class B): Initial: 8 mg daily (AUC increased by 145%) in adult patients with hypertension. There are no dosage adjustments provided in the manufacturer's labeling for pediatric patients.

Severe impairment (Child-Pugh class C): There are no dosage adjustments provided in manufacturer's labeling (has not been studied); however, systemic exposure increases significantly in moderate impairment.

Canadian labeling:

Adults:

Mild to moderate impairment: No dosage adjustment necessary.

Severe impairment: Limited experience; consider initial dose of 4 mg once daily in adult patients with hypertension.

Children: There are no dosage adjustments provided in the manufacturer's labeling (has not been studied).

Administration Administer without regard to meals. An oral suspension may be prepared for children unable to swallow tablets (refer to Extemporaneous Preparations information).

Monitoring Parameters Supine blood pressure, electrolytes, serum creatinine, BUN, urinalysis, symptomatic hypotension, and tachycardia; in heart failure, serum potassium during dose escalation and periodically thereafter

2013 ACCF/AHA Heart Failure guideline recommendations: Within 1-2 weeks after initiation, reassess blood pressure (including postural blood pressure changes), renal function, and serum potassium; follow closely after dose changes. Patients with systolic blood pressure <80 mm Hg, low serum sodium, diabetes mellitus, and impaired renal function should be closely monitored (ACCF/AHA [Yancy, 2013]).

Additional Information May have an advantage over losartan due to minimal metabolism requirements and consequent use in mild-to-moderate hepatic impairment

Dosage Forms Excipient information presented when available (limited, particularly for generics); consult specific product labeling.

Tablet, Oral, as cilexetil:
Atacand: 4 mg, 8 mg, 16 mg, 32 mg [scored]
Generic: 4 mg, 8 mg, 16 mg, 32 mg

Extemporaneous Preparations Oral suspension may be made in concentrations ranging from 0.1 to 2 mg/mL; typically 1 mg/mL oral suspension suitable for majority of prescribed doses; any strength tablet may be used. A 1 mg/mL (total volume: 160 mL) oral suspension may be made with tablets and a 1:1 mixture of Ora-Plus® and Ora-Sweet SF®. Prepare the vehicle by adding 80 mL of Ora-Plus® and 80 mL of Ora-Sweet SF® or, alternatively, use 160 mL of Ora-Blend SF®. Add a small amount of vehicle to five 32 mg tablets and grind into a smooth paste using a mortar and pestle. Transfer the paste to a calibrated amber PET bottle, rinse the mortar and pestle clean using the vehicle, add this to the bottle, and then add a quantity of vehicle sufficient to make 160 mL. The suspension is stable at room temperature for 100 days unopened or 30 days after the first opening; do not freeze; label "shake well before use." (Atacand prescribing information, 2013).

Candesartan and Hydrochlorothiazide
(kan de SAR tan & hye droe klor oh THYE a zide)

Brand Names: US Atacand HCT

Brand Names: Canada Apo-Candesartan HCTZ; Atacand Plus; Candesartan HCT; Candesartan-HCTZ; Mylan-Candesartan HCTZ; PMS-Candesartan HCTZ; Sandoz-Candesartan Plus; Teva-Candesartan/HCTZ

Index Terms Candesartan Cilexetil and Hydrochlorothiazide; Hydrochlorothiazide and Candesartan

Pharmacologic Category Angiotensin II Receptor Blocker; Antihypertensive; Diuretic, Thiazide

Use Hypertension: Treatment of hypertension; combination product should not be used for initial therapy

Dosing

Adult Hypertension, replacement therapy: Oral: Combination product can be substituted for individual agents; maximum therapeutic effect would be expected within 4 weeks

Usual dosage range:

Candesartan: 8 to 32 mg daily, given once daily or twice daily in divided doses

Hydrochlorothiazide: 12.5 to 50 mg once daily

Geriatric No initial dosage adjustment is recommended. Refer to adult dosing.

Renal Impairment

CrCl ≥30 mL/minute: No dosage adjustment necessary.

CrCl <30 mL/minute: No dosage adjustment provided in manufacturer's labeling (safety and efficacy not established); however, AUC and serum levels of candesartan are increased, and the half-life of hydrochlorothiazide is prolonged in severe renal impairment. Use is contraindicated in anuric patients. The Canadian labeling also contraindicates use if CrCl <30 mL/minute/1.73 m^2.

Hepatic Impairment

US labeling:

Mild impairment (Child-Pugh class A): No dosage adjustment necessary.

Moderate to severe impairment (Child-Pugh classes B and C): Not recommended for initiation since an appropriate adjusted dose is not commercially available.

Canadian labeling:

Mild or moderate impairment: Titrate individual components cautiously.

Severe impairment and/or cholestasis: Use is contraindicated.

Additional Information Complete prescribing information should be consulted for additional detail.

Dosage Forms Excipient information presented when available (limited, particularly for generics); consult specific product labeling.

Tablet, oral: 16/12.5: Candesartan cilexetil 16 mg and hydrochlorothiazide 12.5 mg; 32/12.5: Candesartan cilexetil 32 mg and hydrochlorothiazide 12.5 mg; 32/25: Candesartan cilexetil 32 mg and hydrochlorothiazide 25 mg

Atacand HCT:
16/12.5: Candesartan cilexetil 16 mg and hydrochlorothiazide 12.5 mg
32/12.5: Candesartan cilexetil 32 mg and hydrochlorothiazide 12.5 mg
32/25: Candesartan cilexetil 32 mg and hydrochlorothiazide 25 mg

◆ Candesartan Cilexetil see Candesartan on page 294

◆ Candesartan Cilexetil and Hydrochlorothiazide see Candesartan and Hydrochlorothiazide on page 296

◆ Candesartan HCT (Can) *see* Candesartan and Hydrochlorothiazide *on page 296*

◆ Candesartan-HCTZ (Can) *see* Candesartan and Hydrochlorothiazide *on page 296*

◆ CanesOral (Can) *see* Fluconazole *on page 775*

◆ Canesten Topical (Can) *see* Clotrimazole (Topical) *on page 428*

◆ Canesten Vaginal (Can) *see* Clotrimazole (Topical) *on page 428*

Cangrelor (KAN grel or)

Brand Names: US Kengreal
Index Terms Cangrelor Tetrasodium
Pharmacologic Category Antiplatelet Agent; Antiplatelet Agent, Non-thienopyridine
Use Percutaneous coronary intervention (PCI): Adjunct to PCI to reduce the risk of periprocedural myocardial infarction (MI), repeat coronary revascularization, and stent thrombosis in patients who have not been treated with a $P2Y_{12}$ platelet inhibitor and are not being given a glycoprotein IIb/IIIa inhibitor
Pregnancy Considerations Adverse events were observed in some animal reproduction studies.
Breast-Feeding Considerations It is not known if cangrelor is excreted in breast milk
Contraindications Known hypersensitivity (eg, anaphylaxis) to cangrelor or any component of the formulation; significant active bleeding
Warnings/Precautions Similar to other $P2Y_{12}$ antagonists, the use of cangrelor increases the risk of bleeding; however, due to the short elimination half-life, no antiplatelet effect is observed an hour after discontinuation. Although rare, serious cases of hypersensitivity (eg, anaphylaxis, anaphylactic shock, bronchospasm, angioedema, stridor) have been reported with cangrelor. If clopidogrel or prasugrel are administered prior to discontinuation of the cangrelor infusion, no antiplatelet effect will occur until the next dose is administered. Therefore, do not administer until after the cangrelor infusion is discontinued.
Adverse Reactions
Hematologic & oncologic: Hemorrhage (GUSTO: 16%; TIMI: <1%)
Renal: Renal insufficiency (3%; severe; creatinine clearance <30 mL/minute)
Respiratory: Dyspnea (1%)
<1%, (Limited to important or life threatening): Hypersensitivity reaction
Drug Interactions
Metabolism/Transport Effects None known.
Avoid Concomitant Use
Avoid concomitant use of Cangrelor with any of the following: Urokinase
Increased Effect/Toxicity
Cangrelor may increase the levels/effects of: Agents with Antiplatelet Properties; Anticoagulants; Apixaban; Collagenase (Systemic); Dabigatran Etexilate; Deoxycholic Acid; Edoxaban; Ibritumomab; Obinutuzumab; Rivaroxaban; Salicylates; Thrombolytic Agents; Tositumomab and Iodine I 131 Tositumomab; Urokinase

The levels/effects of Cangrelor may be increased by: Dasatinib; Glucosamine; Herbs (Anticoagulant/Antiplatelet Properties); Ibrutinib; Limaprost; Multivitamins/Fluoride (with ADE); Multivitamins/Minerals (with ADEK, Folate, Iron); Multivitamins/Minerals (with AE, No Iron); Omega-3 Fatty Acids; Pentosan Polysulfate Sodium; Pentoxifylline; Prostacyclin Analogues; Tipranavir; Vitamin E; Vitamin E (Oral)
Decreased Effect
Cangrelor may decrease the levels/effects of: Clopidogrel; Prasugrel
Preparation for Administration Reconstitute 50 mg vial by adding 5 mL of Sterile Water for Injection. Swirl gently until dissolved (should be clear and colorless to pale yellow). Avoid vigorous mixing. Allow any foam to settle. Must be diluted prior to administration. Immediately after reconstitution, add the contents of one vial to 250 mL of NS or D_5W; mix thoroughly. Resultant concentration of solution for infusion: 200 mcg/mL.
Patients ≥100 kg will require a minimum of 2 bags.
Storage/Stability Store at controlled room temperature between 20°C and 25°C (68°F and 77°F); excursions are permitted to 15°C to 30°C (59°F and 86°F). Solutions diluted for infusion are stable for up to 12 hours in D_5W or 24 hours in NS at room temperature.
Mechanism of Action Cangrelor, a nonthienopyridine adenosine triphosphate analogue, is a direct $P2Y_{12}$ platelet receptor inhibitor that blocks adenosine diphosphate (ADP)-induced platelet activation and aggregation.

Cangrelor binds selectively and reversibly to the $P2Y_{12}$ receptor, preventing further signaling and platelet activation.
Pharmacodynamics/Kinetics
Onset of action: Platelet inhibition occurs within 2 minutes
Duration of action: Antiplatelet effect is maintained throughout duration of infusion. After discontinuation, platelet function returns to normal within 1 hour
Distribution: Volume of distribution: 3.9 L
Protein binding: ~97% to 98%
Metabolism: Rapidly inactivated in the circulation by dephosphorylation to its primary metabolite, a nucleoside, which has negligible anti-platelet activity
Half-life elimination: ~3 to 6 minutes
Time to peak: Within 2 minutes
Excretion: Urine (58%); feces (35%)
Dosing
Adult
Percutaneous coronary intervention (PCI): IV: 30 mcg/kg bolus prior to PCI followed immediately by an infusion of 4 mcg/kg/minute continued for at least 2 hours or for the duration of the PCI, whichever is longer.
Transitioning patients to oral $P2Y_{12}$ antagonist therapy:
Conversion to clopidogrel: Administer 600 mg of clopidogrel immediately after discontinuing cangrelor infusion. Do not administer clopidogrel prior to cangrelor discontinuation.
Conversion to prasugrel: Administer 60 mg of prasugrel immediately after discontinuing cangrelor infusion. Do not administer prasugrel prior to cangrelor discontinuation.
Conversion to ticagrelor: Administer 180 mg of ticagrelor at any time during cangrelor infusion or immediately after discontinuing cangrelor infusion.
Geriatric Refer to adult dosing
Renal Impairment No dosage adjustment necessary
Hepatic Impairment No dosage adjustment necessary
Administration
IV: Vial must be diluted prior to infusion. Administer via a dedicated IV line.
Obtain bolus volume from the prepared bag and administer rapidly over <1 minute via manual IV push or the infusion pump. Ensure the bolus is completely administered before the start of PCI. Start the infusion immediately after administration of the bolus.
Monitoring Parameters Monitor for signs/symptoms of bleeding.
Dosage Forms Excipient information presented when available (limited, particularly for generics); consult specific product labeling.
Solution Reconstituted, Intravenous:
Kengreal: 50 mg (1 ea)

◆ Cangrelor Tetrasodium *see* Cangrelor *on page 297*
◆ CAPE *see* Capecitabine *on page 297*

Capecitabine (ka pe SITE a been)

Brand Names: US Xeloda
Brand Names: Canada Teva-Capecitabine; Xeloda
Index Terms CAPE
Pharmacologic Category Antineoplastic Agent, Antimetabolite; Antineoplastic Agent, Antimetabolite (Pyrimidine Analog)
Use
Breast cancer, metastatic:
Monotherapy: Treatment of metastatic breast cancer resistant to both paclitaxel and an anthracycline-containing regimen or resistant to paclitaxel in patients for whom further anthracycline therapy is not indicated
Combination therapy: Treatment of metastatic breast cancer (in combination with docetaxel) after failure of a prior anthracycline-containing regimen
Colorectal cancer: First-line treatment of metastatic colorectal cancer when treatment with a fluoropyrimidine alone is preferred; adjuvant therapy of Dukes' C colon cancer after complete resection of the primary tumor when fluoropyrimidine therapy alone is preferred
Pregnancy Considerations Adverse effects were observed in animal reproduction studies. Fetal harm may occur if administered during pregnancy. Women of childbearing potential should use effective contraceptives to avoid pregnancy during treatment.
Breast-Feeding Considerations It is not known if capecitabine is excreted in breast milk. Due to the potential for serious adverse reactions in the nursing infant, the decision to discontinue capecitabine or to discontinue breast-feeding should take into account the importance of treatment to the mother.

◄

Contraindications Known hypersensitivity to capecitabine, fluorouracil, or any component of the formulation; severe renal impairment (CrCl <30 mL/minute)

Warnings/Precautions Hazardous agent - use appropriate precautions for handling and disposal (NIOSH 2014 [group 1]). Bone marrow suppression may occur, hematologic toxicity is more common when used in combination therapy; use with caution; dosage adjustments may be required. Product labeling recommends that patients with baseline platelets <100,000/mm^3 and/or neutrophils <1,500/mm^3 not receive capecitabine therapy and also to withhold for grade 3 or 4 hematologic toxicity during treatment. Patients with certain homozygous or heterozygous mutations of the dihydropyrimidine dehydrogenase (DPD) enzyme are at increased risk for acute early-onset (potentially severe, life-threatening, or fatal) toxicity due to total or near total absence of DPD activity. Toxicity may include mucositis/stomatitis, diarrhea, neutropenia, and neurotoxicity. Patients with partial DPD activity are also at risk for severe, life-threatening, or fatal toxicity. May require therapy interruption or permanent discontinuation, depending on the onset, duration, and severity of toxicity observed. No capecitabine dose has been shown to be safe in patients with complete DPD deficiency; data is insufficient to recommend a dose in patients with partial DPD activity.

Capecitabine may cause diarrhea (may be severe); median time to first occurrence of grade 2 to 4 diarrhea was 34 days; median duration of grades 3 or 4 diarrhea was 5 days. Withhold treatment for grades 2 to 4 diarrhea; subsequent doses should be reduced after grade 3 or 4 diarrhea or recurrence of grade 2 diarrhea. Antidiarrheal therapy (eg, loperamide) is recommended. Necrotizing enterocolitis (typhlitis) has been reported. Dehydration may occur rapidly in patients with diarrhea, nausea, vomiting, anorexia, and/or weakness; adequately hydrate prior to treatment initiation. Elderly patients may be a higher risk for dehydration. **Note:** Canadian labeling recommends treatment interruption for dehydration requiring IV hydration lasting <24 hours and dosage reduction if IV hydration required for ≥24 hours; correct precipitating factors and ensure rehydration prior to resuming therapy.

Hand-and-foot syndrome is characterized by numbness, dysesthesia/paresthesia, tingling, painless or painful swelling, erythema, desquamation, blistering, and severe pain; median onset is 79 days (range: 11 to 360 days). If grade 2 or 3 hand-and-foot syndrome occurs, interrupt administration of capecitabine until decreases to grade 1. Following grade 3 hand-and-foot syndrome, decrease subsequent doses of capecitabine. Stevens-Johnson syndrome and toxic epidermal necrolysis (TEN) have been reported (some fatal); permanently discontinue capecitabine if a severe dermatologic or mucocutaneous reaction occurs. In patients with colorectal cancer, treatment with capecitabine immediately following 6 weeks of fluorouracil/leucovorin (FU/LV) therapy has been associated with an increased incidence of grade ≥3 toxicity, when compared to patients receiving the reverse sequence, capecitabine (two 3-week courses) followed by FU/LV (Hennig, 2008).

Grade 3 and 4 hyperbilirubinemia have been observed in patients with and without hepatic metastases at baseline (median onset: 64 days). Transaminase and alkaline phosphatase elevations have also been reported. If capecitabine-related grade 3 or 4 hyperbilirubinemia occurs, interrupt treatment until bilirubin ≤3 times ULN. Use with caution in patients with mild to moderate hepatic impairment due to liver metastases; effect of severe hepatic impairment has not been studied. Dehydration may occur, resulting in acute renal failure (may be fatal); concomitant use with nephrotoxic agents and baseline renal dysfunction may increase the risk. Use with caution in patients with mild to moderate renal impairment; reduce dose with moderate impairment (exposure to capecitabine and metabolites is increased) and carefully monitor and reduce subsequent dose (with any grade 2 or higher adverse effect) with mild to moderate impairment; use is contraindicated in severe impairment. Use with caution in patients ≥60 years of age, the incidence of treatment-related adverse events may be higher.

Cardiotoxicity has been observed with capecitabine, including myocardial infarction, ischemia, angina, dysrhythmias, cardiac arrest, cardiac failure, sudden death, ECG changes, and cardiomyopathy; may be more common in patients with a history of coronary artery disease. **[US Boxed Warning]: Capecitabine may increase the anticoagulant effects of warfarin; bleeding events, including death, have occurred with concomitant use. Clinically significant increases in prothrombin time (PT) and INR have occurred within several days to months after capecitabine initiation (in patients previously stabilized on anticoagulants), and may continue up to 1 month after capecitabine discontinuation; may occur in patients with or without liver metastases. Monitor PT and INR frequently and adjust anticoagulation dosing accordingly. An increased risk of coagulopathy is correlated with a cancer diagnosis and age >60 years.** Other potentially significant drug-drug interactions may exist, requiring dose or frequency adjustment, additional monitoring, and/or selection of alternative therapy.

An investigational uridine prodrug, uridine triacetate (formerly called vistonuridine), has been studied in a limited number of cases of fluoropyrimidine overdose. Of 17 patients receiving uridine triacetate beginning within 8 to 96 hours after fluorouracil overdose, all patients fully recovered (von Borstel, 2009). Updated data has described a total of 28 patients treated with uridine triacetate for fluorouracil overdose (including overdoses related to continuous infusions delivering fluorouracil at rates faster than prescribed), all of whom recovered fully (Bamat, 2010). An additional case report describes accidental capecitabine ingestion by a 22 month old child; uridine triacetate was initiated approximately 7 hours after exposure. The patient received uridine triacetate every 6 hours for a total of 20 doses through nasogastric tube administration; he was asymptomatic throughout his course and was discharged with normal laboratory values (Kanie, 2011). Refer to Uridine Triacetate monograph.

Adverse Reactions Frequency listed derived from monotherapy trials. Incidence reported for all indications and usage, unless otherwise noted. Frequency not always defined.

>10%:

Cardiovascular: Edema (≤15%)

Central nervous system: Fatigue (≤42%), paresthesia (stage IV breast cancer: 21%; grades 3/4: 1%), pain (≤12%)

Dermatologic: Palmar-plantar erythrodysesthesia (54% to 60%; grades ≥3: 11% to 17%), dermatitis (27% to 37%, grades ≥3: 1%)

Gastrointestinal: Diarrhea (47% to 57%, grades 3/4: 2% to 13%), nausea (34% to 43%; stage IV breast cancer: 53%), vomiting (metastatic colorectal cancer, stage IV breast cancer: 27% to 37%; Dukes' C colon cancer: 15%), abdominal pain (metastatic colorectal cancer: 35%; stage IV breast cancer: 20%; Dukes' C colon cancer: 14%), decreased appetite (26%), stomatitis (22% to 25%), anorexia (stage IV breast cancer: 23%; Dukes' C colon cancer: 9%), constipation (9% to 15%)

Hematologic & oncologic: Lymphocytopenia (stage IV breast cancer: 94%; stage IV breast cancer, grades 3/4: 15% to 44%), anemia (72% to 80%, grades 3/4: ≤3%), neutropenia (≤26%, grades 3/4: ≤3%), thrombocytopenia (stage IV breast cancer: 24%; all: grades 3/4: 1% to 3%)

Hepatic: Hyperbilirubinemia (Metastatic colorectal cancer: 48%; stage IV breast cancer: 22%; all: grades 3/4: 2% to 23%)

Neuromuscular & skeletal: Weakness (≤42%)

Ophthalmic: Eye irritation (13% to 15%)

Miscellaneous: Fever (7% to 18%)

1% to 10%:

Cardiovascular: Venous thrombosis (8%), chest pain (≤6%), atrial fibrillation (<5%), bradycardia (<5%), collapse (<5%), extrasystoles (<5%), pericardial effusion (<5%), ventricular premature contractions (<5%), angina pectoris, cardiac arrest, cardiac arrhythmia, cardiac failure, cardiomyopathy, ECG changes, ischemic heart disease, myocardial infarction

Central nervous system: Lethargy (10%), peripheral sensory neuropathy (10%), headache (5% to 10%), insomnia (≤8%), dizziness (6% to 8%), ataxia (<5%), depression (≤5%), mood changes (5%), abnormal gait (<5%), brain disease (<5%), dysarthria (<5%), dysphasia (<5%), equilibrium disturbance (<5%), irritability (<5%), myasthenia (<5%), sedation (<5%), vertigo (<5%)

Dermatologic: Nail disease (≤7%), skin discoloration (7%), skin rash (7%), alopecia (6%), erythema (6%), dermal ulcer (<5%), pruritus (<5%)

Endocrine & metabolic: Dehydration (7%), hot flash (<5%), hypokalemia (<5%), hypomagnesemia (<5%), increased thirst (<5%), weight gain (<5%), decreased serum calcium (Dukes' C colon cancer: grades 3/4: 2%), increased serum calcium (Dukes' C colon cancer: grades 3/4: 1%)

Gastrointestinal: Gastrointestinal motility disorder (10%), GI inflammation (upper: 8%), oral discomfort (grades 3/4: 10%), dyspepsia (6% to 8%), upper abdominal pain (7%), intestinal obstruction (≤6%), dysgeusia (6%), gastrointestinal hemorrhage (6%), abdominal distention (<5%), dysphagia (<5%), rectal pain (<5%), toxic dilation of intestine (<5%), increased serum alanine

aminotransferase (Dukes' C colon cancer: grades 3/4: 2%), sore throat (2%), necrotizing enterocolitis

Hematologic & oncologic: Hemorrhage (<5%), lymphedema (<5%), granulocytopenia (Dukes' C colon cancer: grades 3/4: 3%), immune thrombocytopenia (1%)

Hepatic: Abnormal hepatic function tests (<5%)

Hypersensitivity: Drug-induced hypersensitivity (<5%)

Infection: Viral infection (metastatic colorectal cancer: 5%)

Neuromuscular & skeletal: Back pain (10%), myalgia (≤9%), arthralgia (8%), limb pain (stage IV breast cancer: 6%), tremor (<5%)

Ophthalmic: Visual disturbance (metastatic colorectal cancer: 5%), conjunctivitis (≤5%), keratoconjunctivitis (<5%)

Respiratory: Cough (≤7%), chest mass (<5%), dyspnea (<5%), flu-like symptoms (<5%), hemoptysis (<5%), hoarseness (<5%), pharyngeal disease (metastatic colorectal cancer: 5%), epistaxis (≤3%), laryngitis (1%)

<1% (limited to important or life-threatening): Acute renal failure, ascites, blood coagulation disorder, bronchitis, bronchospasm, cachexia, cerebrovascular accident, cholestatic hepatitis, confusion, cutaneous lupus erythematosus, ecchymoses, esophagitis, fibrosis, fungal infection, gastric ulcer, gastroenteritis, gastrointestinal perforation, hemorrhage, hepatic failure, hepatic fibrosis, hepatitis, hypersensitivity, hypertension, hypertriglyceridemia, hypotension, keratitis, lacrimal stenosis, leukoencephalopathy, loss of consciousness, myocarditis, nocturia, ostealgia, pancytopenia, phlebitis (venous), photophobia, pneumonia, pulmonary embolism, radiation recall phenomenon, respiratory distress, sepsis, Stevens-Johnson syndrome, syncope, tachycardia, toxic epidermal necrolysis

Drug Interactions

Metabolism/Transport Effects Inhibits CYP2C9 (strong)

Avoid Concomitant Use

Avoid concomitant use of Capecitabine with any of the following: BCG (Intravesical); Deferiprone; Dipyrone; Gimeracil; Natalizumab; Pimecrolimus; Tacrolimus (Topical); Tofacitinib; Vaccines (Live)

Increased Effect/Toxicity

Capecitabine may increase the levels/effects of: Bosentan; Carvedilol; CloZAPine; CYP2C9 Substrates; Deferiprone; Diclofenac (Systemic); Dronabinol; Fingolimod; Fosphenytoin; Lacosamide; Leflunomide; Natalizumab; Ospemifene; Parecoxib; Phenytoin; Ramelteon; Tetrahydrocannabinol; Tofacitinib; Vaccines (Live); Vitamin K Antagonists

The levels/effects of Capecitabine may be increased by: Cannabis; Cimetidine; Denosumab; Dipyrone; Gimeracil; Leucovorin Calcium-Levoleucovorin; MetroNIDAZOLE (Systemic); Pimecrolimus; Roflumilast; Tacrolimus (Topical); Trastuzumab

Decreased Effect

Capecitabine may decrease the levels/effects of: BCG (Intravesical); Coccidioides immitis Skin Test; Sipuleucel-T; Vaccines (Inactivated); Vaccines (Live)

The levels/effects of Capecitabine may be decreased by: Echinacea

Food Interactions Food reduced the rate and extent of absorption of capecitabine. Management: Administer within 30 minutes after a meal.

Storage/Stability Store at room temperature of 25°C (77°F); excursions permitted between 15°C and 30°C (59°F and 86°F). Keep bottle tightly closed.

Mechanism of Action Capecitabine is a prodrug of fluorouracil. It undergoes hydrolysis in the liver and tissues to form fluorouracil which is the active moiety. Fluorouracil is a fluorinated pyrimidine antimetabolite that inhibits thymidylate synthetase, blocking the methylation of deoxyuridylic acid to thymidylic acid, interfering with DNA, and to a lesser degree, RNA synthesis. Fluorouracil appears to be phase specific for the G_1 and S phases of the cell cycle.

Pharmacodynamics/Kinetics

Absorption: Rapid and extensive (rate and extent reduced by food)

Protein binding: <60%; ~35% to albumin

Metabolism:

Hepatic: Inactive metabolites: 5'-deoxy-5-fluorocytidine, 5'-deoxy-5-fluorouridine

Tissue: Enzymatically metabolized to fluorouracil, which is then metabolized to active metabolites, 5-fluoroxyuridine monophosphate (F-UMP) and 5-5-fluoro-2'-deoxyuridine-5'-O-monophosphate (F-dUMP)

Half-life elimination: ~0.75 hour

Time to peak: 1.5 hours; Fluorouracil: 2 hours

Excretion: Urine (96%, 57% as α-fluoro-β-alanine; <3% as unchanged drug); feces (<3%)

Dosing

Adult

Breast cancer, metastatic: Oral: 1,250 mg/m² twice daily for 2 weeks, every 21 days (as either monotherapy or in combination with docetaxel)

Breast cancer, metastatic (off-label dosing): Oral: 1,000 mg/m² twice daily (in combination with ixabepilone) on days 1 to 14 of a 3-week cycle until disease progression or unacceptable toxicity (Thomas, 2007)

Breast cancer, metastatic, HER2+ (off-label dosing): Oral: 1,000 mg/m² twice daily (in combination with lapatinib) on days 1 to 14 of a 3-week cycle until disease progression or unacceptable toxicity (Geyer, 2006) or 1,250 mg/m² twice daily (in combination with trastuzumab) on days 1 to 14 of a 3-week cycle (Bartsch, 2007)

Breast cancer, metastatic, HER2+ with brain metastases, first-line therapy (off-label dosing): Oral: 1,000 mg/m2 twice daily (in combination with lapatinib) on days 1 to 14 of a 3-week cycle until disease progression or unacceptable toxicity (Bachelot, 2012)

Colorectal cancer, metastatic: Oral: 1,250 mg/m² twice daily for 2 weeks, every 21 days. **Note:** Capecitabine toxicities, particularly hand-foot syndrome, may be higher in North American populations; therapy initiation at doses of 1,000 mg/m² twice daily (for 2 weeks every 21 days) may be considered (Haller, 2008).

Colorectal cancer (off-label dosing): Oral: 1,000 mg/m² twice daily (in combination with oxaliplatin) on days 1 to 14 of a 3-week cycle for 8 or 16 cycles (Cassidy, 2008; Haller, 2011; Schmoll, 2007)

Dukes' C colon cancer, adjuvant therapy: Oral: 1,250 mg/m² twice daily for 2 weeks, every 21 days, for a recommended total duration of 24 weeks (8 cycles of 2 weeks of drug administration and 1 week rest period).

Esophageal and gastric cancers (off-label uses): Oral:

Preoperative or definitive chemoradiation: 800 mg/m² twice daily (in combination with cisplatin and radiation) on days 1 to 5 weekly for 5 weeks (Lee, 2007) or 625 mg/m² twice daily (in combination with oxaliplatin and radiation) on days 1 to 5 weekly for 5 weeks (Javle, 2009)

Postoperative chemoradiation: 625 to 825 mg/m² twice daily during radiation therapy (Lee, 2006)

Locally advanced or metastatic (chemoradiation not indicated): 1,000 to 1,250 mg/m² twice daily (monotherapy or in combination with cisplatin with or without trastuzumab) on days 1 to 14 of a 3-week cycle (Bang, 2010; Hong, 2004; Kang, 2009) or 625 mg/m² twice daily (in combination with epirubicin and cisplatin or oxaliplatin) on days 1 to 21 of a 3-week cycle for up to 8 cycles (Cunningham, 2008; Sumpter, 2005)

Hepatobiliary cancers, advanced (off-label use): Oral: 650 mg/m² twice daily (in combination with gemcitabine) on days 1 to 14 of a 3-week cycle (Knox, 2005) or 1,000 mg/m² twice daily (in combination with oxaliplatin) on days 1 to 14 of a 3-week cycle (Nehls, 2008) or 1,250 mg/m² twice daily (in combination with cisplatin) on days 1 to 14 of a 3-week cycle (Kim, 2003); all regimens continued until disease progression or unacceptable toxicity

Neuroendocrine (pancreatic/islet cell) tumors, metastatic or unresectable (off label use): Oral: 750 mg/m² twice daily (in combination with temozolomide) on days 1 to 14 of a 4-week cycle (Strosberg, 2011)

Ovarian, fallopian tube, or peritoneal cancer, platinum-refractory (off label use): Oral: 1,000 mg/m² twice daily on days 1 to 14 of a 3-week cycle until disease progression or unacceptable toxicity (Wolf, 2006)

Pancreatic cancer, metastatic (off-label use): Oral: 1,250 mg/m² twice daily on days 1 to 14 of a 3-week cycle (Cartwright, 2002) or 830 mg/m² twice daily (in combination with gemcitabine) on days 1 to 21 of a 4-week cycle until disease progression or unacceptable toxicity (Cunningham, 2009)

Unknown primary cancer (off-label use): Oral: 1,000 mg/m² twice daily (in combination with oxaliplatin) on days 1 to 14 of a 3-week cycle for up to 6 cycles or until disease progression (Hainsworth, 2010) or 800 mg/m² twice daily (in combination with carboplatin and gemcitabine) on days 1 to 14 of a 3-week cycle for up to 8 cycles or until disease progression or unacceptable toxicity (Schneider, 2007)

Geriatric The elderly may be more sensitive to the toxic effects of fluorouracil. Insufficient data are available to provide dosage modifications.

Renal Impairment Note: Renal function may be estimated using the Cockcroft-Gault formula for dosage adjustment purposes.

Renal impairment at treatment initiation:
CrCl ≥51 mL/minute: Initial: No dosage adjustment necessary.
CrCl 30 to 50 mL/minute: Initial: Administer 75% of usual dose (Cassidy, 2002; Poole, 2002; Xeloda prescribing information, 2015)
CrCl <30 mL/minute: Use is contraindicated (Poole, 2002; Xeloda prescribing information, 2015)
Renal toxicity during treatment: Refer to Dosage Adjustment for Toxicity.

Hepatic Impairment
Hepatic impairment at treatment initiation:
Mild to moderate impairment: No starting dose adjustment necessary (Ecklund, 2005; Superfin, 2007); however, carefully monitor patients.
Severe hepatic impairment: There are no dosage adjustments provided in the manufacturer's labeling (has not been studied).
Hepatotoxicity during treatment: Hyperbilirubinemia, grade 3 or 4: Interrupt treatment until bilirubin ≤3 times ULN; refer to Dosage Adjustment for Toxicity for dosage recommendations.

Obesity *ASCO Guidelines for appropriate chemotherapy dosing in obese adults with cancer:* Utilize patient's actual body weight (full weight) for calculation of body surface area- or weight-based dosing, particularly when the intent of therapy is curative; manage regimen-related toxicities in the same manner as for nonobese patients; if a dose reduction is utilized due to toxicity, consider resumption of full weight-based dosing with subsequent cycles, especially if cause of toxicity (eg, hepatic or renal impairment) is resolved (Griggs, 2012).

Adjustment for Toxicity See table (**Note:** Capecitabine dosing recommendations apply to both monotherapy and when used in combination therapy with docetaxel).

Monitor carefully for toxicity and adjust dose as necessary. Doses reduced for toxicity should not be increased at a later time. For combination therapy, also refer to docetaxel product labeling for docetaxel dose modifications. If treatment delay is required for either capecitabine or docetaxel, withhold both agents until appropriate to resume combination treatment.

Recommended Capecitabine Dose Modifications

Toxicity Grades	During a Course of Therapy	Dose Adjustment for Next Cycle (% of starting dose)
Grade 1	Maintain dose level	Maintain dose level
Grade 2		
1st appearance	Interrupt until resolved to grade 0 or 1	100%
2nd appearance	Interrupt until resolved to grade 0 or 1	75%
3rd appearance	Interrupt until resolved to grade 0 or 1	50%
4th appearance	Discontinue treatment permanently	
Grade 3		
1st appearance	Interrupt until resolved to grade 0 or 1	75%
2nd appearance	Interrupt until resolved to grade 0 or 1	50%
3rd appearance	Discontinue treatment permanently	
Grade 4		
1st appearance	Discontinue permanently	
	or	
	If in the patient's best interest to continue, interrupt until resolved to grade 0 to 1	50%

Dosage adjustments for hematologic toxicity in combination therapy with ixabepilone:
Neutrophils <500/mm^3 for ≥7 days or neutropenic fever: Hold for concurrent diarrhea or stomatitis until neutrophils recover to >1000/mm^3, then continue at same dose
Platelets <25,000/mm^3 (or <50,000/mm^3 with bleeding): Hold for concurrent diarrhea or stomatitis until platelets recover to >50,000/mm^3, then continue at same dose

Administration Usually administered in 2 divided doses taken 12 hours apart. Doses should be taken with water within 30 minutes after a meal. Swallow tablets whole; do not cut or crush.

Hazardous agent; use appropriate precautions for handling and disposal (NIOSH 2014 [group 1]). If it is necessary to manipulate the tablets (eg, to prepare an oral solution), it is recommended to double glove, wear a protective gown, and prepare in a controlled device (NIOSH, 2014).

Monitoring Parameters Renal function should be estimated at baseline to determine initial dose. During therapy, CBC with differential, hepatic function, and renal function should be monitored. Monitor INR closely if receiving concomitant warfarin. Monitor for diarrhea, dehydration, hand-foot syndrome, Stevens-Johnson syndrome, toxic epidermal necrolysis, stomatitis, and cardiotoxicity.

Dosage Forms Excipient information presented when available (limited, particularly for generics); consult specific product labeling.
Tablet, Oral:
Xeloda: 150 mg, 500 mg
Generic: 150 mg, 500 mg

Extemporaneous Preparations Hazardous agent: Use appropriate precautions for handling and disposal (NIOSH 2014 [group 1]). When manipulating tablets, NIOSH recommends double gloving, a protective gown, and preparation in a controlled device; if not prepared in a controlled device, respiratory and eye protection as well as ventilated engineering controls are recommended (NIOSH, 2014).

A 10 mg/mL oral solution may be made with tablets. Crush four 500 mg tablets in a mortar and reduce to a fine powder; add to 200 mL water. Capecitabine tablets are water soluble (data on file from Roche). Administer immediately after preparation, 30 minutes after a meal.
Judson IR, Beale PJ, Trigo JM, et al, "A Human Capecitabine Excretion Balance and Pharmacokinetic Study After Administration of a Single Oral Dose of ^{14}C-Labelled Drug," *Invest New Drugs*, 1999, 17 (1):49-56.

◆ **Capex** *see* Fluocinolone (Topical) *on page 781*
◆ **Capex® (Can)** *see* Fluocinolone (Topical) *on page 781*
◆ **Capital/Codeine** *see* Acetaminophen and Codeine *on page 28*
◆ **Capmist DM [OTC]** *see* Guaifenesin, Pseudoephedrine, and Dextromethorphan *on page 864*
◆ **Capoten** *see* Captopril *on page 300*
◆ **Capozide** *see* Captopril and Hydrochlorothiazide *on page 303*
◆ **Caprelsa** *see* Vandetanib *on page 1873*

Captopril (KAP toe pril)

Brand Names: Canada Apo-Capto; Dom-Captopril; Mylan-Captopril; PMS-Captopril
Index Terms Capoten
Pharmacologic Category Angiotensin-Converting Enzyme (ACE) Inhibitor; Antihypertensive
Additional Appendix Information
Hypertension *on page 1996*
Use
Diabetic nephropathy: Treatment of diabetic nephropathy (proteinuria more than 500 mg daily) in patients with type 1 insulin-dependent diabetes mellitus and retinopathy
Heart failure: Treatment of congestive heart failure
Hypertension: Management of hypertension
Left ventricular dysfunction after myocardial infarction: To improve survival following myocardial infarction in clinically stable patients with left ventricular dysfunction manifested as an ejection fraction of 40% or less, and to reduce the incidence of overt heart failure and subsequent hospitalizations for congestive heart failure in these patients.

Guideline recommendations:
Heart failure: The American College of Cardiology Foundation/American Heart Association (ACCF/AHA) 2013 heart failure guidelines recommend the use of angiotensin-converting enzyme (ACE) inhibitors, along with other guideline directed medical therapies, to prevent heart failure in patients with a reduced ejection fraction who have a history of myocardial infarction (stage B heart failure), to prevent heart failure in any patient with a reduced ejection fraction (stage B heart failure), or to treat those with heart failure and reduced ejection fraction (stage C heart failure) (Yancy, 2013).
Hypertension: The 2014 guideline for the management of high blood pressure in adults (Eighth Joint National Committee [JNC 8]) recommends initiation of pharmacologic treatment to lower blood pressure for the following patients:
• Patients ≥60 years of age with systolic blood pressure (SBP) ≥150 mm Hg or diastolic blood pressure (DBP) ≥90 mm Hg. Goal of therapy is SBP <150 mm Hg and DBP <90 mm Hg.

• Patients <60 years of age with SBP ≥140 mm Hg or DBP is ≥90 mm Hg. Goal of therapy is SBP <140 mm Hg and DBP <90 mm Hg.

• Patients ≥18 years of age with diabetes and SBP ≥140 mm Hg or DBP ≥90 mm Hg. Goal of therapy is SBP <140 mm Hg and DBP <90 mm Hg.

• Patients ≥18 years of age with chronic kidney disease (CKD) and SBP ≥140 mm Hg or DBP ≥90 mm Hg. Goal of therapy is SBP <140 mm Hg and DBP <90 mm Hg.

Chronic kidney disease (CKD) and hypertension: Regardless of race or diabetes status, the use of an ACE inhibitor (ACEI) or angiotensin receptor blocker (ARB) as initial therapy is recommended to improve kidney outcomes. In the general nonblack population (without CKD) including those with diabetes, initial antihypertensive treatment should consist of a thiazide-type diuretic, calcium channel blocker, ACEI, or ARB. In the general black population (without CKD) including those with diabetes, initial antihypertensive treatment should consist of a thiazide-type diuretic or a calcium channel blocker **instead of** an ACEI or ARB.

Coronary artery disease (CAD) and hypertension: The American Heart Association, American College of Cardiology and American Society of Hypertension (AHA/ACC/ASH) 2015 scientific statement for the treatment of hypertension in patients with CAD recommends the use of an ACE inhibitor (or an ARB) as part of a regimen in patients with hypertension and chronic stable angina if there is prior MI, LV systolic dysfunction, diabetes mellitus, or CKD. A BP target of <140/90 mm Hg is reasonable for the secondary prevention of cardiovascular events. A lower target BP (<130/80 mm Hg) may be appropriate in some individuals with CAD, previous MI, stroke or transient ischemic attack, or CAD risk equivalents (AHA/ACC/ASH [Rosendorff 2015]).

STEMI: The 2013 American College of Cardiology Foundation/American Heart Association guidelines for the management of patients with ST-elevation myocardial infarction (STEMI) states that an ACE inhibitor (eg, captopril) should be initiated within the first 24 hours after STEMI in patients with anterior MI, heart failure, or left ventricular ejection fraction ≤40%. It is also reasonable to initiate an ACE inhibitor in all patients with STEMI (ACCF/AHA [O'Gara, 2013]).

Pregnancy Considerations [U.S. Boxed Warning]: Drugs that act on the renin-angiotensin system can cause injury and death to the developing fetus. Discontinue as soon as possible once pregnancy is detected. Captopril crosses the placenta (Hurault de Lingy 1987). Drugs that act on the renin-angiotensin system are associated with oligohydramnios. Oligohydramnios, due to decreased fetal renal function, may lead to fetal lung hypoplasia and skeletal malformations. Their use in pregnancy is also associated with anuria, hypotension, renal failure, skull hypoplasia, and death in the fetus/neonate. Teratogenic effects may occur following maternal use of an ACE inhibitor during the first trimester, although this finding may be confounded by maternal disease. Because adverse fetal events are well documented with exposure later in pregnancy, ACE inhibitor use in pregnant women is not recommended (Seely 2014; Weber 2014). Infants exposed to an ACE inhibitor in utero should be monitored for hyperkalemia, hypotension, and oliguria. Oligohydramnios may not appear until after irreversible fetal injury has occurred. Exchange transfusions or dialysis may be required to reverse hypotension or improve renal function, although data related to the effectiveness in neonates is limited.

Chronic maternal hypertension itself is also associated with adverse events in the fetus/infant and mother. ACE inhibitors are not recommended for the treatment of uncomplicated hypertension in pregnancy (ACOG 2013) and they are specifically contraindicated for the treatment of hypertension and chronic heart failure during pregnancy by some guidelines (Regitz-Zagrosek 2011). In addition, ACE inhibitors should generally be avoided in women of reproductive age (ACOG 2013). If treatment for hypertension or chronic heart failure in pregnancy is needed, other agents should be used (ACOG 2013; Regitz-Zagrosek 2011).

Breast-Feeding Considerations Captopril is excreted in breast milk. According to the manufacturer, the decision to continue or discontinue breast-feeding during therapy should take into account the risk of exposure to the infant and the benefits of treatment to the mother. Some guidelines consider captopril to be acceptable for use in breast-feeding women. Monitoring of the nursing child's weight for the first 4 weeks is recommended (Regitz-Zagrosek 2011).

Contraindications Hypersensitivity to captopril, any other ACE inhibitor, or any component of the formulation; angioedema related to previous treatment with an ACE inhibitor; concomitant use with aliskiren in patients with diabetes mellitus

Warnings/Precautions Anaphylactic reactions may occur rarely with ACE inhibitors. At any time during treatment (especially following first dose) angioedema may occur rarely with ACE inhibitors; may involve the head and neck (potentially compromising airway) or the intestine (presenting with abdominal pain). African-Americans and patients with idiopathic or hereditary angioedema may be at an increased risk. Risk may also be increased with concomitant use of mTOR inhibitor (eg, everolimus) therapy. Prolonged frequent monitoring may be required especially if tongue, glottis, or larynx are involved as they are associated with airway obstruction. Patients with a history of airway surgery may have a higher risk of airway obstruction. Aggressive early and appropriate management is critical. Use in patients with previous angioedema associated with ACE inhibitor therapy is contraindicated. Severe anaphylactoid reactions may be seen during hemodialysis (eg, CVVHD) with high-flux dialysis membranes (eg, AN69), and rarely, during low density lipoprotein apheresis with dextran sulfate cellulose. Rare cases of anaphylactoid reactions have been reported in patients undergoing sensitization treatment with hymenoptera (bee, wasp) venom while receiving ACE inhibitors.

Symptomatic hypotension with or without syncope can occur with ACE inhibitors (usually with the first several doses); effects are most often observed in volume depleted patients; close monitoring of patient is required especially with initial dosing and dosing increases; blood pressure must be lowered at a rate appropriate for the patient's clinical condition. Initiation of therapy in patients with ischemic heart disease or cerebrovascular disease warrants close observation due to the potential consequences posed by falling blood pressure (eg, MI, stroke). Use with caution in hypertrophic cardiomyopathy with outflow tract obstruction and severe aortic stenosis. In patients on chronic ACE inhibitor therapy, intraoperative hypotension may occur with induction and maintenance of general anesthesia; use with caution before, during, or immediately after major surgery. Cardiopulmonary bypass, intraoperative blood loss, or vasodilating anesthesia increases endogenous renin release. Use of ACE inhibitors perioperatively will blunt angiotensin II formation and may result in hypotension. However, discontinuation of therapy prior to surgery is controversial. If continued preoperatively, avoidance of hypotensive agents during surgery is prudent (Hillis, 2011). Extemporaneous preparations of liquid formulations may vary; this may affect the rate and extent of absorption causing intrapatient variability regarding dosing and safety profile for the patient; use with caution and monitor closely if dosage formulations are changed (Bhatt, 2011; Mulla, 2007). **[U.S. Boxed Warning]: Drugs that act on the renin-angiotensin system can cause injury and death to the developing fetus. Discontinue as soon as possible once pregnancy is detected.**

Hyperkalemia may occur with ACE inhibitors; risk factors include renal dysfunction, diabetes mellitus, concomitant use of potassium-sparing diuretics, potassium supplements and/or potassium containing salts. Use cautiously, if at all, with these agents and monitor potassium closely. Cough may occur with ACE inhibitors. Other causes of cough should be considered (eg, pulmonary congestion in patients with heart failure) and excluded prior to discontinuation.

May be associated with deterioration of renal function and/or increases in BUN and serum creatinine, particularly in patients with low renal blood flow (eg, renal artery stenosis, heart failure) whose glomerular filtration rate (GFR) is dependent on efferent arteriolar vasoconstriction by angiotensin II; deterioration may result in oliguria, acute renal failure, and progressive azotemia. Small benign increases in serum creatinine may occur following initiation; consider discontinuation only in patients with progressive and/or significant deterioration in renal function (Bakris, 2000). Use with caution in patients with unstented unilateral/bilateral renal artery stenosis. When unstented bilateral renal artery stenosis is present, use is generally avoided due to the elevated risk of deterioration in renal function unless possible benefits outweigh risks. ACE inhibitors effectiveness is less in black patients than in non-blacks. In addition, ACE inhibitors cause a higher rate of angioedema in black than in non-black patients. Potentially significant drug-drug interactions may exist, requiring dose or frequency adjustment, additional monitoring, and/or selection of alternative therapy.

Rare toxicities associated with ACE inhibitors include cholestatic jaundice (which may progress to fulminant hepatic necrosis, some fatal), agranulocytosis, neutropenia with myeloid hypoplasia; anemia and thrombocytopenia have also occurred. If neutropenia develops (neutrophil count <1,000/mm^3), discontinue therapy. Patients with collagen vascular diseases (especially with concomitant renal impairment) or renal impairment alone may be at increased risk for hematologic toxicity; closely monitor CBC with differential for the first 3 months of therapy and periodically thereafter in these patients. Total urinary proteins greater than 1 g per day have been reported (<1%); nephrotic syndrome occurred in about one-fifth of proteinuric patients. In most cases, proteinuria subsided or cleared within six months (whether or not captopril was continued).

Adverse Reactions

Frequency not defined:

Cardiovascular: Angina pectoris, cardiac arrest, cardiac arrhythmia, cardiac failure, flushing, myocardial infarction, orthostatic hypotension, Raynaud's phenomenon, syncope

Central nervous system: Ataxia, cerebrovascular insufficiency, confusion, depression, drowsiness, myasthenia, nervousness

Dermatologic: Bullous pemphigoid, erythema multiforme, exfoliative dermatitis, pallor, Stevens-Johnson syndrome

Endocrine & metabolic: Gynecomastia, hyponatremia (symptomatic)

Gastrointestinal: Cholestasis, dyspepsia, glossitis, pancreatitis

Genitourinary: Impotence, nephrotic syndrome, oliguria, urinary frequency

Hematologic & oncologic: Agranulocytosis, anemia, pancytopenia, thrombocytopenia

Hepatic: Hepatic necrosis (rare), hepatitis, increased serum alkaline phosphatase, increased serum bilirubin, increased serum transaminases, jaundice

Hypersensitivity: Anaphylactoid reaction, angioedema

Neuromuscular & skeletal: Myalgia, weakness

Ophthalmic: Blurred vision

Renal: Polyuria, renal failure, renal insufficiency

Respiratory: Bronchospasm, eosinophilic pneumonitis, rhinitis

1% to 10%:

Cardiovascular: Hypotension (1% to 3%), chest pain (1%), palpitations (1%), tachycardia (1%)

Dermatologic: Skin rash (maculopapular or urticarial [4% to 7%]; in patients with rash, a positive ANA and/or eosinophilia has been noted in 7% to 10%), pruritus (2%)

Endocrine & metabolic: Hyperkalemia (1% to 11%)

Gastrointestinal: Dysgeusia (2% to 4%; loss of taste or diminished perception)

Genitourinary: Proteinuria (1%)

Hematologic & oncologic: Neutropenia (≤4%; in patients with renal insufficiency or collagen-vascular disease)

Hypersensitivity: Hypersensitivity reaction (rash, pruritus, fever, arthralgia, and eosinophilia: 4% to 7%; depending on dose and renal function)

Renal: Increased serum creatinine, renal insufficiency (worsening; may occur in patients with bilateral renal artery stenosis or hypovolemia)

Respiratory: Cough (<1% to 2%)

Miscellaneous: Hypersensitivity reactions (rash, pruritus, fever, arthralgia, and eosinophilia) have occurred in 4% to 7% of patients (depending on dose and renal function); dysgeusia - loss of taste or diminished perception (2% to 4%)

<1% (Limited to important or life-threatening): Alopecia, angina pectoris, anorexia, aphthous stomatitis, aplastic anemia, cholestatic jaundice, eosinophilia, glomerulonephritis, Guillain-Barre syndrome, hemolytic anemia, Huntington's chorea (exacerbation), hyperthermia, increased erythrocyte sedimentation rate, insomnia, interstitial nephritis, Kaposi's sarcoma, peptic ulcer, pericarditis, psoriasis, seizure (in premature infants), systemic lupus erythematosus, vasculitis, visual hallucination (Doane, 2013)

Drug Interactions

Metabolism/Transport Effects Substrate of CYP2D6 (major); **Note:** Assignment of Major/Minor substrate status based on clinically relevant drug interaction potential

Avoid Concomitant Use

Avoid concomitant use of Captopril with any of the following: Sacubitril

Increased Effect/Toxicity

Captopril may increase the levels/effects of: Allopurinol; Amifostine; Antipsychotic Agents (Second Generation [Atypical]); AzaTHIOprine; Ciprofloxacin (Systemic); Drospirenone; DULoxetine; Ferric Gluconate; Gold Sodium Thiomalate; Grass Pollen Allergen Extract (5 Grass Extract); Hypotension-Associated Agents; Iron Dextran Complex; Levodopa; Lithium; Nonsteroidal Anti-Inflammatory Agents; Pregabalin; Sacubitril; Sodium Phosphates

The levels/effects of Captopril may be increased by: Abiraterone Acetate; Alfuzosin; Aliskiren; Angiotensin II Receptor Blockers; Barbiturates; Brimonidine (Topical); Canagliflozin; Cobicistat; CYP2D6 Inhibitors (Moderate); CYP2D6 Inhibitors (Strong); Dapoxetine; Darunavir; Diazoxide; DPP-IV Inhibitors; Eplerenone; Everolimus; Heparin; Heparin (Low Molecular Weight); Herbs (Hypotensive Properties); Loop Diuretics; Molsidomine; Nicorandil; Obinutuzumab; Panobinostat; Peginterferon Alfa-2b; Pentoxifylline; Phosphodiesterase 5 Inhibitors; Potassium Salts; Potassium-Sparing Diuretics; Prostacyclin Analogues; Salicylates; Sirolimus; Temsirolimus; Thiazide Diuretics; TiZANidine; Tolvaptan; Trimethoprim

Decreased Effect

The levels/effects of Captopril may be decreased by: Amphetamines; Antacids; Aprotinin; Herbs (Hypertensive Properties); Icatibant; Lanthanum; Methylphenidate; Nonsteroidal Anti-Inflammatory Agents; Peginterferon Alfa-2b; Salicylates; Yohimbine

Food Interactions Captopril serum concentrations may be decreased if taken with food. Long-term use of captopril may lead to a zinc deficiency which can result in altered taste perception. Management: Take on an empty stomach 1 hour before or 2 hours after meals.

Storage/Stability Store at 20°C to 25°C (68°F to 77°F); protect from moisture.

Mechanism of Action Competitive inhibitor of angiotensin-converting enzyme (ACE); prevents conversion of angiotensin I to angiotensin II, a potent vasoconstrictor; results in lower levels of angiotensin II which causes an increase in plasma renin activity and a reduction in aldosterone secretion

Pharmacodynamics/Kinetics

Onset of action: Within 15 minutes; Peak effect: Blood pressure reduction: 1 to 1.5 hours after dose

Maximum effect: Antihypertensive: 60-90 minutes; may require several weeks of therapy before full hypotensive effect is seen

Duration: Dose related, may require several weeks of therapy before full hypotensive effect

Absorption: 60% to 75%; rapid

Distribution: V_{dss}: 0.7 L/kg (Duchun, 1982)

Bioavailability: ~60% to 75% (Cody, 1985); reduced 30% to 40% by food

Protein binding: 25% to 30%

Metabolism: 50% metabolized

Half-life elimination:

Infants with CHF: 3.3 hours; range: 1.2 to 12.4 hours (Pereira 1991)

Children: 1.5 hours; range: 0.98 to 2.3 hours (Levy 1991)

Adults, healthy volunteers: ~1.7 hours (Duchin 1982). In two studies, patients with chronic renal failure demonstrated approximately 2-fold longer half-lives as compared to normal subjects (Giudicelli 1984; Onoyama 1981). Half-life was up to 21 hours in patients with severe renal impairment and up to 32 hours in patients on chronic hemodialysis in another study (Duchin 1984)

Time to peak: Within 1 to 2 hours

Excretion: Urine (>95%) within 24 hours (40% to 50% as unchanged drug)

Dosing

Adult Note: Titrate dose according to patient's response; use lowest effective dose.

Acute hypertension (urgency/emergency): Oral, sublingual: 25 mg, may repeat as needed; consider alternative therapy if blood pressure is nonresponsive within 20 to 30 minutes (Angeli, 1991; Castro del Castillo, 1988; Ceyhan, 1990; Damasceno, 1997; Tschollar, 1985). **Note:** May be given sublingually, but therapeutic advantage has not been demonstrated over oral administration (Karakilic, 2012).

Heart failure with reduced ejection fraction (HFrEF) (ACCF/AHA [Yancy, 2013]): Oral:

Initial dose: 6.25 mg 3 times daily

Target dose: 50 mg 3 times daily

Hypertension: Oral: Initial dose: 25 mg 2 to 3 times daily (a lower initial dose of 12.5 mg 3 times daily may also be considered [VA Cooperative Study Group, 1984]); may increase at 1- to 2-week intervals up to 50 mg 3 times daily; add thiazide diuretic, unless severe renal impairment coexists then consider loop diuretic, before further dosage increases or consider other treatment options; maximum dose: 150 mg 3 times daily

Target dose (JNC 8 [James, 2013]): 75 to 100 mg twice daily

Usual dose range (7ASH/ISH [Weber, 2014]): 50 to 100 mg twice daily

LV dysfunction following MI: Oral: Initial: 6.25 mg; if tolerated, follow with 12.5 mg 3 times daily; then increase to 25 mg 3 times daily during next several days and then gradually increase over next several weeks to target dose of 50 mg 3 times daily (some dose schedules are more aggressive to achieve an increased goal dose within the first few days of initiation). **Note:** In those patients with STEMI in the anterior location, heart failure, or LV ejection fraction ≤0.4, an ACE inhibitor (eg, captopril) should be initiated within the first 24 hours after MI (ACCF/AHA [O'Gara, 2013]).

Diabetic nephropathy: Oral: Initial: 25 mg 3 times daily. May be taken with other antihypertensive therapy if required to further lower blood pressure.

Geriatric Refer to adult dosing. In the management of hypertension, consider lower initial doses and titrate to response (Aronow, 2011).

Pediatric Note: Titrate dose according to patient's response; use lowest effective dose.

Hypertension: Children ≤1 year and Adolescents ≤17 years: Oral: Initial: 0.3 to 0.5 mg/kg/dose every 8 hours; titrate upward to maximum of 6 mg/kg/day in 2 to 4 divided doses (NHBPEP, 2004; NHLBI, 2011); maximum daily dose: 450 mg daily.

Renal Impairment
Manufacturers recommendations: Reduce initial daily dose and titrate slowly (1- to 2-week intervals) with smaller increments. Slowly back titrate to determine the minimum effective dose once the desired therapeutic effect has been reached.

Alternative recommendations (Aronoff, 2007):
Adults:
CrCl 10 to 50 mL/minute: Administer at 75% of normal dose every 12-18 hours.
CrCl <10 mL/minute: Administer at 50% of normal dose every 24 hours.
Intermittent hemodialysis (IHD): Administer after hemodialysis on dialysis days
Peritoneal dialysis: Dose for CrCl 10-50 mL/minute; supplemental dose is not necessary
Infants, Children, and Adolescents: **Note:** Renally adjusted dose recommendations are based on doses of 0.1 to 0.5 mg/kg/dose every 6 to 8 hours; maximum daily dose: 6 mg/kg/day.
GFR 10 to 50 mL/minute/1.73 m^2: Administer 75% of dose
GFR <10 mL/minute/1.73 m^2: Administer 50% of dose
Intermittent hemodialysis: Administer 50% of dose
Peritoneal dialysis (PD): Administer 50% of dose

Hepatic Impairment There are no dosage adjustments provided in the manufacturer's labeling (has not been studied).

Dietary Considerations Should be taken at least 1 hour before eating.

Administration Administer at least 1 hour before meals. Unstable in aqueous solutions; to prepare solution for oral administration, mix prior to administration and use within 10 minutes (Allen, 1996).

Monitoring Parameters BUN, electrolytes, serum creatinine; blood pressure. In patients with renal impairment and/or collagen vascular disease, closely monitor CBC with differential for the first 3 months of therapy and periodically thereafter.

2013 ACCF/AHA Heart Failure guideline recommendations: Within 1-2 weeks after initiation and periodically thereafter, reassess renal function and serum potassium especially in patients with preexisting hypotension, hyponatremia, diabetes mellitus, azotemia, or those taking potassium supplements (ACCF/AHA [Yancy, 2013]).

Test Interactions Positive Coombs' [direct]; may cause false-positive results in urine acetone determinations using sodium nitroprusside reagent

Dosage Forms Excipient information presented when available (limited, particularly for generics); consult specific product labeling.
Tablet, Oral:
Generic: 12.5 mg, 25 mg, 50 mg, 100 mg

Dosage Forms: Canada Note: Also refer to Dosage Forms. Excipient information presented when available (limited, particularly for generics); consult specific product labeling.
Tablet, Oral: 6.25 mg

Extemporaneous Preparations A 1 mg/mL oral solution may be made by allowing two 50 mg tablets to dissolve in 50 mL of distilled water. Add the contents of one 500 mg sodium ascorbate injection ampul or one 500 mg ascorbic acid tablet and allow to dissolve. Add quantity of distilled water sufficient to make 100 mL. Label "shake well" and "refrigerate". Stable for 56 days refrigerated.
Nahata MC, Pai VB, and Hipple TF, *Pediatric Drug Formulations*, 5th ed, Cincinnati, OH: Harvey Whitney Books Co, 2004.

Captopril and Hydrochlorothiazide (KAP toe pril & hye droe klor oh THYE a zide)

Index Terms Capozide; Hydrochlorothiazide and Captopril
Pharmacologic Category Angiotensin-Converting Enzyme (ACE) Inhibitor; Antihypertensive; Diuretic, Thiazide
Use Management of hypertension
Dosing
Adult & Geriatric Hypertension, CHF: May be substituted for previously titrated dosages of the individual components; alternatively, may initiate as follows: Oral: Initial: Captopril 25 mg and hydrochlorothiazide 15 mg once daily; titrate to response; may administer in one or more divided doses. Maximum daily dose: Captopril 150 mg and hydrochlorothiazide 50 mg.
Renal Impairment Reduce initial daily dose and titrate slowly (1- to 2-week intervals) with smaller increments. Slowly back titrate to determine the minimum effective dose once the desired therapeutic effect has been reached. Hydrochlorothiazide is contraindicated in patients with anuria.
Hepatic Impairment There are no dosage adjustments provided in the manufacturer's labeling. Use with caution; hydrochlorothiazide may precipitate hepatic coma.
Additional Information Complete prescribing information should be consulted for additional detail.
Dosage Forms Excipient information presented when available (limited, particularly for generics); consult specific product labeling.
Tablet, oral: 25/15: Captopril 25 mg and hydrochlorothiazide 15 mg; 25/25: Captopril 25 mg and hydrochlorothiazide 25 mg; 50/15: Captopril 50 mg and hydrochlorothiazide 15 mg; 50/25: Captopril 50 mg and hydrochlorothiazide 25 mg

- ◆ Carac *see* Fluorouracil (Topical) *on page 786*
- ◆ Carafate *see* Sucralfate *on page 1704*

Carbachol (KAR ba kole)

Brand Names: US Isopto Carbachol; Miostat
Brand Names: Canada Isopto® Carbachol; Miostat®
Index Terms Carbacholine; Carbamylcholine Chloride
Pharmacologic Category Cholinergic Agonist; Ophthalmic Agent, Antiglaucoma; Ophthalmic Agent, Miotic
Use Lowers intraocular pressure in the treatment of glaucoma; cause miosis during surgery
Dosing
Adult & Geriatric
Glaucoma: Ophthalmic: Instill 1-2 drops up to 3 times/day
Ophthalmic surgery (miosis): Intraocular: 0.5 mL instilled into anterior chamber before or after securing sutures
Renal Impairment No dosage adjustment provided in manufacturer's labeling.
Hepatic Impairment No dosage adjustment provided in manufacturer's labeling.
Additional Information Complete prescribing information should be consulted for additional detail.
Dosage Forms Excipient information presented when available (limited, particularly for generics); consult specific product labeling.
Solution, Intraocular:
Miostat: 0.01% (1.5 mL)
Solution, Ophthalmic:
Isopto Carbachol: 1.5% (15 mL); 3% (15 mL)

- ◆ Carbacholine *see* Carbachol *on page 303*
- ◆ Carbaglu *see* Carglumic Acid *on page 317*

CarBAMazepine (kar ba MAZ e peen)

Brand Names: US Carbatrol; Epitol; Equetro; TEGretol; TEGretol-XR
Brand Names: Canada Apo-Carbamazepine; Dom-Carbamazepine; Mapezine; Mylan-Carbamazepine CR; Nu-Carbamazepine; PMS-Carbamazepine; Sandoz-Carbamazepine; Taro-Carbamazepine Chewable; Tegretol; Teva-Carbamazepine
Index Terms CBZ; SPD417
Pharmacologic Category Anticonvulsant, Miscellaneous
Use
Carbatrol, Tegretol, Tegretol-XR: Partial seizures with complex symptomatology (psychomotor, temporal lobe), generalized tonic-clonic seizures (grand mal), mixed seizure patterns, trigeminal neuralgia, glossopharyngeal neuralgia

Equetro: Acute manic or mixed episodes associated with bipolar 1 disorder

Pregnancy Considerations Studies in pregnant women have demonstrated a risk to the fetus. Carbamazepine and its metabolites can be found in the fetus and may be associated with teratogenic effects, including spina bifida, craniofacial defects, cardiovascular malformations, and hypospadias. The risk of teratogenic effects is higher with anticonvulsant polytherapy than monotherapy.

Developmental delays have also been observed following *in utero* exposure to carbamazepine (per manufacturer); however, socioeconomic factors, maternal and paternal IQ, and polytherapy may contribute to these findings. Pregnancy may cause small decreases of carbamazepine plasma concentrations in the second and third trimesters; monitoring should be considered. When used for the treatment of bipolar disorder, use of carbamazepine should be avoided during the first trimester of pregnancy if possible. The use of a single medication for the treatment of bipolar disorder or epilepsy in pregnancy is preferred. Carbamazepine may decrease plasma concentrations of hormonal contraceptives; breakthrough bleeding or unintended pregnancy may occur and alternate or back-up methods of contraception should be considered.

Patients exposed to carbamazepine during pregnancy are encouraged to enroll themselves into the AED Pregnancy Registry by calling 1-888-233-2334. Additional information is available at www.aedpregnancyregistry.org.

Breast-Feeding Considerations Carbamazepine and its active epoxide metabolite are found in breast milk. Carbamazepine can also be detected in the serum of nursing infants. Transient hepatic dysfunction has been observed in some case reports. Nursing should be discontinued if adverse events are observed. According to the manufacturer, the decision to continue or discontinue breast-feeding during therapy should take into account the risk of exposure to the infant and the benefits of treatment to the mother. Respiratory depression, seizures, nausea, vomiting, diarrhea, and/or decreased feeding have been observed in neonates exposed to carbamazepine *in utero* and may represent a neonatal withdrawal syndrome.

Medication Guide Available Yes

Contraindications Hypersensitivity to carbamazepine, tricyclic antidepressants, or any component of the formulation; bone marrow depression; with or within 14 days of MAO inhibitor use; concurrent use of nefazodone; concomitant use of delavirdine or other non-nucleoside reverse transcriptase inhibitors

Warnings/Precautions Hazardous agent - use appropriate precautions for handling and disposal (NIOSH 2014 [group 2]).

[US Boxed Warning]: The risk of developing aplastic anemia or agranulocytosis is increased during treatment. Monitor CBC, platelets, and differential prior to and during therapy; discontinue if significant bone marrow suppression occurs. A spectrum of hematologic effects has been reported with use (eg, agranulocytosis, aplastic anemia, neutropenia, leukopenia, thrombocytopenia, pancytopenia, and anemias); patients with a previous history of adverse hematologic reaction to any drug may be at increased risk. Early detection of hematologic change is important; advise patients of early signs and symptoms including fever, sore throat, mouth ulcers, infections, easy bruising, and petechial or purpuric hemorrhage.

[US Boxed Warning]: Severe and sometimes fatal dermatologic reactions, including toxic epidermal necrolysis (TENS) and Stevens-Johnson syndrome (SJS), may occur during therapy. The risk is increased in patients with the variant *HLA-B*1502* allele, found almost exclusively in patients of Asian ancestry. Patients of Asian descent should be screened prior to initiating therapy. Avoid use in patients testing positive for the allele; discontinue therapy in patients who have a serious dermatologic reaction. The risk of SJS or TENS may also be increased if carbamazepine is used in combination with other antiepileptic drugs associated with these reactions. Presence of the *HLA-B*1502* allele has not been found to predict the risk of less serious dermatologic reactions such as anticonvulsant hypersensitivity syndrome or nonserious rash. The risk of developing a hypersensitivity reaction may be increased in patients with the variant *HLA-A*3101* allele. These hypersensitivity reactions include SJS/TEN, maculopapular eruptions, and drug reaction with eosinophilia and systemic symptoms (DRESS/multiorgan hypersensitivity). The *HLA-A*3101* allele may occur more frequently in patients of African-American, Arabic, Asian, European, Indian, Latin American, and Native American ancestry. Hypersensitivity has also been reported in patients experiencing reactions to other anticonvulsants; the history of hypersensitivity reactions in the patient or their immediate family members should be reviewed. Approximately 25% to 30% of patients allergic to carbamazepine will also have reactions with oxcarbazepine. Potentially serious, sometimes fatal multiorgan hypersensitivity reactions (also known as drug reaction with eosinophilia and systemic symptoms [DRESS]) have been reported with some antiepileptic drugs including carbamazepine; monitor for signs and symptoms of possible disparate manifestations associated with lymphatic, hepatic, renal, and/or hematologic organ systems; gradual discontinuation and conversion to alternate therapy may be required.

Antiepileptics are associated with an increased risk of suicidal behavior/thoughts with use (regardless of indication); patients should be monitored for signs/symptoms of depression, suicidal tendencies, and other unusual behavior changes during therapy and instructed to inform their healthcare provider immediately if symptoms occur.

Administer carbamazepine with caution to patients with history of cardiac damage, ECG abnormalities (or at risk for ECG abnormalities), hepatic or renal disease. Rare cases of a hepatic failure and vanishing bile duct syndrome involving destruction and disappearance of the intrahepatic bile ducts have been reported. Clinical courses of vanishing bile duct syndrome have been variable ranging from fulminant to indolent. Some cases have also had features associated with other immunoallergenic syndromes such as multiorgan hypersensitivity (DRESS syndrome) and serious dermatologic reactions including Stevens-Johnson syndrome. May activate latent psychosis and/or cause confusion or agitation; elderly patients may be at an increased risk for psychiatric effects.

Carbamazepine is not effective in absence, myoclonic, or akinetic seizures; exacerbation of certain seizure types have been seen after initiation of carbamazepine therapy in children with mixed seizure disorders. Abrupt discontinuation is not recommended in patients being treated for seizures. Dizziness or drowsiness may occur; caution should be used when performing tasks which require alertness until the effects are known. Potentially significant interactions may exist, requiring dose or frequency adjustment, additional monitoring, and/or selection of alternative therapy. Carbamazepine has mild anticholinergic activity; use with caution in patients with increased intraocular pressure, or sensitivity to anticholinergic effects. Hyponatremia caused by the syndrome of inappropriate antidiuretic hormone secretion (SIADH) may occur during therapy. Risk may be increased in the elderly or in patients also taking diuretics and may be dose-dependent.

Administration of the suspension will yield higher peak and lower trough serum levels than an equal dose of the tablet form; consider a lower starting dose given more frequently (same total daily dose) when using the suspension. The suspension may contain sorbitol; avoid use in patents with hereditary fructose intolerance.

Adverse Reactions Frequency not defined, unless otherwise specified.

Cardiovascular: Hypertension (3%), aggravation of coronary artery disease, atrioventricular block, cardiac arrhythmia, cardiac failure, edema, hypotension, syncope, thromboembolism, thrombophlebitis

Central nervous system: Dizziness (44%), drowsiness (32%), headache (22%), ataxia (15%), speech disturbance (6%), abnormality in thinking (2%), paresthesia (2%), twitching (2%), vertigo (2%), agitation, amnesia, chills, confusion, depression, fatigue, hallucination, hyperacusis, neuroleptic malignant syndrome (NMS), peripheral neuritis, slurred speech, talkativeness

Dermatologic: Pruritus (8%), skin rash (7%), acute generalized exanthematous pustulosis, alopecia, diaphoresis, dyschromia, erythema multiforme, erythema nodosum, exfoliative dermatitis, onychomadesis, skin photosensitivity, Stevens-Johnson syndrome, toxic epidermal necrolysis, urticaria

Endocrine & metabolic: Abnormal thyroid function test, albuminuria, glycosuria, hypocalcemia, hyponatremia, porphyria, SIADH

Gastrointestinal: Nausea (29%), vomiting (18%), constipation (10%), xerostomia (8%), abdominal pain, anorexia, diarrhea, gastric distress, glossitis, pancreatitis, stomatitis, vanishing bile duct syndrome

Genitourinary: Azotemia, impotence, oliguria, urinary frequency, urinary retention

Hematologic & oncologic: Agranulocytosis, anemia, aplastic anemia, bone marrow depression, eosinophilia, leukocytosis, leukopenia, lymphadenopathy, pancytopenia, purpura, thrombocytopenia

Hepatic: Abnormal hepatic function tests, hepatic failure, hepatitis, jaundice

Hypersensitivity: Hypersensitivity reaction, multi-organ hypersensitivity

Neuromuscular & skeletal: Weakness (8%), tremor (3%), arthralgia, exacerbation of systemic lupus erythematosus, leg cramps, myalgia, osteoporosis

Ophthalmic: Blurred vision (6%), cataract, conjunctivitis, diplopia, increased intraocular pressure, nystagmus, oculomotor disturbance

Otic: Tinnitus

Renal: Increased blood urea nitrogen, renal failure

Respiratory: Dry throat, pneumonia

Miscellaneous: Fever

Postmarketing and/or case reports (Limited to important or life-threatening): Aseptic meningitis, defective spermatogenesis, hepatotoxicity (idiosyncratic) (Chalasani, 2014), hirsutism, lupus-like syndrome, maculopapular rash, paralysis, reduced fertility (male), suicidal ideation

Drug Interactions

Metabolism/Transport Effects Substrate of CYP2C8 (minor), CYP3A4 (major); **Note:** Assignment of Major/Minor substrate status based on clinically relevant drug interaction potential; **Induces** CYP1A2 (strong), CYP2B6 (strong), CYP2C19 (strong), CYP2C8 (strong), CYP2C9 (strong), CYP3A4 (strong), P-glycoprotein, UGT1A1

Avoid Concomitant Use

Avoid concomitant use of CarBAMazepine with any of the following: Abiraterone Acetate; Antihepaciviral Combination Products; Apixaban; Apremilast; Aprepitant; Artemether; Axitinib; Azelastine (Nasal); BCG (Intravesical); Bedaquiline; Boceprevir; Bortezomib; Bosutinib; Cabozantinib; Cariprazine; Ceritinib; CloZAPine; Cobicistat; Cobimetinib; Conivaptan; Crizotinib; Dabigatran Etexilate; Dabrafenib; Daclatasvir; Deferiprone; Dienogest; Dipyrone; Dronedarone; Eliglustat; Elvitegravir; Enzalutamide; Everolimus; Flibanserin; Fusidic Acid (Systemic); Ibrutinib; Idelalisib; Irinotecan Products; Isavuconazonium Sulfate; Itraconazole; Ivabradine; Ivacaftor; Ixazomib; Lapatinib; Ledipasvir; Lumefantrine; Lurasidone; Macitentan; MAO Inhibitors; Mifepristone; Naloxegol; Nefazodone; Netupitant; NIFEdipine; Nilotinib; NiMODipine; Nintedanib; Nisoldipine; Olaparib; Ombitasvir, Paritaprevir, Ritonavir, and Dasabuvir; Orphenadrine; Osimertinib; Palbociclib; Panobinostat; Paraldehyde; PAZOPanib; Pirfenidone; PONATinib; Praziquantel; Ranolazine; Regorafenib; Reverse Transcriptase Inhibitors (Non-Nucleoside); Rivaroxaban; Roflumilast; RomiDEPsin; Simeprevir; Sofosbuvir; Sonidegib; SORAfenib; Stiripentol; Suvorexant; Tasimelteon; Telaprevir; Thalidomide; Ticagrelor; Tofacitinib; Tolvaptan; Toremifene; Trabectedin; TraMADol; Ulipristal; Vandetanib; Vemurafenib; VinCRIStine (Liposomal); Vorapaxar; Voriconazole

Increased Effect/Toxicity

CarBAMazepine may increase the levels/effects of: Adenosine; Alcohol (Ethyl); Azelastine (Nasal); Buprenorphine; Clarithromycin; ClomiPRAMINE; CloZAPine; CNS Depressants; Cyclophosphamide; Deferiprone; Desmopressin; Eslicarbazepine; Fosphenytoin; Hydrocodone; Lacosamide; Lithium; MAO Inhibitors; Methotrimeprazine; Metyrosine; Orphenadrine; Paraldehyde; Phenytoin; Pramipexole; Rotigotine; Thalidomide

The levels/effects of CarBAMazepine may be increased by: Allopurinol; Brimonidine (Topical); Calcium Channel Blockers (Nondihydropyridine); Cannabis; Carbonic Anhydrase Inhibitors; Cimetidine; Ciprofloxacin (Systemic); Clarithromycin; Conivaptan; CYP3A4 Inhibitors (Moderate); CYP3A4 Inhibitors (Strong); Danazol; Darunavir; Dipyrone; Doxylamine; Dronabinol; Droperidol; Fluconazole; Fusidic Acid (Systemic); Grapefruit Juice; HydrOXYzine; Idelalisib; Isoniazid; Kava Kava; LamoTRIgine; Loxapine; Luliconazole; Macrolide Antibiotics; Magnesium Sulfate; Methotrimeprazine; Minocycline; Nabilone; Nefazodone; Protease Inhibitors; QUEtiapine; QuiNINE; Resveratrol; Selective Serotonin Reuptake Inhibitors; Sodium Oxybate; Stiripentol; Tapentadol; Telaprevir; Tetrahydrocannabinol; Thiazide Diuretics; TraMADol; Valproate Products; Zolpidem

Decreased Effect

CarBAMazepine may decrease the levels/effects of: Abiraterone Acetate; Acetaminophen; Afatinib; Albendazole; Antihepaciviral Combination Products; Apixaban; Apremilast; Aprepitant; ARIPiprazole; ARIPiprazole Lauroxil; Artemether; Axitinib; Bazedoxifene; BCG (Intravesical); Bedaquiline; Bendamustine; Boceprevir; Bortezomib; Bosutinib; Brentuximab Vedotin; Brexpiprazole; Cabozantinib; Calcium Channel Blockers (Dihydropyridine); Calcium Channel Blockers (Nondihydropyridine); Canagliflozin; Cannabidiol; Cannabis; Cariprazine; Caspofungin; Ceritinib; Clarithromycin; CloZAPine; Cobicistat; Cobimetinib; Contraceptives (Estrogens); Contraceptives (Progestins); Corticosteroids (Systemic); Crizotinib; CycloSPORINE (Systemic); CYP1A2 Substrates; CYP2B6 Substrates; CYP2C19 Substrates; CYP2C8 Substrates; CYP2C9 Substrates; CYP3A4 Substrates; Dabigatran Etexilate; Dabrafenib; Daclatasvir; Dasatinib; Dexamethasone (Systemic); Diclofenac (Systemic); Dienogest; Dolutegravir; DOXOrubicin (Conventional); Doxycycline; Dronabinol; Dronedarone; Eliglustat; Elvitegravir; Enzalutamide; Erlotinib; Eslicarbazepine; Etoposide; Etoposide Phosphate; Everolimus; Exemestane; Ezogabine; Felbamate; FentaNYL; Fingolimod; Flibanserin; Flunarizine; Fosphenytoin; Gefitinib; GuanFACINE; Haloperidol; Hydrocortisone (Systemic); Ibrutinib; Idelalisib; Imatinib; Irinotecan Products; Isavuconazonium Sulfate; Itraconazole; Ivabradine; Ivacaftor; Ixabepilone; Ixazomib; Lacosamide; LamoTRIgine; Lapatinib; Ledipasvir; Linagliptin; Lopinavir; Lumefantrine; Lurasidone; Macitentan; Maraviroc; Mebendazole; Methadone; MethylPREDNISolone; Mianserin; Mifepristone; Naloxegol; Nefazodone; Netupitant; NIFEdipine; Nilotinib; NiMODipine; Nintedanib; Nisoldipine; Olaparib; Ombitasvir, Paritaprevir, Ritonavir, and Dasabuvir; Osimertinib; OXcarbazepine; Palbociclib; Paliperidone; Panobinostat; PAZOPanib; Perampanel; P-glycoprotein/ABCB1 Substrates; Phenytoin; Pirfenidone; PONATinib; Praziquantel; PrednisoLONE (Systemic); PredniSONE; Propacetamol; Propafenone; Protease Inhibitors; QUEtiapine; QuiNINE; Ranolazine; Regorafenib; Reverse Transcriptase Inhibitors (Non-Nucleoside); RisperiDONE; Rivaroxaban; Roflumilast; Rolapitant; RomiDEPsin; Rufinamide; Saxagliptin; Selective Serotonin Reuptake Inhibitors; Simeprevir; Sofosbuvir; Sonidegib; SORAfenib; SUNItinib; Suvorexant; Tadalafil; Tasimelteon; Telaprevir; Temsirolimus; Tetrahydrocannabinol; Theophylline Derivatives; Thyroid Products; Ticagrelor; Tofacitinib; Tolvaptan; Topiramate; Toremifene; Trabectedin; TraMADol; Treprostinil; Tricyclic Antidepressants; Ulipristal; Valproate Products; Vandetanib; Vecuronium; Vemurafenib; Vilazodone; VinCRIStine (Liposomal); Vitamin K Antagonists; Vorapaxar; Voriconazole; Vortioxetine; Zaleplon; Ziprasidone; Zolpidem; Zuclopenthixol

The levels/effects of CarBAMazepine may be decreased by: Bosentan; CYP3A4 Inducers (Moderate); CYP3A4 Inducers (Strong); Deferasirox; Felbamate; Fosphenytoin; Mefloquine; Methylfolate; Mianserin; Mitotane; Orlistat; Phenytoin; Reverse Transcriptase Inhibitors (Non-Nucleoside); Rufinamide; Siltuximab; St Johns Wort; Theophylline Derivatives; Tocilizumab; TraMADol

Food Interactions Carbamazepine serum levels may be increased if taken with food and/or grapefruit juice. Management: Avoid concurrent ingestion of grapefruit juice. Maintain adequate hydration, unless instructed to restrict fluid intake.

Storage/Stability

Carbatrol, Equetro: Store at controlled room temperature (25°C [77°F]); excursions permitted to 15°C to 30°C (59°F to 86°F); protect from light and moisture.

Tegretol-XR: Store at controlled room temperature, 15°C to 30°C (59°F to 86°F); protect from moisture.

Tegretol tablets and chewable tablets: Store at ≤30°C (86°F); protect from light and moisture.

Tegretol suspension: Store at ≤30°C (86°F); shake well before using.

Mechanism of Action In addition to anticonvulsant effects, carbamazepine has anticholinergic, antineuralgic, antidiuretic, muscle relaxant, antimanic, antidepressive, and antiarrhythmic properties; may depress activity in the nucleus ventralis of the thalamus or decrease synaptic transmission or decrease summation of temporal stimulation leading to neural discharge by limiting influx of sodium ions across cell membrane or other unknown mechanisms; stimulates the release of ADH and potentiates its action in promoting reabsorption of water; chemically related to tricyclic antidepressants

Pharmacodynamics/Kinetics

Absorption: Slowly from the GI tract

Distribution: V_d: Neonates: 1.5 L/kg; Children: 1.9 L/kg; Adults: 0.59 to 2 L/kg; carbamazepine and its active epoxide metabolite distribute into breast milk

Protein binding: Carbamazepine: 75% to 90%, bound to alpha$_1$-acid glycoprotein and nonspecific binding sites on albumin; may be decreased in newborns; Epoxide metabolite: 50%

Metabolism: Induces liver enzymes to increase metabolism and shorten half-life over time; metabolized in the liver by cytochrome P450 3A4 to active epoxide metabolite; epoxide metabolite is metabolized by epoxide hydrolase to the trans-diol metabolite; ratio of serum epoxide to carbamazepine concentrations may be higher in patients receiving polytherapy (vs monotherapy) and in infants (vs older children); boys may have faster carbamazepine clearances and may, therefore, require higher mg/kg/day doses of carbamazepine compared to girls of similar age and weight

Bioavailability: Oral: 75% to 85%; relative bioavailability of extended release tablet to suspension: 89%

Half-life elimination: **Note:** Half-life is variable because of autoinduction which is usually complete 3 to 5 weeks after initiation of a fixed carbamazepine regimen.

Carbamazepine: Initial: 25 to 65 hours; Extended release: 35 to 40 hours; Multiple doses: Children: 8 to 14 hours; Adults: 12 to 17 hours

Epoxide metabolite: Initial: 34 ± 9 hours

Time to peak, serum: Unpredictable:

Immediate release: Multiple doses: Suspension: 1.5 hour; tablet: 4 to 5 hours

Extended release: Carbatrol, Equetro: 12 to 26 hours (single dose), 4 to 8 hours (multiple doses); Tegretol-XR: 3 to 12 hours

Excretion: Urine 72% (1% to 3% as unchanged drug); feces (28%)

Dosing

Adult & Geriatric Dosage must be adjusted according to patient's response and serum concentrations. Administer tablets (chewable or conventional) in 2-3 divided doses daily and suspension in 4 divided doses daily.

Epilepsy: Oral: Initial: 400 mg/day in 2 divided doses (tablets or extended release tablets) or 4 divided doses (oral suspension); increase by up to 200 mg/day at weekly intervals using a twice daily regimen of extended release tablets or capsules, or a 3-4 times/day regimen of other formulations until optimal response and therapeutic levels are achieved; usual dose: 800-1200 mg/day

Maximum recommended dose: 1600 mg/day; however, some patients have required up to 1.6-2.4 g/day

Trigeminal or glossopharyngeal neuralgia: Oral: Initial: 200 mg/day in 2 divided doses (tablets, extended release tablets, or extended release capsules) or 4 divided doses (oral suspension) with food, gradually increasing in increments of 200 mg/day as needed.

Maintenance: Usual: 400-800 mg daily in 2 divided doses (tablets, extended release tablets, or extended release capsules) or 4 divided doses (oral suspension); maximum dose: 1200 mg/day

Bipolar disorder: Oral: Initial: 400 mg/day in 2 divided doses (tablets, extended release tablets, or extended release capsules) or 4 divided doses (oral suspension), may adjust by 200 mg/day increments; maximum dose: 1600 mg/day.

Note: Equetro® is the only formulation specifically approved by the FDA for the management of bipolar disorder.

Neuropathic pain, critically-ill patients (off-label use): Oral: Initial: 50-100 mg twice daily in combination with IV opioids; Maintenance: 100-200 mg every 4-6 hours; maximum dose: 1200 mg daily (Barr 2013)

Pediatric Dosage must be adjusted according to patient's response and serum concentrations. Administer tablets (chewable or conventional) in 2-3 divided doses daily and suspension in 4 divided doses daily.

Epilepsy: Oral:

Children <6 years: Initial: 10-20 mg/kg/day divided twice or 3 times daily as tablets or 4 times/day as suspension; increase dose every week until optimal response and therapeutic levels are achieved

Maintenance dose: Divide into 3-4 doses daily (tablets or suspension); maximum recommended dose: 35 mg/kg/day

Children 6-12 years: Initial: 200 mg/day in 2 divided doses (tablets or extended release tablets) or 4 divided doses (oral suspension); increase by up to 100 mg/day at weekly intervals using a twice daily regimen of extended release tablets or 3-4 times daily regimen of other formulations until optimal response and therapeutic levels are achieved

Maintenance: Usual: 400-800 mg/day; maximum recommended dose: 1000 mg/day

Note: Children <12 years who receive ≥400 mg/day of carbamazepine may be converted to extended release capsules (Carbatrol) using the same total daily dosage divided twice daily

Children >12 years: Refer to adult dosing.

Maximum recommended doses:

Children 12-15 years: 1000 mg/day

Children >15 years: 1200 mg/day

Renal Impairment Dosage adjustments are not required or recommended in the manufacturer's labeling; however, the following guidelines have been used by some clinicians (Aronoff 2007):

Children and Adults:

GFR <10 mL/minute: Administer 75% of dose

Hemodialysis, peritoneal dialysis: Administer 75% of dose (postdialysis)

Continuous renal replacement therapy (CRRT):

Adults: No dosage adjustment recommended

Children: Administer 75% of dose

Hepatic Impairment Use with caution in hepatic impairment; metabolized primarily in the liver.

Dietary Considerations Drug may cause GI upset, take with large amount of water or food to decrease GI upset. May need to split doses to avoid GI upset.

Administration

Suspension: Must be given on a 3-4 times/day schedule versus tablets which can be given 2-4 times/day. Since a given dose of suspension will produce higher peak and lower trough levels than the same dose given as the tablet form, patients given the suspension should be started on lower doses given more frequently (same total daily dose) and increased slowly to avoid unwanted side effects. When carbamazepine suspension has been combined with chlorpromazine or thioridazine solutions, a precipitate forms which may result in loss of effect. Therefore, it is recommended that the carbamazepine suspension dosage form not be administered at the same time with other liquid medicinal agents or diluents. Should be administered with meals.

Extended release capsule (Carbatrol, Equetro): Consists of three different types of beads: Immediate release, extended-release, and enteric release. The bead types are combined in a ratio to allow twice daily dosing. May be opened and contents sprinkled over food such as a teaspoon of applesauce; may be administered with or without food; do not crush or chew.

Extended release tablet: Should be inspected for damage. Damaged extended release tablets (without release portal) should not be administered. Should be administered with meals; swallow whole, do not crush or chew.

Hazardous agent; use appropriate precautions for handling and disposal (NIOSH 2014 [group 2]).

Monitoring Parameters CBC with platelet count and differential, reticulocytes, serum iron, lipid panel, liver function tests, urinalysis, BUN, serum carbamazepine levels, thyroid function tests, serum sodium; pregnancy test; ophthalmic exams (intraocular pressure, pupillary reflexes); observe patient for excessive sedation, especially when instituting or increasing therapy; signs of rash; *HLA-B*1502* genotype screening prior to therapy initiation in patients of Asian descent; suicidality (eg, suicidal thoughts, depression, behavioral changes)

Reference Range

Timing of serum samples: Absorption is slow, peak levels occur 8-65 hours after ingestion of the first dose; the half-life ranges from 8-60 hours, therefore, steady-state is achieved in 2-5 days

Epilepsy: Therapeutic levels: 4-12 mcg/mL (SI: 17-51 micromole/L)

Toxic concentration: >15 mcg/mL; patients who require higher levels of 8-12 mcg/mL (SI: 34-51 micromole/L) should be watched closely. Side effects including CNS effects occur commonly at higher dosage levels. If other anticonvulsants are given therapeutic range is 4-8 mcg/mL.

Test Interactions May cause false-positive serum TCA screen; may interact with some pregnancy tests

Dosage Forms Excipient information presented when available (limited, particularly for generics); consult specific product labeling. [DSC] = Discontinued product

Capsule Extended Release 12 Hour, Oral:

Carbatrol: 100 mg [contains fd&c blue #2 (indigotine)]

Carbatrol: 200 mg, 300 mg

Equetro: 100 mg, 200 mg, 300 mg [contains fd&c blue #2 (indigotine)]

Generic: 100 mg, 200 mg, 300 mg

Suspension, Oral:

TEGretol: 100 mg/5 mL (450 mL) [contains fd&c yellow #6 (sunset yellow), propylene glycol; citrus-vanilla flavor]

Generic: 100 mg/5 mL (450 mL)

Tablet, Oral:

Epitol: 200 mg [scored]

TEGretol: 200 mg [scored; contains fd&c red #40]

Generic: 200 mg

Tablet Chewable, Oral:

TEGretol: 100 mg [DSC]

Generic: 100 mg

Tablet Extended Release 12 Hour, Oral:

TEGretol-XR: 100 mg, 200 mg, 400 mg

Generic: 200 mg, 400 mg

Extemporaneous Preparations Hazardous agent: Use appropriate precautions for handling and disposal (NIOSH 2014 [group 2]).

Note: Commercial oral suspension is available (20 mg/mL)

A 40 mg/mL oral suspension may be made with tablets. Crush twenty 200 mg tablets in a mortar and reduce to a fine powder. Add small portions of Simple Syrup, NF and mix to a uniform paste; mix while adding the vehicle in incremental proportions to **almost** 100 mL; transfer to a calibrated bottle, rinse mortar with vehicle, and add sufficient quantity of vehicle to make 100 mL. Label "shake well" and "refrigerate". Stable for 90 days.

Nahata MC, Pai VB, and Hipple TF, *Pediatric Drug Formulations,* 5th ed, Cincinnati, OH: Harvey Whitney Books Co, 2004.

◆ **Carbamide** *see* Urea *on page 1853*

Carbamide Peroxide (KAR ba mide per OKS ide)

Brand Names: US Auraphene-B [OTC]; Debrox [OTC]; E-R-O Ear Drops [OTC]; E-R-O Ear Wax Removal System [OTC]; Ear Drops Earwax Aid [OTC]; Ear Wax Remover [OTC] [DSC]; Earwax Treatment Drops [OTC]; Gly-Oxide [OTC]; Oral Peroxide [OTC] [DSC]; Thera-Ear [OTC]

Index Terms Urea Peroxide

Pharmacologic Category Anti-inflammatory, Locally Applied; Otic Agent, Cerumenolytic

Use

Oral: Temporary use in cleansing of canker sore and minor wounds or gum inflammation due to minor dental procedures, dentures, orthodontic appliances, accidental injury, or other irritations of mouth and gums; aids in removal of phlegm, mucus, or other secretions associated with occasional sore mouth.

Otic: Aid to soften, loosen, and remove excessive earwax.

Dosing

Adult & Geriatric

Ear wax removal: Otic: Instill 5 to 10 drops twice daily up to 4 days.

Mouth, gum, or dental irritation: Oral: Use up to 4 times daily after meals and at bedtime. For direct application, place several drops undiluted on affected area then expectorate after 2 to 3 minutes **or** for use as an oral rinse, place 10 to 20 drops onto tongue, mix with saliva, swish for ≥1 minute, then expectorate.

Pediatric

Ear wax removal: Otic:

Children <12 years: Individualize the dose according to patient size; 3 drops (range: 1 to 5 drops) twice daily for up to 4 days.

Children ≥12 years and Adolescents: Refer to adult dosing.

Mouth, gum, or dental irritation: Children ≥2 years and Adolescents: Refer to adult dosing.

Additional Information Complete prescribing information should be consulted for additional detail.

Dosage Forms Excipient information presented when available (limited, particularly for generics); consult specific product labeling. [DSC] = Discontinued product

Solution, Mouth/Throat:

Gly-Oxide: 10% (15 mL, 60 mL) [contains propylene glycol]

Oral Peroxide: 10% (60 mL [DSC])

Solution, Otic:

Auraphene-B: 6.5% (15 mL)

Debrox: 6.5% (15 mL) [contains propylene glycol]

E-R-O Ear Drops: 6.5% (15 mL) [contains glycerin]

E-R-O Ear Wax Removal System: 6.5% (15 mL)

Ear Drops Earwax Aid: 6.5% (15 mL) [contains propylene glycol, trolamine (triethanolamine)]

Ear Wax Remover: 6.5% (15 mL [DSC]) [contains propylene glycol]

Earwax Treatment Drops: 6.5% (15 mL) [contains propylene glycol, trolamine (triethanolamine)]

Thera-Ear: 6.5% (15 mL)

◆ **Carbamylcholine Chloride** *see* Carbachol *on page 303*
◆ **Carbatrol** *see* CarBAMazepine *on page 303*

Carbidopa (kar bi DOE pa)

Brand Names: US Lodosyn

Pharmacologic Category Anti-Parkinson's Agent, Decarboxylase Inhibitor

Use Given with carbidopa-levodopa in the treatment of parkinsonism to enable a lower dosage of levodopa to be used and a more rapid response to be obtained and to decrease side effects; use with carbidopa-levodopa in patients requiring additional carbidopa; has no effect without levodopa

Dosing

Adult & Geriatric Parkinson's disease: Oral: **Note:** Optimal daily dosage determined by careful titration; generally if carbidopa is ≥70 mg/day, a 1:10 proportion of carbidopa:levodopa provides the most patient response.

Carbidopa augmentation in patients receiving carbidopa-levodopa:

Patients receiving Sinemet® 10/100: 25 mg carbidopa daily with first daily dose of Sinemet® 10/100; if necessary, 12.5-25 carbidopa mg may be given with each subsequent dose of Sinemet® 10/100; maximum: 200 mg carbidopa/day (including carbidopa from Sinemet®)

Patients receiving Sinemet® 25/250 or Sinemet® 25/100: 25 mg carbidopa with any dose of Sinemet® 25/250 or Sinemet® 25/100 throughout the day; maximum: 200 mg carbidopa/day (including carbidopa from Sinemet®)

Individual titration of carbidopa and levodopa: Initial: 25 mg carbidopa 3-4 times/day; administer at the same time as levodopa, initial dose of levodopa should be 20% to 25% of the previous levodopa dose in carbidopa-naive patients; first dose of carbidopa should be taken ≥12 hours after the last dose of levodopa in carbidopa-naive patients; increase or decrease dose by 1/2 or 1 tablet/day

Additional Information Complete prescribing information should be consulted for additional detail.

Dosage Forms Excipient information presented when available (limited, particularly for generics); consult specific product labeling. [DSC] = Discontinued product

Tablet, Oral:

Lodosyn: 25 mg [DSC] [contains fd&c yellow #6 (sunset yellow)]

Lodosyn: 25 mg [scored; contains fd&c yellow #6 (sunset yellow)]

Generic: 25 mg

Carbidopa and Levodopa
(kar bi DOE pa & lee voe DOE pa)

Brand Names: US Duopa; Parcopa [DSC]; Rytary; Sinemet; Sinemet CR

Brand Names: Canada Apo-Levocarb; Apo-Levocarb CR; Dom-Levo-Carbidopa; Duodopa; Levocarb CR; PMS-Levocarb CR; PRO-Levocarb; Sinemet; Sinemet CR; Teva-Levocarbidopa

Index Terms Levodopa and Carbidopa

Pharmacologic Category Anti-Parkinson's Agent, Decarboxylase Inhibitor; Anti-Parkinson's Agent, Dopamine Precursor

Additional Appendix Information

Oral Dosages That Should Not Be Crushed *on page 2003*

Use Parkinson disease: Treatment of Parkinson disease, postencephalitic parkinsonism, and symptomatic parkinsonism that may follow carbon monoxide and/or manganese intoxication; treatment of motor fluctuations in advanced Parkinson disease (intestinal suspension [Duopa] only).

Pregnancy Considerations Adverse events have been observed in some animal reproduction studies using this combination. Carbidopa can be detected in the umbilical cord, but absorption in fetal tissue is minimal. Levodopa crosses the placenta and can be metabolized by the fetus and detected in fetal tissue (Merchant, 1995). The incidence of Parkinson disease in pregnancy is relatively rare, and information related to the use of carbidopa/levodopa in pregnant women is limited (Ball, 1995; Cook, 1985; Golbe, 1987; Serikawa, 2011; Shulman, 2000). Current guidelines note that the available information is insufficient to make a recommendation for the treatment of restless legs syndrome in pregnant women (Aurora, 2012).

Breast-Feeding Considerations Levodopa is excreted in breast milk. A study was done in one lactating woman at 4.5 months postpartum who had been taking carbidopa/levodopa for several years. Regardless of the formulation (sustained release or immediate release) peak levodopa concentrations in the breast milk were found ~3 hours after the maternal dose and returned to baseline ~6 hours after the dose. The highest milk concentration (3.47 nmol/L) was found following the immediate-release tablet and this was 27% of the peak maternal plasma concentration (occurring 30 minutes after the dose) and ~40% of the simultaneous plasma concentration. Carbidopa was not evaluated (Thulin, 1998). The manufacturer recommends that caution be exercised when administering carbidopa/levodopa to nursing women.

Prescribing and Access Restrictions Duodopa intestinal gel [Canadian product]: In Canada, the Duodopa Education Program is a risk mitigation program established to provide safe and effective use of Duodopa in advanced Parkinson patients. The program involves:

- Education of prescribing neurologists and other health care providers on suitable candidates for treatment, surgical procedures (PEG tube placement), and follow-up care including infusion device education.

- Distribution of educational materials to patients and care-givers describing Duodopa intestinal gel and its proper use, PEG tube placement, and complications associated with the mode of administration and/or PEG tube placement.

Contraindications

Hypersensitivity to levodopa, carbidopa, or any component of the formulation; concurrent use with nonselective monoamine oxidase inhibitors (MAOIs) or use within the last 14 days

Tablets: Additional contraindications: Narrow angle glaucoma

Canadian labeling: Additional contraindications: Clinical or laboratory evidence of uncompensated cardiovascular, endocrine, hepatic, hematologic or pulmonary disease (eg, including bronchial asthma), or renal disease; when administration of a sympathomimetic amine (eg, epinephrine, norepinephrine, isoproterenol) is contraindicated; in the presence of a suspicious, undiagnosed skin lesion or history of melanoma; intestinal gel therapy in patients with any condition preventing the required placement of a PEG tube for administration (ie, pathological changes of gastric wall, inability to bring gastric and abdominal wall together, blood coagulation disorders, peritonitis, acute pancreatitis, paralytic ileus).

Warnings/Precautions

Use with caution in patients with history of cardiovascular disease (including a history of myocardial infarction who have residual atrial, nodal, or ventricular arrhythmias), pulmonary diseases (such as asthma), psychosis, glaucoma, endocrine disease, and in severe renal and hepatic dysfunction. Use oral products with caution in patients with peptic ulcer disease. Use with caution when interpreting plasma/urine catecholamine levels; falsely diagnosed pheochromocytoma has been rarely reported. Dopaminergic agents have been associated with a syndrome resembling neuroleptic malignant syndrome on abrupt withdrawal, rapid dose reduction, significant dosage reduction after long-term use, or changes in dopaminergic therapy. Avoid sudden discontinuation or rapid dose reduction; taper dose to reduce the risk of hyperpyrexia and confusion. Elderly patients may be more sensitive to CNS effects (eg, hallucinations) of levodopa. May cause or exacerbate dyskinesias. May cause orthostatic hypotension; Parkinson disease patients appear to have an impaired capacity to respond to a postural challenge; use with caution in patients at risk of hypotension (such as those receiving antihypertensive drugs) or where transient hypotensive episodes would be poorly tolerated (cardiovascular disease or cerebrovascular disease). Observe patients closely for development of depression with concomitant suicidal tendencies.

Dopamine agonists have been associated with compulsive behaviors and/or loss of impulse control, which has manifested as pathological gambling, increased sexual urges, intense urges to spend money, binge or compulsive eating; and/or other intense urges. Dose reduction or discontinuation of therapy has been reported to reverse these behaviors in some, but not all cases. Risk for melanoma development is increased in Parkinson disease patients; drug causation or factors contributing to risk have not been established. Patients should be monitored closely and periodic skin examinations should be performed. A symptom complex resembling neuroleptic malignant syndrome (NMS) has been reported in association with rapid dose reduction, or abrupt withdrawal. Identification of more severe NMS-like reactions (eg, altered consciousness, hyperthermia, involuntary movements, muscle rigidity, autonomic instability, mental status changes) can be complex; monitor patients closely for this reaction and when the dosage of levodopa is reduced abruptly or discontinued. Discontinue treatment immediately if signs/symptoms arise. Protein in the diet should be distributed throughout the day to avoid fluctuations in levodopa absorption. A high-protein diet may reduce the effectiveness of the enteral formulations. Urine, saliva, or sweat may appear dark in color (red, brown, black) during therapy.

Abnormal thinking and behavior changes have been reported and may include aggressive behavior, agitation, confusion, delirium, delusions, disorientation, paranoid ideation, and psychotic-like behavior. Hallucinations may occur and be accompanied by confusion and to a lesser extent sleep disorder and excessive dreaming; typically presents shortly after initiation of therapy and may require dose reduction. Somnolence and falling asleep while engaged in activities of daily living (including operation of motor vehicles) have been reported; some cases reported that there were no warning signs for the onset of symptoms. Symptom onset may occur well after initiation of treatment; some events have occurred more than 1 year after start of therapy. Prior to treatment initiation, evaluate for factors that may increase these risks such as concomitant sedating medications, and the presence of sleep disorders. Monitor for drowsiness or sleepiness. If significant daytime sleepiness or episodes of falling asleep during activities that require active participation occurs (eg, driving, conversations, eating), discontinue the medication. There is insufficient information to suggest that dose reductions will eliminate these symptoms. Peripheral neuropathy has been reported with use; prior to initiation, evaluate patients for history of neuropathy and known risk factors (eg, deficiency of vitamin B_6 and/or B_{12}, diabetes mellitus, hypothyroidism). Assess patients for peripheral neuropathy periodically during therapy. Potentially significant interactions may exist, requiring dose or frequency adjustment, additional monitoring, and/or selection of alternative therapy.

Intestinal suspension (Duopa): GI complications (eg, bezoar, ileus, implant site erosion/ulcer, intestinal hemorrhage, intestinal ischemia, intestinal obstruction, intestinal perforation, pancreatitis, peritonitis, pneumoperitoneum, postoperative wound infection) may occur (may be fatal). Patients should notify their health care provider immediately if abdominal pain, prolonged constipation, nausea, vomiting, fever, and/or melanotic stool occur.

Intestinal gel (Duodopa [Canadian product]): Product should be prescribed only by neurologists experienced in the treatment of Parkinson disease and who have completed the Duodopa Education Program. Response to levodopa/carbidopa intestinal gel therapy should be assessed with a short term test period of administration via a temporary nasojejunal tube prior to placement of a percutaneous endoscopic gastrostomy-jejunostomy (PEG-J) tube for permanent access and administration. Sudden deterioration in therapy response with recurring motor symptoms may indicate PEG-J tube complications (eg, displacement) or obstruction of the infusion device. Tube or infusion device complications may require initiation of oral levodopa/carbidopa therapy until complications are resolved.

Adverse Reactions

Frequency not always defined.

Cardiovascular: Orthostatic hypotension (≤73%), peripheral edema (Duopa 8%), hypertension (≤8%), ischemia (≤2%), cardiac arrhythmia, chest pain, edema, flushing, hypotension, myocardial infarction, palpitations, phlebitis, syncope

Central nervous system: Dizziness (6% to 19%), headache (13% to 17%; oral 1% to 5%), depression (with or without suicidal tendencies; Duopa 11%), insomnia (6% to 9%), anxiety (2% to 8%), confusion (2% to 8%), abnormal dreams (2% to 6%), polyneuropathy (Duopa 5%), sleep disorder (Duopa 5%), hallucination (1% to 5%), psychosis (1% to 5%), abnormal behavior, abnormal gait, abnormality in thinking, agitation, ataxia, decreased mental acuity, delirium, delusions, disorientation, drowsiness, euphoria, extrapyramidal reaction, falling, fatigue, glossopyrosis, Horner syndrome (reactivation), impulse control disorder, malaise, memory impairment, narcolepsy, nervousness, neuroleptic malignant syndrome, nightmares, numbness, on-off phenomenon, paranoia, paresthesia, pathological gambling, peripheral neuropathy, seizure (causal relationship not established), trismus

Dermatologic: Excessive granulation tissue (Duopa, 5%), skin rash (≤5%), alopecia, diaphoresis, discoloration of sweat

Endocrine & metabolic: Abnormal alanine aminotransferase, abnormal alkaline phosphatase, abnormal aspartate transaminase, abnormal lactate dehydrogenase, glycosuria, hot flash, hyperglycemia, hypokalemia, increased libido (including hypersexuality), increased uric acid, weight gain, weight loss

Gastrointestinal: Nausea (3% to 30%), constipation (≤22%), hiatal hernia (6% to 8%), xerostomia (7%), intestinal obstruction (Duopa 5%), diarrhea (≤5%), dyspepsia (≤5%), ileus (≤5%), vomiting (≤5%), abdominal distress, abdominal pain, anorexia, bruxism, discoloration of saliva, duodenal ulcer, dysgeusia, dysphagia, flatulence, gastrointestinal hemorrhage, heartburn, hiccups, sialorrhea, sore throat

Genitourinary: Bacteriuria (1% to 5%), difficulty in micturition, priapism, proteinuria, urinary frequency, urinary incontinence, urinary retention, urinary tract infection, urine discoloration

Hematologic & oncologic: Leukocyturia (1% to 5%), agranulocytosis, anemia, decreased hematocrit, decreased hemoglobin, hemolytic anemia, IgA vasculitis, leukopenia, malignant melanoma

Hepatic: Abnormal bilirubin levels

Hypersensitivity: Hypersensitivity reaction (angioedema, bullous lesions [including pemphigus-like reactions], pruritus, urticaria)

Immunologic: Abnormal Coombs test

Local: Erythema at injection site (Duopa 19%), application site discharge (Duopa 11%)

Neuromuscular & skeletal: Dyskinesia (12% to 17%; Rytary 2% to 5%; including choreiform, dystonic and other involuntary movements), increased creatine phosphokinase (≤17%), back pain, excessive tremors, leg pain, muscle cramps, muscle twitching, shoulder pain, weakness

Ophthalmic: Blepharospasm, blurred vision, diplopia, glaucoma, increased intraocular pressure, mydriasis, oculogyric crisis (may be associated with acute dystonic reactions)

Renal: Increased blood urea nitrogen (≤13%)

Respiratory: Atelectasis (Duopa 8%), oropharyngeal pain (Duopa 8%), upper respiratory tract infection (Duopa 8%; Sinemet and Sinemet CR ≤2%), cough, dyspnea, hoarseness

Miscellaneous: Procedural complications (from device insertion: Duopa 57%), fever (≤5%)

Drug Interactions

Metabolism/Transport Effects None known.

Avoid Concomitant Use

Avoid concomitant use of Carbidopa and Levodopa with any of the following: Amisulpride; Sulpiride

Increased Effect/Toxicity

Carbidopa and Levodopa may increase the levels/effects of: Amifostine; BuPROPion; Droxidopa; DULoxetine; MAO Inhibitors

The levels/effects of Carbidopa and Levodopa may be increased by: Alfuzosin; Barbiturates; Blood Pressure Lowering Agents; Brimonidine (Topical); Diazoxide; Herbs (Hypotensive Properties); Methylphenidate; Molsidomine; Nicorandil; Obinutuzumab; Papaverine; Pentoxifylline; Phosphodiesterase 5 Inhibitors; Prostacyclin Analogues; Sapropterin

Decreased Effect

Carbidopa and Levodopa may decrease the levels/effects of: Amisulpride; Antipsychotic Agents (First Generation [Typical]); Droxidopa; Sulpiride

The levels/effects of Carbidopa and Levodopa may be decreased by: Amisulpride; Antipsychotic Agents (First Generation [Typical]); Antipsychotic Agents (Second Generation [Atypical]); Fosphenytoin; Glycopyrrolate; Glycopyrrolate (Systemic); Iron Salts; Isoniazid; Methionine; Metoclopramide; Multivitamins/Fluoride (with ADE); Multivitamins/Minerals (with ADEK, Folate, Iron); Multivitamins/Minerals (with AE, No Iron); Papaverine; Phenytoin; Pyridoxine; Sulpiride

Food Interactions High protein diets have the potential to impair levodopa absorption; levodopa competes with certain amino acids for transport across the gut wall or across the blood-brain barrier. Management: Avoid high protein diets.

Preparation for Administration Intestinal suspension (Duopa): Fully thaw in refrigerator prior to use. To ensure controlled thawing, take the cartons containing the seven individual cassettes out of the transport box and separate the cartons from each other. Assign a 12-week, use-by date based on the time the cartons are put into the refrigerator to thaw (may take up to 96 hours to thaw). Once thawed, the individual cartons may be packed in a closer configuration within the refrigerator. Remove one cassette from refrigerator 20 minutes prior to administration (failure to use at room temperature may result in inaccurate dosage).

Storage/Stability

Oral formulations: Store at 25°C (77°F); excursions permitted between 15°C to 30°C (59°F to 86°F). Protect from light and moisture.

Intestinal suspension (Duopa): Store in freezer at -20°C (-4°F). Fully thaw in refrigerator at 2°C to 8°C (36°F to 46°F) prior to use; protect from light. To ensure controlled thawing, remove the cartons containing the seven individual cassettes from the transport box and separate the cartons from each other. Assign a 12-week, use-by date based on the time the cartons are put in the refrigerator to thaw (may take up to 96 hours to thaw). Once thawed, the individual cartons may be packed in a closer configuration within the refrigerator. Cassettes are for single use only and should be discarded daily following infusion (up to 16 hours). Do not re-use opened cassettes.

Intestinal gel (Duodopa [Canadian product]): Store in refrigerator at 2°C to 8°C (36°F to 46°F). Keep in outer carton to protect from light. Cassettes are for single use only and should be discarded daily following infusion (up to 16 hours).

Mechanism of Action Parkinson disease symptoms are due to a lack of striatal dopamine; levodopa circulates in the plasma to the blood-brain-barrier (BBB), where it crosses, to be converted by striatal enzymes to dopamine; carbidopa inhibits the peripheral plasma breakdown of levodopa by inhibiting its decarboxylation, and thereby increases available levodopa at the BBB

Pharmacodynamics/Kinetics

Absorption: Absorption of levodopa may be decreased with high-fat, high-calorie or high-protein meal.

Distribution: Levodopa: 0.9 to 1.6 L/kg (in presence of carbidopa), crosses the blood-brain barrier; Carbidopa: Does not cross the blood-brain barrier

Metabolism: Levodopa has two major pathways (decarboxylation and O-methylation) and two minor pathways (transamination and oxidation) of metabolism; Carbidopa inhibits the decarboxylation of levodopa to dopamine in the peripheral tissue to allow greater levodopa distribution into the CNS

Bioavailability:

Controlled and extended release: Levodopa: Bioavailability is ~70% to 75% relative to availability from immediate release formulation; Carbidopa: Bioavailability is ~50% to 58% relative to availability from immediate release formulation

Intestinal gel [Canadian product]: Levodopa: Similar bioavailability relative to oral administration of tablet formulations (81% to 98%)

Intestinal suspension: Levodopa: 97% relative to oral immediate release tablets

Half-life elimination: Immediate release: Levodopa (in presence of carbidopa): 1.5 hours; Half-life may be prolonged with controlled and extended release formulations due to continuous absorption

Time to peak: Immediate release: 0.5 hours; Controlled and extended release: 2 hours; Intestinal gel [Canadian product]: Therapeutic plasma levels reached 10 to 30 minutes following morning bolus dose; Intestinal suspension: 2.5 hours

Excretion: Urine

Dosing

Adult & Geriatric

Parkinson disease:

Oral:

Immediate release tablet, orally disintegrating tablet:

Note: Carbidopa/levodopa tablets are available in a 1:4 ratio of carbidopa to levodopa as well as 1:10 ratio. Tablets of the two ratios may be given separately or combined as needed to provide the optimum dosage.

Initial: Carbidopa 25 mg/levodopa 100 mg 3 times daily (preferred) or carbidopa 10 mg/levodopa 100 mg 3 to 4 times daily (typically does not provide an adequate amount of carbidopa for most patients)

Patients previously treated with levodopa <1,500 mg daily: Carbidopa 25 mg/levodopa 100 mg 3 or 4 times daily

Patients previously treated with levodopa >1,500 mg daily: Carbidopa 25 mg/levodopa 250 mg 3 or 4 times daily

Note: Discontinue levodopa at least 12 hours before starting therapy with carbidopa/levodopa. Substitute the combination drug at a dosage that will provide approximately 25% (~20% [Canadian labeling]) of the previous levodopa dosage.

Dosage adjustment: Alternate tablet strengths may be substituted according to individual carbidopa/levodopa requirements. Use of more than 1 dosage strength or dosing 4 times daily may be required (maximum: 8 tablets of any strength daily or 200 mg of carbidopa and 2,000 mg of levodopa)

Carbidopa 10 mg/levodopa 100 mg:

U.S. labeling: Increase by 1 tablet daily or every other day, as necessary, to 2 tablets 4 times daily

Canadian labeling: Increase by 1 tablet every 3 days

Carbidopa 25 mg/levodopa 100 mg:

U.S. labeling: Increase by 1 tablet daily or every other day

Canadian labeling: Increase by 1 tablet every 3 days

Carbidopa 25 mg/levodopa 250 mg:

U.S. labeling: Increase by 1/2 or 1 tablet daily or every other day

Canadian labeling: Increase by 1 tablet every day or every other day

Controlled-release tablet:

Patients not currently receiving levodopa: Initial:

U.S. labeling: Carbidopa 50 mg/levodopa 200 mg 2 times daily, at intervals not <6 hours

Canadian labeling: Carbidopa 25 to 50 mg/levodopa 100 to 200 mg 2 times daily, at intervals not <6 hours; initial dosing should not exceed levodopa 600 mg daily

Patients currently receiving levodopa: **Note:** Discontinue levodopa at least 12 hours (at least 8 hours [Canadian labeling]) before starting carbidopa/levodopa therapy. Initial: Substitute at a dosage that will

provide approximately 25% of the previous levodopa dosage; usual initial dose in mild to moderate disease is carbidopa 50 mg/levodopa 200 mg 2 times daily

Patients converting from immediate-release formulation to controlled release: Initial: Dosage should be substituted at an amount that provides ~10% more of levodopa/day; total calculated dosage is administered in divided doses 2 to 3 times/day (or ≥3 times/day for patients maintained on levodopa ≥700 mg). Intervals between doses should be 4 to 8 hours while awake; when divided doses are not equal, smaller doses should be given toward the end of the day. Depending on clinical response, dosage may need to be increased to provide up to 30% more levodopa/day.

Dosage adjustment: May adjust every 3 days; intervals should be >4 hours during the waking day (maximum dose: 8 tablets/day)

Extended-release capsule: **Note:** Carbidopa/levodopa extended-release capsules are **not** interchangeable with other carbidopa/levodopa products.

Patients not currently receiving levodopa: Initial: Carbidopa 23.75 mg/levodopa 95 mg 3 times daily for 3 days; on day 4, increase to carbidopa 36.25 mg/levodopa 145 mg 3 times daily. May increase dose up to carbidopa 97.5 mg/levodopa 390 mg 3 times a day; frequency of dosing may be increased to a maximum of 5 times daily if needed and tolerated (maximum: carbidopa 612.5 mg/levodopa 2,450 mg per day).

Patients converting from immediate-release formulation to extended-release capsules: Initial: Initial dose based off of total current daily dose of levodopa in immediate-release carbidopa/levodopa as follows (frequency of dosing may be increased to a maximum of 5 times daily if needed and tolerated):

If total daily dose of levodopa is between 400 mg to 549 mg: 3 capsules of carbidopa 23.75 mg/levodopa 95 mg 3 times daily (levodopa total daily dose: 855 mg).

If total daily dose of levodopa is between 550 mg to 749 mg: 4 capsules of carbidopa 23.75 mg/levodopa 95 mg 3 times daily (levodopa total daily dose: 1,140 mg).

If total daily dose of levodopa is between 750 mg to 949 mg: 3 capsules of carbidopa 36.25 mg/levodopa 145 mg 3 times daily (levodopa total daily dose: 1,305 mg).

If total daily dose of levodopa is between 950 mg to 1249 mg: 3 capsules of carbidopa 48.75 mg/levodopa 195 mg 3 times daily (levodopa total daily dose: 1,755 mg).

If total daily dose of levodopa is ≥1,250 mg: 4 capsules of carbidopa 48.75 mg/levodopa 195 mg 3 times daily (levodopa total daily dose: 2,340 mg) or 3 capsules of carbidopa 61.25/levodopa 245 mg 3 times daily (levodopa total daily dose: 2,205 mg).

Dosage adjustment: Adjust dose as needed (maximum dose: carbidopa 612.5 mg/levodopa 2,450 mg per day).

Concomitant therapy: For patients currently treated with carbidopa/levodopa plus catechol-O-methyl transferase (COMT) inhibitors (eg, entacapone), the initial total daily dose of carbidopa/levodopa may need to be increased. Use of carbidopa/levodopa extended-release capsules in combination with other levodopa products has not been studied.

Intestinal infusion via PEG-J tube:

Intestinal suspension (Duopa): Initial: **Note:** Prior to initiation of therapy, convert patients from all forms of levodopa to oral immediate-release carbidopa/levodopa tablets (1:4 ratio). Total daily dose (expressed in terms of levodopa) consists of a morning dose, a continuous dose and extra doses. Maximum dose is 2,000 mg of the levodopa component (ie, one cassette per day) over 16 hours. Patients should receive their routine night-time dosage of oral immediate-release carbidopa/levodopa after discontinuation of daily infusion.

Morning dose and continuous dose: Refer to manufacturer's labeling for morning dose and continuous dose calculations and titration instructions.

Extra doses: Can be used to manage acute "off" symptoms that are not controlled by the morning and continuous dose. Set extra dose function at 1 mL (20 mg of levodopa) initially; adjust in 0.2 mL increments if needed. Maximum: One extra dose every 2 hours. **Note:** Frequent extra doses may cause or worsen dyskinesias.

Discontinuation: Avoid sudden discontinuation or rapid dose reduction; taper dose or switch patients to oral immediate-release carbidopa-levodopa.

Intestinal gel (Duodopa [Canadian product]): **Note:** Conversion to/from oral levodopa tablet formulations and the intestinal gel formulation can be done on a 1:1 ratio. Total daily dose (expressed in terms of levodopa) consists of a morning bolus dose, a continuous maintenance dose, and additional bolus doses when necessary. Nighttime dosing may be necessary in certain rare situations (eg, nocturnal akinesia). Dosage adjustments should be carried out over a period of a few weeks. Patients should receive their routine night-time dosage of oral levodopa/carbidopa after discontinuation of daily infusion

Morning bolus dose:

Day 1: Based on a percentage of the previous morning levodopa intake and volume to fill intestinal tubing:

Previous morning dose of levodopa ≤200 mg: Administer Duodopa at 80% of dose

Previous morning dose of levodopa 201 to 399 mg: Administer Duodopa at 70% of dose

Previous morning dose of levodopa ≥400 mg: Administer Duodopa at 60% of dose

Day 2 and beyond till dose is stable: Adjust dose based on response to the previous morning levodopa intake and volume to fill intestinal tubing): Usual: Levodopa 100 to 200 mg (5 to 10 mL); Maximum: Levodopa 300 mg (15 mL)

Continuous maintenance dose: Adjustable in increments of 2 mg/hour (0.1 mL/hour) and based on previous daily intake of levodopa: Usual: Levodopa 40 to 120 mg/hour (2 to 6 mL/hour) infused up to 16 hours; Range: Levodopa 20 to 200 mg/hour (1 to 10 mL/hour). Higher doses may be necessary in exceptional cases.

Additional bolus doses: Usual: Levodopa: 10 to 40 mg (0.5 to 2 mL), if needed for rapid deterioration of motor functions (eg, hypokinesia); may give additional doses hourly until stable dose is established then give every 2 hours as needed. In patients requiring >5 additional boluses/day, consider increasing the maintenance dose

Restless legs syndrome (RLS) (off-label use; Silber, 2004): Oral:

Immediate-release tablet: Carbidopa 25 mg/levodopa 100 mg (0.5 to 1 tablet) given in the evening, at bedtime, or upon waking during the night with RLS symptoms

Controlled-release tablet: Carbidopa 25 mg/levodopa 100 mg (1 tablet) before bedtime for RLS symptoms that awaken patient during the night

Renal Impairment

U.S. labeling: There are no dosage adjustments provided in the manufacturer's labeling; use with caution.

Canadian labeling: There are no dosage adjustments provided in the manufacturer's labeling; titrate dose cautiously in severe impairment. Use is contraindicated in uncompensated renal disease.

Hepatic Impairment

U.S. labeling: There are no dosage adjustments provided in the manufacturer's labeling; use with caution.

Canadian labeling: There are no dosage adjustments provided in the manufacturer's labeling; titrate dose cautiously in severe impairment. Use is contraindicated in uncompensated hepatic disease.

Adjustment for Toxicity Intestinal suspension (Duopa): Dyskinesias or levodopa-related adverse reactions within 1 hour of morning dose on preceding day: Decrease morning dose by 1 mL.

Dyskinesias or adverse reactions lasting ≥1 hour on the preceding day: Decrease the continuous dose by 0.3 mL per hour.

Dyskinesias or adverse reactions lasting for 2 or more periods of ≥1 hour on the preceding day: Decrease the continuous dose by 0.6 mL per hour.

Dietary Considerations Avoid high protein diets (>2 g/kg) which may decrease the efficacy of levodopa via competition with amino acids in crossing the blood-brain barrier. Some products may contain phenylalanine.

Administration

Intestinal suspension (Duopa): Remove one cassette from refrigerator 20 minutes prior to use (failure to use at room temperature may result in inaccurate dosage). Administer as a 16-hour infusion through either a naso-jejunal tube (temporary administration) or through a percutaneous endoscopic gastrostomy-jejunostomy (PEG-J) tube (long-term administration) connected to the CADD-Legacy 1400 pump. At the end of administration, disconnect the tube from the pump at the end of the infusion and flush with room-temperature drinking water with a

syringe. Following discontinuation of the daily infusion, patients should administer their routine night-time dosage of oral immediate-release carbidopa/levodopa.

Intestinal gel (Duodopa [Canadian product]): Gel is administered directly to the jejunum via a portable infusion pump (CADD-legacy Duodopa pump). Administer through a temporary nasojejunal tube for a short-term test period to evaluate patient response and for dose optimization. Long-term administration requires placement of PEG-J tube for intestinal infusion. Continuous maintenance dose is infused throughout the day for up to 16 hours if necessary, may administer at night (eg, nocturnal akinesia). Disconnect PEG-J tube from infusion pump at end of infusion and flush with room temperature water to prevent occlusion of tubing. Following discontinuation of the daily infusion, patients should administer their routine night-time dosage of oral levodopa/carbidopa.

Extended-release capsule: Administer with or without food; a high-fat, high-calorie meal may delay the absorption of levodopa by ~2 hours. Swallow capsules whole; do not chew, divide, or crush capsules. Patients who have difficulty swallowing intact capsules may open the capsule, sprinkle entire contents on a small amount of applesauce (1 to 2 tablespoons) and consume immediately (do not store for future use).

Oral tablet formulations: Space doses evenly over the waking hours. Administer with meals to decrease GI upset. Controlled release product should not be chewed or crushed. Orally disintegrating tablets do not require water; the tablet should disintegrate on the tongue's surface before swallowing.

Monitoring Parameters Signs and symptoms of Parkinson disease; periodic hepatic function tests, BUN, creatinine, and CBC; periodic skin examinations; blood pressure, standing and sitting/supine; symptoms of dyskinesias, mental status changes; cardiac function (particularly during initial dosage adjustment), IOP (in patients with glaucoma); signs and symptoms of neuroleptic malignant syndrome if abrupt discontinuation required (as with surgery); drowsiness or sleepiness; signs of depression (including suicidal thoughts); signs and symptoms of peripheral neuropathy prior to therapy and periodically during therapy.

Additional Canadian labeling recommendations include vitamin B_{12}, vitamin B_6, folic acid, homocysteine, and methylmalonic acid levels prior to initiation and regularly thereafter (Duodopa Canadian product monograph, 2014).

Test Interactions False-positive reaction for urinary glucose; false-negative reaction using glucose-oxidase tests for glucosuria; false-positive urine ketones; false diagnosis for pheochromocytoma (rare) based on plasma and urine levels of catecholamines

Additional Information To block the peripheral conversion of levodopa to dopamine, ≥70 mg/day of carbidopa is needed. "On-off" (a clinical syndrome characterized by sudden periods of drug activity/inactivity), can be managed by giving smaller, more frequent doses of Sinemet or adding a dopamine agonist or selegiline; when adding a new agent, doses of Sinemet can usually be decreased. Protein in the diet should be distributed throughout the day to avoid fluctuations in levodopa absorption. Levodopa is the drug of choice when rigidity is the predominant presenting symptom.

Conversion from levodopa to carbidopa/levodopa: **Note:** Levodopa must be discontinued at least 12 hours prior to initiation of levodopa/carbidopa:

Initial dose: Levodopa portion of carbidopa/levodopa should be at least 25% of previous levodopa therapy.

Levodopa <1,500 mg/day: Sinemet or Parcopa (levodopa 25 mg/carbidopa 100 mg) 3-4 times/day

Levodopa ≥1,500 mg/day: Sinemet or Parcopa (levodopa 25 mg/carbidopa 250 mg) 3-4 times/day

Conversion from immediate release carbidopa/levodopa (Sinemet or Parcopa) to Sinemet CR (50/200):

Sinemet or Parcopa [total daily dose of levodopa]/Sinemet CR:

Sinemet or Parcopa (levodopa 300-400 mg/day): Sinemet CR (50/200) 1 tablet twice daily

Sinemet or Parcopa (levodopa 500-600 mg/day): Sinemet CR (50/200) 1½ tablets twice daily or 1 tablet 3 times/day

Sinemet or Parcopa (levodopa 700-800 mg/day): Sinemet CR (50/200) 4 tablets in 3 or more divided doses

Sinemet or Parcopa (levodopa 900-1,000 mg/day): Sinemet CR (50/200) 5 tablets in 3 or more divided doses

Intervals between doses of Sinemet CR should be 4-8 hours while awake; when divided doses are not equal, smaller doses should be given toward the end of the day

Dosage Forms Excipient information presented when available (limited, particularly for generics); consult specific product labeling. [DSC] = Discontinued product

Capsule Extended Release, Oral:

Rytary:

23.75/95: Carbidopa 23.75 mg and levodopa 95 mg

36.25/145: Carbidopa 36.25 mg and levodopa 145 mg

48.75/195: Carbidopa 48.75 mg and levodopa 195 mg

61.25/245: Carbidopa 61.25 mg and levodopa 245 mg

Suspension, Enteral:

Duopa: Carbidopa 4.63 mg and levodopa 20 mg per 1 mL (100 mL)

Tablet, Oral:

Sinemet:

10/100: Carbidopa 10 mg and levodopa 100 mg

25/100: Carbidopa 25 mg and levodopa 100 mg

25/250: Carbidopa 25 mg and levodopa 250 mg

Generic: 10/100: Carbidopa 10 mg and levodopa 100 mg; 25/100: Carbidopa 25 mg and levodopa 100 mg; 25/250: Carbidopa 25 mg and levodopa 250 mg

Tablet Extended Release, Oral:

Sinemet CR:

25/100: Carbidopa 25 mg and levodopa 100 mg

50/200: Carbidopa 50 mg and levodopa 200 mg

Generic: 25/100: Carbidopa 25 mg and levodopa 100 mg; 50/200: Carbidopa 50 mg and levodopa 200 mg

Tablet, orally disintegrating:

Parcopa:

10/100: Carbidopa 10 mg and levodopa 100 mg [contains phenylalanine 3.4 mg/tablet; mint flavor] [DSC]

25/100: Carbidopa 25 mg and levodopa 100 mg [contains phenylalanine 3.4 mg/tablet; mint flavor] [DSC]

25/250: Carbidopa 25 mg and levodopa 250 mg [contains phenylalanine 8.4 mg/tablet; mint flavor] [DSC]

Generic: 10/100: Carbidopa 10 mg and levodopa 100 mg; 25/100: Carbidopa 25 mg and levodopa 100 mg; 25/250: Carbidopa 25 mg and levodopa 250 mg

Dosage Forms: Canada Excipient information presented when available (limited, particularly for generics); consult specific product labeling.

Intestinal gel:

Duodopa: Carbidopa 5 mg and levodopa 20 mg/1 mL (100 mL)

Extemporaneous Preparations An oral suspension containing carbidopa 1.25 mg and levodopa 5 mg per mL may be made with tablets. Crush ten tablets each containing carbidopa 25 mg and levodopa 100 mg and reduce to a fine powder. Add small portions of a 1:1 mixture of Ora-Sweet® and Ora-Plus® and mix to a uniform paste; mix while adding the vehicle in equal proportions to almost 200 mL; transfer to a calibrated bottle, rinse mortar with vehicle, and add sufficient quantity of vehicle to make 200 mL. Label "shake well" and "refrigerate". Stable 42 days under refrigeration. Also stable 28 days at room temperature.

Nahata MC, Morosco RS, and Leguire LE, "Development of Two Stable Oral Suspensions of Levodopa-Carbidopa for Children With Amblyopia," *J Pediatr Ophthalmol Strabismus*, 2000, 37(6):333-7.

◆ Carbidopa, Entacapone, and Levodopa see Levodopa, Carbidopa, and Entacapone on page 1060

◆ Carbidopa, Levodopa, and Entacapone see Levodopa, Carbidopa, and Entacapone on page 1060

Carbinoxamine (kar bi NOKS a meen)

Brand Names: US Arbinoxa; Karbinal ER; Palgic [DSC]

Index Terms Carbinoxamine Maleate

Pharmacologic Category Ethanolamine Derivative; Histamine H_1 Antagonist; Histamine H_1 Antagonist, First Generation

Use Allergies: For the symptomatic treatment of seasonal and perennial allergic rhinitis; vasomotor rhinitis; allergic conjunctivitis caused by inhalant allergens and foods; mild, uncomplicated allergic skin manifestations of urticaria and angioedema; dermatographism; as therapy for anaphylactic reactions adjunctive to epinephrine and other standard measures after the acute manifestations have been controlled; amelioration of the severity of allergic reactions to blood or plasma.

Dosing

Adult Allergies: Oral:

Extended release: 6-16 mg every 12 hours.

Immediate release: 4-8 mg 3-4 times daily

Geriatric Use caution and initiate at lower end of dosing range. Refer to adult dosing.

Pediatric Allergies: Oral:

Extended release:

Children 2 to <4 years: 3-4 mg every 12 hours.

Children 4 to <6 years: 3-8 mg every 12 hours.

Children 6 to <12 years: 6-12 mg every 12 hours.

Children ≥12 years and Adolescents: Refer to adult dosing.

Immediate release:

Children 2 to <6 years: 0.2-0.4 mg/kg/day divided into 3-4 doses (weight-based dosing preferred) **or** 1-2 mg 3-4 times daily.

Children 6 to <12 years: 2-4 mg 3-4 times daily.

Children ≥12 years and Adolescents: Refer to adult dosing.

Renal Impairment No dosage adjustment provided in manufacturer's labeling.

Hepatic Impairment No dosage adjustment provided in manufacturer's labeling.

Additional Information Complete prescribing information should be consulted for additional detail.

Dosage Forms Excipient information presented when available (limited, particularly for generics); consult specific product labeling. [DSC] = Discontinued product

Liquid Extended Release, Oral, as maleate:

Karbinal ER: 4 mg/5 mL (480 mL) [contains methylparaben, polysorbate 80, propylparaben, sodium metabisulfite; strawberry-banana flavor]

Solution, Oral, as maleate:

Arbinoxa: 4 mg/5 mL (473 mL) [contains methylparaben, propylene glycol, propylparaben; bubble-gum flavor]

Palgic: 4 mg/5 mL (480 mL [DSC]) [contains methylparaben, propylene glycol, propylparaben; bubble-gum flavor]

Generic: 4 mg/5 mL (118 mL, 473 mL)

Tablet, Oral, as maleate:

Arbinoxa: 4 mg [scored]

Palgic: 4 mg [DSC] [scored]

Generic: 4 mg

CARBOplatin (KAR boe pla tin)

Brand Names: Canada Carboplatin Injection; Carboplatin Injection BP

Index Terms CBDCA; Paraplatin

Pharmacologic Category Antineoplastic Agent, Alkylating Agent; Antineoplastic Agent, Platinum Analog

Use Ovarian cancer: Initial treatment of advanced ovarian cancer in combination with other established chemotherapy agents; palliative treatment of recurrent ovarian cancer after prior chemotherapy, including cisplatin-based treatment

Pregnancy Considerations Embryotoxicity and teratogenicity have been observed in animal reproduction studies. May cause fetal harm if administered during pregnancy. Women of childbearing potential should avoid becoming pregnant during treatment.

Breast-Feeding Considerations It is not known if carboplatin is excreted in breast milk. Due to the potential for toxicity in nursing infants, breast-feeding is not recommended.

Contraindications History of severe allergic reaction to carboplatin, cisplatin, other platinum-containing formulations, mannitol, or any component of the formulation; should not be used in patients with severe bone marrow depression or significant bleeding

Warnings/Precautions Hazardous agent - use appropriate precautions for handling and disposal (NIOSH 2014 [group 1]). High doses have resulted in severe abnormalities of liver function tests. **[US Boxed Warning]: Bone marrow suppression, which may be severe, is dose related; may result in infection (due to neutropenia) or bleeding (due to thrombocytopenia); anemia may require blood transfusion;** reduce dosage in patients with bone marrow suppression; cycles should be delayed until WBC and platelet counts have recovered. Patients who have received prior myelosuppressive therapy and patients with renal dysfunction are at increased risk for bone marrow suppression. Anemia is cumulative.

When calculating the carboplatin dose using the Calvert formula and an estimated glomerular filtration rate (GFR), the laboratory method used to measure serum creatinine may impact dosing. Compared to other methods, standardized isotope dilution mass spectrometry (IDMS) may underestimate serum creatinine values in patients with low creatinine values (eg, ≤0.7 mg/dL) and may overestimate GFR in patients with normal renal function. This may result in higher calculated carboplatin doses and increased toxicities. If using IDMS, the Food and Drug Administration (FDA) recommends that clinicians consider capping estimated GFR at a maximum of 125 mL/minute to avoid potential toxicity.

[US Boxed Warning]: Anaphylactic-like reactions have been reported with carboplatin; may occur within minutes of administration. Epinephrine, corticosteroids and antihistamines have been used to treat symptoms. The risk of allergic reactions (including anaphylaxis) is increased in patients previously exposed to platinum therapy. Skin testing and desensitization protocols have been reported (Confina-Cohen, 2005; Lee, 2004; Markman, 2003). When administered as sequential infusions, taxane derivatives (docetaxel, paclitaxel) should be administered before the platinum derivatives (carboplatin, cisplatin) to limit myelosuppression and to enhance efficacy. Ototoxicity may occur when administered concomitantly with aminoglycosides. Clinically significant hearing loss has been reported to occur in pediatric patients when carboplatin was administered at higher than recommended doses in combination with other ototoxic agents (eg, aminoglycosides). In a study of children receiving carboplatin for the treatment of retinoblastoma, those <6 months of age at treatment initiation were more likely to experience ototoxicity; long-term audiology monitoring is recommended (Qaddoumi, 2012). Loss of vision (usually reversible within weeks of discontinuing) has been reported with higher than recommended doses.

Peripheral neuropathy occurs infrequently, the incidence of peripheral neuropathy is increased in patients >65 years of age and those who have previously received cisplatin treatment. Patients >65 years of age are more likely to develop severe thrombocytopenia.

Limited potential for nephrotoxicity unless administered concomitantly with aminoglycosides. **[US Boxed Warning]: Vomiting may occur.** Carboplatin is associated with a moderate emetic potential in adult patients and a high emetic potential in pediatric patients; antiemetics are recommended to prevent nausea and vomiting (Basch, 2011; Dupuis, 2011; Roila, 2010). May be severe in patients who have received prior emetogenic therapy. **[US Boxed Warning]: Should be administered under the supervision of an experienced cancer chemotherapy physician.**

Adverse Reactions Percentages reported with single-agent therapy.

>10%:

Central nervous system: Pain (23%)

Endocrine & metabolic: Hyponatremia (29% to 47%), hypomagnesemia (29% to 43%), hypocalcemia (22% to 31%), hypokalemia (20% to 28%)

Gastrointestinal: Vomiting (65% to 81%), abdominal pain (17%), nausea (without vomiting: 10% to 15%)

Hematologic & oncologic: Bone marrow depression (dose related and dose limiting; nadir at ~21 days with single-agent therapy), anemia (71% to 90%; grades 3/4: 21%), leukopenia (85%; grades 3/4: 15% to 26%), neutropenia (67%; grades 3/4: 16% to 21%), thrombocytopenia (62%; grades 3/4: 25% to 35%)

Hepatic: Increased serum alkaline phosphatase (24% to 37%), increased serum AST (15% to 19%)

Hypersensitivity: Hypersensitivity (2% to 16%)

Neuromuscular & skeletal: Weakness (11%)

Renal: Decreased creatinine clearance (27%), increased blood urea nitrogen (14% to 22%)

1% to 10%:

Central nervous system: Peripheral neuropathy (4% to 6%), neurotoxicity (5%)

Dermatologic: Alopecia (2% to 3%)

Gastrointestinal: Constipation (6%), diarrhea (6%), dysgeusia (1%), mucositis (≤1%), stomatitis (≤1%)

Hematologic & oncologic: Bleeding complications (5%), hemorrhage (5%)

Hepatic: Increased serum bilirubin (5%)

Infection: Infection (5%)

Ophthalmic: Visual disturbance (1%)

Otic: Ototoxicity (1%)

Renal: Increased serum creatinine (6% to 10%)

<1% (Limited to important or life-threatening): Anaphylaxis, anorexia, bronchospasm, cardiac failure, cerebrovascular accident, dehydration, embolism, erythema, febrile neutropenia, hemolytic anemia (acute), hemolytic-uremic syndrome, hypertension, hypotension, injection site reaction (pain, redness, swelling), limb ischemia (acute), malaise, metastases, pruritus, skin rash, tissue necrosis (associated with extravasation), urticaria, vision loss

Drug Interactions

Metabolism/Transport Effects None known.

Avoid Concomitant Use

Avoid concomitant use of CARBOplatin with any of the following: BCG (Intravesical); Deferiprone; Dipyrone; Natalizumab; Pimecrolimus; SORAfenib; Tacrolimus (Topical); Tofacitinib; Vaccines (Live)

Increased Effect/Toxicity

CARBOplatin may increase the levels/effects of: Bexarotene (Systemic); CloZAPine; Deferiprone; Fingolimod; Leflunomide; Natalizumab; Taxane Derivatives; Tofacitinib; Topotecan; Vaccines (Live)

The levels/effects of CARBOplatin may be increased by: Aminoglycosides; Denosumab; Dipyrone; Pimecrolimus; Roflumilast; SORAfenib; Tacrolimus (Topical); Trastuzumab

Decreased Effect

CARBOplatin may decrease the levels/effects of: BCG (Intravesical); Coccidioides immitis Skin Test; Fosphenytoin-Phenytoin; Sipuleucel-T; Vaccines (Inactivated); Vaccines (Live)

The levels/effects of CARBOplatin may be decreased by: Echinacea

Preparation for Administration Hazardous agent; use appropriate precautions for handling and disposal (NIOSH 2014 [group 1]).

Solution for injection: Manufacturer's labeling states solution can be further diluted to concentrations as low as 0.5 mg/mL in NS or D_5W; however, most clinicians generally dilute dose in either 100 mL or 250 mL of NS or D_5W.

Concentrations used for desensitization vary based on protocol.

Needles or IV administration sets that contain aluminum should not be used in the preparation or administration of carboplatin; aluminum can react with carboplatin resulting in precipitate formation and loss of potency.

Storage/Stability Store intact vials at room temperature at 25°C (77°F); excursions permitted to 15°C to 30°C (59°F to 86°F). Protect from light. Further dilution to a concentration as low as 0.5 mg/mL is stable at room temperature (25°C) for 8 hours in NS or D_5W. Stability has also been demonstrated for dilutions in D_5W in PVC bags at room temperature for 9 days (Benaji, 1994); however, the manufacturer recommends use within 8 hours due to lack of preservative. Multidose vials are stable for up to 14 days after opening when stored at 25°C (77°F) following multiple needle entries.

Mechanism of Action Carboplatin is a platinum compound alkylating agent which covalently binds to DNA; interferes with the function of DNA by producing inter-strand DNA cross-links

Pharmacodynamics/Kinetics

Distribution: V_d: 16 L (based on a dose of 300 to 500 mg/m²); into liver, kidney, skin, and tumor tissue

Protein binding: Carboplatin: 0%; Platinum (from carboplatin): Irreversibly binds to plasma proteins

Metabolism: Minimally hepatic to aquated and hydroxylated compounds

Half-life elimination: CrCl >60 mL/minute: Carboplatin: 2.6 to 5.9 hours (based on a dose of 300 to 500 mg/m²); Platinum (from carboplatin): ≥5 days

Excretion: Urine (~70% as carboplatin within 24 hours; 3% to 5% as platinum within 1 to 4 days)

Dosing

Adult Note: Doses for adults are commonly calculated by the target AUC using the Calvert formula, where **Total dose (mg) = Target AUC x (GFR + 25)**. If estimating glomerular filtration rate (GFR) instead of a measured GFR, the Food and Drug Administration (FDA) recommends that clinicians consider capping estimated GFR at a maximum of 125 mL/minute to avoid potential toxicity. Carboplatin is associated with a moderate emetic potential in adult patients; antiemetics are recommended to prevent nausea and vomiting (Basch, 2011; Roila, 2010).

Ovarian cancer, advanced: *Manufacturer's labeling:* IV: 360 mg/m² every 4 weeks (as a single agent) or 300 mg/m² every 4 weeks (in combination with cyclophosphamide) or Target AUC 4 to 6 (single agent; in previously-treated patients)

Off-label dosing for advanced ovarian cancer: IV: Target AUC 5 to 7.5 every 3 weeks (in combination with paclitaxel) (Ozols, 2003; Parmar, 2003) **or** Target AUC 5 every 3 weeks (in combination with docetaxel) (Vasey, 2004)

Bladder cancer (off-label use): IV: Target AUC 5 every 3 weeks (in combination with gemcitabine) (Bamias, 2006) **or** Target AUC 6 every 3 weeks (in combination with paclitaxel) (Vaughn, 2002)

Breast cancer, metastatic (off-label use): IV: Target AUC 6 every 3 weeks (in combination with trastuzumab and paclitaxel) (Robert, 2006) **or** Target AUC 6 every 3 weeks (in combination with trastuzumab and docetaxel) (Pegram, 2004; Valero, 2011)

Cervical cancer, recurrent or metastatic (off-label use): IV: Target AUC 5 every 3 weeks (in combination with paclitaxel) (Pectasides, 2009) **or** Target AUC 5 to 6 every 4 weeks (in combination with paclitaxel) (Tinker, 2005) **or** 400 mg/m² every 28 days (as a single agent) (Weiss, 1990)

Endometrial cancer (off-label use): IV: Target AUC 5 every 3 weeks (in combination with paclitaxel) (Pectasides, 2008) **or** Target AUC 2 on days 1, 8, and 15 every 28 days (in combination with paclitaxel) (Secord, 2007)

Esophageal cancer (off-label use): IV: Target AUC 2 on days 1, 8, 15, 22, and 29 for 1 cycle (in combination with paclitaxel) (van Meerten, 2006) **or** Target AUC 5 every 3 weeks (in combination with paclitaxel) (El-Rayes, 2004)

Head and neck cancer (off-label use): IV: Target AUC 5 every 3 weeks (in combination with cetuximab) (Chan, 2005) **or** Target AUC 5 every 3 weeks (in combination with cetuximab and fluorouracil) (Vermorken, 2008) **or** 300 mg/m² every 4 weeks (in combination with fluorouracil) (Forastiere, 1992) **or** Target AUC 6 every 3 weeks (in combination with paclitaxel) (Clark, 2001)

Hodgkin lymphoma, relapsed or refractory (off-label use): IV: Target AUC 5 (maximum dose: 800 mg) for 2 cycles (in combination with ifosfamide and etoposide) (Moskowitz, 2001)

Malignant pleural mesothelioma (off-label use): IV: Target AUC 5 every 3 weeks (in combination with pemetrexed) (Castagneto, 2008; Ceresoli, 2006)

Melanoma, advanced or metastatic (off-label use): IV: Target AUC 2 days on 1, 8, and 15 every 4 weeks (in combination with paclitaxel) (Rao, 2006)

Non-Hodgkin lymphomas, relapsed or refractory (off-label use): IV: Target AUC 5 (maximum dose: 800 mg) per cycle for 3 cycles (in combination with rituximab, ifosfamide and etoposide) (Kewalramani, 2004)

Non-small cell lung cancer (off-label use): IV: Target AUC 6 every 3 to 4 weeks (in combination with paclitaxel) (Ramalingam, 2008; Schiller, 2002; Strauss, 2008) **or** Target AUC 6 every 3 weeks (in combination with bevacizumab and paclitaxel) (Sandler, 2006) **or** Target AUC 5 every 3 weeks (in combination with pemetrexed) (Gronberg, 2009) **or** in combination with radiation therapy and paclitaxel (Belani, 2005):
Target AUC 6 every 3 weeks for 2 cycles **or**
Target AUC 6 every 3 weeks for 2 cycles; then target AUC 2 weekly for 7 weeks **or**
Target AUC 2 every week for 7 weeks; then target AUC 6 every 3 weeks for 2 cycles

Sarcomas: Ewing sarcoma, osteosarcoma (off-label uses): IV: 400 mg/m²/day for 2 days every 21 days (in combination with ifosfamide and etoposide) (van Winkle, 2005)

Small cell lung cancer (off-label use): IV: Target AUC 6 every 3 weeks (in combination with etoposide) (Skarlos, 2001) **or** Target AUC 5 every 3 weeks (in combination with irinotecan) (Hermes, 2008) **or** Target AUC 5 every 28 days (in combination with irinotecan) (Schmittel, 2006)

Testicular cancer (off-label use): IV: Target AUC 7 as a one-time dose (Oliver, 2011) **or** 700 mg/m²/day for 3 days beginning 5 days prior to peripheral stem cell infusion (in combination with etoposide) for 2 cycles (Einhorn, 2007)

Thymic malignancies (off-label use): IV: Target AUC 5 every 3 weeks (in combination with paclitaxel) (Lemma, 2008)

Unknown primary adenocarcinoma (off-label use): IV: Target AUC 6 every 3 weeks (in combination with paclitaxel) (Briasoulis, 2000) **or** Target AUC 6 every 3 weeks (in combination with docetaxel) (Greco, 2000) **or** Target AUC 6 every 3 weeks (in combination with paclitaxel and etoposide) (Hainsworth, 2006) **or** Target AUC 5 every 3 weeks (in combination with paclitaxel and gemcitabine) (Greco, 2002)

Geriatric The Calvert formula should be used to calculate dosing for elderly patients. Refer to adult dosing.

Pediatric Carboplatin is associated with a high emetic potential in pediatric patients; antiemetics are recommended to prevent nausea and vomiting (Dupuis, 2011).

Central nervous system tumors (off-label use):
Glioma: IV: 175 mg/m² weekly for 4 weeks every 6 weeks, with a 2-week recovery period between courses (in combination with vincristine) (Packer, 1997)
Neuroblastoma, localized and unresectable: IV: Children ≥10 kg: 200 mg/m²/day days 1, 2, and 3 every 21 days for 2 cycles (in combination with etoposide for 2 cycles then followed by cyclophosphamide, doxorubicin and vincristine) (Rubie, 1998) **or** Children <1 year: 6.6 mg/kg/day days 1, 2, and 3 (in combination with etoposide for 2 cycles, then followed by cyclophosphamide, doxorubicin, and vincristine) (Rubie, 2001)
Sarcomas: Ewing sarcoma, osteosarcoma (off-label uses): IV: 400 mg/m²/day for 2 days every 21 days (in combination with ifosfamide and etoposide) (van Winkle, 2005)

Renal Impairment Note: Dose determination with Calvert formula uses GFR and, therefore, inherently adjusts for renal dysfunction.

The manufacturer's labeling recommends the following dosage adjustments for single-agent therapy: Adults:
Baseline CrCl 41 to 59 mL/minute: Initiate at 250 mg/m² and adjust subsequent doses based on bone marrow toxicity
Baseline CrCl 16 to 40 mL/minute: Initiate at 200 mg/m² and adjust subsequent doses based on bone marrow toxicity
Baseline CrCl ≤15 mL/minute: There are no dosage adjustments provided in the manufacturer's labeling.

The following dosage adjustments have also been recommended:
Aronoff, 2007:
Adults (**Note:** For dosing based on **mg/m²**):
GFR >50 mL/minute: No dosage adjustment is necessary
GFR 10 to 50 mL/minute: Administer 50% of the dose
GFR <10 mL/minute: Administer 25% of the dose
Hemodialysis: Administer 50% of dose
Continuous ambulatory peritoneal dialysis (CAPD): Administer 25% of dose
Continuous renal replacement therapy (CRRT): 200 mg/m²
Children:
GFR <50 mL/minute: Use Calvert formula incorporating patient's GFR
Hemodialysis, peritoneal dialysis, continuous renal replacement therapy (CRRT): Use Calvert formula incorporating patient's GFR
Janus, 2010: Hemodialysis: Carboplatin dose (mg) = Target AUC x 25; administer on a nondialysis day, hemodialysis should occur between 12-24 hours after carboplatin dose

Hepatic Impairment There are no dosage adjustments provided in the manufacturer's labeling; however, carboplatin undergoes minimal hepatic metabolism therefore dosage adjustment may not be needed.

Obesity
American Society of Clinical Oncology (ASCO) Guidelines for appropriate chemotherapy dosing in obese adults with cancer: Dosing based on GFR should be considered in obese patients; GFR should not exceed 125 mL/minute (Griggs, 2012).

American Society for Blood and Marrow Transplantation (ASBMT) practice guideline committee position statement on chemotherapy dosing in obesity: Utilize actual body weight (full weight) for calculation of body surface area (when applicable) in carboplatin dosing for hematopoietic stem cell transplant conditioning regimens in adults. Based on the literature, there is no consensus for carboplatin dosing based on AUC in transplant conditioning regimens or dosing adjustments during transplant for obese patients (Bubalo, 2014).

Adjustment for Toxicity Platelets <50,000 cells/mm³ or ANC <500 cells/mm³: Administer 75% of dose

Administration Carboplatin is associated with a moderate emetic potential in adult patients and a high emetic potential in pediatric patients; antiemetics are recommended to prevent nausea and vomiting (Basch, 2011; Dupuis, 2011; Roila, 2010).

Infuse over at least 15 minutes; usually infused over 15 to 60 minutes, although some protocols may require infusions up to 24 hours. When administered as a part of a combination chemotherapy regimen, sequence of administration may vary by regimen; refer to specific protocol for sequence recommendation.

Needles or IV administration sets that contain aluminum should not be used in the preparation or administration of carboplatin; aluminum can react with carboplatin resulting in precipitate formation and loss of potency.

Hazardous agent; use appropriate precautions for handling and disposal (NIOSH 2014 [group 1]).

Monitoring Parameters CBC (with differential and platelet count), serum electrolytes, serum creatinine and BUN, creatinine clearance, liver function tests; audiology evaluations (children <6 months of age)

Dosage Forms Excipient information presented when available (limited, particularly for generics); consult specific product labeling.
Solution, Intravenous:
Generic: 50 mg/5 mL (5 mL); 150 mg/15 mL (15 mL); 450 mg/45 mL (45 mL); 600 mg/60 mL (60 mL)
Solution, Intravenous [preservative free]:
Generic: 50 mg/5 mL (5 mL); 150 mg/15 mL (15 mL); 450 mg/45 mL (45 mL); 600 mg/60 mL (60 mL)
Solution Reconstituted, Intravenous:
Generic: 150 mg (1 ea)

◆ Carboplatin Injection (Can) *see* CARBOplatin *on page 312*

◆ Carboplatin Injection BP (Can) *see* CARBOplatin *on page 312*

◆ Carboprost *see* Carboprost Tromethamine *on page 314*

Carboprost Tromethamine
(KAR boe prost tro METH a meen)

Brand Names: US Hemabate
Brand Names: Canada Hemabate
Index Terms Carboprost; Prostaglandin F₂ Alpha Analog; Prostaglandin F₂ Analog
Pharmacologic Category Abortifacient; Prostaglandin

Use
Termination of pregnancy: For aborting pregnancy between week 13 and 20 of gestation as calculated from the first day of the last normal menstrual period and in the following conditions related to second trimester abortion: Failure of expulsion of the fetus during the course of treatment by another method; premature rupture of membranes in intrauterine methods with loss of drug and insufficient or absent uterine activity; requirement of a repeat intrauterine instillation of drug for expulsion of the fetus; inadvertent or spontaneous rupture of membranes in the presence of a previable fetus and absence of adequate activity for expulsion.

Refractory postpartum uterine hemorrhage: Treatment of postpartum hemorrhage due to uterine atony that has not responded to conventional methods of management. Prior treatment should include the use of intravenously (IV) administered oxytocin, manipulative techniques such as uterine massage and, unless contraindicated, intramuscular ergot preparations.

Dosing
Adult & Geriatric
Refractory postpartum uterine bleeding: IM: Initial: 250 mcg; if needed, may repeat at 15- to 90-minute intervals; maximum total dose: 2 mg (8 doses)
Termination of pregnancy: IM: 250 mcg, then 250 mcg at 1.5- to 3.5-hour intervals, depending on uterine response; a 500 mcg dose may be given if uterine response is not adequate after several 250 mcg doses; do not exceed 12 mg total dose or continuous administration for >2 days. **Note:** A 100 mcg test dose may be considered.

Renal Impairment Use with caution in patients with a history of renal disease; use is contraindicated in patients with active renal impairment.

Hepatic Impairment Use with caution in patients with a history of hepatic disease; use is contraindicated in patients with active hepatic impairment.

Additional Information Complete prescribing information should be consulted for additional detail.

Dosage Forms Excipient information presented when available (limited, particularly for generics); consult specific product labeling.
Solution, Intramuscular [strength expressed as base]:
Hemabate: 250 mcg/mL (1 mL) [contains benzyl alcohol]

◆ Carboxypeptidase-G2 *see* Glucarpidase *on page 847*

◆ Cardec [OTC] *see* Chlorpheniramine and Phenylephrine *on page 376*

◆ Cardec™ DM [OTC] *see* Chlorpheniramine, Phenylephrine, and Dextromethorphan *on page 378*

◆ Cardene *see* NiCARdipine *on page 1275*

◆ Cardene IV *see* NiCARdipine *on page 1275*

◆ Cardene SR [DSC] *see* NiCARdipine *on page 1275*

Carfilzomib (kar FILZ oh mib)

Brand Names: US Kyprolis
Index Terms CFZ; PR-171
Pharmacologic Category Antineoplastic Agent, Proteasome Inhibitor
Use Multiple myeloma, relapsed/refractory: Treatment (monotherapy) of multiple myeloma in patients who have received at least 2 prior therapies (including bortezomib and an immunomodulatory agent) and have demonstrated disease progression on or within 60 days of completion of the last therapy; treatment of multiple myeloma (in combination with lenalidomide and dexamethasone) in patients who have received 1 to 3 prior therapies.

Pregnancy Considerations Adverse events were observed in animal reproduction studies. Based on the mechanism of action, adverse fetal events would be expected to occur with use in pregnant women. Females of reproductive potential are advised to avoid pregnancy during therapy; effective contraception should be used during treatment and for at least 2 weeks following therapy completion.

Breast-Feeding Considerations It is not known if carfilzomib is excreted in breast milk. Due to the potential for serious adverse reactions in the breast-feeding infant, the manufacturer recommends against breast-feeding while on carfilzomib; a decision should be made to discontinue breast-feeding or to discontinue the drug, taking into account the importance of treatment to the mother and the health benefits of breast-feeding. The appropriate timing to restart breast-feeding after treatment discontinuation should be determined with the health care provider.

Contraindications There are no contraindications listed in the manufacturer's labeling.

Warnings/Precautions Hazardous agent - use appropriate precautions for handling and disposal (meets NIOSH 2014 criteria). Thrombocytopenia (including grade 4) was observed in patients receiving carfilzomib, with platelet nadirs occurring between day 8 and day 15 of each 28-day treatment cycle, and recovery to baseline by the start of the next cycle. Monitor platelets closely and adjust dose or withhold therapy if necessary. Anemia, lymphopenia, leukopenia, and neutropenia were also observed. Death caused by cardiac arrest has occurred within 24 hours of drug administration. Carfilzomib has been associated with new-onset or worsening of heart failure (HF), pulmonary edema, decreased left ventricular ejection fraction (LVEF), restrictive cardiomyopathy, myocardial ischemia, and myocardial infarction (including fatalities). Cardiac events typically were observed early in therapy (<5 cycles). Patients 75 years of age or older have an increased risk of heart failure. Monitor closely for cardiac complications and for volume overload (due to pretreatment hydration), particularly in patients at risk for heart failure; withhold carfilzomib therapy for grade 3 or 4 cardiac events until recovery. Patients with New York Heart Association Class III and IV heart failure, recent myocardial infarction (within 3 to 6 months), and conduction abnormalities not managed by medication were excluded from clinical trials and may be at increased risk for cardiac complications. Hypertension has occurred with use; hypertensive crisis and hypertensive emergency have also been reported (some events were fatal). Monitor blood pressure throughout therapy; if hypertension cannot be adequately controlled, interrupt carfilzomib therapy and evaluate; assess risks versus benefits when determining to restart treatment.

Acute respiratory distress syndrome (ARDS), acute respiratory failure, and acute diffuse-infiltrative pulmonary disease (eg, pneumonitis and interstitial lung disease) have occurred in a small number of patients (some events were fatal); discontinue therapy if any of these drug-induced pulmonary toxicities occur. Pulmonary arterial hypertension (PAH) was observed (including grade 3 or higher events) in studies; perform cardiac imaging or other testing as appropriate, and withhold carfilzomib until PAH is resolved or returns to baseline. Dyspnea (including grade 3 or higher events) has been reported; monitor closely. Withhold carfilzomib until pulmonary symptom resolution or return to baseline. Renal toxicity (eg, renal impairment, acute renal failure, renal failure) has been reported with

carfilzomib. Acute renal failure was observed more frequently in patients receiving carfilzomib monotherapy for advanced relapsed/refractory multiple myeloma; renal failure risk is greater when patients have a baseline reduced creatinine clearance. Monitor renal function closely; may require therapy interruption or dose reduction.

Thrombocytopenic thrombotic purpura/hemolytic uremic syndrome (TTP/HUS) has been reported (some fatal); monitor for signs/symptoms. Interrupt therapy if TTP/HUS diagnosis is suspected and manage appropriately (eg, plasma exchange as clinically necessary). If TTP/HUS diagnosis is excluded, may consider reinitiating therapy; the safety of restarting carfilzomib after a TTP/HUS diagnosis is not known. Posterior reversible encephalopathy syndrome (PRES) has been reported rarely with use; symptoms include seizure, headache, lethargy, confusion, blindness, altered consciousness, hypertension, and other visual/neurological disturbances. Discontinue therapy if PRES diagnosis is suspected; the safety of reinitiating therapy after PRES diagnosis is not known. Venous thromboembolism (eg, deep vein thrombosis and pulmonary embolism) has been observed, particularly when used as part of combination therapy with lenalidomide and dexamethasone. Thromboprophylaxis is recommended when appropriate, based on patients' underlying risk factors, treatment regimen, and clinical status.

Infusion reactions such as chills, fever, arthralgia, myalgia, shortness of breath, hypotension, facial flushing, facial edema, vomiting, weakness, syncope, chest tightness, or angina may occur immediately following or within 24 hours of carfilzomib infusion (may be life-threatening). To lessen the incidence and intensity of infusion reactions, administer dexamethasone prior to drug administration. Tumor lysis syndrome (TLS), including fatalities has been observed. TLS risk is increased in multiple myeloma patients with a high tumor burden. Adequately hydrate patients prior to carfilzomib therapy and monitor closely for signs and symptoms of TLS; consider use of antihyperuricemic agents. If TLS occurs, interrupt treatment until resolved.

Hepatic failure, including fatal cases, has been reported rarely (<1%); increased transaminases and hyperbilirubinemia have also been observed. Interrupt carfilzomib therapy in patients with grade 3 or higher hepatic toxicity until resolved or recovered to baseline (may require dose reduction if appropriate to reinitiate); monitor liver enzymes regularly.

Potentially significant interactions may exist, requiring dose or frequency adjustment, additional monitoring, and/or selection of alternative therapy. Consult drug interactions database for more detailed information. Vials contain the excipient cyclodextrin (sulfobutyl ether beta-cyclodextrin), which may accumulate in patients with renal insufficiency, although the clinical significance of this finding is uncertain (Luke 2010).

Adverse Reactions
>10%:
Cardiovascular: Peripheral edema (24%), hypertension (14%), chest wall pain (11%)
Central nervous system: Fatigue (56%), fever (30%), headache (28%), insomnia (18%), chills (16%), dizziness (13%), hypoesthesia (12%), pain (12%)
Endocrine & metabolic: Hypokalemia (14%), hypomagnesemia (14%), hyperglycemia (12%), hypercalcemia (11%), hypophosphatemia (11%)
Gastrointestinal: Nausea (45%), diarrhea (33%), vomiting (22%), constipation (21%), anorexia (12%)
Hematologic: Anemia (47%; grade 3: 21%; grade 4: 1%), thrombocytopenia (36%; grade 3: 13%; grade 4: 10%), lymphopenia (24%; grade 3: 16%; grade 4: 2%), neutropenia (21%; grade 3: 10%; grade 4: 1%), leukopenia (14%; grade 3: 5%; grade 4:<1%)
Hepatic: AST increased (13%; grade 3: 3%; grade 4: <1%)
Neuromuscular & skeletal: Back pain (20%), arthralgia (16%), muscle spasms (14%), peripheral neuropathy (14%; grade 3: 1%), weakness (14%), limb pain (13%)
Renal: Creatinine increased (24%; grade 3: 3%; grade 4: <1%)
Respiratory: Dyspnea (35%; grade 3: 5%; grade 4: <1%), upper respiratory tract infection (28%), cough (26%), pneumonia (13%; grade 3: 10%; grade 4: <1%)
1% to 10%:
Cardiovascular: Cardiac failure (7%; includes CHF, pulmonary edema, ejection fraction decrease)
Endocrine & metabolic: Hyponatremia (10%)
Renal: Renal failure (9%)
Respiratory: Pulmonary arterial hypertension (2%)
Miscellaneous: Herpes zoster reactivation (2%)

◄

<1% (Limited to important or life-threatening): Bilirubin increased, hepatic failure, infusion reaction, intracranial hemorrhage, multiorgan failure, myocardial ischemia, neutropenic fever, sepsis, tumor lysis syndrome

Drug Interactions

Metabolism/Transport Effects Substrate of P-glycoprotein; **Inhibits** P-glycoprotein

Avoid Concomitant Use

Avoid concomitant use of Carfilzomib with any of the following: BCG (Intravesical); Deferiprone; Dipyrone

Increased Effect/Toxicity

Carfilzomib may increase the levels/effects of: CloZA-Pine; Deferiprone

The levels/effects of Carfilzomib may be increased by: Dipyrone; Lumacaftor; P-glycoprotein/ABCB1 Inhibitors; Ranolazine

Decreased Effect

Carfilzomib may decrease the levels/effects of: BCG (Intravesical)

The levels/effects of Carfilzomib may be decreased by: Lumacaftor; P-glycoprotein/ABCB1 Inducers

Preparation for Administration Hazardous agent; use appropriate precautions for handling and disposal (meets NIOSH 2014 criteria). Reconstitute with 29 mL sterile water for injection to a concentration of 2 mg/mL (directing solution onto the inside wall of the vial to avoid foaming). Gently invert and/or swirl vial slowly for ~1 minute to mix; do not shake. If foaming results, allow solution to sit for 2 to 5 minutes until foaming resolves. Reconstituted solution should be clear and colorless. May further dilute dose in 50 mL D$_5$W. The amount contained in each vial may exceed the prescribed dose; use care with dosage and volume calculations. Discard unused portion of the vial.

Storage/Stability Store intact vials refrigerated at 2°C to 8°C (36°F to 46°F). Store in original carton until use to protect from light. Reconstituted drug (in the vial or in a syringe) and preparations diluted for infusion are stable for 4 hours at room temperature or for 24 hours refrigerated at 2°C to 8°C (36°F to 46°F).

Mechanism of Action Carfilzomib inhibits proteasomes, which are responsible for intracellular protein homeostasis. Specifically, it is a potent, selective, and irreversible inhibitor of chymotrypsin-like activity of the 20S proteasome, leading to cell cycle arrest and apoptosis.

Pharmacodynamics/Kinetics

Distribution: V$_{dss}$: 28 L; penetrates all tissues extensively except the brain (Kortuem 2013)

Protein binding: 97%

Metabolism: Rapid and extensive; peptidase cleavage and epoxide hydrolysis; minimal metabolism through cytochrome P450-mediated mechanisms

Half-life elimination: Doses ≥15 mg/m^2: <1 hour on day 1 of cycle 1

Excretion: Urine (25%, primarily as metabolites)

Dosing

Adult & Geriatric Note: Hydrate with oral fluids (30 mL/kg) at least 48 hours prior to initiating cycle 1, as well as with 250 to 500 mL normal saline (or other appropriate IV fluid) before dosing (recommended) and after (if needed) administration during cycle 1 (continue oral and/or IV hydration in subsequent cycles if necessary; monitor for evidence of volume overload and adjust hydration based on individual needs. Premedicate with dexamethasone (4 mg orally or IV, or the recommended dexamethasone dose when used in combination therapy) 30 minutes to 4 hours prior to all doses in cycle 1, and as needed with future cycles to reduce the incidence and severity of infusion reaction. Consider antiviral prophylaxis for patients with a history of herpes zoster infection. Thromboprophylaxis is recommended when administering in combination with lenalidomide and dexamethasone.

Multiple myeloma, relapsed/refractory (single-agent):

IV: **Note:** Patients with a body surface area (BSA) >2.2 m^2 should be dosed based upon a maximum BSA of 2.2 m^2. Dose adjustments for weight changes of ≤20% are not necessary, per manufacturer labeling. Continue until disease progression or unacceptable toxicity.

Cycle 1: 20 mg/m^2 on days 1 and 2; if tolerated, increase dose to 27 mg/m^2 on days 8, 9, 15, and 16 of a 28-day treatment cycle

Cycles 2 to 12: 27 mg/m^2 days 1, 2, 8, 9, 15, and 16 of a 28-day treatment cycle

Cycle 13 and beyond: 27 mg/m^2 on days 1, 2, 15, and 16 of a 28-day treatment cycle

Multiple myeloma, relapsed/refractory (combination therapy [with lenalidomide and dexamethasone]) (Stewart 2015): IV:

Cycle 1: 20 mg/m^2 on days 1 and 2 followed by 27 mg/m^2 on days 8, 9, 15, and 16.

Cycles 2 to 12: 27 mg/m^2 on days 1, 2, 8, 9, 15, and 16.

Cycles 13 to 18: 27 mg/m^2 on days 1, 2, 15, and 16; lenalidomide and dexamethasone may be continued (until disease progression or unacceptable toxicity)

Renal Impairment

Preexisting renal impairment: There are no dosage adjustments provided in the manufacturer's labeling; however, results from a phase 2 study in patients with renal impairment indicate that the pharmacokinetics and safety of carfilzomib were unchanged in this patient population; no dosage adjustment is necessary in patients with baseline dysfunction, including patients on hemodialysis (Badros 2013). **Note:** Dialysis clearance of carfilzomib has not been studied; per manufacturer labeling, administer postdialysis.

Renal toxicity during treatment: Serum creatinine ≥2 times baseline, CrCl <15 mL/minute or CrCl decreases to ≤50% of baseline, or patient requires dialysis: Withhold dose and monitor renal function. If renal toxicity is due to carfilzomib, resume dosing when renal function has improved to within 25% of baseline; resume with a reduced dose by 1 dose level (from 27 mg/m^2 to 20 mg/m^2 or from 20 mg/m^2 to 15 mg/m^2). If toxicity is not due to carfilzomib, restart at the discretion of the prescriber.

Hepatic Impairment

Preexisting hepatic impairment: There are no dosage adjustments provided in the manufacturer's labeling (has not been studied; patients with ALT or AST ≥3 times ULN and bilirubin ≥2 times ULN were excluded from clinical trials).

Hepatotoxicity during treatment: Grade 3 or 4 elevation of bilirubin, transaminases, or other liver abnormalities: Withhold dose until resolved or at baseline. After resolution, if appropriate to reinitiate, consider restarting at a reduced dose level (from 27 mg/m^2 to 20 mg/m^2 or from 20 mg/m^2 to 15 mg/m^2) with frequent monitoring of hepatic function.

Obesity *ASCO Guidelines for appropriate chemotherapy dosing in obese adults with cancer:* In general, utilize patient's actual body weight (full weight) for calculation of body surface area- or weight-based dosing, particularly when the intent of therapy is curative; manage regimen-related toxicities in the same manner as for nonobese patients; if a dose reduction is utilized due to toxicity, consider resumption of full weight-based dosing with subsequent cycles, especially if cause of toxicity (eg, hepatic or renal impairment) is resolved (Griggs 2012). **Note:** According to the manufacturer, patients with a body surface area (BSA) >2.2 m^2 should be dosed based upon a maximum BSA of 2.2 m^2; dose adjustments for weight changes of ≤20% are not necessary.

Adjustment for Toxicity

Hematologic toxicity:

ANC <500/mm^3: Withhold dose; continue at same dose level if ANC recovers to ≥500/mm^3. For subsequent ANC levels <500/mm^3, withhold dose and consider reducing dose by one dose level (from 27 mg/m^2 to 20 mg/m^2 or from 20 mg/m^2 to 15 mg/m^2) if ANC ≥500/mm^3 when restarting.

Platelets: <10,000/mm^3 or evidence of bleeding with thrombocytopenia: Withhold dose; continue at same dose level if platelets recover to ≥10,000/mm^3 and bleeding is controlled. For subsequent platelet levels <10,000/mm^3, withhold dose and consider reducing dose by one dose level (from 27 mg/m^2 to 20 mg/m^2 or from 20 mg/m^2 to 15 mg/m^2) if platelets ≥10,000/mm^3 when restarting..

Nonhematologic toxicity:

Cardiac: Grade 3 or 4, new-onset or worsening of heart failure, decreased left ventricular function, or myocardial ischemia: Withhold dose until resolved or at baseline. After resolution, if appropriate to reinitiate, consider restarting at a reduced dose level (from 27 mg/m^2 to 20 mg/m^2 or from 20 mg/m^2 to 15 mg/m^2).

Hypertension, severe or life-threatening: If hypertension cannot be adequately controlled, withhold dose and evaluate. After resolution, if appropriate to reinitiate (if risk versus benefit ratio is acceptable), consider restarting at a reduced dose level (from 27 mg/m^2 to 20 mg/m^2 or from 20 mg/m^2 to 15 mg/m^2).

Pulmonary toxicity

Acute respiratory distress syndrome, acute respiratory failure, and acute diffuse infiltrative pulmonary disease (drug-induced): Discontinue therapy.

Pulmonary hypertension: Withhold dose until resolved or at baseline. After resolution, if appropriate to reinitiate after severe or life-threatening pulmonary hypertension (if risk versus benefit ratio is acceptable), consider restarting at a reduced dose level (from 27 mg/m^2 to 20 mg/m^2 or from 20 mg/m^2 to 15 mg/m^2).

Grade 3 or 4 dyspnea: Withhold dose until resolved or at baseline. After resolution, if appropriate to reinitiate (if risk versus benefit ratio is acceptable), consider restarting (at next scheduled treatment) at a reduced dose level (from 27 mg/m^2 to 20 mg/m^2 or from 20 mg/m^2 to 15 mg/m^2).

Tumor lysis syndrome: Interrupt treatment until resolved.

Other grade 3 or 4 nonhematologic toxicities: Withhold dose until resolved or at baseline. After resolution, consider restarting (at next scheduled treatment) at a reduced dose level (from 27 mg/m^2 to 20 mg/m^2 or from 20 mg/m^2 to 15 mg/m^2).

Administration IV: Administer over 10 minutes. Do not administer as an IV bolus. Hydrate with oral fluids (30 mL/kg) at least 48 hours prior to initiating cycle 1, as well as with 250 to 500 mL NS (or other appropriate IV fluid) prior to (recommended) and after (if needed) each dose in cycle 1; continue oral and/or IV hydration in subsequent cycles (if necessary). Flush line before and after carfilzomib with NS or D$_5$W. Do not administer with other medications. Premedicate with dexamethasone (4 mg orally or IV, or the recommended dexamethasone dose when used in combination therapy) 30 minutes to 4 hours prior to all doses in cycle 1, and as needed with future cycles to reduce the incidence and severity of infusion reaction. Hazardous agent; use appropriate precautions for handling and disposal (meets NIOSH 2014 criteria).

Monitoring Parameters CBC with differential and platelets (monitor frequently throughout therapy); renal function, pulmonary function (with new or worsening pulmonary symptoms), liver function tests, blood pressure. Signs/symptoms of infusion-related reactions, congestive heart failure, tumor lysis syndrome, peripheral neuropathy, posterior reversible encephalopathy syndrome, thrombocytopenic thrombotic purpura/hemolytic uremic syndrome, and venous thromboembolic events. Monitor for evidence of volume overload due to pre- and posthydration.

Dosage Forms Excipient information presented when available (limited, particularly for generics); consult specific product labeling.

Solution Reconstituted, Intravenous:

Kyprolis: 60 mg (1 ea)

Carglumic Acid (kar GLU mik AS id)

Brand Names: US Carbaglu
Brand Names: Canada Carbaglu
Index Terms N-Carbamoyl-L-Glutamic Acid; N-Carbamyl-glutamate
Pharmacologic Category Antidote; Metabolic Alkalosis Agent; Urea Cycle Disorder (UCD) Treatment Agent
Use Hyperammonemia: Adjunctive treatment of acute hyperammonemia and maintenance therapy of chronic hyperammonemia due to the deficiency of the hepatic enzyme N-acetylglutamate synthase (NAGS) in adult and pediatric patients
Prescribing and Access Restrictions Carbaglu is not available through pharmaceutical wholesalers or retail pharmacies, but only through direct shipping from the Accredo specialty pharmacy. Prescribers must contact Accredo Health Group at 888-454-8860 or refer to www.accredo.com to initiate patients on this product.
Dosing
Adult
Acute hyperammonemia: Oral: 100 to 250 mg/kg/day given in 2 or 4 divided doses (rounded to the nearest 100 mg); titrate to age-appropriate plasma ammonia levels. Concomitant adjunctive ammonia-lowering therapy recommended.
Note: Prior to initiating long-term therapy the Canadian labeling recommends a test dose to determine responsiveness; an example of test dosing includes:
Moderate hyperammonemia: 100 to 200 mg/kg/day in 2 to 4 divided doses for 3 days with a consistent protein intake; measure plasma ammonia levels before and 1 hour after a meal; dose should be adjusted to maintain normal ammonia levels
Chronic hyperammonemia: Oral:
US labeling: Usual dose (based on limited data): <100 mg/kg/day given in 2 or 4 divided doses; titrate to age-appropriate normal plasma ammonia levels
Canadian labeling: Dosing range: 10 mg/kg to 100 mg/kg/day in 2 to 4 divided doses; titrate to age-appropriate normal plasma ammonia levels.

Pediatric
Acute hyperammonemia: Infants, Children, and Adolescents: Oral: 100 to 250 mg/kg/day given in 2 or 4 divided doses; titrate to age-appropriate plasma ammonia levels. Concomitant adjunctive ammonia-lowering therapy recommended.
Note: Prior to initiating long-term therapy the Canadian labeling recommends a test dose to determine responsiveness; examples of test dosing include:
Comatose child: 100 to 250 mg/kg/day in 2 to 4 divided doses; measure plasma ammonia levels at least prior to each administration; ammonia levels should normalize within a few hours of therapy initiation
Moderate hyperammonemia: 100 to 200 mg/kg/day in 2 to 4 divided doses for 3 days with a consistent protein intake; measure plasma ammonia levels before and 1 hour after a meal; dose should be adjusted to maintain normal ammonia levels
Chronic hyperammonemia: Infants, Children, and Adolescents: Oral: Refer to adult dosing.
Renal Impairment There are no dosage adjustments provided in the manufacturer's labeling (has not been studied).
Hepatic Impairment There are no dosage adjustments provided in the manufacturer's labeling (has not been studied).
Additional Information Complete prescribing information should be consulted for additional detail.
Dosage Forms Excipient information presented when available (limited, particularly for generics); consult specific product labeling.
Tablet, Oral:
Carbaglu: 200 mg [scored]

◆ Carimune NF see Immune Globulin *on page 927*

Cariprazine (kar IP ra zeen)

Index Terms Cariprazine Hydrochloride; Vraylar
Pharmacologic Category Second Generation (Atypical) Antipsychotic
Use
Schizophrenia: Treatment of schizophrenia
Bipolar I disorder: Acute treatment of manic or mixed episodes associated with bipolar I disorder
Pregnancy Considerations Antipsychotic use during the third trimester of pregnancy has a risk for abnormal muscle movements (extrapyramidal symptoms [EPS]) and/or withdrawal symptoms in newborns following delivery. Symptoms in the newborn may include agitation, feeding disorder, hypertonia, hypotonia, respiratory distress, somnolence, and tremor; these effects may be self-limiting or require hospitalization.

The ACOG recommends that therapy during pregnancy be individualized; treatment with psychiatric medications during pregnancy should incorporate the clinical expertise of the mental health clinician, obstetrician, primary health care provider, and pediatrician. Safety data related to atypical antipsychotics during pregnancy are limited and routine use is not recommended. However, if a woman is inadvertently exposed to an atypical antipsychotic while pregnant, continuing therapy may be preferable to switching to a typical antipsychotic that the fetus has not yet been exposed to; consider risk:benefit (ACOG 2008).

Health care providers are encouraged to enroll women exposed to cariprazine during pregnancy in the National Pregnancy Registry for Atypical Antipsychotics (866-961-2388 or http://www.womensmentalhealth.org/clinical-and-research-programs/pregnancyregistry/).
Breast-Feeding Considerations It is not known if cariprazine is excreted in breast milk. The manufacturer recommends the development and health benefits of breast-feeding be considered along with the mother's clinical need for therapy and any potential adverse effects on the breast-fed infant.
Contraindications Hypersensitivity to cariprazine or any component of the formulation
Warnings/Precautions [US Boxed Warning]: Elderly patients with dementia-related psychosis treated with antipsychotics are at an increased risk of death compared to placebo. Most deaths appeared to be either cardiovascular (eg, heart failure, sudden death) or infectious (eg, pneumonia) in nature. Cariprazine is not approved for the treatment of dementia-related psychosis.

Leukopenia, neutropenia, and agranulocytosis (sometimes fatal) have been reported in clinical trials and postmarketing reports with antipsychotic use; presence of risk factors (eg, preexisting low WBC/ANC or history of drug-induced leuko-/neutropenia) should prompt periodic blood count

assessment. Discontinue therapy at first signs of blood dyscrasias or if absolute neutrophil count <1,000/mm³.

May cause extrapyramidal symptoms (EPS), including pseudoparkinsonism, acute dystonic reactions, akathisia, and tardive dyskinesia. Risk of dystonia (and possibly other EPS) may be greater with increased doses, use of conventional antipsychotics, males, and younger patients. Factors associated with greater vulnerability to tardive dyskinesia include older in age, female gender combined with postmenopausal status, Parkinson disease, pseudoparkinsonism symptoms, affective disorders (particularly major depressive disorder), concurrent medical diseases such as diabetes, previous brain damage, alcoholism, poor treatment response, and use of high doses of antipsychotics (APA [Lehman 2004]; Soares-Weiser 2007). Consider therapy discontinuation with signs/symptoms of tardive dyskinesia. Use may be associated with neuroleptic malignant syndrome (NMS); monitor for mental status changes, fever, muscle rigidity, autonomic instability, increased creatine phosphokinase, rhabdomyolysis, and/or acute renal failure. If NMS is suspected, discontinue immediately, provide symptomatic treatment, and monitor patient. NMS can recur. Following recovery from NMS, reintroduction of drug therapy should be carefully considered; if an antipsychotic agent is resumed, monitor closely for NMS (APA [Lehman 2004]).

May cause CNS depression, which may impair physical or mental abilities; patients must be cautioned about performing tasks that require mental alertness (eg, operating machinery, driving). May cause orthostatic hypotension; risk is increased at initial dose titration and when increasing the dose. Use with caution in patients at risk of this effect or in those who would not tolerate transient hypotensive episodes (patients who are antipsychotic-naive or have cerebrovascular disease, cardiovascular disease, hypovolemia, dehydration, or are taking concurrent medication use which may predispose to hypotension/bradycardia. Consider using lower starting dosages and slower titrations in these patients.

Use with caution in patients with Parkinson disease; antipsychotics may aggravate motor disturbances (APA [Lehman 2004; Rabins 2007]). Use with caution in patients at risk of seizures or with conditions that potentially lower the seizure threshold. Elderly patients may be at increased risk of seizures due to an increased prevalence of predisposing factors. Antipsychotic use has been associated with esophageal dysmotility and aspiration; use with caution in patients at risk for aspiration pneumonia (eg, Alzheimer dementia) (Maddalena 2004). Impaired core body temperature regulation may occur; caution with strenuous exercise, heat exposure, dehydration, and concomitant medication possessing anticholinergic effects.

Atypical antipsychotics have been associated with metabolic changes including loss of glucose control, lipid changes, and weight gain (risk profile varies between agents). Development of hyperglycemia; in some cases, may be extreme and associated with ketoacidosis, hyperosmolar coma, or death. All patients should be monitored for symptoms of hyperglycemia (eg, polydipsia, polyuria, polyphagia, weakness). Use with caution in patients with diabetes or other disorders of glucose regulation; monitor for worsening of glucose control.

Plasma levels of cariprazine and its major metabolites accumulate over time. Adverse reactions may not appear until several weeks after initiation of treatment. Monitor response and for adverse reactions several weeks after the patient has begun treatment and after each dose increase. With treatment discontinuation the plasma concentration of cariprazine and active metabolites declines by 50% in ~1 week, therefore the decline of plasma concentrations of active drug and metabolite may not be immediately reflected in the patients' clinical symptoms. Potentially significant interactions may exist, requiring dose or frequency adjustment, additional monitoring, and/or selection of alternative therapy.

Adverse Reactions Note: Reactions reported with doses up to 6 mg daily as doses greater than this do not result in significant therapeutic benefit but do increase adverse reactions.

>10%:
  Central nervous system: Drug-induced extrapyramidal reaction (excluding akathisia and restlessness: 15% to 26%), Parkinsonian-like syndrome (13% to 21%), akathisia (9% to 20%), headache (14%), insomnia (9% to 13%)
  Gastrointestinal: Nausea (7% to 13%)
1% to 10%:
  Cardiovascular: Hypertension (2% to 5%), tachycardia (2%)

Central nervous system: Drowsiness (7% to 8%), restlessness (4% to 7%), dizziness (3% to 7%), anxiety (5% to 6%), agitation (5%), dystonia (2% to 5%), fatigue (3% to 4%)
Dermatologic: Skin rash (2%)
Endocrine & metabolic: Weight gain (2% to 3%)
Gastrointestinal: Vomiting (4% to 10%), dyspepsia (5% to 7%), abdominal pain (6%), constipation (6%), diarrhea (4%), toothache (4%), decreased appetite (3%), xerostomia (3%)
Hepatic: Increased liver enzymes (1%)
Neuromuscular & skeletal: Leg pain (4%), back pain (3%), musculoskeletal stiffness (2% to 3%), arthralgia (2%), increased creatine phosphokinase (2%)
Ophthalmic: Blurred vision (4%)

Drug Interactions
Metabolism/Transport Effects Substrate of CYP2D6 (minor), CYP3A4 (major); **Note:** Assignment of Major/Minor substrate status based on clinically relevant drug interaction potential

Avoid Concomitant Use
Avoid concomitant use of Cariprazine with any of the following: Amisulpride; Azelastine (Nasal); Conivaptan; CYP3A4 Inducers (Strong); Fusidic Acid (Systemic); Idelalisib; Metoclopramide; Orphenadrine; Paraldehyde; Sulpiride; Thalidomide

Increased Effect/Toxicity
Cariprazine may increase the levels/effects of: Alcohol (Ethyl); Amisulpride; Azelastine (Nasal); Buprenorphine; CNS Depressants; Hydrocodone; Mequitazine; Methotrimeprazine; Methylphenidate; Metyrosine; Mirtazapine; Orphenadrine; Paraldehyde; Selective Serotonin Reuptake Inhibitors; Serotonin Modulators; Sulpiride; Suvorexant; Thalidomide; Zolpidem

The levels/effects of Cariprazine may be increased by: Acetylcholinesterase Inhibitors (Central); Aprepitant; Blood Pressure Lowering Agents; Brimonidine (Topical); Cannabis; Conivaptan; CYP3A4 Inhibitors (Moderate); CYP3A4 Inhibitors (Strong); Dasatinib; Doxylamine; Dronabinol; Droperidol; Fosaprepitant; Fusidic Acid (Systemic); HydrOXYzine; Idelalisib; Ivacaftor; Kava Kava; Lithium; Luliconazole; Magnesium Sulfate; Methotrimeprazine; Methylphenidate; Metoclopramide; Metyrosine; Mifepristone; Minocycline; Nabilone; Netupitant; Osimertinib; Palbociclib; Perampanel; Rufinamide; Serotonin Modulators; Simeprevir; Sodium Oxybate; Stiripentol; Tapentadol; Tetrabenazine; Tetrahydrocannabinol

Decreased Effect
Cariprazine may decrease the levels/effects of: Amphetamines; Antidiabetic Agents; Anti-Parkinson's Agents (Dopamine Agonist); Quinagolide

The levels/effects of Cariprazine may be decreased by: Bosentan; CYP3A4 Inducers (Moderate); CYP3A4 Inducers (Strong); Dabrafenib; Deferasirox; Lithium; Osimertinib; Siltuximab; St Johns Wort; Tocilizumab

Storage/Stability Store at 20°C to 25°C (68°F to 77°F); excursions permitted between 15°C and 30°C (59°F and 86°F). Protect 3 mg and 4.5 mg capsules from light to prevent color fading.

Mechanism of Action Cariprazine is a second generation antipsychotic which displays partial agonist activity at dopamine D_2 and serotonin 5-HT_{1A} receptors and antagonist activity at serotonin 5-HT_{2A} receptors. It exhibits high affinity for dopamine (D_2 and D_3) and serotonin (5-HT_{1A}) receptors and has low affinity for serotonin 5-HT_{2C} and alpha$_{1A}$-adrenergic receptors. Cariprazine functions as an antagonist for 5-HT_{2B} (high affinity) and 5-HT_{2A} receptors (moderate affinity), binds to histamine H_1 receptors, and has no affinity for muscarinic (cholinergic) receptors.

Pharmacodynamics/Kinetics
Protein binding: 91% to 97%
Metabolism: Extensively metabolized by CYP3A4 and, to a lesser extent, by CYP2D6 to active metabolites (desmethyl cariprazine [DCAR] and didesmethyl cariprazine [DDCAR]). DCAR is further metabolized into DDCAR by CYP3A4 and CYP2D6. DDCAR is then metabolized by CYP3A4 to a hydroxylated metabolite.
Half-life elimination: Cariprazine: 2 to 4 days; DDCAR: 1 to 3 weeks
Time to peak, plasma: Cariprazine: 3 to 6 hours
Excretion: Urine (21%; 1.2% as unchanged drug cariprazine)
Note: After multiple dose administration of cariprazine, mean cariprazine and desmethyl cariprazine (DCAR) reached steady state at around week 1 to week 2 and mean didesmethyl cariprazine (DDCAR) appeared to be approaching steady state around week 4 to week 8. After discontinuation, mean cariprazine and DCAR concentration decreased by about 50% in a day and mean DDCAR concentrations decreased by ~50% in 1 week after the last dose. There was an approximately 90% decline in

plasma exposure within 1 week for cariprazine and DCAR and at about 4 weeks for DDCAR. Following a single dose of 1 mg of cariprazine, DDCAR remained detectable 8 weeks post-dose.

Dosing

Adult & Geriatric Note: Due to the long half-life of cariprazine and its active metabolites, changes in dose will not be fully reflected in plasma for several weeks.

Bipolar I disorder: Oral: Initial: 1.5 mg once daily; adjust dose based on response and tolerability to 3 mg on day 2 and make further adjustments in increments of 1.5 or 3 mg. Recommended dosing range: 3 mg to 6 mg once daily. Maximum dose: 6 mg daily

Schizophrenia: Oral: Initial: 1.5 mg once daily; adjust dose based on response and tolerability to 3 mg on day 2 and make further adjustments in increments of 1.5 or 3 mg. Recommended dosing range: 1.5 mg to 6 mg once daily. Maximum dose: 6 mg daily

Dosage adjustment with concurrent CYP450 inducer or inhibitor therapy:

Strong CYP3A4 *inhibitor* initiated while on stable dose of cariprazine: Reduce the current dose of cariprazine by 50%. For patients taking 4.5 mg daily, reduce the dose to 1.5 mg or 3 mg daily. For patients taking 1.5 mg daily, adjust the dose to every other day. The cariprazine dose may need to be increased if the CYP3A4 inhibitor is withdrawn.

Initiating cariprazine therapy while already on a strong CYP3A4 *inhibitor*: Administer cariprazine 1.5 mg on day 1 and day 3 (no dose administered on day 2). Administer 1.5 mg daily starting on day 4 and increase to a maximum of 3 mg daily. The cariprazine dose may need to be increased if the CYP3A4 inhibitor is withdrawn.

Concomitant use of cariprazine and CYP3A4 *inducers*: Use is not recommended.

Renal Impairment

CrCl ≥30 mL/minute: No dosage adjustment necessary.

CrCl <30 mL/minute: Use not recommended (has not been studied).

Hepatic Impairment

Mild to moderate impairment (Child-Pugh class A or B): No dosage adjustment necessary.

Severe impairment (Child-Pugh class C): Use not recommended (has not been studied).

Administration Oral: Administer with or without food.

Monitoring Parameters Mental status; vital signs (as clinically indicated); blood pressure (baseline; repeat 3 months after antipsychotic initiation, then yearly); weight, height, BMI, waist circumference (baseline; repeat at 4, 8, and 12 weeks after initiating or changing therapy, then quarterly; consider switching to a different antipsychotic for a weight gain ≥5% of initial weight); CBC (as clinically indicated; monitor frequently during the first few months of therapy in patients with preexisting low WBC or history of drug-induced leukopenia/neutropenia); electrolytes and liver function (annually and as clinically indicated); personal and family history of obesity, diabetes, dyslipidemia, hypertension, or cardiovascular disease (baseline; repeat annually); fasting plasma glucose level/HbA$_{1c}$ (baseline; repeat 3 months after starting antipsychotic, then yearly); fasting lipid panel (baseline; repeat 3 months after initiation of antipsychotic; if LDL level is normal repeat at 2- to 5-year intervals or more frequently if clinically indicated); changes in menstruation, libido, development of galactorrhea, erectile and ejaculatory function (yearly); abnormal involuntary movements or parkinsonian signs (baseline; repeat weekly until dose stabilized for at least 2 weeks after introduction and for 2 weeks after any significant dose increase); tardive dyskinesia (every 12 months; high-risk patients every 6 months); ocular examination (yearly in patients >40 years; every 2 years in younger patients) (ADA, 2004; APA [Lehman, 2004]; Marder, 2004).

Product Availability Vraylar: FDA approved September 2015: anticipated availability is currently undetermined.

◆ Cariprazine Hydrochloride *see* Cariprazine on page 317

◆ Caripul (Can) *see* Epoprostenol on page 657

◆ Carisoprodate *see* Carisoprodol on page 319

Carisoprodol (kar eye soe PROE dole)

Brand Names: US Soma
Index Terms Carisoprodate; Isobamate
Pharmacologic Category Skeletal Muscle Relaxant
Use Short-term (2-3 weeks) treatment of acute musculoskeletal pain

Pregnancy Considerations Adverse events have been observed in animal reproduction studies. Limited postmarketing data with meprobamate (the active metabolite) do not show a consistent association between maternal use and an increased risk for congenital malformations.

Breast-Feeding Considerations Carisoprodol and its active metabolite, meprobamate are excreted in breast milk. The manufacturer recommends that caution be exercised when administering carisoprolol to nursing women. Carisoprodol levels in breast milk may be 2 to 4 times that of maternal plasma levels. The estimated dose to the infant was reported as 6.9% of the weight-adjusted maternal dose in one case report (Briggs 2008) and ~4% of the weight-adjusted maternal dose in another (Nordeng 2001). In both cases, breast milk production was decreased requiring supplemental formula or cessation of breast-feeding. Other than slight sedation reported in one infant, no symptoms of withdrawal or other adverse events were noted in these two cases. Effects on long-term development are not known.

Contraindications Hypersensitivity to carisoprodol, carbamates (eg, meprobamate), or any component of the formulation; history of acute intermittent porphyria

Warnings/Precautions Can cause CNS depression, which may impair physical or mental abilities. Concomitant use of other CNS depressants may enhance these effects. Patients must be cautioned about performing tasks which require mental alertness (eg, operating machinery or driving); postmarketing reports of motor vehicle accidents have been associated with use. Effects with other CNS-depressant drugs or ethanol may be potentiated. Use with caution in patients with hepatic/renal dysfunction. Tolerance or drug dependence may result from extended use. Limit use to 2-3 weeks; use caution in patients who may be prone to addiction. May precipitate withdrawal after abrupt cessation of prolonged use. Has been associated (rarely) with seizures in patients with and without seizure history.

Carisoprodol should be used with caution in patients who are poor CYP2C19 metabolizers; poor metabolizers have been shown to have a fourfold increase in exposure to carisoprodol and a 50% reduced exposure to the metabolite meprobamate compared to normal metabolizers. Prevalence of poor metabolizers in the Asian population is ~15% to 20% while that of Caucasians and African-Americans is ~3% to 5%. Potentially significant drug-drug interactions may exist, requiring dose or frequency adjustment, additional monitoring, and/or selection of alternative therapy. Muscle relaxants are poorly tolerated by the elderly due to potent anticholinergic effects, sedation, and risk of fracture. Efficacy is questionable at dosages tolerated by elderly patients; avoid use (Beers Criteria).

Adverse Reactions

>10%: Central nervous system: Drowsiness (13% to 17%)

1% to 10%: Central nervous system: Dizziness (7% to 8%), headache (3% to 5%)

Postmarketing and/or case reports (Limited to important or life-threatening): Abdominal cramps, agitation, allergic dermatitis, anaphylaxis, angioedema, ataxia, burning sensation of eyes, depression, drug dependence, dyspnea, epigastric pain, eosinophilia, erythema multiforme, exacerbation of asthma, fixed drug eruption, hallucination, headache, hiccups, hypersensitivity reaction, idiosyncratic reaction (symptoms may include agitation, ataxia, confusion, diplopia, disorientation, dysarthria, euphoria, extreme weakness, muscle twitching, mydriasis, temporary vision loss, and/or transient quadriplegia); insomnia, irritability, leukopenia, nausea, orthostatic hypotension, pancytopenia, paradoxical central nervous system stimulation, pruritus, psychosis, seizure, skin rash, syncope, tachycardia, transient flushing of face, tremor, urticaria, vertigo, vomiting, weakness, withdrawal syndrome (abdominal cramps, headache, insomnia, nausea, seizure)

Drug Interactions

Metabolism/Transport Effects Substrate of CYP2C19 (major); **Note:** Assignment of Major/Minor substrate status based on clinically relevant drug interaction potential

Avoid Concomitant Use

Avoid concomitant use of Carisoprodol with any of the following: Azelastine (Nasal); Orphenadrine; Paraldehyde; Thalidomide

Increased Effect/Toxicity

Carisoprodol may increase the levels/effects of: Alcohol (Ethyl); Azelastine (Nasal); Buprenorphine; CNS Depressants; Hydrocodone; Methotrimeprazine; Metyrosine; Mirtazapine; Orphenadrine; Paraldehyde; Pramipexole; ROPINIRole; Rotigotine; Selective Serotonin Reuptake Inhibitors; Suvorexant; Thalidomide; Zolpidem

The levels/effects of Carisoprodol may be increased by: Aspirin; Brimonidine (Topical); Cannabis; CYP2C19 Inhibitors (Moderate); CYP2C19 Inhibitors (Strong);

Doxylamine; Dronabinol; Droperidol; HydrOXYzine; Kava Kava; Luliconazole; Magnesium Sulfate; Methotrimeprazine; Minocycline; Nabilone; Perampanel; Rufinamide; Sodium Oxybate; St Johns Wort; Tapentadol; Tetrahydrocannabinol

Decreased Effect

The levels/effects of Carisoprodol may be decreased by: Aspirin; CYP2C19 Inducers (Strong); Dabrafenib; Enzalutamide; Lumacaftor; St Johns Wort

Storage/Stability Store at 20°C to 25°C (68°F to 77°F).

Mechanism of Action Precise mechanism is not yet clear, but many effects have been ascribed to its central depressant actions. In animals, carisoprodol blocks interneuronal activity and depresses polysynaptic neuron transmission in the spinal cord and reticular formation of the brain. It is also metabolized to meprobamate, which has anxiolytic and sedative effects.

Pharmacodynamics/Kinetics

Onset of action: Rapid

Duration: 4-6 hours

Protein binding: Carisoprodol: <70%; Meprobamate: <25% (Olsen, 1994)

Metabolism: Hepatic, via CYP2C19 to active metabolite (meprobamate)

Half-life elimination: Carisoprodol: ~2 hours; Meprobamate: ~10 hours

Time to peak, plasma: 1.5-2 hours

Excretion: Urine, as metabolite

Dosing

Adult Note: Carisoprodol should only be used for short periods (2-3 weeks) due to lack of evidence of effectiveness with prolonged use.

Acute musculoskeletal pain: Oral: 250-350 mg 3 times daily and at bedtime

Geriatric Not recommended for use in the elderly.

Pediatric Adolescents ≥16 years: Refer to adult dosing.

Renal Impairment No dosage adjustment provided in manufacturer's labeling (has not been studied); carisoprodol undergoes renal excretion and should be used with caution.

Dialysis: Removed by hemo- and peritoneal dialysis

Hepatic Impairment No dosage adjustment provided in manufacturer's labeling (has not been studied); carisoprodol undergoes hepatic metabolism and should be used with caution.

Dietary Considerations May be taken with or without food.

Administration Administer with or without food.

Monitoring Parameters CNS effects (eg, mental status, excessive drowsiness); relief of pain and/or muscle spasm; signs of misuse, abuse, and addiction

Dosage Forms Excipient information presented when available (limited, particularly for generics); consult specific product labeling.

Tablet, Oral:

Soma: 250 mg, 350 mg

Generic: 250 mg, 350 mg

Controlled Substance C-IV

Carisoprodol and Aspirin

(kar eye soe PROE dole & AS pir in)

Index Terms Aspirin and Carisoprodol; Soma Compound

Pharmacologic Category Skeletal Muscle Relaxant

Use Relief of discomfort associated with acute, painful skeletal muscle conditions

Dosing

Adult Acute skeletal muscle pain: Oral: 1-2 tablets 4 times/day for 2-3 weeks (maximum: 8 tablets/24 hours)

Geriatric Avoid use in the elderly due to risk of orthostatic hypotension and CNS depression.

Pediatric Children ≥16 years: Refer to adult dosing.

Renal Impairment Use in renal impairment has not been studied; use with caution.

Hepatic Impairment Use in hepatic impairment has not been studied; use with caution.

Additional Information Complete prescribing information should be consulted for additional detail.

Dosage Forms Excipient information presented when available (limited, particularly for generics); consult specific product labeling.

Tablet: Carisoprodol 200 mg and aspirin 325 mg

Controlled Substance C-IV

Carisoprodol, Aspirin, and Codeine

(kar eye soe PROE dole, AS pir in, and KOE deen)

Index Terms Aspirin, Carisoprodol, and Codeine; Codeine, Aspirin, and Carisoprodol; Soma Compound w/Codeine

Pharmacologic Category Skeletal Muscle Relaxant

Use Skeletal muscle relaxant

Dosing

Adult & Geriatric Skeletal muscle relaxant, analgesic: Oral: 1 or 2 tablets 4 times daily (maximum: 8 tablets per day); treatment should be temporary (2-3 weeks)

Renal Impairment No dosage adjustment provided in manufacturer's labeling.

Hepatic Impairment No dosage adjustment provided in manufacturer's labeling.

Additional Information Complete prescribing information should be consulted for additional detail.

Dosage Forms Excipient information presented when available (limited, particularly for generics); consult specific product labeling. [DSC] = Discontinued product

Tablet: Carisoprodol 200 mg, aspirin 325 mg, and codeine phosphate 16 mg

Controlled Substance C-III

- ◆ Carmol [OTC] *see* Urea *on page 1853*
- ◆ Carmol 10 [OTC] *see* Urea *on page 1853*
- ◆ Carmol 20 [OTC] *see* Urea *on page 1853*
- ◆ Carmol-HC® [DSC] *see* Urea and Hydrocortisone *on page 1854*

Carmustine (kar MUS teen)

Brand Names: US BiCNU; Gliadel Wafer

Brand Names: Canada BiCNU; Gliadel Wafer

Index Terms BCNU; Becenum; bis(chloroethyl) nitrosourea; bis-chloronitrosourea; Carmustine Polymer Wafer; Carmustine Sustained-Release Implant Wafer; Carmustinum; WR-139021

Pharmacologic Category Antineoplastic Agent, Alkylating Agent; Antineoplastic Agent, Alkylating Agent (Nitrosourea)

Use

Brain tumors:

Injection: Palliative treatment of brain tumors including glioblastoma, brainstem glioma, medulloblastoma, astrocytoma, ependymoma, and metastatic brain tumors

Wafer (implant): Treatment of newly-diagnosed high-grade malignant glioma (as an adjunct to surgery and radiation); treatment of recurrent glioblastoma multiforme (as adjunct to surgery)

Hodgkin lymphoma, relapsed/refractory: Injection: Palliative treatment (secondary) of Hodgkin lymphoma (in combination with other antineoplastics) that has relapsed with or was refractory to primary therapy

Multiple myeloma: Injection: Palliative treatment of multiple myeloma (in combination with prednisone)

Non-Hodgkin lymphomas, relapsed/refractory: Injection: Palliative treatment (secondary) of non-Hodgkin lymphoma (in combination with other antineoplastics) that has relapsed with or was refractory to primary therapy

Pregnancy Considerations Adverse events have been observed in animal reproduction studies. Carmustine may cause fetal harm if administered to a pregnant woman. Women of childbearing potential should use effective contraception to avoid becoming pregnant while on treatment. May impair fertility. Advise males of potential risk of infertility and to seek fertility/family planning counseling prior to receiving carmustine wafer implants.

Breast-Feeding Considerations It is not known if carmustine is excreted in breast milk. Due to the potential for serious adverse reactions in the nursing infant, the manufacturer recommends breast-feeding be discontinued during treatment.

Contraindications

IV: Hypersensitivity to carmustine or any component of the formulation

Implant: There are no contraindications listed in the manufacturer's labeling.

Warnings/Precautions Hazardous agent - use appropriate precautions for handling and disposal (NIOSH 2014 [group 1]).

Injection:

[US Boxed Warning]: Bone marrow suppression, primarily thrombocytopenia (which may lead to bleeding) and leukopenia (which may lead to infection), is the most common and severe toxicity. Hematologic toxicity is generally delayed; monitor blood counts for at least 6 weeks following treatment. The manufacturer suggests not administering more frequently than every 6 weeks for approved doses/uses. Myelosuppression is cumulative; consider nadir blood counts from prior dose for dosage adjustment. Patients must have platelet counts >100,000/mm³ and leukocytes >4,000/mm³ for a repeat dose. Myelosuppression generally occurs 4 to 6 weeks after administration;

thrombocytopenia occurs at ~4 weeks and persists for 1 to 2 weeks; leukopenia occurs at 5 to 6 weeks and persists for 1 to 2 weeks. Anemia may occur (less common and less severe than leukopenia or thrombocytopenia). Long-term use is associated with the development of secondary malignancies (acute leukemias and bone marrow dysplasias).

[US Boxed Warnings]: Dose-related pulmonary toxicity may occur; patients receiving cumulative doses >1,400 mg/m² are at higher risk. Delayed onset of pulmonary fibrosis may occur years after treatment (may be fatal), particularly in children. Pulmonary toxicity has occurred in children up to 17 years after treatment; this occurred in ages 1 to 16 for the treatment of intracranial tumors; cumulative doses ranged from 770 to 1,800 mg/m² (in combination with cranial radiotherapy). Pulmonary toxicity is characterized by pulmonary infiltrates and/or fibrosis and has been reported from 9 days to 43 months after nitrosourea treatment (including carmustine). Although pulmonary toxicity generally occurs in patients who have received prolonged treatment, pulmonary fibrosis has been reported with cumulative doses <1,400 mg/m². In addition to high cumulative doses, other risk factors for pulmonary toxicity include history of lung disease and baseline predicted forced vital capacity (FVC) or carbon monoxide diffusing capacity (DL$_{CO}$) <70%. Baseline and periodic pulmonary function tests are recommended. For high-dose treatment (transplant; off-label dose), acute lung injury may occur ~1 to 3 months post transplant; advise patients to contact their transplant physician for dyspnea, cough, or fever; interstitial pneumonia may be managed with a course of corticosteroids. Children are at higher risk of delayed pulmonary toxicity with IV carmustine.

Reversible increases in transaminases, bilirubin, and alkaline phosphatase have been reported (rare). Monitor liver function tests periodically during treatment. Renal failure, progressive azotemia, and decreased kidney size have been reported in patients who have received large cumulative doses or prolonged treatment. Renal toxicity has also been reported in patients who have received lower cumulative doses. Monitor renal function tests periodically during treatment.

Carmustine is associated with a moderate to high emetic potential (dose-related); antiemetics are recommended to prevent nausea and vomiting (Basch, 2011; Dupuis, 2011). Injection site burning and local tissue reactions, including swelling, pain, erythema, and necrosis have been reported. Monitor infusion site closely for infiltration or injection site reactions. Off-label administration (intra-arterial intracarotid route) has been associated with ocular toxicity. Consider initiating IV treatment at the lower end of the dose range in elderly patients. The diluent for IV carmustine contains ethanol.

Wafer implant:
Seizures occurred in patients who received carmustine wafer implants, including new or worsening seizures and treatment-emergent seizures. Just over half of treatment-emergent seizures occurred within 5 days of surgery; the median onset of first new or worsened post-operative seizure was 4 days. Optimal anti-seizure therapy should be initiated prior to surgery. Monitor for seizures. Brain edema has been reported in patients with newly diagnosed glioma, including one report of intracranial mass effect unresponsive to corticosteroids which led to brain herniation. Monitor closely for intracranial hypertension related to brain edema, inflammation, or necrosis of brain tissue surrounding resection. Re-operation to remove wafers (or remnants) may be necessary for refractory cases. Cases of meningitis have occurred in patients with recurrent glioma receiving wafer implants. Two cases were bacterial (one patient required removal of implants 4 days after implantation and the other developed meningitis following reoperation for recurrent tumor). Another case was determined to be chemical meningitis and resolved with corticosteroids. Monitor postoperatively for signs/symptoms of meningitis and CNS infection.

Monitor closely for known craniotomy-related complications (seizure, intracranial infection, abnormal wound healing, brain edema). Wafer migration may occur; avoid communication between the resection cavity and the ventricular system to prevent wafer migration; communications larger than the wafer should be closed prior to implantation; wafer migration into the ventricular system may cause obstructive hydrocephalus. Monitor for signs/symptoms of obstructive hydrocephalus.

Impaired neurosurgical wound healing, including would dehiscence, delayed healing, and subdural, subgleal or wound effusions may occur with carmustine wafer implant treatment; cerebrospinal fluid leaks have also been reported. Monitor post-operatively for impaired neurosurgical wound healing.

[US Boxed Warning]: Should be administered under the supervision of an experienced cancer chemotherapy physician. Potentially significant drug-drug interactions may exist, requiring dose or frequency adjustment, additional monitoring, and/or selection of alternative therapy.

Adverse Reactions
IV: Frequency not defined:
Cardiovascular: Cardiac arrhythmia (with high doses), chest pain, flushing (with rapid infusion), hypotension, tachycardia
Central nervous system: Dizziness, headache
Dermatologic: Burning sensation of skin (after skin contact), hyperpigmentation (after skin contact)
Gastrointestinal: Nausea (common; dose related), vomiting (common; dose related)
Hematologic & oncologic: Leukopenia (common; onset: 5 to 6 weeks; recovery: After 1 to 2 weeks), thrombocytopenia (common; onset: ~4 weeks; recovery: After 1 to 2 weeks), anemia, febrile neutropenia, malignant neoplasm (secondary; acute leukemia, bone marrow dysplasias)
Hepatic: Increased serum alkaline phosphatase, increased serum bilirubin, increased serum transaminases
Hypersensitivity: Hypersensitivity reaction
Infection: Infection (with high doses)
Local: Burning sensation at injection site, erythema at injection site, pain at injection site, swelling at injection site, tissue necrosis at injection site, venous thrombosis at injection site (rare)
Ophthalmic: Neuroretinitis, suffusion of the conjunctiva (with rapid infusion)
Renal: Azotemia (progressive; with long-term therapy), nephron atrophy (with long-term therapy), nephrotoxicity, renal failure (with long-term therapy)
Respiratory: Interstitial pneumonitis (with high doses), lung hypoplasia, pulmonary fibrosis (occurring up to 17 years after treatment), pulmonary infiltrates
Wafer:
>10%:
Central nervous system: Seizure (37%; new or worsening: 20%), cerebral edema (4% to 23%), depression (16%)
Dermatologic: Skin rash (5% to 12%)
Gastrointestinal: Nausea (22%), vomiting (21%), constipation (19%)
Genitourinary: Urinary tract infection (21%)
Neuromuscular & skeletal: Weakness (22%)
Miscellaneous: Wound healing impairment (14% to 16%), fever (12%)
1% to 10%:
Cardiovascular: Chest pain (5%)
Central nervous system: Intracranial hypertension (9%), cerebral hemorrhage (6%), meningitis (4%)
Gastrointestinal: Abdominal pain (8%)
Infection: Abscess (local 6%)
Neuromuscular & skeletal: Back pain (7%)
<1% (Limited to important or life-threatening): Sepsis
Drug Interactions
Metabolism/Transport Effects None known.
Avoid Concomitant Use
Avoid concomitant use of Carmustine with any of the following: BCG (Intravesical); Deferiprone; Dipyrone; Natalizumab; Pimecrolimus; Tacrolimus (Topical); Tofacitinib; Vaccines (Live)
Increased Effect/Toxicity
Carmustine may increase the levels/effects of: CloZAPine; Deferiprone; Fingolimod; Leflunomide; Natalizumab; Tofacitinib; Vaccines (Live)

The levels/effects of Carmustine may be increased by: Cimetidine; Denosumab; Dipyrone; Melphalan; Pimecrolimus; Roflumilast; Tacrolimus (Topical); Trastuzumab
Decreased Effect
Carmustine may decrease the levels/effects of: BCG (Intravesical); Coccidioides immitis Skin Test; Sipuleucel-T; Vaccines (Inactivated); Vaccines (Live)

The levels/effects of Carmustine may be decreased by: Echinacea

Preparation for Administration Hazardous agent; use appropriate precautions for handling and disposal (NIOSH 2014 [group 1]).

Injection: Reconstitute initially with 3 mL of supplied diluent (dehydrated alcohol injection, USP); then further dilute with SWFI (27 mL), this provides a concentration of 3.3 mg/mL in ethanol 10%; protect from light; further dilute for infusion with D_5W using a non-PVC container (eg, glass or polyolefin).

Implant: Each wafer is packaged within 2 nested aluminum foil pouches; the inner pouch is sterile and is designed to maintain sterility and protect from moisture; the outer wrap is not sterile. Deliver to the operating room in the unopened outer aluminum foil pouch. Do not open until the wafers are ready to be implanted. Follow manufacturer's instructions for opening the pouch, being careful not to apply pressure to the wafer.

Storage/Stability
Injection: Store intact vials and provided diluent under refrigeration at 2°C to 8°C (36°F to 46°F). Carmustine has a low melting point (30.5°C to 32°C [86.9°F to 89.6°F]); exposure to temperature at or above the melting point will cause the drug to liquefy and appear as an oil film on the vials. If drug liquefies, discard the vials as this is a sign of decomposition.

Reconstituted solutions are stable for 24 hours refrigerated (2°C to 8°C) and protected from light. Examine reconstituted vials for crystal formation prior to use. If crystals are observed, they may be redissolved by warming the vial to room temperature with agitation.

Solutions diluted to a concentration of 0.2 mg/mL in D_5W are stable for 8 hours at room temperature (25°C) in glass and protected from light. Although the manufacturer recommends only glass containers be used, stability of a 1 mg/mL solution in D_5W has also been demonstrated for up to 6 hours (with a 6% to 7% loss of potency) in polyolefin containers (Trissel, 2006).

Wafer: Store at or below -20°C (-4°F). Unopened outer foil pouches may be kept at room temperature for up to 6 hours at a time for up to 3 cycles within a 30-day period.

Mechanism of Action Interferes with the normal function of DNA and RNA by alkylation and cross-linking the strands of DNA and RNA, and by possible protein modification; may also inhibit enzyme processes by carbamylation of amino acids in protein

Pharmacodynamics/Kinetics
Distribution: IV: 3.3 L/kg; readily crosses blood-brain barrier producing CSF levels >50% of blood plasma levels; highly lipid soluble

Metabolism: Rapidly hepatic; forms active metabolites

Half-life elimination: IV: Biphasic: Initial: 1.4 minutes; Secondary: 22 minutes (active metabolites: Plasma half-life of 67 hours)

Excretion: IV: Urine (~60% to 70%) within 96 hours; lungs (~10% as CO_2)

Dosing
Adult & Geriatric Note: Carmustine (IV) is associated with a moderate to high emetic potential (dose-related); antiemetics are recommended to prevent nausea and vomiting (Basch, 2011; Dupuis, 2011).

Brain tumors, Hodgkin lymphoma, multiple myeloma, non-Hodgkin lymphoma (per manufacturer labeling): IV: 150 to 200 mg/m² every 6 weeks or 75 to 100 mg/m²/day for 2 days every 6 weeks

Glioblastoma multiforme (recurrent), glioma (malignant, newly-diagnosed high-grade): Implantation (wafer): 8 wafers (7.7 mg each) implanted intracranially into in the resection cavity (total dose 61.6 mg); should the size and shape not accommodate 8 wafers, the maximum number of wafers feasible (up to 8) should be placed

Indication-specific dosing:
Brain tumor, primary (off-label doses): IV:
80 mg/m²/day for 3 days every 8 weeks for 6 cycles (Brandes, 2004)
200 mg/m² every 8 weeks [maximum cumulative dose: 1500 mg/m²] (Selker, 2002)

Hodgkin lymphoma, relapsed or refractory (off-label dose): IV: Mini-BEAM regimen: 60 mg/m² day 1 every 4 to 6 weeks (in combination with etoposide, cytarabine, and melphalan) (Colwill, 1995; Martin, 2001)

Multiple myeloma, relapsed, refractory (off-label dose): IV: VBMCP regimen: 20 mg/m² day 1 every 35 days (in combination with vincristine, melphalan, cyclophosphamide, and prednisone) (Kyle, 2006; Oken, 1997)

Mycosis fungoides, early stage (off-label use; Zackheim, 2003): Topical:
Ointment (10 mg/100 grams petrolatum): Apply (with gloves) once daily to affected areas

Solution (0.2% solution in alcohol; dilute 5 mL in 60 mL water): Apply (with gloves) once daily to affected areas

Stem cell or bone marrow transplant, autologous (off-label use): IV:
BEAM regimen: 300 mg/m² 6 days prior to transplant (in combination with etoposide, cytarabine, and melphalan) (Chopra, 1993; Linch, 2010)
CBV regimen: 600 mg/m² 3 days prior to transplant (in combination with cyclophosphamide and etoposide) (Reece, 1991)

Renal Impairment
IV: There are no dosage adjustments provided in the manufacturer's labeling. The following dosage adjustments have been reported (Kintzel, 1995):
CrCl 46 to 60 mL/minute: Administer 80% of dose
CrCl 31 to 45 mL/minute: Administer 75% of dose
CrCl ≤30 mL/minute: Consider use of alternative drug.
Wafer implant: There are no dosage adjustments provided in the manufacturer's labeling.

Hepatic Impairment
IV: Dosage adjustment may be necessary; however, no specific guidelines are available.
Wafer implant: There are no dosage adjustments provided in the manufacturer's labeling.

Obesity
*American Society of Clinical Oncology (ASCO) Guidelines for appropriate chemotherapy dosing in obese adults with cancer (**Note:** Excludes HSCT dosing):* Utilize patient's actual body weight (full weight) for calculation of body surface area- or weight-based dosing, particularly when the intent of therapy is curative; manage regimen-related toxicities in the same manner as for nonobese patients; if a dose reduction is utilized due to toxicity, consider resumption of full weight-based dosing with subsequent cycles, especially if cause of toxicity (eg, hepatic or renal impairment) is resolved (Griggs, 2012).

American Society for Blood and Marrow Transplantation (ASBMT) practice guideline committee position statement on chemotherapy dosing in obesity: Utilize actual body weight (full weight) for calculation of body surface area in carmustine dosing for hematopoietic stem cell transplant conditioning regimens in adult patients weighing ≤120% of their ideal body weight (IBW). In patients weighing >120% IBW, utilize adjusted body weight 25% (ABW25) to calculate BSA (Bubalo, 2014). ABW25: Adjusted wt (kg) = Ideal body weight (kg) + 0.25 [actual wt (kg) - ideal body weight (kg)]

Adjustment for Toxicity Hematologic toxicity: Based on nadir counts with previous dose (manufacturer's labeling). IV:
If leukocytes ≥3,000/mm³ and platelets ≥75,000/mm³: Administer 100% of dose
If leukocytes 2,000 to 2,999/mm³ or platelets 25,000 to 74,999/mm³: Administer 70% of dose
If leukocytes <2,000/mm³ or platelets <25,000/mm³: Administer 50% of dose

Administration
Carmustine (IV) is associated with a moderate to high emetic potential (dose-related); antiemetics are recommended to prevent nausea and vomiting (Basch, 2011; Dupuis, 2011).

Injection: Irritant (alcohol-based diluent). Significant absorption to PVC containers; should be prepared in either glass or polyolefin containers. Infuse over at least 2 hours (infusions <2 hours may lead to injection site pain or burning); infuse through a free-flowing saline or dextrose infusion, or administer through a central catheter to alleviate venous pain/irritation.

High-dose carmustine (transplant dose; off-label use): Infuse over a least 2 hours to avoid excessive flushing, agitation, and hypotension; was infused over 1 hour in some trials (Chopra, 1993). **High-dose carmustine may be fatal if not followed by stem cell rescue.** Monitor vital signs frequently during infusion; patients should be supine during infusion and may require the Trendelenburg position, fluid support, and vasopressor support.

Implant: Double glove before handling; outer gloves should be discarded as chemotherapy waste after handling wafers. Any wafer or remnant that is removed upon repeat surgery should be discarded as chemotherapy waste. The outer surface of the external foil pouch is not sterile. Open pouch gently; avoid pressure on the wafers to prevent breakage. Wafers that are broken in half may be used, however, wafers broken into more than 2 pieces should be discarded in a biohazard container. Slight overlapping of wafers during placement is acceptable. Oxidized regenerated cellulose (Surgicel) may be placed over the wafer to secure; irrigate cavity prior to closure.

Topical (off-label use): Apply solution with brush or gauze pads; ointment and solution should be applied while wearing gloves to involved areas only; avoid contact with eyes or mouth (Zackheim, 2003).

Hazardous agent; use appropriate precautions for handling and disposal (NIOSH 2014 [group 1]).

Monitoring Parameters

Injection: CBC with differential and platelet count (weekly for at least 6 weeks after a dose), pulmonary function tests (FVC, DL_{CO}; at baseline and frequently during treatment), liver function (periodically), renal function tests (periodically); monitor blood pressure and vital signs during administration, monitor infusion site for possible infiltration

Wafer: Monitor postoperatively for seizures, impaired neurosurgical wound healing, and signs/symptoms of meningitis, CNS infection, and obstructive hydrocephalus; monitor closely for intracranial hypertension related to brain edema, inflammation, or necrosis of brain tissue surrounding resection.

Dosage Forms Excipient information presented when available (limited, particularly for generics); consult specific product labeling.

Solution Reconstituted, Intravenous:
BiCNU: 100 mg (1 ea) [contains alcohol, usp]
Wafer, Implant:
Gliadel Wafer: 7.7 mg (8 ea) [contains polifeprosan 20]

◆ **Carmustine Polymer Wafer** see Carmustine on page 320

◆ **Carmustine Sustained-Release Implant Wafer** see Carmustine on page 320

◆ **Carmustinum** see Carmustine on page 320

◆ **Caroguard [OTC]** see Beta-Carotene on page 221

◆ **Carrington Antifungal [OTC]** see Miconazole (Topical) on page 1201

◆ **Carter's Little Pills [OTC] (Can)** see Bisacodyl on page 231

◆ **Cartia XT** see Diltiazem on page 553

Carvedilol (KAR ve dil ole)

Brand Names: US Coreg; Coreg CR

Brand Names: Canada Apo-Carvedilol; Auro-Carvedilol; Dom-Carvedilol; JAMP-Carvedilol; Mylan-Carvedilol; Novo-Carvedilol; PMS-Carvedilol; RAN-Carvedilol; ratio-Carvedilol

Pharmacologic Category Antihypertensive; Beta-Blocker With Alpha-Blocking Activity

Use

Hypertension: Management of hypertension.

The 2014 guideline for the management of high blood pressure in adults (Eighth Joint National Committee [JNC 8]) recommends initiation of pharmacologic treatment to lower blood pressure for the following patients (JNC 8 [James, 2013]):

• Patients ≥60 years of age, with systolic blood pressure (SBP) ≥150 mm Hg or diastolic blood pressure (DBP) ≥90 mm Hg. Goal of therapy is SBP <150 mm Hg and DBP <90 mm Hg.

• Patients <60 years of age, with SBP ≥140 mm Hg or DBP ≥90 mm Hg. Goal of therapy is SBP <140 mm Hg and DBP <90 mm Hg.

• Patients ≥18 years of age with diabetes, with SBP ≥140 mm Hg or DBP ≥90 mm Hg. Goal of therapy is SBP <140 mm Hg and DBP <90 mm Hg.

• Patients ≥18 years of age with chronic kidney disease (CKD), with SBP ≥140 mm Hg or DBP ≥90 mm Hg. Goal of therapy is SBP <140 mm Hg and DBP <90 mm Hg.

In patients with CKD, regardless of race or diabetes status, the use of an ACE inhibitor (ACEI) or angiotensin receptor blocker (ARB) as initial therapy is recommended to improve kidney outcomes. In the general non-black population (without CKD) including those with diabetes, initial antihypertensive treatment should consist of a thiazide-type diuretic, calcium channel blocker, ACEI, or ARB. In the general black population (without CKD) including those with diabetes, initial antihypertensive treatment should consist of a thiazide-type diuretic or a calcium channel blocker **instead of** an ACEI or ARB.

Heart failure: Mild to severe chronic heart failure of ischemic or cardiomyopathic origin (usually in addition to standard therapy [eg, diuretics, ACE inhibitors]).

The ACCF/AHA 2013 heart failure guidelines recommend the use of 1 of the 3 beta blockers (ie, bisoprolol, carvedilol, or extended-release metoprolol succinate)

for all patients with recent or remote history of MI or ACS and reduced ejection fraction (rEF) to reduce mortality, for all patients with rEF to prevent symptomatic HF (even if no history of MI), and for all patients with current or prior symptoms of HF with reduced ejection fraction (HFrEF), unless contraindicated, to reduce morbidity and mortality (Yancy, 2013).

Left ventricular dysfunction following myocardial infarction (MI): Left ventricular dysfunction following MI (clinically stable with LVEF ≤40%)

Pregnancy Considerations Adverse events have been observed in animal reproduction studies. In a cohort study, an increased risk of cardiovascular defects was observed following maternal use of beta-blockers during pregnancy (Lennestål, 2009). Intrauterine growth restriction (IUGR), small placentas, as well as fetal/neonatal bradycardia, hypoglycemia, and/or respiratory depression have been observed following in utero exposure to beta-blockers as a class. Adequate facilities for monitoring infants at birth should be available. Untreated chronic maternal hypertension and pre-eclampsia are also associated with adverse events in the fetus, infant, and mother. Carvedilol is not currently recommended for the initial treatment of maternal hypertension during pregnancy (ACOG, 2001; ACOG, 2002).

Breast-Feeding Considerations It is not known if carvedilol is excreted in breast milk. Due to the potential for serious adverse reactions in the nursing infant, the manufacturer recommends a decision be made whether to discontinue nursing or to discontinue the drug, taking into account the importance of treatment to the mother.

Contraindications

Serious hypersensitivity to carvedilol or any component of the formulation; decompensated cardiac failure requiring intravenous inotropic therapy; bronchial asthma or related bronchospastic conditions; second- or third-degree AV block, sick sinus syndrome, and severe bradycardia (except in patients with a functioning artificial pacemaker); cardiogenic shock; severe hepatic impairment

Documentation of allergenic cross-reactivity for drugs alpha/beta adrenergic blocking agents is limited. However, because of similarities in chemical structure and/or pharmacologic actions, the possibility of cross-sensitivity cannot be ruled out with certainty.

Warnings/Precautions Heart failure patients may experience a worsening of renal function (rare); risk factors include ischemic heart disease, diffuse vascular disease, underlying renal dysfunction, and/or systolic BP <100 mm Hg. Initiate cautiously and monitor for possible deterioration in patient status (eg, symptoms of HF). Worsening heart failure or fluid retention may occur during upward titration; dose reduction or temporary discontinuation may be necessary. Adjustment of other medications (ACE inhibitors and/or diuretics) may also be required. Bradycardia may occur; reduce dosage if heart rate drops to <55 beats/minute. Bradycardia may be observed more frequently in elderly patients (>65 years of age); dosage reductions may be necessary.

Symptomatic hypotension with or without syncope may occur with carvedilol (usually within the first 30 days of therapy); close monitoring of patient is required especially with initial dosing and dosing increases; blood pressure must be lowered at a rate appropriate for the patient's clinical condition. Initiation with a low dose, gradual up-titration, and administration with food may help to decrease the occurrence of hypotension or syncope. Advise patients to avoid driving or other hazardous tasks during initiation of therapy due to the risk of syncope. Beta-blocker therapy should not be withdrawn abruptly (particularly in patients with CAD), but gradually tapered to avoid acute tachycardia, hypertension, and/or ischemia. Chronic beta-blocker therapy should not be routinely withdrawn prior to major surgery.

In general, patients with bronchospastic disease should not receive beta-blockers; if used at all, should be used cautiously with close monitoring. May precipitate or aggravate symptoms of arterial insufficiency in patients with PVD; use with caution and monitor for progression of arterial obstruction. Use with caution in patients with diabetes; may potentiate hypoglycemia and/or mask signs and symptoms (eg, sweating, anxiety, tachycardia). In patients with heart failure and diabetes, use of carvedilol may worsen hyperglycemia; may require adjustment of antidiabetic agents. May mask signs of hyperthyroidism (eg, tachycardia); if hyperthyroidism is suspected, carefully manage and monitor; abrupt withdrawal may exacerbate symptoms of hyperthyroidism or precipitate thyroid storm. May induce or exacerbate psoriasis. Use with caution in patients suspected of having Prinzmetal variant angina. Use with caution in patients with myasthenia gravis. Use

with caution in patients with mild to moderate hepatic impairment; use is contraindicated in patients with severe impairment. Use with caution in patients with pheochromocytoma; adequate alpha-blockade is required prior to use. Use caution with history of severe anaphylaxis to allergens; patients taking beta-blockers may become more sensitive to repeated challenges. Treatment of anaphylaxis (eg, epinephrine) in patients taking beta-blockers may be ineffective or promote undesirable effects.

Intraoperative floppy iris syndrome has been observed in cataract surgery patients who were on or were previously treated with alpha₁-blockers; there appears to be no benefit in discontinuing alpha-blocker therapy prior to surgery. Instruct patients to inform ophthalmologist of carvedilol use when considering eye surgery. Potentially significant interactions may exist, requiring dose or frequency adjustment, additional monitoring, and/or selection of alternative therapy.

Some dosage forms may contain polysorbate 80 (also known as Tweens). Hypersensitivity reactions, usually a delayed reaction, have been reported following exposure to pharmaceutical products containing polysorbate 80 in certain individuals (Isaksson, 2002; Lucente 2000; Shelley, 1995). Thrombocytopenia, ascites, pulmonary deterioration, and renal and hepatic failure have been reported in premature neonates after receiving parenteral products containing polysorbate 80 (Alade, 1986; CDC, 1984). See manufacturer's labeling.

Adverse Reactions Note: Frequency ranges include data from hypertension and heart failure trials. Higher rates of adverse reactions have generally been noted in patients with heart failure. However, the frequency of adverse effects associated with placebo is also increased in this population.

>10%:
Cardiovascular: Hypotension (9% to 20%)
Central nervous system: Dizziness (2% to 32%), fatigue (4% to 24%)
Endocrine & metabolic: Hyperglycemia (5% to 12%)
Gastrointestinal: Diarrhea (1% to 12%), weight gain (10% to 12%)
Neuromuscular & skeletal: Weakness (7% to 11%)
1% to 10%:
Cardiovascular: Bradycardia (2% to 10%), syncope (3% to 8%), peripheral edema (1% to 7%), generalized edema (5% to 6%), angina (1% to 6%), dependent edema (≤4%), AV block, cerebrovascular accident, hypertension, hyper-/hypovolemia, orthostatic hypotension, palpitation
Central nervous system: Headache (5% to 8%), depression, fever, hypoesthesia, hypotonia, insomnia, malaise, somnolence, vertigo
Endocrine & metabolic: Hypercholesterolemia (1% to 4%), hypertriglyceridemia (1%), diabetes mellitus, gout, hyperkalemia, hyperuricemia, hypoglycemia, hyponatremia
Gastrointestinal: Nausea (2% to 9%), vomiting (1% to 6%), abdominal pain, melena, periodontitis, weight loss
Genitourinary: Impotence
Hematologic: Anemia, prothrombin decreased, purpura, thrombocytopenia
Hepatic: Alkaline phosphatase increased (1% to 3%), GGT increased, transaminases increased
Neuromuscular & skeletal: Back pain (2% to 7%), arthralgia (1% to 6%), arthritis, muscle cramps, paresthesia
Ocular: Blurred vision (1% to 5%)
Renal: BUN increased (≤6%), nonprotein nitrogen increased (6%), albuminuria, creatinine increased, glycosuria, hematuria, renal insufficiency
Respiratory: Cough (5% to 8%), nasopharyngitis (4%), rales (4%), dyspnea (>3%), pulmonary edema (>3%), rhinitis (2%), nasal congestion (1%), sinus congestion (1%)
Miscellaneous: Injury (3% to 6%), allergy, flu-like syndrome, sudden death
<1% (Limited to important or life-threatening): Anaphylactoid reaction, alopecia, angioedema, aplastic anemia, amnesia, asthma, bronchospasm, bundle branch block, cholestatic jaundice, concentration decreased, diaphoresis, erythema multiforme, exfoliative dermatitis, GI hemorrhage, HDL decreased, hearing decreased, hyperbilirubinemia, hypersensitivity reaction, hypokalemia, hypokinesia, interstitial pneumonitis, leukopenia, libido decreased, migraine, myocardial ischemia, nervousness, neuralgia, nightmares, pancytopenia, paresis, peripheral ischemia, photosensitivity, pruritus, rash (erythematous, maculopapular, and psoriaform), respiratory alkalosis, seizure, Stevens-Johnson syndrome, tachycardia, tinnitus, toxic epidermal necrolysis, urinary incontinence, urticaria, xerostomia

Drug Interactions

Metabolism/Transport Effects Substrate of CYP1A2 (minor), CYP2C9 (minor), CYP2D6 (major), CYP2E1 (minor), CYP3A4 (minor), P-glycoprotein); **Note:** Assignment of Major/Minor substrate status based on clinically relevant drug interaction potential; **Inhibits** P-glycoprotein

Avoid Concomitant Use
Avoid concomitant use of Carvedilol with any of the following: Beta2-Agonists; Bosutinib; Ceritinib; Floctafenine; Methacholine; PAZOPanib; Rivastigmine; Silodosin; Topotecan; VinCRIStine (Liposomal)

Increased Effect/Toxicity
Carvedilol may increase the levels/effects of: Afatinib; Alpha-/Beta-Agonists (Direct-Acting); Alpha1-Blockers; Alpha2-Agonists; Amifostine; Antipsychotic Agents (Phenothiazines); Antipsychotic Agents (Second Generation [Atypical]); Bosutinib; Bradycardia-Causing Agents; Brentuximab Vedotin; Bupivacaine; Cardiac Glycosides; Ceritinib; Cholinergic Agonists; Colchicine; CycloSPORINE (Systemic); Dabigatran Etexilate; Digoxin; Disopyramide; DOXOrubicin (Conventional); DULoxetine; Edoxaban; Ergot Derivatives; Everolimus; Fingolimod; Grass Pollen Allergen Extract (5 Grass Extract); Hypotension-Associated Agents; Insulin; Ivabradine; Lacosamide; Ledipasvir; Levodopa; Lidocaine (Systemic); Lidocaine (Topical); Mepivacaine; Methacholine; Midodrine; Naloxegol; PAZOPanib; P-glycoprotein/ABCB1 Substrates; Prucalopride; Ranolazine; Rifaximin; Silodosin; Sulfonylureas; Topotecan; VinCRIStine (Liposomal)

The levels/effects of Carvedilol may be increased by: Abiraterone Acetate; Acetylcholinesterase Inhibitors; Alpha2-Agonists; Aminoquinolines (Antimalarial); Amiodarone; Anilidopiperidine Opioids; Antipsychotic Agents (Phenothiazines); Barbiturates; Bretylium; Brimonidine (Topical); Calcium Channel Blockers (Nondihydropyridine); Cimetidine; Cobicistat; CYP2C9 Inhibitors (Moderate); CYP2C9 Inhibitors (Strong); CYP2D6 Inhibitors (Moderate); CYP2D6 Inhibitors (Strong); Darunavir; Diazoxide; Digoxin; Dipyridamole; Disopyramide; Dronedarone; Floctafenine; Herbs (Hypotensive Properties); Lumacaftor; Molsidomine; NiCARdipine; Nicorandil; NIFEdipine; Obinutuzumab; Panobinostat; Peginterferon Alfa-2b; Pentoxifylline; P-glycoprotein/ABCB1 Inhibitors; Phosphodiesterase 5 Inhibitors; Propafenone; Prostacyclin Analogues; Ranolazine; Regorafenib; Reserpine; Rivastigmine; Ruxolitinib; Selective Serotonin Reuptake Inhibitors; Tofacitinib

Decreased Effect
Carvedilol may decrease the levels/effects of: Beta2-Agonists; Theophylline Derivatives

The levels/effects of Carvedilol may be decreased by: Amphetamines; Barbiturates; Herbs (Hypertensive Properties); Lumacaftor; Methylphenidate; Nonsteroidal Anti-Inflammatory Agents; Peginterferon Alfa-2b; P-glycoprotein/ABCB1 Inducers; Rifamycin Derivatives; Yohimbine

Food Interactions Food decreases rate but not extent of absorption. Management: Administration with food minimizes risks of orthostatic hypotension.

Storage/Stability
Coreg: Store at <30°C (<86°F). Protect from moisture.
Coreg CR: Store at 25°C (77°F); excursions permitted to 15°C to 30°C (59°F to 86°F). Protect from light.

Mechanism of Action As a racemic mixture, carvedilol has nonselective beta-adrenoreceptor and alpha-adrenergic blocking activity. No intrinsic sympathomimetic activity has been documented. Associated effects in hypertensive patients include reduction of cardiac output, exercise- or beta-agonist-induced tachycardia, reduction of reflex orthostatic tachycardia, vasodilation, decreased peripheral vascular resistance (especially in standing position), decreased renal vascular resistance, reduced plasma renin activity, and increased levels of atrial natriuretic peptide. In CHF, associated effects include decreased pulmonary capillary wedge pressure, decreased pulmonary artery pressure, decreased heart rate, decreased systemic vascular resistance, increased stroke volume index, and decreased right atrial pressure (RAP).

Pharmacodynamics/Kinetics
Onset of action: Antihypertensive effect: Alpha-blockade: Within 30 minutes; Beta-blockade: Within 1 hour
Peak antihypertensive effect: ~1 to 2 hours
Absorption: Oral: Rapid and extensive, but with large first pass effect; first pass effect is stereoselective with R(+) enantiomer achieving plasma concentrations 2 to 3 times higher than S(-) enantiomer; delayed with food
Distribution: V_d: 115 L; distributes into extravascular tissues
Protein binding: >98%, primarily to albumin

Metabolism: Extensively (98%) hepatic, via CYP2C9, 2D6, 3A4, 2C19, 1A2, and 2E1 (2% excreted unchanged); metabolized predominantly by aromatic ring oxidation and glucuronidation; oxidative metabolites undergo conjugation via glucuronidation and sulfation; three active metabolites (4-hydroxyphenyl metabolite is 13 times more potent than parent drug for beta-blockade, however, active metabolites achieve plasma concentrations of only 1/10 of those for carvedilol); first-pass effect; plasma concentrations in the elderly and those with cirrhotic liver disease are 50% and 4 to 7 times higher, respectively. Metabolism is subject to genetic polymorphism; CYP2D6 poor metabolizers have a 2- to 3-fold higher plasma concentration of the R(+) enantiomer and a 20% to 25% increase in the S(-) enantiomer compared to extensive metabolizers.

Bioavailability: Immediate release: ~25% to 35% (due to significant first-pass metabolism); Extended release: ~85% of immediate release; high-fat meal increases AUC and C_{max} ~20%; bioavailability is increased in patients with CHF

Half-life elimination:
Infants and Children 6 weeks to 3.5 years (n=8): 2.2 hours (Laer 2002)
Children and Adolescents 5.5 to 19 years (n=7): 3.6 hours (Laer 2002)
Adults 7 to 10 hours; some have reported lower values: Adults 24 to 37 years (n=9): 5.2 hours (Laer 2002)
R(+)-carvedilol: 5 to 9 hours
S(-)-carvedilol: 7 to 11 hours
Time to peak, plasma: Extended release: ~5 hours
Excretion: Primarily feces; urine (<2%, unchanged)

Dosing
Adult Reduce dosage if heart rate drops to <55 beats/minute.
Hypertension: Oral:
Immediate release: 6.25 mg twice daily; if tolerated, dose should be maintained for 1 to 2 weeks, then increased to 12.5 mg twice daily. If necessary, dosage may be increased to a maximum of 25 mg twice daily after 1 to 2 weeks. Usual dosage range (ASH/ISH [Weber, 2014]): 6.25 to 25 mg twice daily.
Extended release: Initial: 20 mg once daily, if tolerated, dose should be maintained for 1 to 2 weeks increased to 40 mg once daily if necessary; if this dose is tolerated, maintain for 1 to 2 weeks then, if necessary, increase to 80 mg once daily; maximum dose: 80 mg once daily
Heart failure: Oral: **Note:** Initiate only in stable patients or hospitalized patients after volume status has been optimized and IV diuretics, vasodilators, and inotropic agents have all been successfully discontinued. Caution should be used when initiating in patients who required inotropes during their hospital course. Increase dose gradually and monitor for congestive signs and symptoms of HF making every effort to achieve target dose shown to be effective (HFSA [Lindenfeld, 2010]; Packer, 1996; ACCF/AHA [Yancy, 2013])
Immediate release: 3.125 mg twice daily for 2 weeks; if this dose is tolerated, may increase to 6.25 mg twice daily. Double the dose every 2 weeks to the highest dose tolerated by patient. (Prior to initiating therapy, other heart failure medications should be stabilized and fluid retention minimized.)
Maximum recommended dose:
Mild-to-moderate heart failure:
<85 kg: 25 mg twice daily
>85 kg: 50 mg twice daily
Severe heart failure: 25 mg twice daily (Packer, 2001)
Extended release: Initial: 10 mg once daily for 2 weeks; if the dose is tolerated, increase dose to 20 mg, 40 mg, and 80 mg over successive intervals of at least 2 weeks. Maintain on lower dose if higher dose is not tolerated. **Note:** The 2013 ACCF/AHA heart failure guidelines recommend a maximum dose of 80 mg once daily (Yancy, 2013).
Left ventricular dysfunction following MI: Oral: **Note:** Should be initiated only after patient is hemodynamically stable and fluid retention has been minimized.
Immediate release: Initial 3.125 to 6.25 mg twice daily; increase dosage incrementally (ie, from 6.25 to 12.5 mg twice daily) at intervals of 3 to 10 days, based on tolerance, to a target dose of 25 mg twice daily. **Note:** The 2013 ACCF/AHA heart failure guidelines recommend a maximum dose of 50 mg twice daily (Yancy, 2013).
Extended release: Initial: Extended release: Initial: 10 to 20 mg once daily; increase dosage incrementally at intervals of 3 to 10 days, based on tolerance, to a target dose of 80 mg once daily.

Angina pectoris (off-label use): Oral: *Immediate release:* 25 to 50 mg twice daily
Atrial fibrillation (rate control) (off-label use): Usual maintenance dose: 3.125 to 25 mg twice daily (AHA/ACC/HRS [January, 2014]). In patients with heart failure, the initial dose of 3.125 mg twice daily may be increased at 2-week intervals to a target dose of 25 mg twice daily (50 mg twice daily for patients weighing >85 kg) (Khand, 2003)

Conversion from immediate release to extended release (Coreg CR):
Current dose immediate release tablets 3.125 mg twice daily: Convert to extended release capsules 10 mg once daily
Current dose immediate release tablets 6.25 mg twice daily: Convert to extended release capsules 20 mg once daily
Current dose immediate release tablets 12.5 mg twice daily: Convert to extended release capsules 40 mg once daily
Current dose immediate release tablets 25 mg twice daily: Convert to extended release capsules 80 mg once daily
Geriatric Refer to adult dosing. In the management of hypertension, consider lower initial doses and titrate to response (Aronow, 2011).
Renal Impairment No dosage adjustment necessary; not significantly cleared by hemodialysis
Hepatic Impairment
Mild to moderate impairment: There are no dosage adjustments provided in the manufacturer's labeling.
Severe impairment: Use is contraindicated.
Dietary Considerations Should be taken with food to minimize the risk of orthostatic hypotension.
Administration Administer with food to minimize the risk of orthostatic hypotension. Extended-release capsules and its contents should not be crushed, chewed, or divided. Capsules may be opened and its contents sprinkled on applesauce for immediate use.
Monitoring Parameters Heart rate, blood pressure (base need for dosage increase on trough blood pressure measurements and for tolerance on standing systolic pressure 1 hour after dosing); renal studies, BUN, liver function; blood glucose in diabetics; in patients with increased risk for developing renal dysfunction, monitor during dosage titration.
Dosage Forms Excipient information presented when available (limited, particularly for generics); consult specific product labeling.
Capsule Extended Release 24 Hour, Oral, as phosphate:
Coreg CR: 10 mg, 20 mg, 40 mg, 80 mg
Tablet, Oral:
Coreg: 3.125 mg, 6.25 mg, 12.5 mg, 25 mg
Generic: 3.125 mg, 6.25 mg, 12.5 mg, 25 mg
Dosage Forms: Canada Note: Refer to Dosage Forms. Extended-release capsules are not available in Canada.
Extemporaneous Preparations A 1.25 mg/mL carvedilol oral suspension may be made with tablets and one of two different vehicles (Ora-Blend or 1:1 mixture of Ora-Sweet and Ora-Plus). Crush five 25 mg tablets in a mortar and reduce to a fine powder; add 15 mL of purified water and mix to a uniform paste. Mix while adding chosen vehicle in incremental proportions to almost 100 mL; transfer to a calibrated amber bottle, rinse mortar with vehicle, and add quantity of vehicle sufficient to make 100 mL. Label "shake well". Stable for 84 days when stored in amber prescription bottles at room temperature (Loyd, 2006).

Carvedilol oral liquid suspensions (0.1 mg/mL and 1.67 mg/mL) made from tablets, water, Ora-Plus, and Ora-Sweet were stable for 12 weeks when stored in glass amber bottles at room temperature (25°C). Use one 3.125 mg tablet for the 0.1 mg/mL suspension or two 25 mg tablets for the 1.67 mg/mL suspension; grind the tablet(s) and compound a mixture with 5 mL of water, 15 mL Ora-Plus, and 10 mL Ora-Sweet. Final volume of each suspension: 30 mL; label "shake well" (data on file, GlaxoSmithKline, Philadelphia, PA: DOF #132 [**Note:** Manufacturer no longer disseminates this document]).
Loyd A Jr, "Carvedilol 1.25 mg/mL Oral Suspension," *Int J Pharm Compounding,* 2006, 10(3):220.

♦ Casodex *see* Bicalutamide *on page 230*

Caspofungin (kas poe FUN jin)

Brand Names: US Cancidas
Brand Names: Canada Cancidas
Index Terms Caspofungin Acetate
Pharmacologic Category Antifungal Agent, Parenteral; Echinocandin

◄ **Use** Treatment of invasive *Aspergillus* infections in patients who are refractory or intolerant of other therapies; treatment of candidemia and other *Candida* infections (intra-abdominal abscesses, peritonitis, pleural space); treatment of esophageal candidiasis; empirical treatment for presumed fungal infections in febrile neutropenic patients

Pregnancy Considerations Adverse events have been observed in animal reproduction studies. When treatment of invasive *Aspergillus* or *Candida* infections is needed during pregnancy, other agents are preferred (DHHS [adult] 2014; Pappas 2009). Use may be considered in HIV-infected pregnant women with invasive *Aspergillus* or *Candida* infections when refractory to other agents (DHHS [adult] 2014)

Breast-Feeding Considerations It is not known if caspofungin is excreted in breast milk. The manufacturer recommends that caution be exercised when administering caspofungin to nursing women.

Contraindications Hypersensitivity to caspofungin or any component of the formulation

Warnings/Precautions Anaphylaxis and histamine-related reactions (eg, angioedema, facial swelling, bronchospasm, rash, sensation of warmth) have been reported. Discontinue if anaphylaxis occurs; consider discontinuation if histamine-related reactions occur. Administer supportive treatment if needed. Concurrent use of cyclosporine should be limited to patients for whom benefit outweighs risk, due to a high frequency of hepatic transaminase elevations observed during concurrent use. Potentially significant drug-drug interactions may exist, requiring dose or frequency adjustment, additional monitoring, and/or selection of alternative therapy. Use caution in hepatic impairment; increased transaminases and rare cases of liver impairment (including failure and hepatitis) have been reported in pediatric and adult patients. Monitor liver function tests during therapy; if tests become abnormal or worsen, consider discontinuation. Dosage reduction required in adults with moderate hepatic impairment; safety and efficacy have not been established in children with any degree of hepatic impairment and adults with severe hepatic impairment.

Adverse Reactions

>10%:
Cardiovascular: Hypotension (3% to 20%), peripheral edema (6% to 11%), tachycardia (4% to 11%)
Central nervous system: Chills (9% to 23%), headache (5% to 15%)
Dermatologic: Skin rash (4% to 23%)
Endocrine & metabolic: Hypokalemia (5% to 23%)
Gastrointestinal: Diarrhea (6% to 27%), vomiting (6% to 17%), nausea (4% to 15%)
Hematologic & oncologic: Decreased hemoglobin (18% to 21%), decreased hematocrit (13% to 18%), decreased white blood cell count (12%), anemia (2% to 11%)
Hepatic: Increased serum alkaline phosphatase (9% to 22%), increased serum ALT (4% to 18%), increased serum AST (2% to 16%), increased serum bilirubin (5% to 13%)
Local: Localized phlebitis (18%)
Renal: Increased serum creatinine (3% to 11%)
Respiratory: Respiratory failure (2% to 20%), cough (6% to 11%), pneumonia (4% to 11%)
Miscellaneous: Infusion related reaction (20% to 35%), fever (6% to 30%), septic shock (11% to 14%)
5% to 10%:
Cardiovascular: Hypertension (5% to 10%)
Dermatologic: Erythema (4% to 9%), pruritus (6% to 7%)
Endocrine & metabolic: Hypomagnesemia (7%), hyperglycemia (6%)
Gastrointestinal: Gastric irritation (4% to 10%), abdominal pain (4% to 9%)
Hepatic: Decreased serum albumin (7%)
Immunologic: Graft versus host disease (infants, children, and adolescents 1% to 4%)
Infection: Sepsis (5% to 7%)
Local: Catheter infection (infants, children, and adolescents 1% to 9%)
Renal: Hematuria (10%), increased blood urea nitrogen (4% to 9%)
Respiratory: Dyspnea (9%), pleural effusion (9%), respiratory distress (≤8%), rales (7%)
<5% (Limited to important or life-threatening): Abdominal distention, adult respiratory distress syndrome, anaphylaxis, anorexia, anxiety, arthralgia, atrial fibrillation, back pain, bacteremia, blood coagulation disorder, cardiac arrest, confusion, constipation, decreased appetite, decubitus ulcer, depression, dizziness, drowsiness, dyspepsia, dystonia, edema, epistaxis, erythema multiforme, fatigue, febrile neutropenia, flushing, hepatic failure, hepatitis, hepatomegaly, hepatotoxicity, histamine release (including facial swelling, bronchospasm, sensation of

warmth), hypercalcemia, hyperkalemia, hypervolemia, hypoxia, increased gamma-glutamyl transferase, infusion site reaction (pain/pruritus/swelling), insomnia, limb pain, myocardial infarction, nephrotoxicity (serum creatinine ≥2 x baseline value or ≥1 mg/dL in patients with serum creatinine above ULN range), pancreatitis, pulmonary edema, pulmonary infiltrates, renal failure, seizure, Stevens-Johnson syndrome, tachypnea, thrombocytopenia, tremor, urinary tract infection, urticaria, weakness

Drug Interactions

Metabolism/Transport Effects None known.

Avoid Concomitant Use
Avoid concomitant use of Caspofungin with any of the following: Saccharomyces boulardii

Increased Effect/Toxicity
The levels/effects of Caspofungin may be increased by: CycloSPORINE (Systemic)

Decreased Effect
Caspofungin may decrease the levels/effects of: Saccharomyces boulardii; Tacrolimus (Systemic)

The levels/effects of Caspofungin may be decreased by: Inducers of Drug Clearance; Rifampin

Preparation for Administration Bring refrigerated vial to room temperature. Reconstitute vials using 10.8 mL 0.9% sodium chloride for injection, SWFI, or bacteriostatic water for injection, resulting in a concentration of 5 mg/mL for the 50 mg vial, and 7 mg/mL for the 70 mg vial (vials contain overfill). Mix gently to dissolve until clear solution is formed; do not use if cloudy or contains particles. Solution should be further diluted with 0.9%, 0.45%, or 0.225% sodium chloride or LR (do not exceed final concentration of 0.5 mg/mL).

Storage/Stability Store intact vials at 2°C to 8°C (36°F to 46°F). Reconstituted solution may be stored at ≤25°C (≤77°F) for 1 hour prior to preparation of infusion solution. Solutions diluted for infusion should be used within 24 hours when stored at ≤25°C (≤77°F) or within 48 hours when stored at 2°C to 8°C (36°F to 46°F).

Mechanism of Action Inhibits synthesis of β(1,3)-D-glucan, an essential component of the cell wall of susceptible fungi. Highest activity is in regions of active cell growth. Mammalian cells do not require β(1,3)-D-glucan, limiting potential toxicity.

Pharmacodynamics/Kinetics
Distribution: CSF concentrations: Nondetectable [<10 ng/mL (n=1)] (Sáez-Llorens 2009)
Protein binding: ~97% to albumin
Metabolism: Slowly, via hydrolysis and *N*-acetylation as well as by spontaneous degradation, with subsequent metabolism to component amino acids. Overall metabolism is extensive.
Half-life elimination: Beta (distribution): 9 to 11 hours (~8 hours in children <12 years); Terminal: 40 to 50 hours; beta phase half-life is 32% to 43% lower in pediatric patients than in adult patients
Excretion: Urine (41%; primarily as metabolites, ~1% of total dose as unchanged drug); feces (35%; primarily as metabolites)

Dosing

Adult & Geriatric Note: Duration of caspofungin treatment should be determined by patient status and clinical response.

Aspergillosis (invasive): IV: Initial dose: 70 mg on day 1; subsequent dosing: 50 mg once daily. Duration of therapy should be a minimum of 6 to 12 weeks or throughout period of immunosuppression and until lesions have resolved (Walsh 2008). Salvage treatment with 70 mg once daily (off-label dosing) has been reported (Maertens 2006).

Aspergillosis (invasive) in HIV-infected patients (off-label use): Adolescents and Adults: IV: Initial dose: 70 mg on day 1; subsequent dosing: 50 mg once daily. Continue until infection resolution and CD4 count >200 cells/mm³ (HHS [OI adult 2015]).

Candidemia: IV: Initial dose: 70 mg on day 1; subsequent dosing: 50 mg once daily; generally continue for at least 14 days after the last positive culture or longer if neutropenia warrants. Higher doses (150 mg once daily infused over ~2 hours) compared to the standard adult dosing regimen (50 mg once daily) have not demonstrated additional benefit or toxicity in patients with invasive candidiasis (Betts 2009).

Esophageal candidiasis: IV: 50 mg once daily; continue for 7 to 14 days after symptom resolution. **Note:** The majority of patients studied for this indication also had oropharyngeal involvement.

Esophageal candidiasis in HIV-infected patients (off-label use): Adolescents and Adults: IV: 50 mg once daily; continue for 14 to 21 days (HHS [OI adult 2015]).

Preparation for Administration Powder for suspension: Refer to manufacturer's product labeling for reconstitution instructions. Shake vigorously until suspended.

Storage/Stability Store capsules, tablets and un-reconstituted oral suspension at 20°C to 25°C (68°F to 77F); excursions are permitted to 15°C to 30°C (59°F to 86°F). After reconstitution, oral suspension may be stored for 14 days under refrigeration (4°C).

Mechanism of Action Inhibits bacterial cell wall synthesis by binding to one or more of the penicillin-binding proteins (PBPs) which in turn inhibits the final transpeptidation step of peptidoglycan synthesis in bacterial cell walls, thus inhibiting cell wall biosynthesis. Bacteria eventually lyse due to ongoing activity of cell wall autolytic enzymes (autolysins and murein hydrolases) while cell wall assembly is arrested.

Pharmacodynamics/Kinetics

Absorption: Rapid and well absorbed from GI tract

Distribution: V_d: 0.31 L/kg

Protein binding: 20%

Half-life elimination: 1 to 2 hours; 20 to 24 hours in renal failure

Time to peak serum concentration: Within 70 to 90 minutes

Excretion: Urine (>90% as unchanged drug within 24 hours)

Dosing

Adult & Geriatric

Susceptible infections: Oral: 1-2 g daily in a single dose or 2 divided doses

Pharyngitis, group A streptococci (IDSA guidelines): Oral: 30 mg/kg once daily (maximum: 1 g daily) for 10 days (Shulman, 2012). **Note:** Recommended as an alternative agent in penicillin-allergic patients; however, avoid in patients with immediate type hypersensitivity to penicillin.

Prosthetic joint infection, chronic oral antimicrobial suppression, staphylococci (oxacillin-susceptible) (preferred) (off-label use): 500 mg every 12 hours (Osmon, 2013)

Skin and skin structure infections: Oral: 1 g daily in a single or 2 divided doses

Tonsillitis: Oral: 1 g daily in a single or 2 divided doses for 10 days

Urinary tract infections: Oral: 1 g twice daily. For uncomplicated infections: 1 or 2 g daily in a single or 2 divided doses

Pediatric

Tonsillitis/Impetigo: Oral: 30 mg/kg/day in a single dose or divided every 12 hours

Urinary tract infections/Skin and skin structure infections (except impetigo): Oral: 30 mg/kg/day divided every 12 hours (maximum: 2000 mg daily)

Pharyngitis, group A streptococci (IDSA guidelines): Oral: Refer to adult dosing.

Renal Impairment

CrCl 25 to 50 mL/minute: Administer every 12 hours.

CrCl 10 to 25 mL/minute: Administer every 24 hours.

CrCl <10 mL/minute: Administer every 36 hours.

Hepatic Impairment No dosage adjustment provided in manufacturer's labeling.

Administration Administer around-the-clock to promote less variation in peak and trough serum levels. Administer without regards to meals; administration with food may diminish GI complaints.

Monitoring Parameters Monitor renal function. Observe for signs and symptoms of anaphylaxis during first dose.

Test Interactions Positive direct Coombs', false-positive urinary glucose test using cupric sulfate (Benedict's solution, Clinitest®, Fehling's solution), false-positive serum or urine creatinine with Jaffé reaction

Dosage Forms Excipient information presented when available (limited, particularly for generics); consult specific product labeling.

Capsule, Oral:

Generic: 500 mg

Suspension Reconstituted, Oral:

Generic: 250 mg/5 mL (100 mL); 500 mg/5 mL (75 mL, 100 mL)

Tablet, Oral:

Generic: 1 g

◆ Cefadroxil Monohydrate see Cefadroxil on page 328

CeFAZolin (sef A zoe lin)

Brand Names: Canada Cefazolin For Injection; Cefazolin For Injection, USP

Index Terms Ancef; Cefazolin Sodium; Kefzol

Pharmacologic Category Antibiotic, Cephalosporin (First Generation)

Use

Biliary tract infections: Due to *Escherichia coli*, various strains of streptococci, *Proteus mirabilis*, *Klebsiella* species and *Staphylococcus aureus*.

Bone and joint infections: Due to *S. aureus*.

Endocarditis: Due to *S. aureus* (penicillin-sensitive and penicillin-resistant) and group A beta-hemolytic streptococci.

Genital infections (ie, prostatitis, epididymitis): Due to *E. coli*, *P. mirabilis*, and *Klebsiella* species.

Perioperative prophylaxis: The prophylactic administration of cefazolin preoperatively, intraoperatively, and postoperatively may reduce the incidence of certain postoperative infections in patients undergoing surgical procedures.

Respiratory tract infections: Due to *S. pneumoniae*, *Klebsiella* species, *Haemophilus influenzae*, *S. aureus* (penicillin-sensitive and penicillin-resistant) and group A beta-hemolytic streptococci.

Septicemia: Due to *Streptococcus pneumoniae*, *S. aureus* (penicillin-sensitive and penicillin-resistant), *P. mirabilis*, *E. coli* and *Klebsiella* species.

Skin and skin structure infections: Due to *S. aureus* (penicillin-sensitive and penicillin-resistant), group A beta-hemolytic streptococci and other strains of streptococci.

Urinary tract infections: Due to *E. coli*, *P. mirabilis*, *Klebsiella* species and some strains of enterobacter.

Pregnancy Considerations Adverse effects were not observed in animal reproduction studies. Cefazolin crosses the placenta. Adverse events have not been reported in the fetus following administration of cefazolin prior to cesarean section. Cefazolin is recommended for group B streptococcus prophylaxis in pregnant patients with a nonanaphylactic penicillin allergy. It is also one of the antibiotics recommended for prophylactic use prior to cesarean delivery and may be used in certain situations prior to vaginal delivery in women at high risk for endocarditis.

Due to pregnancy-induced physiologic changes, the pharmacokinetics of cefazolin are altered. The half-life is shorter, the AUC is smaller, and the clearance and volume of distribution are increased.

Breast-Feeding Considerations Small amounts of cefazolin are excreted in breast milk. The manufacturer recommends that caution be exercised when administering cefazolin to nursing women. Nondose-related effects could include modification of bowel flora.

Contraindications Known allergy to the cephalosporin group of antibiotics

Warnings/Precautions Modify dosage in patients with severe renal impairment. Use with caution in patients with a history of penicillin allergy, especially IgE-mediated reactions (eg, anaphylaxis, angioedema, urticaria). Prolonged use may result in fungal or bacterial superinfection, including *C. difficile*-associated diarrhea (CDAD) and pseudomembranous colitis; CDAD has been observed >2 months postantibiotic treatment. May be associated with increased INR, especially in nutritionally-deficient patients, prolonged treatment, hepatic or renal disease. Use with caution in patients with a history of seizure disorder; high levels, particularly in the presence of renal impairment, may increase risk of seizures. Potentially significant drug-drug interactions may exist, requiring dose or frequency adjustment, additional monitoring, and/or selection of alternative therapy.

Adverse Reactions Frequency not defined.

Cardiovascular: Localized phlebitis

Central nervous system: Seizure

Dermatologic: Pruritus, skin rash, Stevens-Johnson syndrome

Gastrointestinal: Abdominal cramps, anorexia, diarrhea, nausea, oral candidiasis, pseudomembranous colitis, vomiting

Genitourinary: Vaginitis

Hepatic: Hepatitis, increased serum transaminases

Hematologic: Eosinophilia, leukopenia, neutropenia, thrombocythemia, thrombocytopenia

Hypersensitivity: Anaphylaxis

Local: Pain at injection site

Renal: Increased blood urea nitrogen, increased serum creatinine, renal failure

Miscellaneous: Fever

Drug Interactions

Metabolism/Transport Effects None known.

Avoid Concomitant Use

Avoid concomitant use of CeFAZolin with any of the following: BCG (Intravesical)

Increased Effect/Toxicity

CeFAZolin may increase the levels/effects of: Fosphenytoin; Phenytoin; Vitamin K Antagonists

The levels/effects of CeFAZolin may be increased by: Probenecid

Decreased Effect

CeFAZolin may decrease the levels/effects of: BCG (Intravesical); BCG Vaccine (Immunization); Sodium Picosulfate; Typhoid Vaccine

Preparation for Administration Dilute 500 mg vial with 2 mL SWFI and 1 g vial with 2.5 mL SWFI; reconstituted solution may be directly injected after further dilution with 5 mL SWFI or further diluted for IV administration in 50-100 mL compatible solution; 10 g vial may be diluted with 45 mL to yield 1 g/5 mL or 96 mL to yield 1 g/10 mL.

Storage/Stability Store intact vials at room temperature and protect from temperatures exceeding 40°C. Reconstituted solutions of cefazolin are light yellow to yellow. Protection from light is recommended for the powder and for the reconstituted solutions. Reconstituted solutions are stable for 24 hours at room temperature and for 10 days under refrigeration. Stability of parenteral admixture at room temperature (25°C) is 48 hours. Stability of parenteral admixture at refrigeration temperature (4°C) is 14 days.

DUPLEX: Store at 20°C to 25°C (68°F to 77°F); excursions permitted to 15°C to 30°C (59°F to 86°F) prior to activation. Following activation, stable for 24 hours at room temperature and for 7 days under refrigeration.

Mechanism of Action Inhibits bacterial cell wall synthesis by binding to one or more of the penicillin-binding proteins (PBPs) which in turn inhibits the final transpeptidation step of peptidoglycan synthesis in bacterial cell walls, thus inhibiting cell wall biosynthesis. Bacteria eventually lyse due to ongoing activity of cell wall autolytic enzymes (autolysins and murein hydrolases) while cell wall assembly is arrested.

Pharmacodynamics/Kinetics

Distribution: Widely into most body tissues and fluids including gallbladder, liver, kidneys, bone, sputum, bile, pleural, and synovial; CSF penetration is poor

Protein binding: 74% to 86%

Metabolism: Minimally hepatic

Half-life elimination: IM or IV: Neonates: 3 to 5 hours; Adults: 90 to 150 minutes (prolonged with renal impairment)

Time to peak, serum: IM: 0.5 to 2 hours; IV: Within 5 minutes

Excretion: Urine (80% to 100% as unchanged drug)

Dosing

Adult & Geriatric

Usual dosage range: IM, IV: 1-1.5 g every 8 hours, depending on severity of infection; maximum: 12 g daily

Cholecystitis, mild-to-moderate: IV: 1-2 g every 8 hours for 4-7 days (provided source controlled)

Endocarditis due to MSSA (without prosthesis) (off-label use): IV: 2 g every 8 hours for 6 weeks with or without gentamicin for the initial 3-5 days; **Note:** Recommended for penicillin-allergic (nonanaphylactoid) patients (Baddour 2005)

Group B streptococcus (neonatal prophylaxis): IV: 2 g once, then 1 g every 8 hours until delivery (CDC 2010)

Intra-abdominal infection, complicated, community-acquired, mild-to-moderate (in combination with metronidazole): IV: 1-2 g every 8 hours for 4-7 days (provided source controlled)

Moderate-to-severe infections: IV: 500 mg to 1 g every 6-8 hours

Mild infection with gram-positive cocci: IV: 250-500 mg every 8 hours

Perioperative prophylaxis:

Manufacturer's labeling: IM, IV: 1 g initiated 30-60 minutes prior to surgery; may repeat after 2 hours if procedure is lengthy with 500 mg to 1 g intraoperatively, followed by 500 mg to 1 g every 6-8 hours for 24 hours postoperatively.

Guideline recommendations (off-label): IV: **Note:** For most surgical procedures, joint clinical practice guidelines from the American Society of Health-System Pharmacists, Infectious Diseases Society of America, Surgical Infection Society, and Society for Healthcare Epidemiology of America (ASHP/IDSA/SIS/SHEA) recommend a dose of 2 g within 60 minutes prior to surgical incision (for nonobese patients weighing <120 kg). For procedures requiring anaerobic coverage (eg, appendectomy, small bowel surgery with intestinal obstruction, colon procedures), combine cefazolin with metronidazole as an alternative to a second generation cephalosporin with anaerobic activity (eg, cefoxitin or cefotetan). Cefazolin doses may be repeated intraoperatively in 4 hours if procedure is lengthy or if there is excessive blood loss (Bratzler 2013).

Obesity: The ASHP/IDSA/SIS/SHEA guidelines recommend that for patients weighing ≥120 kg, a dose of 3 g within 60 minutes prior to surgical incision should be administered (Bratzler 2013). Alternatively, for patients with BMI >40 kg/m², a single 2 g dose may be sufficient for common general surgical procedures lasting <5 hours; patients enrolled in this multigroup study had a BMI up to a group mean of 55.7 kg/m² (Ho 2012).

Cardiothoracic surgery: IV: 1 g (see **"Note"**) initiated 30-60 minutes prior to surgery (usually at the time of anesthetic induction); repeat dose if the duration of operation exceeds 3 hours (Hillis 2011). The ASHP/IDSA/SIS/SHEA guidelines recommend the use of 2 g (single dose) administered within 60 minutes prior to surgical incision (Bratzler 2013). May either continue for ≤48 hours postoperatively or administer as a single dose preoperatively (may be preferred due to reduced cost and potential for antimicrobial resistance) (Bratzler 2013; Bucknell 2000; Douglas 2011; Edwards 2006; Hillis 2011).

Note: For patients weighing >60 kg, the Society of Thoracic Surgeons recommends a preoperative dose of 2 g administered within 60 minutes of skin incision. If the surgical incision remains open in the operating room, follow with 1 g every 3-4 hours unless cardiopulmonary bypass is to be discontinued within 4 hours then delay administration (Engelman 2007).

Peritonitis, treatment (off-label route; Li 2010): Intraperitoneal:

Intermittent exchange: 15 mg/kg per exchange every 24 hours in the long dwell (≥6 hours)

Continuous exchange: Loading dose: 500 mg per liter of dialysate. Maintenance: 125 mg per liter of dialysate.

Note: If patient has residual renal function (eg, >100 mL/day urine output), empirically increase each dose by 25%

Automated peritoneal dialysis: 20 mg/kg every 24 hours in the long day dwell; **Note:** Guidelines suggest nighttime levels of intraperitoneal cefazolin may fall below the MIC of most organisms and adding cefazolin to each exchange may be warranted

Pneumococcal pneumonia: IV: 500 mg every 12 hours

Prophylaxis against infective endocarditis (off-label use): IM, IV: 1 g 30-60 minutes before procedure. Intramuscular injections should be avoided in patients who are receiving anticoagulant therapy. In these circumstances, orally administered regimens should be given whenever possible. Intravenously administered antibiotics should be used for patients who are unable to tolerate or absorb oral medications.

Note: American Heart Association (AHA) guidelines now recommend prophylaxis only in patients undergoing invasive procedures and in whom underlying cardiac conditions may predispose to a higher risk of adverse outcomes should infection occur. As of April 2007, routine prophylaxis for GI/GU procedures is no longer recommended by the AHA.

Prophylaxis in total joint replacement patients undergoing dental procedures which produce bacteremia (off-label use): IM, IV: 1 g 1 hour prior to procedure (ADA/AAOS 2003). **Note:** In general, patients with prosthetic joint implants do not require prophylactic antibiotics prior to dental procedures. In planning an invasive oral procedure, dental consultation with the patient's orthopedic surgeon may be advised to review the risks of infection (Sollecito 2015).

Prosthetic joint infection, *Staphylococcal* (oxacillin-susceptible): IV: 1-2 g every 8 hours for 2-6 weeks (in combination with rifampin) followed by oral antibiotic treatment and suppressive regimens (Osmon 2013)

Severe infection: IV: 1-1.5 g every 6 hours

Skin and soft tissue infection due to MSSA, including pyomyositis: IV: 1 g every 8 hours for 7 to 14 days; treat pyomyositis for 14 to 21 days (IDSA [Stevens 2014])

Skin and soft tissue necrotizing infection due to MSSA (off-label use): IV: 1 g every 8 hours; continue until further debridement is not necessary, patient has clinically improved, and patient is afebrile for 48 to 72 hours (IDSA [Stevens 2014])

Streptococcal skin infections: IV: 1 g every 8 hours (IDSA [Stevens 2014])

Empiric therapy: IV: Initial dose: 70 mg on day 1; subsequent dosing: 50 mg once daily; continue until resolution of neutropenia; if fungal infection confirmed, continue for a minimum of 14 days (continue for at least 7 days after resolution of both neutropenia and clinical symptoms); if clinical response inadequate, may increase up to 70 mg once daily if tolerated, but increased efficacy not demonstrated.

Dosage adjustment with concomitant use of an enzyme inducer:
Patients receiving rifampin: 70 mg caspofungin once daily
Patients receiving carbamazepine, dexamethasone, efavirenz, nevirapine, or phenytoin (and possibly other enzyme inducers): May require an increased dose of caspofungin 70 mg once daily.

Pediatric

Aspergillosis (invasive), candidemia, esophageal candidiasis, empiric therapy: Infants ≥3 months, Children, and Adolescents ≤17 years: IV: Initial dose: 70 mg/m² on day 1, subsequent dosing: 50 mg/m² once daily, if clinical response inadequate, may increase to 70 mg/m² once daily if tolerated, but increased efficacy not demonstrated (maximum dose, loading or maintenance: 70 mg). Duration of caspofungin treatment should be determined by patient status and clinical response; refer to adult dosing for indication-specific recommended durations.

Aspergillosis (invasive) in HIV-infected patients (off-label use): Adolescents: IV: Refer to adult dosing.

Esophageal candidiasis in HIV-infected patients (off-label use): Adolescents: IV: Refer to adult dosing.

Dosage adjustment with concomitant use of an enzyme inducer: *Patients receiving carbamazepine, dexamethasone, efavirenz, nevirapine, phenytoin, or rifampin (and possibly other enzyme inducers):* Consider 70 mg/m² once daily (maximum: 70 mg daily)

Renal Impairment No dosage adjustment necessary.
End-stage renal disease (ESRD) requiring hemodialysis: Poorly dialyzed; no supplemental dose or dosage adjustment necessary, including patients on intermittent hemodialysis (IHD), peritoneal dialysis, or continuous renal replacement therapy (eg, CVVHD).

Hepatic Impairment
Adults:
Mild insufficiency (Child-Pugh class A): No dosage adjustment necessary.
Moderate insufficiency (Child-Pugh class B): 70 mg on day 1 (where recommended), followed by 35 mg once daily
Severe insufficiency (Child-Pugh class C): No dosage adjustment provided in manufacturer's labeling (has not been studied).
Children: Mild-to-severe insufficiency (Child-Pugh classes A, B, or C): No dosage adjustment provided in manufacturer's labeling (has not been studied).

Administration Infuse slowly, over ~1 hour. Monitor during infusion; isolated cases of possible histamine-related reactions have occurred during clinical trials (rash, flushing, pruritus, facial edema).

Monitoring Parameters Liver function; anaphylaxis or histamine-related reactions (eg, facial swelling, bronchospasm, sensation of warmth)

Dosage Forms Excipient information presented when available (limited, particularly for generics); consult specific product labeling.
Solution Reconstituted, Intravenous, as acetate:
Cancidas: 50 mg (1 ea); 70 mg (1 ea)

◆ Caspofungin Acetate *see* Caspofungin *on page 325*
◆ Castor Oil, Trypsin, and Balsam Peru *see* Trypsin, Balsam Peru, and Castor Oil *on page 1849*
◆ Cataflam *see* Diclofenac (Systemic) *on page 540*
◆ Cataflam [DSC] *see* Diclofenac (Systemic) *on page 540*
◆ Catapres *see* CloNIDine *on page 421*
◆ Catapres-TTS-1 *see* CloNIDine *on page 421*
◆ Catapres-TTS-2 *see* CloNIDine *on page 421*
◆ Catapres-TTS-3 *see* CloNIDine *on page 421*
◆ Cathflo Activase *see* Alteplase *on page 80*
◆ Caverject *see* Alprostadil *on page 78*
◆ Caverject Impulse *see* Alprostadil *on page 78*
◆ CaviRinse *see* Fluoride *on page 782*
◆ Cayston *see* Aztreonam (Oral Inhalation) *on page 195*
◆ Caziant *see* Ethinyl Estradiol and Desogestrel *on page 701*
◆ CB-1348 *see* Chlorambucil *on page 370*
◆ CB7630 *see* Abiraterone Acetate *on page 21*

◆ CBDCA *see* CARBOplatin *on page 312*
◆ CBZ *see* CarBAMazepine *on page 303*
◆ CC-4047 *see* Pomalidomide *on page 1469*
◆ CC-5013 *see* Lenalidomide *on page 1042*
◆ CC-10004 *see* Apremilast *on page 142*
◆ CCI-779 *see* Temsirolimus *on page 1752*
◆ ccIIV3 [Flucelvax] *see* Influenza Virus Vaccine (Inactivated) *on page 945*
◆ CCNU *see* Lomustine *on page 1096*
◆ 2-CdA *see* Cladribine *on page 401*
◆ CDB-2914 *see* Ulipristal *on page 1851*
◆ CDCA *see* Chenodiol *on page 369*
◆ CDDP *see* CISplatin *on page 395*
◆ CDP870 *see* Certolizumab Pegol *on page 362*
◆ CDX *see* Bicalutamide *on page 230*
◆ CE *see* Estrogens (Conjugated/Equine, Systemic) *on page 690*
◆ CE *see* Estrogens (Conjugated/Equine, Topical) *on page 693*
◆ Ceclor *see* Cefaclor *on page 327*
◆ Cedax *see* Ceftibuten *on page 348*
◆ CEE *see* Estrogens (Conjugated/Equine, Systemic) *on page 690*
◆ CEE *see* Estrogens (Conjugated/Equine, Topical) *on page 693*
◆ CeeNU *see* Lomustine *on page 1096*
◆ CeeNU [DSC] *see* Lomustine *on page 1096*

Cefaclor (SEF a klor)

Brand Names: Canada Apo-Cefaclor; Ceclor; Novo-Cefaclor; Nu-Cefaclor; PMS-Cefaclor
Index Terms Ceclor; Raniclor
Pharmacologic Category Antibiotic, Cephalosporin (Second Generation)
Use
Acute bacterial exacerbations of chronic bronchitis (extended-release tablets only): Treatment of acute bacterial exacerbations of chronic bronchitis due to *Haemophilus influenzae* (non-beta-lactamase-producing strains only), *Moraxella catarrhalis* (including beta-lactamase-producing strains) or *Streptococcus pneumoniae*.
Lower respiratory tract infections (capsules and oral suspension only): Treatment of lower respiratory tract infections, including pneumonia, caused by *S. pneumoniae*, *H. influenzae*, and *Streptococcus pyogenes*.
Otitis media (capsules and oral suspension only): Treatment of otitis media caused by *S. pneumoniae, H. influenzae,* staphylococci, and *S. pyogenes*.
Pharyngitis and tonsillitis: Treatment of pharyngitis and tonsillitis due to *S. pyogenes*.
Secondary bacterial infections of acute bronchitis (extended-release tablets only): Treatment of secondary bacterial infections of acute bronchitis due to *H. influenzae* (non-beta-lactamase-producing strains only), *M. catarrhalis* (including β-lactamase-producing strains), or *S. pneumoniae*.
Skin and skin structure infections, uncomplicated: Treatment of uncomplicated skin and skin structure infections due to *Staphylococcus aureus* (methicillin-susceptible) or *S. pyogenes* (capsules and oral suspension only).
Urinary tract infections (capsules and oral suspension only): Treatment of urinary tract infections, including pyelonephritis and cystitis, caused by *Escherichia coli*, *Proteus mirabilis*, *Klebsiella* spp, and coagulase-negative staphylococci.
Dosing
Adult & Geriatric
Treatment of susceptible infections: Oral:
Immediate-release: 250 to 500 mg every 8 hours
Extended-release: 500 mg every 12 hours

Indication-specific dosing: Note: An extended-release tablet dose of 500 mg twice daily is clinically equivalent to an immediate-release capsule dose of 250 mg 3 times daily; an extended-release tablet dose of 500 mg twice daily is **NOT** clinically equivalent to 500 mg 3 times daily of other cefaclor formulations.
Acute bacterial exacerbations of chronic bronchitis:
Oral: Extended-release: 500 mg every 12 hours for 7 days
Secondary bacterial infection of acute bronchitis:
Oral: Extended-release: 500 mg every 12 hours for 7 days

Pediatric

Treatment of susceptible infections: Usual dosage range:
Infants ≥1 month, Children, and Adolescents: Oral: Immediate-release: 20 to 40 mg/kg/day divided every 8 to 12 hours; maximum dose: 1,000 mg/day
Adolescents ≥16 years: Oral: Extended-release: 500 mg every 12 hours

Indication-specific dosing:
Infants >1 month, Children, and Adolescents:

Lower respiratory tract infections: Oral: Immediate-release: 20 to 40 mg/kg/day divided every 8 hours (maximum dose: 1,000 mg/day). If beta-hemolytic streptococcus/S. pyogenes suspected, treat for at least 10 days.

Otitis media: Oral: Immediate-release: 40 mg/kg/day divided every 12 hours (maximum dose: 1,000 mg/day). If beta-hemolytic streptococcus/S. pyogenes suspected, treat for at least 10 days.

Pharyngitis/tonsillitis: Oral: Immediate-release: 20 mg/kg/day divided every 12 hours (maximum dose: 1,000 mg/day). If beta-hemolytic streptococcus/S. pyogenes confirmed, treat for at least 10 days. **Note:** Not a preferred drug (Shulman 2012).

Skin and skin structure infections, uncomplicated: Oral: Immediate-release: 20 to 40 mg/kg/day divided every 8 hours (maximum dose: 1,000 mg/day). If due to beta-hemolytic streptococcus/S. pyogenes, treat for at least 10 days.

Urinary tract infections: Oral: Immediate-release: 20 to 40 mg/kg/day divided every 8 hours (maximum dose: 1,000 mg/day).

Adolescents ≥16 years: **Note:** An extended-release tablet dose of 500 mg twice daily is clinically equivalent to an immediate-release capsule dose of 250 mg 3 times daily; an extended-release tablet dose of 500 mg twice daily is **NOT** clinically equivalent to 500 mg 3 times daily of other cefaclor formulations.

Acute bacterial exacerbations of chronic bronchitis: Oral: Extended-release: 500 mg every 12 hours for 7 days

Secondary bacterial infection of acute bronchitis: Oral: Extended-release: 500 mg every 12 hours for 7 days

Renal Impairment

Manufacturer's labeling:
Oral, immediate-release: There are no dosage adjustments provided in the manufacturer's labeling; however, half-life is increased in anuric patients; use with caution.
Oral, extended-release: There are no dosage adjustments provided in the manufacturer's labeling.
Dialysis: Moderately dialyzable (20% to 50%)

Alternative recommendations (off-label dosing) (Aronoff 2007):
Adults: Oral, immediate-release:
Mild to severe impairment: No dosage adjustment necessary.
End-stage renal disease (ESRD) on intermittent hemodialysis (IHD) (administer after hemodialysis on dialysis days): Supplement with 250 to 500 mg after dialysis.
Peritoneal dialysis: Administer 250 to 500 mg every 8 hours.
Infants, Children and Adolescents: Oral, immediate-release:
GFR ≥10 mL/minute: No dosage adjustment necessary.
GFR <10 mL/minute: Administer 50% of the recommended dose (based on indication)
End-stage renal disease (ERD) on intermittent hemodialysis (IHD) (supplemental dose post-hemodialysis needed): Administer 50% of the recommended dose (based on indication).
Peritoneal dialysis: Administer 50% of the recommended dose (based on indication).

Hepatic Impairment There are no dosage adjustments provided in the manufacturer's labeling.

Additional Information Complete prescribing information should be consulted for additional detail.

Dosage Forms Excipient information presented when available (limited, particularly for generics); consult specific product labeling.
Capsule, Oral:
Generic: 250 mg, 500 mg
Suspension Reconstituted, Oral:
Generic: 125 mg/5 mL (150 mL); 250 mg/5 mL (150 mL); 375 mg/5 mL (100 mL)
Tablet Extended Release 12 Hour, Oral:
Generic: 500 mg

Cefadroxil (sef a DROKS il)

Brand Names: Canada Apo-Cefadroxil; PRO-Cefadroxil; Teva-Cefadroxil

Index Terms Cefadroxil Monohydrate; Duricef

Pharmacologic Category Antibiotic, Cephalosporin (First Generation)

Use

Pharyngitis and/or tonsillitis: Treatment of pharyngitis and/or tonsillitis caused by Streptococcus pyogenes (group A beta-hemolytic streptococci).

Skin and skin structure infections: Treatment of skin and skin structure infections caused by staphylococci and/or streptococci.

Urinary tract infection: Treatment of urinary tract infections caused by Escherichia coli, Proteus mirabilis, and Klebsiella species.

Pregnancy Considerations Adverse events have not been observed in animal reproduction studies. Cefadroxil crosses the placenta. Limited data is available concerning the use of cefadroxil in pregnancy; however, adverse fetal effects were not noted in a small clinical trial.

Breast-Feeding Considerations Very small amounts of cefadroxil are excreted in breast milk. The manufacturer recommends that caution be exercised when administering cefadroxil to nursing women. Nondose-related effects could include modification of bowel flora.

Contraindications Hypersensitivity to cefadroxil, any component of the formulation, or other cephalosporins

Warnings/Precautions Modify dosage in patients with renal impairment (CrCl <50 mL/minute/1.73 m^2). Use with caution in patients with a history of penicillin allergy, especially IgE-mediated reactions (eg, anaphylaxis, angioedema, urticaria). Use with caution in patients with a history of gastrointestinal disease, particularly colitis. Prolonged use may result in fungal or bacterial superinfection, including C. difficile-associated diarrhea (CDAD) and pseudomembranous colitis; CDAD has been observed >2 months postantibiotic treatment. Only IM penicillin has been shown to be effective in the prophylaxis of rheumatic fever. Cefadroxil is generally effective in the eradication of streptococci from the oropharynx; efficacy data for cefadroxil in the prophylaxis of subsequent rheumatic fever episodes are not available.

Suspension may contain sulfur dioxide (sulfite); hypersensitivity reactions, including anaphylaxis and/or asthmatic exacerbations, may occur (may be life threatening).

Benzyl alcohol and derivatives: Some dosage forms may contain sodium benzoate/benzoic acid; benzoic acid (benzoate) is a metabolite of benzyl alcohol; large amounts of benzyl alcohol (≥99 mg/kg/day) have been associated with a potentially fatal toxicity ("gasping syndrome") in neonates; the "gasping syndrome" consists of metabolic acidosis, respiratory distress, gasping respirations, CNS dysfunction (including convulsions, intracranial hemorrhage), hypotension, and cardiovascular collapse (AAP ["Inactive" 1997]; CDC, 1982); some data suggests that benzoate displaces bilirubin from protein binding sites (Ahlfors, 2001); avoid or use dosage forms containing benzyl alcohol derivative with caution in neonates. See manufacturer's labeling.

Adverse Reactions

1% to 10%: Gastrointestinal: Diarrhea
<1% (Limited to important or life-threatening): Agranulocytosis, anaphylaxis, angioedema, cholestasis, Clostridium difficile associated diarrhea, dyspepsia, erythema multiforme, erythematous rash, genital candidiasis, hepatic failure, increased serum transaminases, maculopapular rash, neutropenia, pseudomembranous colitis, serum sickness, Stevens-Johnson syndrome, thrombocytopenia, vaginitis

Drug Interactions

Metabolism/Transport Effects None known.

Avoid Concomitant Use
Avoid concomitant use of Cefadroxil with any of the following: BCG (Intravesical)

Increased Effect/Toxicity
Cefadroxil may increase the levels/effects of: Vitamin K Antagonists

The levels/effects of Cefadroxil may be increased by: Probenecid

Decreased Effect
Cefadroxil may decrease the levels/effects of: BCG (Intravesical); BCG Vaccine (Immunization); Sodium Picosulfate; Typhoid Vaccine

Food Interactions Concomitant administration with food, infant formula, or cow's milk does **not** significantly affect absorption.

Preparation for Administration Powder for suspension: Refer to manufacturer's product labeling for reconstitution instructions. Shake vigorously until suspended.

Storage/Stability Store capsules, tablets and un-reconstituted oral suspension at 20°C to 25°C (68°F to 77F); excursions are permitted to 15°C to 30°C (59°F to 86°F). After reconstitution, oral suspension may be stored for 14 days under refrigeration (4°C).

Mechanism of Action Inhibits bacterial cell wall synthesis by binding to one or more of the penicillin-binding proteins (PBPs) which in turn inhibits the final transpeptidation step of peptidoglycan synthesis in bacterial cell walls, thus inhibiting cell wall biosynthesis. Bacteria eventually lyse due to ongoing activity of cell wall autolytic enzymes (autolysins and murein hydrolases) while cell wall assembly is arrested.

Pharmacodynamics/Kinetics
Absorption: Rapid and well absorbed from GI tract
Distribution: V_d: 0.31 L/kg
Protein binding: 20%
Half-life elimination: 1 to 2 hours; 20 to 24 hours in renal failure
Time to peak serum concentration: Within 70 to 90 minutes
Excretion: Urine (>90% as unchanged drug within 24 hours)

Dosing

Adult & Geriatric

Susceptible infections: Oral: 1-2 g daily in a single dose or 2 divided doses

Pharyngitis, group A streptococci (IDSA guidelines): Oral: 30 mg/kg once daily (maximum: 1 g daily) for 10 days (Shulman, 2012). **Note:** Recommended as an alternative agent in penicillin-allergic patients; however, avoid in patients with immediate type hypersensitivity to penicillin.

Prosthetic joint infection, chronic oral antimicrobial suppression, staphylococci (oxacillin-susceptible) (preferred) (off-label use): 500 mg every 12 hours (Osmon, 2013)

Skin and skin structure infections: Oral: 1 g daily in a single or 2 divided doses

Tonsillitis: Oral: 1 g daily in a single or 2 divided doses for 10 days

Urinary tract infections: Oral: 1 g twice daily. For uncomplicated infections: 1 or 2 g daily in a single or 2 divided doses

Pediatric

Tonsillitis/Impetigo: Oral: 30 mg/kg/day in a single dose or divided every 12 hours

Urinary tract infections/Skin and skin structure infections (except impetigo): Oral: 30 mg/kg/day divided every 12 hours (maximum: 2000 mg daily)

Pharyngitis, group A streptococci (IDSA guidelines): Oral: Refer to adult dosing.

Renal Impairment
CrCl 25 to 50 mL/minute: Administer every 12 hours.
CrCl 10 to 25 mL/minute: Administer every 24 hours.
CrCl <10 mL/minute: Administer every 36 hours.

Hepatic Impairment No dosage adjustment provided in manufacturer's labeling.

Administration Administer around-the-clock to promote less variation in peak and trough serum levels. Administer without regards to meals; administration with food may diminish GI complaints.

Monitoring Parameters Monitor renal function. Observe for signs and symptoms of anaphylaxis during first dose.

Test Interactions Positive direct Coombs', false-positive urinary glucose test using cupric sulfate (Benedict's solution, Clinitest®, Fehling's solution), false-positive serum or urine creatinine with Jaffé reaction

Dosage Forms Excipient information presented when available (limited, particularly for generics); consult specific product labeling.
Capsule, Oral:
Generic: 500 mg
Suspension Reconstituted, Oral:
Generic: 250 mg/5 mL (100 mL); 500 mg/5 mL (75 mL, 100 mL)
Tablet, Oral:
Generic: 1 g

◆ Cefadroxil Monohydrate see Cefadroxil on page 328

CeFAZolin (sef A zoe lin)

Brand Names: Canada Cefazolin For Injection; Cefazolin For Injection, USP
Index Terms Ancef; Cefazolin Sodium; Kefzol
Pharmacologic Category Antibiotic, Cephalosporin (First Generation)

Use

Biliary tract infections: Due to *Escherichia coli*, various strains of streptococci, *Proteus mirabilis*, *Klebsiella* species and *Staphylococcus aureus*.

Bone and joint infections: Due to *S. aureus*.

Endocarditis: Due to *S. aureus* (penicillin-sensitive and penicillin-resistant) and group A beta-hemolytic streptococci.

Genital infections (ie, prostatitis, epididymitis): Due to *E. coli*, *P. mirabilis*, and *Klebsiella* species.

Perioperative prophylaxis: The prophylactic administration of cefazolin preoperatively, intraoperatively, and postoperatively may reduce the incidence of certain postoperative infections in patients undergoing surgical procedures.

Respiratory tract infections: Due to *S. pneumoniae*, *Klebsiella* species, *Haemophilus influenzae*, *S. aureus* (penicillin-sensitive and penicillin-resistant) and group A beta-hemolytic streptococci.

Septicemia: Due to *Streptococcus pneumoniae*, *S. aureus* (penicillin-sensitive and penicillin-resistant), *P. mirabilis*, *E. coli* and *Klebsiella* species.

Skin and skin structure infections: Due to *S. aureus* (penicillin-sensitive and penicillin-resistant), group A beta-hemolytic streptococci and other strains of streptococci.

Urinary tract infections: Due to *E. coli*, *P. mirabilis*, *Klebsiella* species and some strains of enterobacter.

Pregnancy Considerations Adverse effects were not observed in animal reproduction studies. Cefazolin crosses the placenta. Adverse events have not been reported in the fetus following administration of cefazolin prior to cesarean section. Cefazolin is recommended for group B streptococcus prophylaxis in pregnant patients with a nonanaphylactic penicillin allergy. It is also one of the antibiotics recommended for prophylactic use prior to cesarean delivery and may be used in certain situations prior to vaginal delivery in women at high risk for endocarditis.

Due to pregnancy-induced physiologic changes, the pharmacokinetics of cefazolin are altered. The half-life is shorter, the AUC is smaller, and the clearance and volume of distribution are increased.

Breast-Feeding Considerations Small amounts of cefazolin are excreted in breast milk. The manufacturer recommends that caution be exercised when administering cefazolin to nursing women. Nondose-related effects could include modification of bowel flora.

Contraindications Known allergy to the cephalosporin group of antibiotics

Warnings/Precautions Modify dosage in patients with severe renal impairment. Use with caution in patients with a history of penicillin allergy, especially IgE-mediated reactions (eg, anaphylaxis, angioedema, urticaria). Prolonged use may result in fungal or bacterial superinfection, including *C. difficile*-associated diarrhea (CDAD) and pseudomembranous colitis; CDAD has been observed >2 months postantibiotic treatment. May be associated with increased INR, especially in nutritionally-deficient patients, prolonged treatment, hepatic or renal disease. Use with caution in patients with a history of seizure disorder; high levels, particularly in the presence of renal impairment, may increase risk of seizures. Potentially significant drug-drug interactions may exist, requiring dose or frequency adjustment, additional monitoring, and/or selection of alternative therapy.

Adverse Reactions Frequency not defined.
Cardiovascular: Localized phlebitis
Central nervous system: Seizure
Dermatologic: Pruritus, skin rash, Stevens-Johnson syndrome
Gastrointestinal: Abdominal cramps, anorexia, diarrhea, nausea, oral candidiasis, pseudomembranous colitis, vomiting
Genitourinary: Vaginitis
Hepatic: Hepatitis, increased serum transaminases
Hematologic: Eosinophilia, leukopenia, neutropenia, thrombocythemia, thrombocytopenia
Hypersensitivity: Anaphylaxis
Local: Pain at injection site
Renal: Increased blood urea nitrogen, increased serum creatinine, renal failure
Miscellaneous: Fever

Drug Interactions

Metabolism/Transport Effects None known.

Avoid Concomitant Use
Avoid concomitant use of CeFAZolin with any of the following: BCG (Intravesical)

Increased Effect/Toxicity
CeFAZolin may increase the levels/effects of: Fosphenytoin; Phenytoin; Vitamin K Antagonists

The levels/effects of CeFAZolin may be increased by: Probenecid

Decreased Effect
CeFAZolin may decrease the levels/effects of: BCG (Intravesical); BCG Vaccine (Immunization); Sodium Picosulfate; Typhoid Vaccine

Preparation for Administration Dilute 500 mg vial with 2 mL SWFI and 1 g vial with 2.5 mL SWFI; reconstituted solution may be directly injected after further dilution with 5 mL SWFI or further diluted for IV administration in 50-100 mL compatible solution; 10 g vial may be diluted with 45 mL to yield 1 g/5 mL or 96 mL to yield 1 g/10 mL.

Storage/Stability Store intact vials at room temperature and protect from temperatures exceeding 40°C. Reconstituted solutions of cefazolin are light yellow to yellow. Protection from light is recommended for the powder and for the reconstituted solutions. Reconstituted solutions are stable for 24 hours at room temperature and for 10 days under refrigeration. Stability of parenteral admixture at room temperature (25°C) is 48 hours. Stability of parenteral admixture at refrigeration temperature (4°C) is 14 days.

DUPLEX: Store at 20°C to 25°C (68°F to 77°F); excursions permitted to 15°C to 30°C (59°F to 86°F) prior to activation. Following activation, stable for 24 hours at room temperature and for 7 days under refrigeration.

Mechanism of Action Inhibits bacterial cell wall synthesis by binding to one or more of the penicillin-binding proteins (PBPs) which in turn inhibits the final transpeptidation step of peptidoglycan synthesis in bacterial cell walls, thus inhibiting cell wall biosynthesis. Bacteria eventually lyse due to ongoing activity of cell wall autolytic enzymes (autolysins and murein hydrolases) while cell wall assembly is arrested.

Pharmacodynamics/Kinetics
Distribution: Widely into most body tissues and fluids including gallbladder, liver, kidneys, bone, sputum, bile, pleural, and synovial; CSF penetration is poor

Protein binding: 74% to 86%

Metabolism: Minimally hepatic

Half-life elimination: IM or IV: Neonates: 3 to 5 hours; Adults: 90 to 150 minutes (prolonged with renal impairment)

Time to peak, serum: IM: 0.5 to 2 hours; IV: Within 5 minutes

Excretion: Urine (80% to 100% as unchanged drug)

Dosing
Adult & Geriatric

Usual dosage range: IM, IV: 1-1.5 g every 8 hours, depending on severity of infection; maximum: 12 g daily

Cholecystitis, mild-to-moderate: IV: 1-2 g every 8 hours for 4-7 days (provided source controlled)

Endocarditis due to MSSA (without prosthesis) (off-label use): IV: 2 g every 8 hours for 6 weeks with or without gentamicin for the initial 3-5 days; **Note:** Recommended for penicillin-allergic (nonanaphylactoid) patients (Baddour 2005)

Group B streptococcus (neonatal prophylaxis): IV: 2 g once, then 1 g every 8 hours until delivery (CDC 2010)

Intra-abdominal infection, complicated, community-acquired, mild-to-moderate (in combination with metronidazole): IV: 1-2 g every 8 hours for 4-7 days (provided source controlled)

Moderate-to-severe infections: IV: 500 mg to 1 g every 6-8 hours

Mild infection with gram-positive cocci: IV: 250-500 mg every 8 hours

Perioperative prophylaxis:

Manufacturer's labeling: IM, IV: 1 g initiated 30-60 minutes prior to surgery; may repeat after 2 hours if procedure is lengthy with 500 mg to 1 g intraoperatively, followed by 500 mg to 1 g every 6-8 hours for 24 hours postoperatively.

Guideline recommendations (off-label): IV: **Note:** For most surgical procedures, joint clinical practice guidelines from the American Society of Health-System Pharmacists, Infectious Diseases Society of America, Surgical Infection Society, and Society for Healthcare Epidemiology of America (ASHP/IDSA/SIS/SHEA) recommend a dose of 2 g within 60 minutes prior to surgical incision (for nonobese patients weighing <120 kg). For procedures requiring anaerobic coverage (eg, appendectomy, small bowel surgery with intestinal obstruction, colon procedures), combine cefazolin with metronidazole as an alternative to a second generation cephalosporin with anaerobic activity (eg, cefoxitin or cefotetan). Cefazolin doses may be repeated intraoperatively in 4 hours if procedure is lengthy or if there is excessive blood loss (Bratzler 2013).

Obesity: The ASHP/IDSA/SIS/SHEA guidelines recommend that for patients weighing ≥120 kg, a dose of 3 g within 60 minutes prior to surgical incision should be administered (Bratzler 2013). Alternatively, for patients with BMI >40 kg/m² , a single 2 g dose may be sufficient for common general surgical procedures lasting <5 hours; patients enrolled in this multigroup study had a BMI up to a group mean of 55.7 kg/m² (Ho 2012).

Cardiothoracic surgery: IV: 1 g (see **"Note"**) initiated 30-60 minutes prior to surgery (usually at the time of anesthetic induction); repeat dose if the duration of operation exceeds 3 hours (Hillis 2011). The ASHP/IDSA/SIS/SHEA guidelines recommend the use of 2 g (single dose) administered within 60 minutes prior to surgical incision (Bratzler 2013). May either continue for ≤48 hours postoperatively or administer as a single dose preoperatively (may be preferred due to reduced cost and potential for antimicrobial resistance) (Bratzler 2013; Bucknell 2000; Douglas 2011; Edwards 2006; Hillis 2011).

Note: For patients weighing >60 kg, the Society of Thoracic Surgeons recommends a preoperative dose of 2 g administered within 60 minutes of skin incision. If the surgical incision remains open in the operating room, follow with 1 g every 3-4 hours unless cardiopulmonary bypass is to be discontinued within 4 hours then delay administration (Engelman 2007).

Peritonitis, treatment (off-label route; Li 2010): Intraperitoneal:

Intermittent exchange: 15 mg/kg per exchange every 24 hours in the long dwell (≥6 hours)

Continuous exchange: Loading dose: 500 mg per liter of dialysate. Maintenance: 125 mg per liter of dialysate.

Note: If patient has residual renal function (eg, >100 mL/day urine output), empirically increase each dose by 25%

Automated peritoneal dialysis: 20 mg/kg every 24 hours in the long day dwell; **Note:** Guidelines suggest nighttime levels of intraperitoneal cefazolin may fall below the MIC of most organisms and adding cefazolin to each exchange may be warranted

Pneumococcal pneumonia: IV: 500 mg every 12 hours

Prophylaxis against infective endocarditis (off-label use): IM, IV: 1 g 30-60 minutes before procedure. Intramuscular injections should be avoided in patients who are receiving anticoagulant therapy. In these circumstances, orally administered regimens should be given whenever possible. Intravenously administered antibiotics should be used for patients who are unable to tolerate or absorb oral medications.

Note: American Heart Association (AHA) guidelines now recommend prophylaxis only in patients undergoing invasive procedures and in whom underlying cardiac conditions may predispose to a higher risk of adverse outcomes should infection occur. As of April 2007, routine prophylaxis for GI/GU procedures is no longer recommended by the AHA.

Prophylaxis in total joint replacement patients undergoing dental procedures which produce bacteremia (off-label use): IM, IV: 1 g 1 hour prior to procedure (ADA/AAOS 2003). **Note:** In general, patients with prosthetic joint implants do not require prophylactic antibiotics prior to dental procedures. In planning an invasive oral procedure, dental consultation with the patient's orthopedic surgeon may be advised to review the risks of infection (Sollecito 2015).

Prosthetic joint infection, Staphylococcal (oxacillin-susceptible): IV: 1-2 g every 8 hours for 2-6 weeks (in combination with rifampin) followed by oral antibiotic treatment and suppressive regimens (Osmon 2013)

Severe infection: IV: 1-1.5 g every 6 hours

Skin and soft tissue infection due to MSSA, including pyomyositis: IV: 1 g every 8 hours for 7 to 14 days; treat pyomyositis for 14 to 21 days (IDSA [Stevens 2014])

Skin and soft tissue necrotizing infection due to MSSA (off-label use): IV: 1 g every 8 hours; continue until further debridement is not necessary, patient has clinically improved, and patient is afebrile for 48 to 72 hours (IDSA [Stevens 2014])

Streptococcal skin infections: IV: 1 g every 8 hours (IDSA [Stevens 2014])

Surgical site infection (trunk or extremity [away from axilla or perineum]) (off-label use): IV: 500 mg to 1 g every 8 hours (IDSA [Stevens 2014])

UTI (uncomplicated): IM, IV: 1 g every 12 hours

Pediatric

Usual dosage range: IM, IV: Children >1 month: 25-100 mg/kg/day divided every 6-8 hours; maximum: 6 **g** daily

Community-acquired pneumonia (CAP) (IDSA/PIDS 2011), moderate-to-severe infection, *S. aureus* (methicillin-susceptible) (preferred): Infants >3 months and Children: IM, IV: 150 mg/kg/day divided every 8 hours

Perioperative prophylaxis (off-label use): Children ≥1 year: IV: **Note:** For most surgical procedures, joint clinical practice guidelines from the American Society of Health-System Pharmacists, Infectious Diseases Society of America, Surgical Infection Society, and Society for Healthcare Epidemiology of America (ASHP/IDSA/SIS/SHEA) recommend a dose of 30 mg/kg (maximum dose: 2000 mg) administered within 60 minutes prior to surgical incision. For procedures requiring anaerobic coverage (eg, appendectomy, small bowel surgery with intestinal obstruction, colon procedures), combine cefazolin with metronidazole as an alternative to a second generation cephalosporin with anaerobic activity (eg, cefoxitin or cefotetan). Cefazolin doses may be repeated intraoperatively in 4 hours if procedure is lengthy or if there is excessive blood loss (Bratzler 2013).

Peritonitis, treatment (off-label route; Warady 2012): Infants, Children, and Adolescents: Intraperitoneal:

Intermittent exchange: 20 mg/kg every 24 hours in the long dwell

Continuous exchange: Loading dose: 500 mg per liter of dialysate. Maintenance: 125 mg per liter of dialysate.

Prophylaxis against infective endocarditis (off-label use): Infants and Children: IM, IV: 50 mg/kg 30-60 minutes before procedure; maximum dose: 1000 mg. Intramuscular injections should be avoided in patients who are receiving anticoagulant therapy. In these circumstances, orally administered regimens should be given whenever possible. Intravenously administered antibiotics should be used for patients who are unable to tolerate or absorb oral medications.

Note: American Heart Association (AHA) guidelines now recommend prophylaxis only in patients undergoing invasive procedures and in whom underlying cardiac conditions may predispose to a higher risk of adverse outcomes should infection occur. As of April 2007, routine prophylaxis for GI/GU procedures is no longer recommended by the AHA.

Skin and soft tissue infection due to MSSA, including pyomyositis: Infants and Children: IV: 50 mg/kg/day divided every 8 hours for 7 to 14 days; treat pyomyositis for 14 to 21 days (IDSA [Stevens 2014])

Skin and soft tissue necrotizing infections due to MSSA (off-label use): Infants and Children: IV: 33 mg/kg every 8 hours; continue until further debridement is not necessary, patient has clinically improved, and patient is afebrile for 48 to 72 hours (IDSA [Stevens 2014])

Streptococcal skin infections: Infants and Children: IV: 33 mg/kg every 8 hours (IDSA [Stevens 2014])

Renal Impairment

Adults:

CrCl 35 to 54 mL/minute: Administer full dose in intervals of ≥8 hours

CrCl 11 to 34 mL/minute: Administer 50% of usual dose every 12 hours

CrCl ≤10 mL/minute: Administer 50% of usual dose every 18 to 24 hours

Intermittent hemodialysis (IHD) (administer after hemodialysis on dialysis days): Dialyzable (20% to 50%): 500 mg to 1 g every 24 hours **or** use 1 to 2 g every 48 to 72 hours (Heintz 2009) **or** 15 to 20 mg/kg (maximum dose: 2 g) after dialysis 3 times weekly (Ahern 2003; Sowinski 2001) **or** 2 g after dialysis if next dialysis expected in 48 hours or 3 g after dialysis if next dialysis is expected in 72 hours (Stryjewski 2007).

Note: Dosing dependent on the assumption of 3 times weekly, complete IHD sessions.

Peritoneal dialysis (PD): IV: 500 mg every 12 hours

Continuous renal replacement therapy (CRRT) (Heintz 2009; Trotman 2005): Drug clearance is highly dependent on the method of renal replacement, filter type, and flow rate. Appropriate dosing requires close monitoring of pharmacologic response, signs of adverse reactions due to drug accumulation, as well as drug concentrations in relation to target trough (if appropriate). The following are general recommendations only (based on dialysate flow/ultrafiltration rates of 1 to 2 L/hour and minimal residual renal function) and should not supersede clinical judgment:

CVVH: Loading dose of 2 g followed by 1 to 2 g every 12 hours

CVVHD/CVVHDF: Loading dose of 2 g followed by either 1 g every 8 hours **or** 2 g every 12 hours. **Note:** Dosage of 1 g every 8 hours results in similar steady-state concentrations as 2 g every 12 hours and is more cost effective (Heintz 2009).

Infants >1 month, Children, and Adolescents:

CrCl >70 mL/minute: No dosage adjustment necessary.

CrCl 40 to 70 mL/minute: 60% of usual daily dose divided every 12 hours

CrCl 20 to 40 mL/minute: 25% of usual daily dose divided every 12 hours

CrCl 5 to 20 mL/minute: 10% of usual daily dose every 24 hours

Intermittent hemodialysis (IHD): 25 mg/kg per dose every 24 hours (Aronoff 2007)

Peritoneal dialysis (PD): 25 mg/kg per dose every 24 hours (Aronoff 2007)

Continuous renal replacement therapy (CRRT): 25 mg/kg per dose every 8 hours (Aronoff 2007)

Hepatic Impairment No dosage adjustment provided in manufacturer's labeling.

Obesity Refer to indication-specific dosing for obesity-related information (may not be available for all indications).

Dietary Considerations Some products may contain sodium.

Administration

IM: Inject deep IM into large muscle mass.

IV: Inject direct IV over 5 minutes or may infuse as an intermittent infusion over 30-60 minutes.

Some penicillins (eg, carbenicillin, ticarcillin and piperacillin) have been shown to inactivate aminoglycosides *in vitro*. This has been observed to a greater extent with tobramycin and gentamicin, while amikacin has shown greater stability against inactivation. Concurrent use of these agents may pose a risk of reduced antibacterial efficacy *in vivo*, particularly in the setting of profound renal impairment. However, definitive clinical evidence is lacking. If combination penicillin/aminoglycoside therapy is desired in a patient with renal dysfunction, separation of doses (if feasible), and routine monitoring of aminoglycoside levels, CBC, and clinical response should be considered.

Monitoring Parameters Renal function periodically when used in combination with other nephrotoxic drugs, hepatic function tests, CBC; monitor for signs of anaphylaxis during first dose

Test Interactions Positive direct Coombs', false-positive urinary glucose test using cupric sulfate (Benedict's solution, Clinitest, Fehling's solution), false-positive serum or urine creatinine with Jaffé reaction.

Some penicillin derivatives may accelerate the degradation of aminoglycosides *in vitro*, leading to a potential underestimation of aminoglycoside serum concentration.

Dosage Forms Excipient information presented when available (limited, particularly for generics); consult specific product labeling.

Solution, Intravenous:

Generic: 1 g (50 mL); 2 g (100 mL)

Solution Reconstituted, Injection:

Generic: 500 mg (1 ea); 1 g (1 ea); 10 g (1 ea); 20 g (1 ea); 100 g (1 ea); 300 g (1 ea)

Solution Reconstituted, Injection [preservative free]:

Generic: 500 mg (1 ea); 1 g (1 ea); 10 g (1 ea); 20 g (1 ea)

Solution Reconstituted, Intravenous:

Generic: 1 g (1 ea); 2 g (1 ea)

◆ Cefazolin For Injection (Can) *see* CeFAZolin *on page 329*

◆ Cefazolin For Injection, USP (Can) *see* CeFAZolin *on page 329*

◆ Cefazolin Sodium *see* CeFAZolin *on page 329*

Cefdinir (SEF di ner)

Index Terms CFDN; Omnicef

Pharmacologic Category Antibiotic, Cephalosporin (Third Generation)

Use

Acute bacterial otitis media: Treatment of acute bacterial otitis media in pediatric patients caused by *Haemophilus influenzae* (including beta-lactamase-producing strains), *Streptococcus pneumoniae* (penicillin-susceptible strains only) and *Moraxella catarrhalis* (including beta-lactamase-producing strains).

Acute exacerbations of chronic bronchitis: Treatment of acute exacerbations of chronic bronchitis in adults and adolescents caused by *H. influenzae* (including beta-lactamase producing strains), *H. parainfluenzae* (including beta-lactamase-producing strains), *S. pneumoniae* (penicillin-susceptible strains only) and *M. catarrhalis* (including beta-lactamase-producing strains).

Acute maxillary sinusitis: Treatment of acute maxillary sinusitis in adults and adolescents caused by *H. influenzae* (including beta-lactamase-producing strains), *S. pneumoniae* (penicillin-susceptible strains only) and *M. catarrhalis* (including beta-lactamase-producing strains). **Note:** Limitations of use: According to the IDSA guidelines for acute bacterial rhinosinusitis, cefdinir is no longer recommended as monotherapy for initial empiric treatment (Chow, 2012).

Community-acquired pneumonia: Treatment of community-acquired pneumonia in adults and adolescents caused by *H. influenzae* (including beta-lactamase-producing strains), *H. parainfluenzae* (including beta-lactamase-producing strains), *S. pneumoniae* (penicillin-susceptible strains only) and *M. catarrhalis* (including beta-lactamase-producing strains).

Pharyngitis/Tonsillitis: Treatment of pharyngitis/tonsillitis in adults, adolescents, and pediatric patients caused by *S. pyogenes*.

Uncomplicated skin and skin structure infections: Treatment of uncomplicated skin and skin structure infections in adults, adolescents, and pediatric patients caused by *Staphylococcus aureus* (including beta-lactamase-producing strains) and *S. pyogenes*.

Pregnancy Considerations Teratogenic events have not been observed in animal reproduction studies. An increase in most types of birth defects was not found following first trimester exposure to cephalosporins.

Breast-Feeding Considerations Cefdinir is not detectable in breast milk following a single cefdinir 600 mg dose. If present in breast milk, nondose-related effects could include modification of bowel flora.

Contraindications Hypersensitivity to cefdinir, any component of the formulation, or other cephalosporins.

Warnings/Precautions Administer cautiously to penicillin-sensitive patients, especially IgE-mediated reactions (eg, anaphylaxis, urticaria). Prolonged use may result in fungal or bacterial superinfection, including *C. difficile*-associated diarrhea (CDAD) and pseudomembranous colitis; CDAD has been observed >2 months postantibiotic treatment. Use with caution in patients with a history of colitis. Use caution with renal dysfunction (CrCl <30 mL/minute); dose adjustment may be required. Potentially significant drug-drug interactions may exist, requiring dose or frequency adjustment, additional monitoring, and/or selection of alternative therapy.

Adverse Reactions

>10%: Gastrointestinal: Diarrhea (8% to 15%)

1% to 10%:

Central nervous system: Headache (2%)

Dermatologic: Skin rash (≤3%)

Endocrine & metabolic: Decreased serum bicarbonate (≤1%), glycosuria (≤1%), hyperglycemia (≤1%), hyperphosphatemia (≤1%), increased gamma-glutamyl transferase (≤1%), increased lactate dehydrogenase (≤1%)

Gastrointestinal: Nausea (≤3%), abdominal pain (≤1%), vomiting (≤1%)

Genitourinary: Vulvovaginal candidiasis (≤4%), proteinuria (1% to 2%), occult blood in urine (≤1%), urine alkalinization (≤1%), vaginitis (≤1%)

Hematologic & oncologic: Elevated urine leukocytes (≤2%), lymphocytosis (≤2%), eosinophilia (1%), lymphocytopenia (1%), functional disorder of polymorphonuclear neutrophils (≤1%), thrombocythemia (≤1%), change in WBC count (≤1%)

Hepatic: Increased serum alkaline phosphatase (≤1%), increased serum ALT (≤1%)

Renal: Increased urine specific gravity (≤1%)

<1% (Limited to important or life-threatening): Abnormal stools, anaphylaxis, anorexia, asthma, blood coagulation disorder, bloody diarrhea, candidiasis, cardiac failure, chest pain, cholestasis, conjunctivitis, constipation, cutaneous candidiasis, decreased hemoglobin, decreased urine specific gravity, disseminated intravascular coagulation, dizziness, drowsiness, dyspepsia, enterocolitis (acute), eosinophilic pneumonitis, erythema multiforme, erythema nodosum, exfoliative dermatitis, facial edema, fever, flatulence, fulminant hepatitis, granulocytopenia, hemolytic anemia, hemorrhagic colitis, hemorrhagic diathesis, hepatic failure, hepatitis (acute), hyperkalemia, hyperkinesia, hypersensitivity angiitis, hypertension, hypocalcemia, hypophosphatemia, immune thrombocytopenia, increased amylase, increased blood urea nitrogen, increased monocytes, increased serum AST, increased serum bilirubin, insomnia, interstitial pneumonitis (idiopathic), intestinal obstruction, involuntary body movements, jaundice, laryngeal edema, leukopenia, leukorrhea, loss of consciousness, maculopapular rash, melena, myocardial infarction, pancytopenia, peptic ulcer, pneumonia (drug-induced), pruritus, pseudomembranous colitis, renal disease, renal failure (acute), respiratory failure (acute), rhabdomyolysis, serum sickness, shock, Stevens-Johnson syndrome, stomatitis, thrombocytopenia, toxic epidermal necrolysis, upper gastrointestinal hemorrhage, weakness, xerostomia

Drug Interactions

Metabolism/Transport Effects None known.

Avoid Concomitant Use

Avoid concomitant use of Cefdinir with any of the following: BCG (Intravesical)

Increased Effect/Toxicity

Cefdinir may increase the levels/effects of: Aminoglycosides; Vitamin K Antagonists

The levels/effects of Cefdinir may be increased by: Probenecid

Decreased Effect

Cefdinir may decrease the levels/effects of: BCG (Intravesical); BCG Vaccine (Immunization); Sodium Picosulfate; Typhoid Vaccine

The levels/effects of Cefdinir may be decreased by: Iron Salts; Multivitamins/Minerals (with ADEK, Folate, Iron)

Preparation for Administration Refer to manufacturer's product labeling for reconstitution instructions.

Storage/Stability Store at 20°C to 25°C (68°F to 77°F). Store reconstituted suspension at room temperature 20°C to 25°C (68°F to 77°F) for 10 days.

Mechanism of Action Inhibits bacterial cell wall synthesis by binding to one or more of the penicillin-binding proteins (PBPs) which in turn inhibits the final transpeptidation step of peptidoglycan synthesis in bacterial cell walls, thus inhibiting cell wall biosynthesis. Bacteria eventually lyse due to ongoing activity of cell wall autolytic enzymes (autolysins and murein hydrolases) while cell wall assembly is arrested.

Pharmacodynamics/Kinetics

Distribution: Penetrates into blister fluid, middle ear fluid, tonsils, sinus, and lung tissues; V_d:

Children 6 months to 12 years: 0.67 ± 0.38 L/kg

Adults: 0.35 ± 0.29 L/kg

Protein binding: 60% to 70%

Metabolism: Minimal

Bioavailability: Capsule: 16% to 21%; suspension 25%

Half-life elimination: 1.7 (± 0.6) hours with normal renal function

Time to peak, plasma: 2 to 4 hours

Excretion: Primarily urine (~12% to 18% as unchanged drug)

Dosing

Adult & Geriatric

Acute exacerbations of chronic bronchitis, pharyngitis/tonsillitis: Oral: 300 mg twice daily for 5 to 10 days **or** 600 mg once daily for 10 days

Acute maxillary sinusitis: Oral: 300 mg twice daily **or** 600 mg once daily for 10 days. **Note:** According to the IDSA guidelines for acute bacterial rhinosinusitis, cefdinir is no longer recommended as monotherapy for initial empiric treatment (Chow, 2012).

Community-acquired pneumonia, uncomplicated skin and skin structure infections: Oral: 300 mg twice daily for 10 days

Pediatric

Infants ≥6 months and Children:

Acute bacterial otitis media, pharyngitis/tonsillitis: Oral: 7 mg/kg/dose twice daily for 5 to 10 days **or** 14 mg/kg/dose once daily for 10 days (maximum: 600 mg/day)

Acute maxillary sinusitis: Oral: 7 mg/kg/dose twice daily **or** 14 mg/kg/dose once daily for 10 days (maximum: 600 mg/day). **Note:** According to the IDSA guidelines for acute bacterial rhinosinusitis, cefdinir is no longer recommended as monotherapy for initial empiric treatment (Chow, 2012).

Uncomplicated skin and skin structure infections: Oral: 7 mg/kg/dose twice daily for 10 days (maximum: 600 mg/day).

Adolescents: Refer to adult dosing.

Renal Impairment
CrCl ≥30 mL/minute: No dosage adjustment necessary.
CrCl <30 mL/minute:
Adolescents and Adults: 300 mg once daily
Infants ≥6 months and Children: 7 mg/kg once daily (maximum: 300 mg/day)

ESRD requiring intermittent hemodialysis (IHD): Dialyzable: (63%): Initial dose: 300 mg (or 7 mg/kg/dose) every other day. Postdialysis, 300 mg (or 7 mg/kg/dose) should be given. Subsequent doses (300 mg or 7 mg/kg/dose) should be administered every other day.

Hepatic Impairment No dosage adjustment necessary.

Administration Twice daily doses should be given every 12 hours. May be administered with or without food. Manufacturer recommends administering at least 2 hours before or after antacids or iron supplements. Shake suspension well before use.

Monitoring Parameters Monitor renal function. Observe for signs and symptoms of anaphylaxis during first dose.

Test Interactions False-positive reaction for urinary ketones may occur with nitroprusside- but not nitroferricyanide-based tests. False-positive urine glucose results may occur when using Clinitest®, Benedict's solution, or Fehling's solution; glucose-oxidase-based reaction systems (eg, Clinistix®, Tes-Tape®) are recommended. May cause positive direct Coombs' test.

Dosage Forms Excipient information presented when available (limited, particularly for generics); consult specific product labeling.
Capsule, Oral:
Generic: 300 mg
Suspension Reconstituted, Oral:
Generic: 125 mg/5 mL (60 mL, 100 mL); 250 mg/5 mL (60 mL, 100 mL)

Cefditoren (sef de TOR en)

Brand Names: US Spectracef
Index Terms Cefditoren Pivoxil
Pharmacologic Category Antibiotic, Cephalosporin (Third Generation)
Use Treatment of acute bacterial exacerbation of chronic bronchitis or community-acquired pneumonia (due to susceptible organisms including *Haemophilus influenzae*, *Haemophilus parainfluenzae*, *Streptococcus pneumoniae*-penicillin susceptible only, *Moraxella catarrhalis*); pharyngitis or tonsillitis (*Streptococcus pyogenes*); and uncomplicated skin and skin-structure infections (*Staphylococcus aureus* - not MRSA, *Streptococcus pyogenes*)

Dosing
Adult & Geriatric
Acute bacterial exacerbation of chronic bronchitis: Oral: 400 mg twice daily for 10 days
Community-acquired pneumonia: Oral: 400 mg twice daily for 14 days
Pharyngitis, tonsillitis, uncomplicated skin and skin structure infections: Oral: 200 mg twice daily for 10 days
Pediatric Children ≥12 years and Adolescents: Refer to adult dosing.

Renal Impairment
CrCl >50 mL/minute/1.73 m^2: No dosage adjustment necessary.
CrCl 30 to 49 mL/minute/1.73 m^2: Maximum dose: 200 mg twice daily
CrCl <30 mL/minute/1.73 m^2: Maximum dose: 200 mg once daily
End-stage renal disease (ESRD): There are no specific dosage adjustments provided in the manufacturer's labeling; safety and efficacy have not been established.

Hepatic Impairment
Mild-to-moderate impairment (Child-Pugh class A or B): No dosage adjustment necessary.
Severe impairment (Child-Pugh class C): There are no dosage adjustments provided in the manufacturer's labeling (has not been studied).

Additional Information Complete prescribing information should be consulted for additional detail.

Dosage Forms Excipient information presented when available (limited, particularly for generics); consult specific product labeling.
Tablet, Oral:
Spectracef: 200 mg, 400 mg [contains sodium caseinate]
Generic: 200 mg, 400 mg

◆ Cefditoren Pivoxil *see* Cefditoren *on page 333*

Cefepime (SEF e pim)

Brand Names: US Maxipime
Brand Names: Canada Maxipime
Index Terms Cefepime Hydrochloride
Pharmacologic Category Antibiotic, Cephalosporin (Fourth Generation)
Use
Febrile neutropenia: Treatment (empiric monotherapy) of febrile neutropenic patients.
Intra-abdominal infections: Treatment of complicated intra-abdominal infections, in combination with metronidazole, caused by *Escherichia coli*, viridans group streptococci, *Pseudomonas aeruginosa*, *Klebsiella pneumoniae*, *Enterobacter* species, or *Bacteroides fragilis*.
Pneumonia (moderate to severe): Treatment of moderate to severe pneumonia caused by *Streptococcus pneumoniae*, including cases associated with concurrent bacteremia, *P. aeruginosa*, *K. pneumoniae*, or *Enterobacter* species.
Skin and skin structure infections: Treatment of moderate to severe uncomplicated skin and skin structure infections caused by *Staphylococcus aureus* (methicillin-susceptible isolates only) or *Streptococcus pyogenes*.
Urinary tract infections (including pyelonephritis): Treatment of complicated and uncomplicated urinary tract infections (UTIs), including pyelonephritis, caused by *E. coli* or *K. pneumoniae*, when the infection is severe, or caused by *E. coli*, *K. pneumoniae*, or *Proteus mirabilis*, when the infection is mild to moderate, including cases associated with concurrent bacteremia with these microorganisms.

Pregnancy Considerations Adverse events were not observed in animal reproduction studies. Cefepime crosses the placenta.

Breast-Feeding Considerations Small amounts of cefepime are excreted in breast milk. The manufacturer recommends that caution be exercised when administering cefepime to nursing women. Nondose-related effects could include modification of bowel flora.

Contraindications Hypersensitivity (eg, anaphylaxis, serious skin reactions) to cefepime, other cephalosporins, penicillins, other beta-lactam antibiotics, or any component of the formulation

Warnings/Precautions Severe neurological reactions (some fatal) have been reported, including encephalopathy, myoclonus, seizures, and nonconvulsive status epilepticus; risk may be increased in the presence of renal impairment (CrCl ≤60 mL/minute); ensure dose adjusted for renal function or discontinue therapy if patient develops neurotoxicity; effects are often reversible upon discontinuation of cefepime. Serious adverse reactions have occurred in elderly patients with renal insufficiency given unadjusted doses of cefepime, including life-threatening or fatal occurrences of the following: encephalopathy, myoclonus, and seizures. Hypersensitivity reactions may occur; use with caution in patients with a history of any allergy (particularly drugs), penicillin allergy or beta-lactam sensitivity. If a hypersensitivity reaction occurs, discontinue therapy and institute supportive emergency measures. penicillin allergy or beta-lactam sensitivity. If a hypersensitivity reaction occurs, discontinue therapy and institute supportive emergency measures. Prolonged use may result in fungal or bacterial superinfection, including *C. difficile*-associated diarrhea (CDAD) and pseudomembranous colitis; CDAD has been observed >2 months post-antibiotic treatment. Use with caution in patients with a history of gastrointestinal disease, especially colitis. May be associated with increased INR, especially in nutritionally-deficient patients, prolonged treatment, hepatic or renal disease. Use with caution in patients with a history of seizure disorder; high levels, particularly in the presence of renal impairment, may increase risk of seizures.

Adverse Reactions
>10%: Hematologic & oncologic: Positive direct Coombs test (without hemolysis; 16%)
1% to 10%:
Cardiovascular: Localized phlebitis (1%)
Central nervous system: Headache (1%)
Dermatologic: Skin rash (1% to 4%), pruritus (1%)
Endocrine & metabolic: Hypophosphatemia (3%)

Gastrointestinal: Diarrhea (≤3%), nausea (≤2%), vomiting (≤1%)

Hematologic & oncologic: Eosinophilia (2%)

Hepatic: Increased serum ALT (3%), abnormal partial thromboplastin time (2%), increased serum AST (2%), abnormal prothrombin time (1%)

Local: Local pain (1%)

Miscellaneous: Fever (1%)

<1% (Limited to important or life-threatening): Agranulocytosis, anaphylactic shock, anaphylaxis, brain disease, colitis, coma, confusion, decreased hematocrit, hallucination, hypercalcemia, hyperkalemia, hyperphosphatemia, hypocalcemia, increased blood urea nitrogen, increased serum alkaline phosphatase, increased serum bilirubin, increased serum creatinine, leukopenia, neutropenia, oral candidiasis, pseudomembranous colitis, seizure, status epilepticus (nonconvulsive), stupor, thrombocytopenia, urticaria, vaginitis

Drug Interactions

Metabolism/Transport Effects None known.

Avoid Concomitant Use

Avoid concomitant use of Cefepime with any of the following: BCG (Intravesical)

Increased Effect/Toxicity

Cefepime may increase the levels/effects of: Aminoglycosides; Vitamin K Antagonists

The levels/effects of Cefepime may be increased by: Probenecid

Decreased Effect

Cefepime may decrease the levels/effects of: BCG (Intravesical); BCG Vaccine (Immunization); Sodium Picosulfate; Typhoid Vaccine

Preparation for Administration

IV: Reconstitute 1 or 2 g vial with 10 mL of a compatible diluent (resulting concentration of 100 mg/mL for 1 g vial and 160 mg/mL for 2 g vial) and further dilute in a compatible IV infusion fluid.

IM: Reconstitute 1 g vial with 2.4 mL of SWFI, NS, D5W, lidocaine 0.5% or 1%, or bacteriostatic water for injection; resulting concentration is 280 mg/mL.

Storage/Stability

Vials: Store intact vials at 20°C to 25°C (68°F to 77°F). Protect from light. After reconstitution, stable in NS and D5W for 24 hours at room temperature and 7 days refrigerated. Refer to the manufacturer's product labeling for other acceptable reconstitution solutions.

Dual chamber containers: Store unactivated containers at 20°C to 25°C (68°F to 77°F); excursions permitted to 15°C to 30°C (59°F to 85°F). Do not freeze. Following reconstitution, use within 12 hours if stored at room temperature or within 5 days if stored under refrigeration.

Premixed solution: Store frozen at -20°C (-4°F). Thawed solution is stable for 24 hours at room temperature or 7 days under refrigeration; do not refreeze.

Mechanism of Action Inhibits bacterial cell wall synthesis by binding to one or more of the penicillin-binding proteins (PBPs) which in turn inhibits the final transpeptidation step of peptidoglycan synthesis in bacterial cell walls, thus inhibiting cell wall biosynthesis. Bacteria eventually lyse due to ongoing activity of cell wall autolytic enzymes (autolysis and murein hydrolases) while cell wall assembly is arrested.

Pharmacodynamics/Kinetics

Absorption: IM: Rapid and complete

Distribution: V_d:

Neonates (Capparelli, 2005):

PMA <30 weeks: 0.51 L/kg

PMA >30 weeks: 0.39 L/kg

Infants and Children 2 months to 11 years: 0.3 L/kg

Adults:18 L, 0.26 L/kg; penetrates into inflammatory fluid at concentrations ~80% of serum concentrations and into bronchial mucosa at concentrations ~60% of plasma concentrations; crosses the blood-brain barrier

Protein binding, plasma: ~20%

Metabolism: Minimally hepatic

Half-life elimination:

Neonates: 4 to 5 hours (Lima-Rogel 2008)

Children 2 months to 6 years: 1.77 to 1.96 hours

Adults: 2 hours

Hemodialysis: 13.5 hours

Continuous peritoneal dialysis: 19 hours

Time to peak: IM: 1 to 2 hours; IV: 0.5 hours

Excretion: Urine (85% as unchanged drug)

Dosing

Adult & Geriatric

Febrile neutropenia, monotherapy: IV: 2 g every 8 hours for 7 days or until the neutropenia resolves

Intra-abdominal infections, complicated, severe (in combination with metronidazole): IV: **Note:** 2010 IDSA guidelines recommend a duration of 4 to 7 days (provided source controlled). Not recommended for hospital-acquired intra-abdominal infections (IAI) associated with multidrug-resistant gram negative organisms or in mild-to-moderate community-acquired IAIs due to risk of toxicity and the development of resistant organisms (Solomkin, [IDSA] 2010).

Due to *P. aeruginosa*: 2 g every 8 hours for 7 to 10 days

Not due to *P. aeruginosa*: 2 g every 8 to 12 hours for 7 to 10 days

Pneumonia: IV: **Note:** Duration of therapy may vary considerably for healthcare associated pneumonia (7 to 21 days). In absence of *Pseudomonas*, and if appropriate empiric treatment used and patient responsive, it may be clinically appropriate to reduce duration of therapy to 7 to 10 days (American Thoracic Society Guidelines, 2005).

Due to *P. aeruginosa*: 1 to 2 g every 8 hours for 10 days; **Note:** Longer courses (eg, 14 to 21 days) may be required (American Thoracic Society Guidelines, 2005).

Not due to *P. aeruginosa*: 1 to 2 g every 8 to 12 hours for 10 days

Skin and skin structure infection, uncomplicated: IV: 2 g every 12 hours for 10 days

Urinary tract infections, complicated and uncomplicated:

Mild-to-moderate: IM, IV: 0.5 to 1 g every 12 hours for 7 to 10 days

Severe: IV: 2 g every 12 hours for 10 days

Brain abscess, postneurosurgical prevention (off-label use): IV: 2 g every 8 hours with vancomycin (Tunkel, 2004)

Prosthetic joint infection, *Enterobacter spp.* or *Pseudomonas aeruginosa* (off-label use): IV: 2 g every 12 hours for 4 to 6 weeks; **Note:** When treating *P. aeruginosa*, consider addition of an aminoglycoside (Osmon, 2013)

Pediatric

Infants ≥2 months, Children, and Adolescents ≤16 years (≤40 kg):

Febrile neutropenia: IV: 50 mg/kg/dose every 8 hours for 7 days or until neutropenia resolves (maximum: 2 g/dose)

Pneumonia: IV:

Due to *P. aeruginosa*: 50 mg/kg/dose every 8 hours for 10 days (maximum: 2 g/dose)

Not due to *P. aeruginosa*: 50 mg/kg/dose every 12 hours for 10 days (maximum: 2 g/dose)

Skin and skin structure infections (uncomplicated): IV: 50 mg/kg/dose every 12 hours for 10 days (maximum: 2 g/dose)

Urinary tract infections, complicated and uncomplicated: IV, IM: 50 mg/kg/dose every 12 hours for 7 to 10 days (maximum: 1 g/dose); **Note:** IM may be considered for mild-to-moderate infection only.

Intra-abdominal infection, complicated (off-label use): IV: **Note:** IDSA 2010 guidelines recommend duration of 4 to 7 days (provided source controlled): 50 mg/kg/dose every 12 hours in combination with metronidazole (Solomkin [IDSA], 2010)

Children >40 kg and Adolescents >16 years:

Febrile neutropenia, monotherapy: IV: 2 g every 8 hours for 7 days or until the neutropenia resolves

Intra-abdominal infections, complicated, severe (in combination with metronidazole): IV: **Note:** IDSA 2010 guidelines recommend duration of 4 to 7 days (provided source controlled) (Solomkin, [IDSA] 2010).

Due to *P. aeruginosa*: 2 g every 8 hours for 7 to 10 days

Not due to *P. aeruginosa*: 2 g every 8 to 12 hours for 7 to 10 days

Pneumonia: IV:

Due to *P. aeruginosa*: 1 to 2 g every 8 hours for 10 days

Not due to *P. aeruginosa*: 1 to 2 g every 8 to 12 hours for 10 days

Skin and skin structure infections, uncomplicated: IV: 2 g every 12 hours for 10 days

Urinary tract infections, complicated and uncomplicated:

Mild-to-moderate: IM, IV: 0.5 to 1 g every 12 hours for 7 to 10 days

Severe: IV: 2 g every 12 hours for 10 days

Renal Impairment

Adults: Recommended maintenance schedule based on creatinine clearance (may be estimated using the Cockcroft-Gault formula), compared to normal dosing schedule: See table.

Cefepime Hydrochloride

Creatinine Clearance (mL/minute)	Recommended Maintenance Schedule			
>60 (normal recommended dosing schedule)	500 mg every 12 hours	1 g every 12 hours	2 g every 12 hours	2 g every 8 hours
30-60	500 mg every 24 hours	1 g every 24 hours	2 g every 24 hours	2 g every 12 hours
11-29	500 mg every 24 hours	500 mg every 24 hours	1 g every 24 hours	2 g every 24 hours
<11	250 mg every 24 hours	250 mg every 24 hours	500 mg every 24 hours	1 g every 24 hours

Intermittent hemodialysis (IHD) (administer after hemodialysis on dialysis days): IV: Initial: 1 g (single dose) on day 1. Maintenance: 0.5-1 g every 24 hours **or** 1-2 g every 48-72 hours (Heintz, 2009) **or** 2 g 3 times weekly after dialysis (Perez, 2012). **Note:** Dosing dependent on the assumption of 3 times weekly, complete IHD sessions.

Peritoneal dialysis (PD): Removed to a lesser extent than hemodialysis; administer normal recommended dose every 48 hours

Continuous renal replacement therapy (CRRT) (Heintz, 2009; Trotman, 2005): Drug clearance is highly dependent on the method of renal replacement, filter type, and flow rate. Appropriate dosing requires close monitoring of pharmacologic response, signs of adverse reactions due to drug accumulation, as well as drug concentrations in relation to target trough (if appropriate). The following are general recommendations only (based on dialysate flow/ultrafiltration rates of 1-2 L/hour and minimal residual renal function) and should not supersede clinical judgment:

CVVH: Loading dose of 2 g followed by 1-2 g every 12 hours

CVVHD/CVVHDF: Loading dose of 2 g followed by either 1 g every 8 hours **or** 2 g every 12 hours. **Note:** Dosage of 1 g every 8 hours results in similar steady-state concentrations as 2 g every 12 hours and is more cost effective (Heintz, 2009).

Note: Consider higher dosage of 4 g/day if treating *Pseudomonas* or life-threatening infections in order to maximize time above MIC (Trotman, 2005). Dosage of 2 g every 8 hours may be needed for gram-negative rods with MIC ≥4 mg/L (Heintz, 2009).

Children: No dosage adjustment provided in the manufacturer's labeling; however, similar dosage adjustments to adults would be anticipated based on comparable pharmacokinetics between children and adults.

Hepatic Impairment No dosage adjustment necessary.

Administration May be administered either IM or IV

Inject deep IM into large muscle mass. Inject direct IV over 5 minutes (Garrelts, 1999). Infuse intermittent infusion over 30 minutes.

Monitoring Parameters Monitor renal function. Observe for signs and symptoms of anaphylaxis during first dose.

Test Interactions Positive direct Coombs', false-positive urinary glucose test using cupric sulfate (Benedict's solution, Clinitest®, Fehling's solution), false-positive serum or urine creatinine with Jaffé reaction, false-positive urinary proteins and steroids

Dosage Forms Excipient information presented when available (limited, particularly for generics); consult specific product labeling.

Solution, Intravenous, as hydrochloride:
Generic: 1 g/50 mL (50 mL); 2% (100 mL)
Solution Reconstituted, Injection, as hydrochloride:
Maxipime: 1 g (1 ea); 2 g (1 ea)
Generic: 1 g (1 ea); 2 g (1 ea)
Solution Reconstituted, Intravenous, as hydrochloride:
Maxipime: 1 g (1 ea); 2 g (1 ea)
Generic: 1 g/50 mL (1 ea); 2 g/50 mL (1 ea)

◆ Cefepime Hydrochloride see Cefepime on page 333

Cefixime (sef IKS eem)

Brand Names: US Suprax
Brand Names: Canada Auro-Cefixime; Suprax
Index Terms Cefixime Trihydrate

Pharmacologic Category Antibiotic, Cephalosporin (Third Generation)

Use Treatment of uncomplicated urinary tract infections (due to *Escherichia coli* and *Proteus mirabilis*), otitis media (due to *Haemophilus influenzae*, *Moraxella catarrhalis*, and *Streptococcus pyogenes*), pharyngitis and tonsillitis (due to *Streptococcus pyogenes*), acute exacerbations of chronic bronchitis (due to *Streptococcus pneumoniae* and *Haemophilus influenzae*); uncomplicated cervical/urethral gonorrhea (due to *N. gonorrhoeae* [penicillinase- and non-penicillinase-producing])

Note: Due to concerns of resistance, the CDC no longer recommends use of cefixime as a first-line regimen in the treatment of uncomplicated gonorrhea in the U.S.; ceftriaxone is the preferred cephalosporin (CDC, 2012).

Pregnancy Considerations Teratogenic effects were not observed in animal reproduction studies. Cefixime crosses the placenta and can be detected in the amniotic fluid (Ozyüncü 2010).

Breast-Feeding Considerations It is not known if cefixime is excreted in breast milk. The manufacturer recommends that consideration be given to discontinuing nursing temporarily during treatment. If present in breast milk, nondose-related effects could include modification of bowel flora.

Contraindications Hypersensitivity to cefixime, any component of the formulation, or other cephalosporins

Warnings/Precautions Prolonged use may result in fungal or bacterial superinfection, including *C. difficile*-associated diarrhea (CDAD) and pseudomembranous colitis; CDAD has been observed >2 months postantibiotic treatment. Modify dosage in patients with renal impairment. Use with caution in patients with a history of penicillin allergy, especially IgE-mediated reactions (eg, anaphylaxis, urticaria).

Chewable tablets contain phenylalanine.

Benzyl alcohol and derivatives: Some dosage forms may contain sodium benzoate/benzoic acid; benzoic acid (benzoate) is a metabolite of benzyl alcohol; large amounts of benzyl alcohol (≥99 mg/kg/day) have been associated with a potentially fatal toxicity ("gasping syndrome") in neonates; the "gasping syndrome" consists of metabolic acidosis, respiratory distress, gasping respirations, CNS dysfunction (including convulsions, intracranial hemorrhage), hypotension, and cardiovascular collapse (AAP ["Inactive" 1997]; CDC, 1982); some data suggests that benzoate displaces bilirubin from protein binding sites (Ahlfors, 2001); avoid or use dosage forms containing benzyl alcohol derivative with caution in neonates. See manufacturer's labeling.

Adverse Reactions

>10%: Gastrointestinal: Diarrhea (16%)

2% to 10%: Gastrointestinal: Abdominal pain, nausea, dyspepsia, flatulence, loose stools

<2% (Limited to important or life-threatening): Acute renal failure, anaphylactoid reaction, anaphylaxis, angioedema, candidiasis, dizziness, drug fever, eosinophilia, erythema multiforme, facial edema, fever, headache, hepatitis, hyperbilirubinemia, increased blood urea nitrogen, increased serum creatinine, increased serum transaminases, jaundice, leukopenia, neutropenia, prolonged prothrombin time, pruritus, pseudomembranous colitis, seizure, serum sickness-like reaction, skin rash, Stevens-Johnson syndrome, thrombocytopenia, toxic epidermal necrolysis, urticaria, vaginitis, vomiting

Drug Interactions

Metabolism/Transport Effects None known.

Avoid Concomitant Use

Avoid concomitant use of Cefixime with any of the following: BCG (Intravesical)

Increased Effect/Toxicity

Cefixime may increase the levels/effects of: Aminoglycosides; Vitamin K Antagonists

The levels/effects of Cefixime may be increased by: Probenecid

Decreased Effect

Cefixime may decrease the levels/effects of: BCG (Intravesical); BCG Vaccine (Immunization); Sodium Picosulfate; Typhoid Vaccine

Food Interactions Food delays cefixime absorption. Management: May administer with or without food.

Preparation for Administration Powder for suspension: Refer to manufacturer's product labeling for reconstitution instructions.

Storage/Stability
Capsule, chewable tablet, tablet: Store at 20°C to 25°C (68°F to 77°F).

Powder for suspension: Prior to reconstitution, store at 20°C to 25°C (68°F to 77°F). After reconstitution, suspension may be stored for 14 days at room temperature or under refrigeration.

Mechanism of Action Inhibits bacterial cell wall synthesis by binding to one or more of the penicillin-binding proteins (PBPs); which in turn inhibits the final transpeptidation step of peptidoglycan synthesis in bacterial cell walls, thus inhibiting cell wall biosynthesis. Bacteria eventually lyse due to ongoing activity of cell wall autolytic enzymes (autolysins and murein hydrolases) while cell wall assembly is arrested.

Pharmacodynamics/Kinetics Note: Chewable tablets and oral suspension are bioequivalent. However, oral suspension and tablet (nonchewable)/capsule formulations are **not** considered bioequivalent (oral suspension AUC ~10% to 25% greater compared with tablet after doses of 100-400 mg in normal adult volunteers).

Absorption: 40% to 50%; **Note:** Capsule AUC reduced by ~15% and C_{max} by ~25% when taken with food.

Distribution: Widely throughout the body and reaches therapeutic concentration in most tissues and body fluids, including synovial, pericardial, pleural, peritoneal; bile, sputum, and urine; bone, myocardium, gallbladder, and skin and soft tissue

Protein binding: 65%

Half-life elimination: Normal renal function: 3 to 4 hours; Moderate impairment (CrCl 20 to 40 mL/minute): 6.4 hours; Renal failure: Up to 11.5 hours

Time to peak, serum: Tablet, suspension: 2 to 6 hours; Capsule: 3 to 8 hours; Delayed with food

Excretion: Urine (50% of absorbed dose as active drug); feces (10%)

Dosing
Adult & Geriatric Note: Suprax 400 mg tablets have been discontinued in the US for more than 1 year.

Susceptible infections: Oral: 400 mg daily divided every 12-24 hours

Gonococcal infection, uncomplicated cervical/urethral/rectal (rectal off-label use) gonorrhea due to N. gonorrhoeae: Oral: 400 mg as a single dose in combination with oral azithromycin (preferred) or oral doxycycline (CDC, 2010). **Note:** CDC no longer recommends cefixime as a first-line agent (ceftriaxone is the preferred cephalosporin), if cefixime is used as an alternative agent, test-of-cure follow up in 7 days is recommended; in addition, cefixime is **not** an option for the treatment of uncomplicated gonorrhea of the pharynx (CDC, 2012). In Canada, due to increased antimicrobial resistance, the Public Health Agency of Canada recommends 800 mg as a single dose (off-label dose) for treatment of uncomplicated gonococcal infections.

Gonococcal infection, expedited partner therapy: Oral: 400 mg as a single dose in combination with oral azithromycin (CDC, 2012). **Note:** Only used if a heterosexual partner cannot be linked to evaluation and treatment in a timely manner; dose delivered to partner by patient, collaborating pharmacy, or disease investigation specialist.

S. pyogenes infections: Oral: 400 mg daily divided every 12-24 hours for ≥10 days

Typhoid fever (off-label use): Oral: 15-20 mg/kg/day in 2 divided doses for 7-14 days (Parry, 2002; WHO, 2003)

Pediatric Note: Suprax 400 mg tablets have been discontinued in the US for more than 1 year.

Susceptible infections: Oral: **Note:** Otitis media should be treated using the chewable tablets or suspension **only**. Chewable tablets and suspension achieve higher peak blood levels compared to an equivalent dose using the tablet or capsule.

Children ≥6 months and ≤45 kg: 8 mg/kg/day divided every 12-24 hours (maximum: 400 mg daily)

Dosing recommendations based on body weight (doses are rounded for use of oral suspension or chewable tablet):
5 to <7.6 kg: 50 mg daily
7.6 to <10.1 kg: 80 mg daily
10.1 to <12.6 kg: 100 mg daily
12.6 to <20.6 kg: 150 mg daily
20.6 to <28.1 kg: 200 mg daily
28.1 to <33.1 kg: 250 mg daily
33.1 to <40.1 kg: 300 mg daily
40.1 to ≤45 kg: 350 mg daily

Children >45 kg or >12 years and Adolescents: Refer to adult dosing.

Acute bacterial rhinosinusitis (off-label use): Oral: 8 mg/kg/day divided every 12 hours with concomitant clindamycin for 10-14 days. **Note:** Recommended in patients with non-type I penicillin allergy, after failure of initial therapy or in patients at risk for antibiotic resistance (eg, daycare attendance, age <2 years, recent hospitalization, antibiotic use within the past month) (Chow, 2012).

Gonococcal infection, uncomplicated: Oral: Children >45 kg: 400 mg as a single dose in combination with oral azithromycin (preferred) or oral doxycycline (CDC, 2010). **Note:** CDC no longer recommends cefixime as a first-line agent, only use as an alternative agent with test-of-cure follow up in 7 days (CDC, 2012). In Canada, due to increased antimicrobial resistance, the Public Health Agency of Canada recommends 800 mg as a single dose (off-label dose) for treatment of uncomplicated gonococcal infections in children ≥9 years of age.

S. pyogenes infections: Oral:
Children ≥6 months and ≤45 kg: 8 mg/kg/day divided every 12-24 hours for ≥10 days (maximum: 400 mg daily)

Children >45 kg or >12 years and Adolescents: 400 mg daily divided every 12-24 hours for ≥10 days

Typhoid fever (off-label use): Oral: 15-20 mg/kg/day divided every 12 hours for 7-14 days; maximum 400 mg daily (Girgis, 1995; Stephens, 2002)

Renal Impairment Adults:
CrCl ≥60 mL/minute: No dosage adjustment necessary.
CrCl 21 to 59 mL/minute: 260 mg once daily
CrCl ≤20 mL/minute:
Chewable tablet, tablet: 200 mg once daily
100 mg/5 mL suspension: 172 mg once daily
200 mg/5 mL suspension: 176 mg once daily
500 mg/5 mL suspension: 180 mg once daily
Intermittent hemodialysis (not significantly removed by hemodialysis): 260 mg once daily
CAPD (not significantly removed by peritoneal dialysis):
Chewable tablet, tablet: 200 mg once daily
100 mg/5 mL suspension: 172 mg once daily
200 mg/5 mL suspension: 176 mg once daily
500 mg/5 mL suspension: 180 mg once daily

Hepatic Impairment No dosage adjustment provided in manufacturer's labeling.

Dietary Considerations Chewable tablets contain phenylalanine.

Administration May be administered with or without food. Shake oral suspension well before use. Chewable tablets must be chewed or crushed before swallowing.

Monitoring Parameters Renal function; with prolonged therapy, monitor renal and hepatic function periodically. Observe for signs and symptoms of anaphylaxis during first dose. When used as part of alternative treatment for gonococcal infection, test-of-cure 7 days after dose (CDC, 2012).

Test Interactions Positive direct Coombs', false-positive urinary glucose test using cupric sulfate (Benedict's solution, Clinitest®, Fehling's solution), may cause false-positive serum or urine creatinine with the alkaline picrate-based Jaffé reaction for measuring creatinine; false-positive urine ketones using tests with nitroprusside (but not those using nitroferricyanide).

Product Availability Suprax 400 mg tablets have been discontinued in the US for more than 1 year.

Dosage Forms Excipient information presented when available (limited, particularly for generics); consult specific product labeling. [DSC] = Discontinued product
Capsule, Oral:
Suprax: 400 mg
Suspension Reconstituted, Oral:
Suprax: 100 mg/5 mL (50 mL) [strawberry flavor]
Suprax: 200 mg/5 mL (50 mL, 75 mL); 500 mg/5 mL (10 mL, 20 mL) [contains sodium benzoate; strawberry flavor]
Generic: 100 mg/5 mL (50 mL); 200 mg/5 mL (50 mL, 75 mL)
Tablet, Oral:
Suprax: 400 mg [DSC] [scored]
Tablet Chewable, Oral:
Suprax: 100 mg, 200 mg [contains aspartame, fd&c red #40 aluminum lake; tutti-frutti flavor]

◆ Cefixime Trihydrate see Cefixime on page 335
◆ Cefotan see CefoTEtan on page 339

Cefotaxime (sef oh TAKS eem)

Brand Names: US Claforan; Claforan in D5W
Brand Names: Canada Cefotaxime Sodium For Injection; Claforan
Index Terms Cefotaxime Sodium
Pharmacologic Category Antibiotic, Cephalosporin (Third Generation)

Use

Bacteremia/Septicemia: Treatment of bacteremia/septicemia caused by *Escherichia coli*, *Klebsiella* species, and *Serratia marcescens*, *Staphylococcus aureus* and *Streptococcus* species (including *Streptococcus pneumoniae*).

Bone or joint infections: Treatment of bone or joint infections caused by *S. aureus* (penicillinase and nonpenicillinase producing strains), *Streptococcus* species (including *Streptococcus pyogenes*), *Pseudomonas* species (including *Pseudomonas aeruginosa*), and *Proteus mirabilis*.

CNS infections: Treatment of CNS infections (eg, meningitis, ventriculitis) caused by *Neisseria meningitidis*, *Haemophilus influenzae*, *S. pneumoniae*, *Klebsiella pneumoniae*, and *E. coli*.

Genitourinary infections: Treatment of genitourinary infections, including urinary tract infections (UTIs), caused by *Enterococcus* species, *Staphylococcus epidermidis*, *S. aureus* (penicillinase and nonpenicillinase producing), *Citrobacter* species, *Enterobacter* species, *E. coli*, *Klebsiella* species, *P. mirabilis*, *Proteus vulgaris*, *Providencia stuartii*, *Morganella morganii*, *Providencia rettgeri*, *S. marcescens*, and *Pseudomonas* species (including *P. aeruginosa*). Also, uncomplicated gonorrhea (cervical/urethral and rectal) caused by *Neisseria gonorrhoeae*, including penicillinase-producing strains.

Gynecologic infections: Treatment of gynecologic infections, including pelvic inflammatory disease, endometritis, and pelvic cellulitis, caused by *S. epidermidis*, *Streptococcus* species, *Enterococcus* species, *Enterobacter* species, *Klebsiella* species, *E. coli*, *P. mirabilis*, *Bacteroides* species (including *Bacteroides fragilis*), *Clostridium* species, and anaerobic cocci (including *Peptostreptococcus* and *Peptococcus* species) and *Fusobacterium* species (including *Fusobacterium nucleatum*).

Intra-abdominal infections: Treatment of intra-abdominal infections, including peritonitis caused by *Streptococcus* species, *E. coli*, *Klebsiella* species, *Bacteroides* species, and anaerobic cocci (including *Peptostreptococcus* species and *Peptococcus* species), *P. mirabilis*, and *Clostridium* species.

Lower respiratory tract infections: Treatment of lower respiratory tract infections, including pneumonia, caused by *S. pneumoniae*, *S. pyogenes* (group A streptococci) and other streptococci (excluding enterococci, [eg, *Enterococcus faecalis*]), *S. aureus* (penicillinase and nonpenicillinase producing), *E. coli*, *Klebsiella* species, *H. influenzae* (including ampicillin-resistant strains), *H. parainfluenzae*, *P. mirabilis*, *S. marcescens*, *Enterobacter* species, and indole-positive *Proteus* and *Pseudomonas* species (including *P. aeruginosa*).

Skin and skin structure infections: Treatment of skin and skin structure infections caused by *S. aureus* (penicillinase and nonpenicillinase producing), *S. epidermidis*, *S. pyogenes* (group A streptococci) and other streptococci, *Enterococcus* species, *Acinetobacter* species, *E. coli*, *Citrobacter* species (including *Citrobacter freundii*), *Enterobacter* species, *Klebsiella* species, *P. mirabilis*, *P. vulgaris*, *M. morganii*, *P. rettgeri*, *Pseudomonas* species, *S. marcescens*, *Bacteroides* species, and anaerobic cocci (including *Peptostreptococcus* species and *Peptococcus* species).

Surgical prophylaxis: Reduce the incidence of certain infections in patients undergoing surgical procedures (eg, abdominal or vaginal hysterectomy, GI and GU tract surgery) that may be classified as contaminated or potentially contaminated; reduce the incidence of certain postoperative infections in patients undergoing cesarean section.

Pregnancy Considerations Adverse events have not been observed in animal reproduction studies. Cefotaxime crosses the human placenta and can be found in fetal tissue. An increase in most types of birth defects was not found following first trimester exposure to cephalosporins. During pregnancy, peak cefotaxime serum concentrations are decreased and the serum half-life is shorter. Cefotaxime is approved for use in women undergoing cesarean section (consult current guidelines for appropriate use).

Breast-Feeding Considerations Low concentrations of cefotaxime are found in breast milk. The manufacturer recommends that caution be exercised when administering cefotaxime to nursing women. Nondose-related effects could include modification of bowel flora. The pregnancy-related changes in cefotaxime pharmacokinetics continue into the early postpartum period.

Contraindications Hypersensitivity to cefotaxime, any component of the formulation, or other cephalosporins

Warnings/Precautions A potentially life-threatening arrhythmia has been reported in patients who received a rapid (<1 minute) bolus injection via central venous catheter. Granulocytopenia and more rarely agranulocytosis may develop during prolonged treatment (>10 days). Minimize tissue inflammation by changing infusion sites when needed. Use with caution in patients with a history of penicillin allergy, especially IgE-mediated reactions (eg, anaphylaxis, urticaria). Prolonged use may result in fungal or bacterial superinfection, including *C. difficile*-associated diarrhea (CDAD) and pseudomembranous colitis; CDAD has been observed >2 months postantibiotic treatment. Use with caution in patients with renal impairment; dosage adjustment may be required. Use with caution in patients with a history of colitis. Potentially significant drug-drug interactions may exist, requiring dose or frequency adjustment, additional monitoring, and/or selection of alternative therapy.

Adverse Reactions

1% to 10%:

Dermatologic: Pruritus (≤2%), skin rash (≤2%)

Gastrointestinal: Colitis (≤1%), diarrhea (≤1%), nausea (≤1%), vomiting (≤1%)

Hematologic & oncologic: Eosinophilia (≤2%)

Local: Induration at injection site (IM ≤4%), inflammation at injection site (IV ≤4%), pain at injection site (IM ≤4%), tenderness at injection site (IM ≤4%)

Miscellaneous: Fever (≤2%)

<1% (Limited to important or life-threatening): Acute generalized exanthematous pustulosis, acute renal failure, agranulocytosis, anaphylaxis, bone marrow failure, brain disease, candidiasis, cardiac arrhythmia (after rapid IV injection via central catheter), cholestasis, *Clostridium difficile* associated diarrhea, erythema multiforme, granulocytopenia, hemolytic anemia, hepatitis, increased blood urea nitrogen, increased gamma-glutamyl transferase, increased lactate dehydrogenase, increased serum alkaline phosphatase, increased serum ALT, increased serum AST, increased serum bilirubin, increased serum creatinine, injection site phlebitis, interstitial nephritis, jaundice, leukopenia, neutropenia, pancytopenia, positive direct Coombs test, pseudomembranous colitis, Stevens-Johnson syndrome, thrombocytopenia, toxic epidermal necrolysis, vaginitis

Drug Interactions

Metabolism/Transport Effects None known.

Avoid Concomitant Use

Avoid concomitant use of Cefotaxime with any of the following: BCG (Intravesical)

Increased Effect/Toxicity

Cefotaxime may increase the levels/effects of: Aminoglycosides; Vitamin K Antagonists

The levels/effects of Cefotaxime may be increased by: Probenecid

Decreased Effect

Cefotaxime may decrease the levels/effects of: BCG (Intravesical); BCG Vaccine (Immunization); Sodium Picosulfate; Typhoid Vaccine

Preparation for Administration

IM: Reconstitute vials with SWFI or bacteriostatic water for injection; dilute with 2 mL for the 500 mg vial (resulting concentration ~230 mg/mL), 3 mL for the 1 g vial (resulting concentration ~300 mg/mL), and 5 mL for the 2 g vial (resulting concentration 330 mg/mL). Shake to dissolve.

IV: Reconstitute vials with ≥10 mL SWFI; resulting concentration: 50 mg/mL (500 mg vial), 95 mg/mL (1 g vial), or 180 mg/mL (2 g vial). Shake to dissolve. May be further diluted up to 1000 mL with NS, D$_5$W, D$_{10}$W, D$_5$NS, D$_5$$\frac{1}{2}NS, D_5$$\frac{1}{4}$NS, or LR.

Storage/Stability Store intact vials below 30°C (86°F). Protect from light. Reconstituted solution is stable for 12 to 24 hours at room temperature, 7 to 10 days when refrigerated, for 13 weeks when frozen. For IV infusion in NS or D$_5$W, solution is stable for 24 hours at room temperature, 5 days when refrigerated, or 13 weeks when frozen in Viaflex plastic containers. Thawed solutions of frozen premixed bags are stable for 24 hours at room temperature or 10 days when refrigerated.

Mechanism of Action Inhibits bacterial cell wall synthesis by binding to one or more of the penicillin-binding proteins (PBPs) which in turn inhibits the final transpeptidation step of peptidoglycan synthesis in bacterial cell walls, thus inhibiting cell wall biosynthesis. Bacteria eventually lyse due to ongoing activity of cell wall autolytic enzymes (autolysins and murein hydrolases) while cell wall assembly is arrested. Cefotaxime has activity in the presence of some beta-lactamases, both penicillinases and cephaolosporinases, of gram-negative and gram-positive bacteria. *Enterococcus* species may be intrinsically resistant to cefotaxime. Most extended-spectrum beta-lactamase (ESBL)-producing and carbapenemase-producing isolates are resistant to cefotaxime.

Pharmacodynamics/Kinetics

Distribution: Widely to body tissues and fluids including aqueous humor, ascitic and prostatic fluids, bone; penetrates CSF best when meninges are inflamed

Protein binding: 31% to 50%

Metabolism: Partially hepatic to active metabolite, desacetylcefotaxime

Half-life elimination:

Cefotaxime: Infants ≤1500 g: 4.6 hours; Infants >1500 g: 3.4 hours; Children: 1.5 hours; Adults: 1 to 1.5 hours; prolonged with renal and/or hepatic impairment

Desacetylcefotaxime: 1.3 to 1.9 hours; prolonged with renal impairment (Ings 1982)

Time to peak, serum: IM: Within 30 minutes

Excretion: Urine (~60% as unchanged drug and metabolites)

Dosing

Adult & Geriatric

Usual dosage range: IM, IV:

Uncomplicated infections: IM, IV: 1 g every 12 hours

Moderate-to-severe infections: IM, IV: 1 to 2 g every 8 hours

Life-threatening infections: IV: 2 g every 4 hours

Acute bacterial rhinosinusitis, severe infection requiring hospitalization: IV: 2 g every 4 to 6 hours for 5 to 7 days (Chow 2012)

Arthritis (septic): IV: 1 g every 8 hours

Bacterial enteric infections in HIV-infected patients (empiric treatment) (off-label use): IV: 1 g every 8 hours (HHS [OI adult 2015])

Bite wounds (animal) (off-label use): IV: 1 to 2 g every 6 to 8 hours in combination with clindamycin or metronidazole for anaerobic coverage (IDSA [Stevens 2014])

Brain abscess, meningitis: IV: 2 g every 4 to 6 hours in combination with other antimicrobial therapy as warranted (Kowlessar 2006; Tunkel 2004)

Cesarean section: IM, IV: 1 g IV as soon as the umbilical cord is clamped, then 1 g IV or IM at 6 and 12 hours after the first dose

Complicated community-acquired intra-abdominal infection of mild-to-moderate severity, including hepatic abscess (in combination with metronidazole): IV: 1 to 2 g every 6 to 8 hours for 4 to 7 days (provided source controlled). **Note:** For severe infections consider other antimicrobial agents (Bradley, 1987; Kim 2010; Solomkin 2010).

Gonorrhea (CDC 2010) (as an alternative to ceftriaxone):

Uncomplicated gonorrhea of the cervix, urethra, or rectum (off-label regimen): IM: 0.5 g as a single dose in combination with oral azithromycin (preferred) or oral doxycycline (alternative to preferred)

Note: May also administer 1 g as a single dose for rectal gonorrhea in adult males (per the manufacturer)

Disseminated: IV: 1 g every 8 hours continue for 24 to 48 hours after improvement begins then switch to oral therapy. Total duration of therapy at least 7 days

Lyme disease (as an alternative to ceftriaxone):

Cardiac manifestations: IV: 2 g every 8 hours for 14 to 21 days (Wormser 2006)

CNS manifestations: IV: 2 g every 8 hours for 10 to 28 days (Halperin 2007; Wormser 2006)

Surgical (perioperative) prophylaxis (off-label use): IV: 1 g within 60 minutes prior to surgical incision. Doses may be repeated in 3 hours if procedure is lengthy or if there is excessive blood loss. **Note:** preferred agent (with ampicillin) in liver transplantation (Bratzler 2013).

Obesity: The ASHP/IDSA/SIS/SHEA guidelines recommend that for patients weighing ≥120 kg (or alternatively defined as BMI >30 kg/m^2), a dose of 2 g within 60 minutes prior to surgical incision should be administered (Bratzler 2013).

Peritonitis (spontaneous): IV: 2 g every 8 hours, unless life-threatening then 2 g every 4 hours (Gilbert 2011; Runyon 2009)

Sepsis: IV: 2 g every 6 to 8 hours

Skin and soft tissue necrotizing infections (off-label use):

Polymicrobial infection: IV: 2 g every 6 hours, in combination with metronidazole or clindamycin for empiric therapy of polymicrobial infections. Continue until further debridement is not necessary, patient has clinically improved, and patient is afebrile for 48 to 72 hours (IDSA [Stevens 2014]).

Necrotizing infection due to Vibrio vulnificus: IV: 2 g every 8 hours, in combination with doxycycline. Continue until further debridement is not necessary, patient has clinically improved, and patient is afebrile for 48 to 72 hours (IDSA [Stevens 2014]).

Pediatric

Usual dosage range for susceptible infections:

Infants, Children, and Adolescents:

Manufacturer's labeling:

<50 kg: IM, IV: 50 to 180 mg/kg/day in divided doses every 4 to 6 hours (maximum dose: 12 g daily)

≥50 kg: Refer to adult dosing

Alternate recommendations (Red Book [AAP] 2012): IM, IV:

Mild to moderate infection: 50 to 180 mg/kg/day in divided doses every 6 to 8 hours (maximum dose: 6 g daily)

Severe infection: 200 to 225 mg/kg/day in divided doses every 4 to 6 hours; up to 300 mg/kg per day has been used for meningitis (maximum dose: 12 g daily)

Indication-specific dosing:

Acute bacterial rhinosinusitis, severe infection requiring hospitalization (off-label use): Children: IV: 100 to 200 mg/kg/day divided every 6 hours for 10 to 14 days (Chow 2012)

Arthritis (septic): Children ≥50 kg or Adolescents: Refer to adult dosing.

Bacterial enteric infections in HIV-infected patients (empiric treatment) (off-label use): Adolescents: IV: Refer to adult dosing.

Brain abscess: Children ≥50 kg or Adolescents: Refer to adult dosing.

Cesarean section: Children ≥50 kg or Adolescents: Refer to adult dosing.

Community-acquired pneumonia (CAP) (IDSA/PIDS 2011): Infants >3 months and Children: IV: **Note:** May consider addition of vancomycin or clindamycin to empiric therapy if community-acquired MRSA suspected. In children ≥5 years, a macrolide antibiotic should be added if atypical pneumonia cannot be ruled out.

Empiric treatment, *Haemophilus influenzae*, group A *Streptococcus*, or *S. pneumoniae* (MICs to penicillin ≤2.0 mcg/mL), patient fully immunized for *H. influenzae* type b and *S. pneumoniae*, or minimal local resistance to penicillin in invasive pneumococcal strains (alternative to ampicillin or penicillin): 50 mg/kg/dose every 8 hours

Moderate-to-severe infection, patient not fully immunized for *H. influenzae* type b and *S. pneumoniae*, or significant local resistance to penicillin in invasive pneumococcal strains (preferred): 50 mg/kg/dose every 8 hours

Moderate-to-severe infection, *H. influenzae* (beta-lactamase producing) (preferred): 50 mg/kg/dose every 8 hours

Complicated community-acquired intra-abdominal infection (in combination with metronidazole): Infants and Children: IV: 150 to 200 mg/kg/day divided every 6 to 8 hours (Solomkin 2010)

Gonorrhea (CDC 2010) (as an alternative to ceftriaxone): Children ≥45 kg and Adolescents ≥45 kg: Refer to adult dosing.

Lyme disease (as an alternative to ceftriaxone):

Cardiac or CNS manifestations: Infants and Children: IV: 150 to 200 mg/kg/day in divided doses every 6 to 8 hours for 14 to 28 days; maximum daily dose: 6 g daily (Halperin 2007; Wormser 2006)

Meningitis (in combination with vancomycin): Infants and Children: IV: 225 to 300 mg/kg/day in divided doses every 6 to 8 hours (Tunkel 2004)

Peritonitis (spontaneous): Children ≥50 kg or Adolescents: Refer to adult dosing.

Sepsis:

Infants and Children ≤12 years: IV: 150 mg/kg/day divided every 8 hours

Children ≥50 kg or Adolescents: Refer to adult dosing.

Skin and soft tissue necrotizing infections (off-label use): Infants and Children: IV: 50 mg/kg every 6 hours, in combination with metronidazole or clindamycin for empiric therapy of polymicrobial infections. Continue until further debridement is not necessary, patient has clinically improved, and patient is afebrile for 48 to 72 hours (IDSA [Stevens 2014])

Surgical (perioperative) prophylaxis (off-label use): Children ≥1 year: IV: 50 mg/kg within 60 minutes prior to surgical incision (maximum: 1000 mg per dose). Doses may be repeated in 3 hours if procedure is lengthy or if there is excessive blood loss. **Note:** preferred agent (with ampicillin) in liver transplantation (Bratzler 2013).

Typhoid fever: Infants and Children ≤12 years: IM, IV: 150 to 200 mg/kg/day in 3 to 4 divided doses (maximum: 12 g daily); fluoroquinolone resistant: 80 mg/kg/day in 3 to 4 divided doses (maximum: 12 g daily)

Renal Impairment

Manufacturer's labeling: **Note:** Renal function may be estimated using Cockcroft-Gault formula for dosage adjustment purposes.

CrCl <20 mL/minute/1.73 m²: Dose should be decreased by 50%.

Dialysis: Moderately dialyzable (20% to 50%)

Alternate recommendations:

Adults: The following dosage adjustments have been used by some clinicians (Aronoff 2007; Heintz 2009; Trotman 2005):

GFR >50 mL/minute: Administer every 6 hours (Aronoff 2007)

GFR 10 to 50 mL/minute: Administer every 6 to 12 hours (Aronoff 2007)

GFR <10 mL/minute: Administer every 24 hours **or** decrease the dose by 50% (and administer at usual intervals) (Aronoff 2007)

Intermittent hemodialysis (IHD): Administer 1 to 2 g every 24 hours (on dialysis days, administer after hemodialysis). **Note:** Dosing dependent on the assumption of 3 times/week, complete IHD sessions (Heintz 2009).

Peritoneal dialysis (PD): 1 g every 24 hours (Aronoff 2007)

Continuous renal replacement therapy (CRRT) (Heintz 2009; Trotman 2005): Drug clearance is highly dependent on the method of renal replacement, filter type, and flow rate. Appropriate dosing requires close monitoring of pharmacologic response, signs of adverse reactions due to drug accumulation, as well as drug concentrations in relation to target trough (if appropriate). The following are general recommendations only (based on dialysate flow/ultrafiltration rates of 1 to 2 L/hour and minimal residual renal function) and should not supersede clinical judgment:

CVVH: 1 to 2 g every 8 to 12 hours

CVVHD: 1 to 2 g every 8 hours

CVVHDF: 1 to 2 g every 6 to 8 hours

Children: **Note:** Glomerular filtration rate (GFR) should be estimated using an acceptable pediatric method (eg, Schwartz equation, Traub-Johnson equation, or a height/weight nomogram):

The following dosage adjustments have been used by some clinicians (Aronoff 2007):

GFR 30 to 50 mL/minute/1.73 m²: 35 to 70 mg/kg/dose every 8 to 12 hours

GFR 10 to 29 mL/minute/1.73 m²: 35 to 70 mg/kg/dose every 12 hours

GFR <10 mL/minute/1.73 m²: 35 to 70 mg/kg/dose every 24 hours

Intermittent hemodialysis (IHD): 35 to 70 mg/kg/dose every 24 hours

Peritoneal dialysis: 35 to 70 mg/kg/dose every 24 hours

Continuous renal replacement therapy (CRRT): 35 to 70 mg/kg/dose every 12 hours

Hepatic Impairment There are no dosage adjustments provided in the manufacturer's labeling.

Obesity Refer to indication-specific dosing for obesity-related information (may not be available for all indications).

Dietary Considerations Some products may contain sodium.

Administration

IM: Inject deep IM into large muscle mass. Individual doses of 2 g may be given if the dose is divided and administered in different IM sites.

IV: Can be administered IV bolus over at least 3 to 5 minutes or as an IV intermittent infusion over 15 to 30 minutes.

Monitoring Parameters Observe for signs and symptoms of anaphylaxis during first dose; CBC with differential (especially with long courses [>10 days]); renal function

Test Interactions Positive direct Coombs', false-positive urinary glucose test using cupric sulfate (Benedict's solution, Clinitest®, Fehling's solution), false-positive serum or urine creatinine with Jaffé reaction

Dosage Forms Excipient information presented when available (limited, particularly for generics); consult specific product labeling.

Solution, Intravenous:

Claforan in D5W: 1 g/50 mL (50 mL); 2 g/50 mL (50 mL)

Solution Reconstituted, Injection:

Claforan: 500 mg (1 ea); 1 g (1 ea); 2 g (1 ea); 10 g (1 ea)

Generic: 500 mg (1 ea); 1 g (1 ea); 2 g (1 ea); 10 g (1 ea)

Solution Reconstituted, Intravenous:

Claforan: 1 g (1 ea); 2 g (1 ea)

◆ Cefotaxime Sodium *see* Cefotaxime *on page 336*

◆ Cefotaxime Sodium For Injection (Can) *see* Cefotaxime *on page 336*

CefoTEtan (SEF oh tee tan)

Index Terms Cefotan; Cefotetan Disodium

Pharmacologic Category Antibiotic, Cephalosporin (Second Generation)

Use Surgical (perioperative) prophylaxis; intra-abdominal infections and other mixed infections; respiratory tract, skin and skin structure, bone and joint, urinary tract and gynecologic infections as well as septicemia; active against gram-negative enteric bacilli including *E. coli*, *Klebsiella*, and *Proteus*; less active against staphylococci and streptococci than first generation cephalosporins, but active against anaerobes including *Bacteroides fragilis*

Pregnancy Considerations Adverse events have not been observed in animal reproduction studies. Cefotetan crosses the placenta and produces therapeutic concentrations in the amniotic fluid and cord serum. Cefotetan is one of the antibiotics recommended for prophylactic use prior to cesarean delivery.

Breast-Feeding Considerations Very small amounts of cefotetan are excreted in human milk. The manufacturer recommends caution when giving cefotetan to a breast-feeding mother. Nondose-related effects could include modification of bowel flora.

Contraindications Hypersensitivity to cefotetan, any component of the formulation, or other cephalosporins; previous cephalosporin-associated hemolytic anemia

Warnings/Precautions Modify dosage in patients with severe renal impairment. Although cefotetan contains the methyltetrazolethiol side chain, bleeding has not been a significant problem. Use with caution in patients with a history of penicillin allergy, especially IgE-mediated reactions (eg, anaphylaxis, urticaria). Cefotetan has been associated with a higher risk of hemolytic anemia relative to other cephalosporins (approximately threefold); monitor carefully during use and consider cephalosporin-associated immune anemia in patients who have received cefotetan within 2-3 weeks (either as treatment or prophylaxis). Prolonged use may result in fungal or bacterial superinfection, including *C. difficile*-associated diarrhea (CDAD) and pseudomembranous colitis; CDAD has been observed >2 months postantibiotic treatment. May be associated with increased INR, especially in nutritionally-deficient patients, prolonged treatment, hepatic or renal disease.

Adverse Reactions

1% to 10%:

Gastrointestinal: Diarrhea (1%)

Hepatic: Transaminases increased (1%)

Miscellaneous: Hypersensitivity reactions (1%)

<1%: Anaphylaxis, urticaria, rash, pruritus, pseudomembranous colitis, nausea, vomiting, eosinophilia, thrombocytosis, agranulocytosis, hemolytic anemia, leukopenia, thrombocytopenia, prolonged PT, bleeding, BUN increased, creatinine increased, nephrotoxicity, phlebitis, fever

Reactions reported with other cephalosporins: Seizure, Stevens-Johnson syndrome, toxic epidermal necrolysis, renal dysfunction, toxic nephropathy, cholestasis, aplastic anemia, hemolytic anemia, hemorrhage, pancytopenia, agranulocytosis, colitis, superinfection

Drug Interactions

Metabolism/Transport Effects None known.

Avoid Concomitant Use

Avoid concomitant use of CefoTEtan with any of the following: BCG (Intravesical)

Increased Effect/Toxicity

CefoTEtan may increase the levels/effects of: Alcohol (Ethyl); Aminoglycosides; Carbocisteine; Vitamin K Antagonists

The levels/effects of CefoTEtan may be increased by: Probenecid

Decreased Effect

CefoTEtan may decrease the levels/effects of: BCG (Intravesical); BCG Vaccine (Immunization); Sodium Picosulfate; Typhoid Vaccine

Food Interactions Concurrent use with ethanol may cause a disulfiram-like reaction. Management: Monitor patients.

Storage/Stability Reconstituted solution is stable for 24 hours at room temperature and 96 hours when refrigerated. For IV infusion in NS or D₅W solution and after freezing, thawed solution is stable for 24 hours at room temperature or 96 hours when refrigerated. Frozen solution is stable for 12 weeks. Thawed solutions of the commercially available frozen cefotetan injections are stable for 48 hours at room temperature or 21 days when refrigerated.

◀ **Mechanism of Action** Inhibits bacterial cell wall synthesis by binding to one or more of the penicillin-binding proteins (PBPs) which in turn inhibits the final transpeptidation step of peptidoglycan synthesis in bacterial cell walls, thus inhibiting cell wall biosynthesis. Bacteria eventually lyse due to ongoing activity of cell wall autolytic enzymes (autolysins and murein hydrolases) while cell wall assembly is arrested.

Pharmacodynamics/Kinetics
Absorption: IM: Completely absorbed
Distribution: Widely to body tissues and fluids including bile, gallbladder, kidney, skin, tonsils, uterus, sputum, prostatic and peritoneal fluids; poor penetration into CSF
Protein binding: 76% to 90%
Half-life elimination: 3 to 4.6 hours, prolonged in patients with moderately impaired renal function (up to 10 hours)
Time to peak, serum: IM: 1.5 to 3 hours
Excretion: Primarily urine (51% to 81%, as unchanged drug); feces (20%)

Dosing
Adult & Geriatric
Susceptible infections: IM, IV: 1-6 g daily in divided doses every 12 hours; usual dose: 1-2 g every 12 hours for 5-10 days; 1-2 g may be given every 24 hours for urinary tract infection; **Note:** Due to high rates of *B. fragilis* group resistance, not recommended for the treatment of community-acquired intra-abdominal infections (Solomkin, 2010)
Orbital cellulitis, odontogenic infections: IV: 2 g every 12 hours (Bailey, 2007; Quayle, 1987)
Pelvic inflammatory disease: IV: 2 g every 12 hours; used in combination with doxycycline (CDC, 2010)
Surgical (perioperative) prophylaxis:
Manufacturer's labeling: IV: 1-2 g 30-60 minutes prior to surgery. **Note:** When used for cesarean section, dose should be given as soon as umbilical cord is clamped.
Alternative recommendations: IV: 2 g within 60 minutes prior to surgery. Doses may be repeated in 6 hours if procedure is lengthy or if there is excessive blood loss (Bratzler, 2013).
Urinary tract infection: IM, IV: 500 mg every 12 hours or 1-2 g every 12-24 hours
Pediatric
Severe infections (off-label use): IM, IV: 20-40 mg/kg/dose every 12 hours (maximum: 6 **g** daily)
Surgical (perioperative) prophylaxis (off-label use): Children ≥1 year: IV: 40 mg/kg 30-60 minutes prior to surgery (maximum 2000 mg/dose). Doses may be repeated in 6 hours if procedure is lengthy or if there is excessive blood loss (Bratzler, 2013).
Pelvic inflammatory disease: Adolescents: IV: Refer to adult dosing.
Renal Impairment IM, IV:
CrCl 10 to 30 mL/minute: Administer every 24 hours
CrCl <10 mL/minute: Administer every 48 hours
Hemodialysis: Dialyzable (5% to 20%); administer ¼ the usual dose every 24 hours on days between dialysis; administer ½ the usual dose on the day of dialysis.
Continuous arteriovenous or venovenous hemodiafiltration effects: Administer 750 mg every 12 hours
Hepatic Impairment No dosage adjustment provided in manufacturer's labeling.
Dietary Considerations Some products may contain sodium.
Administration
IM: Inject deep IM into large muscle mass.
IV: Inject direct IV over 3-5 minutes. Infuse intermittent infusion over 30 minutes.
Monitoring Parameters Monitor renal, hepatic, and hematologic function periodically with prolonged therapy. Monitor prothrombin time in patients at risk of prolongation during cephalosporin therapy (nutritionally-deficient, prolonged treatment, renal or hepatic disease). Monitor for signs and symptoms of hemolytic anemia, including hematologic parameters where appropriate.
Test Interactions Positive direct Coombs', false-positive urinary glucose test using cupric sulfate (Benedict's solution, Clinitest®, Fehling's solution), false-positive serum or urine creatinine with Jaffé reaction
Dosage Forms Excipient information presented when available (limited, particularly for generics); consult specific product labeling.
Solution Reconstituted, Injection:
Generic: 1 g (1 ea); 2 g (1 ea); 10 g (1 ea)
Solution Reconstituted, Intravenous:
Generic: 1 g (1 ea); 2 g (1 ea)

◆ Cefotetan Disodium *see* CefoTEtan *on page 339*

CefOXitin (se FOKS i tin)

Brand Names: US Mefoxin

Brand Names: Canada Cefoxitin For Injection
Index Terms Cefoxitin Sodium
Pharmacologic Category Antibiotic, Cephalosporin (Second Generation)
Use
Bone and joint infections: Treatment of bone and joint infections caused by *Staphylococcus aureus* (including penicillinase-producing strains).
Gynecological infections: Treatment of endometritis, pelvic cellulitis, and pelvic inflammatory disease caused by *Escherichia coli*, *Neisseria gonorrhoeae* (including penicillinase-producing strains), *Bacteroides* species including *Bacteroides fragilis*, *Clostridium* species, *P. niger*, *Peptostreptococcus* species, and *Streptococcus agalactiae*.
Intra-abdominal infections: Treatment of peritonitis and intra-abdominal infections or abscess, caused by *E. coli*, *Klebsiella* species, *Bacteroides* species (including *B. fragilis*), and *Clostridium* species.
Lower respiratory tract infections: Treatment of pneumonia and lung abscess, caused by *Streptococcus pneumoniae*, other streptococci (excluding enterococci; eg, *Enterococcus faecalis* [formerly *Streptococcus faecalis*]), *S. aureus* (including penicillinase-producing strains), *E. coli*, *Klebsiella* species, *Haemophilus influenzae*, and *Bacteroides* species.
Perioperative prophylaxis: Prophylaxis of infection in patients undergoing uncontaminated GI surgery, abdominal or vaginal hysterectomy, or cesarean section.
Septicemia: Treatment of septicemia caused by *S. pneumoniae*, *S. aureus* (including penicillinase-producing strains), *E. coli*, *Klebsiella* species, and *Bacteroides* species including *B. fragilis*.
Skin and skin structure infections: Treatment of skin and skin structure infections caused by *S. aureus* (including penicillinase-producing strains), *Staphylococcus epidermidis*, *Streptococcus pyogenes* and other streptococci (excluding enterococci [eg, *E. faecalis*] [formerly *S. faecalis*]), *E. coli*, *Proteus mirabilis*, *Klebsiella* species, *Bacteroides* species including *B. fragilis*, *Clostridium* species, *P. niger*, and *Peptostreptococcus* species.
Urinary tract infections: Treatment of UTIs caused by *E. coli*, *Klebsiella* species, *P. mirabilis*, *Morganella morganii*, *Proteus vulgaris*, and *Providencia* species (including *Providencia rettgeri*).

Limitations of use: Cefoxitin does not have activity against *Chlamydia trachomatis*. When cefoxitin is used to treat pelvic inflammatory disease, add appropriate antichlamydial coverage.

Pregnancy Considerations Adverse events have not been observed in animal reproduction studies. Cefoxitin crosses the placenta and reaches the cord serum and amniotic fluid.

Peak serum concentrations of cefoxitin during pregnancy may be similar to or decreased compared to nonpregnant values. Maternal half-life may be shorter at term. Pregnancy-induced hypertension increases trough concentrations in the immediate postpartum period. Cefoxitin is one of the antibiotics recommended for prophylactic use prior to cesarean delivery.

Breast-Feeding Considerations Very small amounts of cefoxitin are excreted in breast milk. The manufacturer recommends that caution be exercised when administering cefoxitin to nursing women. Nondose-related effects could include modification of bowel flora. Cefoxitin pharmacokinetics may be altered immediately postpartum.

Contraindications Hypersensitivity to cefoxitin, any component of the formulation, or other cephalosporins

Warnings/Precautions Modify dosage in patients with severe renal impairment. Prolonged use may result in superinfection. Use with caution in patients with a history of penicillin allergy, especially IgE-mediated hypersensitivity reactions (eg, anaphylaxis, urticaria). If a hypersensitivity reaction occurs, discontinue immediately. Use with caution in patients with a history of seizures or gastrointestinal disease (particularly colitis). Prolonged use may result in fungal or bacterial superinfection, including *C. difficile*-associated diarrhea (CDAD) and pseudomembranous colitis; CDAD has been observed >2 months postantibiotic treatment. For group A beta-hemolytic streptococcal infections, antimicrobial therapy should be given for at least 10 days to guard against the risk of rheumatic fever or glomerulonephritis. In pediatric patients ≥3 months of age, higher doses have been associated with an increased incidence of eosinophilia and elevated AST. Elderly patients are more likely to have decreased renal function; use care in dose selection and monitor renal function.

Adverse Reactions

1% to 10%: Gastrointestinal: Diarrhea

<1% (Limited to important or life-threatening): Anaphylaxis, angioedema, bone marrow depression, dyspnea, eosinophilia, exacerbation of myasthenia gravis, exfoliative dermatitis, fever, hemolytic anemia, hypotension, increased blood urea nitrogen, increased serum creatinine, increased serum transaminases, interstitial nephritis, jaundice, leukopenia, nausea, nephrotoxicity (increased; with aminoglycosides), phlebitis, prolonged prothrombin time, pruritus, pseudomembranous colitis, skin rash, thrombocytopenia, thrombophlebitis, toxic epidermal necrolysis, urticaria, vomiting

Drug Interactions

Metabolism/Transport Effects None known.

Avoid Concomitant Use

Avoid concomitant use of CefOXitin with any of the following: BCG (Intravesical)

Increased Effect/Toxicity

CefOXitin may increase the levels/effects of: Aminoglycosides; Vitamin K Antagonists

The levels/effects of CefOXitin may be increased by: Probenecid

Decreased Effect

CefOXitin may decrease the levels/effects of: BCG (Intravesical); BCG Vaccine (Immunization); Sodium Picosulfate; Typhoid Vaccine

Preparation for Administration Reconstitute vials with SWFI, bacteriostatic water for injection, NS, or D$_5$W. For IV infusion, solutions may be further diluted in NS, D$_5$¼NS, D$_5$½NS, D$_5$NS, D$_5$W, D$_{10}$W, LR, D$_5$LR, mannitol 5% or 10%, or sodium bicarbonate 5%.

Storage/Stability Prior to reconstitution store between 2°C and 25°C (36°F and 77°F). Avoid exposure to temperatures >50°C (122°F). Cefoxitin tends to darken depending on storage conditions; however, product potency is not adversely affected.

Reconstituted solutions of 1 g per 10 mL in sterile water for injection, bacteriostatic water for injection, sodium chloride 0.9% injection, or dextrose 5% injection are stable for 6 hours at room temperature or for 7 days under refrigeration (<5°C [43°F]).

DUPLEX container: Store unactivated container at 20°C to 25°C (68°F to 77°F); excursions permitted to 15°C to 30°C (59°F to 86°F); do not freeze. Following activation, solution is stable for 12 hours at room temperature and 7 days refrigerated.

Mechanism of Action Inhibits bacterial cell wall synthesis by binding to one or more of the penicillin-binding proteins (PBPs) which in turn inhibits the final transpeptidation step of peptidoglycan synthesis in bacterial cell walls, thus inhibiting cell wall biosynthesis. Bacteria eventually lyse due to ongoing activity of cell wall autolytic enzymes (autolysins and murein hydrolases) while cell wall assembly is arrested.

Pharmacodynamics/Kinetics

Distribution: Widely to body tissues and fluids including ascitic, pleural, synovial, bile; poorly penetrates into CSF even with inflammation of the meninges (Landesman 1981)

Protein binding: 65% to 79%

Half-life elimination: Neonates and Infants (PNA: 10-53 days): 1.4 hours (Regazzi 1983); Adults: 41-59 minutes; prolonged with renal impairment

Time to peak, serum: IM: Within 20-30 minutes

Excretion: Urine (85% as unchanged drug)

Dosing

Adult & Geriatric

Susceptible infections: IV: 1 to 2 g every 6 to 8 hours (IM injection is painful); up to 12 g daily

Bite wounds (animal) (off-label use): IV: 1 g every 6 to 8 hours (IDSA [Stevens 2014])

Gas gangrene: IV: 2 g every 4 hours or 3 g every 6 hours (maximum daily dosage: 12 g daily)

Intra-abdominal infection, complicated, community acquired, mild-to-moderate (Solomkin 2010): IV: 2 g every 6 hours for 4 to 7 days (provided source controlled)

Moderately severe or severe infections: IV: 1 g every 4 hours or 2 g every 6 to 8 hours (maximum daily dosage: 8 g daily)

Mycobacterium abscessus , not MTB or MAI (off-label use; Griffith 2007): IV: 12 g daily in divided doses with concomitant amikacin for ≥14 days

Pelvic inflammatory disease (CDC 2010):

Inpatients: IV: 2 g every 6 hours **plus** doxycycline for at least 24 hours after clinical improvement, followed by doxycycline to complete 14 days

Outpatients: IM: 2 g **plus** oral probenecid, followed by doxycycline (with or without concomitant metronidazole) for 14 days

Surgical (perioperative) prophylaxis:

Manufacturer's labeling (procedures other than Cesarian section): IV: 2 g 30 to 60 minutes prior to surgical incision, followed by 2 g every 6 hours for no more than 24 hours after surgery depending on the procedure

Cesarean section: IV: 2 g as soon as umbilical cord is clamped as a single dose **or** 2 g as soon as umbilical cord is clamped followed by 2 g at 4 and 8 hours after the initial dose.

Alternative recommendations: 2 g within 60 minutes prior to surgical incision. Doses may be repeated in 2 hours if procedure is lengthy or if there is excessive blood loss (Bratzler 2013).

Uncomplicated cutaneous, urinary tract, lung infections: IV: 1 g every 6–8 hours (maximum daily dosage: 4 g daily)

Pediatric Note: For group A beta-hemolytic streptococcal infections, antimicrobial therapy should be given for at least 10 days to guard against the risk of rheumatic fever or glomerulonephritis

Infants >3 months, Children, and Adolescents:

Manufacturer's labeling: IV: 80 to 160 mg/kg/day divided every 4 to 6 hours (maximum daily dose: 12 **g daily**)

Alternative recommendations (Red Book [AAP] 2012):

Mild-to-moderate infection: IV: Infants >3 months and Children: 80 mg/kg/day in divided doses every 6 to 8 hours (maximum daily dose: 4000 mg daily)

Severe infection: IV: Infants >3 months and Children: 160 mg/kg/day in divided doses every 4 to 6 hours (maximum daily dose: 12 **g daily**)

Infants >3 months and Children:

Surgical (perioperative) prophylaxis:

Manufacturer's labeling: IV: 30 to 40 mg/kg 30 to 60 minutes prior to surgical incision followed by 30 to 40 mg/kg/dose every 6 hours for no more than 24 hours after surgery depending on the procedure

Alternative recommendations: Children ≥1 year: IV: 40 mg/kg within 60 minutes prior to surgical incision (maximum: 2000 mg per dose). Doses may be repeated in 2 hours if procedure is lengthy or if there is excessive blood loss (Bratzler 2013).

Adolescents:

Surgical (perioperative) prophylaxis: Refer to adult dosing.

Renal Impairment IV:

CrCl 30 to 50 mL/minute: 1 to 2 g every 8 to 12 hours

CrCl 10 to 29 mL/minute: 1 to 2 g every 12 to 24 hours

CrCl 5 to 9 mL/minute: 0.5 to 1 g every 12 to 24 hours

CrCl <5 mL/minute: 0.5 to 1 g every 24 to 48 hours

Hemodialysis: Loading dose: 1 to 2 g after each hemodialysis; maintenance dose as noted above based on creatinine clearance

Hepatic Impairment There are no dosage adjustments provided in manufacturer's labeling.

Dietary Considerations Some products may contain sodium.

Administration

IM: Inject deep IM into large muscle mass. **Note:** IM injection is painful and this route of administration is not described in the prescribing information.

IV: Can be administered IVP over 3 to 5 minutes or by IV intermittent infusion over 10 to 60 minutes

Monitoring Parameters Monitor renal function periodically when used in combination with other nephrotoxic drugs; prothrombin time. Observe for signs and symptoms of anaphylaxis during first dose.

Test Interactions Positive direct Coombs', false-positive urinary glucose test using cupric sulfate (Benedict's solution, Clinitest®, Fehling's solution), false-positive serum or urine creatinine with Jaffé reaction

Dosage Forms Excipient information presented when available (limited, particularly for generics); consult specific product labeling.

Solution, Intravenous:

Mefoxin: 1 g (50 mL); 2 g (50 mL)

Solution Reconstituted, Injection:

Generic: 10 g (1 ea)

Solution Reconstituted, Injection [preservative free]:

Generic: 10 g (1 ea)

Solution Reconstituted, Intravenous:

Generic: 1 g (1 ea); 2 g (1 ea)

Solution Reconstituted, Intravenous [preservative free]:

Generic: 1 g (1 ea); 2 g (1 ea)

◆ Cefoxitin For Injection (Can) see CefOXitin on page 340

◆ Cefoxitin Sodium see CefOXitin on page 340

Cefpodoxime (sef pode OKS eem)

Index Terms Cefpodoxime Proxetil; Vantin
Pharmacologic Category Antibiotic, Cephalosporin (Third Generation)
Use
Chronic bronchitis, acute bacterial exacerbation: Treatment of acute bacterial exacerbation of chronic bronchitis caused by *Streptococcus pneumoniae*, *Haemophilus influenzae* (non-beta-lactamase-producing strains only), or *Moraxella catarrhalis*.
Gonorrhea:
Acute, uncomplicated anorectal infections in women: Treatment of acute, uncomplicated anorectal infections in women due to *N. gonorrhoeae* (including penicillinase-producing strains). **Note:** Due to issues of resistance, cefpodoxime is no longer recommended for the treatment of acute, uncomplicated anorectal infections in women.
Acute, uncomplicated urethral and cervical: Treatment of acute, uncomplicated urethral and cervical gonorrhea caused by *Neisseria gonorrhoeae* (including penicillinase-producing strains). **Note:** Due to issues of resistance, cefpodoxime is no longer recommended for the treatment of acute, uncomplicated urethral and cervical gonorrhea.
Otitis media, acute: Treatment of acute otitis media caused by *S. pneumoniae*, (excluding penicillin-resistant strains), *Streptococcus pyogenes*, *H. influenzae* (including beta-lactamase-producing strains), or *M. catarrhalis* (including beta-lactamase producing strains).
Pharyngitis or tonsillitis: Treatment of pharyngitis or tonsillitis caused by *S. pyogenes*.
Pneumonia, community-acquired: Treatment of community-acquired pneumonia caused by *S. pneumoniae* or *H. influenzae* (including beta-lactamase-producing strains).
Sinusitis, acute maxillary: Treatment of acute maxillary sinusitis caused by *H. influenzae* (including beta-lactamase producing strains), *S. pneumoniae*, and *M. catarrhalis*. **Note:** According to the Infectious Diseases Society of America (IDSA) guidelines for acute bacterial rhinosinusitis, cefpodoxime is no longer recommended as monotherapy for initial empiric treatment.
Skin and skin structure infections, uncomplicated: Treatment of uncomplicated skin and skin structure infections caused by *S. aureus* (including penicillinase-producing strains) or *S. pyogenes*.
Urinary tract infections (cystitis), uncomplicated: Treatment of cystitis caused by *Escherichia coli*, *Klebsiella pneumoniae*, *Proteus mirabilis*, or *Staphylococcus saprophyticus*.
Pregnancy Considerations Teratogenic events were not observed in animal reproduction studies. An increase in most types of birth defects was not found following first trimester exposure to cephalosporins.
Breast-Feeding Considerations Cefpodoxime is excreted in breast milk. The manufacturer recommends discontinuing nursing or discontinuing the medication in breast-feeding women. Nondose-related effects could include modification of bowel flora.
Contraindications Hypersensitivity to cefpodoxime, any component of the formulation, or other cephalosporins
Warnings/Precautions Modify dosage in patients with severe renal impairment. Prolonged use may result in fungal or bacterial superinfection, including *C. difficile*-associated diarrhea (CDAD) and pseudomembranous colitis; CDAD has been observed >2 months postantibiotic treatment. Use with caution in patients with a history of beta-lactam allergy, especially IgE-mediated reactions (eg, anaphylaxis, urticaria).

Potentially significant drug-drug interactions may exist, requiring dose or frequency adjustment, additional monitoring, and/or selection of alternative therapy.

Benzyl alcohol and derivatives: Some dosage forms may contain sodium benzoate/benzoic acid; benzoic acid (benzoate) is a metabolite of benzyl alcohol; large amounts of benzyl alcohol (≥99 mg/kg/day) have been associated with a potentially fatal toxicity ("gasping syndrome") in neonates; the "gasping syndrome" consists of metabolic acidosis, respiratory distress, gasping respirations, CNS dysfunction (including convulsions, intracranial hemorrhage), hypotension, and cardiovascular collapse (AAP ["Inactive" 1997]; CDC 1982); some data suggests that benzoate displaces bilirubin from protein binding sites (Ahlfors 2001); avoid or use dosage forms containing benzyl alcohol derivative with caution in neonates. See manufacturer's labeling.

Adverse Reactions
>10%:
Dermatologic: Diaper rash (12%)
Gastrointestinal: Diarrhea (infants and toddlers 15%)
1% to 10%:
Central nervous system: Headache (1%)
Dermatologic: Skin rash (1%)
Gastrointestinal: Diarrhea (7%), nausea (4%), abdominal pain (2%), vomiting (1% to 2%)
Genitourinary: Vaginal infection (3%)
<1% (Limited to important or life-threatening): Anaphylaxis, anxiety, chest pain, cough, decreased appetite, dizziness, dysgeusia, epistaxis, eye pruritus, fatigue, fever, flatulence, flushing, fungal skin infection, hypotension, insomnia, malaise, nightmares, pruritus, pseudomembranous colitis, purpuric nephritis, tinnitus, vulvovaginal candidiasis, weakness, xerostomia
Drug Interactions
Metabolism/Transport Effects None known.
Avoid Concomitant Use
Avoid concomitant use of Cefpodoxime with any of the following: BCG (Intravesical)
Increased Effect/Toxicity
Cefpodoxime may increase the levels/effects of: Aminoglycosides; Vitamin K Antagonists

The levels/effects of Cefpodoxime may be increased by: Probenecid
Decreased Effect
Cefpodoxime may decrease the levels/effects of: BCG (Intravesical); BCG Vaccine (Immunization); Sodium Picosulfate; Typhoid Vaccine

The levels/effects of Cefpodoxime may be decreased by: Antacids; H2-Antagonists
Food Interactions Food increases extent of absorption and peak concentration of tablets. Management: Take tablets with food.
Preparation for Administration Suspension: Refer to manufacturer's product labeling for reconstitution instructions.
Storage/Stability
Suspension: Store at 20°C to 25°C (68°F to 77°F); after reconstitution, suspension may be stored in refrigerator for 14 days.
Tablet: Store at 20°C to 25°C (68°F to 77°F); protect from light.
Mechanism of Action Inhibits bacterial cell wall synthesis by binding to one or more of the penicillin-binding proteins (PBPs) which in turn inhibits the final transpeptidation step of peptidoglycan synthesis in bacterial cell walls, thus inhibiting cell wall biosynthesis. Bacteria eventually lyse due to ongoing activity of cell wall autolytic enzymes (autolysins and murein hydrolases) while cell wall assembly is arrested.
Pharmacodynamics/Kinetics
Absorption: Rapid and well absorbed (50%); tablet AUC increased 21% to 33% with food
Distribution: Good tissue penetration, including lung and tonsils; penetrates into pleural fluid
Protein binding: Serum: 22% to 33%; Plasma: 21% to 29%
Metabolism: De-esterified in GI tract to active metabolite, cefpodoxime
Bioavailability: Oral: 50%
Half-life elimination: ~2 to 3 hours; prolonged with renal impairment (~10 hours for CrCl <30 mL/minute)
Time to peak: Tablets: Within 2 to 3 hours; Oral suspension: Slower in presence of food, 48% increase in Tmax
Excretion: Urine (~29% to 33% as unchanged drug) in 12 hours
Dosing
Adult & Geriatric
Bronchitis (chronic), bacterial exacerbation: Oral: 200 mg every 12 hours for 10 days
Pharyngitis/tonsillitis: Oral: 100 mg every 12 hours for 5 to 10 days
Pneumonia, acute community acquired: Oral: 200 mg every 12 hours for 14 days
Rhinosinusitis, acute maxillary: Oral: 200 mg every 12 hours for 10 days
Skin and skin structure: Oral: 400 mg every 12 hours for 7 to 14 days
Urinary tract infection, uncomplicated: Oral: 100 mg every 12 hours for 7 days
Pediatric
Usual dosage range:
Infants ≥2 months and Children <12 years: Oral: 10 mg/kg/day divided every 12 hours (maximum: 200 mg/dose).
Children ≥12 years and Adolescents: Oral: 100 to 400 mg every 12 hours.

Indication-specific dosing:

Bronchitis (chronic), bacterial exacerbation: Children ≥12 years and Adolescents: Oral: Refer to adult dosing.

Otitis media, acute: Infants ≥2 months and Children <12 years: Oral: 5 mg/kg/dose (maximum: 200 mg/dose) every 12 hours for 5 days. **Note:** AAP guidelines recommend duration based on patient age: If <2 years of age or severe symptoms (any age): 10-day course; if 2 to 5 years of age with mild to moderate symptoms: 7-day course; if ≥6 years of age with mild to moderate symptoms: 5- to 7-day course (AAP [Lieberthal 2013]).

Pharyngitis/tonsillitis:
Infants ≥2 months and Children <12 years: Oral: 5mg/kg/dose every 12 hours (maximum: 100 mg/dose) for 5 to 10 days.
Children ≥12 years and Adolescents: Oral: Refer to adult dosing.

Pneumonia, acute community acquired: Children ≥12 years and Adolescents: Oral: Refer to adult dosing.

Rhinosinusitis, acute maxillary:
Infants ≥2 months and Children <12 years: Oral: 5 mg/kg/dose (maximum: 200 mg/dose) every 12 hours for 10 days. **Note:** IDSA recommends use in combination with clindamycin for 10 to 14 days in patients with non-type 1 penicillin allergy, after failure of initial therapy or in patients at risk for antibiotic resistance (eg, daycare attendance, age <2 years, recent hospitalization, antibiotic use within the past month) (Chow 2012).
Children ≥12 years and Adolescents: Oral: Refer to adult dosing.

Skin and skin structure: Children ≥12 years and Adolescents: Oral: Refer to adult dosing.

Urinary tract infection, uncomplicated: Children ≥12 years and Adolescents: Oral: Refer to adult dosing.

Renal Impairment
CrCl ≥30 mL/minute: No dosage adjustment necessary.
CrCl <30 mL/minute: Administer every 24 hours.
Hemodialysis: Dose 3 times/week following dialysis.

Hepatic Impairment Cirrhosis (with or without ascites): No dosage adjustment necessary.

Dietary Considerations Take tablets with food.

Administration Oral: Administer around-the-clock to promote less variation in peak and trough serum levels. Administer tablets with food; suspension may be administered without regard to food. Shake suspension well before using.

Monitoring Parameters Monitor renal function. Observe for signs and symptoms of anaphylaxis during first dose.

Test Interactions Positive direct Coombs', false-positive urinary glucose test using cupric sulfate (Benedict's solution, Clinitest®, Fehling's solution), false-positive serum or urine creatinine with Jaffé reaction

Dosage Forms Excipient information presented when available (limited, particularly for generics); consult specific product labeling.

Suspension Reconstituted, Oral:
Generic: 50 mg/5 mL (50 mL, 100 mL); 100 mg/5 mL (50 mL, 100 mL)
Tablet, Oral:
Generic: 100 mg, 200 mg

◆ **Cefpodoxime Proxetil** *see* Cefpodoxime *on page 342*

Cefprozil (sef PROE zil)

Brand Names: Canada Apo-Cefprozil; Auro-Cefprozil; Ava-Cefprozil; Cefzil; RAN-Cefprozil; Sandoz-Cefprozil
Index Terms Cefzil
Pharmacologic Category Antibiotic, Cephalosporin (Second Generation)
Use

Pharyngitis/tonsillitis: Treatment of mild to moderate pharyngitis/tonsillitis caused by *Streptococcus pyogenes*. Limitations of use: Cefprozil is generally effective in the eradication of *S. pyogenes* from the nasopharynx; however, substantial data establishing the efficacy of cefprozil in the subsequent prevention of rheumatic fever are not available at present.

Otitis media: Treatment of mild to moderate infection caused by *S. pneumoniae, Haemophilus influenzae* (including beta-lactamase-producing strains), and *Moraxella (Branhamella) catarrhalis* (including beta-lactamase-producing strains).

Secondary bacterial infection of acute bronchitis and acute bacterial exacerbation of chronic bronchitis: Treatment of secondary bacterial infections in acute bronchitis and acute bacterial exacerbations of chronic bronchitis caused by *S. pneumoniae, H. influenzae*

(including beta-lactamase-producing strains), and *M. catarrhalis* (including beta-lactamase-producing strains).

Skin and skin-structure infections, uncomplicated: Treatment of uncomplicated skin and skin-structure infections caused by *Staphylococcus aureus* (including penicillinase-producing strains) and *S. pyogenes*.

Pregnancy Considerations Adverse events were not observed in animal reproduction studies.

Breast-Feeding Considerations Small amounts of cefprozil are excreted in breast milk. The manufacturer recommends that caution be exercised when administering cefprozil to nursing women. Nondose-related effects could include modification of bowel flora.

Contraindications Hypersensitivity to cefprozil, any component of the formulation, or other cephalosporins

Warnings/Precautions Modify dosage in patients with severe renal impairment. Hypersensitivity reactions have been reported; if hypersensitivity, occurs, discontinue and institute emergency supportive measures, including airway management and treatment (eg, epinephrine, antihistamines and/or corticosteroids). Use with caution in patients with a history of penicillin allergy. Use with caution in patients with a history of gastrointestinal disease, particularly colitis. Prolonged use may result in fungal or bacterial superinfection, including *C. difficile*-associated diarrhea (CDAD) and pseudomembranous colitis; CDAD has been observed >2 months postantibiotic treatment. Potentially significant interactions may exist, requiring dose or frequency adjustment, additional monitoring, and/or selection of alternative therapy. Some products may contain phenylalanine.

Benzyl alcohol and derivatives: Some dosage forms may contain sodium benzoate/benzoic acid; benzoic acid (benzoate) is a metabolite of benzyl alcohol; large amounts of benzyl alcohol (≥99 mg/kg/day) have been associated with a potentially fatal toxicity ("gasping syndrome") in neonates; the "gasping syndrome" consists of metabolic acidosis, respiratory distress, gasping respirations, CNS dysfunction (including convulsions, intracranial hemorrhage), hypotension, and cardiovascular collapse (AAP ["Inactive" 1997]; CDC, 1982). Some data suggest that benzoate displaces bilirubin from protein-binding sites (Ahlfors, 2001); avoid or use dosage forms containing benzyl alcohol derivative with caution in neonates. See manufacturer's labeling.

Some dosage forms may contain polysorbate 80 (also known as Tweens). Hypersensitivity reactions, usually a delayed reaction, have been reported following exposure to pharmaceutical products containing polysorbate 80 in certain individuals (Isaksson, 2002; Lucente 2000; Shelley, 1995). Thrombocytopenia, ascites, pulmonary deterioration, and renal and hepatic failure have been reported in premature neonates after receiving parenteral products containing polysorbate 80 (Alade, 1986; CDC, 1984). See manufacturer's labeling.

Adverse Reactions
1% to 10%:
Central nervous system: Dizziness (1%)
Dermatologic: Diaper rash (1.5%)
Gastrointestinal: Diarrhea (2.9%), nausea (3.5%), vomiting (1%), abdominal pain (1%)
Genitourinary: Vaginitis, genital pruritus (1.6%)
Hepatic: Transaminases increased (2%)
Miscellaneous: Superinfection
<1% (Limited to important or life-threatening): Anaphylaxis, angioedema, arthralgia, BUN increased, cholestatic jaundice, confusion, creatinine increased, eosinophilia, erythema multiforme, fever, headache, hyperactivity, insomnia, leukopenia, pseudomembranous colitis, rash, serum sickness, somnolence, Stevens-Johnson syndrome, thrombocytopenia, urticaria
Reactions reported with other cephalosporins: Agranulocytosis, aplastic anemia, colitis, hemolytic anemia, hemorrhage, interstitial nephritis, pancytopenia, renal dysfunction, seizure, superinfection, toxic epidermal necrolysis, toxic nephropathy, vaginitis

Drug Interactions
Metabolism/Transport Effects None known.
Avoid Concomitant Use
Avoid concomitant use of Cefprozil with any of the following: BCG (Intravesical)
Increased Effect/Toxicity
Cefprozil may increase the levels/effects of: Aminoglycosides; Vitamin K Antagonists

The levels/effects of Cefprozil may be increased by: Probenecid
Decreased Effect
Cefprozil may decrease the levels/effects of: BCG (Intravesical); BCG Vaccine (Immunization); Sodium Picosulfate; Typhoid Vaccine

◄ **Food Interactions** Food delays cefprozil absorption. Management: May administer with food.

Preparation for Administration Oral suspension: Refer to manufacturer's product labeling for reconstitution instructions. Shake well.

Storage/Stability Store at 20°C to 25°C (68°F to 77°F); excursions permitted to 15°C to 30°C (59°F to 86°F). Refrigerate suspension after reconstitution; discard after 14 days.

Mechanism of Action Inhibits bacterial cell wall synthesis by binding to one or more of the penicillin-binding proteins (PBPs) which in turn inhibits the final transpeptidation step of peptidoglycan synthesis in bacterial cell walls, thus inhibiting cell wall biosynthesis. Bacteria eventually lyse due to ongoing activity of cell wall autolytic enzymes (autolysins and murein hydrolases) while cell wall assembly is arrested.

Pharmacodynamics/Kinetics
Absorption: Well absorbed (95%)
Distribution: V_d: 0.23 L/kg
Protein binding: ~36%
Bioavailability: 95%
Half-life elimination:
Infants and Children (6 months to 12 years): 1.5 hours
Adults:
Normal hepatic and renal function: 1.3 hours
Renal impairment: 5.2 hours
Renal failure: 5.9 hours
Hepatic impairment: 2 hours
Time to peak, serum: Fasting: 1.5 hours
Excretion: Urine (~60% as unchanged drug)

Dosing
Adult & Geriatric
Pharyngitis/tonsillitis: Oral: 500 mg every 24 hours for 10 days (administer for ≥10 days if due to *S. pyogenes*)
Secondary bacterial infection of acute bronchitis or acute bacterial exacerbation of chronic bronchitis: Oral: 500 mg every 12 hours for 10 days
Skin and skin-structure infections, uncomplicated: Oral: 250 to 500 mg every 12 hours, or 500 mg every 24 hours for 10 days

Pediatric
Otitis media: Oral: Infants ≥6 months and Children: 15 mg/kg/dose every 12 hours for 10 days (maximum: 500 mg/dose)
Pharyngitis/tonsillitis:
Children 2 to 12 years: Oral: 7.5 mg/kg/dose every 12 hours for 10 days (administer for ≥10 days if due to *S. pyogenes*) (maximum: 500 mg/day)
Children >12 years and Adolescents: Refer to adult dosing.
Secondary bacterial infection of acute bronchitis or acute bacterial exacerbation of chronic bronchitis: Children >12 years and Adolescents: Refer to adult dosing.
Skin and skin-structure infections, uncomplicated:
Children 2 to 12 years: Oral: 20 mg/kg/day once every 24 hours for 10 days (maximum: 1,000 mg/day)
Children >12 years and Adolescents: Refer to adult dosing.
Urinary tract infection (off-label use): Infants and Children 2 to 24 months: Oral: 15 mg/kg/dose twice daily for 7 to 14 days (AAP, 2011)

Renal Impairment
Manufacturer's labeling: Infants, Children, Adolescents, and Adults: Oral:
CrCl ≥30 mL/minute: No dosage adjustment necessary.
CrCl <30 mL/minute: Reduce dose by 50%.
End-stage renal disease (ESRD) on hemodialysis: Give dose after dialysis on dialysis days.
Alternative recommendations (Aronoff, 2007):
Adults: Oral:
CrCl >50 mL/minute: No dosage adjustment necessary
CrCl <50 mL/minute: Administer 50% of usual dose every 12 hours
Intermittent hemodialysis (IHD): Supplement with 250 mg after dialysis on dialysis days
Peritoneal dialysis: Administer 50% of usual dose every 12 hours
Infants, Children, and Adolescents: Oral:
Recommendations based on 30 mg/kg/day divided every 12 hours in patients with normal renal function:
GFR ≥30 mL/minute/1.73 m^2: No dosage adjustment necessary.
GFR <29 mL/minute/1.73 m^2: 7.5 mg/kg/dose every 12 hours
ESRD on hemodialysis: 7.5 mg/kg/dose every 12 hours; supplement with 5 mg/kg/dose after dialysis on dialysis days
Peritoneal dialysis: 7.5 mg/kg/dose every 12 hours

Hepatic Impairment No dosage adjustment necessary.

Dietary Considerations Oral suspension may contain phenylalanine; consult product labeling.

Administration Oral: Administer without regard to meals. Administer around the clock to promote less variation in peak and trough serum levels.

Monitoring Parameters Monitor renal function at baseline and as clinically indicated. Monitor for signs of anaphylaxis during first dose.

Test Interactions Positive direct Coombs, false-positive urinary glucose test using cupric sulfate (Benedict's solution, Clinitest, Fehling's solution), but not with enzyme-based tests for glycosuria (eg, Clinistix). A false-negative reaction may occur in the ferricyanide test for blood glucose.

Dosage Forms Excipient information presented when available (limited, particularly for generics); consult specific product labeling.
Suspension Reconstituted, Oral:
Generic: 125 mg/5 mL (50 mL, 75 mL, 100 mL); 250 mg/5 mL (50 mL, 75 mL, 100 mL)
Tablet, Oral:
Generic: 250 mg, 500 mg

Ceftaroline Fosamil (sef TAR oh leen FOS a mil)

Brand Names: US Teflaro
Index Terms PPI-0903; PPI-0903M; T-91825; TAK-599
Pharmacologic Category Antibiotic, Cephalosporin (Fifth Generation)
Use
Acute bacterial skin and skin structure infections: Treatment of acute bacterial skin and skin structure infections caused by susceptible isolates of the following gram-positive and gram-negative microorganisms: *Staphylococcus aureus* (including methicillin-susceptible and methicillin-resistant isolates), *Streptococcus pyogenes*, *Streptococcus agalactiae*, *Escherichia coli*, *Klebsiella pneumoniae*, and *Klebsiella oxytoca*.
Community-acquired bacterial pneumonia: Treatment of community-acquired bacterial pneumonia caused by susceptible isolates of the following gram-positive and gram-negative microorganisms: *Streptococcus pneumoniae* (including cases with concurrent bacteremia), *S. aureus* (methicillin-susceptible isolates only), *Haemophilus influenzae*, *K. pneumoniae*, *K. oxytoca*, and *E. coli*.

Pregnancy Considerations Adverse events have been observed in some animal reproduction studies.

Breast-Feeding Considerations It is not known if ceftaroline fosamil is excreted in breast milk. The manufacturer recommends that caution be exercised when administering ceftaroline fosamil to nursing women.

Contraindications Known serious hypersensitivity to ceftaroline, other members of the cephalosporin class, or any component of the formulation

Warnings/Precautions Serious hypersensitivity (anaphylactic) and skin reactions have occurred with ceftaroline. Use with caution in patients with a history of penicillin, cephalosporin, or carbapenem allergy, especially IgE-mediated reactions (eg, anaphylaxis, angioedema, urticaria). Maintain clinical supervision if given to penicillin or beta-lactam allergic patients. Seroconversion from a negative to a positive direct Coombs' test has been reported. Hemolytic anemia was not reported in clinical studies; however, if anemia develops during or after treatment, diagnostic tests should include a direct Coombs' test. If drug-induced hemolytic anemia is considered, discontinue the drug and institute supportive care as clinically indicated. Prolonged use may result in fungal or bacterial superinfection, including *C. difficile*-associated diarrhea (CDAD) and pseudomembranous colitis (including fatalities); CDAD has been observed >2 months postantibiotic treatment. Use with caution in patients with renal impairment (CrCl ≤50 mL/minute); dosage adjustments recommended. Use with caution in the elderly; dosage adjustment should be based on renal function. Potentially significant drug-drug interactions may exist, requiring dose or frequency adjustment, additional monitoring, and/or selection of alternative therapy.

Adverse Reactions
>10%: Hematologic & oncologic: Positive direct Coombs' test (10% to 11%; without hemolysis)
1% to 10%:
Cardiovascular: Phlebitis (2%), bradycardia (<2%), palpitations (<2%)
Central nervous system: Headache (3% to 5% [Steed 2010]), insomnia (3% to 4% [Steed 2010]), convulsions (<2%), dizziness (<2%)
Dermatologic: Pruritus (3% to 4% [Steed 2010]), skin rash (3%), urticaria (<2%)
Endocrine & metabolic: Hypokalemia (2%), hyperglycemia (<2%), hyperkalemia (<2%)

Gastrointestinal: Diarrhea (5%), nausea (4%), constipation (2%), vomiting (2%), abdominal pain (<2%), *Clostridium difficile* associated diarrhea (<2%)

Hematologic & oncologic: Anemia (<2%), eosinophilia (<2%), neutropenia (<2%), thrombocytopenia (<2%)

Hepatic: Increased serum transaminases (2%), hepatitis (<2%)

Hypersensitivity: Anaphylaxis (<2%), hypersensitivity (<2%)

Renal: Renal failure (<2%)

Miscellaneous: Fever (<2%)

<1% (Limited to important or life-threatening): Agranulocytosis

Drug Interactions

Metabolism/Transport Effects None known.

Avoid Concomitant Use

Avoid concomitant use of Ceftaroline Fosamil with any of the following: BCG (Intravesical)

Increased Effect/Toxicity

Ceftaroline Fosamil may increase the levels/effects of: Vitamin K Antagonists

The levels/effects of Ceftaroline Fosamil may be increased by: Probenecid

Decreased Effect

Ceftaroline Fosamil may decrease the levels/effects of: BCG (Intravesical); BCG Vaccine (Immunization); Sodium Picosulfate; Typhoid Vaccine

Preparation for Administration Reconstitute 400 mg or 600 mg vial with 20 mL SWFI, NS, D$_5$W, or LR. Mix gently to reconstitute (<2 minutes). Reconstituted solution should be further diluted for IV administration in 50 to 250 mL of a compatible solution. Prior to dilution for use in a 50 mL bag, withdraw 20 mL of diluent from IV bag; inject the entire contents of the ceftaroline vial (also 20 mL) to achieve a total volume of 50 mL. Use the same solution as used for reconstitution (**Note:** If SWFI was used for reconstitution, then appropriate infusion solutions include NS, $^{1}/_{2}$NS, D$_5$W, D$_{2.5}$W, or LR). Color of infusion solutions ranges from clear and light to dark yellow depending on concentration and storage conditions; potency is not affected.

Storage/Stability Store unused vials at 25°C (77°F); excursions permitted between 15°C and 30°C (59°F and 86°F). Diluted solutions (in infusion bags or Mini-Bag Plus) should be used within 6 hours when stored at room temperature or within 24 hours if refrigerated at 2°C to 8°C (36°F to 46°F).

Mechanism of Action Inhibits bacterial cell wall synthesis by binding to penicillin-binding proteins (PBPs) 1 through 3. This action blocks the final transpeptidation step of peptidoglycan synthesis in bacterial cell walls and inhibits cell wall biosynthesis. Bacteria eventually lyse due to ongoing activity of cell wall autolytic enzymes (autolysis and murein hydrolases) while cell wall assembly is arrested. Ceftaroline has a strong affinity for PBP2a, a modified PBP in MRSA, and PBP2x in *S. pneumoniae*, contributing to its spectrum of activity against these bacteria.

Pharmacodynamics/Kinetics

Distribution: V$_d$: 18.3 to 21.6 L

Protein binding: ~20%

Metabolism: Ceftaroline fosamil (inactive prodrug) undergoes rapid conversion to bioactive ceftaroline in plasma by phosphatase enzyme; ceftaroline is hydrolyzed to form inactive ceftaroline M-1 metabolite

Half-life elimination: ~1.6 hours (single dose); ~2.7 hours (multiple dose)

Time to peak: ~1 hour

Excretion: Urine (~88%); feces (~6%)

Dosing

Adult & Geriatric

Usual dosage range: IV: 600 mg every 12 hours

Indication-specific dosage: IV:

Pneumonia, community-acquired: 600 mg every 12 hours for 5 to 7 days

Skin and skin structure, complicated: 600 mg every 12 hours for 5 to 14 days

Renal Impairment Note: Renal function may be estimated using the Cockcroft-Gault formula for dosage adjustment purposes.

CrCl >50 mL/minute: No dosage adjustment necessary.

CrCl >30 to ≤50 mL/minute: 400 mg every 12 hours

CrCl ≥15 to ≤30 mL/minute: 300 mg every 12 hours

CrCl <15 mL/minute: 200 mg every 12 hours

ESRD patients receiving hemodialysis: 200 mg every 12 hours; dose should be given after hemodialysis on dialysis days

Hepatic Impairment No dosage adjustment provided in manufacturer's labeling (has not been studied). However, ceftaroline is primarily renally eliminated.

Administration Administer by slow IV infusion over 5 to 60 minutes.

Monitoring Parameters Obtain specimen for culture and susceptibility prior to the first dose. Monitor for signs of anaphylaxis during first dose. Monitor renal function.

Additional Information Considered to be ineffective against *Pseudomonas aeruginosa*, *Enterococcus* species (including vancomycin-susceptible and -resistant isolates), extended-spectrum beta-lactamase (ESBL) producing or AmpC overexpressing Enterobacteriaceae.

Dosage Forms Excipient information presented when available (limited, particularly for generics); consult specific product labeling.

Solution Reconstituted, Intravenous:

Teflaro: 400 mg (1 ea); 600 mg (1 ea)

CefTAZidime (SEF tay zi deem)

Brand Names: US Fortaz; Fortaz in D5W; Tazicef

Brand Names: Canada Ceftazidime For Injection; Fortaz

Index Terms Tazidime

Pharmacologic Category Antibiotic, Cephalosporin (Third Generation)

Use

Bacterial septicemia: Treatment of septicemia caused by *Pseudomonas aeruginosa*, *Klebsiella* spp., *Haemophilus influenzae*, *Escherichia coli*, *Serratia* spp., *Streptococcus pneumoniae*, and *Staphylococcus aureus* (methicillin-susceptible strains).

Bone and joint infections: Treatment of bone and joint infections caused by *Pseudomonas aeruginosa*, *Klebsiella* spp., *Enterobacter* spp., and *Staphylococcus aureus* (methicillin-susceptible strains).

CNS infections: Treatment of meningitis caused by *Haemophilus influenzae* and *Neisseria meningitidis*. Ceftazidime has also been used successfully in cases of meningitis due to *Pseudomonas aeruginosa* and *Streptococcus pneumoniae*.

Empiric therapy in the immunocompromised patient: Empiric treatment of infections in immunocompromised patients.

Gynecologic infections: Treatment of endometritis, pelvic cellulitis, and other infections of the female genital tract caused by *Escherichia coli*.

Intra-abdominal infections: Treatment of peritonitis caused by *Escherichia coli*, *Klebsiella* spp., and *Staphylococcus aureus* (methicillin-susceptible strains) and polymicrobial intra-abdominal infections caused by aerobic and anaerobic organisms and some *Bacteroides* spp. (many strains of *Bacteroides fragilis* are resistant).

Lower respiratory tract infections: Treatment of lower respiratory tract infections, including pneumonia, caused by *Pseudomonas aeruginosa* and other *Pseudomonas* spp.; *Haemophilus influenzae*, including ampicillin-resistant strains; *Klebsiella* spp.; *Enterobacter* spp.; *Proteus mirabilis*; *Escherichia coli*; *Serratia* spp.; *Citrobacter* spp.; *Streptococcus pneumoniae*; and *Staphylococcus aureus* (methicillin-susceptible strains).

Skin and skin-structure infections: Treatment of skin and skin-structure infections caused by *Pseudomonas aeruginosa*; *Klebsiella* spp.; *Escherichia coli*; *Proteus* spp.; including *Proteus mirabilis* and indole-positive *Proteus*; *Enterobacter* spp.; *Serratia* spp.; *Staphylococcus aureus* (methicillin-susceptible strains); and *Streptococcus pyogenes* (group A beta-hemolytic streptococci).

Urinary tract infections (UTI): Treatment of complicated and uncomplicated UTIs caused by *Pseudomonas aeruginosa*; *Enterobacter* spp.; *Proteus* spp., including *Proteus mirabilis* and indole-positive *Proteus*; *Klebsiella* spp.; and *Escherichia coli*.

Pregnancy Considerations Adverse events have not been observed in animal reproduction studies. Ceftazidime crosses the placenta and reaches the cord serum and amniotic fluid. An increase in most types of birth defects was not found following first trimester exposure to cephalosporins. Maternal peak serum concentration is unchanged in the first trimester. After the first trimester, serum concentrations decrease by approximately 50% of those in nonpregnant patients. Renal clearance is increased during pregnancy.

Breast-Feeding Considerations Very small amounts of ceftazidime are excreted in breast milk. The manufacturer recommends that caution be exercised when administering ceftazidime to nursing women. Ceftazidime in not absorbed when given orally; therefore, any medication that is distributed to human milk should not result in systemic concentrations in the nursing infant. Nondose-related effects could include modification of bowel flora.

Contraindications Clinically significant hypersensitivity to ceftazidime, other cephalosporins, penicillins, other beta-lactam antibiotics, or any component of the formulation

◄ **Warnings/Precautions** Modify dosage in patients with severe renal impairment. Use with caution in patients with a history of penicillin allergy, especially IgE-mediated reactions (eg, anaphylaxis, urticaria). High ceftazidime levels in patients with renal insufficiency can lead to seizures, encephalopathy, coma, asterixis, myoclonia, and neuromuscular excitability. Reduce total daily dosage. Prolonged use may result in fungal or bacterial super-infection, including *C. difficile*-associated diarrhea (CDAD) and pseudomembranous colitis; CDAD has been observed >2 months postantibiotic treatment. May be associated with increased INR, especially in nutritionally-deficient patients, prolonged treatment, hepatic or renal disease. Use with caution in patients with a history of seizure disorder; high levels may increase risk of seizures.

Adverse Reactions

1% to 10%:

Cardiovascular: Phlebitis (1%)

Endocrine & metabolic: Increased lactate dehydrogenase (6%), increased gamma-glutamyl transferase (5%)

Gastrointestinal: Diarrhea (1%)

Hematologic & oncologic: Eosinophilia (8%), positive direct Coombs test (4%; without hemolysis), thrombo-cythemia (2%)

Hepatic: Increased serum ALT (7%), increased serum AST (6%), increased serum alkaline phosphatase (4%)

Hypersensitivity: Hypersensitivity reactions (2%)

Local: Inflammation at injection site (1%), pain at injection site (1%)

<1% (Limited to important or life-threatening): Agranulocytosis, anaphylaxis, angioedema, asterixis, brain disease, candidiasis, *Clostridium difficile* associated diarrhea, erythema multiforme, hemolytic anemia, hyperbilirubine-mia, increased lactate dehydrogenase, leukopenia, lymphocytosis, myoclonus, nausea, neuromuscular excitability, neutropenia, paresthesia, pseudomembra-nous colitis, renal disease (may be severe, including renal failure), renal insufficiency, seizure, skin rash, Stevens-Johnson syndrome, thrombocytopenia, toxic epidermal necrolysis, vaginitis

Drug Interactions

Metabolism/Transport Effects None known.

Avoid Concomitant Use

Avoid concomitant use of CefTAZidime with any of the following: BCG (Intravesical)

Increased Effect/Toxicity

CefTAZidime may increase the levels/effects of: Amino-glycosides; Vitamin K Antagonists

The levels/effects of CefTAZidime may be increased by: Probenecid

Decreased Effect

CefTAZidime may decrease the levels/effects of: BCG (Intravesical); BCG Vaccine (Immunization); Sodium Picosulfate; Typhoid Vaccine

The levels/effects of CefTAZidime may be decreased by: Chloramphenicol

Preparation for Administration

IM: Using SWFI, bacteriostatic water, lidocaine 0.5%, or lidocaine 1%, reconstitute the 500 mg vials with 1.5 mL or the 1 g vials with 3 mL; final concentration of ~280 mg/mL

IV: Reconstitute intact vials as follows (**Note:** After reconstitution, may dilute further with a compatible solution to administer via IV infusion):

Fortaz, Tazicef:

~100 mg/mL solution:

500 mg vial: 5.3 mL SWFI (withdraw 5 mL from the reconstituted vial to obtain a 500 mg dose)

1 g vial: 10 mL SWFI (withdraw 10 mL from the reconstituted vial to obtain a 1 g dose)

6 g vial: 56 mL SWFI (withdraw 10 mL from the reconstituted vial to obtain a 1 g dose)

~170 mg/mL solution: 2 g vial: 10 mL SWFI (withdraw 11.5 mL from the reconstituted vial to obtain a 2 g dose)

~200 mg/mL solution: 6 g vial: 26 mL SWFI (withdraw 5 mL from the reconstituted vial to obtain a 1 g dose)

Duplex container: Unlatch side tab, unfold, remove foil strip from drug chamber. Point set port in downward direction, fold container just below the diluent meniscus, and squeeze the diluent chamber until the seal between the diluent and drug powder opens. Agitate until dissolved.

Storage/Stability

Vials: Store intact vials at 20°C to 25°C (68°F to 77°F). Protect from light. Reconstituted solution and solution further diluted for IV infusion are stable for 24 weeks when immediately frozen at -20°C (-4°F). After freezing, thawed solution in NS in a Viaflex small volume container for IV administration is stable for 24 hours at room temperature or for 7 days when refrigerated. Do not refreeze the thawed solution. Ceftazidime solutions (concentrations 1 to 40 mg/mL) in NS, D_5W, D_5NS, LR, $D_{10}W$, Ringer's injection, or SWFI are stable for 24 hours at room temperature (20°C to 25°C [68°F to 77°F]) and for 7 days if refrigerated (4°C [39°F]). Consult detailed reference regarding stability of ceftazidime in other solutions.

Duplex container: Store unactivated containers at 20°C to 25°C (68°F to 77°F); excursions permitted to 15°C to 30°C (59°F to 86°F). Protect from light. Do not freeze. Unactivated duplex containers with foil strip removed from the drug chamber must be protected from light and used within 7 days at room temperature. Once activated, must be used within 12 hours if stored at room temperature or within 3 days if stored under refrigeration.

Premixed frozen solution: Store at -20°C (-4°F). Thawed solution is stable for 8 hours at room temperature or for 3 days under refrigeration; do not refreeze.

Mechanism of Action Inhibits bacterial cell wall synthesis by binding to one or more of the penicillin-binding proteins (PBPs), which in turn inhibits the final transpeptidation step of peptidoglycan synthesis in bacterial cell walls, thus inhibiting cell wall biosynthesis. Bacteria eventually lyse due to ongoing activity of cell wall autolytic enzymes (autolysins and murein hydrolases) while cell wall assembly is arrested.

Pharmacodynamics/Kinetics

Distribution: Widely throughout the body including bone, bile, skin, CSF (higher concentrations achieved when meninges are inflamed); endometrium, heart, pleural and lymphatic fluids

Protein binding: <10%

Half-life elimination: 1 to 2 hours, prolonged with renal impairment

Time to peak, serum: IM: ~1 hour

Excretion: Urine (80% to 90% as unchanged drug)

Dosing

Adult & Geriatric

Bacterial arthritis (gram negative bacilli): IV: 1-2 g every 8 hours

Cystic fibrosis: IV:

Manufacturer's labeling: 90 to 150 mg/kg/day every 8 hours (maximum: 6 g daily)

Alternative recommendations: Intermittent IV infusion: 200 to 400 mg/kg/day divided every 6 to 8 hours (maximum: 8 to 12 g daily); **or** by continuous IV infusion: 100 to 200 mg/kg/day (maximum: 12 g daily) (Zobell, 2013)

Empiric therapy in immunocompromised patients: IV: 2 g every 8 hours

Endophthalmitis, bacterial (off-label use): Intravitreal: 2 to 2.25 mg/0.1 mL NS in combination with vancomycin (Jackson, 2003; Roth, 1997)

Intra-abdominal infection, severe (in combination with metronidazole): IV: 2 g every 8 hours for 4 to 7 days (provided source controlled). Not recommended for hospital-acquired intra-abdominal infections (IAI) associated with multidrug-resistant gram negative organisms or in mild-to-moderate community-acquired IAIs due to risk of toxicity and the development of resistant organisms (Solomkin, 2010).

Melioidosis (off-label use): IV: Note: Switching to mer-openem therapy is indicated if patient condition worsens (eg, organ failure, new infection focus development, repeat blood cultures remained positive). Oral eradication therapy is recommended after the intensive (acute) phase treatment is complete (Lipsitz, 2012).

Severe, acute phase: 50 mg/kg/dose every 8 hours (maximum dose: 2 g) or 2 g for one dose, followed by 6 g daily by continuous infusion for ≥10 days with or without TMP/SMX (Lipsitz, 2012).

Peritonitis (CAPD) (off-label route; Li, 2010): Intraperitoneal:

Intermittent: 1 to 1.5 g every 24 hours per exchange in the long dwell (≥6 hours)

Continuous (per liter exchange): Loading dose: 500 mg; maintenance dose: 125 mg. **Note:** If patient has residual renal function (eg, >100 mL/day urine output), empirically increase each dose by 25%.

Pneumonia:

Uncomplicated: IM, IV: 500 mg to 1 g every 8 hours

Hospital-acquired pneumonia (off-label dose): IV: 2 g every 8 hours (ATS/IDSA, 2005)

Prosthetic joint infection, *Pseudomonas aeruginosa* (alternative to cefepime or meropenem): IV: 2 g every 8 hours for 4 to 6 weeks (consider addition of an aminoglycoside) (Osmon, 2013)

Skin and soft tissue infections: IV, IM: 500 mg to 1 g every 8 hours

Severe infections, including meningitis, CNS infection, osteomyelitis, gynecological: IV: 2 g every 8 hours

Urinary tract infections: IV, IM:
Uncomplicated: 250 mg every 12 hours
Complicated: 500 mg every 8 to 12 hours
Pediatric
Susceptible infections: IV:
Children 1 month to 12 years: 30 to 50 mg/kg/dose every 8 hours; maximum dose: 6 g/day (higher doses reserved for immunocompromised patients, cystic fibrosis, or meningitis)
Children ≥12 years: Refer to adult dosing.

Indication-specific dosing:
Cystic fibrosis: Infants, Children, and Adolescents: IV:
Manufacturer's labeling: 150 mg/kg/day divided every 8 hours (maximum: 6 g daily)
Alternative recommendations: 200 to 300 mg/kg/day divided every 8 hours (maximum: 6 g daily) (*Red Book* [AAP], 2012)
Melioidosis (off-label use): IV: Note: Switching to meropenem therapy is indicated if patient condition worsens (eg, organ failure, new infection focus development, repeat blood cultures remained positive). Oral eradication therapy is recommended after the intensive (acute) phase treatment is complete (Lipsitz, 2012).
Severe, acute phase: Infants >3 months, Children, and Adolescents: 50 mg/kg/dose every 8 hours (maximum dose: 2 g) or 2 g for one dose, followed by 6 g daily by continuous infusion for ≥10 days with or without TMP/SMX (Lipsitz, 2012). **Note:** Depending on infection severity, the dose for patients ≥3 months can be ≤40 mg/kg (maximum dose: 2 g) (Lipsitz, 2012).
Renal Impairment Note: If the dose recommended in the dosing section is lower than that recommended for patients with renal insufficiency as outlined below, the lower dose should be used. In severe infections, when the usual dose would be ceftazidime 6 g/day in patients without renal impairment, consider increasing the doses below by 50% or increase the dosing frequency. Further dosage adjustments should be determined by infection severity, susceptibility and patient response to therapy.
CrCl 31 to 50 mL/minute: 1 g every 12 hours
CrCl 16 to 30 mL/minute: 1 g every 24 hours
CrCl 6 to 15 mL/minute: 500 mg every 24 hours
CrCl <5 mL/minute: 500 mg every 48 hours
Intermittent hemodialysis (IHD) (administer after hemodialysis on dialysis days): Dialyzable (50% to 100%): 500 mg to 1 g every 24 hours **or** 1 to 2 g every 48 to 72 hours (Heintz, 2009). **Note:** Dosing dependent on the assumption of 3 times per week, complete IHD sessions.
Peritoneal dialysis (PD): IV:
Intermittent: Loading dose of 1 g, followed by 500 mg every 24 hours
Continuous: Loading dose of 1 g, followed by 500 mg every 24 hours. **Note:** an additional 125 mg per liter of exchange fluid may be added to the dialysate if clinically warranted.
Continuous renal replacement therapy (CRRT) (Heintz, 2009; Trotman, 2005): Drug clearance is highly dependent on the method of renal replacement, filter type, and flow rate. Appropriate dosing requires close monitoring of pharmacologic response, signs of adverse reactions due to drug accumulation, as well as drug concentrations in relation to target trough (if appropriate). The following are general recommendations only (based on dialysate flow/ultrafiltration rates of 1 to 2 L/hour and minimal residual renal function) and should not supersede clinical judgment:
CVVH: Loading dose of 2 g followed by 1 to 2 g every 12 hours
CVVHD/CVVHDF: Loading dose of 2 g followed by either 1 g every 8 hours **or** 2 g every 12 hours. **Note:** Dosage of 1 g every 8 hours results in similar steady-state concentrations as 2 g every 12 hours and is more cost effective. Dosage of 2 g every 8 hours may be needed for gram-negative rods with MIC ≥4 mg/L (Heintz, 2009).
Note: For patients receiving CVVHDF, some recommend giving a loading dose of 2 g followed by 3 g over 24 hours as a continuous IV infusion to maintain concentrations ≥4 times the MIC for susceptible pathogens (Heintz, 2009).
Hepatic Impairment No dosage adjustment necessary.
Dietary Considerations Some products may contain sodium.
Administration Administer around-the-clock to promote less variation in peak and trough serum levels. Ceftazidime can be administered deep IM into large mass muscle, IVP over 3 to 5 minutes, or IV intermittent infusion over 15 to 30 minutes. Do not admix with aminoglycosides in same bottle/bag. Ceftazidime may be administered intravitreally

as 2 to 2.25 mg/0.1 mL NS in combination with vancomycin (separate syringes) (Jackson, 2003; Roth, 1997).

Intraperitoneal administration may be used **in conjunction with** IV use for systemic infections if continuous peritoneal dialysis is used (added to the dialysate in each exchange). Intraperitoneal administration alone may also be used for the treatment of peritonitis and added to the dialysate in intermittent (added to the longest dwell time per day) or continuous (loading dose, followed by a maintenance dose per liter of exchange) peritoneal dialysis.

Monitoring Parameters Monitor renal function. Observe for signs and symptoms of anaphylaxis during first dose.

Test Interactions Positive direct Coombs', false-positive urinary glucose test using cupric sulfate (Benedict's solution, Clinitest®, Fehling's solution), false-positive serum or urine creatinine with Jaffé reaction

Additional Information With some organisms, resistance may develop during treatment (including *Enterobacter* spp and *Serratia* spp). Consider combination therapy or periodic susceptibility testing for organisms with inducible resistance.

Dosage Forms Excipient information presented when available (limited, particularly for generics); consult specific product labeling.
Solution, Intravenous, as sodium [strength expressed as base]:
Fortaz in D5W: 1 g (50 mL); 2 g (50 mL)
Tazicef: 1 g/50 mL (50 mL)
Solution Reconstituted, Injection:
Fortaz: 500 mg (1 ea); 1 g (1 ea); 2 g (1 ea); 6 g (1 ea)
Tazicef: 1 g (1 ea); 2 g (1 ea); 6 g (1 ea)
Generic: 1 g (1 ea); 2 g (1 ea); 6 g (1 ea); 100 g (1 ea)
Solution Reconstituted, Injection [preservative free]:
Generic: 1 g (1 ea); 2 g (1 ea); 6 g (1 ea)
Solution Reconstituted, Intravenous:
Fortaz: 1 g (1 ea); 2 g (1 ea)
Tazicef: 1 g (1 ea); 2 g (1 ea)
Generic: 1 g/50 mL (1 ea); 2 g/50 mL (1 ea)

Ceftazidime and Avibactam
(SEF tay zi deem & a vi BAK tam)

Brand Names: US Avycaz
Index Terms Avibactam and Ceftazidime
Pharmacologic Category Cephalosporin Combination
Use
Intra-abdominal infections, complicated: Treatment of complicated intra-abdominal infections (cIAI) in adults, in combination with metronidazole, caused by *Enterobacter cloacae, Escherichia coli, Klebsiella oxytoca, K. pneumoniae, Proteus mirabilis, Providencia stuartii,* and *Pseudomonas aeruginosa.*
Urinary tract infections, complicated (including pyelonephritis): Treatment of complicated urinary tract infections (cUTI) (including pyelonephritis) in adults, caused by *Citrobacter freundii, C. koseri, Enterobacter aerogenes, E. cloacae, Escherichia coli, Klebsiella pneumoniae, Proteus* spp, and *Pseudomonas aeruginosa.*
Pregnancy Considerations Adverse events have not been observed in animal reproduction studies conducted with ceftazidime; adverse events have been observed in some animal reproduction studies conducted with avibactam.
Breast-Feeding Considerations Ceftazidime is excreted in breast milk. It is not known if avibactam is excreted in breast milk. The manufacturer recommends that caution be exercised when administering ceftazidime and avibactam to breast-feeding women.
Contraindications Serious hypersensitivity to ceftazidime, avibactam, other cephalosporins, or any component of the formulation
Warnings/Precautions Serious and occasionally severe or fatal hypersensitivity (anaphylactic) reactions and serious skin reactions have been reported in patients receiving beta-lactam drugs. Before initiating therapy, carefully investigate previous penicillin, cephalosporin, or carbapenem hypersensitivity. Use caution if given to a patient with a penicillin or other beta-lactam allergy because cross sensitivity among beta-lactam antibacterial drugs has been established. If an allergic reaction occurs, discontinue and institute appropriate therapy. Severe neurological reactions have been reported with ceftazidime, including asterixis, coma, encephalopathy, myoclonus, neuromuscular excitability, seizures, and nonconvulsive status epilepticus. Risk may be increased in the presence of renal impairment; ensure dose adjusted for renal function. Discontinue therapy if patient develops neurotoxicity. Prolonged use may result in fungal or bacterial superinfection, including *C. difficile*-associated diarrhea (CDAD) and pseudomembranous colitis; CDAD has been observed >2 months postantibiotic treatment. In clinical trials, patients with a ▶

CrCl of 30 to 50 mL/minute had lower clinical cure rates than those with CrCl >50 mL/minute; however, these patients received a daily dose that was 33% lower than what is currently recommended for patients with this degree of renal impairment. Monitor renal function at baseline and at least daily in patients with changing renal function. Adjust the dose accordingly. Potentially significant drug-drug interactions may exist, requiring dose or frequency adjustment, additional monitoring, and/or selection of alternative therapy.

Adverse Reactions Frequency not always defined.

1% to 10%:

Central nervous system: Anxiety (10%), dizziness (6%)

Dermatologic: Skin rash (<5%)

Endocrine & metabolic: Hypokalemia (<5%), increased gamma-glutamyl transferase (<5%)

Gastrointestinal: Constipation (10%), abdominal pain (7%), upper abdominal pain (7%), nausea (2%), *Clostridium difficile* associated diarrhea

Hematologic & oncologic: Eosinophilia (<5%), prolonged prothrombin time (<5%), thrombocytopenia (<5%), positive direct coombs test (2%; no hemolytic anemia reactions reported)

Hepatic: Increased serum alkaline phosphatase (3%), increased serum ALT (3%)

Renal: Acute renal failure (<5%), renal impairment (<5%)

Drug Interactions

Metabolism/Transport Effects Refer to individual components.

Avoid Concomitant Use

Avoid concomitant use of Ceftazidime and Avibactam with any of the following: BCG (Intravesical); Probenecid

Increased Effect/Toxicity

Ceftazidime and Avibactam may increase the levels/effects of: Aminoglycosides; Vitamin K Antagonists

The levels/effects of Ceftazidime and Avibactam may be increased by: Probenecid; Teriflunomide

Decreased Effect

Ceftazidime and Avibactam may decrease the levels/effects of: BCG (Intravesical); BCG Vaccine (Immunization); Sodium Picosulfate; Typhoid Vaccine

The levels/effects of Ceftazidime and Avibactam may be decreased by: Chloramphenicol

Preparation for Administration IV: Reconstitute vial with 10 mL of NS, D₅W, SWFI or other compatible solution listed in the manufacturer's labeling (resulting approximate concentration: ceftazidime 167 mg/mL and avibactam 42 mg/mL) and further dilute in 50 to 250 mL of a compatible IV infusion fluid; mix gently. Solution ranges in color from clear to light yellow.

Storage/Stability

Vials: Store intact vials at 25°C (77°F). Protect from light.

Intermittent IV infusion: Admixed solutions are stable up to 12 hours at 20°C to 25°C (68°F to 77°F) and 24 hours at 2°C to 8°C (36°F to 46°F). Use solutions previously stored at 2°C to 8°C (36°F to 46°F) within 12 hours of subsequent storage at 20°C to 25°C (68°F to 77°F).

Mechanism of Action

Ceftazidime inhibits bacterial cell wall synthesis by binding to one or more of the penicillin-binding proteins (PBPs) which in turn inhibits the final transpeptidation step of peptidoglycan synthesis in bacterial cell walls, thus inhibiting cell wall biosynthesis. Bacteria eventually lyse due to ongoing activity of cell wall autolytic enzymes (autolysins and murein hydrolases) while cell wall assembly is arrested.

Avibactam inactivates some beta-lactamases and protects ceftazidime from degradation.

Pharmacodynamics/Kinetics

Distribution: V_d: Ceftazidime: ~17 to 18 L; Avibactam: ~22 to 23 L

Protein binding: Ceftazidime: <10%; Avibactam: ~6% to 8%

Metabolism: Ceftazidime: 80% to 90% of dose eliminated as unchanged drug; Avibactam: Not metabolized

Half-life elimination: Ceftazidime: ~3 hours; Avibactam: ~2.5 hours

Excretion: Ceftazidime: Urine (80% to 90% as unchanged drug); Avibactam: Urine (97%)

Dosing

Adult & Geriatric Note: Dosage recommendations are expressed as total grams of the ceftazidime/avibactam combination.

Intra-abdominal infections, complicated: IV: 2.5 g every 8 hours in combination with metronidazole for 5 to 14 days.

Urinary tract infections, complicated (including pyelonephritis): IV: 2.5 g every 8 hours for 7 to 14 days.

Renal Impairment Note: Estimation of renal function for the purpose of drug dosing should be done using the Cockcroft-Gault formula. Dosage recommendations are expressed as total grams of the ceftazidime/avibactam combination:

CrCl >50 mL/minute: No dosage adjustment necessary.

CrCl 31 to 50 mL/minute: 1.25 g every 8 hours

CrCl 16 to 30 mL/minute: 0.94 g every 12 hours

CrCl 6 to 15 mL/minute: 0.94 g every 24 hours

CrCl ≤5 mL/minute: 0.94 g every 48 hours

End stage renal disease (ESRD) on intermittent hemodialysis (IHD): Administer after hemodialysis on dialysis days; base dose upon patient's estimated renal function (eg, CrCl 6 to 15 mL/minute or CrCl ≤5 mL/minute).

Hepatic Impairment No dosage adjustment necessary.

Administration IV: Administer by intermittent infusion over 2 hours.

Monitoring Parameters Monitor for signs of anaphylaxis during first dose. Monitor renal function at baseline in all patients, and at least daily in patients with renal impairment.

Test Interactions Ceftazidime: Positive direct Coomb. False-positive reaction for urine glucose with certain methods; use glucose tests based on enzymatic glucose oxidase reactions.

Dosage Forms Excipient information presented when available (limited, particularly for generics); consult specific product labeling.

Solution Reconstituted, Intravenous:

Avycaz: 2.5 g: Ceftazidime 2 g and avibactam 0.5 g (1 ea)

◆ Ceftazidime For Injection (Can) *see* CefTAZidime *on page 345*

Ceftibuten (sef TYE byoo ten)

Brand Names: US Cedax

Pharmacologic Category Antibiotic, Cephalosporin (Third Generation)

Use Treatment of acute exacerbations of chronic bronchitis, acute bacterial otitis media, and pharyngitis/tonsillitis

Dosing

Adult & Geriatric Susceptible infections: Oral: 400 mg once daily for 10 days

Pediatric Susceptible infections: Oral:

6 months to <12 years: 9 mg/kg/day for 10 days; maximum daily dose: 400 mg

≥12 years: Refer to adult dosing.

Renal Impairment

CrCl ≥50 mL//minute: No adjustment needed

CrCl 30 to 49 mL//minute: Administer 4.5 mg/kg or 200 mg every 24 hours.

CrCl 5 to 29 mL/minute: Administer 2.25 mg/kg or 100 mg every 24 hours.

Hemodialysis: 39% to 65% removed by a 2 to 4 hour hemodialysis; Administer 400 mg or 9 mg/kg (maximum: 400 mg) after each hemodialysis session.

Hepatic Impairment No dosage adjustment provided in manufacturer's labeling.

Additional Information Complete prescribing information should be consulted for additional detail.

Dosage Forms Excipient information presented when available (limited, particularly for generics); consult specific product labeling.

Capsule, Oral:

Cedax: 400 mg [contains butylparaben, edetate calcium disodium, methylparaben, propylparaben]

Generic: 400 mg

Suspension Reconstituted, Oral:

Cedax: 90 mg/5 mL (60 mL, 90 mL, 120 mL) [contains polysorbate 80, sodium benzoate; cherry flavor]

Cedax: 180 mg/5 mL (30 mL, 60 mL) [contains sodium benzoate; cherry flavor]

Generic: 180 mg/5 mL (60 mL)

◆ Ceftin *see* Cefuroxime *on page 353*

Ceftolozane and Tazobactam
(sef TOL oh zane & taz oh BAK tam)

Brand Names: US Zerbaxa

Index Terms CXA 201; Tazobactam and Ceftolozane

Pharmacologic Category Cephalosporin Combination

Use

Intra-abdominal infections: Treatment of complicated intra-abdominal infections in adults, in combination with metronidazole, caused by *Enterobacter cloacae*, *Escherichia coli*, *Klebsiella oxytoca*, *K. pneumoniae*, *Proteus mirabilis*, *Pseudomonas aeruginosa*, *Bacteroides fragilis*, *Streptococcus anginosus*, *Streptococcus constellatus*, and *Streptococcus salivarius*.

Urinary tract infections: Treatment of complicated urinary tract infections, including pyelonephritis, in adults caused by *Escherichia coli*, *Klebsiella pneumoniae*, *Proteus mirabilis*, and *Pseudomonas aeruginosa*.

Pregnancy Considerations Adverse events were observed in some animal reproduction studies. Tazobactam crosses the placenta (Bourget, 1998).

Breast-Feeding Considerations It is not known if ceftolozane or tazobactam are excreted into breast milk. The manufacturer recommends that caution be used if administered to a nursing woman.

Contraindications Serious hypersensitivity to ceftolozane/tazobactam, piperacillin/tazobactam, other members of the beta-lactam class, or any component of the formulation.

Warnings/Precautions Hypersensitivity and anaphylaxis (serious and sometimes fatal) have been reported in patients receiving beta-lactam drugs. Question patient about previous hypersensitivity reactions to other cephalosporins, penicillins or other beta-lactams. Cross-sensitivity has been established. If administered, use with caution and if anaphylaxis occurs, discontinue and institute appropriate supportive therapy. Use may result in fungal or bacterial superinfection, including *C. difficile*-associated diarrhea (CDAD) and pseudomembranous colitis; CDAD has been observed >2 months postantibiotic treatment. Exposure to ceftolozane is increased with increasing degrees of renal impairment; monitor creatinine clearance (CrCl) at least daily in patients with changing renal function and adjust the dose. In clinical trials, cure rates were lower in patients with a baseline CrCl of 30 to 50 mL/minute.

Adverse Reactions

1% to 10%:
Cardiovascular: Hypotension (<1% to 2%), atrial fibrillation (≤1%)
Central nervous system: Headache (3% to 6%), insomnia (complicated intra-abdominal infections: 4%; complicated UTIs: 1%), anxiety (<1% to 2%), dizziness (≤1%)
Dermatologic: Skin rash (<1% to 2%)
Endocrine: Hypokalemia (complicated intra-abdominal infections: 3%; complicated UTIs: <1%)
Gastrointestinal: Nausea (3% to 8%), diarrhea (2% to 6%), constipation (2% to 4%), vomiting (complicated intra-abdominal infections: 3%, complicated UTIs: 1%), abdominal pain (≤1%)
Hematologic & oncologic: Anemia (<1% to 2%), thrombocythemia (<1% to 2%)
Hepatic: Increased serum ALT (2%), increased serum AST (1% to 2%)
Miscellaneous: Fever (complicated intra-abdominal infections: 6%; complicated UTIs: 2%)
<1% (Limited to important or life-threatening): Abdominal distention, angina pectoris, candidiasis, *Clostridium difficile* associated diarrhea, dyspnea, dyspepsia, flatulence, fungal urinary tract infection, gastritis, hyperglycemia, hypomagnesemia, hypophosphatemia, increased gamma-glutamyl transferase, increased serum alkaline phosphatase, infusion site reaction, intestinal obstruction, nonhemorrhagic stroke, oropharyngeal candidiasis, paralytic ileus, positive direct Coombs test, renal failure, renal insufficiency, tachycardia, urticaria, venous thrombosis

Drug Interactions

Metabolism/Transport Effects None known.

Avoid Concomitant Use
Avoid concomitant use of Ceftolozane and Tazobactam with any of the following: BCG (Intravesical)

Increased Effect/Toxicity
Ceftolozane and Tazobactam may increase the levels/effects of: Vitamin K Antagonists

The levels/effects of Ceftolozane and Tazobactam may be increased by: Probenecid

Decreased Effect
Ceftolozane and Tazobactam may decrease the levels/effects of: BCG (Intravesical); BCG Vaccine (Immunization); Sodium Picosulfate; Typhoid Vaccine

Preparation for Administration
Constitute the vial with 10 mL SWFI or NS and gently shake to dissolve. The final volume is approximately 11.4 mL and contains ceftolozane/tazobactam 1.5 g (ceftolozane 1 g and tazobactam 500 mg).
To prepare the required dose, withdraw the appropriate volume from the reconstituted vial. Add the withdrawn volume to an infusion bag containing 100 mL of NS or D₅W.
Infusions range from clear, colorless solutions to solutions that are clear and slightly yellow. Variations in color within this range do not affect the potency of the product.

Storage/Stability Store intact vials at 2°C to 8°C (36°F to 46°F); protect from light. Reconstituted solution may be held for 1 hour prior to transfer and further dilution in an infusion bag. Diluted solution may be stored for 24 hours at room temperature or for 7 days at 2°C to 8°C (36°F to 46°F); do not freeze.

Mechanism of Action Ceftolozane inhibits bacterial cell wall synthesis by binding to one or more of the penicillin-binding proteins (PBPs); which in turn inhibits the final transpeptidation step of peptidoglycan synthesis in bacterial cell walls, thus inhibiting cell wall biosynthesis. Ceftolozane is an inhibitor of PBPs of *Pseudomonas aeruginosa* (eg, PBP1b, PBP1c, and PBP3) and *Escherichia coli* (eg, PBP3). Tazobactam irreversibly inhibits many beta-lactamases (eg, certain penicillinases and cephalosporinases), and can covalently bind to some plasmid-mediated and chromosomal bacterial beta-lactamases.

Pharmacodynamics/Kinetics
Distribution: V_d: Ceftolozane: 13.5 L; Tazobactam: 18.2 L
Protein binding: Ceftolozane: 16% to 20%; Tazobactam: 30%
Metabolism: Ceftolozane: Not metabolized; Tazobactam: Hydrolyzed to inactive metabolite
Half-life elimination: Ceftolozane: ~3 hours; Tazobactam: ~1 hour
Time to peak, plasma: Immediately following completion of 60-minute infusion
Excretion: Ceftolozane: Urine (>95% as unchanged drug); Tazobactam: urine (>80% as unchanged drug)

Dosing

Adult & Geriatric Note: Zerbaxa (ceftolozane/tazobactam) is a combination product. Dosage recommendations are expressed as grams of ceftolozane/tazobactam combination.

Intra-abdominal infections (complicated): IV: 1.5 g every 8 hours for 4 to 14 days in combination with metronidazole

Urinary tract infections (complicated, includes pyelonephritis): IV: 1.5 g every 8 hours for 7 days

Renal Impairment Note: Estimation of renal function for the purpose of drug dosing should be done using the Cockcroft-Gault formula.
CrCl >50 mL/minute: No dosage adjustment necessary.
CrCl 30 to 50 mL/minute: 750 mg every 8 hours
CrCl 15 to 29 mL/minute: 375 mg every 8 hours
CrCl <15 mL/minute not on dialysis: There are no dosage adjustments provided in the manufacturer's labeling (has not been studied)
End-stage renal disease (ESRD) requiring intermittent hemodialysis (IHD): Dialyzable (~66%). Initial: 750 mg for one dose, followed by 150 mg every 8 hours. Administer dose immediately after dialysis on dialysis days.

Hepatic Impairment No dosage adjustment necessary.

Dietary Considerations Some products may contain sodium.

Administration Intravenous: Administer by intermittent infusion over 60 minutes.

Monitoring Parameters Serum creatinine and CrCl at baseline and daily in patients with changing renal function,

Dosage Forms Excipient information presented when available (limited, particularly for generics); consult specific product labeling.
Solution Reconstituted, Intravenous [preservative free]:
Zerbaxa: 1.5 g: Ceftolozane 1 g and tazobactam 0.5 g (1 ea)

CefTRIAXone (sef trye AKS one)

Brand Names: US Rocephin
Brand Names: Canada Ceftriaxone for Injection; Ceftriaxone for Injection USP; Ceftriaxone Sodium for Injection; Ceftriaxone Sodium for Injection BP
Index Terms Ceftriaxone Sodium
Pharmacologic Category Antibiotic, Cephalosporin (Third Generation)

Use

Bacterial infections:
Treatment: Treatment of lower respiratory tract infections, acute bacterial otitis media, skin and skin structure infections, bone and joint infections, intra-abdominal and urinary tract infections, pelvic inflammatory disease (PID), uncomplicated gonorrhea, bacterial septicemia, and meningitis
Prophylaxis: Used in surgical (perioperative) prophylaxis

Pregnancy Considerations Teratogenic effects have not been observed in animal reproduction studies. Ceftriaxone crosses the placenta and distributes to amniotic fluid. An increase in most types of birth defects was not found following first trimester exposure to cephalosporins. Pregnancy was found to influence the single dose

pharmacokinetics of ceftriaxone when administered prior to delivery. The pharmacokinetics of ceftriaxone following multiple doses in the third trimester are similar to those of nonpregnant patients. Ceftriaxone is recommended for use in pregnant women for the treatment of gonococcal infections, Lyme disease, and may be used in certain situations prior to vaginal delivery in women at high risk for endocarditis (consult current guidelines).

Breast-Feeding Considerations Low concentrations of ceftriaxone are excreted in breast milk. The manufacturer recommends that caution be exercised when administering ceftriaxone to nursing women. Nondose-related effects could include modification of bowel flora.

Contraindications Hypersensitivity to ceftriaxone, any component of the formulation, or other cephalosporins; **do not use in hyperbilirubinemic neonates**, particularly those who are premature since ceftriaxone is reported to displace bilirubin from albumin binding sites; concomitant use with intravenous calcium-containing solutions/products in neonates (≤28 days); IV use of ceftriaxone solutions containing lidocaine.

Warnings/Precautions Serious and sometimes fatal hypersensitivity has been reported. Use caution in patients with a history of any allergy (particularly drugs), penicillin allergy or beta-lactam sensitivity. If severe hypersensitivity occurs, discontinue immediately and institute supportive emergency measures.

Gall bladder pseudolithiasis has been reported, possibly due to cetriaxone-calcium precipitates; probability more likely in pediatric patients; discontinue in patients who develop signs and symptoms of gallbladder disease. Secondary to biliary obstruction, pancreatitis has been reported rarely. Most patients had biliary stasis or sludge risk factors (eg, preceding major surgery, sever illness, TPN). Use with caution in patients with a history of GI disease, especially colitis. Severe cases (including some fatalities) of immune-related hemolytic anemia have been reported in patients receiving cephalosporins, including ceftriaxone. Prolonged use may result in fungal or bacterial superinfection, including *C. difficile*-associated diarrhea (CDAD) and pseudomembranous colitis; CDAD has been observed >2 months postantibiotic treatment.

Potentially significant interactions may exist, requiring dose or frequency adjustment, additional monitoring, and/or selection of alternative therapy. May be associated with increased INR (rarely), especially in nutritionally-deficient patients, prolonged treatment, hepatic or renal disease. Monitor INR during treatment if patient has impaired synthesis or low stores of vitamin K; supplementation may be needed if clinically indicated.

No adjustment is generally necessary in patients with renal impairment; use with caution in patients with concurrent hepatic dysfunction and significant renal disease, dosage should not exceed 2 g/day. Use extreme caution in neonates due to risk of hyperbilirubinemia, particularly in premature infants (contraindicated in hyperbilirubinemic neonates and neonates <41 weeks postmenstrual age). Ceftriaxone may complex with calcium causing precipitation. Fatal lung and kidney damage associated with calcium-ceftriaxone precipitates has been observed in premature and term neonates. Do not reconstitute, admix, or coadminister with calcium-containing solutions, even via separate infusion lines/sites or at different times in any neonatal patient. Ceftriaxone should not be diluted or administered simultaneously with any calcium-containing solution via a Y-site in any patient. However, ceftriaxone and calcium-containing solution may be administered sequentially of one another for use in patients **other than** neonates if infusion lines are thoroughly flushed, with a compatible fluid, between infusions.

Adverse Reactions

>10%:
Dermatologic: Skin tightness (IM: ≤5% to ≤17%; local)
Local: Induration at injection site (≤5% to ≤17%; incidence higher with IM), warm sensation at injection site (IM: ≤5% to ≤17%)

1% to 10%:
Dermatologic: Skin rash (2%)
Gastrointestinal: Diarrhea (3%)
Hematologic & oncologic: Eosinophilia (6%), thrombocythemia (5%), leukopenia (2%)
Hepatic: Increased serum transaminases (3%)
Local: Tenderness at injection site (≤1%), pain at injection site (≤1%)
Renal: Increased blood urea nitrogen (1%)

<1% (Limited to important or life-threatening): Abdominal pain, acute generalized exanthematous pustulosis, acute renal failure (post-renal), agranulocytosis, allergic dermatitis, anaphylactoid reaction, anaphylaxis, anemia, basophilia, blood coagulation disorder, bronchospasm, candidiasis, casts in urine, choledocholithiasis, cholelithiasis, clostridium difficile associated diarrhea, colitis, convulsions, decreased prothrombin time, dysgeusia, dyspepsia, edema, epistaxis, erythema multiforme, fever, flushing, gallbladder sludge, glossitis, glycosuria, granulocytopenia, headache, hematuria, hemolytic anemia, hypersensitivity pneumonitis, increased monocytes, increased serum alkaline phosphatase, increased serum bilirubin, increased serum creatinine, jaundice, kernicterus, leukocytosis, lymphocytopenia, lymphocytosis, nephrolithiasis, neutropenia, oliguria, palpitations, pancreatitis, phlebitis, prolonged prothrombin time, pseudomembranous colitis, seizure, serum sickness, Stevens-Johnson syndrome, stomatitis, thrombocytopenia, toxic epidermal necrolysis, ureteral obstruction, urogenital fungal infection, vaginitis

Drug Interactions

Metabolism/Transport Effects None known.

Avoid Concomitant Use
Avoid concomitant use of CefTRIAXone with any of the following: BCG (Intravesical)

Increased Effect/Toxicity
CefTRIAXone may increase the levels/effects of: Aminoglycosides; Vitamin K Antagonists

The levels/effects of CefTRIAXone may be increased by: Calcium Salts (Intravenous); Probenecid; Ringer's Injection (Lactated)

Decreased Effect
CefTRIAXone may decrease the levels/effects of: BCG (Intravesical); BCG Vaccine (Immunization); Sodium Picosulfate; Typhoid Vaccine

Preparation for Administration

IM injection: Vials should be reconstituted with appropriate volume of diluent (including D_5W, NS, SWFI, bacteriostatic water, or 1% lidocaine) to make a final concentration of 250 mg/mL or 350 mg/mL.
Volume to add to create a **250 mg/mL** solution:
250 mg vial: 0.9 mL
500 mg vial: 1.8 mL
1 g vial: 3.6 mL
2 g vial: 7.2 mL
Volume to add to create a **350 mg/mL** solution:
500 mg vial: 1.0 mL
1 g vial: 2.1 mL
2 g vial: 4.2 mL
IV infusion: Infusion is prepared in two stages: Initial reconstitution of powder, followed by dilution to final infusion solution.
Vials: Reconstitute powder with appropriate IV diluent (including SWFI, D_5W, $D_{10}W$, NS) to create an initial solution of ~100 mg/mL. Recommended volume to add:
250 mg vial: 2.4 mL
500 mg vial: 4.8 mL
1 g vial: 9.6 mL
2 g vial: 19.2 mL
Note: After reconstitution of powder, further dilution into a volume of compatible solution (eg, 50-100 mL of D_5W or NS) is recommended.
Piggyback bottle: Reconstitute powder with appropriate IV diluent (D_5W or NS) to create a resulting solution of ~100 mg/mL. Recommended initial volume to add:
1 g bottle: 10 mL
2 g bottle: 20 mL
Note: After reconstitution, to prepare the final infusion solution, further dilution to 50 mL or 100 mL volumes with the appropriate IV diluent (including D_5W or NS) is recommended.

Storage/Stability

Powder for injection: Prior to reconstitution, store at ≤25°C (≤77°F). Protect from light.
Premixed solution (manufacturer premixed): Store at -20°C; once thawed, solutions are stable for 3 days at 25°C (77°F) or for 21 days at 5°C (41°F). Do not refreeze.
Stability of reconstituted solutions:
10 to 40 mg/mL: Reconstituted in D_5W, $D_{10}W$, NS, or SWFI: Stable for 2 days at room temperature of 25°C (77°F) or for 10 days when refrigerated at 4°C (39°F). Stable for 26 weeks when frozen at -20°C when reconstituted with D_5W or NS. Once thawed (at room temperature), solutions are stable for 2 days at room temperature of 25°C (77°F) or for 10 days when refrigerated at 4°C (39°F); does not apply to manufacturer's premixed bags. Do not refreeze. If D_5NS or $D_51/2NS$ are used, solutions are only stable for 2 days at of 25°C (77°F).
100 mg/mL:
Reconstituted in D_5W, SWFI, or NS: Stable for 2 days at room temperature of 25°C (77°F) or for 10 days when refrigerated at 4°C (39°F).
Reconstituted in lidocaine 1% solution or bacteriostatic water: Stable for 24 hours at room temperature of 25°C (77°F) or for 10 days when refrigerated at 4°C (39°F).

250 to 350 mg/mL: Reconstituted in D_5W, NS, lidocaine 1% solution, bacteriostatic water, or SWFI: Stable for 24 hours at room temperature of 25°C (77°F) or for 3 days when refrigerated at 4°C (39°F).

Mechanism of Action Inhibits bacterial cell wall synthesis by binding to one or more of the penicillin-binding proteins (PBPs) which in turn inhibits the final transpeptidation step of peptidoglycan synthesis in bacterial cell walls, thus inhibiting cell wall biosynthesis. Bacteria eventually lyse due to ongoing activity of cell wall autolytic enzymes (autolysins and murein hydrolases) while cell wall assembly is arrested.

Pharmacodynamics/Kinetics

Absorption: IM: Well absorbed

Distribution: Widely throughout the body including gallbladder, lungs, bone, bile, CSF (higher concentrations achieved when meninges are inflamed); V_d:

Neonates: 0.34 to 0.55 L/kg (Richards 1984)

Infants and Children: 0.3 to 0.4 L/kg (Richards 1984)

Adults: ~6 to 14 L

Protein binding: 85% to 95%

Half-life elimination:

Neonates (Martin 1984): 1 to 4 days: 16 hours; 9 to 30 days: 9 hours

Children (age not specified): 4.1 to 6.6 hours (Richards 1984)

Adults: Normal renal and hepatic function: ~5 to 9 hours

Adults: Renal impairment (mild-to-severe): ~12 to 16 hours

Time to peak, serum: IM: 2 to 3 hours

Excretion: Urine (33% to 67% as unchanged drug); feces (as inactive drug)

Dosing

Adult & Geriatric

Dosage range: IM, IV: Usual dose: 1 to 2 g every 12 to 24 hours, depending on the type and severity of infection

Acute bacterial rhinosinusitis, severe infection requiring hospitalization (off-label use): IV: 1 to 2 g every 12 to 24 hours for 5 to 7 days (Chow 2012)

Arthritis, septic (off-label use): IV: 1 to 2 g once daily (Coiffier 2014; Dalla Vestra 2008; Harwood 2008; Raad 2004). Additional data may be necessary to further define the role of ceftriaxone in this condition.

Bacterial enteric infections in HIV-infected patients (empiric treatment) (off-label use): Adolescents: IV: 1 g every 24 hours (HHS [OI adult 2015])

Bite wounds (animal) (off-label use): IV: 1 g every 12 hours in combination with clindamycin or metronidazole for anaerobic coverage

Brain abscess (off-label use):

Empiric: IV: 2 g every 12 hours with metronidazole (Brouwer 2014; Louvois 2000). Additional data may be necessary to further define the role of ceftriaxone in this condition.

Enterobacteriaceae or Haemophilus spp.: IV: 2 g every 12 hours; **Note:** Often isolated in mixed infection, combination therapy may be needed (Brouwer 2014).

Chancroid (off-label use): IM: 250 mg as single dose (CDC 2010)

Cholecystitis, mild-to-moderate: IV: 1 to 2 g every 12 to 24 hours for 4 to 7 days (provided source controlled) (Solomkin 2010)

Gonococcal infections:

Uncomplicated cervicitis, pharyngitis, proctitis, urethritis, vulvovaginitis (off-label dose): IM: 250 mg in a single dose with oral azithromycin (preferred) or oral doxycycline (alternative) (CDC 2012)

Conjunctivitis (off-label use): IM: 1 g in a single dose (CDC 2010)

Disseminated (off-label use): IM, IV: 1 g once daily for 24 to 48 hours may switch to cefixime (after improvement noted) to complete a total of 7 days of therapy (CDC 2010)

Endocarditis (off-label use): IV: 1 to 2 g every 12 hours for at least 28 days (CDC 2010)

Epididymitis, acute (off-label use): IM: 250 mg in a single dose with doxycycline (CDC 2010)

Meningitis (off-label use): IV: 1 to 2 g every 12 hours for 10 to 14 days (CDC 2010)

Infective endocarditis (off-label use): IM, IV:

Native valve: 2 g once daily for 2 to 4 weeks; **Note:** If using 2-week regimen or for relatively penicillin-resistant streptococcus, concurrent gentamicin is recommended; for HACEK organisms, duration of therapy is 4 weeks (Baddour 2005).

Prosthetic valve: 2 g once daily for 6 weeks (with or without gentamicin [dependent on penicillin MIC]); for HACEK organisms, duration of therapy is 4 weeks (Baddour 2005).

Enterococcus faecalis (resistant to penicillin, aminoglycoside, and vancomycin), native or prosthetic valve: 2 g twice daily for ≥8 weeks administered concurrently with ampicillin (Baddour 2005)

Prophylaxis: 1 g 30 to 60 minutes before procedure (Wilson 2007). Intramuscular injections should be avoided in patients who are receiving anticoagulant therapy. In these circumstances, orally administered regimens should be given whenever possible. Intravenously administered antibiotics should be used for patients who are unable to tolerate or absorb oral medications.

Note: American Heart Association (AHA) guidelines now recommend prophylaxis only in patients undergoing invasive procedures and in whom underlying cardiac conditions may predispose to a higher risk of adverse outcomes should infection occur. As of April 2007, routine prophylaxis for GI/GU procedures is no longer recommended by the AHA.

Intra-abdominal infection, complicated, community-acquired, mild-to-moderate (in combination with metronidazole): IV: 1 to 2 g every 12 to 24 hours for 4 to 7 days (provided source controlled) (Solomkin 2010)

Lyme neuroborreliosis (off-label use): IV: 2 g once daily for 14 days (Halperin 2007)

Meningitis (empiric treatment): IV: 2 g every 12 hours for 7 to 14 days (longer courses may be necessary for selected organisms)

Meningococcal disease, invasive, high-risk patient contacts (chemoprophylaxis) (off-label use): IM: 250 mg in a single dose (CDC 2005; Red Book [AAP 2012])

Pelvic inflammatory disease: IM: 250 mg in a single dose plus doxycycline (with or without metronidazole) (CDC 2010)

Prophylaxis against sexually-transmitted diseases following sexual assault: IM: 250 mg as a single dose (in combination with azithromycin and metronidazole) (CDC 2010)

Prosthetic joint infection: IV:

Staphylococci, oxacillin-susceptible: 1 to 2 g every 24 hours for 2 to 6 weeks (in combination with rifampin) followed by oral antibiotic treatment and suppressive regimens (Osmon 2013)

Streptococci, beta-hemolytic: 2 g every 24 hours for 4 to 6 weeks (Osmon 2013)

Pyelonephritis (acute, uncomplicated): Females: IV: 1 to 2 g once daily (Stamm 1993). Many physicians administer a single parenteral dose before initiating oral therapy (Warren 1999).

Septic/toxic shock (off-label use): IV: 2 g once daily; with clindamycin for toxic shock

Skin and soft tissue necrotizing infection (off-label use) (IDSA [Stevens 2014]): Note: Continue until further debridement is not necessary, patient has clinically improved, and patient is afebrile for 48 to 72 hours.

Due to Aeromonas hydrophilia: IV: 1 to 2 g once daily in combination with doxycycline

Due to Vibrio vulnificus: IV: 1 g once daily in combination with doxycycline

Surgical (perioperative) prophylaxis: IV: 1 g 30 minutes to 2 hours before surgery

Manufacturer's labeling: 1 g 30 minutes to 2 hours before surgery

Alternate dosing: 1 to 2 g within 60 minutes prior to surgery (Bratzler 2013)

Alternate dosing for colorectal procedures: 2 g within 60 minutes prior to surgery with concomitant metronidazole (Bratzler 2013)

Cholecystectomy: 1 to 2 g every 12 to 24 hours, discontinue within 24 hours unless infection outside gallbladder suspected (Solomkin 2010)

Surgical site infections (intestinal or genitourinary tract surgery, surgery of axilla, or perineum) (off-label use): IV: 1 g every 24 hours, in combination with metronidazole (IDSA [Stevens 2014])

Syphilis (off-label use): IM, IV: 1 g once daily for 10 to 14 days; **Note:** Alternative treatment for early syphilis, optimal dose, and duration have not been defined (CDC 2010).

Typhoid fever (off-label use): IV: 2 g every 12 to 24 hours for 10 to 14 days; **Note:** Usually reserved for fluoroquinolone resistant disease (WHO 2003).

Whipple disease (off-label use): IV: Initial: 2 g once daily for 10 to 14 days, then oral therapy (sulfamethoxazole and trimethoprim preferred) (Feurle 2010; Feurle 2013)

Pediatric

Dosage range: Infants, Children, and Adolescents: Usual dose: IM, IV:

Mild-to-moderate infections: 50 to 75 mg/kg/day in 1 to 2 divided doses every 12 to 24 hours (maximum: 2,000 mg daily); continue until at least 2 days after signs and symptoms of infection have resolved

Serious infections: 80-100 mg/kg/day in 1 to 2 divided doses (maximum: 4,000 mg daily)

Acute bacterial rhinosinusitis, severe infection requiring hospitalization (off-label use): IV: 50 mg/kg/day divided every 12 hours for 10 to 14 days (Chow 2012)

Bacterial enteric infections in HIV-infected patients (empiric treatment) (off-label use): Adolescents: IV: Refer to adult dosing.

Community-acquired pneumonia (CAP) (IDSA/PIDS [Bradley 2011]) (off-label dose): Infants >3 months and Children: IV: 50 to 100 mg/kg/day once daily or divided every 12 hours (maximum: 2,000 mg daily). **Note:** May consider addition of vancomycin or clindamycin to empiric therapy if community-acquired MRSA suspected. Use the higher end of the range for penicillin-resistant *S. pneumoniae*; in children ≥5 years, a macrolide antibiotic should be added if atypical pneumonia cannot be ruled out; preferred in patients not fully immunized for *H. influenzae* type b and *S. pneumoniae*, or significant local resistance to penicillin in invasive pneumococcal strains.

Epididymitis, acute (off-label use): Children >8 years (and ≥45 kg) and Adolescents: IM: 250 mg in a single dose with a concomitant doxycycline regimen (CDC 2010; Red Book [AAP 2012])

Epiglottis (off-label use): IV: 100 mg/kg/day as a single dose on day 1, then 50 mg/kg as a single dose on day 2 (Sawyer 1994) or 75 mg/kg once daily for 10 to 14 days (Low 2003). Additional data may be necessary to further define the role of ceftriaxone in this condition.

Gonococcal infections:

Arthritis (CDC 2010): IM, IV:

≤45 kg: 50 mg/kg/dose once daily (maximum: 1,000 mg) for 7 days

>45 kg: 50 mg/kg/dose once daily (maximum: 2,000 mg) for 7 days

Bacteremia (CDC 2010): IM, IV:

≤45 kg: 50 mg/kg/dose once daily (maximum: 1,000 mg) for 7 days

>45 kg: 50 mg/kg/dose once daily (maximum: 2,000 mg) for 7 days

Conjunctivitis (off-label use): IM, IV:

<45 kg: 50 mg/kg in a single dose (maximum: 1,000 mg) (Red Book [AAP 2012])

≥45 kg: Refer to adult dosing.

Disseminated (off-label use): IM, IV:

Infants: 25 to 50 mg/kg/dose once daily for 7 days (10 to 14 days for meningitis) (CDC 2010); **Note:** Use contraindicated in hyperbilirubinemic neonates.

Children <45 kg: 25 to 50 mg/kg/dose once daily (maximum: 1,000 mg) for 7 days (CDC 2010)

Children >45 kg: Refer to adult dosing.

Endocarditis (off-label use):

≤45 kg: IM, IV: 50 mg/kg/day divided every 12 hours (maximum: 2,000 mg daily) for at least 28 days (Red Book [AAP 2012])

>45 kg: IV: Refer to adult dosing.

Meningitis: IV:

≤45 kg: 50 mg/kg/day divided every 12 hours (maximum: 2,000 mg daily); usual duration of treatment is 10 to 14 days (Red Book [AAP 2012])

>45 kg: Refer to adult dosing.

Prophylaxis (due to maternal gonococcal infection): IM, IV: 25 to 50 mg/kg as a single dose (maximum: 125 mg) (CDC 2010)

Uncomplicated cervicitis, pharyngitis, proctitis, urethritis, vulvovaginitis (off-label use) (CDC 2010):

≤45 kg: IM: 125 mg as a single dose (with or without azithromycin or erythromycin) (Red Book [AAP 2012])

>45 kg: Refer to adult dosing.

Infective endocarditis (off-label use): IM, IV:

Native valve: 100 mg/kg once daily (maximum: 2,000 mg daily) for 2 to 4 weeks; **Note:** If using 2-week regimen or for relatively penicillin-resistant streptococcus, concurrent gentamicin is recommended; for HACEK organisms, duration of therapy is 4 weeks (Baddour 2005)

Prosthetic valve: 100 mg/kg once daily (maximum: 2,000 mg daily) for 6 weeks (with or without gentamicin [dependent on penicillin MIC]); for HACEK organisms, duration of therapy is 4 weeks (Baddour 2005)

Enterococcus faecalis (resistant to penicillin, aminoglycoside, and vancomycin), native or prosthetic valve: 100 mg/kg/day divided every 12 hours for ≥8 weeks administered concurrently with ampicillin (Baddour 2005)

Prophylaxis: 50 mg/kg 30 to 60 minutes before procedure; maximum dose: 1,000 mg (Red Book [AAP 2012]; Wilson 2007). Intramuscular injections should be avoided in patients who are receiving anticoagulant therapy. In these circumstances, orally administered regimens should be given whenever possible. Intravenously administered antibiotics should be used for patients who are unable to tolerate or absorb oral medications.

Note: American Heart Association (AHA) guidelines now recommend prophylaxis only in patients undergoing invasive procedures and in whom underlying cardiac conditions may predispose to a higher risk of adverse outcomes should infection occur. As of April 2007, routine prophylaxis for GI/GU procedures is no longer recommended by the AHA.

Lyme disease (off-label use): IM, IV:

Atrioventricular heart block or carditis: 50 to 75 mg/kg once daily (maximum: 2,000 mg) for 2 to 3 weeks (Red Book [AAP 2012])

Encephalitis or other late neurologic disease: 50 to 75 mg/kg once daily (maximum: 2,000 mg) for 2 to 4 weeks (Red Book [AAP 2012])

Neuroborreliosis: 50 to 75 mg/kg once daily (maximum: 2,000 mg) for 14 days (Halperin 2007)

Meningitis: 50 to 75 mg/kg once daily (maximum: 2,000 mg) for 2 weeks (Red Book [AAP 2012])

Persistent or recurrent arthritis: 50 to 75 mg/kg once daily (maximum: 2,000 mg) for 2 to 4 weeks (Red Book [AAP 2012])

Meningitis (empiric treatment): IM, IV: Loading dose of 100 mg/kg (maximum: 4,000 mg), followed by:

Manufacturer's labeling: 100 mg/kg/day divided every 12 to 24 hours (maximum: 4,000 mg daily); usual duration of treatment is 7 to 14 days

Alternate dosing: 80 to 100 mg/kg/day divided every 12 to 24 hours (maximum: 4,000 mg daily) (Tunkel 2004)

Meningococcal disease, invasive, high-risk patient contacts (chemoprophylaxis) (off-label use):

Children and Adolescents <15 years: IM: 125 mg in a single dose (CDC 2005; Red Book [AAP 2012]).

Adolescents ≥15 years: Refer to adult dosing.

Otitis media: IM:

Acute: 50 mg/kg in a single dose (maximum: 1,000 mg)

Persistent or relapsing (off-label dose): 50 mg/kg once daily for 3 days (AAP 2014; Lieberthal 2013)

Pneumonia: IV: 50 to 75 mg/kg once daily

Prophylaxis against sexually-transmitted diseases following sexual assault (off-label use):

≤45 kg: IM: 125 mg in a single dose (in combination with azithromycin and metronidazole) (CDC 2010)

>45 kg: Refer to adult dosing.

Shigella dysentery type 1 (off-label dose): IM: 50 to 100 mg/kg/day for 2 to 5 days (WHO 2005)

Skin/skin structure infections: IM, IV: 50 to 75 mg/kg/day in 1 to 2 divided doses (maximum: 2,000 mg daily)

Surgical (perioperative) prophylaxis (off-label dose): Children ≥1 year: IV: 50 to 75 mg/kg within 60 minutes prior to surgery (maximum: 2,000 mg) (Bratzler 2013)

Typhoid fever (off-label use): IV: 80 mg/kg once daily for 14 days (Stephens 2002)

Renal Impairment There are no dosage adjustments provided in the manufacturer's labeling; however, in patients with concurrent renal and hepatic impairment, maximum daily dose should not exceed 2 g.

ESRD requiring dialysis: Poorly dialyzed; no supplemental dose or dosage adjustment necessary, including patients on intermittent hemodialysis, peritoneal dialysis, or continuous renal replacement therapy (eg, CVVHD) (Aronoff 2007).

Hepatic Impairment There are no dosage adjustments provided in the manufacturer's labeling; however, in patients with concurrent renal and hepatic impairment, maximum daily dose should not exceed 2 g.

Dietary Considerations Some products may contain sodium.

Administration Do not coadminister with calcium-containing solutions.

IM: Inject deep IM into large muscle mass; a concentration of 250 mg/mL or 350 mg/mL is recommended for all vial sizes except the 250 mg size (250 mg/mL is suggested); can be diluted with 1:1 water or 1% lidocaine for IM administration only.

IV: Infuse as an intermittent infusion over 30 minutes. IV push administration over 1 to 4 minutes has been reported in children ≥12 years, adolescents, and adults (concentration: 100 mg/mL), primarily in patients outside the hospital setting (Baumgartner 1983; Garrelts 1988; Poole 1999), although a 2 g dose administered IV push over 5 minutes resulted in tachycardia, restlessness, diaphoresis, and palpitations in one patient (Lossos 1994). IV push administration in young infants may also have been a contributing factor in risk of cardiopulmonary events occurring from interactions between ceftriaxone and calcium (Bradley 2009).

Monitoring Parameters Prothrombin time/INR. Observe for signs and symptoms of anaphylaxis.

Test Interactions Positive direct Coombs', false-positive urinary glucose test using nonenzymatic methods, false-positive galactosemia tests.

Dosage Forms Excipient information presented when available (limited, particularly for generics); consult specific product labeling.

Solution, Intravenous:
Generic: 20 mg/mL (50 mL); 40 mg/mL (50 mL)
Solution Reconstituted, Injection:
Rocephin: 500 mg (1 ea); 1 g (1 ea)
Generic: 250 mg (1 ea); 500 mg (1 ea); 1 g (1 ea); 2 g (1 ea); 100 g (1 ea)
Solution Reconstituted, Intravenous:
Generic: 1 g (1 ea); 2 g (1 ea); 10 g (1 ea)

◆ Ceftriaxone for Injection (Can) *see* CefTRIAXone *on page 349*

◆ Ceftriaxone for Injection USP (Can) *see* CefTRIAXone *on page 349*

◆ Ceftriaxone Sodium *see* CefTRIAXone *on page 349*

◆ Ceftriaxone Sodium for Injection (Can) *see* CefTRIAXone *on page 349*

◆ Ceftriaxone Sodium for Injection BP (Can) *see* CefTRIAXone *on page 349*

Cefuroxime (se fyoor OKS eem)

Brand Names: US Ceftin; Zinacef; Zinacef in Sterile Water
Brand Names: Canada Apo-Cefuroxime; Auro-Cefuroxime; Ceftin; Cefuroxime For Injection; Cefuroxime For Injection, USP; PRO-Cefuroxime; ratio-Cefuroxime
Index Terms Cefuroxime Axetil; Cefuroxime Sodium
Pharmacologic Category Antibiotic, Cephalosporin (Second Generation)
Use

Acute bacterial maxillary sinusitis (tablets and oral suspension only): Treatment of mild-to-moderate acute bacterial maxillary sinusitis in infants ≥3 months, children, adolescents, and adults caused by *S. pneumoniae, H. influenzae* (non-beta-lactamase producing strains).

Note: According to the IDSA guidelines for acute bacterial rhinosinusitis, cefuroxime is no longer recommended as monotherapy for initial empiric treatment (Chow 2012).

Acute otitis media (tablets and oral suspension only): Treatment of infants ≥3 months and children with acute bacterial otitis media caused by *S. pneumoniae, H. influenzae* (including beta-lactamase-producing strains), *Moraxella catarrhalis* (including beta-lactamase-producing strains), or *S. pyogenes*

Bone and joint infections (injection only): Treatment of bone and joint infections caused by *Staphylococcus aureus* (penicillinase- and non-penicillinase-producing strains).

Bronchitis (acute bacterial and secondary bacterial) (tablets only): Treatment of acute bacterial exacerbations of chronic bronchitis and secondary bacterial infections of acute bronchitis in adolescents and adults caused by *Streptococcus pneumoniae, Haemophilus influenzae* (beta-lactamase negative strains), or *Haemophilus parainfluenzae* (beta-lactamase negative strains).

Lower respiratory tract infections (injection only): Treatment of lower respiratory tract infections, including pneumonia, caused by *S. pneumoniae, H. influenzae* (including ampicillin-resistant strains), *Klebsiella* spp., *S. aureus* (penicillinase- and non-penicillinase-producing strains), *Streptococcus pyogenes*, and *Escherichia coli*.

Lyme disease (early) (tablets only): Treatment of patients ≥13 years with early Lyme disease caused by *Borrelia burgdorferi*.

Pharyngitis/tonsillitis (tablets and oral suspension only): Treatment of mild-to-moderate pharyngitis and tonsillitis caused by *S. pyogenes*

Septicemia (injection only): Treatment of septicemia caused by *S. aureus* (penicillinase- and non-penicillinase-producing strains), *S. pneumoniae, E. coli, H. influenzae* (including ampicillin-resistant strains), and *Klebsiella* spp.

Skin and skin structure infection (impetigo) (oral suspension only): Treatment of pediatric patients 3 months to 12 years of age with skin or skin structure infections (impetigo) caused by *S. aureus* (including beta-lactamase-producing strains) or *S. pyogenes*.

Skin and skin structure infection (uncomplicated) (tablets only): Treatment of skin and skin-structure infections (including impetigo) caused by *S. aureus* (penicillinase- and non-penicillinase-producing strains), *S. pyogenes, E. coli, Klebsiella* spp., and *Enterobacter* spp.

Surgical (perioperative) prophylaxis (injection only): Prophylaxis of infection in patients undergoing surgical procedures (eg, vaginal hysterectomy) that are classified as clean-contaminated or potentially contaminated procedures.

Urinary tract infections (tablets and injection only): Treatment of urinary tract infections caused by *E. coli* and *Klebsiella* spp.

Pregnancy Considerations Adverse events were not observed in animal reproduction studies. Cefuroxime crosses the placenta and reaches the cord serum and amniotic fluid. Placental transfer is decreased in the presence of oligohydramnios. Several studies have failed to identify an increased teratogenic risk to the fetus following maternal cefuroxime use.

During pregnancy, mean plasma concentrations of cefuroxime are 50% lower, the AUC is 25% lower, and the plasma half-life is shorter than nonpregnant values. At term, plasma half-life is similar to nonpregnant values and peak maternal concentrations after IM administration are slightly decreased. Pregnancy does not alter the volume of distribution. Cefuroxime is one of the antibiotics recommended for prophylactic use prior to cesarean delivery.

Breast-Feeding Considerations Cefuroxime is excreted in breast milk. Manufacturer recommendations vary; caution is recommended if cefuroxime IV is given to a nursing woman and it is recommended to consider discontinuing nursing temporarily during treatment following oral cefuroxime. Nondose-related effects could include modification of bowel flora.

Contraindications Hypersensitivity to cefuroxime, any component of the formulation, or other beta-lactam antibacterial drugs (eg, penicillins and cephalosporins)

Warnings/Precautions Serious and occasionally severe or fatal hypersensitivity (anaphylactic) reactions have been reported in patients receiving beta-lactam drugs. Before initiating therapy, carefully investigate previous penicillin, cephalosporin, or other allergen hypersensitivity. Use caution if given to a patient with a penicillin or other beta-lactam allergy because cross sensitivity among beta-lactam antibacterial drugs has been established. If an allergic reaction occurs, discontinue and institute appropriate therapy. Modify dosage in patients with severe renal impairment. Use with caution in patients with a history of penicillin allergy, especially IgE-mediated reactions (eg, anaphylaxis, urticaria). Prolonged use may result in fungal or bacterial superinfection, including *C. difficile*-associated diarrhea (CDAD) and pseudomembranous colitis; CDAD has been observed >2 months postantibiotic treatment. Use with caution in patients with a history of colitis. Use with caution in patients with a history of seizure disorder; cephalosporins have been associated with seizure activity, particularly in patients with renal impairment not receiving dose adjustments. Discontinue if seizures occur. May be associated with increased INR, especially in nutritionally deficient patients, prolonged treatment, hepatic or renal disease. Tablets and oral suspension are not bioequivalent (do not substitute on a mg-per-mg basis). Tablets should not be crushed or chewed due to a strong, persistent bitter taste. Patients unable to swallow whole tablets should be prescribed the oral suspension. Potentially significant drug-drug interactions may exist, requiring dose or frequency adjustment, additional monitoring, and/or selection of alternative therapy.

Benzyl alcohol and derivatives: Some dosage forms may contain sodium benzoate/benzoic acid; benzoic acid (benzoate) is a metabolite of benzyl alcohol; large amounts of benzyl alcohol (≥99 mg/kg/day) have been associated with a potentially fatal toxicity ("gasping syndrome") in neonates; the "gasping syndrome" consists of metabolic acidosis, respiratory distress, gasping respirations, CNS dysfunction (including convulsions, intracranial

hemorrhage), hypotension, and cardiovascular collapse (AAP ["Inactive" 1997]; CDC 1982); some data suggests that benzoate displaces bilirubin from protein binding sites (Ahlfors 2001); avoid or use dosage forms containing benzyl alcohol derivative with caution in neonates. See manufacturer's labeling.

Phenylalanine: Some products may contain phenylalanine.

Adverse Reactions

>10%: Gastrointestinal: Diarrhea (4% to 11%, duration dependent)

1% to 10%:

Cardiovascular: Local thrombophlebitis (2%)

Dermatologic: Diaper rash (children 3%)

Endocrine & metabolic: Increased lactate dehydrogenase (1%)

Gastrointestinal: Nausea and vomiting (3% to 7%), unpleasant taste (children 5%)

Genitourinary: Vaginitis (≤5%)

Hematologic & oncologic: Decreased hematocrit (≤10%), decreased hemoglobin (≤10%), eosinophilia (1% to 7%)

Hepatic: Increased serum transaminases (2% to 4%), increased serum alkaline phosphatase (2%)

Immunologic: Jarisch-Herxheimer reaction (6%)

<1% (Limited to important or life-threatening): Anaphylaxis, angioedema, anorexia, brain disease, candidiasis, chest tightness, cholestasis, Clostridium difficile associated diarrhea, colitis, decreased creatinine clearance, drug fever, dyspepsia, dysuria, erythema, erythema multiforme, gastrointestinal hemorrhage, gastrointestinal infection, glossitis, headache, hearing loss, hemolytic anemia, hepatitis, hyperactivity, hyperbilirubinemia, hypersensitivity, hypersensitivity angiitis, increased blood urea nitrogen, increased liver enzymes, increased serum creatinine, increased thirst, interstitial nephritis, irritability, joint swelling, leukopenia, muscle cramps, muscle rigidity, muscle spasm (neck), neutropenia, oral mucosa ulcer, pancytopenia, positive direct Coombs test, prolonged prothrombin time, pseudomembranous colitis, renal insufficiency, renal pain, seizure, serum sickness-like reaction, sialorrhea, sinusitis, Stevens-Johnson syndrome, swollen tongue, tachycardia, thrombocytopenia (rare), toxic epidermal necrolysis, trismus, upper respiratory tract infection, urethral bleeding, urethral pain, urinary tract infection, vaginal discharge, vaginal irritation, viral infection, vulvovaginal candidiasis, vulvovaginal pruritus

Drug Interactions

Metabolism/Transport Effects None known.

Avoid Concomitant Use

Avoid concomitant use of Cefuroxime with any of the following: BCG (Intravesical)

Increased Effect/Toxicity

Cefuroxime may increase the levels/effects of: Aminoglycosides; Vitamin K Antagonists

The levels/effects of Cefuroxime may be increased by: Probenecid

Decreased Effect

Cefuroxime may decrease the levels/effects of: BCG (Intravesical); BCG Vaccine (Immunization); Sodium Picosulfate; Typhoid Vaccine

The levels/effects of Cefuroxime may be decreased by: Antacids; H2-Antagonists

Food Interactions Bioavailability is increased with food; cefuroxime serum levels may be increased if taken with food or dairy products. Management: Administer tablet without regard to meals; suspension must be administered with food.

Preparation for Administration

Oral suspension: Refer to manufacturer's product labeling for reconstitution instructions.

Duplex container: Unlatch side tab, unfold, and remove foil strip from drug chamber. Point set port in downward direction, fold container just below the diluent meniscus, and squeeze the diluent chamber until the seal between the diluent and drug powder opens. Shake until dissolved.

Storage/Stability

Injection: Store intact vials at 15°C to 30°C (59°F to 86°F); protect from light. Reconstituted solution is stable for 24 hours at room temperature and 48 hours when refrigerated. IV infusion in NS or D₅W solution is stable for 24 hours at room temperature, 7 days when refrigerated, or 26 weeks when frozen. After freezing, thawed solution is stable for 24 hours at room temperature or 21 days when refrigerated.

Duplex container: Store unactivated units at 20°C to 25°C (68°F to 77°F). Unactivated units with foil strip removed from the drug chamber must be protected from light and used within 7 days. Once activated, may be stored for up to 24 hours at room temperature or for 7 days under refrigeration. Do not freeze.

ADD-Vantage vials: Joined, but not activated, vials are stable for 14 days. Once activated, stable for 24 hours at room temperature and 7 days refrigerated. Do not freeze.

Premix Galaxy plastic containers: Store frozen at -20°C. Thaw container at room temperature or under refrigeration; do not force thaw. Thawed solution is stable for 24 hours at room temperature and 28 days refrigerated; do not refreeze.

Oral suspension: Prior to reconstitution, store at 2°C to 30°C (36°F to 86°F). Reconstituted suspension is stable for 10 days at 2°C to 8°C (36°F to 46°F).

Tablet: Store at 15°C to 30°C (59°F to 86°F).

Mechanism of Action Inhibits bacterial cell wall synthesis by binding to one or more of the penicillin-binding proteins (PBPs) which in turn inhibits the final transpeptidation step of peptidoglycan synthesis in bacterial cell walls, thus inhibiting cell wall biosynthesis. Bacteria eventually lyse due to ongoing activity of cell wall autolytic enzymes (autolysins and murein hydrolases) while cell wall assembly is arrested.

Pharmacodynamics/Kinetics

Absorption: Oral tablet: Increases with food

Distribution: Widely to body tissues and fluids including bronchial secretions, synovial and pericardial fluid, kidneys, heart, liver, bone and bile; crosses blood-brain barrier; therapeutic concentrations achieved in CSF even when meninges are not inflamed

Protein binding: 33% to 50%

Metabolism: Cefuroxime axetil (oral) is hydrolyzed in the intestinal mucosa and blood to cefuroxime

Bioavailability: Tablet: Fasting: 37%; Following food: 52%; cefuroxime axetil suspension is less bioavailable than the tablet (91% of the AUC for tablets)

Half-life elimination:

Premature neonates:

PNA ≤3 days: Median: 5.8 hours (de Louvois 1982)

PNA ≥8 days: Median: 1.6-3.8 hours (de Louvois 1982)

Children and Adolescents: 1.4-1.9 hours

Adults: ~1 to 2 hours; prolonged with renal impairment

Time to peak, serum: IM: ~15 to 60 minutes; IV: 2 to 3 minutes; Oral: Children: ~3 to 4 hours; Adults: ~2 to 3 hours

Excretion: Urine (66% to 100% as unchanged drug)

Dosing

Adult & Geriatric Note: Cefuroxime axetil film-coated tablets and oral suspension are not bioequivalent and are not substitutable on a mg/mg basis. All oral doses listed are for tablet formulation:

Acute bacterial maxillary sinusitis: Oral: 250 mg twice daily for 10 days

Bronchitis, acute (and exacerbations of chronic bronchitis):

Oral: 250 to 500 mg every 12 hours for 10 days

IV: 500 to 750 mg every 8 hours (complete therapy with oral dosing)

Cholecystitis, mild-to-moderate: IV: 1.5 g every 8 hours for 4 to 7 days (provided source controlled) (Solomkin 2010)

Intra-abdominal infection, complicated, community-acquired, mild-to-moderate (in combination with metronidazole): IV: 1.5 g every 8 hours for 4 to 7 days (provided source controlled) (Solomkin 2010)

Lyme disease (early): Oral: 500 mg twice daily for 20 days

Pharyngitis/tonsillitis: Oral: 250 mg twice daily for 10 days

Pneumonia, uncomplicated: IM, IV: 750 mg every 8 hours. **Note:** Cefuroxime is considered an **alternate** therapy for lower respiratory tract infections in adults caused by Streptococcus pneumoniae (with MICs <2 mcg/mL for penicillin) (Mandell 2007).

Severe or complicated infections: IM, IV: 1.5 g every 8 hours (up to 1.5 g every 6 hours in life-threatening infections)

Skin/skin structure infection, uncomplicated:

Oral: 250 to 500 mg every 12 hours for 10 days

IM, IV: 750 mg every 8 hours

Surgical (perioperative) prophylaxis: IV:

Manufacturer's labeling: 1.5 g 30 minutes to 1 hour prior to procedure (if procedure is prolonged can give 750 mg every 8 hours IV or IM)

Open heart: IV: 1.5 g every 12 hours for a total of 4 doses starting at anesthesia induction

Alternative recommendation: 1.5 g within 60 minutes prior to surgical incision. Doses may be repeated in 4 hours if procedure is lengthy or if there is excessive blood loss (Bratzler 2013).

Urinary tract infection, uncomplicated:
Oral: 250 mg twice daily for 7 to 10 days
IV, IM: 750 mg every 8 hours

Bite wounds (animal) (off-label use) (IDSA [Stevens 2014]): Oral: 500 mg twice daily in combination with clindamycin or metronidazole for anaerobic coverage

Pediatric Note: Cefuroxime axetil film-coated tablets and oral suspension are not bioequivalent and are not substitutable on a mg/mg basis.

Children ≥1 year:

Surgical (perioperative) prophylaxis: IV: 50 mg/kg within 60 minutes prior to surgical incision (maximum dose: 1,500 mg). Doses may be repeated in 4 hours if procedure is lengthy or if there is excessive blood loss (Bratzler 2013).

Infants and Children ≥3 months and ≤12 years:

Acute bacterial maxillary sinusitis, acute otitis media:
Oral: Suspension: 30 mg/kg/day in 2 divided doses for 10 days (maximum dose: 1,000 mg/day); tablet: 250 mg twice daily for 10 days
IM, IV: 75 to 150 mg/kg/day divided every 8 hours (maximum dose: 6 g/day)

Pharyngitis/tonsillitis:
Oral: Suspension: 20 mg/kg/day (maximum: 500 mg/day) in 2 divided doses for 10 days
IM, IV: 75 to 150 mg/kg day divided every 8 hours (maximum: 6 g/day)

Skin and skin structure infection (impetigo): Oral: Suspension: 30 mg/kg/day in 2 divided doses for 10 days (maximum dose: 1,000 mg/day)

Urinary tract infection, uncomplicated (off-label dosing):
Infants and Children ≥2 months to 2 years: Oral: 20 to 30 mg/kg/day divided twice daily for 7 to 14 days (AAP 2011)
Children ≥2 years: Moderate to severe disease (possible pyelonephritis): Oral: 20 to 30 mg/kg/day divided twice daily (maximum dose: 1,000 mg/day) (Bradley 2012; *Red Book* [AAP 2012])

Children >12 years and Adolescents: Refer to adult dosing.

Renal Impairment
Oral:
Manufacturer's labeling:
Adults:
CrCl ≥30 mL/minute: No dosage adjustment necessary
CrCl 10 to <30 mL/minute: Administer recommended dose based on indication every 24 hours
CrCl <10 mL/minute: Administer recommended dose based on indication every 48 hours
ESRD requiring intermittent hemodialysis (IHD): Additional recommended dose based on indication should be given at the end of each dialysis session.

Pediatric: There are no dosage adjustments provided in the manufacturer's labeling; however, the following adjustments have been reported in the literature (Aronoff 2007): **Note:** Renally adjusted dose recommendations are based on doses of 30 mg/kg/day divided every 12 hours:
CrCl ≥30 mL/minute/1.73 m^2: No dosage adjustment necessary.
CrCl 10 to 29 mL/minute/1.73 m^2: 15 mg/kg/dose every 12 hours.
CrCl <10 mL/minute/1.73 m^2: 15 mg/kg/dose every 24 hours.
Hemodialysis: Dialyzable: 15 mg/kg/dose every 24 hours
Peritoneal dialysis: 15 mg/kg/dose every 24 hours

IV: Children and Adults:
Manufacturer's labeling:
CrCl >20 mL/minute: No dosage adjustment necessary
CrCl 10 to 20 mL/minute: Administer recommended dose based on indication every 12 hours
CrCl <10 mL/minute: Administer recommended dose based on indication every 24 hours
Hemodialysis: Administer additional recommended dose based on indication at the end of dialysis
Alternate dosing (Aronoff 2007):
Peritoneal dialysis:
Adults: Administer full dose every 24 hours
Children: 25 to 50 mg/kg dose every 24 hours
Continuous renal replacement therapy (CRRT):
Adults: 1 g every 12 hours
Children: 25 to 50 mg/kg every 8 hours

Hepatic Impairment There are no dosage adjustments provided in the manufacturer's labeling.

Dietary Considerations Some products may contain phenylalanine and/or sodium.
Oral suspension: Should be taken with food.

Administration
Oral suspension: Administer with food. Shake well before use.
Oral tablet: May administer with or without food. Swallow tablet whole (crushed tablet has strong, persistent, bitter taste).
IM: Inject deep IM into large muscle mass.
IV: Inject direct IV over 3 to 5 minutes. Infuse intermittent infusion over 15 to 30 minutes.

Monitoring Parameters Monitor renal, hepatic, and hematologic function periodically with prolonged therapy. Monitor prothrombin time in patients at risk of prolongation during cephalosporin therapy (nutritionally-deficient, prolonged treatment, renal or hepatic disease). Observe for signs and symptoms of anaphylaxis during first dose.

Test Interactions Positive direct Coombs', false-positive urinary glucose test using cupric sulfate (Benedict's solution, Clinitest®, Fehling's solution); false-negative may occur with ferricyanide test. Glucose oxidase or hexokinase-based methods should be used.

Dosage Forms Excipient information presented when available (limited, particularly for generics); consult specific product labeling.
Solution, Intravenous, as sodium [strength expressed as base]:
Zinacef in Sterile Water: 1.5 g (50 mL)
Solution Reconstituted, Injection, as sodium [strength expressed as base]:
Zinacef: 750 mg (1 ea); 1.5 g (1 ea); 7.5 g (1 ea)
Generic: 750 mg (1 ea); 1.5 g (1 ea); 7.5 g (1 ea); 75 g (1 ea); 225 g (1 ea)
Solution Reconstituted, Intravenous, as sodium [strength expressed as base]:
Zinacef: 750 mg (1 ea); 1.5 g (1 ea)
Generic: 750 mg (1 ea); 1.5 g (1 ea); 7.5 g (1 ea)
Suspension Reconstituted, Oral, as axetil [strength expressed as base]:
Ceftin: 125 mg/5 mL (100 mL); 250 mg/5 mL (50 mL, 100 mL) [contains aspartame; tutti-frutti flavor]
Generic: 125 mg/5 mL (100 mL)
Tablet, Oral, as axetil [strength expressed as base]:
Ceftin: 250 mg, 500 mg
Generic: 250 mg, 500 mg

Celecoxib (se le KOKS ib)

Brand Names: US CeleBREX
Brand Names: Canada ACCEL-Celecoxib; ACT Celecoxib; Apo-Celecoxib; Bio-Celecoxib; Celebrex; GD-Celecoxib; JAMP-Celecoxib; Mar-Celecoxib; Mint-Celecoxib; Mylan-Celecoxib; PMS-Celecoxib; Priva-Celecoxib; RAN-Celecoxib; Riva-Celecoxib; Sandoz-Celecoxib; Teva-Celecoxib

Pharmacologic Category Nonsteroidal Anti-inflammatory Drug (NSAID), COX-2 Selective
Use
Acute pain: Management of acute pain.
Ankylosing spondylitis: Relief of the signs/symptoms of ankylosing spondylitis.
Juvenile idiopathic arthritis: Relief of the signs/symptoms of juvenile idiopathic arthritis (JIA) in patients 2 years and older.
Osteoarthritis: Relief of the signs/symptoms of osteoarthritis.
Primary dysmenorrhea: Treatment of primary dysmenorrhea.
Rheumatoid arthritis: Relief of the signs/symptoms of rheumatoid arthritis.
Pregnancy Considerations Teratogenic effects have been observed in some animal studies; therefore, celecoxib is classified as pregnancy category C. Celecoxib is a NSAID that primarily inhibits COX-2 whereas other currently available NSAIDs are nonselective for COX-1 and COX-2. The effects of this selective inhibition to the fetus have not been well studied and limited information is

available specific to celecoxib. NSAID exposure during the first trimester is not strongly associated with congenital malformations; however, cardiovascular anomalies and cleft palate have been observed following NSAID exposure in some studies. The use of a NSAID close to conception may be associated with an increased risk of miscarriage. Nonteratogenic effects have been observed following NSAID administration during the third trimester including: Myocardial degenerative changes, prenatal constriction of the ductus arteriosus, fetal tricuspid regurgitation, failure of the ductus arteriosus to close postnatally; renal dysfunction or failure, oligohydramnios; gastrointestinal bleeding or perforation, increased risk of necrotizing enterocolitis; intracranial bleeding (including intraventricular hemorrhage), platelet dysfunction with resultant bleeding; pulmonary hypertension. Because it may cause premature closure of the ductus arteriosus, the use of celecoxib is not recommended ≥30 weeks gestation. The chronic use of NSAIDs in women of reproductive age may be associated with infertility that is reversible upon discontinuation of the medication. A registry is available for pregnant women exposed to autoimmune medications including celecoxib. For additional information contact the Organization of Teratology Information Specialists, OTIS Autoimmune Diseases Study, at 877-311-8972.

Breast-Feeding Considerations Small amounts of celecoxib are found in breast milk. The manufacturer recommends that caution be exercised when administering celecoxib to nursing women.

Medication Guide Available Yes

Contraindications

Hypersensitivity to celecoxib, sulfonamides, aspirin, other NSAIDs, or any component of the formulation; patients who have demonstrated allergic-type reactions to sulfonamides; patients who have experienced asthma, urticaria, or allergic-type reactions after taking aspirin or other NSAIDs; treatment of perioperative pain in the setting of CABG surgery; active gastrointestinal bleeding.

Note: Although the FDA approved product labeling states this medication is contraindicated with other sulfonamide-containing drug classes, the scientific basis of this statement has been challenged. See "Warnings/Precautions" for more detail.

Canadian labeling: Additional contraindications (not in US labeling): Pregnancy (third trimester); women who are breast-feeding; severe, uncontrolled heart failure; active gastrointestinal ulcer (gastric, duodenal, peptic); inflammatory bowel disease; cerebrovascular bleeding; severe liver impairment or active hepatic disease; severe renal impairment (CrCl <30 mL/minute) or deteriorating renal disease; known hyperkalemia; use in patients <18 years of age

Warnings/Precautions [US Boxed Warning]: NSAIDs are associated with an increased risk of serious (and potentially fatal) adverse cardiovascular thrombotic events, including MI and stroke. Risk may be increased with duration of use or preexisting cardiovascular risk factors or disease. Carefully evaluate individual cardiovascular risk profiles prior to prescribing. New-onset or exacerbation of hypertension may occur (NSAIDs may impair response to thiazide or loop diuretics); may contribute to cardiovascular events; monitor blood pressure; use with caution in patients with hypertension. May cause sodium and fluid retention; use with caution in patients with edema, cerebrovascular disease, or ischemic heart disease. Avoid use in patients with heart failure (ACCF/AHA [Yancy, 2013]). Long-term cardiovascular risk in children has not been evaluated.

[US Boxed Warning]: Celecoxib is contraindicated for treatment of perioperative pain in the setting of coronary artery bypass graft (CABG) surgery. Risk of MI and stroke may be increased with use following CABG surgery.

[US Boxed Warning]: NSAIDs may increase risk of serious gastrointestinal ulceration, bleeding, and perforation (may be fatal). These events may occur at any time during therapy and without warning. Use is contraindicated with active GI bleeding. Use caution with a history of GI ulcers, concurrent therapy with aspirin, anticoagulants and/or corticosteroids, smoking, use of alcohol, the elderly or debilitated patients. When used concomitantly with aspirin, a substantial increase in the risk of gastrointestinal complications (eg, ulcer) occurs; concomitant gastroprotective therapy (eg, proton pump inhibitors) is recommended (Bhatt, 2008).

Use the lowest effective dose for the shortest duration of time, consistent with individual patient goals, to reduce risk of cardiovascular or GI adverse events. Alternate therapies should be considered for patients at high risk.

NSAIDs may cause serious skin adverse events including exfoliative dermatitis, Stevens-Johnson syndrome (SJS), and toxic epidermal necrolysis (TEN); may occur without warning and in patients without prior known sulfa allergy. Anaphylactoid reactions may occur, even without prior exposure; patients with "aspirin triad" (bronchial asthma, aspirin intolerance, rhinitis) may be at increased risk. Do not use in patients who have experienced an anaphylactic reaction with NSAID or aspirin therapy. The manufacturer's labeling states to not administer to patients with aspirin-sensitive asthma due to severe and potentially fatal bronchospasm that has been reported in such patients having received aspirin and the potential for cross reactivity with other NSAIDs. The manufacturer also states to use with caution in patients with other forms of asthma. However, in patients with known aspirin-exacerbated respiratory disease (AERD), the use of celecoxib initiated at a low dose with gradual titration in patients with stable, mild-to-moderate persistent asthma has been used without incident (Morales, 2013).

Use with caution in patients with decreased hepatic (dosage adjustments are recommended for moderate hepatic impairment; not recommended for patients with severe hepatic impairment) or renal function. Transaminase elevations have been reported with use; closely monitor patients with any abnormal LFT. Severe hepatic reactions (eg, fulminant hepatitis, liver failure) have occurred with NSAID use, rarely; discontinue if signs or symptoms of liver disease develop, if systemic manifestations occur, or with persistent or worsening abnormal hepatic function tests. NSAID use may compromise existing renal function; dose-dependent decreases in prostaglandin synthesis may result from NSAID use, causing a reduction in renal blood flow which may cause renal decompensation (usually reversible). Patients with impaired renal function, dehydration, heart failure, liver dysfunction, those taking diuretics, ACE inhibitors, angiotensin II receptor blockers, and the elderly are at greater risk for renal toxicity. Rehydrate patient before starting therapy; monitor renal function closely. Not recommended for use in patients with advanced renal disease or severe renal insufficiency; discontinue use with persistent or worsening abnormal renal function tests. Long-term NSAID use may result in renal papillary necrosis. Should not be considered a treatment or replacement of corticosteroid-dependent diseases.

Anaphylactoid reactions may occur, even with no prior exposure to celecoxib. Use with caution in patients with known or suspected deficiency of cytochrome P450 isoenzyme 2C9; poor metabolizers may have higher plasma levels due to reduced metabolism; consider reduced initial doses. Alternate therapies should be considered in patients with JIA who are poor metabolizers of CYP2C9.

Anemia may occur with use; monitor hemoglobin or hematocrit in patients on long-term treatment. Celecoxib does not affect PT, PTT or platelet counts; does not inhibit platelet aggregation at approved doses. Potentially significant drug-drug interactions may exist, requiring dose or frequency adjustment, additional monitoring, and/or selection of alternative therapy.

Use with caution in pediatric patients with systemic-onset juvenile idiopathic arthritis (JIA); serious adverse reactions, including disseminated intravascular coagulation, may occur. The Canadian labeling contraindicates use in patients <18 years of age.

Sulfonamide ("sulfa") allergy: The FDA-approved product labeling for many medications containing a sulfonamide chemical group includes a broad contraindication in patients with a prior allergic reaction to sulfonamides. There is a potential for cross-reactivity between members of a specific class (eg, two antibiotic sulfonamides). However, concerns for cross-reactivity have previously extended to all compounds containing the sulfonamide structure (SO_2NH_2). An expanded understanding of allergic mechanisms indicates cross-reactivity between antibiotic sulfonamides and nonantibiotic sulfonamides may not occur or at the very least this potential is extremely low (Brackett 2004; Johnson 2005; Slatore 2004; Tornero 2004). In particular, mechanisms of cross-reaction due to antibody production (anaphylaxis) are unlikely to occur with nonantibiotic sulfonamides. T-cell-mediated (type IV) reactions (eg, maculopapular rash) are less well understood and it is not possible to completely exclude this potential based on current insights. In cases where prior reactions were severe (Stevens-Johnson syndrome/TEN), some clinicians choose to avoid exposure to these classes.

Adverse Reactions

≥2%:

Cardiovascular: Peripheral edema

Central nervous system: Dizziness, headache, insomnia

Dermatologic: Skin rash

Gastrointestinal: Abdominal pain, diarrhea, dyspepsia, flatulence, nausea, vomiting

Neuromuscular & skeletal: Arthralgia, back pain

Respiratory: Cough, nasopharyngitis, pharyngitis, rhinitis, sinusitis, upper respiratory tract infection

Miscellaneous: Fever

0.1% to 1.9%:

Cardiovascular: Angina pectoris, aortic insufficiency, chest pain, coronary artery disease, edema, facial edema, hypertension (aggravated), myocardial infarction, palpitations, sinus bradycardia, tachycardia, ventricular hypertrophy

Central nervous system: Anxiety, depression, drowsiness, fatigue, hypertonia, hypoesthesia, migraine, nervousness, pain, paresthesia, vertigo

Dermatologic: Alopecia, cellulitis, dermatitis, diaphoresis, erythematous rash, maculopapular rash, pruritus, skin photosensitivity, urticaria, xeroderma

Endocrine & metabolic: Albuminuria, decreased plasma testosterone, hot flash, hypercholesterolemia, hyperglycemia, hypokalemia, increased nonprotein nitrogen, ovarian cyst, weight gain

Gastrointestinal: Anorexia, constipation, diverticulitis, dysphagia, eructation, esophagitis, gastritis, gastroenteritis, gastroesophageal reflux disease, gastrointestinal ulcer, hemorrhoids, hiatal hernia, increased appetite, melena, stomatitis, tenesmus, xerostomia

Genitourinary: Cystitis, dysuria, hematuria, urinary frequency

Hematologic & oncologic: Anemia, bruise, thrombocythemia

Hepatic: Increased serum alkaline phosphatase, increased serum transaminases

Hypersensitivity: Hypersensitivity exacerbation, hypersensitivity reaction

Neuromuscular & skeletal: Increased creatine phosphokinase, leg cramps, myalgia, osteoarthritis, synovitis, tendonitis

Ophthalmic: Conjunctival hemorrhage, vitreous opacity

Otic: Deafness, labyrinthitis, tinnitus

Renal: Increased blood urea nitrogen, increased serum creatinine, nephrolithiasis

Respiratory: Bronchitis, bronchospasm, dyspnea, epistaxis, flu-like symptoms, laryngitis, pneumonia

Miscellaneous: Cyst

<0.1% (Limited to important or life-threatening): Acute renal failure, agranulocytosis, anaphylactoid reaction, angioedema, anosmia, aplastic anemia, aseptic meningitis, cardiac failure, cerebrovascular accident, cholelithiasis, colitis, deep vein thrombosis, dysgeusia, erythema multiforme, esophageal perforation, exfoliative dermatitis, gangrene of skin or other tissue, gastrointestinal hemorrhage, hepatic failure, hepatic necrosis, hepatitis (including fulminant), hypoglycemia, hyponatremia, interstitial nephritis, intestinal obstruction, intestinal perforation, intracranial hemorrhage, jaundice, leukopenia, pancreatitis, pancytopenia, pulmonary embolism, renal papillary necrosis, sepsis, Stevens-Johnson syndrome, syncope, thrombocytopenia, thrombophlebitis, toxic epidermal necrolysis, vasculitis, ventricular fibrillation

Drug Interactions

Metabolism/Transport Effects Substrate of CYP2C9 (major), CYP3A4 (minor); **Note:** Assignment of Major/Minor substrate status based on clinically relevant drug interaction potential; **Inhibits** CYP2C8 (moderate), CYP2D6 (moderate)

Avoid Concomitant Use

Avoid concomitant use of Celecoxib with any of the following: Amodiaquine; Dexketoprofen; Floctafenine; Ketorolac (Nasal); Ketorolac (Systemic); Mecamylamine; Morniflumate; Nonsteroidal Anti-Inflammatory Agents; NSAID (COX-2 Inhibitor); Omacetaxine; Talniflumate; Thioridazine

Increased Effect/Toxicity

Celecoxib may increase the levels/effects of: 5-ASA Derivatives; Aliskiren; Aminoglycosides; Amodiaquine; Anticoagulants; ARIPiprazole; Bisphosphonate Derivatives; Brexpiprazole; CycloSPORINE (Systemic); CYP2C8 Substrates; CYP2D6 Substrates; Deferasirox; Desmopressin; Digoxin; DOXOrubicin (Conventional); Drospirenone; Eliglustat; Eplerenone; Estrogen Derivatives; Fesoterodine; Haloperidol; Lithium; Mecamylamine; Methotrexate; Metoprolol; Nebivolol; NSAID (COX-2 Inhibitor); Omacetaxine; Porfimer; Potassium-Sparing Diuretics; PRALAtrexate; Prilocaine; Quinolone Antibiotics; Sodium Nitrite; Tacrolimus (Systemic); Tenofovir Products; Thioridazine; Vancomycin; Verteporfin; Vitamin K Antagonists

The levels/effects of Celecoxib may be increased by: ACE Inhibitors; Alcohol (Ethyl); Angiotensin II Receptor Blockers; Antidepressants (Tricyclic, Tertiary Amine); Aspirin; Ceritinib; Corticosteroids (Systemic); CycloSPORINE (Systemic); CYP2C9 Inhibitors (Moderate); CYP2C9 Inhibitors (Strong); Dapsone (Topical); Dexketoprofen; Floctafenine; Herbs (Anticoagulant/Antiplatelet Properties); Ketorolac (Nasal); Ketorolac (Systemic); Loop Diuretics; Lumacaftor; Mifepristone; Morniflumate; Nitric Oxide; Nonsteroidal Anti-Inflammatory Agents; Probenecid; Propafenone; Selective Serotonin Reuptake Inhibitors; Sodium Phosphates; Talniflumate; Thiazide Diuretics; Treprostinil

Decreased Effect

Celecoxib may decrease the levels/effects of: ACE Inhibitors; Aliskiren; Angiotensin II Receptor Blockers; Beta-Blockers; Codeine; Eplerenone; HydrALAZINE; Loop Diuretics; Potassium-Sparing Diuretics; Prostaglandins (Ophthalmic); Selective Serotonin Reuptake Inhibitors; Tamoxifen; Thiazide Diuretics; TraMADol

The levels/effects of Celecoxib may be decreased by: Bile Acid Sequestrants; CYP2C9 Inducers (Strong); Dabrafenib; Enzalutamide; Lumacaftor

Food Interactions Peak concentrations are delayed and AUC is increased by 10% to 20% when taken with a high-fat meal. Management: Administer without regard to meals.

Storage/Stability Store at 25°C (77°F); excursions permitted to 15°C to 30°C (59°F to 86°F).

Mechanism of Action Inhibits prostaglandin synthesis by decreasing the activity of the enzyme, cyclooxygenase-2 (COX-2), which results in decreased formation of prostaglandin precursors; has antipyretic, analgesic, and anti-inflammatory properties. Celecoxib does not inhibit cyclooxygenase-1 (COX-1) at therapeutic concentrations.

Pharmacodynamics/Kinetics

Absorption: Prolonged due to low solubility

Distribution: V_d (apparent): Children and Adolescents ~7-16 years (steady-state): 8.3 ± 5.8 L/kg (Stempak 2002); Adults: ~400 L

Protein binding: ~97% primarily to albumin; binds to alpha$_1$-acid glycoprotein to a lesser extent

Metabolism: Hepatic via CYP2C9; forms inactive metabolites (a primary alcohol, corresponding carboxylic acid, and its glucuronide conjugate)

Bioavailability: Absolute: Unknown

Half-life elimination: Children and Adolescents ~7-16 years (steady-state): 6 ± 2.7 hours (range: 3-10 hours) (Stempak 2002); Adults: ~11 hours (fasted)

Time to peak: Children: Median: 3 hours (range: 1-5.8 hours) (Stempak 2002); Adults: ~3 hours

Excretion: Feces (~57% as metabolites, <3% as unchanged drug); urine (27% as metabolites, <3% as unchanged drug); primary metabolites in feces and urine: Carboxylic acid metabolite (73% of dose); low amounts of glucuronide metabolite appear in urine

Dosing

Adult Note: Use the lowest effective dose for the shortest duration of time, consistent with individual patient treatment goals.

Osteoarthritis: Oral: 200 mg/day as a single dose or in divided doses twice daily

Ankylosing spondylitis: Oral: 200 mg/day as a single dose or in divided doses twice daily; if no effect after 6 weeks, may increase to 400 mg/day. If no response following 6 weeks of treatment with 400 mg/day, consider discontinuation and alternative treatment.

Canadian labeling; Recommended maximum dose: 200 mg/day

Rheumatoid arthritis: Oral: 100-200 mg twice daily

Acute pain or primary dysmenorrhea: Oral: Initial dose: 400 mg, followed by an additional 200 mg if needed on day 1; maintenance dose: 200 mg twice daily as needed

Canadian labeling; Recommended maximum dose for treatment of acute pain: 400 mg/day up to 7 days

Acute gout (off-label use): 800 mg once followed by 400 mg on day 1; then 400 mg twice daily for one week (ACR guidelines [Khanna, 2012]; Schumacker, 2012)

Dosing adjustment in poor CYP2C9 metabolizers (eg, CYP2C9*3/*3): Consider reducing initial dose by 50%; consider alternative treatment in patients with JIA who are poor CYP2C9 metabolizers.

Canadian labeling; Recommended maximum dose: 100 mg/day.

Geriatric Refer to adult dosing. No specific adjustment based on age is recommended. However, the AUC in elderly patients may be increased by 50% as compared to younger subjects. Initiate at the lowest recommended dose in patients weighing <50 kg.

Pediatric Note: Use the lowest effective dose for the shortest duration of time, consistent with individual patient treatment goals. Use in patients <18 years of age is not approved in the Canadian labeling.

Juvenile idiopathic arthritis (JIA): Oral: Children ≥2 years:

≥10 kg to ≤25 kg: 50 mg twice daily
>25 kg: 100 mg twice daily

Dosing adjustment in poor CYP2C9 metabolizers (eg, CYP2C9*3/*3): Consider alternative therapy.

Renal Impairment
US labeling:
Mild or moderate impairment: There are no dosage adjustments provided in the manufacturer's labeling; AUC was ~40% lower in patients with chronic renal insufficiency (GFR 35 to 60 mL/minute) compared with subjects with normal renal function.
Severe impairment: Use is not recommended.
Advanced renal disease: Use is not recommended; however, if celecoxib treatment cannot be avoided, monitor renal function closely.
Abnormal renal function tests (persistent or worsening): Discontinue use.
Canadian labeling:
CrCl ≥30 mL/minute: No dosage adjustment necessary.
CrCl <30 mL/minute: Use is contraindicated.
Abnormal renal function tests (persistent or worsening): Discontinue use.

Hepatic Impairment
Mild impairment (Child-Pugh class A):
US labeling: No dosage adjustment necessary; AUC increased ~40% in mild hepatic impairment compared with healthy subjects.
Canadian labeling: Initiate at the lowest dose.
Moderate impairment (Child-Pugh class B): Reduce dose by 50%.
Severe impairment (Child-Pugh class C):
US labeling: Use is not recommended.
Canadian labeling: Use is contraindicated.
Abnormal liver function tests (persistent or worsening): Discontinue use.

Dietary Considerations May be taken without regard to meals.

Administration May be administered without regard to meals. Capsules may be swallowed whole or the entire contents emptied onto a teaspoon of cool or room temperature applesauce and administered immediately with water. The contents of the capsules sprinkled onto applesauce may be stored under refrigeration for up to 6 hours.

Monitoring Parameters CBC; blood chemistry profile; occult blood loss and periodic liver function tests; monitor renal function (urine output, serum BUN and creatinine); monitor response (pain, range of motion, grip strength, mobility, ADL function), inflammation; blood pressure (baseline and during treatment); observe for weight gain, edema; observe for bleeding, bruising; evaluate gastrointestinal effects (abdominal pain, bleeding, dyspepsia)

JIA: Monitor for development of abnormal coagulation tests with systemic onset JIA

Dosage Forms Excipient information presented when available (limited, particularly for generics); consult specific product labeling.
Capsule, Oral:
CeleBREX: 50 mg, 100 mg, 200 mg, 400 mg
Generic: 50 mg, 100 mg, 200 mg, 400 mg

◆ Celestoderm V (Can) *see* Betamethasone (Topical) on page 224
◆ Celestoderm V/2 (Can) *see* Betamethasone (Topical) on page 224
◆ Celestone [DSC] *see* Betamethasone (Systemic) on page 222
◆ Celestone Soluspan *see* Betamethasone (Systemic) on page 222
◆ CeleXA *see* Citalopram on page 398
◆ Celexa (Can) *see* Citalopram on page 398
◆ CellCept *see* Mycophenolate on page 1240
◆ CellCept Intravenous *see* Mycophenolate on page 1240
◆ CellCept I.V. (Can) *see* Mycophenolate on page 1240
◆ Cell Culture Inactivated Influenza Vaccine, Trivalent [Flucelvax] *see* Influenza Virus Vaccine (Inactivated) on page 945
◆ Celontin *see* Methsuximide on page 1176
◆ Celontin® (Can) *see* Methsuximide on page 1176
◆ Celsentri (Can) *see* Maraviroc on page 1127
◆ Cemill [OTC] *see* Ascorbic Acid on page 155
◆ Cemill SR [OTC] *see* Ascorbic Acid on page 155
◆ CEM-Urea *see* Urea on page 1853
◆ CenFol *see* Folic Acid, Cyanocobalamin, and Pyridoxine on page 805
◆ Centany *see* Mupirocin on page 1239
◆ Centany AT *see* Mupirocin on page 1239
◆ Centuroides Immune FAB2 (Equine) *see* Centuroides Immune F(ab')₂ (Equine) on page 358

Centuroides Immune F(ab')₂ (Equine)
(sen tra ROY dez i MYUN fab too E kwine)

Brand Names: US Anascorp
Index Terms Centuroides Immune FAB2 (Equine); Antivenin (*Centuroides*) Immune F(ab')₂ (Equine); Antivenin Scorpion; Antivenom (*Centuroides*) Immune F(ab')₂ (Equine); Antivenom Scorpion; Scorpion Antivenin; Scorpion Antivenom
Pharmacologic Category Antivenin
Use Treatment of scorpion envenomation
Dosing
Adult Scorpion envenomation: IV: **Note:** Initiate therapy as soon as possible after scorpion sting. Initial: 3 vials (containing ≤360 mg total protein and ≥450 LD50 [mouse] neutralizing units); may administer additional vials in 1-vial increments every 30-60 minutes as needed.
Pediatric Scorpion envenomation: IV: Refer to adult dosing.
Renal Impairment There are no dosage adjustments provided in manufacturer's labeling.
Hepatic Impairment There are no dosage adjustments provided in manufacturer's labeling.
Additional Information Complete prescribing information should be consulted for additional detail.
Dosage Forms Excipient information presented when available (limited, particularly for generics); consult specific product labeling.
Solution Reconstituted, Intravenous [preservative free]:
Anascorp: (1 ea)

◆ Cepacol Dual Relief [OTC] *see* Benzocaine on page 217
◆ Cepacol Sensations Hydra [OTC] *see* Benzocaine on page 217
◆ Cepacol Sensations Warming [OTC] *see* Benzocaine on page 217

Cephalexin (sef a LEKS in)

Brand Names: US Keflex
Brand Names: Canada Apo-Cephalex; Dom-Cephalexin; Keflex; PMS-Cephalexin; Teva-Cephalexin
Index Terms Cephalexin Monohydrate
Pharmacologic Category Antibiotic, Cephalosporin (First Generation)
Use Treatment of susceptible bacterial infections including respiratory tract infections, otitis media, skin and skin structure infections, bone infections, and genitourinary tract infections, including acute prostatitis; alternative therapy for acute infective endocarditis prophylaxis
Pregnancy Considerations Adverse events were not observed in animal reproduction studies. Cephalexin crosses the placenta and produces therapeutic concentrations in the fetal circulation and amniotic fluid. An increased risk of teratogenic effects has not been observed following maternal use of cephalexin. Peak concentrations in pregnant patients are similar to those in nonpregnant patients. Prolonged labor may decrease oral absorption.
Breast-Feeding Considerations Small amounts of cephalexin are excreted in breast milk. The manufacturer recommends that caution be exercised when administering cephalexin to nursing women. Maximum milk concentration occurs ~4 hours after a single oral dose and gradually disappears by 8 hours after administration. Non-dose-related effects could include modification of bowel flora.
Contraindications Hypersensitivity to cephalexin, any component of the formulation, or other cephalosporins
Warnings/Precautions Modify dosage in patients with severe renal impairment. Use with caution in patients with a history of penicillin allergy, especially IgE-mediated reactions (eg, anaphylaxis, urticaria). Prolonged use may result in fungal or bacterial superinfection, including *C. difficile*-associated diarrhea (CDAD) and pseudomembranous colitis; CDAD has been observed >2 months

postantibiotic treatment. May be associated with increased INR, especially in nutritionally-deficient patients, prolonged treatment, hepatic or renal disease.

Adverse Reactions Frequency not defined.

Central nervous system: Agitation, confusion, dizziness, fatigue, hallucination, headache

Dermatologic: Erythema multiforme (rare), genital pruritus, skin rash, Stevens-Johnson syndrome (rare), toxic epidermal necrolysis (rare), urticaria

Gastrointestinal: Abdominal pain, diarrhea, dyspepsia, gastritis, nausea (rare), pseudomembranous colitis, vomiting (rare)

Genitourinary: Genital candidiasis, vaginal discharge, vaginitis

Hematologic & oncologic: Eosinophilia, hemolytic anemia, neutropenia, thrombocytopenia

Hepatic: Cholestatic jaundice (rare), hepatitis (transient, rare), increased serum ALT, increased serum AST

Hypersensitivity: Anaphylaxis, angioedema, hypersensitivity reaction

Neuromuscular & skeletal: Arthralgia, arthritis, arthropathy

Renal: Interstitial nephritis (rare)

Drug Interactions

Metabolism/Transport Effects None known.

Avoid Concomitant Use

Avoid concomitant use of Cephalexin with any of the following: BCG (Intravesical)

Increased Effect/Toxicity

Cephalexin may increase the levels/effects of: MetFORMIN; Vitamin K Antagonists

The levels/effects of Cephalexin may be increased by: Probenecid

Decreased Effect

Cephalexin may decrease the levels/effects of: BCG (Intravesical); BCG Vaccine (Immunization); Sodium Picosulfate; Typhoid Vaccine

The levels/effects of Cephalexin may be decreased by: Multivitamins/Minerals (with ADEK, Folate, Iron); Multivitamins/Minerals (with AE, No Iron); Zinc Salts

Food Interactions Peak antibiotic serum concentration is lowered and delayed, but total drug absorbed is not affected. Cephalexin serum levels may be decreased if taken with food. Management: Administer without regard to food.

Storage/Stability

Capsule: Store at 15°C to 30°C (59°F to 86°F).

Powder for oral suspension: Refrigerate suspension after reconstitution; discard after 14 days.

Tablet: Store at 20°C to 25°C (68°F to 77°F).

Mechanism of Action Inhibits bacterial cell wall synthesis by binding to one or more of the penicillin-binding proteins (PBPs) which in turn inhibits the final transpeptidation step of peptidoglycan synthesis in bacterial cell walls, thus inhibiting cell wall biosynthesis. Bacteria eventually lyse due to ongoing activity of cell wall autolytic enzymes (autolysins and murein hydrolases) while cell wall assembly is arrested.

Pharmacodynamics/Kinetics

Absorption: Rapid (90%); delayed in young children and may be decreased up to 50% in neonates

Distribution: Widely into most body tissues and fluids, including gallbladder, liver, kidneys, bone, sputum, bile, and pleural and synovial fluids; CSF penetration is poor

Protein binding: 6% to 15%

Half-life elimination: Neonates: 5 hours; Children 3-12 months: 2.5 hours; Adults: 0.5 to 1.2 hours (prolonged with renal impairment)

Time to peak, serum: ~1 hour

Excretion: Urine (80% to 100% as unchanged drug) within 8 hours

Dosing

Adult & Geriatric

Dosing range: Oral: 250 to 1000 mg every 6 hours (maximum: 4 g/day)

Indication-specific dosing:

Cellulitis and mastitis: Oral 500 mg every 6 hours

Furunculosis/skin abscess: Oral: 250 mg 4 times/day

Impetigo: Oral: 250 mg every 6 hours; continue for 7 days, depending upon clinical response (IDSA [Stevens 2014])

Prophylaxis against infective endocarditis (dental, oral, or respiratory tract procedures): Oral: 2 g 30 to 60 minutes prior to procedure. **Note:** American Heart Association (AHA) guidelines now recommend prophylaxis only in patients undergoing invasive procedures and in whom underlying cardiac conditions may predispose to a higher risk of adverse outcomes should infection occur.

Prophylaxis in patients with prosthetic joint implants undergoing dental procedures which produce bacteremia: Oral: 2 g 1 hour prior to

procedure (ADA/AAOS 2003). **Note:** In general, patients with prosthetic joint implants do not require prophylactic antibiotics prior to dental procedures. In planning an invasive oral procedure, dental consultation with the patient's orthopedic surgeon may be advised to review the risks of infection (Sollecito 2015).

Prosthetic joint infection, chronic oral antimicrobial suppression (off-label use): Oral:

Propionibacterium spp (alternative to penicillin or amoxicillin): 500 mg every 6 to 8 hours (Osmon 2013)

Staphylococci, oxacillin-susceptible (preferred): 500 mg every 6 to 8 hours (Osmon 2013)

Streptococci, beta-hemolytic (alternative to penicillin or amoxicillin): 500 mg every 6 to 8 hours (Osmon 2013)

Skin and skin structure infections: Oral:

Manufacturer's labeling: 500 mg every 12 hours

Alternate recommendations: 500 mg every 6 hours (IDSA [Stevens 2014])

Streptococcal pharyngitis: Oral: 500 mg every 12 hours. **Note:** Recommended by the Infectious Disease Society of America (IDSA) as an alternative agent for group A streptococcal pharyngitis in penicillin-allergic patients (avoid in patients with immediate-type hypersensitivity to penicillin) with a duration of 10 days (Shulman 2012).

Streptococcal skin infections: 500 mg every 6 hours (IDSA [Stevens 2014])

Surgical site infection (trunk or extremity [away from axilla or perineum]) (off-label use): Oral: 500 mg every 6 hours (IDSA [Stevens 2014])

Uncomplicated cystitis: Oral: 500 mg every 12 hours for 7 to 14 days

Pediatric

Usual dose: Children >1 year: Oral: Dosing range: 25 to 100 mg/kg/day in divided doses every 6 to 8 hours (maximum: 4 g/day)

Indication-specific dosing:

Cellulitis and mastitis: Adolescents >15 years: Refer to adult dosing.

Community-acquired pneumonia (CAP) (IDSA/PIDS 2011), *S. aureus* (methicillin-susceptible), mild infection or step-down therapy (preferred): Infants >3 months and Children: Oral: 75 to 100 mg/kg/day in 3 to 4 divided doses

Furunculosis:

Children: Oral: 25 to 50 mg/kg/day in 4 divided doses

Adolescents >15 years: Refer to adult dosing.

Impetigo: Children: Oral: 25 to 50 mg/kg/day in 3 to 4 divided doses; continue for 7 days, depending upon clinical response (IDSA [Stevens 2014])

Otitis media: Children: 75 to 100 mg/kg/day in 4 divided doses

Prophylaxis against infective endocarditis (dental, oral, or respiratory tract procedures):

Children >1 to 15 years: 50 mg/kg 30 to 60 minutes prior to procedure (maximum: 2 g). **Note:** American Heart Association (AHA) guidelines now recommend prophylaxis only in patients undergoing invasive procedures and in whom underlying cardiac conditions may predispose to a higher risk of adverse outcomes should infection occur.

Adolescents >15 years: Refer to adult dosing.

Prophylaxis in total joint replacement patients undergoing dental procedures which produce bacteremia: Adolescents >15 years: Refer to adult dosing.

Severe infections: Children: Oral: 50 to 100 mg/kg/day in divided doses every 6 to 8 hours

Skin abscess:

Children: Oral: 50 mg/kg/day in 4 divided doses (maximum: 4 g)

Adolescents >15 years: Refer to adult dosing.

Skin and skin structure infections:

Manufacturer's labeling:

Children >1 year: Oral: 25 to 50 mg/kg/day divided every 12 hours

Adolescents >15 years: Refer to adult dosing.

Alternate recommendations: Children: 25 to 50 mg/kg/day divided every 6 hours (IDSA [Stevens 2014])

Streptococcal pharyngitis: Children >1 year: Oral: 25 to 50 mg/kg/day divided every 12 hours. **Note:** Recommended by the Infectious Disease Society of America (IDSA) as an alternative agent for group A streptococcal pharyngitis in penicillin-allergic patients (avoid in patients with immediate-type hypersensitivity to penicillin) at a dose of 40 mg/kg/day divided twice daily (maximum: 1000 mg daily) for 10 days (Shulman 2012).

Uncomplicated cystitis: Adolescents >15 years: Refer to adult dosing.

Renal Impairment Adults:
CrCl 10 to 50 mL/minute: 500 mg every 8 to 12 hours
CrCl <10: 250 to 500 mg every 12 to 24 hours
Hemodialysis: 250 mg every 12 to 24 hours; moderately dialyzable (20% to 50%); give dose after dialysis session

Hepatic Impairment No dosage adjustment provided in manufacturer's labeling.

Dietary Considerations Take without regard to food. If GI distress, take with food.

Administration Take without regard to food. If GI distress, take with food. Give around-the-clock to promote less variation in peak and trough serum levels.

Monitoring Parameters With prolonged therapy monitor renal, hepatic, and hematologic function periodically; monitor for signs of anaphylaxis during first dose.

Test Interactions Positive direct Coombs', false-positive urinary glucose test using cupric sulfate (Benedict's solution, Clinitest®, Fehling's solution), false-positive serum or urine creatinine with Jaffé reaction, false-positive urinary proteins and steroids

Dosage Forms Excipient information presented when available (limited, particularly for generics); consult specific product labeling.
Capsule, Oral:
Keflex: 250 mg, 500 mg, 750 mg [contains brilliant blue fcf (fd&c blue #1), fd&c yellow #10 (quinoline yellow), fd&c yellow #6 (sunset yellow)]
Generic: 250 mg, 500 mg, 750 mg
Suspension Reconstituted, Oral:
Generic: 125 mg/5 mL (100 mL, 200 mL); 250 mg/5 mL (100 mL, 200 mL)
Tablet, Oral:
Generic: 250 mg, 500 mg

◆ Cephalexin Monohydrate see Cephalexin on page 358
◆ Ceprotin see Protein C Concentrate (Human) on page 1524
◆ CERA see Methoxy Polyethylene Glycol-Epoetin Beta on page 1176
◆ Cerdelga see Eliglustat on page 624
◆ Cerebyx see Fosphenytoin on page 816
◆ Cerefolin® NAC see Methylfolate, Methylcobalamin, and Acetylcysteine on page 1179
◆ Cerezyme see Imiglucerase on page 923

Ceritinib (se RI ti nib)

Brand Names: US Zykadia
Brand Names: Canada Zykadia
Index Terms LDK378
Pharmacologic Category Antineoplastic Agent, Anaplastic Lymphoma Kinase Inhibitor; Antineoplastic Agent, Tyrosine Kinase Inhibitor

Use
US labeling: **Non-small cell lung cancer, metastatic:** Treatment of patients with anaplastic lymphoma kinase (ALK)-positive metastatic non-small cell lung cancer (NSCLC) who have progressed on or are intolerant to crizotinib.
Canadian labeling: **Non-small cell lung cancer, locally advanced or metastatic:** Treatment of patients with ALK-positive locally advanced (not amenable to curative therapy) or metastatic NSCLC who have progressed on or are intolerant to crizotinib.

Pregnancy Considerations Adverse events were observed in animal reproduction studies. Based on its mechanism of action, ceritinib may cause fetal harm if administered to a pregnant woman. Women of reproductive potential should use effective contraception during and for at least 2 weeks following therapy discontinuation. The Canadian labeling recommends women and men of reproductive potential use effective contraception during and for up to 3 months following therapy discontinuation.

Breast-Feeding Considerations It is not known if ceritinib is excreted in breast milk. Due to the potential for serious adverse reactions in the nursing infant, breast-feeding is not recommended by the manufacturer.

Contraindications
There are no contraindications listed in the manufacturer's US labeling.
Canadian labeling: Hypersensitivity to ceritinib or any component of the formulation; congenital long QT syndrome or persistent Fridericia-corrected electrocardiogram interval (QTcF) of >500 msec.

Warnings/Precautions Hazardous agent – use appropriate precautions for handling and disposal (meets NIOSH 2014 criteria). Symptomatic bradycardia may occur; heart rate <50 beats/minute has occurred. If possible, avoid concurrent use with other agents known to cause bradycardia (eg, beta blockers, nondihydropyridine calcium channel blockers, clonidine, digoxin). Monitor heart rate and blood pressure regularly. If symptomatic bradycardia (not life-threatening) occurs, withhold treatment until recovery to asymptomatic bradycardia or to a heart rate of ≥60 beats/minute, evaluate concurrent medications, and adjust ceritinib dose. Permanently discontinue for life-threatening bradycardia due to ceritinib; if life-threatening bradycardia occurs and concurrent medications associated with bradycardia can be discontinued or dose adjusted, restart ceritinib at a reduced dose (with frequent monitoring). QTc interval prolongation has occurred in clinical studies, and may be concentration-dependent. QT prolongation may lead to an increased risk for ventricular tachyarrhythmias (eg, torsades de pointes) or sudden death. Correct electrolyte abnormalities prior to initiating therapy. Periodically monitor ECG and electrolytes in patients with heart failure, bradyarrhythmias, electrolyte abnormalities, or who are taking medications known to prolong the QTc interval. May require treatment interruption, dosage reduction, or discontinuation. Avoid use in patients with congenital long QTc syndrome. The Canadian labeling contraindicates use in patients with congenital long QTc syndrome or persistent QTcF of >500 msec. Permanently discontinue in patients who develop QTc interval prolongation in combination with torsades de pointes or polymorphic ventricular tachycardia or signs/symptoms of serious arrhythmia.

Diarrhea, nausea, vomiting, or abdominal pain occurred in the majority of patients in clinical trials; over one-third of patients required dose reductions due to severe or persistent gastrointestinal toxicity. Manage symptoms medically with appropriate therapy (eg, antidiarrheals, antiemetics, fluid replacement) as indicated. May require therapy interruption and dosage reduction. Ceritinib is associated with a moderate emetic potential; antiemetics may be needed to prevent nausea and vomiting. If vomiting occurs, do not administer an additional dose; continue with the next scheduled dose. Hepatotoxicity has been observed in patients treated with ceritinib in clinical trials, including ALT levels >5 times ULN in over one-quarter of patients. Concurrent ALT elevations >3 times ULN with total bilirubin >2 times ULN (with normal alkaline phosphatase) occurred rarely. Monitor liver function tests (eg, ALT, AST, total bilirubin) monthly and as clinically necessary, more frequently in patients who develop transaminase abnormalities. May require therapy interruption, dosage reduction, and/or discontinuation. Use with caution in patients with hepatic impairment (has not been studied in patients with moderate or severe impairment). Ceritinib is metabolized and eliminated hepatically; systemic exposure and toxicities may be increased in patients with hepatic dysfunction. Although rare, pancreatitis (with fatality) has been reported. Grade 3 to 4 lipase and amylase elevations occurred in clinical trials. Monitor lipase and amylase prior to treatment and periodically during treatment as clinically necessary. May require treatment interruption and dose reduction.

Hyperglycemia, including grade 3 and 4 toxicity, has been observed in ceritinib-treated patients. The risk of grade 3 or 4 hyperglycemia increases significantly in diabetic patients or those with glucose intolerance; risk is also increased in patients receiving corticosteroids. Monitor fasting blood glucose levels at baseline and as clinically necessary, particularly in patients with diabetes. May require initiation or optimization of antihyperglycemic therapy. Temporarily interrupt therapy for hyperglycemia until adequately controlled; reduce dose upon recovery. If adequate glycemic control is not possible with medical management, permanently discontinue ceritinib. Severe and life-threatening interstitial lung disease (ILD)/pneumonitis (some fatal) may occur. Monitor for signs/symptoms of pulmonary toxicity; permanently discontinue in patients diagnosed with treatment-related ILD/pneumonitis. Potentially significant interactions may exist, requiring dose or frequency adjustment, additional monitoring, and/or selection of alternative therapy. In vitro studies indicate that ceritinib solubility and bioavailability may be decreased at higher pH; concurrent use with proton pump inhibitors, H₂-receptor antagonists, or antacids has not been evaluated.

Adverse Reactions
>10%:
Central nervous system: Fatigue (52%), neuropathy (17%; including paresthesia, muscular weakness, gait disturbance, peripheral neuropathy, hypoesthesia, peripheral sensory neuropathy, dysesthesia, neuralgia, peripheral motor neuropathy, hypotonia, polyneuropathy)
Dermatologic: Skin rash (16%; including maculopapular rash, acneiform dermatitis)

Endocrine & metabolic: Increased serum glucose (49%; grades 3/4: 13%), decreased serum phosphate (36%)

Gastrointestinal: Diarrhea (86%; grades 3/4: 6%), nausea (80%; grades 3/4: 4%), vomiting (60%; grades 3/4: 4%), abdominal pain (54%), decreased appetite (34%), constipation (29%), increased serum lipase (28%), disease of esophagus (16%; including dyspepsia, gastroesophageal reflux disease, dysphagia)

Hematologic & oncologic: Decreased hemoglobin (84%)

Hepatic: Increased serum ALT (80%; grades 3/4: 27%), increased serum AST (75%; grades 3/4: 13%), increased serum bilirubin (15%; grades 3/4: 1%)

Renal: Increased serum creatinine (58%)

1% to 10%:

Cardiovascular: Prolonged Q-T interval on ECG (4%; >60 msec increase from baseline: 3%; >500 msec: <1%), bradycardia (3%), sinus bradycardia (1%)

Ophthalmic: Visual disturbance (9%; including vision impairment, blurred vision, photopsia, accommodation disorder, presbyopia, reduced visual acuity)

Respiratory: Interstitial pulmonary disease (4%; grades 3/4: 3%)

Drug Interactions

Metabolism/Transport Effects Substrate of CYP3A4 (major), P-glycoprotein; **Note:** Assignment of Major/Minor substrate status based on clinically relevant drug interaction potential; **Inhibits** CYP2C9 (moderate), CYP3A4 (strong)

Avoid Concomitant Use

Avoid concomitant use of Ceritinib with any of the following: Ado-Trastuzumab Emtansine; Alfuzosin; Aprepitant; Astemizole; Avanafil; Axitinib; Barnidipine; Bosutinib; Bradycardia-Causing Agents; Bromocriptine; Cabozantinib; Cobimetinib; Conivaptan; Crizotinib; CYP3A4 Inducers (Strong); CYP3A4 Inhibitors (Strong); Dabrafenib; Dapoxetine; Domperidone; Dronedarone; Eletriptan; Eplerenone; Everolimus; Flibanserin; Fusidic Acid (Systemic); Grapefruit Juice; Halofantrine; Highest Risk QTc-Prolonging Agents; Ibrutinib; Idelalisib; Irinotecan Products; Isavuconazonium Sulfate; Ivabradine; Lapatinib; Lercanidipine; Lomitapide; Lovastatin; Lurasidone; Macitentan; Mifepristone; Naloxegol; Nilotinib; NiMODipine; Nisoldipine; Olaparib; Osimertinib; Palbociclib; Pimozide; Ranolazine; Red Yeast Rice; Regorafenib; Salmeterol; Silodosin; Simeprevir; Simvastatin; Sonidegib; St Johns Wort; Suvorexant; Tamsulosin; Terfenadine; Ticagrelor; Tolvaptan; Toremifene; Trabectedin; Ulipristal; Vemurafenib; VinCRIStine (Liposomal); Vorapaxar

Increased Effect/Toxicity

Ceritinib may increase the levels/effects of: Ado-Trastuzumab Emtansine; Alfuzosin; Alitretinoin (Systemic); Almotriptan; Alosetron; Apixaban; Aprepitant; ARIPiprazole; ARIPiprazole Lauroxil; Astemizole; Avanafil; Axitinib; Barnidipine; Bedaquiline; Bortezomib; Bosentan; Bosutinib; Brentuximab Vedotin; Brexpiprazole; Brinzolamide; Bromocriptine; Budesonide (Nasal); Budesonide (Oral Inhalation); Budesonide (Systemic); Budesonide (Topical); Cabazitaxel; Cabozantinib; Cannabis; Cariprazine; Cilostazol; Cobimetinib; Colchicine; Conivaptan; Crizotinib; CYP2C9 Substrates; CYP3A4 Substrates; Dabrafenib; Daclatasvir; Dapoxetine; Dasatinib; Dienogest; Domperidone; DOXOrubicin (Conventional); Dronabinol; Dronedarone; Drospirenone; Dutasteride; Eletriptan; Eplerenone; Erlotinib; Estazolam; Etizolam; Everolimus; FentaNYL; Fesoterodine; Flibanserin; Fluticasone (Nasal); Fluticasone (Oral Inhalation); Gefitinib; Halofantrine; Highest Risk QTc-Prolonging Agents; Hydrocodone; Ibrutinib; Imatinib; Imidafenacin; Irinotecan Products; Isavuconazonium Sulfate; Ivabradine; Ivacaftor; Ixabepilone; Lacosamide; Lapatinib; Lercanidipine; Levobupivacaine; Levomilnacipran; Lomitapide; Lovastatin; Lurasidone; Macitentan; Maraviroc; MedroxyPROGESTERone; MethylPREDNISolone; Moderate Risk QTc-Prolonging Agents; Naloxegol; Nilotinib; NiMODipine; Nisoldipine; Olaparib; Osimertinib; Ospemifene; Oxybutynin; OxyCODONE; Palbociclib; Panobinostat; Parecoxib; Paricalcitol; PAZOPanib; Pimecrolimus; Pimozide; PONATinib; Pranlukast; PrednisoLONE (Systemic); PredniSONE; Ramelteon; Ranolazine; Red Yeast Rice; Regorafenib; Repaglinide; Retapamulin; Rilpivirine; RomiDEPsin; Ruxolitinib; Salmeterol; Saxagliptin; Sildenafil; Silodosin; Simeprevir; Simvastatin; Sonidegib; SORAfenib; Suvorexant; Tacrolimus (Systemic); Tadalafil; Tamsulosin; Tasimelteon; Terfenadine; Tetrahydrocannabinol; Ticagrelor; Tofacitinib; Tolterodine; Tolvaptan; Toremifene; Trabectedin; TraMADol; Ulipristal; Vardenafil; Vemurafenib; Vilazodone; VinCRIStine (Liposomal); Vindesine; Vinorelbine; Vorapaxar; Zopiclone

The levels/effects of Ceritinib may be increased by: Bradycardia-Causing Agents; Bretylium; Conivaptan; Corticosteroids; CYP3A4 Inhibitors (Moderate); CYP3A4 Inhibitors (Strong); Fusidic Acid (Systemic); Grapefruit Juice; Idelalisib; Ivabradine; Luliconazole; Mifepristone; Netupitant; P-glycoprotein/ABCB1 Inhibitors; QTc-Prolonging Agents (Indeterminate Risk and Risk Modifying); Stiripentol

Decreased Effect

Ceritinib may decrease the levels/effects of: Antidiabetic Agents; Ifosfamide; Prasugrel; Ticagrelor

The levels/effects of Ceritinib may be decreased by: Bosentan; CYP3A4 Inducers (Moderate); CYP3A4 Inducers (Strong); Deferasirox; P-glycoprotein/ABCB1 Inducers; Siltuximab; St Johns Wort; Tocilizumab

Food Interactions

A high-fat meal increases AUC and C$_{max}$ by 73% and 41%, respectively and a low-fat meal increases AUC and C$_{max}$ by 58% and 43%, respectively; systemic exposure when administered with a meal may exceed that of a typical dose, and may result in increased toxicity. Management: Administer on an empty stomach, at least 2 hours before or after a meal.

Grapefruit and grapefruit juice may inhibit the metabolism of ceritinib and increase its systemic exposure. Management: Avoid grapefruit juice during therapy.

Storage/Stability
Store at 25°C (77°F); excursions are permitted between 15°C and 30°C (59°F and 86°F).

Mechanism of Action
Potent inhibitor of anaplastic lymphoma kinase (ALK), a tyrosine kinase involved in the pathogenesis of non-small cell lung cancer. ALK gene abnormalities due to mutations or translocations may result in expression of oncogenic fusion proteins (eg, ALK fusion protein) which alter signaling and expression and result in increased cellular proliferation and survival in tumors which express these fusion proteins. ALK inhibition reduces proliferation of cells expressing the genetic alteration. Ceritinib also inhibits insulin-like growth factor 1 receptor (IGF-1R), insulin receptor (InsR), and ROS1. Ceritinib has demonstrated activity in crizotinib-resistant tumors in NSCLC xenograft models.

Pharmacodynamics/Kinetics

Absorption: AUC and C$_{max}$ increased 73% and 41%, respectively, when administered with a high-fat meal, and 58% and 43%, respectively when taken with a low-fat meal (when compared to fasting)

Distribution: 4,230 L (following a single dose), with a small preferential distribution to red blood cells versus plasma

Protein binding: 97% to human plasma proteins

Metabolism: Primarily hepatic via CYP3A

Half-life elimination: 41 hours

Time to peak: ~4 to 6 hours

Excretion: Feces (~92% with 68% as unchanged drug); urine (~1%)

Dosing

Adult & Geriatric Note: Ceritinib is associated with a moderate emetic potential; antiemetics may be needed to prevent nausea and vomiting.

Non-small cell lung cancer (ALK-positive), metastatic: Oral: 750 mg once daily; continue until disease progression or unacceptable toxicity.

Missed doses: If a dose is missed, take the missed dose unless the next dose is due within 12 hours. If vomiting occurs, do not administer an additional dose, patients should continue with the next scheduled dose.

Dosage adjustment for concomitant therapy:

Strong CYP3A4 inhibitors:

US labeling: Avoid concomitant use of strong CYP3A inhibitors; if concurrent administration cannot be avoided, reduce ceritinib dose by approximately one-third (rounded to the nearest multiple of the 150 mg strength). After discontinuation of the strong CYP3A inhibitor, resume ceritinib therapy at the dose used prior to initiation of the CYP3A4 inhibitor.

Canadian labeling: Avoid concomitant use of strong CYP3A inhibitors.

Strong CYP3A4 inducers: Avoid concurrent use of strong CYP3A inducers (eg, carbamazepine, phenytoin, rifampin, and St John's wort) during treatment with ceritinib.

Renal Impairment

CrCl ≥30 to 90 mL/minute: No dosage adjustment is necessary.

CrCl <30 mL/minute: There are no dosage adjustments provided in the manufacturer's labeling (has not been studied).

Hepatic Impairment

Preexisting mild impairment (total bilirubin ≤ULN and AST >ULN **or** total bilirubin >1 to 1.5 times ULN and any AST): No dosage adjustment is necessary.

Preexisting moderate or severe impairment: There are no dosage adjustments provided in the manufacturer's labeling (has not been studied). Ceritinib is primarily metabolized and eliminated hepatically; exposure is likely increased in patients with hepatic impairment.

Hepatotoxicity during treatment:

ALT or AST >5 times ULN with total bilirubin ≤2 times ULN (US labeling) or ≤1.5 times ULN (Canadian labeling): Interrupt therapy until recovery to baseline or ALT/AST ≤3 times ULN, then resume with a 150 mg dose reduction.

ALT or AST >3 times ULN with total bilirubin >2 times ULN (US labeling) or >1.5 times ULN (Canadian labeling) in the absence of cholestasis or hemolysis: Permanently discontinue therapy.

Adjustment for Toxicity Note: Over half of patients initiating treatment required at least 1 dose reduction; the median time to the first dose reduction was 7 weeks. Discontinue if patients are unable to tolerate 300 mg daily.

Cardiac:

Bradycardia (heart rate <50 beats per minute [US labeling] or <60 beats per minute [Canadian labeling]):

US labeling: Symptomatic bradycardia (not life-threatening): Interrupt therapy and evaluate concomitant medications known to cause bradycardia. Upon recovery to asymptomatic bradycardia or to a heart rate ≥60 beats per minute, adjust the dose.

Canadian labeling: Interrupt therapy and evaluate for concomitant medication known to cause bradycardia. Upon recovery to asymptomatic bradycardia or to a heart rate ≥60 beats per minute:

If concomitant medication is identified and discontinued or its dose adjusted, reinitiate ceritinib at its previous dose.

If no concomitant medication is identified or if it is identified but not discontinued or not dose-adjusted, reinitiate ceritinib with a 150 mg dose reduction.

Symptomatic bradycardia (life-threatening or requiring intervention) in patients taking concomitant medications known to cause bradycardia/hypotension:

US labeling: Interrupt therapy until recovery to asymptomatic bradycardia or to a heart rate ≥60 beats per minute. If the concomitant medication can be adjusted or discontinued, resume ceritinib therapy with the dose reduced by 150 mg.

Canadian labeling: Interrupt therapy until recovery to asymptomatic bradycardia or to a heart rate ≥60 beats per minute. If concomitant medication can be discontinued or its dose adjusted, resume ceritinib with the dose reduced by 300 mg; monitor frequently; permanently discontinue ceritinib for recurrence.

Symptomatic bradycardia (life-threatening) in patients not taking concomitant medications known to cause bradycardia/hypotension: Permanently discontinue therapy.

QTc prolongation:

QTc interval >500 msec on at least 2 separate ECGs: Interrupt therapy until QTc interval is <481 msec or recovers to baseline if baseline QTc is ≥481 msec, then resume therapy with a 150 mg dose reduction.

QTc prolongation in combination with torsades de pointes, polymorphic ventricular tachycardia, or signs/symptoms of serious arrhythmia: Permanently discontinue therapy.

Gastrointestinal:

Severe or intolerable nausea, vomiting, or diarrhea (despite appropriate management): Interrupt therapy until improved, then resume treatment with a 150 mg dose reduction.

Lipase or amylase elevation >2 times ULN: Interrupt therapy and monitor serum lipase and amylase; upon recovery to <1.5 times ULN, resume treatment with a 150 mg dose reduction.

Metabolic: Persistent hyperglycemia >250 mg/dL (despite optimal antihyperglycemic therapy): Interrupt therapy until hyperglycemia is adequately controlled, then resume therapy with a 150 mg dose reduction. If hyperglycemia cannot be controlled, discontinue ceritinib permanently.

Pulmonary: Treatment-related interstitial lung disease/pneumonitis (any grade): Permanently discontinue therapy.

Dietary Considerations Avoid grapefruit and grapefruit juice.

Administration

Ceritinib is associated with a moderate emetic potential; antiemetics may be needed to prevent nausea and vomiting.

Administer orally on an empty stomach (at least 2 hours before or 2 hours after a meal). Hazardous agent; use appropriate precautions for handling and disposal (meets NIOSH 2014 criteria).

The Canadian labeling recommends that the capsule not be crushed or chewed.

Monitoring Parameters ALK positivity; CBC, renal function, liver function, fasting blood glucose (baseline and as clinically necessary); lipase and amylase (baseline and periodically as clinically necessary); electrolytes (baseline and periodically thereafter); cardiac monitoring (heart rate and QTc interval); blood pressure; signs/symptoms of gastrointestinal and pulmonary toxicity; signs/symptoms of pancreatitis.

Dosage Forms Excipient information presented when available (limited, particularly for generics); consult specific product labeling.

Capsule, Oral:

Zykadia: 150 mg [contains fd&c blue #2 (indigotine)]

◆ Cerovel see Urea on page 1853

Certolizumab Pegol (cer to LIZ u mab PEG ol)

Brand Names: US Cimzia; Cimzia Prefilled; Cimzia Starter Kit

Brand Names: Canada Cimzia

Index Terms CDP870

Pharmacologic Category Antirheumatic, Disease Modifying; Gastrointestinal Agent, Miscellaneous; Tumor Necrosis Factor (TNF) Blocking Agent

Use

Ankylosing spondylitis: Treatment of adults with active ankylosing spondylitis (AS)

Crohn disease: Treatment of moderately to severely active Crohn disease in patients who have inadequate response to conventional therapy

Psoriatic arthritis: Treatment of adult patients with active psoriatic arthritis

Rheumatoid arthritis: Treatment of adults with moderately to severely active rheumatoid arthritis (RA) (as monotherapy or in combination with nonbiological disease-modifying antirheumatic drugs [DMARDS])

Pregnancy Considerations Adverse effects were not observed in animal reproduction studies. Certolizumab pegol was found to cross the human placenta. Serum concentrations in 12 infants of 10 mothers were ≥75% lower than the maternal serum at delivery (last maternal dose of 400 mg given 5-42 days prior to birth). Although placental transfer was low, infants may have a slower rate of elimination than adults. In one infant, certolizumab pegol serum concentrations decreased from 1.02 to 0.84 mcg/mL over 4 weeks. Adverse events were not reported. The safety of administering live or live-attenuated vaccines to exposed infants is not known. If a biologic agent such as certolizumab pegol is needed to treat inflammatory bowel disease during pregnancy, it is recommended to hold therapy after 30 weeks gestation (Habal, 2012).

Healthcare providers are encouraged to enroll women exposed to certolizumab pegol during pregnancy in the MotherToBaby Autoimmune Diseases Study by contacting the Organization of Teratology Information Specialists (OTIS) (877-311-8972). The Canadian labeling recommends that women of childbearing potential use reliable contraception during therapy and for at least 5 months after the last dose of certolizumab.

Breast-Feeding Considerations It is not known if certolizumab pegol is excreted in breast milk. Due to the potential for serious adverse reactions in the nursing infant, the manufacturer recommends a decision be made whether to discontinue nursing or to discontinue the drug, taking into account the importance of treatment to the mother.

Medication Guide Available Yes

Contraindications There are no contraindications listed within the manufacturer's U.S. labeling.

Canadian labeling: Hypersensitivity to certolizumab pegol or any component of the formulation; active tuberculosis or other severe infections (eg, sepsis, abscesses, opportunistic infections); moderate to severe heart failure (NYHA Class III/IV)

Warnings/Precautions [U.S. Boxed Warning]: Patients receiving certolizumab are at increased risk for serious infections which may result in hospitalization and/or fatality; infections usually developed in patients receiving concomitant immunosuppressive agents (eg, methotrexate or corticosteroids) and may present as disseminated (rather than local) disease. Active tuberculosis (or reactivation of latent tuberculosis), invasive fungal (including aspergillosis, blastomycosis, candidiasis, coccidioidomycosis, histoplasmosis, and pneumocystosis) and bacterial, viral or other opportunistic infections (including legionellosis and listeriosis) have been reported in patients receiving TNF-blocking agents, including certolizumab. Monitor closely for signs/symptoms of infection. Discontinue for serious infection or sepsis. Consider risks versus

benefits prior to use in patients with a history of chronic or recurrent infection. Consider empiric anti-fungal therapy in patients who are at risk for invasive fungal infection and develop severe systemic illness. Caution should be exercised when considering use in the elderly or in patients with conditions that predispose them to infections (eg, diabetes) or residence/travel from areas of endemic mycoses (blastomycosis, coccidioidomycosis, histoplasmosis), or with latent or localized infections. Do not initiate certolizumab therapy with active infection, including clinically important localized infection. Patients who develop a new infection while undergoing treatment should be monitored closely. **[U.S. Boxed Warning]: Lymphoma and other malignancies (some fatal) have been reported in children and adolescent patients receiving other TNF-blocking agents.** Approximately half of the malignancies reported in children were lympho-mas (Hodgkin and non-Hodgkin) while other cases varied and included malignancies not typically observed in this population. The onset of malignancy was after a median of 30 months (range: 1-84 months) after the initiation of the TNF-blocking agent. Use of TNF blockers may affect defenses against malignancies; impact on the develop-ment and course of malignancies is not fully defined. Chronic immunosuppressant therapy use may be a pre-disposing factor for malignancy development; rheumatoid arthritis alone has been previously associated with an increased rate of lymphoma. Hepatosplenic T-cell lym-phoma (HSTCL), a rare T-cell lymphoma, has also been associated with TNF-blocking agents, primarily reported in adolescent and young adult males with Crohn disease or ulcerative colitis, most of whom had received concurrent treatment with azathioprine and/or 6-mercaptopurine. Mel-anoma and Merkel cell carcinoma have been reported with TNF-blocking agents including certolizumab. Perform peri-odic skin examinations in all patients during therapy, particularly those at increased risk for skin cancer.

Tuberculosis has been reported with certolizumab treat-ment. **[U.S. Boxed Warnings]: Patients should be eval-uated for tuberculosis risk factors and for latent tuberculosis infection (with a tuberculin skin test) prior to therapy. Treatment of latent tuberculosis should be initiated before use. Patients with initial negative tuberculin skin tests should receive continued mon-itoring for tuberculosis throughout treatment;** active tuberculosis has developed in this population during treat-ment. Use with caution in patients who have resided in regions where tuberculosis is endemic. Consider antitu-berculosis treatment (prior to certolizumab treatment) in patients with a history of latent or active tuberculosis if adequate treatment course cannot be confirmed, and for patients with risk factors for tuberculosis despite a negative test. Carefully consider benefits and risks of initiating certolizumab treatment in patients who have been exposed to tuberculosis.

Rare reactivation of hepatitis B virus (HBV) has occurred in chronic carriers of the virus, usually in patients receiving concomitant immunosuppressants; evaluate for HBV prior to initiation in all patients. Patients who test positive for HBV surface antigen should be referred for hepatitis B evaluation/treatment prior to certolizumab initiation. Mon-itor for clinical and laboratory signs of active infection during and for several months following discontinuation of treatment in HBV carriers; interrupt therapy if reactiva-tion occurs and treat appropriately with antiviral therapy; if resumption of therapy is deemed necessary, exercise caution and monitor patient closely.

Hypersensitivity reactions, including angioedema, dysp-nea, hypotension, rash, serum sickness and urticaria have been reported (rarely) with treatment; discontinue and do not resume therapy if hypersensitivity occurs. Some of these reactions have occurred after the first dose. Use with caution in patients who have experienced hypersen-sitivity with other TNF blockers. Use with caution in heart failure patients; worsening heart failure and new onset heart failure have been reported with TNF blockers, includ-ing certolizumab pegol; monitor closely. The Canadian labeling contraindicates use in moderate-to-severe heart failure (NYHA Class III/IV).

Rare cases of pancytopenia and other significant cytope-nias, including aplastic anemia and have been reported with TNF-blocking agents. Leukopenia and thrombocyto-penia have occurred with certolizumab; use with caution in patients with underlying hematologic disorders; consider discontinuing therapy with significant hematologic abnor-malities. Autoantibody formation may develop; rarely resulting in autoimmune disorder, including lupus-like syn-drome; monitor and discontinue if symptoms develop. A small number of patients (8%) develop antibodies to certolizumab during therapy. Antibody-positive patients

may have an increased incidence of adverse events (including injection site pain/erythema, abdominal pain and erythema nodosum). Use with caution in patients with preexisting or recent-onset CNS demyelinating disorders; rare cases of optic neuritis, seizure, peripheral neuropathy, and demyelinating disease (eg, multiple sclerosis, Guillain-Barré syndrome; new onset or exacerbation) have been reported.

Potentially significant drug-drug interactions may exist, requiring dose or frequency adjustment, additional mon-itoring, and/or selection of alternative therapy. Use caution when switching between biological disease modifying anti-rheumatic drugs (DMARDs); overlapping of biological activity may increase the risk for infection.

Patients should be up to date with all immunizations before initiating therapy; patients may receive vaccines other than live or live attenuated vaccines during therapy. There is no data available concerning the effects of therapy on vacci-nation or secondary transmission of live vaccines in patients receiving therapy. Use has not been studied in patients with renal impairment; however, the pharmacoki-netics of the pegylated (polyethylene glycol) component may be dependent on renal function. Use with caution in the elderly, may be at higher risk for infections.

Adverse Reactions

>10%:
Gastrointestinal: Nausea (≤11% [Schreiber, 2005])
Infection: Infection (38%; serious: 3%)
Respiratory: Upper respiratory tract infection (6% to 20%)

1% to 10%:
Cardiovascular: Hypertension (≤5%), angina pectoris (<5%), atrial fibrillation (<5%), cardiac arrhythmia (<5%), cardiac failure (<5%; new or worsening), cere-brovascular accident (<5%), hypertensive heart disease (<5%), ischemic heart disease (<5%), myocardial infarction (<5%), pericardial effusion (<5%), pericarditis (<5%), transient ischemic attacks (<5%), vasculi-tis (<5%)
Central nervous system: Headache (5%), anxiety (<5%), bipolar mood disorder (<5%), suicidal tendencies (<5%), fatigue (≤3%)
Dermatologic: Skin rash (≤9%), alopecia (<5%), derma-titis (<5%), erythema nodosum (<5%), urticaria (<5%)
Endocrine & metabolic: Menstrual disease (<5%)
Genitourinary: Urinary tract infection (≤8%), nephrotic syndrome (<5%)
Hematologic & oncologic: Anemia (<5%), hemorrhage (<5%), hypercoagulability state (<5%), leukopenia (<5%), lymphadenopathy (<5%), pancytopenia (<5%), thrombophlebitis (<5%), positive ANA titer (≤4%)
Hepatic: Hepatitis (<5%), increased serum transami-nases (<5%)
Immunologic: Antibody development (7% to 8%)
Neuromuscular & skeletal: Arthralgia (6% to 7%), back pain (≤4%)
Ophthalmic: Optic neuritis (<5%), retinal hemorrhage (<5%), uveitis (<5%)
Renal: Renal failure (<5%)
Respiratory: Cough (≤6%), nasopharyngitis (5%), tuber-culosis (<5%; peritoneal, pulmonary, and dissemi-nated), bronchitis (≤3%), pharyngitis (≤3%)
Miscellaneous: Fever (3%)

<1% (Limited to important or life-threatening): Aplastic anemia, cytopenia, demyelinating disease (exacerba-tion), fistula, hepatosplenic T-cell lymphoma, hepatotox-icity (idiosyncratic) (Chalasani, 2014), herpes virus infection, hypersensitivity reaction (eg, dyspnea, hot flush, hypotension, malaise, serum sickness, syncope), intestinal obstruction, leukemia, lupus erythematosus, lupus-like syndrome, lymphoma, malignant melanoma, malignant neoplasm, Merkel cell carcinoma, opportunis-tic infection (rare), peripheral edema, peripheral neuro-pathy, pneumonia, psoriasis (including new onset, palmoplantar, pustular, or exacerbation), pyelonephritis, reactivation of HBV, sarcoidosis, seizure, thrombocyto-penia, viral infection

Drug Interactions

Metabolism/Transport Effects None known.

Avoid Concomitant Use

Avoid concomitant use of Certolizumab Pegol with any of the following: Abatacept; Anakinra; Anti-TNF Agents; BCG (Intravesical); Canakinumab; Natalizumab; Pime-crolimus; Rilonacept; RiTUXimab; Tacrolimus (Topical); Tocilizumab; Tofacitinib; Vaccines (Live); Vedolizumab

Increased Effect/Toxicity

Certolizumab Pegol may increase the levels/effects of: Abatacept; Anakinra; Canakinumab; Fingolimod; Leflu-nomide; Natalizumab; Rilonacept; Tofacitinib; Vaccines (Live); Vedolizumab

The levels/effects of Certolizumab Pegol may be increased by: Anti-TNF Agents; Denosumab; Pimecrolimus; RiTUXimab; Roflumilast; Tacrolimus (Topical); Tocilizumab; Trastuzumab

Decreased Effect

Certolizumab Pegol may decrease the levels/effects of: BCG (Intravesical); Coccidioides immitis Skin Test; Sipuleucel-T; Vaccines (Inactivated); Vaccines (Live)

The levels/effects of Certolizumab Pegol may be decreased by: Echinacea; Pegloticase

Preparation for Administration Vials: Allow to reach room temperature prior to reconstitution. Using aseptic technique, reconstitute each vial with 1 mL sterile water for injection (provided) to a concentration of ~200 mg/mL; the manufacturer recommends using a 20-gauge needle (provided). Gently swirl to facilitate wetting of powder; do not shake. Allow vials to set undisturbed (may take up to 30 minutes) until fully reconstituted. Reconstituted solutions should not contain visible particles or gels in the solution.

Storage/Stability

Store intact vials and syringes at 2°C to 8°C (36°F to 46°F); do not freeze. Do not separate contents of carton prior to use. Protect from light. Bring to room temperature prior to administration.

Reconstituted vials may be retained at room temperature for up to 2 hours or refrigerated (do not freeze) for up to 24 hours prior to administration. Discard unused portion of vial or syringe.

Mechanism of Action Certolizumab pegol is a pegylated humanized antibody Fab' fragment of tumor necrosis factor alpha (TNF-alpha) monoclonal antibody. Certolizumab pegol binds to and selectively neutralizes human TNF-alpha activity. (Elevated levels of TNF-alpha have a role in the inflammatory process associated with Crohn disease and in joint destruction associated with rheumatoid arthritis.) Since it is not a complete antibody (lacks Fc region), it does not induce complement activation, antibody-dependent cell-mediated cytotoxicity, or apoptosis. Pegylation of certolizumab allows for delayed elimination and therefore an extended half-life.

Pharmacodynamics/Kinetics

Distribution: V_{ss}: 6-8 L
Bioavailability: SubQ: ~80% (range: 76% to 88%)
Half-life elimination: ~14 days
Time to peak, plasma: 54-171 hours

Dosing

Adult & Geriatric Note: Each 400 mg dose should be administered as 2 injections of 200 mg each

Ankylosing spondylitis: SubQ: Initial: 400 mg, repeat dose 2 and 4 weeks after initial dose; Maintenance: 200 mg every 2 weeks or 400 mg every 4 weeks

Crohn disease: SubQ: Initial: 400 mg, repeat dose 2 and 4 weeks after initial dose; Maintenance: 400 mg every 4 weeks

Psoriatic arthritis: SubQ: Initial: 400 mg, repeat dose 2 and 4 weeks after initial dose; Maintenance: 200 mg every other week. May consider maintenance dose of 400 mg every 4 weeks.

Rheumatoid arthritis: SubQ: Initial: 400 mg, repeat dose 2 and 4 weeks after initial dose; Maintenance: 200 mg every other week. May consider maintenance dose of 400 mg every 4 weeks. May be administered alone or in combination with methotrexate.

Renal Impairment There are no dosage adjustments provided in the manufacturer's labeling (has not been studied); pharmacokinetics of the pegylated (polyethylene glycol) component of certolizumab pegol is expected to be dependent on renal function.

Hepatic Impairment There are no dosage adjustments provided in the manufacturer's labeling.

Adjustment for Toxicity Hypersensitivity, lupus-like syndrome, serious infection, sepsis, or hepatitis B reactivation: Discontinue treatment.

Administration SubQ: Bring to room temperature prior to administration. After reconstitution (of vials), draw each vial into separate syringes (using 20-gauge needles).

Administer each syringe subcutaneously (using provided 23-gauge needle) to separate sites on abdomen or thigh. Rotate injections sites; do not administer to areas where skin is tender, bruised, red, or hard.

Missed doses (Canadian labeling): Wait until the next scheduled dose if within 1 week; if the next scheduled dose is ≥1 week administer as soon as possible then follow with next scheduled dose.

Monitoring Parameters Monitor improvement of symptoms and physical function assessments. Latent TB screening prior to initiating and during therapy; signs/symptoms of infection (prior to, during, and following therapy); CBC with differential; signs/symptoms/worsening of heart failure; HBV screening prior to initiating (all

patients), HBV carriers (during and for several months following therapy); signs and symptoms of hypersensitivity reaction; symptoms of lupus-like syndrome; signs/symptoms of malignancy (eg, splenomegaly, hepatomegaly, abdominal pain, persistent fever, night sweats, weight loss) including periodic skin examinations.

Test Interactions Tests for latent tuberculosis may be falsely negative while on certolizumab pegol treatment. Falsely elevated aPTT assays have been reported with PTT-Lupus Anticoagulant (LA) and Standard Target Activated Partial Thromboplastin time (STA-PTT) tests from Diagnostica Stago, and with HemosIL APTT-SP liquid and HemosIL lyophilized silica tests from Instrumentation Laboratories.

Dosage Forms Excipient information presented when available (limited, particularly for generics); consult specific product labeling.

Kit, Subcutaneous [preservative free]:
Cimzia: 200 mg
Cimzia Prefilled: 200 mg/mL
Cimzia Starter Kit: 6 X 200 mg/mL

Cetirizine (se TI ra zeen)

Brand Names: US All Day Allergy Childrens [OTC]; All Day Allergy [OTC]; Cetirizine HCl Allergy Child [OTC]; Cetirizine HCl Childrens Alrgy [OTC]; Cetirizine HCl Childrens [OTC]; Cetirizine HCl Hives Relief [OTC]; ZyrTEC Allergy Childrens [OTC]; ZyrTEC Allergy [OTC]; ZyrTEC Childrens Allergy [OTC]; ZyrTEC Childrens Hives Relief [OTC]; ZyrTEC Hives Relief [OTC]

Brand Names: Canada Aller-Relief [OTC]; Apo-Cetirizine [OTC]; Extra Strength Allergy Relief [OTC]; PMS-Cetirizine; Reactine; Reactine [OTC]

Index Terms Cetirizine Hydrochloride; P-071; UCB-P071

Pharmacologic Category Histamine H_1 Antagonist; Histamine H_1 Antagonist, Second Generation; Piperazine Derivative

Use

Upper respiratory allergies: Temporarily relieves symptoms of upper respiratory allergies.

Urticaria: Relieves itching due to urticaria.

Pregnancy Considerations Maternal use of cetirizine has not been associated with an increased risk of major malformations. The use of antihistamines for the treatment of rhinitis during pregnancy is generally considered to be safe at recommended doses. Although safety data is limited, cetirizine may be a preferred second generation antihistamine for the treatment of rhinitis during pregnancy.

Breast-Feeding Considerations Cetirizine is excreted into breast milk.

Contraindications Hypersensitivity to cetirizine, hydroxyzine, or any component of the formulation

Warnings/Precautions Cetirizine should be used cautiously in patients with hepatic or renal impairment; consider dosage adjustment in patients with renal impairment. Use with caution in elderly patients; may be more sensitive to adverse effects. May cause drowsiness; use caution performing tasks which require alertness (eg, operating machinery or driving). Potentially significant drug-drug interactions may exist, requiring dose or frequency adjustment, additional monitoring, and/or selection of alternative therapy. Effects may be potentiated when used with other sedative drugs or ethanol.

Adverse Reactions

>10%: Central nervous system: Drowsiness (adults 14%; children 2% to 4%), headache (children 11% to 14%, placebo 12%)

2% to 10%:
Central nervous system: Insomnia (children 9%; adults <2%), fatigue (adults 6%), malaise (4%), dizziness (adults 2%)

Gastrointestinal: Abdominal pain (children 4% to 6%), xerostomia (adults 5%), diarrhea (children 2% to 3%), nausea (children 2% to 3%; placebo 2%), vomiting (children 2% to 3%)

Respiratory: Pharyngitis (children 3% to 6%; placebo 3%), epistaxis (children 2% to 4%; placebo 3%), bronchospasm (children 2% to 3%; placebo 2%)

<2% (Limited to important or life-threatening; as reported in adults and/or children): Aggressive behavior, anaphylaxis, angioedema, ataxia, chest pain, confusion, convulsions, depersonalization, depression, dysgeusia, edema, fussiness, hallucination, hemolytic anemia, hepatic insufficiency, hepatitis, hypertension, hypotension (severe), irritability, nervousness, ototoxicity, palpitations, paralysis, paresthesia, skin photosensitivity, skin rash, suicidal ideation, tongue discoloration, tongue edema, tremor, visual field defect, weakness

Drug Interactions

Metabolism/Transport Effects Substrate of CYP3A4 (minor), P-glycoprotein; **Note:** Assignment of Major/Minor substrate status based on clinically relevant drug interaction potential

Avoid Concomitant Use

Avoid concomitant use of Cetirizine with any of the following: Aclidinium; Azelastine (Nasal); Cimetropium; Eluxadoline; Glucagon; Glycopyrrolate; Glycopyrrolate (Oral Inhalation); Ipratropium (Oral Inhalation); Levosulpiride; Orphenadrine; Paraldehyde; Potassium Chloride; Thalidomide; Tiotropium; Umeclidinium

Increased Effect/Toxicity

Cetirizine may increase the levels/effects of: AbobotulinumtoxinA; Alcohol (Ethyl); Analgesics (Opioid); Anticholinergic Agents; Azelastine (Nasal); Buprenorphine; Cimetropium; CNS Depressants; Eluxadoline; Glucagon; Glycopyrrolate; Glycopyrrolate (Oral Inhalation); Hydrocodone; Methotrimeprazine; Metyrosine; Mirabegron; Mirtazapine; OnabotulinumtoxinA; Orphenadrine; Paraldehyde; Potassium Chloride; Pramipexole; Ramosetron; RimabotulinumtoxinB; ROPINIRole; Rotigotine; Selective Serotonin Reuptake Inhibitors; Suvorexant; Thalidomide; Thiazide Diuretics; Tiotropium; Topiramate; Zolpidem

The levels/effects of Cetirizine may be increased by: Aclidinium; Brimonidine (Topical); Cannabis; Doxylamine; Dronabinol; Droperidol; HydrOXYzine; Ipratropium (Oral Inhalation); Kava Kava; Lumacaftor; Magnesium Sulfate; Methotrimeprazine; Mianserin; Minocycline; Nabilone; Perampanel; P-glycoprotein/ABCB1 Inhibitors; Pramlintide; Ranolazine; Rufinamide; Sodium Oxybate; Tapentadol; Tetrahydrocannabinol; Umeclidinium

Decreased Effect

Cetirizine may decrease the levels/effects of: Acetylcholinesterase Inhibitors; Benzylpenicilloyl Polylysine; Betahistine; Gastrointestinal Agents (Prokinetic); Hyaluronidase; Itopride; Levosulpiride; Secretin

The levels/effects of Cetirizine may be decreased by: Acetylcholinesterase Inhibitors; Amphetamines; Lumacaftor; P-glycoprotein/ABCB1 Inducers

Food Interactions Cetirizine's absorption and maximal concentration are reduced when taken with food. Management: May be taken without regard to meals.

Storage/Stability Store at 20°C to 25°C (68°F to 77°F); excursions are permitted between 15°C and 30°C (59°F and 86°F).

Mechanism of Action Competes with histamine for H_1-receptor sites on effector cells in the gastrointestinal tract, blood vessels, and respiratory tract

Pharmacodynamics/Kinetics

Onset of action: Suppression of skin wheal and flare: 0.7 hours (Simons 1999)

Duration of action: Suppression of skin wheal and flare: ≥24 hours (Simons 1999)

Absorption: Rapid

Distribution: Children: 0.7 L/kg; Adults: 0.56 L/kg (Simons 1999)

Protein binding, plasma: Mean: 93%

Metabolism: Limited hepatic

Half-life elimination: Children: 6.2 hours; Adults: 8 hours

Time to peak, serum: 1 hour

Excretion: Urine (70%; 50% as unchanged drug); feces (10%)

Dosing

Adult Upper respiratory allergies, urticaria: Oral: 5 to 10 mg once daily, depending upon symptom severity (maximum dose: 10 mg daily)

Geriatric Upper respiratory allergies, urticaria: Oral: 5 mg once daily (maximum dose: 5 mg daily). The previously available prescription product recommended a maximum dose of 10 mg once daily in patients <77 years of age or 5 mg once daily in patients ≥77 years of age (Zyrtec Prescribing Information, 2006).

Pediatric Upper respiratory allergies, urticaria: Oral:

Infants 6 to <12 months: 2.5 mg once daily

Children 12 months to <2 years: 2.5 mg once daily; may increase to a maximum dose of 2.5 mg every 12 hours if needed

Children 2 to 5 years: Initial: 2.5 mg once daily; may be increased to a maximum dose of 2.5 mg every 12 hours **or** 5 mg once daily

Children ≥6 years and Adolescents: Refer to adult dosing.

Renal Impairment There are no dosage adjustments provided in the manufacturer's labeling; however, the following adjustments have been recommended (Aronoff, 2007):

Adults:

GFR >50 mL/minute: No dosage adjustment necessary.

GFR ≤50 mL/minute: 5 mg once daily

Intermittent hemodialysis: 5 mg once daily; 5 mg 3 times per week may also be effective.

Peritoneal dialysis: 5 mg once daily.

Infants, Children, and Adolescents:

GFR ≥30 mL/minute/1.73 m^2: No dosage adjustment necessary.

GFR 10 to 29 mL/minute/1.73 m^2: Decrease dose by 50%.

GFR <10 mL/minute/1.73 m^2: Not recommended.

Intermittent hemodialysis or peritoneal dialysis: Decrease dose by 50%.

Hepatic Impairment There are no dosage adjustments provided in the manufacturer's labeling.

Administration

May be administered with or without food.

Chewable tablet: Chew tablet before swallowing; may be taken with or without water.

Monitoring Parameters Relief of symptoms, sedation and anticholinergic effects

Test Interactions May cause false-positive serum TCA screen. May suppress the wheal and flare reactions to skin test antigens.

Dosage Forms Excipient information presented when available (limited, particularly for generics); consult specific product labeling. [DSC] = Discontinued product

Capsule, Oral, as hydrochloride:

ZyrTEC Allergy: 10 mg

Solution, Oral, as hydrochloride:

All Day Allergy Childrens: 5 mg/5 mL (118 mL) [contains methylparaben, propylene glycol, propylparaben]

All Day Allergy Childrens: 5 mg/5 mL (118 mL) [dye free, gluten free; contains methylparaben, propylene glycol, propylparaben]

All Day Allergy Childrens: 1 mg/mL (118 mL [DSC]) [dye free, gluten free, sugar free; contains propylene glycol, sodium benzoate; grape flavor]

Cetirizine HCl Allergy Child: 5 mg/5 mL (120 mL) [alcohol free, dye free, gluten free, sugar free; contains methylparaben, propylene glycol, propylparaben; grape flavor]

Cetirizine HCl Allergy Child: 5 mg/5 mL (120 mL) [alcohol free, sugar free; contains methylparaben, propylene glycol, propylparaben]

Cetirizine HCl Childrens: 1 mg/mL (118 mL) [contains methylparaben, propylene glycol, propylparaben]

Cetirizine HCl Hives Relief: 5 mg/5 mL (120 mL) [alcohol free, sugar free; contains methylparaben, propylene glycol, propylparaben; grape flavor]

Generic: 1 mg/mL (120 mL, 473 mL)

Syrup, Oral, as hydrochloride:

Cetirizine HCl Childrens Alrgy: 1 mg/mL (118 mL, 120 mL) [contains methylparaben, propylene glycol, propylparaben; grape flavor]

Cetirizine HCl Childrens Alrgy: 5 mg/5 mL (120 mL [DSC]) [contains methylparaben, propylene glycol, propylparaben]

ZyrTEC Childrens Allergy: 1 mg/mL (118 mL) [contains methylparaben, propylene glycol, propylparaben; banana-grape flavor]

ZyrTEC Childrens Allergy: 1 mg/mL (118 mL) [dye free, sugar free; contains propylene glycol, sodium benzoate]

ZyrTEC Childrens Allergy: 1 mg/mL (118 mL) [dye free, sugar free; contains propylene glycol, sodium benzoate; bubble-gum flavor]

ZyrTEC Childrens Allergy: 5 mg/5 mL (5 mL, 118 mL) [dye free, sugar free; contains propylene glycol, sodium benzoate; grape flavor]

ZyrTEC Childrens Hives Relief: 1 mg/mL (118 mL) [grape flavor]

Generic: 1 mg/mL (120 mL, 473 mL [DSC], 480 mL); 5 mg/5 mL (5 mL, 120 mL [DSC])

Tablet, Oral, as hydrochloride:

All Day Allergy: 10 mg

ZyrTEC Allergy: 10 mg

ZyrTEC Hives Relief: 10 mg

Generic: 5 mg, 10 mg

Tablet Chewable, Oral, as hydrochloride:
All Day Allergy Childrens: 5 mg [DSC]
All Day Allergy Childrens: 10 mg [tutti-frutti flavor]
ZyrTEC Childrens Allergy: 5 mg [grape flavor]
ZyrTEC Childrens Allergy: 10 mg [contains fd&c blue #2 aluminum lake; grape flavor]
Generic: 5 mg, 10 mg
Tablet Dispersible, Oral, as hydrochloride:
ZyrTEC Allergy: 10 mg
ZyrTEC Allergy Childrens: 10 mg
ZyrTEC Allergy Childrens: 10 mg [citrus flavor]

◆ Cetirizine HCl Allergy Child [OTC] see Cetirizine on page 364

◆ Cetirizine HCl Childrens [OTC] see Cetirizine on page 364

◆ Cetirizine HCl Childrens Alrgy [OTC] see Cetirizine on page 364

◆ Cetirizine HCl Hives Relief [OTC] see Cetirizine on page 364

◆ Cetirizine Hydrochloride see Cetirizine on page 364

◆ Cetraxal see Ciprofloxacin (Otic) on page 393

Cetrorelix (set roe REL iks)

Brand Names: US Cetrotide
Brand Names: Canada Cetrotide®
Index Terms Cetrorelix Acetate
Pharmacologic Category Gonadotropin Releasing Hormone Antagonist
Use Inhibits premature luteinizing hormone (LH) surges in women undergoing controlled ovarian stimulation
Dosing
Adult Controlled ovarian stimulation in conjunction with gonadotropins (FSH, hMG): Female: SubQ:
Single-dose regimen: 3 mg given when serum estradiol levels show appropriate stimulation response, usually stimulation day 7 (range: days 5-9). If hCG is not administered within 4 days, continue cetrorelix at 0.25 mg/day until hCG is administered.
Multiple-dose regimen: 0.25 mg morning or evening of stimulation day 5, or morning of stimulation day 6; continue until hCG is administered.
Geriatric Not intended for use in women ≥65 years of age (Phase 2 and Phase 3 studies included women 19-40 years of age).
Renal Impairment
Severe impairment: Use is contraindicated.
Mild-to-moderate impairment: No dosage adjustment provided in manufacturer's labeling.
Hepatic Impairment No dosage adjustment provided in manufacturer's labeling.
Additional Information Complete prescribing information should be consulted for additional detail.
Dosage Forms Excipient information presented when available (limited, particularly for generics); consult specific product labeling. [DSC] = Discontinued product
Kit, Subcutaneous:
Cetrotide: 0.25 mg, 3 mg [DSC] [contains mannitol]

◆ Cetrorelix Acetate see Cetrorelix on page 366

◆ Cetrotide see Cetrorelix on page 366

◆ Cetrotide® (Can) see Cetrorelix on page 366

Cetuximab (se TUK see mab)

Brand Names: US Erbitux
Brand Names: Canada Erbitux
Index Terms C225; IMC-C225; MOAB C225
Pharmacologic Category Antineoplastic Agent, Epidermal Growth Factor Receptor (EGFR) Inhibitor; Antineoplastic Agent, Monoclonal Antibody
Use
Colorectal cancer, metastatic: Treatment of *KRAS* wild-type (without mutation), epidermal growth factor receptor (EGFR)-expressing metastatic colorectal cancer as determined by approved tests (in combination with FOL-FIRI [irinotecan, fluorouracil, and leucovorin] as first-line treatment, in combination with irinotecan [in patients refractory to irinotecan-based chemotherapy], or as a single agent in patients who have failed irinotecan- and oxaliplatin-based chemotherapy or who are intolerant to irinotecan).
Limitation of use: Cetuximab is not indicated for the treatment of *RAS*-mutant colorectal cancer or when results of the *RAS* mutation tests are unknown.
Head and neck cancer, squamous cell: Treatment of squamous cell cancer of the head and neck (as a single agent for recurrent or metastatic disease after platinum-based chemotherapy failure; in combination with radiation therapy as initial treatment of locally or regionally advanced disease; in combination with platinum and fluorouracil-based chemotherapy as first-line treatment of locoregional or metastatic disease).

Pregnancy Considerations Adverse events were observed in animal reproduction studies. Human IgG is known to cross the placenta. Because cetuximab inhibits epidermal growth factor (EGF), a component of fetal development, adverse effects on pregnancy would be expected. The manufacturer recommends that males and females use effective contraception during therapy and for 6 months following the last dose of cetuximab.

Breast-Feeding Considerations It is not known if cetuximab is excreted in breast milk. IgG antibodies can be detected in breast milk. Due to the potential for serious adverse reactions in the nursing infant, the manufacturer recommends that the decision to discontinue cetuximab or discontinue breast-feeding should take into account the benefits of treatment to the mother. If breast-feeding is interrupted for cetuximab treatment, based on the half-life, breast-feeding should not be resumed for at least 60 days following the last cetuximab dose.

Contraindications
There are no contraindications listed in the manufacturer's US labeling.
Canadian labeling: Known severe hypersensitivity to cetuximab or any component of the formulation

Warnings/Precautions [US Boxed Warning]: In clinical trials, serious infusion reactions have been reported in approximately 3% of patients; fatal outcome has been reported rarely (less than 1 in 1,000); interrupt infusion promptly and permanently discontinue for serious infusion reactions. Reactions have included airway obstruction (bronchospasm, stridor, hoarseness), hypotension, loss of consciousness, shock, myocardial infarction (MI), and/or cardiac arrest. Premedicate with an intravenous (IV) H_1 antagonist 30 to 60 minutes prior to the first dose; premedication for subsequent doses is based on clinical judgment and with consideration of prior reaction to the initial infusion. The use of nebulized albuterol-based premedication to prevent infusion reaction has been reported (Tra, 2008). Approximately 90% of reactions occur with the first infusion despite the use of prophylactic antihistamines. Immediate treatment for anaphylactic/anaphylactoid reactions should be available during administration. The manufacturer recommends monitoring patients for at least 1 hour following completion of infusion, or longer if a reaction occurs. Mild to moderate infusion reactions are managed by slowing the infusion rate (by 50%) and administering antihistamines. Patients with pre-existing IgE antibody against cetuximab (specific for galactose-α-1,3-galactose) are reported to have a higher incidence of severe hypersensitivity reaction. Severe hypersensitivity reaction has been reported more frequently in patients living in the middle south area of the United States, including North Carolina and Tennessee (Chung, 2008; O'Neil, 2007).

[US Boxed Warning]: In patients with squamous cell head and neck cancer, cardiopulmonary arrest and/or sudden death has occurred in 2% of patients receiving radiation therapy in combination with cetuximab and in 3% of patients receiving combination chemotherapy (platinum and fluorouracil-based) with cetuximab. Closely monitor serum electrolytes (magnesium, potassium, calcium) during and after cetuximab treatment (monitor for at least 8 weeks after treatment). Use with caution in patients with history of coronary artery disease, heart failure, and arrhythmias; fatalities have been reported. Interstitial lung disease has been reported; use with caution in patients with preexisting lung disease; interrupt treatment for acute onset or worsening of pulmonary symptoms; permanently discontinue with confirmed interstitial lung disease.

Acneiform rash has been reported in 76% to 88% of patients (severe in 1% to 17%), usually developing within the first 2 weeks of therapy; may require dose modification; generally resolved after discontinuation in most patients, although persisted beyond 28 days in some patients. Acneiform rash should be treated with topical and/or oral antibiotics; topical corticosteroids are not recommended. In colorectal cancer, the presence of acneiform rash correlates with treatment response and prolonged survival (Cunningham, 2004). Life-threatening and fatal bullous mucocutaneous disease (with blisters, erosions, and skin sloughing) has been observed with cetuximab; etiology is not determined; may be due to EGFR inhibition or to idiosyncratic immune-related effects (eg, Stevens-Johnson syndrome, toxic epidermal necrolysis). Other dermatologic toxicities, including dry skin, fissures, hypertrichosis, paronychial inflammation, and skin infections, have been reported; related ocular toxicities (blepharitis,

conjunctivitis, keratitis, ulcerative keratitis with decreased visual acuity) may also occur. Monitor closely for dermatologic toxicities and potential infectious sequelae. Sunlight may exacerbate skin reactions (limit sun exposure).

Hypomagnesemia is common (may be severe); the onset of electrolyte disturbance may occur within days to months after initiation of treatment; monitor magnesium, calcium, and potassium during treatment and for at least 8 weeks after completion; may require electrolyte replacement. Non-neutralizing anti-cetuximab antibodies were detected in 5% of evaluable patients. In a study of radiation therapy **and** cisplatin with or without cetuximab in patients with squamous cell head and neck cancer, an increase in the incidence of adverse reactions (eg, grade 3/4 mucositis, radiation recall, acneiform rash, electrolyte abnormalities, cardiac events including ischemia) was noted in patients receiving cetuximab, including fatal reactions; there was no improvement in the primary end point of progression-free survival.

In patients with colorectal cancer, cetuximab is only indicated for EGFR-expressing metastatic colorectal cancer without *RAS* (*KRAS* or *NRAS*) mutations. Determine *RAS* mutation status prior to treatment (with an approved test). Patients with a codon 12 and 13 (exon 2), codon 59 and 61 (exon 3), and codon 117 and 146 (exon 4) *RAS* mutation are unlikely to benefit from EGFR inhibitor therapy (while experiencing toxicities) and should not receive cetuximab treatment; cetuximab is not effective for colorectal cancer with RAS mutations. Cetuximab is also reported to be ineffective in patients with *BRAF* V600E mutation (Di Nicolantonio, 2008). The American Society of Clinical Oncology (ASCO) provisional clinical opinion (Allegra 2009) recommends genotyping tumor tissue for KRAS mutation in all patients with metastatic colorectal cancer (genotyping may be done on archived specimens). In trials for colorectal cancer, evidence of EGFR expression was required, although the response rate did not correlate with either the percentage of cells positive for EGFR or the intensity of expression. EGFR expression has been detected in nearly all patients with head and neck cancer; therefore laboratory evidence of EGFR expression is not necessary for head and neck cancers.

Adverse Reactions
>10%:
Central nervous system: Fatigue (91%), malaise (≤73%), pain (59%), peripheral sensory neuropathy (45%; grades 3/4: 1%), headache (19% to 38%), insomnia (27%), confusion (18%), chills (≤16%), rigors (≤16%), anxiety (14%), depression (14%)

Dermatologic: Desquamation (95%), acneiform eruption (15% to 88%; grades 3/4: 1% to 18%), radiodermatitis (86%), xeroderma (14% to 57%), pruritus (14% to 47%), skin rash (28% to 44%), changes in nails (31%), acne vulgaris (14% to 22%), paronychia (20%), palmar-plantar erythrodysesthesia (19%), skin fissure (19%), alopecia (12%)

Endocrine & metabolic: Weight loss (15% to 84%), hypomagnesemia (6% to 55%), dehydration (13% to 25%), hypocalcemia (12%), hypokalemia (12%)

Gastrointestinal: Diarrhea (19% to 72%), nausea (49% to 64%), abdominal pain (59%), constipation (53%), vomiting (40%), stomatitis (31% to 32%), anorexia (25% to 30%), dyspepsia (14% to 16%), xerostomia (12%)

Hematologic & oncologic: Neutropenia (49%; grades 3/4: 31%), leukopenia (grades 3/4: 17%)

Hepatic: Increased serum alanine aminotransferase (43%), increased serum aspartate aminotransferase (38%), increased serum alkaline phosphatase (33%)

Infection: Infection (13% to 44%), infection without neutropenia (38%)

Local: Application site reaction (18%)

Neuromuscular & skeletal: Weakness (≤73%), ostealgia (15%), arthralgia (14%)

Ophthalmic: Conjunctivitis (10% to 18%)

Respiratory: Dyspnea (49%), cough (30%), pharyngitis (26%)

Miscellaneous: Fever (22% to 29%), infusion related reaction (10% to 18%; grades 3/4: 2% to 5%)

1% to 10%:
Cardiovascular: Cardiorespiratory arrest (2% to 3%), ischemic heart disease (2%)

Dermatologic: Hypertrichosis

Gastrointestinal: Dysgeusia (10%)

Immunologic: Antibody development (5%)

Infection: Sepsis (1% to 4%)

Renal: Renal failure (1%: colorectal cancer patients; frequency not defined in other populations)

<1% (Limited to important or life-threatening; all studies): Abscess, aseptic meningitis, blepharitis, cardiac arrhythmia, cellulitis, cheilitis, corneal ulcer, hypotension, interstitial pulmonary disease, keratitis, leukopenia, loss of consciousness, myocardial infarction, pulmonary embolism, shock, stridor

Drug Interactions
Metabolism/Transport Effects None known.

Avoid Concomitant Use There are no known interactions where it is recommended to avoid concomitant use.

Increased Effect/Toxicity There are no known significant interactions involving an increase in effect.

Decreased Effect There are no known significant interactions involving a decrease in effect.

Preparation for Administration Reconstitution is not required. Appropriate dose should be added to empty sterile container (may contain a small amount of visible white, amorphous cetuximab particles); do not shake or dilute. Discard unused portion of the vial; discard any remaining solution in infusion container after 8 hours at room temperature or after 12 hours refrigerated.

Storage/Stability Store intact vials refrigerated at 2°C to 8°C (36°F to 46°F); do not freeze. Preparations in infusion containers are stable for up to 12 hours refrigerated at 2°C to 8°C (36°F to 46°F) and up to 8 hours at room temperature of 20°C to 25°C (68°F to 77°F).

Mechanism of Action Recombinant human/mouse chimeric monoclonal antibody which binds specifically to the epidermal growth factor receptor (EGFR, HER1, c-ErbB-1) and competitively inhibits the binding of epidermal growth factor (EGF) and other ligands. Binding to the EGFR blocks phosphorylation and activation of receptor-associated kinases, resulting in inhibition of cell growth, induction of apoptosis, and decreased matrix metalloproteinase and vascular endothelial growth factor production. EGFR signal transduction results in *RAS* wild-type activation; cells with *RAS* mutations appear to be unaffected by EGFR inhibition.

Pharmacodynamics/Kinetics
Distribution: V_d: ~2 to 3 L/m²

Half-life elimination: ~112 hours (range: 63 to 230 hours)

Dosing
Adult & Geriatric Note: Premedicate with an H_1 antagonist (eg, diphenhydramine) IV 30 to 60 minutes prior to the first dose; premedication for subsequent doses is based on clinical judgment.

Colorectal cancer, metastatic, KRAS wild-type (without mutation): IV:

Initial loading dose: 400 mg/m² infused over 120 minutes

Maintenance dose: 250 mg/m² infused over 60 minutes weekly until disease progression or unacceptable toxicity

Note: If given in combination with FOLFIRI (irinotecan, fluorouracil, and leucovorin), complete cetuximab infusion 1 hour prior to FOLFIRI.

Head and neck cancer (squamous cell): IV:

Initial loading dose: 400 mg/m² infused over 120 minutes

Maintenance dose: 250 mg/m² infused over 60 minutes weekly

Note: If given in combination with radiation therapy, administer loading dose 1 week prior to initiation of radiation course; weekly maintenance dose should be completed 1 hour prior to radiation for the duration of radiation therapy (6 to 7 weeks). If given in combination with chemotherapy, administer loading dose on the day of initiation of platinum and fluorouracil-based chemotherapy, cetuximab infusion should be completed 1 hour prior to initiation of chemotherapy; weekly maintenance dose should be completed 1 hour prior to chemotherapy; continue until disease progression or unacceptable toxicity. Monotherapy weekly doses should be continued until disease progression or unacceptable toxicity

Colorectal cancer, advanced, biweekly administration (off-label dosing): IV: 500 mg/m² every 2 weeks (initial dose infused over 120 minutes, subsequent doses infused over 60 minutes) in combination with irinotecan (Pfeiffer 2008)

Non-small cell lung cancer (NSCLC), EGFR-expressing, advanced (off-label use): IV: Initial loading dose: 400 mg/m², followed by maintenance dose: 250 mg/m² weekly in combination with cisplatin and vinorelbine for up to 6 cycles, then as monotherapy until disease progression or unacceptable toxicity (Pirker 2009; Pirker 2012)

Squamous cell skin cancer, unresectable (off-label use): IV: Initial loading dose: 400 mg/m², followed by maintenance dose: 250 mg/m² weekly until disease progression (Maubec 2011)

Renal Impairment There are no dosage adjustments provided in the manufacturer's labeling.

Hepatic Impairment There are no dosage adjustments provided in the manufacturer's labeling.

Adjustment for Toxicity

Infusion reactions, grade 1 or 2 and nonserious grade 3: Reduce the infusion rate by 50% and continue to use prophylactic antihistamines

Infusion reactions, severe: Immediately and permanently discontinue treatment

Pulmonary toxicity:

Acute onset or worsening pulmonary symptoms: Hold treatment

Interstitial lung disease: Permanently discontinue

Skin toxicity, mild to moderate: No dosage modification required

Acneiform rash, severe (grade 3 or 4):

First occurrence: Delay cetuximab infusion 1 to 2 weeks

If improvement, continue at 250 mg/m^2

If no improvement, discontinue therapy

Second occurrence: Delay cetuximab infusion 1 to 2 weeks

If improvement, continue at reduced dose of 200 mg/m^2

If no improvement, discontinue therapy

Third occurrence: Delay cetuximab infusion 1 to 2 weeks

If improvement, continue at reduced dose of 150 mg/m^2

If no improvement, discontinue therapy

Fourth occurrence: Discontinue therapy

Administration Administer via IV infusion; loading dose over 2 hours, weekly maintenance dose over 1 hour. Do not administer as IV push or bolus. Do not shake or dilute. Administer via infusion pump or syringe pump. Following the infusion, an observation period (1 hour) is recommended; longer observation time (following an infusion reaction) may be required. Premedication with an H$_1$ antagonist prior to the initial dose is recommended. The maximum infusion rate is 10 mg/minute. Administer through a low protein-binding 0.22 micrometer in-line filter.

For biweekly administration (off-label frequency and dose), the initial dose was infused over 120 minutes and subsequent doses infused over 60 minutes (Pfeiffer 2007; Pfeiffer 2008).

Monitoring Parameters Vital signs during infusion and observe for at least 1 hour postinfusion. Patients developing dermatologic toxicities should be monitored for the development of complications. Periodic monitoring of serum magnesium, calcium, and potassium are recommended to continue over an interval consistent with the half-life (8 weeks); monitor closely (during and after treatment) for cetuximab plus radiation therapy. *KRAS* genotyping of tumor tissue in patients with colorectal cancer

Dosage Forms Excipient information presented when available (limited, particularly for generics); consult specific product labeling.

Solution, Intravenous [preservative free]:

Erbitux: 100 mg/50 mL (50 mL); 200 mg/100 mL (100 mL) [contains galactose-alpha-1,3-galactose]

Cevimeline (se vi ME leen)

Brand Names: US Evoxac

Brand Names: Canada Evoxac®

Index Terms Cevimeline Hydrochloride

Pharmacologic Category Cholinergic Agonist

Use Treatment of symptoms of dry mouth in patients with Sjögren's syndrome

Dosing

Adult Xerostomia (in Sjögren's syndrome): Oral: 30 mg 3 times/day

Geriatric Refer to adult dosing. No specific dosage adjustment is recommended; however, use caution when initiating due to potential for increased sensitivity.

Renal Impairment No dosage adjustment provided in the manufacturer's labeling.

Hepatic Impairment No dosage adjustment provided in the manufacturer's labeling.

Additional Information Complete prescribing information should be consulted for additional detail.

Dosage Forms Excipient information presented when available (limited, particularly for generics); consult specific product labeling.

Capsule, Oral, as hydrochloride:

Evoxac: 30 mg

Generic: 30 mg

◆ Cevimeline Hydrochloride see Cevimeline on page 368

◆ CFDN see Cefdinir on page 332

◆ CFZ see Carfilzomib on page 315

◆ CG see Chorionic Gonadotropin (Human) on page 382

◆ CG5503 see Tapentadol on page 1736

◆ CGP 33101 see Rufinamide on page 1625

◆ CGP-39393 see Desirudin on page 519

◆ CGP-42446 see Zoledronic Acid on page 1934

◆ CGP-57148B see Imatinib on page 919

◆ CGS-20267 see Letrozole on page 1048

◆ CGX-625 see Omacetaxine on page 1324

◆ ch14.18 see Dinutuximab on page 559

◆ Champix® (Can) see Varenicline on page 1877

◆ Chantix see Varenicline on page 1877

◆ Chantix Continuing Month Pak see Varenicline on page 1877

◆ Chantix Starting Month Pak see Varenicline on page 1877

◆ Charac-25 [OTC] (Can) see Charcoal, Activated on page 368

◆ Charac-50 [OTC] (Can) see Charcoal, Activated on page 368

◆ Charactol-25 [OTC] (Can) see Charcoal, Activated on page 368

◆ Charactol-50 [OTC] (Can) see Charcoal, Activated on page 368

Charcoal, Activated (CHAR kole AK tiv ay ted)

Brand Names: US Actidose-Aqua [OTC]; Actidose/Sorbitol [OTC]; Char-Flo with Sorbitol [OTC]; EZ Char [OTC]; Kerr Insta-Char in Sorbitol [OTC]; Kerr Insta-Char [OTC]

Brand Names: Canada Charac-25 [OTC]; Charac-50 [OTC]; Charactol-25 [OTC]; Charactol-50 [OTC]; Charcodote Susp [OTC]; Charcodote TFS [OTC]; Charcodote-Aqueous Sus; Premium Activated Charcoal [OTC]

Index Terms Activated Carbon; Activated Charcoal; Adsorbent Charcoal; Liquid Antidote; Medicinal Carbon; Medicinal Charcoal

Pharmacologic Category Antidote

Use

Suspension: Activated charcoal is a nonabsorbable adsorbent that may be considered in the management of poisonings when gastrointestinal decontamination of drugs or chemicals is indicated (eg, presentation to a treatment facility within 1 hour of ingestion). Activated charcoal is generally an effective adsorbent of drugs and chemicals with a molecular weight range of 100-1000 daltons. Multidose activated charcoal may be considered if a patient has ingested a life-threatening amount of carbamazepine, dapsone, phenobarbital, quinine, or theophylline (Vale, 1999).

Capsules, tablets: Digestive aid

Pregnancy Considerations Activated charcoal is not absorbed systemically following oral administration. Use during pregnancy is not expected to result in significant exposure to the fetus. In general, medications used as antidotes should take into consideration the health and prognosis of the mother; antidotes should be administered to pregnant women if there is a clear indication for use and should not be withheld because of fears of teratogenicity (Bailey, 2003).

Breast-Feeding Considerations Activated charcoal is not absorbed systemically following oral administration. Breast-feeding is not expected to result in significant exposure to a nursing child.

Contraindications There are no absolute contraindications listed within the manufacturer's labeling.

Note: The American Academy of Clinical Toxicology (AACT) and European Association of Poisons Centres and Clinical Toxicologists (EAPCCT) consider the following to be contraindications to the use of charcoal (Chyka, 2005; Vale, 1999): Presence of intestinal obstruction or GI tract not anatomically intact; patients at risk of GI hemorrhage or perforation; patients with an unprotected airway (eg, CNS depression without intubation); if use would increase the risk and severity of aspiration

Warnings/Precautions Charcoal may cause vomiting; the risk appears to be greater when charcoal is administered with sorbitol (Chyka, 2005). IV antiemetics may be required to reduce the risk of vomiting or to control vomiting to facilitate administration (Vale, 1999). Due to the risk of vomiting, avoid the use of charcoal in hydrocarbon and caustic ingestions. Use caution with decreased peristalsis. Some products may contain sorbitol. Coadministration of a cathartic is **not** recommended; cathartics (eg, sorbitol, mannitol, magnesium sulfate) have not been demonstrated to change patient outcome and have no role in

the management of the poisoned patient. Cathartics subject the patient to the risk of developing significant fluid and electrolyte abnormalities (AACT, 2004a). Do not use products containing sorbitol in persons with a genetic intolerance to fructose or in patients who are dehydrated; may cause excessive diarrhea. Ipecac should not be administered routinely in the management of poisoned patients (AACT, 2004b).

Not effective in the treatment of poisonings due to the ingestion of low molecular weight compounds such as cyanide, iron, ethanol, methanol, or lithium. Most effective when administered within 30-60 minutes of ingestion. Based on experimental and clinical studies, multidose activated charcoal, in most acute poisonings, has not been shown to reduce morbidity or mortality (Vale, 1999). It may be considered if a patient has ingested a life-threatening amount of carbamazepine, dapsone, phenobarbital, quinine, or theophylline, although no controlled studies have demonstrated clinical benefit.

Benzyl alcohol and derivatives: Some dosage forms may contain sodium benzoate/benzoic acid; benzoic acid (benzoate) is a metabolite of benzyl alcohol; large amounts of benzyl alcohol (≥99 mg/kg/day) have been associated with a potentially fatal toxicity ("gasping syndrome") in neonates; the "gasping syndrome" consists of metabolic acidosis, respiratory distress, gasping respirations, CNS dysfunction (including convulsions, intracranial hemorrhage), hypotension, and cardiovascular collapse (AAP ["Inactive" 1997]; CDC, 1982); some data suggests that benzoate displaces bilirubin from protein binding sites (Ahlfors, 2001); avoid or use dosage forms containing benzyl alcohol derivative with caution in neonates. See manufacturer's labeling.

Some dosage forms may contain propylene glycol; large amounts are potentially toxic and have been associated hyperosmolality, lactic acidosis, seizures and respiratory depression; use caution (AAP ["Inactive" 1997]; Zar, 2007). Capsules and tablets should not be used for the treatment of poisoning.

Adverse Reactions Frequency not defined.
Gastrointestinal: Abdominal distention, appendicitis, bowel obstruction, constipation, vomiting
Ocular: Corneal abrasion (with direct contact)
Respiratory: Aspiration, respiratory failure
Miscellaneous: Fecal discoloration (black)

Drug Interactions
Metabolism/Transport Effects None known.
Avoid Concomitant Use There are no known interactions where it is recommended to avoid concomitant use.
Increased Effect/Toxicity There are no known significant interactions involving an increase in effect.
Decreased Effect
Charcoal, Activated may decrease the levels/effects of: Leflunomide; Teriflunomide

Food Interactions The addition of some flavoring agents (eg, milk, ice cream, sherbet, marmalade) are known to reduce the adsorptive capacity, and therefore the efficacy, of activated charcoal and should be avoided in preference to activated charcoal-water slurries; nevertheless, these flavoring agents do not completely compromise the effectiveness of activated charcoal and may be necessary in some circumstances (eg, administration in pediatric patients) to enhance compliance (Cooney, 1995; Dagnone, 2002).

Preparation for Administration Powder: Dilute with at least 8 mL of water per 1 g of charcoal, or mix in a charcoal to water ratio of 1:4 to 1:8; mix vigorously to form a slurry (eg, mix 25 g with sufficient tap water to create a 4-ounce slurry or mix 50 g with sufficient tap water to create an 8-ounce slurry).

Storage/Stability Adsorbs gases from air, store in a closed container.

Mechanism of Action Adsorbs toxic substances, thus inhibiting GI absorption and preventing systemic toxicity. Administration of multiple doses of charcoal may interrupt enteroenteric, enterohepatic, and enterogastric circulation of some drugs; may also adsorb any unabsorbed drug which remains in the gut.

Pharmacodynamics/Kinetics
Note: In studies using adult human volunteers: Mean **reduction** in drug absorption following a single dose of ≥50 g activated charcoal (AACT [Chyka 2005]):
Given within 30 minutes after ingestion: 47.3% reduction
Given at 60 minutes after ingestion: 40.07% reduction
Given at 120 minutes after ingestion: 16.5% reduction
Given at 180 minutes after ingestion: 21.13% reduction
Given at 240 minutes after ingestion: 32.5% reduction
Absorption: Not absorbed from the GI tract
Excretion: Feces (as charcoal)

Dosing
Adult & Geriatric Acute poisoning: Oral, NG: **Note:** Some products may contain sorbitol; coadministration of a cathartic, including sorbitol, is **not** recommended. Some clinicians still recommend dosing activated charcoal in a 10:1 (charcoal:poison) ratio for optimal efficacy (Gude, 2009); however, the amount of poison ingested is commonly unknown, which makes this approach challenging and often impractical (Chyka, 2005).
Single dose (Chyka, 2005): 25-100 g
Multidose: Initial dose: 50-100 g followed by 25-50 g every 4 hours
Pediatric Acute poisoning: Oral, NG: **Note:** Some products may contain sorbitol; coadministration of a cathartic, including sorbitol, is **not** recommended. Some clinicians still recommend dosing activated charcoal in a 10:1 (charcoal:poison) ratio for optimal efficacy (Gude, 2009); however, the amount of poison ingested is commonly unknown, which makes this approach challenging and often impractical (Chyka, 2005).
Single dose (Chyka, 2005):
Infants <1 year: 10-25 g; **Note:** Although dosing by body weight is reported in children (0.5-1 g/kg) and published in many resources, there are no data or scientific rationale to support this recommendation.
Children 1-12 years: 25-50 g
Children >12 years: Refer to adult dosing.
Multidose: Initial dose: 25-50 g; followed by multiple doses of 10-25 g every 4 hours

Administration Flavoring agents (eg, chocolate syrup, concentrated fruit juice) or thickening agents (eg, bentonite, carboxymethylcellulose) can enhance charcoal's palatability. Check for the presence of bowel sounds before administration. IV antiemetics may be required to reduce the risk of vomiting. The activated charcoal container should be agitated thoroughly before administration. The container should be rinsed with a small quantity of water to insure that the patient has received all of the activated charcoal (Krenzelok, 1991).

Capsules and tablets should not be used for the treatment of poisoning.

Dosage Forms Excipient information presented when available (limited, particularly for generics); consult specific product labeling.
Liquid, Oral:
Actidose-Aqua: 15 g/72 mL (72 mL); 25 g/120 mL (120 mL); 50 g/240 mL (240 mL) [sweet flavor]
Actidose/Sorbitol: 25 g/120 mL (120 mL); 50 g/240 mL (240 mL) [sweet flavor]
Kerr Insta-Char: 25 g/120 mL (120 mL); 50 g/240 mL (240 mL) [contains fd&c red #40, methylparaben sodium, propylene glycol, propylparaben sodium, sodium benzoate; cherry flavor]
Kerr Insta-Char: 50 g/240 mL (240 mL) [contains propylene glycol]
Kerr Insta-Char in Sorbitol: 25 g/120 mL (120 mL); 50 g/240 mL (240 mL) [contains fd&c red #40, methylparaben sodium, propylene glycol, propylparaben sodium, sodium benzoate; cherry flavor]
Suspension, Oral:
Char-Flo with Sorbitol: 25 g (120 mL)
Suspension Reconstituted, Oral:
EZ Char: 25 g (1 ea) [contains bentonite]

◆ Charcodote-Aqueous Sus (Can) *see* Charcoal, Activated *on page 368*

◆ Charcodote Susp [OTC] (Can) *see* Charcoal, Activated *on page 368*

◆ Charcodote TFS [OTC] (Can) *see* Charcoal, Activated *on page 368*

◆ Char-Flo with Sorbitol [OTC] *see* Charcoal, Activated *on page 368*

◆ Chateal *see* Ethinyl Estradiol and Levonorgestrel *on page 703*

◆ Chemet *see* Succimer *on page 1702*

◆ Chenodal *see* Chenodiol *on page 369*

◆ Chenodeoxycholic Acid *see* Chenodiol *on page 369*

Chenodiol (kee noe DYE ole)

Brand Names: US Chenodal
Index Terms CDCA; Chenodeoxycholic Acid
Pharmacologic Category Bile Acid
Use Oral dissolution of radiolucent cholesterol gallstones in selected patients as an alternative to surgery
Prescribing and Access Restrictions Prescriptions are only dispensed by a specialty pharmacy, Centric Health Resources, which may be contacted at 866-758-7068.

Dosing

Adult

Cerebrotendinous xanthomatosis (off-label use): Oral: 750 mg daily in 3 divided doses (Beringer, 1984)

Gallstone dissolution (monotherapy): Oral: Initial: 250 mg twice daily for the first 2 weeks and increasing by 250 mg daily each week thereafter until the recommended or maximum tolerated dose is achieved; maintenance: 13-16 mg/kg/day in 2 divided doses. **Note:** Dosages <10 mg/kg are usually ineffective and may increase the risk of cholecystectomy.

Gallstone dissolution (combination therapy; off-label dose): Oral: 5-7.5 mg/kg/day once daily at bedtime, in combination with ursodeoxycholic acid, with or without adjuvant lithotripsy (Jazrawi, 1992; Pereira, 1997; Petroni, 2001)

Renal Impairment No dosage adjustment provided in manufacturer's labeling.

Hepatic Impairment Use extreme caution; contraindicated for use in presence of known hepatocyte dysfunction or bile duct abnormalities.

Additional Information Complete prescribing information should be consulted for additional detail.

Dosage Forms Excipient information presented when available (limited, particularly for generics); consult specific product labeling.

Tablet, Oral:
  Chenodal: 250 mg

Chlorambucil (klor AM byoo sil)

Brand Names: US Leukeran

Brand Names: Canada Leukeran®

Index Terms CB-1348; Chlorambucilum; Chloraminophene; Chlorbutinum; WR-139013

Pharmacologic Category Antineoplastic Agent, Alkylating Agent; Antineoplastic Agent, Alkylating Agent (Nitrogen Mustard)

Use

Chronic lymphocytic leukemia (CLL): Management of CLL

Lymphomas: Management of Hodgkin lymphoma and non-Hodgkin lymphomas (NHL)

Canadian labeling: Additional uses (not in U.S. labeling): Management of Waldenström's macroglobulinemia

Pregnancy Considerations Animal reproduction studies have demonstrated teratogenicity. Chlorambucil crosses the human placenta. Following exposure during the first trimester, case reports have noted adverse renal effects (unilateral agenesis). Women of childbearing potential should avoid becoming pregnant while receiving treatment. **[U.S. Boxed Warning]: Affects human fertility; probably mutagenic and teratogenic as well**; chromosomal damage has been documented. Reversible and irreversible sterility (when administered to prepubertal and pubertal males), azoospermia (in adult males) and amenorrhea (in females) have been observed. Fibrosis, vasculitis and depletion of primordial follicles have been noted on autopsy of the ovaries.

Breast-Feeding Considerations It is not known if chlorambucil is excreted in breast milk. Due to the potential for serious adverse reactions in the nursing infant, the decision to discontinue chlorambucil or to discontinue breast-feeding should take into account the benefits of treatment to the mother.

Contraindications Hypersensitivity to chlorambucil or any component of the formulation; hypersensitivity to other alkylating agents (may have cross-hypersensitivity); prior (demonstrated) resistance to chlorambucil

Canadian labeling: Additional contraindications (not in U.S. labeling): Use within 4 weeks of a full course of radiation or chemotherapy

Warnings/Precautions Hazardous agent - use appropriate precautions for handling and disposal (NIOSH 2014 [group 1]). Seizures have been observed; use with caution in patients with seizure disorder or head trauma; history of nephrotic syndrome and high pulse doses are at higher risk of seizures. **[U.S. Boxed Warning]: May cause severe bone marrow suppression;** neutropenia may be severe. Reduce initial dosage if patient has received myelosuppressive or radiation therapy within the previous 4 weeks, or has a depressed baseline leukocyte or platelet count. Irreversible bone marrow damage may occur with total doses approaching 6.5 mg/kg. Progressive lymphopenia may develop (recovery is generally rapid after discontinuation). Avoid administration of live vaccines to immunocompromised patients. Rare instances of severe skin reactions (eg, erythema multiforme, Stevens-Johnson syndrome, toxic epidermal necrolysis) have been reported; discontinue promptly if skin reaction occurs.

Chlorambucil is primarily metabolized in the liver. Dosage reductions should be considered in patients with hepatic impairment. **[U.S. Boxed Warning]: Affects human fertility; carcinogenic in humans and probably mutagenic and teratogenic as well;** chromosomal damage has been documented. Reversible and irreversible sterility (when administered to prepubertal and pubertal males), azoospermia (in adult males) and amenorrhea (in females) have been observed. **[U.S. Boxed Warning]: Carcinogenic;** acute myelocytic leukemia and secondary malignancies may be associated with chronic therapy. Duration of treatment and higher cumulative doses are associated with a higher risk for development of leukemia. Potentially significant drug-drug interactions may exist, requiring dose or frequency adjustment, additional monitoring, and/or selection of alternative therapy.

Adverse Reactions Frequency not always defined.

Central nervous system: Agitation (rare), ataxia (rare), confusion (rare), drug fever, fever, focal/generalized seizure (rare), hallucinations (rare)

Dermatologic: Angioneurotic edema, erythema multiforme (rare), rash, skin hypersensitivity, Stevens-Johnson syndrome (rare), toxic epidermal necrolysis (rare), urticaria

Endocrine & metabolic: Amenorrhea, infertility, SIADH (rare)

Gastrointestinal: Diarrhea (infrequent), nausea (infrequent), oral ulceration (infrequent), vomiting (infrequent)

Genitourinary: Azoospermia, cystitis (sterile)

Hematologic: Neutropenia (onset: 3 weeks; recovery: 10 days after last dose), bone marrow failure (irreversible), bone marrow suppression, anemia, leukemia (secondary), leukopenia, lymphopenia, pancytopenia, thrombocytopenia

Hepatic: Hepatotoxicity, jaundice

Neuromuscular & skeletal: Flaccid paresis (rare), muscular twitching (rare), myoclonia (rare), peripheral neuropathy, tremor (rare)

Respiratory: Interstitial pneumonia, pulmonary fibrosis

Miscellaneous: Allergic reactions, malignancies (secondary)

Drug Interactions

Metabolism/Transport Effects None known.

Avoid Concomitant Use

Avoid concomitant use of Chlorambucil with any of the following: BCG (Intravesical); Deferiprone; Dipyrone; Natalizumab; Pimecrolimus; Tacrolimus (Topical); Tofacitinib; Vaccines (Live)

Increased Effect/Toxicity

Chlorambucil may increase the levels/effects of: CloZAPine; Deferiprone; Fingolimod; Leflunomide; Natalizumab; Tofacitinib; Vaccines (Live)

The levels/effects of Chlorambucil may be increased by: Denosumab; Dipyrone; Pimecrolimus; Roflumilast; Tacrolimus (Topical); Trastuzumab

Decreased Effect

Chlorambucil may decrease the levels/effects of: BCG (Intravesical); Coccidioides immitis Skin Test; Sipuleucel-T; Vaccines (Inactivated); Vaccines (Live)

The levels/effects of Chlorambucil may be decreased by: Echinacea

Food Interactions Absorption is decreased when administered with food. Management: Administer preferably on an empty stomach.

Storage/Stability Store in refrigerator at 2°C to 8°C (36°F to 46°F).

Mechanism of Action Alkylating agent; interferes with DNA replication and RNA transcription by alkylation and cross-linking the strands of DNA

Pharmacodynamics/Kinetics

Absorption: Rapid and complete (>70%) from GI tract; reduced with food

Distribution: V_d: ~0.3 L/kg

Protein binding: ~99%; primarily to albumin

Metabolism: Hepatic (extensively); primarily to active metabolite, phenylacetic acid mustard

Half-life elimination: ~1.5 hours; Phenylacetic acid mustard: ~1.8 hours

Time to peak, plasma: Within 1 hour; Phenylacetic acid mustard: Within 1.9 ± 0.7 hours

Excretion: Urine (~20% to 60% within 24 hours, primarily as inactive metabolites, <1% as unchanged drug or phenylacetic acid mustard)

Dosing

Adult Note: With bone marrow lymphocytic infiltration involvement (in CLL, Hodgkin lymphoma, or NHL), the maximum dose is 0.1 mg/kg/day. While short treatment courses are preferred, if maintenance therapy is required, the maximum dose is 0.1 mg/kg/day.

Chronic lymphocytic leukemia (CLL): Oral:

U.S. labeling: 0.1 mg/kg/day for 3-6 weeks **or** 0.4 mg/kg pulsed doses administered intermittently, biweekly, or monthly (increased by 0.1 mg/kg/dose until response/toxicity observed)

Canadian labeling: Initial: 0.15 mg/kg/day until WBC is 10,000/mm³; interrupt treatment for 4 weeks, then may resume at 0.1 mg/kg/day until response (generally ~2 years)/toxicity observed

Off-label dosing for CLL: 0.4 mg/kg day 1 every 2 weeks; if tolerated may increase by 0.1 mg/kg with each treatment course to a maximum dose of 0.8 mg/kg and maximum of 24 cycles (Eichhorst, 2009) **or** 30 mg/m² day 1 every 2 weeks (in combination with prednisone) (Raphael, 1991) **or** 40 mg/m² day 1 every 4 weeks until disease progression or complete remission or response plateau for up to a maximum of 12 cycles (Rai, 2000)

Hodgkin lymphoma: Oral:

U.S. labeling: 0.2 mg/kg/day for 3-6 weeks

Canadian labeling: 0.2 mg/kg/day for 4-8 weeks

Non-Hodgkin lymphomas (NHL): Oral:

U.S. labeling: 0.1 mg/kg/day for 3-6 weeks

Canadian labeling: Initial: 0.1-0.2 mg/kg/day for 4-8 weeks; for maintenance treatment, reduce dose or administer intermittently

Waldenström's macroglobulinemia (U.S. off-label use): Oral: 0.1 mg/kg/day (continuously) for at least 6 months **or** 0.3 mg/kg/day for 7 days every 6 weeks for at least 6 months (Kyle, 2000)

Geriatric Refer to adult dosing. Begin at the lower end of dosing range(s)

Pediatric Nephrotic syndrome, steroid sensitive (off-label use): Oral: 0.2 mg/kg once daily for ~8 weeks (Hodson, 2010)

Renal Impairment No dosage adjustment provided in manufacturer's labeling; however, renal elimination of unchanged chlorambucil and active metabolite (phenylacetic acid mustard) is minimal and renal impairment is not likely to affect elimination. The following adjustments have been recommended: Adults:

Aronoff, 2007:

CrCl >50 mL/minute: No adjustment necessary.

CrCl 10-50 mL/minute: Administer 75% of dose.

CrCl <10 mL/minute: Administer 50% of dose.

Peritoneal dialysis (PD): Administer 50% of dose.

Kintzel, 1995: Based on the pharmacokinetics, dosage adjustment is not indicated

Hepatic Impairment Chlorambucil undergoes extensive hepatic metabolism. Although dosage reduction should be considered in patients with hepatic impairment, no dosage adjustment is provided in the manufacturer's labeling (data is insufficient).

Obesity *ASCO Guidelines for appropriate chemotherapy dosing in obese adults with cancer:* Utilize patient's actual body weight (full weight) for calculation of body surface area- or weight-based dosing, particularly when

the intent of therapy is curative; manage regimen-related toxicities in the same manner as for nonobese patients; if a dose reduction is utilized due to toxicity, consider resumption of full weight-based dosing with subsequent cycles, especially if cause of toxicity (eg, hepatic or renal impairment) is resolved (Griggs, 2012). **Note:** The manufacturer recommends the maximum dose should not exceed 0.1 mg/kg/day if maintenance therapy is required and with bone marrow infiltration.

Adjustment for Toxicity

Skin reactions: Discontinue treatment

Hematologic:

WBC or platelets below normal: Reduce dose.

Severely depressed WBC or platelet counts: Discontinue.

Persistently low neutrophil or platelet counts or peripheral lymphocytosis: May be suggestive of bone marrow infiltration; if infiltration confirmed, do not exceed 0.1 mg/kg/day.

Concurrent or within 4 weeks (before or after) of chemotherapy/radiotherapy: Initiate treatment cautiously; reduce dose; monitor closely.

Administration May be administered as a single daily dose; preferably on an empty stomach.

Hazardous agent; use appropriate precautions for handling and disposal (NIOSH 2014 [group 1]).

Monitoring Parameters Liver function tests, CBC with differential (weekly, with WBC monitored twice weekly during the first 3-6 weeks of treatment)

Dosage Forms Excipient information presented when available (limited, particularly for generics); consult specific product labeling.

Tablet, Oral:

Leukeran: 2 mg

Extemporaneous Preparations Hazardous agent: Use appropriate precautions for handling and disposal (NIOSH 2014 [group 1]).

A 2 mg/mL oral suspension may be prepared with tablets. Crush sixty 2 mg tablets in a mortar and reduce to a fine powder. Add small portions of methylcellulose 1% and mix to a uniform paste (total methylcellulose: 30 mL); mix while adding simple syrup in incremental proportions to **almost** 60 mL; transfer to a graduated cylinder, rinse mortar and pestle with simple syrup, and add quantity of vehicle sufficient to make 60 mL. Transfer contents of graduated cylinder to an amber prescription bottle. Label "shake well", "refrigerate", and "protect from light". Stable for 7 days refrigerated.

Dressman JB and Poust RI, "Stability of Allopurinol and of Five Antineoplastics in Suspension," *Am J Hosp Pharm*, 1983, 40(4):616-8.

Nahata MC, Pai VB, and Hipple TF, *Pediatric Drug Formulations*, 5th ed, Cincinnati, OH: Harvey Whitney Books Co, 2004.

◆ Chlorambucilum *see* Chlorambucil *on page 370*

◆ Chloraminophene *see* Chlorambucil *on page 370*

Chloramphenicol (klor am FEN i kole)

Brand Names: Canada Chloromycetin®; Chloromycetin® Succinate; Diochloram®; Pentamycetin®

Pharmacologic Category Antibiotic, Miscellaneous

Use Treatment of serious infections due to organisms resistant to other less toxic antibiotics or when its penetrability into the site of infection is clinically superior to other antibiotics to which the organism is sensitive; useful in infections caused by *Bacteroides*, *H. influenzae*, *Neisseria meningitidis*, *Salmonella*, and *Rickettsia*; active against many vancomycin-resistant enterococci

Pregnancy Considerations Chloramphenicol crosses the placenta producing cord concentrations approaching maternal serum concentrations. An increased risk of teratogenic effects has not been associated with the use of chloramphenicol in pregnancy (Czeizel, 2000; Heinonen, 1977). "Gray Syndrome" has occurred in premature infants and newborns receiving chloramphenicol. The manufacturer recommends caution if used in a pregnant patient near term or during labor. Chloramphenicol may be used for the treatment of Rocky Mountain spotted fever in pregnant women although caution should be used when administration occurs during the third trimester (CDC, 2006).

Breast-Feeding Considerations Chloramphenicol and its inactive metabolites are excreted in breast milk. Chloramphenicol is well absorbed following oral administration; however, metabolism and excretion are highly variable in infants and children. The half-life is also significantly prolonged in low birth weight infants (Powell, 1982). Due to the potential for serious adverse reactions in the nursing infant, the manufacturer recommends that caution be exercised when administering chloramphenicol to nursing women. Other sources recommended avoiding use while

breast-feeding, especially infants <34 weeks postconceptual age or when unusually large doses are needed (Atkinson, 1988; Matsuda, 1984; Plomp, 1983). Non-dose-related effects could include modification of bowel flora.

Contraindications Hypersensitivity to chloramphenicol or any component of the formulation; treatment of trivial or viral infections; bacterial prophylaxis

Warnings/Precautions Hazardous agent - use appropriate precautions for handling and disposal (NIOSH 2014 [group 2]).

Use in neonates (including premature) has resulted in "gray-baby syndrome" characterized by circulatory collapse, cyanosis, acidosis, abdominal distention (with or without emesis), myocardial depression, coma, and death; progression of symptoms is rapid; prompt termination of therapy required. Reaction result from drug accumulation possibly caused by the impaired neonatal hepatic or renal function. Reduce dose with impaired liver function. Use with care in patients with glucose 6-phosphate dehydrogenase deficiency. **[U.S. Boxed Warning]: Serious and fatal blood dyscrasias (aplastic anemia, hypoplastic anemia, thrombocytopenia, and granulocytopenia) have occurred after both short-term and prolonged therapy. Monitor CBC frequently in all patients;** discontinue if evidence of myelosuppression. Irreversible bone marrow suppression may occur weeks or months after therapy. Avoid repeated courses of treatment. Should not be used for minor infections or when less potentially toxic agents are effective. Prolonged use may result in fungal or bacterial superinfection, including *C. difficile*-associated diarrhea (CDAD) and pseudomembranous colitis; CDAD has been observed >2 months postantibiotic treatment.

Adverse Reactions Frequency not defined.

Central nervous system: Confusion, delirium, depression, fever, headache

Dermatologic: Angioedema, rash, urticaria

Gastrointestinal: Diarrhea, enterocolitis, glossitis, nausea, stomatitis, vomiting

Hematologic: Aplastic anemia, bone marrow suppression, granulocytopenia, hypoplastic anemia, pancytopenia, thrombocytopenia

Ocular: Optic neuritis

Miscellaneous: Anaphylaxis, hypersensitivity reactions, Gray syndrome

Drug Interactions

Metabolism/Transport Effects Inhibits CYP2C19 (strong), CYP2C9 (weak)

Avoid Concomitant Use

Avoid concomitant use of Chloramphenicol with any of the following: BCG (Intravesical); Deferiprone; Dipyrone

Increased Effect/Toxicity

Chloramphenicol may increase the levels/effects of: Alcohol (Ethyl); Barbiturates; Carbocisteine; Cilostazol; Citalopram; CloZAPine; CycloSPORINE (Systemic); CYP2C19 Substrates; Deferiprone; Flibanserin; Fosphenytoin; Phenytoin; Sulfonylureas; Tacrolimus (Systemic); Vitamin K Antagonists; Voriconazole

The levels/effects of Chloramphenicol may be increased by: Dipyrone; Fosphenytoin; Phenytoin

Decreased Effect

Chloramphenicol may decrease the levels/effects of: BCG (Intravesical); BCG Vaccine (Immunization); CefTAZidime; Clopidogrel; Sodium Picosulfate; Typhoid Vaccine; Vitamin B12

The levels/effects of Chloramphenicol may be decreased by: Barbiturates; Fosphenytoin; Phenytoin; Rifampin

Storage/Stability Store at room temperature prior to reconstitution. Reconstituted solutions remain stable for 30 days. Use only clear solutions. Frozen solutions remain stable for 6 months.

Mechanism of Action Reversibly binds to 50S ribosomal subunits of susceptible organisms preventing amino acids from being transferred to growing peptide chains thus inhibiting protein synthesis

Pharmacodynamics/Kinetics

Distribution: To most tissues and body fluids; good CSF and brain penetration

CSF concentration with uninflamed meninges: 21% to 50% of plasma concentration

CSF concentration with inflamed meninges: 45% to 89% of plasma concentration

Chloramphenicol: V_d: 0.5-1 L/kg

Chloramphenicol succinate: V_d: 0.2-3.1 L/kg; decreased with hepatic or renal dysfunction

Protein binding: Chloramphenicol: ~60%; decreased with hepatic or renal dysfunction and 30% to 40% in newborn infants

Metabolism:

Chloramphenicol: Hepatic to metabolites (inactive)

Chloramphenicol succinate: Hydrolyzed in the liver, kidney, and lungs to chloramphenicol (active)

Bioavailability:

Chloramphenicol: Oral: ~80%

Chloramphenicol succinate: IV: ~70%; highly variable, dependent upon rate and extent of metabolism to chloramphenicol

Half-life elimination:

Neonates: 1-2 days: 24 hours; 10-16 days: 10 hours

Normal renal function:

Chloramphenicol: Infants: Significantly prolonged; Children 4-6 hours; Adults: ~4 hours

Chloramphenicol succinate: Adults: ~3 hours

End-stage renal disease: Chloramphenicol: 3-7 hours

Hepatic disease: Prolonged

Excretion: Urine (~30% as unchanged chloramphenicol succinate in adults, 6% to 80% in children; 5% to 15% as chloramphenicol)

Dosing

Adult & Geriatric Systemic infections: IV: 50-100 mg/kg/day in divided doses every 6 hours; maximum daily dose: 4 g/day.

Pediatric

Other infections: Children: Usual dosing range: IV: 50-100 mg/kg/day in divided doses every 6 hours; maximum daily dose: 4 g/day

Meningitis: IV: Infants >30 days and Children: 75-100 mg/kg/day divided every 6 hours

Renal Impairment Use with caution; monitor serum concentrations.

Hepatic Impairment Use with caution; monitor serum concentrations.

Dietary Considerations May have increased dietary need for riboflavin, pyridoxine, and vitamin B$_{12}$. Some products may contain sodium.

Administration Do not administer IM; can be administered IVP over at least 1 minute at a concentration of 100 mg/mL, or IV intermittent infusion over 15-30 minutes at a final concentration for administration of ≤20 mg/mL.

Hazardous agent; use appropriate precautions for handling and disposal (NIOSH 2014 [group 2]).

Monitoring Parameters CBC with differential (baseline and every 2 days during therapy), periodic liver and renal function tests, serum drug concentration

Reference Range

Therapeutic levels:

Meningitis:

Peak: 15-25 mcg/mL; toxic concentration: >40 mcg/mL

Trough: 5-15 mcg/mL

Other infections:

Peak: 10-20 mcg/mL

Trough: 5-10 mcg/mL

Timing of serum samples: Draw levels 0.5-1.5 hours after completion of IV dose

Test Interactions May cause false-positive results in urine glucose tests when using cupric sulfate (Benedict's solution, Clinitest®).

Dosage Forms Excipient information presented when available (limited, particularly for generics); consult specific product labeling.

Solution Reconstituted, Intravenous:

Generic: 1 g (1 ea)

◆ **ChloraPrep One Step [OTC]** *see* Chlorhexidine Gluconate *on page* 373

◆ **Chlorax (Can)** *see* Clidinium and Chlordiazepoxide *on page* 405

◆ **Chlorbutinum** *see* Chlorambucil *on page* 370

ChlordiazePOXIDE (klor dye az e POKS ide)

Index Terms Librium; Methaminodiazepoxide Hydrochloride

Pharmacologic Category Benzodiazepine

Use Management of anxiety disorder or for the short-term relief of symptoms of anxiety; withdrawal symptoms of acute alcoholism; preoperative apprehension and anxiety

Dosing

Adult

Anxiety: Oral:

Mild-moderate anxiety: Usual daily dose: 5-10 mg 3-4 times daily

Severe anxiety: Usual daily dose: 20-25 mg 3-4 times daily

Preoperative anxiety: Oral: 5-10 mg 3-4 times daily on the days preceding surgery

Ethanol withdrawal symptoms: Oral: Initial dose: 50-100 mg; dose may be repeated as necessary to a maximum of 300 mg per 24 hours. **Note:** Frequency of

repeat doses is often based on institution-specific protocols. Once agitation is under control, maintain therapy at lowest effective dose.

Geriatric Oral: 5 mg 2-4 times daily. Avoid use if possible due to long-acting metabolite.

Pediatric Anxiety: Oral:

Children <6 years: Not recommended

Children ≥6 years and Adolescents: Anxiety: Usual daily dose: 5 mg 2-4 times daily. Dose may be increased to 10 mg 2-3 times daily in some patients, if necessary.

Renal Impairment Dosage adjustments are not provided in the manufacturer's labeling; however, the following guidelines have been used by some clinicians (Aronoff, 2007): Adults: CrCl <10 mL/minute: Administer 50% of dose.

Peritoneal dialysis: Administer 50% of the dose (Aronoff, 2007).

Hepatic Impairment There are no specific hepatic dosage adjustments provided in the manufacturer's labeling; however, chlordiazepoxide undergoes hepatic metabolism and should be used with caution.

Additional Information Complete prescribing information should be consulted for additional detail.

Dosage Forms Excipient information presented when available (limited, particularly for generics); consult specific product labeling.

Capsule, Oral, as hydrochloride:

Generic: 5 mg, 10 mg, 25 mg

Controlled Substance C-IV

◆ **Chlordiazepoxide and Amitriptyline Hydrochloride** see Amitriptyline and Chlordiazepoxide on page 100

◆ **Chlordiazepoxide and Clidinium** see Clidinium and Chlordiazepoxide on page 405

◆ **Chlorethazine** see Mechlorethamine (Systemic) on page 1130

◆ **Chlorethazine Mustard** see Mechlorethamine (Systemic) on page 1130

Chlorhexidine Gluconate
(klor HEKS i deen GLOO koe nate)

Brand Names: US Betasept Surgical Scrub [OTC]; ChloraPrep One Step [OTC]; Dyna-Hex 2 [OTC]; Hibiclens [OTC]; Hibistat [OTC]; Paroex; Peridex; Periogard; Tegaderm CHG Dressing [OTC]

Brand Names: Canada Apo-Chlorhexidine Oral Rinse; Denti-Care Chlorhexidine Gluconate Oral Rinse; GUM Paroex; ORO-Clense; Perichlor; Peridex Oral Rinse; Periogard; X-Pur Chlorhexidine

Index Terms 3M Avagard [OTC]; CHG

Pharmacologic Category Antibiotic, Oral Rinse; Antibiotic, Topical

Use

Topical: Skin cleanser for preoperative skin preparation, skin wound and general skin cleanser for patients; surgical scrub and antiseptic hand rinse for healthcare personnel

Oral rinse: Antibacterial dental rinse for gingivitis treatment

Periodontal chip: Adjunctive therapy to reduce pocket depth in patients with periodontitis

Dosing

Adult & Geriatric

Treatment of gingivitis: *Oral rinse:* Swish for 30 seconds with 15 mL (one capful) of undiluted oral rinse after toothbrushing, then expectorate; repeat twice daily (morning and evening). Therapy should be initiated immediately following a dental prophylaxis. Patient should be reevaluated and given a dental prophylaxis at intervals no longer than every 6 months.

Periodontitis: *Periodontal chip:* One chip is inserted into a periodontal pocket with a probing pocket depth ≥5 mm. Up to 8 chips may be inserted in a single visit. Treatment is recommended every 3 months in pockets with a remaining depth ≥5 mm. If dislodgment occurs 7 days or more after placement, the subject is considered to have had the full course of treatment. If dislodgment occurs within 48 hours, a new chip should be inserted. The chip biodegrades completely and does not need to be removed. Patients should avoid dental floss at the site of periodontal chip insertion for 10 days after placement because flossing might dislodge the chip.

Insertion of periodontal chip: Pocket should be isolated and surrounding area dried prior to chip insertion. The chip should be grasped using forceps with the rounded edges away from the forceps. The chip should be inserted into the periodontal pocket to its maximum depth. It may be maneuvered into position using the tips of the forceps or a flat instrument.

Skin cleanser for preoperative skin preparation, skin wound and general skin cleanser for patients; surgical scrub and antiseptic hand rinse for healthcare personnel: *Topical:*

Surgical scrub: Scrub hands and forearms for 3 minutes paying close attention to nails, cuticles, and interdigital spaces, and rinse thoroughly, wash for an additional 3 minutes, rinse, and dry thoroughly.

Surgical hand antiseptic: Lotion: Dispense 1 pumpful in palm of 1 hand; dip fingertips of opposite hand into solution and work it under nails. Spread remainder evenly over hand and just above elbow, covering all surfaces. Repeat on other hand. Dispense another pumpful in each hand and reapply to each hand up to the wrist. Allow to dry before gloving.

Healthcare personnel hand antiseptic:

Liquid or solution: Wash with ~5 mL for 15 seconds; rinse thoroughly with water and dry

Lotion: Apply to clean, dry hands and nails. Dispense 1 pumpful (2 mL) into the palm of 1 hand; apply evenly to cover both hands up to the wrists; allow to dry without wiping.

Towelette: Rub 15 seconds paying close attention to nails and interdigital spaces; no watering or toweling necessary

Preoperative skin preparation:

Solution: Apply liberally to surgical site and swab for at least 2 minutes. Dry with sterile towel. Repeat procedure (swab for additional 2 minutes and dry with sterile towel).

Applicator (ChloraPrep One-Step):

Dry surgical sites (eg, abdomen, arm): Completely wet treatment area; use gentle back and forth strokes for ~30 seconds. Allow solution to air dry for ~30 seconds. If using an ignition source (eg, electrocautery), allow solution to completely dry for a minimum of 3 minutes for hairless skin and up to 1 hour in hair; do not blot or wipe away. **Note:** Prior to use with electrocautery procedures, consult specific product labeling to determine if the ChloraPrep product may be used near an ignition source.

Moist surgical sites (eg, inguinal area): Completely wet treatment area; use gentle back and forth strokes for ~2 minutes. Allow solution to air dry for ~1 minute. If using an ignition source (eg, electrocautery), allow solution to completely dry for a minimum of 3 minutes for hairless skin and up to 1 hour in hair; do not blot or wipe away. **Note:** Prior to use with electrocautery procedures, consult specific product labeling to determine if the ChloraPrep product may be used near an ignition source.

Preparation of skin prior to an injection: Swab: Apply swab to procedure site for 15 seconds; allow to air dry for 30 seconds (do not blot or wipe dry). **Note:** Maximum treatment area for 1 swab is ~2.5 inches x 2.5 inches.

Wound care and general skin cleansing: Rinse area with water, then apply minimum amount necessary to cover skin or wound area and wash gently. Rinse again thoroughly.

Additional Information Complete prescribing information should be consulted for additional detail.

Dosage Forms Excipient information presented when available (limited, particularly for generics); consult specific product labeling.

Liquid, External:

Betasept Surgical Scrub: 4% (118 mL, 237 mL, 473 mL, 946 mL, 3780 mL)

Hibiclens: 4% (15 mL, 118 mL, 236 mL, 473 mL, 946 mL, 3790 mL) [contains fd&c red #40, isopropyl alcohol]

Generic: 2% (118 mL); 4% (118 mL, 237 mL, 473 mL, 946 mL, 3800 mL)

Miscellaneous, External:

Hibistat: 0.5% (50 ea) [contains isopropyl alcohol]

Tegaderm CHG Dressing: (Dressing) (1 ea)

Pad, External:

Generic: 2% (2 ea, 6 ea)

Solution, External:

ChloraPrep One Step: 2% (3 mL, 10.5 mL) [latex free]

Dyna-Hex 2: 2% (473 mL) [contains isopropyl alcohol]

Solution, Mouth/Throat:

Paroex: 0.12% (473 mL) [alcohol free; contains fd&c red #40, propylene glycol]

Peridex: 0.12% (118 mL, 473 mL) [contains alcohol, usp, brilliant blue fcf (fd&c blue #1), saccharin sodium]

Periogard: 0.12% (473 mL) [mint flavor]

Generic: 0.12% (15 mL, 473 mL)

◆ **Chlormeprazine** see Prochlorperazine on page 1507

◆ **2-Chlorodeoxyadenosine** see Cladribine on page 401

◆ **Chloromag** see Magnesium Chloride on page 1119

◆ Chloromycetin® (Can) see Chloramphenicol on page 371

◆ Chloromycetin® Succinate (Can) see Chloramphenicol on page 371

Chloroprocaine (klor oh PROE kane)

Brand Names: US Nesacaine; Nesacaine-MPF
Index Terms Chloroprocaine Hydrochloride
Pharmacologic Category Local Anesthetic
Use

Local anesthesia: Production of local anesthesia by infiltration and peripheral nerve block (chloroprocaine with preservatives); production of local anesthesia by infiltration and peripheral and central nerve block, including lumbar and caudal epidural blocks (chloroprocaine without preservatives).

Limitations of use: Do not use chloroprocaine with or without preservatives for subarachnoid administration. Do not use chloroprocaine with preservatives for lumbar or caudal epidural anesthesia.

Dosing

Adult Injectable local anesthetic: Use the smallest dose and concentration required to produce the desired result. Dosage varies with anesthetic procedure, the vascularity of the tissues, depth of anesthesia required, degree of muscle relaxation required, duration of anesthesia, and physical condition of the patient. Use reduced doses in debilitated patients and patients with cardiac disease.

Maximum single dose (without epinephrine): 11 mg/kg; maximum total dose: 800 mg

Maximum single dose (with epinephrine 1:200,000): 14 mg/kg; maximum total dose: 1,000 mg

Caudal block: Preservative free: 2% or 3%: 15 to 25 mL; may repeat at 40- to 60-minute intervals

Infiltration and peripheral nerve block:

Brachial plexus: 2%; 30 to 40 mL; total dose 600 to 800 mg

Digital (without epinephrine): 1%; 3 to 4 mL; total dose: 30 to 40 mg

Infraorbital: 2%: 0.5 to 1 mL; total dose 10 to 20 mg

Mandibular: 2%: 2 to 3 mL; total dose 40 to 60 mg

Paracervical: 1%; 3 mL per each of four sites; total dose: up to 120 mg

Pudendal: 2%; 10 mL each side; total dose: 400 mg

Lumbar epidural block: Preservative-free: 2% or 3%: 2 to 2.5 mL per segment; usual total volume: 15 to 25 mL; may repeat with doses that are 2 to 6 mL less than initial dose every 40 to 50 minutes.

Geriatric Dosage should be reduced; refer to adult dosing.

Pediatric Injectable local anesthetic: Use the smallest dose and concentration required to produce the desired result. Dosage varies with anesthetic procedure, the vascularity of the tissues, depth of anesthesia required, degree of muscle relaxation required, duration of anesthesia, and physical condition of the patient. Use reduced doses in debilitated patients and patients with cardiac disease.

Children >3 years (normally developed) and Adolescents: Maximum dose (without epinephrine): 11 mg/kg; for infiltration, concentrations of 0.5% to 1% are recommended; for nerve block, concentrations of 1% to 1.5% are recommended

Renal Impairment There are no dosage adjustments provided in the manufacturer's labeling. Use with caution due to increased risk of adverse effects.

Hepatic Impairment There are no specific dosage adjustments provided in the manufacturer's labeling; however, dosage should be reduced. Use with caution due to increased risk of adverse effects.

Additional Information Complete prescribing information should be consulted for additional detail.

Dosage Forms Excipient information presented when available (limited, particularly for generics); consult specific product labeling. [DSC] = Discontinued product

Solution, Injection, as hydrochloride:
Nesacaine: 1% (30 mL); 2% (30 mL) [contains disodium edta, methylparaben]
Generic: 2% (30 mL [DSC]); 3% (30 mL [DSC])

Solution, Injection, as hydrochloride [preservative free]:
Nesacaine-MPF: 2% (20 mL); 3% (20 mL) [methylparaben free]
Generic: 2% (20 mL); 3% (20 mL)

◆ Chloroprocaine Hydrochloride see Chloroprocaine on page 374

Chloroquine (KLOR oh kwin)

Brand Names: US Aralen
Brand Names: Canada Aralen; Novo-Chloroquine
Index Terms Chloroquine Phosphate
Pharmacologic Category Aminoquinoline (Antimalarial); Antimalarial Agent
Use

Malaria: Suppressive treatment and acute attacks of malaria due to *Plasmodium vivax*, *P. malariae*, *P. ovale*, and susceptible strains of *P. falciparum*.

Extraintestinal amebiasis: Treatment of extraintestinal amebiasis.

Pregnancy Considerations In animal reproduction studies, drug accumulated in fetal ocular tissues and remained for several months following drug elimination from the rest of the body. Chloroquine and its metabolites cross the placenta and can be detected in the cord blood and urine of the newborn infant (Akintonwa, 1988; Essien, 1982; Law, 2008). In one study, chloroquine and its metabolites were measurable in the cord blood 89 days (mean) after the last maternal dose (Law, 2008).

Malaria infection in pregnant women may be more severe than in nonpregnant women and has a high risk of maternal and perinatal morbidity and mortality. Therefore, pregnant women and women who are likely to become pregnant are advised to avoid travel to malaria-risk areas. Chloroquine is recommended for the treatment of pregnant women for uncomplicated malaria in chloroquine-sensitive regions; when caused by chloroquine-sensitive *P. vivax* or *P. ovale*, pregnant women should be maintained on chloroquine prophylaxis for the duration of their pregnancy (refer to current guidelines) (CDC, 2011; CDC, 2012).

Breast-Feeding Considerations Chloroquine and its metabolite can be detected in breast milk. Per product labeling, 11 lactating women with malaria were given a single oral dose of chloroquine 600 mg. The maximum daily dose to the breast-feeding infant was calculated to be 0.7% of the maternal dose. Additional information has been published and results are variable. In one study, the relative dose to the nursing infant was calculated to be 2.3% (chloroquine) and 1% (metabolite) of the weight-adjusted maternal dose with the samples obtained a median of 17 days after the last dose. Women in this study received chloroquine phosphate 750 mg daily for 3 days. This report also provides data from other studies, listing relative infant doses of chloroquine ranging from 0.9% to 9.5% of the maternal dose (Law, 2008). Due to the potential for serious adverse reactions in the nursing infant, the manufacturer recommends a decision be made whether to discontinue nursing or to discontinue the drug, taking into account the importance of treatment to the mother. Other sources consider the amount of chloroquine exposure to the nursing infant to be safe when normal maternal doses for malaria are used. However, the amount of chloroquine obtained by a nursing infant from breast milk would not provide adequate protection if therapy for malaria in the infant is needed (CDC, 2012).

Contraindications Hypersensitivity to 4-aminoquinoline compounds or any component of the formulation; the presence of retinal or visual field changes either attributable to 4-aminoquinoline compounds or to any other etiology

Warnings/Precautions Use with caution in patients with hepatic impairment, alcoholism or in conjunction with hepatotoxic drugs. May exacerbate psoriasis or porphyria. Use caution in patients with seizure disorders. Use caution in G6PD deficiency; 4-aminoquinolines such as chloroquine has been associated with hemolysis and renal impairment. Use with caution in patients with preexisting auditory damage; discontinue immediately if hearing defects are noted. Retinopathy, maculopathy, and macular degeneration have occurred; irreversible retinal damage has occurred with prolonged or high dose 4-aminoquinoline therapy; risk factors include age, duration of therapy, and/or high doses. Monitoring is required, especially with prolonged therapy. Discontinue immediately if signs/symptoms occur; visual changes may progress even after therapy is discontinued. Use has been associated with ECG changes, AV block, and cardiomyopathy. May cause QT prolongation and subsequent torsade de pointes; avoid use in patients with diagnosed or suspected congenital long QT syndrome. Rare hematologic reactions including agranulocytosis, aplastic anemia, neutropenia, pancytopenia, and thrombocytopenia; monitor CBC during prolonged therapy. Consider discontinuation if severe blood disorders occur that are unrelated to disease. Acute extrapyramidal disorders may occur, usually resolving after discontinuation of therapy and/or symptomatic treatment. Skeletal muscle myopathy or neuromyopathy, leading to progressive weakness and atrophy of proximal muscle groups

have been reported; muscle strength (especially proximal muscles) should be assessed periodically during prolonged therapy; discontinue therapy if weakness occurs. Potentially significant drug-drug interactions may exist, requiring dose or frequency adjustment, additional monitoring, and/or selection of alternative therapy.

Certain strains of *P. falciparum* are resistant to 4-aminoquinoline compounds. Prior to initiation of therapy, it should be determined if chloroquine is appropriate for use in the region to be visited; do not use for the treatment of *P. falciparum* acquired in areas of chloroquine resistance or where chloroquine prophylaxis has failed. Patients should be treated with another antimalarial if patient is infected with a resistant strain of plasmodia. Chloroquine does not prevent relapses in patients with vivax or malariae malaria; will not prevent vivax or malariae infection when administered as a prophylactic. Also consult current CDC guidelines for treatment recommendations.

Adverse Reactions Frequency not defined.

Cardiovascular: Cardiomyopathy, ECG changes (rare; including prolonged QRS and QTc intervals, T wave inversion or depression), hypotension (rare), torsades de pointes (rare)

Central nervous system: Agitation, anxiety, confusion, decreased deep tendon reflex, delirium, depression, extrapyramidal reaction (dystonia, dyskinesia, protrusion of the tongue, torticollis), hallucination, headache, insomnia, personality changes, polyneuropathy, psychosis, seizure

Dermatologic: Alopecia, bleaching of hair, blue gray skin pigmentation, erythema multiforme (rare), exacerbation of psoriasis, exfoliative dermatitis (rare), lichen planus, pleomorphic rash, pruritus, skin photosensitivity, Stevens-Johnson syndrome (rare), toxic epidermal necrolysis (rare), urticaria

Gastrointestinal: Abdominal cramps, anorexia, diarrhea, nausea, vomiting

Hematologic & oncologic: Agranulocytosis (rare; reversible), aplastic anemia, neutropenia, pancytopenia, thrombocytopenia

Hepatic: Hepatitis, increased liver enzymes

Hypersensitivity: Anaphylactoid reaction, anaphylaxis, angioedema

Immunologic: DRESS syndrome

Neuromuscular & skeletal: Myopathy, neuromuscular disease, proximal myopathy

Ophthalmic: Accommodation disturbances, blurred vision, corneal opacity (reversible), macular degeneration (may be irreversible), maculopathy (may be irreversible), nocturnal amblyopia, retinopathy (including irreversible changes in some patients long-term or high-dose therapy), visual field defects

Otic: Deafness (nerve), hearing loss (risk increased in patients with preexisting auditory damage), tinnitus

Drug Interactions

Metabolism/Transport Effects Substrate of CYP2D6 (major), CYP3A4 (major); **Note:** Assignment of Major/Minor substrate status based on clinically relevant drug interaction potential; **Inhibits** CYP2D6 (moderate)

Avoid Concomitant Use

Avoid concomitant use of Chloroquine with any of the following: Agalsidase Alfa; Agalsidase Beta; Artemether; Conivaptan; Fusidic Acid (Systemic); Highest Risk QTc-Prolonging Agents; Idelalisib; Ivabradine; Lumefantrine; Mefloquine; Mifepristone; Thioridazine

Increased Effect/Toxicity

Chloroquine may increase the levels/effects of: Antipsychotic Agents (Phenothiazines); ARIPiprazole; Beta-Blockers; Brexpiprazole; Cardiac Glycosides; CYP2D6 Substrates; Dapsone (Systemic); Dapsone (Topical); DOXOrubicin (Conventional); Fesoterodine; Highest Risk QTc-Prolonging Agents; Lumefantrine; Mefloquine; Metoprolol; Moderate Risk QTc-Prolonging Agents; Nebivolol; Prilocaine; Sodium Nitrite; Thioridazine

The levels/effects of Chloroquine may be increased by: Abiraterone Acetate; Aprepitant; Artemether; Conivaptan; CYP2D6 Inhibitors (Moderate); CYP2D6 Inhibitors (Strong); CYP3A4 Inhibitors (Moderate); CYP3A4 Inhibitors (Strong); Dapsone (Systemic); Dasatinib; Fosaprepitant; Fusidic Acid (Systemic); Idelalisib; Ivabradine; Ivacaftor; Luliconazole; Mefloquine; Mifepristone; Netupitant; Nitric Oxide; Palbociclib; Panobinostat; Peginterferon Alfa-2b; QTc-Prolonging Agents (Indeterminate Risk and Risk Modifying); Simeprevir; Stiripentol

Decreased Effect

Chloroquine may decrease the levels/effects of: Agalsidase Alfa; Agalsidase Beta; Ampicillin; Anthelmintics; Codeine; Rabies Vaccine; Tamoxifen; TraMADol

The levels/effects of Chloroquine may be decreased by: Antacids; Bosentan; CYP3A4 Inducers (Moderate); CYP3A4 Inducers (Strong); Dabrafenib; Deferasirox; Enzalutamide; Kaolin; Lanthanum; Mitotane; Peginterferon Alfa-2b; Siltuximab; St Johns Wort; Tocilizumab

Storage/Stability Store at 25°C (77°F); excursions are permitted between 15°C and 30°C (59°F and 86°F); protect from light.

Mechanism of Action Binds to and inhibits DNA and RNA polymerase; interferes with metabolism and hemoglobin utilization by parasites; inhibits prostaglandin effects; chloroquine concentrates within parasite acid vesicles and raises internal pH resulting in inhibition of parasite growth; may involve aggregates of ferriprotoporphyrin IX acting as chloroquine receptors causing membrane damage; may also interfere with nucleoprotein synthesis

Pharmacodynamics/Kinetics

Absorption: Rapid and almost complete

Distribution: Widely in body tissues including eyes, heart, kidneys, liver, leukocytes, and lungs where retention is prolonged

Protein binding: 50% to 65%

Metabolism: Partially hepatic to main metabolite, desethylchloroquine

Half-life: 3-5 days

Time to peak serum concentration: Oral: Within 1-2 hours

Excretion: Urine (~70%; ~35% as unchanged drug); acidification of urine increases elimination; small amounts of drug may be present in urine months following discontinuation of therapy

Dosing

Adult & Geriatric Note: Each 250 mg of chloroquine phosphate is equivalent to 150 mg of chloroquine base

Malaria chemoprophylaxis: Oral: 500 mg (300 mg base) weekly on the same day each week; begin 1-2 weeks prior to exposure; continue while in endemic area and for 4 weeks after leaving endemic area (CDC, 2014)

Malaria treatment: Oral: 1 g (600 mg base) on day 1, followed by 500 mg (300 mg base) 6-, 24-, and 48 hours after first dose (CDC, 2009)

Extraintestinal amebiasis: Oral: 1 g (600 mg base) daily for 2 days followed by 500 mg daily (300 mg base) for at least 2-3 weeks; may be combined with an intestinal amebicide.

Lupus erythematosus (off-label use): 250 mg (150 mg base) once daily for ≥3 months. **Note:** Not considered first-line agent (Bezerra, 2005; Lesiak, 2008)

Rheumatoid arthritis (off-label use): 250 mg (150 mg base) once daily for ≥1 year. **Note:** Not considered first-line agent (Fowler, 1984; Freedman, 1960)

Pediatric Note: Each 250 mg of chloroquine phosphate is equivalent to 150 mg of chloroquine base

Malaria chemoprophylaxis: Oral: 8.3 mg/kg/week (5 mg/kg base) on the same day each week (not to exceed 500 mg/dose [300 mg base/dose]); begin 1-2 weeks prior to exposure; continue while in endemic area and for 4 weeks after leaving endemic area (CDC, 2014)

Malaria treatment: Oral: 16.6 mg/kg (10 mg/kg base) on day 1 (maximum: 1000 mg [600 mg base]), followed by 8.3 mg/kg (5 mg/kg base) (maximum: 500 mg [300 mg base]) 6-, 24-, and 48 hours after first dose (CDC, 2009)

Renal Impairment The FDA-approved labeling does not contain renal dosing adjustment guidelines; the following guidelines have been used by some clinicians (Aronoff, 2007):

CrCl ≥10 mL/minute: No dosage adjustment necessary.

CrCl <10 mL/minute: Administer 50% of dose.

Hemodialysis effects: Minimally removed by hemodialysis.

Hemodialysis, peritoneal dialysis: Administer 50% of dose.

Continuous renal replacement therapy (CRRT): No dosage adjustment necessary.

Hepatic Impairment No dosage adjustment provided in manufacturer's labeling; use with caution.

Monitoring Parameters Ophthalmic exams at baseline and periodically thereafter during prolonged therapy; visual acuity, expert slit-lamp, fundoscopic and visual field tests are recommended. Evaluate neuromuscular function periodically during prolonged therapy. Periodic CBC in patients receiving prolonged therapy

Dosage Forms Excipient information presented when available (limited, particularly for generics); consult specific product labeling.

Tablet, Oral, as phosphate:

Aralen: 500 mg [equivalent to chloroquine base 300 mg]

Generic: 250 mg [equivalent to chloroquine base 150 mg], 500 mg [equivalent to chloroquine base 300 mg]

◀ **Extemporaneous Preparations** A 15 mg chloroquine phosphate/mL oral suspension (equivalent to 9 mg chloroquine base/mL) may be made from tablets and a 1:1 mixture of Ora-Sweet® and Ora-Plus®. Crush three 500 mg chloroquine phosphate tablets (equivalent to 300 mg base/tablet) in a mortar and reduce to a fine powder. Add 15 mL of the vehicle and mix to a uniform paste; mix while adding the vehicle in incremental proportions to **almost** 100 mL; transfer to a calibrated bottle, rinse mortar with vehicle, and add quantity of vehicle sufficient to make 100 mL. Label "shake well before using" and "protect from light". Stable for up to 60 days when stored in the dark at room temperature or refrigerated (preferred).

Allen LV Jr and Erickson MA 3rd, "Stability of Alprazolam, Chloroquine Phosphate, Cisapride, Enalapril Maleate, and Hydralazine Hydrochloride in Extemporaneously Compounded Oral Liquids," *Am J Health Syst Pharm*, 1998, 55(18):1915-20.

◆ **Chloroquine Phosphate** see Chloroquine on page 374

Chlorothiazide (klor oh THYE a zide)

Brand Names: US Diuril; Sodium Diuril
Pharmacologic Category Antihypertensive; Diuretic, Thiazide
Use Management of hypertension; adjunctive treatment of edema

Guideline recommendations:
Hypertension: The 2014 guideline for the management of high blood pressure in adults (Eighth Joint National Committee [JNC 8]) recommends initiation of pharmacologic treatment to lower blood pressure for the following patients:
• Patients ≥60 years of age with systolic blood pressure (SBP) ≥150 mm Hg or diastolic blood pressure (DBP) ≥90 mm Hg. Goal of therapy is SBP <150 mm Hg and DBP <90 mm Hg.
• Patients <60 years of age with SBP ≥140 mm Hg or DBP is ≥90 mm Hg. Goal of therapy is SBP <140 mm Hg and DBP <90 mm Hg.
• Patients ≥18 years of age with diabetes and SBP ≥140 mm Hg or DBP ≥90 mm Hg. Goal of therapy is SBP <140 mm Hg and DBP <90 mm Hg.
• Patients ≥18 years of age with chronic kidney disease (CKD) and SBP ≥140 mm Hg or DBP ≥90 mm Hg. Goal of therapy is SBP <140 mm Hg and DBP <90 mm Hg.
Chronic kidney disease (CKD) and hypertension: Regardless of race or diabetes status, the use of an ACE inhibitor (ACEI) or angiotensin receptor blocker (ARB) as initial therapy is recommended to improve kidney outcomes. In the general nonblack population (without CKD) including those with diabetes, initial antihypertensive treatment should consist of a thiazide-type diuretic, calcium channel blocker, ACEI, or ARB. In the general black population (without CKD), including those with diabetes, initial antihypertensive treatment should consist of a thiazide-type diuretic or a calcium channel blocker **instead of** an ACEI or ARB.
Coronary artery disease (CAD) and hypertension: The American Heart Association, American College of Cardiology and American Society of Hypertension (AHA/ACC/ASH) 2015 scientific statement for the treatment of hypertension in patients with coronary artery disease (CAD) recommends the use of a thiazide (or thiazide-like diuretic) as part of a regimen in patients with hypertension and chronic stable angina. A BP target of <140/90 mm Hg is reasonable for the secondary prevention of cardiovascular events. A lower target BP (<130/80 mm Hg) may be appropriate in some individuals with CAD, previous MI, stroke or transient ischemic attack, or CAD risk equivalents (AHA/ACC/ASH [Rosendorff 2015]).

Dosing
Adult & Geriatric Note: The manufacturer states that IV and oral dosing are equivalent. Some clinicians may use lower IV doses; however, because of chlorothiazide's poor oral absorption.

Hypertension: Oral: 500 to 2000 mg daily divided in 1 to 2 doses
Edema: Oral, IV: 500 to 1000 mg once or twice daily; intermittent treatment (eg, therapy on alternative days) may be appropriate for some patients
ACCF/AHA 2013 heart failure guidelines:
Oral: 250 to 500 mg once or twice daily (maximum daily dose: 1000 mg)
IV: 500 to 1000 mg once daily in combination with a loop diuretic for sequential nephron blockade
Pediatric Note: The manufacturer states that IV and oral dosing are equivalent. Some clinicians may use lower IV

doses; however, because of chlorothiazide's poor oral absorption. IV dosing in infants and children has not been well established.

Infants <6 months: Oral: 10 to 30 mg/kg/day in 2 divided doses (maximum dose: 375 mg daily)
Infants >6 months and Children: Oral: 10 to 20 mg/kg/day in 1 or 2 divided doses (maximum dose: 375 mg daily in children <2 years or 1000 mg daily in children 2 to 12 years)
Infants and Children: IV (off-label): 5 to 10 mg/kg/day in 2 divided doses (Costello, 2007)
Renal Impairment CrCl <10 mL/minute: Avoid use. Ineffective with CrCl <30 mL/minute unless in combination with a loop diuretic (Aronoff, 2007).
Hepatic Impairment No dosage adjustments provided in manufacturer's labeling; use with caution.
Additional Information Complete prescribing information should be consulted for additional detail.
Dosage Forms Excipient information presented when available (limited, particularly for generics); consult specific product labeling.
Solution Reconstituted, Intravenous, as sodium [strength expressed as base]:
Sodium Diuril: 500 mg (1 ea)
Generic: 500 mg (1 ea)
Solution Reconstituted, Intravenous, as sodium [strength expressed as base, preservative free]:
Generic: 500 mg (1 ea)
Suspension, Oral:
Diuril: 250 mg/5 mL (237 mL) [contains alcohol, usp, benzoic acid, fd&c yellow #10 (quinoline yellow), methylparaben, propylparaben, saccharin sodium]
Tablet, Oral:
Generic: 250 mg, 500 mg

Chlorpheniramine and Acetaminophen
(klor fen IR a meen & a seet a MIN oh fen)

Brand Names: US Coricidin HBP® Cold and Flu [OTC]
Index Terms Acetaminophen and Chlorpheniramine
Pharmacologic Category Alkylamine Derivative; Analgesic, Miscellaneous; Histamine H_1 Antagonist; Histamine H_1 Antagonist, First Generation
Use Cold and flu symptoms: Symptomatic relief of headache, sneezing, runny nose, fever, and minor aches and pains of colds and flu
Dosing
Adult
Cold and flu symptoms: Oral: Two tablets (chlorpheniramine 4 mg/acetaminophen 650 mg) every 4 to 6 hours (maximum: 12 tablets in 24 hours [chlorpheniramine 24 mg/acetaminophen 3,900 mg])
Geriatric Refer to adult dosing. Use with caution.
Pediatric
Cold and flu symptoms: Oral:
Children 6 to <12 years: One tablet (chlorpheniramine 2 mg/acetaminophen 325 mg) every 4 to 6 hours (maximum: 5 tablets in 24 hours [chlorpheniramine 10 mg/acetaminophen 1,625 mg])
Children ≥12 years and Adolescents: Oral: Refer to adult dosing.
Renal Impairment There are no dosage adjustments provided in the manufacturer's labeling.
Hepatic Impairment There are no dosage adjustments provided in the manufacturer's labeling; use with caution. Limited, low-dose therapy is usually well tolerated in hepatic disease/cirrhosis; however, cases of hepatotoxicity at daily acetaminophen dosages <4 g/day have been reported. Avoid chronic use in hepatic impairment.
Additional Information Complete prescribing information should be consulted for additional detail.
Dosage Forms Excipient information presented when available (limited, particularly for generics); consult specific product labeling.
Tablet: Chlorpheniramine maleate 2 mg and acetaminophen 325 mg

◆ **Chlorpheniramine and Dextromethorphan** see Dextromethorphan and Chlorpheniramine on page 534

Chlorpheniramine and Phenylephrine
(klor fen IR a meen & fen il EF rin)

Brand Names: US AccuHist Drops [OTC] [DSC]; Actifed Cold/Allergy [OTC]; Cardec [OTC]; Dallergy [OTC]; Ed A-Hist [OTC]; Ed ChlorPed D [OTC]; LoHist [OTC] [DSC]; Nasohist [OTC] [DSC]; NoHist [OTC] [DSC]; NoHist-LQ [OTC]; Rescon-Jr [DSC]; Sudafed PE Sinus/Allergy [OTC]; Triaminic Cold/Allergy Child [OTC]; Trigofen [OTC] [DSC]; Virdec [OTC] [DSC]

Index Terms Chlorpheniramine Maleate and Phenylephrine Hydrochloride; Phenylephrine and Chlorpheniramine

Pharmacologic Category Alkylamine Derivative; Alpha-Adrenergic Agonist; Decongestant; Histamine H₁ Antagonist; Histamine H₁ Antagonist, First Generation

Use Upper respiratory tract conditions: Temporary relief of symptoms (nasal congestion; runny nose; sneezing; itching of the eyes, nose, or throat) associated with the common cold, sinusitis, allergic rhinitis, and other upper respiratory tract conditions.

Dosing

Adult & Geriatric Upper respiratory tract conditions: Oral: **Note:** Chlorpheniramine dosing in terms of chlorpheniramine maleate; phenylephrine dosing in terms of phenylephrine hydrochloride:

Liquid:
Chlorpheniramine 1 mg and phenylephrine 2.5 mg per 1 mL: 4 mL every 4 hours (maximum: 24 mL/24 hours)
Chlorpheniramine 4 mg and phenylephrine 10 mg per 5 mL: 5 mL every 4 to 6 hours (maximum: 30 mL/24 hours)

Tablet:
Chlorpheniramine 4 mg and phenylephrine 10 mg: One tablet every 4 to 6 hours (maximum: 6 tablets/24 hours)
Chlorpheniramine 4 mg and phenylephrine 20 mg (sustained-release): 1 or 2 tablets every 12 hours (maximum: 4 tablets/24 hours)

Pediatric Upper respiratory tract conditions: Oral: **Note:** Chlorpheniramine dosing in terms of chlorpheniramine maleate; phenylephrine dosing in terms of phenylephrine hydrochloride:

Children 2 to 5 years:
Liquid:
Chlorpheniramine 2 mg and phenylephrine 5 mg per 1 mL: 0.5 mL every 4 hours (maximum: 3 mL/24 hours)

Children 6 to 11 years:
Liquid:
Chlorpheniramine 1 mg and phenylephrine 2 to 2.5 mg per 1 mL: 2 mL every 4 to 6 hours (maximum: 12 mL/24 hours)
Chlorpheniramine 1 to 2 mg and phenylephrine 3.5 to 5 mg per 1 mL: 1 mL every 4 to 6 hours (maximum: 6 mL/24 hours)
Chlorpheniramine 1 mg and phenylephrine 2.5 mg per 5 mL: 10 mL every 4 hours (maximum: 60 mL/24 hours)
Chlorpheniramine 4 mg and phenylephrine 10 mg per 5 mL: 2.5 mL every 4 to 6 hours (maximum: 15 mL/24 hours)

Tablet:
Chlorpheniramine 4 mg and phenylephrine 10 mg: One-half tablet every 4 to 6 hours (maximum: 3 tablets/24 hours)
Chlorpheniramine 4 mg and phenylephrine 20 mg (sustained-release): 1 tablet every 12 hours (maximum: 2 tablets/24 hours)

Children ≥12 years and Adolescents: Refer to adult dosing:

Renal Impairment There are no dosage adjustments provided in the manufacturer's labeling.

Hepatic Impairment There are no dosage adjustments provided in the manufacturer's labeling.

Additional Information Complete prescribing information should be consulted for additional detail.

Dosage Forms Excipient information presented when available (limited, particularly for generics); consult specific product labeling. [DSC] = Discontinued product

Liquid, Oral:
AccuHist Drops: Chlorpheniramine maleate 1 mg and phenylephrine hydrochloride 2.5 mg per 1 mL (59.2 mL [DSC]) [alcohol free, dye free, sugar free; contains sodium benzoate]
Cardec: Chlorpheniramine maleate 1 mg and phenylephrine hydrochloride 3.5 mg per 1 mL (30 mL) [alcohol free, gluten free, sugar free; contains brilliant blue fcf (fd&c blue #1), fd&c red #40, methylparaben, propylene glycol, propylparaben; grape flavor]
Dallergy: Chlorpheniramine maleate 1 mg and phenylephrine hydrochloride 2 mg per 1 mL (30 mL [DSC]) [peach-tangerine flavor]
Dallergy: Chlorpheniramine maleate 1 mg and phenylephrine hydrochloride 2.5 mg per 1 mL (30 mL) [alcohol free, sugar free; contains fd&c yellow #6 (sunset yellow), propylene glycol, saccharin sodium; peach flavor]
Ed A-Hist: Chlorpheniramine maleate 4 mg and phenylephrine hydrochloride 10 mg per 5 mL (473 mL) [gluten free, sugar free; contains alcohol, usp, brilliant blue fcf (fd&c blue #1), propylene glycol, saccharin sodium, sodium benzoate; grape flavor]

Ed ChlorPed D: Chlorpheniramine maleate 2 mg and phenylephrine hydrochloride 5 mg per 1 mL (60 mL) [alcohol free, gluten free, sugar free; contains brilliant blue fcf (fd&c blue #1), fd&c yellow #6 (sunset yellow), methylparaben, propylene glycol, propylparaben; apple sauce flavor]
LoHist: Chlorpheniramine maleate 1 mg and phenylephrine hydrochloride 2.5 mg per 1 mL (59.2 mL [DSC]) [alcohol free, dye free, gluten free, sugar free; contains methylparaben, propylene glycol, propylparaben]
Nasohist: Chlorpheniramine maleate 1 mg and phenylephrine hydrochloride 2 mg per 1 mL (30 mL [DSC]) [alcohol free, dye free, sugar free; contains propylene glycol, saccharin sodium]
NoHist-LQ: Chlorpheniramine maleate 4 mg and phenylephrine hydrochloride 10 mg per 5 mL (473 mL) [alcohol free, sugar free; contains edetate disodium, methylparaben, propylene glycol, propylparaben, saccharin calcium; bubble-gum flavor]
Trigofen: Chlorpheniramine maleate 1 mg and phenylephrine hydrochloride 2 mg per 1 mL (30 mL [DSC]) [alcohol free, dye free, sugar free; contains methylparaben, propylene glycol, propylparaben; orange-vanilla flavor]
Virdec: Chlorpheniramine maleate 1 mg and phenylephrine hydrochloride 3.5 mg per 1 mL (30 mL [DSC]) [alcohol free, gluten free, sugar free; contains brilliant blue fcf (fd&c blue #1), fd&c red #40, methylparaben, propylene glycol, propylparaben; raspberry flavor]

Syrup, Oral:
Triaminic Cold/Allergy Child: Chlorpheniramine maleate 1 mg and phenylephrine hydrochloride 2.5 mg per 5 mL (118 mL) [alcohol free; contains benzoic acid, edetate disodium, fd&c yellow #6 (sunset yellow)]

Tablet, Oral:
Actifed Cold/Allergy: Chlorpheniramine maleate 4 mg and phenylephrine hydrochloride 10 mg [scored; pseudoephedrine free]
Ed A-Hist: Chlorpheniramine maleate 4 mg and phenylephrine hydrochloride 10 mg [scored; contains fd&c blue #2 (indigotine), fd&c yellow #6 (sunset yellow), tartrazine (fd&c yellow #5)]
NoHist: Chlorpheniramine maleate 3 mg and phenylephrine hydrochloride 10 mg [DSC]
Sudafed PE Sinus/Allergy: Chlorpheniramine maleate 4 mg and phenylephrine hydrochloride 10 mg [scored; pseudoephedrine free]

Tablet Extended Release 12 Hour, Oral:
Rescon-Jr: Chlorpheniramine maleate 4 mg and phenylephrine hydrochloride 20 [DSC] [scored]

Chlorpheniramine and Pseudoephedrine
(klor fen IR a meen & soo doe e FED rin)

Brand Names: US Dicel® Chewable [OTC]; LoHist-D [OTC]; Maxichlor PSE [OTC]; Neutrahist Pediatric [OTC]; SudoGest™ Sinus & Allergy [OTC]

Brand Names: Canada Triaminic® Cold & Allergy

Index Terms Allerest; Chlorpheniramine Maleate and Pseudoephedrine Hydrochloride; Chlorpheniramine Tannate and Pseudoephedrine Tannate; Pseudoephedrine and Chlorpheniramine

Pharmacologic Category Alkylamine Derivative; Alpha/Beta Agonist; Decongestant; Histamine H₁ Antagonist; Histamine H₁ Antagonist, First Generation

Use Relief of nasal congestion associated with the common cold, hay fever, allergic rhinitis, and other allergies

Dosing

Adult & Geriatric Rhinitis/decongestant: Oral: **Note:** All dosing is presented in terms of chlorpheniramine maleate and pseudoephedrine hydrochloride.

Liquid: Chlorpheniramine 2 mg and pseudoephedrine 30 mg per 5 mL: 10 mL every 4-6 hours (maximum: 60 mL/24hours)

Tablet:
Chlorpheniramine 2 mg and pseudoephedrine 30 mg: Two tablets every 4-6 hours (maximum: 8 tablets/24 hours)
Chlorpheniramine 4 mg and pseudoephedrine 60 mg: One tablet every 4-6 hours (maximum: 4 tablets/24 hours)

Pediatric Rhinitis/decongestant: Oral: **Note:** All dosing is presented in terms of chlorpheniramine maleate and pseudoephedrine hydrochloride.

Children: 6-11 years:
Liquid:
Chlorpheniramine 0.8 mg and pseudoephedrine 9 mg per 1 mL: 2 mL every 4-6 hours (maximum: 8 mL/24 hours)
Chlorpheniramine 2 mg and pseudoephedrine 30 mg per 5 mL: 5 mL every 4-6 hours (maximum: 30 mL/24 hours)

Tablet:

Chlorpheniramine 2 mg and pseudoephedrine 30 mg: One tablet every 4-6 hours (maximum: 4 tablets/24 hours)

Chlorpheniramine 4 mg and pseudoephedrine 60 mg: One-half tablet every 4-6 hours (maximum: 2 tablets/24 hours)

Children ≥12 years: Refer to adult dosing.

Additional Information Complete prescribing information should be consulted for additional detail.

Dosage Forms Excipient information presented when available (limited, particularly for generics); consult specific product labeling. [DSC] = Discontinued product

Liquid, oral:

LoHist-D: Chlorpheniramine maleate 2 mg and pseudoephedrine hydrochloride 30 mg per 5 mL (473 mL) [dye free, ethanol free, sugar free; cherry flavor]

Liquid, oral [drops]:

Neutrahist Pediatric: Chlorpheniramine maleate 0.8 mg and pseudoephedrine hydrochloride 9 mg per 1 mL (30 mL) [ethanol free, sugar free; contains propylene glycol; cherry flavor]

Tablet, oral: Chlorpheniramine maleate 4 mg and pseudoephedrine hydrochloride 60 mg

Maxichlor PSE: Chlorpheniramine maleate 4 mg and pseudoephedrine hydrochloride 60 mg

SudoGest™ Sinus & Allergy: Chlorpheniramine maleate 4 mg and pseudoephedrine hydrochloride 60 mg

Tablet, chewable, oral:

Dicel® Chewables: Chlorpheniramine maleate 2 mg and pseudoephedrine hydrochloride 30 mg [ethanol free; contains sodium 17 mg/tablet, soy lecithin; strawberry-banana cream flavor]

Chlorpheniramine, Phenylephrine, and Dextromethorphan

(klor fen IR a meen, fen il EF rin, & deks troe meth OR fan)

Brand Names: US Cardec™ DM [OTC]; Corfen-DM [OTC]; De-Chlor DM [OTC]; Ed A-Hist DM [OTC]; Father John's® Plus [OTC]; Maxichlor PEH DM [OTC] [DSC]; nasohist™ DM pediatric [OTC] [DSC]; Neo DM [OTC] [DSC]; NoHist DM [OTC]; Norel CS [OTC]; Trigofen DM [OTC]; Virdec DM [OTC] [DSC]

Index Terms Dextromethorphan, Chlorpheniramine, and Phenylephrine; Phenylephrine, Chlorpheniramine, and Dextromethorphan

Pharmacologic Category Alkylamine Derivative; Alpha-Adrenergic Agonist; Antitussive; Decongestant; Histamine H_1 Antagonist; Histamine H_1 Antagonist, First Generation

Use Temporary relief of cough and upper respiratory symptoms associated with allergies or the common cold

Dosing

Adult & Geriatric Note: All dosing is presented in terms of chlorpheniramine maleate, phenylephrine hydrochloride, and dextromethorphan hydrobromide.

Relief of cough and cold symptoms: Oral:

Liquid:

Chlorpheniramine 2 mg, phenylephrine 5 mg, and dextromethorphan 5 mg per 15 mL: 30 mL every 4 hours (maximum: 180 mL/24 hours)

Chlorpheniramine 2-4 mg, phenylephrine 5-10 mg, and dextromethorphan 15 mg per 5 mL: 5 mL every 4-6 hours (maximum: 30 mL/24 hours)

Tablet: Chlorpheniramine 4 mg, phenylephrine 10 mg, and dextromethorphan 20 mg: One tablet every 4-6 hours (maximum: 6 tablets/24 hours)

Pediatric Note: All dosing is presented in terms of chlorpheniramine maleate, phenylephrine hydrochloride, and dextromethorphan hydrobromide.

Relief of cough and cold symptoms: Oral:

Children: 2-5 years: Liquid: Chlorpheniramine 1 mg, phenylephrine 2.5 mg, and dextromethorphan 2.5 mg per 1 mL: 1 mL every 4-6 hours (maximum: 4 mL/24 hours)

Children: 6-11 years:

Liquid:

Chlorpheniramine 0.75 mg, phenylephrine 1.75 mg, and dextromethorphan 2.75 mg per 1 mL: 2 mL every 4-6 hours (maximum: 12 mL/24 hours)

Chlorpheniramine 1 mg, phenylephrine 2-2.5 mg, and dextromethorphan 2.5-3 mg per 1 mL: 2 mL every 4-6 hours (maximum: 8 mL/24 hours)

Chlorpheniramine 1 mg, phenylephrine 3.5 mg, and dextromethorphan 3 mg per 1 mL: 1 mL every 4-6 hours (maximum: 6 mL/24 hours)

Chlorpheniramine 2-4 mg, phenylephrine 5-10 mg, and dextromethorphan 15 mg per 5 mL: 2.5 mL every 4-6 hours (maximum: 15 mL/24 hours)

Tablet: Chlorpheniramine 4 mg, phenylephrine 10 mg, and dextromethorphan 20 mg: One-half tablet every 4-6 hours (maximum: 3 tablets/24 hours)

Children ≥12 years: Refer to adult dosing.

Additional Information Complete prescribing information should be consulted for additional detail.

Dosage Forms Excipient information presented when available (limited, particularly for generics); consult specific product labeling. [DSC] = discontinued product.

Liquid, oral:

Corfen-DM: Chlorpheniramine maleate 4 mg, phenylephrine hydrochloride 10 mg, and dextromethorphan hydrobromide 15 mg per 5 mL (473 mL) [dye free, ethanol free, sugar free; contains propylene glycol; grape flavor]

De-Chlor DM: Chlorpheniramine maleate 2 mg, phenylephrine hydrochloride 10 mg, and dextromethorphan hydrobromide 15 mg per 5 mL (473 mL) [dye free, ethanol free, sugar free; contains propylene glycol; strawberry flavor]

Ed A-Hist DM: Chlorpheniramine maleate 4 mg, phenylephrine hydrochloride 10 mg, and dextromethorphan hydrobromide 15 mg per 5 mL (473 mL) [gluten free, sugar free; contains propylene glycol; banana flavor]

Father John's® Plus: Chlorpheniramine maleate 2 mg, phenylephrine hydrochloride 5 mg, and dextromethorphan hydrobromide 5 mg per 15 mL (118 mL) [ethanol free]

NoHist DM: Chlorpheniramine maleate 4 mg, phenylephrine hydrochloride 10 mg, and dextromethorphan hydrobromide 15 mg per 5 mL (473 mL) [dye free, ethanol free, sugar free; contains propylene glycol; grape flavor]

Norel CS: Chlorpheniramine maleate 4 mg, phenylephrine hydrochloride 10 mg, and dextromethorphan hydrobromide 12.5 mg per 5 mL (473 mL) [dye free, ethanol free, sugar free; contains propylene glycol; grape flavor]

Liquid, oral [drops]:

Cardec™ DM: Chlorpheniramine maleate 1 mg, phenylephrine hydrochloride 3.5 mg, and dextromethorphan hydrobromide 3 mg per 1 mL (30 mL) [ethanol free, gluten free, sugar free; contains propylene glycol, sodium benzoate; grape flavor]

nasohist™ DM pediatric: Chlorpheniramine maleate 1 mg, phenylephrine hydrochloride 2 mg, and dextromethorphan hydrobromide 3 mg per 1 mL (30 mL) [dye free, ethanol free, sugar free; contains propylene glycol; orange-vanilla flavor] [DSC]

Neo DM: Chlorpheniramine maleate 0.75 mg, phenylephrine hydrochloride 1.75 mg, and dextromethorphan hydrobromide 2.75 mg per 1 mL (30 mL) [ethanol free, sugar free; contains propylene glycol; black cherry flavor] [DSC]

Trigofen DM: Chlorpheniramine maleate 1 mg, phenylephrine hydrochloride 2 mg, and dextromethorphan hydrobromide 3 mg per 1 mL (30 mL) [dye free, ethanol free, sugar free; contains propylene glycol]

Virdec DM: Chlorpheniramine maleate 1 mg, phenylephrine hydrochloride 3.5 mg, and dextromethorphan hydrobromide 3 mg per 1 mL (30 mL) [ethanol free, gluten free, sugar free; contains propylene glycol; grape flavor] [DSC]

Tablet, oral:

Ed A-Hist: Chlorpheniramine maleate 4 mg, phenylephrine hydrochloride 10 mg, and dextromethorphan hydrobromide 10 mg

Maxichlor PEH DM: Chlorpheniramine maleate 4 mg, phenylephrine hydrochloride 10 mg, and dextromethorphan hydrobromide 20 mg [scored] [DSC]

Chlorpheniramine, Pseudoephedrine, and Dextromethorphan

(klor fen IR a meen, soo doe e FED rin, & deks troe meth OR fan)

Brand Names: US Dicel® DM Chewables [OTC]; Kidkare Children's Cough/Cold [OTC]; M-END DM [OTC] [DSC]; Maxichlor PSE DM [OTC] [DSC]; Neutrahist PDX [OTC] [DSC]; Pedia Relief™ Cough-Cold [OTC]; Pediatric Cough & Cold [OTC]; Rescon DM [OTC]

Index Terms Chlorpheniramine Maleate, Pseudoephedrine Hydrochloride, and Dextromethorphan Hydrobromide; Chlorpheniramine Tannate, Pseudoephedrine Tannate, and Dextromethorphan Tannate; Chlorpheniramine, Dextromethorphan, and Pseudoephedrine; Dexchlorpheniramine Tannate, Pseudoephedrine Tannate, and Dextromethorphan Tannate; Dextromethorphan, Chlorpheniramine, and Pseudoephedrine; Pseudoephedrine, Chlorpheniramine, and Dextromethorphan

Pharmacologic Category Alkylamine Derivative; Alpha/Beta Agonist; Antitussive; Decongestant; Histamine H_1 Antagonist; Histamine H_1 Antagonist, First Generation

Use Temporarily relieves nasal congestion, runny nose, cough, and sneezing due to the common cold, hay fever, or allergic rhinitis

Dosing

Adult & Geriatric Relief of cold symptoms: Oral: **Note:** All dosing is presented in terms of chlorpheniramine maleate, pseudoephedrine hydrochloride, and dextromethorphan hydrobromide.

Liquid:

Chlorpheniramine 2 mg, pseudoephedrine 15 mg, and dextromethorphan 15 mg per 5 mL: 10 mL every 6 hours (maximum: 40 mL/24 hours)

Chlorpheniramine 2 mg, pseudoephedrine 30 mg, and dextromethorphan 10 mg per 5 mL: 10 mL every 4-6 hours (maximum: 40 mL/24 hours)

Chlorpheniramine 4 mg, pseudoephedrine 20 mg, and dextromethorphan 20 mg per 5 mL: 5 mL every 4-6 hours (maximum: 30 mL/24 hours)

Tablet:

Chlorpheniramine 2 mg, pseudoephedrine 30 mg, and dextromethorphan 10 mg: Two tablets every 4-6 hours (maximum: 8 tablets/24 hours)

Chlorpheniramine 4 mg, pseudoephedrine 60 mg, and dextromethorphan 20 mg: One tablet every 4-6 hours (maximum: 4 tablets/24 hours)

Pediatric Relief of cold symptoms: Oral: **Note:** All dosing is presented in terms of chlorpheniramine maleate, pseudoephedrine hydrochloride, and dextromethorphan hydrobromide.

Children 6-11 years:

Liquid:

Chlorpheniramine 0.8 mg, pseudoephedrine 9 mg, and dextromethorphan 3 mg per 1 mL: 2 mL every 4-6 hours (maximum: 8 mL/24 hours)

Chlorpheniramine 1 mg, pseudoephedrine 15 mg, and dextromethorphan 5 mg per 5 mL: 10 mL every 4-6 hours (maximum: 40 mL/24 hours)

Chlorpheniramine 2 mg, pseudoephedrine 15 mg, and dextromethorphan 15 mg per 5 mL: 5 mL every 6 hours (maximum: 20 mL/24 hours)

Chlorpheniramine 2 mg, pseudoephedrine 30 mg, and dextromethorphan 10 mg per 5 mL: 5 mL every 4-6 hours (maximum: 20 mL/24 hours)

Chlorpheniramine 4 mg, pseudoephedrine 20 mg, and dextromethorphan 20 mg per 5 mL: 2.5 mL every 4-6 hours (maximum: 15 mL/24 hours)

Tablet:

Chlorpheniramine 2 mg, pseudoephedrine 30 mg, and dextromethorphan 10 mg: One tablet every 4-6 hours (maximum: 4 tablets/24 hours)

Chlorpheniramine 4 mg, pseudoephedrine 60 mg, and dextromethorphan 20 mg: One-half tablet every 4-6 hours (maximum: 2 tablets/24 hours)

Children ≥12 years: Refer to adult dosing.

Additional Information Complete prescribing information should be consulted for additional detail.

Dosage Forms Excipient information presented when available (limited, particularly for generics); consult specific product labeling. [DSC] = discontinued product

Liquid, oral:

Kidkare Children's Cough/Cold: Chlorpheniramine maleate 1 mg, pseudoephedrine hydrochloride 15 mg, and dextromethorphan hydrobromide 5 mg per 5 mL (118 mL) [ethanol free; contains propylene glycol and sodium benzoate; cherry flavor]

Maxichlor PSE DM: Chlorpheniramine maleate 4 mg, pseudoephedrine hydrochloride 20 mg, and dextromethorphan hydrobromide 20 mg per 5 mL (473 mL) [sugar free; contains propylene glycol; vanilla flavor]

M-END DM: Chlorpheniramine maleate 2 mg, pseudoephedrine hydrochloride 15 mg, and dextromethorphan hydrobromide 15 mg per 5 mL (30 mL) [ethanol free, sugar free; contains propylene glycol; orange flavor] [DSC]

Pedia Relief™ Cough-Cold: Chlorpheniramine maleate 1 mg, pseudoephedrine hydrochloride 15 mg, and dextromethorphan hydrobromide 5 mg per 5 mL (120 mL) [ethanol free; contains propylene glycol and sodium benzoate; cherry flavor]

Pediatric Cough & Cold: Chlorpheniramine maleate 1 mg, pseudoephedrine hydrochloride 15 mg, and dextromethorphan hydrobromide 5 mg per 5 mL (120 mL) [ethanol free; contains propylene glycol, sodium benzoate; wild cherry flavor]

Rescon DM: Chlorpheniramine maleate 2 mg, pseudoephedrine hydrochloride 30 mg, and dextromethorphan hydrobromide 10 mg per 5 mL (120 mL, 480 mL) [dye free, ethanol free, sugar free; cherry flavor]

Liquid, oral [drops]:

Neutrahist PDX: Chlorpheniramine maleate 0.8 mg, pseudoephedrine hydrochloride 9 mg, and dextromethorphan hydrobromide 3 mg per 1 mL (30 mL) [ethanol free, sugar free; contains propylene glycol; grape flavor] [DSC]

Tablet, oral: Chlorpheniramine maleate 4 mg, pseudoephedrine hydrochloride 60 mg, and dextromethorphan hydrobromide 20 mg

Maxichlor PSE DM: Chlorpheniramine maleate 4 mg, pseudoephedrine hydrochloride 60 mg, and dextromethorphan hydrobromide 20 mg [DSC]

Tablet, chewable, oral:

Dicel® DM Chewables: Chlorpheniramine maleate 2 mg, pseudoephedrine hydrochloride 30 mg, and dextromethorphan hydrobromide 10 mg [ethanol free; contains sodium 19 mg/tablet, soy lecithin; cotton candy flavor]

◆ Chlorpheniramine Tannate and Pseudoephedrine Tannate see Chlorpheniramine and Pseudoephedrine on page 377

◆ Chlorpheniramine Tannate, Pseudoephedrine Tannate, and Dextromethorphan Tannate see Chlorpheniramine, Pseudoephedrine, and Dextromethorphan on page 379

ChlorproMAZINE (klor PROE ma zeen)

Brand Names: Canada Chlorpromazine Hydrochloride Inj; Teva-Chlorpromazine

Index Terms Chlorpromazine Hydrochloride; CPZ; Thorazine

Pharmacologic Category Antimanic Agent; First Generation (Typical) Antipsychotic

Use

Behavioral problems: Treatment of severe behavioral problems in children 1 to 12 years of age marked by combativeness and/or explosive hyperexcitable behavior (out of proportion to immediate provocations).

Bipolar disorder: Treatment of manic episodes associated with bipolar disorder.

Hiccups: Treatment of intractable hiccups.

Hyperactivity: Short-term treatment of hyperactive children who show excessive motor activity with accompanying conduct disorders consisting of some or all of the following symptoms: impulsivity, difficulty sustaining attention, aggressiveness, mood lability, and poor frustration tolerance.

Nausea/Vomiting: Management of nausea and vomiting.

Porphyria, acute intermittent: Treatment of acute intermittent porphyria.

Schizophrenia/Psychotic disorders: Treatment of schizophrenia and psychotic disorders.

Surgery: Management of restlessness and apprehension prior to surgery.

Tetanus: Adjunctive therapy in the treatment of tetanus.

Dosing

Adult

Bipolar disorder/psychotic disorders/schizophrenia:

Oral: Range: 30 to 800 mg daily in 2 to 4 divided doses, initiate at lower doses and titrate as needed; usual dose: 200 to 800 mg daily; some patients may require 1 to 2 g daily, however, therapeutic gain is limited at doses >1 g daily

IM: Initial: 25 mg, may repeat (25 to 50 mg) in 1 to 4 hours, gradually increase to a maximum of 400 mg/dose every 4 to 6 hours until patient is controlled; usual dose: 200 to 800 mg daily

Intractable hiccups:

Oral, IM: 25 to 50 mg 3 to 4 times/day

IV (refractory to oral or IM treatment): 25 to 50 mg via slow IV infusion

Nausea and vomiting:

Oral: 10 to 25 mg every 4 to 6 hours as needed

IM: 25 to 50 mg every 3 to 4 hours as needed

IV (during surgery): 2 mg per fractional injection at 2 minute intervals using a 1 mg/mL solution; do not exceed 25 mg

Porphyria, acute intermittent:

Oral: 25 to 50 mg 3 to 4 times daily; usually may be discontinued after several weeks although maintenance therapy may be necessary

IM: 25 mg 3 or 4 times daily (until patient can tolerate oral administration)

Presurgical apprehension:

Oral: 25 to 50 mg 2 to 3 hours prior to surgery

IM: 12.5 to 25 mg 1 to 2 hours prior to surgery

Tetanus: IM, IV: 25 to 50 mg 3 or 4 times daily; titrate to response

Geriatric

Manufacturer's labeling: Oral, IM, IV: Dosages in the lower range of recommended adult dosing are generally sufficient. Titrate dosage slowly and monitor carefully.

Alternate dosing: Psychotic disorders: Oral: Routine use is not recommended; however, if used, the following doses have been used: Initial: 10 to 25 mg 3 times daily (Denham 1980; Gareri 2003; Salzman 2005); titrate dose slowly. Usual dosage range: 50 to 200 mg daily in divided doses (Salzman 2005). Mean dosage range: 25 to 75 mg daily in divided doses (Gareri 2003). Doses greater than 300 to 400 mg/day are rarely necessary (Denham 1980). **Note:** IM administration may be used in the very acutely disturbed patient (Denham 1980). IM doses are approximately 4 times more potent than comparable oral doses (Salzman 2005).

Pediatric

Behavior problems; severe: Note: Begin with low doses and gradually titrate as needed to lowest effective dose; route of administration should be determined by severity of symptoms.

Infants ≥6 months, Children, and Adolescents weighing ≤45.5 kg:

Oral: Initial: 0.55 mg/kg/dose every 4 to 6 hours as needed; may titrate as required; in severe cases, higher doses may be required (50 to 100 mg daily); in older children, higher daily doses (200 mg daily or higher) may be necessary; maximum daily dose: 500 mg/**day**; daily doses >500 mg have not been shown to further improve behavior in pediatric patients with severe mental impairment

IM, IV (off-label): Initial: 0.55 mg/kg/dose every 6-8 hours as needed; may titrate as required in severe cases (Kliegman, 2007)

Maximum recommended daily doses:

Children <5 years or weighing <22.7 kg: 40 mg/**day**

Children ≥5 years and Adolescents or weighing 22.7 to 45.5 kg: 75 mg/**day**

Adolescents weighing >45.5 kg:

Oral: Range: 30 to 800 mg daily in 2 to 4 divided doses, initiate at lower doses and titrate as needed; usual dose is 200 mg daily

IM, IV (off-label): 25 mg initially, may repeat (25 to 50 mg) in 1 to 4 hours, gradually increase to a maximum of 400 mg/dose every 4 to 6 hours until patient controlled; usual dose 200 to 800 mg daily (Kliegman, 2007)

Nausea and vomiting, treatment (non-CINV):

Infants ≥6 months, Children, and Adolescents weighing ≤45.5 kg: Oral, IM, IV: 0.55 mg/kg/dose every 6 to 8 hours as needed; in severe cases, higher doses may be needed; usual maximum daily dose: IM, IV:

Children <5 years or weighing <22.7 kg: 40 mg/**day**

Children ≥5 years and Adolescents or weighing 22.7 to 45.5 kg: 75 mg/**day**

Adolescents weighing >45.5 kg:

Oral: 10 to 25 mg every 4 to 6 hours as needed

IM, IV: Initial: 25 mg; if tolerated (no hypotension), then may give 25 to 50 mg every 4 to 6 hours as needed

Prevention of chemotherapy-associated nausea and vomiting (Pediatric Oncology Group of Ontario [POGO] dosing recommendation): Highly or moderately emetogenic chemotherapy (patients who cannot receive corticosteroids): Infants ≥6 months, Children, and Adolescents: IV: 0.5 mg/kg/dose every 6 hours (in combination with ondansetron or granisetron); if not controlled, may increase up to 1 mg/kg/dose; monitor for sedation, maximum dose: 50 mg (Dupuis, 2013)

Presurgical apprehension: Infants ≥6 months, Children, and Adolescents:

Oral: 0.55 mg/kg 2 to 3 hours prior to surgery; maximum dose 50 mg

IM: 0.55 mg/kg/dose 1 to 2 hours prior to surgery; maximum dose 25 mg

Tetanus:

Infants ≥6 months, Children, and Adolescents weighing ≤45.5 kg: IM, IV: 0.55 mg/kg/dose every 6 to 8 hours; in severe cases higher doses may be needed

Usual maximum daily dose:

Children <5 years or weighing <22.7 kg: 40 mg/**day**

Children ≥5 years and Adolescents or weighing 22.7 to 45.5 kg: 75 mg/**day**

Adolescents weighing ≥45.5 kg: IM, IV: 25 to 50 mg every 6 to 8 hours; begin with low dose titrate to response

Renal Impairment There are no dosage adjustments provided in the manufacturer's labeling; use with caution. Not dialyzable (0% to 5%)

Hepatic Impairment There are no dosage adjustments provided in the manufacturer's labeling; use with caution.

Additional Information Complete prescribing information should be consulted for additional detail.

Dosage Forms Excipient information presented when available (limited, particularly for generics); consult specific product labeling.

Solution, Injection, as hydrochloride:

Generic: 25 mg/mL (1 mL); 50 mg/2 mL (2 mL)

Tablet, Oral, as hydrochloride:

Generic: 10 mg, 25 mg, 50 mg, 100 mg, 200 mg

◆ Chlorpromazine Hydrochloride *see* ChlorproMAZINE *on page 379*

◆ Chlorpromazine Hydrochloride Inj (Can) *see* ChlorproMAZINE *on page 379*

ChlorproPAMIDE (klor PROE pa mide)

Brand Names: Canada Apo-Chlorpropamide®

Pharmacologic Category Antidiabetic Agent, Sulfonylurea

Use Management of blood sugar in type 2 diabetes mellitus (noninsulin dependent, NIDDM) as an adjunct to diet and exercise to lower blood glucose

Dosing

Adult Type 2 diabetes: Oral: The dosage of chlorpropamide is variable and should be individualized based upon the patient's response

Initial dose: 250 mg daily in mild-to-moderate diabetes in middle-aged, stable diabetic patients

Titration: After 5-7 days of initiation, subsequent daily dosages may be increased or decreased by 50-125 mg at 3- to 5-day intervals

Maintenance dose: 100-250 mg daily; severe patients with diabetes may require 500 mg daily; avoid doses >750 mg daily

Geriatric Refer to adult dosing. Reduce initial dose to 100-125 mg/day in older patients; after 5-7 days of initiation, subsequent daily dosages may be increased or decreased by 50-125 mg at 3- to 5-day intervals (slower upward titration may be appropriate in older patients)

Renal Impairment No specific dosage adjustment provided in manufacturer's labeling; conservative initial and maintenance doses are recommended.

Alternate recommendations (Aronoff, 2007):

CrCl >50 mL/minute: Reduce dose by 50%.

CrCl <50 mL/minute: Avoid use.

Hemodialysis: Avoid use.

Peritoneal dialysis: Avoid use.

Continuous renal replacement therapy (CRRT): Avoid use.

Hepatic Impairment No specific dosage adjustment provided in manufacturer's labeling; conservative initial and maintenance doses are recommended in patients with liver impairment since chlorpropamide undergoes extensive hepatic metabolism.

Additional Information Complete prescribing information should be consulted for additional detail.

Dosage Forms Excipient information presented when available (limited, particularly for generics); consult specific product labeling.

Tablet, Oral:

Generic: 100 mg, 250 mg

Chlorthalidone (klor THAL i done)

Brand Names: US Thalitone [DSC]

Brand Names: Canada Apo-Chlorthalidone

Index Terms Hygroton

Pharmacologic Category Antihypertensive; Diuretic, Thiazide-Related

Use Management of mild-to-moderate hypertension when used alone or in combination with other agents; treatment of edema associated with heart failure, renal dysfunction, hepatic cirrhosis, or corticosteroid and estrogen therapy.

Guideline recommendations:
Hypertension: The 2014 guideline for the management of high blood pressure in adults (Eighth Joint National Committee [JNC 8]) recommends initiation of pharmacologic treatment to lower blood pressure for the following patients:
• Patients ≥60 years of age with systolic blood pressure (SBP) ≥150 mm Hg or diastolic blood pressure (DBP) ≥90 mm Hg. Goal of therapy is SBP <150 mm Hg and DBP <90 mm Hg.
• Patients <60 years of age with SBP ≥140 mm Hg or DBP is ≥90 mm Hg. Goal of therapy is SBP <140 mm Hg and DBP <90 mm Hg.
• Patients ≥18 years of age with diabetes and SBP ≥140 mm Hg or DBP ≥90 mm Hg. Goal of therapy is SBP <140 mm Hg and DBP <90 mm Hg.
• Patients ≥18 years of age with chronic kidney disease (CKD) and SBP ≥140 mm Hg or DBP ≥90 mm Hg. Goal of therapy is SBP <140 mm Hg and DBP <90 mm Hg.
Chronic kidney disease (CKD) and hypertension: In patients with CKD, regardless of race or diabetes status, the use of an ACE inhibitor (ACEI) or angiotensin receptor blocker (ARB) as initial therapy is recommended to improve kidney outcomes. In the general nonblack population (without CKD) including those with diabetes, initial antihypertensive treatment should consist of a thiazide-type diuretic, calcium channel blocker, ACEI, or ARB. In the general black population (without CKD), including those with diabetes, initial antihypertensive treatment should consist of a thiazide-type diuretic or a calcium channel blocker **instead of** an ACEI or ARB.
Coronary artery disease (CAD) and hypertension: The American Heart Association, American College of Cardiology and American Society of Hypertension (AHA/ACC/ASH) 2015 scientific statement for the treatment of hypertension in patients with coronary artery disease (CAD) recommends the use of a thiazide (or thiazide-like diuretic) as part of a regimen in patients with hypertension and chronic stable angina. A BP target of <140/90 mm Hg is reasonable for the secondary prevention of cardiovascular events. A lower target BP (<130/80 mm Hg) may be appropriate in some individuals with CAD, previous MI, stroke or transient ischemic attack, or CAD risk equivalents (AHA/ACC/ASH [Rosendorff 2015]).

Dosing
Adult
Edema: Initial: 50 to 100 mg once daily or 100 mg on alternate days; maximum dose: 200 mg daily
Heart failure-associated edema: Initial: 12.5 to 25 mg once daily; maximum daily dose: 100 mg (ACCF/AHA [Yancy 2013])
Hypertension: Oral: Initial: 25 mg once daily **or** 12.5 mg once daily (JNC 8 [James, 2013]); may increase after a suitable trial to 50 mg once daily; maximum: 100 mg daily; usual dosage range (ASH/ISH [Weber, 2014]): 12.5 to 25 mg daily. Target dose range (JNC 8 [James, 2013]): 12.5 to 25 mg daily.
Calcium nephrolithiasis (off-label use): 25 mg once daily (AUA Guidelines [Pearle, 2014])
Geriatric Oral: Initial: 12.5 to 25 mg once daily or every other day; there is little advantage to using doses >25 mg daily.
Pediatric Hypertension (off-label use): Children and Adolescents: Oral: Initial: 0.3 mg/kg once daily, up to 2 mg/kg/day; maximum: 50 mg daily (NHBPEP, 2004; NHLBI, 2011)
Renal Impairment
CrCl ≥10 mL/minute: No dosage adjustment necessary (Aronoff, 2007)
CrCl <10 mL/minute: Avoid use. Ineffective with low GFR (Aronoff, 2007)
Hepatic Impairment There are no dosage adjustments provided in manufacturer's labeling; use with caution.
Additional Information Complete prescribing information should be consulted for additional detail.
Dosage Forms Excipient information presented when available (limited, particularly for generics); consult specific product labeling. [DSC] = Discontinued product
Tablet, Oral:
Thalitone: 15 mg [DSC]
Generic: 25 mg, 50 mg, 100 mg

◆ Chlorthalidone and Azilsartan *see* Azilsartan and Chlorthalidone *on page 190*
◆ Chlor-Tripolon ND® (Can) *see* Loratadine and Pseudoephedrine *on page 1102*

Chlorzoxazone (klor ZOKS a zone)

Brand Names: US Lorzone; Parafon Forte DSC
Pharmacologic Category Skeletal Muscle Relaxant
Use Symptomatic treatment of muscle spasm and pain associated with acute musculoskeletal conditions
Dosing
Adult Muscle spasm: Oral: 500 mg 3-4 times daily, may increase up to 750 mg 3-4 times daily. May consider dose reductions as symptoms improve.
Geriatric In general, avoid use or use cautiously at lower doses. Refer to adult dosing.
Renal Impairment No dosage adjustment provided in manufacturer's labeling.
Hepatic Impairment No dosage adjustment provided in manufacturer's labeling.
Additional Information Complete prescribing information should be consulted for additional detail.
Dosage Forms Excipient information presented when available (limited, particularly for generics); consult specific product labeling.
Tablet, Oral:
Lorzone: 375 mg [contains sodium benzoate]
Lorzone: 750 mg [scored; contains sodium benzoate]
Parafon Forte DSC: 500 mg [scored; contains brilliant blue fcf (fd&c blue #1), fd&c yellow #10 (quinoline yellow), sodium benzoate]
Generic: 500 mg

◆ Cholbam *see* Cholic Acid *on page 381*
◆ Cholecalciferol and Alendronate *see* Alendronate and Cholecalciferol *on page 68*

Cholestyramine Resin (koe LES teer a meen REZ in)

Brand Names: US Prevalite; Questran; Questran Light
Brand Names: Canada Novo-Cholamine; Novo-Cholamine Light; Olestyr; PMS-Cholestyramine; Questran; Questran Light Sugar Free; ZYM-Cholestyramine-Light; ZYM-Cholestyramine-Regular
Pharmacologic Category Antilipemic Agent, Bile Acid Sequestrant
Use Adjunct in the management of primary hypercholesterolemia; pruritus associated with elevated levels of bile acids; regression of arteriolosclerosis
Dosing
Adult & Geriatric Dosages are expressed in terms of anhydrous resin:
Dyslipidemia: Oral: Initial: 4 g 1-2 times/day; increase gradually over ≥1-month intervals; maintenance: 8-16 g/day divided in 2 doses; maximum: 24 g/day
Pediatric Dosages are expressed in terms of anhydrous resin:
Dyslipidemia (off-label use): Oral: 240 mg/kg/day in 2-3 divided doses; titrate dose to response and tolerance; maximum: 8 g/day
Renal Impairment No dosage adjustment provided in manufacturer's labeling; however, use with caution in renal impairment; may cause hyperchloremic acidosis.
Hepatic Impairment No dosage adjustment provided; not absorbed from the gastrointestinal tract.
Additional Information Complete prescribing information should be consulted for additional detail.
Dosage Forms Excipient information presented when available (limited, particularly for generics); consult specific product labeling. [DSC] = Discontinued product
Packet, Oral:
Prevalite: 4 g (1 ea, 42 ea, 60 ea) [contains aspartame; orange flavor]
Questran: 4 g (1 ea, 60 ea) [orange flavor]
Questran Light: 4 g (1 ea [DSC], 60 ea [DSC]) [sugar free; contains aspartame; orange flavor]
Generic: 4 g (1 ea, 60 ea)
Powder, Oral:
Prevalite: 4 g/dose (231 g) [contains aspartame; orange flavor]
Questran: 4 g/dose (378 g) [orange flavor]
Questran Light: 4 g/dose (210 g) [sugar free; contains aspartame; orange flavor]
Generic: 4 g/dose (210 g, 239.4 g, 378 g)

Cholic Acid (KOE lik AS id)

Brand Names: US Cholbam
Pharmacologic Category Bile Acid
Use
Bile acid synthesis disorders: Treatment of bile acid synthesis disorders due to single enzyme defects (SEDs).

Peroxisomal disorders: Treatment (adjunctive) of peroxisomal disorders (PDs), including Zellweger spectrum disorders, in patients who exhibit manifestations of hepatic disease, steatorrhea, or complications from decreased fat soluble vitamin absorption.

Limitations of use: The safety and effectiveness of cholic acid on extrahepatic manifestations of bile acid synthesis disorders due to SEDs or PDs, including Zellweger spectrum disorders, have not been established.

Prescribing and Access Restrictions Cholbam is only available through an exclusive pharmacy provider, Dohmen Life Science Services, Inc. For additional information, call 844.CHOLBAM (844.246.5226) or visit http://www.cholbam.com/support-and-resources/cholbam-4-u/.

Dosing

Adult Bile acid synthesis disorders, peroxisomal disorders: Oral: 10 to 15 mg/kg (once daily or in 2 divided doses); administer 11 to 17 mg/kg (once daily or in 2 divided doses) in patients with concomitant familial hypertriglyceridemia.

Pediatric Neonates ≥3 weeks, Infants, Children, and Adolescents: Oral: Refer to adult dosing.

Renal Impairment There are no dosage adjustments provided in the manufacturer's labeling.

Hepatic Impairment There are no dosage adjustments provided in the manufacturer's labeling. Discontinue if hepatic function does not improve within 3 months of starting treatment, if complete biliary obstruction develops, or if there are persistent clinical or laboratory indicators of worsening hepatic function or cholestasis; continue to monitor hepatic function and consider restarting a lower dose when parameters return to baseline.

Additional Information Complete prescribing information should be consulted for additional detail.

Dosage Forms Excipient information presented when available (limited, particularly for generics); consult specific product labeling.

Capsule, Oral:
Cholbam: 50 mg, 250 mg

◆ **Choline Fenofibrate** see Fenofibrate and Derivatives on page 746

Choline Magnesium Trisalicylate
(KOE leen mag NEE zhum trye sa LIS i late)

Index Terms Tricosal; Trilisate
Pharmacologic Category Salicylate
Use

Acute painful shoulder: Management of acute painful shoulder

Analgesia: Relief of mild to moderate pain

Antipyresis: Management of pyrexia

Arthritis: Relief of signs/symptoms of osteoarthritis, rheumatoid arthritis, and other arthritis (long-term management and acute flares)

Juvenile rheumatoid arthritis: Anti-inflammatory or analgesic management (in children) of juvenile rheumatoid arthritis and other appropriate conditions

Dosing

Adult Note: Dosing is based on salicylate content. Individualize dose based on response; may require 2 to 3 weeks to achieve optimal effect.

Acute painful shoulder, osteoarthritis, rheumatoid arthritis, or other severe arthritis: Oral: Initial: 1500 mg twice daily or 3000 mg once daily at bedtime

Analgesia (mild to moderate pain) or pyrexia: Oral: 2000 mg to 3000 mg daily in 2 or 3 divided doses; adjust dose to obtain optimal therapeutic response.

Geriatric Usual dose: 750 mg 3 times daily; adjust dose to obtain optimum therapeutic response.

Pediatric Note: Dosing is based on salicylate content. Individualize dose based on response; may require 2 to 3 weeks to achieve optimal effect.

Juvenile rheumatoid arthritis: Oral:
Children and Adolescents ≤37 kg: 50 mg/kg daily in 2 divided doses
Children and Adolescents >37 kg: 2250 mg daily in 2 divided doses

Renal Impairment There are no dosage adjustments provided in the manufacturer's labeling; use with caution in acute or chronic renal impairment. Avoid use in severe renal impairment; monitor salicylate levels and adjust dose accordingly.

Hepatic Impairment There are no dosage adjustments provided in the manufacturer's labeling; use with caution in acute or chronic hepatic impairment; monitor salicylate levels and adjust dose accordingly.

Additional Information Complete prescribing information should be consulted for additional detail.

Dosage Forms Excipient information presented when available (limited, particularly for generics); consult specific product labeling.

Liquid, Oral:
Generic: 500 mg/5 mL (240 mL)
Tablet, Oral:
Generic: 1000 mg

◆ **Chondroitin Sulfate and Sodium Hyaluronate** see Sodium Chondroitin Sulfate and Sodium Hyaluronate on page 1673

◆ **Choriogonadotropin Alfa** see Chorionic Gonadotropin (Recombinant) on page 382

◆ **Chorionic Gonadotropin for Injection (Can)** see Chorionic Gonadotropin (Human) on page 382

Chorionic Gonadotropin (Human)
(kor ee ON ik goe NAD oh troe pin, HYU man)

Brand Names: US Novarel; Pregnyl
Brand Names: Canada Chorionic Gonadotropin for Injection; Pregnyl
Index Terms CG; hCG
Pharmacologic Category Gonadotropin; Ovulation Stimulator
Use

Hypogonadotrophic hypogonadism: Treatment of hypogonadism secondary to a pituitary deficiency in males.

Ovulation induction: Induction of ovulation and pregnancy in the anovulatory, infertile woman in whom the cause of anovulation is secondary and not caused by primary ovarian failure, and who has been appropriately pretreated with human menotropins.

Prepubertal cryptorchidism: Treatment of prepubertal cryptorchidism not caused by anatomic obstruction.

Dosing

Adult & Geriatric

Ovulation induction: Females: IM: 5000 to 10,000 units 1 day following last dose of menotropins

Hypogonadotropic hypogonadism: Males: IM:
US labeling: Various regimens:
500 to 1,000 units 3 times/week for 3 weeks, followed by the same dose twice weekly for 3 weeks **or**
4,000 units 3 times/week for 6 to 9 months, then reduce dosage to 2000 units 3 times/week for additional 3 months
Canadian labeling: 4,000 to 5,000 units 3 times/week for 6 to 8 weeks with a rest of period of 2 to 3 weeks between courses of therapy

Spermatogenesis induction associated with hypogonadotropic hypogonadism (off-label use): IM: Males: 1,000 to 2,000 units 2 to 3 times/week. Administer hCG until serum testosterone levels are normal (may require 2 to 3 months of therapy), then may add menopausal gonadotropin of FSH if needed to induce spermatogenesis; continue hCG at the dose required to maintain testosterone levels (AACE 2002).

Pediatric

Prepubertal cryptorchidism: Children ≥4 years and Adolescents (males): IM:
US labeling: **Note:** Therapy is usually instituted between the ages of 4 and 9:
4,000 units 3 times/week for 3 weeks **or**
5,000 units every second day for 4 injections **or**
500 units 3 times/week for 4 to 6 weeks **or**
15 injections of 500 to 1,000 units administered over 6 weeks
Canadian labeling: **Note:** Therapy is instituted at various ages ranging from early childhood to immediately before expected puberty (appropriate age: 12 years):
4,000 units 3 times/week for 2 to 3 weeks **or**
1,000 units 3 times/week for 6 to 8 weeks

Renal Impairment There are no dosage adjustments provided in the manufacturer's labeling; use with caution.

Hepatic Impairment There are no dosage adjustments provided in the manufacturer's labeling.

Additional Information Complete prescribing information should be consulted for additional detail.

Dosage Forms Excipient information presented when available (limited, particularly for generics); consult specific product labeling.

Solution Reconstituted, Intramuscular:
Novarel: 10,000 units (1 ea) [contains benzyl alcohol]
Pregnyl: 10,000 units (1 ea) [contains benzyl alcohol, sodium chloride]
Generic: 10,000 units (1 ea)

Chorionic Gonadotropin (Recombinant)
(kor ee ON ik goe NAD oh troe pin ree KOM be nant)

Brand Names: US Ovidrel

Brand Names: Canada Ovidrel®

Index Terms Choriogonadotropin Alfa; r-hCG

Pharmacologic Category Gonadotropin; Ovulation Stimulator

Use As part of an assisted reproductive technology (ART) program, induces ovulation in infertile females who have been pretreated with follicle stimulating hormones (FSH); induces ovulation and pregnancy in infertile females when the cause of infertility is functional

Dosing

Adult Assisted reproductive technologies (ART) and ovulation induction in females: SubQ: 250 mcg given 1 day following the last dose of follicle stimulating agent. Use only after adequate follicular development has been determined. Hold treatment when there is an excessive ovarian response.

Geriatric Safety and efficacy have not been established.

Renal Impairment Safety and efficacy have not been established.

Hepatic Impairment Safety and efficacy have not been established.

Additional Information Complete prescribing information should be consulted for additional detail.

Dosage Forms Excipient information presented when available (limited, particularly for generics); consult specific product labeling.

Injectable, Subcutaneous:

Ovidrel: 250 mcg/0.5 mL (0.5 mL)

◆ CI-1008 *see* Pregabalin *on page 1500*

◆ Cialis *see* Tadalafil *on page 1730*

Ciclesonide (Systemic) (sye KLES oh nide)

Brand Names: US Alvesco

Brand Names: Canada Alvesco

Pharmacologic Category Corticosteroid, Inhalant (Oral)

Use

Bronchial asthma: Prophylactic management of bronchial asthma

Guideline recommendations: A low-dose inhaled corticosteroid *(in addition to an as-needed short acting beta₂-agonist)* is the initial preferred long term control medication for children, adolescents, and adult patients with persistent asthma who are candidates for treatment according to a step-wise treatment approach (GINA 2015; NAEPP 2007).

Dosing

Adult & Geriatric Asthma: Oral inhalation (Alvesco): **Note:** Titrate to the lowest effective dose once asthma stability is achieved:

US labeling:

Prior therapy with bronchodilators alone: Initial: 80 mcg twice daily (maximum dose: 320 mcg/day)

Prior therapy with inhaled corticosteroids: Initial: 80 mcg twice daily (maximum dose: 640 mcg/day)

Prior therapy with oral corticosteroids: Initial: 320 mcg twice daily (maximum dose: 640 mcg/day)

Canadian labeling: Initial: 400 mcg once daily; maintenance: 100-800 mcg/day (1-2 puffs once daily; more severe asthma may require 400 mcg twice daily). **Note:** Canadian Thoracic Society 2010 Asthma Management guidelines recommendation: Doses >200 mcg/day may provide minimal additional benefit while increasing risks for adverse events; add-on therapy should be considered prior to dose increases >200 mcg/day (Lougheed 2010).

Asthma guidelines: Global Initiative for Asthma guidelines (GINA 2015): HFA inhaler (refers to Alvesco 80 mcg and 160 mcg strengths available in the US):

"Low" dose: 80 to 160 mcg daily

"Medium" dose: >160 to 320 mcg daily

"High" dose: >320 mcg daily

Conversion: *Conversion from oral to orally-inhaled steroid:* Initiation of oral inhalation therapy should begin in patients who have previously been stabilized on oral corticosteroids (OCS). A gradual dose reduction of OCS should begin ~7-10 days after starting inhaled therapy. U.S. labeling recommends reducing prednisone dose no more rapidly than ≤2.5 mg/day on a weekly basis. The Canadian labeling recommends decreasing the daily dose of prednisone by 1 mg (or equivalent of other OCS) every 7 days in closely monitored patients, and every 10 days in patients whom close monitoring is not possible. In the presence of withdrawal symptoms, resume previous OCS dose for 1 week before attempting further dose reductions.

Pediatric Asthma: Oral inhalation (Alvesco): **Note:** Titrate to the lowest effective dose once asthma stability is achieved:

US labeling: Children ≥12 years and Adolescents: Refer to adult dosing.

Canadian labeling:

Children 6 to 11 years: Initial: 100-200 mcg once daily; maintenance: 100-200 mcg/day (1-2 puffs once daily). **Note:** Canadian Thoracic Society 2010 Asthma Management guidelines recommend dose titration in children 6-11 years who fail to achieve an adequate response in spite of adherence to therapy and/or lack of alternative factors (eg, environmental triggers) which might impair response (Lougheed 2010).

Children ≥12 years and Adolescents: Refer to adult dosing.

Asthma guidelines: Global Initiative for Asthma guidelines (GINA 2015): HFA inhaler (refers to Alvesco 80 mcg and 160 mcg strengths available in the US):

Children ≤5 years: "Low" dose: 160 mcg daily

Children 6 to 11 years:

"Low" dose: 80 mcg daily

"Medium" dose: >80 to 160 mcg daily

"High" dose: >160 mcg daily

Children ≥12 years and Adolescents: Refer to adult dosing.

Renal Impairment There are no dosage adjustments provided in the manufacturer labeling (has not been studied); however, dose adjustments may not be necessary as ≤20% of drug is eliminated renally.

Hepatic Impairment Dosage adjustments are not necessary.

Additional Information Complete prescribing information should be consulted for additional detail.

Dosage Forms Considerations Alvesco 6.1 g canisters contain 60 inhalations.

Dosage Forms Excipient information presented when available (limited, particularly for generics); consult specific product labeling.

Aerosol Solution, Inhalation:

Alvesco: 80 mcg/actuation (6.1 g); 160 mcg/actuation (6.1 g)

Dosage Forms: Canada Excipient information presented when available (limited, particularly for generics); consult specific product labeling.

Aerosol for oral inhalation:

Alvesco: 100 mcg/inhalation [30-, 60-, and 120 metered actuations]; 200 mcg/inhalation [30-, 60-, and 120 metered actuations]

Ciclesonide (Nasal) (sye KLES oh nide)

Brand Names: US Omnaris; Zetonna

Brand Names: Canada Drymira; Omnaris; Omnaris HFA

Pharmacologic Category Corticosteroid, Nasal

Use Management of seasonal and perennial allergic rhinitis

Dosing

Adult & Geriatric Perennial allergic rhinitis, seasonal allergic rhinitis:

Omnaris®: 2 sprays (50 mcg/spray) per nostril once daily; maximum: 200 mcg/day

Zetonna™: 1 spray (37 mcg/spray) per nostril once daily; maximum: 74 mcg/day

Pediatric

Perennial allergic rhinitis: Children ≥12 years: Refer to adult dosing:

Seasonal allergic rhinitis:

U.S. labeling: Children ≥6 year: Refer to adult dosing.

Canadian labeling: Children ≥12 years: Refer to adult dosing.

Renal Impairment No dosage adjustment provided in manufacturer's labeling (has not been studied).

Hepatic Impairment No dosage adjustment necessary.

Additional Information Complete prescribing information should be consulted for additional detail.

Dosage Forms Considerations

Omnaris 12.5 g bottles contain 120 actuations.

Zetonna 6.1 g canisters contain 60 actuations.

Dosage Forms Excipient information presented when available (limited, particularly for generics); consult specific product labeling.

Aerosol Solution, Nasal:

Zetonna: 37 mcg/actuation (6.1 g)

Suspension, Nasal:

Omnaris: 50 mcg/actuation (12.5 g) [contains edetate sodium (tetrasodium)]

◆ Ciclodan *see* Ciclopirox *on page 384*

◆ Ciclodan Cream *see* Ciclopirox *on page 384*

◆ Ciclodan Solution *see* Ciclopirox *on page 384*

Ciclopirox (sye kloe PEER oks)

Brand Names: US Ciclodan; Ciclodan Cream; Ciclodan Solution; Ciclopirox Treatment; CNL8 Nail; Loprox; Pedipirox-4 Nail [DSC]; Penlac

Brand Names: Canada Apo-Ciclopirox; Loprox; Penlac; PMS-Ciclopirox; Stieprox; Taro-Ciclopirox

Index Terms Ciclopirox Olamine

Pharmacologic Category Antifungal Agent, Topical

Use

Cream/suspension: Treatment of tinea pedis (athlete's foot), tinea cruris (jock itch), tinea corporis (ringworm), cutaneous candidiasis, and tinea versicolor (pityriasis)

Gel: Treatment of tinea pedis (athlete's foot), tinea corporis (ringworm); seborrheic dermatitis of the scalp

Lacquer (solution): Topical treatment of mild-to-moderate onychomycosis of the fingernails and toenails due to *Trichophyton rubrum* (not involving the lunula) and the immediately-adjacent skin

Shampoo: Treatment of seborrheic dermatitis of the scalp

Dosing

Adult & Geriatric

Tinea pedis, tinea corporis: Topical:

Cream and suspension: Apply twice daily, gently massage into affected areas; if no improvement after 4 weeks of treatment, re-evaluate the diagnosis.

Gel: Apply twice daily, gently massage into affected areas and surrounding skin; if no improvement after 4 weeks of treatment, re-evaluate diagnosis

Tinea cruris, cutaneous candidiasis, and tinea versicolor: Topical: *Cream and suspension:* Apply twice daily, gently massage into affected areas; if no improvement after 4 weeks of treatment, re-evaluate the diagnosis.

Onychomycosis of the fingernails and toenails: Topical: *Lacquer (solution):* Apply to adjacent skin and affected nails daily (as a part of a comprehensive management program for onychomycosis). Remove with alcohol every 7 days.

Seborrheic dermatitis of the scalp: Topical:

Gel: Apply twice daily, gently massage into affected areas and surrounding skin; if no improvement after 4 weeks of treatment, re-evaluate diagnosis.

Shampoo: Apply ~5 mL to wet hair; lather, and leave in place ~3 minutes; rinse. May use up to 10 mL for longer hair. Repeat twice weekly for 4 weeks; allow a minimum of 3 days between applications; if no improvement after 4 weeks of treatment, re-evaluate diagnosis.

Pediatric

Tinea pedis, tinea corporis: Topical:

Cream and suspension: Children >10 years: Refer to adult dosing.

Gel: Children >16 years: Refer to adult dosing.

Tinea cruris, cutaneous candidiasis, and tinea versicolor: Topical: *Cream and suspension:* Children >10 years: Refer to adult dosing.

Onychomycosis of the fingernails and toenails: Topical: *Lacquer (solution):* Children ≥12 years: Refer to adult dosing.

Seborrheic dermatitis of the scalp: Topical: *Gel and shampoo:* Children >16 years: Refer to adult dosing.

Renal Impairment No dosage adjustment provided in manufacturer's labeling.

Hepatic Impairment No dosage adjustment provided in manufacturer's labeling.

Additional Information Complete prescribing information should be consulted for additional detail.

Dosage Forms Excipient information presented when available (limited, particularly for generics); consult specific product labeling. [DSC] = Discontinued product

Cream, External, as olamine:

Ciclodan: 0.77% (90 g) [contains benzyl alcohol, cetyl alcohol]

Generic: 0.77% (15 g, 30 g, 90 g)

Gel, External:

Loprox: 0.77% (30 g [DSC], 45 g [DSC], 100 g [DSC]) [contains isopropyl alcohol]

Generic: 0.77% (30 g, 45 g, 100 g)

Kit, External:

Ciclodan Cream: 0.77% [contains benzyl alcohol, cetyl alcohol, edetate disodium, propylene glycol]

Ciclodan Solution: 8% [contains edetate disodium, isopropyl alcohol, menthol]

Ciclopirox Treatment: 8% [contains edetate disodium, isopropyl alcohol, menthol]

CNL8 Nail: 8% [contains isopropyl alcohol]

Pedipirox-4 Nail: 8% [DSC] [contains isopropyl alcohol]

Generic: 8%

Shampoo, External:

Loprox: 1% (120 mL)

Generic: 1% (120 mL)

Solution, External:

Ciclodan: 8% (6.6 mL) [contains isopropyl alcohol]

Penlac: 8% (6.6 mL) [contains ethyl acetate, isopropyl alcohol]

Generic: 8% (6.6 mL)

Suspension, External, as olamine:

Generic: 0.77% (30 mL, 60 mL)

◆ **Ciclopirox Olamine** see Ciclopirox on page 384
◆ **Ciclopirox Treatment** see Ciclopirox on page 384
◆ **Ciclosporin** see CycloSPORINE (Ophthalmic) on page 465
◆ **Ciclosporin** see CycloSPORINE (Systemic) on page 459
◆ **CidalEaze** see Lidocaine (Topical) on page 1074
◆ **Cidecin** see DAPTOmycin on page 490

Cidofovir (si DOF o veer)

Brand Names: US Vistide

Pharmacologic Category Antiviral Agent

Use

Cytomegalovirus retinitis: Treatment of cytomegalovirus (CMV) retinitis in patients with AIDS.

Limitations of use: Safety and efficacy have not been established for treatment of other CMV infections (eg, pneumonitis, gastroenteritis), congenital or neonatal CMV disease, or CMV disease in non-HIV infected individuals.

Pregnancy Considerations

[US Boxed Warning]: Possibly carcinogenic and teratogenic based on animal data. May cause hypospermia. Women of childbearing potential should use effective contraception during therapy and for 1 month following treatment. Males should use a barrier contraceptive during therapy and for 3 months following treatment.

The indications for treating CMV retinitis during pregnancy are the same as in nonpregnant HIV infected woman; however systemic therapy should be avoided during the first trimester when possible. When therapy is needed to treat maternal infection, agents other than cidofovir are recommended (DHHS [Adult OI 2014]).

Breast-Feeding Considerations It is not known if cidofovir is excreted in breast milk. Due to the potential for serious adverse reactions in the nursing infant, breast-feeding is not recommended. In addition, HIV-infected mothers are discouraged from breast-feeding to decrease the potential transmission of HIV.

Contraindications Hypersensitivity to cidofovir or any component of the formulation; history of clinically-severe hypersensitivity to probenecid or other sulfa-containing medications; serum creatinine >1.5 mg/dL; CrCl ≤55 mL/minute; urine protein ≥100 mg/dL (≥2+ proteinuria); use with or within 7 days of nephrotoxic agents; direct intraocular injection.

Warnings/Precautions Hazardous agent - use appropriate precautions for handling and disposal (NIOSH 2014 [group 2]).

[US Boxed Warning]: Acute renal failure resulting in dialysis and/or contributing to death has occurred with as few as 1 or 2 doses of cidofovir. Renal function (serum creatinine and urine protein) must be monitored within 48 hours prior to each dose of cidofovir and the dose of cidofovir modified as appropriate. Administration must be accompanied by oral probenecid and intravenous saline prehydration. Contraindicated in patients with a baseline serum creatinine >1.5 mg/dL, CrCl ≤55 mL/minute, or urine protein ≥100 mg/dL (≥2+ proteinuria); dosage adjustment or discontinuation of therapy may be required for changes in renal function during treatment. **[US Boxed Warning]: Neutropenia has been reported; monitor neutrophil counts during therapy.** Monitor for signs of metabolic acidosis; decreased sodium bicarbonate with proximal tubule injury and renal wasting syndrome (including Fanconi syndrome), as well as metabolic acidosis with hepatic impairment and pancreatitis (including some fatal cases) have been reported. **[US Boxed Warning]: Possibly carcinogenic and teratogenic based on animal data. May cause hypospermia. [US Boxed Warning]: Indicated only for CMV retinitis treatment in patients with AIDS.** For intravenous use only, **not** for direct intraocular injection; iritis, ocular hypotony, and permanent impairment of vision may occur. Decreased intraocular pressure, sometimes associated with decreased visual acuity, uveitis, or iritis may occur; monitor intraocular pressure for and

signs of iritis/uveitis during therapy. If uveitis or iritis occurs, consider treatment with topical corticosteroids with or without topical cycloplegic agents.

Adverse Reactions

>10%:

Central nervous system: Chills, fever, headache, pain

Dermatologic: Alopecia, rash

Gastrointestinal: Nausea, vomiting, diarrhea, anorexia

Hematologic: Anemia, neutropenia

Neuromuscular & skeletal: Weakness

Ocular: Intraocular pressure decreased, iritis, ocular hypotony, uveitis

Renal: Creatinine increased, proteinuria, renal toxicity

Respiratory: Cough, dyspnea

Miscellaneous: Infection, oral moniliasis, serum bicarbonate decreased

1% to 10%:

Renal: Fanconi syndrome

Respiratory: Pneumonia

<1%: Hepatic failure, metabolic acidosis, pancreatitis

Frequency not defined (limited to important or life-threatening reactions):

Cardiovascular: Cardiomyopathy, cardiovascular disorder, CHF, edema, orthostatic hypotension, shock, syncope, tachycardia

Central nervous system: Agitation, amnesia, anxiety, confusion, convulsion, dizziness, hallucinations, insomnia, malaise, vertigo

Dermatologic: Photosensitivity reaction, skin discoloration, urticaria

Endocrine & metabolic: Adrenal cortex insufficiency

Gastrointestinal: Abdominal pain, aphthous stomatitis, colitis, constipation, dysphagia, fecal incontinence, gastritis, GI hemorrhage, gingivitis, melena, proctitis, splenomegaly, stomatitis, tongue discoloration

Genitourinary: Urinary incontinence

Hematologic: Hypochromic anemia, leukocytosis, leukopenia, lymphadenopathy, lymphoma-like reaction, pancytopenia, thrombocytopenia, thrombocytopenic purpura

Hepatic: Hepatomegaly, hepatosplenomegaly, jaundice, liver function tests abnormal, liver damage, liver necrosis

Local: Injection site reaction

Neuromuscular & skeletal: Tremor

Ocular: Amblyopia, blindness, cataract, conjunctivitis, corneal lesion, diplopia, vision abnormal

Otic: Hearing loss

Miscellaneous: Allergic reaction, sepsis

Drug Interactions

Metabolism/Transport Effects None known.

Avoid Concomitant Use There are no known interactions where it is recommended to avoid concomitant use.

Increased Effect/Toxicity

Cidofovir may increase the levels/effects of: Tenofovir Products

The levels/effects of Cidofovir may be increased by: Tenofovir Products

Decreased Effect There are no known significant interactions involving a decrease in effect.

Preparation for Administration Hazardous agent; use appropriate precautions for handling and disposal (NIOSH 2014 [group 2]).

Dilute dose in NS 100 mL prior to infusion.

Storage/Stability Store intact vials at 20°C to 25°C (68°F to 77°F). Admixtures may be stored for ≤24 hours under refrigeration; however, admixtures must be administered within 24 hours of preparation.

Mechanism of Action Cidofovir is converted to cidofovir diphosphate (the active intracellular metabolite); cidofovir diphosphate suppresses CMV replication by selective inhibition of viral DNA synthesis. Incorporation of cidofovir diphosphate into growing viral DNA chain results in viral DNA synthesis rate reduction.

Pharmacodynamics/Kinetics The following pharmacokinetic data are based on a combination of cidofovir administered with probenecid:

Distribution: V_d: 0.41 L/kg; does not cross significantly into CSF

Protein binding: <6%

Metabolism: Minimal; phosphorylation occurs intracellularly to the active metabolite cidofovir diphosphate

Half-life elimination, plasma: ~2.6 hours; intracellular elimination half-lives of metabolites are longer (range: 24 to 87 hours) (Lea 1996)

Excretion: Urine (70% to 85% as unchanged drug)

Clearance:

Renal clearance without probenecid: 150 ± 26.9 mL/minute/1.73 m²

Renal clearance with probenecid: 98.6 ± 27.9 mL/minute/1.73 m²

Dosing

Adult & Geriatric CMV retinitis: IV:

Induction treatment: 5 mg/kg/dose with concomitant probenecid once weekly for 2 consecutive weeks

Maintenance treatment: 5 mg/kg/dose with concomitant probenecid once every 2 weeks

Concomitant therapy:

Probenecid: 2 g 3 hours prior to cidofovir dose, then 1 g at 2 hours and 8 hours after completion of the infusion

Hydration: Patients should also receive 1 L of NS intravenously infused over 1 to 2 hours immediately prior to each cidofovir infusion. If tolerated, a second liter may be administered over 1 to 3 hours at the start of cidofovir infusion or immediately following infusion.

Renal Impairment

Preexisting renal impairment: Serum creatinine >1.5 mg/dL, CrCl ≤55 mL/minute, or urine protein ≥100 mg/dL (≥2+ proteinuria): Use is contraindicated.

Changes in renal function during therapy:

Serum creatinine increases by 0.3 to 0.4 mg/dL: Reduce dose to 3 mg/kg.

Serum creatinine increases ≥0.5 mg/dL or development of ≥3+ proteinuria: Discontinue therapy.

Hepatic Impairment There are no dosage adjustments provided in the manufacturer's labeling.

Administration For IV infusion only. Infuse over 1 hour. Administer with concomitant probenecid. Hydrate with 1 L of NS IV over 1 to 2 hours immediately prior to cidofovir infusion. If tolerated, a second liter may be administered over a 1- to 3-hour period at the start of or immediately following cidofovir infusion.

Hazardous agent; use appropriate precautions for handling and disposal (NIOSH 2014 [group 2]).

Monitoring Parameters Serum creatinine and urine protein (at baseline and within 48 hours of each dose), WBC with differential (prior to each dose); intraocular pressure and visual acuity, signs and symptoms of uveitis/iritis; metabolic acidosis.

Dosage Forms Excipient information presented when available (limited, particularly for generics); consult specific product labeling.

Solution, Intravenous:

Vistide: 75 mg/mL (5 mL)

Solution, Intravenous [preservative free]:

Generic: 75 mg/mL (5 mL)

◆ Cilastatin and Imipenem *see* Imipenem and Cilastatin *on page 923*

Cilostazol (sil OH sta zol)

Brand Names: US Pletal

Index Terms OPC-13013

Pharmacologic Category Antiplatelet Agent; Phosphodiesterase-3 Enzyme Inhibitor; Vasodilator

Additional Appendix Information

Oral Antiplatelet Comparison Chart *on page 1963*

Use Intermittent claudication: Reduction of symptoms of intermittent claudication, as indicated by an increased walking distance.

Pregnancy Considerations Adverse events have been observed in animal reproduction studies.

Breast-Feeding Considerations It is not known if cilostazol is excreted in human milk. Due to the potential for serious adverse reactions in the nursing infant, the manufacturer recommends a decision be made whether to discontinue nursing or to discontinue the drug, taking into account the importance of treatment to the mother.

Contraindications Hypersensitivity to cilostazol or any component of the formulation; heart failure of any severity

Warnings/Precautions [US Boxed Warning]: The use of this drug is contraindicated in patients with heart failure. Phosphodiesterase inhibitors have decreased survival rates in patients with class III-IV heart failure. Patients with history of ischemic heart disease may be at increased risk for exacerbation of angina pectoris or myocardial infarction. May induce tachycardia, palpitation, tachyarrhythmia, and/or hypotension. Cases of thrombocytopenia or leukopenia progressing to agranulocytosis, reversible upon discontinuation, have been reported when not immediately discontinued; monitor platelets and white blood cell counts periodically. Time required to recover adequate platelet function is ~2 days (Hill, 2011). Of note, bleeding times were not significantly altered by cilostazol after 3 to 14 days of treatment (Kim, 2004; Wilhite, 2003). Use caution in moderate to severe hepatic impairment (has not been studied). Use cautiously in severe renal impairment (CrCl <25 mL/minute). Potentially significant drug-drug interactions may exist, requiring dose or frequency adjustment, additional monitoring, and/or selection of alternative therapy. Cilostazol has not been studied in

patients with active pathological bleeding or hemostatic disorders; avoid use in these patients.

Adverse Reactions

>10%:
Central nervous system: Headache (27% to 34%)
Gastrointestinal: Diarrhea (12% to 19%), abnormal stools (12% to 15%)
Infection: Infection (10% to 14%)
Respiratory: Rhinitis (7% to 12%)

1% to 10%:
Cardiovascular: Palpitations (5% to 10%), peripheral edema (7% to 9%), tachycardia (4%), atrial fibrillation (<2%), atrial flutter (<2%), cardiac arrest (<2%), cardiac failure (<2%), cerebral infarction (<2%), edema (<2%), hypotension (<2%), myocardial infarction (<2%), nodal arrhythmia (<2%), orthostatic hypotension (<2%), supraventricular tachycardia (<2%), syncope (<2%), varicose veins (<2%), ventricular premature contractions (<2%), ventricular tachycardia (<2%)
Central nervous system: Dizziness (9% to 10%), vertigo (3%), chills (<2%), insomnia (<2%), malaise (<2%), neuralgia (<2%)
Dermatologic: Ecchymoses (<2%), skin hypertrophy (<2%), urticarial (<2%), xeroderma (<2%)
Endocrine & metabolic: Albuminuria (<2%), gout (<2%), hyperlipidemia (<2%), hyperuricemia (<2%), increased gamma-glutamyl transferase (<2%)
Gastrointestinal: Nausea (7%), dyspepsia (6%), abdominal pain (4% to 5%), flatulence (3%), anorexia (<2%), cholelithiasis (<2%), colitis (<2%), duodenal ulcer (<2%), duodenitis (<2%), esophageal hemorrhage (<2%), esophagitis (<2%), gastritis (<2%), gastroenteritis (<2%), gingival hemorrhage (<2%), hematemesis (<2%), melena (<2%), peptic ulcer (<2%), periodontal abscess (<2%)
Genitourinary: Cystitis (<2%), urinary frequency (<2%), vaginal hemorrhage (<2%), vaginitis (<2%)
Hematologic & oncologic: Anemia (<2%), hemorrhage (<2%), hemorrhage (eye, <2%), iron deficiency anemia (<2%), polycythemia (<2%), purpura (<2%), rectal hemorrhage (<2%), retroperitoneal hemorrhage (<2%)
Hypersensitivity: Tongue edema (<2%)
Neuromuscular & skeletal: Back pain (7%), myalgia (3%), arthralgia (<2%), bursitis (<2%), neck stiffness (<2%), osteaglgia (<2%)
Ophthalmic: Blindness (<2%), conjunctivitis (<2%), diplopia (<2%), retinal hemorrhage (<2%)
Otic: Otalgia (<2%), tinnitus (<2%)
Renal: Increased serum creatinine (<2%)
Respiratory: Pharyngitis (10%), cough (3% to 4%), asthma (<2%), epistaxis (<2%), hemoptysis (<2%), pneumonia (<2%), sinusitis (<2%)
Miscellaneous: Fever (<2%)
<2% (Limited to important or life-threatening): Agranulocytosis, anaphylaxis, aplastic anemia, cerebral hemorrhage, cerebrovascular accident, coronary thrombosis (stent), gastrointestinal hemorrhage, granulocytopenia, hematoma (extradural), hepatic insufficiency, hyperglycemia, hypersensitivity, hypertension, interstitial pneumonitis, intracranial hemorrhage, jaundice, leukopenia, prolonged Q-T interval on ECG, pancytopenia, pulmonary hemorrhage, Stevens-Johnson syndrome, subcutaneous hemorrhage, subdural hematoma, thrombocytopenia, thrombosis, torsades de pointes

Drug Interactions

Metabolism/Transport Effects Substrate of CYP1A2 (minor), CYP2C19 (major), CYP2D6 (minor), CYP3A4 (major); **Note:** Assignment of Major/Minor substrate status based on clinically relevant drug interaction potential; **Inhibits** CYP3A4 (weak)

Avoid Concomitant Use
Avoid concomitant use of Cilostazol with any of the following: Conivaptan; Fusidic Acid (Systemic); Idelalisib; Pimozide; Urokinase

Increased Effect/Toxicity
Cilostazol may increase the levels/effects of: Agents with Antiplatelet Properties; Anticoagulants; Apixaban; ARIPiprazole; Collagenase (Systemic); Dabigatran Etexilate; Deoxycholic Acid; Dofetilide; Edoxaban; Flibanserin; Hydrocodone; Ibritumomab; Lomitapide; NiMODipine; Obinutuzumab; Pimozide; Riociguat; Rivaroxaban; Salicylates; Thrombolytic Agents; Tositumomab and Iodine I 131 Tositumomab; Urokinase

The levels/effects of Cilostazol may be increased by: Anagrelide; Conivaptan; CYP2C19 Inhibitors; CYP3A4 Inhibitors (Moderate); CYP3A4 Inhibitors (Strong); Dasatinib; Fosaprepitant; Fusidic Acid (Systemic); Glucosamine; Herbs (Anticoagulant/Antiplatelet Properties); Ibrutinib; Idelalisib; Ivacaftor; Limaprost; Luliconazole; Mifepristone; Multivitamins/Fluoride (with ADE); Multivitamins/Minerals (with ADEK, Folate, Iron); Multivitamins/Minerals (with AE, No Iron); Omega-3 Fatty Acids; Osimertinib; Palbociclib; Pentosan Polysulfate Sodium; Pentoxifylline; Prostacyclin Analogues; Simeprevir; Stiripentol; Tipranavir; Vitamin E; Vitamin E (Oral)

Decreased Effect
The levels/effects of Cilostazol may be decreased by: Bosentan; CYP3A4 Inducers (Moderate); CYP3A4 Inducers (Strong); Dabrafenib; Deferasirox; Enzalutamide; Mitotane; Osimertinib; Siltuximab; St Johns Wort; Tocilizumab

Food Interactions Taking cilostazol with a high-fat meal may increase peak concentration by 90% and increase AUC by 25%. Grapefruit juice may increase serum levels of cilostazol and enhance toxic effects. Management: Administer cilostazol on an empty stomach 30 minutes before or 2 hours after meals. Avoid concurrent ingestion of grapefruit juice.

Storage/Stability Store at 25°C (77°F); excursions are permitted between 15°C and 30°C (59°F and 86°F).

Mechanism of Action Cilostazol and its metabolites are inhibitors of phosphodiesterase III. As a result, cyclic AMP is increased leading to reversible inhibition of platelet aggregation, vasodilation, and inhibition of vascular smooth muscle cell proliferation.

Pharmacodynamics/Kinetics

Onset of action: Effect on walking distance: 2 to 4 weeks; may require up to 12 weeks
Protein binding: Cilostazol 95% to 98%; active metabolites: 66% to 97%
Metabolism: Hepatic; CYP1A2 (minor), CYP2C19 (major), CYP2D6 (minor), CYP3A4 (major).
Half-life elimination: ~11 to 13 hours
Excretion: Urine (74%) and feces (20%) as metabolites

Dosing

Adult & Geriatric

Intermittent claudication: Oral: 100 mg twice daily. The American College of Chest Physicians recommends use when refractory to exercise therapy and smoking cessation; use in combination with either aspirin or clopidogrel (ACCP [Guyatt, 2012]). **Note:** Discontinue treatment if symptoms are not improved after 3 months of therapy

PCI (following elective stent placement) (off-label use): Oral: 100 mg twice daily in combination with aspirin or clopidogrel. **Note:** Only recommended in patients with an allergy or intolerance to either aspirin or clopidogrel (ACCP [Guyatt, 2012]).

Secondary prevention of noncardioembolic stroke or TIA (off-label use): Oral: 100 mg twice daily. **Note:** Clopidogrel or aspirin/extended release dipyridamole recommended over the use of cilostazol (ACCP [Guyatt, 2012]).

Dosage adjustment with concomitant medications:
CYP2C19 inhibitors (eg, fluconazole, omeprazole, ticlopidine): Reduce cilostazol to 50 mg twice daily
Strong or moderate CYP3A4 inhibitors (eg, diltiazem, erythromycin, itraconazole, ketoconazole): Reduce cilostazol to 50 mg twice daily

Renal Impairment
CrCl ≥25 mL/minute: No dosage adjustment necessary (Mallikaarjun, 1999).
CrCl <25 mL/minute: No dosage adjustment necessary (Mallikaarjun, 1999). Severe renal impairment increases metabolite concentrations; use with caution.
End-stage renal disease (ESRD) on dialysis: There are no dosage adjustments provided in the manufacturer's labeling (has not been studied); however, high protein binding makes removal by dialysis unlikely.

Hepatic Impairment
Mild impairment: No dosage adjustment necessary (Bramer, 1999).
Moderate to severe impairment: There are no dosage adjustments provided in the manufacturer's labeling (has not been studied); use with caution.

Administration Oral: Administer 30 minutes before or 2 hours after meals (breakfast and dinner).

Monitoring Parameters Platelets and WBC counts periodically

Dosage Forms Excipient information presented when available (limited, particularly for generics); consult specific product labeling.
Tablet, Oral:
Pletal: 50 mg, 100 mg
Generic: 50 mg, 100 mg

◆ Ciloxan see Ciprofloxacin (Ophthalmic) on page 393

Cimetidine (sye MET i deen)

Brand Names: US Cimetidine Acid Reducer [OTC]; Heartburn Relief [OTC] [DSC]; Tagamet HB [OTC]

Brand Names: Canada Apo-Cimetidine; Dom-Cimetidine; Mylan-Cimetidine; Novo-Cimetidine; Nu-Cimet; PMS-Cimetidine

Pharmacologic Category Histamine H₂ Antagonist

Use

Duodenal ulcer: Short-term treatment of active duodenal ulcer and maintenance therapy after the healing of active ulcer.

Gastric ulcer: Short-term treatment of active, benign gastric ulcer.

Gastroesophageal reflux disease: Treatment of erosive gastroesophageal reflux disease (GERD).

Pathological hypersecretory conditions: Treatment of pathological hypersecretory conditions (eg, Zollinger-Ellison syndrome, systemic mastocytosis, multiple endocrine adenomas).

Heartburn (OTC only): Relief and prevention of heartburn associated with acid indigestion and sour stomach.

Dosing

Adult & Geriatric

Duodenal ulcer, active: Oral: 300 mg 4 times daily or 800 mg at bedtime or 400 mg twice daily for up to 8 weeks

Note: Higher doses of 1600 mg at bedtime for 4 weeks may be beneficial for a subpopulation of patients with larger duodenal ulcers (>1 cm defined endoscopically) who are also heavy smokers (≥1 pack/day).

Duodenal ulcer, prophylaxis: 400 mg at bedtime

Gastric ulcer, active: 300 mg 4 times daily or 800 mg at bedtime for up to 8 weeks

Gastroesophageal reflux disease: 400 mg 4 times daily or 800 mg twice daily for 12 weeks

Pathological hypersecretory conditions: 300 mg 4 times daily; adjust dose to patient response; maximum 2.4 g/day

Interstitial cystitis (bladder pain syndrome) (off-label use): 200 mg 3 times daily or 300 to 400 mg twice daily (Dasgupta 2001; Seshadri 1994; Thilagarajah 2001)

Peptic ulcer disease eradication of Helicobacter pylori (off-label use): 400 mg twice daily; requires combination therapy with antibiotics

Heartburn (OTC labeling):

Prevention: 200 mg daily up to 30 minutes prior to eating foods or beverages that cause heartburn (maximum: 400 mg/24 hours).

Relief of symptoms: 200 mg daily; maximum: 400 mg/24 hours.

Pediatric

Children and Adolescents <16 years: Oral: 20 to 40 mg/kg/day (limited experience)

Heartburn (prevention or relief) (OTC labeling): Children ≥12 years and Adolescents: Oral: Refer to adult dosing.

Renal Impairment

Manufacturer's labeling:

Mild to moderate renal impairment: There are no dosage adjustments provided in the manufacturer's labeling; use with caution.

Severe renal impairment: 300 mg every 12 hours; may increase frequency with caution. When hepatic impairment is also present, further reductions in dosage may be necessary.

Alternate recommendations (Aronoff 2007):

GFR >50 mL/minute: No dosage adjustment necessary.

GFR 10 to 50 mL/minute: Administer 50% of normal dose

GFR <10 mL/minute: 300 mg every 8 to 12 hours

Hemodialysis: Dose after dialysis

CCRT: Administer 50% of normal dose

Peritoneal dialysis: 300 mg every 8 to 12 hours

Hepatic Impairment There are no dosage adjustments provided in the manufacturer's labeling; use with caution. Dosage adjustments may be needed in patients with both renal and hepatic impairment.

Additional Information Complete prescribing information should be consulted for additional detail.

Dosage Forms Excipient information presented when available (limited, particularly for generics); consult specific product labeling. [DSC] = Discontinued product

Solution, Oral, as hydrochloride [strength expressed as base]:

Generic: 300 mg/5 mL (237 mL, 240 mL, 473 mL [DSC])

Tablet, Oral:

Cimetidine Acid Reducer: 200 mg

Heartburn Relief: 200 mg [DSC] [contains polysorbate 80]

Tagamet HB: 200 mg

Generic: 200 mg, 300 mg, 400 mg, 800 mg

◆ Cimetidine Acid Reducer [OTC] see Cimetidine on page 386

◆ Cimzia see Certolizumab Pegol on page 362

◆ Cimzia Prefilled see Certolizumab Pegol on page 362

◆ Cimzia Starter Kit see Certolizumab Pegol on page 362

Cinacalcet (sin a KAL cet)

Brand Names: US Sensipar

Brand Names: Canada Sensipar

Index Terms AMG 073; Cinacalcet Hydrochloride

Pharmacologic Category Calcimimetic

Use

Hyperparathyroidism, primary: Treatment of severe hypercalcemia in adult patients with primary hyperparathyroidism for whom parathyroidectomy would be indicated on the basis of serum calcium levels, but who are unable to undergo parathyroidectomy

Hyperparathyroidism, secondary: Treatment of secondary hyperparathyroidism in adult patients with chronic kidney disease (CKD) on dialysis.

Limitation of use: Not indicated for use in patients with CKD who are not on dialysis (due to the increased risk of hypocalcemia)

Parathyroid carcinoma: Treatment of hypercalcemia in adult patients with parathyroid carcinoma

Pregnancy Considerations Adverse events have been observed in animal reproduction studies. Women who become pregnant during cinacalcet treatment are encouraged to enroll in Amgen's Pregnancy Surveillance Program (1-800-772-6436).

Breast-Feeding Considerations It is not known if cinacalcet is excreted in breast milk. Due to the potential for clinically significant adverse reactions in the nursing infant, the manufacturer recommends a decision be made whether to discontinue nursing or the drug, taking into account the importance of treatment to the mother. Women who choose to continue nursing during cinacalcet treatment are encouraged to enroll in Amgen's Lactation Surveillance Program (1-800-772-6436).

Contraindications

Serum calcium lower than the lower limit of normal range

Canadian labeling: Additional contraindications (not in U.S. labeling): Hypersensitivity to any component of the formulation

Warnings/Precautions Life-threatening and fatal events associated with hypocalcemia have occurred. Use is contraindicated if the serum calcium is less than the lower limit of the normal range. Monitor serum calcium and for symptoms of hypocalcemia (eg, muscle cramps, myalgia, paresthesia, seizure, tetany); may require treatment interruption, dose reduction, or initiation (or dose increases) of calcium-based phosphate binder and/or vitamin D to raise serum calcium depending on calcium levels or symptoms of hypocalcemia. Use with caution in patients with a seizure disorder (seizure threshold is lowered by significant serum calcium reductions); monitor calcium levels closely. Adynamic bone disease may develop if intact parathyroid hormone (iPTH) levels are suppressed <100 pg/mL; reduce dose or discontinue use of cinacalcet and/or vitamin D if iPTH levels decrease below 150 pg/mL.

Use caution in patients with moderate-to-severe hepatic impairment (Child-Pugh classes B and C); monitor serum calcium, serum phosphorus and iPTH closely. In the U.S., the long-term safety and efficacy of cinacalcet has not been evaluated in chronic kidney disease (CKD) patients with hyperparathyroidism not requiring dialysis. Not indicated for CKD patients not receiving dialysis. Although possibly related to lower baseline calcium levels, clinical studies have shown an increased incidence of hypocalcemia (<8.4 mg/dL) in patients not requiring dialysis. Cases of idiosyncratic hypotension, worsening of heart failure, and/or arrhythmia have been reported in patients with impaired cardiovascular function; may correlate with decreased serum calcium. QT prolongation and ventricular arrhythmia secondary to hypocalcemia have also been reported. Potentially significant interactions may exist, requiring dose or frequency adjustment, additional monitoring, and/or selection of alternative therapy.

Adverse Reactions

>10%:

Cardiovascular: Hypotension (12%)

Central nervous system: Paresthesia (14% to 29%), headache (≤21%), fatigue (12% to 21%), depression (10% to 18%)

Endocrine & metabolic: Hypocalcemia (<8.4 mg/dL: 6% to 75%; <7.5 mg/dL: 29% to 33%), dehydration (≤24%), hypercalcemia (12% to 21%), hypoparathyroidism (intact parathyroid hormone <100 pg/mL: ≤11%)

Gastrointestinal: Nausea (30% to 66%), vomiting (26% to 52%), diarrhea (21%), anorexia (6% to 21%), constipation (5% to 18%), abdominal pain (11%)

Hematologic & oncologic: Anemia (6% to 17%)

Neuromuscular & skeletal: Bone fracture (12% to 21%), muscle spasm (11% to 18%), arthralgia (6% to 17%), weakness (5% to 17%), myalgia (15%), back pain (12%), limb pain (10% to 12%)

Respiratory: Dyspnea (13%), cough (12%), upper respiratory tract infection (8% to 12%)

1% to 10%:

Cardiovascular: Hypertension (7%)

Central nervous system: Dizziness (7% to 10%), non-cardiac chest pain (6%), seizure (≤3%)

Endocrine & metabolic: Hyperkalemia (8%)

Gastrointestinal: Upper abdominal pain (8%), dyspepsia (7%), decreased appetite (6%)

Hypersensitivity: Hypersensitivity reaction (9%)

Infection: Localized infection (dialysis access site; 5%)

Postmarketing and/or case reports (Limited to important or life-threatening): Adynamic bone disease, cardiac arrhythmia, cardiac failure, hypotension (idiosyncratic), prolonged Q-T interval on ECG (secondary to hypocalcemia), ventricular arrhythmia (secondary to hypocalcemia)

Drug Interactions

Metabolism/Transport Effects Substrate of CYP1A2 (minor), CYP2D6 (minor), CYP3A4 (major); **Note:** Assignment of Major/Minor substrate status based on clinically relevant drug interaction potential; **Inhibits** CYP2D6 (strong)

Avoid Concomitant Use

Avoid concomitant use of Cinacalcet with any of the following: Conivaptan; Fusidic Acid (Systemic); Idelalisib; Mequitazine; Pimozide; Tamoxifen; Thioridazine

Increased Effect/Toxicity

Cinacalcet may increase the levels/effects of: ARIPiprazole; ARIPiprazole Lauroxil; AtoMOXetine; Brexpiprazole; CYP2D6 Substrates; Dapoxetine; DOXOrubicin (Conventional); DULoxetine; Eliglustat; Fesoterodine; Iloperidone; Mequitazine; Metoprolol; Nebivolol; Pimozide; Propafenone; Tamsulosin; Tetrabenazine; Thioridazine; TraMADol; Tricyclic Antidepressants; Vortioxetine

The levels/effects of Cinacalcet may be increased by: Aprepitant; Conivaptan; CYP3A4 Inhibitors (Moderate); CYP3A4 Inhibitors (Strong); Dasatinib; Fosaprepitant; Fusidic Acid (Systemic); Idelalisib; Ivacaftor; Luliconazole; Mifepristone; Netupitant; Osimertinib; Palbociclib; Simeprevir; Stiripentol

Decreased Effect

Cinacalcet may decrease the levels/effects of: Codeine; Hydrocodone; Iloperidone; Tacrolimus (Systemic); Tamoxifen; TraMADol

The levels/effects of Cinacalcet may be decreased by: Osimertinib

Food Interactions Food increases bioavailability. Management: Administer with food or shortly after a meal.

Storage/Stability Store at 25°C (77°F); excursions permitted to 15°C to 30°C (59°F to 86°F).

Mechanism of Action Increases the sensitivity of the calcium-sensing receptor on the parathyroid gland thereby, concomitantly lowering parathyroid hormone (PTH), serum calcium, and serum phosphorus levels, preventing progressive bone disease and adverse events associated with mineral metabolism disorders.

Pharmacodynamics/Kinetics

Distribution: V_d: ~1,000 L

Protein binding: ~93% to 97%

Metabolism: Hepatic (extensive) via CYP3A4, 2D6, 1A2; forms inactive metabolites

Half-life elimination: Terminal: 30 to 40 hours; moderate hepatic impairment: 65 hours; severe hepatic impairment: 84 hours

Time to peak, plasma: ~2 to 6 hours; increased with food.

Excretion: Urine ~80% (as metabolites); feces ~15%

Dosing

Adult & Geriatric Note: Do not titrate dose more frequently than every 2 to 4 weeks. May be used alone or in combination with vitamin D and/or phosphate binders. Dosage adjustment may be required in patients on concurrent CYP3A4 inhibitors.

Hyperparathyroidism, primary: Oral: Initial: 30 mg twice daily; increase dose incrementally (to 60 mg twice daily, 90 mg twice daily, and 90 mg 3 or 4 times daily) as necessary to normalize serum calcium levels.

Hyperparathyroidism, secondary: Oral: Initial: 30 mg once daily; increase dose incrementally (to 60 mg once daily, 90 mg once daily, 120 mg once daily, and 180 mg once daily) as necessary to maintain intact parathyroid hormone (iPTH) level between 150 to 300 pg/mL.

Parathyroid carcinoma: Oral: Initial: 30 mg twice daily; increase dose incrementally (to 60 mg twice daily, 90 mg twice daily, and 90 mg 3 to 4 times daily) as necessary to normalize serum calcium levels.

Renal Impairment No dosage adjustment necessary.

Hepatic Impairment

Mild impairment (Child-Pugh class A): No dosage adjustment necessary.

Moderate to severe impairment (Child-Pugh class B or C); may have an increased exposure to cinacalcet and increased half-life. Dosage adjustments may be necessary based on serum calcium, serum phosphorus, and/or iPTH.

Adjustment for Toxicity Dosage adjustment for hypocalcemia:

If serum calcium >7.5 mg/dL but <8.4 mg/dL **or** if hypocalcemia symptoms occur: Use calcium-containing phosphate binders and/or vitamin D to raise calcium levels.

If serum calcium <7.5 mg/dL **or** if hypocalcemia symptoms persist and the dose of vitamin D cannot be increased: Withhold cinacalcet until serum calcium ≥8 mg/dL and/or symptoms of hypocalcemia resolve. Reinitiate cinacalcet at the next lowest dose.

If iPTH <150 pg/mL: Reduce dose or discontinue cinacalcet and/or vitamin D.

Administration Administer with food or shortly after a meal. Do not break or divide tablet; should be taken whole.

Monitoring Parameters

Monitor for signs/symptoms of hypocalcemia. Monitor serum calcium and iPTH concentrations closely in patients on concurrent CYP3A4 inhibitors, with hepatic impairment or with seizure disorders.

Hyperparathyroidism, secondary: Serum calcium and phosphorus levels prior to initiation and within a week of initiation and frequently during dose titration; iPTH should be measured 1 to 4 weeks after initiation or dosage adjustment (wait at least 12 hours after dose before drawing iPTH levels). After the maintenance dose is established, obtain serum calcium levels monthly.

Parathyroid carcinoma and hyperparathyroidism, primary: Serum calcium levels prior to initiation and within a week of initiation or dosage adjustment; once maintenance dose is established, obtain serum calcium every 2 months.

Reference Range

CKD K/DOQI guidelines definition of stages; chronic disease is kidney damage or GFR <60 mL/minute/1.73 m^2 for ≥3 months:

Stage 2: GFR 60 to 89 mL/minute/1.73 m^2 (kidney damage with mild decrease GFR)

Stage 3: GFR 30 to 59 mL/minute/1.73 m^2 (moderate decrease GFR)

Stage 4: GFR 15 to 29 mL/minute/1.73 m^2 (severe decrease GFR)

Stage 5: GFR <15 mL/minute/1.73 m^2 or dialysis (kidney failure)

Target range for iPTH: Adults:

Stage 3 CKD: 35 to 70 pg/mL

Stage 4 CKD: 70 to 110 pg/mL

Stage 5 CKD: 150 to 300 pg/mL

Serum phosphorus: Adults:

Stage 3 and 4 CKD: ≥2.7 to <4.6 mg/dL

Stage 5 CKD: 3.5 to 5.5 mg/dL

Serum calcium-phosphorus product: Adults: Stage 3 to 5 CKD: <55 mg^2/dL^2

Dosage Forms Excipient information presented when available (limited, particularly for generics); consult specific product labeling.

Tablet, Oral:

Sensipar: 30 mg, 60 mg, 90 mg

◆ Cinacalcet Hydrochloride *see* Cinacalcet *on page 387*

◆ Cinryze *see* C1 Inhibitor (Human) *on page 276*

◆ Cipralex (Can) *see* Escitalopram *on page 673*

◆ Cipralex MELTZ (Can) *see* Escitalopram *on page 673*

◆ Cipro *see* Ciprofloxacin (Systemic) *on page 388*

◆ Cipro XL (Can) *see* Ciprofloxacin (Systemic) *on page 388*

◆ Ciprodex *see* Ciprofloxacin and Dexamethasone *on page 393*

Ciprofloxacin (Systemic) (sip roe FLOKS a sin)

Brand Names: US Cipro; Cipro in D5W; Cipro XR

Brand Names: Canada ACT Ciprofloxacin; Apo-Ciproflox; Auro-Ciprofloxacin; Cipro; Cipro XL; Ciprofloxacin Injection; Ciprofloxacin Injection USP; Ciprofloxacin Intravenous Infusion; Ciprofloxacin Intravenous Infusion BP; Dom-Ciprofloxacin; JAMP-Ciprofloxacin; Mar-Ciprofloxacin; Mint-Ciprofloxacin; Mint-Ciprofloxacin; Mylan-Ciprofloxacin; PHL-Ciprofloxacin; PMS-Ciprofloxacin; PMS-Ciprofloxacin XL; PRO-Ciprofloxacin; RAN-Ciproflox;

ratio-Ciprofloxacin; Riva-Ciprofloxacin; Sandoz-Ciprofloxacin; Septa-Ciprofloxacin; Taro-Ciprofloxacin; Teva-Ciprofloxacin

Index Terms Ciprofloxacin Hydrochloride; Proquin XR
Pharmacologic Category Antibiotic, Fluoroquinolone
Use

Children: Complicated urinary tract infections and pyelonephritis due to *E. coli*. **Note:** Although effective, ciprofloxacin is not the drug of first choice in children.

Children and Adults: To reduce incidence or progression of disease following exposure to aerolized *Bacillus anthracis*; prophylaxis and treatment of plague, including pneumonic and septicemic plague, due to *Yersinia pestis*.

Adults: Treatment of the following infections when caused by susceptible bacteria: Urinary tract infections; acute uncomplicated cystitis in females; chronic bacterial prostatitis; lower respiratory tract infections (including acute exacerbations of chronic bronchitis); acute sinusitis; skin and skin structure infections; bone and joint infections; complicated intra-abdominal infections (in combination with metronidazole); infectious diarrhea; typhoid fever due to *Salmonella typhi* (eradication of chronic typhoid carrier state has not been proven); uncomplicated cervical and urethra gonorrhea (due to *N. gonorrhoeae*); nosocomial pneumonia; empirical therapy for febrile neutropenic patients (in combination with piperacillin)

Note: As of April 2007, the CDC no longer recommends the use of fluoroquinolones for the treatment of gonococcal disease.

Pregnancy Considerations Adverse events have been observed in some animal reproduction studies. Ciprofloxacin crosses the placenta and produces measurable concentrations in the amniotic fluid and cord serum (Ludlam 1997). Based on available data, an increased risk of teratogenic effects has not been observed following ciprofloxacin use during pregnancy (Bar-Oz 2009; Padberg 2014). Ciprofloxacin is recommended for prophylaxis and treatment of pregnant women exposed to anthrax (Meaney-Delman 2014). Serum concentrations of ciprofloxacin may be lower during pregnancy than in nonpregnant patients (Giamarellou 1989).

Breast-Feeding Considerations Ciprofloxacin is excreted in breast milk. Due to the potential for serious adverse reactions in the nursing infant, the manufacturer recommends a decision be made whether to discontinue nursing or to discontinue the drug, taking into account the importance of treatment to the mother. However infant serum levels were undetectable (<0.03 mcg/mL) in one report (Gardner 1992). There has been a single case report of perforated pseudomembranous colitis in a breast-feeding infant whose mother was taking ciprofloxacin (Harmon 1992). Ciprofloxacin is recommended for the prophylaxis and treatment of *Bacillus anthracis* in lactating women (Meaney-Delman 2014).

Medication Guide Available Yes
Contraindications Hypersensitivity to ciprofloxacin, any component of the formulation, or other quinolones; concurrent administration of tizanidine

Warnings/Precautions [US Boxed Warning]: There have been reports of tendon inflammation and/or rupture with quinolone antibiotics in all ages; risk may be increased with concurrent corticosteroids, solid organ transplant recipients, and in patients >60 years of age. Rupture of the Achilles tendon sometimes requiring surgical repair has been reported more frequently; but other tendon sites (eg, rotator cuff, biceps) have also been reported. Strenuous physical activity, rheumatoid arthritis, and renal impairment may be an independent risk factor for tendonitis. Inflammation and rupture may occur bilaterally. Cases have been reported within the first 48 hours, during, and up to several months after discontinuation of therapy. Discontinue at first sign of tendon inflammation or pain. Use with caution in patients with rheumatoid arthritis; may increase risk of tendon rupture. Use with caution in patients with a history of tendon disorders.

CNS effects may occur (tremor, restlessness, confusion, and hallucinations, increased intracranial pressure [including pseudotumor cerebri] or seizures). Reactions may occur following the first dose. Use with caution in patients with known or suspected CNS disorder or consider discontinuation if CNS effects develop. Potential for seizures, although very rare, may be increased with concomitant NSAID therapy. Use with caution in individuals at risk of seizures (CNS disorders or concurrent therapy with medications which may lower seizure threshold; status epilepticus has occurred) or if clinically appropriate, consider alternative antimicrobial therapy. Discontinue if seizures occur.

Fluoroquinolones may prolong QTc interval; avoid use in patients with a history of or at risk for QTc prolongation, torsade de pointes, uncorrected hypokalemia,

hypomagnesemia, cardiac disease (heart failure, myocardial infarction, bradycardia) or concurrent administration of other medications known to prolong the QT interval (including Class Ia and Class III antiarrhythmics, cisapride, erythromycin, antipsychotics, and tricyclic antidepressants). Hepatocellular, cholestatic, or mixed liver injury has been reported, including hepatic necrosis, life-threatening hepatic events, and fatalities. Acute liver injury can be rapid onset (range: 1-39 days), often associated with hypersensitivity. Most fatalities occurred in patients >55 years of age. Discontinue immediately if signs/symptoms of hepatitis (abdominal tenderness, dark urine, jaundice, pruritus) occur. Additionally, temporary increases in transaminases or alkaline phosphatase or cholestatic jaundice may occur (highest risk in patients with previous liver damage).

Prolonged use may result in fungal or bacterial superinfection, including *C. difficile*-associated diarrhea (CDAD) and pseudomembranous colitis; CDAD has been observed >2 months postantibiotic treatment. Rarely crystalluria has occurred; urine alkalinity may increase the risk. Ensure adequate hydration during therapy. Adverse effects, including those related to joints and/or surrounding tissues, are increased in pediatric patients and therefore, ciprofloxacin should not be considered as drug of choice in children (exception is anthrax treatment). Peripheral neuropathy has been reported (rare); may occur soon after initiation of therapy and may be irreversible; discontinue if symptoms of sensory or sensorimotor neuropathy occur.

Fluoroquinolones have been associated with the development of serious, and sometimes fatal, hypoglycemia, most often in elderly diabetics but also in patients without diabetes. This occurred most frequently with gatifloxacin (no longer available systemically), but may occur at a lower frequency with other quinolones.

Severe hypersensitivity reactions, including anaphylaxis, have occurred with quinolone therapy. Reactions may present as typical allergic symptoms after a single dose, or may manifest as severe idiosyncratic dermatologic, vascular, pulmonary, renal, hepatic, and/or hematologic events, usually after multiple doses. Prompt discontinuation of drug should occur if skin rash or other symptoms arise. **[US Boxed Warning]: Quinolones may exacerbate myasthenia gravis; avoid use (rare, potentially life-threatening weakness of respiratory muscles may occur).** Use caution in renal impairment. Avoid excessive sunlight and take precautions to limit exposure (eg, loose fitting clothing, sunscreen); may cause moderate-to-severe photosensitivity/phototoxicity reactions. Discontinue use if photosensitivity occurs. Since ciprofloxacin is ineffective in the treatment of syphilis and may mask symptoms, all patients should be tested for syphilis at the time of gonorrheal diagnosis and 3 months later. Hemolytic reactions may (rarely) occur with quinolone use in patients with latent or actual glucose-6-phosphate dehydrogenase (G6PD) deficiency.

Potentially significant interactions may exist, requiring dose or frequency adjustment, additional monitoring, and/or selection of alternative therapy. Serious and fatal reactions including seizures, status epilepticus, cardiac arrest and respiratory failure have been reported with concomitant administration of theophylline. If concurrent use is unavoidable, monitor serum theophylline levels and adjust theophylline dose as warranted.

Adverse Reactions
1% to 10%:
  Central nervous system: Neurological signs and symptoms (children 2%; includes dizziness, insomnia, nervousness, somnolence), headache (IV administration), restlessness (IV administration)
  Dermatologic: Skin rash (children 2%, adults 1%)
  Gastrointestinal: Diarrhea (children 5%; adults 2%), vomiting (children 5%; adults 1%), abdominal pain (children 3%; adults <1%), dyspepsia (children 3%; adults <1%), nausea (3%)
  Hepatic: Increased serum AST (adults 1%), increased serum ALT
  Local: Injection site reactions (IV administration)
  Respiratory: Rhinitis (children 3%)
  Miscellaneous: Fever (children 2%; adults <1%)
<1% (Limited to important or life-threatening): Abnormal gait, acute generalized exanthematous pustulosis, acute gout attack, acute renal failure, ageusia, agitation, agranulocytosis, albuminuria, anaphylactic shock, anaphylaxis, anemia, angina pectoris, angioedema, anorexia, anosmia, anxiety, arthralgia, ataxia, atrial flutter, bone marrow depression (life-threatening), bronchospasm, candidiasis, candiduria, cardiorespiratory arrest, casts in urine, cerebral thrombosis, chills, cholestatic jaundice, chromatopsia, *Clostridium difficile*-associated diarrhea,

confusion, constipation, crystalluria (particularly in alkaline urine), decreased hematocrit, decreased hemoglobin, decreased prothrombin time, delirium, depersonalization, depression (including self-injurious behavior), dizziness, drowsiness, dyspepsia (adults), dysphagia, dysphasia, dyspnea, edema, eosinophilia, erythema multiforme, erythema nodosum, exacerbation of myasthenia gravis, exfoliative dermatitis, fixed drug eruption, flatulence, gastrointestinal hemorrhage, hallucination, headache (oral), hematuria, hemolytic anemia, hepatic failure, hepatic necrosis, hepatotoxicity (idiosyncratic) (Chalasani, 2014), hyperesthesia, hyperglycemia, hyperpigmentation, hypersensitivity reaction, hypertension, hypertonia, hypoglycemia, hypotension, increased blood urea nitrogen, increased creatine phosphokinase, increased INR (in patients treated with vitamin K antagonists), increased intracranial pressure, increased lactate dehydrogenase, increased serum alkaline phosphatase, increased serum bilirubin, increased serum cholesterol, increased serum creatinine, increased serum glucose, increased serum lipase, increased serum triglycerides, increased uric acid, insomnia, interstitial nephritis, intestinal perforation, irritability, jaundice, laryngeal edema, lethargy, lymphadenopathy, malaise, manic behavior, mastalgia, methemoglobinemia, migraine, myalgia, myocardial infarction, myoclonus, nephritis, nephrolithiasis, nightmares, nystagmus, orthostatic hypotension, palpitations, pancreatitis, pancytopenia (life-threatening), paranoia, paresthesia, peripheral neuropathy, petechia, phobia, phototoxicity, pneumonitis, polyneuropathy, prolonged prothrombin time (in patients treated with vitamin K antagonists), pseudotumor cerebri, pulmonary edema, rupture of tendon, seizure (including grand mal), serum sickness-like reaction, skin photosensitivity, status epilepticus, Stevens-Johnson syndrome, suicidal ideation, suicidal tendencies, syncope, tachycardia, tendonitis, thrombocythemia, thrombocytopenia, thrombophlebitis, tinnitus, torsades de pointes, toxic epidermal necrolysis, toxic psychosis, tremor, twitching, unresponsive to stimuli, urethral bleeding, vaginitis, vasculitis, ventricular arrhythmia, ventricular ectopy, visual disturbance, vulvovaginal candidiasis, weakness

Drug Interactions

Metabolism/Transport Effects Substrate of OAT3, P-glycoprotein; **Inhibits** CYP1A2 (strong), CYP3A4 (weak)

Avoid Concomitant Use

Avoid concomitant use of Ciprofloxacin (Systemic) with any of the following: Agomelatine; BCG (Intravesical); CloZAPine; DULoxetine; Highest Risk QTc-Prolonging Agents; Ivabradine; Mifepristone; Pimozide; Pomalidomide; Strontium Ranelate; Tasimelteon; TiZANidine

Increased Effect/Toxicity

Ciprofloxacin (Systemic) may increase the levels/effects of: Agomelatine; ARIPiprazole; Bendamustine; Blood Glucose Lowering Agents; Caffeine; CarBAMazepine; CloZAPine; CYP1A2 Substrates; DULoxetine; Erlotinib; Flibanserin; Highest Risk QTc-Prolonging Agents; Hydrocodone; Kola Nut; Lomitapide; Methotrexate; Moderate Risk QTc-Prolonging Agents; NiMODipine; Pentoxifylline; Pimozide; Pirfenidone; Pomalidomide; Porfimer; Rasagiline; Roflumilast; ROPINIRole; Ropivacaine; Tasimelteon; Theophylline Derivatives; TiZANidine; Varenicline; Verteporfin; Vitamin K Antagonists

The levels/effects of Ciprofloxacin (Systemic) may be increased by: ACE Inhibitors; Angiotensin II Receptor Blockers; Corticosteroids (Systemic); Fosphenytoin; Ivabradine; Lumacaftor; Mifepristone; Nonsteroidal Anti-Inflammatory Agents; P-glycoprotein/ABCB1 Inhibitors; Probenecid; QTc-Prolonging Agents (Indeterminate Risk and Risk Modifying); Ranolazine; Spironolactone; Teriflunomide

Decreased Effect

Ciprofloxacin (Systemic) may decrease the levels/effects of: BCG (Intravesical); BCG Vaccine (Immunization); Blood Glucose Lowering Agents; Didanosine; Fosphenytoin; Mycophenolate; Phenytoin; Sodium Picosulfate; Thyroid Products; Typhoid Vaccine

The levels/effects of Ciprofloxacin (Systemic) may be decreased by: Antacids; Calcium Salts; Didanosine; Iron Salts; Lanthanum; Lumacaftor; Magnesium Salts; Multivitamins/Minerals (with ADEK, Folate, Iron); Multivitamins/Minerals (with AE, No Iron); P-glycoprotein/ABCB1 Inducers; Quinapril; Sevelamer; Strontium Ranelate; Sucralfate; Zinc Salts

Food Interactions Food decreases rate, but not extent, of absorption. Ciprofloxacin serum levels may be decreased if taken with divalent or trivalent cations. Rarely, crystalluria may occur. Enteral feedings may decrease plasma concentrations of ciprofloxacin probably by >30% inhibition of absorption. Management: May administer with food to minimize GI upset. Avoid or take ciprofloxacin 2 hours before or 6 hours after antacids, dairy products, or calcium-fortified juices alone or in a meal containing >800 mg calcium, oral multivitamins, or mineral supplements containing divalent and/or trivalent cations. Ensure adequate hydration during therapy. Ciprofloxacin should not be administered with enteral feedings. The feeding would need to be discontinued for 1-2 hours prior to and after ciprofloxacin administration. Nasogastric administration produces a greater loss of ciprofloxacin bioavailability than does nasoduodenal administration.

Preparation for Administration Injection, vial: May be diluted with NS, D$_5$W, SWFI, D$_{10}$W, D$_5$¹/₄NS, D$_5$¹/₂NS, LR.

Storage/Stability

Injection:

Premixed infusion: Store between 5°C to 25°C (41°F to 77°F); avoid freezing. Protect from light.

Vial: Store between 5°C to 30°C (41°F to 86°F); avoid freezing. Protect from light. Diluted solutions of 0.5-2 mg/mL are stable for up to 14 days refrigerated or at room temperature.

Microcapsules for oral suspension: Prior to reconstitution, store below 25°C (77°F). Protect from freezing. Following reconstitution, store below 30°C (86°F) for up to 14 days. Protect from freezing.

Tablet:

Immediate release: Store between 20°C to 25°C (68°F to 77°F); excursions are permitted between 15°C and 30°C (59°F and 86°F).

Extended release: Store at 25°C (77°F); excursions are permitted between 15°C and 30°C (59°F and 86°F).

Mechanism of Action Inhibits DNA-gyrase in susceptible organisms; inhibits relaxation of supercoiled DNA and promotes breakage of double-stranded DNA

Pharmacodynamics/Kinetics

Absorption: Oral: Well-absorbed; 500 mg orally every 12 hours produces an equivalent AUC to that produced by 400 mg IV over 60 minutes every 12 hours

Distribution: V$_d$: 2.1 to 2.7 L/kg; tissue concentrations often exceed serum concentrations especially in kidneys, gallbladder, liver, lungs, gynecological tissue, and prostatic tissue; CSF concentrations: 10% of serum concentrations (noninflamed meninges), 14% to 37% (inflamed meninges)

Protein binding: 20% to 40%

Metabolism: Partially hepatic; forms 4 metabolites (limited activity)

Bioavailability: Oral: 50% to 85%; younger CF patients have a lower bioavailability of 68% vs CF patients >13 years of age with bioavailability of 95%

Half-life elimination: Children: 4 to 5 hours; Adults: Normal renal function: 3 to 5 hours

Time to peak: Oral:

Immediate release tablet: 0.5 to 2 hours

Extended release tablet: Cipro XR: 1 to 2.5 hours

Excretion: Urine (30% to 50% as unchanged drug); feces (15% to 43%; <1% as unchanged drug)

Clearance: After IV: CF children: 0.84 L/hour/kg; Adults: 0.5 to 0.6 L/hour/kg

Dosing

Adult Note: Extended release tablets and immediate release formulations are not interchangeable. Unless otherwise specified, oral dosing reflects the use of immediate release formulations.

Anthrax:

Inhalational (postexposure prophylaxis):

Oral: 500 mg every 12 hours for 60 days

IV: 400 mg every 12 hours for 60 days

Cutaneous (treatment, CDC guidelines): Oral: Immediate release formulation: 500 mg every 12 hours for 60 days. **Note:** In the presence of systemic involvement, extensive edema, lesions on head/neck, refer to IV dosing for treatment of inhalational/gastrointestinal/oropharyngeal anthrax.

Inhalational/gastrointestinal/oropharyngeal (treatment, CDC guidelines): IV: 400 mg every 12 hours. **Note:** Initial treatment should include two or more agents predicted to be effective (per CDC recommendations). Continue combined therapy for 60 days.

Bacterial enteric infections in HIV-infected patients (empiric treatment) (off-label use; HHS [OI adult 2015]):

Oral: 500 to 750 mg every 12 hours

IV: 400 mg every 12 hours

Bite wounds (animal, human) (off-label use) (IDSA [Stevens 2014]): Note: Recommended as an alternative therapy for human bite wound in patients hypersensitive to beta-lactams.

Oral: 500 to 750 mg twice daily; in combination with metronidazole

IV: 400 mg every 12 hours; in combination with metronidazole

Bone/joint infections:
Oral: 500 to 750 mg twice daily for 4 to 8 weeks
IV:
 Mild/moderate: 400 mg every 12 hours for 4 to 8 weeks
 Severe/complicated: 400 mg every 8 hours for 4 to 8 weeks

Chancroid (off-label use): Oral: 500 mg twice daily for 3 days (CDC 2010)

Cystitis, acute uncomplicated:
Oral, immediate release: 250 mg every 12 hours for 3 days
Oral, extended release (Cipro XR): 500 mg every 24 hours for 3 days

Endocarditis due to HACEK organisms (off-label use) (Baddour 2005): Note: Not first-line option; use only if intolerant of beta-lactam therapy:
Oral: 500 mg every 12 hours for 4 weeks (native valve) or 6 weeks (prosthetic valve)
IV: 400 mg every 12 hours for 4 weeks (native valve) or 6 weeks (prosthetic valve)

Epididymitis, chlamydial (off-label use): Oral: 500 mg single dose (Canadian STI Guidelines 2008)

Febrile neutropenia: IV: 400 mg every 8 hours for 7 to 14 days (combination therapy with piperacillin generally recommended)

Gonococcal infections:
Urethral/cervical gonococcal infections: Oral: 250 to 500 mg as a single dose (CDC recommends concomitant doxycycline or azithromycin due to possible coinfection with *Chlamydia*); **Note:** As of April 2007, the CDC no longer recommends the use of fluoroquinolones for the treatment of uncomplicated gonococcal disease.

Granuloma inguinale (donovanosis) (off-label use):
Oral: 750 mg twice daily for at least 3 weeks (and until lesions have healed) (CDC 2010)

Infectious diarrhea: Oral:
Salmonella: 500 mg twice daily for 5 to 7 days
Shigella (including Shigella dysentery type 1) (off-label regimen): 500 mg twice daily for 3 days (IDSA 2001)
Traveler's diarrhea (off-label regimen): Mild: 750 mg as a single dose (CDC 2012; de la Cabada Bauch 2011); Severe: 500 mg twice daily for 3 days (IDSA 2001)
Vibrio cholerae (off-label regimen): 1 g as a single (CDC 2011)

Infectious diarrhea due to *Salmonella, Shigella, or Campylobacter* in HIV-infected patients (off-label use; HHS [OI adult 2015]): Note: Patients with bacteremia due to *Campylobacter* should receive additional therapy with an aminoglycoside
Oral: 500 to 750 mg every 12 hours
IV: 400 mg every 12 hours)
Duration of therapy: Oral, IV:
 Salmonella: Without bacteremia: 7 to 14 days (CD4 count ≥200 cells/mm^3) or 2 to 6 weeks (CD4 count <200 cells/mm^3); With bacteremia: 14 days or longer based on clinical condition (CD4 count ≥200 cells/mm^3) or 2 to 6 weeks (CD4 count <200 cells/mm^3)
 Shigella or *Campylobacter:* Gastroenteritis: 7 to 10 days; Bacteremia: ≥14 days; Recurrent infections: *Campylobacter:* 2 to 6 weeks; *Shigella:* ≤6 weeks

Intra-abdominal, complicated, community-acquired (in combination with metronidazole): Note: Avoid using in settings where *E. coli* susceptibility to fluoroquinolones is <90%:
Oral: 500 mg every 12 hours for 7 to 14 days
IV: 400 mg every 12 hours for 7 to 14 days; **Note:** 2010 IDSA guidelines recommend treatment duration of 4 to 7 days (provided source controlled)

Lower respiratory tract:
Oral: 500 to 750 mg twice daily for 7 to 14 days
IV: 400 mg every 8 to 12 hours for 7 to 14 days

Meningococcal meningitis prophylaxis (off-label use): Oral: 500 mg as a single dose (CDC 2005)

Nosocomial pneumonia: IV: 400 mg every 8 hours for 10 to 14 days

Periodontitis (off-label use): Oral: 500 mg every 12 hours for 8 to 10 days (Rams 1992)

Plague:
Manufacturer's labeling:
 Oral: 500 to 750 mg every 12 hours for 14 days
 IV: 400 mg every 8 to 12 hours for 14 days
Alternate dosing:
 Contained casualty management: IV: 400 mg twice daily for 10 days. Can switch to oral administration when clinically indicated (Bossi 2004; CDC [plague] 2012; Inglesby 2000).
 Mass casualty management: Oral: 500 mg twice daily for 10 days (Inglesby 2000)

Mass casualty postexposure prophylaxis: Oral: 500 mg twice daily for 7 days (Bossi 2004; CDC [plague] 2012; Inglesby 2000).

Prostatitis (chronic, bacterial):
Oral: 500 mg every 12 hours for 28 days
IV: 400 mg every 12 hours for 28 days

Sinusitis (acute):
Oral: 500 mg every 12 hours for 10 days
IV: 400 mg every 12 hours for 10 days

Skin/skin structure infections:
Oral: 500 to 750 mg twice daily for 7 to 14 days
IV: Mild to moderate: 400 mg every 12 hours for 7 to 14 days; Severe/complicated: 400 mg every 8 hours for 7 to 14 days

Skin and soft tissue necrotizing infection due to *Aeromonas hydrophila* (off-label use): IV: 400 mg every 12 hours; in combination with doxycycline. Continue treatment until further debridement is not necessary, patient has clinically improved, and patient is afebrile for 48 to 72 hours (IDSA [Stevens 2014]).

Spontaneous bacterial peritonitis (prevention) (off-label use): Oral: Long-term prophylaxis: 500 mg once daily (preferred) (Terg 2008). Weekly dosing of 750 mg orally for long-term prophylaxis has been studied, but concerns regarding quinolone bacterial resistance limit use (AASLD [Runyon 2012]; Roulachon 1995). American Association for the Study of Liver Diseases (AASLD) guidelines note that intermittent dosing (ie, 5 days/week, weekly) of antibiotics, although shown to be effective in SBP prevention, may be inferior to daily dosing due to development of bacterial resistance. Daily dosing regimens are preferred (AASLD [Runyon 2012]).

Surgical (preoperative) prophylaxis (off-label use): IV: 400 mg within 120 minutes prior to surgical incision (Bratzler 2013)

Surgical site infection (intestinal or GU tract, perineum, or axilla) (off-label use) (IDSA [Stevens 2014]):
Oral: 750 mg every 12 hours, in combination with metronidazole
IV: 400 mg every 12 hours, in combination with metronidazole

Tularemia (off-label use):
Contained casualty management: IV: 400 mg twice daily for 10 days. Can switch to oral administration when clinically indicated (Dennis 2001).
Mass casualty management or postexposure prophylaxis: Oral: 500 or 750 mg twice daily for 14 days. At least 14 days of therapy is recommended in oral regimens (Bossi [tularemia] 2004; Dennis 2001; Stevens 2014).

Typhoid fever: Oral: 500 mg every 12 hours for 10 days

Urinary tract infection:
Oral, immediate release: 250 to 500 mg every 12 hours for 7 to 14 days
IV: 200 to 400 mg every 8 to 12 hours for 7 to 14 days

Urinary tract infection, complicated (including pyelonephritis): Oral, extended release (Cipro XR): 1000 mg every 24 hours for 7 to 14 days

Geriatric Refer to adult dosing. Adjust dose carefully based on renal function.

Pediatric See Warnings/Precautions. **Note:** Extended release tablets and immediate release formulations are not interchangeable. Unless otherwise specified, oral dosing reflects the use of immediate release formulations.

Anthrax:
Inhalational (postexposure prophylaxis):
 Oral: 15 mg/kg/dose every 12 hours for 60 days; maximum: 500 mg/dose
 IV: 10 mg/kg/dose every 12 hours for 60 days; do **not** exceed 400 mg/dose (800 mg/day)
Cutaneous (treatment, CDC guidelines): Oral: 10 to 15 mg/kg every 12 hours for 60 days (maximum: 1000 mg/day); amoxicillin 80 mg/kg/day divided every 8 hours is an option for completion of treatment after clinical improvement. **Note:** In the presence of systemic involvement, extensive edema, lesions on head/neck, refer to IV dosing for treatment of inhalational/gastrointestinal/oropharyngeal anthrax.
Inhalational/gastrointestinal/oropharyngeal (treatment, CDC guidelines): IV: Initial: 10 to 15 mg/kg every 12 hours for 60 days (maximum: 500 mg/dose); switch to oral therapy when clinically appropriate; refer to adult dosing for notes on combined therapy and duration

Bacterial enteric infections in HIV-infected patients (empiric treatment) (off-label use): Adolescents: Refer to adult dosing

Community-acquired pneumonia (CAP) (IDSA/PIDS 2011): *H. influenzae*, moderate-to-severe infection (alternative to ampicillin, ceftriaxone, or cefotaxime): Infants >3 months and Children: IV: 30 mg/kg/day divided every 12 hours

Cystic fibrosis (off-label use): Children 5 to 17 years: Oral: 40 mg/kg/day divided every 12 hours administered following 1 week of IV therapy has been reported in a clinical trial; total duration of therapy: 10 to 21 days (Rubio 1997)

IV: 30 mg/kg/day divided every 8 hours for 1 week, followed by oral therapy, has been reported in a clinical trial (Rubio 1997)

Infectious diarrhea due to *Salmonella, Shigella,* or *Campylobacter* in HIV-infected patients (off-label dose): Adolescents: Refer to adult dosing.

Shigella dysentery type 1 (off-label use): Oral: 30 mg/kg/day in 2 divided doses for 3 days (WHO 2005)

Plague:

Manufacturer's labeling: Infants, Children, and Adolescents:

Oral: 15 mg/kg/dose every 8 to 12 hours for 10 to 21 days; maximum: 500 mg/dose

IV: 10 mg/kg/dose every 8 to 12 hours for 10 to 21 days; maximum: 400 mg/dose

Alternate dosing: Children and Adolescents:

Contained casualty management: IV: 15 mg/kg twice daily for 10 days (maximum: 1000 mg/day). Can switch to oral administration when clinically indicated (CDC [plague] 2014; Inglesby 2000).

Mass casualty management: Oral: 20 mg/kg twice daily for 10 days (maximum: 1000 mg/day) (Inglesby 2000)

Mass casualty postexposure prophylaxis: Oral: 20 mg/kg twice daily for 7 days (maximum: 1000 mg/day) (CDC [plague] 2014; Inglesby 2000)

Surgical (preoperative) prophylaxis (off-label use): Children ≥1 year: IV: 10 mg/kg within 120 minutes prior to surgical incision (maximum: 400 mg/dose) (Bratzler 2013)

Urinary tract infection (complicated) or pyelonephritis: Children 1 to 17 years:

Oral: 20 to 40 mg/kg/day in 2 divided doses (every 12 hours) for 10 to 21 days; maximum: 1,500 mg/day. **Note:** 30 to 40 mg/kg/day reserved for severe infections (*Red Book* 2012).

IV: 6 to 10 mg/kg every 8 hours for 10 to 21 days (maximum: 400 mg/dose)

Renal Impairment Adults:

Manufacturer's labeling:

Oral, immediate release:

CrCl >50 mL/minute: No dosage adjustment necessary.

CrCl 30 to 50 mL/minute: 250 to 500 mg every 12 hours

CrCl 5 to 29 mL/minute: 250 to 500 mg every 18 hours

ESRD on intermittent hemodialysis (IHD)/peritoneal dialysis (PD) (administer after dialysis on dialysis days): 250 to 500 mg every 24 hours

Oral, extended release:

CrCl ≥30 mL/minute: No dosage adjustment necessary.

CrCl <30 mL/minute: 500 mg every 24 hours

ESRD on intermittent hemodialysis (IHD)/peritoneal dialysis (PD) (administer after dialysis on dialysis days): 500 mg every 24 hours

IV:

CrCl ≥30 mL/minute: No dosage adjustment necessary.

CrCl 5 to 29 mL/minute: 200 to 400 mg every 18 to 24 hours

Alternate recommendations: Oral (immediate release), IV:

CrCl >50 mL/minute: No dosage adjustment necessary (Aronoff 2007).

CrCl 10 to 50 mL/minute: Administer 50% to 75% of usual dose every 12 hours (Aronoff 2007).

CrCl <10 mL/minute: Administer 50% of usual dose every 12 hours (Aronoff 2007).

Intermittent hemodialysis (IHD) (administer after hemodialysis on dialysis days): Minimally dialyzable (<10%): Oral: 250 to 500 mg every 24 hours **or** IV: 200 to 400 mg every 24 hours (Heintz 2009). **Note:** Dosing dependent on the assumption of 3 times weekly, complete IHD sessions.

Continuous renal replacement therapy (CRRT) (Heintz 2009; Trotman 2005): Drug clearance is highly dependent on the method of renal replacement, filter type, and flow rate. Appropriate dosing requires close monitoring of pharmacologic response, signs of adverse reactions due to drug accumulation, as well as drug concentrations in relation to target trough (if appropriate). The following are general recommendations only (based on dialysate flow/ultrafiltration rates of 1 to 2 L/hour and minimal residual renal function) and should not supersede clinical judgment:

CVVH/CVVHD/CVVHDF: IV: 200 to 400 mg every 12 to 24 hours

Hepatic Impairment There are no dosage adjustments provided in manufacturer's labeling. Use with caution in severe impairment.

Dietary Considerations Food: Drug may cause GI upset; take without regard to meals (manufacturer prefers that immediate release tablet is taken 2 hours after meals). Extended release tablet may be taken with meals that contain dairy products (calcium content <800 mg), but not with dairy products alone.

Dairy products, calcium-fortified juices, oral multivitamins, and mineral supplements: Absorption of ciprofloxacin is decreased by divalent and trivalent cations. The manufacturer states that the usual dietary intake of calcium (including meals which include dairy products) has not been shown to interfere with ciprofloxacin absorption. Immediate release ciprofloxacin and Cipro XR may be taken 2 hours before or 6 hours after any of these products.

Caffeine: Patients consuming regular large quantities of caffeinated beverages may need to restrict caffeine intake if excessive cardiac or CNS stimulation occurs.

Administration

Oral: May administer with food to minimize GI upset; avoid antacid use; maintain proper hydration and urine output. Administer immediate release ciprofloxacin and Cipro XR at least 2 hours before or 6 hours after antacids or other products containing calcium, iron, or zinc (including dairy products or calcium-fortified juices). Separate oral administration from drugs which may impair absorption (see Drug Interactions).

Oral suspension: Should not be administered through feeding tubes (suspension is oil-based and adheres to the feeding tube). Patients should avoid chewing on the microcapsules.

Nasogastric/orogastric tube: Crush immediate-release tablet and mix with water. Flush feeding tube before and after administration. Hold tube feedings at least 1 hour before and 2 hours after administration.

Tablet, extended release: Do not crush, split, or chew. May be administered with meals containing dairy products (calcium content <800 mg), but not with dairy products alone.

Parenteral: Administer by slow IV infusion over 60 minutes into a large vein (reduces risk of venous irritation).

Monitoring Parameters CBC, renal and hepatic function during prolonged therapy

Reference Range Therapeutic: 2.6 to 3 mcg/mL; Toxic: >5 mcg/mL

Test Interactions Some quinolones may produce a false-positive urine screening result for opioids using commercially-available immunoassay kits. This has been demonstrated most consistently for levofloxacin and ofloxacin, but other quinolones have shown cross-reactivity in certain assay kits. Confirmation of positive opioid screens by more specific methods should be considered.

Additional Information Although the systemic use of ciprofloxacin is only FDA-approved in children for the treatment of complicated UTI and postexposure treatment of inhalation anthrax, use of the fluoroquinolones in pediatric patients is increasing. Current recommendations by the American Academy of Pediatrics note that the systemic use of these agents in children should be restricted to infections caused by multidrug resistant pathogens with no safe or effective alternative, and when parenteral therapy is not feasible or other oral agents are not available.

Dosage Forms Excipient information presented when available (limited, particularly for generics); consult specific product labeling.

Solution, Intravenous:

Cipro in D5W: 200 mg/100 mL (100 mL) [latex free]

Generic: 200 mg/100 mL (100 mL); 400 mg/200 mL (200 mL); 200 mg/20 mL (20 mL); 400 mg/40 mL (40 mL)

Solution, Intravenous [preservative free]:

Cipro in D5W: 200 mg/100 mL (100 mL); 400 mg/200 mL (200 mL) [latex free]

Generic: 200 mg/100 mL (100 mL); 400 mg/200 mL (200 mL); 200 mg/20 mL (20 mL); 400 mg/40 mL (40 mL)

Suspension Reconstituted, Oral:
Cipro: 250 mg/5 mL (100 mL); 500 mg/5 mL (100 mL) [strawberry flavor]
Generic: 250 mg/5 mL (100 mL); 500 mg/5 mL (100 mL)
Tablet, Oral, as hydrochloride [strength expressed as base]:
Cipro: 250 mg, 500 mg
Generic: 100 mg, 250 mg, 500 mg, 750 mg
Tablet Extended Release 24 Hour, Oral, as base and hydrochloride [strength expressed as base]:
Cipro XR: 500 mg, 1000 mg
Generic: 500 mg, 1000 mg

Extemporaneous Preparations A 50 mg/mL oral suspension may be made using 2 different vehicles (a 1:1 mixture of Ora-Sweet and Ora-Plus or a 1:1 mixture of Methylcellulose 1% and Simple Syrup, NF). Crush twenty 500 mg tablets and reduce to a fine powder. Add a small amount of vehicle and mix to a uniform paste; mix while adding the vehicle in geometric proportions to **almost** 200 mL; transfer to a calibrated bottle, rinse mortar with vehicle, and add quantity of vehicle sufficient to make 200 mL. Label "shake well" and "refrigerate". Stable 91 days refrigerated and 70 days at room temperature. **Note:** Microcapsules for oral suspension available (50 mg/mL; 100 mg/mL); not for use in feeding tubes.

Nahata MC, Pai VB, and Hipple TF, *Pediatric Drug Formulations,* 5th ed, Cincinnati, OH: Harvey Whitney Books Co, 2004.

Ciprofloxacin (Ophthalmic) (sip roe FLOKS a sin)

Brand Names: US Ciloxan
Brand Names: Canada Ciloxan
Index Terms Ciprofloxacin Hydrochloride
Pharmacologic Category Antibiotic, Fluoroquinolone; Antibiotic, Ophthalmic
Use Treatment of superficial ocular infections (corneal ulcers, conjunctivitis) due to susceptible strains
Dosing
Adult & Geriatric
Bacterial conjunctivitis:
Ophthalmic solution: Instill 1-2 drops into the conjunctival sac every 2 hours while awake for 2 days and 1-2 drops every 4 hours while awake for the next 5 days
Ophthalmic ointment: Apply a 1/2 inch ribbon into the conjunctival sac 3 times/day for the first 2 days, followed by a 1/2 inch ribbon applied twice daily for the next 5 days
Corneal ulcer: *Ophthalmic solution:* Instill 2 drops into affected eye every 15 minutes for the first 6 hours, then 2 drops into the affected eye every 30 minutes for the remainder of the first day. On day 2, instill 2 drops into the affected eye hourly. On days 3-14, instill 2 drops into affected eye every 4 hours. Treatment may continue after day 14 if re-epithelialization has not occurred.
Pediatric
Bacterial conjunctivitis:
Ophthalmic solution: Children ≥1 year: Refer to adult dosing.
Ophthalmic ointment: Children ≥2 years: Refer to adult dosing.
Corneal ulcer: *Ophthalmic solution:* Children ≥1 year: Refer to adult dosing.
Renal Impairment No dosage adjustment provided in manufacturer's labeling.
Hepatic Impairment No dosage adjustment provided in manufacturer's labeling.
Additional Information Complete prescribing information should be consulted for additional detail.
Dosage Forms Excipient information presented when available (limited, particularly for generics); consult specific product labeling.
Ointment, Ophthalmic, as hydrochloride:
Ciloxan: 0.3% (3.5 g)
Solution, Ophthalmic, as hydrochloride:
Ciloxan: 0.3% (5 mL) [contains benzalkonium chloride, edetate disodium]
Generic: 0.3% (2.5 mL, 5 mL, 10 mL)

Ciprofloxacin (Otic) (sip roe FLOKS a sin)

Brand Names: US Cetraxal
Index Terms Ciprofloxacin Hydrochloride; Otiprio
Pharmacologic Category Antibiotic, Fluoroquinolone; Antibiotic, Otic
Use Treatment of acute otitis externa due to susceptible strains of *Pseudomonas aeruginosa* or *Staphylococcus aureus*
Dosing
Adult & Geriatric Acute otitis externa: Otic solution: Instill 0.25 mL (contents of 1 single-dose container) into affected ear twice daily for 7 days

Pediatric Acute otitis externa: Otic solution: Children ≥1 year: Refer to adult dosing.
Additional Information Complete prescribing information should be consulted for additional detail.
Product Availability Otiprio: FDA approved December 2015; availability anticipated in the first quarter 2016. Otiprio is indicated for the treatment of pediatric patients with bilateral otitis media with effusion undergoing tympanostomy tube placement. Information pertaining to this product within the monograph is pending revision.
Dosage Forms Excipient information presented when available (limited, particularly for generics); consult specific product labeling.
Solution, Otic, as hydrochloride [preservative free]:
Cetraxal: 0.2% (1 ea)
Generic: 0.2% (1 ea)

Ciprofloxacin and Dexamethasone (sip roe FLOKS a sin & deks a METH a sone)

Brand Names: US Ciprodex
Brand Names: Canada Ciprodex
Index Terms Ciprofloxacin Hydrochloride and Dexamethasone; Dexamethasone and Ciprofloxacin
Pharmacologic Category Antibiotic, Otic; Antibiotic/Corticosteroid, Otic; Corticosteroid, Otic
Use
Acute otitis media: Treatment of acute otitis media in pediatric patients ≥6 months of age with tympanostomy tubes due to susceptible isolates of *Staphylococcus aureus*, *Streptococcus pneumoniae*, *Haemophilus influenza*, *Moraxella catarrhalis*, and *Pseudomonas aeruginosa*.
Acute otitis externa: Treatment of acute otitis externa in pediatric patients ≥6 months of age and adults due to susceptible isolates of *Staphylococcus aureus* and *Pseudomonas aeruginosa*.
Dosing
Adult & Geriatric Acute otitis externa: Otic: Instill 4 drops into affected ear(s) twice daily for 7 days
Pediatric
Acute otitis externa: Infants ≥6 months of age, Children, and Adolescents: Otic: Refer to adult dosing.
Acute otitis media in patients with tympanostomy tubes: Infants ≥6 months of age, Children, and Adolescents: Otic: Instill 4 drops into affected ear(s) twice daily for 7 days
Renal Impairment There are no dosage adjustments provided in the manufacturer's labeling.
Hepatic Impairment There are no dosage adjustments provided in the manufacturer's labeling.
Additional Information Complete prescribing information should be consulted for additional detail.
Dosage Forms Excipient information presented when available (limited, particularly for generics); consult specific product labeling.
Suspension, otic:
Ciprodex: Ciprofloxacin 0.3% and dexamethasone 0.1% (7.5 mL) [contains benzalkonium chloride]

Ciprofloxacin and Hydrocortisone (sip roe FLOKS a sin & hye droe KOR ti sone)

Brand Names: US Cipro® HC
Brand Names: Canada Cipro® HC
Index Terms Ciprofloxacin Hydrochloride and Hydrocortisone; Hydrocortisone and Ciprofloxacin
Pharmacologic Category Antibiotic, Otic; Antibiotic/Corticosteroid, Otic; Corticosteroid, Otic
Use Treatment of acute otitis externa, sometimes known as "swimmer's ear"
Dosing
Adult & Geriatric Otitis externa: Otic: The recommended dosage for all patients is three drops of the suspension in the affected ear twice daily for 7 days; twice-daily dosing schedule is more convenient for patients than that of existing treatments with hydrocortisone, which are typically administered 3 or 4 times a day; a twice-daily dosage schedule may be especially helpful for parents and caregivers of young children
Pediatric Children ≥1 year: Refer to adult dosing.
Renal Impairment No dosage adjustment provided in manufacturer's labeling.
Hepatic Impairment No dosage adjustment provided in manufacturer's labeling.
Additional Information Complete prescribing information should be consulted for additional detail.

Dosage Forms Excipient information presented when available (limited, particularly for generics); consult specific product labeling.

Suspension, otic:
Cipro® HC: Ciprofloxacin hydrochloride 0.2% and hydrocortisone 1% (10 mL) [contains benzyl alcohol]

Cisatracurium (sis a tra KYOO ree um)

Brand Names: US Nimbex

Brand Names: Canada Cisatracurium Besylate Injection; Cisatracurium Omega; Nimbex

Index Terms Cisatracurium Besylate

Pharmacologic Category Neuromuscular Blocker Agent, Nondepolarizing

Use Adjunct to general anesthesia to facilitate endotracheal intubation and to relax skeletal muscles during surgery; to facilitate mechanical ventilation in ICU patients; does not relieve pain or produce sedation

Pregnancy Considerations Adverse events have not been observed in animal reproduction studies.

Breast-Feeding Considerations It is not known if cisatracurium is excreted in breast milk. The manufacturer recommends that caution be exercised when administering cisatracurium to nursing women.

Contraindications Hypersensitivity to cisatracurium besylate or any component of the formulation; use of the 10 mL multiple-dose vials in premature infants (formulation contains benzyl alcohol)

Warnings/Precautions Maintenance of an adequate airway and respiratory support is critical; certain clinical conditions may result in potentiation or antagonism of neuromuscular blockade:

Antagonism: Respiratory alkalosis, hypercalcemia, demyelinating lesions, peripheral neuropathies, denervation, and muscle trauma

Potentiation: Electrolyte abnormalities (eg, severe hypocalcemia, severe hypokalemia, hypermagnesemia), neuromuscular diseases, metabolic acidosis, metabolic alkalosis, respiratory acidosis, Eaton-Lambert syndrome and myasthenia gravis

Hypothermia may slow Hoffmann elimination thereby prolonging the duration of activity (Greenberg, 2013). Resistance may occur in burn patients (≥20% of total body surface area), usually several days after the injury, and may persist for several months after wound healing. Resistance may occur in patients who are immobilized. Cross-sensitivity with other neuromuscular-blocking agents may occur; use extreme caution in patients with previous anaphylactic reactions to other neuromuscular-blocking agents. Bradycardia may be more common with cisatracurium than with other neuromuscular blocking agents since it has no clinically significant effects on heart rate to counteract the bradycardia produced by anesthetics. Use caution in the elderly. Should be administered by adequately trained individuals familiar with its use.

Benzyl alcohol and derivatives: Some dosage forms may contain benzyl alcohol; large amounts of benzyl alcohol (≥99 mg/kg/day) have been associated with a potentially fatal toxicity ("gasping syndrome") in neonates; the "gasping syndrome" consists of metabolic acidosis, respiratory distress, gasping respirations, CNS dysfunction (including convulsions, intracranial hemorrhage), hypotension and cardiovascular collapse (AAP ["Inactive" 1997]; CDC, 1982); some data suggests that benzoate displaces bilirubin from protein binding sites (Ahlfors, 2001); avoid or use dosage forms containing benzyl alcohol with caution in neonates. See manufacturer's labeling.

Adverse Reactions Effects are minimal and transient.

<1% (Limited to important or life-threatening): Bradycardia, bronchospasm, flushing, hypotension, muscle calcification (prolonged use), myopathy (acute quadriplegic syndrome; prolonged use), pruritus, skin rash

Drug Interactions

Metabolism/Transport Effects None known.

Avoid Concomitant Use

Avoid concomitant use of Cisatracurium with any of the following: QuiNINE

Increased Effect/Toxicity

Cisatracurium may increase the levels/effects of: Cardiac Glycosides; Corticosteroids (Systemic); OnabotulinumtoxinA; RimabotulinumtoxinB

The levels/effects of Cisatracurium may be increased by: AbobotulinumtoxinA; Aminoglycosides; Calcium Channel Blockers; Capreomycin; Clindamycin (Topical); Colistimethate; CycloSPORINE (Systemic); Fosphenytoin-Phenytoin; Inhalational Anesthetics; Ketorolac (Nasal); Ketorolac (Systemic); Lincosamide Antibiotics; Lithium; Loop Diuretics; Magnesium Salts; Minocycline; Polymyxin B; Procainamide; QuiNIDine; QuiNINE; Spironolactone; Tetracycline Derivatives; Vancomycin

Decreased Effect

The levels/effects of Cisatracurium may be decreased by: Acetylcholinesterase Inhibitors; Fosphenytoin-Phenytoin; Loop Diuretics

Storage/Stability Refrigerate intact vials at 2°C to 8°C (36°F to 46°F). Use vials within 21 days upon removal from the refrigerator to room temperature of 25°C (77°F). Per the manufacturer, dilutions of 0.1 mg/mL in 0.9% sodium chloride (NS), dextrose 5% in water (D5W), or D5NS are stable for up to 24 hours at room temperature or under refrigeration; dilutions of 0.1-0.2 mg/mL in D5LR are stable for up to 24 hours in the refrigerator. *Additional stability data:* Dilutions of 0.1, 2, and 5 mg/mL in D5W or NS are stable in the refrigerator for up to 30 days; at room temperature (23°C), dilutions of 0.1 and 2 mg/mL began exhibiting substantial drug loss between 7-14 days; dilutions of 5 mg/mL in D5W or NS are stable for up to 30 days at room temperature (23°C) (Xu, 1998). Usual concentration: 0.1-0.4 mg/mL.

Mechanism of Action Blocks neural transmission at the myoneural junction by binding with cholinergic receptor sites

Pharmacodynamics/Kinetics

Onset of action: IV: 2-3 minutes
Peak effect: 3-5 minutes

Duration: Dose dependent, 35 to 45 minutes after a single 0.1 mg/kg dose; recovery begins in 20-35 minutes when anesthesia is balanced; recovery is attained in 90% of patients in 25-93 minutes

Distribution: V_{dss}: 145 mL/kg (21% larger V_{dss} when receiving inhalational anesthetics)

Protein binding: Not studied due to rapid degradation at physiologic pH

Metabolism: Undergoes rapid nonenzymatic degradation in the bloodstream (Hofmann elimination) to laudanosine and inactive metabolites; laudanosine may cause CNS stimulation (association not established in humans) and has less accumulation with prolonged use than atracurium due to lower requirements for clinical effect

Half-life elimination: 22-29 minutes

Excretion: Urine (95%; <10% as unchanged drug); feces (4%)

Clearance: Children: 5.89 mL/kg/minute; Adults: 4.57 mL/kg/minute

Dosing

Adult & Geriatric Neuromuscular blockade: IV (not to be used IM):

Operating room administration:

Intubating dose: 0.15-0.2 mg/kg as components of propofol/nitrous oxide/oxygen induction-intubation technique. (**Note:** May produce generally good or excellent conditions for tracheal intubation in 1.5-2 minutes with clinically effective duration of action during propofol anesthesia of 55-61 minutes.) Initial dose after succinylcholine for intubation: 0.1 mg/kg; maintenance dose: 0.03 mg/kg 40-60 minutes after initial dose, then at ~20-minute intervals based on clinical criteria.

Continuous infusion: After an initial bolus, a diluted solution can be given by continuous infusion for maintenance of neuromuscular blockade during extended surgery; adjust the rate of administration according to the patient's response as determined by peripheral nerve stimulation. An initial infusion rate of 3 **mcg/kg/minute** (0.18 **mg/kg/hour**) may be required to rapidly counteract the spontaneous recovery of

neuromuscular function; thereafter, a rate of 1-2 mcg/kg/**minute** (0.06-0.12 **mg**/kg/**hour**) should be adequate to maintain continuous neuromuscular block in the 89% to 99% range in most pediatric and adult patients. Consider reduction of the infusion rate by 30% to 40% when administering during stable isoflurane, enflurane, sevoflurane, or desflurane anesthesia. Spontaneous recovery from neuromuscular blockade following discontinuation of infusion of cisatracurium may be expected to proceed at a rate comparable to that following single bolus administration.

Intensive care unit administration:
Manufacturer's labeling: Loading dose: 0.15-0.2 mcg/kg; at initial signs of recovery from bolus dose, begin the infusion at a dose of 3 mcg/kg/**minute** (0.18 **mg**/kg/**hour**) and adjust rate accordingly (follow the principles for infusion in the operating room); dosage ranges of 0.5-10 mcg/kg/**minute** (0.03-0.6 **mg**/kg/**hour**) have been reported. If patient is allowed to recover from neuromuscular blockade, readministration of a bolus dose may be necessary to quickly re-establish neuromuscular block prior to reinstituting the infusion.
or
Loading dose: 0.1 mg/kg (additional boluses of 0.05 mg/kg until train-of-four response is ³/₄ or less can be used); then initiate an infusion at 2.5-3 mcg/kg/**minute** (0.15-0.18 **mg**/kg/**hour**) and adjust rate accordingly (Baumann, 2004; Lagneau, 2002).
or
Loading dose: 0.1 to 0.2 mg/kg; immediately following loading dose administration, begin an infusion at 1-3 mcg/kg/**minute** (0.06-0.18 **mg**/kg/**hour**) and adjust rate accordingly (Greenberg, 2013).

Pediatric Neuromuscular blockade: IV (not to be used IM):
Operating room administration:
Infants 1-23 months: *Intubating dose:* 0.15 mg/kg over 5-10 seconds
Children 2-12 years: *Intubating dose:* 0.1-0.15 mg/kg over 5-10 seconds (**Note:** When given during stable opioid/nitrous oxide/oxygen anesthesia, 0.1 mg/kg produces maximum neuromuscular block in an average of 2.8 minutes and clinically effective block for 28 minutes.)
Children ≥2 years: *Continuous infusion:* Refer to adult dosing.
Intensive care unit administration: Refer to adult dosing.

Renal Impairment Because slower times to onset of complete neuromuscular block were observed in renal dysfunction patients, extending the interval between the administration of cisatracurium and intubation attempt may be required to achieve adequate intubation conditions.

Hepatic Impairment No dosage adjustment provided in manufacturer's labeling. The time to onset of action was ~1 minute faster in patients with end-stage liver disease, but was not associated with clinically significant changes in recovery time.

Usual Infusion Concentrations: Adult IV infusion: 100 mg in 250 mL (total volume) (concentration: 400 mcg/mL) of D₅W or NS

Administration Administer IV only; give undiluted as bolus injection over 5-10 seconds. Continuous infusion requires the use of an infusion pump. The use of a peripheral nerve stimulator will permit the most advantageous use of cisatracurium, minimize the possibility of overdosage or underdosage and assist in the evaluation of recovery.

Do not administer IM (excessive tissue irritation).

Monitoring Parameters Peripheral nerve stimulator measuring twitch response (when appropriate); vital signs (heart rate, blood pressure, respiratory rate)

Additional Information Cisatracurium is classified as an intermediate-duration neuromuscular-blocking agent. It does not appear to have a cumulative effect on the duration of blockade. Neuromuscular-blocking potency is 3 times that of atracurium; maximum block is up to 2 minutes longer than for equipotent doses of atracurium.

Dosage Forms Excipient information presented when available (limited, particularly for generics); consult specific product labeling.
Solution, Intravenous:
Nimbex: 10 mg/5 mL (5 mL)
Nimbex: 20 mg/10 mL (10 mL) [contains benzyl alcohol]
Nimbex: 10 mg/mL (20 mL)
Generic: 20 mg/10 mL (10 mL)
Solution, Intravenous [preservative free]:
Generic: 10 mg/5 mL (5 mL); 10 mg/mL (20 mL)

◆ Cisatracurium Besylate *see* Cisatracurium *on page 394*
◆ Cisatracurium Besylate Injection (Can) *see* Cisatracurium *on page 394*

◆ Cisatracurium Omega (Can) *see* Cisatracurium *on page 394*
◆ cis-DDP *see* CISplatin *on page 395*
◆ cis-Diamminedichloroplatinum *see* CISplatin *on page 395*

CISplatin (SIS pla tin)

Brand Names: Canada Cisplatin Injection; Cisplatin Injection BP; Cisplatin Injection, Mylan STD
Index Terms CDDP; cis-DDP; cis-Diamminedichloroplatinum; cis-platinum; DDP; Platinol; Platinol-AQ
Pharmacologic Category Antineoplastic Agent, Alkylating Agent; Antineoplastic Agent, Platinum Analog
Use
Bladder cancer, advanced: Treatment (as a single agent) of advanced bladder cancer (transitional cell) in patients who are no longer candidates for local therapy including surgery and/or radiation therapy
Ovarian cancer, metastatic: Treatment of metastatic ovarian cancer (in combination with other chemotherapy agents) in patients who have previously received appropriate surgery and/or radiation therapy, or as a single agent for refractory tumors in patients who have not previously received cisplatin
Testicular cancer, metastatic: Treatment of metastatic testicular cancer (in combination with other chemotherapy agents) in patients who have previously received appropriate surgery and/or radiation therapy
Pregnancy Considerations Adverse effects have been observed in animal reproduction studies. Women of childbearing potential should be advised to avoid pregnancy during treatment. May case fetal harm if administered during pregnancy.
Breast-Feeding Considerations Cisplatin is excreted in breast milk. Breast-feeding is not recommended by the manufacturer.
Contraindications History of allergic reactions to cisplatin, other platinum-containing compounds, or any component of the formulation; preexisting renal impairment; myelosuppressed patients; hearing impairment
Warnings/Precautions Hazardous agent - use appropriate precautions for handling and disposal (NIOSH 2014 [group 1]). **[US Boxed Warning]: Doses >100 mg/m²/cycle (once every 3 to 4 weeks) are rare; verify with the prescriber.** Exercise caution to avoid inadvertent overdose due to potential sound-alike/look-alike confusion between CISplatin and CARBOplatin or prescribing practices that fail to differentiate daily doses from the total dose per cycle. At the approved dose, cisplatin should not be administered more frequently than once every 3 to 4 weeks. Patients should receive adequate hydration, with or without diuretics, prior to and for 24 hours after cisplatin administration. **[US Boxed Warning]: Cumulative renal toxicity associated with cisplatin is severe.** Monitor serum creatinine, blood urea nitrogen, creatinine clearance, and serum electrolytes (calcium, magnesium, potassium, and sodium) closely. According to the manufacturer's labeling, use is contraindicated in patients with preexisting renal impairment and renal function must return to normal prior to administering subsequent cycles; some literature recommends reduced doses with renal impairment. Nephrotoxicity may be potentiated by aminoglycosides.

Use caution in the elderly; may cause or exacerbate syndrome of inappropriate antidiuretic hormone secretion or hyponatremia; monitor sodium closely with initiation or dosage adjustments in older adults (Beers Criteria). Elderly patients may be more susceptible to nephrotoxicity and peripheral neuropathy; select dose cautiously and monitor closely.

[US Boxed Warning]: Dose-related toxicities include myelosuppression, nausea, and vomiting. Cisplatin is associated with a high emetic potential; antiemetics are recommended to prevent nausea and vomiting (Basch, 2011; Dupuis, 2011; Roila, 2010). Nausea and vomiting are dose-related and may be immediate and/or delayed. Diarrhea may also occur. **[US Boxed Warning]: Ototoxicity, which may be more pronounced in children, is manifested by tinnitus and/or loss of high frequency hearing and occasionally, deafness; may be significant.** Ototoxicity is cumulative and may be severe. Audiometric testing should be performed at baseline and prior to each dose. Certain genetic variations in the thiopurine S-methyltransferase (TPMT) gene may be associated with an increased risk of ototoxicity in children administered conventional cisplatin doses (Pussegoda, 2013). Controversy may exist regarding the role of TPMT variants in cisplatin ototoxicity (Ratain, 2013; Yang, 2013); the association has not been consistent across populations and

studies. Children without the TPMT gene variants may still be at risk for ototoxicity. Cumulative dose, prior or concurrent exposure to other ototoxic agents (eg, aminoglycosides, carboplatin), prior cranial radiation, younger age, and type of cancer may also increase the risk for ototoxicity in children (Knight, 2005; Landier, 2014). Pediatric patients should receive audiometric testing at baseline, prior to each dose, and for several years after discontinuing therapy. An international grading scale (SIOP Boston scale) has been developed to assess ototoxicity in children (Brock, 2012). Severe (and possibly irreversible) neuropathies (including stocking-glove paresthesias, areflexia, and loss of proprioception/vibratory sensation) may occur with higher than recommended doses or more frequent administration; may require therapy discontinuation. Seizures, loss of motor function, loss of taste, leukoencephalopathy, and posterior reversible leukoencephalopathy syndrome (PRES [formerly RPLS]) have also been described. Serum electrolytes, particularly magnesium and potassium, should be monitored and replaced as needed during and after cisplatin therapy.

[US Boxed Warning]: Anaphylactic-like reactions have been reported; may include facial edema, bronchoconstriction, tachycardia, and hypotension and may occur within minutes of administration; symptoms may be managed with epinephrine, corticosteroids, and/or antihistamines. Hyperuricemia has been reported with cisplatin use, and is more pronounced with doses >50 mg/m^2; consider antihyperuricemic therapy to reduce uric acid levels. Local infusion site reactions may occur; monitor infusion site during administration; avoid extravasation. Secondary malignancies have been reported with cisplatin in combination with other chemotherapy agents. Potentially significant drug-drug interactions may exist, requiring dose or frequency adjustment, additional monitoring, and/or selection of alternative therapy. [US Boxed Warning]: Should be administered under the supervision of an experienced cancer chemotherapy physician. Adequate diagnostic and treatment facilities and appropriate management of potential complications should be readily available. Cisplatin is a vesicant at higher concentrations, and an irritant at lower concentrations; ensure proper needle or catheter placement prior to and during infusion; avoid extravasation. Local infusion site reactions may occur; monitor infusion site during administration.

Adverse Reactions

>10%:
Central nervous system: Neurotoxicity (peripheral neuropathy is dose and duration dependent)
Gastrointestinal: Nausea and vomiting (76% to 100%)
Genitourinary: Nephrotoxicity (28% to 36%; acute renal failure and chronic renal insufficiency)
Hematologic & oncologic: Anemia (≤40%), leukopenia (25% to 30%; nadir: Day 18 to 23; recovery: By day 39; dose related), thrombocytopenia (25% to 30%; nadir: Day 18 to 23; recovery: By day 39; dose related)
Hepatic: Increased liver enzymes
Otic: Ototoxicity (children 40% to 60%; adults 10% to 31%; as tinnitus, high frequency hearing loss)
1% to 10%: Local: Local irritation
<1% (Limited to important or life-threatening): Alopecia (mild), ageusia, anaphylaxis, aortic thrombosis (Fernandes, 2011), autonomic neuropathy, bradycardia (Schlumbrecht, 2015), cardiac arrhythmia, cardiac failure, cerebrovascular accident, extravasation, hemolytic anemia (acute), hemolytic-uremic syndrome, hiccups, hypercholesterolemia, hyperuricemia, hypocalcemia, hypokalemia, hypomagnesemia, hyponatremia, hypophosphatemia, increased serum amylase, leukoencephalopathy, myocardial infarction, neutropenic enterocolitis (Furonaka, 2005), optic neuritis, pancreatitis (Trivedi, 2005), papilledema, peripheral ischemia (acute), phlebitis (Tokuda, 2014), SIADH, tachycardia, thrombotic thrombocytopenic purpura

Drug Interactions

Metabolism/Transport Effects None known.

Avoid Concomitant Use
Avoid concomitant use of CISplatin with any of the following: BCG (Intravesical); Deferiprone; Dipyrone; Natalizumab; Pimecrolimus; Tacrolimus (Topical); Tofacitinib; Vaccines (Live)

Increased Effect/Toxicity
CISplatin may increase the levels/effects of: Aminoglycosides; CloZAPine; Deferiprone; Fingolimod; Leflunomide; Natalizumab; Taxane Derivatives; Tofacitinib; Topotecan; Vaccines (Live); Vinorelbine

The levels/effects of CISplatin may be increased by: Denosumab; Dipyrone; Loop Diuretics; Pimecrolimus; Roflumilast; Tacrolimus (Topical); Trastuzumab

Decreased Effect
CISplatin may decrease the levels/effects of: BCG (Intravesical); Coccidioides immitis Skin Test; Fosphenytoin-Phenytoin; Sipuleucel-T; Vaccines (Inactivated); Vaccines (Live)

The levels/effects of CISplatin may be decreased by: Alpha-Lipoic Acid; Echinacea

Preparation for Administration Hazardous agent; use appropriate precautions for handling and disposal (NIOSH 2014 [group 1]). Must be diluted prior to infusion; dilute in NS, D$_5$/0.45% NaCl or D$_5$/NS to a concentration of 0.05 to 2 mg/mL. The infusion solution should have a final sodium chloride concentration ≥0.2%. Do **NOT** dilute in D$_5$W. Needles or IV administration sets that contain aluminum should not be used in the preparation or administration; aluminum can react with cisplatin resulting in precipitate formation and loss of potency.

Storage/Stability Store intact vials at 15°C to 25°C (59°F to 77°F). Protect from light. Do not refrigerate solution (precipitate may form). Further dilution **stability is dependent on the chloride ion concentration** and should be mixed in solutions of NS (at least 0.3% NaCl). According to the manufacturer, after initial entry into the vial, solution is stable for 28 days protected from light or for at least 7 days under fluorescent room light at room temperature.
Further dilutions in NS, D$_5$/0.45% NaCl or D$_5$/NS to a concentration of 0.05 to 2 mg/mL are stable for 72 hours at 4°C to 25°C.

Mechanism of Action Inhibits DNA synthesis by the formation of DNA cross-links; denatures the double helix; covalently binds to DNA bases and disrupts DNA function; may also bind to proteins; the cis-isomer is 14 times more cytotoxic than the trans-isomer; both forms cross-link DNA but cis-platinum is less easily recognized by cell enzymes and, therefore, not repaired. Cisplatin can also bind two adjacent guanines on the same strand of DNA producing intrastrand cross-linking and breakage.

Pharmacodynamics/Kinetics

Distribution: IV: Rapidly into tissue; high concentrations in kidneys, liver, ovaries, uterus, and lungs
Protein binding: >90% (O'Dwyer 2000)
Metabolism: Nonenzymatic; inactivated (in both cell and bloodstream) by sulfhydryl groups; covalently binds to glutathione and thiosulfate
Half-life elimination:
Children: Free drug: 1.3 hours; Total platinum: 44 hours
Adults: Initial: 14 to 49 minutes; Beta: 0.7 to 4.6 hours; Gamma: 24 to 127 hours (O'Dwyer 2000)
Excretion: Urine (>90%); feces (minimal)

Dosing

Adult VERIFY ANY CISPLATIN DOSE EXCEEDING 100 mg/m^2 PER COURSE. Pretreatment hydration with 1 to 2 L of IV fluid is recommended. Cisplatin is associated with a high emetic potential; antiemetics are recommended to prevent nausea and vomiting (Basch 2011; Roila 2010).

Bladder cancer, advanced: IV: 50 to 70 mg/m^2 every 3 to 4 weeks; heavily pretreated patients: 50 mg/m^2 every 4 weeks

Ovarian cancer, metastatic: IV:
Single agent: 100 mg/m^2 every 4 weeks
Combination therapy: 75 to 100 mg/m^2 every 4 weeks or (off-label dosing) 75 mg/m^2 every 3 weeks (Ozols 2003)
Intraperitoneal (off-label route): 100 mg/m^2 on day 2 of a 21-day treatment cycle (in combination with IV and intraperitoneal paclitaxel) for 6 cycles (Armstrong 2006)

Testicular cancer, metastatic: IV: 20 mg/m^2/day for 5 days repeated every 3 weeks (in combination with bleomycin and etoposide) (Cushing 2004; Saxman 1998)
Testicular germ cell tumor, malignant (off-label dosing): IV: 25 mg/m^2 on days 2 to 5 every 3 weeks (in combination with paclitaxel and ifosfamide) for 4 cycles (Kondagunta 2005) or 20 mg/m^2 on days 1 to 5 every 3 weeks (in combination with bleomycin and etoposide) for 4 cycles (Nichols 1998) or 20 mg/m^2 on days 1 to 5 every 3 weeks (in combination with etoposide and ifosfamide) for 4 cycles (Nichols 1998)

Breast cancer, triple-negative (off-label use): IV: Neoadjuvant therapy (single agent): 75 mg/m^2 on day 1 every 3 weeks for 4 cycles (Silver 2010). Additional data may be necessary to further define the role of cisplatin in this setting.

Cervical cancer (off-label use): IV: 75 mg/m^2 on day 1 every 3 weeks (in combination with fluorouracil and radiation) for 3 cycles (Morris 1999) **or** 70 mg/m^2 on day 1 every 3 weeks for 4 cycles (in combination with fluorouracil; cycles 1 and 2 given concurrently with radiation) (Peters 2000) **or** 50 mg/m^2 on day 1 every 4 weeks (in combination with radiation and fluorouracil) for 2 cycles (Whitney 1999)

Endometrial carcinoma, recurrent, metastatic, or high-risk (off-label use): IV: 50 mg/m^2 on day 1 every 3 weeks (in combination with doxorubicin ± paclitaxel) for 7 cycles or until disease progression or unacceptable toxicity (Fleming 2004)

Esophageal and gastric cancers (off-label uses): IV:
CF regimen: 100 mg/m^2 over 30 minutes on days 1 and 29 (preoperative chemoradiation; in combination with fluorouracil) (Tepper 2008)

ECF, ECX regimens: 60 mg/m^2 on day 1 every 21 days for up to 8 cycles in combination with epirubicin (E) and either fluorouracil (F) or capecitabine (X) (Cunningham 2008) **or**

ECF regimen: 60 mg/m^2 on day 1 every 21 days for 3 preoperative and 3 postoperative cycles in combination with epirubicin and fluorouracil (Cunningham 2006)

TCF or DCF regimen: 75 mg/m^2 on day 1 every 3 weeks (in combination with docetaxel and fluorouracil) until disease progression or unacceptable toxicity (Ajani 2007; Van Cutsem 2006)

Head and neck cancer (off-label use): IV:
Locally-advanced disease: 100 mg/m^2 every 3 weeks for 3 doses (with concurrent radiation) (Bernier 2004; Cooper 2004) **or** 75 mg/m^2 every 3 weeks (in combination with docetaxel and fluorouracil) for 4 cycles or until disease progression or unacceptable toxicity (if no disease progression after 4 cycles, chemotherapy was followed by radiation) (Vermorken 2007) **or** 100 mg/m^2 every 3 weeks (in combination with docetaxel and fluorouracil) for 3 cycles or until disease progression or unacceptable toxicity (chemotherapy was followed by chemoradiation) (Posner 2007)

Metastatic disease: 100 mg/m^2 every 3 weeks (in combination with fluorouracil and cetuximab) until disease progression or unacceptable toxicity or a maximum of 6 cycles (Vermorken 2008)

Hodgkin lymphoma, relapsed/refractory (off-label use): IV:
DHAP regimen: 100 mg/m^2 continuous infusion over 24 hours on day 1 for 2 cycles; median duration between cycle 1 and 2 was 16 days (in combination with dexamethasone and cytarabine) (Josting 2002)

ESHAP regimen: 25 mg/m^2/day on days 1 to 4 (in combination with etoposide, methylprednisolone, and cytarabine) every 3 to 4 weeks for 3 or 6 cycles (Aparicio 1999)

Malignant pleural mesothelioma (off-label use): IV: 75 mg/m^2 on day 1 of each 21-day cycle (in combination with pemetrexed) (Vogelzang 2003) **or** 100 mg/m^2 on day 1 of a 28-day cycle (in combination with gemcitabine) (Nowak 2002) **or** 80 mg/m^2 on day 1 of a 21-day cycle (in combination with gemcitabine) (van Haarst 2002)

Multiple myeloma (off-label use): IV: VDT-PACE regimen: 10 mg/m^2/day administered as a continuous infusion on days 1 to 4 of each cycle; repeat every 4 to 6 weeks (in combination with bortezomib, dexamethasone, thalidomide, doxorubicin, cyclophosphamide, and etoposide) (Lee 2003; Pineda-Roman 2008)

Non-Hodgkin lymphoma, relapsed/refractory: IV:
DHAP regimen: 100 mg/m^2 continuous infusion over 24 hours on day 1 every 3 to 4 weeks for 6 to 10 cycles (in combination with dexamethasone and cytarabine) (Velasquez 1988)

ESHAP regimen: 25 mg/m^2/day continuous infusion over 24 hours on days 1 to 4 every 3 to 4 weeks for 6 to 8 cycles (in combination with etoposide, methylprednisolone, and cytarabine) (Velasquez 1994)

Non-small cell lung cancer (NSCLC; off-label use): IV:
Note: There are multiple cisplatin-containing regimens for the treatment of NSCLC. Listed below are several commonly used regimens:

100 mg/m^2 on day 1 every 4 weeks (in combination with etoposide) for 3 to 4 cycles; (Arriagada 2007), or

100 mg/m^2 on day 1 every 4 weeks (in combination with vinorelbine) (Kelly 2001; Wozniak 1998), or

100 mg/m^2 on day 1 every 4 weeks (in combination with gemcitabine) (Comella 2000), or

80 mg/m^2 on day 1 every 3 weeks (in combination with gemcitabine) (Ohe 2007), or

75 mg/m^2 on day 1 every 3 weeks (in combination with pemetrexed) for up to 6 cycles or until disease progression or unacceptable toxicity (Scagliotti 2008)

Osteosarcoma (off-label use; combination chemotherapy): Adults <30 years: IV: 60 mg/m^2/day for 2 days on weeks 2, 7, 25, and 28 (neoadjuvant) or weeks 5, 10, 25, and 28 (adjuvant) in combination with methotrexate, leucovorin, doxorubicin, cyclophosphamide, bleomycin, and dactinomycin (Goorin 2003)

Penile cancer, metastatic (off-label use): IV: 25 mg/m^2 over 2 hours on days 1, 2, and 3 every 3 to 4 weeks (in combination with paclitaxel and ifosfamide) for 4 cycles (Pagliaro 2010)

Small cell lung cancer (SCLC; off-label use): IV:
Limited-stage disease: 60 mg/m^2 on day 1 every 3 weeks for 4 cycles (in combination with etoposide and concurrent radiation) (Turrisi 1999)

Extensive-stage disease: 80 mg/m^2 on day 1 every 3 weeks (in combination with etoposide) for 4 cycles (Lara 2009) or a maximum of 8 cycles (Ihde 1994) **or** 60 mg/m^2 on day 1 every 4 weeks for 4 cycles (in combination with irinotecan) (Lara 2009)

Geriatric Refer to adult dosing. Select dose cautiously and monitor closely in the elderly; may be more susceptible to nephrotoxicity and peripheral neuropathy.

Pediatric VERIFY ANY CISPLATIN DOSE EXCEEDING **100 mg/m^2 PER COURSE.** Pretreatment hydration is recommended. Cisplatin is associated with a high emetic potential; antiemetics are recommended to prevent nausea and vomiting (Dupuis 2011).

Germ cell tumors (off-label use; combination chemotherapy): IV: 20 mg/m^2/day on days 1 to 5 or 100 mg/m^2 on day 1 of a 21-day treatment cycle (Pinkerton 1986)

Hepatoblastoma (off-label use; combination chemotherapy): IV: 80 mg/m^2 continuous infusion over 24 hours on day 1 of a 21-day treatment cycle (Pritchard 2000)

Medulloblastoma (off-label use; combination chemotherapy): IV: 75 mg/m^2 on either day 0 or day 1 of each chemotherapy cycle (Packer 2006)

Neuroblastoma, high-risk (off-label use; combination chemotherapy): IV: 50 mg/m^2/day on days 0 to 3 of a 21-day cycle (cycles 3 and 5) (Naranjo 2011) **or** 50 mg/m^2/day on days 1 to 4 (cycles 3, 5, and 7) (Kushner 1994)

Osteosarcoma (off-label use; combination chemotherapy): IV: 60 mg/m^2/day for 2 days on weeks 2, 7, 25, and 28 (neoadjuvant) or weeks 5, 10, 25, and 28 (adjuvant) in combination with methotrexate, leucovorin, doxorubicin, cyclophosphamide, bleomycin, and dactinomycin (Goorin 2003)

Renal Impairment Note: The manufacturer(s) recommend that repeat courses of cisplatin should not be given until serum creatinine is <1.5 mg/dL and/or BUN is <25 mg/dL and use is contraindicated in preexisting renal impairment. The following adjustments have been recommended.

Aronoff 2007:
CrCl 10 to 50 mL/minute: Administer 75% of dose
CrCl <10 mL/minute: Administer 50% of dose
Hemodialysis: Partially cleared by hemodialysis
  Administer 50% of dose posthemodialysis
  Continuous ambulatory peritoneal dialysis (CAPD): Administer 50% of dose
  Continuous renal replacement therapy (CRRT): Administer 75% of dose
Janus 2010: Hemodialysis: Reduce initial dose by 50%; administer post hemodialysis or on nondialysis days.
Kintzel 1995:
CrCl 46 to 60 mL/minute: Administer 75% of dose
CrCl 31 to 45 mL/minute: Administer 50% of dose
CrCl <30 mL/minute: Consider use of alternative drug

Hepatic Impairment There are no dosage adjustments provided in the manufacturer's labeling. However, cisplatin undergoes nonenzymatic metabolism and predominantly renal elimination; therefore, dosage adjustment is likely not necessary.

Obesity *ASCO Guidelines for appropriate chemotherapy dosing in obese adults with cancer:* Utilize patient's actual body weight (full weight) for calculation of body surface area- or weight-based dosing, particularly when the intent of therapy is curative; manage regimen-related toxicities in the same manner as for nonobese patients; if a dose reduction is utilized due to toxicity, consider resumption of full weight-based dosing with subsequent cycles, especially if cause of toxicity (eg, hepatic or renal impairment) is resolved (Griggs 2012).

Dietary Considerations Some products may contain sodium.

Administration Cisplatin is associated with a high emetic potential; antiemetics are recommended to prevent nausea and vomiting (Basch 2011; Dupuis 2011; Roila 2010). Pretreatment hydration with 1 to 2 L of fluid is recommended prior to cisplatin administration; adequate post

hydration and urinary output (>100 mL/hour) should be maintained for 24 hours after administration.

IV: Infuse over 6 to 8 hours (according to the manufacturer's labeling); has also been infused (off-label rates) over 30 minutes to 3 hours, at a rate of 1 mg/minute, or as a continuous infusion; infusion rate varies by protocol (refer to specific protocol for infusion details). Do not administer as a rapid IV injection. Also refer to specific protocol for information regarding recommended concomitant hydration and diuretics.

Intraperitoneal (off-label route): Solution was prepared in warmed saline and infused as rapidly as possible through an implantable intraperitoneal catheter (Armstrong 2006).

Needles or IV administration sets that contain aluminum should not be used in the preparation or administration; aluminum may react with cisplatin resulting in precipitate formation and loss of potency.

Vesicant (at higher concentrations); ensure proper needle or catheter placement prior to and during infusion; avoid extravasation.

Extravasation management: If extravasation occurs, stop infusion immediately and disconnect (leave cannula/needle in place); gently aspirate extravasated solution (do **NOT** flush the line); initiate sodium thiosulfate antidote; elevate extremity.

Sodium thiosulfate 1/6 M solution: Inject 2 mL into existing IV line for each 100 mg of cisplatin extravasated; then consider also injecting 1 mL as 0.1 mL subcutaneous injections (clockwise) around the area of extravasation, may repeat subcutaneous injections several times over the next 3 to 4 hours (Ener 2004).

Dimethyl sulfoxide (DMSO) may also be considered an option: Apply to a region covering twice the affected area every 8 hours for 7 days; begin within 10 minutes of extravasation; do not cover with a dressing (Perez Fidalgo 2012).

Hazardous agent; use appropriate precautions for handling and disposal (NIOSH 2014 [group 1]).

Monitoring Parameters Renal function (serum creatinine, BUN, CrCl [baseline and before each cycle]); electrolytes (particularly calcium, magnesium, potassium, and sodium [baseline and before each cycle]); CBC with differential and platelet count (weekly); liver function tests (periodic); urine output, urinalysis; audiography (baseline and prior to each subsequent dose, and following treatment in children), neurologic exam (with high dose); monitor infusion site during infusion

Dosage Forms Excipient information presented when available (limited, particularly for generics); consult specific product labeling.

Solution, Intravenous:
  Generic: 50 mg/50 mL (50 mL); 100 mg/100 mL (100 mL)
Solution, Intravenous [preservative free]:
  Generic: 50 mg/50 mL (50 mL); 100 mg/100 mL (100 mL); 200 mg/200 mL (200 mL)

◆ Cisplatin Injection (Can) *see* CISplatin *on page 395*
◆ Cisplatin Injection BP (Can) *see* CISplatin *on page 395*
◆ Cisplatin Injection, Mylan STD (Can) *see* CISplatin *on page 395*
◆ cis-platinum *see* CISplatin *on page 395*
◆ *Cis*-Retinoic Acid *see* ISOtretinoin *on page 996*
◆ 13-*cis*-Retinoic Acid *see* ISOtretinoin *on page 996*
◆ 13-*cis*-Vitamin A Acid *see* ISOtretinoin *on page 996*

Citalopram (sye TAL oh pram)

Brand Names: US CeleXA

Brand Names: Canada Abbott-Citalopram; Accell-Citalopram; ACT Citalopram; AG-Citalopram; Apo-Citalopram; Auro-Citalopram; Celexa; Citalopram-Odan; CTP 30; Dom-Citalopram; ECL-Citalopram; JAMP-Citalopram; Mar-Citalopram; Mint-Citalopram; Mylan-Citalopram; Nat-Citalopram; PHL-Citalopram; PMS-Citalopram; Q-Citalopram; RAN-Citalo; Riva-Citalopram; Sandoz-Citalopram; Septa-Citalopram; Teva-Citalopram

Index Terms Citalopram Hydrobromide; Nitalapram

Pharmacologic Category Antidepressant, Selective Serotonin Reuptake Inhibitor

Use Treatment of depression

Pregnancy Considerations Adverse events have been observed in animal reproduction studies. Citalopram and its metabolites cross the human placenta. An increased risk of teratogenic effects, including cardiovascular defects, may be associated with maternal use of citalopram or other SSRIs; however, available information is conflicting. Nonteratogenic effects in the newborn following SSRI/SNRI exposure late in the third trimester include respiratory distress, cyanosis, apnea, seizures, temperature instability, feeding difficulty, vomiting, hypoglycemia, hypo- or hypertonia, hyper-reflexia, jitteriness, irritability, constant crying, and tremor. Symptoms may be due to the toxicity of the SSRIs/SNRIs or a discontinuation syndrome and may be consistent with serotonin syndrome associated with SSRI treatment. Persistent pulmonary hypertension of the newborn (PPHN) has also been reported with SSRI exposure. The long-term effects of *in utero* SSRI exposure on infant development and behavior are not known.

Due to pregnancy-induced physiologic changes, women who are pregnant may require adjusted doses of citalopram to achieve euthymia. The ACOG recommends that therapy with SSRIs or SNRIs during pregnancy be individualized; treatment of depression during pregnancy should incorporate the clinical expertise of the mental health clinician, obstetrician, primary healthcare provider, and pediatrician. According to the American Psychiatric Association (APA), the risks of medication treatment should be weighed against other treatment options and untreated depression. For women who discontinue antidepressant medications during pregnancy and who may be at high risk for postpartum depression, the medications can be restarted following delivery. Treatment algorithms have been developed by the ACOG and the APA for the management of depression in women prior to conception and during pregnancy.

Breast-Feeding Considerations Citalopram and its metabolites are excreted in breast milk. According to the manufacturer, the decision to continue or discontinue breast-feeding during therapy should take into account the risk of exposure to the infant and the benefits of treatment to the mother. Excessive somnolence, decreased feeding, colic, irritability, restlessness, and weight loss have been reported in breast-fed infants. The long-term effects on development and behavior have not been studied; therefore, citalopram should be prescribed to a mother who is breast-feeding only when the benefits outweigh the potential risks. Maternal use of an SSRI during pregnancy may cause delayed milk secretion.

Medication Guide Available Yes

Contraindications

Hypersensitivity to citalopram or any component of the formulation; use of MAO inhibitors intended to treat psychiatric disorders (concurrently or within 14 days of discontinuing either citalopram or the MAO inhibitor); initiation of citalopram in a patient receiving linezolid or intravenous methylene blue; concomitant use with pimozide

Canadian labeling: Additional contraindications (not in US labeling): Known QT interval prolongation or congenital long QT syndrome

Warnings/Precautions [US Boxed Warning]: Antidepressants increase the risk of suicidal thinking and behavior in children, adolescents, and young adults (18 to 24 years of age) with major depressive disorder (MDD) and other psychiatric disorders; consider risk prior to prescribing. Short-term studies did not show an increased risk in patients >24 years of age and showed a decreased risk in patients ≥65 years. Closely monitor patients for clinical worsening, suicidality, or unusual changes in behavior, particularly during the initial 1-2 months of therapy or during periods of dosage adjustments (increases or decreases); the patient's family or caregiver should be instructed to closely observe the patient and communicate condition with healthcare provider. A medication guide concerning the use of antidepressants should be dispensed with each prescription. **Citalopram is not FDA approved for use in children.**

The possibility of a suicide attempt is inherent in major depression and may persist until remission occurs. Use caution in high-risk patients. Worsening depression and severe abrupt suicidality that are not part of the presenting symptoms may require discontinuation or modification of drug therapy. The patient's family or caregiver should be alerted to monitor patients for the emergence of suicidality and associated behaviors (such as agitation, irritability, hostility, impulsivity, and hypomania) and call healthcare provider.

May worsen psychosis in some patients or precipitate a shift to mania or hypomania in patients with bipolar disorder. Patients presenting with depressive symptoms should be screened for bipolar disorder. Monotherapy in patients with bipolar disorder should be avoided. **Citalopram is not FDA approved for the treatment of bipolar depression.**

Potentially life-threatening serotonin syndrome (SS) has occurred with serotonergic agents (eg, SSRIs, SNRIs), particularly when used in combination with other serotonergic agents (eg, triptans, TCAs, fentanyl, lithium,

tramadol, buspirone, St. John's wort, tryptophan) or agents that impair metabolism of serotonin (eg, MAO inhibitors intended to treat psychiatric disorders, other MAO inhibitors [ie, linezolid and intravenous methylene blue]). Discontinue treatment (and any concomitant serotonergic agent) immediately if signs/symptoms arise. May increase the risks associated with electroconvulsive therapy. Has a low potential to impair cognitive or motor performance; caution operating hazardous machinery or driving. Bone fractures have been associated with antidepressant treatment. Consider the possibility of a fragility fracture if an antidepressant-treated patient presents with unexplained bone pain, point tenderness, swelling, or bruising (Rabenda 2013; Rizzoli 2012).

Citalopram causes dose-dependent QTc prolongation; torsade de pointes, ventricular tachycardia, and sudden death have been reported. Use is not recommended in patients with congenital long QT syndrome, bradycardia, recent MI, uncompensated heart failure, hypokalemia, and/or hypomagnesemia, or patients receiving concomitant medications which prolong the QT interval; if use is essential and cannot be avoided in these patients, ECG monitoring is recommended. Discontinue therapy in any patient with persistent QTc measurements >500 msec. Serum electrolytes, particularly potassium and magnesium, should be monitored prior to initiation and periodically during therapy in any patient at increased risk for significant electrolyte disturbances; hypokalemia and/or hypomagnesemia should be corrected prior to use. Due to the QT prolongation risk, doses >40 mg/day are not recommended. Additionally, the maximum daily dose should not exceed 20 mg/day in certain populations (eg, CYP2C19 poor metabolizers, patients with hepatic impairment, elderly patients). Potentially significant interactions may exist, requiring dose or frequency adjustment, additional monitoring, and/or selection of alternative therapy. Consult drug interactions database for more detailed information.

Use with caution in patients with a previous seizure disorder or condition predisposing to seizures such as brain damage or alcoholism. May cause or exacerbate sexual dysfunction. Use caution in elderly patients; may be potentially inappropriate in patients with a history of falls or fractures, and may cause hyponatremia/SIADH (elderly at increased risk); volume depletion and diuretics may increase risk. Monitor sodium closely with initiation or dosage adjustments in older adults (Beers Criteria). May cause mild pupillary dilation which in susceptible individuals can lead to an episode of narrow-angle glaucoma. Consider evaluating patients who have not had an iridectomy for narrow-angle glaucoma risk factors. Citalopram is not FDA-approved for use in children; however, if used, monitor weight and growth regularly during therapy due to the potential for decreased appetite and weight loss with SSRI use.

Abrupt discontinuation or interruption of antidepressant therapy has been associated with a discontinuation syndrome. Symptoms arising may vary with antidepressant however commonly include nausea, vomiting, diarrhea, headaches, light-headedness, dizziness, diminished appetite, sweating, chills, tremors, paresthesias, fatigue, somnolence, and sleep disturbances (eg, vivid dreams, insomnia). Greater risks for developing a discontinuation syndrome have been associated with antidepressants with shorter half-lives, longer durations of treatment, and abrupt discontinuation. For antidepressants of short or intermediate half-lives, symptoms may emerge within 2-5 days after treatment discontinuation and last 7-14 days (APA 2010; Fava 2006; Haddad 2001; Shelton 2001; Warner 2006).

Adverse Reactions

>10%:

Central nervous system: Drowsiness (18%; dose related), insomnia (15%; dose related)

Dermatologic: Diaphoresis (11%; dose related)

Gastrointestinal: Nausea (21%), xerostomia (20%)

1% to 10%:

Cardiovascular: Prolonged Q-T interval on ECG (2%), hypotension (≥1%), orthostatic hypotension (≥1%), tachycardia (≥1%), bradycardia (1%)

Central nervous system: Fatigue (5%; dose related), anxiety (4%), agitation (3%), yawning (2%; dose related), amnesia (≥1%), apathy (≥1%), confusion (≥1%), depression (≥1%), lack of concentration (≥1%), migraine (≥1%), paresthesia (≥1%)

Dermatologic: Skin rash (≥1%), pruritus (≥1%)

Endocrine & metabolic: Decreased libido (1% to 4%), amenorrhea (≥1%), weight gain (≥1%), weight loss (≥1%)

Gastrointestinal: Diarrhea (8%), dyspepsia (5%), anorexia (4%), vomiting (4%), abdominal pain (3%), dysgeusia (≥1%), flatulence (≥1%), increased appetite (≥1%), sialorrhea (≥1%)

Genitourinary: Ejaculatory disorder (6%), dysmenorrhea (3%), impotence (3%; dose related)

Neuromuscular & skeletal: Tremor (8%), arthralgia (2%), myalgia (2%)

Ophthalmic: Accommodation disturbance (≥1%)

Renal: Polyuria (≥1%)

Respiratory: Rhinitis (5%), upper respiratory tract infection (5%), sinusitis (3%), cough (≥1%)

Miscellaneous: Fever (2%)

<1% (Limited to important or life threatening): Abnormal serum prolactin levels, acute renal failure, alopecia, anaphylaxis, anemia, angina pectoris, angioedema, angle-closure glaucoma, arthritis, asthma, atrial fibrillation, bronchitis, bundle branch block, bursitis, cardiac arrest, cardiac failure, cataract, catatonia, cerebrovascular accident, cholelithiasis, delirium, delusions, depersonalization, diplopia, diverticulitis, drug dependence, duodenal ulcer, eczema, erythema multiforme, extrapyramidal reaction, extrasystoles, galactorrhea, gastric ulcer, gastrointestinal hemorrhage, granulocytopenia, gynecomastia, hallucination, heavy eyelids, hemolytic anemia, hepatic necrosis, hepatitis, hypersensitivity reaction, hypertension, hypertrichosis, hypoglycemia, hypokalemia, hyponatremia, hypoprothrombinemia, hypothyroidism, ischemic heart disease, leukocytosis, leukopenia, lymphadenopathy, lymphocytopenia, lymphocytosis, melanosis, myasthenia, myocardial infarction, nephrolithiasis, neuroleptic malignant syndrome (Stevens, 2008), obesity, osteoporosis, pancreatitis, phlebitis, pneumonia, priapism, psoriasis, psychosis, pulmonary embolism, rhabdomyolysis, seizure, serotonin syndrome, skin photosensitivity, syncope, thrombocytopenia, thrombosis, tonic-clonic seizures, torsades de pointes, toxic epidermal necrolysis, transient ischemic attacks, urinary incontinence, urinary retention, vaginal hemorrhage, ventricular arrhythmia, withdrawal syndrome

Drug Interactions

Metabolism/Transport Effects Substrate of CYP2C19 (major), CYP2D6 (minor), CYP3A4 (major); **Note:** Assignment of Major/Minor substrate status based on clinically relevant drug interaction potential; **Inhibits** CYP1A2 (weak), CYP2B6 (weak), CYP2C19 (weak), CYP2D6 (weak)

Avoid Concomitant Use

Avoid concomitant use of Citalopram with any of the following: Conivaptan; Dapoxetine; Dosulepin; Fluconazole; Fusidic Acid (Systemic); Highest Risk QTc-Prolonging Agents; Idelalisib; Iobenguane I 123; Ivabradine; Linezolid; MAO Inhibitors; Methylene Blue; Mifepristone; Moderate Risk QTc-Prolonging Agents; Pimozide; Tryptophan; Urokinase

Increased Effect/Toxicity

Citalopram may increase the levels/effects of: Agents with Antiplatelet Properties; Anticoagulants; Antidepressants (Serotonin Reuptake Inhibitor/Antagonist); Antipsychotic Agents; Apixaban; Aspirin; Blood Glucose Lowering Agents; BusPIRone; CarBAMazepine; Collagenase (Systemic); Dabigatran Etexilate; Deoxycholic Acid; Desmopressin; Dextromethorphan; Dosulepin; Edoxaban; Highest Risk QTc-Prolonging Agents; Ibritumomab; Methylene Blue; Mexiletine; NSAID (COX-2 Inhibitor); NSAID (Nonselective); Obinutuzumab; Pimozide; Rivaroxaban; Salicylates; Serotonin Modulators; Thiazide Diuretics; Thrombolytic Agents; TiZANidine; Tositumomab and Iodine I 131 Tositumomab; TraMADol; Tricyclic Antidepressants; Urokinase; Vitamin K Antagonists

The levels/effects of Citalopram may be increased by: Alcohol (Ethyl); Analgesics (Opioid); Antiemetics (5HT3 Antagonists); Antipsychotic Agents; Aprepitant; BuPROPion; BusPIRone; Cimetidine; CNS Depressants; Conivaptan; CYP2C19 Inhibitors (Moderate); CYP2C19 Inhibitors (Strong); CYP3A4 Inhibitors (Moderate); CYP3A4 Inhibitors (Strong); Dapoxetine; Fluconazole; Fosaprepitant; Fusidic Acid (Systemic); Glucosamine; Herbs (Anticoagulant/Antiplatelet Properties); Ibrutinib; Idelalisib; Ivabradine; Ivacaftor; Limaprost; Linezolid; Lithium; Luliconazole; MAO Inhibitors; Metaxalone; Metoclopramide; Metyrosine; Mifepristone; Moderate Risk QTc-Prolonging Agents; Multivitamins/Fluoride (with ADE); Multivitamins/Minerals (with ADEK, Folate, Iron); Multivitamins/Minerals (with AE, No Iron); Netupitant; Omega-3 Fatty Acids; Palbociclib; Pentosan Polysulfate Sodium; Pentoxifylline; Prostacyclin Analogues; QTc-Prolonging Agents (Indeterminate Risk and Risk Modifying); Simeprevir; Stiripentol; Tedizolid; Tipranavir; TraMADol; Tricyclic Antidepressants; Tryptophan; Vitamin E; Vitamin E (Oral)

Decreased Effect

Citalopram may decrease the levels/effects of: Iobenguane I 123; Ioflupane I 123; Thyroid Products

The levels/effects of Citalopram may be decreased by: Bosentan; CarBAMazepine; CYP2C19 Inducers (Strong); CYP3A4 Inducers (Moderate); CYP3A4 Inducers (Strong); Cyproheptadine; Dabrafenib; Deferasirox; Enzalutamide; Mitotane; NSAID (COX-2 Inhibitor); NSAID (Nonselective); Rifampin; Siltuximab; St Johns Wort; Tocilizumab

Storage/Stability Store at 25°C (77°F); excursions permitted to 15°C to 30°C (59°F to 86°F). Protect from moisture.

Mechanism of Action A racemic bicyclic phthalane derivative, citalopram selectively inhibits serotonin reuptake in the presynaptic neurons and has minimal effects on norepinephrine or dopamine. Uptake inhibition of serotonin is primarily due to the *S*-enantiomer of citalopram. Displays little to no affinity for serotonin, dopamine, adrenergic, histamine, GABA, or muscarinic receptor subtypes.

Pharmacodynamics/Kinetics

Onset of action: Depression: The onset of action is 1-4 weeks; however, individual response varies greatly and full response may not be seen until 8-12 weeks after initiation of treatment.

Duration: 1-2 days

Distribution: V_d: 12 L/kg

Protein binding, plasma: ~80%

Metabolism: Extensively hepatic, via CYP3A4 and 2C19 (major pathways), and 2D6 (minor pathway); metabolized to demethylcitalopram (DCT), didemethylcitalopram (DDCT), citalopram-N-oxide, and a deaminated propionic acid derivative, which are at least eight times less potent than citalopram

Bioavailability: 80%; tablets and oral solution are bioequivalent

Half-life elimination: 24-48 hours (average: 35 hours); doubled with hepatic impairment and increased by 30% (following multiple doses) to 50% (following single dose) in elderly patients (≥60 years)

Time to peak, serum: 1-6 hours, average within 4 hours

Excretion: Urine (Citalopram 10% and DCT 5%)

Note: Clearance was decreased, while half-life was significantly increased in patients with hepatic impairment. Mild-to-moderate renal impairment may reduce clearance (17%) and prolong half-life of citalopram. No pharmacokinetic information is available concerning patients with severe renal impairment. AUC and half-life were significantly increased in elderly patients (≥60 years), and in poor CYP2C19 metabolizers, steady state C_{max} and AUC was increased by 68% and 107%, respectively.

Dosing

Adult Note: Doses >40 mg daily are not recommended due to the risk of QT prolongation.

Depression: Adults <60 years: Oral: Initial: 20 mg once daily; increase the dose by 20 mg at an interval of ≥1 week to a maximum dose of 40 mg daily. Additional efficacy with doses >40 mg daily has not been demonstrated in clinical trials.

Poor metabolizers of CYP2C19 or concurrent use of moderate-to-strong CYP2C19 inhibitors (eg, cimetidine, omeprazole): Maximum dose: 20 mg daily

Panic disorder (off-label use): Initial: 10 mg daily for 7 days, then increase dose to 20 mg daily (Perna 2003; Stahl 2003). Consider further dosage adjustments based on response and tolerability. Mean dose in flexible-dose clinical trials was 20 to 40 mg daily; doses up to 60 mg daily have been evaluated (Leinonen 2000; Perna 2003; Seedat 2003; Stahl 2003; Wade 1997).

Discontinuation of therapy: Upon discontinuation of antidepressant therapy, gradually taper the dose to minimize the incidence of withdrawal symptoms and allow for the detection of re-emerging symptoms. Evidence supporting ideal taper rates is limited. APA and NICE guidelines suggest tapering therapy over at least several weeks with consideration to the half-life of the antidepressant; antidepressants with a shorter half-life may need to be tapered more conservatively. In addition for long-term treated patients, WFSBP guidelines recommend tapering over 4-6 months. If intolerable withdrawal symptoms occur following a dose reduction, consider resuming the previously prescribed dose and/or decrease dose at a more gradual rate (APA 2010; Bauer 2002; Haddad 2001; NCCMH 2010; Schatzberg 2006; Shelton 2001; Warner 2006).

MAO inhibitor recommendations:

Switching to or from an MAO inhibitor intended to treat psychiatric disorders:

Allow 14 days to elapse between discontinuing an MAO inhibitor intended to treat psychiatric disorders and initiation of citalopram.

Allow 14 days to elapse between discontinuing citalopram and initiation of an MAO inhibitor intended to treat psychiatric disorders.

Use with other MAO inhibitors (linezolid or IV methylene blue):

Do not initiate citalopram in patients receiving linezolid or IV methylene blue; consider other interventions for psychiatric condition.

If urgent treatment with linezolid or IV methylene blue is required in a patient already receiving citalopram and potential benefits outweigh potential risks, discontinue citalopram promptly and administer linezolid or IV methylene blue. Monitor for serotonin syndrome for 2 weeks or until 24 hours after the last dose of linezolid or IV methylene blue, whichever comes first. May resume citalopram 24 hours after the last dose of linezolid or IV methylene blue.

Geriatric Depression: Elderly ≥60 years: Oral: Initial: 20 mg once daily; maximum dose in adults ≥60 years: 20 mg daily due to increased exposure and the risk of QT prolongation. Refer to adult dosing.

Discontinuation of therapy: Refer to adult dosing.

MAO inhibitor recommendations: Refer to adult dosing.

Pediatric Obsessive-compulsive disorder (off-label use): Children and Adolescents: Oral: 10-40 mg/day (Mukaddes 2003; Thomsen 1997; Thomsen 2001)

Discontinuation of therapy: Refer to adult dosing.

MAO inhibitor recommendations: Refer to adult dosing.

Renal Impairment

Mild-to-moderate impairment: No dosage adjustment necessary.

Severe impairment: CrCl <20 mL/minute: No dosage adjustment provided in manufacturer's labeling (has not been studied); use caution.

Hepatic Impairment Initial: 20 mg once daily; maximum recommended dose: 20 mg daily due to decreased clearance and the risk of QT prolongation

Dietary Considerations May be taken without regard to food.

Administration May be administered without regard to food.

Monitoring Parameters ECG (patients at increased risk for QT-prolonging effects due to certain conditions); electrolytes (potassium and magnesium concentrations [prior to initiation and periodically during therapy in patients at increased risk for electrolyte abnormalities]); signs/symptoms of arrhythmias (eg, dizziness, palpitations, syncope); liver function tests and CBC with continued therapy; monitor patient periodically for symptom resolution; signs/symptoms of serotonin syndrome; mental status for depression, suicidal ideation (especially at the beginning of therapy or when doses are increased or decreased), anxiety, social functioning, mania, panic attacks; akathisia

Dosage Forms Excipient information presented when available (limited, particularly for generics); consult specific product labeling.

Solution, Oral:
Generic: 10 mg/5 mL (240 mL)

Tablet, Oral:
CeleXA: 10 mg
CeleXA: 20 mg, 40 mg [scored]
Generic: 10 mg, 20 mg, 40 mg

Citric Acid, Sodium Citrate, and Potassium Citrate

(SIT rik AS id, SOW dee um SIT rate, & poe TASS ee um SIT rate)

Brand Names: US Cytra-3; Virtrate-3

Index Terms Polycitra; Potassium Citrate, Citric Acid, and Sodium Citrate; Sodium Citrate, Citric Acid, and Potassium Citrate

Pharmacologic Category Alkalinizing Agent

Use Conditions where long-term maintenance of an alkaline urine is desirable as in control and dissolution of uric acid and cystine calculi of the urinary tract

Dosing

Adult & Geriatric Alkalinizing agent/bicarbonate precursor/potassium supplement: Oral: 15-30 mL diluted in water after meals and at bedtime

Pediatric Alkalinizing agent/bicarbonate precursor/potassium supplement: Oral: Children: 5-15 mL diluted in water after meals and at bedtime

Additional Information Complete prescribing information should be consulted for additional detail.

Dosage Forms Excipient information presented when available (limited, particularly for generics); consult specific product labeling.

Solution, Oral:

Virtrate-3: Citric acid 334 mg, sodium citrate 500 mg, and potassium citrate 550 mg per 5 mL (473 mL) [sugar free; contains fd&c yellow #6 (sunset yellow), polyethylene glycol, propylene glycol, saccharin sodium, sodium benzoate; raspberry flavor]

Generic: Citric acid 334 mg, sodium citrate 500 mg, and potassium citrate 550 mg per 5 mL (473 mL)

Syrup, Oral:

Cytra-3: Citric acid 334 mg, sodium citrate 500 mg, and potassium citrate 550 mg per 5 mL (473 mL) [alcohol free, sugar free; contains fd&c yellow #6 (sunset yellow), polyethylene glycol, propylene glycol, saccharin sodium, sodium benzoate; vanilla flavor]

Cladribine (KLA dri been)

Brand Names: US Leustatin [DSC]
Brand Names: Canada Cladribine Injection
Index Terms 2-CdA; 2-Chlorodeoxyadenosine; Leustatin
Pharmacologic Category Antineoplastic Agent, Antimetabolite; Antineoplastic Agent, Antimetabolite (Purine Analog)
Use Treatment of active hairy cell leukemia
Dosing

Adult & Geriatric Details concerning dosing in combination regimens should also be consulted.

Hairy cell leukemia: IV: 0.09 mg/kg/day continuous infusion for 7 days for 1 cycle **or** (off-label dosing) 0.1 mg/kg/day continuous infusion for 7 days for 1 cycle (Goodman, 2003; Saven, 1998)

Acute myeloid leukemia, induction (off-label use): IV: CLAG or CLAG-M regimen: 5 mg/m²/day over 2 hours for 5 days; a second induction may be administered if needed (Robak, 2000; Wierzbowska, 2008; Wrzesień-Kuś, 2003)

Chronic lymphocytic leukemia (off-label use): IV: 0.1 mg/kg/day continuous infusion for 7 days every 4-5 weeks (Saven, 1995) **or** 0.14 mg/kg/day over 2 hours for 5 days every 28 days for 3-6 cycles (Byrd, 2003)

Mantle cell lymphoma (off-label use): IV: 5 mg/m²/day over 2 hours for 5 days every 4 weeks for 2-6 cycles (Inwards, 2008; Rummel, 1999) **or** 5 mg/m²/day over 2 hours for 5 days every 4 weeks for 2-6 cycles (in combination with rituximab) (Inwards, 2008)

Waldenström's macroglobulinemia (off-label use):
IV: 0.1 mg/kg/day continuous infusion for 7 days every 4 weeks for 2 cycles (Dimopoulos, 1994)
SubQ: 0.1 mg/kg/day for 5 consecutive days every month for 4 cycles (in combination with rituximab) (Laszlo, 2010)

Pediatric

Acute myeloid leukemia (off-label use): IV: 8.9 mg/m²/day continuous infusion for 5 days for 1 or 2 courses (Krance, 2001) **or** 9 mg/m²/day over 30 minutes for 5 days for 1 course (in combination with cytarabine) (Crews, 2002; Rubnitz, 2009)

Langerhans cell histiocytosis, refractory (off-label use): IV: 5 mg/m²/day over 2 hours for 5 days every 21 days for up to 6 cycles (Weitzman, 2009)

Renal Impairment No dosage adjustment provided in the manufacturer's labeling (due to inadequate data); use with caution. The following adjustments have been used (Aronoff, 2007):

Adults:
CrCl 10-50 mL/minute: Administer 75% of dose
CrCl <10 mL/minute: Administer 50% of dose
Continuous ambulatory peritoneal dialysis (CAPD): Administer 50% of dose

Children:
CrCl 10-50 mL/minute: Administer 50% of dose
CrCl <10 mL/minute: Administer 30% of dose
Hemodialysis: Administer 30% of dose
Continuous renal replacement therapy (CRRT): Administer 50% of dose

Hepatic Impairment No dosage adjustment provided in the manufacturer's labeling (due to inadequate data); use with caution.

Obesity ASCO Guidelines for appropriate chemotherapy dosing in obese adults with cancer: Utilize patient's actual body weight (full weight) for calculation of body surface area- or weight-based dosing, particularly when the intent of therapy is curative; manage regimen-related toxicities in the same manner as for nonobese patients; if a dose reduction is utilized due to toxicity, consider resumption of full weight-based dosing with subsequent cycles, especially if cause of toxicity (eg, hepatic or renal impairment) is resolved (Griggs, 2012).

Additional Information Complete prescribing information should be consulted for additional detail.

Dosage Forms Excipient information presented when available (limited, particularly for generics); consult specific product labeling. [DSC] = Discontinued product

Solution, Intravenous:
Leustatin: 1 mg/mL (10 mL [DSC])
Generic: 1 mg/mL (10 mL [DSC])
Solution, Intravenous [preservative free]:
Generic: 1 mg/mL (10 mL)

Clarithromycin (kla RITH roe mye sin)

Brand Names: US Biaxin; Biaxin XL; Biaxin XL Pac
Brand Names: Canada Accel-Clarithromycin; Apo-Clarithromycin; Apo-Clarithromycin XL; Biaxin; Biaxin BID; Biaxin XL; Dom-Clarithromycin; Mylan-Clarithromycin; PMS-Clarithromycin; RAN-Clarithromycin; Riva-Clarithromycin; Sandoz-Clarithromycin; Teva-Clarithromycin
Pharmacologic Category Antibiotic, Macrolide
Use

Infants and Children 6 months and older:
Acute maxillary sinusitis due to susceptible *H. influenzae*, *S. pneumoniae*, or *Moraxella catarrhalis*
Acute otitis media due to susceptible *H. influenzae*, *M. catarrhalis*, or *S. pneumoniae*
Community-acquired pneumonia due to susceptible *Mycoplasma pneumoniae*, *S. pneumoniae*, or *Chlamydophila* (also known as *Chlamydia*) *pneumoniae* (TWAR)
Disseminated mycobacterial infections due to *M. avium* or *M. intracellulare*
Pharyngitis/tonsillitis due to susceptible *S. pyogenes*
Prevention of disseminated mycobacterial infections due to *M. avium* complex (MAC) disease in patients with advanced HIV infection (20 months of age and older)
Uncomplicated skin/skin structure infection due to susceptible *S. aureus* or *S. pyogenes*

Adults:
Pharyngitis/tonsillitis due to susceptible *S. pyogenes*
Acute maxillary sinusitis due to susceptible *H. influenzae*, *M. catarrhalis*, or *S. pneumoniae*
Acute exacerbation of chronic bronchitis due to susceptible *H. influenzae*, *H. parainfluenzae*, *M. catarrhalis*, or *S. pneumoniae*
Community-acquired pneumonia due to susceptible *H. influenzae*, *H. parainfluenzae*, *M. catarrhalis*,

Mycoplasma pneumoniae, S. pneumoniae, or *Chlamydophila* (also known as *Chlamydia*) *pneumoniae* (TWAR)

Uncomplicated skin/skin structure infections due to susceptible *S. aureus* or *S. pyogenes*

Disseminated mycobacterial infections due to *M. avium* or *M. intracellulare*

Prevention of disseminated mycobacterial infections due to MAC disease in patients with advanced HIV infection

Duodenal ulcer disease due to *H. pylori* in regimens with other drugs including amoxicillin and lansoprazole or omeprazole, or in combination with omeprazole or ranitidine bismuth citrate (no longer marketed in the U.S.). **Note:** Regimens that contain clarithromycin as the single antimicrobial agent are more likely to be associated with the development of clarithromycin resistance.

Pregnancy Considerations Adverse events have been documented in some animal reproduction studies. Clarithromycin crosses the placenta (Witt 2003). The manufacturer recommends that clarithromycin not be used in a pregnant woman unless there are no alternative therapies. Clarithromycin is generally not recommended for the treatment or prophylaxis of *Mycobacterium avium* complex (MAC) or bacterial respiratory disease in HIV-infected pregnant patients (DHHS 2013).

Breast-Feeding Considerations Clarithromycin and its active metabolite (14-hydroxy clarithromycin) are excreted into breast milk. The manufacturer recommends that caution be used if administered to nursing women. Decreased appetite, diarrhea, rash, and somnolence have been noted in nursing infants exposed to macrolide antibiotics (Goldstein 2009).

Contraindications Hypersensitivity to clarithromycin, erythromycin, any of the macrolide antibiotics, or any component of the formulation; history of cholestatic jaundice/hepatic dysfunction associated with prior use of clarithromycin; history of QT prolongation or ventricular cardiac arrhythmia, including torsade de pointes; concomitant use with cisapride, pimozide, ergotamine, dihydroergotamine, HMG-CoA reductase inhibitors extensively metabolized by CYP3A4 (eg, lovastatin, simvastatin), astemizole or terfenadine (not available in the U.S.); concomitant use with colchicine in patients with renal or hepatic impairment

Warnings/Precautions Use has been associated with QT prolongation and infrequent cases of arrhythmias, including torsade de pointes; use is contraindicated in patients with a history of QT prolongation and ventricular arrhythmias, including torsade de pointes. Systemic exposure is increased in the elderly; may be at increased risk of torsade de pointes, particularly if concurrent severe renal impairment. Use with caution in patients at risk of prolonged cardiac repolarization. Use with caution in patients with uncorrected hypokalemia or hypomagnesemia, clinically significant bradycardia, and patients receiving Class IA (eg, quinidine, procainamide) or Class III (eg, amiodarone, dofetilide, sotalol) antiarrhythmic agents. Use caution in patients with coronary artery disease.

Elevated liver function tests and hepatitis (hepatocellular and/or cholestatic with or without jaundice) have been reported; usually reversible after discontinuation of clarithromycin. May lead to hepatic failure or death (rarely), especially in the presence of preexisting diseases and/or concomitant use of medications. Discontinue immediately if symptoms of hepatitis occur. Dosage adjustment needed in severe renal impairment. Use with caution in patients with myasthenia gravis.

Potentially significant drug-drug interactions may exist, requiring dose or frequency adjustment, additional monitoring, and/or selection of alternative therapy. Colchicine toxicity (including fatalities) has been reported with concomitant use; concomitant use is contraindicated in patients with renal or hepatic impairment. Clarithromycin in combination with ranitidine bismuth citrate should not be used in patients with a history of acute porphyria. Prolonged use may result in fungal or bacterial superinfection, including *C. difficile*-associated diarrhea (CDAD) and pseudomembranous colitis; CDAD has been observed >2 months postantibiotic treatment. Decreased *H. pylori* eradication rates have been observed with short-term (≤7 days) combination therapy. Current guidelines recommend 10 to 14 days of therapy (triple or quadruple) for eradication of *H. pylori* in pediatric and adult patients (Chey 2007; NASPHGAN [Koletzko 2011]).

Severe acute reactions have (rarely) been reported, including anaphylaxis, Stevens-Johnson syndrome (SJS), toxic epidermal necrolysis (TEN), drug rash with eosinophilia and systemic symptoms (DRESS), and Henoch-Schönlein purpura (IgA vasculitis); discontinue therapy and initiate treatment immediately for severe acute hypersensitivity reactions. The presence of extended release tablets in the stool has been reported, particularly in patients with anatomic (eg, ileostomy, colostomy) or functional GI disorders with decreased transit times. Consider alternative dosage forms (eg, suspension) or an alternative antimicrobial for patients with tablet residue in the stool and no signs of clinical improvement. Some dosage forms may contain propylene glycol; large amounts are potentially toxic and have been associated hyperosmolality, lactic acidosis, seizures, and respiratory depression; use caution (AAP, 1997; Zar 2007).

Adverse Reactions

1% to 10%:

Central nervous system: Headache (2%), insomnia

Dermatologic: Skin rash (children 3%)

Gastrointestinal: Dysgeusia (adults 3% to 7%), vomiting (children 6%), diarrhea (3% to 6%), nausea (adults 3%), abdominal pain (2% to 3%), dyspepsia (adults 2%)

Hematologic & oncologic: Prolonged prothrombin time (adults 1%)

Hepatic: Abnormal hepatic function tests

Hypersensitivity: Anaphylactoid reaction

Infection: Candidiasis (including oral)

Renal: Increased blood urea nitrogen (4%)

<1% (Limited to important or life-threatening): Acne vulgaris, ageusia, altered sense of smell, anxiety, asthma, atrial fibrillation, behavioral changes, cardiac arrest, cellulitis, cholestatic hepatitis, *Clostridium difficile* associated diarrhea, *Clostridium difficile* (colitis), dental discoloration (reversible with dental cleaning), depression, disorientation, DRESS syndrome, drowsiness, dyskinesia, epistaxis, esophagitis, extrasystoles, gastritis, gastroesophageal reflux disease, glossitis, hallucination, hearing loss (reversible), hemorrhage, hepatic failure, hepatotoxicity (idiosyncratic) (Chalasani, 2014), hyperhidrosis, hypersensitivity, hypoglycemia, IgA vasculitis, increased gamma-glutamyl transferase, increased INR, increased lactate dehydrogenase, interstitial nephritis, leukopenia, loss of consciousness, malaise, manic behavior, neck stiffness, neutropenia, pancreatitis, parasominas, paresthesia, prolonged QT interval on ECG, pruritus, pseudomembranous colitis, pulmonary embolism, renal failure, rhabdomyolysis, seizure, Stevens-Johnson syndrome, stomatitis, thrombocytopenia, tinnitus, tongue discoloration, torsades de pointes, vaginal infection, ventricular arrhythmia, ventricular tachycardia

Drug Interactions

Metabolism/Transport Effects Substrate of CYP3A4 (major); **Note:** Assignment of Major/Minor substrate status based on clinically relevant drug interaction potential; **Inhibits** CYP1A2 (weak), CYP3A4 (strong), P-glycoprotein

Avoid Concomitant Use

Avoid concomitant use of Clarithromycin with any of the following: Ado-Trastuzumab Emtansine; Alfuzosin; Aprepitant; Astemizole; Avanafil; Axitinib; Barnidipine; BCG (Intravesical); Bosutinib; Bromocriptine; Cabozantinib; Ceritinib; Cisapride; Cobimetinib; Conivaptan; Crizotinib; Dabrafenib; Dapoxetine; Dihydroergotamine; Disopyramide; Domperidone; Dronedarone; Eletriptan; Eplerenone; Ergotamine; Everolimus; Flibanserin; FLUoxetine; Fusidic Acid (Systemic); Halofantrine; Highest Risk QTc-Prolonging Agents; Ibrutinib; Idelalisib; Irinotecan Products; Isavuconazonium Sulfate; Ivabradine; Lapatinib; Lercanidipine; Lomitapide; Lopinavir; Lovastatin; Lurasidone; Macitentan; Mifepristone; Naloxegol; Nilotinib; NiMODipine; Nisoldipine; Olaparib; Osimertinib; Palbociclib; PAZOPanib; Pimozide; QUEtiapine; QuiNINE; Ranolazine; Red Yeast Rice; Regorafenib; Salmeterol; Silodosin; Simeprevir; Simvastatin; Sonidegib; Suvorexant; Tamsulosin; Terfenadine; Ticagrelor; Tolvaptan; Topotecan; Toremifene; Trabectedin; Ulipristal; Vemurafenib; VinCRIStine (Liposomal); Vorapaxar

Increased Effect/Toxicity

Clarithromycin may increase the levels/effects of: Ado-Trastuzumab Emtansine; Afatinib; Alfentanil; Alfuzosin; Alitretinoin (Systemic); Almotriptan; Alosetron; ALPRAZolam; Antineoplastic Agents (Vinca Alkaloids); Apixaban; Aprepitant; ARIPiprazole; ARIPiprazole Lauroxil; Astemizole; AtorvaSTATin; Avanafil; Axitinib; Barnidipine; Bedaquiline; Boceprevir; Bortezomib; Bosentan; Bosutinib; Brentuximab Vedotin; Brexpiprazole; Brinzolamide; Bromocriptine; Budesonide (Nasal); Budesonide (Oral Inhalation); Budesonide (Systemic); Budesonide (Topical); BusPIRone; Cabazitaxel; Cabergoline; Cabozantinib; Calcium Channel Blockers; Cannabis; CarBAMazepine; Cardiac Glycosides; Cariprazine; Ceritinib; Cilostazol; Cisapride; CloZAPine; Cobicistat; Cobimetinib; Colchicine; Conivaptan; Corticosteroids (Orally Inhaled); Corticosteroids (Systemic); Crizotinib; CYP3A4 Inducers (Strong); CYP3A4 Substrates; Dabigatran Etexilate; Dabrafenib; Daclatasvir; Dapoxetine; Dasatinib;

Dienogest; Dihydroergotamine; Disopyramide; Domperidone; DOXOrubicin (Conventional); Dronabinol; Dronedarone; Drospirenone; Dutasteride; Edoxaban; Eletriptan; Eplerenone; Ergot Derivatives; Ergotamine; Erlotinib; Estazolam; Etizolam; Everolimus; FentaNYL; Fesoterodine; Flibanserin; FLUoxetine; Fluticasone (Nasal); Fluticasone (Oral Inhalation); Gefitinib; GlipiZIDE; GlyBURIDE; GuanFACINE; Halofantrine; Highest Risk QTc-Prolonging Agents; Hydrocodone; Ibrutinib; Imatinib; Imidafenacin; Irinotecan Products; Isavuconazonium Sulfate; Ivabradine; Ivacaftor; Ixabepilone; Lacosamide; Lapatinib; Ledipasvir; Lercanidipine; Levobupivacaine; Levomilnacipran; Lomitapide; Lopinavir; Lovastatin; Lurasidone; Macitentan; Maraviroc; MedroxyPROGESTERone; MethylPREDNISolone; Midazolam; Moderate Risk QTc-Prolonging Agents; Naloxegol; Nilotinib; NiMODipine; Nintedanib; Nisoldipine; Olaparib; Osimertinib; Ospemifene; Oxybutynin; OxyCODONE; Palbociclib; Panobinostat; Parecoxib; Paricalcitol; PARoxetine; PAZOPanib; P-glycoprotein/ABCB1 Substrates; Pimecrolimus; Pimozide; Pitavastatin; PONATinib; Pranlukast; Pravastatin; PredniSOLONE (Systemic); PredniSONE; Protease Inhibitors; Prucalopride; QUEtiapine; QuiNINE; Ramelteon; Ranolazine; Red Yeast Rice; Regorafenib; Repaglinide; Retapamulin; Rifaximin; Rilpivirine; Rivaroxaban; RomiDEPsin; Ruxolitinib; Salmeterol; Saxagliptin; SIldenafil; Silodosin; Simeprevir; Simvastatin; Sirolimus; Sonidegib; SORAfenib; Suvorexant; Tacrolimus (Systemic); Tacrolimus (Topical); Tadalafil; Tamsulosin; Tasimelteon; Telaprevir; Temsirolimus; Terfenadine; Tetrahydrocannabinol; Theophylline Derivatives; Ticagrelor; TiZANidine; Tofacitinib; Tolterodine; Tolvaptan; Topotecan; Toremifene; Trabectedin; TraMADol; TraZODone; Triazolam; Uliprisal; Vardenafil; Vemurafenib; Vilazodone; VinCRIStine (Liposomal); Vitamin K Antagonists; Vorapaxar; Zidovudine; Zopiclone

The levels/effects of Clarithromycin may be increased by: Antihepaciviral Combination Products; Boceprevir; Bosentan; Cobicistat; Conivaptan; CYP3A4 Inducers (Moderate); CYP3A4 Inducers (Strong); CYP3A4 Inhibitors (Moderate); CYP3A4 Inhibitors (Strong); Fusidic Acid (Systemic); Idelalisib; Ivabradine; Lopinavir; Luliconazole; Mifepristone; Netupitant; Protease Inhibitors; QTc-Prolonging Agents (Indeterminate Risk and Risk Modifying); Stiripentol; Telaprevir; TraZODone

Decreased Effect

Clarithromycin may decrease the levels/effects of: BCG (Intravesical); BCG Vaccine (Immunization); Clopidogrel; Ifosfamide; Prasugrel; Sodium Picosulfate; Ticagrelor; Typhoid Vaccine; Zidovudine

The levels/effects of Clarithromycin may be decreased by: Bosentan; CYP3A4 Inducers (Moderate); CYP3A4 Inducers (Strong); Deferasirox; Efavirenz; Enzalutamide; Etravirine; Lopinavir; Mitotane; Protease Inhibitors; Siltuximab; St Johns Wort; Tocilizumab

Food Interactions Immediate release: Food delays rate, but not extent of absorption; Extended release: Food increases clarithromycin AUC by ~30% relative to fasting conditions. Management: Administer immediate release products without regard to meals. Administer extended release products with food.

Storage/Stability

Extended release tablets: Store at 20°C to 25°C (68°F to 77°F); excursions are permitted between 15°C and 30°C (59°F and 86°F).

Immediate release tablets:

250 mg: Store at 15°C to 30°C (59°F to 86°F). Protect from light.

500 mg: Store at 20°C to 25°C (68°F to 77°F).

Granules for suspension: Store at 15°C to 30°C (59°F to 86°F) prior to and following reconstitution. Do not refrigerate. Use within 14 days of reconstitution.

Mechanism of Action Exerts its antibacterial action by binding to 50S ribosomal subunit resulting in inhibition of protein synthesis. The 14-OH metabolite of clarithromycin is twice as active as the parent compound against certain organisms.

Pharmacodynamics/Kinetics

Absorption:

Immediate release: Rapid; food delays rate, but not extent of absorption

Extended-release: Fasting is associated with ~30% lower AUC relative to administration with food

Distribution: Widely into most body tissues; manufacturer reports no data in regards to CNS penetration

Protein binding: 42% to 70% (Peters, 1992)

Metabolism: Partially hepatic via CYP3A4; converted to 14-OH clarithromycin (active metabolite); undergoes extensive first-pass metabolism

Bioavailability: ~50%

Half-life elimination: Immediate release: Clarithromycin: 3-7 hours; 14-OH-clarithromycin: 5-9 hours

Time to peak: Immediate release: 2-3 hours; Extended release: 5-8 hours

Excretion: Urine (20% to 40% as unchanged drug; additional 10% to 15% as metabolite); feces (29% to 40% mostly as metabolites) (Ferrero, 1990)

Clearance: Approximates normal GFR

Dosing

Adult

Usual dosage range: Oral: 250-500 mg every 12 hours **or** 1000 mg (two 500 mg extended release tablets) once daily for 7-14 days

Acute exacerbation of chronic bronchitis: Oral:

M. catarrhalis and *S. pneumoniae*: 250 mg every 12 hours for 7-14 days **or** 1000 mg (two 500 mg extended release tablets) once daily for 7 days

H. influenzae: 500 mg every 12 hours for 7-14 days **or** 1000 mg (two 500 mg extended release tablets) once daily for 7 days

H. parainfluenzae: 500 mg every 12 hours for 7 days **or** 1000 mg (two 500 mg extended release tablets) once daily for 7 days

Acute maxillary sinusitis: Oral: 500 mg every 12 hours for 14 days **or** 1000 mg (two 500 mg extended release tablets) once daily for 14 days

Bartonellosis in HIV-infected patients (excluding CNS infections and endocarditis) (off-label use; HHS [OI adult 2015]): Oral:

Treatment (alternative to preferred): 500 mg twice daily for at least 3 months

Long-term suppressive therapy: 500 mg twice daily; may discontinue if completed 3 to 4 months therapy and CD4 >200 cells/mm³ for at least 6 months Note: Some clinicians would discontinue only if Bartonella titers have also decreased four-fold

Lyme disease (off-label use): Oral: 500 mg twice daily for 14-21 days (not recommended for pregnant women) (Wormser 2006)

Mycobacterial infection, disseminated (prevention and treatment): Oral:

Manufacturer's labeling: 500 mg twice daily (use with other antimycobacterial drugs, eg, ethambutol or rifampin). Continue therapy if clinical response is observed; may discontinue when patient is considered at low risk of disseminated infection.

Alternate dosing: *Mycobacterium avium* complex disease (MAC) in HIV-infected patients (HHS [OI adult 2015]):

Primary prophylaxis: 500 mg twice daily; may discontinue when CD4 count >100 cells/mm³ for ≥3 months in response to ART

Treatment and chronic maintenance therapy: 500 mg twice daily plus ethambutol; consider additional agents (eg, rifabutin, aminoglycoside, fluoroquinolone) for CD4 <50 cells/mm³, high mycobacterial load, or ineffective antiretroviral therapy; may discontinue chronic maintenance if no signs/symptoms of MAC disease, have maintained a CD4 count >100 cells/mm³ for >6 months in response to ART, and completed at least 12 months of therapy

Peptic ulcer disease: Eradication of *Helicobacter pylori*: Dual or triple combination regimens with bismuth subsalicylate, amoxicillin, an H₂-receptor antagonist, or proton-pump inhibitor: Oral: 500 mg every 8-12 hours for 10-14 days

Pertussis (off-label use): Oral: 500 mg twice daily for 7 days (CDC 2005)

Pharyngitis, tonsillitis: Oral: 250 mg every 12 hours for 10 days. **Note:** Recommended by the Infectious Disease Society of America (IDSA) as an alternative agent for group A streptococcal pharyngitis in penicillin-allergic patients (Shulman 2012).

Pneumonia: Oral:

C. pneumoniae, *M. pneumoniae*, and *S. pneumoniae*: 250 mg every 12 hours for 7-14 days **or** 1000 mg (two 500 mg extended release tablets) once daily for 7 days

H. influenzae: 250 mg every 12 hours for 7 days **or** 1000 mg (two 500 mg extended release tablets) once daily for 7 days

H. parainfluenzae and *M. catarrhalis*: 1000 mg (two 500 mg extended release tablets) once daily for 7 days

Prophylaxis against infective endocarditis (off-label use): Oral: 500 mg 30-60 minutes prior to procedure. **Note:** American Heart Association (AHA) guidelines now recommend prophylaxis only in patients undergoing invasive procedures and in whom underlying cardiac conditions may predispose to a higher risk of adverse outcomes should infection occur. As of April

2007, routine prophylaxis for GI/GU procedures is no longer recommended by the AHA (Wilson 2007).

Skin and skin structure infection, uncomplicated: Oral: 250 mg every 12 hours for 7-14 days

Geriatric Refer to adult dosing. May make age-related reductions in renal function; monitor and adjust dose if necessary.

Pediatric

Usual dosage range: Note: All pediatric dosing recommendations based on immediate release product formulations (tablet and oral suspension):

Infants ≥6 months, Children, and Adolescents: Oral: 7.5 mg/kg every 12 hours (maximum: 500 mg/dose) for 10 days

Acute otitis media: Infants ≥6 months, Children, and Adolescents: Oral: 7.5 mg/kg/dose (maximum: 500 mg/dose) every 12 hours for 10 days. **Note:** Due to increased *S. pneumoniae* and *H. influenzae* resistance, macrolides are not routinely recommended as a treatment option (Lieberthal 2013)

Bartonellosisin (treatment/long-term suppressive therapy) HIV-infected patients (excluding CNS infections and endocarditis) (off-label use): Adolescents: Oral: Refer to adult dosing.

Community-acquired pneumonia (CAP): Infants >3 months and Children: Oral: **Note:** A beta-lactam antibiotic should be added if typical bacterial pneumonia cannot be ruled out.

Presumed atypical *(M. pneumoniae, C. pneumoniae, C. trachomatis)* infection, mild-to-severe atypical infection or step-down therapy (alternative to azithromycin): 7.5 mg/kg/dose (maximum dose: 500 mg) every 12 hours (Bradley 2011)

Lyme disease (off-label use): Infants, Children, and Adolescents: Oral: 7.5 mg/kg/dose (maximum dose: 500 mg) twice daily for 14-21 days (Wormser 2006)

Mycobacterial infection, disseminated (prevention and treatment): Oral:

Manufacturer's labeling: 7.5 mg/kg/dose (maximum: 500 mg/dose) twice daily; use in combination with other antimycobacterial agents for the treatment of disseminated MAC. **Note:** Safety of clarithromycin for MAC not studied in children <20 months.

Alternative recommendations: Disseminated *Mycobacterium avium* complex (MAC) disease in HIV-exposed/-positive patients:

Infants and children (CDC 2009):

Primary prophylaxis: 7.5 mg/kg/dose (maximum: 500 mg/dose) twice daily

Secondary prophylaxis: 7.5 mg/kg/dose (maximum: 500 mg/dose) twice daily, plus ethambutol, with or without rifabutin

Treatment: 7.5-15 mg/kg/dose (maximum: 500 mg/dose) twice daily plus ethambutol, plus rifabutin (for severe disease)

Adolescents: Refer to adult dosing.

Pertussis (off-label use): Infants ≥1 month, Children, and Adolescents: Oral: 7.5 mg/kg/dose (maximum: 500 mg/dose) every 12 hours for 7 days (CDC 2005)

Pharyngitis/tonsillitis: Oral: 7.5 mg/kg/dose (maximum: 250 mg/dose) every 12 hours for 10 days. **Note:** Recommended by the Infectious Disease Society of America (IDSA) as an alternative agent for group A streptococcal pharyngitis in penicillin-allergic patients (Shulman 2012).

Prophylaxis against infective endocarditis (off-label use): Children and Adolescents: Oral: 15 mg/kg/dose (maximum: 500 mg/dose) 30-60 minutes before procedure (maximum: 500 mg). **Note:** American Heart Association (AHA) guidelines now recommend prophylaxis only in patients undergoing invasive procedures and in whom underlying cardiac conditions may predispose to a higher risk of adverse outcomes should infection occur. As of April 2007, routine prophylaxis for GI/GU procedures is no longer recommended by the AHA (Wilson 2007).

Sinusitis: Infants ≥6 months, Children, and Adolescents: Oral: 7.5 mg/kg/dose (maximum: 500 mg/dose) every 12 hours for 10 days

Skin/skin structure infections, uncomplicated: Infants ≥6 months, Children, and Adolescents: Oral: 7.5 mg/kg/dose (maximum: 250 mg dose) every 12 hours for 10 days

Renal Impairment

CrCl <30 mL/minute: Decrease clarithromycin dose by 50%

Hemodialysis: Administer after HD session is completed (Aronoff 2007).

In combination with atazanavir or ritonavir:

CrCl 30-60 mL/minute: Decrease clarithromycin dose by 50%.

CrCl <30 mL/minute: Decrease clarithromycin dose by 75%.

Hepatic Impairment No dosing adjustment is needed as long as renal function is normal.

Dietary Considerations Extended release tablets should be taken with food.

Administration Immediate release tablets and granules for suspension: Administer with or without meals. Administer every 12 hours rather than twice daily to avoid peak and trough variation. Shake suspension well before each use.

Extended release tablets: Administer with food. Do not crush or chew.

Monitoring Parameters CBC with differential, BUN, creatinine; perform culture and sensitivity studies prior to initiating drug therapy as appropriate

Dosage Forms Excipient information presented when available (limited, particularly for generics); consult specific product labeling.

Suspension Reconstituted, Oral:

Biaxin: 250 mg/5 mL (50 mL, 100 mL) [fruit punch flavor]

Generic: 125 mg/5 mL (50 mL, 100 mL); 250 mg/5 mL (50 mL, 100 mL)

Tablet, Oral:

Biaxin: 250 mg [contains brilliant blue fcf (fd&c blue #1), fd&c yellow #10 (quinoline yellow)]

Biaxin: 500 mg [contains fd&c yellow #10 (quinoline yellow)]

Generic: 250 mg, 500 mg

Tablet Extended Release 24 Hour, Oral:

Biaxin XL: 500 mg [contains fd&c yellow #10 (quinoline yellow)]

Biaxin XL Pac: 500 mg [contains fd&c yellow #10 (quinoline yellow)]

Generic: 500 mg

Clemastine (KLEM as teen)

Brand Names: US Dayhist Allergy 12 Hour Relief [OTC]; Tavist Allergy [OTC]

Index Terms Clemastine Fumarate

Pharmacologic Category Ethanolamine Derivative; Histamine H_1 Antagonist; Histamine H_1 Antagonist, First Generation

Use

Allergic rhinitis: Relief of symptoms associated with allergic rhinitis or other upper respiratory allergies (eg, sneezing, rhinorrhea, pruritus, and lacrimation) in children ≥12 years of age and adults (tablets and syrup) and in children 6 to 12 years (syrup only)

Urticaria/angioedema: Relief of mild, uncomplicated allergic skin manifestations of urticaria and angioedema

in children ≥12 years of age and adults (tablets and syrup) and in children 6 to 12 years (syrup only)

OTC Labeling:

Common cold/hay fever/upper respiratory allergies: Relief of symptoms associated with the common cold (eg, rhinorrhea, sneezing, throat/nose pruritus, lacrimation) in children ≥12 years of age and adults

Dosing

Adult & Geriatric

Allergic rhinitis: Oral: Clemastine fumarate 1.34 mg (1 mg base) twice daily; may be increased as needed. Maximum daily dose: Clemastine fumarate 8.04 mg/**day** (6 mg/**day** base)

Common cold/hay fever/upper respiratory allergies (OTC labeling): Oral: Clemastine fumarate 1.34 mg (1 mg base) twice daily. Maximum daily dose: Clemastine fumarate 2.68 mg/**day** (2 mg/**day** base)

Urticaria/angioedema: Oral: Clemastine fumarate 2.68 mg (2 mg base) twice daily; may be increased as needed to a maximum daily dose of clemastine fumarate 8.04 mg/**day** (6 mg/**day** base)

Pediatric

Allergic rhinitis: Oral:

Children 6 to <12 years: Syrup: Clemastine fumarate 0.67 mg (0.5 mg base) twice daily; dosage may be increased as required; single doses up to clemastine fumarate 3 mg (2.25 mg base) have been tolerated. Maximum daily dose: Clemastine fumarate 4.02 mg/**day** (3 mg/**day** base)

Children ≥12 years and Adolescents: Syrup, tablets: Clemastine fumarate 1.34 mg (1 mg base) twice daily; dosage may be increased as required. Maximum daily dose: Clemastine fumarate 8.04 mg/**day** (6 mg/**day** base)

Common cold/hay fever/upper respiratory allergies (OTC labeling): Children ≥12 years and Adolescents: Oral: Clemastine fumarate 1.34 mg (1 mg base) twice daily. Maximum daily dose: Clemastine fumarate 2.68 mg/**day** (2 mg/**day** base)

Urticaria/angioedema: Oral:

Children 6 to <12 years: Syrup: Clemastine fumarate 1.34 mg (1 mg base) twice daily. Maximum daily dose: Clemastine fumarate 4.02 mg/**day** (3 mg/**day** base)

Children ≥12 years and Adolescents: Syrup, tablets: Clemastine fumarate 2.68 mg (2 mg base) twice daily; may be increased as needed to a maximum daily dose of clemastine fumarate 8.04 mg/**day** (6 mg/**day** base)

Renal Impairment There are no dosage adjustments provided in the manufacturer's labeling.

Hepatic Impairment There are no dosage adjustments provided in the manufacturer's labeling.

Additional Information Complete prescribing information should be consulted for additional detail.

Dosage Forms Excipient information presented when available (limited, particularly for generics); consult specific product labeling. [DSC] = Discontinued product

Syrup, Oral, as fumarate:

Generic: 0.67 mg/5 mL (120 mL [DSC])

Tablet, Oral, as fumarate:

Dayhist Allergy 12 Hour Relief: 1.34 mg [scored; sodium free]

Tavist Allergy: 1.34 mg [scored; sodium free]

Generic: 1.34 mg, 2.68 mg

♦ Clemastine Fumarate *see* Clemastine *on page 404*

♦ Clenia [DSC] *see* Sulfur and Sulfacetamide *on page 1716*

♦ Cleocin *see* Clindamycin (Systemic) *on page 405*

♦ Cleocin *see* Clindamycin (Topical) *on page 409*

♦ Cleocin in D5W *see* Clindamycin (Systemic) *on page 405*

♦ Cleocin Phosphate *see* Clindamycin (Systemic) *on page 405*

♦ Cleocin-T *see* Clindamycin (Topical) *on page 409*

Clevidipine (klev ID i peen)

Brand Names: US Cleviprex

Index Terms Clevidipine Butyrate

Pharmacologic Category Antihypertensive; Calcium Channel Blocker; Calcium Channel Blocker, Dihydropyridine

Additional Appendix Information

Hypertension *on page 1996*

Use Management of hypertension

Dosing

Adult Management of hypertension: IV: Initial: 1-2 mg/hour

Titration: Initial: dose may be doubled at 90-second intervals toward blood pressure goal. As blood pressure

approaches goal, dose may be increased by less than double every 5-10 minutes. **Note:** For every 1-2 mg/hour increase in dose, an approximate reduction of 2-4 mm Hg in systolic blood pressure may occur.

Usual maintenance: 4-6 mg/hour; maximum: 21 mg/hour (1000 mL within a 24-hour period due to lipid load restriction). There is limited short-term experience with doses up to 32 mg/hour. Data is limited beyond 72 hours.

Geriatric Refer to adult dosing. Initiate at the low end of the dosage range.

Renal Impairment No adjustment required with initial infusion rate.

Hepatic Impairment No adjustment required with initial infusion rate.

Additional Information Complete prescribing information should be consulted for additional detail.

Dosage Forms Excipient information presented when available (limited, particularly for generics); consult specific product labeling.

Emulsion, Intravenous:

Cleviprex: 0.5 mg/mL (50 mL, 100 mL) [contains edetate disodium, egg yolk phospholipids, soybean oil]

♦ Clevidipine Butyrate *see* Clevidipine *on page 405*

♦ Cleviprex *see* Clevidipine *on page 405*

Clidinium and Chlordiazepoxide
(kli DI nee um & klor dye az e POKS ide)

Brand Names: US Librax

Brand Names: Canada Chlorax; Librax

Index Terms Chlordiazepoxide and Clidinium

Pharmacologic Category Antispasmodic Agent, Gastrointestinal; Benzodiazepine

Use

Irritable bowel syndrome: Possibly effective for treatment of irritable bowel syndrome (eg, irritable colon, spastic colon, mucous colitis) and acute enterocolitis

Peptic ulcer: Possibly effective as adjunct treatment of peptic ulcer

Dosing

Adult

Irritable bowel syndrome: Oral: 1 to 2 capsules 3 to 4 times daily

Peptic ulcer: Oral: 1 to 2 capsules 3 to 4 times daily

Debilitated patients: Initial dose should not exceed 2 capsules per day, to be increased gradually as needed and tolerated.

Discontinuation of therapy: Do not abruptly discontinue after prolonged use; taper dose gradually.

Geriatric Initial dosage should not exceed 2 capsules per day, to be increased gradually as needed and tolerated; refer to adult dosing.

Renal Impairment There are no dosage adjustments provided in the manufacturer's labeling; use with caution.

Hepatic Impairment There are no dosage adjustments provided in the manufacturer's labeling; use with caution.

Additional Information Complete prescribing information should be consulted for additional detail.

Dosage Forms Excipient information presented when available (limited, particularly for generics); consult specific product labeling.

Capsule: Clidinium bromide 2.5 mg and chlordiazepoxide hydrochloride 5 mg

Librax: Clidinium bromide 2.5 mg and chlordiazepoxide hydrochloride 5 mg

Controlled Substance C-IV or nonscheduled (DEA exemption status dependent)

♦ Climara *see* Estradiol (Systemic) *on page 681*

♦ ClimaraPro *see* Estradiol and Levonorgestrel *on page 686*

♦ Clindacin ETZ *see* Clindamycin (Topical) *on page 409*

♦ Clindacin-P *see* Clindamycin (Topical) *on page 409*

♦ Clindacin Pac *see* Clindamycin (Topical) *on page 409*

♦ Clindagel *see* Clindamycin (Topical) *on page 409*

♦ ClindaMax *see* Clindamycin (Topical) *on page 409*

♦ Clindamycin IV Infusion (Can) *see* Clindamycin (Systemic) *on page 405*

Clindamycin (Systemic) (klin da MYE sin)

Brand Names: US Cleocin; Cleocin in D5W; Cleocin Phosphate; CLIN Single Use

Brand Names: Canada Apo-Clindamycin; Auro-Clindamycin; Ava-Clindamycin; Clindamycin Injection; Clindamycin Injection SDZ; Clindamycin Injection, USP; Clindamycin IV Infusion; Clindamycine; Dalacin C;

Mylan-Clindamycin; PMS-Clindamycin; Riva-Clindamycin; Teva-Clindamycin

Index Terms Clindamycin Hydrochloride; Clindamycin Palmitate

Pharmacologic Category Antibiotic, Lincosamide

Use

Treatment of infections: Treatment of infections due to susceptible organisms:

Bone and joint infections: Including acute hematogenous osteomyelitis caused by *Staphylococcus aureus* and as adjunctive therapy in the surgical treatment of chronic bone and joint infections caused by susceptible organisms.

Gynecological infections: Including endometritis, nongonococcal tubo-ovarian abscess, pelvic cellulitis, and postsurgical vaginal cuff infection caused by susceptible anaerobes.

Intra-abdominal infections: Including peritonitis and intra-abdominal abscess caused by susceptible anaerobic organisms.

Lower respiratory tract infections: Including pneumonia, empyema, and lung abscess caused by anaerobes, *Streptococcus pneumoniae*, other streptococci (except *Enterococcus faecalis*), and *S. aureus*.

Septicemia: Caused by *S. aureus*, streptococci (except *E. faecalis*), and susceptible anaerobes.

Serious infections: Caused by susceptible strains of streptococci, pneumococci, and staphylococci.

Skin and skin structure infections: Caused by *Streptococcus pyogenes*, *S. aureus*, and anaerobes.

Pregnancy Considerations Adverse events were not observed in animal reproduction studies. Clindamycin crosses the placenta and can be detected in the cord blood and fetal tissue (Philipson 1973; Weinstein 1976). Clindamycin injection contains benzyl alcohol which may also cross the placenta. Clindamycin pharmacokinetics are not affected by pregnancy (Philipson 1976; Weinstein 1976). Clindamycin is recommended for use in pregnant women for the prophylaxis of group B streptococcal disease in newborns (alternative therapy) (ACOG 485, 2011); prophylaxis and treatment of *Toxoplasma gondii* encephalitis (alternative therapy), or *Pneumocystis pneumonia* (PCP) (alternative therapy) (HHS [OI adult 2015]); bacterial vaginosis (CDC [Workowski 2015]); anthrax (Meaney-Delman 2014); or malaria (CDC 2013). Clindamycin is also one of the antibiotics recommended for prophylactic use prior to cesarean delivery and may be used in certain situations prior to vaginal delivery in women at high risk for endocarditis (ACOG 120, 2011).

Breast-Feeding Considerations Clindamycin can be detected in breast milk; reported concentrations range from 0.7 to 3.8 mcg/mL following maternal doses of 150 mg orally to 600 mg IV. Due to the potential for serious adverse reactions in neonates, breast-feeding is not recommended by the manufacturer. Nondose-related effects could include modification of bowel flora. One case of bloody stools in an infant occurred after a mother received clindamycin while breast-feeding; however, a causal relationship was not confirmed (Mann 1980).

Contraindications Hypersensitivity to preparations containing clindamycin, lincomycin, or any component of the formulation.

Warnings/Precautions Dosage adjustment may be necessary in patients with severe hepatic dysfunction. **[U.S. Boxed Warning]: Can cause severe and possibly fatal colitis.** Should be reserved for serious infections where less toxic antimicrobial agents are inappropriate. It should not be used in patients with nonbacterial infections such as most upper respiratory tract infections. Hypertoxin producing strains of *C. difficile* cause increased morbidity and mortality, as these infections can be refractory to antimicrobial therapy and may require colectomy. *C. difficile*-associated diarrhea (CDAD) must be considered in all patients who present with diarrhea following antibiotic use. CDAD has been observed >2 months postantibiotic treatment. Use with caution in patients with a history of gastrointestinal disease, particularly colitis. Discontinue drug if significant diarrhea, abdominal cramps, or passage of blood and mucus occurs. Use may result in overgrowth of nonsusceptible organisms, particularly yeast. Should superinfection occur, appropriate measures should be taken as indicated by the clinical situation. May cause hypersensitivity. Serious anaphylactoid reactions require immediate emergency treatment with epinephrine. Oxygen and IV corticosteroids should also be administered as indicated. Severe or fatal reactions such as toxic epidermal necrolysis (TEN) have been reported. Discontinue if severe skin reaction occurs. Premature and low birth weight infants may be more likely to develop toxicity. Some products may contain tartrazine (FD&C yellow no. 5), which may cause allergic reactions in certain individuals. Allergy is frequently seen in patients who also have an aspirin hypersensitivity. Use caution in atopic patients. A subgroup of older patients with associated severe illness may tolerate diarrhea less well. Monitor carefully for changes in bowel frequency. Not appropriate for use in the treatment of meningitis due to inadequate penetration into the CSF. Do not inject IV undiluted as a bolus. Product should be diluted in compatible fluid and infused over 10 to 60 minutes. Potentially significant interactions may exist, requiring dose or frequency adjustment, additional monitoring, and/or selection of alternative therapy.

Benzyl alcohol and derivatives: Some dosage forms may contain benzyl alcohol; large amounts of benzyl alcohol (≥99 mg/kg/day) have been associated with a potentially fatal toxicity ("gasping syndrome") in neonates; the "gasping syndrome" consists of metabolic acidosis, respiratory distress, gasping respirations, CNS dysfunction (including convulsions, intracranial hemorrhage), hypotension and cardiovascular collapse (AAP ["Inactive" 1997]; CDC, 1982); some data suggests that benzoate displaces bilirubin from protein binding sites (Ahlfors, 2001); avoid or use dosage forms containing benzyl alcohol with caution in neonates. See manufacturer's labeling.

Adverse Reactions Frequency not defined.

Cardiovascular: Cardiac arrest (rare; IV administration), hypotension (rare; IV administration), thrombophlebitis (IV)

Central nervous system: Metallic taste

Dermatologic: Acute generalized exanthematous pustulosis, erythema multiforme (rare), exfoliative dermatitis (rare), maculopapular rash, pruritus, skin rash, Stevens-Johnson syndrome (rare), toxic epidermal necrolysis, urticaria, vesiculobullous dermatitis

Gastrointestinal: Abdominal pain, antibiotic-associated colitis, *Clostridium difficile* associated diarrhea, diarrhea, esophageal ulcer, esophagitis, nausea, pseudomembranous colitis, unpleasant taste, vomiting

Genitourinary: Azotemia, oliguria, proteinuria, vaginitis

Hematologic & oncologic: Agranulocytosis, eosinophilia (transient), neutropenia (transient), thrombocytopenia

Hepatic: Abnormal hepatic function tests, jaundice

Hypersensitivity: Anaphylactoid reaction (rare)

Immunologic: DRESS syndrome

Local: Abscess at injection site (IM), induration at injection site (IM), irritation at injection site (IM), pain at injection site (IM)

Neuromuscular & skeletal: Polyarthritis (rare)

Renal: Renal insufficiency (rare)

Drug Interactions

Metabolism/Transport Effects Substrate of CYP3A4 (minor); **Note:** Assignment of Major/Minor substrate status based on clinically relevant drug interaction potential

Avoid Concomitant Use

Avoid concomitant use of Clindamycin (Systemic) with any of the following: BCG (Intravesical); Erythromycin (Systemic); Mecamylamine

Increased Effect/Toxicity

Clindamycin (Systemic) may increase the levels/effects of: Mecamylamine; Neuromuscular-Blocking Agents

Decreased Effect

Clindamycin (Systemic) may decrease the levels/effects of: BCG (Intravesical); BCG Vaccine (Immunization); Erythromycin (Systemic); Sodium Picosulfate; Typhoid Vaccine

The levels/effects of Clindamycin (Systemic) may be decreased by: Kaolin

Food Interactions Peak concentrations may be delayed with food. Management: May administer with food.

Preparation for Administration Never administer undiluted as bolus. For IV infusion, dilute vials with 50 to 100 mL of compatible diluent; concentration of clindamycin for IV infusion should not exceed 18 mg/mL.

Storage/Stability

Capsule: Store at room temperature of 20°C to 25°C (68°F to 77°F).

IV: Infusion solution in NS or D_5W solution is stable for 16 days at room temperature, 32 days refrigerated, or 8 weeks frozen. Prior to use, store vials and premixed bags at controlled room temperature 20°C to 25°C (68°F to 77°F). After initial use, discard any unused portion of vial after 24 hours.

Oral solution: Do not refrigerate reconstituted oral solution (it will thicken). Following reconstitution, oral solution is stable for 2 weeks at room temperature of 20°C to 25°C (68°F to 77°F).

Mechanism of Action Reversibly binds to 50S ribosomal subunits preventing peptide bond formation thus inhibiting bacterial protein synthesis; bacteriostatic or bactericidal depending on drug concentration, infection site, and organism

Pharmacodynamics/Kinetics

Absorption: Oral, hydrochloride: Rapid (90%); clindamycin palmitate must be hydrolyzed in the GI tract before it is active

Distribution: Distributed in body fluids and tissues including saliva, ascites fluid, pleural fluid, bone, and bile; no significant levels in CSF, even with inflamed meninges

Protein binding: 94%

Metabolism: Clindamycin phosphate is converted to clindamycin HCl (active)

Bioavailability: Oral: ~90%

Half-life elimination:
Neonates: Premature: 8.7 hours; Full-term: 3.6 hours
Infants 1 month to 1 year: 3 hours
Children: ~2.5 hours
Adults: 3 hours
Elderly (oral) 4 hours (range: 3.4 to 5.1 hours)

Time to peak, serum: Oral: Within 60 minutes; IM: 1 to 3 hours

Excretion: Urine (10%) and feces (~4%) as active drug and metabolites

Dosing

Adult & Geriatric

Usual dose:
Oral: 150 to 450 mg/dose every 6 hours
IM, IV: 600 to 2,700 mg daily in 2 to 4 divided doses; up to 4,800 mg IV daily may be used in life-threatening infections

Amnionitis: IV: 450 to 900 mg every 8 hours

Anthrax (off-label use) (Hendricks 2014):
Postexposure prophylaxis: Oral: 600 mg every 8 hours for 60 days after exposure
Cutaneous, treatment: Oral: 600 mg every 8 hours for 7 to 10 days after naturally acquired infection; 60 days following biological weapon related event
Systemic, treatment: IV: 900 mg every 8 hours; use in combination with a bactericidal antimicrobial (eg, fluoroquinolone, penicillin G); if meningitis is suspected or cannot be ruled out, use in combination with 2 bactericidal antimicrobials (eg, fluoroquinolone **and** beta-lactam). Duration of therapy is 2 weeks when meningitis has been excluded; ≥2 to 3 weeks for possible/confirmed meningitis. Patients exposed to aerosolized spores require prophylaxis to complete an antimicrobial course of 60 days from illness onset.
Injectional: IV: 600 mg every 8 hours in combination with ciprofloxacin and other antibiotics (eg, a 5-drug combination) (Hicks 2012)

Babesiosis (off-label use):
Oral: 600 mg 3 times daily for 7 to 10 days with quinine (Vannier 2012; Wormser 2006)
IV: 300 to 600 mg every 6 hours for 7 to 10 days with quinine (Vannier 2012; Wormser 2006)
Note: Relapsing infection may require at least 6 weeks of therapy (Vannier 2012)

Bacterial vaginosis (off-label use): Oral: 300 mg twice daily for 7 days (CDC 2010)

Bite wounds (animal) (off-label use):
Oral: 300 mg 3 times daily; in combination with a second- or third-generation cephalosporin, levofloxacin, or sulfamethoxazole and trimethoprim (IDSA [Stevens 2014])
IV: 600 mg every 6 to 8 hours; in combination with a second- or third-generation cephalosporin, levofloxacin, or sulfamethoxazole and trimethoprim (IDSA [Stevens 2014])

Gangrenous pyomyositis: IV: 900 mg every 8 hours with penicillin G (Brook, 1999; Hassel 2004; Wong 2013)

Group B streptococcus (neonatal prophylaxis) (off-label use): IV: 900 mg every 8 hours until delivery (CDC 2010)

Impetigo: Oral: 300 to 450 mg 4 times daily for 7 days, depending on response (IDSA [Stevens 2014])

Malaria, severe (off-label use): IV: Load: 10 mg/kg followed by 15 mg/kg/day divided every 8 hours *plus* IV quinidine gluconate; switch to oral therapy (clindamycin *plus* quinine) when able for total clindamycin treatment duration of 7 days (**Note:** Quinine duration is region specific, consult CDC for current recommendations) (CDC 2013)

Malaria, uncomplicated treatment (off-label use): Oral: 20 mg/kg/day divided every 8 hours for 7 days *plus* quinine (CDC 2013)

Osteomyelitis due to MRSA (off-label use): IV, Oral: 600 mg 3 times daily for a minimum of 8 weeks (some experts combine with rifampin) (Liu 2011)

Pelvic inflammatory disease: IV: 900 mg every 8 hours with gentamicin (conventional or single daily dosing); 24 hours after clinical improvement may convert to oral doxycycline 100 mg twice daily **or** clindamycin 450 mg 4 times daily to complete 14 days of total

therapy. Avoid doxycycline if tubo-ovarian abscess is present (CDC 2010).

Pharyngitis, group A streptococci (IDSA recommendations): Oral:
Acute treatment in penicillin-allergic patients: 21 mg/kg/day divided every 8 hours (maximum: 300 mg per dose) for 10 days (Shulman 2012)
Chronic carrier treatment: 20 to 30 mg/kg/day divided every 8 hours (maximum: 300 mg per dose) for 10 days (Shulman 2012)

***Pneumocystis* pneumonia (PCP) in HIV-infected patients (alternative to preferred therapy) (off-label use):**
IV: 600 mg every 6 hours or 900 mg every 8 hours with primaquine for 21 days (HHS [OI adult 2015])
Oral: 450 mg every 6 hours or 600 mg every 8 hours with primaquine for 21 days (HHS [OI adult 2015])

Pneumonia due to MRSA (off-label use): IV, Oral: 600 mg 3 times daily for 7 to 21 days (Liu 2011)

Prophylaxis against infective endocarditis (off-label use):
Oral: 600 mg 30 to 60 minutes before procedure with no follow-up dose needed (Wilson 2007)
IM, IV: 600 mg 30 to 60 minutes before procedure. Intramuscular injections should be avoided in patients who are receiving anticoagulant therapy. In these circumstances, orally administered regimens should be given whenever possible. Intravenously administered antibiotics should be used for patients who are unable to tolerate or absorb oral medications (Wilson 2007).
Note: American Heart Association (AHA) guidelines now recommend prophylaxis only in patients undergoing invasive procedures and in whom underlying cardiac conditions may predispose to a higher risk of adverse outcomes should infection occur. As of April 2007, routine prophylaxis for GI/GU procedures is no longer recommended by the AHA.

Prophylaxis in total joint replacement patients undergoing dental procedures which produce bacteremia (off-label use): Note: In general, patients with prosthetic joint implants do not require prophylactic antibiotics prior to dental procedures. In planning an invasive oral procedure, dental consultation with the patient's orthopedic surgeon may be advised to review the risks of infection (Sollecito 2015).
Oral: 600 mg 1 hour prior to procedure (ADA 2003)
IV: 600 mg 1 hour prior to procedure (for patients unable to take oral medication) (ADA 2003)

Prosthetic joint infection:
Chronic antimicrobial suppression, Staphylococci (oxacillin-susceptible) (alternative to cephalexin or cefadroxil) (off-label use): Oral: 300 mg every 6 hours (Osmon 2013)
Propionibacterium acnes, treatment (alternative to penicillin G or ceftriaxone):
Oral: 300 to 450 mg every 6 hours for 4 to 6 weeks (Osmon 2013)
IV: 600 to 900 mg every 8 hours for 4 to 6 weeks (Osmon 2013)

Septic arthritis due to MRSA (off-label use): IV, Oral: 600 mg 3 times daily for 3 to 4 weeks (Liu 2011)

Skin and soft tissue infections due to MSSA:
Oral: 300 to 450 mg 4 times daily for 7 to 14 days (IDSA [Stevens 2014])
IV: 600 mg every 8 hours for 7 to 14 days (IDSA [Stevens 2014])

Skin and soft tissue infections due to MRSA (off-label use):
Oral: 300 to 450 mg 4 times daily for 7 to 14 days (IDSA [Stevens 2014])
IV: 600 mg every 8 hours for 7 to 14 days (IDSA [Stevens 2014])
Complicated infections: IV, Oral: 600 mg 3 times daily for 7 to 14 days (IDSA [Liu 2011])
Cellulitis: Oral: 300 to 450 mg 3 times daily for 5 to 10 days (Liu 2011)

Skin and soft tissue necrotizing infections (off-label use): IV: 600 to 900 mg every 8 hours, in combination with cefotaxime for empiric therapy of polymicrobial infections **or** in combination with penicillin IV for the treatment of group A streptococcal or *Clostridium* species necrotizing infections. May give as monotherapy for MSSA. Continue until further debridement is not necessary, patient has clinically improved, and patient is afebrile for 48 to 72 hours (IDSA [Stevens 2014])

Streptococcal skin infections: IV: 600 to 900 mg every 8 hours (IDSA [Stevens 2014])

Surgical (perioperative) prophylaxis (off-label use): IV: 900 mg within 60 minutes prior to surgical incision. Doses may be repeated in 6 hours if procedure is lengthy (Bratzler 2013).

CLINDAMYCIN (SYSTEMIC)

Toxic shock syndrome: IV: 900 mg every 8 hours with additional concomitant therapy (Lappin 2009; Wong 2013)

***Toxoplasma gondii* encephalitis in HIV-infected patients (off label use):**

Treatment (alternative to preferred regimen): IV, Oral: 600 mg every 6 hours in combination with pyrimethamine and leucovorin. Continue therapy for at least 6 weeks; longer duration may be required if incomplete response or extensive disease (HHS [OI adult 2015]).

Chronic maintenance therapy (alternative to preferred regimen): Oral: 600 mg every 8 hours in combination with pyrimethamine and leucovorin; may discontinue when asymptomatic and CD4 count >200 cells/mm^3 for 6 months in response to ART (HHS [OI adult 2015])

Pediatric
Usual dose:
Infants and Children:

Oral: 8 to 40 mg/kg/day in 3 to 4 divided doses; Manufacturer's labeling: 8 to 20 mg/kg/day (as hydrochloride) or 8 to 25 mg/kg/day (as palmitate) in 3 to 4 divided doses; minimum dose of palmitate: 37.5 mg 3 times daily

IM, IV: Manufacturer's labeling: 20 to 40 mg/kg/day in 3 to 4 divided doses

Acute bacterial rhinosinusitis (off-label use): Oral: 30 to 40 mg/kg/day divided every 8 hours with concomitant cefixime or cefpodoxime for 10 to 14 days. **Note:** Recommended in patients with non-type I penicillin allergy, after failure of initial therapy or in patients at risk for antibiotic resistance (eg, daycare attendance, age <2 years, recent hospitalization, antibiotic use within the past month) (Chow 2012).

Anthrax (off-label use) (Bradley 2014):

Postexposure prophylaxis: Oral: 30 mg/kg/day divided every 8 hours for 60 days after exposure (maximum: 900 mg/dose)

Cutaneous, treatment: Oral: 30 mg/kg/day divided every 8 hours for 7 to 10 days after naturally acquired infection; up to 60 days following biological weapon related event (maximum: 900 mg/dose)

Systemic, treatment: IV: 40 mg/kg/day divided every 8 hours for ≥14 days (maximum: 900 mg/dose); use in combination with a bactericidal antimicrobial (eg, fluoroquinolone, penicillin G); if meningitis is suspected or cannot be ruled out, use in combination with 2 bactericidal antimicrobials (eg, fluoroquinolone **and** beta-lactam or glycopeptide). Continue with prophylaxis therapy for up to 60 days from onset of illness.

Babesiosis (off-label use): Oral: 20 to 40 mg/kg divided every 8 hours for 7 to 10 days *plus* quinine (*Medical Letter* 2007)

Impetigo: Oral: 20 mg/kg/day divided every 8 hours for 7 days, depending on response (IDSA [Stevens 2014])

Malaria, severe (off-label use): IV: Load: 10 mg/kg followed by 15 mg/kg/day divided every 8 hours *plus* IV quinidine gluconate; switch to oral therapy (clindamycin *plus* quinine) when able for total clindamycin treatment duration of 7 days (**Note:** Quinine duration is region specific, consult CDC for current recommendations) (CDC 2013)

Malaria, uncomplicated treatment (off-label use): Oral: 20 mg/kg/day divided every 8 hours for 7 days *plus* quinine (CDC 2013)

Osteomyelitis due to MRSA (off-label use): IV, Oral: 10 to 13 mg/kg/dose every 6 to 8 hours for a minimum of 4 to 6 weeks (maximum: 40 mg/kg/day) (Liu 2011)

Pharyngitis, group A streptococci (IDSA recommendations): Oral:

Acute treatment in penicillin-allergic patients: 21 mg/kg/day divided every 8 hours (maximum: 300 mg per dose) for 10 days (Shulman 2012).

Chronic carrier treatment: 20 to 30 mg/kg/day divided every 8 hours (maximum: 300 mg per dose) for 10 days (Shulman 2012).

Pneumocystis pneumonia (PCP) in HIV-infected patients (alternative to preferred therapy) (off-label use): Adolescents: Refer to adult dosing.

Pneumonia:

Community-acquired pneumonia (CAP) (IDSA/PIDS 2011): Infants >3 months and Children: **Note:** In children ≥5 years, a macrolide antibiotic should be added if atypical pneumonia cannot be ruled out.

Group A *Streptococcus:*

Moderate-to-severe infection (alternative to ampicillin/penicillin): IV: 40 mg/kg/day divided every 6 to 8 hours

Mild infection, step-down therapy (alternative to amoxicillin/penicillin): Oral: 40 mg/kg/day divided every 8 hours

Presumed bacterial (in addition to recommended antibiotic therapy), *S. pneumoniae* moderate-to-severe (MICs to penicillin ≤2.0 mcg/mL) (alternative to ampicillin/penicillin): IV: 40 mg/kg/day divided every 6-8 hours

S. pneumoniae:

Moderate-to-severe infection (MICs to penicillin ≥4.0 mcg/mL) (alternative to ceftriaxone): IV: 40 mg/kg/day divided every 6-8 hours

Mild infection, step-down therapy (MICs to penicillin ≥4.0 mcg/mL) (alternative to levofloxacin or linezolid): Oral: 30 to 40 mg/kg/day divided every 8 hours

S. aureus (methicillin-susceptible):

Moderate-to-severe infection (alternative to cefazolin or oxacillin): IV: 40 mg/kg/day divided every 6 to 8 hours

Mild infection, step-down therapy (alternative to cephalexin): Oral: 30 to 40 mg/kg/day divided every 6 to 8 hours

S. aureus (methicillin-resistant/clindamycin-susceptible):

Moderate-to-severe infection (preferred): IV: 40 mg/kg/day divided every 6 to 8 hours; recommended duration: 7 to 21 days (Liu 2011)

Mild infection, step-down therapy (preferred): Oral: 30 to 40 mg/kg/day divided every 6 to 8 hours; recommended duration: 7 to 21 days (Liu 2011)

Healthcare-associated pneumonia (HAP) (methicillin-resistant/clindamycin-susceptible): Children: Oral, IV: 30 to 40 mg/kg/day divided every 6 to 8 hours for 7 to 21 days (Liu 2011)

Prophylaxis against infective endocarditis (off-label use):

Oral: 20 mg/kg 30 to 60 minutes before procedure (Wilson 2007)

IM, IV: 20 mg/kg 30 to 60 minutes before procedure. Intramuscular injections should be avoided in patients who are receiving anticoagulant therapy. In these circumstances, orally administered regimens should be given whenever possible. Intravenously administered antibiotics should be used for patients who are unable to tolerate or absorb oral medications (Wilson 2007).

Note: American Heart Association (AHA) guidelines now recommend prophylaxis only in patients undergoing invasive procedures and in whom underlying cardiac conditions may predispose to a higher risk of adverse outcomes should infection occur. As of April 2007, routine prophylaxis for GI/GU procedures is no longer recommended by the AHA.

Septic arthritis due to MRSA (off-label use): IV, Oral: 10 to 13 mg/kg/dose every 6 to 8 hours for minimum of 3 to 4 weeks (maximum: 40 mg/kg/day) (Liu 2011)

Skin and soft tissue infections due to MSSA:

Oral: 25 to 30 mg/kg/day divided every 8 hours for 7 to 14 days (IDSA [Stevens 2014])

IV: 25 to 40 mg/kg/day divided every 8 hours for 7 to 14 days (IDSA [Stevens 2014])

Skin and soft tissue infections due to MRSA (off-label use):

Oral: 30 to 40 mg/kg/day divided every 8 hours for 7 to 14 days (IDSA [Stevens 2014])

IV: 25 to 40 mg/kg/day divided every 8 hours for 7 to 14 days (IDSA [Stevens 2014])

Complicated infections: Oral, IV: 10 to 13 mg/kg/dose every 6 to 8 hours for 7 to 14 days (maximum: 40 mg/kg/day) (Liu 2011)

Cellulitis: Oral: 10 to 13 mg/kg/dose every 6 to 8 hours for 5 to 10 days (maximum: 40 mg/kg/day) (Liu 2011)

Skin and soft tissue necrotizing infections (off-label use): IV: 10 to 13 mg/kg/dose every 8 hours, in combination with cefotaxime for empiric therapy of polymicrobial infections **or** in combination with penicillin IV for the treatment of group A streptococcal or *Clostridium* species necrotizing infections. May give as monotherapy for MSSA. Continue until further debridement is not necessary, patient has clinically improved, and patient is afebrile for 48 to 72 hours (IDSA [Stevens 2014])

Streptococcal skin infections: IV: 10 to 13 mg/kg/dose every 8 hours (IDSA [Stevens 2014])

Surgical (perioperative) prophylaxis (off-label use): IV: 10 mg/kg within 60 minutes prior to surgical incision. Doses may be repeated in 6 hours if procedure is lengthy (maximum single dose: 900 mg) (Bratzler 2013).

***Toxoplasma gondii* encephalitis in HIV-exposed/-positive patients (off-label use):**

Children:

Treatment: IV, Oral: 5 to 7.5 mg/kg/dose (maximum dose: 600 mg) every 6 hours (plus pyrimethamine and leucovorin) (DHHS [OI Children 2013])

Secondary prevention: Oral: 7 to 10 mg/kg/dose (maximum dose: 600 mg) every 8 hours (plus pyrimethamine and leucovorin) (DHHS [OI Children 2013])

Adolescents: Refer to adult dosing.

Renal Impairment Mild to moderate impairment: No dosage adjustment necessary

End stage renal disease (ESRD) on hemodialysis or peritoneal dialysis: Not removed from serum (eg, poorly dialyzed); no supplemental dose or dosage adjustment necessary

Continuous renal replacement therapy (CRRT) (eg, CVVH, CVVHD, CVVHDF): No supplemental dose or dosage adjustment necessary (Heintz 2009).

Hepatic Impairment Mild impairment: There are no dosage adjustments provided in the manufacturer's labeling.

Moderate to severe impairment: There are no dosage adjustments provided in the manufacturer's labeling; in studies of patients with moderate or severe liver disease, half-life is prolonged, however, when administered on an every 8 hour schedule, accumulation should rarely occur. In severe liver disease, use caution and monitor liver enzymes periodically during therapy.

Dietary Considerations May be taken with food.

Administration

IM: Deep IM sites, rotate sites; do not exceed 600 mg in a single injection.

IV: **Never administer undiluted as bolus**; administer by IV intermittent infusion over at least 10-60 minutes, at a maximum rate of 30 mg/minute (do not exceed 1200 mg/hour).

Oral: Administer with a full glass of water to minimize esophageal ulceration; give around-the-clock to promote less variation in peak and trough serum levels.

Monitoring Parameters Observe for changes in bowel frequency. Monitor for colitis and resolution of symptoms. In severe liver disease monitor liver function tests periodically; during prolonged therapy monitor CBC, liver and renal function tests periodically.

Additional Information *In vitro* susceptibility rates to clindamycin are higher in community acquired versus hospital acquired MRSA, although this may vary by geographic region. The D-zone test is recommended for detection of inducible resistance to clindamycin in erythromycin-resistant but clindamycin-susceptible isolates (Liu, 2011).

Dosage Forms Excipient information presented when available (limited, particularly for generics); consult specific product labeling. [DSC] = Discontinued product

Capsule, Oral, as hydrochloride [strength expressed as base]:

Cleocin: 75 mg, 150 mg [contains brilliant blue fcf (fd&c blue #1), tartrazine (fd&c yellow #5)]

Cleocin: 300 mg [contains brilliant blue fcf (fd&c blue #1)]

Generic: 75 mg, 150 mg, 300 mg

Kit, Injection, as phosphate [strength expressed as base]:

CLIN Single Use: 300 mg/2 mL [contains benzyl alcohol, edetate disodium]

Solution, Injection, as phosphate [strength expressed as base]:

Cleocin Phosphate: 300 mg/2 mL (2 mL) [contains benzyl alcohol]

Cleocin Phosphate: 300 mg/2 mL (2 mL); 600 mg/4 mL (4 mL) [contains benzyl alcohol, edetate disodium]

Cleocin Phosphate: 900 mg/6 mL (6 mL) [contains benzyl alcohol]

Cleocin Phosphate: 900 mg/6 mL (6 mL); 9 g/60 mL (60 mL) [contains benzyl alcohol, edetate disodium]

Generic: 300 mg/2 mL (2 mL); 600 mg/4 mL (4 mL); 900 mg/6 mL (6 mL); 9000 mg/60 mL (60 mL); 9 g/60 mL (60 mL)

Solution, Intravenous, as phosphate [strength expressed as base]:

Cleocin in D5W: 300 mg/50 mL (50 mL); 600 mg/50 mL (50 mL); 900 mg/50 mL (50 mL) [contains edetate disodium]

Cleocin Phosphate: 600 mg/4 mL (4 mL) [contains benzyl alcohol, edetate disodium]

Cleocin Phosphate: 900 mg/6 mL (6 mL) [contains benzyl alcohol]

Generic: 300 mg/50 mL (50 mL); 600 mg/50 mL (50 mL); 900 mg/50 mL (50 mL); 150 mg/mL (2 mL); 300 mg/2 mL (2 mL [DSC]); 600 mg/4 mL (4 mL [DSC]); 900 mg/6 mL (6 mL)

Solution Reconstituted, Oral, as palmitate hydrochloride [strength expressed as base]:

Cleocin: 75 mg/5 mL (100 mL) [contains ethylparaben]

Generic: 75 mg/5 mL (100 mL)

Clindamycin (Topical) (klin da MYE sin)

Brand Names: US Cleocin; Cleocin-T; Clindacin ETZ; Clindacin Pac; Clindacin-P; Clindagel; ClindaMax; Clindesse; Evoclin

Brand Names: Canada Clinda-T; Clindasol; Clindets; Dalacin T; Dalacin Vaginal; Taro-Clindamycin

Index Terms Clindamycin Phosphate

Pharmacologic Category Antibiotic, Lincosamide; Topical Skin Product, Acne

Use Treatment of bacterial vaginosis (vaginal cream, vaginal suppository); topically in treatment of severe acne

Dosing

Adult & Geriatric

Acne: *Topical:*

Gel (Cleocin T®, ClindaMax®), pledget, lotion, solution: Apply a thin film twice daily

Gel (Clindagel®), foam (Evoclin®): Apply once daily

Bacterial vaginosis: *Intravaginal:*

Suppositories: Insert one ovule (100 mg clindamycin) daily into vagina at bedtime for 3 days

Cream:

Cleocin®: One full applicator inserted intravaginally once daily before bedtime for 3 or 7 consecutive days in nonpregnant patients or for 7 consecutive days in pregnant patients

Clindesse®: One full applicator inserted intravaginally as a single dose at anytime during the day in nonpregnant patients

Pediatric Acne: *Topical:* Children ≥12 years: Refer to adult dosing.

Additional Information Complete prescribing information should be consulted for additional detail.

Dosage Forms Excipient information presented when available (limited, particularly for generics); consult specific product labeling. [DSC] = Discontinued product

Cream, Vaginal, as phosphate [strength expressed as base]:

Cleocin: 2% (40 g) [contains benzyl alcohol]

Clindesse: 2% (5 g, 5.8 g [DSC]) [contains disodium edta, methylparaben, propylparaben]

Generic: 2% (40 g)

Foam, External, as phosphate [strength expressed as base]:

Evoclin: 1% (50 g, 100 g) [contains cetyl alcohol, propylene glycol]

Generic: 1% (50 g, 100 g)

Gel, External, as phosphate [strength expressed as base]:

Cleocin-T: 1% (30 g, 60 g) [contains methylparaben, propylene glycol]

Clindagel: 1% (40 mL [DSC], 75 mL) [contains methylparaben, polyethylene glycol, propylene glycol]

ClindaMax: 1% (30 g, 60 g)

Generic: 1% (30 g, 60 g)

Kit, External, as phosphate [strength expressed as base]:

Clindacin ETZ: 1% [contains cetyl alcohol, isopropyl alcohol, propylene glycol]

Clindacin Pac: 1% [contains cetyl alcohol, isopropyl alcohol, propylene glycol]

Lotion, External, as phosphate [strength expressed as base]:

Cleocin-T: 1% (60 mL) [contains cetostearyl alcohol, methylparaben]

ClindaMax: 1% (60 mL)

Generic: 1% (60 mL)

Solution, External, as phosphate [strength expressed as base]:

Cleocin-T: 1% (30 mL, 60 mL) [contains isopropyl alcohol, propylene glycol]

Generic: 1% (30 mL, 60 mL)

◄ Suppository, Vaginal, as phosphate [strength expressed as base]:
Cleocin: 100 mg (3 ea)
Swab, External, as phosphate [strength expressed as base]:
Cleocin-T: 1% (60 ea) [contains isopropyl alcohol, propylene glycol]
Clindacin ETZ: 1% (60 ea) [contains isopropyl alcohol, propylene glycol]
Clindacin-P: 1% (69 ea) [contains isopropyl alcohol, propylene glycol]
Generic: 1% (60 ea)

Clindamycin and Tretinoin
(klin da MYE sin & TRET i noyn)

Brand Names: US Veltin; Ziana
Index Terms Clindamycin Phosphate and Tretinoin; Tretinoin and Clindamycin; Veltin
Pharmacologic Category Acne Products; Retinoic Acid Derivative; Topical Skin Product; Topical Skin Product, Acne
Use Acne: For the treatment of acne vulgaris in patients ≥12 years.
Dosing
Adult Acne: Topical: Apply once daily in the evening or at bedtime
Pediatric Acne: Topical: Children ≥12 years and Adolescents: Refer to adult dosing.
Renal Impairment There are no dosage adjustments provided in the manufacturer's labeling; however, dosage adjustment unlikely due to low systemic absorption.
Hepatic Impairment There are no dosage adjustments provided in the manufacturer's labeling; however, dosage adjustment unlikely due to low systemic absorption.
Additional Information Complete prescribing information should be consulted for additional detail.
Dosage Forms Excipient information presented when available (limited, particularly for generics); consult specific product labeling.
Gel, topical:
Veltin™: Clindamycin phosphate 1.2% and tretinoin 0.025% (30 g, 60 g)
Ziana®: Clindamycin phosphate 1.2% and tretinoin 0.025% (30 g, 60 g)

◆ Clindamycine (Can) see Clindamycin (Systemic) on page 405
◆ Clindamycin Hydrochloride see Clindamycin (Systemic) on page 405
◆ Clindamycin Injection (Can) see Clindamycin (Systemic) on page 405
◆ Clindamycin Injection SDZ (Can) see Clindamycin (Systemic) on page 405
◆ Clindamycin Injection, USP (Can) see Clindamycin (Systemic) on page 405
◆ Clindamycin Palmitate see Clindamycin (Systemic) on page 405
◆ Clindamycin Phosphate see Clindamycin (Topical) on page 409
◆ Clindamycin Phosphate and Tretinoin see Clindamycin and Tretinoin on page 410
◆ Clindasol (Can) see Clindamycin (Topical) on page 409
◆ Clinda-T (Can) see Clindamycin (Topical) on page 409
◆ Clindesse see Clindamycin (Topical) on page 409
◆ Clindets (Can) see Clindamycin (Topical) on page 409
◆ Clinolipid see Fat Emulsion (Plant Based) on page 743
◆ Clinoril see Sulindac on page 1717
◆ Clinoril [DSC] see Sulindac on page 1717
◆ Clinpro 5000 see Fluoride on page 782
◆ CLIN Single Use see Clindamycin (Systemic) on page 405

CloBAZam (KLOE ba zam)

Brand Names: US Onfi
Brand Names: Canada Apo-Clobazam; Clobazam-10; Dom-Clobazam; Frisium; Novo-Clobazam; PMS-Clobazam
Pharmacologic Category Benzodiazepine
Use
US labeling: **Lennox-Gastaut syndrome:** Adjunctive treatment of seizures associated with Lennox-Gastaut syndrome in patients ≥2 years
Canadian labeling: **Epilepsy:** Adjunctive treatment of epilepsy

Pregnancy Considerations Adverse events were observed in animal reproduction studies. Clobazam crosses the placenta. An increased risk of fetal malformations may be associated with first trimester exposure. The Canadian labeling contraindicates use in the first trimester. Exposure to benzodiazepines immediately prior to or during birth may result in hypothermia, hypotonia, respiratory depression, and difficulty feeding in the neonate; neonates exposed to benzodiazepines late in pregnancy may develop dependence and withdrawal. The incidence of premature birth and low birth weights may be increased following maternal use of benzodiazepines; hypoglycemia and respiratory problems in the neonate may occur following exposure late in pregnancy. Neonatal withdrawal symptoms may occur within days to weeks after birth and "floppy infant syndrome" (which also includes withdrawal symptoms) has been reported with some benzodiazepines (Bergman, 1992; Iqbal, 2002; Wikner, 2007). A combination of factors influences the potential teratogenicity of anticonvulsant therapy. When treating women with epilepsy, monotherapy with the lowest effective dose and avoidance medications known to have a high incidence of teratogenic effects is recommended (Harden, 2009; Wlodarczyk, 2012).

Patients exposed to clobazam during pregnancy are encouraged to enroll themselves into the North American Antiepileptic Drug (NAAED) Pregnancy Registry by calling 1-888-233-2334. Additional information is available at www.aedpregnancyregistry.org.

Breast-Feeding Considerations Clobazam is excreted into breast milk. Due to the potential for serious adverse reactions in the nursing infant, the U.S. manufacturer recommends a decision be made whether to discontinue nursing or to discontinue the drug, taking into account the importance of treatment to the mother. Use in nursing women is contraindicated in the Canadian labeling. Drowsiness, lethargy, or weight loss in nursing infants have been observed in case reports following maternal use of some benzodiazepines (Iqbal, 2002).

Medication Guide Available Yes
Contraindications Hypersensitivity to clobazam or any component of the formulation.
Canadian labeling (not in US labeling): Myasthenia gravis; narrow-angle glaucoma; severe hepatic or respiratory disease; sleep apnea; history of substance abuse; use in the first trimester of pregnancy; breast-feeding

Warnings/Precautions Serious reactions, including Stevens-Johnson syndrome (SJS) and toxic epidermal necrolysis (TEN), have been reported. Monitor patients closely for signs and symptoms especially during the first 8 weeks or when reintroducing therapy. Permanently discontinue if SJS/TEN suspected.

Rebound or withdrawal symptoms may occur following abrupt discontinuation or large decreases in dose (more common with prolonged treatment). Cautiously taper dose if drug discontinuation is required. In the elderly, lower doses are recommended. Use with caution in patients with mild-to-moderate hepatic impairment or with preexisting muscle weakness or ataxia (may cause muscle weakness). The Canadian labeling contraindicates use in patients with severe hepatic impairment or with myasthenia gravis. Concentrations of the active metabolite are 3 to 5 times higher in patients who are known CYP2C19 poor metabolizers compared to CYP2C19 extensive metabolizers; dose adjustment is needed in patients who are poor CYP2C19 metabolizers.

Causes CNS depression (dose related) resulting in sedation, dizziness, confusion, or ataxia which may impair physical and mental capabilities. Patients must be cautioned about performing tasks which require mental alertness (eg, operating machinery or driving). Use with caution in patients with respiratory disease. The Canadian labeling contraindicates use in severe respiratory insufficiency or sleep apnea syndrome.

Tolerance, psychological and physical dependence may occur with prolonged use. Where possible, avoid use in patients with drug abuse, alcoholism, or psychiatric disease (eg, depression, psychosis). May increase risk of suicidal thoughts/behavior.

Acute withdrawal, including seizures, may be precipitated in patients after administration of flumazenil to patients receiving long-term benzodiazepine therapy. Potentially significant drug-drug interactions may exist, requiring dose or frequency adjustment, additional monitoring, and/or selection of alternative therapy.

Benzodiazepines have been associated with anterograde amnesia. Paradoxical reactions, including hyperactive or aggressive behavior, have been reported with benzodiazepines, particularly in adolescent/pediatric or psychiatric patients. Does not have analgesic, antidepressant, or antipsychotic properties.

Adverse Reactions

>10%:

Central nervous system: Drowsiness (16% to 25%), lethargy (10% to 15%), agressive behavior (8% to 14%), irritability (3% to 11%)

Gastrointestinal: Sialorrhea (13% to 14%)

Respiratory: Upper respiratory tract infection (13% to 14%)

Miscellaneous: Fever (10% to 17%)

1% to 10%:

Central nervous system: Ataxia (10%), sedation (9%), insomnia (5% to 7%), psychomotor agitation (5%), fatigue (3% to 5%), dysarthria (2% to 5%), dysarthria (2% to 5%)

Gastrointestinal: Constipation (2% to 10%), vomiting (7% to 9%), decreased appetite (7%), increased appetite (2% to 5%), dysphagia (5%)

Genitourinary: Urinary tract infection (2% to 5%)

Respiratory: Cough (3% to 7%), pneumonia (3% to 7%), bronchitis (2% to 5%)

Postmarketing and/or case reports (Limited to important or life-threatening): Angioedema, aspiration, behavioral changes, blurred vision, confusion, delirium, delusions, depression, diplopia, eosinophilia, hallucination, hypothermia, leukopenia, lip edema, mood changes, respiratory depression, Stevens-Johnson syndrome, suicidal ideation, suicidal tendencies, thrombocytopenia, toxic epidermal necrolysis, urinary retention, withdrawal syndrome

Drug Interactions

Metabolism/Transport Effects Substrate of CYP2B6 (minor), CYP2C19 (major), CYP3A4 (minor), P-glycoprotein; **Note:** Assignment of Major/Minor substrate status based on clinically relevant drug interaction potential; **Inhibits** CYP2D6 (moderate); **Induces** CYP3A4 (weak)

Avoid Concomitant Use

Avoid concomitant use of CloBAZam with any of the following: Azelastine (Nasal); Methadone; OLANZapine; Orphenadrine; Paraldehyde; Sodium Oxybate; Thalidomide; Thioridazine

Increased Effect/Toxicity

CloBAZam may increase the levels/effects of: Azelastine (Nasal); Brexpiprazole; Buprenorphine; CloZAPine; CNS Depressants; CYP2D6 Substrates; DOXOrubicin (Conventional); Eliglustat; Fesoterodine; Hydrocodone; Methadone; Methotrimeprazine; Metoprolol; Metyrosine; Mirtazapine; Nebivolol; Orphenadrine; Paraldehyde; Pramipexole; ROPINIRole; Rotigotine; Selective Serotonin Reuptake Inhibitors; Sodium Oxybate; Stiripentol; Suvorexant; Thalidomide; Thioridazine; Zolpidem

The levels/effects of CloBAZam may be increased by: Alcohol (Ethyl); Brimonidine (Topical); Cannabis; CYP2C19 Inhibitors (Moderate); CYP2C19 Inhibitors (Strong); Doxylamine; Dronabinol; Droperidol; HydrOXYzine; Kava Kava; Luliconazole; Magnesium Sulfate; Methotrimeprazine; Minocycline; Nabilone; OLANZapine; Perampanel; Propafenone; Rufinamide; Stiripentol; Tapentadol; Teduglutide; Tetrahydrocannabinol

Decreased Effect

CloBAZam may decrease the levels/effects of: ARIPiprazole; Codeine; Contraceptives (Estrogens); Contraceptives (Progestins); NiMODipine; Saxagliptin; Tamoxifen; TraMADol

The levels/effects of CloBAZam may be decreased by: CYP2C19 Inducers (Strong); Dabrafenib; Enzalutamide; Lumacaftor; Theophylline Derivatives; Yohimbine

Food Interactions Ethanol: Concomitant administration may increase bioavailability of clobazam by 50%. Management: Monitor for increased effects with coadministration.

Storage/Stability Tablets and suspension: Store at 20°C to 25°C (68°F to 77°F). Dispose of unused suspension 90 days after opening bottle.

Mechanism of Action Clobazam is a 1,5 benzodiazepine which binds to stereospecific benzodiazepine receptors on the postsynaptic GABA neuron at several sites within the central nervous system, including the limbic system, reticular formation. Enhancement of the inhibitory effect of GABA on neuronal excitability results by increased neuronal membrane permeability to chloride ions. This shift in chloride ions results in hyperpolarization (a less excitable state) and stabilization. Benzodiazepine receptors and effects appear to be linked to the GABA-A receptors. Benzodiazepines do not bind to GABA-B receptors.

Pharmacodynamics/Kinetics

Onset: Maximum effect: 5-9 days

Absorption: Rapid and extensive; not affected by food or crushing tablet

Distribution: 100 L

Protein binding: Clobazam: 80% to 90%; N-desmethylclobazam (NCLB): 70%

Metabolism: Hepatic via CYP3A4 and to a lesser extent via CYP2C19 and 2B6 (N-demethylation to active metabolite [N-desmethyl] with ~20% activity of clobazam). CYP2C19 primarily mediates subsequent hydroxylation of the N-desmethyl metabolite; metabolic rate increased in children (53% to 69%) (Ng, 2007). Plasma concentrations of NCLB are 5 times higher in CYP2C19 poor metabolizers versus extensive metabolizers.

Bioavailability: 87% (Ng, 2007)

Half-life elimination: Children: Clobazam: 16 hours (Ng, 2007); Adults: Clobazam: 36 to 42 hours; N-desmethyl (active): 71 to 82 hours

Time to peak: Tablet: 0.5 to 4 hours; Oral suspension: 0.5 to 2 hours

Excretion: Urine (~82%; unchanged drug: 2%, NCLB and other metabolites: ~94%); feces (~11%; 1% unchanged drug)

Dosing

Adult

US labeling:

Lennox-Gastaut (adjunctive): Oral: **Note:** Dose should be titrated according to patient tolerability and response.

≤30 kg: Initial: 5 mg once daily for ≥1 week, then increase to 5 mg twice daily for ≥1 week, then increase to 10 mg twice daily thereafter

>30 kg: Initial: 5 mg twice daily for ≥1 week, then increase to 10 mg twice daily for ≥1 week, then increase to 20 mg twice daily thereafter

CYP2C19 poor metabolizers:

≤30 kg: Initial: 5 mg once daily for ≥2 weeks, then increase to 5 mg twice daily; after ≥1 week may increase to 10 mg twice daily

>30 kg: Initial: 5 mg once daily for ≥1 week, then increase to 5 mg twice daily for ≥1 week, then increase to 10 mg twice daily; after ≥1 week may increase to 20 mg twice daily

Canadian labeling:

Epilepsy (adjunctive): Oral: Initial: 5 to 15 mg/day; dosage may be gradually adjusted (based on tolerance and seizure control) to a maximum of 80 mg/day. **Note:** Daily doses of up to 30 mg may be taken as a single dose at bedtime; higher doses should be divided.

CYP2C19 poor metabolizers: Initiate at lowest recommended doses; titrate slowly as tolerated to half of usual recommended maximum dose. If needed, dose may be further increased as tolerated to usual recommended maximum dose beginning day 21.

Catamenial epilepsy (off-label use): Oral: 20 to 30 mg daily for 10 days during the perimenstrual period (Feely, 1984)

Geriatric

US labeling:

Lennox-Gastaut (adjunctive): Oral:

≤30 kg: Initial: 5 mg once daily for ≥2 weeks, then increase to 5 mg twice daily; after ≥1 week may increase to 10 mg twice daily based on patient tolerability and response

>30 kg: Initial: 5 mg once daily for ≥1 week, then increase to 5 mg twice daily for ≥1 week, then increase to 10 mg twice daily; after ≥1 week may increase to 20 mg twice daily based on patient tolerability and response

Canadian labeling.

Epilepsy (adjunctive): Oral: Refer to adult dosing. Initiate therapy at lowest possible dose and titrate slowly; monitor closely.

Pediatric

US labeling:

Lennox-Gastaut (adjunctive): Children ≥2 years and Adolescents: Oral: Refer to adult dosing.

Canadian labeling:

Epilepsy (adjunctive):

Children <2 years: Oral: Initial 0.5 to 1 mg/kg/day

Children 2 to 16 years: Oral: Initial: 5 mg daily; may be increased (no more frequently than every 5 days) to a maximum of 40 mg daily. **Note:** Daily doses of up to 30 mg may be taken as a single dose at bedtime; higher doses should be divided.

CYP2C19 poor metabolizers: Initiate at lowest recommended doses; titrate slowly as tolerated to half of usual recommended age-based maximum dose. If needed, dose may be further increased as tolerated to recommended age-based maximum dose beginning day 21.

Epilepsy (monotherapy) (off-label use): Children 2 to 16 years: Oral: Initial: Titrate slowly over 1 to 3 weeks to target dose of ~0.5 mg/kg/day in 2 divided doses (Canadian Study Group, 1998)

Renal Impairment

US labeling:

CrCl ≥30 mL/minute: No dosage adjustment necessary.

CrCl <30 mL/minute: There are no dosage adjustments provided in the manufacturer's labeling (has not been studied); use with caution.

Canadian labeling: There are no specific dosage adjustments provided in the manufacturer's labeling; however, a reduced dosage is recommended.

Hepatic Impairment

US labeling:

Mild to moderate impairment:

≤30 kg: Initial: 5 mg once daily for ≥2 weeks, then increase to 5 mg twice daily; after ≥1 week may increase to 10 mg twice daily based on patient tolerability and response

>30 kg: Initial: 5 mg once daily for ≥1 week, then increase to 5 mg twice daily for ≥1 week, then increase to 10 mg twice daily; after ≥1 week may increase to 20 mg twice daily based on patient tolerability and response

Severe impairment: There are no dosage adjustments provided in the manufacturer's labeling (has not been studied). Use with caution; undergoes extensive hepatic metabolism.

Canadian labeling:

Mild to moderate impairment: Initiate at lowest recommended doses; titrate slowly as tolerated to half of usual recommended age-based maximum dose. If needed, dose may be further increased as tolerated to usual recommended age-based maximum dose beginning day 21.

Severe impairment: Use is contraindicated.

Administration Oral: May be administered with or without food. Tablets can be crushed and mixed in applesauce. Shake suspension well before using; only use the oral dosing syringe supplied with the suspension. Daily doses greater than 5 mg should be divided and administered twice daily.

Monitoring Parameters Respiratory and mental status/suicidality (eg, suicidal thoughts, depression, behavioral changes). The Canadian labeling recommends periodic CBC, liver function, renal function and thyroid function tests.

Dosage Forms Excipient information presented when available (limited, particularly for generics); consult specific product labeling. [DSC] = Discontinued product

Suspension, Oral:

Onfi: 2.5 mg/mL (120 mL) [contains methylparaben, polysorbate 80, propylene glycol, propylparaben; berry flavor]

Tablet, Oral:

Onfi: 5 mg [DSC]

Onfi: 10 mg, 20 mg [scored]

Dosage Forms: Canada Excipient information presented when available (limited, particularly for generics); consult specific product labeling.

Tablet, Oral: 10 mg

Controlled Substance C-IV

◆ Clobazam-10 (Can) *see* CloBAZam *on page 410*

Clobetasol (kloe BAY ta sol)

Brand Names: US Clobetasol Propionate E; Clobex; Clobex Spray; Clodan; Cormax Scalp Application; Cormax [DSC]; Olux; Olux-E; Temovate; Temovate E

Brand Names: Canada Clobex; Dermovate; Mylan-Clobetasol; Novo-Clobetasol; Olux-E; PMS-Clobetasol; ratio-Clobetasol; Taro-Clobetasol

Index Terms Clobetasol Propionate

Pharmacologic Category Corticosteroid, Topical

Additional Appendix Information

Topical Corticosteroids *on page 1952*

Use Steroid-responsive dermatoses: Short-term relief of inflammation and pruritic manifestations of moderate to severe corticosteroid-responsive dermatoses

Dosing

Adult & Geriatric Note: Discontinue when control achieved; if improvement not seen within 2 weeks, reassessment of diagnosis may be necessary.

Oral mucosal inflammation (off-label use): Topical: *Cream:* Apply twice daily for up to 2 weeks (maximum dose: 50 g/week); discontinue application when control is achieved; if no improvement is seen, reassessment of diagnosis may be necessary

Steroid-responsive dermatoses: Topical: *Cream, emollient cream, foam, gel, lotion, ointment, solution:* Apply twice daily for up to 2 weeks (maximum dose: 50 g/week or 50 mL/week)

Mild to moderate plaque-type psoriasis of nonscalp areas: Topical: *Foam:* Apply twice daily for up to 2 weeks (maximum dose: 50 g/week)

Moderate to severe plaque-type psoriasis: Topical:

Emollient cream, lotion: Apply twice daily for up to 2 weeks; can be used for up to 4 weeks when application is <10% of body surface area (maximum dose: 50 g/week or 50 mL/week). Treatment with lotion beyond 2 weeks should be limited to localized lesions (<10% body surface area) which have not improved sufficiently.

Spray: Apply by spraying directly onto affected area twice daily and gently rub into skin. Limit treatment to 4 consecutive weeks; treatment beyond 2 weeks should be limited to localized lesions which have not improved sufficiently. Maximum total dose: 50 g/week or 59 mL/week. Do not use more than 26 sprays per application or 52 sprays per day.

Scalp psoriasis, moderate to severe: Topical:

Foam: Apply twice daily for up to 2 weeks (maximum dose: 50 g/week)

Shampoo: Apply thin film to dry scalp once daily (maximum dose: 50 g/week or 50 mL/week); leave in place for 15 minutes, then add water, lather; rinse thoroughly. Limit treatment to 4 consecutive weeks.

Pediatric Note: Discontinue when control achieved; if improvement not seen within 2 weeks, reassessment of diagnosis may be necessary. Use in children <12 years is not recommended.

Mild to moderate plaque-type psoriasis of nonscalp areas: Topical: *Foam:* Children ≥12 years and Adolescents: Refer to adult dosing.

Moderate to severe plaque-type psoriasis: Topical:

Emollient cream: Adolescents ≥16 years: Refer to adult dosing.

Lotion, spray: Adolescents ≥18 years: Refer to adult dosing.

Scalp psoriasis, moderate to severe: Topical:

Foam: Children ≥12 years and Adolescents: Refer to adult dosing.

Shampoo: Adolescents ≥18 years: Refer to adult dosing.

Steroid-responsive dermatoses: Topical:

Cream, emollient cream, foam, gel, ointment, solution: Children ≥12 years and Adolescents: Refer to adult dosing.

Lotion: Adolescents ≥18 years: Refer to adult dosing.

Oral mucosal inflammation (off-label use): Topical: *Cream:* Children ≥12 years and Adolescents: Refer to adult dosing.

Renal Impairment There are no dosage adjustments provided in the manufacturer's labeling.

Hepatic Impairment There are no dosage adjustments provided in the manufacturer's labeling.

Additional Information Complete prescribing information should be consulted for additional detail.

Dosage Forms Excipient information presented when available (limited, particularly for generics); consult specific product labeling. [DSC] = Discontinued product

Cream, External, as propionate:

Clobetasol Propionate E: 0.05% (15 g, 30 g, 60 g) [contains cetostearyl alcohol, propylene glycol]

Clobetasol Propionate E: 0.05% (15 g, 30 g, 60 g) [contains propylene glycol]

Temovate: 0.05% (30 g, 60 g) [contains cetostearyl alcohol, chlorocresol (chloro-m-cresol), propylene glycol]

Temovate E: 0.05% (60 g)

Generic: 0.05% (15 g, 30 g, 45 g, 60 g)

Foam, External, as propionate:

Olux: 0.05% (50 g, 100 g) [contains cetyl alcohol, propylene glycol]

Olux-E: 0.05% (50 g, 100 g) [contains cetyl alcohol, propylene glycol]

Generic: 0.05% (50 g, 100 g)

Gel, External, as propionate:

Temovate: 0.05% (60 g) [contains propylene glycol]

Generic: 0.05% (15 g, 30 g, 60 g)

Kit, External, as propionate:

Clodan: 0.05% [contains alcohol, usp, cetyl alcohol, edetate disodium, propylene glycol]

Liquid, External, as propionate:

Clobex Spray: 0.05% (59 mL, 125 mL) [contains alcohol, usp]

Generic: 0.05% (59 mL, 125 mL)

Lotion, External, as propionate:

Clobex: 0.05% (59 mL, 118 mL)

Generic: 0.05% (59 mL, 118 mL)

Ointment, External, as propionate:
Cormax: 0.05% (15 g [DSC], 45 g [DSC]) [contains propylene glycol]
Temovate: 0.05% (15 g, 30 g) [contains propylene glycol]
Generic: 0.05% (15 g, 30 g, 45 g, 60 g)
Shampoo, External, as propionate:
Clobex: 0.05% (118 mL) [contains alcohol, usp]
Clodan: 0.05% (118 mL) [contains alcohol, usp]
Generic: 0.05% (118 mL)
Solution, External, as propionate:
Cormax: 0.05% (25 mL [DSC], 50 mL [DSC]) [contains isopropyl alcohol]
Cormax Scalp Application: 0.05% (50 mL) [contains isopropyl alcohol]
Temovate: 0.05% (50 mL)
Generic: 0.05% (25 mL, 50 mL)

◆ Clobetasol Propionate see Clobetasol on page 412
◆ Clobetasol Propionate E see Clobetasol on page 412
◆ Clobex see Clobetasol on page 412
◆ Clobex Spray see Clobetasol on page 412

Clocortolone (kloe KOR toe lone)

Brand Names: US Cloderm; Cloderm Pump
Brand Names: Canada Cloderm
Index Terms Clocortolone Pivalate
Pharmacologic Category Corticosteroid, Topical
Additional Appendix Information
Topical Corticosteroids on page 1952
Use Steroid-responsive dermatoses: Treatment of inflammation and pruritus of corticosteroid-responsive dermatoses (intermediate-potency topical corticosteroid)
Dosing
Adult & Geriatric
Steroid-responsive dermatoses: Topical: Apply sparingly and gently; rub into affected area 3 times/day. Therapy should be discontinued when control is achieved; if no improvement is seen, reassessment of diagnosis may be necessary.
Note: May use occlusive dressings for the management of psoriasis or recalcitrant conditions. If infection develops, discontinue occlusive dressing and institute appropriate antimicrobial therapy.
Renal Impairment There are no dosage adjustments provided in the manufacturer's labeling.
Hepatic Impairment There are no dosage adjustments provided in the manufacturer's labeling.
Additional Information Complete prescribing information should be consulted for additional detail.
Dosage Forms Excipient information presented when available (limited, particularly for generics); consult specific product labeling. [DSC] = Discontinued product
Cream, External, as pivalate:
Cloderm: 0.1% (45 g, 90 g) [contains edetate disodium, methylparaben, propylparaben]
Cloderm: 0.1% (45 g [DSC], 90 g [DSC]) [contains methylparaben, propylparaben]
Cloderm Pump: 0.1% (30 g, 75 g) [contains edetate disodium, methylparaben, propylparaben]
Cloderm Pump: 0.1% (30 g [DSC], 75 g [DSC]) [contains methylparaben, propylparaben]
Generic: 0.1% (45 g, 75 g, 90 g)

◆ Clocortolone Pivalate see Clocortolone on page 413
◆ Clodan see Clobetasol on page 412
◆ Cloderm see Clocortolone on page 413
◆ Cloderm Pump see Clocortolone on page 413

Clofarabine (klo FARE a been)

Brand Names: US Clolar
Brand Names: Canada Clolar
Index Terms CAFdA; Clofarex
Pharmacologic Category Antineoplastic Agent, Antimetabolite; Antineoplastic Agent, Antimetabolite (Purine Analog)
Use Acute lymphoblastic leukemia: Treatment of relapsed or refractory acute lymphoblastic leukemia (ALL) in patients 1 to 21 years of age (after at least 2 prior regimens)
Pregnancy Considerations Adverse events were observed in animal reproduction studies. May cause fetal harm if administered to a pregnant woman. Women of childbearing potential should be advised to use effective contraception and avoid becoming pregnant during therapy.
Breast-Feeding Considerations It is not known if clofarabine is excreted in breast milk. Due to the potential for serious adverse reactions in the nursing infant, breast-feeding should be avoided during clofarabine treatment.
Contraindications
There are no contraindications listed in the manufacturer's U.S. labeling.
Canadian labeling: Hypersensitivity to clofarabine or any component of the formulation; symptomatic CNS involvement; history of serious heart, liver, kidney, or pancreas disease; severe hepatic impairment (AST and/or ALT >5 x ULN, and/or bilirubin >3 x ULN); severe renal impairment (CrCl <30 mL/minute)
Warnings/Precautions Hazardous agent - use appropriate precautions for handling and disposal (NIOSH 2014 [group 1]). Cytokine release syndrome (eg, tachypnea, tachycardia, hypotension, pulmonary edema) may develop into capillary leak syndrome, systemic inflammatory response syndrome (SIRS), and organ dysfunction; discontinue with signs/symptoms of SIRS or capillary leak syndrome (rapid onset respiratory distress, hypotension, pleural/pericardial effusion, and multiorgan failure) and consider supportive treatment with diuretics, corticosteroids, and/or albumin. Prophylactic corticosteroids may prevent or diminish the signs/symptoms of cytokine release. May require dosage reduction. Monitor blood pressure during 5 days of treatment; discontinue if hypotension develops. Monitor if on concurrent medications known to affect blood pressure. Dose-dependent, reversible myelosuppression (neutropenia, thrombocytopenia, and anemia) is common; may be severe and prolonged. Monitor blood counts and platelets. May be at increased risk for infection due to neutropenia; opportunistic infection or sepsis (may be severe or fatal), is increased due to prolonged neutropenia and immunocompromised state; monitor for signs and symptoms of infection and treat promptly if infection develops. May require therapy discontinuation. Serious and fatal hemorrhages (including cerebral, gastrointestinal, and pulmonary hemorrhage) have occurred, usually associated with thrombocytopenia. Monitor and manage coagulation parameters.

Serious and fatal cases of Stevens-Johnson syndrome (SJS) and toxic epidermal necrolysis (TEN) have been reported. Discontinue clofarabine for exfoliative or bullous rash, or if SJS or TEN are suspected. Clofarabine is associated with a moderate emetic potential; antiemetics are recommended to prevent nausea and vomiting (Basch, 2011; Dupuis, 2011; Roila, 2010). Serious and fatal enterocolitis (including neutropenic colitis, cecitis, and *C. difficile* colitis) has been reported, usually occurring within 30 days of treatment, and when used in combination with other chemotherapy. May lead to complication including necrosis, perforation, hemorrhage or sepsis. Monitor for signs/symptoms of enterocolitis and manage promptly.

Has not been studied in patients with hepatic impairment; use with caution (per manufacturer's labeling). Canadian labeling contraindicates use in severe impairment or in patients with a history of serious hepatic disease. Transaminases and bilirubin may be increased during treatment; transaminase elevations generally occur within 10 days of administration and persist for ≤15 days. In some cases, hepatotoxicity was severe and fatal. The risk for hepatotoxicity, including hepatic sinusoidal obstruction syndrome (SOS; formerly called veno-occlusive disease), is increased in patients who have previously undergone a hematopoietic stem cell transplant. Monitor liver function closely; may require therapy interruption or discontinuation; discontinue if SOS is suspected. Elevated creatinine, acute renal failure, and hematuria were observed in clinical studies. Monitor renal function closely; may require dosage reduction or therapy discontinuation. A pharmacokinetic study demonstrated that systemic exposure increases as creatinine clearance decreases (CrCl <60 mL/minute) (Bonate, 2011). Dosage reduction required for moderate renal impairment (CrCl 30-60 mL/minute); use with caution in patients with CrCl <30 mL/minute (has not been studied). Canadian labeling contraindicates use in severe impairment or in patients with a history of serious kidney disease. Minimize the use of drugs known to cause renal toxicity during the 5-day treatment period; avoid concomitant hepatotoxic medications. Tumor lysis syndrome/hyperuricemia may occur as a consequence of leukemia treatment, including treatment with clofarabine, usually occurring in the first treatment cycle. May lead to life-threatening acute renal failure; adequate hydration and prophylactic antihyperuricemic therapy throughout treatment will reduce the risk/effects of tumor lysis syndrome; monitor closely. Potentially significant drug-drug interactions may exist, requiring dose or frequency adjustment, additional monitoring, and/or selection of alternative therapy.

Adverse Reactions

>10%:

Cardiovascular: Tachycardia (35%), hypotension (29%; grade 3: 11%; grade 4: 8%), flushing (19%), hypertension (13%), edema (12%)

Central nervous system: Headache (43%), chills (34%), fatigue (34%), anxiety (21%), pain (15%)

Dermatologic: Pruritus (43%), skin rash (38%), palmar-plantar erythrodysesthesia (16%), erythema (11%)

Gastrointestinal: Vomiting (78%; grades 3/4: 9%), nausea (73%; grades 3/4: 15%), diarrhea (56%), abdominal pain (8% to 35%), anorexia (30%), gingival bleeding (17%), mucosal inflammation (16%), oral candidiasis (11%)

Genitourinary: Hematuria (13%)

Hematologic & oncologic: Leukopenia (grades 3/4: 88%), anemia (83%; grades 3/4: 75%), lymphocytopenia (grades 3/4: 82%), thrombocytopenia (81%; grades 3/4: 80%), neutropenia (grades 3/4: 10% to 64%), febrile neutropenia (55%; grades 3/4: 54%), petechia (26%)

Hepatic: Increased serum ALT (81%; grades 3/4: 43% to 44%), increased serum AST (74%; grades 3/4: 36%), increased bilirubin (45%; grades 3/4: 13%)

Infection: Infection (83%; includes bacterial, fungal, and viral), sepsis (including septic shock; 17%)

Local: Catheter infection (12%)

Neuromuscular & skeletal: Limb pain (30%), myalgia (14%)

Renal: Creatinine increased (50%; grades 3/4: 8%)

Respiratory: Epistaxis (27%), dyspnea (13%), pleural effusion (12%)

Miscellaneous: Fever (39%)

1% to 10%:

Cardiovascular: Pericardial effusion (8%), capillary leak syndrome (4%), hepatic veno-occlusive disease (2%)

Central nervous system: Drowsiness (10%), irritability (10%), lethargy (10%), agitation (5%), mental status changes (1% to 4%)

Dermatologic: Cellulitis (8%), pruritic rash (8%)

Gastrointestinal: Rectal pain (8%), pseudomembranous colitis (7%), stomatitis (7%), pancreatitis (1% to 4%), typhlitis (1% to 4%)

Hematologic & oncologic: Tumor lysis syndrome (grade 3: 6%), oral mucosal petechiae (5%)

Hepatic: Jaundice (8%), hyperbilirubinemia (1% to 4%; grade 4: 2%)

Hypersensitivity: Hypersensitivity (1% to 4%)

Infection: Herpes simplex infection (10%), bacteremia (9%), candidiasis (7%), herpes zoster (7%), staphylococcal bacteremia (6%), staphylococcal sepsis (5%), sepsis syndrome (2%)

Neuromuscular & skeletal: Back pain (10%), ostealgia (10%), weakness (10%), arthralgia (9%)

Respiratory: Pneumonia (10%), respiratory distress (10%), tachypnea (9%), upper respiratory tract infection (5%), pulmonary edema (1% to 4%)

<1% (Limited to important or life-threatening): Bone marrow failure, enterocolitis (occurs more frequently within 30 days of treatment and with combination chemotherapy), exfoliative dermatitis, gastrointestinal hemorrhage, hallucination (Jeha, 2006), hepatomegaly (Jeha, 2006), hypokalemia (Jeha, 2006), hyponatremia, hypophosphatemia, increased right ventricular pressure (Jeha, 2006), left ventricular systolic dysfunction (Jeha, 2006), major hemorrhage (including cerebral and pulmonary; majority of cases associated with thrombocytopenia), pancytopenia, Stevens-Johnson syndrome, syncope, toxic epidermal necrolysis

Drug Interactions

Metabolism/Transport Effects None known.

Avoid Concomitant Use

Avoid concomitant use of Clofarabine with any of the following: BCG (Intravesical); Deferiprone; Dipyrone; Natalizumab; Pimecrolimus; Tacrolimus (Topical); Tofacitinib; Vaccines (Live)

Increased Effect/Toxicity

Clofarabine may increase the levels/effects of: Amifostine; Antipsychotic Agents (Second Generation [Atypical]); CloZAPine; Deferiprone; DULoxetine; Fingolimod; Hypotension-Associated Agents; Leflunomide; Levodopa; Natalizumab; Tofacitinib; Vaccines (Live)

The levels/effects of Clofarabine may be increased by: Alfuzosin; Barbiturates; Blood Pressure Lowering Agents; Brimonidine (Topical); Denosumab; Diazoxide; Dipyrone; Herbs (Hypotensive Properties); Molsidomine; Nicorandil; Obinutuzumab; Pentoxifylline; Phosphodiesterase 5 Inhibitors; Pimecrolimus; Prostacyclin Analogues; Roflumilast; Tacrolimus (Topical); Trastuzumab

Decreased Effect

Clofarabine may decrease the levels/effects of: BCG (Intravesical); Coccidioides immitis Skin Test; Sipuleucel-T; Vaccines (Inactivated); Vaccines (Live)

The levels/effects of Clofarabine may be decreased by: Echinacea

Preparation for Administration Hazardous agent; use appropriate precautions for handling and disposal (NIOSH 2014 [group 1]). Clofarabine should be diluted with NS or D₅W to a final concentration of 0.15 to 0.4 mg/mL. Manufacturer recommends the product be filtered through a 0.2 micron filter prior to dilution.

Storage/Stability Store intact vials at room temperature of 25°C (77°F); excursions permitted to 15°C to 30°C (59°F to 86°F). Solutions diluted for infusion in D₅W or NS may be stored for 24 hours at room temperature.

Mechanism of Action Clofarabine, a purine (deoxyadenosine) nucleoside analog, is metabolized to clofarabine 5'-triphosphate. Clofarabine 5'-triphosphate decreases cell replication and repair as well as causing cell death. To decrease cell replication and repair, clofarabine 5'-triphosphate competes with deoxyadenosine triphosphate for the enzymes ribonucleotide reductase and DNA polymerase. Cell replication is decreased when clofarabine 5'-triphosphate inhibits ribonucleotide reductase from reacting with deoxyadenosine triphosphate to produce deoxynucleotide triphosphate which is needed for DNA synthesis. Cell replication is also decreased when clofarabine 5'-triphosphate competes with DNA polymerase for incorporation into the DNA chain; when done during the repair process, cell repair is affected. To cause cell death, clofarabine 5'-triphosphate alters the mitochondrial membrane by releasing proteins, an inducing factor and cytochrome C.

Pharmacodynamics/Kinetics

Distribution: V_d: Decreased with increasing age, based on pharmacokinetic simulations: 5.8 L/kg (3 years old); 3.1 L/kg (30 years old); 2.7 L/kg (82 years old) (Bonate 2011); Children and Adolescents 2 to 19 years: 172 L/m²

Protein binding: 47%, primarily to albumin

Metabolism: Intracellular by deoxycytidine kinase and mono- and diphosphokinases to active metabolite clofarabine 5'-triphosphate; limited hepatic metabolism (0.2%)

Half-life elimination: Children and Adolescents 2 to 19 years: 5.2 hours; Children and Adults: 7 hours; may be prolonged in in the elderly and in patients with renal impairment (Bonate, 2011)

Excretion: Urine (49% to 60%, as unchanged drug)

Dosing

Adult Note: Consider prophylactic corticosteroids (hydrocortisone 100 mg/m² on days 1 to 3) to prevent signs/symptoms of capillary leak syndrome or systemic inflammatory response syndrome (SIRS), and hydration and antihyperuricemic therapy (to reduce the risk of tumor lysis syndrome/hyperuricemia). Calculate body surface area (BSA) prior to each cycle, utilizing actual body weight. Clofarabine is associated with a moderate emetic potential; antiemetics are recommended to prevent nausea and vomiting (Basch, 2011; Roila, 2010).

Acute lymphoblastic leukemia (ALL) relapsed or refractory: Adults ≤21 years: IV: 52 mg/m²/day days 1 through 5; repeat every 2 to 6 weeks; subsequent cycles should begin no sooner than 14 days from day 1 of the previous cycle (subsequent cycles may be administered when ANC ≥750/mm³)

Acute lymphoblastic leukemia, relapsed/refractory (ALL; off-label population): IV:

Induction: 40 mg/m² once daily for 5 days; may repeat induction cycle once in 3 to 6 weeks if needed (depending on marrow response and recovery) (Kantarjian, 2003)

Consolidation: 30 mg/m² once daily for 5 days (or last tolerated induction dose, whichever is lower); repeat every 4 weeks for up to a maximum of 6 consolidation cycles (Kantarjian, 2003)

Acute myeloid leukemia (AML), refractory (off-label use): Adults <70 years: IV:

Induction: 25 mg/m²/day for 5 days (in combination with cytarabine and filgrastim) may repeat one time after 21 days if needed (Becker, 2011)

Consolidation: 20 mg/m²/day for 5 days (in combination with cytarabine and filgrastim) for 1 or 2 cycles (Becker, 2011)

Pediatric Note: Consider prophylactic corticosteroids (hydrocortisone 100 mg/m² on days 1 to 3) to prevent signs/symptoms of capillary leak syndrome or systemic inflammatory response syndrome (SIRS), and hydration and antihyperuricemic therapy (to reduce the risk of tumor lysis syndrome/hyperuricemia). Calculate body surface area (BSA) prior to each cycle, utilizing actual body weight. Clofarabine is associated with a moderate emetic potential; antiemetics are recommended to prevent nausea and vomiting (Dupuis, 2011).

Acute lymphoblastic leukemia (ALL), relapsed or refractory: Children ≥1 year and Adolescents: IV: 52 mg/m²/day days 1 through 5; repeat every 2 to 6 weeks; subsequent cycles should begin no sooner than 14 days from day 1 of the previous cycle (subsequent cycles may be administered when ANC ≥750/mm³)

Langerhans cell histiocytosis, refractory (off-label use): Children 1 to 18 years: IV: 25 mg/m²/day days 1 through 5; repeat every 28 days for 2 to 8 cycles (Simko, 2014). Additional data may be necessary to further define the role of clofarabine in this condition.

Renal Impairment Clofarabine undergoes renal elimination and exposure is increased as creatinine clearance decreases (Bonate 2011).

Renal impairment at baseline:

U.S. labeling:

CrCl 30-60 mL/minute: Reduce dose by 50%

CrCl <30 mL/minute: There are no dosage adjustments provided in the manufacturer's labeling; use with caution (has not been studied).

Canadian labeling:

CrCl ≥30 mL/minute: There are no dosage adjustments provided in the manufacturer's labeling; use with caution (has not been studied).

CrCl <30 mL/minute: Use is contraindicated.

Renal toxicity during treatment: Grade 3 or higher increase in serum creatinine: Discontinue clofarabine; may reinitiate with a 25% dose reduction after patient is stable and organ function recovers to baseline

Hepatic Impairment

Hepatic impairment at baseline: There are no dosage adjustments provided in the manufacturer's labeling; use with caution (has not been studied). Canadian labeling contraindicates use in severe impairment.

Hepatotoxicity during treatment: Grade 3 or higher increase in bilirubin: Discontinue clofarabine; may reinitiate with a 25% dose reduction after patient is stable and organ function recovers to baseline.

Obesity *American Society for Blood and Marrow Transplantation (ASBMT) practice guideline committee position statement on chemotherapy dosing in obesity:* Utilize actual body weight (full weight) for calculation of body surface area in clofarabine dosing for hematopoietic stem cell transplant conditioning regimens in pediatrics and adults (Bubalo, 2014).

Adjustment for Toxicity

Hematologic toxicity: ANC <500/mm³ lasting ≥4 weeks: Reduce dose by 25% for next cycle

Nonhematologic toxicity:

Clinically significant infection: Withhold treatment until infection is under control, then restart at full dose

Grade 3 toxicity excluding infection, nausea and vomiting, and transient elevations in transaminases and bilirubin: Withhold treatment; may reinitiate with a 25% dose reduction with resolution or return to baseline

Grade ≥3 increase in creatinine or bilirubin: Discontinue; may reinitiate with 25% dosage reduction when creatinine or bilirubin return to baseline and patient is stable; administer antihyperuricemic therapy for elevated uric acid.

Grade 4 toxicity (noninfectious): Discontinue treatment.

Capillary leak or systemic inflammatory response syndrome (SIRS) early signs/symptoms (eg, hypotension, tachycardia, tachypnea, pulmonary edema): Discontinue clofarabine; institute supportive measures. May consider reinitiating with a 25% dose reduction after patient is stable and organ function recovers to baseline.

Dermatologic toxicity: Exfoliative or bullous rash, or suspected Stevens-Johnson syndrome or toxic epidermal necrolysis: Discontinue clofarabine.

Hypotension (during the 5 days of infusion): Discontinue clofarabine. If hypotension is transient and resolves (without pharmacologic intervention), may reinitiate with 25% dosage reduction (Canadian labeling).

Administration

Clofarabine is associated with a moderate emetic potential; antiemetics are recommended to prevent nausea and vomiting (Basch, 2011; Dupuis, 2011; Roila, 2010).

IV infusion: Infuse over 2 hours for relapsed/refractory ALL. May be infused over 1 hour for some off-label protocols (Becker, 2011; Kantarjian, 2003). Continuous IV fluids are encouraged to decrease adverse events and tumor lysis effects. Hypotension may be a sign of capillary leak syndrome or systemic inflammatory response syndrome (SIRS). Discontinue if the patient becomes hypotensive during administration; may consider therapy reinitiation with a 25% dose reduction after return to baseline. Do not administer any other medications through the same intravenous line.

Hazardous agent; use appropriate precautions for handling and disposal (NIOSH 2014 [group 1]).

Monitoring Parameters CBC with differential and platelets (daily during treatment, then 1 to 2 times weekly or as necessary); liver and kidney function (during 5 days of clofarabine administration); coagulation parameters, blood pressure, cardiac function, and respiratory status during infusion; signs and symptoms of tumor lysis syndrome, infection, hepatic sinusoidal obstruction syndrome, enterocolitis, and cytokine release syndrome (tachypnea, tachycardia, hypotension, pulmonary edema); hydration status

Dosage Forms Excipient information presented when available (limited, particularly for generics); consult specific product labeling.

Solution, Intravenous [preservative free]:

Clolar: 1 mg/mL (20 mL)

◆ **Clofarex** see Clofarabine on page *413*
◆ **Clolar** see Clofarabine on page *413*
◆ **Clomid [DSC]** see ClomiPHENE on page *415*
◆ **Clomid (Can)** see ClomiPHENE on page *415*

ClomiPHENE (KLOE mi feen)

Brand Names: US Clomid [DSC]; Serophene

Brand Names: Canada Clomid; Serophene

Index Terms Clomiphene Citrate

Pharmacologic Category Ovulation Stimulator; Selective Estrogen Receptor Modulator (SERM)

Use Treatment of ovulatory dysfunction in women desiring pregnancy

Pregnancy Considerations Adverse events were observed in animal reproduction studies. The incidence of adverse fetal effects following maternal use of clomiphene for ovulation induction is similar to those seen in the general population. Clomiphene is not indicated for use in women who are already pregnant.

Breast-Feeding Considerations It is not known if clomiphene is excreted into breast milk. The manufacturer recommends that caution be used if administered to nursing women. Clomiphene may decrease lactation.

Contraindications Hypersensitivity to clomiphene citrate or any of its components; liver disease or history of liver disease; abnormal uterine bleeding; enlargement or development of ovarian cyst (not due to polycystic ovarian syndrome); uncontrolled thyroid or adrenal dysfunction; presence of an organic intracranial lesion such as pituitary tumor; pregnancy

Warnings/Precautions Use with caution in patients unusually sensitive to pituitary gonadotropins (eg, polycystic ovarian syndrome [PCOS]); a lower dose may be necessary. Use caution in patients with uterine fibroids, may cause further enlargement. Blurring or other visual symptoms can occur; symptoms may increase with higher doses or duration of therapy and in some cases may be irreversible. Patients with visual disturbances should discontinue therapy and receive prompt ophthalmic evaluation. Prolonged use may increase the risk of borderline or invasive ovarian cancer. Multiple births may result from the use of this medication; advise patient of the potential risk of multiple births before starting the treatment. Use should be supervised by physicians who are thoroughly familiar with infertility problems and their management.

Ovarian enlargement may be accompanied by abdominal distention or abdominal pain and generally regresses without treatment within a few days or weeks after therapy discontinuation. If ovaries are abnormally enlarged, withhold therapy until ovaries return to pretreatment size; reduce clomiphene dose and duration of future cycles. Ovarian hyperstimulation syndrome (OHSS), an exaggerated response to ovulation induction therapy, is characterized by an increase in vascular permeability which causes a fluid shift from intravascular space to third space compartments (eg, peritoneal cavity, thoracic cavity) (ASRM 2008; SOGC-CFAS 2011). This syndrome may begin within 24 hours of treatment, but may become most severe 7 to 10 days after therapy (SOGC-CFAS 2011). OHSS is typically self-limiting with spontaneous resolution, although it may be more severe and protracted if pregnancy occurs (ASRM 2008). Symptoms of mild/moderate OHSS may include abdominal distention/discomfort, diarrhea, nausea, and/or vomiting. Severe OHSS symptoms may include abdominal pain that is severe, acute respiratory distress syndrome, anuria/oliguria, ascites, dyspnea, hypotension, nausea/vomiting (intractable), pericardial effusions, tachycardia, or thromboembolism. Decreased creatinine clearance, hemoconcentration, hypoproteinemia, elevated liver enzymes, elevated WBC, and electrolyte imbalances may also be present (ASRM 2008; Fiedler 2012; SOGC-CFAS 2011). If severe OHSS occurs, stop ▶

treatment and consider hospitalizing the patient (ASRM 2008; SOGC-CFAS 2011). Treatment is primarily symptomatic and includes fluid and electrolyte management, analgesics, and prevention of thromboembolic complications (ASRM 2008; SOGC-CFAS 2011). The ascitic, pleural, and pericardial fluids may be removed if needed to relieve symptoms (eg, pulmonary distress or cardiac tamponade) (ASRM 2008; SOGC-CFAS 2011). Women with OHSS should avoid pelvic examination and/or intercourse (ASRM 2008; SOGC-CFAS 2011).

Appropriate use: To minimize risks, use only at the lowest effective dose for the shortest duration of therapy (especially for the first course of therapy). Women with PCOS, amenorrhea-galactorrhea syndrome, psychogenic amenorrhea, post oral contraceptive amenorrhea, and some cases of secondary amenorrhea of undetermined cause may most likely benefit from clomiphene therapy.

Adverse Reactions

>10%: Endocrine & metabolic: Ovarian enlargement (14%)
1% to 10%:
Central nervous system: Headache (1%)
Endocrine & metabolic: Hot flashes (10%), breast discomfort (2%), abnormal uterine bleeding (1%)
Gastrointestinal: Distention/bloating/discomfort (6%), nausea (2%), vomiting (2%)
Ocular: Visual symptoms (2%, includes blurred vision, diplopia, floaters, lights, phosphenes, photophobia, scotomata, waves)
<1% (Limited to important or life-threatening): Abnormal accommodation, acne, allergic reaction, arrhythmia, chest pain, depression, dizziness, dyspnea, edema, endometriosis, erythema multiforme, erythema nodosum, eye pain, fatigue, fever, hepatitis, hypertension, hypertrichosis, leukocytosis, macular edema, migraine, mood changes, neoplasms, optic neuritis, ovarian cyst, ovarian hemorrhage, palpitation, PE, phlebitis, posterior vitreous detachment, pruritus, psychosis, retinal hemorrhage, retinal thrombosis, retinal vascular spasm, seizure, stroke, syncope, tachycardia, thrombophlebitis, thyroid disorder, tinnitus, transaminase increased, tubal pregnancy, uterine hemorrhage, vision loss (temporary/prolonged)

Drug Interactions

Metabolism/Transport Effects None known.

Avoid Concomitant Use
Avoid concomitant use of ClomiPHENE with any of the following: Ospemifene

Increased Effect/Toxicity
ClomiPHENE may increase the levels/effects of: Ospemifene

Decreased Effect
ClomiPHENE may decrease the levels/effects of: Ospemifene

Storage/Stability Store at room temperature of 15°C to 30°C (59°F to 86°F). Protect from light, heat, and excessive humidity.

Mechanism of Action Clomiphene is a racemic mixture consisting of zuclomiphene (~38%) and enclomiphene (~62%), each with distinct pharmacologic properties. Clomiphene acts at the level of the hypothalamus, occupying cell surface and intracellular estrogen receptors (ERs) for longer durations than estrogen. This interferes with receptor recycling, effectively depleting hypothalamic ERs and inhibiting normal estrogenic negative feedback. Impairment of the feedback signal results in increased pulsatile GnRH secretion from the hypothalamus and subsequent pituitary gonadotropin (FSH, LH) release, causing growth of the ovarian follicle, followed by follicular rupture (ASRM 2013; Dickey, 1996).

Pharmacodynamics/Kinetics

Onset of action: Ovulation: 5 to 10 days following course of treatment
Duration: Effects are cumulative; ovulation may occur in the cycle following the last treatment (Dickey, 1996)
Absorption: Readily absorbed
Metabolism: Hepatic; undergoes enterohepatic recirculation (Goldstein 2000)
Half-life elimination: ~5 days (Goldstein 2000)
Time to peak, plasma: ~6 hours (Goldstein 2000)
Excretion: Primarily feces (42%); urine (8%); some excretion may occur for up to 6 weeks after therapy is discontinued

Dosing

Adult Ovulation induction: Oral: Females: **Note:** Intercourse should be timed to coincide with the expected time of ovulation (usually 5 to 10 days after a clomiphene course).
Initial course: 50 mg once daily for 5 days. Begin on or about the fifth day of cycle if progestin-induced bleeding is scheduled or spontaneous uterine bleeding occurs prior to therapy. Therapy may be initiated at anytime in patients with no recent uterine bleeding.

Dose adjustment: Subsequent doses may be increased to 100 mg once daily for 5 days only if ovulation does not occur at the initial dose. Lower doses (12.5 to 25 mg daily) may be used in women sensitive to clomiphene or who consistently develop large ovarian cysts (ASRM 2013).
Repeat courses: If needed, the 5-day cycle may be repeated as early as 30 days after the previous one. Exclude the presence of pregnancy. The lowest effective dose should be used.
Maximum dose: 100 mg once daily for 5 days for up to 6 cycles. Discontinue if ovulation does not occur after 3 courses of treatment; or if 3 ovulatory responses occur but pregnancy is not achieved. Long-term therapy (>6 cycles) is not recommended. Re-evaluate if menses does not occur following ovulatory response. Doses have ranged from 50 to 250 mg daily, although doses >100 mg daily have not been shown to increase pregnancy rates (ASRM 2013). The maximum recommended dose in women with PCOS is 150 mg daily (ESHRE/ASRM 2008).

Renal Impairment There are no dosage adjustments provided in the manufacturer's labeling.

Hepatic Impairment Use is contraindicated in patients with a history of liver disease or dysfunction.

Administration The total daily dose should be taken at one time to maximize effectiveness (Dickey, 1996).

Monitoring Parameters

Prior to therapy: serum estrogen. Rule out primary pituitary or ovarian failure, endometriosis/endometrial carcinoma, adrenal disorders, thyroid disorders, hyperprolactinemia, and male infertility.
Pelvic exam prior to each course of therapy; pregnancy test prior to repeat courses; ovulation (may include serum estradiol, progesterone, urinary luteinizing hormone; ultrasound) (ASRM 2013).
OHSS: Monitoring of hospitalized patients should include abdominal circumference, albumin, cardiorespiratory status, electrolytes, fluid balance, hematocrit, hemoglobin, serum creatinine, urine output, urine specific gravity, vital signs, weight (daily or as necessary) and liver enzymes (weekly) (ASRM 2008; SOGC-CFAS 2011).

Dosage Forms Excipient information presented when available (limited, particularly for generics); consult specific product labeling. [DSC] = Discontinued product
Tablet, Oral, as citrate:
Clomid: 50 mg [DSC]
Serophene: 50 mg [scored]
Generic: 50 mg

◆ Clomiphene Citrate see ClomiPHENE on page 415

ClomiPRAMINE (kloe MI pra meen)

Brand Names: US Anafranil
Brand Names: Canada Anafranil; Apo-Clomipramine; CO Clomipramine; Dom-Clomipramine; Novo-Clomipramine
Index Terms Clomipramine Hydrochloride
Pharmacologic Category Antidepressant, Tricyclic (Tertiary Amine)
Use Treatment of obsessive-compulsive disorder (OCD)
Pregnancy Considerations Adverse events were observed in some animal reproduction studies. Clomipramine and its metabolite desmethylclomipramine cross the placenta and can be detected in cord blood and neonatal serum at birth (Loughhead, 2006; ter Horst, 2011). Data from five newborns found the half-life for clomipramine in the neonate to be 42 ± 16 hours following *in utero* exposure. Serum concentrations were not found to correlate to withdrawal symptoms (ter Horst, 2011). Withdrawal symptoms (including jitteriness, tremor, and seizures) have been observed in neonates whose mothers took clomipramine up to delivery.

The ACOG recommends that therapy for depression during pregnancy be individualized; treatment should incorporate the clinical expertise of the mental health clinician, obstetrician, primary healthcare provider, and pediatrician (ACOG, 2008). According to the American Psychiatric Association (APA), the risks of medication treatment should be weighed against other treatment options and untreated depression. For women who discontinue antidepressant medications during pregnancy and who may be at high risk for postpartum depression, the medications can be restarted following delivery (APA, 2010). Treatment algorithms have been developed by the ACOG and the APA for the management of depression in women prior to conception and during pregnancy (Yonkers, 2009).

Breast-Feeding Considerations Clomipramine is excreted in breast milk. Based on information from three mother-infant pairs, following maternal use of clomipramine 75-150 mg/day, the estimated exposure to the

breast-feeding infant would be 0.4% to 4% of the weight-adjusted maternal dose. Adverse events have not been reported in nursing infants (information from seven cases). Infants should be monitored for signs of adverse events; routine monitoring of infant serum concentrations is not recommended (Fortinguerra, 2009). Due to the potential for serious adverse reactions in the nursing infant, the decision to continue or discontinue breast-feeding during therapy should take into account the risk of exposure to the infant and the benefits of treatment to the mother.

Medication Guide Available Yes

Contraindications Hypersensitivity to clomipramine, other tricyclic agents, or any component of the formulation; use of MAO inhibitors intended to treat psychiatric disorders (concurrently or within 14 days of discontinuing either clomipramine or the MAO inhibitor); initiation of clomipramine in a patient receiving linezolid or intravenous methylene blue; use in a patient during the acute recovery phase of MI

Warnings/Precautions [U.S. Boxed Warning]: Antidepressants increase the risk of suicidal thinking and behavior in children, adolescents, and young adults (18 to 24 years of age) with major depressive disorder (MDD) and other psychiatric disorders; consider risk prior to prescribing. Short-term studies did not show an increased risk in patients >24 years of age and showed a decreased risk in patients ≥65 years. Closely monitor patients for clinical worsening, suicidality, or unusual changes in behavior, particularly during the initial 1 to 2 months of therapy or during periods of dosage adjustments (increases or decreases); the patient's family or caregiver should be instructed to closely observe the patient and communicate condition with health care provider. A medication guide should be dispensed with each prescription. **Clomipramine is FDA approved for the treatment of OCD in children ≥10 years of age.**

The possibility of a suicide attempt is inherent in major depression and may persist until remission occurs. Use caution in high-risk patients. Worsening depression and severe abrupt suicidality that are not part of the presenting symptoms may require discontinuation or modification of drug therapy. The patient's family or caregiver should be alerted to monitor patients for the emergence of suicidality and associated behaviors (such as agitation, irritability, hostility, impulsivity, and hypomania) and notify the healthcare provider.

May worsen psychosis in some patients or precipitate a shift to mania or hypomania in patients with bipolar disorder. Patients presenting with depressive symptoms should be screened for bipolar disorder. Monotherapy in patients with bipolar disorder should be avoided. **Clomipramine is not FDA approved for bipolar depression.**

Potentially life-threatening serotonin syndrome (SS) has occurred with serotonergic agents (eg, SSRIs, SNRIs), particularly when used in combination with other serotonergic agents (eg, triptans, TCAs, fentanyl, lithium, tramadol, buspirone, St John's wort, tryptophan) or agents that impair metabolism of serotonin (eg, MAO inhibitors intended to treat psychiatric disorders, other MAO inhibitors [ie, linezolid and intravenous methylene blue]). Discontinue treatment (and any concomitant serotonergic agent) immediately if signs/symptoms arise. TCAs may rarely cause bone marrow suppression; monitor for any signs of infection and obtain CBC if symptoms (eg, fever, sore throat) evident. May cause seizures (relationship to dose and/or duration of therapy) - do not exceed maximum doses. Use caution in patients with a previous seizure disorder or condition predisposing to seizures such as brain damage, alcoholism, or concurrent therapy with other drugs which lower the seizure threshold. May increase the risks associated with electroconvulsive therapy. Bone fractures have been associated with antidepressant treatment. Consider the possibility of a fragility fracture if an antidepressant-treated patient presents with unexplained bone pain, point tenderness, swelling, or bruising (Rabenda, 2013; Rizzoli, 2012). Use with caution in patients with tumors of the adrenal medulla (eg, pheochromocytoma, neuroblastoma); may cause hypertensive crises. Has been associated with a high incidence of sexual dysfunction. Weight gain may occur.

May cause CNS depression, which may impair physical or mental abilities; patients must be cautioned about performing tasks that require mental alertness (eg, operating machinery or driving). The degree of sedation, anticholinergic effects, and conduction abnormalities are high relative to other antidepressants. The risk of orthostasis is moderate to high relative to other antidepressants. Use with caution in patients with a history of cardiovascular disease (including previous MI, stroke, tachycardia, or conduction abnormalities). Use with caution in patients

with urinary retention, benign prostatic hyperplasia, narrow-angle glaucoma, xerostomia, visual problems, constipation, or a history of bowel obstruction. Potentially significant drug-drug interactions may exist, requiring dose or frequency adjustment, additional monitoring, and/or selection of alternative therapy.

Recommended by the manufacturer to discontinue prior to elective surgery; risks exist for drug interactions with anesthesia and for cardiac arrhythmias. However, definitive drug interactions have not been widely reported in the literature and continuation of tricyclic antidepressants is generally recommended as long as precautions are taken to reduce the significance of any adverse events that may occur (Pass, 2004). Use with caution in patients with hepatic impairment; increases in ALT/AST have occurred, including rare reports of severe hepatic injury (some fatal); monitor hepatic transaminases periodically in patients with hepatic impairment. Use with caution in patients with renal dysfunction. May cause mild pupillary dilation which in susceptible individuals can lead to an episode of narrow-angle glaucoma. Consider evaluating patients who have not had an iridectomy for narrow-angle glaucoma risk factors.

Abrupt discontinuation or interruption of antidepressant therapy has been associated with a discontinuation syndrome. Symptoms arising may vary with antidepressant however commonly include nausea, vomiting, diarrhea, headaches, light-headedness, dizziness, diminished appetite, sweating, chills, tremors, paresthesias, fatigue, somnolence, and sleep disturbances (eg, vivid dreams, insomnia). Greater risks for developing a discontinuation syndrome have been associated with antidepressants with shorter half-lives, longer durations of treatment, and abrupt discontinuation. For antidepressants of short or intermediate half-lives, symptoms may emerge within 2-5 days after treatment discontinuation and last 7-14 days (APA, 2010; Fava, 2006; Haddad, 2001; Shelton, 2001; Warner, 2006).

Adverse Reactions Data shown for children reflects both children and adolescents studied in clinical trials.

>10%:

Cardiovascular: Orthostatic hypotension (20%; adults, children, and adolescents 4% to 6%), tachycardia (20%; adults, children, and adolescents 2% to 4%)

Central nervous system: Dizziness (adults 54%; children & adolescents 41%), drowsiness (46% to 54%), headache (adults 52%), fatigue (35% to 39%), insomnia (adults 25%; children & adolescents 11%), nervousness (adults 18%; children & adolescents 4%), myoclonus (adults 13%; children & adolescents 2%)

Dermatologic: Diaphoresis (adults 29%; children & adolescents 9%)

Endocrine & metabolic: Change in libido (adults 21%), weight gain (adults 18%; children & adolescents 2%)

Gastrointestinal: Xerostomia (adults 84%, children & adolescents 63%), constipation (adults 47%; children & adolescents 22%), nausea (adults 33%), dyspepsia (13% to 22%), anorexia (12% to 22%), diarrhea (7% to 13%), abdominal pain (adults 11%), increased appetite (adults 11%)

Genitourinary: Ejaculation failure (adults 42%, children & adolescents 6%), impotence (adults 20%), difficulty in micturition (adults 14%; children & adolescents 4%)

Neuromuscular & skeletal: Tremor (adults 54%; children & adolescents 33%), myalgia (adults 13%)

Ophthalmic: Visual disturbance (adults 18%; children & adolescents 7%)

Respiratory: Pharyngitis (adults 14%), rhinitis (adults 12%)

1% to 10%:

Cardiovascular: Flushing (7% to 8%), chest pain (children & adolescents 7%), palpitations (4%), ECG abnormality (2%), syncope (children & adolescents 2%)

Central nervous system: Anxiety (adults 9%; children & adolescents 2%), paresthesia (adults 9%), memory impairment (7% to 9%), sleep disorder (4% to 9%), twitching (adults 7%), depression (adults 5%), lack of concentration (adults 5%), pain (3% to 4%), hypertonia (2% to 4%), abnormal dreams (adults 3%), agitation (adults 3%), confusion (adults 3%; children & adolescents 2%), migraine (adults 3%), psychosomatic disorder (adults 3%), speech disturbance (adults 3%), yawning (adults 3%), aggressive behavior (children & adolescents 2%), chills (adults 2%), depersonalization (2%), emotional lability (adults 2%), irritability (children & adolescents 2%), paresis (children & adolescents 2%), myasthenia (1% to 2%), panic attack (1% to 2%), abnormality in thinking (≥1%), vertigo (≥1%)

Dermatologic: Skin rash (4% to 8%), pruritus (adults 6%), body odor (children & adolescents 2%), dermatitis (adults 2%), xeroderma (adults 2%), urticaria (adults 1%)

Endocrine & metabolic: Weight loss (children & adolescents 7%), hot flash (2% to 5%), menstrual disease (adults 4%), amenorrhea (adults 1%)

Gastrointestinal: Dysgeusia (4% to 8%), vomiting (7%), flatulence (adults 6%), aphthous stomatitis (children & adolescents 2%), dysphagia (adults 2%), gastrointestinal disease (adults 2%), halitosis (children & adolescents 2%), esophagitis (adults 1%)

Genitourinary: Urinary retention (children & adolescents 7%; adults 2%), urinary tract infection (adults 6%), urinary frequency (adults 5%), lactation (nonpuerperal; adults 4%), breast hypertrophy (adults 2%), cystitis (adults 2%), leukorrhea (adults 2%), vaginitis (adults 2%), mastalgia (adults 1%)

Hematologic & oncologic: Purpura (adults 3%)

Hepatic: Increased serum ALT (>3 x ULN: 3%), increased serum AST (>3 x ULN: 1%)

Hypersensitivity: Hypersensitivity reaction (children & adolescents 7%)

Neuromuscular & skeletal: Weakness (children & adolescents 2%; adults 1%)

Ophthalmic: Abnormal lacrimation (adults 3%), anisocoria (children & adolescents 2%), blepharospasm (children & adolescents 2%), mydriasis (adults 2%), ocular allergy (children & adolescents 2%), conjunctivitis (adults 1%)

Otic: Tinnitus (4% to 6%)

Respiratory: Bronchospasm (children & adolescents 7%; adults 2%), sinusitis (adults 6%), dyspnea (children & adolescents 2%), epistaxis (adults 2%), laryngitis (children & adolescents 2%)

Miscellaneous: Fever (adults 4%)

<1% (Limited to important or life-threatening): Abnormal electroencephalogram, accommodation disturbance, agranulocytosis, albuminuria, alopecia, anemia, aneurysm, angle-closure glaucoma, anticholinergic syndrome, aphasia, apraxia, ataxia, atrial flutter, blepharitis, bloody stools, bone marrow depression, bradycardia, brain disease, breast fibroadenosis, bronchitis, bundle branch block, cardiac arrest, cardiac arrhythmia, cardiac failure, catalepsy, cellulitis, cerebral hemorrhage, cervical dysplasia, cheilitis, chloasma, cholinergic syndrome, choreoathetosis, chromatopsia, chronic enteritis, colitis, coma, conjunctival hemorrhage, cyanosis, deafness, dehydration, delirium, delusions, dental caries, dermal ulcer, diabetes mellitus, diplopia, duodenitis, dyskinesia, dystonia, edema, edema (oral), endometrial hyperplasia, endometriosis, enlargement of salivary glands, epididymitis, erythematous rash, exophthalmos, exostosis, extrapyramidal reaction, extrasystoles, gastric dilation, gastric ulcer, gastroesophageal reflux disease, glycosuria, goiter, gout, gynecomastia, hallucination, heart block, hematuria, hemiparesis, hemoptysis, hepatic injury (severe), hepatitis, hostility, hyperacusis, hypercholesterolemia, hyperesthesia, hyperglycemia, hyperkinesia, hyperreflexia, hyperthermia, hyperthyroidism, hyperuricemia, hyperventilation, hypnogenic hallucinations, hypoesthesia, hypokalemia, hypokinesia, hypothyroidism, hypoventilation, intestinal obstruction, irritable bowel syndrome, ischemic heart disease, keratitis, laryngismus, leukemoid reaction, leukopenia, lupus erythematous-like rash, lymphadenopathy, maculopapular rash, manic reaction, muscle spasm, mutism, myocardial infarction, myopathy, myositis, nephrolithiasis, neuralgia, neuropathy, nocturnal amblyopia, oculogyric crisis, oculomotor nerve paralysis, ovarian cyst, pancytopenia, paralytic ileus, paranoia, peptic ulcer, periarteritis nodosa, peripheral ischemia, pharyngeal edema, phobia, photophobia, pneumonia, premature ejaculation, pseudolymphoma, psoriasis, psychosis, pyelonephritis, pyuria, rectal hemorrhage, renal cyst, schizophrenic reaction, scleritis, seizure, sensory disturbance, serotonin syndrome, skin hypertrophy, skin photosensitivity, somnambulism, strabismus, stupor, suicidal ideation, thrombocytopenia, thrombophlebitis, tongue ulcer, torticollis, urinary incontinence, uterine hemorrhage, uterine inflammation, vaginal hemorrhage, vasospasm, ventricular tachycardia, visual field defect, voice disorder, withdrawal syndrome

Drug Interactions

Metabolism/Transport Effects Substrate of CYP1A2 (major), CYP2C19 (major), CYP2D6 (major), CYP3A4 (minor); **Note:** Assignment of Major/Minor substrate status based on clinically relevant drug interaction potential; **Inhibits** CYP2D6 (moderate)

Avoid Concomitant Use

Avoid concomitant use of ClomiPRAMINE with any of the following: Aclidinium; Azelastine (Nasal); Cimetropium; Dapoxetine; Dronedarone; Eluxadoline; Glucagon; Glycopyrrolate; Glycopyrrolate (Oral Inhalation); Iobenguane I 123; Ipratropium (Oral Inhalation); Levosulpiride; Linezolid; MAO Inhibitors; Methylene Blue; Moxonidine;

Orphenadrine; Paraldehyde; Potassium Chloride; Thalidomide; Thioridazine; Tiotropium; Umeclidinium

Increased Effect/Toxicity

ClomiPRAMINE may increase the levels/effects of: AbobotulinumtoxinA; Alcohol (Ethyl); Alpha-/Beta-Agonists (Direct-Acting); Alpha1-Agonists; Amifostine; Amphetamines; Analgesics (Opioid); Anticholinergic Agents; Antipsychotic Agents; Antipsychotic Agents (Second Generation [Atypical]); ARIPiprazole; Aspirin; Azelastine (Nasal); Beta2-Agonists; Brexpiprazole; Buprenorphine; Cimetropium; Citalopram; CNS Depressants; CYP2D6 Substrates; Desmopressin; DOXOrubicin (Conventional); Dronedarone; Eliglustat; Eluxadoline; Escitalopram; Fesoterodine; Glucagon; Glycopyrrolate; Glycopyrrolate (Oral Inhalation); Highest Risk QTc-Prolonging Agents; Hydrocodone; Hypotension-Associated Agents; Levodopa; Methotrimeprazine; Methylene Blue; Metoprolol; Metyrosine; Milnacipran; Mirabegron; Moderate Risk QTc-Prolonging Agents; Nebivolol; Nicorandil; NSAID (COX-2 Inhibitor); NSAID (Nonselective); OnabotulinumtoxinA; Orphenadrine; Paraldehyde; Potassium Chloride; Pramipexole; QuiNIDine; Ramosetron; RimabotulinumtoxinB; ROPINIRole; Rotigotine; Serotonin Modulators; Sodium Phosphates; Sulfonylureas; Suvorexant; Thalidomide; Thiazide Diuretics; Thioridazine; Tiotropium; Topiramate; TraMADol; Vitamin K Antagonists; Yohimbine; Zolpidem

The levels/effects of ClomiPRAMINE may be increased by: Abiraterone Acetate; Aclidinium; Alfuzosin; Altretamine; Antiemetics (5HT3 Antagonists); Antipsychotic Agents; Blood Pressure Lowering Agents; Brimonidine (Topical); BuPROPion; Cannabis; CarBAMazepine; Cimetidine; Cinacalcet; Citalopram; Cobicistat; CYP1A2 Inhibitors (Moderate); CYP1A2 Inhibitors (Strong); CYP2C19 Inhibitors (Moderate); CYP2C19 Inhibitors (Strong); CYP2D6 Inhibitors (Moderate); CYP2D6 Inhibitors (Strong); Dapoxetine; Darunavir; Deferasirox; Dexmethylphenidate; Diazoxide; Doxylamine; Dronabinol; Droperidol; DULoxetine; Escitalopram; FLUoxetine; FluvoxaMINE; Grapefruit Juice; Herbs (Hypotensive Properties); HydrOXYzine; Ipratropium (Oral Inhalation); Kava Kava; Linezolid; Lithium; Luliconazole; Magnesium Sulfate; MAO Inhibitors; Metaxalone; Methotrimeprazine; Methylphenidate; Metoclopramide; Metyrosine; Mianserin; Mifepristone; Minocycline; Molsidomine; Nabilone; Nicorandil; Obinutuzumab; Panobinostat; PARoxetine; Peginterferon Alfa-2b; Pentoxifylline; Perampanel; Phosphodiesterase 5 Inhibitors; Pramlintide; Propafenone; Prostacyclin Analogues; Protease Inhibitors; QuiNIDine; Rufinamide; Sertraline; Sodium Oxybate; Tapentadol; Tedizolid; Tetrahydrocannabinol; Thyroid Products; TraMADol; Umeclidinium; Valproate Products; Vemurafenib

Decreased Effect

ClomiPRAMINE may decrease the levels/effects of: Acetylcholinesterase Inhibitors; Alpha1-Agonists; Alpha2-Agonists; Alpha2-Agonists (Ophthalmic); Codeine; Gastrointestinal Agents (Prokinetic); Iobenguane I 123; Itopride; Levosulpiride; Moxonidine; Secretin; Tamoxifen

The levels/effects of ClomiPRAMINE may be decreased by: Acetylcholinesterase Inhibitors; Barbiturates; Cannabis; CYP1A2 Inducers (Strong); CYP2C19 Inducers (Strong); Cyproterone; Dabrafenib; Enzalutamide; Lumacaftor; Osimertinib; Peginterferon Alfa-2b; St Johns Wort; Teriflunomide

Food Interactions Serum concentrations/toxicity may be increased by grapefruit juice. Management: Avoid grapefruit juice.

Storage/Stability Store at controlled room temperature at 20°C to 25°C (68°F to 77°F).

Mechanism of Action Clomipramine appears to affect serotonin uptake while its active metabolite, desmethylclomipramine, affects norepinephrine uptake

Pharmacodynamics/Kinetics

Onset of action: 1-2 weeks; maximum effect: 8-12 weeks

Duration of action: 1-2 days

Absorption: Rapid

Distribution: Distributes into CSF and brain, active metabolite (desmethylclomipramine) also distributes into CSF with average CSF to plasma ratio: 2.6

Protein binding: 97%, primarily to albumin

Metabolism: Hepatic to desmethylclomipramine (DMI; active); extensive first-pass effect; metabolites undergo glucuronide conjugation; metabolism of clomipramine and DMI may be capacity limited (ie, may display nonlinear pharmacokinetics); with multiple dosing, plasma concentrations of DMI are greater than clomipramine

Half-life elimination: Adults (following a 150 mg dose): Clomipramine 19-37 hours (mean: 32 hours); DMI: 54-77 hours (mean: 69 hours)

Time to peak, plasma: 2-6 hours

Excretion: Urine (50% to 60%; 0.8% to 1.3% as parent drug and active metabolite (combined amount); feces (24% to 32%)

Dosing

Adult & Geriatric

Obsessive-compulsive disorder (OCD), treatment:
Oral:

Initial: 25 mg daily; may gradually increase as tolerated over the first 2 weeks to ~100 mg daily in divided doses

Maintenance: May further increase over next several weeks up to a maximum of 250 mg daily; after titration, may give as a single once daily dose at bedtime

Panic attacks (off-label use): Oral: Initial: 10-25 mg daily; titrate gradually (usually weekly) to an effective dose (usual dosage range: 50-150 mg daily); in some studies dose was titrated up to a maximum dose of 200-250 mg daily, if needed (Bakker, 1999; Cassano, 1988; McTavish, 1990; Modigh 1992; Stein, 2010)

Discontinuation of therapy: Upon discontinuation of antidepressant therapy, gradually taper the dose to minimize the incidence of withdrawal symptoms and allow for the detection of re-emerging symptoms. Evidence supporting ideal taper rates is limited. APA and NICE guidelines suggest tapering therapy over at least several weeks with consideration to the half-life of the antidepressant; antidepressants with a shorter half-life may need to be tapered more conservatively. In addition for long-term treated patients, WFSBP guidelines recommend tapering over 4-6 months. If intolerable withdrawal symptoms occur following a dose reduction, consider resuming the previously prescribed dose and/or decrease dose at a more gradual rate (APA, 2007; APA, 2010; Bauer, 2002; Haddad, 2001; NCCMH, 2010; Schatzberg, 2006; Shelton, 2001; Warner, 2006).

MAO inhibitor recommendations:

Switching to or from an MAO inhibitor intended to treat psychiatric disorders:

Allow 14 days to elapse between discontinuing an MAO inhibitor intended to treat psychiatric disorders and initiation of clomipramine.

Allow 14 days to elapse between discontinuing clomipramine and initiation of an MAO inhibitor intended to treat psychiatric disorders.

Use with other MAO inhibitors (linezolid or IV methylene blue):

Do not initiate clomipramine in patients receiving linezolid or IV methylene blue; consider other interventions for psychiatric condition.

If urgent treatment with linezolid or IV methylene blue is required in a patient already receiving clomipramine and potential benefits outweigh potential risks, discontinue clomipramine promptly and administer linezolid or IV methylene blue. Monitor for serotonin syndrome for 2 weeks or until 24 hours after the last dose of linezolid or IV methylene blue, whichever comes first. May resume clomipramine 24 hours after the last dose of linezolid or IV methylene blue.

Pediatric Obsessive-compulsive disorder (OCD), treatment: Children ≥10 years and Adolescents: Oral:

Initial: 25 mg daily; gradually increase as tolerated over the first 2 weeks to 3 mg/kg/day or 100 mg daily (whichever is less) in divided doses

Maintenance: May further increase over next several weeks up to maximum of 3 mg/kg/day or 200 mg daily (whichever is less); after titration, may give as a single once daily dose at bedtime

Discontinuation of therapy: Refer to adult dosing.

MAO inhibitor recommendations: Refer to adult dosing.

Renal Impairment No dosage adjustment provided in manufacturer's labeling (has not been studied). Use with caution in patients with significantly impaired renal function.

Hepatic Impairment No dosage adjustment provided in manufacturer's labeling (has not been studied). Use with caution in patients with hepatic impairment.

Administration During titration, may divide doses and administer with meals to decrease gastrointestinal side effects. After titration, may administer total daily dose at bedtime to decrease daytime sedation.

Monitoring Parameters Pulse rate and blood pressure prior to and during therapy; ECG/cardiac status in older adults and patients with cardiac disease; suicidal ideation (especially at the beginning of therapy, after initiation, or when doses are increased or decreased); signs/symptoms of serotonin syndrome; hepatic transaminases (periodically during therapy in patients with preexisting hepatic impairment)

Test Interactions Increased glucose; may interfere with urine detection of methadone (false-positive)

Dosage Forms Excipient information presented when available (limited, particularly for generics); consult specific product labeling.

Capsule, Oral, as hydrochloride:
Anafranil: 25 mg, 50 mg, 75 mg
Generic: 25 mg, 50 mg, 75 mg

Dosage Forms: Canada Excipient information presented when available (limited, particularly for generics); consult specific product labeling.

Tablet, Oral, as hydrochloride: 10 mg, 25 mg, 50 mg

♦ Clomipramine Hydrochloride *see* ClomiPRAMINE *on page 416*

♦ Clonapam (Can) *see* ClonazePAM *on page 419*

ClonazePAM (kloe NA ze pam)

Brand Names: US KlonoPIN

Brand Names: Canada Apo-Clonazepam; Clonapam; Clonazepam-R; CO Clonazepam; Dom-Clonazepam; Dom-Clonazepam-R; Mylan-Clonazepam; PHL-Clonazepam; PHL-Clonazepam-R; PMS-Clonazepam; PMS-Clonazepam-R; PRO-Clonazepam; ratio-Clonazepam; Riva-Clonazepam; Rivotril; Sandoz-Clonazepam; Teva-Clonazepam; ZYM-Clonazepam

Pharmacologic Category Benzodiazepine

Use

Panic disorder: Treatment of panic disorder, with or without agoraphobia.

Seizure disorders: Mono- or adjunctive therapy in the treatment of the Lennox-Gastaut syndrome (petit mal variant), akinetic, and myoclonic seizures; absence seizures (petit mal) unresponsive to succinimides.

Pregnancy Considerations Adverse events have been observed in some animal reproduction studies. Clonazepam crosses the placenta. Teratogenic effects have been observed with some benzodiazepines; however, additional studies are needed. The incidence of premature birth and low birth weights may be increased following maternal use of benzodiazepines; hypoglycemia and respiratory problems in the neonate may occur following exposure late in pregnancy. Neonatal withdrawal symptoms may occur within days to weeks after birth and "floppy infant syndrome" (which also includes withdrawal symptoms) has been reported with some benzodiazepines, including clonazepam (Bergman 1992; Iqbal 2002; Wikner 2007). A combination of factors influences the potential teratogenicity of anticonvulsant therapy. When treating women with epilepsy, monotherapy with the lowest effective dose and avoidance medications known to have a high incidence of teratogenic effects is recommended (Harden 2009; Wlodarczyk 2012).

Patients exposed to clonazepam during pregnancy are encouraged to enroll themselves into the AED Pregnancy Registry by calling 1-888-233-2334. Additional information is available at www.aedpregnancyregistry.org.

Breast-Feeding Considerations Clonazepam is excreted in breast milk. Drowsiness, lethargy, or weight loss in nursing infants have been observed in case reports following maternal use of some benzodiazepines (Iqbal 2002). Breast-feeding is not recommended by the manufacturer.

Medication Guide Available Yes

Contraindications Hypersensitivity to clonazepam, other benzodiazepines, or any component of the formulation; significant liver disease; acute narrow-angle glaucoma

Warnings/Precautions Pooled analysis of trials involving various antiepileptics (regardless of indication) showed an increased risk of suicidal thoughts/behavior (incidence rate: 0.43% treated patients compared to 0.24% of patients receiving placebo); risk observed as early as 1 week after initiation and continued through duration of trials (most trials ≤24 weeks). Monitor all patients for notable changes in behavior that might indicate suicidal thoughts or depression; notify healthcare provider immediately if symptoms occur. Use caution in patients with depression, particularly if suicidal risk may be present.

Benzodiazepines have been associated with anterograde amnesia (Nelson 1999). May cause CNS depression, which may impair physical or mental abilities; patients must be cautioned about performing tasks which require mental alertness (eg, operating machinery or driving. Paradoxical reactions, including hyperactive or aggressive behavior, have been reported with benzodiazepines, particularly in adolescent/pediatric or psychiatric patients (Mancuso 2004). Clonazepam may cause respiratory depression and may produce an increase in salivation; use with caution in patients with respiratory disease and

in patients who have difficulty handling secretions. May be used in patients with open angle glaucoma who are receiving appropriate therapy; contraindicated in acute narrow angle glaucoma. Use with caution in patients with a history of drug abuse or acute alcoholism; potential for drug dependency exists. Tolerance, psychological and physical dependence may occur with prolonged use. Use with caution in patients with hepatic impairment; accumulation likely to occur. Contraindicated in patients with significant hepatic impairment. Use with caution in patients with renal impairment; clonazepam metabolites are renally eliminated. Use with caution in debilitated patients. Use with extreme caution in patients who are at risk of falls; benzodiazepines have been associated with falls and traumatic injury.

Does not have analgesic, antidepressant, or antipsychotic properties. Worsening of seizures may occur when added to patients with multiple seizure types. Periodically reevaluate the long-term usefulness of clonazepam for the individual patient. Clonazepam is a long half-life benzodiazepine. Duration of action after a single dose is determined by redistribution rather than metabolism. Tolerance develops to the anticonvulsant effects. It does not develop to the anxiolytic effects (Vinkers 2012). Chronic use of this agent may increase the perioperative benzodiazepine dose needed to achieve desired effect. Rebound or withdrawal symptoms may occur following abrupt discontinuation or large decreases in dose. Use caution when reducing dose or withdrawing therapy; decrease slowly and monitor for withdrawal symptoms. Flumazenil may cause withdrawal in patients receiving long-term benzodiazepine therapy (Brogden 1988). Potentially significant drug-drug interactions may exist, requiring dose or frequency adjustment, additional monitoring, and/or selection of alternative therapy. Use appropriate precautions for handling and disposal (NIOSH 2014 [group 3]).

Adverse Reactions Reactions reported in patients with seizure and/or panic disorder. Frequency not always defined.

Cardiovascular: Edema (ankle or facial), palpitation

Central nervous system: Amnesia, ataxia (seizure disorder ~30%; panic disorder 5%), behavior problems (seizure disorder ~25%), coma, confusion, coordination impaired, depression, dizziness, drowsiness (seizure disorder ~50%), emotional lability, fatigue, fever, hallucinations, headache, hysteria, insomnia, intellectual ability reduced, memory disturbance, nervousness; paradoxical reactions (including aggressive behavior, agitation, anxiety, excitability, hostility, irritability, nervousness, nightmares, sleep disturbance, vivid dreams), psychosis, slurred speech, somnolence (panic disorder 37%), vertigo

Dermatologic: Hair loss, hirsutism, skin rash

Endocrine & metabolic: Dysmenorrhea, libido increased/decreased

Gastrointestinal: Abdominal pain, anorexia, appetite increased/decreased, coated tongue, constipation, dehydration, diarrhea, encopresis, gastritis, gum soreness, nausea, weight changes (loss/gain), xerostomia

Genitourinary: Colpitis, dysuria, ejaculation delayed, enuresis, impotence, micturition frequency, nocturia, urinary retention, urinary tract infection

Hematologic: Anemia, eosinophilia, leukopenia, thrombocytopenia

Hepatic: Alkaline phosphatase increased (transient), hepatomegaly, transaminases increased (transient)

Neuromuscular & skeletal: Choreiform movements, coordination abnormal, dysarthria, hypotonia, muscle pain, muscle weakness, myalgia, tremor

Ocular: Blurred vision, eye movements abnormal, diplopia, nystagmus

Respiratory: Bronchitis, chest congestion, cough, hypersecretions, pharyngitis, respiratory depression, respiratory tract infection, rhinitis, rhinorrhea, shortness of breath, sinusitis

Miscellaneous: Allergic reaction, aphonia, dysdiadochokinesis, "glassy-eyed" appearance, hemiparesis, flu-like syndrome, lymphadenopathy

<1% (Limited to important or life-threatening): Apathy, burning skin, chest pain, depersonalization, dyspnea, excessive dreaming, hyperactivity, hypoesthesia, hypotension postural, infection, migraine, organic disinhibition, pain, paresthesia, paresis, periorbital edema, polyuria, suicidal attempt, suicide ideation, thick tongue, twitching, visual disturbance, xerophthalmia

Drug Interactions

Metabolism/Transport Effects Substrate of CYP3A4 (major); **Note:** Assignment of Major/Minor substrate status based on clinically relevant drug interaction potential

Avoid Concomitant Use

Avoid concomitant use of ClonazePAM with any of the following: Azelastine (Nasal); Conivaptan; Fusidic Acid (Systemic); Idelalisib; Methadone; OLANZapine; Orphenadrine; Paraldehyde; Sodium Oxybate; Thalidomide

Increased Effect/Toxicity

ClonazePAM may increase the levels/effects of: Alcohol (Ethyl); Azelastine (Nasal); Buprenorphine; CloZAPine; CNS Depressants; Hydrocodone; Methadone; Methotrimeprazine; Metyrosine; Mirtazapine; Orphenadrine; Paraldehyde; Pramipexole; ROPINIRole; Rotigotine; Selective Serotonin Reuptake Inhibitors; Sodium Oxybate; Suvorexant; Thalidomide; Zolpidem

The levels/effects of ClonazePAM may be increased by: Aprepitant; Brimonidine (Topical); Cannabis; Cobicistat; Conivaptan; Cosyntropin; CYP3A4 Inhibitors (Moderate); CYP3A4 Inhibitors (Strong); Dasatinib; Doxylamine; Dronabinol; Droperidol; Fosaprepitant; Fusidic Acid (Systemic); HydrOXYzine; Idelalisib; Ivacaftor; Kava Kava; Luliconazole; Magnesium Sulfate; Methotrimeprazine; Mifepristone; Minocycline; Nabilone; Netupitant; OLANZapine; Osimertinib; Palbociclib; Perampanel; Rufinamide; Simeprevir; Stiripentol; Tapentadol; Teduglutide; Tetrahydrocannabinol; Vigabatrin

Decreased Effect

The levels/effects of ClonazePAM may be decreased by: Bosentan; CYP3A4 Inducers (Moderate); CYP3A4 Inducers (Strong); Dabrafenib; Deferasirox; Enzalutamide; Mitotane; Osimertinib; Siltuximab; St Johns Wort; Theophylline Derivatives; Tocilizumab; Yohimbine

Storage/Stability

Tablets: Store at 20°C to 25°C (68°F to 77°F).

Orally disintegrating tablets: Store at 25°C (77°F); excursions permitted between 15°C and 30°C (59°F and 80°F)

Mechanism of Action The exact mechanism is unknown, but believed to be related to its ability to enhance the activity of GABA; suppresses the spike-and-wave discharge in absence seizures by depressing nerve transmission in the motor cortex.

Pharmacodynamics/Kinetics

Onset of action: ~20 to 40 minutes (Hanson 1972)

Duration: Infants and young children: 6 to 8 hours (Hanson 1972); Adults: ≤12 hours (Hanson 1972)

Absorption: Rapidly and completely absorbed

Distribution: Children: V_d: 1.5 to 3 L/kg (Walson 1996); Adults: V_d: 1.5 to 64.4 L/kg (Walson 1996)

Protein binding: ~85%

Metabolism: Extensively hepatic via glucuronide and sulfate conjugation; undergoes nitroreduction to 7-aminoclonazepam, followed by acetylation to 7-acetamidoclonazepam; nitroreduction and acetylation are via cytochrome P450 enzyme system; metabolites undergo glucuronide and sulfate conjugation

Bioavailability: ~90%

Half-life elimination: Children: 22 to 33 hours (Walson 1996); Adults: 17 to 60 hours (Walson 1996)

Time to peak, serum: 1 to 4 hours

Excretion: Urine (<2% as unchanged drug); metabolites excreted as glucuronide or sulfate conjugates

Dosing

Adult

Panic disorder: Oral: 0.25 mg twice daily; increase in increments of 0.125 to 0.25 mg twice daily every 3 days; target dose: 1 mg daily (maximum: 4 mg daily)

Discontinuation of treatment: To discontinue, treatment should be withdrawn gradually. Decrease dose by 0.125 mg twice daily every 3 days until medication is completely withdrawn.

Seizure disorders: Oral:

Initial daily dose not to exceed 1.5 mg given in 3 divided doses; may increase by 0.5 to 1 mg every third day until seizures are controlled or adverse effects seen (maximum: 20 mg daily)

Usual maintenance dose: 2 to 8 mg daily in 1 to 2 divided doses (Brodie 1997); do not exceed 20 mg daily

Burning mouth syndrome (off-label use):

Oral: Initial: 0.25 at bedtime for 1 week; increase dose by ≤0.25 mg every week; maximum dose: 3 mg daily in 3 divided doses. **Note:** Use should be limited (Buchanan 2008; Grushka 1998).

Topical: May administer topically with 1 mg 3 times daily (after each meal). **Note:** Patient should be instructed to suck on the tablet, retain saliva in mouth near the pain sites without swallowing for 3 minutes, and then expectorate saliva (Gremeau-Richard 2004).

Essential tremor (off-label use): Oral: Initial: 0.5 mg at bedtime; increase dose by 0.5 mg every 3 to 4 days; maximum dose: 6 mg daily (Biary 1987; Thompson 1984; Zesiewicz 2005; Zesiewicz 2011).

REM sleep behavior disorder (off-label use): 0.25 to 2 mg 30 minutes prior to bedtime (maximum: 4 mg 30 minutes prior to bedtime). **Note:** Use with caution in patients with dementia, gait disorders, or obstructive sleep apnea (Aurora 2010).

Tardive dyskinesia (off-label use): Oral: Initial: 1 mg/day; adjust dosage based on response and tolerability by 1 mg/day every 3 to 4 days up to a maximum dose of 4.5 mg/day (Thaker 1990)

Tic disorders (off-label use): Oral: Initial: 0.5 mg at bedtime; adjust dose by 0.5 mg every 2 weeks based on response and tolerability. Dosing range in clinical studies was 1 to 12 mg/day (Merikangas 1985; Troung 1988).

Geriatric Refer to adult dosing. Initiate with low doses and observe closely.

Pediatric

Seizure disorders: Oral:

Children <10 years or <30 kg:

Initial daily dose: 0.01 to 0.03 mg/kg/day (maximum: 0.05 mg/kg/day) given in 2 to 3 divided doses; increase by no more than 0.25 to 0.5 mg every third day until seizures are controlled or adverse effects seen.

Usual maintenance dose: 0.1 to 0.2 mg/kg/day divided 3 times daily; not to exceed 0.2 mg/kg/day.

Children >10 years or ≥30 kg and Adolescents: Refer to adult dosing.

Renal Impairment There are no dosage adjustments provided in the manufacturer's labeling; use with caution. Clonazepam metabolites may accumulate in patients with renal impairment.

Hepatic Impairment There are no dosage adjustments provided in the manufacturer's labeling; use with caution. Clonazepam undergoes hepatic metabolism. Contraindicated in patients with significant hepatic impairment.

Administration To reduce somnolence, administration of one dose at bedtime may be desirable.

Orally-disintegrating tablet: Open pouch and peel back foil on the blister; do not push tablet through foil. Use dry hands to remove tablet and place in mouth. May be swallowed with or without water. Use immediately after removing from package.

Tablet: Swallow whole with water.

Hazardous agent; use appropriate precautions for handling and disposal (NIOSH 2014 [group 3]).

Monitoring Parameters CBC, liver and renal function tests (periodically with long-term therapy) suicidality (eg, suicidal thoughts, depression, behavioral changes)

Reference Range Relationship between serum concentration and seizure control is not well established. Therapeutic doses have been associated with serum concentrations of ~15 to 70 ng/mL (Pataslos 2008)

Additional Information Ethosuximide or valproic acid may be preferred for treatment of absence (petit mal) seizures. Clonazepam-induced behavioral disturbances may be more frequent in mentally handicapped patients. Abrupt discontinuation after sustained use (generally >10 days) may cause withdrawal symptoms. Flumazenil, a competitive benzodiazepine antagonist at the CNS receptor site, reverses benzodiazepine-induced CNS depression.

Dosage Forms Excipient information presented when available (limited, particularly for generics); consult specific product labeling.

Tablet, Oral:

KlonoPIN: 0.5 mg [scored]

KlonoPIN: 1 mg [contains fd&c blue #1 aluminum lake, fd&c blue #2 aluminum lake]

KlonoPIN: 2 mg

Generic: 0.5 mg, 1 mg, 2 mg

Tablet Dispersible, Oral:

Generic: 0.125 mg, 0.25 mg, 0.5 mg, 1 mg, 2 mg

Controlled Substance C-IV

Extemporaneous Preparations Hazardous agent: Use appropriate precautions for handling and disposal (NIOSH 2014 [group 3]).

A 0.1 mg/mL oral suspension may be made with tablets and one of three different vehicles (cherry syrup; a 1:1 mixture of Ora-Sweet® and Ora-Plus®; or a 1:1 mixture of Ora-Sweet® SF and Ora-Plus®). Crush six 2 mg tablets in a mortar and reduce to a fine powder. Add 10 mL of the chosen vehicle and mix to a uniform paste; mix while adding the vehicle in incremental proportions to **almost** 120 mL; transfer to a calibrated bottle, rinse mortar with vehicle, and add quantity of vehicle sufficient to make 120 mL. Label "shake well" and "protect from light". Stable for 60 days when stored in amber prescription bottles in the dark at room temperature or refrigerated.

Allen LV Jr and Erickson MA 3rd, "Stability of Acetazolamide, Allopurinol, Azathioprine, Clonazepam, and Flucytosine in Extemporaneously Compounded Oral Liquids," *Am J Health Syst Pharm* 1996, 53(16):1944-9.

◆ Clonazepam-R (Can) see ClonazePAM *on page 419*

CloNIDine (KLON i deen)

Brand Names: US Catapres; Catapres-TTS-1; Catapres-TTS-2; Catapres-TTS-3; Duraclon; Kapvay; Nexiclon XR [DSC]

Brand Names: Canada Apo-Clonidine; Catapres; Dixarit; Dom-Clonidine; Novo-Clonidine

Index Terms Clonidine Hydrochloride

Pharmacologic Category Alpha$_2$-Adrenergic Agonist; Antihypertensive

Additional Appendix Information

Hypertension *on page 1996*

Use

Oral:

Immediate release: Management of hypertension (monotherapy or as adjunctive therapy)

Extended release (Kapvay): Treatment of attention-deficit/hyperactivity disorder (ADHD) (monotherapy or as adjunctive therapy)

Epidural (Duraclon): For continuous epidural administration as adjunctive therapy with opioids for treatment of severe cancer pain in patients tolerant to or unresponsive to opioids alone; epidural clonidine is generally more effective for neuropathic pain and less effective (or possibly ineffective) for somatic or visceral pain

Transdermal patch: Management of hypertension (monotherapy or as adjunctive therapy)

Note: According to the Eighth Joint National Committee (JNC 8) guidelines, clonidine is **not** recommended for the initial treatment of hypertension (James 2013). According to the AHA/ACC/ASH 2015 scientific statement for the treatment of hypertension in patients with coronary artery disease (CAD), clonidine should be avoided for the treatment of hypertension in patients with heart failure (with reduced ejection fraction) of ischemic origin (AHA/ACC/ASH [Rosendorff 2015]).

Pregnancy Considerations Adverse events have been observed in some animal reproduction studies. Clonidine crosses the placenta; concentrations in the umbilical cord plasma are similar to those in the maternal serum and concentrations in the amniotic fluid may be 4 times those in the maternal serum. The pharmacokinetics of clonidine may be altered during pregnancy (Buchanan 2009). Untreated chronic maternal hypertension is associated with adverse events in the fetus, infant, and mother. If treatment for hypertension during pregnancy is needed, other agents are preferred (ACOG 2012). **[U.S. Boxed Warning]: Epidural clonidine is not recommended for obstetrical or postpartum pain** due to risk of hemodynamic instability.

Breast-Feeding Considerations Clonidine is excreted in breast milk. Concentrations have been noted as ~7% to 8% of those in the maternal plasma following oral dosing (Atkinson 1988; Bunjes 1993) and twice those in the maternal serum following epidural administration. The manufacturer recommends caution be used if administered to nursing women. Another source recommends avoiding use when nursing infants born <34 weeks gestation or when large maternal doses are needed (Atkinson 1988).

Contraindications Hypersensitivity to clonidine hydrochloride or any component of the formulation

Epidural administration: Injection site infection; concurrent anticoagulant therapy; bleeding diathesis; administration above the C4 dermatome

Warnings/Precautions May cause CNS depression, which may impair physical or mental abilities; patients must be cautioned about performing tasks which require mental alertness (eg, operating machinery or driving). Sedating effects may be potentiated when used with other CNS-depressant drugs or ethanol. Use with caution in patients with severe coronary insufficiency; conduction disturbances; recent MI, CVA, or chronic renal insufficiency. The hemodynamic effects may be prolonged in those with renal impairment; elimination half-life significantly prolonged (up to 41 hours) in patients with severe renal impairment. May cause dose dependent reductions in heart rate; use with caution in patients with preexisting bradycardia or those predisposed to developing bradycardia. Caution in sinus node dysfunction. Use with caution in patients concurrently receiving agents known to reduce SA node function and/or AV nodal conduction (eg, digoxin, diltiazem, metoprolol, verapamil). May cause significant xerostomia. Clonidine may cause eye dryness in patients who wear contact lenses.

[US Boxed Warning]: Must dilute concentrated epidural injectable (500 mcg/mL) solution prior to use. Epidural clonidine is not recommended for perioperative, obstetrical, or postpartum pain due to risk of ▶

◀ **hemodynamic instability.** Clonidine injection should be administered via a continuous epidural infusion device. Monitor closely for catheter-related infection such as meningitis or epidural abscess. Epidural clonidine is not recommended for use in patients with severe cardiovascular disease or hemodynamic instability; may lead to cardiovascular instability (hypotension, bradycardia). Symptomatic hypotension may occur with use; in all patients, use epidural clonidine with caution due to the potential for severe hypotension especially in women and those of low body weight. Most hypotensive episodes occur within the first 4 days of initiation; however, episodes may occur throughout the duration of therapy.

Gradual withdrawal is needed (taper oral immediate release or epidural dose gradually over 2 to 4 days to avoid rebound hypertension) if drug needs to be stopped. Patients should be instructed about abrupt discontinuation (causes rapid increase in BP and symptoms of sympathetic overactivity). In patients on both a beta-blocker and clonidine where withdrawal of clonidine is necessary, withdraw the beta-blocker first and several days before clonidine withdrawal, then slowly decrease clonidine. In children and adolescents, extended release formulation (Kapvay) should be tapered in decrements of no more than 0.1 mg every 3 to 7 days. Discontinue oral immediate release formulations within 4 hours of surgery then restart as soon as possible afterwards. Discontinue oral extended release formulations up to 28 hours prior to surgery, then restart the following day.

Oral formulations of clonidine (immediate release versus extended release) are not interchangeable on a mg:mg basis due to different pharmacokinetic profiles.

Transdermal patch may contain conducting metal (eg, aluminum); remove patch prior to MRI. Due to the potential for altered electrical conductivity, remove transdermal patch before cardioversion or defibrillation. Localized contact sensitization to the transdermal system has been reported; in these patients, allergic reactions (eg, generalized rash, urticaria, angioedema) have also occurred following subsequent substitution of oral therapy.

In pediatric patients, epidural clonidine should be reserved for cancer patients with severe intractable pain, unresponsive to other analgesics or epidural or spinal opioids. Use oral formulations with caution in pediatric patients since children commonly have gastrointestinal illnesses with vomiting and are susceptible to hypertensive episodes due to abrupt inability to take oral medication.

Adverse Reactions Frequency not always defined.

Oral, Transdermal: Incidence of adverse events may be less with transdermal compared to oral due to the lower peak/trough ratio.

>10%:

Central Nervous System: Drowsiness (2% to 38%), headache (1% to 29%), fatigue (4% to 16%), dizziness (2% to 16%)

Dermatologic: Transient skin rash (localized; characterized by pruritus and erythema; transdermal 15% to 50%), contact dermatitis (transdermal 8% to 34%)

Gastrointestinal: Xerostomia (≤40%), upper abdominal pain (15%)

1% to 10%:

Cardiovascular: Bradycardia (≤4%), edema (3%), localized blanching (transdermal 1%), palpitations (1%), tachycardia (≤3%), atrioventricular block, cardiac arrhythmia, cardiac failure, cerebrovascular accident, chest pain, ECG abnormality, flushing, orthostatic hypotension, prolonged Q-T Interval on ECG, Raynaud's phenomenon, syncope

Central Nervous System: Sedation (3% to 10%), irritability (5% to 9%), nightmares (4% to 9%), insomnia (≤6%), emotional disturbance (4%), lethargy (3%), nervousness (1% to 3%), depression (1%), throbbing (transdermal 1%), withdrawal syndrome (1%), aggressive behavior, agitation, anxiety, behavioral changes, delirium, delusions, hallucination (visual and auditory), malaise, numbness (localized; transdermal), paresthesia, parotid pain (oral), restlessness, vivid dream

Dermatologic: Localized vesiculation (transdermal 7%), allergic contact sensitivity (transdermal 5%), hyperpigmentation (transdermal 5%), burning sensation of skin (transdermal 3%), excoriation (transdermal 3%), macular eruption (1%), papule (transdermal 1%), alopecia, hypopigmentation (localized; transdermal), pallor, skin rash, urticaria

Endocrine & metabolic: Gynecomastia (1%), weight gain (<1%), decreased libido, hyperglycemia (transient; oral), increased thirst

Gastrointestinal: Constipation (1% to 10%), viral gastrointestinal infection (5%), anorexia (1%), abdominal pain (oral), diarrhea, gastrointestinal pseudo-obstruction (oral), nausea, parotitis (oral), sore throat, vomiting

Genitourinary: Urinary incontinence (4%), sexual disorder (3%), erectile dysfunction (2% to 3%), nocturia (1%), pollakiuria, urinary retention

Hematologic & oncologic: Thrombocytopenia (oral)

Hepatic: Abnormal hepatic function tests (mild transient abnormalities; <1%), hepatitis

Hypersensitivity: Angioedema

Neuromuscular & skeletal: Weakness (10%), tremor (1% to 4%), arthralgia (1%), myalgia (1%), leg cramps (<1%), increased creatine phosphokinase (transient; oral), limb pain

Ophthalmic: Accommodation disturbance, blurred vision, burning sensation of eyes, decreased lacrimation, dry eye syndrome, increased lacrimation

Otic: Otitis media (≤3%), otalgia

Respiratory: Asthma, dry nose, epistaxis, flu-like symptoms, nasal congestion, nasopharyngitis, respiratory tract infection, rhinorrhea

Miscellaneous: Crying (1% to 3%), fever

Epidural: Note: The following adverse events occurred more often than placebo in cancer patients with intractable pain being treated with concurrent epidural morphine.

>10%:

Cardiovascular: Hypotension (45%), orthostatic hypotension (32%)

Central nervous system: Confusion (13%), dizziness (13%)

Gastrointestinal: Xerostomia (13%)

1% to 10%:

Cardiovascular: Chest pain (5%)

Central nervous system: Hallucination (5%)

Dermatologic: Diaphoresis (5%)

Gastrointestinal: Nausea and vomiting (8%)

Otic: Tinnitus (5%)

Drug Interactions

Metabolism/Transport Effects None known.

Avoid Concomitant Use

Avoid concomitant use of CloNIDine with any of the following: Azelastine (Nasal); Ceritinib; Iobenguane I 123; Orphenadrine; Paraldehyde; Thalidomide

Increased Effect/Toxicity

CloNIDine may increase the levels/effects of: Alcohol (Ethyl); Amifostine; Antipsychotic Agents (Second Generation [Atypical]); Azelastine (Nasal); Beta-Blockers; Bradycardia-Causing Agents; Buprenorphine; Calcium Channel Blockers (Nondihydropyridine); Cardiac Glycosides; Ceritinib; CNS Depressants; DULoxetine; Hydrocodone; Hypotension-Associated Agents; Ivabradine; Lacosamide; Levodopa; Methotrimeprazine; Metyrosine; Orphenadrine; Paraldehyde; Pramipexole; ROPINIRole; Rotigotine; Selective Serotonin Reuptake Inhibitors; Suvorexant; Thalidomide; Zolpidem

The levels/effects of CloNIDine may be increased by: Alfuzosin; Barbiturates; Beta-Blockers; Bretylium; Brimonidine (Topical); Cannabis; Diazoxide; Doxylamine; Dronabinol; Droperidol; Herbs (Hypotensive Properties); HydrOXYzine; Kava Kava; Magnesium Sulfate; Methotrimeprazine; Methylphenidate; Minocycline; Molsidomine; Nabilone; Nicorandil; Obinutuzumab; Pentoxifylline; Perampanel; Phosphodiesterase 5 Inhibitors; Prostacyclin Analogues; Rufinamide; Ruxolitinib; Sodium Oxybate; Tapentadol; Tetrahydrocannabinol; Tofacitinib

Decreased Effect

CloNIDine may decrease the levels/effects of: Iobenguane I 123

The levels/effects of CloNIDine may be decreased by: Amphetamines; Herbs (Hypertensive Properties); Mirtazapine; Serotonin/Norepinephrine Reuptake Inhibitors; Tricyclic Antidepressants; Yohimbine

Preparation for Administration Epidural formulation: Prior to administration, the 500 mcg/mL concentration must be diluted in 0.9% sodium chloride for injection (preservative-free) to a final concentration of 100 mcg/mL.

Storage/Stability

Epidural formulation: Store at 25°C (77°F); excursions permitted to 15°C to 30°C (59°F to 86°F). **Preservative free;** discard unused portion.

Tablets: Store at 25°C (77°F); excursions permitted to 15°C to 30°C (59°F to 86°F). Protect from light.

Extended release tablets: Store at 20°C to 25°C (68°F to 77°F). Protect from light.

Transdermal patches: Store below 30°C (86°F).

Mechanism of Action Stimulates alpha$_2$-adrenoceptors in the brain stem, thus activating an inhibitory neuron, resulting in reduced sympathetic outflow from the CNS, producing a decrease in peripheral resistance, renal vascular resistance, heart rate, and blood pressure; epidural clonidine may produce pain relief at spinal presynaptic and postjunctional alpha$_2$-adrenoceptors by preventing pain signal transmission; pain relief occurs only for the body regions innervated by the spinal segments where analgesic concentrations of clonidine exist. For the treatment of ADHD, the mechanism of action is unknown; it has been proposed that postsynaptic alpha$_2$-agonist stimulation regulates subcortical activity in the prefrontal cortex, the area of the brain responsible for emotions, attentions, and behaviors and causes reduced hyperactivity, impulsiveness, and distractibility.

Pharmacodynamics/Kinetics

Onset of action:

Antihypertensive effect: Oral: Immediate release: 0.5 to 1 hour (maximum reduction in blood pressure: 2 to 4 hours); Transdermal: Initial application: 2 to 3 days

Attention-deficit/hyperactivity disorder: Oral: Extended release: Onset of action: 1 to 2 weeks (AAP 2011)

Duration: Oral: Immediate release: 6 to 10 hours

Absorption: Oral: Extended release tablets (Kapvay) are not bioequivalent with immediate release formulations; peak plasma concentrations are 50% lower compared to immediate release formulations

Distribution: V$_d$: Adults: 2.9 L/kg; highly lipid soluble; distributes readily into extravascular sites

Note: Epidurally administered clonidine readily distributes into plasma via the epidural veins and attains clinically significant systemic concentrations.

Protein binding: 20% to 40%

Metabolism: Extensively hepatic to inactive metabolites; undergoes enterohepatic recirculation

Bioavailability: Oral: Immediate release: 70% to 80%; Extended release (Kapvay): ~89% (relative to immediate release formulation); Transdermal: ~60%

Half-life elimination:

Neonates: 44 to 72 hours

Children: 8 to 12 hours

Adults: Normal renal function: 12 to 16 hours; Renal impairment: ≤41 hours

Epidural administration: CSF half-life elimination: 1.3 ± 0.5 hours

Transdermal: Half-life elimination (after patch removal): ~20 hours (due to skin depot effect; increase in plasma clonidine concentrations may occur after patch removal [MacGregor 1985])

Time to peak, plasma: Oral: Immediate release: 1 to 3 hours; Extended release: 7 to 8 hours

Excretion: Urine (40% to 60% as unchanged drug)

Dosing

Adult Note: Dosing is expressed as the salt (clonidine hydrochloride) unless otherwise noted. Formulations of clonidine (immediate release versus extended release) are not interchangeable on a mg:mg basis due to different pharmacokinetic profiles. Compounded oral suspensions may be available in multiple concentrations (up to 10-times more concentrated); precautions should be taken to verify and avoid confusion between the different concentrations; dose should be clearly presented as mcg or mg as appropriate.

Hypertension:

Oral: Immediate release: Initial dose: 0.1 mg twice daily (maximum recommended dose: 2.4 mg/day); usual dose range (ASH/ISH [Weber 2014]): 0.1 to 0.2 mg twice daily

Transdermal: Initial: 0.1 mg/24 hour patch applied once every 7 days and increase by 0.1 mg at 1- to 2-week intervals (dosages >0.6 mg/24 hours do not improve efficacy); usual dose range (ASH/ISH [Weber 2014]): 0.1 to 0.3 mg/24 hour patch applied once every 7 days

Acute hypertension (urgency) (off-label use): Oral: Initial 0.1 to 0.2 mg; may be followed by additional doses of 0.1 mg every hour, if necessary, to a maximum total dose of 0.7 mg (Atkin 1992; Jaker 1989)

Off-label route of administration: Sublingual: Initial: 0.1 to 0.2 mg; followed by 0.05 to 0.1 mg every hour until blood pressure controlled or a cumulative dose of 0.7 mg is reached (Cunningham 1994; Matuschka 1999)

Clozapine-induced sialorrhea (off-label use):

Oral: Initial: 0.05 mg at bedtime; if no improvement after 2 weeks, may increase to 0.1 mg at bedtime (Praharaj 2005)

Transdermal: 0.1 to 0.2 mg/24 hour patch applied once weekly (Grabowski 1992).

Note: Additional data may be necessary to further define the role of clonidine in this condition.

Nicotine withdrawal symptoms (off-label use) (Fiore 2008):

Oral: Initial: 0.1 mg twice daily; titrate by 0.1 mg/day every 7 days if needed; dosage range used in clinical trials: 0.15 to 0.75 mg/day; duration of therapy ranged from 3 to 10 weeks in clinical trials

Transdermal: Initial: 0.1 mg/24 hour patch applied once every 7 days and increase by 0.1 mg at 1-week intervals if necessary; dosage range used in clinical trials: 0.1 to 0.2 mg/24 hour patch applied once every 7 days; duration of therapy ranged from 3 to 10 weeks in clinical trials

Tourette syndrome (off-label use): Oral: Immediate release: Initial: 0.025 to 0.05 mg once daily; gradually increase dose based on response and tolerability up to a usual dosage of 0.1 to 0.6 mg/day in 3 to 4 divided doses (Murphy 2013; Pringsheim 2012; Roessner 2011).

Pain management: Epidural infusion: Reserved for cancer patients with severe intractable pain, unresponsive to other opioid analgesics: Starting dose: 30 mcg/hour; titrate as required for relief of pain or presence of side effects; experience with doses >40 mcg/hour is limited; should be considered an adjunct to opioid therapy

Conversion from oral to transdermal: **Note:** If transitioning from oral to transdermal therapy, overlap oral regimen for 1 to 2 days; transdermal route takes 2 to 3 days to achieve therapeutic effects. An example transition is below:

Day 1: Place Catapres-TTS 1; administer 100% of oral dose.

Day 2: Administer 50% of oral dose.

Day 3: Administer 25% of oral dose.

Day 4: Patch remains, no further oral supplement necessary.

Conversion from transdermal to oral: After transdermal patch removal, therapeutic clonidine levels persist for ~8 hours and then slowly decrease over several days. Consider starting oral clonidine no sooner than 8 hours after patch removal.

Geriatric Hypertension: Oral: Immediate release: Initial: 0.1 mg once daily at bedtime, increase gradually as needed.

Pediatric Note: Dosing is expressed as the salt (clonidine hydrochloride) unless otherwise noted. Formulations of clonidine (immediate release versus extended release) are not interchangeable on a mg:mg basis due to different pharmacokinetic profiles. Compounded oral suspensions may be available in multiple concentrations (up to 10-times more concentrated); precautions should be taken to verify and avoid confusion between the different concentrations; dose should be clearly presented as mcg or mg as appropriate.

Hypertension (off-label use): Oral: Children ≥12 years: Immediate release: Initial: 0.2 mg/day in 2 divided doses; increase gradually, if needed, in 0.1 mg/day increments at weekly intervals; maximum: 2.4 mg/day (rarely required) (NHBPEP, Fourth Report)

Severe hypertension (off-label use): Oral: Children: Immediate release: 0.05 to 0.1 mg/dose; may repeat up to a maximum total dose of 0.8 mg (NHBPEP, Fourth Report)

Clonidine tolerance test (test of growth hormone release from pituitary) (off-label use): Oral: Immediate release:

0.15 mg/m^2 as a single dose (Lanes 1982)

or

5 mcg/kg as a single dose; maximum dose: 250 mcg (Richmond 2008)

ADHD: Oral: **Note:** May be used alone or as an adjunct to stimulants.

Immediate release (off-label indication; Pliszka 2007):

Children ≤45 kg: Initial: 0.05 mg at bedtime; sequentially increase every 3 to 7 days by 0.05 mg increments as twice daily, then 3 times daily, then 4 times daily; maximum daily dose: 0.2 mg/day for patients weighing 27 to 40.5 kg; 0.3 mg/day for patients weighing 40.5 to 45 kg. When discontinuing therapy, taper gradually over 1 to 2 weeks.

Children >45 kg: Initial: 0.1 mg at bedtime; sequentially increase every 3 to 7 days by 0.1 mg increments as twice daily, then 3 times daily, then 4 times daily; maximum daily dose: 0.4 mg/day. When discontinuing therapy, taper gradually over 1 to 2 weeks.

Extended release (Kapvay): Children ≥6 years: Initial: 0.1 mg at bedtime; increase in 0.1 mg/day increments every 7 days until desired response, doses should be administered twice daily in the morning and at bedtime (either split equally or with the higher split dosage given at bedtime); maximum daily dose: 0.4 mg/day. ▶

Note: When discontinuing therapy, taper daily dose by ≤0.1 mg every 3 to 7 days.

Conduct/oppositional-defiant disorder with or without ADHD (off-label use): Children ≥5 years and Adolescents: Oral: Immediate release: Initial: 0.05 mg/day; gradual titration every 3 to 7 days in 0.05 mg increments to 2 to 3 times daily schedule has been used most frequently, some patients may require 4 daily doses; usual final dose range: 0.2 to 0.3 mg/day in 2-3 divided doses, reported overall range: 0.15 to 0.4 mg/day in divided doses; most reported experience in patients with ADHD comorbidity (Connor 2000; Kemph 1993; Palumbo 2008). Additional data may be necessary to further define the role of clonidine in this condition.

Tourette syndrome (off-label use): Children ≥7 years and Adolescents: Oral: Immediate release: Initial: 0.025 to 0.05 mg once daily; gradually increase dose based on response and tolerability using small increments (0.025 mg) up to a usual dosage of 0.1 to 0.4 mg/day in 3 to 4 divided doses (Murphy 2013; Pringsheim 2012; Roessner 2011; The Tourette's Syndrome Study Group 2002). **Note:** Greater efficacy shown in patients with ADHD comorbidity (Weisman 2013).

Pain management: Epidural infusion: Reserved for cancer patients with severe intractable pain, unresponsive to other opioid analgesics: Initial: 0.5 mcg/kg/**hour**; adjust with caution, based on clinical effect

Renal Impairment

Adults: Oral (immediate release), transdermal, epidural: The manufacturer recommends dosage adjustment according to degree of renal impairment; however, no specific dosage adjustment provided in manufacturer's labeling. Bradycardia, sedation, and hypotension may be more likely to occur in patients with renal failure; half-life significantly prolonged in patients with severe renal failure; consider use of lower initial doses and monitor closely.

Children: Oral (extended release), epidural: The manufacturer recommends dosage adjustment according to degree of renal impairment; however, no specific dosage adjustment provided (has not been studied).

Hemodialysis: Not dialyzable (0% to 5%); supplemental dose is not necessary. Oral antihypertensive drugs given preferentially at night may reduce the nocturnal surge of blood pressure and minimize the intradialytic hypotension that may occur when taken the morning before a dialysis session (K/DOQI 2005).

Hepatic Impairment No dosage adjustment provided in manufacturer's labeling.

Administration

Epidural: Specialized techniques are required for continuous epidural administration; administration via this route should only be performed by qualified individuals familiar with the techniques of epidural administration and patient management problems associated with this route. Familiarization of the epidural infusion device is essential. Do not discontinue clonidine abruptly; if needed, gradually reduce dose over 2 to 4 days to avoid withdrawal symptoms.

Oral: May be taken with or without food. Do not discontinue clonidine abruptly. If needed, gradually reduce dose over 2-4 days to avoid rebound hypertension.

Extended release tablet: Kapvay: Swallow whole; do not crush, split, or chew.

Transdermal patch: Patches should be applied weekly at a consistent time to a clean, hairless area of the upper outer arm or chest. Rotate patch sites weekly. Redness under patch may be reduced if a topical corticosteroid spray is applied to the area before placement of the patch (Tom 1994). Dispose of any used or unused patches by folding adhesive ends together, replace in pouch or sealed container, and discard properly in trash away from children and pets.

Monitoring Parameters Blood pressure, standing and sitting/supine, mental status, heart rate

When used for the treatment of ADHD, thoroughly evaluate for cardiovascular risk. Monitor heart rate, blood pressure (when started and weaned), and consider obtaining ECG prior to initiation (Vetter 2008).

Clonidine tolerance test: In addition to growth hormone concentrations, monitor blood pressure and blood glucose (Huang 2001).

Epidural: Carefully monitor infusion pump; inspect catheter tubing for obstruction or dislodgement to reduce risk of inadvertent abrupt withdrawal of infusion. Monitor closely for catheter-related infection (eg, meningitis or epidural abscess).

Test Interactions Positive Coombs' test

Additional Information Each 0.1 mg of clonidine hydrochloride (salt form) is equivalent to 0.087 mg of the free base.

Transdermal clonidine should only be used in patients unable to take oral medication. The transdermal product is much more expensive than oral clonidine and produces no better therapeutic effects.

When used for ADHD treatment, clonidine is recommended to be used as part of a comprehensive treatment program (eg, psychological, educational, and social) for attention-deficit disorder.

Dosage Forms Excipient information presented when available (limited, particularly for generics); consult specific product labeling. [DSC] = Discontinued product

Liquid Extended Release, Oral, as base:
Nexiclon XR: 0.09 mg/mL (118 mL [DSC]) [contains methylparaben, polysorbate 80, propylparaben; strawberry-banana flavor]

Miscellaneous, Oral, as hydrochloride:
Kapvay: 0.1 mg AM dose, 0.2 mg PM dose (60 ea [DSC])

Patch Weekly, Transdermal:
Catapres-TTS-1: 0.1 mg/24 hr (4 ea)
Catapres-TTS-2: 0.2 mg/24 hr (4 ea)
Catapres-TTS-3: 0.3 mg/24 hr (4 ea)
Generic: 0.1 mg/24 hr (1 ea, 4 ea); 0.2 mg/24 hr (1 ea, 4 ea); 0.3 mg/24 hr (1 ea, 4 ea)

Solution, Epidural, as hydrochloride:
Duraclon: 100 mcg/mL (10 mL)
Generic: 100 mcg/mL (10 mL); 500 mcg/mL (10 mL)

Solution, Epidural, as hydrochloride [preservative free]:
Duraclon: 100 mcg/mL (10 mL)
Duraclon: 500 mcg/mL (10 mL) [pyrogen free]
Generic: 100 mcg/mL (10 mL); 500 mcg/mL (10 mL)

Tablet, Oral, as hydrochloride:
Catapres: 0.1 mg [scored; contains brilliant blue fcf (fd&c blue #1), fd&c yellow #6 (sunset yellow)]
Catapres: 0.2 mg, 0.3 mg [scored; contains fd&c yellow #6 (sunset yellow)]
Generic: 0.1 mg, 0.2 mg, 0.3 mg

Tablet Extended Release 12 Hour, Oral, as hydrochloride:
Kapvay: 0.1 mg
Generic: 0.1 mg

Tablet Extended Release 24 Hour, Oral, as base:
Nexiclon XR: 0.17 mg [DSC] [scored]

Dosage Forms: Canada Note: Also refer to Dosage Forms. Epidural solution and extended-release tablets are not available in Canada.

Excipient information presented when available (limited, particularly for generics); consult specific product labeling.

Tablet, Oral, as hydrochloride: 0.025 mg

Extemporaneous Preparations

0.01 mg/mL concentration

A **0.01** mg/mL oral suspension may be made from tablets. Crush twenty 0.1 mg tablets in a glass mortar and reduce to a fine powder. Slowly add Ora-Blend in ~15 mL increments while mixing to form a uniform paste until approximately half of the total volume (~100 mL) is added. Transfer the suspension to a graduated cylinder. Rinse the mortar and pestle with the remaining vehicle and add quantity to fill the volume within the graduated cylinder to 200 mL. Transfer this amount to a calibrated bottle. Label "shake well". When stored in clear plastic syringes, the suspension is stable for at least 91 days at room temperature (25°C) or refrigerated (4°C).

Ma C, Decarie D, Ensom MHH. Stability of clonidine oral suspension in oral plastic syringes. *Am J Health-Syst Pharm.* 2014;71:657-661.

0.1 mg/mL concentration

A **0.1** mg/mL oral suspension may be made from tablets. Crush thirty 0.2 mg tablets in a glass mortar and reduce to a fine powder. Slowly add 2 mL Purified Water USP and mix to a uniform paste. Slowly add Simple Syrup, NF in 15 mL increments; transfer to a calibrated bottle, rinse mortar with vehicle, and add quantity of vehicle sufficient to make 60 mL. Label "shake well" and "refrigerate". Stable for 28 days when stored in amber glass bottles and refrigerated.

Levinson ML and Johnson CE. Stability of an extemporaneously compounded clonidine hydrochloride oral liquid. *Am J Hosp Pharm.* 1992;49(1):122-125.

◆ **Clonidine Hydrochloride** see CloNIDine on page 421

Clopidogrel (kloh PID oh grel)

Brand Names: US Plavix
Brand Names: Canada Abbott-Clopidogrel; Accel-Clopidogrel; ACT Clopidogrel; Apo-Clopidogrel; Auro-Clopidogrel; Dom-Clopidogrel; JAMP-Clopidogrel; Mar-Clopidogrel; Mint-Clopidogrel; Mylan-Clopidogrel; Plavix; PMS-Clopidogrel; RAN-Clopidogrel; Riva-Clopidogrel; Sandoz-Clopidogrel; Teva-Clopidogrel

Index Terms Clopidogrel Bisulfate

Pharmacologic Category Antiplatelet Agent; Antiplatelet Agent, Thienopyridine

Additional Appendix Information

Oral Antiplatelet Comparison Chart *on page 1963*

Use

Unstable angina/non-ST-segment elevation myocardial infarction: To decrease the rate of a combined end point of cardiovascular death, MI, or stroke, as well as the rate of a combined end point of cardiovascular death, MI, stroke, or refractory ischemia in patients with non-ST-segment elevation acute coronary syndrome (unstable angina/non-ST-elevation myocardial infarction [UA/NSTEMI]), including patients who are to be managed medically and those who are to be managed with coronary revascularization.

ST-segment elevation acute myocardial infarction: To reduce the rate of death from any cause and the rate of a combined end point of death, reinfarction, or stroke in patients with ST-elevation MI (STEMI).

Recent myocardial infarction, recent stroke, or established peripheral arterial disease: To reduce the rate of a combined end point of new ischemic stroke (fatal or nonfatal), new MI (fatal or nonfatal), and other vascular death in patients with a history of recent MI, recent stroke, or established peripheral arterial disease.

Canadian labeling: Additional use (not in U.S. labeling): Prevention of atherothrombotic and thromboembolic events, including stroke, in patients with atrial fibrillation with at least 1 risk factor for vascular events who are not suitable for treatment with an anticoagulant and are at a low risk for bleeding.

Pregnancy Considerations Adverse events were not observed in animal reproduction studies. Information related to use during pregnancy is limited (Bauer, 2012; DeSantis, 2011; Myers, 2011).

Breast-Feeding Considerations It is not known if clopidogrel is excreted into breast milk. Due to the potential for serious adverse reactions in the nursing infant, the manufacturer recommends a decision be made whether to discontinue nursing or to discontinue the drug, taking into account the importance of treatment to the mother.

Medication Guide Available Yes

Contraindications Hypersensitivity to clopidogrel or any component of the formulation; active pathological bleeding such as peptic ulcer or intracranial hemorrhage

Canadian labeling: Additional contraindications (not in U.S. labeling): Significant liver impairment or cholestatic jaundice

Warnings/Precautions [U.S. Boxed Warning]: Patients with one or more copies of the variant *CYP2C19*2* and/ or *CYP2C19*3* alleles (and potentially other reduced-function variants) may have reduced conversion of clopidogrel to its active thiol metabolite. Lower active metabolite exposure may result in reduced platelet inhibition and, thus, a higher rate of cardiovascular events following MI or stent thrombosis following PCI. Although evidence is insufficient to recommend routine genetic testing, tests are available to determine CYP2C19 genotype and may be used to determine therapeutic strategy; alternative treatment or treatment strategies may be considered if patient is identified as a CYP2C19 poor metabolizer. Genetic testing may be considered prior to initiating clopidogrel in patients at moderate or high risk for poor outcomes (eg, PCI in patients with extensive and/ or very complex disease). The optimal dose for CYP2C19 poor metabolizers has yet to be determined. After initiation of clopidogrel, functional testing (eg, VerifyNow® P2Y12 assay) may also be done to determine clopidogrel responsiveness (Holmes, 2010).

Use with caution in patients who may be at risk of increased bleeding, including patients with PUD, trauma, or surgery. In patients with coronary stents, premature interruption of therapy may result in stent thrombosis with subsequent fatal and nonfatal MI. Duration of therapy, in general, is determined by the type of stent placed (bare metal or drug eluting) and whether an ACS event was ongoing at the time of placement. Consider discontinuing 5 days before elective surgery (except in patients with cardiac stents that have not completed their full course of dual antiplatelet therapy; patient-specific situations need to be discussed with cardiologist; AHA/ACC/SCAI/ACS/ ADA Science Advisory provides recommendations). Discontinue at least 5 days before elective CABG; when urgent CABG is necessary, the ACCF/AHA CABG guidelines recommend discontinuation for at least 24 hours prior to surgery (ACCF/AHA [Hillis, 2011]). The ACCF/AHA STEMI guidelines recommend discontinuation for at least 24 hours prior to *on-pump* CABG if possible; *off-pump* CABG may be performed within 24 hours of clopidogrel administration if the benefits of prompt revascularization outweigh the risks of bleeding (ACCF/AHA [O'Gara, 2013]).

Because of structural similarities, cross-reactivity has been reported among the thienopyridines (clopidogrel, prasugrel, and ticlopidine); use with caution or avoid in patients with hypersensitivity or hematologic reactions to previous thienopyridine use. Use of clopidogrel is contraindicated in patients with hypersensitivity to clopidogrel, although desensitization may be considered for mild-to-moderate hypersensitivity.

Use caution in concurrent treatment with anticoagulants (eg, heparin, warfarin) or other antiplatelet drugs; bleeding risk is increased. Concurrent use with drugs known to inhibit CYP2C19 (eg, proton pump inhibitors) may reduce levels of active metabolite and subsequently reduce clinical efficacy and increase the risk of cardiovascular events; if possible, avoid concurrent use of moderate-to-strong CYP2C19 inhibitors. In patients requiring antacid therapy, consider use of an acid-reducing agent lacking (eg, ranitidine/famotidine) or with less CYP2C19 inhibition. According to the manufacturer, avoid concurrent use of omeprazole (even when scheduled 12 hours apart) or esomeprazole; if a PPI is necessary, the use of an agent with comparatively less effect on the antiplatelet activity of clopidogrel is recommended. Of the PPIs, pantoprazole has the lowest degree of CYP2C19 inhibition *in vitro* (Li, 2004) and has been shown to have has less effect on conversion of clopidogrel to its active metabolite compared to omeprazole (Angiolillo, 2011). Although lansoprazole exhibits the most potent CYP2C19 inhibition *in vitro* (Li, 2004; Ogilvie, 2012), an *in vivo* study of extensive CYP2C19 metabolizers showed less reduction of the active metabolite of clopidogrel by lansoprazole/dexlansoprazole compared to esomeprazole/omeprazole (Frelinger, 2012). Avoidance of rabeprazole appears prudent due to potent *in vitro* CYP2C19 inhibition and lack of sufficient comparative *in vivo* studies with other PPIs. In contrast to these warnings, others have recommended the continued use of PPIs, regardless of the degree of inhibition, in patients with multiple risk factors for GI bleeding who are also receiving clopidogrel since no evidence has established clinically meaningful differences in outcome; however, a clinically-significant interaction cannot be excluded in those who are poor metabolizers of clopidogrel. Staggering PPIs with clopidogrel is not recommended until further evidence is available (Abraham, 2010). Concurrent use of aspirin and clopidogrel is not recommended for secondary prevention of ischemic stroke or TIA in patients unable to take oral anticoagulants due to hemorrhagic risk (Furie, 2011).

Use with caution in patients with severe liver or renal disease (experience is limited). Cases of TTP (usually occurring within the first 2 weeks of therapy), resulting in some fatalities, have been reported; urgent plasmapheresis is required. Use in patients with severe hepatic impairment or cholestatic jaundice is contraindicated in the Canadian labeling. Cases of TTP (usually occurring within the first 2 weeks of therapy), resulting in some fatalities, have been reported; urgent plasmapheresis is required. In patients with recent lacunar stroke (within 180 days), the use of clopidogrel in addition to aspirin did not significantly reduce the incidence of the primary outcome of stroke recurrence (any ischemic stroke or intracranial hemorrhage) compared to aspirin alone; the use of clopidogrel in addition to aspirin did however increase the risk of major hemorrhage and the rate of all-cause mortality (SPS3 Investigators, 2012).

Assess bleeding risk carefully prior to initiating therapy in patients with atrial fibrillation (Canadian labeling; not an approved use in U.S. labeling); in clinical trials, a significant increase in major bleeding events (including intracranial hemorrhage and fatal bleeding events) was observed in patients receiving clopidogrel plus aspirin versus aspirin alone. Vitamin K antagonist (VKA) therapy (in suitable patients) has demonstrated a greater benefit in stroke reduction than aspirin (with or without clopidogrel).

Adverse Reactions As with all drugs that may affect hemostasis, bleeding is associated with clopidogrel. Hemorrhage may occur at virtually any site. Risk is dependent on multiple variables, including the concurrent use of multiple agents that alter hemostasis and patient susceptibility. Frequency not always defined.

Dermatologic: Pruritus

Gastrointestinal: Gastrointestinal hemorrhage (2%)

Hematologic & oncologic: Hematoma

Respiratory: Epistaxis

<1%, postmarketing, and/or case reports (Limited to important or life-threatening): Abdominal pain, abnormal hepatic function tests, acute generalized exanthematous

pustulosis, acute hepatic failure, agranulocytosis, anasarca, aplastic anemia, arthralgia, bullous rash, chronic gastric ulcer with perforation, colitis (including ulcerative or lymphocytic), confusion, decreased neutrophils, decreased platelet count, dermal hemorrhage, DRESS syndrome, drug-induced hypersensitivity (to other thienopyridines [eg, ticlopidine, prasugrel]), duodenal ulcer, eczema, eosinophilia, eosinophilic pneumonitis, erythema multiforme, erythematous rash, exfoliative dermatitis, gastric ulcer, gastritis, glomerulopathy, granulocytopenia, gynecomastia, hallucination, hemarthrosis, hematuria, hemophilia A (acquired), hemophthalmos (including conjunctival and retinal), hemoptysis, hemothorax, hepatitis (noninfectious), hepatitis A, hyperbilirubinemia, hypermenorrhea, hypersensitivity reaction, hypochromic anemia, hypotension, IgA vasculitis, increased serum creatinine, interstitial pneumonitis, intracranial hemorrhage, ischemic necrosis, leukopenia, lichen planus, liver steatosis, maculopapular rash, musculoskeletal disease (bleeding), myalgia, pancreatitis, pancytopenia, paresthesia, prolonged bleeding time, pulmonary embolism, pulmonary hemorrhage, purpura, respiratory tract hemorrhage, retroperitoneal hemorrhage, serum sickness, Stevens-Johnson syndrome, stomatitis, thrombotic thrombocytopenic purpura, toxic epidermal necrolysis, upper gastrointestinal tract ulcer (hemorrhagic), vasculitis, wound hemorrhage

Drug Interactions

Metabolism/Transport Effects Substrate of CYP2C19 (major), CYP3A4 (minor); **Note:** Assignment of Major/Minor substrate status based on clinically relevant drug interaction potential; **Inhibits** CYP2B6 (moderate), CYP2C8 (strong), CYP2C9 (weak), SLCO1B1

Avoid Concomitant Use

Avoid concomitant use of Clopidogrel with any of the following: Amodiaquine; Dabrafenib; Enzalutamide; Esomeprazole; Ombitasvir, Paritaprevir, Ritonavir, and Dasabuvir; Omeprazole; Selexipag; Urokinase

Increased Effect/Toxicity

Clopidogrel may increase the levels/effects of: Agents with Antiplatelet Properties; Amodiaquine; Anticoagulants; Apixaban; BuPROPion; Collagenase (Systemic); CYP2B6 Substrates; CYP2C8 Substrates; Dabigatran Etexilate; Dabrafenib; Deoxycholic Acid; Edoxaban; Enzalutamide; Ibritumomab; Obinutuzumab; Ombitasvir, Paritaprevir, Ritonavir, and Dasabuvir; Pioglitazone; Repaglinide; Rivaroxaban; Rosuvastatin; Salicylates; Selexipag; Thrombolytic Agents; Tositumomab and Iodine I 131 Tositumomab; Treprostinil; Urokinase; Warfarin

The levels/effects of Clopidogrel may be increased by: Dasatinib; FluvoxaMINE; Glucosamine; Herbs (Anticoagulant/Antiplatelet Properties); Ibrutinib; Limaprost; Luliconazole; Multivitamins/Fluoride (with ADE); Multivitamins/Minerals (with ADEK, Folate, Iron); Multivitamins/Minerals (with AE, No Iron); Omega-3 Fatty Acids; Pentosan Polysulfate Sodium; Pentoxifylline; Prostacyclin Analogues; Rifamycin Derivatives; Tipranavir; Vitamin E; Vitamin E (Oral)

Decreased Effect

Clopidogrel may decrease the levels/effects of: Cyclophosphamide

The levels/effects of Clopidogrel may be decreased by: Amiodarone; Calcium Channel Blockers; Cangrelor; CYP2C19 Inhibitors (Moderate); CYP2C19 Inhibitors (Strong); Dexlansoprazole; Esomeprazole; FluvoxaMINE; Grapefruit Juice; Lansoprazole; Macrolide Antibiotics; Morphine (Liposomal); Morphine (Systemic); Omeprazole; Pantoprazole; RABEprazole

Food Interactions Consumption of three 200 mL glasses of grapefruit juice a day may substantially reduce clopidogrel antiplatelet effects. Management: Avoid or minimize the consumption of grapefruit or grapefruit juice (Holmberg, 2013).

Storage/Stability Store at 25°C (77°F); excursions permitted to 15°C to 30°C (59°F to 86°F).

Mechanism of Action Clopidogrel requires *in vivo* biotransformation to an active thiol metabolite. The active metabolite irreversibly blocks the $P2Y_{12}$ component of ADP receptors on the platelet surface, which prevents activation of the GPIIb/IIIa receptor complex, thereby reducing platelet aggregation. Platelets blocked by clopidogrel are affected for the remainder of their lifespan (~7-10 days).

Pharmacodynamics/Kinetics

Onset of action: Inhibition of platelet aggregation (IPA): Dose-dependent:
300-600 mg loading dose: Detected within 2 hours
50-100 mg/day: Detected by the second day of treatment

Peak effect: Time to maximal IPA: Dose-dependent: **Note:** Degree of IPA based on adenosine diphosphate (ADP) concentration used during light aggregometry:
300-600 mg loading dose:
ADP 5 micromole/L: 20% to 30% IPA at 6 hours post administration (Montelescot, 2006)
ADP 20 micromole/L: 30% to 37% IPA at 6 hours post administration (Montelescot, 2006)
50-100 mg/day: ADP 5 micromole/L: 50% to 60% IPA at 5-7 days (Herbert, 1993)
Duration of action: Platelet aggregation and bleeding time gradually return to baseline after ~5 days after discontinuation.
Absorption: Rapid, well absorbed
Protein binding: Parent drug: 98%; Inactive metabolite (carboxylic acid derivative): 94%
Metabolism: Extensively hepatic via esterase-mediated hydrolysis to a carboxylic acid derivative (inactive) and via CYP450-mediated (CYP2C19 primarily) oxidation to a thiol metabolite (active)
Half-life elimination: Parent drug: ~6 hours; Thiol derivative (active metabolite): ~30 minutes; carboxylic acid derivative (inactive; main circulating metabolite): ~8 hours; **Note:** A clopidogrel radiolabeled study has shown that covalent binding to platelets accounts for 2% of radiolabel and has a half-life of 11 days.
Time to peak, serum: ~0.75 hours
Excretion: Following administration of a single ^{14}C-labeled clopidogrel oral dose; radioactivity measured over 5 days: Urine (50%); feces (46%)

Dosing

Adult & Geriatric

Recent MI, recent stroke, or established peripheral arterial disease (PAD): Oral: 75 mg once daily. **Note:** The ACCF/AHA guidelines for PAD recommend clopidogrel as an alternative to aspirin (Class Ib recommendation) or in conjunction with aspirin for those who are not at an increased risk of bleeding but are of high cardiovascular risk (Class Ib recommendation). These recommendations also pertain to those with intermittent claudication or critical limb ischemia, prior lower extremity revascularization, or prior amputation for lower extremity ischemia (Rooke 2011).

Acute coronary syndrome (ACS): Oral:
Unstable angina, non-ST-segment elevation myocardial infarction (UA/NSTEMI): Initial: 300 mg loading dose, followed by 75 mg once daily for up to 12 months (in combination with aspirin indefinitely) (ACCF/AHA [Anderson 2013]). The American College of Chest Physicians recommends combination aspirin dose of 75-100 mg (Guyatt 2012). **Note:** If patient is to undergo PCI, see *Percutaneous coronary intervention (PCI) for acute coronary syndrome* dosing.
ST-segment elevation myocardial infarction (STEMI): receiving fibrinolytic therapy (in combination with aspirin and appropriate anticoagulant) (ACCF/AHA [O'Gara 2013]): **Note:** If patient is to undergo primary PCI, see *Percutaneous coronary intervention (PCI) for acute coronary syndrome* dosing.
Age ≤75 years: Loading dose of 300 mg followed by 75 mg once daily for at least 14 days up to 1 year (in the absence of bleeding)
Age >75 years: 75 mg once daily (no loading dose) for at least 14 days up to 1 year (in the absence of bleeding)
Percutaneous coronary intervention (PCI) for acute coronary syndrome (eg, UA/NSTEMI or STEMI) (off-label use): 600 mg (loading dose) given as early as possible before or at the time of PCI, followed by 75 mg once daily for at least 12 months (in combination with aspirin 81 mg/day) (ACCF/AHA [Anderson 2013]; ACCF/AHA/SCAI [Levine 2011]; ACCF/AHA [O'Gara 2013]).
PCI after fibrinolytic therapy (ACCF/AHA [O'Gara 2013]):
Fibrinolytic administered **with** a loading dose of clopidogrel: Continue 75 mg once daily and do not administer an additional loading dose.
Fibrinolytic administered within previous 24 hours **without** a loading dose of clopidogrel: Administer 300 mg loading dose before or at the time of PCI.
Fibrinolytic administered more than 24 hours ago without a loading dose of clopidogrel: Administer 600 mg loading dose before or at the time of PCI.
Higher versus standard maintenance dosing: May consider a maintenance dose of 150 mg once daily for 6 days, then 75 mg once daily thereafter in patients not at high risk for bleeding (ACCF/AHA [Anderson 2013]; CURRENT-OASIS 7 Investigators 2010); however, in another study, in patients with high on-treatment platelet reactivity, the use of 150 mg once daily for 6 months did not demonstrate

a difference in 6-month incidence of death from cardiovascular causes, nonfatal MI, or stent thrombosis compared to standard dose therapy (Price 2011).

Duration of clopidogrel (in combination with aspirin) after stent placement for ACS and non-ACS indications: **Premature interruption of therapy may result in stent thrombosis with subsequent fatal and nonfatal MI.** According to the ACCF/AHA/SCAI PCI guidelines, at least 12 months of clopidogrel is recommended for those with ACS receiving either stent type (bare metal [BMS] or drug eluting stent [DES]) or those receiving a DES for a non-ACS indication (ie, elective PCI) (ACCF/AHA [Anderson 2013]; ACCF/AHA/SCAI [Levine 2011]). The ACCF/AHA guidelines for the management of UA/NSTEMI recommend up to 12 months of clopidogrel in patients with ACS who receive a BMS (ACCF/AHA [Anderson 2013]). A duration >12 months may be considered in patients with DES placement. Recent data has demonstrated that continued dual antiplatelet therapy for a total of 30 months (compared to 12 months) significantly reduced the risk of stent thrombosis and major adverse cardiovascular/cerebrovascular events but was associated with a higher risk of bleeding (Mauri 2014). Those receiving a BMS for a non-ACS indication should be given clopidogrel for at least 1 month and ideally up to 12 months; if patient is at increased risk of bleeding, give for a minimum of 2 weeks (ACCF/AHA/SCAI [Levine 2011]).

CYP2C19 poor metabolizers (ie, CYP2C19*2 or *3 carriers): Although routine genetic testing is not recommended in patients treated with clopidogrel undergoing PCI, testing may be considered to identify poor metabolizers who would be at risk for poor outcomes while receiving clopidogrel; if identified, these patients may be considered for an alternative P2Y$_{12}$ inhibitor (Levine 2011). An appropriate regimen for this patient population has not been established in clinical outcome trials. Although a 600 mg loading dose, followed by 150 mg once daily produced greater active metabolite exposure and antiplatelet response compared to the 300 mg/75 mg regimen, it does not appear that this dosing strategy improves outcomes for this patient population (Price 2011; Simon 2011).

Atrial fibrillation (in patients not candidates for warfarin and at a low risk of bleeding) (Canadian labeling; ACTIVE Investigators 2009; off-label use in U.S.): Oral: 75 mg once daily (in combination with aspirin 75-100 mg once daily). **Note:** Combination may also be used as an alternative for patients with atrial fibrillation and mitral stenosis (Guyatt 2012).

Carotid artery stenosis, symptomatic (including recent carotid endarterectomy) (off-label use): Oral: 75 mg once daily (Guyatt 2012)

Coronary artery bypass graft surgery (secondary prevention) (off-label use) (AHA [Kulik 2015]):
Following off-pump CABG: 75 mg once daily (in combination with aspirin) for 1 year
Aspirin-allergic or -intolerant patients: 75 mg once daily; continue indefinitely

Coronary artery disease (CAD), established (off-label use): Oral: 75 mg once daily. **Note:** Established CAD defined as patients 1-year post ACS, with prior revascularization, coronary stenosis >50% by angiogram, and/or evidence for cardiac ischemia on diagnostic testing (includes patients after the first year post-ACS and/or with prior CABG surgery) (Guyatt 2012).

Peripheral artery percutaneous transluminal angioplasty (with or without stenting) or peripheral artery bypass graft surgery, postprocedure (off-label use): Oral: 75 mg once daily. **Note:** For below-knee bypass graft surgery with prosthetic grafts, combine with aspirin 75-100 mg/day (Guyatt 2012).

Secondary prevention of cardioembolic stroke (patient not candidate for oral anticoagulation) (off-label use): Oral: 75 mg once daily (in combination with aspirin) (Guyatt 2012)

Renal Impairment No dosage adjustment necessary (Basra 2011). **Note:** GFR stage 5 (ie, ESRD or an eGFR <15 mL/minute) is associated with higher residual platelet reactivity with maintenance dosing (Muller 2012).

Hepatic Impairment Use with caution; experience is limited. **Note:** Inhibition of ADP-induced platelet aggregation and mean bleeding time prolongation were similar in patients with severe hepatic impairment compared to healthy subjects after repeated doses of 75 mg once daily for 10 days.

Dietary Considerations May be taken without regard to meals. Avoid grapefruit juice (Holmberg, 2013).

Administration May be administered without regard to meals.

Monitoring Parameters Signs of bleeding; hemoglobin and hematocrit periodically. May consider platelet function testing to determine platelet inhibitory response or genotyping for CYP2C19 loss of function variant if results of testing may alter management (ACCF/AHA [Anderson, 2013]).

Dosage Forms Excipient information presented when available (limited, particularly for generics); consult specific product labeling.
Tablet, Oral:
Plavix: 75 mg, 300 mg
Generic: 75 mg, 300 mg

Extemporaneous Preparations A 5 mg/mL oral suspension may be made using tablets. Crush four 75 mg tablets and reduce to a fine powder. Add a small amount of a 1:1 mixture of Ora-Sweet® and Ora-Plus® and mix to a uniform paste; mix while adding the vehicle in geometric proportions to **almost** 60 mL; transfer to a calibrated bottle, rinse mortar with vehicle, and add quantity of vehicle sufficient to make 60 mL. Label "shake well". Stable 60 days at room temperature or under refrigeration.
Skillman KL, Caruthers RL, and Johnson CE, "Stability of an Extemporaneously Prepared Clopidogrel Oral Suspension," *Am J Health Syst Pharm*, 2010, 67(7):559-61.

◆ Clopidogrel Bisulfate see Clopidogrel on page 424

Clorazepate (klor AZ e pate)

Brand Names: US Tranxene-T
Brand Names: Canada Apo-Clorazepate; Novo-Clopate
Index Terms Clorazepate Dipotassium; Tranxene T-Tab
Pharmacologic Category Benzodiazepine
Use Treatment of generalized anxiety disorder; management of ethanol withdrawal; adjunct anticonvulsant in management of partial seizures
Medication Guide Available Yes
Dosing
Adult
Anxiety: Oral: 7.5-15 mg 2-4 times/day
Ethanol withdrawal: Oral: Initial: 30 mg, then 15 mg 2-4 times/day on first day; maximum daily dose: 90 mg; gradually decrease dose over subsequent days.
Seizures (anticonvulsant): Oral: Initial: Up to 7.5 mg/dose 2-3 times/day; increase dose by 7.5 mg at weekly intervals; not to exceed 90 mg/day
Geriatric Oral: Anxiety: 7.5 mg 1-2 times/day; use is not recommended in the elderly.
Pediatric
Seizures (anticonvulsant): Oral:
Children 9-12 years: Initial: 3.75-7.5 mg/dose twice daily; increase dose by 3.75 mg at weekly intervals, not to exceed 60 mg/day in 2-3 divided doses.
Children >12 years: Refer to adult dosing.
Renal Impairment No dosage adjustment provided in manufacturer's labeling; use with caution.
Hepatic Impairment No dosage adjustment provided in manufacturer's labeling; use with caution.
Additional Information Complete prescribing information should be consulted for additional detail.
Dosage Forms Excipient information presented when available (limited, particularly for generics); consult specific product labeling.
Tablet, Oral, as dipotassium:
Tranxene-T: 3.75 mg [scored; contains fd&c blue #2 (indigotine)]
Tranxene-T: 7.5 mg [scored; contains fd&c yellow #6 (sunset yellow)]
Tranxene-T: 15 mg [scored]
Generic: 3.75 mg, 7.5 mg, 15 mg
Controlled Substance C-IV

◆ Clorazepate Dipotassium see Clorazepate on page 427
◆ Clotrimaderm (Can) see Clotrimazole (Topical) on page 428
◆ Clotrimazole 3 Day [OTC] see Clotrimazole (Topical) on page 428

Clotrimazole (Oral) (kloe TRIM a zole)

Index Terms Mycelex
Pharmacologic Category Antifungal Agent, Imidazole Derivative; Antifungal Agent, Oral Nonabsorbed
Use
Oropharyngeal candidiasis (treatment): Local treatment of oropharyngeal candidiasis.

Oropharyngeal candidiasis (prophylaxis): To reduce the incidence of oropharyngeal candidiasis in immunocompromised patients undergoing chemotherapy, radiotherapy, or steroid therapy utilized in the treatment of leukemia, solid tumors, or renal transplantation.

Dosing

Adult & Geriatric

Oropharyngeal candidiasis (prophylaxis): Oral: 10 mg dissolved slowly 3 times daily for the duration of chemotherapy or until steroids are reduced to maintenance levels.

Oropharyngeal candidiasis (treatment): Oral: 10 mg dissolved slowly 5 times daily for 14 consecutive days. Note: When used for initial treatment in patients with HIV-1, duration of therapy is 7 to 14 days (DHHS [adult] 2014; DHHS [pediatric] 2013).

Pediatric Oropharyngeal candidiasis (treatment): Children ≥3 years and Adolescents: Refer to adult dosing.

Renal Impairment There are no dosage adjustments provided in the manufacturer's labeling.

Hepatic Impairment There are no dosage adjustments provided in the manufacturer's labeling.

Additional Information Complete prescribing information should be consulted for additional detail.

Dosage Forms Excipient information presented when available (limited, particularly for generics); consult specific product labeling.

Lozenge, Mouth/Throat:
Generic: 10 mg (70 ea, 140 ea)
Troche, Mouth/Throat:
Generic: 10 mg

Clotrimazole (Topical) (kloe TRIM a zole)

Brand Names: US 3 Day Vaginal [OTC]; Alevazol [OTC]; Clotrimazole 3 Day [OTC]; Clotrimazole Anti-Fungal [OTC]; Clotrimazole GRx [OTC]; Desenex [OTC]; Gyne-Lotrimin 3 [OTC]; Gyne-Lotrimin [OTC]; Lotrimin AF For Her [OTC]; Lotrimin AF [OTC]; Pro-Ex Antifungal [OTC]; Shopko Athletes Foot [OTC]

Brand Names: Canada Canesten Topical; Canesten Vaginal; Clotrimaderm; Trivagizole-3

Pharmacologic Category Antifungal Agent, Imidazole Derivative; Antifungal Agent, Topical; Antifungal Agent, Vaginal

Use Treatment of susceptible fungal infections, including dermatophytoses, superficial mycoses, and cutaneous candidiasis, as well as vulvovaginal candidiasis

Dosing

Adult & Geriatric

Dermatophytosis, cutaneous candidiasis: Topical (cream, solution): Apply twice daily; if no improvement occurs after 4 weeks of therapy, re-evaluate diagnosis.

Vulvovaginal candidiasis: Intravaginal:
Cream (1%): Insert 1 applicatorful of 1% vaginal cream daily (preferably at bedtime) for 7 consecutive days.
Cream (2%): Insert 1 applicatorful of 2% vaginal cream daily (preferably at bedtime) for 3 consecutive days.

Dermatologic infection (superficial): Topical (cream, solution): Apply to affected area twice daily (morning and evening) for 7 consecutive days.

Pediatric Vaginal, topical infections: Children >12 years: Refer to adult dosing.

Additional Information Complete prescribing information should be consulted for additional detail.

Dosage Forms Excipient information presented when available (limited, particularly for generics); consult specific product labeling.

Cream, External:
Clotrimazole Anti-Fungal: 1% (14.17 g, 28.35 g) [contains benzyl alcohol, cetyl alcohol]
Clotrimazole GRx: 1% (14 g) [contains benzyl alcohol, cetyl alcohol, polysorbate 80]
Desenex: 1% (15 g, 30 g)
Lotrimin AF: 1% (12 g, 24 g)
Lotrimin AF For Her: 1% (24 g)
Pro-Ex Antifungal: 1% (42 g) [contains cetyl alcohol, edetate trisodium, methylparaben, trolamine (triethanolamine)]
Shopko Athletes Foot: 1% (28.4 g) [contains benzyl alcohol, cetostearyl alcohol]
Generic: 1% (15 g, 30 g, 45 g)
Cream, Vaginal:
3 Day Vaginal: 2% (21 g) [contains benzyl alcohol, cetyl alcohol]
Clotrimazole 3 Day: 2% (22.2 g)
Gyne-Lotrimin: 1% (45 g) [contains benzyl alcohol]
Gyne-Lotrimin 3: 2% (21 g) [contains benzyl alcohol, cetyl alcohol]
Generic: 1% (45 g)

Ointment, External:
Alevazol: 1% (56.7 g)
Solution, External:
Generic: 1% (10 mL, 30 mL)

◆ **Clotrimazole and Betamethasone** see Betamethasone and Clotrimazole on page 225

◆ **Clotrimazole Anti-Fungal [OTC]** see Clotrimazole (Topical) on page 428

◆ **Clotrimazole GRx [OTC]** see Clotrimazole (Topical) on page 428

CloZAPine (KLOE za peen)

Brand Names: US Clozaril; FazaClo; Versacloz

Brand Names: Canada Apo-Clozapine; Clozaril; Gen-Clozapine

Pharmacologic Category Second Generation (Atypical) Antipsychotic

Use

Schizophrenia, treatment resistant: Treatment of severely ill patients with schizophrenia who fail to respond adequately to antipsychotic treatment.

Suicidal behavior in schizophrenia or schizoaffective disorder: To reduce the risk of suicidal behavior in patients with schizophrenia or schizoaffective disorder who are judged to be at chronic risk for reexperiencing suicidal behavior, based on history and recent clinical state.

Pregnancy Considerations Adverse events were not observed in animal reproduction studies. Clozapine crosses the placenta and can be detected in the fetal blood and amniotic fluid (Barnas, 1994). Antipsychotic use during the third trimester of pregnancy has a risk for abnormal muscle movements (extrapyramidal symptoms [EPS]) and/or withdrawal symptoms in newborns following delivery. Symptoms in the newborn may include agitation, feeding disorder, hypertonia, hypotonia, respiratory distress, somnolence, and tremor; these effects may be self-limiting or require hospitalization.

Clozapine may theoretically cause agranulocytosis in the fetus and should not routinely be used in pregnancy (NICE, 2007). The American College of Obstetricians and Gynecologists recommends that therapy during pregnancy be individualized; treatment with psychiatric medications during pregnancy should incorporate the clinical expertise of the mental health clinician, obstetrician, primary healthcare provider, and pediatrician. Safety data related to atypical antipsychotics during pregnancy is limited and routine use is not recommended. However, if a woman is inadvertently exposed to an atypical antipsychotic while pregnant, continuing therapy may be preferable to switching to a typical antipsychotic that the fetus has not yet been exposed to; consider risk:benefit (ACOG, 2008). An increased risk of exacerbation of psychosis should be considered when discontinuing or changing treatment during pregnancy and postpartum.

Healthcare providers are encouraged to enroll women 18 to 45 years of age exposed to clozapine during pregnancy in the Atypical Antipsychotics Pregnancy Registry (1-866-961-2388 or http://www.womensmentalhealth.org/pregnancyregistry).

Women with amenorrhea associated with use of other antipsychotic agents may return to normal menstruation when switching to clozapine therapy. Reliable contraceptive measures should be employed by women of childbearing potential switching to clozapine therapy.

Breast-Feeding Considerations Clozapine was found to accumulate in breast milk in concentrations higher than the maternal plasma (Barnas, 1994). Breast-feeding is not recommended by the manufacturer. Clozapine may theoretically cause agranulocytosis in the nursing infant and should not routinely be used in women who are breast-feeding (NICE, 2007).

Prescribing and Access Restrictions

US: Clozapine is only available through the Clozapine REM Program because of the risk of severe neutropenia. Health care professionals must be certified with the program by enrolling and completing training in order to prescribe clozapine. Patients must be enrolled in the program and comply with ANC testing and monitoring requirements in order to receive clozapine. Pharmacies must be certified with the program by enrolling and completing training in order to dispense to patients who are eligible to receive clozapine.

Further information is available at http://www.clozapinerems.com or 1-844-267-8678.

Canada: Currently, there are multiple manufacturers that distribute clozapine and each manufacturer has its own registry and distribution system. Patients must be registered in a database that includes their location, prescribing physician, testing laboratory, and dispensing pharmacist before using clozapine. Patients may not be switched from one brand of clozapine to another without completion of a new registry-specific patient registration form by signed by the prescribing physician. Information specific to each monitoring program is available from the individual manufacturers.

Contraindications

Serious hypersensitivity to clozapine or any component of the formulation (eg, photosensitivity, vasculitis, erythema multiforme, or Stevens-Johnson syndrome [SJS])

Canadian labeling: Additional contraindications (not in US labeling): Myeloproliferative disorders; history of toxic or idiosyncratic agranulocytosis or severe granulocytopenia (unless due to previous chemotherapy); concomitant use with other agents that suppress bone marrow function; active hepatic disease associated with nausea, anorexia, or jaundice; progressive hepatic disease or hepatic failure; paralytic ileus; uncontrolled epilepsy; severe CNS depression or comatose states; severe renal impairment; severe cardiac disease (eg, myocarditis); patients unable to undergo blood testing

Warnings/Precautions Clozapine treatment has caused severe neutropenia, defined as an absolute neutrophil count (ANC) less than 500/mcL. Severe neutropenia can lead to serious infection and death. Prior to initiating treatment, a baseline ANC must be ≥1,500/mcL for the general population and must be ≥1,000/mcL for patients with documented Benign Ethnic Neutropenia. During treatment, patients must have regular ANC monitoring. Advise patients to immediately report symptoms consistent with severe neutropenia or infection (eg, fever, weakness, lethargy, sore throat). Risk is greatest within the first 18 weeks of therapy. The mechanism of clozapine-induced neutropenia is unknown and is not dose-dependent. Because of the risk of severe neutropenia, clozapine is available only through a restricted program under a Risk Evaluation Mitigation Strategy (REMS) called the Clozapine REMS Program. Canadian labeling recommends all patients be screened for a history of neutropenia and agranulocytosis associated with clozapine use (ie, are not in the non-rechallengeable databases of any clozapine suppliers).In addition, Canadian labeling contraindicates use in patients with a history of myeloproliferative disorder, toxic or idiosyncratic agranulocytosis, or severe granulocytopenia (unless due to previous chemotherapy). Patients with benign ethic neutropenia (BEN), a condition observed in certain ethnic groups whose average absolute neutrophil count (ANC) values are lower than standard laboratory ranges for neutrophils, have different ANC monitoring parameters due to their lower baseline ANC levels. BEN is most commonly observed in individuals of African descent, some Middle Eastern ethic group, in other non-Caucasian ethnic groups with darker skin, and in men. BEN patients are not at increased risk for developing clozapine-induced neutropenia. Consider hematology consultation prior to initiation. Eosinophilia, defined as a blood eosinophil count of >700/mcL, has been reported to occur with clozapine and usually occurs within the first month of treatment. If eosinophilia develops, evaluate for signs or symptoms of systemic reactions (eg, rash or other allergic symptoms), myocarditis, or organ-specific disease. If systemic disease is suspected, discontinue clozapine immediately. If an eosinophilia cause unrelated to clozapine is identified treat the underlying cause and continue clozapine. In the absence of organ involvement continue clozapine under careful monitoring. If the total eosinophil count continues to increase over several weeks in the absence of systemic disease, base interruption of treatment and rechallenge (after eosinophil count decreases) on overall clinical assessment and consultation with internist or hematologist (**Note:** The Canadian labeling recommends discontinuing therapy for eosinophil count >3,000/mm³; may resume therapy when eosinophil count <1,000/mm³).

[US Boxed Warning]: Elderly patients with dementia-related psychosis treated with antipsychotics are at an increased risk of death compared to placebo. Most deaths appeared to be either cardiovascular (eg, heart failure, sudden death) or infectious (eg, pneumonia) in nature. Clozapine is not approved for the treatment of dementia-related psychosis. The elderly are more susceptible to adverse effects (including agranulocytosis, cardiovascular, anticholinergic, and tardive dyskinesia). An increased incidence of cerebrovascular effects (eg, transient ischemic attack, stroke), including fatalities, has been reported in placebo-controlled trials of atypical antipsychotics in elderly patients with dementia-related psychosis.

May cause CNS depression, which may impair physical or mental abilities; patients must be cautioned about performing tasks that require mental alertness (eg, operating machinery or driving); use caution in patients receiving general anesthesia. **[US Boxed Warning]: Seizures have been associated with clozapine use in a dose-dependent manner. Initiate treatment with no more than 12.5 mg, titrate gradually using divided dosing. Use with caution in patients at risk of seizures, including those with a history of seizures, head trauma, brain damage, alcoholism, or concurrent therapy with medications which may lower seizure threshold. Patients should be warned that a sudden loss of consciousness may occur with seizures.** Benign transient temperature elevation (>38°C or 100.4°F) may occur; peaking within the first 3 weeks of treatment. May be associated with an increase or decrease in WBC count. Rule out infection, severe neutropenia, and neuroleptic malignant syndrome (NMS) in patients presenting with fever. However, clozapine may also be associated with severe febrile reactions, including neuroleptic malignant syndrome (NMS). Impaired core body temperature regulation may occur; caution with strenuous exercise, heat exposure, dehydration, and concomitant medication possessing anticholinergic effects (Kerwin, 2004; Safferman, 1991). Clozapine's potential for extrapyramidal symptoms (including tardive dyskinesia) appears to be extremely low. Risk of dystonia (and probably other EPS) may be greater with increased doses, use of conventional antipsychotics, males, and younger patients.

[US Boxed Warning]: Fatalities due to myocarditis and cardiomyopathy have been reported. Upon suspicion of these reactions discontinue clozapine and obtain a cardiac evaluation. Symptoms may include chest pain, tachycardia, palpitations, dyspnea, fever, flu-like symptoms, hypotension, or ECG changes. Patients with Clozaril-related myocarditis or cardiomyopathy should generally not be rechallenged with clozapine. If the benefit of treatment is judged to outweigh the potential risks of recurrent myocarditis or cardiomyopathy, rechallenge may be considered in consultation with a cardiologist, after a complete cardiac evaluation, and under close monitoring. Myocarditis and cardiomyopathy may occur at any period during clozapine treatment; however, typically myocarditis presents within the first 2 months and cardiomyopathy after 8 weeks of treatment. Cases of thromboembolism, including pulmonary embolism and stroke resulting in fatalities, have been associated with clozapine. Clozapine is associated with QT prolongation and ventricular arrhythmias including torsade de pointes; cardiac arrest and sudden death may occur. Use caution in patients with conditions that may increase the risk of QT prolongation, including history of QT prolongation, long QT syndrome, family history of long QT syndrome or sudden cardiac death, significant cardiac arrhythmia, recent myocardial infarction, uncompensated heart failure, treatment with other medications that cause QT prolongation, treatment with medications that inhibit the metabolism of clozapine, hypokalemia, and hypomagnesemia. Consider obtaining a baseline ECG and serum chemistry panel. Correct electrolyte abnormalities prior to initiating therapy. Discontinue clozapine if QTc interval >500 msec. Undesirable changes in lipids have been observed with antipsychotic therapy; incidence varies with product. Periodically monitor total serum cholesterol, triglycerides, LDL, and HDL concentrations.

Potentially significant drug-drug interactions may exist, requiring dose or frequency adjustment, additional monitoring, and/or selection of alternative therapy. Use caution when converting from brand to generic formulation; poor tolerability, including relapse, has been reported usually soon after product switch (1 to 3 months); monitor closely during this time (Bobo, 2010).

May cause anticholinergic effects; use with caution in patients with urinary retention, benign prostatic hyperplasia, narrow-angle glaucoma, xerostomia, visual problems, constipation, or history of bowel obstruction. Because of its potential to significantly decreased GI motility, use is associated with increased risk of paralytic ileus, bowel obstruction, fecal impaction, bowel perforation, and in rare cases death. Bowel regimens and monitoring are recommended. Sialorrhea and drooling may occur with clozapine use; symptoms may be more profound during sleep and may be dose-related. As a result of excessive saliva, patients may initially experience choking sensations that cause nighttime awakening, hoarseness or dysphonia of the voice, and a chronic cough. Skin irritation and infections, aspiration pneumonia, chronic sleep disturbances with daytime fatigue and somnolence, painful swelling of the salivary glands, and symptomatic aerophagia with resultant gas bloating, pain, and flatus may also develop. ▶

May cause hyperglycemia; in some cases may be extreme and associated with ketoacidosis, hyperosmolar coma, or death. In some cases, hyperglycemia resolved after discontinuation of the antipsychotic; however, some patients have required continuation of antidiabetic treatment. Monitor for symptoms of hyperglycemia including polydipsia, polyuria, polyphagia, and weakness. Use with caution in patients with diabetes or other disorders of glucose regulation; monitor for worsening of glucose control. Antipsychotic use has been associated with esophageal dysmotility and aspiration; use with caution in patients at risk of aspiration pneumonia (eg, Alzheimer disease). Use with caution in patients with hepatic disease or impairment; monitor hepatic function regularly. Hepatitis has been reported as a consequence of therapy. Use with caution in patients with renal disease.

Use caution with cardiovascular or pulmonary disease; gradually increase dose. **[US Boxed Warning]: Orthostatic hypotension, bradycardia, syncope, and cardiac arrest have been reported with clozapine treatment. Risk is highest during the initial titration period and with rapid dose increases. Symptoms can develop with the first dose and with doses as low as 12.5 mg per day. Initiate treatment with no more than 12.5 mg once daily or twice daily, titrate slowly, and use divided doses. Use with caution in patients at risk for these effects (eg, cerebrovascular disease, cardiovascular disease) or with predisposing conditions for hypotensive episodes (eg, hypovolemia, concurrent antihypertensive medication);** reactions can be fatal. Consider dose reduction if hypotension occurs. May cause tachycardia; tachycardia is not limited to a reflex response to orthostatic hypotension.

The possibility of a suicide attempt is inherent in psychotic illness or bipolar disorder; use caution in high-risk patients during initiation of therapy. Prescriptions should be written for the smallest quantity consistent with good patient care. Medication should not be stopped abruptly; taper off over 1 to 2 weeks. If conditions warrant abrupt discontinuation (eg, severe neutropenia, myocarditis, cardiomyopathy), monitor patient for psychosis and cholinergic rebound (eg, headache, nausea, vomiting, diarrhea, profuse diaphoresis). Significant weight gain has been observed with antipsychotic therapy; incidence varies with product. Monitor waist circumference and BMI. Clozapine levels may be lower in patients who smoke. Smokers may require twice the daily dose as nonsmokers in order to obtain an equivalent clozapine concentration (Tsuda, 2014). Smoking cessation may cause toxicity in a patient stabilized on clozapine. Monitor change in smoking. Consider baseline serum clozapine levels and/or empiric dosage adjustments (30% to 40% reduction) in patients expected to have a prolonged hospital stay with forced smoking cessation. Case reports suggest symptoms from increasing clozapine concentrations may develop 2 to 4 weeks after smoking cessation (Lowe 2010). Clozapine concentrations may be increased in CYP2D6 poor metabolizers; dose reduction may be necessary. FazaClo oral disintegrating tablets contain phenylalanine.

Adverse Reactions

>10%:
Cardiovascular: Tachycardia (25%)
Central nervous system: Drowsiness (39% to 46%), dizziness (19% to 27%), insomnia (2% to 20%)
Gastrointestinal: Sialorrhea (31% to 48%), weight gain (4% to 31%), constipation (14% to 25%), nausea/vomiting (3% to 17%), abdominal discomfort/heartburn (4% to 14%)

1% to 10%:
Cardiovascular: Hypotension (9%), syncope (6%), hypertension (4%), angina pectoris (1%), ECG changes (1%)
Central nervous system: Headache (7%), fever (5%), agitation (4%), akinesia (4%), nightmares (4%), restlessness (4%), akathisia (3%), confusion (3%), seizure (3%; dose related), fatigue (2%), anxiety (1%), ataxia (1%), depression (1%), lethargy (1%), myoclonic seizures (1%), pain (1%), slurred speech (1%)
Dermatologic: Skin rash (2%)
Gastrointestinal: Xerostomia (6%), diarrhea (2%), anorexia (1%), sore throat (1%)
Genitourinary: Genitourinary complaint (abnormal ejaculation, retention, urgency, incontinence; 1% to 2%)
Hematologic: Leukopenia (3%)
Hepatic: Abnormal hepatic function tests (1%)
Neuromuscular & skeletal: Tremor (6%), hypokinesia (4%), muscle rigidity (3%), hyperkinesia (1%), muscle spasm (1%), weakness (1%)
Ocular: Visual disturbance (5%)
Respiratory: Dyspnea (1%), nasal congestion (1%)
Miscellaneous: Diaphoresis (6%), numbness of tongue (1%)

<1%, postmarketing, and/or case reports (Limited to important or life-threatening): Abnormal electrocardiogram, agranulocytosis, amnesia, anemia, aspiration, bronchitis, cardiac failure, cataplexy, cerebrovascular accident, cholestasis, colitis, deep vein thrombosis, delirium, dermatitis, difficult micturition, dyschromia, edema, eosinophilia, erythema multiforme, fecal impaction, gastric ulcer, gastroenteritis, granulocytopenia, hallucinations, hematemesis, hepatotoxicity, hyperglycemia, hyperosmolar coma, hypersensitivity reaction, hyperuricemia, hypothermia, impotence, increased erythrocyte sedimentation rate, liver steatosis, lower respiratory tract infection, mental retardation, mitral valve insufficiency, myasthenia syndrome, mydriasis, myocarditis, myoclonus, neuroleptic malignant syndrome, obsessive compulsive disorder, orthostatic hypotension, pancreatitis (acute), paralytic ileus, parkinsonian like-syndrome, pheochromocytoma (pseudo), pericardial effusion, pericarditis, periorbital edema, phlebitis, pleural effusion, priapism, prolonged QT interval on ECG, psychosis exacerbated, pulmonary embolism, rectal hemorrhage, renal failure, respiratory arrest, rhabdomyolysis, sialadentitis, sepsis, skin photosensitivity, speech disturbance, status epilepticus, Stevens-Johnson syndrome, syncope, systemic lupus erythematosus, tardive dyskinesia, thrombocytopenia, thrombocytosis, thrombophlebitis, torsade de pointes, weight loss

Drug Interactions

Metabolism/Transport Effects Substrate of CYP1A2 (major), CYP2A6 (minor), CYP2C19 (minor), CYP2C9 (minor), CYP2D6 (minor), CYP3A4 (minor); **Note:** Assignment of Major/Minor substrate status based on clinically relevant drug interaction potential; **Inhibits** CYP1A2 (weak), CYP2C19 (weak), CYP2C9 (weak), CYP2D6 (moderate), CYP2E1 (weak)

Avoid Concomitant Use

Avoid concomitant use of CloZAPine with any of the following: Aclidinium; Amisulpride; Azelastine (Nasal); CarBAMazepine; Cimetropium; Ciprofloxacin (Systemic); CYP3A4 Inducers (Strong); Eluxadoline; Glucagon; Glycopyrrolate; Glycopyrrolate (Oral Inhalation); Highest Risk QTc-Prolonging Agents; Ipratropium (Oral Inhalation); Ivabradine; Levosulpiride; Metoclopramide; Mifepristone; Orphenadrine; Paraldehyde; Potassium Chloride; St Johns Wort; Sulpiride; Thalidomide; Thioridazine; Tiotropium; Umeclidinium

Increased Effect/Toxicity

CloZAPine may increase the levels/effects of: AbobotulinumtoxinA; Alcohol (Ethyl); Amifostine; Amisulpride; Analgesics (Opioid); Anticholinergic Agents; Antipsychotic Agents (Second Generation [Atypical]); ARIPiprazole; Azelastine (Nasal); Brexpiprazole; Cimetropium; CNS Depressants; CYP2D6 Substrates; DOXOrubicin (Conventional); DULoxetine; Eluxadoline; Fesoterodine; Glucagon; Glycopyrrolate; Glycopyrrolate (Oral Inhalation); Highest Risk QTc-Prolonging Agents; Hydrocodone; Hypotension-Associated Agents; Mequitazine; Methotrimeprazine; Methylphenidate; Metoprolol; Metyrosine; Mirabegron; Mirtazapine; Moderate Risk QTc-Prolonging Agents; Nebivolol; OnabotulinumtoxinA; Orphenadrine; Paraldehyde; Potassium Chloride; Ramosetron; RimabotulinumtoxinB; Serotonin Modulators; Sulpiride; Suvorexant; Thalidomide; Thiazide Diuretics; Thioridazine; Tiotropium; TiZANidine; Topiramate; Zolpidem

The levels/effects of CloZAPine may be increased by: Abiraterone Acetate; Acetylcholinesterase Inhibitors (Central); Aclidinium; Alfuzosin; Barbiturates; Benzodiazepines; Blood Pressure Lowering Agents; Brimonidine (Topical); Cannabis; CarBAMazepine; Cimetidine; Ciprofloxacin (Systemic); CYP1A2 Inhibitors (Moderate); CYP1A2 Inhibitors (Strong); Deferasirox; Diazoxide; Doxylamine; Dronabinol; Droperidol; Herbs (Hypotensive Properties); HydrOXYzine; Ipratropium (Oral Inhalation); Ivabradine; Kava Kava; Lithium; Macrolide Antibiotics; Magnesium Sulfate; Methotrimeprazine; Methylphenidate; Metoclopramide; Metyrosine; Mianserin; Mifepristone; Minocycline; Molsidomine; Myelosuppressive Agents; Nabilone; Nefazodone; Nicorandil; Obinutuzumab; Omeprazole; Peginterferon Alfa-2b; Pentoxifylline; Perampanel; Phosphodiesterase 5 Inhibitors; Pramlintide; Prostacyclin Analogues; QTc-Prolonging Agents (Indeterminate Risk and Risk Modifying); Rufinamide; Selective Serotonin Reuptake Inhibitors; Serotonin Modulators; Sodium Oxybate; Tapentadol; Tetrahydrocannabinol; Umeclidinium

Decreased Effect

CloZAPine may decrease the levels/effects of: Acetylcholinesterase Inhibitors; Amphetamines; Antidiabetic Agents; Anti-Parkinson's Agents (Dopamine Agonist); Codeine; Gastrointestinal Agents (Prokinetic); Itopride; Levosulpiride; Quinagolide; Secretin; Tamoxifen; TraMADol

The levels/effects of CloZAPine may be decreased by: Acetylcholinesterase Inhibitors; Cannabis; CarBAMazepine; CYP3A4 Inducers (Strong); Cyproterone; Lithium; Omeprazole; St Johns Wort; Teriflunomide

Storage/Stability

Suspension: Store at ≤25°C (77°F). Protect from light. Do not refrigerate or freeze. Suspension is stable for 100 days after initial bottle opening.

Tablet: Store at ≤30°C (86°F).

Tablet, dispersible: Store at 20°C to 25°C (68°F to 77°F); excursions permitted to 15°C to 30°C (59°F to 86°F). Protect from moisture; do not remove from package until ready to use.

Mechanism of Action The therapeutic efficacy of clozapine (dibenzodiazepine antipsychotic) is proposed to be mediated through antagonism of the dopamine type 2 (D_2) and serotonin type 2A (5-HT_{2A}) receptors. In addition, it acts as an antagonist at alpha-adrenergic, histamine H_1, cholinergic, and other dopaminergic and serotonergic receptors.

Pharmacodynamics/Kinetics

Onset of action: Within 1 week for sedation, improvement in sleep; 6-12 weeks for antipsychotic effects; Adequate trial: 6-12 weeks at a therapeutic dose and blood level; Maximum effect: 6-12 months; improvement may continue 6-12 months after clozapine initiation (Meltzer 2003)

Duration of action: Variable

Protein binding: 97% to serum proteins

Metabolism: Extensively hepatic; forms metabolites with limited (desmethyl metabolite) or no activity (hydroxylated and N-oxide derivative derivatives). **Note:** A pediatric pharmacokinetic study (n=6; age: 9-16 years) found higher concentrations of the desmethyl metabolite in comparison to clozapine (especially in females) when compared to data from adult studies; the authors suggest that both the parent drug and desmethyl metabolite contribute to the efficacy and adverse effect profile in children and adolescents (Frazier 2003).

Bioavailability: 12% to 81% (not affected by food); orally disintegrating tablets are bioequivalent to the regular tablets

Half-life elimination: Steady state: 12 hours (range: 4-66 hours)

Time to peak: Suspension: 2.2 hours (range: 1 to 3.5 hours); Tablets: 2.5 hours (range: 1 to 6 hours); Dispersible tablets: 2.3 hours (range: 1 to 6 hours)

Excretion: Urine (~50%) and feces (30%) with trace amounts of unchanged drug

Dosing

Adult

Note:

US labeling: Prior to initiating treatment, obtain a baseline CBC, including the ANC; the ANC must be ≥1,500/mcL for the general population and ≥1,000/mcL for patients with documented Benign Ethnic Neutropenia (BEN) in order to initiate treatment. To continue treatment, the ANC must be monitored regularly.

Canadian labeling: Prior to initiating treatment, obtain a baseline WBC and ANC; the WBC must be ≥3,500/mm³ and the ANC must be ≥2,000/mm³ in order to initiate treatment. To continue treatment, the WBC and ANC must be monitored regularly.

Schizophrenia: Oral: Initial: 12.5 mg once or twice daily; increase, as tolerated, in increments of 25 to 50 mg daily to a target dose of 300 to 450 mg daily (administered in divided doses) by the end of 2 weeks; may further titrate in increments not exceeding 100 mg and no more frequently than once or twice weekly. Maximum total daily dose: 900 mg. **Note:** In some efficacy studies, total daily dosage was administered in 3 divided doses.

Suicidal behavior in schizophrenia or schizoaffective disorder: Oral: Initial: 12.5 mg once or twice daily; increased, as tolerated, in increments of 25 to 50 mg daily to a target dose of 300 to 450 mg daily (administered in divided doses) by the end of 2 weeks; may further titrate in increments not exceeding 100 mg and no more frequently than once or twice weekly. Mean dose is ~300 mg daily; maximum total daily dose: 900 mg. **Note:** If no longer a suicide risk, may resume prior antipsychotic therapy after gradually tapering off clozapine over 1 to 2 weeks (Meltzer 2003; Wagstaff 2003).

Bipolar disorder (off-label use): Oral: Initial: 25 mg daily; increased, as tolerated in increments of 25 mg daily to a maximum dose of 550 mg daily. Average daily dose ~300 mg daily (Green, 2000).

Schizoaffective disorder (off-label use): Oral: Initial: 25 mg daily; increased, as tolerated to a maximum dose of 600 mg daily. Average daily dose: ~200 mg daily (Ciapparelli, 2003).

Dosage adjustment with concomitant therapy:

Strong CYP1A2 inhibitors (eg, fluvoxamine, ciprofloxacin):

Initiating clozapine with concomitant medication or adding a concomitant medication while taking clozapine: Use one-third of the clozapine dose.

Discontinuing concomitant medication while continuing clozapine: Increase clozapine dose based on clinical response.

Moderate or weak CYP1A2 inhibitors (eg, oral contraceptives, caffeine), CYP2D6 or CYP3A4 inhibitors (eg, cimetidine, escitalopram, erythromycin, paroxetine, bupropion, fluoxetine, quinidine, duloxetine, terbinafine, sertraline):

Initiating clozapine with concomitant medication or adding a concomitant medication while taking clozapine: Monitor for adverse reactions and if necessary, consider reducing the clozapine dose.

Discontinuing concomitant medication while continuing clozapine: Monitor for lack of effectiveness and if necessary, consider increasing the clozapine dose.

Strong CYP3A4 inducers (eg, phenytoin, carbamazepine, St John's wort, rifampin):

Initiating clozapine with concomitant medication or adding a concomitant medication while taking clozapine: Concomitant use is not recommended. However, if the CYP3A4 inducer is necessary, monitor for decreased effectiveness and if necessary, consider increasing the clozapine dose.

Discontinuing concomitant medication while continuing clozapine: Reduce clozapine dose based on clinical response.

Moderate or weak CYP1A2 (eg, tobacco smoke) or CYP3A4 inducers:

Initiating clozapine with concomitant medication or adding a concomitant medication while taking clozapine: Monitor for decreased effectiveness and if necessary, consider increasing the clozapine dose.

Discontinuing concomitant medication while continuing clozapine: Monitor for adverse reactions and if necessary, consider reducing the clozapine dose.

Reinitiation of therapy: If dosing is interrupted for ≥48 hours, therapy must be reinitiated at 12.5 mg once or twice daily to minimize the risk of hypotension, bradycardia, and syncope; if dose is well tolerated, may be increased more rapidly than with initial titration, unless cardiopulmonary arrest occurred during initial titration, then retitrate with extreme caution.

Discontinuation of therapy: In the event of planned discontinuation of clozapine, gradual reduction in dose over a 1- to 2-week period is recommended. If conditions warrant abrupt discontinuation (eg, severe neutropenia), monitor patient for psychosis and cholinergic rebound (eg, headache, nausea, vomiting, diarrhea, profuse diaphoresis).

Geriatric

Note:

US labeling: Prior to initiating treatment, obtain a baseline CBC, including the ANC; the ANC must be ≥1,500/mcL for the general population and ≥1,000/mcL for patients with documented Benign Ethnic Neutropenia (BEN) in order to initiate treatment. To continue treatment, the ANC must be monitored regularly.

Canadian labeling: Prior to initiating treatment, obtain a baseline WBC and ANC; the WBC must be ≥3,500/mm³ and the ANC must be ≥2,000/mm³ in order to initiate treatment. To continue treatment, the WBC and ANC must be monitored regularly.

Schizophrenia: Oral: Experience in the elderly is limited; may initiate with 12.5 mg once daily for 3 days, then increase to 25 mg once daily for 3 days as tolerated; may further increase, as tolerated, in increments of 12.5 to 25 mg daily every 3 days to desired response; maximum total daily dosage: 300 mg (Howanitz, 1999). Mean recommended dosage range: 25 to 150 mg (in divided doses) (Gareri, 2000).

Psychosis/agitation related to Alzheimer dementia (off-label use): Oral: Initial: 12.5 mg once daily; if necessary, gradually increase as tolerated not to exceed 75 to 100 mg daily (Rabins, 2007)

Renal Impairment

US labeling: There are no dosage adjustments provided in the manufacturer's labeling; however, labeling suggests that dose reductions may be necessary with significant impairment but does not provide specific dosing recommendations.

Canadian labeling:

Mild to moderate impairment: Initial dose: 12.5 mg once daily

Severe impairment: Use is contraindicated

Hepatic Impairment

US labeling: There are no dosage adjustments provided in the manufacturer's labeling; however, labeling suggests that dose reductions may be necessary with significant impairment.

Canadian labeling: Contraindicated in active liver disease associated with nausea, anorexia, or jaundice; progressive liver disease; or hepatic failure. There is no dosage adjustment provided in the manufacturer's labeling for stable preexisting hepatic disorders; use with caution.

Dietary Considerations Some products may contain phenylalanine.

Administration May be taken without regard to food. Total daily dose may be divided into uneven doses with larger dose administered at bedtime. The Canadian labeling suggests that maintenance doses ≤200 mg daily may be administered as single dose in the evening.

Orally disintegrating tablet: Remove from foil blister by peeling apart (do not push tablet through the foil). Remove immediately prior to use. Place tablet in mouth and chew or allow to dissolve; swallow with saliva. If dosing requires splitting tablet, throw unused portion away.

Suspension: Shake bottle prior to use. Using syringe adaptor and oral syringe provided withdrawal dose from bottle. Administer immediately after preparation using the oral syringe provided.

Monitoring Parameters Mental status; CBC (see monitoring recommendations based on ANC); vital signs (as clinically indicated); ECG (as clinically indicated); blood pressure (baseline; repeat 3 months after antipsychotic initiation, then yearly); signs and symptoms of myocarditis and cardiomyopathy; weight, height, body mass index, waist circumference (baseline; repeat at 4, 8, and 12 weeks after initiating or changing therapy, then yearly; consider switching to a different antipsychotic for a weight gain 5% or more of initial weight); electrolytes and liver function (annually and as clinically indicated); personal and family history of obesity, diabetes, dyslipidemia, hypertension, or cardiovascular disease (baseline; repeat annually); fasting plasma glucose level/HbA$_{1c}$ (baseline; repeat 3 months after starting antipsychotic, then yearly); lipid panel (baseline; repeat 3 months after initiation of antipsychotic; if low-density lipoprotein level is normal, repeat at 2- to 5-year intervals or more frequently if clinical indicated); changes in menstruation, libido, development of galactorrhea, and erectile and ejaculatory function (yearly); abnormal involuntary movements or parkinsonian signs (baseline; repeat weekly until dose stabilized for at least 2 weeks after introduction and for 2 weeks after any significant dose increase); tardive dyskinesia (every 12 months; high-risk patients every 6 months); ocular examination (yearly in patients older than 40 years; every 2 years in younger patients) (ADA, 2004; Lehman, 2004; Marder, 2004).

US labeling:

General population: Prior to initiating treatment, obtain a baseline CBC, including the ANC; the ANC must be ≥1,500/mcL for the general population in order to initiate treatment. During the first 6 months of treatment, monitor the ANC weekly. If the ANC remains ≥1,500/mcL, the monitoring frequency can be reduced to every 2 weeks for the next 6 months. If the ANC remains ≥1,500/mcL for the second 6 months of continuous therapy, the ANC monitoring frequency can be reduced to once every 4 weeks.

Treatment interruption: If ANC is ≥1,500/mcL and treatment is interrupted for <30 days, continue monitoring as before, if ≥30 days monitor as if a new patient.

Treatment discontinuation: For abrupt clozapine discontinuation for a reason unrelated to neutropenia in the general population, continuation of ANC monitoring is recommended until the ANC is ≥1,500/mcL. Additional ANC monitoring is required for any patient reporting onset of fever, defined as a temperature of 38.5°C (101.3°F) or greater, during the 2 weeks after discontinuation.

Monitor patients for psychosis and cholinergic rebound (eg, headache, nausea, vomiting, diarrhea, profuse diaphoresis).

Hematologic toxicity monitoring: Confirm all initial reports of ANC <1,500/mcL with a repeat ANC within 24 hours.

Fever: Interrupt clozapine as a precautionary measure in any patient who develops a fever, defined as a temperature of 38.5°C (101.3°F) or greater, and obtain an ANC level. Fever is often the first sign of neutropenic infection.

Mild neutropenia (1,000 to 1,499/mcL): Continue treatment; monitor ANC 3 times weekly until ≥1,500/mcL and then return to previous monitoring schedule.

Moderate neutropenia (500 to 999/mcL): Interrupt therapy, recommend hematology consultation, and begin daily ANC monitoring until ANC ≥1,000/mcL and then may consider restarting therapy. Follow with 3 times weekly monitoring until ANC ≥1,500/mcL. Once ANC ≥1,500/mcL, check ANC weekly for 4 weeks and then return to previous monitoring schedule.

If fever occurs in any patient with an ANC <1,000/mcL, initiate appropriate workup and treatment for infection.

Severe neutropenia (<500/mcL): Interrupt therapy, recommend hematology consultation, and begin daily ANC monitoring until ANC ≥1,000/mcL. Follow with 3 times weekly monitoring until ANC ≥1,500/mcL. Do not rechallenge unless prescriber determines benefits outweigh risks. If rechallenged, resume treatment as a new patient once ANC ≥1,500/mcL.

Benign Ethnic Neutropenia (BEN): Prior to initiating treatment, obtain at least 2 baseline CBC levels, including the ANC; the ANC must be ≥1,000/mcL for patients with documented Benign Ethnic Neutropenia (BEN) in order to initiate treatment. During the first 6 months of treatment, monitor the ANC weekly. If the ANC remains ≥1,000/mcL, the monitoring frequency can be reduced to every 2 weeks for the next 6 months. If the ANC remains ≥1,000/mcL for the second 6 months of continuous therapy, the ANC monitoring frequency can be reduced to once every 4 weeks.

Treatment interruption: If ANC is ≥1,000/mcL and treatment is interrupted for <30 days, continue monitoring as before, if ≥30 days monitor as if a new patient.

Treatment discontinuation: For abrupt clozapine discontinuation for a reason unrelated to neutropenia in BEN patients, continuation of ANC monitoring is recommended until the ANC is ≥1,000/mcL or above their baseline. Additional ANC monitoring is required for any patient reporting onset of fever, defined as a temperature of 38.5°C (101.3°F) or greater, during the 2 weeks after discontinuation.

Monitor patients for psychosis and cholinergic rebound (eg, headache, nausea, vomiting, diarrhea, profuse diaphoresis).

Hematologic toxicity monitoring: Confirm all initial reports of ANC <1,500/mcL with a repeat ANC within 24 hours.

Fever: Interrupt clozapine as a precautionary measure in any patient who develops a fever, defined as a temperature of 38.5°C (101.3°F) or greater, and obtain an ANC level. Fever is often the first sign of neutropenic infection.

BEN neutropenia (500 to 999/mcL): Continue therapy, recommend hematology consultation, and begin 3 times weekly ANC monitoring until ANC ≥1,000/mcL or greater than or equal to patients known baseline. Once ANC ≥1,000/mcL or patient's known baseline, check ANC weekly for 4 weeks and then return to previous monitoring schedule.

If fever occurs in any patient with an ANC <1,000/mcL, initiate appropriate workup and treatment for infection.

BEN severe neutropenia (<500/mcL): Interrupt therapy, recommend hematology consultation, and begin daily ANC monitoring until ANC ≥500/mcL. Follow with 3 times weekly monitoring until ANC greater than or equal to patients baseline. Do not rechallenge unless prescriber determines benefits outweigh risks. If rechallenged, resume treatment as a new patient once ANC ≥1,000/mcL.

Hospice patients: For hospice patients (ie, terminally ill patients with an estimated life expectancy of ≤6 months), ANC monitoring may be reduced to a frequency of once every 6 months after a discussion with the patient and caregiver. Base ANC monitoring on individual treatment needs to control psychiatric symptoms and terminal illness.

Concurrent use of other drugs associated with neutropenia: If clozapine is used concurrently with an agent known to cause neutropenia (eg, some chemotherapeutic agents), consider monitoring patients more closely. Consult with treating oncologist in patients receiving concomitant chemotherapy.

Canadian labeling:
Prior to initiating treatment, obtain a baseline WBC and ANC; the WBC must be ≥3,500/mm^3 and the ANC must be ≥2,000/mm^3 in order to initiate treatment. Initiate treatment in an inpatient setting or an outpatient setting with medical supervision and monitor of vital signs for at least 6 to 8 hours after the first few doses. During the first 6 months (26 weeks) of treatment WBC and ANC should be obtained at baseline and at least weekly. If counts remain acceptable (WBC ≥3,500/mm^3, ANC ≥2,000/mm^3) during this time period, then they may be monitored every other week for the next 6 months (26 weeks). If WBC/ANC continue to remain within these acceptable limits after the second 6 months (26 weeks) of therapy, monitoring can be decreased to every 4 weeks. If clozapine is discontinued, a weekly WBC should be conducted for an additional 4 weeks or until WBC is ≥3,500/mm^3 and ANC is ≥2,000/mm^3.

Special populations: Patients with low WBC counts because of benign ethnic neutropenia should be given special consideration and may be started on clozapine after consultation with a hematologist. Patients with a history of bone marrow disorders should be evaluated by a hematologist prior to starting clozapine; therapy may be initiated if the benefit outweighs the risk.

Treatment interruption: **Note:** Only applies to patients with WBC ≥3,500/mm^3 and the ANC ≥2,000/mm^3. If treatment is interrupted for **<3 days**, continue monitoring as before. If **≥3 days** of therapy interruption, resume weekly hematologic monitoring for an additional 6 weeks, then resume previous monitoring schedule. If treatment is interrupted for >4 weeks, monitor as if a new patient.

Hematologic toxicity monitoring:
Flu-like complaints or other symptoms which might suggest infection: Continue treatment; monitor WBC and ANC twice weekly.

Substantial drop in WBC or ANC (single drop or cumulative drop within 4 weeks of WBC ≥3,000/mm^3, reaching a value <4,000/mm^3, or ANC ≥1,500/mm^3, reaching a value <2,500/mm^3): Repeat WBC and ANC; if repeat values are WBC 3,000 to 3,500/mm^3 and ANC <2,000/mm^3, then monitor twice weekly. Continue treatment; monitor WBC and ANC twice weekly until WBC >3,500/mm^3 and ANC >2,000/mm^3 then return to previous monitoring schedule.

WBC 2,000 to 3,500/mm^3 and/or ANC 1,500 to 2,000/mm^3: Continue treatment; monitor WBC and ANC twice weekly until WBC >3,500/mm^3 and ANC >2,000/mm^3, then return to previous monitoring schedule.

WBC <2,000/mm^3 and/or ANC <1,500/mm^3: Discontinue treatment and do not rechallenge patient; continue to monitor WBC/ANC closely and monitor for signs of infection. If WBC falls <1,000/mm^3 or ANC falls <500/mm^3, place patient in protective isolation with close observation.

Eosinophilia (eosinophil count >3,000/mm^3): Discontinue treatment and restart only after the eosinophil count is <1,000/mm^3. Patients with both eosinophilia and clozapine-induced myocarditis should not be reexposed to clozapine.

Thrombocytopenia (platelet count <50,000/mm^3): Discontinue treatment.

Reference Range Clozapine levels >350 ng/mL may be associated with an increased likelihood of clinical response. However, increases of serum concentrations above this have not been shown to confer greater improvements and may increase the risk of adverse events (Remington 2013).

Dosage Forms Excipient information presented when available (limited, particularly for generics); consult specific product labeling.
Suspension, Oral:
  Versacloz: 50 mg/mL (100 mL) [contains methylparaben sodium, propylparaben sodium]
Tablet, Oral:
  Clozaril: 25 mg, 100 mg [scored]
  Generic: 25 mg, 50 mg, 100 mg, 200 mg
Tablet Dispersible, Oral:
  FazaClo: 12.5 mg, 25 mg, 100 mg, 150 mg, 200 mg [contains aspartame]
  Generic: 12.5 mg, 25 mg, 100 mg, 150 mg, 200 mg

Dosage Forms: Canada Note: Refer to Dosage Forms. Dispersible tablet and oral suspension are not available in Canada.

- Clozaril *see* CloZAPine *on page 428*
- CMA-676 *see* Gemtuzumab Ozogamicin *on page 836*
- C-Met/Hepatocyte Growth Factor Receptor Tyrosine Kinase Inhibitor PF-02341066 *see* Crizotinib *on page 450*
- C-Met/HGFR Tyrosine Kinase Inhibitor PF-02341066 *see* Crizotinib *on page 450*
- CMV Hyperimmune Globulin *see* Cytomegalovirus Immune Globulin (Intravenous-Human) *on page 472*
- CMV-IGIV *see* Cytomegalovirus Immune Globulin (Intravenous-Human) *on page 472*
- CNJ-016 *see* Vaccinia Immune Globulin (Intravenous) *on page 1857*
- CNL8 Nail *see* Ciclopirox *on page 384*
- CNTO-148 *see* Golimumab *on page 852*
- CNTO 328 *see* Siltuximab *on page 1655*
- CNTO 1275 *see* Ustekinumab *on page 1856*
- Coagulant Complex Inhibitor *see* Anti-inhibitor Coagulant Complex (Human) *on page 134*
- Coagulation Factor I *see* Fibrinogen Concentrate (Human) *on page 765*
- Coagulation Factor VIIa *see* Factor VIIa (Recombinant) *on page 733*
- CO Alendronate (Can) *see* Alendronate *on page 66*
- Co-Amoxiclav *see* Amoxicillin and Clavulanate *on page 111*
- Coartem *see* Artemether and Lumefantrine *on page 154*
- CO Atenolol (Can) *see* Atenolol *on page 166*

Cobicistat (koe BIK i stat)

Brand Names: US Tybost
Pharmacologic Category Cytochrome P-450 Inhibitor
Use
HIV-1 infection: Treatment of HIV-1 infection to increase systemic exposure of atazanavir or darunavir (once-daily dosing regimen) in combination with other antiretroviral agents
Limitations of use: Cobicistat is **not** interchangeable with ritonavir to increase systemic exposure of darunavir 600 mg twice daily, fosamprenavir, saquinavir, or tipranavir due to lack of exposure data. The use of cobicistat is not recommended with darunavir 600 mg twice daily, fosamprenavir, saquinavir, or tipranavir.

Pregnancy Considerations Adverse events were not observed in animal reproduction studies. The HHS Perinatal HIV Guidelines note there are insufficient data to recommend use in pregnancy.

Regardless of CD4 count or HIV RNA copy number, all HIV-infected pregnant women should receive a combination antiretroviral (ARV) drug regimen. A combination of antepartum, intrapartum, and infant ARV prophylaxis is recommended. ARV therapy should be started as soon as possible in women with symptomatic infection. Although earlier initiation may be more effective in reducing the perinatal transmission of HIV, initiation may be delayed until after 12 weeks gestation in women who do not require immediate treatment after careful consideration of maternal conditions (eg, nausea and vomiting) and the potential risks of first trimester fetal exposure for specific agents. A scheduled cesarean delivery at 38 weeks gestation is recommended for all women with HIV RNA >1000 copies/mL or unknown concentrations near delivery in order to decrease transmission. If ARV therapy must be interrupted for <24 hours during the peripartum period, stop then restart all medications simultaneously in order to decrease the chance of developing resistance. Long-term follow-up is recommended for all infants exposed to ARV medications. In couples who want to conceive, the HIV-infected partner should attain maximum viral suppression prior to conception.

Health care providers are encouraged to enroll pregnant women exposed to antiretroviral medications in the Antiretroviral Pregnancy Registry (1-800-258-4263 or www.APRegistry.com). Health care providers caring for HIV-infected women and their infants may contact the National Perinatal HIV Hotline (888-448-8765) for clinical consultation (HHS [perinatal], 2014).

Breast-Feeding Considerations It is not known if cobicistat is excreted into breast milk. Maternal or infant antiretroviral therapy does not completely eliminate the risk of postnatal HIV transmission. In addition, multiclass-resistant virus has been detected in breast-feeding infants despite maternal therapy. Therefore, in the United States, where formula is accessible, affordable, safe, and sustainable, and the risk of infant mortality due to diarrhea and respiratory infections is low, complete avoidance of breast-feeding by HIV-infected women is recommended to decrease potential transmission of HIV (HHS [perinatal], 2014).

Contraindications Concomitant use of cobicistat with atazanavir or darunavir with alfuzosin, carbamazepine, cisapride, dronedarone, ergot derivatives (eg, dihydroergotamine, ergotamine, methylergonovine), indinavir, irinotecan, lovastatin, midazolam (oral), nevirapine, phenobarbital, phenytoin, pimozide, rifampin, sildenafil (when used for pulmonary arterial hypertension), simvastatin, St John's wort, triazolam

Warnings/Precautions Patients may develop immune reconstitution syndrome resulting in the occurrence of an inflammatory response to an indolent or residual opportunistic infection during initial HIV treatment or activation of autoimmune disorders (eg, Graves' disease, polymyositis, Guillain-Barré syndrome) later in therapy; further evaluation and treatment may be required. May inhibit tubular secretion of creatinine without affecting actual renal glomerular function; use caution when interpreting serum creatinine values in patients with medical conditions or receiving drugs needing to be monitored with estimated creatinine clearance (CrCl). Patients who experience a confirmed increase in serum creatinine >0.4 mg/dL from baseline should have renal function monitored closely. Assess estimated CrCl prior to initiating therapy; consider alternative medications that do not require dosage adjustments in patients with renal impairment. When used with concomitant tenofovir disoproxil fumarate, may cause renal toxicity (acute renal failure and/or Fanconi syndrome); avoid use with concurrent or recent nephrotoxic therapy. In patients receiving concomitant tenofovir disoproxil fumarate, assess creatinine clearance, urine glucose, and urine protein prior to and periodically during treatment; assess serum phosphorus in patients with or at risk for renal impairment. Do not initiate therapy in combination with tenofovir disoproxil fumarate in patients with CrCl <70 mL/minute.

Use with HIV-1 protease inhibitors other than atazanavir or darunavir administered once daily is not recommended; use with more than one antiretroviral that requires pharmacokinetic enhancement (eg, two protease inhibitors or elvitegravir in combination with a protease inhibitor) is not recommended. Avoid concurrent use with other cobicistat-containing products or ritonavir-containing products. Potentially significant drug-drug interactions may exist, requiring dose or frequency adjustment, additional monitoring, and/or selection of alternative therapy. Complex or unknown mechanisms of drug interactions preclude extrapolation of ritonavir drug interactions to certain cobicistat interactions. Cobicistat and ritonavir when administered with either atazanavir or darunavir may result in different drug interactions when used with concomitant medications.

Adverse Reactions All adverse reactions are from trials using cobicistat coadministered with atazanavir, emtricitabine + tenofovir unless otherwise noted.

Frequency not always defined.

Central nervous system: Abnormal dreams (<2%), depression (<2%), fatigue (<2%), headache (<2%), insomnia (<2%)

Dermatologic: Skin rash (5%)

Endocrine & metabolic: Glycosuria (≥1000 mg/dL: 3%), increased gamma-glutamyl transferase (>5.0 x ULN: 2%), Fanconi's syndrome (<2%), increased HDL cholesterol, increased LDL cholesterol, increased serum cholesterol, increased serum triglycerides

Gastrointestinal: Nausea (2% to 12%), increased serum lipase (9%), increased serum amylase (>2.0 x ULN: 4%), diarrhea (<2%), upper abdominal pain (<2%), vomiting (<2%)

Genitourinary: Hematuria (>75 RBC/HPF: 3%)

Hepatic: Hyperbilirubinemia (>2.5 x ULN: 65%), jaundice (5% to 13%), increased serum ALT (>5.0 x ULN: 3%), increased serum AST (>5.0 x ULN: 3%)

Neuromuscular & skeletal: Increased creatine phosphokinase (≥10.0 x ULN: 5%), rhabdomyolysis (<2%)

Ophthalmic: Ocular icterus (3% to 15%)

Renal: Nephrolithiasis (<2%), renal disease (<2%), decreased creatinine clearance (no effect on renal glomerular function in patients with normal renal function), increased serum creatinine, renal insufficiency

Drug Interactions

Metabolism/Transport Effects Substrate of CYP3A4 (major); **Note:** Assignment of Major/Minor substrate status based on clinically relevant drug interaction potential; **Inhibits** BCRP, CYP2D6 (weak), CYP3A4 (strong), P-glycoprotein, SLCO1B1, SLCO1B3

Avoid Concomitant Use

Avoid concomitant use of Cobicistat with any of the following: Ado-Trastuzumab Emtansine; Alfuzosin; Aprepitant; Astemizole; Avanafil; Axitinib; Barnidipine; Boceprevir; Bosutinib; Bromocriptine; Cabozantinib; CarBAMazepine; Ceritinib; Cisapride; Cobimetinib; Conivaptan; Crizotinib; Dabrafenib; Dapoxetine; Dihydroergotamine; Domperidone; Dronedarone; Eletriptan; Eplerenone; Ergotamine; Everolimus; Flibanserin; Fluticasone (Oral Inhalation); Fosphenytoin-Phenytoin; Halofantrine; Ibrutinib; Irinotecan Products; Isavuconazonium Sulfate; Ivabradine; Lapatinib; Lercanidipine; Lomitapide; Lovastatin; Lurasidone; Macitentan; Methylergonovine; Midazolam; Naloxegol; Nilotinib; NiMODipine; Nisoldipine; Olaparib; Osimertinib; Palbociclib; PAZOPanib; PHENobarbital; Pimozide; Primidone; Ranolazine; Red Yeast Rice; Regorafenib; Rifampin; Rifapentine; Rivaroxaban; Salmeterol; Silodosin; Simeprevir; Simvastatin; Sonidegib; St Johns Wort; Suvorexant; Tamsulosin; Telaprevir; Terfenadine; Ticagrelor; Tolvaptan; Topotecan; Toremifene; Trabectedin; Triazolam; Ulipristal; Vemurafenib; VinCRIStine (Liposomal); Vorapaxar

Increased Effect/Toxicity

Cobicistat may increase the levels/effects of: Ado-Trastuzumab Emtansine; Afatinib; Alfuzosin; Alitretinoin (Systemic); Almotriptan; Alosetron; Amiodarone; Apixaban; Aprepitant; ARIPiprazole; ARIPiprazole Lauroxil; Astemizole; AtorvaSTATin; Avanafil; Axitinib; Barnidipine; Bedaquiline; Boceprevir; Bortezomib; Bosentan; Bosutinib; Brentuximab Vedotin; Brexpiprazole; Brinzolamide; Bromocriptine; Budesonide (Nasal); Budesonide (Oral Inhalation); Budesonide (Systemic); Budesonide (Topical); Buprenorphine; Cabazitaxel; Cabozantinib; Cannabis; Cariprazine; Ceritinib; Cilostazol; Cisapride; Clarithromycin; ClonazePAM; Cobimetinib; Colchicine; Conivaptan; Contraceptives (Progestins); Corticosteroids (Orally Inhaled); Corticosteroids (Systemic); Crizotinib; CYP2D6 Substrates; CYP3A4 Substrates; Dabigatran Etexilate; Dabrafenib; Daclatasvir; Dapoxetine; Dasatinib; Dihydroergotamine; Dofetilide; Domperidone; DOXOrubicin (Conventional); Dronabinol; Dronedarone; Dutasteride; Edoxaban; Eletriptan; Eliglustat; Eplerenone; Ergotamine; Erlotinib; Estazolam; Ethosuximide; Etizolam; Everolimus; FentaNYL; Fesoterodine; Flibanserin; Fluticasone (Nasal); Fluticasone (Oral Inhalation); Gefitinib; GuanFACINE; Halofantrine; Hydrocodone; Ibrutinib; Idelalisib; Iloperidone; Imatinib; Imidafenacin; Irinotecan Products; Isavuconazonium Sulfate; Itraconazole; Ivabradine; Ivacaftor; Ixabepilone; Ketoconazole (Systemic); Lacosamide; Lapatinib; Ledipasvir; Lercanidipine; Levobupivacaine; Levomilnacipran; Lomitapide; Lovastatin; Lumefantrine; Lurasidone; Macitentan; Maraviroc; Methadone; Methylergonovine; MethylPREDNISolone; Midazolam; Mifepristone; Naloxegol; Nilotinib; NiMODipine; Nintedanib; Nisoldipine; Olaparib; Osimertinib; Ospemifene; Oxybutynin; OxyCODONE; Palbociclib; Panobinostat; Parecoxib; Paricalcitol; PAZOPanib; P-glycoprotein/ABCB1 Substrates; Pimecrolimus; Pimozide; PONATinib; Pranlukast; PredniSOLONE (Systemic); PredniSONE; Propafenone; Prucalopride; QUEtiapine; QuiNIDine; Ramelteon; Ranolazine; Red Yeast Rice; Regorafenib; Repaglinide; Retapamulin; Rifaximin; Rilpivirine; Riociguat; Rivaroxaban; RomiDEPsin; Ruxolitinib; Salmeterol; Saxagliptin; Sildenafil; Silodosin; Simeprevir; Simvastatin; Sonidegib; SORAfenib; Suvorexant; Tacrolimus (Systemic); Tadalafil; Tamsulosin; Tasimelteon; Telaprevir; Telithromycin; Tenofovir Products; Terfenadine; Tetrahydrocannabinol; Ticagrelor; Tofacitinib; Tolterodine; Tolvaptan; Topotecan; Toremifene; Trabectedin; TraMADol; Triazolam; Ulipristal; Vardenafil; Vemurafenib; Vilazodone; VinCRIStine (Liposomal); Vindesine; Vinorelbine; Vorapaxar; Voriconazole; Warfarin; Zopiclone; Zuclopenthixol

The levels/effects of Cobicistat may be increased by: Clarithromycin; Itraconazole; Ketoconazole (Systemic); Telithromycin; Voriconazole

Decreased Effect

Cobicistat may decrease the levels/effects of: Contraceptives (Estrogens); Ifosfamide; Prasugrel; Ticagrelor

The levels/effects of Cobicistat may be decreased by: CarBAMazepine; CYP3A4 Inducers (Moderate); CYP3A4 Inducers (Strong); Deferasirox; Dexamethasone (Systemic); Enzalutamide; Fosphenytoin-Phenytoin; Mitotane; OXcarbazepine; PHENobarbital;

Primidone; Rifampin; Rifapentine; Siltuximab; St Johns Wort; Tocilizumab

Storage/Stability Store at 25°C (77°F); excursions are permitted between 15°C and 30°C (59°F and 86°F). Keep tightly closed. Dispense only in original container.

Mechanism of Action Cobicistat is a mechanism-based inhibitor of cytochrome P450 3A (CYP3A). Inhibition of CYP3A-mediated metabolism by cobicistat and increases the systemic exposure of CYP3A substrates atazanavir and darunavir.

Pharmacodynamics/Kinetics

Protein binding: 97% to 98%

Metabolism: Via CYP3A enzymes and to a minor extent by CYP2D6 enzymes and does not undergo glucuronidation

Half-life: Terminal: ~3 to 4 hours

Time to peak, plasma: 3.5 hours

Excretion: Feces (~86%), urine (~8%)

Dosing

Adult

HIV-1 infection: Oral: **Note:** Must be administered with concomitant atazanavir or darunavir and other antiretroviral drugs. See individual agents. Cobicistat is a component (as a pharmacokinetic enhancer) of a recommended initial regimen (with elvitegravir/tenofovir disoproxil fumarate/emtricitabine) in ART-naïve patients with a pre-ART CrCl >70 mL/minute (HHS [adult] 2015). *Treatment-naive or experienced:* 150 mg once daily with concomitant atazanavir

Treatment-naive or experienced with no darunavir resistance-associated substitutions: 150 mg once daily with concomitant darunavir

Renal Impairment

When **not** used with concomitant tenofovir disoproxil fumarate: No dosage adjustment necessary.

When used with concomitant tenofovir disoproxil fumarate:

CrCl ≥70 mL/minute: No dosage adjustment necessary.

CrCl <70 mL/minute: Use is not recommended.

Hepatic Impairment

Mild-to-moderate hepatic impairment (Child-Pugh class A or B): No dosage adjustment necessary.

Severe hepatic impairment (Child-Pugh class C): There are no dosage adjustments provided in the manufacturer's labeling (has not been studied).

Dietary Considerations Take with food

Administration Oral: Administer with food

Monitoring Parameters CBC with differential, reticulocyte count, CD4 count, HIV RNA plasma levels, and serum creatinine at baseline and when clinically indicated during therapy; when coadministered with tenofovir disoproxil fumarate, serum creatinine, urine glucose and urine protein prior to initiation and as clinically indicated during therapy; assess serum phosphorus in patients with or at risk for renal impairment. Patients who experience a confirmed increase in serum creatinine >0.4 mg/dL from baseline should have renal function monitored closely. Testing for HBV is recommended prior to the initiation of antiretroviral therapy.

Test Interactions May inhibit tubular secretion of creatinine without affecting actual renal glomerular function. Patients who experience a confirmed increase in serum creatinine >0.4 mg/dL from baseline should have renal function monitored closely.

Dosage Forms Excipient information presented when available (limited, particularly for generics); consult specific product labeling.

Tablet, Oral:

Tybost: 150 mg [contains fd&c yellow #6 aluminum lake]

◆ Cobicistat and Darunavir *see* Darunavir and Cobicistat *on page 499*

◆ Cobicistat, Emtricitabine, Tenofovir Alafenamide, and Elvitegravir *see* Elvitegravir, Cobicistat, Emtricitabine, and Tenofovir Alafenamide *on page 632*

◆ Cobicistat, Emtricitabine, Tenofovir Disoproxil Fumarate, and Elvitegravir *see* Elvitegravir, Cobicistat, Emtricitabine, and Tenofovir Disoproxil Fumarate *on page 632*

Cobimetinib (koe bi ME ti nib)

Brand Names: US Cotellic

Index Terms Cobimetinib Fumarate; Cotellic; GDC-0973; XL518

Pharmacologic Category Antineoplastic Agent, MEK Inhibitor

Use

Melanoma, unresectable or metastatic: Treatment of unresectable or metastatic melanoma in patients with a BRAF V600E or V600K mutation (in combination with vemurafenib)

Limitations of use: Not indicated for treatment of patients with wild-type BRAF melanoma

Pregnancy Considerations Adverse events were observed in animal reproduction studies. Based on the mechanism of action, cobimetinib would be expected to cause fetal harm. Women of reproductive potential should use effective contraception during therapy and for 2 weeks after the final dose.

Breast-Feeding Considerations It is not known if cobimetinib is excreted in breast milk. The manufacturer does not recommend breast-feeding during therapy or for 2 weeks after the final dose.

Prescribing and Access Restrictions Available through specialty pharmacies. Further information may be obtained from the manufacturer, Genentech, at 1-888-249-4918, or at http://www.cotellic.com.

Contraindications There are no contraindications listed in the manufacturer's labeling.

Warnings/Precautions Hazardous agent – Use appropriate precautions for handling and disposal (meets NIOSH 2014 criteria).

New primary cutaneous malignancies may occur. Malignancies included cutaneous squamous cell carcinoma (cuSCC) or keratoacanthoma (KA), basal cell carcinoma (BCC), and second primary melanoma. The median time to detection of first cuSCC or KA was 4 months (range: 2 to 11 months); the median time to first detection of BCC was 4 months (range: 1 to 13 months). Dermatologic exams should be performed prior to initiation, every 2 months during treatment, and for 6 months following discontinuation of cobimetinib/vemurafenib combination therapy. Suspicious lesions should be managed with excision and dermatopathologic evaluation. Dosage adjustment is not recommended for new cutaneous malignancies. Vemurafenib may be associated with the development of noncutaneous malignancy; monitor for signs/symptoms of noncutaneous malignancy during combination treatment.

Hemorrhage, including major symptomatic bleeding in a critical area/organ, may occur with cobimetinib. Grade 3 to 4 bleeding has occurred. Cerebral hemorrhage, gastrointestinal bleeding, reproductive system hemorrhage, and hematuria have been reported. May require treatment interruption, dose reduction, and/or discontinuation. Symptomatic or asymptomatic declines in left ventricular ejection fraction (LVEF) may occur with cobimetinib. Safety has not been established in patients with baseline LVEF below the institutional lower limit of normal (LLN) or below 50%. Assess LVEF (by echocardiogram or MUGA scan) prior to therapy initiation, 1 month after initiation, and every 3 months thereafter until cobimetinib is discontinued. May require treatment interruption, dose reduction and/or discontinuation. Also assess LVEF at ~2 weeks, 4 weeks, 10 weeks, 16 weeks, and then as clinically indicated after a dose reduction or treatment interruption. The median time to first onset of LVEF decline was 4 months (range: 23 days to 13 months). Decreased LVEF resolved to >LLN or within 10% of baseline at nearly two-thirds of patients with a median time to resolution of 3 months (range: 4 days to 12 months).

Severe rash and other skin reactions (including grades 3 and 4) may occur; some events required hospitalization. The median time to onset of grade 3 and 4 rash events was 11 days (range: 3 days to ~3 months); most patients with grades 3 and 4 rash experienced complete resolution at a median time of 21 days (range: 4 days to 17 months). May require treatment interruption, dose reduction and/or discontinuation. Photosensitivity was reported in nearly one-half of patients (may be severe). The median time to first onset of photosensitivity was 2 months (range: 1 day to 14 months); the median duration was 3 months (range: 2 days to 14 months). Photosensitivity resolved in nearly two-thirds of patients. Advise patients to avoid sun exposure, wear protective clothing, and use a broad-spectrum UVA/UVB sunscreen and lip balm (SPF 30 or higher) when outdoors. Photosensitivity may require treatment interruption, dose reduction, and/or discontinuation. Ocular toxicities may occur, including serous retinopathy (fluid accumulation under retina layers). Chorioretinopathy and retinal detachment have been reported; retinal vein occlusion has also been reported (case report). The time to first onset of serous retinopathy ranged between 2 days to 9 months with a duration of 1 day to 15 months. Perform ophthalmic examinations regularly during treatment, and with reports of new or worsening visual disturbances. If serous retinopathy is diagnosed, interrupt treatment until visual symptoms improve; may require treatment interruption, dose reduction, and/or discontinuation.

Hepatotoxicity (including grades 3 or 4 transaminase, total bilirubin, or alkaline phosphatase elevations) may occur with cobimetinib. Monitor liver function test at baseline and monthly during treatment, or as clinically necessary. Grade 3 and 4 elevations may require treatment interruption, dose reduction, and/or discontinuation. Rhabdomyolysis and creatine phosphokinase (CPK) elevations may occur with cobimetinib. The median time to first occurrence of grade 3 or 4 CPK elevations was 16 days (range: 12 days to 11 months), with a median time to resolution of 15 days (range: 9 days to 11 months). Obtain baseline serum CPK and creatinine levels at baseline, periodically during treatment and as clinically indicated. If CPK is elevated, evaluate for signs/symptoms of rhabdomyolysis or other etiology. Depending on severity, may require treatment interruption, dose reduction, and/or discontinuation.

Prior to initiating therapy, confirm BRAF V600K or V600E mutation status with an approved test; approved for use in patients with BRAF V600K and BRAF V600E mutations. Not indicated for use in patients with wild-type BRAF melanoma. Potentially significant drug-drug interactions may exist, requiring dose or frequency adjustment, additional monitoring, and/or selection of alternative therapy.

Adverse Reactions Percentages reported as part of combination chemotherapy regimens.

>10%:
Cardiovascular: Decreased left ventricular ejection fraction (grades 2/3: 26%), hypertension (15%)
Dermatologic: Skin photosensitivity (46% to 47%, grades 3/4: 4%; includes solar dermatitis and sunburn), acneiform eruption (16%, grades 3/4: 2%)
Endocrine & metabolic: Hypophosphatemia (68%), increased gamma-glutamyl transferase (65%; grades 3/4: 21%), hypoalbuminemia (42%), hyponatremia (38%), hyperkalemia (26%), hypokalemia (25%), hypocalcemia (24%)
Gastrointestinal: Diarrhea (60%), nausea (41%), vomiting (24%), stomatitis (14%; includes aphthous stomatitis, mucositis, and oral mucosa ulcer)
Hematologic & oncologic: Lymphocytopenia (73%, grades 3/4: 10%), anemia (69%; grades 3/4: 3%), thrombocytopenia (18%), hemorrhage (13%, grades 3/4: 1%; includes bruise, ecchymoses, epistaxis, gingival hemorrhage, hematemesis, hematochezia, hemoptysis, hemorrhoidal bleeding, hypermenorrhea, melena, menometrorrhagia, nail bed bleeding, pulmonary hemorrhage, purpura, rectal hemorrhage, rupture of ovarian cyst, subarachnoid hemorrhage, subgaleal hematoma, traumatic hematoma, uterine hemorrhage, and vaginal hemorrhage)
Hepatic: Increased serum AST (73%, grades 3/4: 7% to 8%), increased serum alkaline phosphatase (71%, grades 3/4: 7%), increased serum ALT (68%, grades 3/4: 11%)
Neuromuscular & skeletal: Increased creatine phosphokinase (79%, grades 3/4: 12% to 14%)
Ophthalmic: Visual impairment (15%, grades 3/4: <1%; includes blurred vision, decreased visual acuity), chorioretinopathy (13%, grades 3/4: <1%), retinal detachment (12%, grades 3/4: 2%; includes detachment of macular retinal pigment epithelium and retinal pigment epithelium detachment)
Renal: Increased serum creatinine (100%; grades 3/4: 3%)
Miscellaneous: Fever (28%)
1% to 10%:
Central nervous system: Chills (10%)
Dermatologic: Skin rash (grades 3/4: 16%; grade 4: 2%; rash resulting in hospitalization: 3%)
Gastrointestinal: Gastrointestinal hemorrhage (4%)
Genitourinary: Genitourinary tract hemorrhage (2%), hematuria (2%)
Hematologic & oncologic: Keratoacanthoma (≤6%), squamous cell carcinoma of skin (≤6%), basal cell carcinoma (5%)
Hepatic: Abnormal bilirubin levels (grades 3/4: 2%)
<1% (Limited to important or life-threatening): Cerebral hemorrhage, malignant melanoma (second primary), malignant neoplasm (non-cutaneous)

Drug Interactions
Metabolism/Transport Effects Substrate of CYP3A4 (major), P-glycoprotein; **Note:** Assignment of Major/Minor substrate status based on clinically relevant drug interaction potential

Avoid Concomitant Use
Avoid concomitant use of Cobimetinib with any of the following: Conivaptan; CYP3A4 Inducers (Moderate); CYP3A4 Inducers (Strong); CYP3A4 Inhibitors (Moderate); CYP3A4 Inhibitors (Strong); Fusidic Acid (Systemic); Idelalisib

Increased Effect/Toxicity
Cobimetinib may increase the levels/effects of: Porfimer; Verteporfin

The levels/effects of Cobimetinib may be increased by: Conivaptan; CYP3A4 Inhibitors (Moderate); CYP3A4 Inhibitors (Strong); Dasatinib; Fosaprepitant; Fusidic Acid (Systemic); Idelalisib; Ivacaftor; Luliconazole; Osimertinib; Palbociclib; Simeprevir; Stiripentol

Decreased Effect
The levels/effects of Cobimetinib may be decreased by: CYP3A4 Inducers (Moderate); CYP3A4 Inducers (Strong); Deferasirox; Osimertinib; Siltuximab; Tocilizumab

Storage/Stability Store below 30°C (86°F).
Mechanism of Action Cobimetinib is a potent and selective inhibitor of the mitogen-activated extracellular kinase (MEK) pathway (Larkin 2014); it reversibly inhibits MEK1 and MEK2, which are upstream regulators of the extracellular signal-related kinase (ERK) pathway. The ERK pathway promotes cellular proliferation. MEK1 and MEK2 are part of the BRAF pathway, which is activated by BRAF V600E and K mutations. Vemurafenib targets a different kinase in the RAS/RAF/MEK/ERK pathway; when cobimetinib and vemurafenib are used in combination, increased apoptosis and reduced tumor growth occurs.

Pharmacodynamics/Kinetics
Distribution: 806 L
Protein binding: 95%; to plasma proteins
Metabolism: Hepatic; via CYP3A4 oxidation and UGT2B7 glucuronidation
Bioavailability, absolute: 46%
Half-life elimination, mean: 44 hours (range: 23 to 70 hours)
Time to peak, median: 2.4 hours (range: 1 to 24 hours)
Excretion: Feces (76%; ~7 as unchanged drug); Urine (~18%; ~2% as unchanged drug)

Dosing
Adult & Geriatric
Melanoma, unresectable or metastatic (with BRAF V600E or V600K mutations): Oral: 60 mg once daily days 1 to 21 of each 28-day treatment cycle (in combination with vemurafenib); continue until disease progression or unacceptable toxicity (Larkin 2014).
Missed doses: If a dose is missed or if vomiting occurs after a dose is taken, resume with the next scheduled dose (do not take an additional dose).
Dosage adjustment for concurrent CYP3A4 inhibitors: Avoid concurrent use of strong or moderate CYP3A4 inhibitors with cobimetinib. If concurrent short-term use (≤14 days) of a moderate CYP3A4 inhibitor cannot be avoided, reduce the cobimetinib dose from 60 mg to 20 mg; after the moderate CYP3A4 inhibitor is discontinued, resume the previous dose of 60 mg. If the current dose is 40 or 20 mg daily, alternatives to the strong or moderate CYP3A4 inhibitor should be used.

Renal Impairment
CrCl 30 to 89 mL/minute: No dosage adjustment is necessary.
CrCl <30 mL/minute: There is no dosage adjustment provided in the manufacturer's labeling (has not been established).

Hepatic Impairment
Hepatic impairment prior to treatment:
Mild impairment (total bilirubin ≤ULN and AST >ULN **or** total bilirubin >ULN to ≤1.5 times ULN and any AST): No dosage adjustment is necessary.
Moderate to severe impairment: There is no dosage adjustment provided in the manufacturer's labeling (has not been studied); however, exposure may be increased.
Hepatotoxicity during treatment:
First occurrence of grade 4 lab abnormality (ALT, AST, or alkaline phosphatase >20 times ULN or total bilirubin >10 times ULN) or hepatotoxicity: Withhold cobimetinib for up to 4 weeks; if improves to grades 0 or 1, resume at the next lower dose level. Permanently discontinue if not improved to grade 0 or 1 within 4 weeks.
Recurrent grade 4 lab abnormality or hepatotoxicity: Permanently discontinue.

Adjustment for Toxicity
Recommended cobimetinib dose reductions for toxicity (vemurafenib may also require dosage adjustment):
First dose reduction: 40 mg once daily
Second dose reduction: 20 mg once daily
Subsequent modification (if unable to tolerate 20 mg once daily): Permanently discontinue

Cardiotoxicity:

Asymptomatic cardiomyopathy (absolute decrease in LVEF >10% [from baseline] and less than the institutional lower limit of normal [LLN]): Withhold cobimetinib for 2 weeks and repeat LVEF. If LVEF ≥ LLN **and** absolute decrease from baseline is ≤10%, resume at the next lower dose level. Permanently discontinue if LVEF < LLN **or** absolute decrease from baseline is >10%.

Symptomatic cardiomyopathy (symptomatic LVEF decrease from baseline): Withhold cobimetinib for up to 4 weeks and repeat LVEF. If symptoms resolve **and** LVEF ≥ LLN **and** absolute decrease from baseline is ≤10%, resume at the next lower dose level. Permanently discontinue if symptoms persist **or** LVEF < LLN **or** absolute decrease from baseline is >10%.

CPK elevation or rhabdomyolysis:

Grade 4 CPK elevation (>10 times ULN) or any CPK elevation with myalgia: Withhold cobimetinib for up to 4 weeks; if improves to grade 3 or lower, resume at the next lower dose level. Permanently discontinue if not improved within 4 weeks.

Dermatologic toxicity:

Grade 2 (intolerable) or grade 3 or 4: Withhold or reduce dose.

New primary cutaneous or noncutaneous malignancies: No cobimetinib dosage modification is necessary.

Hemorrhage:

Grade 3: Withhold cobimetinib for up to 4 weeks; if improves to grades 0 or 1, resume at the next lower dose level. Permanently discontinue if not improved within 4 weeks.

Grade 4: Permanently discontinue.

Ocular:

Serous retinopathy: Withhold cobimetinib for up to 4 weeks; if signs/symptoms improve, resume at the next lower dose level. Permanently discontinue if not improved or symptoms recur within 4 weeks at the lower dose.

Retinal vein occlusion: Permanently discontinue.

Photosensitivity:

Grade 2 (intolerable), grade 3 or 4: Withhold cobimetinib for up to 4 weeks; if improves to grades 0 or 1, resume at the next lower dose level. Permanently discontinue if not improved within 4 weeks.

Other toxicities:

Grade 2 (intolerable), or any grade 3: Withhold cobimetinib for up to 4 weeks; if improves to grades 0 or 1, resume at the next lower dose level. Permanently discontinue if not improved within 4 weeks.

Grade 4, first occurrence: Withhold cobimetinib until adverse reaction improves to grade 0 or 1 and then resume at the next lower dose level or permanently discontinue.

Grade 4, recurrent: Permanently discontinue.

Administration Oral: May be administered with or without food.

Hazardous agent; use appropriate precautions for handling and disposal (meets NIOSH 2014 criteria). NIOSH recommends single gloving for administration of intact tablets (NIOSH 2014).

Monitoring Parameters

BRAF V600K or V600E mutation status (prior to treatment); liver function tests (baseline and monthly during treatment, more frequently if clinically indicated); creatine phosphokinase and serum creatinine (baseline and periodically during treatment, more frequently if clinically indicated). Assess left ventricular ejection fraction (LVEF) by echocardiogram or MUGA prior to therapy initiation, 1 month after initiation, and every 3 months thereafter until cobimetinib is discontinued; also assess LVEF at ~2 weeks, 4 weeks, 10 weeks, 16 weeks, and then as clinically indicated after a dose reduction or treatment interruption.

Dermatologic exams (baseline, every 2 months during treatment, and for 6 months following discontinuation); ophthalmic examinations (regularly during treatment and with reports of new or worsening visual disturbances); monitor for signs/symptoms of dermatologic toxicity, hemorrhage, noncutaneous malignancy, photosensitivity, and rhabdomyolysis.

Dosage Forms Excipient information presented when available (limited, particularly for generics); consult specific product labeling.

Tablet, Oral:

Cotellic: 20 mg

♦ Cobimetinib Fumarate *see* Cobimetinib *on page 435*

Cocaine (koe KANE)

Index Terms Cocaine Hydrochloride

Pharmacologic Category Local Anesthetic

Use Topical anesthesia (and vasoconstriction) for mucous membranes of the oral, laryngeal, or nasal cavities.

Dosing

Adult Anesthesia: Topical: Dosage depends on the area to be anesthetized, tissue vascularity, technique of anesthesia, and individual patient tolerance; the lowest dose necessary to produce adequate anesthesia should be used; concentrations of 1% to 10% may be used, with 4% being the most frequently used concentration (maximum total dose: 3 mg/kg **or** 200 mg) (Liao 1999; McGee 2010). Lasts for 30 minutes or longer depending on concentration and vascularity of anesthetized tissue. Use reduced dosages for children, elderly, or debilitated patients.

Geriatric Refer to adult dosing; use with caution.

Pediatric Children and Adolescents: Refer to adult dosing.

Renal Impairment There are no dosage adjustments provided in the manufacturer's labeling.

Hepatic Impairment There are no dosage adjustments provided in the manufacturer's labeling.

Additional Information Complete prescribing information should be consulted for additional detail.

Dosage Forms Excipient information presented when available (limited, particularly for generics); consult specific product labeling.

Solution, External, as hydrochloride:

Generic: 4% (4 mL, 10 mL); 10% (4 mL)

Controlled Substance C-II

♦ Cocaine Hydrochloride *see* Cocaine *on page 437*

♦ CO Candesartan (Can) *see* Candesartan *on page 294*

♦ CO Clomipramine (Can) *see* ClomiPRAMINE *on page 416*

♦ CO Clonazepam (Can) *see* ClonazePAM *on page 419*

♦ Codar GF *see* Guaifenesin and Codeine *on page 861*

Codeine (KOE deen)

Brand Names: Canada Codeine Contin; PMS-Codeine; ratio-Codeine

Index Terms Codeine Phosphate; Codeine Sulfate; Methylmorphine

Pharmacologic Category Analgesic, Opioid; Antitussive

Use

Pain: Management of mild-to-moderately-severe pain

Cough: *Canadian labeling:* Additional use (not in US labeling): Relief of exhausting, nonproductive cough which does not respond to nonopioid antitussives

Pregnancy Considerations Adverse events have been observed in animal reproduction studies. Opioid analgesics cross the placenta. In humans, birth defects (including some heart defects) have been associated with maternal use of codeine during the first trimester of pregnancy (Broussard 2011). If chronic opioid exposure occurs in pregnancy, adverse events in the newborn (including withdrawal) may occur; monitoring of the neonate is recommended. The minimum effective dose should be used if opioids are needed (Chou 2009). Neonatal abstinence syndrome following opioid exposure may present with autonomic (eg, fever, temperature instability), gastrointestinal (eg, diarrhea, vomiting, poor feeding/weight gain), or neurologic (eg, high pitched crying, increased muscle tone, irritability, seizure, tremor) symptoms (Dow 2012; Hudak 2012).

Breast-Feeding Considerations Codeine and its metabolite (morphine) are found in breast milk and can be detected in the serum of nursing infants. The relative dose to a nursing infant has been calculated to be ~1% of the weight-adjusted maternal dose (Spigset 2000). Higher levels of morphine may be found in the breast milk of lactating mothers who are "ultrarapid metabolizers" of codeine; patients with two or more copies of the variant CYP2D6*2 allele may have extensive conversion to morphine and thus increased opioid-mediated effects. In one case, excessively high serum concentrations of morphine were reported in a breast-fed infant following maternal use of acetaminophen with codeine. The mother was later found to be an "ultrarapid metabolizer" of codeine; symptoms in the infant included feeding difficulty and lethargy, followed by death. Caution should be used since most persons are not aware if they have the genotype resulting in "ultra-rapid metabolizer" status. When codeine is used in breast-feeding women, it is recommended to use the lowest dose for the shortest duration of time and observe the infant for increased sleepiness, difficulty in feeding or breathing, or limpness (FDA 2007; Koren 2006). The US labeling recommends that caution be used if administered to a nursing woman. Codeine Contin [Canadian product] is

contraindicated in nursing women. According to other guidelines, when treatment is needed for pain in nursing women, other agents should be used; if codeine cannot be avoided it should not be used for >4 days (Kahan 2011; Wong 2011).

Medication Guide Available Yes

Contraindications

Hypersensitivity to codeine or any component of the formulation; respiratory depression in the absence of resuscitative equipment; acute or severe bronchial asthma or hypercarbia; presence or suspicion of paralytic ileus; postoperative pain management in children who have undergone tonsillectomy and/or adenoidectomy

Canadian labeling: Additional contraindications (not in US labeling): Hypersensitivity to other opioid analgesics; cor pulmonale; acute alcoholism; delirium tremens; severe CNS depression; convulsive disorders; increased cerebrospinal or intracranial pressure; head injury; obstructive airway disease (in addition to asthma); known or suspected mechanical GI obstruction or any disease that affects bowel transit; suspected surgical abdomen (eg, acute appendicitis or pancreatitis); use with or within 14 days of MAO inhibitors; pregnancy and during labor and delivery; children <12 years of age; Additional product specific contraindications: Codeine Contin: acute pain; intermittent or short duration pain that can be managed with alternative pain medication; breast-feeding

Warnings/Precautions Note: Recommendations between US and Canadian labeling may vary (eg, use of codeine in certain patients/conditions may be contraindicated in the Canadian labeling only; refer to Contraindications).

[US Boxed Warning]: Respiratory depression and death have occurred in children who received codeine following tonsillectomy and/or adenoidectomy and were found to have evidence of being ultra-rapid metabolizers of codeine due to a CYP2D6 polymorphism. Deaths have also occurred in nursing infants after being exposed to high concentrations of morphine because the mothers were ultra-rapid metabolizers. Use is contraindicated in the postoperative pain management of children who have undergone tonsillectomy and/or adenoidectomy. The Canadian labeling contraindicates use in children <12 years of age. Use caution in patients with two or more copies of the variant CYP2D6*2 allele; may have extensive conversion to morphine and thus increased opioid-mediated effects. Avoid the use of codeine in these patients; consider alternative analgesics such as morphine or a nonopioid agent (Crews 2012). The occurrence of this phenotype is seen in 0.5% to 1% of Chinese and Japanese, 0.5% to 1% of Hispanics, 1% to 10% of Caucasians, 3% of African-Americans, and 16% to 28% of North Africans, Ethiopians, and Arabs.

May cause dose-related respiratory depression. The risk is increased in elderly patients, debilitated patients, and patients with conditions associated with hypoxia, hypercapnia, or upper airway obstruction. Use with caution in patients with preexisting respiratory compromise (hypoxia), COPD or other obstructive pulmonary disease, and kyphoscoliosis or other skeletal disorder which may alter respiratory function; critical respiratory depression may occur, even at therapeutic dosages.

After chronic maternal exposure to opioids, neonatal withdrawal syndrome may occur in the newborn; monitor neonate closely. Signs and symptoms include irritability, hyperactivity and abnormal sleep pattern, high pitched cry, tremor, vomiting, diarrhea and failure to gain weight. Onset, duration and severity depend on the drug used, duration of use, maternal dose, and rate of drug elimination by the newborn. Opioid withdrawal syndrome in the neonate, unlike in adults, may be life-threatening and should be treated according to protocols developed by neonatology experts.

Use may cause or aggravate constipation; chronic use may result in obstructive bowel disease, particularly in those with underlying intestinal motility disorders. Constipation may also be problematic in patients with unstable angina or those patients post-myocardial infarction. Avoid use in patients with gastrointestinal obstruction, particularly paralytic ileus. May cause hypotension; use with caution in patients with hypovolemia, cardiovascular disease (including acute MI), or drugs which may exaggerate hypotensive effects (including phenothiazines or general anesthetics). May cause CNS depression, which may impair physical or mental abilities; patients must be cautioned about performing tasks which require mental alertness (eg, operating machinery or driving).

Use with extreme caution in patients with head injury, intracranial lesions, or elevated intracranial pressure;

exaggerated elevation of ICP may occur. Use with caution in patients with hypersensitivity reactions to other phenanthrene-derivative opioid agonists (hydrocodone, hydromorphone, levorphanol, oxycodone, oxymorphone), adrenal insufficiency (including Addison's disease), biliary tract dysfunction, pancreatitis, thyroid dysfunction, morbid obesity, prostatic hyperplasia and/or urinary stricture, or severe hepatic or renal impairment. Use may obscure diagnosis or clinical course of patients with acute abdominal conditions. May induce or aggravate seizures; use with caution in patients with seizure disorders. Avoid use in patients with CNS depression or coma as these patients are susceptible to intracranial effects of CO_2 retention.

Use with caution in patients with a history of drug abuse or acute alcoholism; potential for drug dependency exists. Tolerance, psychological and physical dependence may occur with prolonged use. Potentially significant drug interactions may exist, requiring dose or frequency adjustment, additional monitoring, and/or selection of alternative therapy. Effects may be potentiated when used with other sedative drugs or ethanol. Concurrent use of agonist/antagonist analgesics may precipitate withdrawal symptoms and/or reduced analgesic efficacy in patients following prolonged therapy with mu opioid agonists. Abrupt discontinuation following prolonged use may also lead to withdrawal symptoms.

Some preparations contain sulfites which may cause allergic reactions. Healthcare provider should be alert to the potential for abuse, misuse, and diversion.

Adverse Reactions Frequency not defined.

Cardiovascular: Bradycardia, cardiac arrest, circulatory depression, flushing, hypertension, hypotension, palpitations, shock, syncope, tachycardia

Central nervous system: Abnormal dreams, agitation, anxiety, apprehension, ataxia, chills, depression, disorientation, dizziness, drowsiness, dysphoria, euphoria, fatigue, hallucination, headache, increased intracranial pressure, insomnia, nervousness, paresthesia, sedation, shakiness, taste disorder, vertigo

Dermatologic: Diaphoresis, pruritus, skin rash, urticaria

Gastrointestinal: Abdominal cramps, abdominal pain, anorexia, biliary tract spasm, constipation, diarrhea, nausea, pancreatitis, vomiting, xerostomia

Genitourinary: Urinary hesitancy, urinary retention

Hypersensitivity: Hypersensitivity reaction

Neuromuscular & skeletal: Laryngospasm, muscle rigidity, tremor, weakness

Ophthalmic: Blurred vision, diplopia, miosis, nystagmus, visual disturbance

Respiratory: Bronchospasm, dyspnea, respiratory arrest, respiratory depression

<1% (Limited to important or life-threatening): Hypogonadism (Brennan, 2013; Debono, 2011)

Drug Interactions

Metabolism/Transport Effects Substrate of CYP2D6 (major); **Note:** Assignment of Major/Minor substrate status based on clinically relevant drug interaction potential

Avoid Concomitant Use

Avoid concomitant use of Codeine with any of the following: Azelastine (Nasal); Eluxadoline; Mixed Agonist / Antagonist Opioids; Orphenadrine; Paraldehyde; Thalidomide

Increased Effect/Toxicity

Codeine may increase the levels/effects of: Alcohol (Ethyl); Alvimopan; Azelastine (Nasal); CNS Depressants; Desmopressin; Diuretics; Eluxadoline; Hydrocodone; Methotrimeprazine; Metyrosine; Mirtazapine; Orphenadrine; Paraldehyde; Pramipexole; Ramosetron; ROPINIRole; Rotigotine; Selective Serotonin Reuptake Inhibitors; Suvorexant; Thalidomide; Zolpidem

The levels/effects of Codeine may be increased by: Amphetamines; Anticholinergic Agents; Antipsychotic Agents (Phenothiazines); Brimonidine (Topical); Cannabis; Doxylamine; Dronabinol; Droperidol; HydrOXYzine; Kava Kava; Magnesium Sulfate; Methotrimeprazine; Minocycline; Nabilone; Perampanel; Rufinamide; Sodium Oxybate; Somatostatin Analogs; Succinylcholine; Tapentadol; Tetrahydrocannabinol

Decreased Effect

Codeine may decrease the levels/effects of: Pegvisomant

The levels/effects of Codeine may be decreased by: Ammonium Chloride; CYP2D6 Inhibitors (Moderate); CYP2D6 Inhibitors (Strong); Mixed Agonist / Antagonist Opioids; Naltrexone

Storage/Stability

Immediate release tablet, oral solution: Store at 15°C to 30°C (59°F to 86°F). Protect from moisture and light.

Controlled release tablet [Canadian product]: Store at 15°C to 30°C (59°F to 86°F).

Mechanism of Action Binds to opioid receptors in the CNS, causing inhibition of ascending pain pathways, altering the perception of and response to pain; causes cough suppression by direct central action in the medulla; produces generalized CNS depression

Pharmacodynamics/Kinetics

Onset of action: Oral: Immediate release: 0.5-1 hour

Peak effect: Oral: Immediate release: 1-1.5 hours

Duration: Immediate release: 4-6 hours

Absorption: Oral: Adequate

Distribution: ~3-6 L/kg

Protein binding: ~7% to 25%

Metabolism: Hepatic via UGT2B7 and UGT2B4 to codeine-6-glucuronide, via CYP2D6 to morphine (active), and via CYP3A4 to norcodeine. Morphine is further metabolized via glucuronidation to morphine-3-glucuronide and morphine-6-glucuronide (active).

Bioavailability: 53%

Half-life elimination: 2.5-3.5 hours

Time to peak, plasma: Immediate release: 1 hour; Controlled release [Canadian product]: 3.3 hours

Excretion: Urine (~90%, ~10% of the total dose as unchanged drug); feces

Dosing

Adult

Cough: Oral:

Canadian labeling:

Immediate release tablet: 15 mg to 30 mg every 6 to 8 hours as needed (maximum: 120 mg/day).

Oral solution: 5 mL (25 mg) every 6 to 8 hours as needed.

Alternative recommendation (off-label use in US): Reported doses vary; range: 7.5 to 120 mg/day as a single dose or in divided doses (Bolser 2006; Smith 2010); **Note:** The American College of Chest Physicians does not recommend the routine use of codeine as an antitussive in patients with upper respiratory infections (Bolser 2006).

Pain management (analgesic): Oral: **Note:** These are guidelines and do not represent the maximum doses that may be required in all patients. Doses should be titrated to pain relief/prevention.

Immediate release (tablet, oral solution): Initial: 15 to 60 mg every 4 hours as needed; maximum total daily dose: 360 mg/day; patients with prior opioid exposure may require higher initial doses. **Note:** The American Pain Society recommends an initial dose of 30 to 60 mg for adults with moderate pain (American Pain Society 2008).

Controlled release: Codeine Contin [Canadian product]: **Note:** Titrate at intervals of ≥48 hours until adequate analgesia has been achieved. Daily doses >600 mg/day should not be used; patients requiring higher doses should be switched to an opioid approved for use in severe pain. In patients who receive both Codeine Contin and an immediate release or combination product for breakthrough pain, the rescue dose of immediate release codeine product should be ≤12.5% of the total daily Codeine Contin dose.

Opioid-naive patients: Initial: 50 mg every 12 hours

Conversion from immediate release codeine preparations: Immediate release codeine preparations contain ~75% codeine base. Therefore, patients who are switching from immediate release codeine preparations may be transferred to a ~25% lower total daily dose of Codeine Contin, equally divided into 2 daily doses every 12 hours.

*Conversion from a combination codeine product (eg, codeine with acetaminophen **or** aspirin):* See table:

Number of 30 mg Codeine Combination Tablets Daily	Initial Dose of Codeine Contin	Maintenance Dose of Codeine Contin
≤6	50 mg every 12 h	100 mg every 12 h
7-9	100 mg every 12 h	150 mg every 12 h
10-12	150 mg every 12 h	200 mg every 12 h
>12	200 mg every 12 h	200-300 every 12 h (maximum: 300 mg every 12 h)

Conversion from another opioid analgesic: Using the patient's current opioid dose, calculate an equivalent daily dose of immediate release codeine. A ~25% lower dose of Codeine Contin should then be initiated, equally divided into 2 daily doses.

Discontinuation of therapy: **Note:** Gradual dose reduction is recommended if clinically appropriate. Initially reduce the total daily dose by 50% and administer equally divided into 2 daily doses for 2 days followed by a 25% reduction every 2 days thereafter.

Geriatric Refer to adult dosing. Use with caution and consider initiation at the low end of the dosing range; reduced initial dosages may be necessary.

Pediatric

Cough: Canadian labeling: Children ≥12 years and Adolescents: Oral: Refer to adult dosing.

Pain management (analgesic): Oral: **Note:** These are guidelines and do not represent the maximum doses that may be required in all patients. Doses should be titrated to pain relief/prevention.)

Canadian labeling: Children ≥12 years and Adolescents:

Immediate release (tablet, oral solution): Refer to adult dosing.

Controlled release: Use is not recommended (has not been studied)

Alternative recommendations (off-label use in US): Immediate release (tablet, oral solution): Initial: 0.5 to 1 mg/kg/dose every 4 hours as needed; maximum: 60 mg/dose (American Pain Society 2008)

Renal Impairment

US labeling: There are no specific dosage adjustments provided in the manufacturers labeling; however, clearance may be reduced; active metabolites may accumulate. Initiate at lower doses or longer dosing intervals followed by careful titration.

Canadian labeling:

Immediate release (tablet, oral solution):

CrCl >50 mL/minute: No dosage adjustment necessary.

CrCl 10 to 50 mL/minute: Administer 75% of dose and titrate carefully as needed.

CrCl <10 mL/minute: Administer 50% of dose and titrate carefully as needed.

Controlled release: There are no dosage adjustments provided in the manufacturer labeling; however, a reduced dosage is recommended

Alternate recommendations: The following guidelines have been used by some clinicians (Aronoff 2007):

CrCl 10 to 50 mL/minute: Administer 75% of dose

CrCl <10 mL/minute: Administer 50% of dose

Hepatic Impairment There are no dosage adjustments provided in the manufacturer's labeling (has not been studied); however, initial lower doses or longer dosing intervals followed by careful titration are recommended.

Administration May administer without regard to meals. Take with food or milk to decrease adverse GI effects.

Controlled release tablets: Codeine Contin [Canadian product]: Tablets should be swallowed whole; do not chew, dissolve, or crush. All strengths may be halved, **except** the 50 mg tablets; half tablets should also be swallowed intact.

Monitoring Parameters Pain relief, respiratory and mental status, blood pressure, heart rate; signs or symptoms of hypogonadism or hypoadrenalism (Brennan 2013)

Test Interactions Some quinolones may produce a false-positive urine screening result for opioids using commercially-available immunoassay kits. This has been demonstrated most consistently for levofloxacin and ofloxacin, but other quinolones have shown cross-reactivity in certain assay kits. Confirmation of positive opioid screens by more specific methods should be considered.

Dosage Forms Excipient information presented when available (limited, particularly for generics); consult specific product labeling. [DSC] = Discontinued product

Solution, Oral, as sulfate:

Generic: 30 mg/5 mL (500 mL [DSC])

Tablet, Oral, as sulfate:

Generic: 15 mg, 30 mg, 60 mg

Dosage Forms: Canada Excipient information presented when available (limited, particularly for generics); consult specific product labeling.

Solution, Oral, as phosphate: 25 mg/5 mL

Tablet, Controlled Release:

Codeine Contin: 50 mg, 100 mg, 150 mg, 200 mg

Controlled Substance C-II

Extemporaneous Preparations A 3 mg/mL oral suspension may be made with codeine phosphate powder, USP. Add 600 mg of powder to a 400 mL beaker. Add 2.5 mL of Sterile Water for Irrigation, USP, and stir to dissolve the powder. Mix for 10 minutes while adding Ora-Sweet to make 200 mL; transfer to a calibrated bottle. Stable 98 days at room temperature.

Dentinger PJ and Swenson CF, "Stability of Codeine Phosphate in an Extemporaneously Compounded Syrup," *Am J Health Syst Pharm*, 2007, 64(24):2569-73.

◆ Codeine and Acetaminophen see Acetaminophen and Codeine on page 28

◆ Codeine and Guaifenesin see Guaifenesin and Codeine on page 861

Colchicine (KOL chi seen)

Brand Names: US Colcrys; Mitigare

Brand Names: Canada Jamp-Colchicine; PMS-Colchicine

Pharmacologic Category Antigout Agent

Use

Familial Mediterranean fever (Colcrys only): Treatment of familial Mediterranean fever in adults and children 4 years and older.

Gout flares: Prophylaxis and the treatment of acute gout flares when taken at the first sign of a flare. **Note:** Mitigare is only approved for prophylaxis of gout flares.

Pregnancy Considerations Adverse events were observed in animal reproduction studies. Colchicine crosses the human placenta. Use during pregnancy in the treatment of familial Mediterranean fever has not shown an increase in miscarriage, stillbirth, or teratogenic effects (limited data).

Breast-Feeding Considerations Colchicine enters breast milk; exclusively breast-fed infants are expected to receive <10% of the weight-adjusted maternal dose (limited data). The manufacturer recommends that caution be used if administered to a nursing woman.

Medication Guide Available Yes

Contraindications Concomitant use of a P-glycoprotein (P-gp) or strong CYP3A4 inhibitor in presence of renal or hepatic impairment

Mitigare: Patients with both renal and hepatic impairment.

Canadian labeling: Additional contraindications (not in US labeling): Hypersensitivity to colchicine; serious gastrointestinal, hepatic, renal, and cardiac disease

Warnings/Precautions Hazardous agent - use appropriate precautions for handling and disposal (NIOSH 2014 [group 3]). Myelosuppression (eg, thrombocytopenia, leukopenia, granulocytopenia, pancytopenia) and aplastic anemia have been reported in patients receiving therapeutic doses. Neuromuscular toxicity (including rhabdomyolysis) has been reported in patients receiving therapeutic doses; patients with renal dysfunction and elderly patients are at increased risk. Concomitant use of cyclosporine, diltiazem, verapamil, fibrates, and statins may increase the risk of myopathy. Clearance is decreased in renal or hepatic impairment; monitor closely for adverse effects/toxicity. Dosage adjustments may be required depending on degree of impairment or indication, and may be affected by the use of concurrent medication (CYP3A4 or P-gp inhibitors). Concurrent use of P-gp or strong CYP3A4 inhibitors is contraindicated in renal impairment; fatal toxicity has been reported. Colchicine is not an analgesic and should not be used to treat pain from other causes. Potentially significant interactions may exist, requiring dose or frequency adjustment, additional monitoring, and/or selection of alternative therapy.

Adverse Reactions Frequency not always defined.

>10%: Gastrointestinal: Gastrointestinal disease (26% to 77%), diarrhea (23% to 77%), vomiting (17%), nausea (4% to 17%)

1% to 10%:

Central nervous system: Fatigue (1% to 4%), headache (1% to 2%)

Endocrine & metabolic: Gout (4%)

Gastrointestinal: Abdominal cramps, abdominal pain

Respiratory: Pharyngolaryngeal pain (2% to 3%)

<1% (Limited to important or life-threatening): Alopecia, bone marrow depression, dermatitis, disseminated intravascular coagulation, hepatotoxicity, hypersensitivity reaction, increased creatine phosphokinase, lactose intolerance, myalgia, myasthenia, oligospermia, purpura, rhabdomyolysis, toxic neuromuscular disease

Drug Interactions

Metabolism/Transport Effects Substrate of CYP3A4 (major), P-glycoprotein; **Note:** Assignment of Major/Minor substrate status based on clinically relevant drug interaction potential

Avoid Concomitant Use

Avoid concomitant use of Colchicine with any of the following: Antihepaciviral Combination Products; Conivaptan; Fusidic Acid (Systemic); Idelalisib

Increased Effect/Toxicity

Colchicine may increase the levels/effects of: HMG-CoA Reductase Inhibitors

The levels/effects of Colchicine may be increased by: Antihepaciviral Combination Products; Conivaptan; CYP3A4 Inhibitors (Moderate); CYP3A4 Inhibitors (Strong); Dasatinib; Digoxin; Fibric Acid Derivatives; Fosamprenavir; Fosaprepitant; Fusidic Acid (Systemic); Idelalisib; Luliconazole; Lumacaftor; Mifepristone; Osimertinib; Palbociclib; P-glycoprotein/ABCB1 Inhibitors; Stiripentol; Telaprevir; Tipranavir

Decreased Effect

Colchicine may decrease the levels/effects of: Choline C 11; Cyanocobalamin; Multivitamins/Fluoride (with ADE); Multivitamins/Minerals (with ADEK, Folate, Iron); Multivitamins/Minerals (with AE, No Iron)

The levels/effects of Colchicine may be decreased by: Lumacaftor; Osimertinib; P-glycoprotein/ABCB1 Inducers

Food Interactions Grapefruit juice may increase colchicine serum concentrations. Management: Administer orally with water and maintain adequate fluid intake. Dose adjustment may be required based on indication if ingesting grapefruit juice. Avoid grapefruit juice with hepatic or renal impairment.

Storage/Stability Store at 20°C to 25°C (68°F to 77°F). Protect from light and moisture.

Mechanism of Action Disrupts cytoskeletal functions by inhibiting β-tubulin polymerization into microtubules, preventing activation, degranulation, and migration of neutrophils associated with mediating some gout symptoms. In familial Mediterranean fever, may interfere with intracellular assembly of the inflammasome complex present in neutrophils and monocytes that mediate activation of interleukin-1β.

Pharmacodynamics/Kinetics

Onset of action: Oral: Pain relief: ~18 to 24 hours

Distribution: Concentrates in leukocytes, kidney, spleen, and liver; does not distribute in heart, skeletal muscle, and brain

V_d: 5 to 8 L/kg

Protein binding: ~39%

Metabolism: Hepatic via CYP3A4; 3 metabolites (2 primary, 1 minor)

Bioavailability: ~45%

Half-life elimination: 27 to 31 hours (multiple oral doses; young, healthy volunteers)

Time to peak, serum: Oral: 0.5 to 3 hours

Excretion: Urine (40% to 65% as unchanged drug); enterohepatic recirculation and biliary excretion also possible

Dosing

Adult

Familial Mediterranean fever (FMF): Oral: Colcrys: 1.2 to 2.4 mg daily in 1 to 2 divided doses. Titration: Increase or decrease dose in 0.3 mg daily increments based on efficacy or adverse effects

Gout: Oral:

US labeling:

Flare treatment (Colcrys): Initial: 1.2 mg at the first sign of flare, followed in 1 hour with a single dose of 0.6 mg (maximum: 1.8 mg within 1 hour). Patients receiving prophylaxis therapy may receive treatment dosing; wait 12 hours before resuming prophylaxis dose. **Note:** Current FDA-approved dose for gout flare is substantially lower than what has been historically used clinically. Doses larger than the currently recommended dosage for gout flare have not been proven to be more effective.

Prophylaxis (Colcrys and Mitigare): 0.6 mg once or twice daily; maximum: 1.2 mg daily. The duration of prophylaxis is 6 months or 3 months (patients without tophi) to 6 months (≥1 tophi) after achieving target serum uric acid levels (ACR guidelines [Khanna 2012]).

Canadian labeling:

Flare treatment: Initial: 1.2 mg at the first sign of flare, followed in 1 hour with a single dose of 0.6 mg (maximum: 1.8 mg within 1 hour). Do not repeat treatment for at least 3 days. Wait at least 12 hours to resume prophylactic dose.

Prophylaxis: 0.6 mg once or twice daily; maximum: 1.2 mg per 24 hours

Pericarditis, acute (off-label use): Note: The 0.5 mg tablets are not available in the US or Canada. However, the 0.6 mg tablets are used empirically in place of 0.5 mg tablets in countries where they are not available:

Patients >70 kg: 0.5 mg twice daily for 3 months (Imazio 2013)

Patients ≤70 kg or unable to tolerate higher dosing regimen: 0.5 mg once daily for 3 months (Imazio 2013)

Note: Loading doses of colchicine used in earlier studies may not be necessary in the treatment of acute pericarditis according to newer data; lower doses are proposed to improve patient compliance and reduce adverse effects (Adler 2015; Imazio 2010b; Imazio 2013).

Concomitant therapy: Use in combination with high-dose aspirin or ibuprofen for 7 to 14 days, followed by a gradual tapering of the dose over 3 to 4 weeks (ESC [Adler 2015]). In patients with contraindications to NSAIDS/aspirin, glucocorticoid therapy has been used (eg, prednisone for 2 weeks with gradual tapering) (Imazio 2013). Concurrent gastroduodenal prophylaxis with a proton pump inhibitor has been used and is recommended (ESC [Adler 2015]; Imazio 2005a; Imazio 2013)

Pericarditis, recurrent (off-label use): Note: The 0.5 mg or 1 mg tablets are not available in the US or Canada. However, the 0.6 mg tablets are used empirically in place of 0.5 mg tablets in countries where they are not available:

Regimens with loading dose:

Patients ≥70 kg: 0.5 to 1 mg every 12 hours on day 1, followed by 0.25 to 0.5 mg every 12 hours for 6 months (Imazio 2005b; Imazio 2011).

Patients <70 kg or unable to tolerate higher dosing regimen: 0.5 mg every 12 hours on day 1, followed by 0.5 mg once daily for 6 months (Imazio 2005b; Imazio 2011).

Regimens without loading dose:

Patients >70 kg: 0.5 mg twice daily for 6 months (Imazio 2014a).

Patients ≤70 kg or unable to tolerate higher dosing regimen: 0.5 mg once daily for 6 months (Imazio 2014a).

Note: Weight-based dosing without loading doses may improve compliance and reduce GI adverse effects according to expert opinion (ESC [Adler 2015]; Imazio 2010b; Imazio 2013). Recent data demonstrated comparable beneficial outcomes to studies that used loading doses (Imazio 2005b; Imazio 2011, Imazio 2014a).

Concomitant therapy: Use in combination with high-dose aspirin, ibuprofen, or indomethacin based on initial regimen used for the acute episode and type of pericarditis (eg, idiopathic, viral, autoimmune, or post-myocardial infarction). Coadministration with corticosteroids (prednisone) is reserved for refractory cases or patients with contraindications to NSAID therapy (ESC [Adler 2015]). Proton pump inhibitors have been administered during aspirin or NSAID therapy as gastroduodenal prophylaxis (Imazio 2005b; Imazio 2011; Imazio 2014a).

Postpericardiotomy syndrome (prevention) (off-label use): Note: Regimens without a loading dose may improve patient compliance and reduce side effects (Imazio 2014b). The 0.5 mg or 1 mg tablets are not available in the US or Canada. However, the 0.6 mg tablets are used empirically in place of 0.5 mg tablets in countries where they are not available:

Regimens with loading dose:

Patients ≥70 kg: 1 mg twice daily given on post-operative day 3, followed by 0.5 mg twice daily for 1 month (Imazio 2010a).

Patients <70 kg or unable to tolerate higher dosing regimen: 0.5 mg twice daily given on post-operative day 3, followed by 0.5 mg once daily for 1 month (Imazio 2010a).

Regimens without loading dose:

Patients ≥70 kg: 0.5 mg twice daily initiated 48 to 72 hours prior to surgery and continued for 1 month (Imazio 2014b).

Patients <70 kg: 0.5 mg once daily initiated 48 to 72 hours prior to surgery and continued for 1 month (Imazio 2014b).

Dosage adjustment for concomitant therapy with CYP3A4 or P-glycoprotein (P-gp) inhibitors: Note: Colcrys labeling recommends dosage adjustments in patients receiving CYP3A4 or P-gp inhibitors up to 14 days prior to initiation of colchicine. Treatment of gout flare with colchicine is not recommended in patients receiving prophylactic colchicine and CYP3A4 inhibitors.

Coadministration of **strong** CYP3A4 inhibitor (eg, atazanavir, clarithromycin, darunavir/ritonavir, indinavir, itraconazole, ketoconazole, lopinavir/ritonavir, nefazodone, nelfinavir, ritonavir, saquinavir, telithromycin, tipranavir/ritonavir):

FMF: Maximum dose: 0.6 mg daily (0.3 mg twice daily)

Gout prophylaxis:

US labeling:

Colcrys:

If original dose is 0.6 mg twice daily, adjust dose to 0.3 mg once daily

If original dose is 0.6 mg once daily, adjust dose to 0.3 mg every other day

Mitigare: Avoid concomitant use; if coadministration is necessary, reduce daily dosage or dose frequency and monitor closely.

Canadian labeling:

If original dose is 0.6 mg twice daily, adjust dose to 0.3 mg once daily

If original dose is 0.6 mg once daily, adjust dose to 0.3 mg every other day

Gout flare treatment:

US labeling: Initial: 0.6 mg, followed in 1 hour by a single dose of 0.3 mg; do not repeat for at least 3 days

Canadian labeling: Initial: 0.6 mg, followed in 1 hour by a single dose of 0.3 mg; do not repeat for at least 3 days

Coadministration of **moderate** CYP3A4 inhibitor (eg, aprepitant, diltiazem, erythromycin, fluconazole, fosamprenavir, grapefruit juice, verapamil):

FMF: Maximum dose: 1.2 mg daily (0.6 mg twice daily)

Gout prophylaxis:

US labeling:

Colcrys:

If original dose is 0.6 mg twice daily, adjust dose to 0.3 mg twice daily **or** 0.6 mg once daily

If original dose is 0.6 mg once daily, adjust dose to 0.3 mg once daily

Mitigare: Avoid concomitant use; if coadministration is necessary, reduce daily dosage or dose frequency and monitor closely.

Canadian labeling:

If original dose is 0.6 mg twice daily, adjust dose to 0.3 mg twice daily **or** 0.6 mg once daily

If original dose is 0.6 mg once daily, adjust dose to 0.3 mg once daily

Gout flare treatment: 1.2 mg as a single dose; do not repeat for at least 3 days

Coadministration of P-gp inhibitor (eg, cyclosporine, ranolazine):

FMF: Maximum dose: 0.6 mg daily (0.3 mg twice daily)

Gout prophylaxis:

US labeling:

Colcrys:

If original dose is 0.6 mg twice daily, adjust dose to 0.3 mg once daily

If original dose is 0.6 mg once daily, adjust dose to 0.3 mg every other day

Mitigare: Avoid concomitant use; if coadministration is necessary, reduce daily dosage or dose frequency and monitor closely.

Canadian labeling:

If original dose is 0.6 mg twice daily, adjust dose to 0.3 mg once daily

If original dose is 0.6 mg once daily, adjust dose to 0.3 mg every other day

Gout flare treatment: Initial: 0.6 mg as a single dose; do not repeat for at least 3 days

Geriatric Use caution; reduce prophylactic daily dose by 50% in individuals >70 years (Terkeltaub 2009)

Pediatric
Familial Mediterranean fever (FMF): Oral:
US labeling: Colcrys only:
Children 4 to 6 years: 0.3 to 1.8 mg daily in 1 to 2 divided doses
Children 6 to 12 years: 0.9 to 1.8 mg daily in 1 to 2 divided doses
Adolescents >12 years: Refer to adult dosing.
Canadian labeling: Children >12 years and Adolescents: Refer to adult dosing.
Gout prophylaxis/treatment: Oral: Adolescents >16 years: Refer to adult dosing.
Renal Impairment Concurrent use of colchicine and P-gp or strong CYP3A4 inhibitors is **contraindicated** in renal impairment. Fatal toxicity has been reported. Use of colchicine to treat gout flares is not recommended in patients with renal impairment receiving prophylactic colchicine.
FMF:
CrCl 30 to 80 mL/minute: Monitor closely for adverse effects; dose reduction may be necessary.
CrCl <30 mL/minute: Initial dose: 0.3 mg daily; use caution if dose titrated; monitor for adverse effects.
Dialysis: 0.3 mg as a single dose; use caution if dose titrated; dosing can be increased with close monitoring; monitor for adverse effects. Not removed by dialysis.
Gout prophylaxis:
CrCl 30 to 80 mL/minute:
Colcrys: Dosage adjustment not required; monitor closely for adverse effects.
Mitigare: There are no dosage adjustments provided in the manufacturer's labeling (has not been studied).
CrCl <30 mL/minute:
Colcrys: Initial dose: 0.3 mg daily; use caution if dose titrated; monitor for adverse effects.
Mitigare: There is no specific dosage adjustment provided in the manufacturer's labeling; dosage reduction or alternative therapy should be considered
Dialysis:
Colcrys: 0.3 mg twice weekly; monitor closely for adverse effects.
Mitigare: There are no dosage adjustments provided in the manufacturer's labeling; monitor closely.
Gout flare treatment: Colcrys: **Note:** Treatment of gout flares is not recommended in patients with renal impairment who are receiving colchicine for prophylaxis.
CrCl 30 to 80 mL/minute: Dosage adjustment not required; monitor closely for adverse effects.
CrCl <30 mL/minute: Dosage reduction not required but may be considered; treatment course should not be repeated more frequently than every 14 days.
Dialysis: 0.6 mg as a single dose; treatment course should not be repeated more frequently than every 14 days. Not removed by dialysis.

Hemodialysis: Not dialyzable (0% to 5%); avoid chronic use of colchicine.
Hepatic Impairment Concurrent use of colchicine and P-glycoprotein or strong CYP3A4 inhibitors is **contraindicated** in hepatic impairment. Fatal toxicity has been reported. Treatment of gout flare with colchicine is not recommended in patients with hepatic impairment receiving prophylactic colchicine.
FMF:
Mild to moderate impairment: Use caution; monitor closely for adverse effects.
Severe impairment: There is no specific dosage adjustment provided in the manufacturer's labeling; dosage adjustment should be considered.
Gout prophylaxis:
Mild to moderate impairment:
Colcrys: Dosage adjustment not required; monitor closely for adverse effects.
Mitigare: There are no dosage adjustments provided in the manufacturer's labeling (has not been studied).
Severe impairment: Colcrys and Mitigare: There is no specific dosage adjustment provided in the manufacturer's labeling; dosage adjustment should be considered.
Gout flare treatment: **Note:** Treatment of gout flares is not recommended in patients with hepatic impairment who are receiving colchicine for prophylaxis.
Mild to moderate impairment: Dosage adjustment not required; monitor closely for adverse effects.
Severe impairment: Dosage reduction not required but may be considered; treatment course should not be repeated more frequently than every 14 days.

Dietary Considerations May be taken without regard to meals. May need to supplement with vitamin B_{12}. Avoid grapefruit juice.

Administration Administer orally with water and maintain adequate fluid intake. May be administered without regard to meals.

Hazardous agent; use appropriate precautions for handling and disposal (NIOSH 2014 [group 3]).
Monitoring Parameters CBC, renal and hepatic function tests
Test Interactions May cause false-positive results in urine tests for erythrocytes or hemoglobin
Additional Information Oral colchicine had been available as an unapproved medication without FDA-approved prescribing information. In August 2009, the FDA approved prescribing information for a brand name colchicine product. The currently approved prescribing information recommends a lower than historically used dosage for the treatment of acute gout. This recommendation is based on data from the AGREE trial. In this trial, low-dose colchicine (1.8 mg total) had similar efficacy to high dose colchicine (4.8 mg total). Additionally, the low dosage regimen was associated with a lower incidence (26% vs 77%) of GI adverse events. Parenteral formulation of colchicine is no longer available in the US; serious life-threatening complications (eg, neutropenia, acute renal failure, thrombocytopenia, heart failure) associated with intravenous colchicine have occurred prior to market withdrawal. The risks associated with oral colchicine are believed to be lower compared to intravenous use.
Dosage Forms Excipient information presented when available (limited, particularly for generics); consult specific product labeling. [DSC] = Discontinued product
Capsule, Oral:
Mitigare: 0.6 mg [contains brilliant blue fcf (fd&c blue #1), fd&c yellow #10 (quinoline yellow)]
Generic: 0.6 mg
Tablet, Oral:
Colcrys: 0.6 mg [DSC] [contains fd&c blue #2 (indigotine), fd&c red #40]
Colcrys: 0.6 mg [scored; contains fd&c blue #2 (indigotine), fd&c red #40]
Generic: 0.6 mg

Colchicine and Probenecid
(KOL chi seen & proe BEN e sid)

Index Terms ColBenemid; Probenecid and Colchicine
Pharmacologic Category Anti-inflammatory Agent; Antigout Agent; Uricosuric Agent
Use Treatment of chronic gouty arthritis when complicated by frequent, recurrent acute attacks of gout
Dosing
Adult & Geriatric Gout: Oral: One tablet/day for 1 week, then 1 tablet twice daily thereafter
Note: Current prescribing information states a maximum dose of 4 tablets per day; however this exceeds the usual maximum dose of colchicine for gout prophylaxis (1.2 mg per day).
Renal Impairment CrCl <30 mL/minute: Probenecid may not be effective in patients with chronic renal insufficiency.
Hepatic Impairment No dosage adjustment provided in manufacturer's labeling; use with caution.
Additional Information Complete prescribing information should be consulted for additional detail.
Dosage Forms Excipient information presented when available (limited, particularly for generics); consult specific product labeling.
Tablet: Colchicine 0.5 mg and probenecid 0.5 g

◆ **Colcrys** see Colchicine on page 440

Colesevelam (koh le SEV a lam)

Brand Names: US Welchol
Brand Names: Canada Lodalis
Pharmacologic Category Antilipemic Agent, Bile Acid Sequestrant
Use
Diabetes mellitus, type 2: Improve glycemic control in adults with type 2 diabetes mellitus (noninsulin dependent, NIDDM) in conjunction with diet and exercise
Heterozygous familial hypercholesterolemia: Management of heterozygous familial hypercholesterolemia (heFH) in adolescent patients (males and postmenarcheal females 10-17 years of age) used alone or in combination with a 3-hydroxy-3-methylglutaryl coenzyme A (HMG-CoA) reductase inhibitor when after an adequate trial of dietary therapy patient continues to have low-density lipoprotein-cholesterol (LDL-C) ≥190 mg/dL or LDL-C ≥160 mg/dL with positive family history of premature cardiovascular disease (CVD) or with two or more CVD risk factors.

Hyperlipidemia:
U.S. labeling: Management of elevated LDL-C in adults with primary hyperlipidemia (Fredrickson type IIa) when used alone or in combination with an HMG-CoA reductase inhibitor in conjunction with diet and exercise
Canadian labeling (Lodalis): Adjunct to diet and lifestyle modifications in the management of primary hypercholesterolemia (Fredrickson type IIa) as monotherapy or in combination with an HMG-CoA reductase inhibitor

Limitations of use: Should not be used for the treatment of type 1 diabetes or diabetic ketoacidosis. Colesevelam has not been studied in Fredrickson Type I, III, IV, and V dyslipidemias; type 2 diabetes in combination with a dipeptidyl peptidase 4 inhibitor; pediatric patients with type 2 diabetes; children <10 years of age or in premenarchal girls. No effect on cardiovascular morbidity and mortality has been established. There is no evidence of macrovascular disease risk reduction with colesevelam use.

Dosing
Adult & Geriatric *U.S. labeling:* **Hyperlipidemia, type 2 diabetes mellitus:** Oral:
Once-daily dosing: 3.75 g (oral suspension or 6 tablets)
Twice-daily dosing: 1.875 g (3 tablets)
Canadian labeling: **Hyperlipidemia:** Oral:
Combination therapy: 2.5 to 3.75 g (4 to 6 tablets) daily; maximum dose: 3.75 g (6 tablets) given once daily or 1.875 g (3 tablets) given twice daily
Monotherapy: Initial: 1.875 g (3 tablets) twice daily or 3.75 g (6 tablets) once daily; maximum dose: 4.375 g (7 tablets) daily

Pediatric Heterozygous familial hypercholesterolemia: Children 10 to 17 years (males and postmenarchal females): Oral: 3.75 g once daily (oral suspension). **Note:** Due to large tablet size, oral suspension is recommended in pediatric patients.

Renal Impairment No dosage adjustments necessary; not absorbed from the gastrointestinal tract.

Hepatic Impairment No dosage adjustments necessary; not absorbed from the gastrointestinal tract.

Additional Information Complete prescribing information should be consulted for additional detail.

Dosage Forms Considerations Welchol contains phenylalanine 27 mg per 3.75 gram packet

Dosage Forms Excipient information presented when available (limited, particularly for generics); consult specific product labeling.
Packet, Oral, as hydrochloride:
Welchol: 3.75 g (30 ea) [sugar free; contains aspartame]
Tablet, Oral, as hydrochloride:
Welchol: 625 mg

Dosage Forms: Canada Excipient information presented when available (limited, particularly for generics); consult specific product labeling.
Tablet, oral, as hydrochloride:
Lodalis: 625 mg

◆ Colestid see Colestipol on page 443
◆ Colestid Flavored see Colestipol on page 443

Colestipol (koe LES ti pole)

Brand Names: US Colestid; Colestid Flavored; Micronized Colestipol HCl
Brand Names: Canada Colestid
Index Terms Colestipol Hydrochloride
Pharmacologic Category Antilipemic Agent, Bile Acid Sequestrant
Use Primary hypercholesterolemia: Adjunctive therapy to diet in patients with primary hypercholesterolemia
Dosing
Adult & Geriatric Primary hypercholesterolemia: Oral:
Granules: Initial: 5 g once or twice daily; increase by 5 g per day at 1- to 2-month intervals. In patients with preexisting constipation, initiate at 5 g once daily for 5 to 7 days, then increase to 5 g twice daily. Maintenance: 5 to 30 g per day, once daily or in divided doses.
Tablets: Initial: 2 g once or twice daily; increase by 2 g once or twice daily at 1- to 2-month intervals. Maintenance: 2 to 16 g per day, once daily or in divided doses.

Renal Impairment There are no dosage adjustments provided in the manufacturer's labeling; however, dosage adjustment is unlikely because not absorbed from the gastrointestinal tract.

Hepatic Impairment There are no dosage adjustments provided in the manufacturer's labeling; however, dosage adjustment is unlikely because not absorbed from the gastrointestinal tract.

Additional Information Complete prescribing information should be consulted for additional detail.

Dosage Forms Considerations Colestid tablets contain micronized colestipol. Generic tablets are available in micronized and non-micronized formulations.

Dosage Forms Excipient information presented when available (limited, particularly for generics); consult specific product labeling.
Granules, Oral, as hydrochloride:
Colestid: 5 g (300 g, 500 g) [unflavored flavor]
Colestid Flavored: 5 g (450 g) [contains aspartame; orange flavor]
Generic: 5 g (500 g)
Packet, Oral, as hydrochloride:
Colestid: 5 g (30 ea, 90 ea) [unflavored flavor]
Colestid Flavored: 5 g (60 ea) [contains aspartame; orange flavor]
Generic: 5 g (30 ea, 90 ea)
Tablet, Oral, as hydrochloride:
Colestid: 1 g
Micronized Colestipol HCl: 1 g
Generic: 1 g

◆ Colestipol Hydrochloride see Colestipol on page 443
◆ Colidrops [DSC] see Hyoscyamine on page 899

Colistimethate (koe lis ti METH ate)

Brand Names: US Coly-Mycin M
Brand Names: Canada Coly-Mycin M
Index Terms Colistimethate Sodium; Colistin Methanesulfonate; Colistin Methanesulphonate; Colistin Sulfomethate; Pentasodium Colistin Methanesulfonate; Polymyxin E
Pharmacologic Category Antibiotic, Miscellaneous
Use Treatment of acute or chronic infections due to sensitive strains of certain gram-negative bacilli (particularly *Pseudomonas aeruginosa*) which are resistant to other antibacterials or in patients allergic to other antibacterials

Pregnancy Considerations Adverse events have been observed in animal reproduction studies. Colistimethate crosses the placenta in humans.

Breast-Feeding Considerations Colistin (the active form of colistimethate sodium) and colistin sulphate (another form of colistin) are excreted in human milk. The manufacturer recommends caution if giving colistimethate sodium to a breast-feeding woman. Nondose-related effects could include modification of bowel flora.

Contraindications Hypersensitivity to colistimethate, colistin, or any component of the formulation

Warnings/Precautions Use only to prevent or treat infections strongly suspected or proven to be caused by susceptible bacteria to minimize development of bacterial drug resistance. Nephrotoxicity has been reported; use with caution in patients with preexisting renal disease; dosage adjustments may be required. Withhold treatment if signs of renal impairment occur during treatment. Respiratory arrest has been reported with use; impaired renal function may increase the risk for neuromuscular blockade and apnea. Transient, reversible neurological disturbances (eg, dizziness, numbness, paresthesia, generalized pruritus, slurred speech, tingling, vertigo) may occur. Patients must be cautioned about performing tasks which require mental alertness (eg, operating machinery or driving). Dose reduction may reduce neurologic symptoms; monitor closely. Use of inhaled colistimethate cause bronchoconstriction. Use with caution in patients with hyperactive airways; consider administration of a bronchodilator 15 minutes prior to administration. Colistimethate solutions change to bioactive colistin, a component of which may result in severe pulmonary toxicity. Solutions for inhalation must be mixed immediately prior to administration and used within 24 hours.

Prolonged use may result in fungal or bacterial superinfection, including *C. difficile*-associated diarrhea (CDAD) and pseudomembranous colitis; CDAD has been observed >2 months postantibiotic treatment.

Potentially significant drug-drug interactions may exist, requiring dose or frequency adjustment, additional monitoring, and/or selection of alternative therapy. Use caution when prescribing or dispensing; potential for dosing errors due to lack of standardization in literature when referring to product and dose; colistimethate (inactive prodrug) and colistin base strengths are not interchangeable; verify prescribed dose is expressed in terms of colistin base activity prior to dispensing.

Adverse Reactions Frequency not always defined.
Central nervous system: Neurotoxicity (7%; higher incidence with high-dose IV use in cystic fibrosis [Boss 1991; Koch-Weser 1970]), dizziness, headache, oral paresthesia, peripheral paresthesia, slurred speech, vertigo
Dermatologic: Pruritus, skin rash, urticaria

Gastrointestinal: Gastric distress

Genitourinary: Decreased urine output, nephrotoxicity (18% to 26% [Dalfino 2012; Oliveira 2009]), proteinuria

Neuromuscular & skeletal: Lower extremity weakness

Renal: Acute renal failure (33% to 60% [Akajagbor 2013; Deryke 2010]), increased blood urea nitrogen, increased serum creatinine

Respiratory: Apnea, respiratory distress

Miscellaneous: Fever

<1% (Limited to important or life-threatening): Pulmonary toxicity (acute respiratory tract failure following inhalation, bronchoconstriction, bronchospasm, chest tightness, respiratory distress)

Drug Interactions

Metabolism/Transport Effects None known.

Avoid Concomitant Use

Avoid concomitant use of Colistimethate with any of the following: Bacitracin (Systemic); BCG (Intravesical); Mecamylamine

Increased Effect/Toxicity

Colistimethate may increase the levels/effects of: Bacitracin (Systemic); Mecamylamine; Neuromuscular-Blocking Agents

The levels/effects of Colistimethate may be increased by: Aminoglycosides; Amphotericin B; Capreomycin; Cefazedone; Polymyxin B; Vancomycin

Decreased Effect

Colistimethate may decrease the levels/effects of: BCG (Intravesical); BCG Vaccine (Immunization); Sodium Picosulfate; Typhoid Vaccine

Preparation for Administration

IV or IM use: Reconstitute each vial containing 150 mg of colistin base activity with 2 mL of SWFI resulting in a concentration of 75 mg colistin base activity/mL; swirl gently to avoid frothing. May further dilute in D$_5$W or NS for IV infusion.

Intrathecal/intraventricular use (off-label route): Reconstitute with preservative-free diluent (SWFI or NS) only; use promptly after preparation; discard unused portion of vial (Quinn 2005).

Nebulized inhalation (off-label route): Reconstitute vial containing 150 mg of colistin base activity with 2 mL SWFI, resulting in a concentration of 75 mg colistin base activity/mL; further dilute dose to a total volume of 3-4 mL in NS (Michalopoulos 2008); alternatively, further dilute 150 mg colistin base activity to a total volume of 10 mL in SWFI (concentration: 15 mg colistin base activity/mL) (Lu 2012). Storing for >24 hours may increase the risk for potential lung toxicity; preparation immediately prior to administration is recommended (FDA 2007; Le 2010, Wallace 2008).

Storage/Stability Store intact vials (prior to reconstitution) at 20°C to 25°C (68°F to 77°F); excursions permitted to 15°C to 30°C (59°F to 86°F). Reconstituted vials may be refrigerated at 2°C to 8°C (36°F to 46°F) or stored at 20°C to 25°C (68°F to 77°F) for up to 7 days. Solutions for infusion should be freshly prepared; do not use beyond 24 hours.

Mechanism of Action Colistimethate (or the sodium salt [colistimethate sodium]) is the inactive prodrug which is hydrolyzed to colistin, which acts as a cationic detergent and damages the bacterial cytoplasmic membrane causing leaking of intracellular substances and cell death

Pharmacodynamics/Kinetics

Absorption: Not absorbed from the GI tract, mucous membranes, or intact skin (Note: GI absorption has been observed in infants).

Distribution: Distributes widely, except for CNS, synovial, pleural, and pericardial fluids

Healthy volunteer: IV: Colistimethate: V$_d$: 8.92 L; Colistin: V$_d$: 12.4 L (Couet 2012)

Critically ill: IV: Colistimethate: V$_d$: 5.3 to 13.5 L; Colistin: V$_d$: 7.2 to 189 L (Couet 2012)

Cystic fibrosis: Adolescents and Adults: IV: Colistimethate: V$_{dss}$: 0.09 ± 0.03 L/kg (Reed 2001)

Protein binding: 50%

Metabolism: Colistimethate sodium (inactive prodrug) is hydrolyzed to colistin (active form). **Note:** Only ~30% of colistimethate sodium is converted to colistin (Couet 2011)

Half-life elimination: IM, IV: Colistimethate: 2 to 3 hours

Critically ill: Infants (including premature infants), Children, Adolescents, and Adults: IV: Colistimethate: 2.3 hours; Colistin: 14.4 hours (Plachouras 2009)

Cystic fibrosis: IV: Colistin: ~4 hours (Li 2003)

ESRD patients receiving CAPD: IV: Colistin: 13.2 hours (Koomanachai 2014)

Time to peak:

Healthy volunteers: IV: Colistin: 2 hours (range: 1 to 4 hours) (Couet 2011)

Critically ill: IV: Colistin: ~7 hours (Plachouras 2009)

Excretion: Primarily urine (as unchanged drug); most colistin recovered in the urine is from postexcretion hydrolysis of colistimethate sodium (Couet 2011).

Dosing

Adult & Geriatric Note: Dosage expressed in terms of **colistin base activity**. **Colistimethate sodium** 1 mg is equivalent to ~12,500 units of **colistimethate sodium**; **Colistimethate sodium** ~2.67 mg is equivalent to 1 mg of **colistin base activity** (Li 2006; Nation 2014).

Susceptible infections: IM, IV: 2.5 to 5 mg/kg/day in 2 to 4 divided doses; maximum: 5 mg/kg/day

Severe infections (due to multidrug-resistant organisms susceptible to colistin in the critically ill) (off-label dosing): IV: Loading dose: 270 mg followed by 135 mg twice daily (Dalfino 2012; Plachouras 2009). Additional trials may be necessary to further evaluate the use of this dosing in critically ill patients with this condition.

May also consider using the following calculations; however, although derived from critically ill patients, the use of this algorithm has not been prospectively evaluated in the critically ill (Garonzik 2011):

Loading dose of colistin base activity (mg) = Target average colistin steady-state plasma concentration (in mg/L) x 2 x weight (in kg). For patient weight, use the lower of ideal or actual body weight expressed in kg. In obese patients, application of these equations has not been evaluated.

Daily maintenance dose of colistin base activity (mg) = Target average colistin steady-state plasma concentration (in mg/L) x ([1.5 x CrCl] + 30). **See Dosing in Renal Impairment for frequency of administration based on CrCl.**

Note: Do not exceed a total daily dose of 300 mg (according to this algorithm). Unless it is appropriate to target a low colistin steady-state plasma concentration (C$_{ss,avg}$), the authors do not recommended the use of these calculations in patients with CrCl >70 mL/minute/1.73 m^2, in which case the loading dose or the daily maintenance dose may be substantially greater than 300 mg. Use caution with loading doses >300 mg. Target C$_{ss,avg}$ is typically 2.5 mg/L (range: 2 to 4 mg/L [Couet 2012]) and should be based on MIC, site, and severity of infection. CrCl is expresssed in mL/minute/1.73 m^2.

Bronchiectasis, pulmonary colonization/infection with susceptible organisms in patients with cystic fibrosis and noncystic fibrosis (off-label use/route): Inhalation: 30 to 150 mg in NS (3 to 4 mL total) via nebulizer 1 to 3 times daily (maximum dose: 150 mg 2 times daily) (Le 2010; Sabuda 2008; Steinfort 2007). **Note:** Lower doses have been used in noncystic fibrosis patients with bronchiectasis (Steinfort 2007); the most commonly used dose is 150 mg twice daily (Le 2010).

Meningitis (susceptible gram-negative organisms): Intrathecal/Intraventricular (off-label route): 10 mg/day (IDSA 2004); **Note:** Dosage in clinical reports has ranged from 1.6 to 20 mg/day in 1 or 2 divided doses (maximum single dose: 10 mg) (administered with concomitant systemic antimicrobial therapy) (Guardado 2008; Kasiakou 2005; Katragkou 2005)

Cystic fibrosis (off-label use): IV: 3 mg/kg/day in 3 divided doses (Young 2013)

Ventilator-associated pneumonia due to susceptible multidrug-resistant *Pseudomonas aeruginosa, Acinetobacter baumannii,* or *Klebsiella pneumoniae* (off-label use/route): Nebulization (via ventilator circuit): 150 mg every 8 hours delivered over 60 minutes for 14 days or until successful wean from mechanical ventilation (treatment duration range: 7 to 19 days) (Lu 2012). May consider using as an adjunct in patients receiving IV colistin; may improve clinical outcomes (Doshi 2013; Tumbarello 2013; Valachis 2015).

Pediatric Note: Dosage expressed in terms of **colistin base activity**. **Colistimethate sodium** 1 mg is equivalent to ~12,500 units of **colistimethate sodium**; **Colistimethate sodium** ~2.67 mg is equivalent to 1 mg of **colistin base activity** (Li 2006; Nation 2014).

Susceptible infections: IM, IV: 2.5 to 5 mg/kg/day in 2 to 4 divided doses; maximum: 5 mg/kg/day

Renal Impairment Note: Dosage expressed in terms of **colistin base activity**.

IM, IV: Adults:

Manufacturer's labeling:

CrCl ≥80 mL/minute: No dosage adjustment necessary; maximum: 5 mg/kg/day

CrCl 50 to 79 mL/minute: 2.5 to 3.8 mg/kg/day in 2 divided doses

CrCl 30 to 49 mL/minute: 2.5 mg/kg/day once daily or in 2 divided doses

CrCl 10 to 29 mL/minute: 1.5 mg/kg every 36 hours

Alternative recommendations:

Severe infections (due to multidrug-resistant organisms susceptible to colistin in the critically ill) (Dalfino 2012): **Note:** CrCl calculated using the Cockcroft-Gault equation. IV:

CrCl ≥50 mL/minute: Loading dose of 270 mg followed by 135 mg twice daily.

CrCl 20 to 50 mL/minute: Loading dose of 270 mg followed by 135 mg once daily.

CrCl <20 mL/minute: Loading dose of 270 mg followed by 135 mg every 48 hours.

May also consider using the following calculations; however, although derived from critically ill patients, the use of this algorithm has not been prospectively evaluated in the critically ill (Garonzik 2011):

Loading dose of colistin base activity (mg) = Target average colistin steady-state plasma concentration (in mg/L) x 2 x weight (in kg). For patient weight, use the lower of ideal or actual body weight expressed in kg. In obese patients, application of these equations has not been evaluated.

Daily maintenance dose of colistin base activity (mg) = Target average colistin steady-state plasma concentration (in mg/L) x ([1.5 x CrCl] + 30)

Note: Use caution with loading doses >300 mg. Do not exceed a total daily dose of 300 mg (according to this algorithm). Target $C_{ss,avg}$ is typically 2.5 mg/L but may range from 2 to 4 mg/L (Couet 2012). Calculate CrCl using the Jellife method mL/minute/1.73 m^2 or the Cockcroft-Gault method (normalized to BSA of 1.73 m^2).

CrCl >70 mL/minute/1.73 m^2: Administer calculated daily maintenance dose in 2 to 3 divided doses every 12 or 8 hours, respectively. **Note:** Unless it is appropriate to target a low colistin $C_{ss,avg}$, the authors do not recommended the use of these calculations in patients with CrCl >70 mL/minute/1.73 m^2.

CrCl 10 to 70 mL/minute/1.73 m^2: Administer calculated daily maintenance dose in 2 to 3 divided doses every 12 or 8 hours, respectively.

CrCl <10 mL/minute/1.73 m^2: Administer calculated daily maintenance dose in divided doses every 12 hours.

Intermittent hemodialysis (IHD) (administer after hemodialysis on dialysis days): IV: 1.5 mg/kg every 24 to 48 hours (Heintz 2009). **Note:** Dosing dependent on the assumption of 3 times/week, complete IHD sessions. Alternatively, may administer a daily dose of 30 mg for every 1 mg/L colistin $C_{ss,avg}$ target given in divided doses every 12 hours on nonhemodialysis days. For example, if the $C_{ss,avg}$ target is 2.5 mg/L, then administer 37.5 mg every 12 hours on nonhemodialysis days. On hemodialysis days (ideally performed at the end of the colistin dosage interval), administer a supplemental dose of 50% of the total daily dose if the supplemental dose is administered during the last half hour of the hemodialysis session **or** 30% of the total daily dose if the supplemental dose is administered after the hemodialysis session. These recommendations, although derived from critically ill patients, have not been prospectively evaluated in the critically ill (Garonzik 2011).

Continuous renal replacement therapy (CRRT) (Heintz 2009; Trotman 2005): Drug clearance is highly dependent on the method of renal replacement, filter type, and flow rate. Appropriate dosing requires close monitoring of pharmacologic response, signs of adverse reactions due to drug accumulation, as well as drug concentrations in relation to target trough (if appropriate). The following are general recommendations only (based on dialysate flow/ultrafiltration rates of 1 to 2 L/hour and minimal residual renal function) and should not supersede clinical judgment:

CVVH/CVVHD/CVVHDF: IV: 2.5 mg/kg every 24 to 48 hours (frequency dependent upon site or severity of infection or susceptibility of pathogen). Alternatively, in patients receiving CVVH or CVVHD, may administer a daily dose of 192 mg for every 1 mg/L colistin $C_{ss,avg}$ target given 2 to 3 equally divided doses every 12 or 8 hours, respectively (Garonzik 2011).

Note: A single case report has demonstrated that the use of 2.5 mg/kg every 48 hours with a dialysate flow rate of 1 L/hour may be inadequate and that dosing every 24 hours was well-tolerated. Based on pharmacokinetic analysis, the authors recommend dosing as frequent as every 12 hours in patients receiving CVVHDF (Li 2005).

Hepatic Impairment No dosage adjustment provided in manufacturer's labeling.

Obesity Doses should be based on ideal body weight in obese patients.

Adjustment for Toxicity

CNS toxicity: Dose reduction may reduce neurologic symptoms.

Nephrotoxicity: Withhold treatment if signs of renal impairment occur during treatment.

Administration

Parenteral: Administer by IM, direct IV injection over 3 to 5 minutes, intermittent infusion over 30 minutes (Beringer 2001; Conway, 1997), or by continuous IV infusion (according to the manufacturer). For continuous IV infusion, one-half of the total daily dose is administered by direct IV injection over 3 to 5 minutes followed 1 to 2 hours later by the remaining one-half of the total daily dose diluted in a compatible IV solution infused over 22 to 23 hours. The final concentration for continuous infusion administration should be based on the patient's fluid needs; infusion should be completed within 24 hours of preparation.

Inhalation (off-label route): Administer solution via nebulizer (vibrating plate nebulizer may be preferred [Lu 2012]) promptly following preparation to decrease possibility of high concentrations of colistin from forming which may lead to potentially life-threatening lung toxicity. Consider use of a bronchodilator (eg, albuterol) within 15 minutes prior to administration (Le 2010). If patient is on a ventilator, place medicine in a T-piece at the midinspiratory circuit of the ventilator. One study in adult patients with VAP administered colistimethate (150 mg colistin base activity/10 mL SWFI) using a vibrating plate nebulizer over 60 minutes (Lu 2012).

Note: A case report of fatal lung toxicity implicated *in vitro* colistin formation from an inhalation solution as a potential etiology, but data regarding the concentration, formulation and storage of the inhaled colistin administered to the patient were not reported (FDA 2007; McCoy 2007; Wallace 2008). An acceptable limit of *in vitro* colistin formation to prevent potential toxicity is unknown. Limited stability data are available regarding the storage of colistin solution for inhaled administration (Healan 2012; Wallace 2008). Storing for >24 hours may increase the risk for potential lung toxicity; preparation immediately prior to administration is recommended (FDA 2007; Le 2010, Wallace 2008).

Intrathecal/intraventricular (off-label route): Administer only preservative-free solutions via intrathecal/intraventricular routes. Administer promptly after preparation. Discard unused portion of vial.

Monitoring Parameters Serum creatinine, BUN; urine output; signs of neurotoxicity; signs of bronchospasm (inhalation [off-label route])

Dosage Forms Excipient information presented when available (limited, particularly for generics); consult specific product labeling.

Solution Reconstituted, Injection [strength expressed as base]:

Coly-Mycin M: 150 mg (1 ea)

Generic: 150 mg (1 ea)

Solution Reconstituted, Injection [strength expressed as base, preservative free]:

Generic: 150 mg (1 ea)

◆ Colistimethate Sodium *see* Colistimethate *on page 443*

◆ Colistin, Hydrocortisone, Neomycin, and Thonzonium *see* Neomycin, Colistin, Hydrocortisone, and Thonzonium *on page 1266*

◆ Colistin Methanesulfonate *see* Colistimethate *on page 443*

◆ Colistin Methanesulphonate *see* Colistimethate *on page 443*

◆ Colistin Sulfomethate *see* Colistimethate *on page 443*

Collagenase (Systemic) (KOL la je nase)

Brand Names: US Xiaflex

Brand Names: Canada Xiaflex

Index Terms Collagenase Clostridium Histolyticum

Pharmacologic Category Enzyme

Use

Dupuytren contracture: Treatment of adults with Dupuytren contracture with a palpable cord

Peyronie disease: Treatment of adult men with Peyronie disease with a palpable plaque and curvature deformity of at least 30 degrees at the start of therapy

Prescribing and Access Restrictions As a requirement of the Risk Evaluation and Mitigation Strategy (REMS) program, access to this medication is restricted. Because of the risks of corporal rupture or other serious penile

injury, collagenase (for the treatment of Peyronie disease) is available only through a restricted program under a REMS called the XIAFLEX REMS Program. Prescribers and healthcare sites must be certified with the program. Call 1-877-313-1235 or visit www.Xiaflexrems.com for more information.

Medication Guide Available Yes

Dosing

Adult & Geriatric

Dupuytren contracture: Intralesional: Inject 0.58 mg per cord affecting a metacarpophalangeal (MP) joint or a proximal interphalangeal (PIP) joint. If contracture persists, finger extension procedure should be performed 24 to 72 hours following injection to facilitate cord disruption. If MP or PIP contracture remains, may reinject cord with a single dose of 0.58 mg 4 weeks following initial injection; injections and finger extension procedures may be administered up to 3 times per cord separated by ~4 week intervals. **Note:** Up to 2 injections per hand may be used during a treatment; 2 palpable cords affecting 2 joints or 1 palpable cord affecting 2 joints in the same finger may be injected at 2 locations during a treatment. Other palpable cords with contractures of MP or PIP joints may be injected at other treatment visits ~4 weeks apart.

Peyronie disease: Intralesional: Males: Inject 0.58 mg into a Peyronie plaque; repeat injection 1 to 3 days later. A penile modeling procedure should be performed 1 to 3 days after the second injection. Administer a second treatment cycle (two 0.58 mg injections and a penile modeling procedure) in ~6 weeks if needed (maximum, 4 treatment cycles [a total of 8 injection procedures and 4 penile modeling procedures]); subsequent treatment cycles should not be administered if the curvature deformity is <15 degrees after a treatment cycle or health care provider determines further treatment is not indicated. The safety of more than 1 treatment course (ie, 4 treatment cycles) is not known. **Note:** If more than 1 plaque is present, inject into the plaque causing the curvature deformity.

Renal Impairment There are no dosage adjustments provided in the manufacturer's labeling. However, dosage adjustment unlikely due to low systemic absorption.

Hepatic Impairment There are no dosage adjustments provided in the manufacturer's labeling. However, dosage adjustment unlikely due to low systemic absorption.

Additional Information Complete prescribing information should be consulted for additional detail.

Dosage Forms Excipient information presented when available (limited, particularly for generics); consult specific product labeling.

Solution Reconstituted, Injection:
Xiaflex: 0.9 mg (1 ea)

Collagenase (Topical) (KOL la je nase)

Brand Names: US Santyl
Brand Names: Canada Santyl
Pharmacologic Category Enzyme, Topical Debridement
Use Dermal ulcers: Debriding chronic dermal ulcers and severely burned areas.

Dosing

Adult & Geriatric Dermal ulcers: Topical: Apply once daily (or more frequently if the dressing becomes soiled) until debridement of necrotic tissue is complete and granulation tissue is well established. If infection is present, apply an appropriate topical antibiotic prior to the application of collagenase. If the infection persists despite treatment, discontinue use of collagenase until remission of the infection.

Renal Impairment There are no dosage adjustments provided in the manufacturer's labeling; it is not known if collagenase is absorbed systemically following topical application.

Hepatic Impairment There are no dosage adjustments provided in the manufacturer's labeling; it is not known if collagenase is absorbed systemically following topical application.

Additional Information Complete prescribing information should be consulted for additional detail.

Dosage Forms Excipient information presented when available (limited, particularly for generics); consult specific product labeling.

Ointment, External:
Santyl: 250 units/g (30 g, 90 g)

Conivaptan (koe NYE vap tan)

Brand Names: US Vaprisol
Index Terms Conivaptan Hydrochloride; YM087
Pharmacologic Category Vasopressin Antagonist
Use Treatment of euvolemic and hypervolemic hyponatremia in hospitalized patients

Pregnancy Considerations Adverse events were observed in animal reproduction studies.

Breast-Feeding Considerations It is not known if conivaptan is excreted in breast milk. Due to the potential for serious adverse reactions in the nursing infant, the manufacturer recommends a decision should be made whether to discontinue nursing or to discontinue the drug, taking into account the importance of treatment to the mother.

Contraindications Hypersensitivity to conivaptan, corn or corn products, or any component of the formulation; use in hypovolemic hyponatremia; concurrent use with strong CYP3A4 inhibitors (eg, ketoconazole, itraconazole, ritonavir, indinavir, and clarithromycin); anuria

Warnings/Precautions Monitor closely for rate of serum sodium increase and neurological status; overly rapid serum sodium correction (>12 mEq/L/24 hours) can lead to seizures, permanent neurological damage, coma, or death. Discontinue use if rate of serum sodium increase is undesirable; may reinitiate infusion (at reduced dose) if hyponatremia persists in the absence of neurological symptoms typically associated with rapid sodium rise. Of note, raising serum sodium concentrations with conivaptan has not demonstrated symptomatic benefit. Discontinue if hypovolemia or hypotension occurs. Safety and efficacy in patients with hypervolemic hyponatremia associated with heart failure have not been established. Use in small numbers of hypervolemic, hyponatremic heart failure patients led to increased adverse events. In other heart failure studies, conivaptan did not show significant

improvements in outcomes over placebo. Coadministration with digoxin may increase digoxin concentrations; monitor digoxin concentrations. Use with caution in patients with hepatic impairment; dosage adjustment may be required. May cause injection-site reactions.

Adverse Reactions

>10%:
Cardiovascular: Orthostatic hypotension (6% to 14%)
Central nervous system: Fever (5% to 11%)
Endocrine & metabolic: Hypokalemia (10% to 22%)
Local: Injection site reactions including pain, erythema, phlebitis, swelling (63% to 73%)

1% to 10%:
Cardiovascular: Hypertension (6% to 8%), hypotension (5% to 8%), peripheral edema (3% to 8%), phlebitis (5%), atrial fibrillation (2% to 5%), ECG abnormality (≤5%)
Central nervous system: Headache (8% to 10%), insomnia (4% to 5%), confusion (≤5%), pain (2%)
Dermatologic: Pruritus (1% to 5%), erythema (3%)
Endocrine & metabolic: Hyponatremia (6% to 8%), hypomagnesemia (2% to 5%), hyper-/hypoglycemia (3%)
Gastrointestinal: Constipation (6% to 8%), vomiting (5% to 7%), diarrhea (≤7%), nausea (3% to 5%), dry mouth (4%), dehydration (2%), oral candidiasis (2%)
Genitourinary: Urinary tract infection (4% to 5%)
Hematologic: Anemia (5% to 6%)
Renal: Polyuria (5% to 6%), hematuria (2%)
Respiratory: Pneumonia (2% to 5%), pharyngolaryngeal pain (1% to 5%)
Miscellaneous: Thirst (3% to 6%)
<1%, postmarketing, and/or case reports (limited to important or life-threatening): Atrial arrhythmias, sepsis

Drug Interactions

Metabolism/Transport Effects Substrate of CYP3A4 (major); **Note:** Assignment of Major/Minor substrate status based on clinically relevant drug interaction potential; **Inhibits** CYP3A4 (moderate)

Avoid Concomitant Use

Avoid concomitant use of Conivaptan with any of the following: Antifungal Agents (Azole Derivatives, Systemic); Aprepitant; Bosutinib; Cobimetinib; CYP3A4 Inhibitors (Strong); CYP3A4 Substrates; Domperidone; Flibanserin; Fusidic Acid (Systemic); Ibrutinib; Idelalisib; Ivabradine; Lomitapide; Naloxegol; Olaparib; Pimozide; Simeprevir; Tolvaptan; Trabectedin; Ulipristal

Increased Effect/Toxicity

Conivaptan may increase the levels/effects of: Amifostine; Antipsychotic Agents (Second Generation [Atypical]); Apixaban; Aprepitant; Bosentan; Bosutinib; Budesonide (Topical); Cannabis; Cobimetinib; CYP3A4 Substrates; Digoxin; Dofetilide; Domperidone; Dronabinol; DULoxetine; Flibanserin; Hypotension-Associated Agents; Ibrutinib; Imatinib; Ivabradine; Levodopa; Lomitapide; Naloxegol; Olaparib; Pimecrolimus; Pimozide; Propafenone; Simeprevir; Tetrahydrocannabinol; Tolvaptan; Trabectedin; Ulipristal; Vilazodone; Vindesine; Zuclopenthixol

The levels/effects of Conivaptan may be increased by: Antifungal Agents (Azole Derivatives, Systemic); Barbiturates; Blood Pressure Lowering Agents; Brimonidine (Topical); CYP3A4 Inhibitors (Moderate); CYP3A4 Inhibitors (Strong); Diazoxide; Fusidic Acid (Systemic); Herbs (Hypotensive Properties); Idelalisib; Luliconazole; Molsidomine; Netupitant; Nicorandil; Obinutuzumab; Osimertinib; Pentoxifylline; Prostacyclin Analogues

Decreased Effect

Conivaptan may decrease the levels/effects of: Ifosfamide

The levels/effects of Conivaptan may be decreased by: Bosentan; CYP3A4 Inducers (Moderate); CYP3A4 Inducers (Strong); Deferasirox; Enzalutamide; Mitotane; Osimertinib; Siltuximab; St Johns Wort; Tocilizumab

Storage/Stability Store at 25°C (77°F); brief excursions permitted up to 40°C (104°F). Protect from light and freezing. Do not remove protective overwrap until ready for use.

Mechanism of Action Conivaptan is an arginine vasopressin (AVP) receptor antagonist with affinity for AVP receptor subtypes V_{1A} and V_2. The antidiuretic action of AVP is mediated through activation of the V_2 receptor, which functions to regulate water and electrolyte balance at the level of the collecting ducts in the kidney. Serum levels of AVP are commonly elevated in euvolemic or hypervolemic hyponatremia, which results in the dilution of serum sodium and the relative hyponatremic state. Antagonism of the V_2 receptor by conivaptan promotes the excretion of free water (without loss of serum electrolytes) resulting in net fluid loss, increased urine output, decreased urine osmolality, and subsequent restoration of normal serum sodium concentrations.

Pharmacodynamics/Kinetics

Protein binding: 99%
Metabolism: Hepatic via CYP3A4 to four minimally-active metabolites
Half-life elimination: ~5-8 hours
Excretion: Feces (83%); urine (12%, primarily as metabolites)

Dosing

Adult & Geriatric Euvolemic or hypervolemic hyponatremia: IV: 20 mg infused over 30 minutes as a loading dose, followed by a continuous infusion of 20 mg over 24 hours (0.83 mg/hour) for 2-4 days; may increase to a maximum dose of 40 mg over 24 hours (1.7 mg/hour) if serum sodium not rising sufficiently; total duration of therapy not to exceed 4 days. **Note:** If patient requires 40 mg/24 hours, may administer two consecutive 20 mg/100 mL premixed solutions over 24 hours (ie, 20 mg over 12 hours followed by 20 mg over 12 hours).

Renal Impairment

CrCl ≥30mL/minute: No dosage adjustment necessary.
CrCl <30 mL/minute: Use not recommended; clinical response reduced; contraindicated in anuria (no benefit expected).

Hepatic Impairment

Mild impairment: No dosage adjustment necessary.
Moderate impairment: 10 mg infused over 30 minutes as a loading dose, followed by a continuous infusion of 10 mg over 24 hours (0.42 mg/hour) for 2-4 days; may increase to a maximum dose of 20 mg over 24 hours (0.83 mg/hour) if serum sodium not rising sufficiently; total duration of therapy not to exceed 4 days.
Severe impairment: Use not recommended (not studied).

Usual Infusion Concentrations: Adult Note: Premixed solutions available.
IV infusion: 20 mg in 100 mL (concentration: 0.2 mg/mL) of D_5W

Administration For intravenous use only; infuse into large veins and change infusion site every 24 hours to minimize vascular irritation. Do not administer with any other product in the same intravenous line or container.

Monitoring Parameters Rate of serum sodium increase, blood pressure, volume status, urine output

Dosage Forms Excipient information presented when available (limited, particularly for generics); consult specific product labeling.
Solution, Intravenous, as hydrochloride:
Vaprisol: 20 mg (100 mL)

- Conventional Vincristine *see* VinCRIStine *on page 1897*
- ConZip *see* TraMADol *on page 1821*
- CO Olopatadine (Can) *see* Olopatadine (Ophthalmic) *on page 1323*
- CO Paroxetine (Can) *see* PARoxetine *on page 1399*
- Copaxone *see* Glatiramer Acetate *on page 840*
- Copegus *see* Ribavirin (Systemic) *on page 1574*
- Copolymer-1 *see* Glatiramer Acetate *on page 840*

Copper (KOP er)

Brand Names: US Coppermin [OTC]; Cu-5 [OTC]
Index Terms Cupric Chloride; Cupric Chloride Dihydrate
Pharmacologic Category Trace Element, Parenteral
Use Supplement to intravenous solutions given for total parenteral nutrition (TPN) to maintain copper serum levels and to prevent depletion of endogenous stores and subsequent deficiency symptoms
Dosing
Adult Supplementation: IV (incorporated into parenteral nutrition): 0.3-0.5 mg/day (ASPEN, 2002); 0.5-1.5 mg/day (manufacturer's product labeling)
High output intestinal fistula: Some clinicians may use twice the recommended daily allowance (ASPEN, 2002).
Geriatric Use caution. Start at the low end of dosing range.
Pediatric Supplementation: Infants and Children: IV (incorporated into parenteral nutrition): 20 mcg/kg/day
Renal Impairment Use caution; contains aluminum.
Hepatic Impairment Use caution; dosage reduction may be required.
Additional Information Complete prescribing information should be consulted for additional detail.
Dosage Forms Excipient information presented when available (limited, particularly for generics); consult specific product labeling.
Capsule, Oral [preservative free]:
Cu-5: 5 mg [dye free]
Solution, Intravenous:
Generic: 0.4 mg/mL (10 mL)
Tablet, Oral:
Coppermin: 5 mg [corn free, rye free, wheat free]

- Coppermin [OTC] *see* Copper *on page 448*
- Cordarone *see* Amiodarone *on page 94*
- Cordran *see* Flurandrenolide *on page 791*
- Coreg *see* Carvedilol *on page 323*
- Coreg CR *see* Carvedilol *on page 323*
- Corfen-DM [OTC] *see* Chlorpheniramine, Phenylephrine, and Dextromethorphan *on page 378*
- Corgard *see* Nadolol *on page 1245*
- Coricidin HBP Chest Congestion and Cough [OTC] *see* Guaifenesin and Dextromethorphan *on page 861*
- Coricidin HBP® Cold and Flu [OTC] *see* Chlorpheniramine and Acetaminophen *on page 376*
- Coricidin® HBP Cough & Cold [OTC] *see* Dextromethorphan and Chlorpheniramine *on page 534*
- Corifact *see* Factor XIII Concentrate (Human) *on page 739*
- Corlanor *see* Ivabradine *on page 1002*
- Corlopam *see* Fenoldopam *on page 749*
- Cormax [DSC] *see* Clobetasol *on page 412*
- Cormax Scalp Application *see* Clobetasol *on page 412*
- Correct [OTC] *see* Bisacodyl *on page 231*
- Cortaid Maximum Strength [OTC] *see* Hydrocortisone (Topical) *on page 886*
- CortAlo *see* Hydrocortisone (Topical) *on page 886*
- Cortamed (Can) *see* Hydrocortisone (Topical) *on page 886*
- Cortef *see* Hydrocortisone (Systemic) *on page 886*
- Cortenema *see* Hydrocortisone (Topical) *on page 886*
- Corticool [OTC] *see* Hydrocortisone (Topical) *on page 886*

Corticorelin (kor ti koe REL in)

Brand Names: US Acthrel
Index Terms Corticorelin Ovine Triflutate; Human Corticotrophin-Releasing Hormone, Analogue; Ovine Corticotrophin-Releasing Hormone (oCRH)
Pharmacologic Category Diagnostic Agent

Use Cushing syndrome, differential diagnosis: Used as a diagnostic aid to differentiate between pituitary and ectopic production of ACTH in patients with ACTH-dependent disease
Dosing
Adult
Cushing syndrome, differential diagnosis: IV: 1 mcg/kg

Interpretation of results: Note: Basal and peak responses differ depending on AM or PM administration; therefore, any repeat evaluations on the same patient are recommended to be done at the same time of day as the initial testing.
Increased plasma ACTH and cortisol concentrations following administration: Patients with Cushing disease will exhibit high basal plasma ACTH plus high basal plasma cortisol (20 to 40 mcg/dL). Corticorelin administration will result in increased plasma ACTH and cortisol concentrations. This response pattern indicates an impairment of the negative feedback of cortisol on the pituitary.
Little or no response of plasma ACTH and cortisol concentrations following administration: Patients with ectopic production of ACTH will exhibit high basal plasma ACTH (may be very high) plus high basal plasma cortisol (20 to 40 mcg/dL). Corticorelin administration will result in little or no response of plasma ACTH and cortisol concentrations. Clinicians should note that there have been rare instances of patients with ectopic sources of ACTH that have responded to the corticorelin test.
Pediatric Cushing syndrome, differential diagnosis: Children and Adolescents: Refer to adult dosing.
Renal Impairment There are no dosage adjustments provided in the manufacturer's labeling.
Hepatic Impairment There are no dosage adjustments provided in the manufacturer's labeling.
Additional Information Complete prescribing information should be consulted for additional detail.
Dosage Forms Excipient information presented when available (limited, particularly for generics); consult specific product labeling.
Solution Reconstituted, Intravenous, as trifluoroacetate:
Acthrel: 100 mcg (1 ea)

- Corticorelin Ovine Triflutate *see* Corticorelin *on page 448*
- Cortifoam *see* Hydrocortisone (Topical) *on page 886*
- Cortimyxin (Can) *see* Neomycin, Polymyxin B, and Hydrocortisone (Ophthalmic) *on page 1267*
- Cortimyxin (Can) *see* Neomycin, Polymyxin B, and Hydrocortisone (Otic) *on page 1267*
- Cortimyxin (Can) *see* Neomycin, Polymyxin B, and Hydrocortisone (Topical) *on page 1268*
- Cortisol *see* Hydrocortisone (Systemic) *on page 886*
- Cortisol *see* Hydrocortisone (Topical) *on page 886*

Cortisone (KOR ti sone)

Index Terms Compound E; Cortisone Acetate
Pharmacologic Category Corticosteroid, Systemic
Additional Appendix Information
Corticosteroids Systemic Equivalencies *on page 1950*
Use
Allergic states: Control of severe or incapacitating allergic conditions intractable to adequate trials of conventional treatment of atopic dermatitis, bronchial asthma, contact dermatitis, drug hypersensitivity reactions, seasonal or perennial allergic rhinitis, and serum sickness.
Dermatologic diseases: Bullous dermatitis herpetiformis, exfoliative dermatitis, mycosis fungoides, pemphigus, severe erythema multiforme (Stevens-Johnson syndrome), severe psoriasis, severe seborrheic dermatitis.
Endocrine disorders: Congenital adrenal hyperplasia, hypercalcemia associated with cancer, nonsuppurative thyroiditis, primary or secondary adrenocortical insufficiency (hydrocortisone or cortisone is the first choice; synthetic analogs may be used in conjunction with mineralocorticoids when applicable; in infancy, mineralocorticoid supplementation is of particular importance).
Gastrointestinal diseases: To tide the patient over a critical period of the disease in regional enteritis and ulcerative colitis.
Hematologic disorders: Acquired (autoimmune) hemolytic anemia, congenital (erythroid) hypoplastic anemia, erythroblastopenia (red blood cell [RBC] anemia), idiopathic thrombocytopenic purpura in adults, secondary thrombocytopenia in adults.

Neoplastic diseases: Palliative management of leukemias and lymphomas in adults; acute leukemia of childhood.

Ophthalmic diseases: Severe acute and chronic allergic and inflammatory processes involving the eye and its adnexa (eg, allergic conjunctivitis, allergic corneal marginal ulcers, anterior segment inflammation, chorioretinitis, diffuse posterior uveitis and choroiditis, keratitis, herpes zoster ophthalmicus, iritis and iridocyclitis, optic neuritis, sympathetic ophthalmia).

Renal diseases: To induce diuresis or remission of proteinuria in nephrotic syndrome, without uremia, of the idiopathic type or that is caused by lupus erythematosus.

Respiratory diseases: Aspiration pneumonitis, berylliosis, fulminating or disseminated pulmonary tuberculosis when used concurrently with appropriate antituberculosis chemotherapy, Loeffler syndrome not manageable by other means, symptomatic sarcoidosis.

Rheumatic disorders: Adjunctive therapy for short-term administration (to tide the patient over an acute episode or exacerbation) in acute and subacute bursitis; acute gouty arthritis; acute nonspecific tenosynovitis; ankylosing spondylitis; epicondylitis; posttraumatic osteoarthritis; psoriatic arthritis; rheumatoid arthritis (RA), including juvenile RA (select cases may require low-dose maintenance therapy); and synovitis of osteoarthritis. During an exacerbation or as maintenance therapy in select cases of acute rheumatic carditis, systemic dermatomyositis (polymyositis), and systemic lupus erythematosus.

Miscellaneous: Tuberculous meningitis with subarachnoid block or impending block when used concurrently with appropriate antituberculous chemotherapy; trichinosis with neurologic or myocardial involvement.

Dosing
Adult & Geriatric Note: Dosing depends on the condition being treated and the response of the patient. Temporary supplemental doses may be warranted during times of stress (ie, trauma, surgery, severe infection). Discontinuation of therapy requires gradual withdrawal by tapering the dose.

Anti-inflammatory/immunosuppressive/endocrine disorders: Oral: Initial: 25 to 300 mg/day; adjust dose to patient response.

Physiologic replacement: Oral: 25 to 35 mg/day

Pediatric Note: Dosing depends on the condition being treated and the response of the patient. Temporary supplemental doses may be warranted during times of stress (ie, trauma, surgery, severe infection). Discontinuation of therapy requires gradual withdrawal by tapering the dose.

Anti-inflammatory or immunosuppressive: Oral: 2.5 to 10 mg/kg/day **or** 20 to 300 mg/m²/day in divided doses every 6 to 8 hours

Physiologic replacement: Oral: 0.5 to 0.75 mg/kg/day **or** 20 to 25 mg/m²/day in divided doses every 8 hours

Renal Impairment There are no dosage adjustments provided in the manufacturer's labeling; use with caution.

Hepatic Impairment There are no dosage adjustments provided in the manufacturer's labeling; use with caution.

Additional Information Complete prescribing information should be consulted for additional detail.

Dosage Forms Excipient information presented when available (limited, particularly for generics); consult specific product labeling.

Tablet, Oral, as acetate:
  Generic: 25 mg

Cosyntropin (koe sin TROE pin)

Brand Names: US Cortrosyn
Brand Names: Canada Cortrosyn; Synacthen Depot
Index Terms Synacthen; Tetracosactide; Tetracosactrin
Pharmacologic Category Corticosteroid, Systemic; Diagnostic Agent
Use Diagnostic test to differentiate primary adrenal from secondary (pituitary) adrenocortical insufficiency

Synacthen Depot [Canadian product]: Additional indications: Treatment of various disease states (eg, collagen, dermatologic, endocrine, ocular, hemolytic). Consult manufacturer labeling for detailed list.

Dosing
Adult & Geriatric
Diagnostic use: Screening of adrenocortical insufficiency:
Cosyntropin **powder** for injection (IM, IV) **or** cosyntropin **solution** for injection (IV only [manufacturer labeling does not recommend IM administration of solution for injection]):
Conventional dose: 0.25 mg; **Note:** Doses in the range of 0.25-0.75 mg have been used in clinical studies; however, maximal response is seen with 0.25 mg dose. When greater cortisol stimulation is needed, an IV infusion may be used: 0.25 mg administered at 0.04 mg/hour over 6 hours
Low-dose protocol (off-label dose): 1 mcg (Abdu, 1999); **Note:** The use of the low-dose protocol has been advocated by some clinicians, particularly in mild or secondary adrenal insufficiency. The low-dose protocol is not recommended in critically-ill patients (Marik, 2008).

Synacthen Depot [Canadian product]: IM: 1 mg administered as a single dose or once daily for 3 or 4 days (depending on method of testing; refer to manufacturer labeling for detailed information). **Note:** For patients with severe adrenal insufficiency, some clinicians administer dexamethasone on days that Synacthen Depot is administered to provide steroid coverage.

Therapeutic use: Synacthen Depot [Canadian product]: IM (**Note:** Titrate to lowest effective dose at the longest effective dosing interval): Initial for acute treatment: 1 mg daily for 3 days; maintenance dose is individualized: 0.5-1 mg every 2-3 days or twice weekly or 2 mg once weekly or less frequently

Transferring from corticosteroids: Synacthen Depot [Canadian product]: IM: Initial: 1 mg daily; gradually reduce steroid by 25% of original dose on successive days. Upon withdrawal from steroid adjust Synacthen® Depot dose as needed.

Transferring from animal-derived ACTH: Synacthen Depot [Canadian product]: IM: Conversion varies depending on product previously used. Manufacturer suggests that patients previously receiving ACTH gel 40 units daily should receive Synacthen® Depot 0.5 mg every other day; adjust dose based on response, preferably by extending the dosing interval.

Pediatric
Diagnostic use: Screening of adrenocortical insufficiency:
Cosyntropin **powder** for injection (IM, IV) **or** cosyntropin **solution** for injection (IV only [manufacturer labeling does not recommend IM administration of solution for injection]):
Children ≤2 years: 0.125 mg
Children >2 years: Refer to adult dosing.
Synacthen Depot [Canadian product]: IM: Children >3 years: Refer to adult dosing.

Therapeutic use: Synacthen Depot [Canadian product]: IM: **Note:** Titrate to lowest effective dose at the longest effective dosing interval.
Children 3-6 years: Initial: 0.25-0.5 mg daily; maintenance: 0.25-0.5 mg every 2-8 days
Children 7-15 years: Initial: 0.25-1 mg daily; maintenance: 0.25-1 mg every 2-8 days
Children ≥16 years: Refer to adult dosing.

Transferring from corticosteroids: Synacthen Depot [Canadian product]: IM: Children >3 years: Refer to adult dosing.

Transferring from animal-derived ACTH: Synacthen Depot [Canadian product]: IM: Children >3 years: Refer to adult dosing.

Renal Impairment No dosage adjustment provided in manufacturer's labeling (has not been studied).

◀

Hepatic Impairment No dosage adjustment provided in manufacturer's labeling (has not been studied).

Additional Information Complete prescribing information should be consulted for additional detail.

Dosage Forms Excipient information presented when available (limited, particularly for generics); consult specific product labeling.

Solution, Intravenous:
Generic: 0.25 mg/mL (1 mL)
Solution Reconstituted, Injection:
Cortrosyn: 0.25 mg (1 ea)
Generic: 0.25 mg (1 ea)
Solution Reconstituted, Injection [preservative free]:
Generic: 0.25 mg (1 ea)

Dosage Forms: Canada Excipient information presented when available (limited, particularly for generics); consult specific product labeling.

Injection, suspension:
Synacthen Depot: 1 mg/mL (1 mL) [contains benzyl alcohol]

Crizotinib (kriz OH ti nib)

Brand Names: US Xalkori

Brand Names: Canada Xalkori

Index Terms C-Met/Hepatocyte Growth Factor Receptor Tyrosine Kinase Inhibitor PF-02341066; C-Met/HGFR Tyrosine Kinase Inhibitor PF-02341066; MET Tyrosine Kinase Inhibitor PF-02341066; PF-02341066

Pharmacologic Category Antineoplastic Agent, Anaplastic Lymphoma Kinase Inhibitor; Antineoplastic Agent, Tyrosine Kinase Inhibitor

Use Non-small cell lung cancer, metastatic: Treatment of patients with metastatic non-small cell lung cancer (NSCLC) whose tumors are anaplastic lymphoma kinase (ALK)-positive (as detected by an approved test)

Pregnancy Considerations Adverse events have been observed in animal reproduction studies. Based on the mechanism of action, crizotinib may cause fetal harm if administered during pregnancy. Women of childbearing potential should use adequate contraception during treatment and for at least 45 days after the last crizotinib dose; men of reproductive potential should use adequate contraception methods during and for at least 90 days after treatment. The Canadian labeling recommends adequate contraception during treatment and for at least 90 days after the last dose for both males and females.

Breast-Feeding Considerations It is not known if crizotinib is excreted in breast milk. Due to the potential for serious adverse reactions in the nursing infant, the manufacturer recommends against breast-feeding during treatment and for 45 days after the final dose.

Prescribing and Access Restrictions Available through specialty pharmacies. Further information may be obtained from the manufacturer, Pfizer, at 1-877-744-5675, or at http://www.pfizerpro.com

Contraindications

U.S. labeling: There are no contraindications listed in the manufacturer's labeling.

Canadian labeling: Hypersensitivity to crizotinib or any component of the formulation; congenital long QT syndrome or with persistent Fridericia-corrected QT interval (QTcF) ≥500 msec

Warnings/Precautions Hazardous agent - use appropriate precautions for handling and disposal (NIOSH 2014 [group 1]). Approved for use only in patients with metastatic non-small cell lung cancer (NSCLC) who test positive for the abnormal anaplastic lymphoma kinase (ALK) gene. The Vysis ALK break-apart FISH probe kit is approved to test for the gene abnormality.

Fatalities due to crizotinib-induced hepatotoxicity have occurred. Grade 3 or 4 ALT increases (usually asymptomatic and reversible) have been observed in clinical trials. May require dosage interruption and/or reduction; permanent discontinuation was necessary in some cases; elevations in ALT or AST >5 x ULN were observed; concurrent ALT or AST elevations ≥3 x ULN and total bilirubin elevations ≥2 x ULN (without alkaline phosphatase elevations) occurred rarely. Transaminase elevation onset generally was within 2 months of treatment initiation. Monitor liver function tests, including ALT and total bilirubin every 2 weeks during the first 2 months of therapy, then monthly and as clinically necessary. Use with caution in patients with hepatic impairment (has not been studied); crizotinib is extensively metabolized in the liver and liver impairment is likely to increase crizotinib levels.

Severe, life-threatening, and potentially fatal interstitial lung disease (ILD)/pneumonitis has been associated with crizotinib. Onset was generally within 3 months of treatment initiation. Monitor for pulmonary symptoms which may indicate ILD/pneumonitis; exclude other potential causes (eg, disease progression, infection, other pulmonary disease, or radiation therapy). Permanently discontinue if treatment-related ILD/pneumonitis is confirmed.

Symptomatic bradycardia may occur; heart rate <50 beats/minute has occurred. If possible, avoid concurrent use with other agents known to cause bradycardia (eg, beta blockers, nondihydropyridine calcium channel blockers, clonidine, digoxin). Monitor heart rate and blood pressure regularly. If symptomatic bradycardia (not life-threatening) occurs, withhold treatment until recovery to asymptomatic bradycardia or to a heart rate of ≥60 beats/minute, evaluate concurrent medications, and potentially reduce crizotinib dose. Permanently discontinue for life-threatening bradycardia due to crizotinib; if life-threatening bradycardia occurs and concurrent medications associated with bradycardia can be discontinued or dose adjusted, restart crizotinib at a reduced dose (with frequent monitoring). QTc prolongation has been observed; consider periodic monitoring of ECG and electrolytes in patients with heart failure, bradyarrhythmias, electrolyte abnormalities, or who are taking medications known to prolong the QT interval. May require treatment interruption, dosage reduction, or discontinuation. Avoid use in patients with congenital long QT syndrome. Canadian labeling contraindicates use in patients with congenital long QT syndrome or persistent QTcF ≥500 msec.

Ocular toxicities (eg, blurred vision, diplopia, photophobia, photopsia, visual acuity decreased, visual brightness, visual field defect, visual impairment, and/or vitreous floaters) commonly occur. Onset is generally within 1 week of treatment initiation. Grade 4 visual field defect with vision loss had been reported (rare); optic atrophy and optic nerve disorder have been reported as potential causes of vision loss. Discontinue with new onset of severe visual loss (best corrected vision less than 20/200 in one or both eyes). Obtain ophthalmic evaluation (including best corrected visual acuity, retinal photographs, visual fields, optical coherence tomography, and other evaluations as appropriate). The risks of re-starting crizotinib after severe vision loss have not been evaluated; the decision to resume therapy should consider the potential benefits of treatment. Reduce initial dose in patients with severe renal impairment not requiring dialysis. Potentially significant drug-drug and drug-food interactions may exist, requiring dose or frequency adjustment, additional monitoring, and/or selection of alternative therapy. Avoid concomitant use with strong CYP3A4 inhibitors and inducers and with CYP3A4 substrates. Crizotinib is associated with a

moderate emetic potential; antiemetics may be needed to prevent nausea and vomiting.

Adverse Reactions Frequency not always defined.

Cardiovascular: Edema (31% to 49%), bradycardia (5% to 15%; grades 3/4: 1%), pulmonary embolism (6%), prolonged Q-T interval on ECG (5% to 6%; grades 3/4: 2% to 3%), syncope (1% to 3%), cardiac arrhythmia, septic shock

Central nervous system: Fatigue (27% to 29%), neuropathy (19% to 25%; includes dysesthesia, gait disturbance, hypoesthesia, muscular weakness, neuralgia, peripheral neuropathy, parasthesia, peripheral sensory neuropathy, polyneuropathy, burning sensation in skin), headache (22%), dizziness (18% to 22%)

Dermatologic: Skin rash (9% to 11%)

Endocrine & metabolic: Hypophosphatemia (28% to 32%), hypokalemia (18%), weight loss (10%), weight gain (8%), diabetic ketoacidosis (≤2%)

Gastrointestinal: Diarrhea (60% to 61%), nausea (55% to 56%), vomiting (46% to 47%), constipation (42% to 43%), decreased appetite (30%), abdominal pain (26%), dysgeusia (26%), dyspepsia (8% to 14%), dysphagia (10%)

Hematologic & oncologic: Neutropenia (49% to 52%; grades 3/4: 11% to 12%), lymphocytopenia (48% to 51%; grades 3/4: 7% to 9%)

Hepatic: Increased serum ALT (76% to 79%; grades 3/4: 11% to 17%), increased serum AST (61% to 66%; grades 3/4: 6% to 9%), hepatic failure (1%)

Infection: Sepsis (≤5%)

Neuromuscular & skeletal: Limb pain (16%), muscle spasm (8%)

Ophthalmic: Visual disturbance (60% to 71%; grades 3/4: <1%; grade 4: <1%; onset: <2 weeks; includes blurred vision, diplopia, photophobia, photopsia, visual acuity decreased, visual brightness, visual field defect, visual impairment, vitreous floaters)

Renal: Renal cyst (3% to 5%)

Respiratory: Upper respiratory tract infection (26% to 32%), adult respiratory distress syndrome (≤5%), interstitial pulmonary disease (≤5%; grades 3/4: 1%; includes acute respiratory distress syndrome, pneumonitis), pneumonia (≤5%), respiratory failure (≤5%), dyspnea (2%)

Miscellaneous: Fever (19%)

<1% (Limited to important or life-threatening): Hepatotoxicity

Drug Interactions

Metabolism/Transport Effects Substrate of CYP3A4 (major), P-glycoprotein; **Note:** Assignment of Major/Minor substrate status based on clinically relevant drug interaction potential; **Inhibits** CYP2B6 (moderate), CYP3A4 (moderate), OCT1, OCT2, P-glycoprotein

Avoid Concomitant Use

Avoid concomitant use of Crizotinib with any of the following: Alfentanil; Aprepitant; Bosutinib; Ceritinib; Cobimetinib; Conivaptan; CycloSPORINE (Systemic); CYP3A4 Inducers (Strong); CYP3A4 Inhibitors (Strong); Dihydroergotamine; Domperidone; Ergotamine; FentaNYL; Flibanserin; Fusidic Acid (Systemic); Grapefruit Juice; Highest Risk QTc-Prolonging Agents; Ibrutinib; Idelalisib; Ivabradine; Lomitapide; Mifepristone; Naloxegol; Olaparib; PAZOPanib; Pimozide; QuiNIDine; Silodosin; Simeprevir; Sirolimus; St Johns Wort; Tacrolimus (Systemic); Tolvaptan; Topotecan; Trabectedin; Ulipristal; VinCRIStine (Liposomal)

Increased Effect/Toxicity

Crizotinib may increase the levels/effects of: Afatinib; Alfentanil; Apixaban; Aprepitant; ARIPiprazole; Avanafil; Bosentan; Bosutinib; Bradycardia-Causing Agents; Brentuximab Vedotin; Brexpiprazole; Bromocriptine; Budesonide (Systemic); Budesonide (Topical); BuPROPion; Cannabis; Ceritinib; Cilostazol; Cobimetinib; Colchicine; CycloSPORINE (Systemic); CYP2B6 Substrates; CYP3A4 Substrates; Dabigatran Etexilate; Dapoxetine; Dihydroergotamine; Domperidone; DOXOrubicin (Conventional); Dronabinol; Edoxaban; Eletriptan; Eplerenone; Ergotamine; Everolimus; FentaNYL; Flibanserin; Highest Risk QTc-Prolonging Agents; Hydrocodone; Ibrutinib; Imatinib; Ivabradine; Ivacaftor; Lacosamide; Ledipasvir; Lomitapide; Lurasidone; Moderate Risk QTc-Prolonging Agents; Naloxegol; NiMODipine; Nintedanib; Olaparib; OxyCODONE; PAZOPanib; P-glycoprotein/ABCB1 Substrates; Pimecrolimus; Pimozide; Prucalopride; QuiNIDine; Ranolazine; Rifaximin; Rivaroxaban; Salmeterol; Saxagliptin; Silodosin; Simeprevir; Sirolimus; Sonidegib; Suvorexant; Tacrolimus (Systemic); Tetrahydrocannabinol; Tolvaptan; Topotecan; Trabectedin; Ulipristal; Vilazodone; VinCRIStine (Liposomal); Vindesine; Zopiclone

The levels/effects of Crizotinib may be increased by: Bretylium; Conivaptan; CYP3A4 Inhibitors (Moderate); CYP3A4 Inhibitors (Strong); Dasatinib; Fosaprepitant; Fusidic Acid (Systemic); Grapefruit Juice; Idelalisib; Ivabradine; Luliconazole; Mifepristone; Netupitant; Palbociclib; P-glycoprotein/ABCB1 Inhibitors; QTc-Prolonging Agents (Indeterminate Risk and Risk Modifying); Ruxolitinib; Stiripentol; Tofacitinib

Decreased Effect

Crizotinib may decrease the levels/effects of: Cyclophosphamide; Ifosfamide

The levels/effects of Crizotinib may be decreased by: Bosentan; CYP3A4 Inducers (Moderate); CYP3A4 Inducers (Strong); Dabrafenib; Deferasirox; P-glycoprotein/ABCB1 Inducers; Siltuximab; St Johns Wort; Tocilizumab

Food Interactions Grapefruit juice may increase serum crizotinib levels. Management: Avoid grapefruit and grapefruit juice.

Storage/Stability Store between 20°C and 25°C (68°F and 77°F); excursions are permitted between 15°C and 30°C (59°F and 86°F).

Mechanism of Action Tyrosine kinase receptor inhibitor, which inhibits anaplastic lymphoma kinase (ALK), Hepatocyte Growth Factor Receptor (HGFR, c-MET), and Recepteur d'Origine Nantais (RON). ALK gene abnormalities due to mutations or translocations may result in expression of oncogenic fusion proteins (eg, ALK fusion protein) which alter signaling and expression and result in increased cellular proliferation and survival in tumors which express these fusion proteins. Approximately 2% to 7% of patients with NSCLC have the abnormal echinoderm microtubule-associated protein-like 4, or EML4-ALK gene (which has a higher prevalence in never smokers or light smokers and in patients with adenocarcinoma). Crizotinib selectively inhibits ALK tyrosine kinase, which reduces proliferation of cells expressing the genetic alteration.

Pharmacodynamics/Kinetics

Distribution: V_{ss}: 1772 L

Protein binding: 91%

Metabolism: Hepatic, via CYP3A4/5

Bioavailability: 43% (range: 32% to 66%); bioavailability is reduced 14% with a high-fat meal

Half-life elimination: Terminal: 42 hours

Time to peak: 4 to 6 hours

Excretion: Feces (63%; 53% as unchanged drug); urine (22%; 2% as unchanged drug)

Dosing

Adult & Geriatric Note: Crizotinib is associated with a moderate emetic potential; antiemetics may be needed to prevent nausea and vomiting.

Non-small cell lung cancer (NSCLC), metastatic (ALK-positive): Oral: 250 mg twice daily, continue treatment until disease progression or unacceptable toxicity

Missed doses: If a dose is missed, take as soon as remembered unless it is <6 hours prior to the next scheduled dose (skip the dose if <6 hours before the next dose); do not take 2 doses at the same time to make up for a missed dose. If vomiting occurs after dose, administer the next dose at the regularly scheduled time.

Renal Impairment

Mild to moderate impairment (CrCl 30-89 mL/minute): No dosage adjustment necessary.

Severe impairment (CrCl <30 mL/minute) not requiring dialysis: Initial: 250 mg once daily.

Hepatic Impairment

Hepatotoxicity **prior to** treatment: No dosage adjustment provided in manufacturer's labeling (has not been studied); crizotinib undergoes extensive hepatic metabolism and systemic exposure may be increased with impairment; use with caution.

Hepatotoxicity **during** treatment:

Grade 3 or 4 ALT or AST elevation (ALT or AST >5 x ULN) with ≤ grade 1 total bilirubin elevation (total bilirubin ≤1.5 x ULN): Withhold treatment until recovery to baseline or ≤ grade 1 (<3 x ULN), then resume at a reduced dose (200 mg twice daily).

Recurrent grade 3 or 4 ALT or AST elevation with ≤ grade 1 total bilirubin elevation: Withhold treatment until recovery to baseline or ≤ grade 1, then resume at the next lower reduced dose (250 mg once daily).

Recurrent grade 3 or 4 ALT or AST elevation on 250 mg once daily: Permanently discontinue.

Grade 2, 3, or 4 ALT or AST elevation (ALT or AST >3 x ULN) with concurrent grade 2, 3, or 4 total bilirubin elevation (>1.5 x ULN) in the absence of cholestasis or hemolysis: Permanently discontinue.

Adjustment for Toxicity Note: If dose reduction is necessary, reduce dose to 200 mg orally twice daily; if necessary, further reduce to 250 mg once daily. If unable to tolerate 250 mg once daily, permanently discontinue therapy.

Hematologic toxicity (except lymphopenia, unless lymphopenia is associated with clinical events such as opportunistic infection):

Grade 3 toxicity (WBC 1,000 to 2,000/mm^3, ANC 500 to 1,000/mm^3, platelets 25,000 to 50,000/mm^3), grade 3 anemia: Withhold treatment until recovery to ≤ grade 2, then resume at the same dose and schedule.

Grade 4 toxicity (WBC <1,000/mm^3, ANC <500/mm^3, platelets <25,000/mm^3), grade 4 anemia: Withhold treatment until recovery to ≤ grade 2, then resume at 200 mg twice daily.

Recurrent grade 4 toxicity on 200 mg twice daily: Withhold treatment until recovery to ≤ grade 2, then resume at 250 mg once daily.

Recurrent grade 4 toxicity on 250 mg once daily: Permanently discontinue.

Nonhematologic toxicities:

Cardiovascular toxicities:

QTc prolongation:

Grade 3 QTc prolongation (QTc >500 msec without life-threatening signs or symptoms) on at least 2 separate ECGs: Withhold treatment until recovery to baseline or to ≤ grade 1 (QTc ≤480 msec), then resume at 200 mg twice daily.

Recurrent grade 3 QTc prolongation at 200 mg twice daily: Withhold treatment until recovery to baseline or to ≤ grade 1, then resume at 250 mg once daily.

Recurrent grade 3 QTc prolongation at 250 mg once daily: Permanently discontinue.

Grade 4 QTc prolongation (QTc >500 msec or ≥60 msec change from baseline with life-threatening symptoms): Permanently discontinue.

Bradycardia:

Grade 2 bradycardia (symptomatic with medical intervention indicated) or grade 3 bradycardia (severe/medically significant with intervention indicated): Withhold until recovery to asymptomatic bradycardia or to a heart rate of ≥60 beats/minute and evaluate concomitant medications. If contributing concomitant medication is identified and discontinued (or dose adjusted), then resume crizotinib at the previous dose. If no contributing concomitant medication is identified (or cannot be discontinued or dose adjusted), resume crizotinib at a reduced dose.

Grade 4 bradycardia (life-threatening with urgent intervention indicated): Withhold until recovery to asymptomatic bradycardia or to a heart rate of ≥60 beats/minute and evaluate concomitant medications. If contributing concomitant medication is identified and discontinued (or dose adjusted), then resume crizotinib at 250 mg once daily with frequent monitoring. If no contributing concomitant medication is identified, permanently discontinue crizotinib. Permanently discontinue for recurrence.

Hepatotoxicity: Refer to Dosage Adjustment in Hepatic Impairment.

Ocular toxicity: Visual loss (grade 4 visual disorder) or new onset of severe visual loss (best corrected vision less than 20/200 in one or both eyes): Discontinue during evaluation of severe vision loss.

Pulmonary toxicity: Interstitial lung disease (ILD)/pneumonitis (any grade; not attributable to disease progression, infection, other pulmonary disease or radiation therapy): Permanently discontinue.

Dietary Considerations Avoid grapefruit and grapefruit juice.

Administration

Crizotinib is associated with a moderate emetic potential; antiemetics may be needed to prevent nausea and vomiting.

Swallow capsules whole (do not crush, dissolve, or open capsules). Administer with or without food. If vomiting occurs after dose, administer the next dose at the regularly scheduled time.

Hazardous agent; use appropriate precautions for handling and disposal (NIOSH 2014 [group 1]).

Monitoring Parameters ALK positivity; CBC with differential monthly and as clinically appropriate (monitor more frequently if grades 3 or 4 abnormalities observed or with fever or infection), liver function tests every 2 weeks for the first 2 months, then monthly and as clinically appropriate (monitor more frequently if grades 2, 3, or 4 abnormalities observed); renal function (baseline and periodic). Monitor pulmonary symptoms (for interstitial lung disease [ILD]/pneumonitis). Monitor heart rate and blood pressure; consider monitoring ECG and electrolytes in patients with heart failure, bradycardia, bradyarrhythmias, electrolyte abnormalities, or who are taking medications known to prolong the QT interval. Obtain ophthalmic evaluation (including best corrected visual acuity, retinal photographs, visual fields, optical coherence tomography, and other evaluations as appropriate) if severe visual loss occurs.

Dosage Forms Excipient information presented when available (limited, particularly for generics); consult specific product labeling.

Capsule, Oral:

Xalkori: 200 mg, 250 mg

Crofelemer (kroe FEL e mer)

Brand Names: US Fulyzaq

Index Terms *Croton lechleri*; Provir; SP-303

Pharmacologic Category Antidiarrheal

Use Symptomatic relief of noninfectious diarrhea in patients with HIV/AIDS on antiretroviral therapy

Dosing

Adult Diarrhea, noninfectious (associated with antiretroviral therapy for HIV/AIDS): Oral: 125 mg twice daily

Renal Impairment No dosage adjustment provided in the manufacturer's labeling.

Hepatic Impairment No dosage adjustment provided in the manufacturer's labeling.

Additional Information Complete prescribing information should be consulted for additional detail.

Dosage Forms Excipient information presented when available (limited, particularly for generics); consult specific product labeling.

Tablet Delayed Release, Oral:

Fulyzaq: 125 mg [contains methylparaben, propylparaben]

◆ *Crotalidae Immune F(ab')2 (Equine) see Crotalidae Immune F(ab')$_2$ (Equine) on page 452*

Crotalidae Immune F(ab')$_2$ (Equine)
(kroe TAL ih die i MYUN fab two EE kwine)

Index Terms Crotalidae Immune F(ab')2 (Equine); Anavip; Antivenin; Antivenin (*Crotalidae*) Immune F(ab')2 (Equine); Antivenom (*Crotalidae*) Immune F(ab')2 (Equine); Crotalidae Immune F(ab')2 (Equine); Crotalidae Immune Fab2 (Equine); Crotaline Antivenin Immune F(ab')2 (Equine); Crotaline Antivenom Immune F(ab')2 (Equine); Snake Antivenin F(ab')2 (Equine); Snake Antivenom F(ab')2 (Equine)

Pharmacologic Category Antivenin

Use Rattlesnake envenomation: Management of adult and pediatric patients with North American rattlesnake envenomation

Dosing

Adult

Rattlesnake envenomation: IV: **Note:** Initiate therapy as soon as possible after a rattlesnake bite in patients exhibiting any signs of envenomation.

Initial: Ten vials; may repeat every hour as needed until local signs of envenomation are not progressing, systemic symptoms are resolved and coagulation parameters have normalized or are trending toward normal. There is no known maximum dose.

Maintenance: Four vials as needed; may administer for any re-emerging symptoms, including coagulopathies

Geriatric Refer to adult dosing

Pediatric Rattlesnake envenomation: Infants, Children, and Adolescents: IV: Refer to adult dosing.

Renal Impairment There are no dosage adjustments provided in the manufacturer's labeling.

Hepatic Impairment There are no dosage adjustments provided in the manufacturer's labeling.

Additional Information Complete prescribing information should be consulted for additional detail.

Product Availability Anavip: FDA approved May 2015; availability anticipated in October 2018

◆ *Crotaline Antivenin Immune F(ab')2 (Equine) see Crotalidae Immune F(ab')$_2$ (Equine) on page 452*

◆ *Crotaline Antivenom Immune F(ab')2 (Equine) see Crotalidae Immune F(ab')$_2$ (Equine) on page 452*

Crotamiton (kroe TAM i tonn)

Brand Names: US Eurax

Brand Names: Canada Eurax Cream

Pharmacologic Category Scabicidal Agent

Use Treatment of scabies (*Sarcoptes scabiei*) and symptomatic treatment of pruritus

Dosing

Adult & Geriatric

Pruritus: Topical: Massage into affected areas until medication is completely absorbed; repeat as necessary

Scabies: Topical: Apply a thin layer and massage drug onto skin of the entire body from the neck to the toes (with special attention to skin folds, creases, and interdigital spaces). Repeat application in 24 hours. May retreat if new lesions appear or itching persists more than 2 to 4 weeks after initial treatment (CDC 2010).

Additional Information Complete prescribing information should be consulted for additional detail.

Dosage Forms Excipient information presented when available (limited, particularly for generics); consult specific product labeling.

Cream, External:
Eurax: 10% (60 g)
Lotion, External:
Eurax: 10% (60 g, 454 g)

Cyanocobalamin (sye an oh koe BAL a min)

Brand Names: US B-12 Compliance Injection; Nascobal; Physicians EZ Use B-12
Index Terms CaloMist; Vitamin B$_{12}$
Pharmacologic Category Vitamin, Water Soluble
Use Treatment of pernicious anemia; vitamin B$_{12}$ deficiency due to dietary deficiencies or malabsorption diseases, inadequate secretion of intrinsic factor, and inadequate utilization of B$_{12}$ (eg, during neoplastic treatment); increased B$_{12}$ requirements due to pregnancy, thyrotoxicosis, hemorrhage, malignancy, liver or kidney disease

Dosing
Adult & Geriatric
Recommended intake (IOM, 1998): 2.4 mcg daily
Pregnancy: 2.6 mcg daily
Lactation: 2.8 mcg daily
Vitamin B$_{12}$ deficiency:
Intranasal (Nascobal): 500 mcg in one nostril once weekly
Oral: 1000-2000 mcg daily for 1-2 weeks; maintenance: 1000 mcg daily (Langan, 2011; Oh, 2003)
IM, deep SubQ: May use initial treatment similar to that for pernicious anemia depending on severity of deficiency: 100 mcg daily for 6-7 days; if improvement, administer same dose on alternate days for 7 doses, then every 3-4 days for 2-3 weeks; once hematologic values have returned to normal, maintenance dosage: 100 mcg monthly.
Note: Given the lack of toxicity associated with cyanocobalamin, higher doses may be preferred, especially in cases of severe deficiency. Alternate dosing regimens exist with initial doses ranging from 100-1000 mcg every day or every other day for 1-2 weeks and maintenance doses of 100-1000 mcg every 1-3 months (Oh, 2003).

Pernicious anemia: IM, deep SubQ (administer concomitantly with folic acid if needed, 1 mg daily for 1 month): 100 mcg daily for 6-7 days; if improvement, administer same dose on alternate days for 7 doses, then every 3-4 days for 2-3 weeks; once hematologic values have returned to normal, maintenance dosage: 100 mcg monthly.
Note: Given the lack of toxicity associated with cyanocobalamin, higher doses may be preferred, especially in cases of severe deficiency. Alternate dosing regimens exist with initial doses ranging from 100-1000 mcg every day or every other day for 1-2 weeks and maintenance doses of 100-1000 mcg every 1-3 months (Oh, 2003).
Hematologic remission (without evidence of nervous system involvement):
Intranasal (Nascobal): 500 mcg in one nostril once weekly
Oral: 1000-2000 mcg daily
IM, SubQ: 100-1000 mcg monthly
Pediatric
Adequate intake (IOM, 1998):
Children:
0-6 months: 0.4 mcg daily
7-12 months: 0.5 mcg daily
Recommended intake (IOM, 1998):
Children:
1-3 years: 0.9 mcg daily
4-8 years: 1.2 mcg daily
9-13 years: 1.8 mcg daily
Adolescents >14 years: Refer to adult dosing.
Vitamin B$_{12}$ deficiency: IM, deep SubQ: Dosage in children is not well established: 0.2 mcg/kg for 2 days, followed by 1000 mcg daily for 2-7 days, followed by 100 mcg weekly for 1 month; for malabsorptive causes of B$_{12}$ deficiency, monthly maintenance doses of 100 mcg have been recommended **or** as an alternative 100 mcg daily for 10-15 days, then once or twice weekly for several months (Rasmussen, 2001).
Pernicious anemia: IM, deep SubQ (administer concomitantly with folic acid if needed, 1 mg daily for 1 month): 30-50 mcg daily for 2 or more weeks (to a total dose of 1000-5000 mcg), then follow with 100 mcg monthly as maintenance dosage
Renal Impairment There are no dosage adjustments provided in the manufacturer's labeling. Use with caution; some formulations may also contain aluminum, which may accumulate in renal impairment.
Hepatic Impairment There are no dosage adjustments provided in the manufacturer's labeling.
Additional Information Complete prescribing information should be consulted for additional detail.
Dosage Forms Excipient information presented when available (limited, particularly for generics); consult specific product labeling. [DSC] = Discontinued product
Kit, Injection:
B-12 Compliance Injection: 1000 mcg/mL [contains benzyl alcohol]
Physicians EZ Use B-12: 1000 mcg/mL [contains benzyl alcohol]
Liquid, Sublingual:
Generic: 3000 mcg/mL (52 mL)
Lozenge, Oral:
Generic: 50 mcg (100 ea); 100 mcg (100 ea); 250 mcg (100 ea, 250 ea); 500 mcg (100 ea, 250 ea)
Solution, Injection:
Generic: 1000 mcg/mL (1 mL, 10 mL, 30 mL)
Solution, Nasal:
Nascobal: 500 mcg/0.1 mL (1 ea, 1.3 mL [DSC]) [contains benzalkonium chloride]
Tablet, Oral:
Generic: 100 mcg, 250 mcg, 500 mcg, 1000 mcg
Tablet, Oral [preservative free]:
Generic: 100 mcg, 500 mcg, 1000 mcg
Tablet Extended Release, Oral:
Generic: 1000 mcg
Tablet Sublingual, Sublingual:
Generic: 2500 mcg
Tablet Sublingual, Sublingual [preservative free]:
Generic: 2500 mcg

◆ **Cyclessa** see Ethinyl Estradiol and Desogestrel
on page 701

Cyclobenzaprine (sye kloe BEN za preen)

Brand Names: US Active-Cyclobenzaprine; Amrix; EnovaRX-Cyclobenzaprine HCl; Fexmid; Flexeril [DSC]; Tabradol FusePaq

Brand Names: Canada Apo-Cyclobenzaprine; Auro-Cyclobenzaprine; Ava-Cyclobenzaprine; Dom-Cyclobenzaprine; JAMP-Cyclobenzaprine; Mylan-Cyclobenzaprine; Novo-Cycloprine; PHL-Cyclobenzaprine; PMS-Cyclobenzaprine; Q-Cyclobenzaprine; ratio-Cyclobenzaprine; Riva-Cycloprine; ZYM-Cyclobenzaprine

Index Terms Cyclobenzaprine Hydrochloride; Flexeril

Pharmacologic Category Skeletal Muscle Relaxant

Use Short-term (2-3 weeks) treatment of muscle spasm associated with acute, painful musculoskeletal conditions

Pregnancy Considerations Adverse events have not been observed in animal reproduction studies. The manufacturer recommends avoiding use during pregnancy unless clearly needed.

Breast-Feeding Considerations It is not known if cyclobenzaprine is excreted in breast milk. The manufacturer recommends that caution be exercised when administering cyclobenzaprine to nursing women.

Contraindications Hypersensitivity to cyclobenzaprine or any component of the formulation; during or within 14 days of MAO inhibitors; hyperthyroidism; congestive heart failure; arrhythmias; heart block or conduction disturbances; acute recovery phase of MI

Warnings/Precautions May cause CNS depression, which may impair physical or mental abilities; ethanol and/or other CNS depressants may enhance these effects. Patients must be cautioned about performing tasks which require mental alertness (eg, operating machinery or driving). Cyclobenzaprine shares the toxic potentials of the tricyclic antidepressants (including arrhythmias, tachycardia, and conduction time prolongation) and the usual precautions of tricyclic antidepressant therapy should be observed; use with caution in patients with urinary hesitancy or retention, angle-closure glaucoma or increased intraocular pressure, hepatic impairment, or in the elderly.

Potentially life-threatening serotonin syndrome has occurred with cyclobenzaprine when used in combination with other serotonergic agents (eg, SSRIs, SNRIs, TCAs, meperidine, tramadol, buspirone, MAO inhibitors), bupropion, and verapamil. Monitor patients closely especially during initiation/dose titration for signs/symptoms of serotonin syndrome such as mental status changes (eg, agitation, hallucinations); autonomic instability (eg, tachycardia, labile blood pressure, diaphoresis); neuromuscular changes (eg, tremor, rigidity, myoclonus); GI symptoms (eg, nausea, vomiting, diarrhea); and/or seizures. Discontinue cyclobenzaprine and any concomitant serotonergic agent immediately if signs/symptoms arise. Concomitant use or use within 14 days of discontinuing an MAO inhibitor is contraindicated.

Muscle relaxants are poorly tolerated by the elderly due to potent anticholinergic effects, sedation, and risk of fracture. Efficacy is questionable at dosages tolerated by elderly patients; avoid use (Beers Criteria). Extended release capsules not recommended for use in mild-to-severe hepatic impairment or in the elderly. Potentially significant drug-drug interactions may exist, requiring dose or frequency adjustment, additional monitoring, and/or selection of alternative therapy. Effects may be potentiated when used with other CNS depressants or ethanol.

Adverse Reactions

>10%:

Central nervous system: Drowsiness (1% to 39%), dizziness (1% to 11%)

Gastrointestinal: Xerostomia (6% to 32%)

1% to 10%:

Central nervous system: Fatigue (1% to 6%), headache (1% to 5%), confusion (1% to 3%), decreased mental acuity (1% to 3%), irritability (1% to 3%), nervousness (1% to 3%)

Gastrointestinal: Dyspepsia (≤4%), abdominal pain (1% to 3%), acid regurgitation (1% to 3%), constipation (1% to 3%), diarrhea (1% to 3%), nausea (1% to 3%), unpleasant taste (1% to 3%)

Neuromuscular & skeletal: Weakness (1% to 3%)

Ophthalmic: Blurred vision (1% to 3%)

Respiratory: Pharyngitis (1% to 3%), upper respiratory tract infection (1% to 3%)

<1% (Limited to important or life-threatening): Anaphylaxis, angioedema, cardiac arrhythmia, convulsions, hepatitis (rare), hypertonia, hypotension, paresthesia, psychosis, seizure, serotonin syndrome, skin rash, syncope, tachycardia

Drug Interactions

Metabolism/Transport Effects Substrate of CYP1A2 (major), CYP2D6 (minor), CYP3A4 (minor); **Note:** Assignment of Major/Minor substrate status based on clinically relevant drug interaction potential

Avoid Concomitant Use

Avoid concomitant use of Cyclobenzaprine with any of the following: Aclidinium; Azelastine (Nasal); Cimetropium; Dapoxetine; Eluxadoline; Glucagon; Glycopyrrolate; Glycopyrrolate (Oral Inhalation); Ipratropium (Oral Inhalation); Levosulpiride; MAO Inhibitors; Orphenadrine; Paraldehyde; Potassium Chloride; Thalidomide; Tiotropium; Umeclidinium

Increased Effect/Toxicity

Cyclobenzaprine may increase the levels/effects of: AbobotulinumtoxinA; Alcohol (Ethyl); Analgesics (Opioid); Anticholinergic Agents; Antipsychotic Agents; Azelastine (Nasal); Buprenorphine; Cimetropium; CNS Depressants; Eluxadoline; Glucagon; Glycopyrrolate; Glycopyrrolate (Oral Inhalation); Hydrocodone; MAO Inhibitors; Methotrimeprazine; Metoclopramide; Metyrosine; Mirabegron; OnabotulinumtoxinA; Orphenadrine; Paraldehyde; Potassium Chloride; Pramipexole; Ramosetron; RimabotulinumtoxinB; ROPINIRole; Rotigotine; Serotonin Modulators; Suvorexant; Thalidomide; Thiazide Diuretics; Tiotropium; Topiramate; TraMADol; Zolpidem

The levels/effects of Cyclobenzaprine may be increased by: Abiraterone Acetate; Aclidinium; Antiemetics (5HT3 Antagonists); Antipsychotic Agents; Brimonidine (Topical); Cannabis; CYP1A2 Inhibitors (Moderate); CYP1A2 Inhibitors (Strong); Dapoxetine; Deferasirox; Doxylamine; Dronabinol; Droperidol; HydrOXYzine; Ipratropium (Oral Inhalation); Kava Kava; Magnesium Sulfate; Metaxalone; Methotrimeprazine; Mianserin; Minocycline; Nabilone; Peginterferon Alfa-2b; Perampanel; Pramlintide; Rufinamide; Sodium Oxybate; Tapentadol; Tetrahydrocannabinol; Umeclidinium; Vemurafenib

Decreased Effect

Cyclobenzaprine may decrease the levels/effects of: Acetylcholinesterase Inhibitors; Gastrointestinal Agents (Prokinetic); Itopride; Levosulpiride; Secretin

The levels/effects of Cyclobenzaprine may be decreased by: Acetylcholinesterase Inhibitors

Food Interactions Food increases bioavailability (peak plasma concentrations increased by 35% and area under the curve by 20%) of the extended release capsule. Management: Monitor for increased effects if taken with food.

Storage/Stability

Amrix, Flexeril: Store at 25°C (77°F); excursions permitted to 15°C to 30°C (59°F to 86°F). Protect from light.

Fexmid: Store at 20°C to 25°C (68°F to 77°F).

Mechanism of Action Centrally-acting skeletal muscle relaxant pharmacologically related to tricyclic antidepressants; reduces tonic somatic motor activity influencing both alpha and gamma motor neurons

Pharmacodynamics/Kinetics

Onset of action: Immediate release tablet: Within 1 hour

Duration of action: Immediate release tablet: 12 to 24 hours

Metabolism: Hepatic via CYP3A4, 1A2, and 2D6; may undergo enterohepatic recirculation

Bioavailability: 33% to 55%

Half-life elimination: Normal hepatic function: Range: 8-37 hours; immediate release tablet: 18 hours; extended release capsule: 32 hours; impaired hepatic function: 46.2 hours (range: 22.4 to 188 hours) (Winchell 2002)

Time to peak, serum: Immediate release tablet: ~4 hours (Winchell 2002); Extended release capsule: 7-8 hours

Excretion: Urine (primarily as glucuronide metabolites); feces (as unchanged drug; Hucker 1978)

Clearance: 0.7 L/minute

Dosing

Adult Muscle spasm: Oral: **Note:** Do not use longer than 2-3 weeks

Capsule, extended release: Usual: 15 mg once daily; some patients may require up to 30 mg once daily

Tablet, immediate release: Initial: 5 mg 3 times daily; may increase up to 10 mg 3 times daily if needed

Geriatric

Capsule, extended release: Use not recommended

Tablet, immediate release: Initial: 5 mg; titrate dose slowly and consider less frequent dosing

Pediatric Muscle spasm: Oral: Tablet, immediate release: Children ≥15 years: Refer to adult dosing.

Renal Impairment No dosage adjustment provided in manufacturer's labeling.

Hepatic Impairment

Capsule, extended release: Mild-to-severe impairment: Use not recommended.

Tablet, immediate release:

Mild impairment: Initial: 5 mg; use with caution; titrate slowly and consider less frequent dosing

Moderate-to-severe impairment: Use not recommended

Administration Oral: Extended release capsules: Administer at the same time each day. Do not crush or chew.

Monitoring Parameters Signs/symptoms of serotonin syndrome (patients receiving other serotonergic drugs)

Test Interactions May cause false-positive serum TCA screen (Wong, 1995)

Dosage Forms Considerations

EnovaRX-Cyclobenzaprine and Active-Cyclobenzaprine creams are compounded from kits. Refer to manufacturer's labeling for compounding instructions.

Tabradol FusePaq is a compounding kit for the preparation of an oral suspension in a vehicle containing methylsulfonylmethane. Refer to manufacturer's labeling for compounding instructions.

Dosage Forms Excipient information presented when available (limited, particularly for generics); consult specific product labeling. [DSC] = Discontinued product

Capsule Extended Release 24 Hour, Oral, as hydrochloride:

Amrix: 15 mg

Amrix: 30 mg [contains brilliant blue fcf (fd&c blue #1), fd&c blue #2 (indigotine), fd&c red #40, fd&c yellow #6 (sunset yellow)]

Cream, Transdermal, as hydrochloride:

Active-Cyclobenzaprine: 5% (120 g) [contains chlorocresol (chloro-m-cresol)]

EnovaRX-Cyclobenzaprine HCl: 20 mg/g (120 g) [contains cetearyl alcohol]

Suspension, Oral, as hydrochloride:

Tabradol FusePaq: 1 mg/mL (250 mL) [contains saccharin sodium, sodium benzoate]

Tablet, Oral, as hydrochloride:

Fexmid: 7.5 mg

Flexeril: 5 mg [DSC], 10 mg [DSC]

Generic: 5 mg, 7.5 mg, 10 mg

◆ Cyclobenzaprine Hydrochloride see Cyclobenzaprine on page 454

◆ Cyclogyl see Cyclopentolate on page 455

◆ Cyclomen® (Can) see Danazol on page 486

◆ Cyclomydril® see Cyclopentolate and Phenylephrine on page 455

Cyclopentolate (sye kloe PEN toe late)

Brand Names: US AK-Pentolate [DSC]; Cyclogyl

Brand Names: Canada AK Pentolate Oph Soln; Cyclogyl; Diopentolate; Minims Cyclopentolate; PMS-Cyclopentolate

Index Terms Cyclopentolate Hydrochloride

Pharmacologic Category Anticholinergic Agent, Ophthalmic

Use Mydriasis/Cycloplegia: Produce mydriasis and cycloplegia.

Dosing

Adult & Geriatric

Mydriasis, cycloplegia: Ophthalmic: Instill 1 or 2 drops of 0.5%, 1%, or 2% solution; may repeat in 5 to 10 minutes; heavily pigmented irides may require use of higher strengths.

Anterior uveitis (off-label use): Ophthalmic: Instill 1 drop of 1% solution 3 times daily (AOA [Alexander, 2004]).

Pediatric

Mydriasis, cycloplegia: Note: Cyclopentolate and phenylephrine combination formulation is the preferred agent for use in infants due to lower cyclopentolate concentration and reduced risk for systemic reactions (Chew, 2005).

Infants: Ophthalmic: Instill 1 drop of 0.5% solution as a single dose.

Children and Adolescents: Ophthalmic: Instill 1 or 2 drops of 0.5%, 1%, or 2% solution; may repeat with 0.5% or 1% solution in 5 to 10 minutes.

Renal Impairment There are no dosage adjustments provided in the manufacturer's labeling.

Hepatic Impairment There are no dosage adjustments provided in the manufacturer's labeling.

Additional Information Complete prescribing information should be consulted for additional detail.

Dosage Forms Excipient information presented when available (limited, particularly for generics); consult specific product labeling. [DSC] = Discontinued product

Solution, Ophthalmic, as hydrochloride:

AK-Pentolate: 1% (2 mL [DSC])

Cyclogyl: 0.5% (15 mL); 1% (2 mL, 5 mL, 15 mL); 2% (2 mL, 5 mL, 15 mL)

Generic: 1% (2 mL, 15 mL); 2% (2 mL, 5 mL, 15 mL)

Cyclopentolate and Phenylephrine
(sye kloe PEN toe late & fen il EF rin)

Brand Names: US Cyclomydril®

Index Terms Phenylephrine and Cyclopentolate

Pharmacologic Category Ophthalmic Agent, Mydriatic

Use Mydriasis: For the production of mydriasis.

Dosing

Adult & Geriatric Diagnostic aid (mydriasis): Ophthalmic: Instill 1 drop into the eye every 5 to 10 minutes.

Pediatric Diagnostic aid (mydriasis): Infants, Children, and Adolescents: Ophthalmic: Refer to adult dosing.

Additional Information Complete prescribing information should be consulted for additional detail.

Dosage Forms Excipient information presented when available (limited, particularly for generics); consult specific product labeling.

Solution, ophthalmic:

Cyclomydril: Cyclopentolate hydrochloride 0.2% and phenylephrine hydrochloride 1% (2 mL, 5 mL) [contains benzalkonium chloride]

◆ Cyclopentolate Hydrochloride see Cyclopentolate on page 455

Cyclophosphamide (sye kloe FOS fa mide)

Brand Names: Canada Procytox

Index Terms CPM; CTX; CYT; Cytoxan; Neosar

Pharmacologic Category Antineoplastic Agent, Alkylating Agent; Antineoplastic Agent, Alkylating Agent (Nitrogen Mustard); Antirheumatic Miscellaneous; Immunosuppressant Agent

Use

Oncology uses: Treatment of acute lymphoblastic leukemia (ALL), acute myelocytic leukemia (AML), breast cancer, chronic lymphocytic leukemia (CLL), chronic myeloid leukemia (CML), Hodgkin lymphoma, mycosis fungoides, multiple myeloma, neuroblastoma, non-Hodgkin lymphomas (including Burkitt lymphoma), ovarian adenocarcinoma, and retinoblastoma

Limitations of use: Although potentially effective as a single-agent in susceptible malignancies, cyclophosphamide is more frequently used in combination with other chemotherapy drugs

Canadian labeling: Additional use (not in US labeling): Treatment of lung cancer

Nononcology uses: US labeling: Nephrotic syndrome: Treatment of minimal change nephrotic syndrome (biopsy proven) in children who are unresponsive or intolerant to corticosteroid therapy

Limitations of use: The safety and efficacy for the treatment of nephrotic syndrome in adults or in other renal diseases has not been established.

Pregnancy Considerations Cyclophosphamide crosses the placenta and can be detected in amniotic fluid (D'Incalci 1982). Based on the mechanism of action, cyclophosphamide may cause fetal harm if administered during pregnancy. Adverse events (including ectrodactylia) were observed in human studies following exposure to cyclophosphamide. Women of childbearing potential should avoid pregnancy while receiving cyclophosphamide and for up to 1 year after completion of treatment. Males with female partners who are or may become pregnant should use a condom during and for at least 4 months after cyclophosphamide treatment. Cyclophosphamide may cause sterility in males and females (may be irreversible) and amenorrhea in females. When treatment is needed for lupus nephritis, cyclophosphamide should be avoided in women who are pregnant or those who wish to preserve their fertility (Hahn 2012). Chemotherapy, if indicated, may be administered to pregnant women with breast cancer as part of a combination chemotherapy regimen (common regimens administered during pregnancy include doxorubicin (or epirubicin), cyclophosphamide, and fluorouracil); chemotherapy should not be administered during the first trimester, after 35 weeks gestation, or within 3 weeks of planned delivery (Amant 2010; Loibl 2006).

Breast-Feeding Considerations Cyclophosphamide is excreted into breast milk. Leukopenia and thrombocytopenia were noted in an infant exposed to cyclophosphamide while nursing. The mother was treated with one course of cyclophosphamide 6 weeks prior to delivery then ▶

cyclophosphamide IV 6 mg/kg (300 mg) once daily for 3 days beginning 20 days postpartum. Complete blood counts were obtained in the breast-feeding infant on each day of therapy; WBC and platelets decreased by day 3 (Durodola 1979). Due to the potential for serious adverse effects in the nursing infant, a decision should be made to discontinue cyclophosphamide or to discontinue breast-feeding, taking into account the importance of treatment to the mother.

Contraindications

US labeling: Hypersensitivity to cyclophosphamide or any component of the formulation; urinary outflow obstruction

Canadian labeling: Hypersensitivity to cyclophosphamide or its metabolites, urinary outflow obstructions, severe myelosuppression, severe renal or hepatic impairment, active infection (especially varicella zoster), severe immunosuppression

Warnings/Precautions Hazardous agent - use appropriate precautions for handling and disposal (NIOSH 2014 [group 1]).

Cyclophosphamide is associated with the development of hemorrhagic cystitis, pyelitis, ureteritis, and hematuria. Hemorrhagic cystitis may rarely be severe or fatal. Bladder fibrosis may also occur, either with or without cystitis. Urotoxicity is due to excretion of cyclophosphamide metabolites in the urine and appears to be dose- and treatment duration-dependent, although may occur with short-term use. Increased hydration and frequent voiding is recommended to help prevent cystitis; some protocols utilize mesna to protect against hemorrhagic cystitis. Monitor urinalysis for hematuria or other signs of urotoxicity. Severe or prolonged hemorrhagic cystitis may require medical or surgical treatment. While hematuria generally resolves within a few days after treatment is withheld, it may persist in some cases. Discontinue cyclophosphamide with severe hemorrhagic cystitis. Exclude or correct any urinary tract obstructions prior to treatment initiation (use is contraindicated with bladder outlet obstruction). Use with caution (if at all) in patients with active urinary tract infection. Use with caution in patients with renal impairment; dosage adjustment may be needed. Decreased renal excretion and increased serum levels (cyclophosphamide and metabolites) may occur in patients with severe renal impairment (CrCl 10 to 24 mL/minute; monitor for signs/symptoms of toxicity. Use is contraindicated in severe impairment in the Canadian labeling. Cyclophosphamide and metabolites are dialyzable; differences in amount dialyzed may occur due to dialysis system used. If dialysis is required, maintain a consistent interval between administration and dialysis.

Leukopenia, neutropenia, thrombocytopenia, and anemia may commonly occur; may be dose related. Bone marrow failure has been reported. Bone marrow failure and severe immunosuppression may lead to serious (and fatal) infections, including sepsis and septic shock, or may reactive latent infections. Antimicrobial prophylaxis may be considered in appropriate patients. Initiate antibiotics for neutropenic fever; antifungal and antiviral medications may also be necessary. Monitor blood counts during treatment. Avoid use if neutrophils are ≤1,500/mm^3 and platelets are <50,000/mm^3. Consider growth factors (primary or secondary prophylaxis) in patients at increased risk for complications due to neutropenia. Platelet and neutrophil nadirs are usually at weeks 1 and 2 of treatment and recovery is expected after ~20 days. Severe myelosuppression may be more prevalent in heavily pretreated patients or in patients receiving concomitant chemotherapy and/or radiation therapy. Monitor for infections; immunosuppression and serious infections may occur; serious infections may require dose reduction, or interruption or discontinuation of treatment.

Cardiotoxicity has been reported (some fatal), usually with high doses associated with transplant conditioning regimens, although may rarely occur with lower doses. Cardiac abnormalities do not appear to persist. Cardiotoxicities reported have included arrhythmias (supraventricular and ventricular [some with QT prolongation]), congestive heart failure, heart block, hemopericardium (secondary to hemorrhagic myocarditis and myocardial necrosis), myocarditis (including hemorrhagic), pericarditis, pericardial effusion including cardiac tamponade, and tachyarrhythmias. Cardiotoxicity is related to endothelial capillary damage; symptoms may be managed with diuretics, ACE inhibitors, beta-blockers, or inotropics (Floyd 2005). The risk for cardiotoxicity may be increased with higher doses, advanced age, and in patients with prior radiation to the cardiac region, and in patients who have received prior or concurrent cardiotoxic medication. Use with caution in patients with preexisting cardiovascular disease or those at risk for cardiotoxicity. For patients with cardiac risk factors or preexisting cardiac disease, monitor during treatment.

Pulmonary toxicities, including pneumonitis, pulmonary fibrosis, pulmonary veno-occlusive disease, and acute respiratory distress syndrome, have been reported. Monitor for signs/symptoms of pulmonary toxicity. Consider pulmonary function testing to assess the severity of pneumonitis (Morgan 2011). Cyclophosphamide-induced pneumonitis is rare and may present as early (within 1 to 6 months) or late onset (several months to years). Early onset may be reversible with discontinuation; late onset is associated with pleural thickening and may persist chronically (Malik 1996). In addition, late onset pneumonitis (>6 months after therapy initiation) may be associated with increased mortality.

Hepatic sinusoidal obstruction syndrome (SOS), formerly called veno-occlusive liver disease (VOD), has been reported in patients receiving chemotherapy regimens containing cyclophosphamide. A major risk factor for SOS is cytoreductive conditioning transplantation regimens with cyclophosphamide used in combination with total body irradiation or busulfan (or other agents). Other risk factors include preexisting hepatic dysfunction, prior radiation to the abdominal area, and low performance status. Children <3 years of age are reported to be at increased risk for hepatic SOS; monitor for signs or symptoms of hepatic SOS, including bilirubin >1.4 mg/dL, unexplained weight gain, ascites, hepatomegaly, or unexplained right upper quadrant pain (Arndt 2004). SOS has also been reported in patients receiving long-term lower doses for immunosuppressive indications. Use with caution in patients with hepatic impairment; dosage adjustment may be needed. Use is contraindicated in severe impairment in the Canadian labeling. The conversion between cyclophosphamide to the active metabolite may be reduced in patients with severe hepatic impairment, potentially reducing efficacy.

Nausea and vomiting commonly occur. Cyclophosphamide is associated with a moderate to high emetic potential (depending on dose, regimen, or administration route); antiemetics are recommended to prevent nausea and vomiting (Basch 2011; Dupuis 2011; Roila 2010). Stomatitis/mucositis may also occur. Anaphylactic reactions have been reported; cross-sensitivity with other alkylating agents may occur. Hyponatremia associated with increased total body water, acute water intoxication, and a syndrome resembling SIADH (syndrome of inappropriate secretion of antidiuretic hormone) has been reported; some have been fatal. May interfere with wound healing. May impair fertility; interferes with oogenesis and spermatogenesis. Effect on fertility is generally dependent on dose and duration of treatment and may be irreversible. The age at treatment initiation and cumulative dose were determined to be risk factors for ovarian failure in cyclophosphamide use for the treatment of systemic lupus erythematosus (SLE) (Mok 1998). Potentially significant drug-drug interactions may exist, requiring dose or frequency adjustment, additional monitoring, and/or selection of alternative therapy. Secondary malignancies (bladder cancer, myelodysplasia, acute leukemias, lymphomas, thyroid cancer, and sarcomas) have been reported with both single-agent and with combination chemotherapy regimens; onset may be delayed (up to several years after treatment). Bladder cancer usually occurs in patients previously experiencing hemorrhagic cystitis; risk may be reduced by preventing hemorrhagic cystitis.

Adverse Reactions Frequency not defined.

Dermatologic: Alopecia (reversible; onset: 3-6 weeks after start of treatment)

Endocrine & metabolic: Amenorrhea, azoospermia, gonadal suppression, oligospermia, oogenesis impaired, sterility

Gastrointestinal: Abdominal pain, anorexia, diarrhea, mucositis, nausea/vomiting (dose-related), stomatitis

Genitourinary: Hemorrhagic cystitis

Hematologic: Anemia, leukopenia (dose-related; recovery: 7-10 days after cessation), myelosuppression, neutropenia, neutropenic fever, thrombocytopenia

Postmarketing and/or case reports: Acute respiratory distress syndrome, anaphylactic reactions, anaphylaxis, arrhythmias (with high-dose [HSCT] therapy), bladder/urinary fibrosis, blurred vision, cardiac tamponade (with high-dose [HSCT] therapy), cardiotoxicity, confusion, dyspnea, ejection fraction decreased, erythema multiforme, gastrointestinal hemorrhage, hearing disorders, heart block, heart failure (with high-dose [HSCT] therapy), hematuria, hemopericardium, hemorrhagic colitis, hemorrhagic myocarditis (with high-dose [HSCT] therapy), hemorrhagic ureteritis, hepatic sinusoidal obstruction syndrome (SOS; formerly called veno-occlusive liver disease), hepatitis, hepatotoxicity, hypersensitivity

reactions, hyperuricemia, hypokalemia, hyponatremia, interstitial pneumonitis, interstitial pulmonary fibrosis (with high doses), jaundice, latent infection reactivation, mesenteric ischemia (acute), methemoglobinemia (with high-dose [HSCT] therapy), multiorgan failure, myocardial necrosis (with high-dose [HSCT] therapy), neurotoxicity, neutrophilic eccrine hidradenitis, ovarian fibrosis, pancreatitis, pericarditis, pigmentation changes (skin/fingernails), pneumonia, pulmonary hypertension, pulmonary infiltrates, pulmonary veno-occlusive disease, pyelonephritis, radiation recall, renal tubular necrosis, reversible posterior leukoencephalopathy syndrome (RPLS), rhabdomyolysis, secondary malignancy, septic shock, sepsis, SIADH, Stevens-Johnson syndrome, testicular atrophy, thrombocytopenia (immune mediated), thrombotic disorders (arterial and venous), toxic epidermal necrolysis, toxic megacolon, tumor lysis syndrome, wound healing impaired

Drug Interactions

Metabolism/Transport Effects Substrate of CYP2A6 (minor), CYP2B6 (major), CYP2C19 (minor), CYP2C9 (minor), CYP3A4 (minor); **Note:** Assignment of Major/Minor substrate status based on clinically relevant drug interaction potential; **Induces** CYP2B6 (weak/moderate), CYP2C9 (weak/moderate)

Avoid Concomitant Use

Avoid concomitant use of Cyclophosphamide with any of the following: BCG (Intravesical); Belimumab; Deferiprone; Dipyrone; Etanercept; Natalizumab; Pimecrolimus; Tacrolimus (Topical); Tofacitinib; Vaccines (Live)

Increased Effect/Toxicity

Cyclophosphamide may increase the levels/effects of: Amiodarone; Antineoplastic Agents (Anthracycline, Systemic); CloZAPine; CycloSPORINE (Systemic); Deferiprone; Fingolimod; Leflunomide; Natalizumab; Sargramostim; Succinylcholine; Tofacitinib; Vaccines (Live)

The levels/effects of Cyclophosphamide may be increased by: Allopurinol; AzaTHIOprine; Belimumab; CYP2B6 Inducers (Strong); Denosumab; Dipyrone; Etanercept; Filgrastim; Pentostatin; Pimecrolimus; Protease Inhibitors; Quazepam; Roflumilast; Tacrolimus (Topical); Thiazide Diuretics; Trastuzumab

Decreased Effect

Cyclophosphamide may decrease the levels/effects of: BCG (Intravesical); Coccidioides immitis Skin Test; CycloSPORINE (Systemic); Sipuleucel-T; Vaccines (Inactivated); Vaccines (Live)

The levels/effects of Cyclophosphamide may be decreased by: CYP2B6 Inhibitors (Moderate); Dabrafenib; Echinacea; Lumacaftor

Preparation for Administration Hazardous agent; use appropriate precautions for handling and disposal (NIOSH 2014 [group 1]).

Injection powder for reconstitution: Reconstitute with 25 mL for a 500 mg vial, 50 mL for a 1000 mg vial, or 100 mL for a 2000 mg vial to a concentration of 20 mg/mL using NS only for direct IV push, or NS or SWFI for IV infusion; swirl gently to mix. For IV infusion, further dilute for infusion in D5W, 1/2NS, or D5NS, to a minimum concentration of 2 mg/mL.

Storage/Stability

Injection powder for reconstitution: Store intact vials of powder at ≤25°C (77°F). Exposure to excessive temperatures during transport or storage may cause active ingredient to melt (vials with melting may have a clear to yellow viscous liquid which may appear as droplets); do not use vials with signs of melting. Solutions reconstituted in sterile water for injection should be further diluted immediately; do not inject SWFI reconstituted solution directly. Reconstituted solutions in normal saline (NS) are stable for 24 hours at room temperature and for 6 days refrigerated at 2°C to 8°C (36°F to 46°F). Solutions diluted for infusion in 1/2NS or NS are stable for 24 hours at room temperature and for 6 days refrigerated; solutions diluted in D5W or D5NS are stable for 24 hours at room temperature and for 36 hours refrigerated.

Capsules: Store at 20°C to 25°C (68°F to 77°F); excursions are permitted between 15°C and 30°C (59°F and 86°F).

Tablets: Store tablets at ≤25°C (77°F); brief excursions are permitted up to 30°C (86°F); protect from temperatures >30°C (86°F).

Mechanism of Action Cyclophosphamide is an alkylating agent that prevents cell division by cross-linking DNA strands and decreasing DNA synthesis. It is a cell cycle phase nonspecific agent. Cyclophosphamide also possesses potent immunosuppressive activity. Cyclophosphamide is a prodrug that must be metabolized to active metabolites in the liver.

Pharmacodynamics/Kinetics

Absorption: Oral: Well absorbed

Distribution: V_d: 30 to 50 L (approximates total body water); crosses into CSF (not in high enough concentrations to treat meningeal leukemia)

Protein binding: ~20%; some metabolites are bound at >60%

Metabolism: Hepatic to active metabolites acrolein, 4-aldophosphamide, 4-hydroperoxycyclophosphamide, and nor-nitrogen mustard

Bioavailability: >75%

Half-life elimination: IV: 3 to 12 hours; Children: 4 hours; Adults: 6 to 8 hours

Time to peak: Oral: ~1 hour; IV: Metabolites: 2 to 3 hours

Excretion: Urine (10 to 20% as unchanged drug); feces (4%)

Dosing

Adult Cyclophosphamide is associated with a moderate to high emetic potential (depending on dose, regimen, or administration route); antiemetics are recommended to prevent nausea and vomiting (Basch 2011; Roila 2010).

US labeling: **Malignancy:**

IV: 40 to 50 mg/kg in divided doses over 2 to 5 days **or** 10 to 15 mg/kg every 7 to 10 days **or** 3 to 5 mg/kg twice weekly

Oral: 1 to 5 mg/kg/day (initial and maintenance dosing)

Canadian labeling: **Malignancy:**

IV: Initial: 40 to 50 mg/kg (1500 to 1800 mg/m²) administered as 10 to 20 mg/kg/day over 2 to 5 days; Maintenance: 10 to 15 mg/kg (350 to 550 mg/m²) every 7 to 10 days **or** 3 to 5 mg/kg (110 to 185 mg/m²) twice weekly

Oral: Initial 1 to 5 mg/kg/day (depending on tolerance); Maintenance: 1 to 5 mg/kg/day

Indication specific and/or off-label uses/dosing:

Acute lymphoblastic leukemia (off-label dosing): Multiple-agent regimens:

Hyper-CVAD regimen: IV: 300 mg/m² over 3 hours (with mesna) every 12 hours for 6 doses on days 1, 2, and 3 during odd-numbered cycles (cycles 1, 3, 5, 7) of an 8-cycle phase (Kantarjian 2004)

CALGB8811 regimen: IV:

Adults <60 years: Induction phase: 1200 mg/m² on day 1 of a 4-week cycle; Early intensification phase: 1000 mg/m² on day 1 of a 4-week cycle (repeat once); Late intensification phase: 1000 mg/m² on day 29 of an 8-week cycle (Larson 1995)

Adults ≥60 years: Induction phase: 800 mg/m² on day 1 of a 4-week cycle; Early intensification phase: 1000 mg/m² on day 1 of a 4-week cycle (repeat once); Late intensification phase: 1000 mg/m² on day 29 of an 8-week cycle (Larson 1995)

Breast cancer (off-label dosing):

AC regimen: IV: 600 mg/m² on day 1 every 21 days (in combination with doxorubicin) for 4 cycles (Fisher 1990)

CEF regimen: Oral: 75 mg/m²/day days 1 to 14 every 28 days (in combination with epirubicin and fluorouracil) for 6 cycles (Levine 1998)

CMF regimen: Oral: 100 mg/m²/day days 1 to 14 every 28 days (in combination with methotrexate and fluorouracil) for 6 cycles (Levine 1998) **or** IV: 600 mg/m² on day 1 every 21 days (in combination with methotrexate and fluorouracil); Goldhirsch 1998)

Chronic lymphocytic leukemia (off-label dosing): IV: R-FC regimen: 250 mg/m²/day for 3 days every 28 days (in combination with rituximab and fludarabine) for 6 cycles (Robak 2010)

Ewing sarcoma (off-label use): IV: VAC/IE regimen: VAC: 1200 mg/m² (plus mesna) on day 1 of a 21-day treatment cycle (in combination with vincristine and doxorubicin [then dactinomycin when maximum doxorubicin dose reached]), alternates with IE (ifosfamide and etoposide) for a total of 17 cycles (Grier 2003)

Gestational trophoblastic tumors, high-risk (off-label use): IV: EMA/CO regimen: 600 mg/m² on day 8 of 2-week treatment cycle (in combination with etoposide, methotrexate, dactinomycin, and vincristine), continue for at least 2 treatment cycles after a normal hCG level (Escobar 2003; Lurain 2006)

Granulomatosis with polyangiitis (GPA; Wegener granulomatosis) (off-label use; in combination with glucocorticoids):

Low-dose: Oral: 1.5 to 2 mg/kg/day (Jayne 2003; Stone 2010) or 2 mg/kg/day until remission, followed by 1.5 mg/kg/day for 3 additional months (de Groot 2009; Harper 2012)

Pulse: IV: 15 mg/kg (maximum dose: 1200 mg) every 2 weeks for 3 doses, followed by maintenance pulses of either 15 mg/kg IV (maximum dose: 1200 mg) every 3 weeks or 2.5 to 5 mg/kg/day orally on days 1, 2, and 3 every 3 weeks for 3 months after remission achieved (de Groot 2009; Harper 2012)

Hodgkin lymphoma (off-label dosing): IV:

BEACOPP regimen: 650 mg/m^2 on day 1 every 3 weeks (in combination with bleomycin, etoposide, doxorubicin, vincristine, procarbazine, and prednisone) for 8 cycles (Diehl 2003)

BEACOPP escalated regimen: 1200 mg/m^2 on day 1 every 3 weeks (in combination with bleomycin, etoposide, doxorubicin, vincristine, procarbazine, and prednisone) for 8 cycles (Diehl 2003)

Multiple myeloma (off-label dosing): Oral: CyBorD regimen: 300 mg/m^2 on days 1, 8, 15, and 22 every 4 weeks (in combination with bortezomib and dexamethasone) for 4 cycles; may continue beyond 4 cycles (Khan 2012)

Non-Hodgkin lymphoma (off-label dosing): IV:

R-CHOP regimen: 750 mg/m^2 on day 1 every 3 weeks (in combination with rituximab, doxorubicin, vincristine, and prednisone) for 8 cycles (Coiffier 2002)

R-EPOCH (dose adjusted) regimen: 750 mg/m^2 on day 5 every 3 weeks (in combination with rituximab, etoposide, prednisone, vincristine, and doxorubicin) for 6 to 8 cycles (Garcia-Suarez 2007)

CODOX-M/IVAC (Burkitt lymphoma): Cycles 1 and 3 (CODOX-M): 800 mg/m^2 on day 1, followed by 200 mg/m^2 on days 2 to 5 (Magrath 1996) **or** 800 mg/m^2 on days 1 and 2 (Lacasce 2004), in combination with vincristine, doxorubicin, and methotrexate; CODOX-M alternates with IVAC (etoposide, ifosfamide, and cytarabine) for a total of 4 cycles

Lupus nephritis (off-label use): IV: 500 mg once every 2 weeks for 6 doses or 500 to 1000 mg/m^2 once every month for 6 doses (Hahn 2012) **or** 500 to 1000 mg/m^2 every month for 6 months, then every 3 months for a total of at least 2.5 years (Austin 1986; Gourley 1996)

Ovarian germ cell tumors (malignant; off-label use): IV: 150 mg/m^2 on days 1 to 5 every 28 days (in combination with dactinomycin and vincristine) for at least 10 cycles (Slayton 1985)

Small cell lung cancer (SCLC), refractory (off-label use): IV: 1000 mg/m^2 (maximum: 2000 mg) on day 1 every 3 weeks (in combination with doxorubicin and vincristine) until disease progression or unacceptable toxicity (von Pawel 1999)

Stem cell transplant conditioning (off-label use): IV:

Nonmyeloablative transplant (allogeneic): 750 mg/m^2/day for 3 days beginning 5 days prior to transplant (in combination with fludarabine) (Khouri 2008)

Myeloablative transplant:

100 mg/kg (based on IBW, unless actual weight <95% of IBW) as a single dose 2 days prior to transplant (in combination with total body irradiation and etoposide) (Thompson 2008)

50 mg/kg/day for 4 days beginning 5 days before transplant (with or without antithymocyte globulin [equine]) (Champlin 2007)

50 mg/kg/day for 4 days beginning 5 days prior to transplant (in combination with busulfan) (Cassileth 1993)

60 mg/kg/day for 2 days (in combination with busulfan and total body irradiation) (Anderson 1996)

1800 mg/m^2/day for 4 days beginning 7 days prior to transplant (in combination with etoposide and carmustine) (Reece 1991)

Geriatric Refer to adult dosing; adjust for renal clearance.

Pediatric Cyclophosphamide is associated with a moderate to high emetic potential (depending on dose, regimen, or administration route); antiemetics are recommended to prevent nausea and vomiting (Dupuis 2011).

US labeling:

Malignancy:

IV: 40 to 50 mg/kg in divided doses over 2 to 5 days **or** 10 to 15 mg/kg every 7 to 10 days **or** 3 to 5 mg/kg twice weekly

Oral: 1 to 5 mg/kg/day (initial and maintenance dosing)

Nephrotic syndrome, corticosteroid refractory or intolerant, or corticosteroid sparing: Oral: Initial: 2 mg/kg once daily for 8 to 12 weeks (maximum cumulative dose: 168 mg/kg); treatment beyond 90 days may increase the potential for sterility in males; treatment beyond 1 course is not recommended (Lombel 2013)

Canadian labeling: **Malignancy:**

IV: Initial: 2 to 8 mg/kg (60 to 250 mg/m^2) in divided doses for 6 or more days; Maintenance: 10 to 15 mg/kg every 7 to 10 days or 30 mg/kg every 3 to 4 weeks or when bone marrow function recovers

Oral: Initial: 2 to 8 mg/kg (60 to 250 mg/m^2) in divided doses for 6 or more days; Maintenance: 2 to 5 mg/kg (50 to 150 mg/m^2) twice weekly

Indication specific and/or off-label uses/dosing:

Ewing sarcoma (off-label use): IV: VAC/IE regimen: VAC: 1200 mg/m^2 (plus mesna) on day 1 of a 21-day treatment cycle (in combination with vincristine and doxorubicin [then dactinomycin when maximum doxorubicin dose reached]), alternates with IE (ifosfamide and etoposide) for a total of 17 cycles (Grier 2003)

Hodgkin lymphoma (off-label dosing): IV: BEACOPP escalated regimen: 1200 mg/m^2 on day 0 of a 21-day treatment cycle (in combination with bleomycin, etoposide, doxorubicin, vincristine, prednisone, and procarbazine) for 4 cycles (Kelly 2011)

Lupus nephritis (off-label use): IV: 500 to 1000 mg/m^2 every month for 6 months, then every 3 months for a total of 2.5 to 3 years (Austin 1986; Gourley 1996; Lehman 2000)

Ovarian germ cell tumors (malignant; off-label use): IV: 150 mg/m^2 on days 1 to 5 every 28 days (in combination with dactinomycin and vincristine) for at least 10 cycles (Slayton 1985)

Neuroblastoma (off-label dosing): IV: CE-CAdO regimen, courses 3 and 4: 300 mg/m^2 days 1 to 5 every 21 days for 2 cycles (Rubie 1998) **or** 10 mg/kg days 1 to 5 every 21 days for 2 cycles (Rubie 2001). **Note:** Decreased doses may be recommended for newborns or children <10 kg.

Stem cell transplant conditioning (off-label use): Myeloablative transplant: IV: 50 mg/kg/day for 4 days beginning 5 days before transplant (with or without antithymocyte globulin [equine]) (Champlin 2007)

Wilms tumor, relapsed (off-label use): Infants, Children, and Adolescents: IV (in combination with vincristine, doxorubicin, mesna, etoposide, filgrastim, and radiation therapy) (Green 2007):

Pediatrics ≤30 kg: 14.7 mg/kg days 1 to 5 of weeks 3, 9, 15, and 21 and 14.7 mg/kg days 1 to 3 of weeks 6, 12, 18, and 24

Pediatrics >30 kg: 440 mg/m^2 days 1 to 5 of weeks 3, 9, 15, and 21 and 440 mg/m^2 days 1 to 3 of weeks 6, 12, 18, and 24

Renal Impairment

US labeling: There are no dosage adjustments provided in the manufacturer's labeling (use with caution; elevated levels of metabolites may occur).

Canadian labeling:

Mild impairment: There are no dosage adjustments provided in the manufacturer's labeling

Moderate impairment: Dose reduction may be necessary; manufacturer's labeling does not provide specific dosing recommendations

Severe impairment: Use is contraindicated.

The following adjustments have also been recommended:

Aronoff 2007: Children and Adults:

CrCl ≥10 mL/minute: No dosage adjustment required.

CrCl <10 mL/minute: Administer 75% of normal dose.

Hemodialysis: Moderately dialyzable (20% to 50%); administer 50% of normal dose; administer after hemodialysis

Continuous ambulatory peritoneal dialysis (CAPD): Administer 75% of normal dose.

Continuous renal replacement therapy (CRRT): Administer 100% of normal dose.

Janus 2010: Hemodialysis: Administer 75% of normal dose; administer after hemodialysis

Hepatic Impairment The conversion between cyclophosphamide to the active metabolite may be reduced in patients with severe hepatic impairment, potentially reducing efficacy.

US labeling: There are no dosage adjustments provided in the manufacturer's labeling.

Canadian labeling:

Mild-to-moderate impairment: There are no dosage adjustments provided in the manufacturer's labeling.

Severe impairment: Use is contraindicated.

The following adjustments have been recommended (Floyd 2006):

Serum bilirubin 3.1 to 5 mg/dL or transaminases >3 times ULN: Administer 75% of normal dose.

Serum bilirubin >5 mg/mL: Avoid use.

Obesity

American Society of Clinical Oncology (ASCO) Guidelines for appropriate chemotherapy dosing in obese adults with cancer (**Note:** Excludes HSCT dosing): Utilize patient's actual body weight (full weight) for calculation of body surface area- or weight-based dosing, particularly when the intent of therapy is curative; manage regimen-related toxicities in the same manner

as for nonobese patients; if a dose reduction is utilized due to toxicity, consider resumption of full weight-based dosing with subsequent cycles, especially if cause of toxicity (eg, hepatic or renal impairment) is resolved (Griggs 2012).

American Society for Blood and Marrow Transplantation (ASBMT) practice guideline committee position statement on chemotherapy dosing in obesity (Bubalo 2014):
Cy200 (cyclophosphamide total dose of 200 mg/kg): Use the lesser of IBW or actual body weight (ABW).
Cy120 (cyclophosphamide total dose of 120 mg/kg): Use either IBW or ABW for patients ≤120% IBW (preferred method for adults of all body sizes); use ABW25 for patients >120% IBW (preferred for pediatric patients).
ABW25: Adjusted wt (kg) = Ideal body weight (kg) + 0.25 [actual wt (kg) - ideal body weight (kg)]

Adjustment for Toxicity
Hematologic toxicity: May require dose reduction or treatment interruption; Canadian labeling recommends reducing initial dose by 30% to 50% if bone marrow function compromised (due to prior radiation therapy, prior chemotherapy, or tumor infiltration)
Hemorrhagic cystitis, severe: Discontinue treatment

Administration
Cyclophosphamide is associated with a moderate to high emetic potential (depending on dose, regimen, or administration route); antiemetics are recommended to prevent nausea and vomiting (Basch 2011; Dupuis 2011; Roila 2010).

IV: Infusion rate may vary based on protocol (refer to specific protocol for infusion rate). Administer by direct IV injection (if reconstituted in NS), IVPB, or continuous IV infusion

Bladder toxicity: To minimize bladder toxicity, increase normal fluid intake during and for 1 to 2 days after cyclophosphamide dose. Most adult patients will require a fluid intake of at least 2 L/day. High-dose regimens should be accompanied by vigorous hydration with or without mesna therapy. Morning administration may be preferred to ensure adequate hydration throughout the day.

Hematopoietic stem cell transplant: Approaches to reduction of hemorrhagic cystitis include infusion of 0.9% NaCl 3 L/m²/24 hours, infusion of 0.9% NaCl 3 L/m²/ 24 hours with continuous 0.9% NaCl bladder irrigation 300 to 1000 mL/hour, and infusion of 0.9% NaCl 1.5 to 3 L/m²/24 hours with intravenous mesna. Hydration should begin at least 4 hours before cyclophosphamide and continue at least 24 hours after completion of cyclophosphamide. The dose of daily mesna used may be 67% to 100% of the daily dose of cyclophosphamide. Mesna can be administered as a continuous 24-hour intravenous infusion or be given in divided doses every 4 hours. Mesna should begin at the start of treatment, and continue at least 24 hours following the last dose of cyclophosphamide.

Oral: Tablets are not scored and should not be cut, chewed, or crushed. Swallow capsules whole; do not open, crush, or chew. To minimize bladder toxicity, increase normal fluid intake. Morning administration may be preferred to ensure adequate hydration throughout the day; do not administer tablets/capsules at bedtime.

Hazardous agent; use appropriate precautions for handling and disposal (NIOSH 2014 [group 1]). Wear gloves when handling capsules/tablets and container. NIOSH recommends single gloving for administration of intact capsules or tablets (NIOSH 2014). Avoid exposure to broken capsules; if contact occurs, wash hands immediately and thoroughly.

Monitoring Parameters
CBC with differential and platelets, BUN, UA, serum electrolytes, serum creatinine; monitor for signs/symptoms of hemorrhagic cystitis or other urinary/renal toxicity, pulmonary, cardiac, and/or hepatic toxicity

Additional Information
In patients with CYP2B6 G516T variant allele, cyclophosphamide metabolism is markedly increased; metabolism is not influenced by CYP2C9 and CYP2C19 isotypes (Xie 2006).

Dosage Forms
Excipient information presented when available (limited, particularly for generics); consult specific product labeling.
Capsule, Oral:
Generic: 25 mg, 50 mg
Solution Reconstituted, Injection:
Generic: 500 mg (1 ea); 1 g (1 ea); 2 g (1 ea)
Tablet, Oral:
Generic: 25 mg, 50 mg

Dosage Forms: Canada
Additional dosage forms available in Canada. Excipient information presented when available (limited, particularly for generics); consult specific product labeling.
Injection, powder for reconstitution: 200 mg

Extemporaneous Preparations
Hazardous agent: Use appropriate precautions for handling and disposal (NIOSH 2014 [group 1]). When compounding an oral solution or suspension, NIOSH recommends double gloving, a protective gown, and preparation in a controlled device; if not prepared in a controlled device, respiratory and eye protection as well as ventilated engineering controls are recommended (NIOSH 2014).

Liquid solutions for oral administration may be prepared by dissolving cyclophosphamide injection in Aromatic Elixir, N.F. Store refrigerated (in glass container) for up to 14 days.
Cyclophosphamide Prescribing Information, Baxter Healthcare Corporation, Deerfield, Il, May, 2013.

A 10 mg/mL oral suspension may be prepared by reconstituting one 2 g vial for injection with 100 mL of NaCl 0.9%, providing an initial concentration of 20 mg/mL. Mix this solution in a 1:1 ratio with either Simple Syrup, NF or Ora-Plus® to obtain a final concentration of 10 mg/mL. Label "shake well" and "refrigerate". Stable for 56 days refrigerated.
Kennedy R, Groepper D, Tagen M, et al, "Stability of Cyclophosphamide in Extemporaneous Oral Suspensions," *Ann Pharmacother*, 2010, 44(2):295-301.

◆ Cycloset see Bromocriptine *on page 255*
◆ Cyclosporin A see CycloSPORINE (Ophthalmic) *on page 465*
◆ Cyclosporin A see CycloSPORINE (Systemic) *on page 459*

CycloSPORINE (Systemic) (SYE kloe spor een)

Brand Names: US Gengraf; Neoral; SandIMMUNE
Brand Names: Canada Apo-Cyclosporine; Neoral; Sandimmune I.V.; Sandoz-Cyclosporine
Index Terms Ciclosporin; CsA; CyA; Cyclosporin A
Pharmacologic Category Calcineurin Inhibitor; Immunosuppressant Agent

Use
Cyclosporine modified:
Transplant rejection prophylaxis: Prophylaxis of organ rejection in kidney, liver, and heart transplants (has been used with azathioprine and/or corticosteroids)
Rheumatoid arthritis: Treatment of severe, active rheumatoid arthritis (RA) not responsive to methotrexate alone
Psoriasis: Treatment of severe, recalcitrant plaque psoriasis in nonimmunocompromised adults unresponsive to or unable to tolerate other systemic therapy
Cyclosporine non-modified: Transplant rejection (prophylaxis/treatment): Prophylaxis of organ rejection in kidney, liver, and heart transplants (has been used with azathioprine and/or corticosteroids; treatment of chronic organ rejection)

Canadian labeling: Additional uses (not in US labeling):
Cyclosporine modified: Nephrotic syndrome: Induction and maintenance of remission in steroid dependent/resistant nephrotic syndrome due to glomerular disease (eg, minimal change nephropathy, membranous glomerulonephritis, focal and segmental glomerulosclerosis); maintenance of steroid induced remission allowing for steroid dose reduction or withdrawal.
Cyclosporine modified/non-modified: Bone marrow transplantation: Prophylaxis of graft rejection following bone marrow transplantation; prophylaxis or treatment of graft-versus-host disease (GVHD)

Pregnancy Considerations Adverse events were not observed following the use of oral cyclosporine in animal reproduction studies (using doses that were not maternally toxic). In humans, cyclosporine crosses the placenta; maternal concentrations do not correlate with those found in the umbilical cord. Cyclosporine may be detected in the serum of newborns for several days after birth (Claris 1993). Based on clinical use, premature births and low birth weight were consistently observed in pregnant transplant patients (additional pregnancy complications also present). Formulations may contain alcohol; the alcohol content should be taken into consideration in pregnant women.

The pharmacokinetics of cyclosporine may be influenced by pregnancy (Grimer 2007). Cyclosporine may be used in pregnant renal, liver, or heart transplant patients (Cowan 2012; EBPG Expert Group on Renal Transplantation 2002; McGuire 2009; Parhar 2012). If therapy is needed for

psoriasis, other agents are preferred; however, cyclosporine may be used as an alternative agent along with close clinical monitoring; use should be avoided during the first trimester if possible (Bae 2012). If treatment is needed for lupus nephritis, other agents are recommended to be used in pregnant women (Hahn 2012).

Following transplant, normal menstruation and fertility may be restored within months; however, appropriate contraception is recommended to prevent pregnancy until 1-2 years following the transplant to improve pregnancy outcomes (Cowan 2012; EBPG Expert Group on Renal Transplantation 2002; McGuire 2009; Parhar 2012).

A pregnancy registry has been established for pregnant women taking immunosuppressants following any solid organ transplant (National Transplantation Pregnancy Registry, Temple University, 877-955-6877).

A pregnancy registry has also been established for pregnant women taking Neoral for psoriasis or rheumatoid arthritis (Neoral Pregnancy Registry for Psoriasis and Rheumatoid Arthritis, Thomas Jefferson University, 888-522-5581).

Breast-Feeding Considerations Cyclosporine is excreted in breast milk. Concentrations of cyclosporine in milk vary widely and breast-feeding during therapy is generally not recommended (Bae 2012; Cowan 2012). Due to the potential for serious adverse in the breast-feeding infant, a decision should be made to discontinue cyclosporine or to discontinue breast-feeding, taking into account the importance of treatment to the mother. Formulations may contain alcohol which may be present in breast milk and could be absorbed orally by the breast-feeding infant.

Contraindications

Hypersensitivity to cyclosporine or any component of the formulation. IV cyclosporine is contraindicated in hypersensitivity to polyoxyethylated castor oil (Cremophor EL). Rheumatoid arthritis and psoriasis patients with abnormal renal function, uncontrolled hypertension, or malignancies. Concomitant treatment with PUVA or UVB therapy, methotrexate, other immunosuppressive agents, coal tar, or radiation therapy are also contraindications for use in patients with psoriasis.

Canadian labeling: Additional contraindications (not in US labeling): Concurrent use with bosentan; rheumatoid arthritis and psoriasis patients with primary or secondary immunodeficiency excluding autoimmune disease, uncontrolled infection, or malignancy (excluding non-melanoma skin cancer).

Warnings/Precautions Hazardous agent - use appropriate precautions for handling and disposal (NIOSH 2014 [group 2]).

[US Boxed Warning]: Increased risk of lymphomas and other malignancies (including fatal outcomes), **particularly skin cancers;** risk is related to intensity/duration of therapy and the use of more than one immunosuppressive agent; all patients should avoid excessive sun/UV light exposure. **[US Boxed Warning]: May cause hypertension; risk is increased with increasing doses/duration.** Use caution when changing dosage forms.

[US Boxed Warning]: Renal impairment, including structural kidney damage has occurred (when used at high doses); risk is increased with increasing doses/duration; monitor renal function closely. Elevations in serum creatinine and BUN generally respond to dosage reductions. Use caution with other potentially nephrotoxic drugs (eg, acyclovir, aminoglycoside antibiotics, amphotericin B, ciprofloxacin); monitor renal function closely with concomitant use. If significant renal impairment occurs, reduce the dose of the coadministered medication or consider alternative treatment. Elevations in serum creatinine and BUN associated with nephrotoxicity generally respond to dosage reductions. In renal transplant patients with rapidly rising BUN and creatinine, carefully evaluate to differentiate between cyclosporine-associated nephrotoxicity and renal rejection episodes. In cases of severe rejection that fail to respond to pulse steroids and monoclonal antibodies, switching to an alternative immunosuppressant agent may be preferred to increasing cyclosporine to excessive blood concentrations.

[US Boxed Warning]: Increased risk of infection with use; serious and fatal infections have been reported. Bacterial, viral, fungal, and protozoal infections (including opportunistic infections) have occurred. Polyoma virus infections, such as the JC virus and BK virus, may result in serious and sometimes fatal outcomes. The JC virus is associated with progressive multifocal leukoencephalopathy (PML), and PML has been reported in patients receiving cyclosporine. PML may be fatal and presents with hemiparesis, apathy, confusion, cognitive deficiencies, and ataxia; consider neurologic consultation as indicated. The BK virus is associated with nephropathy, and polyoma virus-associated nephropathy (PVAN) has been reported in patients receiving cyclosporine. PVAN is associated with serious adverse effects including renal dysfunction and renal graft loss. If PML or PVAN occur in transplant patients, consider reducing immunosuppression therapy as well as the risk that reduced immunosuppression poses to grafts.

Hepatotoxicity (transaminase and bilirubin elevations) and liver injury, including cholestasis, jaundice, hepatitis, and liver failure, has been reported. These events were mainly in patients with confounding factors including infections, coadministration with other potentially hepatotoxic medications, underlying conditions, and significant comorbidities. Fatalities have also been reported rarely, primarily in transplant patients. Increased hepatic enzymes and bilirubin have occurred, usually in the first month and when used at high doses; improvement is usually seen with dosage reduction.

Should be used initially with corticosteroids in transplant patients. Significant hyperkalemia (with or without hyperchloremic metabolic acidosis) and hyperuricemia have occurred with therapy. Syndromes of microangiopathic hemolytic anemia and thrombocytopenia have occurred and may result in graft failure; it is accompanied by platelet consumption within the graft. Syndrome may occur without graft rejection. Although management of the syndrome is unclear, discontinuation or reduction of cyclosporine, in addition to streptokinase and heparin administration or plasmapheresis, has been associated with syndrome resolution. However, resolution seems to be dependent upon early detection of the syndrome via indium 111 labeled platelet scans.

May cause seizures, particularly if used with high-dose corticosteroids. Encephalopathy (including posterior reversible encephalopathy syndrome [PRES]) has also been reported; predisposing factors include hypertension, hypomagnesemia, hypocholesterolemia, high-dose corticosteroids, high cyclosporine serum concentration, and graft-versus-host disease (GVHD). Encephalopathy may be more common in patients with liver transplant compared to kidney transplant. Other neurotoxic events, such as optic disc edema (including papilloedema and potential visual impairment), have been rarely reported primarily in transplant patients.

[US Boxed Warning]: The modified/non-modified formulations are not bioequivalent; cyclosporine (modified) has increased bioavailability as compared to cyclosporine (non-modified) and the products cannot be used interchangeably without close monitoring. Cyclosporine (modified) refers to the oral solution and capsule dosage formulations of cyclosporine in an aqueous dispersion (previously referred to as "microemulsion"). Potentially significant drug-drug/drug-food interactions may exist, requiring dose or frequency adjustment, additional monitoring, and/or selection of alternative therapy. Gingival hyperplasia may occur; avoid concomitant nifedipine in patients who develop gingival hyperplasia (may increase frequency of hyperplasia). Monitor cyclosporine concentrations closely following the addition, modification, or deletion of other medication. Live, attenuated vaccines may be less effective; vaccination should be avoided. Make dose adjustments based on cyclosporine blood concentrations. **[US Boxed Warning]: Cyclosporine non-modified absorption is erratic; monitor blood concentrations closely. [US Boxed Warning]: Prescribing and dosage adjustment should only be under the direct supervision of an experienced physician. Adequate laboratory/medical resources and follow-up are necessary.** Anaphylaxis has been reported with IV use; reserve for patients who cannot take oral form. **[US Boxed Warning]: Risk of skin cancer may be increased in transplant patients.** Due to the increased risk for nephrotoxicity in renal transplantation, avoid using standard doses of cyclosporine in combination with everolimus; reduced cyclosporine doses are recommended; monitor cyclosporine concentrations closely. Cyclosporine and everolimus combination therapy may increase the risk for proteinuria. Cyclosporine combined with either everolimus or sirolimus may increase the risk for thrombotic microangiopathy/thrombotic thrombocytopenic purpura/hemolytic uremic syndrome (TMA/TTP/HUS). Cyclosporine has extensive hepatic metabolism and exposure is increased in patients with severe hepatic impairment; may require dose reduction.

Patients with psoriasis should avoid excessive sun exposure. **[US Boxed Warning]: Risk of skin cancer may be increased with a history of PUVA and possibly methotrexate or other immunosuppressants, UVB, coal tar, or radiation.**

Rheumatoid arthritis: If receiving other immunosuppressive agents, radiation or UV therapy, concurrent use of cyclosporine is not recommended.

Products may contain corn oil, ethanol (consider alcohol content in certain patient populations, including pregnant or breast-feeding women, patients with liver disease, seizure disorders, alcohol dependency, or pediatrics), or propylene glycol; injection also contains the vehicle Cremophor EL (polyoxyethylated castor oil), which has been associated with hypersensitivity (anaphylactic) reactions. Due to the risk for anaphylaxis, IV cyclosporine should be reserved for use in patients unable to take an oral formulation. Some dosage forms may contain propylene glycol; large amounts are potentially toxic and have been associated hyperosmolality, lactic acidosis, seizures, and respiratory depression; use caution (AAP 1997; Zar 2007).

Adverse Reactions Adverse reactions reported with systemic use, including rheumatoid arthritis, psoriasis, and transplantation (kidney, liver, and heart). Percentages noted include the highest frequency regardless of indication/dosage. Frequencies may vary for specific conditions or formulation.

>10%:
Cardiovascular: Hypertension (8% to 53%), edema (5% to 14%)
Central nervous system: Headache (2% to 25%), paresthesia (1% to 11%)
Dermatologic: Hypertrichosis (5% to 19%)
Endocrine & metabolic: Hirsutism (21% to 45%), increased serum triglycerides (15%), female genital tract disease (9% to 11%)
Gastrointestinal: Nausea (2% to 23%), diarrhea (3% to 13%), gingival hyperplasia (2% to 16%), abdominal distress (<1% to 15%), dyspepsia (2% to 12%)
Genitourinary: Urinary tract infection (kidney transplant: 21%)
Infection: Increased susceptibility to infection (3% to 25%), viral infection (kidney transplant: 16%)
Neuromuscular & skeletal: Tremor (7% to 55%), leg cramps (2% to 12%)
Renal: Increased serum creatinine (16% to ≥50%), renal insufficiency (10% to 38%)
Respiratory: Upper respiratory tract infection (1% to 14%)

Kidney, liver, and heart transplant only (≤2% unless otherwise noted):
Cardiovascular: Chest pain (≤4%), flushing (<1% to 4%), glomerular capillary thrombosis, myocardial infarction
Central nervous system: Convulsions (1% to 5%), anxiety, confusion, lethargy, tingling sensation
Dermatologic: Skin infection (7%), acne vulgaris (1% to 6%), nail disease (brittle fingernails), hair breakage, night sweats, pruritus
Endocrine & metabolic: Gynecomastia (<1% to 4%), hyperglycemia, hypomagnesemia, weight loss
Gastrointestinal: Vomiting (2% to 10%), anorexia, aphthous stomatitis, constipation, dysphagia, gastritis, hiccups, pancreatitis
Genitourinary: Hematuria
Hematologic & oncologic: Leukopenia (<1% to 6%), lymphoma (<1% to 6%), anemia, thrombocytopenia, upper gastrointestinal hemorrhage
Hepatic: Hepatotoxicity (<1% to 7%)
Infection: Localized fungal infection (8%), cytomegalovirus disease (5%), septicemia (5%), abscess (4%), fungal infection (systemic: 2%)
Neuromuscular & skeletal: Arthralgia, myalgia, weakness
Ophthalmic: Conjunctivitis, visual disturbance
Otic: Hearing loss, tinnitus
Respiratory: Sinusitis (<1% to 7%), pneumonia (6%)
Miscellaneous: Fever

Rheumatoid arthritis only (1% to <3% unless otherwise noted):
Cardiovascular: Chest pain (4%), cardiac arrhythmia (2%), abnormal heart sounds, cardiac failure, myocardial infarction, peripheral ischemia
Central nervous system: Dizziness (8%), pain (6%), insomnia (4%), depression (3%), migraine (2% to 3%), anxiety, drowsiness, emotional lability, hypoesthesia, lack of concentration, malaise, neuropathy, nervousness, paranoia, vertigo
Dermatologic: Cellulitis, dermatological reaction, dermatitis, diaphoresis, dyschromia, eczema, enanthema, folliculitis, nail disease, pruritus, urticaria, xeroderma

Endocrine & metabolic: Menstrual disease (3%), decreased libido, diabetes mellitus, goiter, hot flash, hyperkalemia, hyperuricemia, hypoglycemia, increased libido, weight gain, weight loss
Gastrointestinal: Vomiting (9%), flatulence (5%), gingivitis (4%), constipation, dysgeusia, dysphagia, enlargement of salivary glands, eructation, esophagitis, gastric ulcer, gastritis, gastroenteritis, gingival hemorrhage, glossitis, peptic ulcer, tongue disease, xerostomia
Genitourinary: Leukorrhea (1%), breast fibroadenosis, hematuria, mastalgia, nocturia, urine abnormality, urinary incontinence, urinary urgency, uterine hemorrhage
Hematologic & oncologic: Purpura (3% to 4%), anemia, carcinoma, leukopenia, lymphadenopathy
Hepatic: Hyperbilirubinemia
Infection: Abscess (including renal), bacterial infection, candidiasis, fungal infection, herpes simplex infection, herpes zoster, viral infection
Neuromuscular & skeletal: Arthralgia, bone fracture, dislocation, myalgia, stiffness, synovial cyst, tendon disease, weakness
Ophthalmic: Cataract, conjunctivitis, eye pain, visual disturbance
Otic: Tinnitus, deafness, vestibular disturbance
Renal: Abscess (renal), increased blood urea nitrogen, polyuria, pyelonephritis
Respiratory: Cough (5%), dyspnea (5%), sinusitis (4%), abnormal breath sounds, bronchospasm, epistaxis, tonsillitis

Psoriasis only (1% to <3% unless otherwise noted):
Cardiovascular: Chest pain, flushing
Central nervous system: Psychiatric disturbance (4% to 5%), pain (3% to 4%), dizziness, insomnia, nervousness, vertigo
Dermatologic: Acne vulgaris, folliculitis, hyperkeratosis, pruritus, skin rash, xeroderma
Endocrine & metabolic: Hot flash
Gastrointestinal: Abdominal distention, constipation, gingival hemorrhage, increased appetite
Genitourinary: Urinary frequency
Hematologic & oncologic: Abnormal erythrocytes, altered platelet function, blood coagulation disorder, carcinoma, hemorrhagic diathesis
Hepatic: Hyperbilirubinemia
Neuromuscular & skeletal: Arthralgia (1% to 6%)
Ophthalmic: Visual disturbance
Respiratory: Flu-like symptoms (8% to 10%), bronchospasm (5%), cough (5%), dyspnea (5%), rhinitis (5%), respiratory tract infection
Miscellaneous: Fever

Postmarketing and/or case reports (Limited to important or life-threatening; any indication): Anaphylaxis/anaphylactoid reaction (possibly associated with Cremophor EL vehicle in injection formulation), brain disease, central nervous system toxicity, cholestasis, cholesterol increased, exacerbation of psoriasis (transformation to erythrodermic or pustular psoriasis), gout, haemolytic uremic syndrome, hepatic insufficiency, hepatitis, hyperbilirubinemia, hyperkalemia, hyperlipidemia, hypertrichosis, hyperuricemia, hypomagnesemia, impaired consciousness, increased susceptibility to infection (including JC virus and BK virus), jaundice, leg pain (possibly a manifestation of Calcineurin-Inhibitor Induced Pain Syndrome), malignant lymphoma, migraine, myalgia, myopathy, myositis, papilledema, progressive multifocal leukoencephalopathy, pseudotumor cerebri, pulmonary edema (noncardiogenic), renal disease (polyoma virus-associated), reversible posterior leukoencephalopathy syndrome, rhabdomyolysis, thrombotic microangiopathy

Drug Interactions

Metabolism/Transport Effects Substrate of CYP3A4 (major), P-glycoprotein; **Note:** Assignment of Major/Minor substrate status based on clinically relevant drug interaction potential; **Inhibits** BSEP, CYP2C9 (weak), CYP3A4 (weak), P-glycoprotein, SLCO1B1

Avoid Concomitant Use

Avoid concomitant use of CycloSPORINE (Systemic) with any of the following: Aliskiren; AtorvaSTATin; BCG (Intravesical); Bosentan; Bosutinib; Cholic Acid; Conivaptan; Crizotinib; Dronedarone; Enzalutamide; Eplerenone; Foscarnet; Fusidic Acid (Systemic); Idelalisib; Lercanidipine; Lovastatin; Mifepristone; Natalizumab; PAZOPanib; Pimecrolimus; Pimozide; Pitavastatin; Potassium-Sparing Diuretics; Silodosin; Simeprevir; Simvastatin; Sitaxentan; Tacrolimus (Systemic); Tacrolimus (Topical); Tofacitinib; Topotecan; Vaccines (Live); VinCRIStine (Liposomal)

◀

Increased Effect/Toxicity

CycloSPORINE (Systemic) may increase the levels/ effects of: Afatinib; Aliskiren; Ambrisentan; ARIPiprazole; AtorvaSTATin; Boceprevir; Bosentan; Bosutinib; Brentuximab Vedotin; Calcium Channel Blockers (Dihydropyridine); Calcium Channel Blockers (Nondihydropyridine); Caspofungin; Cholic Acid; Colchicine; Dabigatran Etexilate; Dexamethasone (Systemic); Digoxin; Dofetilide; DOXOrubicin (Conventional); Dronedarone; Edoxaban; Eluxadoline; Etoposide; Etoposide Phosphate; Everolimus; Ezetimibe; Fibric Acid Derivatives; Fimasartan; Fingolimod; Flibanserin; Fluvastatin; Hydrocodone; Imipenem; Ledipasvir; Leflunomide; Lercanidipine; Lomitapide; Loop Diuretics; Lovastatin; Methotrexate; MethylPREDNISolone; Minoxidil (Systemic); Minoxidil (Topical); MitoXANtrone; Naloxegol; Natalizumab; Neuromuscular-Blocking Agents; NiMODipine; Nonsteroidal Anti-Inflammatory Agents; PAZOPanib; P-glycoprotein/ ABCB1 Substrates; Pimozide; Pitavastatin; Pravastatin; PredniSOLONE (Systemic); PredniSONE; Protease Inhibitors; Prucalopride; Ranolazine; Repaglinide; Rifaximin; Rosuvastatin; Silodosin; Simeprevir; Simvastatin; Sirolimus; Sitaxentan; Tacrolimus (Systemic); Tacrolimus (Topical); Ticagrelor; Tofacitinib; Topotecan; Vaccines (Live); VinCRIStine (Liposomal)

The levels/effects of CycloSPORINE (Systemic) may be increased by: AcetaZOLAMIDE; Aminoglycosides; Amiodarone; Amphotericin B; Androgens; Angiotensin II Receptor Blockers; Antifungal Agents (Azole Derivatives, Systemic); Aprepitant; Boceprevir; Bromocriptine; Calcium Channel Blockers (Nondihydropyridine); Carvedilol; Chloramphenicol; Conivaptan; Crizotinib; Cyclophosphamide; CYP3A4 Inhibitors (Moderate); CYP3A4 Inhibitors (Strong); Dasatinib; Denosumab; Dexamethasone (Systemic); Eplerenone; Ezetimibe; Fluconazole; Fosaprepitant; Foscarnet; Fusidic Acid (Systemic); GlyBURIDE; Grapefruit Juice; Idelalisib; Imatinib; Imipenem; Ivacaftor; Lercanidipine; Luliconazole; Macrolide Antibiotics; Melphalan; Methotrexate; MethylPREDNISolone; Metoclopramide; Metreleptin; Mifepristone; Netupitant; Nonsteroidal Anti-Inflammatory Agents; Norfloxacin; Ombitasvir, Paritaprevir, and Ritonavir; Ombitasvir, Paritaprevir, Ritonavir, and Dasabuvir; Omeprazole; Osimertinib; Palbociclib; P-glycoprotein/ABCB1 Inhibitors; Pimecrolimus; Potassium-Sparing Diuretics; Pravastatin; PredniSOLONE (Systemic); PredniSONE; Protease Inhibitors; Pyrazinamide; Quinupristin; Ranolazine; Ritonavir; Roflumilast; Simeprevir; Sirolimus; Stiripentol; Sulfonamide Derivatives; Tacrolimus (Systemic); Tacrolimus (Topical); Telaprevir; Temsirolimus; Trastuzumab

Decreased Effect

CycloSPORINE (Systemic) may decrease the levels/ effects of: BCG (Intravesical); Coccidioides immitis Skin Test; GlyBURIDE; Mycophenolate; Sipuleucel-T; Vaccines (Inactivated); Vaccines (Live)

The levels/effects of CycloSPORINE (Systemic) may be decreased by: Adalimumab; Armodafinil; Ascorbic Acid; Barbiturates; Bosentan; CarBAMazepine; Colesevelam; Cyclophosphamide; CYP3A4 Inducers (Moderate); CYP3A4 Inducers (Strong); Dabrafenib; Deferasirox; Dexamethasone (Systemic); Echinacea; Efavirenz; Enzalutamide; Fibric Acid Derivatives; Fosphenytoin; Griseofulvin; Imipenem; MethylPREDNISolone; Metreleptin; Mitotane; Modafinil; Multivitamins/Fluoride (with ADE); Multivitamins/Minerals (with ADEK, Folate, Iron); Multivitamins/Minerals (with AE, No Iron); Nafcillin; Orlistat; Osimertinib; P-glycoprotein/ABCB1 Inducers; Phenytoin; PredniSOLONE (Systemic); PredniSONE; Rifamycin Derivatives; Sevelamer; Siltuximab; Somatostatin Analogs; St Johns Wort; Sulfinpyrazone; Sulfonamide Derivatives; Tocilizumab; Vitamin E; Vitamin E (Oral)

Food Interactions
Grapefruit juice increases cyclosporine serum concentrations. Management: Avoid grapefruit juice.

Preparation for Administration
Hazardous agent - use appropriate precautions for handling and disposal (NIOSH 2014 [group 2]).

Injection: To minimize leaching of DEHP, non-PVC containers and sets should be used for preparation and administration.

Sandimmune injection: Injection should be further diluted (1 mL [50 mg] of concentrate in 20-100 mL of D_5W or NS) for administration by intravenous infusion.

Oral solution: Should be mixed in glass containers (not in plastic).

Storage/Stability
Capsules (modified): Store in the original unit-dose container at 20°C to 25°C (68°F to 77°F).

Capsules (non-modified): Store at 25°C (77°F); excursions are permitted between 15°C and 30°C (59°F and 86°F). An odor may be detected upon opening the unit-dose container, which will dissipate shortly thereafter. This odor does not affect the quality of the product.

Injection: Store below 30°C (86°F) or at controlled room temperature (product dependent). Protect from light. Stability of injection of parenteral admixture at room temperature (25°C) is 6 hours in PVC; 12 to 24 hours in Excel, PAB containers, or glass. The manufacturer recommends discarding diluted infusion solutions after 24 hours.

Oral solution (modified): Store in the original container at 20°C to 25°C (68°F to 77°F). Do not store in the refrigerator. Once opened, use within 2 months. At temperatures below 20°C (68°F), the solution may gel; light flocculation or the formation of a light sediment also may occur. There is no impact on product performance or dosing using the syringe provided. Allow to warm to room temperature (25°C [77°F]) to reverse these changes.

Oral solution (non-modified): Store in the original container at temperatures below 30°C (86°F). Do not store in the refrigerator. Protect from freezing. Once opened, use within 2 months.

Mechanism of Action
Inhibition of production and release of interleukin II and inhibits interleukin II-induced activation of resting T-lymphocytes.

Pharmacodynamics/Kinetics

Absorption: Oral:

Cyclosporine (non-modified): Erratic and incomplete; dependent on presence of food, bile acids, and GI motility; larger oral doses are needed in pediatrics due to shorter bowel length and limited intestinal absorption

Cyclosporine (modified): Erratic and incomplete; increased absorption, up to 30% when compared to cyclosporine (non-modified); less dependent on food, bile acids, or GI motility when compared to cyclosporine (non-modified)

Distribution: Widely in tissues and body fluids including the liver, pancreas, and lungs

V_{dss}: 4-6 L/kg in renal, liver, and marrow transplant recipients (slightly lower values in cardiac transplant patients; children <10 years have higher values); ESRD: 3.49 L/kg

Protein binding: 90% to 98% to lipoproteins

Metabolism: Extensively hepatic via CYP3A4; forms at least 25 metabolites; extensive first-pass effect following oral administration

Bioavailability: Oral:

Cyclosporine (non-modified): Dependent on patient population and transplant type (<10% in adult liver transplant patients and as high as 89% in renal transplant patients); bioavailability of Sandimmune capsules and oral solution are equivalent; bioavailability of oral solution is ~30% of the IV solution

Children: 28% (range: 17% to 42%); gut dysfunction common in BMT patients and oral bioavailability is further reduced

Cyclosporine (modified): Bioavailability of Neoral capsules and oral solution are equivalent:

Children: 43% (range: 30% to 68%)

Adults: 23% greater than with cyclosporine (non-modified) in renal transplant patients; 50% greater in liver transplant patients

Half-life elimination: Oral: May be prolonged in patients with hepatic impairment and shorter in pediatric patients due to the higher metabolism rate

Cyclosporine (non-modified): Biphasic: Alpha: 1.4 hours; Terminal: 19 hours (range: 10-27 hours)

Cyclosporine (modified): Biphasic: Terminal: 8.4 hours (range: 5-18 hours)

Time to peak, serum: Oral:

Cyclosporine (non-modified): 2-6 hours; some patients have a second peak at 5-6 hours

Cyclosporine (modified): Renal transplant: 1.5-2 hours

Excretion: Primarily feces; urine (6%, 0.1% as unchanged drug and metabolites)

Dosing

Adult Neoral/Gengraf and Sandimmune are not bioequivalent and cannot be used interchangeably.

Psoriasis: Oral: Cyclosporine (modified): Initial dose: 2.5 mg/kg daily, divided twice daily

Titration:

US labeling: Increase by 0.5 mg/kg daily if insufficient response is seen after 4 weeks of treatment. Additional dosage increases may be made every 2 weeks if needed (maximum dose: 4 mg/kg daily)

Canadian labeling: Increase by 0.5 to 1 mg/kg daily if insufficient response is seen after 4 weeks of treatment. Additional dosage increases may be made every 4 weeks if needed (maximum dose: 5 mg/kg daily)

Discontinue if no benefit is seen by 6 weeks of therapy at the maximum dose. Once patients are adequately controlled, the dose should be decreased to the lowest effective dose. Doses lower than 2.5 mg/kg daily may be effective. The Canadian labeling recommends attempting to wean patients off therapy if no relapse occurs within 6 months of achieving remission. Treatment longer than 1 year is not recommended.

Note: Increase the frequency of blood pressure monitoring after each alteration in dosage of cyclosporine. Cyclosporine dosage should be decreased by 25% to 50% in patients with no history of hypertension who develop sustained hypertension during therapy and, if hypertension persists, treatment with cyclosporine should be discontinued.

Rheumatoid arthritis: Oral: Cyclosporine (modified): Initial dose: 2.5 mg/kg daily, divided twice daily; salicylates, NSAIDs, and oral glucocorticoids may be continued (refer to Drug Interactions)

Titration:

US labeling: Dose may be increased by 0.5 to 0.75 mg/kg daily if insufficient response is seen after 8 weeks of treatment; additional dosage increases may be made again at 12 weeks (maximum dose: 4 mg/kg daily). Discontinue if no benefit is seen by 16 weeks of therapy.

Canadian labeling: If insufficient response to initial dose after 6 weeks, may increase dose gradually as tolerated (maximum dose: 5 mg/kg daily); maintenance therapy should be individualized to the lowest effective and tolerable dose; may take up to 12 weeks before full effect is achieved.

Note: Increase the frequency of blood pressure monitoring after each alteration in dosage of cyclosporine. Cyclosporine dosage should be decreased by 25% to 50% in patients with no history of hypertension who develop sustained hypertension during therapy and, if hypertension persists, treatment with cyclosporine should be discontinued.

Solid organ transplant (newly transplanted patients): Adjunct therapy with corticosteroids is recommended. Initial dose should be given 4 to 12 hours prior to transplant or may be given postoperatively; adjust initial dose to achieve desired plasma concentration.

Oral: Dose is dependent upon type of transplant and formulation:

Cyclosporine (modified):

Renal: 9 ± 3 mg/kg daily, in 2 divided doses

Liver: 8 ± 4 mg/kg daily, in 2 divided doses

Heart: 7 ± 3 mg/kg daily, in 2 divided doses

Cyclosporine (non-modified): Initial doses of 10 to 14 mg/kg daily have been used for renal transplants (the manufacturer's labeling includes dosing from initial clinical trials of 15 mg/kg daily [range: 14 to 18 mg/kg daily]; however, this higher dosing level is rarely used any longer). Continue initial dose daily for 1 to 2 weeks; taper by 5% per week to a maintenance dose of 5 to 10 mg/kg daily; some renal transplant patients may be dosed as low as 3 mg/kg daily

Note: When using the non-modified formulation, cyclosporine levels may increase in liver transplant patients when the T-tube is closed; dose may need decreased

IV: Cyclosporine (non-modified): Manufacturer's labeling: Initial dose: 5 to 6 mg/kg daily or one-third of the oral dose as a single dose, infused over 2 to 6 hours; use should be limited to patients unable to take capsules or oral solution; patients should be switched to an oral dosage form as soon as possible.

Note: Many transplant centers administer cyclosporine as "divided dose" infusions (in 2 to 3 doses daily) or as a continuous (24-hour) infusion; dosages range from 3 to 7.5 mg/kg daily. Specific institutional protocols should be consulted.

Note: Conversion to cyclosporine (modified) from cyclosporine (non-modified): Start with daily dose previously used and adjust to obtain preconversion cyclosporine trough concentration. Plasma concentrations should be monitored every 4 to 7 days and dose adjusted as necessary, until desired trough level is obtained. When transferring patients with previously poor absorption of cyclosporine (non-modified), monitor trough levels at least twice weekly (especially if initial dose exceeds 10 mg/kg daily); high plasma levels are likely to occur.

Acute graft versus host disease (GVHD), prevention (off-label use in the US): IV followed by oral:

Initial: IV: 3 mg/kg daily 1 day prior to transplant; may convert to oral therapy when tolerated; titrate dose to appropriate cyclosporine trough concentration (in combination with methotrexate); taper per protocol (refer to specific references for tapering and target trough details); discontinue 6 months post-transplant in the absence of acute GVHD (Ratanatharathorn 1998; Ruutu 2013; Storb 1986a; Storb 1986b)

or

Initial: IV: 5 mg/kg (continuous infusion over 20 hours) each day for 6 days (loading dose) starting 2 days prior to transplant, then 3 mg/kg over 20 hours each day for 11 days starting on post-transplant day 4, then 3.75 mg/kg over 20 hours each day for 21 days starting on day 15, then **oral** (in 2 divided daily doses): 10 mg/kg daily days 36 to 83, then 8 mg/kg daily days 84 to 97, then 6 mg/kg daily days 98 to 119, then 4 mg/kg daily days 120 to 180, then discontinue (in combination with methotrexate +/- corticosteroid) (Chao 1993; Chao 2000)

Bone marrow transplantation *(Canadian labeling):*

Note: IV administration is preferred for initial therapy.

Oral: Cyclosporine (modified): Initial: 12.5 to 15 mg/kg daily in 2 divided doses beginning 1 day prior to transplant; Maintenance: ~12.5 mg/kg daily in 2 divided doses every 12 hours for at least 3 to 6 months (higher doses may be required in patients with gastrointestinal conditions which may decrease absorption); decrease dose gradually to zero by 1 year following transplant. Patients who develop GVHD after discontinuation of cyclosporine may be reinitiated on therapy with a loading dose of 10 to 12.5 mg/kg followed by the previously established maintenance dose. Patients with mild, chronic GVHD should be treated with lowest effective dose.

IV: Cyclosporine (non-modified): Initial: 3 to 5 mg/kg daily or one-third of the oral dose as a single dose (infused over 2 to 6 hours) beginning 1 day prior to transplant; Maintenance: May continue initial dose for up to 2 weeks; however, patients should be switched to an oral dosage form as soon as possible.

Focal segmental glomerulosclerosis (off-label use in the US): Oral: Initial: 3.5 to 5 mg/kg daily divided every 12 hours (in combination with oral prednisone) (Braun 2008; Cattran 1999)

Interstitial cystitis (bladder pain syndrome) (off-label use): Oral: Initial: 2 to 3 mg/kg/day in 2 divided doses (maximum of 300 mg daily). Once symptom relief is established, the dose can be tapered as tolerated (to as low as 1 mg/kg as a single daily dose) and in some cases can be stopped with continued benefit. Treatment duration was at least 6 months to more than 1 year in some patients (Forrest 2012; Sairanen 2004; Sairanen 2005; Sairanen 2008).

Nephrotic syndrome *(Canadian labeling):* Oral: Cyclosporine (modified):

Initial: 3.5 mg/kg daily in 2 divided doses every 12 hours; titrate for induction of remission and renal function. Adjunct therapy with low-dose oral corticosteroids is recommended for patients with an inadequate response to cyclosporine (particularly if steroid-resistant).

Maintenance: Dose is individualized based on proteinuria, serum creatinine, and tolerability but should be maintained at lowest effective dose; maximum dose: 5 mg/kg daily. Discontinue if no improvement is observed after 3 months.

Lupus nephritis (off-label use): Oral: Cyclosporine (modified): Initial: 4 mg/kg daily for 1 month (reduce dose if trough concentrations >200 ng/mL); reduce dose by 0.5 mg/kg every 2 weeks to a maintenance dose of 2.5 to 3 mg/kg daily (Moroni 2006)

Ulcerative colitis, severe (steroid-refractory) (off-label use):

IV: Cyclosporine (non-modified): 2 to 4 mg/kg daily, infused continuously over 24 hours. (Lichtiger 1994; Van Assche 2003). **Note:** Some studies suggest no therapeutic difference between low-dose (2 mg/kg) and high-dose (4 mg/kg) cyclosporine regimens (Van Assche 2003).

Oral: Cyclosporine (modified): 2.3 to 3 mg/kg every 12 hours (De Saussure 2005; Weber 2006)

Note: Patients responsive to IV therapy should be switched to oral therapy when possible.

Geriatric Refer to adult dosing. **Sandimmune and Neoral/Gengraf are not bioequivalent and cannot be used interchangeably.**

Pediatric

Bone marrow transplantation *(Canadian labeling)*:

Note: IV administration is preferred for initial therapy.

Oral: Cyclosporine (modified): Initial: 12.5 to 15 mg/kg daily in 2 divided doses beginning 1 day prior to transplant; Maintenance: ~12.5 mg/kg daily in 2 divided doses every 12 hours for at least 3 to 6 months (higher doses may be required in patients with gastrointestinal conditions which may decrease absorption); decrease dose gradually to zero by 1 year following transplant. Patients who develop graft versus host disease (GVHD) after discontinuation of cyclosporine may be reinitiated on therapy with a loading dose of 10 to 12.5 mg/kg followed by the previously established maintenance dose. Patients with mild, chronic GVHD should be treated with lowest effective dose.

IV: Cyclosporine (non-modified): Initial: 3 to 5 mg/kg daily or one-third of the oral dose as a single dose (infused over 2 to 6 hours) beginning 1 day prior to transplant; Maintenance: may continue initial dose for up to 2 weeks; however, patients should be switched to an oral dosage form as soon as possible.

Nephrotic syndrome *(Canadian labeling)*: Oral: Cyclosporine (modified):

Initial: 4.2 mg/kg daily in 2 divided doses every 12 hours; titrate for induction of remission and renal function. Adjunct therapy with low-dose oral corticosteroids is recommended for patients with an inadequate response to cyclosporine (particularly if steroid-resistant).

Maintenance: Dose is individualized based on proteinuria, serum creatinine, and tolerability but should be maintained at lowest effective dose; maximum dose: 6 mg/kg daily. Discontinue if no improvement is observed after 3 months.

Solid organ transplant: Refer to adult dosing. Children may require, and are able to tolerate, larger doses than adults.

Renal Impairment

Nephrotic syndrome: *Canadian labeling:* Initial: 2.5 mg/kg daily

Serum creatinine levels >30% above pretreatment levels: Take another sample within 2 weeks; if the level remains >30% above pretreatment levels, decrease dosage of cyclosporine (modified) by 25% to 50%.

Psoriasis (severe):

Abnormal renal function prior to treatment: Use is contraindicated.

Abnormal renal function during treatment:

US labeling:

Serum creatinine levels ≥25% above pretreatment levels: Take another sample within 2 weeks; if the level remains ≥25% above pretreatment levels, decrease dosage of cyclosporine (modified) by 25% to 50%. If two dosage adjustments do not reverse the increase in serum creatinine levels, treatment should be discontinued.

Serum creatinine levels ≥50% above pretreatment levels: Decrease cyclosporine dosage by 25% to 50%. If two dosage adjustments do not reverse the increase in serum creatinine levels, treatment should be discontinued.

Canadian labeling: Serum creatinine levels >30% above pretreatment levels: Decrease dosage of cyclosporine (modified) by 25% to 50%. If dosage adjustment does not reverse the increase in serum creatinine levels within 30 days, discontinue treatment.

Rheumatoid arthritis:

Abnormal renal function prior to treatment: Use is contraindicated.

Abnormal renal function during treatment: *Canadian labeling:*

Serum creatinine levels >30% above pretreatment levels: Take another sample within 2 weeks; if the level remains ≥30% above pretreatment levels, manufacturer labeling recommends reducing dose but does not provide specific dosing recommendation. If dosage adjustment does not reverse the increase in serum creatinine levels within 30 days, discontinue treatment.

Serum creatinine levels >50% above pretreatment levels: Reduce dose by 50%; if dosage adjustment does not reverse the increase in serum creatinine levels within 30 days, discontinue treatment.

Hemodialysis: Supplemental dose is not necessary.

Peritoneal dialysis: Supplemental dose is not necessary.

Hepatic Impairment

Mild-to-moderate impairment: There are no dosage adjustments provided in the manufacturer's labeling; monitor blood concentrations.

Severe impairment: There are no dosage adjustments provided in the manufacturer's labeling; however, metabolism is extensively hepatic (exposure is increased). Monitor blood concentrations; may require dose reduction.

Dietary Considerations Avoid grapefruit juice with oral cyclosporine use.

Administration

Oral solution: Do not administer liquid from plastic or styrofoam cup. May dilute Neoral oral solution with orange juice or apple juice. May dilute Sandimmune oral solution with milk, chocolate milk, or orange juice. Avoid changing diluents frequently. Mix thoroughly and drink at once. Use syringe provided to measure dose. Mix in a glass container and rinse container with more diluent to ensure total dose is taken. Do not rinse syringe before or after use (may cause dose variation).

Administer this medication consistently with relation to time of day and meals.

Combination therapy with renal transplantation:

Everolimus: Administer cyclosporine at the same time as everolimus

Sirolimus: Administer cyclosporine 4 hours prior to sirolimus

IV: The manufacturer recommends that following dilution, intravenous admixture be administered over 2-6 hours. However, many transplant centers administer as divided doses (2-3 doses/day) or as a 24-hour continuous infusion. Discard solution after 24 hours. Anaphylaxis has been reported with IV use; reserve for patients who cannot take oral form. Patients should be under continuous observation for at least the first 30 minutes of the infusion, and should be monitored frequently thereafter. Maintain patent airway; other supportive measures and agents for treating anaphylaxis should be present when IV drug is given. To minimize leaching of DEHP, non-PVC sets should be used for administration.

Hazardous agent - use appropriate precautions for handling and disposal (NIOSH 2014 [group 2]).

Monitoring Parameters Monitor plasma concentrations periodically and following the addition, modification, or deletion of other medications. Monitor renal function (serum creatinine and BUN) after any cyclosporine dosage changes or addition, modification, or deletion of other medications. Monitor blood pressure after any cyclosporine dosage changes or addition, modification, or deletion of other medications. Monitor for hypersensitivity reactions (IV cyclosporine). Monitor for signs/symptoms of hepatotoxicity, secondary malignancy, infection.

Nephrotic syndrome (Canadian labeling): Baseline blood pressure (2 readings within 2 weeks), fasting serum creatinine (at least 3 levels within 2 weeks), creatinine clearance, urinalysis, CBC, liver function, serum uric acid, serum potassium, and malignancy screening (eg, skin, mouth, lymph nodes). Biweekly monitoring of blood pressure for initial 3 months and then monthly thereafter, frequent monitoring of renal function and periodic cyclosporine trough levels are recommended during therapy. Consider renal biopsy in patients with steroid-dependent minimal change neuropathy who have been maintained on therapy >1 year.

Transplant patients: Cyclosporine trough levels, serum electrolytes, renal function, hepatic function, blood pressure, lipid profile

Psoriasis therapy: Baseline blood pressure, serum creatinine (2 levels each), BUN, CBC, serum magnesium, potassium, uric acid, lipid profile. Biweekly monitoring of blood pressure, complete blood count, serum creatinine, and levels of BUN, uric acid, potassium, lipids, and magnesium during the first 3 months of treatment for psoriasis. Monthly monitoring is recommended after this initial period. (**Note:** The Canadian labeling recommends bimonthly monitoring of serum creatinine after the initial period if serum creatinine remains stable and cyclosporine dose is ≤2.5 mg/kg daily, and monthly monitoring for higher doses). Also evaluate any atypical skin lesions prior to therapy. Increase the frequency of blood pressure monitoring after each alteration in dosage of cyclosporine.

Rheumatoid arthritis: Baseline blood pressure, and serum creatinine (2 levels each); serum creatinine every 2 weeks for first 3 months, then monthly if patient is stable. Increase the frequency of blood pressure monitoring after each alteration in dosage of cyclosporine. Additional Canadian labeling recommendations include CBC, hepatic function, urinalysis, serum potassium and uric acid (baseline and periodic thereafter).

Reference Range Reference ranges are method dependent and specimen dependent; use the same analytical method consistently

Method-dependent and specimen-dependent: Trough levels should be obtained:

Oral: 12-18 hours after dose (chronic usage)

IV: 12 hours after dose **or** immediately prior to next dose

Therapeutic range: Not absolutely defined, dependent on organ transplanted, time after transplant, organ function and CsA toxicity:

General range of 100-400 ng/mL

Toxic level: Not well defined, nephrotoxicity may occur at any level

Recommended cyclosporine therapeutic ranges when administered in combination with everolimus for renal transplant (Zortress product labeling 2013):

Month 1 post-transplant: 100-200 ng/mL

Months 2 and 3 post-transplant: 75-150 ng/mL

Months 4 and 5 post-transplant: 50-100 ng/mL

Months 6-12 post-transplant: 25-50 ng/mL

Test Interactions Specific whole blood assay for cyclosporine may be falsely elevated if sample is drawn from the same central venous line through which dose was administered (even if flush has been administered and/or dose was given hours before); cyclosporine metabolites cross-react with radioimmunoassay and fluorescence polarization immunoassay

Dosage Forms Considerations

Cyclosporine (modified): Gengraf and Neoral

Cyclosporine (non-modified): SandIMMUNE

Cyclosporine injection contains polyoxyethylated castor oil (Cremophor EL)

Dosage Forms Excipient information presented when available (limited, particularly for generics); consult specific product labeling.

Capsule, Oral:

Gengraf: 25 mg, 100 mg [contains cremophor el, fd&c blue #2 (indigotine)]

Neoral: 25 mg, 100 mg [contains alcohol, usp]

SandIMMUNE: 25 mg, 100 mg

Generic: 25 mg, 50 mg, 100 mg

Solution, Intravenous:

SandIMMUNE: 50 mg/mL (5 mL) [contains alcohol, usp, cremophor el]

Generic: 50 mg/mL (5 mL)

Solution, Oral:

Gengraf: 100 mg/mL (50 mL) [contains propylene glycol]

Neoral: 100 mg/mL (50 mL) [contains alcohol, usp]

SandIMMUNE: 100 mg/mL (50 mL) [contains alcohol, usp]

Generic: 100 mg/mL (50 mL)

Dosage Forms: Canada Excipient information presented when available (limited, particularly for generics); consult specific product labeling.

Capsule, Oral:

Neoral: 10 mg, 25 mg, 50 mg, 100 mg [contains alcohol]

Solution, Intravenous:

SandIMMUNE IV: 50 mg/mL (1 mL, 5 mL) [contains alcohol, cremophor el]

Solution, Oral:

Neoral: 100 mg/mL (50 mL) [contains alcohol, propylene glycol]

CycloSPORINE (Ophthalmic)
(SYE kloe spor een)

Brand Names: US Restasis

Brand Names: Canada Restasis®

Index Terms Ciclosporin; CsA; CyA; Cyclosporin A

Pharmacologic Category Calcineurin Inhibitor; Immunosuppressant Agent

Use Increase tear production when suppressed tear production is presumed to be due to keratoconjunctivitis sicca-associated ocular inflammation (in patients not already using topical anti-inflammatory drugs or punctal plugs)

Dosing

Adult & Geriatric Keratoconjunctivitis sicca: Ophthalmic: Instill 1 drop in each eye every 12 hours

Pediatric Keratoconjunctivitis sicca: Ophthalmic: Adolescents ≥16 years: Refer to adult dosing.

Renal Impairment No dosage adjustment provided in manufacturer's labeling. However, dosage adjustment unlikely due to low systemic absorption.

Hepatic Impairment No dosage adjustment provided in manufacturer's labeling. However, dosage adjustment unlikely due to low systemic absorption.

Additional Information Complete prescribing information should be consulted for additional detail.

Dosage Forms Excipient information presented when available (limited, particularly for generics); consult specific product labeling.

Emulsion, Ophthalmic [preservative free]:

Restasis: 0.05% (1 ea) [contains polysorbate 80]

◆ Cyklokapron *see* Tranexamic Acid *on page 1827*

◆ Cymbalta *see* DULoxetine *on page 610*

Cyproheptadine (si proe HEP ta deen)

Brand Names: Canada Euro-Cyproheptadine; PMS-Cyproheptadine

Index Terms Cyproheptadine Hydrochloride; Periactin

Pharmacologic Category Histamine H$_1$ Antagonist; Histamine H$_1$ Antagonist, First Generation; Piperidine Derivative

Use Perennial and seasonal allergic rhinitis and other allergic symptoms including urticaria

Pregnancy Considerations Adverse events have been observed in some animal reproduction studies. Maternal antihistamine use has generally not resulted in an increased risk of birth defects; however, information specific to cyproheptadine is limited. Antihistamines are recommended for the treatment of rhinitis, urticaria, and pruritus with rash in pregnant women (although second generation antihistamines may be preferred). Antihistamines are not recommended for treatment of pruritus associated with intrahepatic cholestasis in pregnancy.

Breast-Feeding Considerations It is not known if cyproheptadine is excreted into breast milk. Premature infants and newborns have a higher risk of intolerance to antihistamines. Use while breast-feeding is contraindicated by the manufacturer. Antihistamines may decrease maternal serum prolactin concentrations when administered prior to the establishment of nursing.

Contraindications Hypersensitivity to cyproheptadine or any component of the formulation; narrow-angle glaucoma; bladder neck obstruction; pyloroduodenal obstruction; symptomatic prostatic hyperplasia; stenosing peptic ulcer; concurrent use of MAO inhibitors; use in debilitated elderly patients; use in premature and term newborns due to potential association with SIDS; breast-feeding

Warnings/Precautions May cause CNS depression, which may impair physical or mental abilities; patients must be cautioned about performing tasks which require mental alertness (eg, operating machinery or driving). Effects may be potentiated when used with other sedative drugs or ethanol. Use with caution in patients with cardiovascular disease; increased intraocular pressure; respiratory disease; or thyroid dysfunction. In the elderly, avoid use of this potent anticholinergic agent due to increased risk of confusion, dry mouth, constipation, and other anticholinergic effects; clearance decreases in patients of advanced age (Beers Criteria). Antihistamines may cause excitation in young children.

Adverse Reactions Frequency not defined.

Cardiovascular: Extrasystoles, hypotension, palpitations, tachycardia

Central nervous system: Ataxia, chills, confusion, dizziness, drowsiness, euphoria, excitement, fatigue, hallucination, headache, hysteria, insomnia, irritability, nervousness, neuritis, paresthesia, restlessness, sedation, seizure, vertigo

Dermatologic: Diaphoresis, skin photosensitivity, skin rash, urticaria

Gastrointestinal: Abdominal pain, anorexia, cholestasis, constipation, diarrhea, increased appetite, nausea, vomiting, xerostomia

Genitourinary: Difficulty in micturition, urinary frequency, urinary retention

Hematologic & oncologic: Agranulocytosis, hemolytic anemia, leukopenia, thrombocytopenia

Hepatic: Hepatic failure, hepatitis, jaundice

Hypersensitivity: Anaphylactic shock, angioedema, hypersensitivity reaction

Neuromuscular & skeletal: Tremor

Ophthalmic: Blurred vision, diplopia

Otic: Labyrinthitis (acute), tinnitus

Respiratory: Nasal congestion, pharyngitis, thickening of bronchial secretions

Drug Interactions

Metabolism/Transport Effects None known.

Avoid Concomitant Use

Avoid concomitant use of Cyproheptadine with any of the following: Aclidinium; Azelastine (Nasal); Cimetropium; Eluxadoline; Glucagon; Glycopyrrolate; Glycopyrrolate (Oral Inhalation); Ipratropium (Oral Inhalation); Levosulpiride; MAO Inhibitors; Orphenadrine; Paraldehyde; Potassium Chloride; Thalidomide; Tiotropium; Umeclidinium

Increased Effect/Toxicity

Cyproheptadine may increase the levels/effects of: Abobotulinumtoxin A; Alcohol (Ethyl); Analgesics (Opioid); Anticholinergic Agents; Azelastine (Nasal); Buprenorphine; Cimetropium; CNS Depressants; Eluxadoline; Glucagon; Glycopyrrolate; Glycopyrrolate (Oral Inhalation); Hydrocodone; Methotrimeprazine; Metyrosine; Mirabegron; Mirtazapine; OnabotulinumtoxinA; Orphenadrine; Paraldehyde; Potassium Chloride; Pramipexole; Ramosetron; RimabotulinumtoxinB; ROPINIRole; Rotigotine; Suvorexant; Thalidomide; Thiazide Diuretics; Tiotropium; Topiramate; Zolpidem

The levels/effects of Cyproheptadine may be increased by: Aclidinium; Brimonidine (Topical); Cannabis; Doxylamine; Dronabinol; Droperidol; HydrOXYzine; Ipratropium (Oral Inhalation); Kava Kava; Magnesium Sulfate; MAO Inhibitors; Mianserin; Minocycline; Nabilone; Perampanel; Pramlintide; Rufinamide; Sodium Oxybate; Tapentadol; Tetrahydrocannabinol; Umeclidinium

Decreased Effect

Cyproheptadine may decrease the levels/effects of: Acetylcholinesterase Inhibitors; Benzylpenicilloyl Polylysine; Betahistine; Gastrointestinal Agents (Prokinetic); Hyaluronidase; Itopride; Levosulpiride; MAO Inhibitors; Secretin; Selective Serotonin Reuptake Inhibitors

The levels/effects of Cyproheptadine may be decreased by: Acetylcholinesterase Inhibitors; Amphetamines

Storage/Stability

Oral solution: Store at 15°C to 30°C (59°F to 86°F); protect from light.

Oral syrup: Store at 20°C to 25°C (68°F to 77°F); excursions permitted to 15°C to 30°C (59°F to 86°F); protect from light.

Oral tablets: Store at 20°C to 25°C (68°F to 77°F).

Mechanism of Action A potent antihistamine and serotonin antagonist, competes with histamine for H_1-receptor sites on effector cells in the gastrointestinal tract, blood vessels, and respiratory tract

Pharmacodynamics/Kinetics

Absorption: Well absorbed

Metabolism: Primarily by hepatic glucuronidation via UGT1A (Walker, 1996)

Half-life elimination: Metabolites: ~16 hours (Paton, 1985)

Time to peak, plasma: 6-9 hours (Paton, 1985)

Excretion: Urine (~40% primarily as metabolites); feces (2% to 20%, <6% as unchanged drug)

Dosing

Adult

Allergic conditions: Oral: 4-20 mg daily divided every 8 hours (not to exceed 0.5 mg/kg/day); some patients may require up to 32 mg daily for adequate control of symptoms

Migraine headache prophylaxis (off-label use): Oral: 2 mg every 12 hours (with or without propranolol) (Holland, 2012; Rao, 2000)

Serotonin syndrome (off-label use): Oral: Initial: 12 mg followed by 2 mg every 2 hours or 4-8 mg every 6 hours as needed for symptom control (Boyer, 2005; Sun-Edelstein, 2008)

Spasticity associated with spinal cord damage (off-label use): Oral: Initial: 2-4 mg every 8 hours; maximum: 8 mg every 8 hours (Barbeau, 1982; Wainberg, 1990)

Geriatric Refer to adult dosing. Initiate therapy at the lower end of the dosage range.

Pediatric

Allergic conditions: Oral: 0.25 mg/kg/day or 8 mg/m²/day in 2-3 divided doses **or**

Children 2-6 years: 2 mg every 8-12 hours (not to exceed 12 mg daily)

Children 7-14 years: 4 mg every 8-12 hours (not to exceed 16 mg daily)

Migraine headache prophylaxis (off-label use): Oral: 4 mg every 8-12 hours

Renal Impairment No dosage adjustment provided in manufacturer's labeling. However, elimination is diminished in renal insufficiency.

Hepatic Impairment No dosage adjustment provided in manufacturer's labeling.

Test Interactions Diagnostic antigen skin test results may be suppressed; false positive serum TCA screen

Dosage Forms Excipient information presented when available (limited, particularly for generics); consult specific product labeling.

Syrup, Oral, as hydrochloride:

Generic: 2 mg/5 mL (10 mL, 473 mL)

Tablet, Oral, as hydrochloride:

Generic: 4 mg

◆ Cyproheptadine Hydrochloride *see* Cyproheptadine *on page* 465

◆ Cyramza *see* Ramucirumab *on page* 1554

◆ Cyred *see* Ethinyl Estradiol and Desogestrel *on page* 701

◆ Cystadane *see* Betaine *on page* 221

◆ Cystagon *see* Cysteamine (Systemic) *on page* 466

◆ Cystaran *see* Cysteamine (Ophthalmic) *on page* 467

Cysteamine (Systemic) (sis TEE a meen)

Brand Names: US Cystagon; Procysbi

Index Terms Cysteamine Bitartrate; Mercaptamine

Pharmacologic Category Anticystine Agent; Urinary Tract Product

Use Nephropathic cystinosis: Treatment of nephropathic cystinosis in adults and pediatric patients

Dosing

Adult & Geriatric Nephropathic cystinosis: Oral: **Note:** Begin therapy as soon as the diagnosis of nephropathic cystinosis has been confirmed.

Initial: Initiate therapy with 1/6 to 1/4 of maintenance dose; titrate slowly upward over 4 to 6 weeks.

Maintenance dose: Dosage adjustments should be made based on target WBC cystine levels (<1 nmol half-cystine/mg protein) and/or plasma cysteamine concentrations. If the patient is tolerating therapy, the target WBC cystine level should be <1 nmol half-cystine/mg protein; patients with poorer tolerability may still receive benefit when WBC cystine levels are kept at <2 nmol half-cystine/mg protein. If the WBC cystine level is >1 nmol half-cystine/mg protein but plasma cysteamine is >0.1 mg/L, confirm that the patient is compliant with regard to administration (including proper dosing interval and relationship between administration of medication and food).

Immediate release: 2 g daily in 4 divided doses; maximum dose: 1.95 g/m²/day or 90 mg/kg/day (off-label dose) (Gahl 2002).

Missed doses: Administer missed dose as soon as possible. If the next scheduled dose is due in <2 hours, skip the missed dose and resume the regular dosing schedule.

Switching from cysteamine hydrochloride or phosphocysteamine solutions: Initiate immediate-release cysteamine bitartrate at an equimolar dose to the cysteamine hydrochloride or phosphocysteamine dose; monitor WBC cystine levels 2 weeks after the switch, then every 3 months thereafter.

Delayed release:

Initial: 0.2 to 0.3 g/m²/day divided every 12 hours; titrate slowly upward over 4 to 6 weeks to target maintenance dose.

Maintenance: 1.3 g/m²/day divided every 12 hours; may increase as needed in 10% increments (maximum dose: 1.95 g/m²/day).

Missed doses: Administer missed dose as soon as possible up to 8 hours after the scheduled dose. If the next scheduled dose is due in <4 hours, skip the missed dose and resume the regular dosing schedule. Do not take 2 doses at one time to make up for the missed dose.

Switching from immediate-release cysteamine bitartrate to delayed-release cysteamine bitartrate: Initiate delayed-release cysteamine bitartrate at a total daily dose equal to the total daily dose of the immediate-release formulation; monitor WBC cystine levels and/or plasma cysteamine concentration 2 weeks after the switch, then quarterly for 6 months, then a minimum of 2 times annually thereafter. Titrate the dose as needed to achieve target WBC cystine concentrations (maximum 1.95 g/m²/day)

Pediatric Nephropathic cystinosis: Oral: **Note:** Begin therapy as soon as the diagnosis of nephropathic cystinosis has been confirmed.

Initial: Initiate therapy with 1/6 to 1/4 of maintenance dose; titrate slowly upward over 4-6 weeks.

Maintenance dose: Dosage adjustments should be made based on target WBC cystine levels (<1 nmol half-cystine/mg protein) and/or plasma cysteamine concentrations. If the patient is tolerating therapy, the target WBC cystine level should be <1 nmol half-cystine/mg protein; patients with poorer tolerability may still receive benefit when WBC cystine levels are kept at <2 nmol half-cystine/mg protein. If the WBC cystine level is >1 nmol half-cystine/mg protein but plasma cysteamine is >0.1 mg/L, confirm that the patient is compliant with regard to administration (including proper dosing interval and relationship between administration of medication and food).

Children and Adolescents weighing ≤50 kg: 1.3 g/m^2/day or 60 mg/kg/day (off-label dose) (Gahl 2002) divided into 4 doses; maximum dose: 1.95 g/m^2/day or 90 mg/kg/day (off-label dose) (Gahl 2002).

Adolescents weighing >50 kg: Refer to adult dosing.

Missed doses: Refer to adult dosing

Switching from cysteamine hydrochloride or phospho-cysteamine solutions: Refer to adult dosing.

Delayed release:

Children ≥2 years and Adolescents: Refer to adult dosing.

Missed doses: Refer to adult dosing.

Switching from immediate-release cysteamine bitartrate to delayed-release cysteamine bitartrate: Refer to adult dosing.

Renal Impairment There are no dosage adjustments provided in the manufacturer's labeling.

Hepatic Impairment There are no dosage adjustments provided in the manufacturer's labeling.

Adjustment for Toxicity

Gastrointestinal symptoms, (gastrointestinal bleeding, nausea, vomiting, anorexia, or abdominal pain), transient skin rashes, CNS symptoms (eg, seizures, lethargy, somnolence, depression, encephalopathy):

Immediate release: Temporarily discontinue therapy. Reinitiate at a lower dose; titrate slowly.

Delayed release: Decrease dose. May temporarily discontinue therapy and reinitiate at a lower dose; titrate slowly.

Severe skin rashes (eg, erythema multiforme bullosa, toxic epidermal necrolysis): Permanently discontinue therapy.

Additional Information Complete prescribing information should be consulted for additional detail.

Dosage Forms Excipient information presented when available (limited, particularly for generics); consult specific product labeling.

Capsule, Oral:

Cystagon: 50 mg, 150 mg

Capsule Delayed Release, Oral:

Procysbi: 25 mg, 75 mg

Cysteamine (Ophthalmic) (sis TEE a meen)

Brand Names: US Cystaran

Index Terms Cysteamine Hydrochloride

Pharmacologic Category Anticystine Agent; Ophthalmic Agent

Use Treatment of corneal cystine crystal accumulation in patients with cystinosis

Dosing

Adult & Geriatric Ocular cystinosis: Ophthalmic: Instill 1 drop in each eye every hour while awake

Renal Impairment No dosage adjustment provided in manufacturer's labeling. However, dosage adjustment unlikely due to low systemic absorption.

Hepatic Impairment No dosage adjustment provided in manufacturer's labeling. However, dosage adjustment unlikely due to low systemic absorption.

Additional Information Complete prescribing information should be consulted for additional detail.

Dosage Forms Excipient information presented when available (limited, particularly for generics); consult specific product labeling.

Solution, Ophthalmic:

Cystaran: 0.44% (15 mL) [contains benzalkonium chloride]

◆ Cysteamine Bitartrate see Cysteamine (Systemic) on page 466

◆ Cysteamine Hydrochloride see Cysteamine (Ophthalmic) on page 467

◆ Cystistat (Can) see Hyaluronate and Derivatives on page 879

◆ Cystospaz-M see Hyoscyamine on page 899

◆ CYT see Cyclophosphamide on page 455

◆ Cytarabine see Cytarabine (Conventional) on page 467

Cytarabine (Conventional)
(sye TARE a been con VEN sha nal)

Brand Names: Canada Cytarabine Injection; Cytosar

Index Terms Ara-C; Arabinosylcytosine; Conventional Cytarabine; Cytarabine; Cytarabine Hydrochloride; Cytosar-U; Cytosine Arabinosine Hydrochloride

Pharmacologic Category Antineoplastic Agent, Antimetabolite; Antineoplastic Agent, Antimetabolite (Pyrimidine Analog)

Use

Acute myeloid leukemia: Remission induction (in combination with other chemotherapy medications) in acute myeloid leukemia (AML)

Acute lymphocytic leukemia: Treatment of acute lymphocytic leukemia (ALL)

Chronic myeloid leukemia: Treatment of chronic myeloid leukemia (CML; blast phase)

Meningeal leukemia: Prophylaxis and treatment of meningeal leukemia

Pregnancy Considerations Adverse effects were demonstrated in animal reproduction studies. Limb and ear defects have been noted in case reports of cytarabine exposure during the first trimester of pregnancy. The following have also been noted in the neonate: Pancytopenia, WBC depression, electrolyte abnormalities, prematurity, low birth weight, decreased hematocrit or platelets. Risk to the fetus is decreased if treatment can be avoided during the first trimester; however, women of childbearing potential should be advised of the potential risks.

Breast-Feeding Considerations It is not known if cytarabine is excreted in breast milk. Due to the potential for serious adverse reactions in the nursing infant, the decision to discontinue cytarabine or to discontinue breast-feeding should take into account the importance of treatment to the mother.

Contraindications Hypersensitivity to cytarabine or any component of the formulation

Warnings/Precautions Hazardous agent - use appropriate precautions for handling and disposal (NIOSH 2014 [group 1]). **[U.S. Boxed Warning]: Myelosuppression (leukopenia, thrombocytopenia and anemia) is the major toxicity of cytarabine.** Use with caution in patients with prior drug-induced bone marrow suppression. Monitor blood counts frequently; once blasts are no longer apparent in the peripheral blood, bone marrow should be monitored frequently. Monitor for signs of infection or neutropenic fever due to neutropenia or bleeding due to thrombocytopenia. **[U.S. Boxed Warning]: Toxicities (less serious) include nausea, vomiting, diarrhea, abdominal pain, oral ulcerations and hepatic dysfunction.** In adults, doses >1000 mg/m^2 are associated with a moderate emetic potential (Basch, 2011; Roila, 2010). In pediatrics, doses >200 mg/m^2 are associated with a moderate emetic potential and 3000 mg/m^2 is associated with a high emetic potential (Dupuis, 2011); antiemetics are recommended to prevent nausea and vomiting.

High-dose regimens are associated with CNS, gastrointestinal, ocular (reversible corneal toxicity and hemorrhagic conjunctivitis; prophylaxis with ophthalmic corticosteroid drops is recommended), pulmonary toxicities and cardiomyopathy. Neurotoxicity associated with high-dose treatment may present as acute cerebellar toxicity (with or without cerebral impairment), personality changes, or may be severe with seizure and/or coma; may be delayed, occurring up to 3 to 8 days after treatment has begun. Risk factors for neurotoxicity include cumulative cytarabine dose, prior CNS disease and renal impairment; high-dose therapy (>18 g/m^2 per cycle) and age >50 years also increase the risk for cerebellar toxicity (Herzig, 1987). Tumor lysis syndrome and subsequent hyperuricemia may occur; monitor, consider antihyperuricemic therapy and hydrate accordingly. Potentially significant drug-drug interactions may exist, requiring dose or frequency adjustment, additional monitoring, and/or selection of alternative therapy. There have been case reports of fatal cardiomyopathy when high dose cytarabine was used in combination with cyclophosphamide as a preparation regimen for transplantation.

Use with caution in patients with impaired renal and hepatic function; may be at higher risk for CNS toxicities; dosage adjustments may be necessary. Sudden respiratory distress, rapidly progressing to pulmonary edema and cardiomegaly has been reported with high dose cytarabine. May present as severe dyspnea with a rapid onset and refractory hypoxia with diffuse pulmonary infiltrates, leading to respiratory failure; may be fatal (Morgan, 2011). Cytarabine (ARA-C) syndrome is characterized by fever, myalgia, bone pain, chest pain (occasionally), maculopapular rash, conjunctivitis, and malaise; generally occurs 6 to 12 hours following administration; may be managed with corticosteroids. Anaphylaxis resulting in acute cardiopulmonary arrest has been reported (rare). There have been reports of acute pancreatitis in patients receiving continuous infusion cytarabine and in patients receiving cytarabine who were previously treated with L-asparaginase. **[U.S. Boxed Warning]: Should be administered under the supervision of an experienced cancer chemotherapy physician. Due to the potential toxicities, induction treatment with cytarabine should be in a facility with sufficient laboratory and supportive resources.** Some

products may contain benzyl alcohol; do not use products containing benzyl alcohol or products reconstituted with bacteriostatic diluent intrathecally or for high-dose cytarabine regimens. Benzyl alcohol is associated with gasping syndrome in premature infants. Delayed progressive ascending paralysis has been reported in two children who received combination chemotherapy with IV and intrathecal cytarabine at conventional doses for the treatment of acute myeloid leukemia (was fatal in one patient). When used for intrathecal administration, should not be prepared during the preparation of any other agents; after preparation, store intrathecal medications in an isolated location or container clearly marked with a label identifying as "intrathecal" use only; delivery of intrathecal medications to the patient should only be with other medications also intended for administration into the central nervous system (Jacobson, 2009).

Adverse Reactions

Frequent:

Central nervous system: Fever

Dermatologic: Rash

Gastrointestinal: Anal inflammation, anal ulceration, anorexia, diarrhea, mucositis, nausea, vomiting

Hematologic: Myelosuppression, neutropenia (onset: 1 to 7 days; nadir [biphasic]: 7 to 9 days and at 15 to 24 days; recovery [biphasic]: 9 to 12 days and at 24 to 34 days), thrombocytopenia (onset: 5 days; nadir: 12 to 15 days; recovery 15 to 25 days), anemia, bleeding, leukopenia, megaloblastosis, reticulocytes decreased

Hepatic: Hepatic dysfunction, transaminases increased (acute)

Local: Thrombophlebitis

Less frequent:

Cardiovascular: Chest pain, pericarditis

Central nervous system: Dizziness, headache, neural toxicity, neuritis

Dermatologic: Alopecia, pruritus, skin freckling, skin ulceration, urticaria

Gastrointestinal: Abdominal pain, bowel necrosis, esophageal ulceration, esophagitis, pancreatitis, sore throat

Genitourinary: Urinary retention

Hepatic: Jaundice

Local: Injection site cellulitis

Ocular: Conjunctivitis

Renal: Renal dysfunction

Respiratory: Dyspnea

Miscellaneous: Allergic edema, anaphylaxis, sepsis

Infrequent and/or case reports: Acute respiratory distress syndrome, amylase increased, angina, aseptic meningitis, cardiopulmonary arrest (acute), cerebral dysfunction, cytarabine syndrome (bone pain, chest pain, conjunctivitis, fever, maculopapular rash, malaise, myalgia); exanthematous pustulosis, hepatic sinusoidal obstruction syndrome (SOS; veno-occlussive disease), hyperuricemia, injection site inflammation (SubQ injection), injection site pain (SubQ injection), interstitial pneumonitis, lipase increased, paralysis (intrathecal and IV combination therapy), reversible posterior leukoencephalopathy syndrome (RPLS), rhabdomyolysis, toxic megacolon

Adverse events associated with high-dose cytarabine (CNS, gastrointestinal, ocular, and pulmonary toxicities are more common with high-dose regimens):

Cardiovascular: Cardiomegaly, cardiomyopathy (in combination with cyclophosphamide)

Central nervous system: Cerebellar toxicity, coma, neurotoxicity (up to 55% in patients with renal impairment), personality change, somnolence

Dermatologic: Alopecia (complete), desquamation, rash (severe)

Gastrointestinal: Gastrointestinal ulcer, pancreatitis, peritonitis, pneumatosis cystoides intestinalis

Hepatic: Hyperbilirubinemia, liver abscess, liver damage, necrotizing colitis

Neuromuscular & skeletal: Peripheral neuropathy (motor and sensory)

Ocular: Corneal toxicity, hemorrhagic conjunctivitis

Respiratory: Pulmonary edema, syndrome of sudden respiratory distress

Miscellaneous: Sepsis

Adverse events associated with intrathecal cytarabine administration:

Central nervous system: Accessory nerve paralysis, fever, necrotizing leukoencephalopathy (with concurrent cranial irradiation, intrathecal methotrexate, and intrathecal hydrocortisone), neurotoxicity, paraplegia

Gastrointestinal: Dysphagia, nausea, vomiting

Ocular: Blindness (with concurrent systemic chemotherapy and cranial irradiation), diplopia

Respiratory: Cough, hoarseness

Miscellaneous: Aphonia

Drug Interactions

Metabolism/Transport Effects None known.

Avoid Concomitant Use

Avoid concomitant use of Cytarabine (Conventional) with any of the following: BCG (Intravesical); Deferiprone; Dipyrone; Natalizumab; Pimecrolimus; Tacrolimus (Topical); Tofacitinib; Vaccines (Live)

Increased Effect/Toxicity

Cytarabine (Conventional) may increase the levels/effects of: CloZAPine; Deferiprone; Fingolimod; Leflunomide; Natalizumab; Tofacitinib; Vaccines (Live)

The levels/effects of Cytarabine (Conventional) may be increased by: Denosumab; Dipyrone; Pimecrolimus; Roflumilast; Tacrolimus (Topical); Trastuzumab

Decreased Effect

Cytarabine (Conventional) may decrease the levels/effects of: BCG (Intravesical); Coccidioides immitis Skin Test; Flucytosine; Sipuleucel-T; Vaccines (Inactivated); Vaccines (Live)

The levels/effects of Cytarabine (Conventional) may be decreased by: Echinacea

Preparation for Administration Hazardous agent; use appropriate precautions for handling and disposal (NIOSH 2014 [group 1]). **Note:** Solutions containing bacteriostatic agents may be used for SubQ and standard-dose (100 to 200 mg/m^2) IV cytarabine preparations, but should not be used for the preparation of either intrathecal doses or high-dose IV therapies.

IV:

Powder for reconstitution: Reconstitute with bacteriostatic water for injection (for standard-dose).

For IV infusion: Further dilute in 250 to 1000 mL 0.9% NaCl or D$_5$W.

Intrathecal: Powder for reconstitution: Reconstitute with preservative free sodium chloride 0.9%; may further dilute to preferred final volume (volume generally based on institution or practitioner preference; may be up to 12 mL) with Elliott's B solution, sodium chloride 0.9% or lactated Ringer's. Intrathecal medications should not be prepared during the preparation of any other agents.

Triple intrathecal therapy (TIT): Cytarabine 30 to 50 mg with hydrocortisone sodium succinate 15 to 25 mg and methotrexate 12 mg are reported to be compatible together in a syringe (Cheung, 1984) and cytarabine 18 to 36 mg with hydrocortisone 12 to 24 mg and methotrexate 6 to 12 mg, prepared to a final volume of 6 to 12 mL, is reported compatible as well (Lin, 2008). Intrathecal preparations should be administered as soon as possible after preparation because intrathecal preparations are preservative free.

Storage/Stability Store intact vials of powder for reconstitution at 20°C to 25°C (68°F to 77°F); store intact vials of solution at 15°C to 30°C (59°F to 86°F).

IV:

Powder for reconstitution: Reconstituted solutions should be stored at room temperature and used within 48 hours.

For IV infusion: Solutions for IV infusion diluted in D$_5$W or NS are stable for 8 days at room temperature, although the manufacturer recommends administration as soon as possible after preparation.

Intrathecal: Administer as soon as possible after preparation. After preparation, store intrathecal medications in an isolated location or container clearly marked with a label identifying as "intrathecal" use only.

Mechanism of Action Inhibits DNA synthesis. Cytarabine gains entry into cells by a carrier process, and then must be converted to its active compound, aracytidine triphosphate. Cytarabine is a pyrimidine analog and is incorporated into DNA; however, the primary action is inhibition of DNA polymerase resulting in decreased DNA synthesis and repair. The degree of cytotoxicity correlates linearly with incorporation into DNA; therefore, incorporation into the DNA is responsible for drug activity and toxicity. Cytarabine is specific for the S phase of the cell cycle (blocks progression from the G$_1$ to the S phase).

Pharmacodynamics/Kinetics

Absorption: Not effective when administered orally; less than 20% absorbed orally

Distribution: V$_d$: 3 ± 11.9 L/kg; total body water; widely and rapidly since it enters the cells readily; crosses blood-brain barrier with CSF levels of 40% to 50% of plasma level

Protein binding: 13%

Metabolism: Primarily hepatic; metabolized by deoxycytidine kinase and other nucleotide kinases to aracytidine triphosphate (active); about 86% to 96% of dose is metabolized to inactive uracil arabinoside (ARA-U); intrathecal administration results in little conversion to ARA-U due to the low levels of deaminase in the cerebral spinal fluid

Half-life elimination: IV: Initial: 7 to 20 minutes; Terminal: 1 to 3 hours; Intrathecal: 2 to 6 hours

Time to peak, plasma: SubQ: 20 to 60 minutes

Excretion: Urine (~80%; 90% as metabolite ARA-U) within 24 hours

Dosing

Adult & Geriatric Note: Doses >1000 mg/m^2 are associated with a moderate emetic potential in adults (Basch, 2011; Roila, 2010); antiemetics are recommended to prevent nausea and vomiting.

Acute myeloid leukemia (AML) remission induction: IV: Standard-dose (manufacturer's labeling; in combination with other chemotherapy agents): 100 mg/m^2/day continuous infusion for 7 days **or** 200 mg/m^2/day continuous infusion (as 100 mg/m^2 over 12 hours every 12 hours) for 7 days

Indication-specific dosing:

AML induction: IV:

7 + 3 regimens (a second induction course may be administered if needed; refer to specific references): 100 mg/m^2/day continuous infusion for 7 days (in combination with daunorubicin **or** idarubicin **or** mitoxantrone) (Arlin, 1990; Dillman, 1991; Fernandez, 2009; Vogler, 1992; Wiernik, 1992) **or** (Adults <60 years) 200 mg/m^2/day continuous infusion for 7 days (in combination with daunorubicin) (Dillman, 1991)

Low intensity therapy (off-label dosing): Adults ≥65 years: SubQ: 20 mg/m^2/day for 14 days out of every 28-day cycle for at least 4 cycles (Fenaux, 2010) **or** 10 mg/m^2 every 12 hours for 21 days; if complete response not achieved, may repeat a second course after 15 days (Tilly, 1990)

AML consolidation (off-label use): IV:

5 + 2 regimens: 100 mg/m^2/day continuous infusion for 5 days (in combination with daunorubicin **or** idarubicin **or** mitoxantrone) (Arlin, 1990; Wiernik, 1992)

5 + 2 + 5 regimen: 100 mg/m^2/day continuous infusion for 5 days (in combination with daunorubicin **and** etoposide) (Bishop, 1996)

Single-agent: Adults ≤60 years: 3000 mg/m^2 over 3 hours every 12 hours on days 1, 3, and 5 (total of 6 doses); repeat every 28 to 35 days for 4 courses (Mayer, 1994)

AML salvage treatment (off-label use): IV:

CLAG regimen: 2000 mg/m^2/day over 4 hours for 5 days (in combination with cladribine and G-CSF); may repeat once if needed (Wrzesień -Kuś, 2003)

CLAG-M regimen: 2000 mg/m^2/day over 4 hours for 5 days (in combination with cladribine, G-CSF, and mitoxantrone); may repeat once if needed (Wierzbowska, 2008)

FLAG regimen: 2000 mg/m^2/day over 4 hours for 5 days (in combination with fludarabine and G-CSF); may repeat once if needed (Montillo, 1998)

GCLAC regimen: Adults 18 to 70 years (Becker, 2011):

Induction: 2,000 mg/m^2 over 2 hours once daily for 5 days (in combination with clofarabine and filgrastim; administer 4 hours after initiation of clofarabine); may repeat induction once if needed.

Consolidation: 1,000 mg/m^2 over 2 hours once daily for 5 days (in combination with clofarabine and filgrastim; administer 4 hours after initiation of clofarabine) for 1 or 2 cycles

HiDAC (high-dose cytarabine) ± an anthracycline: 3000 mg/m^2 over 1 hour every 12 hours for 6 days (total of 12 doses) (Herzig, 1985)

MEC regimen: 1000 mg/m^2/day over 6 hours for 6 days (in combination with mitoxantrone and etoposide) (Amadori, 1991) **or**

Adults <60 years: 500 mg/m^2/day continuous infusion days 1, 2, and 3 and days 8, 9, and 10 (in combination with mitoxantrone and etoposide); may administer a second course if needed (Archimbaud, 1991; Archimbaud, 1995)

Acute promyelocytic leukemia (APL) induction (off-label dosing): IV: 200 mg/m^2/day continuous infusion for 7 days beginning on day 3 of treatment (in combination with tretinoin and daunorubicin) (Ades, 2006; Ades, 2008; Powell, 2010)

APL consolidation (off-label use): IV:

In combination with idarubicin and tretinoin: High-risk patients (WBC ≥10,000/mm^3) (Sanz, 2010): Adults ≤60 years:

First consolidation course: 1000 mg/m^2/day for 4 days

Third consolidation course: 150 mg/m^2 every 8 hours for 4 days

In combination with idarubicin, tretinoin, and thioguanine: High-risk patients (WBC >10,000/mm^3) (Lo Coco, 2010): Adults ≤61 years:

First consolidation course: 1000 mg/m^2/day for 4 days

Third consolidation course: 150 mg/m^2 every 8 hours for 5 days

In combination with daunorubicin (Ades, 2006; Ades, 2008):

First consolidation course: 200 mg/m^2/day for 7 days

Second consolidation course:

Age ≤60 years and low risk (WBC <10,000/mm^3): 1000 mg/m^2 every 12 hours for 4 days (8 doses)

Age <50 years and high risk (WBC ≥10,000/mm^3): 2000 mg/m^2 every 12 hours for 5 days (10 doses)

Age 50 to 60 years and high risk (WBC ≥10,000/mm^3): 1500 mg/m^2 every 12 hours for 5 days (10 doses) (Ades, 2008)

Age >60 years and high risk (WBC ≥10,000/mm^3): 1000 mg/m^2 every 12 hours for 4 days (8 doses)

Acute lymphocytic leukemia (ALL; off-label dosing):

Induction regimen, relapsed or refractory: IV: 3000 mg/m^2 over 3 hours daily for 5 days (in combination with idarubicin [day 3]) (Weiss, 2002)

Dose-intensive regimen: IV: 3000 mg/m^2 over 2 hours every 12 hours days 2 and 3 (4 doses/cycle) of even numbered cycles (in combination with methotrexate; alternates with Hyper-CVAD) (Kantarjian, 2000)

CALGB 8811 regimen (Larson, 1995): SubQ

Early intensification phase: 75 mg/m^2/dose days 1 to 4 and 8 to 11 (4-week cycle; repeat once)

Late intensification phase: 75 mg/m^2/dose days 29 to 32 and 36 to 39

Linker protocol: Adults <50 years: IV: 300 mg/m^2/day days 1, 4, 8, and 11 of even numbered consolidation cycles (in combination with teniposide) (Linker, 1991)

Chronic lymphocytic leukemia (CLL; off-label use):

OFAR regimen: IV: 1000 mg/m^2/dose over 2 hours days 2 and 3 every 4 weeks for up to 6 cycles (in combination with oxaliplatin, fludarabine, and rituximab) (Tsimberidou, 2008)

Primary central nervous system (CNS) lymphoma (off-label use): IV: 2000 mg/m^2 over 1 hour every 12 hours days 2 and 3 (total of 4 doses) every 3 weeks (in combination with methotrexate and followed by whole brain irradiation) for a total of 4 courses (Ferreri, 2009)

Hodgkin lymphoma, relapsed or refractory (off-label use): IV:

DHAP regimen: 2000 mg/m^2 over 3 hours every 12 hours day 2 (total of 2 doses/cycle) for 2 cycles (in combination with dexamethasone and cisplatin) (Josting, 2002)

ESHAP regimen: 2000 mg/m^2 day 5 (in combination with etoposide, methylprednisolone, and cisplatin) every 3 to 4 weeks for 3 or 6 cycles (Aparicio, 1999)

Mini-BEAM regimen: 100 mg/m^2 every 12 hours days 2 to 5 (total of 8 doses) every 4 to 6 weeks (in combination with carmustine, etoposide, and melphalan) (Colwill, 1995; Martin, 2001)

BEAM regimen (transplant preparative regimen): 200 mg/m^2 twice daily for 4 days beginning 5 days prior to transplant (in combination with carmustine, etoposide, and melphalan) (Chopra, 1993)

Non-Hodgkin lymphomas (off-label use): IV:

CALGB 9251 regimen: Cycles 2, 4, and 6: 150 mg/m^2/day continuous infusion days 4 and 5 (Lee, 2001; Rizzieri, 2004)

CODOX-M/IVAC regimen:

Adults ≤60 years: Cycles 2 and 4 (IVAC): 2000 mg/m^2 every 12 hours days 1 and 2 (total of 4 doses/cycle) (IVAC is combination with ifosfamide, mesna, and etoposide; IVAC alternates with CODOX-M) (Magrath, 1996)

Adults ≤65 years: Cycles 2 and 4 (IVAC): 2000 mg/m^2 over 3 hours every 12 hours days 1 and 2 (total of 4 doses/cycle) (IVAC is combination with ifosfamide, mesna, and etoposide; IVAC alternates with CODOX-M) (Mead, 2008)

Adults >65 years: Cycles 2 and 4 (IVAC): 1000 mg/m^2 over 3 hours every 12 hours days 1 and 2 (total of 4 doses/cycle) (IVAC is combination with ifosfamide, mesna, and etoposide; IVAC alternates with CODOX-M) (Mead, 2008)

DHAP regimen:

Adults ≤70 years: 2000 mg/m^2 over 3 hours every 12 hours day 2 (total of 2 doses/cycle) every 3 to 4 weeks for 6 to 10 cycles (in combination with dexamethasone and cisplatin) (Velasquez, 1988)

Adults >70 years: 1000 mg/m^2 over 3 hours every 12 hours day 2 (total of 2 doses/cycle) every 3 to 4 weeks for 6 to 10 cycles (in combination with dexamethasone and cisplatin) (Velasquez, 1988)

ESHAP regimen: 2000 mg/m^2 over 2 hours day 5 every 3 to 4 weeks for 6 to 8 cycles (in combination with etoposide, methylprednisolone, and cisplatin) (Velasquez, 1994)

◀

BEAM regimen (transplant preparative regimen): 200 mg/m^2 twice daily for 3 days beginning 4 days prior to transplant (in combination with carmustine, etoposide, and melphalan) (Linch, 2010) **or** 100 mg/m^2 over 1 hour every 12 hours for 4 days beginning 5 days prior to transplant (in combination with carmustine, etoposide, and melphalan) (van Imhoff, 2005)

Meningeal leukemia: Intrathecal: **Note:** Optimal intrathecal chemotherapy dosing should be based on age rather than on body surface area (BSA); CSF volume correlates with age and not to BSA (Bleyer, 1983; Kerr, 2001). Dosing provided in the manufacturer's labeling is BSA-based (usual dose 30 mg/m^2 every 4 days; range: 5 to 75 mg/m^2 once daily for 4 days or once every 4 days until CNS findings normalize, followed by 1 additional treatment).

Off-label uses or doses for intrathecal therapy: Intrathecal:

CNS prophylaxis (ALL): 100 mg weekly for 8 doses, then every 2 weeks for 8 doses, then monthly for 6 doses (high-risk patients) **or** 100 mg on day 7 or 8 with each chemotherapy cycle for 4 doses (low risk patients) **or** 16 doses (high-risk patients) (Cortes, 1995)

or as part of intrathecal triple therapy (TIT): 40 mg days 0 and 14 during induction, days 1, 4, 8, and 11 during CNS therapy phase, every 18 weeks during intensification and maintenance phases (Storring, 2009)

CNS prophylaxis (APL, as part of TIT): 50 mg per dose; administer 1 dose prior to consolidation and 2 doses during each of 2 consolidation phases (total of 5 doses) (Ades, 2006; Ades, 2008)

CNS leukemia treatment (ALL, as part of TIT): 40 mg twice weekly until CSF cleared (Storring, 2009)

CNS lymphoma treatment: 50 mg twice a week for 4 weeks, then weekly for 4-8 weeks, then every other week for 4 weeks, then every 4 weeks for 4 doses (Glantz, 1999)

Leptomeningeal metastases treatment: 25 to 100 mg twice weekly for 4 weeks, then once weekly for 4 weeks, then a maintenance regimen of once a month (Chamberlain, 2010) **or** 40 to 60 mg per dose (DeAngelis, 2005)

Pediatric Note: Doses >200 mg/m^2 are associated with a moderate emetic potential and 3000 mg/m^2 is associated with a high emetic potential (Dupuis, 2011); antiemetics are recommended to prevent nausea and vomiting.

Acute myeloid leukemia (AML) remission induction: IV: Standard-dose (manufacturer's labeling labeling; in combination with other chemotherapy agents): 100 mg/m^2/day continuous infusion for 7 days **or** 200 mg/m^2/day continuous infusion (as 100 mg/m^2 over 12 hours every 12 hours) for 7 days

Indication-specific dosing:
AML induction: *7 + 3 regimen:* IV:

Children <3 years (off-label dosing): 3.3 mg/kg/day continuous infusion for 7 days; minimum of 2 courses (in combination with daunorubicin) (Woods, 1990)

Children ≥3 years: 100 mg/m^2/day continuous infusion for 7 days; minimum of 2 courses (in combination with daunorubicin) (Woods, 1990)

AML consolidation (off-label use): *5 + 2 + 5 regimen:* IV: Adolescents ≥15 years: 100 mg/m^2/day continuous infusion for 5 days for 2 consolidation courses (in combination with daunorubicin and etoposide) (Bishop, 1996)

AML salvage treatment (off-label use):

Clofarabine/Cytarabine regimen: Induction: IV: Children ≥1 year and Adolescents: 1,000 mg/m^2/day over 2 hours for 5 days (in combination with clofarabine; cytarabine is administered 4 hours after initiation of clofarabine) for up to 2 induction cycles (Cooper, 2014)

FLAG regimen: IV: Children ≥11 years: 2,000 mg/m^2/day over 4 hours for 5 days (in combination with fludarabine and G-CSF); may repeat once if needed (Montillo, 1998)

MEC regimen: IV:

Children ≥5 years: 1,000 mg/m^2/day over 6 hours for 6 days (in combination with etoposide and mitoxantrone) (Amadori, 1991)

Adolescents ≥15 years: 500 mg/m^2/day continuous infusion days 1, 2, and 3 and days 8, 9, and 10 (in combination with mitoxantrone and etoposide); may administer a second course if needed (Archimbaud, 1991; Archimbaud, 1995)

Acute lymphocytic leukemia (ALL; off-label dosing): *POG 8602/PVA regimen, intensification phase:* IV: Children ≥1 year: 1,000 mg/m^2 continuous infusion over 24 hours day 1 (beginning 12 hours after start of methotrexate) every 3 weeks or every 12 weeks for 6 cycles (Land, 1994)

Non-Hodgkin lymphomas (off-label use):

CODOX-M/IVAC regimen: IV: Children ≥3 years: Cycles 2 and 4 (IVAC): 2,000 mg/m^2 every 12 hours days 1 and 2 (total of 4 doses/cycle) (IVAC is combination with ifosfamide, mesna and etoposide; IVAC alternates with CODOX-M) (Magrath, 1996)

High-dose cytarabine: IV: Children >1 year and Adolescents: 3,000 mg/m^2 over 3 hours every 12 hours on days 2 and 3 (secondary phase; total of 4 doses) in combination with methotrexate and intrathecal methotrexate/cytarabine (Bowman, 1996)

Meningeal leukemia: Intrathecal: **Note:** Optimal intrathecal chemotherapy dosing should be based on age rather than on body surface area (BSA); CSF volume correlates with age and not to BSA (Bleyer, 1983; Kerr, 2001). Dosing provided in the manufacturer's labeling is BSA-based (usual dose 30 mg/m^2 every 4 days; range: 5 to 75 mg/m^2 once daily for 4 days or once every 4 days until CNS findings normalize, followed by 1 additional treatment).

Age-based intrathecal dosing (off-label; Woods, 1990): Intrathecal:

CNS prophylaxis:
<1 year: 20 mg per dose
1 to 1.99 years: 30 mg per dose
2 to 2.99 years: 50 mg per dose
≥3 years: 70 mg per dose

ALL CNS prophylaxis, age-specific doses from literature:

Administer on day 0 of induction therapy (Gaynon, 1993):
1 to <2 years: 30 mg per dose
2 to <3 years: 50 mg per dose
≥3 years: 70 mg per dose

Administer as part of triple intrathecal therapy (TIT) on days 1 and 15 of induction therapy; days 1, 15, 50, and 64 (standard risk patients) or days 1, 15, 29, and 43 (high-risk patients) during consolidation therapy; day 1 of reinduction therapy, and during maintenance therapy (very high-risk patients receive on days 1, 22, 45, and 59 of induction, days 8, 22, 36, and 50 of consolidation therapy, days 8 and 38 of reinduction therapy, and during maintenance) (Lin, 2007):
<1 year: 18 mg per dose
1 to 2 years: 24 mg per dose
2 to 3 years: 30 mg per dose
≥3 years: 36 mg per dose

Administer on day 0 of induction therapy, then as part of TIT on days 7, 14, and 21 during consolidation therapy; as part of TIT on days 0, 28, and 35 for 2 cycles of delayed intensification therapy, and then maintenance treatment as part of TIT on day 0 every 12 weeks for 38 months (boys) or 26 months (girls) from initial induction treatment (Matloub, 2006):
1 to <2 years: 16 mg per dose
2 to <3 years: 20 mg per dose
≥3 years: 24 to 30 mg per dose

Administer on day 15 of induction therapy, days 1 and 15 of reinduction phase; and day 1 of cycle 2 of maintenance 1A phase (Pieters, 2007):
<1 year: 15 mg per dose
≥1 year: 20 mg per dose

Treatment, CNS leukemia (ALL): Intrathecal: Administer as part of TIT weekly until CSF remission, then every 4 weeks throughout continuation treatment (Lin, 2007):
<1 year: 18 mg per dose
1 to 2 years: 24 mg per dose
2 to 3 years: 30 mg per dose
≥3 years: 36 mg per dose

Renal Impairment There are no dosage adjustments provided in the manufacturer's labeling; however, the following adjustments have been recommended:

Aronoff, 2007 (cytarabine 100 to 200 mg/m^2): Children and Adults: No adjustment necessary

Kintzel, 1995 (high-dose cytarabine 1 to 3 g/m^2):
CrCl 46 to 60 mL/minute: Administer 60% of dose
CrCl 31 to 45 mL/minute: Administer 50% of dose
CrCl <30 mL/minute: Consider use of alternative drug

Smith, 1997 (high-dose cytarabine; ≥2 g/m^2/dose):
Serum creatinine 1.5 to 1.9 mg/dL or increase (from baseline) of 0.5 to 1.2 mg/dL: Reduce dose to 1 g/m^2/dose
Serum creatinine ≥2 mg/dL or increase (from baseline) of >1.2 mg/dL: Reduce dose to 0.1 g/m^2/day as a continuous infusion

Hemodialysis: In 4 hour dialysis sessions (with high flow polysulfone membrane) 6 hours after cytarabine 1 g/m^2 over 2 hours, 63% of the metabolite ARA-U was extracted from plasma (based on a single adult case report) (Radeski, 2011)

Hepatic Impairment Dose may need to be adjusted in patients with liver failure since cytarabine is partially detoxified in the liver. There are no dosage adjustments provided in the manufacturer's labeling; however, the following adjustments have been recommended:

Floyd, 2006: Transaminases (any elevation): Administer 50% of dose; may increase subsequent doses in the absence of toxicities

Koren, 1992 (dose level not specified): Bilirubin >2 mg/dL: Administer 50% of dose; may increase subsequent doses in the absence of toxicities

Obesity

American Society of Clinical Oncology (ASCO) Guidelines for appropriate chemotherapy dosing in obese adults with cancer: Utilize patient's actual body weight (full weight) for calculation of body surface area- or weight-based dosing, particularly when the intent of therapy is curative; manage regimen-related toxicities in the same manner as for nonobese patients; if a dose reduction is utilized due to toxicity, consider resumption of full weight-based dosing with subsequent cycles, especially if cause of toxicity is resolved (eg, hepatic or renal impairment) is resolved (Griggs, 2012).

American Society for Blood and Marrow Transplantation (ASBMT) practice guideline committee position statement on chemotherapy dosing in obesity: Utilize actual body weight (full weight) for calculation of body surface area in cytarabine dosing for hematopoietic stem cell transplant conditioning regimens in pediatrics and adults (Bubalo, 2014).

Administration

IV: Infuse standard dose therapy for AML (100 to 200 mg/m^2/day) as a continuous infusion. Infuse high-dose therapy (off-label) over 1 to 3 hours (usually). Other rates have been used; refer to specific reference.

In adults, doses >1000 mg/m^2 are associated with a moderate emetic potential (Basch, 2011; Roila, 2010). In pediatrics, doses >200 mg/m^2 are associated with a moderate emetic potential and 3000 mg/m^2 is associated with a high emetic potential (Dupuis, 2011); antiemetics are recommended to prevent nausea and vomiting.

Intrathecal: Intrathecal doses should be administered as soon as possible after preparation.

May also be administered SubQ.

Hazardous agent; use appropriate precautions for handling and disposal (NIOSH 2014 [group 1]).

Monitoring Parameters Liver function tests, CBC with differential and platelet count, serum creatinine, BUN, serum uric acid

Dosage Forms Excipient information presented when available (limited, particularly for generics); consult specific product labeling.

Solution, Injection:
Generic: 20 mg/mL (25 mL); 100 mg/mL (20 mL)
Solution, Injection [preservative free]:
Generic: 20 mg/mL (5 mL, 50 mL); 100 mg/mL (20 mL)
Solution Reconstituted, Injection:
Generic: 100 mg (1 ea); 500 mg (1 ea); 1 g (1 ea)

◆ Cytarabine Hydrochloride *see* Cytarabine (Conventional) *on page 467*

◆ Cytarabine Injection (Can) *see* Cytarabine (Conventional) *on page 467*

◆ Cytarabine Lipid Complex *see* Cytarabine (Liposomal) *on page 471*

Cytarabine (Liposomal)
(sye TARE a been lye po SO mal)

Brand Names: US DepoCyt
Brand Names: Canada DepoCyt
Index Terms Cytarabine Lipid Complex; Cytarabine Liposome; DepoFoam-Encapsulated Cytarabine; DTC 101; Liposomal Cytarabine
Pharmacologic Category Antineoplastic Agent, Antimetabolite; Antineoplastic Agent, Antimetabolite (Pyrimidine Analog)
Use Lymphomatous meningitis: Intrathecal treatment of lymphomatous meningitis
Pregnancy Considerations Adverse effects were observed in animal reproductive studies with conventional cytarabine. Conventional cytarabine has been associated with fetal malformations when given as a component of systemic combination chemotherapy during the first trimester. Systemic exposure following intrathecal administration of cytarabine liposomal is negligible; however, women of childbearing potential should avoid becoming pregnant during treatment.

Breast-Feeding Considerations It is not known if cytarabine (liposomal) is excreted in breast milk; the systemic exposure following intrathecal administration of cytarabine (liposomal) is negligible. Due to the potential for serious adverse reactions in the nursing infant, a decision should be made to discontinue cytarabine (liposomal) or to discontinue breast-feeding, taking into account the importance of treatment to the mother.

Contraindications Hypersensitivity to cytarabine or any component of the formulation; active meningeal infection

Warnings/Precautions Hazardous agent - use appropriate precautions for handling and disposal (NIOSH 2014 [group 1]). **[US Boxed Warning]: Chemical arachnoiditis (nausea, vomiting, headache, fever) occurs commonly; may be fatal if untreated. Dexamethasone should be administered concomitantly with cytarabine (liposomal) to diminish chemical arachnoid symptoms;** the incidence and severity of chemical arachnoiditis is reduced with dexamethasone. If chemical arachnoiditis is suspected, exclude other possible inflammatory, infectious, or neoplastic conditions. Toxic effects may be related to a single dose or to cumulative administration and usually occur within 5 days, although may occur at any time during treatment. Monitor continuously for development of neurotoxicity; dose reduction or discontinuation may be necessary. Hydrocephalus has been reported and may be precipitated by chemical arachnoiditis.

May cause neurotoxicity (including myelopathy), which may lead to permanent neurologic deficit (rare). The risk for neurotoxicity is increased when administered with other antineoplastic agents or with cranial/spinal irradiation. CSF flow blockage may lead to increased free cytarabine concentrations in the CSF and increases the risk for neurotoxicity; consider assessing CSF flow prior to administration. Persistent (extreme) somnolence, hemiplegia, visual disturbances (including blindness; may be total and permanent), deafness, cranial nerve palsies have been reported. Signs/symptoms of peripheral neuropathy (eg, pain, numbness, paresthesia, weakness, impaired bowel/bladder control) have also been reported. Combined neurologic features (cauda equina syndrome) have been reported in some cases. If neurotoxicity develops, reduce subsequent doses or discontinue treatment. Headache, nausea, and fever are early signs of neurotoxicity. Transient elevations in CSF protein and CSF white blood cell counts have been observed following administration.

For intrathecal use only. Intrathecal medications should not be prepared during the preparation of any other agents. After preparation, store intrathecal medications in an isolated location or container clearly marked with a label identifying as "intrathecal" use only. Delivery of intrathecal medications to the patient should only be with other medications intended for administration into the central nervous system (Jacobson, 2009).

Adverse Reactions

>10%:
Cardiovascular: Peripheral edema (11%)
Central nervous system: Chemical arachnoiditis (without dexamethasone premedication: 100%; with dexamethasone premedication: 33% to 42%; grade 4: 19% to 30%; onset: ≤5 days); headache (56%), confusion (33%), fever (32%), fatigue (25%), seizure (20% to 22%), dizziness (18%), lethargy (16%), insomnia (14%), memory impairment (14%), pain (14%)
Endocrine & metabolic: Dehydration (13%)
Gastrointestinal: Nausea (46%), vomiting (44%), constipation (25%), diarrhea (12%), appetite decreased (11%)
Genitourinary: Urinary tract infection (14%)
Hematologic: Anemia (12%), thrombocytopenia (3% to 11%)
Neuromuscular & skeletal: Weakness (40%), back pain (24%), abnormal gait (23%), limb pain (15%), neck pain (14%), arthralgia (11%), neck stiffness (11%)
Ocular: Blurred vision (11%)

1% to 10%:
Cardiovascular: Tachycardia (9%), hypotension (8%), hypertension (6%), syncope (3%), edema (2%)
Central nervous system: Agitation (10%), hypoesthesia (10%), depression (8%), anxiety (7%), sensory neuropathy (3%)
Dermatologic: Pruritus (2%)
Endocrine & metabolic: Hypokalemia (7%), hyponatremia (7%), hyperglycemia (6%)

Gastrointestinal: Abdominal pain (9%), dysphagia (8%), anorexia (5%), hemorrhoids (3%), mucosal inflammation (3%)

Genitourinary: Incontinence (7%), urinary retention (5%)

Hematologic: Neutropenia (10%), contusion (2%)

Neuromuscular & skeletal: Muscle weakness (10%), tremor (9%), peripheral neuropathy (3% to 4%), abnormal reflexes (3%)

Otic: Hypoacusis (6%)

Respiratory: Dyspnea (10%), cough (7%), pneumonia (6%)

Miscellaneous: Diaphoresis (2%)

1% (Limited to important or life-threatening): Anaphylaxis, bladder control impaired, blindness, bowel control impaired, cauda equine syndrome, cranial nerve palsies, CSF protein increased, CSF WBC increased, deafness, encephalopathy, hemiplegia, hydrocephalus, infectious meningitis, intracranial pressure increased, myelopathy, neurologic deficit, numbness, papilledema, somnolence, visual disturbance

Drug Interactions

Metabolism/Transport Effects None known.

Avoid Concomitant Use

Avoid concomitant use of Cytarabine (Liposomal) with any of the following: BCG (Intravesical); Tofacitinib

Increased Effect/Toxicity

Cytarabine (Liposomal) may increase the levels/effects of: Fingolimod; Tofacitinib

Decreased Effect

Cytarabine (Liposomal) may decrease the levels/effects of: BCG (Intravesical)

Preparation for Administration Hazardous agent; use appropriate precautions for handling and disposal (NIOSH 2014 [group 1]). Gloves should be worn during preparation and administration. Allow vial to warm to room temperature. Particles may settle in diluent over time, and may be resuspended with gentle agitation or inversion immediately prior to withdrawing from the vial. Do not agitate aggressively. Withdraw from the vial immediately prior to administration. No further reconstitution or dilution is required. Do not mix with any other medications. Intrathecal medications should not be prepared during the preparation of any other agents (Jacobson, 2009).

Storage/Stability

Store intact vial at 2°C to 8°C (36°F to 46°F); protect from freezing. Avoid aggressive agitation. Withdraw from the vial immediately prior to administration; solutions should be used within 4 hours of withdrawal from the vial.

After preparation, store intrathecal medications in an isolated location or container clearly marked with a label identifying as "intrathecal" use only (Jacobson, 2009).

Mechanism of Action Cytarabine liposomal is a sustained-release formulation of the active ingredient cytarabine, an antimetabolite which acts through inhibition of DNA synthesis and is cell cycle-specific for the S phase of cell division. Cytarabine is converted intracellularly to its active metabolite cytarabine-5'-triphosphate (ara-CTP). Ara-CTP also appears to be incorporated into DNA and RNA; however, the primary action is inhibition of DNA polymerase, resulting in decreased DNA synthesis and repair. The liposomal formulation allows for gradual release, resulting in prolonged exposure.

Pharmacodynamics/Kinetics

Absorption: Systemic exposure following intrathecal administration is negligible since transfer rate from CSF to plasma is slow

Half-life elimination, CSF: 6 to 82 hours

Time to peak, CSF: Intrathecal: <1 hour

Dosing

Adult & Geriatric Note: Initiate dexamethasone 4 mg twice daily (oral or IV) for 5 days, beginning on the day of cytarabine liposomal administration.

Lymphomatous meningitis: Intrathecal:

Induction: 50 mg every 14 days for a total of 2 doses (weeks 1 and 3)

Consolidation: 50 mg every 14 days for 3 doses (weeks 5, 7, and 9), followed by an additional dose at week 13

Maintenance: 50 mg every 28 days for 4 doses (weeks 17, 21, 25, and 29)

Renal Impairment There are no dosage adjustments provided in the manufacturer's labeling (has not been studied).

Hepatic Impairment There are no dosage adjustments provided in the manufacturer's labeling (has not been studied).

Adjustment for Toxicity If drug-related neurotoxicity develops, reduce dose to 25 mg. If toxicity persists, discontinue treatment.

Administration For intrathecal use only. Dose should be removed from vial immediately before administration (must be administered within 4 hours of removal from the vial).

An in-line filter should **NOT** be used. Administer directly into the CSF via an intraventricular reservoir or by direct injection into the lumbar sac. Injection should be made slowly (over 1 to 5 minutes). Patients should lie flat for 1 hour after lumbar puncture. After administration, observe for immediate toxic reactions.

Hazardous agent; use appropriate precautions for handling and disposal (NIOSH 2014 [group 1]). Gloves should be worn during preparation and administration. If contact with skin occurs, immediately wash with soap and water; if contact with mucous membranes occurs, flush thoroughly with water.

Monitoring Parameters Monitor closely for signs of an immediate reaction; chemical arachnoiditis; neurotoxicity

Dosage Forms Excipient information presented when available (limited, particularly for generics); consult specific product labeling.

Suspension, Intrathecal:

DepoCyt: 50 mg/5 mL (5 mL) [contains cholesterol, dioleoylphosphatidylcholine (dopc), dipalmitoylphosphatidylglycerol (dppg), triolein]

◆ Cytarabine Liposome *see* Cytarabine (Liposomal) *on page 471*

◆ CytoGam® *see* Cytomegalovirus Immune Globulin (Intravenous-Human) *on page 472*

Cytomegalovirus Immune Globulin (Intravenous-Human)

(sye toe meg a low VYE rus i MYUN GLOB yoo lin in tra VEE nus HYU man)

Brand Names: US CytoGam®

Brand Names: Canada CytoGam®

Index Terms CMV Hyperimmune Globulin; CMV-IGIV

Pharmacologic Category Blood Product Derivative; Immune Globulin

Additional Appendix Information

Immunization Administration Recommendations *on page 1974*

Immunization Schedules *on page 1979*

Use Prophylaxis of cytomegalovirus (CMV) disease associated with kidney, lung, liver, pancreas, and heart transplants; concomitant use with ganciclovir should be considered in organ transplants (other than kidney) from CMV seropositive donors to CMV seronegative recipients

Dosing

Adult & Geriatric

Prophylaxis of CMV disease in kidney transplant: IV:

Initial dose (within 72 hours of transplant): 150 mg/kg/dose

2-, 4-, 6-, and 8 weeks after transplant: 100 mg/kg/dose

12- and 16 weeks after transplant: 50 mg/kg/dose

Prophylaxis of CMV disease in liver, lung, pancreas, or heart transplant: IV:

Initial dose (within 72 hours of transplant): 150 mg/kg/dose

2-, 4-, 6-, and 8 weeks after transplant: 150 mg/kg/dose

12- and 16 weeks after transplant: 100 mg/kg/dose

Treatment of severe CMV pneumonitis in hematopoietic stem cell transplant (off-label use; in combination with ganciclovir): IV: 400 mg/kg on days 1, 2, and 7, followed by 200 mg/kg on day 14; if still symptomatic, may administer an additional 200 mg/kg on day 21 (Reed, 1988) **or** 150 mg/kg twice weekly (Alexander, 2010)

Pediatric Prophylaxis of CMV disease in kidney, liver, lung, pancreas, or heart transplant: Children and Adolescents: IV: Refer to adult dosing.

Renal Impairment No dosage adjustment provided in manufacturer's labeling; use with caution. Infuse at minimum rate possible.

Hepatic Impairment No dosage adjustment provided in manufacturer's labeling.

Additional Information Complete prescribing information should be consulted for additional detail.

Dosage Forms Excipient information presented when available (limited, particularly for generics); consult specific product labeling.

Injection, solution [preservative free]:

CytoGam®: 50 mg (± 10 mg)/mL (50 mL) [contains sodium 20-30 mEq/L, human albumin, and sucrose 50 mg/mL]

◆ Cytomel *see* Liothyronine *on page 1083*

◆ Cytosar (Can) *see* Cytarabine (Conventional) *on page 467*

◆ Cytosar-U *see* Cytarabine (Conventional) *on page 467*

◆ Cytosine Arabinosine Hydrochloride *see* Cytarabine (Conventional) *on page 467*

Dabigatran Etexilate (da BIG a tran ett EX ill ate)

Brand Names: US Pradaxa
Brand Names: Canada Pradaxa
Index Terms Dabigatran Etexilate Mesylate
Pharmacologic Category Anticoagulant; Anticoagulant, Direct Thrombin Inhibitor
Additional Appendix Information
Oral Anticoagulant Comparison Chart *on page 1957*
Reversal of Oral Anticoagulants *on page 1959*
Use
Deep venous thrombosis and pulmonary embolism treatment and prevention: Treatment of deep venous thrombosis (DVT) and pulmonary embolism in patients who have been treated with a parenteral anticoagulant for 5 to 10 days; to reduce the risk of recurrence of DVT and pulmonary embolism in patients who have been previously treated.
Nonvalvular atrial fibrillation (to reduce the risk of stroke and systemic embolism): Reduce the risk of stroke and systemic embolism in patients with nonvalvular atrial fibrillation (AF)
   Note: The 2014 American Heart Association/American College of Cardiology/Heart Rhythm Society guidelines for the management of AF recommend oral anticoagulation for patients with nonvalvular AF or atrial flutter with prior stroke, TIA, or a CHA$_2$DS$_2$-VASc score ≥2. As an alternative to warfarin, dabigatran may also be used for 3 weeks prior and 4 weeks after cardioversion in patients with AF or atrial flutter of ≥48 hours duration or when the duration is unknown (January 2014).
Postoperative thromboprophylaxis:
   US labeling: Prophylaxis of deep vein thrombosis (DVT) and pulmonary embolism in patients who have undergone hip replacement surgery.
   Canadian labeling: Postoperative thromboprophylaxis in patients who have undergone total hip or knee replacement procedures
Pregnancy Considerations Adverse events were observed in some animal reproduction studies. An *ex vivo* human placenta dual perfusion model illustrated that dabigatran crossed the placenta at term; dabigatran etexilate mesylate (prodrug) had limited placental transfer (Bapat 2014). Data are insufficient to evaluate the safety of direct thrombin inhibitors during pregnancy; use of oral agents during pregnancy should be avoided (Guyatt 2012). Consider the risks of bleeding and stroke if used during pregnancy.
Breast-Feeding Considerations It is not known if dabigatran etexilate is excreted into breast milk. Due to the potential for serious adverse reactions in the nursing infant, the US labeling recommends a decision be made whether to discontinue nursing or to discontinue the drug, taking into account the importance of treatment to the mother. The Canadian labeling contraindicates use in nursing women. The use of alternative anticoagulants is preferred (Guyatt 2012).
Medication Guide Available Yes
Contraindications
Serious hypersensitivity (eg, anaphylaxis or anaphylactic shock) to dabigatran or any component of the formulation; active pathological bleeding; patients with mechanical prosthetic heart valve(s)
Canadian labeling: Additional contraindications (not in US labeling): Severe renal impairment (CrCl <30 mL/minute); bleeding diathesis, patients with spontaneous or pharmacological hemostatic impairment or clinically significant active bleeding (including GI bleeding); lesions at risk of clinically significant bleeding (eg, hemorrhagic or ischemic cerebral infarction) within previous 6 months; nursing women; concomitant therapy with oral ketoconazole; concomitant use with other anticoagulants including unfractionated heparin (except when used to maintain central venous or arterial catheter patency), low molecular weight heparins, heparin derivatives (eg, fondaparinux), antithrombin agents (eg, bivalirudin), and oral anticoagulants (eg, warfarin, rivaroxaban, apixaban) except during transitioning of therapy from or to dabigatran

Warnings/Precautions [US Boxed Warning]: Upon premature discontinuation, the risk of thrombotic events is increased. If dabigatran must be discontinued for a reason other than pathological bleeding or completion of a course of therapy, consider the use of another anticoagulant during the time of interruption.

[US Boxed Warning]: Spinal or epidural hematomas may occur with neuraxial anesthesia (epidural or spinal anesthesia) or spinal puncture in patients who are anticoagulated; may result in long-term or permanent paralysis. The risk of spinal/epidural hematoma is increased with the use of indwelling epidural catheters, concomitant administration of other drugs that affect hemostasis (eg, NSAIDS, platelet inhibitors, other anticoagulants), in patients with a history of traumatic or repeated epidural or spinal punctures, or a history of spinal deformity or spinal surgery. Placement or removal of an epidural catheter or lumbar puncture is best performed when the anticoagulant effect of dabigatran is low; however, the optimal timing between the administration of dabigatran and neuraxial procedures is not known. Monitor frequently for signs and symptoms of neurologic impairment (eg, midline back pain, numbness/weakness of legs, bowel/bladder dysfunction); prompt diagnosis and treatment are necessary. In patients who are anticoagulated or pharmacologic thromboprophylaxis is anticipated, assess risks versus benefits prior to neuraxial interventions. If possible, discontinue dabigatran 1-2 days (CrCl ≥50 mL/minute) or 3-5 days (CrCl <50 mL/minute) before invasive or surgical procedures due to the increased risk of bleeding; consider longer times for patients undergoing major surgery, spinal puncture, or insertion of a spinal or epidural catheter or port. If surgery cannot be delayed, the risk of bleeding is elevated; weigh risk of bleeding with urgency of procedure. Bleeding risk can be assessed by the ecarin clotting time (ECT) if available; if ECT is not available, use of aPTT may provide an approximation of dabigatran's anticoagulant activity. Use a specific reversal agent (eg, idarucizumab) in case of emergency surgery or urgent procedures when reversal of anticoagulant effect of dabigatran is needed. Following peri-spinal procedures, the Canadian labeling recommends initiating therapy after hemostasis is obtained and no sooner than 2 hours following puncture or catheter removal; use is not recommended in patients undergoing anesthesia with post-operative indwelling epidural catheters.

The most common complication is bleeding, and sometimes fatal bleeding. Risk factors for bleeding include concurrent use of drugs that increase the risk of bleeding (eg, antiplatelet agents, heparin), renal impairment, impairment, and elderly patients (especially if low body weight). Monitor for signs and symptoms of bleeding; discontinue in patients with active pathological bleeding. **Important:** Idarucizumab is commercially available for dabigatran reversal. Dabigatran is dialyzable (~57% removed over 4 hours); however, supporting data are limited for utilizing this method. The use of a PCC (Cofact, not available in the US) has been shown to be **ineffective** for dabigatran reversal (Eerenberg 2011); however, the manufacturer does suggest that PCC or recombinant factor VIIa may be considered, although their use has not been evaluated in clinical trials. FEIBA NF was reported to have been effective in rapidly reversing the anticoagulant effects of dabigatran in one case study (Dager 2013). Platelet concentrates should be considered when thrombocytopenia is present or long-acting antiplatelet drugs have been used. Use in patients with moderate hepatic impairment (Child-Pugh class B) demonstrated large inter-subject variability; however, no consistent change in exposure or pharmacodynamics was seen. Patients with active liver disease were excluded from the Randomized Evaluation of Long-term Anticoagulation Therapy (RE-LY) trial (Connolly 2009). The Canadian labeling recommends avoiding use in patients with severe hepatic impairment (Child-Pugh class C), acute liver disease, or with increased liver enzymes ≥2 times ULN. Use is not recommended in patients with valvular heart disease, including the

presence of a bioprosthetic heart valve (has not been evaluated); use is contraindicated in patients with mechanical prosthetic heart valves. In addition to several case reports (Chu 2012; Price 2012; Stewart 2012), one clinical trial reported significantly more thromboembolic events (valve thrombosis, stroke, TIA, and MI) and an excess of major bleeding (predominantly postoperative pericardial effusions requiring intervention for hemodynamic compromise) in patients with mechanical prosthetic heart valves receiving dabigatran compared with those receiving adjusted-dose warfarin.

Due to an increased risk of bleeding, avoid use, if possible, with other direct thrombin inhibitors (eg, bivalirudin), unfractionated heparin or heparin derivatives, low molecular weight heparins (eg, enoxaparin), fondaparinux, thienopyridines (eg, clopidogrel), GPIIb/IIIa antagonists (eg, eptifibatide), aspirin, coumarin derivatives, sulfinpyrazone, and ticagrelor. NSAIDs should be used cautiously. Appropriate doses of unfractionated heparin may be used to maintain catheter patency. Potentially significant drug interactions may exist, requiring dose or frequency adjustment, additional monitoring, and/or selection of alternative therapy.

Evaluate renal function prior to and during therapy, particularly if used in patients with any degree of preexisting renal impairment or in any condition that may result in a decline in renal function (eg, hypovolemia, dehydration, concomitant use of medications with a potential to affect renal function); dabigatran concentrations may increase in any degree of renal impairment and increase the risk of bleeding. In moderate impairment, serum concentrations may increase 3 times higher than normal compared to concentrations in patients with normal renal function. However, in patients with nonvalvular AF, US labeling only requires dosage reduction in patients with severe renal impairment (CrCl 15-30 mL/minute) and dosing recommendations cannot be provided in patients with CrCl <15 mL/minute due to insufficient evidence. Per the American College of Chest Physicians, dabigatran is considered contraindicated in patients with severe renal impairment (CrCl ≤30 mL/minute) (Guyatt 2012). The Canadian labeling also contraindicates use in severe renal impairment (CrCl <30 mL/minute) and recommends indication-specific dose reductions in patients with moderate impairment (CrCl 30-50 mL/minute). Discontinue therapy in any patient who develops acute renal failure.

In the elderly, use with extreme caution or consider other treatment options. No dosage adjustment is recommended in the US manufacturer's labeling based on age alone (unless renal impairment coexists); however, risk of bleeding increases with age. Numerous reports of excess anticoagulation, including fatalities, have been observed with use in older adults (ISMP [Smetzer 2012]; ISMP [Smetzer 2015]). In particular, an increased risk of GI bleeding has been observed in patients ≥75 years of age despite similar efficacy observed with dabigatran in the elderly as compared to warfarin-treated patients (Graham 2015; Sharma 2015). Dabigatran is associated with more than a 5-fold variation in plasma concentrations in patients receiving the same dose, indicating a wide therapeutic range. Significant factors affecting increased dabigatran plasma concentrations have been found to be increasing age, decreased CrCl, lower body weight and female gender. Renal function was the predominant patient characteristic determining plasma concentrations, with age as the most important covariate (Reilly 2014). Depending on individual patient characteristics, particularly advanced age and potential for renal impairment, consider other treatment options, particularly in the US where lack of other available dosing options exist (ie, 110 mg dose) (Kalbalik 2015). The Canadian labeling includes recommendations for a dose reductions for in elderly patients (refer to Dosing). Per the Beers Criteria, there is a greater risk of bleeding in older adults aged ≥75 years (exceeds warfarin bleeding risk) and therapy should be used with caution in patients ≥75 years of age or in patients with CrCl <30 mL/minute (Beers Criteria).

Adverse Reactions Adverse reactions listed below are reflective of both the U.S. and Canadian product information; frequency may vary by indication. **Important:** No specific antidote exists for dabigatran reversal; protamine and vitamin K do not reverse or impact anticoagulant effects of dabigatran. Dabigatran is dialyzable (~57% removed over 4 hours); however, supporting data are limited for utilizing this method. The use of a PCC (Cofact, not available in the U.S.) has been shown to be **ineffective** for dabigatran reversal (Eerenberg, 2011); however, the manufacturer does suggest that activated PCC (eg, FEIBA NF), recombinant factor VIIa, or concentrates of factors II, IX, or X may be considered, although their use has not been evaluated in clinical trials. FEIBA NF was reported to have been effective in rapidly reversing the anticoagulant effects of dabigatran in one case study (Dager, 2013). Platelet concentrates should be considered when thrombocytopenia is present or long-acting antiplatelet drugs have been used.

>10%:

Gastrointestinal: Gastrointestinal symptoms (eg, dyspepsia, gastritis-like symptoms; 25% to 35%)

Hematologic & oncologic: Hemorrhage (11% to 19%; major hemorrhage: ≤6%; hemorrhage [life-threatening]: 2%)

1% to 10%:

Dermatologic: Wound secretion (5%; postprocedural discharge: 1%; bloody discharge: <1%)

Gastrointestinal: Dyspepsia (8%; includes abdominal pain, abdominal discomfort, epigastric discomfort), gastrointestinal hemorrhage (≤6%; major: ≤2%), gastritis (3%; includes gastroesophageal reflux disease, esophagitis, erosive gastritis, gastrointestinal hemorrhage, hemorrhagic gastritis, gastrointestinal ulcer)

Genitourinary: Hematuria (1%)

Hematologic & oncologic: Anemia (1% to 4%), hematoma (1% to 2%), hemorrhage (postprocedural or wound: 1% to 2%)

Hepatic: Increased serum ALT (≥3 x ULN: 2% to 3%)

<1% (Limited to important or life-threatening): Allergic edema, anaphylactic shock, anaphylaxis, angioedema, catheter site hemorrhage, cerebrovascular accident (in patients with prosthetic heart valve), decreased hematocrit, ecchymoses, epidural hematoma (with spinal puncture or spinal/epidural anesthesia), esophageal ulcer, genitourinary tract hemorrhage, hemarthrosis, hemophthalmos, hemorrhagic death, hemorrhoidal bleeding, hepatic insufficiency, hypersensitivity reaction, incision site hemorrhage, increased serum AST, intracranial hemorrhage (includes hemorrhagic stroke, subarachnoid bleeding, subdural hematoma), muscle hemorrhage, myocardial infarction (in patients with prosthetic heart valve), rectal hemorrhage, retroperitoneal hemorrhage, severe hemorrhagic pericardial effusion (occurred postoperatively in patients with prosthetic heart valve; required intervention for hemodynamic compromise), spinal hematoma (with spinal puncture or spinal/ epidural anesthesia), thrombocytopenia, thromboembolism (in patients with prosthetic heart valve), transient ischemic attacks (in patients with prosthetic heart valve)

Drug Interactions

Metabolism/Transport Effects Substrate of P-glycoprotein

Avoid Concomitant Use

Avoid concomitant use of Dabigatran Etexilate with any of the following: Anticoagulants; Apixaban; Edoxaban; Hemin; Omacetaxine; P-glycoprotein/ABCB1 Inducers; Rivaroxaban; Sulfinpyrazone; Urokinase; Vorapaxar

Increased Effect/Toxicity

Dabigatran Etexilate may increase the levels/effects of: Anticoagulants; Collagenase (Systemic); Deferasirox; Deoxycholic Acid; Ibritumomab; Nintedanib; Obinutuzumab; Omacetaxine; Rivaroxaban; Tositumomab and Iodine I 131 Tositumomab

The levels/effects of Dabigatran Etexilate may be increased by: Agents with Antiplatelet Properties; Amiodarone; Antiplatelet Agents (P2Y12 Inhibitors); Apixaban; Aspirin; Clarithromycin; Dasatinib; Dronedarone; Edoxaban; Hemin; Herbs (Anticoagulant/Antiplatelet Properties); Ketoconazole (Systemic); Limaprost; Lumacaftor; Nonsteroidal Anti-Inflammatory Agents; NSAID (Nonselective); Omega-3 Fatty Acids; Pentosan Polysulfate Sodium; P-glycoprotein/ABCB1 Inhibitors; Prostacyclin Analogues; QuiNIDine; Salicylates; Sugammadex; Sulfinpyrazone; Thrombolytic Agents; Tibolone; Ticagrelor; Urokinase; Verapamil; Vitamin E; Vitamin E (Oral); Vorapaxar

Decreased Effect

The levels/effects of Dabigatran Etexilate may be decreased by: Antacids; AtorvaSTATin; Estrogen Derivatives; Lumacaftor; P-glycoprotein/ABCB1 Inducers; Progestins; Proton Pump Inhibitors

Food Interactions Food has no effect on the bioavailability of dabigatran, but delays the time to peak plasma concentrations by 2 hours. Management: Administer without regard to meals.

Storage/Stability

Blister: Store at 25°C (77°F); excursions permitted between 15°C to 30°C (59°F to 86°F). Dispense and store in original package to protect from moisture.

Bottle: Store at 25°C (77°F); excursions permitted between 15°C to 30°C (59°F to 86°F). Dispense and store in original manufacturer's bottle to protect from moisture; discard 4 months after opening original container.

Mechanism of Action Prodrug lacking anticoagulant activity that is converted *in vivo* to the active dabigatran, a specific, reversible, direct thrombin inhibitor that inhibits both free and fibrin-bound thrombin. Inhibits coagulation by preventing thrombin-mediated effects, including cleavage of fibrinogen to fibrin monomers, activation of factors V, VIII, XI, and XIII, and inhibition of thrombin-induced platelet aggregation.

Pharmacodynamics/Kinetics

Absorption: Rapid; initially slow postoperatively

Distribution: V_d: 50-70 L

Protein binding: 35%

Metabolism: Hepatic; dabigatran etexilate is rapidly and completely hydrolyzed to dabigatran (active form) by plasma and hepatic esterases; dabigatran undergoes hepatic glucuronidation to active acylglucuronide isomers (similar activity to parent compound; accounts for <10% of total dabigatran in plasma)

Bioavailability: 3% to 7%

Half-life elimination: 12-17 hours; Elderly: 14-17 hours; Mild-to-moderate renal impairment: 15-18 hours; Severe renal impairment: 28 hours (Stangier 2010)

Time to peak, plasma: Dabigatran: 1 hour; delayed 2 hours by food (no effect on bioavailability)

Excretion: Urine (80%)

Dosing

Adult

DVT and pulmonary embolism (treatment and prevention): Oral:

US labeling: 150 mg twice daily (after 5 to 10 days of parenteral anticoagulation)

Canadian labeling: 150 mg twice daily (after 5 to 10 days of parenteral anticoagulation); dose reduction to 110 mg twice daily is recommended in patients at increased risk of bleeding, including patients ≥75 years with ≥1 risk factor for bleeding

Nonvalvular atrial fibrillation (to reduce the risk of stroke and systemic embolism): Oral:

US labeling: 150 mg twice daily.

Canadian labeling: 150 mg twice daily; dose reduction to 110 mg twice daily is recommended in patients at increased risk of bleeding, including patients ≥75 years with ≥1 risk factor for bleeding; however, efficacy in stroke prevention may be lessened with this dose.

Postoperative thromboprophylaxis: Oral:

US labeling:

Hip replacement: Initial: 110 mg given 1 to 4 hours after completion of surgery and establishment of hemostasis; if not initiated on the day of surgery, initiate therapy with 220 mg once daily after hemostasis has been achieved; maintenance: 220 mg once daily (total duration of therapy: 28 to 35 days; ACCP recommendation [Guyatt 2012]: Minimum of 10 to 14 days; extended duration of up to 35 days suggested)

Canadian labeling:

Knee replacement: Initial: 110 mg given 1 to 4 hours after completion of surgery and establishment of hemostasis **OR** 220 mg as 1 dose in postoperative patients in whom therapy is not initiated on day of surgery regardless of reason; maintenance: 220 mg once daily (total duration of therapy: 10 days; ACCP recommendation [Guyatt 2012]: Minimum of 10 to 14 days; extended duration of up to 35 days suggested)

Hip replacement: Initial: 110 mg given 1 to 4 hours after completion of surgery and establishment of hemostasis **OR** 220 mg as 1 dose in postoperative patients in whom therapy is not initiated on day of surgery regardless of reason; maintenance: 220 mg once daily (total duration of therapy: 28 to 35 days; ACCP recommendation [Guyatt 2012]: Minimum of 10 to 14 days; extended duration of up to 35 days suggested)

Conversion:

Conversion from a parenteral anticoagulant: Initiate dabigatran ≤2 hours prior to the time of the next scheduled dose of the parenteral anticoagulant (eg, enoxaparin) or at the time of discontinuation for a continuously administered parenteral drug (eg, IV heparin); discontinue parenteral anticoagulant at the time of dabigatran initiation.

Conversion to a parenteral anticoagulant:

US labeling: Wait 12 hours (CrCl ≥30 mL/minute) or 24 hours (CrCl <30 mL/minute) after the last dose of dabigatran before initiating a parenteral anticoagulant.

Canadian labeling: Wait 12 hours (DVT and pulmonary embolism treatment/prevention, nonvalvular atrial fibrillation) or 24 hours (postoperative thromboprophylaxis) after the last dose of dabigatran before initiating a parenteral anticoagulant.

Conversion from warfarin: Discontinue warfarin and initiate dabigatran when INR <2.0

Conversion to warfarin: Since dabigatran contributes to INR elevation, warfarin's effect on the INR will be better reflected only after dabigatran has been stopped for ≥2 days. Start time must be adjusted based on CrCl:

CrCl >50 mL/minute: Initiate warfarin 3 days before discontinuation of dabigatran

CrCl 30 to 50 mL/minute: Initiate warfarin 2 days before discontinuation of dabigatran

CrCl 15 to 30 mL/minute: Initiate warfarin 1 day before discontinuation of dabigatran (dabigatran use is contraindicated in Canadian labeling when CrCl <30 mL/minute).

CrCl <15 mL/minute: There are no recommendations provided in the US manufacturer's labeling.

Dosing adjustment with concomitant medications:

US labeling:

DVT and pulmonary embolism (treatment and prevention):

Any P-glycoprotein inducer (eg, rifampin): Avoid concurrent use.

Any P-glycoprotein inhibitor (eg, amiodarone, clarithromycin, dronedarone, quinidine, verapamil, and others) with CrCl <50 mL/minute: Avoid concurrent use.

Nonvalvular atrial fibrillation (to prevent stroke and systemic embolism):

Dronedarone or ketoconazole (oral) with CrCl 30 to 50 mL/minute: Reduce dabigatran dose to 75 mg twice daily.

Any P-glycoprotein inducer (eg, rifampin): Avoid concurrent use.

Any P-glycoprotein inhibitor (eg, amiodarone, clarithromycin, dronedarone, quinidine, verapamil, and others) with CrCl <30 mL/minute: Avoid concurrent use.

Postoperative thromboprophylaxis (hip replacement):

Any P-glycoprotein inducer (eg, rifampin): Avoid concurrent use.

Any P-glycoprotein inhibitor (eg, amiodarone, clarithromycin, dronedarone, quinidine, verapamil, and others) with CrCl <50 mL/minute: Avoid concurrent use.

Canadian labeling: **Note:** Regardless of indication, avoid simultaneous initiation of verapamil and dabigatran; administer dabigatran at least 2 hours prior to verapamil.

Postoperative thromboprophylaxis: *Strong P-gp inhibitors (eg, amiodarone, quinidine, verapamil):* Use caution and consider reducing dabigatran to 150 mg once daily. In patients with CrCl 30 to 50 mL/minute and receiving verapamil, consider dabigatran dose reduction to 75 mg once daily. Avoid initiation of verapamil in postoperative patients who are already receiving dabigatran. Use with the strong P-gp inhibitor ketoconazole (oral) is contraindicated.

Geriatric

US labeling:

DVT and pulmonary embolism/Nonvalvular atrial fibrillation (to prevent stroke and systemic embolism)/postoperative thromboprophylaxis: Oral:

Patients >65 years: Refer to adult dosing. No dosage adjustment required unless renal impairment exists; however, risk of bleeding increases with age. Numerous reports of excess anticoagulation, including fatalities, have been observed with use in older adults (ISMP [Smetzer 2012]; ISMP [Smetzer 2015]).

Patients ≥75 years: **Use with extreme caution or consider other treatment options (see Warnings/Precautions).** No dosage adjustment provided in manufacturer's labeling based on age alone (unless renal impairment coexists); however, risk of bleeding increases with age. Numerous reports of excess anticoagulation, including fatalities, have been observed with use in older adults (ISMP [Smetzer 2012]; ISMP [Smetzer 2015]).

Canadian labeling:

DVT and pulmonary embolism/Nonvalvular atrial fibrillation (to prevent stroke and systemic embolism): Oral:

Patients <80 years: 150 mg twice daily; **Note:** The manufacturer labeling recommends that a dose reduction to 110 mg twice daily in patients >75 years with at least one other risk factor for bleeding (eg, moderate renal impairment [CrCl 30 to 50 mL/minute], concomitant treatment with strong P-gp inhibitors, or previous GI bleed); however, efficacy in stroke prevention may be lessened with this dose reduction.

Patients ≥80 years: 110 mg twice daily

Postoperative thromboprophylaxis: Oral: Patients >75 years: Use with caution; consider a dose of 150 mg once daily

Renal Impairment Note: Clinical trial evaluating safety and efficacy utilized the Cockcroft-Gault formula with the use of actual body weight (data on file; Boehringer Ingelheim Pharmaceuticals Inc 2012).

DVT and pulmonary embolism (treatment and prevention):

US labeling:

CrCl >30 mL/minute: No dosage adjustment necessary **unless** patient has a CrCl <50 mL/minute and is receiving concomitant P-gp inhibitors, then avoid coadministration.

CrCl ≤30 mL/minute: There are no dosage recommendations provided in the manufacturer's labeling (has not been studied). Patients with CrCl <30 mL/minute (Schulman 2009; Schulman 2011) or CrCl ≤30 mL/minute (Schulman 2013) were excluded from the respective clinical trials.

Hemodialysis: There are no dosage recommendations provided in the manufacturer's labeling (has not been studied). Patients receiving hemodialysis were excluded from clinical trials (Schulman 2009; Schulman 2011; Schulman 2013).

Canadian labeling:

CrCl >50 mL/minute: No dosage adjustment is necessary

CrCl 30 to 50 mL/minute: There are no dosage adjustments provided in the manufacturer's labeling (has not been studied); dose selection should be based on risk/benefit assessment.

CrCl <30 mL/minute: Use is contraindicated.

Nonvalvular atrial fibrillation (to prevent stroke and systemic embolism):

US labeling:

CrCl >50 mL/minute: No dosage adjustment necessary. Use with caution in mild renal impairment (CrCl 50 to 80 mL/minute) due to risk for increased dabigatran exposure (area under the curve may be increased 1.5 times higher than normal).

CrCl 30 to 50 mL/minute: No dosage adjustment necessary **unless** patient receiving concomitant dronedarone or oral ketoconazole, then reduce dabigatran to 75 mg twice daily. Use with caution in moderate renal impairment due to risk for increased dabigatran exposure (area under the curve may be increased 3 times higher than normal), particularly if patient is also of advanced age. In patients with moderate-to-severe chronic kidney disease, dose reduction may be considered although safety and efficacy of this approach has not been established (AHA/ACC/HRS [January 2014]).

CrCl 15 to 30 mL/minute: 75 mg twice daily **unless** patient receiving concomitant P-gp inhibitor, then avoid concurrent use. **Note:** Patients with CrCl <30 mL/minute were excluded from the RE-LY trial (Connolly 2009). Dose based on pharmacokinetic data; safety and efficacy has not been established. Per the American College of Chest Physicians, dabigatran is considered contraindicated in patients with severe renal impairment (CrCl ≤30 mL/minute) (Guyatt 2012).

CrCl <15 mL/minute: There are no dosage recommendations provided in the manufacturer's labeling (has not been studied). Per the American College of Chest Physicians, dabigatran is considered contraindicated in patients with severe renal impairment (CrCl ≤30 mL/minute) (Guyatt 2012). In addition, the AHA/ACC/HRS does not recommend dabigatran for patients with AF and end-stage chronic kidney disease (January 2014).

Hemodialysis: There are no dosage recommendations provided in the manufacturer's labeling (has not been studied). The AHA/ACC/HRS does not recommend dabigatran for patients with AF on hemodialysis (January 2014). **Note:** Hemodialysis removes ~57% over 4 hours

Canadian labeling:

CrCl >50 mL/minute: No dosage adjustment necessary.

CrCl 30 to 50 mL/minute: No dosage adjustment is generally necessary; use with caution in moderate renal impairment due to risk for increased dabigatran exposure (area under the curve may be increased 3 times higher than normal), particularly if patient is also of advanced age. In patients with moderate to severe chronic kidney disease, dose reduction may be considered although safety and efficacy of this approach has not been established (AHA/ACC/HRS [January 2014]).

CrCl <30 mL/minute: Use is contraindicated.

Postoperative thromboprophylaxis:

US labeling:

CrCl >30 mL/minute: No dosage adjustment necessary **unless** patient has a CrCl <50 mL/minute and is receiving concomitant P-gp inhibitors, then avoid coadministration.

CrCl ≤30 mL/minute: There are no dosage recommendations provided in the manufacturer's labeling (has not been studied). Patients with CrCl <30 mL/minute (Eriksson 2007; Eriksson 2011) were excluded from the respective clinical trials.

Hemodialysis: There are no dosage recommendations provided in the manufacturer's labeling (has not been studied).

Canadian labeling:

CrCl >50 mL/minute: No dosage adjustment necessary.

CrCl 30 to 50 mL/minute: Initial: 75 mg given 1 to 4 hours after completion of surgery and establishment of hemostasis; Maintenance: 150 mg once daily **unless** patient receiving concomitant verapamil, then consider reducing dabigatran to 75 mg once daily.

CrCl <30 mL/minute: Use is contraindicated.

Hepatic Impairment

US labeling: There are no dosage adjustments provided in manufacturer's labeling; consistent changes in exposure or pharmacodynamics were not observed in a study of patients with moderate impairment.

Canadian labeling: There are no dosage adjustments provided in manufacturer's labeling; no change in exposure was seen in a study of patients with moderate impairment (Child-Pugh class B). Use is not recommended in patients with severe impairment (Child-Pugh class C), acute liver disease, or with increased liver enzymes ≥2 times ULN.

Administration Oral: Administer with a full glass of water without regard to meals; however, if dyspepsia occurs, consider administration with meals. Do not break, chew, or open capsules, as this will lead to 75% increase in absorption and potentially serious adverse reactions.

Monitoring Parameters Routine monitoring of coagulation tests not required. However, the measurement of activated partial thromboplastin time (aPTT) (values >2.5 x control may indicate overanticoagulation), ecarin clotting test (ECT) if available, or thrombin time (TT; most sensitive) may be useful to determine presence of dabigatran and level of coagulopathy; CBC with differential; renal function prior to initiation and periodically as clinically indicated (ie, situations associated with a decline in renal function) and according to the AHA/ACC/HRS, at least annually in all patients (January 2014)

Reference Range

At therapeutic dabigatran doses, aPTT, ECT (ecarin clotting time), and TT (thrombin time) are prolonged. A median peak aPTT of ~2 x control and a median trough aPTT of 1.5 x control were observed in subjects taking dabigatran 150 mg twice daily in the RE-LY trial

A therapeutic range has not been established for aPTT or for other tests of anticoagulant activity

Dosage Forms Excipient information presented when available (limited, particularly for generics); consult specific product labeling.

Capsule, Oral:

Pradaxa: 75 mg [contains fd&c yellow #6 (sunset yellow)]

Pradaxa: 110 mg [contains fd&c blue #2 (indigotine)]

Pradaxa: 150 mg [contains fd&c blue #2 (indigotine), fd&c yellow #6 (sunset yellow)]

Dosage Forms: Canada Excipient information presented when available (limited, particularly for generics); consult specific product labeling.

Capsule, oral:

Pradax: 75 mg, 110 mg, 150 mg

◆ Dabigatran Etexilate Mesylate *see* Dabigatran Etexilate on page 473

Dabrafenib (da BRAF e nib)

Brand Names: US Tafinlar
Brand Names: Canada Tafinlar
Index Terms GSK2118436
Pharmacologic Category Antineoplastic Agent, BRAF Kinase Inhibitor
Use

Melanoma, metastatic or unresectable:

US labeling: Treatment of unresectable or metastatic melanoma in patients with a BRAF V600E mutation (single agent therapy) or in patients with BRAF V600E or BRAF V600K mutations (in combination with trametinib); confirm BRAF V600E or BRAF V600K mutation status with an approved test prior to treatment.

Canadian labeling: Treatment of unresectable or metastatic melanoma in patients with a BRAF V600 mutation (as detected by a validated test) as single agent therapy or in combination with trametinib.

Limitations of use: Not indicated for treatment of patients with wild-type BRAF melanoma.

Pregnancy Considerations Adverse effects were observed in animal reproduction studies. Based on its mechanism of action, dabrafenib would be expected to cause fetal harm if administered to a pregnant woman. Females of reproductive potential should use a highly effective nonhormonal contraceptive during therapy and for at least 2 weeks [US labeling] or at least 4 weeks [Canadian labeling] (for single-agent therapy) or 4 months (for combination therapy with trametinib) after treatment is complete; hormonal contraceptives may not be effective. Spermatogenesis may be impaired in males (observed in animal studies); family planning and fertility counseling should be considered prior to therapy.

Breast-Feeding Considerations It is not known if dabrafenib is excreted into breast milk. Due to the potential for serious adverse reactions in the nursing infant, breast-feeding is not recommended by the manufacturer during treatment and for 2 weeks (single agent therapy) or 4 months (combination therapy with trametinib) after the last dose.

Medication Guide Available Yes

Contraindications

There are no contraindications listed in the manufacturer's US labeling.

Canadian labeling: Hypersensitivity to dabrafenib or any component of the formulation.

Warnings/Precautions Hazardous agent – use appropriate precautions for handling and disposal (meets NIOSH 2014 criteria). Serious adverse reactions (retinal vein occlusion, interstitial lung disease) that occur with single-agent trametinib may also occur when dabrafenib is administered in combination with trametinib. Cardiomyopathy may be observed when used as a single agent or in combination with trametinib. The median time to onset of cardiomyopathy was ~8 months (range: 28 days to ~25 months) when used in combination with trametinib, and ~4 months (range: 28 days to ~19 months) for single agent therapy. Assess LVEF (by echocardiogram or MUGA scan) prior to combination therapy initiation, at 1 month, and then at 2- to 3-month intervals while on therapy. Cardiac dysfunction may require dabrafenib treatment interruption (see trametinib monograph for dosage modifications). Cardiomyopathy resolved following therapy adjustments and/or interruption. QTcF prolongation >60 msec above baseline or to >500 msec was reported (rare), both as a single agent or when used in combination with trametinib. Hemorrhage, including symptomatic bleeding in a critical area/organ, may occur with dabrafenib either as a single agent or in combination with trametinib. Major bleeding events (some fatal) included intracranial or gastrointestinal hemorrhage. May require treatment interruption and dosage reduction; permanently discontinue dabrafenib (and trametinib) for all grade 4 hemorrhagic events and any grade 3 event that does not improve with therapy interruption. Venous thromboembolism events (some fatal) may occur when dabrafenib is used in combination with trametinib. DVT and PE occurred at an increased incidence with combination therapy. Patients should seek immediate medical attention with symptoms of DVT or PE (shortness of breath, chest pain, arm/leg swelling). Dabrafenib therapy may be continued for uncomplicated DVT or PE; permanently discontinue trametinib for life-threatening PE.

Serious febrile reactions and fever (any severity) complicated by hypotension, rigors or chills, dehydration, or renal failure were observed during dabrafenib single-agent therapy and when used in combination with trametinib. The median time to initial fever (single-agent therapy) was 11 days (range: 1 day to 6.6 months); median duration was 3 days (range: 1 day to 4.2 months). In patients treated with combination therapy, the median time to onset of fever was 1 month (range 1 day to 23.5 months) and the median duration was 3 days (range: 1 day to 11.3 months). Interrupt dabrafenib therapy for fever ≥38.5°C (101.3°F) or for any other serious febrile reaction complicated by hypotension, rigors/chills, dehydration, or renal failure; evaluate promptly for signs/symptoms of infection. Dosage reduction (or discontinuation) may be required; when resuming therapy after a febrile reaction, may require administration of antipyretics as secondary prophylaxis. Administer corticosteroids (eg, prednisone 10 mg daily or equivalent) for at least 5 days for second or subsequent episodes of pyrexia if temperature does not return to baseline within 3 days of fever onset, or for pyrexia associated with complications (eg, dehydration, hypotension, severe chills/rigors with no evidence of active

infection). Hyperglycemia may occur while on therapy (either as a single agent or in combination with trametinib); may require initiation of insulin or oral hypoglycemic agent therapy (or an increased dose if already taking). Monitor serum glucose at baseline and as clinically necessary in patients with preexisting diabetes or hyperglycemia. Instruct patients to report symptoms of severe hyperglycemia (eg, polydipsia, polyuria).

Serious dermatologic toxicity (eg, rash, dermatitis, acneiform rash, palmar-plantar erythrodysesthesia syndrome, erythema) may occur when used in combination with trametinib (known complication of single-agent trametinib therapy); some patients required hospitalization for severe toxicity or for secondary skin infections. The median time to onset and resolution of skin toxicity for combination therapy was 2 months (range: 1 day to 22 months) and 1.2 months (range: 1 day to ~24 months), respectively. Monitor for dermatologic toxicity and signs/symptoms of secondary infections. Treatment interruption, dose reduction, and/or therapy discontinuation may be necessary. Cutaneous squamous cell carcinoma and keratoacanthoma (cuSCC) and new primary melanoma were observed during single agent dabrafenib therapy at an increased incidence compared with control therapy in clinical trials. The median time to first occurrence of cuSCC was 2.1 months (range: 1 to 53 weeks); approximately one-third of patients who developed cuSCC had more than one occurrence (with continued treatment). The median time between diagnosis of the first and second lesions was 6 weeks. When used in combination with trametinib, cuSCC occurred less frequently than with single-agent dabrafenib therapy; time to diagnosis ranged from 1.8 to 16.8 months after the initiation of combination treatment, and from 9 days to ~21 months for single-agent therapy. Basal cell carcinoma (BCC) may also occur with combination or single-agent therapy; the incidence of BCC is ~3% for combination therapy versus 6% for single-agent dabrafenib. The time to BCC diagnosis ranged from ~3 to ~24 months for patients receiving combination therapy. Dermatologic evaluations should be performed prior to initiating therapy, every 2 months during therapy, and for up to 6 months post discontinuation. There are case reports of noncutaneous malignancies, including pancreatic cancer (KRAS mutation-positive), colorectal cancer (recurrent NRAS mutation-positive), hand and neck cancer, and glioblastoma, with combination therapy; monitor for signs/symptoms of noncutaneous malignancies. Dabrafenib should be permanently discontinued if RAS mutation-positive noncutaneous malignancies develop (no trametinib dosage reduction is required).

Retinal pigment epithelial detachments (RPED) were seen in clinical trials when used in combination with trametinib (a known complication of trametinib single-agent therapy). Detachments were typically bilateral and multifocal and occurred in the central macular area of the retina. Promptly (within 24 hours) refer patients for ophthalmological evaluations if loss of vision or other visual disturbances occur; dabrafenib dosage modification is not necessary for RPED (trametinib therapy modification may be required). Ophthalmic exams (including retinal evaluation) should be performed periodically during treatment with combination therapy. Uveitis, including iritis and iridocyclitis, has been reported with dabrafenib single-agent therapy and when used in combination with trametinib; manage symptomatically with local ophthalmic steroid and mydriatic drops. May require dabrafenib treatment interruption or permanent discontinuation (does not require alteration in trametinib therapy). Monitor for signs/symptoms of uveitis (eg, eye pain, photophobia, vision changes).

Potentially significant drug-drug interactions may exist, requiring dose or frequency adjustment, additional monitoring, and/or selection of alternative therapy. Drugs affecting gastric pH (eg, proton pump inhibitors, H2-receptor antagonists, antacids) may alter dabrafenib solubility, resulting in decreased bioavailability. Clinical trials have not been performed to evaluate concomitant administration and its effect on dabrafenib efficacy. Patients with glucose-6-phosphate dehydrogenase (G6PD) deficiency may be at risk for hemolytic anemia when administered dabrafenib; use with caution and closely observe for signs/symptoms of hemolytic anemia. Not indicated for treatment of patients with wild-type BRAF melanoma. Exposing wild-type cells to BRAF inhibitors such as dabrafenib may result in paradoxical activation of MAP-kinase signaling and increased cell proliferation. Prior to initiating therapy, confirm BRAF V600E or BRAF V600K mutations (US labeling) or BRAF V600 mutations (Canadian labeling) status with an approved test. Data regarding single-agent use in patients with BRAF V600K mutation is limited; compared to BRAF V600E mutation, lower response rates have been

observed with BRAF V600K mutation. Data regarding other less common BRAF V600 mutations is lacking.

Adverse Reactions

Monotherapy:

>10%:

Cardiovascular: Peripheral edema (17%)

Central nervous system: Fatigue (40%), headache (28% to 32%), chills (17%)

Dermatologic: Dermatological reaction (68%), skin rash (17% to 53%), hyperkeratosis (37%), alopecia (22%), palmar-plantar erythrodysesthesia (20%), pruritus (13%)

Endocrine & metabolic: Hyperglycemia (49% to 50%; grades 3/4: 2% to 6%), hypophosphatemia (37% to 40%), increased gamma-glutamyl transferase (38%), hyponatremia (8% to 36%), hypoalbuminemia (23%), hypokalemia (23%), hyperkalemia (15%)

Gastrointestinal: Diarrhea (28%), abdominal pain (21%), nausea (21%), decreased appetite (19%), vomiting (15%), constipation (11%)

Hematologic & oncologic: Lymphocytopenia (40%; grades 3/4: 6%), anemia (28%), papilloma (27%), leukopenia (21%), malignant neoplasm of skin (keratoacanthoma and squamous cell carcinoma; 7% to 19%; grades 3/4: 4%)

Hepatic: Increased serum alkaline phosphatase (19% to 26%), increased serum AST (15%), increased serum ALT (11%)

Neuromuscular & skeletal: Arthralgia (27% to 34%), myalgia (11% to 23%), limb pain (19%), back pain (11% to 12%)

Respiratory: Cough (12% to 21%)

Miscellaneous: Fever (26% to 28%; grades 3/4: ≤4%)

1% to 10%:

Cardiovascular: Prolonged Q-T interval on ECG (>60 msec from baseline: 2%; >500 msec: 2%)

Central nervous system: Dizziness (9%), insomnia (8%)

Dermatologic: Actinic keratosis (9%), night sweats (6%), xeroderma (6%), acneiform eruption (4%), erythema (2%)

Endocrine & metabolic: Hypocalcemia (9%), hypomagnesemia (6%), hypercalcemia (4%), dehydration (2%)

Gastrointestinal: Pancreatitis (<10%), xerostomia (6%)

Genitourinary: Urinary tract infection (9%)

Hematologic & oncologic: Neutropenia (9%; grades 3/4: 2%), thrombocytopenia (8%), basal cell carcinoma (2%), hemorrhage (2%), malignant melanoma (2%)

Hypersensitivity: Hypersensitivity (bullous rash, <10%)

Neuromuscular & skeletal: Muscle spasm (4%)

Ophthalmic: Uveitis (including iritis, 1%)

Renal: Interstitial nephritis (<10%), increased serum creatinine (9%)

Respiratory: Nasopharyngitis (10%)

Miscellaneous: Febrile reaction (2%)

Combination therapy with trametanib:

>10%:

Cardiovascular: Peripheral edema (28% to 31%), prolonged Q-T interval on ECG (>60 msec from baseline: 13%; >500 msec: 4%)

Central nervous system: Chills (50% to 58%), fatigue (53% to 57%), headache (29% to 37%), insomnia (11% to 18%), dizziness (13% to 16%)

Dermatologic: Dermatological reaction (65%; 3% required hospitalization), skin rash (43% to 45%), night sweats (15% to 24%), xeroderma (9% to 18%), acneiform eruption (11% to 16%), actinic keratosis (7% to 15%), erythema (6% to 15%), pruritus (11%)

Endocrine & metabolic: Hyperglycemia (58% to 67%; grades 3/4: 5% to 6%), increased gamma-glutamyl transferase (54% to 56%), hyponatremia (48% to 55%), hypoalbuminemia (43% to 53%), hypophosphatemia (41% to 47%), hypokalemia (15% to 29%), hyperkalemia (18% to 22%), hypocalcemia (13% to 20%), hypercalcemia (15% to 19%), hypomagnesemia (2% to 18%), dehydration (6% to 11%)

Gastrointestinal: Nausea (44% to 46%), vomiting (40% to 43%), diarrhea (26% to 36%), abdominal pain (24% to 33%), decreased appetite (22% to 30%), constipation (17% to 22%), xerostomia (11%)

Genitourinary: Urinary tract infection (6% to 13%)

Hematologic & oncologic: Leukopenia (46% to 62%; grades 3/4: 4% to 5%), lymphocytopenia (55% to 59%; grades 3/4: 19% to 22%), anemia (46% to 55%; grades 3/4: 4% to 7%), neutropenia (37% to 55%; grades 3/4: 2% to 13%), thrombocytopenia (31%; grades 3/4: 2% to 4%), hemorrhage (11% to 16%; major hemorrhage [intracranial or gastric]: 5%)

Hepatic: Increased serum alkaline phosphatase (60% to 67%), increased serum AST (54% to 60%), increased serum ALT (35% to 42%), hyperbilirubinemia (7% to 15%)

Neuromuscular & skeletal: Arthralgia (27% to 44%), myalgia (22% to 24%), back pain (11% to 18%), limb pain (11% to 16%), muscle spasm (2% to 16%)

Renal: Increased serum creatinine (20% to 24%)

Respiratory: Cough (11% to 29%), oropharyngeal pain (7% to 13%)

Miscellaneous: Fever (57% to 71%; grades 3/4: 5% to 9%), febrile reaction (25%)

1% to 10%:

Cardiovascular: Hypertension (<10%), cardiomyopathy (≤9%), venous thromboembolism (deep vein thrombosis or pulmonary embolism; 7%)

Dermatologic: Cellulitis (<10%), folliculitis (<10%), hyperhidrosis (<10%), hyperkeratosis (<10%), palmar-plantar erythrodysesthesia (<10%), paronychia (<10%), pustular rash (<10%), secondary skin infection (3%)

Endocrine & metabolic: Hyperglycemia (grade 3: 5% to 6%)

Gastrointestinal: Pancreatitis (<10%), stomatitis (<10%)

Hematologic & oncologic: Cutaneous papilloma (<10%), basal cell carcinoma (9%), malignant neoplasm of skin (keratoacanthoma and squamous cell carcinoma; 7%)

Neuromuscular & skeletal: Weakness (<10%)

Ophthalmic: Blindness (transient; <10%), blurred vision (<10%), retinal detachment (pigment epithelium; 1%), uveitis (1%)

Renal: Renal failure (2% to 7%)

<1% (Limited to important or life-threatening): Glioblastoma, malignant neoplasm of colon and rectum (recurrent NRAS mutation-positive), malignant neoplasm of head and neck, pancreatic adenocarcinoma (KRAS mutation-positive)

Drug Interactions

Metabolism/Transport Effects Substrate of BCRP, CYP2C8 (major), CYP3A4 (major), P-glycoprotein; **Note:** Assignment of Major/Minor substrate status based on clinically relevant drug interaction potential; **Inhibits** BCRP, SLCO1B1; **Induces** CYP2B6 (weak/moderate), CYP2C19 (weak/moderate), CYP2C8 (weak/moderate), CYP2C9 (weak/moderate), CYP3A4 (moderate)

Avoid Concomitant Use

Avoid concomitant use of Dabrafenib with any of the following: Axitinib; Bedaquiline; Bosutinib; Cobimetinib; Conivaptan; CYP2C8 Inducers (Strong); CYP2C8 Inhibitors (Strong); CYP3A4 Inducers (Strong); CYP3A4 Inhibitors (Strong); Flibanserin; Fusidic Acid (Systemic); Idelalisib; Nisoldipine; Olaparib; Palbociclib; PAZOPanib; Ranolazine; Simeprevir; Sonidegib

Increased Effect/Toxicity

Dabrafenib may increase the levels/effects of: Highest Risk QTc-Prolonging Agents; Moderate Risk QTc-Prolonging Agents; PAZOPanib; Topotecan

The levels/effects of Dabrafenib may be increased by: Conivaptan; CYP2C8 Inhibitors (Moderate); CYP2C8 Inhibitors (Strong); CYP3A4 Inhibitors (Moderate); CYP3A4 Inhibitors (Strong); Deferasirox; Fusidic Acid (Systemic); Idelalisib; Luliconazole; Mifepristone; Osimertinib; Trametinib

Decreased Effect

Dabrafenib may decrease the levels/effects of: Antidiabetic Agents; ARIPiprazole; Axitinib; Bedaquiline; Bosutinib; Cobimetinib; Contraceptives (Estrogens); Contraceptives (Progestins); CYP2B6 Substrates; CYP2C19 Substrates; CYP2C8 Substrates; CYP2C9 Substrates; CYP3A4 Substrates; Daclatasvir; FentaNYL; Flibanserin; Ibrutinib; Nisoldipine; Olaparib; Palbociclib; Proton Pump Inhibitors; Ranolazine; Saxagliptin; Simeprevir; Sonidegib

The levels/effects of Dabrafenib may be decreased by: Antacids; CYP2C8 Inducers (Strong); CYP3A4 Inducers (Strong); H2-Antagonists; Osimertinib; Proton Pump Inhibitors; St Johns Wort

Food Interactions Administration with a high-fat meal decreased C_{max} and AUC by 51% and 31%, respectively, and delayed median T_{max} by ~4 hours. Management: Administer 1 hour before or 2 hours after a meal.

Storage/Stability Store at 25°C (77°F); excursions permitted to 15°C to 30°C (59°F to 86°F).

Mechanism of Action Selectively inhibits some mutated forms of the protein kinase B-raf (BRAF). BRAF V600 mutations result in constitutive activation of the BRAF pathway; through BRAF inhibition, dabrafenib inhibits tumor cell growth. The combination of dabrafenib and trametinib allows for greater inhibition of the MAPK pathway, resulting in BRAF V600 melanoma cell death (Flaherty, 2012).

Pharmacodynamics/Kinetics

Absorption: Decreased with a high-fat meal

Distribution: 70.3 L

Protein binding: 99.7% to plasma proteins

Metabolism: Hepatic via CYP2C8 and CYP3A4 to hydroxy-dabrafenib (active) which is further metabolized via CYP3A4 oxidation to desmethyl-dabrafenib (active)

Bioavailability: 95%

Half-life elimination: Parent drug: 8 hours; Hydroxy-dabrafenib (active metabolite): 10 hours; Desmethyl-dabrafenib (active metabolite): 21 to 22 hours

Time to peak: 2 hours; delayed with a high-fat meal

Excretion: Feces (71%); urine (23%; metabolites only)

Dosing

Adult & Geriatric

US labeling:

Melanoma, metastatic or unresectable (with BRAF V600E mutation): Oral: 150 mg twice daily (approximately every 12 hours) until disease progression or unacceptable toxicity (single-agent therapy)

Melanoma, metastatic or unresectable (with BRAF V600E or BRAF V600K mutation): Oral: 150 mg twice daily (approximately every 12 hours) until disease progression or unacceptable toxicity (in combination with trametinib)

Canadian labeling: **Melanoma, metastatic or unresectable (with BRAF V600 mutation):** Oral: 150 mg twice daily (approximately every 12 hours) until disease progression or unacceptable toxicity (single-agent therapy or in combination with trametinib)

Missed doses: A missed dose may be administered up to 6 hours prior to the next dose; do not administer if <6 hours until the next dose.

Renal Impairment

Mild to moderate impairment (GFR ≥30 mL/minute/1.73 m^2): No dosage adjustment necessary.

Severe impairment (GFR <30 mL/minute/1.73 m^2): There are no dosage adjustments provided in the manufacturer's labeling (has not been studied)

Hepatic Impairment

Mild impairment: No dosage adjustment necessary.

Moderate to severe impairment: There are no dosage adjustments provided in the manufacturer's labeling (has not been studied); however, metabolism is primarily hepatic and exposure may be increased in patients with moderate to severe impairment.

Adjustment for Toxicity

Recommended dabrafenib dose reductions for toxicity:

First dose reduction: 100 mg twice daily

Second dose reduction: 75 mg twice daily

Third dose reduction: 50 mg twice daily

Subsequent modifications (if unable to tolerate 50 mg twice daily): Permanently discontinue.

Note: If using combination therapy, refer to Trametinib monograph for recommended trametinib dose reductions.

Cardiac:

>20% absolute decrease in LVEF from baseline and LVEF is below institutional LLN: Interrupt dabrafenib therapy; if improved, may resume at the same dose.

Symptomatic heart failure: Interrupt dabrafenib therapy; if improved, may resume at the same dose.

Dermatologic:

Intolerable grade 2 skin toxicity or grade 3 or 4 skin toxicity: Interrupt dabrafenib therapy for up to 3 weeks. If toxicity improves within 3 weeks, resume at a lower dose level. If toxicity does not improve within 3 weeks following therapy interruption, permanently discontinue dabrafenib.

New primary cutaneous malignancy: No dabrafenib dosage modification is necessary.

Fever:

Fever of 38.5°C to 40°C (101.3°F to 104°F): Interrupt dabrafenib therapy until temperature normalizes. Resume at the same or lower dose level.

Fever >40°C (104°F) and/or fever complicated by rigors, hypotension, dehydration, or renal failure: Interrupt dabrafenib therapy until temperature normalizes. Resume at a lower dose level or permanently discontinue. May require prophylactic antipyretics (secondary prophylaxis) upon resumption. Administer corticosteroids (eg, prednisone 10 mg daily or equivalent) for at least 5 days for second or subsequent pyrexia if temperature does not return to baseline within 3 days of onset of fever, or for fever associated with complications (eg, dehydration, hypotension, severe chills/rigors with no evidence of active infection).

Hemorrhage:

Grade 3 hemorrhage: Interrupt dabrafenib therapy. If hemorrhage improves, resume at a lower dose level. If hemorrhage does not improve following therapy interruption, permanently discontinue dabrafenib.

Grade 4 hemorrhage: Permanently discontinue dabrafenib.

Ocular:

Uveitis including iritis and iridocyclitis: If mild or moderate uveitis does not respond to local ocular therapy (or for severe uveitis), interrupt dabrafenib therapy for up to 6 weeks. If improves to ≤ grade 1 within 6 weeks following therapy interruption, resume at the same dose. If does not improve, or for persistent grade 2 or higher uveitis of >6 week duration, permanently discontinue dabrafenib.

Grade 2 or 3 retinal pigment epithelial detachments (RPED): No dabrafenib dosage modification is necessary.

Retinal vein occlusion: No dabrafenib dosage modification is necessary.

Pulmonary: Interstitial lung disease or pneumonitis: No dabrafenib dosage modification is necessary.

Venous thromboembolism: Uncomplicated DVT or PE: No dabrafenib dosage modification is necessary.

Other toxicity:

Intolerable grade 2 or any grade 3 toxicity: Interrupt dabrafenib therapy until resolution to ≤ grade 1; resume at a lower dose level. If toxicity does not improve following therapy interruption, permanently discontinue dabrafenib.

Grade 4 toxicity (first occurrence): Interrupt dabrafenib therapy until resolution to ≤ grade 1; consider resuming at a lower dose level or permanently discontinue.

Grade 4 toxicity (recurrent after dosage reduction): Permanently discontinue dabrafenib.

New primary noncutaneous malignancy (RAS mutation-positive): Permanently discontinue dabrafenib.

Administration Administer orally at least 1 hour before or 2 hours after a meal; doses should be ~12 hours apart. Do not open, crush, or break capsules. A missed dose may be administered up to 6 hours prior to the next dose. When administered in combination with trametinib, take the once-daily dose of trametinib at the same time each day with either the morning or evening dose of dabrafenib.

Hazardous agent; use appropriate precautions for handling and disposal (meets NIOSH 2014 criteria). NIOSH recommends single gloving for administration of intact capsules (NIOSH 2014).

Monitoring Parameters BRAFV600 mutation status (prior to treatment); serum glucose (particularly in patients with preexisting diabetes mellitus or hyperglycemia); electrolytes; renal function; dermatologic evaluations prior to initiation, every 2 months during therapy, and for up to 6 months following discontinuation to assess for new cutaneous malignancies; monitor for febrile drug reactions and signs/symptoms of infections; signs/symptoms of uveitis (eg, eye pain, photophobia, vision changes), monitor for signs/symptoms of hemolytic anemia.

For patients receiving combination therapy with trametinib: Hepatic function (Canadian labeling recommends approximately every 4 weeks for 6 months after initiation then periodically as clinically indicated); CBC (baseline and periodically during therapy); assess LVEF (by echocardiogram or MUGA scan) at baseline, 1 month after therapy initiation, and then at 2- to 3-month intervals; monitor for signs/symptoms of hemorrhage, venous thromboembolism, interstitial lung disease, and RPED, or retinal vein occlusion.

Dosage Forms Excipient information presented when available (limited, particularly for generics); consult specific product labeling.

Capsule, Oral:

Tafinlar: 50 mg, 75 mg

Dacarbazine (da KAR ba zeen)

Brand Names: Canada Dacarbazine for Injection

Index Terms DIC; Dimethyl Triazeno Imidazole Carboxamide; DTIC; DTIC-Dome; Imidazole Carboxamide; Imidazole Carboxamide Dimethyltriazene; WR-139007

Pharmacologic Category Antineoplastic Agent, Alkylating Agent (Triazene)

Use Treatment of malignant melanoma, Hodgkin lymphoma

Pregnancy Considerations [U.S. Boxed Warning]: This agent is carcinogenic and/or teratogenic when used in animals; adverse effects have been observed in animal studies. There are no adequate and well-controlled trials in pregnant women; use in pregnancy only if the potential benefit outweighs the potential risk to the fetus.

Breast-Feeding Considerations Due to the potential for serious adverse reactions in the nursing infant, breast-feeding is not recommended.

Contraindications Hypersensitivity to dacarbazine or any component of the formulation

Warnings/Precautions Hazardous agent - use appropriate precautions for handling and disposal (NIOSH 2014 [group 1]). **[U.S. Boxed Warnings]: Bone marrow suppression is a common toxicity;** leukopenia and thrombocytopenia may be severe; may result in treatment delays or discontinuation; monitor closely. **Hepatotoxicity with hepatocellular necrosis and hepatic vein thrombosis has been reported (rare),** usually with combination chemotherapy, but may occur with dacarbazine alone. The half-life is increased in patients with renal and/or hepatic impairment; use caution, monitor for toxicity and consider dosage reduction. Anaphylaxis may occur following dacarbazine administration. Extravasation may result in tissue damage and severe pain. **[U.S. Boxed Warnings]: May be carcinogenic and/or teratogenic. Should be administered under the supervision of an experienced cancer chemotherapy physician.** Carefully evaluate the potential benefits of therapy against the risk for toxicity. Dacarbazine is associated with a high emetic potential; antiemetics are recommended to prevent nausea and vomiting (Basch, 2011; Dupuis, 2011; Roila, 2010).

Adverse Reactions Frequency not always defined.

Dermatologic: Alopecia

Gastrointestinal: Nausea and vomiting (>90%), anorexia

Hematologic: Myelosuppression (onset: 5-7 days; nadir: 7-10 days; recovery: 21-28 days), leukopenia, thrombocytopenia

Local: Pain on infusion

Infrequent, postmarketing, and/or case reports: Anaphylactic reactions, anemia, diarrhea, eosinophilia, erythema, facial flushing, facial paresthesia, flu-like syndrome (fever, myalgia, malaise), hepatic necrosis, hepatic vein occlusion, liver enzymes increased (transient), paresthesia, photosensitivity, rash, renal functions test abnormalities, taste alteration, urticaria

Drug Interactions

Metabolism/Transport Effects Substrate of CYP1A2 (major), CYP2E1 (major); **Note:** Assignment of Major/Minor substrate status based on clinically relevant drug interaction potential

Avoid Concomitant Use

Avoid concomitant use of Dacarbazine with any of the following: BCG (Intravesical); Deferiprone; Dipyrone; Natalizumab; Pimecrolimus; Tacrolimus (Topical); Tofacitinib; Vaccines (Live)

Increased Effect/Toxicity

Dacarbazine may increase the levels/effects of: CloZAPine; Deferiprone; Fingolimod; Leflunomide; Natalizumab; Tofacitinib; Vaccines (Live)

The levels/effects of Dacarbazine may be increased by: Abiraterone Acetate; CYP1A2 Inhibitors (Moderate); CYP1A2 Inhibitors (Strong); CYP2E1 Inhibitors (Moderate); CYP2E1 Inhibitors (Strong); Deferasirox; Denosumab; Dipyrone; Peginterferon Alfa-2b; Pimecrolimus; Roflumilast; Tacrolimus (Topical); Trastuzumab; Vemurafenib

Decreased Effect

Dacarbazine may decrease the levels/effects of: BCG (Intravesical); Coccidioides immitis Skin Test; Sipuleucel-T; Vaccines (Inactivated); Vaccines (Live)

The levels/effects of Dacarbazine may be decreased by: Cannabis; CYP1A2 Inducers (Strong); Cyproterone; Echinacea; Osimertinib; SORAfenib; Teriflunomide

Preparation for Administration Hazardous agent; use appropriate precautions for handling and disposal (NIOSH 2014 [group 1]). The manufacturer recommends reconstituting 100 mg and 200 mg vials with 9.9 mL and 19.7 mL SWFI, respectively, to a concentration of 10 mg/mL; some institutions use different standard dilutions (eg, 20 mg/mL).

Standard IV dilution: Dilute in 250-1000 mL D_5W or NS.

Storage/Stability Store intact vials under refrigeration (2°C to 8°C). Protect from light. The following stability information has also been reported: Intact vials are stable for 3 months at room temperature (Cohen, 2007). Reconstituted solution is stable for 24 hours at room temperature (20°C) and 96 hours under refrigeration (4°C) when protected from light, although the manufacturer recommends use within 72 hours if refrigerated and 8 hours at room temperature. Solutions for infusion (in D_5W or NS) are stable for 24 hours at room temperature if protected from light. Decomposed drug turns pink.

Mechanism of Action Alkylating agent which is converted to the active alkylating metabolite MTIC [(methyl-triazene-1-yl)-imidazole-4-carboxamide] via the cytochrome P450 system. The cytotoxic effects of MTIC are manifested through alkylation (methylation) of DNA at the O^6, N^7 guanine positions which lead to DNA double strand breaks and apoptosis. Non-cell cycle specific.

Pharmacodynamics/Kinetics

Distribution: Exceeds total body water; suggesting binding to some tissue (probably liver) (Perry 2012)

Protein binding: ~5%

Metabolism: Extensively hepatic to the active metabolite MTIC [(methyl-triazene-1-yl)-imidazole-4-carboxamide]

Half-life elimination: Biphasic: Initial: 20-40 minutes, Terminal: 5 hours; Patients with renal and hepatic dysfunction: Initial: 55 minutes, Terminal: 7.2 hours

Excretion: Urine (~40% as unchanged drug)

Dosing

Adult & Geriatric Note: Dacarbazine is associated with a high emetic potential; antiemetics are recommended to prevent nausea and vomiting (Basch, 2011; Roila, 2010).

Hodgkin lymphoma (combination chemotherapy): IV: 375 mg/m^2/dose days 1 and 15 every 4 weeks (ABVD regimen)

Metastatic melanoma: IV: 250 mg/m^2/dose days 1-5 every 3 weeks

Metastatic melanoma (off-label dosing; in combination with cisplatin and vinblastine): IV: 800 mg/m^2 on day 1 every 3 weeks (Atkins, 2008; Eton, 2002)

Soft tissue sarcoma (off-label use; MAID regimen): IV: 250 mg/m^2/day continuous infusion for 4 days every 3 weeks (total of 1000 mg/m^2/cycle) (Antman, 1993; Antman, 1998)

Pediatric Note: Dacarbazine is associated with a high emetic potential; antiemetics are recommended to prevent nausea and vomiting (Dupuis, 2011).

Hodgkin lymphoma (combination chemotherapy): IV: 375 mg/m^2/dose days 1 and 15 every 4 weeks (ABVD regimen; Hutchinson, 1998)

Renal Impairment The FDA-approved labeling does not contain dosage adjustment guidelines. The following guidelines have been used by some clinicians (Kintzel, 1995):

CrCl 46-60 mL/minute: Administer 80% of dose

CrCl 31-45 mL/minute: Administer 75% of dose

CrCl <30 mL/minute: Administer 70% of dose

Hepatic Impairment The FDA-approved labeling does not contain adjustment guidelines. May cause hepatotoxicity; monitor closely for signs of toxicity.

Obesity *ASCO Guidelines for appropriate chemotherapy dosing in obese adults with cancer:* Utilize patient's actual body weight (full weight) for calculation of body surface area- or weight-based dosing, particularly when the intent of therapy is curative; manage regimen-related toxicities in the same manner as for nonobese patients; if a dose reduction is utilized due to toxicity, consider resumption of full weight-based dosing with subsequent cycles, especially if cause of toxicity (eg, hepatic or renal impairment) is resolved (Griggs, 2012).

Administration Dacarbazine is associated with a high emetic potential; antiemetics are recommended to prevent nausea and vomiting (Basch, 2011; Dupuis, 2011; Roila, 2010).

Infuse over 30 to 60 minutes; rapid infusion may cause severe venous irritation. May also be administered as a continuous infusion (off-label administration rate) depending on the protocol.

Extravasation management: Local pain, burning sensation, and irritation at the injection site may be relieved by local application of hot packs. If extravasation occurs, apply cold packs. Protect exposed tissue from light following extravasation.

Hazardous agent; use appropriate precautions for handling and disposal (NIOSH 2014 [group 1]).

Monitoring Parameters CBC with differential, liver function

Dosage Forms Excipient information presented when available (limited, particularly for generics); consult specific product labeling.

Solution Reconstituted, Intravenous:

Generic: 100 mg (1 ea); 200 mg (1 ea)

Solution Reconstituted, Intravenous [preservative free]:

Generic: 200 mg (1 ea)

◆ Dacarbazine for Injection (Can) *see* Dacarbazine *on page 479*

Daclatasvir (dak LAT as vir)

Brand Names: US Daklinza

Index Terms Daclatasvir Dihydrochloride

Pharmacologic Category Antihepaciviral, NS5A Inhibitor

Use Chronic hepatitis C (genotype 3): Treatment of chronic hepatitis C virus (HCV) genotype 3 infection in combination with sofosbuvir

Pregnancy Considerations Adverse events were not observed in animal reproduction studies.

Breast-Feeding Considerations It is not known if daclatasvir is excreted into breast milk. According to the manufacturer, the decision to breastfeed during therapy should take into account the risk of exposure to the infant and the benefits of treatment to the mother. Breast-feeding is not linked to the spread of hepatitis C virus; however, if nipples are cracked or bleeding, breast-feeding is not recommended (CDC [Workowski 2015]).

Contraindications Concurrent use of strong CYP3A inducers (eg, carbamazepine, phenytoin, rifampin, St. John's wort)

Warnings/Precautions When used in combination with sofosbuvir and amiodarone, symptomatic bradycardia (eg, near-fainting, dizziness, lightheadedness, malaise, weakness, excessive tiredness, shortness of breath, chest pain, confusion, or memory problems) has been reported; pacemaker intervention may be required. Bradycardia generally occurs within hours or days but has been observed up to 2 weeks after treatment initiation. Risk factors include concomitant beta blocker use, underlying cardiac morbidities, and/or advanced hepatic disease. Patients receiving amiodarone (with no alternate treatment options) and initiating daclatasvir and sofosbuvir treatment, and patients on daclatasvir and sofosbuvir treatment who are initiating amiodarone therapy should have inpatient cardiac monitoring for the first 48 hours of amiodarone coadministration and daily outpatient self-monitoring through at least the first 2 weeks of treatment. Patients discontinuing amiodarone just prior to starting daclatasvir and sofosbuvir treatment should also undergo similar cardiac monitoring procedures. Bradycardia usually resolves after HCV treatment discontinuation. Sustained virologic response rates are reduced in patients with cirrhosis; optimal duration of treatment for patients with cirrhosis has not been established. Safety and efficacy have not been established in patients with decompensated cirrhosis or liver transplant. Do not use as monotherapy; use only in combination with sofosbuvir. Potentially significant drug-drug interactions may exist, requiring dose or frequency adjustment, additional monitoring, and/or selection of alternative therapy.

Adverse Reactions All adverse drug reactions are from combination therapy trials with sofosbuvir.

>10%
Central nervous system: Fatigue (14%), headache (14%)
1% to 10%:
Gastrointestinal: Nausea (8%), diarrhea (5%), increased serum lipase (2%; >3x ULN, transient)

Drug Interactions

Metabolism/Transport Effects Substrate of CYP3A4 (major), P-glycoprotein; **Note:** Assignment of Major/Minor substrate status based on clinically relevant drug interaction potential; **Inhibits** BCRP, P-glycoprotein, SLCO1B1, SLCO1B3

Avoid Concomitant Use
Avoid concomitant use of Daclatasvir with any of the following: Amiodarone; Bosutinib; Conivaptan; CYP3A4 Inducers (Strong); Fusidic Acid (Systemic); Idelalisib; PAZOPanib; Silodosin; St Johns Wort; Topotecan; VinCRIStine (Liposomal)

Increased Effect/Toxicity
Daclatasvir may increase the levels/effects of: Afatinib; Amiodarone; Bosutinib; Brentuximab Vedotin; Colchicine; Dabigatran Etexilate; Digoxin; DOXOrubicin (Conventional); Edoxaban; Everolimus; HMG-CoA Reductase Inhibitors; Ledipasvir; Naloxegol; PAZOPanib; P-glycoprotein/ABCB1 Substrates; Prucalopride; Ranolazine; Rifaximin; Silodosin; Topotecan; VinCRIStine (Liposomal)

The levels/effects of Daclatasvir may be increased by: Aprepitant; Conivaptan; CYP3A4 Inhibitors (Moderate); CYP3A4 Inhibitors (Strong); Dasatinib; Fosaprepitant; Fusidic Acid (Systemic); Idelalisib; Ivacaftor; Luliconazole; Mifepristone; Netupitant; Osimertinib; Palbociclib; Simeprevir; Stiripentol

Decreased Effect
The levels/effects of Daclatasvir may be decreased by: CYP3A4 Inducers (Moderate); CYP3A4 Inducers (Strong); Dabrafenib; Deferasirox; Osimertinib; Siltuximab; St Johns Wort; Tocilizumab

Storage/Stability Store at 25°C (77°F); excursions permitted between 15°C and 30°C (59°F and 86°F)

Mechanism of Action Daclatasvir binds to the N-terminus within Domain 1 of HCV nonstructural protein 5A (NS5A) and inhibits viral RNA replication and virion assembly.

Pharmacodynamics/Kinetics
Distribution: V_{dss}: 47 L
Protein binding: ~99%
Metabolism: Primarily via CYP3A
Bioavailability: 67%
Half-life elimination: 12 to 15 hours
Time to peak: 2 hours

Excretion: Feces (88%, 53% unchanged); urine (6.6%, primarily unchanged)

Dosing

Adult & Geriatric

Chronic hepatitis C (genotype 3): Oral: 60 mg once daily with concomitant sofosbuvir for 12 weeks. **Note:** Discontinue if sofosbuvir is permanently discontinued.

Dosage adjustment with concomitant medications:
Strong inhibitors of CYP3A: 30 mg once daily
Moderate CYP3A inducers: 90 mg once daily
Strong CYP3A inducers: Concomitant use is contraindicated.

Renal Impairment No dosage adjustment necessary.

Hepatic Impairment Child-Pugh class A, B, or C: No dosage adjustment necessary.

Administration Oral: Administer with or without food.

Monitoring Parameters Liver enzymes and serum creatinine at baseline and periodically when clinically indicated. If used in combination with amiodarone or in patients who discontinued amiodarone just prior to initiating sofosbuvir in combination with daclatasvir, inpatient cardiac monitoring for the first 48 hours of coadministration, then outpatient self-monitoring of heart rate daily through at least the first 2 weeks of treatment.

Dosage Forms Excipient information presented when available (limited, particularly for generics); consult specific product labeling.
Tablet, Oral:
Daklinza: 30 mg [contains fd&c blue #2 aluminum lake]
Daklinza: 60 mg

◆ Daclatasvir Dihydrochloride *see* Daclatasvir on page 480

◆ Dacogen *see* Decitabine on page 508

◆ DACT *see* DACTINomycin on page 481

DACTINomycin (dak ti noe MYE sin)

Brand Names: US Cosmegen
Brand Names: Canada Cosmegen
Index Terms ACT-D; Actinomycin; Actinomycin Cl; Actinomycin D; DACT
Pharmacologic Category Antineoplastic Agent, Antibiotic
Use Treatment of Wilms' tumor, childhood rhabdomyosarcoma, Ewing's sarcoma, metastatic testicular tumors (nonseminomatous), gestational trophoblastic neoplasm; regional perfusion (palliative or adjunctive) of locally recurrent or locoregional solid tumors (sarcomas, carcinomas and adenocarcinomas)

Dosing

Adult Note: Medication orders for dactinomycin are commonly written in MICROgrams (eg, 150 mcg) although many regimens list the dose in MILLIgrams (eg, mg/kg or mg/m²). The dose intensity per 2-week cycle should not exceed 15 mcg/kg/day for 5 days or 400-600 mcg/m²/day for 5 days. The manufacturer recommends calculation of the dosage for obese or edematous adult patients on the basis of body surface area in an effort to relate dosage to lean body mass. Dactinomycin is associated with a high emetic potential; antiemetics are recommended to prevent nausea and vomiting (Basch, 2011).

Testicular cancer, metastatic: IV: 1000 mcg/m² on day 1 (in combination with cyclophosphamide, bleomycin, cisplatin, and vinblastine)

Gestational trophoblastic neoplasm: IV: 12 mcg/kg/day for 5 days (as a single agent) **or** 500 mcg/dose on days 1 and 2 (in combination with etoposide, methotrexate, leucovorin, vincristine, cyclophosphamide, and cisplatin) **or** (off-label dosing for low-risk disease) 1.25 mg/m2 every 2 weeks as a single agent (Osborne, 2011)

Wilms tumor, Ewing's sarcoma, rhabdomyosarcoma: IV: 15 mcg/kg/day for 5 days (in various combination regimens and schedules)

Regional perfusion (dosages and techniques may vary by institution; obese patients and patients with prior chemotherapy or radiation therapy may require lower doses): Lower extremity or pelvis: 50 mcg/kg; Upper extremity: 35 mcg/kg

Osteosarcoma (off-label use): IV: 600 mcg/m² on days 1, 2, and 3 of weeks 15, 31, 34, 39, and 42 (as part of a combination chemotherapy regimen) (Goorin, 2003)

Ovarian (germ cell) tumor (off-label use): IV: 500 mcg daily for 5 days every 4 weeks (in combination with vincristine and cyclophosphamide) (Gershenson, 1985) **or** 300 mcg/m²/day for 5 days every 4 weeks (in combination with vincristine and cyclophosphamide) (Slayton, 1985)

Geriatric Refer to adult dosing. Elderly patients are at increased risk of myelosuppression; dosing should begin at the low end of the dosing range.

Pediatric Note: Medication orders for dactinomycin are commonly written in MICROgrams (eg, 150 mcg) although many regimens list the dose in MILLIgrams (eg, mg/kg or mg/m^2). The dose intensity per 2-week cycle should not exceed 15 mcg/kg/day for 5 days or 400-600 mcg/m^2/day for 5 days. Dactinomycin is associated with a high emetic potential; antiemetics are recommended to prevent nausea and vomiting (Dupuis, 2011).

Wilms tumor, rhabdomyosarcoma, Ewing's sarcoma:
Children >6 months: IV: 15 mcg/kg/day for 5 days (in various combination regimens and schedules)

Off-label dosing:
Rhabdomyosarcoma: IV:
VAC regimen:
Children <1 year: 25 mcg/kg every 3 weeks, weeks 0 to 45 (in combination with vincristine and cyclophosphamide, and mesna); dose omission required following radiation therapy (Raney, 2011)
Children ≥1 year: 45 mcg/kg (maximum dose: 2500 mcg) every 3 weeks, weeks 0 to 45 (in combination with vincristine and cyclophosphamide, and mesna); dose omission required following radiation therapy (Raney, 2011)
Wilms tumor: IV:
DD-4A regimen: 45 mcg/kg on day 1 every 6 weeks for 54 weeks (in combination with doxorubicin and vincristine) (Green, 1998)
EE-4A regimen: 45 mcg/kg on day 1 every 3 weeks for 18 weeks (in combination with vincristine) (Green, 1998)
VAD regimen:
Children <1 year: 750 mcg/m^2 every 6 weeks for 1 year (stage III disease) (in combination with vincristine and doxorubicin) (Pritchard, 1995)
Children ≥1 year: 1500 mcg/m^2 every 6 weeks for 1 year (stage III disease) (in combination with vincristine and doxorubicin) (Pritchard, 1995)
Osteosarcoma (off-label use): IV: 600 mcg/m^2 on days 1, 2, and 3 of weeks 15, 31, 34, 39, and 42 (as part of a combination chemotherapy regimen) (Goorin, 2003)

Renal Impairment There are no dosage adjustments provided in the manufacturer's labeling; however, based on the amount of urinary excretion, dosage adjustments may not be necessary.

Hepatic Impairment
U.S. labeling: There are no dosage adjustments provided in manufacturer's labeling.
Canadian labeling:
Mild impairment: There are no dosage adjustments provided.
Moderate-severe impairment: Dose reduction may be considered; 33% to 50% dose reductions for patients with hyperbilirubinemia have been recommended by some clinicians.
Off-label dosing: Any transaminase increase: Reduce dose by 50%; may increase by monitoring toxicities (Floyd, 2006).

Obesity *ASCO Guidelines for appropriate chemotherapy dosing in obese adults with cancer:* Utilize patient's actual body weight (full weight) for calculation of body surface area- or weight-based dosing, particularly when the intent of therapy is curative; manage regimen-related toxicities in the same manner as for nonobese patients; if a dose reduction is utilized due to toxicity, consider resumption of full weight-based dosing with subsequent cycles, especially if cause of toxicity (eg, hepatic or renal impairment) is resolved (Griggs, 2012).

Additional Information Complete prescribing information should be consulted for additional detail.

Dosage Forms Excipient information presented when available (limited, particularly for generics); consult specific product labeling. [DSC] = Discontinued product
Solution Reconstituted, Intravenous:
Cosmegen: 0.5 mg (1 ea)
Solution Reconstituted, Intravenous [preservative free]:
Generic: 0.5 mg (1 ea [DSC])

◆ Daklinza see Daclatasvir *on page 480*

◆ Dalacin C (Can) see Clindamycin (Systemic) *on page 405*

◆ Dalacin T (Can) see Clindamycin (Topical) *on page 409*

◆ Dalacin Vaginal (Can) see Clindamycin (Topical) *on page 409*

Dalbavancin (dal ba VAN sin)

Brand Names: US Dalvance
Index Terms BI 397; Zeven
Pharmacologic Category Glycopeptide
Use Acute bacterial skin and skin structure infections: Treatment of adult patients with acute bacterial skin and skin structure infections (ABSSSI) caused by susceptible isolates of the following gram-positive microorganisms: *Staphylococcus aureus* (including methicillin-susceptible and methicillin-resistant strains), *Streptococcus pyogenes*, *Streptococcus agalactiae* and *Streptococcus anginosus* group (including *S. anginosus*, *S. intermedius*, *S. constellatus*)
Pregnancy Considerations Adverse events were observed in some animal reproduction studies. The long half-life of dalbavancin should be considered when evaluating potential exposure to the fetus.
Breast-Feeding Considerations It is not known of dalbavancin is excreted into breast milk. The manufacturer recommends that caution be used if administered to a nursing woman.
Contraindications Hypersensitivity to dalbavancin or to any component of the formulation
Warnings/Precautions Serious hypersensitivity (anaphylactic) and skin reactions have been reported. Discontinue treatment if an allergic reaction occurs. Dalbavancin cross-sensitivity to other glycopeptides may occur; exercise caution in patients with a history of glycopeptide allergy; carefully screen for previous hypersensitivity reactions to glycopeptides prior to administration. Patients with normal baseline transaminase levels may have alanine aminotransferase (ALT) elevation >3 times the upper limit of normal (ULN) during therapy; in clinical studies, abnormalities in liver tests (ALT, AST, bilirubin) were reported with similar frequency in the dalbavancin and comparator arms. ALT elevations were reversible after discontinuation. Rapid intravenous infusions of dalbavancin (<30 minutes) may cause reactions that resemble "Red-Man Syndrome," (eg, flushing of the upper body, urticaria, pruritus, rash). Stopping or slowing the infusion may result in cessation of these reactions. Use may result in fungal or bacterial superinfection, including *Clostridium difficile*-associated diarrhea (CDAD) and pseudomembranous colitis; CDAD has been observed >2 months postantibiotic treatment.

Adverse Reactions
1% to 10%:
Cardiovascular: Flushing (<2%), phlebitis (<2%)
Central nervous system: Headache (5%), dizziness (<2%)
Dermatologic: Skin rash (3%), pruritus (2%), urticaria (<2%)
Endocrine & Metabolic: Hypoglycemia (<2%)
Gastrointestinal: Nausea (6%), diarrhea (4%), vomiting (3%), abdominal pain (<2%), gastrointestinal hemorrhage (<2%), hematochezia (<2%), melena (<2%), oral candidiasis (<2%), pseudomembranous colitis (<2%)
Hematologic & oncologic: Acute posthemorrhagic anemia (<2%), anemia (<2%), eosinophilia (<2%), hematoma (spontaneous; <2%), increased INR (<2%), leukopenia (<2%), neutropenia (<2%), petechia (<2%), thrombocythemia (<2%), thrombocytopenia (<2%), wound hemorrhage (<2%)
Hepatic: Hepatotoxicity (<2%)
Hepatic: Increased serum alkaline phosphatase (<2%), increased serum transaminases (<2%)
Hypersensitivity: Anaphylactoid reaction (<2%)
Infection: Vulvovaginal infection (mycotic; <2%)
Respiratory: Bronchospasm (<2%)
Miscellaneous: Infusion related reaction (<2%)
<1% (Limited to important or life-threatening): Hypersensitivity reaction, increased serum ALT (>3 x ULN)

Drug Interactions
Metabolism/Transport Effects None known.
Avoid Concomitant Use
Avoid concomitant use of Dalbavancin with any of the following: BCG (Intravesical)
Increased Effect/Toxicity There are no known significant interactions involving an increase in effect.
Decreased Effect
Dalbavancin may decrease the levels/effects of: BCG (Intravesical); BCG Vaccine (Immunization); Sodium Picosulfate; Typhoid Vaccine

Preparation for Administration Reconstitute with 25 mL of SWFI for each 500 mg vial. Alternate between gentle swirling and inversion of the vial until contents are completely dissolved. Do not shake. The reconstituted vial contains 20 mg/mL dalbavancin as a clear, colorless to yellow solution. Dilute for infusion in D$_5$W (final solution concentration 1 to 5 mg/mL).

Storage/Stability Store intact vials at 25°C (77°F); excursions are permitted between 15°C and 30°C (59°F and 86°F). Reconstituted vials and diluted solution may be stored refrigerated at 2°C to 8°C (36°F to 46°F) or at room temperature 20°C to 25°C (68°F to 77°F). Do not freeze. The total time from reconstitution to dilution to administration should be ≤48 hours.

Mechanism of Action Dalbavancin is a lipoglycopeptide which binds to the D-alanyl-D-alanine terminus of the stem pentapeptide in nascent cell wall peptidoglycan prevents cross-linking and interferes with cell wall synthesis. It is bactericidal *in vitro* against *Staphylococcus aureus* and *Streptococcus pyogenes*

Pharmacodynamics/Kinetics
Distribution: V_d: 7 to 13 L (Leighton, 2004)
Protein binding: 93% (primarily to albumin)
Metabolism: Minor metabolite (hydroxy-dalbavancin)
Half-life elimination: 346 hours
Excretion: Urine (33% as unchanged drug, 12% as hydroxy metabolite); feces (20%)

Dosing
Adult Usual dosage range: IV: 1000 mg as a single dose initially, followed by 500 mg as a single dose 1 week later
Indication-specific dosing: Acute bacterial skin and skin structure infections: IV: 1000 mg as a single dose initially, followed by 500 mg as a single dose 1 week later
Geriatric Refer to adult dosing
Renal Impairment
CrCl ≥30 mL/minute: No dosage adjustment necessary.
CrCl <30 mL/minute: 750 mg as a single dose initially, followed by 375 mg as a single dose 1 week later.
ESRD patients receiving intermittent hemodialysis (IHD) (regularly scheduled): No dosage adjustment necessary; administer without regard to hemodialysis.
Hepatic Impairment
Mild hepatic impairment (Child-Pugh class A): No dosage adjustment necessary.
Moderate or severe hepatic impairment (Child-Pugh class B or C): There are no dosage adjustments provided in the manufacturer's labeling (has not been studied); use with caution.
Usual Infusion Concentrations: Adult *IV infusion:* 500 mg or 1000 mg in 100 to 1000 mL (concentration of 1 to 5 mg/mL) of D_5W.
Administration IV: Infuse over 30 minutes. If a common IV line is being used to administer other drugs in addition to dalbavancin, the line should be flushed before and after each infusion with D_5W.
Monitoring Parameters Baseline BUN, serum creatinine, and liver function tests (AST, ALT, bilirubin). Monitor patients for any infusion-related reactions and for super-infection during therapy.
Dosage Forms Excipient information presented when available (limited, particularly for generics); consult specific product labeling.
Solution Reconstituted, Intravenous [preservative free]:
Dalvance: 500 mg (1 ea)

Dalfampridine (dal FAM pri deen)

Brand Names: US Ampyra
Brand Names: Canada Fampyra
Index Terms 4-aminopyridine; 4-AP; EL-970; Fampridine; Fampridine-SR
Pharmacologic Category Potassium Channel Blocker
Use Treatment to improve walking in patients with multiple sclerosis (MS)
Medication Guide Available Yes
Dosing
Adult & Geriatric Multiple sclerosis: Oral: 10 mg every 12 hours (maximum daily dose: 20 mg); no additional benefit seen with doses >20 mg daily
Missed doses: Do not administer double or extra doses if a dose is missed.
Renal Impairment Note: Creatinine clearance is estimated with Cockcroft-Gault formula.
U.S. labeling:
Mild renal impairment (CrCl 51-80 mL/minute): No dosage adjustment recommended by the manufacturer; however, use with extreme caution as risk of seizure may be increased secondary to reduced clearance.
Moderate-to-severe renal impairment (CrCl ≤50 mL/minute): Use is contraindicated.
Canadian labeling:
Mild-to-severe impairment (CrCl ≤80 mL/minute): Use is contraindicated.
Hepatic Impairment No dosage adjustment required; drug undergoes minimal metabolism and is primarily excreted unchanged in the urine.

Additional Information Complete prescribing information should be consulted for additional detail.
Dosage Forms Excipient information presented when available (limited, particularly for generics); consult specific product labeling.
Tablet Extended Release 12 Hour, Oral:
Ampyra: 10 mg
Dosage Forms: Canada Excipient information presented when available (limited, particularly for generics); consult specific product labeling.
Tablet, extended release, oral:
Fampyra™: 10 mg

Dalteparin (dal TE pa rin)

Brand Names: US Fragmin
Brand Names: Canada Fragmin
Index Terms Dalteparin Sodium
Pharmacologic Category Anticoagulant; Anticoagulant, Low Molecular Weight Heparin
Use Prevention of deep vein thrombosis (DVT) which may lead to pulmonary embolism, in patients requiring abdominal surgery who are at risk for thromboembolism complications (eg, patients >40 years of age, obesity, patients with malignancy, history of DVT or pulmonary embolism, and surgical procedures requiring general anesthesia and lasting >30 minutes); prevention of DVT in patients undergoing hip-replacement surgery; patients immobile during an acute illness; prevention of ischemic complications in patients with unstable angina or non-Q-wave myocardial infarction on concurrent aspirin therapy; in patients with cancer, extended treatment (6 months) of acute symptomatic venous thromboembolism (DVT and/or PE) to reduce the recurrence of venous thromboembolism

Canadian labeling: Additional use (off-label use in U.S.): Treatment of acute DVT; prevention of venous thromboembolism (VTE) in patients at risk of VTE undergoing general surgery; anticoagulant in extracorporeal circuit during hemodialysis and hemofiltration
Pregnancy Considerations Adverse effects were not observed in animal reproduction studies. Low molecular weight heparin (LMWH) does not cross the placenta; increased risks of fetal bleeding or teratogenic effects have not been reported (Bates, 2012).

LMWH is recommended over unfractionated heparin for the treatment of acute venous thromboembolism (VTE) in pregnant women. LMWH is also recommended over unfractionated heparin for VTE prophylaxis in pregnant women with certain risk factors. LMWH should be discontinued at least 24 hours prior to induction of labor or a planned cesarean delivery. For women undergoing cesarean section and who have additional risk factors for developing VTE, the prophylactic use of LMWH may be considered. For women who require long-term anticoagulation with warfarin and who are considering pregnancy, LMWH substitution should be done prior to conception when possible. When choosing therapy, fetal outcomes (ie, pregnancy loss, malformations), maternal outcomes (ie, VTE, hemorrhage), burden of therapy, and maternal preference should be considered (Guyatt, 2012). LMWH may also be used in women with mechanical heart valves (consult current guidelines for details) (Bates, 2012; Nishimura, 2014).

Multiple-dose vials contain benzyl alcohol (avoid in pregnant women due to association with gasping syndrome in premature infants); use of preservative-free formulation is recommended.
Breast-Feeding Considerations In lactating women receiving prophylactic doses of dalteparin, small amounts of anti-xa activity was noted in breast milk. The milk/plasma ratio was <0.025 to 0.224. Oral absorption of low molecular weight heparin is extremely low, and is therefore unlikely to cause adverse events in a nursing infant. Use of LMWH may be continued in breast-feeding women (Guyatt, 2012).
Contraindications Hypersensitivity to dalteparin (eg, pruritus, rash, anaphylactic reactions) or any component of the formulation; history of heparin-induced thrombocytopenia (HIT) or HIT with thrombosis; hypersensitivity to heparin or pork products; active major bleeding; patients with unstable angina, non-Q-wave MI, or prolonged venous

thromboembolism prophylaxis undergoing epidural/neuraxial anesthesia

Note: Use of dalteparin in patients with current HIT or HIT with thrombosis is **not** recommended and considered contraindicated due to high cross-reactivity to heparin-platelet factor-4 antibody (Guyatt [ACCP], 2012; Warkentin, 1999).

Canadian labeling: Additional contraindications (not in U.S. labeling): Septic endocarditis, major blood clotting disorders; acute gastroduodenal ulcer; cerebral hemorrhage; severe uncontrolled hypertension; diabetic or hemorrhagic retinopathy; other diseases that increase risk of hemorrhage; injuries to and operations on the CNS, eyes, and ears

Warnings/Precautions [U.S. Boxed Warning]: Spinal or epidural hematomas, including subsequent paralysis, may occur with recent or anticipated neuraxial anesthesia (epidural or spinal) or spinal puncture in patients anticoagulated with LMWH or heparinoids. Consider risk versus benefit prior to spinal procedures; risk is increased by the use of concomitant agents which may alter hemostasis, the use of indwelling epidural catheters for analgesia, a history of spinal deformity or spinal surgery, as well as traumatic or repeated epidural or spinal punctures. Optimal timing between neuraxial procedures and dalteparin administration is not known. Delay placement or removal of catheter for at least 12 hours after administration of 2,500 units once daily, at least 15 hours after the administration of 5,000 units once daily, and at least 24 hours after the administration of higher doses (200 units/kg once daily, 120 units/kg twice daily) and consider doubling these times in patients with creatinine clearance <30 mL/minute; risk of neuraxial hematoma may still exist since antifactor Xa levels are still detectable at these time points. Upon removal of catheter, consider delaying next dose of dalteparin for at least 4 hours. Patient should be observed closely for bleeding, signs and symptoms of neurological impairment, bowel and/or bladder dysfunction if therapy is administered during or immediately following diagnostic lumbar puncture, epidural anesthesia, or spinal anesthesia. If neurological compromise is noted, urgent treatment is necessary. If spinal hematoma is suspected, diagnose and treat immediately; spinal cord decompression may be considered although it may not prevent or reverse neurological sequelae. Use of dalteparin is contraindicated in patients undergoing epidural/neuraxial anesthesia. Patient should be observed closely for bleeding if dalteparin is administered during or immediately following diagnostic lumbar puncture, epidural anesthesia, or spinal anesthesia.

Use with caution in patients with preexisting thrombocytopenia, recent childbirth, subacute bacterial endocarditis, peptic ulcer disease, pericarditis or pericardial effusion, liver or renal function impairment, recent lumbar puncture, vasculitis, concurrent use of aspirin (increased bleeding risk), previous hypersensitivity to heparin, heparin-associated thrombocytopenia. Monitor platelet count closely. Cases of dalteparin-induced thrombocytopenia and thrombosis (similar to heparin-induced thrombocytopenia [HIT]), some complicated by organ infarction, limb ischemia, or death, have been observed. In patients with a history of HIT or HIT with thrombosis, dalteparin is contraindicated. Consider discontinuation of therapy in any patient developing significant thrombocytopenia (eg, <100,000/mm^3) and/or thrombosis related to initiation of dalteparin especially when associated with a positive *in vitro* test for antiplatelet antibodies. Use caution in patients with congenital or drug-induced thrombocytopenia or platelet defects.

Monitor patient closely for signs or symptoms of bleeding. Certain patients are at increased risk of bleeding. Risk factors include bacterial endocarditis; congenital or acquired bleeding disorders; active ulcerative or angiodysplastic GI diseases; severe uncontrolled hypertension; hemorrhagic stroke; or use shortly after brain, spinal, or ophthalmology surgery; in patients treated concomitantly with platelet inhibitors; recent GI bleeding; thrombocytopenia or platelet defects; hypertensive or diabetic retinopathy; or in patients undergoing invasive procedures. Protamine may be considered as a partial reversal agent in overdose situations (consult Protamine monograph for dosing recommendations).

Use with caution in patients with severe renal impairment or severe hepatic impairment; accumulation may occur with repeated dosing increasing the risk for bleeding. Heparin can cause hyperkalemia by affecting aldosterone. Similar reactions could occur with dalteparin. Monitor for hyperkalemia. Do **not** administer intramuscularly. Not to be used interchangeably (unit for unit) with heparin or any other low molecular weight heparins.

Benzyl alcohol and derivatives: Some dosage forms may contain benzyl alcohol and should not be used in pregnant women. In neonates, large amounts of benzyl alcohol (≥99 mg/kg/day) have been associated with a potentially fatal toxicity ("gasping syndrome"); the "gasping syndrome" consists of metabolic acidosis, respiratory distress, gasping respirations, CNS dysfunction (including convulsions, intracranial hemorrhage), hypotension, and cardiovascular collapse (AAP ["Inactive" 1997]; CDC, 1982); some data suggests that benzoate displaces bilirubin from protein binding sites (Ahlfors, 2001); avoid or use dosage forms containing benzyl alcohol with caution in neonates. See manufacturer's labeling.

There is no consensus for adjusting/correcting the weight-based dosage of LMWH for patients who are morbidly obese (BMI ≥40 kg/m^2). The American College of Chest Physicians Practice Guidelines suggest consulting with a pharmacist regarding dosing in bariatric surgery patients and other obese patients who may require higher doses of LMWH (Gould, 2012).

Adverse Reactions Note: As with all anticoagulants, bleeding is the major adverse effect of dalteparin. Hemorrhage may occur at virtually any site. Risk is dependent on multiple variables.

>10%: Hematologic & oncologic: Hemorrhage (3% to 14%), thrombocytopenia (including heparin-induced thrombocytopenia, <1%; cancer clinical trials: ~11%)

1% to 10%:
Hematologic & oncologic: Major hemorrhage (≤6%), wound hematoma (3%)
Hepatic: Increased serum ALT (>3 x ULN: 4% to 10%), increased serum AST (>3 x ULN: 5% to 9%)
Local: Pain at injection site (≤12%), hematoma at injection site (≤7%)

<1% (Limited to important or life-threatening): Alopecia, anaphylactoid reaction, gastrointestinal hemorrhage, hemoptysis, hypersensitivity reaction (fever, pruritus, rash, injections site reaction, bullous eruption), postoperative wound bleeding, skin necrosis, subdural hematoma, thrombosis (associated with heparin-induced thrombocytopenia). Spinal or epidural hematomas can occur following neuraxial anesthesia or spinal puncture, resulting in paralysis.

Drug Interactions

Metabolism/Transport Effects None known.

Avoid Concomitant Use

Avoid concomitant use of Dalteparin with any of the following: Apixaban; Dabigatran Etexilate; Edoxaban; Hemin; Omacetaxine; Rivaroxaban; Urokinase; Vorapaxar

Increased Effect/Toxicity

Dalteparin may increase the levels/effects of: ACE Inhibitors; Aliskiren; Angiotensin II Receptor Blockers; Anticoagulants; Canagliflozin; Collagenase (Systemic); Deferasirox; Deoxycholic Acid; Eplerenone; Ibritumomab; Nintedanib; Obinutuzumab; Omacetaxine; Palifermin; Potassium Salts; Potassium-Sparing Diuretics; Rivaroxaban; Tositumomab and Iodine I 131 Tositumomab

The levels/effects of Dalteparin may be increased by: 5-ASA Derivatives; Agents with Antiplatelet Properties; Apixaban; Dabigatran Etexilate; Dasatinib; Edoxaban; Hemin; Herbs (Anticoagulant/Antiplatelet Properties); Ibrutinib; Limaprost; Nonsteroidal Anti-Inflammatory Agents; Omega-3 Fatty Acids; Pentosan Polysulfate Sodium; Pentoxifylline; Prostacyclin Analogues; Salicylates; Sugammadex; Thrombolytic Agents; Tibolone; Tipranavir; Urokinase; Vitamin E; Vitamin E (Oral); Vorapaxar

Decreased Effect

Dalteparin may decrease the levels/effects of: Factor X (Human)

The levels/effects of Dalteparin may be decreased by: Estrogen Derivatives; Progestins

Preparation for Administration Canadian labeling: If necessary, may dilute in isotonic sodium chloride or dextrose solutions to a concentration of 20 units/mL. Use within 24 hours of mixing.

Storage/Stability Store at 20°C to 25°C (68°F to 77°F). Multidose vials may be stored for up to 2 weeks at room temperature after entering.

Mechanism of Action Low molecular weight heparin analog with a molecular weight of 4000-6000 daltons; the commercial product contains 3% to 15% heparin with a molecular weight <3000 daltons, 65% to 78% with a molecular weight of 3000-8000 daltons and 14% to 26% with a molecular weight >8000 daltons; while dalteparin has been shown to inhibit both factor Xa and factor IIa

(thrombin), the antithrombotic effect of dalteparin is characterized by a higher ratio of antifactor Xa to antifactor IIa activity (ratio = 4)

Pharmacodynamics/Kinetics
Onset of action: Anti-Xa activity: Within 1-2 hours

Duration: >12 hours

Distribution: V_d: 40-60 mL/kg

Protein binding: Low affinity for plasma proteins (Howard, 1997)

Bioavailability: SubQ: 81% to 93%

Half-life elimination (route dependent): Anti-Xa activity: 2-5 hours; prolonged in chronic renal insufficiency: 3.7-7.7 hours (following a single 5000 unit dose)

Time to peak, serum: Anti-Xa activity: ~4 hours

Excretion: Primarily renal (Howard, 1997)

Dosing
Adult & Geriatric Note: Each 2500 units of anti-Xa activity is equal to 16 mg of dalteparin.

Anticoagulant for hemodialysis and hemofiltration:
IV: Canadian labeling (not in U.S. labeling):

Chronic renal failure with no other bleeding risks:

Hemodialysis/filtration ≤4 hours: IV bolus: 5,000 units

Hemodialysis/filtration >4 hours: IV bolus: 30-40 units/kg, followed by an infusion of 10-15 units/kg/hour (typically produces plasma concentrations of 0.5-1 units anti-Xa/mL)

Acute renal failure and high bleeding risk: IV bolus: 5-10 units/kg, followed by an infusion of 4-5 units/kg/hour (typically produces plasma concentrations of 0.2-0.4 units anti-Xa/mL)

DVT prophylaxis: Note: In morbidly obese patients (BMI ≥40 kg/m²), increasing the prophylactic dose by 30% may be appropriate (Nutescu, 2009):

Abdominal surgery:

Low-to-moderate DVT risk: SubQ: 2500 units 1-2 hours prior to surgery, then once daily for 5-10 days postoperatively

High DVT risk: SubQ: 5000 units the evening prior to surgery and then once daily for 5-10 days postoperatively. Alternatively in patients with malignancy: 2500 units 1-2 hours prior to surgery, 2500 units 12 hours later, then 5000 units once daily for 5-10 days postoperatively.

General surgery with risk factors for VTE: Canadian labeling (not in U.S. labeling): 2500 units 1-2 hours preoperatively followed by 2500-5000 units every morning (may administer 2500 units no sooner than 4 hours after surgery and 8 hours after previous dose provided hemostasis has been achieved) or if other risk factors are present (eg, malignancy, heart failure), then may administer 5000 units the evening prior to surgery followed by 5000 units every evening postoperatively; continue treatment until patient is mobilized (approximately ≥5-7 days)

Total hip replacement surgery: SubQ: **Note:** Three treatment options are currently available. Dose is given for 5-10 days, although up to 14 days of treatment have been tolerated in clinical trials. The American College of Chest Physicians (ACCP) recommends a minimum duration of at least 10-14 days; extended duration of up to 35 days is suggested (Guyatt, 2012).

Postoperative regimen:

Initial: 2500 units 4-8 hours after surgery (or later if hemostasis not achieved). The ACCP recommends initiation ≥12 hours after surgery if postoperative regimen chosen (Guyatt, 2012).

Maintenance: 5000 units once daily; allow at least 6 hours to elapse after initial postsurgical dose (adjust administration time accordingly)

Preoperative regimen (starting day of surgery):

Initial: 2500 units within 2 hours **before** surgery. The ACCP recommends initiation ≥12 hours before surgery if preoperative regimen chosen (Guyatt, 2012). At 4-8 hours **after** surgery (or later if hemostasis not achieved), administer 2500 units.

Maintenance: 5000 units once daily; allow at least 6 hours to elapse after initial postsurgical dose (adjust administration time accordingly)

Preoperative regimen (starting evening prior to surgery):

Initial: 5000 units 10-14 hours **before** surgery. The ACCP recommends initiation ≥12 hours before surgery if preoperative regimen chosen (Guyatt, 2012). At 4-8 hours **after** surgery (or later if hemostasis not achieved), administer 5000 units.

Maintenance: 5000 units once daily, allowing 24 hours between doses

Immobility during acute illness: 5000 units once daily

Unstable angina or non-Q-wave myocardial infarction: SubQ: 120 units/kg body weight (maximum dose: 10,000 units) every 12 hours for up to 5-8 days with concurrent aspirin therapy. Discontinue dalteparin once patient is clinically stable.

Obesity: Use actual body weight to calculate dose; dose capping at 10,000 units recommended (Nutescu, 2009)

Venous thromboembolism, extended treatment in cancer patients: SubQ:

Initial (month 1): 200 units/kg (maximum dose: 18,000 units) once daily for 30 days

Maintenance (months 2-6): ~150 units/kg (maximum dose: 18,000 units) once daily. If platelet count between 50,000-100,000/mm³, reduce dose by 2,500 units until platelet count recovers to ≥100,000/mm³. If platelet count <50,000/mm³, discontinue dalteparin until platelet count recover to >50,000/mm³.

Obesity: Use actual body weight to calculate dose; dose capping is not recommended (Nutescu, 2009). However, the manufacturer recommends a maximum dose of 18,000 units per day for the treatment of VTE in cancer patients.

DVT (with or without PE) treatment in noncancer patients (off-label use in U.S.): SubQ: 200 units/kg once daily (Feissinger, 1996; Jaff, 2011; Wells, 2005) **or** 100 units/kg twice daily (Jaff, 2011). Use of once daily administration is suggested (Guyatt, 2012).

Canadian labeling: SubQ: 200 units/kg once daily (maximum dose: 18,000 units/day) **or** alternatively, may adapt dose as follows (SubQ):

46-56 kg: 10,000 units once daily

57-68 kg: 12,500 units once daily

69-82 kg: 15,000 units once daily

≥83 kg: 18,000 units once daily

Note: If increased bleeding risk, may give 100 units/kg SubQ twice daily. Concomitant treatment with a vitamin-K antagonist is usually initiated immediately.

Obesity: Use actual body weight to calculate dose; dose capping is not recommended (Nutescu, 2009). One study demonstrated similar anti-Xa levels after 3 days of therapy in obese patients (>40% above IBW; range: 82-190 kg) compared to those ≤20% above IBW or between 20% to 40% above IBW (Wilson, 2001).

Pregnant women (off-label use): 200 units/kg/dose once daily or 100 units/kg/dose every 12 hours. Discontinue ≥24 hours prior to the induction of labor or cesarean section. Dalteparin therapy may be substituted with heparin near term. Continue anticoagulation therapy for ≥6 weeks postpartum (minimum duration of therapy: 3 months). LMWH or heparin therapy is preferred over warfarin during pregnancy (Bates, 2012).

Mechanical heart valve (aortic or mitral position) to bridge anticoagulation (off-label use): 100 units/kg/dose every 12 hours (ACCP [Douketis, 2012]). **Note:** If used in pregnant patients, target anti-Xa level of 0.8 to 1.2 units/mL, 4 to 6 hours postdose (AHA/ACC [Nishimura, 2014]).

Prevention of recurrent venous thromboembolism in pregnancy (off-label use): SubQ: 5000 units once daily. Therapy should continue for 6 weeks postpartum in high-risk women (Bates, 2012).

Renal Impairment Half-life is increased in patients with chronic renal failure, use with caution, accumulation can be expected; specific dosage adjustments have not been recommended. Accumulation was not observed in critically ill patients with severe renal insufficiency (CrCl <30 mL/minute) receiving prophylactic doses (5000 units) for a median of 7 days (Douketis, 2008). In cancer patients, receiving treatment for venous thromboembolism, if CrCl <30 mL/minute, manufacturer recommends monitoring anti-Xa levels to determine appropriate dose.

Hepatic Impairment No dosage adjustment provided in manufacturer's labeling; use with caution.

Obesity Refer to indication-specific dosing for obesity-related information (may not be available for all indications).

Administration
For deep SubQ injection; may be injected in a U-shape to the area surrounding the navel, the upper outer side of the thigh, or the upper outer quadrangle of the buttock. Use thumb and forefinger to lift a fold of skin when injecting dalteparin to the navel area or thigh. Insert needle at a 45- to 90-degree angle. The entire length of needle should be inserted. Do not expel air bubble from fixed-dose syringe prior to injection. Air bubble (and extra solution, if applicable) may be expelled from graduated syringes. In order to minimize bruising, do not rub injection site.

To convert from IV unfractionated heparin (UFH) infusion to SubQ dalteparin (Nutescu, 2007): Calculate specific dose for dalteparin based on indication, discontinue UFH and begin dalteparin within 1 hour

To convert from SubQ dalteparin to IV UFH infusion (Nutescu, 2007): Discontinue dalteparin; calculate specific dose for IV UFH infusion based on indication; omit heparin bolus/loading dose

Converting from SubQ dalteparin dosed every 12 hours: Start IV UFH infusion 10-11 hours after last dose of dalteparin

Converting from SubQ dalteparin dosed every 24 hours: Start IV UFH infusion 22-23 hours after last dose of dalteparin

IV (Canadian labeling; not an approved route in U.S. labeling): Administer as bolus IV injection or as continuous infusion. Recommended concentration for infusion: 20 units/mL.

Monitoring Parameters Periodic CBC including platelet count; stool occult blood tests; monitoring of PT and PTT is not necessary. Once patient has received 3-4 doses, anti-Xa levels, drawn 4-6 hours after dalteparin administration, may be used to monitor effect in patients with severe renal dysfunction or if abnormal coagulation parameters or bleeding should occur. For patients >190 kg, if anti-Xa monitoring is available, adjusting dose based on anti-Xa levels is recommended; if anti-Xa monitoring is unavailable, reduce dose if bleeding occurs (Nutescu, 2009).

Reference Range

Recurrent VTE prophylaxis in pregnant women: Peak anti-Xa concentrations: 0.2-0.6 units/mL (Bates, 2012)

Treatment of venous thromboembolism: Peak anti-Xa concentration target (measured 4 hours after administration): *Once-daily dosing:* 1.05 anti-Xa units/mL (Garcia, 2012); per the manufacturer, target anti-Xa range is 0.5-1.5 units/mL (measured 4-6 hours after administration and after patient received 3-4 doses)

Dosage Forms Excipient information presented when available (limited, particularly for generics); consult specific product labeling. [DSC] = Discontinued product

Solution, Subcutaneous:

Fragmin: 25,000 units/mL (3.8 mL [DSC]); 95,000 units/3.8 mL (3.8 mL) [contains benzyl alcohol]

Solution, Subcutaneous [preservative free]:

Fragmin: 10,000 units/mL (1 mL); 2500 units/0.2 mL (0.2 mL); 5000 units/0.2 mL (0.2 mL); 7500 units/0.3 mL (0.3 mL); 12,500 units/0.5 mL (0.5 mL); 15,000 units/0.6 mL (0.6 mL); 18,000 units/0.72 mL (0.72 mL)

♦ Dalteparin Sodium *see* Dalteparin *on page 483*

♦ Dalvance *see* Dalbavancin *on page 482*

Danazol (DA na zole)

Brand Names: Canada Cyclomen®
Index Terms Danocrine
Pharmacologic Category Androgen
Use Treatment of endometriosis, fibrocystic breast disease, and hereditary angioedema
Dosing
Adult & Geriatric
Endometriosis (females): Oral:
Mild disease: Initial: 200-400 mg/day in 2 divided doses
Moderate-to-severe disease: Initial: 800 mg/day in 2 divided doses
Maintenance: Mild-severe disease: Dosage should be individualized. Continue therapy uninterrupted for 3-6 months (up to 9 months).
Fibrocystic breast disease (females): Oral: Range: 100-400 mg/day in 2 divided doses. Pain and tenderness may be eliminated in 2-3 months; elimination of nodularity may require therapy for 4-6 months.
Hereditary angioedema (males/females): Oral: Initial: 200 mg 2-3 times/day; after favorable response, decrease the dosage by 50% or less at intervals of 1-3 months or longer if the frequency of attacks dictates. If an attack occurs, increase the dosage by up to 200 mg/day.
Renal Impairment Use is contraindicated in patients with markedly impaired renal function.
Hepatic Impairment Use is contraindicated in patients with markedly impaired hepatic function.
Additional Information Complete prescribing information should be consulted for additional detail.
Dosage Forms Excipient information presented when available (limited, particularly for generics); consult specific product labeling.
Capsule, Oral:
Generic: 50 mg, 100 mg, 200 mg

♦ Dandrex [OTC] *see* Selenium Sulfide *on page 1647*

♦ Danocrine *see* Danazol *on page 486*

♦ Dantrium *see* Dantrolene *on page 486*

Dantrolene (DAN troe leen)

Brand Names: US Dantrium; Revonto; Ryanodex
Brand Names: Canada Dantrium
Index Terms Dantrolene Sodium
Pharmacologic Category Skeletal Muscle Relaxant
Use
IV: Management of malignant hyperthermia (MH); prevention of MH in susceptible individuals (preoperative/postoperative administration)
Oral: Treatment of spasticity associated with upper motor neuron disorders (eg, spinal cord injury, stroke, cerebral palsy, or multiple sclerosis); management of MH; prevention of MH in susceptible individuals (preoperative/postoperative administration)
Note: Dantrolene prophylaxis is not recommended for most MH-susceptible patients, provided nontriggering anesthetics are used and an adequate supply of dantrolene is available.
Pregnancy Considerations Adverse events have been observed in animal reproduction studies. Dantrolene crosses the human placenta. Cord blood concentrations are similar to those in the maternal plasma at term. and dantrolene can be detected in the newborn serum at delivery. Adverse events were not observed in the newborn following maternal doses of 100 mg/day administered orally prior to delivery (Shime, 1988). Uterine atony has been reported following dantrolene injection after delivery; however, this may be due in part to the mannitol contained in the IV preparation (Shin, 1995; Weingarten, 1987). Prophylactic use of dantrolene is not routinely recommended in pregnant women susceptible to MH prior to obstetric surgery, if use is needed, close monitoring of the mother and newborn is recommended (Krause, 2004; Norman, 1995).
Breast-Feeding Considerations Low amounts of dantrolene are excreted into breast milk. Due to the potential for serious adverse reactions in the nursing infant, the manufacturer recommends that a decision be made whether to discontinue nursing or to discontinue the drug, taking into account the importance of treatment to the mother. In a case report, the half-life of dantrolene in breast milk was calculated to be 9 hours; the highest milk concentration was 1.2 mcg/mL following a maternal IV dose; however, the maternal serum concentrations were not reported (Fricker, 1998).
Contraindications
IV: There are no contraindications listed within the manufacturer's labeling.
Oral: Active hepatic disease; should not be used when spasticity is used to maintain posture/balance during locomotion or to obtain/maintain increased function
Warnings/Precautions [U.S. Boxed Warning]: Oral: Has potential for hepatotoxicity. Higher doses (ie, ≥800 mg/day), even sporadic short courses, may increase the risk of severe hepatic injury although hepatic injury may occur at doses <400 mg/day. Overt hepatitis has been most frequently observed between the third and twelfth month of therapy. Hepatic injury appears to be greater in females, in patients >35 years of age, and those taking concurrent medications. A higher incidence of fatal hepatic events have been reported in the elderly, although concurrent disease states and concurrent use of hepatotoxic drugs may have contributed. Idiosyncratic and hypersensitivity reactions (sometimes fatal) of the liver have also occurred. Monitor hepatic function at baseline and as clinically indicated during treatment. Discontinue therapy if abnormal liver function tests occur or benefits are not observed within 45 days when utilized for chronic spasticity.

Loss of grip strength, weakness in the legs, dyspnea, respiratory muscle weakness, dysphagia, and decreased inspiratory capacity has occurred with IV dantrolene. Patients should not ambulate without assistance until they have normal strength and balance. Monitor patients for the adequacy of ventilation and for difficulty swallowing/choking.

Use oral therapy with caution in patients with impaired cardiac, hepatic, or pulmonary function (particularly in obstructive pulmonary disease). Oral therapy may cause photosensitivity. Lightheadedness, dizziness, somnolence, and vertigo may occur and may persist for 48-hours postdose; patients must be cautioned about performing tasks which require mental alertness (eg, operating machinery or driving).

Injection may contain mannitol. In addition to IV dantrolene, supportive measures must also be utilized for management of malignant hyperthermia; administer diuretics to prevent late kidney injury due to myoglobinuria. Alkaline

solution; may cause tissue necrosis if extravasated (vesicant); ensure proper needle or catheter placement prior to and during infusion; avoid extravasation.

Some dosage forms may contain polysorbate 80 (also known as Tweens). Hypersensitivity reactions, usually a delayed reaction, have been reported following exposure to pharmaceutical products containing polysorbate 80 in certain individuals (Isaksson, 2002; Lucente 2000; Shelley, 1995). Thrombocytopenia, ascites, pulmonary deterioration, and renal and hepatic failure have been reported in premature neonates after receiving parenteral products containing polysorbate 80 (Alade, 1986; CDC, 1984). See manufacturer's labeling.

Potentially significant interactions may exist, requiring dose or frequency adjustment, additional monitoring, and/ or selection of alternative therapy.

Adverse Reactions Frequency not always defined.

Cardiovascular: Flushing (intravenous: 27%), atrioventricular block (intravenous: 3%), tachycardia (3%), cardiac failure, phlebitis, variable blood pressure

Central nervous system: Drowsiness (17%; drowsiness may persist for 48 hours post dose), voice disorder (intravenous: 13%), feeling abnormal (intravenous: 10%), dizziness (3%), headache (3%), myasthenia (3%), chills, choking sensation, confusion, depression, fatigue, insomnia, malaise, nervousness, seizure, speech disturbance

Dermatologic: Acneiform eruption (capsules), diaphoresis, eczematous rash, erythema (intravenous), hair disease (abnormal growth), pruritus, urticaria

Gastrointestinal: Dysphagia (10%; use caution at meal time on day of administration as swallowing may be difficult), nausea (10%), vomiting (3%), abdominal cramps, anorexia, constipation, diarrhea, dysgeusia, gastric irritation, gastrointestinal hemorrhage, sialorrhea

Genitourinary: Crystalluria, difficulty in micturition, erectile dysfunction, hematuria, nocturia, urinary frequency, urinary incontinence, urinary retention

Hematologic & oncologic: Anemia, aplastic anemia, leukopenia, lymphocytic lymphoma, thrombocytopenia

Hepatic: Hepatitis

Hypersensitivity: Anaphylaxis

Local: Injection site reaction (intravenous: 3%; pain, erythema, swelling), local tissue necrosis (with extravasation due to high product pH)

Neuromuscular & skeletal: Limb pain (intravenous: 3%), back pain, myalgia

Ophthalmic: Blurred vision (intravenous: 3%), diplopia, epiphora, visual disturbance

Respiratory: Dyspnea (intravenous), pleural effusion (with pericarditis), pulmonary edema (rare), respiratory depression

Miscellaneous: Fever

<1% (Limited to important or life-threatening): Decrease in forced vital capacity (intravenous), dyspnea (intravenous), hepatic disease, hepatotoxicity (oral), increased liver enzymes (oral), respiratory muscle failure (intravenous)

Drug Interactions

Metabolism/Transport Effects Substrate of CYP3A4 (major); **Note:** Assignment of Major/Minor substrate status based on clinically relevant drug interaction potential

Avoid Concomitant Use

Avoid concomitant use of Dantrolene with any of the following: Azelastine (Nasal); Calcium Channel Blockers (Nondihydropyridine); Conivaptan; Fusidic Acid (Systemic); Idelalisib; Orphenadrine; Paraldehyde; Thalidomide

Increased Effect/Toxicity

Dantrolene may increase the levels/effects of: Alcohol (Ethyl); Azelastine (Nasal); Buprenorphine; Calcium Channel Blockers (Nondihydropyridine); CNS Depressants; Hydrocodone; Methotrimeprazine; Metyrosine; Mirtazapine; Orphenadrine; Paraldehyde; Pramipexole; ROPINIRole; Rotigotine; Selective Serotonin Reuptake Inhibitors; Suvorexant; Thalidomide; Vecuronium; Zolpidem

The levels/effects of Dantrolene may be increased by: Aprepitant; Brimonidine (Topical); Cannabis; Conivaptan; CYP3A4 Inhibitors (Moderate); CYP3A4 Inhibitors (Strong); Dasatinib; Dexketoprofen; Doxylamine; Dronabinol; Droperidol; Fosaprepitant; Fusidic Acid (Systemic); HydrOXYzine; Idelalisib; Ivacaftor; Kava Kava; Lacidipine; Luliconazole; Magnesium Sulfate; Methotrimeprazine; Mifepristone; Minocycline; Nabilone; Netupitant; Osimertinib; Palbociclib; Perampanel; Rufinamide; Simeprevir; Sodium Oxybate; Stiripentol; Tapentadol; Tetrahydrocannabinol

Decreased Effect

The levels/effects of Dantrolene may be decreased by: Bosentan; CYP3A4 Inducers (Moderate); CYP3A4 Inducers (Strong); Dabrafenib; Deferasirox; Enzalutamide; Mitotane; Osimertinib; Siltuximab; St Johns Wort; Tocilizumab

Preparation for Administration Injection, powder for reconstitution:

Dantrium, Revonto: Reconstitute vial by adding 60 mL of sterile water for injection only (**not bacteriostatic water for injection**); avoid glass bottles for IV infusion due to potential for precipitate formation.

Ryanodex: Reconstitute vial by adding 5 mL of sterile water for injection only (**not bacteriostatic water for injection**); shake well (suspension is an orange color). Do not dilute or transfer the suspension to another container to infuse the product.

Storage/Stability

Capsules: Store at 20°C to 25°C (68°F to 77°F).

Injection, powder for reconstitution: Protect from light. Use reconstituted solution within 6 hours of preparation.

Dantrium: Store unreconstituted vials and reconstituted solutions at 15°C to 30°C (59°F to 86°F).

Revonto: Store unreconstituted vials and reconstituted solutions at 20°C to 25°C (68°F to 77°F).

Ryanodex: Store unreconstituted vials at 20°C to 25°C (68°F to 77°F); excursions are permitted between 15°C and 30°C (59°F and 86°F). Store reconstituted solutions at 20°C to 25°C (68°F to 77°F).

Mechanism of Action Acts directly on skeletal muscle by interfering with release of calcium ion from the sarcoplasmic reticulum; prevents or reduces the increase in myoplasmic calcium ion concentration that activates the acute catabolic processes associated with malignant hyperthermia

Pharmacodynamics/Kinetics

Absorption: Oral: 70% (Allen 1988)

Distribution: V_d: 36.4 ± 11.7 L

Metabolism: Hepatic; major metabolites are 5-hydroxy dantrolene and an acetylamino metabolite of dantrolene.

Half-life elimination:

Neonates (at birth): ~20 hours (Shime 1988)

Children 2 to 7 years: 10 hours (range: 8.1 to 14.8 hours) (Lerman 1989)

Adults: 4 to 11 hours

Time to peak: IV: 1 minute post-dose (dantrolene); 24 hours post-dose (5-hydroxy dantrolene)

Excretion: Feces (45% to 50%); urine (25% as unchanged drug and metabolites)

Dosing

Adult & Geriatric

Spasticity: Oral:

Note: Dose should be titrated and individualized for maximum effect; use the lowest dose compatible with optimal response. Some patients may not respond until a higher daily dosage is achieved; each dose level should be maintained for 7 days to determine patient response. If no further benefit observed with the higher dose level, then decrease dosage to previous dose level. Because of the potential for hepatotoxicity, stop therapy if benefits are not evident within 45 days.

Initial: 25 mg once daily for 7 days; increase to 25 mg 3 times daily for 7 days, increase to 50 mg 3 times daily for 7 days, and then increase to 100 mg 3 times daily; some patients may require 100 mg 4 times daily; maximum dose: 400 mg daily

Malignant hyperthermia (MH):

Preoperative prophylaxis: **Note:** Dantrolene prophylaxis is not recommended for most MH-susceptible patients, provided nontriggering anesthetics are used and an adequate supply of dantrolene is available.

Oral: 4 to 8 mg/kg/day in 3 to 4 divided doses, begin 1 to 2 days prior to surgery with last dose 3 to 4 hours prior to surgery

IV: 2.5 mg/kg ~1¼ hours prior to anesthesia and infused over at least 1 minute (Ryanodex) or 1 hour (Dantrium, Revonto) with additional doses as needed and individualized

Crisis: IV: 2.5 mg/kg (MHAUS recommendation, available at www.mhaus.org); continuously repeat dose until symptoms subside or a cumulative dose of 10 mg/kg is reached (rarely, some patients may require up to 30 mg/kg for initial treatment). **Note:** Manufacturer's labeling suggests an initial minimum dose of 1 mg/kg.

24-hour MH Hotline (for emergencies only):

United States: 1-800-644-9737

Outside the U.S.: 00-1-209-417-3722

Postcrisis follow-up:

MHAUS protocol suggestion: 1 mg/kg every 4 to 6 hours (route not specified) **or** a continuous IV infusion of 0.25 mg/kg/hour for at least 24 hours; further doses may be indicated

Manufacturer's labeling: Oral: 4 to 8 mg/kg/day in 4 divided doses for 1 to 3 days; IV dantrolene may be used to prevent or attenuate recurrence of MH signs when oral therapy is not practical; individualize dosage beginning with 1 mg/kg or more as the clinical situation dictates

Neuroleptic malignant syndrome (off-label use): IV: 1 to 2.5 mg/kg, may repeat dose up to maximum cumulative dose of 10 mg/kg/day, then switch to oral dosage (Strawn, 2007; Susman, 2001)

Pediatric

Spasticity: Oral:

Note: Dose should be titrated and individualized for maximum effect; use the lowest dose compatible with optimal response. Some patients may not respond until a higher daily dosage is achieved; each dose level should be maintained for 7 days to determine patient response. If no further benefit observed with the higher dose level, then decrease dosage to previous dose level. Because of the potential for hepatotoxicity, stop therapy if benefits are not evident within 45 days.

Initial: 0.5 mg/kg/dose once daily for 7 days; increase to 0.5 mg/kg/dose 3 times daily for 7 days, increase to 1 mg/kg/dose 3 times daily for 7 days, and then increase to 2 mg/kg/dose 3 times daily; some patients may require 2 mg/kg/dose 4 times daily; maximum dose: 400 mg daily

Malignant hyperthermia (MH): Refer to adult dosing.

Renal Impairment There are no dosage adjustments provided in the manufacturer's labeling.

Hepatic Impairment There are no dosage adjustments provided in the manufacturer's labeling; use of oral dantrolene in patients with active liver disease (eg, hepatitis and cirrhosis) is contraindicated.

Administration IV: Therapeutic or emergency dose can be administered with rapid continuous IV push. Follow-up doses should be administered over at least 1 minute (Ryanodex) or 1 hour (Dantrium, Revonto).

Vesicant; ensure proper needle or catheter placement prior to and during infusion; avoid extravasation.

Extravasation management: If extravasation occurs, stop infusion immediately and disconnect (leave cannula/needle in place); gently aspirate extravasated solution (do **NOT** flush the line); remove needle/cannula; elevate extremity.

Monitoring Parameters Motor performance should be monitored for therapeutic outcomes; nausea, vomiting, and liver function tests (baseline and at appropriate intervals thereafter) should be monitored for potential hepatotoxicity; intravenous administration requires cardiac, blood pressure, and respiratory monitoring.

Malignant hyperthermia: During and post-acute phase: Per MHAUS protocol, patient should be observed in an ICU for at least 24 hours since recrudescence may occur; monitor for arrhythmias; monitor vital signs (including core temperature), electrolytes, ABG, CK, end tidal CO_2 ($EtCO_2$)/capnography, urine output, urine myoglobin

Dosage Forms Excipient information presented when available (limited, particularly for generics); consult specific product labeling. [DSC] = Discontinued product

Capsule, Oral, as sodium:
Dantrium: 25 mg, 50 mg, 100 mg [DSC] [contains fd&c yellow #6 (sunset yellow)]
Generic: 25 mg, 50 mg, 100 mg
Solution Reconstituted, Intravenous, as sodium:
Dantrium: 20 mg (1 ea)
Revonto: 20 mg (1 ea)
Suspension Reconstituted, Intravenous, as sodium:
Ryanodex: 250 mg (1 ea) [contains polysorbate 80]

Extemporaneous Preparations A 5 mg/mL oral suspension may be made with dantrolene capsules, a citric acid solution, and either simple syrup or syrup BP (containing 0.15% w/v methylhydroxybenzoate). Add the contents of five 100 mg dantrolene capsules to a citric acid solution (150 mg citric acid powder in 10 mL water); mix while adding the chosen vehicle in incremental proportions to almost 100 mL. Transfer to a calibrated bottle and add quantity of vehicle sufficient to make 100 mL. Label "shake well" and "refrigerate". Simple syrup suspension is stable for 2 days refrigerated; syrup BP suspension is stable for 30 days refrigerated.

Nahata MC, Pai VB, and Hipple TF, *Pediatric Drug Formulations*, 5th ed, Cincinnati, OH: Harvey Whitney Books Co, 2004.

◆ Dantrolene Sodium *see* Dantrolene *on page 486*

Dapagliflozin and Metformin
(dap a gli FLOE zin & met FOR min)

Brand Names: US Xigduo XR

Index Terms Metformin and Dapagliflozin; Metformin Hydrochloride and Dapagliflozin

Pharmacologic Category Antidiabetic Agent, Biguanide; Antidiabetic Agent, Sodium-Glucose Cotransporter 2 (SGLT2) Inhibitor; Sodium-Glucose Cotransporter 2 (SGLT2) Inhibitor

Use

Diabetes mellitus, type 2: As an adjunct to diet and exercise to improve glycemic control in adults with type 2 diabetes mellitus (noninsulin dependent, NIDDM) when treatment with both dapagliflozin and metformin is appropriate.

Limitations of use: Not indicated in patients with type 1 diabetes (insulin dependent, IDDM) or for the treatment of diabetic ketoacidosis.

Dosing

Adult Note: If converting from a metformin extended release product that is being taken in the evening, skip the last dose before starting the dapagliflozin/metformin combination product.

Diabetes mellitus, type 2: Oral: Initial: Individualize based on patient's current antidiabetic regimen. May gradually increase dose based on effectiveness and tolerability; range: dapagliflozin 5 mg/metformin 500 mg once daily to dapagliflozin 10 mg/metformin 2,000 mg once daily. Maximum: dapagliflozin 10 mg/metformin 2,000 mg once daily.

Geriatric Diabetes mellitus, type 2: Oral: The initial and maintenance dosing should be conservative, due to the potential for decreased renal function. Generally, elderly patients should not be titrated to the maximum dose of metformin. Do not use in patients ≥80 years of age unless normal renal function has been established.

Renal Impairment

eGFR ≥60 mL/minute/1.73 m²: No dosage adjustment necessary.

eGFR <60 mL/minute/1.73 m² or CrCl <60 mL/minute: Use is contraindicated.

Hepatic Impairment The manufacturer recommends to avoid metformin since liver disease is considered a risk factor for the development of lactic acidosis during metformin therapy. However, continued use of metformin in diabetics with liver dysfunction, including cirrhosis, has been used successfully and may be associated with a survival benefit in carefully selected patients; use cautiously in patients at risk for lactic acidosis (eg, renal impairment, alcohol use) (Brackett, 2010; Zhang, 2014). No dosage adjustment is necessary for dapagliflozin in patients with mild to severe hepatic impairment according to the manufacturer's labeling for dapagliflozin.

Additional Information Complete prescribing information should be consulted for additional detail.

Dosage Forms Excipient information presented when available (limited, particularly for generics); consult specific product labeling.

Tablet Extended Release 24 Hour, Oral:
Xigduo XR: Dapagliflozin 10 mg and metformin hydrochloride 500 mg, Dapagliflozin 10 mg and metformin hydrochloride 1000 mg, Dapagliflozin 5 mg and metformin hydrochloride 1000 mg
Xigduo XR: Dapagliflozin 5 mg and metformin hydrochloride 500 mg [contains fd&c yellow #6 aluminum lake]

◆ Dapcin *see* DAPTOmycin *on page 490*

Dapsone (Systemic) (DAP sone)

Index Terms Diaminodiphenylsulfone

Pharmacologic Category Antibiotic, Miscellaneous

Use Treatment of leprosy (due to susceptible strains of *Mycobacterium leprae*) and dermatitis herpetiformis

Pregnancy Considerations Adverse events were observed in some animal reproduction studies. Dapsone crosses the placenta (Brabin, 2004). Per the manufacturer, dapsone has not shown an increased risk of congenital anomalies when given during all trimesters of pregnancy. Several reports have described adverse effects in the newborn after *in utero* exposure to dapsone, including neonatal hemolytic disease, methemoglobinemia, and hyperbilirubinemia (Hocking, 1968; Kabra, 1998; Thornton, 1989). Dapsone may be used in pregnant women requiring maintenance therapy of either leprosy or dermatitis herpetiformis. Dapsone may be used as an alternative agent for prophylaxis of *Pneumocystis jirovecii* pneumonia (PCP) in pregnant, HIV-infected patients (DHHS [OI], 2013).

Breast-Feeding Considerations Dapsone is excreted in breast milk and can be detected in the serum of nursing infants. Hemolytic anemia has been reported in a breast-fed infant (Sanders, 1982). Due to the potential for serious adverse reactions in the nursing infant, the manufacturer recommends a decision be made whether to discontinue nursing or to discontinue the drug, taking into account the importance of treatment to the mother.

Contraindications Hypersensitivity to dapsone or any component of the formulation

Warnings/Precautions Use with caution in patients with severe anemia, G6PD, methemoglobin reductase deficiency or hemoglobin M deficiency; hypersensitivity to other sulfonamides; aplastic anemia, agranulocytosis and other severe blood dyscrasias have resulted in death; monitor carefully; serious dermatologic reactions (including toxic epidermal necrolysis) are rare but potential occurrences; sulfone reactions may also occur as potentially fatal hypersensitivity reactions; these, but not leprosy reactional states, require drug discontinuation. Motor loss and muscle weakness have been reported with use. Prolonged use may result in fungal or bacterial superinfection, including *C. difficile*-associated diarrhea and pseudomembranous colitis.

Adverse Reactions Frequency not always defined.

>10%: Hematologic: Reticulocyte increase (2% to 12%), hemolysis (>10%; dose related; seen in patients with and without G6PD deficiency), hemoglobin decrease (>10%; 1-2 g/dL; almost all patients), methemoglobinemia (>10%), red cell life span shortened (>10%), Agranulocytosis, anemia, leukopenia, pure red cell aplasia (case report)

Cardiovascular: Tachycardia

Central nervous system: Fever, headache, insomnia, psychosis, vertigo

Dermatologic: Bullous and exfoliative dermatitis, erythema nodosum, exfoliative dermatitis, morbilliform and scarlatiniform reactions, phototoxicity, Stevens-Johnson syndrome, toxic epidermal necrolysis, urticaria

Endocrine & metabolic: Hypoalbuminemia (without proteinuria), male infertility

Gastrointestinal: Abdominal pain, nausea, pancreatitis, vomiting

Hepatic: Cholestatic jaundice, hepatitis

Neuromuscular & skeletal: Drug-induced lupus erythematosus, lower motor neuron toxicity (prolonged therapy), peripheral neuropathy (rare, nonleprosy patients)

Ocular: Blurred vision

Otic: Tinnitus

Renal: Albuminuria, nephrotic syndrome, renal papillary necrosis

Respiratory: Interstitial pneumonitis, pulmonary eosinophilia

Miscellaneous: Infectious mononucleosis-like syndrome (rash, fever, lymphadenopathy, hepatic dysfunction)

Drug Interactions

Metabolism/Transport Effects Substrate of CYP2C19 (minor), CYP2C8 (minor), CYP2C9 (major), CYP2E1 (minor), CYP3A4 (major); **Note:** Assignment of Major/Minor substrate status based on clinically relevant drug interaction potential

Avoid Concomitant Use

Avoid concomitant use of Dapsone (Systemic) with any of the following: BCG (Intravesical)

Increased Effect/Toxicity

Dapsone (Systemic) may increase the levels/effects of: Antimalarial Agents; Atazanavir; Prilocaine; Sodium Nitrite; Trimethoprim

The levels/effects of Dapsone (Systemic) may be increased by: Antimalarial Agents; Ceritinib; CYP2C9 Inhibitors (Moderate); CYP2C9 Inhibitors (Strong); Dapsone (Topical); Mifepristone; Nitric Oxide; Osimertinib; Probenecid; Trimethoprim

Decreased Effect

Dapsone (Systemic) may decrease the levels/effects of: BCG (Intravesical); BCG Vaccine (Immunization); Sodium Picosulfate; Typhoid Vaccine

The levels/effects of Dapsone (Systemic) may be decreased by: Bosentan; CYP2C9 Inducers (Strong); CYP3A4 Inducers (Moderate); CYP3A4 Inducers (Strong); Dabrafenib; Deferasirox; Enzalutamide; Mitotane; Osimertinib; Rifamycin Derivatives; Siltuximab; St Johns Wort; Tocilizumab

Storage/Stability Store at 20°C to 25°C (68°F to 76°F). Protect from light.

Mechanism of Action Competitive antagonist of para-aminobenzoic acid (PABA) and prevents normal bacterial utilization of PABA for the synthesis of folic acid

Pharmacodynamics/Kinetics

Absorption: Rapid and almost complete

Protein binding: Dapsone: 70% to 90%; Metabolite: ~99%

Distribution: V_d: 1.5 L/kg; throughout total body water and present in all tissues, especially liver and kidney

Metabolism: Hepatic (acetylation and hydroxylation); forms multiple metabolites

Half-life elimination: Children: 15.1 hours (Mirochnick 1993); Adults: 28 hours (range: 10 to 50 hours)

Time to peak: Within 4-8 hours

Excretion: Urine (~85% as metabolites)

Dosing

Adult & Geriatric

Leprosy: Oral: 100 mg daily, in combination with other antileprosy agents; duration of therapy is variable

Dermatitis herpetiformis: Oral: Start at 50 mg daily, increase to 300 mg daily, or higher to achieve full control, reduce dosage to minimum level as soon as possible

Aphthous ulcers, severe (off-label use): Oral:

Initial: 25 mg daily for 3 days; increase dose in increments of 25 mg daily every 3 days up to 100 mg daily for 3 days, then increase by 25 mg daily every 7 days up to 150 mg daily. Administer in 2 divided doses (75 mg dose is administered in 3 divided doses).

Maintenance: 100 to 150 mg daily in 2 divided doses with or without concomitant colchicine (Rogers, 1982; Lynde 2009)

Bullous systemic lupus erythematosus (off-label use): Oral: 100 mg once daily with or without prednisone (Fabbri, 2003).

Pemphigus vulgaris (off-label use): Oral: 25 mg daily for 7 days, then increase dose in increments of 25 mg daily every 7 days up to 100 mg daily for 7 days (4 weeks total therapy) with concomitant prednisone. Administer in 2 divided doses (a 75 mg dose is administered in 3 divided doses) (Azizi, 2008). **Note:** If patient becomes lesion free, taper and discontinue gradually by decreasing dose 25 mg daily over 7 days. If no new lesions are seen, gradual taper is continued. If lesions recur, dose is increased by 25 mg daily at 7-day intervals until the patient develops no new lesions. Taper is usually ~4 weeks total.

***Pneumocystis* pneumonia (PCP) in HIV-infected patients (off-label use; HHS [OI adult 2015]):** Oral:

Prophylaxis (primary or secondary; alternative to preferred therapy): 100 mg daily once daily or in 2 divided doses as monotherapy **or** 50 mg daily in combination with weekly pyrimethamine and leucovorin **or** 200 mg weekly in combination with weekly pyrimethamine and leucovorin

Treatment (mild to moderate disease; alternative to preferred therapy): 100 mg once daily in combination with trimethoprim for 21 days

***Toxoplasma gondii* encephalitis in HIV-infected patients (alternative to preferred therapy) (off-label use):** *Primary prophylaxis:* Oral: 50 mg daily, in combination with weekly pyrimethamine and leucovorin **or** 200 mg weekly in combination with weekly pyrimethamine and leucovorin (HHS [OI adult 2015])

Pediatric

Leprosy: Oral: Children: 1 to 2 mg/kg/24 hours, up to a maximum of 100 mg/day, in combination with other antileprosy agents; duration of therapy is variable

***Pneumocystis* pneumonia (PCP) in HIV-exposed/-positive patients (off-label use):** Oral:

Prophylaxis (primary or secondary; alternative to preferred therapy):

Infants and Children: 2 mg/kg/day once daily (maximum dose: 100 mg daily) or 4 mg/kg/dose once weekly (maximum dose: 200 mg) (CDC, 2009)

Adolescents: Refer to adult dosing.

Treatment (alternative to preferred therapy):

Infants and Children: 2 mg/kg/day once daily (maximum dose: 100 mg daily) in combination with trimethoprim for 21 days (CDC, 2009)

Adolescents: Refer to adult dosing.

***Toxoplasma gondii* encephalitis in HIV-exposed/-positive patients (alternative to preferred therapy) (off-label use):** *Primary prophylaxis:* Oral:

Infants and Children: 2 mg/kg or 15 mg/m² up to a maximum of 25 mg once daily, in combination with pyrimethamine and leucovorin (CDC, 2009)

Adolescents (mild to moderate disease): Refer to adult dosing.

Renal Impairment No guidelines are available.

Dietary Considerations Do not give with antacids, alkaline foods, or drugs.

Administration May administer with meals if GI upset occurs.

Monitoring Parameters Check G6PD levels (prior to initiation); CBC (weekly for first month, monthly for 6 months and semiannually thereafter); reticulocyte counts; liver function tests. Monitor patients for signs of jaundice and hemolysis.

Dosage Forms Excipient information presented when available (limited, particularly for generics); consult specific product labeling.

Tablet, Oral:

Generic: 25 mg, 100 mg

Extemporaneous Preparations A 2 mg/mL oral suspension may be made with tablets and a 1:1 mixture of Ora-Sweet® and Ora-Plus®. Crush eight 25 mg tablets in a mortar and reduce to a fine powder. Add small portions of vehicle and mix to a uniform paste; mix while adding the vehicle in incremental proportions to **almost** 100 mL; transfer to a calibrated bottle, rinse mortar with vehicle, and add quantity of vehicle sufficient to make 100 mL. Label "shake well". Stable for 90 days at room temperature or refrigerated.

Jacobus Pharmaceutical Company makes a 2 mg/mL proprietary liquid formulation available under an IND for the prophylaxis of *Pneumocystis jirovecii* pneumonia.

Nahata MC, Morosco RS, and Trowbridge JM, "Stability of Dapsone in Two Oral Liquid Dosage Forms," *Ann Pharmacother*, 2000, 34 (7-8):848-50.

◆ **Daptacel** *see* Diphtheria and Tetanus Toxoids, and Acellular Pertussis Vaccine *on page 567*

DAPTOmycin (DAP toe mye sin)

Brand Names: US Cubicin

Brand Names: Canada Cubicin

Index Terms Cidecin; Dapcin; LY146032

Pharmacologic Category Antibiotic, Cyclic Lipopeptide

Use

Skin and skin structure infections, complicated: For the treatment of complicated skin and skin structure infections caused by susceptible isolates of the following gram-positive bacteria: *Staphylococcus aureus* (including methicillin-resistant isolates), *Streptococcus pyogenes*, *Streptococcus agalactiae*, *Streptococcus dysgalactiae* subspecies *equisimilis*, and *Enterococcus faecalis* (vancomycin-susceptible strains only).

S. aureus bloodstream infections:

For the treatment of *S. aureus* bloodstream infections (bacteremia), including those with right-sided infective endocarditis, caused by methicillin-susceptible and methicillin-resistant isolates.

Patients with persisting or relapsing *S. aureus* infection or poor clinical response should have repeat blood cultures. If a culture is positive for *S. aureus*, perform minimum inhibitory concentration (MIC) susceptibility testing of the isolate using a standardized procedure and diagnostic evaluation to rule out sequestered foci of infection.

General information: Daptomycin is not indicated for the treatment of pneumonia.

Pregnancy Considerations Adverse events were not observed in animal reproduction studies. Successful use of daptomycin during the second and third trimesters of pregnancy has been described; however, only limited information is available from case reports.

Breast-Feeding Considerations Low concentrations of daptomycin have been detected in breast milk; however, daptomycin is poorly absorbed orally. The manufacturer recommends caution if daptomycin is used during breast-feeding. Per the Canadian product labeling, daptomycin should be discontinued while breast-feeding. Nondose-related effects could include modification of bowel flora.

Contraindications Hypersensitivity to daptomycin

Warnings/Precautions May be associated with an increased incidence of myopathy; discontinue in patients with signs and symptoms of myopathy in conjunction with an increase in CPK (>5 times ULN or 1,000 units/L) or in asymptomatic patients with a CPK ≥10 times ULN. Myopathy may occur more frequently at dose and/or frequency in excess of recommended dosages. Consider temporarily interrupting therapy with other agents associated with an increased risk of myopathy (eg, HMG-CoA reductase inhibitors) during daptomycin therapy. Not indicated for the treatment of pneumonia (inactivation by pulmonary surfactant). Use caution in renal impairment (dosage adjustment required severe renal impairment [CrCl <30 mL/minute]). Limited data (eg, subgroup analysis) from cSSSI and endocarditis trials suggest possibly reduced clinical efficacy (relative to comparators) in patients with baseline moderate renal impairment (<50 mL/minute).

Symptoms suggestive of peripheral neuropathy have been observed with treatment; monitor for new-onset or worsening neuropathy. Prolonged use may result in fungal or bacterial superinfection, including *C. difficile*-associated diarrhea (CDAD) and pseudomembranous colitis; CDAD has been observed >2 months postantibiotic treatment. Repeat blood cultures in patients with persisting or relapsing *S. aureus* bacteremia/endocarditis or poor clinical response. If culture is positive for *S. aureus*, perform minimum inhibitory concentration (MIC) susceptibility testing of the isolate and diagnostic evaluation of the patient to rule out sequestered foci of infection. Appropriate surgical intervention (eg, debridement, removal of prosthetic devices, valve replacement surgery) and/or consideration of a change in antibacterial therapy may be necessary. Hypersensitivity reactions and anaphylaxis (including angioedema, and drug rash with eosinophilia and systemic symptoms [DRESS]) have been reported with use; discontinue use immediately with signs/symptoms of hypersensitivity and initiate appropriate treatment. Use has been associated with eosinophilic pneumonia; generally develops 2 to 4 weeks after therapy initiation. Monitor for signs/symptoms of eosinophilic pneumonia, including new onset or worsening fever, dyspnea, difficulty breathing, new infiltrates on chest imaging studies, and/or >25% eosinophils present in bronchoalveolar lavage. Discontinue use immediately with signs/symptoms of eosinophilic pneumonia and initiate appropriate treatment (ie, corticosteroids). May reoccur with re-exposure. Although not approved for use in children, the manufacturer recommends to avoid use in pediatric patients <12 months due to risk of potential muscular, neuromuscular, and/or nervous systems effects observed in neonatal canines.

Adverse Reactions

>10%:

Gastrointestinal: Diarrhea (5% to 12%), vomiting (3% to 12%), constipation (6% to 11%)

Hematologic & oncologic: Anemia (2% to 13%)

1% to 10%:

Cardiovascular: Chest pain (7%), peripheral edema (7%), hypertension (1% to 6%), hypotension (2% to 5%)

Central nervous system: Insomnia (5% to 9%), headache (5% to 7%), dizziness (2% to 6%), anxiety (5%)

Dermatologic: Skin rash (4% to 7%), pruritus (3% to 6%), diaphoresis (5%), erythema (5%)

Endocrine & metabolic: Hypokalemia (9%), hyperkalemia (5%), hyperphosphatemia (3%)

Gastrointestinal: Nausea (6% to 10%), abdominal pain (6%), dyspepsia (1% to 4%), loose stools (4%), gastrointestinal hemorrhage (2%)

Genitourinary: Urinary tract infection (2% to 7%)

Hematologic & oncologic: Eosinophilia (2%), increased INR (2%)

Hepatic: Increased serum transaminases (2% to 3%), increased serum alkaline phosphatase (2%)

Infection: Gram-negative organism infection (8%), bacteremia (5%), sepsis (5%), fungal infection (2% to 3%)

Local: Injection site reaction (3% to 6%)

Neuromuscular & skeletal: Increased creatine phosphokinase (3% to 9%), limb pain (2% to 9%), back pain (7%), osteomyelitis (6%), weakness (5%), arthralgia (1% to 3%)

Renal: Renal failure (2% to 3%)

Respiratory: Pharyngolaryngeal pain (8%), pleural effusion (6%), cough (3%), pneumonia (3%), dyspnea (2% to 3%)

Miscellaneous: Fever (2% to 7%)

<1% (Limited to important or life-threatening): Atrial fibrillation, atrial flutter, candidiasis, cardiac arrest, *Clostridium difficile* associated diarrhea, coma (post anaesthesia/surgery), eczema, eosinophilic pneumonitis, hallucination, hypomagnesemia, hypersensitivity, jaundice, increased lactate dehydrogenase, lymphadenopathy, mental status changes, neutropenia (Knoll 2013), oral candidiasis, peripheral neuropathy, proteinuria, prolonged prothrombin time, renal insufficiency, rhabdomyolysis, increased serum bicarbonate, Stevens-Johnson syndrome, stomatitis, supraventricular cardiac arrhythmia, thrombocytopenia, thrombocythemia

Drug Interactions

Metabolism/Transport Effects None known.

Avoid Concomitant Use There are no known interactions where it is recommended to avoid concomitant use.

Increased Effect/Toxicity

The levels/effects of DAPTOmycin may be increased by: HMG-CoA Reductase Inhibitors

Decreased Effect There are no known significant interactions involving a decrease in effect.

Preparation for Administration Reconstitute vial with 10 mL NS to a concentration of 50 mg/mL. Add NS to vial and rotate gently to wet powder. Allow to stand for 10 minutes, then gently swirl to obtain completely reconstituted solution. Do not shake or agitate vial vigorously. If administering via IVPB, further dilute in 50 mL NS prior to administration.

Storage/Stability

Store original packages at 2°C to 8°C (36°F to 46°F); avoid excessive heat. Daptomycin vials are for single use only.

US labeling: Reconstituted solution is stable in the vial for 12 hours at room temperature or up to 48 hours if refrigerated at 2°C to 8°C (36°F to 46°F). The diluted solution is stable in the infusion bag for 12 hours at room temperature or 48 hours if refrigerated. The combined time (reconstituted solution in vial and diluted solution in infusion bag) should not exceed 12 hours at room temperature or 48 hours refrigerated. Extended storage information for reconstituted vial and diluted solution may be available; contact product manufacturer to obtain current recommendations.

Canadian labeling: Reconstituted solution is stable in the vial or infusion solution for 12 hours at 25°C (77°F) or up to 10 days if refrigerated at 2°C to 8°C (36°F to 46°F) under normal lighting. The manufacturer recommends using reconstituted solution within 72 hours if stored under refrigeration. The combined time (reconstituted solution in vial and diluted solution in infusion bag) should not exceed 12 hours at up to 25°C (77°F) or 10 days at 2°C to 8°C (36°F to 46°F).

Mechanism of Action Daptomycin binds to components of the cell membrane of susceptible organisms and causes rapid depolarization, inhibiting intracellular synthesis of DNA, RNA, and protein. Daptomycin is bactericidal in a concentration-dependent manner.

Pharmacodynamics/Kinetics

Distribution: V_{ss}:
Neonates and Infants <3 months: Median: 0.21 L/kg (range: 0.11 to 0.34 L/kg) (Cohen-Wolkowiez 2012)
Children 2 to 6 years: 0.14 L/kg (Abdel-Rahman 2008; Abdel-Rahman 2011)
Children 7 to 17 years: 0.11 ± 0.02 L/kg (Abdel-Rahman 2008)
Adults: 0.1 L/kg; Critically-ill patients: V_{ss}: 0.23 ± 0.14 L/kg (Vilay 2010)

Protein binding: 90% to 93%; 84% to 88% in patients with CrCl <30 mL/minute

Metabolism: Minor amounts of oxidative metabolites have been detected; does not induce or inhibit cytochrome P450 enzymes

Half-life elimination:
Neonates and Infants <3 months: Median: 6.2 hours (range: 3.7 to 9 hours) (Cohen-Wolkowiez 2012)
Children 2 to 6 years: Mean range: 5.3 to 5.7 hours (Abdel-Rahman 2008; Abdel-Rahman 2011)
Children 7 to 11 years: 5.6 ± 2.2 hours (Abdel-Rahman 2008)
Children 12 to 17 years: 6.7 ± 2.2 hours (Abdel-Rahman 2008)
Adults: 8 to 9 hours (up to 28 hours in renal impairment)

Excretion: Urine (78%; primarily as unchanged drug); feces (6%)

Clearance:
Neonates and Infants <3 months: Median: 21 mL/hour/kg (range: 16 to 34 mL/hour/kg) (Cohen-Wolkowiez 2012)
Children 2 to 6 years: 19 to 20 mL/hour/kg (Abdel-Rahman 2008; Abdel-Rahman 2011)
Children 7 to 11 years: 17 mL/hour/kg (Abdel-Rahman 2008)
Children 12 to 17 years: 11 mL/hour/kg (Abdel-Rahman 2008)
Adults: 8.3 to 9 mL/hour/kg

Dosing

Adult & Geriatric

Infective endocarditis (left-sided, native or prosthetic valve) (off-label use): 6 to 8 mg/kg once daily (Carugati 2013; Das 2011; Dohmen 2013; Kaya 2013). **Note:** Some experts use up to 8 to 10 mg/kg; additional studies are necessary (IDSA [Liu 2011]).

Infective endocarditis (right-sided, native valve) due to S. aureus: Note: Clinical trial demonstrating noninferiority to standard therapy for *S. aureus* right-sided endocarditis included only patients with native valve infective endocarditis (Fowler 2006)
Manufacturer labeling:
U.S. labeling: 6 mg/kg once daily for 2 to 6 weeks
Canadian labeling: 6 mg/kg once daily for 10 days to 6 weeks; may consider an additional 2 weeks of therapy
Alternate recommendation: 8 to 10 mg/kg once daily (IDSA [Liu 2011])

Osteomyelitis (off-label use): IV: 6 mg/kg once daily for a minimum of 8 weeks (some experts combine with rifampin) (Liu 2011)

Prosthetic joint infection (off-label use): IV:
Enterococcus spp (penicillin-susceptible or -resistant) (alternative treatment): 6 mg/kg every 24 hours for 4 to 6 weeks (consider adding an aminoglycoside) followed by an oral antibiotic suppressive regimen (Osmon 2013)

Staphylococci (oxacillin-susceptible or -resistant) (alternative treatment): 6 mg/kg every 24 hours for 2 to 6 weeks used in combination with rifampin followed by oral antibiotic treatment and suppressive regimens (Osmon 2013)

S. aureus bloodstream infections:
Manufacturer labeling:
U.S. labeling: 6 mg/kg once daily for 2 to 6 weeks
Canadian labeling: 6 mg/kg once daily for 10 days to 6 weeks; may consider an additional 2 weeks of therapy
Alternate recommendation: 8 to 10 mg/kg once daily for complicated bacteremia (IDSA [Liu 2011])

Septic arthritis (off-label use): IV: 6 mg/kg once daily for 3 to 4 weeks (Liu 2011)

Skin and skin structure infections, complicated: 4 mg/kg once daily for 7 to 14 days

Renal Impairment

CrCl ≥30 mL/minute: No dosage adjustment necessary.
CrCl <30 mL/minute:
Skin and soft tissue infections: 4 mg/kg every 48 hours
Staphylococcal bacteremia: 6 mg/kg every 48 hours

Intermittent hemodialysis or peritoneal dialysis (PD): Dose as in CrCl <30 mL/minute (administer after hemodialysis on dialysis days) or (off-label dosing) may administer 6 mg/kg after hemodialysis 3 times weekly (Salama 2010)
Note: Hemodialysis: Dialyzable: 15% (removed by 4-hour hemodialysis session); 50% (removed by 4-hour high permeability intermittent hemodialysis session) (Salama 2010).

Continuous renal replacement therapy (CRRT) (Heintz 2009; Trotman 2005): Drug clearance is highly dependent on the method of renal replacement, filter type, and flow rate. Appropriate dosing requires close monitoring of pharmacologic response, signs of adverse reactions due to drug accumulation, as well as drug concentrations in relation to target trough (if appropriate). The following are general recommendations only (based on dialysate flow/ultrafiltration rates of 1 to 2 L/hour and minimal residual renal function) and should not supersede clinical judgment:
Continuous veno-venous hemodialysis (CVVHD): 8 mg/kg every 48 hours (Vilay 2010)
Note: For other forms of CRRT (eg, CVVH or CVVHDF), dosing as with CrCl <30 mL/minute may result in low C_{max}. May consider 4 to 6 mg/kg every 24 hours (or 8 mg/kg every 48 hours) depending on site or severity of infection or if not responding to standard dosing; therapeutic drug monitoring and/or more frequent serum CPK levels may be necessary (Heintz 2009).

Slow extended daily dialysis (or extended dialysis): 6 mg/kg every 24 hours (Kielstein 2010); **Note:** Dialysis should be initiated within 8 hours of administering daptomycin dose to avoid dose accumulation.

Hepatic Impairment No dosage adjustment necessary for mild-to-moderate impairment (Child-Pugh class A or B). Not evaluated in severe hepatic impairment (Child-Pugh class C).

Administration May administer IV push over 2 minutes or infuse IVPB over 30 minutes. Do not use in conjunction with ReadyMED® elastomeric infusion pumps (Cardinal Health, Inc) due to an impurity (2-mercaptobenzothiazole) leaching from the pump system into the daptomycin solution.

Monitoring Parameters Monitor signs and symptoms of infection. CPK should be monitored at least weekly during therapy; more frequent monitoring if current or prior statin therapy, unexplained CPK increases, and/or renal impairment. Monitor for muscle pain or weakness, especially if noted in distal extremities. Monitor for new onset or worsening peripheral neuropathy. Canadian labeling recommends CPK monitoring every 48 hours with unexplained muscle pain, tenderness, weakness or cramps. Monitor for signs/symptoms of eosinophilic pneumonia.

Reference Range
Trough concentrations at steady-state:
4 mg/kg once daily: 5.9 ± 1.6 mcg/mL
6 mg/kg once daily: 6.7 ± 1.6 mcg/mL
Note: Trough concentrations are not predictive of efficacy/toxicity. Drug exhibits concentration-dependent bactericidal activity, so C_{max}:MIC ratios may be a more useful parameter.

Test Interactions Daptomycin may cause false prolongation of the PT and increase of INR with certain recombinant thromboplastin reagents. This appears to be a dose-dependent phenomenon. If PT/INR is elevated, repeat PT/INR immediately prior to next daptomycin dose (eg, trough). If PT/INR remains elevated, repeat PT/INR using alternate reagents (if available) and evaluate for other causes of elevated PT/INR.

Dosage Forms Excipient information presented when available (limited, particularly for generics); consult specific product labeling.

Solution Reconstituted, Intravenous [preservative free]:

Cubicin: 500 mg (1 ea)

◆ Daraprim *see* Pyrimethamine *on page 1534*

◆ Daraprim [DSC] (Can) *see* Pyrimethamine *on page 1534*

Daratumumab (dar a TOOM ue mab)

Brand Names: US Darzalex

Index Terms JNJ-54767414

Pharmacologic Category Antineoplastic Agent, Anti-CD38; Antineoplastic Agent, Monoclonal Antibody

Use Multiple myeloma, relapsed/refractory: Treatment of multiple myeloma in patients who have received at least 3 prior lines of therapy including a proteasome inhibitor (PI) and an immunomodulatory agent or who are double-refractory to a PI and an immunomodulatory agent.

Pregnancy Considerations Animal reproduction studies have not been conducted. Daratumumab is a monoclonal antibody; monoclonal antibodies are known to cross the placenta. Based on the mechanism of action, daratumumab may cause myeloid or lymphoid cell depletion and decreased bone density in the fetus. Females of reproduction potential should use effective contraception during therapy and for 3 months after treatment is complete. The administration of live vaccines should be deferred for neonates and infants exposed to daratumumab in utero until a hematology evaluation can be completed.

Breast-Feeding Considerations It is not known if daratumumab is excreted into breast milk. Daratumumab is a monoclonal antibody; monoclonal antibodies can be detected in breast milk and are not expected to enter the neonatal or infant circulation in substantial amounts. According to the manufacturer, the decision to breast-feed during therapy should take into account the risk of exposure to the infant and the benefits of treatment to the mother.

Contraindications There are no contraindications listed in the manufacturer's labeling.

Warnings/Precautions Severe infusion reactions may occur (including bronchospasm, hypoxia, dyspnea, and hypertension), mostly during the first infusion. Other signs and symptoms include cough, wheezing, larynx and throat tightness/irritation, laryngeal edema, pulmonary edema, nasal congestion, and allergic rhinitis. Less commonly reported symptoms include hypotension, headache, rash urticarial, pruritus, nausea, vomiting, and chills. Infusion reactions were reported in approximately 50% of patients in clinical trials. Reactions may also be seen during subsequent infusions, and generally occur either during the infusion or within 4 hours of completion (median onset was 1.5 hours [range: up to ~9 hours]; some reactions occurred up to 48 hours after the infusion. Premedication with antihistamines, antipyretics, and corticosteroids is required; interrupt infusion for any reaction and manage as appropriate. Reduce the infusion rate for grade 1, 2, or 3 reaction; permanently discontinue therapy for grade 4 infusion reaction. Administer in a facility with immediate access to resuscitative measures (ie, glucocorticoids, epinephrine, bronchodilators, and/or oxygen). Administer oral corticosteroids on the first and second day after infusion to reduce the risk of delayed infusion reactions. Consider short- and long-acting bronchodilators and inhaled corticosteroids for patients with obstructive pulmonary disorders; monitor closely.

Lymphopenia, neutropenia, thrombocytopenia, and anemia (including grade 3 and 4 toxicity) were commonly reported as treatment emergent adverse reactions in clinical trials. Monitor complete blood counts as clinically necessary. Daratumumab (a human IgG kappa monoclonal antibody) may be detected on serum protein electrophoresis and immunofixation assays which monitor for endogenous M-protein. Interference with these assays by daratumumab may affect the determination of complete response and disease progression in some patients with IgG kappa myeloma protein. Through binding to CD38 on red blood cells, daratumumab use may result in a positive indirect antiglobulin test (Coombs test). Daratumumab-mediated Coombs test positivity may persist for up to 6 months after the last infusion. In addition, daratumumab (bound to red blood cells) masks antibody detection to minor antigens in the patient's serum; ABO and Rh blood type determination are not affected. Notify blood transfusion centers and blood banks that a patient has received daratumumab, and type and screen patients prior to therapy initiation.

Adverse Reactions

Cardiovascular: Hypertension (10%)

Central nervous system: Fatigue (39%), headache (12%), chills (10%)

Gastrointestinal: Nausea (27%), diarrhea (16%), constipation (15%), decreased appetite (15%), vomiting (14%)

Hematologic & oncologic: Lymphocytopenia (72%; grade: 3: 30%; grade 4: 10%), neutropenia (60%; grade 3: 17%; grade 4: 3%), thrombocytopenia (48%; grade 3: 10%; grade 4: 8%), anemia (45%; grade 3: 19%)

Infection: Herpes zoster (3%)

Local: Infusion site reaction (first infusion: 46% to 48%; grade 3: 3%; second infusion: 5%; subsequent infusions: 4%)

Neuromuscular & skeletal: Back pain (23%), arthralgia (17%), leg pain (15%), musculoskeletal chest pain (12%)

Respiratory: Cough (21%), upper respiratory (20%), nasal congestion (17%), dyspnea (15%), nasopharyngitis (15%), pneumonia (6% to 11%)

Miscellaneous: Fever (3% to 21%), physical health deterioration (3%)

Drug Interactions

Metabolism/Transport Effects None known.

Avoid Concomitant Use There are no known interactions where it is recommended to avoid concomitant use.

Increased Effect/Toxicity There are no known significant interactions involving an increase in effect.

Decreased Effect There are no known significant interactions involving a decrease in effect.

Preparation for Administration Determine the appropriate dose and volume of daratumumab required (based on patient's actual body weight); daratumumab should be colorless to pale yellow (do not use if opaque particles, discoloration, or other foreign particles are observed). Remove the volume of 0.9% sodium chloride injection from the infusion bag that is equal to the required volume of the daratumumab dose. Add the appropriate daratumumab volume to a 1,000 mL (first infusion) or 500 mL (subsequent infusions) 0.9% sodium chloride bag; gently invert to mix (do not shake). Infusion bags/containers must be made of polyvinylchloride (PVC), polypropylene (PP), polyethylene (PE) or polyolefin blend (PP+PE). If the diluted solution is refrigerated prior to use, allow to come to room temperature before administration. After dilution, may develop very small translucent to white proteinaceous particles; do not use if discolored or if visibly opaque or foreign particles are observed.

Storage/Stability Store intact vials at 2°C to 8°C (36°F to 46°F). Do not freeze or shake; protect from light. Solutions diluted for infusion may be stored for up to 24 hours at 2°C to 8°C (36°F to 46°F) if protected from light; do not freeze. Use immediately after coming to room temperature; infusion should be completed within 15 hours. Discard any unused portion of the solution.

Mechanism of Action Daratumumab is an IgG1κ human monoclonal antibody directed against CD38. CD38 is a cell surface glycoprotein which is highly expressed on myeloma cells, yet is expressed at low levels on normal lymphoid and myeloid cells (Lokhorst 2015). By binding to CD38, daratumumab inhibits the growth of CD38 expressing tumor cells by inducing apoptosis directly through Fc mediated cross linking as well as by immune-mediated tumor cell lysis through complement dependent cytotoxicity, antibody dependent cell mediated cytotoxicity, and antibody dependent cellular phagocytosis.

Pharmacodynamics/Kinetics

Distribution: Central: 4.7 ± 1.3 L

Half-life elimination: 18 ± 9 days

Dosing

Adult & Geriatric Note: Premedicate approximately 1 hour prior to infusion with an IV corticosteroid, an oral antipyretic, and an oral or IV antihistamine. Post-infusion, administer an oral corticosteroid on the first and second day after each infusion to reduce the risk of delayed infusion reactions. To prevent herpes zoster reactivation, initiate antiviral prophylaxis within 1 week of starting daratumumab and continue for 3 months following completion of treatment. Per the manufacturer, daratumumab dosing should be based on actual body weight.

Multiple myeloma, relapsed/refractory: Adults: IV:

Weeks 1 to 8: 16 mg/kg once weekly

Weeks 9 to 24: 16 mg/kg once every 2 weeks

Weeks 25 and beyond: 16 mg/kg once every 4 weeks until disease progression

Missed dose: If a dose is missed, administer as soon as possible and adjust the schedule accordingly (maintain the treatment interval).

Premedications:

Corticosteroid: IV: Methylprednisolone 100 mg or equivalent intermediate- or long-acting corticosteroid; following the second infusion, the dose may be decreased (eg, methylprednisolone 60 mg or equivalent) **plus**

Antipyretic: Oral: Acetaminophen 650 to 1000 mg **plus** *Antihistamine:* IV or Oral: Diphenhydramine 25 to 50 mg or equivalent

Post-infusion medication: Administer an oral corticosteroid (eg, methylprednisolone 20 mg or equivalent) on the first and second day after all infusions. In patients with a history of obstructive pulmonary disorder, consider short and long-acting bronchodilators and inhaled corticosteroids post-infusion. If no major infusion reactions occur during the first 4 infusions, these additional inhaled post-infusion medications may be discontinued.

Renal Impairment Preexisting impairment: No dosage adjustment is necessary.

Hepatic Impairment

Mild impairment (total bilirubin 1 to 1.5 times ULN or AST >ULN): No dosage adjustment necessary.

Moderate to severe impairment (total bilirubin >1.5 times ULN and any AST): There are no dosage adjustments provided in the manufacturer's labeling (has not been studied).

Adjustment for Toxicity

Infusion reactions: Immediately interrupt infusion for reaction of any severity. Manage symptoms as clinically appropriate.

Grade 1 or 2 (mild to moderate) infusion reaction: Once symptoms resolve, resume the infusion at no more than 50% of the rate at which the reaction occurred. If no further reactions are observed, may escalate the infusion rate as appropriate (see Administration).

Grade 3 (severe) infusion reaction: If symptoms improve to grade 2 or lower, consider resuming the infusion at no more than 50% of the rate at which the reaction occurred. If no further reactions are observed, may escalate the infusion rate as appropriate (see Administration). If a grade 3 reaction recurs, repeat the steps above. Permanently discontinue if a grade 3 infusion reaction occurs for the third time.

Grade 4 (life-threatening) infusion reaction: Permanently discontinue.

Administration For IV infusion only. Do not administer IV push or as a bolus. Premedicate with an IV corticosteroid, acetaminophen, and an IV or oral antihistamine (see Dosing) approximately 60 minutes prior to administration. Infuse in an environment equipped to monitor for and manage infusion reactions. Administer with an infusion set fitted with a flow regulator and with an inline, sterile, non-pyrogenic, low protein-binding polyethersulfone filter (0.22 or 0.2 micrometer). Polyurethane, polybutadiene, polyvinylchloride, polypropylene, or polyethylene administration sets are required. Do not exceed infusion rates below. Do not mix with or infuse with other medications. Begin infusion immediately after infusion bag reaches room temperature (if refrigerated). Infusion should be completed within 15 hours. Interrupt infusion for any severity of infusion reaction; if the reaction resolves or improves to ≤ grade 2, may resume infusion (see Dosage Adjustment for Toxicity). If infusion cannot be completed, do not save unused portion for reuse. Post-infusion, administer an oral corticosteroid on the first and second day after all infusions to reduce the risk of delayed infusion reactions. In patients with a history of obstructive pulmonary disorder, consider short and long-acting bronchodilators and inhaled corticosteroids post-infusion.

Infusion rate:

First infusion (1,000 mL volume): Infuse at 50 mL/hour for the first hour. If no infusion reactions occur, may increase the rate by 50 mL/hour every hour (maximum rate: 200 mL/hour).

Second infusion (500 mL volume): Infuse at 50 mL/hour for the first hour. Escalate the rate only if there were no grade 1 or greater infusion reactions during the first 3 hours of the first infusion. If no infusion reactions occur, may increase the rate by 50 mL/hour every hour (maximum rate: 200 mL/hour).

Subsequent infusions (500 mL volume): Escalate the rate only if there were no grade 1 or greater infusion reactions during a final infusion rate of ≥100 mL/hour in the first 2 infusions. Infuse at 100 mL/hour for the first hour. If no infusion reactions occur, may increase the rate by 50 mL/hour every hour (maximum rate: 200 mL/hour).

Monitoring Parameters Complete blood cell counts as clinically necessary; type and screen (blood type) prior to initiating therapy; signs/symptoms of infusion reactions.

Test Interactions Daratumumab binds to CD38 on red blood cells and results in a positive indirect antiglobulin test (Coombs test), which may persist for up to 6 months after the last infusion. Daratumumab may also mask antibody detection to minor antigens in the patient's serum. Mitigation methods include treating reagent red blood cells with dithiothreitol (DTT) to disrupt daratumumab binding or genotyping. As the Kell blood group system is also sensitive to DTT, K-negative units should be supplied after ruling out or identifying alloantibodies using DTT-treated red blood cells.

Daratumumab may be detected on both serum protein electrophoresis and immunofixation assays used for multiple myeloma endogenous M-protein monitoring, and may affect the determination of complete response and disease progression of some patients with IgG kappa myeloma protein. In patients with persistent very good partial response, consider other methods to evaluate the depth of treatment response.

Dosage Forms Excipient information presented when available (limited, particularly for generics); consult specific product labeling.

Solution, Intravenous [preservative free]:

Darzalex: 100 mg/5 mL (5 mL); 400 mg/20 mL (20 mL) [contains mouse protein (murine) (hamster)]

Darbepoetin Alfa (dar be POE e tin AL fa)

Brand Names: US Aranesp (Albumin Free)

Brand Names: Canada Aranesp

Index Terms Darbepoetin Alfa Polysorbate; Erythropoiesis-Stimulating Agent (ESA); Erythropoiesis-Stimulating Protein; NESP; Novel Erythropoiesis-Stimulating Protein

Pharmacologic Category Colony Stimulating Factor; Erythropoiesis-Stimulating Agent (ESA); Hematopoietic Agent

Use

Anemia: Treatment of anemia due to concurrent myelosuppressive chemotherapy in patients with cancer (non-myeloid malignancies) receiving chemotherapy (palliative intent) for a planned minimum of 2 additional months of chemotherapy; treatment of anemia due to chronic kidney disease (including patients on dialysis and not on dialysis)

Limitations of use: In clinical trials, darbepoetin alfa has not demonstrated improved quality of life, fatigue, or well-being. Darbepoetin alfa is **not** indicated for use under the following conditions:

- Cancer patients receiving hormonal therapy, therapeutic biologic products, or radiation therapy unless also receiving concurrent myelosuppressive chemotherapy

- Cancer patients receiving myelosuppressive chemotherapy when the expected outcome is curative

- As a substitute for red blood cell (RBC) transfusion in patients requiring immediate correction of anemia

Pregnancy Considerations Adverse events were observed in animal reproduction studies. Women who become pregnant during treatment with darbepoetin alfa are encouraged to enroll in Amgen's Pregnancy Surveillance Program (800-772-6436).

Breast-Feeding Considerations It is not known if darbepoetin alfa is excreted in breast milk. The manufacturer recommends that caution be exercised when administering darbepoetin alfa to nursing women.

Prescribing and Access Restrictions As a requirement of the REMS program, access to this medication is restricted. Healthcare providers and hospitals must be enrolled in the ESA APPRISE (Assisting Providers and Cancer Patients with Risk Information for the Safe use of ESAs) Oncology Program (866-284-8089; http://www.esa-apprise.com) to prescribe or dispense ESAs (ie, darbepoetin alfa, epoetin alfa) to patients with cancer.

Medication Guide Available Yes

Contraindications Serious allergic reaction to darbepoetin alfa or any component of the formulation; uncontrolled hypertension; pure red cell aplasia (PRCA) that begins after treatment with darbepoetin alfa or other erythropoietin protein drugs

Warnings/Precautions [US Boxed Warning]: Erythropoiesis-stimulating agents (ESAs) increased the risk of serious cardiovascular events, myocardial infarction, stroke, venous thromboembolism, vascular access thrombosis, and/or tumor progression in clinical studies when administered to target hemoglobin levels >11 g/dL (and provide no additional benefit); a rapid rise in hemoglobin (>1 g/dL over 2 weeks) may also contribute to these risks. **[US Boxed Warning]: A shortened overall survival and/or increased risk of tumor progression or recurrence has been reported in studies with breast, cervical, head and neck, lymphoid, and non-small cell lung cancer patients.** It is of note that in these studies, patients received ESAs to a target

hemoglobin of ≥12 g/dL; although risk has not been excluded when dosed to achieve a target hemoglobin of <12 g/dL. **[US Boxed Warnings]: To decrease these risks, and risk of cardio- and thrombovascular events, use ESAs in cancer patients only for the treatment of anemia related to concurrent myelosuppressive chemotherapy and use the lowest dose needed to avoid red blood cell transfusions. Discontinue ESA following completion of the chemotherapy course. ESAs are not indicated for patients receiving myelosuppressive therapy when the anticipated outcome is curative.** A dosage modification is appropriate if hemoglobin levels rise >1 g/dL per 2-week time period during treatment (Rizzo 2010). Use of ESAs has been associated with an increased risk of venous thromboembolism (VTE) without a reduction in transfusions in patients >65 years of age with cancer (Hershman 2009). Improved anemia symptoms, quality of life, fatigue, or well-being have not been demonstrated in controlled clinical trials. **[US Boxed Warning]: Because of the risks of decreased survival and increased risk of tumor growth or progression, health care providers and hospitals must enroll and comply with the ESA APPRISE (Assisting Providers and Cancer Patients with Risk Information for the Safe use of ESAs) Oncology Program to prescribe or dispense ESAs to cancer patients.** Prescribers and patients will have to provide written documentation of discussed risks prior to each course.

[US Boxed Warning]: An increased risk of death, serious cardiovascular events, and stroke was reported in patients with chronic kidney disease (CKD) administered ESAs to target hemoglobin levels ≥11 g/dL; use the lowest dose sufficient to reduce the need for RBC transfusions. An optimal target hemoglobin level, dose or dosing strategy to reduce these risks has not been identified in clinical trials. Hemoglobin rising >1 g/dL in a 2-week period may contribute to the risk (dosage reduction recommended). The American College of Physicians recommends against the use of ESAs in patients with mild to moderate anemia and heart failure or coronary heart disease (ACP [Qaseem 2013]). The American College of Cardiology Foundation/American Heart Association (ACCF/AHA) 2013 Heart Failure Guidelines do not provide a clear recommendation on the use of ESAs in anemic heart failure patients. The effects of ESAs on quality of life measures, morbidity, and mortality are potentially modest and still unclear. The authors declined to provide an official recommendation regarding the use of ESAs pending the completion of ongoing randomized trials (ACCF/AHA [Yancy 2013]).

CKD patients who exhibit an inadequate hemoglobin response to ESA therapy may be at a higher risk for cardiovascular events and mortality compared to other patients. ESA therapy may reduce dialysis efficacy (due to increase in red blood cells and decrease in plasma volume); adjustments in dialysis parameters may be needed. Patients treated with epoetin may require increased heparinization during dialysis to prevent clotting of the extracorporeal circuit. CKD patients not requiring dialysis may have a better response to darbepoetin alfa and may require lower doses. Increased mortality was observed in patients undergoing coronary artery bypass surgery who received epoetin; these deaths were associated with thrombotic events. An increased risk of deep vein thrombosis (DVT) has been observed in patients treated with epoetin undergoing surgical orthopedic procedures. Darbepoetin alfa is **not** approved for reduction in allogeneic red blood cell transfusions in patients scheduled for surgical procedures. The risk for seizures is increased with darbepoetin alfa use in patients with CKD; use with caution in patients with a history of seizures. Monitor closely for neurologic symptoms during the first several months of therapy. Use with caution in patients with hypertension; hypertensive encephalopathy has been reported. Use is contraindicated in patients with uncontrolled hypertension. If hypertension is difficult to control, reduce or hold darbepoetin alfa. Due to the delayed onset of erythropoiesis, darbepoetin alfa is **not** recommended for acute correction of severe anemia or as a substitute for emergency transfusion.

Prior to treatment, correct or exclude deficiencies of iron, vitamin B$_{12}$, and/or folate, as well as other factors that may impair erythropoiesis (inflammatory conditions, infections, bleeding). Prior to and during therapy, iron stores must be evaluated. Supplemental iron is recommended if serum ferritin <100 mcg/L or serum transferrin saturation <20%; most patients with CKD will require iron supplementation. Poor response should prompt evaluation of these potential factors, as well as possible malignant processes and hematologic disease (thalassemia, refractory anemia, myelodysplastic disorder), occult blood loss, hemolysis,

osteitis fibrosa cystic, and/or bone marrow fibrosis. Severe anemia and pure red cell aplasia (PRCA) with associated neutralizing antibodies to erythropoietin has been reported, predominantly in patients with CKD receiving SubQ darbepoetin alfa (the intravenous (IV) route is preferred for hemodialysis patients). Cases have also been reported in patients with hepatitis C who were receiving ESAs, interferon, and ribavirin. Patients with a sudden loss of response to darbepoetin alfa (with severe anemia and a low reticulocyte count) should be evaluated for PRCA with associated neutralizing antibodies to erythropoietin; discontinue treatment (permanently) in patients with PRCA secondary to neutralizing antibodies to erythropoietin. Antibodies may cross-react; do not switch to another ESA in patients who develop antibody-mediated anemia.

The American Society of Clinical Oncology (ASCO) and American Society of Hematology (ASH) 2010 updates to the clinical practice guidelines for the use of ESAs in patients with cancer indicate that ESAs are appropriate when used according to the parameters identified within the Food and Drug Administration (FDA)-approved labeling for epoetin and darbepoetin alfa (Rizzo 2010). ESAs are an option for chemotherapy-associated anemia when the hemoglobin has fallen to <10 g/dL to decrease the need for RBC transfusions. ESAs should only be used in conjunction with concurrent chemotherapy. Although the FDA label now limits ESA use to the palliative setting, the ASCO/ASH guidelines suggest using clinical judgment in weighing risks versus benefits as formal outcomes studies of ESA use defined by intent of chemotherapy treatment have not been conducted.

Potentially serious allergic reactions have been reported (rarely), including anaphylactic reactions, angioedema, bronchospasm, rash, and urticaria. Discontinue immediately (and permanently) in patients who experience serious allergic/anaphylactic reactions. Some products may contain latex. Some dosage forms may contain polysorbate 80 (also known as Tweens). Hypersensitivity reactions, usually a delayed reaction, have been reported following exposure to pharmaceutical products containing polysorbate 80 in certain individuals (Isaksson 2002; Lucente 2000; Shelley 1995). Thrombocytopenia, ascites, pulmonary deterioration, and renal and hepatic failure have been reported in premature neonates after receiving parenteral products containing polysorbate 80 (Alade 1986; CDC 1984). See manufacturer's labeling.

Adverse Reactions

>10%:
Cardiovascular: Hypertension (31%), peripheral edema (17%), edema (6% to 13%)
Gastrointestinal: Abdominal pain (10% to 13%)
Respiratory: Dyspnea (17%), cough (12%)

1% to 10%:
Cardiovascular: Angina pectoris, hypotension, myocardial infarction, pulmonary embolism, thromboembolism, thrombosis of vascular graft (arteriovenous), vascular injury (vascular access complications)
Central nervous system: Cerebrovascular disease
Dermatologic: Erythema, skin rash
Endocrine & metabolic: Hypervolemia

<1% (Limited to important or life-threatening): Anaphylaxis, anemia (associated with neutralizing antibodies; severe; with or without other cytopenias), angioedema, bronchospasm, cerebrovascular accident, hypersensitivity reaction, hypertensive encephalopathy, pure red cell aplasia, seizure, tumor growth (progression/recurrence; cancer patients), urticaria

Drug Interactions

Metabolism/Transport Effects None known.

Avoid Concomitant Use There are no known interactions where it is recommended to avoid concomitant use.

Increased Effect/Toxicity

Darbepoetin Alfa may increase the levels/effects of: Lenalidomide; Thalidomide

The levels/effects of Darbepoetin Alfa may be increased by: Nandrolone

Decreased Effect There are no known significant interactions involving a decrease in effect.

Storage/Stability Store at 2°C to 8°C (36°F to 46°F); do not freeze. Do not shake. Protect from light. Store in original carton until use. The following stability information has also been reported: May be stored at room temperature for up to 7 days (Cohen 2007).

Mechanism of Action Induces erythropoiesis by stimulating the division and differentiation of committed erythroid progenitor cells; induces the release of reticulocytes from the bone marrow into the bloodstream, where they mature to erythrocytes. There is a dose-response relationship with this effect. This results in an increase in reticulocyte counts followed by a rise in hematocrit and hemoglobin levels.

When administered SubQ or IV, darbepoetin alfa's half-life is ~3 times that of epoetin alfa concentrations.

Pharmacodynamics/Kinetics

Onset of action: Increased hemoglobin levels not generally observed until 2 to 6 weeks after initiating treatment

Absorption: SubQ: Slow

Distribution: V_d: 0.06 L/kg

Bioavailability: CKD: SubQ: Adults: ~37% (range: 30% to 50%); Children: 54% (range: 32% to 70%)

Half-life elimination:

CKD: Adults:

IV: 21 hours

SubQ: Nondialysis patients: 70 hours (range: 35 to 139 hours); Dialysis patients: 46 hours (range: 12 to 89 hours)

Cancer: Adults: SubQ: 74 hours (range: 24 to 144 hours); Children: 49 hours

Note: Darbepoetin alfa half-life is approximately 3-fold longer than epoetin alfa following IV administration

Time to peak: SubQ:

CKD: Adults: 48 hours (range: 12 to 72 hours; independent of dialysis); Children: 36 hours (range: 10 to 58 hours)

Cancer: Adults: 71 to 90 hours (range: 28 to 123 hours); Children: 71 hours (range: 21 to 143 hours)

Dosing

Adult & Geriatric Note: Evaluate iron status in all patients before and during treatment and maintain iron repletion.

Anemia associated with chronic kidney disease (CKD): Individualize dosing and use the lowest dose necessary to reduce the need for red blood cell (RBC) transfusions.

Chronic kidney disease patients ON dialysis (IV route is preferred for hemodialysis patients; initiate treatment when hemoglobin is <10 g/dL; reduce dose or interrupt treatment if hemoglobin approaches or exceeds 11 g/dL): IV, SubQ: Initial: 0.45 mcg/kg once weekly **or** 0.75 mcg/kg once every 2 weeks **or** conversion from epoetin alfa: Epoetin alfa doses of <1,500 to ≥90,000 units per week may be converted to darbepoetin alfa doses ranging from 6.25 to 200 mcg per week (see adult column in conversion table below).

Chronic kidney disease patients NOT on dialysis (consider initiating treatment when hemoglobin is <10 g/dL; use only if rate of hemoglobin decline would likely result in RBC transfusion and desire is to reduce risk of alloimmunization or other RBC transfusion-related risks; reduce dose or interrupt treatment if hemoglobin exceeds 10 g/dL): IV, SubQ: Initial: 0.45 mcg/kg once every 4 weeks

Dosage adjustments for chronic kidney disease patients (either on dialysis or not on dialysis): Do not increase dose more frequently than every 4 weeks (dose decreases may occur more frequently).

If hemoglobin increases >1 g/dL in any 2-week period: Decrease dose by ≥25%

If hemoglobin does not increase by >1 g/dL after 4 weeks: Increase dose by 25%

Inadequate or lack of response: If adequate response is not achieved over 12 weeks, further increases are unlikely to be of benefit and may increase the risk for adverse events; use the minimum effective dose that will maintain a hemoglobin level sufficient to avoid RBC transfusions **and** evaluate patient for other causes of anemia; discontinue treatment if responsiveness does not improve

Anemia due to chemotherapy in cancer patients: Initiate treatment only if hemoglobin <10 g/dL and anticipated duration of myelosuppressive chemotherapy is at least 2 additional months. Titrate dosage to use the minimum effective dose that will maintain a hemoglobin level sufficient to avoid RBC transfusions. Discontinue darbepoetin alfa following completion of chemotherapy.

SubQ: Initial: 2.25 mcg/kg once weekly **or** 500 mcg once every 3 weeks until completion of chemotherapy

Dosage adjustments:

Increase dose: If hemoglobin does not increase by 1 g/dL **and** remains below 10 g/dL after initial 6 weeks (for patients receiving weekly therapy only), increase dose to 4.5 mcg/kg once weekly (no dosage adjustment if using every-3-week dosing).

Reduce dose by 40% if hemoglobin increases >1 g/dL in any 2-week period **or** hemoglobin reaches a level sufficient to avoid RBC transfusion.

Withhold dose if hemoglobin exceeds a level needed to avoid RBC transfusion. Resume treatment with a 40% dose reduction when hemoglobin approaches a level where transfusions may be required.

Discontinue: On completion of chemotherapy or if after 8 weeks of therapy there is no hemoglobin response or RBC transfusions still required

Symptomatic anemia associated with MDS (off-label use): SubQ: 150 to 300 mcg once weekly (Giraldo 2006; Stasi 2005) **or** 500 mcg once every 2 to 3 weeks (Gabrilove 2008)

Conversion from epoetin alfa to darbepoetin alfa in CKD (on dialysis): See table

Conversion From Epoetin Alfa to Darbepoetin Alfa in Chronic Kidney Disease (Estimated Initial Dose)

Previous Dosage of Epoetin Alfa (units/week)	Children Darbepoetin Alfa Dosage (mcg/week)	Adults Darbepoetin Alfa Dosage (mcg/week)
<1,500	Not established	6.25
1,500 to 2,499	6.25	6.25
2,500 to 4,999	10	12.5
5,000 to 10,999	20	25
11,000 to 17,999	40	40
18,000 to 33,999	60	60
34,000 to 89,999	100	100
≥90,000	200	200

Note: In patients receiving epoetin alfa 2 to 3 times per week, darbepoetin alfa is administered once weekly. In patients receiving epoetin alfa once weekly, darbepoetin alfa is administered once every 2 weeks. The darbepoetin alfa dose to be administered every 2 weeks is derived by adding together 2 weekly epoetin alfa doses and then converting to the appropriate darbepoetin alfa dose. Titrate dose to hemoglobin response thereafter. The dose conversion in this table does not accurately estimate the once-monthly dose in chronic kidney disease (CKD) patients not on dialysis.

Pediatric Note: Evaluate iron status in all patients before and during treatment and maintain iron repletion.

Anemia associated with chronic kidney disease (CKD): Individualize dosing and use the lowest dose necessary to reduce the need for red blood cell (RBC) transfusions.

Chronic kidney disease patients ON dialysis (IV route is preferred for hemodialysis patients; initiate treatment when hemoglobin is <10 g/dL; reduce dose or interrupt treatment if hemoglobin approaches or exceeds 12 g/dL): IV, SubQ: Initial: 0.45 mcg/kg once weekly or conversion from epoetin alfa: Initial dose: Epoetin alfa doses of 1,500 to ≥90,000 units per week may be converted to darbepoetin alfa doses ranging from 6.25 to 200 mcg per week (see conversion table in adult dosing).

Chronic kidney disease patients NOT on dialysis (consider initiating treatment when hemoglobin is <10 g/dL; use only if rate of hemoglobin decline would likely result in RBC transfusion and desire is to reduce risk of alloimmunization or other RBC transfusion-related risks; reduce dose or interrupt treatment if hemoglobin exceeds 12 g/dL): IV, SubQ: Initial: 0.45 mcg/kg once weekly or 0.75 mcg/kg once every 2 weeks

Dosage adjustments for chronic kidney disease patients: Do not increase dose more frequently than every 4 weeks (dose decreases may occur more frequently).

If hemoglobin increases >1 g/dL in any 2-week period: Decrease dose by ≥25%

If hemoglobin does not increase by >1 g/dL after 4 weeks: Increase dose by 25%

Inadequate or lack of response: If adequate response is not achieved over 12 weeks, further increases are unlikely to be of benefit and may increase the risk for adverse events; use the minimum effective dose that will maintain a hemoglobin level sufficient to avoid RBC transfusions **and** evaluate patient for other causes of anemia; discontinue treatment if responsiveness does not improve

Renal Impairment No dosage adjustment necessary.

Hepatic Impairment There are no dosage adjustments provided in the manufacturer's labeling.

Dietary Considerations Supplemental iron intake may be required in patients with low iron stores.

Administration May be administered by SubQ or IV injection. The IV route is recommended in hemodialysis patients. Do not shake; vigorous shaking may denature darbepoetin alfa, rendering it biologically inactive. Do not dilute or administer in conjunction with other drug solutions. Discard any unused portion of the vial; do not pool unused portions.

Monitoring Parameters Hemoglobin (at least once per week until maintenance dose established and after dosage changes; monitor less frequently once hemoglobin is stabilized); CKD patients should be also be monitored at least

monthly following hemoglobin stability); iron stores (transferrin saturation and ferritin) prior to and during therapy; serum chemistry (CKD patients); blood pressure; fluid balance (CKD patients); seizures (CKD patients following initiation for first few months, includes new-onset or change in seizure frequency or premonitory symptoms)

Cancer patients: Examinations recommended by the ASCO/ASH guidelines (Rizzo 2010) prior to treatment include peripheral blood smear (in some situations a bone marrow exam may be necessary), assessment for iron, folate, or vitamin B_{12} deficiency, reticulocyte count, renal function status, and occult blood loss; during ESA treatment, assess baseline and periodic iron, total iron-binding capacity, and transferrin saturation or ferritin levels.

Dosage Forms Excipient information presented when available (limited, particularly for generics); consult specific product labeling. [DSC] = Discontinued product

Solution, Injection [preservative free]:
Aranesp (Albumin Free): 10 mcg/0.4 mL (0.4 mL); 25 mcg/mL (1 mL); 40 mcg/mL (1 mL); 60 mcg/mL (1 mL); 100 mcg (1 mL); 150 mcg/0.75 mL (0.75 mL [DSC]); 200 mcg/mL (1 mL); 300 mcg/mL (1 mL) [albumin free; contains mouse protein (murine) (hamster), polysorbate 80]

Solution Prefilled Syringe, Injection [preservative free]:
Aranesp (Albumin Free): 25 mcg/0.42 mL (0.42 mL); 40 mcg/0.4 mL (0.4 mL); 60 mcg/0.3 mL (0.3 mL); 100 mcg/0.5 mL (0.5 mL); 150 mcg/0.3 mL (0.3 mL); 200 mcg/0.4 mL (0.4 mL); 300 mcg/0.6 mL (0.6 mL); 500 mcg/mL (1 mL) [albumin free; contains mouse protein (murine) (hamster), polysorbate 80]

♦ **Darbepoetin Alfa Polysorbate** see Darbepoetin Alfa on page 493

Darifenacin (dar i FEN a sin)

Brand Names: US Enablex
Brand Names: Canada Enablex®
Index Terms Darifenacin Hydrobromide; UK-88,525
Pharmacologic Category Anticholinergic Agent
Use Management of symptoms of bladder overactivity (urge incontinence, urgency, and frequency)
Pregnancy Considerations Adverse events have been observed in animal reproduction studies.
Breast-Feeding Considerations It is not known if darifenacin is excreted in breast milk. The manufacturer recommends that caution be exercised when administering darifenacin to nursing women.
Contraindications Hypersensitivity to darifenacin or any component of the formulation; uncontrolled narrow-angle glaucoma; urinary retention, paralytic ileus, GI or GU obstruction
Warnings/Precautions Cases of angioedema involving the face, lips, tongue, and/or larynx have been reported during treatment; some cases have occurred after the first dose. May be life-threatening. Immediately discontinue and institute supportive care if tongue, hypopharynx, or larynx is involved. Central nervous system effects have been reported (eg, headache, confusion, hallucinations, somnolence); monitor, particularly at treatment initiation or dose increase, reduce dose or discontinue if necessary. May cause drowsiness and/or blurred vision, which may impair physical or mental abilities; patients must be cautioned about performing tasks which require mental alertness (eg, operating machinery or driving). May occur in the presence of increased environmental temperature; use caution in hot weather and/or exercise. Use with caution with hepatic impairment; dosage limitation is required in moderate hepatic impairment (Child-Pugh class B). Not recommended for use in severe hepatic impairment (Child-Pugh class C). Use with caution in patients with clinically-significant bladder outlet obstruction or prostatic hyperplasia (nonobstructive). Use caution in patients with decreased GI motility, constipation, hiatal hernia, reflux esophagitis, and ulcerative colitis. Use caution in patients with myasthenia gravis. In patients with controlled narrow-angle glaucoma, darifenacin should be used with extreme caution and only when the potential benefit outweighs risks of treatment. Use with caution in patients taking strong CYP3A4 inhibitors (see Drug Interactions); dosage limitation of darifenacin is required. This medication is associated with potent anticholinergic properties which may be inappropriate in older adults depending on comorbidities (eg, dementia, delirium) (Beers Criteria).

Adverse Reactions
>10%: Gastrointestinal: Xerostomia (19% to 35%), constipation (15% to 21%)
1% to 10%:
Cardiovascular: Hypertension (≥1%), peripheral edema (≥1%)

Central nervous system: Headache (7%), dizziness (<2%), pain (≥1%)
Dermatological: Pruritus (≥1%), skin rash (≥1%), xeroderma (≥1%)
Endocrine & metabolic: Weight gain (≥1%)
Gastrointestinal: Dyspepsia (3% to 8%), abdominal pain (2% to 4%), nausea (2% to 4%), vomiting (≥1%)
Genitourinary: Urinary tract infection (4% to 5%), vaginitis (≥1%), urinary retention (acute)
Neuromuscular & skeletal: Weakness (<3%), arthralgia (≥1%), back pain (≥1%)
Ophthalmic: Dry eye syndrome (2%), visual disturbance (≥1%)
Respiratory: Flu-like symptoms (1% to 3%), bronchitis (≥1%), pharyngitis (≥1%), rhinitis (≥1%), sinusitis (≥1%)
Postmarketing and/or case reports (Limited to important or life-threatening): Anaphylaxis, angioedema, confusion, erythema multiforme, granuloma (annulare), hallucination, hypersensitivity reaction

Drug Interactions
Metabolism/Transport Effects Substrate of CYP2D6 (minor), CYP3A4 (major); **Note:** Assignment of Major/Minor substrate status based on clinically relevant drug interaction potential; **Inhibits** CYP2D6 (moderate)
Avoid Concomitant Use
Avoid concomitant use of Darifenacin with any of the following: Aclidinium; Cimetropium; Conivaptan; Eluxadoline; Fusidic Acid (Systemic); Glucagon; Glycopyrrolate; Glycopyrrolate (Oral Inhalation); Idelalisib; Ipratropium (Oral Inhalation); Levosulpiride; Potassium Chloride; Thioridazine; Tiotropium; Umeclidinium
Increased Effect/Toxicity
Darifenacin may increase the levels/effects of: AbobotulinumtoxinA; Analgesics (Opioid); Anticholinergic Agents; ARIPiprazole; Brexpiprazole; Cannabinoid-Containing Products; Cimetropium; CYP2D6 Substrates; DOXOrubicin (Conventional); Eliglustat; Eluxadoline; Fesoterodine; Glucagon; Glycopyrrolate; Glycopyrrolate (Oral Inhalation); Metoprolol; Mirabegron; Nebivolol; OnabotulinumtoxinA; Potassium Chloride; Ramosetron; RimabotulinumtoxinB; Thiazide Diuretics; Thioridazine; Tiotropium; Topiramate

The levels/effects of Darifenacin may be increased by: Aclidinium; Aprepitant; Conivaptan; CYP3A4 Inhibitors (Moderate); CYP3A4 Inhibitors (Strong); Dasatinib; Fosaprepitant; Fusidic Acid (Systemic); Idelalisib; Ipratropium (Oral Inhalation); Ivacaftor; Luliconazole; Mianserin; Mifepristone; Netupitant; Osimertinib; Palbociclib; Pramlintide; Propafenone; Simeprevir; Stiripentol; Umeclidinium
Decreased Effect
Darifenacin may decrease the levels/effects of: Acetylcholinesterase Inhibitors; Codeine; Gastrointestinal Agents (Prokinetic); Itopride; Levosulpiride; Secretin; Tamoxifen; TraMADol

The levels/effects of Darifenacin may be decreased by: Acetylcholinesterase Inhibitors; Bosentan; CYP3A4 Inducers (Moderate); CYP3A4 Inducers (Strong); Dabrafenib; Deferasirox; Enzalutamide; Mitotane; Osimertinib; Siltuximab; St Johns Wort; Tocilizumab
Storage/Stability Store at 25°C (77°F); excursions permitted to 15°C to 30°C (59°F to 86°F). Protect from light.
Mechanism of Action Selective antagonist of the M3 muscarinic (cholinergic) receptor subtype. Blockade of the receptor limits bladder contractions, reducing the symptoms of bladder irritability/overactivity (urge incontinence, urgency and frequency).
Pharmacodynamics/Kinetics
Distribution: V_{dss}: ~163 L
Protein binding: ~98% (primarily alpha₁-acid glycoprotein)
Metabolism: Hepatic, via CYP3A4 (major) and CYP2D6 (minor)
Bioavailability: 15% to 19%
Half-life elimination: ~13-19 hours
Time to peak, plasma: ~7 hours
Excretion: As metabolites (inactive); urine (60%), feces (40%)
Dosing
Adult & Geriatric
Symptoms of bladder overactivity: Oral: Initial: 7.5 mg once daily. If response is not adequate after a minimum of 2 weeks, dosage may be to 15 mg once daily.
Dosage adjustment with concomitant potent CYP3A4 inhibitors (eg, ketoconazole, itraconazole, ritonavir, nelfinavir, clarithromycin, nefazodone): Daily dosage should not exceed 7.5 mg daily
Renal Impairment No dosage adjustment necessary.
Hepatic Impairment
Mild impairment (Child-Pugh class A): No dosage adjustment necessary.

Moderate impairment (Child-Pugh class B): Daily dosage should not exceed 7.5 mg daily

Severe impairment (Child-Pugh class C): Has not been evaluated; use is not recommended

Dietary Considerations May be taken without regard to meals, with or without food.

Administration Tablet should be taken with liquid and swallowed whole; do not chew, crush, or split tablet. May be taken without regard to food.

Dosage Forms Excipient information presented when available (limited, particularly for generics); consult specific product labeling. [DSC] = Discontinued product

Tablet Extended Release 24 Hour, Oral:

Enablex: 7.5 mg, 15 mg

Enablex: 15 mg [DSC] [contains fd&c yellow #6 aluminum lake]

♦ **Darifenacin Hydrobromide** see Darifenacin on page 496

Darunavir (dar OO na veer)

Brand Names: US Prezista

Brand Names: Canada Prezista

Index Terms Darunavir Ethanolate; DRV; TMC-114

Pharmacologic Category Antiretroviral, Protease Inhibitor (Anti-HIV)

Use HIV infection: Treatment of HIV-1 infection, coadministered with ritonavir and other antiretroviral agents, in adults and pediatric patients 3 years and older

Pregnancy Considerations Teratogenic effects have not been observed in animal reproduction studies. Darunavir has a low level of transfer across the human placenta. Serum concentrations are decreased during pregnancy; therefore, once-daily dosing is not recommended; twice-daily dosing should be used. The DHHS Perinatal HIV Guidelines consider darunavir to be an alternative protease inhibitor (PI) for use in antiretroviral-naive pregnant patients when combined with low-dose ritonavir boosting. A small increased risk of preterm birth has been associated with maternal use of protease inhibitor-based combination antiretroviral (ARV) therapy during pregnancy; however, the benefits of use generally outweigh this risk and PIs should not be withheld if otherwise recommended. Hyperglycemia, new onset of diabetes mellitus, or diabetic ketoacidosis have been reported with PIs; it is not clear if pregnancy increases this risk.

Regardless of CD4 count or HIV RNA copy number, all HIV-infected pregnant women should receive an ARV drug regimen combination of antepartum, intrapartum, and infant ARV prophylaxis. ARV therapy should be started as soon as possible in women with symptomatic infection. Although earlier initiation may be more effective in reducing the perinatal transmission of HIV, initiation may be delayed until after 12 weeks gestation in women who do not require immediate treatment after careful consideration of maternal conditions (eg, nausea and vomiting) and the potential risks of first trimester fetal exposure for specific agents. A scheduled cesarean delivery at 38 weeks gestation is recommended for all women with HIV RNA >1000 copies/mL or unknown concentrations near delivery in order to decrease transmission. If ARV therapy must be interrupted for <24 hours during the peripartum period, stop then restart all medications simultaneously in order to decrease the chance of developing resistance. Long-term follow-up is recommended for all infants exposed to ARV medications. In couples who want to conceive, the HIV-infected partner should attain maximum viral suppression prior to conception.

Healthcare providers are encouraged to enroll pregnant women exposed to antiretroviral medications in the Antiretroviral Pregnancy Registry (1-800-258-4263 or www.-APRegistry.com). Healthcare providers caring for HIV-infected women and their infants may contact the National Perinatal HIV Hotline (888-448-8765) for clinical consultation (HHS [perinatal], 2014).

Breast-Feeding Considerations It is not known if darunavir is excreted into breast milk. Maternal or infant antiretroviral therapy does not completely eliminate the risk of postnatal HIV transmission. In addition, multiclass-resistant virus has been detected in breast-feeding infants despite maternal therapy. Therefore, in the United States, where formula is accessible, affordable, safe, and sustainable, and the risk of infant mortality due to diarrhea and respiratory infections is low, complete avoidance of breast-feeding by HIV-infected women is recommended to decrease potential transmission of HIV (HHS [perinatal], 2014).

Contraindications

Coadministration with drugs that are highly dependent on CYP3A for clearance and drugs for which elevated plasma concentrations are associated with serious and/or life-threatening events (narrow therapeutic index) (eg, alfuzosin, dronedarone, colchicine, ranolazine, ergot derivatives [dihydroergotamine, ergonovine, ergotamine, methylergonovine], cisapride, pimozide, midazolam (oral), triazolam, St John's wort, lovastatin, simvastatin, rifampin, sildenafil [for the treatment of pulmonary hypertension]). Must be coadministered with ritonavir; refer to individual monograph for ritonavir for additional contraindication information.

Canadian labeling: Additional contraindications: Hypersensitivity to darunavir or any component of the formulation; coadministration with amiodarone, apixaban, astemizole (not available in Canada), bepridil (not available in Canada), colchicine (in patients with renal and/or hepatic impairment), lidocaine (systemic), quinidine, rivaroxaban, terfenadine (not available in Canada); severe (Child-Pugh class C) hepatic impairment

Warnings/Precautions Darunavir has a high potential for drug interactions requiring dose or frequency adjustment, additional monitoring, and/or selection of alternative therapy.

Use with caution in patients with hepatic impairment, including active chronic hepatitis; consider interruption or discontinuation with worsening hepatic function. Not recommended in severe hepatic impairment (contraindicated in Canadian labeling). Infrequent cases of drug-induced hepatitis (including acute and cytolytic) have been reported. Liver injury has been reported with use (including some fatalities), though generally in patients on multiple medications, with advanced HIV disease, hepatitis B/C coinfection, and/or immune reconstitution syndrome. Monitor patients closely; consider interrupting or discontinuing therapy if signs/symptoms of liver impairment occur.

May cause fat redistribution (buffalo hump, increased abdominal girth, breast engorgement, facial atrophy). Patients may develop immune reconstitution syndrome resulting in the occurrence of an inflammatory response to an indolent or residual opportunistic infection during initial HIV treatment or activation of autoimmune disorders (eg, Graves disease, polymyositis, Guillain-Barré syndrome) later in therapy; further evaluation and treatment may be required. May increase cholesterol and/or triglycerides. Pancreatitis has been observed with use. Risk for pancreatitis may be increased in patients with elevated triglycerides, advanced HIV disease, or history of pancreatitis. Protease inhibitors have been associated with glucose dysregulation; use caution in patients with diabetes. Initiation or dose adjustments of antidiabetic agents may be required. Use with caution in patients with hemophilia A or B; increased bleeding during protease inhibitor (PI) therapy has been reported. In some patients, additional factor VIII was administered. In more than half the cases, PI therapy was continued or reintroduced if it had been discontinued. Use with caution in patients with sulfonamide allergy (contains sulfa moiety) or hemophilia. Protease inhibitors have been associated with a variety of hypersensitivity events (some severe), including rash, anaphylaxis (rare), angioedema, bronchospasm, erythema multiforme, Stevens-Johnson syndrome (rare), acute generalized exanthematous pustulosis, toxic epidermal necrolysis, and/or drug rash with eosinophilia and systemic symptoms (DRESS). Discontinue treatment if severe skin reactions develop. Severe skin reactions may be accompanied by fever, malaise, fatigue, arthralgias, hepatitis, oral lesion, blisters, conjunctivitis, and/or eosinophilia. Mild-to-moderate rash may occur early in treatment and resolve with continued therapy. Treatment history and resistance data should guide use of darunavir with ritonavir. Darunavir/ritonavir plus raltegravir should not be used in adolescent and adult HIV-1 patients with CD4 count <200 cells/mm³ and/or HIV RNA >100,000 copies/mL (HHS [adult] 2015). Do not administer darunavir with ritonavir in pediatric patients younger than 3 years (toxicity and mortality observed in animal studies).

Adverse Reactions As a class, protease inhibitors potentially cause dyslipidemias which includes elevated cholesterol and triglycerides and a redistribution of body fat centrally to cause increased abdominal girth, buffalo hump, facial atrophy, and breast enlargement. These agents also cause hyperglycemia. Frequency of adverse events is reported for darunavir/ritonavir. See also Ritonavir monograph.

>10%:

Dermatologic: Skin rash (children: 5% to 19%; adults: 6% to 7%)

Endocrine & metabolic: Hypercholesterolemia (adults: grade 2: 23% to 25%; grade 3: 1% to 10%; children: grade 3: 1%), increased LDL cholesterol (adults: grade 2: 14%; grade 3: 8% to 9%; children: grade 3: 3%), hyperglycemia (grade 2: 10% to 11%; grade 3: 1%; grade 4: <1%)

Gastrointestinal: Vomiting (children: 13% to 33%; adults: 2% to 5%), nausea (children: 4% to 25%; adults: 4% to 7%), diarrhea (children: 11% to 24%; adults: 8% to 14%)

2% to 10%:

Central nervous system: Headache (children: 9%; adults: 3% to 7%), fatigue (children: 3%; adults: ≤2%)

Dermatologic: Pruritus (children: 8%; adults: <2%)

Endocrine & metabolic: Increased serum triglycerides (grade 2: 3% to 10%; grade 3: 2% to 7%; grade 4: 1% to 3%), increased amylase (adults: grade 2: 5% to 6%; grade 3: 5% to 7%; children: grade 3: 4%, grade 4: 1%), diabetes mellitus (2%)

Gastrointestinal: Abdominal pain (children: 5% to 10%; adults: 5% to 6%), decreased appetite (children: 8%; adults: 2%), anorexia (children: 5%; adults: 2%), increased serum lipase (adults: grade 2: 3%; grade 3: ≤2%; grade 4: <1%; children: grade 3: 1%), abdominal distention (2%), dyspepsia (2%)

Hepatic: Increased serum ALT (adults: grade 2: 7%; grade 3: 2% to 3%; grade 4: ≤1%; children: grade 3: 3%; grade 4: 1%), increased serum AST (adults: grade 2: 6%; grade 3: 2% to 4%; grade 4: ≤1%; children: grade 3: 1%)

Neuromuscular & skeletal: Weakness (≤3%)

<2% (Limited to important or life-threatening): Acute renal failure, alopecia, arthritis, bradycardia, cerebrovascular accident, depression, dermatitis (including dermatitis medicamentosa), DRESS syndrome, facial paralysis, folliculitis, gynecomastia, hematuria, hepatic failure, hepatic neoplasm (malignant), hepatitis (acute and cytolytic), hepatotoxicity, hyperlipidemia, hypersensitivity, hyperthermia, immune reconstitution syndrome, impaired consciousness, infection (including clostridium infection, parasitic infection [cryptosporidiosis], cytomegalovirus disease [encephalitis], hepatitis B, esophageal candidiasis), malignant lymphoma, myocardial infarction, nephrolithiasis, neutropenia, obesity, oropharyngeal ulcer, osteoporosis, pancreatitis, pancytopenia, peripheral neuropathy, pneumothorax, progressive multifocal leukoencephalopathy, pulmonary edema, rectal hemorrhage, redistribution of body fat (eg, buffalo hump, increased abdominal girth, breast engorgement, facial atrophy), respiratory failure, rhabdomyolysis (coadministration with HMG-CoA reductase inhibitors), seizure, sepsis, skin rash (toxic), tachycardia, uveitis

Drug Interactions

Metabolism/Transport Effects **Substrate** of CYP3A4 (major), P-glycoprotein; **Note:** Assignment of Major/Minor substrate status based on clinically relevant drug interaction potential; **Inhibits** CYP2D6 (weak), CYP3A4 (strong), P-glycoprotein

Avoid Concomitant Use

Avoid concomitant use of Darunavir with any of the following: Ado-Trastuzumab Emtansine; Alfuzosin; Aprepitant; Astemizole; Avanafil; Axitinib; Barnidipine; Bosutinib; Bromocriptine; Cabozantinib; Ceritinib; Cisapride; Cobimetinib; Conivaptan; Crizotinib; Dabrafenib; Dapoxetine; Domperidone; Dronedarone; Eletriptan; Eplerenone; Ergot Derivatives; Everolimus; Flibanserin; Fosphenytoin; Fusidic Acid (Systemic); Halofantrine; Ibrutinib; Idelalisib; Irinotecan Products; Isavuconazonium Sulfate; Ivabradine; Lapatinib; Lercanidipine; Lomitapide; Lopinavir; Lovastatin; Lurasidone; Macitentan; Midazolam; Naloxegol; Nilotinib; NiMODipine; Nisoldipine; Olaparib; Ombitasvir, Paritaprevir, Ritonavir, and Dasabuvir; Osimertinib; Palbociclib; PAZOPanib; Pimozide; Ranolazine; Red Yeast Rice; Regorafenib; Rifampin; Rifapentine; Rivaroxaban; Salmeterol; Saquinavir; Silodosin; Simeprevir; Simvastatin; Sonidegib; St Johns Wort; Suvorexant; Tamsulosin; Telaprevir; Terfenadine; Ticagrelor; Tipranavir; Tolvaptan; Topotecan; Toremifene; Trabectedin; Triazolam; Ulipristal; Vemurafenib; VinCRIStine (Liposomal); Vorapaxar; Voriconazole

Increased Effect/Toxicity

Darunavir may increase the levels/effects of: Ado-Trastuzumab Emtansine; Afatinib; Alfuzosin; Alitretinoin (Systemic); Almotriptan; Alosetron; ALPRAZolam; Amiodarone; Apixaban; Aprepitant; ARIPiprazole; ARIPiprazole Lauroxil; Astemizole; AtorvaSTATin; Avanafil; Axitinib; Barnidipine; Bedaquiline; Bortezomib; Bosentan; Bosutinib; Brentuximab Vedotin; Brexpiprazole; Brinzolamide; Bromocriptine; Budesonide (Nasal); Budesonide (Oral Inhalation); Budesonide (Systemic); Budesonide (Topical); Buprenorphine; Cabazitaxel; Cabozantinib; Calcium Channel Blockers (Nondihydropyridine);

Cannabis; CarBAMazepine; Cariprazine; Ceritinib; Cilostazol; Cisapride; Clarithromycin; Cobimetinib; Colchicine; Conivaptan; Corticosteroids (Orally Inhaled); Corticosteroids (Systemic); Crizotinib; Cyclophosphamide; CycloSPORINE (Systemic); CYP2D6 Substrates; CYP3A4 Substrates; Dabigatran Etexilate; Dabrafenib; Daclatasvir; Dapoxetine; Dasatinib; Digoxin; Dofetilide; Domperidone; DOXOrubicin (Conventional); Dronabinol; Dronedarone; Dutasteride; Edoxaban; Efavirenz; Eletriptan; Eliglustat; Elvitegravir; Enfuvirtide; Eplerenone; Ergot Derivatives; Erlotinib; Estazolam; Estazolam; Everolimus; FentaNYL; Fesoterodine; Flibanserin; Fluticasone (Nasal); Fluticasone (Oral Inhalation); Gefitinib; GuanFACINE; Halofantrine; Hydrocodone; Ibrutinib; Iloperidone; Imatinib; Imidafenacin; Irinotecan Products; Isavuconazonium Sulfate; Itraconazole; Ivabradine; Ivacaftor; Ixabepilone; Ketoconazole (Systemic); Lacosamide; Lapatinib; Ledipasvir; Lercanidipine; Levobupivacaine; Levomilnacipran; Lomitapide; Lovastatin; Lumefantrine; Lurasidone; Macitentan; Maraviroc; Meperidine; MethylPREDNISolone; Midazolam; Mifepristone; Naloxegol; Nefazodone; Nevirapine; Nilotinib; NiMODipine; Nintedanib; Nisoldipine; Olaparib; Osimertinib; Ospemifene; Oxybutynin; OxyCODONE; Palbociclib; Panobinostat; Parecoxib; Paricalcitol; PAZOPanib; P-glycoprotein/ABCB1 Substrates; Pimecrolimus; Pimozide; PONATinib; Pranlukast; Pravastatin; PrednisoLONE (Systemic); PredniSONE; Propafenone; Protease Inhibitors; Prucalopride; QUEtiapine; QuiNIDine; Ramelteon; Ranolazine; Red Yeast Rice; Regorafenib; Repaglinide; Retapamulin; Rifabutin; Rifaximin; Rilpivirine; Riociguat; Rivaroxaban; RomiDEPsin; Rosuvastatin; Ruxolitinib; Salmeterol; Saxagliptin; Sildenafil; Silodosin; Simeprevir; Simvastatin; Sonidegib; SORAfenib; Suvorexant; Tacrolimus (Systemic); Tacrolimus (Topical); Tadalafil; Tamsulosin; Tasimelteon; Temsirolimus; Tenofovir Disoproxil Fumarate; Terfenadine; Tetrahydrocannabinol; Ticagrelor; Tofacitinib; Tolterodine; Tolvaptan; Topotecan; Toremifene; Trabectedin; TraMADol; TraZODone; Triazolam; Tricyclic Antidepressants; Ulipristal; Vardenafil; Vemurafenib; Vilazodone; VinCRIStine (Liposomal); Vindesine; Vinorelbine; Vorapaxar; Zopiclone; Zuclopenthixol

The levels/effects of Darunavir may be increased by: Clarithromycin; Conivaptan; CycloSPORINE (Systemic); CYP3A4 Inhibitors (Moderate); CYP3A4 Inhibitors (Strong); Delavirdine; Enfuvirtide; Fusidic Acid (Systemic); Idelalisib; Itraconazole; Ketoconazole (Systemic); Luliconazole; Mifepristone; Netupitant; Nevirapine; Rifabutin; Simeprevir; Stiripentol; Tenofovir Disoproxil Fumarate

Decreased Effect

Darunavir may decrease the levels/effects of: Abacavir; Antidiabetic Agents; Boceprevir; Clarithromycin; Contraceptives (Estrogens); Contraceptives (Progestins); Delavirdine; Didanosine; Etravirine; Ifosfamide; Meperidine; Methadone; Norethindrone; PARoxetine; PHENobarbital; Phenytoin; Prasugrel; Sertraline; Telaprevir; Ticagrelor; Valproate Products; Voriconazole; Warfarin; Zidovudine

The levels/effects of Darunavir may be decreased by: Boceprevir; Bosentan; CYP3A4 Inducers (Moderate); CYP3A4 Inducers (Strong); Deferasirox; Efavirenz; Enzalutamide; Fosphenytoin; Garlic; Lopinavir; Mitotane; Ombitasvir, Paritaprevir, and Ritonavir; Ombitasvir, Paritaprevir, Ritonavir, and Dasabuvir; Rifampin; Rifapentine; Saquinavir; Siltuximab; St Johns Wort; Telaprevir; Tipranavir; Tocilizumab

Food Interactions Absorption and bioavailability are increased when administered with food. Management: Take with meals.

Storage/Stability

Tablets: Store at 25°C (77°F); excursions are permitted between 15°C and 30°C (59°F and 86°F).

Suspension: Store at 25°C (77°F); excursions are permitted between 15°C and 30°C (59°F and 86°F). Do not refrigerate or freeze.

Mechanism of Action Binds to the site of HIV-1 protease activity and inhibits cleavage of viral Gag-Pol polyprotein precursors into individual functional proteins required for infectious HIV. This results in the formation of immature, noninfectious viral particles.

Pharmacodynamics/Kinetics All kinetic parameters derived in the presence of ritonavir coadministration; pharmacokinetic data in pediatric patients (6 to 18 years) reported to be similar to adult data.

Absorption: Increased ~40% with food

Protein binding: ~95%; primarily to alpha$_1$ acid glycoprotein (AAG)

Metabolism: Hepatic, via CYP3A to minimally active metabolites

Bioavailability: Absolute oral: 82% (darunavir 600 mg single dose with ritonavir twice daily); bioavailability is increased 30% to 40% with food

Half-life elimination: ~15 hours

Time to peak, plasma: 2.5 to 4 hours

Excretion: Feces (~80%, 41% as unchanged drug); urine (~14%, 8% as unchanged drug)

Dosing

Adult & Geriatric Treatment of HIV infection: Oral:

Treatment-naive: 800 mg once daily; coadministration with ritonavir 100 mg **or** cobicistat 150 mg once daily is required. **Note:** Darunavir/ritonavir is a component of a recommended initial regimen (with tenofovir/emtricitabine) in ART naive patients (HHS [adult] 2015).

Treatment-experienced: Note: Genotypic testing is recommended in therapy experienced patients.

With no darunavir resistance-associated substitutions: 800 mg once daily; coadministration with ritonavir 100 mg **or** cobicistat 150 mg once daily is required

With ≥1 darunavir resistance-associated substitution: 600 mg twice daily; coadministration with ritonavir 100 mg twice daily is required

If genotypic testing is not possible: 600 mg twice daily, coadministered with ritonavir 100 mg twice daily

Pediatric Treatment of HIV infection: Children ≥3 years and Adolescents: Oral: **Note:** Coadministration with ritonavir is required; do not exceed the maximum recommended darunavir adult dose (800 mg to 1200 mg daily depending upon indication). Genotypic testing is recommended in therapy-experienced patients.

Treatment-naive patients or treatment-experienced with no darunavir resistance-associated substitutions: Note: Guidelines do not recommend once-daily dosing in any patient <12 years, patients 12 to18 years who are treatment experienced with prior treatment failure, or patients ≥18 years with darunavir resistance-associated viral mutations. (HHS [pediatric], 2014). Use in treatment-naive pediatric patients is not approved in the Canadian labeling.

Dosing recommendations based on body weight using the oral suspension:

≥10 kg to <11 kg: 350 mg once daily with ritonavir 64 mg once daily. **Note:** The 350 mg darunavir (tablet) dose for this weight group is rounded up to 360 mg (3.6 mL) for suspension dosing convenience.

≥11 kg to <12 kg: 385 mg once daily with ritonavir 64 mg once daily. **Note:** The 385 mg darunavir (tablet) dose for this weight group is rounded up to 400 mg (4 mL) for suspension dosing convenience.

≥12 kg to <13 kg: 420 mg once daily with ritonavir 80 mg once daily

≥13 kg to <14 kg: 455 mg once daily with ritonavir 80 mg once daily. **Note:** The 455 mg darunavir (tablet) dose for this weight group is rounded up to 460 mg (4.6 mL) for suspension dosing convenience.

≥14 kg to <15 kg: 490 mg once daily with ritonavir 96 mg once daily. **Note:** The 490 mg darunavir (tablet) dose for this weight group is rounded up to 500 mg (5 mL) for suspension dosing convenience.

Dosing recommendations based on body weight using the oral suspension or tablets:

≥15 kg to <30 kg: 600 mg once daily with ritonavir 100 mg once daily

≥30 kg to <40 kg: 675 mg once daily with ritonavir 100 mg once daily. **Note:** The 675 mg dose using darunavir tablets for this weight group is rounded up to 680 mg (6.8 mL) for suspension dosing convenience.

≥40 kg: 800 mg once daily with ritonavir 100 mg once daily

Treatment-experienced patients with at ≥1 darunavir resistance-associated substitution. Darunavir resistance-associated viral mutations include: V11I, V32I, L33F, I47V, I50V, I54L, I54M, T74P, L76V, I84V, and L89V. **Note:** Guidelines recommend this twice daily dosing for all patients <12 years (HHS [pediatric], 2014).

Dosing recommendations based on body weight using the oral suspension:

≥10 kg to <11 kg: 200 mg twice daily with ritonavir 32 mg twice daily

≥11 kg to <12 kg: 220 mg twice daily with ritonavir 32 mg twice daily

≥12 kg to <13 kg: 240 mg twice daily with ritonavir 40 mg twice daily

≥13 kg to <14 kg: 260 mg twice daily with ritonavir 40 mg twice daily

≥14 kg to <15 kg: 280 mg twice daily with ritonavir 48 mg twice daily

Dosing recommendations based on body weight using the oral suspension or tablets:

≥15 kg to <30 kg: 375 mg twice daily with ritonavir 48 mg twice daily. **Note:** The 375 mg darunavir (tablet) dose for this weight group is rounded up to 380 mg (3.8 mL) for suspension dosing convenience.

≥30 kg to <40 kg: 450 mg twice daily with ritonavir 60 mg twice daily. **Note:** The 450 mg darunavir (tablet) dose for this weight group is rounded up to 460 mg (4.6 mL) for suspension dosing convenience.

≥40 kg: 600 mg twice daily with ritonavir 100 mg twice daily

Renal Impairment

US labeling:

Mild or moderate impairment (CrCl ≥30 mL/minute): There are no dosage adjustments provided in the manufacturer's labeling; however, need for adjustment not expected based on pharmacokinetic data.

Severe impairment (CrCl <30 mL/minute): There are no dosage adjustments provided in the manufacturer's labeling (has not been studied).

Canadian labeling: Mild, moderate, or severe impairment: No dosage adjustment necessary.

Hepatic Impairment

Mild to moderate impairment (Child-Pugh class A or B): No dosage adjustments necessary

Severe impairment (Child-Pugh class C): Use not recommended (contraindicated in Canadian labeling).

Adjustment for Toxicity

Severe rash: Discontinue treatment.

New or worsening liver dysfunction: Consider interrupting or discontinuing treatment.

Dietary Considerations Absorption increased with food. Take with meals.

Administration Coadministration with ritonavir and food is required (bioavailability is increased). Shake suspension prior to each dose; use provided oral dosing syringe to measure dose. In patients taking darunavir once daily, if a dose of darunavir or ritonavir is missed by >12 hours, the next dose should be taken at the regularly scheduled time. If a dose of darunavir or ritonavir is missed by <12 hours, the dose should be taken immediately, and then the next dose should be taken at the regularly scheduled time. In patients taking darunavir twice daily, if a dose of darunavir or ritonavir is missed by >6 hours, the next dose should be taken at the regularly scheduled time. If a dose of darunavir or ritonavir is missed by <6 hours, the dose should be taken immediately, and then the next dose should be taken at the regularly scheduled time.

Monitoring Parameters Viral load, CD4, baseline genotyping in treatment-experienced patients (if possible); serum glucose; transaminase levels prior to and during therapy (increase monitoring in patients at risk for liver impairment), cholesterol, triglycerides

Dosage Forms Excipient information presented when available (limited, particularly for generics); consult specific product labeling. [DSC] = Discontinued product

Suspension, Oral:

Prezista: 100 mg/mL (200 mL) [contains methylparaben sodium; strawberry cream flavor]

Tablet, Oral:

Prezista: 75 mg, 150 mg

Prezista: 400 mg [DSC], 600 mg [contains fd&c yellow #6 (sunset yellow)]

Prezista: 800 mg

Darunavir and Cobicistat

(dar OO na veer & koe BIK i stat)

Brand Names: US Prezcobix

Brand Names: Canada Prezcobix

Index Terms Cobicistat and Darunavir

Pharmacologic Category Antiretroviral, Protease Inhibitor (Anti-HIV); Cytochrome P-450 Inhibitor

Use

HIV infection: Treatment of HIV-1 infection, coadministered with other antiretroviral agents, in treatment-naive and in treatment-experienced patients without darunavir resistant-associated substitutions (V11I, V32I, L33F, I47V, I50V, I54L, I54M, T74P, L76V, I84V, L89V)

Note: For treatment-experienced patients, the Canadian labeling indicates use in patients without any darunavir resistant-associated substitutions

Pregnancy Considerations Adverse events have not been observed in animal reproduction studies using the individual agents. The HHS Perinatal HIV Guidelines note there are insufficient data to recommend use of cobicistat in pregnancy. Darunavir has a low level of transfer across the human placenta.

Health care providers are encouraged to enroll pregnant women exposed to antiretroviral medications in the Antiretroviral Pregnancy Registry (1-800-258-4263 or www.-APRegistry.com). Health care providers caring for HIV-infected women and their infants may contact the National Perinatal HIV Hotline (888-448-8765) for clinical consultation (HHS [perinatal], 2014).

Breast-Feeding Considerations It is not known if darunavir or cobicistat are excreted into breast milk. Maternal or infant antiretroviral therapy does not completely eliminate the risk of postnatal HIV transmission. In addition, multiclass-resistant virus has been detected in breast-feeding infants despite maternal therapy. Therefore, in the United States, where formula is accessible, affordable, safe, and sustainable, and the risk of infant mortality because of diarrhea and respiratory infections is low, complete avoidance of breast-feeding by HIV-infected women is recommended to decrease potential transmission of HIV (HHS [perinatal], 2014).

Contraindications
Coadministration with alfuzosin, dronedarone, lurasidone, colchicine (in patients with renal or hepatic impairment), rifampin, ergot derivatives (eg, dihydroergotamine, ergonovine, ergotamine, methylergonovine), cisapride (not available in Canada), St John's wort, lovastatin, simvastatin, pimozide, ranolazine, sildenafil (for treatment of pulmonary arterial hypertension), oral midazolam, triazolam

Canadian labeling: Additional contraindications (not in US labeling): Hypersensitivity to darunavir, cobicistat, or any component of the formulation; severe hepatic impairment (Child-Pugh class C). Coadministration with amiodarone, bepridil (not available in Canada), lidocaine (systemic), quinidine, salmeterol, astemizole (not available in Canada), or terfenadine (not available in Canada)

Warnings/Precautions Protease inhibitors have been associated with a variety of hypersensitivity events (some severe); discontinue treatment if severe skin reactions develop. May cause redistribution of fat (eg, buffalo hump, peripheral wasting with increased abdominal girth, cushingoid appearance). Patients may develop immune reconstitution syndrome resulting in the occurrence of an inflammatory response to an indolent or residual opportunistic infection during initial HIV treatment or activation of autoimmune disorders (eg, Graves disease, polymyositis, Guillain-Barré syndrome) later in therapy; further evaluation and treatment may be required. Increases in total cholesterol and triglycerides have been reported with darunavir; screening should be done prior to therapy and periodically throughout treatment. Pancreatitis has been observed during therapy with darunavir; use caution in patients at risk for pancreatitis.

Cobicistat may inhibit tubular secretion of creatinine without affecting actual renal glomerular function; use caution when interpreting serum creatinine values. Patients who experience a confirmed increase in serum creatinine >0.4 mg/dL from baseline should have renal function monitored closely. Concomitant use of cobicistat and tenofovir may cause renal toxicity (acute renal failure and/or Fanconi syndrome); avoid use with concurrent or recent nephrotoxic therapy. Calculate estimated creatinine clearance (CrCl) prior to initiation of therapy and monitor renal function during therapy. In patients receiving concomitant tenofovir, assess urine glucose and urine protein prior to and periodically during treatment; assess serum phosphorus in patients with or at risk for renal impairment. Do not initiate therapy in combination with tenofovir in patients with CrCl <70 mL/minute.

Darunavir may exacerbate preexisting hepatic dysfunction; use with caution in patients with advanced HIV disease or preexisting liver disease, hepatitis B/C coinfection, and/or immune reconstitution syndrome. Monitor LFTs closely at baseline and during treatment in all patients; in patients with baseline elevations, consider increased monitoring, especially in the first few months of therapy. Consider interrupting or discontinuing therapy if signs/symptoms of new or worsening liver impairment (eg, clinically significant LFT elevations, fatigue, anorexia, nausea, jaundice, dark urine, liver tenderness, hepatomegaly) occur. Use in severe liver impairment (Child-Pugh class C) is not recommended (US labeling) or contraindicated (Canadian labeling).

Changes in glucose tolerance, hyperglycemia, exacerbation of diabetes, DKA, and new-onset diabetes mellitus have been reported in patients receiving protease inhibitors. Initiation or dose adjustments of antidiabetic agents may be required. Use with caution in patients with hemophilia A or B; increased bleeding (eg, spontaneous skin hematomas and hemarthroses) has been reported during protease inhibitor therapy. Some patients receive additional factor VIII. In more than half of the cases, protease inhibitor treatment was continued or reintroduced if treatment was discontinued. Use with caution in patients with sulfonamide allergy (darunavir contains sulfa moiety).

Potentially significant drug-drug interactions may exist, requiring dose or frequency adjustment, additional monitoring, and/or selection of alternative therapy.

Adverse Reactions Adverse reactions listed below are reflective of both the US and Canadian product information. Frequency not always defined. Reactions reported with combination product: Also see individual agents.
1% to 10%:
Central nervous system: Headache (3%)
Dermatologic: Skin rash (5% to 16%)
Gastrointestinal: Diarrhea (5%), nausea (4%), vomiting (2%), abdominal pain (1%), flatulence (1%)
Hepatic: Increased liver enzymes (1%)
Hypersensitivity: Drug-induced hypersensitivity (2%)
Immunologic: Immune reconstitution syndrome
<1% (Limited to important or life-threatening): Abnormal dreams, absence seizures, acute respiratory distress, anemia, anorexia, anxiety, arthropathy, biliary obstruction, blurred vision, breast hypertrophy, cerebral infarction, clostridium infection, conjunctivitis, convulsions, cryptosporidiosis, cytomegalovirus disease, dehydration, depression, diabetes mellitus, diabetic ketoacidosis, dizziness, drug toxicity, dyspepsia, encephalitis, eosinophilia, esophageal candidiasis, exacerbation of diabetes mellitus, Fanconi's syndrome, feeling of heaviness, gastritis, Graves disease, Guillain-Barré syndrome, hemarthrosis, hematoma, hematuria, hepatic cirrhosis, hepatic neoplasm, hepatitis, hepatomegaly, hypercholesterolemia, hypersensitivity, hypertriglyceridemia, impaired consciousness, increased serum bilirubin, increased serum transaminases, limb pain, lipoatrophy, lipodystrophy, lipohypertrophy, maculopathy, malaise, malignant lymphoma, metabolic acidosis, myocarditis, myositis, neoplasm, neuromuscular disease, oral lesion, ostealgia, osteonecrosis, pancreatitis, pancytopenia, paralysis, peripheral neuropathy, pneumothorax, polymyositis, progressive multifocal leukoencephalopathy, pulmonary edema, rectal hemorrhage, renal failure, renal insufficiency, renal tubular necrosis, respiratory failure, rhabdomyolysis, sepsis, Stevens-Johnson syndrome, swelling of eye, uveitis, weakness

Drug Interactions
Metabolism/Transport Effects Refer to individual components.

Avoid Concomitant Use
Avoid concomitant use of Darunavir and Cobicistat with any of the following: Ado-Trastuzumab Emtansine; Alfuzosin; Aprepitant; Astemizole; Avanafil; Axitinib; Barnidipine; Boceprevir; Bosutinib; Bromocriptine; Cabozantinib; CarBAMazepine; Ceritinib; Cisapride; Cobimetinib; Conivaptan; Crizotinib; Dabrafenib; Dapoxetine; Dihydroergotamine; Domperidone; Dronedarone; Eletriptan; Eplerenone; Ergot Derivatives; Ergotamine; Everolimus; Flibanserin; Fluticasone (Oral Inhalation); Fosphenytoin; Fosphenytoin-Phenytoin; Fusidic Acid (Systemic); Halofantrine; Ibrutinib; Idelalisib; Irinotecan Products; Isavuconazonium Sulfate; Ivabradine; Lapatinib; Lercanidipine; Lomitapide; Lopinavir; Lovastatin; Lurasidone; Macitentan; Methylergonovine; Midazolam; Naloxegol; Nilotinib; NiMODipine; Nisoldipine; Olaparib; Ombitasvir, Paritaprevir, Ritonavir, and Dasabuvir; Osimertinib; Palbociclib; PAZOPanib; PHENobarbital; Pimozide; Primidone; Ranolazine; Red Yeast Rice; Regorafenib; Rifampin; Rifapentine; Rivaroxaban; Salmeterol; Saquinavir; Silodosin; Simeprevir; Simvastatin; Sonidegib; St Johns Wort; Suvorexant; Tamsulosin; Telaprevir; Terfenadine; Ticagrelor; Tipranavir; Tolvaptan; Topotecan; Toremifene; Trabectedin; Triazolam; Ulipristal; Vemurafenib; VinCRIStine (Liposomal); Vorapaxar; Voriconazole

Increased Effect/Toxicity
Darunavir and Cobicistat may increase the levels/effects of: Ado-Trastuzumab Emtansine; Afatinib; Alfuzosin; Alitretinoin (Systemic); Almotriptan; Alosetron; ALPRAZolam; Amiodarone; Apixaban; Aprepitant; ARIPiprazole; ARIPiprazole Lauroxil; Astemizole; AtorvaSTATin; Avanafil; Axitinib; Barnidipine; Bedaquiline; Boceprevir; Bortezomib; Bosentan; Bosutinib; Brentuximab Vedotin; Brexpiprazole; Brinzolamide; Bromocriptine; Budesonide (Nasal); Budesonide (Oral Inhalation); Budesonide (Systemic); Budesonide (Topical); Buprenorphine; Cabazitaxel; Cabozantinib; Calcium Channel Blockers (Nondihydropyridine); Cannabis; Cariprazine; Ceritinib; Cilostazol; Cisapride; Clarithromycin; Cobimetinib; Colchicine; Conivaptan; Contraceptives (Progestins); Corticosteroids (Orally Inhaled); Corticosteroids (Systemic); Crizotinib; Cyclophosphamide; CycloSPORINE (Systemic); CYP2D6 Substrates; CYP3A4 Substrates; Dabigatran Etexilate; Dabrafenib; Daclatasvir; Dapoxetine;

Dasatinib; Digoxin; Dihydroergotamine; Dofetilide; Domperidone; DOXOrubicin (Conventional); Dronabinol; Dronedarone; Dutasteride; Edoxaban; Efavirenz; Eletriptan; Eliglustat; Elvitegravir; Enfuvirtide; Eplerenone; Ergot Derivatives; Ergotamine; Erlotinib; Estazolam; Etizolam; Everolimus; FentaNYL; Fesoterodine; Flibanserin; Fluticasone (Nasal); Fluticasone (Oral Inhalation); Gefitinib; GuanFACINE; Halofantrine; Hydrocodone; Ibrutinib; Iloperidone; Imatinib; Imidafenacin; Irinotecan Products; Isavuconazonium Sulfate; Itraconazole; Ivabradine; Ivacaftor; Ixabepilone; Ketoconazole (Systemic); Lacosamide; Lapatinib; Ledipasvir; Lercanidipine; Levobupivacaine; Levomilnacipran; Lomitapide; Lovastatin; Lumefantrine; Lurasidone; Macitentan; Maraviroc; Meperidine; Methadone; Methylergonovine; Methyl-PREDNISolone; Midazolam; Mifepristone; Naloxegol; Nefazodone; Nevirapine; Nilotinib; NiMODipine; Nintedanib; Nisoldipine; Olaparib; Osimertinib; Ospemifene; Oxybutynin; OxyCODONE; Palbociclib; Panobinostat; Parecoxib; Paricalcitol; PAZOPanib; P-glycoprotein/ABCB1 Substrates; Pimecrolimus; Pimozide; PONATinib; Pranlukast; Pravastatin; PrednisoLONE (Systemic); PredniSONE; Propafenone; Protease Inhibitors; Prucalopride; QUEtiapine; QuiNIDine; Ramelteon; Ranolazine; Red Yeast Rice; Regorafenib; Repaglinide; Retapamulin; Rifabutin; Rifaximin; Rilpivirine; Riociguat; Rivaroxaban; RomiDEPsin; Rosuvastatin; Ruxolitinib; Salmeterol; Saxagliptin; Sildenafil; Silodosin; Simeprevir; Simvastatin; Sonidegib; SORAfenib; Suvorexant; Tacrolimus (Systemic); Tacrolimus (Topical); Tadalafil; Tamsulosin; Tasimelteon; Telaprevir; Telithromycin; Temsirolimus; Tenofovir Disoproxil Fumarate; Tenofovir Products; Terfenadine; Tetrahydrocannabinol; Ticagrelor; Tofacitinib; Tolterodine; Tolvaptan; Topotecan; Toremifene; Trabectedin; TraMADol; TraZODone; Triazolam; Tricyclic Antidepressants; Ulipristal; Vardenafil; Vemurafenib; Vilazodone; VinCRIStine (Liposomal); Vindesine; Vinorelbine; Vorapaxar; Warfarin; Zopiclone; Zuclopenthixol

The levels/effects of Darunavir and Cobicistat may be increased by: Clarithromycin; Conivaptan; CycloSPORINE (Systemic); CYP3A4 Inhibitors (Moderate); CYP3A4 Inhibitors (Strong); Delavirdine; Enfuvirtide; Fusidic Acid (Systemic); Idelalisib; Itraconazole; Ketoconazole (Systemic); Luliconazole; Mifepristone; Netupitant; Nevirapine; Rifabutin; Simeprevir; Stiripentol; Telithromycin; Tenofovir Disoproxil Fumarate

Decreased Effect

Darunavir and Cobicistat may decrease the levels/effects of: Abacavir; Antidiabetic Agents; Contraceptives (Estrogens); Contraceptives (Progestins); Delavirdine; Didanosine; Etravirine; Ifosfamide; Meperidine; Methadone; Norethindrone; PARoxetine; Prasugrel; Sertraline; Telaprevir; Ticagrelor; Valproate Products; Voriconazole; Warfarin; Zidovudine

The levels/effects of Darunavir and Cobicistat may be decreased by: Bosentan; CarBAMazepine; CYP3A4 Inducers (Moderate); CYP3A4 Inducers (Strong); Deferasirox; Dexamethasone (Systemic); Efavirenz; Enzalutamide; Fosphenytoin; Fosphenytoin-Phenytoin; Garlic; Lopinavir; Mitotane; Ombitasvir, Paritaprevir, and Ritonavir; Ombitasvir, Paritaprevir, Ritonavir, and Dasabuvir; OXcarbazepine; PHENobarbital; Primidone; Rifampin; Rifapentine; Saquinavir; Siltuximab; St Johns Wort; Telaprevir; Tipranavir; Tocilizumab

Food Interactions Absorption and bioavailability of darunavir are increased when administered with food. Management: Take with meals.

Storage/Stability Store at 20°C to 25°C (68°F to77°F); excursions are permitted between 15°C and 30°C (59°F and 86°F).

Mechanism of Action Darunavir binds to the site of HIV-1 protease activity and inhibits cleavage of viral Gag-Pol polyprotein precursors into individual functional proteins required for infectious HIV. This results in the formation of immature, noninfectious viral particles.

Cobicistat is a mechanism-based inhibitor of cytochrome P450 3A (CYP3A). Inhibition of CYP3A-mediated metabolism by cobicistat and increases the systemic exposure of CYP3A substrates (eg, darunavir).

Pharmacodynamics/Kinetics Refer to individual monographs.

Dosing

Adult Note: Genotype testing is advised prior to therapy initiation; if testing is not feasible, use is recommended in protease-inhibitor naïve patients only. Dosage modifications are not possible with darunavir/cobicistat combination tablet.

HIV-1 infection (treatment-naive or treatment-experienced without darunavir resistance-associated substitutions; **Note:** For treatment-experienced patients, the

Canadian labeling indicates use in patients without any darunavir resistant-associated substitutions): Oral: One tablet (darunavir 800 mg/cobicistat 150 mg) once daily.

Note: Administer with other antiretroviral agents

Missed dose: If <12 hours, take dose as soon as possible; if >12 hours resume at next regularly scheduled time.

Geriatric Refer to adult dosing. Use with caution.

Renal Impairment

US labeling: There are no dosage adjustments provided in the manufacturer's labeling. If CrCl <70 mL/minute, do not coadminister as part of a regimen that includes tenofovir disoproxil fumarate.

Canadian labeling: No dosage adjustment necessary. If CrCl <70 mL/minute, do not coadminister as part of regimens that include emtricitabine, lamivudine, tenofovir disoproxil fumarate, or adefovir.

Hepatic Impairment

Mild to moderate impairment (Child-Pugh class A or B): There are no dosage adjustments provided in the manufacturer's labeling (has not been studied); pharmacokinetic data with darunavir and cobicistat (as individual agents) suggest that dosage adjustment is not necessary.

Severe impairment (Child-Pugh class C):

US labeling: Use is not recommended.

Canadian labeling (not in US labeling): Use is contraindicated.

Dietary Considerations Take with meals.

Administration Administer with food. The Canadian labeling indicates that the tablet should be swallowed whole and not be crushed or broken.

Monitoring Parameters Viral load, baseline genotyping in treatment-experienced patients (if possible); serum glucose; liver function prior to and during therapy (increase monitoring in patients at risk for liver impairment), cholesterol, triglycerides; CBC with differential, reticulocyte count, CD4 count, serum creatinine at baseline and when clinically indicated during therapy; when coadministered with tenofovir, serum creatinine, urine glucose, and urine protein prior to initiation and as clinically indicated during therapy; assess serum phosphorus in patients with or at risk for renal impairment. Patients who experience a confirmed increase in serum creatinine >0.4 mg/dL from baseline should have renal function monitored closely. Testing for HBV is recommended prior to the initiation of antiretroviral therapy.

Dosage Forms Excipient information presented when available (limited, particularly for generics); consult specific product labeling.

Tablet, Oral:

Prezcobix: Darunavir 800 mg and cobicistat 150 mg

◆ Darunavir Ethanolate *see* Darunavir *on page 497*

◆ Darzalex *see* Daratumumab *on page 492*

◆ Dasabuvir, Ombitasvir, Paritaprevir, and Ritonavir *see* Ombitasvir, Paritaprevir, Ritonavir, and Dasabuvir *on page 1327*

Dasatinib (da SA ti nib)

Brand Names: US Sprycel
Brand Names: Canada Sprycel
Index Terms BMS-354825
Pharmacologic Category Antineoplastic Agent, BCR-ABL Tyrosine Kinase Inhibitor; Antineoplastic Agent, Tyrosine Kinase Inhibitor

Use

Acute lymphoblastic leukemia: Treatment of Philadelphia chromosome-positive (Ph+) acute lymphoblastic leukemia (ALL) with resistance or intolerance to prior therapy.

Chronic myeloid leukemia: Treatment of newly diagnosed Ph+ chronic myeloid leukemia (CML) in chronic phase; treatment of chronic, accelerated, or myeloid or lymphoid blast phase Ph+ CML with resistance or intolerance to prior therapy, including imatinib.

Pregnancy Considerations Dasatinib crosses the placenta, with fetal plasma and amniotic concentrations comparable to maternal concentrations. Adverse effects, including hydrops fetalis and fetal leukopenia and thrombocytopenia have been reported following maternal exposure to dasatinib. Women of reproductive potential should use effective contraception during and for 30 days after the final dose to avoid becoming pregnant. Pregnant women are advised to avoid contact with crushed or broken tablets.

Breast-Feeding Considerations It is not known if dasatinib is excreted in breast milk. According to the manufacturer, due to the potential for serious adverse reactions in

the nursing infant, breast-feeding is not recommended during treatment and for 2 weeks following the final dose.

Contraindications

US labeling: There are no contraindications listed in the manufacturer's labeling.

Canadian labeling: Hypersensitivity to dasatinib or any other component of the formulation); breast-feeding

Warnings/Precautions Hazardous agent - use appropriate precautions for handling and disposal (NIOSH 2014 [group 1]). Severe dose-related bone marrow suppression (thrombocytopenia, neutropenia, anemia) is associated with treatment (usually reversible); dosage adjustment and/or temporary interruption may be required for severe myelosuppression; the incidence of myelosuppression is higher in patients with advanced chronic myeloid leukemia (CML) and Ph+ acute lymphoblastic leukemia (ALL). Monitor blood counts every 2 weeks for 12 weeks and then every 3 months thereafter or as clinically indicated (for chronic phase CML) or weekly for the first 2 months, then monthly thereafter or as clinically necessary (for accelerated or blast phase CML or for ALL). Fatal intracranial and GI hemorrhage have been reported in association with dasatinib use. Severe hemorrhage (including CNS, GI) may occur due to thrombocytopenia; in addition to thrombocytopenia, dasatinib may also cause platelet dysfunction. Concomitant medications that inhibit platelet function or anticoagulants may increase the risk of bleeding. Potentially significant drug-drug interactions may exist, requiring dose or frequency adjustment, additional monitoring, and/or selection of alternative therapy. Use caution with patients taking anticoagulants or medications interfering with platelet function; not studied in clinical trials. Avoid concomitant use with CYP3A4 inducers and inhibitors; if concomitant use cannot be avoided, consider dasatinib dosage adjustments. Elevated gastric pH may reduce dasatinib bioavailability; avoid concomitant use with proton pump inhibitors and H_2 blockers. If needed, may consider antacid administration at least 2 hours before or 2 hours after the dasatinib dose.

Cardiomyopathy, diastolic dysfunction, heart failure (congestive), left ventricular dysfunction, and MI have been reported; monitor for signs and symptoms of cardiac dysfunction. Dasatinib may cause fluid retention, including pleural and pericardial effusions, pulmonary hypertension, and generalized or superficial edema. A prompt chest x-ray (or other appropriate diagnostic imaging) is recommended for signs suggestive of effusion (new or worsening dyspnea on exertion or at rest, pleuritic chest pain, or dry cough). Fluid retention may be managed with supportive care (diuretics or corticosteroids); thoracentesis and oxygen therapy may be necessary for severe fluid retention; consider dose reduction or treatment interruption. Utilizing once-daily dosing is associated with a decreased frequency of fluid retention. The risk for pleural effusion is increased in patients with hypertension, prior cardiac history and a twice a day administration schedule; interrupt treatment for grade ≥2 effusion; may consider reinitiating at a reduced dose after resolution (Quintás-Cardama, 2007). Use caution in patients where fluid accumulation may be poorly tolerated, such as in cardiovascular disease (HF or hypertension) and pulmonary disease. Patients 65 years of age and older are more likely to experience toxicity (compared with younger patients). Dasatinib may increase the risk for pulmonary arterial hypertension (PAH). PAH may occur at any time after starting treatment, including after >12 months of therapy. Evaluate for underlying cardiopulmonary disease prior to therapy initiation and during therapy; evaluate and rule out alternative etiologies in patients with symptoms suggestive of PAH (eg, dyspnea, fatigue, hypoxia, fluid retention) and interrupt therapy if symptoms are severe. Discontinue permanently with confirmed PAH diagnosis (may be reversible upon discontinuation).

May prolong QT interval; there are reports of patients with QTcF >500 msec. Use caution in patients at risk for QT prolongation, including patients with long QT syndrome, patients taking antiarrhythmic medications or other medications that lead to QT prolongation or potassium-wasting diuretics, patients with cumulative high-dose anthracycline therapy, and conditions which cause hypokalemia or hypomagnesemia. Correct hypokalemia and hypomagnesemia prior to and during dasatinib therapy. Cases of severe mucocutaneous dermatologic reactions (including Stevens-Johnson syndrome and erythema multiforme) have been reported with dasatinib. Discontinue dasatinib if severe mucocutaneous reaction occurs and other etiologies have been ruled out. Use caution with hepatic impairment due to extensive hepatic metabolism. Tumor lysis syndrome (TLS) has been reported in patients with resistance to imatinib therapy, usually in patients with advanced phase disease. Risk for TLS is higher in patients with advanced stage disease and/or a high tumor burden; monitor patients at risk more frequently. Maintain adequate hydration and correct uric acid levels prior to treatment; monitor electrolyte levels.

Adverse Reactions

≥10%:

Cardiovascular: Facial edema, peripheral edema

Central nervous system: Headache (12% to 33%), fatigue (8% to 26%), pain (11%)

Dermatologic: Skin rash (11% to 21%; includes drug eruption, erythema, erythema multiforme, erythematous rash, erythrosis, exfoliative rash, follicular rash, heat rash, macular rash, maculopapular rash, milia, papular rash, pruritic rash, pustular rash, skin exfoliation, skin irritation, urticaria vesiculosa, vesicular rash), pruritus (12%)

Endocrine & metabolic: Fluid retention (19% to 48%; grades 3/4: 1% to 8%; cardiac-related: 9%)

Gastrointestinal: Diarrhea (17% to 31%), nausea (8% to 24%), vomiting (5% to 16%), abdominal pain (7% to 12%)

Hematologic & oncologic: Thrombocytopenia (grades 3/4: 22% to 85%), neutropenia (grades 3/4: 29% to 79%), anemia (grades 3/4: 13% to 74%), hemorrhage (8% to 26%; grades 3/4: 1% to 9%), febrile neutropenia (4% to 12%; grades 3/4: 4% to 12%)

Infection: Infection (9% to 14%; includes bacterial, fungal, viral)

Local: Localized edema (3% to 22%; grades 3/4: ≤1%; superficial)

Neuromuscular & skeletal: Musculoskeletal pain (<22%), myalgia (7% to 13%), arthralgia (≤13%)

Respiratory: Pleural effusion (5% to 28%; grades 3/4: ≤7%), dyspnea (3% to 24%)

Miscellaneous: Fever (6% to 18%)

1% to <10%:

Cardiovascular: Cardiac conduction disturbance (7%), ischemic heart disease (4%), cardiac disease (≤4%; includes cardiac failure, cardiomyopathy, diastolic dysfunction, ejection fraction decreased, left ventricular dysfunction, ventricular failure), edema (≤4%; generalized), pericardial effusion (≤4%; grades 3/4: ≤1%), prolonged Q-T interval on ECG (≤1%), cardiac arrhythmia, chest pain, flushing, hypertension, palpitations, tachycardia

Central nervous system: Chills, depression, dizziness, drowsiness, insomnia, myasthenia, neuropathy, peripheral neuropathy

Dermatologic: Acne vulgaris, alopecia, dermatitis, eczema, hyperhidrosis, urticaria, xeroderma

Endocrine & metabolic: Hyperuricemia, weight gain, weight loss

Gastrointestinal: Constipation (10%), gastrointestinal hemorrhage (2% to 9%; grades 3/4: 1% to 7%), abdominal distention, change in appetite, colitis (including neutropenic colitis), dysgeusia, dyspepsia, enterocolitis, gastritis, mucositis, stomatitis

Hematologic & oncologic: CNS hemorrhage (≤3%; grades 3/4: ≤3%), bruise

Hepatic: Increased serum bilirubin (grades 3/4: ≤6%), increased serum ALT (grades 3/4: ≤5%), increased serum AST (grades 3/4: ≤4%), ascites (≤1%)

Infection: Herpes virus infection, sepsis

Neuromuscular & skeletal: Muscle spasm (5%), stiffness, weakness

Ophthalmic: Blurred vision, decreased visual acuity, dry eye syndrome, visual disturbance

Otic: Tinnitus

Renal: Increased serum creatinine (grades 3/4: ≤8%)

Respiratory: Pulmonary hypertension (≤5%; grades 3/4: ≤1%), pulmonary edema (≤4%; grades 3/4: ≤3%), cough, pneumonia (bacterial, viral, or fungal), pneumonitis, pulmonary infiltrates, upper respiratory tract infection

Miscellaneous: Soft tissue injury (oral)

<1% (Limited to important or life-threatening): Abnormal platelet aggregation, abnormal T waves on ECG, acute coronary syndrome, acute respiratory distress, amnesia, anal fissure, angina pectoris, arthritis, asthma, ataxia, atrial fibrillation, atrial flutter, bullous skin disease, cardiac arrest, cardiomegaly, cerebrovascular accident, cholecystitis, cholestasis, conjunctivitis, convulsions, coronary artery disease, cor pulmonale, cranial nerve palsy (facial), decreased libido, deep vein thrombosis, dementia, dermal ulcer, diabetes mellitus, dyschromia, dysphagia, embolism, equilibrium disturbance, erythema nodosum, esophagitis, fibrosis (dermal), fistula (anal), gastroesophageal reflux disease, gynecomastia, hearing loss, hepatitis, hypercholesterolemia, hypersensitivity, hypersensitivity angiitis, hyperthyroidism, hypoalbuminemia, hypotension, hypothyroidism, increased gamma-glutamyl transferase, increased lacrimation, increased

pulmonary artery pressure, increased troponin, inflammation (panniculitis), interstitial pulmonary disease, intestinal obstruction, livedo reticularis, lymphadenopathy, lymphocytopenia, myocardial infarction, myocarditis, optic neuritis, osteonecrosis, palmar-plantar erythrodysesthesia, pancreatitis, pericarditis, photophobia, pleuropericarditis, prolongation P-R interval on ECG, proteinuria, pulmonary embolism, pure red cell aplasia, renal failure, renal insufficiency, rhabdomyolysis, skin photosensitivity, Stevens-Johnson syndrome, Sweet's syndrome, syncope, tendonitis, thrombophlebitis, thrombosis, thyroiditis, transient ischemic attacks, tumor lysis syndrome, upper gastrointestinal tract ulcer, urinary frequency, ventricular arrhythmia, ventricular tachycardia, voice disorder

Drug Interactions

Metabolism/Transport Effects Substrate of CYP3A4 (major); **Note:** Assignment of Major/Minor substrate status based on clinically relevant drug interaction potential; **Inhibits** CYP3A4 (weak)

Avoid Concomitant Use
Avoid concomitant use of Dasatinib with any of the following: BCG (Intravesical); Conivaptan; Deferiprone; Dipyrone; Fusidic Acid (Systemic); H2-Antagonists; Idelalisib; Natalizumab; Pimecrolimus; Pimozide; Proton Pump Inhibitors; St Johns Wort; Tacrolimus (Topical); Tofacitinib; Vaccines (Live)

Increased Effect/Toxicity
Dasatinib may increase the levels/effects of: Acetaminophen; Agents with Antiplatelet Properties; Anticoagulants; ARIPiprazole; CloZAPine; CYP3A4 Substrates; Deferiprone; Fingolimod; Flibanserin; Highest Risk QTc-Prolonging Agents; Hydrocodone; Leflunomide; Lomitapide; Moderate Risk QTc-Prolonging Agents; Natalizumab; NiMODipine; Pimozide; Propacetamol; Tofacitinib; Vaccines (Live)

The levels/effects of Dasatinib may be increased by: Acetaminophen; Aprepitant; Conivaptan; CYP3A4 Inhibitors (Moderate); CYP3A4 Inhibitors (Strong); Denosumab; Dipyrone; Fosaprepitant; Fusidic Acid (Systemic); Idelalisib; Ivacaftor; Luliconazole; Mifepristone; Netupitant; Osimertinib; Palbociclib; Pimecrolimus; Roflumilast; Simeprevir; Stiripentol; Tacrolimus (Topical); Trastuzumab; Voriconazole

Decreased Effect
Dasatinib may decrease the levels/effects of: BCG (Intravesical); Coccidioides immitis Skin Test; Sipuleucel-T; Vaccines (Inactivated); Vaccines (Live)

The levels/effects of Dasatinib may be decreased by: Antacids; Bosentan; CYP3A4 Inducers (Moderate); CYP3A4 Inducers (Strong); Dabrafenib; Deferasirox; Dexamethasone (Systemic); Echinacea; Enzalutamide; H2-Antagonists; Mitotane; Osimertinib; Proton Pump Inhibitors; Siltuximab; St Johns Wort; Tocilizumab

Food Interactions Dasatinib serum concentrations may be increased when taken with grapefruit or grapefruit juice. Management: Avoid concurrent use.

Storage/Stability Store at 20°C to 25°C (68°F to 77°F); excursions permitted to 15°C to 30°C (59°F to 86°F).

Mechanism of Action BCR-ABL tyrosine kinase inhibitor; targets most imatinib-resistant BCR-ABL mutations (except the T315I and F317V mutants) by distinctly binding to active and inactive ABL-kinase. Kinase inhibition halts proliferation of leukemia cells. Also inhibits SRC family (including SRC, LKC, YES, FYN); c-KIT, EPHA2 and platelet derived growth factor receptor (PDGFRβ)

Pharmacodynamics/Kinetics
Distribution: 2505 L

Protein binding: Dasatinib: 96%; metabolite (active): 93%

Metabolism: Hepatic (extensive); metabolized by CYP3A4 (primarily), flavin-containing mono-oxygenase-3 (FOM-3) and uridine diphosphate-glucuronosyltransferase (UGT) to an active metabolite and other inactive metabolites (the active metabolite plays only a minor role in the pharmacology of dasatinib)

Half-life elimination: Terminal: 3 to 5 hours

Time to peak, plasma: 0.5 to 6 hours

Excretion: Feces (~85%, 19% as unchanged drug); urine (~4%, 0.1% as unchanged drug)

Dosing
Adult & Geriatric Note: The effect of discontinuation on long-term disease outcome after achieving cytogenetic response (including complete cytogenetic response) or major molecular response is not known.

Chronic myelogenous leukemia (CML), Philadelphia chromosome-positive (Ph+), newly diagnosed in chronic phase: Oral: 100 mg once daily until disease progression or unacceptable toxicity. In clinical studies, a dose escalation to 140 mg once daily was allowed in patients not achieving hematologic or cytogenetic response at recommended initial dosage.

CML, Ph+, resistant or intolerant: Oral:
Chronic phase: 100 mg once daily until disease progression or unacceptable toxicity. In clinical studies, a dose escalation to 140 mg once daily was allowed in patients not achieving hematologic or cytogenetic response at recommended initial dosage.

Accelerated or blast phase: 140 mg once daily until disease progression or unacceptable toxicity. In clinical studies, a dose escalation to 180 mg once daily was allowed in patients not achieving hematologic or cytogenetic response at recommended initial dosage.

Acute lymphoblastic leukemia (ALL), Ph+: Oral: 140 mg once daily until disease progression or unacceptable toxicity. In clinical studies, a dose escalation to 180 mg once daily was allowed in patients not achieving hematologic or cytogenetic response at recommended initial dosage.

Gastrointestinal stromal tumors (GIST; off-label use): Oral: 70 mg twice daily (Montemurro, 2012; Trent, 2011).

Missed doses: If a dose is missed, take the next regularly scheduled dose; 2 doses should not be taken at the same time.

Dosage adjustment for concomitant CYP3A4 inhibitors: Avoid concomitant administration with strong CYP3A4 inhibitors (eg, clarithromycin, itraconazole, ketoconazole, nefazodone, protease inhibitors, telithromycin, voriconazole, grapefruit juice); if concomitant administration with a strong CYP3A4 inhibitor cannot be avoided, consider reducing dasatinib from 100 mg once daily to 20 mg once daily **or** from 140 mg once daily to 40 mg once daily, with careful monitoring. If reduced dose is not tolerated, the strong CYP3A4 inhibitor must be discontinued or dasatinib therapy temporarily held until concomitant inhibitor use has ceased. When a strong CYP3A4 inhibitor is discontinued, allow a washout period (~1 week) prior to adjusting dasatinib dose upward.

Dosage adjustment for concomitant CYP3A4 inducers: Avoid concomitant administration with strong CYP3A4 inducers (eg, carbamazepine, dexamethasone, phenobarbital, phenytoin, rifabutin, rifampin, St John's wort); if concomitant administration with a strong CYP3A4 inducer cannot be avoided, consider increasing the dasatinib dose with careful monitoring.

Renal Impairment There are no dosage adjustments provided in the manufacturer's labeling. However, <4% of dasatinib and metabolites are renally excreted.

Hepatic Impairment No initial dosage adjustment is necessary; use with caution. Transaminase or bilirubin elevations during treatment may be managed with treatment interruption or dose reduction.

Adjustment for Toxicity
Hematologic toxicity: Note: Growth factor support may be considered in patients with resistant myelosuppression.

Chronic phase CML (100 mg daily starting dose): For ANC <500/mm^3 or platelets <50,000/mm^3, withhold treatment until ANC ≥1000/mm^3 and platelets ≥50,000/mm^3; then resume treatment at the original starting dose if recovery occurs in ≤7 days. If platelets <25,000/mm^3 or recurrence of ANC <500/mm^3 for >7 days, withhold treatment until ANC ≥1000/mm^3 and platelets ≥50,000/mm^3; then resume treatment at 80 mg once daily (second episode). For third episode, further reduce dose to 50 mg once daily (for newly diagnosed patients) or discontinue (for patients resistant or intolerant to prior therapy)

Accelerated or blast phase CML and Ph+ ALL (140 mg once daily starting dose): For ANC <500/mm^3 or platelets <10,000/mm^3, if cytopenia unrelated to leukemia, withhold treatment until ANC ≥1000/mm^3 and platelets ≥20,000/mm^3; then resume treatment at the original starting dose. If cytopenia recurs, withhold treatment until ANC ≥1000/mm^3 and platelets ≥20,000/mm^3; then resume treatment at 100 mg once daily (second episode) or 80 mg once daily (third episode). For cytopenias related to leukemia (confirm with marrow aspirate or biopsy), consider dose escalation to 180 mg once daily.

Nonhematologic toxicity: Withhold treatment until toxicity improvement or resolution; if appropriate, resume treatment at a reduced dose based on the event severity and recurrence.

Dermatologic toxicities: Manage rash with antihistamines or topical or systemic steroids (Khoury, 2009), or treatment interruption, dose reduction, or discontinuation. Discontinue if dasatinib-related severe mucocutaneous reaction occurs.

Fluid retention: Manage with diuretics, short courses of corticosteroids, and/or supportive care. Severe pleural effusions may require thoracentesis and oxygen

therapy; consider dose reduction or treatment interruption. For grade 3 pleural effusion, withhold treatment until resolves to grade 1 or lower and consider corticosteroids (eg, prednisone 20 to 40 mg/day for 3 to 4 days), diuretics, thoracentesis and/or pleurodesis; may resume dasatinib at a decreased dose when effusion resolves (Khoury, 2009).

Pulmonary arterial hypertension: Discontinue with confirmed pulmonary arterial hypertension.

Dietary Considerations Avoid grapefruit juice.

Administration Administer once daily (morning or evening). May be taken without regard to food. Swallow whole; do not break, crush, or chew tablets. Take with a meal if GI upset occurs (Khoury, 2009).

Hazardous agent; use appropriate precautions for handling and disposal (NIOSH 2014 [group 1]). Avoid exposure to crushed tablets. Although crushing of the tablets is not recommended, if it is necessary to manipulate the tablets (eg, to prepare an oral suspension), it is recommended to double glove, wear a protective gown, and prepare in a controlled device (NIOSH 2014).

Monitoring Parameters CBC with differential every 2 weeks for 12 weeks and then every 3 months thereafter or as clinically indicated (for chronic phase chronic myeloid leukemia [CML]) **or** weekly for 2 months, then monthly or as clinically necessary (for accelerated or blast phase CML or for acute lymphoblastic leukemia [ALL]); bone marrow biopsy; liver function tests, electrolytes including calcium, phosphorus, magnesium; monitor for fluid retention; monitor for signs/symptoms of cardiac dysfunction; ECG monitoring if at risk for QTc prolongation; chest x-ray is recommended for symptoms suggestive of pleural effusion (eg, cough, dyspnea); signs/symptoms of tumor lysis syndrome and dermatologic reactions.

Thyroid function testing recommendations (Hamnvik, 2011):

Preexisting levothyroxine therapy: Obtain baseline TSH levels, then monitor every 4 weeks until levels and levothyroxine dose are stable, then monitor every 2 months

Without preexisting thyroid hormone replacement: TSH at baseline, then monthly for 4 months, then every 2 to 3 months

Dosage Forms Excipient information presented when available (limited, particularly for generics); consult specific product labeling.

Tablet, Oral:

Sprycel: 20 mg, 50 mg, 70 mg, 80 mg, 100 mg, 140 mg

Extemporaneous Preparations Hazardous agent: Use appropriate precautions for handling and disposal (NIOSH 2014 [group 1]). When manipulating tablets, NIOSH recommends double gloving, a protective gown, and preparation in a controlled device; if not prepared in a controlled device, respiratory and eye protection as well as ventilated engineering controls are recommended (NIOSH 2014).

An oral suspension may be prepared by dissolving dasatinib tablet(s) for one dose in 30 mL chilled orange or apple juice (without preservatives). After 5 minutes, swirl the contents for 3 seconds and repeat the process every 5 minutes for a total of 20 minutes following addition of tablet(s). Minimize time between end of 20 minutes and administration since suspension will taste more bitter if allowed to stand longer. Swirl contents of container one last time, then administer immediately. To ensure the full dose is administered, rinse container with 15 mL juice and administer residue. May be administered orally (or by nasogastric tube). Discard any unused portion after 60 minutes.

Sprycel data on file, Bristol-Myers Squibb

DAUNOrubicin (Conventional)

(daw noe ROO bi sin con VEN sha nal)

Brand Names: Canada Cerubidine; Daunorubicin Hydrochloride for Injection

Index Terms Cerubidine; Conventional Daunomycin; Daunomycin; DAUNOrubicin Hydrochloride; Rubidomycin Hydrochloride

Pharmacologic Category Antineoplastic Agent, Anthracycline; Antineoplastic Agent, Topoisomerase II Inhibitor

Use

Acute lymphocytic leukemia: Treatment (remission induction) of acute lymphocytic leukemia (ALL) in children and adults (in combination with other chemotherapy)

Acute myeloid leukemia: Treatment (remission induction) of acute myeloid leukemia (AML) in adults (in combination with other chemotherapy)

Pregnancy Considerations Adverse events have been observed in animal reproduction studies. Daunorubicin crosses the placenta. Women of reproductive potential should avoid pregnancy.

Breast-Feeding Considerations It is not known if daunorubicin is excreted into breast milk. Due to the potential for serious adverse reactions in the nursing infant, the manufacturer recommends a decision be made whether to discontinue nursing or to discontinue the drug, taking into account the importance of treatment to the mother.

Contraindications Hypersensitivity to daunorubicin or any component of the formulation

Warnings/Precautions Hazardous agent - use appropriate precautions for handling and disposal (NIOSH 2014 [group 1]). **[U.S. Boxed Warning]: Potent vesicant; if extravasation occurs, severe local tissue damage leading to ulceration and necrosis, and pain may occur. For IV administration only. NOT for IM or SubQ administration. Administer through a rapidly flowing IV line.** Ensure proper needle or catheter placement prior to and during infusion. Avoid extravasation. **[U.S. Boxed Warning]: Severe bone marrow suppression may occur when used at therapeutic doses; may lead to infection or hemorrhage.** Use with caution in patients with drug-induced bone marrow suppression (preexisting), unless the therapy benefit outweighs the toxicity risk. Monitor blood counts at baseline and frequently during therapy.

[U.S. Boxed Warning]: May cause cumulative, dose-related myocardial toxicity; may lead to heart failure. May occur either during treatment or may be delayed (months to years after cessations of treatment). The incidence of irreversible myocardial toxicity increases as the total cumulative (lifetime) dosages approach 550 mg/m^2 in adults, 400 mg/m^2 in adults receiving chest radiation, 300 mg/m^2 in children >2 years of age, or 10 mg/kg in children <2 years of age. Total cumulative dose should take into account prior treatment with other anthracyclines or anthracenediones, previous or concomitant treatment with cardiotoxic agents or irradiation of chest. Although the risk increases with cumulative dose, irreversible cardiotoxicity may occur at any dose level. Patients with preexisting heart disease, hypertension, concurrent administration of other antineoplastic agents, prior or concurrent chest irradiation, advanced age; and infants and children are at increased risk. Monitor left ventricular (LV) function (baseline and periodic) with ECHO or MUGA scan; monitor ECG. Cardiotoxicity may occur more frequently in elderly patients. Use with caution in patients with impaired renal function and/or poor marrow reserve due to advanced age; dosage adjustment may be necessary. Infants and children are at increased risk for developing delayed cardiotoxicity; long-term periodic cardiac function monitoring is recommended.

[U.S. Boxed Warning]: Dosage reductions are recommended in patients with renal or hepatic impairment; significant impairment may result in increased toxicities. May cause tumor lysis syndrome and hyperuricemia. Urinary alkalinization and prophylaxis with an antihyperuricemic agent may be necessary. Monitor electrolytes, renal function, and hydration status. Use with caution in patients who have received radiation therapy; reduce dosage in patients who are receiving radiation therapy simultaneously. Secondary leukemias may occur when used with combination chemotherapy or radiation therapy. **[U.S. Boxed Warning]: Should be administered under the supervision of an experienced cancer chemotherapy physician.** Use caution when selecting product for preparation and dispensing; indications, dosages, and adverse event profiles differ between conventional daunorubicin hydrochloride solution and daunorubicin liposomal. Potentially significant drug-drug interactions may exist, requiring dose or frequency adjustment, additional monitoring, and/or selection of alternative therapy.

Adverse Reactions

>10%:

Cardiovascular: Transient ECG abnormalities (supraventricular tachycardia, S-T wave changes, atrial or ventricular extrasystoles); generally asymptomatic and self-limiting. CHF, dose related, may be delayed for 7-8 years after treatment.

Dermatologic: Alopecia (reversible), radiation recall

Gastrointestinal: Mild nausea or vomiting, stomatitis

Genitourinary: Discoloration of urine (red)

Hematologic: Myelosuppression (onset: 7 days; nadir: 10-14 days; recovery: 21-28 days), primarily leukopenia; thrombocytopenia and anemia

1% to 10%:

Dermatologic: Skin "flare" at injection site; discoloration of saliva, sweat, or tears

Endocrine & metabolic: Hyperuricemia

Gastrointestinal: Abdominal pain, GI ulceration, diarrhea

<1% (Limited to important or life-threatening): Anaphylactoid reaction, arrhythmia, bilirubin increased, cardiomyopathy, hepatitis, infertility; local (cellulitis, pain, thrombophlebitis at injection site); MI, myocarditis, neutropenic typhlitis, pericarditis, secondary leukemia, skin rash, sterility, systemic hypersensitivity (including urticaria, pruritus, angioedema, dysphagia, dyspnea); transaminases increased

Drug Interactions

Metabolism/Transport Effects Substrate of P-glycoprotein

Avoid Concomitant Use

Avoid concomitant use of DAUNOrubicin (Conventional) with any of the following: BCG (Intravesical); Deferiprone; Dipyrone; Natalizumab; Pimecrolimus; Tacrolimus (Topical); Tofacitinib; Vaccines (Live)

Increased Effect/Toxicity

DAUNOrubicin (Conventional) may increase the levels/ effects of: CloZAPine; Deferiprone; Fingolimod; Leflunomide; Natalizumab; Tofacitinib; Vaccines (Live)

The levels/effects of DAUNOrubicin (Conventional) may be increased by: Bevacizumab; Cyclophosphamide; Denosumab; Dipyrone; Lumacaftor; P-glycoprotein/ ABCB1 Inhibitors; Pimecrolimus; Ranolazine; Roflumilast; Tacrolimus (Topical); Taxane Derivatives; Trastuzumab

Decreased Effect

DAUNOrubicin (Conventional) may decrease the levels/ effects of: BCG (Intravesical); Cardiac Glycosides; Coccidioides immitis Skin Test; Sipuleucel-T; Vaccines (Inactivated); Vaccines (Live)

The levels/effects of DAUNOrubicin (Conventional) may be decreased by: Cardiac Glycosides; Echinacea; Lumacaftor; P-glycoprotein/ABCB1 Inducers

Preparation for Administration Hazardous agent; use appropriate precautions for handling and disposal (NIOSH 2014 [group 1]). Dilute vials of powder for injection [Canadian product] with 4 mL SWFI for a final concentration of 5 mg/mL. May further dilute solution or reconstituted daunorubicin solution in D_5W or NS for infusion.

Storage/Stability

Solution: Store intact vials at 2°C to 8°C (36°F to 46°F). Protect from light. Retain in carton until time of use. Solution prepared for infusion may be stored at 20°C to 25°C (68°F to 77°F) for up to 24 hours. Discard unused portion.

Lyophilized powder [Canadian product]: Store intact vials of powder at 15°C to 30°C (59°F to 86°F). Protect from light. Retain in carton until time of use. Reconstituted daunorubicin is stable for 24 hours at room temperature or 48 hours when refrigerated at 2°C to 8°C (36°F to 46°F). Protect reconstituted solution from light.

Mechanism of Action Inhibits DNA and RNA synthesis by intercalation between DNA base pairs and by steric obstruction. Daunomycin intercalates at points of local uncoiling of the double helix. Although the exact mechanism is unclear, it appears that direct binding to DNA (intercalation) and inhibition of DNA repair (topoisomerase II inhibition) result in blockade of DNA and RNA synthesis and fragmentation of DNA.

Pharmacodynamics/Kinetics

Distribution: Distributes widely into tissues, particularly the liver, kidneys, lung, spleen, and heart; does not distribute into the CNS

Metabolism: Primarily hepatic to daunorubicinol (active), then to inactive aglycones, conjugated sulfates, and glucuronides

Half-life elimination: Initial: 45 minutes; Terminal: 18.5 hours; Daunorubicinol plasma half-life: ~27 hours

Excretion: Feces (40%); urine (~25% as unchanged drug and metabolites)

Dosing

Adult & Geriatric Daunorubicin is associated with a moderate emetic potential; antiemetics are recommended to prevent nausea and vomiting (Basch, 2011; Roila, 2010).

Manufacturer's labeling: **Note:** Cumulative doses above 550 mg/m^2 in adults without risk factors for cardiotoxicity and above 400 mg/m^2 in adults receiving chest irradiation are associated with an increased risk of cardiomyopathy.

Acute lymphocytic leukemia (ALL):

IV: 45 mg/m^2 on days 1, 2, and 3 (in combination with vincristine, prednisone, and asparaginase)

Acute myeloid leukemia (AML):

Adults <60 years: Induction: IV: 45 mg/m^2 on days 1, 2, and 3 of the first course of induction therapy; subsequent courses: 45 mg/m^2 on days 1 and 2 (in combination with cytarabine)

Adults ≥60 years: Induction: IV: 30 mg/m^2 on days 1, 2, and 3 of the first course of induction therapy; subsequent courses: 30 mg/m^2 on days 1 and 2 (in combination with cytarabine)

Indication-specific dosing (off-label dosing):

ALL:

CALGB 8811 regimen: IV: 45 mg/m^2 (in patients <60 years) or 30 mg/m^2 (in patients ≥60 years) on days 1, 2, and 3 of induction (Course I; 4 week cycle), in combination with cyclophosphamide, prednisone, vincristine, and asparaginase (Larson, 1995)

CCG 1961: Adults ≤21 years: Induction: 25 mg/m^2 once weekly for 4 weeks (in combination with vincristine, prednisone, and asparaginase) (Nachman, 2009)

GRAALL-2003: Adults ≤60 years: IV:

Induction: 50 mg/m^2 on days 1, 2, and 3 **and** 30 mg/m^2 on days 15 and 16 (in combination with prednisone, vincristine, asparaginase, cyclophosphamide, and G-CSF support) (Huguet, 2009)

Late intensification: 30 mg/m^2 on days 1, 2, and 3 (in combination with prednisone, vincristine, asparaginase, cyclophosphamide, and G-CSF support) (Huguet, 2009)

MRC UKALLXII/ECOG E2993: Adults <60 years: IV: Induction (Phase I): 60 mg/m^2 on days 1, 8, 15, and 22 (in combination with vincristine, asparaginase, and prednisone) (Rowe, 2005)

PETHEMA ALL-96: Adults ≤30 years: IV:

Induction: 30 mg/m^2 on days 1, 8, 15, and 22 (in combination with vincristine, prednisone, asparaginase, and cyclophosphamide) (Ribera, 2008)

Consolidation-2/Reinduction: 30 mg/m^2 on days 1, 2, 8, and 9 (in combination with vincristine, dexamethasone, asparaginase, and cyclophosphamide) (Ribera, 2008)

Protocol 8707: Adults ≤60 years: IV: Induction and Consolidation 2A cycles: 60 mg/m^2 on days 1, 2, and 3 (in combination with vincristine, prednisone, and asparaginase). An additional 60 mg/m^2 daunorubicin dose may be administered on day 15 of induction if bone marrow biopsy on day 14 shows residual disease (Linker, 2002).

AML: Induction:

CCG 2891: Adults <21 years: IV: 20 mg/m^2/day continuous infusion on days 0 to 4 and 10 to 14 (in combination with dexamethasone, cytarabine, thioguanine, and etoposide) (Woods, 1996)

Adults <60 years: IV: 90 mg/m^2 on days 1, 2, and 3 (in combination with cytarabine). If residual disease was observed on day 12 to day 14 bone marrow biopsy, 45 mg/m^2 for 3 days was administered (in combination with cytarabine) (Fernandez, 2009).

Adults <60 years: IV: 60 mg/m^2 on days 1, 2, and 3 (in combination with cytarabine and cladribine); may repeat if partial remission occurs (Holowiecki, 2012).

Adults ≥60 years: IV: 45 or 90 mg/m^2 on days 1, 2, and 3 (in combination with cytarabine); the escalated 90 mg/m^2 dose was associated with increased remission rates and overall survival in the subgroup of patients 60 to 65 years of age as compared to patients >65 years (Lowenberg, 2009)

Acute promyelocytic leukemia (APL):

Induction: Adults: IV: 50 mg/m^2 on days 3, 4, 5, and 6 (in combination with ATRA and cytarabine) (Powell, 2010) **or** 60 mg/m^2 on days 1, 2, and 3 (in combination with ATRA and cytarabine) (Ades, 2008)

Consolidation: Adults: IV: 50 mg/m^2 on days 1, 2, and 3 for 2 cycles (in combination with ATRA; arsenic trioxide was administered for 2 cycles prior to daunorubicin and ATRA) (Powell, 2010) **or** 60 mg/m^2 on days 1, 2, and 3 during cycle 1 of consolidation (in combination with cytarabine), followed by 45 mg/m^2 on days 1, 2, and 3 during cycle 2 of consolidation (in combination with cytarabine) (Ades, 2008)

Pediatric Daunorubicin is associated with a moderate emetic potential; antiemetics are recommended to prevent nausea and vomiting (Dupuis, 2011).

Manufacturer's labeling: **Note:** Cumulative doses above 300 mg/m^2 in children >2 years or 10 mg/kg in children <2 years of age are associated with an increased risk of cardiomyopathy.

Acute lymphocytic leukemia (ALL):

Children <2 years or BSA <0.5 m^2: Remission induction: IV: 1 mg/kg/dose on day 1 every week for up to 4 to 6 cycles (in combination with vincristine and prednisone)

Children ≥2 years and BSA ≥0.5 m^2: Remission induction: IV: 25 mg/m^2 on day 1 every week for up to 4 to 6 cycles (in combination with vincristine and prednisone)

Indication-specific dosing (off-label dosing):
ALL:

CCG 1961: Children ≥10 years and Adolescents: IV: Induction: 25 mg/m^2 once weekly for 4 weeks (in combination with vincristine, prednisone, and asparaginase) (Nachman, 2009)

GRAALL-2003: Adolescents ≥15 years: IV: Induction: 50 mg/m^2 on days 1, 2, and 3 **and** 30 mg/m^2 on days 15 and 16 (in combination with prednisone, vincristine, asparaginase, cyclophosphamide, and G-CSF support) (Huguet, 2009)

Late intensification: 30 mg/m^2 on days 1, 2, and 3 (in combination with prednisone, vincristine, asparaginase, cyclophosphamide, and G-CSF support) (Huguet, 2009)

MRC UKALLXII/ECOG E2993: Adolescents ≥15 years: IV: Induction (Phase I): 60 mg/m^2 on days 1, 8, 15, and 22 (in combination with vincristine, asparaginase, and prednisone) (Rowe, 2005)

PETHEMA ALL-96: Adolescents ≥15 years: IV: Induction: 30 mg/m^2 on days 1, 8, 15, and 22 (in combination with vincristine, prednisone, asparaginase, and cyclophosphamide) (Ribera, 2008)

Consolidation-2/Reinduction: 30 mg/m^2 on days 1, 2, 8, and 9 (in combination with vincristine, dexamethasone, asparaginase, and cyclophosphamide) (Ribera, 2008)

Acute myeloid leukemia (AML): Induction:

CCG 2891:

Children <3 years: IV: 0.67 mg/kg/day continuous infusion on days 0 to 4 and 10 to 14 (in combination with dexamethasone, cytarabine, thioguanine, and etoposide) (Woods, 1996)

Children ≥3 years and Adolescents: IV: 20 mg/m^2/day continuous infusion on days 0 to 4 and 10 to 14 (in combination with dexamethasone, cytarabine, thioguanine, and etoposide) (Woods, 1996)

MRC AML 10/12: Children ≤14 years: IV: 50 mg/m^2 on days 1, 3, and 5 for 2 cycles (in combination with cytarabine and etoposide) (Gibson, 2005)

Renal Impairment The manufacturer's labeling recommends the following adjustment: S_{cr} >3 mg/dL: Administer 50% of normal dose

The following adjustments have also been recommended (Aronoff, 2007):

Adults: No dosage adjustment necessary.

Children:

CrCl <30 mL/minute: Administer 50% of dose

Hemodialysis/continuous ambulatory peritoneal dialysis (CAPD): Administer 50% of dose

Hepatic Impairment

The manufacturer's labeling recommends the following adjustments:

Serum bilirubin 1.2 to 3 mg/dL: Administer 75% of dose

Serum bilirubin >3 mg/dL: Administer 50% of dose

The following adjustments have also been recommended (Floyd, 2006):

Serum bilirubin 1.2 to 3 mg/dL: Administer 75% of dose

Serum bilirubin 3.1 to 5 mg/dL: Administer 50% of dose

Serum bilirubin >5 mg/dL: Avoid use

Administration Daunorubicin is associated with a moderate emetic potential; antiemetics are recommended to prevent nausea and vomiting (Basch, 2011; Dupuis, 2011; Roila, 2010).

For IV administration only. Do not administer IM or SubQ. Administer as slow IV push over 1 to 5 minutes into the tubing of a rapidly infusing IV solution of D$_5$W or NS or may dilute further and infuse over 15 to 30 minutes.

Vesicant; ensure proper needle or catheter placement prior to and during infusion; avoid extravasation.

Extravasation management: If extravasation occurs, stop infusion immediately and disconnect (leave cannula/needle in place); gently aspirate extravasated solution (do **NOT** flush the line); remove needle/cannula; elevate extremity. Initiate antidote (dexrazoxane or dimethyl sulfate [DMSO]). Apply dry cold compresses for 20 minutes 4 times daily for 1 to 2 days (Perez Fidalgo, 2012); withhold cooling beginning 15 minutes before dexrazoxane infusion; continue withholding cooling until 15 minutes after infusion is completed. Topical DMSO should not be administered in combination with dexrazoxane; may lessen dexrazoxane efficacy.

Dexrazoxane: Adults: 1000 mg/m^2 (maximum dose: 2000 mg) IV (administer in a large vein remote from site of extravasation) over 1 to 2 hours days 1 and 2, then 500 mg/m^2 (maximum dose: 1000 mg) IV over 1-2 hours day 3; begin within 6 hours of extravasation. Day 2 and day 3 doses should be administered at approximately the same time (± 3 hours) as the dose on day 1 (Mouridsen, 2007; Perez Fidalgo, 2012). **Note:** Reduce dexrazoxane dose by 50% in patients with moderate to severe renal impairment (CrCl <40 mL/minute).

DMSO: Children and Adults: Apply topically to a region covering twice the affected area every 8 hours for 7 days; begin within 10 minutes of extravasation; do not cover with a dressing (Perez Fidalgo, 2012).

Hazardous agent; use appropriate precautions for handling and disposal (NIOSH 2014 [group 1]).

Monitoring Parameters CBC with differential and platelet count, liver function test, ECG, left ventricular ejection function (echocardiography [ECHO] or multigated radionuclide angiography [MUGA] scan), renal function test, signs/symptoms of extravasation

Dosage Forms Excipient information presented when available (limited, particularly for generics); consult specific product labeling.

Injectable, Intravenous:

Generic: 5 mg/mL (4 mL)

Injectable, Intravenous [preservative free]:

Generic: 5 mg/mL (4 mL, 10 mL)

◆ **DAUNOrubicin Hydrochloride** see DAUNOrubicin (Conventional) on page 504

◆ **Daunorubicin Hydrochloride for Injection (Can)** see DAUNOrubicin (Conventional) on page 504

DAUNOrubicin (Liposomal)
(daw noe ROO bi sin lye po SO mal)

Brand Names: US DaunoXome

Index Terms DAUNOrubicin Citrate; DAUNOrubicin Citrate (Liposomal); DAUNOrubicin Citrate Liposome; Liposomal DAUNOrubicin

Pharmacologic Category Antineoplastic Agent, Anthracycline; Antineoplastic Agent, Topoisomerase II Inhibitor

Use

Kaposi sarcoma: First-line treatment of advanced HIV-associated Kaposi sarcoma

Limitation of use: Daunorubicin (liposomal) is not recommended in HIV-related Kaposi sarcoma which is less than advanced.

Pregnancy Considerations Adverse events were observed in animal reproduction studies. May cause fetal harm if administered during pregnancy. Women of childbearing potential should avoid becoming pregnant while receiving treatment.

Breast-Feeding Considerations Based on information from daunorubicin (conventional), it is not known if daunorubicin (liposomal) is excreted into breast milk. Daunorubicin (liposomal) is indicated for advanced HIV-associated Kaposi sarcoma. In the United States, where formula is accessible, affordable, safe, and sustainable, and the risk of infant mortality due to diarrhea and respiratory infections is low, complete avoidance of breast-feeding by HIV-infected women is recommended to decrease potential transmission of HIV (DHHS [perinatal], 2012).

Contraindications

Hypersensitivity to daunorubicin (liposomal) or any component of the formulation

Documentation of allergenic cross-reactivity for drugs in this class is limited. However, because of similarities in chemical structure and/or pharmacologic actions, the possibility of cross-sensitivity cannot be ruled out with certainty.

Warnings/Precautions Hazardous agent - use appropriate precautions for handling and disposal (NIOSH 2014 [group 1]). **[US Boxed Warning]: Due to the potential for cardiac toxicity and heart failure, monitor cardiac function regularly, especially in patients with previous therapy with anthracyclines, thoracic radiation, or who have preexisting cardiac disease.** Cardiomyopathy is usually associated with a decrease left in ventricular ejection fraction (LVEF). Although the risk increases with cumulative dose, irreversible cardiotoxicity may occur with anthracycline treatment at any dose level. Patients who have received prior anthracycline therapy (DOXOrubicin >300 mg/m^2 or equivalent), with preexisting heart disease, hypertension, concurrent administration of other antineoplastic agents, prior or concurrent chest irradiation, and advanced age are at increased risk. Evaluate LVEF prior to treatment and periodically during treatment (at cumulative doses of daunorubicin liposomal 320 mg/m^2 and every 160 mg/m^2 thereafter or every 160 mg/m^2 in patients at higher risk).

[US Boxed Warning]: May cause bone marrow suppression, particularly neutropenia (may be severe). Monitor blood counts. Monitor closely for infections (including opportunistic infections). **[US Boxed Warning]: Reduce dosage in patients with hepatic impairment.** Use caution with renal impairment; may require dose adjustment. **[US Boxed Warning]: The lipid component is associated with infusion-related reactions (back pain, flushing, chest tightness) usually within the first 5 minutes of infusion and subsides with interruption of the infusion, and generally does not recur if the infusion is resumed at a lower rate.** Monitor for infusion reactions; interrupt infusion if reaction occurs, and resume at reduced infusion rate.

Although not reported with daunorubicin (liposomal), daunorubicin (conventional) is associated with local tissue necrosis if extravasated. Potentially significant drug-drug interactions may exist, requiring dose or frequency adjustment, additional monitoring, and/or selection of alternative therapy. **[US Boxed Warning]: Should be administered under the supervision of an experienced cancer chemotherapy physician.**

Adverse Reactions Frequency not always defined.

Cardiovascular: Edema (11%), chest pain (10%), angina pectoris (≤5%), atrial fibrillation (≤5%), cardiac arrest (≤5%), cardiac tamponade (≤5%), hypertension (≤5%), myocardial infarction (≤5%), palpitations (≤5%), pericardial effusion (≤5%), pulmonary hypertension (≤5%), sinus tachycardia (≤5%), supraventricular tachycardia (≤5%), syncope (≤5%), tachycardia (≤5%), ventricular premature contractions (≤5%), decreased left ventricular ejection fraction (3%; reduction of 20% to 25%), cardiomyopathy (cumulative, dose-related; total dose above 300 mg/m^2)

Central nervous system: Fatigue (49%), headache (25%), rigors (19%), neuropathy (13%), depression (10%), malaise (10%), dizziness (8%), insomnia (6%), abnormality in thinking (≤5%), amnesia (≤5%), anxiety (≤5%), ataxia (≤5%), confusion (≤5%), drowsiness (≤5%), emotional lability (≤5%), hallucination (≤5%), hypertonia (≤5%), meningitis (≤5%), seizure (≤5%)

Dermatologic: Diaphoresis (14%), alopecia (8%), pruritus (7%), folliculitis (≤5%), seborrhea (≤5%), xeroderma (≤5%)

Endocrine & metabolic: Dehydration (≤5%), hot flash (≤5%), increased thirst (≤5%)

Gastrointestinal: Nausea (54%), diarrhea (38%), abdominal pain (23%), anorexia (23%), vomiting (23%), stomatitis (10%), constipation (7%), tenesmus (5%), dental caries (≤5%), dysgeusia (≤5%), dysphagia (≤5%), gastritis (≤5%), gastrointestinal hemorrhage (≤5%), gingival hemorrhage (≤5%), hemorrhoids (≤5%), hiccups (≤5%), increased appetite (≤5%), melena (≤5%), xerostomia (≤5%)

Genitourinary: Dysuria (≤5%), nocturia (≤5%)

Hematologic & oncologic: Neutropenia (<1,000 cells/mm^3: 36%; grade 4: 15%), lymphadenopathy (≤5%), splenomegaly (≤5%), bone marrow depression (especially granulocytes; platelets and erythrocytes less effected), severe granulocytopenia (may be associated with fever and result in infection)

Hepatic: Hepatomegaly (≤5%)

Hypersensitivity: Hypersensitivity reaction (24%)

Infection: Opportunistic infection (40%; median time to first infection/illness: 214 days)

Local: inflammation at injection site (≤5%)

Neuromuscular & skeletal: Back pain (16%), arthralgia (7%), myalgia (7%), abnormal gait (≤5%), hyperkinesia (≤5%), tremor (≤5%)

Ophthalmic: Visual disturbance (5%), conjunctivitis (≤5%), eye pain (≤5%)

Otic: Deafness (≤5%), otalgia (≤5%), tinnitus (≤5%)

Renal: Polyuria (≤5%)

Respiratory: Cough (28%), dyspnea (26%), rhinitis (12%), sinusitis (8%), flu-like symptoms (5%), hemoptysis (≤5%), increased bronchial secretions (≤5%), pulmonary infiltrates (≤5%)

Miscellaneous: Fever (47%), infusion-related reaction (14%; includes back pain, flushing, chest tightness)

Drug Interactions

Metabolism/Transport Effects Substrate of P-glycoprotein

Avoid Concomitant Use

Avoid concomitant use of DAUNOrubicin (Liposomal) with any of the following: BCG (Intravesical); Deferiprone; Dipyrone; Natalizumab; Pimecrolimus; Tacrolimus (Topical); Tofacitinib; Vaccines (Live)

Increased Effect/Toxicity

DAUNOrubicin (Liposomal) may increase the levels/effects of: CloZAPine; Deferiprone; Fingolimod; Leflunomide; Natalizumab; Tofacitinib; Vaccines (Live)

The levels/effects of DAUNOrubicin (Liposomal) may be increased by: Bevacizumab; Cyclophosphamide; Denosumab; Dipyrone; Lumacaftor; P-glycoprotein/ABCB1 Inhibitors; Pimecrolimus; Ranolazine; Roflumilast; Tacrolimus (Topical); Taxane Derivatives; Trastuzumab

Decreased Effect

DAUNOrubicin (Liposomal) may decrease the levels/effects of: BCG (Intravesical); Cardiac Glycosides; Coccidioides immitis Skin Test; Sipuleucel-T; Vaccines (Inactivated); Vaccines (Live)

The levels/effects of DAUNOrubicin (Liposomal) may be decreased by: Cardiac Glycosides; Echinacea; Lumacaftor; P-glycoprotein/ABCB1 Inducers

Preparation for Administration Hazardous agent; use appropriate precautions for handling and disposal (NIOSH 2014 [group 1]). The only fluid that may be mixed with daunorubicin (liposomal) is D$_5$W. Dilute with an equivalent volume of D$_5$W to a 1:1 solution (to a concentration of 1 mg daunorubicin liposomal/mL). Must **not** be mixed with saline, bacteriostatic agents (such as benzyl alcohol), or any other solution. Do not mix with other medications.

Storage/Stability Store intact vials at 2°C to 8°C (36°F to 46°F); do not freeze. Protect from light. Diluted daunorubicin liposomal for infusion may be refrigerated at 2°C to 8°C (36°F to 46°F) for a maximum of 6 hours (if not used immediately).

Mechanism of Action Liposomal preparation of daunorubicin; liposomes have been shown to penetrate solid tumors more effectively, possibly because of their small size and longer circulation time. Once in tissues, daunorubicin is released (over time). Daunorubicin inhibits DNA and RNA synthesis by intercalation between DNA base pairs and by steric obstruction; and intercalates at points of local uncoiling of the double helix. Although the exact mechanism is unclear, it appears that direct binding to DNA (intercalation) and inhibition of DNA repair (topoisomerase II inhibition) result in blockade of DNA and RNA synthesis and fragmentation of DNA.

Pharmacodynamics/Kinetics

Distribution: V$_d$: ~5 to 8 L

Metabolism: Daunorubicinol (major active metabolite) is detected at low levels in plasma

Half-life elimination: Distribution: 4.4 hours

Excretion: Primarily feces; some urine

Dosing

Adult & Geriatric Note: DAUNOrubicin (liposomal) is different from the conventional DAUNOrubicin formulation; do **NOT** substitute (indications and doses are different).

Kaposi sarcoma: IV: 40 mg/m^2 once every 2 weeks; continue until disease progression.

Renal Impairment Serum creatinine >3 mg/dL: Administer 50% of normal dose.

Hepatic Impairment

Bilirubin 1.2 to 3 mg/dL: Administer 75% of normal dose.

Bilirubin >3 mg/dL: Administer 50% of normal dose.

Obesity *ASCO Guidelines for appropriate chemotherapy dosing in obese adults with cancer:* Utilize patient's actual body weight (full weight) for calculation of body surface area- or weight-based dosing, particularly when the intent of therapy is curative; manage regimen-related toxicities in the same manner as for nonobese patients; if a dose reduction is utilized due to toxicity, consider resumption of full weight-based dosing with subsequent cycles, especially if cause of toxicity (eg, hepatic or renal impairment) is resolved (Griggs 2012).

Adjustment for Toxicity

ANC <750/mm^3: Withhold treatment.

Infusion reactions (back pain, flushing, chest tightness): Temporarily interrupt infusion; may resume at a slower rate.

Administration Infuse over 1 hour; do not mix with other drugs. Do NOT administer with an in-line filter. Avoid extravasation.

Hazardous agent; use appropriate precautions for handling and disposal (NIOSH 2014 [group 1]).

Monitoring Parameters CBC with differential and platelets (prior to each dose), liver function tests, renal function tests; evaluate cardiac function (baseline left ventricular ejection fraction [LVEF] prior to treatment initiation; repeat LVEF at total cumulative doses of 320 mg/m², and every 160 mg/m² thereafter; patients with preexisting cardiac disease, history of prior chest irradiation, or history of prior anthracycline treatment should have baseline LVEF and every 160 mg/m² thereafter); signs and symptoms of infection or disease progression; monitor closely for infusion reactions

Dosage Forms Considerations Daunorubicin (liposomal) injection contains sucrose 2,125 mg/25 mL

Dosage Forms Excipient information presented when available (limited, particularly for generics); consult specific product labeling.

Injectable, Intravenous [preservative free]:
DaunoXome: 2 mg/mL (25 mL) [pyrogen free]

Decitabine (de SYE ta been)

Brand Names: US Dacogen

Index Terms 5-Aza-2'-deoxycytidine; 5-Aza-dCyd; Deoxyazacytidine; Dezocitidine

Pharmacologic Category Antineoplastic Agent, Antimetabolite; Antineoplastic Agent, DNA Methylation Inhibitor

Use Myelodysplastic syndromes: Treatment of myelodysplastic syndromes (MDS), including previously treated and untreated, de novo and secondary MDS of all French-American-British (FAB) subtypes (refractory anemia, refractory anemia with ringed sideroblasts, refractory anemia with excess blasts, refractory anemia with excess blasts in transformation, and chronic myelomonocytic leukemia) and intermediate-1, intermediate-2, and high-risk International Prognostic Scoring System (IPSS) groups

Pregnancy Considerations Adverse events were observed in animal reproduction studies. Based on the mechanism of action, decitabine may cause fetal harm if administered during pregnancy. Women of childbearing potential should be advised to use effective contraception to avoid pregnancy during treatment and for 1 month after treatment. In addition, males should be advised to avoid fathering a child while on decitabine therapy and for 2 months after treatment.

Breast-Feeding Considerations Because of the potential for serious adverse reactions in the nursing infant, a decision should be made to discontinue breast-feeding or the drug, taking into account the importance of treatment to the mother.

Contraindications There are no contraindications listed in the manufacturer's labeling.

Warnings/Precautions Hazardous agent - use appropriate precautions for handling and disposal (NIOSH 2014 [group 1]). Neutropenia and thrombocytopenia commonly

occur; anemia and neutropenic fever have also been reported. Myelosuppression and worsening neutropenia are more common in first two treatment cycles and may not correlate with progression of underlying MDS. Hematologic toxicity may require dosage adjustment (after the first cycle), growth factor support, and/or antimicrobial agents. Monitor for infection. Potentially significant drug-drug interactions may exist, requiring dose or frequency adjustment, additional monitoring, and/or selection of alternative therapy.

Adverse Reactions

>10%:

Cardiovascular: Peripheral edema (25% to 27%), pallor (23%), edema (5% to 18%), cardiac murmur (16%), hypotension (6% to 11%)

Central nervous system: Fever (6% to 53%), fatigue (46%), headache (23% to 28%), insomnia (14% to 28%), dizziness (18% to 21%), chills (16%), pain (5% to 13%), confusion (8% to 12%), lethargy (12%), anxiety (9% to 11%), hypoesthesia (11%)

Dermatologic: Petechiae (12% to 39%), bruising (9% to 22%), rash (11% to 19%), erythema (5% to 14%), cellulitis (9% to 12%), lesions (5% to 11%), pruritus (9% to 11%)

Endocrine & metabolic: Hyperglycemia (6% to 33%), hypoalbuminemia (7% to 24%), hypomagnesemia (5% to 24%), hypokalemia (12% to 22%), hyperkalemia (13%), hyponatremia (19%)

Gastrointestinal: Nausea (40% to 42%), constipation (30% to 35%), diarrhea (28% to 34%), vomiting (16% to 25%), anorexia/appetite decreased (8% to 23%), abdominal pain (5% to 14%), oral mucosal petechiae (13%), stomatitis (11% to 12%), dyspepsia (10% to 12%)

Hematologic: Neutropenia (38% to 90%; grades 3/4: 37% to 87%; recovery 28-50 days), thrombocytopenia (27% to 89%; grades 3/4: 24% to 85%), anemia (31% to 82%; grades 3/4: 22%), febrile neutropenia (20% to 29%; grades 3/4: 23%), leukopenia (6% to 28%; grades 3/4: 22%), lymphadenopathy (12%)

Hepatic: Hyperbilirubinemia (6% to 14%), alkaline phosphatase increased (11%)

Local: Tenderness (11%)

Neuromuscular & skeletal: Rigors (22%), arthralgia (17% to 20%), limb pain (18% to 19%), back pain (17% to 18%), weakness (15%)

Respiratory: Cough (27% to 40%), dyspnea (29%), pneumonia (20% to 22%), pharyngitis (16%), lung crackles (14%), epistaxis (13%)

5% to 10%:

Cardiovascular: Tachycardia (8%), chest pain/discomfort (6% to 7%), facial edema (6%), hypertension (6%), heart failure (5%)

Central nervous system: Depression (9%), malaise (5%)

Dermatologic: Alopecia (8%), dry skin (8%), urticaria (6%)

Endocrine & metabolic: Hyperuricemia (10%), LDH increased (8%), bicarbonate increased (6%), dehydration (6% to 8%), hypochloremia (6%), bicarbonate decreased (5%), hypoproteinemia (5%)

Gastrointestinal: Mucosal inflammation (9%), weight loss (9%), gingival bleeding (8%), hemorrhoids (8%), loose stools (7%), tongue ulceration (7%), dysphagia (5% to 6%), oral candidiasis (6%), toothache (6%), abdominal distension (5%), gastroesophageal reflux (5%), glossodynia (5%), lip ulceration (5%), oral pain (5%), tooth abscess (5%)

Genitourinary: Urinary tract infection (7%), dysuria (6%), polyuria (5%)

Hematologic: Bacteremia (5% to 8%), hematoma (5%), pancytopenia (5%), thrombocythemia (5%)

Hepatic: Ascites (10%), AST increased (10%), hypobilirubinemia (5%)

Local: Catheter infection (8%), catheter site erythema (5%), catheter site pain (5%), injection site swelling (5%)

Neuromuscular & skeletal: Myalgia (5% to 9%), falling (8%), chest wall pain (7%), muscle spasm (7%), bone pain (6%), musculoskeletal pain/discomfort (5% to 6%), crepitation (5%)

Ocular: Blurred vision (6%)

Otic: Ear pain (6%)

Respiratory: Breath sounds abnormal (5% to 10%), hypoxia (10%), upper respiratory tract infection (10%), pharyngolaryngeal pain (8%), rales (8%), pulmonary edema (6%), sinusitis (5% to 6%), pleural effusion (5%), postnasal drip (5%), sinus congestion (5%)

Miscellaneous: Candidal infection (10%), staphylococcal infection (7%), transfusion reaction (7%), night sweats (5%)

<5% (Limited to important or life-threatening): Anaphylactic reaction, atrial fibrillation, bronchopulmonary aspergillosis, cardiomyopathy, cardiorespiratory arrest/failure, catheter site hemorrhage, cholecystitis, fungal infection, gastrointestinal hemorrhage, gingival pain, hemoptysis, hypersensitivity, intracranial hemorrhage, mental status change, MI, mycobacterium avium complex infection, peridiverticular abscess, pseudomonal lung infection, pulmonary embolism, pulmonary infiltrates, pulmonary mass, renal failure, respiratory arrest, sepsis, splenomegaly, supraventricular tachycardia, Sweet's syndrome (acute febrile neutrophilic dermatosis), urethral hemorrhage

Drug Interactions

Metabolism/Transport Effects None known.

Avoid Concomitant Use

Avoid concomitant use of Decitabine with any of the following: BCG (Intravesical); Deferiprone; Dipyrone

Increased Effect/Toxicity

Decitabine may increase the levels/effects of: CloZAPine; Deferiprone

The levels/effects of Decitabine may be increased by: Dipyrone

Decreased Effect

Decitabine may decrease the levels/effects of: BCG (Intravesical)

Preparation for Administration Hazardous agent; use appropriate precautions for handling and disposal (NIOSH 2014 [group 1]). Vials should be reconstituted with 10 mL SWFI to a concentration of 5 mg/mL. Immediately further dilute with NS, D$_5$W, or lactated Ringer's to a final concentration of 0.1 to 1 mg/mL. Use appropriate precautions for handling and disposal. Solutions not administered within 15 minutes of preparation should be prepared with cold (2°C to 8°C [36°F to 46°F]) infusion solutions.

Storage/Stability Store intact vials at 25°C (77°F); excursions permitted to 15°C to 30°C (59°F to 86°F). Solutions diluted for infusion may be stored for up to 4 hours prior to infusion refrigerated at 2°C to 8°C (36°F to 46°F) **if** prepared with cold infusion fluids. Infusion should begin within 15 minutes of preparation if room temperature infusion solutions are utilized.

Mechanism of Action After phosphorylation, decitabine is incorporated into DNA and inhibits DNA methyltransferase causing hypomethylation and subsequent cell death (within the S-phase of the cell cycle).

Pharmacodynamics/Kinetics

Distribution: ~63 to 89 L/m^2 (Cashen 2008)

Metabolism: Possibly via deamination by cytidine deaminase

Half-life elimination: ~30 to 35 minutes

Dosing

Adult & Geriatric

Myelodysplastic syndromes (MDS): IV:

15 mg/m^2 over 3 hours every 8 hours (45 mg/m^2/day) for 3 days (135 mg/m^2/cycle) every 6 weeks; treatment is recommended for at least 4 cycles and may continue until the patient no longer benefits.

Adjustment for prolonged hematologic toxicity (ANC <1,000/mm^3 and platelets <50,000/mm^3):

>6 weeks but <8 weeks: Delay dose for up to 2 weeks and temporarily reduce dose to 11 mg/m^2 every 8 hours (33 mg/m^2/day) for 3 days (99 mg/m^2/cycle)

>8 weeks but <10 weeks: Assess for disease progression; if no disease progression, delay dose for up to 2 weeks and reduce dose to 11 mg/m^2 every 8 hours (33 mg/m^2/day) for 3 days (99 mg/m^2/cycle); maintain or increase dose with subsequent cycles if clinically indicated

or

20 mg/m^2 over 1 hour daily for 5 days every 28 days (delay subsequent treatment cycles until hematologic recovery [ANC ≥1,000/mm^3 and platelets ≥50,000/mm^3]); treatment is recommended for at least 4 cycles and may continue until the patient no longer benefits.

Acute myeloid leukemia (AML) (off-label use): Adults ≥60 years: IV: 20 mg/m^2 over 1 hour daily for 5 days every 28 days until relapse, disease progression, or unacceptable toxicity (Cashen 2010; Kantarjian 2012)

Renal Impairment

Preexisting impairment: There are no dosage adjustments provided in the manufacturer's labeling (has not been studied); use with caution.

Renal toxicity during treatment: Serum creatinine ≥2 mg/dL: Temporarily hold treatment until resolution.

Hepatic Impairment

Preexisting impairment: There are no dosage adjustments provided in the manufacturer's labeling (has not been studied); use with caution.

Hepatotoxicity during treatment: ALT and/or bilirubin ≥2 times ULN: Temporarily hold treatment until resolution.

Adjustment for Toxicity

Hematologic toxicity (ANC <1,000/mm^3 and platelets <50,000/mm^3): Delay and/or reduce dose; refer to adult dosing for recommendations specific to each MDS dosing regimen

Nonhematologic toxicity: Temporarily hold treatment until resolution for any of the following toxicities:

Serum creatinine ≥2 mg/dL

ALT, bilirubin ≥2 times ULN

Active or uncontrolled infection

Administration Infuse over 1 to 3 hours. For the treatment of myelodysplastic syndromes, administer by IV infusion over 3 hours (15 mg/m^2 dose) or over 1 hour (20 mg/m^2 dose). For the treatment of acute myeloid leukemia (off-label use), administer by IV infusion over 1 hour (Cashen 2010; Kantarjian 2012). Premedication with antiemetics is recommended according to the manufacturer.

Hazardous agent; use appropriate precautions for handling and disposal (NIOSH 2014 [group 1]).

Monitoring Parameters CBC with differential and platelets (with each cycle and more frequently if needed); liver enzymes (prior to treatment initiation and periodically); serum creatinine (prior to treatment initiation and periodically)

Dosage Forms Excipient information presented when available (limited, particularly for generics); consult specific product labeling.

Solution Reconstituted, Intravenous:

Dacogen: 50 mg (1 ea)

Generic: 50 mg (1 ea)

◆ **Declomycin** *see* Demeclocycline *on page 515*

◆ **Decongestant [OTC] [DSC]** *see* Pseudoephedrine *on page 1527*

◆ **Decongestant 12Hour Max St [OTC]** *see* Pseudoephedrine *on page 1527*

◆ **Deep Sea Nasal Spray [OTC]** *see* Sodium Chloride *on page 1671*

Deferasirox (de FER a sir ox)

Brand Names: US Exjade; Jadenu

Brand Names: Canada Exjade

Index Terms ICL670

Pharmacologic Category Chelating Agent

Use

Chronic iron overload due to transfusions: Treatment of chronic iron overload caused by blood transfusions (transfusional hemosiderosis) in patients 2 years and older.

Chronic iron overload in nontransfusion-dependent thalassemia syndromes: Treatment of chronic iron overload in patients 10 years and older with nontransfusion-dependent thalassemia syndromes and with a liver iron concentration (LIC) of at least 5 mg of iron per gram of liver dry weight (mg Fe/g dw) and a serum ferritin greater than 300 mcg/L (US labeling) or serum ferritin consistently above 800 mcg/L (Canadian labeling).

Limitations of use: Safety and efficacy of deferasirox in combination with other iron chelation therapies have not been established. Controlled studies of deferasirox in myelodysplastic syndromes and chronic iron overload due to transfusions have not been conducted.

Pregnancy Considerations Adverse events were observed in animal reproduction studies. Information related to the use of deferasirox in pregnant women is limited (Vini 2011).

Breast-Feeding Considerations It is not known if deferasirox is excreted in breast milk. Due to the potential for serious adverse reactions in the nursing infant, the manufacturer recommends a decision be made to discontinue breast-feeding or to discontinue the drug, taking into account the importance of treatment to the mother.

Prescribing and Access Restrictions Deferasirox (Exjade) is only available through a restricted distribution program called EPASS Complete Care. Prescribers must enroll patients in this program in order to obtain the medication. For patient enrollment, contact 1-888-90-EPASS (1-888-903-7277).

Contraindications

Known hypersensitivity to deferasirox or any component of the formulation; CrCl <40 mL/minute or serum creatinine >2 times the age-appropriate ULN; poor performance status; high-risk myelodysplastic syndromes; advanced malignancies; platelet counts <50,000/mm^3

Canadian labeling: Additional contraindications (not in US labeling): MDS patients with <1 year life expectancy; CrCl <60 mL/minute

◀ **Warnings/Precautions [US Boxed Warning]: Acute renal failure (including fatalities and cases requiring dialysis) may occur; observed more frequently in patients with comorbid conditions and advanced hematologic malignancies. Obtain serum creatinine and calculate creatinine clearance in duplicate at baseline prior to initiation, and monitor at least monthly thereafter; in patients with underlying renal dysfunction or at risk for acute renal failure, monitor creatinine weekly during the first month then at least monthly thereafter. Dose reduction, interruption, or discontinuation should be considered for serum creatinine elevations.** Monitor serum creatinine and/or CrCl more frequently if creatinine levels are increasing. Use with caution in renal impairment; dosage modification or treatment discontinuation may be required; reductions in initial dose are recommended for patients with CrCl 40 to 60 mL/minute; use is contraindicated in patients with CrCl <40 mL/minute (US labeling) or <60 mL/minute (Canadian labeling) or serum creatinine >2 times age-appropriate ULN. May cause proteinuria; monitor monthly. Renal tubular damage, including Fanconi syndrome, has also been reported, primarily in pediatric/adolescent patients with beta-thalassemia and serum ferritin levels <1,500 mcg/L.

[US Boxed Warning]: Hepatic injury and failure (including fatalities) may occur. Monitor transaminases and bilirubin at baseline, every 2 weeks for 1 month, then at least monthly thereafter. Hepatitis and elevated transaminases have also been reported. Hepatotoxicity is more common in patients >55 years of age and in patients with significant comorbidities (eg, cirrhosis, multiorgan failure). Reduce dose or temporarily interrupt treatment for severe or persistent increases in transaminases/bilirubin. **[US Boxed Warning]: Avoid use in patients with severe (Child-Pugh class C) hepatic impairment; a dose reduction is required in patients with moderate (Child-Pugh class B) hepatic impairment.** Monitor patients with mild (Child-Pugh class A) or moderate (Child-Pugh class B) impairment closely for efficacy and for adverse reactions requiring dosage reduction.

[US Boxed Warning]: Gastrointestinal (GI) hemorrhage (including fatalities) may occur; observed more frequently in elderly patients with advanced hematologic malignancies and/or low platelet counts; discontinue treatment for suspected GI hemorrhage or ulceration. Other GI effects including irritation and ulceration (sometimes complicated with GI perforation, including fatalities) have been reported. Use caution with concurrent medications that may increase risk of adverse GI effects (eg, NSAIDs, corticosteroids, anticoagulants, oral bisphosphonates). Monitor patients closely for signs/symptoms of GI ulceration/bleeding.

May cause skin rash (dose-related), including erythema multiforme; mild to moderate rashes may resolve without treatment interruption; for severe rash, interrupt and consider restarting at a lower dose with dose escalation and oral steroids; discontinue if erythema multiforme is suspected. Severe skin reactions, including Stevens-Johnson syndrome (SJS) and erythema multiforme, have also been reported; if suspected, discontinue immediately and evaluate. Do not reintroduce therapy. Hypersensitivity reactions, including severe reactions (anaphylaxis and angioedema) have been reported, onset is usually within the first month of treatment; discontinue if severe. Auditory (decreased hearing and high-frequency hearing loss) or ocular disturbances (lens opacities, cataracts, intraocular pressure elevation, and retinal disorders) have been reported (rare); monitor and consider dose reduction or treatment interruption. Bone marrow suppression (including agranulocytosis, neutropenia, thrombocytopenia, and worsening anemia) has been reported, risk may be increased in patients with preexisting hematologic disorders; monitor blood counts regularly; interrupt treatment in patients who develop cytopenias; may reinitiate once cause of cytopenia has been determined; use contraindicated if platelet count <50,000/mm³. Potentially significant drug-drug interactions may exist, requiring dose or frequency adjustment, additional monitoring, and/or selection of alternative therapy. For transfusion-related iron overload, treatment should be initiated with evidence of chronic iron overload (ie, transfusion of ≥100 mL/kg of packed RBCs [eg, ≥20 units for a 40 kg individual] and serum ferritin consistently >1,000 mcg/L). For non-transfusion-dependent iron overload, initiate with liver iron concentration ≥5 mg Fe/g dry liver weight and serum ferritin >300 mcg/L. Prior to use, consider risk versus anticipated benefit with respect to individual patient's life expectancy and prognosis. Use with caution in elderly patients due to the higher incidence of toxicity (eg, hepatotoxicity) and fatal events during use. Overchelation of iron may increase development of toxicity; consider temporary interruption of treatment in transfusional iron overload when serum ferritin <500 mcg/L; in non-transfusion-dependent thalassemia when serum ferritin <300 mcg/L or hepatic iron concentration <3 mg Fe/g dry weight. May contain lactose; Canadian product labeling recommends avoiding use in patients with galactose intolerance, Lapp lactase deficiency, or glucose-galactose malabsorption syndromes. Deferasirox has a low affinity for binding with zinc and copper, may cause variable decreases in the serum concentration of these trace minerals.

Adverse Reactions Frequency not always defined.

>10%:

Central nervous system: Headache (Phatak 2010, Vichinsky 2007)

Dermatologic: Skin rash (dose related; 2% to 11%)

Gastrointestinal: Abdominal pain (dose related; 21% to 28%), nausea (dose related; 2% to 23%), vomiting (dose related; 10% to 21%), diarrhea (dose related; 5% to 20%)

Genitourinary: Proteinuria (19%)

Infection: Viral infection (Vichinsky 2007)

Renal: Increased serum creatinine (dose related; 2% to 38%)

Respiratory: Cough (Vichinsky 2007), nasopharyngitis (Vichinsky 2007)

1% to 10%:

Central nervous system: Fatigue (≤1%)

Hepatic: Increased serum ALT (2% to 8%)

Neuromuscular & skeletal: Arthralgia (Vichinsky 2007), back pain (Vichinsky 2007)

Respiratory: Pharyngolaryngeal pain (≤1%), respiratory tract infection (Vichinsky 2007), pharyngitis (Vichinsky 2007)

<1% (Limited to important or life-threatening): Abnormal hepatic function tests, acute renal failure, agranulocytosis, alopecia, anaphylaxis, anemia (worsening), angioedema, cataract, cholelithiasis, cytopenia, drug fever, duodenal ulcer, dyschromia, edema, erythema multiforme, Fanconi's syndrome, gastric ulcer, gastritis, gastrointestinal hemorrhage, gastrointestinal perforation, glycosuria, hearing loss (including high frequency), hematuria, fever, hepatic failure, hepatic insufficiency, hepatitis, hyperactivity, hypersensitivity angiitis, hypersensitivity reaction, hypocalcemia, IgA vasculitis, increased intraocular pressure, increased serum bilirubin (Vichinsky 2007), interstitial nephritis, maculopathy, neutropenia, nontuberculous mycobacterial infection, optic neuritis, pancreatitis (associated with gallstones), purpura, renal tubular disease, renal tubular necrosis, retinopathy, sleep disorder, Stevens-Johnson syndrome, thrombocytopenia, visual disturbance

Drug Interactions

Metabolism/Transport Effects Substrate of UGT1A1; **Inhibits** CYP1A2 (moderate), CYP2C8 (moderate)

Avoid Concomitant Use

Avoid concomitant use of Deferasirox with any of the following: Aluminum Hydroxide; Amodiaquine; Theophylline; TiZANidine

Increased Effect/Toxicity

Deferasirox may increase the levels/effects of: Agomelatine; Amodiaquine; CYP1A2 Substrates; CYP2C8 Substrates; Pirfenidone; Repaglinide; Theophylline; TiZANidine

The levels/effects of Deferasirox may be increased by: Anticoagulants; Bisphosphonate Derivatives; Corticosteroids; Corticosteroids (Systemic); Nonsteroidal Anti-Inflammatory Agents

Decreased Effect

Deferasirox may decrease the levels/effects of: CYP3A4 Substrates

The levels/effects of Deferasirox may be decreased by: Aluminum Hydroxide; Bile Acid Sequestrants; Fosphenytoin; PHENobarbital; Phenytoin; Rifampin; Ritonavir

Food Interactions

Tablets for oral suspension: Bioavailability is increased variably when taken with food. Management: Take on an empty stomach at the same time each day at least 30 minutes before food. Maintain adequate hydration, unless instructed to restrict fluid intake.

Tablets: Bioavailability decreased slightly (not clinically meaningful) after a low-fat meal and increased after a high-fat meal. Management: Take on an empty stomach or with a light meal (containing ~250 calories and <7% fat content).

Storage/Stability Store at 25°C (77°F); excursions permitted to 15°C and 30°C (59°F and 86°F). Protect from moisture.

Mechanism of Action Selectively binds iron, forming a complex that is excreted primarily through the feces.

Pharmacodynamics/Kinetics
Distribution: Adults: 14.4 ± 2.7L

Protein binding: ~99% to serum albumin

Metabolism: Hepatic via glucuronidation by UGT1A1(primarily) and UGT1A3; minor oxidation by CYP450; undergoes enterohepatic recirculation

Bioavailability: Tablets for oral suspension: 70%; Tablets: 36% greater than tablets for oral suspension

Half-life elimination: 8 to 16 hours

Time to peak, plasma: Tablets and tablets for oral suspension: ~1.5 to 4 hours

Excretion: Feces (84%); urine (8%)

Clearance: Moderately lower (by 17.5%) in women than in men.

Dosing
Adult & Geriatric Note: Calculate dose to the nearest whole tablet size.

Conversion from Exjade to Jadenu: The dose for Jadenu should be ~30% lower (rounded to the nearest whole tablet).

Chronic iron overload due to transfusions: Oral:

Note: Treatment should only be initiated with evidence of chronic iron overload (ie, transfusion of ≥100 mL/kg of packed red blood cells [eg, ≥20 units for a 40 kg individual] and serum ferritin consistently >1,000 mcg/L).

US labeling:

Exjade:

Initial: 20 mg/kg once daily

Maintenance: **Note:** Consider interrupting therapy for serum ferritin <500 mcg/L (risk of toxicity may be increased). Adjust dose every 3 to 6 months based on serum ferritin trends; adjust by 5 or 10 mg/kg/day; titrate to individual response and treatment goals. In patients not adequately controlled with 30 mg/kg/day, doses up to 40 mg/kg/day may be considered for serum ferritin levels persistently >2,500 mcg/L and not decreasing over time (doses above 40 mg/kg/day are not recommended).

Jadenu:

Initial: 14 mg/kg once daily

Maintenance: **Note:** Consider interrupting therapy for serum ferritin <500 mcg/L (risk of toxicity may be increased). Adjust dose every 3 to 6 months based on serum ferritin trends; adjust by 3.5 or 7 mg/kg/day; titrate to individual response and treatment goals. In patients not adequately controlled with 21 mg/kg/day, doses up to 28 mg/kg/day may be considered for serum ferritin levels persistently >2,500 mcg/L and not decreasing over time (doses above 28 mg/kg/day are not recommended).

Canadian labeling: Dosing based on treatment goal and patient's individual transfusion rate:

Exjade:

Treatment goal: Maintenance of acceptable body iron levels:

Initial: 10 mg/kg once daily if transfused packed red blood cells (pRBCs) <7 mL/kg/month (approximately <2 units per month for an adult)

Initial: 20 mg/kg once daily if transfused pRBCs ≥7 mL/kg/month (approximately >2 units per month for an adult)

Treatment goal: Iron overload reduction:

Initial: 20 mg/kg once daily if transfused pRBCs <14 mL/kg/month (approximately <4 units per month for an adult)

Initial: 30 mg/kg once daily if transfused pRBCs ≥14 mL/kg/month (approximately >4 units per month for an adult)

Maintenance: **Note:** Consider interrupting therapy for serum ferritin <500 mcg/L (risk of toxicity may be increased).

Adjust dose every 3 to 6 months based on serum ferritin trends; adjust by 5 or 10 mg/kg/day; titrate to individual response and treatment goals. In patients with beta-thalassemia not adequately controlled with 30 mg/kg/day, doses up to 40 mg/kg/day may be considered. Do not exceed 30 mg/kg/day in non-beta-thalessemic patients.

Chronic iron overload in non-transfusion-dependent thalassemia syndromes: Oral:

US labeling: **Note:** Treatment should only be initiated with evidence of chronic iron overload (hepatic iron concentration ≥5 mg Fe/g dry weight and serum ferritin >300 mcg/L).

Exjade:

Initial: 10 mg/kg once daily. Consider increasing to 20 mg/kg once daily after 4 weeks if baseline hepatic iron concentration is >15 mg Fe/g dry weight.

Maintenance: Monitor serum ferritin monthly; if serum ferritin is <300 mcg/L, interrupt therapy and obtain hepatic iron concentration. Monitor hepatic iron concentration every 6 months; interrupt therapy if hepatic iron concentration <3 mg Fe/g dry weight. After 6 months of therapy, consider dose adjustment to a maximum of 20 mg/kg/day if hepatic iron concentration >7 mg Fe/g dry weight. Reduce dose to ≤10 mg/kg when hepatic iron concentration is 3 to 7 mg Fe/g dry weight. Do not exceed 20 mg/kg/day. After interruption, resume treatment when hepatic iron concentration >5 mg Fe/g dry weight.

Jadenu:

Initial: 7 mg/kg once daily. Consider increasing to 14 mg/kg once daily after 4 weeks if baseline hepatic iron concentration is >15 mg Fe/g dry weight.

Maintenance: Monitor serum ferritin monthly; if serum ferritin is <300 mcg/L, interrupt therapy and obtain hepatic iron concentration. Monitor hepatic iron concentration every 6 months; interrupt therapy if hepatic iron concentration <3 mg Fe/g dry weight. After 6 months of therapy, consider dose adjustment to a maximum of 14 mg/kg/day if hepatic iron concentration >7 mg Fe/g dry weight. Reduce dose to ≤7 mg/kg when hepatic iron concentration is 3 to 7 mg Fe/g dry weight. Do not exceed 14 mg/kg/day. After interruption, resume treatment when hepatic iron concentration >5 mg Fe/g dry weight.

Canadian labeling: **Note:** Treatment should only be initiated with evidence of chronic iron overload (hepatic iron concentration ≥5 mg Fe/g dry weight and serum ferritin consistently >800 mcg/L).

Exjade:

Initial: 10 mg/kg/day

Maintenance: Do not exceed 10 mg/kg/day in patients whose hepatic iron concentration was not evaluated and if serum ferritin ≤2,000 mcg/L. Monitor serum ferritin monthly; consider dose adjustment by 5 or 10 mg/kg/day every 3 to 6 months if hepatic iron concentration ≥7 mg Fe/g dry weight or serum transferrin levels consistently >2,000 mcg/L. Patients receiving >10 mg/kg should have their dose reduced to ≤10 mg/kg when hepatic iron concentration <7 mg Fe/g dry weight or serum ferritin <2,000 mcg/L. Interrupt therapy when hepatic iron concentration <3 mg Fe/g dry weight or serum ferritin <300 mcg/L. Doses above 20 mg/kg/day are not recommended.

Dosage adjustment with concomitant bile acid sequestrants (eg, cholestyramine, colesevelam, colestipol) or potent UGT inducers (eg, rifampin, phenytoin, phenobarbital, ritonavir): Avoid concomitant use; if coadministration necessary, consider increasing the initial dose of deferasirox dose by 50%; monitor serum ferritin and clinical response.

Pediatric Note: Calculate dose to the nearest whole tablet size. When calculating dose, consider changes in weight over time.

Chronic iron overload due to transfusions: Children ≥2 years and Adolescents: Refer to adult dosing.

Chronic iron overload in non-transfusion-dependent thalassemia syndromes: Children ≥10 years and Adolescents: Refer to adult dosing.

Conversion from Exjade to Jadenu: The dose for Jadenu should be ~30% lower (rounded to the nearest whole tablet).

Renal Impairment Creatinine clearance should be estimated using the Cockcroft-Gault formula.

Renal impairment at treatment initiation:

CrCl >60 mL/minute: No dosage adjustment necessary.

CrCl 40 to 60 mL/minute:

US labeling: Reduce initial dose by 50%.

Canadian labeling: Use is contraindicated.

CrCl <40 mL/minute or serum creatinine >2 times age-appropriate ULN: Use is contraindicated.

Renal toxicity during treatment:

US labeling:

Transfusional iron overload:

Adolescents ≥16 years and Adults: For increase in serum creatinine ≥33% above the average baseline, repeat within 1 week; if still elevated by ≥33%: Reduce daily dose by 10 mg/kg (for Exjade) **or** 7 mg/kg (for Jadenu)

Children ≥2 years to Adolescents 15 years: For increase in serum creatinine >33% above the average baseline level and above the age-appropriate ULN: Reduce daily dose by 10 mg/kg (for Exjade) **or** 7 mg/kg (for Jadenu)

All patients: CrCl <40 mL/minute or serum creatinine >2 times age-appropriate ULN: Discontinue treatment.

Non-transfusion-dependent thalassemia syndromes:
Adolescents ≥16 years and Adults: For increase in serum creatinine ≥33% above the average baseline, repeat within 1 week; if still elevated by ≥33%:

Exjade: Interrupt therapy if the dose is 5 mg/kg; reduce dose by 50% if the dose is 10 or 20 mg/kg

Jadenu: Interrupt therapy if the dose is 3.5 mg/kg; reduce dose by 50% if the dose is 7 or 14 mg/kg

Children ≥10 years to Adolescents 15 years: For increase in serum creatinine >33% above the average baseline level and above the age-appropriate ULN: Reduce daily dose by 5 mg/kg (for Exjade) **or** 3.5 mg/kg (for Jadenu)

All patients: CrCl <40 mL/minute or serum creatinine >2 times age-appropriate ULN: Discontinue treatment.

Canadian labeling:
Adolescents ≥16 years and Adults: For increase in serum creatinine >33% above the average pretreatment level for 2 consecutive weekly levels, reduce daily dose by 10 mg/kg.

Children ≥2 years and Adolescents <16 years: For increase in serum creatinine above the age-appropriate ULN for 2 consecutive levels, reduce daily dose by 10 mg/kg.

All patients: Progressive increase serum creatinine beyond ULN: Withhold treatment.

Hepatic Impairment

Hepatic impairment at treatment initiation:

Mild impairment (Child-Pugh class A): No dosage adjustment necessary; monitor closely for efficacy and for adverse reactions requiring dosage reduction.

Moderate impairment (Child-Pugh class B): Initial: Reduce dose by 50%; monitor closely for efficacy and for adverse reactions requiring dosage reduction.

Severe impairment (Child-Pugh class C): Avoid use.

Hepatic toxicity during treatment: Severe or persistent increases in transaminases/bilirubin: Reduce dose or temporarily interrupt treatment.

Adjustment for Toxicity

Bone marrow suppression: Interrupt treatment; may reinitiate once cause of cytopenia has been determined; use contraindicated if platelet count <50,000/mm³

Dermatologic toxicity:

Rash (severe): Interrupt treatment; may reintroduce at a lower dose (with future dose escalation) and short-term oral corticosteroids.

Severe skin reaction (Stevens-Johnson syndrome, erythema multiforme): Discontinue and evaluate.

Gastrointestinal: Discontinue treatment for suspected GI ulceration or hemorrhage.

Hearing loss or visual disturbance: Consider dose reduction or treatment interruption.

Dietary Considerations

Tablets for oral suspension: Bioavailability increased variably when taken with food; take on empty stomach 30 minutes before a meal.

Tablets: Bioavailability decreased slightly (not clinically meaningful) after a low-fat meal and increased after a high fat meal; take on an empty stomach or with a light meal (containing ~250 calories and <7% fat content).

Administration Oral:

Tablets (Jadenu): Swallow with water or other liquids at the same time each day. Take on an empty stomach or with a light meal (contains less than 7% fat content and ~250 calories). For patients who have difficulty swallowing whole tablets, may crush tablets and mix with soft foods (eg, yogurt, applesauce); consume entire mixture immediately after preparation (do not store for future use). Commercial crushers with serrated surfaces should be avoided for crushing a single 90 mg tablet.

Tablets for suspension (Exjade): Administer tablets by making an oral suspension; **do not chew or swallow tablets whole.** Completely disperse tablets in water, orange juice, or apple juice (use 3.5 ounces for total doses <1 g; 7 ounces for doses ≥1 g); stir to form a fine suspension and drink entire contents. Rinse remaining residue with more fluid; drink. Avoid dispersion of tablets in milk (due to slowed dissolution) or carbonated drinks (due to foaming) (Séchaud, 2008). Administer at same time each day on an empty stomach, at least 30 minutes before food. Do not take simultaneously with aluminum-containing antacids.

Do not take simultaneously with aluminum-containing antacids.

Monitoring Parameters Serum ferritin (baseline, monthly thereafter), iron levels (baseline), CBC with differential, serum creatinine and creatinine clearance (2 baseline assessments then monthly thereafter; in patients who are at increased risk of complications [eg, preexisting renal conditions, elderly, comorbid conditions, or receiving other potentially nephrotoxic medications]: weekly for the first month then at least monthly thereafter); hepatic iron concentration (non-transfusion-dependent thalassemia; baseline, every 6 months); urine protein (monthly); monitor serum creatinine and/or creatinine clearance more frequently if creatinine levels are increasing; serum transaminases (ALT/AST) and bilirubin (baseline, every 2 weeks for the first month, then monthly); baseline and annual auditory and ophthalmic examination (including slit lamp examinations and dilated fundoscopy); performance status (in patients with hematologic malignancies); signs/symptoms of GI ulcers or hemorrhage; cumulative number of RBC units received

Canadian labeling also recommends monitoring growth and body weight every 12 months in pediatric patients.

Dosage Forms Excipient information presented when available (limited, particularly for generics); consult specific product labeling.

Tablet, Oral:
Jadenu: 90 mg, 180 mg, 360 mg

Tablet Soluble, Oral:
Exjade: 125 mg, 250 mg, 500 mg

Deferiprone (de FER i prone)

Brand Names: US Ferriprox
Index Terms APO-066
Pharmacologic Category Chelating Agent
Use

Transfusional iron overload: Treatment of transfusional iron overload due to thalassemia syndromes with inadequate response to other chelation therapy.

Limitation of use: Safety and effectiveness have not been established for the treatment of transfusional iron overload in patients with other chronic anemias.

Medication Guide Available Yes
Dosing

Adult Note: Round dose to the nearest 250 mg (or ½ tablet) or 2.5 mL (oral solution). If serum ferritin falls consistently below 500 mcg/L, consider temporary treatment interruption.

Transfusional iron overload: Oral: Initial: 25 mg/kg 3 times/day (75 mg/kg/day); individualize dose based on response and therapeutic goal; maximum dose: 33 mg/kg 3 times/day (99 mg/kg/day)

Geriatric Refer to adult dosing. Begin at the low end of dosing range.

Renal Impairment There are no dosage adjustments provided in the manufacturer's labeling.

Hepatic Impairment There are no dosage adjustments provided in the manufacturer's labeling (has not been studied in patients with severe impairment).

Adjustment for Toxicity

ANC <1,500/mm³ and >500/mm³: Interrupt treatment immediately and monitor until recovery; do not rechallenge unless the potential benefit outweighs the risk.

ANC <500/mm³: In addition to treatment interruption, consider hospitalization (and other clinically-appropriate management); do not resume unless the potential benefits outweigh potential risks

Infection: Interrupt treatment; monitor ANC more frequently

Additional Information Complete prescribing information should be consulted for additional detail.

Dosage Forms Excipient information presented when available (limited, particularly for generics); consult specific product labeling.

Solution, Oral:
Ferriprox: 100 mg/mL (500 mL) [contains fd&c yellow #6 (sunset yellow); cherry-peppermint flavor]

Tablet, Oral:
Ferriprox: 500 mg [scored]

Deferoxamine (de fer OKS a meen)

Brand Names: US Desferal
Brand Names: Canada Deferoxamine Mesylate for Injection; Desferal; PMS-Deferoxamine
Index Terms Deferoxamine Mesylate; Desferrioxamine; DFM
Pharmacologic Category Antidote; Chelating Agent
Use Adjunct in the treatment of acute iron intoxication; treatment of chronic iron overload secondary to multiple transfusions

Canadian labeling (off-label use in the U.S.): Diagnosis of aluminum overload; treatment of chronic aluminum overload in patients with end-stage renal failure undergoing maintenance dialysis

Dosing

Adult

Acute iron toxicity: Note: The IV route is used when severe toxicity is evidenced by cardiovascular collapse or systemic symptoms (coma, shock, metabolic acidosis, or gastrointestinal bleeding) or potentially severe intoxications (peak serum iron level >500 mcg/dL) (Perrone, 2011). When severe symptoms are not present, the IM route may be used (per the manufacturer).

IM, IV: Initial: 1,000 mg, may be followed by 500 mg every 4 hours for 2 doses; subsequent doses of 500 mg have been administered every 4 to 12 hours based on clinical response (maximum recommended dose: 6,000 mg/day [per manufacturer])

Canadian labeling:

IM: Initial: 90 mg/kg/dose (maximum/dose: 2,000 mg) followed by 45 mg/kg every 4 to 12 hours as needed (maximum: 6000 mg/24 hours)

IV: 15 mg/kg/hour up to a maximum of 80 mg/kg/dose or maximum of 6,000 mg/24 hours

Chronic iron overload:

IM: 500 to 1,000 mg/day (maximum: 1000 mg/day)

IV: 40 to 50 mg/kg/day (maximum: 60 mg/kg/day) over 8 to 12 hours for 5 to 7 days per week

SubQ: 1,000 to 2,000 mg/day or 20 to 40 mg/kg/day over 8 to 24 hours

Off-label dosing: IV, SubQ: 25 to 50 mg/kg over 8 to 10 hours 5 to 7 days per week (Brittenham, 2011)

Canadian labeling: IV, SubQ: 1,000 to 4,000 mg/day (20 to 60 mg/kg/day) over ~12 hours (may further increase iron excretion with infusion at the same dose over 24 hours). SubQ infusions are administered 4 to 7 days per week based on the degree of iron overload.

Diagnosis of aluminum-induced toxicity with CKD (off-label use; K/DOQI guidelines, 2003): IV: Test dose: 5 mg/kg during the last hour of dialysis if serum aluminum levels are 60 to 200 mcg/L, or clinical signs/symptoms of toxicity, or aluminum exposure prior to parathyroid surgery. Measure aluminum just prior to deferoxamine; remeasure 2 days later (test is positive if serum aluminum is ≥50 mcg/L. Do not use if aluminum serum levels are >200 mcg/L.

Canadian labeling: **Note:** Measure serum aluminum levels prior to and after administration of deferoxamine. IV: Test dose: 5 mg/kg/dose (infusion rate not to exceed 15 mg/kg/hour) following hemodialysis (preferred) or during the last hour of dialysis if serum aluminum levels are >60 mcg/L in association with serum ferritin levels >100 mcg/L; continuous rise in serum aluminum over the next 24 to 48 hours suggests overload. Remeasure serum aluminum levels prior to next hemodialysis, test is considered positive if serum aluminum levels increase >150 mcg/L above baseline.

Treatment of aluminum toxicity with CKD (off-label use; K/DOQI guidelines, 2003): IV:

Administer after diagnostic deferoxamine test dose. **Note:** The risk for deferoxamine-associated neurotoxicity is increased if aluminum serum levels are >200 mcg/L; withhold deferoxamine and administer intensive dialysis until <200 mcg/L.

Aluminum rise ≥300 mcg/L: 5 mg/kg once a week 5 hours before dialysis for 4 months

Aluminum rise <300 mcg/L: 5 mg/kg once a week during the last hour of dialysis for 2 months

Canadian labeling: Treatment should be considered for symptomatic patients with serum aluminum levels >60 mcg/L and a positive deferoxamine test dose.

Hemodialysis: IV: 5 mg/kg/dose (infusion rate not to exceed 15 mg/kg/hour) once weekly for 3 months following hemodialysis (preferred) or during the last hour of dialysis administered. Withhold treatment for 1 month then perform deferoxamine test. Further treatment is not recommended if 2 consecutive tests (performed 1 month apart) yield an increase in serum aluminum levels <75 mcg/L.

Continuous ambulatory or cyclic peritoneal dialysis: Intraperitoneal (preferred), IM, SubQ infusion (slow), or IV infusion (slow): 5 mg/kg/dose once weekly prior to final daily exchange

Geriatric Refer to adult dosing. May initiate at the lower end of the dosing range.

Pediatric

Acute iron toxicity: Children and Adolescents: **Note:** The IV route is used when severe toxicity is evidenced by cardiovascular collapse or systemic symptoms (coma, shock, metabolic acidosis, or gastrointestinal bleeding) or potentially severe intoxications (peak serum iron level >500 mcg/dL) (Perrone, 2011). When severe symptoms are not present, the IM route may be used (per the manufacturer).

IM: 90 mg/kg/dose every 8 hours (maximum: 6,000 mg/24 hours)

IV: 15 mg/kg/hour (maximum: 6,000 mg/24 hours)

Canadian labeling:

IM: Initial: 90 mg/kg/dose (maximum/dose: 1,000 mg) followed by 45 mg/kg every 4 to 12 hours as needed (maximum: 6,000 mg/24 hours)

IV: 15 mg/kg/hour up to a maximum of 80 mg/kg/dose or maximum of 6,000 mg/24 hours

Chronic iron overload: Children ≥3 years and Adolescents:

IV: 20 to 40 mg/kg/day over 8 to 12 hours for 5 to 7 days per week; dose should not exceed 40 mg/kg/day until growth has ceased

SubQ: 20 to 40 mg/kg/day over 8 to 12 hours (maximum: 1,000 to 2,000 mg/day)

Off-label dosing: IV, SubQ: 25 to 30 mg/kg over 8 to 10 hours 5 to 7 days per week (Brittenham, 2011)

Diagnosis of aluminum induced toxicity with CKD (off-label use; K/DOQI guidelines, 2003): Children and Adolescents: IV: Test dose: 5 mg/kg during the last hour of dialysis if serum aluminum levels are 60 to 200 mcg/L, or clinical signs/symptoms of toxicity, or aluminum exposure prior to parathyroid surgery. Measure aluminum just prior to deferoxamine; remeasure 2 days later (test is positive if serum aluminum is ≥50 mcg/L). Do not use if aluminum serum levels are >200 mcg/L.

Treatment of aluminum toxicity with CKD (off-label use; K/DOQI guidelines, 2003): Children and Adolescents: IV: Administer after diagnostic deferoxamine test dose. **Note:** The risk for deferoxamine-associated neurotoxicity is increased if aluminum serum levels are >200 mcg/L; withhold deferoxamine and administer intensive dialysis until <200 mcg/L.

Aluminum rise ≥300 mcg/L: 5 mg/kg once a week 5 hours before dialysis for 4 months

Aluminum rise <300 mcg/L: 5 mg/kg once a week during the last hour of dialysis for 2 months

Renal Impairment Severe renal disease or anuria: Use is contraindicated in the manufacturer's U.S. labeling.

The following adjustments have been used by some clinicians (Aronoff, 2007): Adults:

CrCl >50 mL/minute: No adjustment required

CrCl 10 to 50 mL/minute, CRRT: Administer 25% to 50% of normal dose

CrCl<10 mL/minute, hemodialysis, peritoneal dialysis: Avoid use

Hepatic Impairment There are no dosage adjustments provided in the manufacturer's labeling (has not been studied).

Additional Information Complete prescribing information should be consulted for additional detail.

Dosage Forms Excipient information presented when available (limited, particularly for generics); consult specific product labeling. [DSC] = Discontinued product

Solution Reconstituted, Injection, as mesylate:

Desferal: 500 mg (1 ea); 2 g (1 ea [DSC])

Generic: 500 mg (1 ea); 2 g (1 ea)

◆ Deferoxamine Mesylate *see* Deferoxamine *on page 512*

◆ Deferoxamine Mesylate for Injection (Can) *see* Deferoxamine *on page 512*

Degarelix (deg a REL ix)

Brand Names: US Firmagon

Brand Names: Canada Firmagon

Index Terms Degarelix Acetate; FE200486

Pharmacologic Category Antineoplastic Agent, Gonadotropin-Releasing Hormone Antagonist; Gonadotropin Releasing Hormone Antagonist

Use Prostate cancer, advanced: Treatment of advanced prostate cancer

Dosing

Adult & Geriatric Prostate cancer, advanced: SubQ:

Loading dose: 240 mg administered as two 120 mg (3 mL) injections

Maintenance dose: 80 mg administered as one 4 mL injection every 28 days (beginning 28 days after initial loading dose)

Renal Impairment

CrCl 50 to 80 mL/minute: No dosage adjustment necessary.

CrCl <50 mL/minute: There are no dosage adjustments provided in the manufacturer's labeling; use with caution.

Hepatic Impairment

Mild-to-moderate hepatic impairment: No dosage adjustment necessary; monitor serum testosterone levels.

Severe hepatic impairment: There are no dosage adjustments provided in the manufacturer's labeling (has not been studied); use with caution.

Additional Information Complete prescribing information should be consulted for additional detail.

Dosage Forms Excipient information presented when available (limited, particularly for generics); consult specific product labeling.

Solution Reconstituted, Subcutaneous, as acetate:
Firmagon: 80 mg (1 ea); 120 mg (1 ea)

◆ Degarelix Acetate see Degarelix on page 513
◆ Dehydrobenzperidol see Droperidol on page 607
◆ Delatestryl see Testosterone on page 1766

Delavirdine (de la VIR deen)

Brand Names: US Rescriptor
Brand Names: Canada Rescriptor
Index Terms DLV; U-90152S
Pharmacologic Category Antiretroviral, Reverse Transcriptase Inhibitor, Non-nucleoside (Anti-HIV)
Use Treatment of HIV-1 infection in combination with at least two additional antiretroviral agents
Pregnancy Considerations Adverse events were observed in some animal reproduction studies. Hypersensitivity reactions (including hepatic toxicity and rash) are more common in women on NNRTI therapy; it is not known if pregnancy increases this risk.

Regardless of CD4 count or HIV RNA copy number, all HIV-infected pregnant women should receive a combination antiretroviral (ARV) drug regimen. A combination of antepartum, intrapartum, and infant ARV prophylaxis is recommended. ARV therapy should be started as soon as possible in women with symptomatic infection. Although earlier initiation may be more effective in reducing the perinatal transmission of HIV, initiation may be delayed until after 12 weeks gestation in women who do not require immediate treatment after careful consideration of maternal conditions (eg, nausea and vomiting) and the potential risks of first trimester fetal exposure for specific agents. A scheduled cesarean delivery at 38 weeks gestation is recommended for all women with HIV RNA >1000 copies/mL or unknown concentrations near delivery in order to decrease transmission. If ARV therapy must be interrupted for <24 hours during the peripartum period, stop then restart all medications simultaneously in order to decrease the chance of developing resistance. Long-term follow-up is recommended for all infants exposed to ARV medications. In couples who want to conceive, the HIV-infected partner should attain maximum viral suppression prior to conception.

Health care providers are encouraged to enroll pregnant women exposed to antiretroviral medications in the Antiretroviral Pregnancy Registry (1-800-258-4263 or www.-APRegistry.com). Health care providers caring for HIV-infected women and their infants may contact the National Perinatal HIV Hotline (888-448-8765) for clinical consultation (HHS [perinatal] 2014).

Breast-Feeding Considerations It is not known if delavirdine is excreted into breast milk. Maternal or infant antiretroviral therapy does not completely eliminate the risk of postnatal HIV transmission. In addition, multiclass-resistant virus has been detected in breast-feeding infants despite maternal therapy. Therefore, in the United States, where formula is accessible, affordable, safe, and sustainable, and the risk of infant mortality due to diarrhea and respiratory infections is low, complete avoidance of breast-feeding by HIV-infected women is recommended to decrease potential transmission of HIV (HHS [perinatal] 2014).

Contraindications Hypersensitivity to delavirdine or any component of the formulation; concurrent use of alprazolam, astemizole, cisapride, ergot alkaloids, midazolam, pimozide, rifampin, terfenadine, or triazolam

Warnings/Precautions Use with caution in patients with hepatic or renal dysfunction; due to rapid emergence of resistance, delavirdine should not be used as monotherapy or as a component of an initial antiretroviral regimen; cross-resistance may be conferred to other non-nucleoside reverse transcriptase inhibitors, although potential for cross-resistance with protease inhibitors is low. Long-term effects of delavirdine are not known. May cause redistribution of fat (eg, buffalo hump, peripheral wasting with increased abdominal girth, cushingoid appearance). Patients may develop immune reconstitution syndrome resulting in the occurrence of an inflammatory response to an indolent or residual opportunistic infection during initial HIV treatment or activation of autoimmune disorders (eg, Graves' disease, polymyositis, Guillain-Barré syndrome) later in therapy; further evaluation and treatment may be required. Safety and efficacy have not been established in children. Rash, which occurs frequently,

may require discontinuation of therapy; usually occurs within 1-3 weeks and lasts <2 weeks. Most patients may resume therapy following a treatment interruption. Use with caution in patients taking strong CYP3A4 inhibitors, moderate or strong CYP3A4 inducers and major CYP3A4 substrates (see Drug Interactions); consider alternative agents that avoid or lessen the potential for CYP-mediated interactions.

Adverse Reactions Frequency of adverse reactions reported from occurrence in clinical trials with delavirdine when used as part of combination antiretroviral therapy.

>10%:
Central nervous system: Headache (19% to 20%), depressive symptoms (10% to 15%), fever (4% to 12%)
Dermatologic: Rash (16% to 32%)
Gastrointestinal: Nausea (20% to 25%), vomiting (3% to 11%)
1% to 10%:
Central nervous system: Anxiety (6% to 8%)
Endocrine & metabolic: Transaminases increased (2% to 5%), amylase increased (3%), bilirubin increased (2%)
Gastrointestinal: Diarrhea, vomiting, abdominal pain (4% to 6%)
Hematologic: Prothrombin time increased (2%), hemoglobin decreased (1% to 3%)
Respiratory: Bronchitis (6% to 8%)
Frequency not defined (limited to important or life threatening): Abscess, adenopathy, alkaline phosphatase increased, allergic reaction, angioedema, anorexia, arrhythmia, bloody stool, bone pain, bruising, cardiac insufficiency, cardiac rate abnormal, cardiomyopathy, chest congestion, cognitive impairment, colitis, confusion, conjunctivitis, dermal leukocytoclastic vasculitis, desquamation, diverticulitis, dyspnea, emotional lability, eosinophilia, erythema multiforme, fecal incontinence, fungal dermatitis, gamma glutamyl transpeptidase increased, gastroenteritis, gastrointestinal bleeding, granulocytosis, gum hemorrhage, hallucination, hematuria, hepatomegaly, hyperglycemia, hyperkalemia, hypertension, hypertriglyceridemia, hyperuricemia, hypocalcemia, hyponatremia, hypophosphatemia, infection, jaundice, kidney pain, leukopenia, lipase increased, menstrual irregularities, moniliasis (oral/vaginal), orthostatic hypotension, pancreatitis, pancytopenia, paralysis, peripheral vascular disorder, pneumonia, purpura, redistribution of body fat, renal calculi, serum creatinine increased, spleen disorder, Stevens-Johnson syndrome, tetany, thrombocytopenia, urinary tract infection, vertigo
Postmarketing and/or case reports: Acute renal failure, hemolytic anemia, hepatic failure, immune reconstitution syndrome, rhabdomyolysis

Drug Interactions

Metabolism/Transport Effects Substrate of CYP2D6 (minor), CYP3A4 (major); **Note:** Assignment of Major/Minor substrate status based on clinically relevant drug interaction potential; **Inhibits** CYP1A2 (weak), CYP2C19 (strong), CYP2C9 (strong), CYP2D6 (strong), CYP3A4 (weak)

Avoid Concomitant Use

Avoid concomitant use of Delavirdine with any of the following: Astemizole; CarBAMazepine; Efavirenz; Etravirine; Fosamprenavir; Fosphenytoin; H2-Antagonists; Mequitazine; Phenytoin; Pimozide; Proton Pump Inhibitors; Rifamycin Derivatives; Rilpivirine; St Johns Wort; Tamoxifen; Terfenadine; Thioridazine

Increased Effect/Toxicity

Delavirdine may increase the levels/effects of: ARIPiprazole; ARIPiprazole Lauroxil; Astemizole; AtoMOXetine; Bosentan; Brexpiprazole; Cilostazol; Citalopram; CYP2C19 Substrates; CYP2C9 Substrates; CYP2D6 Substrates; Dapoxetine; Diclofenac (Systemic); Dofetilide; DOXOrubicin (Conventional); Dronabinol; DULoxetine; Efavirenz; Eliglustat; Etravirine; Fesoterodine; Flibanserin; Fosamprenavir; Fosphenytoin; Hydrocodone; Iloperidone; Lacosamide; Lomitapide; Mequitazine; Metoprolol; Nebivolol; NiMODipine; Ospemifene; Parecoxib; Phenytoin; Pimozide; Propafenone; Protease Inhibitors; Ramelteon; Rifamycin Derivatives; Rilpivirine; Tamsulosin; Terfenadine; Tetrabenazine; Tetrahydrocannabinol; Thioridazine; TiZANidine; TraMADol; Vortioxetine

The levels/effects of Delavirdine may be increased by: Cannabis; Osimertinib

Decreased Effect

Delavirdine may decrease the levels/effects of: CarBAMazepine; Clopidogrel; Codeine; Efavirenz; Etravirine; Hydrocodone; Iloperidone; Rilpivirine; Tamoxifen; TraMADol

The levels/effects of Delavirdine may be decreased by: Antacids; Bosentan; CarBAMazepine; CYP3A4 Inducers (Moderate); CYP3A4 Inducers (Strong); Dabrafenib;

Deferasirox; Enzalutamide; Fosamprenavir; Fospheny-
toin; H2-Antagonists; Mitotane; Osimertinib; Phenytoin;
Protease Inhibitors; Proton Pump Inhibitors; Rifamycin
Derivatives; Siltuximab; St Johns Wort; Tocilizumab

Storage/Stability Store at 20°C to 25°C (68°F to 77°F).
Protect from humidity.

Mechanism of Action Delavirdine binds directly to
reverse transcriptase, blocking RNA-dependent and
DNA-dependent DNA polymerase activities

Pharmacodynamics/Kinetics

Absorption: Rapid

Distribution: Low concentration in saliva and semen; CSF
0.4% concurrent plasma concentration

Protein binding: ~98%, primarily albumin

Metabolism: Hepatic via CYP3A4 and 2D6 (**Note:** May
reduce CYP3A activity and inhibit its own metabolism.)

Bioavailability: Tablet: 85% as tablet; ~100% as oral slurry

Half-life elimination: 5.8 hours (range: 2-11 hours)

Time to peak, plasma: 1 hour

Excretion: Urine (51%, <5% as unchanged drug); feces
(44%); nonlinear kinetics exhibited

Dosing

**Adult & Geriatric HIV-1 infection (part of combina-
tion):** Oral: 400 mg 3 times/day

Pediatric HIV-1 infection (part of combination): Adolescents ≥16 years: Refer to adult dosing.

Renal Impairment No dosage adjustment provided in
manufacturer's labeling (has not been studied). Guidelines state that no dosage adjustment is necessary in
renal impairment (HHS [adult] 2015).

Hepatic Impairment No dosage adjustment provided in
manufacturer's labeling (has not been studied). However,
delavirdine is primarily metabolized by the liver, use with
caution.

Dietary Considerations May be taken without regard to
meals.

Administration Patients with achlorhydria should take the
drug with an acidic beverage; antacids and delavirdine
should be separated by 1 hour. A dispersion of delavirdine
may be prepared by adding four 100 mg tablets to at least
3 oz of water. Allow to stand for a few minutes and stir until
uniform dispersion. Drink immediately. Rinse glass and
mouth, then swallow the rinse to ensure total dose administered. The 200 mg tablets should be taken intact.

Monitoring Parameters Liver function tests if administered with saquinavir

Additional Information Potential compliance problems,
frequency of administration, and adverse effects should be
discussed with patients before initiating therapy to help
prevent the emergence of resistance.

Dosage Forms Excipient information presented when
available (limited, particularly for generics); consult specific
product labeling.

Tablet, Oral, as mesylate:

Rescriptor: 100 mg, 200 mg

Extemporaneous Preparations A dispersion of delavirdine may be made with tablets. Add four 100 mg tablets to
at least 3 oz of water; allow to stand for a few minutes and
stir until uniform dispersion. Administer immediately. To
ensure full dose is administered, rinse glass and drink
liquid; also rinse mouth and swallow following ingestion.

♦ Delestrogen *see* Estradiol (Systemic) *on page 681*

♦ Delsym Cough + Chest Congestion DM [OTC] *see*
Guaifenesin and Dextromethorphan *on page 861*

♦ Delta-9-tetrahydro-cannabinol *see* Dronabinol
on page 606

♦ Delta-9 THC *see* Dronabinol *on page 606*

♦ Deltacortisone *see* PredniSONE *on page 1496*

♦ Deltadehydrocortisone *see* PredniSONE *on page 1496*

♦ Deltasone *see* PredniSONE *on page 1496*

♦ Delyla *see* Ethinyl Estradiol and Levonorgestrel
on page 703

♦ Delzicol *see* Mesalamine *on page 1151*

♦ Demadex *see* Torsemide *on page 1816*

Demeclocycline (dem e kloe SYE kleen)

Index Terms Declomycin; Demeclocycline Hydrochloride;
Demethylchlortetracycline

Pharmacologic Category Antibiotic, Tetracycline Derivative

Use Treatment of susceptible bacterial infections (eg, acne,
urinary tract infections, respiratory infections) caused by
both gram-negative and gram-positive organisms

Note: Use of demeclocycline as an antibacterial agent is
uncommon; alternative tetracycline agents (eg, doxycycline, minocycline, tetracycline) are generally preferred.

Dosing

Adult & Geriatric

Susceptible infections: Manufacturer's labeling: Oral:
150 mg 4 times/day or 300 mg twice daily

SIADH (off-label use): Oral: 600 to 1,200 mg/day (Goh,
2004; Gross, 2008, Verbalis, 2013). **Note:** Limited high
quality evidence exists to define the clinical role, if any,
of demeclocycline in this condition. European clinical
practice guidelines recommend against the use of
demeclocycline for the management of hyponatremia
in patients with SIADH (Spasovski, 2014).

Pediatric Susceptible infections: Manufacturer's labeling: Oral: Children >8 years: 7-13 mg/kg/day (maximum:
600 mg/day) divided every 6-12 hours

Renal Impairment Use with caution; dosage adjustment
and/or increase in time interval between doses recommended in manufacturer's labeling; no specific adjustment recommendations provided.

Hepatic Impairment Use with caution; dosage adjustment and/or increase in time interval between doses
recommended in manufacturer's labeling; no specific
adjustment recommendations provided.

Additional Information Complete prescribing information
should be consulted for additional detail.

Dosage Forms Excipient information presented when
available (limited, particularly for generics); consult specific
product labeling.

Tablet, Oral, as hydrochloride:

Generic: 150 mg, 300 mg

♦ Demeclocycline Hydrochloride *see* Demeclocycline
on page 515

♦ Demerol *see* Meperidine *on page 1144*

♦ 4-Demethoxydaunorubicin *see* IDArubicin *on page 910*

♦ Demethylchlortetracycline *see* Demeclocycline
on page 515

♦ Demser *see* Metyrosine *on page 1200*

♦ Demulen *see* Ethinyl Estradiol and Ethynodiol Diacetate
on page 702

♦ Demulen 30 (Can) *see* Ethinyl Estradiol and Ethynodiol
Diacetate *on page 702*

♦ Denavir *see* Penciclovir *on page 1418*

Denosumab (den OH sue mab)

Brand Names: US Prolia; Xgeva

Brand Names: Canada Prolia; Xgeva

Index Terms AMG-162

Pharmacologic Category Bone-Modifying Agent; Monoclonal Antibody

Use

Hypercalcemia of malignancy (Xgeva): Treatment of
hypercalcemia of malignancy refractory to bisphosphonate therapy

Osteoporosis/bone loss (Prolia): Treatment of osteoporosis in postmenopausal women at high risk of fracture;
treatment of osteoporosis (to increase bone mass) in
men at high risk of fracture; treatment of bone loss in
men receiving androgen-deprivation therapy (ADT) for
nonmetastatic prostate cancer; treatment of bone loss
in women receiving aromatase inhibitor (AI) therapy for
breast cancer

Tumors (Xgeva): Prevention of skeletal-related events
(eg, fracture, spinal cord compression, bone pain requiring surgery/radiation therapy) in patients with bone metastases from solid tumors; treatment of giant cell tumor of
the bone in adults and skeletally mature adolescents that
is unresectable or where surgical resection is likely to
result in severe morbidity

Limitation of use: Denosumab is NOT indicated for prevention of skeletal-related events in patients with multiple
myeloma

Pregnancy Considerations Use of Prolia is contraindicated in pregnant women. Adverse events were observed
in animal reproduction studies. Specifically, increased fetal
loss, stillbirths, postnatal mortality, absent lymph nodes,
abnormal bone growth, and decreased neonatal growth
was observed in cynomolgus monkeys exposed to denosumab throughout pregnancy. Denosumab was measurable in the offspring at one month of age. Fetal exposure to
monoclonal antibodies is expected to increase as pregnancy progresses. Women of reproductive potential
should be advised to use effective contraception during
denosumab treatment and for at least 5 months following
the last dose. Studies of denosumab when used for
osteoporosis/bone loss in men demonstrated that it is
unlikely that a female partner or fetus would be exposed
during unprotected sex to pharmacologically relevant
denosumab concentrations via seminal fluid; however,
exposure from seminal fluid of men receiving denosumab

for other indications and higher doses is unknown and therefore their pregnant partners should be counseled regarding this potential risk.

Women exposed to denosumab during pregnancy should contact the Amgen Pregnancy Surveillance Program (800-772-6436).

Breast-Feeding Considerations It is not known if denosumab is excreted in breast milk. According to the manufacturer, the decision to discontinue denosumab or discontinue breast-feeding should take into account the benefits of treatment to the mother. In some animal studies, mammary gland development was impaired following exposure to denosumab during pregnancy, resulting in impaired lactation postpartum.

Medication Guide Available Yes

Contraindications Hypersensitivity to denosumab or any component of the formulation; preexisting hypocalcemia; pregnancy (Prolia only)

Warnings/Precautions Clinically significant hypersensitivity (including anaphylaxis) has been reported. May include throat tightness, facial edema, upper airway edema, lip swelling, dyspnea, pruritus, rash, urticaria, and hypotension. If anaphylaxis or clinically significant hypersensitivity occurs, initiate appropriate management and permanently discontinue. Denosumab may cause or exacerbate hypocalcemia; severe symptomatic cases (including fatalities) have been reported. An increased risk has been observed with increasing renal dysfunction, most commonly severe dysfunction (creatinine clearance <30 mL/minute and/or on dialysis), and with inadequate/no calcium supplementation. Monitor calcium levels; correct preexisting hypocalcemia prior to therapy. Monitor levels more frequently when denosumab is administered with other drugs that can also lower calcium levels. Use caution in patients with a history of hypoparathyroidism, thyroid surgery, parathyroid surgery, malabsorption syndromes, excision of small intestine, severe renal impairment/dialysis, or other conditions which would predispose the patient to hypocalcemia; monitor calcium, phosphorus, and magnesium closely during therapy (the manufacturer recommends monitoring within 14 days of injection [Prolia] or during the first weeks of therapy initiation [Xgeva]). Hypocalcemia lasting weeks to months (and requiring frequent monitoring) has been reported in postmarketing analyses. Administer calcium, vitamin D, and magnesium as necessary. Patients with severe renal impairment (CrCl <30 mL/minute) or those on dialysis may also develop marked elevations of serum parathyroid hormone (PTH). Incidence of infections may be increased, including serious skin infections, abdominal, urinary, ear, or periodontal infections. Endocarditis has also been reported following use. Patients should be advised to contact their healthcare provider if signs or symptoms of severe infection or cellulitis develop. Use with caution in patients with impaired immune systems or using concomitant immunosuppressive therapy; may be at increased risk for serious infections. Evaluate the need for continued treatment with serious infection.

Atypical femur fractures have been reported in patients receiving denosumab. The fractures may occur anywhere along the femoral shaft (may be bilateral) and commonly occur with minimal to no trauma to the area. Some patients experience prodromal pain weeks or months before the fracture occurs. Because these fractures also occur in osteoporosis patients not treated with denosumab, it is unclear if denosumab therapy is the cause for the fractures; concomitant glucocorticoids may contribute to fracture risk. Advise patients to report new/unusual hip, thigh, or groin pain; and if so, evaluate for atypical/incomplete fracture. Contralateral limb should be assessed if atypical fracture occurs. Consider interrupting therapy in patients who develop an atypical femoral fracture. Osteonecrosis of the jaw (ONJ) has been reported in patients receiving denosumab. ONJ may manifest as jaw pain, osteomyelitis, osteitis, bone erosion, tooth/periodontal infection, toothache, gingival ulceration/erosion. Risk factors include invasive dental procedures (eg, tooth extraction, dental implants, boney surgery); a diagnosis of cancer, concomitant chemotherapy, corticosteroids, immunosuppressive therapy, or angiogenesis inhibitors, poor oral hygiene, ill-fitting dentures; and comorbid disorders (anemia, coagulopathy, diabetes, infection, gingival infections, and other preexisting dental disease). Concomitant use with other medications associated with this condition may increase the risk of developing ONJ. In studies of patients with osseous metastasis, a longer duration of denosumab exposure was associated with a higher incidence of ONJ. Patients should maintain good oral hygiene during treatment. A dental exam and preventive dentistry is recommended prior to therapy initiation. The risk:benefit

must be assessed by the treating physician and/or dentist/surgeon prior to any invasive dental procedure; avoid invasive procedures in patients with bone metastases receiving therapy for prevention of skeletal-related events. Patients developing ONJ while on denosumab therapy should receive care by a dentist or oral surgeon; extensive dental surgery to treat ONJ may exacerbate ONJ; evaluate individually and consider interrupting or discontinuing therapy if extensive dental surgery is necessary. Severe and occasionally incapacitating bone, joint, and/or muscle pain has been reported (time to onset of symptoms has varied from one day to several months after initiating therapy). Consider discontinuing use if severe symptoms develop.

Postmenopausal osteoporosis: For use in women at high risk for fracture which is defined as a history of osteoporotic fracture or multiple risk factors for fracture. May also be used in women who failed or did not tolerate other therapies.

Bone metastases: Denosumab is not indicated for the prevention of skeletal-related events in patients with multiple myeloma. In trials of with multiple myeloma patients, denosumab was noninferior to zoledronic acid in delaying time to first skeletal-related event and mortality was increased in a subset of the denosumab-treated group.

Breast cancer: The American Society of Clinical Oncology (ASCO) updated guidelines on the role of bone-modifying agents (BMAs) in the prevention and treatment of skeletal-related events for metastatic breast cancer patients (Van Poznak 2011). The guidelines recommend initiating a BMA (denosumab, pamidronate, zoledronic acid) in patients with metastatic breast cancer to the bone. There is currently no literature indicating the superiority of one particular BMA. Optimal duration is not defined; however, the guidelines recommend continuing therapy until substantial decline in patient's performance status. The ASCO guidelines are in alignment with package insert guidelines for dosing, renal dose adjustments, infusion times, prevention and management of osteonecrosis of the jaw, and monitoring of laboratory parameter recommendations. BMAs are not the first-line therapy for pain. BMAs are to be used as adjunctive therapy for cancer-related bone pain associated with bone metastasis, demonstrating a modest pain control benefit. BMAs should be used in conjunction with agents such as NSAIDs, opioid and nonopioid analgesics, corticosteroids, radiation/surgery, and interventional procedures.

Denosumab therapy results in significant suppression of bone turnover; the long term effects of treatment are not known but may contribute to adverse outcomes such as ONJ, atypical fractures, or delayed fracture healing; monitor. Use with caution in patients with renal impairment (CrCl <30 mL/minute) or patients on dialysis; risk of hypocalcemia is increased. Dose adjustment is not needed when administered at 60 mg every 6 months (Prolia); once-monthly dosing has not been evaluated in patients with renal impairment (Xgeva). Dermatitis, eczema, and rash (which are not necessarily specific to the injection site) have been reported; consider discontinuing if severe symptoms occur. Packaging may contain natural latex rubber. May impair bone growth in children with open growth plates or inhibit eruption of dentition. In pediatrics, indicated only for the treatment of giant cell tumor of the bone in adolescents who are skeletally mature. Do not administer Prolia and Xgeva to the same patient for different indications. Denosumab is intended for subcutaneous route only and should not be administered intravenously, intramuscularly, or intradermally.

Adverse Reactions A postmarketing safety program for Prolia is available to collect information on adverse events; more information is available at http://www.proliasafety.com. To report adverse events for either Prolia or Xgeva, prescribers may also call Amgen at 800-772-6436 or FDA at 800-332-1088.

Percentages noted with Prolia (60 mg every 6 months) unless specified as Xgeva (120 mg every 4 weeks):
>10%:
Cardiovascular: Hypertension (11%, Lewiecki 2007)
Central nervous system: Fatigue (Xgeva: ≤45%), headache (Xgeva: 13% to 24%), peripheral edema (5%; Xgeva: 24%)
Dermatologic: Dermatitis (4% to 11%), eczema (4% to 11%), skin rash (3% to 11%)
Endocrine & metabolic: Hypophosphatemia (Xgeva: 32%; grade 3: 10% to 15%), hypocalcemia (2%; Xgeva: 3% to 18%; grade 3: 3%)
Gastrointestinal: Nausea (Xgeva: 31%), decreased appetite (Xgeva: 24%), vomiting (Xgeva: 24%), constipation (Xgeva: 21%), diarrhea (Xgeva: 20%)
Hematologic & oncologic: Anemia (Xgeva: 21%)
Infection: Influenza (11%, Lewiecki 2007)

Neuromuscular & skeletal: Weakness (Xgeva: ≤45%), arthralgia (7% to 14%), limb pain (10% to 12%), back pain (8% to 12%)

Respiratory: Dyspnea (Xgeva: 21% to 27%), cough (Xgeva: 15%)

1% to 10%:

Cardiovascular: Angina pectoris (3%)

Central nervous system: Sciatica (5%)

Endocrine & metabolic: Hypercholesterolemia (7%)

Gastrointestinal: Flatulence (2%)

Hematologic & oncologic: Malignant neoplasm (new; 3% to 5%)

Infection: Serious infection (4%)

Neuromuscular & skeletal: Musculoskeletal pain (6%), ostealgia (4%), myalgia (3%), osteonecrosis (jaw; ≤2%; Xgeva ≤2%)

Ophthalmic: Cataract (≤5%)

Respiratory: Nasopharyngitis (7%), upper respiratory tract infection (5%)

<1% (Limited to important or life-threatening): Antibody development (both formulations), endocarditis, femur fracture (both formulations; diaphyseal, subtrochanteric), hypersensitivity (both formulations), hypotension, pancreatitis

Drug Interactions

Metabolism/Transport Effects None known.

Avoid Concomitant Use

Avoid concomitant use of Denosumab with any of the following: Belimumab

Increased Effect/Toxicity

Denosumab may increase the levels/effects of: Belimumab; Immunosuppressants

Decreased Effect There are no known significant interactions involving a decrease in effect.

Storage/Stability Store in original carton under refrigeration at 2°C to 8°C (36°F to 46°F). Do not freeze. Prior to use, bring to room temperature of 25°C (77°F) in original container (usually takes 15 to 30 minutes); do not use any other methods for warming. Use within 14 days once at room temperature. Protect from direct heat and light; do not expose to temperatures >25°C (77°F). Avoid vigorous shaking.

Mechanism of Action Denosumab is a monoclonal antibody with affinity for nuclear factor-kappa ligand (RANKL). Osteoblasts secrete RANKL; RANKL activates osteoclast precursors and subsequent osteolysis which promotes release of bone-derived growth factors, such as insulin-like growth factor-1 (IGF1) and transforming growth factor-beta (TGF-beta), and increases serum calcium levels. Denosumab binds to RANKL, blocks the interaction between RANKL and RANK (a receptor located on osteoclast surfaces), and prevents osteoclast formation, leading to decreased bone resorption and increased bone mass in osteoporosis. In solid tumors with bony metastases, RANKL inhibition decreases osteoclastic activity leading to decreased skeletal related events and tumor-induced bone destruction. In giant cell tumors of the bone (which express RANK and RANKL), denosumab inhibits tumor growth by preventing RANKL from activating its receptor (RANK) on the osteoclast surface, osteoclast precursors, and osteoclast-like giant cells.

Pharmacodynamics/Kinetics

Onset of action: Decreases markers of bone resorption by ~85% within 3 days; maximal reductions observed within 1 month

Hypercalcemia of malignancy: Time to response (median): 9 days; Time to complete response (median): 23 days (Hu 2014)

Duration: Markers of bone resorption return to baseline within 12 months of discontinuing therapy

Hypercalcemia of malignancy: Duration of response (median): 104 days; Duration of complete response (median): 34 days (Hu 2014)

Bioavailability: SubQ: 62%

Half-life elimination: ~25 to 28 days

Time to peak, serum: 10 days (range: 3 to 21 days)

Dosing

Adult & Geriatric Note: Administer calcium and vitamin D as necessary to prevent or treat hypocalcemia

Hypercalcemia of malignancy (Xgeva): SubQ: 120 mg every 4 weeks; during the first month, give an additional 120 mg on days 8 and 15 (Hu 2014)

Prevention of skeletal-related events in bone metastases from solid tumors (Xgeva): SubQ: 120 mg every 4 weeks (Fizazi 2011; Henry 2011; Stopeck 2010)

Treatment of androgen deprivation-induced bone loss in men with prostate cancer (Prolia): SubQ: 60 mg as a single dose, once every 6 months (Smith 2009)

Treatment of aromatase inhibitor-induced bone loss in women with breast cancer (Prolia): SubQ: 60 mg as a single dose, once every 6 months (Ellis 2008)

Treatment of giant cell tumor of the bone (Xgeva): SubQ: 120 mg once every 4 weeks; during the first month, give an additional 120 mg on days 8 and 15 (Blay 2011; Thomas 2010)

Treatment of osteoporosis in men or postmenopausal women (Prolia): SubQ: 60 mg as a single dose, once every 6 months

Pediatric Note: Administer calcium and vitamin D as necessary to prevent or treat hypocalcemia

Treatment of giant cell tumor of the bone (Xgeva): Adolescents (skeletally mature) 13 to 17 years: SubQ: 120 mg once every 4 weeks; during the first month, give an additional 120 mg on days 8 and 15

Renal Impairment Monitor patients with severe impairment (CrCl <30 mL/minute or on dialysis) due to increased risk of hypocalcemia.

Prolia: No dosage adjustment is necessary.

Xgeva:

US labeling: There are no dosage adjustments provided in the manufacturer's labeling. However, in studies of patients with varying degrees of renal impairment, the degree of renal impairment had no effect on denosumab pharmacokinetics or pharmacodynamics.

Canadian labeling: No dosage adjustment is necessary.

Hepatic Impairment There are no dosage adjustments provided in the manufacturer's labeling (has not been studied).

Dietary Considerations Ensure adequate calcium and vitamin D intake to prevent or treat hypocalcemia. Calcium 1000 mg/day and vitamin D ≥400 units/day is recommended in product labeling (Prolia). If dietary intake is inadequate, dietary supplementation is recommended. Women and men should consume:

Calcium: 1000 mg/day (men: 50 to 70 years) **or** 1200 mg/day (women ≥51 years and men ≥71 years) (IOM 2011; NOF 2014)

Vitamin D: 800 to 1000 units/day (men and women ≥50 years) (NOF 2014). Recommended Dietary Allowance (RDA): 600 units/day (men and women ≤70 years) **or** 800 units/day (men and women ≥71 years) (IOM 2011).

Administration SubQ: Denosumab is intended for subcutaneous route only and should not be administered intravenously, intramuscularly, or intradermally. Prior to administration, bring to room temperature in original container (allow to stand ~15 to 30 minutes); do not warm by any other method. Solution may contain trace amounts of translucent to white protein particles; do not use if cloudy, discolored (normal solution should be clear and colorless to pale yellow), or contains excessive particles or foreign matter. Avoid vigorous shaking. Administer via SubQ injection in the upper arm, upper thigh, or abdomen.

Prolia: If a dose is missed, administer as soon as possible, then continue dosing every 6 months from the date of the last injection.

Monitoring Parameters Recommend monitoring of serum creatinine, serum calcium, phosphorus and magnesium (especially within the first 14 days of therapy [Prolia] or during the first weeks of therapy initiation [Xgeva]), signs and symptoms of hypocalcemia, especially in patients predisposed to hypocalcemia (severe renal impairment, thyroid/parathyroid surgery, malabsorption syndromes, hypoparathyroidism); infection, or dermatologic reactions; routine oral exam (prior to treatment); dental exam if risk factors for ONJ; monitor for sings/symptoms of hypersensitivity

Osteoporosis: Bone mineral density (BMD) should be re-evaluated every 2 years (or more frequently) after initiating therapy (NOF 2014); annual measurements of height and weight, assessment of chronic back pain; serum calcium and 25(OH)D; may consider monitoring biochemical markers of bone turnover

Reference Range

Calcium (total): Adults: 9.0 to 11.0 mg/dL (2.05 to 2.54 mmol/L), may slightly decrease with aging

Phosphorus: 2.5 to 4.5 mg/dL (0.81 to 1.45 mmol/L)

Vitamin D: There is no clear consensus on a reference range for total serum 25(OH)D concentrations or the validity of this level as it relates clinically to bone health. In addition, there is significant variability in the reporting of serum 25(OH)D levels as a result of different assay types in use; however, the following ranges have been suggested:

Adults (IOM 2011): Sufficient levels in practically all persons: ≥20 ng/mL (50 nmol/L); concern for risk of toxicity: >50 ng/mL (125 nmol/L)

Osteoporosis patients (NOF 2014): Recommended level to reach and maintain: ~30 ng/mL (75 nmol/L)

Dosage Forms Excipient information presented when available (limited, particularly for generics); consult specific product labeling.

Solution, Subcutaneous [preservative free]:

Prolia: 60 mg/mL (1 mL) [contains mouse protein (murine) (hamster)]

Xgeva: 120 mg/1.7 mL (1.7 mL)

Deoxycholic Acid (dee ox i KOE lik AS id)

Index Terms ATX-101; Kybella
Pharmacologic Category Lipolytic
Use

Submental convexity/fullness: Improvement in the appearance of moderate to severe convexity or fullness associated with submental fat in adults.

Limitations of use: The safe and effective use for the treatment of subcutaneous fat outside the submental region has not been established and is not recommended.

Pregnancy Considerations Adverse events have been observed in some animal reproduction studies. Pregnant women and women of reproductive potential not using effective contraception were excluded from initial studies (McDiarmid, 2014; Rzany, 2014).

Breast-Feeding Considerations It is not known if deoxycholic acid from this preparation is excreted in breast milk. According to the manufacturer, the decision to breast-feed during therapy should consider the benefits of breast-feeding, the risk of exposure to the infant, and the benefits of treatment to the mother. Breast-feeding women were excluded from initial studies (McDiarmid 2014; Rzany 2014).

Contraindications Presence of infection at the injection sites

Warnings/Precautions Marginal mandibular nerve injury (eg, asymmetric smile or facial muscle paresis) has been reported. All injuries resolved spontaneously (median 44 days; range 1 to 298 days). Do not inject into or in close proximity to the marginal mandibular branch of the facial nerve. To avoid injury to the marginal mandibular nerve, do not inject above the inferior border of the mandible; do not inject within a region defined by a 1 to 1.5 cm line below the inferior border (from the angle of the mandible to the mentum); and only inject within the target submental fat treatment area. Dysphagia has occurred in the setting of administration site reactions (eg, pain, swelling, and submental area induration). All occurrences resolved spontaneously (median 34 days; range 1 to 81 days). Also avoid use in patients with current or prior history of dysphagia; condition may be exacerbated. Injection site hematoma or bruising has been reported. Use with caution in patients with bleeding abnormalities or who are currently taking antiplatelet or anticoagulant therapy. Excessive bleeding or bruising in treatment area may occur. Screen patients for other causes of submental convexity/fullness (eg, thyromegaly, cervical adenopathy). Use caution in patients with prior submental surgical or aesthetic treatments; changes in anatomy or landmarks, presence of scar tissue may impact safe administration or aesthetic result. Carefully consider use in patients with excessive skin laxity or prominent platysmal bands or other conditions for which reduction of submental fat may be aesthetically undesirable. For subcutaneous use only. Do not inject into or in close proximity (1 to 1.5 cm) of salivary glands, lymph nodes, or muscles.

Adverse Reactions Frequency not always defined.

Cardiovascular: Hypertension (3%), presyncope, syncope

Central nervous system: Paresthesia (14%), headache (8%), nerve damage (4%, marginal mandibular)

Dermatologic: Injection site pruritus (12%), skin tightness (5% injection site), skin discoloration at injection site, urticaria at injection site

Gastrointestinal: Dysphagia (2%), nausea (2%)

Hematologic & oncologic: Lymphadenopathy

Local: Injection site reaction (96%), swelling at injection site (20% to 87%), bruising at injection site (72%), hematoma at injection site (72%), pain at injection site (16% to 70%), injection site numbness (42% to 66%), erythema at injection site (27%), induration at injection site (23%), injection site nodule (13%), warm sensation at injection site (4%), bleeding at injection site

Neuromuscular & skeletal: Neck pain

Respiratory: Oropharyngeal pain (3%)

Drug Interactions

Metabolism/Transport Effects None known.

Avoid Concomitant Use There are no known interactions where it is recommended to avoid concomitant use.

Increased Effect/Toxicity

The levels/effects of Deoxycholic Acid may be increased by: Agents with Antiplatelet Properties; Anticoagulants

Decreased Effect There are no known significant interactions involving a decrease in effect.

Preparation for Administration Do not dilute.

Storage/Stability Store intact vials at 20°C to 25°C (68°F to 77°F); excursions are permitted between 15°C and 30°C (59°F and 86°F).

Mechanism of Action Deoxycholic acid is a cytolytic drug that physically destroys the cell membrane causing lysis when injected into tissue.

Pharmacodynamics/Kinetics

Duration: Post treatment deoxycholic plasma levels return to endogenous range within 24 hours

Absorption: Rapid after subcutaneous injection

Protein binding: 98%

Metabolism: Not metabolized to any significant extent

Time to peak: 18 minutes

Excretion: Feces (as intact drug)

Dosing

Adult Submental convexity/fullness: SubQ: Inject into submental subcutaneous fat tissue at an area-adjusted dose of 2 mg/cm^2 (maximum per treatment: 50 injections spaced 1 cm apart [0.2 mL each; total 10 mL]). Maximum number of treatments: 6 treatments spaced at ≥1-month intervals.

Renal Impairment There are no dosage adjustments provided in the manufacturer's labeling.

Hepatic Impairment There are no dosage adjustments provided in the manufacturer's labeling (has not been studied); however, doses administered are ~3% of total body acid pool and are unlikely to be affected by hepatic impairment.

Administration Subcutaneous: Prior to each treatment, palpate the submental area to ensure sufficient submental fat in the target treatment area. Outline the planned treatment area with a surgical pen and apply a 1 cm injection grid to mark the injection sites; do not inject outside the defined parameters. Using a large bore needle, draw 1 mL into a sterile 1 mL syringe. Have the patient tense the platysma. Pinch the submental fat and, using a 30 gauge (or smaller) 0.5 inch needle, inject 0.2 mL into the pre-platysmal fat next to each of the marked injection sites by advancing the needle perpendicular to the skin. Inject into fat tissue at the depth of approximately mid-way into the subcutaneous fat layer; avoid injection into the postplatysmal fat. Upon needle withdrawal, pressure may be applied to each injection site as necessary to minimize bleeding; an adhesive dressing may be applied. Ice/cold packs, topical and/or injectable local anesthesia (eg, lidocaine) may be used. Discard any remaining solution after use.

Monitoring Parameters Monitor postinjection for submental area induration, pain or swelling or marginal mandibular nerve injury.

Desipramine (des IP ra meen)

Brand Names: US Norpramin
Brand Names: Canada Dom-Desipramine; Novo-Desipramine; Nu-Desipramine; PMS-Desipramine
Index Terms Desipramine Hydrochloride; Desmethylimipramine Hydrochloride
Pharmacologic Category Antidepressant, Tricyclic (Secondary Amine)
Use Depression: Treatment of depression
Medication Guide Available Yes
Dosing
  Adult
  Depression: Oral: Initial dose: 25 to 50 mg once daily or in divided doses (APA, 2010; WFSBP 2013); increase based on tolerance and response; usual maintenance dose: 100 to 200 mg once daily or in divided doses; doses up to 300 mg daily may be necessary in severely depressed patients (maximum: 300 mg daily)
  Neuropathic pain (off-label use): Oral: Initial: 25 mg at bedtime; increase dose in increments of 25 mg daily every 3 to 7 days as necessary until the desired effect is obtained; maximum dose: 150 mg daily (Dworkin, 2007; Max, 1992).

  Discontinuation of therapy: Upon discontinuation of antidepressant therapy, gradually taper the dose to minimize the incidence of withdrawal symptoms and allow for the detection of re-emerging symptoms. Evidence supporting ideal taper rates is limited. APA and NICE guidelines suggest tapering therapy over at least several weeks with consideration to the half-life of the antidepressant; antidepressants with a shorter half-life may need to be tapered more conservatively. In addition for long-term treated patients, WFSBP guidelines recommend tapering over 4-6 months. If intolerable withdrawal symptoms occur following a dose reduction, consider resuming the previously prescribed dose and/or decrease dose at a more gradual rate (APA, 2010; Bauer, 2002; Haddad, 2001; NCCMH, 2010; Schatzberg, 2006; Shelton, 2001; Warner 2006).

MAO inhibitor recommendations:
Switching to or from an MAO inhibitor intended to treat psychiatric disorders:
  Allow 14 days to elapse between discontinuing an MAO inhibitor intended to treat psychiatric disorders and initiation of desipramine.
  Allow 14 days to elapse between discontinuing desipramine and initiation of an MAO inhibitor intended to treat psychiatric disorders.
Use with other MAO inhibitors (linezolid or IV methylene blue):
  Do not initiate desipramine in patients receiving linezolid or IV methylene blue; consider other interventions for psychiatric condition.
  If urgent treatment with linezolid or IV methylene blue is required in a patient already receiving desipramine and potential benefits outweigh potential risks, discontinue desipramine promptly and administer linezolid or IV methylene blue. Monitor for serotonin syndrome for 2 weeks or until 24 hours after the last dose of linezolid or IV methylene blue, whichever comes first. May resume desipramine 24 hours after the last dose of linezolid or IV methylene blue.
Geriatric
  Depression: Oral: Initial dose: Start at a lower dosage level and increase based on tolerance and response to a usual maximum of 100 mg daily; usual maintenance dose: 25 to 100 mg mg once daily or in divided doses; doses up to 150 mg daily may be necessary in severely depressed patients (maximum: 150 mg daily)

  Discontinuation of therapy: Refer to adult dosing.
  MAO inhibitor recommendations: Refer to adult dosing.
Pediatric
  Depression: Note: Not FDA approved for use in pediatric patients; controlled clinical trials have not shown tricyclic antidepressants to be superior to placebo for the treatment of depression in children and adolescents (Dopheide, 2006; Wagner, 2005).
  Children 6 to 12 years (off-label use): Oral: 1 to 3 mg/kg/day in divided doses; monitor carefully with doses >3 mg/kg/day; maximum dose: 5 mg/kg/day (Kliegman, 2007).
  Adolescents: Oral: Initial dose: Start at a lower dosage level and increase based on tolerance and response to a usual maximum of 100 mg daily; usual maintenance dose: 25 to 100 mg once daily or in divided doses; doses up to 150 mg daily may be necessary in severely depressed patients (maximum: 150 mg daily)

  Discontinuation of therapy: Refer to adult dosing.
  MAO inhibitor recommendations: Refer to adult dosing.
  Renal Impairment There are no dosage adjustments provided in the manufacturer's labeling; use with caution.
  Hepatic Impairment There are no dosage adjustments provided in the manufacturer's labeling.
  Additional Information Complete prescribing information should be consulted for additional detail.
  Dosage Forms Excipient information presented when available (limited, particularly for generics); consult specific product labeling.
  Tablet, Oral, as hydrochloride:
  Norpramin: 10 mg, 25 mg, 50 mg, 75 mg, 100 mg, 150 mg
  Generic: 10 mg, 25 mg, 50 mg, 75 mg, 100 mg, 150 mg

Desirudin (des i ROO din)

Brand Names: US Iprivask
Index Terms CGP-39393; Desulfato-Hirudin; Desulfatohirudin; Desulphatohirudin; r-Hirudin; Recombinant Desulfatohirudin; Recombinant Hirudin
Pharmacologic Category Anticoagulant; Anticoagulant, Direct Thrombin Inhibitor
Use Deep vein thrombosis, prophylaxis: Prophylaxis of deep vein thrombosis (DVT) in patients undergoing hip-replacement surgery
Dosing
  Adult & Geriatric Note: Initial dose may be given up to 5 to 15 minutes prior to surgery (after induction of regional anesthesia, if used); has been administered for up to 12 days (average: 9 to 12 days) in clinical trials

  DVT prophylaxis: SubQ: 15 mg every 12 hours; interrupt therapy if aPTT exceeds 2 times control; resume at a reduced dose (based on the degree of aPTT abnormality) when aPTT is <2 times control

Renal Impairment

Moderate impairment (CrCl ≥31 to 60 mL/minute/1.73 m²): Initial dose: 5 mg every 12 hours. Interrupt therapy if aPTT exceeds 2 times control; resume at a reduced dose (based on the degree of aPTT abnormality) when aPTT is <2 times control.

Severe impairment (CrCl <31 mL/minute/1.73 m²): Initial dose: 1.7 mg every 12 hours. Interrupt therapy if aPTT exceeds 2 times control; resume at a reduced dose (based on the degree of aPTT abnormality) when aPTT is <2 times control.

Hepatic Impairment There are no dosage adjustments provided in the manufacturer's labeling (has not been studied); use with caution.

Additional Information Complete prescribing information should be consulted for additional detail.

Dosage Forms Excipient information presented when available (limited, particularly for generics); consult specific product labeling.

Solution Reconstituted, Subcutaneous:

Iprivask: 15 mg (1 ea)

◆ **Desitin Maximum Strength Original [OTC]** see Zinc Oxide on page 1929

◆ **Desitin Rapid Relief [OTC]** see Zinc Oxide on page 1929

Desloratadine (des lor AT a deen)

Brand Names: US Clarinex; Clarinex Reditabs

Brand Names: Canada Aerius; Aerius Kids; Desloratadine Allergy Control

Pharmacologic Category Histamine H₁ Antagonist; Histamine H₁ Antagonist, Second Generation; Piperidine Derivative

Use Relief of nasal and non-nasal symptoms of seasonal allergic rhinitis (SAR) and perennial allergic rhinitis (PAR); treatment of chronic idiopathic urticaria (CIU)

Dosing

Adult & Geriatric

Chronic idiopathic urticaria: Oral: 5 mg once daily. In one clinical trial, the titrated use of higher doses (up to 10 mg twice daily) in adults demonstrated clinical improvement (Staevska, 2010).

Seasonal or perennial allergic rhinitis: Oral: 5 mg once daily

Pediatric

Perennial allergic rhinitis, chronic idiopathic urticaria: Oral:

Children:

6 to 11 months: 1 mg once daily

12 months to 5 years: 1.25 mg once daily

6 to 11 years: 2.5 mg once daily

Children ≥12 years and Adolescents: Refer to adult dosing.

Seasonal allergic rhinitis: Oral:

Children:

2 to 5 years: 1.25 mg once daily

6 to 11 years: 2.5 mg once daily

Children ≥12 years and Adolescents: Refer to adult dosing.

Renal Impairment

Adults: Mild to severe impairment: 5 mg every other day.

Children: There are no dosage adjustments provided in manufacturer's labeling (has not been studied).

Hepatic Impairment

Adults: Mild to severe impairment: 5 mg every other day.

Children: There are no dosage adjustments provided in manufacturer's labeling (has not been studied).

Additional Information Complete prescribing information should be consulted for additional detail.

Dosage Forms Excipient information presented when available (limited, particularly for generics); consult specific product labeling.

Syrup, Oral:

Clarinex: 0.5 mg/mL (473 mL) [contains edetate disodium, fd&c yellow #6 (sunset yellow), propylene glycol, sodium benzoate; bubble-gum flavor]

Tablet, Oral:

Clarinex: 5 mg [contains fd&c blue #2 aluminum lake]

Generic: 5 mg

Tablet Dispersible, Oral:

Clarinex Reditabs: 2.5 mg, 5 mg [contains aspartame; tutti-frutti flavor]

Generic: 2.5 mg, 5 mg

◆ **Desloratadine Allergy Control (Can)** see Desloratadine on page 520

Desloratadine and Pseudoephedrine (des lor AT a deen & soo doe e FED rin)

Brand Names: US Clarinex-D 12 Hour; Clarinex-D 24 Hour [DSC]

Index Terms Pseudoephedrine and Desloratadine

Pharmacologic Category Alpha/Beta Agonist; Decongestant; Histamine H₁ Antagonist; Histamine H₁ Antagonist, Second Generation; Piperidine Derivative

Use Seasonal allergic rhinitis: Relief of nasal and non-nasal symptoms of seasonal allergic rhinitis, including nasal congestion, in adults and adolescents 12 years and older

Dosing

Adult & Geriatric Note: Clarinex-D 24 Hour has been discontinued in the US for more than 1 year.

Seasonal or allergic rhinitis: Oral:

Clarinex-D 12 Hour: Desloratadine 2.5 mg/pseudoephedrine 120 mg every 12 hours; Maximum: Desloratadine 5 mg/pseudoephedrine 240 mg daily

Clarinex-D 24 Hour: Desloratadine 5 mg/pseudoephedrine 240 mg once daily; Maximum: Desloratadine 5 mg/pseudoephedrine 240 mg once daily

Pediatric Note: Clarinex-D 24 Hour has been discontinued in the US for more than 1 year.

Seasonal or allergic rhinitis: Oral: Adolescents ≥12 years: Refer to adult dosing.

Renal Impairment Use is not recommended.

Hepatic Impairment Use is not recommended.

Additional Information Complete prescribing information should be consulted for additional detail.

Product Availability Clarinex-D 24 Hour has been discontinued in the US for more than 1 year.

Dosage Forms Excipient information presented when available (limited, particularly for generics); consult specific product labeling. [DSC] = Discontinued product

Tablet Extended Release 12 Hour, Oral:

Clarinex-D 12 Hour: Desloratadine 2.5 mg and pseudoephedrine sulfate 120 mg [contains fd&c blue #2 aluminum lake]

Tablet Extended Release 24 Hour, Oral:

Clarinex-D 24 Hour: Desloratadine 5 mg and pseudoephedrine sulfate 240 mg [DSC] [contains fd&c blue #2 aluminum lake]

◆ **Desmethylimipramine Hydrochloride** see Desipramine on page 519

Desmopressin (des moe PRES in)

Brand Names: US DDAVP; DDAVP Rhinal Tube; Stimate

Brand Names: Canada Apo-Desmopressin; DDAVP; DDAVP Melt; DDAVP Rhinyle; Nocdurna; Octostim; PMS-Desmopressin; Teva-Desmopressin

Index Terms 1-Deamino-8-D-Arginine Vasopressin; Desmopressin Acetate

Pharmacologic Category Antihemophilic Agent; Hemostatic Agent; Hormone, Posterior Pituitary; Vasopressin Analog, Synthetic

Use

Injection:

Diabetes insipidus: Antidiuretic replacement therapy in the management of central (cranial) diabetes insipidus; management of the temporary polyuria and polydipsia following head trauma or surgery in the pituitary region. Limitations of use: Desmopressin is ineffective for the treatment of nephrogenic diabetes insipidus.

Hemophilia A: For use in patients with hemophilia A with factor VIII coagulant activity levels >5% to maintain hemostasis during surgical procedures and postoperatively when administered 30 minutes prior to the scheduled procedure and to also stop bleeding due to spontaneous or trauma-induced injuries, such as hemarthroses, intramuscular hematomas, or mucosal bleeding.

Limitations of use: Not indicated for the treatment of hemophilia A with factor VIII coagulant activity levels ≤5%, for the treatment of hemophilia B, or in patients who have factor VIII antibodies. In certain clinical situations, it may be justified to try desmopressin with careful monitoring in patients with factor VIII levels between 2% and 5%.

Von Willebrand disease (type 1): For use in patients with mild to moderate classic von Willebrand disease (type 1) with factor VIII coagulant activity levels >5% to maintain hemostasis during surgical procedures and postoperatively when administered 30 minutes prior to the scheduled procedure and to stop bleeding due to spontaneous or trauma-induced injuries, such as hemarthroses, intramuscular hematomas, or mucosal bleeding.

Limitations of use: Patients with von Willebrand disease who are least likely to respond are those with severe homozygous von Willebrand disease with factor VIII coagulant activity and factor VIII von Willebrand factor antigen levels <1%; other patients may respond (variable) depending on the type of molecular defect they have. Check bleeding time and factor VIII coagulant activity, ristocetin cofactor activity, and von Willebrand factor antigen during administration of desmopressin to ensure that adequate levels are being achieved. Not indicated for the treatment of severe classic von Willebrand disease (type I) or when there is evidence of an abnormal molecular form of factor VIII antigen.

Intranasal:

Diabetes insipidus (DDAVP Rhinal tube): Antidiuretic replacement therapy in the management of central (cranial) diabetes insipidus; management of the temporary polyuria and polydipsia following head trauma or surgery in the pituitary region.

Limitation of use: Desmopressin is ineffective for the treatment of nephrogenic diabetes insipidus.

Hemophilia A (Stimate): For use in patients with hemophilia A with factor VIII coagulant activity levels >5% and to stop bleeding due to spontaneous or trauma-induced injuries, such as hemarthroses, intramuscular hematomas, or mucosal bleeding.

Limitations of use: Not indicated for the treatment of hemophilia A with factor VIII coagulant activity levels ≤5%, for the treatment of hemophilia B, or in patients who have factor VIII antibodies.

von Willebrand disease (type 1) (Stimate): For use in patients with mild to moderate classic von Willebrand disease (type 1) with factor VIII coagulant activity levels >5% and to stop bleeding due to spontaneous or trauma-induced injuries, such as hemarthroses, intramuscular hematomas, mucosal bleeding, or menorrhagia.

Limitations of use: Not indicated for the treatment of severe classic von Willebrand disease (type 1) or when there is evidence of an abnormal molecular form of factor VIII antigen.

Tablets:

Diabetes insipidus: Antidiuretic replacement therapy in the management of central diabetes insipidus; management of the temporary polyuria and polydipsia following head trauma or surgery in the pituitary region.

Limitation of use: Desmopressin is ineffective for the treatment of nephrogenic diabetes insipidus.

Primary nocturnal enuresis: Management of primary nocturnal enuresis, either alone or as an adjunct to behavioral conditioning or other nonpharmacologic intervention.

Pregnancy Considerations Adverse events were not observed in animal reproduction studies. Anecdotal reports suggest congenital anomalies and low birth weight. However, causal relationship has not been established. Desmopressin has been used safely throughout pregnancy for the treatment of diabetes insipidus (Brewster, 2005; Schrier, 2010). The use of desmopressin is limited for the treatment of von Willebrand disease in pregnant women (NHLBI, 2007).

Breast-Feeding Considerations It is not known if desmopressin is excreted in breast milk. The manufacturer recommends that caution be exercised when administering desmopressin to nursing women.

Contraindications Known hypersensitivity to desmopressin acetate or any component of the formulations; hyponatremia or a history of hyponatremia; moderate-to-severe renal impairment (CrCl <50 mL/minute). There are no contraindications listed in the Stimate prescribing information.

Canadian labeling: Additional contraindications (not in US labeling): Type 2B or platelet-type (pseudo) von Willebrand's disease (injection, intranasal, oral, sublingual); known hyponatremia, habitual or psychogenic polydipsia, cardiac insufficiency or other conditions requiring diuretic therapy (intranasal, sublingual); nephrosis, severe hepatic dysfunction (sublingual); primary nocturnal enuresis (intranasal)

Warnings/Precautions Severe allergic reactions have been reported with desmopressin; anaphylactic reactions have only occurred rarely with IV and intranasal administration. Desmopressin use may rarely lead to hyponatremia with associated signs and symptoms (eg, nausea/vomiting, headache, depressed reflexes, disorientation, irritability, muscle weakness/spasms/cramps) and extreme decreases in plasma osmolality, resulting in seizures, coma, respiratory arrest, and death. Risk factors for hyponatremia with desmopressin use include cystic fibrosis, renal dysfunction, heart failure, young age, advanced age, inappropriate high fluid intake, a higher than recommended dose, and concomitant use of medications known to either increase thirst or cause syndrome of inappropriate ADH secretion (SIADH). Fluid restriction during use is recommended. Monitor for signs/symptoms of hyponatremia Fluid intake should be adjusted downward in the elderly and in very young patients to decrease the possibility of water intoxication and hyponatremia. Use with caution in patients with habitual or psychogenic polydipsia. Patients consuming excessive amounts of water are at greater risk of hyponatremia. Use in these patients is contraindicated in Canadian labeling. Patients should be instructed to restrict fluid intake from 1 hour before to 8 hours after taking desmopressin tablets.

Acute cerebrovascular thrombosis and acute myocardial infarction have occurred (rare) with desmopressin injection; use with caution in patients predisposed to thrombus formation. Patients with type 2B von Willebrand disease requiring hemostasis should not be treated with desmopressin since may result in platelet aggregation, thrombocytopenia, and possibly thrombosis. Injection and intranasal desmopressin may cause a slight increase or transient decrease in blood pressure, and a compensatory increase in heart rate. Use with caution in patients with coronary artery insufficiency and/or hypertensive cardiovascular disease.

When using desmopressin for primary nocturnal enuresis, treatment should be interrupted if the patient experiences an acute illness (eg, fever, recurrent vomiting or diarrhea), vigorous exercise, or any condition associated with an increase in water consumption to prevent hyponatremia.

Consider alternative route of administration if changes in the nasal mucosa due to intranasal use (scarring, edema) occur leading to unreliable absorption. Some patients may demonstrate a change in response after long-term therapy (>6 months) characterized as decreased response or a shorter duration of response. Consider alternative route of administration (IV or intranasal) with inadequate therapeutic response at maximum recommended oral doses.

Adverse Reactions Frequency may not be defined (may be dose or route related).

Cardiovascular: Decreased blood pressure (IV), increased blood pressure (IV), flushing (facial)

Central nervous system: Headache (2% to 5%), dizziness (intranasal; ≤3%), chills (intranasal; 2%), nostril pain (intranasal; ≤2%)

Dermatologic: Skin rash

Endocrine & metabolic: Hyponatremia, water intoxication

Gastrointestinal: Abdominal pain (intranasal; 2%) gastrointestinal disease (intranasal; ≤2%), nausea (intranasal; ≤2%), abdominal cramps, sore throat

Hepatic: Increased serum transaminases (transient; associated primarily with tablets)

Local: Burning sensation at injection site, erythema at injection site, swelling at injection site

Neuromuscular & Skeletal: Weakness (intranasal; ≤2%)

Ophthalmic: Abnormal lacrimation (intranasal; ≤2%), conjunctivitis (intranasal; ≤2%), ocular edema (intranasal; ≤2%)

Respiratory: Rhinitis (intranasal; 3% to 8%), epistaxis (intranasal; ≤3%), cough, nasal congestion, upper respiratory tract infection

<1% (Limited to important or life-threatening): Abnormality in thinking, agitation, anaphylaxis (rare), balanitis, cerebral thrombosis (IV; acute), chest pain, coma, diarrhea, drowsiness, dyspepsia, edema, eye pruritus, hypersensitivity reaction (rare), insomnia, localized warm feeling, myocardial infarction (IV), pain, palpitations, photophobia, seizure, tachycardia, vomiting, vulvar pain

Drug Interactions

Metabolism/Transport Effects None known.

Avoid Concomitant Use

Avoid concomitant use of Desmopressin with any of the following: Tolvaptan

Increased Effect/Toxicity

Desmopressin may increase the levels/effects of: Lithium

The levels/effects of Desmopressin may be increased by: Analgesics (Opioid); CarBAMazepine; ChlorproMAZINE; LamoTRIgine; Nonsteroidal Anti-Inflammatory Agents; Selective Serotonin Reuptake Inhibitors; Tricyclic Antidepressants

Decreased Effect

The levels/effects of Desmopressin may be decreased by: Demeclocycline; Lithium; Tolvaptan

Preparation for Administration

DDAVP injection: Hemophilia A and von Willebrand disease (type 1): Dilute solution for injection in 10 or 50 mL NS for IV infusion (10 mL for children ≤10 kg; 50 mL for adults and children >10 kg).

Stimate nasal spray: Press pump down 4 times to prime prior to initial use.

◄ **Storage/Stability**

DDAVP:

Nasal spray: Store at controlled room temperature of 20°C to 25°C (68°F to 77°F). Keep nasal spray in upright position.

Rhinal Tube solution: Store refrigerated at 2°C to 8°C (36°F to 46°F). May store at controlled room temperature of 20°C to 25°C (68°F to 77°F) for up to 3 weeks.

Solution for injection: Store refrigerated at 2°C to 8°C (36°F to 46°F).

Tablet: Store at controlled room temperature of 20°C to 25°C (68°F to 77°F). Avoid excessive heat. Protect from light.

DDAVP Melt (CAN; not available in US): Store at 15°C to 25°C (59°F to 77°F) in original container. Protect from moisture.

Stimate nasal spray: Store at room temperature not to exceed 25°C (77°F). Discard 6 months after opening bottle. Store bottle in upright position.

Mechanism of Action Synthetic analogue of the antidiuretic hormone arginine vasopressin. In a dose dependent manner, desmopressin increases cyclic adenosine monophosphate (cAMP) in renal tubular cells which increases water permeability resulting in decreased urine volume and increased urine osmolality; increases plasma levels of von Willebrand factor, factor VIII, and t-PA contributing to a shortened activated partial thromboplastin time (aPTT) and bleeding time.

Pharmacodynamics/Kinetics

Onset of action:

Intranasal: Antidiuretic: 15 to 30 minutes; Increased factor VIII and von Willebrand factor (vWF) activity (dose related): 30 minutes

Peak effect: Antidiuretic: 1 hour; Increased factor VIII and vWF activity: 1.5 hours

IV infusion: Increased factor VIII and vWF activity: 30 minutes (dose related)

Peak effect: 1.5 to 2 hours

Oral tablet: Antidiuretic: ~1 hour

Peak effect: 4 to 7 hours

Duration: Intranasal, Injection, Oral tablet: ~6 to 14 hours

Absorption: Sublingual: Rapid

Bioavailability: Intranasal: ~3.5%; Oral tablet: 5% compared to intranasal, 0.16% compared to IV

Half-life elimination: 2 to 4 hours; Renal impairment: 9 hours

Excretion: Urine (primarily)

Dosing

Adult & Geriatric

Diabetes insipidus: Note: Fluid restriction should be observed. Dosing should be individualized to response.

IV, SubQ: U.S. labeling: 2 to 4 mcg daily (0.5 to 1 mL) in 2 divided doses or one-tenth ($^1/_{10}$) of the maintenance intranasal dose. Fluid restriction should be observed.

IM, IV, SubQ: Canadian labeling: 1 to 4 mcg (0.25 to 1 mL) once daily or one-tenth ($^1/_{10}$) of the maintenance intranasal dose. Fluid restriction should be observed.

Intranasal (100 mcg/mL nasal solution): Usual dose range: 10 to 40 mcg daily (0.1 to 0.4 mL) as a single dose or divided 2 to 3 times daily; adjust morning and evening doses separately for an adequate diurnal rhythm of water turnover. Most adults require 10 mcg (0.1 mL) twice daily. **Note:** The nasal spray pump can only deliver doses of 10 mcg (0.1 mL) or multiples of 10 mcg (0.1 mL); if doses other than this are needed, the rhinal tube delivery system is preferred. Fluid restriction should be observed.

Oral:

US labeling: Initial: 0.05 mg twice daily; total daily dose should be increased or decreased as needed to obtain adequate antidiuresis (range: 0.1 to 1.2 mg divided 2 to 3 times daily). Fluid restriction should be observed.

Canadian labeling: Initial: 0.1 mg 3 times daily; total daily dose should be increased or decreased as needed to obtain adequate antidiuresis (range: 0.3 to 1.2 mg divided 3 times daily). Fluid restriction should be observed.

Sublingual formulation [Canadian product]: Initial: 60 mcg 3 times daily; total daily dose should be increased or decreased as needed to obtain adequate antidiuresis. Usual maintenance: 120 to 720 mcg equally divided 2 or 3 times daily. Fluid restriction should be observed.

Nocturnal enuresis: *Oral:* Initial: 0.2 mg at bedtime; dose may be titrated up to 0.6 mg to achieve desired response.

Hemophilia A and von Willebrand disease (type 1):

IV: 0.3 mcg/kg by slow infusion; may repeat dose if needed (based on clinical response and laboratory results); if used preoperatively, administer 30 minutes before procedure

Canadian labeling (not in US labeling): Maximum IV dose: 20 mcg

Intranasal (using high concentration spray [1.5 mg/mL] [eg, Stimate]): <50 kg: 150 mcg (1 spray in a single nostril); ≥50 kg: 300 mcg (1 spray each nostril); repeat use is determined by the patient's clinical condition and laboratory work. If using preoperatively, administer 2 hours before surgery.

Uremic bleeding associated with acute or chronic renal failure (off-label use): IV: 0.4 mcg/kg over 10 minutes (Watson, 1984)

Prevention of surgical bleeding in patients with uremia (off-label use): IV: 0.3 mcg/kg over 30 minutes (Mannucci, 1983)

Pediatric

Diabetes insipidus: Note: Fluid restriction should be observed in these patients; younger patients more susceptible to plasma osmolality shifts and possible hyponatremia. Dosing should be individualized to response.

Parenteral:

US labeling: Children ≥12 years and Adolescents: IV, SubQ: Refer to adult dosing.

Alternative recommendations (off-label): Infants and Children <12 years: IV, SubQ: No definitive dosing available. Adult dosing should **not** be used in this age group; adverse events such as hyponatremia-induced seizures may occur. Dose should be reduced. Some have suggested an initial dosage range of 0.1 to 1 mcg daily in 1 or 2 divided doses (Cheetham, 2002). Initiate at low dose and increase as necessary. Closely monitor serum sodium levels and urine output; fluid restriction is recommended.

Canadian labeling: IM, IV, SubQ: Children and Adolescents: 0.4 mcg (0.1 mL) once daily or one-tenth ($^1/_{10}$) of the maintenance intranasal dose. Fluid restriction should be observed.

Intranasal (using 100 mcg/mL nasal solution [eg, DDAVP]):

Infants ≥3 months and Children ≤12 years: Usual dose range: 5 to 30 mcg daily (0.05 to 0.3 mL daily) as a single dose or divided 2 times daily; adjust morning and evening doses separately for an adequate diurnal rhythm of water turnover. **Note:** The nasal spray pump can only deliver doses of 10 mcg (0.1 mL) or multiples of 10 mcg (0.1 mL); if doses other than this are needed, the rhinal tube delivery system is preferred. Fluid restriction should be observed.

Adolescents: Refer to adult dosing.

Oral:

US labeling: Children ≥4 years and Adolescents: Refer to adult dosing.

Canadian labeling:

Children: Initial: 0.1 mg 3 times daily; total daily dose should be increased or decreased as needed to obtain adequate antidiuresis (range: 0.3 to 1.2 mg divided 3 times daily). Divide daily doses so that the evening dose is 2 times higher than the morning or afternoon dose to ensure adequate antidiuresis during the night. Fluid restriction should be observed.

Adolescents: Refer to adult dosing.

Sublingual formulation [Canadian product]:

Children: Initial: 60 mcg 3 times daily; total daily dose should be increased or decreased as needed to obtain adequate antidiuresis. Usual maintenance: 120 to 720 mcg equally divided 2 to 3 times daily; divide daily doses so that the evening dose is 2 times higher than the morning or afternoon dose to ensure adequate antidiuresis during the night. Fluid restriction should be observed.

Adolescents: Refer to adult dosing.

Hemophilia A and von Willebrand disease (type 1):

IV: Infants ≥3 months, Children, and Adolescents: Refer to adult dosing.

Note: Adverse events such as hyponatremia-induced seizures have been reported especially in young children using this dosing regimen (Das, 2005; Molnar, 2005; Smith, 1989; Thumfart, 2005; Weinstein, 1989). Fluid restriction and careful monitoring of serum sodium levels and urine output are necessary.

Intranasal (using high concentration spray [1.5 mg/mL] [eg, Stimate]): Infants ≥11 months, Children, and Adolescents: Refer to adult dosing.

Nocturnal enuresis:
Oral:
Children ≥6 years and Adolescents (US labeling) or Children ≥5 years and Adolescents (Canadian labeling): Initial: 0.2 mg at bedtime. Dose may be titrated up to 0.6 mg to achieve desired response. Fluid intake should be limited 1 hour prior to dose until the next morning, or at least 8 hours after administration.

Sublingual [Canadian product]: Children ≥5 years and Adolescents: Initial: 120 mcg administered 1 hour before bedtime; dose may be titrated up to a maximum of 360 mcg to achieve desired response. Fluid intake should be limited 1 hour prior to dose until the next morning, or at least 8 hours after administration.

Renal Impairment CrCl <50 mL/minute: Use is contraindicated according to the manufacturers (except 1.5 mg/mL nasal spray); however, has been used in acute and chronic renal failure patients experiencing uremic bleeding or for prevention of surgical bleeding (off-label uses) (Mannucci, 1983; Watson, 1984).

Hepatic Impairment There are no dosage adjustments provided in the manufacturer's labeling.

Administration
IM (Canadian labeling; not in US labeling), IV push, SubQ injection: Central diabetes insipidus: Withdraw dose from ampul into appropriate syringe size (eg, insulin syringe). Further dilution is not required. Administer as direct injection.

IV infusion:
Hemophilia A, von Willebrand disease (type 1), and prevention of surgical bleeding in patients with uremia (off-label) (Mannucci, 1983): Infuse over 15 to 30 minutes

Acute uremic bleeding (off-label) (Watson, 1984a): May infuse over 10 minutes

Intranasal: Ensure that nasal passages are intact, clean, and free of obstruction prior to administration.

DDAVP: Nasal pump spray: Delivers 0.1 mL (10 mcg); for doses <10 mcg or for other doses which are not multiples, use rhinal tube. DDAVP Nasal spray delivers fifty 10 mcg doses. For 10 mcg dose, administer in one nostril. Any solution remaining after 50 doses should be discarded. Pump must be primed prior to first use.

DDAVP Rhinal tube: Insert top of dropper into tube (arrow marked end) in downward position. Squeeze dropper until solution reaches desired calibration mark. Disconnect dropper. Grasp the tube ¾ inch from the end and insert tube into nostril until the fingertips reach the nostril. Place opposite end of tube into the mouth (holding breath). Tilt head back and blow with a strong, short puff into the nostril (for very young patients, an adult should blow solution into the child's nose). Reseal dropper after use.

Oral:
Diabetes insipidus: Fluid restriction should be observed.
Primary nocturnal enuresis: Minimize fluid intake beginning 1 hour prior to administration and continue until the morning (for at least 8 hours).

May administer with or without food. Food may reduce/delay absorption although does not affect antidiuretic activity (Rittig, 1998).

Monitoring Parameters Blood pressure and pulse should be monitored during IV infusion

Note: For all indications, fluid intake, urine volume, and signs and symptoms of hyponatremia should be closely monitored especially in high-risk patient subgroups (eg, young children, elderly, patients with heart failure).

Diabetes insipidus: Urine specific gravity, plasma and urine osmolality, serum electrolytes

Hemophilia A: Factor VIII coagulant activity, factor VIII ristocetin cofactor activity, and factor VIII antigen levels, aPTT

von Willebrand disease: Factor VIII coagulant activity, factor VIII ristocetin cofactor activity, and factor VIII von Willebrand antigen levels, bleeding time

Nocturnal enuresis: Serum electrolytes if used for >7 days

Additional Information 10 mcg of desmopressin acetate is equivalent to 40 units

Dosage Forms Considerations
DDAVP and Minirin 5 mL bottles contain 50 sprays.
Stimate 2.5 mL bottles contain 25 sprays.

Dosage Forms Excipient information presented when available (limited, particularly for generics); consult specific product labeling. [DSC] = Discontinued product
Solution, Injection, as acetate:
DDAVP: 4 mcg/mL (1 mL)
DDAVP: 4 mcg/mL (10 mL) [contains chlorobutanol (chlorobutol)]
Generic: 4 mcg/mL (1 mL, 10 mL)

Solution, Nasal, as acetate:
DDAVP: 0.01% (5 mL) [contains benzalkonium chloride]
DDAVP Rhinal Tube: 0.01% (2.5 mL) [contains chlorobutanol (chlorobutol)]
Stimate: 1.5 mg/mL (2.5 mL) [contains benzalkonium chloride]
Generic: 0.01% (2.5 mL, 5 mL)
Tablet, Oral, as acetate:
DDAVP: 0.1 mg
DDAVP: 0.1 mg [DSC], 0.2 mg [scored]
Generic: 0.1 mg, 0.2 mg

Dosage Forms: Canada Excipient information presented when available (limited, particularly for generics); consult specific product labeling.
Tablet, Sublingual, as acetate:
DDAVP® Melt: 60 mcg, 120 mcg, 240 mcg

◆ Desmopressin Acetate see Desmopressin on page 520
◆ Desocort (Can) see Desonide on page 523
◆ Desogen see Ethinyl Estradiol and Desogestrel on page 701
◆ Desogestrel and Ethinyl Estradiol see Ethinyl Estradiol and Desogestrel on page 701
◆ Desonate see Desonide on page 523

Desonide (DES oh nide)

Brand Names: US Desonate; DesOwen; DesOwen Cream w/Cetaphil Lot [DSC]; DesOwen Lot w/Cetaphil Cream [DSC]; DesOwen Oint w/Cetaphil Lot [DSC]; LoKara; Verdeso

Brand Names: Canada Desocort; PDP-Desonide; Tridesilon; Verdeso

Pharmacologic Category Corticosteroid, Topical

Additional Appendix Information
Topical Corticosteroids on page 1952

Use
Atopic dermatitis (foam and gel): Treatment of mild to moderate atopic dermatitis in patients 3 months and older

Corticosteroid-responsive dermatoses (cream, ointment, and lotion): Relief of the inflammatory and pruritic manifestations of corticosteroid-responsive dermatoses.

Dosing
Adult & Geriatric
Atopic dermatitis: Topical: Foam, gel: Apply 2 times daily sparingly. Therapy should be discontinued when control is achieved. If no improvement is seen within 4 weeks, reassessment of diagnosis may be necessary; treatment should not exceed 4 consecutive weeks.

Corticosteroid responsive dermatoses: Topical: Cream, ointment, lotion: Apply 2 to 3 times daily sparingly. Therapy should be discontinued when control is achieved. If no improvement is seen within 2 weeks, reassessment of diagnosis may be necessary.

Pediatric Atopic dermatitis: Infants ≥3 months, Children, and Adolescents: Foam, gel: Refer to adult dosing.

Renal Impairment There are no dosage adjustments provided in the manufacturer's labeling.

Hepatic Impairment There are no dosage adjustments provided in the manufacturer's labeling.

Additional Information Complete prescribing information should be consulted for additional detail.

Dosage Forms Excipient information presented when available (limited, particularly for generics); consult specific product labeling. [DSC] = Discontinued product
Cream, External:
DesOwen: 0.05% (60 g)
Generic: 0.05% (15 g, 60 g)
Foam, External:
Verdeso: 0.05% (50 g [DSC], 100 g) [contains cetyl alcohol, propylene glycol]
Gel, External:
Desonate: 0.05% (60 g) [contains edetate disodium dihydrate, methylparaben, propylene glycol, propylparaben]
Kit, External:
DesOwen Cream w/Cetaphil Lot: 0.05% [DSC] [contains benzyl alcohol, propylene glycol]
DesOwen Lot w/Cetaphil Cream: 0.05% [DSC] [contains benzyl alcohol, cetyl alcohol, edetate sodium (tetrasodium), methylparaben, peg-30 glyceryl stearate, propylene glycol, propylparaben]
DesOwen Oint w/Cetaphil Lot: 0.05% [DSC] [contains benzyl alcohol]
Lotion, External:
DesOwen: 0.05% (59 mL, 118 mL) [contains cetyl alcohol, edetate disodium, methylparaben, propylene glycol, propylparaben]
LoKara: 0.05% (59 mL, 118 mL)
Generic: 0.05% (59 mL, 118 mL)

◀ Ointment, External:
DesOwen: 0.05% (60 g)
Generic: 0.05% (15 g, 60 g)

◆ DesOwen *see* Desonide *on page 523*
◆ DesOwen Cream w/Cetaphil Lot [DSC] *see* Desonide *on page 523*
◆ DesOwen Lot w/Cetaphil Cream [DSC] *see* Desonide *on page 523*
◆ DesOwen Oint w/Cetaphil Lot [DSC] *see* Desonide *on page 523*
◆ Desoxicream (Can) *see* Desoximetasone *on page 524*

Desoximetasone (des oks i MET a sone)

Brand Names: US Topicort; Topicort Spray
Brand Names: Canada Desoxicream; Topicort®; Topicort® Gel; Topicort® Mild; Topicort® Ointment
Index Terms Desoxymethasone
Pharmacologic Category Corticosteroid, Topical
Additional Appendix Information
Topical Corticosteroids *on page 1952*
Use
Cream, gel, ointment: Relief of inflammation and pruritic symptoms of corticosteroid-responsive dermatosis
Spray: Plaque psoriasis treatment
Dosing
Adult & Geriatric Note: Therapy should be discontinued when control is achieved; if no improvement is seen within 4 weeks, reassessment of diagnosis may be necessary.
Corticosteroid-responsive dermatoses: Topical: Cream, gel, ointment: Apply a thin film to affected area twice daily
Plaque psoriasis treatment: Topical: Spray: Apply a thin film to affected area twice daily
Pediatric Note: Therapy should be discontinued when control is achieved; if no improvement is seen within 4 weeks, reassessment of diagnosis may be necessary.
Corticosteroid-responsive dermatoses: Children and Adolescents: Topical: Cream, gel, ointment: Refer to adult dosing.
Renal Impairment No dosage adjustment provided in manufacturer's labeling.
Hepatic Impairment No dosage adjustment provided in manufacturer's labeling; use caution.
Additional Information Complete prescribing information should be consulted for additional detail.
Dosage Forms Excipient information presented when available (limited, particularly for generics); consult specific product labeling. [DSC] = Discontinued product
Cream, External:
Topicort: 0.05% (15 g [DSC], 60 g, 100 g [DSC]) [contains cetostearyl alcohol, edetate disodium]
Topicort: 0.25% (15 g [DSC], 60 g, 100 g [DSC]) [contains cetostearyl alcohol]
Generic: 0.05% (15 g, 60 g, 100 g); 0.25% (15 g, 60 g, 100 g)
Gel, External:
Topicort: 0.05% (15 g [DSC], 60 g) [contains alcohol, usp, edetate disodium, trolamine (triethanolamine)]
Generic: 0.05% (15 g, 60 g)
Liquid, External:
Topicort Spray: 0.25% (100 mL) [contains isopropyl alcohol, levomenthol]
Ointment, External:
Topicort: 0.05% (15 g [DSC], 60 g, 100 g); 0.25% (15 g [DSC], 60 g, 100 g [DSC])
Generic: 0.05% (60 g, 100 g); 0.25% (15 g, 60 g, 100 g)

◆ Desoxyephedrine Hydrochloride *see* Methamphetamine *on page 1164*
◆ Desoxymethasone *see* Desoximetasone *on page 524*
◆ Desoxyn *see* Methamphetamine *on page 1164*
◆ Desoxyphenobarbital *see* Primidone *on page 1503*
◆ Desulfato-Hirudin *see* Desirudin *on page 519*
◆ Desulphatohirudin *see* Desirudin *on page 519*

Desvenlafaxine (des ven la FAX een)

Brand Names: US Khedezla; Pristiq
Brand Names: Canada Pristiq
Index Terms O-desmethylvenlafaxine; ODV
Pharmacologic Category Antidepressant, Serotonin/Norepinephrine Reuptake Inhibitor
Use Major depressive disorder: Treatment of major depressive disorder (MDD)
Medication Guide Available Yes

Dosing
Adult & Geriatric Major depressive disorder (MDD):
Oral: 50 mg once daily; doses up to 400 mg once daily have been studied and have shown to be effective; however, the manufacturer states there is no additional benefit at doses >50 mg per day. The Canadian labeling recommends a maximum dose of 100 mg daily.

Discontinuation of therapy: Upon discontinuation of antidepressant therapy, gradually taper the dose to minimize the incidence of withdrawal symptoms and allow for the detection of re-emerging symptoms. The 25 mg tablet is intended for a gradual reduction in dose when discontinuing treatment. Evidence supporting ideal taper rates is limited. APA and NICE guidelines suggest tapering therapy over at least several weeks with consideration to the half-life of the antidepressant; antidepressants with a shorter half-life may need to be tapered more conservatively. In addition for long-term treated patients, WFSBP guidelines recommend tapering over 4 to 6 months. If intolerable withdrawal symptoms occur following a dose reduction, consider resuming the previously prescribed dose and/or decrease dose at a more gradual rate (APA, 2010; Bauer, 2002; Haddad, 2001; NCCMH, 2010; Schatzberg, 2006; Shelton, 2001; Warner, 2006).

MAO inhibitor recommendations:
Switching to or from an MAO inhibitor intended to treat psychiatric disorders:
Allow 14 days to elapse between discontinuing an MAO inhibitor intended to treat psychiatric disorders and initiation of desvenlafaxine.
Allow 7 days to elapse between discontinuing desvenlafaxine and initiation of an MAO inhibitor intended to treat psychiatric disorders.
Use with other MAO inhibitors (linezolid or IV methylene blue):
Do not initiate desvenlafaxine in patients receiving linezolid or IV methylene blue; consider other interventions for psychiatric condition.
If urgent treatment with linezolid or IV methylene blue is required in a patient already receiving desvenlafaxine and potential benefits outweigh potential risks, discontinue desvenlafaxine promptly and administer linezolid or IV methylene blue. Monitor for serotonin syndrome for 7 days (US labeling) or 14 days (Canadian labeling) or until 24 hours after the last dose of linezolid or IV methylene blue, whichever comes first. May resume desvenlafaxine 24 hours after the last dose of linezolid or IV methylene blue.
Renal Impairment
US labeling:
CrCl >50 mL/minute: No dosage adjustment necessary.
CrCl 30 to 50 mL/minute: 50 mg once daily (maximum)
CrCl <30 mL/minute: 25 mg once daily or 50 mg every other day (maximum)
End-stage renal disease (ESRD) requiring hemodialysis (HD): 25 mg once daily or 50 mg every other day (maximum). Supplemental doses should not be given after HD.
Canadian labeling:
CrCl ≥30 mL/minute: There are no dosage adjustments provided in the manufacturer's labeling.
CrCl <30 mL/minute: 50 mg every other day (maximum)
ESRD requiring hemodialysis (HD): 50 mg every other day (maximum). Supplemental doses should not be given after HD.
Hepatic Impairment
US labeling:
Mild impairment: No dosage adjustment necessary.
Moderate-to-severe impairment: Initial: 50 mg once daily; maximum dose: 100 mg once daily
Canadian labeling: No dosage adjustment necessary.
Additional Information Complete prescribing information should be consulted for additional detail.
Dosage Forms Excipient information presented when available (limited, particularly for generics); consult specific product labeling.
Tablet Extended Release 24 Hour, Oral:
Khedezla: 50 mg
Khedezla: 100 mg [contains fd&c yellow #6 (sunset yellow)]
Generic: 50 mg, 100 mg
Tablet Extended Release 24 Hour, Oral, as fumarate [strength expressed as base]:
Generic: 50 mg, 100 mg
Tablet Extended Release 24 Hour, Oral, as succinate [strength expressed as base]:
Pristiq: 25 mg, 50 mg, 100 mg

◆ Desyrel *see* TraZODone *on page 1834*
◆ Detemir Insulin *see* Insulin Detemir *on page 955*

Dexamethasone (Systemic)
(deks a METH a sone)

Brand Names: US Baycadron [DSC]; Dexamethasone Intensol; DexPak 10 Day; DexPak 13 Day; DexPak 6 Day; DoubleDex

Brand Names: Canada Apo-Dexamethasone; Dexasone; Dom-Dexamethasone; PHL-Dexamethasone; PMS-Dexamethasone; PRO-Dexamethasone; ratio-Dexamethasone

Index Terms Decadron; Dexamethasone Sodium Phosphate

Pharmacologic Category Anti-inflammatory Agent; Antiemetic; Corticosteroid, Systemic

Additional Appendix Information

Corticosteroids Systemic Equivalencies on page 1950

Use Primarily as an anti-inflammatory or immunosuppressant agent in the treatment of a variety of diseases including those of allergic, dermatologic, gastrointestinal, endocrine, hematologic, inflammatory, neoplastic, nervous system, ophthalmic, renal, respiratory, rheumatic, and autoimmune origin; management of cerebral edema, chronic swelling, as a diagnostic agent, diagnosis of Cushing syndrome, antiemetic

Pregnancy Considerations Adverse events have been observed with corticosteroids in animal reproduction studies. Betamethasone crosses the placenta (Brownfoot 2013); and is partially metabolized by placental enzymes to an inactive metabolite (Murphy 2007). Some studies have shown an association between first trimester systemic corticosteroid use and oral clefts (Park-Wyllie 2000; Pradat 2003). Systemic corticosteroids may have an effect on fetal growth (decreased birth weight); however, information is conflicting (Lunghi 2010). Hypoadrenalism may occur in newborns following maternal use of corticosteroids during pregnancy; monitor.

Because antenatal corticosteroid administration may reduce the incidence of intraventricular hemorrhage, necrotizing enterocolitis, neonatal mortality, and respiratory distress syndrome, the injection is often used in patients with preterm premature rupture of membranes (membrane rupture between 24 0/7 weeks and 34 0/7 weeks of gestation) who are at risk of preterm delivery (ACOG 2013). When systemic corticosteroids are needed in pregnancy, it is generally recommended to use the lowest effective dose for the shortest duration of time, avoiding high doses during the first trimester (Leachman 2006; Lunghi 2010; Makol 2011; Østensen 2009).

Women exposed to dexamethasone during pregnancy for the treatment of an autoimmune disease may contact the OTIS Autoimmune Diseases Study at 877-311-8972.

Breast-Feeding Considerations Corticosteroids are excreted in human milk; information specific to dexamethasone has not been located. The manufacturer notes that when used systemically, maternal use of corticosteroids have the potential to cause adverse events in a nursing infant (eg, growth suppression, interfere with endogenous corticosteroid production). Due to the potential for serious adverse reactions in the nursing infant, the manufacturer recommends a decision be made whether to discontinue nursing or to discontinue the drug, taking into account the importance of treatment to the mother. If there is concern about exposure to the infant, some guidelines recommend waiting 4 hours after the maternal dose of an oral systemic corticosteroid before breast-feeding in order to decrease potential exposure to the nursing infant (based on a study using prednisolone) (Bae 2011; Leachman 2006; Makol 2011; Ost 1985).

Contraindications Hypersensitivity to dexamethasone or any component of the formulation, including sulfites; systemic fungal infections, cerebral malaria

Warnings/Precautions Corticosteroids are not approved for epidural injection. Serious neurologic events (eg, spinal cord infarction, paraplegia, quadriplegia, cortical blindness, stroke), some resulting in death, have been reported with epidural injection of corticosteroids, with and without use of fluoroscopy. Intra-articular injection may produce systemic as well as local effects. Appropriate examination of any joint fluid present is necessary to exclude a septic process. Avoid injection into an infected site. Do not inject into unstable joints. Patients should not overuse joints in which symptomatic benefit has been obtained as long as the inflammatory process remains active. Frequent intra-articular injection may result in damage to joint tissues.

Use with caution in patients with thyroid disease, hepatic impairment, renal impairment, cardiovascular disease, diabetes, glaucoma, cataracts, myasthenia gravis, osteoporosis, seizures, or GI diseases (diverticulitis, intestinal anastomoses, peptic ulcer, ulcerative colitis) due to perforation risk. Avoid ethanol may enhance gastric mucosal irritation. Use caution following acute MI (corticosteroids have been associated with myocardial rupture). Because of the risk of adverse effects, systemic corticosteroids should be used cautiously in the elderly in the smallest possible effective dose for the shortest duration. May affect growth velocity; growth should be routinely monitored in pediatric patients. Withdraw therapy with gradual tapering of dose.

May cause hypercorticism or suppression of hypothalamic-pituitary-adrenal (HPA) axis, particularly in younger children or in patients receiving high doses for prolonged periods. HPA axis suppression may lead to adrenal crisis. Withdrawal and discontinuation of a corticosteroid should be done slowly and carefully. Particular care is required when patients are transferred from systemic corticosteroids to inhaled products due to possible adrenal insufficiency or withdrawal from steroids, including an increase in allergic symptoms. Adult patients receiving >20 mg per day of prednisone (or equivalent) may be most susceptible. Fatalities have occurred due to adrenal insufficiency in asthmatic patients during and after transfer from systemic corticosteroids to aerosol steroids; aerosol steroids do not provide the systemic steroid needed to treat patients having trauma, surgery, or infections. Dexamethasone does not provide adequate mineralocorticoid activity in adrenal insufficiency (may be employed as a single dose while cortisol assays are performed). The lowest possible dose should be used during treatment; discontinuation and/or dose reductions should be gradual. Rare cases of anaphylactoid reactions have been observed in patients receiving corticosteroids. Patients may require higher doses when subject to stress (ie, trauma, surgery, severe infection).

Acute myopathy has been reported with high dose corticosteroids, usually in patients with neuromuscular transmission disorders; may involve ocular and/or respiratory muscles; monitor creatine kinase; recovery may be delayed. Perineal burning, tingling, pain and pruritus have been reported with IV administration. May occur more commonly in females, with higher doses, and with rapid administration. Symptom onset is sudden and usually resolves in <1 minute (Allan 1986; Neff 2002; Perron 2003; Singh 2011). Corticosteroid use may cause psychiatric disturbances, including depression, euphoria, insomnia, mood swings, and personality changes. Preexisting psychiatric conditions may be exacerbated by corticosteroid use. Prolonged use of corticosteroids may increase the incidence of secondary infection, mask acute infection (including fungal infections), prolong or exacerbate viral infections, or limit response to vaccines. Exposure to chickenpox or measles should be avoided; corticosteroids should not be used to treat ocular herpes simplex. Corticosteroids should not be used for cerebral malaria, fungal infections, or viral hepatitis. Close observation is required in patients with latent tuberculosis and/or TB reactivity; restrict use in active TB (only fulminating or disseminated TB in conjunction with antituberculosis treatment). Amebiasis should be ruled out in any patient with recent travel to tropic climates or unexplained diarrhea prior to initiation of corticosteroids.

Prolonged treatment with corticosteroids has been associated with the development of Kaposi sarcoma (case reports); if noted, discontinuation of therapy should be considered. High-dose corticosteroids should not be used to manage acute head injury. Some products may contain sodium sulfite, a sulfite that may cause allergic-type reactions including anaphylaxis and life-threatening or less severe asthmatic episodes in susceptible patients. Potentially significant drug-drug interactions may exist, requiring dose or frequency adjustment, additional monitoring, and/or selection of alternative therapy. Some dosage forms may contain propylene glycol; large amounts are potentially toxic and have been associated hyperosmolality, lactic acidosis, seizures, and respiratory depression; use caution (AAP ["Inactive" 1997]; Zar 2007).

Benzyl alcohol and derivatives: Some dosage forms may contain sodium benzoate/benzoic acid; benzoic acid (benzoate) is a metabolite of benzyl alcohol; large amounts of benzyl alcohol (≥99 mg/kg/day) have been associated with a potentially fatal toxicity ("gasping syndrome") in neonates; the "gasping syndrome" consists of metabolic acidosis, respiratory distress, gasping respirations, CNS dysfunction (including convulsions, intracranial hemorrhage), hypotension, and cardiovascular collapse (AAP

["Inactive" 1997]; CDC 1982); some data suggests that benzoate displaces bilirubin from protein binding sites (Ahlfors 2001); avoid or use dosage forms containing benzyl alcohol derivative with caution in neonates. See manufacturer's labeling.

Adverse Reactions Frequency not defined.

Cardiovascular: Arrhythmia, bradycardia, cardiac arrest, cardiomyopathy, CHF, circulatory collapse, edema, hypertension, myocardial rupture (post-MI), syncope, thromboembolism, vasculitis

Central nervous system: Depression, emotional instability, euphoria, headache, intracranial pressure increased, insomnia, malaise, mood swings, neuritis, personality changes, pseudotumor cerebri (usually following discontinuation), psychic disorders, seizure, vertigo

Dermatologic: Acne, allergic dermatitis, alopecia, angioedema, bruising, dry skin, erythema, fragile skin, hirsutism, hyper-/hypopigmentation, hypertrichosis, perianal pruritus (following IV injection), petechiae, rash, skin atrophy, skin test reaction impaired, striae, urticaria, wound healing impaired

Endocrine & metabolic: Adrenal suppression, carbohydrate tolerance decreased, Cushing's syndrome, diabetes mellitus, glucose intolerance decreased, growth suppression (children), hyperglycemia, hypokalemic alkalosis, menstrual irregularities, negative nitrogen balance, pituitary-adrenal axis suppression, protein catabolism, sodium retention

Gastrointestinal: Abdominal distention, appetite increased, gastrointestinal hemorrhage, gastrointestinal perforation, nausea, pancreatitis, peptic ulcer, ulcerative esophagitis, weight gain

Genitourinary: Altered (increased or decreased) spermatogenesis

Hepatic: Hepatomegaly, transaminases increased

Local: Postinjection flare (intra-articular use), thrombophlebitis

Neuromuscular & skeletal: Arthropathy, aseptic necrosis (femoral and humoral heads), fractures, muscle mass loss, myopathy (particularly in conjunction with neuromuscular disease or neuromuscular-blocking agents), neuropathy, osteoporosis, parasthesia, tendon rupture, vertebral compression fractures, weakness

Ocular: Cataracts, exophthalmos, glaucoma, intraocular pressure increased

Renal: Glucosuria

Respiratory: Pulmonary edema

Miscellaneous: Abnormal fat deposition, anaphylactoid reaction, anaphylaxis, avascular necrosis, diaphoresis, hiccups, hypersensitivity, impaired wound healing, infections, Kaposi's sarcoma, moon face, secondary malignancy

Drug Interactions

Metabolism/Transport Effects Substrate of CYP3A4 (major), P-glycoprotein; **Note:** Assignment of Major/Minor substrate status based on clinically relevant drug interaction potential; **Inhibits** P-glycoprotein; **Induces** CYP2A6 (weak/moderate), CYP2B6 (weak/moderate), CYP2C9 (weak/moderate), CYP3A4 (weak), P-glycoprotein, UGT1A1

Avoid Concomitant Use

Avoid concomitant use of Dexamethasone (Systemic) with any of the following: Aldesleukin; BCG (Intravesical); Cabozantinib; Conivaptan; Fusidic Acid (Systemic); Idelalisib; Indium 111 Capromab Pendetide; Lapatinib; Mifepristone; Natalizumab; Nilotinib; Pimecrolimus; Rilpivirine; RomiDEPsin; Tacrolimus (Topical); Ticagrelor; Tofacitinib; VinCRIStine (Liposomal)

Increased Effect/Toxicity

Dexamethasone (Systemic) may increase the levels/ effects of: Acetylcholinesterase Inhibitors; Amphotericin B; Androgens; CycloSPORINE (Systemic); Deferasirox; Fingolimod; Fosphenytoin; Leflunomide; Lenalidomide; Loop Diuretics; Natalizumab; Nicorandil; NSAID (COX-2 Inhibitor); NSAID (Nonselective); Phenytoin; Quinolone Antibiotics; Thalidomide; Thiazide Diuretics; Tofacitinib; Vaccines (Live); Warfarin

The levels/effects of Dexamethasone (Systemic) may be increased by: Aprepitant; Asparaginase (E. coli); Asparaginase (Erwinia); Conivaptan; CycloSPORINE (Systemic); CYP3A4 Inhibitors (Moderate); CYP3A4 Inhibitors (Strong); Denosumab; Estrogen Derivatives; Fosamprenavir; Fosaprepitant; Fusidic Acid (Systemic); Idelalisib; Indacaterol; Ivacaftor; Luliconazole; Mifepristone; Netupitant; Neuromuscular-Blocking Agents (Nondepolarizing); Osimertinib; Palbociclib; P-glycoprotein/ ABCB1 Inhibitors; Pimecrolimus; Ranolazine; Roflumilast; Salicylates; Simeprevir; Stiripentol; Tacrolimus (Topical); Telaprevir; Trastuzumab

Decreased Effect

Dexamethasone (Systemic) may decrease the levels/ effects of: Aldesleukin; Antidiabetic Agents; ARIPiprazole; BCG (Intravesical); Cabozantinib; Calcitriol (Systemic); Caspofungin; Cobicistat; Coccidioides immitis Skin Test; Corticorelin; CycloSPORINE (Systemic); Dasatinib; Elvitegravir; Fosamprenavir; Fosphenytoin; Hyaluronidase; Hydrocodone; Imatinib; Indium 111 Capromab Pendetide; Isoniazid; Ixabepilone; Lapatinib; Nilotinib; NiMODipine; Phenytoin; Rilpivirine; RomiDEPsin; Salicylates; Saxagliptin; Sipuleucel-T; SUNItinib; Telaprevir; Ticagrelor; Triazolam; Urea Cycle Disorder Agents; Vaccines (Inactivated); Vaccines (Live); VinCRIStine (Liposomal)

The levels/effects of Dexamethasone (Systemic) may be decreased by: Antacids; Bile Acid Sequestrants; Bosentan; CYP3A4 Inducers (Moderate); CYP3A4 Inducers (Strong); Dabrafenib; Deferasirox; Echinacea; Enzalutamide; Fosphenytoin; Mifepristone; Mitotane; Osimertinib; P-glycoprotein/ABCB1 Inducers; Phenytoin; Siltuximab; St Johns Wort; Tocilizumab

Preparation for Administration

Oral: Oral administration of dexamethasone for croup may be prepared using a parenteral dexamethasone formulation and mixing it with an oral flavored syrup (Bjornson 2004).

IV: May be given undiluted or further diluted in NS or D_5W. Use preservative-free product when used in neonates, especially premature infants.

Storage/Stability

Elixir: Store at 15°C to 30°C (59°F to 86°F); avoid freezing.

Injection: Store intact vials at 20°C to 25°C (68°F to 77°F); excursions permitted to 15°C to 30°C (59°F to 86°F). Protect from light, heat, and freezing. Diluted solutions should be used within 24 hours.

Oral concentrated solution (Intensol): Store at 20°C to 25°C (68°F to 77°F); do not freeze; do not use if precipitate is present; dispense only in original bottle and only with manufacturer-supplied calibrated dropper; discard open bottle after 90 days.

Oral solution: Store at 20°C to 25°C (68°F to 77°F).

Tablets: Store at 20°C to 25°C (68°F to 77°F); protect from moisture.

Mechanism of Action A long acting corticosteroid with minimal sodium-retaining potential. Decreases inflammation by suppression of neutrophil migration, decreased production of inflammatory mediators, and reversal of increased capillary permeability; suppresses normal immune response. Dexamethasone's mechanism of antiemetic activity is unknown.

Pharmacodynamics/Kinetics

Onset of action: IV: Prompt

Duration: Metabolic effects can last for 72 hours

Absorption: Oral: 61% to 86%

Metabolism: Hepatic

Half-life elimination:

Extremely low birth-weight infants with BPD: 9.3 hours

Children 3 months to 16 years: 4.3 hours

Adults: Oral: ~4 hours (Czock 2005); IV: ~1 to 5 hours (Hochhaus 2001; Miyabo 1991; Rohdewald 1987; Toth 1999)

Time to peak, serum: Oral: 1 to 2 hours (Czock 2005); IM: ~30 to 120 minutes (Egerman 1997; Hochhaus 2001); IV: 5 to 10 minutes (free dexamethasone) (Miyabo 1991; Rohdewald 1987)

Excretion: Urine (~10%) (Duggan 1975; Miyabo 1991)

Dosing

Adult

Anti-inflammatory:

Oral, IM, IV: 0.75 to 9 mg/day in divided doses every 6 to 12 hours

Intra-articular, intralesional, or soft tissue: 0.4 to 6 mg/day

Extubation or airway edema: Oral, IM, IV: 0.5 to 2 mg/kg/day in divided doses every 6 hours beginning 24 hours prior to extubation and continuing for 4 to 6 doses afterwards

Cerebral edema: IV: 10 mg stat, 4 mg IM/IV (should be given as sodium phosphate) every 6 hours until response is maximized, then switch to oral regimen, then taper off if appropriate; dosage may be reduced after 2 to 4 days and gradually discontinued over 5 to 7 days

Dexamethasone suppression test (depression/suicide indicator) (off-label use): Oral: 1 mg at 11 PM, draw blood at 8 AM the following day for plasma cortisol determination

Cushing syndrome, diagnostic: Oral: 1 mg at 11 PM, draw blood at 8 AM; greater accuracy for Cushing's syndrome may be achieved by the following:

Dexamethasone 0.5 mg by mouth every 6 hours for 48 hours (with 24-hour urine collection for 17-hydroxycorticosteroid excretion)

Differentiation of Cushing syndrome due to ACTH excess from Cushing due to other causes: Oral: Dexamethasone 2 mg every 6 hours for 48 hours (with 24-hour urine collection for 17-hydroxycorticosteroid excretion)

Multiple sclerosis (acute exacerbation): Oral: 30 mg/day for 1 week, followed by 4 to 12 mg/day for 1 month

Treatment of shock:

Addisonian crisis/shock (eg, adrenal insufficiency/responsive to steroid therapy): IV: 4 to 10 mg as a single dose, which may be repeated if necessary

Unresponsive shock (eg, unresponsive to steroid therapy): IV: 1 to 6 mg/kg as a single IV dose or up to 40 mg initially followed by repeat doses every 2 to 6 hours while shock persists

Physiological replacement: Oral, IM, IV (should be given as sodium phosphate): 0.03 to 0.15 mg/kg/day **or** 0.6 to 0.75 mg/m^2/day in divided doses every 6 to 12 hours

Acute mountain sickness (AMS)/high altitude cerebral edema (HACE) (off-label use):

Prevention: Oral: 2 mg every 6 hours **or** 4 mg every 12 hours starting on the day of ascent; may be discontinued after staying at the same elevation for 2 to 3 days or if descent is initiated; do not exceed a 10 day duration (Luks 2010). **Note:** In situations of rapid ascent to altitudes >3500 meters (such as rescue or military operations), 4 mg every 6 hours may be considered (Luks 2010).

Treatment: Oral, IM, IV:

AMS: 4 mg every 6 hours (Luks 2010)

HACE: Initial: 8 mg as a single dose; Maintenance: 4 mg every 6 hours until symptoms resolve (Luks 2010)

Antenatal fetal maturation (off-label use): IM: In women with preterm premature rupture of membranes (membrane rupture between 24 0/7 weeks and 34 0/7 weeks of gestation), a single course of corticosteroids is recommended if there is a risk of preterm delivery (ACOG 2013). Although the optimal corticosteroid and dose have not been determined, dexamethasone 6 mg every 12 hours for a total of 4 doses has been used in most studies (Brownfoot 2013).

Chemotherapy-associated nausea and vomiting, prevention (off-label use):

High emetic potential chemotherapy: Oral, IV: 12 mg on day 1 prior to chemotherapy (in combination with aprepitant or fosaprepitant and a 5HT$_3$ antagonist on day 1) followed by 8 mg on days 2 to 3 or days 2 to 4 (with aprepitant on days 2 and 3 if aprepitant used on day 1) (Basch 2011; Roila 2010) **or** (if aprepitant/fosaprepitant not used): 20 mg day 1 (in combination with a 5HT$_3$ antagonist on day 1) followed by 8 mg twice daily for 3 to 4 days (MASCC 2013)

Moderate emetic potential chemotherapy: Oral, IV: 8 mg on day 1 prior to chemotherapy (in combination with a 5HT$_3$ antagonist on day 1) and 8 mg on days 2 and 3 (Basch 2011; Roila 2010)

Low emetic potential chemotherapy: Oral, IV: 8 mg prior to chemotherapy (Basch 2011; Roila 2010)

Multiple myeloma (off-label use): Oral: 40 mg once daily on days 1 to 4, 9 to 12, and 17 to 20 (as induction therapy) in combination with bortezomib and doxorubicin for 3 cycles (Sonneveld 2012) **or** 40 mg once weekly on days 1, 8, 15, and 22 every 28 days (in combination with lenalidomide) until disease progression (Rajkumar 2010) or 40 mg once weekly on days 1, 8, 15, and 22 every 28 days (in combination with pomalidomide) until disease progression or unacceptable toxicity (San Miguel 2013) **or** 40 mg once weekly on days 1, 8, 15, and 22 every 28 days (in combination with ixazomib and lenalidomide) until disease progression or unacceptable toxicity (Moreau 2015) **or** 28 mg orally plus 8 mg IV (prior to elotuzumab) on days 1, 8, 15, and 22 every 28 days for 2 cycles, followed by 28 mg orally plus 8 mg IV (prior to elotuzumab) on days 1 and 15 and 40 mg orally on days 8 and 22 every 28 days thereafter until disease progression or unacceptable toxicity (in combination with elotuzumab and lenalidomide) (Lonial 2015). **Note:** Multiple dexamethasone-containing regimens are available for the treatment of multiple myeloma. Refer to appropriate literature/guidelines for additional details.

Geriatric Refer to adult dosing. Use cautiously in the elderly in the smallest possible dose.

Pediatric

Anti-inflammatory and/or immunosuppressant: Oral, IM, IV: 0.08 to 0.3 mg/kg/day **or** 2.5 to 10 mg/m^2/day in divided doses every 6 to 12 hours

Extubation or airway edema: Oral, IM, IV: 0.5 to 2 mg/kg/day in divided doses every 6 hours beginning 24 hours prior to extubation and continuing for 4 to 6 doses afterwards

Cerebral edema: IV: Loading dose: 1 to 2 mg/kg/dose as a single dose; maintenance: 1 to 1.5 mg/kg/day (maximum: 16 mg/day) in divided doses every 4 to 6 hours, taper off over 1 to 6 weeks

Croup (laryngotracheobronchitis): Oral, IM, IV: 0.6 mg/kg once; usual maximum dose: 16 mg (doses as high as 20 mg have been used) (Bjornson 2004; Hegenbarth 2008; Rittichier 2000); a single oral dose of 0.15 mg/kg has been shown effective in children with mild to moderate croup (Russell 2004; Sparrow 2006)

Bacterial meningitis: Infants and Children >6 weeks: IV: 0.15 mg/kg/dose every 6 hours for the first 2 to 4 days of antibiotic treatment; start dexamethasone 10 to 20 minutes before or with the first dose of antibiotic

Physiologic replacement: Oral, IM, IV: 0.03 to 0.15 mg/kg/day **or** 0.6 to 0.75 mg/m^2/day in divided doses every 6 to 12 hours

Acute mountain sickness (AMS)/high altitude cerebral edema (HACE) (off-label use): Oral, IM, IV: 0.15 mg/kg/dose every 6 hours; consider using for high altitude pulmonary edema because of associated HACE with this condition (Luks 2010; Pollard 2001)

Chemotherapy-associated nausea and vomiting, prevention (off-label use): Pediatric Oncology Group of Ontario guideline recommendations (Dupuis, 2013): Infants, Children, and Adolescents:

High emetic potential chemotherapy: Oral, IV: 6 mg/m^2/dose every 6 hours (in combination with a 5HT$_3$ antagonist and aprepitant [if no interaction with aprepitant and if ≥12 years]); reduce dexamethasone dose by 50% if administered concomitantly with aprepitant

Moderate emetic potential chemotherapy: Oral, IV:

BSA ≤0.6 m^2: 2 mg every 12 hours (in combination with a 5HT$_3$ antagonist)

BSA >0.6 m^2: 4 mg every 12 hours (in combination with a 5HT$_3$ antagonist)

Renal Impairment There are no dosage adjustments provided in the manufacturer's labeling; use with caution. Hemodialysis or peritoneal dialysis: Supplemental dose is not necessary.

Hepatic Impairment There are no dosage adjustments provided in the manufacturer's labeling.

Dietary Considerations May be taken with meals to decrease GI upset. May need diet with increased potassium, pyridoxine, vitamin C, vitamin D, folate, calcium, and phosphorus.

Administration

Oral: Administer with meals to decrease GI upset.

IV: May administer the 4 mg/mL or 10 mg/mL concentration undiluted over ≤1 minute (Gahart 2015). Rapid administration may be associated with perineal irritation (especially with higher doses); consider further dilution and administration by IV intermittent infusion over 5 to 15 minutes (Allan 1986; Neff 2002; Perron 2003; Singh 2011).

IM: Administer the 4 mg/mL or 10 mg/mL concentration deep IM.

Intra-articular: Administer into affected joint using the 4 mg/mL concentration only.

Intralesional injection: Administer into affected area using the 4 mg/mL concentration only.

Soft tissue injection: Administer into affected tissue using the 4 mg/mL concentration only.

Monitoring Parameters Hemoglobin, occult blood loss, serum potassium, glucose, growth in children

Reference Range Dexamethasone suppression test, overnight: 8 AM cortisol <6 mcg/100 mL (dexamethasone 1 mg); plasma cortisol determination should be made on the day after giving dose

Test Interactions May suppress the wheal and flare reactions to skin test antigens

Additional Information Effects of inhaled/intranasal steroids on growth have been observed in the absence of laboratory evidence of HPA axis suppression, suggesting that growth velocity is a more sensitive indicator of systemic corticosteroid exposure in pediatric patients than some commonly used tests of HPA axis function. The long-term effects of this reduction in growth velocity associated with orally-inhaled and intranasal corticosteroids, including the impact on final adult height, are unknown. The potential for "catch up" growth following discontinuation of treatment with inhaled corticosteroids has not been adequately studied.

Withdrawal/tapering of therapy: Corticosteroid tapering following short-term use is limited primarily by the need to control the underlying disease state; tapering may be accomplished over a period of days. Following longer-term use, tapering over weeks to months may be necessary to avoid signs and symptoms of adrenal insufficiency and to allow recovery of the HPA axis. Testing of HPA axis responsiveness may be of value in selected patients. Subtle deficits in HPA response may persist for months after discontinuation of therapy, and may require supplemental dosing during periods of acute illness or surgical stress.

Dosage Forms Excipient information presented when available (limited, particularly for generics); consult specific product labeling. [DSC] = Discontinued product
Concentrate, Oral:
  Dexamethasone Intensol: 1 mg/mL (30 mL) [contains alcohol, usp; unflavored flavor]
Elixir, Oral:
  Baycadron: 0.5 mg/5 mL (237 mL [DSC]) [contains alcohol, usp, benzoic acid, fd&c red #40, propylene glycol; raspberry flavor]
  Generic: 0.5 mg/5 mL (237 mL)
Kit, Injection, as sodium phosphate:
  DoubleDex: 10 mg/mL
Solution, Oral:
  Generic: 0.5 mg/5 mL (240 mL, 500 mL)
Solution, Injection, as sodium phosphate:
  Generic: 4 mg/mL (1 mL, 5 mL, 30 mL); 20 mg/5 mL (5 mL); 120 mg/30 mL (30 mL); 10 mg/mL (1 mL, 10 mL [DSC]); 100 mg/10 mL (10 mL)
Solution, Injection, as sodium phosphate [preservative free]:
  Generic: 4 mg/mL (1 mL); 10 mg/mL (1 mL)
Tablet, Oral:
  DexPak 10 Day: 1.5 mg [scored; contains fd&c red #40 aluminum lake]
  DexPak 13 Day: 1.5 mg [scored; contains fd&c red #40 aluminum lake]
  DexPak 6 Day: 1.5 mg [scored; contains fd&c red #40 aluminum lake]
  Generic: 0.5 mg, 0.75 mg, 1 mg, 1.5 mg, 2 mg, 4 mg, 6 mg

Dexamethasone (Ophthalmic)
(deks a METH a sone)

Brand Names: US Maxidex; Ozurdex
Brand Names: Canada Diodex; Maxidex; Ozurdex
Index Terms Dexamethasone Sodium Phosphate
Pharmacologic Category Anti-inflammatory Agent, Ophthalmic; Corticosteroid, Ophthalmic; Corticosteroid, Otic
Use
  Management of steroid-responsive inflammatory conditions such as allergic conjunctivitis, iritis, or cyclitis; symptomatic treatment of corneal injury from chemical, radiation, or thermal burns, or penetration of foreign bodies. The ophthalmic solution is also indicated for otic use to treat steroid-responsive inflammatory conditions of the external auditory meatus.
  Ophthalmic intravitreal implant (Ozurdex): Treatment of macular edema following branch retinal vein occlusion (BRVO) or central retinal vein occlusion (CRVO); treatment of noninfective uveitis affecting the posterior segment of the eye; treatment of diabetic macular edema
Dosing
  Adult
    Anti-inflammatory:
    Ophthalmic:
      Solution: Instill 1 to 2 drops into conjunctival sac every hour during the day and every other hour during the night; gradually reduce dose to 1 drop every 4 hours, then to 3 to 4 times/day
      Suspension: Instill 1 to 2 drops into conjunctival sac up to 4 to 6 times/day; may use hourly in severe disease; taper prior to discontinuation
    Otic: Solution: Initial: Instill 3 to 4 drops into the aural canal 2 to 3 times a day; reduce dose gradually once a favorable response is obtained. Alternately, may pack the aural canal with a gauze wick saturated with the solution; remove from the ear after 12 to 24 hours. Repeat as necessary.
    Diabetic macular edema (pseudophakic or phakic patients scheduled for cataract surgery) or macular edema (following BRVO or CRVO): Ocular implant: Intravitreal injection: 0.7 mg implant injected in affected eye
    Noninfective uveitis: Ocular implant: Intravitreal injection: 0.7 mg implant injected in affected eye
  Geriatric Refer to adult dosing. Solution/suspension: Use cautiously in the elderly in the smallest possible dose.

Renal Impairment There are no dosage adjustment provided in the manufacturer's labeling.
Hepatic Impairment There are no dosage adjustment provided in the manufacturer's labeling.
Additional Information Complete prescribing information should be consulted for additional detail.
Dosage Forms Excipient information presented when available (limited, particularly for generics); consult specific product labeling.
Implant, Intraocular [preservative free]:
  Ozurdex: 0.7 mg (1 ea)
Solution, Ophthalmic, as phosphate:
  Generic: 0.1% (5 mL)
Suspension, Ophthalmic:
  Maxidex: 0.1% (5 mL)

◆ Dexamethasone and Ciprofloxacin *see* Ciprofloxacin and Dexamethasone *on page 393*
◆ Dexamethasone and Tobramycin *see* Tobramycin and Dexamethasone *on page 1802*
◆ Dexamethasone Intensol *see* Dexamethasone (Systemic) *on page 525*
◆ Dexamethasone, Neomycin, and Polymyxin B *see* Neomycin, Polymyxin B, and Dexamethasone *on page 1267*
◆ Dexamethasone Sodium Phosphate *see* Dexamethasone (Ophthalmic) *on page 528*
◆ Dexamethasone Sodium Phosphate *see* Dexamethasone (Systemic) *on page 525*
◆ Dexasone (Can) *see* Dexamethasone (Systemic) *on page 525*

Dexchlorpheniramine (deks klor fen EER a meen)

Index Terms Dexchlorpheniramine Maleate
Pharmacologic Category Alkylamine Derivative; Histamine H_1 Antagonist; Histamine H_1 Antagonist, First Generation
Use Hypersensitivity reactions: For the treatment of perennial and seasonal allergic rhinitis; vasomotor rhinitis; allergic conjunctivitis; mild, uncomplicated allergic skin manifestations of urticaria and angioedema; amelioration of allergic reactions to blood or plasma; dermatographism; adjunctive therapy for the management of anaphylactic reactions.
Dosing
  Adult & Geriatric Allergy symptoms: Oral: 2 mg every 4 to 6 hours
  Pediatric Allergy symptoms: Oral:
    Children 2 to 5 years: 0.5 mg every 4 to 6 hours
    Children 6 to 11 years: 1 mg every 4 to 6 hours
    Children ≥12 years and Adolescents: Refer to adult dosing.
  Renal Impairment There are no dosage adjustments provided in the manufacturer's labeling.
  Hepatic Impairment There are no dosage adjustments provided in the manufacturer's labeling.
  Additional Information Complete prescribing information should be consulted for additional detail.
  Dosage Forms Excipient information presented when available (limited, particularly for generics); consult specific product labeling. [DSC] = Discontinued product
  Syrup, Oral, as maleate:
    Generic: 2 mg/5 mL (473 mL [DSC])

◆ Dexchlorpheniramine Maleate *see* Dexchlorpheniramine *on page 528*
◆ Dexchlorpheniramine Tannate, Pseudoephedrine Tannate, and Dextromethorphan Tannate *see* Chlorpheniramine, Pseudoephedrine, and Dextromethorphan *on page 379*
◆ Dexedrine *see* Dextroamphetamine *on page 532*
◆ Dexferrum [DSC] *see* Iron Dextran Complex *on page 986*
◆ Dexilant *see* Dexlansoprazole *on page 528*
◆ Dexiron (Can) *see* Iron Dextran Complex *on page 986*

Dexlansoprazole (deks lan SOE pra zole)

Brand Names: US Dexilant
Brand Names: Canada Dexilant
Index Terms Kapidex; TAK-390MR
Pharmacologic Category Proton Pump Inhibitor; Substituted Benzimidazole

Use

Erosive esophagitis: Healing of all grades of erosive esophagitis for up to 8 weeks; to maintain healing of erosive esophagitis and relief of heartburn for up to 6 months.

Gastroesophageal reflux disease: Treatment of heartburn associated with symptomatic nonerosive gastroesophageal reflux disease (GERD) for 4 weeks.

Medication Guide Available Yes

Dosing

Adult & Geriatric

Erosive esophagitis (EE): Oral: Short-term treatment: 60 mg once daily for up to 8 weeks; maintenance of healed EE and symptomatic relief of heartburn: 30 mg once daily for up to 6 months. **Note:** Doses >30 mg do not provide additional benefit during maintenance phase.

Symptomatic GERD: Oral: Short-term treatment: 30 mg once daily for 4 weeks. **Note:** Doses >30 mg do not provide additional benefit during maintenance phase.

Renal Impairment No dosage adjustment necessary

Hepatic Impairment

Mild hepatic impairment (Child-Pugh class A): No dosage adjustment necessary

Moderate hepatic impairment (Child-Pugh class B): Consider a maximum dose of 30 mg once daily

Severe hepatic impairment (Child-Pugh class C): There are no dosage adjustments provided in the manufacturer's labeling (has not been studied).

Additional Information Complete prescribing information should be consulted for additional detail.

Dosage Forms Excipient information presented when available (limited, particularly for generics); consult specific product labeling.

Capsule Delayed Release, Oral:

Dexilant: 30 mg, 60 mg [contains fd&c blue #2 aluminum lake]

Dexmedetomidine (deks MED e toe mi deen)

Brand Names: US Precedex

Brand Names: Canada Precedex

Index Terms Dexmedetomidine Hydrochloride

Pharmacologic Category Alpha$_2$-Adrenergic Agonist; Sedative

Use

Intensive care unit sedation: Sedation of initially-intubated and mechanically-ventilated patients during treatment in an intensive care setting.

Procedural sedation: Procedural sedation prior to and/or during awake fiberoptic intubation; sedation prior to and/or during surgical or other procedures of nonintubated patients

Pregnancy Considerations Adverse effects were observed in some animal reproduction studies. Dexmedetomidine is expected to cross the placenta. Information related to use during pregnancy is limited (El-Tahan, 2012).

Breast-Feeding Considerations It is not known if dexmedetomidine is excreted in breast milk. The manufacturer recommends that caution be exercised when administering dexmedetomidine to nursing women.

Contraindications

There are no contraindications listed in the U.S. manufacturer's labeling.

Canadian labeling: Hypersensitivity to dexmedetomidine or any component of the formulation.

Warnings/Precautions Should be administered only by persons skilled in management of patients in intensive care setting or operating room. Patients should be continuously monitored. Episodes of bradycardia, hypotension, and sinus arrest have been associated with dexmedetomidine. At low concentrations, mean arterial pressure (MAP) may be reduced without changes in other hemodynamic parameters (eg, pulmonary artery occlusion pressure [PAOP]); however, at higher concentrations (>1.9 ng/mL), MAP, CVP, PAOP, PVR, and SVR increase (Ebert, 2000). Use caution in patients with heart block, severe ventricular dysfunction, hypovolemia, diabetes, chronic hypertension, and elderly. Use with caution in patients with hepatic impairment; dosage reductions recommended. Use with caution in patients receiving vasodilators or drugs which decrease heart rate. If medical intervention is required, treatment may include stopping or decreasing the infusion; increasing the rate of IV fluid administration, use of pressor agents, and elevation of the lower extremities. Transient hypertension has been primarily observed during the loading dose administration and is associated with the initial peripheral vasoconstrictive effects of dexmedetomidine. Treatment is generally unnecessary; however, reduction of infusion rate may be required. Patients

may be arousable and alert when stimulated. This alone should not be considered as lack of efficacy in the absence of other clinical signs/symptoms. When withdrawn abruptly in patients who have received >24 hours of therapy, withdrawal symptoms similar to clonidine withdrawal may result (eg, hypertension, tachycardia, nervousness, nausea, vomiting, agitation, headaches). Use for >24 hours is not recommended by the manufacturer. Use of infusions >24 hours has been associated with tolerance and tachyphylaxis and dose-related increase in adverse reactions.

Adverse Reactions Frequency dependent upon dose, duration, and indication.

>10%:

Cardiovascular: Hypotension (24% to 56%), bradycardia (5% to 42%), systolic hypertension (28%), tachycardia (25%), hypertension (diastolic; 12%), hypertension (11%)

Central nervous system: Agitation (5% to 14%)

Gastrointestinal: Constipation (6% to 14%), nausea (3% to 11%)

Respiratory: Respiratory depression (37%; placebo 32%)

1% to 10%:

Cardiovascular: Atrial fibrillation (2% to 9%), peripheral edema (3% to 7%), hypovolemia (3%), edema (2%)

Central nervous system: Anxiety (5% to 9%)

Endocrine & metabolic: Hypokalemia (9%), hyperglycemia (7%), hypoglycemia (5%), increased thirst (2%), hypocalcemia (1%), hypomagnesemia (1%)

Gastrointestinal: Xerostomia (3% to 4%)

Genitourinary: Oliguria (2%)

Hematologic & oncologic: Anemia (3%)

Renal: Acute renal failure (2% to 3%), decreased urine output (1%)

Respiratory: Respiratory failure (2% to 10%), adult respiratory distress syndrome (1% to 9%), pleural effusion (2%), wheezing (≤1%)

Miscellaneous: Fever (5% to 7%), withdrawal syndrome (ICU sedation; 3% to 5%)

Postmarketing and/or case reports (Limited to important or life-threatening): Acidosis, apnea, atrioventricular block, bronchospasm, cardiac arrest, cardiac disease, chills, confusion, convulsions, decreased visual acuity, delirium, drug tolerance (use >24 hours), extrasystoles, hallucination, heart block, hemorrhage, hepatic insufficiency, hyperbilirubinemia, hypercapnia, hyperkalemia, hyperpyrexia, hypoxia, increased blood urea nitrogen, increased gamma-glutamyl transferase, increased serum alkaline phosphatase, increased serum ALT, increased serum AST, inversion T wave on ECG, myocardial infarction, neuralgia, neuritis, oliguria, photopsia, pulmonary congestion, respiratory acidosis, rigors, seizure, sinoatrial arrest, speech disturbance, supraventricular tachycardia, tachyphylaxis (use >24 hours), variable blood pressure, ventricular arrhythmia, ventricular tachycardia, visual disturbance

Drug Interactions

Metabolism/Transport Effects Substrate of CYP2A6 (major); **Note:** Assignment of Major/Minor substrate status based on clinically relevant drug interaction potential; **Inhibits** CYP1A2 (weak), CYP2C9 (weak)

Avoid Concomitant Use

Avoid concomitant use of Dexmedetomidine with any of the following: Ceritinib; Iobenguane I 123

Increased Effect/Toxicity

Dexmedetomidine may increase the levels/effects of: Amifostine; Antipsychotic Agents (Second Generation [Atypical]); Beta-Blockers; Bradycardia-Causing Agents; Ceritinib; DULoxetine; Hypotension-Associated Agents; Ivabradine; Lacosamide; Levodopa; TiZANidine

The levels/effects of Dexmedetomidine may be increased by: Alfuzosin; Barbiturates; Beta-Blockers; Blood Pressure Lowering Agents; Bretylium; Brimonidine (Topical); CYP2A6 Inhibitors (Moderate); CYP2A6 Inhibitors (Strong); Diazoxide; Herbs (Hypotensive Properties); Molsidomine; Nicorandil; Obinutuzumab; Pentoxifylline; Phosphodiesterase 5 Inhibitors; Prostacyclin Analogues; Ruxolitinib; Tofacitinib

Decreased Effect

Dexmedetomidine may decrease the levels/effects of: Iobenguane I 123

The levels/effects of Dexmedetomidine may be decreased by: Mirtazapine; Serotonin/Norepinephrine Reuptake Inhibitors; Tricyclic Antidepressants

Preparation for Administration Dexmedetomidine injection concentrate (100 mcg/mL) must be diluted in sodium chloride 0.9% solution to achieve the required concentration (4 mcg/mL) prior to administration. Add 2 mL (200 mcg) of dexmedetomidine to 48 mL of sodium chloride 0.9% for a total volume of 50 mL (4 mcg/mL). Shake gently to mix.

◄ **Storage/Stability** Store at controlled room temperature of 25°C (77°F); excursions permitted to 15°C to 30°C (59°F to 86°F). The Canadian labeling indicates that following dilution of dexmedetomidine concentrate (100 mcg/mL) in sodium chloride 0.9% to a concentration of 4 mcg/mL, the resultant solution is stable for 25 hours at 15°C to 30°C (59°F to 86°F).

Mechanism of Action Selective alpha$_2$-adrenoceptor agonist with anesthetic and sedative properties thought to be due to activation of G-proteins by alpha$_{2a}$-adrenoceptors in the brainstem resulting in inhibition of norepinephrine release; peripheral alpha$_{2b}$-adrenoceptors are activated at high doses or with rapid IV administration resulting in vasoconstriction.

Pharmacodynamics/Kinetics

Onset of action: IV Bolus: 5 to 10 minutes
Peak effect: 15 to 30 minutes
Duration (dose dependent): 60 to 120 minutes
Distribution: V_{ss}: ~118 L; rapid
Protein binding: ~94%
Metabolism: Hepatic via N-glucuronidation, N-methylation, and CYP2A6
Half-life elimination: Distribution: ~6 minutes; Terminal: ~up to 3 hours (Venn, 2002); significantly prolonged in patients with severe hepatic impairment (Cunningham, 1999)
Excretion: Urine (95%); feces (4%)
Clearance: Adults: 39 L/hour; hepatic impairment (Child-Pugh Class A, B, or C): mean clearance values were 74%, 64%, and 53% respectively, of those observed in healthy adults; clearance at birth is approximately 30% of adults, reaching adult values between 6-12 months of age

Dosing

Adult Note: Errors have occurred due to misinterpretation of dosing information. Maintenance dose expressed as mcg/**hour**. Individualized and titrated to desired clinical effect. At recommended doses, dexmedetomidine does not provide adequate and reliable amnesia (when necessary); therefore, use of additional agents with amnestic properties (eg, benzodiazepines) may be necessary (Ebert, 2000).

ICU sedation: IV: Initial: Loading infusion (optional; see **"Note"** below) of 1 mcg/kg over 10 minutes (U.S. labeling) or 20 minutes (Canadian labeling), followed by a maintenance infusion (see **"Note"** below) of 0.2 to 0.7 mcg/kg/**hour**; adjust rate to desired level of sedation; titration no more frequently than every 30 minutes may reduce the incidence of hypotension (Gerlach, 2009)
Note: *Loading infusion:* The loading dose may be omitted for this indication if patient is either being converted from another sedative and patient is adequately sedated or there are concerns for hemodynamic compromise. *Maintenance infusion:* Dosing ranges between 0.2 to 1.4 mcg/kg/**hour** have been reported during randomized controlled clinical trials (Pandharipande, 2007; Riker, 2009). Although infusion rates as high as 2.5 mcg/kg/**hour** have been used, it is thought that doses >1.5 mcg/kg/**hour** do not add to clinical efficacy (Venn, 2003). Manufacturer recommends duration of infusion should not exceed 24 hours; however, randomized clinical trials have demonstrated efficacy and safety comparable to lorazepam and midazolam with longer-term infusions of up to ~5 days (Pandharipande, 2007; Riker, 2009).
Procedural sedation: IV: Initial: Loading infusion of 1 mcg/kg (or 0.5 mcg/kg for less invasive procedures [eg, ophthalmic]) over 10 minutes, followed by a maintenance infusion of 0.6 mcg/kg/**hour**, titrate to desired effect; usual range: 0.2 to 1 mcg/kg/**hour**
Fiberoptic intubation (awake): IV: Initial: Loading infusion of 1 mcg/kg over 10 minutes, followed by a maintenance infusion of 0.7 mcg/kg/**hour** until endotracheal tube is secured (Bergese, 2010).
Craniotomy (awake) (off-label use): IV: Initial: Loading infusion of 1 mcg/kg over 10 minutes, followed by a maintenance infusion of 0.5 mcg/kg/**hour**, titrate to desired effect (Bekker, 2008); usual range: 0.1 to 0.7 mcg/kg/**hour** (Piccioni, 2008)

Geriatric
ICU sedation: IV: Refer to adult dosing. Consider dosage reduction. No specific guidelines available. Dose selections should be cautious, at the low end of dosage range; titration should be slower, allowing adequate time to evaluate response.
Procedural sedation: IV: Refer to adult dosing: Initial: Loading infusion of 0.5 mcg/kg over 10 minutes; Maintenance infusion: Dosage reduction should be considered.

Renal Impairment There are no dosage adjustments provided in the manufacturer's labeling; however, dexmedetomidine pharmacokinetics were not significantly different in patients with severe renal impairment compared to those with normal renal function.

Hepatic Impairment The manufacturer labeling recommends considering a dose reduction but does not provide specific dosing recommendations. Clearance is reduced in varying degrees based on the level of impairment.

Usual Infusion Concentrations: Pediatric IV infusion: 4 mcg/mL

Usual Infusion Concentrations: Adult IV infusion: 200 mcg in 50 mL (concentration: 4 mcg/mL) of NS

Administration Administer using a controlled infusion device. Advisable to use administration components made with synthetic or coated natural rubber gaskets. Parenteral products should be inspected visually for particulate matter and discoloration prior to administration. If loading dose used, administer over 10 minutes; may extend to 20 minutes to further reduce vasoconstrictive effects. Titration no more frequently than every 30 minutes may reduce the incidence of hypotension when used for ICU sedation (Gerlach, 2009).

Monitoring Parameters Level of sedation; heart rate, respiration, rhythm, blood pressure; pain control. **Note:** Dexmedetomidine causes minimal respiratory depression, inhibits salivation, and is analgesic-sparing.

Critically-ill mechanically ventilated patients: Monitor depth of sedation with either the Richmond Agitation-Sedation Scale (RASS) or Sedation-Agitation Scale (SAS) (Barr, 2013)

Dosage Forms Excipient information presented when available (limited, particularly for generics); consult specific product labeling.
Solution, Intravenous [preservative free]:
Precedex: 200 mcg/2 mL (2 mL) [additive free]
Precedex: 200 mcg/50 mL (50 mL); 400 mcg/100 mL (100 mL) [latex free]
Precedex: 80 mcg/20 mL (20 mL)
Generic: 200 mcg/2 mL (2 mL)

◆ **Dexmedetomidine Hydrochloride** *see* Dexmedetomidine *on page 529*

Dexmethylphenidate (dex meth il FEN i date)

Brand Names: US Focalin; Focalin XR
Index Terms Dexmethylphenidate Hydrochloride
Pharmacologic Category Central Nervous System Stimulant
Use Attention-deficit/hyperactivity disorder: Treatment of attention-deficit/hyperactivity disorder (ADHD) in patients ≥6 years
Medication Guide Available Yes
Dosing
Adult & Geriatric
ADHD: Patients not currently taking methylphenidate or who are on other stimulants: Oral:
Immediate release: Initial: 2.5 mg twice daily; dosage may be adjusted in increments of 2.5 to 5 mg at weekly intervals (maximum dose: 20 mg/day)
Extended release: Initial: 10 mg once daily; dosage may be adjusted in increments of 10 mg at weekly intervals (maximum dose: 40 mg/day)

Conversion to dexmethylphenidate from methylphenidate: *Immediate release and extended release:* Initial: One-half the total daily dose of racemic methylphenidate

Conversion from dexmethylphenidate immediate release to dexmethylphenidate extended release: Patients currently using dexmethylphenidate immediate-release may be switched to the same daily dose of dexmethylphenidate extended-release.

Dose reductions and discontinuation: Reduce dose or discontinue in patients with paradoxical aggravation of symptoms. Discontinue if no improvement is seen after one month of treatment.

Pediatric
ADHD: Children ≥6 years and Adolescents: Patients not currently taking methylphenidate or who are on other stimulants: Oral:
Immediate release: Initial: 2.5 mg twice daily; dosage may be adjusted in increments of 2.5 to 5 mg at weekly intervals (maximum dose: 20 mg/day)
Extended release: Initial: 5 mg once daily; dosage may be adjusted in increments of 5 mg at weekly intervals (maximum dose: 30 mg/day)

Conversion to dexmethylphenidate from methylphenidate: *Immediate release and extended release:* Initial: Refer to adult dosing.

Conversion from dexmethylphenidate immediate release to dexmethylphenidate extended release: Refer to adult dosing.

Dose reductions and discontinuation: Refer to adult dosing.

Renal Impairment There are no dosage adjustments provided in the manufacturer's labeling (has not been studied). However, considering extensive metabolism to inactive compounds, renal insufficiency expected to have minimal effect on kinetics of dexmethylphenidate.

Hepatic Impairment There are no dosage adjustments provided in the manufacturer's labeling (has not been studied).

Additional Information Complete prescribing information should be consulted for additional detail.

Dosage Forms Excipient information presented when available (limited, particularly for generics); consult specific product labeling.

Capsule Extended Release 24 Hour, Oral, as hydrochloride:
Focalin XR: 5 mg [contains fd&c blue #2 (indigotine)]
Focalin XR: 10 mg
Focalin XR: 15 mg [contains fd&c blue #2 (indigotine)]
Focalin XR: 20 mg
Focalin XR: 25 mg [contains fd&c blue #2 (indigotine)]
Focalin XR: 30 mg
Focalin XR: 35 mg, 40 mg [contains fd&c blue #2 (indigotine)]
Generic: 5 mg, 10 mg, 15 mg, 20 mg, 30 mg, 40 mg
Tablet, Oral, as hydrochloride:
Focalin: 2.5 mg, 5 mg, 10 mg
Generic: 2.5 mg, 5 mg, 10 mg

Controlled Substance C-II

◆ **Dexmethylphenidate Hydrochloride** see Dexmethylphenidate on page 530

◆ **DexPak 6 Day** see Dexamethasone (Systemic) on page 525

◆ **DexPak 10 Day** see Dexamethasone (Systemic) on page 525

◆ **DexPak 13 Day** see Dexamethasone (Systemic) on page 525

Dexpanthenol (deks PAN the nole)

Index Terms Pantothenyl Alcohol

Pharmacologic Category Gastrointestinal Agent, Stimulant; Topical Skin Product

Use Prophylactic use to minimize paralytic ileus; treatment of postoperative distention; topical to relieve itching and to aid healing of minor dermatoses

Dosing
Adult & Geriatric
Prevention of postoperative ileus: IM: 250-500 mg stat, repeat in 2 hours, followed by doses every 6 hours until danger passes
Paralytic ileus: IM: 500 mg stat, repeat in 2 hours, followed by doses every 6 hours, if needed
Renal Impairment No dosage adjustment provided in manufacturer's labeling.
Hepatic Impairment No dosage adjustment provided in manufacturer's labeling.

Additional Information Complete prescribing information should be consulted for additional detail.

Dosage Forms Excipient information presented when available (limited, particularly for generics); consult specific product labeling. [DSC] = Discontinued product
Solution, Injection:
Generic: 250 mg/mL (2 mL [DSC])

Dexrazoxane (deks ray ZOKS ane)

Brand Names: US Totect; Zinecard
Brand Names: Canada Zinecard
Index Terms ICRF-187
Pharmacologic Category Antidote; Antidote, Extravasation; Chemoprotective Agent
Use
Prevention of cardiomyopathy associated with doxorubicin (Zinecard, generic products): To reduce the incidence and severity of cardiomyopathy associated with doxorubicin administration in women with metastatic breast cancer who have received a cumulative doxorubicin dose of 300 mg/m^2 and will benefit from continuing doxorubicin therapy to maintain tumor control. Not recommended for use with initial doxorubicin therapy.
Extravasation of anthracyclines (Totect): Treatment of extravasation resulting from intravenous anthracycline chemotherapy.

Dosing
Adult & Geriatric
Prevention of doxorubicin cardiomyopathy: IV: A 10:1 ratio of dexrazoxane:doxorubicin (dexrazoxane 500 mg/m^2:doxorubicin 50 mg/m^2). **Note:** Cardiac monitoring should continue during dexrazoxane therapy; doxorubicin/dexrazoxane should be discontinued in patients who develop a decline in LVEF or clinical CHF.
Treatment of anthracycline extravasation: IV: 1000 mg/m^2 on days 1 and 2 (maximum dose: 2000 mg), followed by 500 mg/m^2 on day 3 (maximum dose: 1000 mg); begin treatment as soon as possible, within 6 hours of extravasation
Pediatric Prevention of doxorubicin cardiomyopathy associated with acute lymphoblastic leukemia treatment (high-risk patients; off-label use): IV: A 10:1 ratio of dexrazoxane:doxorubicin (eg, dexrazoxane 300 mg/m^2:doxorubicin 30 mg/m^2) was used in patients with high-risk acute lymphoblastic leukemia; dexrazoxane is administered immediately prior to the doxorubicin dose (Lipshultz, 2010; Moghrabi, 2007; Silverman, 2010)
Renal Impairment Note: Renal function may be estimated using the Cockcroft-Gault formula.
Mild (CrCl ≥40 mL/minute) impairment: No dosage adjustment necessary.
Moderate-to-severe (CrCl <40 mL/minute) impairment:
Prevention of cardiomyopathy: Reduce dose by 50%, using a 5:1 dexrazoxane:doxorubicin ratio (dexrazoxane 250 mg/m^2:doxorubicin 50 mg/m^2)
Anthracycline extravasation: Reduce dose by 50%
Hepatic Impairment
Prevention of cardiomyopathy: Since doxorubicin dosage is reduced in hyperbilirubinemia, a proportional reduction in dexrazoxane dosage is recommended (maintain a 10:1 ratio of dexrazoxane:doxorubicin)
Anthracycline extravasation: There are no dosage adjustments provided in the manufacturer's labeling (has not been studied).
Additional Information Complete prescribing information should be consulted for additional detail.
Dosage Forms Excipient information presented when available (limited, particularly for generics); consult specific product labeling.
Solution Reconstituted, Intravenous:
Totect: 500 mg (1 ea) [pyrogen free]
Zinecard: 250 mg (1 ea); 500 mg (1 ea) [pyrogen free]
Generic: 250 mg (1 ea); 500 mg (1 ea)

Dextran (DEKS tran)

Brand Names: US LMD in D5W; LMD in NaCl
Index Terms 10% LMD; Dextran 40; Dextran, Low Molecular Weight
Pharmacologic Category Plasma Volume Expander, Colloid
Use Blood volume expander used in treatment of shock or impending shock when blood or blood products are not available; also used as a priming fluid in pump oxygenators during cardiopulmonary bypass and for prophylaxis of venous thrombosis and pulmonary embolism in surgical procedures associated with a high risk of thromboembolic complications
Dosing
Adult & Geriatric
Volume expansion/shock: IV: Dextran 40: Infuse 500-1000 mL (~10 mL/kg) as rapidly as possible (maximum: 20 mL/kg/day for first 24 hours; 10 mL/kg/day thereafter); therapy should not be continued beyond 5 days
Pump prime: Dextran 40: Varies with the volume of the pump oxygenator; generally, the solution is added in a dose of 10-20 mL/kg (or 1-2 g/kg); usual maximum total dose: 20 mL/kg (or 2 g/kg)
Postoperative prophylaxis of venous thrombosis/pulmonary embolism: Dextran 40: **Note:** Current ACCP guidelines for the prevention of venous thromboembolism in surgical patients do not recommend the use of dextran; consider the use of other anticoagulants (Falck-Ytter, 2012; Gould, 2012). Per the manufacturer, begin during surgical procedure and give 500-1000 mL (~10 mL/kg); continue treatment with 500 mL once daily for 2-3 additional days. Additional 500 mL doses may be administered every 2-3 days during the period of risk (up to 2 weeks postoperatively).
Pediatric Treatment of shock or impending shock (when blood or blood products are not available): IV: Dextran 40: Infuse 10 mL/kg as rapidly as possible (maximum: 20 mL/kg/day for the first 24 hours; 10 mL/kg/day thereafter); therapy should not be continued beyond 5 days
Renal Impairment Use with extreme caution.

Hepatic Impairment Use with extreme caution.
Additional Information Complete prescribing information should be consulted for additional detail.
Dosage Forms Excipient information presented when available (limited, particularly for generics); consult specific product labeling.
Solution, Intravenous:
LMD in D5W: 10% Dextran 40 (500 mL) [latex free]
LMD in NaCl: 10% Dextran 40 (500 mL) [latex free]

◆ Dextran 40 *see* Dextran *on page 531*

◆ Dextran, Low Molecular Weight *see* Dextran *on page 531*

◆ Dextrin *see* Wheat Dextrin *on page 1921*

Dextroamphetamine (deks troe am FET a meen)

Brand Names: US Dexedrine; ProCentra; Zenzedi
Brand Names: Canada Dexedrine
Index Terms Dextroamphetamine Sulfate
Pharmacologic Category Central Nervous System Stimulant
Use
Attention-deficit/hyperactivity disorder: Treatment of attention-deficit/hyperactivity disorder (ADHD) as part of a total treatment program that typically includes other remedial measures (psychological, educational, social) for a stabilizing effect in children 3 to 16 years of age.
Narcolepsy: Treatment of narcolepsy.
Pregnancy Considerations Adverse effects have been observed in animal reproduction studies. The majority of human data is based on illicit amphetamine/methamphetamine exposure and not from therapeutic maternal use (Golub, 2005). Use of amphetamines during pregnancy may lead to an increased risk of premature birth and low birth weight; newborns may experience symptoms of withdrawal. Behavioral problems may also occur later in childhood (LaGasse, 2012).
Breast-Feeding Considerations The majority of human data is based on illicit amphetamine/methamphetamine exposure and not from therapeutic maternal use (Golub, 2005). Amphetamines are excreted into breast milk and use may decrease milk production. Increased irritability, agitation, and crying have been reported in nursing infants (ACOG, 2011). The manufacturer recommends that mothers taking dextroamphetamine refrain from nursing.
Medication Guide Available Yes
Contraindications
Hypersensitivity or idiosyncrasy to dextroamphetamine, other sympathomimetic amines, or any component of the formulation; advanced arteriosclerosis, symptomatic cardiovascular disease, moderate-to-severe hypertension; hyperthyroidism; glaucoma; agitated states; patients with a history of drug abuse; during or within 14 days following MAO inhibitor therapy.
Documentation of allergenic cross-reactivity for amphetamines is limited. However, because of similarities in chemical structure and/or pharmacologic actions, the possibility of cross-sensitivity cannot be ruled out with certainty.
Warnings/Precautions [U.S. Boxed Warning]: Use has been associated with serious cardiovascular events including sudden death in patients with preexisting structural cardiac abnormalities or other serious heart problems (sudden death in children and adolescents; sudden death, stroke and MI in adults. These products should be avoided in the patients with known serious structural cardiac abnormalities, cardiomyopathy, serious heart rhythm abnormalities, or other serious cardiac problems that could increase the risk of sudden death that these conditions alone carry. Patients should be carefully evaluated for cardiac disease prior to initiation of therapy. Patients who develop symptoms such as exertional chest pain, unexplained syncope, or other symptoms suggestive of cardiac disease during treatment should undergo a prompt cardiac evaluation. Use with caution in patients with hypertension and other cardiovascular conditions that might be exacerbated by increases in blood pressure or heart rate. Amphetamines may impair the ability to engage in potentially hazardous activities. May cause visual disturbances. Stimulants are associated with peripheral vasculopathy, including Raynaud's phenomenon; signs/symptoms are usually mild and intermittent, and generally improve with dose reduction or discontinuation. Digital ulceration and/or soft tissue breakdown have been observed rarely; monitor for digital changes during therapy and seek further evaluation (eg, rheumatology) if necessary.

Limited information exists regarding amphetamine use in seizure disorder (Cortese, 2013). The manufacturer recommends use with caution in patients with a history of seizure disorder; may lower seizure threshold leading to new onset or breakthrough seizure activity. Use with caution in patients with preexisting psychosis or bipolar disorder. May exacerbate symptoms of behavior and thought disorder or induce mixed/manic episode, respectively. New onset psychosis or mania may also occur with stimulant use. Observe for symptoms of aggression and/or hostility. Stimulants may exacerbate tics (motor and phonic) and Tourette syndrome. Evaluate for tics and Tourette syndrome prior to therapy initiation. **[U.S. Boxed Warning]: Potential for drug dependency exists; prolonged use may lead to drug dependency.** Use is contraindicated in patients with history of ethanol or drug abuse. Prescriptions should be written for the smallest quantity consistent with good patient care to minimize possibility of overdose. Abrupt discontinuation following high doses or for prolonged periods may result in symptoms for withdrawal.

Use caution in the elderly due to CNS stimulant adverse effects. Appetite suppression may occur, particularly in children. Use of stimulants has been associated with weight loss and slowing of growth rate; monitor growth rate and weight during treatment. Treatment interruption may be necessary in patients who are not increasing in height or gaining weight as expected.

Benzyl alcohol and derivatives: Some dosage forms may contain sodium benzoate/benzoic acid; benzoic acid (benzoate) is a metabolite of benzyl alcohol; large amounts of benzyl alcohol (≥99 mg/kg/day) have been associated with a potentially fatal toxicity ("gasping syndrome") in neonates; the "gasping syndrome" consists of metabolic acidosis, respiratory distress, gasping respirations, CNS dysfunction (including convulsions, intracranial hemorrhage), hypotension, and cardiovascular collapse (AAP ["Inactive" 1997]; CDC, 1982); some data suggests that benzoate displaces bilirubin from protein binding sites (Ahlfors, 2001); avoid or use dosage forms containing benzyl alcohol derivative with caution in neonates. See manufacturer's labeling.
Adverse Reactions Frequency not defined.
Cardiovascular: Cardiomyopathy, hypertension, palpitations, tachycardia
Central nervous system: Aggressive behavior, dizziness, dysphoria, euphoria, exacerbation of tics, Gilles de la Tourette's syndrome, headache, insomnia, mania, over-stimulation, psychosis, restlessness
Dermatologic: Urticaria
Endocrine & metabolic: Change in libido, weight loss
Gastrointestinal: Anorexia, constipation, diarrhea, unpleasant taste, xerostomia
Genitourinary: Frequent erections, impotence, prolonged erection
Neuromuscular & skeletal: Dyskinesia, rhabdomyolysis, tremor
Ophthalmic: Accommodation disturbances, blurred vision
Drug Interactions
Metabolism/Transport Effects Substrate of CYP2D6 (minor); **Note:** Assignment of Major/Minor substrate status based on clinically relevant drug interaction potential
Avoid Concomitant Use
Avoid concomitant use of Dextroamphetamine with any of the following: Iobenguane I 123; MAO Inhibitors
Increased Effect/Toxicity
Dextroamphetamine may increase the levels/effects of: Analgesics (Opioid); Doxofylline; Sympathomimetics

The levels/effects of Dextroamphetamine may be increased by: Alkalinizing Agents; Antacids; AtoMOXetine; Cannabinoid-Containing Products; Carbonic Anhydrase Inhibitors; Linezolid; MAO Inhibitors; Proton Pump Inhibitors; Tedizolid; Tricyclic Antidepressants
Decreased Effect
Dextroamphetamine may decrease the levels/effects of: Antihistamines; Antihypertensive Agents; Ethosuximide; Iobenguane I 123; Ioflupane I 123; PHENobarbital; Phenytoin

The levels/effects of Dextroamphetamine may be decreased by: Ammonium Chloride; Antipsychotic Agents; Ascorbic Acid; Gastrointestinal Acidifying Agents; Lithium; Methenamine; Multivitamins/Fluoride (with ADE); Multivitamins/Minerals (with ADEK, Folate, Iron); Multivitamins/Minerals (with AE, No Iron); Urinary Acidifying Agents
Food Interactions Amphetamine serum levels may be reduced if taken with acidic food, juices, or vitamin C. Management: Monitor response when taken concurrently.
Storage/Stability Store at 20°C to 25°C (68°F to 77°F). Protect from light.
Mechanism of Action Amphetamines are noncatecholamine, sympathomimetic amines that promote release of catecholamines (primarily dopamine and norepinephrine)

from their storage sites in the presynaptic nerve terminals. A less significant mechanism may include their ability to block the reuptake of catecholamines by competitive inhibition.

Pharmacodynamics/Kinetics
Duration of action: Immediate release: 4 to 6 hours; extended release: 8 hours (Dopheide 2009)
Metabolism: Hepatic via CYP monooxygenase and glucuronidation
Half-life elimination: Adults: 10 to 12 hours
Time to peak, serum: Immediate release: ~3 hours; Sustained release: ~8 hours
Excretion: Urine; urinary excretion is pH dependent and is increased with acid urine (low pH)

Dosing
Adult
Narcolepsy: Oral: Initial: 10 mg once daily; may increase in increments of 10 mg at weekly intervals until optimal response is obtained; usual dosage: 5 to 60 mg daily in divided doses.
Geriatric Refer to adult dosing; start at lowest dose. Use with caution.

Pediatric
Attention-deficit/hyperactivity disorder (ADHD):
Children 3 to 5 years: Oral: Immediate release tablets and oral solution: Initial: 2.5 once daily; may increase in increments of 2.5 mg at weekly intervals until optimal response is obtained; maximum dose: 40 mg daily (Dopheide 2009). Note: Although FDA approved, current guidelines do not recommend use in children ≤5 years due to insufficient evidence (AAP, 2011).
Children ≥6 years and Adolescents: Oral:
Immediate release tablets and oral solution: Initial: 5 mg once or twice daily; may increase in increments of 5 mg at weekly intervals until optimal response is reached; maximum dose: 40 mg daily (Dopheide 2009).
Extended release capsules: Initial: 5 mg once or twice daily; may increase in increments of 5 mg at weekly intervals until optimal response is reached. Maximum dose: 40 mg daily (Dopheide 2009); a maximum daily dose of 60 mg in divided doses has been used in children >50 kg (Dopheide, 2009; Pliszka 2007).
Narcolepsy:
Children 6 to 12 years: Oral: Initial: 5 mg once daily; may increase in increments of 5 mg at weekly intervals until optimal response is obtained; usual dosage: 5 to 60 mg daily in divided doses.
Children >12 years and Adolescents: Refer to adult dosing.
Renal Impairment There are no dosage adjustments provided in the manufacturer's labeling.
Hepatic Impairment There are no dosage adjustments provided in the manufacturer's labeling.
Administration Administer initial dose upon awakening; do not administer doses late in the evening due to potential for insomnia.
Immediate release tablets and oral solution: If needed, 1 to 2 additional doses may be administered at intervals of 4 to 6 hours.
Extended release and sustained release capsules: Do not crush sustained release drug products. Formulations may be used for once-daily administration, if appropriate.
Monitoring Parameters Cardiac evaluation should be completed on any patient who develops exertional chest pain, unexplained syncope, and any symptom of cardiac disease during treatment with stimulants; behavioral changes; signs of peripheral vasculopathy (eg, digital changes); growth and weight in children; CNS activity in all patients; signs of misuse, abuse, or addiction.

When used for the treatment of ADHD, thoroughly evaluate for cardiovascular risk. Monitor heart rate, blood pressure, and consider obtaining ECG prior to initiation (Vetter, 2008).
Test Interactions Amphetamines may elevate plasma corticosteroid levels; may interfere with urinary steroid determinations.
Dosage Forms Excipient information presented when available (limited, particularly for generics); consult specific product labeling.
Capsule Extended Release 24 Hour, Oral, as sulfate:
Dexedrine: 5 mg, 10 mg, 15 mg [contains brilliant blue fcf (fd&c blue #1), fd&c blue #1 aluminum lake, fd&c red #40, fd&c yellow #10 (quinoline yellow), fd&c yellow #6 (sunset yellow)]
Generic: 5 mg, 10 mg, 15 mg
Solution, Oral, as sulfate:
ProCentra: 5 mg/5 mL (473 mL) [contains benzoic acid, saccharin sodium; bubble-gum flavor]
Generic: 5 mg/5 mL (473 mL)

Tablet, Oral, as sulfate:
Dexedrine: 5 mg, 10 mg [scored]
Zenzedi: 2.5 mg
Zenzedi: 5 mg [scored; contains fd&c yellow #6 (sunset yellow)]
Zenzedi: 7.5 mg [contains brilliant blue fcf (fd&c blue #1), fd&c yellow #10 (quinoline yellow)]
Zenzedi: 10 mg [scored; contains fd&c blue #2 (indigotine), fd&c red #40, fd&c yellow #6 (sunset yellow)]
Zenzedi: 15 mg [contains brilliant blue fcf (fd&c blue #1), fd&c blue #2 (indigotine), fd&c red #40]
Zenzedi: 20 mg [contains brilliant blue fcf (fd&c blue #1)]
Zenzedi: 30 mg [contains fd&c yellow #10 (quinoline yellow)]
Generic: 5 mg, 10 mg
Controlled Substance C-II

Dextroamphetamine and Amphetamine
(deks troe am FET a meen & am FET a meen)

Brand Names: US Adderall; Adderall XR
Brand Names: Canada Adderall XR
Index Terms Amphetamine and Dextroamphetamine
Pharmacologic Category Central Nervous System Stimulant
Use Attention-deficit/hyperactivity disorder (ADHD); narcolepsy
Medication Guide Available Yes
Dosing
Adult & Geriatric Note: Use lowest effective individualized dose; administer first dose as soon as awake.
ADHD: Oral:
Adderall: Initial: 5 mg once or twice daily; increase daily dose in 5 mg increments at weekly intervals until optimal response is obtained; usual maximum dose: 40 mg daily given in 1 to 3 divided doses per day. Use intervals of 4 to 6 hours between additional doses.
Adderall XR: Initial: 20 mg once daily in the morning; higher doses (up to 60 mg once daily) have been evaluated; however, there is not adequate evidence that higher doses afforded additional benefit. The Canadian labeling recommends a maximum dose of 30 mg/day.
Conversion from immediate release to extended release formulation: Patients may be switched from the immediate release formulation to the extended release formulation using the same total daily dose once daily.
Narcolepsy: Adderall: Oral: Initial: 10 mg daily; increase daily dose in 10 mg increments at weekly intervals until optimal response is obtained; maximum dose: 60 mg daily given in 1 to 3 divided doses per day with intervals of 4 to 6 hours between doses.
Pediatric Note: Use lowest effective individualized dose; administer first dose as soon as awake.
ADHD: Oral:
Children: <3 years: Not recommended.
Children: 3 to 5 years (Adderall): Initial: 2.5 mg once daily given every morning; increase daily dose in 2.5 mg increments at weekly intervals until optimal response is obtained; maximum dose: 40 mg daily given in 1 to 3 divided doses per day. Use intervals of 4 to 6 hours between additional doses.
Children: 6 to 12 years:
Adderall: Initial: 5 mg once or twice daily; increase daily dose in 5 mg increments at weekly intervals until optimal response is obtained; usual maximum dose: 40 mg daily given in 1 to 3 divided doses per day. Use intervals of 4 to 6 hours between additional doses.
Adderall XR: 5 to 10 mg once daily in the morning; if needed, may increase daily dose in 5 to 10 mg increments at weekly intervals (maximum dose: 30 mg daily)
Conversion from immediate release to extended release formulation: Patients may be switched from the immediate release formulation to the extended release formulation using the same total daily dose once daily.
Adolescents 13 to 17 years:
Adderall: Initial: 5 mg once or twice daily; increase daily dose in 5 mg increments at weekly intervals until optimal response is obtained (usual maximum dose: 40 mg daily given in 1 to 3 divided doses); use intervals of 4 to 6 hours between additional doses.
Adderall XR: 10 mg once daily in the morning; maybe increased to 20 mg daily after 1 week if symptoms are not controlled; higher doses (up to 60 mg)/day have been evaluated; however, there is not adequate evidence that higher doses afforded additional benefit. The Canadian labeling recommends a maximum dose of 30 mg/day.

Conversion from immediate release to extended release formulation: Patients may be switched from the immediate release formulation to the extended release formulation using the same total daily dose once daily.

Narcolepsy: *Adderall:* Oral:

Children: 6 to 12 years: Initial: 5 mg daily; increase daily dose in 5 mg increments at weekly intervals until optimal response is obtained; maximum dose: 60 mg daily given in 1 to 3 divided doses per day with intervals of 4 to 6 hours between doses.

Children >12 years: Refer to adult dosing.

Renal Impairment

US labeling: There are no dosage adjustments provided in the manufacturer's labeling.

Canadian labeling:

Mild or moderate impairment: There are no dosage adjustments provided in the manufacturer's labeling.

Severe impairment: (GFR 15 to <30 mL/minute/1.73 m²): Maximum dose: 20 mg/day.

Hemodialysis: There are no specific dosage adjustments provided in the manufacturer's labeling; however, the manufacturer recommends considering further dosage reductions (compared to that recommended for severe impairment). Dextroamphetamine is not dialyzable.

Hepatic Impairment There are no dosage adjustments provided in the manufacturer's labeling.

Additional Information Complete prescribing information should be consulted for additional detail.

Dosage Forms Excipient information presented when available (limited, particularly for generics); consult specific product labeling.

Capsule, extended release, oral:

Adderall XR:

5 mg [dextroamphetamine sulfate 1.25 mg, dextroamphetamine saccharate 1.25 mg, amphetamine aspartate monohydrate 1.25 mg, amphetamine sulfate 1.25 mg (equivalent to amphetamine base 3.1 mg)]

10 mg [dextroamphetamine sulfate 2.5 mg, dextroamphetamine saccharate 2.5 mg, amphetamine aspartate monohydrate 2.5 mg, amphetamine sulfate 2.5 mg (equivalent to amphetamine base 6.3 mg)]

15 mg [dextroamphetamine sulfate 3.75 mg, dextroamphetamine saccharate 3.75 mg, amphetamine aspartate monohydrate 3.75 mg, amphetamine sulfate 3.75 mg (equivalent to amphetamine base 9.4 mg)]

20 mg [dextroamphetamine sulfate 5 mg, dextroamphetamine saccharate 5 mg, amphetamine aspartate monohydrate 5 mg, amphetamine sulfate 5 mg (equivalent to amphetamine base 12.5 mg)]

25 mg [dextroamphetamine sulfate 6.25 mg, dextroamphetamine saccharate 6.25 mg, amphetamine aspartate monohydrate 6.25 mg, amphetamine sulfate 6.25 mg (equivalent to amphetamine base 15.6 mg)]

30 mg [dextroamphetamine sulfate 7.5 mg, dextroamphetamine saccharate 7.5 mg, amphetamine aspartate monohydrate 7.5 mg, amphetamine sulfate 7.5 mg (equivalent to amphetamine base 18.8 mg)]

Generic:

5 mg [dextroamphetamine sulfate 1.25 mg, dextroamphetamine saccharate 1.25 mg, amphetamine aspartate monohydrate 1.25 mg, amphetamine sulfate 1.25 mg (equivalent to amphetamine base 3.1 mg)]

10 mg [dextroamphetamine sulfate 2.5 mg, dextroamphetamine saccharate 2.5 mg, amphetamine aspartate monohydrate 2.5 mg, amphetamine sulfate 2.5 mg (equivalent to amphetamine base 6.3 mg)]

15 mg [dextroamphetamine sulfate 3.75 mg, dextroamphetamine saccharate 3.75 mg, amphetamine aspartate monohydrate 3.75 mg, amphetamine sulfate 3.75 mg (equivalent to amphetamine base 9.4 mg)]

20 mg [dextroamphetamine sulfate 5 mg, dextroamphetamine saccharate 5 mg, amphetamine aspartate monohydrate 5 mg, amphetamine sulfate 5 mg (equivalent to amphetamine base 12.5 mg)]

25 mg [dextroamphetamine sulfate 6.25 mg, dextroamphetamine saccharate 6.25 mg, amphetamine aspartate monohydrate 6.25 mg, amphetamine sulfate 6.25 mg (equivalent to amphetamine base 15.6 mg)]

30 mg [dextroamphetamine sulfate 7.5 mg, dextroamphetamine saccharate 7.5 mg, amphetamine aspartate monohydrate 7.5 mg, amphetamine sulfate 7.5 mg (equivalent to amphetamine base 18.8 mg)]

Tablet, oral:

Adderall:

5 mg [dextroamphetamine sulfate 1.25 mg, dextroamphetamine saccharate 1.25 mg, amphetamine aspartate monohydrate 1.25 mg, amphetamine sulfate 1.25 mg (equivalent to amphetamine base 3.13 mg)]

7.5 mg [dextroamphetamine sulfate 1.875 mg, dextroamphetamine saccharate 1.875 mg, amphetamine aspartate monohydrate 1.875 mg, amphetamine sulfate 1.875 mg (equivalent to amphetamine base 4.7 mg)]

10 mg [dextroamphetamine sulfate 2.5 mg, dextroamphetamine saccharate 2.5 mg, amphetamine aspartate monohydrate 2.5 mg, amphetamine sulfate 2.5 mg (equivalent to amphetamine base 6.3 mg)]

12.5 mg [dextroamphetamine sulfate 3.125 mg, dextroamphetamine saccharate 3.125 mg, amphetamine aspartate monohydrate 3.125 mg, amphetamine sulfate 3.125 mg (equivalent to amphetamine base 7.8 mg)]

15 mg [dextroamphetamine sulfate 3.75 mg, dextroamphetamine saccharate 3.75 mg, amphetamine aspartate monohydrate 3.75 mg, amphetamine sulfate 3.75 mg (equivalent to amphetamine base 9.4 mg)]

20 mg [dextroamphetamine sulfate 5 mg, dextroamphetamine saccharate 5 mg, amphetamine aspartate monohydrate 5 mg, amphetamine sulfate 5 mg (equivalent to amphetamine base 12.6 mg)]

30 mg [dextroamphetamine sulfate 7.5 mg, dextroamphetamine saccharate 7.5 mg, amphetamine aspartate monohydrate 7.5 mg, amphetamine sulfate 7.5 mg (equivalent to amphetamine base 18.8 mg)]

Generic:

5 mg [dextroamphetamine sulfate 1.25 mg, dextroamphetamine saccharate 1.25 mg, amphetamine aspartate monohydrate 1.25 mg, amphetamine sulfate 1.25 mg (equivalent to amphetamine base 3.13 mg)]

7.5 mg [dextroamphetamine sulfate 1.875 mg, dextroamphetamine saccharate 1.875 mg, amphetamine aspartate monohydrate 1.875 mg, amphetamine sulfate 1.875 mg (equivalent to amphetamine base 4.7 mg)]

10 mg [dextroamphetamine sulfate 2.5 mg, dextroamphetamine saccharate 2.5 mg, amphetamine aspartate monohydrate 2.5 mg, amphetamine sulfate 2.5 mg (equivalent to amphetamine base 6.3 mg)]

12.5 mg [dextroamphetamine sulfate 3.125 mg, dextroamphetamine saccharate 3.125 mg, amphetamine aspartate monohydrate 3.125 mg, amphetamine sulfate 3.125 mg (equivalent to amphetamine base 7.8 mg)]

15 mg [dextroamphetamine sulfate 3.75 mg, dextroamphetamine saccharate 3.75 mg, amphetamine aspartate monohydrate 3.75 mg, amphetamine sulfate 3.75 mg (equivalent to amphetamine base 9.4 mg)]

20 mg [dextroamphetamine sulfate 5 mg, dextroamphetamine saccharate 5 mg, amphetamine aspartate monohydrate 5 mg, amphetamine sulfate 5 mg (equivalent to amphetamine base 12.6 mg)]

30 mg [dextroamphetamine sulfate 7.5 mg, dextroamphetamine saccharate 7.5 mg, amphetamine aspartate monohydrate 7.5 mg, amphetamine sulfate 7.5 mg (equivalent to amphetamine base 18.8 mg)]

Controlled Substance C-II

♦ Dextroamphetamine Sulfate *see* Dextroamphetamine on page 532

Dextromethorphan and Chlorpheniramine

(deks troe meth OR fan & klor fen IR a meen)

Brand Names: US Coricidin® HBP Cough & Cold [OTC]; Dimetapp® Children's Long Acting Cough Plus Cold [OTC]; Robitussin® Children's Cough & Cold Long-Acting [OTC]; Scot-Tussin® DM Maximum Strength [OTC]; Triaminic® Children's Softchews® Cough & Runny Nose [OTC]

Index Terms Chlorpheniramine and Dextromethorphan; Chlorpheniramine Maleate and Dextromethorphan Hydrobromide; Dextromethorphan Hydrobromide and Chlorpheniramine Maleate

Pharmacologic Category Alkylamine Derivative; Antitussive; Histamine H_1 Antagonist; Histamine H_1 Antagonist, First Generation

Use Symptomatic relief of runny nose, sneezing, itchy/watery eyes, cough, and other upper respiratory symptoms associated with hay fever, common cold, or upper respiratory allergies

Dosing

Adult & Geriatric General dosing guidelines; consult specific product labeling.

Cough, cold symptoms: Oral: Dextromethorphan 30 mg and chlorpheniramine 4 mg every 6 hours as needed (maximum: 120 mg dextromethorphan and 16 mg chlorpheniramine/24 hours)

Pediatric General dosing guidelines; consult specific product labeling.

Cough, cold symptoms: Oral:

Children 6-11 years:

Liquid: Dextromethorphan 15 mg and chlorpheniramine 2 mg every 6 hours as needed (maximum: 60 mg dextromethorphan and 8 mg chlorpheniramine/24 hours)

Chewable tablet: Dextromethorphan 10 mg and chlorpheniramine 2 mg every 4-6 hours as needed (maximum: 50 mg dextromethorphan and 10 mg chlorpheniramine/24 hours)

Children ≥12 years: Refer to adult dosing.

Additional Information Complete prescribing information should be consulted for additional detail.

Dosage Forms Excipient information presented when available (limited, particularly for generics); consult specific product labeling.

Syrup, oral:

Dimetapp® Children's Long Acting Cough Plus Cold: Dextromethorphan hydrobromide 7.5 mg and chlorpheniramine maleate 1 mg per 5 mL (118 mL) [ethanol free, sugar free; contains sodium 3 mg/5 mL, sodium benzoate, propylene glycol; grape flavor]

Robitussin® Children's Cough and Cold Long-Acting: Dextromethorphan hydrobromide 7.5 mg and chlorpheniramine maleate 1 mg per 5 mL (118 mL) [ethanol free; contains sodium 3 mg/5 mL, sodium benzoate, propylene glycol; fruit punch flavor]

Scot-Tussin® DM Maximum Strength: Dextromethorphan hydrobromide 15 mg and chlorpheniramine maleate 2 mg per 5 mL (118 mL) [ethanol free, dye free, sugar free; cherry-strawberry flavor]

Tablet, oral:

Coricidin® HBP Cough and Cold: Dextromethorphan hydrobromide 30 mg and chlorpheniramine maleate 4 mg

Tablet, softchew, oral:

Triaminic® Children's Softchews® Cough & Runny Nose: Dextromethorphan hydrobromide 5 mg and chlorpheniramine maleate 1 mg [contains coconut oil, phenylalanine 17.6 mg/softchew, sodium 5 mg/softchew; cherry flavor]

◆ Dextromethorphan and Guaifenesin *see* Guaifenesin and Dextromethorphan *on page 861*

Dextromethorphan and Phenylephrine
(deks troe meth OR fan & fen il EF rin)

Brand Names: US PediaCare® Children's Multi-Symptom Cold [OTC]; Safetussin® CD [OTC]; Sudafed PE® Children's Cold & Cough [OTC]; Triaminic® Day Time Cold & Cough [OTC]

Index Terms Dextromethorphan Hydrobromide and Phenylephrine Hydrochloride; Phenylephrine and Dextromethorphan

Pharmacologic Category Antitussive; Decongestant

Use Temporary relief of symptoms of hay fever, the common cold, and upper respiratory allergies including sinus/nasal congestion, minor bronchial/throat irritation, and cough

Dosing

Adult & Geriatric Relief of nasal/sinus congestion and cough: Oral (Safetussin® CD): 10 mL every 6 hours as needed (maximum: 40 mL/24 hours)

Pediatric Relief of nasal/sinus congestion and cough: Oral:

Children 4-6 years: PediaCare® Children's Multi-Symptom Cold, Sudafed PE® Children's Cold & Cough, Triaminic® Day Time Cold & Cough: 5 mL every 4 hours as needed (maximum: 30 mL/24 hours)

Children 6-12 years:

PediaCare® Children's Multi-Symptom Cold, Sudafed PE® Children's Cold & Cough, Triaminic® Day Time Cold & Cough: 10 mL every 4 hours as needed (maximum: 60 mL/24 hours)

Safetussin® CD: 5 mL every 6 hours as needed (maximum: 20 mL/24 hours)

Children ≥12 years: Refer to adult dosing.

Additional Information Complete prescribing information should be consulted for additional detail.

Dosage Forms Excipient information presented when available (limited, particularly for generics); consult specific product labeling.

Liquid, oral:

Sudafed PE® Children's Cold & Cough: Dextromethorphan hydrobromide 5 mg and phenylephrine hydrochloride 2.5 mg per 5 mL (118 mL) [ethanol free, sugar free; contains sodium 15 mg/5 mL, sodium benzoate; grape flavor]

Syrup:

PediaCare® Children's Multi-Symptom Cold: Dextromethorphan hydrobromide 5 mg and phenylephrine hydrochloride 2.5 mg per 5 mL (118 mL) [contains sodium 15 mg/5 mL; sodium benzoate; grape flavor]

Safetussin® CD: Dextromethorphan hydrobromide 15 mg and phenylephrine hydrochloride 2.5 mg per 5 mL (120 mL), [alcohol free; sugar free; contains menthol, propylene glycol; orange flavor]

Triaminic® Day Time Cold & Cough: Dextromethorphan hydrobromide 5 mg and phenylephrine hydrochloride 2.5 mg per 5 mL (120 mL, 240 mL) [contains benzoic acid; sodium 2 mg/5 mL; propylene glycol; cherry flavor]

◆ Dextromethorphan and Promethazine *see* Promethazine and Dextromethorphan *on page 1513*

◆ Dextromethorphan and Pseudoephedrine *see* Pseudoephedrine and Dextromethorphan *on page 1528*

Dextromethorphan and Quinidine
(deks troe meth OR fan & KWIN i deen)

Brand Names: US Nuedexta

Index Terms Dextromethorphan Hydrobromide and Quinidine Sulfate; Quinidine and Dextromethorphan

Pharmacologic Category N-Methyl-D-Aspartate Receptor Antagonist

Use Pseudobulbar affect: Treatment of pseudobulbar affect (PBA)

Pregnancy Considerations Adverse events were observed in animal reproduction studies using this combination. See individual agents.

Breast-Feeding Considerations Quinidine is excreted in breast milk; excretion of dextromethorphan is not known. The manufacturer recommends that caution be exercised when administering this combination to nursing women. See individual agents.

Contraindications Hypersensitivity to dextromethorphan, quinidine, quinine, mefloquine, or any component of the formulation; concomitant use with quinidine or other medications containing quinidine, quinine, or mefloquine; history of quinine-, mefloquine-, or quinidine-induced thrombocytopenia, hepatitis, bone marrow depression, or lupus-like syndrome; concurrent administration with or within 2 weeks of discontinuing an MAO inhibitor; patients with prolonged QT interval, congenital QT syndrome, or history of torsade de pointes; patients with heart failure; concurrent use of drugs that prolong the QT interval and are metabolized by CYP2D6 (eg, pimozide, thioridazine); patients with complete atrioventricular (AV) block without an implanted pacemaker or patients at high risk of complete AV block

Warnings/Precautions Immune-mediated thrombocytopenia (severe or fatal) may be associated with quinidine use. Unless clearly not drug related, discontinue immediately; continued use may be associated with an increase in fatal hemorrhage. Thrombocytopenia generally resolves within a few days of discontinuation. Therapy should not be restarted in sensitized patients. Agranulocytosis, angioedema, bronchospasm, hemolytic anemia, increased skeletal muscle enzymes, lymphadenopathy, myalgia, pneumonitis, rash, sicca syndrome, uveitis, vasculitis, may be associated with use. Lupus-like syndrome, with polyarthritis and sometimes a positive antinuclear antibody test, may occur with quinidine. Use is contraindicated in patients with quinidine-, quinine-, or mefloquine-induced lupus-like syndrome. Quinidine has also been associated with hepatitis, including granulomatous hepatitis, occurring generally during the first few weeks of therapy. Most cases resolve when quinidine is discontinued. Use is contraindicated in patients with prior history of immune-mediated thrombocytopenia associated with structurally related drugs (eg, quinine, mefloquine) and in patients with quinidine-, quinine-, or mefloquine-induced lupus-like syndrome.

Concomitant use of moderate or strong CYP3A4 inhibitors may increase quinidine levels and prolong the QTc interval. Quinidine inhibits CYP2D6; concomitant use with CYP2D6 substrates may cause an accumulation of concomitantly administered drug and/or reduce active metabolite formation, decreasing their safety and/or efficacy. Use with caution in patients who are poor metabolizers of CYP2D6 metabolized drugs. Quinidine in this combination product is used to inhibit CYP2D6 in order to increase plasma concentrations of dextromethorphan. In patients who are poor metabolizers, this effect would not be significant; however, adverse events related to quinidine may still be observed. Genotyping should be considered in patients considered to be at risk of quinidine toxicity prior to therapy. Symptoms associated with serotonin syndrome such as agitation, confusion, hallucinations, hyper-reflexia,

myoclonus, shivering, and tachycardia may occur with concomitant proserotonergic drugs (ie, SSRIs/SNRIs or triptans); especially with higher dextromethorphan doses. Discontinue therapy if such reaction occurs. Effects with other sedative drugs or ethanol may be potentiated.

Use caution in patients with left ventricular hypertrophy or left ventricular dysfunction which are more common in patients with chronic hypertension, coronary artery disease or history of stroke; risk of QTc prolongation may be increased. Use is contraindicated in patients with prolonged QT interval, congenital QT syndrome, or history of torsade de pointes, patients with heart failure, complete AV block without an implanted pacemaker or patients at high risk of complete AV block. Correct hypokalemia or hypomagnesemia prior to therapy. Use caution with medications which may further prolong the QT interval or cause cardiac arrhythmias. Dose dependent QTc prolongation may occur. Monitor patients at risk following the first dose. Discontinue if arrhythmia occurs.

May cause anticholinergic effects; use caution in patients with myasthenia gravis or other conditions which may be affected. May cause dizziness; use caution in patients with motor impairment or history of falls. Safety and efficacy have not been established with severe hepatic or renal impairment; increased serum concentrations may occur. Has not shown to be safe or effective in other types of commonly occurring emotional liabilities (eg, neurological disease or injury). Patients with a history of drug abuse should be monitored closely for signs of abuse/misuse (eg, development of tolerance, increase in dose, or drug-seeking behavior). Abuse of dextromethorphan may cause brain damage, cardiac arrhythmia, loss of consciousness, or death. Periodically reassess the need for treatment; spontaneous improvement of PBA may occur.

Adverse Reactions Also see individual agents.
>10%: Gastrointestinal: Diarrhea (13%)
1% to 10%:
Cardiovascular: Peripheral edema (5%)
Central nervous system: Dizziness (10%)
Gastrointestinal: Vomiting (5%), flatulence (3%)
Genitourinary: Urinary tract infection (4%)
Hepatic: GGT increased (3%)
Neuromuscular & skeletal: Weakness (5%)
Respiratory: Cough (5%)
Miscellaneous: Influenza (4%)

Drug Interactions
Metabolism/Transport Effects Refer to individual components.

Avoid Concomitant Use
Avoid concomitant use of Dextromethorphan and Quinidine with any of the following: Amiodarone; Antifungal Agents (Azole Derivatives, Systemic); Bosutinib; Conivaptan; Crizotinib; Dapoxetine; Enzalutamide; Erythromycin (Systemic); Fingolimod; Fusidic Acid (Systemic); Haloperidol; Highest Risk QTc-Prolonging Agents; Idelalisib; Ivabradine; Lopinavir; MAO Inhibitors; Mefloquine; Mequitazine; Mifepristone; Moderate Risk QTc-Prolonging Agents; Nelfinavir; PAZOPanib; Pimozide; Propafenone; Ritonavir; Saquinavir; Silodosin; Tamoxifen; Thioridazine; Tipranavir; Topotecan; VinCRIStine (Liposomal)

Increased Effect/Toxicity
Dextromethorphan and Quinidine may increase the levels/effects of: Afatinib; Antipsychotic Agents; ARIPiprazole; ARIPiprazole Lauroxil; AtoMOXetine; Bosutinib; Brentuximab Vedotin; Brexpiprazole; Calcium Channel Blockers (Dihydropyridine); Cardiac Glycosides; Colchicine; CYP2D6 Substrates; Dabigatran Etexilate; Dalfampridine; Dextromethorphan; DOXOrubicin (Conventional); Edoxaban; Everolimus; Fesoterodine; Flibanserin; Haloperidol; Highest Risk QTc-Prolonging Agents; Ledipasvir; Lomitapide; Mefloquine; Memantine; Mequitazine; Metoprolol; Naloxegol; Nebivolol; Neuromuscular-Blocking Agents; NiMODipine; PAZOPanib; P-glycoprotein/ABCB1 Substrates; Pimozide; Propafenone; Propranolol; Prucalopride; Rifaximin; Serotonin Modulators; Silodosin; Tamsulosin; Thioridazine; Topotecan; Tricyclic Antidepressants; Verapamil; VinCRIStine (Liposomal); Vitamin K Antagonists; Vortioxetine

The levels/effects of Dextromethorphan and Quinidine may be increased by: Abiraterone Acetate; Amiodarone; Antacids; Antiemetics (5HT3 Antagonists); Antifungal Agents (Azole Derivatives, Systemic); Antipsychotic Agents; Aprepitant; Atazanavir; Boceprevir; Calcium Channel Blockers (Dihydropyridine); Carbonic Anhydrase Inhibitors; Cimetidine; Cobicistat; Conivaptan; Crizotinib; CYP2D6 Inhibitors (Moderate); CYP2D6 Inhibitors (Strong); CYP3A4 Inhibitors (Moderate); CYP3A4 Inhibitors (Strong); Dapoxetine; Darunavir; Diltiazem; Erythromycin (Systemic); Fingolimod; Fosamprenavir; Fosaprepitant; Fosphenytoin; Fusidic Acid

(Systemic); Haloperidol; Idelalisib; Indinavir; Ivabradine; Ivacaftor; Lopinavir; Luliconazole; Lurasidone; MAO Inhibitors; Metaxalone; Mifepristone; Moderate Risk QTc-Prolonging Agents; Nelfinavir; Netupitant; Ombitasvir, Paritaprevir, and Ritonavir; Ombitasvir, Paritaprevir, Ritonavir, and Dasabuvir; Palbociclib; Parecoxib; Peginterferon Alfa-2b; P-glycoprotein/ABCB1 Inhibitors; PHENobarbital; QTc-Prolonging Agents (Indeterminate Risk and Risk Modifying); QuiNIDine; Reserpine; Ritonavir; Saquinavir; Selective Serotonin Reuptake Inhibitors; Simeprevir; Stiripentol; Telaprevir; Tipranavir; Tricyclic Antidepressants; Verapamil

Decreased Effect
Dextromethorphan and Quinidine may decrease the levels/effects of: Codeine; Dihydrocodeine; Hydrocodone; Tamoxifen

The levels/effects of Dextromethorphan and Quinidine may be decreased by: Bosentan; Calcium Channel Blockers (Dihydropyridine); CYP3A4 Inducers (Moderate); CYP3A4 Inducers (Strong); Dabrafenib; Deferasirox; Enzalutamide; Etravirine; Fosphenytoin; Kaolin; Mitotane; Peginterferon Alfa-2b; P-glycoprotein/ABCB1 Inducers; PHENobarbital; Phenytoin; Potassium-Sparing Diuretics; Primidone; Rifamycin Derivatives; Siltuximab; St Johns Wort; Sucralfate; Tocilizumab

Food Interactions Grapefruit juice may increase levels of quinidine. Tonic water contains quinine. Management: Avoid grapefruit juice. Avoid tonic water.

Storage/Stability Store at 25°C (77°F); excursions permitted to 15°C to 30°C (59°F to 86°F).

Mechanism of Action Dextromethorphan may relieve the symptoms of PBA by binding to sigma-1 receptors in the brain which may be involved in behavior, however the exact mechanism of action is not known. Quinidine is used to block the rapid metabolism of dextromethorphan, thereby increasing serum concentrations. The dose of quinidine in this combination product provides serum concentrations 1% to 3% of those needed to treat cardiac arrhythmias.

Pharmacodynamics/Kinetics
Absorption: Bioavailability of dextromethorphan increased ~20-fold when administered with quinidine.
Protein binding: Dextromethorphan: 60% to 70%; Quinidine: 80% to 89%
Metabolism: Dextromethorphan: Hepatic via CYP2D6 to dextrorphan (active); Quinidine: Hepatic via CYP3A4 to 3-hydroxyquinidine (active) and other metabolites
Half-life elimination: Dextromethorphan: 13 hours in extensive metabolizers; Quinidine: 7 hours in extensive metabolizers
Time to peak: Dextromethorphan: 3 to 4 hours; Quinidine: 1 to 2 hours
Excretion: Urine (~20% as unchanged)

Dosing
Adult
Pseudobulbar affect: Oral: Dextromethorphan 20 mg/quinidine 10 mg once daily for 7 days, then increase to dextromethorphan 20 mg/quinidine 10 mg every 12 hours; reassess patient periodically to determine if continued use is necessary. Do not exceed dextromethorphan 40 mg/quinidine 20 mg in a 24-hour period.

Renal Impairment
Mild to moderate impairment (CrCl 30 to 80 mL/minute): No dosage adjustment necessary.
Severe impairment (CrCl <30 mL/minute): There are no dosage adjustments provided in the manufacturer's labeling (has not been studied); however, increases in dextromethorphan/quinidine levels are likely to be observed.

Hepatic Impairment
Mild to moderate impairment (Child-Pugh class A or B): No dosage adjustment necessary; however, an increase in adverse reactions is observed with moderate impairment.
Severe impairment (Child-Pugh class C): There are no dosage adjustments provided in the manufacturer's labeling (has not been studied); however, increases in dextromethorphan/quinidine levels are likely to be observed.

Dietary Considerations Avoid grapefruit juice.
Administration May be administered with or without food. Administer twice-daily doses every 12 hours.

Monitoring Parameters QT interval at baseline and 3 to 4 hours after the first dose in patients at risk for QTc prolongation; potassium and magnesium prior to and during therapy; CBC, liver and renal function tests; periodically assess risk factors for arrhythmias during treatment; periodically reassess the need for treatment (spontaneous improvement of PBA may occur); worsening myasthenia gravis or other sensitive conditions due to anticholinergic effects.

Test Interactions See individual agents.

Dosage Forms Excipient information presented when available (limited, particularly for generics); consult specific product labeling.

Capsule, oral:

Nuedexta: Dextromethorphan hydrobromide 20 mg and quinidine sulfate 10 mg

♦ Dextromethorphan, Chlorpheniramine, and Phenylephrine see Chlorpheniramine, Phenylephrine, and Dextromethorphan on page 378

♦ Dextromethorphan, Chlorpheniramine, and Pseudoephedrine see Chlorpheniramine, Pseudoephedrine, and Dextromethorphan on page 379

♦ Dextromethorphan, Guaifenesin, and Pseudoephedrine see Guaifenesin, Pseudoephedrine, and Dextromethorphan on page 864

♦ Dextromethorphan Hydrobromide and Chlorpheniramine Maleate see Dextromethorphan and Chlorpheniramine on page 534

♦ Dextromethorphan Hydrobromide and Phenylephrine Hydrochloride see Dextromethorphan and Phenylephrine on page 535

♦ Dextromethorphan Hydrobromide and Quinidine Sulfate see Dextromethorphan and Quinidine on page 535

♦ Dex-Tuss see Guaifenesin and Codeine on page 861

♦ Dezocitidine see Decitabine on page 508

♦ dFdC see Gemcitabine on page 832

♦ dFdCyd see Gemcitabine on page 832

♦ DFM see Deferoxamine on page 512

♦ DFMO see Eflornithine on page 621

♦ D-Forte (Can) see Ergocalciferol on page 663

♦ DHAD see MitoXANtrone on page 1221

♦ DHAQ see MitoXANtrone on page 1221

♦ DHE see Dihydroergotamine on page 552

♦ D.H.E. 45 see Dihydroergotamine on page 552

♦ DHPG Sodium see Ganciclovir (Systemic) on page 828

♦ Diabeta see GlyBURIDE on page 847

♦ DiaBeta (Can) see GlyBURIDE on page 847

♦ Diabetic Siltussin DAS-Na [OTC] see GuaiFENesin on page 860

♦ Diabetic Siltussin-DM DAS-Na [OTC] see Guaifenesin and Dextromethorphan on page 861

♦ Diabetic Siltussin-DM DAS-Na Maximum Strength [OTC] see Guaifenesin and Dextromethorphan on page 861

♦ Diabetic Tussin [OTC] see GuaiFENesin on page 860

♦ Diabetic Tussin DM [OTC] see Guaifenesin and Dextromethorphan on page 861

♦ Diabetic Tussin DM Maximum Strength [OTC] see Guaifenesin and Dextromethorphan on page 861

♦ Diabetic Tussin Mucus Relief [OTC] see GuaiFENesin on page 860

♦ DiaB Klenz [OTC] see Sodium Chloride on page 1671

♦ Dialyvite Omega-3 Concentrate [OTC] see Omega-3 Fatty Acids on page 1329

♦ Diaminocyclohexane Oxalatoplatinum see Oxaliplatin on page 1349

♦ Diaminodiphenylsulfone see Dapsone (Systemic) on page 488

♦ Diamode [OTC] see Loperamide on page 1097

♦ Diamox® (Can) see AcetaZOLAMIDE on page 30

♦ Diamox Sequels see AcetaZOLAMIDE on page 30

♦ Diarr-Eze (Can) see Loperamide on page 1097

♦ Diastat (Can) see Diazepam on page 537

♦ Diastat AcuDial see Diazepam on page 537

♦ Diastat Pediatric see Diazepam on page 537

♦ Diazemuls (Can) see Diazepam on page 537

Diazepam (dye AZ e pam)

Brand Names: US Diastat AcuDial; Diastat Pediatric; Diazepam Intensol; Valium

Brand Names: Canada Apo-Diazepam; Bio-Diazepam; Diastat; Diazemuls; Diazepam Auto Injector; Diazepam Injection SDZ; Diazepam Injection USP; Novo-Dipam; PMS-Diazepam; Valium

Pharmacologic Category Benzodiazepine

Use

Acute ethanol withdrawal (oral and injection): May be useful in symptomatic relief of acute agitation, tremor, impending or acute delirium, tremens, and hallucinosis.

Anxiety (oral and injection): Management of anxiety disorders; short-term relief of the symptoms of anxiety.

Muscle spasm (oral and injection): As an adjunct for the relief of skeletal muscle spasm due to reflex spasm caused by local pathology (eg, inflammation of muscles or joints, secondary to trauma); spasticity caused by upper motor neuron disorders (eg, cerebral palsy, paraplegia); athetosis; stiff-man syndrome; tetanus.

Preoperative (injection): Relief of anxiety and tension in patients undergoing surgical procedures; prior to cardioversion for the relief of anxiety and tension and to diminish patient's recall (IV only); as an adjunct prior to endoscopic procedures for apprehension, anxiety, or acute stress reactions and to diminish patient's recall.

Note: Use of diazepam in patients undergoing cardioversion or endoscopic procedures has been superseded by agents with a more pharmacokinetically favorable profile (eg, midazolam) (Thomas 2014; Triantafillidis 2013)

Seizures: Adjunct in convulsive disorders (oral); management of select, refractory epilepsy patients on stable regimens of antiepileptic drugs requiring intermittent use of diazepam to control episodes of increased seizure activity (rectal); adjunct in severe recurrent convulsive seizures (injection).

Status epilepticus (injection): Adjunct in status epilepticus.

Pregnancy Considerations Adverse events have been observed in animal reproduction studies. In humans, diazepam and its metabolites (N-desmethyldiazepam, temazepam, and oxazepam) cross the placenta. Teratogenic effects have been observed with diazepam; however, additional studies are needed. The incidence of premature birth and low birth weights may be increased following maternal use of benzodiazepines; hypoglycemia and respiratory problems in the neonate may occur following exposure late in pregnancy. Neonatal withdrawal symptoms may occur within days to weeks after birth and "floppy infant syndrome" (which also includes withdrawal symptoms) has been reported with some benzodiazepines (including diazepam) (Bergman 1992; Iqbal 2002; Wikner 2007). A combination of factors influences the potential teratogenicity of anticonvulsant therapy. When treating women with epilepsy, monotherapy with the lowest effective dose and avoidance of medications known to have a high incidence of teratogenic effects is recommended (Harden 2009; Wlodarczyk 2012).

Breast-Feeding Considerations Diazepam and its metabolites are excreted in breast milk in concentrations approximately one-tenth of those in maternal plasma (days 3 to 9 postpartum). Drowsiness, lethargy, or weight loss in breast-feeding infants have been observed in case reports following maternal use of some benzodiazepines, including diazepam (Iqbal 2002). Breast-feeding is not recommended (Iqbal 2002). Because diazepam and its metabolites may be present in breast milk for prolonged periods following administration of the rectal gel, the manufacturer recommends discontinuing breast-feeding for an appropriate period of time.

Contraindications

Hypersensitivity to diazepam or any component of the formulation; acute narrow-angle glaucoma; untreated open-angle glaucoma; infants <6 months of age (oral); myasthenia gravis, severe respiratory impairment, severe hepatic impairment, sleep apnea syndrome (oral tablet).

Documentation of allergenic cross-reactivity for benzodiazepines is limited. However, because of similarities in chemical structure and/or pharmacologic actions, the possibility of cross-sensitivity cannot be ruled out with certainty.

Warnings/Precautions When used as an adjunct in treating convulsive disorders, an increase in frequency/severity of tonic-clonic seizures may occur and require dose adjustment of anticonvulsant. Abrupt withdrawal may result in a temporary increase in the frequency and/or severity of seizures. Use with caution in debilitated patients, obese patients, patients with hepatic disease, or renal impairment. Oral tablet is contraindicated in patients with severe hepatic impairment, severe respiratory impairment, or sleep apnea syndrome. Use with caution in patients with respiratory disease or impaired gag reflex.

Use caution in patients with depression or anxiety associated with depression, particularly if suicidal risk may be present. Use with extreme caution in patients with a history of drug abuse or acute alcoholism; potential for drug dependency exists. Tolerance and psychological and physical dependence may occur with prolonged use (generally >10 days). Use with extreme caution in patients who are at risk of falls; benzodiazepines have been associated with falls and traumatic injury. Rebound or withdrawal symptoms may occur following abrupt discontinuation or large decreases in dose. Use caution when reducing dose or withdrawing therapy; decrease slowly and monitor for withdrawal symptoms. The benzodiazepine receptor antagonist flumazenil may cause withdrawal in patients receiving long-term benzodiazepine therapy. Diazepam is a long half-life benzodiazepine. Tolerance develops to the sedative, hypnotic, and anticonvulsant effects. It does not develop to the anxiolytic or skeletal muscle relaxing effects (Vinkers 2012). Chronic use of this agent may increase the perioperative benzodiazepine dose needed to achieve desired effect.

Benzodiazepines have been associated with anterograde amnesia. Paradoxical reactions, including hyperactive or aggressive behavior, hallucinations, and psychoses, have been reported with benzodiazepines, particularly in adolescent/pediatric or elderly patients. Diazepam should be discontinued if such reactions occur. Does not have analgesic, antidepressant, or antipsychotic properties. May be used in patients with open-angle glaucoma who are receiving appropriate therapy; contraindicated in acute narrow-angle glaucoma and untreated open-angle glaucoma. Potentially significant interactions may exist, requiring dose or frequency adjustment, additional monitoring, and/or selection of alternative therapy.

May cause CNS depression, which may impair physical or mental abilities; patients must be cautioned about performing tasks that require mental alertness (eg, operating machinery, driving). In older adults, benzodiazepines increase the risk of impaired cognition, delirium, falls, fractures, and motor vehicle accidents. Due to increased sensitivity in this age group and slower metabolism of long-acting agents (such as diazepam), avoid use for treatment of insomnia, agitation, or delirium (Beers Criteria).

Parenteral: Vesicant; ensure proper needle or catheter placement prior to and during administration; avoid extravasation. Acute hypotension, muscle weakness, apnea, and/or cardiac arrest have occurred with parenteral administration. Acute effects may be more prevalent in patients receiving concurrent barbiturates, opioids, or ethanol. Appropriate resuscitative equipment and qualified personnel should be available during administration and monitoring. Avoid use of the injection in patients in shock, coma, or in acute ethanol intoxication with depression of vital signs. Intra-arterial injection should be avoided. Tonic status epilepticus has been precipitated in patients treated with diazepam IV for absence status or absence variant status.

Rectal gel: Administration of rectal gel should only be performed by individuals trained to recognize characteristic seizure activity and monitor response. Not recommended for chronic, daily use. Use with caution in patients with neurologic damage.

Some dosage forms may contain benzyl alcohol and/or sodium benzoate/benzoic acid; benzoic acid (benzoate) is a metabolite of benzyl alcohol; large amounts of benzyl alcohol ($\geq$99 mg/kg/day) have been associated with a potentially fatal toxicity ("gasping syndrome") in neonates; the "gasping syndrome" consists of metabolic acidosis, respiratory distress, gasping respirations, CNS dysfunction (including convulsions, intracranial hemorrhage), hypotension, and cardiovascular collapse (AAP 1997; CDC 1982); some data suggest that benzoate displaces bilirubin from protein binding sites (Ahlfors 2001); avoid or use dosage forms containing benzyl alcohol and/or benzyl alcohol derivative with caution in neonates. See manufacturer's labeling.

Some dosage forms may contain propylene glycol; large amounts are potentially toxic and have been associated with hyperosmolality, lactic acidosis, seizures, and respiratory depression; use caution (AAP 1997; Zar 2007).

Adverse Reactions Frequency not defined. Adverse reactions may vary by route of administration.

Cardiovascular: Hypotension, localized phlebitis, vasodilatation

Central nervous system: Amnesia, ataxia, confusion, depression, drowsiness, dysarthria, fatigue, headache, slurred speech, vertigo

Dermatologic: Skin rash

Endocrine & metabolic: Change in libido

Gastrointestinal: Altered salivation (dry mouth or hypersalivation), constipation, diarrhea, nausea

Genitourinary: Urinary incontinence, urinary retention

Hepatic: Jaundice

Local: Pain at injection site

Neuromuscular & skeletal: Tremor, weakness

Ophthalmic: Blurred vision, diplopia

Respiratory: Apnea, asthma, bradypnea

Miscellaneous: Paradoxical reaction (eg, aggressiveness, agitation, anxiety, delusions, hallucinations, inappropriate behavior, increased muscle spasms, insomnia, irritability, psychoses, rage, restlessness, sleep disturbances, stimulation)

Drug Interactions

Metabolism/Transport Effects Substrate of CYP1A2 (minor), CYP2B6 (minor), CYP2C19 (major), CYP2C9 (minor), CYP3A4 (major); **Note:** Assignment of Major/Minor substrate status based on clinically relevant drug interaction potential; **Inhibits** CYP2C19 (weak)

Avoid Concomitant Use

Avoid concomitant use of Diazepam with any of the following: Azelastine (Nasal); Conivaptan; Fusidic Acid (Systemic); Idelalisib; Methadone; OLANZapine; Orphenadrine; Paraldehyde; Sodium Oxybate; Thalidomide

Increased Effect/Toxicity

Diazepam may increase the levels/effects of: Alcohol (Ethyl); Alfentanil; Azelastine (Nasal); Buprenorphine; CloZAPine; CNS Depressants; Hydrocodone; Methadone; Methotrimeprazine; Metyrosine; Mirtazapine; Orphenadrine; Paraldehyde; Pramipexole; ROPINIRole; Rotigotine; Selective Serotonin Reuptake Inhibitors; Sodium Oxybate; Suvorexant; Thalidomide; Zolpidem

The levels/effects of Diazepam may be increased by: Aprepitant; Brimonidine (Topical); Cannabis; Conivaptan; Cosyntropin; CYP2C19 Inhibitors (Moderate); CYP2C19 Inhibitors (Strong); CYP3A4 Inhibitors (Moderate); CYP3A4 Inhibitors (Strong); Dasatinib; Disulfiram; Doxylamine; Dronabinol; Droperidol; Etravirine; Fosamprenavir; Fosaprepitant; Fusidic Acid (Systemic); HydrOXYzine; Idelalisib; Ivacaftor; Kava Kava; Luliconazole; Magnesium Sulfate; Methotrimeprazine; Mifepristone; Minocycline; Nabilone; Netupitant; OLANZapine; Osimertinib; Palbociclib; Perampanel; Ritonavir; Rufinamide; Saquinavir; Simeprevir; Stiripentol; Tapentadol; Teduglutide; Tetrahydrocannabinol

Decreased Effect

The levels/effects of Diazepam may be decreased by: Bosentan; CYP2C19 Inducers (Strong); CYP3A4 Inducers (Moderate); CYP3A4 Inducers (Strong); Dabrafenib; Deferasirox; Enzalutamide; Etravirine; Mitotane; Osimertinib; Siltuximab; St Johns Wort; Theophylline Derivatives; Tocilizumab; Yohimbine

Food Interactions Diazepam serum concentrations may be decreased if taken with food. Grapefruit juice may increase diazepam serum concentrations. Management: Avoid concurrent use of grapefruit juice. Maintain adequate hydration, unless instructed to restrict fluid intake.

Storage/Stability

Injection: Store at 20°C to 25°C (68°F to 77°F). Protect from light. Do not refrigerate autoinjector.

Oral solution: Store at 25°C (77°F); excursions permitted to 15°C to 30°C (59°F to 86°F). Protect from light. Discard opened bottle of concentrated oral solution after 90 days.

Rectal gel: Store at 25°C (77°F); excursion permitted to 15°C to 30°C (59°F to 86°F).

Tablet: Store at 15°C to 30°C (59°F to 86°F).

Mechanism of Action Binds to stereospecific benzodiazepine receptors on the postsynaptic GABA neuron at several sites within the central nervous system, including the limbic system, reticular formation. Enhancement of the inhibitory effect of GABA on neuronal excitability results by increased neuronal membrane permeability to chloride ions. This shift in chloride ions results in hyperpolarization (a less excitable state) and stabilization. Benzodiazepine receptors and effects appear to be linked to the GABA-A receptors. Benzodiazepines do not bind to GABA-B receptors.

Pharmacodynamics/Kinetics

Onset of action:

Sedation: Pediatric patients: IV: 4 to 5 minutes (Krauss 2006)

Status epilepticus: IV: 1 to 3 minutes; Rectal: 2 to 10 mintues

Duration of action:

Sedation: Pediatric patients: 60 to 120 minutes (Krauss 2006)

Status epilepticus: 15 to 30 minutes

Absorption:
Oral: Well absorbed (>90%); delayed and decreased when administered with a moderate fat meal
Rectal: Well absorbed
Distribution: V_d:
IV: 1.2 L/kg (range: 0.6 to 2 L/kg) (Greenblatt 1989a)
Oral: 1.1 L/kg (range: 0.6 to 1.8 L/kg (Greenblatt 1989b)
Rectal: 1 L/kg
Protein binding:
Oral: 98%
Rectal: 95% to 98%
Metabolism: Hepatic; diazepam is N-demethylated by CYP3A4 and 2C19 to the active metabolite N-desme-thyldiazepam, and is hydroxylated by CYP3A4 to the active metabolite temazepam. N-desmethyldiazepam and temazepam are both further metabolized to oxaze-pam. Temazepam and oxazepam are largely eliminated by glucuronidation.
Bioavailability:
IM: >90% (Lamson 2011)
Oral: >90%
Rectal: 90%
Half-life elimination: **Note:** Diazepam accumulates upon multiple dosing and the terminal elimination half-life is slightly prolonged.
IM:
Premature neonates (GA: 28 to 34 weeks): 54 hours
Infants: ~30 hours (Moreselli 1972)
Children 3 to 8 years: 18 hours (Morselli 1972)
Adults: Parent: ~60 to 72 hours; Desmethyldiazepam: ~152 to 174 hours (Lamson 2011)
IV: Parent: 33 to 45 hours; Desmethyldiazepam: 87 hours (Cloyd 1998; Greenblatt 1989a)
Oral: Parent: 44 to 48 hours; Desmethyldiazepam: 100 hours (Greenblatt 1989b)
Rectal: Parent: 45 to 46 hours; Desmethyldiazepam: 71 to 99 hours (Cloyd 1998)
Time to peak:
IM: 1 hour (Lamson 2011)
IV: 0.01 hours (Cloyd 1998)
Oral: 15 minutes to 2.5 hours (1.25 hours when fasting; 2.5 hours with food) (Greenblatt 1989b)
Rectal: 1.5 hours
Excretion: Urine (predominantly as glucuronide conjugates)

Dosing

Adult Note: Oral absorption is more reliable than IM
Acute ethanol withdrawal:
IV, IM: 10 mg initially; may administer 5 to 10 mg 3 to 4 hours later, if needed
Oral: 10 mg 3 to 4 times during first 24 hours, then decrease to 5 mg 3 to 4 times daily as needed
Anxiety (symptoms/disorders):
Oral: 2 to 10 mg 2 to 4 times daily if needed
IM, IV: 2 to 10 mg; may repeat in 3 to 4 hours, if needed
Muscle spasm:
Oral: 2 to 10 mg 3 or 4 times daily
IV, IM: Initial: 5 to 10 mg; then 5 to 10 mg in 3 to 4 hours, if necessary. Larger doses may be required if associated with tetanus.
Preoperative: Anxiety: IM: 10 mg prior to surgery
Sedation in the ICU patient: *IV:* Loading dose: 5 to 10 mg; Maintenance dose: 0.03 to 0.1 mg/kg every 30 minutes to 6 hours (Barr 2013)
Seizures:
Adjunctive maintenance therapy: Oral: 2 to 10 mg 2 to 4 times daily.
Intermittent management of seizures: Rectal gel (Diastat): 0.2 mg/kg; may be repeated in 4 to 12 hours if needed; do not use for more than 5 episodes per month or more than one episode every 5 days. **Note:** Round dose to the nearest 2.5 mg increment.
Status epilepticus:
IV:
Manufacturer's labeling: 5 to 10 mg; may repeat every 10 to 15 minutes (maximum total dose: 30 mg). If necessary, may repeat in 2 to 4 hours.
Neurocritical Care Society recommendations: 0.15 mg/kg (maximum dose: 10 mg) given at a rate of ≤5 mg/minute; may repeat in 5 minutes (NCS [Brophy 2012]).
Rectal (formulation not specified): **Note:** Diazepam may be administered rectally when there is no IV access and IM administration of midazolam (drug of choice for IM administration during status epilepticus) is contra-indicated (NCS [Brophy 2012]). The parenteral formu-lation of diazepam may be given rectally if rectal gel (Diastat) is not available (Arif 2008).
Premonitory/Out-of-hospital treatment: 10 mg once; may repeat once if necessary (Kälviäinen 2007)
Skeletal muscle relaxant (adjunct therapy): *Oral:* 2 to 10 mg 3 to 4 times daily

Geriatric Oral absorption is more reliable than IM
Elderly and/or debilitated patients:
Oral: 2 to 2.5 mg 1 to 2 times daily initially; increase gradually as needed and tolerated.
Rectal gel: Due to the increased half-life in elderly and debilitated patients, consider reducing dose.

Pediatric

Conscious sedation for procedures:
Oral:
Children: 0.2 to 0.3 mg/kg (maximum dose: 10 mg) 45 to 60 minutes prior to procedure
Adolescents: 10 mg
IV: Adolescents: 5 mg; may repeat with 2.5 mg if needed
Febrile seizure prophylaxis: *Oral:* Children: 1 mg/kg/day divided every 8 hours; initiate therapy at first sign of fever and continue for 24 hours after fever is gone
Muscle spasm associated with tetanus: *IV, IM:*
Infants >30 days and Children <5 years: 1 to 2 mg/dose every 3 to 4 hours as needed
Children ≥5 years: 5 to 10 mg/dose every 3 to 4 hours as needed
Sedation or muscle relaxation or anxiety:
Oral: Children: 0.12 to 0.8 mg/kg/day in divided doses every 6 to 8 hours
IM, IV: Children: 0.04 to 0.3 mg/kg/dose every 2 to 4 hours to a maximum of 0.6 mg/kg within an 8-hour period if needed
Seizures: *Rectal gel (Diastat):* Round dose to the near-est 2.5 mg increment; dose may be repeated in 4 to 12 hours if needed; do not use for more than 5 episodes per month or more than one episode every 5 days.
Children 2 to 5 years: 0.5 mg/kg (maximum dose: 20 mg)
Children 6 to 11 years: 0.3 mg/kg (maximum dose: 20 mg)
Children ≥12 years and Adolescents: 0.2 mg/kg (max-imum dose: 20 mg)
Status epilepticus:
IV: American Academy of Pediatrics and Neurocritical Care Society recommendations: 0.1 to 0.3 mg/kg (maximum dose: 10 mg) given over ~2 minutes; may repeat dose after 5 to 10 minutes (AAP [Hegenbarth 2008]) or 0.15 mg/kg (maximum dose: 10 mg) given at a rate of ≤5 mg/minute; may repeat in 5 minutes (NCS [Brophy 2012])
Rectal (formulation not specified): **Note:** According to the Neurocritical Care Society, diazepam may be administered rectally when there is no IV access and IM administration of midazolam (drug of choice for IM administration during status epilepticus) is contraindi-cated (NCS [Brophy 2012]). The parenteral formula-tion of diazepam may be given rectally if rectal gel (Diastat) is not available (Arif 2008; Dieckmann 1994). Maximum recommended dose according to the man-ufacturer: 20 mg/dose
Children 2 to 5 years: 0.5 mg/kg
Children 6 to 11 years: 0.3 mg/kg
Children >12 years and Adolescents: 0.2 mg/kg
American Academy of Pediatrics recommendations (AAP [Hegenbarth 2008]): Initial: 0.5 mg/kg (maximum dose: 20 mg).
Spasticity in cerebral palsy (off-label use): *Oral:* Dose should be individualized:
Children ≤5 years: <8.5 kg: 0.5 to 1 mg at bedtime; 8.5 to 15 kg: 1 to 2 mg at bedtime (Mathew 2005)
Children 5 to 16 years: 1.25 mg 3 times daily to 5 mg 4 times daily (Engle 1966)

Renal Impairment There are no dosage adjustments provided in the manufacturer's labeling; use with caution. Hemodialysis: Not dialyzable (0% to 5%); supplemental dose is not necessary.

Hepatic Impairment There are no dosage adjustments provided in the manufacturer's labeling; use with caution. The oral tablets are contraindicated in severe hepatic impairment.

Administration

Oral: Administer with food or water. Dilute or mix oral concentrate with water, juice, soda, applesauce, or pud-ding before use; measure dose only with calibrated dropper provided.
IV: Administer undiluted by slow IV push; do not mix with other solutions or medications. Rapid injection may cause respiratory depression or hypotension. In infants and children, do not exceed 1 to 2 mg/minute IV push; in adults, maximum infusion rate is 5 mg/minute. Do not administer through small veins (eg, dorsum of hand/wrist). Avoid intra-arterial administration. Continuous infu-sion is not recommended because of precipitation in IV fluids and absorption of drug into infusion bags and tubing.

Vesicant; ensure proper needle or catheter placement prior to and during infusion; avoid extravasation.

Extravasation management: If extravasation occurs, stop IV administration immediately and disconnect (leave cannula/needle in place); gently aspirate extravasated solution (do **NOT** flush the line); remove needle/cannula; elevate extremity. Apply dry cold compresses (Hurst 2004).

Rectal gel: Prior to administration, confirm that prescribed dose is visible and correct, and that the green "ready" band is visible. Place patient on side (facing person responsible for monitoring), with top leg bent forward. Insert rectal tip (lubricated) gently into rectum until rim fits snug against rectal opening; push plunger gently over 3 seconds. After additional 3 seconds, remove syringe; hold buttocks together while slowly counting to 3 to prevent leakage; keep patient on side, facing towards you and continue to observe patient; discard any unused medication, syringe, and all used materials; do not reuse; see manufacturer's Administration and Disposal Instructions.

Monitoring Parameters Heart rate, respiratory rate, blood pressure, and mental status; liver enzymes and CBC with long-term therapy.

Critically-ill mechanically-ventilated patients: Monitor depth of sedation with either the Richmond Agitation-Sedation Scale (RASS) or Sedation-Agitation Scale (SAS) (Barr 2013)

Test Interactions False-negative urinary glucose determinations when using Clinistix® or Diastix®

Additional Information Diazepam does not have any analgesic effects.

Diastat AcuDial: When dispensing, consult package information for directions on setting patient's dose; confirm green "ready" band is visible prior to dispensing product.

Dosage Forms Excipient information presented when available (limited, particularly for generics); consult specific product labeling.

Concentrate, Oral:
Diazepam Intensol: 5 mg/mL (30 mL) [contains alcohol, usp; unflavored flavor]
Generic: 5 mg/mL (30 mL)

Device, Intramuscular:
Generic: 10 mg/2 mL (2 mL)

Gel, Rectal:
Diastat AcuDial: 10 mg (1 ea); 20 mg (1 ea) [contains alcohol, usp, benzoic acid, sodium benzoate]
Diastat Pediatric: 2.5 mg (1 ea) [contains benzoic acid, benzyl alcohol, propylene glycol, sodium benzoate]
Generic: 2.5 mg (1 ea); 10 mg (1 ea); 20 mg (1 ea)

Solution, Injection:
Generic: 5 mg/mL (2 mL, 10 mL)

Solution, Oral:
Generic: 1 mg/mL (5 mL, 500 mL)

Tablet, Oral:
Valium: 2 mg, 5 mg, 10 mg [scored]
Generic: 2 mg, 5 mg, 10 mg

Controlled Substance C-IV

◆ Diazepam Auto Injector (Can) see Diazepam on page 537

◆ Diazepam Injection SDZ (Can) see Diazepam on page 537

◆ Diazepam Injection USP (Can) see Diazepam on page 537

◆ Diazepam Intensol see Diazepam on page 537

Diazoxide (dye az OKS ide)

Brand Names: US Proglycem
Brand Names: Canada Proglycem
Pharmacologic Category Antidote, Hypoglycemia; Vasodilator, Direct-Acting

Use

Hyperinsulinemic hypoglycemia: Management of hypoglycemia due to hyperinsulinism due to the following conditions in adults (ie, inoperable islet cell adenoma or carcinoma, or extrapancreatic malignancy) and infants and children (ie, leucine sensitivity, islet cell hyperplasia, nesidioblastosis, extrapancreatic malignancy, islet cell adenoma, or adenomatosis; may be used preoperatively as a temporary measure, and postoperatively, if hypoglycemia persists).

Note: Consider treatment with diazoxide when other specific medical therapy or surgical management for hypoglycemia due to the above conditions either has been unsuccessful or is not feasible.

Dosing

Adult & Geriatric Hyperinsulinemic hypoglycemia:
Oral: Initial dose: 3 mg/kg/day divided into 3 equal doses every 8 hours; dosing range: 3 to 8 mg/kg/day divided into 2 or 3 equal doses every 8 to 12 hours. Adjust dose until the desired clinical and laboratory effects are produced. **Note:** In certain instances, patients with refractory hypoglycemia may require higher doses. Discontinue if no effect after 2 to 3 weeks.

Pediatric Hyperinsulinemic hypoglycemia: Oral:
Neonates and Infants: Initial dose: 10 mg/kg/day divided into 3 equal doses every 8 hours; dosing range: 8 to 15 mg/kg/day divided into 2 or 3 equal doses every 8 to 12 hours. Adjust dose until the desired clinical and laboratory effects are produced. Discontinue if no effect after 2 to 3 weeks.
Children and Adolescents: Refer to adult dosing.

Renal Impairment There are no dosage adjustments provided in the manufacturer's labeling; a reduced dose should be considered (half-life may be prolonged).

Hepatic Impairment There are no dosage adjustments provided in the manufacturer's labeling.

Additional Information Complete prescribing information should be consulted for additional detail.

Dosage Forms Excipient information presented when available (limited, particularly for generics); consult specific product labeling.
Suspension, Oral:
Proglycem: 50 mg/mL (30 mL) [chocolate mint flavor]

Dosage Forms: Canada Excipient information presented when available (limited, particularly for generics); consult specific product labeling.
Capsule, oral:
Proglycem: 100 mg

◆ Dibenzyline see Phenoxybenzamine on page 1440

◆ DIC see Dacarbazine on page 479

◆ Dicel® Chewable [OTC] see Chlorpheniramine and Pseudoephedrine on page 377

◆ Dicel® DM Chewables [OTC] see Chlorpheniramine, Pseudoephedrine, and Dextromethorphan on page 379

◆ Diclectin® (Can) see Doxylamine and Pyridoxine on page 606

◆ Diclegis® see Doxylamine and Pyridoxine on page 606

Diclofenac (Systemic) (dye KLOE fen ak)

Brand Names: US Cambia; Cataflam [DSC]; Dyloject; Voltaren-XR [DSC]; Zipsor; Zorvolex
Brand Names: Canada Apo-Diclo; Apo-Diclo Rapide; Apo-Diclo SR; Cambia; Diclofenac EC; Diclofenac ECT; Diclofenac K; Diclofenac SR; Diclofenac-SR; Dom-Diclofenac; Dom-Diclofenac SR; PMS-Diclofenac; PMS-Diclofenac K; PMS-Diclofenac-SR; PRO-Diclo-Rapide; Sandoz-Diclofenac; Sandoz-Diclofenac Rapide; Sandoz-Diclofenac SR; Teva-Diclofenac; Teva-Diclofenac EC; Teva-Diclofenac K; Teva-Diclofenac SR; Voltaren; Voltaren Rapide; Voltaren SR
Index Terms Cataflam; Diclofenac Potassium; Diclofenac Sodium; Voltaren; Zorvolex
Pharmacologic Category Nonsteroidal Anti-inflammatory Drug (NSAID); Nonsteroidal Anti-inflammatory Drug (NSAID), Oral

Use

Analgesia
Capsules/immediate-release tablets only: Relief of mild to moderate acute pain
Injection only: Management of mild to moderate acute pain and moderate to severe acute pain (alone or in combination with opioid analgesics) in adults

Ankylosing spondylitis (delayed-release tablets only): Acute or long-term use in the relief of signs and symptoms of ankylosing spondylitis

Dysmenorrhea (immediate-release tablets only): Treatment of primary dysmenorrhea

Migraine (powder for oral solution only): Acute treatment of migraine attacks with or without aura in adults

Osteoarthritis (immediate-release, extended-release, and delayed-release tablets; capsules [Zorvolex]; and suppositories [Canadian product] only): Relief of signs and symptoms of osteoarthritis.

Rheumatoid arthritis (immediate-release, extended-release, and delayed-release tablets; and suppositories [Canadian product] only): Relief of signs and symptoms of rheumatoid arthritis.

Pregnancy Considerations Adverse events were not observed in the initial animal reproduction studies; therefore, manufacturers classify most dosage forms of diclofenac as pregnancy category C (oral, injection: Category D ≥30 weeks gestation). Diclofenac crosses the placenta and

can be detected in fetal tissue and amniotic fluid. NSAID exposure during the first trimester is not strongly associated with congenital malformations; however, cardiovascular anomalies and cleft palate have been observed following NSAID exposure in some studies. The use of a NSAID close to conception may be associated with an increased risk of miscarriage. Nonteratogenic effects have been observed following NSAID administration during the third trimester including: Myocardial degenerative changes, prenatal constriction of the ductus arteriosus, fetal tricuspid regurgitation, failure of the ductus arteriosus to close postnatally; renal dysfunction or failure, oligohydramnios; gastrointestinal bleeding or perforation, increased risk of necrotizing enterocolitis; intracranial bleeding (including intraventricular hemorrhage), platelet dysfunction with resultant bleeding; pulmonary hypertension. Because they may cause premature closure of the ductus arteriosus, use of NSAIDs in pregnancy (particularly late pregnancy) should be avoided. Product labeling for Cambia, Zipsor, and Zorvolex specifically notes that use at ≥30 weeks' gestation should be avoided. Use in the third trimester is contraindicated in the Canadian labeling. The chronic use of NSAIDs in women of reproductive age may be associated with infertility that is reversible upon discontinuation of the medication. A registry is available for pregnant women exposed to autoimmune medications including diclofenac. For additional information contact the Organization of Teratology Information Specialists, OTIS Autoimmune Diseases Study, at 877-311-8972

Breast-Feeding Considerations Low concentrations of diclofenac can be found in breast milk. Breast-feeding is not recommended by most manufacturers. The manufacturers of the injection recommend that caution be exercised when administering diclofenac to breast-feeding women. Use while breast-feeding is contraindicated in Canadian labeling.

Medication Guide Available Yes

Contraindications

Hypersensitivity to diclofenac (eg, anaphylactoid reactions, serious skin reactions) or bovine protein (Zipsor only) or any component of the formulation; patients who have experienced asthma, urticaria, or other allergic-type reactions after taking aspirin or other NSAIDs; treatment of perioperative pain in the setting of CABG surgery; patients with moderate to severe renal impairment in the perioperative period and who are at risk for volume depletion (injection only)

Canadian labeling: Additional contraindications (not in U.S. labeling): Severe uncontrolled heart failure, active gastric/duodenal/peptic ulcer; active GI bleed or perforation; regional ulcer, gastritis, or ulcerative colitis; cerebrovascular bleeding or other bleeding disorders; inflammatory bowel disease; severe hepatic impairment; active hepatic disease; severe renal impairment (CrCl <30 mL/minute) or deteriorating renal disease; known hyperkalemia; patients <16 years of age; breast-feeding; pregnancy (third trimester); use of diclofenac suppository if recent history of bleeding or inflammatory lesions of rectum/anus

Warnings/Precautions [U.S. Boxed Warning]: NSAIDs are associated with an increased risk of adverse cardiovascular thrombotic events, including MI and stroke. Risk may increase with dose and duration of use or preexisting cardiovascular risk factors or disease. Carefully evaluate individual cardiovascular risk profiles (eg, hypertension, ischemic heart disease, diabetes, smoking) and consider alternative agents if appropriate) prior to prescribing. May cause new-onset hypertension or worsening of existing hypertension. Monitor blood pressure closely. Use caution with fluid retention. Avoid use in heart failure (ACCF/AHA [Yancy, 2013]). Concurrent administration of ibuprofen, and potentially other nonselective NSAIDs, may interfere with aspirin's cardioprotective effect. **[U.S. Boxed Warning]: Use is contraindicated for treatment of perioperative pain in the setting of coronary artery bypass graft (CABG) surgery.** Risk of MI and stroke may be increased with use following CABG surgery.

NSAID use may compromise existing renal function; dose-dependent decreases in prostaglandin synthesis may result from NSAID use, reducing renal blood flow which may cause renal decompensation. NSAID use may increase the risk for hyperkalemia (Canadian labeling contraindicates use with known hyperkalemia). Patients with impaired renal function, dehydration, heart failure, liver dysfunction, those taking diuretics and ACEI, and the elderly are at greater risk of renal toxicity and hyperkalemia. Rehydrate patient before starting therapy; monitor renal function closely. Not recommended for use in patients with advanced renal disease. Injection is not recommended in patients with moderate to severe renal impairment and is contraindicated in patients with

moderate to severe renal impairment in the perioperative period and who are at risk for volume depletion. Long-term NSAID use may result in renal papillary necrosis while persistent urinary symptoms (eg, dysuria, bladder pain), cystitis, or hematuria may occur any time after initiating NSAID therapy. Discontinue therapy with symptom onset and evaluate for origin.

[U.S. Boxed Warning]: NSAIDs may increase risk of gastrointestinal irritation, inflammation, ulceration, bleeding, and perforation. These events may occur at any time during therapy and without warning. Use caution with a history of GI disease (bleeding or ulcers), concurrent therapy with aspirin, anticoagulants and/or corticosteroids, smoking, use of alcohol, the elderly or debilitated patients. When used concomitantly with aspirin, a substantial increase in the risk of gastrointestinal complications (eg, ulcer) occurs; concomitant gastroprotective therapy (eg, proton pump inhibitors) is recommended (Bhatt, 2008).

Use the lowest effective dose for the shortest duration of time, consistent with individual patient goals, to reduce risk of cardiovascular or GI adverse events. Alternate therapies should be considered for patients at high risk. Canadian labeling contraindicates use in patients with active gastric/duodenal/peptic ulcer; active GI bleed or perforation; or regional ulcer, gastritis, or ulcerative colitis.

NSAIDs may cause photosensitivity or serious skin adverse events including exfoliative dermatitis, Stevens-Johnson syndrome (SJS), and toxic epidermal necrolysis (TEN); discontinue use at first sign of skin rash or hypersensitivity. Anaphylactoid reactions may occur, even without prior exposure; patients with "aspirin triad" (bronchial asthma, aspirin intolerance, rhinitis) may be at increased risk. Do not use in patients who experience bronchospasm, asthma, rhinitis, or urticaria with NSAID or aspirin therapy. Use caution in other forms of asthma. Platelet adhesion and aggregation may be decreased; may prolong bleeding time; patients with coagulation disorders or who are receiving anticoagulants should be monitored closely. Anemia may occur; patients on long-term NSAID therapy should be monitored for anemia. Rarely, NSAID use may cause severe blood dyscrasias (eg, agranulocytosis, aplastic anemia, thrombocytopenia).

Use with caution in patients with impaired hepatic function (Canadian labeling contraindicates use in severe hepatic impairment or active hepatic disease). Closely monitor patients with any abnormal LFT. Transaminase elevations have been observed with use, generally within the first 2 months of therapy, but may occur at any time. Risk may be higher with diclofenac than other NSAIDS (Laine, 2009; Rostom, 2005). Significant elevations in transaminases (eg, >3 x ULN) occur before patients become symptomatic; initiate monitoring 4 to 8 weeks into therapy. Rarely, severe hepatic reactions (eg, fulminant hepatitis, liver failure) have occurred; discontinue all formulations if signs or symptoms of liver disease develop, or if systemic manifestations occur. Use with caution in hepatic porphyria (may trigger attack; Jose, 2008).

NSAIDS may cause drowsiness, dizziness, blurred vision, and other neurologic effects which may impair physical or mental abilities; patients must be cautioned about performing tasks which require mental alertness (eg, operating machinery or driving). Discontinue use with blurred or diminished vision and perform ophthalmologic exam. Monitor vision with long-term therapy. May increase the risk of aseptic meningitis, especially in patients with systemic lupus erythematosus (SLE) and mixed connective tissue disorders. In the elderly, avoid chronic use (unless alternative agents ineffective and patient can receive concomitant gastroprotective agent); nonselective oral NSAID use is associated with an increased risk of GI bleeding and peptic ulcer disease in older adults in high risk category (eg, >75 years or age or receiving concomitant oral/parenteral corticosteroids, anticoagulants, or antiplatelet agents) (Beers Criteria).

Withhold for at least 4 to 6 half-lives prior to surgical or dental procedures.

Different formulations of oral diclofenac are not bioequivalent, even if the milligram strength is the same; do not interchange products. Zipsor (capsule) contains gelatin; use is contraindicated in patients with history of hypersensitivity to bovine protein. Oral solution is only indicated for the acute treatment of migraine; not indicated for migraine prophylaxis or cluster headache; contains phenylalanine. Injection is not indicated for long-term use. ▶

Adverse Reactions

Injection: Frequency not always defined.

Cardiovascular: Edema (≤10%), cerebrovascular accident, hypertension, myocardial infarction, significant cardiovascular event

Central Nervous System: Headache (≤10%), dizziness (8%)

Dermatologic: Pruritus (≤10%), skin rash (≤10%), exfoliative dermatitis, Stevens-Johnson syndrome, toxic epidermal necrolysis

Endocrine & Metabolic: Fluid retention

Gastrointestinal: Constipation (13%), abdominal pain (≤10%), diarrhea (≤10%), dyspepsia (≤10%), esophageal perforation (≤10%), flatulence (≤10%), gastrointestinal ulcer (≤10%; including gastric/duodenal), heartburn (≤10%), intestinal perforation (≤10%), nausea (≤10%), vomiting (≤10%)

Hematologic & Oncologic: Anemia (≤10%), hemorrhage (≤10%), prolonged bleeding time (≤10%)

Hepatic: Increased liver enzymes (≤10%), increased serum transaminases (15%), increased serum ALT (≤4%; >8X ULN: ≤1%), increased serum AST (2% to ≤4%; >8X ULN: ≤1%)

Hypersensitivity: Anaphylactoid reaction

Local: Infusion site reaction (10%), extravasation (3%)

Otic: Tinnitus (≤10%)

Renal: Renal insufficiency (≤10%)

Miscellaneous: Wound healing impairment (8%), gastrointestinal inflammation

<1% (Limited to important or life-threatening): Abnormal Dreams, agranulocytosis, alopecia, anaphylaxis, angioedema, anxiety, aplastic anemia, asthma, auditory impairment, blurred vision, cardiac arrhythmia, change in appetite, colitis, coma, confusion, congestive heart failure, conjunctivitis, convulsions, cystitis, depression, diaphoresis, drowsiness, dyspnea, dysuria, ecchymoses, eosinophilia, eructation, erythema multiforme, esophagitis, exfoliative dermatitis, fever, fulminant hepatitis, gastritis, gastrointestinal hemorrhage, glossitis, hallucination, hematemesis, hematuria, hemolytic anemia, hepatic failure, hepatic necrosis, hepatitis, hepatotoxicity, hyperglycemia, hypertension, hypotension, infection, insomnia, interstitial nephritis, jaundice, leukopenia, lymphadenopathy, malaise, melena, meningitis, nervousness, oliguria, palpitations, pancreatitis, pancytopenia, paresthesia, pneumonia, polyuria, proteinuria, purpura, rectal hemorrhage, renal failure, respiratory depression, sepsis, skin photosensitivity, stomatitis, syncope, tachycardia, thrombocytopenia, toxic epidermal necrolysis, tremor, urticaria, vasculitis, vertigo, weakness, weight changes

Oral: Frequency not always defined.

>10%:

Cardiovascular: Edema (33%)

Hepatic: Increased serum transaminases (≤3 x ULN; 15%)

1% to 10%:

Cardiovascular: Hypertension (2% to 3%)

Central nervous system: Headache (4% to 8%), procedural pain (3%), dizziness (2%), falling (2%)

Dermatologic: Pruritus (7%), skin rash

Gastrointestinal: Constipation (5% to 8%), nausea (6% to 7%), diarrhea (6%), GI adverse effects (gastric ulcer, hemorrhage, and perforation; ≤4%, risk increases with therapy duration), abdominal pain (2% to 3%), vomiting (3%), dyspepsia (2% to 3%), flatulence (2% to 3%), heartburn, abdominal discomfort (2%), duodenal ulcer

Genitourinary: Urinary tract infection (7%)

Hematologic & oncologic: Bruise (3%), anemia, prolonged bleeding time

Hepatic: Increased serum ALT (>3 x ULN: ≤4%; >8 x ULN: ≤1%), increased serum AST (>3 x ULN; ≤4%; >8 x ULN: ≤1%)

Infection: Influenza (3%)

Neuromuscular & skeletal: Osteoarthritis (5%), arthralgia (3%), back pain (3%), limb pain (3%)

Renal: Renal function abnormality

Otic: Tinnitus

Renal: Increased serum creatinine (2%), renal function abnormality

Respiratory: Upper respiratory tract infection (8%), nasopharyngitis (6%), sinusitis (3% to 5%), cough (4%), bronchitis (3%)

<1% (Limited to important or life-threatening): Agranulocytosis, alopecia, anaphylactoid reaction, aplastic anemia, aseptic meningitis, asthma, cardiac arrhythmia, cardiac failure, cerebrovascular accident, colitis, coma, conjunctivitis, cystitis, decreased hemoglobin, depression, diplopia, eosinophilia, erythema multiforme, esophageal ulcer, esophagitis, gastritis, hearing loss, hemolytic anemia, hepatic failure, hepatitis, hyperglycemia, hypotension, interstitial nephritis, intestinal perforation, lymphadenopathy, memory impairment, meningitis, myocardial

infarction, pancreatitis, pancytopenia, peptic ulcer, pneumonia, psychotic reaction, purpura, rectal hemorrhage, renal failure, respiratory depression, seizure, sepsis, skin photosensitivity, Stevens-Johnson syndrome, tachycardia, toxic epidermal necrolysis, vasculitis

Rectal suppository [Canadian product]:

Also refer to adverse reactions associated with oral formulations.

<1% (Limited to important or life-threatening): Hemorrhoids (exacerbation), local hemorrhage, proctitis

Drug Interactions

Metabolism/Transport Effects Substrate of CYP1A2 (minor), CYP2B6 (minor), CYP2C19 (minor), CYP2C8 (minor), CYP2C9 (minor), CYP2D6 (minor), CYP3A4 (minor); **Note:** Assignment of Major/Minor substrate status based on clinically relevant drug interaction potential; **Inhibits** CYP1A2 (weak), CYP2C9 (weak), CYP2E1 (weak), UGT1A6

Avoid Concomitant Use

Avoid concomitant use of Diclofenac (Systemic) with any of the following: Dexketoprofen; Floctafenine; Ketorolac (Nasal); Ketorolac (Systemic); Morniflumate; NSAID (COX-2 Inhibitor); Omacetaxine; Talniflumate; Urokinase

Increased Effect/Toxicity

Diclofenac (Systemic) may increase the levels/effects of: 5-ASA Derivatives; Agents with Antiplatelet Properties; Aliskiren; Aminoglycosides; Anticoagulants; Apixaban; Bisphosphonate Derivatives; Collagenase (Systemic); CycloSPORINE (Systemic); Dabigatran Etexilate; Deferasirox; Deferiprone; Deoxycholic Acid; Desmopressin; Digoxin; Drospirenone; Edoxaban; Eplerenone; Haloperidol; Ibritumomab; Lithium; Methotrexate; Nonsteroidal Anti-Inflammatory Agents; NSAID (COX-2 Inhibitor); Obinutuzumab; Omacetaxine; PEMEtrexed; Porfimer; Potassium-Sparing Diuretics; PRALAtrexate; Quinolone Antibiotics; Rivaroxaban; Salicylates; Tacrolimus (Systemic); Tenofovir Products; Thrombolytic Agents; TIZANidine; Tositumomab and Iodine I 131 Tositumomab; Urokinase; Vancomycin; Verteporfin; Vitamin K Antagonists

The levels/effects of Diclofenac (Systemic) may be increased by: ACE Inhibitors; Alcohol (Ethyl); Angiotensin II Receptor Blockers; Antidepressants (Tricyclic, Tertiary Amine); Corticosteroids (Systemic); CycloSPORINE (Systemic); CYP2C9 Inhibitors (Strong); Dasatinib; Dexketoprofen; Floctafenine; Glucosamine; Herbs (Anticoagulant/Antiplatelet Properties); Ibrutinib; Ketorolac (Nasal); Ketorolac (Systemic); Limaprost; Loop Diuretics; Morniflumate; Multivitamins/Fluoride (with ADE); Multivitamins/Minerals (with ADEK, Folate, Iron); Multivitamins/Minerals (with AE, No Iron); Omega-3 Fatty Acids; Pentosan Polysulfate Sodium; Pentoxifylline; Probenecid; Prostacyclin Analogues; Selective Serotonin Reuptake Inhibitors; Serotonin/Norepinephrine Reuptake Inhibitors; Sodium Phosphates; Talniflumate; Thiazide Diuretics; Tipranavir; Treprostinil; Vitamin E; Vitamin E (Oral); Voriconazole

Decreased Effect

Diclofenac (Systemic) may decrease the levels/effects of: ACE Inhibitors; Aliskiren; Angiotensin II Receptor Blockers; Beta-Blockers; Eplerenone; HydrALAZINE; Loop Diuretics; Potassium-Sparing Diuretics; Prostaglandins (Ophthalmic); Salicylates; Selective Serotonin Reuptake Inhibitors; Thiazide Diuretics

The levels/effects of Diclofenac (Systemic) may be decreased by: Bile Acid Sequestrants; CYP2C9 Inducers (Strong); Salicylates

Preparation for Administration Oral solution: Empty contents of packet into 1-2 ounces (30-60 mL) of water (do not use other liquids); mix well and administer immediately.

Storage/Stability

Capsule, powder for oral solution: Store at 25°C (77°F); excursions permitted to 15°C to 30°C (59°F to 86°F). Protect from moisture.

Injection: Store at 20°C to 25°C (68°F to 77°F). Do not freeze. Protect from light.

Suppository [Canadian product]: Store at 15°C to 30°C (59°F to 86°F); protect from heat.

Tablet: Store immediate-release and ER tablets below 30°C (86°F); store delayed-release tablets at 20°C to 25°C (68°F to 77°F). Protect from moisture.

Mechanism of Action Reversibly inhibits cyclooxygenase-1 and 2 (COX-1 and 2) enzymes, which results in decreased formation of prostaglandin precursors; has antipyretic, analgesic, and anti-inflammatory properties

Other proposed mechanisms not fully elucidated (and possibly contributing to the anti-inflammatory effect to varying degrees), include inhibiting chemotaxis, altering lymphocyte activity, inhibiting neutrophil aggregation/activation, and decreasing proinflammatory cytokine levels.

Pharmacodynamics/Kinetics

Onset of action:

Cataflam (potassium salt) is more rapid than the sodium salt because it dissolves in the stomach instead of the duodenum

Suppository [Canadian product]: More rapid onset, but slower rate of absorption when compared to enteric coated tablet

Distribution: ~1.4 L/kg

Protein binding: >99%, primarily to albumin

Metabolism: Hepatic; undergoes first-pass metabolism; forms several metabolites (1 with weak activity)

Bioavailability: 55%

Half-life elimination: Oral: ~2 hours; Injection: ~1 to 2 hours

Time to peak, serum: **Note:** Fasted values reported for oral products; may be delayed with food

Cambia: ~0.25 hours

Cataflam, Zorvolex: ~1 hour

Voltaren XR ~5 hours

Zipsor: ~0.5 hour

Injection: ~5 minutes

Suppository [Canadian product]: ≤1 hour; **Note:** Suppository: C_{max}: Approximately two-thirds of that observed with enteric coated tablet (equivalent 50 mg dose)

Tablet, delayed release (diclofenac sodium): ~2 hours

Excretion: Urine (~65%); feces (~35%)

Dosing

Adult

Analgesia:

Oral:

Immediate-release tablet: 50 mg 3 times daily; may administer 100 mg loading dose, followed by 50 mg every 8 hours

Canadian labeling: 50 mg every 6 to 8 hours for up to 7 days (maximum: 100 mg daily)

Immediate-release capsule:

Zipsor (diclofenac potassium): 25 mg 4 times daily

Zorvolex (diclofenac acid): 18 mg or 35 mg 3 times daily

IV: 37.5 mg every 6 hours as needed (maximum: 150 mg daily).

Primary dysmenorrhea: Oral: Immediate-release tablet: 50 mg 3 times daily; may administer 100 mg loading dose, followed by 50 mg every 8 hours

Canadian labeling: Immediate release tablet: Day 1: Initial: 100 mg then 50 mg every 6 to 8 hours (maximum: 200 mg daily); Day 2 and beyond (up to 7 days): 50 mg every 6 to 8 hours (maximum: 100 mg daily)

Rheumatoid arthritis:

Oral: Immediate-release tablet: 150 to 200 mg daily in 3 to 4 divided doses; Delayed-release tablet: 150 to 200 mg daily in 2 to 4 divided doses; Extended-release tablet: 100 mg daily (may increase dose to 200 mg daily in 2 divided doses)

Canadian labeling: Enteric-coated tablet: 50 mg every 8 hours (maximum: 100 mg daily); Slow-release tablet: 75 to 100 mg daily (maximum: 100 mg daily)

Rectal suppository [Canadian product]: Insert 50 mg or 100 mg rectally as single dose to substitute for final oral daily dose (maximum combined dose [rectal and oral]: 100 mg daily)

Osteoarthritis:

Oral:

Immediate-release tablet: 150 to 200 mg daily in 3 to 4 divided doses; Delayed-release tablet: 150 to 200 mg daily in 2 to 4 divided doses; Extended-release tablet: 100 mg daily; may increase dose to 200 mg daily in 2 divided doses

Canadian labeling: Enteric-coated tablet: 50 mg every 8 hours (maximum: 100 mg daily); Slow-release tablet: 75 to 100 mg daily (maximum: 100 mg daily)

Immediate-release capsule: Zorvolex (diclofenac acid): 35 mg 3 times daily.

Rectal suppository [Canadian product]: Insert 50 mg or 100 mg rectally as single dose to substitute for final oral daily dose (maximum combined dose [rectal and oral]: 100 mg daily)

Ankylosing spondylitis: Oral: Delayed-release tablet: 100 to 125 mg daily in 4 to 5 divided doses

Migraine: Oral: Oral solution: 50 mg (one packet) as a single dose at the time of migraine onset; safety and efficacy of a second dose have not been established.

Geriatric Refer to adult dosing. Use lowest recommended dose and frequency in elderly to initiate therapy for indications listed in adult dosing.

Pediatric Juvenile idiopathic arthritis (off-label use): Children ≥3 years and Adolescents: Oral: Delayed-release tablet (diclofenac sodium): 2 to 3 mg/kg/day in divided doses (Haapasaari, 1983; Hashkes, 2005)

Renal Impairment

U.S. labeling: There are no dosage adjustments provided in the manufacturer's labeling; not recommended in patients with advanced renal disease or significant renal impairment; use of injection is contraindicated in patients with moderate to severe renal impairment in the perioperative period and who are at risk for volume depletion.

Canadian labeling: There are no dosage adjustments provided in the manufacturer's labeling; however, the manufacturer recommends that reduced dosages should be considered. Use in severe renal impairment (CrCl <30 mL/minute) or deteriorating renal disease is contraindicated.

Hepatic Impairment

Hepatic impairment at treatment initiation:

U.S. labeling: May require dosage adjustment due to extensive hepatic metabolism. Additional product-specific recommendations:

Cambia: Use in patients with hepatic impairment only if benefits outweigh risks

Zorvolex: Initial: Initiate treatment at the lowest dose; if efficacy is not achieved with the lowest dose, discontinue use.

Injection:

Mild impairment: No dosage adjustment necessary.

Moderate to severe impairment: Use is not recommended (has not been studied).

Canadian labeling: There are no dosage adjustments provided in the manufacturer's labeling; however, the manufacturer recommends that reduced dosages should be considered. Use is contraindicated in severe liver impairment or active liver disease.

Hepatic impairment during treatment: Persistent or worsening abnormal liver function tests, clinical signs/symptoms consistent with liver disease, or systemic manifestations of liver disease (eg, eosinophilia, rash, abdominal pain, diarrhea, dark urine): Discontinue immediately.

Dietary Considerations Oral formulations may be taken with food to decrease GI distress. Food may reduce effectiveness of oral solution. Some products may contain phenylalanine.

Administration

Injection: Administer as an IV bolus over 15 seconds.

Oral: Do not crush delayed- or extended-release tablets. Administer with food or milk to avoid gastric distress.

Cambia, Zorvolex: Taking with food may cause a reduction in effectiveness.

Rectal suppository [Canadian product]: Remove entire plastic wrapping prior to inserting rectally.

Monitoring Parameters

Monitor CBC, liver enzymes (periodically during chronic therapy starting 4 to 8 weeks after initiation), electrolytes, BUN/serum creatinine; monitor urine output; occult blood loss; blood pressure

Canadian labeling also recommends periodic ophthalmic evaluation during extended therapy or with onset of vision changes.

Dosage Forms Excipient information presented when available (limited, particularly for generics); consult specific product labeling. [DSC] = Discontinued product

Capsule, Oral, as base:

Zorvolex: 18 mg, 35 mg [contains brilliant blue fcf (fd&c blue #1), fd&c blue #2 (indigotine)]

Capsule, Oral, as potassium:

Zipsor: 25 mg [contains gelatin (bovine)]

Packet, Oral, as potassium:

Cambia: 50 mg (1 ea, 9 ea) [contains aspartame, saccharin sodium; anise-mint flavor]

Solution, Intravenous, as sodium:

Dyloject: 37.5 mg/mL (1 mL)

Tablet, Oral, as potassium:

Cataflam: 50 mg [DSC]

Generic: 50 mg

Tablet Delayed Release, Oral, as sodium:

Generic: 25 mg, 50 mg, 75 mg

Tablet Extended Release 24 Hour, Oral, as sodium:

Voltaren-XR: 100 mg [DSC]

Generic: 100 mg

Dosage Forms: Canada Note: Refer also to Dosage Forms; Zipsor and Zorvolex capsules are not currently available in Canada. Excipient information presented when available (limited, particularly for generics); consult specific product labeling.

Suppository:

Voltaren: 50 mg, 100 mg

Diclofenac (Ophthalmic) (dye KLOE fen ak)

Brand Names: US Voltaren [DSC]
Brand Names: Canada Voltaren Ophtha
Index Terms Diclofenac Sodium
Pharmacologic Category Nonsteroidal Anti-inflammatory Drug (NSAID); Nonsteroidal Anti-inflammatory Drug (NSAID), Ophthalmic
Use
US labeling:
Ocular pain/photophobia: Temporary relief of pain and photophobia in patients undergoing corneal refractive surgery
Postoperative ocular inflammation: Treatment of postoperative inflammation following cataract extraction

Canadian labeling:
Ocular pain/photophobia: Treatment of nonchronic posttraumatic inflammation in nonpenetrating wounds
Postoperative ocular inflammation: Treatment of postoperative inflammation following cataract surgery
Dosing
Adult & Geriatric
US labeling:
Postoperative ocular inflammation: Cataract surgery: Ophthalmic: Instill 1 drop into affected eye 4 times/day beginning 24 hours after cataract surgery and continuing for 2 weeks.
Ocular pain/photophobia: Corneal refractive surgery: Ophthalmic: Instill 1 to 2 drops into affected eye within the hour prior to surgery, within 15 minutes following surgery, and then continue for 4 times/day, up to 3 days.
Canadian labeling:
Postoperative ocular inflammation: Cataract surgery: Instill 1 drop into affected eye up to 5 times during the 3 hours preceding surgery, at 15, 30, and 45 minutes following surgery, then 1 drop 3 to 5 times/day for up to 4 weeks.
Nonchronic post-traumatic ocular inflammation (nonpenetrating wounds): Note: Obtain wound culture prior to initiation then instill 1 drop 4 to 5 times/day, based on disease severity.
Renal Impairment There are no dosage adjustments provided in the manufacturer's labeling. However, dosage adjustment unlikely due to low systemic absorption.
Hepatic Impairment There are no dosage adjustments provided in the manufacturer's labeling. However, dosage adjustment unlikely due to low systemic absorption.
Additional Information Complete prescribing information should be consulted for additional detail.
Dosage Forms Excipient information presented when available (limited, particularly for generics); consult specific product labeling. [DSC] = Discontinued product
Solution, Ophthalmic, as sodium:
Voltaren: 0.1% (5 mL [DSC]) [contains cremophor el, edetate disodium]
Generic: 0.1% (2.5 mL, 5 mL)

Diclofenac and Misoprostol
(dye KLOE fen ak & mye soe PROST ole)

Brand Names: US Arthrotec
Brand Names: Canada ACT Diclo-Miso; Arthrotec; GD-Diclofenac/Misoprostol
Index Terms Misoprostol and Diclofenac
Pharmacologic Category Nonsteroidal Anti-inflammatory Drug (NSAID), Oral; Prostaglandin
Use
Osteoarthritis: Treatment of the signs and symptoms of osteoarthritis in patients at high risk for NSAID-induced gastric and duodenal ulceration
Rheumatoid arthritis: Treatment of the signs and symptoms of rheumatoid arthritis in patients at high risk for NSAID-induced gastric and duodenal ulceration
Medication Guide Available Yes
Dosing
Adult
US labeling:
Osteoarthritis: Oral: Diclofenac 50 mg/misoprostol 200 mcg: One tablet 3 times daily
Rheumatoid arthritis: Oral: Diclofenac 50 mg/misoprostol 200 mcg: One tablet 3 or 4 times daily
Note: For both indications, may administer diclofenac 50 mg/misoprostol 200 mcg or diclofenac 75 mg/misoprostol 200 mcg one tablet twice daily if recommended dose is not tolerated; however, these options are less effective in preventing GI ulceration. May adjust dose using individual agents in combination with diclofenac/misoprostol. The maximum daily dose of misoprostol is 800 mcg and the maximum

single dose of misoprostol is 200 mcg. The maximum daily dose of diclofenac is 150 mg daily (osteoarthritis) or 225 mg daily (rheumatoid arthritis).
Canadian labeling: **Osteoarthritis, Rheumatoid arthritis:** Diclofenac 50 mg/misoprostol 200 mcg: One tablet 2 times daily (maximum diclofenac dose: 100 mg daily)
Geriatric May require reduced dosage due to lower body weight; monitor renal function
Renal Impairment
US labeling: There are no dosage adjustments provided in the manufacturer's labeling; not recommended in patients with advanced renal disease.
Canadian labeling:
Mild to moderate impairment: Consider lowest dose and monitor closely.
Severe impairment (CrCl <30 mL/minute) or deteriorating renal disease: Use is contraindicated.
Hepatic Impairment
US labeling: There are no dosage requirements in the manufacturer's labeling; however, the bioavailability of misoprostol may be increased in patients with hepatic impairment.
Canadian labeling:
Mild to moderate impairment: There are no dosage adjustments provided in the manufacturer's labeling (monitor closely).
Significant impairment or active hepatic disease: Use is contraindicated.
Additional Information Complete prescribing information should be consulted for additional detail.
Dosage Forms Excipient information presented when available (limited, particularly for generics); consult specific product labeling.
Tablet, oral: Diclofenac sodium 50 mg and misoprostol 200 mcg; Diclofenac sodium 75 mg and misoprostol 200 mcg
Arthrotec 50: Diclofenac sodium 50 mg and misoprostol 200 mcg
Arthrotec 75: Diclofenac sodium 75 mg and misoprostol 200 mcg

◆ Diclofenac EC (Can) *see* Diclofenac (Systemic) *on page 540*

◆ Diclofenac ECT (Can) *see* Diclofenac (Systemic) *on page 540*

◆ Diclofenac K (Can) *see* Diclofenac (Systemic) *on page 540*

◆ Diclofenac Potassium *see* Diclofenac (Systemic) *on page 540*

◆ Diclofenac Sodium *see* Diclofenac (Ophthalmic) *on page 544*

◆ Diclofenac Sodium *see* Diclofenac (Systemic) *on page 540*

◆ Diclofenac SR (Can) *see* Diclofenac (Systemic) *on page 540*

Dicloxacillin (dye kloks a SIL in)

Index Terms Dicloxacillin Sodium
Pharmacologic Category Antibiotic, Penicillin
Use Treatment of systemic infections such as pneumonia, skin and soft tissue infections, and osteomyelitis caused by penicillinase-producing staphylococci
Dosing
Adult & Geriatric
Susceptible infections: Oral: 125 to 500 mg every 6 hours
Erysipelas, furunculosis, mastitis, otitis externa, septic bursitis, skin abscess: Oral: 500 mg every 6 hours
Prosthetic joint infection: Chronic suppression therapy: Staphylococci (oxacillin-susceptible) (off-label regimen): Oral: 500 mg every 6 to 8 hours (Osmon 2013)
Skin and soft tissue infection due to MSSA: Oral: 500 mg every 6 hours for 7 to 14 days (IDSA [Stevens 2014])
***Staphylococcus aureus*, methicillin susceptible infection if no IV access:** Oral: 500 to 1000 mg every 6 to 8 hours
Bite wounds (animal) (off-label use): Oral: 500 mg 4 times daily; in combination with penicillin (IDSA [Stevens 2014])
Impetigo (off-label use): Oral: 250 mg 4 times daily for 7 days, depending on response (IDSA [Stevens 2014])
Pediatric Use in newborns is not recommended.
Susceptible infections: Oral:
Children <40 kg: 12.5 to 25 mg/kg/day divided every 6 hours; doses of 50 to 100 mg/kg/day in divided doses every 6 hours have been used for therapy of osteomyelitis
Children >40 kg: 125 to 250 mg every 6 hours

Furunculosis: Oral: 25 to 50 mg/kg/day divided every 6 hours

Osteomyelitis: Oral: 50 to 100 mg/kg/day in divided doses every 6 hours

Skin and soft tissue infection due to MSSA: 25 to 50 mg/kg/day divided every 6 hours for 7 to 14 days (IDSA [Stevens 2014])

Renal Impairment

No specific adjustment provided in manufacturer's labeling; a reduction in total dosage should be considered in renal impairment.

Not dialyzable (0% to 5%); supplemental dose is not necessary.

Peritoneal dialysis effects: Supplemental dose is not necessary.

Continuous arteriovenous or venovenous hemofiltration: Supplemental dose is not necessary.

Hepatic Impairment No dosage adjustment provided in manufacturer's labeling.

Additional Information Complete prescribing information should be consulted for additional detail.

Dosage Forms Excipient information presented when available (limited, particularly for generics); consult specific product labeling.

Capsule, Oral:

Generic: 250 mg, 500 mg

◆ Dicloxacillin Sodium *see* Dicloxacillin *on page 544*

◆ Dicopanol FusePaq *see* DiphenhydrAMINE (Systemic) *on page 561*

Dicyclomine (dye SYE kloe meen)

Brand Names: US Bentyl

Brand Names: Canada Bentylol; Dicyclomine Hydrochloride Injection; Formulex; Jamp-Dicyclomine; Protylol; Riva-Dicyclomine

Index Terms Dicyclomine Hydrochloride; Dicycloverine Hydrochloride

Pharmacologic Category Anticholinergic Agent

Use Treatment of functional bowel/irritable bowel syndrome

Dosing

Adult Gastrointestinal motility disorders/irritable bowel:

Oral: Initial: 20 mg 4 times daily for 7 days; after 1 week, may increase to 40 mg 4 times daily. If efficacy not achieved in 2 weeks or if adverse effects require a dose <80 mg/day, therapy should be discontinued. Safety data are not available for doses >80 mg daily for a duration that exceeds 2 weeks.

IM **(should not be used IV):** 10-20 mg 4 times daily for 1-2 days; convert to oral therapy as soon as possible

Geriatric Refer to adult dosing. Use caution; lower dosages may be required.

Renal Impairment No dosage adjustment provided in the manufacturer's labeling (has not been studied); use with caution.

Hepatic Impairment No dosage adjustment provided in the manufacturer's labeling (has not been studied); use with caution.

Additional Information Complete prescribing information should be consulted for additional detail.

Dosage Forms Excipient information presented when available (limited, particularly for generics); consult specific product labeling. [DSC] = Discontinued product

Capsule, Oral, as hydrochloride:

Bentyl: 10 mg [contains brilliant blue fcf (fd&c blue #1), fd&c red #40]

Generic: 10 mg

Solution, Intramuscular, as hydrochloride:

Bentyl: 10 mg/mL (2 mL) [pyrogen free]

Solution, Oral, as hydrochloride:

Generic: 10 mg/5 mL (473 mL)

Syrup, Oral, as hydrochloride:

Bentyl: 10 mg/5 mL (480 mL [DSC]) [contains brilliant blue fcf (fd&c blue #1), fd&c red #40, fd&c yellow #6 (sunset yellow), methylparaben, propylene glycol, propylparaben, saccharin sodium]

Tablet, Oral, as hydrochloride:

Bentyl: 20 mg

Generic: 20 mg

◆ Dicyclomine Hydrochloride *see* Dicyclomine *on page 545*

◆ Dicyclomine Hydrochloride Injection (Can) *see* Dicyclomine *on page 545*

◆ Dicycloverine Hydrochloride *see* Dicyclomine *on page 545*

◆ Di-Dak-Sol [OTC] *see* Sodium Hypochlorite *on page 1675*

Didanosine (dye DAN oh seen)

Brand Names: US Videx; Videx EC

Brand Names: Canada Videx; Videx EC

Index Terms ddI; Dideoxyinosine

Pharmacologic Category Antiretroviral, Reverse Transcriptase Inhibitor, Nucleoside (Anti-HIV)

Use HIV infection: Treatment of HIV-1 infection in combination with other antiretroviral agents.

Medication Guide Available Yes

Dosing

Adult Treatment of HIV infection: Oral:

Dosing based on patient weight:

Pediatric powder for oral solution (Videx):

<60 kg: 125 mg twice daily (preferred) or 250 mg once daily

≥60 kg: 200 mg twice daily (preferred) or 400 mg once daily

Delayed release capsule (Videx EC):

25 kg to <60 kg: 250 mg once daily

≥60 kg: 400 mg once daily

Dosage adjustment for concomitant therapy:

When taken with tenofovir:

<60 kg and CrCl ≥60 mL/minute: 200 mg once daily

≥60 kg and CrCl ≥60 mL/minute: 250 mg once daily

Geriatric Refer to adult dosing. Elderly patients have a higher frequency of pancreatitis (10% versus 5% in younger patients); monitor renal function and dose accordingly.

Pediatric Treatment of HIV infection: Oral:

Pediatric powder for oral solution (Videx): **Note:** Once-daily dosing of the oral solution is not FDA approved in children.

Infants: 2 weeks to 8 months: 100 mg/m^2 twice daily is recommended by the manufacturer; 50 mg/m^2 may be considered in infants 2 weeks to <3 months (HHS [pediatric], 2014)

Infants and Children >8 months: 120 mg/m^2 twice daily, not to exceed adult dose, is recommended by the manufacturer.

Adolescents: Dosing based on patient weight: Refer to adult dosing.

Children 3 to 21 years (off-label dose): Treatment-naive: 240 mg/m^2/dose once daily (maximum: 400 mg/dose) (HHS [pediatric], 2014)

Delayed release capsule (Videx EC):

Children ≥6 years:

20 kg to <25 kg: 200 mg once daily

25 kg to <60 kg: 250 mg once daily

≥60 kg: 400 mg once daily

Children 3 to 21 years (off-label dose): Treatment-naive: 240 mg/m^2/dose once daily (maximum: 400 mg/dose) (HHS [pediatric], 2014)

Renal Impairment

Adults: Dosing based on patient weight, creatinine clearance, and dosage form: See table.

Recommended Dose (mg) of Didanosine by Body Weight – Adults

Creatinine Clearance (mL/min)	≥60 kg		<60 kg	
	Powder for Oral Solution	Delayed Release Capsule	Powder for Oral Solution	Delayed Release Capsule
≥60	400 mg daily or 200 mg twice daily	400 mg daily	250 mg daily or 125 mg twice daily	250 mg daily
30-59	200 mg daily or 100 mg twice daily	200 mg daily	150 mg daily or 75 mg twice daily	125 mg daily
10-29	150 mg daily	125 mg daily	100 mg daily	125 mg daily
<10	100 mg daily	125 mg daily	75 mg daily	See **Note**

Note: Per manufacturer, not suitable for use in patients <60 kg with CrCr <10 mL/minute; use alternate formulation.

Patients requiring hemodialysis or CAPD: Dose per CrCl <10 mL/minute. Didanosine is not removed via CAPD and minimal amount of dose (≤7%) is removed by hemodialysis; no supplemental dosing necessary.

Children: No specific guidelines available; consider dosage reduction using adjustments for adults.

Hepatic Impairment No dosage adjustment necessary.

Additional Information Complete prescribing information should be consulted for additional detail.

Dosage Forms Excipient information presented when available (limited, particularly for generics); consult specific product labeling.

Capsule Delayed Release, Oral:

Videx EC: 125 mg, 200 mg, 250 mg, 400 mg

Generic: 125 mg, 200 mg, 250 mg, 400 mg
Solution Reconstituted, Oral:
Videx: 2 g (100 mL); 4 g (200 mL)

- Dideoxyinosine *see* Didanosine *on page 545*
- Didronel *see* Etidronate *on page 713*
- Didronel [DSC] *see* Etidronate *on page 713*
- Dienogest and Estradiol *see* Estradiol and Dienogest *on page 686*
- Dietary Fiber Laxative [OTC] *see* Psyllium *on page 1529*

Diethylpropion (dye eth il PROE pee on)

Index Terms Amfepramone; Diethylpropion Hydrochloride; Tenuate; Tenuate Dospan
Pharmacologic Category Anorexiant; Central Nervous System Stimulant; Sympathomimetic
Use Short-term (few weeks) adjunct in the management of exogenous obesity

Pharmacotherapy for weight loss is recommended only for obese patients with a body mass index ≥30 kg/m², or ≥27 kg/m² in the presence of other risk factors such as hypertension, diabetes, and/or dyslipidemia or a high waist circumference; therapy should be used in conjunction with a comprehensive weight management program.
Dosing
Adult & Geriatric Obesity (short-term adjunct): Oral:
Immediate release: 25 mg 3 times daily
Controlled release: 75 mg once daily at midmorning
Pediatric Children >16 years: Refer to adult dosing.
Renal Impairment No dosage adjustment provided in manufacturer's labeling; use with caution.
Hepatic Impairment No dosage adjustment provided in manufacturer's labeling.
Additional Information Complete prescribing information should be consulted for additional detail.
Dosage Forms Excipient information presented when available (limited, particularly for generics); consult specific product labeling.
Tablet, Oral, as hydrochloride:
Generic: 25 mg
Tablet Extended Release 24 Hour, Oral, as hydrochloride:
Generic: 75 mg
Controlled Substance C-IV

- Diethylpropion Hydrochloride *see* Diethylpropion *on page 546*
- Differin *see* Adapalene *on page 44*
- Differin® (Can) *see* Adapalene *on page 44*
- Differin® XP (Can) *see* Adapalene *on page 44*
- Dificid *see* Fidaxomicin *on page 765*
- Dificid™ (Can) *see* Fidaxomicin *on page 765*
- Difimicin *see* Fidaxomicin *on page 765*

Diflorasone (dye FLOR a sone)

Brand Names: US ApexiCon; ApexiCon E; Psorcon
Index Terms Diflorasone Diacetate
Pharmacologic Category Corticosteroid, Topical
Additional Appendix Information
Topical Corticosteroids *on page 1952*
Use Dermatoses: Treatment of inflammation and pruritic symptoms of corticosteroid-responsive dermatoses (high to very high potency topical corticosteroid)
Dosing
Adult & Geriatric Corticosteroid-responsive dermatosis: Topical: Apply sparingly 1 to 3 times daily. Therapy should be discontinued when control is achieved; if no improvement is seen, reassessment of diagnosis may be necessary.
Renal Impairment There are no dosage adjustments provided in the manufacturer's labeling.
Hepatic Impairment There are no dosage adjustments provided in the manufacturer's labeling.
Additional Information Complete prescribing information should be consulted for additional detail.
Dosage Forms Excipient information presented when available (limited, particularly for generics); consult specific product labeling.
Cream, External, as diacetate:
ApexiCon E: 0.05% (60 g)
ApexiCon E: 0.05% (30 g, 60 g) [contains cetyl alcohol, propylene glycol]
Psorcon: 0.05% (60 g) [contains cetyl alcohol, propylene glycol]
Generic: 0.05% (15 g, 30 g, 60 g)

Ointment, External, as diacetate:
ApexiCon: 0.05% (30 g, 60 g)
Generic: 0.05% (15 g, 30 g, 60 g)

- Diflorasone Diacetate *see* Diflorasone *on page 546*
- Diflucan *see* Fluconazole *on page 775*
- Diflucan injection (Can) *see* Fluconazole *on page 775*
- Diflucan One (Can) *see* Fluconazole *on page 775*
- Diflucan PWS (Can) *see* Fluconazole *on page 775*

Diflunisal (dye FLOO ni sal)

Brand Names: Canada Apo-Diflunisal; Novo-Diflunisal
Index Terms Dolobid
Pharmacologic Category Nonsteroidal Anti-inflammatory Drug (NSAID), Oral
Use
Mild to moderate pain: For acute or long-term use for symptomatic treatment of mild to moderate pain
Osteoarthritis/Rheumatoid arthritis (RA): For acute or long-term use for symptomatic relief of osteoarthritis and RA
Medication Guide Available Yes
Dosing
Adult
Mild to moderate pain: Oral: Initial: 1 g, followed by 500 mg every 12 hours; maintenance doses of 500 mg every 8 hours may be necessary in some patients; maximum daily dose: 1.5 g
Dosage adjustments: A lower dosage may be appropriate depending on pain severity, patient response, or weight; Initial: 500 mg, followed by 250 mg every 8-12 hours; maximum daily dose: 1.5 g
Arthritis: Oral: 500 mg to 1 g daily in 2 divided doses; maximum daily dose: 1.5 g
Geriatric
Mild to moderate pain: Oral: Initial: 500 mg, followed by 250 mg every 8-12 hours; maximum daily dose: 1.5 g
Arthritis: Refer to adult dosing.
Renal Impairment No dosage adjustment provided in the manufacturer's labeling; however the following adjustments have been used by some clinicians (Aronoff, 2007):
CrCl <50 mL/minute: Administer 50% of normal dose.
Hemodialysis: No supplement required.
CAPD: No supplement required.
Hepatic Impairment No dosage adjustment provided in manufacturer's labeling; use with caution.
Additional Information Complete prescribing information should be consulted for additional detail.
Dosage Forms Excipient information presented when available (limited, particularly for generics); consult specific product labeling.
Tablet, Oral:
Generic: 500 mg
Dosage Forms: Canada Excipient information presented when available (limited, particularly for generics); consult specific product labeling.
Tablet, Oral: 250 mg

- Difluorodeoxycytidine Hydrochlorothiazide *see* Gemcitabine *on page 832*

Difluprednate (dye floo PRED nate)

Brand Names: US Durezol
Pharmacologic Category Corticosteroid, Ophthalmic
Use
Inflammation/pain: Treatment of inflammation and pain following ocular surgery.
Uveitis: Treatment of endogenous anterior uveitis.
Dosing
Adult & Geriatric
Endogenous anterior uveitis: Ophthalmic: Instill 1 drop into conjunctival sac of the affected eye(s) 4 times daily for 14 days, then taper as clinically indicated
Inflammation/pain associated with ocular surgery: Ophthalmic:
US labeling: Instill 1 drop in conjunctival sac of the affected eye(s) 4 times daily beginning 24 hours after surgery, continue for 2 weeks, then decrease to 2 times daily for 1 week, then taper based on response
Canadian labeling: Instill 1 drop in conjunctival sac of the affected eye(s) 4 times daily beginning 24 hours after surgery, continue for 2 weeks, then taper based on response

Pediatric Inflammation/pain associated with ocular surgery: Infants, Children, and Adolescents: Refer to adult dosing. **Note:** Canadian labeling does not approve use in pediatric patients.

Renal Impairment There are no dosage adjustments provided in the manufacturer's labeling; however, systemic absorption is limited.

Hepatic Impairment There are no dosage adjustments provided in the manufacturer's labeling; however, systemic absorption is limited.

Additional Information Complete prescribing information should be consulted for additional detail.

Dosage Forms Excipient information presented when available (limited, particularly for generics); consult specific product labeling.

Emulsion, Ophthalmic:
Durezol: 0.05% (5 mL) [contains edetate sodium (tetrasodium), polysorbate 80]

◆ Digestive Enzyme see Pancrelipase on page 1384
◆ Digibind see Digoxin Immune Fab on page 550
◆ DigiFab see Digoxin Immune Fab on page 550
◆ Digitalis see Digoxin on page 547
◆ Digitek see Digoxin on page 547
◆ Digox see Digoxin on page 547

Digoxin (di JOKS in)

Brand Names: US Digitek; Digox; Lanoxin; Lanoxin Pediatric
Brand Names: Canada Apo-Digoxin; Digoxin Injection CSD; Lanoxin; Pediatric Digoxin CSD; PMS-Digoxin; Toloxin
Index Terms Digitalis; Lanoxicaps
Pharmacologic Category Antiarrhythmic Agent, Miscellaneous; Cardiac Glycoside
Use
Atrial fibrillation: For the control of ventricular response rate in adults with chronic atrial fibrillation.
Heart failure: For the treatment of mild-to-moderate (or stage C as recommended by the ACCF/AHA) heart failure (HF) in adults; to increase myocardial contractility in pediatric patients with heart failure
Note: In treatment of atrial fibrillation (AF), use is not considered first-line in patients with AF; digoxin may be considered for rate control in patients with heart failure with reduced ejection fraction (HFrEF) without pre-excitation or in sedentary patients (AHA/ACC/HRS [January, 2014]). In the treatment of heart failure, digoxin should be considered for use only in HF with reduced ejection fraction (HFrEF) when symptoms remain despite guideline-directed medical therapy or as initial therapy in patients with severe symptoms yet to respond to guideline-directed medical therapy (ACCF/AHA [Yancy, 2013]).
Pregnancy Considerations Animal reproduction studies have not been conducted. Digoxin crosses the placenta and serum concentrations are similar in the mother and fetus at delivery. Digoxin is recommended as first-line in the treatment of fetal tachycardia determined to be SVT. In pregnant women with SVT, use of digoxin is recommended (Blomström-Lundqvist, 2003).
Breast-Feeding Considerations Digoxin is excreted into breast milk and similar concentrations are found within mother's serum and milk. The manufacturer recommends that caution be used when administered to nursing women.
Contraindications Hypersensitivity to digoxin (rare) or other forms of digitalis, or any component of the formulation; ventricular fibrillation
Warnings/Precautions Watch for proarrhythmic effects (especially with digoxin toxicity). Withdrawal in clinically stable patients with HF may lead to recurrence of HF symptoms. During an episode of atrial fibrillation or flutter in patients with an accessory bypass tract (eg, Wolff-Parkinson-White syndrome) or pre-excitation syndrome, use has been associated with increased anterograde conduction down the accessory pathway leading to ventricular fibrillation; avoid use in such patients (ACLS [Neumar, 2010]; AHA/ACC/HRS [January, 2014]). Because digoxin slows sinoatrial and AV conduction, the drug commonly prolongs the PR interval. Digoxin may cause severe sinus bradycardia or sinoatrial block in patients with preexisting sinus node disease. Avoid use in patients with second- or third-degree heart block (except in patients with a functioning artificial pacemaker) (Yancy, 2013); incomplete AV block (eg, Stokes-Adams attack) may progress to complete block with digoxin administration. Digoxin should be considered for use only in heart failure (HF) with reduced ejection fraction (HFrEF) when symptoms remain despite guideline-directed medical therapy. It may also be considered in patients with both HF and atrial fibrillation;

however, beta blockers may offer better ventricular rate control than digoxin (ACCF/AHA [Yancy, 2013]). When used for rate control in patients with atrial fibrillation or heart failure, monitor serum concentrations closely; may be associated with an increased risk of mortality especially when serum concentrations are not properly controlled (Vamos 2015). Avoid use in patients with hypertrophic cardiomyopathy (HCM) and outflow tract obstruction unless used to control ventricular response with atrial fibrillation; outflow obstruction may worsen due to the positive inotropic effects of digoxin. Digoxin is potentially harmful in the treatment of dyspnea in patients with HCM in the absence of atrial fibrillation (Gersh, 2011). In a murine model of viral myocarditis, digoxin in high doses was shown to be detrimental (Matsumori, 1999). If used in humans, therefore, digoxin should be used with caution and only at low doses (Frishman, 2007). The manufacturer recommends avoiding the use of digoxin in patients with myocarditis.

Use with caution in patients with hyperthyroidism (increased digoxin clearance) and hypothyroidism (reduced digoxin clearance). Atrial arrhythmias associated with hypermetabolic (eg, hyperthyroidism) or hyperdynamic (hypoxia, arteriovenous shunt) states are very difficult to treat; treat underlying condition first. Use with caution in patients with an acute MI; may increase myocardial oxygen demand. During an acute coronary syndrome, digoxin administered IV may be used to slow a rapid ventricular response and improve left ventricular (LV) function in the acute treatment of atrial fibrillation associated with severe LV function and heart failure or hemodynamic instability (AHA/ACC/HRS [January, 2014]). Reduce dose with renal impairment and when amiodarone, propafenone, quinidine, or verapamil are added to a patient on digoxin; use with caution in patients taking strong inducers or inhibitors of P-glycoprotein (eg, cyclosporine). Avoid rapid IV administration of calcium in digitalized patients; may produce serious arrhythmias.

Atrial arrhythmias associated with hypermetabolic states are very difficult to treat; treat underlying condition first; if digoxin is used, ensure digoxin toxicity does not occur. Patients with beri beri heart disease may fail to adequately respond to digoxin therapy; treat underlying thiamine deficiency concomitantly. Correct electrolyte disturbances, especially hypokalemia or hypomagnesemia, prior to use and throughout therapy; toxicity may occur despite therapeutic digoxin concentrations. Hypercalcemia may increase the risk of digoxin toxicity; maintain normocalcemia. It is not necessary to routinely reduce or hold digoxin therapy prior to elective electrical cardioversion for atrial fibrillation; however, exclusion of digoxin toxicity (eg, clinical and ECG signs) is necessary prior to cardioversion. If signs of digoxin excess exist, withhold digoxin and delay cardioversion until toxicity subsides (AHA/ACC/HRS [January, 2014]). IV administration: Vesicant; ensure proper needle or catheter placement prior to and during administration; avoid extravasation. Some dosage forms may contain propylene glycol; large amounts are potentially toxic and have been associated hyperosmolality, lactic acidosis, seizures, and respiratory depression; use caution (AAP, 1997; Zar, 2007). Use with caution in the elderly; decreases in renal clearance may result in toxic effects; in general, avoid doses >0.125 mg/day; in heart failure, higher doses may increase the risk of potential toxicity and have not been shown to provide additional benefit (Beers Criteria).

Adverse Reactions Incidence not always reported.
Cardiovascular: Accelerated junctional rhythm, asystole, atrial tachycardia with or without block, AV dissociation, first-, second- (Wenckebach), or third-degree heart block, facial edema, PR prolongation, PVCs (especially bigeminy or trigeminy), ST segment depression, ventricular tachycardia or ventricular fibrillation
Central nervous system: Dizziness (6%), mental disturbances (5%), headache (4%), apathy, anxiety, confusion, delirium, depression, fever, hallucinations
Dermatologic: Rash (erythematous, maculopapular [most common], papular, scarlatiniform, vesicular or bullous), pruritus, urticaria, angioneurotic edema
Gastrointestinal: Nausea (4%), vomiting (2%), diarrhea (4%), abdominal pain, anorexia
Neuromuscular & skeletal: Weakness
Ocular: Visual disturbances (blurred or yellow vision)
Respiratory: Laryngeal edema
<1% (Limited to important or life-threatening): Asymmetric chorea, gynecomastia, thrombocytopenia, palpitation, intestinal ischemia, hemorrhagic necrosis of the intestines, vaginal cornification, eosinophilia, sexual dysfunction, diaphoresis

◀

Drug Interactions
Metabolism/Transport Effects Substrate of CYP3A4 (minor), P-glycoprotein; **Note:** Assignment of Major/Minor substrate status based on clinically relevant drug interaction potential

Avoid Concomitant Use
Avoid concomitant use of Digoxin with any of the following: Ceritinib

Increased Effect/Toxicity
Digoxin may increase the levels/effects of: Adenosine; Bradycardia-Causing Agents; Carvedilol; Ceritinib; Colchicine; Dronedarone; Ivabradine; Lacosamide; Midodrine

The levels/effects of Digoxin may be increased by: Aminoquinolines (Antimalarial); Amiodarone; Amphotericin B; Antithyroid Agents; AtorvaSTATin; Barnidipine; Beta-Blockers; Boceprevir; Bretylium; Brimonidine (Topical); Calcium Channel Blockers (Nondihydropyridine); Calcium Polystyrene Sulfonate; Calcium Salts; Carvedilol; CloNIDine; Conivaptan; CycloSPORINE (Systemic); Daclatasvir; Dronedarone; Edrophonium; Eliglustat; Eprostenol; Etravirine; Flecainide; Flibanserin; Glycopyrrolate; Glycopyrrolate (Systemic); Isavuconazonium Sulfate; Itraconazole; Lenalidomide; Levosulpiride; Licorice; Loop Diuretics; Lumacaftor; Macrolide Antibiotics; Mifepristone; Milnacipran; Mirabegron; Multivitamins/Fluoride (with ADE); Multivitamins/Minerals (with ADEK, Folate, Iron); Multivitamins/Minerals (with AE, No Iron); Nefazodone; Neuromuscular-Blocking Agents; NIFEdipine; Nonsteroidal Anti-Inflammatory Agents; Ombitasvir, Paritaprevir, and Ritonavir; Parathyroid Hormone; Paricalcitol; P-glycoprotein/ABCB1 Inhibitors; Posaconazole; Potassium-Sparing Diuretics; Propafenone; Protease Inhibitors; QuiNIDine; QuiNINE; Ranolazine; Regorafenib; Reserpine; Ruxolitinib; Simeprevir; SitaGLIPtin; Sodium Polystyrene Sulfonate; Spironolactone; Telaprevir; Telmisartan; Thiazide Diuretics; Ticagrelor; Tofacitinib; Tolvaptan; Trimethoprim; Vandetanib; Vemurafenib; Vilazodone; Vitamin D Analogs

Decreased Effect
Digoxin may decrease the levels/effects of: Antineoplastic Agents (Anthracycline, Systemic)

The levels/effects of Digoxin may be decreased by: 5-ASA Derivatives; Acarbose; Aminoglycosides; Antineoplastic Agents (Anthracycline, Systemic); Bile Acid Sequestrants; Kaolin; Lumacaftor; PenicillAMINE; P-glycoprotein/ABCB1 Inducers; Polyethylene Glycol 3350; Polyethylene Glycol 4000; Potassium-Sparing Diuretics; St Johns Wort; Sucralfate

Food Interactions Digoxin peak serum concentrations may be decreased if taken with food. Meals containing increased fiber (bran) or foods high in pectin may decrease oral absorption of digoxin.

Preparation for Administration
IM: No dilution required.

IV: May be administered undiluted or diluted fourfold in D$_5$W, NS, or SWFI for direct injection. Less than fourfold dilution may lead to drug precipitation.

Storage/Stability Store at 25°C (77°F); excursions permitted to 15°C to 30°C (59°F to 86°F). Protect elixir, injection, and tablets from light.

Mechanism of Action
Heart failure: Inhibition of the sodium/potassium ATPase pump in myocardial cells results in a transient increase of intracellular sodium, which in turn promotes calcium influx via the sodium-calcium exchange pump leading to increased contractility. May improve baroreflex sensitivity (Gheorghiade, 1991).

Supraventricular arrhythmias: Direct suppression of the AV node conduction to increase effective refractory period and decrease conduction velocity - positive inotropic effect, enhanced vagal tone, and decreased ventricular rate to fast atrial arrhythmias. Atrial fibrillation may decrease sensitivity and increase tolerance to higher serum digoxin concentrations.

Pharmacodynamics/Kinetics
Onset of action: Heart rate control: Oral: 1 to 2 hours; IV: 5 to 60 minutes

Peak effect: Heart rate control: Oral: 2 to 8 hours; IV: 1 to 6 hours; **Note:** In patients with atrial fibrillation, median time to ventricular rate control in one study was 6 hours (range: 3 to 15 hours) (Siu, 2009)

Duration: Adults: 3 to 4 days

Absorption: By passive nonsaturable diffusion in the upper small intestine; food may delay, but does not affect extent of absorption

Distribution:

Normal renal function: 6 to 7 L/kg

V$_d$: Extensive to peripheral tissues, with a distinct distribution phase which lasts 6 to 8 hours; concentrates in heart, liver, kidney, skeletal muscle, and intestines.

Heart/serum concentration is 70:1. Pharmacologic effects are delayed and do not correlate well with serum concentrations during distribution phase.

Hyperthyroidism: Increased V$_d$

Hyperkalemia, hyponatremia: Decreased digoxin distribution to heart and muscle

Hypokalemia: Increased digoxin distribution to heart and muscles

Concomitant quinidine therapy: Decreased V$_d$

Chronic renal failure: 4 to 6 L/kg

Decreased sodium/potassium ATPase activity - decreased tissue binding

Neonates, full-term: 7.5 to 10 L/kg

Children: 16 L/kg

Adults: 7 L/kg, decreased with renal disease

Protein binding: ~25%; in uremic patients, digoxin is displaced from plasma protein binding sites

Metabolism: Via sequential sugar hydrolysis in the stomach or by reduction of lactone ring by intestinal bacteria (in ~10% of population, gut bacteria may metabolize up to 40% of digoxin dose); once absorbed, only ~16% is metabolized to 3-beta-digoxigenin, 3-keto-digoxigenin, and glucuronide and sulfate conjugates; metabolites may contribute to therapeutic and toxic effects of digoxin; metabolism is reduced with decompensated HF

Bioavailability: Oral (formulation dependent): Elixir: 70% to 85%; Tablet: 60% to 80%

Half-life elimination (age, renal and cardiac function dependent):

Neonates: Premature: 61 to 170 hours; Full-term: 35 to 45 hours

Infants: 18 to 25 hours

Children: 18 to 36 hours

Adults: 36 to 48 hours

Adults, anephric: 3.5 to 5 days

Half-life elimination: Parent drug: 38 hours; Metabolites: Digoxigenin: 4 hours; Monodigitoxoside: 3 to 12 hours

Time to peak, serum: Oral: 1 to 3 hours

Excretion: Urine (50% to 70% as unchanged drug)

Dosing
Adult Note: When changing from oral (tablets or liquid) or IM to IV therapy, dosage should be reduced by 20% to 25%.

Atrial fibrillation (rate control) (off-label dose):

Total digitalizing dose (TDD): IV: 8 to 12 **mcg**/kg; administer half of TDD over 5 minutes with the remaining portion as 25% fractions at 4 to 8 hour intervals (ACLS [Neumar, 2010]) **or** may administer 0.25 mg with repeat dosing to a maximum of 1.5 mg over 24 hours followed by an oral maintenance regimen (AHA/ACC/HRS [January, 2014])

Maintenance: Oral: 0.125 to 0.25 mg once daily (AHA/ACC/HRS [January, 2014])

Heart failure: Daily maintenance dose (**Note:** Loading dose not recommended): Oral: 0.125 to 0.25 mg once daily; higher daily doses (eg, 0.375 to 0.5 mg daily) are rarely necessary. If patient is >70 years of age, has impaired renal function, or has a low lean body mass, low doses (eg, 0.125 mg daily or every other day) should be used initially (ACCF/AHA [Yancy, 2013]). **Note:** IV digoxin may be used to control ventricular response in patients with atrial fibrillation and heart failure with reduced ejection fraction (HFrEF) who do not have an accessory pathway or pre-excitation syndrome (AHA/ACC/HRS [January, 2014]). The addition of a beta-blocker to digoxin is usually more effective in controlling ventricular response, particularly during exercise (ACCF/AHA [Yancy, 2013]).

Supraventricular tachyarrhythmias (rate control):

Initial: Total digitalizing dose:

Oral: 0.75 to 1.5 mg

IV, IM: 0.5 to 1 mg (**Note:** IM not preferred due to severe injection site pain.)

Give ¹/₂ (one-half) of the total digitalizing dose (TDD) as the initial dose, then give ¹/₄ (one-quarter) of the TDD in each of 2 subsequent doses at 6- to 8-hour intervals. Obtain ECG 6 hours after each dose to assess potential toxicity.

Daily maintenance dose:

Oral: 0.125 to 0.5 mg once daily

IV, IM: 0.1 to 0.4 mg once daily (**Note:** IM not preferred due to severe injection site pain.)

Geriatric Dose is based on assessment of lean body mass and renal function. Elderly patients with low lean body mass may experience higher digoxin concentrations due to reduced volume of distribution (Cheng, 2010). Decrease dose in patients with decreased renal function (see Dosing in Renal Impairment).

Heart failure: If patient is >70 years of age, low doses (eg, 0.125 mg daily or every other day) should be used (ACCF/AHA [Yancy, 2013]).

Pediatric Atrial dysrhythmias (rate control), HF: When changing from oral (tablets or liquid) or IM to IV therapy, dosage should be reduced by 20% to 25%. See table.

Dosage Recommendations for Digoxin[1]

Age	Total Digitalizing Dose[2,3] (mcg/kg)		Daily Maintenance Dose[3,4] (mcg/kg)	
	Oral	IV or IM[5]	Oral	IV or IM[5]
Preterm infant	20-30	15-25	5-7.5	4-6
Full-term infant	25-35	20-30	6-10	5-8
1 mo - 2 y	35-60	30-50	10-15	7.5-12
2-5 y	30-40	25-35	7.5-10	6-9
5-10 y	20-35	15-30	5-10	4-8
>10 y	10-15	8-12	2.5-5	2-3

[1]**Heart failure:** A lower serum digoxin concentration may be adequate to treat heart failure (compared to cardiac arrhythmias); consider doses at the lower end of the recommended range for treatment of heart failure; a digitalizing dose (loading dose) may not be necessary when treating heart failure (Ross, 2001).

[2]**Do not give full total digitalizing dose (TDD) at once.** Give one-half of the total digitalizing dose (TDD) in the initial dose, then give one-quarter of the TDD in each of two subsequent doses at 6- to 8-hour intervals. Obtain ECG 6 hours after each dose to assess potential toxicity.

[3]Based on lean body weight and normal renal function for age. Decrease dose in patients with decreased renal function; digitalizing dose often not recommended in infants and children.

[4]Divided every 12 hours in infants and children <10 years of age. Given once daily to children >10 years of age and adults.

[5]IM not preferred due to severe injection site pain. If IM route is necessary, administer as deep injection followed by massage of injection site.

Renal Impairment

Adults: Oral, IV:
Loading dose: There are no dosage adjustments provided in the manufacturer's labeling, however, 50% to 70% of a digoxin dose is excreted unchanged in the urine. The following adjustments have been recommended:
ESRD: If loading dose necessary, reduce dose by 50% (Aronoff, 2007)
Acute renal failure: Based on expert opinion, if patient in acute renal failure requires ventricular rate control (eg, in atrial fibrillation), consider alternative therapy. If loading digoxin becomes necessary, patient volume of distribution may be increased and reduction in loading dose may not be necessary; however, maintenance dosing will require adjustment as long as renal failure persists.
Maintenance dose:
Manufacturer's labeling: Dosage reductions and close monitoring recommended; see product labeling for specific dosage recommendations based on CrCl.
Alternate dosing (Golightly, 2014):
GFR >50 mL/minute: No dosage adjustment necessary.
GFR 10 to 50 mL/minute: 0.0625 mg every 24 to 36 hours (25% to 75% of the usual dose every 24 to 36 hours).
GFR <10 mL/minute: 0.0625 mg every 48 hours (10% to 25% of the usual dose every 48 hours).
Hemodialysis: Nondialyzable (due to extensive binding to skeletal muscle and myocardium): 0.0625 mg every 48 hours (10% to 25% of the usual dose every 48 hours). No supplemental dose necessary (Mooradian, 1988).
CAPD: 0.0625 mg every 48 hours (10% to 25% of the usual dose every 48 hours).
Continuous renal replacement therapy (CRRT): 0.0625 mg every 48 hours (10% to 25% of the usual dose every 48 hours).
Heart failure: Initial maintenance dose (Bauman, 2006; Jusko, 1974; Koup, 1975): **Note:** The following suggested dosing recommendations are intended to achieve a target digoxin concentration of 0.7 ng/mL. Renal function estimated using Cockcroft-Gault formula.
CrCl >120 mL/minute: 0.25 mg once daily
CrCl 80 to 120 mL/minute: Alternate between doses of 0.25 mg and 0.125 mg once daily
CrCl 30 to 80 mL/minute: 0.125 mg once daily
CrCl <30 mL/minute: 0.125 mg every 48 hours
Note: A contemporary digoxin dosing nomogram using creatinine clearance and ideal body weight or height has been published for determining the initial maintenance dose in patients with heart failure to achieve a target digoxin concentration of 0.7 ng/mL (Bauman, 2006).

Pediatric: Oral, IV:
Loading dose: There are no dosage adjustments provided in the manufacturer's labeling; however, 50% to 70% of a digoxin dose is excreted unchanged in the urine.
Maintenance dose: Dosage reductions and close monitoring recommended; see product labeling for specific dosage recommendations based on CrCl.
Hepatic Impairment No dosage adjustment provided in manufacturer's labeling.

Dietary Considerations Maintain adequate amounts of potassium in diet to decrease risk of hypokalemia (hypokalemia may increase risk of digoxin toxicity).

Administration

IM: IV route preferred. If IM injection necessary, administer by deep injection followed by massage at the injection site. Inject no more than 2 mL per injection site. May cause intense pain.
IV: May be administered undiluted or diluted. Inject slowly over ≥5 minutes.
Vesicant; ensure proper needle or catheter placement prior to and during administration; avoid extravasation.
Extravasation management: If extravasation occurs, stop IV administration immediately and disconnect (leave cannula/needle in place); gently aspirate extravasated solution (do **NOT** flush the line); remove needle/cannula; elevate extremity.

Monitoring Parameters

Heart rate and rhythm should be monitored along with periodic ECGs to assess desired effects and signs of toxicity; baseline and periodic serum creatinine. Periodically monitor serum potassium, magnesium, and calcium especially if on medications where these electrolyte disturbances can occur (eg, diuretics), or if patient has a history of hypokalemia or hypomagnesemia. Observe patients for noncardiac signs of toxicity, confusion, and depression.
When to draw serum digoxin concentrations: Digoxin serum concentrations are monitored because digoxin possesses a narrow therapeutic serum range; the therapeutic endpoint is difficult to quantify and digoxin toxicity may be life-threatening. Digoxin serum concentrations should be drawn **at least 6 to 8 hours after last dose, regardless of route of administration (optimally 12 to 24 hours after a dose). Note:** Serum digoxin concentrations may decrease in response to exercise due to increased skeletal muscle uptake; a period of rest (eg, ~2 hours) after exercise may be necessary prior to drawing serum digoxin concentrations.
Initiation of therapy:
If a loading dose is given: Digoxin serum concentration may be drawn within 12 to 24 hours after the initial loading dose administration. Concentrations drawn this early may confirm the relationship of digoxin plasma concentrations and response but are of little value in determining maintenance doses.
If a loading dose is not given: Digoxin serum concentration should be obtained after 3 to 5 days of therapy.
Maintenance therapy:
Trough concentrations should be followed just prior to the next dose or at a minimum of 6 to 8 hours after last dose.
Digoxin serum concentrations should be obtained within 5 to 7 days (approximate time to steady-state) after any dosage changes. Continue to obtain digoxin serum concentrations 7 to 14 days after any change in maintenance dose. **Note:** In patients with end-stage renal disease, it may take 15 to 20 days to reach steady-state.
Patients who are receiving electrolyte-depleting medications such as diuretics, serum potassium, magnesium, and calcium should be monitored closely.
Digoxin serum concentrations should be obtained whenever any of the following conditions occur:
Questionable patient compliance or to evaluate clinical deterioration following an initial good response
Changing renal function
Suspected digoxin toxicity
Initiation or discontinuation of therapy with drugs (eg, amiodarone, quinidine, verapamil) which potentially interact with digoxin.
Any disease changes (eg, thyroid disease)

Reference Range

Digoxin therapeutic serum concentrations:
Heart failure: 0.5 to 0.9 ng/mL (ACCF/AHA [Yancy, 2013])
Adults: <0.5 ng/mL; probably indicates underdigitalization unless there are special circumstances
Toxic: >2 ng/mL
Digoxin-like immunoreactive substance (DLIS) may cross-react with digoxin immunoassay. DLIS has been found in patients with renal and liver disease, heart failure, neonates, and pregnant women (3rd trimester).

Test Interactions Spironolactone may interfere with digoxin radioimmunoassay.

Dosage Forms Excipient information presented when available (limited, particularly for generics); consult specific product labeling. [DSC] = Discontinued product

Solution, Injection:

Lanoxin: 0.25 mg/mL (2 mL) [contains alcohol, usp, propylene glycol]

Lanoxin Pediatric: 0.1 mg/mL (1 mL) [contains alcohol, usp, propylene glycol]

Generic: 0.25 mg/mL (1 mL, 2 mL)

Solution, Oral:

Generic: 0.05 mg/mL (60 mL)

Tablet, Oral:

Digitek: 125 mcg [scored; contains fd&c yellow #10 aluminum lake]

Digitek: 250 mcg [scored]

Digox: 125 mcg [scored; contains fd&c yellow #10 aluminum lake]

Digox: 250 mcg [scored]

Lanoxin: 62.5 mcg [contains fd&c yellow #6 (sunset yellow)]

Lanoxin: 125 mcg [scored; contains fd&c yellow #10 (quinoline yellow), fd&c yellow #6 (sunset yellow)]

Lanoxin: 125 mcg [DSC] [contains fd&c yellow #10 aluminum lake, fd&c yellow #6 aluminum lake]

Lanoxin: 125 mcg [DSC] [contains fd&c yellow #10 aluminum lake, fd&c yellow #6 aluminum lake]

Lanoxin: 187.5 mcg

Lanoxin: 250 mcg [scored]

Generic: 125 mcg, 250 mcg

Dosage Forms: Canada Excipient information presented when available (limited, particularly for generics); consult specific product labeling.

Tablet, oral:

Apo-Digoxin: 62.5 mcg, 125 mcg, 250 mcg

Digoxin Immune Fab (di JOKS in i MYUN fab)

Brand Names: US DigiFab
Brand Names: Canada DigiFab
Index Terms Antidigoxin Fab Fragments, Ovine; Digibind
Pharmacologic Category Antidote

Use Digoxin toxicity: Treatment of life-threatening or potentially life-threatening digoxin intoxication, including:

- Acute digoxin ingestion (≥10 mg in adults; 4 mg [>0.1 mg/kg] in children); resulting in serum concentration ≥10 ng/mL)

- Chronic ingestion leading to steady state digoxin concentrations >6 ng/mL in adults or >4 ng/mL in children

- Manifestations of life-threatening digoxin toxicity due to overdose (severe ventricular arrhythmias, progressive bradycardia, second or third degree heart block not responsive to atropine, serum potassium concentration >5.5 mEq/L in adults or >6 mEq/L in children)

Pregnancy Considerations Animal reproduction studies have not been conducted. In general, medications used as antidotes should take into consideration the health and prognosis of the mother; antidotes should be administered to pregnant women if there is a clear indication for use and should not be withheld because of fears of teratogenicity (Bailey, 2003).

Breast-Feeding Considerations It is not known if digoxin immune fab is excreted in breast milk. The manufacturer recommends caution be exercised when administering to nursing women.

Contraindications There are no contraindications listed in the manufacturer's labeling.

Warnings/Precautions Digoxin immune Fab is derived from ovine (sheep) Fab immunoglobulin fragments; hypersensitivity reactions (eg, anaphylactic or anaphylactoid reactions, delayed allergic reactions) are possible. Patients with allergies to sheep proteins and patients with prior exposure to ovine antibodies or ovine Fab may be at a higher risk for anaphylactic reactions. In patients who develop an anaphylactic reaction, discontinue the infusion immediately and administer emergency care; balance the need for epinephrine against its potential risk in the setting of digitalis toxicity. Processed with papain and may cause hypersensitivity reactions in patients allergic to papaya, other papaya extracts, papain, chymopapain, or the pineapple-enzyme bromelain. There may also be cross allergenicity with dust mite and latex allergens.

Patients experiencing acute digitalis toxicity may present with significant hyperkalemia due to shifting of potassium into the extracellular space. Upon treatment with digoxin immune Fab, potassium shifts back into the intracellular space and may result in hypokalemia. Monitor potassium closely, especially during the first few hours after administration; treat hypokalemia cautiously when clinically indicated.

In patients chronically maintained on digoxin for HF, administration of digoxin immune Fab may result in exacerbation of HF symptoms due to a reduction in digoxin serum concentration. If reinitiation is required, consider postponing until Fab fragments have been eliminated completely; elimination may take several days or longer, especially in patients with renal impairment. Use with caution in patients with renal failure (experience limited); the Fab-digoxin complex will be eliminated more slowly. Toxicity may recur; prolonged monitoring for recurrence of symptoms and evaluation of free (unbound) digoxin concentrations (if test available) may be warranted in this patient population.

Adverse Reactions Frequency not defined.

Cardiovascular: Heart failure exacerbation (due to withdrawal of digoxin), orthostatic hypotension, rapid ventricular response (patients with atrial fibrillation; due to withdrawal of digoxin)

Endocrine & metabolic: Hypokalemia

Local: Phlebitis

Miscellaneous: Allergic reactions, serum sickness

Drug Interactions

Metabolism/Transport Effects None known.

Avoid Concomitant Use There are no known interactions where it is recommended to avoid concomitant use.

Increased Effect/Toxicity There are no known significant interactions involving an increase in effect.

Decreased Effect There are no known significant interactions involving a decrease in effect.

Preparation for Administration Reconstitute each vial to a concentration of 10 mg/mL by adding 4 mL SWFI; gently mix. Add reconstituted digoxin immune fab to an appropriate volume of NS. For very small doses, the reconstituted vial can be further diluted by adding an additional 36 mL NS to achieve a final concentration of 1 mg/mL. Infants and small children who require very small doses may be administered reconstituted digoxin immune undiluted using a tuberculin syringe.

Storage/Stability Store vials at 2°C to 8°C (36°F to 46°F); do not freeze. Reconstituted solutions are stable for 4 hours when stored at 2°C to 8°C (36°F to 46°F). The following stability information has also been reported: May be stored at room temperature for up to 30 days (Cohen, 2007).

Mechanism of Action Digoxin immune antigen-binding fragments (Fab) are specific antibodies for the treatment of digitalis intoxication in carefully selected patients; binds with molecules of digoxin or DIGIToxin and is then excreted by the kidneys and removed from the body

Pharmacodynamics/Kinetics

Onset of action: IV: Digitalis toxicity: Improvement may be seen within 20 to 90 minutes (Betten, 2006)

Distribution: V_d: 0.3 L/kg

Half-life elimination: 15 to 20 hours; may be increased up to 10-fold in patient with renal impairment

Excretion: Urine (concentrations declining within 5 to 7 days)

Dosing

Adult & Geriatric Each vial of digoxin immune Fab 40 mg will bind ~0.5 mg of digoxin or DIGIToxin.

Digoxin toxicity: Note: Estimation of the dose is based on the body burden of digitalis. This may be calculated if the amount ingested is known or the post-distribution serum drug level is known (round the dose up to the nearest whole vial). If the amount ingested is unknown, general dosing guidelines should be used.

Acute ingestion of unknown amount: IV: Initial: 10 vials; if needed, administer a second dose of 10 vials (20 vials total is adequate to treat most life-threatening ingestions).

Acute ingestion of known amount: IV:

Based on number of tablets or capsules ingested:

Step 1: Calculate total body load (mg)

Digoxin capsules or DIGIToxin:

Total body load (mg) = Amount (mg) digoxin capsules **or** DIGIToxin ingested

Digoxin tablets:

Total body load (mg) = 0.8 x (amount [mg] digoxin tablets ingested)

Step 2: Calculate number of vials needed

Digoxin Immune Fab Dose (vials) = Total body load (mg) / (0.5)

Alternatively, the following table gives an estimation of the number of vials needed based on the number of **digoxin** tablets or capsules ingested.

Approximate Dose of Digoxin Immune Fab (in vials) for Reversal of a Single Large Digoxin Overdose

Number of Digoxin Tablets or Capsules Ingested[1]	Dose of Digoxin Immune Fab (# of Vials)
25	10
50	20
75	30
100	40
150	60
200	80

[1]250 mcg tablets with 80% bioavailability or 200 mcg capsules with 100% bioavailability.

Based on steady-state serum digoxin concentration:

Adults:

Digoxin Immune Fab Dose (vials) = (serum digoxin concentration [ng/mL] x weight [kg]) / **100**

Alternatively, the following table gives an estimation of the number of vials needed based on the steady-state serum digoxin concentration.

Adult Dose Estimates of Digoxin Immune Fab (in # of Vials) From Steady-State Serum Digoxin Concentration

Patient Weight (kg)	Serum Digoxin Concentration (ng/mL)						
	1	2	4	8	12	16	20
40	0.5 vial	1 vial	2 vials	3 vials	5 vials	7 vials	8 vials
60	0.5 vial	1 vial	3 vials	5 vials	7 vials	10 vials	12 vials
70	1 vial	2 vials	3 vials	6 vials	9 vials	11 vials	14 vials
80	1 vial	2 vials	3 vials	7 vials	10 vials	13 vials	16 vials
100	1 vial	2 vials	4 vials	8 vials	12 vials	16 vials	20 vials

Based on steady-state DIGIToxin concentration: If the calculated dose based on the DIGIToxin concentration is different from the estimated dose based on the known ingested amount (if available), use the higher dose.

Digoxin Immune Fab Dose (vials) = [serum **DIGIToxin** concentration (ng/mL) x weight (kg)] / **1000**

Chronic toxicity (serum digoxin concentration unavailable): IV: Adults: 6 vials is adequate to reverse most cases of toxicity

Pediatric Each vial of digoxin immune Fab 40 mg will bind ~0.5 mg of digoxin or DIGIToxin.

Digoxin toxicity: Note: Estimation of the dose is based on the body burden of digitalis. This may be calculated if the amount ingested is known or the post-distribution serum drug level is known (round the dose up to the nearest whole vial). If the amount ingested is unknown, general dosing guidelines should be used.

Acute ingestion of unknown amount: IV: Refer to adult dosing.

Acute ingestion of known amount: IV: Refer to adult dosing.

Based on steady-state serum digoxin concentration:

Infants and Children ≤20 kg: May require smaller doses; calculate the dose in milligrams (mg).

Digoxin Immune Fab Dose (mg) = [(serum digoxin concentration [ng/mL] x weight [kg]) / **100**] x (digoxin immune Fab amount per vial [mg/vial])

Note: Digoxin immune Fab amount per vial: 40 mg/vial.

Alternatively, the following table gives an estimation of the amount of digoxin immune Fab needed based on the steady-state serum digoxin concentration.

Infants and Small Children Dose Estimates of Digoxin Immune Fab (in mg) From Steady-State Serum Digoxin Concentration

Patient Weight (kg)	Serum Digoxin Concentration (ng/mL)						
	1	2	4	8	12	16	20
1	0.4 mg[1]	1 mg[1]	1.5 mg[1]	3 mg[1]	5 mg	6.5 mg	8 mg
3	1 mg[1]	2.5 mg[1]	5 mg	10 mg	14 mg	19 mg	24 mg
5	2 mg[1]	4 mg	8 mg	16 mg	24 mg	32 mg	40 mg
10	4 mg	8 mg	16 mg	32 mg	48 mg	64 mg	80 mg
20	8 mg	16 mg	32 mg	64 mg	96 mg	128 mg	160 mg

[1]Dilution of reconstituted vial to 1 mg/mL may be desirable.

Children >20 kg and Adolescents: Refer to adult dosing.

Based on steady-state DIGIToxin concentration: Refer to adult dosing.

Chronic toxicity (serum digoxin concentration unavailable): IV:

Infants and Children <20 kg: 1 vial is adequate to reverse most cases of toxicity

Children ≥20 kg and Adolescents: Refer to adult dosing.

Renal Impairment There are no dosage adjustments provided in the manufacturer's labeling; however, use with caution since digoxin-digoxin immune Fab complex is renally eliminated. Patients should undergo prolonged monitoring for recurrence of toxicity.

Hepatic Impairment There are no dosage adjustments provided in the manufacturer's labeling.

Administration Administer by slow IV infusion over at least 30 minutes. May also be given by bolus injection if cardiac arrest is imminent (infusion-related reaction may occur). Infants and small children who require very small doses can be administered reconstituted digoxin immune fab undiluted using a tuberculin syringe. Stopping the infusion and restarting at a slower rate may help if an infusion-related reaction occurs.

Monitoring Parameters Prior to the first dose of digoxin immune Fab evaluate serum potassium, serum digoxin concentration, and serum creatinine; closely monitor serum potassium (eg, hourly for 4-6 hours; at least daily thereafter), temperature, blood pressure, and electrocardiogram after administration. **Total serum digoxin concentrations will rise precipitously following administration of digoxin immune Fab due to the presence of the Fab-digoxin complex; because digoxin bound to Fab fragments cannot result in toxicity, this rise has no clinical meaning.** Therefore, avoid monitoring total serum digoxin concentrations until the Fab fragments have been eliminated completely; this may be several days to weeks in patients with renal impairment (Ujhelyi, 1995). Monitor for volume overload in children <20 kg. Monitor for signs and symptoms of a hypersensitivity reaction.

Patients with renal failure may experience a recurrence of toxicity; prolonged monitoring for recurrence of symptoms and evaluation of free (unbound) digoxin concentrations (if test available) may be warranted in this patient population.

Test Interactions Digoxin immune fab may interfere with digitalis immunoassay measurements, thereby resulting in clinically misleading total serum digoxin concentrations until all Fab fragments are eliminated from the body (may take several days to >1 week after administration). Digoxin serum samples should be obtained before digoxin immune fab administration, if possible.

Dosage Forms Excipient information presented when available (limited, particularly for generics); consult specific product labeling.

Solution Reconstituted, Intravenous [preservative free]:
DigiFab: 40 mg (1 ea)

◆ Digoxin Injection CSD (Can) see Digoxin on page 547
◆ Dihematoporphirin Ether see Porfimer on page 1474
◆ Dihydroartemisinin Hemisuccinate Sodium see Artesunate on page 154

Dihydrocodeine, Aspirin, and Caffeine
(dye hye droe KOE deen, AS pir in, & KAF een)

Brand Names: US Synalgos®-DC

Index Terms Aspirin, Dihydrocodeine, and Caffeine; Caffeine, Dihydrocodeine, and Aspirin; Dihydrocodeine Compound; Dihydrocodeine, Aspirin, and Caffeine

Pharmacologic Category Analgesic, Opioid
Use Pain: Management of moderate to moderately severe pain
Dosing
Adult Pain: Oral: Two capsules (aspirin 712.8 mg/caffeine 60 mg/dihydrocodeine 32 mg) every 4 hours as needed for pain
Geriatric Refer to adult dosing. Initial dosing should be cautious (low end of adult dosing range).
Pediatric Children >12 years and Adolescents: Refer to adult dosing.
Renal Impairment There are no dosage adjustments provided in the manufacturer's labeling.
Hepatic Impairment There are no dosage adjustments provided in the manufacturer's labeling.
Additional Information Complete prescribing information should be consulted for additional detail.
Dosage Forms Excipient information presented when available (limited, particularly for generics); consult specific product labeling.
Capsule, oral:
Synalgos®-DC: Dihydrocodeine bitartrate 16 mg, aspirin 356.4 mg, and caffeine 30 mg
Generic: Dihydrocodeine bitartrate 16 mg, aspirin 356.4 mg, and caffeine 30 mg
Controlled Substance C-III

◆ **Dihydrocodeine, Aspirin, and Caffeine** see Dihydrocodeine, Aspirin, and Caffeine on page 551

◆ **Dihydrocodeine Compound** see Dihydrocodeine, Aspirin, and Caffeine on page 551

Dihydroergotamine (dye hye droe er GOT a meen)

Brand Names: US D.H.E. 45; Migranal
Brand Names: Canada Migranal®
Index Terms DHE; Dihydroergotamine Mesylate
Pharmacologic Category Antimigraine Agent; Ergot Derivative
Use Treatment of migraine headache with or without aura; injection also indicated for treatment of cluster headaches
Pregnancy Considerations Dihydroergotamine is oxytocic and should not be used during pregnancy.
Breast-Feeding Considerations Ergot derivatives inhibit prolactin and it is known that ergotamine is excreted in breast milk (vomiting, diarrhea, weak pulse, and unstable blood pressure have been reported in nursing infants). It is not known if dihydroergotamine would also cause these effects, however, it is likely that it is excreted in human breast milk. Do not use in nursing women.
Contraindications Hypersensitivity to dihydroergotamine or any component of the formulation; uncontrolled hypertension, ischemic heart disease, angina pectoris, history of MI, silent ischemia, or coronary artery vasospasm including Prinzmetal's angina; hemiplegic or basilar migraine; peripheral vascular disease; sepsis; severe hepatic or renal dysfunction; following vascular surgery; avoid use within 24 hours of sumatriptan, zolmitriptan, other serotonin agonists, or ergot-like agents; avoid during or within 2 weeks of discontinuing MAO inhibitors; concurrent use of peripheral and central vasoconstrictors; ergot alkaloids are contraindicated with potent inhibitors of CYP3A4 (includes protease inhibitors, azole antifungals, and some macrolide antibiotics); pregnancy, breast-feeding
Warnings/Precautions [U.S. Boxed Warning]: Ergot alkaloids are contraindicated with potent inhibitors of CYP3A4 (includes protease inhibitors, azole antifungals, and some macrolide antibiotics); concomitant use associated with an increased risk of vasospasm leading to cerebral ischemia and/or ischemia of the extremities. Do not give to patients with risk factors for CAD until a cardiovascular evaluation has been performed; if evaluation is satisfactory, the healthcare provider should administer the first dose and cardiovascular status should be periodically evaluated. May cause vasospastic reactions; persistent vasospasm may lead to gangrene or death in patients with compromised circulation. Discontinue if signs of vasoconstriction develop. Rare reports of increased blood pressure in patients without history of hypertension. Rare reports of adverse cardiac events (acute MI, life-threatening arrhythmias, death) have been reported following use of the injection. Cerebral hemorrhage, subarachnoid hemorrhage, and stroke have also occurred following use of the injection. Not for prolonged use. Pleural and peritoneal fibrosis have been reported with prolonged daily use. Cardiac valvular fibrosis has also been associated with ergot alkaloids. Use with caution in the elderly.

Migranal® Nasal Spray: Local irritation to nose and throat (usually transient and mild-moderate in severity) can occur; long-term consequences on nasal or respiratory mucosa have not been extensively evaluated.
Adverse Reactions
>10%: Nasal spray: Respiratory: Rhinitis (26%)
1% to 10%: Nasal spray:
Central nervous system: Taste disorder (8%), dizziness (4%), drowsiness (3%)
Endocrine & metabolic: Hot flash (1%)
Gastrointestinal: Nausea (10%), vomiting (4%), diarrhea (2%)
Local: Application site reaction (6%)
Neuromuscular & skeletal: Stiffness (1%), weakness (1%)
Respiratory: Pharyngitis (3%)
<1% (Limited to important or life-threatening): Injection and nasal spray: Abdominal pain, anxiety, cerebral hemorrhage, cerebrovascular accident, coronary artery vasospasm, diaphoresis, diarrhea, dizziness, dyspnea, edema, fibrothorax (prolonged use), flushing, headache, hyperkinesia, hypertension, ischemic heart disease, muscle cramps, myalgia, myasthenia, myocardial infarction, palpitations, paresthesia, peripheral cyanosis, peripheral ischemia, retroperitoneal fibrosis (prolonged use), skin rash, subarachnoid hemorrhage, tremor, valvular sclerosis (associated with ergot alkaloids), ventricular fibrillation, ventricular tachycardia (transient)
Drug Interactions
Metabolism/Transport Effects Substrate of CYP3A4 (major); **Note:** Assignment of Major/Minor substrate status based on clinically relevant drug interaction potential
Avoid Concomitant Use
Avoid concomitant use of Dihydroergotamine with any of the following: Alpha-/Beta-Agonists; Alpha1-Agonists; Antihepaciviral Combination Products; Boceprevir; Clarithromycin; Cobicistat; Conivaptan; Crizotinib; Dapoxetine; Enzalutamide; Fusidic Acid (Systemic); Idelalisib; Itraconazole; Ketoconazole (Systemic); Lorcaserin; Mifepristone; Nitroglycerin; Posaconazole; Protease Inhibitors; Serotonin 5-HT1D Receptor Agonists; Telaprevir; Voriconazole
Increased Effect/Toxicity
Dihydroergotamine may increase the levels/effects of: Alpha-/Beta-Agonists; Alpha1-Agonists; Antipsychotic Agents; Metoclopramide; Serotonin 5-HT1D Receptor Agonists; Serotonin Modulators

The levels/effects of Dihydroergotamine may be increased by: Antiemetics (5HT3 Antagonists); Antihepaciviral Combination Products; Antipsychotic Agents; Aprepitant; Beta-Blockers; Boceprevir; Clarithromycin; Cobicistat; Conivaptan; Crizotinib; CYP3A4 Inhibitors (Moderate); CYP3A4 Inhibitors (Strong); Dapoxetine; Dasatinib; Fosaprepitant; Fusidic Acid (Systemic); Idelalisib; Itraconazole; Ivacaftor; Ketoconazole (Systemic); Lorcaserin; Luliconazole; Macrolide Antibiotics; Metaxalone; Mifepristone; Netupitant; Nitroglycerin; Osimertinib; Palbociclib; Posaconazole; Protease Inhibitors; Serotonin 5-HT1D Receptor Agonists; Simeprevir; Stiripentol; Tedizolid; Telaprevir; Voriconazole
Decreased Effect
Dihydroergotamine may decrease the levels/effects of: Nitroglycerin

The levels/effects of Dihydroergotamine may be decreased by: Enzalutamide; Osimertinib
Storage/Stability
Injection: Store below 25°C (77°F); do not refrigerate or freeze; protect from heat. Protect from light.
Nasal spray: Prior to use, store below 25°C (77°F); do not refrigerate or freeze. Once spray applicator has been prepared, use within 8 hours; discard any unused solution.
Mechanism of Action Ergot alkaloid alpha-adrenergic blocker directly stimulates vascular smooth muscle to vasoconstrict peripheral and cerebral vessels; also has effects on serotonin receptors
Pharmacodynamics/Kinetics
Onset of action: IM: 15-30 minutes
Duration: IM: 3-4 hours
Distribution: V_d: ~800 L
Protein binding: 93%
Metabolism: Extensively hepatic (one active metabolite)
Half-life elimination: ~9-10 hours
Time to peak, serum: IM: 24 minutes; IV: 1-2 minutes; Intranasal: 30-60 minutes; SubQ 15-45 minutes
Excretion: Primarily feces; urine (6% to 7% as unchanged drug)
Clearance: 1.5 mL/minute

Dosing

Adult

Migraine, cluster headache:

IM, SubQ: 1 mg at first sign of headache; repeat hourly to a maximum dose of 3 mg/day; maximum dose: 6 mg/week

IV: 1 mg at first sign of headache; repeat hourly up to a maximum dose of 2 mg/day; maximum dose: 6 mg/week

Intranasal: 1 spray (0.5 mg) of nasal spray should be administered into each nostril; if needed, repeat after 15 minutes, up to a total of 4 sprays (2 mg). **Note:** Do not exceed 6 sprays (3 mg) in a 24-hour period and no more than 8 sprays (4 mg) in a week.

Intractable migraine (status migrainosus; >72 hours):

IV: Raskin protocol (off-label dosing): Initial test dose: 0.5 mg (following premedication with metoclopramide); subsequent dosing is titrated (range: 0.2-1 mg) every 8 hours for 2-3 days and administered with or without metoclopramide based on response and tolerance (Raskin, 1986; Raskin, 1990). **Note:** Some clinicians use modified versions of this protocol, with additional adjunctive medications and/or alternate antiemetic agents.

Geriatric Refer to adult dosing. Patients >65 years of age were not included in controlled clinical studies.

Renal Impairment Contraindicated in severe renal impairment

Hepatic Impairment Dosage reductions are probably necessary but specific guidelines are not available; contraindicated in severe hepatic dysfunction.

Administration

Intranasal: Prior to administration of nasal spray, the nasal spray applicator must be primed (pumped 4 times); in order to let the drug be absorbed through the skin in the nose, patients should not inhale deeply through the nose while spraying or immediately after spraying; for best results, treatment should be initiated at the first symptom or sign of an attack; however, nasal spray can be used at any stage of a migraine attack.

IM, SubQ: May administer by intramuscular or subcutaneous injection.

IV: Administer slowly over 2-3 minutes (Raskin protocol)

Reference Range Minimum concentration for vasoconstriction is reportedly 0.06 ng/mL

Dosage Forms Considerations

Migranal nasal solution contains caffeine 10 mg/mL

Dosage Forms Excipient information presented when available (limited, particularly for generics); consult specific product labeling.

Solution, Injection, as mesylate:
D.H.E. 45: 1 mg/mL (1 mL)
Generic: 1 mg/mL (1 mL)
Solution, Nasal, as mesylate:
Migranal: 4 mg/mL (1 mL)
Generic: 4 mg/mL (1 mL)

Diltiazem (dil TYE a zem)

Brand Names: US Cardizem; Cardizem CD; Cardizem LA; Cartia XT; Dilacor XR [DSC]; Dilt-CD [DSC]; Dilt-XR; Diltiazem CD; Diltiazem HCl CD [DSC]; Diltzac [DSC]; Matzim LA; Taztia XT; Tiazac

Brand Names: Canada ACT Diltiazem CD; ACT Diltiazem T; Apo-Diltiaz; Apo-Diltiaz CD; Apo-Diltiaz SR; Apo-Diltiaz TZ; Cardizem CD; Diltiazem Hydrochloride Injection; Diltiazem TZ; Diltiazem-CD; PMS-Diltiazem CD; Sandoz-Diltiazem CD; Sandoz-Diltiazem T; Teva-Diltiazem; Teva-Diltiazem CD; Teva-Diltiazem HCL ER Capsules; Tiazac; Tiazac XC

Index Terms Diltiazem Hydrochloride

Pharmacologic Category Antianginal Agent; Antiarrhythmic Agent, Class IV; Antihypertensive; Calcium Channel Blocker; Calcium Channel Blocker, Nondihydropyridine

Use

Oral: Primary hypertension; chronic stable angina or angina from coronary artery spasm

Guideline recommendations:

Hypertension: The 2014 guideline for the management of high blood pressure in adults (JNC 8) recommends initiation of pharmacologic treatment to lower blood pressure for the following patients (JNC8 [James 2013]):

• Patients ≥60 years of age, with systolic blood pressure (SBP) ≥150 mm Hg or diastolic blood pressure (DBP) ≥90 mm Hg. Goal of therapy is SBP <150 mm Hg and DBP <90 mm Hg.

• Patients <60 years of age, with SBP ≥140 mm Hg or DBP ≥90 mm Hg. Goal of therapy is SBP <140 mm Hg and DBP <90 mm Hg.

• Patients ≥18 years of age with diabetes, with SBP ≥140 mm Hg or DBP ≥90 mm Hg. Goal of therapy is SBP <140 mm Hg and DBP <90 mm Hg.

• Patients ≥18 years of age with chronic kidney disease (CKD), with SBP ≥140 mm Hg or DBP ≥90 mm Hg. Goal of therapy is SBP <140 mm Hg and DBP <90 mm Hg.

Chronic kidney disease (CKD) and hypertension: Regardless of race or diabetes status, the use of an ACE inhibitor (ACEI) or angiotensin receptor blocker (ARB) as initial therapy is recommended to improve kidney outcomes. In the general nonblack population (without CKD) including those with diabetes, initial antihypertensive treatment should consist of a thiazide-type diuretic, calcium channel blocker, ACEI, or ARB. In the general black population (without CKD) including those with diabetes, initial antihypertensive treatment should consist of a thiazide-type diuretic or a calcium channel blocker **instead of** an ACEI or ARB.

Coronary artery disease (CAD) and hypertension: The American Heart Association, American College of Cardiology and American Society of Hypertension (AHA/ACC/ASH) 2015 scientific statement for the treatment of hypertension in patients with coronary artery disease (CAD) recommends that a non-dihydropyridine CCB (verapamil, diltiazem) may be used as a substitute for a beta blocker in patients who have an intolerance or contraindication to beta blockers with ongoing ischemia, hypertension and chronic stable angina, or if angina or hypertension continues to be uncontrolled while receiving standard therapies (eg, beta blocker). However, a non-dihydropyridine CCB (eg, verapamil, diltiazem) should be avoided in patients with LV dysfunction and heart failure (with reduced ejection fraction). A BP target of <140/90 mm Hg is reasonable for the secondary prevention of cardiovascular events. A lower target BP (<130/80 mm Hg) may be appropriate in some individuals with CAD, previous MI, stroke or transient ischemic attack, or CAD risk equivalents (AHA/ACC/ASH [Rosendorff 2015]).

Injection: Control of rapid ventricular rate in patients with atrial fibrillation or atrial flutter; conversion of paroxysmal supraventricular tachycardia (PSVT)

Pregnancy Considerations Adverse events have been observed in animal reproduction studies. Untreated chronic maternal hypertension is associated with adverse events in the fetus, infant, and mother. If treatment for hypertension during pregnancy is needed, other agents are preferred (ACOG 2013). The Canadian labeling contraindicates use in pregnant women or women of childbearing potential. Women with hypertrophic cardiomyopathy who are controlled with diltiazem prior to pregnancy may continue therapy, but increased fetal monitoring is recommended (Gersh 2011).

Breast-Feeding Considerations Diltiazem is excreted into breast milk in concentrations similar to those in the maternal plasma (Okada, 1985). Breast-feeding is not recommended by the manufacturer.

Contraindications

Oral: Hypersensitivity to diltiazem or any component of the formulation; sick sinus syndrome (except in patients with a functioning artificial pacemaker); second- or third-degree AV block (except in patients with a functioning artificial pacemaker); hypotension (systolic <90 mm Hg); acute MI and pulmonary congestion

Intravenous (IV): Hypersensitivity to diltiazem or any component of the formulation; sick sinus syndrome (except in patients with a functioning artificial pacemaker); second- or third-degree AV block (except in patients with a functioning artificial pacemaker); severe hypotension; cardiogenic shock; administration concomitantly or within a few hours of the administration of IV beta-blockers; atrial fibrillation or flutter associated with accessory bypass tract (eg, Wolff-Parkinson-White syndrome, short PR syndrome); ventricular tachycardia (with wide-complex tachycardia [QRS ≥0.12 seconds], must determine whether origin is supraventricular or ventricular)

Canadian labeling: Additional contraindications (not in U.S. labeling): IV and Oral: Pregnancy; use in women of child-bearing potential; concurrent use with intravenous dantrolene

Warnings/Precautions Can cause first-, second-, and third-degree AV block or sinus bradycardia and risk increases with agents known to slow cardiac conduction. The most common side effect is peripheral edema; occurs within 2-3 weeks of starting therapy. Symptomatic hypotension with or without syncope can rarely occur; blood pressure must be lowered at a rate appropriate for the patient's clinical condition. Ethanol may increase risk of hypotension or vasodilation. Advise patients to avoid ethanol. Use caution in left ventricular dysfunction (may exacerbate condition). The ACCF/AHA heart failure guidelines recommend to avoid use in patients with heart failure due to lack of benefit and/or worse outcomes with calcium channel blockers in general (ACCF/AHA [Yancy 2013]). Use with caution in hypertrophic obstructive cardiomyopathy; routine use is currently not recommended due to insufficient evidence (Maron 2003). Use with caution in hepatic or renal dysfunction. Transient dermatologic reactions have been observed with use; if reaction persists, discontinue. May (rarely) progress to erythema multiforme or exfoliative dermatitis. Potentially significant interactions may exist, requiring dose or frequency adjustment, additional monitoring, and/or selection of alternative therapy.

Adverse Reactions Note: Frequencies represent ranges for various dosage forms. Patients with impaired ventricular function and/or conduction abnormalities may have higher incidence of adverse reactions.

>10%:
Cardiovascular: Edema (2% to 15%)
Central nervous system: Headache (5% to 12%)
2% to 10%:
Cardiovascular: Atrioventricular block (2% to 8%; first degree), edema (2% to 8%; lower limb), bradycardia (2% to 6%), hypotension (<2% to 4%), vasodilatation (2% to 3%), extrasystoles (2%), flushing (1% to 2%), palpitations (1% to 2%)
Central nervous system: Dizziness (3% to 10%), pain (6%), nervousness (2%)
Dermatologic: Skin rash (1% to 4%)
Endocrine & metabolic: Gout (1% to 2%)
Gastrointestinal: Dyspepsia (1% to 6%), constipation (<2% to 4%), vomiting (2%), diarrhea (1% to 2%)
Local: Injection site reaction (4%; itching, burning)
Neuromuscular & skeletal: Weakness (1% to 4%), myalgia (2%)
Respiratory: Rhinitis (<2% to 10%), pharyngitis (2% to 6%), dyspnea (1% to 6%), bronchitis (1% to 4%), cough (≤3), sinus congestion (1% to 2%)
<2% (Limited to important or life-threatening): Amblyopia, amnesia, atrioventricular block (second or third degree), bundle branch block, cardiac arrhythmia, cardiac failure, depression, dysgeusia, extrapyramidal reaction, gingival hyperplasia, hemolytic anemia, hypersensitivity reaction, increased serum alkaline phosphatase, increased serum ALT, increased serum AST, petechiae, skin photosensitivity, Stevens-Johnson syndrome, syncope, tachycardia, thrombocytopenia, tremor, toxic epidermal necrolysis

Drug Interactions

Metabolism/Transport Effects Substrate of CYP2C9 (minor), CYP2D6 (minor), CYP3A4 (major), P-glycoprotein; **Note:** Assignment of Major/Minor substrate status based on clinically relevant drug interaction potential; **Inhibits** CYP2C9 (weak), CYP2D6 (weak), CYP3A4 (moderate)

Avoid Concomitant Use

Avoid concomitant use of Diltiazem with any of the following: Aprepitant; Bosutinib; Ceritinib; Cobimetinib; Conivaptan; Dantrolene; Domperidone; Flibanserin; Fusidic Acid (Systemic); Ibrutinib; Idelalisib; Ivabradine; Lomitapide; Naloxegol; Olaparib; Pimozide; Rifampin; Simeprevir; Tolvaptan; Trabectedin; Ulipristal

Increased Effect/Toxicity

Diltiazem may increase the levels/effects of: Alfentanil; Amifostine; Amiodarone; Antipsychotic Agents (Second Generation [Atypical]); Apixaban; Aprepitant; ARIPiprazole; AtorvaSTATin; Atosiban; Avanafil; Beta-Blockers; Bosentan; Bosutinib; Bradycardia-Causing Agents; Brexpiprazole; Bromocriptine; Budesonide (Systemic); Budesonide (Topical); BusPIRone; Calcium Channel Blockers (Dihydropyridine); Cannabis; CarBAMazepine; Cardiac Glycosides; Ceritinib; Cilostazol; Cobimetinib; Colchicine; CycloSPORINE (Systemic); CYP3A4 Substrates; Dapoxetine; Dofetilide; Domperidone; DOXOrubicin (Conventional); Dronabinol; Dronedarone; DULoxetine; Eletriptan; Eliglustat; Eplerenone; Everolimus; FentaNYL; Fingolimod; Flibanserin; Fosaprepitant; Fosphenytoin; Halofantrine; Hydrocodone; Hypotension-Associated Agents; Ibrutinib; Imatinib; Ivabradine; Ivacaftor; Lacosamide; Levodopa; Lithium; Lomitapide; Lovastatin; Lurasidone; Magnesium Salts; Midodrine; Naloxegol; Neuromuscular-Blocking Agents (Nondepolarizing); NiMODipine; Nitroprusside; Olaparib; OxyCODONE; Phenytoin; Pimecrolimus; Pimozide; Propafenone; QuiNIDine; Ranolazine; Red Yeast Rice; Salicylates; Salmeterol; Saxagliptin; Simeprevir; Simvastatin; Sonidegib; Suvorexant; Tacrolimus (Systemic); Tacrolimus (Topical); Tetrahydrocannabinol; Tolvaptan; Trabectedin; Ulipristal; Vilazodone; Vindesine; Zopiclone; Zuclopenthixol

The levels/effects of Diltiazem may be increased by: Alfuzosin; Alpha1-Blockers; Anilidopiperidine Opioids; Antifungal Agents (Azole Derivatives, Systemic); AtorvaSTATin; Barbiturates; Bretylium; Brimonidine (Topical); Calcium Channel Blockers (Dihydropyridine); Cimetidine; CloNIDine; Conivaptan; CycloSPORINE (Systemic); CYP3A4 Inhibitors (Moderate); CYP3A4 Inhibitors (Strong); Dantrolene; Dasatinib; Diazoxide; Dronedarone; Fluconazole; Fosaprepitant; Fusidic Acid (Systemic); Grapefruit Juice; Herbs (Hypotensive Properties); Idelalisib; Ivabradine; Lovastatin; Luliconazole; Macrolide Antibiotics; Magnesium Salts; Mifepristone; Molsidomine; Netupitant; Nicorandil; Obinutuzumab; Osimertinib; Palbociclib; Pentoxifylline; P-glycoprotein/ABCB1 Inhibitors; Phosphodiesterase 5 Inhibitors; Prostacyclin Analogues; Protease Inhibitors; Regorafenib; Ruxolitinib; Simvastatin; Stiripentol; Tofacitinib

Decreased Effect

Diltiazem may decrease the levels/effects of: Clopidogrel; Ifosfamide

The levels/effects of Diltiazem may be decreased by: Amphetamines; Barbiturates; Bosentan; Calcium Salts; CarBAMazepine; Colestipol; CYP3A4 Inducers (Moderate); CYP3A4 Inducers (Strong); Dabrafenib; Deferasirox; Efavirenz; Enzalutamide; Herbs (Hypertensive Properties); Methylphenidate; Mitotane; Nafcillin; Osimertinib; P-glycoprotein/ABCB1 Inducers; Phenytoin; Rifampin; Rifamycin Derivatives; Siltuximab; St Johns Wort; Tocilizumab; Yohimbine

Food Interactions Diltiazem serum levels may be elevated if taken with food. Serum concentrations were not altered by grapefruit juice in small clinical trials.

Preparation for Administration

Solution for injection: Continuous IV infusion: Further dilute with NS, D$_5$W, or D$_5$1/2NS to a maximum final concentration of 1 mg/mL.

Solution reconstituted, IV (ADD-Vantage): Refer to manufacturer's labeling.

Storage/Stability

Capsule, tablet: Store 20°C to 25°C (68°F to 77°F); excursions permitted to 15°C to 30°C (59°F to 86°F). Protect from light. Avoid excessive heat (>30°C) and humidity.

Solution for injection: Store in refrigerator at 2°C to 8°C (36°F to 46°F); do not freeze. May be stored at room temperature for up to 1 month. Following dilution to ≤1 mg/mL with D$_5$1/2NS, D$_5$W, or NS, solution is stable for 24 hours at room temperature (15°C to 30°C (59°F to 86°F) or under refrigeration.

Solution reconstituted, intravenous (ADD-Vantage): Store at 20°C to 25°C (68°F to 77°F); do not freeze. Following reconstitution, solution is stable for 24 hours at room temperature or under refrigeration (2°C to 8°C [36°F to 46°F]).

Mechanism of Action Nondihydropyridine calcium channel blocker which inhibits calcium ion from entering the "slow channels" or select voltage-sensitive areas of vascular smooth muscle and myocardium during depolarization, producing a relaxation of coronary vascular smooth muscle and coronary vasodilation; increases myocardial oxygen delivery in patients with vasospastic angina

Pharmacodynamics/Kinetics

Onset of action: Oral: Immediate release tablet: 30 to 60 minutes; IV: Bolus: 3 minutes

Duration: IV: Bolus: 1 to 3 hours; Continuous infusion (after discontinuation): 0.5 to 10 hours

Absorption: Immediate release tablet: >90%; Extended release capsule: ~93%

Distribution: V_d: 3 to 13 L/kg

Protein binding: 70% to 80%

Metabolism: Hepatic (extensive first-pass effect) via CYP-450 and conjugation; forms metabolites N-monodesmethyldiltiazem, desacetyldiltiazem, desacetyl-Nmonodes-methyldiltiazem, desacetyl-O-desmethyldiltiazem, and desacetyl-N, O-desmethyldiltiazem; following single IV injection, plasma concentrations of N-monodesmethyldiltiazem and desacetyldiltiazem are typically undetectable; however, these metabolites accumulate to detectable concentrations following 24-hour constant rate infusion.

Bioavailability: Oral: ~40% (undergoes extensive first-pass metabolism)

Half-life elimination: Immediate release tablet: 3 to 4.5 hours; Extended release tablet: 6 to 9 hours; Extended release capsules: 5 to 10 hours; IV: single dose: ~3.4 hours; continuous infusion: 4 to 5 hours

Time to peak, serum: Immediate release tablet: 2 to 4 hours; Extended release tablet: 11 to 18 hours; Extended release capsule: 10 to 14 hours

Excretion: Urine (2% to 4% as unchanged drug); feces

Dosing

Adult

Angina: Oral:

Capsule, extended release:

Dilacor XR, Dilt-XR: Initial: 120 mg once daily; titrate over 7 to 14 days; usual dose range (ACC/AHA [Gibbons 2002]): 120 to 320 mg daily; maximum: 480 mg daily

Cardizem CD, Cartia XT: Initial: 120 to 180 mg once daily; titrate over 7 to 14 days; usual dose range (ACC/AHA [Gibbons 2002]): 120 to 320 mg daily; maximum: 480 mg daily

Tiazac, Taztia XT: Initial: 120 to 180 mg once daily; titrate over 7 to 14 days; usual dose range (ACC/AHA [Gibbons 2002]): 120 to 320 mg daily; maximum: 540 mg daily

Tablet, extended release (Cardizem LA, Matzim LA, Tiazac XC [Canadian product]): 180 mg once daily; may increase at 7- to 14-day intervals; usual dose range (ACC/AHA [Gibbons 2002]): 120 to 320 mg/day; maximum: 360 mg daily

Tablet, immediate release (Cardizem): Usual starting dose: 30 mg 4 times daily; titrate dose gradually at 1- to 2-day intervals; usual dose range (ACC/AHA [Gibbons 2002]): 120 to 320 mg daily in 4 divided doses

Hypertension: Oral:

Capsule, extended release (once-daily dosing):

Cardizem CD, Cartia XT: Initial: 180 to 240 mg once daily; dose adjustment may be made after 14 days; usual dose range (ASH/ISH [Weber 2014]): 240 to 360 mg daily; maximum: 480 mg daily

Dilacor XR, Dilt-XR: Initial: 180 to 240 mg once daily; dose adjustment may be made after 14 days; usual dose range (ASH/ISH [Weber 2014]): 240 to 360 mg daily; maximum: 540 mg daily

Tiazac, Taztia XT: Initial: 120 to 240 mg once daily; dose adjustment may be made after 14 days; usual dose range (ASH/ISH [Weber 2014]): 240 to 360 mg daily; maximum: 540 mg daily

Capsule, extended release (twice-daily dosing): Initial: 60 to 120 mg twice daily; dose adjustment may be made after 14 days; usual range: 240 to 360 mg daily

Note: Diltiazem is available as a generic intended for either once- or twice-daily dosing, depending on the formulation; verify appropriate extended release capsule formulation is administered.

Tablet, extended release (Cardizem LA, Matzim LA, Tiazac XC [Canadian product]): Initial: 180 to 240 mg once daily; dose adjustment may be made after 14 days; usual dose range (ASH/ISH [Weber 2014]): 240 to 360 mg daily; maximum: 540 mg daily

Atrial fibrillation, atrial flutter, PSVT: IV:

Initial bolus dose: 0.25 mg/kg actual body weight over 2 minutes (average adult dose: 20 mg); ACLS guideline recommends 15 to 20 mg

Repeat bolus dose (may be administered after 15 minutes if the response is inadequate): 0.35 mg/kg actual body weight over 2 minutes (average adult dose: 25 mg); ACLS guideline recommends 20 to 25 mg

Continuous infusion (infusions >24 hours or infusion rates >15 mg/hour are not recommended): Initial infusion rate of 10 mg/hour; rate may be increased in 5 mg/hour increments up to 15 mg/hour as needed; some patients may respond to an initial rate of 5 mg/hour.

If diltiazem injection is administered by continuous infusion for >24 hours, the possibility of decreased diltiazem clearance, prolonged elimination half-life, and increased diltiazem and/or diltiazem metabolite plasma concentrations should be considered.

Atrial fibrillation (rate control) (off-label use): Oral: Extended release (capsule or tablet): Usual maintenance dose: 120 to 360 mg once daily (AHA/ACC/HRS [January 2014])

Conversion from IV diltiazem to oral diltiazem:

Oral dose (mg daily) is approximately equal to [rate (mg/hour) x 3 + 3] x 10.

3 mg/hour = 120 mg daily

5 mg/hour = 180 mg daily

7 mg/hour = 240 mg daily

11 mg/hour = 360 mg daily

Geriatric Refer to adult dosing. In the management of hypertension, consider lower initial doses (eg, 120 mg once daily using extended release capsule) and titrate to response (Aronow 2011).

Pediatric

Children: Minimal information available; some centers use the following:

Hypertension (off-label use): Oral: Initial: 1.5-2 mg/kg/day in 3 divided doses (maximum: 6 mg/kg/day, up to 360 mg daily) (Flynn 2000)

Adolescents: Refer to adult dosing.

Renal Impairment There are no dosage adjustments provided in the manufacturer's labeling; use with caution.

Dialysis: Not removed by hemo- or peritoneal dialysis; supplemental dose is not necessary.

Hepatic Impairment There are no dosage adjustment provided in the manufacturer's labeling; use with caution; extensively metabolized by the liver; half-life is increased in patients with cirrhosis.

Usual Infusion Concentrations: Adult IV infusion: 125 mg in 125 mL (total volume) (concentration: 1 mg/mL) of D_5W or NS

Administration

Oral:

Immediate release tablet (Cardizem): Administer before meals and at bedtime. The manufacturer recommends to swallow the tablet whole; do not split, crush, or chew. Crushing immediate release tablets may alter pharmacokinetics; film coating is designed to slowly release diltiazem. However, an oral suspension has been made using the immediate release tablets (Allen 1996).

Long acting dosage forms: Do not open, chew, or crush; swallow whole. Administer at same time of day either morning or evening.

Cardizem CD, Cardizem LA, Cartia XT, Matzim LA: Administer without regard to meals.

Dilacor XR: Administer on an empty stomach.

Dilt XR: Administer on an empty stomach in the morning.

Taztia XT, Tiazac: Capsules may be opened and sprinkled on a spoonful of applesauce. Applesauce should not be hot and should be swallowed without chewing, followed by drinking a glass of water.

Tiazac XC [Canadian product]: Administer at bedtime

IV: Bolus doses given over 2 minutes with continuous ECG and blood pressure monitoring. Continuous infusion should be via infusion pump. May increase infusion rate in 5 mg/hour increments as needed (maximum: 15 mg/hour). Response to bolus may require several minutes to reach maximum. Response may persist for several hours after infusion is discontinued.

Monitoring Parameters Liver function tests, kidney function, blood pressure, ECG, heart rate; consult individual institutional policies and procedures. Ventricular rate control in patients with atrial fibrillation or flutter: Patients who respond, usually have at least a 20% decrease in ventricular response rate or a rate <100 beats/minute.

Dosage Forms Excipient information presented when available (limited, particularly for generics); consult specific product labeling. [DSC] = Discontinued product

Capsule Extended Release 12 Hour, Oral, as hydrochloride:
  Generic: 60 mg, 90 mg, 120 mg
Capsule Extended Release 24 Hour, Oral, as hydrochloride:
  Cardizem CD: 120 mg, 180 mg, 240 mg, 300 mg, 360 mg [contains brilliant blue fcf (fd&c blue #1)]
  Cartia XT: 120 mg, 180 mg, 240 mg, 300 mg
  Dilacor XR: 240 mg [DSC]
  Dilt-CD: 120 mg [DSC]
  Dilt-CD: 180 mg [DSC], 240 mg [DSC] [contains brilliant blue fcf (fd&c blue #1)]
  Dilt-CD: 300 mg [DSC]
  Dilt-XR: 120 mg, 180 mg, 240 mg [contains brilliant blue fcf (fd&c blue #1), fd&c red #40, fd&c yellow #10 (quinoline yellow)]
  Diltiazem CD: 120 mg
  Diltiazem CD: 180 mg [contains brilliant blue fcf (fd&c blue #1), fd&c yellow #10 (quinoline yellow)]
  Diltiazem CD: 240 mg [contains fd&c yellow #10 (quinoline yellow)]
  Diltiazem HCl CD: 360 mg [DSC] [contains brilliant blue fcf (fd&c blue #1)]
  Diltzac: 120 mg [DSC] [contains brilliant blue fcf (fd&c blue #1)]
  Diltzac: 180 mg [DSC]
  Diltzac: 240 mg [DSC], 300 mg [DSC] [contains brilliant blue fcf (fd&c blue #1)]
  Diltzac: 360 mg [DSC]
  Taztia XT: 120 mg [contains brilliant blue fcf (fd&c blue #1), fd&c blue #1 aluminum lake, fd&c blue #2 aluminum lake, fd&c red #40, fd&c red #40 aluminum lake, fd&c yellow #10 aluminum lake]
  Taztia XT: 180 mg [contains brilliant blue fcf (fd&c blue #1), fd&c blue #1 aluminum lake, fd&c red #40 aluminum lake, fd&c yellow #10 (quinoline yellow), fd&c yellow #10 aluminum lake, fd&c yellow #6 (sunset yellow)]
  Taztia XT: 240 mg [contains brilliant blue fcf (fd&c blue #1), fd&c blue #1 aluminum lake, fd&c blue #2 aluminum lake, fd&c red #40, fd&c red #40 aluminum lake, fd&c yellow #10 aluminum lake]
  Taztia XT: 300 mg [contains brilliant blue fcf (fd&c blue #1), fd&c blue #1 aluminum lake, fd&c blue #2 aluminum lake, fd&c red #40, fd&c red #40 aluminum lake, fd&c yellow #10 aluminum lake, fd&c yellow #6 (sunset yellow)]
  Taztia XT: 360 mg [contains brilliant blue fcf (fd&c blue #1), fd&c blue #1 aluminum lake, fd&c blue #2 aluminum lake, fd&c red #40 aluminum lake, fd&c yellow #10 aluminum lake]
  Tiazac: 120 mg, 180 mg, 240 mg, 300 mg, 360 mg, 420 mg [contains brilliant blue fcf (fd&c blue #1), fd&c red #40]
  Generic: 120 mg, 180 mg, 240 mg, 300 mg, 360 mg, 420 mg
Solution, Intravenous, as hydrochloride:
  Generic: 25 mg/5 mL (5 mL, 25 mL); 50 mg/10 mL (10 mL); 125 mg/25 mL (25 mL)
Solution, Intravenous, as hydrochloride [preservative free]:
  Generic: 25 mg/5 mL (5 mL [DSC]); 50 mg/10 mL (10 mL); 125 mg/25 mL (25 mL)
Solution Reconstituted, Intravenous, as hydrochloride:
  Generic: 100 mg (1 ea)
Tablet, Oral, as hydrochloride:
  Cardizem: 30 mg
  Cardizem: 30 mg [contains fd&c blue #1 aluminum lake, fd&c yellow #10 aluminum lake]
  Cardizem: 60 mg [DSC] [scored]
  Cardizem: 60 mg [scored; contains fd&c blue #1 aluminum lake, fd&c yellow #10 aluminum lake, fd&c yellow #6 aluminum lake, methylparaben]
  Cardizem: 90 mg [DSC] [scored]
  Cardizem: 120 mg [DSC] [contains fd&c yellow #10 aluminum lake, fd&c yellow #6 aluminum lake, methylparaben]
  Cardizem: 120 mg [scored; contains fd&c yellow #10 aluminum lake, fd&c yellow #6 aluminum lake, methylparaben]
  Generic: 30 mg, 60 mg, 90 mg, 120 mg
Tablet Extended Release 24 Hour, Oral, as hydrochloride:
  Cardizem LA: 120 mg, 180 mg, 240 mg, 300 mg, 360 mg, 420 mg
  Matzim LA: 180 mg, 240 mg, 300 mg, 360 mg, 420 mg
  Generic: 180 mg, 240 mg, 300 mg, 360 mg, 420 mg

Dosage Forms: Canada Note: Also refer to Dosage Forms. Excipient information presented when available (limited, particularly for generics); consult specific product labeling.
Tablet, Extended Release, Oral, as hydrochloride:
  Tiazac XC: 120 mg, 180 mg, 240 mg, 300 mg, 360 mg

Extemporaneous Preparations A 12 mg/mL oral suspension may be made from tablets (regular, not extended release) and one of three different vehicles (cherry syrup, a 1:1 mixture of Ora-Sweet® and Ora-Plus®, or a 1:1 mixture of Ora-Sweet® SF and Ora-Plus®). Crush sixteen 90 mg tablets in a mortar and reduce to a fine powder. Add 10 mL of the chosen vehicle and mix to a uniform paste; mix while adding the vehicle in incremental proportions to **almost** 120 mL; transfer to a calibrated bottle, rinse mortar with vehicle, and add quantity of vehicle sufficient to make 120 mL. Label "shake well" and "protect from light". Stable for 60 days when stored in amber plastic prescription bottles in the dark at room temperature or refrigerated.
Allen LV and Erickson MA, "Stability of Baclofen, Captopril, Diltiazem Hydrochloride, Dipyridamole, and Flecainide Acetate in Extemporaneously Compounded Oral Liquids," *Am J Health Syst Pharm,* 1996, 53(18):2179-84.

- ◆ Diltiazem CD *see* Diltiazem *on page 553*
- ◆ Diltiazem-CD (Can) *see* Diltiazem *on page 553*
- ◆ Diltiazem HCl CD [DSC] *see* Diltiazem *on page 553*
- ◆ Diltiazem Hydrochloride *see* Diltiazem *on page 553*
- ◆ Diltiazem Hydrochloride Injection (Can) *see* Diltiazem *on page 553*
- ◆ Diltiazem TZ (Can) *see* Diltiazem *on page 553*
- ◆ Dilt-XR *see* Diltiazem *on page 553*
- ◆ Diltzac [DSC] *see* Diltiazem *on page 553*

DimenhyDRINATE (dye men HYE dri nate)

Brand Names: US Dramamine [OTC]; Driminate [OTC]; Motion Sickness [OTC]
Brand Names: Canada Apo-Dimenhydrinate [OTC]; Children's Motion Sickness Liquid [OTC]; Dimenhydrinate Injection [OTC]; Dinate [OTC]; Gravol IM; Gravol [OTC]; Jamp-Dimenhydrinate [OTC]; Nauseatol [OTC]; Novo-Dimenate [OTC]; PMS-Dimenhydrinate [OTC]; Sandoz-Dimenhydrinate [OTC]; Travel Tabs [OTC]
Pharmacologic Category Ethanolamine Derivative; Histamine H_1 Antagonist; Histamine H_1 Antagonist, First Generation

Use
  Motion sickness: Treatment and prevention of nausea, vertigo, and vomiting associated with motion sickness.
  Note: In Canada, dimenhydrinate is also approved for the treatment and prevention of radiation sickness, postoperative vomiting, and drug-induced vomiting; and for the treatment of nausea, vomiting, and vertigo due to Mènière disease and other labyrinthine disturbances

Dosing
  Adult & Geriatric
    Motion sickness, nausea/vomiting, or vertigo:
      Oral: 50 to 100 mg every 4 to 6 hours, not to exceed 400 mg daily
      IM, IV: 50 mg every 4 hours; maximum: 100 mg every 4 hours
      Rectal suppository [Canadian product]: 50 to 100 mg 3 to 4 times daily
  Pediatric
    Motion sickness, nausea/vomiting, or vertigo:
      Oral:
        Children 2 to 5 years: 12.5 to 25 mg every 6 to 8 hours, maximum: 75 mg daily
        Children 6 to 12 years: 25 to 50 mg every 6 to 8 hours, maximum: 150 mg daily
      IM: Children: 1.25 mg/kg **or** 37.5 mg/m^2 4 times daily; maximum: 300 mg daily
      Rectal suppository [Canadian product]:
        Children 6 to 8 years: 12.5 to 25 mg 2 to 3 times daily
        Children 9 to 12 years: 25 to 50 mg 2 to 3 times daily
        Adolescents ≥13 years: 50 mg 2 to 3 times daily

Renal Impairment There are no dosage adjustments provided in the manufacturer's labeling.
Hepatic Impairment There are no dosage adjustments provided in the manufacturer's labeling.
Additional Information Complete prescribing information should be consulted for additional detail.
Dosage Forms Excipient information presented when available (limited, particularly for generics); consult specific product labeling. [DSC] = Discontinued product
Solution, Injection:
  Generic: 50 mg/mL (1 mL)

Tablet, Oral:
Dramamine: 50 mg
Dramamine: 50 mg [scored]
Driminate: 50 mg [scored]
Motion Sickness: 50 mg [DSC]
Motion Sickness: 50 mg [scored]
Generic: 50 mg
Tablet Chewable, Oral:
Dramamine: 50 mg [contains aspartame, fd&c yellow #6 aluminum lake]
Dramamine: 50 mg [scored; contains aspartame, fd&c yellow #6 aluminum lake]

Dosage Forms: Canada
Excipient information presented when available (limited, particularly for generics); consult specific product labeling.
Suppository, Rectal:
Sandoz-Dimenhydrinate: 50 mg, 100 mg

◆ Dimenhydrinate Injection (Can) see DimenhyDRINATE on page 556

Dimercaprol (dye mer KAP role)

Brand Names: US Bal in Oil
Index Terms 2,3-Dimercapto-1-Propanol; 2,3-Dimercapto-propan-1-Ol; 2,3-Dimercaptopropanol; BAL; British Anti-Lewisite; Dithioglycerol
Pharmacologic Category Antidote
Use Antidote to gold, arsenic (except arsine), or acute mercury poisoning (except nonalkyl mercury); adjunct to edetate CALCIUM disodium in acute lead poisoning
Dosing
Adult & Geriatric Note: Premedication with a histamine H$_1$ antagonist (eg, diphenhydramine) is recommended.
Arsenic or gold poisoning (acute, mild): Deep IM: 2.5 mg/kg every 6 hours for 2 days, then every 12 hours for 1 day, followed by once daily for 10 days
Arsenic or gold poisoning (acute, severe): Deep IM: 3 mg/kg every 4 hours for 2 days, then every 6 hours for 1 day, followed every 12 hours for 10 days
Mercury poisoning (acute): Deep IM: 5 mg/kg initially, followed by 2.5 mg/kg 1-2 times/day for 10 days
Lead poisoning: Deep IM: **Note:** For the treatment of high blood lead levels in children, the CDC recommends chelation treatment when blood lead levels are >45 mcg/dL (CDC, 2002); however, dimercaprol is only recommended for use (in combination with edetate CALCIUM disodium) in children whose blood lead levels are >70 mcg/dL or in children with lead encephalopathy (AAP, 2005; Chandran, 2010). In adults, available guidelines recommend chelation therapy with blood lead levels >50 mcg/dL and significant symptoms; chelation therapy may also be indicated with blood lead levels ≥100 mcg/dL and/or symptoms (Kosnett, 2007). Blood lead levels ≥70 mcg/dL, symptomatic lead poisoning, or lead encephalopathy (in conjunction with edetate CALCIUM disodium): 4 mg/kg every 4 hours for 2-7 days; duration of therapy of at least 3 days is recommended by some experts (Chandran, 2010). **Note:** Begin treatment with edetate CALCIUM disodium with the second dimercaprol dose.
Pediatric Note: Premedication with a histamine H$_1$ antagonist (eg, diphenhydramine) is recommended. Refer to adult dosing.
Renal Impairment No adjustment provided in manufacturer's labeling. Use with extreme caution or discontinue if acute renal insufficiency develops during therapy.
Hepatic Impairment Use is contraindicated in hepatic insufficiency (except in cases of postarsenical jaundice).
Additional Information Complete prescribing information should be consulted for additional detail.
Dosage Forms Excipient information presented when available (limited, particularly for generics); consult specific product labeling.
Solution, Intramuscular:
Bal in Oil: 100 mg/mL (3 mL) [contains benzyl benzoate, peanut oil]

◆ 2,3-Dimercapto-1-Propanol see Dimercaprol on page 557

◆ 2,3-Dimercaptopropan-1-Ol see Dimercaprol on page 557

◆ 2,3-Dimercaptopropanol see Dimercaprol on page 557

◆ Dimetapp® Children's Long Acting Cough Plus Cold [OTC] see Dextromethorphan and Chlorpheniramine on page 534

◆ Dimetapp® Children's Nighttime Cold & Congestion [OTC] see Diphenhydramine and Phenylephrine on page 564

Dimethyl Fumarate (dye meth il FYOO ma rate)

Brand Names: US Tecfidera
Brand Names: Canada Tecfidera
Index Terms BG-12; Dimethylfumarate; DMF; FAG-201
Pharmacologic Category Fumaric Acid Derivative; Immunomodulator, Systemic
Use Multiple sclerosis: Treatment of patients with relapsing forms of multiple sclerosis
Pregnancy Considerations
Adverse events were observed in animal reproduction studies.
Women exposed to dimethyl fumarate during pregnancy are encouraged to enroll in the Pregnancy Registry by calling 866-810-1462 or visiting www.tecfiderapregnancyregistry.com.
Breast-Feeding Considerations It is not known if dimethyl fumarate is excreted into breast milk. The manufacturer recommends that caution be exercised when administering dimethyl fumarate to nursing women.
Contraindications Hypersensitivity to dimethyl fumarate or any component of the formulation
Warnings/Precautions Dimethyl fumarate should only be prescribed by health care providers who are experienced in the diagnosis and management of multiple sclerosis. Anaphylaxis and angioedema may occur after the first dose or at any time during treatment. Discontinue therapy if signs and symptoms of anaphylaxis or angioedema occur. Progressive multifocal leukoencephalopathy (PML) with fatality has been reported (rare); withhold therapy immediately at the first sign or symptom suggestive of PML (eg, progressive weakness on one side of the body or clumsiness of limbs; vision disturbances; mental status changes).

Decreased lymphocyte counts may occur with use. Obtain a complete blood cell count (CBC), including lymphocyte count, prior to initiation of therapy, after 6 months of treatment, every 6 to 12 months thereafter, and as clinically indicated. Consider therapy interruption in patients with lymphocyte counts <0.5 x 10^9/L persisting >6 months and in patients with signs and symptoms of serious infections. The Canadian labeling recommends additional CBC monitoring prior to switching patients to other therapies known to reduce lymphocyte counts and that dimethyl fumarate treatment not be initiated in patients who are immunocompromised due to other treatments (eg, antineoplastic, immunosuppressive or immune modulating therapies) or disease (eg, immunodeficiency syndrome) or in patients with signs/symptoms of a serious infection.

Use commonly causes GI events (eg, nausea, vomiting, diarrhea, abdominal pain, dyspepsia) and mild to moderate flushing (eg, warmth, redness, itching, burning sensation). GI events generally occur in the first month of use and decrease thereafter. To improve tolerability, administer with food or temporarily reduce the dosage. Flushing generally appears soon after initiation, and improves or resolves with subsequent dosing. Administration with food may decrease flushing incidence. Administration of aspirin (nonenteric coated ≤325 mg) 30 minutes prior to dimethyl fumarate or a temporary dose reduction may also reduce the incidence and severity of flushing. The Canadian labeling does not recommend use of aspirin >4 days for the management of flushing (has not been studied). The Canadian labeling recommends caution be exercised when administering in patients with severe active GI disease.

Transaminase elevations (usually <3 times ULN) were observed, generally occurring in the first 6 months of treatment. Use may cause rash, pruritus, or erythema. There are case reports of contact dermatitis resulting from dimethyl fumarate (DMF) exposure after use as a fungicide and desiccant in the shipping of furniture (Bruze, 2011; Giménez-Arnau, 2011; Ropper, 2012). In clinical trials, proteinuria was reported at a slightly higher incidence than that observed with placebo; significance of these findings is unknown. Potentially significant interactions may exist, requiring dose or frequency adjustment, additional monitoring, and/or selection of alternative therapy.

Adverse Reactions
>10%:
Cardiovascular: Flushing (40%)
Gastrointestinal: Abdominal pain (18%), diarrhea (14%), nausea (12%)
Infection: Infection (60%; placebo: 58%)
1% to 10%:
Dermatologic: Pruritus (8%), skin rash (8%), erythema (5%)
Gastrointestinal: Vomiting (9%), dyspepsia (5%)
Genitourinary: Proteinuria (6%)

Hematologic: Lymphocytopenia (2% to 6%)

Hepatic: Increased serum AST (4%)

<1% (Limited to important or life-threatening: Anaphylaxis, angioedema, eosinophilia (transient), progressive multifocal leukoencephalopathy

Drug Interactions

Metabolism/Transport Effects None known.

Avoid Concomitant Use There are no known interactions where it is recommended to avoid concomitant use.

Increased Effect/Toxicity

Dimethyl Fumarate may increase the levels/effects of: Vaccines (Live)

Decreased Effect

Dimethyl Fumarate may decrease the levels/effects of: Vaccines (Live)

Storage/Stability Store at 15°C to 30°C (50°F to 86°F). Protect capsules from light and store in the original container.

Mechanism of Action DMF and its active metabolite, monomethyl fumarate (MMF), have been shown to activate the nuclear factor (erythroid-derived 2)-like 2 (Nrf2) pathway, which is involved in cellular response to oxidative stress. The mechanism by which dimethyl fumarate (DMF) exerts a therapeutic effect in MS is unknown, although it is believed to result from its anti-inflammatory and cytoprotective properties via activation of the Nrf2 pathway (Fox, 2012; Gold, 2012).

Pharmacodynamics/Kinetics

Distribution: V_d: MMF: 53 to 73 L

Protein binding: MMF: 27% to 45%

Metabolism: Undergoes rapid and extensive presystemic hydrolysis by esterases to its active metabolite, monomethyl fumarate (MMF); MMF is further metabolized via the tricarboxylic acid (TCA) cycle. Major serum metabolites include: MMF, fumaric acid, citric acid, and glucose.

Half-life elimination: MMF: ~1 hour

Time to peak: 2 to 2.5 hours; delayed to 5.5 hours with food

Excretion: CO_2 via exhalation (~60%); urine (16%; trace amounts as unchanged MMF), feces (1%)

Dosing

Adult & Geriatric Multiple sclerosis (relapsing): Oral: Initial: 120 mg twice daily for 7 days; then increase to the maintenance dose: 240 mg twice daily

Renal Impairment No dosage adjustment necessary.

Hepatic Impairment No dosage adjustment necessary.

Adjustment for Toxicity

Flushing, GI intolerance, or intolerance to maintenance dose: Consider temporary dose reduction to 120 mg twice daily (resume recommended maintenance dose of 240 mg twice daily within 4 weeks). Consider discontinuation in patients who cannot tolerate return to the maintenance dose.

Serious infection: Consider withholding treatment until infection resolves.

Dietary Considerations Taking with food may decrease the incidence or severity of flushing.

Administration Swallow capsules whole; do not crush, chew, open the capsule, or sprinkle contents on food. Administer with or without food; administering with food may decrease the incidence of flushing. Administration of aspirin (nonenteric coated ≤325 mg) 30 minutes prior to dimethyl fumarate may also reduce the incidence and severity of flushing. Canadian labeling suggests that missed doses may be taken if ≥4 hours lapse between the morning and evening doses.

Monitoring Parameters CBC including lymphocyte count (obtained prior to initiation of therapy, after 6 months of treatment, then every 6 to 12 months thereafter and as clinically necessary).

Canadian labeling recommends obtaining a CBC, hepatic transaminases, and a urinalysis within 6 months prior to use, after 6 months of therapy, then every 6 to 12 months during therapy and as clinically indicated.

Additional Information Dimethyl fumarate (DMF) has been implicated as the cause of an outbreak of contact dermatitis in Europe resulting from DMF's use as a fungicide and desiccant in the shipping of furniture (Bruze, 2011; Giménez-Arnau, 2011; Ropper, 2012); may be irritating to mucous membranes (do not crush, chew, or open capsule).

Dosage Forms Excipient information presented when available (limited, particularly for generics); consult specific product labeling.

Capsule Delayed Release, Oral:

Tecfidera: 120 mg, 240 mg [contains brilliant blue fcf (fd&c blue #1)]

Miscellaneous, Oral:

Tecfidera: Capsule, delayed release: 120 mg (14s) and Capsule, delayed release: 240 mg (46s) (60 ea) [contains brilliant blue fcf (fd&c blue #1)]

◆ **Dimethylfumarate** *see* Dimethyl Fumarate *on page 557*

◆ **Dimethyl Triazeno Imidazole Carboxamide** *see* Dacarbazine *on page 479*

◆ **Dinate [OTC] (Can)** *see* DimenhyDRINATE *on page 556*

Dinoprostone (dye noe PROST one)

Brand Names: US Cervidil; Prepidil; Prostin E2

Brand Names: Canada Cervidil®; Prepidil®; Prostin E_2®

Index Terms PGE_2; Prostaglandin E_2

Pharmacologic Category Abortifacient; Prostaglandin

Use

Endocervical gel (Prepidil): Promote cervical ripening in patients at or near term in whom there is a medical or obstetrical indication for the induction of labor

Suppositories (Prostin E_2): Terminate pregnancy from 12th through 20th week of gestation; evacuate uterus in cases of missed abortion or intrauterine fetal death up to 28 weeks of gestation; manage benign hydatidiform mole (nonmetastatic gestational trophoblastic disease)

Tablet (oral) (Prostin E_2; [Canadian product]): Elective induction of labor; when indications for induction of labor exist (eg, premature rupture of amniotic membranes, toxemia of pregnancy, Rh incompatibility, diabetes mellitus, hypertension, postmaturity, intrauterine death or fetal growth retardation)

Vaginal gel (Prostin E_2; [Canadian product]): Induction of labor in patients at or near term with singleton pregnancy, vertex presentation, and favorable induction features

Vaginal insert (Cervidil): Initiation and/or continuation of cervical ripening in patients at or near term in whom there is a medical or obstetrical indication for the induction of labor

Dosing

Adult

Abortifacient: *Vaginal suppository:* Insert 20 mg (1 suppository) high in vagina, repeat at 3- to 5-hour intervals until abortion occurs; continued administration for longer than 2 days is not advisable

Cervical ripening:

Endocervical gel: Using catheter supplied with gel, insert 0.5 mg into the cervical canal. May repeat every 6 hours if needed. Maximum cumulative dose: 1.5 mg/24 hours

Tablet (oral) [Canadian product]:

Induction: Initial: 0.5 mg and then repeat 0.5 mg dose 1 hour later; may give additional 0.5 mg dose on an hourly basis as needed for satisfactory uterine response. Maintain patient at the lowest effective dose. **Note:** Failure to induce regular contractions after 8 hours indicates failed induction and alternative management of patient should be considered. If patient vomits an intact tablet during therapy repeat dose. If patient vomits intact tablets following 2 successive doses, withhold therapy until next scheduled dose. If patient vomits a partial tablet or if no tablet is visible, continue at next regularly scheduled dose.

Parity ≥2 times or Bishop Score of ≥6: Administer 0.5 mg hourly throughout induction (discontinue hourly dose for excessive uterine activity)

Nulliparous or multiparous and resistant to induction (Bishop Score <6): If inadequate response after 2 hours of therapy may increase dose in 0.5 mg increments at hourly intervals up to a maximum single dose of 1.5 mg.

Maintenance of labor: 0.5 mg dose hourly; may occasionally withhold hourly dose to assess need for further dosing

Vaginal gel [Canadian product]: Initial: Using prefilled syringe, insert 1 mg into the posterior fornix of the vaginal canal; may give 1 additional dose of 1-2 mg 6 hours later if needed.

Vaginal insert: Insert 10 mg transversely into the posterior fornix of the vagina (to be removed at the onset of active labor or after 12 hours)

Pediatric Females of reproductive age: Refer to adult dosing.

Additional Information Complete prescribing information should be consulted for additional detail.

Dosage Forms Excipient information presented when available (limited, particularly for generics); consult specific product labeling.

Gel, Vaginal:

Prepidil: 0.5 mg/3 g (3 g)

Insert, Vaginal:

Cervidil: 10 mg (1 ea)

Suppository, Vaginal:

Prostin E2: 20 mg (5 ea)

Dosage Forms: Canada Excipient information presented when available (limited, particularly for generics); consult specific product labeling.

Gel, vaginal:

Prostin E$_2$®: 1 mg/3 g (3 g), 2 mg/3 g (3 g)

Tablet, oral:

Prostin E$_2$®: 0.5 mg [contains lactose]

Dinutuximab (din ue TUX i mab)

Brand Names: US Unituxin

Index Terms ch14.18; MOAB Ch14.18

Pharmacologic Category Antineoplastic Agent, Anti-GD2; Antineoplastic Agent, Monoclonal Antibody

Use Neuroblastoma: Treatment of high-risk neuroblastoma (in combination with granulocyte-macrophage colony-stimulating factor [GM-CSF; sargramostim], interleukin-2 [IL-2; aldesleukin] and 13-cis-retinoic acid [RA; isotretinoin]) in pediatric patients who achieve at least a partial response to prior first-line multiagent, multimodality therapy.

Pregnancy Considerations Reproduction studies have not been completed with dinutuximab. Monoclonal antibodies cross the placenta, the largest amount during the third trimester of pregnancy. Based on the mechanism of action, dinutuximab may cause fetal harm. Women of reproductive potential should use effective contraception during therapy and for 2 months after the last dose.

Breast-Feeding Considerations It is not known if dinutuximab is excreted in breast milk. IgG molecules are excreted in breast milk. Due to the potential for serious adverse reactions in the nursing infant, breast-feeding is not recommended by the manufacturer.

Contraindications History of anaphylaxis to dinutuximab

Warnings/Precautions [US Boxed Warning]: Serious and potentially life-threatening infusion reactions occurred in approximately one-fourth of patients treated with dinutuximab. Administer required prehydration and premedication, including antihistamines, prior to each dinutuximab infusion. Monitor patients closely for signs and symptoms of an infusion reaction during and for at least 4 hours following completion of each dinutuximab infusion. Immediately interrupt dinutuximab for severe infusion reactions and permanently discontinue dinutuximab for anaphylaxis. Infusion reactions typically occurred during infusion or within 24 hours of completion and may include facial and upper airway edema, dyspnea, bronchospasm, stridor, urticaria, and hypotension. Infusion reactions may require blood pressure support, bronchodilator therapy, corticosteroids, infusion rate interruption and/or reduction, or permanent therapy discontinuation. Infusion should be in a facility with cardiopulmonary medication/equipment available. Severe capillary leak syndrome was reported in close to one-fourth of patients receiving dinutuximab. Immediately interrupt infusion if capillary leak syndrome develops; infusion rate reduction and/or therapy discontinuation may be necessary. Initiate appropriate management in patients with symptomatic or severe capillary leak syndrome. Severe hypotension occurred more frequently in patients receiving dinutuximab. Intravenous hydration is required prior to each infusion; closely monitor blood pressure during infusion. May require therapy interruption or discontinuation; initiate appropriate medical management in patients with a systolic blood pressure (SBP) less than lower limit of normal for age, or SBP that is decreased by more than 15% compared to baseline. Electrolyte abnormalities (such as hyponatremia, hypokalemia, and hypocalcemia) were reported in at least one-fourth of patients who received dinutuximab, including grade 3 or 4 events. In a study of a related anti-GD2 antibody, syndrome of inappropriate antidiuretic hormone secretion (SIADH) resulting in severe hyponatremia was reported. Monitor electrolytes closely during therapy.

[US Boxed Warning]: Dinutuximab causes severe neuropathic pain in the majority of patients. Administer intravenous opioids prior to, during, and for 2 hours following completion of the dinutuximab infusion. In clinical studies of patients with high-risk neuroblastoma, grade 3 peripheral sensory neuropathy occurred in 2% to 9% of patients. In clinical studies of dinutuximab and related GD2-binding antibodies, severe motor neuropathy was observed in adults. Resolution of motor neuropathy was not documented in all cases. Permanently discontinue dinutuximab for severe unresponsive pain, severe sensory neuropathy, or moderate to severe peripheral motor neuropathy. In patients who experienced peripheral sensory neuropathy of any grade, the median duration was 9 days (range: 3 to 163 days). Most patients experienced pain; severe pain was observed in over 50% of patients treated with dinutuximab;

pain may occur despite analgesic/opioid therapy. Pain typically occurred during infusion and included abdominal, generalized, extremity, or back pain, neuralgia, musculoskeletal chest pain, and arthralgia. Premedication with analgesics, including opioids, is required prior to each dose, during the infusion, and for 2 hours following the infusion. Severe pain may require reduction of the infusion rate or therapy discontinuation.

Severe (grade 3 or 4) anemia, neutropenia, thrombocytopenia, and neutropenic fever were observed in dinutuximab-treated patients. Monitor complete blood counts closely during treatment. Severe (grade 3 or 4) bacteremia was reported more frequently in dinutuximab-treated patients, and required intravenous antibiotics or other urgent interventions. Sepsis was also observed in patients receiving dinutuximab. Monitor closely for signs/symptoms of systemic infection; may require therapy interruption until resolution of infection. Hemolytic uremic syndrome (without documented infection) resulted in renal insufficiency, electrolyte abnormalities, anemia, and hypertension in a small number of patients. Atypical hemolytic uremic syndrome recurred in one patient upon rechallenge. Permanently discontinue if hemolytic uremic syndrome develops; manage supportively. Neurological ocular toxicity such as blurred vision, photophobia, mydriasis, fixed or unequal pupils, optic nerve disorder, and papilledema were reported in clinical trials. In patients who experienced complete resolution of ocular toxicity, the median duration of toxicity was 4 days (range: 0 to 221 days). May require therapy interruption, dosage reduction, or treatment discontinuation. Potentially significant interactions may exist, requiring dose or frequency adjustment, additional monitoring, and/or selection of alternative therapy.

Adverse Reactions Frequency not always defined.

>10%:

Cardiovascular: Hypotension (60%; grades 3/4: 16%), capillary leak syndrome (40%; grades ≥3: 6% to 23%), tachycardia (19%), edema (17%), hypertension (14%)

Central nervous system: Pain (85%; grades 3/4: 51%), peripheral neuropathy (13%; grades 3/4: 6%)

Dermatologic: Urticaria (37%; grades 3/4: 13%)

Endocrine & metabolic: Hyponatremia (58%; grades 3/4: 23%), hypokalemia (43%), hypoalbuminemia (33%), hypocalcemia (27%), hypophosphatemia (20%), hyperglycemia (18%), hypertriglyceridemia (16%), hypomagnesemia (12%)

Gastrointestinal: Increased serum alanine aminotransferase (56%), vomiting (46%), diarrhea (43%), increased serum aspartate aminotransferase (28%), decreased appetite (15%)

Genitourinary: Proteinuria (16%)

Hematologic & oncologic: Thrombocytopenia (66%; grades 3/4: 39%), lymphocytopenia (62%; grades 3/4: 51%), anemia (51%; grades 3/4: 34%), neutropenia (39%; grades 3/4: 34%), hemorrhage (17%; grades 3/4: 6%), febrile neutropenia (grades 3/4: 4%)

Infection: Sepsis (18%; grade 3/4: 16%), infection (device related, 16%; grade 3/4: 16%), bacteremia (grades 3/4: 13%)

Renal: Increased serum creatinine (15%)

Respiratory: Hypoxia (24%)

Miscellaneous: Fever (72%; grades 3/4: 40%), infusion related reaction (60%)

1% to 10%

Central nervous system: Peripheral sensory neuropathy (9%; grade 3: 1%), peripheral motor neuropathy (grade 3: 1%)

Endocrine & metabolic: Weight gain (10%), electrolyte disturbance

Gastrointestinal: Nausea (10%)

Hematologic & oncologic: Hemolytic-uremic syndrome (2%)

Hypersensitivity: Severe infusion related reaction

Ophthalmic: Blurred vision (2%), blepharoptosis, optic nerve damage, papilledema, photophobia

Renal: Renal insufficiency

<1% (Limited to important or life-threatening): Diplopia, fixation of pupils, mydriasis

Drug Interactions

Metabolism/Transport Effects None known.

Avoid Concomitant Use

Avoid concomitant use of Dinutuximab with any of the following: BCG (Intravesical); Belimumab; Deferiprone; Dipyrone; Natalizumab; Pimecrolimus; Tacrolimus (Topical); Tofacitinib; Vaccines (Live)

Increased Effect/Toxicity

Dinuximab may increase the levels/effects of: Amifostine; Antipsychotic Agents (Second Generation [Atypical]); Belimumab; CloZAPine; Deferiprone; DULoxetine; Fingolimod; Hypotension-Associated Agents; Leflunomide; Levodopa; Natalizumab; Tofacitinib; Vaccines (Live)

The levels/effects of Dinutuximab may be increased by: Alfuzosin; Barbiturates; Blood Pressure Lowering Agents; Brimonidine (Topical); Denosumab; Diazoxide; Dipyrone; Herbs (Hypotensive Properties); Molsidomine; Nicorandil; Obinutuzumab; Pentoxifylline; Phosphodiesterase 5 Inhibitors; Pimecrolimus; Prostacyclin Analogues; Roflumilast; Tacrolimus (Topical); Trastuzumab

Decreased Effect

Dinutuximab may decrease the levels/effects of: BCG (Intravesical); Coccidioides immitis Skin Test; Sipuleucel-T; Vaccines (Inactivated); Vaccines (Live)

The levels/effects of Dinutuximab may be decreased by: Echinacea

Preparation for Administration Must be diluted prior to infusion. Withdraw the required dinutuximab volume and inject into a 100 mL bag of NS. Mix by gentle inversion; do not shake. Discard unused vial contents. Initiate infusion within 4 hours of preparation. Do not use if cloudy, discolored (pronounced), or contains particulates.

Storage/Stability Store intact vials at 2°C to 8°C (36°F to 46°F); do not freeze. Do not shake. Keep the vial in the outer carton to protect from light. Solutions diluted for infusion should be stored at 2°C to 8°C (36°F to 46°F). Initiate infusion within 4 hours of preparation. Discard diluted solution 24 hours after preparation.

Mechanism of Action Dinutuximab binds to the disialoganglioside GD2, which is highly expressed in neuroblastoma, most melanomas, and other tumors, as well as on normal tissues such as neurons, skin melanocytes, and peripheral sensory nerve fibers (Yu, 2010). By binding to CD2, dinutuximab induces cell lysis (of GD2-expressing cells) through antibody-dependent cell-mediated cytotoxicity (ADCC) and complement-dependent cytotoxicity (CDC).

Pharmacodynamics/Kinetics

Distribution: Pediatric: 5.4 L

Half-life elimination, terminal: 10 days

Dosing

Pediatric

Neuroblastoma, high-risk: IV: 17.5 mg/m²/day for 4 consecutive days for a maximum of 5 cycles (in combination with GM-CSF [sargramostim], IL-2 [aldesleukin] and 13-cis-retinoic acid [isotretinoin]). Infuse on days 4, 5, 6, and 7 during cycles 1, 3, and 5 (cycles 1, 3, and 5 are 24 days in duration); infuse on days 8, 9, 10, and 11 during cycles 2 and 4 (cycles 2 and 4 are 32 days in duration).

Premedications:

Analgesics: Administer morphine 50 mcg/kg IV immediately prior to dinutuximab infusion initiation; continue as a morphine drip at an infusion rate of 20 to 50 mcg/kg/hour during and for 2 hours following completion of infusion. May administer additional doses of 25 to 50 mcg/kg IV as needed up to once every 2 hours followed by an increase in the drip rate in clinically stable patients. Consider conversion to fentanyl or hydromorphone if morphine is not tolerated; if pain is inadequately controlled with opioids, consider adjunct therapy with gabapentin or lidocaine.

Antihistamine: Administer an antihistamine (eg, diphenhydramine 0.5 to 1 mg/kg/dose; maximum dose 50 mg) IV over 10 to 15 minutes starting 20 minutes prior to dinutuximab infusion and every 4 to 6 hours as tolerated during the infusion.

Antipyretics: Administer acetaminophen (10 to 15 mg/kg/dose; maximum dose 650 mg) 20 minutes prior to each infusion and every 4 to 6 hours as needed for fever and pain. May administer ibuprofen (5 to 10 mg/kg/dose) every 6 hours as needed for control of persistent fever or pain.

IV hydration: Administer NS 10 mL/kg IV over 1 hour just prior to each dinutuximab infusion.

Renal Impairment There are no dosage adjustments provided in the manufacturer's labeling (has not been studied).

Hepatic Impairment There are no dosage adjustments provided in the manufacturer's labeling (has not been studied).

Adjustment for Toxicity

Anaphylaxis, grade 3 or 4: Permanently discontinue therapy.

Capillary leak syndrome:

Moderate to severe, but not life-threatening: Immediately interrupt infusion; upon resolution, resume infusion at 50% of the previous rate.

Life-threatening: Discontinue infusion for the current cycle; in subsequent cycles, infuse at 50% of the previous rate. If life-threatening capillary leak syndrome recurs, permanently discontinue therapy.

Hemolytic uremic syndrome: Permanently discontinue therapy and administer supportive management.

Hyponatremia, grade 4 (despite appropriate fluid management): Permanently discontinue therapy.

Hypotension (symptomatic hypotension, systolic blood pressure [SBP] less than lower limit of normal for age, or SBP decreased by more than 15% compared to baseline): Interrupt infusion; upon resolution, resume infusion at 50% of the previous rate. If blood pressure remains stable for ≥2 hours, increase infusion rate as tolerated up to a maximum rate of 1.75 mg/m²/hour.

Infection (systemic)/sepsis, severe: Discontinue therapy until infection resolves; may resume therapy with subsequent cycles.

Infusion-related reaction:

Mild to moderate reaction (eg, transient rash, fever, rigors, and localized urticaria that respond promptly to symptomatic treatment): Reduce infusion rate by 50%; monitor closely. Upon resolution, gradually increase infusion rate up to a maximum of 1.75 mg/m²/hour.

Severe or prolonged reaction (eg, mild bronchospasm without other symptoms, angioedema that does not affect the airway): Immediately interrupt infusion; if symptoms resolve rapidly, resume infusion at 50% of the previous rate and monitor closely. If reaction recurs, discontinue therapy until the following day. If symptoms resolve and further treatment is warranted, premedicate with IV hydrocortisone 1 mg/kg (maximum 50 mg) and infuse at a rate of 0.875 mg/m²/hour in an intensive care unit. If reaction recurs again, permanently discontinue therapy.

Life-threatening reaction: Permanently discontinue therapy and administer supportive management.

Neuropathy:

Grade 4 sensory neuropathy or grade 3 sensory neuropathy that interferes with daily activities for more than 2 weeks: Permanently discontinue therapy.

Grade 2 peripheral motor neuropathy: Permanently discontinue therapy.

Ocular neurological disorders (eg, blurred vision, photophobia, mydriasis, fixed or unequal pupils, optic nerve disorder, eyelid ptosis, and/or papilledema): Discontinue infusion until symptom resolution; upon resolution, reduce *dose* by 50%. If reaction recurs, or if reaction is accompanied by visual impairment (eg, subtotal or total vision loss), permanently discontinue therapy.

Pain, severe (grade 3): Decrease the infusion rate to 0.875 mg/m²/hour. If pain is not adequately controlled despite rate reduction and use of maximum supportive measures, permanently discontinue therapy.

Serum sickness, grade 3 or 4: Permanently discontinue therapy.

Administration Administer as an IV infusion only; **do not administer as an IV push or bolus.** Administer NS 10 mL/kg IV over 1 hour just prior to each dinutuximab infusion. Premedicate with analgesics, an antihistamine, and an antipyretic prior to administration (see Dosing). Infuse in an environment equipped to monitor for and manage infusion reactions. Interrupt infusion for toxicity (see Dosage Adjustment for Toxicity).

Initiate infusion at a rate of 0.875 mg/m²/hour for 30 minutes. Increase infusion rate gradually as tolerated to a maximum rate of 1.75 mg/m²/hour to infuse over 10 to 20 hours each day. Monitor patients closely for signs and symptoms of an infusion reaction during and for at least 4 hours following completion of each dinutuximab infusion.

Monitoring Parameters CBC with differential, serum electrolytes, renal function, blood pressure; monitor for signs/symptoms of infusion reactions (during and for at least 4 hours after infusion), pain, peripheral neuropathy, capillary leak syndrome, infection/sepsis, hemolytic uremic syndrome, and ocular toxicity

Dosage Forms Excipient information presented when available (limited, particularly for generics); consult specific product labeling.

Solution, Intravenous [preservative free]:

Unituxin: 17.5 mg/5 mL (5 mL) [contains mouse protein (murine) (hamster)]

◆ Diocaine® (Can) *see* Proparacaine *on page 1515*

◆ Diocarpine (Can) *see* Pilocarpine (Ophthalmic) *on page 1452*

DiphenhydrAMINE (Systemic)
(dye fen HYE dra meen)

Brand Names: US Aler-Dryl [OTC]; Allergy Relief Childrens [OTC]; Allergy Relief [OTC]; Altaryl [OTC]; Anti-Hist Allergy [OTC]; Anti-Hist [OTC] [DSC]; Banophen [OTC]; Benadryl Allergy Childrens [OTC]; Benadryl Allergy [OTC]; Benadryl Dye-Free Allergy [OTC]; Benadryl [OTC]; Complete Allergy Medication [OTC]; Complete Allergy Relief [OTC]; Dicopanol FusePaq; Diphen [OTC]; Diphenhist [OTC]; Dytuss [DSC]; Genahist [OTC]; Geri-Dryl [OTC]; GoodSense Allergy Relief [OTC]; Naramin [OTC]; Nighttime Sleep Aid [OTC]; Nytol Maximum Strength [OTC]; Nytol [OTC]; Ormir [OTC]; PediaCare Childrens Allergy [OTC]; Pharbedryl; Pharbedryl [OTC]; Q-Dryl [OTC]; QlearQuil Nighttime Allergy [OTC]; Quenalin [OTC]; Scot-Tussin Allergy Relief [OTC]; Siladryl Allergy [OTC]; Silphen Cough [OTC]; Simply Allergy [OTC]; Simply Sleep [OTC]; Sleep Tabs [OTC]; Sominex Maximum Strength [OTC]; Sominex [OTC]; Tetra-Formula Nighttime Sleep [OTC]; Total Allergy Medicine [OTC]; Total Allergy [OTC]; Triaminic Childrens Allergy [OTC] [DSC]; Triaminic Cough/Runny Nose [OTC]; ZzzQuil [OTC]

Brand Names: Canada Allerdryl; Allernix; Benadryl; Nytol; Nytol Extra Strength; PMS-Diphenhydramine; Simply Sleep; Sominex

Index Terms Benadryl; Diphenhydramine Citrate; Diphenhydramine Hydrochloride; Diphenhydramine Tannate

Pharmacologic Category Ethanolamine Derivative; Histamine H$_1$ Antagonist; Histamine H$_1$ Antagonist, First Generation

Use Symptomatic relief of allergic symptoms caused by histamine release including nasal allergies and allergic dermatosis; adjunct to epinephrine in the treatment of anaphylaxis; insomnia, occasional; prevention or treatment of motion sickness; antitussive; management of Parkinsonian syndrome including drug-induced extrapyramidal symptoms (dystonic reactions) alone or in combination with centrally acting anticholinergic agents

Pregnancy Considerations Adverse events have not been observed in animal reproduction studies. Diphenhydramine crosses the placenta. Maternal diphenhydramine use has generally not resulted in an increased risk of birth defects; however, adverse events (withdrawal symptoms, respiratory depression) have been reported in newborns exposed to diphenhydramine in utero. Antihistamines are recommended for the treatment of rhinitis, urticaria, and pruritus with rash in pregnant women (although second generation antihistamines may be preferred). Antihistamines are not recommended for treatment of pruritus associated with intrahepatic cholestasis in pregnancy.

Breast-Feeding Considerations Diphenhydramine is excreted into breast milk; been reported in a breast-feeding infant. Premature infants and newborns have a higher risk of intolerance to antihistamines. Breast-feeding is contraindicated by the manufacturer. Antihistamines may decrease maternal serum prolactin concentrations when administered prior to the establishment of nursing.

Contraindications Hypersensitivity to diphenhydramine, other structurally related antihistamines, or any component of the formulation; neonates or premature infants; breast-feeding

Additional contraindications: Parenteral: Use as a local anesthetic

OTC labeling: When used for self-medication, do not use in children <6 years, to make a child sleep, or with any other diphenhydramine-containing products (including topical products)

Warnings/Precautions Causes sedation, caution must be used in performing tasks which require alertness (eg, operating machinery or driving). Potentially significant drug-drug interactions may exist, requiring dose or frequency adjustment, additional monitoring, and/or selection of alternative therapy. Sedative effects of CNS depressants or ethanol are potentiated. Antihistamines may cause excitation in young children. Toxicity (overdose) in pediatric patients may result in hallucinations, convulsions, or death; neonates and young children are highly sensitive to depressive effects of diphenhydramine; use is contraindicated in neonates. Use with caution in patients with angle-closure glaucoma, pyloroduodenal obstruction (including stenotic peptic ulcer), urinary tract obstruction (including bladder neck obstruction and symptomatic prostatic hyperplasia), asthma, hyperthyroidism, increased intraocular pressure, and cardiovascular disease (including hypertension and tachycardia).

Some preparations contain soy protein; avoid use in patients with soy protein or peanut allergies. Some products may contain phenylalanine. Some products may contain alcohol. Some dosage forms may contain propylene glycol; large amounts are potentially toxic and have been associated hyperosmolality, lactic acidosis, seizures, and respiratory depression; use caution (AAP ["Inactive" 1997]; Zar, 2007).

Benzyl alcohol and derivatives: Some dosage forms may contain sodium benzoate/benzoic acid; benzoic acid (benzoate) is a metabolite of benzyl alcohol; large amounts of benzyl alcohol (≥99 mg/kg/day) have been associated with a potentially fatal toxicity ("gasping syndrome") in neonates; the "gasping syndrome" consists of metabolic acidosis, respiratory distress, gasping respirations, CNS dysfunction (including convulsions, intracranial hemorrhage), hypotension, and cardiovascular collapse (AAP ["Inactive" 1997]; CDC, 1982); some data suggests that benzoate displaces bilirubin from protein binding sites (Ahlfors, 2001); avoid or use dosage forms containing benzyl alcohol derivative with caution in neonates. See manufacturer's labeling.

Some dosage forms may contain polysorbate 80 (also known as Tweens). Hypersensitivity reactions, usually a delayed reaction, have been reported following exposure to pharmaceutical products containing polysorbate 80 in certain individuals (Isaksson, 2002; Lucente 2000; Shelley, 1995). Thrombocytopenia, ascites, pulmonary deterioration, and renal and hepatic failure have been reported in premature neonates after receiving parenteral products containing polysorbate 80 (Alade, 1986; CDC, 1984). See manufacturer's labeling.

Oral products: In the elderly, avoid use of this potent anticholinergic agent due to increased risk of confusion, dry mouth, constipation, and other anticholinergic effects; clearance decreases in patients of advanced age; tolerance develops to hypnotic effects; when used for severe allergic reaction, use may be appropriate (Beers Criteria). Oral solutions are available in two concentrations (ie, 12.5 mg/5 mL and 50 mg/30 mL [eg, ZzzQuil]); precautions should be taken to verify and avoid confusion between the different concentrations; dose should be clearly presented as "mg"; the 50 mg/30 mL oral solution is indicated for the occasional treatment of insomnia.

Parenteral products: Subcutaneous or intradermal use has been associated with tissue necrosis; administer IV or IM only.

Adverse Reactions Frequency not defined.

Cardiovascular: Chest tightness, extrasystoles, hypotension, palpitations, tachycardia

Central nervous system: Ataxia, chills, confusion, dizziness, drowsiness, euphoria, excitement, fatigue, headache, insomnia, irritability, nervousness, neuritis, paradoxical excitation, paresthesia, restlessness, sedation, seizure, vertigo

Dermatologic: Diaphoresis

Endocrine & metabolic: Menstrual disease (early menses)

Gastrointestinal: Anorexia, constipation, diarrhea, dry mucous membranes, epigastric distress, nausea, vomiting, xerostomia

Genitourinary: Difficulty in micturition, urinary frequency, urinary retention

Hematologic & oncologic: Agranulocytosis, hemolytic anemia, thrombocytopenia

Hypersensitivity: Anaphylactic shock

Neuromuscular & skeletal: Tremor

Ophthalmic: Blurred vision, diplopia

Otic: Labyrinthitis (acute), tinnitus

Respiratory: Constriction of the pharynx, nasal congestion, thickening of bronchial secretions, wheezing

Drug Interactions

Metabolism/Transport Effects Inhibits CYP2D6 (moderate)

Avoid Concomitant Use

Avoid concomitant use of DiphenhydrAMINE (Systemic) with any of the following: Aclidinium; Azelastine (Nasal); Cimetropium; Eluxadoline; Glucagon; Glycopyrrolate; Glycopyrrolate (Oral Inhalation); Ipratropium (Oral Inhalation); Levosulpiride; Orphenadrine; Paraldehyde; Potassium Chloride; Thalidomide; Thioridazine; Tiotropium; Umeclidinium

Increased Effect/Toxicity

DiphenhydrAMINE (Systemic) may increase the levels/effects of: AbobotulinumtoxinA; Alcohol (Ethyl); Analgesics (Opioid); Anticholinergic Agents; ARIPiprazole; Azelastine (Nasal); Brexpiprazole; Buprenorphine; Cimetropium; CNS Depressants; CYP2D6 Substrates; DOXOrubicin (Conventional); Eliglustat; Eluxadoline; Fesoterodine; Glucagon; Glycopyrrolate; Glycopyrrolate (Oral Inhalation); Highest Risk QTc-Prolonging Agents; Hydrocodone; Methotrimeprazine; Metoprolol; Metyrosine; Mirabegron; Mirtazapine; Moderate Risk QTc-Prolonging Agents; Nebivolol; OnabotulinumtoxinA; Orphenadrine; Paraldehyde; Potassium Chloride; Pramipexole; Ramosetron; RimabotulinumtoxinB; ROPINIRole; Rotigotine; Selective Serotonin Reuptake Inhibitors; Suvorexant; Thalidomide; Thiazide Diuretics; Thioridazine; Tiotropium; Topiramate; Zolpidem

The levels/effects of DiphenhydrAMINE (Systemic) may be increased by: Aclidinium; Brimonidine (Topical); Cannabis; Doxylamine; Dronabinol; Droperidol; HydrOXYzine; Ipratropium (Oral Inhalation); Kava Kava; Magnesium Sulfate; Methotrimeprazine; Mianserin; Mifepristone; Minocycline; Nabilone; Perampanel; Pramlintide; Propafenone; Rufinamide; Sodium Oxybate; Tapentadol; Tetrahydrocannabinol; Umeclidinium

Decreased Effect

DiphenhydrAMINE (Systemic) may decrease the levels/effects of: Acetylcholinesterase Inhibitors; Benzylpenicilloyl Polylysine; Betahistine; Codeine; Gastrointestinal Agents (Prokinetic); Hyaluronidase; Itopride; Levosulpiride; Secretin; Tamoxifen; TraMADol

The levels/effects of DiphenhydrAMINE (Systemic) may be decreased by: Acetylcholinesterase Inhibitors; Amphetamines

Storage/Stability

Injection: Store at room temperature of 20°C to 25°C (68°F to 77°F); protect from light and freezing.

Oral: Store at room temperature. Protect capsules and tablets from moisture. Protect oral solution from freezing and light.

Mechanism of Action Competes with histamine for H_1-receptor sites on effector cells in the gastrointestinal tract, blood vessels, and respiratory tract; anticholinergic and sedative effects are also seen

Pharmacodynamics/Kinetics

Duration:

Histamine-induced wheal suppression: ≤10 hours (Simons, 1990)

Histamine-induced flare suppression: ≤12 hours (Simons, 1990)

Distribution: V_d: Children: 22 L/kg (range: 15 to 28 L/kg); Adults: 17 L/kg (range: 13 to 20 L/kg); Elderly: 14 L/kg (range: 7 to 20 L/kg) (Blyden, 1986; Simons, 1990)

Protein binding: 98.5% (Vozeh, 1988)

Metabolism: Extensively hepatic n-demethylation via CYP2D6; minor demethylation via CYP1A2, 2C9 and 2C19; smaller degrees in pulmonary and renal systems; significant first-pass effect (Akutsu, 2007)

Bioavailability: 42% to 62% (Paton, 1985)

Half-life elimination: Children: 5 hours (range: 4 to 7 hours); Adults: 9 hours (range: 7 to 12 hours); Elderly: 13.5 hours (range: 9 to 18 hours) (Blyden, 1986; Simons, 1990)

Time to peak, serum: ~2 hours (Blyden, 1986; Simons, 1990)

Excretion: Urine (as metabolites and unchanged drug) (Albert, 1975; Maurer, 1988)

Dosing

Adult

Allergic reactions:

Oral: 25 to 50 mg every 4 to 8 hours; maximum: 300 mg daily

IM, IV: 10 to 50 mg per dose; single doses up to 100 mg may be used if needed; not to exceed 400 mg daily

Antitussive: Oral: 25 mg every 4 hours; maximum: 150 mg daily

Motion sickness: Note: When used for prophylaxis, administer 30 minutes before motion.

Oral (treatment or prophylaxis): 25 to 50 mg every 6 to 8 hours

IM, IV (treatment): 10 to 50 mg per dose; single doses up to 100 mg may be used if needed; maximum: 400 mg daily

Insomnia, occasional: Oral: 50 mg at bedtime

Parkinsonism:

Oral: 25 to 50 mg 3 or 4 times daily

IM, IV: 10 to 50 mg per dose; single doses up to 100 mg may be used if needed; maximum: 400 mg daily

Rhinitis, sneezing due to common cold: Oral: 25 to 50 mg every 4 to 6 hours; maximum: 300 mg daily

Pediatric

Allergic reactions: Infants, Children, and Adolescents: IM, IV, Oral: 5 mg/kg/day in divided doses every 6 to 8 hours; maximum: 300 mg daily

Alternate dosing by age: Oral:

2 to <6 years (off-label use): 6.25 mg every 4 to 6 hours; maximum: 37.5 mg daily (Kleigman, 2011)

6 to <12 years: 12.5 to 25 mg every 4 to 6 hours; maximum: 150 mg daily

≥12 years: Refer to adult dosing.

Anaphylaxis (adjunct to epinephrine)/allergic reaction (off-label use): Infants, Children, and Adolescents: IM, IV, Oral: 1 to 2 mg/kg/dose; maximum: 50 mg/dose (Hegenbarth, 2008; Kliegman, 2011; Liberman, 2008; Lieberman, 2010; Simons, 2011)

Antitussive: Children ≥12 years: Refer to adult dosing.

Dystonic reactions (off-label use): Infants, Children, and Adolescents: IM, IV: 1 to 2 mg/kg/dose; maximum single dose: 50 mg (Hegenbarth, 2008; Kliegman, 2011)

Insomnia, occasional: Oral:

Children 2 to 12 years, weighing 10 to 50 kg (off-label use): Limited data available: 1 mg/kg administered 30 minutes before bedtime; maximum single dose: 50 mg (Russo, 1976)

Children ≥12 years and Adolescents: Refer to adult dosing.

Motion sickness:

Prophylaxis: Oral:

Manufacturer's labeling: Infants, Children, and Adolescents: **Note:** Administer 30 minutes before motion

Weight-directed dosing: 5 mg/kg/day divided into 3 to 4 doses; maximum: 300 mg daily

Fixed dosing: 12.5 to 25 mg 3 to 4 times daily

Alternate dosing: Children 2 to 12 years: Limited data available: 0.5 to 1 mg/kg/dose every 6 hours; maximum single dose: 25 mg. First dose should be administered 1 hour before travel (CDC, 2014).

Treatment: Infants, Children, and Adolescents:

IV, IM: 5 mg/kg/day divided into 4 doses; maximum: 300 mg daily

Oral:

Weight-directed dosing: 5 mg/kg/day divided into 3 to 4 doses; maximum: 300 mg daily

Fixed dosing: 12.5 to 25 mg 3 to 4 times daily

Rhinitis, sneezing due to common cold: Oral:

Children 6 to <12 years: 12.5 to 25 mg every 4 to 6 hours; maximum: 150 mg daily

Children ≥12 years and Adolescents: Refer to adult dosing.

Renal Impairment There are no dosage adjustments provided in the manufacturer's labeling.

Hepatic Impairment There are no dosage adjustments provided in the manufacturer's labeling.

Dietary Considerations Some products may contain sodium and/or phenylalanine.

Administration When used to prevent motion sickness, first dose should be given 30 minutes prior to exposure. When used for occasional insomnia, dose should be given 30 minutes before bedtime.

Injection solution is for IV or deep IM administration only. For IV administration, inject at a rate ≤25 mg/minute. Local necrosis may result with SubQ or intradermal use.

Monitoring Parameters Relief of symptoms, mental alertness

Test Interactions May interfere with urine detection of methadone and phencyclidine (false-positives); may cause false-positive serum TCA screen; may suppress the wheal and flare reactions to skin test antigens

Dosage Forms Considerations Dicopanol FusePaq is a compounding kit for the preparation of an oral suspension. Refer to manufacturer's labeling for compounding instructions.

Dosage Forms Excipient information presented when available (limited, particularly for generics); consult specific product labeling. [DSC] = Discontinued product

Capsule, Oral, as hydrochloride:
Allergy Relief: 25 mg [contains brilliant blue fcf (fd&c blue #1), butylparaben, edetate calcium disodium, fd&c blue #2 (indigotine), fd&c red #40, fd&c yellow #10 (quinoline yellow), methylparaben, polysorbate 80, propylparaben]
Anti-Hist: 25 mg [DSC]
Banophen: 25 mg [contains brilliant blue fcf (fd&c blue #1), fd&c red #40, fd&c yellow #6 (sunset yellow), methylparaben, propylparaben]
Banophen: 50 mg [contains brilliant blue fcf (fd&c blue #1), fd&c red #40]
Benadryl: 25 mg
Benadryl Allergy: 25 mg [dye free]
Benadryl Dye-Free Allergy: 25 mg [dye free]
Diphenhist: 25 mg [DSC] [contains brilliant blue fcf (fd&c blue #1), butylparaben, fd&c red #40, methylparaben, propylparaben]
Diphenhist: 25 mg [contains brilliant blue fcf (fd&c blue #1), fd&c red #40]
Genahist: 25 mg
Geri-Dryl: 25 mg
GoodSense Allergy Relief: 25 mg [dye free]
Ormir: 50 mg [contains fd&c yellow #10 (quinoline yellow), fd&c yellow #6 (sunset yellow)]
Pharbedryl: 25 mg, 50 mg [contains brilliant blue fcf (fd&c blue #1), fd&c red #40]
Q-Dryl: 25 mg [contains brilliant blue fcf (fd&c blue #1), butylparaben, fd&c red #40, methylparaben, propylparaben]
ZzzQuil: 25 mg [contains brilliant blue fcf (fd&c blue #1), fd&c red #40]
Generic: 25 mg, 50 mg
Elixir, Oral, as hydrochloride:
Altaryl: 12.5 mg/5 mL (120 mL, 480 mL, 3840 mL) [contains alcohol, usp]
Generic: 12.5 mg/5 mL (5 mL, 10 mL)
Liquid, Oral, as hydrochloride:
Allergy Relief Childrens: 12.5 mg/5 mL (118 mL, 480 mL) [alcohol free; contains fd&c red #40, sodium benzoate]
Banophen: 12.5 mg/5 mL (118 mL) [alcohol free; cherry flavor]
Banophen: 12.5 mg/5 mL (473 mL) [alcohol free, sugar free; cherry flavor]
Benadryl Allergy Childrens: 12.5 mg/5 mL (118 mL, 236 mL) [alcohol free; contains fd&c red #40, sodium benzoate]
Benadryl Allergy Childrens: 12.5 mg/5 mL (5 mL, 236 mL) [alcohol free; contains fd&c red #40, sodium benzoate; cherry flavor]
Benadryl Allergy Childrens: 12.5 mg/5 mL (118 mL) [alcohol free, dye free, sugar free; contains saccharin sodium, sodium benzoate]
Diphenhist: 12.5 mg/5 mL (118 mL, 473 mL) [alcohol free; contains fd&c red #40, saccharin sodium, sodium benzoate; fruit flavor]
Naramin: 12.5 mg/5 mL (5 mL) [alcohol free; contains fd&c red #40, sodium benzoate; cherry flavor]
PediaCare Childrens Allergy: 12.5 mg/5 mL (118 mL) [alcohol free; contains fd&c red #40, sodium benzoate]
Q-Dryl: 12.5 mg/5 mL (118 mL, 237 mL, 473 mL) [alcohol free; contains fd&c red #40, saccharin sodium, sodium benzoate; cherry flavor]
Scot-Tussin Allergy Relief: 12.5 mg/5 mL (118.3 mL, 240 mL, 480 mL, 3780 mL) [alcohol free, dye free, saccharin free, sodium free, sorbitol free, sugar free]

Siladryl Allergy: 12.5 mg/5 mL (118 mL, 237 mL, 473 mL) [alcohol free, sugar free; contains fd&c red #40, methylparaben, propylene glycol, propylparaben, saccharin sodium; cherry flavor]
Total Allergy Medicine: 12.5 mg/5 mL (118 mL) [alcohol free]
ZzzQuil: 50 mg/30 mL (177 mL, 354 mL) [contains alcohol, usp, brilliant blue fcf (fd&c blue #1), fd&c red #40, propylene glycol, saccharin sodium, sodium benzoate; berry flavor]
ZzzQuil: 50 mg/30 mL (354 mL) [contains alcohol, usp, brilliant blue fcf (fd&c blue #1), fd&c red #40, propylene glycol, saccharin sodium, sodium benzoate; vanilla cherry flavor]
ZzzQuil: 50 mg/30 mL (177 mL, 354 mL) [alcohol free; contains brilliant blue fcf (fd&c blue #1), propylene glycol, saccharin sodium, sodium benzoate; mango berry flavor]
Solution, Injection, as hydrochloride:
Generic: 50 mg/mL (1 mL, 10 mL)
Solution, Injection, as hydrochloride [preservative free]:
Generic: 50 mg/mL (1 mL)
Strip, Oral, as hydrochloride:
Triaminic Childrens Allergy: 12.5 mg (14 ea [DSC]) [contains alcohol, usp, brilliant blue fcf (fd&c blue #1), fd&c red #40, isopropyl alcohol, propylene glycol]
Triaminic Cough/Runny Nose: 12.5 mg (14 ea) [contains alcohol, usp, brilliant blue fcf (fd&c blue #1), fd&c red #40]
Triaminic Cough/Runny Nose: 12.5 mg (16 ea) [contains alcohol, usp, brilliant blue fcf (fd&c blue #1), fd&c red #40; grape flavor]
Suspension Reconstituted, Oral, as hydrochloride:
Dicopanol FusePaq: 5 mg/mL (150 mL) [contains sodium benzoate]
Syrup, Oral, as hydrochloride:
Altaryl: 12.5 mg/5 mL (120 mL, 480 mL, 3785 mL) [alcohol free; cherry flavor]
Dytuss: 12.5 mg/5 mL (480 mL [DSC])
Quenalin: 12.5 mg/5 mL (120 mL) [fruit flavor]
Silphen Cough: 12.5 mg/5 mL (118 mL, 237 mL, 473 mL) [contains alcohol, usp, fd&c red #40, menthol, methylparaben, propylene glycol, propylparaben; strawberry flavor]
Tablet, Oral, as hydrochloride:
Aler-Dryl: 50 mg
Allergy Relief: 25 mg [contains polysorbate 80]
Anti-Hist Allergy: 25 mg
Banophen: 25 mg
Benadryl: 25 mg
Benadryl Allergy: 25 mg
Benadryl Allergy: 25 mg [contains edetate calcium disodium, fd&c red #40, methylparaben, polysorbate 80, propylparaben]
Complete Allergy Medication: 25 mg
Complete Allergy Relief: 25 mg
Diphen: 25 mg
Diphenhist: 25 mg
Geri-Dryl: 25 mg
Nighttime Sleep Aid: 25 mg [contains fd&c blue #1 aluminum lake, fd&c blue #2 aluminum lake, polysorbate 80]
Nighttime Sleep Aid: 50 mg [DSC] [contains fd&c blue #1 aluminum lake]
Nytol: 25 mg
Nytol Maximum Strength: 50 mg
QlearQuil Nighttime Allergy: 25 mg [contains fd&c blue #1 aluminum lake, fd&c blue #2 aluminum lake]
Simply Allergy: 25 mg
Simply Sleep: 25 mg [contains brilliant blue fcf (fd&c blue #1)]
Sleep Tabs: 25 mg [scored; contains fd&c blue #1 aluminum lake]
Sominex: 25 mg [contains fd&c blue #1 aluminum lake]
Sominex Maximum Strength: 50 mg [contains fd&c blue #1 aluminum lake, polysorbate 80]
Tetra-Formula Nighttime Sleep: 50 mg [contains fd&c blue #1 aluminum lake]
Total Allergy: 25 mg
Generic: 25 mg
Tablet Chewable, Oral, as hydrochloride:
Benadryl Allergy Childrens: 12.5 mg [contains aspartame, fd&c blue #1 aluminum lake; cherry flavor]
Benadryl Allergy Childrens: 12.5 mg [contains aspartame, fd&c blue #1 aluminum lake; grape flavor]

◆ Diphenhydramine and Acetaminophen see Acetaminophen and Diphenhydramine on page 29

◆ Diphenhydramine and ASA see Aspirin and Diphenhydramine on page 162

◆ Diphenhydramine and Aspirin see Aspirin and Diphenhydramine on page 162

Diphenhydramine and Phenylephrine
(dye fen HYE dra meen & fen il EF rin)

Brand Names: US Aldex® CT [DSC]; Benadryl-D® Allergy & Sinus [OTC]; Benadryl-D® Children's Allergy & Sinus [OTC]; Dimetapp® Children's Nighttime Cold & Congestion [OTC]; Triaminic® Children's Night Time Cold & Cough [OTC]

Index Terms Diphenhydramine Hydrochloride and Phenylephrine Hydrochloride; Diphenhydramine Tannate and Phenylephrine Tannate; Phenylephrine and Diphenhydramine; Phenylephrine Hydrochloride and Diphenhydramine Hydrochloride; Phenylephrine Tannate and Diphenhydramine Tannate

Pharmacologic Category Alpha-Adrenergic Agonist; Decongestant; Ethanolamine Derivative; Histamine H$_1$ Antagonist; Histamine H$_1$ Antagonist, First Generation

Use Temporary relief of symptoms of allergic rhinitis, sinusitis, and other upper respiratory conditions, including sinus/nasal congestion, sneezing, stuffy/runny nose, itchy/watery eyes, and cough

Dosing

Adult & Geriatric Allergic symptoms, nasal congestion: Oral:

Aldex® CT: 1-2 tablets every 6 hours

OTC labeling: **Note:** General dosing guidelines; refer to specific product labeling:

10-20 mL every 4 hours as needed (maximum: 6 doses/24 hours) **or** 1 tablet every 4 hours as needed (maximum: 6 doses/24 hours)

Pediatric Allergic symptoms, nasal congestion: Oral:

Aldex® CT:

Children 6-11 years: One-half to 1 tablet every 6 hours
Children ≥12 years: Refer to adult dosing.

OTC labeling:

Children <6 years: Use not recommended
Children 6-11 years:

Benadryl-D® Children's Allergy & Sinus: 5 mL every 4 hours as needed (maximum: 6 doses/24 hours)
Dimetapp® Children's Nighttime Cold and Congestion, Triaminic® Children's Night Time Cold & Cough: 10 mL every 4 hours as needed (maximum: 6 doses/24 hours)

Children ≥12 years: Refer to adult dosing.

Additional Information Complete prescribing information should be consulted for additional detail.

Dosage Forms Excipient information presented when available (limited, particularly for generics); consult specific product labeling. [DSC] = Discontinued product

Liquid, oral:

Benadryl-D® Children's Allergy & Sinus: Diphenhydramine hydrochloride 12.5 mg and phenylephrine hydrochloride 5 mg per 5 mL (118 mL) [ethanol free, sugar free; contains sodium 10 mg/5 mL, sodium benzoate; grape flavor]

Syrup, oral:

Dimetapp® Children's Nighttime Cold and Congestion: Diphenhydramine hydrochloride 6.25 mg and phenylephrine hydrochloride 2.5 mg per 5 mL (120 mL) [ethanol free, sugar free; contains propylene glycol, sodium 4 mg/5 mL, sodium benzoate; grape flavor]
Triaminic® Children's Night Time Cold & Cough: Diphenhydramine hydrochloride 6.25 mg and phenylephrine hydrochloride 2.5 mg per 5 mL (118 mL) [contains ethanol, propylene glycol, sodium 6 mg/5 mL; grape flavor]

Tablet, oral:

Benadryl-D® Allergy & Sinus: Diphenhydramine hydrochloride 25 mg and phenylephrine hydrochloride 10 mg

Tablet, chewable, oral:

Aldex® CT: Diphenhydramine hydrochloride 12.5 mg and phenylephrine hydrochloride 5 mg [contains phenylalanine; strawberry flavor] [DSC]

◆ Diphenhydramine Citrate *see* DiphenhydrAMINE (Systemic) *on page 561*

◆ Diphenhydramine Citrate and Aspirin *see* Aspirin and Diphenhydramine *on page 162*

◆ Diphenhydramine Hydrochloride *see* DiphenhydrAMINE (Systemic) *on page 561*

◆ Diphenhydramine Hydrochloride and Phenylephrine Hydrochloride *see* Diphenhydramine and Phenylephrine *on page 564*

◆ Diphenhydramine Tannate *see* DiphenhydrAMINE (Systemic) *on page 561*

◆ Diphenhydramine Tannate and Phenylephrine Tannate *see* Diphenhydramine and Phenylephrine *on page 564*

Diphenoxylate and Atropine
(dye fen OKS i late & A troe peen)

Brand Names: US Lomotil
Brand Names: Canada Lomotil
Index Terms Atropine and Diphenoxylate
Pharmacologic Category Antidiarrheal
Use Diarrhea: Adjunctive management of diarrhea

Pregnancy Considerations Animal reproduction studies have not been conducted with this combination. Refer to individual agents.

Breast-Feeding Considerations Atropine is excreted in breast milk; diphenoxylic acid may be excreted in breast milk. The manufacturer recommends that caution be exercised when administering diphenoxylate/atropine to nursing women. Refer to individual agents.

Contraindications

Hypersensitivity to diphenoxylate, atropine, or any component of the formulation; obstructive jaundice; diarrhea associated with pseudomembranous enterocolitis or enterotoxin-producing bacteria

Canadian labeling: Additional contraindications (not in US labeling): Jaundice

Warnings/Precautions Do not exceed recommended dosage; overdose may result in severe respiratory depression, coma, and possible permanent brain damage or death. Clinical improvement of acute diarrhea is usually observed within 48 hours. If there is no response within 48 hours in children, diphenoxylate/atropine is unlikely to be effective and should be discontinued; if chronic diarrhea is not improved symptomatically within 10 days at maximum dosage, control is unlikely with further use.

Use in conjunction with fluid and electrolyte therapy when appropriate. In case of severe dehydration or electrolyte imbalance, withhold diphenoxylate/atropine treatment until corrective therapy has been initiated. Inhibiting peristalsis may lead to fluid retention in the intestine aggravating dehydration and electrolyte imbalance. Reduction of intestinal motility may be deleterious in diarrhea resulting from *Shigella, Salmonella*, toxigenic strains of *E. coli*, and pseudomembranous enterocolitis associated with broad-spectrum antibiotics; use is not recommended.

Use with caution in children; not recommended for use in children <2 years of age (US labeling) or <4 years (Canadian labeling). Younger children may be predisposed to delayed toxicity; signs of atropinism may occur even at recommended doses, especially in patients with Down syndrome.

Use caution with acute ulcerative colitis, hepatic or renal dysfunction. Physical and psychological dependence have been reported with higher than recommended dosing. Atropine may be inappropriate in older adults depending on comorbidities (eg, dementia, delirium) due to its potent anticholinergic effects (Beers Criteria). May cause CNS depression, which may impair physical or mental abilities; patients must be cautioned about performing tasks that require mental alertness (eg, operating machinery or driving). Potentially significant interactions may exist, requiring dose or frequency adjustment, additional monitoring, and/or selection of alternative therapy.

Adverse Reactions Frequency not defined.

Cardiovascular: Flushing, tachycardia
Central nervous system: Confusion, depression, dizziness, drowsiness, euphoria, headache, hyperthermia, lethargy, malaise, numbness, restlessness, sedation
Dermatologic: Pruritus, urticaria, xeroderma
Gastrointestinal: Abdominal distress, anorexia, gingival swelling, nausea, pancreatitis, paralytic ileus, toxic megacolon, vomiting, xerostomia
Genitourinary: Urinary retention
Hypersensitivity: Anaphylaxis, angioedema

Drug Interactions

Metabolism/Transport Effects None known.

Avoid Concomitant Use

Avoid concomitant use of Diphenoxylate and Atropine with any of the following: Aclidinium; Azelastine (Nasal); Cimetropium; Eluxadoline; Glucagon; Glycopyrrolate; Glycopyrrolate (Oral Inhalation); Ipratropium (Oral Inhalation); Levosulpiride; Orphenadrine; Paraldehyde; Potassium Chloride; Thalidomide; Tiotropium; Umeclidinium

Increased Effect/Toxicity

Diphenoxylate and Atropine may increase the levels/effects of: AbobotulinumtoxinA; Alcohol (Ethyl); Analgesics (Opioid); Anticholinergic Agents; Azelastine (Nasal); Buprenorphine; Cimetropium; CNS Depressants; Eluxadoline; Glucagon; Glycopyrrolate; Glycopyrrolate (Oral Inhalation); Hydrocodone; Methotrimeprazine; Metyrosine; Mirabegron; Mirtazapine; OnabotulinumtoxinA;

Orphenadrine; Paraldehyde; Potassium Chloride; Pramipexole; Ramosetron; RimabotulinumtoxinB; ROPINIRole; Rotigotine; Selective Serotonin Reuptake Inhibitors; Suvorexant; Thalidomide; Thiazide Diuretics; Tiotropium; Topiramate; Zolpidem

The levels/effects of Diphenoxylate and Atropine may be increased by: Aclidinium; Brimonidine (Topical); Cannabis; Doxylamine; Dronabinol; Droperidol; HydrOXYzine; Ipratropium (Oral Inhalation); Kava Kava; Magnesium Sulfate; Methotrimeprazine; Mianserin; Minocycline; Nabilone; Perampanel; Pramlintide; Rufinamide; Sodium Oxybate; Tapentadol; Tetrahydrocannabinol; Umeclidinium

Decreased Effect

Diphenoxylate and Atropine may decrease the levels/effects of: Acetylcholinesterase Inhibitors; Gastrointestinal Agents (Prokinetic); Itopride; Levosulpiride; Secretin

The levels/effects of Diphenoxylate and Atropine may be decreased by: Acetylcholinesterase Inhibitors

Storage/Stability

Oral solution: Store at 20°C to 25°C (68°F to 77°F). Discard opened bottle after 90 days.

Tablet: Store at 20°C to 25°C (68°F to 77°F); protect from light.

Mechanism of Action Diphenoxylate inhibits excessive GI motility and GI propulsion; commercial preparations contain a subtherapeutic amount of atropine to discourage abuse

Pharmacodynamics/Kinetics

Atropine: See Atropine monograph.

Diphenoxylate:

Onset of action: Within 45 to 60 minutes

Absorption: Well absorbed

Metabolism: Extensively hepatic via ester hydrolysis to diphenoxylic acid (active)

Bioavailability: ~90%

Half-life elimination: Diphenoxylate: 2.5 hours; Diphenoxylic acid: 12 to 14 hours

Time to peak, serum: ~2 hours

Excretion: Primarily feces (49% as unchanged drug and metabolites); urine (~14%, as unchanged drug [<1%] and metabolites)

Dosing

Adult & Geriatric

Diarrhea: Oral: **Note:** If no improvement within 48 hours (acute symptoms) or 10 days at maximum dose (chronic symptoms) therapy is likely to be ineffective.

Initial: Diphenoxylate 5 mg (2 tablets) 3 or 4 times daily until control achieved (maximum: 20 mg/day), then reduce dose as needed; maintenance doses may be as low as 25% of initial daily dose required for control.

Pediatric

Diarrhea: **Note:** If no improvement within 48 hours (acute symptoms) therapy is likely to be ineffective.

US labeling: Children ≥2 years to <13 years (liquid only): Oral:

Initial: Diphenoxylate 0.3 to 0.4 mg/kg/day in 4 divided doses or alternatively:

2 years (11 to 14 kg): 1.5 to 3 mL 4 times daily

3 years (12 to 16 kg): 2 to 3 mL 4 times daily

4 years (14 to 20 kg): 2 to 4 mL 4 times daily

5 years (16 to 23 kg): 2.5 to 4.5 mL 4 times daily

6 to 8 years (17 to 32 kg): 2.5 to 5 mL 4 times daily

9 to 12 years (23 to 55 kg): 3.5 to 5 mL 4 times daily

Maintenance: Doses may be as low as 25% of initial daily dose; reduce dose as soon as possible after symptoms have been controlled

Canadian labeling: ≥4 years and Adolescents: Oral:

Initial: Diphenoxylate 0.3 to 0.4 mg/kg/day in divided doses or alternatively:

4 to 8 years (20 to 27 kg): 2.5 mg 3 times daily

9 to 12 years (27 to 36 kg): 2.5 mg 4 times daily

≥13 years: 5 mg 4 times daily

Renal Impairment There are no specific dosage adjustments provided in the manufacturer's labeling. Use with extreme caution in patients with advanced hepatorenal disease.

Hepatic Impairment There are no specific dosage adjustments provided in the manufacturer's labeling. Use with extreme caution in patients with abnormal hepatic function and in advanced hepatorenal disease.

Administration Use of the liquid preparation is recommended in children <13 years of age; use only plastic dropper provided when measuring liquid. Dropper has a 2 mL (1 mg) capacity and is calibrated in increments of 1/2 mL (0.25 mg).

Monitoring Parameters Watch for signs of atropinism (dryness of skin and mucous membranes, tachycardia, thirst, flushing); monitor number and consistency of stools; observe for signs of toxicity, fluid and electrolyte loss, hypotension, and respiratory depression

Dosage Forms Excipient information presented when available (limited, particularly for generics); consult specific product labeling. [DSC] = Discontinued product

Solution, Oral: Diphenoxylate hydrochloride 2.5 mg and atropine sulfate 0.025 mg per 5 mL (5 mL, 10 mL, 60 mL)

Lomotil: Diphenoxylate hydrochloride 2.5 mg and atropine sulfate 0.025 mg per 5 mL (60 mL) [contains alcohol 15%; cherry flavor] [DSC]

Tablet, Oral: Diphenoxylate hydrochloride 2.5 mg and atropine sulfate 0.025 mg

Lomotil: Diphenoxylate hydrochloride 2.5 mg and atropine sulfate 0.025 mg

Dosage Forms: Canada Excipient information presented when available (limited, particularly for generics); consult specific product labeling.

Tablet, Oral: Diphenoxylate hydrochloride 2.5 mg and atropine sulfate 0.025 mg

Controlled Substance C-V

◆ Diphenylhydantoin see Phenytoin on page 1444

Diphtheria and Tetanus Toxoid
(dif THEER ee a & TET a nus TOKS oyds)

Brand Names: US Tenivac

Brand Names: Canada Td Adsorbed

Index Terms DT; Td; Tetanus and Diphtheria Toxoid

Pharmacologic Category Vaccine; Vaccine, Inactivated (Bacterial)

Additional Appendix Information

Immunization Administration Recommendations *on page 1974*

Immunization Schedules *on page 1979*

Use Diphtheria and tetanus disease prevention:

Diphtheria and tetanus toxoids adsorbed for pediatric use (DT): Infants ≥6 weeks and children through 6 years of age: Active immunization against diphtheria and tetanus when pertussis vaccine is contraindicated

Tetanus and diphtheria toxoids adsorbed for adult use (Td) (Tenivac): Children ≥7 years, adolescents, and adults: Active immunization against diphtheria and tetanus; tetanus prophylaxis in wound management

The Advisory Committee on Immunization Practices (ACIP) recommends routine vaccination for the following:

• Children ≥7 years, adolescents, and adults should receive a booster dose of Td every 10 years; may substitute a single Td booster dose with Tdap (CDC/ACIP 60[1] 2011)

• Children 7 to 10 years, adolescents, adults, and elderly (≥65 years) patients who are wounded in bombings or similar mass casualty events who have penetrating injuries or nonintact skin exposure and who cannot confirm receipt of a tetanus booster within the previous 5 years, may also receive a single dose of Td; children ≥11 years and adults may also receive Td if Tdap is unavailable (CDC [Chapman, 2008])

Medication Guide Available Yes

Dosing

Adult & Geriatric

Primary immunization (Td): IM:

Manufacturer labeling (Tenivac): Patients previously not immunized should receive 2 primary doses of 0.5 mL each, given at an interval of 8 weeks; third (reinforcing) dose of 0.5 mL 6 to 8 months later

ACIP recommendations: Patients previously not immunized should receive 2 primary doses of 0.5 mL each, given at an interval of 4 weeks; third (reinforcing) dose of 0.5 mL 6 to 12 months later. Patients not completely immunized (<3 doses) should receive the remaining doses. For patients who have not received Tdap, a dose should be included as part of primary immunization (in place of one of the Td doses) (CDC/ACIP [Kim 2015]).

Booster immunization (Td): IM: 0.5 mL every 10 years (for routine booster in patients who have completed primary immunization series). The ACIP prefers Tdap for use in in some situations if no contraindications exist; refer to Diphtheria and Tetanus Toxoids, and Acellular Pertussis Vaccine monograph for additional information.

Tetanus prophylaxis in wound management (CDC/ACIP [Broder 2006]): IM: Tetanus prophylaxis in patients with wounds should be based on if the wound is clean or contaminated, the immunization status of the patient. Wound management includes proper use of tetanus toxoid and/or tetanus immune globulin (TIG),

wound cleaning, and (if required) surgical debridement and the proper use of antibiotics. Patients with an uncertain or incomplete tetanus immunization status should have additional follow up to ensure a series is completed. Patients with a history of Arthus reaction following a previous dose of a tetanus toxoid-containing vaccine should not receive a tetanus toxoid-containing vaccine until >10 years after the most recent dose even if they have a wound that is neither clean nor minor. See table.

Tetanus Prophylaxis in Wound Management

History of Tetanus Immunization Doses	Clean, Minor Wounds		All Other Wounds[1]	
	Tetanus Toxoid[2]	TIG	Tetanus Toxoid[2]	TIG
Uncertain or <3 doses	Yes	No	Yes	Yes
3 or more doses	No[3]	No	No[4]	No

[1]Such as, but not limited to, wounds contaminated with dirt, feces, soil, and saliva; puncture wounds; wounds from crushing, tears, burns, and frostbite.

[2]Tetanus toxoid in this chart refers to a tetanus toxoid-containing vaccine. For children ≤6 years of age, DTaP (DT, if pertussis vaccine contraindicated) is preferred to tetanus toxoid alone. For children ≥7 years, adolescents, and adults, Td preferred to tetanus toxoid alone; Tdap may be preferred if the patient has not previously been vaccinated with Tdap.

[3]Yes, if ≥10 years since last dose.

[4]Yes, if ≥5 years since last dose.

Abbreviations: **DT** = Diphtheria and Tetanus Toxoids (formulation for age ≤6 years); **DTaP** = Diphtheria and Tetanus Toxoids, and Acellular Pertussis (formulation for age ≤6 years; Daptacel, Infanrix); **Td** = Diphtheria and Tetanus Toxoids (formulation for age ≥7 years; Tenivac); **TT** = Tetanus toxoid (adsorbed [formulation for age ≥7 years]); **Tdap** = Diphtheria and Tetanus Toxoids, and Acellular Pertussis (Adacel or Boostrix [formulations for age ≥7 years]); **TIG** = Tetanus Immune Globulin.

Pediatric

Primary immunization: IM:

Children 6 weeks to ≤6 years (DT): **Note:** For use when a pertussis-containing vaccine is contraindicated: 0.5 mL per dose, total of 5 doses administered as follows:

Three doses, usually given at 2-, 4-, and 6 months of age; may be given as early as 6 weeks of age and repeated every 4 to 8 weeks

Fourth dose: Given at ~15 to 18 months of age, but at least 6 months after third dose. The fourth dose may be given as early as 12 months of age, but at least 6 months must have elapsed between the third dose and the fourth dose.

Fifth dose: Given at 4 to 6 years of age, prior to starting school or kindergarten; if the fourth dose is given at ≥4 years of age, the fifth dose may be omitted

For children who start primary immunization series ≥4 months of age, refer to current ACIP "Catch-up Immunization Schedule"

Children ≥7 years (Td): Refer to adult dosing.

Booster immunization: IM: For routine booster in patients who have completed primary immunization series. The ACIP prefers Tdap for use in in some situations if no contraindications exist; refer to Diphtheria and Tetanus Toxoids, and Acellular Pertussis Vaccine monograph for additional information.

Children 11 to 12 years (Td): 0.5 mL as a single dose when at least 5 years have elapsed since last dose of toxoid-containing vaccine. If not contraindicated, Tdap is the preferred dose for this dose. Subsequent routine doses are not recommended more often than every 10 years. **Note:** If Tdap is given as part of catch-up dosing at 7 to 10 years of age, the 11 to 12 year booster is not needed. Regular Td booster immunizations should begin 10 years after the last dose of the primary series.

Tetanus prophylaxis in wound management: *Children ≥7 years:* Refer to adult dosing.

Renal Impairment There are no dosage adjustments provided in the manufacturer's labeling.

Hepatic Impairment There are no dosage adjustments provided in the manufacturer's labeling.

Additional Information Complete prescribing information should be consulted for additional detail.

Dosage Forms Excipient information presented when available (limited, particularly for generics); consult specific product labeling. [DSC] = Discontinued product

Injection, suspension [Td, adult; preservative free]: Diphtheria 2 Lf units and tetanus 2 Lf units per 0.5 mL (0.5 mL)

Tenivac: Diphtheria 2 Lf units and tetanus 5 Lf units per 0.5 mL (0.5 mL) [contains aluminum, may contain natural rubber/natural latex in prefilled syringe]

Injection, suspension [DT, pediatric; preservative free]: Diphtheria 6.7 Lf units and tetanus 5 Lf units per 0.5 mL (0.5 mL) [DSC]; Diphtheria 25 Lf units and tetanus 5 Lf units per 0.5 mL (0.5 mL) [contains aluminum]

Diphtheria and Tetanus Toxoids, Acellular Pertussis, and Poliovirus Vaccine

(dif THEER ee a & TET a nus TOKS oyds, ay CEL yoo lar per TUS sis & POE lee oh VYE rus vak SEEN)

Brand Names: US Kinrix; Quadracel

Brand Names: Canada Adacel-Polio; Boostrix-Polio; Infanrix-IPV; Quadracel

Index Terms Diphtheria and Tetanus Toxoids and Acellular Pertussis Adsorbed, and Inactivated Poliovirus Vaccine Combined; Diphtheria, Tetanus Toxoids, Acellular Pertussis (DTaP); DTaP-IPV; Poliovirus, Inactivated (IPV)

Pharmacologic Category Vaccine; Vaccine, Inactivated (Bacterial); Vaccine, Inactivated (Viral)

Additional Appendix Information

Immunization Administration Recommendations *on page 1974*

Immunization Schedules *on page 1979*

Use Diphtheria, tetanus, pertussis, and poliovirus disease prevention:

Kinrix: Active booster immunization against diphtheria, tetanus, pertussis, and poliomyelitis as the fifth dose in the diphtheria, tetanus, and acellular pertussis (DTaP) vaccine series and as the fourth dose in the inactivated poliovirus vaccine (IPV) series in children 4 through 6 years of age whose previous DTaP vaccine doses have been with Infanrix (DTaP) and/or Pediarix (DTaP-hepatitis B-IPV) for the first 3 doses and Infanrix (DTaP) for the fourth dose.

Quadracel:

US labeling: Active booster immunization against diphtheria, tetanus, pertussis, and poliomyelitis as the fifth dose in the diphtheria, tetanus, and acellular pertussis (DTaP) vaccine series and as the fourth or fifth dose in the inactivated poliovirus vaccine (IPV) series in children 4 through 6 years of age whose previous DTaP vaccine doses have been 4 doses of Pentacel (DTaP-IPV/Haemophilus b conjugate [tetanus toxoid conjugate] vaccine) and/or Daptacel (DTaP).

Canadian labeling: Active primary immunization against diphtheria, tetanus, pertussis, and poliomyelitis for infants and children 6 months through 6 years of age.

Adacel-Polio [Canadian product]: Active booster immunization against diphtheria, tetanus, pertussis, and poliomyelitis in patients 4 years and older; alternative to fifth dose of DTaP-IPV in patients 4 to 6 years of age; may be used for wound management when a tetanus toxoid-containing vaccine is needed for wound management [refer to current National Advisory Committee on Immunization (NACI) guidelines]

Boostrix Polio [Canadian product]: Active booster immunization against diphtheria, tetanus, pertussis, and poliomyelitis in patients 4 years and older; may be used for wound management when a tetanus toxoid-containing vaccine is needed for wound management [refer to current National Advisory Committee on Immunization (NACI) guidelines]

Infanrix-IPV [Canadian product]: Active booster immunization against diphtheria, tetanus, pertussis, and poliomyelitis in children ≥15 months through 6 years of age

Dosing

Adult

Booster immunization: Adacel-Polio, Boostrix-Polio [Canadian products]: IM: 0.5 mL as a single dose

Pediatric

Immunization:

US labeling: Kinrix, Quadracel: IM: Children 4 to 6 years: 0.5 mL as a single dose

Canadian labeling:

Adacel-Polio: IM: Children ≥4 years and Adolescents: Refer to adult dosing for booster dose.

Boostrix-Polio: IM: Children ≥4 years, and Adolescents: Refer to adult dosing for booster dose

Infanrix-IPV: Children 15 months to 6 years: IM: 0.5 mL as initial booster dose at 15 to 18 months of age and 0.5 mL as second booster dose between 4 to 6 years (may be administered with monovalent *H. Influenzae* type b vaccine). If primary immunization is delayed, same booster interval can be used prior to seventh birthday.

Quadracel: IM: Infants ≥2 months and Children to 6 years: 0.5 mL administer as a 4 dose primary series, usually given at 2, 4, 6, and 18 months of age; followed by a booster dose at 4 to 6 years of age

Renal Impairment There are no dosage adjustments provided in the manufacturer's labeling.

Hepatic Impairment There are no dosage adjustments provided in the manufacturer's labeling.

Additional Information Complete prescribing information should be consulted for additional detail.

Dosage Forms Excipient information presented when available (limited, particularly for generics); consult specific product labeling.

Injection, suspension [preservative free]:

Kinrix: Diphtheria toxoid 25 Lf, tetanus toxoid 10 Lf, acellular pertussis antigens [inactivated pertussis toxin 25 mcg, filamentous hemagglutinin 25 mcg, pertactin 8 mcg], type 1 poliovirus 40 D-antigen units, type 2 poliovirus 8 D-antigen units, and type 3 poliovirus 32 D-antigen units per 0.5 mL (0.5 mL) [contains aluminum, neomycin sulfate, polymyxin B, polysorbate 80; may contain natural rubber/natural latex in prefilled syringe]

Quadracel: Diphtheria toxoid 15 Lf, tetanus toxoid 5 Lf, acellular pertussis antigens [detoxified pertussis toxin 20 mcg, filamentous hemagglutinin 20 mcg, pertactin 3 mcg, fimbriae (types 2 and 3) 5 mcg], type 1 poliovirus 40 D-antigen units, type 2 poliovirus 8 D-antigen units, and type 3 poliovirus 32 D-antigen units per 0.5 mL (0.5 mL) [contains aluminum, neomycin sulfate, polymyxin B, polysorbate 80]

Dosage Forms: Canada Excipient information presented when available (limited, particularly for generics); consult specific product labeling.

Injection, suspension [preservative free]:

Adacel-Polio: Diphtheria toxoid 2 Lf, tetanus toxoid 5 Lf, acellular pertussis antigens [inactivated pertussis toxoid 2.5 mcg, filamentous hemagglutinin 5 mcg, pertactin 3 mcg, types 2 and 3 fimbriae 5 mcg], type 1 poliovirus 40 D-antigen units, type 2 poliovirus 8 D-antigen units, and type 3 poliovirus 32 D-antigen units per 0.5 mL (0.5 mL) [contains aluminum, neomycin sulfate, polymyxin B, polysorbate 80, streptomycin]

Boostrix-Polio: Diphtheria toxoid 2.5 Lf, tetanus toxoid 5 Lf, acellular pertussis antigens [inactivated pertussis toxoid 8 mcg, filamentous hemagglutinin 8 mcg, pertactin 2.5 mcg], type 1 poliovirus 40 D-antigen units, type 2 poliovirus 8 D-antigen units, and type 3 poliovirus 32 D-antigen units per 0.5 mL (0.5 mL) [contains aluminum, neomycin sulfate, polymyxin B]

Infanrix-IPV: Diphtheria toxoid 25 Lf, tetanus toxoid 10 Lf, acellular pertussis antigens [inactivated pertussis toxoid 25 mcg, filamentous hemagglutinin 25 mcg, pertactin 8 mcg], type 1 poliovirus 40 D-antigen units, type 2 poliovirus 8 D-antigen units, and type 3 poliovirus 32 D-antigen units per 0.5 mL (0.5 mL) [contains aluminum, neomycin sulfate, polymyxin B]

Quadracel: Diphtheria toxoid 15 Lf, tetanus toxoid 5 Lf, acellular pertussis antigens [detoxified pertussis toxin 20 mcg, filamentous hemagglutinin 20 mcg, pertactin 3 mcg, fimbriae (types 2 and 3) 5 mcg], type 1 poliovirus 40 D-antigen units, type 2 poliovirus 8 D-antigen units, and type 3 poliovirus 32 D-antigen units per 0.5 mL (0.5 mL) [contains aluminum, neomycin sulfate, polymyxin B, polysorbate 80]

Diphtheria and Tetanus Toxoids, Acellular Pertussis, Poliovirus and Haemophilus b Conjugate Vaccine

(dif THEER ee a & TET a nus TOKS oyds ay CEL yoo lar per TUS sis POE lee oh VYE rus & hem OF fi lus bee KON joo gate vak SEEN)

Brand Names: US Pentacel

Brand Names: Canada Infanrix-IPV/HIB; Pediacel; Pentacel

Index Terms Haemophilus B Conjugate (Hib); Haemophilus B Polysaccharide; Diphtheria Toxoid; Diphtheria, Tetanus Toxoids, Acellular Pertussis (DTaP); DTaP-IPV/Hib; Pertussis, Acellular (Adsorbed); Poliovirus, Inactivated (IPV); Tetanus Toxoid

Pharmacologic Category Vaccine; Vaccine, Inactivated (Bacterial); Vaccine, Inactivated (Viral)

Additional Appendix Information

Immunization Administration Recommendations on page 1974

Immunization Schedules on page 1979

Use Diphtheria, pertussis, teatunus, poliomyelitis, and haemophilus B disease prevention: Active immunization against diphtheria, tetanus, pertussis, poliomyelitis, and invasive disease caused by H. influenzae type b in children 6 weeks to <5 years of age

Advisory Committee on Immunization Practices (ACIP) recommends that Pentacel (DTaP-IPV/Hib) may be used to provide the recommended DTaP, IPV, and Hib immunization in infants and children ≤4 years of age. Whenever

feasible, the same manufacturer should be used to provide the pertussis component; however, vaccination should not be deferred if a specific brand is not known or is not available. The Hib component in Pentacel contains a tetanus toxoid conjugate. A Hib vaccine containing the PRP-OMP conjugate (PedvaxHIB) may provide a more rapid seroconversion following the first dose and may be preferable to use in certain populations (eg, American Indian or Alaska Native children) (CDC 57[39] 2008).

Dosing

Pediatric

Primary immunization: Infants and Children 6 weeks to <5 years: IM: 0.5 mL per dose administered at 2, 4, 6 and 15-18 months of age (total of 4 doses). The first dose may be administered as early as 6 weeks of age. Following completion of the 4-dose series, children should receive a dose of DTaP vaccine at 4 to 6 years of age (Daptacel recommended due to same pertussis antigen used in both products).

Note: Per the ACIP, polio vaccine is given at 2, 4, and 6 to 18 months of age. Use of the minimum age and minimum intervals during the first 6 months of life should only be done when the vaccine recipient is at risk for imminent exposure to circulating poliovirus (shorter intervals and earlier start dates may lead to lower seroconversion (CDC 58[30] 2009). Pentacel is not indicated for the polio booster dose given at 4 to 6 years of age; Kinrix or IPV should be used.

Use in infants and children previously vaccinated with one or more component, and who are also scheduled to receive all vaccine components:

Previously vaccinated with ≥1 dose of Daptacel or IPV vaccines: Pentacel may be used to complete the first 4 doses of the DTaP or IPV series in children scheduled to receive the other components in the vaccine.

Previously vaccinated with ≥1 dose of Haemophilus b Conjugate vaccine: Pentacel may be used to complete the series in children scheduled to receive the other components in the vaccine; however, if different brands of Haemophilus b Conjugate vaccine are administered to complete the series, 3 primary immunizing doses are needed, followed by a booster dose.

Note: Completion of 3 doses of Pentacel provides primary immunization against diphtheria, tetanus, H. influenzae type B, and poliomyelitis. Completion of the 4-dose series with Pentacel provides primary immunization against pertussis. It also provides a booster vaccination against diphtheria, tetanus, H. influenzae type B, and poliomyelitis.

Renal Impairment There are no dosage adjustments provided in the manufacturer's labeling.

Hepatic Impairment There are no dosage adjustments provided in the manufacturer's labeling.

Additional Information Complete prescribing information should be consulted for additional detail.

Dosage Forms Excipient information presented when available (limited, particularly for generics); consult specific product labeling.

Injection, suspension:

Pentacel®: Diphtheria toxoid 15 Lf, tetanus toxoid 5 Lf, acellular pertussis antigens [pertussis toxin detoxified 20 mcg, filamentous hemagglutinin 20 mcg, pertactin 3 mcg, fimbriae (types 2 and 3) 5 mcg], type 1 poliovirus 40 D-antigen units; type 2 poliovirus 8 D-antigen units; type 3 poliovirus 32 D-antigen units, and Haemophilus b capsular polysaccharide 10 mcg [bound to tetanus toxoid 24 mcg] per 0.5 mL (0.5 mL) [contains albumin, aluminum, neomycin, polymyxin B sulfate, and polysorbate 80; supplied in two vials, one containing DTaP-IPV liquid and one containing Hib powder]

◆ Diphtheria and Tetanus Toxoids and Acellular Pertussis Adsorbed, and Inactivated Poliovirus Vaccine Combined see Diphtheria and Tetanus Toxoids, Acellular Pertussis, and Poliovirus Vaccine on page 566

◆ Diphtheria and Tetanus Toxoids and Acellular Pertussis Adsorbed, Hepatitis B (Recombinant) and Inactivated Poliovirus Vaccine Combined see Diphtheria, Tetanus Toxoids, Acellular Pertussis, Hepatitis B (Recombinant), and Poliovirus (Inactivated) Vaccine on page 569

Diphtheria and Tetanus Toxoids, and Acellular Pertussis Vaccine

(dif THEER ee a & TET a nus TOKS oyds & ay CEL yoo lar per TUS sis vak SEEN)

Brand Names: US Adacel; Boostrix; Daptacel; Infanrix

Brand Names: Canada Adacel; Boostrix

Index Terms DTaP; Tdap; Tetanus Toxoid, Reduced Diphtheria Toxoid, and Acellular Pertussis, Adsorbed; Tripedia

Pharmacologic Category Vaccine; Vaccine, Inactivated (Bacterial)

Additional Appendix Information

Immunization Administration Recommendations *on page 1974*

Immunization Schedules *on page 1979*

Use Diphtheria, tetanus, and pertussis disease prevention:

Daptacel, Infanrix (DTaP): Active immunization against diphtheria, tetanus, and pertussis from age 6 weeks through 6 years of age (prior to seventh birthday)

Adacel, Boostrix (Tdap): Active booster immunization against diphtheria, tetanus, and pertussis in persons 10 years and older (Boostrix) or persons 10 to 64 years of age (Adacel)

The Advisory Committee on Immunization Practices (ACIP) recommends routine vaccination for the following:

Infants and Children 6 weeks to <7 years (DTaP):
- For primary immunization against diphtheria, tetanus and pertussis (Use of diphtheria toxoid [ACIP] 2000)
- Pediatric patients who are wounded in bombings or similar mass casualty events and who have penetrating injuries or nonintact skin exposure, and have an uncertain vaccination history should receive a tetanus booster with DTaP (if no contraindications exist) (CDC [Chapman 2008]).

Children 7 to 10 years (Tdap):
- Children who did not complete a fully primary DTaP series should receive a single dose of Tdap (if no contraindications exist) (CDC/ACIP 60[1] 2011)
- Children never vaccinated against diphtheria, tetanus, or pertussis, or whose vaccination status is not known should receive a series of three vaccinations containing tetanus and diphtheria toxoids and the first dose should be with Tdap (CDC/ACIP 60[1] 2011)

Adolescents 11 to 18 years (Tdap):
- A single dose of Tdap as a booster dose in adolescents who have completed the recommended childhood DTaP vaccination series (preferred age of administration is 11 to 12 years) (CDC/ACIP 60[1] 2011)

Adolescents ≥11 years and adults (Tdap):
- Persons wounded in bombings or similar mass casualty events and who cannot confirm receipt of a tetanus booster within the previous 5 years and who have penetrating injuries or nonintact skin exposure should receive a single dose of Tdap (CDC/ACIP 61[25] 2012; CDC [Chapman 2008])

Pregnant patients: (Tdap): Pregnant females should receive a single dose with each pregnancy, preferably between 27-36 weeks gestation (CDC/ACIP 62[7] 2013)

Adults ≥19 years (including adults ≥65 years) (Tdap): A single dose of Tdap should be given to all patients who have not previously received Tdap or for whom their vaccine status is unknown. Following administration of Tdap, Td vaccine should be used for routine boosters (CDC/ACIP [Kim 2015]). The following patients, who have not yet received Tdap or for whom vaccine status is not known, should receive a single dose of Tdap as soon as feasible:
- Close contacts of children <12 months of age; Tdap should ideally be administered at least 2 weeks prior to beginning close contact (CDC/ACIP 60[41] 2011; CDC/ACIP [Kretsinger 2006]).
- Health care providers with direct patient contact (CDC/ACIP [Kretsinger 2006])

Note: Tdap is currently recommended for a single dose only (all age groups) (CDC/ACIP 60[1] 2011; CDC/ACIP 61[25] 2012), except pregnant females (CDC/ACIP 62[7] 2013)

Medication Guide Available Yes

Dosing

Adult Note: Tdap can be administered regardless of the interval between the last tetanus or diphtheria toxoid containing vaccine. Tdap is currently recommended for a single dose only (CDC/ACIP 60[1] 2011; CDC/ACIP 61[25] 2012), except pregnant females who should receive a Tdap dose during each pregnancy (preferably between 27 and 36 weeks' gestation) (CDCACIP 62[7] 2013).

Booster immunization: ACIP recommendations: IM: Adults ≥19 years: 0.5 mL per dose. A single dose of Tdap should be given to replace a single dose of the 10 year Td booster in patients who have not previously received Tdap or for whom vaccine status is not known. A single dose of Tdap is recommended for health care personnel who have not previously received Tdap and who have direct patient contact (CDC [Kretsinger 2006]). Tdap should be administered regardless of interval since last tetanus- or diphtheria-containing vaccine (CDC/ACIP 61[25] 2012).

Booster immunization: Manufacturer's labeling: IM: Adults (Adacel [≤64 years], Boostrix): 0.5 mL as a single dose, administered 5 years after last dose of tetanus toxoid, diphtheria toxoid, and/or pertussis-containing vaccine

Wound management (CDC/ACIP [Broder 2006]): IM: Adacel or Boostrix may be used as an alternative to Td vaccine when a tetanus toxoid-containing vaccine is needed for wound management, and in whom the pertussis component is also indicated. Tetanus prophylaxis in patients with wounds should be based on if the wound is clean or contaminated, the immunization status of the patient. Wound management includes proper use of tetanus toxoid and/or tetanus immune globulin (TIG), wound cleaning, and (if required) surgical debridement and the proper use of antibiotics. Patients with an uncertain or incomplete tetanus immunization status should have additional follow up to ensure a series is completed. Patients with a history of Arthus reaction following a previous dose of a tetanus toxoid-containing vaccine should not receive a tetanus toxoid-containing vaccine until >10 years after the most recent dose even if they have a wound that is neither clean nor minor. See table.

Tetanus Prophylaxis in Wound Management

History of Tetanus Immunization Doses	Clean, Minor Wounds		All Other Wounds[1]	
	Tetanus Toxoid[2]	TIG	Tetanus Toxoid[2]	TIG
Uncertain or <3 doses	Yes	No	Yes	Yes
3 or more doses	No[3]	No	No[4]	No

[1]Such as, but not limited to, wounds contaminated with dirt, feces, soil, and saliva; puncture wounds; wounds from crushing, tears, burns, and frostbite.

[2]Tetanus toxoid in this chart refers to a tetanus toxoid-containing vaccine. For children ≤6 years of age, DTaP (DT, if pertussis vaccine contraindicated) is preferred to tetanus toxoid alone. For children ≥7 years, adolescents, and adults, Td preferred to tetanus toxoid alone; Tdap may be preferred if the patient has not previously been vaccinated with Tdap.

[3]Yes, if ≥10 years since last dose.

[4]Yes, if ≥5 years since last dose.

Abbreviations: **DT** = Diphtheria and Tetanus Toxoids (formulation for age ≤6 years); **DTaP** = Diphtheria and Tetanus Toxoids, and Acellular Pertussis (formulation for age ≤6 years; Daptacel®, Infanrix®); **Td** = Diphtheria and Tetanus Toxoids (formulation for age ≥7 years; Decavac®,Tenivac™); **TT**= Tetanus toxoid (adsorbed [formulation for age ≥7 years]); **Tdap** = Diphtheria and Tetanus Toxoids, and Acellular Pertussis (Adacel® or Boostrix® [formulations for age ≥7 years]); **TIG** = Tetanus Immune Globulin

Geriatric

Booster Immunization: IM: Adults ≥65 years:

ACIP recommendations: Refer to adult dosing. In adults ≥65 years Boostrix should be used if feasible; however, ACIP has concluded that either Tdap vaccine (Boostrix or Adacel) may be used (CDC/ACIP 61 [25] 2012).

Manufacturer's labeling: Boostrix: 0.5 mL as a single dose, administered 5 years after last dose of tetanus toxoid, diphtheria toxoid, and/or pertussis-containing vaccine.

Wound Management: IM: Refer to adult dosing.

Pediatric

Primary immunization: IM:

Infants and Children 6 weeks to <7 years: **Note:** Whenever possible, the same product should be used for all doses. Interruption of recommended schedule does not require starting the series over; a delay between doses should not interfere with final immunity.

Daptacel, Infanrix: 0.5 mL per dose, total of 5 doses administered as follows:

Three doses, usually given at 2-, 4-, and 6 months of age; may be given as early as 6 weeks of age and repeated every 4 to 8 weeks

Fourth dose: Given at ~15 to 20 months of age, but at least 6 months after third dose. The fourth dose may be given as early as 12 months of age.

Fifth dose: Given at 4 to 6 years of age, prior to starting school or kindergarten; if the fourth dose is given at ≥4 years of age, the fifth dose may be omitted

For children who start primary immunization series ≥4 months of age, refer to current ACIP "Catch-up Immunization Schedule".

Booster immunization: ACIP recommendations:
Note: Tdap can be administered regardless of the interval between the last tetanus or diphtheria toxoid containing vaccine. Tdap is currently recommended for a single dose only (CDC/ACIP 60[1] 2011), except pregnant females who should receive a Tdap dose during each pregnancy (preferably between 27 and 36 weeks' gestation) (CDCACIP 62[7] 2013).

Children ≥10 years and Adolescents to 18 years: IM: 0.5 mL per dose. Tdap should be given as a single booster dose at age 11 or 12 years in adolescents who have completed a childhood DTaP vaccination series, followed by booster doses of Td every 10 years. Adolescents who have not received Tdap at age 11 or 12 should receive a single dose of Tdap in place of a single Td booster dose (CDC [Broder 2006]; CDC/ACIP 60[1] 2011; CDC/ACIP [Strikas 2015]).

Booster immunization: Manufacturer's labeling: IM:
Children ≥10 years and Adolescents (Adacel, Boostrix): 0.5 mL as a single dose, administered 5 years after last dose of tetanus toxoid, diphtheria toxoid, and/or pertussis-containing vaccine
Wound management: Refer to adult dosing.
Renal Impairment There are no dosage adjustments provided in the manufacturer's labeling.
Hepatic Impairment There are no dosage adjustments provided in the manufacturer's labeling.
Additional Information Complete prescribing information should be consulted for additional detail.
Dosage Forms Excipient information presented when available (limited, particularly for generics); consult specific product labeling.
Injection, suspension [Tdap, booster formulation]:
Adacel: Diphtheria 2 Lf units, tetanus 5 Lf units, and acellular pertussis antigens [detoxified pertussis toxin 2.5 mcg, filamentous hemagglutinin 5 mcg, pertactin 3 mcg, fimbriae (types 2 and 3) 5 mcg] per 0.5 mL (0.5 mL) [contains aluminum; may contain natural rubber/natural latex in prefilled syringe]
Boostrix: Diphtheria 2.5 Lf units, tetanus 5 Lf units, and acellular pertussis antigens [inactivated pertussis toxin 8 mcg, filamentous hemagglutinin 8 mcg, pertactin 2.5 mcg] per 0.5 mL (0.5 mL) [contains aluminum and polysorbate 80; may contain natural rubber/natural latex in prefilled syringe]
Injection, suspension [DTaP, active immunization formulation]:
Daptacel: Diphtheria 15 Lf units, tetanus 5 Lf units, and acellular pertussis antigens [detoxified pertussis toxin 10 mcg, filamentous hemagglutinin 5 mcg, pertactin 3 mcg, fimbriae (types 2 and 3) 5 mcg] per 0.5 mL (0.5 mL) [preservative free; contains aluminum]
Infanrix: Diphtheria 25 Lf units, tetanus 10 Lf units, and acellular pertussis antigens [inactivated pertussis toxin 25 mcg, filamentous hemagglutinin 25 mcg, pertactin 8 mcg] per 0.5 mL (0.5 mL) [preservative free; contains aluminum and polysorbate 80]
Infanrix: Diphtheria 25 Lf units, tetanus 10 Lf units, and acellular pertussis antigens [inactivated pertussis toxin 25 mcg, filamentous hemagglutinin 25 mcg, pertactin 8 mcg] per 0.5 mL (0.5 mL) [preservative free; contains aluminum and polysorbate 80; prefilled syringes contain natural rubber/natural latex] [DSC]

◆ Diphtheria, Tetanus Toxoids, Acellular Pertussis (DTaP) *see* Diphtheria and Tetanus Toxoids, Acellular Pertussis, and Poliovirus Vaccine *on page 566*

◆ Diphtheria, Tetanus Toxoids, Acellular Pertussis (DTaP) *see* Diphtheria and Tetanus Toxoids, Acellular Pertussis, Poliovirus and *Haemophilus* b Conjugate Vaccine *on page 567*

Diphtheria, Tetanus Toxoids, Acellular Pertussis, Hepatitis B (Recombinant), and Poliovirus (Inactivated) Vaccine
(dif THEER ee a, TET a nus TOKS oyds, ay CEL yoo lar per TUS sis, hep a TYE tis bee ree KOM be nant, & POE lee oh VYE rus in ak ti VAY ted tod vak SEEN)

Brand Names: US Pediarix
Brand Names: Canada Pediarix
Index Terms Diphtheria and Tetanus Toxoids and Acellular Pertussis Adsorbed, Hepatitis B (Recombinant) and Inactivated Poliovirus Vaccine Combined; Diphtheria, Tetanus Toxoids, Acellular Pertussis, Hepatitis B (Recombinant), and Poliovirus (Inactivated) Vaccine; Diphtheria, Tetanus Toxoids, Acellular Pertussis, Hepatitis B (Recombinant), and Poliovirus (Inactivated) Vaccine; DTaP-HepB-IPV
Pharmacologic Category Vaccine; Vaccine, Inactivated (Bacterial); Vaccine, Inactivated (Viral)

Additional Appendix Information
Immunization Administration Recommendations *on page 1974*
Immunization Schedules *on page 1979*
Use Diphtheria, tetanus, pertussis, poliomyelitis, and hepatitis B prevention: Combination vaccine for the active immunization against diphtheria, tetanus, pertussis, hepatitis B virus (all known subtypes), and poliomyelitis (caused by poliovirus types 1, 2, and 3)

The Advisory Committee on Immunization Practices (ACIP) recommends Pediarix for the following (CDC 52 [10] 2003):
- Primary vaccination for DTaP, Hep B, and IPV in children at 2, 4, and 6 months of age.
- To complete the primary vaccination series in children who have received DTaP (Infanrix) and who are scheduled to receive the other components of the vaccine. Whenever feasible, the same manufacturer should be used to provide the pertussis component; however, vaccination should not be deferred if a specific brand is not known or is not available. HepB and IPV from different manufacturers are interchangeable.

Dosing
Pediatric
Primary immunization: Infants and Children 6 weeks to <7 years: IM: 0.5 mL/dose; administer as a 3-dose series at 2-, 4-, and 6 months of age in 6- to 8-week intervals (preferably 8-week intervals). Vaccination usually begins at 2 months, but may be started as early as 6 weeks of age.
Note: Pediarix is approved for the first 3 doses of polio vaccine. Per the ACIP, polio vaccine is given at 2, 4 and 6 to 18 months of age. Use of the minimum age and minimum intervals during the first 6 months of life should only be done when the vaccine recipient is at risk for imminent exposure to circulating poliovirus (shorter intervals and earlier start dates may lead to lower seroconversion) (CDC 58[30] 2009).
Use in infants and children previously vaccinated with one or more component, and who are also scheduled to receive all vaccine components:
Infants previously vaccinated with hepatitis B vaccine: Infants previously vaccinated with 1 or 2 doses of another hepatitis B vaccine may use Pediarix to complete the 3-dose series. Not for use as birth dose of hepatitis B vaccine. Infants born to HBsAg-positive women should begin dosing with DTaP-HepB-IPV by age 6-8 weeks after receiving the single antigen hepatitis B vaccine at birth (CDC/ACIP [Strikas 2015]).
Infants previously vaccinated with diphtheria and tetanus toxoids, and acellular pertussis vaccine (DTaP): Infants previously vaccinated with 1 or 2 doses of Infanrix may use Pediarix to complete the first 3 doses of the series; use of Pediarix to complete DTaP vaccination started with products other than Infanrix has not been studied.
Infants previously vaccinated with inactivated polio vaccine (IPV): Infants previously vaccinated with 1 or 2 doses of IPV may use Pediarix to complete the first 3 doses of the series.
Renal Impairment There are no dosage adjustment provided in the manufacturer's labeling.
Hepatic Impairment There are no dosage adjustment provided in the manufacturer's labeling.
Additional Information Complete prescribing information should be consulted for additional detail.
Dosage Forms Excipient information presented when available (limited, particularly for generics); consult specific product labeling.
Injection, suspension [preservative free]:
Pediarix: Diphtheria toxoid 25 Lf, tetanus toxoid 10 Lf, acellular pertussis antigens [inactivated pertussis toxin 25 mcg, filamentous hemagglutin 25 mcg, pertactin 8 mcg, HBsAg 10 mcg, type 1 poliovirus 40 D antigen units, type 2 poliovirus 8 D antigen units and type 3 poliovirus 32 D antigen units] per 0.5 mL (0.5 mL) [contains aluminum, neomycin sulfate (trace amounts), polymyxin B (trace amounts), polysorbate 80, and yeast protein ≤5%; may contain natural rubber/natural latex in prefilled syringe]

◆ Diphtheria, Tetanus Toxoids, Acellular Pertussis, Hepatitis B (Recombinant), and Poliovirus (Inactivated) Vaccine *see* Diphtheria, Tetanus Toxoids, Acellular Pertussis, Hepatitis B (Recombinant), and Poliovirus (Inactivated) Vaccine *on page 569*

◆ Diphtheria, Tetanus Toxoids, Acellular Pertussis, Hepatitis B (Recombinant), and Poliovirus Vaccine *see* Diphtheria, Tetanus Toxoids, Acellular Pertussis, Hepatitis B (Recombinant), and Poliovirus (Inactivated) Vaccine *on page 569*

◆ Diphtheria Toxoid see Diphtheria and Tetanus Toxoids, Acellular Pertussis, Poliovirus and *Haemophilus* b Conjugate Vaccine *on page 567*

◆ Dipivalyl Epinephrine see Dipivefrin *on page 570*

Dipivefrin (dye PI ve frin)

Brand Names: Canada Ophtho-Dipivefrin™; PMS-Dipivefrin; Propine®

Index Terms Dipivalyl Epinephrine; Dipivefrin Hydrochloride; DPE

Pharmacologic Category Alpha/Beta Agonist; Ophthalmic Agent, Antiglaucoma; Ophthalmic Agent, Vasoconstrictor

Use Reduces elevated intraocular pressure in chronic open-angle glaucoma; also used to treat ocular hypertension, low tension, and secondary glaucomas

Dosing

Adult & Geriatric Glaucoma: Ophthalmic: Instill 1 drop every 12 hours into the eyes

Renal Impairment No dosage adjustment provided in manufacturer's labeling.

Hepatic Impairment No dosage adjustment provided in manufacturer's labeling.

Additional Information Complete prescribing information should be consulted for additional detail.

Dosage Forms Excipient information presented when available (limited, particularly for generics); consult specific product labeling. [DSC] = Discontinued product

Solution, ophthalmic, as hydrochloride [drops]:

Propine®: 0.1% (10 mL [DSC]) [contains benzalkonium chloride]

◆ Dipivefrin Hydrochloride see Dipivefrin *on page 570*

◆ Diprivan see Propofol *on page 1516*

◆ Diprolene see Betamethasone (Topical) *on page 224*

◆ Diprolene AF see Betamethasone (Topical) *on page 224*

◆ Dipropylacetic Acid see Valproic Acid and Derivatives *on page 1861*

◆ Diprosone (Can) see Betamethasone (Topical) *on page 224*

Dipyridamole (dye peer ID a mole)

Brand Names: US Persantine

Brand Names: Canada Apo-Dipyridamole FC®; Dipyridamole For Injection; Persantine®

Pharmacologic Category Antiplatelet Agent; Vasodilator

Use

Oral: Used with warfarin to decrease thrombosis in patients after artificial heart valve replacement

IV: Diagnostic agent in CAD

Pregnancy Considerations Adverse events have not been observed in animal reproduction studies.

Breast-Feeding Considerations Dipyridamole is excreted in breast milk. The manufacturer recommends that caution be exercised when administering dipyridamole to nursing women.

Contraindications Hypersensitivity to dipyridamole or any component of the formulation

Warnings/Precautions Use with caution in patients with hypotension, unstable angina, and/or recent MI. Use with caution in hepatic impairment. Avoid use of oral dipyridamole in this age group due to risk of orthostatic hypotension and availability of more efficacious alternative agents (Beers Criteria). Use caution in patients on other antiplatelet agents or anticoagulation. Severe adverse reactions have occurred with IV administration (rarely); use the IV form with caution in patients with bronchospastic disease or unstable angina. Aminophylline should be available in case of urgency or emergency with IV use.

Adverse Reactions

Oral: Frequency not always defined.

Central nervous system: Dizziness (14%), headache (2%)

Dermatologic: Skin rash (2%), pruritus

Gastrointestinal: Abdominal distress (6%), diarrhea, vomiting

Hepatic: Hepatic insufficiency

Postmarketing and/or case reports (Limited to important or life-threatening): Alopecia, arthritis, cholelithiasis, dyspepsia, fatigue, hepatitis, hypersensitivity reaction, hypotension, laryngeal edema, malaise, myalgia, nausea, palpitations, paresthesia, tachycardia, thrombocytopenia

IV:

>10%:

Cardiovascular: Exacerbation of angina pectoris (20%)

Central nervous system: Dizziness (12%), headache (12%)

1% to 10%:

Cardiovascular: ECG abnormality (5% to 8%; ST-T changes, extrasystoles), hypotension (5%), flushing (3%), tachycardia (3%), altered blood pressure (2%), hypertension (2%)

Central nervous system: Pain (3%), fatigue (1%), paresthesia (1%)

Gastrointestinal: Nausea (5%)

Respiratory: Dyspnea (3%)

<1% (Limited to important or life-threatening): Abdominal pain, arthralgia, ataxia, back pain, bronchospasm, cardiac arrhythmia (ventricular tachycardia, bradycardia, AV block, SVT, atrial fibrillation, asystole), cardiomyopathy, cough, depersonalization, diaphoresis, dysgeusia, dyspepsia, dysphagia, ECG abnormality (unspecified), edema, eructation, flatulence, hypersensitivity reaction, hypertonia, hyperventilation, increased appetite, increased thirst, injection site reaction, leg cramps (intermittent claudication), malaise, mastalgia, muscle rigidity, myalgia, myocardial infarction, orthostatic hypotension, otalgia, palpitations, perineal pain, pharyngitis, pleuritic chest pain, pruritus, renal pain, rhinitis, skin rash, syncope, tenesmus, tinnitus, tremor, urticaria, vertigo, visual disturbance, vomiting, weakness, xerostomia

Drug Interactions

Metabolism/Transport Effects Inhibits BCRP, P-glycoprotein

Avoid Concomitant Use

Avoid concomitant use of Dipyridamole with any of the following: Bosutinib; PAZOPanib; Riociguat; Silodosin; Topotecan; Urokinase; VinCRIStine (Liposomal)

Increased Effect/Toxicity

Dipyridamole may increase the levels/effects of: Adenosine; Afatinib; Agents with Antiplatelet Properties; Anticoagulants; Apixaban; Beta-Blockers; Bosutinib; Brentuximab Vedotin; Colchicine; Collagenase (Systemic); Dabigatran Etexilate; Deoxycholic Acid; DOXOrubicin (Conventional); Edoxaban; Everolimus; Ibritumomab; Ledipasvir; Naloxegol; Obinutuzumab; PAZOPanib; P-glycoprotein/ABCB1 Substrates; Prucalopride; Ranolazine; Regadenoson; Rifaximin; Riociguat; Rivaroxaban; Salicylates; Silodosin; Thrombolytic Agents; Topotecan; Tositumomab and Iodine I 131 Tositumomab; Urokinase; VinCRIStine (Liposomal)

The levels/effects of Dipyridamole may be increased by: Dasatinib; Glucosamine; Herbs (Anticoagulant/Antiplatelet Properties); Ibrutinib; Limaprost; Multivitamins/Fluoride (with ADE); Multivitamins/Minerals (with ADEK, Folate, Iron); Multivitamins/Minerals (with AE, No Iron); Omega-3 Fatty Acids; Pentosan Polysulfate Sodium; Pentoxifylline; Prostacyclin Analogues; Tipranavir; Vitamin E; Vitamin E (Oral)

Decreased Effect

Dipyridamole may decrease the levels/effects of: Acetylcholinesterase Inhibitors

Preparation for Administration Prior to administration, dilute solution for injection to a ≥1:2 ratio in NS, ½NS, or D₅W. Total volume should be ~20-50 mL.

Storage/Stability IV: Store between 15°C to 25°C (59°F to 77°F); do not freeze. Protect from light.

Mechanism of Action Inhibits the activity of adenosine deaminase and phosphodiesterase, which causes an accumulation of adenosine, adenine nucleotides, and cyclic AMP; these mediators then inhibit platelet aggregation and may cause vasodilation; may also stimulate release of prostacyclin or PGD₂; causes coronary vasodilation

Pharmacodynamics/Kinetics

Absorption: Readily, but variable

Distribution: Adults: V_d: 2-3 L/kg

Protein binding: 91% to 99%

Metabolism: Hepatic to glucuronide conjugate

Half-life elimination: Terminal: 10-12 hours

Time to peak, serum: 2-2.5 hours

Excretion: Feces (as glucuronide conjugates and unchanged drug)

Dosing

Adult & Geriatric

Adjunctive therapy for prophylaxis of thromboembolism with cardiac valve replacement: Oral: 75-100 mg 4 times/day

Evaluation of coronary artery disease: IV: 0.14 mg/kg/minute for 4 minutes; maximum dose: 60 mg

Following dipyridamole infusion, inject thallium-201 within 5 minutes. **Note:** Aminophylline should be available for urgent/emergent use; dosing of 50-100 mg (range: 50-250 mg) IV push over 30-60 seconds.

Pediatric Adjunctive therapy for prophylaxis of thromboembolism with cardiac valve replacement: Oral: Children ≥12 years: Refer to adult dosing.

Renal Impairment No dosage adjustment provided in manufacturer's labeling.

Hepatic Impairment No dosage adjustment provided in manufacturer's labeling.

Dietary Considerations Should be taken with water 1 hour before meals.

Administration

IV: Infuse diluted solution over 4 minutes.

Tablet: Administer with water 1 hour before meals.

Monitoring Parameters Blood pressure, heart rate, ECG (stress test)

Test Interactions Concurrent caffeine or theophylline use may demonstrate a false-negative result with dipyridamole-thallium myocardial imaging.

Dosage Forms Excipient information presented when available (limited, particularly for generics); consult specific product labeling.

Solution, Intravenous:

Generic: 5 mg/mL (2 mL, 10 mL)

Tablet, Oral:

Persantine: 25 mg, 50 mg, 75 mg [contains fd&c yellow #10 aluminum lake, methylparaben, propylparaben, sodium benzoate]

Generic: 25 mg, 50 mg, 75 mg

Extemporaneous Preparations A 10 mg/mL oral suspension may be made with tablets and one of three different vehicles (cherry syrup, a 1:1 mixture of Ora-Sweet® and Ora-Plus®, or a 1:1 mixture of Ora-Sweet® SF and Ora-Plus®). Crush twenty-four 50 mg tablets in a mortar and reduce to a fine powder. Add 20 mL of the chosen vehicle and mix to a uniform paste; mix while adding the vehicle in incremental proportions to **almost** 120 mL; transfer to a calibrated bottle, rinse mortar with vehicle, and add quantity of vehicle sufficient to make 120 mL. Label "shake well" and "protect from light". Stable for 60 days when stored in amber plastic prescription bottles in the dark at room temperature or refrigerated.

Allen LV and Erickson III MA, "Stability of Baclofen, Captopril, Diltiazem, Hydrochloride, Dipyridamole, and Flecainide Acetate in Extemporaneously Compounded Oral Liquids," Am J Health Syst Pharm, 1996, 53:2179-84.

♦ Dipyridamole and Aspirin see Aspirin and Dipyridamole on page 162

♦ Dipyridamole For Injection (Can) see Dipyridamole on page 570

♦ Disalcid see Salsalate on page 1634

♦ Disalicylic Acid see Salsalate on page 1634

♦ DisCoVisc see Sodium Chondroitin Sulfate and Sodium Hyaluronate on page 1673

♦ Disodium Thiosulfate Pentahydrate see Sodium Thiosulfate on page 1682

♦ d-Isoephedrine Hydrochloride see Pseudoephedrine on page 1527

Disopyramide (dye soe PEER a mide)

Brand Names: US Norpace; Norpace CR

Brand Names: Canada Norpace; Rythmodan; Rythmodan-LA

Index Terms Disopyramide Phosphate

Pharmacologic Category Antiarrhythmic Agent, Class Ia

Use Life-threatening ventricular arrhythmias (eg, sustained ventricular tachycardia)

Dosing

Adult

Ventricular arrhythmias: Oral: **Note:** Since newer agents with less toxicity are available, the use of disopyramide for this indication has fallen out of favor. Controlled release formulation not to be used when rapid achievement of disopyramide plasma concentrations is desired. A maximum dose up to 400 mg every 6 hours (immediate release) may be required for patients with severe refractory ventricular tachycardia.

<50 kg:

Immediate release: An initial loading dose of 200 mg may be administered if rapid onset is required. Maintenance dose: 100 mg every 6 hours

Controlled release: Maintenance dose: 200 mg every 12 hours

≥50 kg:

Immediate release: An initial loading dose of 300 mg may be administered if rapid onset is required. Maintenance dose: 150 mg every 6 hours. If rapid control is necessary and no response seen within 6 hours of loading dose, may increase maintenance dose to 200 mg every 6 hours.

Controlled release: Maintenance dose: 300 mg every 12 hours

Atrial fibrillation (maintenance of sinus rhythm) (off-label use; AHA/ACC/HRS [January, 2014]): Oral: **Note:** May be more desirable for patients with vagally-induced AF or hypertrophic cardiomyopathy associated with dynamic outflow tract obstruction; use in combination with a beta blocker or a non-dihydropyridine calcium channel blocker.

Immediate release: Usual dose: 100 to 200 mg every 6 hours

Controlled release: Usual dose: 200 to 400 mg every 12 hours

Hypertrophic cardiomyopathy (obstructive physiology) with or without atrial fibrillation (off-label use): Oral: Initial: *Controlled release:* 200 to 250 mg twice daily. If symptoms do not improve, increase by 100 mg/day at 2-week intervals to a maximum daily dose of 600 mg (Gersh, 2011; Sherrid, 2005).

Geriatric Refer to adult dosing. Dose with caution, starting at the lower end of dosing range.

Pediatric Arrhythmias: Oral: *Immediate release:*

<1 year: 10 to 30 mg/kg/24 hours in 4 divided doses

1 to 4 years: 10 to 20 mg/kg/24 hours in 4 divided doses

4 to 12 years: 10 to 15 mg/kg/24 hours in 4 divided doses

12 to 18 years: 6 to 15 mg/kg/24 hours in 4 divided doses

Renal Impairment

Manufacturer's labeling:

Immediate release:

CrCl >40 mL/minute: 100 mg every 6 hours

CrCl 30 to 40 mL/minute: 100 mg every 8 hours

CrCl 15 to 30 mL/minute: 100 mg every 12 hours

CrCl <15 mL/minute: 100 mg every 24 hours

Controlled release:

CrCl >40 mL/minute: 200 mg every 12 hours

CrCl ≤40 mL/minute: Not recommended for use

Alternative recommendations (Aronoff, 2007): *Immediate release:*

CrCl >50 mL/minute: 100 to 200 mg every 8 hours

CrCl 10 to 50 mL/minute: 100 to 200 mg every 12 to 24 hours

CrCl <10 mL/minute: 100 to 200 mg every 24 to 48 hours

Dialysis: Not dialyzable (0% to 5%) by hemo- or peritoneal methods; supplemental dose is not necessary.

Hepatic Impairment Manufacturer's labeling:

Immediate release: 100 mg every 6 hours

Controlled release: 200 mg every 12 hours

Additional Information Complete prescribing information should be consulted for additional detail.

Dosage Forms Excipient information presented when available (limited, particularly for generics); consult specific product labeling.

Capsule, Oral:

Norpace: 100 mg, 150 mg

Generic: 100 mg, 150 mg

Capsule Extended Release 12 Hour, Oral:

Norpace CR: 100 mg, 150 mg

♦ Disopyramide Phosphate see Disopyramide on page 571

Disulfiram (dye SUL fi ram)

Brand Names: US Antabuse

Pharmacologic Category Aldehyde Dehydrogenase Inhibitor

Use Management of chronic alcoholism

Dosing

Adult & Geriatric Alcoholism: Oral: **Note:** Do not administer until the patient has abstained from ethanol for at least 12 hours.

Initial: 500 mg once daily for 1-2 weeks (maximum daily dose: 500 mg)

Average maintenance dose: 250 mg once daily (range: 125-500 mg; maximum daily dose: 500 mg); duration of therapy is to continue until the patient is fully recovered socially and a basis for permanent self-control has been established; maintenance therapy may be required for months or even years.

Renal Impairment No dosage adjustment provided in manufacturer's labeling. Use with extreme caution in chronic and acute nephritis.

Hepatic Impairment No dosage adjustment provided in manufacturer's labeling. Use with extreme caution in hepatic cirrhosis or insufficiency.

Additional Information Complete prescribing information should be consulted for additional detail.

Dosage Forms Excipient information presented when available (limited, particularly for generics); consult specific product labeling.
Tablet, Oral:
Antabuse: 250 mg
Antabuse: 500 mg [scored]
Generic: 250 mg, 500 mg

- ◆ Dithioglycerol *see* Dimercaprol *on page 557*
- ◆ Dithranol *see* Anthralin *on page 129*
- ◆ Ditropan *see* Oxybutynin *on page 1355*
- ◆ Ditropan XL *see* Oxybutynin *on page 1355*
- ◆ Diuril *see* Chlorothiazide *on page 376*
- ◆ Divalproex Sodium *see* Valproic Acid and Derivatives *on page 1861*
- ◆ Divigel *see* Estradiol (Systemic) *on page 681*
- ◆ Dixarit (Can) *see* CloNIDine *on page 421*
- ◆ 5071-1DL(6) *see* Megestrol *on page 1135*
- ◆ *dl*-Alpha Tocopherol *see* Vitamin E *on page 1906*
- ◆ DLV *see* Delavirdine *on page 514*
- ◆ D-Mannitol *see* Mannitol *on page 1124*
- ◆ 4-DMDR *see* IDArubicin *on page 910*
- ◆ DMF *see* Dimethyl Fumarate *on page 557*
- ◆ DMSA *see* Succimer *on page 1702*
- ◆ D-Natural-5 [OTC] *see* Vitamin A and Vitamin D (Systemic) *on page 1906*
- ◆ Doans Extra Strength [OTC] *see* Magnesium Salicylate *on page 1121*
- ◆ Doans Pills [OTC] *see* Magnesium Salicylate *on page 1121*

DOBUTamine (doe BYOO ta meen)

Brand Names: Canada Dobutamine Injection, USP; Dobutrex
Index Terms Dobutamine Hydrochloride
Pharmacologic Category Adrenergic Agonist Agent; Inotrope
Use
Cardiac decompensation: Short-term management of patients with cardiac decompensation
American College of Cardiology/American Heart Association heart failure (HF) guideline recommendations (ACCF/AHA [Yancy 2013]): To maintain systemic perfusion and preserve end-organ performance in patients with cardiogenic shock; bridge therapy in stage D HF unresponsive to guideline-directed medical therapy and device therapy in patients awaiting heart transplant or mechanical circulatory support; short-term management of hospitalized patients with severe systolic dysfunction presenting with low blood pressure and significantly depressed cardiac output; long-term management (palliative therapy) in select patients with stage D HF unresponsive to guideline-directed medical therapy and device therapy who are not candidates for heart transplant or mechanical circulatory support.
Pregnancy Considerations Adverse events have not been observed in animal reproduction studies. Dobutamine should not be used as a diagnostic agent during stress testing in pregnant women (Regitz-Zagrosek 2011).
Breast-Feeding Considerations It is not known if dobutamine is excreted in breast milk. The manufacturer recommends that caution be exercised when administering dobutamine to nursing women.
Contraindications
Hypersensitivity to dobutamine or sulfites (some contain sodium metabisulfate), or any component of the formulation; Hypertrophic cardiomyopathy with outflow tract obstruction (formerly known as idiopathic hypertrophic subaortic stenosis [IHSS])
Note: When utilized for stress testing, additional contraindications according to the American Society of Nuclear Cardiology (ASNC) include patients with recent (<1 week) MI, unstable angina, severe aortic stenosis, atrial tachyarrhythmias with uncontrolled ventricular response, prior history of ventricular tachycardia, uncontrolled hypertension (>200/110 mm Hg), aortic dissection or large aortic aneurysm, and patients on beta blockers where heart rate and inotropic responses to dobutamine will be attenuated (ASNC [Henzlova 2009])
Warnings/Precautions Ventricular arrhythmias, including nonsustained ventricular tachycardia and supraventricular arrhythmias, have been reported (Tisdale 1995). Observe closely for arrhythmias in patients with acute heart failure; sudden cardiac death has been observed (O'Connor 1999; Pickworth 1992; Young 2000). Ensure that ventricular rate

is controlled in atrial fibrillation/flutter before initiating; may increase ventricular response rate. In heart transplant candidates, institute appropriate measures to protect patient against risks of sudden cardiac death (Young 2000). May cause dose-related increases in heart rate and exacerbate ventricular ectopy (dose-related). An increased risk of hospitalization and death has been observed with prolonged use in NYHA Class III/IV heart failure patients (O'Connor 1999). Correct electrolyte disturbances, especially hypokalemia or hypomagnesemia, prior to use and throughout therapy to minimize the risk of arrhythmias (ACC/AHA/ESC [Zipes 2006]; Tisdale 1995). An increase in blood pressure is more common due to augmented cardiac output, but occasionally a patient may become hypotensive.

If needed, correct hypovolemia first to optimize hemodynamics. Ineffective therapeutically in the presence of mechanical obstruction such as severe aortic stenosis. Use caution in patients with active myocardial ischemia or recent myocardial infarction or recent myocardial infarction (can increase myocardial oxygen demand). Use cautiously in the elderly starting at lower end of the dosage range. Use with extreme caution in patients taking MAO inhibitors. The ACCF/AHA 2013 heart failure guidelines do not recommend long-term use of intravenous inotropic therapy except for palliative purposes in end-stage disease (ACCF/AHA [Yancy 2013]). Product may contain sodium sulfite.
Adverse Reactions Incidence of adverse events is not always reported.
Cardiovascular: Ventricular premature contractions (5%; dose related), angina pectoris (1% to 3%), chest pain (1% to 3%; nonspecific), palpitations (1% to 3%), hypotension, increased blood pressure, increased heart rate, localized phlebitis, ventricular ectopy (increased)
Central nervous system: Headache (1% to 3%), paresthesia
Dermatologic: Skin necrosis (isolated cases)
Endocrine & metabolic: Decreased serum potassium (slight)
Gastrointestinal: Nausea (1% to 3%)
Hematologic & oncologic: Thrombocytopenia (isolated cases)
Local: Local inflammation, local pain (from infiltration)
Neuromuscular & skeletal: Leg cramps (mild)
Respiratory: Dyspnea (1% to 3%)
Miscellaneous: Fever (1% to 3%)
Drug Interactions
Metabolism/Transport Effects Substrate of COMT
Avoid Concomitant Use
Avoid concomitant use of DOBUTamine with any of the following: Iobenguane I 123
Increased Effect/Toxicity
DOBUTamine may increase the levels/effects of: Doxofylline; Sympathomimetics

The levels/effects of DOBUTamine may be increased by: AtoMOXetine; Cannabinoid-Containing Products; COMT Inhibitors; Linezolid; Tedizolid
Decreased Effect
DOBUTamine may decrease the levels/effects of: Iobenguane I 123

The levels/effects of DOBUTamine may be decreased by: Calcium Salts
Storage/Stability Store reconstituted solution under refrigeration for 48 hours or 6 hours at room temperature. Stability of parenteral admixture at room temperature (25°C) is 48 hours; at refrigeration (4°C) stability is 7 days. Remix solution every 24 hours. Pink discoloration of solution indicates slight oxidation but no significant loss of potency.
Mechanism of Action Dobutamine, a racemic mixture, stimulates myocardial beta$_1$-adrenergic receptors primarily by the (+) enantiomer and some alpha$_1$ receptor agonism by the (-) enantiomer, resulting in increased contractility and heart rate, and stimulates both beta$_2$- and alpha$_1$-receptors in the vasculature. Although beta$_2$ and alpha$_1$ adrenergic receptors are also activated, the effects of beta$_2$ receptor activation may equally offset or be slightly greater than the effects of alpha$_1$ stimulation, resulting in some vasodilation in addition to the inotropic and chronotropic actions (Leier 1988; Majerus 1989; Ruffolo 1987). Lowers central venous pressure and wedge pressure, but has little effect on pulmonary vascular resistance (Leier 1977; Leier 1978).
Pharmacodynamics/Kinetics
Onset of action: IV: 1-10 minutes
Peak effect: 10-20 minutes

Metabolism: In tissues and hepatically to inactive metabolites

Half-life elimination: 2 minutes

Excretion: Urine (as metabolites)

Dosing

Adult & Geriatric

Cardiac decompensation: IV infusion:

Initial dose: 0.5 to 1 mcg/kg/minute (per the manufacturer); may also initiate at higher doses (eg, 2.5 mcg/kg/minute) depending on severity of decompensation with titration to desired response (Leier 1977).

Maintenance dose: 2 to 20 mcg/kg/minute. **Note:** In patients with heart failure, lower doses are preferred to minimize adverse effects (ACCF/AHA [Yancy 2013]).

Maximum dose: 40 mcg/kg/minute. The ACCF/AHA 2013 heart failure guidelines and the Surviving Sepsis Campaign recommend a maximum dose of 20 mcg/kg/minute (ACCF/AHA [Yancy 2013]; SCCM [Dellinger 2013]).

Adult Advanced Cardiovascular Life Support (ACLS) guideline recommendation (in the immediate post-cardiac arrest care setting): IV infusion: Initial: 5 to 10 mcg/kg/minute; titrate to effect (AHA [Peberdy 2010])

Stress echocardiography (diagnostic agent) (off-label use): IV infusion: Initial: 5 to 10 mcg/kg/minute; increase at 3-minute intervals to 20 mcg/kg/minute, then 30 mcg/kg/minute, and then 40 mcg/kg/minute. May coadminister atropine in patients who do not achieve target heart rate (ASNC [Henzlova 2009]).

Pediatric

Cardiac decompensation: Refer to adult dosing.

Pediatric Advanced Life Support (PALS) guideline recommendation (to maintain cardiac output and for postresuscitation stabilization): IV or I.O.: Dose range: 2 to 20 mcg/kg/minute (AHA [Kleinman 2010]).

Renal Impairment There are no dosage adjustments provided in the manufacturer's labeling.

Hepatic Impairment There are no dosage adjustments provided in the manufacturer's labeling.

Usual Infusion Concentrations: Pediatric Note: Premixed solutions available.

IV infusion: 1000 **mcg**/mL, 2000 **mcg**/mL, **or** 4000 **mcg**/mL

Usual Infusion Concentrations: Adult Note: Premixed solutions available.

IV infusion: 250 mg in 500 mL (concentration: 500 **mcg**/mL), 500 mg in 250 mL (concentration: 2000 **mcg**/mL), **or** 1000 mg in 250 mL (concentration: 4000 **mcg**/mL) of D$_5$W or NS

Administration Always administer via infusion device; administer into large vein.

Monitoring Parameters Blood pressure, ECG, heart rate, CVP, RAP, MAP; serum glucose, renal function; urine output; if pulmonary artery catheter is in place, monitor CI, PCWP, and SVR; ScvO$_2$ or SvO$_2$

Consult individual institutional policies and procedures.

Dosage Forms Excipient information presented when available (limited, particularly for generics); consult specific product labeling.

Solution, Intravenous, as hydrochloride:

Generic: 1 mg/mL (250 mL); 2 mg/mL (250 mL); 4 mg/mL (250 mL); 250 mg/20 mL (20 mL); 500 mg/40 mL (40 mL)

◆ Dobutamine Hydrochloride see DOBUTamine on page 572

◆ Dobutamine Injection, USP (Can) see DOBUTamine on page 572

◆ Dobutrex (Can) see DOBUTamine on page 572

◆ Docefrez see DOCEtaxel on page 573

DOCEtaxel (doe se TAKS el)

Brand Names: US Docefrez; Taxotere

Brand Names: Canada Docetaxel for Injection; Taxotere

Index Terms RP-6976

Pharmacologic Category Antineoplastic Agent, Antimicrotubular; Antineoplastic Agent, Taxane Derivative

Use

US labeling:

Docefrez:

Breast cancer: Treatment of breast cancer (locally advanced/metastatic) after prior chemotherapy failure

Non-small cell lung cancer: Treatment of locally advanced or metastatic non–small cell lung cancer (NSCLC) after prior platinum-based chemotherapy failure; treatment of previously untreated unresectable locally advanced or metastatic NSCLC (in combination with cisplatin)

Prostate cancer: Treatment of hormone-refractory metastatic prostate cancer (in combination with prednisone)

Taxotere (and various generic brands):

Breast cancer: Treatment of breast cancer (locally advanced/metastatic) after prior chemotherapy failure; adjuvant treatment (in combination with doxorubicin and cyclophosphamide) of operable node-positive breast cancer

Gastric cancer: Treatment of advanced gastric adenocarcinoma, including gastroesophageal junction adenocarcinoma (in combination with cisplatin and fluorouracil) in patients who have not received prior chemotherapy for advanced disease

Head and neck cancer: Treatment (induction) of locally advanced squamous cell head and neck cancer (in combination with cisplatin and fluorouracil)

NSCLC: Treatment of locally advanced or metastatic NSCLC after failure of prior platinum-based chemotherapy; treatment of previously untreated unresectable locally advanced or metastatic NSCLC (in combination with cisplatin)

Prostate cancer: Treatment of androgen-independent (hormone refractory) metastatic prostate cancer (in combination with prednisone)

Canadian labeling:

Breast cancer: Treatment of breast cancer (locally advanced/metastatic [in combination with doxorubicin]; adjuvant treatment of operable node-positive [in combination with doxorubicin and cyclophosphamide]; advanced or metastatic [in combination with capecitabine] after failure of anthracycline-containing chemotherapy)

Head and neck cancer: Treatment (monotherapy) of recurrent and/or metastatic squamous cell head and neck cancer after failure of a prior chemotherapy regimen

NSCLC: Treatment of locally advanced or metastatic NSCLC (as a single-agent or in combination with platinum derivatives)

Ovarian cancer: Treatment of metastatic ovarian cancer following failure of first-line or subsequent chemotherapy

Prostate cancer: Treatment of hormone refractory, metastatic prostate cancer (in combination with prednisone or prednisolone)

Pregnancy Considerations Adverse events have been observed in animal reproduction studies. An *ex vivo* human placenta perfusion model illustrated that docetaxel crossed the placenta at term. Placental transfer was low and affected by the presence of albumin; higher albumin concentrations resulted in lower docetaxel placental transfer (Berveiller, 2012). Some pharmacokinetic properties of docetaxel may be altered in pregnant women (van Hasselt 2014). Women of childbearing potential should avoid becoming pregnant during therapy. A pregnancy registry is available for all cancers diagnosed during pregnancy at Cooper Health (877-635-4499).

Breast-Feeding Considerations It is not known if docetaxel is excreted into breast milk. Due to the potential for serious adverse reactions in nursing the infant, the US labeling recommends a decision be made to discontinue breast-feeding or the drug, taking into account the importance of treatment to the mother. The Canadian labeling contraindicates use in breast-feeding women.

Contraindications

Severe hypersensitivity to docetaxel or any component of the formulation; severe hypersensitivity to other medications containing polysorbate 80; neutrophil count <1500/mm^3

Canadian labeling: Additional contraindications (not in U.S. labeling): Severe hepatic impairment; pregnancy; breast-feeding

Warnings/Precautions Hazardous agent - use appropriate precautions for handling and disposal (NIOSH 2014 [group 1]). **[US Boxed Warning]: Avoid use in patients with bilirubin exceeding upper limit of normal (ULN) or AST and/or ALT >1.5 times ULN in conjunction with alkaline phosphatase >2.5 times ULN. Patients with bilirubin elevations or abnormal transaminases (with concurrent abnormal alkaline phosphatase) are at increased risk for grade 4 neutropenia, neutropenic fever, infections, severe thrombocytopenia, severe stomatitis, severe skin toxicity, and toxic death. Patients with isolated transaminase elevations >1.5 times ULN also had a higher rate of grade 4 neutropenic fever, although no increased incidence of toxic death. Monitor bilirubin, AST or ALT, and alkaline phosphatase prior to each docetaxel cycle.** The alcohol content of the docetaxel formulation should be taken into account when administering to patients with hepatic impairment. Canadian labeling contraindicates use in ▶

severe hepatic impairment. **[US Boxed Warnings]: Severe hypersensitivity reactions, characterized by generalized rash/erythema, hypotension, broncho-spasms, or rare anaphylaxis may occur (may be fatal; has occurred in patients receiving 3-day corticosteroid premedication). Hypersensitivity reactions require immediate discontinuation of the docetaxel infusion and administration of appropriate therapy. Do not administer to patients with a history of severe hyper-sensitivity to docetaxel or polysorbate 80 (component of formulation). Severe fluid retention, characterized by pleural effusion (requiring immediate drainage, ascites with pronounced abdominal distention, periph-eral edema (poorly tolerated), dyspnea at rest, cardiac tamponade, generalized edema, and weight gain, has been reported (despite the use of premedication with 3 days of dexamethasone).** Fluid retention may begin as lower extremity peripheral edema and become generalized with a median weight gain of 2 kg. In patients with breast cancer, the median cumulative dose to onset of moderate or severe fluid retention was 819 mg/m^2; fluid retention resolves in a median of 16 weeks after discontinuation. Minor reactions including flushing or localized skin reac-tions may also occur. Observe for hypersensitivity, espe-cially with the first two infusions. Discontinue for severe reactions; do not rechallenge if severe. Patients should be premedicated with a corticosteroid (starting one day prior to administration) to reduce the incidence and severity of hypersensitivity reactions and fluid retention; severity is reduced with dexamethasone premedication starting one day prior to docetaxel administration. Premedication with oral corticosteroids is recommended to decrease the inci-dence and severity of fluid retention and severity of hyper-sensitivity reactions. The manufacturer recommends dexamethasone 16 mg/day (8 mg twice daily) orally for 3 days, starting the day before docetaxel administration; for prostate cancer, when prednisone is part of the antineo-plastic regimen, dexamethasone 8 mg orally is adminis-tered at 12 hours, 3 hours, and 1 hour prior to docetaxel.

[US Boxed Warning]: Patients with abnormal liver function, those receiving higher doses, and patients with non–small cell lung cancer and a history of prior treatment with platinum derivatives who receive sin-gle-agent docetaxel at a dose of 100 mg/m^2 are at higher risk for treatment-related mortality.

Neutropenia is the dose-limiting toxicity. Patients with increased liver function tests experienced more episodes of neutropenia with a greater number of severe infections. **[US Boxed Warning]: Patients with an absolute neu-trophil count <1,500/mm^3 should not receive doce-taxel. Monitor blood counts frequently to monitor for neutropenia (which may be severe and result in infec-tion).** The dose-limiting toxicity is neutropenia. Platelets should recover to >100,000/mm^3 prior to treatment. Mon-itor liver function tests frequently. Hematologic toxicity may require dose reduction or therapy discontinuation.

Cutaneous reactions including erythema (with edema) and desquamation have been reported; may require dose reduction. Cystoid macular edema (CME) has been reported; if vision impairment occurs, a prompt compre-hensive ophthalmic exam is recommended. If CME is diagnosed, initiate appropriate CME management and discontinue docetaxel (consider non-taxane treatments). In a study of patients receiving docetaxel for the adjuvant treatment of breast cancer, a majority of patients experi-enced tearing, which occurred in patients with and without lacrimal duct obstruction at baseline; onset was generally after cycle 1, but subsided in most patients within 4 months after therapy completion (Chan 2013). Dosage adjustment is recommended with severe neurosensory symptoms (paresthesia, dysesthesia, pain); persistent symptoms may require discontinuation; reversal of symptoms may be delayed after discontinuation. Some docetaxel formu-lations contain alcohol (content varies by formulation), which may affect the central nervous system and cause symptoms of alcohol intoxication. Consider alcohol content and use with caution in patients for whom alcohol intake should be avoided or minimized. Patients should avoid driving or operating machinery immediately after the infu-sion. An FDA-approved non-alcohol generic formulation (20 mg/mL) is available. Treatment-related acute myeloid leukemia or myelodysplasia occurred in patients receiving docetaxel in combination with anthracyclines and/or cyclo-phosphamide. Fatigue and weakness (may be severe) have been reported; symptoms may last a few days up to several weeks; in patients with progressive disease, weakness may be associated with a decrease in perform-ance status. Potentially significant drug-drug interactions may exist, requiring dose or frequency adjustment, addi-tional monitoring, and/or selection of alternative therapy. Docetaxel is an irritant with vesicant-like properties; ensure

proper needle or catheter placement prior to and during infusion; avoid extravasation.

Some dosage forms may contain polysorbate 80 (also known as Tweens). Hypersensitivity reactions, usually a delayed reaction, have been reported following exposure to pharmaceutical products containing polysorbate 80 in certain individuals (Isaksson 2002; Lucente 2000; Shelley 1995). Thrombocytopenia, ascites, pulmonary deteriora-tion, and renal and hepatic failure have been reported in premature neonates after receiving parenteral products containing polysorbate 80 (Alade 1986; CDC 1984). See manufacturer's labeling.

Adverse Reactions Percentages reported for docetaxel monotherapy; frequency may vary depending on diagno-sis, dose, liver function, prior treatment, and premedica-tion. The incidence of adverse events was usually higher in patients with elevated liver function tests.

>10%:
  Central nervous system: Central nervous system toxicity (20% to 58%; severe: 6%; including neuropathy)
  Dermatologic: Alopecia (56% to 76%), dermatological reaction (20% to 48%; severe: ≤5%), nail disease (11% to 41%)
  Endocrine & metabolic: Fluid retention (13% to 60%; severe: 7% to 9%; dose dependent)
  Gastrointestinal: Stomatitis (19% to 53%; severe 1% to 8%), diarrhea (23% to 43%; severe: 5% to 6%), nausea (34% to 42%), vomiting (22% to 23%)
  Hematologic & oncologic: Neutropenia (84% to 99%; grade 4: 75% to 86%; nadir [median]: 7 days, duration [severe neutropenia]: 7 days; dose dependent), leuko-penia (84% to 99%; grade 4: 32% to 44%), anemia (65% to 97%; dose dependent; grades 3/4: 8% to 9%), thrombocytopenia (8% to 14%; grade 4: 1%; dose dependent), febrile neutropenia (5% to 14%; dose dependent)
  Hepatic: Increased serum transaminases (4% to 19%)
  Hypersensitivity: Hypersensitivity (1% to 21%; with pre-medication 15%)
  Infection: Infection (1% to 34%; dose dependent)
  Neuromuscular & skeletal: Weakness (53% to 66%; severe 13% to 18%), myalgia (3% to 23%), neuro-muscular reaction (16%)
  Respiratory: Pulmonary reaction (41%)
  Miscellaneous: Fever (31% to 35%)
1% to 10%:
  Cardiovascular: Decreased left ventricular ejection frac-tion (8% to 10%), hypotension (3%)
  Central nervous system: Peripheral motor neuropathy (4%; severe; mainly distal extremity weakness)
  Gastrointestinal: Dysgeusia (6%)
  Hepatic: Increased serum bilirubin (9%), increased serum alkaline phosphatase (4% to 7%)
  Local: Infusion site reactions (4%, including hyperpig-mentation, inflammation, redness, dryness, phlebitis, extravasation, swelling of the vein)
  Neuromuscular and skeletal: Arthralgia (3% to 9%)
  Ophthalmic: Epiphora (associated with canalicular steno-sis [≤77% with weekly administration; ≤1% with every 3-week administration])
<1% (Limited to important or life-threatening): Acute mye-locytic leukemia, acute respiratory distress, anaphylactic shock, anorexia, ascites, atrial fibrillation, atrial flutter, atrioventricular block, bradycardia, bronchospasm, car-diac arrhythmia, cardiac failure, cardiac tamponade, chest pain, chest tightness, colitis, confusion, conjuncti-vitis, constipation, cystoid macular edema, deep vein thrombosis, dehydration, disease of the lacrimal appara-tus (duct obstruction), disseminated intravascular coagu-lation, drug fever, duodenal ulcer, dyspnea, ECG abnormality, erythema multiforme, esophagitis, gastro-intestinal hemorrhage, gastrointestinal obstruction, gas-trointestinal perforation, hearing loss, hemorrhagic diathesis, hepatitis, hypertension, hyponatremia, intesti-nal obstruction, interstitial pulmonary disease, ischemic colitis, ischemic heart disease, loss of consciousness (transient), lymphedema (peripheral), multiorgan failure, myelodysplastic syndrome, myocardial infarction, neutro-penic enterocolitis, ototoxicity, palmar-plantar erythrody-sesthesia, pericardial effusion, pleural effusion, pneumonia, pneumonitis, pruritus, pulmonary edema, pulmonary embolism, pulmonary fibrosis, radiation pneu-monitis, radiation recall phenomenon, renal failure, renal insufficiency, respiratory failure, skin changes (sclero-derma-like), seizure, sepsis, sinus tachycardia, Ste-vens-Johnson syndrome, subacute cutaneous lupus erythematosus, syncope, toxic epidermal necrolysis, tachycardia, thrombophlebitis, unstable angina pectoris, visual disturbance (transient)

Drug Interactions

Metabolism/Transport Effects Substrate of CYP3A4 (major), P-glycoprotein; **Note:** Assignment of Major/Minor substrate status based on clinically relevant drug interaction potential

Avoid Concomitant Use

Avoid concomitant use of DOCEtaxel with any of the following: BCG (Intravesical); Conivaptan; Deferiprone; Dipyrone; Fusidic Acid (Systemic); Idelalisib; Natalizumab; Pimecrolimus; Tacrolimus (Topical); Tofacitinib; Vaccines (Live)

Increased Effect/Toxicity

DOCEtaxel may increase the levels/effects of: Antineoplastic Agents (Anthracycline, Systemic); CloZAPine; Deferiprone; Fingolimod; Leflunomide; Natalizumab; Tofacitinib; Vaccines (Live)

The levels/effects of DOCEtaxel may be increased by: Antifungal Agents (Azole Derivatives, Systemic); Conivaptan; CYP3A4 Inhibitors (Moderate); CYP3A4 Inhibitors (Strong); Dasatinib; Denosumab; Dipyrone; Dronedarone; Fusidic Acid (Systemic); Idelalisib; Ivacaftor; Luliconazole; Mifepristone; Netupitant; Osimertinib; Palbociclib; P-glycoprotein/ABCB1 Inhibitors; Pimecrolimus; Platinum Derivatives; Ranolazine; Roflumilast; Simeprevir; SORAfenib; Stiripentol; Tacrolimus (Topical); Trastuzumab

Decreased Effect

DOCEtaxel may decrease the levels/effects of: BCG (Intravesical); Coccidioides immitis Skin Test; Sipuleucel-T; Vaccines (Inactivated); Vaccines (Live)

The levels/effects of DOCEtaxel may be decreased by: Bosentan; CYP3A4 Inducers (Moderate); CYP3A4 Inducers (Strong); Dabrafenib; Deferasirox; Echinacea; Enzalutamide; Mitotane; Osimertinib; P-glycoprotein/ABCB1 Inducers; Siltuximab; St Johns Wort; Tocilizumab

Preparation for Administration Hazardous agent; use appropriate precautions for handling and disposal (NIOSH 2014 [group 1]).

Preparation instructions may vary by manufacturer, refer to specific prescribing information. **Note:** Some formulations contain overfill.

Note: Multiple concentrations: Docetaxel is available as a one-vial formulation at concentrations of 10 mg/mL (generic formulation) and 20 mg/mL (concentrate; Taxotere, generic [including a non-alcohol generic formulation]), and as a lyophilized powder (Docefrez) which is reconstituted (with provided diluent) to 20 mg/0.8 mL (20 mg vial) or 24 mg/mL (80 mg vial). Admixture errors have occurred due to the availability of various concentrations. Docetaxel was previously available as a two-vial formulation which included two vials (a concentrated docetaxel vial and a diluent vial), resulting in a reconstituted concentration of 10 mg/mL; the two-vial formulation has been discontinued by the Taxotere manufacturer (available generically).

One-vial formulations: Further dilute for infusion in 250 to 500 mL of NS or D5W in a non-DEHP container (eg, glass, polypropylene, polyolefin) to a final concentration of 0.3 to 0.74 mg/mL. Gently rotate and invert manually to mix thoroughly; avoid shaking or vigorous agitation.

Non-alcohol formulation: Use a 20 gauge needle to withdraw docetaxel from the vial; dilute in 250 mL of NS or D5W to a final concentration of 0.3 to 0.74 mg/mL. If docetaxel dose is >200 mg, use a larger volume of infusion fluid to maintain a final concentration of 0.3 to 0.74 mg/mL. Mix by gentle manual rotation.

Taxotere: Use **only** a 21 gauge needle to withdraw docetaxel from the vial (larger bore needles, such as 18 gauge or 19 gauge needles, may cause stopper coring and rubber precipitates). If intact vials were stored refrigerated, allow to stand at room temperature for 5 minutes prior to dilution. Inspect vials prior to dilution; solution is supersaturated and may crystalize over time; do not use if crystalized.

Lyophilized powder: Dilute with the provided diluent (contains ethanol in polysorbate 80); add 1 mL to each 20 mg vial (resulting concentration is 20 mg/0.8 mL) and 4 mL to each 80 mg vial (resulting concentration is 24 mg/mL). Shake well to dissolve completely. Reconstituted solution is supersaturated and could crystallize over time; if crystals appear, discard the solution (should no longer be used). If air bubbles are present, allow to stand for a few minutes while air bubbles dissipate. Further dilute in 250 mL of NS or D5W in a non-DEHP container (eg, glass, polypropylene, polyolefin) to a final concentration of 0.3 to 0.74 mg/mL (for doses >200 mg, use a larger volume of NS or D5W, not to exceed a final concentration of 0.74 mg/mL). Mix thoroughly by manual agitation.

Two-vial formulation (*generic; concentrate plus diluent formulation*): Vials should be diluted with 13% (w/w) polyethylene glycol 400/water (provided with the drug) to a final concentration of 10 mg/mL. Do not shake. Further dilute for infusion in 250 to 500 mL of NS or D5W in a non-DEHP container (eg, glass, polypropylene, polyolefin) to a final concentration of 0.3 to 0.74 mg/mL. Gently rotate to mix thoroughly. Do not use the two-vial formulation with the one-vial formulation for the same admixture product.

Storage/Stability Storage and stability may vary by manufacturer, refer to specific prescribing information.

Docetaxel 10 mg/mL: Store intact vials between 2°C to 25°C (36°F to 77°F) (actual recommendations may vary by generic manufacturer; consult manufacturer's labeling). Protect from bright light. Freezing does not adversely affect the product. Multi-use vials (80 mg/8 mL and 160 mg/16 mL) are stable for up to 28 days after first entry when stored between 2°C to 8°C (36°F to 46°F) and protected from light. Solutions diluted for infusion should be used within 4 hours of preparation, including infusion time.

Docetaxel 20 mg/mL concentrate:

Taxotere: Store intact vials between 2°C to 25°C (36°F to 77°F). Protect from bright light. Freezing does not adversely affect the product. Solutions diluted for infusion in non-PVC containers should be used within 6 hours of preparation, including infusion time, when stored between 2°C to 25°C (36°F to 77°F) or within 48 hours when stored between 2°C to 8°C (36°F to 46°F).

Generic formulations: Store intact vials at 25°C (77°F); excursions permitted between 15°C to 30°C (59°F to 86°F). Protect from light. Solutions diluted for infusion should be used within 4 hours of preparation, including infusion time.

Non-alcohol formulation: Store intact vials at 20°C to 25°C (68°F to 77°F). Protect from light. After the first use and following multiple needle entries and withdrawals, multi-use vials (80 mg/4 mL and 160 mg/8 mL) are stable for up to 28 days when stored between 2°C to 8°C (36°F to 46°F) and protected from light. Solutions diluted for infusion in NS or D5W are stable for 24 hours when stored between 2°C to 8°C (36°F to 46°F).

Docetaxel lyophilized powder (Docefrez): Store intact vials between 2°C to 8°C (36°F to 46°F). Protect from light. Allow vials (and provided diluent) to stand at room temperature for 5 minutes prior to reconstitution. After reconstitution, may be stored refrigerated or at room temperature for up to 8 hours. Solutions diluted for infusion should be used within 6 hours of preparation, including infusion time. According to the manufacturer, physical and chemical in-use stability of the infusion solution (prepared as recommended) has been demonstrated in non-PVC bags up to 48 hours when stored between 2°C and 8°C (36°F and 46°F).

Two-vial formulation (*generic; concentrate plus diluent formulation*): Reconstituted solutions of the two-vial formulation are stable in the vial for 8 hours at room temperature or under refrigeration. Solutions diluted for infusion in polyolefin containers should be used within 4 hours of preparation, including infusion time.

Mechanism of Action Docetaxel promotes the assembly of microtubules from tubulin dimers, and inhibits the depolymerization of tubulin which stabilizes microtubules in the cell. This results in inhibition of DNA, RNA, and protein synthesis. Most activity occurs during the M phase of the cell cycle.

Pharmacodynamics/Kinetics Exhibits linear pharmacokinetics at the recommended dosage range

Distribution: Extensive extravascular distribution and/or tissue binding; V_{dss}: 113 L (mean steady state)

Protein binding: ~94% to 97%, primarily to alpha$_1$-acid glycoprotein, albumin, and lipoproteins

Metabolism: Hepatic; oxidation via CYP3A4 to metabolites

Half-life elimination: Terminal: ~11 hours

Excretion: Feces (~75%, <8% as unchanged drug); urine (~6%)

Dosing

Adult & Geriatric Note: Premedicate with corticosteroids for 3 days, beginning one day prior to docetaxel administration, to reduce the severity of hypersensitivity reactions and fluid retention. Patients being treated for prostate cancer with concurrent prednisone should be premedicated with oral dexamethasone at 12 hours, 3 hours, and 1 hour prior to docetaxel administration.

◄ *US labeling:*

Breast cancer: IV:

Locally advanced or metastatic: 60 to 100 mg/m^2 every 3 weeks (as a single agent)

Operable, node-positive (adjuvant treatment): TAC regimen: 75 mg/m^2 every 3 weeks for 6 courses (in combination with doxorubicin and cyclophosphamide) (Mackey 2013; Martin 2005)

Adjuvant treatment (off-label dosing): 75 mg/m^2 every 21 days (in combination with cyclophosphamide) for 4 cycles (Jones 2006) **or** 75 mg/m^2 every 21 days (in combination with carboplatin and trastuzumab) for 6 cycles (Slamon 2011)

Neoadjuvant treatment (off-label dosing): 75 mg/m^2 (cycle 1; if tolerated, may increase to 100 mg/m^2 in subsequent cycles) every 21 days for a total of 4 cycles (in combination with trastuzumab and pertuzumab) (Gianni 2012)

Metastatic treatment (off-label dosing):

Every-3-week administration: 75 mg/m^2 (cycle 1; may increase to 100 mg/m^2 in subsequent cycles) every 21 days for at least 6 cycles (in combination with trastuzumab and pertuzumab) (Baselga 2012; Swain 2013) **or** 100 mg/m^2 every 21 days (in combination with trastuzumab) for at least 6 cycles (Marty 2005) **or** 75 mg/m^2 every 21 days (in combination with capecitabine) until disease progression or unacceptable toxicity (O'Shaughnessy 2002) **or** 60 mg/m^2, 75 mg/m^2, or 100 mg/m^2 every 21 days for at least 6 cycles until disease progression, unacceptable toxicity, or discontinuation (Harvey 2006)

Weekly administration: 40 mg/m^2/dose once a week (as a single agent) for 6 weeks followed by a 2-week rest, repeat until disease progression or unacceptable toxicity (Burstein 2000) **or** 35 mg/m^2/dose once weekly for 3 weeks, followed by a 1-week rest, may increase to 40 mg/m^2 once weekly for 3 weeks followed by a 1-week rest with cycle 2 (Rivera 2008) **or** 35 mg/m^2/dose once weekly (in combination with trastuzumab) for 3 weeks followed by a 1-week rest; repeat until disease progression or unacceptable toxicity (Esteva 2002)

Non-small cell lung cancer: IV: 75 mg/m^2 every 3 weeks (as a single agent or in combination with cisplatin)

Prostate cancer: IV: 75 mg/m^2 every 3 weeks (in combination with prednisone)

Gastric adenocarcinoma: IV: 75 mg/m^2 every 3 weeks (in combination with cisplatin and fluorouracil)

Sequential chemotherapy and chemoradiation (off-label dosing): Induction: 75 mg/m^2 on days 1 and 22 (in combination with cisplatin) for 2 cycles, followed by chemoradiation: 20 mg/m^2 weekly for 5 weeks (in combination with cisplatin and radiation) (Ruhstaller 2009)

Locally advanced or metastatic disease (off-label dosing): 50 mg/m^2 on day 1 every 2 weeks (in combination with fluorouracil, leucovorin, and oxaliplatin) until disease progression or unacceptable toxicity up to a maximum of 8 cycles (Al-Batran 2008)

Head and neck cancer: IV: 75 mg/m^2 every 3 weeks (in combination with cisplatin and fluorouracil) for 3 or 4 cycles, followed by radiation therapy

Canadian labeling:

Breast cancer: IV:

Locally advanced or metastatic: 75 mg/m^2 (as combination therapy) **or** 100 mg/m^2 (as a single agent) every 3 weeks

Operable, node-positive (adjuvant treatment): 75 mg/m^2 every 3 weeks for 6 courses (in combination with doxorubicin and cyclophosphamide)

Non-small cell lung cancer (locally advanced or metastatic), ovarian cancer (metastatic), head and neck cancer (recurrent and/or metastatic): IV: 75 mg/m^2 (as combination therapy) **or** 100 mg/m^2 (as a single agent) every 3 weeks

Prostate cancer (hormone-refractory, metastatic): IV: 75 mg/m^2 every 3 weeks (in combination with prednisone or prednisolone)

Off-label uses:

Bladder cancer, metastatic (off-label use): IV: 100 mg/m^2 every 3 weeks (as a single agent) (McCaffrey 1997) **or** 35 mg/m^2 on days 1 and 8 of a 21-day cycle (in combination with gemcitabine and cisplatin) for at least 6 cycles or until disease progression or unacceptable toxicity (Pectasides 2002)

Esophageal cancer (off-label use): IV:

Sequential chemotherapy and chemoradiation: Induction: 75 mg/m^2 on days 1 and 22 (in combination with cisplatin) for 2 cycles, followed by chemoradiation: 20 mg/m^2 weekly for 5 weeks (in combination with cisplatin and radiation) (Ruhstaller 2009)

Definitive chemoradiation: 60 mg/m^2 on days 1 and 22 (in combination with cisplatin and radiation) for 1 cycle (Li 2010)

Locally advanced or metastatic disease: 75 mg/m^2 on day 1 every 3 weeks (in combination with cisplatin and fluorouracil) (Ajani 2007; Van Cutsem 2006) **or** 50 mg/m^2 on day 1 every 2 weeks (in combination with fluorouracil, leucovorin, and oxaliplatin) until disease progression or unacceptable toxicity up to a maximum of 8 cycles (Al-Batran 2008) **or** 35 mg/m^2 on days 1, 8, 15, 29, 36, 43, 50, and 57 (in combination with cisplatin, fluorouracil, and radiotherapy; neoadjuvant setting) (Pasini 2013)

Ewing sarcoma, osteosarcoma (recurrent or progressive; off-label uses): IV: 100 mg/m^2 on day 8 of a 21-day cycle (in combination with gemcitabine) (Navid 2008)

Ovarian cancer (off-label use in US): IV: 60 mg/m^2 every 3 weeks (in combination with carboplatin) for up to 6 cycles (Markman 2001) **or** 75 mg/m^2 every 3 weeks (in combination with carboplatin) for 6 cycles (Vasey 2004) **or** 35 mg/m^2 (maximum dose: 70 mg) weekly for 3 weeks followed by a 1-week rest (in combination with carboplatin) (Kushner 2007)

Small cell lung cancer, relapsed (off-label use): IV: 100 mg/m^2 every 3 weeks (Smyth 1994)

Soft tissue sarcoma (off-label use): IV: 100 mg/m^2 on day 8 of a 3-week treatment cycle (in combination with gemcitabine and filgrastim or pegfilgrastim) (Leu 2004; Maki 2007)

Unknown-primary, adenocarcinoma (off-label use): IV: 65 mg/m^2 every 3 weeks (in combination with carboplatin) (Greco 2000) **or** 75 mg/m^2 on day 8 of a 3-week treatment cycle (in combination with gemcitabine) for up to 6 cycles (Pouessel 2004) **or** 60 mg/m^2 on day 1 of a 3-week treatment cycle (in combination with cisplatin) (Mukai 2010)

Dosing adjustment for concomitant CYP3A4 inhibitors: Avoid the concomitant use of strong CYP3A4 inhibitors with docetaxel. If concomitant use of a strong CYP3A4 inhibitor cannot be avoided, consider reducing the docetaxel dose by 50% (based on limited pharmacokinetic data).

Pediatric Note: Premedicate with corticosteroids for 3 days, beginning one day prior to docetaxel administration, to reduce the severity of hypersensitivity reactions and fluid retention. Dexamethasone (dose not specified) was administered for 3 to 4 days, starting the day before or the day of docetaxel administration and continuing for 2 days afterward in the bone sarcoma study (Navid 2008).

Ewing sarcoma, osteosarcoma (recurrent or progressive; off-label uses): Children ≥8 years and Adolescents: IV: 100 mg/m^2 on day 8 of a 21-day cycle (in combination with gemcitabine) (Navid 2008)

Renal Impairment Renal excretion is minimal (~6%), therefore, the need for dosage adjustments for renal dysfunction is unlikely (Janus 2010; Li 2007). Not removed by hemodialysis, may be administered before or after hemodialysis (Janus 2010).

Hepatic Impairment

US labeling:

Total bilirubin greater than the ULN, or AST and/or ALT >1.5 times ULN concomitant with alkaline phosphatase >2.5 times ULN: Use is not recommended.

Hepatic impairment dosing adjustment specific for gastric or head and neck cancer:

AST/ALT >2.5 to ≤5 times ULN and alkaline phosphatase ≤2.5 times ULN: Administer 80% of dose

AST/ALT >1.5 to ≤5 times ULN and alkaline phosphatase >2.5 to ≤5 times ULN: Administer 80% of dose

AST/ALT >5 times ULN and /or alkaline phosphatase >5 times ULN: Discontinue docetaxel

Canadian labeling:

Serum bilirubin >ULN **or** AST and/or ALT >1.5 times ULN associated with alkaline phosphatase >2.5 times ULN: Avoid use.

Severe hepatic impairment: Use is contraindicated.

The following adjustments have also been used (Floyd 2006):

Transaminases 1.6 to 6 times ULN: Administer 75% of dose.

Transaminases >6 times ULN: Use clinical judgment.

Obesity ASCO Guidelines for appropriate chemotherapy dosing in obese adults with cancer: Utilize patient's actual body weight (full weight) for calculation of body surface area- or weight-based dosing, particularly when the intent of therapy is curative; manage regimen-related toxicities in the same manner as for nonobese patients; if a dose reduction is utilized due to toxicity, consider resumption of full weight-based dosing with subsequent cycles, especially if cause of toxicity (eg, hepatic or renal impairment) is resolved (Griggs 2012).

Adjustment for Toxicity
US labeling:

Note: Toxicity includes febrile neutropenia, neutrophils <500/mm^3 for >1 week, severe or cumulative cutaneous reactions; in non–small cell lung cancer, this may also include platelet nadir <25,000/mm^3 and other grade 3/4 nonhematologic toxicities.

Breast cancer (single agent): Patients dosed initially at 100 mg/m^2; reduce dose to 75 mg/m^2; **Note:** If the patient continues to experience these adverse reactions, the dosage should be reduced to 55 mg/m^2 or therapy should be discontinued; discontinue for peripheral neuropathy ≥ grade 3. Patients initiated at 60 mg/m^2 who do not develop toxicity may tolerate higher doses.

Breast cancer, adjuvant treatment (combination chemotherapy): TAC regimen should be administered when neutrophils are ≥1500/mm^3. Patients experiencing febrile neutropenia should receive G-CSF in all subsequent cycles. Patients with persistent febrile neutropenia (while on G-CSF), patients experiencing severe/cumulative cutaneous reactions, moderate neurosensory effects (signs/symptoms) or grade 3 or 4 stomatitis should receive a reduced dose (60 mg/m^2) of docetaxel. Discontinue therapy with persistent toxicities after dosage reduction.

Non-small cell lung cancer:

Monotherapy: Patients dosed initially at 75 mg/m^2 should have dose held until toxicity is resolved, then resume at 55 mg/m^2; discontinue for peripheral neuropathy ≥ grade 3.

Combination therapy (with cisplatin): Patients dosed initially at 75 mg/m^2 should have the docetaxel dosage reduced to 65 mg/m^2 in subsequent cycles; if further adjustment is required, dosage may be reduced to 50 mg/m^2.

Prostate cancer: Reduce dose to 60 mg/m^2; discontinue therapy if toxicities persist at lower dose.

Gastric cancer, head and neck cancer: Note: Cisplatin may require dose reductions/therapy delays for peripheral neuropathy, ototoxicity, and/or nephrotoxicity. Patients experiencing febrile neutropenia, documented infection with neutropenia or neutropenia >7 days should receive G-CSF in all subsequent cycles. For neutropenic complications despite G-CSF use, further reduce dose to 60 mg/m^2. Dosing with neutropenic complications in subsequent cycles should be further reduced to 45 mg/m^2. Patients who experience grade 4 thrombocytopenia should receive a dose reduction from 75 mg/m^2 to 60 mg/m^2. Discontinue therapy for persistent toxicities.

Gastrointestinal toxicity for docetaxel in combination with cisplatin and fluorouracil for treatment of gastric cancer or head and neck cancer:

Diarrhea, grade 3:
First episode: Reduce fluorouracil dose by 20%
Second episode: Reduce docetaxel dose by 20%
Diarrhea, grade 4:
First episode: Reduce fluorouracil and docetaxel doses by 20%
Second episode: Discontinue treatment
Stomatitis, grade 3:
First episode: Reduce fluorouracil dose by 20%
Second episode: Discontinue fluorouracil for all subsequent cycles
Third episode: Reduce docetaxel dose by 20%
Stomatitis, grade 4:
First episode: Discontinue fluorouracil for all subsequent cycles
Second episode: Reduce docetaxel dose by 20%

Canadian labeling: **Note:** Toxicity includes febrile neutropenia, neutrophils ≤500/mm^3 for >1 week, severe or cumulative cutaneous reactions, or severe neurosensory symptoms.

Patients initially dosed at 100 mg/m^2: Reduce dose to 75 mg/m^2; Patients initially dosed at 75 mg/m^2: Reduce dose to 60 mg/m^2. Discontinue therapy for persistent toxicities after dosage reduction.

Breast cancer, adjuvant treatment (combination chemotherapy): Patients experiencing febrile neutropenia should receive G-CSF in all subsequent cycles. Patients with persistent febrile neutropenia (while on G-CSF), patients experiencing severe/cumulative cutaneous reactions, severe neurosensory symptoms, or grade 3 or 4 stomatitis should have their dose reduced to 60 mg/m^2. Discontinue therapy with persistent toxicities after dosage reduction.

Concomitant use with capecitabine (treatment of metastatic breast cancer):

Grade 2 toxicities:
First episode: Interrupt therapy until resolution to < grade 2, then resume docetaxel and capecitabine at previous dose; consider prophylactic measures if appropriate and/or possible
Second episode of same toxicity: Interrupt therapy until resolution to < grade 2, then resume docetaxel at 55 mg/m^2; reduce capecitabine dose to 75% of original dose
Further episodes of same toxicity: Discontinue docetaxel; interrupt capecitabine until resolution to < grade 2, then resume at 50% of original dose (third episode) or discontinue therapy altogether (fourth episode)

Grade 3 toxicities:
First episode: Occurring at time treatment is due: Interrupt docetaxel until resolution to < grade 2 (maximum delay ≤2 weeks), then resume docetaxel at 55 mg/m^2; reduce capecitabine dose to 75% of original dose (consider prophylactic measure if appropriate); if no resolution to < grade 2 within 2 weeks, discontinue docetaxel but may resume capecitabine at 75% of original dose after resolution to < grade 2. Occurring between cycles and resolves to < grade 2 by time of next treatment: Administer docetaxel at 55 mg/m^2 and reduce capecitabine dose to 75% of original dose; consider prophylactic measures if appropriate and/or possible.
Further episodes of same toxicity: Discontinue docetaxel; interrupt capecitabine until resolution to < grade 2, then resume capecitabine at 50% of original dose (second episode) or discontinue therapy altogether (third episode)

Grade 4 toxicities: First episode: Discontinue docetaxel and capecitabine therapy or if deemed clinically necessary, capecitabine may be continued at 50% of original dose

Administration Administer IV infusion over 1-hour through nonsorbing polyethylene lined (non-DEHP) tubing; in-line filter is not necessary (the use of a filter during administration is not recommended by the manufacturer). Infusion should be completed within 4 hours of final preparation. **Note:** Premedication with corticosteroids for 3 days, beginning the day before docetaxel administration, is recommended to reduce the incidence and severity of hypersensitivity reactions and fluid retention. Some docetaxel formulations contain alcohol (content varies by formulation); use with caution in patients for whom alcohol intake should be avoided or minimized (a non-alcohol generic formulation [20 mg/mL] is also available).

Irritant with vesicant-like properties; avoid extravasation. Assure proper needle or catheter position prior to administration.

Extravasation management: If extravasation occurs, stop infusion immediately and disconnect (leave cannula/needle in place); gently aspirate extravasated solution (do **NOT** flush the line); remove needle/cannula; elevate extremity. Information conflicts regarding the use of warm or cold compresses (Perez Fidalgo 2012; Polovich 2009).

Hazardous agent; use appropriate precautions for handling and disposal (NIOSH 2014 [group 1]).

Monitoring Parameters CBC with differential, liver function tests, bilirubin, alkaline phosphatase, renal function; monitor for hypersensitivity reactions, neurosensory symptoms, gastrointestinal toxicity (eg, diarrhea, stomatitis), cutaneous reactions, visual impairment, fluid retention, epiphora, and canalicular stenosis

Product Availability Docetaxel (non-alcohol formula): FDA approved December 2015; availability anticipated in January 2016.

Dosage Forms Considerations Non-alcohol formulation (Eagle/Teikuku pharmaceuticals): Concentrate, Intravenous [alcohol-free]: Generic: 20 mg/mL (1 mL; single-dose vial); 80 mg/4 mL (4 mL multi-dose vial); 160 mg/8 mL (8 mL; multi-dose vial)

Dosage Forms Excipient information presented when available (limited, particularly for generics); consult specific product labeling. [DSC] = Discontinued product

Concentrate, Intravenous:

Taxotere: 20 mg/mL (1 mL); 80 mg/4 mL (4 mL); 20 mg/0.5 mL (0.5 mL [DSC]) [contains alcohol, usp, polysorbate 80]

Generic: 20 mg/mL (1 mL); 80 mg/4 mL (4 mL); 160 mg/8 mL (8 mL); 20 mg/0.5 mL (0.5 mL); 80 mg/2 mL (2 mL)

Concentrate, Intravenous [preservative free]:

Generic: 20 mg/mL (1 mL); 80 mg/4 mL (4 mL); 140 mg/7 mL (7 mL); 160 mg/8 mL (8 mL)

Solution, Intravenous:

Generic: 20 mg/2 mL (2 mL); 80 mg/8 mL (8 mL); 160 mg/16 mL (16 mL); 200 mg/20 mL (20 mL)

Solution Reconstituted, Intravenous:

Docefrez: 20 mg (1 ea); 80 mg (1 ea) [contains alcohol, usp, polysorbate 80]

◆ Docetaxel for Injection (Can) *see* DOCEtaxel on page 573

◆ Docosahexaenoic Acid *see* Omega-3 Fatty Acids on page 1329

Docosanol (doe KOE san ole)

Brand Names: US Abreva [OTC]

Index Terms n-Docosanol; Behenyl Alcohol

Pharmacologic Category Antiviral Agent, Topical

Use Cold sore/fever blister: Treatment of cold sores/fever blisters on the face or lips.

Dosing

Adult & Geriatric Cold sore/fever blister: Topical: Apply 5 times daily to affected area of face or lips. Start at first sign of cold sore or fever blister and continue until healed. If not healed within 10 days, discontinue use and contact health care provider.

Pediatric Cold sore/fever blister: Children ≥12 years and Adolescents: Refer to adult dosing.

Renal Impairment There are no dosage adjustments provided in the manufacturer's labeling.

Hepatic Impairment There are no dosage adjustments provided in the manufacturer's labeling.

Additional Information Complete prescribing information should be consulted for additional detail.

Dosage Forms Excipient information presented when available (limited, particularly for generics); consult specific product labeling.

Cream, External:

Abreva: 10% (2 g) [contains benzyl alcohol]

◆ Doc-Q-Lace [OTC] [DSC] *see* Docusate on page 578

◆ Doc-Q-Lax [OTC] *see* Docusate and Senna on page 579

◆ Docu [OTC] *see* Docusate on page 578

◆ Docuprene [OTC] *see* Docusate on page 578

Docusate (DOK yoo sate)

Brand Names: US Colace Clear [OTC]; Colace [OTC]; D.O.S. [OTC]; Diocto [OTC]; Doc-Q-Lace [OTC] [DSC]; DocQLace [OTC]; Docu Soft [OTC]; Docu [OTC]; Docuprene [OTC]; Docusil [OTC]; DocuSol Kids [OTC]; DocuSol Mini [OTC]; DOK [OTC]; Dulcolax Stool Softener [OTC]; Enemeez Mini [OTC]; Healthy Mama Move It Along [OTC]; Kao-Tin [OTC]; KS Stool Softener [OTC]; Laxa Basic [OTC]; Pedia-Lax [OTC]; Promolaxin [OTC]; Silace [OTC]; Sof-Lax [OTC]; Stool Softener Laxative DC [OTC] [DSC]; Stool Softener [OTC]; Sur-Q-Lax [OTC]; Vacuant Mini-Enema [OTC] [DSC]

Brand Names: Canada Apo-Docusate Calcium [OTC]; Apo-Docusate Sodium [OTC]; Calax [OTC]; Colace [OTC]; Docusate Sodium Odan [OTC]; Dom-Docusate Sodium [OTC]; Dosolax [OTC]; Dulcocomfort Stool Softener [OTC]; Euro-Docusate C [OTC]; Jamp-Docusate [OTC]; Novo-Docusate Calcium [OTC]; Novo-Docusate Sodium [OTC]; PHL-Docusate Sodium [OTC]; PMS-Docusate Calcium [OTC]; PMS-Docusate Sodium [OTC]; ratio-Docusate Sodium [OTC]; Selax [OTC]; Silace [OTC]; Sirop Docusate De Sodium [OTC]; Soflax C [OTC]; Soflax [OTC]; Taro-Docusate [OTC]; Teva-Docusate Calcium [OTC]; Teva-Docusate Sodium [OTC]

Index Terms Dioctyl Calcium Sulfosuccinate; Dioctyl Sodium Sulfosuccinate; Docusate Calcium; Docusate Potassium; Docusate Sodium; DOSS; DSS

Pharmacologic Category Stool Softener

Use Stool softener: Prevention of straining during defecation and constipation associated with hard, dry stools; relief of occasional constipation

Dosing

Adult & Geriatric Note: The following are general dosing guidelines; refer to specific product labeling for dosing instructions.

Stool softener:

Oral:

Docusate calcium: 240 mg once daily

Docusate sodium: 50 to 360 mg once daily or in divided doses

Rectal: 283 mg per 5 mL: 283 mg (1 enema) 1 to 3 times daily

Ceruminolytic (off-label use): Intra-aural: Administer 1 mL of docusate sodium in 2 mL syringes; if no clearance in 15 minutes, irrigate with 50 or 100 mL lukewarm normal saline (Singer 2000)

Pediatric Note: The following are general dosing guidelines; refer to specific product labeling for dosing instructions.

Stool softener:

Oral:

Docusate calcium: Children ≥12 years and Adolescents: Refer to adult dosing.

Docusate sodium:

Children 2 to <12 years: 50 to 150 mg once daily or in divided doses

Children ≥12 years and Adolescents: Refer to adult dosing.

Rectal:

Children 2 to <12 years:

100 mg per 5 mL: 100 mg (1 enema) once daily

283 mg per 5 mL: 283 mg (1 enema) once daily

Children ≥12 years and Adolescents: 283 mg per 5 mL: Refer to adult dosing.

Ceruminolytic (off-label use): Children and Adolescents: Intra-aural: Administer 1 mL of docusate sodium in 2 mL syringes; if no clearance in 15 minutes, irrigate with 50 or 100 mL lukewarm normal saline (Singer 2000)

Renal Impairment There are no dosage adjustments provided in the manufacturer's labeling

Hepatic Impairment There are no dosage adjustments provided in the manufacturer's labeling

Additional Information Complete prescribing information should be consulted for additional detail.

Dosage Forms Excipient information presented when available (limited, particularly for generics); consult specific product labeling. [DSC] = Discontinued product

Capsule, Oral, as calcium:

Kao-Tin: 240 mg [sodium free; contains brilliant blue fcf (fd&c blue #1), fd&c red #40, fd&c yellow #6 (sunset yellow)]

Kao-Tin: 240 mg [DSC] [sodium free; contains fd&c red #40]

Stool Softener: 240 mg [contains brilliant blue fcf (fd&c blue #1), fd&c red #40, fd&c yellow #6 (sunset yellow)]

Stool Softener Laxative DC: 240 mg [DSC] [contains fd&c red #40]

Sur-Q-Lax: 240 mg

Generic: 240 mg

Capsule, Oral, as sodium:

Colace: 50 mg [DSC]

Colace: 100 mg [contains fd&c red #40, fd&c yellow #6 (sunset yellow)]

Colace Clear: 50 mg [dye free]

D.O.S.: 250 mg

DocQLace: 100 mg [contains fd&c red #40, fd&c yellow #6 (sunset yellow)]

Docu Soft: 100 mg

Docusil: 100 mg

DOK: 100 mg [contains fd&c red #40, fd&c yellow #6 (sunset yellow)]

DOK: 250 mg [DSC]

DOK: 250 mg [contains fd&c red #40, fd&c yellow #6 (sunset yellow)]

Dulcolax Stool Softener: 100 mg [contains fd&c red #40, fd&c yellow #6 (sunset yellow)]

KS Stool Softener: 100 mg [stimulant free; contains brilliant blue fcf (fd&c blue #1), fd&c red #40, methylparaben, propylparaben, tartrazine (fd&c yellow #5)]

Laxa Basic: 100 mg, 250 mg [DSC]

Sof-Lax: 100 mg

Stool Softener: 100 mg

Stool Softener: 100 mg, 250 mg [DSC] [contains fd&c red #40, fd&c yellow #6 (sunset yellow)]

Stool Softener: 100 mg [stimulant free; contains brilliant blue fcf (fd&c blue #1), fd&c red #40, fd&c yellow #6 (sunset yellow)]

Stool Softener: 100 mg, 250 mg [stimulant free; contains fd&c red #40, fd&c yellow #6 (sunset yellow)]

Generic: 100 mg, 250 mg

Enema, Rectal, as sodium:
DocuSol Kids: 100 mg/5 mL (5 ea) [contains polyethylene glycol]
DocuSol Mini: 283 mg (5 ea)
Enemeez Mini: 283 mg (5 mL)
Vacuant Mini-Enema: 283 mg (5 mL [DSC])
Liquid, Oral, as sodium:
Dioto: 50 mg/5 mL (473 mL) [contains fd&c red #40, methylparaben, polyethylene glycol, propylene glycol, propylparaben; vanilla flavor]
Dioto: 50 mg/5 mL (473 mL) [contains parabens, polyethylene glycol]
Doc-Q-Lace: 150 mg/15 mL (473 mL [DSC]) [contains methylparaben, propylene glycol, propylparaben]
Docu: 50 mg/mL (10 mL, 473 mL) [contains methylparaben, polyethylene glycol, propylene glycol, propylparaben, sodium benzoate; vanilla flavor]
Pedia-Lax: 50 mg/15 mL (118 mL) [contains edetate disodium, methylparaben, polyethylene glycol, propylene glycol, propylparaben; fruit punch flavor]
Silace: 150 mg/15 mL (473 mL) [lemon-vanilla flavor]
Generic: 50 mg/5 mL (10 mL, 25 mL [DSC], 473 mL [DSC])
Syrup, Oral, as sodium:
Colace: 60 mg/15 mL (473 mL [DSC]) [alcohol free, sugar free; contains fd&c red #40, propylene glycol, saccharin sodium]
Dioto: 60 mg/15 mL (473 mL) [contains fd&c red #40, menthol, methylparaben, polyethylene glycol, propylparaben, sodium benzoate; peppermint flavor]
Dioto: 60 mg/15 mL (473 mL [DSC]) [contains fd&c red #40, methylparaben, propylene glycol, propylparaben, sodium benzoate; peppermint flavor]
Dioto: 60 mg/15 mL (473 mL) [contains fd&c red #40, propylene glycol, saccharin sodium, sodium benzoate]
Doc-Q-Lace: 60 mg/15 mL (473 mL [DSC]) [contains alcohol, usp, fd&c red #40, methylparaben, propylene glycol, propylparaben, sodium benzoate]
Silace: 60 mg/15 mL (473 mL) [contains alcohol, usp; peppermint flavor]
Generic: 60 mg/15 mL (25 mL [DSC], 473 mL [DSC])
Tablet, Oral, as sodium:
Docuprene: 100 mg [contains sodium benzoate]
DOK: 100 mg [scored]
Healthy Mama Move It Along: 100 mg [scored; stimulant free; contains sodium benzoate]
Promolaxin: 100 mg [scored; contains sodium benzoate]
Stool Softener: 100 mg [contains sodium benzoate]
Generic: 100 mg

Docusate and Senna (DOK yoo sate & SEN na)

Brand Names: US Doc-Q-Lax [OTC]; Dok Plus [OTC]; Geri-Stool [OTC]; Peri-Colace [OTC]; Senexon-S [OTC]; Senna Plus [OTC]; SennaLax-S [OTC]; Senokot-S [OTC]; SenoSol-SS [OTC]
Index Terms Docusate and Sennosides; Senna and Docusate; Senna-S; Sennosides and Docusate
Pharmacologic Category Laxative, Stimulant; Stool Softener
Use Constipation: Relief of occasional constipation
Dosing
Adult Constipation: OTC ranges: Oral: Initial: Two tablets (17.2 mg sennosides plus 100 mg docusate) once daily (maximum: 4 tablets twice daily)
Geriatric Constipation: OTC ranges: Oral: Consider half the initial dose in older, debilitated patients
Pediatric Constipation: OTC ranges: Oral:
2 to 6 years: Initial: 4.3 mg sennosides plus 25 mg docusate (1/2 tablet) once daily (maximum: 1 tablet twice daily)
6 to 12 years: Initial: 8.6 sennosides plus 50 mg docusate (1 tablet) once daily (maximum: 2 tablets twice daily)
≥12 years: Refer to adult dosing.
Additional Information Complete prescribing information should be consulted for additional detail.
Dosage Forms Excipient information presented when available (limited, particularly for generics); consult specific product labeling.
Tablet, oral: Docusate sodium 50 mg and sennosides 8.6 mg
Doc-Q-Lax: Docusate sodium 50 mg and sennosides 8.6 mg
Dok Plus: Docusate sodium 50 mg and sennosides 8.6 mg [contains sodium benzoate]
Geri-Stool: Docusate sodium 50 mg and sennosides 8.6 mg
Peri-Colace: Docusate sodium 50 mg and sennosides 8.6 mg
Senexon-S: Docusate sodium 50 mg and sennosides 8.6 mg [contains calcium 20 mg/tablet, sodium 6 mg/tablet]

SennaLax-S: Docusate sodium 50 mg and sennosides 8.6 mg [contains sodium benzoate]
Senna Plus: Docusate sodium 50 mg and sennosides 8.6 mg
Senokot-S: Docusate sodium 50 mg and sennosides 8.6 mg [sugar free; contains sodium 4 mg/tablet]
SenoSol-SS: Docusate sodium 50 mg and sennosides 8.6 mg [contains sodium 3 mg/tablet]

◆ **Docusate and Sennosides** see Docusate and Senna on page 579
◆ **Docusate Calcium** see Docusate on page 578
◆ **Docusate Potassium** see Docusate on page 578
◆ **Docusate Sodium** see Docusate on page 578
◆ **Docusate Sodium Odan [OTC] (Can)** see Docusate on page 578
◆ **Docusil [OTC]** see Docusate on page 578
◆ **Docu Soft [OTC]** see Docusate on page 578
◆ **DocuSol Kids [OTC]** see Docusate on page 578
◆ **DocuSol Mini [OTC]** see Docusate on page 578

Dofetilide (doe FET il ide)

Brand Names: US Tikosyn
Pharmacologic Category Antiarrhythmic Agent, Class III
Use Maintenance of normal sinus rhythm in patients with chronic atrial fibrillation/atrial flutter of longer than 1-week duration who have been converted to normal sinus rhythm; conversion of atrial fibrillation and atrial flutter to normal sinus rhythm
Pregnancy Considerations Adverse events have been observed in animal reproduction studies.
Breast-Feeding Considerations It is not known if dofetilide is excreted in breast milk. Breast-feeding is not recommended by the manufacturer.
Prescribing and Access Restrictions As a requirement of the REMS program, access to this medication is restricted. Tikosyn® is only available to prescribers and hospitals that have confirmed their participation in a designated Tikosyn® Education Program. The program provides comprehensive education about the importance of in-hospital treatment initiation and individualized dosing.

T.I.P.S. is the Tikosyn® In Pharmacy System designated to allow retail pharmacies to stock and dispense Tikosyn® once they have been enrolled. A participating pharmacy must confirm receipt of the T.I.P.S. program materials and educate its pharmacy staff about the procedures required to fill an outpatient prescription for Tikosyn®. The T.I.P.S. enrollment form is available at www.tikosyn.com. Tikosyn® is only available from a special mail order pharmacy, and enrolled retail pharmacies. Pharmacists must verify that the hospital/prescriber is a confirmed participant before Tikosyn® is provided. For participant verification, the pharmacist may call 1-800-788-7353 or use the web site located at www.tikosynlist.com. Further details and directions on the program are provided at www.tikosyn.com.

Dofetilide therapy must be initiated/adjusted in a hospital setting with proper monitoring under the guidance of experienced personnel.
Medication Guide Available Yes
Contraindications Hypersensitivity to dofetilide or any component of the formulation; patients with congenital or acquired long QT syndromes, do not use if baseline QT interval or QTc is >440 msec (500 msec in patients with ventricular conduction abnormalities); severe renal impairment (CrCl <20 mL/minute [Cockcroft-Gault method]); concurrent use with verapamil, cimetidine, hydrochlorothiazide (alone or in combinations), trimethoprim (alone or in combination with sulfamethoxazole), itraconazole (according to itraconazole prescribing information) ketoconazole, prochlorperazine, dolutegravir, or megestrol
Warnings/Precautions [U.S. Boxed Warning]: Must be initiated (or reinitiated) in a setting with continuous monitoring and staff familiar with the recognition and treatment of life-threatening arrhythmias. Patients must be monitored with continuous ECG for a minimum of 3 days, or for a minimum of 12 hours after electrical or pharmacological cardioversion to normal sinus rhythm, whichever is greater. Patients should be readmitted for continuous monitoring if dosage is later increased.

Reserve for patients who are highly symptomatic with atrial fibrillation/atrial flutter; risk of torsade de pointes (TdP) significantly increases with doses >500 mcg twice daily; hold Class I or Class III antiarrhythmics for at least three half-lives prior to starting dofetilide; use in patients previously on amiodarone therapy only if serum amiodarone level is <0.3 mg/L or if amiodarone was discontinued ≥3 months ago; correct hypokalemia or hypomagnesemia

before initiating dofetilide and maintain within normal limits during treatment. The risk of TdP may be higher in certain patient subgroups (eg, patients with heart failure). Most episodes of TdP occur within the first 3 days of therapy. Risk of hypokalemia and/or hypomagnesemia may be increased by potassium-depleting diuretics, increasing the risk of TdP. Concurrent use with other drugs known to prolong QTc interval is not recommended.

In the treatment of atrial fibrillation in the elderly, avoid antiarrhythmics as first-line treatment. In older adults, data suggests rate control may provide more benefits than risks compared to rhythm control for most patients (Beers Criteria).

Patients with sick sinus syndrome or with second or third-degree heart block should not receive dofetilide unless a functional pacemaker is in place. Defibrillation threshold is reduced in patients with ventricular tachycardia or ventricular fibrillation undergoing implantation of a cardioverter-defibrillator device. Use with caution in renal impairment; **dose adjustment required for patients with CrCl ≤60 mL/minute.** Use with caution in patients with severe hepatic impairment; not studied.

Adverse Reactions Supraventricular arrhythmia patients:

>10%: Central nervous system: Headache (11%)

2% to 10%:

Central nervous system: Dizziness (8%), insomnia (4%)

Cardiovascular: Ventricular tachycardia (2.6% to 3.7%), chest pain (10%), torsade de pointes (3.3% in HF patients and 0.9% in patients with a recent MI; up to 10.5% in patients receiving doses in excess of those recommended). Torsade de pointes occurs most frequently within the first 3 days of therapy.

Dermatologic: Rash (3%)

Gastrointestinal: Nausea (5%), diarrhea (3%), abdominal pain (3%)

Neuromuscular & skeletal: Back pain (3%)

Respiratory: Respiratory tract infection (7%), dyspnea (6%)

Miscellaneous: Flu-like syndrome (4%)

<2%:

Central nervous system: CVA, facial paralysis, flaccid paralysis, migraine, paralysis

Cardiovascular: AV block (0.4% to 1.5%), bundle branch block (0.1% to 0.5%), heart block (0.1% to 0.5%), ventricular fibrillation (0% to 0.4%), bradycardia, cardiac arrest, edema, MI, sudden death, syncope

Dermatologic: Angioedema

Gastrointestinal: Liver damage

Neuromuscular & skeletal: Paresthesia

Respiratory: Cough

Drug Interactions

Metabolism/Transport Effects Substrate of CYP3A4 (minor); **Note:** Assignment of Major/Minor substrate status based on clinically relevant drug interaction potential

Avoid Concomitant Use

Avoid concomitant use of Dofetilide with any of the following: Antifungal Agents (Azole Derivatives, Systemic); Cimetidine; Dolutegravir; Fingolimod; Highest Risk QTc-Prolonging Agents; Ivabradine; LamoTRIgine; Megestrol; Mifepristone; Moderate Risk QTc-Prolonging Agents; Prochlorperazine; Propafenone; Saquinavir; Thiazide Diuretics; Trimethoprim; Verapamil

Increased Effect/Toxicity

Dofetilide may increase the levels/effects of: Highest Risk QTc-Prolonging Agents; Lidocaine (Topical)

The levels/effects of Dofetilide may be increased by: AMILoride; Antifungal Agents (Azole Derivatives, Systemic); Cimetidine; Cobicistat; CYP3A4 Inhibitors (Moderate); CYP3A4 Inhibitors (Strong); CYP3A4 Inhibitors (Weak); Dolutegravir; Fingolimod; Ivabradine; LamoTRIgine; Lidocaine (Topical); Loop Diuretics; Megestrol; MetFORMIN; Mifepristone; Moderate Risk QTc-Prolonging Agents; Prochlorperazine; Propafenone; QTc-Prolonging Agents (Indeterminate Risk and Risk Modifying); Saquinavir; Thiazide Diuretics; Triamterene; Trimethoprim; Verapamil

Decreased Effect There are no known significant interactions involving a decrease in effect.

Mechanism of Action Vaughan Williams Class III antiarrhythmic activity. Blockade of the cardiac ion channel carrying the rapid component of the delayed rectifier potassium current. Dofetilide has no effect on sodium channels, adrenergic alpha-receptors, or adrenergic beta-receptors. It increases the monophasic action potential duration due to delayed repolarization. The increase in the QT interval is a function of prolongation of both effective and functional refractory periods in the His-Purkinje system and the ventricles. Changes in cardiac conduction velocity and sinus node function have not been

observed in patients with or without structural heart disease. PR and QRS width remain the same in patients with preexisting heart block and or sick sinus syndrome.

Pharmacodynamics/Kinetics

Absorption: Well absorbed

Distribution: V_d: 3 L/kg

Protein binding: 60% to 70%

Metabolism: Hepatic via CYP3A4, but low affinity for it; metabolites formed by N-dealkylation and N-oxidation

Bioavailability: >90%

Half-life elimination: ~10 hours; prolonged with renal impairment

Time to peak, serum: Fasting: 2-3 hours

Excretion: Urine (80%; 80% as unchanged drug, 20% as inactive or minimally active metabolites); renal elimination consists of glomerular filtration and active tubular secretion via cationic transport system

Dosing

Adult Note: QT or QTc must be determined prior to first dose. If QTc >440 msec (>500 msec in patients with ventricular conduction abnormalities), dofetilide is contraindicated.

Atrial fibrillation/atrial flutter: Oral:

Initial: 500 mcg twice daily. Initial dosage must be adjusted in patients with estimated CrCl <60 mL/minute (see Dosage Adjustment in Renal Impairment). Dofetilide may be initiated at lower doses than recommended based on physician discretion.

Modification of dosage in response to initial dose: QTc interval should be measured 2 to 3 hours after the initial dose. If the QTc increases to more than 15% above baseline QTc or if the QTc is >500 msec (>550 msec in patients with ventricular conduction abnormalities), dofetilide dose should be reduced. If the starting dose was 500 mcg twice daily, then reduce to 250 mcg twice daily. If the starting dose was 250 mcg twice daily, then reduce to 125 mcg twice daily. If the starting dose was 125 mcg twice daily, then reduce to 125 mcg once daily. If at any time after the second dose is given the QTc is >500 msec (>550 msec in patients with ventricular conduction abnormalities), dofetilide should be discontinued.

Geriatric Refer to adult dosing. No specific dosage adjustments are recommended based on age; however, careful assessment of renal function is particularly important in this population.

Renal Impairment Note: Using the Modification of Diet in Renal Disease (MDRD) equation and subsequent eGFR to determine dose may lead to overestimation of creatinine clearance and overdose of medication; use only the Cockcroft-Gault equation to estimate creatinine clearance (Denetclaw, 2011). Use actual body weight when using the Cockcroft-Gault equation to calculate creatinine clearance (weight range of patients enrolled in clinical trials: 40-134 kg).

CrCl >60 mL/minute: Administer 500 mcg twice daily.

CrCl 40-60 mL/minute: Administer 250 mcg twice daily.

CrCl 20-39 mL/minute: Administer 125 mcg twice daily.

CrCl <20 mL/minute: Contraindicated.

Hepatic Impairment No dosage adjustments required in Child-Pugh class A and B; patients with severe hepatic impairment were not studied.

Monitoring Parameters ECG monitoring with attention to QT (if heart rate <60 beats per minute) or QTc and occurrence of ventricular arrhythmias, baseline serum creatinine and changes in serum creatinine. Upon initiation (or reinitiation) continuous ECG monitoring recommended for a minimum of 3 days, or for at least 12 hours after electrical or pharmacological conversion to normal sinus rhythm, whichever is greater. Check serum potassium and magnesium levels at baseline and throughout therapy especially if on medications where these electrolyte disturbances can occur, or if patient has a history of hypokalemia or hypomagnesemia. QT or QTc must be monitored at baseline prior to the first dose and 2-3 hours afterwards. If at baseline, QTc >440 msec (>500 msec in patients with ventricular conduction abnormalities), dofetilide is contraindicated. If dofetilide initiated, QTc interval must be determined 2-3 hours after each subsequent dose of dofetilide for in-hospital doses 2-5. Thereafter, QT or QTc and creatinine clearance should be evaluated every 3 months. If at any time during therapy after the second dose the measured QTc is >500 msec (>550 msec in patients with ventricular conduction abnormalities), dofetilide should be discontinued.

Consult individual institutional policies and procedures.

Dosage Forms Excipient information presented when available (limited, particularly for generics); consult specific product labeling.

Capsule, Oral:

Tikosyn: 125 mcg, 250 mcg, 500 mcg

◆ DOK [OTC] *see* Docusate *on page 578*

◆ Dok Plus [OTC] *see* Docusate and Senna *on page 579*

Dolasetron (dol A se tron)

Brand Names: US Anzemet
Brand Names: Canada Anzemet
Index Terms Dolasetron Mesylate; MDL 73,147EF
Pharmacologic Category Antiemetic; Selective 5-HT$_3$ Receptor Antagonist
Use

U.S. labeling:

Injection: Prevention and treatment of postoperative nausea and vomiting in adults and children ≥2 years

Oral: Prevention of nausea and vomiting associated with moderately emetogenic cancer chemotherapy (initial and repeat courses) in adults and children ≥2 years

Canadian labeling: Oral: Prevention of nausea and vomiting associated with emetogenic cancer chemotherapy (initial and repeat courses)

Pregnancy Considerations Adverse events have not been observed in animal reproduction studies.

Breast-Feeding Considerations It is not known if dolasetron is excreted in breast milk. The manufacturer recommends that caution be exercised when administering dolasetron to nursing women.

Contraindications

U.S. labeling:

Injection: Hypersensitivity to dolasetron or any component of the formulation; intravenous administration is contraindicated when used for prevention of chemotherapy-associated nausea and vomiting

Tablet: Hypersensitivity to dolasetron or any component of the formulation

Canadian labeling: Hypersensitivity to dolasetron or any component of the formulation; use in children and adolescents <18 years of age; use for the prevention or treatment of postoperative nausea and vomiting; concomitant use with apomorphine

Warnings/Precautions Dolasetron is associated with a number of dose-dependent increases in ECG intervals (eg, PR, QRS duration, QT/QTc, JT), usually occurring 1-2 hours after IV administration and usually lasting 6-8 hours; however, may last ≥24 hours and rarely lead to heart block or arrhythmia. Clinically relevant QT-interval prolongation may occur resulting in torsade de pointes, when used in conjunction with other agents that prolong the QT interval (eg, Class I and III antiarrhythmics). Avoid use in patients at greater risk for QT prolongation (eg, patients with congenital long QT syndrome, medications known to prolong QT interval, electrolyte abnormalities, and cumulative high-dose anthracycline therapy) and/or ventricular arrhythmia. Correct potassium or magnesium abnormalities prior to initiating therapy. IV formulations of 5-HT$_3$ antagonists have more association with ECG interval changes, compared to oral formulations. Reduction in heart rate may also occur with the 5-HT$_3$ antagonists. Use with caution in children and adolescents who have or may develop QTc prolongation; rare cases of supraventricular and ventricular arrhythmias, cardiac arrest, and MI have been reported in this population. ECG monitoring is recommended in patients with renal impairment and in the elderly.

Serotonin syndrome has been reported with 5-HT$_3$ receptor antagonists, predominantly when used in combination with other serotonergic agents (eg, SSRIs, SNRIs, MAOIs, mirtazapine, fentanyl, lithium, tramadol, and/or methylene blue). Some of the cases have been fatal. The majority of serotonin syndrome reports due to 5-HT$_3$ receptor antagonist have occurred in a post-anesthesia setting or in an infusion center. Serotonin syndrome has also been reported following overdose of another 5-HT$_3$ receptor antagonist. Monitor patients for signs of serotonin syndrome, including mental status changes (eg, agitation, hallucinations, delirium, coma); autonomic instability (eg, tachycardia, labile blood pressure, diaphoresis, dizziness, flushing, hyperthermia); neuromuscular changes (eg, tremor, rigidity, myoclonus, hyperreflexia, incoordination); gastrointestinal symptoms (eg, nausea, vomiting, diarrhea); and/or seizures. If serotonin syndrome occurs, discontinue 5-HT$_3$ receptor antagonist treatment and begin supportive management.

Use with caution in patients allergic to other 5-HT$_3$ receptor antagonists; cross-reactivity has been reported with other 5-HT$_3$ receptor antagonists. **For chemotherapy-associated nausea and vomiting, should be used on a scheduled basis, not on an "as needed" (PRN) basis,** since data support the use of this drug only in the prevention of nausea and vomiting (due to antineoplastic therapy) and not in the rescue of nausea and vomiting. Not intended for treatment of nausea and vomiting or for chronic continuous therapy. If the prophylaxis dolasetron dose for postoperative nausea and vomiting has failed, a repeat dose should not be administered as rescue or treatment for postoperative nausea and vomiting. Potentially significant drug-drug interactions may exist, requiring dose or frequency adjustment, additional monitoring, and/or selection of alternative therapy.

Some dosage forms may contain polysorbate 80 (also known as Tweens). Hypersensitivity reactions, usually a delayed reaction, have been reported following exposure to pharmaceutical products containing polysorbate 80 in certain individuals (Isaksson, 2002; Lucente 2000; Shelley, 1995). Thrombocytopenia, ascites, pulmonary deterioration, and renal and hepatic failure have been reported in premature neonates after receiving parenteral products containing polysorbate 80 (Alade, 1986; CDC, 1984). See manufacturer's labeling.

Adverse Reactions Adverse events may vary according to indication and route of administration.

>10%: Central nervous system: Headache (oral: 18% to 23%; IV: 9%)

1% to 10%:

Cardiovascular: Bradycardia (4% to 5%; may be severe after IV administration), tachycardia (≤3%), edema (<2%), facial edema (<2%), flushing (<2%), hypotension (<2%; may be severe after IV administration), orthostatic hypotension (<2%), peripheral edema (<2%), peripheral ischemia (<2%), phlebitis (<2%), sinus arrhythmia (<2%), thrombophlebitis (<2%)

Central nervous system: Fatigue (oral: 3% to 6%), dizziness (1% to 6%), pain (≤3%), abnormal dreams (<2%), agitation (<2%), anxiety (<2%), ataxia (<2%), chills (≤2%), confusion (<2%), depersonalization (<2%), paresthesia (<2%), shivering (≤2%), sleep disorder (<2%), twitching (<2%), vertigo (<2%)

Dermatologic: Diaphoresis (<2%), skin rash (<2%), urticaria (<2%)

Endocrine & metabolic: Increased gamma-glutamyl transferase (<2%)

Gastrointestinal: Diarrhea (oral: 2% to 5%), dyspepsia (≤3%), abdominal pain (<2%), anorexia (<2%), constipation (<2%), dysgeusia (<2%), pancreatitis (<2%)

Genitourinary: Dysuria (<2%), hematuria (<2%)

Hematologic and oncologic: Anemia (<2%), hematoma (<2%), prolonged prothrombin time (<2%), prolonged partial thromboplastin time (<2%), purpura (<2%), thrombocytopenia (<2%)

Hepatic: Hyperbilirubinemia (<2%), increased serum alkaline phosphatase (<2%)

Hypersensitivity: Anaphylaxis (<2%)

Local: Burning sensation at injection site (IV: <2%), pain at injection site (IV: <2%)

Neuromuscular & skeletal: Arthralgia (<2%), myalgia (<2%), tremor (<2%)

Ophthalmic: Photophobia (<2%), visual disturbance (<2%)

Otic: Tinnitus (<2%)

Renal: Acute renal failure (<2%), polyuria (<2%)

Respiratory: Bronchospasm (<2%), dyspnea (<2%), epistaxis (<2%)

<1% (Limited to important or life-threatening): Abnormal T waves on ECG, appearance of U waves on ECG, atrial fibrillation, atrioventricular block, bundle branch block (left and right), chest pain, extrasystoles (APCs or VPCs), increased serum ALT (transient), increased serum AST (transient), ischemic heart disease, nodal arrhythmia, prolongation P-R interval on ECG (dose-dependent), prolonged Q-T interval on ECG, serotonin syndrome, slow R wave progression, ST segment changes on ECG, supraventricular cardiac arrhythmia, syncope (may be severe after IV administration), torsades de pointes, ventricular arrhythmia (may be serious), ventricular fibrillation cardiac arrest (intravenous), wide complex tachycardia (intravenous), widened QRS complex on ECG (dose-dependent)

Drug Interactions

Metabolism/Transport Effects Substrate of CYP2C9 (minor), CYP3A4 (minor); **Note:** Assignment of Major/Minor substrate status based on clinically relevant drug interaction potential; **Inhibits** CYP2D6 (weak)

Avoid Concomitant Use

Avoid concomitant use of Dolasetron with any of the following: Apomorphine; Highest Risk QTc-Prolonging Agents; Ivabradine; Mequitazine; Mifepristone

Increased Effect/Toxicity

Dolasetron may increase the levels/effects of: Apomorphine; ARIPiprazole; Highest Risk QTc-Prolonging Agents; Mequitazine; Moderate Risk QTc-Prolonging Agents; Panobinostat; Serotonin Modulators ▶

The levels/effects of Dolasetron may be increased by: Ivabradine; Mifepristone; QTc-Prolonging Agents (Indeterminate Risk and Risk Modifying)

Decreased Effect

Dolasetron may decrease the levels/effects of: Tapentadol; TraMADol

Food Interactions Food does not affect the bioavailability of oral doses.

Preparation for Administration May be administered undiluted, or diluted in 50 mL of a compatible solution (ie, 0.9% NS, D_5W, $D_5^1/_2NS$, D_5LR, LR, and 10% mannitol injection).

Storage/Stability

Injection: Store intact vials at 20°C to 25°C (68°F to 77°F); excursions are permitted to 15°C to 30°C (59°F to 86°F). Protect from light. Solutions diluted for infusion are stable under normal lighting conditions at room temperature for 24 hours or under refrigeration for 48 hours.

Tablets: Store at 20°C to 25°C (68°F to 77°F). Protect from light.

Mechanism of Action Selective serotonin receptor (5-HT$_3$) antagonist, blocking serotonin both peripherally (primary site of action) and centrally at the chemoreceptor trigger zone

Pharmacodynamics/Kinetics

Absorption: Oral: Rapid and complete

Distribution: Hydrodolasetron: Children: 5.9 to 7.4 L/kg; Adults: 5.8 L/kg

Protein binding: Hydrodolasetron: 69% to 77% (50% bound to alpha$_1$-acid glycoprotein)

Metabolism: Hepatic; rapid reduction by carbonyl reductase to hydrodolasetron (active metabolite); further metabolized by CYP2D6, CYP3A, and flavin monooxygenase

Bioavailability: Oral: Not affected by food; Children: 59% (formulation not specified); Adults: ~75%

Half-life elimination:

Dolasetron: IV: ≤10 minutes

Hydrodolasetron:

Oral: Children: 5.5 hours; Adolescents: 6.4 hours; Adults: 8.1 hours

IV: Children: 4.8 hours; Adults: 7.3 hours

Severe renal impairment: 11 hours

Severe hepatic impairment: 11 hours

Time to peak, plasma: Hydrodolasetron: IV: 0.6 hours; Oral: ~1 hour

Excretion: Urine ~67% (dolasetron: <1% excreted unchanged in urine; hydrodolasetron: 53% to 61% of the total dose); Feces ~33%

Dosing

Adult & Geriatric Note: Use of intravenous dolasetron is contraindicated for the prevention of chemotherapy induced nausea and vomiting. In Canada, use of dolasetron is also contraindicated in the prevention and treatment of postoperative nausea and vomiting in adults.

U.S. labeling:

Prevention of chemotherapy-associated nausea and vomiting (including initial and repeat courses): Oral: 100 mg within 1 hour before chemotherapy

Postoperative nausea and vomiting:

Prevention: IV: 12.5 mg ~15 minutes before cessation of anesthesia (do not exceed the recommended dose)

Treatment: IV: 12.5 mg as soon as nausea or vomiting present (do not exceed the recommended dose)

Canadian labeling: **Prevention of chemotherapy-associated nausea and vomiting (including initial and repeat courses):** Adults: Oral: 100 mg within 1 hour before chemotherapy

Pediatric Note: In Canada, use of dolasetron is contraindicated in children and adolescents <18 years of age.

Prevention of chemotherapy-associated nausea and vomiting (including initial and repeat courses): Children 2-16 years: Oral: 1.8 mg/kg within 1 hour before chemotherapy; maximum: 100 mg/dose

Postoperative nausea and vomiting: Children 2-16 years:

Prevention:

Oral: 1.2 mg/kg within 2 hours before surgery; maximum: 100 mg/dose

IV: 0.35 mg/kg ~15 minutes before cessation of anesthesia; maximum: 12.5 mg/dose

Treatment:

IV: 0.35 mg/kg as soon as nausea or vomiting present; maximum: 12.5 mg/dose

Renal Impairment No dosage adjustment necessary; however, ECG monitoring is recommended in patients with renal impairment.

Hepatic Impairment No dosage adjustment necessary.

Administration

IV injection may be given either undiluted as an IV push over 30 seconds or diluted in 50 mL of compatible fluid and infused over 15 minutes. Flush line before and after dolasetron administration.

Oral: When unable to administer in tablet form, dolasetron injection may be diluted in apple or apple-grape juice and taken orally; this dilution is stable for 2 hours at room temperature (Anzemet prescribing information, 2013).

Monitoring Parameters ECG (in patients with cardiovascular disease, elderly, renally impaired, those at risk of developing hypokalemia and/or hypomagnesemia); potassium, magnesium

Additional Information Efficacy of dolasetron, for chemotherapy treatment, is enhanced with concomitant administration of dexamethasone 20 mg (increases complete response by 10% to 20%). Oral administration of the intravenous solution is equivalent to tablets.

Dosage Forms Excipient information presented when available (limited, particularly for generics); consult specific product labeling.

Solution, Intravenous, as mesylate:

Anzemet: 20 mg/mL (0.625 mL, 5 mL, 25 mL)

Tablet, Oral, as mesylate:

Anzemet: 50 mg, 100 mg

Extemporaneous Preparations Dolasetron injection may be diluted in apple or apple-grape juice and taken orally; this dilution is stable for 2 hours at room temperature (Anzemet prescribing information, 2013).

A 10 mg/mL oral suspension may be prepared with tablets and either a 1:1 mixture of Ora-Plus and Ora-Sweet SF or a 1:1 mixture of strawberry syrup and Ora-Plus. Crush twelve 50 mg tablets in a mortar and reduce to a fine powder. Slowly add chosen vehicle to **almost** 60 mL; transfer to a calibrated bottle, rinse mortar with vehicle, and add quantity of vehicle sufficient to make 60 mL. Label "shake well" and "refrigerate". Stable for 90 days refrigerated.

Anzemet® prescribing information, sanofi-aventis U.S. LLC, Bridgewater, NJ; 2013.

Johnson CE, Wagner DS, and Bussard WE, "Stability of Dolasetron in Two Oral Liquid Vehicles," *Am J Health Syst Pharm*, 2003, 60 (21):2242-4.

Donepezil (doh NEP e zil)

Brand Names: US Aricept; Aricept ODT [DSC]

Brand Names: Canada Accel-Donepezil; ACT-Donepezil; ACT-Donepezil ODT; Apo-Donepezil; Aricept; Aricept RDT; Auro-Donepezil; Bio-Donepezil; JAMP-Donepezil; Mar-Donepezil; Mylan-Donepezil; PMS-Donepezil; RAN-Donepezil; Riva-Donepezil; Sandoz-Donepezil; Sandoz-Donepezil ODT; Septa Donepezil; Teva-Donepezil

Index Terms E2020

Pharmacologic Category Acetylcholinesterase Inhibitor (Central)

Use Alzheimer disease: Treatment of mild, moderate, or severe dementia of the Alzheimer type

Pregnancy Considerations Adverse events have been observed in some animal reproduction studies.

Breast-Feeding Considerations It is not known if donepezil is excreted in breast milk. The manufacturer recommends that caution be used if administered to a nursing woman.

Contraindications

Hypersensitivity to donepezil, piperidine derivatives, or any component of the formulation

Documentation of allergenic cross-reactivity for drugs in this class is limited. However, because of similarities in chemical structure and/or pharmacologic actions, the possibility of cross-sensitivity cannot be ruled out with certainty.

Warnings/Precautions Donepezil may be associated with QTc prolongation and torsades de pointes; use with caution in patients at risk of prolonged cardiac repolarization (Howes, 2014). Cholinesterase inhibitors may have vagotonic effects which may cause bradycardia and/or heart block in patients with or without a history of cardiac disease; syncopal episodes have been associated with donepezil. Use with caution in patients with sick-sinus syndrome, bradycardia, or conduction abnormalities. Alzheimer treatment guidelines consider bradycardia to be a relative contraindication for use of centrally-active cholinesterase inhibitors (APA [Rabins 2007]). Use with caution with COPD or asthma. Use with caution in patients with a history of seizure disorder; cholinomimetics may potentially cause generalized seizures, although seizure activity may also result from Alzheimer disease. Use with caution in patients at risk of ulcer disease (eg, previous history or NSAID use); cholinesterase inhibitors may increase gastric acid secretion; monitor for symptoms of bleeding. Use with caution in patients with bladder outlet obstruction or prostatic hyperplasia; cholinomimetics may cause or worsen outflow obstructions, including possible exacerbation of ▶

BPH symptoms (APA [Rabins 2007]). May cause dose-related diarrhea, nausea, and/or vomiting, which usually resolves in 1 to 3 weeks. May cause anorexia and/or weight loss (dose-related). Patients weighing <55 kg may experience more nausea, vomiting, and weight loss than patients ≥55 kg.

Rare cases of neuroleptic malignant syndrome (NMS) have been reported (Matsumoto 2004; Warwick 2008). Discontinuation of donepezil therapy may be necessary in patients presenting with symptoms of NMS or unexplained high fever without additional symptoms. Rare cases of rhabdomyolysis (including acute renal failure) have been reported after a few months of therapy (Sahin 2014) or in the days following therapy initiation and dose increase (Aricept Canadian product monograph 2014). Use with caution in patients with risk factors for rhabdomyolysis. Discontinuation of therapy may be necessary for marked elevation of CPK levels and/or symptoms (eg, muscle pain, tenderness or weakness, malaise, fever, dark urine) suggesting rhabdomyolysis. Potentially significant interactions may exist, requiring dose or frequency adjustment, additional monitoring, and/or selection of alternative therapy.

Adverse Reactions

>10%:
Central nervous system: Insomnia (2% to 14%)
Gastrointestinal: Nausea (3% to 19%; dose related), diarrhea (5% to 15%; dose related)
Infection: Infection (11%)
Miscellaneous: Accidental injury (7% to 13%)

1% to 10%:
Cardiovascular: Hypertension (3%), chest pain (2%), syncope (2%), atrial fibrillation (≥1%), bradycardia (≥1%), cardiac failure (≥1%), ECG abnormality (≥1%), edema (≥1%), hypotension (≥1%), peripheral edema (≥1%), vasodilation (≥1%)

Central nervous system: Headache (3% to 10%), pain (3% to 9%), dizziness (2% to 8%), fatigue (1% to 8%), abnormal dreams (3%), hallucination (3%), hostility (3%), depression (2% to 3%), nervousness (1% to 3%), confusion (2%), drowsiness (2%), emotional lability (2%), personality disorder (2%), abnormal crying (≥1%), abnormal gait (≥1%), aggressive behavior (≥1%), agitation (≥1%), anxiety (≥1%), aphasia (≥1%), ataxia (≥1%), convulsions (≥1%), delusions (≥1%), irritability (≥1%), paresthesia (≥1%), restlessness (≥1%), vertigo (≥1%), wandering (≥1%)

Dermatologic: Ecchymosis (4% to 5%), eczema (3%), dermal ulcer (≥1%), diaphoresis (≥1%), pruritus (≥1%), skin rash (≥1%), urticaria (≥1%)

Endocrine & metabolic: Weight loss (3% to 5%; dose related), hyperlipidemia (2%), dehydration (1% to 2%), glycosuria (≥1%), hot flash (≥1%), increased lactate dehydrogenase (≥1%), increased libido (≥1%)

Gastrointestinal: Vomiting (3% to 9%; dose related), anorexia (2% to 8%), abdominal pain (≥1%), bloating (≥1%), constipation (≥1%), dyspepsia (≥1%), epigastric pain (≥1%), fecal incontinence (≥1%), gastroenteritis (≥1%), gastrointestinal hemorrhage (≥1%), sore throat (≥1%), toothache (≥1%)

Genitourinary: Urinary incontinence (1% to 3%), urinary frequency (2%), cystitis (≥1%), hematuria (≥1%), nocturia (≥1%), urinary tract infection (≥1%)

Hematologic & oncologic: Bruise (2%), hemorrhage (2%), anemia (≥1%)

Hepatic: Increased serum alkaline phosphatase (≥1%)

Infection: Fungal infection (≥1%), influenza (≥1%)

Neuromuscular & skeletal: Muscle cramps (3% to 8%), back pain (3%), increased creatine phosphokinase (3%), arthritis (1% to 2%), weakness (1% to 2%), bone fracture (≥1%), tremor (≥1%)

Ophthalmic: Blurred vision (≥1%), cataract (≥1%), eye irritation (≥1%)

Respiratory: Bronchitis (≥1%), dyspnea (≥1%), flu-like symptoms (≥1%), increased cough (≥1%), pharyngitis (≥1%), pneumonia (≥1%)

Miscellaneous: Fever (2%)

<1% (Limited to important or life-threatening): Abnormal hepatic function tests, abnormal lacrimation, abnormal vision, abscess, albuminuria, alopecia, angina pectoris, apathy, arteritis, arthralgia, asthma, atelectasis, atrophic striae, benign prostatic hypertrophy, blepharitis, breast fibroadenosis, cachexia, cardiomegaly, cellulitis, cerebral hemorrhage, cerebral infarction, cerebral ischemia, cerebrovascular accident, chills, cholecystitis, cholelithiasis, conjunctival hemorrhage, conjunctivitis, convulsions, decreased libido, deep vein thrombosis, dementia, dermatitis, diverticulitis, duodenal ulcer, dysarthria, dysgeusia, dysphagia, dysphoria, dysuria, eosinophilia, epigastric distress, epistaxis, eructation, erythema, erythrocytopenia, esophagitis, euphoria, extrapyramidal reaction, facial edema, fasciculations, fibrocystic breast

changes, first degree atrioventricular block, fungal dermatitis, gastritis, gastric ulcer, gingivitis, glaucoma, goiter, gout, hearing loss, heart block, hemiplegia, hemolytic anemia, hepatitis, hernia, herpes zoster, hiatal hernia, hirsutism, hyperbilirubinemia, hyperglycemia, hyperkeratosis, hypersensitivity reaction, hypertonia, hypokalemia, hypokinesia, hyponatremia, hypoproteinemia, hypoxia, increased appetite, increased blood urea nitrogen, increased gamma-glutamyl transferase, increased postvoid residual urine volume, increased serum creatinine, intestinal obstruction, intracranial hemorrhage, iron deficiency anemia, irritable bowel syndrome, jaundice, leg cramps, leukocytosis, localized coldness, localized numbness, malaise, mastitis, melena, myalgia, myasthenia, myocardial infarction, neuralgia, neurodermatitis, neuroleptic malignant syndrome, night sweats, nystagmus, orthostatic hypotension, osteoporosis, otitis externa, otitis media, pacing, pancreatitis, paranoia, peptic ulcer disease, periodontal abscess, periodontitis, periorbital edema, peripheral vascular disease, pleurisy, polydipsia, prolonged Q-T interval on ECG, psoriasis, pulmonary congestion, pyelonephritis, pyuria, rectal hemorrhage, renal failure, retinal hemorrhage, rhabdomyolysis, rhinitis, seeing spots, sensation of cold, sepsis, severe depression, sialorrhea, skin discoloration, sleep apnea, supraventricular extrasystole, supraventricular tachycardia, thrombocythemia, thrombocytopenia, tinnitus, tongue edema, tonic-clonic seizures, torsades de pointes, transient ischemic attacks, unsociability, urinary urgency, uterine hemorrhage, vaginitis, vasodilation, ventricular premature contractions, ventricular tachycardia, vertigo, vesiculobullous dermatitis, vitamin B12 deficiency anemia, weight gain, wheezing, xeroderma, xerophthalmia, xerostomia

Drug Interactions

Metabolism/Transport Effects Substrate of CYP2D6 (minor), CYP3A4 (minor); **Note:** Assignment of Major/Minor substrate status based on clinically relevant drug interaction potential

Avoid Concomitant Use
Avoid concomitant use of Donepezil with any of the following: Ceritinib

Increased Effect/Toxicity
Donepezil may increase the levels/effects of: Antipsychotic Agents; Beta-Blockers; Bradycardia-Causing Agents; Ceritinib; Cholinergic Agonists; Ivabradine; Lacosamide; Succinylcholine

The levels/effects of Donepezil may be increased by: Bretylium; Corticosteroids (Systemic); Ruxolitinib; Tofacitinib

Decreased Effect
Donepezil may decrease the levels/effects of: Anticholinergic Agents; Neuromuscular-Blocking Agents (Nondepolarizing)

The levels/effects of Donepezil may be decreased by: Anticholinergic Agents; Dipyridamole

Storage/Stability Store at 15°C to 30°C (59°F to 86°F).

Mechanism of Action Alzheimer's disease is characterized by cholinergic deficiency in the cortex and basal forebrain, which contributes to cognitive deficits. Donepezil reversibly and noncompetitively inhibits centrally-active acetylcholinesterase, the enzyme responsible for hydrolysis of acetylcholine. This appears to result in increased concentrations of acetylcholine available for synaptic transmission in the central nervous system.

Pharmacodynamics/Kinetics

Absorption: Well absorbed
Distribution: V_{dss}: 12 to 16 L/kg
Protein binding: ~96%, primarily to albumin (75%) and alpha$_1$-acid glycoprotein (21%)
Metabolism: Extensive hepatic metabolism via CYP2D6 and 3A4 and glucuronidation to four major metabolites (two are active)
Half-life elimination: 70 hours; time to steady-state: 15 days
Time to peak, plasma: Tablet, 10 mg: 3 hours; Tablet, 23 mg: ~8 hours; **Note:** Peak plasma concentrations almost twofold higher for the 23 mg tablet compared to the 10 mg tablet
Excretion: Urine (57%; 17% as unchanged drug); feces (15%)

Dosing

Adult

Alzheimer dementia: Oral:
Mild-to-moderate: Initial: 5 mg once daily; may increase to 10 mg once daily after 4 to 6 weeks; effective dosage range in clinical studies: 5 to 10 mg/day

Moderate-to-severe: Initial: 5 mg once daily; may increase to 10 mg once daily after 4 to 6 weeks; may increase further to 23 mg once daily after ≥3 months; effective dosage range in clinical studies: 10 to 23 mg/day

Dementia associated with Parkinson disease (off-label use): 5 mg once daily; may increase to 10 mg once daily after 4 to 6 weeks; may increase further to 23 mg once daily after the use of 10 mg once daily ≥3 months (APA [Rabins 2007]); Dubois 2012)

Lewy body dementia (off-label use): Initial: 3 mg once daily for 2 weeks, then increase to 5 mg once daily. After 4 weeks may further increase dose based on response and tolerability up to 10 mg once daily (Ikeda 2013; Mori 2012)

Geriatric Refer to adult dosing. **Note:** The Canadian labeling recommends a maximum dose of 5 mg once daily in elderly women (≥85 years of age) of low body weight.

Renal Impairment There are no dosage adjustments provided in the manufacturer's labeling. Limited data suggest severe renal impairment does not adversely affect donepezil clearance.

Hepatic Impairment There are no dosage adjustments provided in the manufacturer's labeling.

Dietary Considerations May take with or without food.

Administration Administer at bedtime without regard to food.

Aricept 23 mg tablet: Swallow whole with water; do **NOT** crush or chew due to an increased rate of absorption. The 23 mg strength is provided in a unique film-coated formulation different from the 5 mg or 10 mg tablet strengths, which results in an altered pharmacokinetic profile.

Aricept ODT: Allow tablet to dissolve completely on tongue and follow with water.

Monitoring Parameters Mental status, weight, symptoms of GI intolerance, symptoms of active or occult GI bleeding.

Dosage Forms Excipient information presented when available (limited, particularly for generics); consult specific product labeling. [DSC] = Discontinued product

Tablet, Oral, as hydrochloride:
Aricept: 5 mg, 10 mg, 23 mg
Generic: 5 mg, 10 mg, 23 mg
Tablet Dispersible, Oral, as hydrochloride:
Aricept ODT: 5 mg [DSC], 10 mg [DSC]
Generic: 5 mg, 10 mg

◆ Donnatal® see Hyoscyamine, Atropine, Scopolamine, and Phenobarbital on page 900

◆ Donnatal Extentabs® see Hyoscyamine, Atropine, Scopolamine, and Phenobarbital on page 900

DOPamine (DOE pa meen)

Index Terms Dopamine Hydrochloride; Intropin
Pharmacologic Category Adrenergic Agonist Agent; Inotrope
Additional Appendix Information
Adult ACLS Algorithms on page 1993
Use Adjunct in the treatment of shock (eg, MI, open heart surgery, renal failure, cardiac decompensation) that persists after adequate fluid volume replacement

American College of Cardiology/American Heart Association heart failure (HF) guideline recommendations (ACCF/AHA [Yancy 2013]): To maintain systemic perfusion and preserve end-organ performance in patients with cardiogenic shock; bridge therapy in stage D HF unresponsive to guideline-directed medical therapy and device therapy in patients awaiting heart transplant or mechanical circulatory support; short-term management of hospitalized patients with severe systolic dysfunction presenting with low blood pressure and significantly depressed cardiac output; long-term management (palliative therapy) in select patients with stage D HF unresponsive to guideline-directed medical therapy and device therapy who are not candidates for heart transplant or mechanical circulatory support.

Low-dose dopamine may be considered in combination with diuretic therapy to facilitate diuresis and preserve renal function and renal blood flow in those with acute decompensated HF (ACCF/AHA Yancy 2013). Data published after the release of these guidelines confirm prior evidence that the use of low-dose dopamine does not improve renal function or congestive symptoms when used in combination with diuretic therapy in this population (Chen 2013; Triposkiadis 2014).

Pregnancy Considerations Adverse events have been observed in some animal reproduction studies. It is not known if dopamine crosses the placenta. In general, medications used for ACLS in pregnant women are given at the same dose as nonpregnant patients (AHA [Vanden Hoek] 2010).

Breast-Feeding Considerations It is not known if dopamine is excreted in breast milk. The manufacturer recommends that caution be exercised when administering dopamine to nursing women.

Contraindications Hypersensitivity to sulfites (commercial preparation contains sodium bisulfite); pheochromocytoma; uncorrected tachyarrhythmias; ventricular fibrillation

Warnings/Precautions Use with caution in patients with cardiovascular disease or cardiac arrhythmias or patients with occlusive vascular disease. Assure adequate circulatory volume to minimize need for vasoconstrictors when used in hemodynamic support. Avoid hypertension; monitor blood pressure closely and adjust infusion rate. May cause increases in heart rate, increasing the risk of tachycardia and other tachyarrhythmias including ventricular arrhythmias (Tisdale 1995). In heart transplant candidates, institute appropriate measures to protect patient against risks of sudden cardiac death (Young 2000). Correct electrolyte disturbances, especially hypokalemia or hypomagnesemia, prior to use and throughout therapy to minimize the risk of arrhythmias (ACC/AHA/ESC [Zipes 2006]; Tisdale 1995). Use with caution in patients with active myocardial ischemia or recent myocardial infarction; may increase myocardial oxygen consumption. Use has been associated with a higher incidence of adverse events (eg, tachyarrhythmias) in adult patients with shock compared to norepinephrine. Higher 28-day mortality was also seen in patients with septic shock. The 2012 Surviving Sepsis Campaign (SSC) guidelines suggest dopamine use as an alternative to norepinephrine only in patients with low risk of tachyarrhythmias and absolute or relative bradycardia (SCCM [Dellinger 2013]). Use with extreme caution in patients taking MAO inhibitors; prolong hypertension may result from concurrent use. According to the ACCF/AHA 2013 heart failure guidelines, long-term use of intravenous inotropic therapy without a specific indication or for reasons other than palliation is potentially harmful (ACCF/AHA [Yancy 2013]).

Vesicant; ensure proper needle or catheter placement prior to and during infusion. Avoid extravasation; infuse into a large vein if possible. Avoid infusion into leg veins. Watch IV site closely. **[U.S. Boxed Warning]: If extravasation occurs, infiltrate the area with diluted phentolamine (5 to 10 mg in 10 to 15 mL of saline) with a fine hypodermic needle. Phentolamine should be administered as soon as possible after extravasation is noted to prevent sloughing/necrosis.** Product may contain sodium metabisulfite.

Adverse Reactions Frequency not defined.
Cardiovascular: Angina pectoris, atrial fibrillation, bradycardia, ectopic beats, hypertension, hypotension, palpitations, tachycardia, vasoconstriction, ventricular arrhythmia, ventricular conduction, widened QRS complex on ECG
Central nervous system: Anxiety, headache
Dermatologic: Gangrene (high dose), piloerection
Endocrine & metabolic: Increased serum glucose (usually not above normal limits)
Gastrointestinal: Nausea, vomiting
Genitourinary: Azotemia
Ophthalmic: Increased intraocular pressure, mydriasis
Renal: Polyuria
Respiratory: Dyspnea
Miscellaneous: Tissue necrosis
Drug Interactions
Metabolism/Transport Effects Substrate of COMT, OCT2
Avoid Concomitant Use
Avoid concomitant use of DOPamine with any of the following: Ergot Derivatives; Inhalational Anesthetics; Iobenguane I 123; Lurasidone
Increased Effect/Toxicity
DOPamine may increase the levels/effects of: Doxofylline; Lurasidone; Sympathomimetics

The levels/effects of DOPamine may be increased by: AtoMOXetine; Beta-Blockers; BuPROPion; Cannabinoid-Containing Products; COMT Inhibitors; Ergot Derivatives; Hyaluronidase; Inhalational Anesthetics; Linezolid; Serotonin/Norepinephrine Reuptake Inhibitors; Tedizolid; Tricyclic Antidepressants
Decreased Effect
DOPamine may decrease the levels/effects of: Benzylpenicilloyl Polylysine; Iobenguane I 123

The levels/effects of DOPamine may be decreased by: Alpha1-Blockers; Spironolactone

Storage/Stability Protect from light. Solutions that are darker than slightly yellow should not be used.

Mechanism of Action Stimulates both adrenergic and dopaminergic receptors, lower doses are mainly dopaminergic stimulating and produce renal and mesenteric vasodilation; higher doses also are both dopaminergic and beta₁-adrenergic stimulating and produce cardiac stimulation and renal vasodilation; large doses stimulate alpha-adrenergic receptors

Pharmacodynamics/Kinetics Note: Children: Dopamine has exhibited nonlinear kinetics in children; with dose changes, may not achieve steady-state for ~1 hour rather than 20 minutes

Onset of action: Adults: Within 5 minutes

Duration: Adults: <10 minutes

Metabolism: Renal, hepatic, plasma; 75% to inactive metabolites by monoamine oxidase and 25% to norepinephrine (active)

Half-life elimination: ~2 minutes

Excretion: Urine (as metabolites)

Clearance: Neonates: Varies and appears to be age related; clearance is more prolonged with combined hepatic and renal dysfunction

Dosing

Adult & Geriatric

Hemodynamic support: IV infusion:

Manufacturer's labeling: Dosage range: 2 to 20 mcg/kg/minute; titrate to desired response (maximum: 50 mcg/kg/minute; however, doses >20 mcg/kg/minute may not have a beneficial effect on blood pressure and may increase the risk of tachyarrhythmias; infusion may be gradually increased by 5- to 10-mcg/kg/minute increments until optimal response is obtained

ACLS guideline recommendations (to treat hypotension especially if associated with symptomatic bradycardia in the immediate post-cardiac arrest care setting): Initial: 5 to 10 mcg/kg/minute; titrate to effect (AHA [Peberdy 2010])

Note: If dosages >20 to 30 mcg/kg/minute are needed, a more direct-acting vasopressor may be more beneficial (ie, epinephrine, norepinephrine).

Hemodynamic effects of dopamine are dose dependent (however, this is relative and there is overlap of clinical effects between dosing ranges):

Low-dose: 1 to 5 mcg/kg/minute, results in increased renal blood flow and urine output

Intermediate-dose: 5 to 10 mcg/kg/minute, results in increased renal blood flow, heart rate, cardiac contractility, and cardiac output

High-dose: >10 mcg/kg/minute, alpha-adrenergic effects begin to predominate, resulting in vasoconstriction, increased blood pressure, in addition to increased heart rate, cardiac contractility, and cardiac output due to beta-adrenergic effects.

Inotropic support in advanced heart failure: IV infusion: 5 to 15 mcg/kg/minute; lower doses are preferred (ACCF/AHA [Yancy 2013]).

Pediatric

Hemodynamic support: IV infusion:

Manufacturer's labeling: Dosage range: 2 to 20 mcg/kg/minute, titrate to desired response (maximum: 50 mcg/kg/minute; however, doses >20 mcg/kg/minute may not have a beneficial effect on blood pressure and may increase the risk of tachyarrhythmias. Infusion may be gradually increased by 5- to 10-mcg/kg/minute increments until optimal response is obtained.

Pediatric Advanced Life Support (PALS) guideline recommendation (to maintain cardiac output and for postresuscitation stabilization): IV or I.O.: Dose range: 2 to 20 mcg/kg/minute (AHA [Kleinman 2010])

Hemodynamic effects of dopamine are dose dependent (however, this is relative and there is overlap of clinical effects between dosing ranges):

Low-dose: 1 to 5 mcg/kg/minute, results in increased renal blood flow and urine output

Intermediate-dose: 5 to 10 mcg/kg/minute, results in increased renal blood flow, heart rate, cardiac contractility, and cardiac output

High-dose: >10 mcg/kg/minute, alpha-adrenergic effects begin to predominate, resulting in vasoconstriction, increased blood pressure in addition to increased heart rate, cardiac contractility, and cardiac output due to beta-adrenergic effects.

Usual Infusion Concentrations: Pediatric Note: Premixed solutions available.

IV infusion: 1600 mcg/mL or 3200 mcg/mL

Usual Infusion Concentrations: Adult Note: Premixed solutions available.

IV infusion: 400 mg in 250 mL (concentration: 1600 mcg/mL) or 800 mg in 250 mL (concentration: 3200 mcg/mL) of D₅W or NS

Administration Administer as a continuous infusion with the use of an infusion pump. Administer into large vein to prevent the possibility of extravasation (central line administration); monitor continuously for free flow; use infusion device to control rate of flow; administration into an umbilical arterial catheter is not recommended; when discontinuing the infusion, gradually decrease the dose of dopamine (sudden discontinuation may cause hypotension). Vials (concentrated solution) must be diluted prior to use.

Vesicant; ensure proper needle or catheter placement prior to and during infusion; avoid extravasation.

Extravasation management: If extravasation occurs, stop infusion immediately and disconnect (leave cannula/needle in place); gently aspirate extravasated solution (do NOT flush the line); remove needle/cannula; elevate extremity. Initiate phentolamine (or alternative) antidote. Apply dry warm compresses (Hurst 2004).

Phentolamine (no longer available in the US): Dilute 5-10 mg in 10-15 mL NS and administer into extravasation site as soon as possible after extravasation (AHA [Peberdy 2010])

Alternatives to phentolamine:

Nitroglycerin topical 2% ointment (based on limited case reports in neonates/infants): Apply 4 mm/kg as a thin ribbon to the affected areas; may repeat after 8 hours if needed (Wong 1992) or apply a 1-inch strip on the affected site (Denkler 1989)

Terbutaline (based on limited case reports): Infiltrate extravasation area using a solution of terbutaline 1 mg diluted to 10 mL in NS (large extravasation site; administration volume varied from 3-10 mL) or 1 mg diluted in 1 mL NS (small/distal extravasation site; administration volume varied from 0.5-1 mL) (Stier 1999)

Monitoring Parameters Blood pressure, ECG, heart rate, CVP, RAP, MAP; serum glucose, renal function; urine output; if pulmonary artery catheter is in place, monitor CI, PCWP, SVR, and PVR

Consult individual institutional policies and procedures.

Additional Information Dopamine is most frequently used for treatment of hypotension because of its peripheral vasoconstrictor action. In this regard, dopamine is often used together with dobutamine and minimizes hypotension secondary to dobutamine-induced vasodilation. Thus, pressure is maintained by increased cardiac output (from dobutamine) and vasoconstriction (by dopamine). It is critical neither dopamine nor dobutamine be used in patients in the absence of correcting any hypovolemia as a cause of hypotension.

Low-dose dopamine is often used in the intensive care setting for presumed beneficial effects on renal function. However, there is no clear evidence that low-dose dopamine confers any renal or other benefit. Indeed, dopamine may act on dopamine receptors in the carotid bodies causing chemoreflex suppression. In patients with heart failure, dopamine may inhibit breathing and cause pulmonary shunting. Both these mechanisms would act to decrease minute ventilation and oxygen saturation. This could potentially be deleterious in patients with respiratory compromise and patients being weaned from ventilators.

Dosage Forms Excipient information presented when available (limited, particularly for generics); consult specific product labeling. [DSC] = Discontinued product

Solution, Intravenous, as hydrochloride:

Generic: 0.8 mg/mL (250 mL, 500 mL); 1.6 mg/mL (250 mL, 500 mL); 3.2 mg/mL (250 mL); 40 mg/mL (5 mL, 10 mL); 80 mg/mL (5 mL, 10 mL [DSC]); 160 mg/mL (5 mL)

Doripenem (dore i PEN em)

Brand Names: US Doribax

Index Terms S-4661

Pharmacologic Category Antibiotic, Carbapenem

Use Treatment of complicated intra-abdominal infections and complicated urinary tract infections (including pyelonephritis) due to susceptible aerobic gram-positive, aerobic gram-negative (including *Pseudomonas aeruginosa*), and anaerobic bacteria

Pregnancy Considerations Adverse events have not been observed in animal reproduction studies. Information related to use during pregnancy has not been located.

Breast-Feeding Considerations It is not known if doripenem is excreted into breast milk. The manufacturer recommends that caution be exercised when administering doripenem to nursing women.

Contraindications Known serious hypersensitivity to doripenem or other carbapenems (eg, ertapenem, imipenem, meropenem) or any component of the formulation; anaphylactic reactions to beta-lactam antibiotics

Warnings/Precautions Serious hypersensitivity reactions, including anaphylaxis, and skin reactions have been reported in patients receiving beta-lactams. Use may result in fungal or bacterial superinfection, including *C. difficile*-associated diarrhea (CDAD) and pseudomembranous colitis; CDAD has been observed >2 months postantibiotic treatment. Not indicated for the treatment of pneumonia including ventilator-associated pneumonia; decreased efficacy and increased mortality observed in a phase 3 study using a higher dose and fixed 7-day administration (Kollef, 2012). Use with caution in patients with renal impairment; dosage adjustment required in patients with moderate-to-severe renal dysfunction. Carbapenems have been associated with CNS adverse effects, including confusional states and seizures (myoclonic); use caution with CNS disorders (eg, brain lesions, stroke, or history of seizures) and adjust dose in renal impairment to avoid drug accumulation, which may increase seizure risk. Patients receiving doses >500 mg every 8 hours may also be at increased risk of seizures. Potentially significant interactions may exist, requiring dose or frequency adjustment, additional monitoring, and/or selection of alternative therapy. Administer via intravenous infusion only. Per manufacturer's labeling, investigational experience of doripenem via inhalation resulted in pneumonitis.

Adverse Reactions

>10%:

Central nervous system: Headache (3% to 16%)

Gastrointestinal: Diarrhea (6% to 12%), nausea (4% to 12%)

1% to 10%:

Cardiovascular: Phlebitis (2% to 8%)

Dermatologic: Skin rash (2% to 7%; includes allergic/bullous dermatitis, erythema, macular/papular eruptions, urticaria, and erythema multiforme), pruritus (1% to 3%)

Gastrointestinal: Oral candidiasis (1% to 3%), pseudomembranous colitis (≤1%)

Hematologic & oncologic: Anemia (2% to 10%)

Hepatic: Increased serum transaminases (2% to 7%)

Renal: Renal insufficiency (≤1%)

Miscellaneous: Vaginal infection (1% to 2%)

<1% (Limited to important or life-threatening): Anaphylaxis, leukopenia, neutropenia, pneumonia, seizure, Stevens-Johnson syndrome, thrombocytopenia, toxic epidermal necrolysis

Drug Interactions

Metabolism/Transport Effects None known.

Avoid Concomitant Use

Avoid concomitant use of Doripenem with any of the following: BCG (Intravesical); Probenecid

Increased Effect/Toxicity

The levels/effects of Doripenem may be increased by: Probenecid

Decreased Effect

Doripenem may decrease the levels/effects of: BCG (Intravesical); BCG Vaccine (Immunization); Sodium Picosulfate; Typhoid Vaccine; Valproate Products

Preparation for Administration Reconstitute 250 mg vial with 10 mL of SWFI or NS; further dilute for infusion with 50 mL or 100 mL of NS or D$_5$W. Shake gently until clear. Reconstitute 500 mg vial with 10 mL of SWFI or NS; further dilute for infusion with 100 mL of NS or D$_5$W. Shake gently until clear. Reconstituted vial may be stored for up to 1 hour prior to preparation of infusion solution. To prepare a 250 mg dose using a 500 mg vial, reconstitute the 500 mg vial with 10 mL of SWFI or NS and further dilute with 100 mL of compatible solution as above, but remove and discard 55 mL from the infusion bag to leave the remaining solution containing the 250 mg dose.

Storage/Stability Store dry powder vials at 15°C to 30°C (59°F to 86°F). Stability of solution when diluted in NS is 12 hours at room temperature or 72 hours under refrigeration; stability in D$_5$W is 4 hours at room temperature and 24 hours under refrigeration.

Mechanism of Action Inhibits bacterial cell wall synthesis by binding to several of the penicillin-binding proteins (PBP-2, PBP-3, PBP-4), which in turn inhibits the final transpeptidation step of peptidoglycan synthesis in bacterial cell walls, thus inhibiting cell wall biosynthesis; bacteria eventually lyse due to ongoing activity of cell wall autolytic enzymes (autolysins and murein hydrolases) while cell wall assembly is arrested.

Pharmacodynamics/Kinetics Note: As with other time-dependent antibiotics, doripenem shows bacteriostatic effects at T>MIC <40% and bactericidal effects at T>MIC>40%. Of note, prolonged infusion time (over 4 hours) was more effective in increasing T>MIC over 40% to up to 81%. Pharmacokinetics are linear (AUC directly proportional to dose) at doses administered over 1 hour.

Distribution: Penetrates well into body fluids and tissues, including peritoneal and retroperitoneal fluids, gallbladder, bile, and urine

V$_d$: 16.8 L

Protein binding: 8% to 9%

Metabolism: Non-CYP-mediated metabolism via hydrolysis by dehydropeptidase-I to doripenem-M1 (inactive metabolite)

Half-life elimination: ~1 hour

Excretion: Urine (71% as unchanged drug; 15% as doripenem-M1 metabolite); feces (<1%)

Dializable with reduction in systemic levels by 48% to 62%.

Dosing

Adult & Geriatric Note: A switch to appropriate oral antimicrobial therapy may be considered after 3 days of parenteral therapy and demonstrated clinical improvement.

Intra-abdominal infection, complicated, severe: IV: 500 mg every 8 hours for 5-14 days. **Note:** 2010 IDSA guidelines recommend treatment duration of 4-7 days (provided source controlled). Not recommended for mild-to-moderate, community-acquired intra-abdominal infections due to risk of toxicity and the development of resistant organisms (Solomkin, 2010).

Urinary tract infection (complicated) or pyelonephritis: IV: 500 mg every 8 hours for 10-14 days

Intravenous catheter-related bloodstream infection (off-label use): IV: 500 mg every 8 hours for 7-14 days (IDSA, 2009)

Renal Impairment

CrCl >50 mL/minute: No adjustment necessary.

CrCl 30-50 mL/minute: 250 mg every 8 hours

CrCl 11-29 mL/minute: 250 mg every 12 hours

Hemodialysis: Dializable (~52% of dose removed during 4-hour session in ESRD patients)

Intermittent HD: 250 mg every 24 hours; if treating infections caused by *Pseudomonas aeruginosa*, administer 500 mg every 12 hours on day 1, followed by 500 mg every 24 hours (Tanoue, 2011)

CVVHDF: 250 mg every 12 hours (Hidaka, 2010).

Hepatic Impairment There are no dosage adjustments provided in manufacturer's labeling (has not been studied). However, doripenem undergoes minimal hepatic metabolism.

Administration Infuse intravenously over 1 hour. Use of 4-hour infusion has been studied in the treatment of VAP (off-label use) (Chastre, 2008).

Monitoring Parameters Monitor for signs of anaphylaxis during first dose; periodic renal assessment; consider hematologic monitoring during prolonged therapy

Additional Information One mechanism of resistance to doripenem is production of the Ambler's class B metallo-beta-lactamase, a potent carbapenemase produced by *Stenotrophomonas maltophilia*.

Dosage Forms Excipient information presented when available (limited, particularly for generics); consult specific product labeling.

Solution Reconstituted, Intravenous:

Doribax: 250 mg (1 ea); 500 mg (1 ea)

Dornase Alfa (DOOR nase AL fa)

Brand Names: US Pulmozyme

Brand Names: Canada Pulmozyme

Index Terms Recombinant Human Deoxyribonuclease; rhDNase

Pharmacologic Category Enzyme; Mucolytic Agent

Use Cystic fibrosis: Management of cystic fibrosis patients, in conjunction with standard therapies, to improve pulmonary function; reduce the risk of respiratory tract infections requiring parenteral antibiotics in patients with a forced vital capacity (FVC) ≥40% of predicted.

Dosing

Adult & Geriatric

Cystic fibrosis: Inhalation: 2.5 mg daily through selected jet nebulizers in conjunction with a Pulmo-Aide, Pari-Proneb, Mobilaire, or Porta-Neb compressor system or eRapid Nebulizer System

Patients unable to inhale or exhale orally throughout the entire treatment period may use Pari-Baby nebulizer. Some patients may benefit from twice daily administration.

Parapneumonic pleural effusions and empyemas (off-label use): Intrapleural: 5 mg (diluted in 30 mL of sterile water) administered twice daily >2 hours after each intrapleural alteplase dose (with a 1-hour dwell time for each drug) for a total of 3 days (Rahman, 2011). Some clinicians suggest consideration of fibrinolytic use in patients in whom treatment with at least 24 hours of chest tube drainage has failed and who are poor surgical candidates (Hamblin, 2010).

Pediatric Cystic fibrosis: Inhalation:

Infants and Children ≤5 years: Not approved for use; however, studies using this therapy in small numbers of children as young as 3 months of age have reported efficacy and similar side effects.

Children >5 years: Refer to adult dosing.

Renal Impairment There are no dosage adjustment provided in manufacturer's labeling.

Hepatic Impairment There are no dosage adjustment provided in manufacturer's labeling.

Additional Information Complete prescribing information should be consulted for additional detail.

Dosage Forms Excipient information presented when available (limited, particularly for generics); consult specific product labeling.

Solution, Inhalation:
Pulmozyme: 1 mg/mL (2.5 mL)

◆ Doryx see Doxycycline on page 601

Dorzolamide (dor ZOLE a mide)

Brand Names: US Trusopt

Brand Names: Canada Sandoz-Dorzolamide; Trusopt

Index Terms Dorzolamide Hydrochloride

Pharmacologic Category Carbonic Anhydrase Inhibitor (Ophthalmic); Ophthalmic Agent, Antiglaucoma

Use Elevated intraocular pressure: Treatment of elevated intraocular pressure (IOP) in patients with ocular hypertension or open-angle glaucoma

Dosing

Adult & Geriatric

Elevated intraocular pressure: Ophthalmic: Instill 1 drop in the affected eye(s) 3 times daily

Pediatric Refer to adult dosing.

Renal Impairment

CrCl ≥30 mL/minute: There are no dosage adjustments provided in the manufacturer's labeling.

CrCl <30 mL/minute: Use is not recommended (has not been studied).

Hepatic Impairment There are no dosage adjustments provided in the manufacturer's labeling (have not been studied); use with caution.

Additional Information Complete prescribing information should be consulted for additional detail.

Dosage Forms Excipient information presented when available (limited, particularly for generics); consult specific product labeling.

Solution, Ophthalmic:
Trusopt: 2% (10 mL)
Generic: 2% (10 mL)

Dosage Forms: Canada Excipient information presented when available (limited, particularly for generics); consult specific product labeling.

Solution, ophthalmic [drops; preservative free]:
Trusopt: 2% (0.2 mL)

Dorzolamide and Timolol
(dor ZOLE a mide & TYE moe lole)

Brand Names: US Cosopt; Cosopt PF

Brand Names: Canada Apo-Dorzo-Timop; Cosopt; Cosopt Preservative Free; Sandoz-Dorzolamide/Timolol

Index Terms Timolol and Dorzolamide

Pharmacologic Category Beta-Adrenergic Blocker, Nonselective; Carbonic Anhydrase Inhibitor (Ophthalmic); Ophthalmic Agent, Antiglaucoma

Use Elevated intraocular pressure: Reduction of elevated intraocular pressure (IOP) in patients with open-angle glaucoma or ocular hypertension who are insufficiently responsive to beta-blockers

Dosing

Adult & Geriatric Elevated intraocular pressure: Ophthalmic: Instill 1 drop in affected eye(s) twice daily

Pediatric Elevated intraocular pressure: Children ≥2 years and Adolescents: Ophthalmic: Refer to adult dosing.

Renal Impairment

CrCl ≥30 mL/minute: No dosage adjustment necessary.

CrCl <30 mL/minute: Use is not recommended (has not been studied).

Hepatic Impairment There are no dosage adjustments provided in the manufacturer's labeling (has not been studied); use with caution.

Additional Information Complete prescribing information should be consulted for additional detail.

Dosage Forms Considerations Ophthalmic solution contains dorzolamide hydrochloride 2.23% [22.3 mg/mL] and timolol maleate 0.68% [6.8 mg/mL]

Dosage Forms Excipient information presented when available (limited, particularly for generics); consult specific product labeling.

Solution, ophthalmic [drops]: Dorzolamide 2% [20 mg/mL] and timolol 0.5% [5 mg/mL] (10 mL)
Cosopt: Dorzolamide 2% [20 mg/mL] and timolol 0.5% [5 mg/mL] (10 mL) [contains benzalkonium chloride]
Solution, ophthalmic [drops, preservative free]:
Cosopt PF: Dorzolamide 2% [20 mg/mL] and timolol 0.5% [5mg/mL] (0.2 mL)

◆ Dorzolamide Hydrochloride see Dorzolamide on page 588

◆ D.O.S. [OTC] see Docusate on page 578

◆ Dosolax [OTC] (Can) see Docusate on page 578

◆ DOSS see Docusate on page 578

◆ Dostinex see Cabergoline on page 279

◆ Double Antibiotic [OTC] see Bacitracin and Polymyxin B (Topical) on page 196

◆ DoubleDex see Dexamethasone (Systemic) on page 525

◆ Double Tussin DM [OTC] see Guaifenesin and Dextromethorphan on page 861

◆ Dovobet (Can) see Calcipotriene and Betamethasone on page 282

◆ Dovonex see Calcipotriene on page 282

Doxapram (DOKS a pram)

Brand Names: US Dopram

Index Terms Doxapram Hydrochloride

Pharmacologic Category Respiratory Stimulant

Use Respiratory stimulant for respiratory depression secondary to anesthesia, mild-to-moderate drug-induced respiratory and CNS depression; acute hypercapnia secondary to COPD

Note: In general, the use of doxapram as a respiratory stimulant in adults is limited; alternate therapies are preferred.

Dosing

Adult & Geriatric Note: Although manufacturer's dosing recommendations are presented for these FDA-approved indications, use of doxapram has largely been replaced by alternate preferred agents.

Respiratory depression following anesthesia: IV:
Intermittent injection: Initial: 0.5-1 mg/kg; may repeat at 5-minute intervals (only in patients who demonstrate initial response); maximum total dose: 2 mg/kg

IV infusion: Initial: 5 mg/minute until adequate response or adverse effects seen; decrease to 1-3 mg/minute; maximum total dose: 4 mg/kg

Drug-induced CNS depression: IV:
Intermittent injection: Initial: Priming dose of 1-2 mg/kg; repeat after 5 minutes; may repeat at 1-2 hour intervals (until sustained consciousness); maximum: 3000 mg daily. May repeat in 24 hours if necessary.

IV infusion: Initial: Priming dose of 1-2 mg/kg repeated in 5 minutes. If no response, wait 1-2 hours and repeat priming dose. If some stimulation is noted, initiate infusion at 1-3 mg/minute (depending on size of patient/depth of CNS depression); suspend infusion if patient begins to awaken. Infusion should not be continued for >2 hours. May reinstitute infusion as described above, including bolus, after rest interval of 30 minutes to 2 hours; maximum: 3000 mg daily.

Acute hypercapnia secondary to COPD: IV infusion: Initial: Initiate infusion at 1-2 mg/minute (depending on size of patient/depth of CNS depression); may increase to maximum rate of 3 mg/minute; infusion should not be continued for >2 hours. Monitor arterial blood gases prior to initiation of infusion and at 30-minute intervals

during the infusion (to identify possible development of acidosis/CO_2 retention). Additional infusions are not recommended (per manufacturer).

Pediatric Children ≥12 years and Adolescents: Refer to adult dosing.

Renal Impairment No dosage adjustment provided in manufacturer's labeling (has not been studied); however, use caution in severe impairment due to the potential for altered pharmacokinetics.

Hepatic Impairment No dosage adjustment provided in manufacturer's labeling (has not been studied); however, use caution in severe impairment due to the potential for altered pharmacokinetics.

Additional Information Complete prescribing information should be consulted for additional detail.

Dosage Forms Excipient information presented when available (limited, particularly for generics); consult specific product labeling.

Solution, Intravenous, as hydrochloride:
Dopram: 20 mg/mL (20 mL) [contains benzyl alcohol]
Generic: 20 mg/mL (20 mL)

◆ Doxapram Hydrochloride see Doxapram on page 588

Doxazosin (doks AY zoe sin)

Brand Names: US Cardura; Cardura XL

Brand Names: Canada Apo-Doxazosin; Cardura-1; Cardura-2; Cardura-4; Dom-Doxazosin; Doxazosin-1; Doxazosin-2; Doxazosin-4; Mylan-Doxazosin; PMS-Doxazosin; Teva-Doxazosin

Index Terms Doxazosin Mesylate

Pharmacologic Category Alpha$_1$ Blocker; Antihypertensive

Use

Immediate release formulation: Treatment of hypertension as monotherapy or in conjunction with diuretics, ACE inhibitors, beta-blockers, or calcium antagonists; treatment of urinary outflow obstruction and/or obstructive and irritative symptoms associated with benign prostatic hyperplasia (BPH)

Note: The 2014 guideline for the management of high blood pressure in adults (Eighth Joint National Committee [JNC 8] [James 2013]) does **not** recommend the use of doxazosin in the treatment of hypertension (JNC8 [James 2013]). According to the AHA/ACC/ASH 2015 scientific statement for the treatment of hypertension in patients with coronary artery disease (CAD), doxazosin should only be used if other drugs for the management of hypertension and heart failure do not achieve BP control at maximum tolerated doses (AHA/ACC/ASH [Rosendorff 2015]).

Extended release formulation: Treatment of urinary outflow obstruction and/or obstructive and irritative symptoms associated with BPH

Pregnancy Considerations Adverse events were observed in some animal reproduction studies. Untreated chronic maternal hypertension is associated with adverse events in the fetus, infant, and mother. If treatment for hypertension during pregnancy is needed, other agents are generally preferred (ACOG, 2013).

Breast-Feeding Considerations Doxazosin is excreted into breast milk. Information is available from a single case report following a maternal dose of doxazosin 4 mg every 24 hours for 2 doses. Milk samples were obtained at various intervals over 24 hours, beginning ~17 hours after the first dose. Maternal serum samples were obtained at nearly the same times, beginning ~1 hour later. The highest serum and milk concentrations of doxazosin were observed ~1 hour after the dose. Using the highest milk concentration (4.15 mcg/L), the estimated dose to the nursing infant was calculated to be <1% of the weight-adjusted maternal dose (Jensen, 2013). The manufacturer recommends that caution be used if administered to nursing women.

Contraindications Hypersensitivity to quinazolines (prazosin, terazosin), doxazosin, or any component of the formulation

Warnings/Precautions Can cause significant orthostatic hypotension and syncope, especially with first dose; anticipate a similar effect if therapy is interrupted for a few days, if dosage is rapidly increased, or if another antihypertensive drug (particularly vasodilators) or a PDE-5 inhibitor is introduced. Discontinue if symptoms of angina occur or worsen. Patients should be cautioned about performing hazardous tasks when starting new therapy or adjusting dosage upward. Priapism has been associated with use (rarely). Prostate cancer should be ruled out before starting for BPH. Use with caution in mild-to-moderate hepatic impairment; not recommended in severe dysfunction. Intraoperative floppy iris syndrome has been observed in cataract surgery patients who were on or were previously treated with alpha$_1$-blockers. Causality has not been established and there appears to be no benefit in discontinuing alpha-blocker therapy prior to surgery. In the elderly, avoid use as an antihypertensive due to high risk of orthostatic hypotension; alternative agents preferred due to a more favorable risk/benefit profile (Beers Criteria).

The extended release formulation consists of drug within a nondeformable matrix; following drug release/absorption, the matrix/shell is expelled in the stool. The use of nondeformable products in patients with known stricture/narrowing of the GI tract has been associated with symptoms of obstruction. Use caution in patients with increased GI retention (eg, chronic constipation) as doxazosin exposure may be increased. Extended release formulation is not indicated for use in women or for the treatment of hypertension.

Adverse Reactions

>10%: Central nervous system: Dizziness (5% to 19%), malaise (≤12%), fatigue (8% to ≤12%), headache (6% to 10%)

1% to 10%:

Cardiovascular: Edema (3% to 4%), hypotension (1% to 2%), orthostatic hypotension (<1% to 2%), cardiac arrhythmia (1%), facial edema (1%), flushing (1%), palpitations (1%)

Central nervous system: Drowsiness (1% to 5%), vertigo (2% to 4%), pain (2%), anxiety (1%), ataxia (1%), hypertonia (1%), insomnia (1%), movement disorder (1%), myasthenia (1%)

Endocrine & metabolic: Sexual disorder (2%)

Gastrointestinal: Abdominal pain (2%), nausea (1% to 2%), dyspepsia (1%), xerostomia (1%)

Genitourinary: Urinary incontinence (1%), urinary tract infection (1%)

Neuromuscular & skeletal: Weakness (4% to 7%), muscle cramps (1%), myalgia (1%), arthralgia (≤1%), arthritis (≤1%)

Ophthalmic: Visual disturbance (2%)

Otic: Tinnitus (1%)

Renal: Polyuria (2%)

Respiratory: Respiratory tract infection (5%), rhinitis (3%), dyspnea (1% to 3%), epistaxis (1%)

<1% (Limited to important or life-threatening): Abnormal hepatic function tests, abnormal lacrimation, abnormality in thinking, agitation, alopecia, altered sense of smell, amnesia, angina pectoris, anorexia, blurred vision, bradycardia, bronchospasm (aggravated), cerebrovascular accident, cholestasis, cholestatic hepatitis, confusion, decreased libido, depersonalization, dysgeusia, dysuria, emotional lability, fecal incontinence, flu-like symptoms, gastroenteritis, gastrointestinal obstruction, gout, gynecomastia, hematuria, hepatitis, hot flash, hypersensitivity reaction, hypoesthesia, hypokalemia, impotence, increased appetite, increased thirst, infection, intraoperative floppy iris syndrome (cataract surgery), lack of concentration, leukopenia, lymphadenopathy, mastalgia, migraine, myocardial infarction, nephrolithiasis, nervousness, neutropenia, nocturia, orthostatic dizziness, otalgia, paranoia, paresis, paresthesia, peripheral ischemia, photophobia, priapism, purpura, rigors, syncope, tachycardia, thrombocytopenia, tremor, twitching, urinary frequency, urination disorder, xeroderma

Drug Interactions

Metabolism/Transport Effects Substrate of CYP2C19 (minor), CYP2D6 (minor), CYP3A4 (major); **Note:** Assignment of Major/Minor substrate status based on clinically relevant drug interaction potential

Avoid Concomitant Use

Avoid concomitant use of Doxazosin with any of the following: Alpha1-Blockers; Boceprevir; Conivaptan; Fusidic Acid (Systemic); Idelalisib

Increased Effect/Toxicity

Doxazosin may increase the levels/effects of: Alpha1-Blockers; Amifostine; Antipsychotic Agents (Second Generation [Atypical]); Calcium Channel Blockers; DULoxetine; Hypotension-Associated Agents; Levodopa

The levels/effects of Doxazosin may be increased by: Aprepitant; Barbiturates; Beta-Blockers; Boceprevir; Brimonidine (Topical); Conivaptan; CYP3A4 Inhibitors (Moderate); CYP3A4 Inhibitors (Strong); Dapoxetine; Dasatinib; Diazoxide; Fosaprepitant; Fusidic Acid (Systemic); Herbs (Hypotensive Properties); Idelalisib; Ivacaftor; Luliconazole; Mifepristone; Molsidomine; Netupitant; Nicorandil; Obinutuzumab; Osimertinib; Palbociclib; Pentoxifylline; Phosphodiesterase 5 Inhibitors; Prostacyclin Analogues; Simeprevir; Stiripentol

Decreased Effect

Doxazosin may decrease the levels/effects of: Alpha-/Beta-Agonists; Alpha1-Agonists

The levels/effects of Doxazosin may be decreased by: Amphetamines; Bosentan; CYP3A4 Inducers (Moderate); CYP3A4 Inducers (Strong); Dabrafenib; Deferasirox; Enzalutamide; Herbs (Hypertensive Properties); Methylphenidate; Mitotane; Osimertinib; Siltuximab; St Johns Wort; Tocilizumab; Yohimbine

Storage/Stability Store at 25°C (77°F); excursions permitted between 15°C to 30°C (59°F to 86°F).

Mechanism of Action

Hypertension: Competitively inhibits postsynaptic alpha$_1$-adrenergic receptors which results in vasodilation of veins and arterioles and a decrease in total peripheral resistance and blood pressure; ~50% as potent on a weight by weight basis as prazosin.

BPH: Competitively inhibits postsynaptic alpha$_1$-adrenergic receptors in prostatic stromal and bladder neck tissues. This reduces the sympathetic tone-induced urethral stricture causing BPH symptoms.

Pharmacodynamics/Kinetics Note: Not significantly affected by increased age

Duration: >24 hours

Protein binding: ~98%

Metabolism: Extensively hepatic to active metabolites; primarily via CYP3A4; secondary pathways involve CYP2D6 and 2C19

Bioavailability: Immediate release: ~65%; Extended release relative to immediate release: 54% to 59%

Half-life elimination: Immediate release: ~22 hours; Extended release: 15 to 19 hours; prolonged in patients with hepatic impairment

Time to peak, serum: Immediate release: 2-3 hours; Extended release: 8-9 hours

Excretion: Feces (63%, primarily as metabolites); urine (9%, primarily as metabolites)

Dosing

Adult

BPH: Oral:

Immediate release: 1 mg once daily in morning or evening; may be increased to 2 mg once daily. Thereafter titrate upwards, if needed, every 1-2 weeks, balancing therapeutic benefit with doxazosin-induced postural hypotension. Goal: 4-8 mg daily; maximum dose: 8 mg daily

Reinitiation of therapy: If therapy is discontinued for several days, restart at 1 mg dose and titrate as before

Extended release: 4 mg once daily with breakfast; titrate based on response and tolerability every 3-4 weeks to maximum recommended dose of 8 mg daily

Reinitiation of therapy: If therapy is discontinued for several days, restart at 4 mg dose and titrate as before

Note: Conversion to extended release from immediate release: Omit final evening dose of immediate release prior to starting morning dosing with extended release product; initiate extended release product using 4 mg once daily

Hypertension: Oral: *Immediate release:* 1 mg once daily in morning or evening; may be increased to 2 mg once daily. Thereafter titrate upwards, if needed, every 1-2 weeks, balancing therapeutic benefit with doxazosin-induced postural hypotension. Usual dosage range (ASH/ISH [Weber, 2014]): 1-2 mg daily; Maximum dose: 16 mg daily

Reinitiation of therapy: If therapy is discontinued for several days, restart at 1 mg dose and titrate as before

Ureteral calculi (distal) expulsion (off-label use): Oral: *Immediate release:* 4 mg once daily in evening (Gurbuz, 2011; Resorlu, 2011). **Note:** Patients with stones >10 mm were excluded from studies.

Geriatric Refer to adult dosing. In the management of hypertension, consider lower initial doses (eg, immediate release: 0.5 mg once daily) and titrate to response (Aronow, 2011)

Pediatric Hypertension (off-label use): Children and Adolescents 1-17 years: Oral: Immediate release: Initial: 1 mg once daily; maximum: 4 mg daily (NHBPEP, 2004)

Renal Impairment No dosage adjustment provided in the manufacturer's labeling (however, limited data suggest renal impairment does not significantly alter pharmacokinetic parameters).

Hepatic Impairment Use with caution in mild-to-moderate hepatic dysfunction. Do not use with severe impairment.

Dietary Considerations Cardura® XL: Take with morning meal.

Administration Cardura® XL: Tablets should be swallowed whole; do not crush, chew, or divide. Administer with morning meal.

Monitoring Parameters Blood pressure, standing and sitting/supine; syncope may occur usually within 90 minutes of the initial dose or dose increase

Additional Information First-dose hypotension occurs less frequently with doxazosin as compared to prazosin; this may be due to its slower onset of action.

Dosage Forms Excipient information presented when available (limited, particularly for generics); consult specific product labeling.

Tablet, Oral:

Cardura: 1 mg, 2 mg, 4 mg, 8 mg [scored]

Generic: 1 mg, 2 mg, 4 mg, 8 mg

Tablet Extended Release 24 Hour, Oral:

Cardura XL: 4 mg, 8 mg

Dosage Forms: Canada Note: Refer to Dosage Forms. Extended-release capsules are not available in Canada.

♦ Doxazosin-1 (Can) see Doxazosin on page 589
♦ Doxazosin-2 (Can) see Doxazosin on page 589
♦ Doxazosin-4 (Can) see Doxazosin on page 589
♦ Doxazosin Mesylate see Doxazosin on page 589

Doxepin (Systemic) (DOKS e pin)

Brand Names: US Silenor

Brand Names: Canada Apo-Doxepin; Novo-Doxepin; Silenor; Sinequan; Zonalon

Index Terms Doxepin Hydrochloride; Sinequan

Pharmacologic Category Antidepressant, Tricyclic (Tertiary Amine)

Use

Depression and/or anxiety: Treatment of psychoneurotic patients with depression and/or anxiety; depression and/or anxiety associated with alcoholism; depression and/or anxiety associated with organic disease; psychotic depressive disorders with associated anxiety, including involutional depression and manic-depressive disorders.

Insomnia (Silenor only): Treatment of insomnia characterized by difficulty with sleep maintenance.

Pregnancy Considerations Adverse events were observed in animal reproduction studies. Tricyclic antidepressants may be associated with irritability, jitteriness, and convulsions (rare) in the neonate (Yonkers 2009).

The ACOG recommends that therapy for depression during pregnancy be individualized; treatment should incorporate the clinical expertise of the mental health clinician, obstetrician, primary healthcare provider, and pediatrician (ACOG 2008). According to the American Psychiatric Association (APA), the risks of medication treatment should be weighed against other treatment options and untreated depression. For women who discontinue antidepressant medications during pregnancy and who may be at high risk for postpartum depression, the medications can be restarted following delivery (APA 2010). Treatment algorithms have been developed by the ACOG and the APA for the management of depression in women prior to conception and during pregnancy (Yonkers 2009).

Breast-Feeding Considerations Doxepin and N-desmethyldoxepin are excreted into breast milk (Frey, 1999; Kemp, 1985). Drowsiness, vomiting, poor feeding, and muscle hypotonia were noted in a nursing infant following maternal use of doxepin. Symptoms began to resolve 24 hours after feedings with breast milk were discontinued (Frey, 1999). In addition, product labeling notes that drowsiness and apnea have been reported in a nursing infant following maternal use of doxepin for depression. The manufacturer recommends that caution be used if administered to a nursing woman.

Medication Guide Available Yes

Contraindications

Hypersensitivity to doxepin, dibenzoxepins, or any component of the formulation; glaucoma; urinary retention; use of MAO inhibitors within 14 days

Documentation of allergenic cross-reactivity for tricyclic antidepressants is limited. However, because of similarities in chemical structure and/or pharmacologic actions, the possibility of cross-sensitivity cannot be ruled out with certainty.

Warnings/Precautions [US Boxed Warning]: Antidepressants increase the risk of suicidal thinking and behavior in children, adolescents, and young adults (18-24 years of age) with major depressive disorder (MDD) and other psychiatric disorders; consider risk prior to prescribing. Short-term studies did not show an increased risk in patients >24 years of age and showed a decreased risk in patients ≥65 years. Closely monitor for clinical worsening, suicidality, or unusual changes in behavior, particularly during the initial 1 to 2 months of therapy or during periods of dosage adjustments (increases or decreases); the patient's family or caregiver

should be instructed to closely observe the patient and communicate condition with healthcare provider. A medication guide should be dispensed with each prescription. **Doxepin is not approved for use in pediatric patients.**

The possibility of a suicide attempt is inherent in major depression and may persist until remission occurs. Use caution in high-risk patients. Worsening depression and severe abrupt suicidality that are not part of the presenting symptoms may require discontinuation or modification of drug therapy. The patient's family or caregiver should be alerted to monitor patients for the emergence of suicidality and associated behaviors (such as agitation, irritability, hostility, impulsivity, and hypomania) and call healthcare provider.

Risk of suicidal behavior may be increased regardless of doxepin dose; antidepressant doses of doxepin are 10- to 100-fold higher than doses for insomnia.

May precipitate a shift to mania or hypomania in patients with bipolar disorder. Patients presenting with depressive symptoms should be screened for bipolar disorder. Monotherapy in patients with bipolar disorder should be avoided. **Doxepin is not FDA approved for the treatment of bipolar depression.**

Should only be used for insomnia after evaluation of potential causes of sleep disturbance. Failure of sleep disturbance to resolve after 7 to 10 days may indicate psychiatric or medical illness. An increased risk for hazardous sleep-related activities has been noted; discontinue use with any sleep-related episodes. The risks of sedative and anticholinergic effects are high relative to other antidepressant agents. Anxiety, psychosis, and other neuropsychiatric symptoms may occur unpredictably. May cause CNS depression, which may impair physical or mental abilities; patients must be cautioned about performing tasks that require mental alertness (eg, operating machinery or driving). Also use caution in patients with benign prostatic hyperplasia, xerostomia, visual problems, constipation, or history of bowel obstruction.

May cause orthostatic hypotension or conduction disturbances (risks are moderate relative to other antidepressants). Use with caution in patients with a history of cardiovascular disease (including previous MI, stroke, tachycardia, or conduction abnormalities). Use with caution in patients with respiratory compromise or sleep apnea; use of Silenor is generally not recommended with severe sleep apnea.

Use caution in patients with a previous seizure disorder or condition predisposing to seizures such as brain damage, alcoholism, or concurrent therapy with other drugs which lower the seizure threshold (APA 2010). Bone fractures have been associated with antidepressant treatment. Consider the possibility of a fragility fracture if an antidepressant-treated patient presents with unexplained bone pain, point tenderness, swelling, or bruising (Rabenda 2013; Rizzoli 2012). Use with caution in patients with hepatic dysfunction. May cause mild pupillary dilation which in susceptible individuals can lead to an episode of narrow-angle glaucoma. Consider evaluating patients who have not had an iridectomy for narrow-angle glaucoma risk factors. Potentially significant drug-drug interactions may exist, requiring dose or frequency adjustment, additional monitoring, and/or selection of alternative therapy.

May cause confusion and over sedation in the elderly. In the elderly, avoid doses >6 mg/day in this age group due to its potent anticholinergic and sedative properties, and potential to cause orthostatic hypotension; safety of doses ≤6 mg/day is comparable to placebo. In addition, may also cause or exacerbate syndrome of inappropriate antidiuretic hormone secretion or hyponatremia; monitor sodium closely with initiation or dosage adjustments in older adults (Beers Criteria).

Abrupt discontinuation or interruption of antidepressant therapy has been associated with a discontinuation syndrome. Symptoms arising may vary with antidepressant however commonly include nausea, vomiting, diarrhea, headaches, lightheadedness, dizziness, diminished appetite, sweating, chills, tremors, paresthesias, fatigue, somnolence, and sleep disturbances (eg, vivid dreams, insomnia). Greater risks for developing a discontinuation syndrome have been associated with antidepressants with shorter half-lives, longer durations of treatment, and abrupt discontinuation. For antidepressants of short or intermediate half-lives, symptoms may emerge within 2-5 days after treatment discontinuation and last 7 to 14 days (APA 2010; Fava 2006; Haddad 2001; Shelton 2001; Warner 2006).

Adverse Reactions Actual frequency may be dependent on diagnosis.

Cardiovascular: Hypertension (chronic insomnia patients ≤3%), edema, flushing, hypotension, tachycardia

Central nervous system: Sedation (chronic insomnia patients 6% to 9%), dizziness (chronic insomnia patients ≥1%), ataxia, chills, confusion, disorientation, drowsiness, extrapyramidal reaction, fatigue, hallucination, headache, numbness, paresthesia, seizure, tardive dyskinesia

Dermatologic: Alopecia, diaphoresis (excessive), pruritus, skin photosensitivity, skin rash

Endocrine & metabolic: Altered serum glucose, change in libido, galactorrhea, gynecomastia, SIADH, weight gain

Gastrointestinal: Nausea (chronic insomnia patients 2%), gastroenteritis (chronic insomnia patients ≤2%), anorexia, aphthous stomatitis, constipation, diarrhea, dysgeusia, dyspepsia, vomiting, xerostomia

Genitourinary: Breast hypertrophy, testicular swelling, urinary retention

Hematologic & oncologic: Agranulocytosis, eosinophilia, leukopenia, purpura, thrombocytopenia

Hepatic: Jaundice

Neuromuscular & skeletal: Tremor, weakness

Ophthalmic: Blurred vision

Otic: Tinnitus

Respiratory: Upper respiratory tract infection (chronic insomnia patients 4%), exacerbation of asthma

<1% (Limited to important or life-threatening): Adenocarcinoma (lung, stage I), adjustment disorder, anemia, angle-closure glaucoma, atrioventricular block, bone fracture, breast cyst, cerebrovascular accident, chest pain, decreased neutrophils, decreased performance on neuropsychometrics, decreased range of motion (joints), depression, ECG abnormality (ST-T segment, QRS complex, QRS axis), eye infection, fungal infection, gastroesophageal reflux disease, hematochezia, hematoma, hemoglobinuria, hyperbilirubinemia, hyperkalemia, hypermagnesemia, hypersensitivity, hypoacusis, hypokalemia, increased serum ALT, increased serum transaminases, malignant melanoma, migraine, peripheral edema, pneumonia, sleep paralysis, somnambulism (complex sleep-related behavior [sleep-driving, cooking or eating food, making phone calls]), staphylococcal cellulitis, syncope, tenosynovitis, tooth infection, urinary incontinence, urinary tract infection, viral infection

Drug Interactions

Metabolism/Transport Effects Substrate of CYP1A2 (minor), CYP2C19 (minor), CYP2D6 (major), CYP3A4 (minor); **Note:** Assignment of Major/Minor substrate status based on clinically relevant drug interaction potential

Avoid Concomitant Use

Avoid concomitant use of Doxepin (Systemic) with any of the following: Aclidinium; Azelastine (Nasal); Cimetropium; Dapoxetine; Dronedarone; Eluxadoline; Glucagon; Glycopyrrolate; Glycopyrrolate (Oral Inhalation); Iobenguane I 123; Ipratropium (Oral Inhalation); Levosulpiride; Linezolid; MAO Inhibitors; Methylene Blue; Moxonidine; Orphenadrine; Paraldehyde; Potassium Chloride; Thalidomide; Tiotropium; Umeclidinium

Increased Effect/Toxicity

Doxepin (Systemic) may increase the levels/effects of: AbobotulinumtoxinA; Alcohol (Ethyl); Alpha-/Beta-Agonists (Direct-Acting); Alpha1-Agonists; Amphetamines; Analgesics (Opioid); Anticholinergic Agents; Antipsychotic Agents; Aspirin; Azelastine (Nasal); Beta2-Agonists; Buprenorphine; Cimetropium; Citalopram; CNS Depressants; Desmopressin; Dronedarone; Eluxadoline; Escitalopram; Glucagon; Glycopyrrolate; Glycopyrrolate (Oral Inhalation); Highest Risk QTc-Prolonging Agents; Hydrocodone; Methotrimeprazine; Methylene Blue; Metyrosine; Mirabegron; Moderate Risk QTc-Prolonging Agents; Nicorandil; NSAID (COX-2 Inhibitor); NSAID (Nonselective); OnabotulinumtoxinA; Orphenadrine; Paraldehyde; Potassium Chloride; Pramipexole; QuiNIDine; Ramosetron; RimabotulinumtoxinB; ROPINIRole; Rotigotine; Serotonin Modulators; Sodium Phosphates; Sulfonylureas; Suvorexant; Thalidomide; Thiazide Diuretics; Tiotropium; Topiramate; TraMADol; Vitamin K Antagonists; Yohimbine; Zolpidem

The levels/effects of Doxepin (Systemic) may be increased by: Abiraterone Acetate; Aclidinium; Altretamine; Antiemetics (5HT3 Antagonists); Antipsychotic Agents; Brimonidine (Topical); BuPROPion; Cannabis; Cimetidine; Cinacalcet; Citalopram; Cobicistat; CYP2D6 Inhibitors (Moderate); CYP2D6 Inhibitors (Strong); Dapoxetine; Darunavir; Dexmethylphenidate; Doxylamine; Dronabinol; Droperidol; DULoxetine; Escitalopram; FLUoxetine; FluvoxaMINE; HydrOXYzine; Ipratropium (Oral Inhalation); Kava Kava; Linezolid; Lithium; Magnesium Sulfate; MAO Inhibitors; Metaxalone; Methotrimeprazine; Methylphenidate; Metoclopramide; ▶

Metyrosine; Mianserin; Mifepristone; Minocycline; Nabilone; Panobinostat; PARoxetine; Peginterferon Alfa-2b; Perampanel; Pramlintide; Protease Inhibitors; QuiNIDine; Rufinamide; Sertraline; Sodium Oxybate; Tapentadol; Tedizolid; Tetrahydrocannabinol; Thyroid Products; TraMADol; Umeclidinium; Valproate Products

Decreased Effect

Doxepin (Systemic) may decrease the levels/effects of: Acetylcholinesterase Inhibitors; Alpha1-Agonists; Alpha2-Agonists; Alpha2-Agonists (Ophthalmic); Gastrointestinal Agents (Prokinetic); Iobenguane I 123; Itopride; Levosulpiride; Moxonidine; Secretin

The levels/effects of Doxepin (Systemic) may be decreased by: Acetylcholinesterase Inhibitors; Barbiturates; CarBAMazepine; Peginterferon Alfa-2b; St Johns Wort

Food Interactions Administration with a high-fat meal increases the bioavailability of Silenor and delays the peak plasma concentration by ~3 hours. Management: Silenor should not be taken during or within 3 hours of a meal.

Preparation for Administration Concentrate, oral: Must dilute with approximately 120 mL of water, whole or skimmed milk, or orange, grapefruit, tomato, prune or pineapple juice prior to administration. Do not mix with carbonated beverages (physically incompatible). Doxepin concentrate and methadone syrup can be mixed together with Gatorade, lemon or orange juice, sugar water, Tang, or water, but not with grape juice.

Storage/Stability Store at room temperature. Protect from light.

Mechanism of Action

Increases the synaptic concentration of serotonin and norepinephrine in the central nervous system by inhibition of their reuptake by the presynaptic neuronal membrane (Pinder, 1977); antagonizes the histamine (H_1) receptor for sleep maintenance.

Efficacy of doxepin in the off-label use of chronic urticaria is believed to be related to its potent H_1 and H_2 receptor antagonist activity (Kozel 2004).

Pharmacodynamics/Kinetics

Onset of action: Individual responses may vary; 4 to 8 weeks of treatment are needed before determining if a patient with depression is partially or nonresponsive (APA 2010); onset of anxiolytic effects may have a latency of 2 to 6 weeks (Bandelow 2008)

Absorption: Administration with a high-fat meal increases the bioavailability of Silenor and delays the peak plasma concentration by ~3 hours

Distribution: V_d: 20.2 L/kg (Ziegler, 1978); Silenor 11,930 L

Protein binding: ~80%

Metabolism: Hepatic via CYP2C19 and 2D6; primary metabolite is N-desmethyldoxepin (active)

Half-life elimination: Adults: Doxepin: ~15 hours; N-desmethyldoxepin: 31 hours

Time to peak, serum: Fasting: Silenor: 3.5 hours

Excretion: Urine (<3% as unchanged drug or N-desmethyldoxepin)

Dosing

Adult

Depression and/or anxiety: Oral: Initial: 25 to 50 mg as a single dose at bedtime or in divided doses; gradually increase based on response and tolerability to a usual dose of 100-300 mg daily (APA 2010; Bauer 2013)

Insomnia (Silenor): Oral: 3 to 6 mg once daily within 30 minutes of bedtime; maximum dose: 6 mg daily

Chronic urticaria (off-label use): Oral: Adults: 10 mg 3 times daily (Greene, 1985) **or** 10 mg to 30 mg once daily at bedtime (Yadav 2009)

Discontinuation of therapy: Upon discontinuation of antidepressant therapy, gradually taper the dose to minimize the incidence of withdrawal symptoms and allow for the detection of re-emerging symptoms. Evidence supporting ideal taper rates is limited. APA and NICE guidelines suggest tapering therapy over at least several weeks with consideration to the half-life of the antidepressant; antidepressants with a shorter half-life may need to be tapered more conservatively. In addition for long-term treated patients, WFSBP guidelines recommend tapering over 4 to 6 months. If intolerable withdrawal symptoms occur following a dose reduction, consider resuming the previously prescribed dose and/or decrease dose at a more gradual rate (APA, 2010; Bauer 2002; Haddad 2001; NCCMH 2010; Schatzberg 2006; Shelton 2001; Warner 2006).

MAO inhibitor recommendations:

Switching to or from an MAO inhibitor intended to treat psychiatric disorders:

Allow 14 days to elapse between discontinuing an MAO inhibitor intended to treat psychiatric disorders and initiation of doxepin.

Allow 14 days to elapse between discontinuing doxepin and initiation of an MAO inhibitor intended to treat psychiatric disorders.

Use with other MAO inhibitors (such as linezolid or IV methylene blue):

Do not initiate doxepin in patients receiving linezolid or IV methylene blue; consider other interventions for psychiatric condition.

If urgent treatment with linezolid or IV methylene blue is required in a patient already receiving doxepin and potential benefits outweigh potential risks, discontinue doxepin promptly and administer linezolid or IV methylene blue. Monitor for serotonin syndrome for 2 weeks or until 24 hours after the last dose of linezolid or IV methylene blue, whichever comes first. May resume doxepin 24 hours after the last dose of linezolid or IV methylene blue.

Geriatric

Depression and/or anxiety: Oral: Carefully adjust the use of doxepin on a once-a-day dosage regimen in elderly patients based on the patient's condition; elderly patients generally should be started on low doses of doxepin and observed closely

Insomnia: Oral: 3 mg once daily within 30 minutes of bedtime; increase to 6 mg once daily if clinically needed; maximum dose: 6 mg daily

Discontinuation of therapy: Refer to adult dosing.

MAO inhibitor recommendations: Refer to adult dosing.

Renal Impairment There are no dosage adjustments provided in manufacturer's labeling.

Hepatic Impairment Silenor: Initial: 3 mg once daily

Administration

Depression and/or anxiety: Oral: Administer the total daily dosage in divided or once a day dosage schedule. If the once a day schedule is employed the maximum recommended dose is 150 mg once daily at bedtime. The 150 mg capsule strength is intended for maintenance therapy only and is not for initiation of treatment.

Insomnia: Oral: Administer within 30 minutes prior to bedtime; do not take within 3 hours of food.

Monitoring Parameters Evaluate mental status, suicide ideation (especially at the beginning of therapy or when doses are increased or decreased); anxiety, social functioning, mania, panic attacks or other unusual changes in behavior; heart rate, blood pressure and ECG in older adults and patients with preexisting cardiac disease; blood glucose; weight and BMI; blood levels are useful for therapeutic monitoring (APA 2010).

Insomnia: Re-evaluate diagnosis if insomnia does not remit within 7-10 days of treatment.

Reference Range Proposed therapeutic concentration (doxepin plus desmethyldoxepin): 50-250 ng/mL. Utility of serum level monitoring is controversial (Leucht 2001).

Dosage Forms Excipient information presented when available (limited, particularly for generics); consult specific product labeling.

Capsule, Oral:

Generic: 10 mg, 25 mg, 50 mg, 75 mg, 100 mg, 150 mg

Concentrate, Oral:

Generic: 10 mg/mL (118 mL, 120 mL)

Tablet, Oral:

Silenor: 3 mg [contains brilliant blue fcf (fd&c blue #1)]

Silenor: 6 mg [contains brilliant blue fcf (fd&c blue #1), fd&c yellow #10 (quinoline yellow)]

Dosage Forms: Canada Note: Refer to Dosage Forms. Oral concentrate is not available in Canada.

Doxepin (Topical) (DOKS e pin)

Brand Names: US Prudoxin; Zonalon

Brand Names: Canada Zonalon

Index Terms Doxepin Hydrochloride

Pharmacologic Category Topical Skin Product

Use Pruritus: Short-term (≤8 days) management of moderate pruritus in adults with atopic dermatitis or lichen simplex chronicus.

Dosing

Adult

Pruritus: Topical: **Note:** Risk of systemic side effects is greater when applying to over 10% of body surface area. If excessive drowsiness occurs it may be necessary to decrease the BSA treated, decrease the frequency of applications and/or the amount of cream applied or discontinue therapy.

US labeling: Apply a thin film 4 times/day with at least 3- to 4-hour interval between applications; not recommended for use >8 days.

Canadian labeling: Apply a thin film 3 to 4 times/day with at least 3- to 4-hour interval between applications; not recommended for use >8 days.

Neuropathic pain (off-label use): Topical: 3.3% cream (extemporaneous preparation): Apply a thin film to painful area 3 times daily (McCleane 2000).

Geriatric Refer to adult dosing; use with caution.

Pediatric Pruritus: Children ≥12 years and Adolescents (Canadian labeling): Topical: Refer to adult dosing.

Renal Impairment There are no dosage adjustments provided in the manufacturer's labeling (has not been studied); higher doxepin concentrations may occur with renal impairment.

Hepatic Impairment There are no dosage adjustments provided in the manufacturer's labeling.

Additional Information Complete prescribing information should be consulted for additional detail.

Dosage Forms Excipient information presented when available (limited, particularly for generics); consult specific product labeling.

Cream, External, as hydrochloride:
Prudoxin: 5% (45 g) [contains benzyl alcohol, cetyl alcohol]
Zonalon: 5% (30 g, 45 g) [contains benzyl alcohol, cetyl alcohol]

♦ Doxepin Hydrochloride *see* Doxepin (Systemic) *on page 590*

♦ Doxepin Hydrochloride *see* Doxepin (Topical) *on page 592*

Doxercalciferol (doks er kal si fe FEER ole)

Brand Names: US Hectorol
Brand Names: Canada Hectorol
Index Terms 1α-Hydroxyergocalciferol
Pharmacologic Category Vitamin D Analog
Use

Secondary hyperparathyroidism (dialysis): Injection, oral: Treatment of secondary hyperparathyroidism in patients with chronic kidney disease on dialysis
Secondary hyperparathyroidism (predialysis patients): Oral: Treatment of secondary hyperparathyroidism in patients with stage 3 or 4 chronic kidney disease

Dosing

Adult & Geriatric Secondary hyperparathyroidism:
Oral:
Dialysis patients:
Initial dose: iPTH >400 pg/mL: 10 mcg 3 times/week at dialysis for 8 weeks
Dose titration:
iPTH level >300 pg/mL (dose should be titrated to lower iPTH to within the range of 150 to 300 pg/mL): Increase to 12.5 mcg 3 times/week at dialysis for 8 more weeks; this titration process can continue at 8-week intervals in 2.5 mcg/dose increments (maximum: 20 mcg 3 times/week).
iPTH level 150 to 300 pg/mL: Maintain current dose
iPTH level <100 pg/mL: Suspend doxercalciferol for 1 week; resume at a reduced dose; decrease each dose (not weekly dose) by at least 2.5 mcg
Hypercalcemia, hyperphosphatemia, or serum calcium times serum phosphorus product >55 mg^2/dL^2: Decrease or suspend dose and/or adjust dose of phosphate binders; if dose is suspended, resume at a reduced dose; decrease each dose (not weekly dose) by at least 2.5 mcg.
Predialysis patients:
Initial dose: iPTH >70 pg/mL with stage 3 disease or >110 pg/mL with stage 4 disease: 1 mcg/day for 2 weeks
Dose titration:
iPTH level >70 pg/mL with stage 3 disease or >110 pg/mL with stage 4 disease (dose should be titrated to lower iPTH to 35 to 70 pg/mL with stage 3 disease or to 70 to 110 pg/mL with stage 4 disease): Increase dose by 0.5 mcg per day every 2 weeks as necessary (maximum dose: 3.5 mcg/day)
iPTH level 35 to 70 pg/mL with stage 3 disease or 70 to 110 pg/mL with stage 4 disease: Maintain current dose
iPTH level is <35 pg/mL with stage 3 disease or <70 pg/mL with stage 4 disease: Suspend doxercalciferol for 1 week, then resume at a reduced dose (at least 0.5 mcg per day lower)
Hypercalcemia, hyperphosphatemia, or serum calcium times serum phosphorus product >55 mg^2/dL^2: Decrease or suspend dose and/or adjust dose of phosphate binders; if dose is suspended, resume at a reduced dose (at least 0.5 mcg per day lower).

IV:
Dialysis patients:
Initial dose: iPTH level >400 pg/mL: 4 mcg 3 times/week after dialysis for 8 weeks
Dose titration:
iPTH level decreased by <50% and >300 pg/mL (dose should be titrated to lower iPTH to within a range of 150 to 300 pg/mL): Increase by 1 to 2 mcg at 8-week intervals, as necessary (doses >18 mcg/week have not been studied).
iPTH level decreased by >50% and >300 pg/mL: Maintain current dose
iPTH level 150 to 300 pg/mL: Maintain current dose
iPTH level <100 pg/mL: Suspend doxercalciferol for 1 week; resume at a reduced dose (at least 1 mcg lower)
Hypercalcemia, hyperphosphatemia, or serum calcium times serum phosphorus product >55 mg^2/dL^2: Decrease or suspend dose and/or adjust dose of phosphate binders; if dose is suspended, resume at a reduced dose (at least 1 mcg lower)

Renal Impairment No dosage adjustment necessary.

Hepatic Impairment There are no dosage adjustments provided in the manufacturer's labeling. Use with caution and consider more frequent monitoring of iPTH, calcium, and phosphorus levels.

Additional Information Complete prescribing information should be consulted for additional detail.

Dosage Forms Excipient information presented when available (limited, particularly for generics); consult specific product labeling.

Capsule, Oral:
Hectorol: 0.5 mcg [contains alcohol, usp, fd&c red #40, fd&c yellow #10 (quinoline yellow)]
Hectorol: 1 mcg [contains fd&c yellow #6 (sunset yellow)]
Hectorol: 2.5 mcg [contains alcohol, usp, fd&c yellow #10 (quinoline yellow)]
Generic: 0.5 mcg, 1 mcg, 2.5 mcg
Solution, Intravenous:
Hectorol: 2 mcg/mL (1 mL); 4 mcg/2 mL (2 mL) [contains alcohol, usp, disodium edta]
Generic: 4 mcg/2 mL (2 mL)

♦ Doxidan *see* Bisacodyl *on page 231*

♦ Doxil *see* DOXOrubicin (Liposomal) *on page 597*

DOXOrubicin (Conventional) (doks oh ROO bi sin con VEN sha nal)

Brand Names: US Adriamycin
Brand Names: Canada Adriamycin PFS; Doxorubicin Hydrochloride For Injection, USP; Doxorubicin Hydrochloride Injection
Index Terms ADR (error-prone abbreviation); Adria; Conventional Doxorubicin; Doxorubicin HCl; Doxorubicin Hydrochloride; Hydroxydaunomycin Hydrochloride; Hydroxyldaunorubicin Hydrochloride
Pharmacologic Category Antineoplastic Agent, Anthracycline; Antineoplastic Agent, Topoisomerase II Inhibitor
Use

Breast cancer: Treatment component of adjuvant therapy in women with evidence of axillary lymph node involvement following resection of primary breast cancer

Metastatic cancers or disseminated neoplastic conditions: Treatment of acute lymphoblastic leukemia, acute myeloid leukemia, Wilms tumor, neuroblastoma, soft tissue and bone sarcomas, breast cancer, ovarian cancer, transitional cell bladder carcinoma, thyroid carcinoma, gastric carcinoma, Hodgkin lymphoma, non-Hodgkin lymphoma, and bronchogenic carcinoma in which the small cell histologic type is the most responsive compared with other cell types

Pregnancy Considerations Adverse events have been observed in animal reproduction studies. Based on the mechanism of action, doxorubicin may cause fetal harm if administered during pregnancy (according to the manufacturer's labeling). Advise patients (females of reproductive potential and males with female partners of reproductive potential) to use effective nonhormonal contraception during and for 6 months following therapy. Limited information is available from a retrospective study of women who received doxorubicin (in combination with cyclophosphamide) during the second or third (prior to week 35) trimester for the treatment of pregnancy-associated breast cancer (Ring, 2005). Some pharmacokinetic properties of doxorubicin may be altered in pregnant women (van Hasselt, 2014). The European Society for Medical Oncology (ESMO) has published guidelines for diagnosis, treatment, and follow-up of cancer during pregnancy (Peccatori 2013); the guidelines recommend referral to a facility with expertise in cancer during pregnancy and encourage a multidisciplinary team (obstetrician,

neonatologist, oncology team). If chemotherapy is indicated, it should **not** be administered in the first trimester, but may begin in the second trimester. There should be a 3-week time period between the last chemotherapy dose and anticipated delivery, and chemotherapy should not be administered beyond week 33 of gestation.

A pregnancy registry is available for all cancers diagnosed during pregnancy at Cooper Health (877-635-4499).

Breast-Feeding Considerations Doxorubicin and its metabolites are excreted in breast milk. Due to the potential for serious adverse reactions in the nursing infant, the manufacturer recommends a decision be made whether to discontinue nursing or to discontinue the drug, taking into account the importance of treatment to the mother.

Contraindications Hypersensitivity (including anaphylaxis) to doxorubicin, any component of the formulation, or to other anthracyclines or anthracenediones; recent MI (within past 4 to 6 weeks), severe myocardial insufficiency, severe arrhythmia; previous therapy with high cumulative doses of doxorubicin, daunorubicin, idarubicin, or other anthracycline and anthracenediones; severe persistent drug-induced myelosuppression or baseline neutrophil count <1500/mm³; severe hepatic impairment (Child-Pugh class C or bilirubin >5 mg/dL)

Warnings/Precautions Hazardous agent - use appropriate precautions for handling and disposal (NIOSH 2014 [group 1]). **[U.S. Boxed Warning]: May cause cumulative, dose-related, myocardial toxicity (early or delayed, including acute left ventricular failure and HF). The risk of cardiomyopathy increases with cumulative exposure and with concomitant cardiotoxic therapy; the incidence of irreversible myocardial toxicity increases as the total cumulative (lifetime) dosages approach 300 to 500 mg/m². Assess left ventricular ejection fraction (LVEF) with either an echocardiogram or MUGA scan before, during, and after therapy; increase the frequency of assessments as the cumulative dose exceeds 300 mg/m².** Cardiotoxicity is dose-limiting. Delayed cardiotoxicity may occur late in treatment or within months to years after completion of therapy, and is typically manifested by LVEF reduction and/or heart failure (may be life threatening). Subacute effects such as pericarditis and myocarditis may also occur. Early toxicity may consist of tachyarrhythmias, including sinus tachycardia, premature ventricular contractions, and ventricular tachycardia, as well as bradycardia. Electrocardiographic changes including ST-T wave changes, atrioventricular and bundle-branch block have also been reported. These effects are not necessarily predictive of subsequent delayed cardiotoxicity. Total cumulative dose should take into account prior treatment with other anthracyclines or anthracenediones, previous or concomitant treatment with other cardiotoxic agents or irradiation of chest. Although the risk increases with cumulative dose, irreversible cardiotoxicity may occur at any dose level. Patients with active or dominant cardiovascular disease, concurrent administration of cardiotoxic drugs, prior therapy with other anthracyclines or anthracenediones, prior or concurrent chest irradiation, advanced age, and infants and children are at increased risk. Alternative administration schedules (weekly or continuous infusions) have been associated with less cardiotoxicity.

[U.S. Boxed Warning]: Vesicant; if extravasation occurs, severe local tissue damage leading to tissue injury, blistering, ulceration, and necrosis may occur. Discontinue infusion immediately and apply ice to the affected area. For IV administration only. Do not administer IM or SubQ. Ensure proper needle or catheter placement prior to and during infusion. Avoid extravasation.

[U.S. Boxed Warning]: May cause severe myelosuppression, which may result in serious infection, septic shock, transfusion requirements, hospitalization, and death. Myelosuppression may be dose-limiting and primarily manifests as leukopenia and neutropenia; anemia and thrombocytopenia may also occur. The nadir typically occurs 10 to 14 days after administration with cell count recovery around day 21. Monitor blood counts at baseline and regularly during therapy.

[U.S. Boxed Warning]: Secondary acute myelogenous leukemia (AML) and myelodysplastic syndrome (MDS) have been reported following treatment. AML and MDS typically occur within one to three years of treatment; risk factors for development of secondary AML or MDS include treatment with anthracyclines in combination with DNA-damaging antineoplastics (eg, alkylating agents) and/or radiation therapy, heavily pretreated patients, and escalated anthracycline doses. May cause tumor lysis syndrome and hyperuricemia (in patients with rapidly growing tumors). Urinary alkalinization and prophylaxis

with an antihyperuricemic agent may be necessary. Monitor electrolytes, renal function, and hydration status. **[U.S. Boxed Warning]: Dosage modification is recommended in patients with impaired hepatic function;** toxicities may be increased in patients with hepatic impairment. Use is contraindicated in patients with severe impairment (Child-Pugh class C or bilirubin >5 mg/dL). Monitor hepatic function tests (eg, transaminases, alkaline phosphatase, and bilirubin) closely. Use with caution in patients who have received radiation therapy; radiation recall may occur. May increase radiation-induced toxicity to the myocardium, mucosa, skin, and liver. Doxorubicin is associated with a moderate or high emetic potential (depending on dose or regimen); antiemetics are recommended to prevent nausea and vomiting (Basch, 2011; Dupuis, 2011; Roila, 2010). Potentially significant drug-drug interactions may exist, requiring dose or frequency adjustment, additional monitoring, and/or selection of alternative therapy.

In men, doxorubicin may damage spermatozoa and testicular tissue, resulting in possible genetic fetal abnormalities; may also result in oligospermia, azoospermia, and permanent loss of fertility (sperm counts have been reported to return to normal levels in some men, occurring several years after the end of therapy). In females of reproductive potential, doxorubicin may cause infertility and result in amenorrhea; premature menopause can occur. Children are at increased risk for developing delayed cardiotoxicity; long-term cardiac function monitoring is recommended. Doxorubicin may contribute to prepubertal growth failure in children; may also contribute to gonadal impairment (usually temporary). Radiation recall pneumonitis has been reported in children receiving concomitant dactinomycin and doxorubicin. **[U.S. Boxed Warning]: Should be administered under the supervision of an experienced cancer chemotherapy physician.** Use caution when selecting product for preparation and dispensing; indications, dosages and adverse event profiles differ between conventional doxorubicin hydrochloride solution and doxorubicin liposomal. Both formulations are the same concentration. As a result, serious errors have occurred.

Adverse Reactions Frequency not defined.

Cardiovascular:

Acute cardiotoxicity: Atrioventricular block, bradycardia, bundle branch block, ECG abnormalities, extrasystoles (atrial or ventricular), sinus tachycardia, ST-T wave changes, supraventricular tachycardia, tachyarrhythmia, ventricular tachycardia

Delayed cardiotoxicity: LVEF decreased, CHF (manifestations include ascites, cardiomegaly, dyspnea, edema, gallop rhythm, hepatomegaly, oliguria, pleural effusion, pulmonary edema, tachycardia); myocarditis, pericarditis

Central nervous system: Malaise

Dermatologic: Alopecia, itching, photosensitivity, radiation recall, rash; discoloration of saliva, sweat, or tears

Endocrine & metabolic: Amenorrhea, dehydration, infertility (may be temporary), hyperuricemia

Gastrointestinal: Abdominal pain, anorexia, colon necrosis, diarrhea, GI ulceration, mucositis, nausea, vomiting

Genitourinary: Discoloration of urine

Hematologic: Leukopenia/neutropenia (75%; nadir: 10-14 days; recovery: by day 21); thrombocytopenia and anemia

Local: Skin "flare" at injection site, urticaria

Neuromuscular & skeletal: Weakness

Postmarketing and/or case reports: Anaphylaxis, azoospermia, bilirubin increased, coma (when in combination with cisplatin or vincristine), conjunctivitis, fever, gonadal impairment (children), growth failure (prepubertal), hepatitis, hyperpigmentation (nail, skin & oral mucosa), infection, keratitis, lacrimation, myelodysplastic syndrome, neutropenic fever, neutropenic typhlitis, oligospermia, peripheral neurotoxicity (with intra-arterial doxorubicin), phlebosclerosis, radiation recall pneumonitis (children), secondary acute myelogenous leukemia, seizure (when in combination with cisplatin or vincristine), sepsis, shock, Stevens-Johnson syndrome, systemic hypersensitivity (including urticaria, pruritus, angioedema, dysphagia, and dyspnea), toxic epidermal necrolysis, transaminases increased, urticaria

Drug Interactions

Metabolism/Transport Effects Substrate of CYP2D6 (major), CYP3A4 (major), P-glycoprotein; **Note:** Assignment of Major/Minor substrate status based on clinically relevant drug interaction potential; **Inhibits** CYP2B6 (moderate), CYP2D6 (weak); **Induces** P-glycoprotein

Avoid Concomitant Use

Avoid concomitant use of DOXOrubicin (Conventional) with any of the following: BCG (Intravesical); Conivaptan; Deferiprone; Dipyrone; Fusidic Acid (Systemic); Idelalisib; Natalizumab; Pimecrolimus; Tacrolimus (Topical); Tofacitinib; Vaccines (Live)

Increased Effect/Toxicity

DOXOrubicin (Conventional) may increase the levels/effects of: ARIPiprazole; CYP2B6 Substrates; Deferiprone; Fingolimod; Leflunomide; Mercaptopurine; Natalizumab; Tofacitinib; Vaccines (Live); Zidovudine

The levels/effects of DOXOrubicin (Conventional) may be increased by: Abiraterone Acetate; Bevacizumab; Conivaptan; Cyclophosphamide; CycloSPORINE (Systemic); CYP2D6 Inhibitors (Moderate); CYP2D6 Inhibitors (Strong); CYP3A4 Inhibitors (Moderate); CYP3A4 Inhibitors (Strong); Dasatinib; Denosumab; Dipyrone; Fosaprepitant; Fusidic Acid (Systemic); Idelalisib; Luliconazole; Mifepristone; Osimertinib; Palbociclib; Panobinostat; Peginterferon Alfa-2b; P-glycoprotein/ABCB1 Inhibitors; Pimecrolimus; Roflumilast; SORAfenib; Stiripentol; Tacrolimus (Topical); Taxane Derivatives; Trastuzumab

Decreased Effect

DOXOrubicin (Conventional) may decrease the levels/effects of: BCG (Intravesical); Cardiac Glycosides; Coccidioides immitis Skin Test; Cyclophosphamide; Sipuleucel-T; Stavudine; Vaccines (Inactivated); Vaccines (Live); Zidovudine

The levels/effects of DOXOrubicin (Conventional) may be decreased by: Bosentan; Cardiac Glycosides; CYP3A4 Inducers (Moderate); CYP3A4 Inducers (Strong); Dabrafenib; Deferasirox; Dexrazoxane; Echinacea; Enzalutamide; Mitotane; Osimertinib; Peginterferon Alfa-2b; P-glycoprotein/ABCB1 Inducers; Siltuximab; St Johns Wort; Tocilizumab

Preparation for Administration Hazardous agent; use appropriate precautions for handling and disposal (NIOSH 2014 [group 1]). Reconstitute lyophilized powder with NS (using 5 mL for the 10 mg vial; 10 mL for the 20 mg vial; or 25 mL for the 50 mg vial) to a final concentration of 2 mg/mL; gently shake until contents are dissolved. May further dilute doxorubicin solution or reconstituted doxorubicin solution in 50 to 1000 mL D_5W or NS for infusion. Unstable in solutions with a pH <3 or >7.

Storage/Stability

Lyophilized powder: Store powder at 20°C to 25°C (68°F to 77°F). Protect from light. Retain in carton until time of use. Discard unused portion from single-dose vials. Reconstituted doxorubicin is stable for 7 days at room temperature under normal room lighting and for 15 days when refrigerated at 2°C to 8°C (36°F to 46°F). Protect reconstituted solution from light.

Solution: Store refrigerated at 2°C to 8°C (36°F to 46°F). Protect from light. Retain in carton until time of use. Discard unused portion. Storage of vials of solution under refrigeration may result in formation of a gelled product; if gelling occurs, place vials at room temperature for 2 to 4 hours to return the product to a slightly viscous, mobile solution.

Mechanism of Action Inhibition of DNA and RNA synthesis by intercalation between DNA base pairs by inhibition of topoisomerase II and by steric obstruction. Doxorubicin intercalates at points of local uncoiling of the double helix. Although the exact mechanism is unclear, it appears that direct binding to DNA (intercalation) and inhibition of DNA repair (topoisomerase II inhibition) result in blockade of DNA and RNA synthesis and fragmentation of DNA. Doxorubicin is also a powerful iron chelator; the iron-doxorubicin complex can bind DNA and cell membranes and produce free radicals that immediately cleave the DNA and cell membranes.

Pharmacodynamics/Kinetics

Distribution: V_d: 809 to 1,214 L/m²; does not cross the blood-brain barrier

Protein binding, plasma: ~75%

Metabolism: Primarily hepatic to doxorubicinol (active), then to inactive aglycones, conjugated sulfates, and glucuronides

Half-life elimination:
 Distribution: ~5 minutes
 Terminal: 20 to 48 hours
 Male: 54 hours; Female: 35 hours

Excretion: Feces (~40% as unchanged drug); urine (5% to 12% as unchanged drug and metabolites)

Clearance:
 Infants and Children <2 years: 813 mL/minute/m²
 Children and Adolescents >2 years: 1,540 mL/minute/m²
 Adults: 324 to 809 mL/minutes/m² (appears to be higher in men than women)

Dosing

Adult & Geriatric Doxorubicin is associated with a moderate to high emetic potential (depending on dose or regimen); antiemetics are recommended to prevent nausea and vomiting (Basch, 2011; Roila, 2010).

Manufacturer's labeling: **Note:** Lower dosages should be considered for patients with inadequate marrow reserve (due to advanced age, prior treatment, or neoplastic marrow infiltration). Cumulative doses above 550 mg/m² are associated with an increased risk of cardiomyopathy.

Breast cancer: IV: 60 mg/m² on day 1 of a 21-day cycle (in combination with cyclophosphamide) for 4 cycles

Metastatic solid tumors, leukemia, or lymphoma: IV: Single-agent therapy: 60 to 75 mg/m² every 21 days Combination therapy: 40 to 75 mg/m² every 21 to 28 days

Indication-specific dosing (off-label dosing):
Acute lymphoblastic leukemia: IV:
 Hyper-CVAD regimen: 50 mg/m² on day 4 of Courses 1, 3, 5, and 7 (in combination with cyclophosphamide, vincristine, and dexamethasone); alternating cycles with high-dose methotrexate and cytarabine (Kantarjian, 2004)
 CALGB 8811 regimen: 30 mg/m² on days 1, 8 and 15 of late intensification (Course IV; 8-week cycle); in combination with vincristine, dexamethasone, cyclophosphamide, thioguanine, and cytarabine (Larson, 1995)

Bladder cancer, transitional cell: IV: *Dose-dense MVAC regimen:* 30 mg/m² on day 2 every 14 days (in combination with methotrexate, vinblastine, and cisplatin) (Sternberg, 2001)

Breast cancer: IV:
 CAF regimen: 30 mg/m² on days 1 and 8 every 28 days for 6 cycles (in combination with cyclophosphamide and fluorouracil) (Bull, 1978)
 FAC regimen: 50 mg/m² on day 1 (or administered as a 72-hour continuous infusion) every 21 days for 6 cycles (in combination with fluorouracil and cyclophosphamide) (Assikis, 2003)
 TAC regimen: 50 mg/m² on day 1 every 21 days for 6 cycles (in combination with docetaxel and cyclophosphamide) (Martin, 2005)

Ewing sarcoma: IV:
 VAC/IE regimen: Adults ≤30 years: 75 mg/m² on day 1 every 21 days for 5 cycles (in combination with vincristine and cyclophosphamide; after 5 cycles, dactinomycin replaced doxorubicin), alternating cycles with ifosfamide and etoposide for a total of 17 cycles (Grier, 2003)
 VAIA regimen: Adults <35 years: 30 mg/m²/day on days 1 and 2 every 21 days (doxorubicin alternates with dactinomycin; in combination with vincristine and ifosfamide) for14 cycles (Paulussen, 2008)
 VIDE regimen: 20 mg/m²/day over 4 hours on days 1 to 3 every 21 days for 6 cycles (in combination with vincristine, ifosfamide, and etoposide) (Juergens, 2006)

Hodgkin lymphoma: IV:
 ABVD regimen: 25 mg/m² on days 1 and 15 every 28 days (in combination with bleomycin, vinblastine, and dacarbazine) for 2 to 4 cycles (Bonadonna, 2004; Engert, 2010)
 BEACOPP and escalated BEACOPP regimens: 25 mg/m² (BEACOPP) or 35 mg/m² (escalated BEACOPP) on day 1 every 21 days (in combination with bleomycin, etoposide, cyclophosphamide, vincristine, procarbazine, and prednisone) (Engert, 2009)
 Stanford V regimen: 25 mg/m² on weeks 1, 3, 5, 7, 9, and 11 of a 12-week cycle (in combination with mechlorethamine, vinblastine, vincristine, bleomycin, etoposide, and prednisone) (Horning, 2002)

Non-Hodgkin lymphoma: IV:
 CHOP or RCHOP regimen: 50 mg/m² on day 1 every 21 days (in combination with cyclophosphamide, vincristine, and prednisone +/- rituximab) (Coiffier, 2010; McKelvey, 1976)
 Hyper-CVAD + rituximab regimen: 50 mg/m² administered as a continuous infusion over 24 hours on day 4 of Courses 1, 3, 5, and 7 (21-day treatment cycles; in combination with cyclophosphamide, vincristine, dexamethasone, and rituximab); alternating cycles with high-dose methotrexate and cytarabine (Thomas, 2006)

Dose-adjusted EPOCH or REPOCH regimen: 10 mg/m²/day administered as a continuous infusion on days 1 to 4 every 21 days (in combination with etoposide, vincristine, cyclophosphamide, and prednisone +/- rituximab) (Garcia-Suarez, 2007; Wilson, 2002)

Nordic regimen (Maxi-CHOP): 75 mg/m² on day 1 every 21 days (in combination with cyclophosphamide, vincristine, prednisone, and rituximab), alternating cycles with high-dose cytarabine (Geisler, 2008)

Osteosarcoma: IV:

Cisplatin/doxorubicin regimen: Adults ≤40 years: 25 mg/m² (bolus infusion) on days 1 to 3 every 21 days (in combination with cisplatin) (Bramwell, 1992)

High-dose methotrexate/cisplatin/doxorubicin/ifosfamide regimen: Adults <40 years:

Preoperative: 75 mg/m² administered as a continuous infusion over 24 hours on day 3 of weeks 1 and 7 (in combination with methotrexate, cisplatin, and ifosfamide) (Bacci, 2003)

Postoperative: 90 mg/m² administered as a continuous infusion over 24 hours on weeks 13, 22, and 31 (in combination with methotrexate, cisplatin, and ifosfamide) (Bacci, 2003)

High-dose methotrexate/cisplatin/doxorubicin regimen: Adults <40 years:

Preoperative: 60 mg/m² over 8 hours on days 9 and 36 (in combination with methotrexate and cisplatin) (Bacci, 2000)

Postoperative: 45 mg/m²/day over 4 hours for 2 consecutive days (in combination with methotrexate, cisplatin +/- ifosfamide, +/- etoposide; refer to protocol for criteria, frequency, and other specific information) (Bacci, 2000)

Small cell lung cancer, recurrent: IV: *CAV regimen:* 45 mg/m² (maximum dose: 100 mg) on day 1 every 21 days (in combination with cyclophosphamide and vincristine) until disease progression or unacceptable toxicity or for at least 4 or 6 cycles past maximum response (von Pawel, 1999)

Soft tissue sarcoma: IV:

Nonspecific histologies:

AD regimen: 60 mg/m² on day 1 every 21 days (either as a bolus infusion or administered continuously over 96 hours; in combination with dacarbazine) (Zalupski, 1991)

AIM regimen: 30 mg/m² on days 1 and 2 every 21 days (in combination with ifosfamide and mesna) (Edmonson, 1993)

MAID regimen: 20 mg/m²/day as a continuous infusion on days 1 to 3 every 21 days (in combination with ifosfamide, mesna, and dacarbazine) (Elias, 1989)

Single-agent regimen: 75 mg/m² on day 1 every 21 days until disease progression or unacceptable toxicity (Santoro, 1995)

Rhabdomyosarcoma:

VAC/IE regimen: Adults <21 years: 37.5 mg/m² on days 1 and 2 (administered over 18 hours each day) every 6 weeks (in combination with vincristine and cyclophosphamide), alternating cycles with ifosfamide and etoposide (Arndt, 1998)

VAI regimen (based on a limited number of patients): Adults: 25 mg/m²/day on days 1 to 3 every 21 days (in combination with vincristine and ifosfamide) (Ogilvie, 2010)

Off-label uses:

Endometrial carcinoma, advanced: IV: 60 mg/m² on day 1 every 21 days for 8 cycles; maximum cumulative dose: 420 mg/m² (in combination with cisplatin) (Randall, 2006)

Multiple myeloma: IV:

PAD regimen: Induction: 9 mg/m²/day on days 1 to 4 for 3 cycles (in combination with bortezomib and dexamethasone) (Sonneveld, 2012)

VDT-PACE regimen: 10 mg/m²/day administered as a continuous infusion on days 1 to 4 of each cycle (in combination with bortezomib, dexamethasone, thalidomide, cisplatin, cyclophosphamide, and etoposide) (Lee, 2003; Pineda-Roman, 2008)

Thymomas and thymic malignancies: IV:

CAP regimen: 50 mg/m² on day 1 every 21 days for up to 8 cycles (in combination with cisplatin and cyclophosphamide) (Loehrer, 1994)

ADOC regimen: 40 mg/m² on day 1 every 21 days (in combination with cisplatin, vincristine, and cyclophosphamide) (Fornasiero, 1991)

Uterine sarcoma: IV: 60 mg/m² on day 1 every 21 days; maximum cumulative dose: 480 mg/m² (Omura, 1983) **or** 50 mg/m² (over 15 minutes) on day 1 every 21 days; maximum cumulative dose: 450 mg/m² (in combination with ifosfamide/mesna) (Sutton, 1996)

Waldenstrom macroglobulinemia: IV: *R-CHOP regimen:* 50 mg/m² on day 1 every 21 days for 4 to 8 cycles (in combination with cyclophosphamide, vincristine, prednisone, and rituximab) (Buske, 2009)

Pediatric Doxorubicin is associated with a moderate to high emetic potential (depending on dose or regimen); antiemetics are recommended to prevent nausea and vomiting (Dupuis, 2011).

Manufacturer's labeling: Note: Lower dosages should be considered for patients with inadequate marrow reserve (due to advanced age, prior treatment, or neoplastic marrow infiltration). Cumulative doses above 550 mg/m² are associated with an increased risk of cardiomyopathy.

Metastatic solid tumors, leukemia, or lymphoma: Children and Adolescents: IV:

Single-agent therapy: 60 to 75 mg/m² every 21 days Combination therapy: 40 to 75 mg/m² every 21 to 28 days

Indication-specific dosing (off-label dosing):

Acute lymphoblastic leukemia: IV:

DFCI Consortium Protocol 00-01: Children ≥1 year and Adolescents:

Induction: 30 mg/m²/dose on days 0 and 1 of a 4-week cycle (Vrooman, 2013)

CNS therapy: High-risk patients: 30 mg/m² on day 1 of a 3-week cycle (with dexrazoxane) (Vrooman, 2013)

Intensification: High-risk patients: 30 mg/m² on day 1 of every 3-week cycle (with dexrazoxane; cumulative doxorubicin dose: 300 mg/m²) (Vrooman, 2013)

Ewing sarcoma: Children and Adolescents: IV:

VAC/IE regimen: 75 mg/m² on day 1 every 21 days for 5 cycles (in combination with vincristine and cyclophosphamide; after 5 cycles, dactinomycin replaced doxorubicin), alternating cycles with ifosfamide and etoposide for a total of 17 cycles (Grier, 2003)

VAIA regimen: 30 mg/m²/day on days 1 and 2 every 21 days (doxorubicin alternates with dactinomycin; in combination with vincristine and ifosfamide) for 14 cycles (Paulussen, 2008)

VIDE regimen: 20 mg/m²/day over 4 hours on days 1 to 3 every 21 days for 6 cycles (in combination with vincristine, ifosfamide, and etoposide) (Juergens, 2006)

Osteosarcoma: Children and Adolescents: IV:

Cisplatin/doxorubicin regimen: 25 mg/m² (bolus infusion) on days 1 to 3 every 21 days (in combination with cisplatin) (Bramwell, 1992)

High-dose methotrexate/cisplatin/doxorubicin/ifosfamide regimen:

Preoperative: 75 mg/m² administered as a continuous infusion over 24 hours on day 3 of weeks 1 and 7 (in combination with methotrexate, cisplatin, and ifosfamide) (Bacci, 2003)

Postoperative: 90 mg/m² administered as a continuous infusion over 24 hours on weeks 13, 22, and 31 (in combination with methotrexate, cisplatin, and ifosfamide) (Bacci, 2003)

High-dose methotrexate/cisplatin/doxorubicin regimen:

Preoperative: 60 mg/m² over 8 hours on days 9 and 36 (in combination with methotrexate and cisplatin) (Bacci, 2000)

Postoperative: 45 mg/m²/day over 4 hours for 2 consecutive days (in combination with methotrexate, cisplatin +/- ifosfamide, +/- etoposide; refer to protocol for criteria, frequency, and other specific information) (Bacci, 2000)

Rhabdomyosarcoma: Children and Adolescents: IV: *VAC/IE regimen:* 37.5 mg/m² on days 1 and 2 (administered over 18 hours each day) every 6 weeks (in combination with vincristine and cyclophosphamide), alternating cycles with ifosfamide and etoposide (Arndt, 1998)

Renal Impairment

Mild, moderate, or severe impairment: No dosage adjustment provided in the manufacturers' labeling; however, adjustments are likely not necessary given limited renal excretion.

The following adjustments have also been recommended (Aronoff, 2007):

CrCl <50 mL/minute: No dosage adjustment necessary.
Hemodialysis: Supplemental dose is not necessary.

Hepatic Impairment
The manufacturers' labeling recommends the following adjustments:
Serum bilirubin 1.2 to 3 mg/dL: Administer 50% of dose.
Serum bilirubin 3.1 to 5 mg/dL: Administer 25% of dose.
Severe hepatic impairment (Child-Pugh class C or bilirubin >5 mg/dL): Use is contraindicated.
The following adjustments have also been recommended (Floyd, 2006):
Transaminases 2 to 3 times ULN: Administer 75% of dose.
Transaminases >3 times ULN: Administer 50% of dose.

Obesity *ASCO Guidelines for appropriate chemotherapy dosing in obese adults with cancer:* Utilize patient's actual body weight (full weight) for calculation of body surface area- or weight-based dosing, particularly when the intent of therapy is curative; manage regimen-related toxicities in the same manner as for nonobese patients; if a dose reduction is utilized due to toxicity, consider resumption of full weight-based dosing with subsequent cycles, especially if cause of toxicity (eg, hepatic or renal impairment) is resolved (Griggs, 2012).

Adjustment for Toxicity Cardiotoxicity: Discontinue in patients who develop signs/symptoms of cardiomyopathy.

Administration Doxorubicin is associated with a moderate to high emetic potential (depending on dose or regimen); antiemetics are recommended to prevent nausea and vomiting (Basch, 2011; Dupuis, 2011; Roila, 2010).

Administer IV push over at least 3 to 10 minutes or by continuous infusion (infusion via central venous line recommended). Do not administer IM or SubQ. Rate of administration varies by protocol, refer to individual protocol for details. Protect from light until completion of infusion. Avoid contact with alkaline solutions. Monitor for local erythematous streaking along vein and/or facial flushing (may indicate rapid infusion rate); decrease the rate if occurs.

Vesicant; ensure proper needle or catheter placement prior to and during infusion; avoid extravasation.

Extravasation management: If extravasation occurs, stop infusion immediately and disconnect (leave cannula/needle in place); gently aspirate extravasated solution (do **NOT** flush the line); remove needle/cannula; elevate extremity. Initiate antidote (dexrazoxane or dimethyl sulfate [DMSO]). Apply dry cold compresses for 20 minutes 4 times daily for 1 to 2 days (Perez Fidalgo, 2012); withhold cooling beginning 15 minutes before dexrazoxane infusion; continue withholding cooling until 15 minutes after infusion is completed. Topical DMSO should not be administered in combination with dexrazoxane; may lessen dexrazoxane efficacy.
Dexrazoxane: Adults: 1000 mg/m^2 (maximum dose: 2000 mg) IV (administer in a large vein remote from site of extravasation) over 1 to 2 hours days 1 and 2, then 500 mg/m^2 (maximum dose: 1000 mg) IV over 1 to 2 hours day 3; begin within 6 hours of extravasation. Day 2 and day 3 doses should be administered at approximately the same time (± 3 hours) as the dose on day 1 (Mouridsen, 2007; Perez Fidalgo, 2012). **Note:** Reduce dexrazoxane dose by 50% in patients with moderate to severe renal impairment (CrCl <40 mL/minute).
DMSO: Children and Adults: Apply topically to a region covering twice the affected area every 8 hours for 7 days; begin within 10 minutes of extravasation; do not cover with a dressing (Perez Fidalgo, 2012).

Hazardous agent; use appropriate precautions for handling and disposal (NIOSH 2014 [group 1]).

Monitoring Parameters CBC with differential and platelet count; liver function tests (bilirubin, ALT/AST, alkaline phosphatase); serum uric acid, calcium, potassium, phosphate and creatinine; hydration status; cardiac function (baseline, periodic, and followup): ECG, left ventricular ejection fraction (echocardiography [ECHO] or multigated radionuclide angiography [MUGA]); monitor infusion site

Dosage Forms Excipient information presented when available (limited, particularly for generics); consult specific product labeling. [DSC] = Discontinued product
Solution, Intravenous, as hydrochloride:
Adriamycin: 2 mg/mL (5 mL, 10 mL, 25 mL, 100 mL)
Generic: 2 mg/mL (5 mL, 10 mL, 25 mL, 100 mL)
Solution, Intravenous, as hydrochloride [preservative free]:
Generic: 2 mg/mL (5 mL, 10 mL, 25 mL, 75 mL, 100 mL)
Solution Reconstituted, Intravenous, as hydrochloride:
Adriamycin: 10 mg (1 ea); 20 mg (1 ea); 50 mg (1 ea)
Generic: 10 mg (1 ea [DSC]); 50 mg (1 ea)
Solution Reconstituted, Intravenous, as hydrochloride [preservative free]:
Generic: 10 mg (1 ea); 50 mg (1 ea [DSC])

DOXOrubicin (Liposomal)
(doks oh ROO bi sin lye po SO mal)

Brand Names: US Doxil; Lipodox; Lipodox 50
Brand Names: Canada Caelyx; Myocet
Index Terms DOXOrubicin Hydrochloride (Liposomal); DOXOrubicin Hydrochloride Encapsulated Liposomes (Myocet); DOXOrubicin Hydrochloride Liposome; DOXOrubicin Hydrochloride Liposomes (Myocet); Lipodox; Liposomal DOXOrubicin; Pegylated DOXOrubicin Liposomal; Pegylated Liposomal DOXOrubicin; Pegylated Liposomal DOXOrubicin Hydrochloride (Doxil, Caelyx)
Pharmacologic Category Antineoplastic Agent, Anthracycline; Antineoplastic Agent, Topoisomerase II Inhibitor
Use
US labeling:
AIDS-related Kaposi sarcoma: Treatment of AIDS-related Kaposi sarcoma (after failure of or intolerance to prior systemic therapy)
Multiple myeloma: Treatment of multiple myeloma (in combination with bortezomib) in patients who are bortezomib- naïve and have received at least 1 prior therapy
Ovarian cancer, advanced: Treatment of progressive or recurrent ovarian cancer (after platinum-based treatment)
Canadian labeling: Treatment of metastatic breast cancer (as monotherapy [Caelyx] or in combination with cyclophosphamide [Myocet]); advanced ovarian cancer (after failure of first-line treatment [Caelyx]); AIDS-related Kaposi sarcoma (after failure of or intolerance to prior systemic therapy [Caelyx])

Pregnancy Considerations Adverse events were observed in animal reproduction studies. May cause fetal harm if administered during pregnancy. Women and men of reproductive potential should use effective contraception during therapy and for 6 months after treatment. Doxorubicin liposomal may damage spermatozoa and testicular tissue in males and may result in oligospermia, azoospermia, and permanent loss of fertility. May cause amenorrhea, infertility, and premature menopause in females.

Breast-Feeding Considerations It is not known if doxorubicin liposomal is excreted in breast milk. Due to the potential for serious adverse reactions in the nursing infant, breast-feeding should be discontinued during treatment.

Contraindications
Severe hypersensitivity (including anaphylaxis) to doxorubicin liposomal, conventional doxorubicin, or any component of the formulation
Canadian labeling (Caelyx): Additional contraindications (not in US labeling): Breast-feeding

Warnings/Precautions Hazardous agent - use appropriate precautions for handling and disposal (NIOSH 2014 [group 1]).

[US Boxed Warning]: Doxorubicin liposomal may cause myocardial damage (including congestive heart failure) as the total cumulative dose of doxorubicin approaches 550 mg/m^2. In a clinical study of 250 patients with advanced cancer who were treated with doxorubicin liposomal, the risk of cardiotoxicity was 11% when the cumulative anthracycline dose was between 450 to 550 mg/m^2. Prior use of other anthracyclines or anthracenediones should be included in calculations of total cumulative dosage. The risk of cardiomyopathy may be increased at lower cumulative doses in patients with prior mediastinal irradiation. Myocardial damage may manifest as acute left ventricular failure; cardiotoxicity is defined as a >20% decrease in resting left ventricular ejection fraction (LVEF) from baseline (if LVEF remained in the normal range) or a >10% decrease from baseline (where LVEF was less than the institutional lower limit of normal). Some patients developed signs/symptoms of heart failure without documented evidence of cardiotoxicity. The risk of cardiomyopathy with doxorubicin is generally proportional to the cumulative exposure, although the relationship between cumulative doxorubicin liposomal dose and the risk of cardiotoxicity is not known. For Myocet [Canadian product], cardiotoxicity may occur as the cumulative (lifetime) dose approaches 750 mg/m^2. Anthracycline-induced cardiotoxicity may be delayed (after discontinuation of anthracycline treatment). Assess left ventricular function with echocardiogram or MUGA prior to and during treatment to detect acute changes; monitor after treatment to detect delayed cardiotoxicity. Use in patients with a history of cardiovascular disease only if potential benefits outweigh cardiovascular risk.

[US Boxed Warning]: Acute infusion-related reactions consisting of, but not limited to, flushing, shortness of breath, facial swelling, headache, chills, back pain, tightness in the chest or throat, and/or hypotension occurred in 11% of patients with solid tumors treated with doxorubicin liposomal. Serious, life-threatening and fatal infusion reactions have been reported. Infusion reactions have also included chest pain, pruritus, rash, cyanosis, syncope, tachycardia, bronchospasm, asthma, and apnea. Most reactions occurred during the first infusion. Some reactions have resulted in dose interruption. Medication and equipment to manage infusion reactions should be immediately available during infusion. Initiate infusion at a rate of 1 mg/minute, with the rate increased (to complete infusion over 60 minutes) as tolerated. If an infusion reaction occurs, temporarily interrupt infusion until resolved and resume at a reduced rate. Discontinue for serious or life-threatening infusion reactions.

Neutropenia, anemia, and thrombocytopenia may occur. Monitor blood counts. Treatment delay, dosage modification, or discontinuation may be required. Hematologic toxicity may occur at a higher frequency and severity with combination chemotherapy. Palmar-plantar erythrodysesthesia (hand-foot syndrome) has been reported in patients receiving doxorubicin liposomal; it is usually seen after 2 to 3 treatment cycles, although may also occur earlier; dosage modification may be required; in severe or debilitating cases, treatment discontinuation may be required. Pharmacokinetics in patients with hepatic impairment has not been adequately studied. Doxorubicin is predominantly eliminated hepatically; reduce doxorubicin liposomal dose in patients with serum bilirubin ≥1.2 mg/dL.

Cases of secondary oral cancers (primarily squamous cell carcinoma) have been reported with long-term (>1 year) doxorubicin liposomal exposure; these secondary oral malignancies have occurred during treatment and up to 6 years after treatment. The development of oral ulceration or discomfort should be monitored and further evaluated in patients with past or present use of doxorubicin liposomal. Tissue distribution of the liposomal doxorubicin compared to free doxorubicin may play a role in the development of oral secondary malignancies associated with long-term use.

Liposomal vs conventional formulation dosing: Liposomal formulations of doxorubicin should **NOT** be substituted for conventional doxorubicin hydrochloride on a mg-per-mg basis. Potentially significant drug-drug interactions may exist, requiring dose or frequency adjustment, additional monitoring, and/or selection of alternative therapy. Use of Caelyx [Canadian product] in splenectomized patients with AIDS-related Kaposi sarcoma is not recommended (has not been studied).

Adverse Reactions Frequency not always defined.
>10%:
Cardiovascular: Cardiomyopathy (dose related): 11%; Kaposi sarcoma: <1%), cardiotoxicity (11%), chest tightness (11%), flushing (11%), hypotension (1% to 11%)
Central nervous system: Fatigue (>20%), headache (≤11%)
Dermatologic: Palmar-plantar erythrodysesthesia (ovarian cancer: ≤51%; grades 3/4: 24%), skin rash (grades 3/4: 29%, Kaposi sarcoma: 1% to 5%), alopecia (9% to 19%), facial swelling (11%)
Gastrointestinal: Nausea (ovarian cancer: 46%; Kaposi sarcoma: 17% to 18%; grades 3/4: 5%), stomatitis (grades 3/4: 41%, Kaposi sarcoma: 5% to 8%), vomiting (grades 3/4: 33%; Kaposi sarcoma: 8%), constipation (>20%), diarrhea (grades 3/4: 21%; Kaposi sarcoma: 3% to 8%), anorexia (20%; Kaposi sarcoma: 1% to 5%), mucous membrane disease (14%; grades 3/4: 4%), dyspepsia 12%; grades 3/4: <1%)
Hematologic & oncologic: Thrombocytopenia (dose related, Kaposi sarcoma: 1% to 61%), neutropenia (dose related: 4% to 49%), leukopenia (37%), anemia (16% to 58%; dose related <1% to 5%)
Neuromuscular & skeletal: Weakness (grades 3/4: 40%; Kaposi sarcoma: 7% to 10%), back pain (grades 3/4: 11% to 12%; Kaposi sarcoma: 1% to 5%)
Respiratory: Pharyngitis (16%; Kaposi sarcoma <1%), dyspnea (1% to 15%)
Miscellaneous: Fever (21%; Kaposi sarcoma: 8% to 9%; grades 3/4: <1%), infusion related reaction (7% to 11%)
1% to 10%:
Cardiovascular: Cardiac arrest (≤10%), chest pain (Kaposi sarcoma: 1% to 5%), deep thrombophlebitis (ovarian cancer: 1% to 10%), tachycardia (1% to 10%), vasodilation (ovarian cancer: 1% to 10%)
Central nervous system: Depression (ovarian cancer: 1% to 10%), dizziness (1% to 10%), drowsiness (1% to 10%), chills (Kaposi sarcoma: 1% to 5%)
Dermatologic: Acne vulgaris (ovarian cancer: 1% to 10%), ecchymoses (ovarian cancer: 1% to 10%), exfoliative dermatitis (ovarian cancer: 1% to 10%), fungal dermatitis (ovarian cancer: 1% to 10%), furunculosis (ovarian cancer: 1% to 10%), herpes simplex dermatitis (1% to 10%), pruritus (1% to 10%), skin discoloration (ovarian cancer: 1% to 10%), vesiculobullous dermatitis (ovarian cancer: 1% to 10%), xeroderma (ovarian cancer: 1% to 10%), maculopapular rash (≤10%)
Endocrine & metabolic: Hypercalcemia (ovarian cancer: 1% to 10%), hypokalemia (ovarian cancer: 1% to 10%), hyponatremia (ovarian cancer: 1% to 10%), weight loss (1% to 10%), dehydration (≤10%), hyperglycemia (1% to 5%)
Gastrointestinal: Dysphagia (1% to 10%), esophagitis (ovarian cancer: 1% to 10%), intestinal obstruction (ovarian cancer: 1% to 10%), oral candidiasis (1% to 10%), oral mucosa ulcer (1% to 10%), dysgeusia (1% to ≤10%), abdomen enlarged (ovarian cancer 1% to 5%), glossitis (1% to 5%), increased serum alanine aminotransferase (Kaposi sarcoma 1% to 5%), cachexia
Genitourinary: Hematuria (ovarian cancer: 1% to 10%), hemorrhagic cystitis, urinary tract infection (ovarian cancer: 1% to 10%), vulvovaginal candidiasis (ovarian cancer 1% to 10%)
Hematologic & oncologic: Rectal hemorrhage (ovarian cancer: 1% to 10%), hemolysis (1% to 5%), prolonged prothrombin time (1% to 5%), bone marrow depression (Kaposi sarcoma), progression of cancer (Kaposi sarcoma)
Hepatic: Hyperbilirubinemia (1% to 10%), increased serum alkaline phosphatase (Kaposi sarcoma 1% to 8%)
Hypersensitivity: Hypersensitivity reaction (Kaposi sarcoma 1% to 5%)
Infection: Infection (1% to 12%), herpes zoster (≤10%), paresthesia (5%), myalgia (ovarian cancer: 1% to 5%), neuropathy (ovarian cancer 1% to 5%), toxoplasmosis (Kaposi sarcoma)
Ocular: Dry eye syndrome (ovarian cancer: 1% to 10%), conjunctivitis (≤10%), retinitis (Kaposi sarcoma 1% to 5%) optic neuritis (Kaposi sarcoma)
Respiratory: Epistaxis (ovarian cancer: 1% to 10%), pneumonia (1% to 10%), rhinitis (ovarian cancer: 1% to 10%), sinusitis (ovarian cancer: 1% to 10%), increased cough (≤10%), cough (Kaposi sarcoma)
<1% (Limited to important or life-threatening): Abnormal vision albuminuria, abscess, acute brain syndrome, alkaline phosphatase increased, anaphylactic reaction, anxiety, arthralgia, asthma, balanitis, blindness, bone pain, bronchitis, bundle branch block (Kaposi sarcoma), BUN increased, cardiomegaly, cardiomyopathy, cellulitis, CHF, colitis, creatinine increased, cryptococcosis, candidiasis (Kaposi sarcoma), congestive heart failure (Kaposi sarcoma), confusion, cryptococcosis (Kaposi sarcoma), diabetes mellitus, dysuria, edema, emotional lability, erythema multiforme, erythema nodosum, eosinophilia, fecal impaction, flatulence, hemorrhage, hepatic failure, hepatitis (Kaposi sarcoma, hepatosplenomegaly, hyperkalemia, hypernatremia, hyperuricemia, hyperventilation, hypoglycemia, hyperlipidemia, hypomagnesemia, hypophosphatemia, hypoproteinemia, hypothermia, injection site hemorrhage, insomnia, jaundice, ketosis, lactic dehydrogenase increased, lymphadenopathy, lymphangitis, migraine, myositis, muscle spasm, optic neuritis, pain, pallor, palpitations (Kaposi sarcoma), pancreatitis, pericardial effusion, petechia, pneumothorax, peripheral edema, pleural effusion, pulmonary embolism, radiation injury, sclerosing cholangitis, seizure, secondary acute myelocytic leukemia, sepsis (Kaposi sarcoma), skin necrosis, syncope, squamous cell carcinoma, Stevens-Johnson syndrome, tenesmus, thrombophlebitis (Kaposi sarcoma), thromboplastin decreased, thrombosis (Kaposi sarcoma), tinnitus, toxic epidermal necrolysis, urticaria, ventricular arrhythmia (Kaposi sarcoma)

Drug Interactions
Metabolism/Transport Effects Substrate of CYP2D6 (major), CYP3A4 (major); **Note:** Assignment of Major/Minor substrate status based on clinically relevant drug interaction potential; **Inhibits** CYP2B6 (moderate)

Avoid Concomitant Use
Avoid concomitant use of DOXOrubicin (Liposomal) with any of the following: BCG (Intravesical); Conivaptan; Deferiprone; Dipyrone; Fusidic Acid (Systemic); Idelalisib; Natalizumab; Pimecrolimus; Tacrolimus (Topical); Tofacitinib; Vaccines (Live)

Increased Effect/Toxicity

DOXOrubicin (Liposomal) may increase the levels/effects of: CloZAPine; CYP2B6 Substrates; Deferiprone; Fingolimod; Leflunomide; Natalizumab; Tofacitinib; Vaccines (Live); Zidovudine

The levels/effects of DOXOrubicin (Liposomal) may be increased by: Abiraterone Acetate; Aprepitant; Bevacizumab; Conivaptan; Cyclophosphamide; CYP2D6 Inhibitors (Moderate); CYP2D6 Inhibitors (Strong); CYP3A4 Inhibitors (Moderate); CYP3A4 Inhibitors (Strong); Dasatinib; Denosumab; Dipyrone; Fosaprepitant; Fusidic Acid (Systemic); Idelalisib; Ivacaftor; Luliconazole; Mifepristone; Netupitant; Osimertinib; Palbociclib; Panobinostat; Peginterferon Alfa-2b; Pimecrolimus; Roflumilast; Simeprevir; Stiripentol; Tacrolimus (Topical); Taxane Derivatives; Trastuzumab

Decreased Effect

DOXOrubicin (Liposomal) may decrease the levels/effects of: BCG (Intravesical); Cardiac Glycosides; Coccidioides immitis Skin Test; Cyclophosphamide; Sipuleucel-T; Stavudine; Vaccines (Inactivated); Vaccines (Live); Zidovudine

The levels/effects of DOXOrubicin (Liposomal) may be decreased by: Bosentan; Cardiac Glycosides; CYP3A4 Inducers (Moderate); CYP3A4 Inducers (Strong); Dabrafenib; Deferasirox; Echinacea; Enzalutamide; Mitotane; Osimertinib; Peginterferon Alfa-2b; Siltuximab; St Johns Wort; Tocilizumab

Preparation for Administration Hazardous agent; use appropriate precautions for handling and disposal (NIOSH 2014 [group 1]).

Doxil, Caelyx: Dilute doses ≤90 in D_5W 250 mL prior to administration. Dilute doses >90 mg in D_5W 500 mL. Solution is not clear, but has a red, translucent appearance due to the liposomal dispersion. Dilute only in D_5W; do not use bacteriostatic agents; do not mix with other medications.

Myocet: Refer to product labeling for detailed reconstitution and preparation information.

Storage/Stability Store intact vials refrigerated at 2°C to 8°C (36°F to 46°F); avoid freezing.

Doxil, Caelyx: Solutions diluted for infusion should be refrigerated at 2°C to 8°C (36°F to 46°F); administer within 24 hours.

Myocet: Refer to product labeling for detailed reconstitution and preparation information. Following reconstitution, may be stored up to 8 hours at room temperature or up to 72 hours refrigerated at 2°C to 8°C (36°F to 46°F); do not freeze.

Mechanism of Action Doxorubicin inhibits DNA and RNA synthesis by intercalating between DNA base pairs causing steric obstruction and inhibits topoisomerase-II at the point of DNA cleavage. Doxorubicin is also a powerful iron chelator. The iron-doxorubicin complex can bind DNA and cell membranes, producing free hydroxyl (OH) radicals that cleave DNA and cell membranes. Active throughout entire cell cycle. Doxorubicin liposomal is a pegylated formulation which protects the liposomes, and thereby increases blood circulation time.

Pharmacodynamics/Kinetics

Distribution: V_{dss}: ~2.7 to 2.8 L/m²; largely confined to vascular fluid

Protein binding, plasma: Unknown; nonliposomal (conventional) doxorubicin: ~70%

Half-life elimination: Terminal: Distribution: ~4.7 to 5.2 hours, Elimination: ~52 to 55 hours

Metabolism: Hepatic and in plasma to doxorubicinol and the sulfate and glucuronide conjugates of 4-demethyl,7-deoxyaglycones

Dosing

Adult & Geriatric Liposomal formulations of doxorubicin should **NOT** be substituted for conventional doxorubicin hydrochloride on a mg-per-mg basis.

US labeling:

AIDS-related Kaposi sarcoma: IV: 20 mg/m² once every 21 days until disease progression or unacceptable toxicity

Multiple myeloma: IV: 30 mg/m² on day 4 every 21 days (in combination with bortezomib) for 8 cycles or until disease progression or unacceptable toxicity (Orlowski 2007)

Multiple myeloma, newly diagnosed (off-label dosing): IV: 40 mg/m² on day 1 every 4 weeks (in combination with vincristine and dexamethasone) for at least 4 cycles (Rifkin, 2006).

Ovarian cancer, advanced: IV: 50 mg/m² once every 28 days until disease progression or unacceptable toxicity

Ovarian cancer, advanced, recurrent (off-label dosing): IV: 40 mg/m² once every 28 days (as a single agent) until disease progression or unacceptable toxicity (Ferrandina, 2008; Rose, 2001) or 30 mg/m² once every 28 days (in combination with carboplatin) for at least 6 cycles (Pujade-Lauraine, 2010) or 40 mg/m² once every 28 days (in combination with bevacizumab) until disease progression or unacceptable toxicity (Pujade-Lauraine, 2014).

Canadian labeling:

AIDS-related Kaposi sarcoma (Caelyx): IV: 20 mg/m² once every 2 to 3 weeks; continue as long as responding and tolerating

Breast cancer, metastatic: IV:

Caelyx: 50 mg/m² once every 4 weeks until disease progression or unacceptable toxicity

Myocet: 60 to 75 mg/m² once every 3 weeks (in combination with cyclophosphamide)

Ovarian cancer, advanced (Caelyx): IV: 50 mg/m² once every 4 weeks until disease progression or unacceptable toxicity

Off-label uses/doses:

Breast cancer, metastatic (off-label use in US): IV: 50 mg/m² every 4 weeks (Keller, 2004)

Cutaneous T-cell lymphomas (off-label use): IV: 20 mg/m² days 1 and 15 every 4 weeks for 6 cycles (Dummer, 2012) **or** 20 mg/m² every 4 weeks (Wollina, 2003)

Hodgkin lymphoma, salvage treatment (off-label use): IV: GVD regimen: 10 mg/m² (post-transplant patients) or 15 mg/m² (transplant-naive patients) days 1 and 8 every 3 weeks (in combination with gemcitabine and vinorelbine) for 2 to 6 cycles (Bartlett, 2007)

Soft tissue sarcoma, advanced (off-label use): IV: 50 mg/m² every 4 weeks for 6 cycles (Judson, 2001)

Uterine sarcoma, advanced or recurrent (off-label use): IV: 50 mg/m² every 4 weeks until disease progression or unacceptable toxicity (Sutton, 2005)

Renal Impairment There are no dosage adjustments provided in the manufacturer's labeling (has not been studied).

Hepatic Impairment

US labeling: There are no dosage adjustments provided in the manufacturer's labeling. However, doxorubicin is predominantly hepatically eliminated and reduced doxorubicin liposomal doses are recommended in patients with serum bilirubin ≥1.2 mg/dL.

Canadian labeling:

Caelyx: AIDS-related Kaposi sarcoma:

Bilirubin 1.2 to 3 mg/dL: Administer 50% of normal dose

Bilirubin >3 mg/dL: Administer 25% of normal dose

Caelyx: Breast cancer and ovarian cancer:

Bilirubin 1.2 to 3 mg/dL: Initial dose: Administer 75% of normal dose; if tolerated and no change in bilirubin/hepatic enzymes, may increase to full dose with cycle 2

Bilirubin >3 mg/dL: Initial dose: Administer 50% of normal dose; if tolerated and no change in bilirubin/hepatic enzymes, may increase dose to 75% of normal dose for cycle 2; if cycle 2 dose tolerated, may increase to full dose for subsequent cycles.

Myocet: Breast cancer:

Bilirubin 1.2 to 3 mg/dL: Administer 50% of normal dose

Bilirubin >3 mg/dL: Administer 25% of normal dose

Obesity *ASCO Guidelines for appropriate chemotherapy dosing in obese adults with cancer:* Utilize patient's actual body weight (full weight) for calculation of body surface area- or weight-based dosing, particularly when the intent of therapy is curative; manage regimen-related toxicities in the same manner as for nonobese patients; if a dose reduction is utilized due to toxicity, consider resumption of full weight-based dosing with subsequent cycles, especially if cause of toxicity (eg, hepatic or renal impairment) is resolved (Griggs, 2012).

Adjustment for Toxicity

US labeling: Note: Once a dosage reduction due to toxicity has been implemented, the dose should not be increased at a later time.

Recommended Dose Modification Guidelines

Toxicity Grade	Dose Adjustment
HAND-FOOT SYNDROME (HFS)	
1 (Mild erythema, swelling, or desquamation not interfering with daily activities)	No prior Grade 3 or 4 HFS toxicity: No dosage adjustment is necessary. Prior Grade 3 or 4 HFS toxicity: Delay dose up to 2 weeks and decrease dose by 25%.
2 (Erythema, desquamation, or swelling interfering with, but not precluding, normal physical activities; small blisters or ulcerations <2 cm in diameter)	Delay dosing up to 2 weeks or until resolved to Grade 0 or 1. If after 2 weeks there is no resolution, discontinue liposomal doxorubicin. If resolved to Grade 0 or 1 within 2 weeks and no prior Grade 3 or 4 HFS, continue treatment at previous dose. If a prior Grade 3 or 4 HFS has occurred, decrease dose by 25%.
3 (Blistering, ulceration, or swelling interfering with walking or normal daily activities; cannot wear regular clothing)	Delay dosing up to 2 weeks or until resolved to Grade 0 or 1, then decrease dose by 25%. If no resolution after 2 weeks, discontinue liposomal doxorubicin.
4 (Diffuse or local process causing infectious complications, or a bedridden state or hospitalization)	Delay dosing up to 2 weeks or until resolved to Grade 0 or 1, then decrease dose by 25%. If no resolution after 2 weeks, discontinue liposomal doxorubicin.
STOMATITIS	
1 (Painless ulcers, erythema, or mild soreness)	No prior Grade 3 or 4 toxicity: No dosage adjustment is necessary. Prior Grade 3 or 4 toxicity: Delay dose up to 2 weeks and decrease dose by 25%.
2 (Painful erythema, edema, or ulcers, but can eat)	Delay dosing up to 2 weeks or until resolved to Grade 0 or 1. If after 2 weeks there is no resolution, discontinue liposomal doxorubicin. If resolved to Grade 0 or 1 within 2 weeks and no prior Grade 3 or 4 stomatitis, continue treatment at previous dose. If prior Grade 3 or 4 stomatitis, decrease dose by 25%.
3 (Painful erythema, edema, or ulcers, and cannot eat)	Delay dosing up to 2 weeks or until resolved to Grade 0 or 1. Decrease dose by 25% and return to original dosing interval. If after 2 weeks there is no resolution, discontinue liposomal doxorubicin.
4 (Requires parenteral or enteral support)	Delay dosing up to 2 weeks or until resolved to Grade 0 or 1. Decrease dose by 25% and return to original dosing interval. If after 2 weeks there is no resolution, discontinue liposomal doxorubicin.

See table: "Hematologic Toxicity"

Hematologic Toxicity
(see below for multiple myeloma)

Grade	ANC	Platelets	Modification
1	1,500 to 1,900/mm^3	75,000 to 150,000/mm^3	No dosage adjustment is necessary.
2	1,000 to <1,500/mm^3	50,000 to <75,000/mm^3	Delay until ANC ≥1,500/mm^3 and platelets ≥75,000/mm^3; resume treatment at previous dose.
3	500 to 999/mm^3	25,000 to <50,000/mm^3	Delay until ANC ≥1,500/mm^3 and platelets ≥75,000/mm^3; resume treatment at previous dose.
4	<500/mm^3	<25,000/mm^3	Delay until ANC ≥1,500/mm^3 and platelets ≥75,000/mm^3; resume at 25% dose reduction or continue at previous dose with granulocyte growth factor support.

Doxorubicin Liposomal Dosing Adjustment for Toxicity in Treatment with Bortezomib (for Multiple Myeloma) (see Bortezomib monograph for bortezomib dosage reduction with toxicity guidelines):

Fever ≥38°C and ANC <1,000/mm^3: If prior to doxorubicin liposomal treatment (day 4), do not administer (withhold); if after doxorubicin liposomal administered, reduce dose by 25% in next cycle.

ANC <500/mm^3, platelets <25,000/mm^3, hemoglobin <8 g/dL: If prior to doxorubicin liposomal treatment (day 4); do not administer (withhold); if after doxorubicin liposomal administered and if bortezomib dose reduction occurred for hematologic toxicity, reduce dose by 25% in next cycle

Grade 3 or 4 nonhematologic toxicity: Delay dose until resolved to grade <2 and then reduce dose by 25%

Neuropathic pain or peripheral neuropathy: No dose reductions needed for doxorubicin liposomal, refer to Bortezomib monograph for bortezomib dosing adjustment.

Canadian labeling:
Caelyx: Nonhematologic toxicity: Breast cancer, ovarian cancer:

Caelyx: Recommended Dose Modification Guidelines

Toxicity Grade	Week After Prior Caelyx Dose (Breast Cancer or Ovarian Cancer)	
	Weeks 4 and 5	Week 6
HAND-FOOT SYNDROME (HFS)		
1 (Mild erythema, swelling, or desquamation not interfering with daily activities)	Redose unless patient has experienced previous Grade 3 or 4 HFS toxicity. If so, wait an additional week	Decrease dose by 25%; return to 4-week interval
2 (Erythema, desquamation, or swelling interfering with, but not precluding, normal physical activities; small blisters or ulcerations <2 cm in diameter)	Wait an additional week	Decrease dose by 25%; return to 4-week interval
3 (Blistering, ulceration, or swelling interfering with walking or normal daily activities; cannot wear regular clothing)	Wait an additional week	Discontinue therapy
4 (Diffuse or local process causing infectious complications, or a bedridden state or hospitalization)	Wait an additional week	Discontinue therapy
STOMATITIS		
1 (Painless ulcers, erythema, or mild soreness)	Redose unless patient has experienced previous Grade 3 or 4 stomatitis. If so, wait an additional week.	Decrease dose by 25%; return to 4-week interval or if warranted, discontinue therapy
2 (Painful erythema, edema, or ulcers, but can eat)	Wait an additional week	Decrease dose by 25%; return to 4-week interval or if warranted, discontinue therapy
3 (Painful erythema, edema, or ulcers, and cannot eat)	Wait an additional week	Discontinue therapy
4 (Requires parenteral or enteral support)	Wait an additional week	Discontinue therapy

Caelyx: Hematologic toxicity: Breast cancer, ovarian cancer: Refer to US dosage adjustment for hematologic toxicity section.

Caelyx: Nonhematologic toxicity: AIDS-related Kaposi sarcoma:

Caelyx: Recommended Dose Modification Guidelines: Hand-Foot Syndrome (HFS) (AIDS-related Kaposi Sarcoma)

Toxicity Grade	Weeks Since Last Caelyx Dose (AIDS-related Kaposi Sarcoma)	
	3 Weeks	4 Weeks
HAND-FOOT SYNDROME (HFS)		
1 (Mild erythema, swelling, or desquamation not interfering with daily activities)	Redose unless patient has experienced previous Grade 3 or 4 skin toxicity. If so, wait an additional week	Decrease dose by 25%; return to 3-week interval
2 (Erythema, desquamation, or swelling interfering with, but not precluding, normal physical activities; small blisters or ulcerations <2 cm in diameter)	Wait an additional week	Decrease dose by 50%; return to 3-week interval
3 (Blistering, ulceration, or swelling interfering with walking or normal daily activities; cannot wear regular clothing)	Wait an additional week	Discontinue therapy
4 (Diffuse or local process causing infectious complications, or a bedridden state or hospitalization)	Wait an additional week	Discontinue therapy

Caelyx: Recommended Dose Modification Guidelines: Stomatitis (AIDS-related Kaposi Sarcoma)

STOMATITIS Toxicity grade:	Caelyx Dosage Adjustment (AIDS-related Kaposi Sarcoma)
1 (Painless ulcers, erythema, or mild soreness)	No dosage adjustment
2 (Painful erythema, edema, or ulcers, but can eat)	Wait 1 week and if symptoms improve, redose at 100% dose
3 (Painful erythema, edema, or ulcers, and cannot eat)	Wait 1 week and if symptoms improve, redose with a 25% dose reduction
4 (Requires parenteral or enteral support)	Wait 1 week and if symptoms improve, redose with a 50% dose reduction

Caelyx: Hematologic toxicity: AIDS-related Kaposi sarcoma:

Caelyx: Hematologic Toxicity (AIDS-related Kaposi Sarcoma)

Grade	ANC	Platelets	Modification
1	1,500 to 1,900/mm^3	75,000 to 150,000/mm^3	None
2	1,000 to <1,500/mm^3	50,000 to <75,000/mm^3	None
3	500 to 999/mm^3	25,000 to <50,000/mm^3	Wait until ANC ≥1,000/mm^3 and/or platelets ≥50,000/mm^3; redose with a 25% dose reduction.
4	<500/mm^3	<25,000/mm^3	Wait until ANC ≥1,000/mm^3 and/or platelets ≥50,000/mm^3; redose with a 50% dose reduction.

Myocet: Hematologic or gastrointestinal toxicity: Dosage reduction: If initial dose was 75 mg/m^2, reduce dose to 60 mg/m^2; if initial dose was 60 mg/m^2, reduce dose to 50 mg/m^2. If toxicity persists with subsequent cycles, consider reducing dose further (from 60 mg/m^2 to 50 mg/m^2 or from 50 mg/m^2 to 40 mg/m^2).

Neutropenia: If grade 4 neutropenia (ANC <500/mm^3) without fever lasting ≥7 days or grade 4 neutropenia of any duration with concurrent fever (≥38.5°C) occurs, consider reducing dose with subsequent cycles. **Note:** Prior to dose reductions, prophylactic cytokine therapy may be considered.

Thrombocytopenia or anemia: If grade 4 thrombocytopenia or anemia occurs, hold therapy until recovery to ≤ grade 2. Reduce dose with subsequent cycles or consider discontinuing treatment.

Gastrointestinal toxicity or mucositis: Grade 3 mucositis persisting ≥3 days, or grade 4 mucositis of any duration, or grade 3 or 4 gastrointestinal toxicity not responsive to interventions and/or prophylaxis: Consider dose reduction with subsequent cycles.

Administration Monitor for infusion reaction. For IV infusion only; do not administer IV push.

Doxil, Caelyx: Administer IVPB over 60 minutes; the manufacturer recommends infusing the first dose at initial rate of 1 mg/minute to minimize risk of infusion reactions; if no infusion-related reactions are observed, then increase the infusion rate for completion over 1 hour. Do **NOT** administer undiluted. Do **NOT** infuse with in-line filters. Do not mix with other medications. Monitor for local erythematous streaking along vein and/or facial flushing (may indicate rapid infusion rate).

For multiple myeloma, administer doxorubicin liposomal after bortezomib on day 4 of each cycle.

Myocet: Infuse over 1 hour.

Irritant (Perez Fidalgo, 2012); monitor infusion site; avoid extravasation. Assure proper needle or catheter position prior to administration.

Extravasation management: If extravasation, infiltration, or burning/stinging sensation occurs, stop infusion immediately and disconnect (leave cannula/needle in place); gently aspirate extravasated solution (do **NOT** flush the line); remove needle/cannula; elevate extremity (Perez Fidalgo, 2012; Polovich, 2009). Do not apply pressure to the site. Apply ice to the site for 15 minutes 4 times a day for 3 days.

Hazardous agent; use appropriate precautions for handling and disposal (NIOSH 2014 [group 1]). If contact with skin/mucosa occurs, wash immediately with soap and water.

Monitoring Parameters CBC with differential and platelet count, liver function tests (ALT/AST, bilirubin, alkaline phosphatase); monitor infusion site, monitor for infusion reactions, hand-foot syndrome, stomatitis, and oral ulceration/discomfort suggestive of secondary oral malignancy Cardiac function (left ventricular ejection fraction [LVEF]; baseline and periodic); echocardiography, or MUGA scan may be used.

Dosage Forms Excipient information presented when available (limited, particularly for generics); consult specific product labeling.

Injectable, Intravenous, as hydrochloride:
Doxil: 2 mg/mL (10 mL, 25 mL)
Lipodox: 2 mg/mL (10 mL)
Lipodox 50: 2 mg/mL (25 mL)
Generic: 2 mg/mL (10 mL, 25 mL)

Dosage Forms: Canada

Excipient information presented when available (limited, particularly for generics); consult specific product labeling.
Injection, solution, as hydrochloride, pegylated:
Caelyx: 2 mg/mL (10 mL, 25 mL)
Injection, encapsulated liposomes:
Myocet: 3-vial kit (doxorubicin HCl for injection 50 mg/vial, liposomes for injection, and buffer for injection)

- ◆ Doxorubicin HCl *see* DOXOrubicin (Conventional) *on page 593*
- ◆ Doxorubicin Hydrochloride *see* DOXOrubicin (Conventional) *on page 593*
- ◆ DOXOrubicin Hydrochloride Encapsulated Liposomes (Myocet) *see* DOXOrubicin (Liposomal) *on page 597*
- ◆ Doxorubicin Hydrochloride For Injection, USP (Can) *see* DOXOrubicin (Conventional) *on page 593*
- ◆ Doxorubicin Hydrochloride Injection (Can) *see* DOXOrubicin (Conventional) *on page 593*
- ◆ DOXOrubicin Hydrochloride (Liposomal) *see* DOXOrubicin (Liposomal) *on page 597*
- ◆ DOXOrubicin Hydrochloride Liposome *see* DOXOrubicin (Liposomal) *on page 597*
- ◆ DOXOrubicin Hydrochloride Liposomes (Myocet) *see* DOXOrubicin (Liposomal) *on page 597*
- ◆ Doxy 100 *see* Doxycycline *on page 601*
- ◆ Doxycin (Can) *see* Doxycycline *on page 601*

Doxycycline (doks i SYE kleen)

Brand Names: US Acticlate; Adoxa; Adoxa Pak 1/100; Adoxa Pak 1/150; Adoxa Pak 2/100; Alodox Convenience [DSC]; Avidoxy; Doryx; Doxy 100; Mondoxyne NL; Monodox; Morgidox; NicAzelDoxy 30 [DSC]; NicAzelDoxy 60 [DSC]; Ocudox [DSC]; Oracea; TargaDOX; Vibramycin

Brand Names: Canada Apo-Doxy; Apo-Doxy Tabs; Apprilon; Dom-Doxycycline; Doxycin; Doxytab; Periostat; PHL-Doxycycline; PMS-Doxycycline; Teva-Doxycycline; Vibra-Tabs; Vibramycin

Index Terms Doxycycline Calcium; Doxycycline Hyclate; Doxycycline Monohydrate

Pharmacologic Category Antibiotic, Tetracycline Derivative

Use Principally in the treatment of infections caused by susceptible *Rickettsia*, *Chlamydia*, *Chlamydophila*, and *Mycoplasma*; malaria prophylaxis (areas with chloroquine- and/or pyrimethamine-sulfadoxine resistant strains) for short-term travel (<4 months); treatment for syphilis, uncomplicated *Neisseria gonorrhoeae* (alternative agent), *Listeria*, *Actinomyces israelii*, and *Clostridium* infections in penicillin-allergic patients; used for community-acquired pneumonia and other common infections due to susceptible organisms; anthrax due to *Bacillus anthracis*, including inhalational anthrax (postexposure); treatment of infections caused by uncommon susceptible gram-negative and gram-positive organisms including *Borrelia recurrentis*, *Ureaplasma urealyticum*, *Haemophilus ducreyi*, *Yersinia pestis* (plague), *Francisella tularensis* (tularemia due to zoonotic infection), *Vibrio cholerae*, *Campylobacter fetus*, *Brucella* spp, *Bartonella bacilliformis*, and *Klebsiella granulomatis*, Q fever; intestinal amebiasis; severe acne

Oracea (US labeling), Apprilon (Canadian labeling): Treatment of inflammatory lesions associated with rosacea

Periostat (Canadian labeling; not available in the US): Adjunctive periodontitis treatment to scaling and root planing to promote attachment level gain and reduce pocket depth

◄ **Pregnancy Considerations** Tetracyclines cross the placenta and accumulate in developing teeth and long tubular bones. Therapeutic doses of doxycycline during pregnancy are unlikely to produce substantial teratogenic risk, but data are insufficient to say that there is no risk. In general, reports of exposure have been limited to short durations of therapy in the first trimester. Tetracyclines may discolor fetal teeth following maternal use during pregnancy; the specific teeth involved and the portion of the tooth affected depends on the timing and duration of exposure relative to tooth calcification. As a class, tetracyclines are generally considered second-line antibiotics in pregnant women and their use should be avoided. Tetracycline medications should be used during pregnancy only when other medications are contraindicated or ineffective (Mylonas 2011).

Breast-Feeding Considerations Doxycycline is excreted in breast milk (Chung 2002). According to the manufacturer, the decision to continue or discontinue breast-feeding during therapy should take into account the risk of exposure to the infant and the benefits of treatment to the mother. Although nursing is not specifically contraindicated, the effects of long-term exposure via breast milk are not known. Oral absorption of doxycycline is not markedly influenced by simultaneous ingestion of milk; therefore, oral absorption of doxycycline by the breast-feeding infant would not be expected to be diminished by the calcium in the maternal milk. Nondose-related effects could include modification of bowel flora.

Contraindications

US labeling: Hypersensitivity to doxycycline, tetracycline, or any component of the formulation

Canadian labeling: Hypersensitivity to doxycycline, tetracycline, or any component of the formulation; myasthenia gravis

Periostat, Apprilon: Additional contraindications: Use in infants and children <8 years of age or during second or third trimester of pregnancy; breast-feeding

Warnings/Precautions Photosensitivity reaction may occur with this drug; avoid prolonged exposure to sunlight or tanning equipment. Antianabolic effects of tetracyclines can increase BUN (dose-related). Hypersensitivity syndromes have been reported, including drug rash with eosinophilia and systemic symptoms (DRESS), urticaria, angioneurotic edema, anaphylaxis, anaphylactoid purpura, serum sickness, pericarditis, and systemic lupus erythematosus exacerbation. Hepatotoxicity rarely occurs; if symptomatic, conduct LFT and discontinue drug. Intracranial hypertension (headache, blurred vision, diplopia, vision loss, and/or papilledema) has been associated with use. Women of childbearing age who are overweight or have a history of intracranial hypertension are at greater risk. Concomitant use of isotretinoin (known to cause pseudotumor cerebri) and doxycycline should be avoided. Intracranial hypertension typically resolves after discontinuation of treatment; however, permanent visual loss is possible. If visual symptoms develop during treatment, prompt ophthalmologic evaluation is warranted. Intracranial pressure can remain elevated for weeks after drug discontinuation; monitor patients until they stabilize. Prolonged use may result in fungal or bacterial superinfection, including *C. difficile*-associated diarrhea (CDAD) and pseudomembranous colitis; CDAD has been observed >2 months postantibiotic treatment. May cause tissue hyperpigmentation, tooth enamel hypoplasia, or permanent tooth discoloration; use of tetracyclines should be avoided during tooth development (last half of pregnancy, infancy, and children <8 years of age) unless other drugs are not likely to be effective or are contraindicated. However, recommended in treatment of anthrax exposure, tickborne rickettsial diseases, and Q fever. Do not use during pregnancy. In addition to affecting tooth development, tetracycline use has been associated with retardation of skeletal development and reduced bone growth. When used for malaria prophylaxis, does not completely suppress asexual blood stages of *Plasmodium* strains. Doxycycline does not suppress *Plasmodium falciparum*'s sexual blood stage gametocytes. Patients completing a regimen may still transmit the infection to mosquitoes outside endemic areas.

Oracea (US labeling) or Apprilon (Canadian labeling): Additional specific warnings: Should not be used for the treatment or prophylaxis of bacterial infections, since the lower dose of drug per capsule may be subefficacious and promote resistance. Syrup contains sodium metabisulfite. Effectiveness of products intended for use in periodontitis has not been established in patients with coexistent oral candidiasis; use with caution in patients with a history or predisposition to oral candidiasis.

Adverse Reactions Frequency not always defined.

Central nervous system: Headache (2%), bulging fontanel (infants), intracranial hypertension (adults), pericarditis

Dermatologic: Discoloration of thyroid gland (brown/black, no dysfunction reported), erythema multiforme, erythematous rash, exfoliative dermatitis, maculopapular rash, skin hyperpigmentation, skin photosensitivity, Stevens-Johnson syndrome, toxic epidermal necrolysis, urticaria

Endocrine & metabolic: Hypoglycemia

Gastrointestinal: Nausea (13%), vomiting (8%), diarrhea (3%), upper abdominal pain (2%), anorexia, *Clostridium difficile* associated diarrhea, dental discoloration (children), dysphagia, enterocolitis, esophageal ulcer, esophagitis, glossitis

Genitourinary: Vaginitis (bacterial, 3%), vulvovaginal disease (mycotic infection, 2%), inflammatory anogenital lesion

Hematologic & oncologic: Anaphylactoid purpura, eosinophilia, hemolytic anemia, neutropenia, thrombocytopenia

Hepatic: Hepatotoxicity (rare)

Hypersensitivity: Anaphylaxis, angioedema, serum sickness

Neuromuscular & skeletal: Exacerbation of systemic lupus erythematosus

Renal: Increased blood urea nitrogen (dose related)

Note: Additional adverse reactions not listed above that have been reported with Oracea or Periostat (Canadian availability; not available in the U.S.):

Periostat: Arthralgia (6%), dyspepsia (6%), dysmenorrhea (4%), pain (4%), bronchitis (3%)

Oracea: Nasopharyngitis (5%), hypertension (3%), sinusitis (3%), anxiety (2%), fungal infection (2%), increased blood pressure (2%), increased lactate dehydrogenase (2%), increased serum AST (2%), influenza (2%), pain (2%), abdominal pain (1% to 2%), back pain (1%), hyperglycemia (1%), sinus headache (1%), xerostomia (1%)

Drug Interactions

Metabolism/Transport Effects None known.

Avoid Concomitant Use

Avoid concomitant use of Doxycycline with any of the following: BCG (Intravesical); Mecamylamine; Retinoic Acid Derivatives; Strontium Ranelate

Increased Effect/Toxicity

Doxycycline may increase the levels/effects of: Mecamylamine; Mipomersen; Neuromuscular-Blocking Agents; Porfimer; Retinoic Acid Derivatives; Verteporfin; Vitamin K Antagonists

Decreased Effect

Doxycycline may decrease the levels/effects of: BCG (Intravesical); BCG Vaccine (Immunization); Iron Salts; Penicillins; Sodium Picosulfate; Typhoid Vaccine

The levels/effects of Doxycycline may be decreased by: Antacids; Barbiturates; Bile Acid Sequestrants; Bismuth Subcitrate; Bismuth Subsalicylate; Calcium Salts; CarBAMazepine; Fosphenytoin; Iron Salts; Lanthanum; Magnesium Salts; Multivitamins/Minerals (with ADEK, Folate, Iron); Multivitamins/Minerals (with AE, No Iron); Phenytoin; Quinapril; Rifampin; Strontium Ranelate; Sucralfate; Sucroferric Oxyhydroxide

Food Interactions

Ethanol: Chronic ethanol ingestion may reduce the serum concentration of doxycycline.

Food: Doxycycline serum levels may be slightly decreased if taken with food or milk. Administration with iron or calcium may decrease doxycycline absorption. May decrease absorption of calcium, iron, magnesium, zinc, and amino acids. Management: Doryx tablets can be administered without regard to meals.

Preparation for Administration IV infusion: Following reconstitution with sterile water for injection, dilute to a final concentration of 0.1-1 mg/mL using a compatible solution.

Storage/Stability

Capsule, tablet: Store at 20°C to 25°C (68°F to 77°F); excursions are permitted between 15°C and 30°C (59°F and 86°F). Protect from light and moisture.

Syrup, oral suspension: Store below 30°C (86°F); protect from light.

IV infusion: Protect from light. Stability varies based on solution.

Mechanism of Action Inhibits protein synthesis by binding with the 30S and possibly the 50S ribosomal subunit(s) of susceptible bacteria; may also cause alterations in the cytoplasmic membrane

Periostat capsules (Canadian availability; not available in the US): Proposed mechanism: Has been shown to inhibit collagenase activity *in vitro*. Also has been noted to reduce elevated collagenase activity in the gingival crevicular fluid of patients with periodontal disease. Systemic levels do not reach inhibitory concentrations against bacteria.

Pharmacodynamics/Kinetics

Absorption: Oral: Almost completely from the GI tract; absorption can be reduced by food or milk by 20%

Distribution: Widely into body tissues and fluids including synovial, pleural, prostatic, seminal fluids, and bronchial secretions; saliva, aqueous humor, and CSF penetration is poor; Periostat (Canadian availability; not available in the US): ~53-134 L

Protein binding: 90%

Metabolism: Not hepatic; partially inactivated in GI tract by chelate formation

Bioavailability: Reduced at high pH; may be clinically significant in patients with gastrectomy, gastric bypass surgery or who are otherwise deemed achlorhydric

Half-life elimination: Single dose: 12-15 hours (usually increases to 22-24 hours with multiple doses); End-stage renal disease: 18-25 hours

Oracea (US labeling), Apprilon (Canadian labeling): Single dose: 21 hours

Periostat: Single dose: 18 hours

Time to peak, serum: 1.5-4 hours

Excretion: Feces (30%); urine (23%)

Dosing

Adult & Geriatric

Usual dosage range: Oral, IV: 100 to 200 mg/day in 1 to 2 divided doses

Acute bacterial rhinosinusitis (off-label use): Oral: 200 mg/day in 1 to 2 divided doses for 5 to 7 days (Chow 2012)

Anthrax:

Inhalational (postexposure prophylaxis): Oral, IV (use oral route when possible): 100 mg every 12 hours for 60 days (ACIP 2010)

Cutaneous (treatment): Oral: 100 mg every 12 hours for 60 days. **Note:** In the presence of systemic involvement, extensive edema, lesions on head/neck, refer to IV dosing for treatment of inhalational/gastrointestinal/oropharyngeal anthrax

Inhalational/gastrointestinal/oropharyngeal (treatment): IV: Initial: 100 mg every 12 hours; switch to oral therapy when clinically appropriate; some recommend initial loading dose of 200 mg, followed by 100 mg every 8 to 12 hours (Franz 1997). **Note:** Initial treatment should include two or more agents predicted to be effective (CDC 2001). Agents suggested for use in conjunction with doxycycline or ciprofloxacin include rifampin, vancomycin, imipenem, penicillin, ampicillin, chloramphenicol, clindamycin, and clarithromycin. May switch to oral antimicrobial therapy when clinically appropriate. Continue combined therapy for 60 days

Bacillary angiomatosis, cutaneous (off-label use): Oral: 100 mg twice daily. **Note:** Duration of initial therapy should be for 2 weeks to 2 months, although treatment durations are not standardized (IDSA [Stevens 2014])

Bartonella infection in HIV-infected patients (off-label use; HHS [OI adult 2015]): Note: Duration of therapy is at least 3 months; continuation of therapy depends on relapse occurrence and clinical condition

Bacillary Angiomatosis, Peliosis Hepatis, Bacteremia, and Osteomyelitis: Oral, IV: 100 mg every 12 hours

Infections Involving the CNS: Oral, IV: 100 mg every 12 hours; may add rifampin therapy

Confirmed Bartonella Endocarditis: 100 mg IV every 12 hours in combination with gentamicin for 2 weeks, then continue with doxycycline 100 mg IV or orally every 12 hours

Other Severe Infections: Oral, IV: 100 mg every 12 hours in combination with rifampin

Bite wounds (animal/human) (off-label use) (IDSA [Stevens 2014]):

Animal bite: Oral, IV: 100 mg twice daily

Human bite: Oral: 100 mg twice daily

Brucellosis: Oral: 100 mg twice daily for 6 weeks with rifampin or streptomycin

Cellulitis (purulent) due to community-acquired MRSA (off-label use): Oral: 100 mg twice daily for 5 to 10 days (Liu 2011)

Chlamydial infections, uncomplicated: Oral: 100 mg twice daily for ≥7 days

Community-acquired pneumonia, bronchitis: Oral, IV: 100 mg twice daily (Ailani 1999; Mandell 2007)

Epididymitis: Oral: 100 mg twice daily for 10 days (in combination with ceftriaxone) (CDC 2010)

Gonococcal infection, uncomplicated: Oral: **Note:** Azithromycin is preferred over doxycycline as the second antimicrobial in combination with ceftriaxone in uncomplicated infections due to a high prevalence of tetracycline resistance in isolates (CDC 2012).

Cervix, rectum (off-label use), urethra: 100 mg twice daily for 7 days in combination with ceftriaxone (preferred) or cefixime (only if ceftriaxone is not available and test-of-cure follow up in 7 days) (CDC 2010; CDC 2012).

Pharynx: 100 mg twice daily for 7 days in combination with ceftriaxone (CDC 2012).

Alternatively, the manufacturer recommends a single-visit dose administered in nonanorectal infections in men: 300 mg initially, repeat dose in 1 hour (total dose: 600 mg)

Granuloma inguinale (donovanosis): Oral: 100 mg twice daily for at least 3 weeks (and until lesions have healed) (CDC 2010)

Lyme disease (off-label use): Oral (Halperin 2007; Wormser 2006):

Prevention: Initiate within 72 hours of tick removal: 200 mg administered as a single dose

Treatment (early Lyme disease without neurologic manifestations): 100 mg twice daily for 10 to 21 days

Treatment (meningitis or other early neurologic manifestations): 100 to 200 mg twice daily for 14 days (range: 10 to 28 days)

Lymphogranuloma venereum: Oral: 100 mg twice daily for 21 days (CDC 2010)

Malaria chemoprophylaxis: Oral: 100 mg/day. Start 1 to 2 days prior to travel to endemic area; continue daily during travel and for 4 weeks after leaving endemic area

Malaria, severe, treatment (off-label use): Oral, IV: 100 mg every 12 hours for 7 days with quinidine gluconate. **Note:** Quinidine gluconate duration is region specific; consult CDC for current recommendations (CDC 2011).

Malaria, uncomplicated, treatment (off-label use): Oral: 100 mg twice daily for 7 days with quinine sulfate. **Note:** Quinine sulfate duration is region specific; consult CDC for current recommendations (CDC 2011).

Nongonococcal urethritis: Oral: 100 mg twice daily for 7 days (CDC 2010)

Pelvic inflammatory disease:

Treatment, inpatient: Oral, IV: 100 mg twice daily (in combination with cefoxitin or cefotetan); may transition to oral doxycycline (add clindamycin or metronidazole if tubo-ovarian abscess present) to complete 14 days of treatment (CDC 2010)

Treatment, outpatient: Oral: 100 mg twice daily for 14 days (with or without metronidazole); preceded by a single IM dose of cefoxitin (plus oral probenecid) or ceftriaxone (CDC 2010)

Periodontitis: Oral (Periostat [Canadian availability; not available in the US]): 20 mg twice daily as an adjunct following scaling and root planing; may treat for up to 9 months

Periodontitis, refractory (off-label use): Oral: 100 to 200 mg daily (Jolkovsky 2006)

Proctitis: Oral: 100 mg twice daily for 7 days (in combination with ceftriaxone) (CDC 2010)

Q fever: Oral:

Acute: 100 mg every 12 hours for 14 days (CDC 2013); **Note:** In patients who have valvular heart disease, consider increasing the duration of therapy to 1 year and adding hydroxychloroquine to the regimen to prevent endocarditis; consultation with an infectious disease expert is recommended (CDC 2002; Fenollar 2001).

Chronic (CDC 2013):

Endocarditis or vascular infection: 100 mg every 12 hours in combination with hydroxychloroquine for ≥18 months

Noncardiac organ disease: 100 mg every 12 hours in combination with hydroxychloroquine (duration based on serologic response; ID consult recommended)

Postpartum with serologic evidence present >12 months after delivery: 100 mg every 12 hours in combination with hydroxychloroquine for 12 months

Rosacea Oral (Oracea [US labeling], Apprilon [Canadian labeling]): 40 mg once daily in the morning

Sclerosing agent for pleural effusion (off-label use): Intrapleural: 500 mg as a single dose in 100 mL NS (Porcel 2006); may require a repeat dose (Kvale 2007)

Skin and soft tissue infections (off-label use) (IDSA [Stevens 2014]):

Due to MSSA or MRSA: Oral: 100 mg twice daily

Necrotizing infection due to Aeromonas hydrophila or Vibrio vulnificus: IV: 100 mg every 12 hours; in combination with ciprofloxacin or ceftriaxone for Aeromonas hydrophila or in combination with ceftriaxone or cefotaxime for Vibrio vulnificus. Continue treatment until further debridement is not necessary, patient has clinically improved, and patient is afebrile for 48 to 72 hours.

Syphilis:

Primary/secondary syphilis: Oral: 100 mg twice daily for 14 days (CDC 2010)

Latent syphilis: Oral: 100 mg twice daily for 28 days (CDC 2010)

◀

Tickborne rickettsial disease: Oral, IV: 100 mg twice daily for 5 to 7 days; severe or complicated disease may require longer treatment; human granulocytotropic anaplasmosis (HGA) should be treated for 10 to 14 days.

Tularemia:

Mild to moderate infections: Oral: 100 mg twice daily for 14 days (IDSA [Stevens 2014])

Mass casualty management or postexposure prophylaxis (when used as a biological weapon): Oral: 100 mg twice daily for 14 days (Dennis 2001)

Contained casualty management (when used as a biological weapon): IV (may transition to oral if clinically appropriate): 100 mg every 12 hours for 14-21 days (Dennis 2001)

Vibrio cholerae: Oral: 300 mg as a single dose (WHO 2004)

Yersinia pestis **(plague):** Oral, IV: 200 mg initially then 100 mg twice daily **or** 200 mg once daily for 10 to 14 days (Daya 2005; Inglesby 2000; IDSA [Stevens 2014])

Pediatric

Usual dosage range:

Children >8 years (≤45 kg): Oral, IV: 2 to 5 mg/kg/day in 1 to 2 divided doses, not to exceed 200 mg/day

Children >8 years (>45 kg): Oral, IV: Refer to adult dosing.

Anthrax:

Inhalational (postexposure prophylaxis) (ACIP 2010): Oral, IV (use oral route when possible):

≤8 years: 2.2 mg/kg every 12 hours for 60 days

>8 years and ≤45 kg: 2.2 mg/kg every 12 hours for 60 days

>8 years and >45 kg: 100 mg every 12 hours for 60 days

Cutaneous (treatment): Oral: See dosing for "Inhalational (postexposure prophylaxis)"

Note: In the presence of systemic involvement, extensive edema, and/or lesions on head/neck, doxycycline should initially be administered IV

Inhalational/gastrointestinal/oropharyngeal (treatment): IV: Refer to dosing for inhalational anthrax (postexposure prophylaxis); switch to oral therapy when clinically appropriate.

Note: Initial treatment should include two or more agents predicted to be effective (CDC 2001). Agents suggested for use in conjunction with doxycycline or ciprofloxacin include rifampin, vancomycin, imipenem, penicillin, ampicillin, chloramphenicol, clindamycin, and clarithromycin. May switch to oral antimicrobial therapy when clinically appropriate. Continue combined therapy for 60 days

Bartonella **infection in HIV-infected patients (off-label use):** Refer to adult dosing

Community-acquired pneumonia (CAP) (IDSA/PIDS 2011): Children >7 years: Oral: **Note:** A beta-lactam antibiotic should be added if typical bacterial pneumonia cannot be ruled out.

Presumed atypical, mild atypical (*M. pneumoniae, C. pneumoniae, C. trachomatis*) infection or step-down therapy (alternative to azithromycin): 2 to 4 mg/kg/day in 2 divided doses (maximum: 200 mg/day)

Cellulitis (purulent) due to community-acquired MRSA (off-label use): Children >8 years and ≤45 kg: Oral: 2 mg/kg/dose every 12 hours for 5 to 10 days; >45 kg: Refer to adult dosing (Liu 2011)

Chlamydial infections, uncomplicated: Children >8 years (and >45 kg): Oral: *Manufacturer's recommendation:* 100 mg twice daily for 7 days; alternatively, for endocervical or urethral infections, may give 200 mg once daily for 7 days

Localized juvenile periodontitis (LJP) (off-label use): Oral: 50 to 100 mg/day

Lyme disease (off-label use): Children ≥8 years: Oral (Halperin 2007; Wormser 2006):

Prevention: 4 mg/kg (maximum: 200 mg) administered as a single dose; **Note:** Initiate within 72 hours of tick removal

Treatment (early Lyme disease without neurologic manifestations): 1 to 2 mg/kg twice daily for 10 to 21 days (maximum: 100 mg/dose)

Treatment (meningitis and other early neurologic manifestations): 4 to 8 mg/kg/day in 2 divided doses for 10 to 28 days (maximum: 200 mg/dose)

Malaria chemoprophylaxis: Children ≥8 years: Oral:

Manufacturer's labeling: 2 mg/kg/day (maximum: 100 mg daily). Start 1 to 2 days prior to travel to endemic area; continue daily during travel and for 4 weeks after leaving endemic area (CDC 2012)

Alternative recommendation: 2.2 mg/kg/day (maximum: 100 mg daily). Start 1 to 2 days prior to travel to endemic area; continue daily during travel and for 4 weeks after leaving endemic area (CDC 2012)

Malaria, severe, treatment (off-label use): Children ≥8 years: Oral, IV:

<45 kg: 2.2 mg/kg (maximum dose: 100 mg) every 12 hours for 7 days with quinidine gluconate. **Note:** Quinidine gluconate duration is region specific; consult CDC for current recommendations (CDC 2011).

≥45 kg: 100 mg every 12 hours for 7 days with quinidine gluconate. **Note:** Quinidine gluconate duration is region specific; consult CDC for current recommendations (CDC 2011).

Malaria, uncomplicated, treatment (off-label use): Children ≥8 years: Oral: 2.2 mg/kg (maximum dose: 100 mg) every 12 hours for 7 days with quinine sulfate. **Note:** Quinine sulfate duration is region specific, consult CDC for current recommendations (CDC 2011).

Prosthetic joint infection (off-label use): Oral:

Chronic oral antimicrobial suppression:

Propionibacterium spp (alternative to penicillin or amoxicillin): 100 mg twice daily (Osmon 2013)

Staphylococci (oxacillin-resistant): 100 mg twice daily (Osmon 2013)

Staphylococci (oxacillin-sensitive or -resistant) oral phase treatment (after completion of pathogen-specific IV) following 1-stage exchange:

Total ankle, elbow, hip, or shoulder arthroplasty: 100 mg twice daily for 3 months; **Note:** Must be used in combination with rifampin (Osmon 2013).

Total knee arthroplasty: 100 mg twice daily for 6 months; **Note:** Must be used in combination with rifampin (Osmon 2013)

Q fever: Oral:

Acute:

Children <8 years with high-risk criteria (eg, hospitalized or have severe illness, with preexisting heart valvulopathy, immunocompromised, or with delayed Q fever diagnosis who have experienced illness for >14 days without resolution of symptoms): 2.2 mg/kg/dose (maximum: 100 mg per dose) twice daily for 14 days (CDC 2013).

Children <8 years with mild or uncomplicated illness: 2.2 mg/kg/dose (maximum: 100 mg per dose) twice daily for 5 days. If patient remains febrile past 5 days of treatment, switch to sulfamethoxazole and trimethoprim (CDC 2013). **Note:** Some clinicians may recommend initial treatment with sulfamethoxazole and trimethoprim for children <8 years with mild or uncomplicated illness (Hartzell 2008; CDC 2013).

Children ≥8 years and Adolescents: 2.2 mg/kg/dose (maximum: 100 mg per dose) twice daily for 14 days (CDC 2013).

Chronic: ID consult recommended for treatment of chronic Q fever (CDC 2013)

Skin and soft tissue infections due to MSSA or MRSA (off-label use): Children ≥8 years: Oral:

≤45 kg: 2 mg/kg every 12 hours (IDSA [Lui 2011])

>45 kg: 100 mg twice daily (IDSA [Lui 2011]; IDSA [Stevens 2014])

Tickborne rickettsial disease: Note: The American Academy of Pediatrics Committee on Infectious Diseases identifies doxycycline as the drug of choice in children of any age.

Children ≤8 years: Oral, IV: 2.2 mg/kg (maximum dose: 100 mg) every 12 hours for 5 to 7 days

Children >8 years and >45 kg: Oral, IV: 100 mg twice daily for 5 to 7 days; severe or complicated disease may require longer treatment; human granulocytotropic anaplasmosis (HGA) should be treated for 10 to 14 days

Tularemia (when used as a biological weapon) (off-label use) (Dennis 2001):

Mass casualty management or postexposure prophylaxis: Oral:

Children <45 kg: 2.2 mg/kg twice daily for 14 days

Children ≥45 kg: 100 mg twice daily for 14 days

Contained casualty management: IV (may transition to oral if clinically indicated):

Children <45 kg: 2.2 mg/kg twice daily for 14 to 21 days

Children ≥45 kg: 100 mg every 12 hours for 14 to 21 days

Renal Impairment No dosage adjustment necessary.

Poorly dialyzed (0% to 5%); no supplemental dose or dosage adjustment necessary, including patients on intermittent hemodialysis, peritoneal dialysis, or continuous renal replacement therapy (eg, CVVHD).

Hepatic Impairment There are no dosage adjustments provided in the manufacturer's labeling.

Dietary Considerations

Tetracyclines (in general): Take with food if gastric irritation occurs. While administration with food may decrease GI absorption of doxycycline by up to 20%, administration on an empty stomach is not recommended due to GI intolerance. Of currently available tetracyclines, doxycycline has the least affinity for calcium.

Doryx tablets: May be taken without regard to meals; nausea occurs more frequently when taken on an empty stomach.

Oracea (US labeling), Apprilon (Canadian labeling): Take on an empty stomach 1 hour before or 2 hours after meals.

Periostat (Canadian availability; not available in the US): Take at least 1 hour before morning and evening meals. Some products may contain sodium.

Administration Oral administration is preferable unless patient has significant nausea and vomiting; IV and oral routes are bioequivalent.

Oral: May give with meals to decrease GI upset. Capsule and tablet: Administer with at least 8 ounces of water and have patient sit up for at least 30 minutes after taking to reduce the risk of esophageal irritation and ulceration.

Oracea (US labeling), Apprilon (Canadian labeling): Administer on an empty stomach 1 hour before or 2 hours after meals.

Doryx: Administer without regard to meals; nausea occurs more frequently when taken on an empty stomach. May be administered by carefully breaking up the tablet and sprinkling tablet contents on a spoonful of cold applesauce. The delayed release pellets must not be crushed or damaged when breaking up tablet. Should be administered immediately after preparation and without chewing.

Periostat (Canadian availability; not available in the US): Administer 1 hour before breakfast and evening meal.

IV: Infuse IV doxycycline over 1-4 hours. Avoid extravasation. Prolonged IV administration may cause thrombophlebitis. Oral administration is preferable unless patient has significant nausea and vomiting; IV and oral routes are bioequivalent.

Intrapleural (off-label route): Add to 100 mL NS and instill into chest tube (Porcel 2006)

Monitoring Parameters Perform culture and sensitivity testing prior to initiating therapy. CBC, renal and liver function tests periodically with prolonged therapy. When used as part of alternative treatment for gonococcal infection, test of cure 7 days after dose (CDC 2012).

Patients with no risk factors for chronic Q fever should undergo clinical and serological evaluation 6 months after diagnosis of acute Q fever to identify possible progression to chronic disease. Postpartum women treated during pregnancy for acute Q fever, others who are at high risk for progression to chronic disease or when used as part of treatment for chronic Q fever infection unrelated to endocarditis or vascular infection (eg, osteoarticular infections or chronic hepatitis), assess serologic response at 3, 6, 12, 18, and 24 months after diagnosis of acute Q fever (or after delivery in pregnant women) (CDC 2013).

Test Interactions Injectable tetracycline formulations (if they contain large amounts of ascorbic acid) may result in a false-negative urine glucose using glucose oxidase tests (eg, Clinistix, Diastix, Tes-Tape); false elevations of urinary catecholamines with fluorescence

Additional Information Oracea (US labeling) or Apprilon (Canadian labeling) capsules are not bioequivalent to other doxycycline products.

Dosage Forms Considerations

Alodox Convenience kits contain doxycycline tablets 20 mg, plus eyelid cleanser

Morgidox kits contain doxycycline capsules 100 mg, plus AcuWash moisturizing Daily Cleanser

NizAzel Doxy kits contain doxycycline tablets 100 mg, plus NicAzel FORTE dietary supplement tablets

Ocudox kits contain doxycycline capsules 50 mg, plus eyelid cleanser and Tears Again Advanced eyelid spray

Dosage Forms Excipient information presented when available (limited, particularly for generics); consult specific product labeling. [DSC] = Discontinued product

Capsule, Oral, as hyclate [strength expressed as base]:
Morgidox: 100 mg [contains brilliant blue fcf (fd&c blue #1)]
Vibramycin: 100 mg [contains brilliant blue fcf (fd&c blue #1)]
Generic: 50 mg, 100 mg

Capsule, Oral, as monohydrate [strength expressed as base]:
Adoxa: 150 mg [contains fd&c red #40, fd&c yellow #6 (sunset yellow)]
Mondoxyne NL: 50 mg [contains fd&c yellow #10 (quinoline yellow)]
Mondoxyne NL: 75 mg
Mondoxyne NL: 100 mg [contains fd&c yellow #10 (quinoline yellow)]
Monodox: 75 mg, 100 mg
Generic: 50 mg, 75 mg, 100 mg, 150 mg

Capsule Delayed Release, Oral, as monohydrate [strength expressed as base]:
Oracea: 40 mg
Generic: 40 mg

Kit, Combination, as hyclate [strength expressed as base]:
Alodox Convenience: 20 mg [DSC]
Morgidox: 1 x 100 mg, 2 x 100 mg [contains brilliant blue fcf (fd&c blue #1), cetyl alcohol, edetate disodium]
Ocudox: 50 mg [DSC] [contains brilliant blue fcf (fd&c blue #1)]

Kit, Oral, as monohydrate [strength expressed as base]:
NicAzelDoxy 30: 100 mg [DSC] [contains brilliant blue fcf (fd&c blue #1), fd&c yellow #10 aluminum lake, fd&c yellow #6 (sunset yellow), fd&c yellow #6 aluminum lake, tartrazine (fd&c yellow #5)]
NicAzelDoxy 60: 100 mg [DSC] [contains brilliant blue fcf (fd&c blue #1), fd&c yellow #10 aluminum lake, fd&c yellow #6 (sunset yellow), fd&c yellow #6 aluminum lake, tartrazine (fd&c yellow #5)]

Solution Reconstituted, Intravenous, as hyclate [strength expressed as base]:
Generic: 100 mg (1 ea [DSC])

Solution Reconstituted, Intravenous, as hyclate [strength expressed as base, preservative free]:
Doxy 100: 100 mg (1 ea)
Generic: 100 mg (1 ea)

Suspension Reconstituted, Oral, as monohydrate:
Generic: 25 mg/5 mL (60 mL)

Suspension Reconstituted, Oral, as monohydrate [strength expressed as base]:
Vibramycin: 25 mg/5 mL (60 mL) [contains brilliant blue fcf (fd&c blue #1), methylparaben, propylparaben; raspberry flavor]
Generic: 25 mg/5 mL (60 mL)

Syrup, Oral, as calcium [strength expressed as base]:
Vibramycin: 50 mg/5 mL (473 mL) [contains butylparaben, propylene glycol, propylparaben, sodium metabisulfite; raspberry-apple flavor]

Tablet, Oral, as hyclate [strength expressed as base]:
Acticlate: 75 mg [contains brilliant blue fcf (fd&c blue #1), fd&c yellow #6 (sunset yellow)]
Acticlate: 150 mg [scored; contains fd&c blue #2 (indigotine)]
TargaDOX: 50 mg [contains fd&c blue #2 (indigotine), fd&c yellow #6 (sunset yellow)]
Generic: 20 mg, 100 mg

Tablet, Oral, as monohydrate [strength expressed as base]:
Adoxa: 50 mg
Adoxa: 75 mg [contains fd&c yellow #10 aluminum lake, fd&c yellow #6 (sunset yellow)]
Adoxa: 100 mg
Adoxa Pak 1/100: 100 mg [contains fd&c yellow #10 aluminum lake, fd&c yellow #6 (sunset yellow)]
Adoxa Pak 2/100: 100 mg [contains fd&c yellow #10 aluminum lake, fd&c yellow #6 (sunset yellow)]
Adoxa Pak 1/150: 150 mg [scored; contains fd&c yellow #6 (sunset yellow)]
Avidoxy: 100 mg [contains fd&c yellow #10 aluminum lake, fd&c yellow #6 aluminum lake]
Generic: 50 mg, 75 mg, 100 mg, 150 mg

Tablet Delayed Release, Oral, as hyclate [strength expressed as base]:
Doryx: 50 mg
Doryx: 150 mg, 200 mg [scored]
Generic: 75 mg, 100 mg, 150 mg

Dosage Forms: Canada Excipient information presented when available (limited, particularly for generics); consult specific product labeling.

Capsule, oral, as monohydrate [strength expressed as base]:
Apprilon: 40 mg [30 mg (immediate release) and 10 mg (delayed release)]

Capsule, oral, as hyclate [strength expressed as base]:
Periostat: 20 mg

Extemporaneous Preparations If a public health emergency is declared and liquid doxycycline is unavailable for the treatment of anthrax, emergency doses may be prepared for children or adults who cannot swallow tablets.

Add 20 mL of water to one 100 mg tablet. Allow tablet to soak in the water for 5 minutes to soften. Crush into a fine powder and stir until well mixed. Appropriate dose should be taken from this mixture. To increase palatability, mix with food or drink. If mixing with drink, add 15 mL of milk, chocolate milk, chocolate pudding, or apple juice to the appropriate dose of mixture. If using apple juice, also add 4 teaspoons of sugar. Doxycycline and water mixture may be stored at room temperature for up to 24 hours.

US Food and Drug Administration, Center for Drug Evaluation and Research, "Public Health Emergency Home Preparation Instructions for Doxycycline." Available at http://www.fda.gov/Drugs/Emergency-Preparedness/BioterrorismandDrugPreparedness/ucm130996.htm

◆ Doxycycline Calcium see Doxycycline on page 601

◆ Doxycycline Hyclate see Doxycycline on page 601

◆ Doxycycline Monohydrate see Doxycycline on page 601

Doxylamine and Pyridoxine
(dox IL a meen & peer i DOX een)

Brand Names: US Diclegis®
Brand Names: Canada Diclectin®
Index Terms Doxylamine Succinate and Pyridoxine Hydrochloride; Pyridoxine and Doxylamine
Pharmacologic Category Ethanolamine Derivative; Histamine H_1 Antagonist; Histamine H_1 Antagonist, First Generation; Vitamin, Water Soluble
Use Treatment of pregnancy-associated nausea and vomiting
Dosing
Adult & Geriatric Nausea and vomiting associated with pregnancy: Oral:
U.S. labeling: Day 1: Two delayed release tablets (a total of doxylamine 20 mg and pyridoxine 20 mg) at bedtime. If symptoms are controlled the next day, continue taking 2 tablets at bedtime. If symptoms persist into the afternoon of Day 2, take 2 tablets at bedtime, then 1 tablet in the morning of Day 3 and 2 tablets at bedtime. If symptoms are controlled on Day 4, continue with 1 tablet in the morning and 2 tablets at bedtime. If symptoms are **not** controlled on Day 4, increase dose to 1 tablet in the morning, 1 tablet midafternoon, and 2 tablets in the evening. Tablets should be taken as scheduled and not on an as needed basis. Maximum dose: Four tablets daily.
Canadian labeling: Take 2 delayed release tablets (a total of doxylamine 20 mg and pyridoxine 20 mg) at bedtime. One additional tablet may be taken in the morning or midafternoon; dose should be individualized to control symptoms. Tablets should not be taken on an as needed basis. Maximum dose: Four tablets daily. A gradual tapering of the dose is recommended to prevent a sudden onset of symptoms.
Renal Impairment No dosage adjustment provided in manufacturer's labeling (has not been studied).
Hepatic Impairment No dosage adjustment provided in manufacturer's labeling (has not been studied).
Additional Information Complete prescribing information should be consulted for additional detail.
Dosage Forms Excipient information presented when available (limited, particularly for generics); consult specific product labeling.
Tablet, delayed release:
Diclegis®: Doxylamine succinate 10 mg and pyridoxine hydrochloride 10 mg
Dosage Forms: Canada Excipient information presented when available (limited, particularly for generics); consult specific product labeling.
Tablet, delayed release:
Diclectin®: Doxylamine 10 mg and pyridoxine 10 mg

◆ Doxylamine Succinate and Pyridoxine Hydrochloride see Doxylamine and Pyridoxine on page 606

◆ Doxytab (Can) see Doxycycline on page 601

◆ DPA see Valproic Acid and Derivatives on page 1861

◆ DPE see Dipivefrin on page 570

◆ D-Penicillamine see PenicillAMINE on page 1418

◆ DPH see Phenytoin on page 1444

◆ DPM [OTC] see Urea on page 1853

◆ Dramamine [OTC] see DimenhyDRINATE on page 556

◆ Dramamine Less Drowsy [OTC] see Meclizine on page 1131

◆ Dr Gs Clear Nail [OTC] see Tolnaftate on page 1807

◆ Driminate [OTC] see DimenhyDRINATE on page 556

◆ Drisdol see Ergocalciferol on page 663

◆ Dritho-Creme HP see Anthralin on page 129

◆ Dritho-Scalp [DSC] see Anthralin on page 129

◆ Drixoral® ND (Can) see Pseudoephedrine on page 1527

Dronabinol (droe NAB i nol)

Brand Names: US Marinol
Index Terms Delta-9 THC; Delta-9-tetrahydro-cannabinol; Tetrahydrocannabinol; THC
Pharmacologic Category Antiemetic; Appetite Stimulant
Use
Appetite stimulation in AIDS patients: Treatment of anorexia associated with weight loss in patients with AIDS.
Chemotherapy-induced nausea and vomiting: Treatment of nausea and vomiting associated with cancer chemotherapy in patients who have failed to respond adequately to conventional antiemetic treatments.
Pregnancy Considerations Adverse events have been observed in animal reproduction studies.
Breast-Feeding Considerations Dronabinol is excreted in breast milk. Breast-feeding is not recommended by the manufacturer.
Contraindications Hypersensitivity to dronabinol, cannabinoids, sesame oil, or any component of the formulation.
Warnings/Precautions Use with caution in patients with seizure disorders and in the elderly. May cause occasional hypotension, possible hypertension, syncope, or tachycardia; use with caution in patients with cardiac disorders. May cause CNS depression, which may impair physical or mental abilities; patients must be cautioned about performing tasks that require mental alertness (eg, operating machinery, driving).

Administration with phenothiazines (eg, prochlorperazine) for the management of chemotherapy-induced nausea and vomiting may result in improved efficacy (compared to either drug alone) without additional toxicity. Use with caution in patients with a history of substance abuse, including alcohol abuse or dependence; potential for drug dependency exists. Tolerance, psychological and physical dependence may occur with prolonged use. May cause withdrawal symptoms upon abrupt discontinuation. Use with caution in patients with mania, depression, or schizophrenia; careful psychiatric monitoring is recommended.
Adverse Reactions Frequency not always specified.
>1%:
Cardiovascular: Palpitations, tachycardia, vasodilation/ facial flushing
Central nervous system: Euphoria (8% to 24%, dose related), abnormal thinking (3% to 10%), dizziness (3% to 10%), paranoia (3% to 10%), somnolence (3% to 10%), amnesia, anxiety, ataxia, confusion, depersonalization, hallucination
Gastrointestinal: Abdominal pain (3% to 10%), nausea (3% to 10%), vomiting (3% to 10%)
Neuromuscular & skeletal: Weakness
<1% (Limited to important or life-threatening): Conjunctivitis, depression, diarrhea, fatigue, fecal incontinence, flushing, hypotension, myalgia, nightmares, seizure, speech difficulties, tinnitus, vision difficulties
Drug Interactions
Metabolism/Transport Effects Substrate of CYP2C9 (minor), CYP3A4 (minor); **Note:** Assignment of Major/ Minor substrate status based on clinically relevant drug interaction potential
Avoid Concomitant Use There are no known interactions where it is recommended to avoid concomitant use.
Increased Effect/Toxicity
Dronabinol may increase the levels/effects of: Alcohol (Ethyl); CNS Depressants; Sympathomimetics

The levels/effects of Dronabinol may be increased by: Anticholinergic Agents; Cocaine; CYP2C9 Inhibitors (Moderate); CYP2C9 Inhibitors (Strong); CYP3A4 Inhibitors (Moderate); CYP3A4 Inhibitors (Strong); Ritonavir
Decreased Effect
The levels/effects of Dronabinol may be decreased by: CYP3A4 Inducers (Strong)
Storage/Stability Store in a cool environment between 8°C and 15°C (46°F and 59°F) or refrigerated; protect from freezing.
Mechanism of Action Dronabinol (synthetic delta-9-tetrahydrocannabinol [delta-9-THC]), an active cannabinoid and natural occurring component of *Cannabis sativa L.* (marijuana), activates cannabinoid receptors CB_1 and CB_2. Activation of the CB_1 receptor produces marijuana-like effects on psyche and circulation, whereas activation of the CB_2 receptor does not. Dronabinol has approximately equal affinity for the CB_1 and CB_2 receptors; however, efficacy is less at CB_2 receptors. Activation of the cannabinoid system with dronabinol causes psychological effects that can be divided into 4 groups: affective (euphoria and easy laughter); sensory (increased

perception of external stimuli and of the person's own body); somatic (feeling of the body floating or sinking in the bed); and cognitive (distortion of time perception, memory lapses, difficulty in concentration). Most effects (eg, analgesia, appetite enhancement, muscle relaxation, hormonal actions) are mediated by central cannabinoid receptors (CB_1), their distribution reflecting many of the medicinal benefits and adverse effects (Grotenhermen 2003).

Pharmacodynamics/Kinetics
Onset of action: ~0.5 to 1 hour
Peak effect: 2 to 4 hours
Duration: 4 to 6 hours (psychoactive effects); ≥24 hours (appetite stimulation)
Absorption: Oral: 90% to 95%; 10% to 20% of dose gets into systemic circulation
Distribution: V_d: ~10 L/kg; dronabinol is highly lipophilic
Protein binding: ~97%
Metabolism: Extensive first-pass hepatic primarily via microsomal hydroxylation to metabolites, some of which are active; 11-hydroxy-delta-9-tetrahydrocannabinol (11-OH-THC) is the major active metabolite
Half-life elimination: Biphaisc: Alpha: 4 hours; Terminal: 25 to 36 hours
Time to peak, serum: 0.5 to 4 hours
Excretion: Feces (50%, 5% as unchanged drug); Urine (10% to 15%)

Dosing
Adult & Geriatric Note: Use caution when increasing the dose of dronabinol because of the increased frequency of dose-related adverse reactions at higher dosages.
Appetite stimulation in AIDS patients: Oral: Initial: 2.5 mg twice daily (before lunch and dinner); for patients unable to tolerate this dosage, may reduce to 2.5 mg once daily (in the evening or at bedtime). May increase dose gradually based on response and tolerability (maximum: 20 mg per day [in divided doses]).
Chemotherapy-induced nausea and vomiting (manufacturer's labeling): Oral: 5 mg/m² administered 1 to 3 hours before chemotherapy, then give 5 mg/m²/dose every 2 to 4 hours after chemotherapy for a total of 4 to 6 doses/day; increase doses in increments of 2.5 mg/m² based on response and tolerability (maximum: 15 mg/m²/dose). **Note:** Initiate with the lowest recommended dose and titrate to response; most patients respond to 5 mg 3 to 4 times daily; based on initial results, the dose may be escalated during a chemotherapy cycle or with subsequent cycles.
Chemotherapy-induced nausea and vomiting, refractory (off-label dosing): Oral: 2.5 to 10 mg 3 or 4 times daily (Lohr 2008)
Pediatric Chemotherapy-induced nausea and vomiting: Oral: Refer to adult dosing. Use caution when increasing the dose because of the increased frequency of dose-related adverse reactions at higher dosages.
Renal Impairment There are no dosage adjustments provided in the manufacturer's labeling.
Hepatic Impairment There are no dosage adjustments provided in the manufacturer's labeling.
Dietary Considerations Capsules contain sesame oil.
Administration Oral: For appetite stimulation, administer twice-daily doses before lunch and dinner; administer single doses in the evening or at bedtime.
Monitoring Parameters CNS effects, heart rate, blood pressure, behavioral profile
Dosage Forms Excipient information presented when available (limited, particularly for generics); consult specific product labeling.
Capsule, Oral:
Marinol: 2.5 mg, 5 mg, 10 mg [contains sesame oil]
Generic: 2.5 mg, 5 mg, 10 mg
Controlled Substance C-III

Dronedarone (droe NE da rone)

Brand Names: US Multaq
Brand Names: Canada Multaq
Index Terms Dronedarone Hydrochloride; SR33589
Pharmacologic Category Antiarrhythmic Agent, Class III
Use Paroxysmal or persistent atrial fibrillation: To reduce the risk of hospitalization for atrial fibrillation (AF) in patients in sinus rhythm with a history of paroxysmal or persistent AF
Medication Guide Available Yes

Dosing
Adult & Geriatric Note: Prior to initiation of dronedarone, class I or III antiarrhythmics (eg, amiodarone, flecainide, propafenone, quinidine, disopyramide, dofetilide, sotalol) or drugs that are strong inhibitors of CYP3A (eg, ketoconazole) must be stopped.
Paroxysmal or persistent atrial fibrillation: Oral: 400 mg twice daily.
Renal Impairment No dosage adjustment necessary.
Hepatic Impairment
Mild-to-moderate impairment: No dosage adjustment necessary.
Severe impairment: Use is contraindicated.
Additional Information Complete prescribing information should be consulted for additional detail.
Dosage Forms Excipient information presented when available (limited, particularly for generics); consult specific product labeling.
Tablet, Oral:
Multaq: 400 mg

◆ Dronedarone Hydrochloride see Dronedarone on page 607

Droperidol (droe PER i dole)

Brand Names: Canada Droperidol Injection, USP
Index Terms Dehydrobenzperidol; Inapsine
Pharmacologic Category Antiemetic; First Generation (Typical) Antipsychotic
Use Prevention and/or treatment of nausea and vomiting from surgical and diagnostic procedures
Pregnancy Considerations Adverse events were observed in some animal reproduction studies. Although use in pregnancy has been reported, due to cases of QT prolongation and torsade de pointes (some fatal), use of other agents in pregnant women is preferred (ACOG, 2004).
Breast-Feeding Considerations It is not known if droperidol is excreted in breast milk. The manufacturer recommends that caution be exercised when administering droperidol to nursing women.
Contraindications Hypersensitivity to droperidol or any component of the formulation; known or suspected QT prolongation, including congenital long QT syndrome (prolonged QTc is defined as >440 msec in males or >450 msec in females)

Canadian labeling: Additional contraindications (not in U.S. labeling): Not for use in children ≤2 years of age
Warnings/Precautions May alter cardiac conduction. **[U.S. Boxed Warning]: Cases of QT prolongation and torsade de pointes, including some fatal cases, have been reported.** Use extreme caution in patients with bradycardia (<50 bpm); cardiac disease, concurrent MAO inhibitor therapy, Class I and Class III antiarrhythmics or other drugs known to prolong QT interval, and electrolyte disturbances (hypokalemia or hypomagnesemia), including concomitant drugs which may alter electrolytes (diuretics).

Use with caution in patients with seizures or severe liver disease. May be sedating, use with caution in disorders where CNS depression is a feature. Caution in patients with hemodynamic instability, predisposition to seizures, subcortical brain damage, pheochromocytoma or renal disease. Esophageal dysmotility and aspiration have been associated with antipsychotic use - use with caution in patients at risk of pneumonia (ie, Alzheimer's disease). Caution in breast cancer or other prolactin-dependent tumors (may elevate prolactin levels). May alter temperature regulation or mask toxicity of other drugs due to antiemetic effects. May cause orthostatic hypotension - use with caution in patients at risk of this effect or those who would tolerate transient hypotensive episodes (cerebrovascular disease, cardiovascular disease, or other medications which may predispose). Significant hypotension may occur.

May cause anticholinergic effects (confusion, agitation, constipation, xerostomia, blurred vision, urinary retention). Therefore, they should be used with caution in patients with decreased gastrointestinal motility, urinary retention, BPH, xerostomia, visual problems, or narrow-angle glaucoma (screening is recommended). Relative to other neuroleptics, droperidol has a low potency of cholinergic blockade.

May cause extrapyramidal symptoms, including pseudoparkinsonism, acute dystonic reactions, akathisia, and tardive dyskinesia. Risk of dystonia (and possibly other EPS) may be greater with increased doses, use of conventional antipsychotics, males, and younger patients. Risk of

tardive dyskinesia and potential for irreversibility may be increased in elderly patients (particularly women), prolonged therapy, and higher total cumulative dose. May be associated with neuroleptic malignant syndrome (NMS). May mask toxicity of other drugs or conditions (eg, intestinal obstruction, Reye's syndrome, brain tumor) due to antiemetic effects. Use with caution in the elderly; reduce initial dose.

Adverse Reactions Frequency not defined.

Cardiovascular: Cardiac arrest, hypertension, hypotension (especially orthostatic), QTc prolongation (dose dependent), tachycardia, torsade de pointes, ventricular tachycardia

Central nervous system: Anxiety, chills, depression (postoperative, transient), dizziness, drowsiness (postoperative) increased, dysphoria, extrapyramidal symptoms (akathisia, dystonia, oculogyric crisis), hallucinations (postoperative), hyperactivity, neuroleptic malignant syndrome (NMS) (rare), restlessness

Respiratory: Bronchospasm, laryngospasm

Miscellaneous: Anaphylaxis, shivering

Drug Interactions

Metabolism/Transport Effects None known.

Avoid Concomitant Use

Avoid concomitant use of Droperidol with any of the following: Aclidinium; Amisulpride; Azelastine (Nasal); Cimetropium; Eluxadoline; Glucagon; Glycopyrrolate; Glycopyrrolate (Oral Inhalation); Highest Risk QTc-Prolonging Agents; Ipratropium (Oral Inhalation); Ivabradine; Levosulpiride; Metoclopramide; Mifepristone; Orphenadrine; Paraldehyde; Potassium Chloride; Sulpiride; Thalidomide; Tiotropium; Umeclidinium

Increased Effect/Toxicity

Droperidol may increase the levels/effects of: AbobotulinumtoxinA; Alcohol (Ethyl); Amisulpride; Anticholinergic Agents; Azelastine (Nasal); Cimetropium; CNS Depressants; Eluxadoline; Glucagon; Glycopyrrolate; Glycopyrrolate (Oral Inhalation); Highest Risk QTc-Prolonging Agents; Hydrocodone; Mequitazine; Methotrimeprazine; Methylphenidate; Metoclopramide; Mirabegron; Moderate Risk QTc-Prolonging Agents; OnabotulinumtoxinA; Orphenadrine; Paraldehyde; Potassium Chloride; Ramosetron; RimabotulinumtoxinB; Selective Serotonin Reuptake Inhibitors; Serotonin Modulators; Sulpiride; Suvorexant; Thalidomide; Thiazide Diuretics; Tiotropium; Zolpidem

The levels/effects of Droperidol may be increased by: Acetylcholinesterase Inhibitors (Central); Aclidinium; Brimonidine (Topical); Cannabis; Dronabinol; Ipratropium (Oral Inhalation); Ivabradine; Kava Kava; Lithium; Magnesium Sulfate; Methotrimeprazine; Methylphenidate; Metyrosine; Mifepristone; Minocycline; Nabilone; Perampanel; Pramlintide; QTc-Prolonging Agents (Indeterminate Risk and Risk Modifying); Rufinamide; Serotonin Modulators; Sodium Oxybate; Tapentadol; Tetrahydrocannabinol; Umeclidinium

Decreased Effect

Droperidol may decrease the levels/effects of: Acetylcholinesterase Inhibitors; Amphetamines; Anti-Parkinson's Agents (Dopamine Agonist); Gastrointestinal Agents (Prokinetic); Itopride; Levosulpiride; Quinagolide; Secretin

The levels/effects of Droperidol may be decreased by: Acetylcholinesterase Inhibitors; Anti-Parkinson's Agents (Dopamine Agonist); Lithium

Preparation for Administration IV infusion: Dilute in 50-100 mL NS or D5W.

Storage/Stability Store at 20°C to 25°C (68°F to 77°F); excursions permitted to 15°C to 30°C (59°F to 86°F). Protect from light. Solutions diluted in NS or D5W are stable at room temperature for up to 7 days in PVC bags or glass bottles. Solutions diluted in LR are stable at room temperature for 24 hours in PVC bags and up to 7 days in glass bottles.

Mechanism of Action Droperidol is a butyrophenone antipsychotic; antiemetic effect is a result of blockade of dopamine stimulation of the chemoreceptor trigger zone. Other effects include alpha-adrenergic blockade, peripheral vascular dilation, and reduction of the pressor effect of epinephrine resulting in hypotension and decreased peripheral vascular resistance; may also reduce pulmonary artery pressure

Pharmacodynamics/Kinetics

Onset of action: 3-10 minutes

Peak effect: ~30 minutes

Duration: 2-4 hours, may extend to 12 hours

Absorption: IM: Rapid

Distribution: Crosses blood-brain barrier and placenta

V_d: Children: ~0.6 L/kg; Adults: ~1.5 L/kg

Protein binding: 85% to 90%

Metabolism: Hepatic, to *p*-fluorophenylacetic acid, benzimidazolone, *p*-hydroxypiperidine

Half-life elimination: ~2.3 hours

Excretion: Urine (75%, <1% as unchanged drug); feces (22%, 11% as unchanged drug)

Dosing

Adult & Geriatric Note: Titrate carefully to desired effect

Prevention of PONV: IM, IV:

Manufacturer labeling: Maximum initial dose: 2.5 mg; additional doses of 1.25 mg may be administered with caution to achieve desired effect

Consensus guideline recommendations: 0.625-1.25 mg IV administered at the end of surgery (Gan, 2007)

Canadian labeling:

Prevention and treatment of PONV: IV: 0.625-1.25 mg 30 minutes prior to anticipated end of surgery, and then every 6 hours as needed for breakthrough PONV

Pediatric Note: Titrate carefully to desired effect

Prevention of postoperative nausea and vomiting (PONV): IM, IV: Children 2-12 years:

Manufacturer labeling: Maximum dose: 0.1 mg/kg; additional doses may be repeated with caution to achieve desired effect

Consensus guideline recommendations: 0.01-0.015 mg/kg (maximum: 1.25 mg) IV administered at the end of surgery (Gan, 2007)

Canadian labeling:

Prevention and treatment of PONV: IV: Children >2 years and Adolescents: 0.02-0.05 mg/kg (maximum dose: 1.25 mg) 30 minutes prior to anticipated end of surgery, and then every 6 hours as needed for breakthrough PONV

Renal Impairment

U.S. labeling: Specific dosing recommendations are not provided; use with caution.

Canadian labeling: IV: 0.625 mg; additional dosing should be administered with caution.

Hepatic Impairment

U.S. labeling: Specific dosing recommendations are not provided; use with caution.

Canadian labeling: IV: 0.625 mg; additional dosing should be administered with caution.

Administration Administer IM or IV; according to the manufacturer, IV push administration should be slow. For IV infusion, further dilute.

Monitoring Parameters To identify QT prolongation, a 12-lead ECG prior to use is recommended; continued ECG monitoring for 2-3 hours following administration is recommended. Vital signs; serum magnesium and potassium; mental status, abnormal involuntary movement scale (AIMS); observe for dystonias, extrapyramidal side effects, and temperature changes

Dosage Forms Excipient information presented when available (limited, particularly for generics); consult specific product labeling.

Solution, Injection:

Generic: 2.5 mg/mL (2 mL)

◆ DTO (error-prone abbreviation) see Opium Tincture on page 1338

◆ D-Trp(6)-LHRH see Triptorelin on page 1847

◆ Duavee see Estrogens (Conjugated/Equine) and Bazedoxifene on page 693

◆ Ducodyl [OTC] see Bisacodyl on page 231

◆ Duetact see Pioglitazone and Glimepiride on page 1455

Dulaglutide (doo la GLOO tide)

Brand Names: US Trulicity
Index Terms LY2189265
Pharmacologic Category Antidiabetic Agent, Glucagon-Like Peptide-1 (GLP-1) Receptor Agonist
Use Type 2 diabetes mellitus: Adjunct to diet and exercise to improve glycemic control in adults with type 2 diabetes mellitus (noninsulin dependent, NIDDM)
Pregnancy Considerations Adverse events have been observed in some animal reproduction studies.

In women with diabetes, maternal hyperglycemia can be associated with congenital malformations as well as adverse effects in the fetus, neonate, and the mother (ACOG 2005; ADA 2015; Kitzmiller 2008; Metzger 2007). To prevent adverse outcomes, prior to conception and throughout pregnancy maternal blood glucose and HbA$_{1c}$ should be kept as close to target goals as possible but without causing significant hypoglycemia (ACOG 2013; ADA 2015; Blumer 2013; Kitzmiller 2008). Prior to pregnancy, effective contraception should be used until glycemic control is achieved (Kitzmiller 2008). Other agents are currently recommended to treat diabetes in pregnant women (ACOG 2013; Blumer 2013).

Breast-Feeding Considerations It is not known if dulaglutide is excreted in breast milk. Due to the potential for serious adverse reactions in the nursing infant, the manufacturer recommends a decision be made whether to discontinue nursing or to discontinue the drug, taking into account the importance of treatment to the mother.

Medication Guide Available Yes
Contraindications Serious hypersensitivity to dulaglutide or any component of the formulation; personal or family history of medullary thyroid carcinoma (MTC); patients with multiple endocrine neoplasia syndrome type 2 (MEN2)

Warnings/Precautions [US Boxed Warning] Thyroid C-cell tumors have developed in animal studies with glucagon-like peptide-1 (GLP-1) receptor agonists; it is not known if dulaglutide causes thyroid C-cell tumor, including medullary thyroid carcinoma (MTC) in humans. Routine monitoring of serum calcitonin or using thyroid ultrasound monitoring is of uncertain value for early detection of MTC in patients treated with dulaglutide. Patients should be counseled on the potential risk of MTC with the use of dulaglutide and informed them of symptoms of thyroid tumors symptoms (eg, neck mass, dysphagia, dyspnea, persistent hoarseness) of thyroid tumors. Use is contraindicated in patients with a personal or a family history of MTC and in patients with multiple endocrine neoplasia syndrome type 2 (MEN2). Cases of MTC in humans have been reported in patients treated with the GLP-1 receptor agonist liraglutide. Consultation with an endocrinologist is recommended in patients with thyroid nodules on physical examination or neck imaging and in patients who develop elevated calcitonin concentrations.

Use is not recommended in patients with preexisting severe gastrointestinal disease. Hypersensitivity reactions have been reported; discontinue therapy in the event of a hypersensitivity reaction. Cases of pancreatitis have been reported; monitor for signs and symptoms of pancreatitis (eg, persistent severe abdominal pain). If pancreatitis is suspected, discontinue use. Do not resume therapy if pancreatitis is confirmed. Consider antidiabetic therapies other than dulaglutide in patients with a history of pancreatitis.

Use with caution in patients with renal impairment, particularly during initiation of therapy and dose escalation. Acute renal failure and chronic renal failure exacerbation (sometimes requiring hemodialysis) have been reported; some cases have been reported in patients with no known preexisting renal disease. A majority of reported cases occurred in patients with nausea/vomiting/diarrhea or dehydration. Use with caution in patients with hepatic impairment.

Not recommended for first-line therapy in patients inadequately controlled on diet and exercise alone. Do not use in patients with type 1 diabetes mellitus or for the treatment of diabetic ketoacidosis; not a substitute for insulin. Diabetes self-management education (DSME) is essential to

maximize the effectiveness of therapy. Potentially significant drug-drug interactions may exist, requiring dose or frequency adjustment, additional monitoring, and/or selection of alternative therapy.

Adverse Reactions
>10%: Gastrointestinal: Nausea (12% to 21%), diarrhea (9% to 13%), vomiting (6% to 13%), abdominal pain (7% to 10%)
1% to 10%:
Cardiovascular: Sinus tachycardia (3% to 6%), prolongation P-R interval on ECG (3%), first degree atrioventricular block (2%)
Central nervous system: Fatigue (4% to 6%)
Endocrine & metabolic: Hypoglycemia (3% to 6%)
Gastrointestinal: Abdominal pain (7% to 9%), decreased appetite (5% to 9%), dyspepsia (4% to 6%), constipation (4%), flatulence (3%), abdominal distension (2% to 3%), gastroesophageal reflux disease (2%), eructation (1% to 2%)
Immunologic: Antibody development (2%)
<1% (Limited to important or life-threatening): Acute renal failure, chronic renal failure, hypersensitivity reaction, increased serum amylase, increased serum lipase, injection site reaction, pancreatitis

Drug Interactions
Metabolism/Transport Effects None known.
Avoid Concomitant Use There are no known interactions where it is recommended to avoid concomitant use.
Increased Effect/Toxicity
Dulaglutide may increase the levels/effects of: Hypoglycemia-Associated Agents; Insulin; Sulfonylureas

The levels/effects of Dulaglutide may be increased by: Alpha-Lipoic Acid; Androgens; MAO Inhibitors; Pegvisomant; Quinolone Antibiotics; Salicylates; Selective Serotonin Reuptake Inhibitors
Decreased Effect
The levels/effects of Dulaglutide may be decreased by: Hyperglycemia-Associated Agents; Quinolone Antibiotics; Thiazide Diuretics
Storage/Stability Store at 36°F to 46°F (2°C to 8°C). Do not freeze. Protect from light. If needed, each single-dose pen or prefilled syringe can be kept at room temperature, not to exceed 86°F (30°C) for a total of 14 days.
Mechanism of Action Dulaglutide is an agonist of human glucagon-like peptide-1 (GLP-1) receptor and augments glucose dependent insulin secretion and slows gastric emptying.
Pharmacodynamics/Kinetics
Bioavailability: 47% to 65%
Distribution: V$_d$: ~17 to 19 L
Metabolism: Degradation to amino acids by protein catabolism pathways.
Half-life elimination: ~5 days
Time to peak, plasma: 24 to 72 hours
Dosing
Adult & Geriatric
Type 2 diabetes mellitus: SubQ: 0.75 mg once weekly; may increase to 1.5 mg once weekly if inadequate glycemic response; maximum:1.5 mg once weekly
Missed doses: If a dose is missed, administer as soon as possible within 3 days after the missed dose; dosing can then be resumed on the usual day of administration. If there are less than 3 days until next scheduled dose, omit the missed dose and resume administration at the next regularly scheduled weekly dose.
Renal Impairment No dosage adjustment necessary; use caution when initiating or escalating doses.
Hepatic Impairment There are no dosage adjustments provided in the manufacturer's labeling; use with caution
Dietary Considerations Individualized medical nutrition therapy (MNT) based on ADA recommendations is an integral part of therapy.
Administration Do not inject intravenously or intramuscularly. Inject subcutaneously into the upper arm, thigh, or abdomen; when administering within the same body region, use a different injection site each week. Administer once weekly on the same day each week, without regard to meals or time of day. The day of weekly administration may be changed, as long as the last dose was administered ≥3 days before. If using concomitantly with insulin, administer as separate injections (do not mix); may inject in the same body region as insulin, but not adjacent to one another.
Monitoring Parameters Plasma glucose, HbA$_{1c}$, renal function, signs/symptoms of pancreatitis
Reference Range
Recommendations for glycemic control in nonpregnant adults with diabetes (ADA, 2015):
HbA$_{1c}$: <7% (a more aggressive [<6.5%] or less aggressive [<8%] HbA$_{1c}$ goal may be targeted based on patient-specific characteristics)

◄

Preprandial capillary plasma glucose: 80 to 130 mg/dL
Peak postprandial capillary blood glucose: <180 mg/dL

Recommendations for glycemic control in pediatric (all age groups) patients with type 1 diabetes (ADA, 2015):
HbA$_{1c}$: <7.5% (individualization may be appropriate based on patient-specific characteristics; <7% is reasonable if it can be achieved without excessive hypoglycemia)
Preprandial capillary plasma glucose: 90 to 130 mg/dL
Bedtime and overnight capillary blood glucose: 90 to 150 mg/dL

Dosage Forms Excipient information presented when available (limited, particularly for generics); consult specific product labeling.
Solution Pen-injector, Subcutaneous:
Trulicity: 0.75 mg/0.5 mL (0.5 mL); 1.5 mg/0.5 mL (0.5 mL) [contains polysorbate 80]

◆ **Dulcocomfort Stool Softener [OTC] (Can)** see Docusate on page 578

◆ **Dulcolax [OTC]** see Bisacodyl on page 231

◆ **Dulcolax For Women [OTC] (Can)** see Bisacodyl on page 231

◆ **Dulcolax Milk of Magnesia [OTC]** see Magnesium Hydroxide on page 1120

◆ **Dulcolax Stool Softener [OTC]** see Docusate on page 578

◆ **Dulera** see Mometasone and Formoterol on page 1228

DULoxetine (doo LOX e teen)

Brand Names: US Cymbalta; Irenka
Brand Names: Canada Cymbalta
Index Terms (+)-(S)-N-Methyl-γ-(1-naphthyloxy)-2-thiophenepropylamine Hydrochloride; Duloxetine Hydrochloride; LY248686
Pharmacologic Category Antidepressant, Serotonin/Norepinephrine Reuptake Inhibitor
Use
Chronic musculoskeletal pain: Management of chronic musculoskeletal pain.
Diabetic peripheral neuropathic pain: Management of diabetic peripheral neuropathy.
Fibromyalgia (except Irenka): Management of fibromyalgia.
Generalized anxiety disorder: Treatment of generalized anxiety disorder (GAD).
Major depressive disorder: Treatment of major depressive disorder (MDD).
Pregnancy Considerations Adverse events have been observed in animal reproduction studies. Nonteratogenic effects in the newborn following SSRI/SNRI exposure late in the third trimester include respiratory distress, cyanosis, apnea, seizures, temperature instability, feeding difficulty, vomiting, hypoglycemia, hyper- or hypotonia, hyperreflexia, jitteriness, irritability, constant crying, and tremor. Symptoms may be due to the toxicity of the SNRIs/SSRIs or a discontinuation syndrome and may be consistent with serotonin syndrome associated with SSRI treatment. The long-term effects of in utero SNRI/SSRI exposure on infant development and behavior are not known.

The ACOG recommends that therapy with SSRIs or SNRIs during pregnancy be individualized; treatment of depression during pregnancy should incorporate the clinical expertise of the mental health clinician, obstetrician, primary health care provider, and pediatrician. According to the American Psychiatric Association (APA), the risks of medication treatment should be weighed against other treatment options and untreated depression. For women who discontinue antidepressant medications during pregnancy and who may be at high risk for postpartum depression, the medications can be restarted following delivery. Treatment algorithms have been developed by the ACOG and the APA for the management of depression in women prior to conception and during pregnancy.

Health care providers are encouraged to enroll women exposed to duloxetine during pregnancy in the Cymbalta Pregnancy Registry (866-814-6975 or http://cymbaltapregnancyregistry.com).
Breast-Feeding Considerations Duloxetine is excreted in human milk and has been detected in the serum of a nursing infant. The US labeling recommends that caution be exercised when administering duloxetine to nursing women. The Canadian labeling recommends that nursing be avoided during duloxetine therapy. The long-term effects on neurobehavior have not been studied.
Medication Guide Available Yes

Contraindications Use of monoamine oxidase (MAO) inhibitors intended to treat psychiatric disorders (concurrently or within 14 days of discontinuing the MAO inhibitor); initiation of MAO inhibitor intended to treat psychiatric disorders within 5 days of discontinuing duloxetine; initiation of duloxetine in a patient receiving linezolid or intravenous methylene blue.

Canadian labeling: Additional contraindications (not in US labeling): Hypersensitivity to duloxetine or any component of the formulation; hepatic impairment; severe renal impairment (eg, CrCl <30 mL/minute) or end-stage renal disease (ESRD); uncontrolled narrow-angle glaucoma; concomitant use with thioridazine or with CYP1A2 inhibitors.

Warnings/Precautions [US Boxed Warning]: Antidepressants increase the risk of suicidal thinking and behavior in children, adolescents, and young adults (18 to 24 years of age) with major depressive disorder (MDD) and other psychiatric disorders; consider risk prior to prescribing. Short-term studies did not show an increased risk in patients >24 years of age and showed a decreased risk in patients ≥65 years. Closely monitor for clinical worsening, suicidality, or unusual changes in behavior, particularly during the initial 1 to 2 months of therapy or during periods of dosage adjustments (increases or decreases); the patient's family or caregiver should be instructed to closely observe the patient and communicate condition with healthcare provider. A medication guide concerning the use of antidepressants in children and teenagers should be dispensed with each prescription. **Duloxetine is not FDA approved for use in children.**

The possibility of a suicide attempt is inherent in major depression and may persist until remission occurs. Use caution in high-risk patients. Worsening depression and severe abrupt suicidality that are not part of the presenting symptoms may require discontinuation or modification of drug therapy. The patient's family or caregiver should be alerted to monitor patients for the emergence of suicidality and associated behaviors (such as agitation, irritability, hostility, impulsivity, and hypomania) and call healthcare provider.

May worsen psychosis in some patients or precipitate a shift to mania or hypomania in patients with bipolar disorder. Patients presenting with depressive symptoms should be screened for bipolar disorder. Monotherapy in patients with bipolar disorder should be avoided. **Duloxetine is not FDA approved for the treatment of bipolar depression.**

May cause orthostatic hypotension/syncope at therapeutic doses especially within the first week of therapy and after dose increases. Consider dose reduction or discontinuation of duloxetine if orthostatic hypotension or syncope occurs. Monitor blood pressure with initiation of therapy, dose increases (especially in patients receiving >60 mg/day), or with concomitant use of vasodilators, CYP2D6 inhibitors/substrates, or CYP1A2 inhibitors. Use caution in patients with hypertension. May increase blood pressure. Rare cases of hypertensive crisis have been reported; evaluate blood pressure prior to initiating therapy and periodically thereafter; consider dose reduction or gradual discontinuation of therapy in individuals with sustained hypertension during therapy. Falls with serious consequences including bone fractures and hospitalization have been reported in patients receiving therapeutic doses of duloxetine. The risk of falling appears related to the degree of orthostatic decrease in blood pressure. Risks may also be greater in elderly patients, patients taking concomitant medications that induce orthostatic hypotension or are potent CYP1A2 inhibitors, and in patients taking doses >60 mg/day. Consider dose reduction or discontinuation of duloxetine if falls occur.

Modest increases in serum glucose and hemoglobin A$_{1c}$ (HbA$_{1c}$) levels have been observed in some diabetic patients receiving duloxetine therapy for diabetic peripheral neuropathic pain (DPNP). Duloxetine may cause increased urinary resistance; advise patient to report symptoms of urinary hesitation/difficulty. Has a low potential to impair cognitive or motor performance. Use caution in patients with a previous seizure disorder or condition predisposing to seizures such as brain damage or alcoholism (Montgomery, 2005). Avoid use in patients with substantial ethanol intake, evidence of liver disease, or hepatic impairment (contraindicated in Canadian labeling). Rare cases of hepatic failure (including fatalities) have been reported with use. Hepatitis with abdominal pain, hepatomegaly, elevated transaminase levels >20 times the upper limit of normal (ULN) with and without jaundice have all been observed. Discontinue therapy with the presentation of jaundice or other signs of hepatic dysfunction and do not

reinitiate therapy unless another source or cause is identified. Use caution in patients with impaired gastric motility (eg, some diabetics) may affect stability of the capsule's enteric coating.

Severe skin reactions (including Stevens-Johnson syndrome and erythema multiforme) have been reported; discontinue immediately if blisters, peeling rash, mucosal erosions, or any other signs of hypersensitivity reactions are suspected. May cause hyponatremia/SIADH (elderly at increased risk); volume depletion (diuretics may increase risk). May cause mild pupillary dilation which in susceptible individuals can lead to an episode of narrow-angle glaucoma. Consider evaluating patients who have not had an iridectomy for narrow-angle glaucoma risk factors. May cause or exacerbate sexual dysfunction. Use caution with renal impairment; avoid use in patients with CrCl <30 mL/ minute or ESRD (contraindicated in Canadian labeling for severe renal impairment or ESRD). May impair platelet aggregation; use caution with concomitant use of NSAIDs, ASA, or other drugs that affect coagulation; the risk of bleeding may be potentiated. Bone fractures have been associated with antidepressant treatment. Consider the possibility of a fragility fracture if an antidepressant-treated patient presents with unexplained bone pain, point tenderness, swelling, or bruising (Rabenda, 2013; Rizzoli, 2012).

Potentially life-threatening serotonin syndrome (SS) has occurred with serotonergic agents (eg, SSRIs, SNRIs), particularly when used in combination with other serotonergic agents (eg, triptans, tricyclic antidepressants, fentanyl, lithium, tramadol, tryptophan, buspirone, and St John's wort) or drugs that impair serotonin metabolism (eg, MAO inhibitors, specifically linezolid, methylene blue, and others used for psychiatric disorders). Monitor patients closely for signs/symptoms of SS which may include mental status changes (eg, agitation, hallucinations, delirium), seizures, autonomic instability (eg, tachycardia, dizziness, diaphoresis), neuromuscular symptoms (eg, tremor, rigidity, myoclonus), or gastrointestinal symptoms (eg, nausea, vomiting, diarrhea). Discontinue treatment (and any concomitant serotonergic agents) immediately if signs/symptoms of SS arise.

Use caution in elderly patients; may cause or exacerbate syndrome of inappropriate antidiuretic hormone secretion or hyponatremia; monitor sodium closely with initiation or dosage adjustments in older adults (Beers Criteria). Some formulations may contain sucrose; patients with fructose intolerance, glucose-galactose malabsorption, or sucrase-isomaltase deficiency should avoid use.

Abrupt discontinuation or interruption of antidepressant therapy has been associated with a discontinuation syndrome. Symptoms arising may vary with antidepressant however commonly include nausea, vomiting, diarrhea, headaches, lightheadedness, dizziness, diminished appetite, sweating, chills, tremors, paresthesias, fatigue, somnolence, and sleep disturbances (eg, vivid dreams, insomnia). Greater risks for developing a discontinuation syndrome have been associated with antidepressants with shorter half-lives, longer durations of treatment, and abrupt discontinuation. For antidepressants of short or intermediate half-lives, symptoms may emerge within 2 to 5 days after treatment discontinuation and last 7 to 14 days (APA, 2010; Fava, 2006; Haddad, 2001; Shelton, 2001; Warner, 2006).

Adverse Reactions

>10%:

Central nervous system: Headache (13% to 14%), drowsiness (9% to 11%; dose related), fatigue (≤7% to ≤11%; dose related)

Gastrointestinal: Nausea (18% to 23%), xerostomia (adults: 11% to 14%; dose related, children and adolescents: 2%), abdominal pain (children and adolescents: 13%, adults: 5%)

Endocrine & metabolic: Weight loss (children and adolescents: 14%, adults: ≥1%)

Neuromuscular & skeletal: Weakness (≤7% to ≤11%; dose related)

1% to 10%:

Cardiovascular: Flushing (3%), increased blood pressure (2%), palpitations (≥1% to 2%)

Central nervous system: Insomnia (7% to 10%; dose related), dizziness (8% to 9%), agitation (3% to 4%), anxiety (3%), delayed ejaculation (2%; dose related), yawning (≥1% to 2%), abnormal dreams (≥1%), anorgasmia (≥1%), chills (≥1%), hypoesthesia (≥1%), lethargy (≥1%), paresthesia (≥1%), rigors (≥1%), sleep disorder (≥1%), vertigo (≥1%)

Dermatologic: Diaphoresis (6%), pruritus (≥1%)

Endocrine & metabolic: Decreased libido (3%), orgasm abnormal (≥1% to 2%), hot flash (≥1%), weight gain (≥1%)

Gastrointestinal: Constipation (9% to 10%; dose related), diarrhea (6% to 9%), vomiting (adults: 3% to 4%; children and adolescents: 9%), decreased appetite (6% to 10%; dose related), dyspepsia (2%), dysgeusia (≥1%), flatulence (≥1%)

Genitourinary: Erectile dysfunction (4%), ejaculatory disorder (2%), urinary frequency (≥1%)

Hepatic: Increased serum ALT (>3 x ULN: 1%)

Neuromuscular & skeletal: Tremor (2% to 3%; dose related), musculoskeletal pain (≥1%)

Ophthalmic: Blurred vision (≥1% to 3%)

Respiratory: Oropharyngeal pain (children and adolescents: 4%; adults: ≥1%), cough (children and adolescents: 3%)

<1% (Limited to important or life-threatening): Angle-closure glaucoma, apathy, bruxism, cholestatic jaundice, disorientation, dysarthria, dysphagia, dysuria, emotional lability, erythema multiforme, extrapyramidal reaction, falling, gastroenteritis, gastrointestinal hemorrhage, hallucination, hematoma, hepatic failure, hostility, hyperglycemia, hyperkalemia, hyperlipidemia, hypersensitivity, hypokalemia, hypothyroidism, impulsivity, increased serum bicarbonate, menopausal symptoms, menstrual disease, muscle spasm, myocardial infarction, night sweats, orthostatic hypotension, outbursts of anger (particularly early in treatment or after treatment discontinuation), panic attack, restless leg syndrome, seizure, sensation of cold, serotonin syndrome, SIADH, skin photosensitivity, Stevens-Johnson syndrome, suicidal ideation, supraventricular cardiac arrhythmia, syncope, tachycardia, testicular pain, trismus, urinary retention, urinary urgency

Drug Interactions

Metabolism/Transport Effects Substrate of CYP1A2 (major), CYP2D6 (minor); **Note:** Assignment of Major/ Minor substrate status based on clinically relevant drug interaction potential; **Inhibits** CYP2D6 (moderate)

Avoid Concomitant Use

Avoid concomitant use of DULoxetine with any of the following: CYP1A2 Inhibitors (Strong); Dapoxetine; Iobenguane I 123; Linezolid; MAO Inhibitors; Methylene Blue; Thioridazine; Urokinase

Increased Effect/Toxicity

DULoxetine may increase the levels/effects of: Agents with Antiplatelet Properties; Alpha-/Beta-Agonists; Anticoagulants; Antipsychotic Agents; Apixaban; ARIPiprazole; Aspirin; Brexpiprazole; Collagenase (Systemic); CYP2D6 Substrates; Dabigatran Etexilate; Deoxycholic Acid; DOXOrubicin (Conventional); Edoxaban; Eliglustat; Fesoterodine; Ibritumomab; Methylene Blue; Metoprolol; Nebivolol; NSAID (Nonselective); Obinutuzumab; PARoxetine; Rivaroxaban; Salicylates; Serotonin Modulators; Thioridazine; Thrombolytic Agents; Tositumomab and Iodine I 131 Tositumomab; Tricyclic Antidepressants; Urokinase

The levels/effects of DULoxetine may be increased by: Abiraterone Acetate; Alcohol (Ethyl); Antiemetics (5HT3 Antagonists); Antipsychotic Agents; ARIPiprazole; Blood Pressure Lowering Agents; CYP1A2 Inhibitors (Moderate); CYP1A2 Inhibitors (Strong); CYP2D6 Inhibitors (Strong); Dapoxetine; Dasatinib; Deferasirox; Glucosamine; Herbs (Anticoagulant/Antiplatelet Properties); Ibrutinib; Limaprost; Linezolid; MAO Inhibitors; Metaxalone; Metoclopramide; Multivitamins/Fluoride (with ADE); Multivitamins/Minerals (with ADEK, Folate, Iron); Multivitamins/Minerals (with AE, No Iron); Omega-3 Fatty Acids; PARoxetine; Peginterferon Alfa-2b; Pentosan Polysulfate Sodium; Pentoxifylline; Propafenone; Prostacyclin Analogues; Tedizolid; Tipranavir; Vemurafenib; Vitamin E; Vitamin E (Oral)

Decreased Effect

DULoxetine may decrease the levels/effects of: Alpha2-Agonists; Codeine; Iobenguane I 123; Ioflupane I 123; Tamoxifen

The levels/effects of DULoxetine may be decreased by: Cannabis; CYP1A2 Inducers (Strong); Cyproterone; Osimertinib; Teriflunomide

Storage/Stability Store at 25°C (77°F); excursions are permitted between 15°C and 30°C (59°F and 86°F).

Mechanism of Action Duloxetine is a potent inhibitor of neuronal serotonin and norepinephrine reuptake and a weak inhibitor of dopamine reuptake. Duloxetine has no significant activity for muscarinic cholinergic, H_1-histaminergic, or alpha$_2$-adrenergic receptors. Duloxetine does not possess MAO-inhibitory activity.

Pharmacodynamics/Kinetics

Absorption: Well absorbed, 2-hour delay in absorption after ingestion; food decreases extent of absorption ~10% (no effect on C_{max})

Distribution: ~1,640 L

◀

Protein binding: >90%; primarily to albumin and alpha$_1$-acid glycoprotein

Metabolism: Hepatic, via CYP1A2 and CYP2D6; forms multiple metabolites (inactive)

Half-life elimination: ~12 hours (range: 8 to 17 hours); ~4 hours longer in elderly women

Time to peak: 6 hours; 10 hours when ingested with food

Excretion: Urine (~70%; <1% of total dose as unchanged drug); feces (~20%)

Dosing

Adult

Major depressive disorder: Oral:

US labeling: Initial: 40 to 60 mg daily; dose may be divided (ie, 20 or 30 mg twice daily) or given as a single daily dose of 60 mg. For some patients it may be desirable to start at 30 mg once daily for 1 week before increasing to 60 mg once daily. Maintenance: 60 mg once daily; maximum dose: 120 mg daily.

Canadian labeling: Initial: 60 mg once daily. Based on tolerability, it may be desirable to start at 30 mg once daily for 1 to 2 weeks before increasing to maintenance dose of 60 mg once daily; maximum dose: 60 mg daily.

Note: Doses >60 mg daily have not been demonstrated to be more effective than 60 mg daily.

Diabetic neuropathy: Oral:

US labeling: Initial: 60 mg once daily; lower initial doses may be considered in patients where tolerability is a concern and/or renal impairment is present; maximum dose: 60 mg once daily.

Canadian labeling: Initial: 60 mg daily. Based on tolerability, it may be desirable to start at 30 mg once daily for 1 to 2 weeks before increasing to 60 mg once daily; maximum dose: 120 mg daily.

Note: Doses >60 mg/day administered in clinical trials offered no additional benefit and were less well tolerated than dose of 60 mg daily.

Fibromyalgia (excluding Irenka): Oral:

US labeling: Initial: 30 mg once daily for 1 week, then increase to 60 mg once daily as tolerated; maximum dose: 60 mg daily.

Canadian labeling: Intial: 30 to 60 mg once daily (based on tolerability) for 1 to 2 weeks; then increase to 60 mg once daily as tolerated; maximum dose: 60 mg daily.

Note: Doses >60 mg daily administered in clinical trials offered no additional benefit and were less well tolerated than dose of 60 mg daily.

Generalized anxiety disorder: Oral: Initial: 60 mg once daily; for some patients it may be desirable to start at 30 mg once daily for 1 week before increasing to 60 mg once daily. For doses >60 mg once daily, titrate dose in increments of 30 mg once daily over 1 week (US labeling) or 1 to 2 weeks (Canadian labeling) as tolerated; maximum dose: 120 mg once daily. **Note:** Doses >60 mg once daily have not been demonstrated to be more effective than 60 mg once daily.

Chronic musculoskeletal pain: Oral: 30 mg once daily for 1 week (US labeling) or 1 to 2 weeks (Canadian labeling), then increase to 60 mg once daily as tolerated; maximum dose: 60 mg daily. **Note:** Doses >60 mg once daily administered in clinical trials offered no additional benefit and were less well tolerated than dose of 60 mg once daily. The Canadian labeling indicates that a maximum dose of 120 mg daily may be considered for patients with chronic pain associated with osteoarthritis of the knee.

Stress urinary incontinence (women) (off-label use): Oral: 40 mg twice daily (Li, 2013). Lower initial doses have been used to reduce adverse effects: 20 mg twice daily for 2 weeks titrated to or followed by 40 mg twice daily (Castro-Diaz, 2007; Schagen van Leeuwen, 2008).

Discontinuation of therapy: Upon discontinuation of antidepressant therapy, gradually taper the dose to minimize the incidence of withdrawal symptoms and allow for the detection of re-emerging symptoms. Evidence supporting ideal taper rates is limited. APA and NICE guidelines suggest tapering therapy over at least several weeks with consideration to the half-life of the antidepressant; antidepressants with a shorter half-life may need to be tapered more conservatively. In addition for long-term treated patients, WFSBP guidelines recommend tapering over 4-6 months. If intolerable withdrawal symptoms occur following a dose reduction, consider resuming the previously prescribed dose and/or decrease dose at a more gradual rate (APA, 2010; Bauer, 2002; Haddad, 2001; NCCMH, 2010; Schatzberg, 2006; Shelton, 2001; Warner, 2006).

MAO inhibitor recommendations:

Switching to or from an MAO inhibitor intended to treat psychiatric disorders:

Allow 14 days to elapse between discontinuing an MAO inhibitor intended to treat psychiatric disorders and initiation of duloxetine.

Allow ≥5 to 14 days to elapse between discontinuing duloxetine and initiation of an MAO inhibitor intended to treat psychiatric disorders.

Use with other MAO inhibitors (such as linezolid or IV methylene blue):

Do not initiate duloxetine in patients receiving linezolid or IV methylene blue; consider other interventions for psychiatric condition.

If urgent treatment with linezolid or IV methylene blue is required in a patient already receiving duloxetine and potential benefits outweigh potential risks, discontinue duloxetine promptly and administer linezolid or IV methylene blue. Monitor for serotonin syndrome for 5 days or until 24 hours after the last dose of linezolid or IV methylene blue, whichever comes first. May resume duloxetine 24 hours after the last dose of linezolid or IV methylene blue.

Geriatric

Generalized anxiety disorder: Oral: Initial: 30 mg once daily; after 2 weeks may increase to 60 mg once daily; titrate doses >60 mg once daily in increments of 30 mg once daily; maximum dose: 120 mg once daily.

Other indications: Refer to adult dosing.

Discontinuation of therapy: Refer to adult dosing.

MAO inhibitor recommendations: Refer to adult dosing.

Pediatric Generalized anxiety disorder: Children and Adolescents 7 to 17 years: Oral: Initial: 30 mg once daily; after 2 weeks may increase based on response and tolerability to 60 mg once daily; titrate doses >60 mg once daily in increments of 30 mg once daily; maximum dose: 120 mg once daily. **Note:** Use in patients <18 years of age is not approved in the Canadian labeling.

Renal Impairment

CrCl ≥30 mL/minute: There are no dosage adjustments provided in the manufacturer's labeling; however pharmacokinetic studies suggest that mild to moderate renal impairment (CrCl 30 to 80 mL/minute) has no significant effect on duloxetine clearance

CrCl <30 mL/minute: Avoid use (contraindicated in Canadian labeling)

End-stage renal disease (ESRD): Avoid use (contraindicated in Canadian labeling)

Hepatic Impairment Avoid use in hepatic impairment (contraindicated in Canadian labeling).

Administration Swallow capsule whole; do not crush or chew. Although the manufacturer does not recommend opening the capsule to facilitate administration, the contents of capsule may be sprinkled on applesauce or in apple juice and swallowed (without chewing) immediately; do not sprinkle contents on chocolate pudding (Wells, 2008). Administer without regard to meals.

Monitoring Parameters Blood pressure should be checked prior to initiating therapy and then regularly monitored, especially in patients with a high baseline blood pressure; mental status for depression, suicidal ideation (especially at the beginning of therapy or when doses are increased or decreased), anxiety, social functioning, mania, panic attacks or other unusual changes in behavior; glucose levels and HbA$_{1c}$ levels in diabetic patients, creatinine, BUN, transaminases

Dosage Forms Excipient information presented when available (limited, particularly for generics); consult specific product labeling.

Capsule Delayed Release Particles, Oral:

Cymbalta: 20 mg, 30 mg, 60 mg [contains fd&c blue #2 (indigotine)]

Irenka: 40 mg

Generic: 20 mg, 30 mg, 40 mg, 60 mg

◆ Duloxetine Hydrochloride *see* DULoxetine *on page 610*

◆ Duodopa (Can) *see* Carbidopa and Levodopa *on page 307*

◆ Duodote *see* Atropine and Pralidoxime *on page 179*

◆ DuoNeb *see* Ipratropium and Albuterol *on page 978*

◆ Duopa *see* Carbidopa and Levodopa *on page 307*

◆ DuP 753 *see* Losartan *on page 1107*

◆ Duraclon *see* CloNIDine *on page 421*

◆ Duragesic *see* FentaNYL *on page 750*

◆ Duragesic MAT (Can) *see* FentaNYL *on page 750*

◆ Duramorph *see* Morphine (Systemic) *on page 1230*

◆ Durela (Can) *see* TraMADol *on page 1821*

◆ Durezol *see* Difluprednate *on page 546*

- Duricef *see* Cefadroxil *on page 328*
- Durlaza *see* Aspirin *on page 157*
- Durolane (Can) *see* Hyaluronate and Derivatives *on page 879*

Dutasteride (doo TAS teer ide)

Brand Names: US Avodart
Brand Names: Canada ACT-Dutasteride; Apo-Dutasteride; Avodart; Med-Dutasteride; Mint-Dutasteride; PMS-Dutasteride; Riva-Dutasteride; Sandoz-Dutasteride; Teva-Dutasteride
Pharmacologic Category 5 Alpha-Reductase Inhibitor
Use

Benign prostatic hyperplasia: Treatment of symptomatic benign prostatic hyperplasia (BPH) as monotherapy (to improve symptoms, reduce the risk of acute urinary retention, and to reduce the risk of need for BPH-related surgery) or combination therapy with tamsulosin
Limitations of use: Not approved for the prevention of prostate cancer.

Dosing

Adult & Geriatric Benign prostatic hyperplasia (BPH):
Males: Oral: 0.5 mg once daily alone or in combination with tamsulosin
Renal Impairment No dosage adjustment is necessary
Hepatic Impairment There are no dosage adjustments provided in the manufacturer's labeling (has not been studied). Dutasteride is extensively hepatically metabolized and exposure could be increased in hepatic impairment, however, higher doses studied did not generally produce additional adverse effects.
Additional Information Complete prescribing information should be consulted for additional detail.
Dosage Forms Excipient information presented when available (limited, particularly for generics); consult specific product labeling.
Capsule, Oral:
Avodart: 0.5 mg
Generic: 0.5 mg

Dutasteride and Tamsulosin
(doo TAS teer ide & tam SOO loe sin)

Brand Names: US Jalyn
Brand Names: Canada Jalyn
Index Terms Tamsulosin and Dutasteride; Tamsulosin Hydrochloride and Dutasteride
Pharmacologic Category 5 Alpha-Reductase Inhibitor; Alpha₁ Blocker
Use

Benign prostatic hyperplasia: Treatment of symptomatic benign prostatic hyperplasia (BPH) in men with an enlarged prostate.
Limitations of use: Dutasteride-containing products are not approved for the prevention of prostate cancer.

Dosing
Adult & Geriatric
Benign prostatic hyperplasia (BPH): Males: Oral: One capsule (0.5 mg dutasteride/0.4 mg tamsulosin) once daily ~30 minutes after the same meal each day
Renal Impairment
CrCl ≥10 mL/minute/1.73 m²: No dosage adjustment necessary.
CrCl <10 mL/minute/1.73 m²: There are no dosage adjustments provided in the manufacturer's labeling (has not been studied).
Hepatic Impairment There are no dosage adjustments provided in the manufacturer's labeling. See individual agents.
Additional Information Complete prescribing information should be consulted for additional detail.
Dosage Forms Excipient information presented when available (limited, particularly for generics); consult specific product labeling.
Capsule, oral:
Jalyn: Dutasteride 0.5 mg and tamsulosin hydrochloride 0.4 mg
Generic: Dutasteride 0.5 mg and tamsulosin hydrochloride 0.4 mg

- Duvoid (Can) *see* Bethanechol *on page 226*
- DW286 *see* Gemifloxacin *on page 836*
- DX-88 *see* Ecallantide *on page 613*
- Dyanavel XR *see* Amphetamine *on page 115*
- Dyazide *see* Hydrochlorothiazide and Triamterene *on page 884*

Dyclonine (DYE kloe neen)

Brand Names: US Sucrets® Children's [OTC]; Sucrets® Maximum Strength [OTC]; Sucrets® Regular Strength [OTC]
Index Terms Dyclonine Hydrochloride
Pharmacologic Category Local Anesthetic, Oral
Use Temporary relief of pain associated with oral mucosa
Dosing
Adult & Geriatric Temporary relief of pain: Oral topical:
Lozenge: One lozenge every 2 hours as needed (maximum: 10 lozenges/day)
Pediatric Temporary relief of pain: Children ≥2 years: Refer to adult dosing.
Additional Information Complete prescribing information should be consulted for additional information.
Dosage Forms Excipient information presented when available (limited, particularly for generics); consult specific product labeling. [DSC] = Discontinued product
Lozenge, oral, as hydrochloride:
Sucrets® Children's: 1.2 mg (18s) [cherry flavor]
Sucrets® Maximum Strength: 3 mg (18s) [black-cherry flavor]
Sucrets® Maximum Strength: 3 mg (18s) [wintergreen flavor]
Sucrets® Regular Strength: 2 mg (18s)
Sucrets® Regular Strength: 2 mg (18s [DSC]) [wild cherry flavor]

- Dyclonine Hydrochloride *see* Dyclonine *on page 613*
- Dyloject *see* Diclofenac (Systemic) *on page 540*
- Dymista *see* Azelastine and Fluticasone *on page 188*
- Dynacin *see* Minocycline *on page 1211*
- Dynacin [DSC] *see* Minocycline *on page 1211*
- DynaCirc CR [DSC] *see* Isradipine *on page 998*
- Dyna-Hex 2 [OTC] *see* Chlorhexidine Gluconate *on page 373*
- Dyrenium *see* Triamterene *on page 1843*
- Dyspel [OTC] *see* Ibuprofen *on page 905*
- Dysport *see* AbobotulinumtoxinA *on page 23*
- Dysport (Glabellar Lines) *see* AbobotulinumtoxinA *on page 23*
- Dytuss [DSC] *see* DiphenhydrAMINE (Systemic) *on page 561*
- 7E3 *see* Abciximab *on page 20*
- E-400 [OTC] *see* Vitamin E *on page 1906*
- E-400-Clear [OTC] *see* Vitamin E *on page 1906*
- E-400-Mixed [OTC] *see* Vitamin E *on page 1906*
- E2020 *see* Donepezil *on page 583*
- E 2080 *see* Rufinamide *on page 1625*
- E7080 *see* Lenvatinib *on page 1046*
- E7389 *see* Eribulin *on page 664*
- EACA *see* Aminocaproic Acid *on page 93*
- Ear Drops Earwax Aid [OTC] *see* Carbamide Peroxide *on page 307*
- Ear Wax Remover [OTC] [DSC] *see* Carbamide Peroxide *on page 307*
- Earwax Treatment Drops [OTC] *see* Carbamide Peroxide *on page 307*
- Ebixa (Can) *see* Memantine *on page 1139*

Ecallantide (e KAL lan tide)

Brand Names: US Kalbitor
Index Terms DX-88
Pharmacologic Category Kallikrein Inhibitor
Use Hereditary angioedema: Treatment of acute attacks of hereditary angioedema (HAE) in patients 12 years and older
Medication Guide Available Yes
Dosing
Adult & Geriatric Hereditary angioedema (HAE) treatment: SubQ: 30 mg (as three 10 mg [1 mL] injections); if attack persists, may repeat an additional 30 mg within 24 hours
Pediatric Hereditary angioedema (HAE) treatment: Children ≥12 years and Adolescents: Refer to adult dosing
Renal Impairment There are no dosage adjustments provided in the manufacturer's labeling (has not been studied).
Hepatic Impairment There are no dosage adjustments provided in the manufacturer's labeling (has not been studied).

Additional Information Complete prescribing information should be consulted for additional detail.

Dosage Forms Excipient information presented when available (limited, particularly for generics); consult specific product labeling.

Solution, Subcutaneous [preservative free]:

Kalbitor: 10 mg/mL (1 mL)

Echothiophate Iodide
(ek oh THYE oh fate EYE oh dide)

Brand Names: US Phospholine Iodide

Index Terms Ecostigmine Iodide

Pharmacologic Category Acetylcholinesterase Inhibitor; Ophthalmic Agent, Antiglaucoma; Ophthalmic Agent, Miotic

Use

Accommodative esotropia: Concomitant esotropias with a significant accommodative component.

Glaucoma: Treatment of chronic open-angle glaucoma; subacute or chronic angle-closure glaucoma (postiridectomy or where surgery is refused or contraindicated); certain nonuveitic secondary types of glaucoma, especially glaucoma following cataract surgery.

Dosing

Adult & Geriatric

Glaucoma: Ophthalmic:

Initial: Instill 1 drop (0.03%) twice daily into eyes with 1 dose just prior to bedtime

Maintenance: Twice-daily dosing is preferred but some patients have been treated with once-daily or every-other-day dosing (with 1 dose just prior to bedtime).

Conversion from other ophthalmic agents: If IOP control was unsatisfactory, patients may be expected to require higher doses of echothiophate (eg, ≥0.06%); however, patients should be initially started on the 0.03% strength for a short period to better tolerance.

Pediatric

Accommodative esotropia: Ophthalmic:

Diagnosis: Instill 1 drop (0.125%) once daily into both eyes at bedtime for 2 to 3 weeks

Treatment: Usual dose: 1 drop of 0.06% once daily or 0.125% every other day (maximum: 1 drop of 0.125% in both eyes/day). **Note:** Use lowest concentration and frequency that gives satisfactory response; 0.3% has been proven to be effective.

Renal Impairment There are no dosage adjustments provided in the manufacturer's labeling.

Hepatic Impairment There are no dosage adjustments provided in the manufacturer's labeling.

Additional Information Complete prescribing information should be consulted for additional detail.

Dosage Forms Excipient information presented when available (limited, particularly for generics); consult specific product labeling.

Solution Reconstituted, Ophthalmic:

Phospholine Iodide: 0.125% (5 mL)

Econazole (e KONE a zole)

Brand Names: US Ecoza

Index Terms Econazole Nitrate; Ecoza; Spectazole

Pharmacologic Category Antifungal Agent, Imidazole Derivative; Antifungal Agent, Topical

Use Fungal infection:

Cream: Treatment of tinea pedis, tinea cruris, and tinea corporis caused by *Trichophyton rubrum*, *Trichophyton mentagrophytes*, *Trichophyton tonsurans*, *Microsporum canis*, *Microsporum audouini*, *Microsporum gypseum*, and *Epidermophyton floccosum* in the treatment of cutaneous candidiasis, and in the treatment of tinea versicolor.

Foam: Treatment of interdigital tinea pedis caused by *Trichophyton rubrum*, *Trichophyton mentagrophytes*, and *Epidermophyton floccosum* in patients 12 years and older

Dosing

Adult & Geriatric

Tinea pedis: Topical: Cream, Foam: Apply sufficient amount to cover affected areas once daily for 4 weeks

Tinea cruris, tinea corporis, tinea versicolor: Topical: Cream: Apply sufficient amount to cover affected areas once daily for 2 weeks

Cutaneous candidiasis: Topical: Cream: Apply sufficient quantity twice daily (morning and evening) for 2 weeks

Pediatric Tinea pedis: Children ≥12 years and Adolescents: Topical: Foam: Apply sufficient amount to cover affected area once daily for 4 weeks

Additional Information Complete prescribing information should be consulted for additional detail.

Product Availability Ecoza topical foam: FDA approved October 2013; anticipated availability currently unknown

Dosage Forms Excipient information presented when available (limited, particularly for generics); consult specific product labeling.

Cream, External, as nitrate:

Generic: 1% (15 g, 30 g, 85 g)

Foam, External, as nitrate:

Ecoza: 1% (70 g) [contains propylene glycol, trolamine (triethanolamine)]

Eculizumab (e kue LIZ oo mab)

Brand Names: US Soliris

Brand Names: Canada Soliris

Index Terms h5G1.1; Monoclonal Antibody 5G1.1; Monoclonal Antibody Anti-C5

Pharmacologic Category Monoclonal Antibody; Monoclonal Antibody, Complement Inhibitor

Use

Atypical hemolytic uremic syndrome: Treatment of atypical hemolytic uremic syndrome (aHUS) to inhibit complement-mediated thrombotic microangiopathy.

Limitation of use: Eculizumab is not indicated for the treatment of patients with Shiga toxin *Escherichia coli*-related hemolytic uremic syndrome.

Paroxysmal nocturnal hemoglobinuria: Treatment of paroxysmal nocturnal hemoglobinuria (PNH) to reduce hemolysis.

Pregnancy Considerations Adverse events were observed in animal reproduction studies. Eculizumab crosses the placenta and can be detected in cord blood. Pregnant women with PNH and their fetuses have high rates of morbidity and mortality during pregnancy and the postpartum period. Treatment of PNH with eculizumab has been shown to increase fetal survival and decrease maternal complications (Kelly 2015). Use of eculizumab for the treatment of a HUS in pregnancy has also been described (Ardissino 2013).

Breast-Feeding Considerations Excretion of eculizumab into breast milk was not noted in breast milk samples from 10 women. In a separate case report, eculizumab was detected in the initial breast milk sample of a woman, but not subsequent samples (Kelly 2015). The manufacturer recommends that caution be used if administered to nursing women.

Prescribing and Access Restrictions Patients and providers must enroll with Soliris REMS OneSource Safety Program (1-888-765-4747) or at solirisrems.com prior to treatment initiation.

Medication Guide Available Yes

Contraindications Unresolved serious *Neisseria meningitidis* infection; patients not currently vaccinated against *Neisseria meningitidis* (unless risks of treatment delay outweigh risk of developing a meningococcal infection)

Warnings/Precautions [US Boxed Warning]: Meningococcal (*Neisseria meningitides*) infections have occurred in patients receiving eculizumab; may be fatal or life-threatening if not detected and treated promptly. Monitor closely for early signs of meningococcal infection; evaluate and treat promptly if suspected. Follow current meningococcal immunization recommendations for patients with complement deficiencies. Vaccinate with meningococcal vaccine at least 2 weeks prior to initiation of treatment (unless the risks of delaying eculizumab outweigh the risk of developing meningococcal infection); revaccinate according to current guidelines. Polyvalent meningococcal vaccines are recommended. If urgent treatment is

necessary in an unvaccinated patient, administer meningococcal vaccine as soon as possible. Although the risk/benefits of prophylactic meningococcal antibiotic therapy have not been determined, prophylactic antibiotics were administered in clinical studies until at least 2 weeks after vaccination. Meningococcal infections developed in some patients despite vaccination. Discontinue eculizumab during the treatment of serious meningococcal infections. In addition to meningitis, the risk of other infections, especially encapsulated bacteria (eg, *Streptococcus pneumoniae*, *H. influenzae*) is increased with eculizumab treatment (because eculizumab blocks terminal complement activation). Aspergillus infections have occurred in immunocompromised and neutropenic patients. Children should receive vaccination for prevention of *S. pneumoniae*, *H. influenzae* according to current ACIP guidelines. Use caution in patients with concurrent systemic infection. Patients should be up to date with all immunizations before initiating therapy. **[US Boxed Warning]: Access is restricted through a REMS program. Prescribers must be enrolled in the program; enrollment and additional information is available at 1-888-765-4747 or solirisrems.com.** Counsel patients on the risk of meningococcal infection; ensure patients are vaccinated and provide educational materials.

Infusion reactions, including anaphylaxis or hypersensitivity, may occur; interrupt infusion for severe reaction (eg, cardiovascular instability, respiratory compromise). Continue monitoring for 1 hour after completion of infusion. Patients with PNH who discontinue treatment may be at increased risk for serious hemolysis; monitor closely for at least 8 weeks after treatment discontinuation. When used for aHUS, monitor for at least 12 weeks after treatment discontinuation for signs/symptoms of thrombotic microangiopathy (TMA) complications (angina, dyspnea, mental status changes, seizure, or thrombosis; occurrence of two or repeated measurement of any one of the following: Serum creatinine elevation (≥25% from baseline or nadir), serum LDH elevation (≥25% from baseline or nadir), thrombocytopenia (platelet decrease by ≥25% compared to baseline or peak). If TMA complications occur after stopping eculizumab, consider reinitiation of treatment, plasmapheresis, plasma exchange, fresh frozen plasma infusion, and/or appropriate organ-specific measures. In clinical trials, anticoagulant therapy was continued in patients who were receiving these agents (due to history of or risk for thromboembolism) prior to initiation of eculizumab. Potentially significant drug-drug interactions may exist, requiring dose or frequency adjustment, additional monitoring, and/or selection of alternative therapy. The effect of anticoagulant therapy withdrawal is unknown; treatment with eculizumab should not alter anticoagulation management

Adverse Reactions Frequency reported for adolescent and adult patients ≥13 years unless otherwise noted.
>10%:
Cardiovascular: Hypertension (aHUS: 17% to 59%; infants, children, and adolescents 5 months through 17 years: 18%), peripheral edema (20% to 29%), tachycardia (aHUS: children 21%), hypotension (12% to 20%)
Central nervous system: Headache (37% to 50%; serious: 2%; infants, children, and adolescents 5 months through 17 years: 18%), insomnia (10% to 24%), fatigue (7% to 20%)
Dermatologic: Skin rash (infants ≥5 months, children, adolescents, and adults 12% to 18%), pruritus (6% to 15%)
Endocrine & metabolic: Hypokalemia (10% to 18%)
Gastrointestinal: Diarrhea (32% to 47%; infants, children, and adolescents 2 months through 17 years: 32%), vomiting (15% to 47%; infants, children, and adolescents 2 months through 17 years: 21% to 27%), nausea (12% to 40%), abdominal pain (15% to 30%), gastroenteritis (5% to 18%), dyspepsia (infants, children, and adolescents 5 months through 17 years: 14%)
Genitourinary: Urinary tract infection (15% to 35%; infants, children, and adolescents 5 months through 17 years: 18%), uropathy (infants, children, and adolescents 5 months through 17 years: 18%), proteinuria (5% to 12%)
Hematologic & oncologic: Anemia (17% to 35%; serious: 2%), neoplasm (6% to 30%), leukopenia (16% to 24%)
Local: Catheter infection (infants, children, and adolescents 5 months through 17 years: 14%)
Neuromuscular & skeletal: Weakness (15% to 20%), back pain (5% to 19%), arthralgia (6% to 17%), muscle spasm (infants, children, and adolescents 5 months through 17 years: 14%), limb pain (7% to 11%)
Ophthalmic: Eye disease (10% to 29%; infants, children, and adolescents 5 months through 17 years: 14%)
Renal: Renal insufficiency (15% to 29%)

Respiratory: Nasopharyngitis (18% to 55%; infants, children, and adolescents 5 months through 17 years: 27%), upper respiratory tract infection (infants ≥2 months, children, adolescents, and adults 5% to 40%), cough (infants ≥5 months, children, adolescents, and adults 12% to 36%), nasal congestion (aHUS: children 21%), rhinitis (infants, children, and adolescents 5 months through 17 years: 18%), bronchitis (10% to 18%), oropharyngeal pain (infants, children, and adolescents 5 months through 17 years: 14%)
Miscellaneous: Fever (infants, children, and adolescents 2 months through 17 years: 47% to 50%; adults 17% to 25%)
1% to 10%:
Gastrointestinal: Constipation (7%)
Immunologic: Antibody development (2% to 3%; neutralizing: 1%)
Infection: Herpes virus infection (7%), viral infection (serious: 2%), meningococcal infection (≤1%)
Neuromuscular & skeletal: Myalgia (7%)
Respiratory: Respiratory tract infection (7%), sinusitis (7%), flu-like symptoms (5%)
<1% (Limited to important or life-threatening): Aspergillosis, cholangitis, endometritis, hematoma (mild), infusion related reaction, pyelonephritis

Drug Interactions
Metabolism/Transport Effects None known.
Avoid Concomitant Use
Avoid concomitant use of Eculizumab with any of the following: BCG (Intravesical); Belimumab; Natalizumab; Pimecrolimus; Tacrolimus (Topical); Tofacitinib; Vaccines (Live)
Increased Effect/Toxicity
Eculizumab may increase the levels/effects of: Belimumab; Fingolimod; Leflunomide; Natalizumab; Tofacitinib; Vaccines (Live)

The levels/effects of Eculizumab may be increased by: Denosumab; Pimecrolimus; Roflumilast; Tacrolimus (Topical); Trastuzumab
Decreased Effect
Eculizumab may decrease the levels/effects of: BCG (Intravesical); Coccidioides immitis Skin Test; Sipuleucel-T; Vaccines (Inactivated); Vaccines (Live)

The levels/effects of Eculizumab may be decreased by: Echinacea

Preparation for Administration Add eculizumab to an infusion bag and dilute with an equal volume of D_5W, sodium chloride 0.9%, sodium chloride 0.45%, or Ringer's injection to a final concentration of 5 mg/mL (eg, 300 mg to a total volume of 60 mL, 600 mg in a total volume of 120 mL, 900 mg in a total volume of 180 mL, or 1200 mg to a total volume of 240 mL). Gently invert bag to mix thoroughly; do not shake.

Storage/Stability Prior to dilution, store intact vials at 2°C to 8°C (36°F to 46°F); do not freeze. Protect from light; do not shake. Following dilution, store at room temperature or refrigerate; use within 24 hours. If refrigerated, allow admixture to reach room temperature prior to administration (do not use a heat source for warming).

Mechanism of Action Terminal complement-mediated intravascular hemolysis is a key clinical feature of paroxysmal nocturnal hemoglobinuria (PNH); blocking the formation of membrane attack complex (MAC) results in stabilization of hemoglobin and a reduction in the need for RBC transfusions. Impairment of complement activity regulation leads to uncontrolled complement activation in atypical hemolytic uremic syndrome (aHUS). Eculizumab is a humanized monoclonal IgG antibody that binds to complement protein C5, preventing cleavage into C5a and C5b. Blocking the formation of C5b inhibits the subsequent formation of terminal complex C5b-9 or MAC.

Pharmacodynamics/Kinetics
Onset of action: PNH: Reduced hemolysis: ≤1 week
Distribution: PNH: 7.7 L; aHUS: 6.14 L
Half-life elimination: PNH: ~11 days (range: ~8-15 days); aHUS: ~12 days (during plasma exchange the half-life is reduced to 1.26 hours)

Dosing
Adult & Geriatric Note: Patients must receive meningococcal vaccine at least 2 weeks prior to treatment initiation; revaccinate according to current guidelines. Treatment should be administered at the recommended time interval although administration may be varied by ±2 days.
Atypical hemolytic uremic syndrome (aHUS): IV: Induction: 900 mg weekly for 4 doses; Maintenance: 1200 mg at week 5, then 1200 mg every 2 weeks
Supplemental dosing for patients receiving plasmapheresis or plasma exchange: If most recent dose was ≥600 mg, administer 600 mg within 60 minutes after each plasmapheresis or plasma exchange

◄

Supplemental dosing for patients receiving fresh frozen plasma infusion: If most recent dose was ≥300 mg, administer 300 mg within 60 minutes prior to each infusion of fresh frozen plasma

Paroxysmal nocturnal hemoglobinuria (PNH): IV: 600 mg weekly for 4 doses, followed by 900 mg 1 week later; then 900 mg every 2 weeks

Pediatric Note: Patients must receive meningococcal vaccine at least 2 weeks prior to treatment initiation; revaccinate according to current guidelines. Treatment should be administered at the recommended time interval although administration may be varied by ±2 days.

Atypical hemolytic uremic syndrome (aHUS): IV:

Children 5 kg to <10 kg: Induction: 300 mg weekly for 1 dose; Maintenance: 300 mg at week 2, then 300 mg every 3 weeks

Children 10 kg to <20 kg: Induction: 600 mg weekly for 1 dose; Maintenance: 300 mg at week 2, then 300 mg every 2 weeks

Children 20 kg to <30 kg: Induction: 600 mg weekly for 2 doses; Maintenance: 600 mg at week 3, then 600 mg every 2 weeks

Children 30 kg to <40 kg: Induction: 600 mg weekly for 2 doses; Maintenance: 900 mg at week 3, then 900 mg every 2 weeks

Children ≥40 kg: Induction: 900 mg weekly for 4 doses; Maintenance: 1200 mg at week 5, then 1200 mg every 2 weeks

Supplemental dosing for patients receiving plasmapheresis or plasma exchange:

If most recent dose was 300 mg, administer 300 mg within 60 minutes after each plasmapheresis or plasma exchange

If most recent dose was ≥600 mg, administer 600 mg within 60 minutes after each plasmapheresis or plasma exchange

Supplemental dosing for patients receiving fresh frozen plasma infusion: If most recent dose was ≥300 mg, administer 300 mg within 60 minutes prior to each infusion of fresh frozen plasma

Renal Impairment There are no dosage adjustments provided in the manufacturer's labeling (has not been studied).

Hepatic Impairment There are no dosage adjustments provided in the manufacturer's labeling (has not been studied).

Administration IV: Allow to reach room temperature prior to administration. Infuse over 35 minutes in adults and over 1 to 4 hours in pediatric patients; do not administer as an IV push or bolus. Decrease infusion rate or discontinue for infusion reactions; do not exceed a maximum 2-hour duration of infusion in adults. Monitor for at least 1 hour following completion of infusion (for signs/symptoms of infusion reaction).

Monitoring Parameters CBC with differential, lactic dehydrogenase (LDH), serum creatinine, AST, urinalysis; early signs/symptoms of meningococcal infection; signs and symptoms of infusion reaction (during infusion and for 1 hour after infusion complete).

After discontinuation:

aHUS: Signs/symptoms of thrombotic microangiopathy (TMA) complications (monitor for at least 12 weeks after treatment discontinuation), including angina, dyspnea, mental status changes, seizure, or thrombosis; occurrence of two or repeated measurement of any one of the following: Serum creatinine elevation (≥25% from baseline or nadir), serum LDH elevation (≥25% from baseline or nadir), thrombocytopenia (platelet decrease by ≥25% compared to baseline or peak).

PNH: Signs and symptoms of intravascular hemolysis (monitor for at least 8 weeks after discontinuation), including anemia, fatigue, pain, dark urine, dyspnea, or thrombosis.

Dosage Forms Excipient information presented when available (limited, particularly for generics); consult specific product labeling.

Solution, Intravenous [preservative free]:

Soliris: 10 mg/mL (30 mL)

♦ Ed A-Hist [OTC] *see* Chlorpheniramine and Phenylephrine *on page 376*

♦ Ed A-Hist DM [OTC] *see* Chlorpheniramine, Phenylephrine, and Dextromethorphan *on page 378*

♦ Ed A-Hist PSE [OTC] *see* Triprolidine and Pseudoephedrine *on page 1847*

♦ Edarbi *see* Azilsartan *on page 188*

♦ Edarbyclor *see* Azilsartan and Chlorthalidone *on page 190*

♦ Ed Baclofen [DSC] *see* Baclofen *on page 197*

♦ Ed Bron GP [OTC] *see* Guaifenesin and Phenylephrine *on page 862*

♦ Ed ChlorPed D [OTC] *see* Chlorpheniramine and Phenylephrine *on page 376*

♦ Edecrin *see* Ethacrynic Acid *on page 699*

Edetate CALCIUM Disodium

(ED e tate KAL see um dye SOW dee um)

Index Terms CaEDTA; Calcium Disodium Edetate; Calcium Disodiumethylenediaminetetraacetic Acid; Edetate Disodium CALCIUM; EDTA (CALCIUM Disodium) (error-prone abbreviation)

Pharmacologic Category Chelating Agent

Use Treatment of symptomatic acute and chronic lead poisoning

Dosing

Adult & Geriatric

Lead poisoning: Note: Available guidelines recommend chelation therapy with blood lead levels >50 mcg/dL and significant symptoms; chelation therapy may also be indicated with blood lead levels ≥100 mcg/dL and/or symptoms (Kosnett, 2007). Depending upon the blood lead level, additional courses may be necessary; at least 2-4 days should elapse before repeat treatment is initiated.

Blood lead levels <70 mcg/dL and asymptomatic: IM, IV: 1000 mg/m^2/day for 5 days

Blood lead levels ≥70 mcg/dL or symptomatic lead poisoning (in conjunction with dimercaprol): **Note:** Begin treatment with edetate CALCIUM disodium with the second dimercaprol dose: IM, IV: 1000 mg/m^2/day **or** 25-50 mg/kg/day for 5 days; a maximum dose of 3000 mg has been suggested (Howland, 2011)

Lead encephalopathy (in conjunction with dimercaprol): **Note:** Begin treatment with edetate CALCIUM disodium with the second dimercaprol dose: IM, IV: 1500 mg/m^2/day **or** 50-75 mg/kg/day for 5 days; a maximum dose of 3000 mg has been suggested (Howland, 2011)

Lead nephropathy: An alternative dosing regimen reflecting the reduction in renal clearance is based upon the serum creatinine; **Note:** Repeat regimen monthly until lead levels are reduced to an acceptable level: IM, IV:

S_{cr} 2-3 mg/dL: 500 mg/m^2 every 24 hours for 5 days

S_{cr} 3-4 mg/dL: 500 mg/m^2 every 48 hours for 3 doses

S_{cr} >4 mg/dL: 500 mg/m^2 once weekly

Pediatric

Lead poisoning: Note: For the treatment of high blood lead levels in children, the CDC recommends chelation treatment when blood lead levels are >45 mcg/dL (CDC, 2002). The AAP recommends succimer as the drug used for initial management in asymptomatic children when blood lead levels are >45 mcg/dL and <70 mcg/dL. Edetate CALCIUM disodium can be used in children allergic to succimer (AAP, 2005; Chandran, 2010). Combination therapy with edetate CALCIUM disodium and dimercaprol is recommended for use in children whose blood lead levels are ≥70 mcg/dL or in children with lead encephalopathy (AAP, 2005; Chandran, 2010). Depending upon the blood lead level, additional courses may be necessary; at least 2-4 days should elapse before repeat treatment is initiated.

Blood lead levels <70 mcg/dL and asymptomatic: IM, IV: 1000 mg/m^2/day for 5 days or 50 mg/kg/day (maximum: 1000 mg/day) for 5 days (Chandran, 2010)

Blood lead levels ≥70 mcg/dL or symptomatic lead poisoning (in conjunction with dimercaprol): **Note:** Begin treatment with edetate CALCIUM disodium with the second dimercaprol dose: IM, IV: 1000 mg/m^2/day **or** 25-50 mg/kg/day (maximum: 1000 mg/day) for 5 days (Chandran, 2010; Howland, 2011)

Lead encephalopathy (in conjunction with dimercaprol): **Note:** Begin treatment with edetate CALCIUM disodium with the second dimercaprol dose: IM, IV: 1500 mg/m^2/day **or** 50-75 mg/kg/day (maximum: 1000 mg/day) for 5 days (Chandran, 2010; Howland, 2011)

Renal Impairment Dose should be reduced with preexisting mild renal disease. Limiting the daily dose to 1 g in children and 2 g in adults may decrease risk of nephrotoxicity, although larger doses may be needed in the treatment of lead encephalopathy (Howland, 2011).

Additional Information Complete prescribing information should be consulted for additional detail.

Dosage Forms Excipient information presented when available (limited, particularly for generics); consult specific product labeling. [DSC] = Discontinued product

Solution, Injection:

Generic: 500 mg/2.5 mL (2.5 mL [DSC]); 1 g/5 mL (5 mL)

◆ Edetate Disodium CALCIUM *see* Edetate CALCIUM Disodium *on page 616*

◆ Edex *see* Alprostadil *on page 78*

◆ Edluar *see* Zolpidem *on page 1940*

Edoxaban (e DOX a ban)

Brand Names: US Savaysa

Index Terms Edoxaban Tosylate

Pharmacologic Category Anticoagulant; Anticoagulant, Factor Xa Inhibitor

Additional Appendix Information

Oral Anticoagulant Comparison Chart *on page 1957*

Use

Deep vein thrombosis and pulmonary embolism: Treatment of deep vein thrombosis (DVT) and pulmonary embolism (PE) following 5 to 10 days of initial therapy with a parenteral anticoagulant.

Nonvalvular atrial fibrillation: To reduce the risk of stroke and systemic embolism (SE) in patients with nonvalvular atrial fibrillation (NVAF)

Limitations of use: Edoxaban should not be used in NVAF patients with CrCl >95 mL/minute because of an increased risk of ischemic stroke compared to warfarin

Pregnancy Considerations Adverse events were observed in some animal reproduction studies. Ten pregnancies were reported in a study using edoxaban for the treatment of DVT or PE. Estimated exposure occurred during the first trimester with duration of exposure ~6 weeks; outcomes included six live births (two preterm), one first-trimester spontaneous abortion, and three elective terminations of pregnancy.

Breast-Feeding Considerations It is not known if edoxaban is excreted in breast milk. Due to the potential for serious adverse reactions in the nursing infant, the manufacturer recommends a decision be made whether to discontinue nursing or to discontinue the drug, taking into account the importance of treatment to the mother.

Medication Guide Available Yes

Contraindications Active pathological bleeding

Warnings/Precautions May increase the risk of bleeding; serious, potentially fatal bleeding may occur. Concomitant use of drugs that affect hemostasis (eg, aspirin, other antiplatelet agents, other antithrombotic agents, fibrinolytic therapy, chronic NSAID use) increases the risk of bleeding. Monitor for signs and symptoms of bleeding. Discontinue therapy with active pathological hemorrhage and promptly evaluate for bleeding source. No specific antidote exists for edoxaban reversal; hemodialysis does not have a substantial impact on edoxaban clearance. Protamine sulfate, vitamin K, and tranexamic acid are not expected to reverse the anticoagulant effect of edoxaban.

[U.S. Boxed Warning]: Premature discontinuation of any oral anticoagulant, including edoxaban, in the absence of adequate alternative anticoagulation increases the risk of ischemic events. If edoxaban is discontinued for reasons other than pathological bleeding or completion of a course of therapy, consider the use of another anticoagulant.

Use is not recommended in patients with moderate or severe hepatic impairment (Child-Pugh class B and C) or patients with CrCl <15 mL/minute (limited clinical data). In patients with CrCl of 15 to 50 mL/minute or venous thromboembolism (DVT and/or PE) and body weight ≤60 kg, dosage reduction is necessary. Potentially significant interactions may exist, requiring dose or frequency adjustment, additional monitoring, and/or selection of alternative therapy.

[U.S. Boxed Warning]: Do not administer to nonvalvular atrial fibrillation (NVAF) patients with CrCl >95 mL/minute (calculated using the Cockcroft-Gault formula). In clinical trials, these patients had an increased rate of ischemic stroke with edoxaban 60 mg once daily compared with patients treated with warfarin; use another anticoagulant in these patients. Safety and efficacy have not been established in patients with mechanical heart valves or moderate to severe mitral stenosis; use is not recommended. Nonvalvular atrial fibrillation is defined as atrial fibrillation that occurs in the absence of rheumatic mitral valve disease, mitral valve repair, or prosthetic heart valve (AHA/ACC/HRS [January, 2014]).

[U.S. Boxed Warning]: Spinal or epidural hematomas resulting in long-term or permanent paralysis may occur with neuraxial anesthesia (epidural or spinal anesthesia) or spinal/epidural puncture; the risk is increased by the use of indwelling epidural catheters with concomitant administration of other drugs that affect hemostasis (eg, NSAIDS, platelet inhibitors, other anticoagulants), in patients with a history of traumatic or repeated epidural or spinal punctures, a history of spinal deformity or surgery, or if optimal timing between the administration of edoxaban and neuraxial procedures is not known. Consider the potential benefit versus risk prior to neuraxial intervention in patients who are anticoagulated or scheduled to be anticoagulated for thromboprophylaxis. Monitor for signs and symptoms of neurologic impairment (eg, numbness/weakness of legs, bowel/bladder dysfunction). If neurologic impairment is noted, prompt treatment is necessary. In patients who receive both edoxaban and neuraxial anesthesia, avoid removal of epidural or intrathecal catheter for at least 12 hours following last edoxaban dose; avoid edoxaban administration for at least 2 hours following catheter removal.

Discontinue edoxaban at least 24 hours prior to elective surgery or invasive procedures. If surgery cannot be delayed, the risk of bleeding should be weighed against the urgency of intervention. Reinitiate edoxaban when adequate hemostasis has been achieved unless oral therapy cannot be administered, then consider administration of a parenteral anticoagulant.

Adverse Reactions

>10%:

Hematologic and oncologic: Hemorrhage (22%)

1% to 10%:

Dermatologic: Dermal hemorrhage (6%), skin rash (4%)

Gastrointestinal: Gastrointestinal hemorrhage (4%), lower GI bleeding (3%)

Genitourinary: Vaginal hemorrhage (9%), gross hematuria (≤2%), urethral bleeding (≤2%)

Hematologic and oncologic: Major hemorrhage, non-life-threatening (7% to 9%; non-critical organ: 1%; critical organ: <1%), major hemorrhage (1%), oral hemorrhage (≤3%), anemia (2%), decreased hemoglobin (≥2 g/dL: 1%), puncture site bleeding (1%)

Hepatic: Abnormal hepatic function tests (5% to 8%)

Respiratory: Epistaxis (5%), pharyngeal bleeding (≤3%)

<1% (Limited to important or life-threatening): Hemorrhagic stroke, interstitial pulmonary disease (confounded by concomitant amiodarone therapy and infectious pneumonia), intracranial hemorrhage (includes epidural hematoma, nonhemorrhagic stroke with major hemorrhagic conversion, primary hemorrhagic stroke, subarachnoid hemorrhage, subdural hematoma)

Drug Interactions

Metabolism/Transport Effects Substrate of P-glycoprotein

Avoid Concomitant Use

Avoid concomitant use of Edoxaban with any of the following: Anticoagulants; Apixaban; Dabigatran Etexilate; Hemin; Omacetaxine; Rifampin; Rivaroxaban; Urokinase; Vorapaxar

Increased Effect/Toxicity

Edoxaban may increase the levels/effects of: Anticoagulants; Collagenase (Systemic); Deferasirox; Deoxycholic Acid; Ibritumomab; Nintedanib; Obinutuzumab; Omacetaxine; Rivaroxaban; Tositumomab and Iodine I 131 Tositumomab

The levels/effects of Edoxaban may be increased by: Agents with Antiplatelet Properties; Antiplatelet Agents (P2Y12 Inhibitors); Apixaban; Aspirin; Dabigatran Etexilate; Dasatinib; Hemin; Herbs (Anticoagulant/Antiplatelet Properties); Limaprost; Lumacaftor; Nonsteroidal Anti-Inflammatory Agents; NSAID (Nonselective); Omega-3 Fatty Acids; Pentosan Polysulfate Sodium; P-glycoprotein/ABCB1 Inhibitors; Prostacyclin Analogues; Salicylates; Sugammadex; Thrombolytic Agents; Tibolone; Tipranavir; Urokinase; Vitamin E; Vitamin E (Oral); Vorapaxar

Decreased Effect

Edoxaban may decrease the levels/effects of: Factor X (Human)

The levels/effects of Edoxaban may be decreased by: Estrogen Derivatives; Lumacaftor; P-glycoprotein/ABCB1 Inducers; Progestins; Rifampin

Storage/Stability Store at 20°C to 25°C (68°F to 77°F); excursions permitted to 15°C to 30°C (59°F to 86°F).

Mechanism of Action Edoxaban, a selective factor Xa inhibitor, inhibits free factor Xa and prothrombinase activity and inhibits thrombin-induced platelet aggregation. Inhibition of factor Xa in the coagulation cascade reduces thrombin generation and thrombus formation.

Pharmacodynamics/Kinetics

Distribution: V_{dss}: 107 L

Protein binding: ~55%

Metabolism: Minimal via hydrolysis, conjugation and oxidation by CYP3A4; predominant metabolite (M-4) is active (<10% of parent compound)

Bioavailability: 62%
Half-life elimination: 10 to 14 hours
Time to peak: 1 to 2 hours
Excretion: Urine (primarily unchanged); renal clearance: ~50% of total clearance

Dosing

Adult & Geriatric Note: Prior to initiation of edoxaban, assess creatinine clearance (CrCl) using the Cockcroft-Gault equation. For patients with nonvalvular atrial fibrillation, do **not** use edoxaban if CrCl is >95 mL/minute. Dosage reduction necessary in all patients with CrCl 15 to 50 mL/minute.

Deep vein thrombosis and pulmonary embolism: Oral: 60 mg once daily after 5 to 10 days of initial therapy with a parenteral anticoagulant.
Patient weight ≤60 kg: 30 mg once daily
Concomitant therapy with specific P-gp inhibitors (ie, verapamil, quinidine; the short-term use of azithromycin, clarithromycin, erythromycin, oral itraconazole, oral ketoconazole): 30 mg once daily

Nonvalvular atrial fibrillation (NVAF) (to prevent stroke and systemic embolism): Oral: 60 mg once daily

Conversion:

Conversion *from* continuous infusion unfractionated heparin: Discontinue heparin infusion and initiate edoxaban 4 hours later.
Conversion *from* low molecular weight heparin (LMWH): Discontinue LMWH and initiate edoxaban at the time of the next scheduled administration of LMWH.
Conversion *from* oral anticoagulants (other than warfarin and vitamin K antagonists): Discontinue current oral anticoagulant and initiate edoxaban at the time of the next scheduled dose of the other oral anticoagulant.
Conversion *from* warfarin or other vitamin K antagonists: Discontinue warfarin and initiate edoxaban as soon as INR falls to ≤2.5.
Conversion *to* a non-vitamin-K dependent oral anticoagulant: Discontinue edoxaban and initiate the other oral anticoagulant at the time the next dose of edoxaban would have been taken.
Conversion *to* a parenteral anticoagulant: Discontinue edoxaban and initiate the parenteral anticoagulant at the time the next dose of edoxaban would have been taken.
Conversion *to* warfarin:
Oral option: For patients taking edoxaban 60 mg once daily, reduce the dose to 30 mg once daily and begin warfarin concomitantly. For patients taking edoxaban 30 mg once daily, reduce the dose to 15 mg once daily and begin warfarin concomitantly. Measure INR at least weekly and just prior to the daily dose of edoxaban to minimize influence of edoxaban on INR measurements. Discontinue edoxaban once a stable INR ≥2 is achieved; continue warfarin.
Parenteral option: Discontinue edoxaban and initiate a parenteral anticoagulant and warfarin at the time of the next scheduled edoxaban dose. Discontinue the parenteral anticoagulant once a stable INR ≥2 is achieved; continue warfarin.

Renal Impairment Note: Calculate CrCl using the Cockcroft-Gault equation.

Deep vein thrombosis and pulmonary embolism:
CrCl ≥51 mL/minute: No dosage adjustment recommended.
CrCl 15 to 50 mL/minute: 30 mg once daily
CrCl <15 mL/minute: Use is not recommended.
Nonvalvular atrial fibrillation:
CrCl >95 mL/minute: Use is not recommended.
CrCl 51 to 95 mL/minute: No dosage adjustment recommended.
CrCl 15 to 50 mL/minute: 30 mg once daily
CrCl <15 mL/minute: Use is not recommended.
Hemodialysis: Total edoxaban exposure reduced by <7% during a 4-hour dialysis session.

Hepatic Impairment

Mild impairment (Child-Pugh class A): No dosage adjustment necessary.
Moderate to severe impairment (Child-Pugh class B and C): Use is not recommended.

Administration Administer without regard to food. If dose is missed, the dose should be taken as soon as possible on the same day. Dosing should resume the next day according to the normal dosing schedule. Dose should not be doubled.

Monitoring Parameters Routine monitoring of coagulation tests not required; however, edoxaban prolongs the PT and aPTT. Monitor for signs and symptoms of bleeding including neurological impairment.

Dosage Forms Excipient information presented when available (limited, particularly for generics); consult specific product labeling.
Tablet, Oral:
Savaysa: 15 mg, 30 mg, 60 mg

◆ Edoxaban Tosylate *see* Edoxaban *on page 617*

Edrophonium (ed roe FOE nee um)

Brand Names: US Enlon
Brand Names: Canada Enlon; Tensilon
Index Terms Edrophonium Chloride
Pharmacologic Category Acetylcholinesterase Inhibitor; Antidote; Diagnostic Agent
Use Diagnosis of myasthenia gravis; differentiation of cholinergic crises from myasthenia crises; reversal of nondepolarizing neuromuscular blockers
Note: Although the onset of action of neostigmine is delayed, the use of neostigmine (with glycopyrrolate) is usually preferred over edrophonium for the reversal of nondepolarizing neuromuscular blockers due to a longer duration of action (Barash 2009; Morgan 2013).

Dosing

Adult & Geriatric

Diagnosis of myasthenia gravis:
Manufacturer's labeling:
IV: 2 mg test dose administered over 15 to 30 seconds; if no cholinergic reaction occurs after 45 seconds then administer 8 mg. If cholinergic reaction occurs after initial test dose, stop testing; test dose may be repeated after 30 minutes
IM: 10 mg; if cholinergic reaction occurs, administer 2 mg 30 minutes later to rule out false-negative reaction.
Alternate dosing: **Note:** Methods vary in regards to the initial and repeat doses. However, all regimens utilize a maximum cumulative dose of 10 mg and emphasize that the incremental administration is to help avoid excessive muscarinic side effects. Atropine should be available at the bedside during the testing for the rare case in which severe bradycardia, cardiac arrhythmia, or hypotension develops. The following edrophonium dosing strategies have been described:
IV:
2 mg; if after 90 seconds there is *definite* improvement, then test is considered positive and may be terminated. If symptoms recur, then may administer another 2 mg dose. If there is *no definite* improvement with the initial dose, then may administer 3 mg and observe patient for an additional 90 seconds; if test not positive, then may administer the remaining 5 mg and observe patient for 3 to 5 more minutes (Seybold 1986).
Or
1 mg (test dose); if after 60 seconds there are no adverse effects, then administer 3 mg. If after 60 seconds there is no improvement, then administer an additional 3 mg; after an additional 60 seconds, repeat a 3 mg dose if necessary for a total dose of 10 mg (Pascuzzi 2003).

Evaluation of treatment requirements in myasthenia gravis: IV: 1 to 2 mg given 1 hour after oral dose of anticholinesterase; response will be myasthenic in undertreated patients, adequate in the controlled patient, and cholinergic in the overtreated patient; adjust as appropriate.

Differentiation of cholinergic from myasthenic crisis: IV: 1 mg; may repeat after 1 minute. Note: Intubation and controlled ventilation may be required if patient has cholinergic crisis.

Reversal of nondepolarizing neuromuscular blocking agents: Note: Atropine should be administered with edrophonium (or glycopyrrolate administered several minutes prior to edrophonium) to diminish the cholinergic effects, especially bradycardia (Barash 2009; Morgan 2013).
Manufacturer's labeling: IV: 10 mg over 30 to 45 seconds; may repeat as necessary up to a maximum cumulative dose of 40 mg
Alternate dosing: IV: Usual dose: 0.5 to 1 mg/kg (Engbaek 1985; Miller 2010; Morgan 2013)

Pediatric Diagnosis of myasthenia gravis: Note: Usually administered IV; if not possible, IM or SubQ may be used; however, the results are variable and it may take longer for reaction (Kliegman 2015). Atropine should be available at bedside during the testing for the rare case in which severe bradycardia, cardiac arrhythmia, or hypotension develops.

Test dose: Limited data available: Some experts suggest an initial test dose to assess for hypersensitivity or sensitivity to muscarinic effects: IV: 0.01 mg/kg (Kliegman 2015; Swainman 2012)

Diagnostic dose:

Manufacturer's labeling:

Infants: IV: 0.5 mg

Children and Adolescents:

≤34 kg:

IV: 1 mg; if no response after 45 seconds, it may be repeated in 1 mg increments every 30 to 45 seconds to a total of 5 mg

IM: 2 mg

>34 kg:

IV: 2 mg; if no response after 45 seconds, it may be repeated in 1 mg increments every 30 to 45 seconds to a total of 10 mg

IM: 5 mg

Alternate dosing: Weight-directed dosing: Limited data available: Children and Adolescents: IV, IM, SubQ: Initial: 0.01 to 0.02 mg/kg every 30 to 45 seconds up to the maximum dose (Kliegman 2015; Swaiman 2012). **Note:** Typical cumulative dose for a 3 to 5 year old is 5 mg/dose (Kliegman 2011)

Maximum total dose (Kliegman 2015; Swaiman 2012):

Children and Adolescents: <30 kg: 0.1 mg/kg

Children and Adolescents ≥30 kg: 0.2 mg/kg or 10 mg; whichever is less

Renal Impairment There are no dosage adjustments provided in manufacturer's labeling.

Hepatic Impairment There are no dosage adjustments provided in the manufacturer's labeling.

Additional Information Complete prescribing information should be consulted for additional detail.

Dosage Forms Excipient information presented when available (limited, particularly for generics); consult specific product labeling.

Solution, Injection, as chloride:

Enlon: 10 mg/mL (15 mL) [contains phenol]

♦ Edrophonium Chloride *see* Edrophonium *on page 618*

♦ ED-SPAZ *see* Hyoscyamine *on page 899*

♦ Ed-Spaz *see* Hyoscyamine *on page 899*

♦ EDTA (CALCIUM Disodium) (error-prone abbreviation) *see* Edetate CALCIUM Disodium *on page 616*

♦ Edurant *see* Rilpivirine *on page 1586*

♦ EES (Can) *see* Erythromycin (Systemic) *on page 670*

♦ E.E.S. 400 *see* Erythromycin (Systemic) *on page 670*

♦ E.E.S. Granules *see* Erythromycin (Systemic) *on page 670*

Efavirenz (e FAV e renz)

Brand Names: US Sustiva

Brand Names: Canada Mylan-Efavirenz; Sustiva; Teva-Efavirenz

Pharmacologic Category Antiretroviral, Reverse Transcriptase Inhibitor, Non-nucleoside (Anti-HIV)

Use HIV-1 infection: Treatment of HIV-1 infection in combination with other antiretroviral agents in adults and pediatric patients at least 3 months old and weighing at least 3.5 kg

Pregnancy Considerations Teratogenic effects have been observed in primates receiving efavirenz. Efavirenz has a moderate level of transfer across the human placenta. Based on data from the Antiretroviral Pregnancy Registry, an increased risk of overall birth defects has not been observed following first trimester exposure to efavirenz; however, neural tube and other CNS defects have been reported. Due to the low number of first trimester exposures and the low incidence of neural tube defects in the general population, available data are insufficient to evaluate risk. Other antiretroviral agents should strongly be considered for use in women of childbearing potential who are planning to become pregnant or who are sexually active and not using effective contraception. Nonpregnant women of reproductive age should undergo pregnancy testing prior to initiation of efavirenz. Barrier contraception should be used in combination with other (hormonal) methods of contraception during therapy and for 12 weeks after efavirenz is discontinued. Neural tube defects would occur following exposure during the first 5 to 6 weeks of gestation (most pregnancies are not detected before 4 to 6 weeks gestation). For women who present in the first trimester already on an efavirenz-containing regimen and who have adequate viral suppression, efavirenz may be continued; changing regimens may lead to loss of viral control and increase the risk of perinatal transmission. Pharmacokinetic data from available studies do not suggest dose alterations are needed during pregnancy. The DHHS Perinatal HIV Guidelines consider efavirenz to be a preferred NNRTI for use in antiretroviral-naive pregnant women after 8 weeks gestation. Hypersensitivity reactions (including hepatic toxicity and rash) are more common in women on NNRTI therapy; it is not known if pregnancy increases this risk.

Regardless of CD4 count or HIV RNA copy number, all HIV-infected pregnant women should receive a combination antiretroviral (ARV) drug regimen. A combination of antepartum, intrapartum, and infant ARV prophylaxis is recommended. ARV therapy should be started as soon as possible in women with symptomatic infection. Although earlier initiation may be more effective in reducing the perinatal transmission of HIV, initiation may be delayed until after 12 weeks gestation in women who do no require immediate treatment after careful consideration of maternal conditions (eg, nausea and vomiting) and the potential risks of first trimester fetal exposure for specific agents. A scheduled cesarean delivery at 38 weeks gestation is recommended for all women with HIV RNA >1000 copies/mL or unknown concentration near delivery in order to decrease transmission. If ARV therapy must be interrupted for <24 hours during the peripartum period, stop then restart all medications simultaneously in order to decrease the chance of developing resistance. Long-term follow-up is recommended for all infants exposed to ARV medications. In couples who want to conceive, the HIV-infected partner should attain maximum viral suppression prior to conception.

Health care providers are encouraged to enroll pregnant women exposed to antiretroviral medications in the Antiretroviral Pregnancy Registry (1-800-258-4263 or www.APRegistry.com). Health care providers caring for HIV-infected women and their infants may contact the National Perinatal HIV Hotline (888-448-8765) for clinical consultation (HHS [perinatal], 2014).

Breast-Feeding Considerations Efavirenz is excreted into breast milk. Although breast-feeding is not recommended, plasma concentrations of efavirenz in nursing infants have been reported as ~13% of maternal plasma concentrations.

Maternal or infant antiretroviral therapy does not completely eliminate the risk of postnatal HIV transmission. In addition, multiclass-resistant virus has been detected in breast-feeding infants despite maternal therapy. Therefore, in the United States, where formula is accessible, affordable, safe, and sustainable, and the risk of infant mortality due to diarrhea and respiratory infections is low, complete avoidance of breast-feeding by HIV-infected women is recommended to decrease potential transmission of HIV (HHS [perinatal], 2014).

Prescribing and Access Restrictions Efavirenz oral solution is available only through an expanded access (compassionate use) program. Enrollment information may be obtained by calling 877-372-7097.

Contraindications Hypersensitivity (eg, Stevens-Johnson syndrome, erythema multiforme, toxic skin eruptions) to efavirenz or any component of the formulation

Warnings/Precautions Do not use as single-agent therapy. Avoid pregnancy; women of childbearing potential should undergo pregnancy testing prior to initiation of therapy. Use caution with other agents metabolized by cytochrome P450 isoenzyme 3A4 (see Contraindications); concomitant use of other efavirenz-containing products should be avoided (unless needed for dosage adjustment with concomitant rifampin treatment). Use caution with history of mental illness/drug abuse (predisposition to psychological reactions); may cause CNS and psychiatric symptoms, which include impaired concentration, dizziness or drowsiness (avoid potentially hazardous tasks such as driving or operating machinery if these effects are noted); CNS effects may be potentiated when used with other psychoactive drugs or ethanol. Serious psychiatric side effects have been associated with efavirenz, including severe depression, suicidal ideation, nonfatal suicide attempts, paranoia, and mania; instruct patients to contact healthcare provider if serious psychiatric effects occur. May cause mild-to-moderate maculopapular rash; usually occurs within 2 weeks of starting therapy; discontinue if severe rash (involving blistering, desquamation, mucosal involvement, or fever) develops; contraindicated in patients with a history of a severe cutaneous reaction (eg, Stevens-Johnson syndrome). Children are more susceptible.

Caution in patients with known or suspected hepatitis B or C infection or Child-Pugh class A hepatic impairment; not recommended in Child-Pugh class B or C hepatic impairment. Persistent elevations of serum transaminases >5 times the upper limit of normal should prompt evaluation - benefit of continued therapy should be weighed against

possible risk of hepatotoxicity. Hepatic failure has been reported, including patients with no preexisting hepatic disease or other identifiable risk factors. Monitor liver function tests in patients with underlying hepatic disease (eg, hepatitis B or C, marked transaminase elevations or taking concomitant medications that may cause hepatotoxicity). Ethanol may increase hepatotoxic potential; instruct patients to limit or avoid alcohol. Increases in total cholesterol and triglycerides have been reported; screening should be done prior to therapy and periodically throughout treatment. May cause redistribution of fat (eg, buffalo hump, peripheral wasting with increased abdominal girth, cushingoid appearance). Patients may develop immune reconstitution syndrome resulting in the occurrence of an inflammatory response to an indolent or residual opportunistic infection during initial HIV treatment or activation of autoimmune disorders (eg, Graves' disease, polymyositis, Guillain-Barré syndrome) later in therapy; further evaluation and treatment may be required. Use with caution in patients with a history of seizure disorder; seizures have been associated with use. Avoid efavirenz-based regimens if possible in patients with HIV-associated dementia; neuropsychiatric side effects of efavirenz may hinder assessment of the effects of antiretrovirals on the improvement of symptoms associated with HIV-associated dementia (HHS [adult] 2015). Efavirenz administered as monotherapy or added on to a failing regimen may result in rapid viral resistance to efavirenz. Consider cross-resistance when adding antiretroviral agents on to efavirenz therapy. Do not use efavirenz plus abacavir and lamivudine (or emtricitabine) in adolescent and adult HIV-1 patients with a pre-ART HIV RNA >100,000 copies/mL (HHS [adult] 2015).

Adverse Reactions Unless otherwise noted, frequency of adverse events is as reported in adults receiving combination antiretroviral therapy.

>10%:
Central nervous system: Dizziness (2% to 28%; children 16%), fever (children 21%), depression (≤19%; severe: 1% to 2%), insomnia (≤16%), anxiety (2% to 13%), pain (1% to 13%; children 14%), headache (2% to 8%; children 11%)

Dermatologic: Rash (5% to 26%, grade 3/4: <1%; children ≤46%, grade 3/4: 2% to 4%)

Endocrine & metabolic: HDL increased (25% to 35%), total cholesterol increased (20% to 40%), triglycerides increased (≥751 mg/dL: 6% to 11%)

Gastrointestinal: Diarrhea (3% to 14%; children: ≤39%), nausea (2% to 10%; children 12%), vomiting (3% to 6%; children 12%)

Respiratory: Cough (children 16%)

1% to 10%:
Central nervous system: Impaired concentration (≤8%), somnolence (≤7%), fatigue (≤8%), abnormal dreams (1% to 6%), nervousness (2% to 7%), hallucinations (1%)

Dermatologic: Pruritus (≤9%)

Endocrine & metabolic: Hyperglycemia (>250 mg/dL: 2% to 5%)

Gastrointestinal: Dyspepsia (≤4%), abdominal pain (2% to 3%), anorexia (≤2%), amylase increased (grade 3/4: ≤6%)

Hematologic: Neutropenia (grade 3/4: 2% to 10%)

Hepatic: Incidence higher with hepatitis B and/or C coinfection: ALT increased (grades 3/4: 2% to 8%), AST increased (grades 3/4: 5% to 8%)

<1% (Limited to important or life-threatening): Allergic reaction, ataxia, body fat accumulation/redistribution, cerebellar coordination disturbances, delusions, dermatitis (photoallergic), erythema multiforme, gynecomastia, hepatic failure, hepatitis, immune reconstitution syndrome, malabsorption, mania, neuropathy, neurosis, palpitations, pancreatitis, paranoia, psychosis, seizures, Stevens-Johnson syndrome, suicide attempts, suicidal ideation, visual abnormalities

Drug Interactions

Metabolism/Transport Effects Substrate of CYP2B6 (major), CYP3A4 (major); **Note:** Assignment of Major/Minor substrate status based on clinically relevant drug interaction potential; **Inhibits** CYP2C19 (moderate), CYP2C8 (moderate), CYP2C9 (moderate); **Induces** CYP2B6 (weak/moderate), CYP3A4 (moderate), UGT1A1

Avoid Concomitant Use
Avoid concomitant use of Efavirenz with any of the following: Amodiaquine; Antihepaciviral Combination Products; Axitinib; Azelastine (Nasal); Bedaquiline; Boceprevir; Bosutinib; CarBAMazepine; Cobimetinib; Elvitegravir; Etravirine; Flibanserin; Itraconazole; Ketoconazole (Systemic); Nevirapine; Nisoldipine; Olaparib; Orphenadrine; Palbociclib; Paraldehyde; Posaconazole; Ranolazine; Reverse Transcriptase Inhibitors

(Non-Nucleoside); Rilpivirine; Simeprevir; Sonidegib; St Johns Wort; Thalidomide; Ulipristal

Increased Effect/Toxicity
Efavirenz may increase the levels/effects of: Alcohol (Ethyl); Amodiaquine; Azelastine (Nasal); Bosentan; Cannabis; Carvedilol; Cilostazol; Citalopram; CNS Depressants; CYP2C19 Substrates; CYP2C8 Substrates; CYP2C9 Substrates; Dronabinol; Etravirine; Fosphenytoin; Hydrocodone; Ifosfamide; Methotrimeprazine; Metyrosine; Mirtazapine; Nevirapine; Orphenadrine; Paraldehyde; Phenytoin; Pramipexole; Proguanil; Rilpivirine; Ritonavir; ROPINIRole; Rotigotine; Selective Serotonin Reuptake Inhibitors; Suvorexant; Tetrahydrocannabinol; Thalidomide; Vitamin K Antagonists; Zolpidem

The levels/effects of Efavirenz may be increased by: Boceprevir; Brimonidine (Topical); Cannabis; CYP2B6 Inhibitors (Moderate); Darunavir; Doxylamine; Dronabinol; Droperidol; HydrOXYzine; Kava Kava; Magnesium Sulfate; Methotrimeprazine; Mifepristone; Minocycline; Nabilone; Nevirapine; Osimertinib; Perampanel; Quazepam; Reverse Transcriptase Inhibitors (Non-Nucleoside); Ritonavir; Rufinamide; Saquinavir; Sodium Oxybate; Tapentadol; Tetrahydrocannabinol; Voriconazole

Decreased Effect
Efavirenz may decrease the levels/effects of: Alcohol (Ethyl); Antihepaciviral Combination Products; ARIPiprazole; Artemether; Atazanavir; AtorvaSTATin; Atovaquone; Axitinib; Bedaquiline; Boceprevir; Bosutinib; Buprenorphine; BuPROPion; Calcium Channel Blockers; Canagliflozin; CarBAMazepine; Caspofungin; Clarithromycin; Clopidogrel; Cobimetinib; Contraceptives (Progestins); CycloSPORINE (Systemic); CYP3A4 Substrates; Daclatasvir; Darunavir; Diltiazem; Dolutegravir; Elvitegravir; Etonogestrel; Etravirine; Everolimus; FentaNYL; Flibanserin; Fosamprenavir; Ibrutinib; Ifosfamide; Indinavir; Itraconazole; Ketoconazole (Systemic); Lopinavir; Lovastatin; Maraviroc; Methadone; NiMODipine; Nisoldipine; Norgestimate; Olaparib; Palbociclib; Posaconazole; Pravastatin; Proguanil; Ranolazine; Rifabutin; Rilpivirine; Rolapitant; Saquinavir; Saxagliptin; Sertraline; Simeprevir; Simvastatin; Sirolimus; Sonidegib; Tacrolimus (Systemic); Telaprevir; Ulipristal; Vitamin K Antagonists; Voriconazole

The levels/effects of Efavirenz may be decreased by: Bosentan; CarBAMazepine; CYP2B6 Inducers (Strong); CYP3A4 Inducers (Moderate); CYP3A4 Inducers (Strong); Dabrafenib; Deferasirox; Enzalutamide; Fosphenytoin; Ginkgo Biloba; Mitotane; Nevirapine; Osimertinib; Phenytoin; Reverse Transcriptase Inhibitors (Non-Nucleoside); Rifabutin; Rifampin; Siltuximab; St Johns Wort; Telaprevir; Tocilizumab

Food Interactions High-fat/high-caloric meals increase the absorption of efavirenz. CNS effects are possible. Management: Avoid high-fat/high-caloric meals. Administer at or before bedtime on an empty stomach unless using capsule sprinkle method in patients unable to swallow capsules or tablets. If capsule sprinkle method is used, patient should not consume additional food for 2 hours after administration.

Storage/Stability Store at 25°C (77°F); excursion permitted to 15°C to 30°C (59°F to 86°F).

Mechanism of Action As a non-nucleoside reverse transcriptase inhibitor, efavirenz has activity against HIV-1 by binding to reverse transcriptase. It consequently blocks the RNA-dependent and DNA-dependent DNA polymerase activities including HIV-1 replication. It does not require intracellular phosphorylation for antiviral activity.

Pharmacodynamics/Kinetics
Absorption: Increased by high-fat/high-caloric meals

Distribution: CSF concentrations are 0.69% of plasma (range: 0.26% to 1.2%); however, CSF:plasma concentration ratio is 3 times higher than free fraction in plasma

Protein binding: >99%, primarily to albumin

Metabolism: Hepatic via CYP3A and 2B6 to inactive hydroxylated metabolites which then undergo glucuronidation; induces P450 enzymes and its own metabolism

Bioavailability: 42%

Half-life elimination: Single dose: 52 to 76 hours; Multiple doses: 40 to 55 hours

Time to peak: 3 to 5 hours

Excretion: Feces (16% to 61% primarily as unchanged drug); urine (14% to 34% as metabolites; <1% unchanged drug)

Dosing

Adult & Geriatric

HIV infection: Oral: 600 mg once daily.

Dosage adjustment for concomitant rifampin (only if patient weighs ≥50 kg): Increase efavirenz dose to 800 mg once daily.

Dosage adjustment for concomitant voriconazole: Reduce efavirenz dose to 300 mg once daily and increase voriconazole to 400 mg every 12 hours.

Pediatric Dosage is based on body weight.

HIV infection (as part of combination therapy): Children ≥3 months and ≥3.5 kg: Oral:

3.5 kg to <5 kg: 100 mg once daily
5 kg to <7.5 kg: 150 mg once daily
7.5 kg to <15 kg: 200 mg once daily
15 kg to <20 kg: 250 mg once daily
20 kg to <25 kg: 300 mg once daily
25 kg to <32.5 kg: 350 mg once daily
32.5 kg to <40 kg: 400 mg once daily
≥40 kg: 600 mg once daily; **Note:** Dosage adjustments may be necessary if patient receives certain concomitant medications. Refer to adult dosing.

Renal Impairment There are no dosage adjustment provided in manufacturer's labeling (has not been studied); however, undergoes minimal renal excretion.

Hepatic Impairment

Mild impairment (Child-Pugh class A): No dosage adjustment necessary; use with caution.

Moderate-to-severe impairment (Child-Pugh class B or C): No dosage adjustment provided in manufacturer's labeling (has not been adequately studied); use not recommended.

Dietary Considerations Should be taken on an empty stomach unless using capsule sprinkle method in patients unable to swallow capsules or tablets. If capsule sprinkle method is used, do not consume additional food for 2 hours after administration.

Administration Oral: Administer on an empty stomach. Dosing at or before bedtime is recommended to limit central nervous system effects (HHS, [adult] 2014). Tablets must not be broken.

Capsule contents may be sprinkled onto a small amount of soft food (eg, applesauce, grape jelly, yogurt) for pediatric or adult patients who cannot swallow capsules. Place 1-2 teaspoonfuls of food in a small container. Hold capsule horizontally over container and carefully twist in opposite directions to open, sprinkling contents over food. If more than 1 capsule is needed for a dose, add contents of all capsules needed to 1-2 teaspoonfuls of food; do not add more food. Use a small spoon to gently mix capsule contents with food and administer all of mixture to patient. To ensure entire capsule contents are administered, add another 2 teaspoonfuls of food to the container, mix to incorporate any drug residue, and administer.

Capsule contents may also be mixed with infant formula only for pediatric patients who cannot reliably consume solid foods. Combine entire contents of capsule(s) with 10 mL of reconstituted, room temperature infant formula in a 30 mL small container, stir carefully, then draw up mixture in a 10 mL oral syringe for administration. If more than 1 capsule is needed for a dose, add contents of all capsules needed to 10 mL of formula; do not add more formula. To ensure entire capsule contents are administered, add another 10 mL of formula to the cup, stir to incorporate any drug residue, draw up in oral syringe and administer.

Administer within 30 minutes of mixing. Patient should not consume any additional food or administer additional formula for 2 hours after administration.

Monitoring Parameters Serum transaminases (discontinuation of treatment should be considered for persistent elevations >5 times the upper limit of normal); cholesterol and triglycerides (prior to therapy and periodically during); signs and symptoms of infection; psychiatric effects

Test Interactions False-positive tests for cannabinoids have been reported when the CEDIA DAU Multilevel THC assay is used. False-positive results with other assays for cannabinoids have not been observed. False-positive tests for benzodiazepines have been reported and are likely due to the 8-hydroxy-efavirenz major metabolite.

Additional Information Early virologic failure was observed with tenofovir and didanosine delayed release capsules, plus either efavirenz or nevirapine; use caution in treatment-naive patients with high baseline viral loads.

Dosage Forms Excipient information presented when available (limited, particularly for generics); consult specific product labeling.

Capsule, Oral:
Sustiva: 50 mg, 200 mg
Tablet, Oral:
Sustiva: 600 mg

Efavirenz, Emtricitabine, and Tenofovir Disoproxil Fumarate
(e FAV e renz, em trye SYE ta been, & ten OF oh vir dye soe PROX il FUE ma rate)

Brand Names: US Atripla
Brand Names: Canada Atripla
Index Terms Emtricitabine, Efavirenz, and Tenofovir Disoproxil Fumarate; FTC, TDF, and EFV; Tenofovir Disoproxil Fumarate, Efavirenz, and Emtricitabine
Pharmacologic Category Antiretroviral, Reverse Transcriptase Inhibitor, Non-nucleoside (Anti-HIV); Antiretroviral, Reverse Transcriptase Inhibitor, Nucleoside (Anti-HIV); Antiretroviral, Reverse Transcriptase Inhibitor, Nucleotide (Anti-HIV)
Use Treatment of HIV-1 infection
Dosing

Adult & Geriatric Note: Prior to initiation, patients should be tested for hepatitis B infection, and baseline estimated creatinine clearance, serum phosphorus, urine glucose, and urine protein should be assessed in all patients.

HIV infection: Oral: One tablet once daily.

Pediatric Note: Prior to initiation, patients should be tested for hepatitis B infection, and baseline estimated creatinine clearance, serum phosphorus, urine glucose, and urine protein should be assessed in all patients.

HIV infection:
US labeling: Children ≥12 years and ≥40 kg and Adolescents: Oral: Refer to adult dosing.
Canadian labeling: Use is not approved in pediatric patients.

Renal Impairment Moderate-to-severe renal impairment (CrCl <50 mL/minute): Use not recommended.

Hepatic Impairment

Mild hepatic impairment (Child-Pugh class A): Use with caution.

Moderate or severe hepatic impairment (Child-Pugh class B, C): Not recommended.

Additional Information Complete prescribing information should be consulted for additional detail.

Dosage Forms Excipient information presented when available (limited, particularly for generics); consult specific product labeling.

Tablet, oral:
Atripla: Efavirenz 600 mg, emtricitabine 200 mg, and tenofovir disoproxil fumarate 300 mg

◆ **Effer-K** see Potassium Bicarbonate and Potassium Citrate on page 1479

◆ **Effexor XR** see Venlafaxine on page 1886

◆ **Effient** see Prasugrel on page 1490

Efinaconazole (ef in a KON a zole)

Brand Names: US Jublia
Brand Names: Canada Jublia
Pharmacologic Category Antifungal Agent, Topical
Use Onychomycosis: Topical treatment of onychomycosis of the toenail(s) due to *Trichophyton rubrum* and *Trichophyton mentagrophytes*
Dosing

Adult & Geriatric Onychomycosis: Topical: Apply to affected toenail(s) once daily for 48 weeks.

Renal Impairment There are no dosage adjustments provided in the manufacturer's labeling.

Hepatic Impairment There are no dosage adjustments provided in the manufacturer's labeling.

Additional Information Complete prescribing information should be consulted for additional detail.

Dosage Forms Excipient information presented when available (limited, particularly for generics); consult specific product labeling.

Solution, External:
Jublia: 10% (4 mL, 8 mL) [contains edetate disodium]

Eflornithine (ee FLOR ni theen)

Brand Names: US Vaniqa
Brand Names: Canada Vaniqa®
Index Terms DFMO; Eflornithine Hydrochloride
Pharmacologic Category Antiprotozoal; Topical Skin Product
Use Reduce unwanted hair from face and adjacent areas under the chin

Prescribing and Access Restrictions Injectable eflornithine is donated to World Health Organization (WHO) by the manufacturer. Further information may be found on WHO website at http://www.who.int/trypanosomiasis_african/diagnosis/en/index.html or by contacting the CDC Drug Service (404-639-3670).

Dosing

Adult & Geriatric

Unwanted facial hair (females): Topical: Apply thin layer of cream to affected areas of face and areas under the chin twice daily, at least 8 hours apart.

Treatment of infections caused by *Trypanosoma brucei gambiense* **infection (sleeping sickness; off-label use):** IV infusion: 100 mg/kg/dose given every 6 hours for 14 days (Kappagoda, 2011)

Pediatric Unwanted facial hair (females): Children ≥12 years: Refer to adult dosing.

Renal Impairment Injection: Dose should be adjusted although no specific guidelines are available.

Additional Information Complete prescribing information should be consulted for additional detail.

Dosage Forms Excipient information presented when available (limited, particularly for generics); consult specific product labeling. [DSC] = Discontinued product

Cream, External, as hydrochloride:

Vaniqa: 13.9% (30 g [DSC], 45 g) [contains cetearyl alcohol, methylparaben, propylparaben]

♦ Eflornithine Hydrochloride see Eflornithine on page 621

♦ Eformoterol see Formoterol on page 809

♦ Eformoterol and Budesonide see Budesonide and Formoterol on page 260

♦ Eformoterol and Mometasone see Mometasone and Formoterol on page 1228

♦ Efraloctocog Alfa see Antihemophilic Factor (Recombinant) on page 132

♦ Efudex see Fluorouracil (Topical) on page 786

♦ Egrifta see Tesamorelin on page 1766

♦ EHDP see Etidronate on page 713

♦ Eicosapentaenoic Acid see Omega-3 Fatty Acids on page 1329

♦ EL-970 see Dalfampridine on page 483

♦ Elaprase see Idursulfase on page 913

♦ Elavil see Amitriptyline on page 98

♦ Eldepryl see Selegiline on page 1644

♦ Eldopaque [OTC] [DSC] see Hydroquinone on page 893

♦ Eldopaque® (Can) see Hydroquinone on page 893

♦ Eldopaque Forte [DSC] see Hydroquinone on page 893

♦ Eldoquin [OTC] [DSC] see Hydroquinone on page 893

♦ Eldoquin® (Can) see Hydroquinone on page 893

♦ Eldoquin Forte [DSC] see Hydroquinone on page 893

♦ Electrolyte Lavage Solution see Polyethylene Glycol-Electrolyte Solution on page 1466

Electrolyte Solution, Renal Replacement

(ee LEK trow lite soe LOO shun REE nil ree PLASE ment)

Brand Names: US Normocarb HF 25; Normocarb HF 35; Phoxillum; PrismaSol

Index Terms Continuous Renal Replacement Therapy; CRRT; Renal Replacement Solution

Pharmacologic Category Alkalinizing Agent; Electrolyte Supplement

Use Continuous renal replacement circuit: Used as a replacement solution in continuous renal replacement therapy (CRRT) to replace water and to correct electrolyte and acid-base imbalances; in drug poisoning when CRRT is used to remove dialyzable substances (Phoxillum and PrismaSol only)

Dosing

Adult Note: If using Phoxillum or PrismaSol, ensure that compartment A and B are mixed completely.

Continuous renal replacement circuit: Pre- or post-hemofilter or hemodiafilter: Volume of solution administered depends upon the patient's clinical condition and fluid, electrolyte, acid-base, and glucose balance.

Post-filter replacement: Normocarb HF: Volume infused/hour should not be greater than 1/3 of blood flow rate (eg, blood flow rate 100 mL/minute [6,000 mL/hour], post-filter replacement rate ≤2,000 mL/hour)

Pediatric Infants, Children, and Adolescents: Refer to adult dosing.

Renal Impairment No dosage adjustment necessary.

Hepatic Impairment There are no dosage adjustments provided in the manufacturer's labeling.

Additional Information Complete prescribing information should be consulted for additional detail.

Dosage Forms Excipient information presented when available (limited, particularly for generics); consult specific product labeling.

Injection, solution [concentrate; preservative free]:

Normocarb HF® 25: Bicarbonate 25 mEq/L, chloride 116.5 mEq/L, magnesium 1.5 mEq/L, sodium 140 mEq/L (240 mL) [strength represents final solution after mixing; when diluted as directed, makes 3240 mL of infusate]

Normocarb HF® 35: Bicarbonate 35 mEq/L, chloride 106.5 mEq/L, magnesium 1.5 mEq/L, sodium 140 mEq/L (240 mL) [strength represents final solution after mixing; when diluted as directed, makes 3240 mL of infusate]

Injection, solution [preservative free]:

PrismaSol B22GK 2/0: Bicarbonate 22 mEq/L, chloride 118.5 mEq/L, dextrose 100 mg/dL, lactate 3 mEq/L, magnesium 1.5 mEq/L, potassium 2 mEq/L, sodium 140 mEq/L (5000 mL) [strength represents final solution after mixing]

PrismaSol B22GK 4/0: Bicarbonate 22 mEq/L, chloride 120.5 mEq/L, dextrose 100 mg/dL, lactate 3 mEq/L, magnesium 1.5 mEq/L, potassium 4 mEq/L, sodium 140 mEq/L (5000 mL) [strength represents final solution after mixing]

PrismaSol BGK 0/2.5: Bicarbonate 32 mEq/L, calcium 2.5 mEq/L, chloride 109 mEq/L, dextrose 100 mg/dL, lactate 3 mEq/L, magnesium 1.5 mEq/L, sodium 140 mEq/L (5000 mL) [strength represents final solution after mixing]

PrismaSol BGK 2/0: Bicarbonate 32 mEq/L, chloride 108 mEq/L, dextrose 100 mg/dL, lactate 3 mEq/L, magnesium 1 mEq/L, potassium 2 mEq/L, sodium 140 mEq/L (5000 mL) [strength represents final solution after mixing]

PrismaSol BGK 2/3.5: Bicarbonate 32 mEq/L, calcium 3.5 mEq/L, chloride 111.5 mEq/L, dextrose 100 mg/dL, lactate 3 mEq/L, magnesium 1 mEq/L, potassium 2 mEq/L, sodium 140 mEq/L (5000 mL) [strength represents final solution after mixing]

PrismaSol BGK 4/0/1.2: Bicarbonate 32 mEq/L, chloride 110.2 mEq/L, dextrose 100 mg/dL, lactate 3 mEq/L, magnesium 1.2 mEq/L, potassium 4 mEq/L, sodium 140 mEq/L (5000 mL) [strength represents final solution after mixing]

PrismaSol BGK 4/2.5: Bicarbonate 32 mEq/L, calcium 2.5 mEq/L, chloride 113 mEq/L, dextrose 100 mg/dL, lactate 3 mEq/L, magnesium 1.5 mEq/L, potassium 4 mEq/L, sodium 140 mEq/L (5000 mL) [strength represents final solution after mixing]

PrismaSol BK 0/0/1.2: Bicarbonate 32 mEq/L, chloride 106.2 mEq/L, lactate 3 mEq/L, magnesium 1.2 mEq/L, sodium 140 mEq/L (5000 mL) [strength represents final solution after mixing]

♦ Elelyso see Taliglucerase Alfa on page 1733

♦ Elepsia XR see LevETIRAcetam on page 1056

♦ Elestrin see Estradiol (Systemic) on page 681

Eletriptan (el e TRIP tan)

Brand Names: US Relpax

Brand Names: Canada Relpax®

Index Terms Eletriptan Hydrobromide

Pharmacologic Category Antimigraine Agent; Serotonin 5-HT$_{1B, 1D}$ Receptor Agonist

Use Migraines: Acute treatment of migraine, with or without aura in adults

Pregnancy Considerations Adverse events were observed in animal reproduction studies. Information related to eletriptan use in pregnancy is limited (Källén, 2011; Nezvalová-Henriksen, 2010; Nezvalová-Henriksen, 2012). Until additional information is available, other agents are preferred for the initial treatment of migraine in pregnancy (Da Silva, 2012; MacGregor, 2012; Williams, 2012).

Breast-Feeding Considerations Eletriptan is excreted in breast milk. Eight women were given a single dose of eletriptan 80 mg. The amount of drug detected in breast milk over 24 hours was ~0.02% of the maternal dose and the milk-to-plasma ratio was variable. The presence of the active metabolite was not measured. The manufacturer recommends that caution be exercised when administering eletriptan to nursing women.

Contraindications

Ischemic coronary artery disease (eg, angina pectoris, history of myocardial infarction, documented silent ischemia); coronary artery vasospasm, including Prinzmetal's angina; Wolff-Parkinson-White syndrome or arrhythmias

associated with other cardiac accessory conduction pathway disorders; history of stroke, transient ischemic attack, or history or current evidence of hemiplegic or basilar migraine; peripheral vascular disease; ischemic bowel disease; uncontrolled hypertension; recent use (within 24 hours) of treatment with another 5-HT$_1$ agonist, or an ergotamine-containing or ergot-type medication (eg, dihydroergotamine or methysergide); recent use (within at least 72 hours) of the following potent CYP3A4 inhibitors: ketoconazole, itraconazole, nefazodone, troleandomycin, clarithromycin, ritonavir, or nelfinavir; known hypersensitivity to eletriptan or any component of the formulation.

Canadian labeling: Additional contraindications (not in U.S. labeling): Cardiac arrhythmias (especially tachycardias), valvular heart disease, congenital heart disease, atherosclerotic disease; ophthalmoplegic migraine; Raynaud's syndrome; severe hepatic impairment.

Documentation of allergenic cross-reactivity for serotonin 5-HT$_1$ receptor agonists (triptans) in this class is limited. However, because of similarities in chemical structure and/or pharmacologic actions, the possibility of cross-sensitivity cannot be ruled out with certainty.

Warnings/Precautions Only indicated for treatment of acute migraine; not indicated for migraine prophylaxis, or for the treatment of cluster headache, hemiplegic or basilar migraine. If a patient does not respond to the first dose, the diagnosis of migraine should be reconsidered. Acute migraine agents (eg, triptans, opioids, ergotamine, or a combination of the agents) used for 10 or more days per month may lead to worsening of headaches (medication overuse headache); withdrawal treatment may be necessary in the setting of overuse. Do not give to patients with risk factors for CAD until a cardiovascular evaluation has been performed; if evaluation is satisfactory, the health care provider should administer the first dose (consider ECG monitoring) and cardiovascular status should be periodically evaluated. Cardiac events (coronary artery vasospasm, transient ischemia, MI, ventricular tachycardia/fibrillation, cardiac arrest, and death), cerebral/subarachnoid hemorrhage, stroke (some fatal), peripheral vascular ischemia, gastrointestinal vascular ischemia/infarction, and Raynaud's syndrome have been reported with 5-HT$_1$ agonist administration. Patients who experience sensations of chest pain/pressure/tightness or symptoms suggestive of angina following dosing should be evaluated for coronary artery disease or Prinzmetal's angina before receiving additional doses; if dosing is resumed and similar symptoms recur, monitor with ECG. Significant elevation in blood pressure, including hypertensive crisis with acute impairment of organ systems, has been reported on rare occasions in patients with and without a history of hypertension; monitor blood pressure.

Not recommended for use in patients with severe hepatic impairment; the Canadian labeling contraindicates use in patients with severe impairment. Symptoms of agitation, confusion, hallucinations, hyper-reflexia, myoclonus, shivering, and tachycardia (serotonin syndrome) may occur with concomitant proserotonergic drugs (ie, SSRIs/SNRIs or triptans) or agents which reduce eletriptan's metabolism. Concurrent use of serotonin precursors (eg, tryptophan) is not recommended. If concomitant administration with SSRIs is warranted, monitor closely, especially at initiation and with dose increases. Discontinue eletriptan if serotonin syndrome is suspected. Potentially significant drug-drug interactions may exist, requiring dose or frequency adjustment, additional monitoring, and/or selection of alternative therapy. Use is contraindicated within 72 hours of patients taking strong CYP3A4 inhibitors. Anaphylaxis, anaphylactoid, and hypersensitivity reactions (including angioedema) have occurred; may be life-threatening or fatal.

Adverse Reactions

1% to 10%:

Cardiovascular: Chest pain (2% to 4%; chest tightness, pain, and pressure), palpitations

Central nervous system: Dizziness (6% to 7%), drowsiness (6% to 7%), headache (4%), paresthesia (3% to 4%), chills, hypertonia, hypoesthesia, pain, vertigo

Dermatologic: Diaphoresis

Gastrointestinal: Nausea (8%), xerostomia (3% to 4%), abdominal pain (2%; pain, discomfort, stomach pain, cramps, and pressure), dyspepsia (2%), dysphagia (1% to 2%)

Neuromuscular & skeletal: Weakness (4% to 10%), back pain

Respiratory: Pharyngitis

<1% (Limited to important or life-threatening): Abnormal hepatic function tests, anaphylactoid reaction, anaphylaxis, angina pectoris, angioedema, cardiac arrhythmia, confusion, depersonalization, depression, edema, emotional lability, hyperesthesia, hyperkinesia, hypersensitivity reaction, hypertension, impotence, increased creatine phosphokinase, insomnia, ischemic colitis, lacrimation, myalgia, myasthenia, myocardial infarction, peripheral vascular disorder, photophobia, polyuria, Prinzmetal angina, seizure, skin rash, speech disturbance, stupor, tachycardia, thrombophlebitis, vasospasm, ventricular fibrillation, visual disturbance

Drug Interactions

Metabolism/Transport Effects **Substrate** of CYP3A4 (major); **Note:** Assignment of Major/Minor substrate status based on clinically relevant drug interaction potential

Avoid Concomitant Use

Avoid concomitant use of Eletriptan with any of the following: Conivaptan; CYP3A4 Inhibitors (Strong); Dapoxetine; Ergot Derivatives; Fusidic Acid (Systemic); Idelalisib

Increased Effect/Toxicity

Eletriptan may increase the levels/effects of: Antipsychotic Agents; Droxidopa; Ergot Derivatives; Metoclopramide; Serotonin Modulators

The levels/effects of Eletriptan may be increased by: Antiemetics (5HT3 Antagonists); Antipsychotic Agents; Conivaptan; CYP3A4 Inhibitors (Moderate); CYP3A4 Inhibitors (Strong); Dapoxetine; Dasatinib; Ergot Derivatives; Fosaprepitant; Fusidic Acid (Systemic); Idelalisib; Ivacaftor; Luliconazole; Metaxalone; Mifepristone; Osimertinib; Palbociclib; Simeprevir; Stiripentol; Tedizolid

Decreased Effect

The levels/effects of Eletriptan may be decreased by: Osimertinib

Food Interactions A high-fat meal increases bioavailability. Management: Administer without regard to meals.

Storage/Stability Store at 20°C to 25°C (68°F to 77°F); excursions are permitted between 15°C and 30°C (59°F and 86°F).

Mechanism of Action Selective agonist for serotonin (5-HT$_{1B}$, 5-HT$_{1D}$, and 5-HT$_{1F}$ receptors) in cranial arteries; causes vasoconstriction and reduces sterile inflammation associated with antidromic neuronal transmission correlating with relief of migraine

Pharmacodynamics/Kinetics

Absorption: Well absorbed

Distribution: V$_d$: 138 L

Protein binding: ~85%

Metabolism: Hepatic via CYP3A4; forms one metabolite (active)

Bioavailability: ~50%, increased with high-fat meal

Half-life elimination: ~4 hours (Elderly: 4.4-5.7 hours); Metabolite: ~13 hours

Time to peak, plasma: 1.5-2 hours

Dosing

Adult & Geriatric Note: If the first dose is ineffective, diagnosis needs to be re-evaluated. Safety of treating >3 headaches/month has not been established.

Acute migraine: Oral:

U.S. labeling: Initial: 20-40 mg as a single dose (maximum: 40 mg/dose); if the headache improves but returns, dose may be repeated after 2 hours have elapsed since first dose (maximum: 80 mg daily)

Canadian labeling: Initial: 20-40 mg as a single dose (maximum: 40 mg/dose). If after an initial dose of 20 mg, the headache improves but returns a repeat 20 mg dose may be administered after 2 hours have elapsed since first dose. If an initial dose of 40 mg was administered, a repeat dose is not recommended (maximum: 40 mg daily).

Renal Impairment No dosage adjustment provided in manufacturer's labeling; however, adjustment likely not needed based on pharmacokinetic analysis; monitor for increased blood pressure.

Hepatic Impairment

Mild-to-moderate impairment: No dosage adjustment necessary.

Severe impairment:

U.S. labeling: Use is not recommended.

Canadian labeling: Use is contraindicated.

Administration Administer orally as soon as symptoms appear. May take with or without food.

Monitoring Parameters Headache severity; signs/symptoms suggestive of angina; blood pressure, heart rate, and/or ECG with first dose in patients with likelihood of unrecognized coronary disease, such as patients with significant hypertension, hypercholesterolemia, obese patients,

patients with diabetes, smokers with other risk factors or strong family history of coronary artery disease; signs/ symptoms of serotonin syndrome and hypersensitivity reactions

Dosage Forms Excipient information presented when available (limited, particularly for generics); consult specific product labeling.

Tablet, Oral:

Relpax: 20 mg, 40 mg

♦ Eletriptan Hydrobromide see Eletriptan on page 622
♦ Elidel see Pimecrolimus on page 1452
♦ Eligard see Leuprolide on page 1051

Eliglustat (el i GLOO stat)

Brand Names: US Cerdelga
Index Terms Genz-112638
Pharmacologic Category Enzyme Inhibitor; Glucosylcer-amide Synthase Inhibitor

Use

Gaucher disease: Treatment of adult patients with Gaucher disease type 1 (GD1) who are CYP2D6 extensive metabolizers (EMs), intermediate metabolizers (IMs), or poor metabolizers (PMs).

Limitations of use: Patients who are CYP2D6 ultra-rapid metabolizers (URMs) may not achieve adequate concentrations of eliglustat to achieve a therapeutic effect. A specific dosage cannot be recommended for those patients whose CYP2D6 genotype cannot be determined (IMs).

Pregnancy Considerations

Adverse events were observed in some animal reproduction studies.

Uncontrolled type 1 Gaucher disease is associated an increased risk of spontaneous abortion; maternal hepatosplenomegaly and thrombocytopenia may also occur and lead to adverse pregnancy outcomes.

Breast-Feeding Considerations It is not known if eliglustat is excreted into breast milk. Due to the potential for serious adverse reactions in the nursing infant, the manufacturer recommends a decision be made whether to discontinue nursing or to discontinue the drug, taking into account the importance of treatment to the mother.

Contraindications Concomitant use of a moderate or strong CYP2D6 inhibitor with a moderate or strong CYP3A inhibitor in extensive metabolizers (EMs) or intermediate metabolizers (IMs); concomitant use of a strong CYP3A inhibitor in poor metabolizers (PMs) or IMs

Warnings/Precautions May cause increases in ECG intervals (PR, QTc, and QRS) at substantially elevated plasma concentrations; use is not recommended in patients with preexisting cardiac disease (CHF, recent acute MI, eliglustat bradycardia, heart block, ventricular arrhythmia, long QT syndrome, and in combination with Class IA (eg, quinidine, procainamide) and Class III (eg, amiodarone, sotalol) antiarrhythmic medications (has not been studied). Not recommended in hepatic impairment or cirrhosis (has not been studied). Not recommended in patients with moderate-to-severe renal impairment or end-stage renal disease; use with caution in patients with mild renal impairment. Dosing has not been studied in poor metabolizers (PMs); monitor these patients for adverse reactions. Potentially significant drug-drug interactions may exist, requiring dose or frequency adjustment, additional monitoring, and/or selection of alternative therapy. A registry has been established and all patients with Gaucher disease, and health care providers who treat Gaucher disease are encouraged to participate. Information on the International Collaborative Gaucher Group (ICGG) Gaucher Registry may be obtained at https://www.registrynxt.com or by calling 1-800-745-4447 (ext.15500).

Adverse Reactions

>10%:

Central nervous system: Headache (13% to 40%), fatigue (14%)

Gastrointestinal: Diarrhea (12%), nausea (10% to 12%)

Neuromuscular & skeletal: Arthralgia (45%), back pain (12%), limb pain (11%)

1% to 10%:

Cardiovascular: Palpitations (5%)

Central nervous system: Migraine (10%), dizziness (8%)

Dermatologic: Skin rash (5%)

Gastrointestinal: Flatulence (10%), upper abdominal pain (10%), dyspepsia (7%), gastroesophageal reflux disease (7%), constipation (5%)

Neuromuscular & skeletal: Weakness (8%)

Respiratory: Oropharyngeal pain (10%), cough (7%)

Drug Interactions

Metabolism/Transport Effects Substrate of CYP2D6 (major), CYP3A4 (major); **Note:** Assignment of Major/Minor substrate status based on clinically relevant drug interaction potential; **Inhibits** CYP2D6 (moderate), P-glycoprotein

Avoid Concomitant Use

Avoid concomitant use of Eliglustat with any of the following: Bosutinib; Conivaptan; CYP3A4 Inducers (Strong); Fusidic Acid (Systemic); Grapefruit Juice; Highest Risk QTc-Prolonging Agents; Idelalisib; Ivabradine; Mifepristone; Moderate Risk QTc-Prolonging Agents; PAZOPanib; Silodosin; St Johns Wort; Thioridazine; Topotecan; VinCRIStine (Liposomal)

Increased Effect/Toxicity

Eliglustat may increase the levels/effects of: Afatinib; Bosutinib; Brentuximab Vedotin; Brexpiprazole; Colchicine; CYP2D6 Substrates; Dabigatran Etexilate; Digoxin; DOXOrubicin (Conventional); Edoxaban; Everolimus; Fesoterodine; Highest Risk QTc-Prolonging Agents; Ledipasvir; Metoprolol; Naloxegol; Nebivolol; PAZOPanib; P-glycoprotein/ABCB1 Substrates; Prucalopride; Rifaximin; Silodosin; Thioridazine; Topotecan; VinCRIStine (Liposomal)

The levels/effects of Eliglustat may be increased by: Abiraterone Acetate; Conivaptan; CYP2D6 Inhibitors (Moderate); CYP2D6 Inhibitors (Strong); CYP3A4 Inhibitors (Moderate); CYP3A4 Inhibitors (Strong); Fosaprepitant; Fusidic Acid (Systemic); Grapefruit Juice; Idelalisib; Ivabradine; Ivacaftor; Luliconazole; Mifepristone; Moderate Risk QTc-Prolonging Agents; Palbociclib; Peginterferon Alfa-2b; QTc-Prolonging Agents (Indeterminate Risk and Risk Modifying); Simeprevir; Stiripentol

Decreased Effect

Eliglustat may decrease the levels/effects of: Codeine; Tamoxifen; TraMADol

The levels/effects of Eliglustat may be decreased by: Bosentan; CYP3A4 Inducers (Moderate); CYP3A4 Inducers (Strong); Dabrafenib; Deferasirox; Peginterferon Alfa-2b; Siltuximab; St Johns Wort; Tocilizumab

Storage/Stability Store at 20°C to 25°C (68°F to 77°F); excursions are permitted between 15°C and 30°C (59°F and 86°F).

Mechanism of Action Eliglustat inhibits the enzyme needed to produce glycosphingolipids and decreases the rate of glycosphingolipid glucosylceramide formation. Glucosylceramide accumulates in type 1 Gaucher disease, causing complications specific to this disease.

Pharmacodynamics/Kinetics

Absorption: Systemic exposure depends upon the patient's CYP2D6 phenotype; systemic exposure is up to 9-fold higher in poor metabolizers (PMs).

Distribution: V_d: 835 L

Protein binding: 76% to 83%

Metabolism: Extensive by CYP2D6 (major) and CYP3A4

Bioavailability: Extensive metabolizers (EMs): <5%

Half-life elimination: EMs: 6.5 hours; PMs: 8.9 hours

Time to peak: EMs: 1.5 to 2 hours; PMs: 3 hours

Excretion: Urine (41.8%) and feces (51.4%) as inactive metabolites

Dosing

Adult & Geriatric

Gaucher disease: Oral: **Note:** Dosage is based on patient CYP2D6 metabolizer status (extensive metabolizers [EMs], intermediate metabolizers [IMs], or poor metabolizers [PMs]) determined by an FDA-cleared test.

EMs and IMs: 84 mg twice daily

PMs: 84 mg once daily. **Note:** Dosage has not been studied; however the predicted systemic exposures in these patients are within the range of those observed in clinical studies.

Missed dose: If a dose is missed, take the prescribed dose at the next scheduled time; do not double the next dose.

Dosage adjustment for concomitant therapy with strong or moderate CYP2D6 or CYP3A4 inhibitors:

EMs and IMs taking strong or moderate CYP2D6 inhibitors: 84 mg once daily

EMs taking strong or moderate CYP3A inhibitors: 84 mg once daily

Renal Impairment

Mild renal impairment: No dosage adjustment necessary.

Moderate to severe renal impairment: Use is not recommended (has not been studied).

End-stage renal disease (ESRD): Use is not recommended (has not been studied).

Hepatic Impairment Use is not recommended (has not been studied).

Dietary Considerations Avoid grapefruit or grapefruit juice.

Administration Oral: Administer with or without food. Swallow capsules whole with water; do not crush, dissolve, or open. Avoid grapefruit or grapefruit juice.

Monitoring Parameters Adverse reactions (especially in PMs)

Dosage Forms Excipient information presented when available (limited, particularly for generics); consult specific product labeling.

Capsule, Oral:

Cerdelga: 84 mg [contains fd&c blue #2 (indigotine)]

- ◆ Elimite see Permethrin on page 1432
- ◆ Elinest see Ethinyl Estradiol and Norgestrel on page 711
- ◆ Eliphos see Calcium Acetate on page 286
- ◆ Eliquis see Apixaban on page 137
- ◆ Elitek see Rasburicase on page 1563
- ◆ Elixophyllin see Theophylline on page 1780
- ◆ ElixSure Congestion [OTC] see Pseudoephedrine on page 1527
- ◆ Ella see Ulipristal on page 1851
- ◆ Ellence see Epirubicin on page 651
- ◆ Elmiron see Pentosan Polysulfate Sodium on page 1426
- ◆ Elmiron® (Can) see Pentosan Polysulfate Sodium on page 1426
- ◆ Elocom (Can) see Mometasone (Topical) on page 1228
- ◆ Elocon see Mometasone (Topical) on page 1228
- ◆ Eloctate see Antihemophilic Factor (Recombinant) on page 132

Elosulfase Alfa (el oh SUL fase AL fa)

Brand Names: US Vimizim

Index Terms Elosulfase alfa; N-acetylgalactosamine-6-sulfatase

Pharmacologic Category Enzyme

Use Mucopolysaccharidosis type IVA: Treatment of mucopolysaccharidosis type IVA (MPS IVA; Morquio A syndrome)

Dosing

Adult Note: Premedicate with antihistamines with or without antipyretics 30 to 60 minutes prior to infusion.

Mucopolysaccharidosis type IVA (MPS IVA): IV: 2 mg/kg once weekly

Pediatric Note: Premedicate with antihistamines with or without antipyretics 30 to 60 minutes prior to infusion.

Mucopolysaccharidosis type IVA (MPS IVA): Children ≥5 years and Adolescents: IV: 2 mg/kg once weekly

Renal Impairment There are no dosage adjustments provided in manufacturer's labeling.

Hepatic Impairment There are no dosage adjustments provided in manufacturer's labeling.

Additional Information Complete prescribing information should be consulted for additional detail.

Dosage Forms

Excipient information presented when available (limited, particularly for generics); consult specific product labeling.

Solution, Intravenous [preservative free]:

Vimizim: 5 mg/5 mL (5 mL) [contains mouse protein (murine) (hamster)]

- ◆ Elosulfase alfa see Elosulfase Alfa on page 625

Elotuzumab (el oh TOOZ ue mab)

Brand Names: US Empliciti

Index Terms BMS-901608; Empliciti; HuLuc63; PDL-063

Pharmacologic Category Antineoplastic Agent, Anti-SLAMF7; Antineoplastic Agent, Monoclonal Antibody

Use Multiple myeloma, relapsed/refractory: Treatment of multiple myeloma (in combination with lenalidomide and dexamethasone) in patients who have received 1 to 3 prior therapies

Pregnancy Considerations Animal reproduction studies have not been conducted. Elotuzumab is indicted for use in combination with lenalidomide. Due to its potential to cause fetal harm, lenalidomide is only available through a REMS program. Males and females of reproductive potential using this combination must be able to comply with pregnancy testing and contraception requirements for lenalidomide. Refer to the Lenalidomide monograph for additional information.

Breast-Feeding Considerations It is not known if elotuzumab is excreted into breast milk. Due to the potential for serious adverse reactions in the nursing infant, breastfeeding is not recommended by the manufacturer.

Contraindications There are no contraindications listed in the manufacturer's labeling.

Warnings/Precautions Infusion reactions (eg, fever, chills, hypertension) have been reported; all reactions were grade 3 or lower. Bradycardia and hypotension have also occurred during infusion. The majority of infusion reactions (~70%) occurred during the first dose. Premedicate with dexamethasone, H₁- and H₂-blockers, and acetaminophen prior to each dose. Administer in a facility with immediate access to resuscitative measures (eg, glucocorticoids, epinephrine, bronchodilators, and/or oxygen). May require treatment interruption, infusion rate modification, and/or discontinuation.

Infections were reported in the majority of multiple myeloma patients treated in the clinical trial, including fatal infections. Monitor for opportunistic, fungal, herpes zoster, and other infections during therapy; treat promptly if infections occur. Invasive second primary malignancies have been reported. The rate of hematologic malignancies was the same between the elotuzumab/lenalidomide/dexamethasone group versus the lenalidomide/dexamethasone group. Solid tumors and skin cancer were reported more frequently in the elotuzumab arm versus the control group. Monitor for the development of secondary malignancies.

Liver enzyme elevations (AST/ALT more than 3 times ULN, total bilirubin more than 2 times ULN, and alkaline phosphatase less than 2 times ULN) have occurred. Monitor liver function tests periodically; may require treatment interruption and/or discontinuation. Elotuzumab (a human IgG kappa monoclonal antibody) may be detected on serum protein electrophoresis and immunofixation assays which monitor for endogenous M-protein. Interference with these assays by elotuzumab may affect the determination of complete response and disease progression in some patients with IgG kappa myeloma protein. Potentially significant interactions may exist, requiring dose or frequency adjustment, additional monitoring, and/or selection of alternative therapy.

Adverse Reactions All incidences reported in combination with lenalidomide and dexamethasone.

>10%:

Cardiovascular: Decreased heart rate (66%; <60 bpm), increased heart rate (48%; ≥100 bpm), altered blood pressure (systolic ≥160 mmHg: 33%; systolic <90 mmHg: 29%; diastolic ≥100 mmHg: 17%)

Central nervous system: Fatigue (62%), peripheral neuropathy (27%; grades 3/4: 4%), headache (15%)

Endocrine & metabolic: Hyperglycemia (89%), hypocalcemia (78%), hypoalbuminemia (73%), decreased serum bicarbonate (63%), hyperkalemia (32%), weight loss (14%)

Gastrointestinal: Diarrhea (47%), constipation (36%), decreased appetite (21%), vomiting (15%)

Hematologic & oncologic: Lymphocytopenia (13% to 99%; grades 3/4: 9% to 77%), leukopenia (91%; grades 3/4: 32%), thrombocytopenia (84%; grades 3/4: 19%)

Hepatic: Increased serum alkaline phosphatase (39%; grades 3/4: 1%)

Immunologic: Immunogenicity (19%; neutralizing: 6%)

Infection: Infection (81%; grades 3/4: 28%), opportunistic infection (22%), herpes zoster (14%), fungal infection (10%)

Neuromuscular & skeletal: Limb pain (16%)

Ophthalmic: Cataract (12%)

Respiratory: Cough (34%), nasopharyngitis (25%), upper respiratory tract infection (23%), pneumonia (15% to 20%), oropharyngeal pain (10%)

Miscellaneous: Fever (7% to 37%), infusion related reaction (10%; grade 3: 1%)

1% to 10%:

Cardiovascular: Chest pain (≥5%), pulmonary embolism (3%)

Central nervous system: Hypoesthesia (≥5%), mood changes (≥5%)

Dermatologic: Night sweats (≥5%)

Hematologic & oncologic: Second primary malignant neoplasm (9%), malignant neoplasm of skin (4%), solid tumor (4%), anemia (3%), malignant neoplasm (hematologic: 2%)

Hepatic: Hepatotoxicity (3%)

Hypersensitivity: Hypersensitivity (≥5%)

Renal: Acute renal failure (3%)

Respiratory: Respiratory tract infection (3%)

Drug Interactions

Metabolism/Transport Effects None known.

Avoid Concomitant Use

Avoid concomitant use of Elotuzumab with any of the following: BCG (Intravesical); Belimumab; Natalizumab; Pimecrolimus; Tacrolimus (Topical); Tofacitinib; Vaccines (Live)

Increased Effect/Toxicity

Elotuzumab may increase the levels/effects of: Belimumab; Fingolimod; Leflunomide; Natalizumab; Tofacitinib; Vaccines (Live)

The levels/effects of Elotuzumab may be increased by: Denosumab; Pimecrolimus; Roflumilast; Tacrolimus (Topical); Trastuzumab

Decreased Effect

Elotuzumab may decrease the levels/effects of: BCG (Intravesical); Coccidioides immitis Skin Test; Sipuleucel-T; Vaccines (Inactivated); Vaccines (Live)

The levels/effects of Elotuzumab may be decreased by: Echinacea

Preparation for Administration Reconstitute the 300 mg vial with 13 mL of SWFI, and the 400 mg vial with 17 mL of SWFI (to a concentration of 25 mg/mL) with an 18-gauge or smaller needle (eg, 17, 16, or 15). Slight back pressure may occur during reconstitution. Rotate the vial to dissolve the lyophilized powder (holding the vial upright). To dissolve any powder on the stopper or top of the vial, invert the vial several times; avoid vigorous agitation. **Do not shake.** The powder should dissolve in <10 minutes. After dissolution, allow the reconstituted vials to stand for 5 to 10 minutes (solution should be colorless to slightly yellow, clear to slightly opalescent). Discard if any particulate matter or discoloration is observed.

Each vial contains overfill to allow for withdrawal of 12 mL (300 mg vial) and 16 mL (400 mg vial), respectively. Withdraw appropriate dose from each vial (maximum of 12 mL from the 300 mg vial and 16 mL from the 400 mg vial). Further dilute with 230 mL of 0.9% sodium chloride or D5W in a polyvinyl chloride or polyolefin infusion bag; the volume of diluent may be adjusted in order to not exceed 5 mL/kg of body weight. Do not mix with other medications.

Storage/Stability Store intact vials at 2°C to 8°C (36°F to 46°F). Protect from light (store in the original packaging until use); do not freeze or shake. Solutions diluted for infusion may be stored at 2°C to 8°C (36°F to 46°F) for up to 24 hours (protected from light). A maximum of 8 hours of the 24 hour storage time may be at room temperature and room light. Infusion must be completed within 24 hours of lyophilized powder reconstitution.

Mechanism of Action Elotuzumab is a humanized IgG1 immunostimulatory monoclonal antibody directed against signaling lymphocytic activation molecule family member 7 (SLAMF7, also called CS1 [cell surface glycoprotein CD2 subset 1). SLAMF7 is expressed on most myeloma and natural killer cells, but not on normal tissues; more than 95% of bone marrow myeloma cells express SLAMF7 (Lonial, 2015). Elotuzumab directly activates natural killer cells through both the SLAMF7 pathway and Fc receptors. It also targets SLAMF7 on myeloma cells and mediates antibody-dependent cellular cytotoxicity (ADCC) through the CD16 pathway (Lonial, 2015). This immunostimulatory activity, through the increased activation of natural killer cells, increases anti-tumor activity.

Pharmacodynamics/Kinetics Half-life elimination: ~97% of the maximum steady-state concentration is expected to be eliminated with a geometric mean (CV%) of 82.4 days.

Dosing

Adult Note: Premedicate with dexamethasone, an H_1-blocker (eg, diphenhydramine), an H_2-blocker (eg, ranitidine), and acetaminophen ~45 to 90 minutes prior to infusion (see premedications below). Refer to the Lenalidomide and Dexamethasone monographs for dosing information.

Multiple myeloma, relapsed/refractory: IV: Continue until disease progression or unacceptable toxicity (Lonial, 2015)

Cycles 1 and 2: 10 mg/kg once weekly on days 1, 8, 15, and 22 of a 28-day treatment cycle (in combination with lenalidomide and dexamethasone)

Cycle 3 and beyond: 10 mg/kg once every 2 weeks on days 1 and 15 of a 28-day treatment cycle (in combination with lenalidomide and dexamethasone)

Premedications:

Dexamethasone: Oral and IV: On days that elotuzumab is administered, give dexamethasone 28 mg **orally** 3 to 24 hours before elotuzumab infusion **plus** dexamethasone 8 mg **IV** 45 to 90 minutes prior to infusion. On days that elotuzumab is **not** administered but dexamethasone is due (eg, days 8 and 22 of cycle 3 and beyond), administer the standard dexamethasone dose (40 mg orally).

Antipyretic: Oral: Acetaminophen 650 to 1000 mg

H_1-blocker: IV or Oral: Diphenhydramine 25 to 50 mg or equivalent

H_2-blocker: Ranitidine: 50 mg IV or 150 mg orally or equivalent

Geriatric Refer to adult dosing

Renal Impairment There are no dosage adjustments provided in the manufacturer's labeling; however, based on pharmacokinetics, dosage adjustment is not likely necessary.

Hepatic Impairment

Hepatic impairment prior to treatment:

Mild impairment: There are no dosage adjustments provided in the manufacturer's labeling; however, based on pharmacokinetics, dosage adjustment is not likely necessary.

Moderate to severe impairment: There are no dosage adjustments provided in the manufacturer's labeling (has not been studied).

Hepatotoxicity during treatment: Grade 3 or higher transaminase elevations: Withhold treatment; may consider continuing treatment after liver enzymes return to baseline.

Adjustment for Toxicity

Refer to Lenalidomide monograph for dosage modifications for toxicity. If dosing of one drug in the regimen is delayed, interrupted, or discontinued, treatment with the other medications may continue as scheduled. However, if dexamethasone is delayed or discontinued, administer elotuzumab based on clinical judgment (due to hypersensitivity risk).

Infusion reactions: Grade 2 or greater: Interrupt infusion and manage symptoms as clinically appropriate. When symptoms improve to ≤ grade 1, restart elotuzumab infusion at a rate of 0.5 mL/minute and gradually increase the rate by 0.5 mL/minute every 30 minutes as tolerated to the rate at which the infusion reaction occurred. May continue to escalate the rate if there is no recurrence of the infusion reaction (see Administration). Monitor vital signs every 30 minutes during and for 2 hours after the end of the infusion in patients who experience an infusion reaction. If the reaction recurs, discontinue the elotuzumab infusion and do not restart on that day. Severe infusion reactions may require therapy discontinuation and emergency management.

Administration For IV infusion only. Do not administer IV push or as a bolus. Premedicate with dexamethasone, acetaminophen, and an H_1- and H_2-blocker (see Dosing) approximately 45 to 90 minutes prior to administration. Infuse in an environment equipped to monitor for and manage infusion reactions. Administer with an infusion set and a sterile, non-pyrogenic, low protein-binding filter (0.2 to 1.2 micrometer) using an automated infusion pump. Do not mix with or infuse with other medications. Infusion should be completed within 24 hours of reconstitution. Monitor for infusion reaction. Interrupt infusion for grade 2 or higher infusion reactions; if the reaction resolves or improves to ≤ grade 1, may resume infusion (see Dosage Adjustment for Toxicity). Monitor vital signs every 30 minutes during and for 2 hours after the end of the infusion in patients who experience an infusion reaction.

Infusion rate:

First infusion (Cycle 1, Dose 1): Infuse at 0.5 mL/minute for the first 30 minutes. If no infusion reactions occur, may increase the rate to 1 mL/minute for the next 30 minutes. If tolerated, may then increase the rate to 2 mL/minute until infusion completion (maximum rate: 2 mL/minute).

Second infusion (Cycle 1, Dose 2): If no infusion reactions occurred during the prior infusion, initiate at 1 mL/minute for the first 30 minutes. If tolerated, may then increase the rate to 2 mL/minute until infusion completion (maximum rate: 2 mL/minute).

Subsequent infusions (Cycle 1, Doses 3 and 4 and all subsequent infusions): If no infusion reactions occurred during the prior infusion, initiate and infuse at 2 mL/minute until completion. In patients who have received 4 cycles of elotuzumab, the infusion rate may be increased to a maximum of 5 mL/minute.

Monitoring Parameters Liver function tests (periodically); signs/symptoms of infusion reactions (monitor vital signs every 30 minutes during and for 2 hours after the end of the infusion in patients who experience an infusion reaction), infections, and second primary malignancies

Test Interactions Elotuzumab may be detected on both serum protein electrophoresis (SPEP) and immunofixation assays used for multiple myeloma endogenous M-protein monitoring, and may affect the determination of complete response and disease progression of some patients with IgG kappa myeloma protein. A small peak in the early gamma region on SPEP that is IgG kappa on serum immunofixation may be attributed to elotuzumab (especially when endogenous myeloma protein is IgA, IgM, IgD, or lambda light chain restricted).

Dosage Forms Excipient information presented when available (limited, particularly for generics); consult specific product labeling.

Solution Reconstituted, Intravenous:
Empliciti: 300 mg (1 ea); 400 mg (1 ea) [contains mouse protein (murine) (hamster), polysorbate 80]

- ◆ Eloxatin see Oxaliplatin on page 1349
- ◆ Elta Dermal Wound Cleanser [OTC] see Sodium Chloride on page 1671
- ◆ Elta Seal Moisture Barrier [OTC] see Zinc Oxide on page 1929
- ◆ Eltor® (Can) see Pseudoephedrine on page 1527

Eltrombopag (el TROM boe pag)

Brand Names: US Promacta
Brand Names: Canada Revolade
Index Terms Eltrombopag Olamine; Revolade; SB-497115; SB-497115-GR
Pharmacologic Category Colony Stimulating Factor; Hematopoietic Agent; Thrombopoietic Agent
Use
Aplastic anemia, severe: Treatment of severe aplastic anemia in patients who have had an insufficient response to immunosuppressive therapy.
Chronic hepatitis C infection-associated thrombocytopenia: Treatment of thrombocytopenia in patients with chronic hepatitis C (CHC) to allow the initiation and maintenance of interferon-based therapy.
Chronic immune (idiopathic) thrombocytopenia: Treatment of thrombocytopenia in adult and pediatric patients ≥1 year of age (US labeling) or adult patients (Canadian labeling) with chronic immune (idiopathic) thrombocytopenia (ITP) who have had insufficient response to corticosteroids, immune globulin, or splenectomy.
Limitations of use: For ITP, use eltrombopag only if the degree of thrombocytopenia and clinical condition increase the risk for bleeding. For chronic hepatitis C (CHC), use eltrombopag only if the degree of thrombocytopenia prevents initiation of or limits the ability to maintain interferon-based therapy. For CHC, safety and efficacy have not been established when used in combination with direct-acting antiviral agents without interferon for treatment of CHC infection.
Pregnancy Considerations Adverse effects were observed in animal reproduction studies. A Promacta pregnancy registry has been established to monitor outcomes of women exposed to eltrombopag during pregnancy (1-888-825-5249).
Breast-Feeding Considerations It is not known if eltrombopag is excreted in breast milk. Due to the potential for serious adverse effects in the nursing infant, a decision should be made to discontinue therapy or to discontinue breast-feeding, taking into account the importance of treatment to the mother.
Medication Guide Available Yes
Contraindications
US labeling: There are no contraindications listed in the manufacturer's labeling.
Canadian labeling: Hypersensitivity to eltrombopag or any component of the formulation; severe hepatic impairment (Child-Pugh class C)
Warnings/Precautions Liver enzyme elevations may occur; obtain ALT, AST, and bilirubin prior to treatment initiation, every 2 weeks during adjustment phase, then monthly (after stable dose established); obtain fractionation for elevated bilirubin levels. Repeat abnormal liver function tests within 3 to 5 days; if confirmed abnormal, monitor weekly until resolves, stabilizes, or returns to baseline. Discontinue treatment for ALT levels ≥3 times the upper limit of normal (ULN) in patients with normal hepatic function, or ≥3 times baseline in those with preexisting transaminase elevations and which are progressive, or persistent (≥4 weeks), or accompanied by increased direct bilirubin, or accompanied by clinical signs of liver injury or evidence of hepatic decompensation. Hepatotoxicity may reoccur with re-treatment after therapy interruption; however, if the benefit of treatment outweighs the hepatotoxicity risk, initiate carefully, and monitor liver function tests weekly during the dose adjustment phase; permanently discontinue if liver abnormalities persist, worsen, or recur with rechallenge. Use with caution in patients with preexisting hepatic impairment (clearance may be reduced); dosage reductions are recommended in patients with ITP (except children 1 to 5 years) and severe aplastic anemia who have hepatic dysfunction (no initial dose reductions are necessary in patients with chronic hepatitis C-related thrombocytopenia); monitor closely. The Canadian labeling contraindicates use in patients with severe impairment.

[US Boxed Warning]: May increase risk of hepatic decompensation when used in combination with interferon and ribavirin in patients with chronic hepatitis C. In clinical trials, patients with low albumin (<3.5 g/dL) or a Model for End-Stage Liver Disease (MELD) score ≥10 at baseline had an increased risk of hepatic decompensation; closely monitor these patients during therapy. If antiviral therapy is discontinued for hepatic decompensation according to interferon/ribavirin recommendations, eltrombopag should also be discontinued. Indirect hyperbilirubinemia is commonly observed with eltrombopag when used in combination with peginterferon and ribavirin. In addition, ascites, encephalopathy, and thrombotic events were reported more frequently than placebo in chronic hepatitis C trials.

May increase the risk for bone marrow reticulin formation or progression (Canadian labeling). Monitor peripheral blood smear for cellular morphologic abnormalities; analyze CBC monthly; discontinue treatment with onset of new or worsening abnormalities (eg, teardrop and nucleated RBC, immature WBC) or cytopenias and consider bone marrow biopsy (with staining for fibrosis).

Thromboembolism may occur with excessive increases in platelet levels. Use with caution in patients with known risk factors for thromboembolism (eg, Factor V Leiden, ATIII deficiency, antiphospholipid syndrome, chronic liver disease). Thrombotic events, primarily involving the portal venous system, were more commonly seen in eltrombopag-treated chronic hepatitis C patients with thrombocytopenia (when compared to placebo). Thrombotic events (including portal venous thrombosis) were also reported in a study of non-ITP thrombocytopenic patients with chronic liver disease undergoing elective invasive procedures receiving eltrombopag 75 mg once daily. Symptoms of portal vein thrombosis include abdominal pain, nausea, vomiting, and diarrhea. The risk for portal venous thrombosis is increased in thrombocytopenic patients with chronic liver disease receiving 75 mg once daily for 2 weeks as preparation for invasive procedures. Stimulation of cell surface thrombopoietin (TPO) receptors may increase the risk for hematologic malignancies (Canadian labeling).

Cataract formation or worsening was observed in clinical trials. Monitor regularly for signs and symptoms of cataracts; obtain ophthalmic exam at baseline and during therapy. Use with caution in patients at risk for cataracts (eg, advanced age, long-term glucocorticoid use). Potentially significant drug-drug interactions may exist, requiring dose or frequency adjustment, additional monitoring, and/or selection of alternative therapy. Take eltrombopag at least 2 hours before and 4 hours after antacids, minerals (eg, iron, calcium, aluminum, magnesium, selenium, zinc), or foods high in calcium; may reduce eltrombopag levels. Patients of East-Asian ethnicity (eg, Chinese, Japanese, Korean, Taiwanese) may have greater drug exposure (compared to non-East Asians); therapy should be initiated with lower starting doses in ITP and severe aplastic anemia patients. Use with caution in renal impairment (any degree) and monitor closely; initial dosage adjustment is not necessary.

Do not use to normalize platelet counts. *ITP:* Indicated only when the degree of thrombocytopenia and clinical conditions increase the risk for bleeding in patients with chronic immune ITP; use the lowest dose necessary to achieve and maintain platelet count ≥50,000/mm³. Discontinue if platelet count does not respond to a level to avoid clinically important bleeding after 4 weeks at the maximum recommended dose. *Chronic hepatitis C-associated thrombocytopenia:* Use only when thrombocytopenia prevents the initiation and maintenance of interferon-based therapy; discontinue if antiviral therapy is discontinued. Safety and efficacy have not been established when combined with direct acting antiviral medications approved for chronic hepatitis C genotype 1 infection therapy. *Severe aplastic anemia:* Use the lowest dose to achieve and maintain hematologic response. Discontinue if no hematologic response has occurred after 16 weeks of therapy, excessive platelet count responses or important liver test abnormalities. Consider discontinuation if new cytogenetic abnormalities are observed.

Adverse Reactions Adverse reactions and incidences reported are associated with adults unless otherwise indicated.

>10%:

Central nervous system: Fatigue (ITP: 4%; chronic hepatitis C: 28%; aplastic anemia: 28%), headache (ITP: 10%; chronic hepatitis C: 21%; aplastic anemia 21%), insomnia (chronic hepatitis C: 16%), chills (chronic hepatitis C: 14%), dizziness (aplastic anemia: 14%)

Dermatologic: Pruritus (chronic hepatitis C: 15%), ecchymosis (aplastic anemia: 12%)

Gastrointestinal: Nausea (ITP: 4% to 9%; chronic hepatitis C: 19%; aplastic anemia 33%), diarrhea (aplastic anemia: 21%; chronic hepatitis C: 19%; ITP: 9%; children: 9%), appetite decreased (chronic hepatitis C: 18%), abdominal pain (aplastic anemia 12%; children: 8%)

Hematologic & oncologic: Anemia (chronic hepatitis C: 40%), febrile neutropenia (aplastic anemia: 14%)

Hepatic: Hyperbilirubinemia (total bilirubin ≥1.5 x ULN: 76%; ITP and chronic hepatitis C: 6% to 8%), increased serum transaminases (aplastic anemia: 12%), abnormal hepatic function (ITP: 11%), increased serum ALT (children: 6%; ITP: 5% to 6%), increased serum AST (ITP: 4%; children: 4%)

Neuromuscular & skeletal: Limb pain (aplastic anemia: 19%), weakness (chronic hepatitis C: 16%), arthralgia (aplastic anemia: 12%), muscle spasm (aplastic anemia: 12%), myalgia (ITP and chronic hepatitis C: 5% to 12%)

Respiratory: Cough (aplastic anemia: 23%; chronic hepatitis C: 15%; children: 9%), flu-like syndrome (chronic hepatitis C: 18%), upper respiratory infection (children: 17%; ITP: 7%), dyspnea (aplastic anemia: 14%), oropharyngeal pain (aplastic anemia: 14%; children: 8%; ITP: 4%), nasopharyngitis (children: 12%), rhinorrhea (aplastic anemia: 12%, children: 4%)

Miscellaneous: Fever (chronic hepatitis C: 30%; aplastic anemia: 14%; children: 9%)

1% to 10%:

Cardiovascular: Peripheral edema (chronic hepatitis C: 10%), thrombosis (chronic hepatitis C: 3%)

Dermatologic: Alopecia (ITP: 2%; chronic hepatitis C: 10%), skin rash (children: 5%; ITP: 3%)

Gastrointestinal: Toothache (children: 6%), vomiting (ITP: 6%), xerostomia (ITP: 2%)

Genitourinary: Urinary tract infection (ITP: 5%)

Hematologic & oncologic: Thrombocytopenia (chronic hepatitis C: 3%)

Hepatic: Alkaline phosphatase increased (ITP: 2%)

Infection: Influenza (ITP: 3%)

Neuromuscular & skeletal: Back pain (ITP: 3%), paresthesia (ITP: 3%), musculoskeletal pain (ITP: 2%)

Ophthalmic: Cataract (ITP and chronic hepatitis C: 4% to 8%)

Respiratory: Rhinitis (children: 9%), pharyngitis (ITP: 4%)

<1% (Limited to important or life-threatening): Deep vein thrombosis, dysgeusia, dyspepsia, facial swelling, fecal discoloration, hemorrhage, hypokalemia, increased hemoglobin, increased serum albumin, increased serum creatinine, increased serum total protein, lesion (hepatic), malignant neoplasm (rectosigmoid), oropharyngeal blistering, ostealgia, portal vein thrombosis, pulmonary embolism, retinal hemorrhage, sinus tachycardia, superficial thrombophlebitis, tachycardia, thrombotic microangiopathy (with acute renal failure)

Drug Interactions

Metabolism/Transport Effects Substrate of BCRP, CYP1A2 (minor), CYP2C8 (minor), UGT1A1, UGT1A3; **Note:** Assignment of Major/Minor substrate status based on clinically relevant drug interaction potential; **Inhibits** BCRP, SLCO1B1, UGT1A1, UGT1A3, UGT1A4, UGT1A6, UGT1A9, UGT2B15, UGT2B7

Avoid Concomitant Use

Avoid concomitant use of Eltrombopag with any of the following: Irinotecan Products; PAZOPanib

Increased Effect/Toxicity

Eltrombopag may increase the levels/effects of: BCRP/ABCG2 Substrates; Deferiprone; Eluxadoline; Irinotecan Products; OATP1B1/SLCO1B1 Substrates; PAZOPanib; Rosuvastatin; Topotecan

Decreased Effect

The levels/effects of Eltrombopag may be decreased by: Aluminum Hydroxide; Calcium Salts; Iron Salts; Magnesium Salts; Multivitamins/Minerals (with ADEK, Folate, Iron); Multivitamins/Minerals (with AE, No Iron); Selenium; Sucralfate; Zinc Salts

Food Interactions Food, especially dairy products, may decrease the absorption of eltrombopag. Management: Take on an empty stomach at least 1 hour before or 2 hours after a meal. Separate intake from antacids, foods high in calcium, or minerals (eg, iron, calcium, aluminum, magnesium, selenium, zinc) by at least 4 hours.

Preparation for Administration The oral suspension must be reconstituted with cool or cold water only (do not use hot water). Fill the provided oral syringe with 20 mL of drinking water and empty into the mixing bottle. Add the appropriate eltrombopag dose to the mixing bottle; gently and slowly shake the bottle for at least 20 seconds to mix. If not used immediately, suspension may be stored for up to 30 minutes at room temperature; discard any

solution if not used within 30 minutes. Following administration, discard suspension remaining in bottle in trash (do not dispose of in drain); clean supplies by removing plunger from oral syringe, rinse bottle, lid, syringe, and plunger under running water and air-dry (bottle may stain, this is normal); wash hands with soap and water. If powder or suspension spills during preparation or administration, consider wearing disposable gloves during spill clean-up to avoid staining skin.

Storage/Stability

Oral suspension: Store at 20°C to 25°C (68°F to 77°F); excursions permitted to 15°C to 30°C (59°F to 86°F). Once reconstituted (if not used immediately), the suspension may be stored for a maximum of 30 minutes between 20°C and 25°C (68°F to 77°F); excursions permitted to 15°C to 30°C (59°F to 86°F). Discard the mixture if not used within 30 minutes.

Tablets: Store at 20°C to 25°C (68°F to 77°F); excursions are permitted between 15°C and 30°C (59°F and 86°F). If present, do not remove desiccant. Dispense in original bottle.

Mechanism of Action Thrombopoietin (TPO) nonpeptide agonist which increases platelet counts by binding to and activating the human TPO receptor. Activates intracellular signal transduction pathways to increase proliferation and differentiation of marrow progenitor cells. Does not induce platelet aggregation or activation.

Pharmacodynamics/Kinetics

Onset of action: Platelet count increase: Within 1 to 2 weeks

Peak platelet count increase: 14 to 16 days

Duration: Platelets return to baseline: 1 to 2 weeks after last dose

Protein binding: >99%

Metabolism: Extensive hepatic metabolism; via CYP 1A2, 2C8 oxidation and UGT 1A1, 1A3 glucuronidation

Bioavailability: ~52%; in adults, plasma AUC was increased by 22% with the oral suspension versus tablets

Half-life elimination: ~21 to 32 hours in healthy individuals; ~26 to 35 hours in patients with ITP

Time to peak, plasma: 2 to 6 hours

Excretion: Feces (~59%, 20% as unchanged drug, 21% glutathione-related conjugates); urine (31%, 20% glucuronide of the phenylpyrazole moiety)

Dosing

Adult & Geriatric Note: Do not use eltrombopag to normalize platelet counts.

Chronic immune (idiopathic) thrombocytopenia (ITP):

Oral: **Note:** Use the lowest dose to achieve and maintain platelet count ≥50,000/mm³ as needed to reduce the risk of bleeding. Discontinue if platelet count does not respond to a level that avoids clinically important bleeding after 4 weeks at the maximum daily dose of 75 mg.

Initial: 50 mg once daily (25 mg once daily for patients of East-Asian ethnicity [eg, Chinese, Japanese, Korean, Taiwanese]); dose should be titrated based on platelet response. Maximum dose: 75 mg once daily.

Dosage adjustment based on platelet response (US labeling):

Platelet count <50,000/mm³ (≥2 weeks after treatment initiation or a dose increase): Increase daily dose by 25 mg (if taking 12.5 mg once daily, increase dose to 25 mg once daily prior to increasing the dose amount by 25 mg daily); maximum: 75 mg once daily

Platelet count ≥200,000/mm³ and ≤400,000/mm³ (at any time): Reduce daily dose by 25 mg (if taking 25 mg once daily, decrease dose to 12.5 mg once daily); reassess in 2 weeks

Platelet count >400,000/mm³: Withhold dose; assess platelet count twice weekly; when platelet count <150,000/mm³, resume with the daily dose reduced by 25 mg (if taking 25 mg once daily, resume with 12.5 mg once daily)

Platelet count >400,000/mm³ after 2 weeks at the lowest dose: Discontinue treatment

Dosage adjustment based on platelet response (Canadian labeling):

Platelet count <50,000/mm³ (≥2 weeks after treatment initiation or a dose increase): Increase daily dose by 25 mg; maximum: 75 mg once daily

Platelet count ≥200,000/mm³ and ≤300,000/mm³ (at any time): Reduce daily dose by 25 mg; reassess in 2 weeks

Platelet count >300,000/mm³: Withhold dose; assess platelet count twice weekly; when platelet count <150,000/mm³, resume with the daily dose reduced by 25 mg

Platelet count >300,000/mm³ after 2 weeks at the lowest dose: Discontinue treatment

Chronic hepatitis C-associated thrombocytopenia:
Oral: **Note:** Use the lowest dose to achieve the target platelet count necessary to initiate antiviral therapy (peginterferon and ribavirin) or to avoid dose reductions of peginterferon during antiviral therapy. Discontinue when antiviral therapy is stopped.

Initial: 25 mg once daily; dose should be titrated based on platelet response. Maximum dose: 100 mg once daily

Dosage adjustment based on platelet response (US labeling):

Platelet count <50,000/mm^3 (after at least 2 weeks): Increase daily dose by 25 mg every 2 weeks; maximum dose: 100 mg once daily

Platelet count ≥200,000/mm^3 and ≤400,000/mm^3 (at any time): Reduce daily dose by 25 mg; reassess in 2 weeks

Platelet count >400,000/mm^3: Withhold dose; assess platelet count twice weekly; when platelet count <150,000/mm^3, resume with the daily dose reduced by 25 mg (if taking 25 mg once daily, resume with 12.5 mg once daily)

Platelet count >400,000/mm^3 after 2 weeks at the lowest dose: Discontinue treatment

Dosage adjustment based on platelet response (Canadian labeling):

Platelet count <50,000/mm^3 (after at least 2 weeks): Increase daily dose by 25 mg every 2 weeks; maximum dose: 100 mg once daily

Platelet count ≥150,000/mm^3 and ≤200,000/mm^3: Reduce daily dose by 25 mg; reassess in 2 weeks

Platelet count >200,000/mm^3: Withhold dose; assess platelet count twice weekly; when platelet count <150,000/mm^3, resume with the daily dose reduced by 25 mg (if taking 25 mg once daily, consider resuming with 25 mg every other day)

Platelet count >200,000/mm^3 after 2 weeks at the lowest dose: Discontinue treatment

Severe aplastic anemia: Oral: **Note:** Use the lowest dose to achieve and maintain hematologic response. Hematologic response may take up to 16 weeks and requires dose titration. Discontinue therapy if hematologic response is not achieved after 16 weeks of treatment, for excessive platelet responses or for liver function abnormalities. Consider discontinuing if new cytogenetic abnormalities are observed.

Initial: 50 mg once daily (25 mg once daily for patients of East-Asian ethnicity); dose should be titrated based on platelet response. Maximum dose: 150 mg once daily.

Dosage adjustment based on platelet response (US labeling):

Platelet count <50,000/mm^3 (≥2 weeks after treatment initiation or a dose increase): Increase daily dose by 50 mg (if taking 25 mg once daily, increase dose to 50 mg once daily prior to increasing the dose amount by 50 mg daily); maximum: 150 mg once daily

Platelet count ≥200,000/mm^3 and ≤400,000/mm^3 (at any time): Reduce daily dose by 50 mg; reassess in 2 weeks

Platelet count >400,000/mm^3: Withhold dose for 1 week; when platelet count <150,000/mm^3, resume with the daily dose reduced by 50 mg

Platelet count >400,000/mm^3 after 2 weeks at the lowest dose: Discontinue treatment

Dosage adjustment based on platelet response (Canadian labeling):

Platelet count <50,000/mm^3 (≥2 weeks after treatment initiation or a dose increase): Increase daily dose by 50 mg (if taking 25 mg once daily, increase dose to 50 mg once daily prior to increasing the dose amount by 50 mg daily); maximum: 150 mg once daily

Platelet count ≥200,000/mm^3 and ≤300,000/mm^3 (at any time): Reduce daily dose by 50 mg (if taking 50 mg once daily, reduce daily dose by 25 mg); reassess in 2 weeks

Platelet count >300,000/mm^3: Withhold dose for at least 1 week; when platelet count <150,000/mm^3, resume with the daily dose reduced by 50 mg

Platelet count >300,000/mm^3 after 2 weeks at the lowest dose: Discontinue treatment

For patients who achieve tri-lineage response, including transfusion independence, lasting 8 weeks, may reduce the dose by 50%. If counts remain stable after 8 weeks at the reduced dose, discontinue and monitor blood counts. If platelets counts drop to <30,000/mm^3, hemoglobin to <9 g/dL, or ANC to <500/ mm^3, may reinitiate at the prior effective dose.

Pediatric Note: Do not use eltrombopag to normalize platelet counts.

Chronic immune (idiopathic) thrombocytopenia (ITP):
Note: Use the lowest dose to achieve and maintain platelet count ≥50,000/mm^3 as needed to reduce the risk of bleeding. Discontinue if platelet count does not respond to a level that avoids clinically important bleeding after 4 weeks at the maximum daily dose of 75 mg.

Children 1 to 5 years: Oral: Initial: 25 mg once daily; dose should be titrated based on platelet response (no dosage adjustment required for patients of East Asian ancestry). Maximum dose: 75 mg once daily.

Children ≥6 years and Adolescents: Oral: Refer to adult dosing

Renal Impairment

US labeling: No dosage adjustment is necessary.

Canadian labeling:

Mild to moderate impairment (CrCl ≥30 mL/minute): No dosage adjustment is necessary. Use with caution and monitor closely.

Severe impairment (CrCl <30 mL/minute): Use is generally not recommended.

Hepatic Impairment

Adjustment for hepatic impairment prior to initiating treatment:

Chronic ITP: **Note:** In patients with ITP and hepatic impairment, wait 3 weeks (instead of 2 weeks) after therapy initiation or subsequent dosage changes prior to increasing dose.

US labeling:

Mild, moderate, or severe impairment (Child-Pugh classes A, B, or C): Initial: 25 mg once daily

Patients of East-Asian ethnicity with hepatic impairment (Child-Pugh classes A, B, or C): Initial: Consider 12.5 mg once daily

Canadian labeling:

Mild or moderate impairment (Child-Pugh classes A or B): Initial: 25 mg once daily

Severe impairment (Child-Pugh class C): Use is contraindicated

Chronic hepatitis C-associated thrombocytopenia:

US labeling: Initial: No dosage adjustment is necessary

Canadian labeling:

Mild or moderate impairment (Child-Pugh classes A or B): Initial: No dosage adjustment is necessary

Severe impairment (Child-Pugh class C): Use is contraindicated

Severe aplastic anemia:

US labeling: Mild, moderate, or severe impairment (Child-Pugh classes A, B, or C): Initial: 25 mg once daily

Canadian labeling:

Mild or moderate impairment (Child-Pugh classes A or B): Initial: 25 mg once daily

Severe impairment (Child-Pugh class C): Use is contraindicated

Adjustment for hepatic impairment during treatment:

ALT levels ≥3 times the upper limit of normal (ULN) in patients with normal hepatic function or ≥3 times baseline in those with preexisting transaminase elevations **and** which are progressive, persistent (≥4 weeks), accompanied by increased direct bilirubin, or accompanied by clinical signs of liver injury or evidence of hepatic decompensation: Discontinue treatment. Hepatotoxicity may recur with re-treatment after therapy interruption, but if determined to be clinically beneficial, may cautiously resume treatment; monitor ALT weekly during dosage titration; permanently discontinue if liver function test elevations persist, worsen, or recur.

Dietary Considerations Food, especially dairy products, may decrease the absorption of eltrombopag; allow at least 4 hours between dosing of eltrombopag and polyvalent cation intake (eg, dairy products, calcium-rich foods, multivitamins with minerals).

Administration Administer on an empty stomach, 1 hour before or 2 hours after a meal. Swallow tablets whole; do not crush and mix with food or liquids. Prepare the suspension with cool or cold water only (do not use hot water); discard any suspension not administered within 30 minutes after reconstitution. If powder or suspension spills during preparation or administration, consider wearing disposable gloves during spill clean-up to avoid staining skin. Do not administer concurrently with antacids, foods high in calcium, or minerals (eg, iron, calcium, aluminum, magnesium, selenium, zinc); administer eltrombopag at least 2 hours before and 4 hours after. Do not administer more than one dose within 24 hours.

Monitoring Parameters

Thrombocytopenia due to CHC and chronic ITP: Liver function tests, including ALT, AST, and bilirubin (baseline, every 2 weeks during dosage titration, then monthly; evaluate abnormal liver function tests within 3 to 5 days; monitor weekly until abnormalities resolve, stabilize, or return to baseline or if re-treating [not recommended] after therapy interruption for hepatotoxicity); bilirubin fractionation (for elevated bilirubin); CBC with differential and platelet count (weekly at initiation and during dosage titration, then monthly when stable; after cessation, monitor weekly for ≥4 weeks; when switching between the oral suspension and tablet, monitor platelet counts weekly for 2 weeks, then monthly when stable); peripheral blood smear (baseline and monthly when stable), bone marrow biopsy with staining for fibrosis (if peripheral blood smear reveals abnormality); ophthalmic exam (baseline and during treatment)

Severe aplastic anemia: CBC with differential and platelets (regularly throughout therapy), liver function tests (regularly throughout therapy); ophthalmic exam (baseline and during treatment)

Reference Range Target platelet count (with treatment) of 50,000 to 200,000/mm^3; platelet life span: 8 to 11 days

Product Availability Promacta oral suspension: FDA approved August 2015; anticipated availability is currently unknown.

Dosage Forms Excipient information presented when available (limited, particularly for generics); consult specific product labeling.

Tablet, Oral:

Promacta: 12.5 mg

Promacta: 25 mg [contains fd&c yellow #6 aluminum lake]

Promacta: 50 mg [contains fd&c blue #2 aluminum lake]

Promacta: 75 mg

Dosage Forms: Canada Excipient information presented when available (limited, particularly for generics); consult specific product labeling.

Tablet, Oral:

Revolade: 25 mg, 50 mg, 75 mg

♦ Eltrombopag Olamine see Eltrombopag on page 627

♦ Eltroxin (Can) see Levothyroxine on page 1068

Eluxadoline (el ux AD oh leen)

Brand Names: US Viberzi

Pharmacologic Category Gastrointestinal Agent, Miscellaneous

Use Irritable bowel syndrome with diarrhea: Treatment of irritable bowel syndrome with diarrhea (IBS-D) in adults

Pregnancy Considerations Adverse events have not been observed in animal reproduction studies.

Breast-Feeding Considerations It is not known if eluxadoline is excreted in breast milk. According to the manufacturer, the decision to breastfeed during therapy should take into account the risk of exposure to the infant and the benefits of treatment to the mother.

Contraindications Known or suspected biliary duct obstruction or sphincter of Oddi disease or dysfunction; history of pancreatitis or structural diseases of the pancreas, including known or suspected pancreatic duct obstruction; alcoholism, alcohol abuse, or alcohol addiction, or in patients who drink more than 3 alcoholic beverages per day; severe hepatic impairment (Child-Pugh class C); history of chronic or severe constipation or sequelae from constipation, or known or suspected mechanical gastrointestinal obstruction

Warnings/Precautions May cause sphincter of Oddi spasm resulting in pancreatitis or elevated hepatic enzymes; most often occurs during the first week of treatment and resolves with discontinuation of therapy. Discontinue use if patients experience symptoms of sphincter of Oddi spasm such as acute worsening of epigastric- or biliary-type abdominal pain (eg, right upper quadrant pain) that may radiate to the back or shoulder with or without nausea/vomiting, associated with elevations of pancreatic enzymes or hepatic transaminases). Permanently discontinue use in patients who develop biliary duct obstruction or sphincter of Oddi spasm. Use with caution in patients without a gallbladder, as they are at an increased risk for sphincter of Oddi spasm. Consider alternative therapy in these patients; if therapy is initiated, use a lower dose and monitor for signs and symptoms of sphincter of Oddi spasm (eg, acute abdominal pain, elevated hepatic enzymes, pancreatitis), especially during the first few weeks of treatment. May cause pancreatitis (not associated with sphincter of Oddi spasm); the majority of cases were associated with excessive alcohol intake and resolved with discontinuation of treatment. Avoid chronic or acute excessive alcohol use during therapy. Monitor for

signs and symptoms of pancreatitis; discontinue use if new or worsening abdominal pain that may radiate to the back or shoulder (with or without nausea/vomiting) develops.

Plasma concentrations are increased in patients with hepatic impairment; contraindicated in patients with severe hepatic impairment. Use with caution in patients with mild-to-moderate hepatic impairment; dosage adjustment required; monitor these patients for impaired mental or physical abilities needed to perform potentially hazardous activities (eg, driving a car, operating machinery) and for other eluxadoline-related adverse reactions. Current data suggest that eluxadoline has some potential for drug abuse and psychological dependence. Naloxone should be considered in the event of overdose.

The cytochrome P450 (CYP) isoenzymes involved in the metabolism of eluxadoline have not been clearly established. Thus, strong inhibitors of CYP isoenzymes have the potential to increase exposure to eluxadoline. Monitor patients for increased eluxadoline effects and toxicities if combined with a strong CYP inhibitor. Potentially significant interactions may exist, requiring dose or frequency adjustment, additional monitoring, and/or selection of alternative therapy. Consult drug interactions database for more detailed information.

Adverse Reactions

1% to 10%:

Central nervous system: Dizziness (3%), fatigue (3%), drowsiness (≤2%), euphoria (≤2%), intoxicated feeling (≤2%), sedation (≤2%)

Dermatologic: Skin rash (3%)

Gastrointestinal: Constipation (7% to 8%), nausea (7% to 8%), abdominal pain (6% to 7%), vomiting (4%), spasm of sphincter of Oddi (<1%; 1% to 4% in patients without a gallbladder), abdominal distention (3%), flatulence (3%), viral gastroenteritis (3%), gastroesophageal reflux disease (≤2%)

Hepatic: Increased serum ALT (2% to 3%), increased serum AST (≤2%)

Respiratory: Upper respiratory tract infection (5%), nasopharyngitis (4%), bronchitis (3%), asthma (≤2%), bronchospasm (≤2%), respiratory failure (≤2%), wheezing (≤2%)

<1% (Limited to important or life-threatening): Increased liver enzymes, pancreatitis

Drug Interactions

Metabolism/Transport Effects Substrate of BSEP, MRP2, OAT3, SLCO1B1; Inhibits P-glycoprotein, SLCO1B1

Avoid Concomitant Use

Avoid concomitant use of Eluxadoline with any of the following: Alcohol (Ethyl); Alosetron; Analgesics (Opioid); Anticholinergic Agents

Increased Effect/Toxicity

Eluxadoline may increase the levels/effects of: Rosuvastatin

The levels/effects of Eluxadoline may be increased by: Alcohol (Ethyl); Alosetron; Analgesics (Opioid); Anticholinergic Agents; Antihepaciviral Combination Products; Atazanavir; CycloSPORINE (Systemic); Eltrombopag; Gemfibrozil; Lopinavir; Rifampin; Ritonavir; Saquinavir; Teriflunomide; Tipranavir

Decreased Effect There are no known significant interactions involving a decrease in effect.

Food Interactions Administration with a high fat meal decreased the C_{max} by 50% and AUC by 60%; administration under fed conditions decreased the T_{max} to 1.5 hours as compared to 2 hours under fasting conditions. Management: Administer with food.

Storage/Stability Store at 20°C to 25°C (68°F to 77°F); excursions permitted to 15°C to 30°C (59°F to 86°F).

Mechanism of Action Eluxadoline is a mixed mu-opioid receptor agonist, delta opioid receptor antagonist, and kappa opioid receptor agonist which acts locally to reduce abdominal pain and diarrhea in patients with IBS-D without constipating side effects.

Pharmacodynamics/Kinetics

Protein binding: 81%

Metabolism: Not clearly established; there is evidence that glucuronidation can occur to form an acyl glucuronide metabolite

Half-life elimination: 3.7 to 6 hours

Time to peak: 1.5 hours (range: 1 to 8 hours) under fed conditions; 2 hours (range: 0.5 to 6 hours) under fasting conditions

Excretion: Feces (82.2%); urine (<1%)

Dosing

Adult & Geriatric

Irritable bowel syndrome with diarrhea: Oral:

Patients with a gallbladder: 100 mg twice daily; may decrease to 75 mg twice daily in patients unable to tolerate the 100 mg dose.

Patients without a gallbladder: 75 mg twice daily.

Dosage adjustment for concomitant therapy: Coadministration of OATP1B1 inhibitors (eg, cyclosporine, gemfibrozil, atazanavir, lopinavir, ritonavir, saquinavir, tipranavir, rifampin, eltrombopag): 75 mg twice daily.

Renal Impairment There are no dosage adjustments provided in the manufacturer's labeling.

Hepatic Impairment

Mild (Child-Pugh class A) to moderate (Child-Pugh class B) impairment: 75 mg twice daily.

Severe impairment (Child-Pugh class C): Use is contraindicated.

Adjustment for Toxicity

Severe constipation: Discontinue use in patients who develop severe constipation lasting >4 days.

Sphincter of Oddi spasms: Discontinue use in patients with symptoms of sphincter of Oddi spasm (eg, acute worsening of epigastric- or biliary-type abdominal pain, increased pancreatic enzymes, or increased hepatic transaminases). Permanently discontinue use in patients who develop biliary duct obstruction or sphincter of Oddi spasm.

Dietary Considerations Take with food

Administration Oral: Administer with food.

Monitoring Parameters Monitor for new or worsening abdominal pain that may radiate to the back or shoulder, with or without nausea/vomiting and acute biliary pain with hepatic or pancreatic enzyme elevations, especially in patients without a gallbladder during the first few weeks of therapy. Monitor patients with hepatic impairment for impaired mental or physical abilities and other eluxadoline-related adverse reactions.

Dosage Forms Excipient information presented when available (limited, particularly for generics); consult specific product labeling.

Tablet, Oral:

Viberzi: 75 mg, 100 mg

Controlled Substance C-IV

Elvitegravir (el vi TEG ra vir)

Brand Names: US Vitekta

Pharmacologic Category Antiretroviral, Integrase Inhibitor (Anti-HIV)

Use HIV-1 infection: In combination with an HIV protease inhibitor coadministered with ritonavir and with other antiretroviral drug(s) for the treatment of HIV-1 infection in antiretroviral treatment-experienced adults

Pregnancy Considerations Adverse events were not observed in animal reproduction studies. The DHHS Perinatal HIV Guidelines note there are insufficient data to recommend use in pregnancy.

Regardless of CD4 count or HIV RNA copy number, all HIV-infected pregnant women should receive a combination antiretroviral (ARV) drug regimen. A combination of antepartum, intrapartum, and infant ARV prophylaxis is recommended. ARV therapy should be started as soon as possible in women with symptomatic infection. Although earlier initiation may be more effective in reducing the perinatal transmission of HIV, initiation may be delayed until after 12 weeks gestation in women who do not require immediate treatment after careful consideration of maternal conditions (eg, nausea and vomiting) and the potential risks of first trimester fetal exposure for specific agents. A scheduled cesarean delivery at 38 weeks gestation is recommended for all women with HIV RNA >1,000 copies/mL or unknown concentrations near delivery in order to decrease transmission. If ARV therapy must be interrupted for <24 hours during the peripartum period, stop then restart all medications simultaneously in order to decrease the chance of developing resistance. Long-term follow-up is recommended for all infants exposed to ARV medications. In couples who want to conceive, the HIV-infected partner should attain maximum viral suppression prior to conception.

Health care providers are encouraged to enroll pregnant women exposed to antiretroviral medications in the Antiretroviral Pregnancy Registry (1-800-258-4263 or www.APRegistry.com). Health care providers caring for HIV-infected women and their infants may contact the National Perinatal HIV Hotline (888-448-8765) for clinical consultation (DHHS [perinatal], 2014).

Breast-Feeding Considerations It is not known of elvitegravir is excreted in breast milk. Maternal or infant antiretroviral therapy does not completely eliminate the risk of postnatal HIV transmission. In addition, multiclass-resistant virus has been detected in breast-feeding infants despite maternal therapy. Therefore, in the United States, where formula is accessible, affordable, safe, and sustainable, and the risk of infant mortality due to diarrhea and respiratory infections is low, complete avoidance of breast-feeding by HIV-infected women is recommended to decrease potential transmission of HIV (DHHS [perinatal], 2014).

Contraindications There are no contraindications listed in the manufacturer's labeling.

Warnings/Precautions Patients may develop immune reconstitution syndrome resulting in the occurrence of an inflammatory response to an indolent or residual opportunistic infection during initial HIV treatment or activation of autoimmune disorders (eg, Graves' disease, polymyositis, Guillain-Barré syndrome) later in therapy; further evaluation and treatment may be required. Use is not recommended in severe hepatic impairment (Child-Pugh class C); has not been studied in this population. Not recommended in combination with a protease inhibitor and cobicistat due to lack of dosing recommendations, potential suboptimal plasma concentrations, loss of therapeutic effect, or development of resistance. Administration of unboosted elvitegravir is not recommended (HHS [adult] 2015). Avoid concurrent use with other elvitegravir-containing products. Potentially significant interactions may exist, requiring dose or frequency adjustment, additional monitoring, and/or selection of alternative therapy.

Adverse Reactions Percentages are reported for antiretroviral treatment experienced adults.

1% to 10%:

Central nervous system: Headache (3%), depression (<2%), fatigue (<2%), insomnia (<2%), suicidal ideation (<2%)

Dermatologic: Skin rash (<2%)

Gastrointestinal: Diarrhea (7%), nausea (4%), abdominal pain (<2%), dyspepsia (<2%), vomiting (<2%)

Immunologic: Immune reconstitution syndrome

Drug Interactions

Metabolism/Transport Effects Substrate of CYP3A4 (major), UGT1A1, UGT1A3; **Note:** Assignment of Major/Minor substrate status based on clinically relevant drug interaction potential; **Induces** CYP2C9 (weak/moderate)

Avoid Concomitant Use

Avoid concomitant use of Elvitegravir with any of the following: CarBAMazepine; Efavirenz; Fosphenytoin-Phenytoin; Nevirapine; OXcarbazepine; PHENobarbital; Rifabutin; Rifampin; Rifapentine; St Johns Wort

Increased Effect/Toxicity

Elvitegravir may increase the levels/effects of: Rifabutin

The levels/effects of Elvitegravir may be increased by: Atazanavir; Darunavir; Itraconazole; Ketoconazole (Systemic); Lopinavir; Osimertinib; Voriconazole

Decreased Effect

Elvitegravir may decrease the levels/effects of: Contraceptives (Estrogens)

The levels/effects of Elvitegravir may be decreased by: Antacids; Bosentan; CarBAMazepine; CYP3A4 Inducers (Moderate); CYP3A4 Inducers (Strong); Dabrafenib; Deferasirox; Dexamethasone (Systemic); Efavirenz; Enzalutamide; Fosphenytoin-Phenytoin; Mitotane; Nevirapine; Osimertinib; OXcarbazepine; PHENobarbital; Rifabutin; Rifampin; Rifapentine; Siltuximab; St Johns Wort; Tocilizumab

Storage/Stability Store below 30°C (86°F). Dispense only in original container.

Mechanism of Action Integrase is an HIV-1 encoded enzyme that is required for viral replication. Inhibition of integrase prevents the integration of HIV-1 DNA into host genomic DNA, blocking the formation of the HIV-1 provirus and propagation of the viral infection. Elvitegravir does not inhibit human topoisomerases I or II.

Pharmacodynamics/Kinetics

Absorption: AUC increases with food

Protein binding: 99%

Metabolism: Hepatic via CYP3A enzymes and also hepatic glucuronidation mediated by UGT1A1/3

Half-life elimination: Terminal: ~9 hours

Time to peak, plasma: ~4 hours

Excretion: Feces (~95%); urine (~7%)

Dosing

Adult & Geriatric

HIV-1 infection in antiretroviral treatment-experienced patients: Oral: **Note:** Must be administered in combination with a protease inhibitor, ritonavir, and another antiretroviral drug. See individual agents.

Administered with concomitant atazanavir and ritonavir or lopinavir and ritonavir: 85 mg once daily
Administered with concomitant darunavir and ritonavir, fosamprenavir and ritonavir, or tipranavir and ritonavir: 150 mg once daily

Renal Impairment No dosage adjustment necessary.

Hepatic Impairment
Mild-to-moderate hepatic impairment (Child-Pugh class A or B): No dosage adjustment necessary.
Severe hepatic impairment (Child-Pugh class C): Use is not recommended (has not been studied).

Dietary Considerations Take with food.

Administration Oral: Administer once daily with food.

Monitoring Parameters CBC with differential, reticulocyte count, CD4 count, HIV RNA plasma levels, hepatic function tests, testing for HBV is recommended prior to the initiation of antiretroviral therapy.

Dosage Forms Excipient information presented when available (limited, particularly for generics); consult specific product labeling.
Tablet, Oral:
Vitekta: 85 mg, 150 mg [contains fd&c blue #2 aluminum lake]

Elvitegravir, Cobicistat, Emtricitabine, and Tenofovir Alafenamide
(el vi TEG ra vir, koe BIK i stat, em trye SYE ta been, & ten OF oh vir al a FEN a mide)

Brand Names: US Genvoya

Index Terms Cobicistat, Emtricitabine, Tenofovir Alafenamide, and Elvitegravir; Elvitegravir, Cobicistat, Tenofovir Alafenamide, and Emtricitabine; Emtricitabine, Elvitegravir, Cobicistat, and Tenofovir Alafenamide; Tenofovir Alafenamide, Elvitegravir, Cobicistat, and Emtricitabine

Pharmacologic Category Antiretroviral, Integrase Inhibitor (Anti-HIV); Antiretroviral, Reverse Transcriptase Inhibitor, Nucleoside (Anti-HIV); Antiretroviral, Reverse Transcriptase Inhibitor, Nucleotide (Anti-HIV); Cytochrome P-450 Inhibitor

Use HIV-1 infection: Treatment of HIV-1 infection in adults and pediatric patients 12 years of age and older who have no antiretroviral treatment history or to replace the current antiretroviral regimen in those who are virologically-suppressed (HIV-1 RNA less than 50 copies per mL) on a stable antiretroviral regimen for at least 6 months with no history of treatment failure and no known substitutions associated with resistance to elvitegravir, cobicistat, emtricitabine, or tenofovir alafenamide

Dosing

Adult & Geriatric
Note: Prior to initiation, patients should be tested for hepatitis B infection, and baseline estimated creatinine clearance, urine glucose, and urine protein should be assessed in all patients.
HIV-1: Oral: One tablet once daily.

Pediatric
Note: Prior to initiation, patients should be tested for hepatitis B infection, and baseline estimated creatinine clearance, urine glucose, and urine protein should be assessed in all patients.
HIV-1: Children ≥12 years and Adolescents ≥35 kg: Oral: One tablet once daily.

Renal Impairment
CrCl ≥30 mL/minute: No dosage adjustment necessary.
CrCl <30 mL/minute at initiation of therapy: Use is not recommended.

Hepatic Impairment
Mild to moderate impairment (Child-Pugh class A or B): No dosage adjustment necessary.
Severe impairment (Child-Pugh class C): Use is not recommended (has not been studied).

Additional Information Complete prescribing information should be consulted for additional detail.

Dosage Forms Excipient information presented when available (limited, particularly for generics); consult specific product labeling.
Tablet, Oral:
Genvoya: Elvitegravir 150 mg, cobicistat 150 mg, emtricitabine 200 mg, and tenofovir alafenamide 10 mg [contains fd&c blue #2 aluminum lake]

Elvitegravir, Cobicistat, Emtricitabine, and Tenofovir Disoproxil Fumarate
(el vi TEG ra vir, koe BIK i stat, em trye SYE ta been, & ten OF oh vir dye soe PROX il FUE ma rate)

Brand Names: US Stribild
Brand Names: Canada Stribild
Index Terms Cobicistat, Emtricitabine, Tenofovir Disoproxil Fumarate, and Elvitegravir; Elvitegravir, Cobicistat,

Emtricitabine, and Tenofovir Disoproxil Fumarate; Emtricitabine, Tenofovir Disoproxil Fumarate, Elvitegravir, and Cobicistat; EVG/COBI/FTC/TDF; Quad Pill; Tenofovir Disoproxil Fumarate, Elvitegravir, Cobicistat, and Emtricitabine

Pharmacologic Category Antiretroviral, Integrase Inhibitor (Anti-HIV); Antiretroviral, Reverse Transcriptase Inhibitor, Nucleoside (Anti-HIV); Antiretroviral, Reverse Transcriptase Inhibitor, Nucleotide (Anti-HIV); Cytochrome P-450 Inhibitor

Use HIV-1 infection: Treatment of HIV-1 infection in adults who are antiretroviral treatment-naïve; as a replacement for the current antiretroviral regimen in adults who are virologically-suppressed (HIV-1 RNA <50 copies/mL) on a stable antiretroviral regimen for ≥6 months with no history of treatment failure and no known substitutions associated with resistance to elvitegravir, cobicistat, emtricitabine, or tenofovir.

Dosing

Adult & Geriatric Note: Prior to initiation, patients should be tested for hepatitis B infection, and baseline estimated creatinine clearance, urine glucose, and urine protein should be assessed in all patients.

HIV-1: Oral: One tablet once daily. **Note:** This combination is a recommended initial regimen for antiretroviral-naïve patients with CrCl >70 mL/minute (HHS [adult] 2015).

Renal Impairment
CrCl ≥70 mL/minute: No dosage adjustment necessary.
CrCl <70 mL/minute at initiation of therapy: Initial use is not recommended.
CrCl <50 mL/minute during therapy: Continued use is not recommended.
ESRD requiring dialysis: Use is not recommended.

Hepatic Impairment
Mild-to-moderate hepatic impairment (Child-Pugh class A or B): No dosage adjustment necessary.
Severe hepatic impairment (Child-Pugh class C): Use is not recommended (has not been studied).

Additional Information Complete prescribing information should be consulted for additional detail.

Dosage Forms Excipient information presented when available (limited, particularly for generics); consult specific product labeling.
Tablet, oral:
Stribild: Elvitegravir 150 mg, cobicistat 150 mg, emtricitabine 200 mg, and tenofovir disoproxil fumarate 300 mg

♦ **Elvitegravir, Cobicistat, Emtricitabine, and Tenofovir Disoproxil Fumarate** *see* Elvitegravir, Cobicistat, Emtricitabine, and Tenofovir Disoproxil Fumarate *on page 632*

♦ **Elvitegravir, Cobicistat, Tenofovir Alafenamide, and Emtricitabine** *see* Elvitegravir, Cobicistat, Emtricitabine, and Tenofovir Alafenamide *on page 632*

♦ **E-Max-1000 [OTC]** *see* Vitamin E *on page 1906*

♦ **Emcyt** *see* Estramustine *on page 688*

♦ **EMD 68843** *see* Vilazodone *on page 1893*

♦ **Emend** *see* Aprepitant *on page 143*

♦ **Emend** *see* Fosaprepitant *on page 812*

♦ **Emend® IV (Can)** *see* Fosaprepitant *on page 812*

♦ **EMLA** *see* Lidocaine and Prilocaine *on page 1076*

♦ **Emo-Cort (Can)** *see* Hydrocortisone (Topical) *on page 886*

♦ **Emoquette** *see* Ethinyl Estradiol and Desogestrel *on page 701*

Empagliflozin (em pa gli FLOE zin)

Brand Names: US Jardiance
Brand Names: Canada Jardiance
Index Terms BI10773
Pharmacologic Category Antidiabetic Agent, Sodium-Glucose Cotransporter 2 (SGLT2) Inhibitor; Sodium-Glucose Cotransporter 2 (SGLT2) Inhibitor

Use
Diabetes mellitus, type 2: Treatment of type 2 diabetes mellitus (noninsulin dependent, NIDDM) as an adjunct to diet and exercise to improve glycemic control
Limitations of use:
US labeling: Not recommended for patients with type 1 diabetes or for the treatment of diabetic ketoacidosis
Canadian labeling: Concomitant use with insulin mix is not recommended (has not been studied)

Pregnancy Considerations Adverse events were observed in some animal reproduction studies. The manufacturer recommends the use of alternative therapies in pregnant women, especially during the second and third trimesters.

In women with diabetes, maternal hyperglycemia can be associated with congenital malformations as well as adverse effects in the fetus, neonate, and the mother (ACOG 2005; ADA 2015; Kitzmiller 2008; Metzger 2007). To prevent adverse outcomes, prior to conception and throughout pregnancy maternal blood glucose and HbA$_{1c}$ should be kept as close to target goals as possible but without causing significant hypoglycemia (ACOG 2013; ADA 2015; Blumer 2013; Kitzmiller 2008). Prior to pregnancy, effective contraception should be used until glycemic control is achieved (Kitzmiller 2008). Other agents are currently recommended to treat diabetes in pregnant women (ACOG 2013; Blumer 2013).

Breast-Feeding Considerations It is not known if empagliflozin is excreted into breast milk. Due to the potential for serious adverse reactions in the nursing infant, the manufacturer recommends a decision be made whether to discontinue nursing or to discontinue the drug, taking into account the importance of treatment to the mother.

Contraindications

History of serious hypersensitivity to empagliflozin or any component of the formulation; severe renal impairment (eGFR <30 mL/minute/1.73 m^2), end-stage renal disease (ESRD), or dialysis

Canadian labeling: Additional contraindications (not in US labeling): eGFR <45 mL/minute/1.73 m^2

Warnings/Precautions May cause symptomatic hypotension due to intravascular volume depletion especially in patients with renal impairment, the elderly, patients on diuretics, or those with low systolic blood pressure. Assess volume status prior to initiation in patients at risk of hypotension and correct if depleted; monitor signs and symptoms of hypotension after initiation and increase monitoring in clinical situations where volume contraction is expected. Elevated hemoglobin/hematocrit have been observed; use caution in patients with elevated hematocrit at baseline. Abnormalities in renal function (decreased eGFR, increased serum creatinine) may occur; elderly patients and patients with preexisting renal impairment may be at greater risk. Glycemic efficacy may be decreased and risk of adverse reactions (eg, adverse reaction related to volume depletion, renal impairment, UTI) may be increased with worsening renal function. Assess renal function prior to initiation and periodically during treatment; empagliflozin should not be initiated if initial eGFR is <45 mL/minute/1.73 m^2 and should be discontinued when eGFR is persistently <45 mL/minute/1.73 m^2. Use is contraindicated in severe renal impairment (eGFR <30 mL/minute/1.73 m^2), ESRD, and dialysis patients. The Canadian labeling also contraindicates use if eGFR <45 mL/minute/1.73 m^2. Cases of ketoacidosis resulting in urgent hospitalization have been reported in patients with type 1 and type 2 diabetes mellitus receiving sodium glucose co-transporter-2 (SGLT2) inhibitors; before initiating treatment consider risk factors that may predispose to ketoacidosis (eg, pancreatic insulin deficiency from any cause, caloric restriction, and alcohol abuse). Patients presenting with nausea/vomiting, abdominal pain, generalized malaise, and/or shortness of breath should be assessed immediately for ketoacidosis; if indicated, consider interruption or discontinuation of therapy.

May increase the risk of genital mycotic infections (eg, vulvovaginal mycotic infection, vulvovaginal candidiasis, vulvovaginitis, candida balanitis, balanoposthitis). Patients with a history of these infections or uncircumcised males are at greater risk. Serious urinary infections including urosepsis and pyelonephritis requiring hospitalization have been reported; treatment with SGLT2 inhibitors increases the risk for UTI; monitor for signs and symptoms of UTI and treat as needed. May cause low-density lipoprotein cholesterol (LDL-C) elevation; monitor LDL-C and treat as needed. Risk of intravascular volume depletion, renal impairment, and UTI may be increased in elderly patients. Should not be used in patients with type 1 diabetes mellitus (insulin-dependent, IDDM) or for the treatment of DKA. Potentially significant drug-drug interactions may exist, requiring dose or frequency adjustment, additional monitoring, and/or selection of alternative therapy.

Adverse Reactions

>10%:

Endocrine & metabolic: Hypoglycemia (combination therapy with insulin: 28%, severe hypoglycemia: ≤1%; combination therapy with metformin and a sulfonylurea: 12% to 16%; combination therapy with metformin: 1% to 2%)

Genitourinary: Urinary tract infection (9%; females: 18%; males: 4%), increased urine output (includes polyuria, pollakiuria, nocturia: 3%)

1% to 10%:

Endocrine & metabolic: Increased LDL cholesterol (5% to 7%), dyslipidemia (4%), increased thirst (including polydipsia: 2%)

Gastrointestinal: Nausea (2%)

Hematologic & oncologic: Increased hematocrit (3% to 4%)

Infection: Genitourinary fungal infection (4%; females: 5% to 6% [includes bacterial vaginosis, cervicitis, vulvitis, vulvovaginal candidiasis, vulvovaginal infection, vulvovaginitis]; males: 2% to 3% [includes balanitis, balanoposthitis, genitourinary fungal infection, penile infection, scrotal abscess])

<1% (Limited to important or life-threatening): Decreased estimated GFR (eGFR), hypotension, hypovolemia, increased serum creatinine, ketoacidosis (FDA Safety Communication, December 4, 2015), phimosis, pyelonephritis (FDA Safety Communication, December 4, 2015), urosepsis (FDA Safety Communication, December 4, 2015)

Drug Interactions

Metabolism/Transport Effects Substrate of BCRP, OAT3, P-glycoprotein, SLCO1B1, SLCO1B3, UGT1A3, UGT1A8, UGT1A9, UGT2B7

Avoid Concomitant Use There are no known interactions where it is recommended to avoid concomitant use.

Increased Effect/Toxicity

Empagliflozin may increase the levels/effects of: Hypoglycemia-Associated Agents; Insulin; Loop Diuretics; Sulfonylureas

The levels/effects of Empagliflozin may be increased by: Alpha-Lipoic Acid; Androgens; MAO Inhibitors; Pegvisomant; Quinolone Antibiotics; Salicylates; Selective Serotonin Reuptake Inhibitors; Teriflunomide

Decreased Effect

The levels/effects of Empagliflozin may be decreased by: Hyperglycemia-Associated Agents; Quinolone Antibiotics; Thiazide Diuretics

Storage/Stability Store at 25°C (77°F); excursions are permitted between 15°C and 30°C (59°F and 86°F).

Mechanism of Action By inhibiting sodium-glucose cotransporter 2 (SGLT2) in the proximal renal tubules, empagliflozin reduces reabsorption of filtered glucose from the tubular lumen and lowers the renal threshold for glucose (RT$_G$). SGLT2 is the main site of filtered glucose reabsorption; reduction of filtered glucose reabsorption and lowering of RT$_G$ result in increased urinary excretion of glucose, thereby reducing plasma glucose concentrations.

Pharmacodynamics/Kinetics

Distribution: V$_d$: 73.8 L

Protein binding: 86.2%

Metabolism: Primarily through glucuronidation by UGT2B7, UGT1A3, UGT1A8, and UGT1A9 to minor metabolites

Half-life Elimination: 12.4 hours

Time to Peak: 1.5 hours

Excretion: Urine (54.4%; 50% as unchanged drug); feces (41.2%; majority as unchanged drug)

Dosing

Adult & Geriatric Note: If present, correct volume depletion prior to initiation

Diabetes mellitus, type 2: Oral: Initial: 10 mg once daily; may increase to 25 mg once daily

Renal Impairment

US labeling:

eGFR ≥45 mL/minute/1.73 m^2: No dosage adjustment necessary.

eGFR <45 mL/minute/1.73 m^2: Do not initiate therapy; in patients already taking empagliflozin, discontinue therapy when eGFR is persistently <45 mL/minute/1.73 m^2

eGFR <30 mL/minute/1.73 m^2: Use is contraindicated.

ESRD, dialysis: Use is contraindicated.

Canadian labeling:

eGFR ≥60 mL/minute/1.73 m^2: No dosage adjustment necessary.

eGFR 45 to <60 mL/minute/1.73 m^2: Do not initiate therapy; in patients already taking empagliflozin, monitor closely and discontinue therapy if eGFR is reduced to <45 mL/minute/1.73 m^2.

eGFR <45 mL/minute/1.73 m^2: Use is contraindicated.

ESRD, dialysis: Use is contraindicated.

Hepatic Impairment

US labeling: There are no dosage adjustments provided in the manufacturer's labeling; may be used in patients with hepatic impairment.

Canadian labeling:
Mild or moderate impairment: No dosage adjustment is necessary.

Severe impairment: Use is not recommended (limited data).

Dietary Considerations Individualized medical nutrition therapy (MNT) based on ADA recommendations is an integral part of therapy

Administration Administer once daily in the morning, with or without food.

Monitoring Parameters Blood glucose, HbA$_{1c}$; renal function and volume status (baseline and periodically during treatment); LDL-C; monitor for genital mycotic infections and UTI; blood pressure

Reference Range
Recommendations for glycemic control in nonpregnant adults with diabetes (ADA, 2015):

HbA$_{1c}$: <7% (a more aggressive [<6.5%] or less aggressive [<8%] HbA$_{1c}$ goal may be targeted based on patient-specific characteristics)

Preprandial capillary plasma glucose: 80 to 130 mg/dL
Peak postprandial capillary blood glucose: <180 mg/dL

Recommendations for glycemic control in pediatric (all age groups) patients with type 1 diabetes (ADA, 2015):

HbA$_{1c}$: <7.5% (individualization may be appropriate based on patient-specific characteristics; <7% is reasonable if it can be achieved without excessive hypoglycemia)

Preprandial capillary plasma glucose: 90 to 130 mg/dL
Bedtime and overnight capillary blood glucose: 90 to 150 mg/dL

Test Interactions Positive test for glucosuria; may interfere with 1,5-anhydroglucitol (1,5-AG) assay; use alternative methods to monitor glycemic control.

Dosage Forms Excipient information presented when available (limited, particularly for generics); consult specific product labeling.

Tablet, Oral:
Jardiance: 10 mg, 25 mg

◆ **Empliciti** *see* Elotuzumab *on page 625*

◆ **Emsam** *see* Selegiline *on page 1644*

◆ **Emtec** *see* Acetaminophen and Codeine *on page 28*

Emtricitabine (em trye SYE ta been)

Brand Names: US Emtriva
Brand Names: Canada Emtriva
Index Terms BW524W91; Coviracil; FTC
Pharmacologic Category Antiretroviral, Reverse Transcriptase Inhibitor, Nucleoside (Anti-HIV)
Use Treatment of HIV infection in combination with at least two other antiretroviral agents
Pregnancy Considerations Adverse events were not observed in animal studies. Emtricitabine has a high level of transfer across the human placenta; no increased risk of overall birth defects has been observed according to data collected by the antiretroviral pregnancy registry. Cases of lactic acidosis/hepatic steatosis syndrome related to mitochondrial toxicity have been reported in pregnant women with prolonged use of nucleoside analogues. It is not known if pregnancy itself potentiates this known side effect; however, women may be at increased risk of lactic acidosis and liver damage. In addition, these adverse events are similar to other rare but life-threatening syndromes which occur during pregnancy (eg, HELLP syndrome). Hepatic enzymes and electrolytes should be monitored in women receiving nucleoside analogues and clinicians should watch for early signs of the syndrome. In addition, mitochondrial dysfunction may develop in infants following in utero exposure. A pharmacokinetic study shows a slight decrease in emtricitabine serum levels during the third trimester and immediately postpartum; however, there is no clear need to adjust the dose. The DHHS Perinatal HIV Guidelines consider emtricitabine with tenofovir to be a preferred NRTI backbone in antiretroviral-naive pregnant women. The DHHS Perinatal HIV Guidelines consider emtricitabine plus tenofovir a recommended dual NRTI/NtRTI backbone for HIV/HBV coinfected pregnant women.

Regardless of CD4 count or HIV RNA copy number, all HIV-infected pregnant women should receive a combination antiretroviral (ARV) drug regimen. A combination of antepartum, intrapartum, and infant ARV prophylaxis is recommended. ARV therapy should be started as soon as possible in women with symptomatic infection. Although earlier initiation may be more effective in reducing the perinatal transmission of HIV, initiation may be delayed until after 12 weeks gestation in women who do not require immediate treatment after careful consideration of

maternal conditions (eg, nausea and vomiting) and the potential risks of first trimester fetal exposure for specific agents. A scheduled cesarean delivery at 38 weeks gestation is recommended for all women with HIV RNA >1,000 copies/mL or unknown concentrations near delivery in order to decrease transmission. If ARV therapy must be interrupted for <24 hours during the peripartum period, stop then restart all medications simultaneously in order to decrease the chance of developing resistance. Long-term follow-up is recommended for all infants exposed to ARV medications. In couples who want to conceive, the HIV-infected partner should attain maximum viral suppression prior to conception.

Health care providers are encouraged to enroll pregnant women exposed to antiretroviral medications in the Antiretroviral Pregnancy Registry (1-800-258-4263 or www.APRegistry.com). Healthcare providers caring for HIV-infected women and their infants may contact the National Perinatal HIV Hotline (888-448-8765) for clinical consultation (HHS [perinatal], 2014).

Breast-Feeding Considerations Emtricitabine is excreted into breast milk. Maternal or infant antiretroviral therapy does not completely eliminate the risk of postnatal HIV transmission. In addition, multiclass-resistant virus has been detected in breast-feeding infants despite maternal therapy. Therefore, in the United States, where formula is accessible, affordable, safe, and sustainable, and the risk of infant mortality due to diarrhea and respiratory infections is low, complete avoidance of breast-feeding by HIV-infected women is recommended to decrease potential transmission of HIV (HHS [perinatal], 2014).

Contraindications Hypersensitivity to emtricitabine or any component of the formulation

Warnings/Precautions [U.S. Boxed Warning]: Lactic acidosis, severe hepatomegaly with steatosis, and hepatic failure have occurred rarely with emtricitabine (similar to other nucleoside analogues). Some cases have been fatal; stop treatment if lactic acidosis or hepatotoxicity occur. Prior liver disease, obesity, extended duration of therapy, and female gender may represent risk factors for severe hepatic reactions. Testing for hepatitis B is recommended prior to the initiation of therapy; **[U.S. Boxed Warnings]: Hepatitis B may be exacerbated following discontinuation of emtricitabine; not indicated for treatment of chronic hepatitis B; safety and efficacy in HIV/HBV coinfected patients not established.** May be associated with fat redistribution (buffalo hump, increased abdominal girth, breast engorgement, facial atrophy, and dyslipidemia). Immune reconstitution syndrome may develop resulting in the occurrence of an inflammatory response to an indolent or residual opportunistic infection during initial HIV treatment or activation of autoimmune disorders (eg, Graves' disease, polymyositis, Guillain-Barré syndrome) later in therapy; further evaluation and treatment may be required. Use caution in patients with renal impairment (dosage adjustment required). Concomitant use of other emtricitabine-containing products should be avoided. Concomitant use of lamivudine or lamivudine-containing products should be avoided; cross-resistance may develop.

Adverse Reactions Clinical trials were conducted in patients receiving other antiretroviral agents, and it is not possible to correlate frequency of adverse events with emtricitabine alone. The range of frequencies of adverse events is generally comparable to comparator groups, with the exception of hyperpigmentation, which occurred more frequently in patients receiving emtricitabine. Unless otherwise noted, percentages are as reported in adults.

>10%:
Central nervous system: Dizziness (4% to 25%), headache (6% to 22%), fever (children 18%), insomnia (5% to 16%), abnormal dreams (2% to 11%)
Dermatologic: Hyperpigmentation (children 32%; adults 2% to 4%; primarily of palms and/or soles but may include tongue, arms, lip and nails; generally mild and nonprogressive without associated local reactions such as pruritus or rash); rash (17% to 30%; includes pruritus, maculopapular rash, vesiculobullous rash, pustular rash, and allergic reaction)
Gastrointestinal: Diarrhea (children 20%; adults 9% to 23%), vomiting (children 23%; adults 9%), nausea (13% to 18%), abdominal pain (8% to 14%), gastroenteritis (children 11%)
Neuromuscular & skeletal: Weakness (12% to 16%), CPK increased (grades 3/4: 11% to 12%)
Otic: Otitis media (children 23%)
Respiratory: Cough (children 28%; adults 14%), rhinitis (children 20%; adults 12% to 18%), pneumonia (children 15%)
Miscellaneous: Infection (children 44%)

1% to 10%:

Central nervous system: Depression (6% to 9%), neuropathy/neuritis (4%)

Endocrine & metabolic: Serum triglycerides increased (grades 3/4: 4% to 10%), disordered glucose homeostasis (grades 3/4: 2% to 3%), serum amylase increased (grades 3/4: children 9%; adults 2% to 5%), serum lipase increased (grades 3/4: ≤1%)

Gastrointestinal: Dyspepsia (4% to 8%), serum amylase increased (grades 3/4: 8%)

Genitourinary: Hematuria (grades 3/4: 3%)

Hematologic: Anemia (children: 7%), neutropenia (grades 3/4: children 2%; adults 5%)

Hepatic: Transaminases increased (grades 3/4: 2% to 6%), alkaline phosphatase increased (>550 units/L: 1%), bilirubin increased (grades 3/4: 1%)

Neuromuscular & skeletal: Creatinine kinase increased (grades 3/4: 9%), myalgia (4% to 6%), paresthesia (5% to 6%), arthralgia (3% to 5%)

Respiratory: Upper respiratory tract infection (8%), sinusitis (8%), pharyngitis (5%)

<1% (Limited to important or life-threatening): Immune reconstitution syndrome

Drug Interactions

Metabolism/Transport Effects None known.

Avoid Concomitant Use

Avoid concomitant use of Emtricitabine with any of the following: LamiVUDine

Increased Effect/Toxicity

The levels/effects of Emtricitabine may be increased by: Ganciclovir-Valganciclovir; LamiVUDine; Ribavirin (Oral Inhalation); Ribavirin (Systemic)

Decreased Effect There are no known significant interactions involving a decrease in effect.

Food Interactions Food decreases peak plasma concentrations, but does not alter the extent of absorption or overall systemic exposure. Management: Administer without regard to meals.

Storage/Stability

Capsules: Store at 25°C (77°F); excursions permitted to 15°C to 30°C (59°F to 86°F).

Oral solution: Store at 2°C to 8°C (36°F to 46°F). Use within 3 months if stored at 25°C (77°F) with excursions permitted to 15°C to 30°C (59°F to 86°F).

Mechanism of Action Nucleoside reverse transcriptase inhibitor; emtricitabine is a cytosine analogue which is phosphorylated intracellularly to emtricitabine 5'-triphosphate which interferes with HIV viral RNA dependent DNA polymerase resulting in inhibition of viral replication.

Pharmacodynamics/Kinetics

Absorption: Rapid, extensive

Protein binding: <4%

Metabolism: Converted intracellularly to the active triphosphate form; undergoes minimal biotransformation via oxidation and glucuronide conjugation

Bioavailability: Capsule: 93%; solution: 75%; **Note:** Relative bioavailability of solution to capsule: 80%

Half-life elimination: Normal renal function:

Infants, Children, and Adolescents: Elimination half-life (emtricitabine):

Single dose: 11 hours

Multiple dose: 7.9 to 9.5 hours

Infants 0 to 3 months (n=20; median age: 26 days): 12.1 ± 3.1 hours

Infants 3 to 24 months (n=14): 8.9 ± 3.2 hours

Children 25 months to 6 years (n=19): 11.3 ± 6.4 hours

Children 7 to 12 years (n=17): 8.2 ± 3.2 hours

Adolescents 13 to 17 years (n=27): 8.9 ± 3.3 hours

Adults: Emtricitabine: 10 hours; Intracellular half-life (emtricitabine 5'-triphosphate): 39 hours

Time to peak, plasma: 1-2 hours

Excretion: Urine (86% primarily as unchanged drug, 13% as metabolites, 9% of dose as oxidative metabolite; 4% as glucuronide metabolite); feces (14%)

Clearance: Renal clearance is greater than creatinine clearance; thus, emtricitabine may be eliminated by both glomerular filtration and active tubular secretion

Dosing

Adult & Geriatric

HIV infection: Oral: **Note:** Emtricitabine is a component of recommended initial regimens in all treatment-naive patients (coadministered with dolutegravir and tenofovir, with raltegravir and tenofovir, or with darunavir/ritonavir and tenofovir); as a component of a recommended initial regimen only for treatment-naive patients with pre-ART CrCl>70 mL/minute (coadministered with elvitegravir/cobicistat and tenofovir); and as a component of a recommended initial regimen only for treatment-naive patients who are HLA-B*5701 negative (coadministered with dolutegravir and abacavir) (HHS [adult] 2015).

Capsule: 200 mg once daily

Solution: 240 mg once daily

Pediatric HIV infection: Oral:

Children: 0 to 3 months: Solution: 3 mg/kg/day

Children: 3 months to 17 years:

Capsule: Children >33 kg: 200 mg once daily

Solution: 6 mg/kg once daily; maximum: 240 mg/day

Renal Impairment Adults (consider similar adjustments in children):

CrCl 30 to 49 mL/minute: Capsule: 200 mg every 48 hours; solution: 120 mg every 24 hours

CrCl 15 to 29 mL/minute: Capsule: 200 mg every 72 hours; solution: 80 mg every 24 hours

CrCl <15 mL/minute (including hemodialysis patients): Capsule: 200 mg every 96 hours; solution: 60 mg every 24 hours; administer after dialysis

Hepatic Impairment No dosage adjustment required.

Dietary Considerations May be taken with or without food.

Administration May be administered with or without food.

Monitoring Parameters Viral load, CD4, liver function tests; hepatitis B testing is recommended prior to initiation of therapy

Dosage Forms Excipient information presented when available (limited, particularly for generics); consult specific product labeling.

Capsule, Oral:

Emtriva: 200 mg [contains fd&c blue #2 (indigotine)]

Solution, Oral:

Emtriva: 10 mg/mL (170 mL) [contains edetate disodium, fd&c yellow #6 (sunset yellow), methylparaben, propylene glycol, propylparaben; cotton candy flavor]

Emtricitabine and Tenofovir Disoproxil Fumarate

(em trye SYE ta been & ten OF oh vir dye soe PROX il FUE ma rate)

Brand Names: US Truvada

Brand Names: Canada Truvada

Index Terms Tenofovir Disoproxil Fumarate and Emtricitabine

Pharmacologic Category Antiretroviral, Reverse Transcriptase Inhibitor, Nucleoside (Anti-HIV); Antiretroviral, Reverse Transcriptase Inhibitor, Nucleotide (Anti-HIV)

Use

Treatment of HIV-1 infection in combination with other antiretroviral agents in adults and pediatric patients ≥12 years of age

Pre-exposure prophylaxis (PrEP) for prevention of HIV-1 infection in adults who are at high risk for acquiring HIV

High risk individuals include those with partners known to be HIV-1 infected or who engage in sexual activity within a high prevalence area or social network, and one or more of the following:

- Inconsistent or no condom use
- Diagnosis of sexually-transmitted infections
- Exchange of sex for commodities
- Use of illicit drugs or alcohol dependence
- Incarceration
- Partner of unknown HIV-1 status with any of the above risk factors

When prescribing PrEP healthcare providers **MUST:**

- Include PrEP as part of a comprehensive prevention strategy because PrEP alone is not always effective in preventing HIV-1 infection
- Counsel all uninfected patients to strictly adhere to the dosing schedule, because adherence was strongly correlated with effectiveness in clinical trials
- Confirm a negative HIV-1 test prior to starting PrEP; if a candidate has acute viral infection symptoms and unprotected exposure events <1 month prior, delay PrEP for at least 1 month and retest HIV-1 status or use an Food and Drug Administration (FDA) test approved for HIV-1 diagnosis, including acute or primary HIV-1 infection
- Retest for HIV-1 infection at least every 3 months while the patient receives PrEP

Medication Guide Available Yes

Dosing

Adult & Geriatric Note: Avoid concurrent use with adefovir or lamivudine-containing products or other emtricitabine- and/or tenofovir-containing products.

HIV-1 infection: Oral: One tablet (emtricitabine 200 mg and tenofovir 300 mg) once daily in combination with other antiretroviral agents. **Note:** Emtricitabine and tenofovir is a component of recommended initial regimens in all treatment-naive patients (coadministered with dolutegravir, with raltegravir, or with darunavir/ritonavir), and is a component of a recommended initial regimen only for treatment-naive adolescent and adult patients with pre-ART CrCl >70 mL/minute (coadministered with elvitegravir/cobicistat) (HHS [adult] 2015).

Preexposure prophylaxis (PrEP) for prevention of HIV infection in uninfected high-risk individuals: Oral: One tablet (emtricitabine 200 mg and tenofovir 300 mg) once daily

Hepatitis B treatment in patients with antiviral-resistant HBV or coinfection with HIV (off-label use): Oral: One tablet (emtricitabine 200 mg and tenofovir 300 mg) once daily (Lok 2009)

Occupational HIV postexposure, prophylaxis (PEP) (off-label use): Oral: One tablet (emtricitabine 200 mg and tenofovir 300 mg) once daily for 4 weeks with concomitant raltegravir. Recommended as preferred therapy (Kuhar 2013)

PrEP for prevention of HIV infection in injecting drug users (IDU) who are at risk for parenteral acquisition of HIV but not at risk for sexual acquisition of HIV (off-label use): Oral: One tablet (emtricitabine 200 mg and tenofovir 300 mg) once daily (CDC 2013)

Pediatric HIV-1 infection: Children ≥12 years (≥35 kg) and Adolescents (≥35 kg): Oral: Refer to adult dosing.

Renal Impairment

HIV-1 infection: Adults:

Manufacturer's labeling:

CrCl ≥50 mL/minute: No dosage adjustment necessary

CrCl 30 to 49 mL/minute: Increase interval to every 48 hours.

CrCl <30 mL/minute or hemodialysis: Not recommended.

Alternate recommendations (IDSA [Lucas 2014]): CrCl <50 mL/minute (and not on hemodialysis) or GFR <60 mL/minute/1.73 m²: Avoid use of tenofovir

PrEP: Adults:

CrCl ≥60 mL/minute: No dosage adjustment necessary

CrCl <60 mL/minute: Not recommended.

Hepatic Impairment No dosing adjustment necessary for tenofovir in moderate-to-severe hepatic compromise; no specific data available on emtricitabine in hepatic impairment, but given limited hepatic metabolism, dose adjustments are unlikely.

Additional Information Complete prescribing information should be consulted for additional detail.

Dosage Forms Excipient information presented when available (limited, particularly for generics); consult specific product labeling.

Tablet:

Truvada: Emtricitabine 200 mg and tenofovir disoproxil fumarate 300 mg

♦ Emtricitabine, Efavirenz, and Tenofovir Disoproxil Fumarate see Efavirenz, Emtricitabine, and Tenofovir Disoproxil Fumarate on page 621

♦ Emtricitabine, Elvitegravir, Cobicistat, and Tenofovir Alafenamide see Elvitegravir, Cobicistat, Emtricitabine, and Tenofovir Alafenamide on page 632

Emtricitabine, Rilpivirine, and Tenofovir Disoproxil Fumarate

(em trye SYE ta been, ril pi VIR een, & ten OF oh vir dye soe PROX il FUE ma rate)

Brand Names: US Complera

Brand Names: Canada Complera

Index Terms FTC/RPV/TDF; Rilpivirine, Emtricitabine, and Tenofovir Disoproxil Fumarate; Tenofovir Disoproxil Fumarate, Emtricitabine, and Rilpivirine; Tenofovir Disoproxil Fumarate, Rilpivirine, and Emtricitabine

Pharmacologic Category Antiretroviral, Reverse Transcriptase Inhibitor, Non-nucleoside (Anti-HIV); Antiretroviral, Reverse Transcriptase Inhibitor, Nucleoside (Anti-HIV); Antiretroviral, Reverse Transcriptase Inhibitor, Nucleotide (Anti-HIV)

Use HIV-1 infection: Treatment of HIV-1 infection (as a complete regimen) in antiretroviral treatment-naive adult patients with HIV-1 RNA ≤100,000 copies/mL at the start of therapy, and in certain virologically suppressed (HIV-1 RNA <50 copies/mL) adult patients on a stable antiretroviral regimen at start of therapy in order to replace their current antiretroviral treatment regimen.

Dosing

Adult & Geriatric HIV: Oral: One tablet once daily

Dosage adjustment for concomitant therapy with rifabutin: One tablet once daily plus rilpivirine 25 mg

Renal Impairment

CrCl ≥50 mL/minute: No dosage adjustments necessary.

CrCl <50 mL/minute: Use is not recommended.

ESRD requiring dialysis: Use is not recommended.

Hepatic Impairment

Mild-to-moderate impairment (Child-Pugh class A or B): No dosage adjustments necessary.

Severe impairment (Child-Pugh class C): There are no dosage adjustments provided in the manufacturer's labeling (has not been studied).

Additional Information Complete prescribing information should be consulted for additional detail.

Dosage Forms Excipient information presented when available (limited, particularly for generics); consult specific product labeling.

Tablet, oral:

Complera: Emtricitabine 200 mg, rilpivirine 25 mg, and tenofovir disoproxil fumarate 300 mg

♦ Emtricitabine, Tenofovir Disoproxil Fumarate, Elvitegravir, and Cobicistat see Elvitegravir, Cobicistat, Emtricitabine, and Tenofovir Disoproxil Fumarate on page 632

♦ Emtriva see Emtricitabine on page 634

♦ ENA 713 see Rivastigmine on page 1607

♦ Enablex see Darifenacin on page 496

♦ Enablex® (Can) see Darifenacin on page 496

Enalapril (e NAL a pril)

Brand Names: US Epaned; Vasotec

Brand Names: Canada ACT-Enalapril; Apo-Enalapril; Mylan-Enalapril; PMS-Enalapril; PRO-Enalapril; RAN-Enalapril; Riva-Enalapril; Sandoz-Enalapril; Sig-Enalapril; Taro-Enalapril; Teva-Enalapril; Vasotec

Index Terms Enalapril Maleate

Pharmacologic Category Angiotensin-Converting Enzyme (ACE) Inhibitor; Antihypertensive

Use

Asymptomatic left ventricular dysfunction: Treatment of asymptomatic left ventricular dysfunction

Heart failure: Treatment of symptomatic heart failure (HF)

Hypertension: Treatment of hypertension

Guideline recommendations:

Hypertension: The 2014 guideline for the management of high blood pressure in adults (Eighth Joint National Committee [JNC 8]) recommends initiation of pharmacologic treatment to lower blood pressure for the following patients:

• Patients ≥60 years of age with systolic blood pressure (SBP) ≥150 mm Hg or diastolic blood pressure (DBP) ≥90 mm Hg. Goal of therapy is SBP <150 mm Hg and DBP <90 mm Hg.

• Patients <60 years of age with SBP ≥140 mm Hg or DBP is ≥90 mm Hg. Goal of therapy is SBP <140 mm Hg and DBP <90 mm Hg.

• Patients ≥18 years of age with diabetes and SBP ≥140 mm Hg or DBP ≥90 mm Hg. Goal of therapy is SBP <140 mm Hg and DBP <90 mm Hg.

• Patients ≥18 years of age with chronic kidney disease (CKD) and SBP ≥140 mm Hg or DBP ≥90 mm Hg. Goal of therapy is SBP <140 mm Hg and DBP <90 mm Hg.

Chronic kidney disease (CKD) and hypertension: Regardless of race or diabetes status, the use of an ACE inhibitor (ACEI) or angiotensin receptor blocker (ARB) as initial therapy is recommended to improve kidney outcomes. In the general nonblack population (without CKD) including those with diabetes, initial antihypertensive treatment should consist of a thiazide-type diuretic, calcium channel blocker, ACEI, or ARB. In the general black population (without CKD) including those with diabetes, initial antihypertensive treatment should consist of a thiazide-type diuretic or a calcium channel blocker **instead of** an ACEI or ARB.

Coronary artery disease (CAD) and hypertension: The American Heart Association, American College of Cardiology and American Society of Hypertension (AHA/ACC/ASH) 2015 scientific statement for the treatment of hypertension in patients with CAD recommends the use of an ACE inhibitor (or an ARB) as part of a regimen in patients with hypertension and chronic stable angina if there is prior MI, LV systolic dysfunction, diabetes mellitus, or CKD. A BP target of <140/90 mm Hg is reasonable for the secondary prevention of cardiovascular events. A lower target BP (<130/80 mm Hg) may be appropriate in some individuals with CAD, previous MI, stroke or transient ischemic attack, or CAD risk equivalents (AHA/ACC/ASH [Rosendorff 2015]).

Heart failure: The ACCF/AHA 2013 heart failure guidelines recommend the use of ACE inhibitors, along with other guideline directed medical therapies, to prevent heart failure in patients with a reduced ejection fraction who have a history of MI (Stage B HF), to prevent heart failure in any patient with a reduced ejection fraction (Stage B HF), or to treat those with heart failure and reduced ejection fraction (Stage C HFrEF) (ACCF/AHA [Yancy 2013]).

Pregnancy Considerations [U.S. Boxed Warning]: Drugs that act on the renin-angiotensin system can cause injury and death to the developing fetus. Discontinue as soon as possible once pregnancy is detected. Enalapril crosses the placenta; the active metabolite enalaprilat can be detected in the newborn (Schubiger 1988).

Drugs that act on the renin-angiotensin system are associated with oligohydramnios. Oligohydramnios, due to decreased fetal renal function, may lead to fetal lung hypoplasia and skeletal malformations. The use of these drugs in pregnancy is also associated with anuria, hypotension, renal failure, skull hypoplasia, and death in the fetus/neonate. Teratogenic effects may occur following maternal use of an ACE inhibitor during the first trimester, although this finding may be confounded by maternal disease. Because adverse fetal events are well documented with exposure later in pregnancy, ACE inhibitor use in pregnant women is not recommended (Seely 2014; Weber 2014). Infants exposed to an ACE inhibitor in utero should be monitored for hyperkalemia, hypotension, and oliguria. Oligohydramnios may not appear until after irreversible fetal injury has occurred. Exchange transfusions or dialysis may be required to reverse hypotension or improve renal function, although data related to the effectiveness in neonates is limited.

Chronic maternal hypertension itself is also associated with adverse events in the fetus/infant and mother. ACE inhibitors are not recommended for the treatment of uncomplicated hypertension in pregnancy (ACOG 2013) and they are specifically contraindicated for the treatment of hypertension and chronic heart failure during pregnancy by some guidelines (Regitz-Zagrosek 2011). In addition, ACE inhibitors should generally be avoided in women of reproductive age (ACOG 2013). If treatment for hypertension or chronic heart failure in pregnancy is needed, other agents should be used (ACOG 2013; Regitz-Zagrosek 2011).

Breast-Feeding Considerations Enalapril and enalaprilat are excreted in breast milk. Due to the potential for serious adverse reactions in the nursing infant, the manufacturer recommends a decision be made whether to discontinue nursing or to discontinue the drug, taking into account the importance of treatment to the mother. Some guidelines consider enalapril to be acceptable for use in breast-feeding women. Monitoring of the nursing child's weight for the first 4 weeks is recommended (Regitz-Zagrosek 2011).

Contraindications

Hypersensitivity to enalapril or any component of the formulation; angioedema related to previous treatment with an ACE inhibitor; patients with idiopathic or hereditary angioedema; concomitant use with aliskiren in patients with diabetes mellitus

Documentation of allergenic cross-reactivity for ACE inhibitors is limited. However, because of similarities in chemical structure and/or pharmacologic actions, the possibility of cross-sensitivity cannot be ruled out with certainty.

Canadian labeling: Additional contraindications (not in U.S. labeling): Concomitant use with aliskiren-containing drugs in patients with moderate-to-severe renal impairment (GFR <60 mL/minute/1.73 m^2)

Warnings/Precautions Anaphylactic reactions may occur rarely with ACE inhibitors. At any time during treatment (especially following first dose) angioedema may occur rarely with ACE inhibitors; it may involve the head and neck (potentially compromising airway) or the intestine (presenting with abdominal pain). African-Americans may be at an increased risk. Risk may also be increased with concomitant use of mTOR inhibitor (eg, everolimus) therapy. Prolonged frequent monitoring may be required especially if tongue, glottis, or larynx are involved as they are associated with airway obstruction. Patients with a history of airway surgery may have a higher risk of airway obstruction. Aggressive early and appropriate management is critical. Use in patients with idiopathic or hereditary angioedema or previous angioedema associated with ACE inhibitor therapy is contraindicated. Severe anaphylactoid reactions may be seen during hemodialysis (eg, CVVHD) with high-flux dialysis membranes (eg, AN69), and rarely, during low density lipoprotein apheresis with dextran sulfate cellulose. Rare cases of anaphylactoid reactions have been reported in patients undergoing sensitization treatment with hymenoptera (bee, wasp) venom while receiving ACE inhibitors.

Symptomatic hypotension with or without syncope can occur with ACE inhibitors (usually with the first several doses); effects are most often observed in volume depleted patients; correct volume depletion prior to initiation; close monitoring of patient is required especially with initial dosing and dosing increases; blood pressure must be lowered at a rate appropriate for the patient's clinical condition. Initiation of therapy in patients with ischemic heart disease or cerebrovascular disease warrants close observation due to the potential consequences posed by falling blood pressure (eg, MI, stroke). Use with caution in hypertrophic cardiomyopathy with outflow tract obstruction and severe aortic stenosis. In patients on chronic ACE inhibitor therapy, intraoperative hypotension may occur with induction and maintenance of general anesthesia; use with caution before, during, or immediately after major surgery. Cardiopulmonary bypass, intraoperative blood loss, or vasodilating anesthesia increases endogenous renin release. Use of ACE inhibitors perioperatively will blunt angiotensin II formation and may result in hypotension. However, discontinuation of therapy prior to surgery is controversial. If continued preoperatively, avoidance of hypotensive agents during surgery is prudent (Hillis, 2011).

[U.S. Boxed Warning]: Drugs that act on the renin-angiotensin system can cause injury and death to the developing fetus. Discontinue as soon as possible once pregnancy is detected.

Hyperkalemia may occur with ACE inhibitors; risk factors include renal dysfunction, diabetes mellitus, concomitant use of potassium-sparing diuretics, potassium supplements, and/or potassium-containing salts. Use cautiously, if at all, with these agents and monitor potassium closely. Cough may occur with ACE inhibitors. Other causes of cough should be considered (eg, pulmonary congestion in patients with heart failure) and excluded prior to discontinuation.

May be associated with deterioration of renal function and/or increases in serum creatinine, particularly in patients with low renal blood flow (eg, renal artery stenosis, heart failure) whose glomerular filtration rate (GFR) is dependent on efferent arteriolar vasoconstriction by angiotensin II; deterioration may result in oliguria, acute renal failure, and progressive azotemia. Small increases in serum creatinine may occur following initiation; consider discontinuation only in patients with progressive and/or significant deterioration in renal function. Use with caution in patients with unstented unilateral/bilateral renal artery stenosis. When unstented bilateral renal artery stenosis is present, use is generally avoided due to the elevated risk of deterioration in renal function unless possible benefits outweigh risks. Potentially significant drug-drug interactions may exist, requiring dose or frequency adjustment, additional monitoring, and/or selection of alternative therapy.

Rare toxicities associated with ACE inhibitors include cholestatic jaundice (which may progress to fulminant hepatic necrosis), agranulocytosis, neutropenia or leukopenia with myeloid hypoplasia. Patients with collagen vascular diseases (especially with concomitant renal impairment) or renal impairment alone may be at increased risk for hematologic toxicity; periodically monitor CBC with differential in these patients.

Adverse Reactions Note: Frequency ranges include data from hypertension and heart failure trials. Higher rates of adverse reactions have generally been noted in patients with CHF. However, the frequency of adverse effects associated with placebo is also increased in this population.

>10%: Renal: Increased serum creatinine (≤20%)
1% to 10%:
Cardiovascular: Hypotension (1% to 7%), chest pain (2%), orthostatic effect (1% to 2%), orthostatic hypotension (2%), syncope (≤2%)
Central nervous system: Dizziness (4% to 8%), headache (2% to 5%), fatigue (2% to 3%)
Dermatologic: Skin rash (1% to 2%)
Gastrointestinal: Abdominal pain, anorexia, constipation, diarrhea, dysgeusia, nausea, vomiting
Neuromuscular & skeletal: Weakness
Renal: Renal insufficiency (in patients with bilateral renal artery stenosis or hypovolemia)
Respiratory: Bronchitis (1% to 2%), cough (1% to 2%), dyspnea (1% to 2%)
<1%, postmarketing, and/or case reports: Acute generalized exanthematous pustulosis, agranulocytosis, alopecia, anaphylactoid reaction, angina pectoris, angioedema, anosmia, arthritis, asthma, ataxia, atrial fibrillation, atrial tachycardia, bone marrow depression, bradycardia, cardiac arrest, cardiac arrhythmia, cerebrovascular accident, cholestatic jaundice, confusion, conjunctivitis, depression, eosinophilia, eosinophilic pneumonitis, erythema multiforme, exfoliative dermatitis, giant-cell arteritis, gynecomastia, hallucination, hemolysis (with G6PD), herpes zoster, IgA vasculitis, increased erythrocyte sedimentation rate, intestinal obstruction, ▶

insomnia, interstitial nephritis, leukocytosis, lichenoid eruption, melena, myocardial infarction, myositis, neutropenia, ototoxicity, pancreatitis, pemphigus, pemphigus foliaceus, peripheral neuropathy, positive ANA titer, psychosis, pulmonary edema, pulmonary embolism, pulmonary infarct, pulmonary infiltrates, Raynaud's phenomenon, serositis, Sjogren's syndrome, skin photosensitivity, Stevens-Johnson syndrome, stomatitis, systemic lupus erythematosus, thrombocytopenia, toxic epidermal necrolysis, upper respiratory tract infection, vasculitis, visual hallucination (Doane, 2013)

Drug Interactions

Metabolism/Transport Effects None known.

Avoid Concomitant Use

Avoid concomitant use of Enalapril with any of the following: Sacubitril

Increased Effect/Toxicity

Enalapril may increase the levels/effects of: Allopurinol; Amifostine; Antipsychotic Agents (Second Generation [Atypical]); AzaTHIOprine; Ciprofloxacin (Systemic); Drospirenone; DULoxetine; Ferric Gluconate; Gold Sodium Thiomalate; Grass Pollen Allergen Extract (5 Grass Extract); Hypotension-Associated Agents; Iron Dextran Complex; Levodopa; Lithium; Nonsteroidal Anti-Inflammatory Agents; Pregabalin; Sacubitril; Sodium Phosphates

The levels/effects of Enalapril may be increased by: Alfuzosin; Aliskiren; Angiotensin II Receptor Blockers; Barbiturates; Brimonidine (Topical); Canagliflozin; Dapoxetine; Diazoxide; DPP-IV Inhibitors; Eplerenone; Everolimus; Heparin; Heparin (Low Molecular Weight); Herbs (Hypotensive Properties); Loop Diuretics; Molsidomine; Nicorandil; Obinutuzumab; Pentoxifylline; Phosphodiesterase 5 Inhibitors; Potassium Salts; Potassium-Sparing Diuretics; Prostacyclin Analogues; Salicylates; Sirolimus; Temsirolimus; Thiazide Diuretics; TiZANidine; Tolvaptan; Trimethoprim

Decreased Effect

The levels/effects of Enalapril may be decreased by: Amphetamines; Aprotinin; Herbs (Hypertensive Properties); Icatibant; Lanthanum; Methylphenidate; Nonsteroidal Anti-Inflammatory Agents; Salicylates; Yohimbine

Preparation for Administration Epaned: Solution kit (for 150 mL, enalapril solution 1 mg/mL): Kit contains 1 bottle of enalapril powder and 1 bottle of Ora-Sweet SF dilution to be added to the enalapril powder prior to dispensing. Firmly tap the enalapril powder for oral solution bottle on a hard surface 5 times. Add approximately one-half (75 mL) of the Ora-Sweet SF diluent to the enalapril 150 mL oral solution bottle and shake well for 30 seconds. Add the remainder of the Ora-Sweet SF diluent and shake well for an additional 30 seconds. May be used for 60 days after reconstitution.

Storage/Stability

Solution kit: Store at 25°C (77°F); excursions are permitted between 15°C and 30°C (59°F and 86°F). Do not freeze. Protect from moisture. Once reconstituted, the solution should be stored at 15°C to 30°C (59°F to 86°F) and may be stored for up to 60 days.

Tablet: Store at 25°C (77°F); excursions permitted to 15°C to 30°C (59°F to 86°F). Protect from moisture.

Mechanism of Action Competitive inhibitor of angiotensin-converting enzyme (ACE); prevents conversion of angiotensin I to angiotensin II, a potent vasoconstrictor; results in lower levels of angiotensin II which causes an increase in plasma renin activity and a reduction in aldosterone secretion

Pharmacodynamics/Kinetics

Onset of action: ~1 hour

Peak effect: 4 to 6 hours

Duration: 12 to 24 hours

Absorption: 55% to 75%

Protein binding: ~50% (Davies, 1984)

Metabolism: Prodrug, undergoes hepatic biotransformation to enalaprilat

Half-life elimination:

Enalapril: CHF: Neonates (n=3, PNA: 10-19 days): 10.3 hours (range: 4.2-13.4 hours) (Nakamura, 1994); CHF: Infants and Children ≤6.5 years of age (n=11): 2.7 hours (range: 1.3-6.3 hours) (Nakamura, 1994); Adults: Healthy: 2 hours; Congestive heart failure: 3.4 to 5.8 hours

Enalaprilat: CHF: Neonates (n=3, PNA: 10-19 days): 11.9 hours (range: 5.9-15.6 hours) (Nakamura, 1994); CHF: Infants and Children ≤6.5 years of age (n=11): 11.1 hours (range: 5.1-20.8 hours) (Nakamura, 1994); Infants 6 weeks to 8 months of age: 6 to 10 hours (Lloyd, 1989); Adults: ~35 hours (Till, 1984; Ulm, 1982)

Time to peak, serum: Oral: Enalapril: 0.5 to 1.5 hours; Enalaprilat (active metabolite): 3 to 4.5 hours

Excretion: Urine (61%; 18% of which was enalapril, 43% was enalaprilat); feces (33%; 6% of which was enalapril, 27% was enalaprilat) (Ulm, 1982)

Dosing

Adult & Geriatric Use lower listed initial dose in patients with hyponatremia, hypovolemia, severe congestive heart failure, decreased renal function, or in those receiving diuretics.

Asymptomatic left ventricular dysfunction: Oral: 2.5 mg twice daily, titrated as tolerated to 20 mg daily

Heart failure with reduced ejection fraction (HFrEF): Oral: Initial: 2.5 mg twice daily (usual range: 5 to 40 mg daily in 2 divided doses); titrate slowly at 1- to 2-week intervals. Target dose: 10 to 20 mg twice daily (ACCF/AHA [Yancy, 2013])

Hypertension: Oral: 2.5 to 5 mg daily then increase as required, usually at 1- to 2-week intervals; usual dose range (ASH/ISH [Weber, 2014]): 10 to 40 mg daily. Target dose (JNC 8 [James, 2013]): 20 mg daily in 1 or 2 divided doses. **Note:** Initiate with 2.5 mg if patient is taking a diuretic which cannot be discontinued. May add a diuretic if blood pressure cannot be controlled with enalapril alone.

Conversion from IV **enalaprilat** to oral **enalapril** therapy: If not concurrently receiving diuretics, initiate enalapril 5 mg once daily; if concurrently receiving diuretics and responding to enalaprilat 0.625 mg IV every 6 hours, initiate with enalapril 2.5 mg once daily; subsequent titration as needed.

Pediatric

Hypertension: Children ≥1 month and Adolescents: Oral: Initial: 0.08 mg/kg (up to 5 mg) once daily; adjust dosage based on patient response; doses >0.58 mg/kg (40 mg) have not been evaluated in pediatric patients

Heart failure (off-label dosing): Infants and Children: Oral: Initial: 0.1 mg/kg/day in 1 to 2 divided doses; increase as required over 2 weeks to maximum of 0.5 mg/kg/day. **Note:** Mean dose required for CHF improvement in 39 children (9 days to 17 years) was 0.36 mg/kg/day; select individuals have been treated with doses up to 0.94 mg/kg/day (Leversha, 1994).

Renal Impairment Note: Use in infants and children ≤16 years of age with GFR <30 mL/minute/1.73 m² is not recommended (no dosing data exists).

Manufacturer's labeling:

CrCl >30 mL/minute: No dosage adjustment necessary

CrCl ≤30 mL/minute: Administer 2.5 mg day; titrated upward until blood pressure is controlled.

Heart failure patients with sodium <130 mEq/L or serum creatinine >1.6 mg/dL: Initiate dosage with 2.5 mg daily, increasing to twice daily as needed. Increase further in increments of 2.5 mg/dose at >4-day intervals to a maximum daily dose of 40 mg.

Intermittent hemodialysis (IHD): Moderately dialyzable (20% to 50%): Initial: 2.5 mg on dialysis days; adjust dose on nondialysis days depending on blood pressure response.

Conversion from IV **enalaprilat** to oral **enalapril** therapy:

CrCl >30 mL/minute: May initiate enalapril 5 mg once daily.

CrCl ≤30 mL/minute: May initiate enalapril 2.5 mg once daily.

Alternate recommendations (Aronoff, 2007):

CrCl >50 mL/minute: No dosage adjustment necessary

CrCl 10 to 50 mL/minute: Administer 75% to 100% of usual dose

CrCl <10 mL/minute: Administer 50% of usual dose

Peritoneal dialysis: Supplemental dose is not necessary, although some removal of drug occurs.

Hepatic Impairment No dosage adjustment is necessary. Hydrolysis of enalapril to enalaprilat may be delayed and/or impaired in patients with severe hepatic impairment, but the pharmacodynamic effects of the drug do not appear to be significantly altered.

Dietary Considerations Limit salt substitutes or potassium-rich diet.

Monitoring Parameters Blood pressure; serum creatinine and potassium; if patient has collagen vascular disease and/or renal impairment, periodically monitor CBC with differential

2013 ACCF/AHA Heart Failure guideline recommendations: Within 1-2 weeks after initiation and periodically thereafter, reassess renal function and serum potassium especially in patients with preexisting hypotension, hyponatremia, diabetes mellitus, azotemia, or those taking potassium supplements (ACCF/AHA [Yancy, 2013]).

Test Interactions Positive Coombs' [direct]; may cause false-positive results in urine acetone determinations using sodium nitroprusside reagent

Dosage Forms Excipient information presented when available (limited, particularly for generics); consult specific product labeling.

Solution Reconstituted, Oral, as maleate:
Epaned: 1 mg/mL (150 mL) [contains methylparaben, propylparaben, saccharin sodium; berry-citrus flavor]
Tablet, Oral, as maleate:
Vasotec: 2.5 mg, 5 mg, 10 mg, 20 mg [scored]
Generic: 2.5 mg, 5 mg, 10 mg, 20 mg

Dosage Forms: Canada Note: Refer to Dosage Forms. Oral powder for reconstitution is not available in Canada.

Extemporaneous Preparations Note: Commercial oral solution kit is available (1 mg/mL).

A 1 mg/mL oral suspension may be made with tablets, Bicitra [discontinued] or equivalent, and Ora-Sweet SF. Place ten 20 mg tablets in a 200 mL polyethylene terephthalate bottle; add 50 mL of Bicitra [discontinued] or equivalent and shake well for at least 2 minutes. Let stand for 1 hour then shake for 1 additional minute; add 150 mL of Ora-Sweet SF and shake well. Label "shake well" and "refrigerate". Stable for 30 days when stored in a polyethylene terephthalate bottle and refrigerated (Vasotec prescribing information, 2011).

A 1 mg/mL oral suspension may be made with tablets and one of three different vehicles (cherry syrup, a 1:1 mixture of Ora-Sweet and Ora-Plus, or a 1:1 mixture of Ora-Sweet SF and Ora-Plus). Crush six 20 mg tablets in a mortar and reduce to a fine powder. Add 15 mL of the chosen vehicle and mix to a uniform paste; mix while adding the vehicle in incremental proportions to **almost** 120 mL; transfer to a calibrated bottle, rinse mortar with vehicle, and add quantity of vehicle sufficient to make 120 mL. Label "shake well" and "protect from light". Stable for 60 days when stored in amber plastic prescription bottles in the dark at room temperature or refrigerated (Allen, 1998).

A 1 mg/mL oral suspension may be made with tablets and one of three different vehicles (deionized water, citrate buffer solution at pH 5.0, or a 1:1 mixture of Ora-Sweet and Ora-Plus). Crush twenty 10 mg tablets in a mortar and reduce to a fine powder. Add small portions of the chosen vehicle and mix to a uniform paste; mix while adding vehicle in incremental proportions to **almost** 200 mL; transfer to a graduated cylinder, rinse mortar with vehicle, and add quantity of vehicle sufficient to make 200 mL. Label "shake well" and "protect from light". Preparations made in citrate buffer solution at pH 5.0 and the 1:1 mixture of Ora-Sweet and Ora-Plus are stable for 91 days when stored in plastic prescription bottles in the dark at room temperature or refrigerated. Preparation made in deionized water is stable for 91 days refrigerated or 56 days at room temperature when stored in plastic prescription bottles in the dark. **Note:** To prepare the isotonic citrate buffer solution (pH 5.0), see reference (Nahata, 1998).

A more dilute, 0.1 mg/mL oral suspension may be made with tablets and an isotonic buffer solution at pH 5.0. Grind one 20 mg tablet in a glass mortar and reduce to a fine powder; mix with isotonic citrate buffer (pH 5.0) and filter; add quantity of buffer solution sufficient to make 200 mL. Label "shake well", "protect from light", and "refrigerate". Stable for 90 days (Boulton, 1994).

Allen LV Jr and Erickson MA 3rd, "Stability of Alprazolam, Chloroquine Phosphate, Cisapride, Enalapril Maleate, and Hydralazine Hydrochloride in Extemporaneously Compounded Oral Liquids," Am J Health Syst Pharm, 1998, 55(18):1915-20.

Boulton DW, Woods DJ, Fawcett JP, et al, "The Stability of an Enalapril Maleate Oral Solution Prepared From Tablets," Aust J Hosp Pharm, 1994, 24(2):151-6.

Nahata MC, Morosco RS, and Hipple TF, "Stability of Enalapril Maleate in Three Extemporaneously Prepared Oral Liquids," Am J Health Syst Pharm, 1998, 55(11):1155-7.

Vasotec® prescribing information, Valeant Pharmaceuticals North America LLC, Bridgewater, NJ; 2011.

Enalapril and Hydrochlorothiazide
(e NAL a pril & hye droe klor oh THYE a zide)

Brand Names: US Vaseretic
Brand Names: Canada Teva-Enalapril/HCTZ; Vaseretic
Index Terms Enalapril Maleate and Hydrochlorothiazide; Hydrochlorothiazide and Enalapril
Pharmacologic Category Angiotensin-Converting Enzyme (ACE) Inhibitor; Antihypertensive; Diuretic, Thiazide
Use Hypertension: Treatment of hypertension
Dosing
Adult & Geriatric
Hypertension: Oral: Initial: Enalapril 10 mg/hydrochlorothiazide 25 mg once daily; may increase dose based on patient response after 2 to 3 weeks (maximum: enalapril 20 mg/hydrochlorothiazide 50 mg per day)

Renal Impairment
CrCl >30 mL/minute/1.73 m^2: No dosage adjustment required.
CrCl ≤30 mL/minute/1.73 m^2: Avoid use.
Hepatic Impairment There are no dosage adjustments provided in the manufacturer's labeling; use with caution.
Additional Information Complete prescribing information should be consulted for additional detail.
Dosage Forms Excipient information presented when available (limited, particularly for generics); consult specific product labeling.
Tablet:
Vaseretic:
10/25: Enalapril maleate 10 mg and hydrochlorothiazide 25 mg
Generic:
5/12.5: Enalapril maleate 5 mg and hydrochlorothiazide 12.5 mg
10/25: Enalapril maleate 10 mg and hydrochlorothiazide 25 mg

Enfuvirtide (en FYOO vir tide)

Brand Names: US Fuzeon
Brand Names: Canada Fuzeon
Index Terms T-20
Pharmacologic Category Antiretroviral, Fusion Protein Inhibitor (Anti-HIV)
Use HIV-1 infection: Treatment of HIV-1 infection in combination with other antiretroviral agents in treatment-experienced patients with evidence of HIV-1 replication despite ongoing antiretroviral therapy
Dosing
Adult & Geriatric HIV treatment: SubQ: 90 mg twice daily
Pediatric
HIV treatment:
Children and Adolescents 6 to 16 years: SubQ: 2 mg/kg twice daily (maximum dose: 90 mg twice daily)
Adolescents >16 years: SubQ: Refer to adult dosing.
Renal Impairment No dosage adjustment necessary.
Hepatic Impairment No dosage adjustment necessary (has not been studied).
Additional Information Complete prescribing information should be consulted for additional detail.
Dosage Forms Excipient information presented when available (limited, particularly for generics); consult specific product labeling. [DSC] = Discontinued product
Kit, Subcutaneous:
Fuzeon: 90 mg [DSC]
Solution Reconstituted, Subcutaneous:
Fuzeon: 90 mg (1 ea)

Enoxaparin (ee noks a PA rin)

Brand Names: US Lovenox

Brand Names: Canada Lovenox; Lovenox HP; Lovenox With Preservative

Index Terms Enoxaparin Sodium

Pharmacologic Category Anticoagulant; Anticoagulant, Low Molecular Weight Heparin

Use

Acute coronary syndromes: Unstable angina (UA), non-ST-elevation (NSTEMI), and ST-elevation myocardial infarction (STEMI)

DVT prophylaxis: Following hip or knee replacement surgery, abdominal surgery, or in medical patients with severely-restricted mobility during acute illness who are at risk for thromboembolic complications. **Note:** Patients at risk of thromboembolic complications who undergo abdominal surgery include those with one or more of the following risk factors: >40 years of age, obesity, general anesthesia lasting >30 minutes, malignancy, history of deep vein thrombosis or pulmonary embolism

DVT treatment (acute): Inpatient treatment (patients with or without pulmonary embolism) and outpatient treatment (patients without pulmonary embolism)

Pregnancy Considerations Adverse events were not observed in animal reproduction studies. Low molecular weight heparin (LMWH) does not cross the placenta; increased risks of fetal bleeding or teratogenic effects have not been reported (Bates, 2012).

LMWH is recommended over unfractionated heparin for the treatment of acute venous thromboembolism (VTE) in pregnant women. LMWH is also recommended over unfractionated heparin for VTE prophylaxis in pregnant women with certain risk factors (eg, homozygous factor V Leiden, antiphospholipid antibody syndrome with ≥3 previous pregnancy losses). Prophylaxis is not routinely recommended for women undergoing assisted reproduction therapy; however, LMWH therapy is recommended for women who develop severe ovarian hyperstimulation syndrome. LMWH should be discontinued at least 24 hours prior to induction of labor or a planned cesarean delivery. For women undergoing cesarean section and who have additional risk factors for developing VTE, the prophylactic use of LMWH may be considered (Bates, 2012).

LMWH may also be used in women with mechanical heart valves (consult current guidelines for details) (Bates, 2012; Nishimura, 2014). Women who require long-term anticoagulation with warfarin and who are considering pregnancy, LMWH substitution should be done prior to conception when possible. When choosing therapy, fetal outcomes (ie, pregnancy loss, malformations), maternal outcomes (ie, VTE, hemorrhage), burden of therapy, and maternal preference should be considered (Bates, 2012). Monitoring antifactor Xa levels is recommended (Bates, 2012; Nishimura, 2014).

Multiple-dose vials contain benzyl alcohol (avoid in pregnant women due to association with gasping syndrome in premature infants; use of preservative-free formulations is recommended.

Breast-Feeding Considerations Small amounts of LMWH have been detected in breast milk; however, because it has a low oral bioavailability, it is unlikely to cause adverse events in a nursing infant. Enoxaparin product labeling does not recommend use in nursing women; however, antithrombotic guidelines state that use of LMWH may be continued in breast-feeding women (Guyatt, 2012).

Contraindications

Hypersensitivity to enoxaparin, heparin, pork products, or any component of the formulation (including benzyl alcohol in multiple-dose vials); thrombocytopenia associated with a positive *in vitro* test for antiplatelet antibodies in the presence of enoxaparin; active major bleeding

Canadian labeling: Additional contraindications (not in U.S. labeling): Use of multiple-dose vials in newborns or premature neonates; history of confirmed or suspected immunologically-mediated heparin-induced thrombocytopenia; acute or subacute bacterial endocarditis; major blood clotting disorders; active gastric or duodenal ulcer; hemorrhagic cerebrovascular accident (except if there are systemic emboli); severe uncontrolled hypertension; diabetic or hemorrhagic retinopathy; other conditions or diseases involving an increased risk of hemorrhage; injuries to and operations on the brain, spinal cord, eyes, and ears; spinal/epidural anesthesia when repeated dosing of enoxaparin (1 mg/kg every 12 hours or 1.5 mg/kg daily) is required, due to increased risk of bleeding.

Note: Use of enoxaparin in patients with current heparin-induced thrombocytopenia (HIT) or HIT with thrombosis is **not** recommended and considered contraindicated due to high cross-reactivity to heparin-platelet factor-4 antibody (Guyatt [ACCP], 2012; Warkentin, 1999).

Warnings/Precautions [U.S. Boxed Warning]: Spinal or epidural hematomas, including subsequent long-term or permanent paralysis, may occur with recent or anticipated neuraxial anesthesia (epidural or spinal anesthesia) or spinal puncture in patients anticoagulated with LMWH or heparinoids. Consider risk versus benefit prior to spinal procedures; risk is increased by the use of concomitant agents which may alter hemostasis, the use of indwelling epidural catheters, a history of spinal deformity or spinal surgery, as well as a history of traumatic or repeated epidural or spinal punctures. Optimal timing between neuraxial procedures and enoxaparin administration is not known. Delay placement or removal of catheter for at least 12 hours after administration of low-dose enoxaparin (eg, 30 to 60 mg/day) and at least 24 hours after high-dose enoxaparin (eg, 0.75 to 1 mg/kg twice daily or 1.5 mg/kg once daily) and consider doubling these times in patients with creatinine clearance <30 mL/minute; risk of neuraxial hematoma may still exist since antifactor Xa levels are still detectable at these time points. Patients receiving twice daily high-dose enoxaparin should have the second dose withheld to allow a longer time period prior to catheter placement or removal. Upon removal of catheter, consider withholding enoxaparin for at least 4 hours. **Patient should be observed closely for bleeding and signs and symptoms of neurological impairment if therapy is administered during or immediately following diagnostic lumbar puncture, epidural anesthesia, or spinal anesthesia. If neurological compromise is noted, urgent treatment is necessary.** If spinal hematoma is suspected, diagnose and treat immediately; spinal cord decompression may be considered although it may not prevent or reverse neurological sequelae.

Do not administer intramuscularly. Discontinue use 12 to 24 hours prior to CABG and dose with unfractionated heparin per institutional practice (ACCF/AHA [Anderson, 2013]). Not recommended for thromboprophylaxis in patients with prosthetic heart valves (especially pregnant women). Not to be used interchangeably (unit for unit) with heparin or any other low molecular weight heparins. Monitor patient closely for signs or symptoms of bleeding. Certain patients are at increased risk of bleeding. Risk factors include bacterial endocarditis; congenital or acquired bleeding disorders; active ulcerative or angiodysplastic GI diseases; severe uncontrolled hypertension; hemorrhagic stroke; use shortly after brain, spinal, or ophthalmic surgery; patients treated concomitantly with platelet inhibitors; recent GI bleeding or ulceration; renal dysfunction and hemorrhage; thrombocytopenia or platelet defects or history of heparin-induced thrombocytopenia; severe liver disease; hypertensive or diabetic retinopathy; or in patients undergoing invasive procedures. Protamine may be considered as a partial reversal agent in overdose situations (consult Protamine monograph for dosing recommendations). To minimize risk of bleeding following PCI, achieve hemostasis at the puncture site after PCI. If a closure device is used, sheath can be removed immediately. If manual compression is used, remove sheath 6 hours after the last IV/SubQ dose of enoxaparin. Do not administer further doses until 6 to 8 hours after sheath removal; observe for signs of bleeding/hematoma formation. Cases of enoxaparin-induced thrombocytopenia and thrombosis (similar to heparin-induced thrombocytopenia [HIT]), some complicated by organ infarction, limb ischemia, or death, have been observed. Use with extreme caution or avoid in patients with history of HIT, especially if administered within 100 days of HIT episode (Warkentin, 2001); monitor platelet count closely. Use is contraindicated in patients with thrombocytopenia associated with a positive *in vitro* test for antiplatelet antibodies in the presence of enoxaparin. Discontinue therapy and consider alternative treatment if platelets are <100,000/mm^3 and/or thrombosis develops. Use caution in patients with congenital or drug-induced thrombocytopenia or platelet defects. Risk of bleeding may be increased in women <45 kg and in men <57 kg. Use caution in patients with renal failure; dosage adjustment needed if CrCl <30 mL/minute. Use with caution in the elderly (delayed elimination may occur); dosage alteration/adjustment may be required (eg, omission of IV bolus in acute STEMI in patients ≥75 years of age). Monitor for hyperkalemia; can cause hyperkalemia possibly by suppressing aldosterone production.

Benzyl alcohol and derivatives: Some dosage forms may contain benzyl alcohol and should not be used in pregnant women. In neonates, large amounts of benzyl alcohol (≥99 mg/kg/day) have been associated with a potentially fatal toxicity ("gasping syndrome"); the "gasping syndrome" consists of metabolic acidosis, respiratory distress, gasping respirations, CNS dysfunction (including convulsions, intracranial hemorrhage), hypotension, and cardiovascular collapse (AAP ["Inactive" 1997]; CDC, 1982); some data suggests that benzoate displaces bilirubin from protein binding sites (Ahlfors, 2001); avoid or use dosage forms containing benzyl alcohol with caution in neonates. See manufacturer's labeling.

Safety and efficacy of prophylactic dosing of enoxaparin has not been established in patients who are obese (>30 kg/m^2) nor is there a consensus regarding dosage adjustments. The American College of Chest Physicians Practice Guidelines suggest consulting with a pharmacist regarding dosing in bariatric surgery patients and other obese patients who may require higher doses of LMWH (ACCP [Gould, 2012]).

Adverse Reactions As with all anticoagulants, bleeding is the major adverse effect of enoxaparin. Hemorrhage may occur at virtually any site. Risk is dependent on multiple variables. At the recommended doses, single injections of enoxaparin do not significantly influence platelet aggregation or affect global clotting time (ie, PT or aPTT).

1% to 10%:
Central nervous system: Confusion (2%), pain
Gastrointestinal: Nausea (3%), diarrhea (2%)
Hematologic & oncologic: Major hemorrhage (<1% to 4%; includes cases of intracranial, retroperitoneal, or intraocular hemorrhage; incidence varies with indication/population), thrombocytopenia (moderate 1%; severe 0.1%), anemia (<2%), bruise
Hepatic: Increased serum ALT (6%), increased serum AST (6%)
Local: Hematoma at injection site (9%), irritation at injection site, bruising at injection site, erythema at injection site, pain at injection site
Renal: Hematuria (≤2%)
Miscellaneous: Fever (5% to 8%)
<1% (limited to important or life-threatening): Alopecia, anaphylaxis, anaphylactoid reaction, eczematous rash (plaques), eosinophilia, epidural hematoma (spinal; after neuraxial anesthesia or spinal puncture; risk may be increased with indwelling epidural catheter or concomitant use of other drugs affecting hemostasis), headache, hepatic injury (hepatocellular and cholestatic), hyperkalemia, hyperlipidemia (very rare), hypersensitivity angiitis, hypersensitivity reaction, hypertriglyceridemia, intracranial hemorrhage (up to 0.8%), osteoporosis (following long-term therapy), pruritic erythematous rash (patches), pruritus, purpura, retroperitoneal hemorrhage, severe anemia (hemorrhagic), shock, skin necrosis, thrombocythemia, thrombocytopenia, thrombosis (prosthetic value [in pregnant females] or associated with enoxaparin-induced thrombocytopenia; can cause limb ischemia or organ infarction), urticaria, vesicobullous rash

Drug Interactions

Metabolism/Transport Effects None known.

Avoid Concomitant Use
Avoid concomitant use of Enoxaparin with any of the following: Apixaban; Dabigatran Etexilate; Edoxaban; Hemin; Omacetaxine; Rivaroxaban; Urokinase; Vorapaxar

Increased Effect/Toxicity
Enoxaparin may increase the levels/effects of: ACE Inhibitors; Aliskiren; Angiotensin II Receptor Blockers; Anticoagulants; Canagliflozin; Collagenase (Systemic); Deferasirox; Deoxycholic Acid; Eplerenone; Ibrutumomab; Nintedanib; Obinutuzumab; Omacetaxine; Palifermin; Potassium Salts; Potassium-Sparing Diuretics; Rivaroxaban; Tositumomab and Iodine I 131 Tositumomab

The levels/effects of Enoxaparin may be increased by: 5-ASA Derivatives; Agents with Antiplatelet Properties; Apixaban; Dabigatran Etexilate; Dasatinib; Edoxaban; Hemin; Herbs (Anticoagulant/Antiplatelet Properties); Ibrutinib; Limaprost; Nonsteroidal Anti-Inflammatory Agents; Omega-3 Fatty Acids; Pentosan Polysulfate Sodium; Pentoxifylline; Prostacyclin Analogues; Salicylates; Sugammadex; Thrombolytic Agents; Tibolone; Tipranavir; Urokinase; Vitamin E; Vitamin E (Oral); Vorapaxar

Decreased Effect
Enoxaparin may decrease the levels/effects of: Factor X (Human)

The levels/effects of Enoxaparin may be decreased by: Estrogen Derivatives; Progestins

Storage/Stability Store at 25°C (77°F); excursions permitted to 15°C to 30°C (59°F to 86°F); do not freeze. Do not store multiple-dose vials for >28 days after first use.

Mechanism of Action Standard heparin consists of components with molecular weights ranging from 4000 to 30,000 daltons with a mean of 16,000 daltons. Heparin acts as an anticoagulant by enhancing the inhibition rate of clotting proteases by antithrombin III impairing normal hemostasis and inhibition of factor Xa. Low molecular weight heparins have a small effect on the activated partial thromboplastin time and strongly inhibit factor Xa. Enoxaparin is derived from porcine heparin that undergoes benzylation followed by alkaline depolymerization. The average molecular weight of enoxaparin is 4500 daltons which is distributed as (≤20%) 2000 daltons (≥68%) 2000 to 8000 daltons, and (≤15%) >8000 daltons. Enoxaparin has a higher ratio of antifactor Xa to antifactor IIa activity than unfractionated heparin.

Pharmacodynamics/Kinetics
Onset of action: Peak effect: SubQ: Antifactor Xa and antithrombin (antifactor IIa): 3 to 5 hours
Duration: 40 mg dose: Antifactor Xa activity: ~12 hours
Distribution: 4.3 L (based on antifactor Xa activity)
Protein binding: Does not bind to heparin binding proteins
Metabolism: Hepatic, via desulfation and depolymerization to lower molecular weight molecules with very low biological activity
Bioavailability: Adults: SubQ: ~100%
Half-life elimination, plasma: 2 to 4 times longer than standard heparin, independent of dose; based on anti-Xa activity: 4.5 to 7 hours
Excretion: Urine (40% of dose as active and inactive fragments; 10% as active fragments; 8% to 20% of antifactor Xa activity is recovered within 24 hours)
Clearance: Decreased by 30% in patients with CrCl <30 mL/minute

Dosing
Adult Note: One mg of enoxaparin is equal to 100 units of anti-Xa activity (World Health Organization First International Low Molecular Weight Heparin Reference Standard). Weight-based doses (eg, 1 mg/kg) are commonly rounded to the nearest 10 mg; also see institution-specific rounding protocols if available. Most available pre-filled syringes are graduated in 10 mg increments.

DVT prophylaxis: SubQ:
Obesity: Note: In morbidly-obese patients (BMI ≥40 kg/m^2), increasing the prophylactic dose by 30% may be appropriate for some indications (Nutescu, 2009). For bariatric surgery, dose increases may be >30% based on clinical trial data.
Abdominal surgery: 40 mg once daily, with initial dose given 2 hours prior to surgery; continue until risk of DVT has diminished (usually 7 to 10 days).
Hip replacement surgery:
Twice-daily dosing: 30 mg every 12 hours, with initial dose within 12 to 24 hours after surgery, and every 12 hours for at least 10 days or until risk of DVT has diminished or the patient is adequately anticoagulated on warfarin. The American College of Chest Physicians recommends initiation ≥12 hours preoperatively or ≥12 hours postoperatively; extended duration of up to 35 days suggested (Guyatt, 2012).
Once-daily dosing: 40 mg once daily, with initial dose within 9 to 15 hours before surgery, and daily for at least 10 days (or up to 35 days postoperatively) or until risk of DVT has diminished or the patient is adequately anticoagulated on warfarin. The American College of Chest Physicians recommends initiation ≥12 hours preoperatively or ≥12 hours postoperatively; extended duration of up to 35 days suggested (Guyatt, 2012).
Knee replacement surgery: 30 mg every 12 hours, with initial dose within 12 to 24 hours after surgery, and every 12 hours for at least 10 days or until risk of DVT has diminished or the patient is adequately anticoagulated on warfarin. The American College of Chest Physicians recommends initiation ≥12 hours preoperatively or ≥12 hours postoperatively; extended duration of up to 35 days suggested (Guyatt, 2012).
Medical patients with severely-restricted mobility during acute illness: 40 mg once daily; continue until risk of DVT has diminished (usually 6 to 11 days).
Bariatric surgery (off-label use): Roux-en-Y gastric bypass: Appropriate dosing strategies have not been clearly defined (Borkgren-Okonek, 2008; Scholten, 2002):
BMI ≤50 kg/m^2: 40 mg every 12 hours
BMI >50 kg/m^2: 60 mg every 12 hours

Note: The 2013 AACE/TOS/ASMBS bariatric surgery guidelines recommend, along with early ambulation, both sequential compression devices and subcutaneous LMWH or unfractionated heparin administered within 24 hours after surgery with consideration of extended prophylaxis for those who are at high risk for VTE (eg, history of DVT) (AACE/TOS/ASMBS [Mechanick, 2013]).

Prevention of recurrent venous thromboembolism in pregnancy (off-label use): 40 mg once daily. Therapy should continue for 6 weeks postpartum in high-risk women (Bates, 2012).

DVT treatment (acute): SubQ: **Note:** Start warfarin on the first or second treatment day and continue enoxaparin until INR is ≥2 for at least 24 hours (usually 5 to 7 days) (Guyatt, 2012).

Inpatient treatment (with or without pulmonary embolism): 1 mg/kg/dose every 12 hours or 1.5 mg/kg once daily.

Outpatient treatment (without pulmonary embolism): 1 mg/kg/dose every 12 hours.

Obesity: Use actual body weight to calculate dose; dose capping not recommended; use of twice daily dosing preferred (Nutescu, 2009)

Pregnant women (off-label use): 1 mg/kg/dose every 12 hours. Discontinue ≥24 hours prior to the induction of labor or cesarean section. Enoxaparin therapy may be substituted with heparin near term. Continue anticoagulation therapy for ≥6 weeks postpartum (minimum duration of therapy: 3 months). LMWH or heparin therapy is preferred over warfarin during pregnancy (Bates, 2012).

Percutaneous coronary intervention (PCI), adjunctive therapy (off-label dosing) (ACCF/AHA/SCAI [Levine, 2011]): IV:

If patient undergoing PCI has been treated with multiple doses of enoxaparin and PCI occurs within 8 hours after the last SubQ enoxaparin dose: No additional enoxaparin is needed.

If PCI occurs 8 to 12 hours after the last SubQ enoxaparin dose or the patient received only 1 therapeutic SubQ dose (eg, 1 mg/kg): Administer a single IV dose of 0.3 mg/kg.

If PCI occurs >12 hours after the last SubQ dose: May use an established anticoagulation regimen (eg, full-dose unfractionated heparin or bivalirudin).

If patient has not received prior anticoagulant therapy: 0.5 to 0.75 mg/kg IV bolus dose

ST-elevation MI (STEMI):

Patients <75 years of age: Initial: 30 mg IV single bolus plus 1 mg/kg (maximum: 100 mg for the first 2 doses only) SubQ every 12 hours. The first SubQ dose should be administered with the IV bolus. Maintenance: After first 2 doses, administer 1 mg/kg SubQ every 12 hours.

Patients ≥75 years of age: Initial: SubQ: 0.75 mg/kg every 12 hours (**Note:** No IV bolus is administered in this population); a maximum dose of 75 mg is recommended for the first 2 doses. Maintenance: After first 2 doses, administer 0.75 mg/kg SubQ every 12 hours

Obesity: Use weight-based dosing; a maximum dose of 100 mg is recommended for the first 2 doses (Nutescu, 2009)

Additional notes on STEMI treatment: Therapy may be continued for up to 8 days or until revascularization. Unless contraindicated, all patients should receive aspirin (indefinitely) and clopidogrel (ACCF/AHA [O'Gara, 2013]). In patients with STEMI receiving thrombolytics, initiate enoxaparin dosing between 15 minutes before and 30 minutes after fibrinolytic therapy.

Mechanical heart valve (aortic or mitral position) to bridge anticoagulation (off-label use): SubQ: 1 mg/kg every 12 hours (ACCP [Douketis, 2012]). **Note:** If used in pregnant patients, target anti-Xa level of 0.8 to 1.2 units/mL, 4 to 6 hours postdose (AHA/ACC [Nishimura, 2014]).

Unstable angina or non-ST-elevation MI (NSTEMI): SubQ: 1 mg/kg every 12 hours in conjunction with oral aspirin therapy; continue for the duration of hospitalization (a minimum of at least 2 days) or up to 8 days (ACCF/AHA [Anderson, 2013])

Obesity: Use actual body weight to calculate dose; dose capping not recommended (Nutescu, 2009)

Conversion:

Conversion from IV unfractionated heparin (UFH) infusion to SubQ enoxaparin (Nutescu, 2007): Calculate specific dose for enoxaparin based on indication, discontinue UFH and begin enoxaparin within 1 hour.

Conversion from SubQ enoxaparin to IV UFH infusion (Nutescu, 2007): Discontinue enoxaparin, calculate specific dose for IV UFH infusion based on indication, omit heparin bolus/loading dose:

Converting from SubQ enoxaparin dosed every 12 hours: Start IV UFH infusion 10 to 11 hours after last dose of enoxaparin

Converting from SubQ enoxaparin dosed every 24 hours: Start IV UFH infusion 22 to 23 hours after last dose of enoxaparin

Geriatric SubQ: Refer to adult dosing. Increased incidence of bleeding with doses of 1.5 mg/kg/day or 1 mg/kg every 12 hours; injection-associated bleeding and serious adverse reactions are also increased in the elderly. Careful attention should be paid to elderly patients, particularly those <45 kg. **Note:** Dosage alteration/adjustment may be required.

Pediatric Note: One mg of enoxaparin is equal to 100 units of anti-Xa activity (World Health Organization First International Low Molecular Weight Heparin Reference Standard).

Thromboembolism (off-label use; Monagle, 2012): SubQ:

Infants <2 months: Initial:
Prophylaxis: 0.75 mg/kg every 12 hours
Treatment: 1.5 mg/kg every 12 hours

Infants >2 months and Children ≤18 years: Initial:
Prophylaxis: 0.5 mg/kg every 12 hours
Treatment: 1 mg/kg every 12 hours

Maintenance: See **Dosage Titration** table:

Enoxaparin Pediatric Dosage Titration[1]

Anti-Xa Result	Dose Titration	Time to Repeat Anti-Xa Measurement
<0.35 units/mL	Increase dose by 25%	4 h after next dose
0.35-0.49 units/mL	Increase dose by 10%	4 h after next dose
0.5-1 unit/mL	Keep same dosage	Next day, then 1 wk later, then monthly (4 h after dose)
1.1-1.5 units/mL	Decrease dose by 20%	Before next dose
1.6-2 units/mL	Hold dose for 3 h and decrease dose by 30%	Before next dose, then 4 h after next dose
>2 units/mL	Hold all doses until anti-Xa is 0.5 units/mL, then decrease dose by 40%	Before next dose and every 12 h until anti-Xa <0.5 units/mL

[1]Nomogram to be used for treatment dosing.

Modified from Duplaga BA, et al, "Dosing and Monitoring of Low-Molecular-Weight Heparins in Special Populations," *Pharmacotherapy*, 2001, 21(2):218-34.

Renal Impairment

CrCl ≥30 mL/minute: No specific adjustment recommended (per manufacturer); monitor closely for bleeding.

CrCl <30 mL/minute:

DVT prophylaxis in abdominal surgery, hip replacement, knee replacement, or in medical patients during acute illness: SubQ: 30 mg once daily. **Note:** The Canadian labeling recommends 20 to 30 mg once daily (based on risk/benefit assessment) for prophylaxis in abdominal or colorectal surgery or in medical patients during acute illness.

DVT treatment (inpatient or outpatient treatment in conjunction with warfarin): SubQ: 1 mg/kg once daily

STEMI:

<75 years: Initial: IV: 30 mg as a single dose with the first dose of the SubQ maintenance regimen administered at the same time as the IV bolus; Maintenance: SubQ: 1 mg/kg once daily. **Note:** Canadian labeling recommends a maximum dose of 100 mg for the first SubQ dose.

≥75 years of age: Omit IV bolus; Maintenance: SubQ: 1 mg/kg once daily. **Note:** Canadian labeling recommends a maximum dose of 100 mg for the first SubQ dose.

Unstable angina, NSTEMI: SubQ: 1 mg/kg once daily

Dialysis: Enoxaparin has not been FDA approved for use in dialysis patients. Its elimination is primarily via the renal route. Serious bleeding complications have been reported with use in patients who are dialysis dependent or have severe renal failure. LMWH administration at fixed doses without monitoring has greater unpredictable anticoagulant effects in patients with chronic kidney disease. If used, dosages should be reduced and anti-Xa levels frequently monitored, as accumulation may occur with repeated doses. Many clinicians would not use enoxaparin in this population especially without timely anti-Xa levels.

Hemodialysis: Supplemental dose is not necessary.

Peritoneal dialysis: Significant drug removal is unlikely based on physiochemical characteristics.

Hepatic Impairment There are no dosage adjustments provided in the manufacturer's labeling (has not been studied); use with caution.

Obesity Refer to indication-specific dosing for obesity-related information (may not be available for all indications).

Administration Note: Enoxaparin is available in 100 mg/mL and 150 mg/mL concentrations.

SubQ: Administer by deep SubQ injection alternating between the left or right anterolateral and left or right posterolateral abdominal wall. Do not mix with other infusions or injections. In order to minimize bruising, do not rub injection site. To avoid loss of drug from the 30 mg and 40 mg prefilled syringes, do not expel the air bubble from the syringe prior to injection.

IV: STEMI and PCI only: The U.S. labeling recommends using the multiple-dose vial to prepare IV doses. The Canadian labeling recommends either the multiple-dose vial or a prefilled syringe. Do not mix or coadminister with other medications; may be administered with NS or D_5W. Flush IV access site with a sufficient amount of NS or D_5W prior to and following IV bolus administration. When used prior to percutaneous coronary intervention or as part of treatment for ST-elevation myocardial infarction (STEMI), a single dose may be administered IV except when the patient is ≥75 years of age and is experiencing STEMI then only administer by SubQ injection.

Monitoring Parameters Platelets, occult blood, anti-Xa levels, serum creatinine; monitoring of PT and/or aPTT is not necessary. Routine monitoring of anti-Xa levels is not required, but has been utilized in patients with obesity and/or renal insufficiency. Monitoring anti-Xa levels is recommended in pregnant women receiving therapeutic doses of enoxaparin or when receiving enoxaparin for the prevention of thromboembolism with mechanical heart valves (Guyatt, 2012). For patients >190 kg, if anti-Xa monitoring is available, adjusting dose based on anti-Xa levels is recommended; if anti-Xa monitoring is unavailable, reduce dose if bleeding occurs (Nutescu, 2009). Monitor obese patients closely for signs/symptoms of thromboembolism.

Reference Range The following therapeutic ranges for anti-Xa levels have been suggested, but have not been validated in a controlled trial. Anti-Xa level measured 4 hours postdose.

Treatment of venous thromboembolism: Anti-Xa concentration target (Garcia, 2012):

Once-daily dosing: >1 anti-Xa units/mL; the manufacturer recommends a range of 1 to 2 anti-Xa units/mL

Twice-daily dosing: 0.6 to 1 anti-Xa units/mL

Recurrent VTE prophylaxis in pregnant women: Peak anti-Xa concentrations: 0.2 to 0.6 units/mL (Bates, 2012)

Dosage Forms Excipient information presented when available (limited, particularly for generics); consult specific product labeling.

Solution, Injection, as sodium:
Lovenox: 300 mg/3 mL (3 mL) [contains benzyl alcohol, pork (porcine) protein]
Generic: 300 mg/3 mL (3 mL)
Solution, Subcutaneous, as sodium [preservative free]:
Lovenox: 30 mg/0.3 mL (0.3 mL); 40 mg/0.4 mL (0.4 mL); 60 mg/0.6 mL (0.6 mL); 80 mg/0.8 mL (0.8 mL); 100 mg/mL (1 mL); 120 mg/0.8 mL (0.8 mL); 150 mg/mL (1 mL) [contains pork (porcine) protein]
Generic: 30 mg/0.3 mL (0.3 mL); 40 mg/0.4 mL (0.4 mL); 60 mg/0.6 mL (0.6 mL); 80 mg/0.8 mL (0.8 mL); 100 mg/mL (1 mL); 120 mg/0.8 mL (0.8 mL); 150 mg/mL (1 mL)

◆ Enoxaparin Sodium see Enoxaparin on page 640

◆ Enpresse see Ethinyl Estradiol and Levonorgestrel on page 703

◆ Enskyce see Ethinyl Estradiol and Desogestrel on page 701

◆ Enstilar see Calcipotriene and Betamethasone on page 282

Entacapone (en TA ka pone)

Brand Names: US Comtan
Brand Names: Canada Comtan; Mylan-Entacapone; Sandoz-Entacapone; Teva-Entacapone
Pharmacologic Category Anti-Parkinson's Agent, COMT Inhibitor
Use Parkinson disease: Adjunct to levodopa/carbidopa therapy in patients with idiopathic Parkinson disease who experience "wearing-off" symptoms at the end of a dosing interval
Dosing
Adult & Geriatric Parkinson disease: Oral: 200 mg with each dose of levodopa/carbidopa, up to a maximum of 8 times daily (maximum daily dose: 1600 mg daily).

Note: To optimize therapy, the dosage of levodopa may need to be reduced or the dosing interval may need to be extended. Patients taking levodopa ≥800 mg daily or who had moderate-to-severe dyskinesias prior to therapy required an average decrease of 25% in the daily levodopa dose.

Renal Impairment There are no dosage adjustments provided in the manufacturer's labeling; however, renal function was not found to significantly affect the pharmacokinetics of entacapone.

Hepatic Impairment
U.S. labeling: There are no dosage adjustments provided in the manufacturer's labeling. Treat with caution and monitor carefully; AUC and C_{max} may possibly be doubled.
Canadian labeling: Use is contraindicated.

Additional Information Complete prescribing information should be consulted for additional detail.

Dosage Forms Excipient information presented when available (limited, particularly for generics); consult specific product labeling.
Tablet, Oral:
Comtan: 200 mg
Generic: 200 mg

◆ Entacapone, Carbidopa, and Levodopa see Levodopa, Carbidopa, and Entacapone on page 1060

Entecavir (en TE ka veer)

Brand Names: US Baraclude
Brand Names: Canada Apo-Entecavir; Baraclude; PMS-Entecavir
Pharmacologic Category Antihepadnaviral, Reverse Transcriptase Inhibitor, Nucleoside (Anti-HBV)
Use
U.S. labeling: Treatment of chronic hepatitis B virus (HBV) infection in adults and pediatric patients 2 years and older with evidence of active viral replication and either evidence of persistent transaminase elevations or histologically-active disease. **Note:** In adults, indication is based on data in patients with compensated and decompensated liver disease; in children, indication is based on data in patients with compensated liver disease.
Canadian labeling: Treatment of chronic hepatitis B virus (HBV) infection in adults with compensated liver disease and evidence of active viral replication and either evidence of persistent transaminase elevations or histologically-active disease.

Pregnancy Considerations Teratogenic effects have been observed in animal studies. Information related to use in pregnancy is limited; use only if other options are inappropriate (DHHS [OI], 2013). Pregnant women taking entecavir should enroll in the pregnancy registry by calling 1-800-258-4263.

Breast-Feeding Considerations It is not known if entecavir is excreted in breast milk. Due to the potential for serious adverse reactions in the nursing infant, the manufacturer recommends a decision be made whether to discontinue nursing or to discontinue the drug, taking into account the importance of treatment to the mother.

Contraindications There are no contraindications listed in the manufacturer's U.S. labeling.

Canadian labeling: Hypersensitivity to entecavir or any component of the formulation

Warnings/Precautions Hazardous agent - use appropriate precautions for handling and disposal (NIOSH 2014 [group 2]).

[U.S. Boxed Warning]: Lactic acidosis and severe hepatomegaly with steatosis (including fatal cases) have been reported with nucleoside analogue inhibitors; use with caution in patients with risk factors for liver disease (risk may be increased with female gender, decompensated liver disease, obesity, or prolonged nucleoside inhibitor exposure) and suspend treatment in any patient who develops clinical or laboratory findings suggestive of lactic acidosis or hepatotoxicity (transaminase elevation may/may not accompany hepatomegaly and steatosis)

[U.S. Boxed Warning]: Severe, acute exacerbation of hepatitis B may occur upon discontinuation of anti-hepatitis B therapy, including entecavir. Monitor liver function for at least several months after stopping treatment; reinitiation of antihepatitis B therapy may be required. Use caution in patients with renal impairment or in patients receiving concomitant therapy which may reduce renal function; dose adjustment recommended for CrCl <50 mL/minute. Cross-resistance may develop in patients failing previous therapy with lamivudine. There are limited data available on the use of entecavir in

lamivudine-experienced pediatric patients; use in these patients only if the potential benefit justifies the potential risk to the child.

HIV: **[U.S. Boxed Warning]: May cause the development of HIV resistance in chronic hepatitis B patients with unrecognized or untreated HIV infection.** Determine HIV status prior to initiating treatment with entecavir. **Not recommended for HIV/HBV coinfected patients unless also receiving highly active antiretroviral therapy (HAART).** The manufacturer's labeling states that entecavir does not exhibit any clinically-relevant activity against human immunodeficiency virus (HIV type 1). However, a small number of case reports have indicated declines in virus levels during entecavir therapy. HIV resistance to a common HIV drug has been reported in an HIV/HBV-infected patient receiving entecavir as monotherapy for HBV.

Dose adjustment not required in patients with hepatic impairment. Limited data supporting treatment of chronic hepatitis B in patients with decompensated liver disease; observe for increased adverse reactions, including hepatorenal dysfunction.

Some dosage forms may contain polysorbate 80 (also known as Tweens). Hypersensitivity reactions, usually a delayed reaction, have been reported following exposure to pharmaceutical products containing polysorbate 80 in certain individuals (Isaksson, 2002; Lucente 2000; Shelley, 1995). Thrombocytopenia, ascites, pulmonary deterioration, and renal and hepatic failure have been reported in premature neonates after receiving parenteral products containing polysorbate 80 (Alade, 1986; CDC, 1984). See manufacturer's labeling.

Adverse Reactions Adverse reactions are generally similar in adult and pediatric patients.
>10%:
Cardiovascular: Peripheral edema (16% with decompensated liver disease)
Hepatic: Ascites (15% with decompensated liver disease), increased serum ALT (>5 x ULN: 11% to 12%; post-treatment flare [lamivudine refractory]: >10 x ULN and >2 x baseline: 12%)
Renal: Increased serum creatinine (11% with decompensated liver disease; 1% to 2% with compensated liver disease)
Miscellaneous: Fever (14% with decompensated liver disease)
1% to 10%:
Central nervous system: Headache (2% to 4%), fatigue (1% to 3%), dizziness
Dermatologic: Skin rash
Endocrine & metabolic: Glycosuria (4%), hyperglycemia (2% to 3%), decreased serum bicarbonate (2% with decompensated liver disease)
Gastrointestinal: Increased serum lipase (7%), increased serum amylase (2% to 3%), abdominal pain (children and adolescents >1%), diarrhea (children and adolescents >1%; adults ≤1%), unpleasant taste (children and adolescents >1%), vomiting (children and adolescents >1%; adults <1%), dyspepsia (≤1%), nausea
Genitourinary: Hematuria (9%)
Hematologic & oncologic: Hepatic carcinoma (6% with decompensated liver disease)
Hepatic: Hepatic encephalopathy (10% with decompensated liver disease), increased serum bilirubin (2% to 3%), increased serum ALT (>10 x ULN and >2 x baseline: 2%; post-treatment flare [nucleoside-naive]: >10 x ULN and >2 x baseline: 2% to 8%)
Respiratory: Upper respiratory tract infection (10% with decompensated liver disease)
<1% (Limited to important or life-threatening): Alopecia, anaphylactoid reaction, hepatomegaly, insomnia, lactic acidosis, macular edema (Muqit, 2011), renal failure, thrombocytopenia

Drug Interactions
Metabolism/Transport Effects None known.
Avoid Concomitant Use There are no known interactions where it is recommended to avoid concomitant use.
Increased Effect/Toxicity
The levels/effects of Entecavir may be increased by: Ganciclovir-Valganciclovir; Ribavirin (Oral Inhalation); Ribavirin (Systemic)
Decreased Effect There are no known significant interactions involving a decrease in effect.
Food Interactions Food delays absorption and reduces AUC by 18% to 20%. Management: Administer on an empty stomach 2 hours before or after a meal.
Storage/Stability Store at 25°C (77°F); excursions permitted to 15°C to 30°C (59°F to 86°F). Protect from light. After opening, oral solution can be used up to expiration date on the bottle.

Mechanism of Action Entecavir is intracellularly phosphorylated to guanosine triphosphate which competes with natural substrates to effectively inhibit hepatitis B viral polymerase; enzyme inhibition blocks reverse transcriptase activity thereby reducing viral DNA synthesis.
Pharmacodynamics/Kinetics Note: The pharmacokinetics of pediatric patients ≥2 years are similar to adult values.
Absorption: Delayed with food; C_{max} decreased 44% to 46%, AUC decreased 18% to 20%
Distribution: Extensive (V_d in excess of body water)
Protein binding: ~13%
Metabolism: Minor hepatic glucuronide/sulfate conjugation
Bioavailability: Tablet and oral solution are bioequivalent.
Half-life elimination: Terminal: ~5-6 days; accumulation: ~24 hours
Time to peak, plasma: 0.5-1.5 hours
Excretion: Urine (60% to 73% as unchanged drug)

Dosing
Adult & Geriatric
Hepatitis B virus (HBV) infection, treatment: Oral:
U.S. labeling:
Nucleoside treatment naive: 0.5 mg once daily
Lamivudine-refractory or -resistant viremia (or known lamivudine- or telbivudine-resistant mutations): 1 mg once daily
Decompensated liver disease: 1 mg once daily
Canadian labeling:
Nucleoside treatment naive: 0.5 mg once daily
Lamivudine-refractory or known lamivudine-resistance mutations: 1 mg once daily

HBV reinfection prophylaxis, post liver transplant (with or without HBIG) (off-label use): Oral: 0.5 mg once daily (Fung, 2011) or 1 mg once daily (Perrillo, 2012)

HIV/HBV coinfection (off-label use): Oral:
Nucleoside treatment naive: 0.5 mg once daily
Lamivudine refractory or resistant: 1 mg once daily
Note: Only recommended in patients who cannot take tenofovir; must be used in addition to a fully suppressive antiretroviral therapy regimen (DHHS, 2013).

Treatment duration (AASLD Practice Guidelines, 2009):
Hepatitis Be antigen (HBeAg) positive chronic hepatitis: Treat ≥1 year until HBeAg seroconversion and undetectable serum HBV DNA; continue therapy for ≥6 months after HBeAg seroconversion
HBeAg negative chronic hepatitis: Treat >1 year until hepatitis B surface antigen (HBsAg) clearance
Decompensated liver disease: Lifelong treatment is recommended.
Note: Patients not achieving a primary response (<2 log decrease in serum HBV DNA) after at least 6 months of therapy should either receive additional treatment or be switched to an alternative therapy.

Pediatric
Hepatitis B virus (HBV) infection, treatment (nucleoside treatment naïve or lamivudine-refractory or -resistant viremia [or known lamivudine- or telbivudine-resistance mutations]):
U.S. labeling:
Children ≥2 years and Adolescents: Oral: **Note:** Oral solution should be used for patients weighing ≤30 kg.
Treatment-naive:
10 to 11 kg: 0.15 mg once daily (oral solution)
>11 to 14 kg: 0.2 mg once daily (oral solution)
>14 to 17 kg: 0.25 mg once daily (oral solution)
>17 to 20 kg: 0.3 mg once daily (oral solution)
>20 to 23 kg: 0.35 mg once daily (oral solution)
>23 to 26 kg: 0.4 mg once daily (oral solution)
>26 to 30 kg: 0.45 mg once daily (oral solution)
>30 kg: 0.5 mg once daily (oral solution or tablet)
Lamivudine-experienced:
10 to 11 kg: 0.3 mg once daily (oral solution)
>11 to 14 kg: 0.4 mg once daily (oral solution)
>14 to 17 kg: 0.5 mg once daily (oral solution)
>17 to 20 kg: 0.6 mg once daily (oral solution)
>20 to 23 kg: 0.7 mg once daily (oral solution)
>23 to 26 kg: 0.8 mg once daily (oral solution)
>26 to 30 kg: 0.9 mg once daily (oral solution)
>30 kg: 1 mg once daily (oral solution or tablet)
Canadian labeling: Adolescents ≥16 years: Oral:
Nucleoside treatment-naive: 0.5 mg once daily
Lamivudine-refractory or known lamivudine-resistance mutations: 1 mg once daily

Renal Impairment
Adults (Canadian labeling: Adolescents ≥16 years and Adults): Daily-dosage regimen preferred:
CrCl ≥50 mL/minute: No dosage adjustment necessary.
CrCl 30-49 mL/minute: Administer 50% of usual dose daily or administer the normal dose every 48 hours
CrCl 10-29 mL/minute: Administer 30% of usual dose daily or administer the normal dose every 72 hours

CrCl <10 mL/minute (including hemodialysis and CAPD): Administer 10% of usual dose daily or administer the normal dose every 7 days; administer after hemodialysis

Children >2 years and Adolescents: Insufficient data to recommend a specific dose adjustment in pediatric patients with renal impairment; consider a reduction in the dose or an increase in the dosing interval similar to adjustments for adults.

Hepatic Impairment

Adults (Canadian labeling: Adolescents ≥16 years and Adults): No dosage adjustment necessary.

Children >2 years and Adolescents: There are no dosage adjustments provided in the manufacturer's labeling (has not been studied).

Dietary Considerations Take on an empty stomach (2 hours before or after a meal).

Administration Administer on an empty stomach (2 hours before or after a meal). Do not dilute or mix oral solution with water or other beverages; use calibrated oral dosing syringe. Oral solution and tablet are bioequivalent on a mg-to-mg basis.

Hazardous agent - use appropriate precautions for handling and disposal (NIOSH 2014 [group 2]).

Monitoring Parameters HIV status (prior to initiation of therapy); liver function tests, renal function; in HBV/HIV-coinfected patients, monitor HIV viral load and CD4 count; HBeAg, HBV DNA; in patients with lamivudine-refractory or -resistant viremia (or known lamivudine- or telbivudine-resistance mutations) entecavir resistance can develop rapidly. Monitor HBV DNA every 3 months (DHHS, 2013)

Dosage Forms Excipient information presented when available (limited, particularly for generics); consult specific product labeling.

Solution, Oral:

Baraclude: 0.05 mg/mL (210 mL) [contains methylparaben, propylparaben; orange flavor]

Tablet, Oral:

Baraclude: 0.5 mg, 1 mg

Generic: 0.5 mg, 1 mg

Enzalutamide (en za LOO ta mide)

Brand Names: US Xtandi

Brand Names: Canada Xtandi

Index Terms MDV3100

Pharmacologic Category Antineoplastic Agent, Antiandrogen

Use Prostate cancer, metastatic: Treatment of metastatic, castration-resistant prostate cancer

Pregnancy Considerations Adverse effects were observed in animal reproduction studies. Enzalutamide is an androgen receptor inhibitor and would be expected to cause fetal harm based on its mechanism of action. Enzalutamide is not indicated for use in women and is specifically contraindicated for use in women who are or may become pregnant. Men using this medication should use a condom if having intercourse with a pregnant woman. A condom plus another effective method of birth control is recommended during therapy and for 3 months after treatment for men using this medication and who are having intercourse with a woman of reproductive potential.

Breast-Feeding Considerations Enzalutamide is not indicated for use in women.

Contraindications Women who are or may become pregnant

Canadian labeling: Additional contraindications (not in US labeling): Hypersensitivity to enzalutamide or any component of the formulation; women who are lactating

Warnings/Precautions Hazardous agent - use appropriate precautions for handling and disposal (meets NIOSH 2014 criteria). Seizures were observed in clinical trials (onset: ~1 to 20 months after treatment initiation). Therapy was permanently discontinued and patients were not rechallenged; seizures resolved upon therapy cessation. Patients with predisposing factors for seizure were excluded from the trials; factors include seizure history, underlying brain injury with loss of consciousness, transient ischemic attack within the past 12 months, cerebral vascular accident, brain metastases, brain arteriovenous malformation, or (in one study) the use of concomitant medications which may lower the seizure threshold. Enzalutamide should be used with caution in patients with a history of seizure disorders or other predisposing factors. Discontinue permanently if seizures develop during treatment. Posterior reversible encephalopathy syndrome (PRES) has been reported in patients receiving enzalutamide. PRES is a neurological disorder which may present with rapidly evolving symptoms (headache, seizure, lethargy, confusion, blindness, and other visual/neurologic disturbances) with or without associated hypertension. PRES diagnosis may be confirmed with magnetic resonance imagining (MRI). Discontinue enzalutamide in patients who develop PRES.

Enzalutamide may cause hypospermatogenesis and may impair male fertility. Androgen-deprivation therapy may increase the risk of cardiovascular disease (Levine, 2010). An increase in systolic and diastolic blood pressures has been observed (Scher, 2012); may worsen preexisting hypertension.

Potentially significant drug-drug interactions may exist, requiring dose or frequency adjustment, additional monitoring, and/or selection of alternative therapy. May contain sorbitol; Canadian product labeling recommends avoiding use in patients with fructose intolerance.

Adverse Reactions

>10%:

Cardiovascular: Peripheral edema (12% to 15%), hypertension (6% to 14%)

Central nervous system: Fatigue (≤51%), falling (5% to 13%), headache (11% to 12%), dizziness (10% to 11%)

Endocrine & metabolic: Hot flash (18% to 20%), weight loss (12%)

Gastrointestinal: Constipation (23%), diarrhea (17% to 22%), decreased appetite (19%)

Hematologic & oncologic: Neutropenia (15%; grades 3/4: 1%)

Neuromuscular & skeletal: Weakness (≤51%), back pain (26% to 29%), arthralgia (21%), musculoskeletal pain (15%)

Respiratory: Upper respiratory tract infection (11% to 16%), dyspnea (11%)

1% to 10%:

Central nervous system: Myasthenia (10%), insomnia (8% to 9%), anxiety (7%), paresthesia (7%), cauda equina syndrome (≤7%), spinal cord compression (≤7%), altered mental status (4% to 6%), hypoesthesia (4%), hallucination (2%), restless leg syndrome (2%)

Dermatologic: Pruritus (4%), xeroderma (4%)

Endocrine & metabolic: Gynecomastia (3%)

Gastrointestinal: Dysgeusia (8%)

Genitourinary: Hematuria (7% to 9%), pollakiuria (5%)

Hematologic & oncologic: Thrombocytopenia (6%)

Hepatic: Increased serum bilirubin (3%)

Infection: Infection (≤6%; including sepsis)

Neuromuscular & skeletal: Bone fracture (4% to 9%), stiffness (3%)

Respiratory: Lower respiratory tract infection (8% to 9%), epistaxis (3%)

<1% (Limited to important or life-threatening): Reversible posterior leukoencephalopathy syndrome, seizure

Drug Interactions

Metabolism/Transport Effects Substrate of CYP2C8 (major), CYP3A4 (major); **Note:** Assignment of Major/Minor substrate status based on clinically relevant drug interaction potential; **Inhibits** BCRP, MRP2, P-glycoprotein; **Induces** CYP2C19 (weak/moderate), CYP2C9 (weak/moderate), CYP3A4 (strong)

Avoid Concomitant Use

Avoid concomitant use of Enzalutamide with any of the following: Abiraterone Acetate; Alfentanil; Antihepaciviral Combination Products; Apixaban; Apremilast; Aprepitant; Artemether; Axitinib; Bedaquiline; Boceprevir; Bortezomib; Bosutinib; Cabozantinib; Cariprazine; Ceritinib; CloZAPine; Cobimetinib; Crizotinib; CycloSPORINE (Systemic); CYP2C8 Inducers (Strong); CYP2C8 Inhibitors (Strong); CYP3A4 Inducers (Strong); Dabrafenib;

Daclatasvir; Dienogest; Dihydroergotamine; Dronedarone; Eliglustat; Ergotamine; Everolimus; FentaNYL; Flibanserin; Fosphenytoin-Phenytoin; Ibrutinib; Idelalisib; Indium 111 Capromab Pendetide; Irinotecan Products; Isavuconazonium Sulfate; Itraconazole; Ivabradine; Ivacaftor; Ixazomib; Lapatinib; Lumefantrine; Lurasidone; Macitentan; Mifepristone; Naloxegol; Netupitant; NIFEdipine; Nilotinib; NiMODipine; Nisoldipine; Olaparib; Osimertinib; Palbociclib; Panobinostat; PAZOPanib; Perampanel; Pimozide; PONATinib; Praziquantel; QuiNIDine; Ranolazine; Regorafenib; Rivaroxaban; Roflumilast; RomiDEPsin; Simeprevir; Sirolimus; Sonidegib; SORAfenib; St Johns Wort; Suvorexant; Tacrolimus (Systemic); Tasimelteon; Telaprevir; Ticagrelor; Tofacitinib; Tolvaptan; Toremifene; Trabectedin; Uliprital; Vandetanib; Vemurafenib; VinCRIStine (Liposomal); Vorapaxar; Warfarin

Increased Effect/Toxicity

Enzalutamide may increase the levels/effects of: Clarithromycin; Ifosfamide

The levels/effects of Enzalutamide may be increased by: Clarithromycin; CYP2C8 Inhibitors (Moderate); CYP2C8 Inhibitors (Strong); CYP3A4 Inhibitors (Strong); Deferasirox

Decreased Effect

Enzalutamide may decrease the levels/effects of: Abiraterone Acetate; Alfentanil; Antihepaciviral Combination Products; Apixaban; Apremilast; Aprepitant; ARIPiprazole; ARIPiprazole Lauroxil; Artemether; Axitinib; Bedaquiline; Boceprevir; Bortezomib; Bosutinib; Brentuximab Vedotin; Brexpiprazole; Cabozantinib; Cannabidiol; Cannabis; Cariprazine; Ceritinib; Choline C 11; Clarithromycin; CloZAPine; Cobimetinib; Corticosteroids (Systemic); Crizotinib; CycloSPORINE (Systemic); CYP2C19 Substrates; CYP2C9 Substrates; CYP3A4 Substrates; Dabrafenib; Daclatasvir; Dasatinib; Dexamethasone (Systemic); Dienogest; Dihydroergotamine; DOXOrubicin (Conventional); Dronabinol; Dronedarone; Eliglustat; Ergotamine; Erlotinib; Etoposide; Etoposide Phosphate; Everolimus; Exemestane; FentaNYL; Flibanserin; Fosphenytoin-Phenytoin; Gefitinib; GuanFACINE; Hydrocortisone (Systemic); Ibrutinib; Idelalisib; Ifosfamide; Imatinib; Indium 111 Capromab Pendetide; Irinotecan Products; Isavuconazonium Sulfate; Itraconazole; Ivabradine; Ivacaftor; Ixabepilone; Ixazomib; Lapatinib; Linagliptin; Lumefantrine; Lurasidone; Macitentan; Maraviroc; MethylPREDNISolone; Mifepristone; Naloxegol; Netupitant; NIFEdipine; Nilotinib; NiMODipine; Nisoldipine; Olaparib; Osimertinib; Palbociclib; Panobinostat; PAZOPanib; Perampanel; Pimozide; PONATinib; Praziquantel; PrednisoLONE (Systemic); PredniSONE; Propafenone; QUEtiapine; QuiNIDine; Ranolazine; Regorafenib; Rivaroxaban; Roflumilast; Rolapitant; RomiDEPsin; Saxagliptin; Simeprevir; Sirolimus; Sonidegib; SORAfenib; SUNItinib; Suvorexant; Tacrolimus (Systemic); Tadalafil; Tasimelteon; Telaprevir; Tetrahydrocannabinol; Ticagrelor; Tofacitinib; Tolvaptan; Toremifene; Trabectedin; Uliprital; Vandetanib; Vemurafenib; Vilazodone; VinCRIStine (Liposomal); Vorapaxar; Vortioxetine; Warfarin; Zaleplon; Zuclopenthixol

The levels/effects of Enzalutamide may be decreased by: Bosentan; CYP2C8 Inducers (Strong); CYP3A4 Inducers (Moderate); CYP3A4 Inducers (Strong); Deferasirox; Siltuximab; St Johns Wort; Tocilizumab

Storage/Stability Store at 20°C to 25°C (68°F to 77°F); excursions permitted to 15°C to 30°C (59°F to 86°F). Protect from moisture; keep bottle tightly closed.

Mechanism of Action Enzalutamide is a pure androgen receptor signaling inhibitor; unlike other antiandrogen therapies, it has no known agonistic properties. It inhibits androgen receptor nuclear translocation, DNA binding, and coactivator mobilization, leading to cellular apoptosis and decreased prostate tumor volume.

Pharmacodynamics/Kinetics

Absorption: Rapid

Distribution: 110 L

Protein binding: Parent drug: 97% to 98% to primarily albumin; active metabolite: 95% to plasma proteins

Metabolism: Primarily hepatic via CYP2C8 (responsible for formation of active metabolite N-desmethyl enzalutamide) and CYP3A4

Half-life elimination: Parent drug: 5.8 days (range: 2.8 to 10.2 days); N-desmethyl enzalutamide: 7.8 to 8.6 days

Time to peak: 1 hour (range: 0.5 to 3 hours)

Excretion: Urine (71%); feces (14%); primarily as inactive metabolite

Dosing

Adult & Geriatric

Prostate cancer, metastatic, castration-resistant: Oral: 160 mg once daily

Dosage adjustment for concomitant strong CYP2C8 inhibitors: Avoid concomitant use if possible. If coadministration is necessary, reduce enzalutamide dose to 80 mg once daily. If the strong CYP2C8 inhibitor is discontinued, adjust the enzalutamide dose back up to the dose used prior to the initiation of the strong CYP2C8 inhibitor.

Dosage adjustment for concomitant strong CYP3A4 inducers: Avoid concomitant use if possible. If coadministration is necessary, increase the enzalutamide dose to 240 mg once daily. If the strong CYP3A4 inducer is discontinued, adjust the enzalutamide dose back to the dose used prior to the initiation of the strong CYP3A4 inducer.

Renal Impairment

Preexisting mild-to-moderate impairment (CrCl 30-89 mL/minute): No initial dosage adjustment necessary.

Preexisting severe impairment (CrCl <30 mL/minute), including end-stage renal disease: There are no dosage adjustments provided in the manufacturer's labeling (has not been studied).

Hepatic Impairment Preexisting mild, moderate, or severe impairment (Child-Pugh class A, B, or C): No dosage adjustment necessary. Canadian labeling recommends to avoid use in severe impairment.

Adjustment for Toxicity If ≥ grade 3 toxicity or intolerable side effects occur, withhold treatment for 1 week or until symptom(s) improve to ≤ grade 2, then resume at same dose, or reduce dose to 120 mg or 80 mg once daily, if necessary.

Seizures: Permanently discontinue treatment.

Administration May be administered with or without food; take at the same time each day. Swallow capsules whole; do not chew, dissolve, or open the capsules. Hazardous agent; use appropriate precautions for handling and disposal (meets NIOSH 2014 criteria).

Monitoring Parameters Monitor for signs/symptoms of seizure, loss of consciousness, dizziness, and hallucinations; CBC with differential and liver function tests (baseline and periodic); additional INR monitoring (if on warfarin); blood pressure (baseline and periodic), signs/symptoms of posterior reversible encephalopathy syndrome

Dosage Forms Excipient information presented when available (limited, particularly for generics); consult specific product labeling.

Capsule, Oral:

Xtandi: 40 mg

◆ Epaned *see* Enalapril *on page 636*

◆ Epanova *see* Omega-3 Fatty Acids *on page 1329*

◆ EPEG *see* Etoposide *on page 714*

EPHEDrine (Systemic) (e FED rin)

Index Terms Ephedrine Sulfate

Pharmacologic Category Alpha/Beta Agonist

Use Treatment of anesthesia-induced hypotension

Note: The use of ephedrine for the treatment of acute bronchospasm, Stokes-Adams syndrome (ie, presyncope/syncope) with complete heart block, narcolepsy, or depression has fallen out of favor given the availability of more effective agents for these conditions.

Dosing

Adult & Geriatric

Hypotension induced by anesthesia: IV: 5 to 25 mg/dose slow IV push repeated after 5 to 10 minutes as needed to maintain blood pressure

Idiopathic orthostatic hypotension (off-label use): Oral: 25 to 50 mg 3 times daily; maximum: 150 mg daily. **Note:** Not considered first-line for this indication.

Postoperative nausea and vomiting (PONV) refractory to traditional antiemetics (off-label use): IM: 0.5 mg/kg at the end of surgery (SAMBA [Gan 2007]; Hagemann 2000)

Pediatric

Hypotension induced by anesthesia: IV:

Infants, Children, and Adolescents ≤15 years (off-label dose): 0.1 to 0.2 mg/kg/dose slow IV push; administer as needed to maintain blood pressure; maximum: 25 mg (Taguchi, 1996)

Adolescents >15 years: Refer to adult dosing

Additional Information Complete prescribing information should be consulted for additional detail.

Dosage Forms Excipient information presented when available (limited, particularly for generics); consult specific product labeling. [DSC] = Discontinued product

Capsule, Oral, as sulfate:

Generic: 25 mg [DSC]

Solution, Injection, as sulfate:
Generic: 50 mg/mL (1 mL)
Solution, Injection, as sulfate [preservative free]:
Generic: 50 mg/mL (1 mL)

◆ Ephedrine Sulfate *see* EPHEDrine (Systemic) *on page 646*

◆ E-Pherol [OTC] *see* Vitamin E *on page 1906*

◆ Epidoxorubicin *see* Epirubicin *on page 651*

◆ Epiduo *see* Adapalene and Benzoyl Peroxide *on page 44*

◆ Epiduo Forte *see* Adapalene and Benzoyl Peroxide *on page 44*

◆ Epifoam *see* Pramoxine and Hydrocortisone *on page 1489*

EPINEPHrine (Systemic) (ep i NEF rin)

Brand Names: US Adrenaclick; Adrenalin; Auvi-Q [DSC]; EpiPen 2-Pak; EpiPen Jr 2-Pak; EPIsnap; Twinject [DSC]
Brand Names: Canada Adrenalin; Allerject; Anapen; Anapen Junior; EpiPen; EpiPen Jr; Twinject
Index Terms Adrenaline; Adrenaline Bitartrate; Adrenaline Hydrochloride; Epinephrine Bitartrate; Epinephrine Hydrochloride; Primatene Mist
Pharmacologic Category Alpha/Beta Agonist
Additional Appendix Information
Adult ACLS Algorithms *on page 1993*
Pediatric ALS (PALS) Algorithms *on page 1990*
Use
Hypersensitivity: Treatment of type I allergic reactions including anaphylactic reactions
Hypotension/shock: Treatment of hypotension associated with septic shock (increase mean arterial blood pressure)
Mydriasis during intraocular surgery: Induction and maintenance of mydriasis during intraocular surgery
Pregnancy Considerations Adverse events have been observed in animal reproduction studies. Epinephrine crosses the placenta (Sandler 1964). Uterine vasoconstriction, decreased uterine blood flow, and fetal anoxia may occur. Epinephrine is recommended for the treatment of anaphylaxis in pregnant women. Specific dosing is not available; use with caution and monitor hemodynamic response (Hepner 2013). In general, medications used for ACLS in pregnant women are given at the same dose as nonpregnant patients (AHA [Vanden Hoek] 2010).
Breast-Feeding Considerations It is not known if epinephrine is excreted in breast milk. The manufacturer recommends that caution be exercised when administering epinephrine to nursing women.
Contraindications
There are no absolute contraindications to the use of injectable epinephrine (including Adrenaclick, Auvi-Q, EpiPen, EpiPen Jr, Allerject [Canadian product], and Twinject [Canadian product]) in a life-threatening situation. Some products include the following contraindications: Hypersensitivity to sympathomimetic amines; general anesthesia with halogenated hydrocarbons (eg, halothane) or cyclopropane; narrow angle glaucoma; nonanaphylactic shock; in combination with local anesthesia of certain areas such as fingers, toes, and ears; use in situations where vasopressors may be contraindicated (eg, thyrotoxicosis, diabetes, in obstetrics when maternal blood pressure is in excess of 130/80 mm Hg and in hypertension and other cardiovascular disorders) Injectable solution (Adrenalin, Epinephrine injection, USP): There are no contraindications listed in the manufacturer's labeling.
Warnings/Precautions Use with caution in elderly patients, patients with diabetes mellitus, cardiovascular diseases (eg, coronary artery disease, hypertension), thyroid disease, cerebrovascular disease, in patients with prostate enlargement or urinary retention, or Parkinson disease. May induce cardiac arrhythmias; use with caution especially in patients with cardiac disease or those receiving drugs that sensitize the myocardium. Due to peripheral constriction and cardiac stimulation, pulmonary edema may occur. Due to renal blood vessel constriction, decreased urine output may occur. In hypovolemic patients, correct blood volume depletion before administering any vasopressor. Some products contain sulfites as preservatives; the presence of sulfites in some products should not deter administration during a serious allergic or other emergency situation even if the patient is sulfite-sensitive. Potentially significant drug-drug interactions may exist, requiring dose or frequency adjustment, additional monitoring, and/or selection of alternative therapy.

IV administration: Rapid IV administration may cause death from cerebrovascular hemorrhage or cardiac arrhythmias. However, rapid IV administration during pulseless arrest is necessary. Vesicant; ensure proper needle or catheter placement prior to and during infusion; avoid extravasation. Accidental injection into digits, hands, or feet may result in local reactions, including injection site pallor, coldness and hypoesthesia or injury, resulting in bruising, bleeding, discoloration, erythema, or skeletal injury; patient should seek immediate medical attention if this occurs. Rapid IV administration may cause death from cerebrovascular hemorrhage or cardiac arrhythmias; however, rapid IV administration during pulseless arrest is necessary. Prior to intraocular use, must dilute 1:**1000** (1 mg/mL) solution to a concentration of 1:**100,000** to 1:**1,000,000** (10 **mcg**/mL to 1 **mcg**/mL) prior to intraocular use. When used undiluted, has been associated with corneal endothelial damage. Also, products containing chlorobutanol must not be used intraocularly (may be harmful to corneal endothelium).

Adverse Reactions Frequency not defined.
Cardiovascular: Angina pectoris, cardiac arrhythmia, cerebrovascular accident, chest pain, hypertension, ischemic heart disease, limb ischemia, localized blanching, myocardial infarction, palpitations, supraventricular tachycardia, tachycardia, vasoconstriction, ventricular arrhythmia, ventricular ectopy, ventricular fibrillation
Central nervous system: Anxiety, apprehension, disorientation, dizziness, drowsiness, exacerbation of Parkinson's disease, excitability, headache, memory impairment, nervousness, panic, paresthesia, psychomotor agitation, restlessness, tingling sensation
Dermatologic: Diaphoresis, pallor, piloerection, skin necrosis (with extravasation)
Endocrine & metabolic: Hyperglycemia, hypoglycemia, hypokalemia, increased serum glucose (transient), insulin resistance, lactic acidosis
Gastrointestinal: Nausea, vomiting
Hematologic & oncologic: Hemorrhage (CNS)
Local: Extravasation
Neuromuscular & skeletal: Tremor, weakness
Ophthalmic: Burning sensation of eyes
Renal: Renal insufficiency
Respiratory: Dyspnea, pulmonary edema, rales
Drug Interactions
Metabolism/Transport Effects Substrate of COMT
Avoid Concomitant Use
Avoid concomitant use of EPINEPHrine (Systemic) with any of the following: Ergot Derivatives; Iobenguane I 123; Lurasidone
Increased Effect/Toxicity
EPINEPHrine (Systemic) may increase the levels/effects of: Doxofylline; Lurasidone; Sympathomimetics

The levels/effects of EPINEPHrine (Systemic) may be increased by: AtoMOXetine; Beta-Blockers; Cannabinoid-Containing Products; COMT Inhibitors; Ergot Derivatives; Hyaluronidase; Inhalational Anesthetics; Linezolid; MAO Inhibitors; Serotonin/Norepinephrine Reuptake Inhibitors; Tedizolid; Tricyclic Antidepressants
Decreased Effect
EPINEPHrine (Systemic) may decrease the levels/effects of: Antidiabetic Agents; Benzylpenicilloyl Polylysine; Iobenguane I 123

The levels/effects of EPINEPHrine (Systemic) may be decreased by: Alpha1-Blockers; Promethazine; Spironolactone
Preparation for Administration
Endotracheal (off-label route): Dilute in NS or sterile water.
Intraocular: Dilute 1 mL of 1 mg/mL (1:**1000**) solution in 100 mL to 1000 mL of an ophthalmic irrigation fluid for a final concentration of 1:**100,000** to 1:**1,000,000** (10 **mcg**/mL to 1 **mcg**/mL); may use this solution as an irrigation as needed during the procedure. May also prepare a dilution of 1:**100,000** to 1:**400,000** (10 **mcg**/mL to 2.5 **mcg**/mL) for intracameral administration.
Intravenous: Although the manufacturer recommends dilution in dextrose containing solutions (provides protection against significant loss of potency by oxidation) and does not recommend dilution in NS alone, dilution in NS has been reported to be physically compatible (Trissel 2014).
Storage/Stability Epinephrine is sensitive to light and air. Protection from light is recommended. Oxidation turns drug pink, then a brown color. **Solutions should not be used if they are discolored or contain a precipitate.**
Adrenaclick: Store between 20°C to 25°C (68°F to 77°F); excursions permitted to 15°C to 30°C (59°F to 86°F); do not freeze or refrigerate. Protect from light.
Adrenalin: Store between 20°C to 25°C (68°F to 77°F); do not freeze. Protect from light.
Allerject [Canadian product]: Store between 15°C to 30°C (59°F to 86°F); do not refrigerate. Protect from light.

Auvi-Q: Store between 20°C to 25°C (68°F to 77°F); excursions permitted to 15°C to 30°C (59°F to 86°F); do not refrigerate. Protect from light by storing in outer case provided.

Epinephrine injection, USP: Store between 20°C to 25°C (68°F to 77°F); do not refrigerate; protect from freezing. Protect from light until ready for use.

EpiPen and EpiPen Jr: Store at 25°C (77°F); excursions permitted to 15°C to 30°C (59°F to 86°F); do not freeze or refrigerate. Protect from light by storing in carrier tube provided.

Twinject [Canadian product]: Store between 20°C to 25°C (68°F to 77°F); excursions permitted to 15°C to 30°C (59°F to 86°F); do not freeze or refrigerate. Protect from light.

Stability of injection of parenteral admixture at room temperature (25°C) or refrigeration (4°C) is 24 hours.

Mechanism of Action Stimulates alpha-, beta$_1$-, and beta$_2$-adrenergic receptors resulting in relaxation of smooth muscle of the bronchial tree, cardiac stimulation (increasing myocardial oxygen consumption), and dilation of skeletal muscle vasculature; small doses can cause vasodilation via beta$_2$-vascular receptors; large doses may produce constriction of skeletal and vascular smooth muscle

Pharmacodynamics/Kinetics

Onset of action: Bronchodilation: SubQ: ~5 to 10 minutes

Absorption: Orally ingested doses are rapidly metabolized in GI tract and liver; pharmacologically active concentrations are not achieved

Distribution: Does not cross blood-brain barrier

Metabolism: Taken up into the adrenergic neuron and metabolized by monoamine oxidase and catechol-o-methyltransferase; circulating drug hepatically metabolized

Half-life elimination: IV: <5 minutes

Excretion: Urine (as inactive metabolites, metanephrine, and sulfate and hydroxy derivatives of mandelic acid, small amounts as unchanged drug)

Dosing

Adult & Geriatric

Asystole/pulseless arrest, pulseless VT/VF (ACLS [Neumar 2010]):

IV, I.O.: 1 mg every 3 to 5 minutes until return of spontaneous circulation; if this approach fails, higher doses of epinephrine (up to 0.2 mg/kg) have been used for treatment of specific problems (eg, beta-blocker or calcium channel blocker overdose)

Note: High IV dose epinephrine ie, >1 mg per dose) has not been shown to improve survival or neurological outcomes as compared to standard dose epinephrine and is not recommended (ACLS [Neumar, 2010]; ACLS [Neumar 2015]).

Endotracheal: 2 to 2.5 mg every 3 to 5 minutes until IV/I.O. access established or return of spontaneous circulation; dilute in 5 to 10 mL NS or sterile water. **Note:** Absorption may be greater with sterile water (Naganobu 2000). May cause false-negative reading with exhaled CO$_2$ detectors; use second method to confirm tube placement if CO$_2$ is not detected (ACLS [Neumar 2010]).

Bradycardia (symptomatic; unresponsive to atropine or pacing): *IV infusion:* 2 to 10 mcg/minute **or** 0.1 to 0.5 mcg/kg/minute (7 to 35 mcg/minute in a 70 kg patient); titrate to desired effect (ACLS [Neumar 2010]; AHA [Peberdy 2010]).

Bronchodilator: *SubQ: Acute severe asthma unresponsive to inhaled beta-agonist (off-label use):* 0.01 mg/kg divided into 3 doses of approximately 0.3 mg every 20 minutes. **Note:** The **1:1000** (1 mg/mL) concentration is recommended (AHA [Vanden Hoek 2010]).

Hypersensitivity reaction (eg, anaphylaxis): Note: SubQ administration results in slower absorption and is less reliable. IM administration in the anterolateral aspect of the middle third of the thigh is preferred in the setting of anaphylaxis (AHA [Vanden Hoek 2010]; Kemp 2008).

IM, SubQ: 0.2 to 0.5 mg (**1:1000** [1 mg/mL] solution) every 5 to 15 minutes in the absence of clinical improvement (AHA [Vanden Hoek 2010]; Kemp 2008; Lieberman 2010). If clinician deems appropriate, the 5-minute interval between injections may be shortened to allow for more frequent administration (Lieberman 2010).

IV: 0.1 mg (**1:10,000** [0.1 mg/mL] solution) over 5 minutes; may infuse at 1 to 4 mcg/minute to prevent the need to repeat injections frequently **or** may initiate with an infusion at 5 to 15 mcg/minute (with crystalloid administration) (AHA [Vanden Hoek 2010]; Brown 2004). In general, IV administration should only be done in patients who are profoundly hypotensive or are in cardiopulmonary arrest refractory to volume

resuscitation and several epinephrine injections (Lieberman 2010).

Self-administration following severe allergic reactions (eg, insect stings, food): **Note:** The World Health Organization (WHO) and Anaphylaxis Canada recommend the availability of one dose for every 10 to 20 minutes of travel time to a medical emergency facility. If anaphylactic symptoms persist after first dose, may repeat dose in 5 to 15 minutes (AHA [Vanden Hoek 2010]); more than 2 sequential doses should only be administered under direct medical supervision.

Adrenaclick: IM, SubQ: 0.3 mg; if anaphylactic symptoms persist, dose may be repeated using an additional Adrenaclick injector

Allerject [Canadian product]: IM: 0.3 mg; if anaphylactic symptoms persist, dose may be repeated using an additional Allerject injector

Auvi-Q: IM, SubQ: 0.3 mg; if anaphylactic symptoms persist, dose may be repeated

EpiPen: IM, SubQ: 0.3 mg; if anaphylactic symptoms persist, dose may be repeated using an additional EpiPen

Twinject [Canadian product]: IM, SubQ: 0.3 mg; if anaphylactic symptoms persist, dose may be repeated in 5 to 15 minutes using the same device after partial disassembly

Hypotension/septic shock:

Manufacturer's labeling: Septic shock: IV infusion: Initial: 0.05 to 2 mcg/kg/minute (3.5 to 140 mcg/minute in a 70 kg patient); titrate to desired mean arterial pressure (MAP). May adjust dose every 10 to 15 minutes by 0.05 to 0.2 mcg/kg/minute to achieve desired blood pressure goal. After hemodynamic stabilization, may wean incrementally every 30 minutes over 12 to 24 hours.

American Heart Association recommendation: Severe and fluid resistant (off-label dosing): IV infusion: Initial: 0.1 to 0.5 mcg/kg/minute (7 to 35 mcg/minute in a 70 kg patient); titrate to desired response (AHA [Peberdy 2010]).

Mydriasis during intraocular surgery, induction and maintenance: Intraocular: Must dilute 1:**1000** (1 mg/mL) solution to a concentration of 1:**100,000** to 1:**1,000,000** (10 **mcg**/mL to 1 **mcg**/mL) prior to intraocular use: May use as an irrigation solution as needed during the procedure or may administer intracamerally (ie, directly into the anterior chamber of the eye) with a bolus dose of 0.1 mL of a 1:**100,000** to 1:**400,000** (10 **mcg**/mL to 2.5 **mcg**/mL) dilution.

Pediatric

Asystole/pulseless arrest, pulseless VT/VF (after failed defibrillation attempts) (PALS [Kleinman 2010]): Infants, Children, and Adolescents:

IV, I.O.: 0.01 mg/kg (0.1 mL/kg of 1:**10,000** [0.1 mg/mL] solution) (maximum single dose: 1 mg) every 3 to 5 minutes until return of spontaneous circulation

Endotracheal: 0.1 mg/kg (0.1 mL/kg of 1:**1000** [1 mg/mL] solution) (maximum single dose: 2.5 mg) every 3 to 5 minutes until IV/I.O. access established or return of spontaneous circulation. Flush with 5 mL of NS immediately after administration. May cause false-negative reading with exhaled CO$_2$ detectors; use second method to confirm tube placement if CO$_2$ is not detected (ACLS [Neumar 2010]).

Postresuscitation infusion to maintain cardiac output or stabilize: IV, I.O.: 0.1 to 1 mcg/kg/minute; doses <0.3 mcg/kg/minute generally produce beta-adrenergic effects and higher doses (>0.3 mcg/kg/minute) generally produce alpha-adrenergic vasoconstriction; titrate dosage to desired effect

Bradycardia (symptomatic; unresponsive to atropine or pacing) (PALS [Kleinman 2010]): Infants, Children, and Adolescents:

IV, I.O.: 0.01 mg/kg (0.1 mL/kg of 1:**10,000** [0.1 mg/mL] solution) (maximum single dose: 1 mg) every 3 to 5 minutes as needed

Endotracheal: 0.1 mg/kg or (0.1 mL/kg of 1:**1000** [1 mg/mL] solution) (maximum single dose: 2.5 mg) every 3 to 5 minutes as needed until IV/I.O. access established. Flush with 5 mL of NS immediately after administration. May cause false-negative reading with exhaled CO$_2$ detectors; use second method to confirm tube placement if CO$_2$ is not detected (ACLS [Neumar 2010]).

Continuous infusion: IV, I.O.: 0.1 to 1 mcg/kg/minute; doses <0.3 mcg/kg/minute generally produce beta-adrenergic effects and higher doses (>0.3 mcg/kg/minute) generally produce alpha-adrenergic vasoconstriction; titrate dosage to desired effect

Hypersensitivity reaction (eg, anaphylaxis): Infants, Children, and Adolescents: **Note:** SubQ administration results in slower absorption and is less reliable. IM administration in the anterolateral aspect of the middle third of the thigh is preferred in the setting of anaphylaxis (AHA [Vanden Hoek 2010]; Kemp 2008).

IM, SubQ: 0.01 mg/kg (0.01 mL/kg of **1:1000** [1 mg/mL] solution) (maximum single dose: 0.3 mg) every 5 to 15 minutes; larger IM or SubQ doses, use of IV route, or continuous infusion may be needed for severe anaphylactic reactions (Kemp 2008; Lieberman 2010). If clinician deems appropriate, the 5-minute interval between injections may be shortened to allow for more frequent administration (Lieberman 2010).

Self-administration following severe allergic reactions (eg, insect stings, food): **Note:** World Health Organization (WHO) and Anaphylaxis Canada recommend the availability of 1 dose for every 10 to 20 minutes of travel time to a medical emergency facility. If anaphylactic symptoms persist after first dose, may repeat dose in 5 to 15 minutes (AHA [Vanden Hoek 2010]); more than 2 sequential doses should only be administered under direct medical supervision.

Adrenaclick: IM, SubQ:
  Children 15 to 29 kg: 0.15 mg; if anaphylactic symptoms persist, dose may be repeated using an additional Adrenaclick injector
  Children ≥30 kg: 0.3 mg; if anaphylactic symptoms persist, dose may be repeated using an additional Adrenaclick injector

Allerject [Canadian product]: IM:
  Children 15 to 29 kg: 0.15 mg; if anaphylactic symptoms persist, dose may be repeated using an additional Allerject injector
  Children ≥30 kg: 0.3 mg; if anaphylactic symptoms persist, dose may be repeated using an additional Allerject injector

Auvi-Q: IM, SubQ:
  Children 15 to 29 kg: 0.15 mg; if anaphylactic symptoms persist, dose may be repeated
  Children ≥30 kg: 0.3 mg; if anaphylactic symptoms persist, dose may be repeated

EpiPen Jr: IM, SubQ: Children 15 to 29 kg: 0.15 mg; if anaphylactic symptoms persist, dose may be repeated using an additional EpiPen Jr

EpiPen: IM, SubQ: Children ≥30 kg: 0.3 mg; if anaphylactic symptoms persist, dose may be repeated using an additional EpiPen

Twinject [Canadian product]: IM, SubQ:
  Children 15 to 29 kg: 0.15 mg; if anaphylactic symptoms persist, dose may be repeated in 5 to 15 minutes using the same device after partial disassembly
  Children ≥30 kg: 0.3 mg; if anaphylactic symptoms persist, dose may be repeated in 5 to 15 minutes using the same device after partial disassembly

Alternate auto-injector dose: IM (Sicherer 2007):
  Children 10 to 25 kg: 0.15 mg
  Children >25 kg: 0.3 mg

Hypotension/shock, fluid-resistant (off-label use): Continuous IV infusion: 0.1 to 1 mcg/kg/minute; doses up to 5 mcg/kg/minute may rarely be necessary (Hegenbarth 2008)

Mydriasis during intraocular surgery, induction and maintenance: Infants, Children, and Adolescents: Intraocular: Refer to adult dosing.

Renal Impairment There are no dosage adjustment provided in manufacturer's labeling.

Hepatic Impairment There are no dosage adjustment provided in manufacturer's labeling.

Usual Infusion Concentrations: Pediatric IV infusion: 16 **mcg**/mL, 32 **mcg**/mL, or 64 **mcg**/mL

Usual Infusion Concentrations: Adult IV infusion: 1 mg in 250 mL (concentration: 4 **mcg**/mL) **or** 4 mg in 250 mL (concentration: 16 **mcg**/mL) of D$_5$W or NS; 1 mg in 1,000 mL (concentration: 1 **mcg**/mL) in D$_5$W or D$_5$NS

Administration Epinephrine solutions for injection can be administered IM, I.O., endotracheally, IV, or SubQ. **Note:** Adrenaclick, Allerject [Canadian product], Auvi-Q, EpiPen and EpiPen Jr Auto-Injectors contain a single, fixed-dose of epinephrine and may only be administered IM (preferred) or SubQ. Twinject Auto-Injectors [Canadian product] contain two doses; the first fixed-dose is available for auto-injection; the second dose is available for manual injection following partial disassembly of device.

IV: When administering as a continuous infusion, central line administration is preferred. IV infusions require an infusion pump. If central line not available, as a temporary measure, may administer through a large vein. Avoid use of ankle veins (due to potential for gangrene), leg veins in elderly patients, or leg veins in those suffering from occlusive vascular diseases (eg, diabetic endarteritis, Buerger's disease, arteriosclerosis, atherosclerosis). Vesicant; ensure proper needle or catheter placement prior to and during infusion; avoid extravasation.

Extravasation management: If extravasation occurs, stop infusion immediately and disconnect (leave cannula/needle in place); gently aspirate extravasated solution (do **NOT** flush the line); remove needle/cannula; elevate extremity. Initiate phentolamine (or alternative antidote). Apply dry warm compresses (Hurst 2004).

Phentolamine (no longer available in the US): Dilute 5 to 10 mg in 10 to 15 mL NS and administer into extravasation site as soon as possible after extravasation (Peberdy 2010).

Alternatives to phentolamine:
  Nitroglycerin topical 2% ointment (based on limited case reports in neonates/infants): Apply 4 mm/kg as a thin ribbon to the affected areas; may repeat after 8 hours if needed (Wong 1992) **or** apply a 1-inch strip on the affected site (Denkler 1989).
  Terbutaline (based on limited case reports): Infiltrate extravasation area using a solution of terbutaline 1 mg diluted to 10 mL in NS (large extravasation site; administration volume varied from 3 to 10 mL) **or** 1 mg diluted in 1 mL NS (small/distal extravasation site; administration volume varied from 0.5 to 1 mL) (Stier 1999).

Subcutaneous: SubQ administration results in slower absorption and is less reliable.

IM: IM administration in the anterolateral aspect of the middle third of the thigh is preferred in the setting of anaphylaxis (AHA [Vanden Hoek 2010]; Kemp 2008). IM administration into the buttocks should be avoided. Adrenaclick, Allerject [Canadian product], Auvi-Q, EpiPen, EpiPen Jr, and Twinject Auto-Injectors [Canadian product] should only be injected into the anterolateral aspect of the thigh, through clothing if necessary.

Obesity: In overweight or obese children, because skin surface to muscle depth is greater in the upper half of the thigh, administration into the lower half of the thigh may be preferred. In very obese children, injection into the calf will provide an even greater chance of intramuscular administration (Arkwright 2013).

Endotracheal (cardiac arrest): Dilute in NS or sterile water. Absorption may be greater with sterile water (Naganobu 2000). Stop compressions, spray drug quickly down tube. Follow immediately with several quick insufflations and continue chest compressions. May cause false-negative reading with exhaled CO_2 detectors; use second method to confirm tube placement if CO_2 is not detected (ACLS [Neumar 2010]).

Monitoring Parameters Heart rate, blood pressure (invasive blood pressure monitoring and central venous pressure monitoring recommended while receiving continuous infusion); monitor site of infusion for blanching/extravasation; continuous cardiac monitoring required during continuous infusion. If using to treat hypotension, assess intravascular volume prior to and during therapy; support as needed.

Consult individual institutional policies and procedures.

Dosage Forms Excipient information presented when available (limited, particularly for generics); consult specific product labeling. [DSC] = Discontinued product
Device, Injection:
  EpiPen 2-Pak: 0.3 mg/0.3 mL (2 ea) [latex free; contains sodium metabisulfite]
  EpiPen Jr 2-Pak: 0.15 mg/0.3 mL (2 ea) [contains sodium metabisulfite]
Kit, Injection:
  EPIsnap: 1 mg/mL [contains sodium metabisulfite]
Solution, Injection:
  Adrenalin: 30 mg/30 mL (30 mL) [contains chlorobutanol (chlorobutol), sodium metabisulfite]
  Generic: 0.1 mg/mL (10 mL); 1 mg/mL (1 mL)
Solution, Intravenous [preservative free]:
  Generic: 1 mg/mL (1 mL)
Solution, Injection, as hydrochloride:
  Adrenalin: 1 mg/mL (30 mL [DSC]) [contains chlorobutanol (chlorobutol), sodium bisulfite]
  Adrenalin: 1 mg/mL (1 mL [DSC]) [contains sodium bisulfite]
  Adrenalin: 1 mg/mL (1 mL) [contains sodium metabisulfite]
  Generic: 1 mg/mL (1 mL, 30 mL)
Solution Auto-injector, Injection:
  Adrenaclick: 0.15 mg/0.15 mL (2 ea); 0.3 mg/0.3 mL (2 ea) [latex free; contains chlorobutanol (chlorobutol), sodium bisulfite]

Auvi-Q: 0.15 mg/0.15 mL (2 ea [DSC]); 0.3 mg/0.3 mL (2 ea [DSC]) [contains sodium bisulfite]

Twinject: 0.15 mg/0.15 mL (1 ea [DSC], 2 ea [DSC]); 0.3 mg/0.3 mL (1 ea [DSC], 2 ea [DSC]) [latex free; contains chlorobutanol (chlorobutol), sodium bisulfite]

Generic: 0.15 mg/0.15 mL (1 ea, 2 ea); 0.3 mg/0.3 mL (1 ea, 2 ea)

Solution Prefilled Syringe, Injection:
Generic: 0.1 mg/mL (10 mL)

EPINEPHrine (Oral Inhalation) (ep i NEF rin)

Brand Names: US Asthmanefrin Refill [OTC]; Asthmanefrin Starter Kit [OTC]; Micronefrin [OTC] [DSC]; S2 [OTC]

Brand Names: Canada S2

Index Terms Racemic Epinephrine; Racepinephrine; Racepinephrine HCL

Pharmacologic Category Alpha/Beta Agonist

Use OTC labeling: Treatment of bronchospasm associated with bronchial asthma

Pregnancy Considerations Adverse events have been observed in animal reproduction studies. Epinephrine crosses the placenta (Sandler 1964). Uterine vasoconstriction, decreased uterine blood flow, and fetal anoxia may occur. Epinephrine is recommended for the treatment of anaphylaxis in pregnant women. Specific dosing is not available; use with caution and monitor hemodynamic response (Hepner 2013). In general, medications used for ACLS in pregnant women are given at the same dose as nonpregnant patients (AHA [Vanden Hoek 2010]).

Breast-Feeding Considerations It is not known if epinephrine is excreted in breast milk. The manufacturer recommends that caution be exercised when administering epinephrine to nursing women.

Contraindications Oral inhalation (OTC labeling): Concurrent use or within 2 weeks of MAO inhibitors

Warnings/Precautions Use with caution in patients with diabetes mellitus, cardiovascular diseases (eg, arrhythmias, coronary artery disease, hypertension), thyroid disease, cerebrovascular disease, in patients with prostate enlargement or urinary retention, or in patients with seizure disorders.

Self medication (OTC use): Prior to self-medication, patients should contact healthcare provider. The product should only be used in persons with a diagnosis of asthma. If symptoms are not relieved in 20 minutes or become worse do not continue to use the product - seek immediate medical assistance. The product should not be used more frequently or at higher doses than recommended unless directed by a health care provider. This product should not be used in patients who have required hospitalization for asthma or if a patient is taking prescription medication for asthma. Use with caution in patients with prostate enlargement or urinary retention. Do not use if you have taken a MAO inhibitor (certain drugs used for depression, Parkinson disease, or other conditions) within 2 weeks.

Adverse Reactions There are no adverse reactions listed in the manufacturer's labeling.

Drug Interactions

Metabolism/Transport Effects Substrate of COMT

Avoid Concomitant Use

Avoid concomitant use of EPINEPHrine (Oral Inhalation) with any of the following: Ergot Derivatives; Iobenguane I 123; MAO Inhibitors

Increased Effect/Toxicity

EPINEPHrine (Oral Inhalation) may increase the levels/effects of: Doxofylline; Sympathomimetics

The levels/effects of EPINEPHrine (Oral Inhalation) may be increased by: AtoMOXetine; Beta-Blockers; Cannabinoid-Containing Products; COMT Inhibitors; Ergot Derivatives; Inhalational Anesthetics; MAO Inhibitors; Serotonin/Norepinephrine Reuptake Inhibitors; Tricyclic Antidepressants

Decreased Effect

EPINEPHrine (Oral Inhalation) may decrease the levels/effects of: Iobenguane I 123

The levels/effects of EPINEPHrine (Oral Inhalation) may be decreased by: Alpha1-Blockers; Promethazine; Spironolactone

Preparation for Administration Oral inhalation: S2, Asthmanefrin: If using jet nebulizer, must be diluted with 3 to 5 mL NS. If using handheld rubber bulb nebulizer, dilution is not required.

Storage/Stability S2, Asthmanefrin: Store between 2°C to 20°C (36°F to 68°F). Protect from light.

Mechanism of Action Stimulates alpha-, beta1-, and beta2-adrenergic receptors resulting in relaxation of smooth muscle of the bronchial tree, cardiac stimulation (increasing myocardial oxygen consumption), and dilation of skeletal muscle vasculature; small doses can cause vasodilation via beta2-vascular receptors; large doses may produce constriction of skeletal and vascular smooth muscle

Pharmacodynamics/Kinetics

Onset of action: Bronchodilation: Inhalation: ~1 minute

Distribution: Does not cross blood-brain barrier

Metabolism: Taken up into the adrenergic neuron and metabolized by monoamine oxidase and catechol-o-methyltransferase; circulating drug hepatically metabolized

Excretion: Urine (as inactive metabolites, metanephrine, and sulfate and hydroxy derivatives of mandelic acid, small amounts as unchanged drug)

Dosing

Adult & Geriatric

Bronchospasm, relief of mild asthma symptoms: Nebulization: Racemic epinephrine (2.25% solution): OTC labeling: Hand-bulb nebulizer: Add 0.5 mL to nebulizer; 1 to 3 inhalations, may repeat dose after at least 3 hours if needed. Do not exceed 12 inhalations in 24 hours.

Pediatric

Bronchospasm, relief of mild asthma symptoms: Children ≥4 years and Adolescents: Nebulization: Racemic epinephrine (2.25% solution): OTC labeling: Hand-bulb nebulizer: Add 0.5 mL to nebulizer; 1 to 3 inhalations; may repeat dose after at least 3 hours if needed. Do not exceed 12 inhalations in 24 hours. **Note:** Not recommended for routine management and treatment of asthma (GINA 2015; NAEPP 2007)

Croup (laryngotracheobronchitis), airway edema (off-label use): Infants, Children, and Adolescents: Nebulization: **Note:** Typically relief of symptoms occurs within 10 to 30 minutes and lasts 2 to 3 hours; patients should be observed for rapid symptom recurrence and possible repeat treatment.

Racemic epinephrine (2.25% solution): 0.05 to 0.1 mL/kg (maximum dose: 0.5 mL) diluted in 2 mL NS, may repeat dose every 20 minutes; others have reported use of 0.5 mL as a fixed dose for all patients; use lower end of dosing range for younger infants (Hegenbarth 2008; Rosekrans 1998; Rotta 2003; Wright 2002)

L-epinephrine (using parenteral 1:1000 solution): 0.5 mL/kg of **1:1000** solution (maximum dose: 5 mL) diluted in NS, may repeat dose every 20 minutes; **Note:** Racemic epinephrine 10 mg = 5 mg L-epinephrine (Hegenbarth 2008)

Renal Impairment There are no dosage adjustment provided in manufacturer's labeling.

Hepatic Impairment There are no dosage adjustment provided in manufacturer's labeling.

Administration Oral inhalation: If using jet nebulizer: Administer diluted over ~15 minutes. If using handheld rubber bulb nebulizer, dilution is not required.

Monitoring Parameters FEV1, peak flow, and/or other pulmonary function tests; blood pressure, heart rate; CNS stimulation; serum glucose, serum potassium; asthma symptoms

Dosage Forms Excipient information presented when available (limited, particularly for generics); consult specific product labeling. [DSC] = Discontinued product

Nebulization Solution, Inhalation:
Asthmanefrin Refill: 2.25% (1 ea) [contains edetate disodium]

Asthmanefrin Starter Kit: 2.25% (1 ea) [contains edetate disodium]

Micronefrin: 2.25% (15 mL [DSC], 30 mL [DSC])

Nebulization Solution, Inhalation [preservative free]:
S2: 2.25% (1 ea) [sulfite free; contains edetate disodium]

◆ Epinephrine and Lidocaine see Lidocaine and Epinephrine on page 1075

◆ Epinephrine Bitartrate see EPINEPHrine (Systemic) on page 647

◆ Epinephrine Hydrochloride see EPINEPHrine (Systemic) on page 647

◆ EpiPen (Can) see EPINEPHrine (Systemic) on page 647

◆ EpiPen 2-Pak see EPINEPHrine (Systemic) on page 647

◆ EpiPen Jr (Can) see EPINEPHrine (Systemic) on page 647

◆ EpiPen Jr 2-Pak see EPINEPHrine (Systemic) on page 647

◆ Epipodophyllotoxin see Etoposide on page 714

◆ Epipodophyllotoxin see Etoposide Phosphate on page 717

◆ EpiQuin Micro see Hydroquinone on page 893

◆ EpiQuin Micro/Pump [DSC] see Hydroquinone on page 893

Epirubicin (ep i ROO bi sin)

Brand Names: US Ellence
Brand Names: Canada Ellence; Epirubicin for Injection; Epirubicin Hydrochloride Injection; Pharmorubicin
Index Terms Epidoxorubicin; Epirubicin Hydrochloride; Pidorubicin; Pidorubicin Hydrochloride
Pharmacologic Category Antineoplastic Agent, Anthracycline; Antineoplastic Agent, Topoisomerase II Inhibitor
Use Breast cancer, adjuvant treatment: Adjuvant therapy component for primary breast cancer in patients with evidence of axillary node involvement following tumor resection

Dosing

Adult Note: Patients receiving 120 mg/m^2/cycle as part of combination therapy (CEF-120 regimen) should also receive prophylactic antibiotic therapy with sulfamethoxazole/trimethoprim or a fluoroquinolone. Lower starting doses may be necessary for heavily pretreated patients, patients with preexisting myelosuppression, or with bone marrow involvement. If clinically reasonable, delay epirubicin therapy until other cardiotoxic agents with long half-lives (eg, trastuzumab) have been cleared. The recommended lifetime maximum dose is 900 mg/m^2. Epirubicin is associated with a moderate to high emetic potential (depending on dose or regimen); antiemetics are recommended to prevent nausea and vomiting (Basch 2011; Dupuis 2011; Roila 2010).

Breast cancer, adjuvant treatment: IV: Usual dose: 100-120 mg/m^2 per 3- or 4-week treatment cycle as follows:

60 mg/m^2 on days 1 and 8 every 28 days for 6 cycles in combination with cyclophosphamide and fluorouracil (CEF-120 regimen; Levine 2005) **or**
100 mg/m^2 on day 1 every 21 days for 6 cycles in combination with cyclophosphamide and fluorouracil (FEC-100 regimen; Bonneterre 2005) **or**

Breast cancer (off-label regimens): IV:
EC regimen: 100 mg/m^2 on day 1 every 21 days for 8 cycles in combination with cyclophosphamide (Piccart 2001) **or**
EP or EC regimen: 75 mg/m^2 on day 1 every 21 days for up to 6 cycles in combination with either paclitaxel or cyclophosphamide (Langley 2005) **or**
FEC regimen ± paclitaxel: 90 mg/m^2 on day 1 every 21 days for 6 cycles in combination with fluorouracil and cyclophosphamide or for 4 cycles in combination with fluorouracil and cyclophosphamide followed by paclitaxel (Martin 2008) **or**
FEC regimen followed by pertuzumab + trastuzumab + docetaxel: 100 mg/m^2 on day 1 every 21 days for 3 cycles in combination with fluorouracil and cyclophosphamide, followed by 3 cycles of pertuzumab, trastuzumab, and docetaxel (Schneeweiss 2013) **or**
CEF regimen: 50 mg/m^2 on days 1 and 8 every 21 or 28 days for 6 to 9 cycles in combination with cyclophosphamide and fluorouracil (Ackland 2001)

Esophageal cancer (off-label use): IV:
ECF, ECX, EOF, and EOX regimens: 50 mg/m^2 on day 1 every 21 days for up to 8 cycles in combination with cisplatin (C), oxaliplatin (O), fluorouracil (F), and/or capecitabine (X) (Cunningham 2008) **or**
ECF regimen: 50 mg/m^2 on day 1 every 21 days for 3 preoperative and 3 postoperative cycles in combination with cisplatin and fluorouracil (Cunningham 2006)

Gastric cancer (off-label use): IV:
ECF, ECX, EOF, and EOX regimens: 50 mg/m^2 on day 1 every 21 days for up to 8 cycles in combination with cisplatin (C), oxaliplatin (O), fluorouracil (F), and/or capecitabine (X) (Cunningham 2008; Waters 1999) **or**
ECF regimen: 50 mg/m^2 on day 1 every 21 days for 3 preoperative and 3 postoperative cycles in combination with cisplatin and fluorouracil (Cunningham 2006)

Osteosarcoma (off-label use): IV: 90 mg/m^2 on day 1 every 21 days for 3 cycles before surgery and 90 mg/m^2 on day 1 every 28 days for 3 cycles after surgery (in combination with cisplatin, ifosfamide and mesna) (Basaran 2007)

Soft tissue sarcoma (off-label use): IV: 25 mg/m^2 on days 1, 2, and 3 every 28 days for 4 cycles (in combination with ifosfamide and mesna) (Petrioli 2002) **or** 60 mg/m^2 on days 1 and 2 every 21 days for 5 cycles (in combination with ifosfamide, mesna, and filgrastim) (Frustaci 2001)

Dosage adjustment for toxicity (breast cancer; labeled dosing):
Note: Heavily-treated patients, patients with preexisting bone marrow depression or neoplastic bone marrow infiltration: Lower starting doses (75 to 90 mg/m^2) should be considered.

Delay day 1 dose of subsequent cycles until platelets are ≥100,000/mm^3, ANC ≥1500/mm^3, and nonhematologic toxicities have recovered to ≤ grade 1
Reduce day 1 dose in subsequent cycles to 75% of previous day 1 dose if patient experiences nadir platelet counts <50,000/mm^3, ANC <250/mm^3, neutropenic fever, or grade 3/4 nonhematologic toxicity during the previous cycle
For CEF-120 regimen, reduce day 8 dose to 75% of day 1 dose if platelet counts are 75,000 to 100,000/mm^3 and ANC is 1000 to 1499/mm^3; omit day 8 dose if platelets are <75,000/mm^3, ANC <1000/mm^3, or grade 3/4 nonhematologic toxicity

Geriatric Plasma clearance of epirubicin in elderly female patients was noted to be reduced by 35%. Although no initial dosage reduction is specifically recommended, particular care should be exercised in monitoring toxicity and adjusting subsequent dosage in elderly patients (particularly females >70 years of age).

Renal Impairment The manufacturer's labeling recommends lower doses (dose not specified) in patients with severe renal impairment (serum creatinine >5 mg/dL). Other sources (Aronoff 2007) suggest no dosage adjustment is needed for CrCl <50 mL/minute.

Hepatic Impairment The manufacturer's labeling recommends the following adjustments (based on clinical trial information):
Bilirubin 1.2 to 3 mg/dL or AST 2 to 4 times the upper limit of normal: Administer 50% of recommended starting dose
Bilirubin >3 mg/dL or AST >4 times the upper limit of normal: Administer 25% of recommended starting dose
Severe hepatic impairment: Use is not recommended (has not been studied).

Obesity *ASCO Guidelines for appropriate chemotherapy dosing in obese adults with cancer:* Utilize patient's actual body weight (full weight) for calculation of body surface area- or weight-based dosing, particularly when the intent of therapy is curative; manage regimen-related toxicities in the same manner as for nonobese patients; if a dose reduction is utilized due to toxicity, consider resumption of full weight-based dosing with subsequent cycles, especially if cause of toxicity (eg, hepatic or renal impairment) is resolved (Griggs 2012).

Additional Information Complete prescribing information should be consulted for additional detail.

Dosage Forms Excipient information presented when available (limited, particularly for generics); consult specific product labeling. [DSC] = Discontinued product
Solution, Intravenous, as hydrochloride [preservative free]:
Ellence: 50 mg/25 mL (25 mL); 200 mg/100 mL (100 mL)
Generic: 50 mg/25 mL (25 mL); 200 mg/100 mL (100 mL)
Solution Reconstituted, Intravenous, as hydrochloride:
Generic: 50 mg (1 ea); 200 mg (1 ea [DSC])

◆ **Epirubicin for Injection (Can)** *see* Epirubicin *on page 651*
◆ **Epirubicin Hydrochloride** *see* Epirubicin *on page 651*
◆ **Epirubicin Hydrochloride Injection (Can)** *see* Epirubicin *on page 651*
◆ **EPIsnap** *see* EPINEPHrine (Systemic) *on page 647*
◆ **Epitol** *see* CarBAMazepine *on page 303*
◆ **Epival (Can)** *see* Valproic Acid and Derivatives *on page 1861*
◆ **Epivir** *see* LamiVUDine *on page 1024*
◆ **Epivir HBV** *see* LamiVUDine *on page 1024*

Eplerenone (e PLER en one)

Brand Names: US Inspra
Brand Names: Canada Inspra
Pharmacologic Category Antihypertensive; Diuretic, Potassium-Sparing; Mineralocorticoid (Aldosterone) Receptor Antagonists

Use

Heart failure post-myocardial infarction (MI): Treatment of heart failure (HF) (LVEF ≤40%) following acute MI
Note: According to the Eighth Joint National Committee (JNC 8) guidelines, aldosterone antagonists are **not** recommended for the initial treatment of hypertension (James, 2013).
The ACCF/AHA 2013 heart failure guidelines recommend the use of aldosterone antagonists, along with other guideline directed medical therapies, to reduce morbidity and mortality in patients with an LVEF ≤40% following acute MI who develop symptoms of HF or have a history of diabetes mellitus (Yancy, 2013).

According to the 2013 ACCF/AHA guidelines for the management of ST-elevation myocardial infarction (STEMI) and the guidelines for the management of unstable angina/non-STEMI, an aldosterone antagonist should be given to patients who are already on an ACE inhibitor and beta-blocker, who have an LVEF ≤40% and either symptomatic HF or diabetes mellitus (ACCF/AHA [Anderson, 2013]; ACCF/AHA [O'Gara, 2013]).

Hypertension: Treatment of hypertension (may be used alone or in combination with other antihypertensive agents)

Note: According to the Eighth Joint National Committee (JNC 8) guidelines, aldosterone antagonists are **not** recommended for the initial treatment of hypertension (James, 2013).

Canadian labeling: Additional use (not in U.S. labeling):
Heart failure: Treatment of NYHA class II chronic heart failure (HF) with left ventricular systolic dysfunction

Pregnancy Considerations Adverse events were observed in some animal reproduction studies. Information related to eplerenone use in pregnancy is limited (Cabassi, 2012; Morton, 2011). The use of mineralocorticoid receptor antagonists is not recommended to treat chronic uncomplicated hypertension in pregnant women and should generally be avoided in women of reproductive potential (ACOG, 2013).

Breast-Feeding Considerations It is not known if eplerenone is excreted in breast milk. Due to the potential for serious adverse reactions in the nursing infant, the manufacturer recommends a decision be made whether to discontinue nursing or to discontinue the drug, taking into account the importance of treatment to the mother.

Contraindications

U.S. labeling: Serum potassium >5.5 mEq/L at initiation; CrCl ≤30 mL/minute; concomitant use of strong CYP3A4 inhibitors (see Drug Interactions for details)
The following additional contraindications apply to patients with hypertension: Type 2 diabetes mellitus (noninsulin dependent, NIDDM) with microalbuminuria; serum creatinine >2.0 mg/dL in males or >1.8 mg/dL in females; CrCl <50 mL/minute; concomitant use with potassium supplements or potassium-sparing diuretics

Canadian labeling: Hypersensitivity to eplerenone or any component of the formulation; serum potassium >5 mEq/L at initiation; severe hepatic impairment (Child-Pugh class C); severe renal impairment (eGFR <30 mL/minute/1.73 m²); clinically significant hyperkalemia; concomitant use with potassium supplements, potassium-sparing diuretics or strong CYP3A4 inhibitors
The following additional contraindications apply to patients with hypertension: Type 2 diabetes mellitus (noninsulin dependent, NIDDM) with microalbuminuria; serum creatinine >1.5 mg/dL [132 micromole/L] in males or >1.3 mg/dL [115 micromole/L] in females; eGFR <50 mL/minute/1.73 m²

Warnings/Precautions Monitor closely for hyperkalemia; increases in serum potassium were dose related during clinical trials and rates of hyperkalemia also increased with declining renal function. The concurrent use of larger doses of ACE inhibitors (eg, ≥ lisinopril 10 mg daily) also increases the risk of hyperkalemia (ACCF/AHA [Yancy, 2013]). Dose reduction or interruption of therapy may be necessary with development of hyperkalemia. Use is contraindicated in patients with potassium >5.5 mEq/L (U.S. labeling) or >5 mEq/L (Canadian labeling) at initiation of therapy. Safety and efficacy have not been established in patients with severe hepatic impairment (Canadian labeling contraindicates use in severe hepatic impairment). Use with caution in HF patients post-MI with diabetes (especially if patient has proteinuria); risk of hyperkalemia is increased. Risk of hyperkalemia is increased with declining renal function. Based on indication and degree of renal impairment, use may be contraindicated (refer to Contraindications field). Use with caution in patients with mild renal impairment; contraindicated with moderate-severe impairment. Potentially significant drug-drug interactions may exist, requiring dose or frequency adjustment, additional monitoring, and/or selection of alternative therapy. Avoid potassium supplements, potassium-containing salt substitutes, a diet rich in potassium, or other drugs that can cause hyperkalemia (eg, other potassium-sparing diuretics, NSAIDS). Concomitant use of potassium supplements or potassium-sparing diuretics is contraindicated in the treatment of hypertension (U.S. labeling) or in all patients regardless of indication (Canadian labeling).

When evaluating a heart failure patient for eplerenone treatment, eGFR should be >30 mL/minute/1.73 m² or creatinine should be ≤2.5 mg/dL (men) or ≤2 mg/dL (women) with no recent worsening and potassium <5 mEq/L with no history of severe hyperkalemia (ACCF/AHA [Yancy, 2013]). Serum potassium levels require close

monitoring and management if elevated. The manufacturer recommends to withhold therapy if serum potassium >6 mEq/L. The ACCF/AHA recommends considering discontinuation upon the development of serum potassium >5.5 mEq/L or worsening renal function with careful evaluation of the entire medical regimen. Avoid routine triple therapy with the combined use of an ACE inhibitor, ARB, and eplerenone. Instruct patients with heart failure to discontinue use during an episode of diarrhea or dehydration or when loop diuretic therapy is interrupted (ACCF/AHA [Yancy, 2013]).

Adverse Reactions

>10%: Endocrine & metabolic: Hyperkalemia ([HF post-MI: K >5.5 mEq/L: 16%; K ≥6 mEq/L: 6%] [HTN: K >5.5 mEq/L at doses ≤200 mg: ≤1%; dose of 400 mg: 9%]), hypertriglyceridemia (1% to 15%, dose related)

1% to 10%:
Central nervous system: Dizziness (3%), fatigue (2%)
Endocrine & metabolic: Hyponatremia (2%, dose related), breast pain (males <1% to 1%), gynecomastia (males <1% to 1%), hypercholesterolemia (<1% to 1%)
Gastrointestinal: Diarrhea (2%), abdominal pain (1%)
Genitourinary: Abnormal vaginal bleeding (<1% to 2%)
Renal: Creatinine increased (HF post-MI: 6%), albuminuria (1%)
Respiratory: Cough (2%)
Miscellaneous: Flu-like syndrome (2%)
<1%, postmarketing, and/or case reports: Angioneurotic edema, BUN increased, liver function tests increased, rash, uric acid increased

Drug Interactions

Metabolism/Transport Effects Substrate of CYP3A4 (major); **Note:** Assignment of Major/Minor substrate status based on clinically relevant drug interaction potential

Avoid Concomitant Use

Avoid concomitant use of Eplerenone with any of the following: Conivaptan; CycloSPORINE (Systemic); CYP3A4 Inhibitors (Strong); Fusidic Acid (Systemic); Idelalisib; Itraconazole; Ketoconazole (Systemic); Posaconazole; Tacrolimus (Systemic); Voriconazole

Increased Effect/Toxicity

Eplerenone may increase the levels/effects of: ACE Inhibitors; Amifostine; Ammonium Chloride; Angiotensin II Receptor Blockers; Antipsychotic Agents (Second Generation [Atypical]); Cardiac Glycosides; CycloSPORINE (Systemic); DULoxetine; Hypotension-Associated Agents; Levodopa; Lithium; Potassium Salts; Potassium-Sparing Diuretics; Sodium Phosphates; Tacrolimus (Systemic)

The levels/effects of Eplerenone may be increased by: Alfuzosin; Analgesics (Opioid); Barbiturates; Brimonidine (Topical); Canagliflozin; Conivaptan; CYP3A4 Inhibitors (Moderate); CYP3A4 Inhibitors (Strong); Dasatinib; Diazoxide; Drospirenone; Fluconazole; Fosaprepitant; Fusidic Acid (Systemic); Heparin; Heparin (Low Molecular Weight); Herbs (Hypotensive Properties); Idelalisib; Itraconazole; Ivacaftor; Ketoconazole (Systemic); Luliconazole; Mifepristone; Molsidomine; Nicorandil; Nitrofurantoin; Nonsteroidal Anti-Inflammatory Agents; Obinutuzumab; Osimertinib; Palbociclib; Pentoxifylline; Phosphodiesterase 5 Inhibitors; Posaconazole; Prostacyclin Analogues; Simeprevir; Stiripentol; Tolvaptan; Trimethoprim; Voriconazole

Decreased Effect

Eplerenone may decrease the levels/effects of: Cardiac Glycosides; QuiNIDine

The levels/effects of Eplerenone may be decreased by: Amphetamines; Bosentan; CYP3A4 Inducers (Moderate); CYP3A4 Inducers (Strong); Dabrafenib; Deferasirox; Enzalutamide; Herbs (Hypertensive Properties); Methylphenidate; Mitotane; Nonsteroidal Anti-Inflammatory Agents; Osimertinib; Siltuximab; St Johns Wort; Tocilizumab; Yohimbine

Food Interactions Grapefruit juice increases eplerenone AUC ~25%. Management: Dosage adjustments of eplerenone may be needed.

Storage/Stability Store at controlled room temperature of 25°C (77°F); excursions permitted to 15°C to 30°C (59°F to 86°F).

Mechanism of Action Aldosterone, a mineralocorticoid, increases blood pressure primarily by inducing sodium and water retention. Overexpression of aldosterone is thought to contribute to myocardial fibrosis (especially following myocardial infarction) and vascular fibrosis. Mineralocorticoid receptors are located in the kidney, heart, blood vessels, and brain. Eplerenone selectively blocks mineralocorticoid receptors reducing blood pressure in a dose-dependent manner and appears to prevent myocardial and vascular fibrosis.

Pharmacodynamics/Kinetics
Distribution: V_d: 43-90 L

Protein binding: ~50%; primarily to alpha$_1$-acid glycoproteins

Metabolism: Primarily hepatic via CYP3A4; metabolites inactive

Bioavailability: 69%

Half-life elimination: 4-6 hours

Time to peak, plasma: ~1.5 hours; may take up to 4 weeks for full antihypertensive effect

Excretion: Urine (~67%); feces (32%); <5% as unchanged drug in urine and feces

Dosing
Adult & Geriatric
Hypertension: Oral: Initial: 50 mg once daily; may increase to 50 mg twice daily if response is not adequate; may take up to 4 weeks for full therapeutic response. Doses >100 mg/day are associated with increased risk of hyperkalemia and no greater therapeutic effect.

*Dose modification during concurrent use with **moderate** CYP3A4 inhibitors:* Initial: 25 mg once daily

Heart failure:

U.S. labeling:

Heart failure (post MI): Oral: Initial: 25 mg once daily; dosage goal: Titrate to 50 mg once daily within 4 weeks, as tolerated

Dosage adjustment per serum potassium concentrations for HF (post-MI):

<5 mEq/L:

Increase dose from 25 mg every other day to 25 mg daily **or**

Increase dose from 25 mg daily to 50 mg daily

5 to 5.4 mEq/L: No adjustment needed

5.5 to 5.9 mEq/L:

Decrease dose from 50 mg daily to 25 mg daily **or**

Decrease dose from 25 mg daily to 25 mg every other day **or**

Modify dose from 25 mg every other day to withhold medication

≥6 mEq/L: Withhold medication until potassium <5.5 mEq/L, then restart at 25 mg every other day

Alternatively, the ACCF/AHA 2013 HF guidelines recommend withholding treatment if potassium >5.5 mEq/L or renal function worsens; hold doses until potassium is <5 mEq/L and consider restarting with a reduced dose after confirming resolution of hyperkalemia/renal insufficiency for at least 72 hours (ACCF/AHA [Yancy, 2013]).

Heart failure (NYHA class II-IV with LVEF ≤35%) (off-label dose): Initial: 25 mg once daily; may increase to a maximum dose of 50 mg once daily (ACCF/AHA [Yancy, 2013])

Canadian labeling:

Chronic HF (NYHA class II) or HF (post-MI): Oral:

eGFR ≥50 mL/minute/1.73 m^2 and potassium ≤5 mEq/L: Initial: 25 mg once daily; may increase within 4 weeks as tolerated to a target dose of 50 mg once daily (maximum dose). **Note:** Treatment following MI should be initiated 3 to 14 days after MI.

*Concurrent use with **mild-to-moderate** CYP3A4 inhibitors:* Maximum dose: 25 mg once daily

eGFR 30 to 49 mL/minute/1.73 m^2 and potassium ≤5 mEq/L: Initial: 25 mg every other day; may increase within 4 weeks as tolerated to a target dose of 25 mg once daily (maximum dose). **Note:** Treatment following MI should be initiated 3 to 14 days after MI.

*Concurrent use with **mild-to-moderate** CYP3A4 inhibitors:* Avoid concurrent use (target dose <25 mg once daily has not been studied).

Dosage adjustment (after initiation) per serum potassium concentrations:

<5 mEq/L:

Current dose is 25 mg every other day: Increase to 25 mg daily

Current dose is 25 mg daily and eGFR ≥50 mL/minute/1.73 m^2 or **not taking** concurrent mild-to-moderate CYP3A4 inhibitor: Increase to 50 mg daily

Current dose is 25 mg daily and eGFR 30 to 49 mL/minute/1.73 m^2 or **if taking** concurrent mild-to-moderate CYP3A4 inhibitor: Do not increase dose.

5 to 5.4 mEq/L: No adjustment needed

5.5 to 5.9 mEq/L:

Current dose is 50 mg daily: Decrease to 25 mg daily

Current dose is 25 mg daily: Decrease to 25 mg every other day

Current dose is 25 mg every other day: Withhold further doses; reinitiate only if potassium <5 mEq/L

≥6 mEq/L: Withhold further doses until potassium <5 mEq/L, then may temporarily resume therapy at 25 mg every other day (dose efficacy has not been established); reassess potassium levels in 1 week and if within acceptable limits, increase dose to 25 mg once daily; reassess potassium levels again in 1 week to determine whether therapy should be continued or interrupted.

Renal Impairment
U.S. labeling:

Hypertension:

CrCl ≥50 mL/minute: There are no dosage adjustments provided in the manufacturer's labeling.

CrCl <50 mL/minute or serum creatinine >2 mg/dL (males) or >1.8 mg/dL (females): Use is contraindicated; risk of hyperkalemia increases with declining renal function.

Heart failure (post-MI):

CrCl ≥50 mL/minute: There are no dosage adjustments provided in the manufacturer's labeling.

CrCl 31 to 50 mL/minute or serum creatinine >2 mg/dL (males) or >1.8 mg/dL (females): There are no dosage adjustment provided in the manufacturer's labeling; use with caution.

CrCl ≤30 mL/minute: Use is contraindicated.

Heart failure (including post-MI) (ACCF/AHA [Yancy, 2013]:

eGFR ≥50 mL/minute/1.73 m^2: Initial dose: 25 mg once daily; Maintenance dose (after 4 weeks of treatment and potassium ≤5 mEq/L): 50 mg once daily

eGFR 30 to 49 mL/minute/1.73 m^2: Initial dose: 25 mg once every other day; Maintenance dose (after 4 weeks of treatment and potassium ≤5 mEq/L): 25 mg once daily

eGFR <30 mL/minute/1.73 m^2: Not recommended

Canadian labeling:

Hypertension:

eGFR ≥50 mL/minute/1.73 m^2: There are no dosage adjustments provided in the manufacturer's labeling; monitor serum potassium closely.

eGFR <50 mL/minute/1.73 m^2 or serum creatinine >1.5 mg/dL [132 micromole/L] in males or >1.3 mg/dL [115 micromole/L] in females: Use is contraindicated.

Chronic HF (NYHA class II) or HF (post-MI):

eGFR ≥50 mL/minute/1.73 m^2: No dosage adjustment necessary unless receiving concurrent mild-to-moderate CYP3A4 inhibitor, then maximum dose is 25 mg once daily.

eGFR 30 to 49 mL/minute/1.73 m^2: Initial: 25 mg every other day; titrate to 25 mg once daily (maximum dose) within 4 weeks, as tolerated. Avoid concurrent use with mild-to-moderate CYP3A4 inhibitors.

eGFR ≤30 mL/minute/1.73 m^2: Use is contraindicated.

Hepatic Impairment
U.S. labeling:

Mild-to-moderate impairment: No dosage adjustment necessary.

Severe impairment: No dosage adjustment provided in manufacturer's labeling (has not been studied).

Canadian labeling:

Mild-to-moderate impairment: No dosage adjustment necessary.

Severe impairment: Use is contraindicated.

Dietary Considerations May be taken with or without food. Do not use salt substitutes containing potassium.

Administration May be administered with or without food.

Monitoring Parameters Blood pressure; serum potassium (prior to therapy, within the first week, 1 month after start of treatment or dose adjustment, then periodically as clinically indicated); additionally, check serum potassium in 3-7 days after initiating concurrent therapy with moderate CYP3A4 inhibitor; serum creatinine

ACCF/AHA heart failure guideline recommendations (ACCF/AHA [Yancy, 2013]): Serum potassium and renal function should be checked in 3 days after initiation, at 1 week after initiation, at least monthly for the first 3 months of therapy, and every 3 months thereafter. If adding or increasing the dose of concomitant ACE inhibitors or ARBs, a new cycle of monitoring should be done. If serum potassium increases to >5.5 mEq/L or renal function worsens, hold doses until potassium is <5 mEq/L and consider restarting with a reduced dose after confirming resolution of hyperkalemia/renal insufficiency for at least 72 hours.

◄ **Dosage Forms** Excipient information presented when available (limited, particularly for generics); consult specific product labeling.

Tablet, Oral:
Inspra: 25 mg, 50 mg
Generic: 25 mg, 50 mg

◆ EPO see Epoetin Alfa on page 654

Epoetin Alfa (e POE e tin AL fa)

Brand Names: US Epogen; Procrit
Brand Names: Canada Eprex
Index Terms rHuEPO; rHuEPO-α; EPO; Epoetin Alfa, Recombinant; Erythropoiesis-Stimulating Agent (ESA); Erythropoietin
Pharmacologic Category Colony Stimulating Factor; Erythropoiesis-Stimulating Agent (ESA); Hematopoietic Agent

Use

Anemia: Treatment of anemia due to concurrent myelo-suppressive chemotherapy in patients with cancer (non-myeloid malignancies) receiving chemotherapy (palliative intent) for a planned minimum of 2 additional months of chemotherapy; treatment of anemia due to chronic kidney disease (including patients on dialysis and not on dialysis) to decrease the need for RBC transfusion; treatment of anemia associated with HIV (zidovudine) therapy when endogenous erythropoietin levels ≤500 mUnits/mL; reduction of allogeneic RBC transfusion for elective, noncardiac, nonvascular surgery when perioperative hemoglobin is >10 to ≤13 g/dL and there is a high risk for blood loss

Limitations of use: Epoetin alfa has not been shown to improve quality of life, fatigue, or patient well-being. Epoetin alfa is **not** indicated for use under the following conditions:

- Cancer patients receiving hormonal therapy, therapeutic biologic products, or radiation therapy unless also receiving concurrent myelosuppressive chemotherapy
- Cancer patients receiving myelosuppressive chemotherapy when the expected outcome is curative
- Surgery patients who are willing to donate autologous blood
- Surgery patients undergoing cardiac or vascular surgery
- As a substitute for RBC transfusion in patients requiring immediate correction of anemia

Pregnancy Considerations Adverse events were observed in animal reproduction studies. In vitro studies suggest that recombinant erythropoietin does not cross the human placenta (Reisenberger 1997). Polyhydramnios and intrauterine growth retardation have been reported with use in women with chronic kidney disease (adverse effects also associated with maternal disease). Hypospadias and pectus excavatum have been reported with first trimester exposure (case report).

Recombinant erythropoietin alfa has been evaluated as adjunctive treatment for severe pregnancy associated iron deficiency anemia (Breymann 2001; Krafft 2009) and has been used in pregnant women with iron-deficiency anemia associated with chronic kidney disease (CKD) (Furaz-Czerpak 2012; Josephson 2007).

Amenorrheic premenopausal women should be cautioned that menstruation may resume following treatment with recombinant erythropoietin (Furaz-Czerpak 2012). Multidose formulations containing benzyl alcohol are contraindicated for use in pregnant women; if treatment during pregnancy is needed, single dose preparations should be used.

Women who become pregnant during treatment with epoetin alfa are encouraged to enroll in Amgen's Pregnancy Surveillance Program (1-800-772-6436).

Breast-Feeding Considerations Endogenous erythropoietin is found in breast milk (Semba 2002). It is not known if recombinant erythropoietin alfa is excreted into breast milk. The manufacturer recommends caution be used if the single dose vial preparation is administered to nursing women; use of the multiple dose vials containing benzyl alcohol is contraindicated in breast-feeding women. When administered enterally to neonates (mixed with human milk or infant formula), recombinant erythropoietin did not significantly increase serum EPO concentrations. If passage via breast milk does occur, risk to a nursing infant appears low (Juul 2003).

Prescribing and Access Restrictions As a requirement of the REMS program, access to this medication is restricted. Healthcare providers and hospitals must be enrolled in the ESA APPRISE (Assisting Providers and Cancer Patients with Risk Information for the Safe use of ESAs) Oncology Program (866-284-8089; http://www.esa-apprise.com) to prescribe or dispense ESAs (ie, epoetin alfa, darbepoetin alfa) to patients with cancer.

Medication Guide Available Yes

Contraindications Serious allergic reactions to epoetin alfa or any component of the formulation; uncontrolled hypertension; pure red cell aplasia (PRCA) that begins after treatment with epoetin alfa or other epoetin protein drugs; multidose vials contain benzyl alcohol and are contraindicated in neonates, infants, pregnant women, and nursing women

Warnings/Precautions [US Boxed Warning]: Erythropoiesis-stimulating agents (ESAs) increased the risk of serious cardiovascular events, myocardial infarction, stroke, venous thromboembolism, vascular access thrombosis, mortality, and/or tumor progression in clinical studies when administered to target hemoglobin levels >11 g/dL (and provide no additional benefit); a rapid rise in hemoglobin (>1 g/dL over 2 weeks) may also contribute to these risks. **[US Boxed Warning]: A shortened overall survival and/or increased risk of tumor progression or recurrence has been reported in studies with breast, cervical, head and neck, lymphoid, and non-small cell lung cancer patients.** It is of note that in these studies, patients received ESAs to a target hemoglobin of ≥12 g/dL; although risk has not been excluded when dosed to achieve a target hemoglobin of <12 g/dL. **[US Boxed Warnings]: To decrease these risks, and risk of cardio- and thrombovascular events, use the lowest dose needed to avoid red blood cell transfusions. Use ESAs in cancer patients only for the treatment of anemia related to concurrent myelosuppressive chemotherapy; discontinue ESA following completion of the chemotherapy course. ESAs are not indicated for patients receiving myelosuppressive therapy when the anticipated outcome is curative.** A dosage modification is appropriate if hemoglobin levels rise >1 g/dL per 2-week time period during treatment (Rizzo 2010). Use of ESAs has been associated with an increased risk of venous thromboembolism (VTE) without a reduction in transfusions in patients with cancer (Hershman 2009). Improved anemia symptoms, quality of life, fatigue, or well-being have not been demonstrated in controlled clinical trials. **[US Boxed Warning]: Because of the risks of decreased survival and increased risk of tumor growth or progression, health care providers and hospitals must enroll and comply with the ESA APPRISE (Assisting Providers and Cancer Patients with Risk Information for the Safe use of ESAs) Oncology Program to prescribe or dispense ESAs to cancer patients.** Prescribers and patients will have to provide written documentation of discussed risks prior to each new course.

[US Boxed Warning]: An increased risk of death, serious cardiovascular events, and stroke was reported in chronic kidney disease (CKD) patients administered ESAs to target hemoglobin levels ≥11 g/dL; use the lowest dose sufficient to reduce the need for RBC transfusions. An optimal target hemoglobin level, dose or dosing strategy to reduce these risks has not been identified in clinical trials. Hemoglobin rising >1 g/dL in a 2-week period may contribute to the risk (dosage reduction recommended). The American College of Physicians recommends against the use of ESAs in patients with mild to moderate anemia and heart failure or coronary heart disease (ACP [Qaseem 2013]). The ACCF/AHA 2013 Heart Failure Guidelines do not provide a clear recommendation on the use of erythropoiesis-stimulating agents (ESA) in anemic heart failure patients. The effects of ESAs on quality of life measures, morbidity, and mortality are potentially modest and still unclear. Additionally, the safety of epoetin alfa has not been well studied in this population. The authors declined to provide an official recommendation regarding the use of ESAs pending the completion of ongoing randomized trials (ACCF/AHA [Yancy 2013]).

Chronic kidney disease patients who exhibit an inadequate hemoglobin response to ESA therapy may be at a higher risk for cardiovascular events and mortality compared to other patients. ESA therapy may reduce dialysis efficacy (due to increase in red blood cells and decrease in plasma volume); adjustments in dialysis parameters may be needed. Patients treated with epoetin may require increased heparinization during dialysis to prevent clotting of the extracorporeal circuit. **[US Boxed Warning]: DVT prophylaxis is recommended in perisurgery patients due to the risk of DVT.** Increased mortality was also observed in patients undergoing coronary artery bypass surgery who received epoetin alfa; these deaths were associated with thrombotic events. Epoetin alfa is **not** approved for reduction of red blood cell transfusion in

patients undergoing cardiac or vascular surgery and is **not** indicated for surgical patients willing to donate autologous blood.

Use with caution in patients with hypertension (contraindicated in uncontrolled hypertension) or with a history of seizures; hypertensive encephalopathy and seizures have been reported. If hypertension is difficult to control, reduce or hold epoetin alfa. An excessive rate of rise of hemoglobin is associated with hypertension or exacerbation of hypertension; decrease the epoetin alfa dose if the hemoglobin increase exceeds 1 g/dL in any 2-week period. Blood pressure should be controlled prior to start of therapy and monitored closely throughout treatment. The risk for seizures is increased with epoetin alfa use in patients with CKD; monitor closely for neurologic symptoms during the first several months of therapy. Due to the delayed onset of erythropoiesis, epoetin alfa is **not** recommended for acute correction of severe anemia or as a substitute for emergency transfusion.

Prior to treatment, correct or exclude deficiencies of iron, vitamin B_{12}, and/or folate, as well as other factors which may impair erythropoiesis (inflammatory conditions, infections, bleeding). Prior to and periodically during therapy, iron stores must be evaluated. Supplemental iron is recommended if serum ferritin <100 mcg/L or serum transferrin saturation <20%; most patients with chronic kidney disease will require iron supplementation. Poor response should prompt evaluation of these potential factors, as well as possible malignant processes and hematologic disease (thalassemia, refractory anemia, myelodysplastic disorder), occult blood loss, hemolysis, ostetis fibrosa cystic, and/or bone marrow fibrosis. Severe anemia and pure red cell aplasia (PRCA) with associated neutralizing antibodies to erythropoietin has been reported, predominantly in patients with CKD receiving SubQ epoetin alfa (the IV route is preferred for hemodialysis patients). Cases have also been reported in patients with hepatitis C who were receiving ESAs, interferon, and ribavirin. Patients with a sudden loss of response to epoetin alfa (with severe anemia and a low reticulocyte count) should be evaluated for PRCA with associated neutralizing antibodies to erythropoietin; discontinue treatment (permanently) in patients with PRCA secondary to neutralizing antibodies to epoetin alfa. Antibodies may cross-react; do not switch to another ESA in patients who develop antibody-mediated anemia.

The American Society of Clinical Oncology (ASCO) and American Society of Hematology (ASH) 2010 updates to the clinical practice guidelines for the use of ESAs in patients with cancer indicate that ESAs are appropriate when used according to the parameters identified within the FDA-approved labeling for epoetin and darbepoetin afla (Rizzo 2010). ESAs are an option for chemotherapy associated anemia when the hemoglobin has fallen to <10 g/dL to decrease the need for RBC transfusions. ESAs should only be used in conjunction with concurrent chemotherapy. Although the FDA label now limits ESA use to the palliative setting, the ASCO/ASH guidelines suggest using clinical judgment in weighing risks versus benefits as formal outcomes studies of ESA use defined by intent of chemotherapy treatment have not been conducted.

Potentially serious allergic reactions have been reported (rarely), including anaphylactic reactions, angioedema, bronchospasm, rash, and urticaria. Discontinue immediately (and permanently) in patients who experience serious allergic/anaphylactic reactions.

Some dosage forms may contain polysorbate 80 (also known as Tweens). Hypersensitivity reactions, usually a delayed reaction, have been reported following exposure to pharmaceutical products containing polysorbate 80 in certain individuals (Isaksson 2002; Lucente 2000; Shelley 1995). Thrombocytopenia, ascites, pulmonary deterioration, and renal and hepatic failure have been reported in premature neonates after receiving parenteral products containing polysorbate 80 (Alade 1986; CDC 1984). See manufacturer's labeling.

Some products may contain albumin.

Benzyl alcohol and derivatives: Some dosage forms may contain benzyl alcohol; large amounts of benzyl alcohol (≥99 mg/kg/day) have been associated with a potentially fatal toxicity ("gasping syndrome") in neonates; the "gasping syndrome" consists of metabolic acidosis, respiratory distress, gasping respirations, CNS dysfunction (including convulsions, intracranial hemorrhage), hypotension and cardiovascular collapse (AAP ["Inactive" 1997]; CDC 1982); some data suggests that benzoate displaces bilirubin from protein binding sites (Ahlfors 2001); avoid or use dosage forms containing benzyl alcohol with caution in neonates. See manufacturer's labeling.

Adverse Reactions
>10%:
Cardiovascular: Hypertension (3% to 28%)
Central nervous system: Fever (10% to 42%), headache (5% to 18%)
Dermatologic: Pruritus (12% to 21%), rash (2% to 19%)
Gastrointestinal: Nausea (35% to 56%), vomiting (12% to 28%)
Local: Injection site reaction (7% to 13%)
Neuromuscular & skeletal: Arthralgia (10% to 16%)
Respiratory: Cough (4% to 26%)
1% to 10%:
Cardiovascular: Deep vein thrombosis, edema, thrombosis
Central nervous system: Chills, depression, dizziness, insomnia
Dermatologic: Urticaria
Endocrine & metabolic: Hyperglycemia, hypokalemia
Gastrointestinal: Dysphagia, stomatitis, weight loss
Hematologic: Leukopenia
Local: Clotted vascular access
Neuromuscular & skeletal: Bone pain, muscle spasm, myalgia
Respiratory: Pulmonary embolism, respiratory congestion, upper respiratory infection
<1% (Limited to important or life-threatening): Allergic reaction, anaphylactic reaction, angioedema, bronchospasm, erythema, hypersensitivity reactions, hypertensive encephalopathy, microvascular thrombosis, MI, neutralizing antibodies, porphyria, pure red cell aplasia (PRCA), renal vein thrombosis, retinal artery thrombosis, seizure, stroke, tachycardia, temporal vein thrombosis, thrombophlebitis, TIA, tumor progression

Drug Interactions
Metabolism/Transport Effects None known.
Avoid Concomitant Use There are no known interactions where it is recommended to avoid concomitant use.
Increased Effect/Toxicity
Epoetin Alfa may increase the levels/effects of: Lenalidomide; Thalidomide

The levels/effects of Epoetin Alfa may be increased by: Nandrolone
Decreased Effect There are no known significant interactions involving a decrease in effect.
Preparation for Administration Prior to SubQ administration, preservative free solutions may be mixed with bacteriostatic NS containing benzyl alcohol 0.9% in a 1:1 ratio.
Storage/Stability Vials should be stored at 2°C to 8°C (36°F to 46°F); **Do not freeze. Do not shake.** Protect from light.
Single-dose 1 mL vial contains no preservative: Use one dose per vial. Do not re-enter vial; discard unused portions.
Single-dose vials (except 40,000 units/mL vial) are stable for 2 weeks at room temperature (Cohen 2007). Single-dose 40,000 units/mL vial is stable for 1 week at room temperature.
Multidose 1 mL or 2 mL vial contains preservative. Store at 2°C to 8°C after initial entry and between doses. Discard 21 days after initial entry.
Multidose vials (with preservative) are stable for 1 week at room temperature (Cohen 2007).
Prefilled syringes containing the 20,000 units/mL formulation with preservative are stable for 6 weeks refrigerated (2°C to 8°C) (Naughton 2003).
Dilutions of 1:10 and 1:20 (1 part epoetin alfa:19 parts sodium chloride) are stable for 18 hours at room temperature (Ohls 1996).
Prior to SubQ administration, preservative free solutions may be mixed with bacteriostatic NS containing benzyl alcohol 0.9% in a 1:1 ratio (Corbo 1992).
Dilutions of 1:10 in $D_{10}W$ with human albumin 0.05% or 0.1% are stable for 24 hours.
Mechanism of Action Induces erythropoiesis by stimulating the division and differentiation of committed erythroid progenitor cells; induces the release of reticulocytes from the bone marrow into the bloodstream, where they mature to erythrocytes. There is a dose response relationship with this effect. This results in an increase in reticulocyte counts followed by a rise in hematocrit and hemoglobin levels.
Pharmacodynamics/Kinetics Note: While a much higher peak plasma concentration is achieved after IV bolus administration, it declines at a more rapid rate than after subcutaneous administration (McMahon 1990; Salmonson 1990)
Onset of action: Several days
Peak effect: Hemoglobin level: 2 to 6 weeks
Absorption: SubQ: Slow (McMahon, 1990; Salmonson, 1990)

Distribution: V_d: 9 L; rapid in the plasma compartment; concentrated in liver, kidneys, and bone marrow; similar to extracelluar plasma volume in adults (McMahon, 1990; Salmonson, 1990); reported to be higher in premature neonates on body weight basis (Brown 1993)

Metabolism: Some degradation does occur

Bioavailability: SubQ: Premature neonates: 42% (Brown 1993); Adults: 36% (Salmonson 1990); intraperitoneal epoetin alfa: 3% (Macdougall 1989)

Half-life elimination:

Neonates: With high doses, nonlinear kinetics have been observed (Wu, 2012)

Anemia of prematurity:

PMA <32 week (weight: 800 ± 206 grams): IV: 8.1 ± 2.7 hours; SubQ: 7.1 ± 4.1 hours (Brown 1993)

PMA ≥32 weeks (weight range: 1330 ± 1740 g): SubQ: Median: 7.9 hours (range: 5.6 to 19.4 hours) (Krishnan 1996)

Neuroprotective/hypoxic ischemia encephalopathy (HIE) (Wu, 2012): ≥36 weeks GA; IV:

250 units/kg: 7.6 ± 6.9 hours

500 units/kg: 7.2 ± 1.9 hours

1,000 units/kg: 15 ± 4.5 hours

2,500 units/kg: 18.7 ± 4.7 hours

Infants, Children, and Adolescents: Chronic kidney disease: IV: 4 to 13 hours

Adults: Cancer: SubQ: 16 to 67 hours; Chronic kidney disease: IV: 4 to 13 hours

Time to peak, serum: Pediatric patients >1 month and Adults: Chronic kidney disease: SubQ: 5 to 24 hours

Excretion: Feces (majority); urine (small amounts, 10% unchanged in normal volunteers)

Dosing

Adult & Geriatric Note: Evaluate iron status in all patients before and during treatment and maintain iron repletion.

Anemia associated with chronic kidney disease (CKD): Individualize dosing and use the lowest dose necessary to reduce the need for RBC transfusions.

Chronic kidney disease patients ON dialysis (IV route is preferred for hemodialysis patients; initiate treatment when hemoglobin is <10 g/dL; reduce dose or interrupt treatment if hemoglobin approaches or exceeds 11 g/dL): IV, SubQ: Initial dose: 50 to 100 units/kg 3 times a week

Chronic kidney disease patients NOT on dialysis (consider initiating treatment when hemoglobin is <10 g/dL; use only if rate of hemoglobin decline would likely result in RBC transfusion and desire is to reduce risk of alloimmunization and/or other RBC transfusion-related risks; reduce dose or interrupt treatment if hemoglobin exceeds 10 g/dL): IV, SubQ: Initial dose: 50 to 100 units/kg 3 times a week

Dosage adjustments for chronic kidney disease patients (either on dialysis or not on dialysis): Do not increase dose more frequently than every 4 weeks (dose decreases may occur more frequently); avoid frequent dosage adjustments.

If hemoglobin does not increase by >1 g/dL after 4 weeks: Increase dose by 25%

If hemoglobin increases >1 g/dL in any 2-week period: Reduce dose by ≥25%

Inadequate or lack of response over a 12-week escalation period: Further increases are unlikely to improve response and may increase risks; use the minimum effective dose that will maintain a hemoglobin level sufficient to avoid RBC transfusions and evaluate patient for other causes of anemia. Discontinue therapy if responsiveness does not improve.

Anemia due to chemotherapy in cancer patients: Initiate treatment only if hemoglobin <10 g/dL and anticipated duration of myelosuppressive chemotherapy is at least 2 additional months. Titrate dosage to use the minimum effective dose that will maintain a hemoglobin level sufficient to avoid red blood cell transfusions. Discontinue erythropoietin following completion of chemotherapy. SubQ: Initial dose: 150 units/kg 3 times a week or 40,000 units once weekly until completion of chemotherapy

Dosage adjustments:

If hemoglobin does not increase by ≥1 g/dL **and** remains below 10 g/dL after initial 4 weeks: Increase to 300 units/kg 3 times a week or 60,000 units weekly; discontinue after 8 weeks of treatment if RBC transfusions are still required or there is no hemoglobin response

If hemoglobin exceeds a level needed to avoid red blood cell transfusion: Withhold dose; resume treatment with a 25% dose reduction when hemoglobin approaches a level where transfusions may be required.

If hemoglobin increases >1 g/dL in any 2-week period **or** hemoglobin reaches a level sufficient to avoid red blood cell transfusion: Reduce dose by 25%.

Anemia due to zidovudine in HIV-infected patients: Titrate dosage to use the minimum effective dose that will maintain a hemoglobin level sufficient to avoid red blood cell transfusions. Hemoglobin levels should not exceed 12 g/dL.

Serum erythropoietin levels ≤500 mUnits/mL and zidovudine doses ≤4200 mg/week): IV, SubQ: Initial: 100 units/kg 3 times a week; if hemoglobin does not increase after 8 weeks, increase dose by ~50 to 100 units/kg at 4 to 8 week intervals until hemoglobin reaches a level sufficient to avoid RBC transfusion; maximum dose: 300 units/kg. Withhold dose if hemoglobin exceeds 12 g/dL, may resume treatment with a 25% dose reduction once hemoglobin <11 g/dL. Discontinue if hemoglobin increase is not achieved with 300 units/kg for 8 weeks.

Surgery patients (perioperative hemoglobin should be >10 g/dL and ≤13 g/dL; DVT prophylactic anticoagulation is recommended): SubQ: Initial dose:

300 units/kg/day for 15 days total, beginning 10 days before surgery, on the day of surgery, and for 4 days after surgery **or**

600 units/kg once weekly for 4 doses, given 21-, 14-, and 7 days before surgery, and on the day of surgery

Symptomatic anemia associated with myelodysplastic syndrome (off-label use): SubQ: 150 to 300 units/kg once daily (Greenburg 2009) or 450 to 1000 units/kg/week in divided doses, 3 to 7 times a week (Hellström-Lindberg 1995) or 60,000 units once weekly (Park 2008)

Pediatric Note: Evaluate iron status in all patients before and during treatment and maintain iron repletion.

Anemia associated with chronic kidney disease (CKD): Individualize dosing and use the lowest dose necessary to reduce the need for RBC transfusions.

Chronic kidney disease patients ON dialysis (IV route is preferred for hemodialysis patients; initiate treatment when hemoglobin is <10 g/dL; reduce dose or interrupt treatment if hemoglobin approaches or exceeds 11 g/dL):

Pediatrics 1 month to 16 years: IV, SubQ: Initial dose: 50 units/kg 3 times a week

Dosage adjustments for chronic kidney disease patients: Do not increase dose more frequently than every 4 weeks (dose decreases may occur more frequently); avoid frequent dosage adjustments

If hemoglobin does not increase by >1 g/dL after 4 weeks: Increase dose by 25%

If hemoglobin increases >1 g/dL in any 2-week period: Reduce dose by ≥25%

Inadequate or lack of response over a 12-week escalation period: Further increases are unlikely to improve response and may increase risks; use the minimum effective dose that will maintain a hemoglobin level sufficient to avoid RBC transfusions and evaluate patient for other causes of anemia. Discontinue therapy if responsiveness does not improve.

Anemia due to chemotherapy in cancer patients: Initiate treatment only if hemoglobin <10 g/dL and anticipated duration of myelosuppressive chemotherapy is at least 2 additional months. Titrate dosage to use the minimum effective dose that will maintain a hemoglobin level sufficient to avoid red blood cell transfusions. Discontinue erythropoietin following completion of chemotherapy.

Children ≥5 years and Adolescents: IV: Initial dose: 600 units/kg once weekly until completion of chemotherapy.

Dosage adjustments:

If hemoglobin does not increase by ≥1 g/dL **and** remains <10 g/dL after initial 4 weeks: Increase to 900 units/kg (maximum dose: 60,000 units); discontinue after 8 weeks of treatment if RBC transfusions are still required or there is no hemoglobin response.

If hemoglobin exceeds a level needed to avoid red blood cell transfusion: Withhold dose; resume treatment with a 25% dose reduction when hemoglobin approaches a level where transfusions may be required.

If hemoglobin increases >1 g/dL in any 2-week period **or** hemoglobin reaches a level sufficient to avoid red blood cell transfusion: Reduce dose by 25%.

Anemia due to zidovudine in HIV-infected patients: Titrate dosage to use the minimum effective dose that will maintain a hemoglobin level sufficient to avoid red blood cell transfusions. Hemoglobin levels should not exceed 12 g/dL. Children 8 months to 17 years (based on limited data): IV, SubQ: Reported dosing range: 50 to 400 units/kg 2 to 3 times a week

Renal Impairment No dosage adjustment necessary.

Hepatic Impairment There are no dosage adjustments provided in the manufacturer's labeling.

Administration Do not shake.

SubQ is the preferred route of administration **except** in patients with CKD on hemodialysis.; usually administered undiluted, although may use a 1:1 dilution with bacteriostatic NS.

Patients with CKD on hemodialysis: IV route preferred; it may be administered into the venous line at the end of the dialysis procedure

Monitoring Parameters Transferrin saturation and serum ferritin (prior to and during treatment); hemoglobin (weekly after initiation and following dose adjustments until stable and sufficient to minimize need for RBC transfusion, CKD patients should be also be monitored at least monthly following hemoglobin stability); blood pressure; seizures (CKD patients following initiation for first few months, includes new-onset or change in seizure frequency or premonitory symptoms)

Cancer patients: Examinations recommended by the ASCO/ASH guidelines (Rizzo 2010) prior to treatment include: peripheral blood smear (in some situations a bone marrow exam may be necessary), assessment for iron, folate, or vitamin B_{12} deficiency, reticulocyte count, renal function status, and occult blood loss; during ESA treatment, assess baseline and periodic iron, total iron-binding capacity, and transferrin saturation or ferritin levels.

Reference Range Zidovudine-treated HIV patients: Available evidence indicates patients with endogenous serum erythropoietin levels >500 mU/mL are unlikely to respond

Dosage Forms Excipient information presented when available (limited, particularly for generics); consult specific product labeling.

Solution, Injection:

Epogen: 10,000 units/mL (2 mL); 20,000 units/mL (1 mL) [contains benzyl alcohol]

Procrit: 10,000 units/mL (2 mL); 20,000 units/mL (1 mL) [contains benzyl alcohol]

Solution, Injection [preservative free]:

Epogen: 2000 units/mL (1 mL); 3000 units/mL (1 mL); 4000 units/mL (1 mL); 10,000 units/mL (1 mL)

Procrit: 2000 units/mL (1 mL); 3000 units/mL (1 mL); 4000 units/mL (1 mL); 10,000 units/mL (1 mL); 40,000 units/mL (1 mL)

Dosage Forms: Canada Excipient information presented when available (limited, particularly for generics); consult specific product labeling.

Injection, solution [preservative free]:

Eprex: 1000 units/0.5 mL (0.5 mL), 2000 units/0.5 mL (0.5 mL), 3000 units/0.3 mL (0.3 mL), 4000 units/0.4 mL (0.4 mL), 5000 units/0.5 mL (0.5 mL), 6000 units/0.6 mL (0.6 mL), 8000 units/0.8 mL (0.8 mL), 10,000 units/mL (1 mL), 20,000 units/0.5 mL (0.5 mL), 30,000 units/0.75 mL (0.75 mL), 40,000 units/mL (1 mL) [contains polysorbate 80; prefilled syringe, free of human serum albumin]

◆ Epoetin Alfa, Recombinant see Epoetin Alfa on page 654

◆ Epogen see Epoetin Alfa on page 654

Epoprostenol (e poe PROST en ole)

Brand Names: US Flolan; Veletri

Brand Names: Canada Caripul; Flolan

Index Terms Epoprostenol Sodium; PGI_2; PGX; Prostacyclin

Pharmacologic Category Prostacyclin; Prostaglandin; Vasodilator

Use Pulmonary arterial hypertension: Treatment of pulmonary arterial hypertension (PAH) (WHO Group I) in patients with NYHA Class III or IV symptoms to improve exercise capacity. **Note:** According to treatment guidelines from the Fifth World Symposium on Pulmonary Hypertension (WSPH), continuous IV epoprostenol is recommended as first-line therapy in PAH patients with WHO-FC IV symptoms (WSPH [Gaile 2013]).

Pregnancy Considerations Adverse events have not been observed in animal reproduction studies. Women with PAH are encouraged to avoid pregnancy (McLaughlin 2009).

Breast-Feeding Considerations It is not known if epoprostenol is excreted in breast milk. Due to the potential for serious adverse reactions in the nursing infant, the manufacturer of Flolan and of Caripul [Canadian product] recommends a decision be made whether to discontinue nursing or to discontinue the drug, taking into account the importance of treatment to the mother. The manufacturer of Veletri recommends that caution be exercised when administering epoprostenol to nursing women.

Prescribing and Access Restrictions Orders for epoprostenol are distributed by two sources in the United States. Information on orders or reimbursement assistance may be obtained from either Accredo Health, Inc (1-866-344-4874) or CVS Caremark (1-877-242-2738).

Contraindications

US labeling:

Hypersensitivity to epoprostenol, to structurally-related compounds; or any component of the formulation; chronic use in patients with heart failure due to severe left ventricular systolic dysfunction

Veletri: Additional contraindications: Chronic use in patients who develop pulmonary edema during dose initiation

Canadian labeling: Hypersensitivity to epoprostenol, to structurally-related compounds; or any component of the formulation; chronic use in patients with heart failure due to severe left ventricular systolic dysfunction; chronic use in patients who develop pulmonary edema during dose initiation

Warnings/Precautions Epoprostenol is a potent pulmonary and systemic vasodilator and can cause hypotension and other reactions such as flushing, nausea, vomiting, dizziness, and headache. Monitor blood pressure and symptoms regularly during initiation and after dose change. Initiation or transition to epoprostenol requires specialized cardiopulmonary monitoring in a critical care setting where clinicians are experienced in advanced management of pulmonary arterial hypertension. To reduce the risk of thromboembolism during chronic use, anticoagulants should be coadministered unless contraindicated. Avoid abrupt interruptions or large sudden reductions in dosage; may result in rebound pulmonary hypertension (eg, dyspnea, dizziness, asthenia). A fatal case occurred following interruption; immediate access to medication or pump and infusion sets is essential to prevent treatment interruptions. Some patients with PAH have developed pulmonary edema during dosing adjustment and acute vasodilator testing (an off-label use), which may be associated with concomitant heart failure (LV systolic dysfunction with significantly elevated left heart filling pressures) or pulmonary veno-occlusive disease/pulmonary capillary hemangiomatosis. If pulmonary edema develops during therapy initiation, discontinue and do not readminister. Epoprostenol is a potent inhibitor of platelet aggregation; use with caution in patients with other risk factors for bleeding. Chronic continuous IV infusion of epoprostenol via a chronic indwelling central venous catheter (CVC) has been associated with local infections and serious blood stream infections.

Adverse Reactions Note: Adverse events reported during dose initiation and escalation include flushing (58%), headache (49%), nausea/vomiting (32%), hypotension (16%), anxiety/nervousness/agitation (11%), chest pain (11%); dizziness, abdominal pain, bradycardia, musculoskeletal pain, dyspnea, back pain, diaphoresis, dyspepsia, hypoesthesia/paresthesia, and tachycardia are also reported. Although some adverse reactions may be related to the underlying disease state, abdominal pain, anxiety/nervousness/agitation, arthralgia, bleeding, bradycardia, diarrhea, diaphoresis, flu-like syndrome, flushing, headache, hypotension, jaw pain, nausea, pain, pulmonary edema, rash, tachycardia, thrombocytopenia, and vomiting are clearly contributed to epoprostenol. The following adverse events have been reported during chronic administration for idiopathic or heritable PAH:

>10%:

Cardiovascular: Tachycardia (35% to 43%), flushing (23% to 42%), hypotension (13%)

Central nervous system: Dizziness (83%), headache (46% to 83%), chills (25%), fever (25%), flu-like syndrome (25%), sepsis (25%), anxiety (21%), nervousness (21%), tremor (21%), agitation (11%)

Dermatologic: Dermal ulcer (39%), eczema (25%), skin rash (25%), urticaria (25%)

Gastrointestinal: Nausea (≤67%), vomiting (≤67%), anorexia (66%), diarrhea (37% to 50%)

Local: Injection site reactions: Infection (18%), pain (11%)

Neuromuscular & skeletal: Arthralgia (≤84%), neck pain (≤84%), pain (≤84%), jaw pain (54% to 75%), myalgia (44%), musculoskeletal pain (35%), hyperesthesia (≤12%), hypoesthesia (≤12%), paresthesia (≤12%)

<1%, postmarketing, and/or case reports: Abdominal pain, anemia, ascites, dyspnea, fatigue, hemorrhage, hepatic failure, hyperthyroidism, pancytopenia, pulmonary edema, pulmonary embolism, splenomegaly, thrombocytopenia

Drug Interactions

Metabolism/Transport Effects None known.

Avoid Concomitant Use There are no known interactions where it is recommended to avoid concomitant use.

Increased Effect/Toxicity

Epoprostenol may increase the levels/effects of: Agents with Antiplatelet Properties; Amifostine; Anticoagulants; Antipsychotic Agents (Second Generation [Atypical]); Blood Pressure Lowering Agents; Digoxin; DULoxetine; Hypotension-Associated Agents; Levodopa

The levels/effects of Epoprostenol may be increased by: Alfuzosin; Barbiturates; Blood Pressure Lowering Agents; Brimonidine (Topical); Diazoxide; Herbs (Hypotensive Properties); Molsidomine; Nicorandil; Obinutuzumab; Pentoxifylline; Phosphodiesterase 5 Inhibitors; Prostacyclin Analogues; Thrombolytic Agents

Decreased Effect There are no known significant interactions involving a decrease in effect.

Preparation for Administration

Preparation of Epoprostenol Infusion

To make solution with concentration:	Flolan Instructions	Veletri or Caripul Instructions
	Note: Flolan may only be prepared with sterile diluent provided.	**Note:** Veletri or Caripul may only be prepared with sterile water for injection (SWFI) or NS.
3000 ng/mL	Dissolve one 0.5 mg vial with 5 mL supplied diluent, withdraw 3 mL, and add to a sufficient volume of diluent to make a total of 100 mL.	Dissolve one 0.5 mg vial with 5 mL of SWFI or NS, withdraw 3 mL, and add to a sufficient volume of the identical diluent to make a total of 100 mL.
5000 ng/mL	Dissolve one 0.5 mg vial with 5 mL supplied diluent, withdraw entire vial contents, and add to a sufficient volume of supplied diluent to make a total of 100 mL.	Dissolve one 0.5 mg vial with 5 mL of SWFI or NS, withdraw entire vial contents, and add to a sufficient volume of the identical diluent to make a total of 100 mL.
10,000 ng/mL	Dissolve two 0.5 mg vials each with 5 mL supplied diluent, withdraw entire vial contents, and add to a sufficient volume of supplied diluent to make a total of 100 mL.	Dissolve two 0.5 mg vials each with 5 mL of SWFI or NS, withdraw entire vial contents, and add to a sufficient volume of the identical diluent to make a total of 100 mL.
15,000 ng/mL	Dissolve one 1.5 mg vial with 5 mL supplied diluent, withdraw entire vial contents, and add to a sufficient volume of supplied diluent to make a total of 100 mL.	Dissolve one 1.5 mg vial with 5 mL of SWFI or NS, withdraw entire vial contents, and add to a sufficient volume of the identical diluent to make a total of 100 mL.
20,000 ng/mL	Dissolve two 0.5 mg vials each with 5 mL supplied diluent, withdraw entire vial contents, and add to a sufficient volume of supplied diluent to make a total of **50 mL** (DeWet, 2004).	
30,000 ng/mL		Dissolve two 1.5 mg vials each with 5 mL of SWFI or NS, withdraw entire vial contents, and add to a sufficient volume of the identical diluent to make a total of 100 mL.

Storage/Stability

Flolan: Prior to use, store intact vials and diluent at 15°C to 25°C (59°F to 77°F); do not freeze. Protect from light. Following reconstitution, solution must be stored at 2°C to 8°C (36°F to 46°F) if not used immediately; do not freeze. Protect from light. Storage and administration limits for reconstituted solution are dependent on type of diluent use during reconstitution:

Sterile diluent for Flolan: When used at 15°C to 25°C (59°F to 77°F), reconstituted solutions are stable for up to 8 hours following reconstitution or removal from refrigerator. May also be stored for up to 40 hours at 2°C to 8°C (36°F to 46°F) before use. When used with a cold pack, reconstituted solutions are stable for up to 24 hours; may also be stored at 2°C to 8°C (36°F to 46°F) before use as long as the total time of refrigerated storage and infusion does not exceed 48 hours. Change cold packs every 12 hours. The Canadian labeling recommends changing cold pouches every 8 hours if room temperature approaches 30°C (86°F)

pH 12 sterile diluent for Flolan: Freshly prepared reconstituted solutions or reconstituted solutions that have been stored at 2°C to 8°C (36°F to 46°F) for no longer than 8 days can be administered up to 72 hours at up to 25°C (77°F); 48 hours at up to 30°C (86°F); 24 hours at up to 35°C (95°F); 12 hours at up to 40°C (104°F).

Veletri: Prior to use, store intact vials at 20°C to 25°C (68°F to 77°F); do not freeze. Protect from light. Reconstituted vials must be further diluted prior to use.

Caripul [Canadian product]: Prior to use, store intact vials at 15°C to 30°C (59°F to 86°F); do not freeze. Reconstituted vials must be further diluted prior to use.

Reconstituted solutions of Veletri or Caripul immediately diluted to a final concentration within a drug delivery reservoir may be administered immediately or stored at 2°C to 8°C (36°F to 46°F) for up to 8 days; do not freeze. Protect from light.

If administered immediately, the following maximum durations of administration at room temperature (25°C [77°F]) according to solution concentration are recommended:

U.S. labeling (Veletri):
3000 to <15,000 ng/mL: 48 hours
15,000 to <60,000 ng/mL: 48 hours
≥60,000 ng/mL: 72 hours

Canadian labeling (Caripul):
3000 to <15,000 ng/mL: 48 hours
≥15,000: 48 hours

If stored at 2°C to 8°C (36°F to 46°F) for up to 8 days, the following maximum durations of administration at room temperature (25°C [77°F]) according to solution concentration are recommended:
3000 to <15,000 ng/mL: 24 hours
15,000 to <60,000 ng/mL: 48 hours
≥60,000 ng/mL: 48 hours

Short excursions at 40°C (104°F) are permitted as follows:
Solution concentration <15,000 ng/mL: Up to 2 hours
Solution concentration 15,000 to <60,000 ng/mL: Up to 4 hours
Solution concentration ≥60,000 ng/mL: Up to 8 hours

The following maximum durations of administration at temperatures >25°C to 40°C (>77°F up to 104°F) administered either immediately or after up to 8 days storage at 2°C to 8°C (36°F to 46°F) according to solution concentration are recommended:

Use at temperature >25°C to 30°C (>77°F up to 86°F):
U.S. labeling (Veletri):
<60,000 ng/mL: 24 hours
≥60,000 ng/mL: 48 hours

Canadian labeling (Caripul): All concentrations: 24 hours

Use at temperature up to 40°C (104°F):
U.S. labeling (Veletri): ≥60,000 ng/mL: 24 hours (immediately administered after preparation)

Mechanism of Action Epoprostenol is also known as prostacyclin and PGI$_2$. It is a strong vasodilator of all vascular beds. In addition, it is a potent endogenous inhibitor of platelet aggregation. The reduction in platelet aggregation results from epoprostenol's activation of intracellular adenylate cyclase and the resultant increase in cyclic adenosine monophosphate concentrations within the platelets. Additionally, it is capable of decreasing thrombogenesis and platelet clumping in the lungs by inhibiting platelet aggregation.

Pharmacodynamics/Kinetics

Metabolism: Rapidly hydrolyzed; subject to some enzymatic degradation; forms two active metabolites (6-keto-prostaglandin $F_1\alpha$ and 6,15-diketo-13,14-dihydro-prostaglandin $F_1\alpha$) with minimal activity and 14 inactive metabolites

Half-life elimination: ~6 minutes

Excretion: Urine (84%); feces (4%)

Dosing

Adult & Geriatric

Pulmonary arterial hypertension (PAH): IV: Initial: 2 ng/kg/minute; a lower initial dose may be used if patient is intolerant of starting dose. Increase dose in increments of 1 to 2 ng/kg/minute at intervals of ≥15 minutes until dose-limiting side effects (eg, flushing, jaw pain, headache, hypotension, nausea) are noted or response to epoprostenol plateaus. Usual optimal dose (monotherapy): 25 to 40 ng/kg/minute (McLaughlin 2009); significant patient variability in optimal dose exists. Maximum dose with chronic therapy has not been defined; however, doses as high as 195 ng/kg/minute have been described in children (Rosenzweig 1999).

Dose adjustment during chronic phase of treatment:
If PAH symptoms persist or recur following improvement, increase dose in 1 to 2 ng/kg/minute increments at intervals of ≥15 minutes. May also increase dose at intervals of 24 to 48 hours or longer (eg, every 1 to 2 weeks). **Note:** The need for increased doses should be expected with chronic use; incremental increases occur more frequently during the first few months after the drug is initiated.

In case of dose-limiting pharmacologic events (eg, hypotension, severe nausea, vomiting), decrease dose in 2 ng/kg/minute decrements at intervals of ≥15 minutes until dose-limiting effects resolve. Avoid abrupt withdrawal or sudden large dose reductions. **Note:** Adverse event may resolve without dosage adjustment.

Lung transplant: In patients receiving lung transplants, epoprostenol may be tapered after sequential lung transplantation once the allografts have been reperfused. If cardiopulmonary bypass utilized, epoprostenol may be tapered after pump perfusion has been initiated.

Acute vasodilator testing in patients with PAH (off-label use) (McLaughlin 2009): Note: Acute vasodilator testing should only be done in patients who might be considered candidates for calcium channel blocker therapy.

IV: Initial: 2 ng/kg/minute; increase dose in increments of 2 ng/kg/minute every 10 to 15 minutes; dosing range during testing: 2 to 10 ng/kg/minute

Intraoperative pulmonary hypertension during cardiac surgery with cardiopulmonary bypass (CPB) (off-label use): Inhalation (off-label route): **Note:** Institution-specific protocols vary.

Administration after induction of anesthesia before incision: Flolan: 60 mcg (4 mL of 15,000 ng/mL concentration) via jet nebulizer; effect persists for ~25 minutes (Hache 2003)

or

Intraoperative administration: *Nebulization via ventilator circuit:* Flolan: Using a 15,000 ng/mL concentration and an oxygen flow of 8 L/minute, begin administration via jet nebulizer 5 minutes prior to weaning from CPB; discontinue at least 60 minutes after CPB weaned (Fattouch 2006)

Post-cardiothoracic surgery pulmonary hypertension, right ventricular dysfunction, or refractory hypoxemia (off-label use) (DeWet 2004): Flolan: Inhalation (off-label route): **Note:** May need to change ventilator filter every 2 hours due to glycine buffer diluent; may cause ventilator valve malfunction. Tidal volume delivered by ventilator may require adjustment. *Nebulization via ventilator circuit:* Flolan: Using a 20,000 ng/mL concentration, prime nebulizer chamber with 15 mL; administer remainder at a constant rate of 8 mL/hour; delivers ~38 ng/kg/minute (based on a 70 kg patient); set oxygen flow at 2 to 3 L/minute; wean as tolerated. **Note:** Although not achieved with this regimen, in general, doses >50 ng/kg/minute do not provide additional benefit and may increase the risk of hypotension.

or

Nebulization via facemask with Venturi attachment: Flolan: Using a 20,000 ng/mL concentration, prime nebulizer chamber with 15 mL; set oxygen flow at 2 to 3 L/minute; 8 mL/hour will be nebulized; wean as tolerated.

Weaning procedure: Reduce dose by 50% every 2 to 4 hours (ie, 20,000 ng/mL to 10,000 ng/mL to 5,000 ng/mL) until a concentration of 2,500 ng/mL is reached; carefully discontinue once patient remains stable on this concentration for at least 4 hours.

Pediatric Pulmonary arterial hypertension (PAH): Children (off-label use) and Adolescents (off-label use): Refer to adult dosing.

Renal Impairment There are no dosage adjustments provided in the manufacturer's labeling.

Hepatic Impairment There are no dosage adjustments provided in the manufacturer's labeling.

Administration

IV: For IV use via an infusion pump. Use infusion sets with an in-line 0.22 micron filter. When administered on an ongoing basis, must be infused through a central venous catheter. Peripheral infusion may be used temporarily until central line is established. Do not administer as a bolus injection. Avoid abrupt withdrawal (including interruptions in delivery) or sudden large reductions in dosing. The ambulatory infusion pump should be small and lightweight, be able to adjust infusion rates in 2 ng/kg/minute increments, have occlusion, end of infusion, and low battery alarms, have ± 6% accuracy of the programmed rate, and have positive continuous or pulsatile pressure with intervals ≤3 minutes between pulses. The reservoir should be made of polyvinyl chloride, polypropylene, or glass. Immediate access to back up pump, infusion sets and medication is essential to prevent treatment interruptions. Consult manufacturer's labeling for infusion rate example calculations.

Inhalation (off-label route):

Intraoperative administration: Administer via jet nebulizer connected to the inspiratory limb of the ventilator near the endotracheal tube with a bypass oxygen flow of 8 L/minute to achieve administration of a high proportion of small particles (Fattouch 2006; Hache 2003).

Post-cardiothoracic surgery: May also be administered via jet nebulizer connected to the inspiratory limb of the ventilator near the endotracheal tube or via face mask with a Venturi attachment for aerosolization with a bypass oxygen flow of 2 to 3 L/minute (De Wet 2004). **Note:** Glycine buffer diluent may cause ventilator valve malfunction; it has been recommended that filters be changed on the ventilator every 2 hours; may also use a ventilator heating coil (De Wet 2004).

Monitoring Parameters Monitor for improvements in pulmonary function, decreased exertional dyspnea, fatigue, syncope and chest pain, blood pressure, pulmonary vascular resistance, pulmonary arterial pressure and quality of life. Following establishment of a new chronic infusion rate, measure standing and supine blood pressure for several hours. In addition, the pump device and catheters should be monitored frequently to avoid "system" related failure. Monitor arterial pressure; assess all vital functions. Hypoxia, flushing, and tachycardia may indicate overdose.

Dosage Forms Excipient information presented when available (limited, particularly for generics); consult specific product labeling.

Solution Reconstituted, Intravenous:
Flolan: 0.5 mg (1 ea); 1.5 mg (1 ea)
Veletri: 0.5 mg (1 ea); 1.5 mg (1 ea)
Generic: 0.5 mg (1 ea); 1.5 mg (1 ea)

Dosage Forms: Canada Excipient information presented when available (limited, particularly for generics); consult specific product labeling.

Solution Reconstituted, Intravenous:
Caripul: 0.5 mg (1 ea); 1.5 mg (1 ea)
Flolan: 0.5 mg (1 ea); 1.5 mg (1 ea)

◆ **Epoprostenol Sodium** *see* Epoprostenol *on page 657*

◆ **Epothilone B Lactam** *see* Ixabepilone *on page 1006*

◆ **Eprex (Can)** *see* Epoetin Alfa *on page 654*

Eprosartan (ep roe SAR tan)

Brand Names: US Teveten
Brand Names: Canada Teveten
Pharmacologic Category Angiotensin II Receptor Blocker; Antihypertensive

Use

Hypertension: Treatment of hypertension; may be used alone or in combination with other antihypertensives

Guideline recommendations:

Hypertension: The 2014 guideline for the management of high blood pressure in adults (Eighth Joint National Committee [JNC 8; James, 2013]) recommends initiation of pharmacologic treatment to lower blood pressure for the following patients:

• Patients ≥60 years of age with systolic blood pressure (SBP) ≥150 mm Hg or diastolic blood pressure (DBP) ≥90 mm Hg. Goal of therapy is SBP <150 mm Hg and DBP <90 mm Hg.

• Patients <60 years of age with SBP ≥140 mm Hg or DBP ≥90 mm Hg. Goal of therapy is SBP <140 mm Hg and DBP <90 mm Hg.

• Patients ≥18 years of age with diabetes and SBP ≥140 mm Hg or DBP ≥90 mm Hg. Goal of therapy is SBP <140 mm Hg and DBP <90 mm Hg.

• Patients ≥18 years of age with chronic kidney disease (CKD) and SBP ≥140 mm Hg or DBP ≥90 mm Hg. Goal of therapy is SBP <140 mm Hg and DBP <90 mm Hg.

Chronic kidney disease (CKD) and hypertension: Regardless of race or diabetes status, the use of an ACE inhibitor (ACEI) or angiotensin receptor blocker (ARB) as initial therapy is recommended to improve kidney outcomes. In the general nonblack population (without CKD), including those with diabetes, initial antihypertensive treatment should consist of a thiazide-type diuretic, calcium channel blocker, ACEI, or ARB. In the general black population (without CKD), including those with diabetes, initial antihypertensive treatment should consist of a thiazide-type diuretic or a calcium channel blocker instead of an ACEI or ARB.

Coronary artery disease (CAD) and hypertension: The American Heart Association, American College of Cardiology and American Society of Hypertension (AHA/ACC/ASH) 2015 scientific statement for the treatment of hypertension in patients with CAD recommends the use of an ACE inhibitor (or an ARB) as part of a regimen in patients with hypertension and chronic stable angina if

there is prior MI, LV systolic dysfunction, diabetes mellitus, or CKD. A BP target of <140/90 mm Hg is reasonable for the secondary prevention of cardiovascular events. A lower target BP (<130/80 mm Hg) may be appropriate in some individuals with CAD, previous MI, stroke or transient ischemic attack, or CAD risk equivalents (AHA/ACC/ASH [Rosendorff 2015]).

Pregnancy Considerations [U.S. Boxed Warning]: Drugs that act on the renin-angiotensin system can cause injury and death to the developing fetus. Discontinue as soon as possible once pregnancy is detected. The use of drugs which act on the renin-angiotensin system are associated with oligohydramnios. Oligohydramnios, due to decreased fetal renal function, may lead to fetal lung hypoplasia and skeletal malformations. Use is also associated with anuria, hypotension, renal failure, skull hypoplasia, and death in the fetus/neonate. The exposed fetus should be monitored for fetal growth, amniotic fluid volume, and organ formation. Infants exposed *in utero* should be monitored for hyperkalemia, hypotension, and oliguria (exchange transfusions or dialysis may be needed). These adverse events are generally associated with maternal use in the second and third trimesters.

Untreated chronic maternal hypertension is also associated with adverse events in the fetus, infant, and mother. The use of angiotensin II receptor blockers is not recommended to treat chronic uncomplicated hypertension in pregnant women and should generally be avoided in women of reproductive potential (ACOG, 2013).

Breast-Feeding Considerations It is not known if eprosartan is excreted in breast milk. Due to the potential for serious adverse reactions in the nursing infant, the US manufacturer recommends a decision be made whether to discontinue nursing or to discontinue the drug, taking into account the importance of treatment to the mother. Canadian labeling contraindicates use in breast-feeding women.

Contraindications

Hypersensitivity to eprosartan or any component of the formulation; coadministration with aliskiren in patients with diabetes

Documentation of allergenic cross-reactivity for angiotensin II receptor blockers is limited. However, because of similarities in chemical structure and/or pharmacologic actions, the possibility of cross-sensitivity cannot be ruled out with certainty.

Canadian labeling: Additional contraindications (not in US labeling): Hemodynamically significant bilateral renovascular disease or severe stenosis of a solitary functioning kidney; hereditary problems of galactose intolerance, the Lapp lactase deficiency, or glucose-galactose malabsorption; concomitant use with aliskiren in patients with moderate to severe renal impairment (GFR <60 mL/minute/1.73 m^2); concomitant use with angiotensin-converting enzyme (ACE) inhibitors in patients with diabetic nephropathy; pregnancy; breast-feeding

Warnings/Precautions [U.S. Boxed Warning]: Drugs that act on the renin-angiotensin system can cause injury and death to the developing fetus. Discontinue as soon as possible once pregnancy is detected. May cause hyperkalemia; risk factors include renal dysfunction, diabetes mellitus, concomitant use of ACE inhibitors, aliskiren, potassium-sparing diuretics, potassium supplements and/or potassium containing salts. Use cautiously, if at all, with these agents and monitor potassium closely. Avoid ace inhibitors, aliskiren, and potassium supplementation unless specifically required by health care provider. Avoid use or use a smaller dose in patients who are volume depleted; correct depletion first. May be associated with deterioration of renal function and/or increases in serum creatinine, particularly in patients with low renal blood flow (eg, renal artery stenosis, heart failure) whose glomerular filtration rate (GFR) is dependent on efferent arteriolar vasoconstriction by angiotensin II. Use with caution in unstented unilateral/bilateral renal artery stenosis. When unstented bilateral renal artery stenosis is present, use is generally avoided due to the elevated risk of deterioration in renal function unless possible benefits outweigh risks. Use with caution in preexisting renal insufficiency; significant aortic/mitral stenosis. Potentially significant drug-drug interactions may exist, requiring dose or frequency adjustment, additional monitoring, and/or selection of alternative therapy. Concomitant use of an angiotensin-converting enzyme (ACE) inhibitor or renin inhibitor (eg, aliskiren) is associated with an increased risk of hypotension, hyperkalemia, and renal dysfunction; concomitant use with aliskiren should be avoided in patients with GFR <60 mL/minute and is contraindicated in patients with diabetes mellitus (regardless of GFR). In surgical patients on chronic angiotensin receptor blocker (ARB) therapy, intraoperative hypotension may occur with induction and maintenance of general anesthesia.

Angioedema has been reported rarely with some angiotensin II receptor antagonists (ARBs) and may occur at any time during treatment (especially following first dose). It may involve the head and neck (potentially compromising airway) or the intestine (presenting with abdominal pain). Patients with idiopathic or hereditary angioedema or previous angioedema associated with ACE-inhibitor therapy may be at an increased risk. Prolonged frequent monitoring may be required, especially if tongue, glottis, or larynx are involved, as they are associated with airway obstruction. Patients with a history of airway surgery may have a higher risk of airway obstruction. Discontinue therapy immediately if angioedema occurs. Aggressive early management is critical. Intramuscular (IM) administration of epinephrine may be necessary. Do not readminister to patients who have had angioedema with ARBs.

Adverse Reactions

1% to 10%:

Central nervous system: Fatigue (2%), depression (1%)

Endocrine & metabolic: Hypertriglyceridemia (1%)

Gastrointestinal: Abdominal pain (2%)

Genitourinary: Urinary tract infection (1%)

Respiratory: Upper respiratory tract infection (8%), rhinitis (4%), pharyngitis (4%), cough (4%)

Miscellaneous: Viral infection (2%), injury (2%)

<1% (Limited to important or life-threatening): Abnormal ECG, angina, arthritis, asthma, ataxia, bradycardia, BUN increased, creatinine increased, eczema, edema, esophagitis, ethanol intolerance, gingivitis, gout, hypotension, influenza-like symptoms, leg cramps, leukopenia, maculopapular rash, migraine, neuritis, neutropenia, orthostasis, palpitation, paresthesia, peripheral ischemia, purpura, renal calculus, somnolence, tachycardia, tendonitis, thrombocytopenia, tinnitus, tremor, urinary incontinence, vertigo; rhabdomyolysis has been reported (rarely) with angiotensin-receptor antagonists.

Drug Interactions

Metabolism/Transport Effects Inhibits CYP2C9 (weak)

Avoid Concomitant Use There are no known interactions where it is recommended to avoid concomitant use.

Increased Effect/Toxicity

Eprosartan may increase the levels/effects of: ACE Inhibitors; Amifostine; Antipsychotic Agents (Second Generation [Atypical]); Ciprofloxacin (Systemic); CycloSPORINE (Systemic); Drospirenone; DULoxetine; Hypotension-Associated Agents; Levodopa; Lithium; Nonsteroidal Anti-Inflammatory Agents; Potassium-Sparing Diuretics; Sodium Phosphates

The levels/effects of Eprosartan may be increased by: Alfuzosin; Aliskiren; Barbiturates; Brimonidine (Topical); Canagliflozin; Dapoxetine; Diazoxide; Eplerenone; Heparin; Heparin (Low Molecular Weight); Herbs (Hypotensive Properties); Molsidomine; Nicorandil; Obinutuzumab; Pentoxifylline; Phosphodiesterase 5 Inhibitors; Potassium Salts; Prostacyclin Analogues; Tolvaptan; Trimethoprim

Decreased Effect

The levels/effects of Eprosartan may be decreased by: Amphetamines; Herbs (Hypertensive Properties); Methylphenidate; Nonsteroidal Anti-Inflammatory Agents; Yohimbine

Storage/Stability Store at 20°C to 25°C (68°F to 77°F).

Mechanism of Action Angiotensin II is formed from angiotensin I in a reaction catalyzed by angiotensin-converting enzyme (ACE, kininase II). Angiotensin II is the principal pressor agent of the renin-angiotensin system, with effects that include vasoconstriction, stimulation of synthesis and release of aldosterone, cardiac stimulation, and renal reabsorption of sodium. Eprosartan blocks the vasoconstrictor and aldosterone-secreting effects of angiotensin II by selectively blocking the binding of angiotensin II to the AT1 receptor in many tissues, such as vascular smooth muscle and the adrenal gland. Its action is therefore independent of the pathways for angiotensin II synthesis. Blockade of the renin-angiotensin system with ACE inhibitors, which inhibit the biosynthesis of angiotensin II from angiotensin I, is widely used in the treatment of hypertension. ACE inhibitors also inhibit the degradation of bradykinin, a reaction also catalyzed by ACE. Because eprosartan does not inhibit ACE (kininase II), it does not affect the response to bradykinin. Whether this difference has clinical relevance is not yet known. Eprosartan does not bind to or block other hormone receptors or ion channels known to be important in cardiovascular regulation.

Pharmacodynamics/Kinetics

Protein binding: 98%

Metabolism: Minimally hepatic

Bioavailability: 300 mg dose: 13%

Half-life elimination: Terminal: 5 to 9 hours (Bottorff, 1999)

Time to peak, serum: Fasting: 1 to 2 hours

Excretion: Feces (90%); urine (7%, mostly as unchanged drug)

Dosing

Adult

Hypertension: Oral: Dosage must be individualized. Can administer once or twice daily with total daily doses of 400 to 800 mg. Usual starting dose is 600 mg once daily as monotherapy in patients who are euvolemic. Target dose (JNC 8 [James, 2013]): 600 to 800 mg daily in 1 or 2 divided doses. Limited clinical experience with doses >800 mg.

Geriatric

Hypertension: Oral:

U.S. labeling: Refer to adult dosing.

Canadian labeling: Consider decreasing initial dose to 400 mg once daily

Renal Impairment

U.S. labeling:

Mild impairment: No initial dosage adjustment necessary.

Moderate to severe impairment: No initial dosage adjustment necessary; maximum dose: 600 mg daily.

Hemodialysis: There are no dosage adjustments provided in the manufacturer's labeling; eprosartan is poorly removed by hemodialysis (Cl$_{HD}$ <1 L/hour)

Canadian labeling:

CrCl ≥60 mL/minute: No dosage adjustment necessary.

CrCl 30 to 59 mL/minute: No initial dosage adjustment necessary; monitor closely. Maximum dose: 600 mg daily.

CrCl 5 to 29 mL/minute: Consider decreasing initial dose to 400 mg once daily; monitor closely. Maximum dose: 600 mg daily.

Hemodialysis: There are no dosage adjustments provided in the manufacturer's labeling; eprosartan is poorly removed by hemodialysis (Cl$_{HD}$ <1 L/hour)

Hepatic Impairment

U.S. labeling: No dosage adjustment necessary.

Canadian labeling: Consider decreasing initial dose to 400 mg once daily

Administration May be administered with or without food.

Monitoring Parameters Serum potassium, serum creatinine, BUN, urinalysis, blood pressure

Product Availability Teveten 400 mg tablets have been discontinued in the US more than 1 year.

Dosage Forms Excipient information presented when available (limited, particularly for generics); consult specific product labeling. [DSC] = Discontinued product

Tablet, Oral:

Teveten: 400 mg [DSC], 600 mg [contains polysorbate 80]

Generic: 600 mg

Eprosartan and Hydrochlorothiazide

(ep roe SAR tan & hye droe klor oh THYE a zide)

Brand Names: US Teveten HCT

Brand Names: Canada Teveten Plus

Index Terms Eprosartan Mesylate and Hydrochlorothiazide; Hydrochlorothiazide and Eprosartan

Pharmacologic Category Angiotensin II Receptor Blocker; Antihypertensive; Diuretic, Thiazide

Use

Hypertension: Treatment of hypertension

Limitations of use: Not indicated for initial treatment.

Dosing

Adult Hypertension: Oral: Dose is individualized (combination substituted for individual components): Usual recommended dose:

U.S. labeling: Eprosartan 600 mg/hydrochlorothiazide 12.5 mg once daily; may titrate to eprosartan 600 mg/hydrochlorothiazide 25 mg once daily if response is inadequate. If additional blood pressure control is needed or to maintain a twice-daily schedule of monotherapy, eprosartan 300 mg may be added as an evening dose.

Canadian labeling: Eprosartan 600 mg/hydrochlorothiazide 12.5 mg once daily. **Note:** Combination product is only available in one strength and may be used after successful titration of individual agents to corresponding dose. Dose titration is not possible with available dosage form.

Geriatric

Hypertension: Oral:

U.S. labeling: Refer to adult dosing.

Canadian labeling: Consider decreasing initial dose of eprosartan (monotherapy) to 400 mg once daily

Renal Impairment

U.S. labeling:

Mild impairment: No initial dosage adjustment necessary.

Moderate-to-severe impairment: No initial dosage adjustments necessary. Maximum dose of eprosartan: 600 mg daily. Hydrochlorothiazide is ineffective in patients with CrCl <30 mL/minute.

Hemodialysis: There are no dosage adjustments provided in the manufacturer's labeling; eprosartan is poorly removed by hemodialysis (Cl$_{HD}$ <1 L/hour)

Canadian labeling:

CrCl ≥30 mL/minute: No dosage adjustment necessary.

CrCl <30 mL/minute: Use is contraindicated.

Hepatic Impairment

U.S. labeling: No dosage adjustment necessary; use with caution.

Canadian labeling: Use is not recommended (contraindicated in severe impairment)

Additional Information Complete prescribing information should be consulted for additional detail.

Dosage Forms Excipient information presented when available (limited, particularly for generics); consult specific product labeling.

Tablet:

600 mg/12.5 mg: Eprosartan 600 mg and hydrochlorothiazide 12.5 mg

600 mg/25 mg: Eprosartan 600 mg and hydrochlorothiazide 25 mg

---

Eptifibatide (ep TIF i ba tide)

Brand Names: US Integrilin

Brand Names: Canada Eptifibatide Injection; Integrilin

Index Terms Intrifiban

Pharmacologic Category Antiplatelet Agent, Glycoprotein IIb/IIIa Inhibitor

Use

Acute coronary syndrome: Treatment of patients with acute coronary syndrome (unstable angina/non-ST-segment elevation myocardial infarction [UA/NSTEMI]), including patients who are to be managed medically and those undergoing percutaneous coronary intervention (PCI)

Percutaneous coronary intervention: Treatment of patients undergoing PCI, including those undergoing intracoronary stenting.

Pregnancy Considerations Adverse events have not been observed in animal reproduction studies.

Breast-Feeding Considerations It is not known if eptifibatide is excreted in breast milk. The manufacturer recommends that caution be exercised when administering eptifibatide to nursing women.

Contraindications

Hypersensitivity to eptifibatide or any component of the formulation; active abnormal bleeding within the previous 30 days or a history of bleeding diathesis; history of stroke within 30 days or a history of hemorrhagic stroke; severe hypertension (systolic blood pressure >200 mm Hg or diastolic blood pressure >110 mm Hg) not adequately controlled on antihypertensive therapy; major surgery within the preceding 6 weeks; current or planned administration of another parenteral GP IIb/IIIa inhibitor; dependency on hemodialysis

Canadian labeling: Additional contraindications (not in U.S. labeling): PT >1.2 times control or INR ≥2.0; known history of intracranial disease (eg, neoplasm, arteriovenous malformation, aneurysm); severe renal impairment (CrCl <30 mL/minute); thrombocytopenia (<100,000 cells/mm³); clinically significant liver disease

Warnings/Precautions The most common complication is bleeding, including retroperitoneal, pulmonary, and spontaneous GI and/or GU bleeding; monitor closely for bleeding, especially the arterial access site for the cardiac catheterization. Risk factors for bleeding include older age, a history of bleeding disorders, and concomitant use of drugs that increase the risk of bleeding (thrombolytics, oral anticoagulants, NSAIDs, and/or P2Y12 inhibitors). Patients caution with administration of other drugs affecting hemostasis. Minimize invasive procedures, including

arterial and venous punctures, IM injections, and the use of urinary catheters, nasotracheal intubation and nasogastric tubes. Discontinue ≥2 to 4 hours prior to coronary artery bypass graft surgery (Hillis, 2011). Acute, profound thrombocytopenia (immune-mediated and nonimmune mediated) has occurred and may occur within 24 hours of initiation (Cheema, 2006; Coons, 2005; Nagge, 2003; Rezkalla, 2003; Salengro, 2003). Platelet counts should recover rapidly (within 1-5 days) after discontinuation. Use with extreme caution in patients with platelet counts <100,000/mm³ (contraindicated in the Canadian labeling). If platelet count decreases to <100,000/mm³ during therapy, discontinue eptifibatide and heparin if administered concurrently. Specific management guidelines for GP IIb/IIIa induced thrombocytopenia have been published (Huxtable, 2006; Llevadot, 2000).

Prior to sheath removal, heparin should be discontinued for 3 to 4 hours and the aPTT or ACT should be checked (do not remove unless aPTT is <50 seconds or the ACT <180 seconds). Of note, full dose anticoagulation is no longer used after successful PCI procedures (ACCF/AHA/SCAI [Levine, 2011]). Use caution in renal dysfunction (estimated CrCl <50 mL/minute, using Cockcroft-Gault equation); dosage adjustment required. Use is contraindicated in patients dependent upon hemodialysis. Hypersensitivity reactions have occurred, including anaphylaxis and urticaria. Potentially significant drug-drug interactions may exist, requiring dose or frequency adjustment, additional monitoring, and/or selection of alternative therapy.

Adverse Reactions Bleeding is the major drug-related adverse effect. Access site is often primary source of bleeding complications. Incidence of bleeding is also related to heparin intensity. Patients weighing <70 kg may have an increased risk of major bleeding.

>10%: Hematologic: Bleeding (major: 1% to 11%; minor: 3% to 14%; transfusion required: 2% to 13%)
1% to 10%:
Cardiovascular: Hypotension (up to 7%)
Hematologic: Thrombocytopenia (1% to 3%)
Local: Injection site reaction
<1% (Limited to important or life-threatening): Acute profound thrombocytopenia (including immune-mediated thrombocytopenia), fatal bleeding events, GI hemorrhage, pulmonary hemorrhage

Drug Interactions

Metabolism/Transport Effects None known.

Avoid Concomitant Use
Avoid concomitant use of Eptifibatide with any of the following: Urokinase

Increased Effect/Toxicity
Eptifibatide may increase the levels/effects of: Agents with Antiplatelet Properties; Anticoagulants; Apixaban; Collagenase (Systemic); Dabigatran Etexilate; Deoxycholic Acid; Edoxaban; Ibritumomab; Obinutuzumab; Rivaroxaban; Salicylates; Thrombolytic Agents; Tositumomab and Iodine I 131 Tositumomab; Urokinase

The levels/effects of Eptifibatide may be increased by: Dasatinib; Glucosamine; Herbs (Anticoagulant/Antiplatelet Properties); Ibrutinib; Limaprost; Multivitamins/Fluoride (with ADE); Multivitamins/Minerals (with ADEK, Folate, Iron); Multivitamins/Minerals (with AE, No Iron); Omega-3 Fatty Acids; Pentosan Polysulfate Sodium; Pentoxifylline; Prostacyclin Analogues; Tipranavir; Vitamin E; Vitamin E (Oral)

Decreased Effect There are no known significant interactions involving a decrease in effect.

Storage/Stability Vials should be stored refrigerated at 2°C to 8°C (36°F to 46°F). Vials can be kept at room temperature for 2 months, after which they must be discarded. Protect from light until administration. Do not use beyond the expiration date. Discard any unused portion left in the vial.

Mechanism of Action Eptifibatide is a cyclic heptapeptide which blocks the platelet glycoprotein IIb/IIIa receptor, the binding site for fibrinogen, von Willebrand factor, and other ligands. Inhibition of binding at this final common receptor reversibly blocks platelet aggregation and prevents thrombosis.

Pharmacodynamics/Kinetics

Onset of action: Immediate after initial bolus (>80% inhibition of ADP-induced aggregation achieved 5 minutes after bolus dose); maximal effect achieved within 1 hour (Gilchrist, 2001; Tardiff, 2001)
Duration: Platelet function restored ~4 to 8 hours following discontinuation (Tardiff, 2001)
Protein binding: ~25%
Half-life elimination: ~2.5 hours
Excretion: Primarily urine (as eptifibatide and metabolites)
Clearance: Total body: ~55 mL/kg/hour; Renal: ~50% of total body clearance in healthy subjects

Dosing

Adult

Acute coronary syndrome: IV: 180 mcg/kg bolus (maximum: 22.6 mg) administered as soon as possible following diagnosis, followed by a continuous infusion of 2 mcg/kg/minute (maximum: 15 mg/hour) until hospital discharge or initiation of CABG surgery (discontinue ≥2 to 4 hours before surgery (ACCF/AHA [Hillis, 2011]), up to 72 hours. If PCI performed during initial 72 hours, maintain continuous infusion at the time of PCI and continue until hospital discharge or for up to 18 to 24 hours, whichever comes first (total infusion time ≤96 hours). Concurrent aspirin and heparin therapy (target aPTT 50 to 70 seconds) are recommended. **Note:** If UA/NSTEMI, administration ≥12 hours before angiography was shown not to be superior to provisional use at the time of PCI and has a higher incidence of bleeding (Giugliano, 2009).

Percutaneous coronary intervention (PCI) with or without stenting: IV: 180 mcg/kg bolus (maximum: 22.6 mg) administered immediately before the initiation of PCI, followed by a continuous infusion of 2 mcg/kg/minute (maximum: 15 mg/hour). A second 180 mcg/kg bolus (maximum: 22.6 mg) should be administered 10 minutes after the first bolus. Infusion should be continued until hospital discharge or for up to 18 to 24 hours, whichever comes first; shorter infusion durations (ie, <2 hours) may be considered for nonemergent uncomplicated PCI in patients adequately pretreated with clopidogrel (Fung, 2007). Preprocedural aspirin and heparin therapy (ACT 200 to 250 seconds during PCI) and daily aspirin are recommended. Heparin infusion after PCI is discouraged. In patients who undergo CABG surgery, discontinue infusion ≥2 to 4 hours prior to surgery (ACCF/AHA [Hillis, 2011]).

Primary percutaneous coronary intervention (PCI) during ST-elevation myocardial infarction with or without stenting or pretreatment with clopidogrel (off-label use): IV: Bolus of 180 mcg/kg (maximum: 22.6 mg) administered at the time of PCI, followed by a continuous infusion of 2 mcg/kg/minute (maximum: 15 mg/hour) in combination with heparin or bivalirudin. A second 180 mcg/kg bolus (maximum: 22.6 mg) should be administered 10 minutes after the first bolus (ACCF/AHA [O'Gara, 2013]). Infusion was continued for 24 hours in one study (Zeymer, 2010).

Geriatric Refer to adult dosing. No dosing adjustment for the elderly appears to be necessary; adjust carefully to renal function.

Renal Impairment Note: The Cockcroft-Gault equation using actual body weight should be used to estimate renal function.

Acute coronary syndrome:
CrCl ≥50 mL/minute: No dosage adjustment necessary.
CrCl <50 mL/minute: 180 mcg/kg bolus (maximum: 22.6 mg) administered as soon as possible following diagnosis, followed by a continuous infusion of 1 mcg/kg/minute (maximum: 7.5 mg/hour)
End-stage renal disease (ie, dialysis dependent): Use is contraindicated.
Percutaneous coronary intervention (PCI) with or without stenting:
CrCl ≥50 mL/minute: No dosage adjustment necessary.
CrCl <50 mL/minute: 180 mcg/kg bolus (maximum: 22.6 mg) administered immediately before the initiation of PCI and followed by a continuous infusion of 1 mcg/kg/minute (maximum: 7.5 mg/hour). Administer a second 180 mcg/kg (maximum: 22.6 mg) bolus 10 minutes after the first bolus.
End-stage renal disease (ie, dialysis dependent): Use is contraindicated.

Hepatic Impairment There are no dosage adjustments provided in the manufacturer's labeling (has not been studied).

Administration Bolus dose should be withdrawn from the 10 mL vial into a syringe and administered by IV push. Begin continuous infusion (using an IV infusion pump) immediately following bolus administration, administered undiluted directly from the 100 mL vial. The 100 mL vial should be spiked with a vented infusion set.

Monitoring Parameters Coagulation parameters, signs/symptoms of excessive bleeding. Laboratory tests at baseline and monitoring during therapy: hematocrit and hemoglobin, serum creatinine, PT/aPTT (maintain aPTT between 50-70 seconds unless PCI is to be performed), and ACT with PCI (maintain ACT between 200-300 seconds during PCI). Platelet count recommended at 2-4 hours after initiation, and at 24 hours or prior to discharge, whichever is first.

Assess sheath insertion site and distal pulses of affected leg every 15 minutes for the first hour and then every 1 hour for the next 6 hours. Arterial access site care is important to prevent bleeding. Care should be taken when attempting vascular access that only the anterior wall of the femoral artery is punctured, avoiding a Seldinger (through and through) technique for obtaining sheath access. Femoral vein sheath placement should be avoided unless needed. While the vascular sheath is in place, patients should be maintained on complete bedrest with the head of the bed at a 30° angle and the affected limb restrained in a straight position.

Observe patient for mental status changes, hemorrhage, assess nose and mouth mucous membranes, puncture sites for oozing, ecchymosis and hematoma formation, and examine urine, stool and emesis for presence of occult or frank blood; gentle care should be provided when removing dressings.

Dosage Forms Excipient information presented when available (limited, particularly for generics); consult specific product labeling.

Solution, Intravenous:

Integrilin: 0.75 mg/mL (100 mL); 2 mg/mL (10 mL, 100 mL)

Generic: 0.75 mg/mL (100 mL)

Solution, Intravenous [preservative free]:

Generic: 0.75 mg/mL (100 mL); 2 mg/mL (10 mL, 100 mL)

♦ Eptifibatide Injection (Can) *see* Eptifibatide *on page 661*

♦ Epuris (Can) *see* ISOtretinoin *on page 996*

♦ Epzicom *see* Abacavir and Lamivudine *on page 18*

♦ Equanil *see* Meprobamate *on page 1146*

♦ Equetro *see* CarBAMazepine *on page 303*

♦ Equipto-Baclofen *see* Baclofen *on page 197*

♦ Equipto-Naproxen *see* Naproxen *on page 1256*

♦ ER-086526 *see* Eribulin *on page 664*

♦ Eraxis *see* Anidulafungin *on page 129*

♦ Erbitux *see* Cetuximab *on page 366*

♦ Erdol (Can) *see* Ergocalciferol *on page 663*

Ergocalciferol (er goe kal SIF e role)

Brand Names: US Calcidol [OTC]; Calciferol [OTC]; Drisdol; Drisdol [OTC]

Brand Names: Canada D-Forte; Erdol

Index Terms Activated Ergosterol; D2; Viosterol; Vitamin D2

Pharmacologic Category Vitamin D Analog

Use

Dietary supplement: For use as a vitamin D supplement.

Familial hypophosphatemia: Treatment of familial hypophosphatemia.

Hypoparathyroidism: Treatment of hypoparathyroidism.

Rickets: Treatment of refractory rickets, also known as vitamin D-resistant rickets.

Dosing

Adult Note: 1 mcg = 40 units

Dietary Reference Intake for Vitamin D: Oral (IOM, 2011):

Adults 19 to 70 years: RDA: 600 units/day

Pregnancy/Lactating: RDA: 600 units/day

Osteoporosis prevention (off-label use): Adults ≥50 years: 800 to 1000 units/day (NOF guidelines, 2014)

Vitamin D deficiency treatment (off-label dose): (Holick, 2011): Oral: 6000 units daily or 50,000 units once weekly for at least 8 weeks to achieve a 25(OH)D level >30 ng/mL; then maintenance dose of 1500 to 2000 units daily

Special populations (obese patients, patients on medications known to affect vitamin D metabolism, patients with malabsorption syndromes): 6000 to 10,000 units daily to achieve a 25(OH)D level >30 ng/mL; then maintenance dose of 3000 to 6000 units daily

Vitamin D deficiency/insufficiency in patients with CKD stages 3 to 4 (K/DOQI, 2003): **Note:** Dose is based on 25-hydroxyvitamin D serum level (25[OH]D): Oral (treatment duration should be a total of 6 months):

Serum 25(OH)D <5 ng/mL:

50,000 units/week for 12 weeks, then 50,000 units/month

Serum 25(OH)D 5 to 15 ng/mL:

50,000 units/week for 4 weeks, then 50,000 units/month

Serum 25(OH)D 16 to 30 ng/mL:

50,000 units/month

Hypoparathyroidism: Oral: 1.25 to 5 mg/day (50,000 to 200,000 units) with calcium supplements

Vitamin D-*resistant* rickets: Oral: 12,000 to 500,000 units/day

Geriatric Note: 1 mcg = 40 units

Dietary Reference Intake for Vitamin D: Oral (IOM, 2011):

≤70 years: Refer to adult dosing.

>70 years: RDA: 800 units/day

Pediatric Note: 1 mcg = 40 units

Dietary Reference Intake for Vitamin D: Oral:

Infants 0 to 12 months: Adequate intake: 400 units/day (IOM, 2011)

Breast-fed (fully or partially) Infants: Oral: 10 mcg/day (400 units/day) beginning in the first few days of life; continue supplementation until infant is weaned to ≥1 L/day or 1 quart/day of vitamin D-fortified formula or whole milk (after 12 months of age) (Wagner, 2008)

Nonbreast-fed Infants, Older Children ingesting <1000 mL of vitamin D-fortified formula or milk: Oral: 10 mcg/day (400 units/day) (Wagner, 2008)

Children with increased risk of vitamin D deficiency (chronic fat malabsorption, maintained on chronic antiseizure medications): Oral: Higher doses may be required; use laboratory testing [25 (OH)D, PTH, bone mineral status] to evaluate (Wagner, 2008)

Children and Adolescents 1 to 18 years: RDA: 600 units/day (IOM, 2011)

Vitamin D deficiency treatment (off-label use) (Holick, 2011):

Infants 0 to 1 year: 2000 units daily or 50,000 units once weekly for 6 weeks to achieve a 25(OH)D level >30 ng/mL; then maintenance dose of 400 to 1000 units daily.

Children and Adolescents 1 to 18 years: 2000 units daily or 50,000 units once weekly for at least 6 weeks to achieve a 25(OH)D level >30 ng/mL; then maintenance dose of 600 to 1000 units daily.

Vitamin D deficiency/insufficiency in patients with CKD stages 3 to 4 (K/DOQI, 2005): **Note:** Dose is based on 25-hydroxyvitamin D serum level (25[OH]D): Oral (treatment duration should be a total of 3 months):

Serum 25(OH)D <5 ng/mL:

8000 units/day for 4 weeks, then 4000 units/day for 2 months **or**

50,000 units/week for 4 weeks, then 50,000 units twice a month for 2 months

Serum 25(OH)D 5 to 15 ng/mL:

4000 int units/day **or**

50,000 int units every other week

Serum 25(OH)D 16 to 30 ng/mL:

2000 units/day **or**

50,000 units every 4 weeks

Hypoparathyroidism: Oral: 1.25 to 5 mg/day (50,000 to 200,000 units) and calcium supplements

Vitamin D-*resistant* rickets: Oral: 12,000 to 500,000 units/day

Renal Impairment There are no dosage adjustments provided in the manufacturer's labeling.

Hepatic Impairment There are no dosage adjustments provided in the manufacturer's labeling.

Additional Information Complete prescribing information should be consulted for additional detail.

Dosage Forms Excipient information presented when available (limited, particularly for generics); consult specific product labeling.

Capsule, Oral:

Drisdol: 50,000 units [contains brilliant blue fcf (fd&c blue #1), soybean oil, tartrazine (fd&c yellow #5)]

Generic: 50,000 units

Solution, Oral:

Calcidol: 8000 units/mL (60 mL) [contains propylene glycol]

Calciferol: 8000 units/mL (60 mL) [contains propylene glycol]

Drisdol: 8000 units/mL (60 mL) [contains propylene glycol]

Generic: 8000 units/mL (60 mL)

Tablet, Oral:

Generic: 400 units, 2000 units

♦ Ergomar *see* Ergotamine *on page 663*

Ergotamine (er GOT a meen)

Brand Names: US Ergomar

Index Terms Ergotamine Tartrate

Pharmacologic Category Antimigraine Agent; Ergot Derivative

Use Abort or prevent vascular headaches, such as migraine, migraine variants, or so-called "histaminic cephalalgia"

Dosing

Adult Migraine: Sublingual: 2 mg (1 tablet) under tongue at first sign of migraine, then 2 mg every 30 minutes if needed; maximum dose: 6 mg per 24 hours, 10 mg per week

Geriatric Not recommended for use in the elderly.

Renal Impairment Use is contraindicated in patients with impaired renal function.

Hepatic Impairment Use is contraindicated in patients with impaired hepatic function.

Additional Information Complete prescribing information should be consulted for additional detail.

Dosage Forms Excipient information presented when available (limited, particularly for generics); consult specific product labeling.

Tablet Sublingual, Sublingual, as tartrate:
Ergomar: 2 mg [contains fd&c blue #1 aluminum lake, fd&c yellow #10 aluminum lake, saccharin sodium]

◆ Ergotamine Tartrate *see* Ergotamine *on page 663*

Eribulin (er i BUE lin)

Brand Names: US Halaven
Brand Names: Canada Halaven
Index Terms B1939; E7389; ER-086526; Eribulin Mesylate; Halichondrin B Analog
Pharmacologic Category Antineoplastic Agent, Antimicrotubular
Use Breast cancer, metastatic: Treatment of metastatic breast cancer in patients who have received at least 2 prior chemotherapy regimens for the treatment of metastatic disease (prior treatment should have included an anthracycline and a taxane in either the adjuvant or metastatic setting)
Pregnancy Considerations Adverse effects were observed in animal reproduction studies. Based on its mechanism of action, eribulin would be expected to cause fetal harm if administered during pregnancy. Women of childbearing potential should use effective contraception to avoid pregnancy during eribulin treatment; the Canadian labeling recommends continuing effective contraception for at least 3 months after treatment.
Breast-Feeding Considerations It is not known if eribulin is excreted in breast milk. Due to the potential for serious adverse reactions in the nursing infant, a decision should be made to discontinue eribulin or to discontinue breast-feeding, taking into account the importance of treatment to the mother.
Contraindications There are no contraindications listed in the manufacturer's labeling.
Canadian labeling (not in U.S. labeling): Hypersensitivity to eribulin mesylate, halichondrin B, or its chemical derivatives.
Warnings/Precautions Hazardous agent - use appropriate precautions for handling and disposal (NIOSH 2014 [group 1]). Hematologic toxicity, including severe neutropenia, has occurred; may require treatment delay and dosage reduction. A higher incidence of grade 4 neutropenia and neutropenic fever occurred in patients with ALT or AST >3 x ULN or bilirubin >1.5 x ULN. Monitor complete blood counts prior to each dose; more frequently if severe cytopenias develop. Patients with baseline neutrophils <1,500/mm^3 were not included in clinical studies.

Peripheral neuropathy commonly occurs and is the most frequent toxicity leading to discontinuation. Peripheral neuropathy may be prolonged (>1 year in 5% of patients); may require treatment delay. Monitor for signs of peripheral motor or sensory neuropathy. Some patients may have preexisting neuropathy because of prior chemotherapy; monitor closely for worsening.

QT prolongation was observed on day 8 of eribulin therapy (in an uncontrolled study); monitor ECG in patients with heart failure, bradyarrhythmia, with concomitant medication known to prolong the QT interval, or with electrolyte imbalance; correct hypokalemia and hypomagnesemia prior to treatment; monitor electrolytes periodically during treatment. Avoid use in patients with congenital long QT syndrome.

Dosage reduction required in patients with mild to moderate (Child-Pugh class A or B) hepatic impairment; use has not been studied in patients with severe hepatic impairment; transaminase or bilirubin elevations are associated with a higher incidence of grade 4 neutropenia and neutropenic fever. Dosage reduction required in patients with moderate or severe renal impairment (CrCl 15 to 49 mL/minute). Potentially significant drug-drug interactions may exist, requiring dose or frequency adjustment, additional monitoring, and/or selection of alternative therapy. Some products available internationally may have vial strength and dosing expressed as the base (instead of as the salt); refer to prescribing information for specific dosing information.

Adverse Reactions

>10%:
Central nervous system: Fatigue (≤54%), peripheral neuropathy (35%; grades 3/4: ≤8%), headache (19%)
Dermatologic: Alopecia (45%)
Endocrine & metabolic: Weight loss (21%)
Gastrointestinal: Nausea (35%), constipation (25%), anorexia (20%), diarrhea (18%), vomiting (18%)
Hematologic & oncologic: Neutropenia (82%; grades 3: 28%; grade 4: 29%; nadir: 13 days; recovery: 8 days), anemia (58%; grades 3/4: 2%)
Hepatic: Increased serum ALT (18%)
Neuromuscular & skeletal: Weakness (≤54%), arthralgia (≤22%), myalgia (≤22%), back pain (16%), ostealgia (12%), limb pain (11%)
Respiratory: Dyspnea (16%), cough (14%)
Miscellaneous: Fever (21%)

1% to 10%:
Cardiovascular: Peripheral edema (≥5% to <10%)
Central nervous system: Depression (≥5% to <10%), dizziness (≥5% to <10%), insomnia (≥5% to <10%), myasthenia (≥5% to <10%)
Dermatologic: Skin rash (≥5% to <10%)
Endocrine & metabolic: Hypokalemia (≥5% to <10%)
Gastrointestinal: Mucosal inflammation (9%), abdominal pain (≥5% to <10%), dysgeusia (≥5% to <10%), dyspepsia (≥5% to <10%), stomatitis (≥5% to <10%), xerostomia (≥5% to <10%)
Genitourinary: Urinary tract infection (10%)
Hematologic & oncologic: Febrile neutropenia (5%), thrombocytopenia (grades 3/4: 1%)
Neuromuscular & skeletal: Muscle spasm (≥5% to <10%)
Ophthalmic: Increased lacrimation (≥5% to <10%)
Respiratory: Upper respiratory tract infection (≥5% to <10%)

<1% (Limited to important or life-threatening): Dehydration, drug-induced hypersensitivity, hepatotoxicity, hypomagnesemia, interstitial pulmonary disease, lymphocytopenia, pancreatitis, pneumonia, prolonged Q-T interval on ECG, sepsis

Drug Interactions

Metabolism/Transport Effects Substrate of CYP3A4 (minor); **Note:** Assignment of Major/Minor substrate status based on clinically relevant drug interaction potential

Avoid Concomitant Use
Avoid concomitant use of EriBULin with any of the following: BCG (Intravesical); Deferiprone; Dipyrone

Increased Effect/Toxicity
EriBULin may increase the levels/effects of: CloZAPine; Deferiprone; Highest Risk QTc-Prolonging Agents; Moderate Risk QTc-Prolonging Agents

The levels/effects of EriBULin may be increased by: Dipyrone; Mifepristone

Decreased Effect
EriBULin may decrease the levels/effects of: BCG (Intravesical)

Preparation for Administration Hazardous agent; use appropriate precautions for handling and disposal (NIOSH 2014 [group 1]). No dilution required. May prepare by drawing into a syringe for administration or may dilute in 100 mL normal saline. Discard unused portion of vial.

Storage/Stability Store intact vials at 25°C (77°F); excursions permitted between 15°C and 30°C (59°F and 86°F); do not freeze. Store in original carton. Undiluted solutions in a syringe and solutions diluted in normal saline for infusion are stable for up to 4 hours at room temperature or up to 24 hours refrigerated at 4°C (40°F).

Mechanism of Action Eribulin is a non-taxane microtubule inhibitor which is a halichondrin B analog. It inhibits the growth phase of the microtubule by inhibiting formation of mitotic spindles causing mitotic blockage and arresting the cell cycle at the G$_2$/M phase; suppresses microtubule polymerization yet does not affect depolymerization.

Pharmacodynamics/Kinetics

Distribution: V$_d$: 43 to 114 L/m^2
Protein binding: 49% to 65%
Metabolism: Negligible
Half-life, elimination: ~40 hours
Excretion: Feces (82%, predominantly as unchanged drug); urine (9%, primarily as unchanged drug)

Dosing

Adult & Geriatric Note: *International Considerations:* Some products available internationally may have vial strength and dosing expressed as the base (instead of as the salt). Refer to prescribing information for specific dosing information.

Breast cancer, metastatic: IV: Eribulin mesylate: 1.4 mg/m²/dose on days 1 and 8 of a 21-day treatment cycle

Renal Impairment Note: *International Considerations:* Some products available internationally may have vial strength and dosing expressed as the base (instead of as the salt). Refer to prescribing information for specific dosing information.

Mild impairment (CrCl ≥50 mL/minute): No dosage adjustment required.

Moderate impairment (CrCl 30 to 49 mL/minute): Reduce to eribulin mesylate 1.1 mg/m²/dose.

Severe impairment (CrCl 15 to 29 mL/minute): Reduce to eribulin mesylate 1.1 mg/m²/dose.

ESRD (*Canadian labeling*): Use is not recommended.

Hepatic Impairment Note: *International Considerations:* Some products available internationally may have vial strength and dosing expressed as the base (instead of as the salt). Refer to prescribing information for specific dosing information.

Mild hepatic impairment (Child-Pugh class A): Reduce to eribulin mesylate 1.1 mg/m²/dose.

Moderate hepatic impairment (Child-Pugh class B): Reduce to eribulin mesylate 0.7 mg/m²/dose.

Severe hepatic impairment (Child-Pugh class C): There are no dosage adjustments provided in the manufacturer's U.S. labeling (has not been studied); use is not recommended in the Canadian labeling.

Obesity *ASCO Guidelines for appropriate chemotherapy dosing in obese adults with cancer:* Utilize patient's actual body weight (full weight) for calculation of body surface area- or weight-based dosing, particularly when the intent of therapy is curative; manage regimen-related toxicities in the same manner as for nonobese patients; if a dose reduction is utilized due to toxicity, consider resumption of full weight-based dosing with subsequent cycles, especially if cause of toxicity (eg, hepatic or renal impairment) is resolved (Griggs, 2012).

Adjustment for Toxicity Note: *International Considerations:* Some products available internationally may have vial strength and dosing expressed as the base (instead of as the salt). Refer to prescribing information for specific dosing information.

ANC <1,000/mm³ or platelets <75,000/mm³ or grade 3 or 4 nonhematologic toxicity on day 1 or 8: Withhold dose; may delay day 8 dose up to 1 week. If toxicity resolves to ≤ grade 2 by day 15 administer a reduced dose and wait at least 2 weeks before beginning the next cycle. Omit dose if not resolved to ≤ grade 2 by day 15. Do not re-escalate dose after reduction.

Permanently reduce dose from eribulin mesylate 1.4 mg/m² to 1.1 mg/m² for the following:
ANC <500/mm³ for >7 days
ANC <1000/mm³ with fever or infection
Platelets <25,000/mm³
Platelets <50,000/mm³ requiring transfusion
Nonhematologic toxicity of grade 3 or 4
Dose omission or delay due to toxicity on day 8 of prior cycle

Permanently reduce dose from eribulin mesylate 1.1 mg/m² to 0.7 mg/m² for occurrence of any of the above events; discontinue treatment if the above toxicities occur at the 0.7 mg/m² dose level.

Administration IV: Infuse over 2 to 5 minutes. May be administered undiluted or diluted. Do not administer other medications through the same IV line, or through a line containing dextrose.

Hazardous agent; use appropriate precautions for handling and disposal (NIOSH 2014 [group 1]).

Monitoring Parameters CBC with differential prior to each dose; renal and liver function tests; serum electrolytes, including potassium and magnesium. Assess for peripheral neuropathy prior to each dose. Monitor ECG in patients with heart failure, bradyarrhythmia, with concomitant medication known to prolong the QT interval, and electrolyte abnormalities (eg, hypokalemia, hypomagnesemia).

Additional Information *International considerations:* Eribulin mesylate 1.4 mg is equivalent to eribulin (base) 1.23 mg.

Dosage Forms Excipient information presented when available (limited, particularly for generics); consult specific product labeling.
Solution, Intravenous, as mesylate:
Halaven: 1 mg/2 mL (2 mL) [contains alcohol, usp]

Erlotinib (er LOE tye nib)

Brand Names: US Tarceva
Brand Names: Canada Tarceva
Index Terms CP358774; Erlotinib Hydrochloride; OSI-774
Pharmacologic Category Antineoplastic Agent, Epidermal Growth Factor Receptor (EGFR) Inhibitor; Antineoplastic Agent, Tyrosine Kinase Inhibitor

Use
Non-small cell lung cancer (NSCLC): First-line treatment of metastatic non-small cell lung cancer (NSCLC) in tumors with epidermal growth factor receptor (EGFR) exon 19 deletions or exon 21 (L858R) substitution mutations as detected by an approved test; treatment of locally advanced or metastatic NSCLC after failure of at least 1 prior chemotherapy regimen; maintenance treatment of locally advanced or metastatic NSCLC which has not progressed after 4 cycles of first-line platinum-based chemotherapy
Limitations of use: Use in combination with platinum-based chemotherapy is not recommended. First-line treatment in patients with metastatic NSCLC with EGFR mutations other than exon 19 deletion or exon 21 (L858R) substitution has not been evaluated.

Pancreatic cancer (not an approved use in Canada): First-line treatment of locally advanced, unresectable, or metastatic pancreatic cancer (in combination with gemcitabine)

Pregnancy Considerations Adverse events were observed in animal reproduction studies. Based on the mechanism of action, may cause fetal harm if administered in pregnancy. Females of reproductive potential should be advised to avoid pregnancy; highly effective contraception is recommended during treatment and for at least 2 weeks after treatment has been completed.

Breast-Feeding Considerations It is not known if erlotinib is excreted in breast milk. Due to the potential for serious adverse reactions in the nursing infant, the decision to discontinue breast-feeding or discontinue erlotinib should take into account the benefits of treatment to the mother.

Contraindications
There are no contraindications listed in the manufacturer's U.S. labeling.
Canadian labeling: Hypersensitivity to erlotinib or any component of the formulation

Warnings/Precautions Hazardous agent - use appropriate precautions for handling and disposal (NIOSH 2014 [group 1]). Rare, sometimes fatal, interstitial lung disease (ILD) has occurred; symptoms include acute respiratory distress syndrome, interstitial pneumonia, obliterative bronchiolitis, pneumonitis (including radiation and hypersensitivity), pulmonary fibrosis, and pulmonary infiltrates. The onset of symptoms has been within 5 days to more than 9 months after treatment initiation (median: 39 days). Interrupt treatment for unexplained new or worsening pulmonary symptoms (dyspnea, cough, and fever); permanently discontinue for confirmed ILD.

Hepatic failure and hepatorenal syndrome have been reported, particularly in patients with baseline hepatic impairment (although have also been observed in patients with normal hepatic function). Monitor liver function (transaminases, bilirubin, and alkaline phosphatase); patients with any hepatic impairment (total bilirubin >ULN; Child-Pugh class A, B, or C) should be closely monitored, including those with hepatic disease due to tumor burden. Dosage reduction, interruption, or discontinuation may be recommended for changes in hepatic function. Use with extreme caution in patients with total bilirubin >3 times ULN. Interrupt therapy if total bilirubin is >3 times ULN or transaminases are >5 times ULN in patients without pre-existing hepatic impairment. In patients with baseline hepatic dysfunction or biliary obstruction, interrupt therapy if bilirubin doubles or transaminases triple from baseline values. Increased monitoring of liver function is required in patients with preexisting hepatic impairment or biliary obstruction. Acute renal failure, renal insufficiency, and hepatorenal syndrome have been reported, either secondary to hepatic impairment at baseline or due to severe dehydration; use with caution in patients with or at risk for renal impairment. Monitor closely for dehydration; monitor renal function and electrolytes in patients at risk for dehydration. If severe renal impairment develops, interrupt therapy until toxicity resolves. Gastrointestinal perforation has been reported with use; risk for perforation is increased with concurrent anti-angiogenic agents, corticosteroids, NSAIDs, and/or taxane based-therapy, and patients with history of peptic ulcers or diverticular disease; permanently discontinue in patients who develop perforation.

Bullous, blistering, or exfoliating skin conditions, some suggestive of Stevens-Johnson or toxic epidermal necrolysis (TEN) have been reported. An acne-like rash commonly appears on the face, back, and upper chest. Generalized or severe acneiform, erythematous or maculopapular rash may occur. Skin rash may correlate with treatment response and prolonged survival (Saif, 2008); management of skin rashes that are not serious should include alcohol-free lotions, topical antibiotics, or topical corticosteroids, or if necessary, oral antibiotics and systemic corticosteroids; avoid sunlight. Reduce dose or temporarily interrupt treatment for severe skin reactions; discontinue treatment for bullous, blistering or exfoliative skin toxicity. Corneal perforation and ulceration have been reported with use; decreased tear production, abnormal eyelash growth, keratoconjunctivitis sicca, or keratitis have also been reported and are known risk factors for corneal ulceration/perforation. Interrupt or discontinue treatment in patients presenting with eye pain or other acute or worsening ocular symptoms. Consider a baseline ophthalmologic exam and reassess for ocular toxicities at 4 to 8 weeks after treatment initiation (Renouf, 2012).

MI, CVA, and microangiopathic hemolytic anemia with thrombocytopenia have been reported (rarely) with erlotinib in combination with gemcitabine. Elevated INR and bleeding events (including fatal hemorrhage) have been reported; monitor prothrombin time and INR closely. Erlotinib levels may be lower in patients who smoke; advise patients to stop smoking. Smokers treated with 300 mg/day exhibited steady-state erlotinib levels comparable to former- and never-smokers receiving 150 mg/day (Hughes, 2009). Potentially significant drug-drug interactions may exist, requiring dose or frequency adjustment, additional monitoring, and/or selection of alternative therapy. Avoid concomitant use with proton pump inhibitors. If taken with an H$_2$-receptor antagonist (eg, ranitidine), administer erlotinib 10 hours after the H$_2$-receptor antagonist dose and at least 2 hours prior to the next H$_2$-receptor dose. If an antacid is necessary, separate dosing by several hours. In patients with NSCLC, EGFR mutations, specifically exon 19 deletions and exon 21 mutation (L858R), are associated with better response to erlotinib (Riely, 2006); erlotinib treatment is not recommended in patients with K-ras mutations; they are not likely to benefit from erlotinib treatment (Eberhard, 2005; Miller, 2008). Concurrent erlotinib plus platinum-based chemotherapy is not recommended for first line treatment of locally advanced or metastatic NSCLC due to a lack of clinical benefit. The cobas EGFR mutation test has been approved to detect EGFR mutation for first-line NSCLC treatment. Product may contain lactose; avoid use in patients with Lapp lactase deficiency, glucose-galactose malabsorption, or glucose intolerance.

Adverse Reactions

Adverse reactions reported with monotherapy:

>10%:

Cardiovascular: Chest pain (≤18%)

Central nervous system: Fatigue (9% to 52%)

Dermatologic: Skin rash (49% to 85%; grade 3: 5% to 13%; grade 4: <1%; median onset: 8 days), xeroderma (4% to 21%), pruritus (7% to 16%), paronychia (4% to 16%), alopecia (14% to 15%), acne vulgaris (6% to 12%)

Gastrointestinal: Diarrhea (20% to 62%; grade 3: 2% to 6%; grade 4: <1%; median onset: 12 days), anorexia (9% to 52%), nausea (23% to 33%), decreased appetite (≤28%), vomiting (13% to 23%), mucositis (≤18%), stomatitis (11% to 17%), abdominal pain (3% to 11%), constipation (≤8%)

Genitourinary: Urinary tract infection (≤4%)

Hematologic & oncologic: Anemia (≤11%; grade 4: 1%)

Infection: Increased susceptibility to infection (4% to 24%)

Miscellaneous: Fever (≤11%)

Neuromuscular & skeletal: Weakness (≤53%), back pain (19%), arthralgia (≤13%), musculoskeletal pain (11%)

Ophthalmic: Conjunctivitis (12% to 18%), keratoconjunctivitis sicca (12%)

Respiratory: Cough (33% to 48%), dyspnea (41% to 45%; grades 3/4: 8% to 28%)

1% to 10%:

Cardiovascular: Peripheral edema (≤5%)

Central nervous system: Pain (≤9%), headache (≤7%), anxiety (≤5%), dizziness (≤4%), insomnia (≤4%), neurotoxicity (≤4%), paresthesia (≤4%), voice disorder (≤4%)

Dermatologic: Folliculitis (≤8%), nail disease (≤7%), exfoliative dermatitis (5%), hypertrichosis (5%), skin fissure (5%), acneiform eruption (4% to 5%), erythema (≤5%), dermatitis (4%), erythematous rash (≤4%), palmar-plantar erythrodysesthesia (≤4%), bullous dermatitis

Endocrine & metabolic: Weight loss (4% to 5%)

Gastrointestinal: Dyspepsia (≤5%), xerostomia (≤3%), taste disorder (≤1%)

Hematologic & oncologic: Lymphocytopenia (≤4%; grade 3: 1%), leukopenia (≤3%), thrombocytopenia (≤1%)

Hepatic: Hyperbilirubinemia (7%; grade 3: ≤1%), increased serum ALT (grade 2: 2% to 4%; grade 3: 1% to 3%), increased gamma-glutamyl transferase (≤4%), hepatic failure (≤1%)

Neuromuscular & skeletal: Muscle spasm (≤4%), musculoskeletal chest pain (≤4%), ostealgia (≤4%)

Otic: Tinnitus (≤1%)

Renal: Increased serum creatinine (≤1%), renal failure (≤1%),

Respiratory: Nasopharyngitis (≤7%), epistaxis (≤4%), pulmonary embolism (≤4%), respiratory tract infection (≤4%), pneumonitis (3%), pulmonary fibrosis (3%)

<1%: Interstitial pulmonary disease

Adverse reactions reported with combination (erlotinib plus gemcitabine) therapy:

>10%:

Cardiovascular: Edema (37%), thrombosis (grades 3/4: 11%)

Central nervous system: Fatigue (73% to 79%), depression (19%), dizziness (15%), headache (15%), anxiety (13%)

Dermatologic: Skin rash (70%), alopecia (14%)

Gastrointestinal: Nausea (60%), anorexia (52%), diarrhea (48%), abdominal pain (46%), vomiting (42%), weight loss (39%), stomatitis (22%), dyspepsia (17%), flatulence (13%)

Hepatic: Increased serum ALT (grade 2: 31%, grade 3: 13%, grade 4: <1%), increased serum AST (grade 2: 24%, grade 3: 10%, grade 4 <1%), hyperbilirubinemia (grade 2: 17%, grade 3: 10%, grade 4: <1%)

Infection: Increased susceptibility to infection (39%)

Miscellaneous: Fever (36%)

Neuromuscular & skeletal: Ostealgia (25%), myalgia (21%), neuropathy (13%), rigors (12%)

Respiratory: Dyspnea (24%), cough (16%)

1% to 10%:

Cardiovascular: Cardiac arrhythmia (<5%), syncope (<5%), deep vein thrombosis (4%), cerebrovascular accident (3%; including cerebral hemorrhage), myocardial infarction (2%)

Gastrointestinal: Intestinal obstruction (<5%), pancreatitis (<5%)

Hematologic & oncologic: Hemolytic anemia (<5%), microangiopathic hemolytic anemia with thrombocytopenia (1%)

Renal: Renal insufficiency (<5%), renal failure (1%)

Respiratory: Interstitial pulmonary disease (<3%)

<1%: Bullous dermatitis, exfoliative dermatitis, hepatic failure

Mono- or combination therapy: <1% (Limited to important or life-threatening): Acute peptic ulcer with hemorrhage, bronchiolitis, corneal perforation, corneal ulcer, episcleritis, gastritis, gastrointestinal hemorrhage, gastrointestinal perforation, hearing loss, hematemesis, hematochezia, hepatorenal syndrome, hepatotoxicity, hirsutism, hyperpigmentation, hypokalemia, keratitis, melena, myopathy (in combination with statin therapy), peptic ulcer, rhabdomyolysis (in combination with statin therapy), skin photosensitivity, skin rash (acneiform; sparing prior radiation field), Stevens-Johnson syndrome, toxic epidermal necrolysis, tympanic membrane perforation

Drug Interactions

Metabolism/Transport Effects Substrate of CYP1A2 (minor), CYP3A4 (major); Note: Assignment of Major/Minor substrate status based on clinically relevant drug interaction potential; Inhibits UGT1A1

Avoid Concomitant Use

Avoid concomitant use of Erlotinib with any of the following: Conivaptan; Fusidic Acid (Systemic); Idelalisib; Irinotecan Products; Proton Pump Inhibitors

Increased Effect/Toxicity

Erlotinib may increase the levels/effects of: Irinotecan Products; Warfarin

The levels/effects of Erlotinib may be increased by: Aprepitant; Ciprofloxacin (Systemic); Conivaptan; CYP3A4 Inhibitors (Moderate); CYP3A4 Inhibitors (Strong); Dasatinib; FluvoxaMINE; Fosaprepitant; Fusidic Acid (Systemic); Grapefruit Juice; Idelalisib; Ivacaftor; Luliconazole; Mifepristone; Netupitant; Osimertinib; Palbociclib; Simeprevir; Stiripentol

Decreased Effect

The levels/effects of Erlotinib may be decreased by: Antacids; Bosentan; CYP3A4 Inducers (Moderate); CYP3A4 Inducers (Strong); Dabrafenib; Deferasirox; Enzalutamide; H2-Antagonists; Mitotane; Osimertinib; Proton Pump Inhibitors; Siltuximab; St Johns Wort; Tocilizumab

Food Interactions Erlotinib bioavailability is increased with food. Grapefruit or grapefruit juice may decrease metabolism and increase erlotinib plasma concentrations. Management: Take on an empty stomach at least 1 hour before or 2 hours after the ingestion of food. Avoid grapefruit and grapefruit juice. Maintain adequate nutrition and hydration, unless instructed to restrict fluid intake.

Storage/Stability Store at 25°C (77°F); excursions are permitted between 15°C and 30°C (59°F and 86°F).

Mechanism of Action Reversibly inhibits overall epidermal growth factor receptor (HER1/EGFR) - tyrosine kinase activity. Intracellular phosphorylation is inhibited which prevents further downstream signaling, resulting in cell death. Erlotinib has higher binding affinity for EGFR exon 19 deletion or exon 21 L858R mutations than for the wild type receptor.

Pharmacodynamics/Kinetics

Absorption: Oral: 60% on an empty stomach; almost 100% on a full stomach

Distribution: 232 L

Protein binding: ~93% to albumin and alpha$_1$-acid glycoprotein

Metabolism: Hepatic, via CYP3A4 (major), CYP1A1 (minor), CYP1A2 (minor), and CYP1C (minor)

Bioavailability: Almost 100% when given with food; 60% without food

Half-life elimination: 36 hours

Time to peak, plasma: 4 hours

Excretion: Primarily as metabolites: Feces (83%; 1% as unchanged drug); urine (8%; <1% as unchanged drug)

Dosing

Adult & Geriatric

Non-small cell lung cancer (NSCLC), metastatic, first-line therapy in patients with EGFR exon 19 deletions or exon 21 (L858R) substitution mutations: Oral: 150 mg once daily until disease progression or unacceptable toxicity (Rosell, 2012; Zhou, 2011).

NSCLC, refractory: Oral: 150 mg once daily until disease progression or unacceptable toxicity (Shepherd, 2005)

NSCLC, maintenance therapy: Oral: 150 mg once daily until disease progression or unacceptable toxicity (Capuzzo, 2010)

Pancreatic cancer: Oral: 100 mg once daily until disease progression or unacceptable toxicity (in combination with gemcitabine) (Moore, 2007)

Dosage adjustment for concomitant CYP3A4 inhibitors/inducers:

CYP3A4 inhibitors: Avoid concurrent use if possible; consider dose reductions for severe adverse reactions if erlotinib is administered concomitantly with strong CYP3A4 inhibitors (eg, azole antifungals, clarithromycin, erythromycin, nefazodone, protease inhibitors, telithromycin, grapefruit, or grapefruit juice). Dose reduction (if required) should be done in decrements of 50 mg (after toxicity has resolved to baseline or ≤ grade 1).

Concomitant CYP3A4 and CYP1A2 inhibitor (eg, ciprofloxacin): Avoid concurrent use if possible; consider dose reductions in decrements of 50 mg if severe adverse reactions occur (after toxicity has resolved to baseline or ≤ grade 1).

CYP3A4 inducers: Alternatives to the enzyme-inducing agent should be utilized first. Concomitant administration with CYP3A4 inducers (eg, carbamazepine, phenobarbital, phenytoin, rifamycins, and St John's wort) may require increased erlotinib doses (increase as tolerated at 2-week intervals in 50 mg increments to a maximum of 450 mg); doses >150 mg daily should be considered with rifampin (the maximum erlotinib dose studied in combination with rifampin was 450 mg). Immediately reduce erlotinib dose to recommended starting dose when CYP3A4 inducer is discontinued.

Dosage adjustment for concomitant smoking: Increase dose at 2-week intervals in 50 mg increments to a maximum dose of 300 mg (with careful monitoring) in patients who continue to smoke; immediately reduce erlotinib dose to recommended starting dose upon smoking cessation.

Renal Impairment

Renal impairment at treatment initiation: There are no dosage adjustments provided in the manufacturer's labeling (has not been studied), although <9% of a single dose is excreted in the urine.

Renal toxicity during treatment: Withhold treatment for grades 3/4 renal toxicity (consider discontinuing) and for risk of renal failure due to dehydration; may resume after euvolemia re-established (at previous dose). If treatment withheld due to toxicity and therapy is resumed, reinitiate with a 50 mg dose reduction after toxicity has resolved to baseline or ≤ grade 1.

Hepatic Impairment

Hepatic impairment at treatment initiation:

U.S. labeling:

Total bilirubin > ULN or Child-Pugh classes A, B, and C: There are no dosage adjustments provided in the manufacturer's labeling; use with caution and monitor closely during treatment.

Total bilirubin >3 times ULN: Use extreme caution.

Canadian labeling:

Moderate impairment: There are no dosage adjustments provided in the manufacturer's labeling; however, a reduced dose should be considered.

Severe impairment (including total bilirubin >3 times ULN and/or transaminases >5 times ULN): Use is not recommended.

The following adjustments have also been studied: A reduced starting dose (75 mg once daily) has been recommended in patients with hepatic dysfunction (AST ≥3 times ULN or direct bilirubin 1-7 mg/dL), with individualized dosage escalation if tolerated (Miller, 2007); another study determined that pharmacokinetic and safety profiles were similar between patients with normal hepatic function and moderate hepatic impairment (O'Bryant, 2012).

Hepatotoxicity during treatment: U.S. labeling:

Patients with normal hepatic function at baseline: If total bilirubin >3 times ULN and/or transaminases >5 times ULN during use: Interrupt therapy (consider discontinuing); if treatment is resumed, reinitiate with a 50 mg dose reduction after bilirubin and transaminases return to baseline; discontinue treatment if there is no significant improvement or resolution within 3 weeks.

Patients with baseline hepatic impairment or biliary obstruction: If bilirubin doubles or transaminases triple over baseline during use: Interrupt therapy (consider discontinuing); if treatment is resumed, reinitiate with a 50 mg dose reduction after bilirubin and transaminases return to baseline; discontinue treatment if there is no significant improvement or resolution of hepatotoxicity within 3 weeks.

Adjustment for Toxicity

Dermatologic toxicity:

Bullous, blistering, or exfoliative skin toxicity (severe): Discontinue treatment.

Severe rash (unresponsive to medical management): Withhold treatment; may reinitiate with a 50 mg dose reduction after toxicity has resolved to baseline or ≤ grade 1.

Gastrointestinal toxicity:

Diarrhea: Manage with loperamide; in severe diarrhea (unresponsive to loperamide) or dehydration due to diarrhea, withhold treatment; may reinitiate with a 50 mg dose reduction after toxicity has resolved to baseline or ≤ grade 1.

Gastrointestinal perforation: Discontinue treatment.

Ocular toxicities:

Acute or worsening ocular toxicities (eg, eye pain): Interrupt and consider discontinuing treatment. If therapy is resumed, reinitiate with a 50 mg dose reduction after toxicity has resolved to baseline or ≤ grade 1.

Corneal perforation or severe ulceration: Discontinue treatment.

Keratitis (grade 3 or 4 or grade 2 persisting >2 weeks): Withhold treatment; may reinitiate with a 50 mg dose reduction after toxicity has resolved to baseline or ≤ grade 1.

Pulmonary symptoms: Acute onset (or worsening) of pulmonary symptoms (eg, dyspnea, cough, fever): Interrupt treatment and evaluate for drug-induced interstitial lung disease; discontinue permanently with development of interstitial lung disease

Dietary Considerations Take this medicine on an empty stomach, 1 hour before or 2 hours after a meal. Avoid grapefruit juice.

Administration The manufacturer recommends administration on an empty stomach (at least 1 hour before or 2 hours after the ingestion of food). Avoid concomitant use with proton pump inhibitors. If taken with an H$_2$-receptor antagonist (eg, ranitidine), administer erlotinib 10 hours after the H$_2$-receptor antagonist dose and at least 2 hours prior to the next H$_2$- receptor dose. If an antacid is necessary, separate dosing by several hours.

For patients unable to swallow whole, tablets may be dissolved in 100 mL water and administered orally or via feeding tube (silicone-based); to ensure full dose is received, rinse container with 40 mL water, administer residue and repeat rinse (data on file, Genentech [contact product manufacturer to obtain current information]; Siu, 2007; Soulieres, 2004).

Hazardous agent; use appropriate precautions for handling and disposal (NIOSH 2014 [group 1]).

Monitoring Parameters Periodic liver function tests (transaminases, bilirubin, and alkaline phosphatase); monitor more frequently with worsening liver function; periodic renal function tests and serum electrolytes (in patients at risk for dehydration); hydration status; signs/symptoms of pulmonary toxicity; prothrombin time and INR (in patients on concomitant warfarin therapy); consider a baseline ophthalmologic exam and reassess for ocular toxicities at 4 to 8 weeks after treatment initiation (Renouf, 2012); EGFR mutation status in patients with NSCLC adenocarcinoma (Keedy, 2011); the cobas EGFR mutation test has been approved to detect EGFR mutation for first-line NSCLC treatment

Additional Information In patients with NSCLC, some factors which correlate positively with response to EGFR-tyrosine kinase inhibitor (TKI) therapy include patients who have never smoked, EGFR mutation, and patients of Asian origin. EGFR mutations, specifically exon 19 deletions and exon 21 mutation (L858R) correlate with response to tyrosine kinase inhibition (Riely, 2006). K-ras mutations correlated with poorer outcome with EGFR-TKI therapy in patients with NSCLC (Cooley, 2008; Jackman, 2008; Masarelli, 2007; Shepherd, 2005).

Dosage Forms Excipient information presented when available (limited, particularly for generics); consult specific product labeling.

Tablet, Oral:

Tarceva: 25 mg [contains fd&c yellow #6 (sunset yellow)]

Tarceva: 100 mg, 150 mg

Extemporaneous Preparations Hazardous agent; use appropriate precautions for handling and disposal (NIOSH 2014 [group 1]).

A suspension for oral or feeding tube (silicone-based) administration may be prepared by dissolving tablets needed for dose in 100 mL water. To ensure full dose is received, rinse container with 40 mL water, administer residue and repeat rinse. Administer immediately after preparation; stability of solution is unknown (Data on file from Genentech [contact product manufacturer to obtain current information]).

Siu LL, Soulieres D, Chen EX, et al, "Phase I/II Trial of Erlotinib and Cisplatin in Patients With Recurrent or Metastatic Squamous Cell Carcinoma of the Head and Neck: A Princess Margaret Hospital Phase II Consortium and National Cancer Institute of Canada Clinical Trials Group Study," J Clin Oncol, 2007, 25(16):2178-83. [PubMed 17538162]

Soulieres D, Senzer NN, Vokes EE, et al, "Multicenter Phase II Study of Erlotinib, an Oral Epidermal Growth Factor Receptor Tyrosine Kinase Inhibitor, in Patients With Recurrent or Metastatic Squamous Cell Cancer of the Head and Neck," J Clin Oncol, 2004, 22(1):77-85. [PubMed 14701768]

Ertapenem (er ta PEN em)

Brand Names: US INVanz
Brand Names: Canada Invanz
Index Terms Ertapenem Sodium; L-749,345; MK0826
Pharmacologic Category Antibiotic, Carbapenem
Use Moderate-to-severe infections:
Acute pelvic infections: For the treatment of acute pelvic infections, including postpartum endomyometritis, septic abortion, and postsurgical gynecologic infections caused by Streptococcus agalactiae, Escherichia coli, Bacteroides fragilis, Porphyromonas asaccharolytica, Peptostreptococcus spp, or Prevotella bivia.

Community-acquired pneumonia: For the treatment of community-acquired pneumonia (CAP) caused by Streptococcus pneumoniae (penicillin-susceptible isolates only), including cases with concurrent bacteremia; Haemophilus influenzae (beta-lactamase-negative isolates only); or Moraxella catarrhalis.

Complicated intra-abdominal infections: For the treatment of complicated intra-abdominal infections caused by E. coli, Clostridium clostridioforme, Eubacterium lentum, Peptostreptococcus spp, B. fragilis, Bacteroides distasonis, Bacteroides ovatus, Bacteroides thetaiotaomicron, or Bacteroides uniformis.

Complicated skin and skin structure infections: For the treatment of complicated skin and skin structure infections, including diabetic foot infections without osteomyelitis caused by Staphylococcus aureus (methicillin-susceptible isolates only), S. agalactiae, Streptococcus pyogenes, E. coli, Klebsiella pneumoniae, Proteus mirabilis, B. fragilis, Peptostreptococcus spp, P. asaccharolytica, or P. bivia. Ertapenem has not been studied in diabetic foot infections with concomitant osteomyelitis.

Complicated urinary tract infections: For the treatment of complicated urinary tract infections (UTIs), including pyelonephritis caused by E. coli, including cases with concurrent bacteremia or K. pneumoniae.

Prophylaxis of surgical-site infection in colorectal surgery: For the prophylaxis of surgical-site infection in adults following elective colorectal surgery.

Note: Methicillin-resistant Staphylococcus aureus, Enterococcus spp, penicillin-resistant strains of Streptococcus pneumoniae, Acinetobacter, and Pseudomonas aeruginosa, are **resistant** to ertapenem while most extended-spectrum beta-lactamase (ESBL)-producing bacteria remain sensitive to ertapenem.

Pregnancy Considerations Teratogenic effects were not observed in animal reproduction studies. Ertapenem is approved for the treatment of postpartum endomyometritis, septic abortion, and postsurgical infections. Information related to use during pregnancy has not been located.

Breast-Feeding Considerations Ertapenem is excreted in breast milk. The low concentrations in milk and low oral bioavailability suggest minimal exposure risk to the infant. The manufacturer recommends that caution be exercised when administering ertapenem to nursing women. Non-dose-related effects could include modification of bowel flora.

Contraindications Known hypersensitivity to any component of this product or to other drugs in the same class or in patients who have demonstrated anaphylactic reactions to beta-lactams; known hypersensitivity to local anesthetics of the amide type due to the use of lidocaine as a diluent (IM use only).

Warnings/Precautions Use caution with renal impairment. Dosage adjustment required in patients with moderate to severe renal dysfunction; elderly patients often require lower doses (based upon renal function). Use may result in fungal or bacterial superinfection, including C. difficile-associated diarrhea (CDAD) and pseudomembranous colitis; CDAD has been observed >2 months postantibiotic treatment. Carbapenems have been associated with CNS adverse effects, including confusional states and seizures (myoclonic); use caution with CNS disorders (eg, brain lesions and history of seizures) and adjust dose in renal impairment to avoid drug accumulation, which may increase seizure risk. Serious hypersensitivity reactions, including anaphylaxis, have been reported (some without a history of previous allergic reactions to beta-lactams). Doses for IM administration are mixed with lidocaine; consult Lidocaine (Systemic) information for associated Warnings/Precautions. May decrease divalproex sodium/valproic acid concentrations leading to breakthrough seizures; concomitant use not recommended.

Adverse Reactions

>10%: Gastrointestinal: Diarrhea (6% to 12%)

1% to 10%:

Cardiovascular: Edema (3%), chest pain (<2%), phlebitis (<2%), thrombophlebitis (<2%), hypotension (1% to 2%)

Central nervous system: Headache (2% to 7%), altered mental status (eg, agitation, confusion, disorientation, mental acuity decreased, somnolence, stupor) (3% to 5%), insomnia (3%), dizziness (2%), hypothermia (infants, children, and adolescents <2%)

Dermatologic: Diaper rash (infants and children 5%), skin rash (2% to 3%), pruritus (1% to 2%), genital rash (infants, children, and adolescents <2%), skin lesion (infants, children, and adolescents <2%)

Gastrointestinal: Vomiting (2% to 10%), nausea (6% to 9%), abdominal pain (4% to 5%), constipation (2% to 4%), decreased appetite (infants, children, and adolescents <2%)

Genitourinary: Erythrocyturia (1% to 3%), vaginitis (1% to 3%)

Hematologic & oncologic: Thrombocythemia (4% to 7%), decreased neutrophils (3% to 6%), decreased hemoglobin (5%), decreased hematocrit (3%), leukocytosis (2% to 3%), leukopenia (<2%), eosinophilia (1% to 2%)

Hepatic: Increased serum ALT (8% to 9%), increased serum AST (7% to 8%), increased serum alkaline (4% to 7%)

Infection: Herpes simplex infection (infants, children, and adolescents <2%)

Local: Infused vein complication (4% to 7%)

Neuromuscular & skeletal: Arthralgia (infants, children, and adolescents <2%)

Otic: Otic infection (infants, children, and adolescents <2%)

Respiratory: Cough (≤4%), dyspnea (1% to 3%), nasopharyngitis (infants, children, and adolescents <2%), rhinitis (infants, children, and adolescents <2%), rhinorrhea (infants, children, and adolescents <2%), upper respiratory tract infection (infants, children, and adolescents 2%), wheezing (infants, children, and adolescents <2%)

Miscellaneous: Fever (2% to 5%)

≤1% (Limited to important or life-threatening): Anaphylactoid reaction, anaphylaxis, anuria, asthma, asystole, atrial fibrillation, bradycardia, bronchoconstriction, cardiac arrest, cardiac arrhythmia, cardiac failure, cholelithiasis, *Clostridium difficile* associated diarrhea, delirium, DRESS syndrome, extravasation, gastrointestinal hemorrhage, gout, heart murmur, hemoptysis, hyperglycemia, hyperkalemia, hypertension, hypoxemia, impaired consciousness, intestinal obstruction, jaundice, oral candidiasis, oliguria, pancreatitis, pleural effusion, prolonged prothrombin time, renal insufficiency, seizure, septicemia, septic shock, subdural hematoma, tachycardia, thrombocytopenia, tissue necrosis, ventricular tachycardia

Drug Interactions

Metabolism/Transport Effects None known.

Avoid Concomitant Use

Avoid concomitant use of Ertapenem with any of the following: BCG (Intravesical)

Increased Effect/Toxicity

Ertapenem may increase the levels/effects of: Tacrolimus (Systemic)

The levels/effects of Ertapenem may be increased by: Probenecid

Decreased Effect

Ertapenem may decrease the levels/effects of: BCG (Intravesical); BCG Vaccine (Immunization); Sodium Picosulfate; Typhoid Vaccine; Valproate Products

Preparation for Administration

IM: Reconstitute 1 g vial with 3.2 mL of 1% lidocaine HCl injection (without epinephrine). Shake well.

IV: Reconstitute 1 g vial with 10 mL of sterile water for injection, 0.9% sodium chloride injection, or bacteriostatic water for injection. Shake well. For adults, transfer dose to 50 mL of 0.9% sodium chloride injection; for children, dilute dose with NS to a final concentration ≤20 mg/mL.

Storage/Stability Prior to reconstitution, store vials at ≤25°C (77°F). The reconstituted IM solution should be used within 1 hour after preparation. The reconstituted IV solution may be stored at room temperature (25°C [77°F]) and used within 6 hours, or stored for 24 hours under refrigeration (5°C [41°F]) and used within 4 hours after removal from refrigeration. Do not freeze.

Mechanism of Action Inhibits bacterial cell wall synthesis by binding to one or more of the penicillin-binding proteins; which in turn inhibits the final transpeptidation step of peptidoglycan synthesis in bacterial cell walls, thus inhibiting cell wall biosynthesis. Bacteria eventually lyse due to ongoing activity of cell wall autolytic enzymes (autolysins and murein hydrolases) while cell wall assembly is arrested.

Pharmacodynamics/Kinetics

Absorption: IM: Almost complete

Distribution: V_{dss}:

Children 3 months to 12 years: ~0.2 L/kg

Children 13-17 years: ~0.16 L/kg

Adults: ~0.12 L/kg

Protein binding (concentration dependent, primarily to albumin): 85% at 300 mcg/mL, 95% at <100 mcg/mL

Metabolism: Non-CYP-mediated hydrolysis to inactive metabolite

Bioavailability: IM: ~90%

Half-life elimination:

Children 3 months to 12 years: ~2.5 hours

Children ≥13 years and Adults: ~4 hours

Time to peak: IM: ~2.3 hours

Excretion: Urine (~80% as unchanged drug and metabolite); feces (~10%)

Dosing

Adult & Geriatric Note: IV therapy may be administered for up to 14 days; IM for up to 7 days

Community-acquired pneumonia and complicated urinary tract infections (including pyelonephritis): IM, IV: 1 g once daily; duration of total antibiotic treatment: 10-14 days; duration includes possible switch to appropriate oral therapy after at least 3 days of parenteral treatment, once clinical improvement

demonstrated. **Note:** The carbapenems, including ertapenem, are preferred agents for *Enterobacter* spp and *Burkholderia pseudomallei,* and are considered alternative agents for anaerobes in aspiration pneumonia (IDSA, 2007).

Intra-abdominal infection: IM, IV: 1 g once daily for 5-14 days; **Note:** 2010 IDSA guidelines recommend a treatment duration of 4-7 days (provided source controlled) for community-acquired, mild-to-moderate intra-abdominal infections (Solomkin, 2010)

Pelvic infections (acute): IM, IV: 1 g once daily for 3-10 days

Prophylaxis of surgical site following colorectal surgery: IV: 1 g as a single dose given 1 hour preoperatively

Skin and skin structure infections (excluding diabetic foot infections with osteomyelitis): IM, IV: 1 g once daily for 7-14 days. **Notes:** For diabetic foot infections, recommended treatment duration is up to 4 weeks depending on severity of infection and response to therapy (Lipsky, 2012).

Intravenous catheter-related bloodstream infection (off-label use): IV 1 g once daily (**Note:** Carbapenems, including ertapenem, are preferred agents for extended-spectrum β-lactamase [ESBL]-positive *Escherichia coli* and *Klebsiella, Enterobacter,* and *Serratia* [IDSA, 2009].)

Prosthetic joint infection: *Enterobacter* spp (off-label use): IV: 1 g every 24 hours for 4-6 weeks (Osmon, 2013)

Skin and soft tissue necrotizing infections (off-label use): IV: 1 g once daily in combination with an agent effective against MRSA (eg, vancomycin, linezolid, daptomycin) for empiric therapy of polymicrobial (mixed) infections. Continue until further debridement is not necessary, patient has clinically improved, and patient is afebrile for 48 to 72 hours (IDSA [Stevens, 2014]).

Surgical site infection (intestinal or genitourinary tract surgery) (off-label use): IV: 1 g once daily (IDSA [Stevens, 2014]).

Pediatric Note: IV therapy may be administered for up to 14 days; IM therapy for up to 7 days

Infants ≥3 months and Children:

Community-acquired pneumonia and complicated urinary tract infections (including pyelonephritis): IM, IV: 15 **mg**/kg twice daily (maximum: 1 g daily); duration of total antibiotic treatment: 10-14 days (**Note:** Duration includes possible switch to appropriate oral therapy after at least 3 days of parenteral treatment, once clinical improvement demonstrated.)

Intra-abdominal infection: IM, IV: 15 **mg**/kg twice daily (maximum: 1 g daily) for 5-14 days

Pelvic infections (acute): IM, IV: 15 **mg**/kg twice daily (maximum: 1 g daily) for 3-10 days

Skin and skin structure infections: IM, IV: 15 **mg**/kg twice daily (maximum: 1 g daily) for 7-14 days

Skin and soft tissue necrotizing infections (off-label use): IV: 15 mg/kg every 12 hours in combination with an agent effective against MRSA (eg, vancomycin, linezolid, daptomycin) for empiric therapy of polymicrobial (mixed) infections. Continue until further debridement is not necessary, patient has clinically improved, and patient is afebrile for 48 to 72 hours (IDSA [Stevens, 2014]).

Adolescents:

Community-acquired pneumonia, complicated urinary tract infections (including pyelonephritis): Refer to adult dosing.

Intra-abdominal infection: Refer to adult dosing.

Pelvic infections (acute): Refer to adult dosing.

Skin and skin structure infections (excluding diabetic foot infections with osteomyelitis): Refer to adult dosing.

Renal Impairment

Children: No data available for pediatric patients with renal insufficiency.

Adults:

CrCl >30 mL/minute/1.73 m²: No dosage adjustment necessary.

CrCl ≤30 mL/minute/1.73 m² and ESRD: 500 mg/day

Hemodialysis: When the daily dose is given within 6 hours prior to hemodialysis, a supplementary dose of 150 mg is required following hemodialysis. If ertapenem is given at least 6 hours prior to hemodialysis, no supplementary dose is needed.

CAPD: IV: 500 mg daily (Cardone, 2011)

Hepatic Impairment Adjustments cannot be recommended (lack of experience and research in this patient population).

Dietary Considerations Some products may contain sodium.

▶

Administration

IM: Avoid injection into a blood vessel. Make sure patient does not have an allergy to lidocaine or another anesthetic of the amide type. Administer by deep IM injection into a large muscle mass (eg, gluteal muscle or lateral part of the thigh). Do not administer IM preparation or drug reconstituted for IM administration intravenously.

IV: Infuse over 30 minutes

Monitoring Parameters Periodic renal, hepatic, and hematopoietic assessment during prolonged therapy; neurological assessment

Dosage Forms Excipient information presented when available (limited, particularly for generics); consult specific product labeling.

Solution Reconstituted, Injection:
INVanz: 1 g (1 ea)
Solution Reconstituted, Intravenous:
INVanz: 1 g (1 ea)

◆ Ertapenem Sodium *see* Ertapenem *on page 668*
◆ Erwinase (Can) *see* Asparaginase (*Erwinia*) *on page 156*
◆ Erwinaze *see* Asparaginase (*Erwinia*) *on page 156*
◆ Erwinia chrysanthemi *see* Asparaginase (*Erwinia*) *on page 156*
◆ Ery *see* Erythromycin (Topical) *on page 672*
◆ Erybid (Can) *see* Erythromycin (Systemic) *on page 670*
◆ Eryc *see* Erythromycin (Systemic) *on page 670*
◆ Erygel *see* Erythromycin (Topical) *on page 672*
◆ EryPed 200 *see* Erythromycin (Systemic) *on page 670*
◆ EryPed 400 *see* Erythromycin (Systemic) *on page 670*
◆ Erysol (Can) *see* Erythromycin (Topical) *on page 672*
◆ Ery-Tab *see* Erythromycin (Systemic) *on page 670*
◆ Erythrocin Lactobionate *see* Erythromycin (Systemic) *on page 670*
◆ Erythrocin Stearate *see* Erythromycin (Systemic) *on page 670*

Erythromycin (Systemic) (er ith roe MYE sin)

Brand Names: US E.E.S. 400; E.E.S. Granules; Ery-Tab; EryPed 200; EryPed 400; Erythrocin Lactobionate; Erythrocin Stearate; PCE

Brand Names: Canada Apo-Erythro Base; Apo-Erythro E-C; Apo-Erythro-ES; Apo-Erythro-S; EES; Erybid; Eryc; Novo-Rythro Estolate; Novo-Rythro Ethylsuccinate; Nu-Erythromycin-S; PCE

Index Terms Eryc; Erythromycin Base; Erythromycin Ethylsuccinate; Erythromycin Lactobionate; Erythromycin Stearate

Pharmacologic Category Antibiotic, Macrolide

Use

Bacterial infections: Treatment of susceptible bacterial infections, including *S. pyogenes*, some *S. pneumoniae*, some *S. aureus*, *M. pneumoniae*, *Legionella pneumophila*, diphtheria, pertussis, *Chlamydia*, erythrasma, *N. gonorrhoeae*, *E. histolytica*, syphilis and nongonococcal urethritis, and *Campylobacter* gastroenteritis; used in conjunction with neomycin for decontaminating the bowel

Surgical (preoperative) prophylaxis (colorectal): Colorectal decontamination, in conjunction with other agents, prior to surgical intervention

Pregnancy Considerations Adverse events were not observed in animal reproduction studies. Erythromycin crosses the placenta and low concentrations are found in the fetal serum. Cardiovascular anomalies following exposure in early pregnancy have been reported in some observational studies. Serum concentrations of erythromycin may be variable in pregnant women (Kiefer 1955; Philipson 1976).

In patients with acute infections during pregnancy, erythromycin may be given if an antibiotic is required and appropriate based on bacterial sensitivity (ACOG No. 120 2011). Erythromycin is the antibiotic of choice for preterm premature rupture of membranes (with membrane rupture between 24 0/7 to 33 6/7 weeks gestation) (ACOG 2013), the treatment of granuloma inguinale, and lymphogranuloma venereum in pregnancy (CDC [RR-12] 2010), and the treatment of or long-term suppression of *Bartonella* infection in HIV-infected pregnant patients [DHHS 2013]. Erythromycin may be appropriate as an alternative agent for the treatment of chlamydial infections in pregnant women (consult current guidelines) (CDC [RR-12] 2010).

Breast-Feeding Considerations Erythromycin is excreted in breast milk; therefore, the manufacturer recommends that caution be exercised when administering erythromycin to breast-feeding women. Decreased appetite, diarrhea, rash, and somnolence have been reported in nursing infants exposed to macrolide antibiotics (Goldstein 2009).

One case report and a cohort study raise the possibility for a connection with pyloric stenosis in neonates exposed to erythromycin via breast milk and an alternative antibiotic may be preferred for breast-feeding mothers of infants in this age group (Sorensen 2003; Stang 1986).

Contraindications Hypersensitivity to erythromycin, any macrolide antibiotics, or any component of the formulation Concomitant use with pimozide, cisapride, ergotamine or dihydroergotamine, terfenadine, astemizole, lovastatin, or simvastatin

Warnings/Precautions Use caution with hepatic impairment with or without jaundice has occurred, it may be accompanied by malaise, nausea, vomiting, abdominal colic, and fever; discontinue use if these occur. Potentially significant drug-drug interactions may exist, requiring dose or frequency adjustment, additional monitoring, and/or selection of alternative therapy. Use caution with other medication relying on CYP3A4 metabolism; high potential for drug interactions exists. Prolonged use may result in fungal or bacterial superinfection, including *C. difficile*-associated diarrhea (CDAD) and pseudomembranous colitis; CDAD has been observed >2 months postantibiotic treatment. Use in infants has been associated with infantile hypertrophic pyloric stenosis (IHPS). Macrolides have been associated with rare QTc prolongation and ventricular arrhythmias, including torsade de pointes; avoid use in patients with prolonged QT interval, uncorrected hypokalemia or hypomagnesemia, clinically significant bradycardia, or concurrent use of Class IA (eg, quinidine, procainamide) or Class III (eg, amiodarone, dofetilide, sotalol) antiarrhythmic agents. Avoid concurrent use with strong CYP3A inhibitors; may increase the risk of sudden cardiac death (Ray 2004). Use caution in elderly patients, as risk of adverse events may be increased. Use caution in myasthenia gravis patients; erythromycin may aggravate muscular weakness.

Benzyl alcohol and derivatives: Some dosage forms may contain benzyl alcohol; large amounts of benzyl alcohol (≥99 mg/kg/day) have been associated with a potentially fatal toxicity ("gasping syndrome") in neonates; the "gasping syndrome" consists of metabolic acidosis, respiratory distress, gasping respirations, CNS dysfunction (including convulsions, intracranial hemorrhage), hypotension and cardiovascular collapse (AAP ["Inactive" 1997]; CDC 1982); some data suggests that benzoate displaces bilirubin from protein binding sites (Ahlfors 2001); avoid or use dosage forms containing benzyl alcohol with caution in neonates. See manufacturer's labeling.

Adverse Reactions Frequency not defined. Incidence may vary with formulation.

Cardiovascular: Local thrombophlebitis, prolonged Q-T interval on ECG, torsades de pointes, ventricular arrhythmia, ventricular tachycardia

Central nervous system: Seizure

Dermatologic: Erythema multiforme, pruritus, skin rash, Stevens-Johnson syndrome, toxic epidermal necrolysis, urticaria

Gastrointestinal: Abdominal pain, anorexia, diarrhea, nausea, oral candidiasis, pancreatitis, pseudomembranous colitis, pyloric stenosis (infantile hypertrophic), vomiting

Hepatic: Abnormal hepatic function tests, cholestatic jaundice (most common with estolate), hepatitis

Hypersensitivity: Anaphylaxis, hypersensitivity reaction

Local: Injection site phlebitis

Neuromuscular & skeletal: Weakness

Otic: Hearing loss

Renal: Interstitial nephritis

Postmarketing and/or case reports (Limited to important or life-threatening): Hepatotoxicity (idiosyncratic) (Chalasani, 2014)

Drug Interactions

Metabolism/Transport Effects Substrate of CYP2B6 (minor), CYP3A4 (major), P-glycoprotein; **Note:** Assignment of Major/Minor substrate status based on clinically relevant drug interaction potential; **Inhibits** CYP3A4 (moderate), P-glycoprotein

Avoid Concomitant Use

Avoid concomitant use of Erythromycin (Systemic) with any of the following: Aprepitant; Barnidipine; BCG (Intravesical); Bosutinib; Cisapride; Clindamycin (Topical); Cobimetinib; Conivaptan; Disopyramide; Domperidone; Flibanserin; Fluconazole; Fusidic Acid (Systemic); Highest Risk QTc-Prolonging Agents; Ibrutinib; Idelalisib; Ivabradine; Lincosamide Antibiotics; Lomitapide; Lovastatin; Mequitazine; Mifepristone; Naloxegol; Olaparib; PAZOPanib; Pimozide; QuiNIDine; QuiNINE; Silodosin; Simeprevir; Simvastatin; Terfenadine; Tolvaptan; Topotecan; Trabectedin; Ulipristal; VinCRIStine (Liposomal)

Increased Effect/Toxicity

Erythromycin (Systemic) may increase the levels/effects of: Afatinib; Alfentanil; ALPRAZolam; Antineoplastic Agents (Vinca Alkaloids); Apixaban; Aprepitant; ARIPiprazole; AtorvaSTATin; Avanafil; Barnidipine; Bosentan; Bosutinib; Brentuximab Vedotin; Brexpiprazole; Bromocriptine; Budesonide (Systemic); Budesonide (Topical); BusPIRone; Calcium Channel Blockers; Cannabis; CarBAMazepine; Cardiac Glycosides; Cilostazol; Cisapride; CloZAPine; Cobimetinib; Colchicine; CycloSPORINE (Systemic); CYP3A4 Substrates; Dabigatran Etexilate; Dapoxetine; Disopyramide; Domperidone; Doxofylline; DOXOrubicin (Conventional); Dronabinol; Edoxaban; Eletriptan; Eplerenone; Ergot Derivatives; Estazolam; Everolimus; FentaNYL; Fexofenadine; Flibanserin; Highest Risk QTc-Prolonging Agents; Hydrocodone; Ibrutinib; Imatinib; Ivabradine; Ivacaftor; Ledipasvir; Lomitapide; Lovastatin; Lurasidone; Mequitazine; Midazolam; Moderate Risk QTc-Prolonging Agents; Naloxegol; Nintedanib; Olaparib; OxyCODONE; PAZOPanib; P-glycoprotein/ABCB1 Substrates; Pimecrolimus; Pimozide; Pitavastatin; Pravastatin; QuiNIDine; QuiNINE; Ranolazine; Repaglinide; Rifamycin Derivatives; Rifaximin; Rilpivirine; Rivaroxaban; Salmeterol; Saxagliptin; Sertraline; Sildenafil; Silodosin; Simeprevir; Simvastatin; Sirolimus; Sonidegib; Suvorexant; Tacrolimus (Systemic); Tacrolimus (Topical); Telaprevir; Temsirolimus; Terfenadine; Tetrahydrocannabinol; Theophylline Derivatives; Tolvaptan; Topotecan; Trabectedin; Triazolam; Ulipristal; Vardenafil; Vilazodone; VinCRIStine (Liposomal); Vitamin K Antagonists; Zopiclone

The levels/effects of Erythromycin (Systemic) may be increased by: Conivaptan; CYP3A4 Inhibitors (Moderate); CYP3A4 Inhibitors (Strong); Dasatinib; Fluconazole; Fosaprepitant; Fusidic Acid (Systemic); Idelalisib; Ivabradine; Luliconazole; Mifepristone; Netupitant; Palbociclib; P-glycoprotein/ABCB1 Inhibitors; QTc-Prolonging Agents (Indeterminate Risk and Risk Modifying); Stiripentol; Telaprevir

Decreased Effect

Erythromycin (Systemic) may decrease the levels/effects of: BCG (Intravesical); BCG Vaccine (Immunization); Clindamycin (Topical); Clopidogrel; Ifosfamide; Sodium Picosulfate; Typhoid Vaccine; Zafirlukast

The levels/effects of Erythromycin (Systemic) may be decreased by: Bosentan; CYP3A4 Inducers (Moderate); CYP3A4 Inducers (Strong); Dabrafenib; Deferasirox; Enzalutamide; Etravirine; Lincosamide Antibiotics; Mitotane; P-glycoprotein/ABCB1 Inducers; Siltuximab; St Johns Wort; Tocilizumab

Food Interactions

Ethanol: Ethanol may decrease absorption of erythromycin or enhance effects of ethanol. Management: Avoid ethanol.

Food: Erythromycin serum levels may be altered if taken with food (formulation-dependent). GI upset, including diarrhea, is common. Management: May be taken with food to decrease GI upset, otherwise take around-the-clock with a full glass of water. Do not give with milk or acidic beverages (eg, soda, juice).

Preparation for Administration

Erythromycin lactobionate should be reconstituted with sterile water for injection without preservatives to a concentration of 50 mg/mL. No less than 100 mL of IV diluent should be used for an infusion bag. The final diluted solution should be 1 to 5 mg/mL.

Storage/Stability

Injection: Store unreconstituted vials at 20°C to 25°C (68°F to 77°F). Reconstituted solution (50 mg/mL) is stable for 2 weeks when refrigerated or for 24 hours at room temperature. Erythromycin IV infusion solution is stable at pH 6 to 8; stability of lactobionate is pH dependent; IV form has longest stability in NS. Parenteral admixture in NS is stable for 24 hours at 4°C. Admixtures in NS (including Add-Vantage containers) should be infused within 8 hours of preparation.

Oral suspension:
Granules: Prior to mixing, store at <30°C (86°F). After mixing, store under refrigeration and use within 10 days.
Powder: Prior to mixing, store at <30°C (86°F). After mixing, store at ≤25°C (77°F) and use within 35 days.
Tablet and capsule formulations: Store at <30°C (86°F).

Mechanism of Action

Inhibits RNA-dependent protein synthesis at the chain elongation step; binds to the 50S ribosomal subunit resulting in blockage of transpeptidation

Pharmacodynamics/Kinetics

Absorption: Oral: Variable but better with salt forms than with base form; 18% to 45%; ethylsuccinate may be better absorbed with food

Distribution:
V_d: 0.64 L/kg

Relative diffusion from blood into CSF: Minimal even with inflammation

CSF:blood level ratio: Normal meninges: 2% to 13%; Inflamed meninges: 7% to 25%

Protein binding: Base: 73% to 81%

Metabolism: Demethylation primarily via hepatic CYP3A4

Half-life elimination: Neonates (≤15 days of age): 2.1 hours; Adults: Peak: 1.5-2 hours; End-stage renal disease: 5-6 hours

Time to peak, serum: Base: 4 hours; Ethylsuccinate: 0.5-2.5 hours; Stearate: 3 hours; delayed with food due to differences in absorption

Excretion: Primarily feces; urine (2% to 15% as unchanged drug)

Dosing

Adult & Geriatric Note: Due to differences in absorption, 400 mg erythromycin ethylsuccinate produces the same serum levels as 250 mg erythromycin base or stearate.

Usual dosage range:

Oral:
Base: 250 to 500 mg every 6 to 12 hours; maximum: 4 g daily
Ethylsuccinate: 400 to 800 mg every 6 to 12 hours; maximum: 4 g daily

IV: Lactobionate: 15 to 20 mg/kg/day divided every 6 hours or 500 mg to 1 g every 6 hours; maximum: 4 g daily

Indication-specific dosing:

Bartonella spp infections (bacillary angiomatosis [BA], peliosis hepatis [PH]) (off-label use): Oral: 500 mg (base) 4 times daily for 3 months (BA) or 4 months (PH) (Koehler 1992; Rolain 2004; Stevens 2014; Tappero 1993). **Note:** IDSA skin and soft tissue infection guidelines recommend a duration of initial therapy of 2 weeks to 2 months for cutaneous BA, although treatment durations are not standardized (IDSA [Stevens 2014])

Bartonella spp infections in HIV-infected patients (off-label use; HHS [OI adult 2015]): **Note:** Duration of therapy is at least 3 months; continuation of therapy depends on relapse occurrence and clinical condition
Bacillary angiomatosis, peliosis hepatis, bacteremia, and osteomyelitis: Oral, IV: 500 mg every 6 hours
Other severe infections (excluding CNS infections or endocarditis): Oral, IV: 500 mg every 6 hours with rifampin

Chancroid (off-label use): Oral: 500 mg (base) 3 times daily for 7 days; **Note:** Not a preferred agent; isolates with intermediate resistance have been documented (CDC 2010)

Gastroparesis (off-label use):
IV: 3 mg/kg administered over 45 minutes every 8 hours (Camilleri 2013)
Oral: Patients refractory/intolerant to other prokinetic agents (eg, metoclopramide, domperidone): 250 to 500 mg (base) 3 times daily before meals. Limit duration of therapy, tachyphylaxis may occur after 4 weeks (Camilleri 2013).

Granuloma inguinale (donovanosis) (off-label use): Oral: 500 mg (base) 4 times daily for 21 days (CDC 2010)

Impetigo (IDSA [Stevens 2014]): Oral:
Base: 250 mg 4 times daily for 7 days, depending on response
Ethylsuccinate: 400 mg 4 times daily for 7 days, depending on response

Legionnaire disease: Oral: 1.6 to 4 g (ethylsuccinate) daily or 1 to 4 g (base) daily in divided doses for 21 days. **Note:** No longer preferred therapy and only used in nonhospitalized patients.

Lymphogranuloma venereum: Oral: 500 mg (base) 4 times daily for 21 days; **Note:** Preferred therapy for pregnant or lactating women (CDC 2010)

Nongonococcal urethritis (including coinfection with *C. trachomatis*): Oral: 500 mg (base) 4 times daily for 7 days or 800 mg (ethylsuccinate) 4 times daily for 7 days. **Note:** May use 250 mg (base) or 400 mg (ethylsuccinate) 4 times daily for 14 days if gastrointestinal intolerance.

Pertussis: Oral: 500 mg (base) every 6 hours for 14 days

Surgical (preoperative) prophylaxis (colorectal) (off-label dose): Oral: 1 g erythromycin base per dose at 1 PM, 2 PM, and 11 PM on the day before 8 AM surgery combined with mechanical cleansing of the large intestine, oral neomycin. Perioperative IV antibiotics are also given on the day of surgery (Bratzler 2013).

Pediatric Note: Due to differences in absorption, 400 mg erythromycin ethylsuccinate produces the same serum levels as 250 mg erythromycin base or stearate.

Usual dosage range: Infants and Children:

Oral:

Base: 30 to 50 mg/kg/day in 2 to 4 divided doses; maximum: 2 g daily

Ethylsuccinate: 30 to 50 mg/kg/day in 2 to 4 divided doses; maximum: 3.2 g daily

Stearate: 30 to 50 mg/kg/day in 2 to 4 divided doses; maximum: 2 g daily

IV: Lactobionate: 15 to 20 mg/kg/day divided every 6 hours; maximum: 4 g daily

Indication-specific dosing:

Infants and Children:

Bartonella spp infections (bacillary angiomatosis [BA], peliosis hepatis [PH]) (off-label use): Oral: 40 mg/kg/day (ethylsuccinate) in 4 divided doses (maximum: 2 g daily) for 3 months (BA) or 4 months (PH) (Rolain 2004). **Note:** IDSA skin and soft tissue infection guidelines recommend a duration of initial therapy of 2 weeks to 2 months for cutaneous BA, although treatment durations are not standardized (IDSA [Stevens 2014])

Chlamydial infection *(C. trachomatis):* Children <45 kg: Oral: 50 mg/kg/day (base or ethylsuccinate) in 4 divided doses for 14 days (CDC 2010)

Community-acquired pneumonia (CAP) (IDSA/PIDS 2011): Infants >3 months and Children: **Note:** A beta-lactam antibiotic should be added if typical bacterial pneumonia cannot be ruled out.

Presumed atypical *(M. pneumoniae, Chlamydophila* [also known as *Chlamydia*] *pneumoniae, C. trachomatis)* infection, mild atypical infection or step-down therapy (alternative to azithromycin): Oral: 10 mg/kg/dose every 6 hours

Moderate to severe atypical infection (alternative to azithromycin): IV: 5 mg/kg/dose every 6 hours

Impetigo: Oral: 40 mg/kg/day in 3 to 4 divided doses for 7 days, depending on response (IDSA [Stevens 2014])

Mild/moderate infection: Oral: 30 to 50 mg/kg/day in divided doses every 6 to 12 hours

Pertussis: Oral: 40 to 50 mg/kg/day in 4 divided doses for 14 days; maximum: 2 g daily (not preferred agent for infants <1 month due to IHPS)

Pharyngitis, tonsillitis (streptococcal): Oral: 20 mg (base)/kg/day or 40 mg (ethylsuccinate)/kg/day in 2 divided doses for 10 days. **Note:** No longer preferred therapy due to increased organism resistance.

Surgical (preoperative) prophylaxis (colorectal) (off-label use): Children ≥1 year: Oral: 20 mg (base)/kg (maximum dose: 1000 mg) at 1 PM, 2 PM, and 11 PM on the day before 8 AM surgery combined with mechanical cleansing of the large intestine, oral neomycin. Perioperative IV antibiotics are also given on the day of surgery (Bratzler 2013).

Severe infection: IV: 15 to 20 mg/kg/day divided every 6 hours; maximum: 4 g daily

Adolescents:

Bartonella spp infections in HIV-infected patients (off-label use): Refer to adult dosing.

Renal Impairment Slightly dialyzable (5% to 20%); supplemental dose is not necessary in hemo- or peritoneal dialysis or in continuous arteriovenous or venovenous hemofiltration.

Hepatic Impairment There are no dosage adjustments provided in the manufacturer's labeling; use with caution.

Dietary Considerations Drug may cause GI upset; may take with food. Some products may contain sodium.

Administration

Oral: Do not crush enteric coated drug product. GI upset, including diarrhea, is common. May be administered with food to decrease GI upset. Do not give with milk or acidic beverages.

IV: Infuse 1 g over 20 to 60 minutes. IV infusion may be very irritating to the vein; infusion should be sufficiently slow to minimize pain along the vein. Do not administer IV push or bolus.

Test Interactions False-positive urinary catecholamines (fluorometric assay), 17-hydroxycorticosteroids and 17-ketosteroids

Dosage Forms Excipient information presented when available (limited, particularly for generics); consult specific product labeling.

Capsule Delayed Release Particles, Oral, as base:

Generic: 250 mg

Solution Reconstituted, Intravenous, as lactobionate:

Erythrocin Lactobionate: 500 mg (1 ea); 1000 mg (1 ea)

Suspension Reconstituted, Oral, as ethylsuccinate:

E.E.S. Granules: 200 mg/5 mL (100 mL, 200 mL) [cherry flavor]

EryPed 200: 200 mg/5 mL (100 mL) [fruit flavor]

EryPed 400: 400 mg/5 mL (100 mL) [banana flavor]

Tablet, Oral, as base:

Generic: 250 mg, 500 mg

Tablet, Oral, as ethylsuccinate:

E.E.S. 400: 400 mg [contains fd&c red #40, fd&c yellow #10 (quinoline yellow)]

Generic: 400 mg

Tablet, Oral, as stearate:

Erythrocin Stearate: 250 mg

Tablet Delayed Release, Oral, as base:

Ery-Tab: 250 mg, 333 mg, 500 mg

PCE: 333 mg

PCE: 500 mg [dye free, no artificial color(s)]

Erythromycin (Ophthalmic) (er ith roe MYE sin)

Brand Names: US Ilotycin; Romycin [DSC]

Brand Names: Canada Diomycin®; PMS-Erythromycin

Index Terms Erythromycin Base

Pharmacologic Category Antibiotic, Macrolide; Antibiotic, Ophthalmic

Use Treatment of superficial eye infections involving the conjunctiva or cornea

Dosing

Adult & Geriatric Conjunctivitis: Ophthalmic: Instill ½" (1.25 cm) 2-6 times/day depending on the severity of the infection

Pediatric Conjunctivitis: Children: Ophthalmic: Refer to adult dosing.

Additional Information Complete prescribing information should be consulted for additional detail.

Dosage Forms Excipient information presented when available (limited, particularly for generics); consult specific product labeling. [DSC] = Discontinued product

Ointment, Ophthalmic:

Ilotycin: 5 mg/g (1 g)

Romycin: 5 mg/g (3.5 g [DSC])

Generic: 5 mg/g (1 g, 3.5 g)

Dosage Forms: Canada Excipient information presented when available (limited, particularly for generics); consult specific product labeling.

Ointment, ophthalmic: 0.5% (1 g, 3.5 g)

Erythromycin (Topical) (er ith roe MYE sin)

Brand Names: US Akne-Mycin [DSC]; Ery; Erygel

Brand Names: Canada Erysol

Pharmacologic Category Acne Products; Antibiotic, Macrolide; Antibiotic, Topical; Topical Skin Product; Topical Skin Product, Acne

Use Acne: Treatment of acne vulgaris

Dosing

Adult & Geriatric Acne: Topical:

Gel: Apply sparingly as a thin film over the affected area once or twice daily. Therapeutic response may take up to 6-8 weeks; discontinue use if no improvement after 6-8 weeks or if condition worsens.

Ointment, solution: Apply to affected area twice daily (morning and evening); drying and peeling may be controlled by reducing the frequency of application.

Pads: Rub pad over affected areas twice daily (morning and evening); additional pads may be used, if needed.

Erysol [Canadian product]: Apply thin film to affected area twice daily (morning and evening after the skin has been thoroughly washed and patted dry); may decrease to once daily if irritation develops at application site. Therapeutic response may take up to 6-8 weeks; discontinue use if no improvement after 6-8 weeks or if condition worsens. Maximum therapy duration: 3 months.

Pediatric Acne: Children ≥12 years and Adolescents: Topical: Erysol gel [Canadian product]: Apply thin film to affected area twice daily (morning and evening); may decrease to once daily if irritation develops at application site. Therapeutic response may take up to 6-8 weeks; discontinue use if no improvement after 6-8 weeks or if condition worsens. Maximum therapy duration: 3 months.

Renal Impairment There are no dosage adjustments provided in manufacturer's labeling.

Hepatic Impairment There are no dosage adjustments provided in manufacturer's labeling.

Additional Information Complete prescribing information should be consulted for additional detail.

Dosage Forms Excipient information presented when available (limited, particularly for generics); consult specific product labeling. [DSC] = Discontinued product

Gel, External:

Erygel: 2% (30 g, 60 g)

Generic: 2% (30 g, 60 g)

Ointment, External:

Akne-Mycin: 2% (25 g [DSC]) [contains cetostearyl alcohol]

Pad, External:
  Ery: 2% (60 ea) [contains propylene glycol]
  Generic: 2% (60 ea)
Solution, External:
  Generic: 2% (60 mL)
Dosage Forms: Canada Excipient information presented when available (limited, particularly for generics); consult specific product labeling.
Gel, topical:
  Erysol: 2% (25 g) [contains ethanol, octinoxate and avobenzone]

Erythromycin and Benzoyl Peroxide
(er ith roe MYE sin & BEN zoe il per OKS ide)

Brand Names: US Benzamycin; Benzamycin Pak
Brand Names: Canada Benzamycin
Index Terms Benzoyl Peroxide and Erythromycin
Pharmacologic Category Acne Products; Topical Skin Product, Acne
Use Topical control of acne vulgaris
Dosing
  Adult & Geriatric Acne: Topical: Apply twice daily, morning and evening.
  Pediatric Adolescents ≥12 years: Refer to adult dosing.
Additional Information Complete prescribing information should be consulted for additional detail.
Dosage Forms Excipient information presented when available (limited, particularly for generics); consult specific product labeling.
  Gel, topical: Erythromycin 30 mg and benzoyl peroxide 50 mg per g (23 g, 47 g)
  Benzamycin: Erythromycin 30 mg and benzoyl peroxide 50 mg per g (47 g) [contains alcohol 20%]
  Benzamycin Pak: Erythromycin 30 mg and benzoyl peroxide 50 mg per 0.8 g packet (60s) [supplied with diluent containing alcohol]

- ◆ Erythromycin Base *see* Erythromycin (Ophthalmic) *on page 672*
- ◆ Erythromycin Base *see* Erythromycin (Systemic) *on page 670*
- ◆ Erythromycin Ethylsuccinate *see* Erythromycin (Systemic) *on page 670*
- ◆ Erythromycin Lactobionate *see* Erythromycin (Systemic) *on page 670*
- ◆ Erythromycin Stearate *see* Erythromycin (Systemic) *on page 670*
- ◆ Erythropoiesis-Stimulating Agent (ESA) *see* Darbepoetin Alfa *on page 493*
- ◆ Erythropoiesis-Stimulating Agent (ESA) *see* Epoetin Alfa *on page 654*
- ◆ Erythropoiesis-Stimulating Agent (ESA) *see* Methoxy Polyethylene Glycol-Epoetin Beta *on page 1176*
- ◆ Erythropoiesis-Stimulating Protein *see* Darbepoetin Alfa *on page 493*
- ◆ Erythropoietin *see* Epoetin Alfa *on page 654*

Escitalopram (es sye TAL oh pram)

Brand Names: US Lexapro
Brand Names: Canada ACT Escitalopram; Apo-Escitalopram; Cipralex; Cipralex MELTZ; JAMP-Escitalopram; Mar-Escitalopram; Mylan-Escitalopram; PMS-Escitalopram; Priva-Escitalopram; RAN-Escitalopram; Riva-Escitalopram; Sandoz Escitalopram; Teva-Escitalopram
Index Terms Escitalopram Oxalate; Lu-26-054; S-Citalopram
Pharmacologic Category Antidepressant, Selective Serotonin Reuptake Inhibitor
Use Treatment of major depressive disorder; generalized anxiety disorders (GAD)
  Canadian labeling: Additional use (not in US labeling): Treatment of obsessive-compulsive disorder (OCD)
Pregnancy Considerations Adverse events have been observed in animal reproduction studies. Escitalopram crosses the placenta and is distributed into the amniotic fluid. An increased risk of teratogenic effects, including cardiovascular defects, may be associated with maternal use of escitalopram or other SSRIs; however, available information is conflicting. Nonteratogenic effects in the newborn following SSRI/SNRI exposure late in the third trimester include respiratory distress, cyanosis, apnea, seizures, temperature instability, feeding difficulty, vomiting, hypoglycemia, hypo- or hypertonia, hyper-reflexia, jitteriness, irritability, constant crying, and tremor. Symptoms may be due to the toxicity of the SSRIs/SNRIs or a discontinuation syndrome and may be consistent with serotonin syndrome associated with SSRI treatment.

Persistent pulmonary hypertension of the newborn (PPHN) has also been reported with SSRI exposure. The long-term effects of *in utero* SSRI exposure on infant development and behavior are not known. Escitalopram is the S-enantiomer of the racemic derivative citalopram; also refer to the Citalopram monograph.

Due to pregnancy-induced physiologic changes, some pharmacokinetic parameters of escitalopram may be altered. The ACOG recommends that therapy with SSRIs or SNRIs during pregnancy be individualized; treatment of depression during pregnancy should incorporate the clinical expertise of the mental health clinician, obstetrician, primary healthcare provider, and pediatrician. According to the American Psychiatric Association (APA), the risks of medication treatment should be weighed against other treatment options and untreated depression. For women who discontinue antidepressant medications during pregnancy and who may be at high risk for postpartum depression, the medications can be restarted following delivery. Treatment algorithms have been developed by the ACOG and the APA for the management of depression in women prior to conception and during pregnancy.

Breast-Feeding Considerations Escitalopram and its metabolite are excreted into breast milk. Limited data is available concerning the effects escitalopram may have in the nursing infant and the long-term effects on development and behavior have not been studied. Adverse effects have been reported in nursing infants exposed to some SSRIs. According to the manufacturer, the decision to continue or discontinue breast-feeding during therapy should take into account the risk of exposure to the infant and the benefits of treatment to the mother. Maternal use of an SSRI during pregnancy may cause delayed milk secretion. Escitalopram is the S-enantiomer of the racemic derivative citalopram; also refer to the Citalopram monograph.

Medication Guide Available Yes
Contraindications
  Hypersensitivity to escitalopram, citalopram, or any component of the formulation; use of MAO inhibitors intended to treat psychiatric disorders (concurrently or within 14 days of discontinuing either escitalopram or the MAO inhibitor); initiation of escitalopram in a patient receiving linezolid or intravenous methylene blue; concurrent use of pimozide
  Canadian labeling: Additional contraindications (not in US labeling): Known QT-interval prolongation or congenital long QT syndrome
Warnings/Precautions [US Boxed Warning]: Antidepressants increase the risk of suicidal thinking and behavior in children, adolescents, and young adults (18 to 24 years of age) with major depressive disorder (MDD) and other psychiatric disorders; consider risk prior to prescribing. Short-term studies did not show an increased risk in patients >24 years of age and showed a decreased risk in patients ≥65 years. Closely monitor patients for clinical worsening, suicidality, or unusual changes in behavior, particularly during the initial 1-2 months of therapy or during periods of dosage adjustments (increases or decreases); the patient's family or caregiver should be instructed to closely observe the patient and communicate condition with healthcare provider. A medication guide concerning the use of antidepressants should be dispensed with each prescription. **Escitalopram is not FDA approved for use in children <12 years of age.**

The possibility of a suicide attempt is inherent in major depression and may persist until remission occurs. Use caution in high-risk patients. Worsening depression and severe abrupt suicidality that are not part of the presenting symptoms may require discontinuation or modification of drug therapy. The patient's family or caregiver should be alerted to monitor patients for the emergence of suicidality and associated behaviors (such as agitation, irritability, hostility, impulsivity, and hypomania) and call healthcare provider.

May precipitate a shift to mania or hypomania in patients with bipolar disorder. Patients presenting with depressive symptoms should be screened for bipolar disorder. Monotherapy in patients with bipolar disorder should be avoided. Escitalopram is not FDA approved for the treatment of bipolar depression.

Potentially life-threatening serotonin syndrome (SS) has occurred with serotonergic agents (eg, SSRIs, SNRIs), particularly when used in combination with other serotonergic agents (eg, triptans, TCAs, fentanyl, lithium, tramadol, buspirone, St John's wort, tryptophan) or agents that impair metabolism of serotonin (eg, MAO inhibitors intended to treat psychiatric disorders, other MAO inhibitors [ie, linezolid and intravenous methylene blue]). Discontinue treatment (and any concomitant serotonergic ▶

agent) immediately if signs/symptoms arise. May increase the risks associated with electroconvulsive therapy. Has a low potential to impair cognitive or motor performance; caution operating hazardous machinery or driving. Bone fractures have been associated with antidepressant treatment. Consider the possibility of a fragility fracture if an antidepressant-treated patient presents with unexplained bone pain, point tenderness, swelling, or bruising (Rabenda 2013; Rizzoli 2012).

Use with caution in patients with a recent history of MI or unstable heart disease. Use has been associated with dose-dependent QT-interval prolongation with doses of 10 mg and 30 mg/day in healthy subjects (mean change from baseline: 4.3 msec and 10.7 msec, respectively); prolongation of QT interval and ventricular arrhythmia (including torsade de pointes) have been reported, particularly in females with preexisting QT prolongation or other risk factors (eg, hypokalemia, other cardiac disease).

Use caution with a previous seizure disorder or condition predisposing to seizures such as brain damage, alcoholism, or concurrent therapy with other drugs which lower the seizure threshold. May cause hyponatremia/SIADH (elderly at increased risk; volume depletion (diuretics may increase risk) may occur. Use caution in patients with metabolic disease. May cause or exacerbate sexual dysfunction. Use caution in elderly patients; may be potentially inappropriate in patients with a history of falls or fractures, and may cause or exacerbate syndrome of inappropriate antidiuretic hormone secretion or hyponatremia; monitor sodium closely with initiation or dosage adjustments in older adults (Beers Criteria). Bioavailability and half-life are increased by 50% in the elderly. Use caution with severe renal impairment or liver impairment; concomitant CNS depressants. May cause mild pupillary dilation which in susceptible individuals can lead to an episode of narrow-angle glaucoma. Consider evaluating patients who have not had an iridectomy for narrow-angle glaucoma risk factors. Use with caution in patients who are hemodynamically unstable. Potentially significant drug-drug interactions may exist, requiring dose or frequency adjustment, additional monitoring, and/or selection of alternative therapy. Escitalopram systemic exposure may be increased in CYP2C19 poor metabolizers; Canadian labeling recommends a dosage adjustment in this patient population.

Abrupt discontinuation or interruption of antidepressant therapy has been associated with a discontinuation syndrome. Symptoms arising may vary with antidepressant however commonly include nausea, vomiting, diarrhea, headaches, light-headedness, dizziness, diminished appetite, sweating, chills, tremors, paresthesias, fatigue, somnolence, and sleep disturbances (eg, vivid dreams, insomnia). Greater risks for developing a discontinuation syndrome have been associated with antidepressants with shorter half-lives, longer durations of treatment, and abrupt discontinuation. For antidepressants of short or intermediate half-lives, symptoms may emerge within 2-5 days after treatment discontinuation and last 7-14 days (APA 2010; Fava 2006; Haddad 2001; Shelton 2001; Warner 2006). Some dosage forms may contain propylene glycol; large amounts are potentially toxic and have been associated hyperosmolality, lactic acidosis, seizures, and respiratory depression; use caution (AAP, 1997; Zar 2007).

Adverse Reactions

>10%:

Central nervous system: Headache (24%), insomnia (7% to 14%), drowsiness (4% to 13%)

Gastrointestinal: Nausea (15% to 18%), diarrhea (6% to 14%)

Genitourinary: Ejaculatory disorder (9% to 14%)

1% to 10%:

Central nervous system: Fatigue (2% to 8%), dizziness (4% to 7%), anorgasmia (2% to 6%), abnormal dreams (3%), lethargy (3%), paresthesia (2%), yawning (2%)

Dermatologic: Diaphoresis (3% to 8%)

Endocrine & metabolic: Decreased libido (3% to 7%), menstrual disease (2%)

Gastrointestinal: Xerostomia (4% to 9%), constipation (3% to 6%), dyspepsia (2% to 6%), decreased appetite (3%), vomiting (3%), abdominal pain (2%), flatulence (2%), toothache (2%)

Genitourinary: Impotence (2% to 3%), urinary tract infection (children ≥2%)

Neuromuscular & skeletal: Neck pain (≤3%), shoulder pain (≤3%), back pain (children ≥2%)

Respiratory: Flu-like symptoms (5%), rhinitis (5%), sinusitis (3%), nasal congestion (children ≥2%)

<1% (Limited to important or life-threatening): Abdominal cramps, abnormal gait, acute renal failure, aggressive behavior, agitated depression, agitation, agranulocytosis, akathisia, alopecia, amnesia, anaphylaxis, anemia, angioedema, angle-closure glaucoma, anxiety, apathy, aplastic anemia, arthralgia, ataxia, atrial fibrillation, blurred vision, bradycardia, bronchitis, cardiac failure, cerebrovascular accident, chest pain, choreoathetosis, deep vein thrombosis, delirium, delusions, depersonalization, dermatitis, diabetes mellitus, diplopia, dyskinesia, dysmenorrhea, dysphagia, dyspnea, dystonia, dysuria, ecchymoses, edema, epistaxis, erythema multiforme, extrapyramidal reaction, fever, flushing, gastroenteritis, gastroesophageal reflux disease, gastrointestinal hemorrhage, hallucination, heartburn, hemolytic anemia, hepatic failure, hepatic necrosis, hepatitis, hot flash, hypercholesterolemia, hyperglycemia, hypermenorrhea, hyperprolactinemia, hypersensitivity reaction, hypertension, hypertensive crisis, hypoesthesia, hypoglycemia, hypokalemia, hyponatremia, hypoprothrombinemia, hypotension, immune thrombocytopenia, increased appetite, increased INR, increased liver enzymes, increased serum bilirubin, irritability, jaw tightness, lack of concentration, leukopenia, limb pain, migraine, myalgia, myasthenia, mydriasis, myocardial infarction, myoclonus, neuroleptic malignant syndrome (Stevens, 2008), nightmares, nystagmus, orthostatic hypotension, palpitations, pancreatitis, panic, paranoia, Parkinsonian-like syndrome, phlebitis, priapism, prolonged Q-T interval on ECG, psychosis, pulmonary embolism, rectal hemorrhage, rhabdomyolysis, seizure, serotonin syndrome, SIADH, sinus congestion, sinus headache, skin photosensitivity, skin rash, spontaneous abortion, Stevens-Johnson syndrome, suicidal ideation, suicidal tendencies, syncope, tachycardia, tardive dyskinesia, thrombocytopenia, thrombosis, tinnitus, torsades de pointes, toxic epidermal necrolysis, tremor, urinary frequency, urinary retention, urticaria, ventricular arrhythmia, ventricular tachycardia, vertigo, visual disturbance, withdrawal syndrome

Drug Interactions

Metabolism/Transport Effects Substrate of CYP2C19 (major), CYP3A4 (major); **Note:** Assignment of Major/Minor substrate status based on clinically relevant drug interaction potential; **Inhibits** CYP2D6 (weak)

Avoid Concomitant Use

Avoid concomitant use of Escitalopram with any of the following: Conivaptan; Dapoxetine; Dosulepin; Fusidic Acid (Systemic); Highest Risk QTc-Prolonging Agents; Idelalisib; Iobenguane I 123; Ivabradine; Linezolid; MAO Inhibitors; Methylene Blue; Mifepristone; Moderate Risk QTc-Prolonging Agents; Pimozide; Tryptophan; Urokinase

Increased Effect/Toxicity

Escitalopram may increase the levels/effects of: Agents with Antiplatelet Properties; Anticoagulants; Antidepressants (Serotonin Reuptake Inhibitor/Antagonist); Antipsychotic Agents; Apixaban; Aspirin; Blood Glucose Lowering Agents; BusPIRone; CarBAMazepine; Collagenase (Systemic); Dabigatran Etexilate; Deoxycholic Acid; Desmopressin; Dextromethorphan; Dosulepin; Edoxaban; Highest Risk QTc-Prolonging Agents; Ibritumomab; Methylene Blue; Mexiletine; NSAID (COX-2 Inhibitor); NSAID (Nonselective); Obinutuzumab; Pimozide; Rivaroxaban; Salicylates; Serotonin Modulators; Thiazide Diuretics; Thrombolytic Agents; Tositumomab and Iodine I 131 Tositumomab; TraMADol; Tricyclic Antidepressants; Urokinase; Vitamin K Antagonists

The levels/effects of Escitalopram may be increased by: Alcohol (Ethyl); Analgesics (Opioid); Antiemetics (5HT3 Antagonists); Antipsychotic Agents; Aprepitant; BusPIRone; Cimetidine; CNS Depressants; Conivaptan; CYP2C19 Inhibitors (Moderate); CYP2C19 Inhibitors (Strong); CYP3A4 Inhibitors (Moderate); CYP3A4 Inhibitors (Strong); Dapoxetine; Fosaprepitant; Fusidic Acid (Systemic); Glucosamine; Herbs (Anticoagulant/Antiplatelet Properties); Ibrutinib; Idelalisib; Ivabradine; Ivacaftor; Limaprost; Linezolid; Lithium; Luliconazole; MAO Inhibitors; Metaxalone; Metoclopramide; Metyrosine; Mifepristone; Moderate Risk QTc-Prolonging Agents; Multivitamins/Fluoride (with ADE); Multivitamins/Minerals (with ADEK, Folate, Iron); Multivitamins/Minerals (with AE, No Iron); Netupitant; Omega-3 Fatty Acids; Omeprazole; Palbociclib; Pentosan Polysulfate Sodium; Pentoxifylline; Prostacyclin Analogues; QTc-Prolonging Agents (Indeterminate Risk and Risk Modifying); Stiripentol; Tedizolid; Tipranavir; TraMADol; Tricyclic Antidepressants; Tryptophan; Vitamin E; Vitamin E (Oral)

Decreased Effect

Escitalopram may decrease the levels/effects of: Iobenguane I 123; Ioflupane I 123; Simeprevir; Thyroid Products

The levels/effects of Escitalopram may be decreased by: Boceprevir; Bosentan; CarBAMazepine; CYP2C19 Inducers (Strong); CYP3A4 Inducers (Moderate); CYP3A4 Inducers (Strong); Cyproheptadine; Dabrafenib;

Deferasirox; Enzalutamide; Mitotane; NSAID (COX-2 Inhibitor); NSAID (Nonselective); Siltuximab; St Johns Wort; Telaprevir; Tocilizumab

Storage/Stability Store at 25°C (77°F); excursions permitted to 15°C to 30°C (59°F to 86°F). Cipralex MELTZ [Canadian product] should be stored in original package and protected from light.

Mechanism of Action Escitalopram is the S-enantiomer of the racemic derivative citalopram, which selectively inhibits the reuptake of serotonin with little to no effect on norepinephrine or dopamine reuptake. It has no or very low affinity for 5-HT$_{1-7}$, alpha- and beta-adrenergic, D$_{1-5}$, H$_{1-3}$, M$_{1-5}$, and benzodiazepine receptors. Escitalopram does not bind to or has low affinity for Na$^+$, K$^+$, Cl$^-$, and Ca^{++} ion channels.

Pharmacodynamics/Kinetics

Onset of action: Depression: The onset of action is within a week; however, individual response varies greatly and full response may not be seen until 8-12 weeks after initiation of treatment.

Distribution: V$_d$: ~20 L/kg (Søgaard 2005)

Protein binding: ~56% to plasma proteins

Metabolism: Hepatic via CYP2C19 and 3A4 to S-desmethylcitalopram (S-DCT); S-DCT is metabolized to S-didesmethylcitalopram (S-DDCT) via CYP2D6; in vitro data suggest metabolites do not contribute significantly to the antidepressant effects of escitalopram

Bioavailability: 80%; tablets and oral solution are bioequivalent

Half-life elimination: Mean: Adolescents: 19 hours; Adults: ~27 to 32 hours (increased ~50% in the elderly and doubled in patients with hepatic impairment)

Time to peak: Escitalopram: Adolescents: 2.9 hours; Adults: ~5 hours

Excretion: Urine (8% as unchanged drug; S-DCT 10%)

Clearance (citalopram):

Hepatic impairment: Decreased by 37%

Mild to moderate renal impairment: Decreased by 17%

Severe renal impairment (CrCl <20 mL/minute): No information available

Dosing

Adult

US labeling: **Major depressive disorder, generalized anxiety disorder:** Oral: Initial: 10 mg once daily; dose may be increased to a maximum of 20 mg once daily after at least 1 week

Canadian labeling: **Note:** Orodispersible tablets should only be used for doses that can be accommodated with whole tablets (ie, 10 mg or multiples of that):

Major depressive disorder, generalized anxiety disorder (GAD), obsessive compulsive disorder (OCD): Oral: Initial: 10 mg once daily (may consider 5 mg once daily where sensitivity is a concern); dose may be increased as tolerated to a maximum of 20 mg once daily. In poor CYP2C19 metabolizers, initiate at a dose of 5 mg once daily; may increase dose to a maximum of 10 mg once daily. Patients with GAD or OCD who require extended therapy should be maintained at the lowest effective dose and assessed periodically to determine the need for continued therapy.

Hot flashes (off-label use): Oral: Initial: 10 mg once daily, increase to 20 mg once daily after 4 weeks if symptoms not adequately controlled (Carpenter 2012; Freeman 2011).

Panic disorder (off-label use): Initial: 5 mg once daily for 7 days, then increase dose to 10 mg once daily. Consider further dosage adjustments based on response and tolerability up to 20 mg once daily; mean dose in clinical trials was ~10 mg once daily (Stahl 2003).

Discontinuation of therapy: Upon discontinuation of antidepressant therapy, gradually taper the dose to minimize the incidence of withdrawal symptoms and allow for the detection of re-emerging symptoms. Evidence supporting ideal taper rates is limited. APA and NICE guidelines suggest tapering therapy over at least several weeks with consideration to the half-life of the antidepressant; antidepressants with a shorter half-life may need to be tapered more conservatively. In addition for long-term treated patients, WFSBP guidelines recommend tapering over 4-6 months. If intolerable withdrawal symptoms occur following a dose reduction, consider resuming the previously prescribed dose and/or decrease dose at a more gradual rate (APA 2010; Bauer 2002; Haddad 2001; NCCMH 2010; Schatzberg 2006; Shelton 2001; Warner 2006).

MAO inhibitor recommendations: *US labeling:*

Switching to or from an MAO inhibitor intended to treat psychiatric disorders:

Allow 14 days to elapse between discontinuing an MAO inhibitor intended to treat psychiatric disorders and initiation of escitalopram.

Allow 14 days to elapse between discontinuing escitalopram and initiation of an MAO inhibitor intended to treat psychiatric disorders.

Use with other MAO inhibitors (linezolid or IV methylene blue):

Do not initiate escitalopram in patients receiving linezolid or IV methylene blue; consider other interventions for psychiatric condition.

If urgent treatment with linezolid or IV methylene blue is required in a patient already receiving escitalopram and potential benefits outweigh potential risks, discontinue escitalopram promptly and administer linezolid or IV methylene blue. Monitor for serotonin syndrome for 2 weeks or until 24 hours after the last dose of linezolid or IV methylene blue, whichever comes first. May resume escitalopram 24 hours after the last dose of linezolid or IV methylene blue.

Dosage adjustment with concomitant medications: *Canadian labeling:* Escitalopram dose should not exceed 10 mg once daily in patients taking omeprazole or cimetidine.

Geriatric

Major depressive disorder, generalized anxiety disorder: *US labeling:* Oral: 10 mg once daily

Major depressive disorder, generalized anxiety disorder (GAD), obsessive compulsive disorder (OCD): *Canadian labeling:* Oral: Initial: 5 mg once daily; dose may be increased as tolerated to a maximum of 10 mg once daily.

Discontinuation of therapy: Refer to adult dosing.

MAO inhibitor recommendations: Refer to adult dosing.

Pediatric Major depressive disorder Oral: Children ≥12 years: Initial: 10 mg once daily; dose may be increased to a maximum of 20 mg once daily after at least 3 weeks

Discontinuation of therapy: Refer to adult dosing.

MAO inhibitor recommendations: Refer to adult dosing.

Renal Impairment

Mild-to-moderate impairment: No dosage adjustment is necessary

Severe impairment: CrCl <20 mL/minute (US labeling) or CrCl <30 mL/minute (Canadian labeling): Use with caution.

Hepatic Impairment

US labeling: 10 mg once daily

Canadian labeling:

Mild or moderate impairment (Child-Pugh class A or B): Initial: 5 mg once daily; dose may be increased as tolerated to 10 mg once daily (maximum dose)

Severe Impairment (Child-Pugh class C): No dosage adjustment provided in manufacturer's labeling; has not been studied. Use with caution.

Dietary Considerations May be taken with or without food.

Administration Administer once daily (morning or evening), with or without food.

Cipralex MELTZ [Canadian product] should be dissolved on the tongue and swallowed without water.

Monitoring Parameters Administer once daily (morning or evening), with or without food.

Cipralex MELTZ [Canadian product] should be dissolved on the tongue and swallowed without water.

Additional Information The tablet and oral solution dosage forms are bioequivalent. Cipralex MELTZ orodispersible tablets [Canadian product] are considered bioequivalent to Cipralex tablets [Canadian product].

Clinically, escitalopram 20 mg is equipotent to citalopram 40 mg. Do not coadminister with citalopram.

Dosage Forms Excipient information presented when available (limited, particularly for generics); consult specific product labeling.

Solution, Oral:

Lexapro: 5 mg/5 mL (240 mL) [contains methylparaben, propylene glycol, propylparaben; peppermint flavor]

Generic: 5 mg/5 mL (240 mL)

Tablet, Oral:

Lexapro: 5 mg

Lexapro: 10 mg, 20 mg [scored]

Generic: 5 mg, 10 mg, 20 mg

▶

◀ **Dosage Forms: Canada** Excipient information presented when available (limited, particularly for generics); consult specific product labeling.
Tablet, oral, as oxalate [strength expressed as base]:
Cipralex: 10 mg, 20 mg
Tablet, Orodispersible, as base:
Cipralex MELTZ: 10 mg, 20 mg [mint flavor]

Esmolol (ES moe lol)

Brand Names: US Brevibloc; Brevibloc in NaCl
Brand Names: Canada Brevibloc; Brevibloc Premixed
Index Terms Esmolol Hydrochloride
Pharmacologic Category Antiarrhythmic Agent, Class II; Antihypertensive; Beta-Blocker, Beta-1 Selective
Additional Appendix Information
Hypertension on page 1996
Use Treatment of supraventricular tachycardia (SVT) and atrial fibrillation/flutter (control ventricular rate); treatment of intraoperative and postoperative tachycardia and/or hypertension; treatment of noncompensatory sinus tachycardia
Pregnancy Considerations Adverse events were observed in some animal reproduction studies. Esmolol has been shown to decrease fetal heart rate. Adverse fetal/neonatal events have also been observed with the chronic use of beta-blockers during pregnancy. Esmolol is a short-acting beta-blocker and not indicated for the chronic treatment of hypertension. Esmolol has been evaluated for use during intubation as an agent to offset the exaggerated pressor response observed in pregnant women with hypertension undergoing surgery (Bansal, 2002).
Breast-Feeding Considerations It is not known if esmolol is excreted into breast milk. Due to the potential for serious adverse reactions in the nursing infant, the manufacturer recommends a decision be made whether to discontinue nursing or to discontinue the drug, taking into account the importance of treatment to the mother. The short half-life and the fact that it is not intended for chronic use should limit any potential exposure to the nursing infant.
Contraindications Hypersensitivity to esmolol or any component of the formulation; severe sinus bradycardia; heart block greater than first degree (except in patients with a functioning artificial ventricular pacemaker); sick sinus syndrome; cardiogenic shock; decompensated heart failure; IV administration of calcium channel blockers (eg, verapamil) in close proximity to esmolol (ie, while effects of other drug are still present); pulmonary hypertension

Canadian labeling: Additional contraindications (not in U.S. labeling): Patients requiring inotropic agents and/or vasopressors to maintain cardiac output and systolic blood pressure; hypotension; right ventricular failure secondary to pulmonary hypertension; untreated pheochromocytoma
Warnings/Precautions Can cause bradycardia including sinus pause, heart block, severe bradycardia, and cardiac arrest. Consider preexisting conditions such as first degree AV block, sick sinus syndrome, or other conduction disorders before initiating; use is contraindicated in patients with sick sinus syndrome or second- or third-degree AV block (except in patients with a functioning artificial ventricular pacemaker). Bradycardia may be observed more frequently in elderly patients (>65 years of age); dosage reductions may be necessary. Hypotension is common; patients need close blood pressure monitoring. If an unacceptable drop in blood pressure occurs, reduction in dose or discontinuation may reverse hypotension (usually within 30 minutes). Avoid use in patients with hypovolemia; treat hypovolemia first, otherwise, use of esmolol may attenuate reflex tachycardia and further increase the risk of hypotension. Administer cautiously in compensated heart failure and monitor for a worsening of the condition; use is contraindicated in patients with decompensated heart failure.

Esmolol has been associated with elevations in serum potassium and development of hyperkalemia especially in patients with risk factors (eg, renal impairment); monitor serum potassium during therapy. Use with caution in patients with myasthenia gravis. Use caution in patients

with renal dysfunction (active metabolite retained). Adequate alpha-blockade is required prior to use of any beta-blocker for patients with untreated pheochromocytoma; Canadian labeling contraindicates use in this patient population. Use beta-blockers cautiously in patients with bronchospastic disease; monitor pulmonary status closely. Use cautiously in patients with diabetes because it can mask prominent hypoglycemic symptoms. May mask signs of hyperthyroidism (eg, tachycardia); if hyperthyroidism is suspected, carefully manage and monitor; abrupt withdrawal may exacerbate symptoms of hyperthyroidism or precipitate thyroid storm. Use esmolol with caution in patients with hypertension associated with hypothermia; monitor vital signs closely and titrate esmolol slowly. Use caution with history of severe anaphylaxis to allergens; patients taking beta-blockers may become more sensitive to repeated challenges. Treatment of anaphylaxis (eg, epinephrine) in patients taking beta-blockers may be ineffective or promote undesirable effects. Can precipitate or aggravate symptoms of arterial insufficiency in patients with PVD and Raynaud's disease; use with caution and monitor for progression of arterial obstruction.

Use caution with concurrent use of digoxin, verapamil or diltiazem; bradycardia or heart block can occur (may be fatal). Use is contraindicated when IV calcium channel blockers have been administered in close proximity to esmolol (ie, while effects of other drug are still present). Beta-blocker therapy should not be withdrawn abruptly (particularly in patients with CAD), but gradually tapered to avoid acute tachycardia, hypertension, and/or ischemia. Vesicant; ensure proper needle or catheter placement prior to and during infusion; avoid extravasation. Extravasation can lead to skin necrosis and sloughing; avoid infusions into small veins or through a butterfly catheter.

Adverse Reactions
>10%: Cardiovascular: Blood pressure decreased (20% to 50%), asymptomatic hypotension (dose related: 25%), symptomatic hypotension (dose related: 12%)
1% to 10%:
Cardiovascular: Peripheral ischemia (1%)
Central nervous system: Dizziness (3%), somnolence (3%), confusion (2%), headache (2%), agitation (2%)
Gastrointestinal: Nausea (7%), vomiting (1%)
Local: Infusion site reaction (8%; including irritation, inflammation, and severe reactions associated with extravasation [eg, thrombophlebitis, necrosis, and blistering])
<1% (Limited to important or life-threatening): Abdominal discomfort, abnormal thinking, angioedema, anorexia, anxiety, bradycardia, bronchospasm, cardiac arrest, constipation, coronary arteriospasm, decompensated heart failure, depression, dyspepsia, flushing, heart block, hyperkalemia, lightheadedness, pallor, paresthesia, psoriasis, renal tubular acidosis, seizure, severe bradycardia/asystole (rare), syncope, urinary retention, urticaria, xerostomia

Drug Interactions
Metabolism/Transport Effects None known.
Avoid Concomitant Use
Avoid concomitant use of Esmolol with any of the following: Ceritinib; Floctafenine; Methacholine; Rivastigmine
Increased Effect/Toxicity
Esmolol may increase the levels/effects of: Alpha-/Beta-Agonists (Direct-Acting); Alpha1-Blockers; Alpha2-Agonists; Amifostine; Antipsychotic Agents (Phenothiazines); Antipsychotic Agents (Second Generation [Atypical]); Bradycardia-Causing Agents; Bupivacaine; Cardiac Glycosides; Ceritinib; Cholinergic Agonists; Disopyramide; DULoxetine; Ergot Derivatives; Fingolimod; Grass Pollen Allergen Extract (5 Grass Extract); Hypotension-Associated Agents; Insulin; Ivabradine; Lacosamide; Levodopa; Lidocaine (Systemic); Lidocaine (Topical); Mepivacaine; Methacholine; Midodrine; Sulfonylureas

The levels/effects of Esmolol may be increased by: Acetylcholinesterase Inhibitors; Alpha2-Agonists; Aminoquinolines (Antimalarial); Amiodarone; Anilidopiperidine Opioids; Antipsychotic Agents (Phenothiazines); Barbiturates; Bretylium; Brimonidine (Topical); Calcium Channel Blockers (Nondihydropyridine); Diazoxide; Dipyridamole; Disopyramide; Dronedarone; Floctafenine; Herbs (Hypotensive Properties); Molsidomine; Nicorandil; NIFEdipine; Obinutuzumab; Pentoxifylline; Phosphodiesterase 5 Inhibitors; Propafenone; Prostacyclin Analogues; Regorafenib; Reserpine; Rivastigmine; Ruxolitinib; Tofacitinib
Decreased Effect
Esmolol may decrease the levels/effects of: Beta2-Agonists; Theophylline Derivatives

The levels/effects of Esmolol may be decreased by: Amphetamines; Barbiturates; Herbs (Hypertensive Properties); Methylphenidate; Nonsteroidal Anti-Inflammatory Agents; Rifamycin Derivatives; Yohimbine

Storage/Stability Clear, colorless to light yellow solution which should be stored at 25°C (77°F); excursions permitted to 15°C to 30°C (59°F to 86°F); do not freeze. Protect from excessive heat. Stable for at least 24 hours (under refrigeration or at controlled room temperature) at a final concentration of 10 mg/mL.

Mechanism of Action Class II antiarrhythmic: Competitively blocks response to beta$_1$-adrenergic stimulation with little or no effect of beta$_2$-receptors except at high doses, no intrinsic sympathomimetic activity, no membrane stabilizing activity

Pharmacodynamics/Kinetics

Onset of action: Beta-blockade: IV: 2-10 minutes (quickest when loading doses are administered)

Duration of hemodynamic effects: 10-30 minutes; prolonged following higher cumulative doses, extended duration of use

Distribution: V$_d$:

Children ≥2.5 years and Adolescents ≤16 years: 2 ± 1.4 L/kg (range: 0.5 to 3.6 L/kg) (Wiest 1991)

Adults: Esmolol: ~3.4 L/kg; Acid metabolite: ~0.4 L/kg

Protein binding: Esmolol: 55%; Acid metabolite: 10%

Metabolism: In blood by red blood cell esterases; forms acid metabolite (negligible activity; produces no clinically important effects) and methanol (does not achieve concentrations associated with methanol toxicity)

Half-life elimination:

Children ≥18 months and Adolescents ≤16 years: Variable; mean range: 2.7 to 4.8 minutes (reported full range: 0.2 to 9.9 minutes) (Cuneo 1994; Tabbutt 2008; Wiest 1991; Wiest 1998)

Adults: Esmolol: 9 minutes; Acid metabolite: 3.7 hours; elimination of metabolite decreases with end-stage renal disease

Excretion: Urine (~73% to 88% as acid metabolite, <2% unchanged drug)

Dosing

Adult & Geriatric

U.S. labeling:

Intraoperative and postoperative tachycardia and/or hypertension: IV:

Immediate control: Initial bolus: 1 mg/kg over 30 seconds, followed by a 150 mcg/kg/minute infusion, if necessary. Adjust infusion rate as needed to maintain desired heart rate and/or blood pressure (up to 300 mcg/kg/minute).

Gradual control: Initial bolus: 0.5 mg/kg over 1 minute, followed by a 50 mcg/kg/minute infusion for 4 minutes. Infusion may be continued at 50 mcg/kg/minute or, if the response is inadequate, titrated upward in 50 mcg/kg/minute increments (increased no more frequently than every 4 minutes) to a maximum of 300 mcg/kg/minute; may administer an optional loading dose equal to the initial bolus (0.5 mg/kg over 1 minute) prior to each increase in infusion rate.

For control of tachycardia, doses >200 mcg/kg/minute provide minimal additional effect. *For control of postoperative hypertension,* as many as one-third of patients may require higher doses (250-300 mcg/kg/minute) to control blood pressure; the safety of doses >300 mcg/kg/minute has not been studied.

Supraventricular tachycardia (SVT) or noncompensatory sinus tachycardia: IV: Loading dose (optional): 0.5 mg/kg over 1 minute; follow with a 50 mcg/kg/minute infusion for 4 minutes; response to this initial infusion rate may be a rough indication of the responsiveness of the ventricular rate.

Infusion may be continued at 50 mcg/kg/minute or, if the response is inadequate, titrated upward in 50 mcg/kg/minute increments (increased no more frequently than every 4 minutes) to a maximum of 200 mcg/kg/minute.

To achieve more rapid response, following the initial loading dose and 50 mcg/kg/minute infusion, rebolus with a second 0.5 mg/kg loading dose over 1 minute, and increase the maintenance infusion to 100 mcg/kg/minute for 4 minutes. If necessary, a third (and final) 0.5 mg/kg loading dose may be administered, prior to increasing to an infusion rate of 150 mcg/kg/minute. After 4 minutes of the 150 mcg/kg/minute infusion, the infusion rate may be increased to a maximum rate of 200 mcg/kg/minute (without a bolus dose).

Note: If a loading dose is not administered, a continuous infusion at a fixed dose reaches steady-state in ~30 minutes. In general, the usual effective dose is 50-200 mcg/kg/minute; doses as low as 25 mcg/kg/minute may be adequate. Maintenance infusions may be continued for up to 48 hours.

Acute coronary syndromes (when relative contraindications to beta-blockade exist; off-label use): IV: 0.5 mg/kg over 1 minute; follow with a 50 mcg/kg/minute infusion; if tolerated and response inadequate, may titrate upward in 50 mcg/kg/minute increments every 5-15 minutes to a maximum of 300 mcg/kg/minute (Mitchell, 2002); an additional bolus (0.5 mg/kg over 1 minute) may be administered prior to each increase in infusion rate (Mooss, 1994)

Electroconvulsive therapy (off-label use): IV: 1 mg/kg administered 1 minute prior to induction of anesthesia (Weinger, 1991)

Intubation (off-label use): IV: 1-2 mg/kg given 1.5-3 minutes prior to intubation (Kindler 1996; Levitt 2001; Ugur 2007)

Thyrotoxicosis or thyroid storm (off-label use): IV: 50-100 mcg/kg/minute (Bahn, 2011)

Canadian labeling: **Note:** Not recommended for use >24 hours.

Perioperative tachycardia and/or hypertension: IV:

Associated with intubation: Bolus: 1.5 mg/kg (maximum dose: 100 mg) over 30 seconds given 1-2 minutes prior to intubation.

Intraoperative/postoperative tachycardia and/or hypertension: Initial bolus: 1.5 mg/kg (maximum dose: 100 mg) over 30 seconds, followed by 150 mcg/kg/minute infusion. Adjust infusion rate as needed to maintain desired heart rate or blood pressure (up to 300 mcg/kg/minute).

Atrial fibrillation/atrial flutter: IV:

Loading dose: 0.5 mg/kg over 1 minute; follow with a 50 mcg/kg/minute infusion for 4 minutes; response to this initial infusion rate may be a rough indication of the responsiveness of the ventricular rate.

Infusion may be continued at 50 mcg/kg/minute or, if the response is inadequate, rebolus with a second 0.5 mg/kg loading dose over 1 minute, and increase the maintenance infusion to 100 mcg/kg/minute for 4 minutes. If necessary, repeat same procedure (ie, 0.5 mg/kg loading dose and increase maintenance infusion by 50 mcg/kg/minute for 4 minutes) until target heart rate or safety end point (eg, hypotension) begins to occur then omit subsequent loading dose and decrease dosing increment of maintenance infusion to ≤25 mcg/kg/minute or alternatively, the manufacturer labeling suggests that the titration interval may be extended from 5 minutes to 10 minutes. If safety endpoints are exceeded discontinue infusion and when appropriate, resume infusion at reduced dose.

Note: In general, the usual effective dose is 50-200 mcg/kg/minute; doses as low as 25 mcg/kg/minute may be adequate.

Guidelines for transfer to oral therapy (beta-blocker, calcium channel blocker):

Infusion should be reduced by 50% thirty minutes following the first dose of the alternative agent

Manufacturer suggests following the second dose of the alternative drug, patient's response should be monitored and if control is adequate for the first hour, esmolol may be discontinued.

Renal Impairment No dosage adjustment necessary. Not removed by hemo- or peritoneal dialysis. Supplemental dose is not necessary.

Hepatic Impairment No dosage adjustment necessary.

Usual Infusion Concentrations: Pediatric Note: Premixed solutions available.

IV infusion: 10,000 mcg/mL or 20,000 mcg/mL

Usual Infusion Concentrations: Adult Note: Premixed solutions available.

IV infusion: 2500 mg in 250 mL (concentration: 10,000 mcg/mL) **or** 2000 mg in 100 mL (concentration: 20,000 mcg/mL) of D$_5$W or NS

Administration IV: Loading doses (eg, 0.5 mg/kg) may be administered over 30 seconds to 1 minute depending on how urgent the need for effect. Infusion into small veins or through a butterfly catheter should be avoided (can cause thrombophlebitis). Medication port of premixed bags should be used to withdraw only the initial bolus, if necessary (not to be used for withdrawal of additional bolus doses).

Vesicant; ensure proper needle or catheter placement prior to and during infusion; avoid extravasation.

Extravasation management: If extravasation occurs, stop injection immediately and disconnect (leave cannula/needle in place); gently aspirate extravasated solution (do **NOT** flush the line); remove needle/cannula; elevate extremity.

Monitoring Parameters Blood pressure, MAP, heart rate, continuous ECG, respiratory rate, IV site; serum potassium (especially with renal impairment); consult individual institutional policies and procedures

Dosage Forms Excipient information presented when available (limited, particularly for generics); consult specific product labeling.

Solution, Intravenous, as hydrochloride:
Brevibloc: 10 mg/mL (10 mL)
Brevibloc in NaCl: 2000 mg (100 mL); 2500 mg (250 mL)
Generic: 10 mg/mL (10 mL)
Solution, Intravenous, as hydrochloride [preservative free]:
Generic: 10 mg/mL (10 mL); 100 mg/10 mL (10 mL)

♦ Esmolol Hydrochloride *see* Esmolol *on page 676*

Esomeprazole (es oh ME pray zol)

Brand Names: US NexIUM; Nexium 24HR [OTC]; NexIUM I.V.

Brand Names: Canada Apo-Esomeprazole; Mylan-Esomeprazole; Nexium; PMS-Esomeprazole DR

Index Terms Esomeprazole Magnesium; Esomeprazole Sodium; Esomeprazole Strontium; Nexium 24HR

Pharmacologic Category Proton Pump Inhibitor; Substituted Benzimidazole

Use
Oral:
Esomeprazole magnesium and esomeprazole strontium:
Gastroesophageal reflux disease (Rx only):
Healing of erosive esophagitis: Short-term (4 to 8 weeks) treatment of erosive esophagitis
Maintenance of healing of erosive esophagitis: Maintaining symptom resolution and healing of erosive esophagitis
Symptomatic gastroesophageal reflux disease: Short-term (4 to 8 weeks) treatment of symptomatic gastroesophageal reflux disease (GERD)
Helicobacter pylori **eradication (Rx only):** As part of a multidrug regimen for *Helicobacter pylori* eradication in patients with duodenal ulcer disease (active or history of within the past 5 years)
Risk reduction of nonsteroidal anti-inflammatory drug-associated gastric ulcer (Rx only): Prevention of gastric ulcers associated with continuous NSAID therapy in patients at risk (age ≥60 years and/or history of gastric ulcer)
Pathological hypersecretory conditions, including Zollinger-Ellison syndrome (Rx only): Treatment (long-term) of pathological hypersecretory conditions including Zollinger-Ellison syndrome
Canadian labeling: Additional use (not in US labeling): Oral: Treatment of nonerosive reflux disease (NERD); treatment of NSAID-induced gastric ulcers
Esomeprazole magnesium:
Heartburn (OTC labeling): Treatment of frequent heartburn (≥2 days per week).

IV: Esomeprazole sodium:
Gastroesophageal reflux disease (Rx only): Short-term (≤10 days) treatment of gastroesophageal reflux disease (GERD) with erosive esophagitis in pediatric patients 1 month to 17 years of age and adults when oral therapy is not possible or appropriate
Risk reduction of ulcer rebleeding postprocedure (Rx only): Decrease the risk of rebleeding postendoscopy for acute bleeding gastric or duodenal ulcers in adults

Pregnancy Considerations Adverse events have been observed in some animal reproduction studies. An increased risk of hypospadias was reported following maternal use of proton pump inhibitors (PPIs) during pregnancy (Anderka, 2012), but this was based on a small number of exposures and the same association was not found in another study (Erichsen, 2012). An increased risk of major birth defects following maternal use of PPIs during pregnancy was not observed in an additional study (Pasternak, 2010). Esomeprazole is the s-isomer of omeprazole; refer to the Omeprazole monograph for additional information. When treating GERD in pregnancy, PPIs may be used when clinically indicated (Katz, 2013).

Breast-Feeding Considerations Esomeprazole and strontium (limited data) are excreted in breast milk. The manufacturer of esomeprazole recommends that caution be exercised when administering to nursing women. The manufacturer of esomeprazole strontium recommends a decision be made whether to discontinue nursing or to discontinue the drug, taking into account the importance of treatment to the mother. Esomeprazole is the s-isomer of omeprazole and omeprazole is excreted in breast milk; refer to Omeprazole monograph for additional information.

Medication Guide Available Yes

Contraindications Hypersensitivity (eg, anaphylaxis, anaphylactic shock, angioedema, bronchospasm, acute interstitial nephritis, urticaria) to esomeprazole, other substituted benzimidazole proton pump inhibitors, or any component of the formulation

Warnings/Precautions Use of proton pump inhibitors (PPIs) may increase the risk of gastrointestinal infections (eg, *Salmonella*, *Campylobacter*). Relief of symptoms does not preclude the presence of a gastric malignancy. Atrophic gastritis (by biopsy) has been noted with long-term omeprazole therapy; this may also occur with esomeprazole. No reports of enterochromaffin-like (ECL) cell carcinoids, dysplasia, or neoplasia have occurred. Use of PPIs may increase risk of CDAD, especially in hospitalized patients; consider CDAD diagnosis in patients with persistent diarrhea that does not improve. Use the lowest dose and shortest duration of PPI therapy appropriate for the condition being treated. Safety and efficacy of IV therapy for GERD >10 days have not been established; transition from IV to oral therapy as soon possible. Bioavailability may be increased in Asian populations, the elderly, and patients with hepatic dysfunction. Decreased *H. pylori* eradication rates have been observed with short-term (≤7 days) combination therapy. The American College of Gastroenterology recommends 10-14 days of therapy (triple or quadruple) for eradication of *H. pylori* (Chey, 2007).

PPIs may diminish the therapeutic effect of clopidogrel, thought to be due to reduced formation of the active metabolite of clopidogrel. The manufacturer of clopidogrel recommends either avoidance of both omeprazole (even when scheduled 12 hours apart) and esomeprazole or use of a PPI with comparatively less effect on the active metabolite of clopidogrel (eg, pantoprazole). In contrast to these warnings, others have recommended the continued use of PPIs, regardless of the degree of inhibition, in patients with a history of GI bleeding or multiple risk factors for GI bleeding who are also receiving clopidogrel since no evidence has established clinically meaningful differences in outcome; however, a clinically-significant interaction cannot be excluded in those who are poor metabolizers of clopidogrel (Abraham, 2010; Levine, 2011). Additionally, potentially significant drug-drug interactions may exist, requiring dose or frequency adjustment, additional monitoring, and/or selection of alternative therapy.

Increased incidence of osteoporosis-related bone fractures of the hip, spine, or wrist may occur with PPI therapy. Patients on high-dose or long-term therapy should be monitored. Use the lowest effective dose for the shortest duration of time, use vitamin D and calcium supplementation, and follow appropriate guidelines to reduce risk of fractures in patients at risk. Acute interstitial nephritis has been observed in patients taking PPIs; may occur at any time during therapy and is generally due to an idiopathic hypersensitivity reaction. Discontinue if acute interstitial nephritis develops.

Hypomagnesemia, reported rarely, usually with prolonged PPI use of >3 months (most cases >1 year of therapy); may be symptomatic or asymptomatic; severe cases may cause tetany, seizures, and cardiac arrhythmias. Consider obtaining serum magnesium concentrations prior to beginning long-term therapy, especially if taking concomitant digoxin, diuretics, or other drugs known to cause hypomagnesemia; and periodically thereafter. Hypomagnesemia may be corrected by magnesium supplementation, although discontinuation of esomeprazole may be necessary; magnesium levels typically return to normal within 1 week of stopping.

Prolonged treatment (≥2 years) may lead to vitamin B_{12} malabsorption and subsequent vitamin B_{12} deficiency. The magnitude of the deficiency is dose-related and the association is stronger in females and those younger in age (<30 years); prevalence is decreased after discontinuation of therapy (Lam, 2013).

Severe liver dysfunction may require dosage reductions. Dosage adjustments are not necessary for any degree of renal impairment when using esomeprazole magnesium or esomeprazole sodium; however, since pharmacokinetics of the strontium may be reduced in mild to moderate renal impairment, esomeprazole strontium is not recommended for use in severe impairment (has not been studied). Esomeprazole strontium competes with calcium for intestinal absorption and is incorporated into bone; use of esomeprazole strontium in pediatric patients is not recommended. When used for self-medication (OTC), do not use for >14 days.

Serum chromogranin A (CgA) levels increase secondary to drug-induced decreases in gastric acid. May cause false positive results in diagnostic investigations for neuroendocrine tumors. Temporarily stop omeprazole treatment ≥14 days before CgA test; if CgA level high, repeat test to confirm. Use same commercial lab for testing to prevent variable results.

Adverse Reactions Unless otherwise specified, percentages represent adverse reactions identified in clinical trials evaluating the oral formulation.

>10%: Central nervous system: Headache (IV 11%; oral 2% to 8%)

1% to 10%:

Central nervous system: Dizziness (IV 3%; oral <1%), drowsiness (adults <1%; children 2%)

Dermatologic: Pruritus (IV 1%; oral <1%)

Gastrointestinal: Flatulence (IV 10%; oral ≤5%), diarrhea (IV 4%; oral 2% to <7%), abdominal pain (IV 6%; oral 1% to 6%), nausea (IV 6%; oral 2% to 6%), xerostomia (IV 4%; oral 3%), constipation (IV 3%; oral 2%)

Local: Injection site reaction (IV 2%)

<1% (Limited to important or life-threatening): Aggression, agranulocytosis, alopecia, anaphylaxis, anemia, angioedema, anorexia, benign polyps/nodules, blurred vision, bone fracture, cervical lymphadenopathy, chest pain, *Clostridium difficile*-associated diarrhea (CDAD), conjunctivitis, cyanocobalamin deficiency, cystitis, depression, dermatitis, dysgeusia, dysmenorrhea, epistaxis, erythema multiforme, exacerbation of arthritis, exacerbation of asthma, fibromyalgia syndrome, fungal infection, gastric carcinoid tumor, gastroenteritis, GI dysplasia, GI moniliasis, goiter, gynecomastia, hallucinations, hematuria, hepatic encephalopathy, hepatic failure, hepatitis, hepatotoxicity (idiosyncratic) (Chalasani, 2014), hernia, hyperhidrosis, hyperparathyroidism, hypersensitivity reactions, hypertension, hypertonia, hyperuricemia, hypoesthesia, hypokalemia, hypomagnesemia (with or without hypocalcemia and/or hypokalemia), hyponatremia, impotence, increased gastrin, increased serum alkaline phosphatase, increased serum ALT, increased serum AST, increased serum creatinine, increased thyroid-stimulating hormone, insomnia, interstitial nephritis, jaundice, laryngeal edema, leukocytosis, leukopenia, microscopic colitis, migraine, moniliasis, myasthenia, otitis media, pancreatitis, pancytopenia, parosmia, pathological fracture due to osteoporosis, phlebitis, photosensitivity, pneumonia, polymyalgia rheumatica, proteinuria, pruritus ani, rigors, skin rash (erythematous and maculopapular), Stevens-Johnson syndrome, stomatitis, tachycardia, thrombocytopenia, thrombophlebitis, ttoxic epidermal necrolysis, vaginitis, visual field defect, weight changes

Drug Interactions

Metabolism/Transport Effects Substrate of CYP2C19 (major), CYP3A4 (minor); **Note:** Assignment of Major/Minor substrate status based on clinically relevant drug interaction potential; **Inhibits** CYP2C19 (moderate)

Avoid Concomitant Use

Avoid concomitant use of Esomeprazole with any of the following: Clopidogrel; Dasatinib; Delavirdine; Erlotinib; Nelfinavir; PAZOPanib; Rifampin; Rilpivirine; Risedronate; St Johns Wort

Increased Effect/Toxicity

Esomeprazole may increase the levels/effects of: Amphetamine; Cilostazol; Citalopram; CYP2C19 Substrates; Dexmethylphenidate; Dextroamphetamine; Methotrexate; Methylphenidate; Raltegravir; Risedronate; Saquinavir; Tacrolimus (Systemic); Vitamin K Antagonists; Voriconazole

The levels/effects of Esomeprazole may be increased by: Fluconazole; Ketoconazole (Systemic); Voriconazole

Decreased Effect

Esomeprazole may decrease the levels/effects of: Atazanavir; Bisphosphonate Derivatives; Bosutinib; Cefditoren; Clopidogrel; Cysteamine (Systemic); Dabigatran Etexilate; Dabrafenib; Dasatinib; Delavirdine; Erlotinib; Gefitinib; Indinavir; Iron Salts; Itraconazole; Ketoconazole (Systemic); Ledipasvir; Mesalamine; Multivitamins/Minerals (with ADEK, Folate, Iron); Mycophenolate; Nelfinavir; Nilotinib; PAZOPanib; Posaconazole; Rilpivirine; Riociguat; Risedronate

The levels/effects of Esomeprazole may be decreased by: CYP2C19 Inducers (Strong); Dabrafenib; Enzalutamide; Lumacaftor; Rifampin; St Johns Wort; Tipranavir

Food Interactions Prolonged treatment (≥2 years) may lead to malabsorption of dietary vitamin B_{12} and subsequent vitamin B_{12} deficiency (Lam, 2013).

Preparation for Administration

Granules for oral administration: Empty the 2.5 mg or 5 mg packet into a container with 5 mL of water or empty the 10 mg, 20 mg, or 40 mg packet into a container with 15 mL of water and stir; leave 2-3 minutes to thicken.

Powder for injection:

For IV injection (≥3 minutes): Adults: Reconstitute powder with 5 mL NS.

For IV infusion (10 to 30 minutes):

Children: Initially reconstitute powder (20 mg or 40 mg) with 5 mL of NS, LR, or D_5W, then further dilute to a final volume of 50 mL; withdraw the appropriate amount of the final solution to administer the intended dose.

Adults: Initially reconstitute powder with 5 mL of NS, LR, or D_5W, then further dilute to a final volume of 50 mL.

For IV infusion (loading dose and continuous infusion): Prepare the 80 mg loading dose by reconstituting two 40 mg vials with NS (5 mL each); the contents of the two vials should then be further diluted in NS 100 mL. To prepare the continuous infusion, also reconstitute two 40 mg vials with NS (5 mL each); the contents of the two vials should then be further diluted in NS 100 mL.

Storage/Stability

Capsules: Keep container tightly closed.

Esomeprazole magnesium: Store at 25°C (77°F); excursions permitted to 15°C to 30°C (59°F to 86°F).

Esomeprazole strontium: Store at 20°C to 25°C (68°F to 77°F); excursions permitted to 15°C to 30°C (59°F to 86°F).

Granules: Store at 25°C (77°F); excursions permitted to 15°C to 30°C (59°F to 86°F).

Powder for injection: Store at 25°C (77°F); excursions permitted to 15°C to 30°C (59°F to 86°F). Protect from light. Per the manufacturer, following reconstitution, solution for injection prepared in NS, and solution for infusion prepared in NS or LR should be used within 12 hours; solution for infusion prepared in D_5W should be used within 6 hours. Refrigeration is not required following reconstitution.

Additional stability data: Following reconstitution, solutions for infusion prepared in D_5W, NS, or LR in PVC bags are chemically and physically stable for 48 hours at room temperature (25°C) and for at least 120 hours under refrigeration (4°C) (Kupiec, 2008).

Mechanism of Action Proton pump inhibitor suppresses gastric acid secretion by inhibition of the H^+/K^+-ATPase in the gastric parietal cell. Esomeprazole is the S-isomer of omeprazole.

Pharmacodynamics/Kinetics

Distribution: V_{dss}: 16 L

Protein binding: 97%

Metabolism: Hepatic via CYP2C19 primarily and (to a lesser extent) via 3A4 to hydroxy, desmethyl, and sulfone metabolites (all inactive)

Bioavailability: Oral: 64 after a single dose; 90% with repeat dosing

Half-life elimination:

Infants: 0.93 hours

Children 1 to 5 years: 0.42 to 0.74 hours (Zhao 2006)

Children 6 to 11 years: 0.73 to 0.88 hours (Zhao 2006)

Adolescents 12 to 17 years: 0.82 to 1.22 hours (Li 2006)

Adults: ~1 to 1.5 hours

Time to peak: Oral:

Infants: Median: 3 hours

Children 1 to 5 years: 1.33 to 1.44 hours (Zhao 2006)

Children 6 to 11 years: 1.75 to 1.79 hours (Zhao 2006)

Adolescents 12 to 17 years: 1.96 to 2.04 hours (Li 2006)

Adults: 1.5 to 2 hours

Excretion: Urine (80%, primarily as inactive metabolites; <1% as active drug); feces (20%)

Clearance (with repeated dosing):

Children 1 to 5 years: 6 to 19.44 L/hour (Zhao 2006)

Children 6 to 11 years: 7.84 to 9.22 L/hour (Zhao 2006)

Adolescents 12 to 17 years: 8.36 to 15.88 L/hour (Li 2006)

Dosing

Adult & Geriatric Note: All dosing is expressed in terms of esomeprazole base, regardless of the salt associated with the dosing information. Esomeprazole strontium 24.65 mg is equivalent to 20 mg of esomeprazole base; esomeprazole strontium 49.3 mg is equivalent to 40 mg of esomeprazole base.

Erosive esophagitis (healing): Oral: Esomeprazole magnesium, esomeprazole strontium: Initial: 20 to 40 mg once daily for 4 to 8 weeks; if incomplete healing, may continue for an additional 4 to 8 weeks; maintenance: 20 mg once daily (controlled studies did not extend beyond 6 months)

Heartburn (OTC labeling): 20 mg once daily for 14 days (maximum: 20 mg/day); treatment may be repeated after 4 months if needed

◄

Nonerosive reflux disease (NERD) (Canadian labeling): Oral: Esomeprazole magnesium: Initial: 20 mg once daily for 2 to 4 weeks; lack of symptom control after 4 weeks warrants further evaluation; maintenance (in patients with successful initial therapy): 20 mg once daily as needed

Symptomatic gastroesophageal reflux: Oral: Esomeprazole magnesium, esomeprazole strontium: 20 mg once daily for 4 weeks; may consider an additional 4 weeks of treatment if symptoms do not resolve

Treatment of GERD (short-term): IV: 20 mg or 40 mg once daily. **Note:** Indicated only in cases where oral therapy is inappropriate or not possible; safety/efficacy ≥10 days has not been established.

Prevention of recurrent gastric or duodenal ulcer bleeding postendoscopy: IV: 80 mg over 30 minutes, followed by 8 mg/hour continuous infusion for a total of 72 hours, then 40 mg *orally* once daily for 27 additional days (Sung, 2009) or may follow continuous infusion with any single daily-dose oral proton pump inhibitor (PPI) for a duration dictated by the underlying etiology (Barkun, 2010). **Note:** The use of intermittent PPIs was found to be comparable with the use of continuous infusion PPIs in patients with high-risk endoscopic findings and may be preferred (Sachar, 2014).

Helicobacter pylori **eradication:** Oral:

Manufacturer labeling: Esomeprazole magnesium, esomeprazole strontium: 40 mg once daily administered with amoxicillin 1,000 mg *and* clarithromycin 500 mg twice daily for 10 days

American College of Gastroenterology guidelines (Chey, 2007):

Nonpenicillin allergy: 40 mg once daily administered with amoxicillin 1,000 mg *and* clarithromycin 500 mg twice daily for 10 to 14 days

Penicillin allergy: 40 mg once daily administered with clarithromycin 500 mg *and* metronidazole 500 mg twice daily for 10 to 14 days **or** 40 mg once daily administered with bismuth subsalicylate 525 mg *and* metronidazole 250 mg *plus* tetracycline 500 mg 4 times daily for 10 to 14 days

Canadian labeling: Esomeprazole magnesium: 20 mg twice daily for 7 days; requires combination therapy

Prevention of NSAID-induced gastric ulcers: Oral:

US labeling: Esomeprazole magnesium, esomeprazole strontium: 20 to 40 mg once daily for up to 6 months

Canadian labeling: Esomeprazole magnesium: 20 mg once daily for up to 6 months

Note: 40 mg daily did not show additional benefit over 20 mg daily in clinical trials.

Treatment of NSAID-induced gastric ulcers (Canadian labeling; off-label in US): Oral: Esomeprazole magnesium: 20 mg once daily for 4 to 8 weeks (Goldstein, 2007)

Pathological hypersecretory conditions (Zollinger-Ellison syndrome): Oral: Esomeprazole magnesium, esomeprazole strontium: 40 mg twice daily; adjust regimen to individual patient needs; doses up to 240 mg daily have been administered

Pediatric Note: All dosing is expressed in terms of esomeprazole base, regardless of the salt associated with the dosing information. Esomeprazole strontium is not recommended for use in pediatrics.

Symptomatic GERD: Oral: Esomeprazole magnesium:

Children 1 to 11 years: 10 mg once daily for up to 8 weeks; **Note:** Safety and efficacy of doses >1 mg/kg/day and/or therapy beyond 8 weeks have not been established.

Adolescents 12 to 17 years: 20 mg once daily for up to 4 weeks

Treatment of GERD (short-term): IV: **Note:** Indicated only in cases where oral therapy is inappropriate or not possible; safety/efficacy ≥10 days has not been established.

Children 1 month to <1 year: 0.5 mg/kg once daily

Children 1 to 17 years: <55 kg: 10 mg once daily; ≥55 kg: 20 mg once daily

Erosive esophagitis (healing): Oral: Esomeprazole magnesium:

Children 1 month to <1 year: **Note:** Safety and efficacy of doses >1.33 mg/kg/day and/or therapy beyond 6 weeks have not been established.

3 to 5 kg: 2.5 mg once daily for up to 6 weeks

>5 to 7.5 kg: 5 mg once daily for up to 6 weeks

>7.5 to 12 kg: 10 mg once daily for up to 6 weeks

Children 1 to 11 years: **Note:** Safety and efficacy of doses >1 mg/kg/day and/or therapy beyond 8 weeks have not been established.

<20 kg: 10 mg once daily for 8 weeks

≥20 kg: 10 to 20 mg once daily for 8 weeks

Adolescents 12 to 17 years: 20 to 40 mg once daily for 4 to 8 weeks

Nonerosive reflux disease (NERD) (Canadian labeling): Oral: Esomeprazole magnesium:

Children 1 to 11 years: 10 mg once daily for up to 8 weeks. **Note:** Safety and efficacy of doses >1 mg/kg/day and/or therapy beyond 8 weeks have not been established.

Adolescents 12 to 17 years: 20 mg once daily for 2 to 4 weeks; lack of symptom control after 4 weeks warrants further evaluation

Renal Impairment

Oral:

Esomeprazole magnesium: Mild-to-severe impairment: No dosage adjustment necessary.

Esomeprazole strontium:

Mild-to-moderate impairment: No dosage adjustment necessary.

Severe impairment: Use is not recommended (has not been studied).

IV: Mild-to-severe impairment: No dosage adjustment necessary.

Hepatic Impairment

Oral:

Safety and efficacy not established in children with hepatic impairment.

Mild-to-moderate impairment (Child-Pugh class A or B): Treatment of GERD (short-term): No dosage adjustment necessary.

Severe impairment (Child-Pugh class C): Treatment of GERD (short-term): Dose should not exceed 20 mg (esomeprazole base) daily.

IV:

Treatment of GERD (short-term):

Mild to moderate impairment (Child-Pugh class A or B): No dosage adjustment necessary.

Severe impairment (Child-Pugh class C): Dose should not exceed 20 mg daily

Prevention of recurrent gastric or duodenal ulcer bleeding postendoscopy:

Mild to moderate impairment (Child-Pugh class A or B): 80 mg over 30 minutes, followed by a maximum continuous infusion of 6 mg/hour for a total of 72 hours

Severe impairment (Child-Pugh class C): 80 mg over 30 minutes, followed by a maximum continuous infusion of 4 mg/hour for a total of 72 hour

Dietary Considerations Take at least 1 hour before meals; best if taken before breakfast.

Usual Infusion Concentrations: Pediatric IV infusion: 0.4 mg/mL **or** 0.8 mg/mL

Usual Infusion Concentrations: Adult IV infusion: 20 mg in 50 mL (concentration: 0.4 mg/mL) **or** 40 mg in 50 mL (concentration: 0.8 mg/mL) of D_5W, LR, or NS

Administration

Oral:

Capsule: Should be swallowed whole and taken at least 1 hour before eating (best if taken before breakfast). Capsule can be opened and contents mixed with 1 tablespoon of applesauce. Swallow immediately; mixture should not be chewed or warmed. For patients with difficulty swallowing, use of granules may be more appropriate.

Granules: Empty the 2.5 mg or 5 mg packet into a container with 5 mL of water or the 10 mg, 20 mg, or 40 mg packet into a container with 15 mL of water and stir; leave 2 to 3 minutes to thicken. Stir and drink within 30 minutes. If any medicine remains after drinking, add more water, stir and drink immediately.

Tablet (Canadian formulation, not available in US): Swallow whole or may be dispersed in a half a glass of noncarbonated water. Stir until tablets disintegrate, leaving a liquid containing pellets. Drink contents within 30 minutes. Do not chew or crush pellets. After drinking, rinse glass with water and drink.

IV: Flush line prior to and after administration with NS, LR, or D_5W.

Children: Administer by intermittent infusion (10 to 30 minutes); the manufacturer recommends that children receive intravenous esomeprazole by intermittent infusion only.

Adults:

Treatment of GERD: May be administered by injection (≥3 minutes), or intermittent infusion (10 to 30 minutes)

Prevention of recurrent gastric or duodenal ulcer bleeding postendoscopy: Administer the loading dose over 30 minutes, followed by the continuous infusion at a rate of 8 mg/hour over 71.5 hours (adjust rate of continuous infusion in patients with hepatic dysfunction)

Nasogastric tube:

Capsule: Open capsule and place intact granules into a 60 mL catheter-tip syringe; mix with 50 mL of water.

Replace plunger and shake vigorously for 15 seconds. Ensure that no granules remain in syringe tip. Do not administer if pellets dissolve or disintegrate. Use immediately after preparation. After administration, flush nasogastric tube with additional water.

Granules: Delayed release oral suspension granules can also be given by nasogastric or gastric tube. If using a 2.5 mg or 5 mg packet, first add 5 mL of water to a catheter-tipped syringe, then add granules from packet. If using a 10 mg, 20 mg, or 40 mg packet, first add 15 mL of water to a catheter-tipped syringe, then add granules from packet. Shake the syringe, leave 2 to 3 minutes to thicken. Shake the syringe and administer through nasogastric or gastric tube (size 6 French or greater) within 30 minutes. Refill the syringe with equal amount (5 mL or 15 mL) of water, shake and flush nasogastric/gastric tube.

Tablet (Canadian formulation, not available in US): Disperse tablets in 50 mL of noncarbonated water. Stir until tablets disintegrate leaving a liquid containing pellets. After administration, flush with additional 25 to 50 mL of water to clear the syringe and tube.

Monitoring Parameters Susceptibility testing recommended in patients who fail *H. pylori* eradication regimen. Monitor for rebleeding in patients with peptic ulcer bleed. For patients expected to be on prolonged therapy or who take PPIs with medications such as digoxin or drugs that may cause hypomagnesemia (eg, diuretics), consider monitoring magnesium levels prior to initiation of treatment and periodically thereafter.

Test Interactions Esomeprazole may falsely elevate serum chromogranin A (CgA) levels. The increased CgA level may cause false-positive results in the diagnosis of a neuroendocrine tumor. Temporarily stop esomeprazole ≥14 days prior to assessing CgA level; repeat level if initially elevated; use the same laboratory for all testing of CgA levels.

Product Availability Esomeprazole strontium 24.65 mg capsules have been discontinued for more than 1 year.

Dosage Forms Considerations
Esomeprazole strontium 49.3 mg is equivalent to 40 mg of esomeprazole base.

Dosage Forms Excipient information presented when available (limited, particularly for generics); consult specific product labeling. [DSC] = Discontinued product

Capsule Delayed Release, Oral, as magnesium [strength expressed as base]:
NexIUM: 20 mg, 40 mg [contains brilliant blue fcf (fd&c blue #1), fd&c red #40, fd&c yellow #10 (quinoline yellow)]
Nexium 24HR: 20 mg [contains brilliant blue fcf (fd&c blue #1), fd&c red #40]
Generic: 20 mg, 40 mg

Capsule Delayed Release, Oral, as strontium:
Generic: 24.65 mg [DSC], 49.3 mg [DSC]

Packet, Oral, as magnesium [strength expressed as base]:
NexIUM: 2.5 mg (30 ea); 5 mg (30 ea); 10 mg (30 ea); 20 mg (30 ea); 40 mg (30 ea)

Solution Reconstituted, Intravenous, as sodium [strength expressed as base]:
NexIUM I.V.: 20 mg (1 ea [DSC]); 40 mg (1 ea)
Generic: 20 mg (1 ea); 40 mg (1 ea)

Dosage Forms: Canada Excipient information presented when available (limited, particularly for generics); consult specific product labeling.

Note: Strength expressed as base
Granules, for oral suspension, delayed release, as magnesium:
Nexium®: 10 mg/packet (28s)
Tablet, extended release, as magnesium:
Nexium®: 20 mg, 40 mg

Estazolam (es TA zoe lam)

Index Terms ProSom
Pharmacologic Category Benzodiazepine
Use Short-term management of insomnia
Dosing
Adult Insomnia: Oral: 1 mg at bedtime, some patients may require 2 mg
Geriatric Insomnia: Oral: Initial: 0.5-1 mg at bedtime; initiate at lower dose in debilitated or small elderly patients
Renal Impairment No dosage adjustment provided in manufacturer's labeling (has not been studied); use with caution.
Hepatic Impairment No dosage adjustment provided in manufacturer's labeling (has not been studied); use with caution.
Additional Information Complete prescribing information should be consulted for additional detail.
Dosage Forms Excipient information presented when available (limited, particularly for generics); consult specific product labeling.
Tablet, Oral:
Generic: 1 mg, 2 mg
Controlled Substance C-IV

Estradiol (Systemic) (es tra DYE ole)

Brand Names: US Alora; Climara; Delestrogen; Depo-Estradiol; Divigel; Elestrin; Estrace; Estrasorb [DSC]; Estrogel; Evamist; Femring; Menostar; Minivelle; Vivelle-Dot
Brand Names: Canada Climara; Depo-Estradiol; Divigel; Estradot; EstroGel; Menostar; Oesclim; Sandoz-Estradiol Derm 100; Sandoz-Estradiol Derm 50; Sandoz-Estradiol Derm 75
Index Terms Estradiol; Estradiol Acetate; Estradiol Transdermal; Estradiol Valerate; Gynodiol; Vivelle Dot
Pharmacologic Category Estrogen Derivative
Use
Breast cancer, metastatic: Treatment of metastatic breast cancer (palliation) in appropriately selected men and postmenopausal women.
Hypoestrogenism (female): Treatment of hypoestrogenism due to hypogonadism, castration, or primary ovarian failure
Osteoporosis prevention (female): Prevention of postmenopausal osteoporosis
Limitations of use: For use only in women at significant risk of postmenopausal osteoporosis; consider use of nonestrogen medications.
Prostate cancer, advanced: Treatment of androgen dependent advanced prostatic cancer (palliation)
Vasomotor symptoms associated with menopause: Treatment of moderate to severe vasomotor symptoms associated with menopause.
Vulvar and vaginal atrophy associated with menopause: Treatment of moderate to severe vulvar and vaginal atrophy associated with menopause.
Limitations of use: When used solely for the treatment of vulvar and vaginal atrophy, topical vaginal products should be considered.
Pregnancy Considerations In general, the use of estrogen and progestin as in combination hormonal contraceptives has not been associated with teratogenic effects when inadvertently taken early in pregnancy. These products are contraindicated for use during pregnancy.
Breast-Feeding Considerations Estrogens are excreted in breast milk and have been shown to decrease the quantity and quality of human milk. The manufacturer recommends that caution be used if administered to breast-feeding women. Monitor the growth of the infant closely.
Contraindications
Angioedema, anaphylactic reaction, or hypersensitivity to estradiol or any component of the formulation; undiagnosed abnormal genital bleeding; DVT or PE (current or history of); active or history of arterial thromboembolic disease (eg, stroke, MI); breast cancer (known, suspected or history of), except in appropriately selected patients being treated for metastatic disease; estrogen-dependent tumor (known or suspected); hepatic impairment or disease; known protein C, protein S, antithrombin

deficiency or other known thrombophilic disorders; pregnancy.

Documentation of allergenic cross-reactivity for estrogens is limited. However, because of similarities in chemical structure and/or pharmacologic actions, the possibility of cross-sensitivity cannot be ruled out with certainty.

Warnings/Precautions Hazardous agent: Use appropriate precautions for handling and disposal (NIOSH 2014 [group 2]).

Anaphylaxis requiring emergency medical management has been reported and may develop at any time during therapy. Angioedema involving the face, feet, hands, larynx, and tongue has also been reported.

[US Boxed Warning]: Based on data from the Women's Health Initiative (WHI) studies, an increased risk of invasive breast cancer was observed in postmenopausal women using conjugated estrogens (CE) in combination with medroxyprogesterone acetate (MPA). This risk may be associated with duration of use and declines once combined therapy is discontinued (Chlebowski 2009). The risk of invasive breast cancer was decreased in postmenopausal women with a hysterectomy using CE only, regardless of weight. However, the risk was not significantly decreased in women at high risk for breast cancer (family history of breast cancer, personal history of benign breast disease) (Anderson 2012). An increase in abnormal mammogram findings has also been reported with estrogen alone or in combination with progestin therapy. Estrogen use may lead to severe hypercalcemia in patients with breast cancer and bone metastases; discontinue estrogen if hypercalcemia occurs. Postmenopausal estrogens with or without progestins may increase the risk of ovarian cancer; however, the absolute risk to an individual woman is small. Although results from various studies are not consistent, risk does not appear to be significantly associated with the duration, route, or dose of therapy. In one study, the risk decreased after 2 years following discontinuation of therapy (Mørch 2009). Although the risk of ovarian cancer is rare, women who are at an increased risk (eg, family history) should be counseled about the association (NAMS 2012).

[US Boxed Warning]: Estrogens with or without progestin should not be used to prevent cardiovascular disease. Using data from the Women's Health Initiative (WHI) studies, an increased risk of deep vein thrombosis (DVT) and stroke has been reported with CE and an increased risk of DVT, stroke, pulmonary emboli (PE) and myocardial infarction (MI) has been reported with CE with MPA in postmenopausal women 50 to 79 years of age. Additional risk factors include diabetes mellitus, hypercholesterolemia, hypertension, SLE, obesity, tobacco use, and/or history of venous thromboembolism (VTE). Risk factors should be managed appropriately; discontinue use if adverse cardiovascular events occur or are suspected. Use is contraindicated in women with active DVT, PE, active arterial thromboembolic disease or a history of these conditions.

[US Boxed Warning]: Estrogens with or without progestin should not be used to prevent dementia. In the Women's Health Initiative Memory Study (WHIMS), an increased incidence of probable dementia was observed in women ≥65 years of age taking CE alone or in combination with MPA.

[US Boxed Warning]: The use of unopposed estrogen in women with a uterus is associated with an increased risk of endometrial cancer. The addition of a progestin to estrogen therapy may decrease the risk of endometrial hyperplasia, a precursor to endometrial cancer. Adequate diagnostic measures, including endometrial sampling if indicated, should be performed to rule out malignancy in postmenopausal women with undiagnosed abnormal vaginal bleeding. There is no evidence that the use of natural estrogens results in a different endometrial risk profile than synthetic estrogens at equivalent estrogen doses. The risk of endometrial cancer is dose and duration dependent; risk appears to be greatest with use ≥5 years and may persist following discontinuation of therapy. The use of a progestin is not generally required when low doses of estrogen are used locally for vaginal atrophy (NAMS 2012; NAMS 2013). Estrogens may exacerbate endometriosis. Malignant transformation of residual endometrial implants has been reported posthysterectomy with unopposed estrogen therapy. Consider adding a progestin in women with residual endometriosis posthysterectomy.

[US Boxed Warning]: Estrogens with or without progestin should be used for the shortest duration possible at the lowest effective dose consistent with treatment goals and risks for the individual woman.

Patients should be reevaluated as clinically appropriate to determine if treatment is still necessary. Available data related to treatment risks are from Women's Health Initiative (WHI) studies, which evaluated oral CE 0.625 mg with or without MPA 2.5 mg relative to placebo in postmenopausal women. Other combinations and dosage forms of estrogens and progestins were not studied. **Outcomes reported from clinical trials using CE with or without MPA should be assumed to be similar for other doses and other dosage forms of estrogens and progestins until comparable data becomes available.** Women who are early in menopause, who are in good cardiovascular health, and who are at low risk for adverse cardiovascular events can be considered candidates for estrogen with or without progestin therapy for the relief of menopausal symptoms (ACOG 565 2013). Use of a transdermal product should be considered over an oral agent in women requiring systemic therapy who have risk factors for venous thromboembolism or coronary heart disease (ACOG 556 2013; Schenck-Gustafsson 2011; Tremollieres 2011).

Topical estradiol may be transferred to another person following skin-to-skin contact with the application site. **[US Boxed Warning]: Breast budding and breast masses in prepubertal females and gynecomastia and breast masses in prepubertal males have been reported following unintentional contact with application sites of women using topical estradiol (Evamist). Patients should strictly adhere to instructions for use in order to prevent secondary exposure. In most cases, conditions resolved with removal of estradiol exposure.** If unexpected changes in sexual development occur in prepubertal children, the possibility of unintentional estradiol exposure should be evaluated by a health care provider. Discontinue if conditions for the safe use of the topical spray cannot be met.

Women with inherited thrombophilias (eg, protein C or S deficiency) may have increased risk of venous thromboembolism (DeSancho 2010; van Vlijmen 2011). Use is contraindicated in women with protein C, protein S, antithrombin deficiency, or other known thrombophilic disorders. Estrogen compounds are generally associated with lipid effects such as increased HDL-cholesterol and decreased LDL-cholesterol. Triglycerides may also be increased in women with preexisting hypertriglyceridemia; discontinue if pancreatitis occurs. The use of estrogens and/or progestins may change the results of some laboratory tests (eg, coagulation factors, lipids, glucose tolerance, binding proteins). The dose, route, and the specific estrogen/progestin influence these changes. In addition, personal risk factors (eg, cardiovascular disease, smoking, diabetes, age) also contribute to adverse events; use of specific products may be contraindicated in women with certain risk factors. Estrogens may increase thyroid-binding globulin (TBG) levels leading to increased circulating total thyroid hormone levels. Women on thyroid replacement therapy may require higher doses of thyroid hormone while receiving estrogens. Potentially significant interactions may exist, requiring dose or frequency adjustment, additional monitoring, and/or selection of alternative therapy.

Estrogens may cause retinal vascular thrombosis; discontinue if migraine, loss of vision, proptosis, diplopia, or other visual disturbances occur; discontinue permanently if papilledema or retinal vascular lesions are observed on examination. Use caution with asthma, epilepsy, hepatic hemangiomas, migraine, porphyria, SLE; may exacerbate disease. May have adverse effects on glucose tolerance; use caution in women with diabetes. Use caution with diseases which may be exacerbated by fluid retention, including cardiac or renal dysfunction. Use of postmenopausal estrogen may be associated with an increased risk of gallbladder disease requiring surgery. Estrogens are poorly metabolized in patients with hepatic dysfunction. Use caution with a history of cholestatic jaundice associated with prior estrogen use or pregnancy. Discontinue if jaundice develops or if acute or chronic hepatic disturbances occur. Use is contraindicated with hepatic impairment or disease. Exogenous estrogens may exacerbate angioedema symptoms in women with hereditary angioedema. Use caution with hypoparathyroidism; estrogen-induced hypocalcemia may occur.

Whenever possible, estrogens should be discontinued at least 4 to 6 weeks prior to elective surgery associated with an increased risk of thromboembolism or during periods of prolonged immobilization.

Avoid oral and transdermal patch estrogen products (with or without progestins) in the elderly due to potential of increased risk of breast and endometrial cancers, and lack of proven cardioprotection and cognitive protection (Beers Criteria).

Prior to puberty, estrogens may cause premature closure of the epiphyses. Premature breast development, vaginal bleeding and vaginal cornification may be induced in girls. Modification of the normal puberty process may occur in boys.

Osteoporosis use: For use only in women at significant risk of osteoporosis and for who other nonestrogen medications are not considered appropriate.

Vulvar and vaginal atrophy use: Moderate-to-severe symptoms of vulvar and vaginal atrophy include vaginal dryness, dyspareunia, and atrophic vaginitis. When used solely for the treatment of vulvar and vaginal atrophy, topical vaginal products should be considered. Use caution applying topical products to severely atrophic vaginal mucosa. Use of a progestin is normally not required when low-dose estrogen is applied locally and only for this purpose (NAMS 2012; NAMS 2013).

Topical emulsion, gel: Absorption of the topical emulsion (Estrasorb) and topical gel (Elestrin) is increased by application of sunscreen; do not apply sunscreen within close proximity of estradiol. Application of sunscreen or lotion after EstroGel decreases absorption of estradiol; the effect of applying sunscreen or lotion prior to Estrogel has not been studied. Application of Divigel with sunscreen has not been evaluated.

Topical spray: When sunscreen is applied ~1 hour prior to the topical spray (Evamist), no change in absorption was observed (estradiol absorption was decreased when sunscreen is applied 1 hour after Evamist).

Transdermal patch: May contain conducting metal (eg, aluminum); remove patch prior to MRI.

Vaginal ring: Use may not be appropriate in women with narrow vagina, vaginal stenosis, vaginal infections, cervical prolapse, rectoceles, cystoceles, or other conditions which may increase the risk of vaginal irritation, ulceration, or increase the risk of expulsion. Ring should be removed in case of ulceration, erosion, or adherence to vaginal wall; do not reinsert until healing is complete. Ensure proper vaginal placement of the ring to avoid inadvertent urinary bladder insertion.

Some dosage forms may contain benzyl alcohol; large amounts of benzyl alcohol (≥99 mg/kg/day) have been associated with a potentially fatal toxicity ("gasping syndrome") in neonates; the "gasping syndrome" consists of metabolic acidosis, respiratory distress, gasping respirations, CNS dysfunction (including convulsions, intracranial hemorrhage), hypotension and cardiovascular collapse (AAP ["Inactive" 1997]; CDC 1982); some data suggests that benzoate displaces bilirubin from protein binding sites (Ahlfors 2001); avoid or use dosage forms containing benzyl alcohol with caution in neonates. See manufacturer's labeling. Some products may contain chlorobutanol (a chloral derivative) as a preservative, which may be habit forming. Some products may contain tartrazine.

Adverse Reactions Frequency not defined. Some adverse reactions observed with estrogen and/or progestin combination therapy.

Cardiovascular: Edema (10% to 13%), hypertension (3% to 7%), cerebrovascular accident, deep vein thrombosis, local thrombophlebitis, myocardial infarction, pulmonary thromboembolism, retinal thrombosis, thrombophlebitis, venous thromboembolism

Central nervous system: Headache (9% to 50%), pain (6% to 13%), depression (1% to 11%), anxiety (4% to 10%), dizziness (≤8%), migraine (7%), nipple pain (1% to 7%), hypoesthesia (3%), chorea, dementia, exacerbation of epilepsy, irritability, mood disorder, nervousness

Dermatologic: Skin rash (7% to 9%), pruritus (4% to 7%), chloasma, erythema multiforme, erythema nodosum, localized erythema (transdermal patch), loss of scalp hair, skin discoloration (melasma), urticaria

Endocrine & metabolic: Weight gain (4% to 9%), hot flash (6%), hirsutism (≤5%), change in libido, change in menstrual flow (alterations in frequency and flow of bleeding patterns), exacerbation of diabetes mellitus, exacerbation of porphyria, fibrocystic breast changes, fluid retention, galactorrhea, hypocalcemia, increased serum triglycerides, weight loss

Gastrointestinal: Abdominal pain (6% to 16%), dyspepsia (3% to 9%), constipation (4% to 7%), flatulence (3% to 7%), nausea (3% to 7%), gastroenteritis (3% to 4%), diarrhea (3%), abdominal cramps, bloating, carbohydrate intolerance, gallbladder disease, pancreatitis, vomiting

Genitourinary: Mastalgia (5% to 35%), vaginal hemorrhage (33%), breast tenderness (3% to 17%), endometrium disease (15%), breakthrough bleeding (6% to 11%), leukorrhea (2% to 11%), abnormal uterine bleeding (4% to 10%), breast hypertrophy (7%), dysmenorrhea (7%),

cervical polyp (6%), vulvovaginal candidiasis (6%), urinary tract infection (4% to 6%), change in cervical ectropion, change in cervical secretions, endometrial hyperplasia, nipple discharge, spotting, uterine fibroids (size increased), uterine pain, vaginal discomfort (vaginal ring; burning, irritation, itching), vaginitis

Hematologic & oncologic: Hemorrhagic eruption, hypercoagulability state, malignant neoplasm of breast, ovarian cancer

Hepatic: Cholestatic jaundice, exacerbation of hepatic hemangioma

Hypersensitivity: Hypersensitivity reaction (4% to 5%), anaphylactoid reaction, anaphylaxis, angioedema

Infection: Infection (3% to 12%), fungal infection (3% to 10%)

Local: Application site reaction (gel, spray, transdermal patch ≤1%)

Neuromuscular & skeletal: Arthralgia (4% to 12%), back pain (3% to 11%), weakness (8%), limb pain (7% to 8%), myalgia (5% to 6%), neck pain (3% to 6%), arthropathy (4% to 5%), exacerbation of systemic lupus erythematosus, leg cramps

Ophthalmic: Conjunctivitis (3%), change in corneal curvature (steepening), contact lens intolerance

Otic: Otitis media (3%)

Respiratory: Nasopharyngitis (4% to 20%), upper respiratory tract infection (6% to 17%), flu-like symptoms (8% to 13%), sinusitis (4% to 13%), sinus headache (9% to 11%), bronchitis (6% to 8%), sinus congestion (7%), pharyngitis (2% to 7%), rhinitis (2% to 6%), cough (3% to 4%), asthma (3%), exacerbation of asthma

Miscellaneous: Accidental injury (7% to 14%), cyst (7%)

<1% (Limited to important or life-threatening): Bowel obstruction (vaginal ring), genitourinary complaint (inadvertent ring insertion into the bladder should be considered with unexplained urinary complaints), hemorrhage, mechanical complication of genitourinary device (ring adherence to vaginal or bladder wall), portal vein thrombosis, toxic shock syndrome (vaginal ring), unstable angina pectoris

Drug Interactions

Metabolism/Transport Effects Substrate of CYP1A2 (major), CYP2A6 (minor), CYP2B6 (minor), CYP2C19 (minor), CYP2C9 (minor), CYP2D6 (minor), CYP2E1 (minor), CYP3A4 (major), P-glycoprotein; **Note:** Assignment of Major/Minor substrate status based on clinically relevant drug interaction potential; **Inhibits** CYP1A2 (weak), CYP2C8 (weak)

Avoid Concomitant Use

Avoid concomitant use of Estradiol (Systemic) with any of the following: Amodiaquine; Anastrozole; Dehydroepiandrosterone; Exemestane; Hemin; Indium 111 Capromab Pendetide; Ospemifene

Increased Effect/Toxicity

Estradiol (Systemic) may increase the levels/effects of: Amodiaquine; Anthrax Immune Globulin (Human); C1 inhibitors; Corticosteroids (Systemic); Immune Globulin; Lenalidomide; Ospemifene; ROPINIRole; Thalidomide; Theophylline Derivatives; Tipranavir; TiZANidine

The levels/effects of Estradiol (Systemic) may be increased by: Ascorbic Acid; Dehydroepiandrosterone; Herbs (Estrogenic Properties); NSAID (COX-2 Inhibitor); Osimertinib; P-glycoprotein/ABCB1 Inhibitors; Ranolazine

Decreased Effect

Estradiol (Systemic) may decrease the levels/effects of: Anastrozole; Anticoagulants; Antidiabetic Agents; Chenodiol; Exemestane; Hemin; Hyaluronidase; Indium 111 Capromab Pendetide; Ospemifene; Somatropin; Thyroid Products; Ursodiol

The levels/effects of Estradiol (Systemic) may be decreased by: Bosentan; Cannabis; CYP1A2 Inducers (Strong); CYP3A4 Inducers (Moderate); CYP3A4 Inducers (Strong); Cyproterone; Dabrafenib; Deferasirox; Enzalutamide; Mitotane; Osimertinib; P-glycoprotein/ABCB1 Inducers; Siltuximab; St Johns Wort; Teriflunomide; Tipranavir; Tocilizumab

Food Interactions Folic acid absorption may be decreased. Routine use of ethanol increases estrogen level and risk of breast cancer; may also increase the risk of osteoporosis. Management: Avoid ethanol.

Storage/Stability

Store all products at controlled room temperature. In addition:

Depo-Estradiol: Protect from light.

Evamist: Do not freeze.

Femring: Store in pouch.

Transdermal patch (all products): Store in protective pouch.

Climara, Menostar: Do not store >30°C (>86°F).

Mechanism of Action Estrogens are responsible for the development and maintenance of the female reproductive system and secondary sexual characteristics. Estradiol is the principle intracellular human estrogen and is more potent than estrone and estriol at the receptor level; it is the primary estrogen secreted prior to menopause. Following menopause, estrone and estrone sulfate are more highly produced. Estrogens modulate the pituitary secretion of gonadotropins, luteinizing hormone, and follicle-stimulating hormone through a negative feedback system; estrogen replacement reduces elevated levels of these hormones in postmenopausal women.

Pharmacodynamics/Kinetics

Absorption: Well absorbed from the gastrointestinal tract, mucous membranes, and the skin. Average serum estradiol concentrations (C_{avg}) vary by product

Injection: Estradiol valerate and estradiol cypionate are absorbed over several weeks following IM injection

Topical:

Alora: C_{avg}: 41 to 98 pg/mL

Climara: C_{avg}: 22 to 106 pg/mL

Divigel: C_{avg}: 9.8 to 30.5 pg/mL

Elestrin: C_{avg}: 15.4 to 39.2 pg/mL; Exposure increased by 55% with application of sunscreen 10 minutes prior to dose

Estrasorb: Mean serum concentration on day 22 of therapy: ~35 to 65 pg/mL; Exposure increased by ~38% with application of sunscreen 10 minutes prior to estradiol 8.7 mg and exposure increased by ~46% when sunscreen was applied 25 minutes after estradiol application.

Estrogel: C_{avg} on day 14 of therapy: 28.3 pg/mL. C_{max} of estradiol is altered by repeated daily application (for 7 days) of sunscreen (decreased by 16%) or lotion (increased by 73%) when applied 1 hour after the dose.

Evamist: C_{avg}: 19.6 to 30.9 pg/mL

Menostar: C_{avg}: 13.7 pg/mL

Vivelle-Dot: C_{avg}: 34 to 104 pg/mL

Vaginal: Femring: Rapid during the first hour following application, then declines to a steady rate over 3 months; C_{avg}: 40.6 to 76 pg/mL

Distribution: Widely distributed; high concentrations in the sex hormone target organs

Protein binding: Bound to sex hormone-binding globulin and albumin

Metabolism: Hepatic; partial metabolism via CYP3A4 enzymes; estradiol is reversibly converted to estrone and estriol; oral estradiol also undergoes enterohepatic recirculation by conjugation in the liver, followed by excretion of sulfate and glucuronide conjugates into the bile, then hydrolysis in the intestine and estrogen reabsorption. Sulfate conjugates are the primary form found in postmenopausal women. With transdermal application, less estradiol is metabolized leading to higher circulating concentrations of estradiol and lower concentrations of estrone and conjugates.

Excretion: Primarily urine (as estradiol, estrone, estriol and their glucuronide and sulfate conjugates)

Dosing

Adult & Geriatric Note: Estrasorb has been discontinued in the US for more than 1 year.

General dosing guidelines: When treating postmenopausal women, use estrogens for the shortest duration possible at the lowest effective dose consistent with treatment goals. Reevaluate patients as clinically appropriate to determine if treatment is still necessary. Consider use of an estrogen with a progestin in postmenopausal women with a uterus. Women who have had a hysterectomy generally do not need a progestin; however, one may be needed if there is a history of endometriosis. Dosage needs to be adjusted based upon the patient's response.

Breast cancer, metastatic: Oral (Estrace): Males and postmenopausal females: 10 mg 3 times/day or (off-label dosing) postmenopausal women: 2 mg 3 times/day (Ellis 2009)

Hypoestrogenism (female) due to hypogonadism, castration, or primary ovarian failure:

Oral (Estrace): 1 to 2 mg/day; titrate as necessary to control symptoms using minimal effective dose for maintenance therapy

IM: Valerate (Delestrogen): 10 to 20 mg every 4 weeks

Transdermal (Alora, Climara, Vivelle-Dot): Refer to transdermal product-specific dosing (below).

Hypoestrogenism (female) due to hypogonadism: IM: Cypionate (Depo-Estradiol): 1.5 to 2 mg monthly

Osteoporosis prevention (females):

Oral (Estrace): Lowest effective dose has not been determined; doses of 0.5 mg/day in a cyclic regimen for 23 days of a 28-day cycle were used in clinical studies

Transdermal (Alora, Climara, Menostar, Minivelle, Vivelle-Dot): Refer to transdermal product-specific dosing (below).

Prostate cancer, advanced:

IM: Valerate (Delestrogen): 30 mg or more every 1 to 2 weeks

Oral (Estrace): 1 to 2 mg 3 times/day

Vasomotor symptoms associated with menopause:

Note: Attempt to taper or discontinue at 3- to 6-month intervals

Oral (Estrace): 1 to 2 mg daily, adjusted as necessary to limit symptoms; administration should be cyclic (3 weeks on, 1 week off)

IM: Cypionate (Depo-Estradiol): 1 to 5 mg every 3 to 4 weeks

IM: Valerate (Delestrogen): 10 to 20 mg every 4 weeks

Topical emulsion (Estrasorb): 3.48 g applied once daily in the morning

Topical gel:

Divigel: Initial: 0.25 g/day; adjust dose based on patient response.

Elestrin: Initial: 0.87 g/day applied at the same time each day; adjust dose based on patient response.

EstroGel: 1.25 g/day applied at the same time each day

Topical spray (Evamist): Initial: One spray (1.53 mg) per day. Adjust dose based on patient response. Dosing range: 1 to 3 sprays per day.

Transdermal (Alora, Climara, Minivelle, Vivelle-Dot): Refer to transdermal product-specific dosing (below).

Vaginal ring (Femring): Initial: 0.05 mg intravaginally; following insertion, dose is released daily for 3 months. Usual dose: 0.05 mg to 0.1 mg intravaginally every 3 months.

Vulvar and vaginal atrophy associated with menopause:

IM: Valerate (Delestrogen): 10 to 20 mg every 4 weeks. Attempt to taper or discontinue at 3- to 6-month intervals.

Intravaginal: Vaginal ring (Femring): Initial: 0.05 mg intravaginally; following insertion, dose is released daily for 3 months. Usual dose: 0.05 mg to 0.1 mg intravaginally every 3 months. Attempt to taper or discontinue at 3- to 6-month intervals.

Oral (Estrace): 1 to 2 mg/day; administration should be cyclic (3 weeks on, 1 week off). Attempt to taper or discontinue at 3- to 6-month intervals

Topical gel (EstroGel): 1.25 g/day applied at the same time each day

Transdermal (Alora, Climara, Vivelle-Dot): Refer to transdermal product-specific dosing (below).

Transdermal product-specific dosing:

Note: Indicated dose may be used continuously in patients without a uterus. Continuous or cyclic schedules (3 weeks on, 1 week off) may be used in women with a uterus (indication and product specific; refer to manufacturers labeling). When changing patients from oral to transdermal therapy, start transdermal patch 1 week after discontinuing oral hormone (may begin sooner if symptoms reappear within 1 week):

Hypoestrogenism (female) due to hypogonadism, castration, or primary ovarian failure: Adjust dose as necessary to control symptoms.

Alora: Initial: Initial: Apply 0.05 mg/day patch *twice* weekly.

Climara: Initial: Apply 0.025 mg/day patch *once* weekly.

Vivelle-Dot: Initial: Apply 0.025 mg/day patch *twice* weekly.

Osteoporosis prevention (female):

Alora, Minivelle, Vivelle-Dot: Initial: Apply 0.025 mg/day patch *twice* weekly. Adjust dose as necessary

Climara: Initial: Apply 0.025 mg/day patch *once* weekly; adjust dosage based on response to therapy.

Menostar: Apply 0.014 mg/day patch *once* weekly. In women with a uterus, also administer a progestin for 14 days every 6 to 12 months.

Vasomotor symptoms associated with menopause:

Note: Adjust dose as necessary. Attempt to taper or discontinue at 3- to 6-month intervals.

Alora: Initial: Apply 0.05 mg/day patch *twice* weekly.

Climara: Initial: Apply 0.025 mg/day patch *once* weekly.

Minivelle, Vivelle-Dot: Initial: Apply 0.0375 mg/day patch *twice* weekly.

Vulvar and vaginal atrophy associated with menopause: Note: Adjust dose as necessary. Attempt to taper or discontinue at 3- to 6-month intervals.

Alora: Initial: Apply 0.05 mg/day patch *twice* weekly.

Climara: Initial: Apply 0.025 mg/day patch *once* weekly.

Vivelle-Dot: Initial: Apply 0.0375 mg/day patch *twice* weekly.

Renal Impairment For most products, there are no dosage adjustments provided in the manufacturer's labeling (has not been studied).

Hepatic Impairment For most products, there are no dosage adjustments provided in the manufacturer's labeling (has not been studied); use is contraindicated with hepatic dysfunction or disease

Dietary Considerations Ensure adequate calcium and vitamin D intake when used for the prevention of osteoporosis.

Administration The use of a progestin should be considered when administering estrogens to postmenopausal women with a uterus.

Injection formulation: Intramuscular use only.

Estradiol cypionate: Shake or gently warm vial to redissolve crystals that may have formed during storage.

Estradiol valerate: Should be injected into the upper outer quadrant of the gluteal muscle; administer with a dry needle (solution may become cloudy with wet needle).

Emulsion (Estrasorb): For topical use only; not for ophthalmic, oral, or vaginal use. Do not apply to face or breasts. Apply to clean, dry skin while in a sitting position. Contents of two pouches (total 3.48 g) are to be applied individually, once daily in the morning. Apply contents of first pouch to left thigh; massage into skin of left thigh and calf until thoroughly absorbed. Apply contents of second pouch to the right thigh; massage into skin of right thigh and calf until thoroughly absorbed. Wash hands with soap and water after application. Allow skin to dry before covering legs with clothing.

Gel: Apply to clean, dry, unbroken skin at the same time each day. Wash hands after application. Gel is flammable; avoid fire or flame until skin is dry.

Divigel: Do not apply to face, breasts, vaginal area or irritated skin. The entire contents of packet should be applied to right or left upper thigh each day (alternate sites). Apply over an area ~5 x 7 inches. Do not wash application site for 1 hour. Allow gel to dry before dressing.

Elestrin: Do not apply to breasts or vaginal area. The entire dose should be applied to upper arm and shoulder area using two fingers to spread gel. Allow skin to dry for ≥5 minutes prior to dressing. Prior to first use, pump must be primed. After priming, the pump contains 30 metered doses; discard pump after 30 doses even though container may not be empty. If >1 dose is needed, wait 5 seconds before pumping next dose. To avoid secondary exposure, do not allow others to contact the application site for 2 hours after gel is applied. Allow at least 2 hours between applying gel and going swimming. Wait at least 25 minutes before applying sunscreen to application area. When sunscreen and gel are applied to the same site for >7 consecutive days, the absorption of estradiol is increased; do not apply sunscreen to an area where the gel was applied for ≥7 consecutive days.

EstroGel: Do not apply to breasts or vaginal area. Apply dose into the palm of hand and then apply gel to the other arm, from the wrist to the shoulder. Spread gel as thinly as possible over one arm but do not massage or rub in gel. Allow skin to dry for 5 minutes before dressing. Prior to first use, pump must be primed. After priming, the pump contains 32 daily doses (50 g canister) or 14 daily doses (25 g canister). Discard pump after allotted doses even though container may not be empty. To avoid secondary exposure, do not allow others to contact the application site for ≥1 hour after gel is applied. Wait as long as possible between applying gel and going swimming.

Spray: Evamist: Prior to first use, prime pump by spraying 3 sprays with the cover on. To administer dose, hold container upright and vertical and rest the plastic cone flat against the skin while spraying. Spray to the inner surface of the forearm, starting near the elbow. If more than one spray is needed, apply to adjacent but not overlapping areas. Apply at the same time each day. Allow spray to dry for ~2 minutes; do not rub into skin; do not cover with clothing until dry. Do not wash application site for at least 60 minutes. Apply to clean, dry, unbroken skin. Do not apply to skin other than that of the forearm. Make sure that children do not come in contact with any skin area where the drug was applied. If contact with children is unavoidable, wear a garment with long sleeves that covers the site of application. If

direct exposure should occur, wash the child in the area of exposure with soap and water as soon as possible. Solution contained in the spray is flammable; avoid fire, flame, or smoking until spray has dried. If needed, sunscreen should be applied ~1 hour prior to application of Evamist.

Transdermal patch: General administration instructions (also refer to product labeling): Apply patch immediately after removing from protective pouch to lower abdomen or buttocks. Apply to clean, dry, healthy skin that is free of oil, powder, or lotion. Avoid waistline or other areas where tight clothing may rub the patch off; do not apply to breasts. After application, hold patch in place using palm of hand for 10 seconds. Rotate application sites allowing a 1-week interval between applications at a particular site. In general, if patch falls off, the same patch may be reapplied or a new system may be used for the remainder of the dosing interval. When replacing patch, reapply to a new site. Remove patch slowly after use to avoid skin irritation. If any adhesive remains on the skin after removal, first allow skin to dry for 15 minutes, then gently rub area with an oil-based cream or lotion. Dispose of any used or unused patches by folding adhesive ends together, replace in pouch or sealed container, and discard properly in trash away from children and pets.

Climara, Menostar: Swimming, bathing, or wearing patch while in a sauna have not been studied

Vaginal ring: Exact positioning is not critical for efficacy; however, patient should not feel anything once inserted. In case of discomfort, ring should be pushed further into vagina. If ring is expelled prior to 90 days, it may be rinsed off with warm water and reinserted. Ensure proper vaginal placement of the ring to avoid inadvertent urinary bladder insertion. If vaginal infection develops, Femring may remain in place during local treatment of a vaginal infection.

Hazardous agent; use appropriate precautions for handling and disposal (NIOSH 2014 [group 2]).

Monitoring Parameters Routine physical examination that includes blood pressure and Papanicolaou smear, breast exam, mammogram. Monitor for signs of endometrial cancer in female patients with a uterus. Adequate diagnostic measures, including endometrial sampling, if indicated, should be performed to rule out malignancy in all cases of undiagnosed abnormal genital bleeding. Monitor for loss of vision, sudden onset of proptosis, diplopia, migraine; signs and symptoms of thromboembolic disorders; glycemic control in patients with diabetes; lipid profiles in patients being treated for hyperlipidemias; thyroid function in patients on thyroid hormone replacement therapy.

Menostar: When used in a woman with a uterus, endometrial sampling is recommended at yearly intervals or when clinically indicated.

Menopausal symptoms, vulvar and vaginal atrophy: Assess need for therapy at 3- to 6-month intervals

Prevention of osteoporosis: Bone density measurement

Note: Monitoring of FSH and serum estradiol is not useful when managing vasomotor symptoms associated with menopause or vulvar and vaginal atrophy.

Test Interactions Reduced response to metyrapone test.

Product Availability Estrasorb has been discontinued in the US for more than 1 year.

Dosage Forms Excipient information presented when available (limited, particularly for generics); consult specific product labeling. [DSC] = Discontinued product

Emulsion, Transdermal, as hemihydrate:

Estrasorb: 4.35 mg/1.74 g (1.74 g [DSC]) [contains polysorbate 80, soybean oil]

Gel, Transdermal:

Divigel: 0.25 mg/0.25 g (1 ea); 0.5 mg/0.5 g (1 ea); 1 mg/g (1 g) [contains propylene glycol, trolamine (triethanolamine)]

Elestrin: 0.06% (26 g) [contains edetate disodium, propylene glycol, trolamine (triethanolamine)]

Estrogel: 0.06% (50 g) [contains alcohol, usp, trolamine (triethanolamine)]

Oil, Intramuscular, as cypionate:

Depo-Estradiol: 5 mg/mL (5 mL)

Oil, Intramuscular, as valerate:

Delestrogen: 10 mg/mL (5 mL) [contains chlorobutanol (chlorobutol), sesame oil]

Delestrogen: 20 mg/mL (5 mL); 40 mg/mL (5 mL) [contains benzyl alcohol]

Generic: 10 mg/mL (5 mL [DSC]); 20 mg/mL (5 mL); 40 mg/mL (5 mL)

◄

Patch Twice Weekly, Transdermal:
Alora: 0.025 mg/24 hr (1 ea, 8 ea); 0.05 mg/24 hr (1 ea, 8 ea); 0.075 mg/24 hr (1 ea, 8 ea); 0.1 mg/24 hr (1 ea, 8 ea)
Minivelle: 0.025 mg/24 hr (8 ea); 0.0375 mg/24 hr (8 ea); 0.05 mg/24 hr (8 ea); 0.075 mg/24 hr (8 ea); 0.1 mg/24 hr (8 ea)
Vivelle-Dot: 0.025 mg/24 hr (8 ea); 0.0375 mg/24 hr (1 ea, 8 ea); 0.05 mg/24 hr (1 ea, 8 ea); 0.075 mg/24 hr (1 ea, 8 ea); 0.1 mg/24 hr (1 ea, 8 ea)
Generic: 0.025 mg/24 hr (8 ea); 0.0375 mg/24 hr (8 ea); 0.05 mg/24 hr (8 ea); 0.075 mg/24 hr (8 ea); 0.1 mg/24 hr (8 ea)
Patch Weekly, Transdermal:
Climara: 0.025 mg/24 hr (4 ea); 0.0375 mg/24 hr (4 ea); 0.05 mg/24 hr (1 ea, 4 ea); 0.06 mg/24 hr (4 ea); 0.075 mg/24 hr (4 ea); 0.1 mg/24 hr (1 ea, 4 ea)
Menostar: 14 mcg/24 hr (4 ea)
Generic: 0.025 mg/24 hr (4 ea); 0.0375 mg/24 hr (4 ea); 0.05 mg/24 hr (4 ea); 0.06 mg/24 hr (4 ea); 0.075 mg/24 hr (4 ea); 0.1 mg/24 hr (4 ea)
Ring, Vaginal, as acetate:
Femring: 0.05 mg/24 hr (1 ea); 0.1 mg/24 hr (1 ea)
Solution, Transdermal:
Evamist: 1.53 mg/spray (8.1 mL)
Tablet, Oral:
Estrace: 0.5 mg, 1 mg, 2 mg [scored]
Generic: 0.5 mg, 1 mg, 2 mg

Estradiol (Topical) (es tra DYE ole)

Brand Names: US Estrace; Estring; Vagifem
Brand Names: Canada Estrace; Estring; Vagifem; Vagifem10
Index Terms 17β-estradiol
Pharmacologic Category Estrogen Derivative
Use Vulvar and vaginal atrophy associated with menopause: Treatment of moderate-to-severe vulvar and vaginal atrophy associated with menopause
Dosing
Adult & Geriatric *General dosing guidelines:* When treating postmenopausal women, use estrogens for the shortest duration possible at the lowest effective dose consistent with treatment goals. Reevaluate patients as clinically appropriate to determine if treatment is still necessary. Consider use of an estrogen with a progestin in postmenopausal women with a uterus. Women who have had a hysterectomy generally do not need a progestin; however one may be needed if there is a history of endometriosis. Dosage needs to be adjusted based upon the patient's response
Vulvar and vaginal atrophy associated with menopause: Intravaginal:
Vaginal cream (Estrace): Insert 2 to 4 g daily intravaginally for 1 to 2 weeks, then gradually reduce to ½ the initial dose for 1 to 2 weeks, followed by a maintenance dose of 1 g 1 to 3 times per week. Attempt to taper or discontinue at 3- to 6-month intervals.
Vaginal ring (Estring): 2 mg intravaginally; following insertion, ring should remain in place for 90 days
Vaginal tablet (Vagifem): Initial: Insert 1 tablet (10 mcg) once daily for 2 weeks; Maintenance: Insert 1 tablet twice weekly
Renal Impairment There are no dosage adjustments provided in the manufacturer's labeling (has not been studied).
Hepatic Impairment There are no dosage adjustments provided in the manufacturer's labeling (has not been studied); use is contraindicated with hepatic impairment or disease.
Additional Information Complete prescribing information should be consulted for additional detail.
Dosage Forms Excipient information presented when available (limited, particularly for generics); consult specific product labeling.
Cream, Vaginal:
Estrace: 0.1 mg/g (42.5 g)
Ring, Vaginal, as base:
Estring: 2 mg (1 ea)
Tablet, Vaginal, as base:
Vagifem: 10 mcg

◆ Estradiol Acetate *see* Estradiol (Systemic) *on page 681*

Estradiol and Dienogest
(es tra DYE ole & dye EN oh jest)

Brand Names: US Natazia®
Index Terms Dienogest and Estradiol; Estradiol Valerate and Dienogest

Pharmacologic Category Contraceptive; Estrogen and Progestin Combination
Use Prevention of pregnancy; treatment of heavy menstrual bleeding
Dosing
Adult Contraception or treatment of heavy menstrual bleeding: Females: Oral: Take 1 tablet daily in the order presented in the blister pack
Initial dosing: Start on day 1 of menstrual period (first day of bleeding). A nonhormonal contraceptive should be used for the first 9 days.
Switching from another combination oral contraceptive tablet: Take the first dark yellow tablet on the first day of withdrawal bleeding; do not continue taking tablets from previous contraceptive pack. If withdrawal bleeding does not occur, rule-out pregnancy before starting therapy. A nonhormonal contraceptive should be used for the first 9 days.
Switching from a vaginal ring or patch: Take the first dark yellow tablet on the day the ring or patch is removed. A nonhormonal contraceptive should be used for the first 9 days.
Switching from a progestin-only contraceptive: Take the first dark yellow tablet on the day of the next progestin-only tablet would have been given, or the day the progestin implant or IUD is removed, or on the day the next injection would have been given. A nonhormonal contraceptive should be used for the first 9 days.

Missed doses: If ≤12 hours late, take tablet as soon as remembering and take the next tablet at the usual time. If >12 hours late, instructions vary by day of cycle and number of tablets missed:
If missed ONE dose:
Days 1-17: Take missed tablet immediately; take next tablet at usual time; use back-up (nonhormonal) contraception for the next 9 days; continue taking 1 tablet each day for the rest of the cycle
Days 18-24: Do not continue using current blister pack (throw away); take day 1 of new blister pack; use back-up (nonhormonal) contraception for the next 9 days; continue taking 1 tablet each day for the rest of the cycle
Days 25-28: Take missed tablet immediately; take next tablet at usual time; continue taking 1 tablet each day for the rest of the cycle; no backup method of contraception is needed.
If missed TWO doses in a row:
Days 1-17: Do not take missed tablets; start by taking the tablet for the day it was first noticed that the tablet was missed; use back-up (nonhormonal) contraception for the next 9 days; continue taking 1 tablet each day for the rest of the cycle. If tablets were missed on days 17 and 18, follow directions for missed tablets on days 17-25.
Days 17-25: Do not continue using current blister pack (throw away); take day 3 of new blister pack; use back-up (nonhormonal) contraception for the next 9 days; continue taking 1 tablet each day for the rest of the cycle. If tablets were missed on days 25 and 26, follow directions for missed tablets on days 25-28.
Days 25-28: Do not continue using current blister pack (throw away); start a new pack on the same day, or start a new pack the day it would normally be started; continue taking 1 tablet each day for the rest of the cycle; no backup method of contraception is needed.
Pediatric Contraception: Oral: Refer to adult dosing. Not to be used prior to menarche.
Renal Impairment Safety and efficacy have not been evaluated; dose adjustment not expected to be required.
Hepatic Impairment Use is contraindicated with hepatic disease. Discontinue if hepatic dysfunction occurs.
Additional Information Complete prescribing information should be consulted for additional detail.
Dosage Forms Excipient information presented when available (limited, particularly for generics); consult specific product labeling.
Tablet, oral [four-phasic formulation]:
Natazia®:
Days 1-2: Estradiol valerate 3 mg [2 dark yellow tablets]
Days 3-7: Estradiol valerate 2 mg and dienogest 2 mg [5 medium red tablets]
Days 8-24: Estradiol valerate 2 mg and dienogest 3 mg [17 light yellow tablets]
Days 25-26: Estradiol valerate 1 mg [2 dark red tablets]
Days 27-28: 2 white inactive tablets (28s)

Estradiol and Levonorgestrel
(es tra DYE ole & LEE voe nor jes trel)

Brand Names: US ClimaraPro
Index Terms Levonorgestrel and Estradiol

Pharmacologic Category Estrogen and Progestin Combination

Use

Moderate to severe vasomotor symptoms: Treatment of moderate to severe vasomotor symptoms associated with menopause in women with an intact uterus

Osteoporosis prevention: Prevention of postmenopausal osteoporosis in women with an intact uterus

Limitations of use: Osteoporosis: For use only in women at significant risk of osteoporosis and for whom other nonestrogen medications are not considered appropriate

Dosing

Adult & Geriatric Note: Patients should be treated with the lowest effective dose and for the shortest duration, consistent with treatment goals.

Treatment of moderate to severe vasomotor symptoms associated with menopause or prevention of postmenopausal osteoporosis: Adult females with an intact uterus: Transdermal: Estradiol 0.045 mg/levonorgestrel 0.015 mg: Apply one patch weekly. When used for the treatment of vasomotor symptoms associated with menopause, evaluate to see if therapy is still needed/attempt to discontinue every 3-6 months.

Renal Impairment No dosage adjustment provided in manufacturer's labeling. Total estradiol serum concentrations may be excessive in women with end stage renal disease receiving hemodialysis.

Hepatic Impairment Use is contraindicated in women with hepatic impairment or disease.

Additional Information Complete prescribing information should be consulted for additional detail.

Dosage Forms Excipient information presented when available (limited, particularly for generics); consult specific product labeling.

Patch, transdermal:

ClimaraPro: Estradiol 0.045 mg and levonorgestrel 0.015 mg per 24 hours (4s) [22 cm²; contains estradiol 4.4 mg and levonorgestrel 1.39 mg]

Estradiol and Norethindrone

(es tra DYE ole & nor eth IN drone)

Brand Names: US Activella; CombiPatch; Lopreeza; Mimvey; Mimvey Lo

Brand Names: Canada Activelle; Activelle LD; Estalis

Index Terms Norethindrone and Estradiol

Pharmacologic Category Estrogen and Progestin Combination

Use

Hypoestrogenism (female): (patch): Treatment of hypoestrogenism due to hypogonadism, castration, or primary ovarian failure

Osteoporosis prevention (females): (tablet): Prevention of postmenopausal osteoporosis

Vasomotor symptoms associated with menopause: (patch, tablet): Treatment of moderate to severe vasomotor symptoms associated with menopause

Vulvar and vaginal atrophy associated with menopause: (patch, tablet): Treatment of moderate to severe vulvar and vaginal atrophy associated with menopause

Limitations of use: These combination products are indicated for women with a uterus. When used for osteoporosis, use only in women at significant risk of postmenopausal osteoporosis; consider use of nonestrogen medications. When used solely for the treatment of vulvar and vaginal atrophy, topical vaginal products should be considered.

Dosing

Adult & Geriatric *General dosing guidelines:* Females: These combination products are indicated for women with a uterus. When treating postmenopausal women, use for the shortest duration possible at the lowest effective dose consistent with treatment goals. Reevaluate patients as clinically appropriate to determine if treatment is still necessary. Consider use of an estrogen with a progestin in postmenopausal women with a uterus. Women who have had a hysterectomy generally do not need a progestin; however, one may be needed if there is a history of endometriosis. Dosage needs to be adjusted based upon the patient's response.

Hypoestrogenism: Transdermal:

CombiPatch: Estradiol 0.05 mg/norethindrone acetate 0.14 mg per day or estradiol 0.05 mg/norethindrone acetate 0.25 mg per day

Continuous combined regimen: Apply 1 patch twice weekly

Continuous sequential regimen: Apply estradiol-only patch for first 14 days of cycle, followed by 1 CombiPatch applied twice weekly for the remaining 14 days of a 28-day cycle.

Osteoporosis prevention: Oral

Activella, Lopreeza: Estradiol 1 mg/norethindrone 0.5 mg or estradiol 0.5 mg/norethindrone 0.1 mg: One tablet daily

Mimvey: Estradiol 1 mg/norethindrone 0.5 mg: One tablet daily

Mimvey Lo: Estradiol 0.5 mg/norethindrone 0.1 mg: One tablet daily

Vasomotor symptoms associated with menopause: Oral:

Activella, Lopreeza: Estradiol 1 mg/norethindrone 0.5 mg or estradiol 0.5 mg/norethindrone 0.1 mg: One tablet daily

Activelle [Canadian product]: Estradiol 1 mg/norethindrone 0.5 mg: One tablet daily

Activelle LD [Canadian product]: Estradiol 0.5 mg/ norethindrone 0.1 mg: One tablet daily

Mimvey: Estradiol 1 mg/norethindrone 0.5 mg: One tablet daily

Mimvey Lo: Estradiol 0.5 mg/norethindrone 0.1 mg: One tablet daily

Transdermal: Estradiol 0.05 mg/norethindrone acetate 0.14 mg per day or estradiol 0.05 mg/norethindrone acetate 0.25 mg per day

CombiPatch:

Continuous combined regimen: Apply 1 patch twice weekly

Continuous sequential regimen: Apply estradiol-only patch for first 14 days of cycle, followed by 1 CombiPatch applied twice weekly for the remaining 14 days of a 28-day cycle.

Estalis [Canadian product]: Continuous combined regimen: Apply a new patch twice weekly during a 28-day cycle

Vulvar and vaginal atrophy associated with menopause:

Oral: Activella, Activelle [Canadian product], Lopreeza, Mimvey: Estradiol 1 mg/norethindrone 0.5 mg: One tablet daily

Transdermal: Estradiol 0.05 mg/norethindrone acetate 0.14 mg per day or estradiol 0.05 mg/norethindrone acetate 0.25 mg per day

CombiPatch:

Continuous combined regimen: Apply 1 patch twice weekly

Continuous sequential regimen: Apply estradiol-only patch for first 14 days of cycle, followed by 1 CombiPatch applied twice weekly for the remaining 14 days of a 28-day cycle.

Estalis [Canadian product]: Continuous combined regimen: Apply a new patch twice weekly during a 28-day cycle

Renal Impairment There are no dosage adjustments provided in the manufacturer's labeling (has not been studied); use with caution.

Hepatic Impairment Use is contraindicated with hepatic dysfunction or disease.

Additional Information Complete prescribing information should be consulted for additional detail.

Dosage Forms Excipient information presented when available (limited, particularly for generics); consult specific product labeling.

Patch, transdermal:

CombiPatch:

0.05/0.14: Estradiol 0.05 mg and norethindrone acetate 0.14 mg per day (8s) [9 sq cm]

0.05/0.25: Estradiol 0.05 mg and norethindrone acetate 0.25 mg per day (8s) [16 sq cm]

Tablet, oral: 0.5/0.1: Estradiol 0.5 mg and norethindrone acetate 0.1 mg (28s); 1/0.5: Estradiol 1 mg and norethindrone acetate 0.5 mg (28s)

Activella: 0.5/0.1: Estradiol 0.5 mg and norethindrone acetate 0.1 mg (28s)

Activella: 1/0.5: Estradiol 1 mg and norethindrone acetate 0.5 mg (28s)

Lopreeza: 0.5/0.1: Estradiol 0.5 mg and norethindrone acetate 0.1 mg (28s)

Lopreeza: 1/0.5: Estradiol 1 mg and norethindrone acetate 0.5 mg (28s)

Mimvey: 1/0.5: Estradiol 1 mg and norethindrone acetate 0.5 mg (28s)

Mimvey Lo: Estradiol 0.5 mg and norethindrone acetate 0.1 mg (28s)

◄ **Dosage Forms: Canada** Excipient information presented when available (limited, particularly for generics); consult specific product labeling.

Patch, transdermal:

Estalis:

140/50: Norethindrone acetate 140 mcg and estradiol 50 mcg per day (8s) [9 sq cm; total norethindrone acetate 2.7 mg, total estradiol 0.62 mg]

250/50 Norethindrone acetate 250 mcg and estradiol 50 mcg per day (8s) [16 sq cm; total norethindrone acetate 4.8 mg, total estradiol 0.51 mg]

Tablet, oral:

Activelle: Estradiol 1 mg and norethindrone acetate 0.5 mg

Activelle LD: Estradiol 0.5 mg and norethindrone acetate 0.1 mg

◆ **Estradiol Transdermal** see Estradiol (Systemic) on page 681

◆ **Estradiol Valerate** see Estradiol (Systemic) on page 681

◆ **Estradiol Valerate and Dienogest** see Estradiol and Dienogest on page 686

◆ **Estradot (Can)** see Estradiol (Systemic) on page 681

◆ **Estragyn (Can)** see Estrogens (Esterified) on page 693

Estramustine (es tra MUS teen)

Brand Names: US Emcyt
Brand Names: Canada Emcyt
Index Terms Estramustine Phosphate; Estramustine Phosphate Sodium
Pharmacologic Category Antineoplastic Agent, Alkylating Agent; Antineoplastic Agent, Antimicrotubular; Antineoplastic Agent, Hormone (Estrogen/Nitrogen Mustard)

Use

Prostate cancer: Treatment (palliative) of progressive or metastatic prostate cancer

Limitation of use: A clinical practice guideline from the American Society of Clinical Oncology (ASCO) and Cancer Care Ontario recommends that estramustine not be offered to men with metastatic castration-resistant prostate cancer due to a lack of benefit in survival or quality of life (Basch, 2014).

Dosing

Adult & Geriatric Note: Estramustine is associated with a moderate emetic potential; antiemetics are recommended to prevent nausea and vomiting.

Prostate cancer, progressive or metastatic: Males: Oral: 14 mg/kg/day (range: 10-16 mg/kg/day) in 3 or 4 divided doses

Renal Impairment There are no dosage adjustments provided in the manufacturer's labeling; use with caution.

Hepatic Impairment There are no dosage adjustments provided in the manufacturer's labeling; use with caution (may be poorly metabolized).

Obesity *ASCO Guidelines for appropriate chemotherapy dosing in obese adults with cancer:* Utilize patient's actual body weight (full weight) for calculation of body surface area- or weight-based dosing, particularly when the intent of therapy is curative; manage regimen-related toxicities in the same manner as for nonobese patients; if a dose reduction is utilized due to toxicity, consider resumption of full weight-based dosing with subsequent cycles, especially if cause of toxicity (eg, hepatic or renal impairment) is resolved (Griggs, 2012).

Additional Information Complete prescribing information should be consulted for additional detail.

Dosage Forms Excipient information presented when available (limited, particularly for generics); consult specific product labeling.

Capsule, Oral, as phosphate sodium:

Emcyt: 140 mg

◆ **Estramustine Phosphate** see Estramustine on page 688

◆ **Estramustine Phosphate Sodium** see Estramustine on page 688

◆ **Estrasorb [DSC]** see Estradiol (Systemic) on page 681

◆ **Estratab® (Can)** see Estrogens (Esterified) on page 693

◆ **Estring** see Estradiol (Topical) on page 686

◆ **Estrogel** see Estradiol (Systemic) on page 681

◆ **EstroGel (Can)** see Estradiol (Systemic) on page 681

◆ **Estrogenic Substances, Conjugated** see Estrogens (Conjugated/Equine, Systemic) on page 690

◆ **Estrogenic Substances, Conjugated** see Estrogens (Conjugated/Equine, Topical) on page 693

Estrogens (Conjugated B/Synthetic)

(ES troe jenz, KON joo gate ed, bee, sin THET ik)

Brand Names: US Enjuvia
Pharmacologic Category Estrogen Derivative

Use

Vasomotor symptoms associated with menopause: Treatment of moderate to severe vasomotor symptoms associated with menopause

Vulvar and vaginal atrophy associated with menopause: Treatment of moderate to severe vaginal dryness and pain with intercourse, symptoms of vulvar and vaginal atrophy, associated with menopause

Limitations of use: When used solely for the treatment of vulvar and vaginal atrophy, topical vaginal products should be considered.

Pregnancy Considerations Use is contraindicated in pregnant women. In general, the use of estrogen and progestin as in combination hormonal contraceptives have not been associated with teratogenic effects when inadvertently taken early in pregnancy.

Breast-Feeding Considerations Estrogens can be detected in breast milk and have been shown to decrease the quantity and quality of human milk. The manufacturer recommends that caution be used if administered to nursing women.

Contraindications Hypersensitivity to estrogens or any component of the formulation; undiagnosed abnormal genital bleeding; DVT or PE (current or history of); active or history of arterial thromboembolic disease (eg, stroke, MI); breast cancer (known, suspected or history of); estrogen-dependent tumor (known or suspected); liver impairment or disease; known protein C, protein S, antithrombin deficiency or other known thrombophilic disorders; pregnancy

Warnings/Precautions Hazardous agent - use appropriate precautions for handling and disposal (NIOSH 2014 [group 2]).

[U.S. Boxed Warning]: Based on data from the Women's Health Initiative (WHI) studies, an increased risk of invasive breast cancer was observed in postmenopausal women using conjugated estrogens (CE) in combination with medroxyprogesterone acetate (MPA). This risk may be associated with duration of use and declines once combined therapy is discontinued (Chlebowski 2009). The risk of invasive breast cancer was decreased in postmenopausal women with a hysterectomy using CE only, regardless of weight. However, the risk was not significantly decreased in women at high risk for breast cancer (family history of breast cancer, personal history of benign breast disease) (Anderson 2012). An increase in abnormal mammogram findings has also been reported with estrogen alone or in combination with progestin therapy. Estrogen use may also lead to severe hypercalcemia in patients with breast cancer and bone metastases; discontinue estrogen if hypercalcemia occurs. Use is contraindicated in patients with known or suspected breast cancer.

[US Boxed Warning]: Estrogens with or without progestin should not be used to prevent cardiovascular disease. Using data from the Women's Health Initiative (WHI) studies, an increased risk of deep vein thrombosis (DVT) and stroke has been reported with CE and an increased risk of DVT, stroke, pulmonary emboli (PE) and myocardial infarction (MI) has been reported with CE with MPA in postmenopausal women 50 to 79 years of age. Additional risk factors include diabetes mellitus, hypercholesterolemia, hypertension, SLE, obesity, tobacco use, and/or history of venous thromboembolism (VTE). Risk factors should be managed appropriately; discontinue use immediately if adverse cardiovascular events occur or are suspected. Use is contraindicated in women with active DVT or PE (or a history of these conditions) or in women with active or recent arterial thromboembolic disease (stroke and MI), or a history of these conditions. Women with inherited thrombophilias (eg, protein C or S deficiency) may have increased risk of venous thromboembolism (DeSancho 2010; van Vlijmen 2011). Use is contraindicated in women with protein C, protein S, antithrombin deficiency, or other known thrombophilic disorders. Estrogen compounds are generally associated with lipid effects such as increased HDL-cholesterol and decreased LDL-cholesterol. Triglycerides may also be increased in women with preexisting hypertriglyceridemia; discontinue if pancreatitis occurs.

[US Boxed Warning]: Estrogens with or without pro-gestin should not be used to prevent dementia. In the Women's Health Initiative Memory Study (WHIMS), an increased incidence of probable dementia was observed in women ≥65 years of age taking CE alone or in combination with MPA.

[US Boxed Warning]: The use of unopposed estrogen in women with a uterus is associated with an increased risk of endometrial cancer. The addition of a progestin to estrogen therapy may decrease the risk of endometrial hyperplasia, a precursor to endometrial cancer. Adequate diagnostic measures, including endometrial sampling if indicated, should be per-formed to rule out malignancy in postmenopausal women with undiagnosed abnormal vaginal bleeding. There is no evidence that the use of natural estrogens results in a different endometrial risk profile than synthetic estrogens at equivalent estrogen doses. The risk of endo-metrial cancer appears to be dose and duration depend-ent; risk appears to be greatest with use ≥5 years and may persist following discontinuation of therapy. Estrogens may exacerbate endometriosis. Malignant transformation of residual endometrial implants has been reported posthys-terectomy with unopposed estrogen therapy. Consider adding a progestin in women with residual endometriosis posthysterectomy. Postmenopausal estrogens with or without progestins may increase the risk of ovarian cancer; however, the absolute risk to an individual woman is small. Although results from various studies are not consistent, risk does not appear to be significantly associated with the duration, route, or dose of therapy. In one study, the risk decreased after 2 years following discontinuation of ther-apy (Mørch 2009). Although the risk of ovarian cancer is rare, women who are at an increased risk (eg, family history) should be counseled about the association (NAMS 2012).

[US Boxed Warning]: Estrogens with or without pro-gestin should be used for the shortest duration possi-ble at the lowest effective dose consistent with treatment goals and risks for the individual woman. Hormone therapy for menopausal symptoms is generally initiated in healthy symptomatic women within 10 years of menopause or <60 years of age who do not have contra-indications for use (Stuenkel 2015). Patients should be reevaluated as clinically appropriate to determine if treat-ment is still necessary. Available data related to treatment risks are from Women's Health Initiative (WHI) studies, which evaluated oral CE 0.625 mg with or without MPA 2.5 mg relative to placebo in postmenopausal women. Other combinations and dosage forms of estrogens and progestins were not studied. **Outcomes reported from clinical trials using CE with or without MPA should be assumed to be similar for other doses and other dosage forms of estrogens and progestins until com-parable data becomes available.** Women who are early in menopause, who are in good cardiovascular health, and who are at low risk for adverse cardiovascular events can be considered candidates for estrogen with or without progestin therapy for the relief of menopausal symptoms (ACOG 565 2013). Women at high risk of cardiovascular disease or intermediate to high risk of breast cancer should receive nonhormonal therapy to treat vasomotor symp-toms of menopause (Stuenkel 2015). Use of a transdermal product should be considered over an oral agent in women requiring systemic therapy who have moderate risk factors for coronary heart disease (ACOG 556 2013; Schenck-Gustafsson 2011; Stuenkel 2015). Nonoral routes of ther-apy are recommended for women at increased risk for venous thromboembolism (Stuenkel 2015; Tremol-lieres 2011).

Estrogens may cause retinal vascular thrombosis; discon-tinue if migraine, loss of vision, proptosis, diplopia, or other visual disturbances occur; discontinue permanently if pap-illedema or retinal vascular lesions are observed on exami-nation. Use caution in patients with asthma, epilepsy, hepatic hemangiomas, hereditary angioedema, migraine, porphyria or SLE; may exacerbate disease. May have adverse effects on glucose tolerance; use caution in women with diabetes. Use with caution in patients with diseases that may be exacerbated by fluid retention, including cardiac or renal dysfunction. Use of postmeno-pausal estrogen may be associated with an increased risk of gallbladder disease requiring surgery. Estrogens are poorly metabolized in patients with hepatic dysfunction. Use caution with a history of cholestatic jaundice associ-ated with prior estrogen use or pregnancy. Discontinue if jaundice develops or if acute or chronic hepatic disturban-ces occur. Use is contraindicated with hepatic impairment or disease. Use caution with hypoparathyroidism; estro-gen-induced hypocalcemia may occur.

Potentially significant interactions may exist, requiring dose or frequency adjustment, additional monitoring, and/ or selection of alternative therapy. Estrogens may increase thyroid-binding globulin (TBG) levels leading to increased circulating total thyroid hormone levels. Women on thyroid replacement therapy may require higher doses of thyroid hormone while receiving estrogens. The use of estrogens and/or progestins may change the results of some labo-ratory tests (eg, coagulation factors, lipids, glucose toler-ance, binding proteins). The dose, route, and the specific estrogen/progestin influence these changes. In addition, personal risk factors (eg, cardiovascular disease, smoking, diabetes, age) also contribute to adverse events; use of specific products may be contraindicated in women with certain risk factors.

Avoid use of oral estrogen (with or without progestins) in elderly patients due to potential of increased risk of breast and endometrial cancers, and lack of proven cardioprotec-tion and cognitive protection (Beers Criteria). Although hormone therapy is recommended to be initiated in healthy symptomatic women within 10 years of menopause or <60 years of age who do not have contraindications for use, symptoms may continue in women >60 years of age. The continuation of hormone therapy in women >65 years of age should consider the risks and benefits for the individ-ual woman and should not be discontinued only because of the woman's age (NAMS 2015).

Whenever possible, estrogens should be discontinued at least 4 to 6 weeks prior to elective surgery associated with an increased risk of thromboembolism or during periods of prolonged immobilization.

Vulvar and vaginal atrophy use: Moderate to severe symp-toms of vulvar and vaginal atrophy include vaginal dry-ness, dyspareunia, and atrophic vaginitis. [The combined condition of vulvovaginal atrophy and urinary tract dysfunc-tion is also referred to as genitourinary syndrome of menopause (GSM) (Portman 2014; Stuenkel 2015)]. When used solely for the treatment of vulvar and vaginal atrophy, topical vaginal products should be considered (NAMS 2012; NAMS 2013; Stuenkel 2015).

Adverse Reactions

>10%:

Central nervous system: Headache (25%), pain (10% to 19%)

Gastrointestinal: Abdominal pain (4% to 15%), nausea (10% to 12%)

Genitourinary: Mastalgia (13% to 15%)

1% to 10%:

Cardiovascular: Peripheral edema (4%), chest pain (3% to 4%)

Central nervous system: Dizziness (7%), paresthesia (1% to 6%), chills (4%), depression (3% to 4%), emo-tional lability (3% to 4%)

Dermatologic: Pruritus (6%), fungal dermatitis (2% to 4%), acne vulgaris (1% to 4%)

Gastrointestinal: Flatulence (4% to 7%), constipa-tion (4%)

Genitourinary: Dysmenorrhea (8%), vaginitis (7%), breast tenderness (4%)

Neuromuscular & skeletal: Paresthesia (≤6%), back pain (4%), weakness (3% to 4%)

Respiratory: Bronchitis (7%), rhinitis (7%), flu-like symp-toms (6% to 7%), sinusitis (4% to 7%), increased cough (4%), upper respiratory tract infection (4%), pharyngitis (3% to 4%)

Miscellaneous: Accidental injury (9%)

<1% (Limited to important or life-threatening): Abdominal distention, abdominal distress, alopecia, anaphylaxis, deep vein thrombosis, dementia, gallbladder disease, hypercalcemia, hypersensitivity, insomnia, malignant neoplasm, muscle spasm, skin rash, thrombosis, urtica-ria, visual disturbance

Drug Interactions

Metabolism/Transport Effects Substrate of CYP3A4 (major); **Note:** Assignment of Major/Minor substrate sta-tus based on clinically relevant drug interaction potential

Avoid Concomitant Use

Avoid concomitant use of Estrogens (Conjugated B/Syn-thetic) with any of the following: Anastrozole; Dehydroe-piandrosterone; Exemestane; Hemin; Indium 111 Capromab Pendetide; Ospemifene

Increased Effect/Toxicity

Estrogens (Conjugated B/Synthetic) may increase the levels/effects of: Anthrax Immune Globulin (Human); C1 inhibitors; Corticosteroids (Systemic); Immune Globulin; Lenalidomide; Ospemifene; ROPINIRole; Thalidomide; Theophylline Derivatives; Tipranavir

The levels/effects of Estrogens (Conjugated B/Synthetic) may be increased by: Ascorbic Acid; Dehydroepiandrosterone; Herbs (Estrogenic Properties); NSAID (COX-2 Inhibitor); Osimertinib

Decreased Effect

Estrogens (Conjugated B/Synthetic) may decrease the levels/effects of: Anastrozole; Anticoagulants; Antidiabetic Agents; Chenodiol; Exemestane; Hemin; Hyaluronidase; Indium 111 Capromab Pendetide; Ospemifene; Somatropin; Thyroid Products; Ursodiol

The levels/effects of Estrogens (Conjugated B/Synthetic) may be decreased by: Bosentan; CYP3A4 Inducers (Moderate); CYP3A4 Inducers (Strong); Dabrafenib; Deferasirox; Enzalutamide; Mitotane; Osimertinib; Siltuximab; St Johns Wort; Tipranavir; Tocilizumab

Food Interactions Routine use of ethanol increases estrogen level and risk of breast cancer. Management: Avoid ethanol.

Storage/Stability Store at room temperature of 20°C to 25°C (68°F to 77°F).

Mechanism of Action Conjugated B/synthetic estrogens contain a mixture of 10 synthetic estrogen substances, including sodium estrone sulfate, sodium equilin sulfate, sodium 17-alpha-dihydroequilin, sodium 17-alpha-estradiol, and sodium 17-beta-dihydroequilin. Estrogens are responsible for the development and maintenance of the female reproductive system and secondary sexual characteristics. Estradiol is the principle intracellular human estrogen and is more potent than estrone and estriol at the receptor level; it is the primary estrogen secreted prior to menopause. Following menopause, estrone and estrone sulfate are more highly produced. Estrogens modulate the pituitary secretion of gonadotropins, luteinizing hormone, and follicle-stimulating hormone through a negative feedback system; estrogen replacement reduces elevated levels of these hormones in postmenopausal women.

Pharmacodynamics/Kinetics

Absorption: Well absorbed over a period of several hours
Protein-binding: Sex hormone-binding globulin (SHBG) and albumin
Metabolism: Hepatic via CYP3A4; estradiol is converted to estrone and estriol; also undergoes enterohepatic recirculation; estrone sulfate is the main metabolite in postmenopausal women
Half-life elimination: Conjugated estrone: 8-20 hours; conjugated equilin: 5-17 hours
Excretion: Urine (primarily estriol, also as estradiol, estrone, and conjugates)

Dosing

Adult & Geriatric

General dosing guidelines: When treating postmenopausal women, use estrogens for the shortest duration possible at the lowest effective dose consistent with treatment goals. Reevaluate patients as clinically appropriate to determine if treatment is still necessary. Consider use of an estrogen with a progestin in postmenopausal women with a uterus. Women who have had a hysterectomy generally do not need a progestin; however, one may be needed if there is a history of endometriosis. Dosage needs to be adjusted based upon the patient's response.

Vasomotor symptoms associated with menopause: Oral: Initial: 0.3 mg/day

Vulvar and vaginal atrophy associated with menopause: Oral: 0.3 mg/day

Renal Impairment There are no dosage adjustments provided in the manufacturer's labeling (has not been studied).

Hepatic Impairment Use is contraindicated with hepatic impairment or disease.

Administration Administer at the same time each day. May be taken with or without food. Hazardous agent; use appropriate precautions for handling and disposal (NIOSH 2014 [group 2]).

Monitoring Parameters

Routine physical examination that includes blood pressure and Papanicolaou smear, breast exam, mammogram. Monitor for signs of endometrial cancer in female patients with uterus. Adequate diagnostic measures, including endometrial sampling, if indicated, should be performed to rule out malignancy in all cases of undiagnosed abnormal genital bleeding. Monitor for loss of vision, sudden onset of proptosis, diplopia, migraine; signs and symptoms of thromboembolic disorders; glycemic control in patients with diabetes; lipid profiles in patients being treated for hyperlipidemias; thyroid function in patients on thyroid hormone replacement therapy. Assess need for therapy periodically (eg, 3- to 6-month intervals).

Note: Monitoring of FSH and serum estradiol is not useful when managing vasomotor symptoms associated with menopause or vulvar and vaginal atrophy.

Dosage Forms Excipient information presented when available (limited, particularly for generics); consult specific product labeling.

Tablet, Oral:
Enjuvia: 0.3 mg, 0.45 mg, 0.625 mg [contains edetate disodium, polysorbate 80]
Enjuvia: 0.9 mg [contains edetate disodium, fd&c blue #1 aluminum lake, fd&c yellow #10 aluminum lake, fd&c yellow #6 aluminum lake, polysorbate 80]
Enjuvia: 1.25 mg [contains edetate disodium, polysorbate 80]

Estrogens (Conjugated/Equine, Systemic) (ES troe jenz KON joo gate ed, EE kwine)

Brand Names: US Premarin
Brand Names: Canada C.E.S.; Congest; PMS-Conjugated Estrogens C.S.D.; Premarin
Index Terms C.E.S.; CE; CEE; Conjugated Estrogen; Estrogenic Substances, Conjugated
Pharmacologic Category Estrogen Derivative

Use

Abnormal uterine bleeding (injection only): Treatment of abnormal uterine bleeding due to hormonal imbalance in the absence of organic pathology.
Limitations of use: For short term use only to provide a rapid and temporary increase in estrogen levels.

Breast cancer, metastatic: Treatment of breast cancer (palliation) in appropriately selected men and postmenopausal women.

Hypoestrogenism (female): Treatment of hypoestrogenism due to hypogonadism, castration, or primary ovarian failure.

Osteoporosis prevention (female): Prevention of postmenopausal osteoporosis.
Limitations of use: For use only in women at significant risk of osteoporosis; consider use of non-estrogen medications.

Prostate cancer, advanced: Treatment of androgen-dependent prostatic cancer (palliation).

Vasomotor symptoms associated with menopause: Treatment of moderate to severe vasomotor symptoms associated with menopause.

Vulvar and vaginal atrophy associated with menopause: Treatment of moderate to severe vulvar and vaginal atrophy due to menopause.
Limitations of use: When used solely for the treatment of vulvar and vaginal atrophy, topical vaginal products should be considered.

Pregnancy Considerations These products are contraindicated for use during pregnancy. Estrogens are not indicated for use during pregnancy or immediately postpartum. In general, the use of estrogen and progestin as in combination hormonal contraceptives have not been associated with teratogenic effects when inadvertently taken early in pregnancy.

Breast-Feeding Considerations Estrogen has been shown to decrease the quantity and quality of human milk. The manufacturer recommends that caution be used if administered to a nursing woman.

Contraindications

Angioedema or anaphylactic reaction to estrogens or any component of the formulation; undiagnosed abnormal genital bleeding; DVT or PE (current or history of); active or history of arterial thromboembolic disease (eg, stroke, MI); breast cancer (except in appropriately selected patients being treated for metastatic disease); estrogen-dependent tumor (known or suspected); hepatic impairment or disease; known protein C, protein S, antithrombin deficiency or other known thrombophilic disorders; pregnancy

Canadian labeling: Additional contraindications (not in US labeling): Endometrial hyperplasia; partial or complete vision loss due to ophthalmic vascular disease; migraine with or without aura

Warnings/Precautions Hazardous agent - use appropriate precautions for handling and disposal (NIOSH 2014 [group 2]).

Anaphylaxis requiring emergency medical management has been reported within minutes to hours of taking conjugated estrogen (CE) tablets. Angioedema involving the face, feet, hands, larynx, and tongue has also been reported. Exogenous estrogens may exacerbate symptoms in women with hereditary angioedema.

[US Boxed Warning]: Based on data from the Women's Health Initiative (WHI) studies, an increased risk of invasive breast cancer was observed in postmenopausal women using conjugated estrogens (CE) in combination with medroxyprogesterone acetate (MPA). This risk may be associated with duration of use and declines once combined therapy is discontinued (Chlebowski 2009). The risk of invasive breast cancer was decreased in postmenopausal women with a hysterectomy using CE only, regardless of weight. However, the risk was not significantly decreased in women at high risk for breast cancer (family history of breast cancer, personal history of benign breast disease) (Anderson 2012). An increase in abnormal mammogram findings has also been reported with estrogen alone or in combination with progestin therapy. Estrogen use may lead to severe hypercalcemia in patients with breast cancer and bone metastases; discontinue estrogen if hypercalcemia occurs. Postmenopausal estrogens with or without progestins may increase the risk of ovarian cancer; however, the absolute risk to an individual woman is small. Although results from various studies are not consistent, risk does not appear to be significantly associated with the duration, route, or dose of therapy. In one study, the risk decreased after 2 years following discontinuation of therapy (Mørch 2009). Although the risk of ovarian cancer is rare, women who are at an increased risk (eg, family history) should be counseled about the association (NAMS 2012).

[US Boxed Warning]: Estrogens with or without progestin should not be used to prevent cardiovascular disease. Using data from the Women's Health Initiative (WHI) studies, an increased risk of deep vein thrombosis (DVT) and stroke has been reported with CE and an increased risk of DVT, stroke, pulmonary emboli (PE) and myocardial infarction (MI) has been reported with CE with MPA in postmenopausal women 50 to 79 years of age. Additional risk factors include diabetes mellitus, hypercholesterolemia, hypertension, SLE, obesity, tobacco use, and/or history of venous thromboembolism (VTE). Risk factors should be managed appropriately; discontinue use if adverse cardiovascular events occur or are suspected. Use is contraindicated in women with active DVT, PE, active arterial thromboembolic disease or a history of these conditions.

[US Boxed Warning]: Estrogens with or without progestin should not be used to prevent dementia. In the Women's Health Initiative Memory Study (WHIMS), an increased incidence of probable dementia was observed in women ≥65 years of age taking CE alone or in combination with MPA.

[US Boxed Warning]: The use of unopposed estrogen in women with a uterus is associated with an increased risk of endometrial cancer. The addition of a progestin to estrogen therapy may decrease the risk of endometrial hyperplasia, a precursor to endometrial cancer. Adequate diagnostic measures, including endometrial sampling if indicated, should be performed to rule out malignancy in postmenopausal women with undiagnosed abnormal vaginal bleeding. There is no evidence that the use of natural estrogens results in a different endometrial risk profile than synthetic estrogens at equivalent estrogen doses. The risk of endometrial cancer is dose and duration dependent; risk appears to be greatest with use ≥5 years and may persist following discontinuation of therapy. The use of a progestin is not generally required when low doses of estrogen are used locally for vaginal atrophy (NAMS 2012; NAMS 2013). Estrogens may exacerbate endometriosis. Malignant transformation of residual endometrial implants has been reported posthysterectomy with unopposed estrogen therapy. Consider adding a progestin in women with residual endometriosis posthysterectomy.

[US Boxed Warning]: Estrogens with or without progestin should be used for the shortest duration possible at the lowest effective dose consistent with treatment goals and risks for the individual woman. Patients should be reevaluated as clinically appropriate to determine if treatment is still necessary. Available data related to treatment risks are from Women's Health Initiative (WHI) studies, which evaluated oral CE 0.625 mg with or without MPA 2.5 mg relative to placebo in postmenopausal women. Other combinations and dosage forms of estrogens and progestins were not studied. Outcomes reported from clinical trials using CE with or without MPA should be assumed to be similar for other doses and other dosage forms of estrogens and progestins until comparable data becomes available. Women who are early in menopause, who are in good cardiovascular health, and who are at low risk for adverse cardiovascular events can be considered candidates for estrogen with or without progestin therapy for the relief of menopausal symptoms (ACOG 565 2013). Use of a transdermal product should be considered over an oral agent in women requiring systemic therapy who have risk factors for venous thromboembolism or coronary heart disease (ACOG 556 2013; Schenck-Gustafsson 2011; Tremollieres 2011).

Women with inherited thrombophilias (eg, protein C or S deficiency) may have increased risk of venous thromboembolism (DeSancho 2010; van Vlijmen 2011). Use is contraindicated in women with protein C, protein S, antithrombin deficiency, or other known thrombophilic disorders. Estrogen compounds are generally associated with lipid effects such as increased HDL-cholesterol and decreased LDL-cholesterol. Triglycerides may also be increased in women with preexisting hypertriglyceridemia; discontinue if pancreatitis occurs. The use of estrogens and/or progestins may change the results of some laboratory tests (eg, coagulation factors, lipids, glucose tolerance, binding proteins). The dose, route, and the specific estrogen/progestin influence these changes. In addition, personal risk factors (eg, cardiovascular disease, smoking, diabetes, age) also contribute to adverse events; use of specific products may be contraindicated in women with certain risk factors. Estrogens may increase thyroid-binding globulin (TBG) levels leading to increased circulating total thyroid hormone levels. Women on thyroid replacement therapy may require higher doses of thyroid hormone while receiving estrogens. Potentially significant interactions may exist, requiring dose or frequency adjustment, additional monitoring, and/or selection of alternative therapy.

Estrogens may cause retinal vascular thrombosis; discontinue if migraine, loss of vision, proptosis, diplopia, or other visual disturbances occur; discontinue permanently if papilledema or retinal vascular lesions are observed on examination. Use caution with asthma, epilepsy, hepatic hemangiomas, migraine, porphyria, SLE; may exacerbate disease. Canadian labeling contraindicates use in migraine with aura. May have adverse effects on glucose tolerance; use caution in women with diabetes. Use caution with diseases which may be exacerbated by fluid retention, including cardiac or renal dysfunction. Use of postmenopausal estrogen may be associated with an increased risk of gallbladder disease requiring surgery. Estrogens are poorly metabolized in patients with hepatic dysfunction. Use caution with a history of cholestatic jaundice associated with prior estrogen use or pregnancy. Discontinue if jaundice develops or if acute or chronic hepatic disturbances occur. Use is contraindicated with hepatic impairment or disease. Use caution with hypoparathyroidism; estrogen-induced hypocalcemia may occur.

Whenever possible, estrogens should be discontinued at least 4 to 6 weeks prior to elective surgery associated with an increased risk of thromboembolism or during periods of prolonged immobilization.

Avoid oral and transdermal patch estrogen products (with or without progestins) in the elderly due to potential of increased risk of breast and endometrial cancers, and lack of proven cardioprotection and cognitive protection (Beers Criteria).

Prior to puberty, estrogens may cause premature closure of the epiphyses. Premature breast development, vaginal bleeding and vaginal cornification may be induced in girls. Modification of the normal puberty process may occur in boys.

Osteoporosis use: For use only in women at significant risk of osteoporosis and for who other nonestrogen medications are not considered appropriate.

Vulvar and vaginal atrophy use: Moderate-to-severe symptoms of vulvar and vaginal atrophy include vaginal dryness, dyspareunia, and atrophic vaginitis. When used solely for the treatment of vulvar and vaginal atrophy, topical vaginal products should be considered. Use caution applying topical products to severely atrophic vaginal mucosa. Use of a progestin is normally not required when low-dose estrogen is applied locally and only for this purpose (NAMS 2012; NAMS 2013).

Benzyl alcohol and derivatives: Some dosage forms may contain benzyl alcohol; large amounts of benzyl alcohol (≥99 mg/kg/day) have been associated with a potentially fatal toxicity ("gasping syndrome") in neonates; the "gasping syndrome" consists of metabolic acidosis, respiratory distress, gasping respirations, CNS dysfunction (including convulsions, intracranial hemorrhage), hypotension and cardiovascular collapse (AAP ["Inactive" 1997]; CDC, 1982); some data suggests that benzoate displaces bilirubin from protein binding sites (Ahlfors 2001); avoid or use

dosage forms containing benzyl alcohol with caution in neonates. See manufacturer's labeling.

Adverse Reactions Note: Percentages reported in postmenopausal women following oral use.

>10%:

Central nervous system: Headache (26% to 32%; placebo 28%), pain (17% to 20%; placebo 18%)

Endocrine & metabolic: Breast pain (7% to 12%; placebo 9%)

Gastrointestinal: Abdominal pain (15% to 17%), diarrhea (6% to 7%; placebo 6%)

Genitourinary: Vaginal hemorrhage (2% to 14%)

Neuromuscular & skeletal: Back pain (13% to 14%), arthralgia (7% to 14%; placebo 12%)

Respiratory: Pharyngitis (10% to 12%; placebo 11%), sinusitis: (6% to 11%; placebo 7%)

1% to 10%:

Central nervous system: Depression (5% to 8%), dizziness (4% to 6%), nervousness (2% to 5%)

Dermatologic: Pruritus (4% to 5%)

Gastrointestinal: Flatulence (6% to 7%)

Genitourinary: Vaginitis (5% to 7%), leukorrhea (4% to 7%), vaginal moniliasis (5% to 6%)

Neuromuscular & skeletal: Weakness (7% to 8%), leg cramps (3% to 7%)

Respiratory: Cough increased (4% to 7%)

Additional adverse reactions reported with injection; frequency not defined: Local: injection site: Edema, pain, phlebitis

Postmarketing and/or case reports: Alopecia, anaphylaxis, angioedema, asthma exacerbation, benign meningioma (possible growth), bloating, breast cancer, breast discharge/enlargement/tenderness, cervical secretion changes, chloasma, cholestatic jaundice, contact lens intolerance, dementia, deep vein thrombosis (DVT), dysmenorrhea, edema, endometrial cancer, endometrial hyperplasia, epilepsy exacerbation, erythema multiforme, erythema nodosum, fibrocystic breast changes, galactorrhea, gallbladder disease, glucose intolerance, gynecomastia (males), hepatic hemangiomas (enlargement), hirsutism, hypersensitivity reactions, hypertension, irritability, ischemic colitis, libido changes, melasma, MI, migraine, mood disturbances, nausea, ovarian cancer, pancreatitis, pulmonary emboli (PE), pelvic pain, porphyria exacerbation, rash, retinal vascular thrombosis, stroke, superficial venous thrombosis, thrombophlebitis, triglyceride increase, urticaria, uterine bleeding (abnormal), uterine leiomyomata (increase in size), vaginal candidiasis, vomiting, weight changes

Drug Interactions

Metabolism/Transport Effects Substrate of CYP1A2 (major), CYP2A6 (minor), CYP2B6 (minor), CYP2C19 (minor), CYP2C9 (minor), CYP2D6 (minor), CYP2E1 (minor), CYP3A4 (major); **Note:** Assignment of Major/Minor substrate status based on clinically relevant drug interaction potential; **Inhibits** CYP1A2 (weak)

Avoid Concomitant Use

Avoid concomitant use of Estrogens (Conjugated/Equine, Systemic) with any of the following: Anastrozole; Dehydroepiandrosterone; Exemestane; Hemin; Indium 111 Capromab Pendetide; Ospemifene

Increased Effect/Toxicity

Estrogens (Conjugated/Equine, Systemic) may increase the levels/effects of: Anthrax Immune Globulin (Human); C1 inhibitors; Corticosteroids (Systemic); Immune Globulin; Lenalidomide; Ospemifene; ROPINIRole; Thalidomide; Theophylline Derivatives; Tipranavir; TiZANidine

The levels/effects of Estrogens (Conjugated/Equine, Systemic) may be increased by: Ascorbic Acid; Dehydroepiandrosterone; Herbs (Estrogenic Properties); NSAID (COX-2 Inhibitor); Osimertinib

Decreased Effect

Estrogens (Conjugated/Equine, Systemic) may decrease the levels/effects of: Anastrozole; Anticoagulants; Antidiabetic Agents; Chenodiol; Exemestane; Hemin; Hyaluronidase; Indium 111 Capromab Pendetide; Ospemifene; Somatropin; Thyroid Products; Ursodiol

The levels/effects of Estrogens (Conjugated/Equine, Systemic) may be decreased by: Bosentan; Cannabis; CYP1A2 Inducers (Strong); CYP3A4 Inducers (Moderate); CYP3A4 Inducers (Strong); Cyproterone; Dabrafenib; Deferasirox; Enzalutamide; Mitotane; Osimertinib; Siltuximab; St Johns Wort; Teriflunomide; Tipranavir; Tocilizumab

Food Interactions Folic acid absorption may be decreased. Routine use of ethanol increases estrogen level and risk of breast cancer; may also increase the risk of osteoporosis. Management: Avoid ethanol.

Preparation for Administration Injection: Reconstitute with sterile water for injection; slowly inject diluent against side wall of the vial. Agitate gently; do not shake violently.

Hazardous agent; use appropriate precautions for handling and disposal (NIOSH 2014 [group 2]).

Storage/Stability

Injection: Refrigerate at 2°C to 8°C (36°F to 46°F) prior to reconstitution. Use immediately following reconstitution.

Tablets: Store at room temperature 20°C to 25°C (68°F to 77°F).

Mechanism of Action Conjugated estrogens contain a mixture of estrone sulfate, equilin sulfate, 17 alpha-dihydroequilin, 17 alpha-estradiol and 17 beta-dihydroequilin. Estrogens are responsible for the development and maintenance of the female reproductive system and secondary sexual characteristics. Estradiol is the principle intracellular human estrogen and is more potent than estrone and estriol at the receptor level; it is the primary estrogen secreted prior to menopause. Following menopause, estrone and estrone sulfate are more highly produced. Estrogens modulate the pituitary secretion of gonadotropins, luteinizing hormone, and follicle-stimulating hormone through a negative feedback system; estrogen replacement reduces elevated levels of these hormones in postmenopausal women.

Pharmacodynamics/Kinetics

Absorption: Well absorbed

Distribution: Widely distributes throughout the body; sex hormone target organs contain higher concentrations

Protein binding: Binds to sex-hormone-binding globulin and albumin

Metabolism: Hepatic via CYP3A4; estradiol is converted to estrone and estriol; estrone is also converted to estriol and is converted to estradiol (**Note:** A dynamic equilibrium of metabolic interconversions between estrogens exists in the circulation); also undergoes enterohepatic recirculation (avoided with vaginal administration); estrone sulfate is the main metabolite in postmenopausal women

Half-life elimination: Total estrone: 27 hours

Time to peak, plasma: Total estrone: 7 hours

Excretion: Urine (primarily estriol, also as estradiol, estrone, and conjugates)

Dosing

Adult & Geriatric *General dosing guidelines:* When treating postmenopausal women, use estrogens for the shortest duration possible at the lowest effective dose consistent with treatment goals. Reevaluate patients as clinically appropriate to determine if treatment is still necessary. Consider use of an estrogen with a progestin in postmenopausal women with a uterus. Women who have had a hysterectomy generally do not need a progestin; however one may be needed if there is a history of endometriosis. Dosage needs to be adjusted based upon the patient's response

Abnormal uterine bleeding: Acute/heavy bleeding: IM, IV: 25 mg, may repeat in 6-12 hours if needed (manufacturer's labeling) **or** 25 mg IV repeated every 4 to 6 hours for 24 hours (ACOG 557 2013).

Breast cancer, metastatic: Oral: Males and postmenopausal females: 10 mg 3 times/day for at least 3 months

Hypoestrogenism (female) due to castration or primary ovarian failure: Oral: 1.25 mg/day given cyclically*; adjust according to severity of symptoms and patient response. For maintenance, adjust to the lowest effective dose.

Hypoestrogenism (female) due to hypogonadism: Oral: 0.3 or 0.625 mg/day given cyclically*; dose may be titrated in 6- to 12-month intervals; progestin treatment should be added to maintain bone mineral density once skeletal maturity is achieved.

Osteoporosis prevention (females): Oral: Initial: 0.3 mg/day cyclically* or daily, depending on medical assessment of patient. Dose may be adjusted based on bone mineral density and clinical response. The lowest effective dose should be used.

Prostate cancer, advanced: Oral: 1.25 to 2.5 mg 3 times/day

Uremic bleeding (off-label use): IV: 0.6 mg/kg/day for 5 days (Heistinger 1990; Livio 1986; Viganò 1988)

Vasomotor symptoms associated with menopause: Oral: Initial: 0.3 mg/day. May be given cyclically* or daily, depending on medical assessment of patient. Adjust dose based on patient's response. The lowest dose that will control symptoms should be used.

Vulvar and vaginal atrophy associated with menopause: Oral: Initial: 0.3 mg/day. The lowest dose that will control symptoms should be used. May be given cyclically* or daily, depending on medical assessment of patient. Adjust dose based on patient's response.

***Cyclic administration:** Either 3 weeks on, 1 week off **or** 25 days on, 5 days off

Pediatric Adolescents: Refer to adult dosing.

Renal Impairment There are no dosage adjustments provided in the manufacturer's labeling (has not been studied).

Hepatic Impairment There are no dosage adjustments provided in the manufacturer's labeling (has not been studied). Use is contraindicated with hepatic dysfunction or disease.

Dietary Considerations Ensure adequate calcium and vitamin D intake when used for the prevention of osteoporosis. Powder for reconstitution for injection (25 mg) contains lactose 200 mg.

Administration

Injection: May be administered IV or IM; when administered IV, drug should be administered slowly to avoid the occurrence of a flushing reaction

Oral tablet: Administer at the same time each day. May be administered without regard to meals.

Abnormal uterine bleeding: High-dose therapy (eg, 10 to 20 mg/day) may cause nausea; consider concomitant use of an antiemetic

Hazardous agent; use appropriate precautions for handling and disposal (NIOSH 2014 [group 2]).

Monitoring Parameters Routine physical examination that includes blood pressure and Papanicolaou smear, breast exam, mammogram. Monitor for signs of endometrial cancer in female patients with uterus. Adequate diagnostic measures, including endometrial sampling, if indicated, should be performed to rule out malignancy in all cases of undiagnosed abnormal genital bleeding. Monitor for loss of vision, sudden onset of proptosis, diplopia, migraine; signs and symptoms of thromboembolic disorders; glycemic control in patients with diabetes; lipid profiles in patients being treated for hyperlipidemias; thyroid function in patients on thyroid hormone replacement therapy.

Menopausal symptoms: Assess need for therapy at 3- to 6-month intervals

Prevention of osteoporosis: Bone density measurement

Uremic bleeding: Bleeding time

Note: Monitoring of FSH and serum estradiol is not useful when managing vasomotor symptoms associated with menopause or vulvar and vaginal atrophy.

Test Interactions Reduced response to metyrapone test.

Dosage Forms Excipient information presented when available (limited, particularly for generics); consult specific product labeling.

Solution Reconstituted, Injection:

Premarin: 25 mg (1 ea) [contains benzyl alcohol]

Tablet, Oral:

Premarin: 0.3 mg [contains fd&c blue #2 (indigotine), fd&c yellow #10 (quinoline yellow)]

Premarin: 0.45 mg [contains fd&c blue #2 (indigotine)]

Premarin: 0.625 mg [contains fd&c blue #2 (indigotine), fd&c red #40]

Premarin: 0.9 mg

Premarin: 1.25 mg [contains fd&c yellow #10 (quinoline yellow), fd&c yellow #6 (sunset yellow)]

Estrogens (Conjugated/Equine, Topical) (ES troe jenz KON joo gate ed, EE kwine)

Brand Names: US Premarin

Brand Names: Canada Premarin®

Index Terms C.E.S.; CE; CEE; Conjugated Estrogen; Estrogenic Substances, Conjugated

Pharmacologic Category Estrogen Derivative

Use Vulvar and vaginal atrophy associated with menopause: Treatment of atrophic vaginitis and kraurosis vulvae and moderate-to-severe dyspareunia (pain during intercourse) due to vaginal/vulvar atrophy of menopause

Dosing

Adult & Geriatric

General dosing guidelines: When treating postmenopausal women, use estrogens for the shortest duration possible at the lowest effective dose consistent with treatment goals. Reevaluate patients as clinically appropriate to determine if treatment is still necessary. Consider use of an estrogen with a progestin in postmenopausal women with a uterus. Women who have had a hysterectomy generally do not need a progestin; however one may be needed if there is a history of endometriosis. Dosage needs to be adjusted based upon the patient's response.

Vulvar and vaginal atrophy associated with menopause:

Atrophic vaginitis, kraurosis vulvae: Adult females: Intravaginal: 0.5 g/day (range 0.5 to 2 g/day) administered cyclically (21 days on, 7 days off). Adjust dose based on patient response.

Moderate-to-severe dyspareunia due to menopause: Adult females: Intravaginal: 0.5 g twice weekly (eg, Monday and Thursday) **or** once daily cyclically (21 days on, 7 days off)

Renal Impairment There are no dosage adjustments provided in the manufacturer's labeling (has not been studied).

Hepatic Impairment There are no dosage adjustments provided in the manufacturer's labeling (has not been studied). Use is contraindicated with hepatic dysfunction or disease.

Additional Information Complete prescribing information should be consulted for additional detail.

Dosage Forms Excipient information presented when available (limited, particularly for generics); consult specific product labeling. [DSC] = Discontinued product

Cream, Vaginal:

Premarin: 0.625 mg/g (30 g, 42.5 g [DSC]) [contains benzyl alcohol, cetyl alcohol, propylene glycol monostearate]

Estrogens (Conjugated/Equine) and Bazedoxifene (ES troe jenz, KON joo gate ed/EE kwine & ba ze DOX i feen)

Brand Names: US Duavee

Index Terms Bazedoxifene and Estrogens (Conjugated/Equine); Estrogens (Conjugated/Equine) and Bazedoxifene Acetate

Pharmacologic Category Estrogen Derivative; Selective Estrogen Receptor Modulator (SERM); Tissue-Selective Estrogen Complex (TSEC)

Use

Postmenopausal osteoporosis prophylaxis: Prevention of postmenopausal osteoporosis in women with a uterus

Vasomotor symptoms: Treatment of moderate-to-severe vasomotor symptoms associated with menopause in women with a uterus

Dosing

Adult Menopause (moderate-to-severe vasomotor symptoms), prevention of postmenopausal osteoporosis: Females: Oral: One tablet daily

Geriatric Refer to adult dosing. Use in women >75 years of age is not recommended (has not been studied).

Renal Impairment No dosage adjustment provided in manufacturer's labeling (has not been studied). Use is not recommended.

Hepatic Impairment Use is contraindicated with hepatic dysfunction or disease.

Additional Information Complete prescribing information should be consulted for additional detail.

Dosage Forms

Tablet, oral:

Duavee: Conjugated estrogens 0.45 mg and bazedoxifene 20 mg

◆ Estrogens (Conjugated/Equine) and Bazedoxifene Acetate see Estrogens (Conjugated/Equine) and Bazedoxifene on page 693

Estrogens (Esterified) (ES troe jenz, es TER i fied)

Brand Names: US Menest

Brand Names: Canada Estragyn; Estratab®; Menest®

Index Terms Esterified Estrogens

Pharmacologic Category Estrogen Derivative

Use Treatment of moderate-to-severe vasomotor symptoms associated with menopause; treatment of moderate-to-severe vulvar and vaginal atrophy associated with menopause; hypoestrogenism (due to hypogonadism, castration, or primary ovarian failure); advanced prostatic cancer (palliation), metastatic breast cancer (palliation) in men and postmenopausal women

Pregnancy Considerations In general, the use of estrogen and progestin as in combination hormonal contraceptives have not been associated with teratogenic effects when inadvertently taken early in pregnancy. This product is contraindicated for use during pregnancy.

Breast-Feeding Considerations Estrogen has been shown to decrease the quantity and quality of human milk; use only if clearly needed; monitor the growth of the infant closely.

Contraindications Hypersensitivity to estrogens or any component of the formulation; undiagnosed abnormal vaginal bleeding; DVT or PE (current or history of); active or recent (within 1 year) arterial thromboembolic disease (eg, stroke, MI); carcinoma of the breast (known, suspected or history of), except in appropriately selected patients being treated for metastatic disease; estrogen-dependent tumor; hepatic dysfunction or disease; pregnancy

◀ **Warnings/Precautions** Hazardous agent - use appropriate precautions for handling and disposal (NIOSH 2014 [group 2]).

[U.S. Boxed Warning]: Based on data from the Women's Health Initiative (WHI) studies, an increased risk of invasive breast cancer was observed in postmenopausal women using conjugated estrogens (CE) in combination with medroxyprogesterone acetate (MPA). This risk may be associated with duration of use and declines once combined therapy is discontinued (Chlebowski, 2009). The risk of invasive breast cancer was decreased in postmenopausal women with a hysterectomy using CE only, regardless of weight. However, the risk was not significantly decreased in women at high risk for breast cancer (family history of breast cancer, personal history of benign breast disease) (Anderson, 2012). An increase in abnormal mammogram findings has also been reported with estrogen alone or in combination with progestin therapy. Estrogen use may also lead to severe hypercalcemia in patients with breast cancer and bone metastases; discontinue estrogen if hypercalcemia occurs.

[U.S. Boxed Warning]: The use of unopposed estrogen in women with an intact uterus is associated with an increased risk of endometrial cancer. The addition of a progestin to estrogen therapy may decrease the risk of endometrial hyperplasia, a precursor to endometrial cancer. Adequate diagnostic measures, including endometrial sampling if indicated, should be performed to rule out malignancy in postmenopausal women with undiagnosed abnormal vaginal bleeding. Estrogens may exacerbate endometriosis. Malignant transformation of residual endometrial implants has been reported posthysterectomy with unopposed estrogen therapy. Consider adding a progestin in women with residual endometriosis posthysterectomy. Postmenopausal estrogen therapy and combined estrogen/progesterone therapy may increase the risk of ovarian cancer; however, the absolute risk to an individual woman is small. Although results from various studies are not consistent, risk does not appear to be significantly associated with the duration, route, or dose of therapy. In one study, the risk decreased after 2 years following discontinuation of therapy (Mørch, 2009). Although the risk of ovarian cancer is rare, women who are at an increased risk (eg, family history) should be counseled about the association (NAMS, 2012).

[U.S. Boxed Warning]: Estrogens with or without progestin should not be used to prevent cardiovascular disease. Using data from the Women's Health Initiative (WHI) studies, an increased risk of deep vein thrombosis (DVT) and stroke has been reported with CE and an increased risk of DVT, stroke, pulmonary emboli (PE) and myocardial infarction (MI) has been reported with CE with MPA in postmenopausal women. Additional risk factors include diabetes mellitus, hypercholesterolemia, hypertension, SLE, obesity, tobacco use, and/or history of venous thromboembolism (VTE). Adverse cardiovascular events have also been reported in males taking estrogens for prostate cancer. Risk factors should be managed appropriately; discontinue use if adverse cardiovascular events occur or are suspected. Women with inherited thrombophilias (eg, protein C or S deficiency) may have increased risk of venous thromboembolism (DeSancho, 2010; van Vlijmen, 2011).

[U.S. Boxed Warning]: Estrogens with or without progestin should not be used to prevent dementia. In the Women's Health Initiative Memory Study (WHIMS), an increased incidence of dementia was observed in women ≥65 years of age taking CE alone or in combination with MPA.

[U.S. Boxed Warning]: Estrogens with or without progestin should be used for the shortest duration possible at the lowest effective dose consistent with treatment goals. Before prescribing estrogen therapy to postmenopausal women, the risks and benefits must be weighed for each patient. Women should be informed of these risks and benefits, as well as possible effects of progestin when added to estrogen therapy. Patients should be reevaluated as clinically appropriate to determine if treatment is still necessary. Available data related to treatment risks are from Women's Health Initiative (WHI) studies, which evaluated oral CE 0.625 mg with or without MPA 2.5 mg relative to placebo in postmenopausal women. Other combinations and dosage forms of estrogens and progestins were not studied. **Outcomes reported from clinical trials using CE with or without MPA should be assumed to be similar for other doses and other dosage forms of estrogens and progestins until comparable data becomes available.**

Estrogen compounds are generally associated with lipid effects such as increased HDL-cholesterol and decreased LDL-cholesterol. Triglycerides may also be increased; use with caution in patients with familial defects of lipoprotein metabolism. Estrogens may increase thyroid-binding globulin (TBG) levels leading to increased circulating total thyroid hormone levels. Women on thyroid replacement therapy may require higher doses of thyroid hormone while receiving estrogens.

Estrogens may cause retinal vascular thrombosis; discontinue if migraine, loss of vision, proptosis, diplopia or other visual disturbances occur; discontinue permanently if papilledema or retinal vascular lesions are observed on examination. Estrogens are poorly metabolized in patients with hepatic dysfunction. Use caution with a history of cholestatic jaundice associated with prior estrogen use or pregnancy. Discontinue if jaundice develops or if acute or chronic hepatic disturbances occur. Use is contraindicated with hepatic disease. Use caution in patients with asthma, epilepsy, hepatic hemangiomas, migraine, porphyria, or SLE; may exacerbate disease. May have adverse effects on glucose tolerance; use caution in women with diabetes. Use with caution in patients with diseases which may be exacerbated by fluid retention, including cardiac or renal dysfunction. Use of postmenopausal estrogen may be associated with an increased risk of gallbladder disease requiring surgery. Use with caution in patients with severe hypocalcemia. Avoid use of oral estrogen (with or without progestins) in the elderly due to potential of increased risk of breast and endometrial cancers, and lack of proven cardioprotection and cognitive protection (Beers Criteria). Prior to puberty, estrogens may cause premature closure of the epiphyses, premature breast development in girls or gynecomastia in boys. Vaginal bleeding and vaginal cornification may also be induced in girls. Whenever possible, estrogens should be discontinued at least 4-6 weeks prior to elective surgery associated with an increased risk of thromboembolism or during periods of prolonged immobilization. The use of estrogens and/or progestins may change the results of some laboratory tests (eg, coagulation factors, lipids, glucose tolerance, binding proteins). The dose, route, and the specific estrogen/progestin influences these changes. In addition, personal risk factors (eg, cardiovascular disease, smoking, diabetes, age) also contribute to adverse events; use of specific products may be contraindicated in women with certain risk factors.

Adverse Reactions Frequency not defined.

Cardiovascular: Edema, hypertension, MI, stroke, venous thromboembolism

Central nervous system: Dementia exacerbation, dizziness, epilepsy exacerbation, headache, irritability, mental depression, migraine, mood disturbances, nervousness

Dermatologic: Angioedema, chloasma, erythema multiforme, erythema nodosum, hemorrhagic eruption, hirsutism, pruritus, loss of scalp hair, melasma, rash, urticaria

Endocrine & metabolic: Breast cancer, breast enlargement, breast tenderness, carbohydrate intolerance, fibrocystic breast changes, galactorrhea, hypocalcemia, libido (changes in), nipple discharge, premenstrual like syndrome

Gastrointestinal: Abdominal cramps, bloating, gallbladder disease, nausea, pancreatitis, vomiting, weight gain/loss

Genitourinary: Alterations in frequency and flow of menstrual patterns, breakthrough bleeding, changes in cervical secretions, cervical ectropion changes, cystitis-like syndrome, dysmenorrhea, endometrial hyperplasia, endometrial cancer, increased size of uterine leiomyomata, ovarian cancer, vaginal candidiasis, vaginitis

Hematologic: Aggravation of porphyria

Hepatic: Cholestatic jaundice, hemangioma enlargement

Local: Thrombophlebitis

Neuromuscular & skeletal: Arthralgia, chorea, leg cramps

Ocular: Contact lens intolerance, corneal curvature steepening, retinal vascular thrombosis

Respiratory: Asthma exacerbation, pulmonary embolism

Miscellaneous: Anaphylactoid/anaphylactic reactions

Drug Interactions

Metabolism/Transport Effects Substrate of CYP1A2 (major), CYP2B6 (minor), CYP2C9 (minor), CYP2E1 (minor), CYP3A4 (major); **Note:** Assignment of Major/Minor substrate status based on clinically relevant drug interaction potential

Avoid Concomitant Use

Avoid concomitant use of Estrogens (Esterified) with any of the following: Anastrozole; Dehydroepiandrosterone; Exemestane; Hemin; Indium 111 Capromab Pendetide; Ospemifene

Increased Effect/Toxicity

Estrogens (Esterified) may increase the levels/effects of: Anthrax Immune Globulin (Human); C1 inhibitors; Corticosteroids (Systemic); Immune Globulin; Lenalidomide; Ospemifene; ROPINIRole; Thalidomide; Theophylline Derivatives; Tipranavir

The levels/effects of Estrogens (Esterified) may be increased by: Ascorbic Acid; Dehydroepiandrosterone; Herbs (Estrogenic Properties); NSAID (COX-2 Inhibitor); Osimertinib

Decreased Effect

Estrogens (Esterified) may decrease the levels/effects of: Anastrozole; Anticoagulants; Antidiabetic Agents; Chenodiol; Exemestane; Hemin; Hyaluronidase; Indium 111 Capromab Pendetide; Ospemifene; Somatropin; Thyroid Products; Ursodiol

The levels/effects of Estrogens (Esterified) may be decreased by: Bosentan; Cannabis; CYP1A2 Inducers (Strong); CYP3A4 Inducers (Moderate); CYP3A4 Inducers (Strong); Cyproterone; Dabrafenib; Deferasirox; Enzalutamide; Mitotane; Osimertinib; Siltuximab; St Johns Wort; Teriflunomide; Tipranavir; Tocilizumab

Food Interactions Folic acid absorption may be decreased. Routine use of ethanol increases estrogen level and risk of breast cancer; may also increase the risk of osteoporosis. Management: Avoid ethanol.

Mechanism of Action Esterified estrogens contain a mixture of estrogenic substances; the principle component is estrone. Preparations contain 75% to 85% sodium estrone sulfate and 6% to 15% sodium equilin sulfate such that the total is not <90%. Estrogens are responsible for the development and maintenance of the female reproductive system and secondary sexual characteristics. Estradiol is the principle intracellular human estrogen and is more potent than estrone and estriol at the receptor level; it is the primary estrogen secreted prior to menopause. In males and following menopause in females, estrone and estrone sulfate are more highly produced. Estrogens modulate the pituitary secretion of gonadotropins, luteinizing hormone, and follicle-stimulating hormone through a negative feedback system; estrogen replacement reduces elevated levels of these hormones.

Pharmacodynamics/Kinetics

Absorption: Readily

Distribution: Widely distributed; high concentrations in the sex hormone target organs

Protein binding: Bound to sex hormone-binding globulin and albumin

Metabolism: Hepatic; partial metabolism via CYP3A4 enzymes; estradiol is reversibly converted to estrone and estriol; oral estradiol also undergoes enterohepatic recirculation by conjugation in the liver, followed by excretion of sulfate and glucuronide conjugates into the bile, then hydrolysis in the intestine and estrogen reabsorption. Sulfate conjugates are the primary form found in postmenopausal women.

Excretion: Primarily urine (as estradiol, estrone, estriol, and their glucuronide and sulfate conjugates)

Dosing

Adult & Geriatric

Prostate cancer, advanced: Oral: 1.25-2.5 mg 3 times/day

Female hypoestrogenism due to hypogonadism: Oral: 2.5-7.5 mg/day in divided doses for 20 days followed by a 10-day rest period. Administer cyclically (3 weeks on and 1 week off). If bleeding does not occur by the end of the 10-day period, repeat the same dosing schedule; the number of courses dependent upon the responsiveness of the endometrium. If bleeding occurs before the end of the 10-day period, begin an estrogen-progestin cyclic regimen of 2.5-7.5 mg/day in divided doses for 20 days; during the last 5 days of estrogen therapy, give an oral progestin. If bleeding occurs before regimen is concluded, discontinue therapy and resume on the fifth day of bleeding.

Female hypoestrogenism due to castration and primary ovarian failure: Oral: 1.25 mg/day, cyclically. Adjust dosage upward or downward, according to the severity of symptoms and patient response. For maintenance, adjust dosage to lowest level that will provide effective control.

Vasomotor symptoms associated with menopause: Oral: 1.25 mg/day administered cyclically (3 weeks on and 1 week off). If patient has not menstruated within the last 2 months or more, cyclic administration is started arbitrary. If the patient is menstruating, cyclical administration is started on day 5 of the bleeding. For short-term use only and should be discontinued as soon as possible. Re-evaluate at 3- to 6-month intervals for tapering or discontinuation of therapy.

Vulvar and vaginal atrophy associated with menopause: Oral: 0.3 to ≥1.25 mg/day, depending on the tissue response of the individual patient. Administer cyclically. For short-term use only and should be discontinued as soon as possible. Re-evaluate at 3- to 6-month intervals for tapering or discontinuation of therapy.

Breast cancer, metastatic (appropriately selected patients): Males and postmenopausal females: Oral: 10 mg 3 times/day for at least 3 months

Renal Impairment No dosage adjustment provided in manufacturer's labeling; use with caution.

Hepatic Impairment No dosage adjustment provided in manufacturer's labeling; use with caution.

Dietary Considerations Should be taken with food at same time each day.

Administration Administer with food at same time each day.

Hazardous agent; use appropriate precautions for handling and disposal (NIOSH 2014 [group 2]).

Monitoring Parameters Routine physical examination that includes blood pressure and Papanicolaou smear, breast exam, mammogram. Monitor for signs of endometrial cancer in female patients with uterus. Adequate diagnostic measures, including endometrial sampling, if indicated, should be performed to rule out malignancy in all cases of undiagnosed abnormal vaginal bleeding. Monitor for loss of vision, sudden onset of proptosis, diplopia, migraine; signs and symptoms of thromboembolic disorders; glycemic control in patients with diabetes; lipid profiles in patients being treated for hyperlipidemias; thyroid function in patients on thyroid hormone replacement therapy.

Menopausal symptoms; vulvar and vaginal atrophy: Assess need for therapy at 3- to 6-month intervals

Test Interactions Reduced response to metyrapone test.

Dosage Forms Excipient information presented when available (limited, particularly for generics); consult specific product labeling.

Tablet, Oral:

Menest: 0.3 mg, 0.625 mg, 1.25 mg, 2.5 mg

Estropipate (ES troe pih pate)

Brand Names: US Ortho-Est 0.625 [DSC]; Ortho-Est 1.25 [DSC]

Brand Names: Canada Ogen [DSC]

Index Terms Ortho Est; Piperazine Estrone Sulfate

Pharmacologic Category Estrogen Derivative

Use

Hypoestrogenism, female: Treatment of hypoestrogenism due to hypogonadism, castration, or primary ovarian failure.

Osteoporosis prevention: Prevention of postmenopausal osteoporosis.

Vasomotor symptoms associated with menopause: Treatment of moderate to severe vasomotor symptoms associated with menopause.

Vulval and vaginal atrophy associated with menopause: Treatment of moderate to severe symptoms of vulval and vaginal atrophy associated with menopause.

Limitations of use: When used solely for the treatment of vulvar and vaginal atrophy, topical vaginal products should be considered. When used for osteoporosis prevention, use only in women at significant risk of postmenopausal osteoporosis; consider use of non-estrogen medications

Dosing

Adult & Geriatric

Female: General dosing guidelines: When treating postmenopausal women, use estrogens for the shortest duration possible at the lowest effective dose consistent with treatment goals. Reevaluate patients as clinically appropriate to determine if treatment is still necessary. Consider use of an estrogen with a progestin in postmenopausal women with a uterus. Women who have had a hysterectomy generally do not need a progestin; however one may be needed if there is a history of endometriosis. Dosage needs to be adjusted based upon the patient's response

Hypoestrogenism (female) due to castration or primary ovarian failure: Oral: 1.5 to 9 mg daily for the first 3 weeks of a theoretical cycle, followed by a rest period of 8 to 10 days

Hypoestrogenism (female) due to hypogonadism: Oral: 1.5 to 9 mg daily for the first 3 weeks of a theoretical cycle, followed by a rest period of 8 to 10 days. Repeat if bleeding does not occur by the end of the rest period. The duration of therapy necessary to product the withdrawal bleeding will vary according to the responsiveness of the endometrium. If satisfactory withdrawal bleeding does not occur, give an oral progestin in addition to estrogen during the third week of the cycle.

Osteoporosis prevention: Oral: 0.75 mg daily for 25 days of a 31-day cycle

Vasomotor symptoms associated with menopause: Oral: 0.75 to 6 mg daily. If a patient with vasomotor symptoms has not menstruated within the last ≥2 months, start the cyclic administration arbitrarily. If the patient has menstruated, start cyclic administration on day 5 of bleeding.

Vulvar and vaginal atrophy associated with menopause: Oral: 0.75 to 6 mg daily; administer cyclically.

Renal Impairment There are no dosage adjustments provided in the manufacturer's labeling (has not been studied).

Hepatic Impairment Use is contraindicated with hepatic dysfunction or disease.

Additional Information Complete prescribing information should be consulted for additional detail.

Dosage Forms Excipient information presented when available (limited, particularly for generics); consult specific product labeling. [DSC] = Discontinued product
Tablet, Oral:
Ortho-Est 0.625: 0.75 mg [DSC] [scored]
Ortho-Est 1.25: 1.5 mg [DSC] [scored]
Generic: 0.75 mg, 1.5 mg, 3 mg

◆ Estrostep 21 *see* Ethinyl Estradiol and Norethindrone *on page 708*

◆ Estrostep Fe *see* Ethinyl Estradiol and Norethindrone *on page 708*

Eszopiclone (es zoe PIK lone)

Brand Names: US Lunesta
Pharmacologic Category Hypnotic, Miscellaneous
Use Insomnia: Treatment of insomnia

Pregnancy Considerations Adverse effects were observed in animal reproduction studies. Eszopiclone is the S-isomer of the racemic derivative zopiclone. Available data related to zopiclone (not available in the United States) and similar medications note the potential for preterm birth, low birth weight, and/or small for gestational age infants following maternal use. Long-term use of medications in this class is not recommended during pregnancy and a planned discontinuation should be done to prevent rebound insomnia (Okun 2015).

Breast-Feeding Considerations It is not known if eszopiclone is excreted in breast milk. Eszopiclone is the S-isomer of the racemic derivative zopiclone. Zopiclone is excreted in human milk (Matheson 1990).

Medication Guide Available Yes

Contraindications Hypersensitivity to eszopiclone or any component of the formulation.

Warnings/Precautions Symptomatic treatment of insomnia should be initiated only after careful evaluation of potential causes of sleep disturbance. Failure of sleep disturbance to resolve after 7 to 10 days may indicate psychiatric and/or medical illness. Tolerance did not develop over 6 months of use. Daytime function may be impaired in patients taking higher doses (2 mg or 3 mg) even if used as prescribed; patients taking 3 mg must be cautioned about performing tasks which require mental alertness (operating machinery or driving) the day after use. An increased risk of next-day psychomotor impairment may occur if taken with less than a full night of sleep (7 to 8 hours); if higher than recommended dose is taken; if co-administered with other CNS depressants or other drugs that increase blood concentrations of eszopiclone. Dose adjustment may be necessary if taking concomitant CNS depressants; the use of concomitant sedative-hypnotics at bedtime or in the middle of the night is not recommended. Potentially significant drug-drug interactions may exist, requiring dose or frequency adjustment, additional monitoring, and/or selection of alternative therapy.

Use with caution in patients with depression; worsening of depression, including suicidal ideation has been reported with the use of hypnotics. Intentional overdose may be an issue with this population. The minimum dose that will effectively treat the individual patient should be used. Prescriptions should be written for the smallest quantity consistent with good patient care. Use caution in patients with a history of drug dependence. Hypnotics/sedatives have been associated with abnormal thinking and behavior changes including decreased inhibition, aggression, bizarre behavior, agitation, hallucinations, and depersonalization. These changes may occur unpredictably and may indicate previously unrecognized psychiatric disorders; evaluate appropriately. An increased risk for hazardous sleep-related activities such as sleep-driving, cooking and eating food, and making phone calls while asleep has also been noted; amnesia may also occur. The use of alcohol, other CNS depressants, and exceeding the recommended maximum dose may increase the risk of these activities. Discontinue treatment in patients who report any sleep-related episodes. Use caution in patients with respiratory compromise, COPD, sleep apnea, and hepatic dysfunction (dose adjustment recommended with severe impairment). Because of the rapid onset of action, administer immediately prior to bedtime or after the patient has gone to bed and is having difficulty falling asleep. Abrupt discontinuance or rapid dose decreases may lead to withdrawal symptoms. Hypersensitivity reactions including anaphylaxis as well as angioedema have been reported, in some cases following initial dosing. Patients who develop severe reactions should not be rechallenged.

Use with caution in debilitated and elderly patients; dosage adjustment recommended. Closely monitor elderly or debilitated patients for impaired cognitive and/or motor performance, confusion, and potential for falling. Avoid chronic use (>90 days) in older adults; adverse events, including delirium, falls, fractures, have been observed with nonbenzodiazepine hypnotic use in the elderly similar to events observed with benzodiazepines. Data suggests improvements in sleep duration and latency are minimal (Beers Criteria).

Adverse Reactions
>10%:
Central nervous system: Headache (15% to 21%)
Gastrointestinal: Unpleasant taste (8% to 34%)
1% to 10%:
Cardiovascular: Chest pain (≥1%), peripheral edema (≥1%)
Central nervous system: Somnolence (8% to 10%), dizziness (5% to 7%), pain (4% to 5%), nervousness (up to 5%), depression (1% to 4%), confusion (up to 3%), abnormal dreams (1% to 3%), anxiety (1% to 3%), hallucinations (1% to 3%), migraine
Dermatologic: Rash (3% to 4%), pruritus (1% to 4%)
Endocrine & metabolic: Libido decreased (up to 3%), dysmenorrhea (up to 3%), gynecomastia (males up to 3%)
Gastrointestinal: Xerostomia (3% to 7%), dyspepsia (2% to 6%), nausea (4% to 5%), diarrhea (2% to 4%), vomiting (up to 3%)
Genitourinary: Urinary tract infection (up to 3%)
Neuromuscular & skeletal: Neuralgia (up to 3%)
Miscellaneous: Infection (5% to 10%), viral infection (3%), accidental injury (up to 3%)
<1% (Limited to important or life-threatening): Abnormal thinking, alopecia, amenorrhea, anaphylaxis, anemia, anorexia, ataxia, breast enlargement, breast neoplasm, breast pain, bursitis, cholelithiasis, colitis, complex sleep-related behavior (sleep-driving, cooking or eating food, making phone calls), conjunctivitis, contact dermatitis, cystitis, dehydration, dysphagia, emotional lability, epistaxis, gastritis, gout, halitosis, heat stroke, hepatitis, hepatomegaly, herpes zoster, hypercholesterolemia, hypertension, hypokalemia, insomnia, kidney calculus, laryngitis, lymphadenopathy, memory impairment, menorrhagia, myasthenia, mydriasis, myopathy, neck rigidity, neuritis, neuropathy, nystagmus, oliguria, photosensitivity, ptosis, pyelonephritis, rectal hemorrhage, reflexes decreased, skin discoloration, stomach ulcer, thrombophlebitis, ulcerative stomatitis, urethritis, urinary incontinence, vaginal hemorrhage, vaginitis, vesiculobullous rash, vestibular disorder

Drug Interactions
Metabolism/Transport Effects Substrate of CYP2E1 (minor), CYP3A4 (major); **Note:** Assignment of Major/Minor substrate status based on clinically relevant drug interaction potential

Avoid Concomitant Use
Avoid concomitant use of Eszopiclone with any of the following: Azelastine (Nasal); Conivaptan; Fusidic Acid (Systemic); Idelalisib; Orphenadrine; Paraldehyde; Sodium Oxybate; Thalidomide

Increased Effect/Toxicity
Eszopiclone may increase the levels/effects of: Alcohol (Ethyl); Azelastine (Nasal); Buprenorphine; CNS Depressants; Hydrocodone; Methotrimeprazine; Metyrosine; Mirtazapine; Orphenadrine; Paraldehyde; Pramipexole; ROPINIRole; Rotigotine; Selective Serotonin Reuptake Inhibitors; Sodium Oxybate; Suvorexant; Thalidomide; Zolpidem

The levels/effects of Eszopiclone may be increased by: Aprepitant; Brimonidine (Topical); Cannabis; Conivaptan; CYP3A4 Inhibitors (Moderate); CYP3A4 Inhibitors (Strong); Dasatinib; Doxylamine; Dronabinol; Droperidol; Fosaprepitant; Fusidic Acid (Systemic); HydrOXYzine; Idelalisib; Ivacaftor; Kava Kava; Luliconazole; Magnesium Sulfate; Methotrimeprazine; Mifepristone; Minocycline; Nabilone; Netupitant; Osimertinib; Palbociclib; Perampanel; Rufinamide; Simeprevir; Stiripentol; Tapentadol; Tetrahydrocannabinol

Decreased Effect

The levels/effects of Eszopiclone may be decreased by: Bosentan; CYP3A4 Inducers (Moderate); CYP3A4 Inducers (Strong); Dabrafenib; Deferasirox; Enzalutamide; Flumazenil; Mitotane; Osimertinib; Siltuximab; St Johns Wort; Tocilizumab

Food Interactions Onset of action may be reduced if taken with or immediately after a heavy meal. Management: Take immediately prior to bedtime, not with or immediately after a heavy or high-fat meal.

Storage/Stability Store at 25°C (77°F); excursions permitted to 15°C to 30°C (59°F to 86°F).

Mechanism of Action May interact with GABA-receptor complexes at binding domains located close to or allosterically coupled to benzodiazepine receptors.

Pharmacodynamics/Kinetics

Absorption: Rapid; high-fat/heavy meal may delay absorption

Protein binding: 52% to 59%

Metabolism: Hepatic via oxidation and demethylation (CYP2E1, 3A4); (S)-N-desmethyl zopiclone metabolite has less activity than parent compound

Half-life elimination: ~6 hours; Elderly (≥65 years): ~9 hours

Time to peak, plasma: ~1 hour

Excretion: Urine (up to 75%, primarily as metabolites; <10% as parent drug)

Dosing

Adult

Insomnia: Oral: **Note:** The lowest effective dose should be used.

Initial: 1 mg immediately before bedtime; dosing may be increased to 2 mg or 3 mg if clinically necessary (maximum dose: 3 mg daily)

Debilitated patients: Initial: 1 mg immediately before bedtime (maximum dose: 2 mg)

Concurrent use with strong CYP3A4 inhibitor: Initial: 1 mg immediately before bedtime (maximum dose: 2 mg)

Geriatric

Initial: 1 mg immediately before bedtime (maximum dose: 2 mg)

Renal Impairment No dosage adjustment necessary.

Hepatic Impairment

Mild to moderate impairment: No dosage adjustment necessary.

Severe impairment: Initial: 1 mg immediately before bedtime (maximum dose: 2 mg); use with caution; systemic exposure is doubled in severe impairment.

Dietary Considerations Avoid taking after a heavy meal; may delay onset.

Administration Because of the rapid onset of action, eszopiclone should be administered immediately prior to bedtime or after the patient has gone to bed and is having difficulty falling asleep. Do not take with, or immediately following, a high-fat meal (may delay onset).

Dosage Forms Excipient information presented when available (limited, particularly for generics); consult specific product labeling.

Tablet, Oral:

Lunesta: 1 mg [contains fd&c blue #2 (indigotine)]

Lunesta: 2 mg

Lunesta: 3 mg [contains fd&c blue #2 (indigotine)]

Generic: 1 mg, 2 mg, 3 mg

Controlled Substance C-IV

◆ ET-743 *see* Trabectedin *on page 1818*

Etanercept (et a NER sept)

Brand Names: US Enbrel; Enbrel SureClick

Brand Names: Canada Enbrel

Pharmacologic Category Antirheumatic, Disease Modifying; Tumor Necrosis Factor (TNF) Blocking Agent

Use

Ankylosing spondylitis: Reducing signs and symptoms in patients with active ankylosing spondylitis.

Plaque psoriasis: Treatment of adults ≥18 years of age with chronic moderate to severe plaque psoriasis who are candidates for systemic therapy or phototherapy.

Polyarticular juvenile idiopathic arthritis: Reducing signs and symptoms of moderately to severely active polyarticular juvenile idiopathic arthritis in patients ≥2 years of age.

Psoriatic arthritis: Reducing signs and symptoms, inhibiting the progression of structural damage of active arthritis, and improving physical function in patients with psoriatic arthritis. Etanercept can be used with or without methotrexate.

Rheumatoid arthritis: Reducing signs and symptoms, inducing major clinical response, inhibiting the progression of structural damage, and improving physical function in patients with moderately to severely active rheumatoid arthritis (RA). Etanercept can be initiated in combination with methotrexate or used alone.

Pregnancy Considerations Adverse events have not been observed in animal reproduction studies. Etanercept crosses the placenta. Following in utero exposure, concentrations in the newborn at delivery are 3% to 32% of the maternal serum concentration.

A pregnancy registry has been established to monitor outcomes of women exposed to etanercept during pregnancy (800-772-6436).

Breast-Feeding Considerations Etanercept is excreted into breast milk in low concentrations and is minimally absorbed by a nursing infant (limited data). The manufacturer recommends that caution be used if administered to a nursing woman, taking into account the importance of the drug to the mother and potential effects to the nursing infant. A lactation surveillance program has been established to monitor outcomes of breastfed infants exposed to etanercept (800-772-6436).

Medication Guide Available Yes

Contraindications Sepsis

Warnings/Precautions [US Boxed Warning]: Patients receiving etanercept are at increased risk for serious infections which may result in hospitalization and/or fatality; infections usually developed in patients receiving concomitant immunosuppressive agents (eg, methotrexate or corticosteroids) and may present as disseminated (rather than local) disease. Active tuberculosis (or reactivation of latent tuberculosis), invasive fungal (including aspergillosis, blastomycosis, candidiasis, coccidioidomycosis, histoplasmosis, and pneumocystosis) and bacterial, viral or other opportunistic infections (including legionellosis and listeriosis) have been reported in patients receiving TNF-blocking agents, including etanercept. Monitor closely for signs/symptoms of infection. Discontinue for serious infection or sepsis. Consider risks versus benefits prior to use in patients with a history of chronic or recurrent infection. Consider empiric antifungal therapy in patients who are at risk for invasive fungal infection and develop severe systemic illness. Caution should be exercised when considering use in the elderly or in patients with conditions that predispose them to infections (eg, diabetes) or residence/travel from areas of endemic mycoses (blastomycosis, coccidioidomycosis, histoplasmosis), or with latent or localized infections. Do not initiate etanercept therapy with clinically important active infection. Patients who develop a new infection while undergoing treatment should be monitored closely. **[US Boxed Warning]: Tuberculosis (disseminated or extrapulmonary) has been reported in patients receiving etanercept; both reactivation of latent infection and new infections have been reported.** Patients should be evaluated for tuberculosis risk factors and for latent tuberculosis infection with a tuberculin skin test prior to starting therapy. Treatment of latent tuberculosis should be initiated before etanercept therapy; consider antituberculosis treatment if adequate course of treatment cannot be confirmed in patients with a history of latent or active tuberculosis or with risk factors despite negative skin test. Some patients who tested negative prior to therapy have developed active infection; tests for latent tuberculosis infection may be falsely negative while on etanercept therapy. Monitor for signs and symptoms of tuberculosis in all patients. Rare reactivation of hepatitis B virus (HBV) has occurred in chronic virus carriers, usually in patients receiving concomitant immunosuppressants; evaluate for HBV prior to initiation in all patients. Monitor during and for several months following discontinuation of treatment in HBV carriers; interrupt therapy if reactivation occurs and treat appropriately with antiviral therapy; if resumption of therapy is deemed necessary, exercise caution and monitor patient closely. Patients should be brought up to date with all immunizations before initiating therapy. Live vaccines should not be given concurrently with etanercept; there is no data available concerning secondary transmission of live vaccines in patients receiving therapy. Patients with a significant exposure to varicella virus should temporarily discontinue etanercept. Treatment with varicella zoster immune globulin should be considered.

[US Boxed Warning]: Lymphoma and other malignancies have been reported in children and adolescent patients receiving TNF-blocking agents, including etanercept. Half of the malignancies reported in children were lymphomas (Hodgkin and non-Hodgkin) while other cases varied and included malignancies not typically observed in this population. The impact of etanercept on the ▶

development and course of malignancy is not fully defined. Compared to the general population, an increased risk of lymphoma has been noted in clinical trials; however, rheumatoid arthritis alone has been previously associated with an increased rate of lymphoma. Lymphomas and other malignancies were also observed (at rates higher than expected for the general population) in adult patients receiving etanercept. Etanercept is not recommended for use in patients with Wegener's granulomatosis who are receiving immunosuppressive therapy due to higher incidence of noncutaneous solid malignancies. Hepatosplenic T-cell lymphoma (HSTCL), a rare T-cell lymphoma, has also been associated with TNF-blocking agents, primarily reported in adolescent and young adult males with Crohn disease or ulcerative colitis. Melanoma, nonmelanoma skin cancer, and Merkel cell carcinoma have been reported in patients receiving TNF-blocking agents, including etanercept. Perform periodic skin examinations in all patients during therapy, particularly those at increased risk of skin cancer. Positive antinuclear antibody titers have been detected in patients (with negative baselines). Rare cases of autoimmune disorder, including lupus-like syndrome or autoimmune hepatitis, have been reported; monitor and discontinue if symptoms develop.

Allergic reactions may occur; if an anaphylactic reaction or other serious allergic reaction occurs, administration should be discontinued immediately and appropriate therapy initiated. Use with caution in patients with preexisting or recent onset CNS demyelinating disorders; rare cases of new-onset or exacerbation of CNS demyelinating disorders have occurred; may present with mental status changes and some may be associated with permanent disability. Optic neuritis, transverse myelitis, multiple sclerosis, Guillain-Barré syndrome, other peripheral demyelinating neuropathies, and new-onset or exacerbation of seizures have been reported. Use with caution in patients with heart failure or decreased left ventricular function; worsening and new-onset heart failure has been reported, including in patients without known preexisting cardiovascular disease. Use caution in patients with a history of significant hematologic abnormalities; has been associated with pancytopenia and aplastic anemia (rare). Patients must be advised to seek medical attention if they develop signs and symptoms suggestive of blood dyscrasias; discontinue if significant hematologic abnormalities are confirmed. Use with caution in patients with moderate to severe alcoholic hepatitis. Compared to placebo, the mortality rate in patients treated with etanercept was similar at one month but significantly higher after 6 months.

Due to a higher incidence of serious infections, concomitant use with anakinra is not recommended. Hypoglycemia has been reported in patients receiving concomitant therapy with etanercept and antidiabetic medications; dose reduction of antidiabetic medication may be necessary. Use with caution in patient with diabetes; monitor blood glucose as clinically necessary. Some dosage forms may contain dry natural rubber (latex).

Benzyl alcohol and derivatives: Diluent for injection may contain benzyl alcohol; large amounts of benzyl alcohol (≥99 mg/kg/day) have been associated with a potentially fatal toxicity ("gasping syndrome") in neonates; the "gasping syndrome" consists of metabolic acidosis, respiratory distress, gasping respirations, CNS dysfunction (including convulsions, intracranial hemorrhage), hypotension and cardiovascular collapse (AAP ["Inactive"] 1997]; CDC, 1982); some data suggests that benzoate displaces bilirubin from protein binding sites (Ahlfors, 2001); avoid or use dosage forms containing benzyl alcohol with caution in neonates. See manufacturer's labeling.

Adverse Reactions
>10%:
Central nervous system: Headache (17% to 19%)
Dermatologic: Skin rash (3% to 13%)
Gastrointestinal: Abdominal pain (5%; children 19%), diarrhea (3% to 16%), vomiting (3%; children 13%)
Infection: Infection (50% to 81%; children 62%)
Local: Injection site reaction (14% to 43%; bleeding, bruising, erythema, itching, pain, or swelling)
Respiratory: Upper respiratory tract infection (38% to 65%), respiratory tract infection (21% to 54%), rhinitis (12%)
Miscellaneous: Antibody development (positive antidouble-stranded DNA antibodies 15% by RIA, 3% by *Crithidia luciliae* assay), positive ANA titer (11%)
≥3% to 10%:
Central nervous system: Dizziness (7%)
Dermatologic: Pruritus (2% to 5%)
Gastrointestinal: Nausea (children 9%), dyspepsia (4%)
Neuromuscular & skeletal: Weakness (5%)
Respiratory: Pharyngitis (7%), cough (6%), respiratory distress (5%), sinusitis (3%)

Miscellaneous: Fever (2% to 3%)
<3% (Limited to important or life-threatening): Abscess, adenopathy, anemia, angioedema, anorexia, aplastic anemia, appendicitis, aseptic meningitis, aspergillosis, autoimmune hepatitis, blood coagulation disorder, bursitis, cardiac failure, cerebral ischemia, cerebrovascular accident, cholecystitis, cutaneous lupus erythematous, deep vein thrombosis, demyelinating disease of the central nervous system (suggestive of multiple sclerosis, transverse myelitis, or optic neuritis), depression, dermal ulcer, erythema multiforme, gastritis, gastroenteritis, gastrointestinal hemorrhage, glomerulopathy (membranous), hepatotoxicity (idiosyncratic) (Chalasani, 2014), herpes zoster, hydrocephalus (with normal pressure), hypersensitivity, hypersensitivity reaction, hypertension, hypotension, inflammatory bowel disease, interstitial pulmonary disease, intestinal perforation, ischemic heart disease, leukemia, leukopenia, lupus-like syndrome, lymphadenopathy, malignant lymphoma, malignant melanoma, malignant neoplasm, Merkel cell carcinoma, myocardial infarction, multiple sclerosis, nephrolithiasis, neutropenia, optic neuritis, oral mucosa ulcer, pancreatitis, pancytopenia, pneumonia due to *Pneumocystis carinii*, polymyositis, psoriasis (including new onset, palmoplantar, pustular, or exacerbation), pulmonary disease, pulmonary embolism, reactivation of HBV, sarcoidosis, scleritis, seizure, skin carcinoma, Stevens-Johnson syndrome, subcutaneous nodule, thrombocytopenia, thrombophlebitis, toxic epidermal necrolysis, tuberculosis, tuberculous arthritis, urinary tract infection, uveitis, varicella zoster infection, vasculitis (cutaneous and systemic), weight gain

Drug Interactions
Metabolism/Transport Effects None known.
Avoid Concomitant Use
Avoid concomitant use of Etanercept with any of the following: Abatacept; Anakinra; BCG (Intravesical); Belimumab; Canakinumab; Certolizumab Pegol; Cyclophosphamide; InFLIXimab; Natalizumab; Pimecrolimus; Rilonacept; Tacrolimus (Topical); Tocilizumab; Tofacitinib; Vaccines (Live); Vedolizumab
Increased Effect/Toxicity
Etanercept may increase the levels/effects of: Abatacept; Anakinra; Belimumab; Canakinumab; Certolizumab Pegol; Cyclophosphamide; Fingolimod; InFLIXimab; Leflunomide; Natalizumab; Rilonacept; Tofacitinib; Vaccines (Live); Vedolizumab

The levels/effects of Etanercept may be increased by: Denosumab; Pimecrolimus; Roflumilast; Tacrolimus (Topical); Tocilizumab; Trastuzumab
Decreased Effect
Etanercept may decrease the levels/effects of: BCG (Intravesical); Coccidioides immitis Skin Test; Sipuleucel-T; Vaccines (Inactivated); Vaccines (Live)

The levels/effects of Etanercept may be decreased by: Echinacea
Preparation for Administration Reconstitute lyophilized powder aseptically with 1 mL sterile bacteriostatic water for injection, USP (supplied); swirl gently, do not shake. Do not filter reconstituted solution during preparation or administration.
Storage/Stability
Refrigerate at 2°C to 8°C (36°F to 46°F). Do not freeze. Do not store in extreme heat or cold. Store in the original carton to protect from light or physical damage.
Individual autoinjectors, prefilled syringes, or dose trays (containing multi-use vials and diluent syringes) may be stored at room temperature for a maximum single period of 14 days with protection from light and sources of heat, and humidity. Once an autoinjector, prefilled syringe or dose tray has been stored at room temperature, it should not be placed back into the refrigerator; discard after 14 days.
Once the multi-use vial has been reconstituted, use the reconstituted solution immediately or refrigerate at 2°C to 8°C (36°F to 46°F). Reconstituted solution must be used within 14 days; discard after 14 days.
Mechanism of Action Etanercept is a recombinant DNA-derived protein composed of tumor necrosis factor receptor (TNFR) linked to the Fc portion of human IgG1. Etanercept binds tumor necrosis factor (TNF) and blocks its interaction with cell surface receptors. TNF plays an important role in the inflammatory processes and the resulting joint pathology of rheumatoid arthritis (RA), polyarticular-course juvenile idiopathic arthritis (JIA), ankylosing spondylitis (AS), and plaque psoriasis.
Pharmacodynamics/Kinetics
Onset of action: ~2 to 3 weeks; RA: 1 to 2 weeks; Maximum effect: RA: Full effect is usually seen within 3 months
Absorption: Absorbed slowly after SubQ injection

Distribution: V_d: 1.78 to 3.39 L/m²
Bioavailability: SubQ: 60%
Half-life elimination: RA: SubQ: Children: 70 to 94.8 hours; Adults: 102 ± 30 hours
Time to peak: RA: SubQ: 69 ± 34 hours
Clearance: Children and Adolescents 4 to 17 years: 46 mL/hour/m²; Adults: 160 ± 80 mL/hour

Dosing

Adult

Ankylosing spondylitis, psoriatic arthritis, rheumatoid arthritis: SubQ: **Note:** Methotrexate, glucocorticoids, salicylates, NSAIDs, or analgesics may be continued during etanercept therapy: 50 mg once weekly **or** 25 mg given twice weekly (off-label dose; Bathon, 2000; Calin, 2004; Davis, 2003; Genovese, 2002; Mease, 2000; Mease, 2002); maximum dose (rheumatoid arthritis): 50 mg weekly

Plaque psoriasis: SubQ:
Initial: 50 mg twice weekly; maintain initial dose for 3 months (starting doses of 25 or 50 mg once weekly have also been used successfully)
Maintenance dose: 50 mg once weekly

Acute graft-versus-host disease (GVHD), treatment (off-label use): SubQ: 0.4 mg/kg (maximum: 25 mg/dose) twice weekly for 8 weeks (in combination with methylprednisolone) (Levine, 2008)

Geriatric SubQ: Refer to adult dosing.

Pediatric

Juvenile idiopathic arthritis: Children ≥2 years and Adolescents: SubQ: **Note:** Glucocorticoids, NSAIDs, or analgesics may be continued during etanercept therapy: 0.8 mg/kg (maximum: 50 mg/dose) once weekly **or** 0.4 mg/kg (maximum: 25 mg/dose) twice weekly (off-label dose; Lovell, 2006)

Acute graft-versus-host disease (GVHD), treatment (off-label use): Children ≥1 year and Adolescents: SubQ: Refer to adult dosing.

Renal Impairment There are no dosage adjustments provided in the manufacturer's labeling (has not been studied).

Hepatic Impairment There are no dosage adjustments provided in the manufacturer's labeling (has not been studied).

Administration Administer subcutaneously. Rotate injection sites; may inject into the thigh (preferred), abdomen (avoiding the 2-inch area around the navel), or upper arm. New injections should be given at least one inch from an old site and never into areas where the skin is tender, bruised, red, or hard or into any raised thick, red or scaly skin patches or lesions. For a more comfortable injection, allow autoinjectors, prefilled syringes, and dose trays to reach room temperature for 15 to 30 minutes (≥30 minutes for autoinjector) prior to injection; do not remove the needle cover while allowing product to reach room temperature. There may be small white particles of protein in the solution; this is not unusual for proteinaceous solutions. **Note:** If the health care provider determines that it is appropriate, patients may self-inject after proper training in injection technique.

Monitoring Parameters Monitor improvement of symptoms and physical function assessments. Latent TB screening prior to initiating and during therapy; signs/symptoms of infection (prior to, during, and following therapy); CBC with differential; signs/symptoms/worsening of heart failure; HBV screening prior to initiating (all patients), HBV carriers (during and for several months following therapy); signs and symptoms of hypersensitivity reaction; symptoms of lupus-like syndrome; signs/symptoms of malignancy (eg, splenomegaly, hepatomegaly, abdominal pain, persistent fever, night sweats, weight loss).

Dosage Forms Excipient information presented when available (limited, particularly for generics); consult specific product labeling.
Kit, Subcutaneous [preservative free]:
Enbrel: 25 mg [contains benzyl alcohol, tromethamine]
Solution Auto-injector, Subcutaneous [preservative free]:
Enbrel SureClick: 50 mg/mL (0.98 mL)
Solution Prefilled Syringe, Subcutaneous [preservative free]:
Enbrel: 25 mg/0.5 mL (0.51 mL); 50 mg/mL (0.98 mL)

◆ Ethacrynate Sodium see Ethacrynic Acid on page 699

Ethacrynic Acid (eth a KRIN ik AS id)

Brand Names: US Edecrin; Sodium Edecrin
Brand Names: Canada Edecrin; Sodium Edecrin
Index Terms Ethacrynate Sodium
Pharmacologic Category Diuretic, Loop

Use Management of edema associated with congestive heart failure; hepatic cirrhosis or renal disease; short-term management of ascites due to malignancy, idiopathic edema, and lymphedema

Dosing

Adult Note: Dose equivalency for patients with normal renal function (approximate): Ethacrynic acid 50 mg = bumetanide 1 mg = furosemide 40 mg = torsemide 20 mg

Edema:
Oral: 50-200 mg/day in 1-2 divided doses; may increase in increments of 25-50 mg at intervals of several days to a maximum of 400 mg/24 hours.
IV: 0.5-1 mg/kg/dose (maximum: 100 mg/dose); repeat doses not routinely recommended; however, if indicated, repeat doses every 8-12 hours.

Geriatric Oral: Initial: 25-50 mg/day

Pediatric Edema: Oral: Children: 1 mg/kg/dose once daily; increase at intervals of 2-3 days as needed, to a maximum of 3 mg/kg/day.

Renal Impairment
CrCl <10 mL/minute: Avoid use.
Not removed by hemo- or peritoneal dialysis; supplemental dose is not necessary.

Hepatic Impairment No dosage adjustment provided in manufacturer's labeling, use with caution.

Additional Information Complete prescribing information should be consulted for additional detail.

Dosage Forms Excipient information presented when available (limited, particularly for generics); consult specific product labeling. [DSC] = Discontinued product
Solution Reconstituted, Intravenous, as ethacrynate sodium:
Sodium Edecrin: 50 mg (1 ea)
Generic: 50 mg (1 ea)
Tablet, Oral:
Edecrin: 25 mg [DSC]
Edecrin: 25 mg [scored]

Ethambutol (e THAM byoo tole)

Brand Names: US Myambutol
Brand Names: Canada Etibi
Index Terms Ethambutol Hydrochloride
Pharmacologic Category Antitubercular Agent

Use Treatment of pulmonary tuberculosis in conjunction with other antituberculosis agents

Pregnancy Considerations Teratogenic effects have been seen in animals. There are no adequate and well-controlled studies in pregnant women; there have been reports of ophthalmic abnormalities in infants born to women receiving ethambutol as a component of antituberculous therapy. Use only during pregnancy if benefits outweigh risks.

Breast-Feeding Considerations The manufacturer suggests use during breast-feeding only if benefits to the mother outweigh the possible risk to the infant. Some references suggest that exposure to the infant is low and does not produce toxicity, and breast-feeding should not be discouraged. Other references recommend if breast-feeding, monitor the infant for rash, malaise, nausea, or vomiting.

Contraindications Hypersensitivity to ethambutol or any component of the formulation; optic neuritis (risk vs benefit decision); use in young children, unconscious patients, or any other patient who may be unable to discern and report visual changes

Warnings/Precautions May cause optic neuritis (unilateral or bilateral), resulting in decreased visual acuity or other vision changes. Discontinue promptly in patients with changes in vision, color blindness, or visual defects (effects normally reversible, but reversal may require up to a year). Irreversible blindness has been reported. Monitor visual acuity prior to and during therapy. Evaluation of visual acuity changes may be more difficult in patients with cataracts, optic neuritis, diabetic retinopathy, and inflammatory conditions of the eye; consideration should be given to whether or not visual changes are related to disease progression or effects of therapy. Use only in children whose visual acuity can accurately be determined and monitored (not recommended for use in children <13 years of age unless the benefit outweighs the risk). Dosage modification is required in patients with renal insufficiency; monitor renal function prior to and during treatment. Hepatic toxicity has been reported, possibly due to concurrent therapy; monitor liver function prior to and during treatment.

Adverse Reactions Frequency not defined.
Cardiovascular: Myocarditis, pericarditis
Central nervous system: Confusion, disorientation, dizziness, fever, hallucinations, headache, malaise

Dermatologic: Dermatitis, erythema multiforme, exfoliative dermatitis, pruritus, rash

Endocrine & metabolic: Acute gout or hyperuricemia

Gastrointestinal: Abdominal pain, anorexia, GI upset, nausea, vomiting

Hematologic: Eosinophilia, leukopenia, lymphadenopathy, neutropenia, thrombocytopenia

Hepatic: Hepatitis, hepatotoxicity (possibly related to concurrent therapy), LFTs abnormal

Neuromuscular & skeletal: Arthralgia, peripheral neuritis

Ocular: Optic neuritis; symptoms may include decreased acuity, scotoma, color blindness, or visual defects (usually reversible with discontinuation, irreversible blindness has been described)

Renal: Nephritis

Respiratory: Infiltrates (with or without eosinophilia), pneumonitis

Miscellaneous: Anaphylaxis, anaphylactoid reaction; hypersensitivity syndrome (cutaneous reactions, eosinophilia, and organ-specific inflammation)

Drug Interactions

Metabolism/Transport Effects None known.

Avoid Concomitant Use There are no known interactions where it is recommended to avoid concomitant use.

Increased Effect/Toxicity There are no known significant interactions involving an increase in effect.

Decreased Effect
The levels/effects of Ethambutol may be decreased by: Aluminum Hydroxide

Storage/Stability Store at controlled room temperature of 20°C to 25°C (68°F to 77°F).

Mechanism of Action Inhibits arabinosyl transferase resulting in impaired mycobacterial cell wall synthesis

Pharmacodynamics/Kinetics

Absorption: ~80%

Distribution: Widely throughout body; concentrated in kidneys, lungs, saliva, and red blood cells

Relative diffusion from blood into CSF: Adequate with or without inflammation (exceeds usual MICs)

CSF:blood level ratio: Normal meninges: 0%; Inflamed meninges: 25%

Protein binding: 20% to 30%

Metabolism: Hepatic (20%) to inactive metabolite

Half-life elimination: 2.5-3.6 hours; End-stage renal disease: 7-15 hours

Time to peak, serum: 2-4 hours

Excretion: Urine (~50% as unchanged drug, 8% to 15% as metabolites); feces (~20% as unchanged drug)

Dosing

Adult & Geriatric

Disseminated *Mycobacterium avium* (MAC) treatment in patients with advanced HIV infection (off-label use; ATS/IDSA guidelines, 2007): Oral: 15 mg/kg ethambutol in combination with clarithromycin or azithromycin with/without rifabutin

Tuberculosis, active: Oral: FDA-approved labeling: Adolescents ≥13 years and Adults: Initial: 15 mg/kg once daily (maximum dose: 1.5 g); Re-treatment (previous antituberculosis therapy): 25 mg/kg once daily (maximum dose: 2.5 g) for 60 days or until bacteriologic smears and cultures become negative, followed by 15 mg/kg daily.

Suggested doses by lean body weight (CDC, 2003):
Daily therapy: 15-25 mg/kg (maximum dose: 1.6 g)
40-55 kg: 800 mg
56-75 kg: 1200 mg
76-90 kg: 1600 mg
Twice weekly directly observed therapy (DOT): 50 mg/kg (maximum dose: 4 g)
40-55 kg: 2000 mg
56-75 kg: 2800 mg
76-90 kg: 4000 mg
Three times/week DOT: 25-30 mg/kg (maximum dose: 2.4 g)
40-55 kg: 1200 mg
56-75 kg: 2000 mg
76-90 kg: 2400 mg

Note: Used as part of a multidrug regimen. Treatment regimens consist of an initial 2 month phase, followed by a continuation phase of 4 or 7 additional months; frequency of dosing may differ depending on phase of therapy.

Nontuberculous mycobacterium *(M. kansasii)* (off-label use; ATS/IDSA guidelines, 2007): Oral: 15 mg/kg/day ethambutol for duration to include 12 months of culture-negative sputum; typically used in combination with rifampin and isoniazid; **Note:** Previous recommendations stated to use 25 mg/kg/day for the initial 2 months of therapy; however, IDSA guidelines state this may be unnecessary given the success of rifampin-based regimens with ethambutol 15 mg/kg/day or omitted altogether.

Pediatric

***Mycobacterium avium* (MAC), secondary prophylaxis or treatment: HIV-exposed/-infected (off-label use):** Oral: Infants and Children: 15-25 mg/kg/day once daily (maximum 2.5 g/day) with clarithromycin (or azithromycin) with or without rifabutin (CDC, 2009)

Tuberculosis, active: Oral: **Note:** Used as part of a multidrug regimen; treatment regimens consist of an initial 2-month phase, followed by a continuation phase of 4 or 7 additional months; frequency of dosing may differ depending on phase of therapy.
Children:
HIV negative: Daily therapy: 15-20 mg/kg/day (maximum: 1 g/day); Twice weekly directly observed therapy (DOT): 50 mg/kg (maximum: 2.5 g/dose) (*MMWR*, 2003)
HIV-exposed/-infected: Daily therapy: 15-25 mg/kg/day (maximum: 2.5 g/day) (CDC, 2009)
Adolescents ≥13 years: Refer to adult dosing.

Renal Impairment

MMWR, 2003: CrCl <30 mL/minute and hemodialysis: 15-25 mg/kg/dose 3 times weekly
Aronoff, 2007
CrCl 10-50 mL/minute: Administer every 24-36 hours
CrCl <10 mL/minute: Administer every 48 hours
Hemodialysis: Slightly dialyzable (5% to 20%); Administer dose postdialysis
Peritoneal dialysis: Dose for CrCl <10 mL/minute: Administer every 48 hours
Continuous arteriovenous or venovenous hemofiltration: Dose for CrCl 10-50 mL/minute: Administer every 24-36 hours

Hepatic Impairment No dosage adjustment provided in manufacturer's labeling; use with caution.

Dietary Considerations May be taken with food as absorption is not affected, may cause gastric irritation.

Monitoring Parameters Baseline and periodic (monthly) visual testing (each eye individually, as well as both eyes tested together) in patients receiving >15 mg/kg/day; baseline and periodic renal, hepatic, and hematopoietic tests

Dosage Forms Excipient information presented when available (limited, particularly for generics); consult specific product labeling.
Tablet, Oral, as hydrochloride:
Myambutol: 100 mg
Myambutol: 400 mg [scored]
Generic: 100 mg, 400 mg

◆ **Ethambutol Hydrochloride** *see* Ethambutol *on page 699*

◆ **Ethamolin** *see* Ethanolamine Oleate *on page 700*

◆ **Ethanoic Acid** *see* Acetic Acid (Otic) *on page 30*

◆ **Ethanoic Acid** *see* Acetic Acid (Topical) *on page 31*

Ethanolamine Oleate (ETH a nol a meen OH lee ate)

Brand Names: US Ethamolin

Index Terms Monoethanolamine

Pharmacologic Category Sclerosing Agent

Use Esophageal varices: Treatment of esophageal varices that have recently bled, to prevent rebleeding.

Dosing

Adult & Geriatric

Esophageal varices: IV: 1.5 to 5 mL per varix, (maximum: 20 mL per treatment session). Treatments may be made at the time of the acute bleed and then repeated after 1 week, 6 weeks, 3 months, and 6 months as indicated. **Note:** Patients with cardiopulmonary disease should usually receive less than the maximum recommended dose.

Renal Impairment There are no dosage adjustments provided in the manufacturer's labeling.

Hepatic Impairment There are no dosage adjustments provided in the manufacturer's labeling; patients with Child-Pugh class C hepatic impairment should usually receive less than the recommended maximum dosage.

Additional Information Complete prescribing information should be consulted for additional detail.

Dosage Forms Excipient information presented when available (limited, particularly for generics); consult specific product labeling.
Solution, Intravenous:
Ethamolin: 5% (2 mL) [contains benzyl alcohol]

◆ **Etherified Starch** *see* Tetrastarch *on page 1774*

Ethinyl Estradiol and Desogestrel
(ETH in il es tra DYE ole & des oh JES trel)

Brand Names: US Apri; Azurette; Bekyree; Caziant; Cyclessa; Cyred; Desogen; Emoquette; Enskyce; Juleber; Kariva; Kimidess; Mircette; Ortho-Cept [DSC]; Pimtrea; Reclipsen; Solia; Velivet; Viorele

Brand Names: Canada Apri; Freya; Linessa; Marvelon; Ortho-Cept; Reclipsen

Index Terms Desogestrel and Ethinyl Estradiol; Ortho Cept

Pharmacologic Category Contraceptive; Estrogen and Progestin Combination

Use Contraception: Prevention of pregnancy.

Dosing

Adult Females: Contraception: Oral:

Schedule 1 (Sunday starter): Dose begins on first Sunday after onset of menstruation; if the menstrual period starts on Sunday, take first tablet that very same day. **With a Sunday start, an additional method of contraception should be used until after the first 7 days of consecutive administration.**

For 21-tablet package: Dosage is 1 tablet daily for 21 consecutive days, followed by 7 days off of the medication; a new course begins on the 8th day after the last tablet is taken.

For 28-tablet package: Dosage is 1 tablet daily without interruption.

Schedule 2 (Day 1 starter): Dose starts on first day of menstrual cycle taking 1 tablet daily.

For 21-tablet package: Dosage is 1 tablet daily for 21 consecutive days, followed by 7 days off of the medication; a new course begins on the 8th day after the last tablet is taken.

For 28-tablet package: Dosage is 1 tablet daily without interruption.

If all doses have not been taken on schedule and one menstrual period is missed, the possibility of pregnancy should be considered. If two consecutive menstrual periods are missed, pregnancy test is required before new dosing cycle is started.

Missed doses **monophasic formulations** (refer to package insert for complete information):

One dose missed: Take as soon as remembered or take 2 tablets next day

Two consecutive doses missed in the first 2 weeks: Take 2 tablets as soon as remembered or 2 tablets next 2 days. **An additional method of contraception should be used for 7 days after missed dose.**

Two consecutive doses missed in week 3 or three consecutive doses missed at any time:

Schedule 1 (Sunday starter): Continue to take 1 tablet daily until Sunday, then discard the rest of the pack, and a new pack is started that same day. **An additional method of contraception should be used for 7 days after missed dose.**

Schedule 2 (Day 1 starter): Current pack should be discarded, and a new pack started that same day. **An additional method of contraception should be used for 7 days after missed dose.**

Missed doses **biphasic/triphasic formulations** (refer to package insert for complete information):

One dose missed: Take as soon as remembered.

Two consecutive doses missed in week 1 or week 2 of the pack: Take 2 tablets as soon as remembered and 2 tablets the next day. Resume taking 1 tablet daily until the pack is empty. **An additional method of contraception should be used for 7 days after a missed dose.**

Two consecutive doses missed in week 3 of the pack; **an additional method of contraception must be used for 7 days after a missed dose**:

Schedule 1 (Sunday starter): Take 1 tablet every day until Sunday. Discard the remaining pack and start a new pack of pills on the same day.

Schedule 2 (Day 1 starter): Discard the remaining pack and start a new pack the same day.

Three or more consecutive doses missed; **an additional method of contraception must be used for 7 days after a missed dose**:

Schedule 1 (Sunday starter): Take 1 tablet every day until Sunday; on Sunday, discard the pack and start a new pack.

Schedule 2 (Day 1 starter): Discard the remaining pack and begin new pack of tablets starting on the same day.

Pediatric Females: Contraception: Oral: See adult dosing; not to be used prior to menarche.

Renal Impairment No dosage adjustment provided in manufacturer's labeling; use with caution and monitor blood pressure closely. Consider other forms of contraception.

Hepatic Impairment Contraindicated in patients with hepatic impairment.

Additional Information Complete prescribing information should be consulted for additional detail.

Dosage Forms Excipient information presented when available (limited, particularly for generics); consult specific product labeling. [DSC] = Discontinued product

Tablet, oral [low dose formulation]:

Azurette:
Day 1-21: Ethinyl estradiol 0.02 mg and desogestrel 0.15 mg [21 white tablets]
Day 22-23: 2 inactive green tablets
Day 24-28: Ethinyl estradiol 0.01 mg [5 blue tablets] (28s)

Bekyree:
Day 1-21: Ethinyl estradiol 0.02 mg and desogestrel 0.15 mg [21 white tablets]
Day 22-23: 2 inactive green tablets
Day 24-28: Ethinyl estradiol 0.01 mg [5 yellow tablets] (28s)

Kariva:
Day 1-21: Ethinyl estradiol 0.02 mg and desogestrel 0.15 mg [21 white tablets]
Day 22-23: 2 inactive light green tablets
Day 24-28: Ethinyl estradiol 0.01 mg [5 light blue tablets] (28s)

Kimidess:
Day 1-21: Ethinyl estradiol 0.02 mg and desogestrel 0.15 mg [21 white tablets]
Day 22-23: 2 inactive green tablets
Day 24-28: Ethinyl estradiol 0.01 mg [5 yellow tablets] (28s)

Mircette:
Day 1-21: Ethinyl estradiol 0.02 mg and desogestrel 0.15 mg [21 white tablets]
Day 22-23: 2 inactive green tablets
Day 24-28: Ethinyl estradiol 0.01 mg [5 yellow tablets] (28s)

Pimtrea:
Day 1-21: Ethinyl estradiol 0.02 mg and desogestrel 0.15 mg [21 dark blue tablets]
Day 22-23: 2 inactive white tablets
Day 24-28: Ethinyl estradiol 0.01 mg [5 green tablets] (28s)

Viorele:
Day 1-21: Ethinyl estradiol 0.02 mg and desogestrel 0.15 mg [21 white tablets]
Day 22-23: 2 inactive green tablets
Day 24-28: Ethinyl estradiol 0.01 mg [5 yellow tablets] (28s)

Tablet, oral [monophasic formulation]:

Apri 28: Ethinyl estradiol 0.03 mg and desogestrel 0.15 mg [21 rose tablets and 7 white inactive tablets] (28s)

Cyred: Ethinyl estradiol 0.03 mg and desogestrel 0.15 mg [21 active and 7 inactive tablets] (28s)

Desogen: Ethinyl estradiol 0.03 mg and desogestrel 0.15 mg [21 white tablets and 7 green inactive tablets] (28s)

Emoquette: Ethinyl estradiol 0.03 mg and desogestrel 0.15 mg [21 white tablets and 7 light green inactive tablets] (28s)

Enskyce: Ethinyl estradiol 0.03 mg and desogestrel 0.15 mg [21 light orange tablets and 7 green inactive tablets] (28s)

Juleber: Ethinyl estradiol 0.03 mg and desogestrel 0.15 mg [21 yellow tablets and 7 white inactive tablets] (28s)

Ortho-Cept 28: Ethinyl estradiol 0.03 mg and desogestrel 0.15 mg [21 light orange tablets and 7 green inactive tablets] (28s) [DSC]

Reclipsen: Ethinyl estradiol 0.03 mg and desogestrel 0.15 mg [21 white tablets and 7 green inactive tablets] (28s)

Solia: Ethinyl estradiol 0.03 mg and desogestrel 0.15 mg (28s)

Tablet, oral [triphasic formulation]:

Caziant:
Day 1-7: Ethinyl estradiol 0.025 mg and desogestrel 0.1 mg [7 white tablets]
Day 8-14: Ethinyl estradiol 0.025 mg and desogestrel 0.125 mg [7 light blue tablets]
Day 15-21: Ethinyl estradiol 0.025 mg and desogestrel 0.15 mg [7 blue tablets]
Day 22-28: 7 green inactive tablets (28s)

Cyclessa:
Day 1-7: Ethinyl estradiol 0.025 mg and desogestrel 0.1 mg [7 light yellow tablets]
Day 8-14: Ethinyl estradiol 0.025 mg and desogestrel 0.125 mg [7 orange tablets]
Day 15-21: Ethinyl estradiol 0.025 mg and desogestrel 0.15 mg [7 red tablets]
Day 22-28: 7 green inactive tablets (28s)

Velivet:
Day 1-7: Ethinyl estradiol 0.025 mg and desogestrel 0.1 mg [7 beige tablets]
Day 8-14: Ethinyl estradiol 0.025 mg and desogestrel 0.125 mg [7 orange tablets]
Day 15-21: Ethinyl estradiol 0.025 mg and desogestrel 0.15 mg [7 pink tablets]
Day 22-28: 7 white inactive tablets (28s)

Ethinyl Estradiol and Drospirenone

(ETH in il es tra DYE ole & droh SPYE re none)

Brand Names: US Gianvi; Loryna; Nikki; Ocella; Syeda; Vestura; Yasmin; Yaz; Zarah
Brand Names: Canada Mya; Yasmin; Yaz; Zamine; Zarah
Index Terms Drospirenone and Ethinyl Estradiol
Pharmacologic Category Contraceptive; Estrogen and Progestin Combination
Use
Acne vulgaris (Gianvi, Loryna, Nikki, Vestura, Yaz): Treatment of moderate acne vulgaris in women 14 years and older only if the patient desires an oral contraceptive for birth control
Contraception: Prevention of pregnancy
Premenstrual dysphoric disorder (Gianvi, Yaz): Treatment of premenstrual dysphoric disorder (PMDD) for women who choose to use an oral contraceptive for contraception
Dosing
Adult
Acne (Gianvi, Loryna, Nikki, Vestura, Yaz): Females: Oral: Refer to dosing for contraception.
PMDD (Gianvi, Yaz): Females: Oral: Refer to dosing for contraception.
Contraception: Female: Oral: Dosage is 1 tablet daily for 28 consecutive days. Dosing may be started on the first day of menstrual period (Day 1 starter) or on the first Sunday after the onset of the menstrual period (Sunday starter). **With a Sunday start, an additional method of contraception should be used until after the first 7 days of consecutive administration.**
Day 1 starter: Dose starts on first day of menstrual cycle taking 1 tablet daily.
Sunday starter: Dose begins on first Sunday after onset of menstruation; if the menstrual period starts on Sunday, take first tablet that very same day.
Switching from a different contraceptive:
Oral contraceptive: Start on the same day that a new pack of the previous oral contraceptive would have been taken
Transdermal patch, vaginal ring, injection: Start on the day the next dose would have been due
IUD or implant: Start on the day of removal
Use after childbirth (in women who are not breast-feeding) or after second trimester abortion: Therapy may be started ≥4 weeks postpartum. Pregnancy should be ruled out prior to treatment if menstrual periods have not restarted and an additional method of contraception (nonhormonal) should be used until after the first 7 days of consecutive administration.

Missed doses:
If all doses have been taken on schedule and one menstrual period is missed, continue dosing cycle. If two consecutive menstrual periods are missed, pregnancy test is required before new dosing cycle is started.
If doses have been missed during the first 3 weeks and the menstrual period is missed, pregnancy should be ruled out prior to continuing treatment.
Missed doses (monophasic formulations) (refer to package insert for complete information):
One dose missed: Take as soon as remembered or take 2 tablets next day
Two consecutive doses missed in the first 2 weeks: Take 2 tablets as soon as remembered or 2 tablets next 2 days. **An additional method of contraception should be used for 7 days after missed dose.**
Two consecutive doses missed in week 3 or three consecutive doses missed at any time: **An additional method of contraception must be used for 7 days after a missed dose.**

Day 1 starter: Current pack should be discarded, and a new pack should be started that same day.
Sunday starter: Continue dose of 1 tablet daily until Sunday, then discard the rest of the pack, and a new pack should be started that same day.
Any number of doses missed in week 4: Continue taking one pill each day until pack is empty; no back-up method of contraception is needed
Pediatric Note: Not to be used prior to menarche.
Acne (Gianvi, Loryna, Nikki, Vestura, Yaz): Females: Adolescents ≥14 years: Oral: Refer to adult dosing.
PMDD (Gianvi,Yaz): Females: Oral: Refer to adult dosing.
Contraception: Females: Oral: Refer to adult dosing.
Renal Impairment Contraindicated in patients with renal dysfunction.
Hepatic Impairment Contraindicated in patients with hepatic dysfunction.
Additional Information Complete prescribing information should be consulted for additional detail.
Dosage Forms Excipient information presented when available (limited, particularly for generics); consult specific product labeling.
Tablet, oral:
Gianvi: Ethinyl estradiol 0.02 mg and drospirenone 3 mg [24 light pink active tablets and 4 white inactive tablets] (28s)
Loryna: Ethinyl estradiol 0.02 mg and drospirenone 3 mg [24 peach active tablets and 4 white inactive tablets] (28s)
Nikki: Ethinyl estradiol 0.02 mg and drospirenone 3 mg [24 pink active tablets and 4 white inactive tablets] (28s)
Ocella: Ethinyl estradiol 0.03 mg and drospirenone 3 mg [21 yellow active tablets and 7 white inactive tablets] (28s)
Syeda: Ethinyl estradiol 0.03 mg and drospirenone 3 mg [21 yellow active tablets and 7 white inactive tablets] (28s)
Vestura: Ethinyl estradiol 0.02 mg and drospirenone 3 mg [24 pink active tablets and 4 peach inactive tablets] (28s)
Yasmin: Ethinyl estradiol 0.03 mg and drospirenone 3 mg [21 yellow active tablets and 7 white inactive tablets] (28s)
Yaz: Ethinyl estradiol 0.02 mg and drospirenone 3 mg [24 light pink active tablets and 4 white inactive tablets] (28s)
Zarah: Ethinyl estradiol 0.03 mg and drospirenone 3 mg [21 blue active tablets and 7 peach inactive tablets] (28s)
Generic: Ethinyl estradiol 0.02 mg and drospirenone 3 mg [21 active tablets and 7 inactive tablets] (28s); Ethinyl estradiol 0.03 mg and drospirenone 3 mg [21 active tablets and 7 inactive tablets] (28s)

Ethinyl Estradiol and Ethynodiol Diacetate

(ETH in il es tra DYE ole & e thye noe DYE ole dye AS e tate)

Brand Names: US Kelnor; Zovia
Brand Names: Canada Demulen 30
Index Terms Demulen; Ethynodiol Diacetate and Ethinyl Estradiol
Pharmacologic Category Contraceptive; Estrogen and Progestin Combination
Use Contraception: For the prevention of pregnancy
Limitation of use: Products containing the equivalent of estrogen 50 mcg should not be used unless medically indicated.
Dosing
Adult
Females: Contraception: Oral: 1 tablet once daily
Schedule 1 (Sunday starter): Dose begins on first Sunday after onset of menstruation; if the menstrual period starts on Sunday, take first tablet that very same day. **With a Sunday start, an additional method of contraception should be used until after the first 7 days of consecutive administration:**
Schedule 2 (Day 1 starter): Dose starts on first day of menstrual cycle taking 1 tablet/day:
Missed or late doses (CDC, 2013):
If one dose is late (<24 hours since dose should have been taken) or if one dose is missed (24 to <48 hours since dose should have been taken): Take dose as soon as possible. Continue remaining doses at the usual time (even if that means 2 doses on the same day).

If ≥2 consecutive doses are missed (≥48 hours since dose should have been taken): Take the most recently missed dose as soon as possible, discard any other missed doses. Continue remaining doses at the usual time (even if that means taking 2 doses on the same day); use back-up contraception until hormonal doses have been taken for 7 consecutive days. If doses were missed during the last week of hormonal (active) tablets (eg, days 15 to 21 of a 28-day pack), omit the hormone-free interval by finishing the hormonal pills from the current pack and starting a new pack. If unable to start a new pack immediately, back up contraception is needed until hormonal pills from a new pack have been taken for 7 consecutive days. Consider use of emergency contraception in some situations (refer to guidelines for details).

Also refer to package insert for product specific information.

Pediatric Females: Contraception: Oral: Refer to adult dosing; not to be used prior to menarche.

Renal Impairment There are no dosage adjustments provided in the manufacturer's labeling (has not been studied); use with caution and monitor blood pressure closely.

Hepatic Impairment Use is contraindicated.

Additional Information Complete prescribing information should be consulted for additional detail.

Dosage Forms Excipient information presented when available (limited, particularly for generics); consult specific product labeling.

Tablet, oral [monophasic formulation]:

Kelnor 1/35: Ethinyl estradiol 0.035 mg and ethynodiol diacetate 1 mg [21 light yellow tablets and 7 white inactive tablets] (28s)

Zovia 1/35-28: Ethinyl estradiol 0.035 mg and ethynodiol diacetate 1 mg [21 light pink tablets and 7 white inactive tablets] (28s)

Zovia 1/50-28: Ethinyl estradiol 0.05 mg and ethynodiol diacetate 1 mg [21 pink tablets and 7 white inactive tablets] (28s)

Ethinyl Estradiol and Etonogestrel
(ETH in il es tra DYE ole & et oh noe JES trel)

Brand Names: US NuvaRing®

Brand Names: Canada NuvaRing®

Index Terms Etonogestrel and Ethinyl Estradiol

Pharmacologic Category Contraceptive; Estrogen and Progestin Combination

Use Contraception: For the prevention of pregnancy

Dosing

Adult Females: Contraception: Vaginal: One ring, inserted vaginally and left in place for 3 consecutive weeks, then removed for 1 week. A new ring is inserted 7 days after the last was removed (even if bleeding is not complete) and should be inserted at approximately the same time of day the ring was removed the previous week.

Initial treatment should begin as follows (pregnancy should always be ruled out first):

No hormonal contraceptive use in the past month: Insert ring on the first day of menstrual cycle ("Day 1"). May also insert on days 2-5 even if bleeding is not complete, however, **a spermicide or barrier method of contraception should be used for the following 7 days.***

Switching from combination oral contraceptive: Ring can be inserted on any day within 7 days after the last **active** tablet in the cycle was taken and no later than the first day a new cycle of tablets would begin. Additional forms of contraception are not needed.

Switching from progestin-only contraceptive: **A spermicide or barrier method of contraception should be used for the following 7 days with any of the following.***

If previously using a progestin-only mini-pill, insert the ring on any day of the month; insert the vaginal ring on the day after the last mini-pill; do not skip days between the last pill and insertion of the ring.

If previously using an implant, insert the ring on the same day of implant removal.

If previously using a progestin-containing IUD, insert the ring on day of IUD removal.

If previously using a progestin injection, insert the ring on the day the next injection would be given.

Following complete 1st trimester abortion or miscarriage: Insert ring within the first 5 days of abortion or miscarriage. If not inserted within 5 days, follow instructions for "No hormonal contraceptive use within the past month" and instruct patient to use a non-hormonal contraceptive in the interim.

Following delivery or 2nd trimester abortion or miscarriage: Insert ring 4 weeks postpartum (in women who are not breast-feeding) or following 2nd trimester abortion or miscarriage. **A spermicide or barrier method of contraception should be used for the following 7 days.***

If the ring is accidentally removed from the vagina at any time during the 3-week period of use, it may be rinsed with cool or lukewarm water (not hot) and reinserted as soon as possible. If the ring is not reinserted within 3 hours, contraceptive effectiveness will be decreased. If the ring is accidently removed from the vagina for >3 hours during weeks 1 and 2, the ring should be reinserted as soon as the woman remembers and **a spermicide or barrier method of contraception should be used until the ring has been in place for 7 consecutive days.*** If the ring is accidently removed from the vagina for >3 hours during week 3, the ring should be discarded. A new ring may be inserted immediately, restarting a new 3-week cycle, OR a new ring may be inserted ≤7 days from the time the previous ring was removed or expelled (the second option should only be done if a vaginal ring was in continuous use for ≥7 days prior to the inadvertent expulsion/removal). With either option, **a spermicide or barrier method of contraception should be used until the ring has been in place for 7 consecutive days.*** Additional guidelines are available (CDC, 2013).

If the ring has been removed for longer than 1 week, pregnancy must be ruled out prior to restarting therapy. **A spermicide or barrier method of contraception should be used for the following 7 days.***

If the ring has been left in place for >3 weeks, a new ring should be inserted following a 1-week (ring-free) interval. Protection continues during week 4, however, if the ring is left in place >4 weeks, pregnancy must be ruled out prior to insertion and **a spermicide or barrier method of contraception should be used for the following 7 days.***

Disconnected ring: In the event the ring disconnects at the weld joint, discard and replace with a new ring.

*Note: Diaphragms may interfere with proper ring placement, and therefore, are not recommended for use as an additional form of contraception.

Pediatric Females: Contraception: Vaginal: Refer to adult dosing; not to be used prior to menarche.

Renal Impairment No dosage adjustment provided in manufacturer's labeling (has not been studied).

Hepatic Impairment No dosage adjustment provided in manufacturer's labeling (has not been studied). Use is contraindicated in patients with hepatic impairment.

Additional Information Complete prescribing information should be consulted for additional detail.

Dosage Forms Excipient information presented when available (limited, particularly for generics); consult specific product labeling.

Ring, vaginal:

NuvaRing®: Ethinyl estradiol 0.015 mg/day and etonogestrel 0.12 mg/day (3s) [3-week duration]

Ethinyl Estradiol and Levonorgestrel
(ETH in il es tra DYE ole & LEE voe nor jes trel)

Brand Names: US Altavera; Amethia; Amethia Lo; Amethyst; Ashlyna; Aubra; Aviane; camrese; camrese lo; Chateal; Daysee; Delyla; Enpresse; FaLessa Kit; Falmina; Introvale; Jolessa; Kurvelo; Lessina; Levonest; Levora; LoSeasonique; Lutera; Lybrel; Marlissa; Myzilra; Orsythia; Portia; Quartette; Quasense; Seasonique; Setlakin; Sronyx; Trivora; Vienva

Brand Names: Canada Alesse; Alysena; Aviane; Esme; Lutera; Min-Ovral; Ovima; Portia; Seasonale; Seasonique; Triquilar

Index Terms Levonorgestrel and Ethinyl Estradiol; Triphasil

Pharmacologic Category Contraceptive; Estrogen and Progestin Combination

Use Prevention of pregnancy; postcoital contraception

Pregnancy Considerations Pregnancy should be ruled out prior to treatment and discontinued if pregnancy occurs. In general, the use of combination hormonal contraceptives when inadvertently taken early in pregnancy have not been associated with teratogenic effects. Hormonal contraceptives may be less effective in obese patients. An increase in oral contraceptive failure was noted in women with a BMI >27.3 kg/m². Similar findings were noted in patients weighing ≥90 kg (198 lb) using the contraceptive patch.

Due to increased risk of venous thromboembolism (VTE) postpartum, combination hormonal contraceptives should not be started in any woman <21 days following delivery. ▶

Women without risk factors for VTE and who are not breast-feeding may start combination hormonal contraceptives during 21-42 days postpartum. After 42 days postpartum, restrictions for use are not related to postpartum status and should be based on other medical conditions (CDC, 2011). Some manufacturers recommend waiting ≥4 weeks postpartum before starting this combination.

Breast-Feeding Considerations Jaundice and breast enlargement in the nursing infant have been reported following the use of combination hormonal contraceptives. May decrease the quality and quantity of breast milk; alternative form of contraception is recommended (per manufacturer). The theoretical concerns about decreased milk production are greatest early in the postpartum period when milk production is being established. Postpartum risk status for VTE should be considered when initiating combination hormonal contraceptives after delivery. Combined hormonal contraceptives should not be started <21 days postpartum due to increased risk of VTE. Risk of VTE is still elevated in breast-feeding women until ~42 days postpartum and is greater in women with additional risk factors. After 42 days postpartum, restrictions for use are not related to postpartum VTE risk and should be based on other medical conditions (CDC, 2011). Some manufacturers recommend waiting ≥4 weeks postpartum before starting this combination.

Contraindications Breast cancer or other estrogen- or progestin-dependent neoplasms (current or a history of), hepatic tumors or disease, pregnancy, undiagnosed abnormal uterine bleeding

Use is also contraindicated in women at high risk of arterial or venous thrombotic diseases including: Cerebrovascular disease, coronary artery disease, diabetes mellitus with vascular disease, DVT or PE (current or history of), hypercoagulopathies (inherited or acquired), headaches with focal neurological symptoms, hypertension (uncontrolled), migraine headaches if >35 years of age, thrombogenic valvular or rhythm diseases of the heart (eg, subacute bacterial endocarditis with valvular disease or atrial fibrillation), women >35 years of age who smoke.

Canadian-labeling: Additional contraindication: Ocular lesions due to ophthalmic vascular disease including partial or complete loss of vision or defect in visual fields; severe dyslipoproteinemia; hereditary or acquired predisposition for venous or arterial thrombosis

Warnings/Precautions Hazardous agent - use appropriate precautions for handling and disposal (NIOSH 2014 [group 2]).

Combination hormonal contraceptives do not protect against HIV infection or other sexually-transmitted diseases. **[U.S. Boxed Warning]: The risk of cardiovascular side effects is increased in women who smoke cigarettes; risk increases with age (especially women >35 years of age) and the number of cigarettes smoked; women who use combination hormonal contraceptives should be strongly advised not to smoke. Use is contraindicated in patients >35 years of age who smoke.** Use with caution in patients with risk factors for coronary artery disease (eg, hypertension, hypercholesterolemia, morbid obesity, diabetes, or women who smoke); may lead to increased risk of myocardial infarction. May have a dose-related risk of vascular disease and hypertension; women with hypertension should be encouraged to use a nonhormonal form of contraception. Use is contraindicated with uncontrolled hypertension. May increase the risk of thromboembolism; discontinue use of combination hormonal contraceptives if an arterial or venous thrombotic event occurs. Women with inherited thrombophilias (eg, protein C or S deficiency) may have increased risk of venous thromboembolism (DeSancho, 2010; van Vlijmen, 2011). Use is contraindicated in women with hypercoagulopathies (inherited or acquired). Whenever possible, combination hormonal contraceptives should be discontinued at least 4 weeks prior to and for 2 weeks following elective surgery associated with an increased risk of thromboembolism or during periods of prolonged immobilization. Combination hormonal contraceptives may have a dose-related risk of gallbladder disease and may worsen existing gallbladder disease. Women with renal disease should be encouraged to use another form of contraception. May have adverse effects on glucose tolerance; use caution in women with diabetes.

Combination hormonal contraceptives may affect serum triglyceride and lipoprotein levels. Triglycerides may also be increased; use with caution in patients with familial defects of lipoprotein metabolism. The use of combination hormonal contraceptives has been associated with a slight increase in frequency of breast cancer; however, studies are not consistent. Use is contraindicated in women with (or history of) breast cancer. Use caution with conditions that may be aggravated by fluid retention, depression, or history of migraine. Evaluate new, recurrent, severe or persistent headaches. Use with migraine headaches with or without aura if >35 years of age is contraindicated. Not for use prior to menarche. Estrogens may cause retinal vascular thrombosis; discontinue if migraine, loss of vision, proptosis, diplopia or other visual disturbances occur; discontinue permanently if papilledema or retinal vascular lesions are observed on examination. Risk of chloasma may be increased with history of chloasma gravidarum. Women with history of chloasma should avoid exposure to sun or ultraviolet radiation during therapy. May induce or exacerbate symptoms of hereditary angioedema.

Presentation of irregular, unresolving vaginal bleeding warrants further evaluation including endometrial sampling, if indicated, to rule out malignancy; evaluate hypothalamic-pituitary-function in women with persistent (≥6 months) amenorrhea (especially associated with breast secretion) following discontinuation of therapy. Discontinue use with the onset of sudden enlargement, pain, or tenderness of fibroids (leiomyomata). Extremely rare adenomas and focal nodular hyperplasia resulting in fatal intra-abdominal hemorrhage have been reported in association with long-term oral contraceptive use. Presentation of an abdominal mass, acute abdominal pain, or intra-abdominal bleeding warrants further evaluation to rule out source. Combination hormonal contraceptives may be poorly metabolized in women with hepatic impairment. Discontinue if jaundice develops during therapy or if liver function becomes abnormal. Use is contraindicated with preexisting hepatic tumors or disease. Risk of cholestasis may be increased with previous cholestatic jaundice of pregnancy or jaundice with prior oral contraceptive use. Estrogens may increase thyroid-binding globulin (TBG) levels leading to increased circulating total thyroid hormone levels. Women on thyroid replacement therapy may require higher doses of thyroid hormone while receiving estrogens. The use of estrogens and/or progestins may change the results of some laboratory tests (eg, coagulation factors, lipids, glucose tolerance, binding proteins). The dose, route, and the specific estrogen/progestin influences these changes. In addition, personal risk factors (eg, cardiovascular disease, smoking, diabetes, age) also contribute to adverse events; use of specific products may be contraindicated in women with certain risk factors. Some products may contain tartrazine, which may cause allergic reactions in certain individuals.

The minimum dosage combination of estrogen/progestin that will effectively treat the individual patient should be used. New patients should be started on products containing ≤0.035 mg of estrogen per tablet. Extended cycle regimen contraceptives provide more hormonal exposure per year than conventional monthly contraceptives.

Adverse Reactions The following reactions have been associated with oral contraceptive use:
Increased risk or evidence of association with use:
   Cardiovascular: Arterial thromboembolism, cerebral hemorrhage, cerebral thrombosis, hypertension, mesenteric thrombosis, MI, venous thrombosis (with or without embolism)
   Gastrointestinal: Gallbladder disease
   Hepatic: Hepatic adenomas, liver tumors (benign)
   Local: Thrombophlebitis
   Ocular: Retinal thrombosis
   Respiratory: Pulmonary embolism
Adverse reactions considered drug related:
   Cardiovascular: Edema, varicose vein aggravation
   Central nervous system: Depression, migraine, mood changes
   Dermatologic: Chloasma, melasma, rash (allergic)
   Endocrine & metabolic: Amenorrhea, breakthrough bleeding, breast changes (enlargement, pain, secretion, tenderness), carbohydrate tolerance decreased, fluid retention, infertility (temporary), lactation decreased (with use immediately postpartum), menstrual flow changes, spotting
   Gastrointestinal: Abdominal bloating, abdominal cramps, abdominal pain, appetite changes, nausea, weight changes, vomiting
   Genitourinary: Cervical ectropion, cervical secretion/erosion, endocervical hyperplasia, fibroid enlargement, vaginal candidiasis, vaginitis
   Hematologic: Folate decreased, porphyria exacerbation
   Hepatic: Cholestatic jaundice, focal nodular hyperplasia
   Neuromuscular & skeletal: Chorea exacerbation
   Ocular: Contact lens intolerance, corneal curvature changes (steepening)
   Respiratory: Rhinitis

Miscellaneous: Anaphylactic/anaphylactoid reactions (including angioedema, circulatory collapse, respiratory collapse, urticaria), SLE exacerbation

Adverse reactions in which association is not confirmed or denied: Acne, auditory disturbances, Budd-Chiari syndrome, cataracts, cervical smear abnormal, colitis, cystitis-like syndrome, dizziness, dysmenorrhea, erythema multiforme, erythema nodosum, headache, hemolytic uremic syndrome, hemorrhagic eruption, hirsutism, libido changes, nervousness, optic neuritis (with or without partial or complete loss of vision), pancreatitis, premenstrual syndrome, renal function impaired, scalp hair loss

Drug Interactions

Metabolism/Transport Effects Refer to individual components.

Avoid Concomitant Use

Avoid concomitant use of Ethinyl Estradiol and Levonorgestrel with any of the following: Amodiaquine; Anastrozole; Antihepaciviral Combination Products; Dehydroepiandrosterone; Exemestane; Hemin; Indium 111 Capromab Pendetide; Ospemifene; TiZANidine; Tranexamic Acid

Increased Effect/Toxicity

Ethinyl Estradiol and Levonorgestrel may increase the levels/effects of: Agomelatine; Amodiaquine; Anthrax Immune Globulin (Human); Antihepaciviral Combination Products; C1 inhibitors; Corticosteroids (Systemic); CYP1A2 Substrates; Flibanserin; Immune Globulin; Lenalidomide; Ospemifene; Pirfenidone; ROPINIRole; Selegiline; Thalidomide; Theophylline Derivatives; Tipranavir; TiZANidine; Tranexamic Acid; Voriconazole

The levels/effects of Ethinyl Estradiol and Levonorgestrel may be increased by: Ascorbic Acid; Dehydroepiandrosterone; Herbs (Estrogenic Properties); Metreleptin; Mifepristone; NSAID (COX-2 Inhibitor); Osimertinib; Voriconazole

Decreased Effect

Ethinyl Estradiol and Levonorgestrel may decrease the levels/effects of: Anastrozole; Anticoagulants; Antidiabetic Agents; Chenodiol; Exemestane; Hemin; Hyaluronidase; Indium 111 Capromab Pendetide; LamoTRIgine; Ospemifene; Thyroid Products; Ursodiol; Vitamin K Antagonists

The levels/effects of Ethinyl Estradiol and Levonorgestrel may be decreased by: Aprepitant; Armodafinil; Artemether; Barbiturates; Bexarotene (Systemic); Bile Acid Sequestrants; Boceprevir; Bosentan; CarBAMazepine; CloBAZam; Cobicistat; Colesevelam; CYP3A4 Inducers (Moderate); CYP3A4 Inducers (Strong); Dabrafenib; Deferasirox; Elvitegravir; Enzalutamide; Eslicarbazepine; Exenatide; Felbamate; Fosaprepitant; Fosphenytoin; Griseofulvin; Lesinurad; Lumacaftor; Metreleptin; Mifepristone; Mitotane; Modafinil; Mycophenolate; Nafcillin; Nevirapine; Osimertinib; OXcarbazepine; Phenytoin; Protease Inhibitors; Prucalopride; Retinoic Acid Derivatives; Rifamycin Derivatives; Rufinamide; Siltuximab; St Johns Wort; Sugammadex; Telaprevir; Tipranavir; Tocilizumab; Topiramate

Storage/Stability Store at controlled room temperature of 20°C to 25°C (68°F to 77°F).

Mechanism of Action Combination hormonal contraceptives inhibit ovulation via a negative feedback mechanism on the hypothalamus, which alters the normal pattern of gonadotropin secretion of a follicle-stimulating hormone (FSH) and luteinizing hormone by the anterior pituitary. The follicular phase FSH and midcycle surge of gonadotropins are inhibited. In addition, combination hormonal contraceptives produce alterations in the genital tract, including changes in the cervical mucus, rendering it unfavorable for sperm penetration even if ovulation occurs. Changes in the endometrium may also occur, producing an unfavorable environment for nidation. Combination hormonal contraceptive drugs may alter the tubal transport of the ova through the fallopian tubes. Progestational agents may also alter sperm fertility.

Pharmacodynamics/Kinetics

Absorption: Rapid

Distribution: Ethinyl estradiol: 4.3 L/kg; Levonorgestrel: 1.8 L/kg

Protein binding:

Ethinyl estradiol: 95% to 97% to albumin

Levonorgestrel: 97% to 99% primarily to sex hormone binding globulin (SHBG), lesser amounts to albumin

Metabolism:

Ethinyl estradiol: Hepatic via CYP3A4; undergoes first-pass metabolism; forms metabolites

Levonorgestrel: Forms conjugated in unconjugated metabolites

Bioavailability: Ethinyl estradiol: 38% to 48%; Levonorgestrel: 100%

Half-life elimination: Ethinyl estradiol: 12-23 hours; Levonorgestrel: 22-49 hours

Excretion:

Ethinyl estradiol: Urine and feces

Levonorgestrel: Urine (40% to 68%, parent drug and metabolites); feces (16% to 48% as metabolites)

Dosing

Adult Females:

Contraception, 28-day cycle: Oral:

Schedule 1 (Sunday starter): Dose begins on first Sunday after onset of menstruation; if the menstrual period starts on Sunday, take first tablet that very same day. With a Sunday start, an additional method of contraception should be used until after the first 7 days of consecutive administration:

For 21-tablet package: 1 tablet/day for 21 consecutive days, followed by 7 days off of the medication; a new course begins on the 8th day after the last tablet is taken

For 28-tablet package: 1 tablet/day without interruption

Schedule 2 (Day-1 starter): Dose starts on first day of menstrual cycle taking 1 tablet/day:

For 21-tablet package: 1 tablet/day for 21 consecutive days, followed by 7 days off of the medication; a new course begins on the 8th day after the last tablet is taken

For 28-tablet package: 1 tablet/day without interruption

If all doses have been taken on schedule and one menstrual period is missed, continue dosing cycle. If two consecutive menstrual periods are missed, pregnancy test is required before new dosing cycle is started.

Missed doses **monophasic formulations** (refer to package insert for complete information):

One dose missed: Take as soon as remembered or take 2 tablets next day

Two consecutive doses missed in the first 2 weeks: Take 2 tablets as soon as remembered or 2 tablets next 2 days. An additional method of contraception should be used for 7 days after missed dose.

Two consecutive doses missed in week 3 or three consecutive doses missed at any time: An additional method of contraception must be used for 7 days after a missed dose:

Schedule 1 (Sunday starter): Continue dose of 1 tablet daily until Sunday, then discard the rest of the pack, and a new pack should be started that same day.

Schedule 2 (Day-1 starter): Current pack should be discarded, and a new pack should be started that same day.

Missed doses **biphasic/triphasic formulations** (refer to package insert for complete information):

One dose missed: Take as soon as remembered or take 2 tablets next day.

Two consecutive doses missed in week 1 or week 2 of the pack: Take 2 tablets as soon as remembered and 2 tablets the next day. Resume taking 1 tablet daily until the pack is empty. An additional method of contraception should be used for 7 days after a missed dose.

Two consecutive doses missed in week 3 of the pack: An additional method of contraception must be used for 7 days after a missed dose.

Schedule 1 (Sunday starter): Take 1 tablet every day until Sunday. Discard the remaining pack and start a new pack of pills on the same day.

Schedule 2 (Day-1 starter): Discard the remaining pack and start a new pack the same day.

Three or more consecutive doses missed: An additional method of contraception must be used for 7 days after a missed dose.

Schedule 1 (Sunday starter): Take 1 tablet every day until Sunday; on Sunday, discard the pack and start a new pack.

Schedule 2 (Day-1 starter): Discard the remaining pack and begin new pack of tablets starting on the same day.

Contraception, 91-day cycle (extended cycle regimen): Dose begins on first Sunday after onset of menstruation; if the menstrual period starts on Sunday, take first tablet that very same day. An additional method of contraception should be used until after the first 7 days of consecutive administration:

Introvale, Jolessa, Quasense, Seasonale [Canadian product]: One active tablet/day for 84 consecutive days, followed by 1 inactive tablet/day for 7 days; if all doses have been taken on schedule and one menstrual period is missed, pregnancy should be ruled out prior to continuing therapy.

Seasonique, LoSeasonique, Quartette: One active tablet/day for 84 consecutive days, followed by 1 low dose estrogen tablet/day for 7 days; if all doses have been taken on schedule and one menstrual period is missed, pregnancy should be ruled out prior to continuing therapy.

Missed doses:

One dose missed: Take as soon as remembered or take 2 tablets the next day

Two consecutive doses missed: Take 2 tablets as soon as remembered or 2 tablets the next 2 days. An additional nonhormonal method of contraception should be used for 7 consecutive days after the missed dose.

Three or more consecutive doses missed: Do not take the missed doses; continue taking 1 tablet/day until pack is complete. Bleeding may occur during the following week. An additional nonhormonal method of contraception should be used for 7 consecutive days after the missed dose.

Any number of pills during week 13: Throw away the missed pills and keep taking scheduled pills until the pack is finished. A back-up method of contraception is not needed

Contraception, continuous use (extended cycle regimen): Oral: Lybrel: Take one tablet daily, at the same time each day, without a tablet-free interval. Therapy should be initiated as follows:

No previous contraception: Begin on the first day of menstrual cycle. Back-up contraception is not needed.

Previously taking a 21-day or 28-day combination hormonal contraceptive: Begin on day 1 of the withdrawal bleed (at the latest, 7 days after the last active tablet). Back-up contraception is not needed.

Previously using a progestin-only pill: Begin the day after taking a progestin only pill. Back-up contraception is needed for the first 7 days of therapy.

Previously using contraceptive implant: Begin the day of implant removal. Back-up contraception is needed for the first 7 days of therapy.

Previously using contraceptive injection: Begin when the next injection is due. Back-up contraception is needed for the first 7 days of therapy.

Missed doses:

One dose missed: Take as soon as remembered then take the next tablet at the regular time (2 tablets in 1 day). An additional nonhormonal method of contraception should also be used for 7 consecutive days.

Two consecutive doses missed: If remembered the day of the second missed tablet, take 2 tablets as soon as remembered, then 1 tablet the next day. If remembered the day after the second tablet is missed, take 2 tablets the day remembered, then 2 tablets the next day. An additional nonhormonal method of contraception should also be used for 7 consecutive days.

Three or more consecutive doses missed: Take 1 tablet daily and contact healthcare provider; do not take the missed pills. An additional nonhormonal method of contraception should also be used for 7 consecutive days.

Pediatric Females: Contraception or emergency contraception: Oral: Refer to adult dosing; not to be used prior to menarche.

Renal Impairment Specific guidelines not available; use with caution and monitor blood pressure closely. Consider other forms of contraception.

Hepatic Impairment Contraindicated in patients with hepatic impairment.

Dietary Considerations Should be taken at the same time each day.

Administration Administer at the same time each day.

Quartette: If severe diarrhea or vomiting occur within 3-4 hours after taking a light pink, pink, or purple tablet, it should be considered a missed dose; additional contraceptive measures are recommended.

Hazardous agent; use appropriate precautions for handling and disposal (NIOSH 2014 [group 2]).

Monitoring Parameters Before starting therapy, a physical exam with reference to the breasts and pelvis are recommended, including a Papanicolaou smear. Exam may be deferred if appropriate; pregnancy should be ruled out prior to use. Monitor patient closely for loss of vision, sudden onset of proptosis, diplopia, migraine; blood pressure; signs and symptoms of thromboembolic disorders; signs or symptoms of depression; glycemic control in patients with diabetes; lipid profiles in patients being treated for hyperlipidemias. Adequate diagnostic measures, including endometrial sampling, if indicated, should

be performed to rule out malignancy in all cases of undiagnosed abnormal vaginal bleeding.

Dosage Forms Excipient information presented when available (limited, particularly for generics); consult specific product labeling. [DSC] = Discontinued product

Tablet, oral [low-dose formulation]:

Aubra: Ethinyl estradiol 0.02 mg and levonorgestrel 0.1 mg [21 light yellow tablets and 7 brown inactive tablets] (28s)

Aviane: Ethinyl estradiol 0.02 mg and levonorgestrel 0.1 mg [21 orange tablets and 7 light green inactive tablets] (28s)

Delyla: Ethinyl estradiol 0.02 mg and levonorgestrel 0.1 mg [21 white tablets and 7 yellow inactive tablets] (28s)

FaLessa Kit: Ethinyl estradiol 0.02 mg and levonorgestrel 0.1 mg [21 orange tablets and 7 white inactive tablets] (28s) [contains soya lecithin, tartrazine; packaged with Quatrefolic folate tablets]

Falmina: Ethinyl estradiol 0.02 mg and levonorgestrel 0.1 mg [21 orange tablets and 7 white inactive tablets] (28s) [contains soya lecithin, tartrazine]

Lessina: Ethinyl estradiol 0.02 mg and levonorgestrel 0.1 mg [21 pink tablets and 7 white inactive tablets] (28s)

Lutera: Ethinyl estradiol 0.02 mg and levonorgestrel 0.1 mg [21 white tablets and 7 peach inactive tablets] (28s)

Orsythia: Ethinyl estradiol 0.02 mg and levonorgestrel 0.1 mg [21 pink tablets and 7 light green inactive tablets] (28s)

Sronyx: Ethinyl estradiol 0.02 mg and levonorgestrel 0.1 mg [21 white tablets and 7 peach inactive tablets] (28s)

Vienva: Ethinyl estradiol 0.02 mg and levonorgestrel 0.1 mg [21 white tablets and 7 peach inactive tablets] (28s)

Generic: Ethinyl estradiol 0.02 mg and levonorgestrel 0.1 mg [21 tablets and 7 inactive tablets] (28s)

Tablet, oral [monophasic formulation]:

Altavera: Ethinyl estradiol 0.03 mg and levonorgestrel 0.15 mg [21 peach tablets and 7 white inactive tablets] (28s)

Chateal: Ethinyl estradiol 0.03 mg and levonorgestrel 0.15 mg [21 white tablets and 7 green inactive tablets] (28s)

Kurvelo: Ethinyl estradiol 0.03 mg and levonorgestrel 0.15 mg [21 light orange tablets and 7 pink inactive tablets] (28s)

Levora: Ethinyl estradiol 0.03 mg and levonorgestrel 0.15 mg [21 white tablets and 7 peach inactive tablets] (28s)

Marlissa: Ethinyl estradiol 0.03 mg and levonorgestrel 0.15 mg [21 light orange tablets and 7 pink inactive tablets] (28s)

Portia 28: Ethinyl estradiol 0.03 mg and levonorgestrel 0.15 mg [21 pink tablets and 7 white inactive tablets] (28s)

Generic: Ethinyl estradiol 0.03 mg and levonorgestrel 0.15 mg [21 tablets and 7 inactive tablets] (28s)

Tablet, oral [extended cycle regimen]:

Amethia: Ethinyl estradiol 0.03 mg and levonorgestrel 0.15 mg [84 white tablets] and ethinyl estradiol 0.01 mg [7 light blue tablets] (91s)

Amethia Lo: Ethinyl estradiol 0.02 mg and levonorgestrel 0.1 mg [84 white tablets] and ethinyl estradiol 0.01 mg [7 blue tablets] (91s)

Ashlyna: Ethinyl estradiol 0.03 mg and levonorgestrel 0.15 mg [84 blue tablets] and ethinyl estradiol 0.01 mg [7 yellow tablets] (91s)

camrese: Ethinyl estradiol 0.03 mg and levonorgestrel 0.15 mg [84 light blue-green tablets] and ethinyl estradiol 0.01 mg [7 yellow tablets] (91s)

camrese lo: Ethinyl estradiol 0.02 mg and levonorgestrel 0.1 mg [84 orange tablets] and ethinyl estradiol 0.01 mg [7 yellow tablets] (91s)

Daysee: Ethinyl estradiol 0.03 mg and levonorgestrel 0.15 mg [84 light blue tablets] and ethinyl estradiol 0.01 mg [7 mustard tablets] (91s)

Introvale: Ethinyl estradiol 0.03 mg and levonorgestrel 0.15 mg [84 peach tablets and 7 white inactive tablets] (91s)

Jolessa: Ethinyl estradiol 0.03 mg and levonorgestrel 0.15 mg [84 pink tablets and 7 white inactive tablets] (91s)

LoSeasonique: Ethinyl estradiol 0.02 mg and levonorgestrel 0.1 mg [84 orange tablets] and ethinyl estradiol 0.01 mg [7 yellow tablets] (91s)

Quartette:

Day 1-42: Ethinyl estradiol 0.02 mg and levonorgestrel 0.15 mg [42 light pink tablets]

Day 43-63: Ethinyl estradiol 0.025 mg and levonorgestrel 0.15 mg [21 pink tablets]

Day 64-84: Ethinyl estradiol 0.03 mg and levonorgestrel 0.15 mg [21 purple tablets]

Day 85-91: Ethinyl estradiol 0.01 mg [7 yellow tablets] (91s)

Quasense: Ethinyl estradiol 0.03 mg and levonorgestrel 0.15 mg [84 white tablets and 7 peach inactive tablets] (91s)

Seasonique: Ethinyl estradiol 0.03 mg and levonorgestrel 0.15 mg [84 light blue-green tablets] and ethinyl estradiol 0.01 mg [7 yellow tablets] (91s)

Setlakin: Ethinyl estradiol 0.03 mg and levonorgestrel 0.15 mg [84 pink tablets and 7 white inactive tablets] (91s)

Generic: Ethinyl estradiol 0.02 mg and levonorgestrel 0.1 mg [84 tablets] and ethinyl estradiol 0.01 mg [7 tablets] (91s); Ethinyl estradiol 0.03 mg and levonorgestrel 0.15 mg [84 tablets] and ethinyl estradiol 0.01 mg [7 tablets] (91s); Ethinyl estradiol 0.03 mg and levonorgestrel 0.15 mg [84 tablets and 7 inactive tablets] (91s)

Tablet, oral [noncyclic regimen]:

Amethyst: Ethinyl estradiol 0.02 mg and levonorgestrel 0.09 mg [28 white tablets] (28s)

Lybrel: Ethinyl estradiol 0.02 mg and levonorgestrel 0.09 mg [28 yellow tablets] (28s)

Tablet, oral [triphasic formulation]:

Enpresse:

Day 1-6: Ethinyl estradiol 0.03 mg and levonorgestrel 0.05 mg [6 pink tablets]

Day 7-11: Ethinyl estradiol 0.04 mg and levonorgestrel 0.075 mg [5 white tablets]

Day 12-21: Ethinyl estradiol 0.03 mg and levonorgestrel 0.125 mg [10 orange tablets]

Day 22-28: 7 light green inactive tablets (28s)

Levonest:

Day 1-6: Ethinyl estradiol 0.03 mg and levonorgestrel 0.05 mg [6 yellow tablets]

Day 7-11: Ethinyl estradiol 0.04 mg and levonorgestrel 0.075 mg [5 green tablets]

Day 12-21: Ethinyl estradiol 0.03 mg and levonorgestrel 0.125 mg [10 light brown tablets]

Day 22-28: 7 white inactive tablets (28s)

Myzilra:

Day 1-6: Ethinyl estradiol 0.03 mg and levonorgestrel 0.05 mg [6 beige tablets]

Day 7-11: Ethinyl estradiol 0.04 mg and levonorgestrel 0.075 mg [5 white tablets]

Day 12-21: Ethinyl estradiol 0.03 mg and levonorgestrel 0.125 mg [10 light yellow tablets]

Day 22-28: 7 light green inactive tablets (28s)

Trivora:

Day 1-6: Ethinyl estradiol 0.03 mg and levonorgestrel 0.05 mg [6 blue tablets]

Day 7-11: Ethinyl estradiol 0.04 mg and levonorgestrel 0.075 mg [5 white tablets]

Day 12-21: Ethinyl estradiol 0.03 mg and levonorgestrel 0.125 mg [10 pink tablets]

Day 22-28: 7 peach inactive tablets (28s)

Generic:

Day 1-6: Ethinyl estradiol 0.03 mg and levonorgestrel 0.05 mg [6 tablets]

Day 7-11: Ethinyl estradiol 0.04 mg and levonorgestrel 0.075 mg [5 tablets]

Day 12-21: Ethinyl estradiol 0.03 mg and levonorgestrel 0.125 mg [10 tablets]

Day 22-28: 7 inactive tablets (28s)

◆ Ethinyl Estradiol and NGM see Ethinyl Estradiol and Norgestimate on page 710

Ethinyl Estradiol and Norelgestromin

(ETH in il es tra DYE ole & nor el JES troe min)

Brand Names: US Ortho Evra [DSC]; Xulane

Brand Names: Canada Evra

Index Terms Norelgestromin and Ethinyl Estradiol; Ortho-Evra

Pharmacologic Category Contraceptive; Estrogen and Progestin Combination

Use

Contraception: For the prevention of pregnancy

Limitations of use: The topical patch may be less effective in patients weighing ≥90 kg (198 lb).

Dosing

Adult Females: Contraception: Topical:

Apply one patch each week for 3 weeks (21 total days); followed by one week that is patch-free. Each patch should be applied on the same day each week ("patch change day") and only one patch should be worn at a time. No more than 7 days should pass during the patch-free interval.

Schedule 1 (Sunday starter): Dose begins on first Sunday after onset of menstruation; if the menstrual period starts on Sunday, apply one patch that very same day. **With a Sunday start, an additional method of contraception (nonhormonal) must be used until after the first 7 days of consecutive administration unless the menstrual period starts on Sunday.** Each patch change will then occur on Sunday.

Schedule 2 (Day 1 starter): Dose starts on first day of menstrual cycle, applying one patch during the first 24 hours of menstrual cycle. No back-up method of contraception is needed as long as the patch is applied on the first day of cycle. Each patch change will then occur on that same day of the week.

Additional dosing considerations:

No bleeding during patch-free week/missed menstrual period: If patch has been applied as directed, continue treatment on usual "patch change day". If used correctly, no bleeding during patch-free week does not necessarily indicate pregnancy. However, if no withdrawal bleeding occurs for 2 consecutive cycles, pregnancy should be ruled out. If patch has not been applied as directed, and one menstrual period is missed, pregnancy should be ruled out prior to continuing treatment.

If a patch becomes partially or completely detached for <24 hours: Try to reapply to same place, or replace with a new patch immediately. Do not reapply if patch is no longer sticky, if it is sticking to itself or another surface, or if it has material sticking to it.

If a patch becomes partially or completely detached for >24 hours (or time period is unknown): Apply a new patch and use this day of the week as the new "patch change day" from this point on. **An additional method of contraception (nonhormonal) must be used until after the first 7 days of consecutive administration.**

Switching from oral contraceptives or vaginal ring: Complete current cycle and apply the first patch on the day the next pill cycle would be started or ring would be inserted. If there is no menstrual bleeding within 7 days of taking the last active tablet, the patient can initiate the first patch application; however, pregnancy must be ruled out. If patch is applied later than 7 days after the last active pill or removal of the vaginal ring, **an additional method of contraception (nonhormonal) should be used until after the first 7 days of consecutive administration**

Use after childbirth: Therapy should not be started <4 weeks after childbirth. Pregnancy should be ruled out prior to treatment if menstrual periods have not restarted. **An additional method of contraception (nonhormonal) should be used until after the first 7 days of consecutive administration.**

Use after abortion or miscarriage: Therapy may be started immediately if abortion/miscarriage occurs within the first trimester. If therapy is not started within 5 days, follow instructions for first time use. An additional method of contraception (nonhormonal) should be used until after the first 7 days of consecutive administration. If abortion/miscarriage occurs during the second trimester, therapy should not be started for at least 4 weeks. Follow directions for use after childbirth.

Pediatric Females: Contraception: Topical: Refer to adult dosing; not to be used prior to menarche.

Renal Impairment There are no dosage adjustments provided in manufacturers labeling (has not been studied); use with caution and monitor blood pressure closely.

Hepatic Impairment Contraindicated in patients with hepatic impairment.

Additional Information Complete prescribing information should be consulted for additional detail.

Dosage Forms Excipient information presented when available (limited, particularly for generics); consult specific product labeling. [DSC] = Discontinued product

Patch, transdermal:

Ortho Evra: Ethinyl estradiol 0.75 mg and norelgestromin 6 mg [releases ethinyl estradiol 35 mcg and norelgestromin 150 mcg per day] (1s DSC], 3s [DSC])

Xulane: Ethinyl estradiol 0.53 mg and norelgestromin 4.86 mg [releases ethinyl estradiol 35 mcg and norelgestromin 150 mcg per day] (3s)

◀ **Dosage Forms: Canada** Excipient information presented when available (limited, particularly for generics); consult specific product labeling.

Patch, transdermal:

Evra: Ethinyl estradiol 0.6 mg and norelgestromin 6 mg [releases ethinyl estradiol 35 mcg and norelgestromin 200 mcg per day] (1s, 3s)

Ethinyl Estradiol and Norethindrone
(ETH in il es tra DYE ole & nor eth IN drone)

Brand Names: US Alyacen 1/35; Alyacen 7/7/7; Aranelle; Balziva; Blisovi 24 Fe; Blisovi Fe 1/20; Brevicon; Briellyn; Cyclafem 1/35; Cyclafem 7/7/7; Dasetta 1/35; Dasetta 7/7/7; Estrostep Fe; Femcon Fe; femhrt; Generess Fe; Gildagia; Gildess 24 Fe; Gildess FE 1.5/30; Gildess FE 1/20; Jevantique Lo; Jinteli; Junel 1.5/30; Junel 1/20; Junel Fe 1.5/30; Junel Fe 1/20; Junel Fe 24; Larin 1.5/30; Larin 1/20; Larin 24 Fe; Larin Fe 1.5/30; Larin Fe 1/20; Layolis Fe; Leena; Lo Loestrin Fe; Lo Minastrin Fe [DSC]; Loestrin 21 1.5/30; Loestrin 21 1/20; Loestrin 24 Fe; Loestrin Fe 1.5/30; Loestrin Fe 1/20; Lomedia 24 Fe; Microgestin 1.5/30; Microgestin 1/20; Microgestin 24 Fe; Microgestin Fe 1.5/30; Microgestin Fe 1/20; Minastrin 24 Fe; Modicon; Necon 0.5/35; Necon 1/35; Necon 10/11; Necon 7/7/7; Norinyl 1+35; Nortrel 0.5/35; Nortrel 1/35; Nortrel 7/7/7; Ortho-Novum 1/35; Ortho-Novum 7/7/7; Ovcon 35; Philith; Pirmella 1/35; Pirmella 7/7/7; Tarina FE 1/20; Tilia Fe; Tri-Legest Fe; Tri-Norinyl; Vyfemla; Wera; Wymzya Fe; Zenchent; Zenchent Fe

Brand Names: Canada Brevicon 0.5/35; Brevicon 1/35; FemHRT; Loestrin 1.5/30; Minestrin 1/20; Ortho 0.5/35; Ortho 1/35; Ortho 7/7/7; Select 1/35; Synphasic

Index Terms Estrostep 21; Norethindrone Acetate and Ethinyl Estradiol; Ortho Novum; Ovcon-50

Pharmacologic Category Contraceptive; Estrogen and Progestin Combination

Use

Acne vulgaris: For the treatment of moderate acne vulgaris in females at least 15 years of age.

Limitations of Use: When used for acne, use only in females ≥15 years of age who have achieved menarche, who also desire combination hormonal contraceptive therapy, are unresponsive to topical treatments, have no contraindications to combination hormonal contraceptive use, and plan to stay on therapy for ≥6 months.

Contraception: For the prevention of pregnancy.

Moderate to severe vasomotor symptoms: Treatment of moderate to severe vasomotor symptoms associated with menopause.

Osteoporosis prevention: For prevention of postmenopausal osteoporosis.

Limitations of use: For use only in women at significant risk of osteoporosis and for whom other nonestrogen medications are not considered appropriate.

Dosing

Adult & Geriatric

Adolescents ≥15 years and Adults: Females: Acne:
Estrostep Fe: Oral: Refer to dosing for contraception

Moderate-to-severe vasomotor symptoms associated with menopause: Initial: femhrt 0.5/2.5: Oral: 1 tablet daily; patient should be re-evaluated at 3- to 6-month intervals to determine if treatment is still necessary; patient should be maintained on lowest effective dose

Prevention of osteoporosis: Initial: femhrt 0.5/2.5: Oral: 1 tablet daily; patient should be maintained on lowest effective dose

Contraception: Oral:

Schedule 1 (Sunday starter): Dose begins on first Sunday after onset of menstruation; if the menstrual period starts on Sunday, take first tablet that very same day. (This schedule is not preferred for all products [eg, Generess Fe, Lo Loestrin Fe, Lo Minastrin Fe]). With a Sunday start, an additional method of contraception should be used until after the first 7 days of consecutive administration (all products).

For 21-tablet package: Dosage is 1 tablet daily for 21 consecutive days, followed by 7 days off of the medication; a new course begins on the 8th day after the last tablet is taken.

For 28-tablet package: Dosage is 1 tablet daily without interruption.

Schedule 2 (Day 1 starter): Dose starts on first day of menstrual cycle taking 1 tablet daily.

For 21-tablet package: Dosage is 1 tablet daily for 21 consecutive days, followed by 7 days off of the medication; a new course begins on the 8th day after the last tablet is taken.

For 28-tablet package: Dosage is 1 tablet daily without interruption.

If all doses have not been taken on schedule and one menstrual period is missed, the possibility of pregnancy should be considered. If two consecutive menstrual periods are missed, pregnancy test is required before new dosing cycle is started.

Missed doses **monophasic formulations** (refer to package insert for complete information):

One dose missed: Take as soon as remembered. Take the next tablet at your regular time. You may take 2 tablets in 1 day.

Two consecutive doses missed in the first 2 weeks: Take 2 tablets as soon as remembered and 2 tablets the next day. An additional method of contraception should be used for 7 days after missed dose.

Two consecutive doses missed in week 3 (all products) or in week 4 (some products), or three consecutive doses missed at any time (all products): An additional method of contraception must be used for 7 days after a missed dose.

Schedule 1 (Sunday starter): Continue dose of 1 tablet daily until Sunday, then discard the rest of the pack, and a new pack should be started that same day.

Schedule 2 (Day 1 starter): Current pack should be discarded, and a new pack should be started that same day.

Missed doses **biphasic/triphasic formulations** (refer to package insert for complete information):

One dose missed: Take as soon as remembered. Take the next tablet at your regular time. You may take 2 tablets in 1 day.

Two consecutive doses missed in week 1 or week 2 of the pack: Take 2 tablets as soon as remembered and 2 tablets the next day. Resume taking 1 tablet daily until the pack is empty. An additional method of contraception should be used for 7 days after a missed dose.

Two consecutive doses missed in week 3 of the pack: An additional method of contraception must be used for 7 days after a missed dose.

Schedule 1 (Sunday Starter): Take 1 tablet every day until Sunday. Discard the remaining pack and start a new pack of pills on the same day.

Schedule 2 (Day 1 starter): Discard the remaining pack and start a new pack the same day.

Three or more consecutive doses missed: An additional method of contraception must be used for 7 days after a missed dose.

Schedule 1 (Sunday Starter): Take 1 tablet every day until Sunday; on Sunday, discard the pack and start a new pack.

Schedule 2 (Day 1 Starter): Discard the remaining pack and begin new pack of tablets starting on the same day.

Switching from a different contraceptive:

Oral contraceptive: Start on the same day that a new pack of the previous oral contraceptive would have been taken.

Transdermal patch, vaginal ring, injection: Start on the day the next dose would have been due.

IUD or implant: Start on the day of removal. A backup method of contraception may be required following IUD removal.

Use after childbirth (in women who are not breast-feeding) or after second trimester abortion: Therapy may be started ≥4 weeks postpartum. Pregnancy should be ruled out prior to treatment if menstrual periods have not restarted and an additional method of contraception (nonhormonal) should be used until after the first 7 days of consecutive administration.

Pediatric Females:

Acne: Oral (Estrostep Fe): For use in females ≥15 years; refer to adult dosing for contraception

Contraception: Oral: Refer to adult dosing; not to be used prior to menarche.

Renal Impairment No dosage adjustment provided in manufacturer's labeling; use with caution and monitor blood pressure closely. Consider other forms of contraception.

Hepatic Impairment Contraindicated in patients with hepatic impairment.

Additional Information Complete prescribing information should be consulted for additional detail.

Dosage Forms Excipient information presented when available (limited, particularly for generics); consult specific product labeling. [DSC] = Discontinued product

Tablet, oral:

femhrt 0.5/2.5: Ethinyl estradiol 0.0025 mg and norethindrone acetate 0.5 mg [white tablets] (28s)

Jevantique Lo: Ethinyl estradiol 0.0025 mg and norethindrone acetate 0.5 mg [white tablets] (28s)

Jinteli: Ethinyl estradiol 0.005 mg and norethindrone acetate 1 mg [white tablets] (28s, 90s)

Tablet, oral [monophasic formulation]:

Alyacen 1/35: Ethinyl estradiol 0.035 mg and norethindrone 1 mg [21 peach tablets and 7 light green inactive tablets] (28s)

Balziva: Ethinyl estradiol 0.035 mg and norethindrone 0.4 mg [21 light peach tablets and 7 white inactive tablets] (28s)

Blisovi 24 Fe: Ethinyl estradiol 0.02 mg and norethindrone acetate 1 mg [24 white tablets] and ferrous fumarate 75 mg [4 brown tablets] (28s)

Blisovi Fe 1/20: Ethinyl estradiol 0.02 mg and norethindrone acetate 1 mg [21 yellow tablets] and ferrous fumarate 75 mg [7 brown tablets] (28s)

Brevicon: Ethinyl estradiol 0.035 mg and norethindrone 0.5 mg [21 blue tablets and 7 orange inactive tablets] (28s)

Briellyn: Ethinyl estradiol 0.035 mg and norethindrone 0.4 mg [21 light peach tablets and 7 white-off-white inactive tablets] (28s)

Cyclafem 1/35: Ethinyl estradiol 0.035 mg and norethindrone 1 mg [21 pink tablets and 7 light green inactive tablets] (28s)

Dasetta 1/35: Ethinyl estradiol 0.035 mg and norethindrone 1 mg [21 orange tablets and 7 white inactive tablets] (28s) [contains soya lecithin, tartrazine]

Gildagia: Ethinyl estradiol 0.035 mg and norethindrone 0.4 mg [21 peach tablets and 7 light green inactive tablets] (28s)

Gildess FE 1/20: Ethinyl estradiol 0.02 mg and norethindrone acetate 1 mg [21 white tablets] and ferrous fumarate 75 mg [7 white-speckled brown tablets] (28s)

Gildess FE 1.5/30: Ethinyl estradiol 0.03 mg and norethindrone acetate 1.5 mg [21 light green tablets] and ferrous fumarate 75 mg [7 white-speckled brown tablets] (28s)

Gildess 24 Fe: Ethinyl estradiol 0.02 mg and norethindrone acetate 1 mg [24 white tablets] and ferrous fumarate 75 mg [4 white-speckled brown tablets] (28s)

Junel 1/20: Ethinyl estradiol 0.02 mg and norethindrone acetate 1 mg [yellow tablets] (21s)

Junel 1.5/30: Ethinyl estradiol 0.03 mg and norethindrone acetate 1.5 mg [pink tablets] (21s)

Junel Fe 1/20: Ethinyl estradiol 0.02 mg and norethindrone acetate 1 mg [21 yellow tablets] and ferrous fumarate 75 mg [7 brown tablets] (28s)

Junel Fe 1.5/30: Ethinyl estradiol 0.03 mg and norethindrone acetate 1.5 mg [21 pink tablets] and ferrous fumarate 75 mg [7 brown tablets] (28s)

Junel Fe 24: Ethinyl estradiol 0.02 mg and norethindrone acetate 1 mg [24 pale yellow tablets] and ferrous fumarate 75 mg [4 brown tablets] (28s)

Larin 1/20: Ethinyl estradiol 0.02 mg and norethindrone acetate 1 mg [21 pale yellow tablets] (21s) [contains soya lecithin]

Larin 1.5/30: Ethinyl estradiol 0.03 mg and norethindrone acetate 1.5 mg [21 green tablets] (21s) [contains soya lecithin]

Larin Fe 1/20: Ethinyl estradiol 0.02 mg and norethindrone acetate 1 mg [21 pale yellow tablets] and ferrous fumarate 75 mg [7 brown tablets] (28s) [contains soya lecithin]

Larin Fe 1.5/30: Ethinyl estradiol 0.03 mg and norethindrone acetate 1.5 mg [21 green tablets] and ferrous fumarate 75 mg [7 brown tablets] (28s) [contains soya lecithin]

Larin 24 Fe: Ethinyl estradiol 0.02 mg and norethindrone acetate 1 mg [24 pale yellow tablets] and ferrous fumarate 75 mg [4 brown tablets] (28s)

Loestrin 21 1/20: Ethinyl estradiol 0.02 mg and norethindrone acetate 1 mg [light yellow tablets] (21s)

Loestrin 21 1.5/30: Ethinyl estradiol 0.03 mg and norethindrone acetate 1.5 mg [pink tablets] (21s)

Loestrin 24 Fe: Ethinyl estradiol 0.02 mg and norethindrone acetate 1 mg [24 white tablets] and ferrous fumarate 75 mg [4 brown tablets] (28s)

Loestrin Fe 1/20: Ethinyl estradiol 0.02 mg and norethindrone acetate 1 mg [21 light yellow tablets] and ferrous fumarate 75 mg [7 brown tablets] (28s)

Loestrin Fe 1.5/30: Ethinyl estradiol 0.03 mg and norethindrone acetate 1.5 mg [21 pink tablets] and ferrous fumarate 75 mg [7 brown tablets] (28s)

Lomedia 24 Fe: Ethinyl estradiol 0.02 mg and norethindrone acetate 1 mg [24 white tablets] and ferrous fumarate 75 mg [4 brown tablets] (28s)

Microgestin 1/20: Ethinyl estradiol 0.02 mg and norethindrone acetate 1 mg [white tablets] (21s)

Microgestin 1.5/30: Ethinyl estradiol 0.03 mg and norethindrone acetate 1.5 mg [green tablets] (21s)

Microgestin 24 Fe: Ethinyl estradiol 0.02 mg and norethindrone acetate 1 mg [24 white tablets] and ferrous fumarate 75 mg [4 brown tablets] (28s)

Microgestin Fe 1/20: Ethinyl estradiol 0.02 mg and norethindrone acetate 1 mg [21 white tablets] and ferrous fumarate 75 mg [7 brown tablets] (28s)

Microgestin Fe 1.5/30: Ethinyl estradiol 0.03 mg and norethindrone acetate 1.5 mg [21 green tablets] and ferrous fumarate 75 mg [7 brown tablets] (28s)

Modicon: Ethinyl estradiol 0.035 mg and norethindrone 0.5 mg [21 white tablets and 7 green inactive tablets] (28s)

Necon 0.5/35: Ethinyl estradiol 0.035 mg and norethindrone 0.5 mg [21 light yellow tablets and 7 white inactive tablets] (28s)

Necon 1/35: Ethinyl estradiol 0.035 mg and norethindrone 1 mg [21 dark yellow tablets and 7 white inactive tablets] (28s)

Norinyl 1+35: Ethinyl estradiol 0.035 mg and norethindrone 1 mg [21 yellow-green tablets and 7 orange inactive tablets] (28s)

Nortrel 0.5/35: Ethinyl estradiol 0.035 mg and norethindrone 0.5 mg [21 light yellow tablets and 7 white inactive tablets] (28s)

Nortrel 1/35:

Ethinyl estradiol 0.035 mg and norethindrone 1 mg [yellow tablets] (21s)

Ethinyl estradiol 0.035 mg and norethindrone 1 mg [21 yellow tablets and 7 white inactive tablets] (28s)

Ortho-Novum 1/35: Ethinyl estradiol 0.035 mg and norethindrone 1 mg [21 peach tablets and 7 green inactive tablets] (28s)

Ovcon 35: Ethinyl estradiol 0.035 mg and norethindrone 0.4 mg [21 light peach tablets and 7 green inactive tablets] (28s)

Philith: Ethinyl estradiol 0.035 mg and norethindrone 0.4 mg [21 tan tablets and 7 white inactive tablets] (28s)

Pirmella 1/35: Ethinyl estradiol 0.035 mg and norethindrone 1 mg [21 peach tablets and 7 green inactive tablets] (28s)

Tarina FE 1/20: Ethinyl estradiol 0.02 mg and norethindrone acetate 1 mg [21 white tablets] and ferrous fumarate 75 mg [7 brown tablets] (28s)

Vyfemla: Ethinyl estradiol 0.035 mg and norethindrone 0.4 mg [21 light peach tablets and 7 white inactive tablets] (28s)

Wera: Ethinyl estradiol 0.035 mg and norethindrone 0.5 mg [21 light peach tablets and 7 white inactive tablets] (28s)

Zenchent: Ethinyl estradiol 0.035 mg and norethindrone 0.4 mg [21 orange tablets and 7 white inactive tablets] (28s)

Tablet, chewable, oral [monophasic formulation]: Ethinyl estradiol 0.035 mg and norethindrone 0.4 mg [21 tablets] and ferrous fumarate 75 mg [7 tablets] (28s)

Femcon Fe: Ethinyl estradiol 0.035 mg and norethindrone 0.4 mg [21 white tablets] and ferrous fumarate 75 mg [7 brown tablets] [spearmint flavor] (28s)

Generess Fe: Ethinyl estradiol 0.025 mg and norethindrone 0.8 mg [24 light green tablets] and ferrous fumarate 75 mg [4 brown tablets] (28s)

Layolis Fe: Ethinyl estradiol 0.025 mg and norethindrone 0.8 mg [24 light green tablets] and ferrous fumarate 75 mg [4 brown tablets] [spearmint flavor] (28s)

Minastrin 24 Fe: Ethinyl estradiol 0.02 mg and norethindrone 1 mg [24 white tablets] and ferrous fumarate 75 mg [4 brown tablets] [spearmint flavor] (28s)

Wymzya Fe: Ethinyl estradiol 0.035 mg and norethindrone 0.4 mg [21 white tablets] and ferrous fumarate 75 mg [7 brown tablets] (28s)

Zenchent Fe: Ethinyl estradiol 0.035 mg and norethindrone 0.4 mg [21 light yellow tablets] and ferrous fumarate 75 mg [7 brown tablets] [spearmint flavor] (28s)

Tablet, oral [biphasic formulation]:

Lo Loestrin Fe:

Day 1-24: Ethinyl estradiol 0.01 mg and norethindrone acetate 1 mg [24 blue tablets]

Day 25-26: Ethinyl estradiol 0.01 mg [2 white tablets]

Day 27-28: Ferrous fumarate 75 mg [2 brown tablets] (28s)

◄

Lo Minastrin Fe:
Day 1-24: Ethinyl estradiol 0.01 mg and norethindrone acetate 1 mg [24 blue chewable tablets]
Day 25-26: Ethinyl estradiol 0.01 mg [2 white tablets]
Day 27-28: Ferrous fumarate 75 mg [2 brown tablets] (28s) [DSC]

Necon 10/11:
Day 1-10: Ethinyl estradiol 0.035 mg and norethindrone 0.5 mg [10 light yellow tablets]
Day 11-21: Ethinyl estradiol 0.035 mg and norethindrone 1 mg [11 dark yellow tablets]
Day 22-28: 7 white inactive tablets (28s)

Tablet, oral [triphasic formulation]:

Alyacen 7/7/7:
Day 1-7: Ethinyl estradiol 0.035 mg and norethindrone 0.5 mg [7 white-off-white tablets]
Day 8-14: Ethinyl estradiol 0.035 mg and norethindrone 0.75 mg [7 light peach tablets]
Day 15-21: Ethinyl estradiol 0.035 mg and norethindrone 1 mg [7 peach tablets]
Day 22-28: 7 light green inactive tablets (28s)

Aranelle:
Day 1-7: Ethinyl estradiol 0.035 mg and norethindrone 0.5 mg [7 light yellow tablets]
Day 8-16: Ethinyl estradiol 0.035 mg and norethindrone 1 mg [9 white tablets]
Day 17-21: Ethinyl estradiol 0.035 mg and norethindrone 0.5 mg [5 light yellow tablets]
Day 22-28: 7 peach inactive tablets (28s)

Cyclafem 7/7/7:
Day 1-7: Ethinyl estradiol 0.035 mg and norethindrone 0.5 mg [7 white tablets]
Day 8-14: Ethinyl estradiol 0.035 mg and norethindrone 0.75 mg [7 light pink tablets]
Day 15-21: Ethinyl estradiol 0.035 mg and norethindrone 1 mg [7 pink tablets]
Day 22-28: 7 light green inactive tablets (28s)

Dasetta 7/7/7:
Day 1-7: Ethinyl estradiol 0.035 mg and norethindrone 0.5 mg [7 light peach tablets]
Day 8-14: Ethinyl estradiol 0.035 mg and norethindrone 0.75 mg [7 peach tablets]
Day 15-21: Ethinyl estradiol 0.035 mg and norethindrone 1 mg [7 orange tablets]
Day 22-28: 7 white inactive tablets (28s)

Estrostep Fe:
Day 1-5: Ethinyl estradiol 0.02 mg and norethindrone acetate 1 mg [5 white triangular tablets]
Day 6-12: Ethinyl estradiol 0.03 mg and norethindrone acetate 1 mg [7 white square tablets]
Day 13-21: Ethinyl estradiol 0.035 mg and norethindrone acetate 1 mg [9 white round tablets]
Day 22-28: Ferrous fumarate 75 mg [7 brown tablets] (28s)

Leena:
Day 1-7: Ethinyl estradiol 0.035 mg and norethindrone 0.5 mg [7 light blue tablets]
Day 8-16: Ethinyl estradiol 0.035 mg and norethindrone 1 mg [9 light yellow-green tablets]
Day 17-21: Ethinyl estradiol 0.035 mg and norethindrone 0.5 mg [5 light blue tablets]
Day 22-28: 7 orange inactive tablets (28s)

Necon 7/7/7, Ortho-Novum 7/7/7:
Day 1-7: Ethinyl estradiol 0.035 mg and norethindrone 0.5 mg [7 white tablets]
Day 8-14: Ethinyl estradiol 0.035 mg and norethindrone 0.75 mg [7 light peach tablets]
Day 15-21: Ethinyl estradiol 0.035 mg and norethindrone 1 mg [7 peach tablets]
Day 22-28: 7 green inactive tablets (28s)

Nortrel 7/7/7:
Day 1-7: Ethinyl estradiol 0.035 mg and norethindrone 0.5 mg [7 light yellow tablets]
Day 8-14: Ethinyl estradiol 0.035 mg and norethindrone 0.75 mg [7 blue tablets]
Day 15-21: Ethinyl estradiol 0.035 mg and norethindrone 1 mg [7 peach tablets]
Day 22-28: 7 white inactive tablets (28s)

Pirmella 7/7/7:
Day 1-7: Ethinyl estradiol 0.035 mg and norethindrone 0.5 mg [7 white tablets]
Day 8-14: Ethinyl estradiol 0.035 mg and norethindrone 0.75 mg [7 light peach tablets]
Day 15-21: Ethinyl estradiol 0.035 mg and norethindrone 1 mg [7 peach tablets]
Day 22-28: 7 green inactive tablets (28s)

Tilia Fe:
Day 1-5: Ethinyl estradiol 0.02 mg and norethindrone acetate 1 mg [5 white triangular tablets]
Day 6-12: Ethinyl estradiol 0.03 mg and norethindrone acetate 1 mg [7 white square tablets]
Day 13-21: Ethinyl estradiol 0.035 mg and norethindrone acetate 1 mg [9 white round tablets]
Day 22-28: Ferrous fumarate 75 mg [7 brown tablets] (28s)

Tri-Legest Fe:
Day 1-5: Ethinyl estradiol 0.02 mg and norethindrone acetate 1 mg [5 light pink tablets]
Day 6-12: Ethinyl estradiol 0.03 mg and norethindrone acetate 1 mg [7 light yellow tablets]
Day 13-21: Ethinyl estradiol 0.035 mg and norethindrone acetate 1 mg [9 light blue tablets]
Day 22-28: Ferrous fumarate 75 mg [7 brown tablets] (28s)

Tri-Norinyl:
Day 1-7: Ethinyl estradiol 0.035 mg and norethindrone 0.5 mg [7 blue tablets]
Day 8-16: Ethinyl estradiol 0.035 mg and norethindrone 1 mg [9 yellow-green tablets]
Day 17-21: Ethinyl estradiol 0.035 mg and norethindrone 0.5 mg [5 blue tablets]
Day 22-28: 7 orange inactive tablets (28s)

Ethinyl Estradiol and Norgestimate

(ETH in il es tra DYE ole & nor JES ti mate)

Brand Names: US Estarylla; Mono-Linyah; MonoNessa; Ortho Tri-Cyclen; Ortho Tri-Cyclen Lo; Ortho-Cyclen; Previfem; Sprintec; Tri-Estarylla; Tri-Linyah; Tri-Lo-Estarylla; Tri-Lo-Sprintec; Tri-Previfem; Tri-Sprintec; TriNessa; Tri-Nessa Lo

Brand Names: Canada Cyclen; Tri-Cyclen; Tri-Cyclen Lo; Tricira Lo

Index Terms Ethinyl Estradiol and NGM; Norgestimate and Ethinyl Estradiol; Ortho Cyclen; Ortho Tri Cyclen

Pharmacologic Category Contraceptive; Estrogen and Progestin Combination

Use

Acne vulgaris: For the treatment of moderate acne vulgaris in females at least 15 years of age
Limitations of use: When used for acne, use only in females ≥15 years of age who achieved menarche, who also desire combination hormonal contraceptive therapy, and have no contraindications to combination hormonal contraceptive use.

Contraception: For the prevention of pregnancy.

Dosing

Adult Females:
Acne (Ortho Tri-Cyclen, Tri-Estarylla, TriNessa, Tri-Previfem, Tri-Sprintec): Oral: Refer to dosing for contraception

Contraception: Oral: 1 tablet once daily
Schedule 1 (Sunday starter): Dose begins on first Sunday after onset of menstruation; if the menstrual period starts on Sunday, take first tablet that very same day. **With a Sunday start, an additional method of contraception should be used until after the first 7 days of consecutive administration.**
Schedule 2 (Day 1 starter): Dose starts on first day of menstrual cycle taking 1 tablet daily.
Additional contraceptive dosing considerations:
Switching from a different contraceptive:
Oral contraceptive: Start on the same day that a new pack of the previous oral contraceptive would have been taken.
Transdermal patch, vaginal ring, injection: Start on the day the next dose would have been due.
IUD or implant: Start on the day of removal. A backup method of contraception should be used for the first 7 days if IUD is not removed on the first day of the menstrual cycle.
Use after first trimester abortion or miscarriage: Therapy may be started immediately. If not started within 5 days, a back-up method of contraception should be used for the first 7 days.
Use after childbirth (in women who are not breastfeeding) or after second trimester abortion or miscarriage: Therapy may be started ≥4 weeks postpartum. Pregnancy should be considered prior to treatment if menstrual periods have not restarted. An additional method of contraception (nonhormonal) should be used until after the first 7 days of consecutive administration.

Missed or late doses (CDC 2013):

If one dose is late (<24 hours since dose should have been taken) or if one dose is missed (24 to <48 hours since dose should have been taken): Take dose as soon as possible. Continue remaining doses at the usual time (even if that means 2 doses on the same day).

If ≥2 consecutive doses are missed (≥48 hours since dose should have been taken): Take the most recently missed dose as soon as possible, discard any other missed doses. Continue remaining doses at the usual time (even if that means taking 2 doses on the same day); use back-up contraception until hormonal pills have been taken for 7 consecutive days. If doses were missed during the last week of hormonal (active) tablets (eg, days 15 to 21 of a 28 day pack), omit the hormone free interval by finishing the current pack and starting a new pack. If unable to start a new pack immediately, back up contraception is needed until hormonal pills from a new pack have been taken for 7 consecutive days. Consider use of emergency contraception in some situations (refer to guidelines for details).

Also refer to package insert for product specific information.

Pediatric Females:

Acne: Oral: Children ≥15 years; refer to adult dosing for contraception; not to be used prior to menarche.

Contraception: Oral: Refer to adult dosing; not to be used prior to menarche.

Renal Impairment There are no dosage adjustments provided in manufacturer's labeling (has not been studied); use with caution and monitor blood pressure closely.

Hepatic Impairment Use is contraindicated in patients with hepatic impairment.

Additional Information Complete prescribing information should be consulted for additional detail.

Dosage Forms Excipient information presented when available (limited, particularly for generics); consult specific product labeling.

Tablet, oral [monophasic formulation]:

Estarylla: Ethinyl estradiol 0.035 mg and norgestimate 0.25 mg [21 blue tablets and 7 green inactive tablets] (28s)

MonoNessa, Ortho-Cyclen: Ethinyl estradiol 0.035 mg and norgestimate 0.25 mg [21 blue tablets and 7 dark green inactive tablets] (28s)

Previfem: Ethinyl estradiol 0.035 mg and norgestimate 0.25 mg [21 blue tablets and 7 light green inactive tablets] (28s)

Mono-Linya, Sprintec: Ethinyl estradiol 0.035 mg and norgestimate 0.25 mg [21 blue tablets and 7 white inactive tablets] (28s)

Tablet, oral [triphasic formulation]:

Ortho Tri-Cyclen:

Day 1 to 7: Ethinyl estradiol 0.035 mg and norgestimate 0.18 mg [7 white tablets]

Day 8 to 14: Ethinyl estradiol 0.035 mg and norgestimate 0.215 mg [7 light blue tablets]

Day 15 to 21: Ethinyl estradiol 0.035 mg and norgestimate 0.25 mg [7 blue tablets]

Day 22 to 28: 7 dark green inactive tablets (28s)

Ortho Tri-Cyclen Lo:

Day 1 to 7: Ethinyl estradiol 0.025 mg and norgestimate 0.18 mg [7 white tablets]

Day 8 to 14: Ethinyl estradiol 0.025 mg and norgestimate 0.215 mg [7 light blue tablets]

Day 15 to 21: Ethinyl estradiol 0.025 mg and norgestimate 0.25 mg [7 dark blue tablets]

Day 22 to 28: 7 dark green inactive tablets (28s)

Tri-Estarylla:

Day 1 to 7: Ethinyl estradiol 0.035 mg and norgestimate 0.18 mg [7 white tablets]

Day 8 to 14: Ethinyl estradiol 0.035 mg and norgestimate 0.215 mg [7 light blue tablets]

Day 15 to 21: Ethinyl estradiol 0.035 mg and norgestimate 0.25 mg [7 blue tablets]

Day 22 to 28: 7 green inactive tablets (28s)

Tri-Linyah:

Day 1 to 7: Ethinyl estradiol 0.035 mg and norgestimate 0.18 mg [7 green tablets]

Day 8 to 14: Ethinyl estradiol 0.035 mg and norgestimate 0.215 mg [7 light blue tablets]

Day 15 to 21: Ethinyl estradiol 0.035 mg and norgestimate 0.25 mg [7 blue tablets]

Day 22 to 28: 7 white inactive tablets (28s)

Tri-Lo-Estarylla:

Day 1 to 7: Ethinyl estradiol 0.025 mg and norgestimate 0.18 mg [7 white tablets]

Day 8 to 14: Ethinyl estradiol 0.025 mg and norgestimate 0.215 mg [7 light blue tablets]

Day 15 to 21: Ethinyl estradiol 0.025 mg and norgestimate 0.25 mg [7 blue tablets]

Day 22 to 28: 7 green inactive tablets (28s)

Tri-Lo-Sprintec:

Day 1 to 7: Ethinyl estradiol 0.025 mg and norgestimate 0.18 mg [7 gray tablets]

Day 8 to 14: Ethinyl estradiol 0.025 mg and norgestimate 0.215 mg [7 light blue tablets]

Day 15 to 21: Ethinyl estradiol 0.025 mg and norgestimate 0.25 mg [7 blue tablets]

Day 22 to 28: 7 white inactive tablets (28s)

Tri-Previfem:

Day 1 to 7: Ethinyl estradiol 0.035 mg and norgestimate 0.18 mg [7 white tablets]

Day 8 to 14: Ethinyl estradiol 0.035 mg and norgestimate 0.215 mg [7 light blue tablets]

Day 15 to 21: Ethinyl estradiol 0.035 mg and norgestimate 0.25 mg [7 blue tablets]

Day 22 to 28: 7 light green inactive tablets (28s)

Tri-Sprintec:

Day 1 to 7: Ethinyl estradiol 0.035 mg and norgestimate 0.18 mg [7 gray tablets]

Day 8 to 14: Ethinyl estradiol 0.035 mg and norgestimate 0.215 mg [7 light blue tablets]

Day 15 to 21: Ethinyl estradiol 0.035 mg and norgestimate 0.25 mg [7 blue tablets]

Day 22 to 28: 7 white inactive tablets (28s)

TriNessa:

Day 1 to 7: Ethinyl estradiol 0.035 mg and norgestimate 0.18 mg [7 white tablets]

Day 8 to 14: Ethinyl estradiol 0.035 mg and norgestimate 0.215 mg [7 light blue tablets]

Day 15 to 21: Ethinyl estradiol 0.035 mg and norgestimate 0.25 mg [7 blue tablets]

Day 22 to 28: 7 dark green inactive tablets (28s)

TriNessa Lo:

Day 1 to 7: Ethinyl estradiol 0.025 mg and norgestimate 0.18 mg [7 white tablets]

Day 8 to 14: Ethinyl estradiol 0.025 mg and norgestimate 0.215 mg [7 light blue tablets]

Day 15 to 21: Ethinyl estradiol 0.025 mg and norgestimate 0.25 mg [7 blue tablets]

Day 22 to 28: 7 dark green inactive tablets (28s)

Ethinyl Estradiol and Norgestrel

(ETH in il es tra DYE ole & nor JES trel)

Brand Names: US Cryselle 28; Elinest; Low-Ogestrel; Ogestrel

Index Terms Lo Ovral; Lo/Ovral; Morning After Pill; Norgestrel and Ethinyl Estradiol

Pharmacologic Category Contraceptive; Estrogen and Progestin Combination

Use Contraception: Prevention of pregnancy

Dosing

Adult

Females: Contraception: Oral: 1 tablet once daily

Schedule 1 (Sunday starter): Dose begins on first Sunday after onset of menstruation; if the menstrual period starts on Sunday, take first tablet that very same day. **With a Sunday start, an additional method of contraception should be used until after the first 7 days of consecutive administration.**

Schedule 2 (Day 1 starter): Dose starts on first day of menstrual cycle taking 1 tablet daily.

Missed or late doses (CDC, 2013):

If one dose is late (<24 hours since dose should have been taken) or if one dose is missed (24 to <48 hours since dose should have been taken): Take dose as soon as possible. Continue remaining doses at the usual time (even if that means 2 doses on the same day).

If ≥2 consecutive doses are missed (≥48 hours since dose should have been taken): Take the most recently missed dose as soon as possible, discard any other missed doses. Continue remaining doses at the usual time (even if that means taking 2 doses on the same day); use back-up contraception until hormonal pills have been taken for 7 consecutive days. If doses were missed during the last week of hormonal (active) tablets (eg, days 15 to 21 of a 28 day pack), omit the hormone free interval by finishing the current pack and starting a new pack. If unable to start a new pack immediately, back up contraception is needed until hormonal pills from a new pack have been taken for 7 consecutive days. Consider use of emergency contraception in some situations (refer to guidelines for details).

Also refer to package insert for product specific information.

Females: Emergency contraception: (off-label use; Federal Register, 1997): Oral:

Ethinyl estradiol 0.03 mg and norgestrel 0.3 mg formulation: 4 tablets within 72 hours of unprotected intercourse followed by 4 additional tablets 12 hours after first dose

Ethinyl estradiol 0.05 mg and norgestrel 0.5 mg formulation: 2 tablets within 72 hours of unprotected intercourse followed by 2 additional tablets 12 hours after first dose

Pediatric Females: Contraception or emergency contraception: Oral: See adult dosing; not to be used prior to menarche.

Renal Impairment There are no dosage adjustments provided in the manufacturer's labeling (has not been studied); use with caution and monitor blood pressure closely.

Hepatic Impairment Use is contraindicated in patients with hepatic impairment.

Additional Information Complete prescribing information should be consulted for additional detail.

Dosage Forms Excipient information presented when available (limited, particularly for generics); consult specific product labeling.

Tablet, oral [monophasic formulation]: Ethinyl estradiol 0.03 mg and norgestrel 0.3 mg [21 tablets and 7 inactive tablets] (28s)

Cryselle 28: Ethinyl estradiol 0.03 mg and norgestrel 0.3 mg [21 white tablets and 7 light green inactive tablets] (28s)

Elinest: Ethinyl estradiol 0.03 mg and norgestrel 0.3 mg [21 pale pink tablets and 7 white inactive tablets] (28s) [contains soy products]

Low-Ogestrel: Ethinyl estradiol 0.03 mg and norgestrel 0.3 mg [21 white tablets and 7 peach inactive tablets] (28s)

Ogestrel: Ethinyl estradiol 0.05 mg and norgestrel 0.5 mg [21 white tablets and 7 peach inactive tablets] (28s)

Ethinyl Estradiol, Drospirenone, and Levomefolate

(ETH in il es tra DYE ole, droh SPYE re none, & lee voe me FOE late)

Brand Names: US Beyaz; Safyral
Brand Names: Canada Yaz Plus
Index Terms Drospirenone, Ethinyl Estradiol, and Levomefolate Calcium; Ethinyl Estradiol, Drospirenone, and Levomefolate Calcium; Levomefolate Calcium, Drospirenone, and Ethinyl Estradiol; Levomefolate, Drospirenone, and Ethinyl Estradiol
Pharmacologic Category Contraceptive; Estrogen and Progestin Combination
Use Prevention of pregnancy; treatment of premenstrual dysphoric disorder (PMDD); treatment of acne; folate supplementation
Dosing
Adult
Acne, PMDD: Oral: Females: (Beyaz): Refer to dosing for contraception
Contraception: Oral: Females: (Beyaz, Safyral): Dosage is 1 tablet daily

Beyaz: One pink tablet daily for 24 consecutive days, then one light orange tablet daily on days 25-28

Safyral: One orange tablet daily for 21 consecutive days, then one light orange tablet daily on days 22-28

Dose should be taken at the same time each day, either after the evening meal or at bedtime. Dosing may be started on the first day of menstrual period (Day 1 starter) or on the first Sunday after the onset of the menstrual period (Sunday starter).

Day 1 starter: Dose starts on first day of menstrual cycle taking 1 tablet daily. If first dose is taken later than the first day of the menstrual cycle, **an additional method of contraception should be used until after the first 7 days of consecutive administration.**

Sunday starter: Dose begins on first Sunday after onset of menstruation; if the menstrual period starts on Sunday, take first tablet that very same day. **With a Sunday start, an additional method of contraception should be used until after the first 7 days of consecutive administration.**

Switching from a different contraceptive:

Oral contraceptive: Start on the same day that a new pack of the previous oral contraceptive would have been taken

Transdermal patch, vaginal ring, injection: Start on the day the next dose would have been due

IUD or implant: Start on the day of removal

Use after childbirth (in women who are not breast-feeding) or after second trimester abortion: Therapy may be started ≥4 weeks postpartum. Pregnancy should be ruled out prior to treatment if menstrual periods have not restarted and an additional method of contraception (nonhormonal) should be used until after the first 7 days of consecutive administration.

Missed doses:

If all doses have been taken on schedule and one menstrual period is missed, continue dosing cycle. If two consecutive menstrual periods are missed, rule out pregnancy and discontinue if pregnancy is confirmed.

If doses have been missed during the first 3 weeks or if active tablets (pink tablets) were started later than as directed and the menstrual period is missed, pregnancy should be ruled out prior to continuing treatment.

Missed doses (monophasic formulations) (refer to package insert for complete information):

One dose missed: Take as soon as remembered or take 2 tablets next day

Two consecutive doses missed in the first 2 weeks: Take 2 tablets as soon as remembered or 2 tablets next 2 days. **An additional method of contraception should be used for 7 days after missed dose.**

Two consecutive doses missed in week 3 or three consecutive doses missed at any time: **An additional method of contraception must be used for 7 days after a missed dose.**

Day 1 starter: Current pack should be discarded, and a new pack should be started that same day.

Sunday starter: Continue dose of 1 tablet daily until Sunday, then discard the rest of the pack, and a new pack should be started that same day.

Any number of doses missed in week 4: Throw away the pills that were missed. Continue taking one pill each day until pack is empty; no back-up method of contraception is needed

Pediatric

Acne: Females: Children ≥14 years: Oral: Refer to adult dosing.

Contraception, PMDD: Females: Oral: Refer to adult dosing; not to be used prior to menarche.

Renal Impairment Contraindicated in patients with renal dysfunction.

Hepatic Impairment Contraindicated in patients with hepatic disease. Exposure to drospirenone is ~3 times higher with moderate liver impairment; information not available for severe impairment.

Additional Information Complete prescribing information should be consulted for additional detail.

Dosage Forms Excipient information presented when available (limited, particularly for generics); consult specific product labeling.

Tablet, oral:

Beyaz: Ethinyl estradiol 0.02 mg, drospirenone 3 mg, and levomefolate calcium 0.451 mg [24 pink tablets] and levomefolate calcium 0.451 mg [4 light orange tablets] (28s)

Safyral: Ethinyl estradiol 0.03 mg, drospirenone 3 mg, and levomefolate calcium 0.451 mg [21 orange tablets] and levomefolate calcium 0.451 mg [7 light orange tablets] (28s)

◆ Ethinyl Estradiol, Drospirenone, and Levomefolate Calcium see Ethinyl Estradiol, Drospirenone, and Levomefolate on page 712

◆ Ethiofos see Amifostine on page 90

Ethosuximide (eth oh SUKS i mide)

Brand Names: US Zarontin
Brand Names: Canada Zarontin®
Pharmacologic Category Anticonvulsant, Succinimide
Use Management of absence (petit mal) seizures
Medication Guide Available Yes>
Dosing
Adult & Geriatric Management of absence (petit mal) seizures: Oral: Initial: 500 mg/day; increase by 250 mg as needed every 4-7 days up to 1.5 g/day in divided doses
Pediatric
Absence (petit mal) seizures: Oral:
Children 3-6 years: Initial: 250 mg/day; increase every 4-7 days; usual maintenance dose: 20 mg/kg/day; maximum dose: 1.5 g/day in divided doses.
Children ≥6 years: Refer to adult dosing.

Renal Impairment
No dosage adjustment provided in manufacturer's labeling; use with caution.
Dialysis: Removed by hemodialysis and peritoneal dialysis
Hepatic Impairment No dosage adjustment provided in manufacturer's labeling; use with caution.
Additional Information Complete prescribing information should be consulted for additional detail.
Dosage Forms Excipient information presented when available (limited, particularly for generics); consult specific product labeling.
Capsule, Oral:
Zarontin: 250 mg [contains fd&c yellow #10 (quinoline yellow)]
Generic: 250 mg
Solution, Oral:
Zarontin: 250 mg/5 mL (474 mL) [raspberry flavor]
Generic: 250 mg/5 mL (473 mL, 474 mL)

◆ Ethoxynaphthamido Penicillin Sodium *see* Nafcillin *on page 1246*

◆ Ethyl Aminobenzoate *see* Benzocaine *on page 217*

◆ Ethyl Eicosapentaenoate *see* Omega-3 Fatty Acids *on page 1329*

◆ Ethyl-Eicosapentaenoic Acid *see* Omega-3 Fatty Acids *on page 1329*

◆ Ethyl-EPA *see* Omega-3 Fatty Acids *on page 1329*

◆ Ethyl Esters of Omega-3 Fatty Acids *see* Omega-3 Fatty Acids *on page 1329*

◆ Ethyl Icosapentate *see* Omega-3 Fatty Acids *on page 1329*

◆ Ethynodiol Diacetate and Ethinyl Estradiol *see* Ethinyl Estradiol and Ethynodiol Diacetate *on page 702*

◆ Ethyol *see* Amifostine *on page 90*

◆ Etibi (Can) *see* Ethambutol *on page 699*

Etidronate (e ti DROE nate)

Brand Names: US Didronel [DSC]
Brand Names: Canada ACT Etidronate; Mylan-Etidronate
Index Terms Didronel; EHDP; Etidronate Disodium; Sodium Etidronate
Pharmacologic Category Bisphosphonate Derivative
Use Symptomatic treatment of Paget's disease; prevention and treatment of heterotopic ossification due to spinal cord injury or after total hip replacement
Dosing
Adult & Geriatric Patients should receive supplemental calcium and vitamin D if dietary intake is inadequate.
Paget's disease:
Initial: 5-10 mg/kg/day (not to exceed 6 months) or 11-20 mg/kg/day (not to exceed 3 months). The recommended initial dose is 5 mg/kg/day (not to exceed 6 months). Higher doses should be used only when lower doses are ineffective or there is a need to suppress rapid bone turnover (ie, potential for irreversible neurologic damage) or reduce elevated cardiac output. Doses >20 mg/kg/day are **not** recommended.
Re-treatment: Initiate only after etidronate-free period ≥90 days. Monitor patients every 3-6 months. Re-treatment regimens are the same as for initial treatment.
Heterotopic ossification: Oral:
Caused by spinal cord injury: 20 mg/kg/day for 2 weeks, then 10 mg/kg/day for 10 weeks; total treatment period: 12 weeks
Complicating total hip replacement: 20 mg/kg/day for 1 month preoperatively then 20 mg/kg/day for 3 months postoperatively; total treatment period is 4 months
Renal Impairment Manufacturer's labeling recommends decreasing the dose when GFR is reduced; however, no specific dosage adjustments are provided. Use with caution and monitor closely; etidronate is eliminated intact via the kidneys.
Hepatic Impairment No dosage adjustment provided in manufacturer's labeling.
Additional Information Complete prescribing information should be consulted for additional detail.
Dosage Forms Excipient information presented when available (limited, particularly for generics); consult specific product labeling. [DSC] = Discontinued product
Tablet, Oral, as disodium:
Didronel: 400 mg [DSC] [scored]
Generic: 200 mg, 400 mg

◆ Etidronate Disodium *see* Etidronate *on page 713*

Etodolac (ee toe DOE lak)

Brand Names: Canada Taro-Etodolac
Index Terms Etodolic Acid; Lodine
Pharmacologic Category Nonsteroidal Anti-inflammatory Drug (NSAID), Oral
Use
Acute pain: Management of acute pain (immediate release only).
Arthritis: Relief of the signs and symptoms of osteoarthritis, rheumatoid arthritis, juvenile arthritis (ER only).
Medication Guide Available Yes
Dosing
Adult Note: For chronic conditions, response is usually observed within 1 to 2 weeks.
Acute pain: Oral: Immediate release: 200 to 400 mg every 6 to 8 hours, as needed (doses of >1,000 mg/day have not been adequately evaluated).
Rheumatoid arthritis, osteoarthritis: Oral:
Immediate release: 400 mg 2 times daily **or** 300 mg 2 to 3 times daily **or** 500 mg 2 times daily (doses >1,000 mg/day have not been adequately evaluated). Extended release: Initial: 400 to 1,000 mg once daily.
Geriatric Refer to adult dosing, use with caution. The elderly are more sensitive to antiprostaglandin effects and may need dosage adjustments.
Pediatric Note: For chronic conditions, response is usually observed within 1 to 2 weeks.
Juvenile arthritis: Oral: Extended release: Children ≥6 years and Adolescents ≤16 years:
20 to 30 kg: 400 mg once daily
31 to 45 kg: 600 mg once daily
46 to 60 kg: 800 mg once daily
Children >60 kg: 1,000 mg once daily
Renal Impairment
CrCl >88 mL/minute: No dosage adjustment necessary.
CrCl 37 to 88 mL/minute: No dosage adjustment necessary; however, use with caution.
CrCl <37 mL/minute: Use not recommended; if use must be initiated, use with caution.
Hepatic Impairment No dosage adjustment necessary. However, clearance may be reduced in severe hepatic failure.
Additional Information Complete prescribing information should be consulted for additional detail.
Dosage Forms Excipient information presented when available (limited, particularly for generics); consult specific product labeling.
Capsule, Oral:
Generic: 200 mg, 300 mg
Tablet, Oral:
Generic: 400 mg, 500 mg
Tablet Extended Release 24 Hour, Oral:
Generic: 400 mg, 500 mg, 600 mg
Dosage Forms: Canada Refer to Dosage Forms. **Note:** Tablets and Extended Release tablets are not available in Canada.

◆ Etodolic Acid *see* Etodolac *on page 713*

Etomidate (e TOM i date)

Brand Names: US Amidate
Pharmacologic Category General Anesthetic
Use General anesthesia: Induction of general anesthesia; as a supplement to subpotent anesthetic agents during maintenance of anesthesia for short operative procedures (eg, dilation and curettage, cervical conization).
Pregnancy Considerations Adverse events have been observed in animal reproduction studies.
Breast-Feeding Considerations It is not known if etomidate is excreted in breast milk. The manufacturer recommends that caution be exercised when administering etomidate to nursing women.
Contraindications Hypersensitivity to etomidate or any component of the formulation
Warnings/Precautions Etomidate inhibits 11-B-hydroxylase, an enzyme important in adrenal steroid production. A single induction dose blocks the normal stress-induced increase in adrenal cortisol production for 6 to 8 hours, up to 24 hours in elderly and debilitated patients. Continuous infusion of etomidate for sedation in the ICU may increase mortality because patients may not be able to respond to stress. Administration by continuous infusion is not recommended by the manufacturer. No increase in mortality has been identified with a single dose for induction of anesthesia (McPhee 2013). Consider exogenous corticosteroid replacement in patients undergoing severe stress.

May induce cardiac depression in elderly patients, especially those with hypertension; may require lower doses. Risk of toxicity is greater in patients with renal impairment; use with caution and monitor renal function. When considering use, weigh etomidate hemodynamic properties against the high frequency of transient skeletal muscle movements. According to the manufacturer, etomidate should only be administered by experienced personnel trained in the administration of general anesthetics and in the management of complications encountered during the conduct of general anesthesia. Consult local regulations and individual institutional policies and procedures.

Adverse Reactions
>10%:
Gastrointestinal: Nausea, vomiting on emergence from anesthesia
Local: Pain at injection site (30% to 80%)
Neuromuscular & skeletal: Myoclonus (33%), transient skeletal movements, uncontrolled eye movements
1% to 10%: Hiccups
<1% (Limited to important or life-threatening): Apnea, arrhythmia, bradycardia, decreased cortisol synthesis, hypertension, hyperventilation, hypotension, hypoventilation, laryngospasm, tachycardia

Drug Interactions
Metabolism/Transport Effects None known.
Avoid Concomitant Use There are no known interactions where it is recommended to avoid concomitant use.
Increased Effect/Toxicity There are no known significant interactions involving an increase in effect.
Decreased Effect There are no known significant interactions involving a decrease in effect.
Storage/Stability Store at 20°C to 25°C (68°F to 77°F).
Mechanism of Action Ultrashort-acting nonbarbiturate hypnotic (benzylimidazole) used for rapid induction of anesthesia with minimal cardiovascular effects; produces EEG burst suppression at high doses

Pharmacodynamics/Kinetics
Onset of action: 30 to 60 seconds
Peak effect: 1 minute
Duration: Dose dependent: 2-3 minutes (0.15 mg/kg dose); 4-10 minutes (0.3 mg/kg dose); rapid recovery is due to rapid redistribution
Distribution: V_d: 2 to 4.5 L/kg
Protein binding: 76%; decreased protein binding resulting in an increased percentage of "free" etomidate in patients with renal failure or hepatic cirrhosis
Metabolism: Hepatic and plasma esterases
Half-life elimination: Terminal: 2.6-3.5 hours
Time to peak, serum: 7 minutes
Excretion: Urine ~75% (80% as metabolite; 2% as unchanged drug)

Dosing
Adult
General anesthesia: IV: Initial: 0.3 mg/kg (range: 0.2 to 0.6 mg/kg) over 30 to 60 seconds for induction of anesthesia; maintenance:10 to 20 mcg/kg/minute (Barash 2009; Miller 2010)
Supplementation to subpotent anesthetic agents: IV: Administer smaller increments during short operative procedures to supplement subpotent anesthetic agents, such as nitrous oxide; individualize dosage (usually smaller than the original induction dose).
Procedural sedation (off-label use): IV: Initial: 0.1 to 0.2 mg/kg, followed by 0.05 mg/kg every 3 to 5 minutes as needed (Bahn, 2005; Miner, 2007; Vinson, 2002)
Geriatric Refer to adult dosing; reduced doses may be required.
Pediatric General anesthesia: IV: Children >10 years and Adolescents: Initial: 0.3 mg/kg (range: 0.2 to 0.6 mg/kg) over 30 to 60 seconds for induction of anesthesia; maintenance:10 to 20 mcg/kg/minute (Barash 2009; Miller 2010)
Renal Impairment There are no dosage adjustments provided in the manufacturer's labeling; use with caution, risk of toxicity is greater in patients with renal impairment.
Hepatic Impairment There are no dosage adjustments provided in the manufacturer's labeling.
Administration Administer IV push over 30 to 60 seconds. Solution is highly irritating; avoid administration into small vessels; in some cases, preadministration of lidocaine may be considered. May also administer as a short term continuous infusion after an induction dose to maintain general anesthesia (Barash 2009; Miller 2010)
Monitoring Parameters Cardiac monitoring; blood pressure; renal function (in renal impairment)
Additional Information Etomidate decreases cerebral metabolism and cerebral blood flow while maintaining perfusion pressure. Premedication with opioids or benzodiazepines can decrease myoclonus. Etomidate can enhance somatosensory evoked potential recordings.

Dosage Forms Excipient information presented when available (limited, particularly for generics); consult specific product labeling.
Solution, Intravenous:
Amidate: 2 mg/mL (10 mL, 20 mL) [contains propylene glycol]
Generic: 2 mg/mL (10 mL, 20 mL)
Solution, Intravenous [preservative free]:
Generic: 2 mg/mL (10 mL, 20 mL)

♦ **Etonogestrel and Ethinyl Estradiol** see Ethinyl Estradiol and Etonogestrel on page 703

♦ **ETOP** see Etoposide Phosphate on page 717

♦ **Etopophos** see Etoposide Phosphate on page 717

Etoposide (e toe POE side)

Brand Names: US Toposar
Brand Names: Canada Etoposide Injection; Etoposide Injection USP; Vepesid
Index Terms EPEG; Epipodophyllotoxin; VePesid; VP-16; VP-16-213; VP16
Pharmacologic Category Antineoplastic Agent, Podophyllotoxin Derivative; Antineoplastic Agent, Topoisomerase II Inhibitor

Use
Small cell lung cancer (oral and IV): Treatment (first-line) of small cell lung cancer (SCLC)
Testicular cancer (IV): Treatment of refractory testicular tumors (injectable formulation)

Canadian labeling: Treatment of small cell lung cancer (SCLC; first- and second-line); treatment of non-small cell lung cancer (NSCLC); treatment of non-Hodgkin lymphomas (first-line); treatment of testicular cancer (first-line [injectable formulation] and refractory)

Pregnancy Considerations Adverse events were observed in animal reproduction studies. Fetal growth restriction and newborn myelosuppression have been observed following maternal use of regimens containing etoposide during pregnancy (NTP 2013; Peccatori 2013). The European Society for Medical Oncology has published guidelines for diagnosis, treatment, and follow-up of cancer during pregnancy. The guidelines recommend referral to a facility with expertise in cancer during pregnancy and encourage a multidisciplinary team (obstetrician, neonatologist, oncology team). In general, if chemotherapy is indicated, it should be avoided during in the first trimester, there should be a 3-week time period between the last chemotherapy dose and anticipated delivery, and chemotherapy should not be administered beyond week 33 of gestation. Guidelines for the treatment of SCLC are not provided (Peccatori 2013).

In women of reproductive potential, product labeling for etoposide phosphate notes that it may cause amenorrhea, infertility, or premature menopause; effective contraception should be used during therapy and for ≥6 months after the last dose. In males, azoospermia, oligospermia, or permanent loss of fertility may occur. In addition, spermatozoa and testicular tissue may be damaged. Males with female partners of reproductive potential should use condoms during therapy and for ≥4 months after the last dose.

Breast-Feeding Considerations Etoposide is excreted in breast milk. Based on data from one case report, concentrations are below the limit of detection 24 hours after the last dose (Azuno 1995). Due to the potential for serious adverse reactions in the nursing infant, the manufacturer recommends a decision be made whether to discontinue nursing or to discontinue the drug, taking into account the importance of treatment to the mother.

Contraindications Hypersensitivity to etoposide or any component of the formulation
Canadian labeling: Additional contraindications (not in U.S. labeling): Severe leukopenia or thrombocytopenia; severe hepatic impairment; severe renal impairment

Warnings/Precautions Hazardous agent - use appropriate precautions for handling and disposal (NIOSH 2014 [group 1]). **[U.S. Boxed Warning]: Severe dose-limiting and dose-related myelosuppression with resulting infection or bleeding may occur.** Treatment should be withheld for platelets <50,000/mm³ or absolute neutrophil count (ANC) <500/mm³. May cause anaphylactic-like reactions manifested by chills, fever, tachycardia, bronchospasm, dyspnea, and hypotension. In addition, facial/tongue swelling, coughing, chest tightness, cyanosis, laryngospasm, diaphoresis, hypertension, back pain, loss of consciousness, and flushing have also been reported less commonly. Incidence is primarily associated with intravenous administration (up to 2%) compared to oral administration (<1%). Infusion should be interrupted and medications for the treatment of anaphylaxis should be

available for immediate use. High drug concentration and rate of infusion, as well as presence of benzyl alcohol in the etoposide intravenous formulation have been suggested as contributing factors to the development of hypersensitivity reactions. Etoposide intravenous formulations may contain benzyl alcohol, while etoposide phosphate (the water soluble prodrug of etoposide) intravenous formulation does not contain benzyl alcohol. Case reports have suggested that etoposide phosphate has been used successfully in patients with previous hypersensitivity reactions to etoposide (Collier, 2008; Siderov, 2002). The use of concentrations higher than recommended were associated with higher rates of anaphylactic-like reactions in children.

Secondary acute leukemias have been reported with etoposide, either as monotherapy or in combination with other chemotherapy agents. Must be diluted; do not give IV push, infuse over at least 30 to 60 minutes; hypotension is associated with rapid infusion. If hypotension occurs, interrupt infusion and administer IV hydration and supportive care; decrease infusion upon reinitiation. Etoposide is an irritant; tissue irritation and inflammation have occurred following extravasation. Do not administer IM or SubQ. Dosage should be adjusted in patients with hepatic or renal impairment (Canadian labeling contraindicates use in severe hepatic and/or renal impairment). Use with caution in patients with low serum albumin; may increase risk for toxicities. Use with caution in elderly patients; may be more likely to develop severe myelosuppression and/or GI effects (eg, nausea/vomiting). **[U.S. Boxed Warning]: Should be administered under the supervision of an experienced cancer chemotherapy physician.**

Oral etoposide is associated with a low (adults) or moderate (children) emetic potential; antiemetics may be recommended to prevent nausea and vomiting (Dupuis, 2011; Roila, 2010). Potentially significant drug-drug interactions may exist, requiring dose or frequency adjustment, additional monitoring, and/or selection of alternative therapy.

Benzyl alcohol and derivatives: Some dosage forms may contain benzyl alcohol; large amounts of benzyl alcohol (≥99 mg/kg/day) have been associated with a potentially fatal toxicity ("gasping syndrome") in neonates; the "gasping syndrome" consists of metabolic acidosis, respiratory distress, gasping respirations, CNS dysfunction (including convulsions, intracranial hemorrhage), hypotension, and cardiovascular collapse (AAP ["Inactive" 1997]; CDC, 1982); some data suggests that benzoate displaces bilirubin from protein binding sites (Ahlfors, 2001); avoid or use dosage forms containing benzyl alcohol with caution in neonates. See manufacturer's labeling.

Injectable formulation contains alcohol (~33% v/v); may contribute to adverse reactions, especially with higher etoposide doses.

Polysorbate 80: Some dosage forms may contain polysorbate 80 (also known as Tweens). Hypersensitivity reactions, usually a delayed reaction, have been reported following exposure to pharmaceutical products containing polysorbate 80 in certain individuals (Isaksson, 2002; Lucente 2000; Shelley, 1995). Thrombocytopenia, ascites, pulmonary deterioration, and renal and hepatic failure have been reported in premature neonates after receiving parenteral products containing polysorbate 80 (Alade, 1986; CDC, 1984). See manufacturer's labeling.

Adverse Reactions Note: The following may occur with higher doses used in stem cell transplantation: Alopecia, ethanol intoxication, hepatitis, hypotension (infusion-related), metabolic acidosis, mucositis, nausea and vomiting (severe), secondary malignancy, skin lesions (resembling Stevens-Johnson syndrome).

>10%:

Dermatologic: Alopecia (8% to 66%)

Gastrointestinal: Nausea/vomiting (31% to 43%), anorexia (10% to 13%), diarrhea (1% to 13%)

Hematologic: Leukopenia (60% to 91%; grade 4: 3% to 17%; nadir: 7-14 days; recovery: By day 20), thrombocytopenia (22% to 41%; grades 3/4: 1% to 20%; nadir: 9-16 days; recovery: By day 20), anemia (≤33%)

1% to 10%:

Cardiovascular: Hypotension (1% to 2%; due to rapid infusion)

Gastrointestinal: Stomatitis (1% to 6%), abdominal pain (up to 2%)

Hepatic: Hepatic toxicity (up to 3%)

Neuromuscular & skeletal: Peripheral neuropathy (1% to 2%)

Miscellaneous: Anaphylactic-like reaction (IV infusion 1% to 2%; oral capsules <1%; including chills, fever, tachycardia, bronchospasm, dyspnea)

<1% (Limited to important or life-threatening): Amenorrhea, blindness (transient/cortical), cyanosis, extravasation (induration/necrosis), facial swelling, hypersensitivity, hypersensitivity-associated apnea, interstitial pneumonitis, laryngospasm, maculopapular rash, metabolic acidosis, MI, mucositis, myocardial ischemia, optic neuritis, perivasculitis, pruritus, pulmonary fibrosis, radiation-recall dermatitis, rash, reversible posterior leukoencephalopathy syndrome (RPLS), seizure, Stevens-Johnson syndrome, tongue swelling, toxic epidermal necrolysis, toxic megacolon, vasospasm

Drug Interactions

Metabolism/Transport Effects Substrate of CYP1A2 (minor), CYP2E1 (minor), CYP3A4 (major), P-glycoprotein; **Note:** Assignment of Major/Minor substrate status based on clinically relevant drug interaction potential; **Inhibits** CYP2C9 (weak)

Avoid Concomitant Use

Avoid concomitant use of Etoposide with any of the following: BCG (Intravesical); Conivaptan; Deferiprone; Dipyrone; Fusidic Acid (Systemic); Idelalisib; Natalizumab; Pimecrolimus; Tacrolimus (Topical); Tofacitinib; Vaccines (Live)

Increased Effect/Toxicity

Etoposide may increase the levels/effects of: CloZAPine; Deferiprone; Fingolimod; Leflunomide; Natalizumab; Tofacitinib; Vaccines (Live); Vitamin K Antagonists

The levels/effects of Etoposide may be increased by: Aprepitant; Atovaquone; Conivaptan; CycloSPORINE (Systemic); CYP3A4 Inhibitors (Moderate); CYP3A4 Inhibitors (Strong); Dasatinib; Denosumab; Dipyrone; Fosaprepitant; Fusidic Acid (Systemic); Idelalisib; Ivacaftor; Luliconazole; Mifepristone; Netupitant; Osimertinib; Palbociclib; P-glycoprotein/ABCB1 Inhibitors; Pimecrolimus; Ranolazine; Roflumilast; Simeprevir; Stiripentol; Tacrolimus (Topical); Trastuzumab

Decreased Effect

Etoposide may decrease the levels/effects of: BCG (Intravesical); Coccidioides immitis Skin Test; Sipuleucel-T; Vaccines (Inactivated); Vaccines (Live)

The levels/effects of Etoposide may be decreased by: Bosentan; CYP3A4 Inducers (Moderate); CYP3A4 Inducers (Strong); Dabrafenib; Deferasirox; Enzalutamide; Mitotane; Osimertinib; P-glycoprotein/ABCB1 Inducers; Siltuximab; St Johns Wort; Tocilizumab

Preparation for Administration Hazardous agent; use appropriate precautions for handling and disposal (NIOSH 2014 [group 1]). Etoposide should be diluted to a concentration of 0.2 to 0.4 mg/mL in D_5W or NS for administration. Diluted solutions have concentration-dependent stability: More concentrated solutions have shorter stability times. Precipitation may occur with concentrations >0.4 mg/mL.

Storage/Stability

Capsules: Store oral capsules at 2°C to 8°C (36°F to 46°F); do not freeze. Dispense in a light-resistant container.

Injection: Store intact vials of injection at 20°C to 25°C (68°F to 77°F; do not freeze. According to the manufacturer's labeling, stability for solutions diluted for infusion in D_5W or NS (in glass or plastic containers) varies based on concentration; 0.2 mg/mL solutions are stable for 96 hours at room temperature and 0.4 mg/mL solutions are stable for 24 hours at room temperature (precipitation may occur at concentrations above 0.4 mg/mL).

Etoposide injection contains polysorbate 80 which may cause leaching of diethylhexyl phthalate (DEHP), a plasticizer contained in polyvinyl chloride (PVC) bags and tubing. Higher concentrations and longer storage time after preparation in PVC bags may increase DEHP leaching. Preparation in glass or polyolefin containers will minimize patient exposure to DEHP. When undiluted etoposide injection is stored in acrylic or ABS (acrylonitrile, butadiene and styrene) plastic containers, the containers may crack and leak.

Mechanism of Action Etoposide has been shown to delay transit of cells through the S phase and arrest cells in late S or early G_2 phase. The drug may inhibit mitochondrial transport at the NADH dehydrogenase level or inhibit uptake of nucleosides into HeLa cells. It is a topoisomerase II inhibitor and appears to cause DNA strand breaks. Etoposide does not inhibit microtubular assembly.

Pharmacodynamics/Kinetics

Absorption: Oral: Significant inter- and intrapatient variation

Distribution: Average V_d: Children: 10 L/m²; Adults: 7 to 17 L/m²; poor penetration across the blood-brain barrier; CSF concentrations <5% of plasma concentrations

Protein binding: 94% to 98%

◄

Metabolism: Hepatic, via CYP3A4 and 3A5, to various metabolites; in addition, conversion of etoposide to the O-demethylated metabolites (catechol and quinine) via prostaglandin synthases or myeloperoxidase occurs, as well as glutathione and glucuronide conjugation via GSTT1/GSTP1 and UGT1A1 (Yang, 2009)

Bioavailability: Oral: ~50% (range: 25% to 75%)

Half-life elimination: Terminal: IV: Normal renal/hepatic function: Children: 6 to 8 hours: Adults: 4 to 11 hours

Excretion:

Children: IV: Urine (~55% as unchanged drug) in 24 hours

Adults: IV: Urine (56%; 45% as unchanged drug) within 120 hours; feces (44%) within 120 hours

Dosing

Adult & Geriatric

U.S. labeling:

Small cell lung cancer (combination chemotherapy):

IV: 35 mg/m^2/day for 4 days, up to 50 mg/m^2/day for 5 days every 3 to 4 weeks

Oral: Due to poor bioavailability, oral doses should be twice the IV dose (and rounded to the nearest 50 mg)

Testicular cancer (combination chemotherapy): IV: 50 to 100 mg/m^2/day for days 1 to 5 **or** 100 mg/m^2/day on days 1, 3, and 5 repeated every 3 to 4 weeks

Canadian labeling: Non-Hodgkin lymphoma (in combination with other agents), non-small cell lung cancer (alone or in combination), small cell lung cancer (first-line in combination; second-line alone or in combination), testicular cancer (in combination; oral therapy for refractory disease):

IV: 50 to 100 mg/m^2/day for 5 days

Oral: 100 to 200 mg/m^2/day for 5 days; administer daily doses >200 mg in 2 divided doses.

Adult off-label uses and/or dosing:

Hematopoietic stem cell transplant conditioning regimen, lymphoid malignancies: IV: 60 mg/kg over 4 hours as a single dose 3 or 4 days prior to transplantation (Horning, 1994; Snyder, 1993; Weaver, 1994)

Non-small cell lung cancer: IV: 100 mg/m^2 days 1, 2, and 3 every 3 weeks for 4 cycles or every 4 weeks for 3 to 4 cycles (in combination with cisplatin) (Arriagada, 2004) **or** 50 mg/m^2 days 1 to 5 and days 29 to 33 (in combination with cisplatin and radiation therapy) (Albain, 2009)

Ovarian cancer, refractory: Oral: 50 mg/m^2 once daily for 21 days every 4 weeks until disease progression or unacceptable toxicity (Rose, 1998)

Small cell lung cancer, limited stage (combination chemotherapy): IV: 120 mg/m^2/day on days 1, 2, and 3 every 3 weeks for 4 courses (Turrisi, 1999) **or** 100 mg/m^2/day on days 1, 2, and 3 for induction therapy, followed by consolidation chemotherapy (Saito, 2006) **or** 100 mg/m^2/day on days 1, 2, and 3 every 3 weeks up to a maximum of 6 cycles (Skarlos, 2001) **or** 100 mg/m^2/day IV on day 1, followed by 200 mg/m^2/day **orally** on days 2 through 4 every 3 weeks for a maximum of 5 courses (Sundstrom, 2002)

Small cell lung cancer, extensive stage (combination chemotherapy): 100 mg/m^2/day IV on days 1, 2, and 3 every 3 weeks for 4 cycles (Lara, 2009) **or** 100 mg/m^2/day IV on day 1, followed by 200 mg/m^2/day **orally** on days 2 through 4 every 3 weeks for a maximum of 5 courses (Sundstrom, 2002) **or** IV: 80 mg/m^2/day on days 1, 2, and 3 every 3 weeks up to 8 cycles (Ihede, 1994)

Testicular cancer (combination chemotherapy):

Nonseminoma: IV: 100 mg/m^2/day on days 1 through 5 every 21 days for 3 to 4 courses (Saxman, 1998)

Nonseminoma, metastatic (high-dose regimens): IV: 750 mg/m^2/day administered 5, 4, and 3 days before peripheral blood stem cell infusion, repeat for a second cycle after recovery of granulocyte and platelet counts (Einhorn, 2007) **or** 400 mg/m^2/day (beginning on cycle 3) on days 1, 2, and 3, with peripheral blood stem cell support, administered at 14- to 21-day intervals for 3 cycles (Kondagunta, 2007)

Thymoma, locally advanced or metastatic: IV: 120 mg/m^2 days 1, 2, and 3 every 3 weeks (in combination with cisplatin) for up to 8 cycles (Giaccone, 1996)

Unknown primary adenocarcinoma: Oral: 50 mg once daily on days 1, 3, 5, 7, and 9 alternating with 100 mg once daily on days 2, 4, 6, 8, and 10 every 3 weeks (in combination with paclitaxel and carboplatin) (Greco, 2000; Hainsworth, 2006)

Pediatric Note: Oral etoposide is associated with a moderate emetic potential; antiemetics may be recommended to prevent nausea and vomiting (Dupuis, 2011).

Acute myeloid leukemia (AML) induction (off-label use; combination chemotherapy) (Woods, 1996): IV:

<3 years: 3.3 mg/kg/day continuous infusion for 4 days

≥3 years: 100 mg/m^2/day continuous infusion for 4 days

Central nervous system tumors (off-label use; combination chemotherapy): IV:

<3 years: 6.5 mg/kg/dose days 3 and 4 of each 28-day "B" treatment cycle (Duffner, 1993)

≥3 years: 100 mg/m^2/day on days 1, 2, and 3 of a 3-week treatment cycle (Taylor, 2003)

≥6 years: 150 mg/m^2/day on days 3 and 4 of a 3-week treatment course (Kovnar, 1990)

Hematopoietic stem cell transplantation conditioning regimen: IV: 60 mg/kg/dose over 4 hours as a single dose 3 or 4 days prior to transplantation (Horning, 1994; Snyder, 1993)

Hodgkin lymphoma (off-label use): IV: 200 mg/m^2/day on days 1, 2, and 3 every 3 weeks (Kelly, 2002)

Neuroblastoma (off-label use): IV:

Induction: 100 mg/m^2/day on days 1 to 5 of each cycle (Kaneko, 2002)

Hematopoietic stem cell transplantation conditioning regimen: 200 mg/m^2/day for 4 days beginning 8 or 9 days prior to transplantation (Kaneko, 2002)

Sarcoma, refractory (off-label use): IV: 100 mg/m^2/day on days 1 to 5 of cycle; repeat cycle every 21 days (Van Winkle, 2005)

Renal Impairment Oral, IV:

The manufacturer's U.S. labeling recommends the following adjustments:

CrCl >50 mL/minute: No adjustment required.

CrCl 15 to 50 mL/minute: Administer 75% of dose

CrCl <15 mL minute: Data not available; consider further dose reductions

The following adjustments have also been recommended:

Aronoff, 2007:

Adults:

CrCl 10 to 50 mL/minute: Administer 75% of dose.

CrCl <10 mL minute: Administer 50% of dose.

Hemodialysis: Administer 50% of dose; supplemental posthemodialysis dose is not necessary.

Peritoneal dialysis: Administer 50% of dose; supplemental dose is not necessary.

Continuous renal replacement therapy (CRRT): Administer 75% of dose.

Children:

CrCl 10 to 50 mL/minute/1.73 m^2: Administer 75% of dose.

CrCl <10 mL minute/1.73 m^2: Administer 50% of dose.

Hemodialysis: Administer 50% of dose.

Peritoneal dialysis: Administer 50% of dose.

Continuous renal replacement therapy (CRRT): Administer 75% of dose and reduce for hyperbilirubinemia.

Janus, 2010: Hemodialysis: Reduce dose by 50%; not removed by hemodialysis so may be administered before or after dialysis

Kintzel, 1995:

CrCl 46 to 60 mL/minute: Administer 85% of dose

CrCl 31 to 45 mL/minute: Administer 80% of dose

CrCl ≤30 mL/minute: Administer 75% of dose

Hepatic Impairment

Manufacturer's U.S. labeling: There are no dosage adjustments provided in the manufacturer's labeling.

Canadian labeling:

Mild-to-moderate impairment: There are no dosage adjustments provided in the manufacturer's labeling.

Severe impairment: Use is contraindicated.

The following adjustments have also been recommended:

Donelli, 1998: Liver dysfunction may reduce the metabolism and increase the toxicity of etoposide. Normal doses of IV etoposide should be given to patients with liver dysfunction (dose reductions may result in subtherapeutic concentrations); however, use caution with concomitant liver dysfunction (severe) and renal dysfunction as the decreased metabolic clearance cannot be compensated by increased renal clearance.

Floyd, 2006: Bilirubin 1.5 to 3 mg/dL or AST >3 times ULN: Administer 50% of dose

King, 2001; Koren, 1992: Bilirubin 1.5 to 3 mg/dL or AST >180 units/L: Administer 50% of dose

Obesity

American Society of Clinical Oncology (ASCO) Guidelines for appropriate chemotherapy dosing in obese adults with cancer (Note: Excludes HSCT dosing): Utilize patient's actual body weight (full weight) for calculation of body surface area- or weight-based dosing, particularly when the intent of therapy is curative; manage regimen-related toxicities in the same manner as for nonobese patients; if a dose reduction is utilized due to toxicity, consider resumption of full weight-based dosing with subsequent cycles, especially if cause of toxicity (eg, hepatic or renal impairment) is resolved (Griggs, 2012).

American Society for Blood and Marrow Transplantation (ASBMT) practice guideline committee position statement on chemotherapy dosing in obesity: Utilize actual body weight (full weight) for calculation of body surface area (BSA) for BSA-based dosing and utilize adjusted body weight 25% (ABW25) for mg/kg dosing for hematopoietic stem cell transplant conditioning regimens in adults (Bubalo, 2014).

ABW25: Adjusted wt (kg) = Ideal body weight (kg) + 0.25 [actual wt (kg) - ideal body weight (kg)]

Adjustment for Toxicity Oral, IV:

Infusion (hypersensitivity) reactions: Interrupt infusion.

ANC <500/mm^3 or platelets <50,000/mm^3: Withhold treatment until recovery.

Severe adverse reactions (nonhematologic): Reduce dose or discontinue treatment.

WBC 2000-3000/mm^3 or platelets 75,000-100,000/mm^3: Canadian labeling (not in U.S. labeling): Reduce dose by 50%

Administration

Oral etoposide is associated with a low (adults) or moderate (children) emetic potential; antiemetics may be recommended to prevent nausea and vomiting (Dupuis, 2011; Roila, 2010).

Oral: Doses ≤200 mg/day as a single once daily dose; doses >200 mg should be given in 2 divided doses. If necessary, the injection may be used for oral administration (see Extemporaneous Preparations). Canadian labeling recommends administering capsule on an empty stomach.

IV: Administer standard doses over at least 30 to 60 minutes to minimize the risk of hypotension. Higher (off-label) doses used in transplantation may be infused over longer time periods depending on the protocol. Etoposide injection contains polysorbate 80 which may cause leaching of diethylhexyl phthalate (DEHP), a plasticizer contained in polyvinyl chloride (PVC) tubing. Administration through non-PVC (low sorbing) tubing will minimize patient exposure to DEHP. Etoposide is an irritant; tissue irritation and inflammation have occurred following extravasation; avoid extravasation.

Concentrations >0.4 mg/mL are very unstable and may precipitate within a few minutes. For large doses, where dilution to ≤0.4 mg/mL is not feasible, consideration should be given to slow infusion of the undiluted drug through a running normal saline, dextrose or saline/dextrose infusion; or use of etoposide phosphate. Due to the risk for precipitation, an inline filter may be used; etoposide solutions of 0.1 to 0.4 mg/mL may be filtered through a 0.22 micron filter without damage to the filter; etoposide solutions of 0.2 mg/mL may be filtered through a 0.22 micron filter without significant loss of drug.

Hazardous agent; use appropriate precautions for handling and disposal (NIOSH 2014 [group 1]).

Monitoring Parameters CBC with differential; liver function (bilirubin, ALT, AST), albumin, renal function tests; vital signs (blood pressure); signs of an infusion reaction

Dosage Forms
Excipient information presented when available (limited, particularly for generics); consult specific product labeling.

Capsule, Oral:

Generic: 50 mg

Solution, Intravenous:

Toposar: 100 mg/5 mL (5 mL); 500 mg/25 mL (25 mL); 1 g/50 mL (50 mL) [contains alcohol, usp, polyethylene glycol 300, polysorbate 80]

Generic: 100 mg/5 mL (5 mL); 500 mg/25 mL (25 mL); 1 g/50 mL (50 mL)

Extemporaneous Preparations
Hazardous agent: Use appropriate precautions for handling and disposal (NIOSH 2014 [group 1]).

Etoposide 10 mg/mL oral solution: Dilute etoposide for injection 1:1 with normal saline to a concentration of 10 mg/mL. This solution is stable in plastic oral syringes for 22 days at room temperature. Prior to oral administration, further mix with fruit juice (orange, apple, or lemon; **NOT** grapefruit juice) to a concentration of <0.4 mg/mL; once mixed with fruit juice, use within 3 hours.

McLeod HL and Relling MV, "Stability of Etoposide Solution for Oral Use," *Am J Hosp Pharm*, 1992, 49(11):2784-5.

◆ Etoposide Injection (Can) *see* Etoposide *on page 714*

◆ Etoposide Injection USP (Can) *see* Etoposide *on page 714*

Etoposide Phosphate (e toe POE side FOS fate)

Brand Names: US Etopophos

Index Terms Epipodophyllotoxin; ETOP

Pharmacologic Category Antineoplastic Agent, Podophyllotoxin Derivative; Antineoplastic Agent, Topoisomerase II Inhibitor

Use

Small cell lung cancer: First-line treatment of small cell lung cancer (in combination with other chemotherapy agents)

Testicular cancer, refractory: Treatment of refractory testicular tumors (in combination with other chemotherapy agents) in patients who have already received appropriate therapy with surgery, chemotherapy, and radiation

Pregnancy Considerations Adverse events were observed in animal reproduction studies. Fetal growth restriction and newborn myelosuppression have been observed following maternal use of regimens containing etoposide during pregnancy (NTP 2013; Peccatori 2013). The European Society for Medical Oncology has published guidelines for diagnosis, treatment, and follow-up of cancer during pregnancy. The guidelines recommend referral to a facility with expertise in cancer during pregnancy and encourage a multidisciplinary team (obstetrician, neonatologist, oncology team). In general, if chemotherapy is indicated, it should be avoided during in the first trimester, there should be a 3-week time period between the last chemotherapy dose and anticipated delivery, and chemotherapy should not be administered beyond week 33 of gestation. Guidelines for the treatment of SCLC are not provided (Peccatori 2013).

In women of reproductive potential, etoposide phosphate may cause amenorrhea, infertility, or premature menopause; effective contraception should be used during therapy and for ≥6 months after the last dose. In males, azoospermia, oligospermia, or permanent loss of fertility may occur. In addition, spermatozoa and testicular tissue may be damaged. Males with female partners of reproductive potential should use condoms during therapy and for ≥4 months after the last dose.

Breast-Feeding Considerations Etoposide is excreted in breast milk (Azuno 1995). Due to the potential for serious adverse reactions in the nursing infant, the manufacturer recommends a decision be made whether to discontinue nursing or to discontinue the drug, taking into account the importance of treatment to the mother.

Contraindications Hypersensitivity to etoposide, etoposide phosphate, or any component of the formulation

Warnings/Precautions Hazardous agent - use appropriate precautions for handling and disposal (NIOSH 2014 [group 1]). **[US Boxed Warning]: Severe myelosuppression with resulting infection or bleeding may occur.** Myelosuppression is dose-limiting; fatalities due to myelosuppression have been reported following etoposide administration. Hematologic toxicity may occur both during or after therapy; the leukocyte nadir occurs at days 15 to 22; ANC nadir occurs at days 12 to 19, and the platelet nadir occurs at days 10 to 15. Marrow recovery usually occurs by day 21, although may be delayed. Treatment should be withheld for platelets <50,000/mm^3 or absolute neutrophil count (ANC) <500/mm^3. Monitor blood counts prior to therapy initiation and before each cycle of etoposide phosphate. May cause anaphylactic-like reactions manifested by chills, fever, tachycardia, bronchospasm, dyspnea, and hypotension. In addition, facial/tongue swelling, coughing, throat tightness, cyanosis, laryngospasm, diaphoresis, back pain, hypertension, flushing, apnea and loss of consciousness have also been reported less commonly. Anaphylactic-type reactions have occurred with the first infusion. Infusion should be interrupted and medications for the treatment of anaphylaxis should be available for immediate use. Underlying mechanisms behind

the development of hypersensitivity reactions is unknown, but have been attributed to high drug concentration and rate of infusion. Another possible mechanism may be due to the differences between available etoposide intravenous formulations. Etoposide intravenous formulation contains polysorbate 80 and benzyl alcohol, while etoposide phosphate (the water soluble prodrug of etoposide) intravenous formulation does not contain either vehicle. Case reports have suggested that etoposide phosphate has been used successfully in patients with previous hypersensitivity reactions to etoposide (Collier 2008; Siderov 2002).

Secondary acute leukemias have been reported with etoposide, either as monotherapy or in combination with other chemotherapy agents. Dosage should be adjusted in patients with hepatic or renal impairment. Use with caution in patients with low serum albumin; may increase risk for toxicities. Doses of etoposide phosphate >175 mg/m^2 have not been evaluated. Each 100 mg vial of etoposide phosphate is equivalent to 100 mg of etoposide. Equivalent doses should be used when converting from etoposide to etoposide phosphate. Use caution in elderly patients (may be more likely to develop severe myelosuppression and/or GI effects. Etoposide phosphate may result in infertility in male and female patients. In addition, spermatozoa and testicular tissue damage may occur in males; amenorrhea and premature menopause may also occur in women. Males with female partners of childbearing potential should use condoms during therapy and for at least 4 months after the last dose; females of childbearing potential should use effective contraception during therapy and for 6 months after the last dose. Administer by slow IV infusion; hypotension has been reported with etoposide phosphate administration, generally associated with rapid IV infusion. Injection site reactions may occur; monitor infusion site closely. Potentially significant drug-drug interactions may exist, requiring dose or frequency adjustment, additional monitoring, and/or selection of alternative therapy. **[US Boxed Warning]: Should be administered under the supervision of an experienced cancer chemotherapy physician.**

Adverse Reactions Note: Also see adverse reactions for **etoposide**; etoposide phosphate is converted to etoposide, adverse reactions experienced with etoposide would also be expected with etoposide phosphate.

>10%:

Central nervous system: Chills/fever (24%)

Dermatologic: Alopecia (33% to 44%)

Gastrointestinal: Nausea/vomiting (37%), anorexia (16%), mucositis (11%)

Hematologic: Leukopenia (91%; grade 4: 17%; nadir: day 15-22; recovery: usually by day 21), neutropenia (88%; grade 4: 37%; nadir: day 12-19; recovery: usually by day 21), anemia (72%; grades 3/4: 19%), thrombocytopenia (23%; grade 4: 9%; nadir: day 10-15; recovery: usually by day 21)

Neuromuscular & skeletal: Weakness/malaise (39%)

1% to 10%:

Cardiovascular: Hypotension (1% to 5%), hypertension (3%), facial flushing (2%)

Central nervous system: Dizziness (5%)

Dermatologic: Skin rash (3%)

Gastrointestinal: Constipation (8%), abdominal pain (7%), diarrhea (6%), taste perversion (6%)

Local: Extravasation/phlebitis (5%; including swelling, pain, cellulitis, necrosis, and/or skin necrosis at site of infiltration)

Miscellaneous: Anaphylactic-type reactions (3%; including chills, diaphoresis, fever, rigor, tachycardia, bronchospasm, dyspnea, pruritus)

<1% (Limited to important or life-threatening): Acute leukemia (with/without preleukemia phase), anaphylactic-like reactions, blindness (transient, cortical), cyanosis, dysphagia, erythema, facial swelling, hepatic toxicity, hyperpigmentation, hypersensitivity-associated apnea, infection, interstitial pneumonitis, laryngospasm, maculopapular rash, neutropenic fever, optic neuritis, perivasculitis, pruritus, pulmonary fibrosis, radiation recall dermatitis, seizure, Stevens-Johnson syndrome, tongue swelling, toxic epidermal necrolysis, urticaria

Drug Interactions

Metabolism/Transport Effects Substrate of CYP1A2 (minor), CYP2E1 (minor), CYP3A4 (major), P-glycoprotein; **Note:** Assignment of Major/Minor substrate status based on clinically relevant drug interaction potential; **Inhibits** CYP2C9 (weak)

Avoid Concomitant Use

Avoid concomitant use of Etoposide Phosphate with any of the following: BCG (Intravesical); Conivaptan; Deferiprone; Dipyrone; Fusidic Acid (Systemic); Idelalisib; Natalizumab; Pimecrolimus; Tacrolimus (Topical); Tofacitinib; Vaccines (Live)

Increased Effect/Toxicity

Etoposide Phosphate may increase the levels/effects of: CloZAPine; Deferiprone; Fingolimod; Leflunomide; Natalizumab; Tofacitinib; Vaccines (Live); Vitamin K Antagonists

The levels/effects of Etoposide Phosphate may be increased by: Aprepitant; Conivaptan; CycloSPORINE (Systemic); CYP3A4 Inhibitors (Moderate); CYP3A4 Inhibitors (Strong); Dasatinib; Denosumab; Dipyrone; Fosaprepitant; Fusidic Acid (Systemic); Idelalisib; Ivacaftor; Luliconazole; Mifepristone; Netupitant; Osimertinib; Palbociclib; P-glycoprotein/ABCB1 Inhibitors; Pimecrolimus; Ranolazine; Roflumilast; Simeprevir; Stiripentol; Tacrolimus (Topical); Trastuzumab

Decreased Effect

Etoposide Phosphate may decrease the levels/effects of: BCG (Intravesical); Coccidioides immitis Skin Test; Sipuleucel-T; Vaccines (Inactivated); Vaccines (Live)

The levels/effects of Etoposide Phosphate may be decreased by: Bosentan; CYP3A4 Inducers (Moderate); CYP3A4 Inducers (Strong); Dabrafenib; Deferasirox; Enzalutamide; Mitotane; Osimertinib; P-glycoprotein/ABCB1 Inducers; Siltuximab; St Johns Wort; Tocilizumab

Preparation for Administration Hazardous agent; use appropriate precautions for handling and disposal (NIOSH 2014 [group 1]). Reconstitute vials with 5 mL or 10 mL SWFI, D5W, NS, bacteriostatic water for injection with benzyl alcohol, or bacteriostatic sodium chloride for injection with benzyl alcohol to a concentration of 20 mg/mL or 10 mg/mL etoposide equivalent. These solutions may be administered without further dilution or may be diluted in D5W or NS to a concentration as low as 0.1 mg/mL.

Storage/Stability Store intact vials under refrigeration at 2°C to 8°C (36°F to 46°F). Protect from light. Reconstituted solution is stable refrigerated at 2°C to 8°C (36°F to 46°F) for 7 days. At room temperature of 20°C to 25°C (68°F to 77°F), reconstituted solutions are stable for 24 hours when reconstituted with SWFI, D$_5$W, or NS, or for 48 hours when reconstituted with bacteriostatic water for injection with benzyl alcohol or bacteriostatic sodium chloride for injection with benzyl alcohol. Further diluted solutions for infusion are stable at room temperature 20°C to 25°C (68°F to 77°F) or under refrigeration 2°C to 8°C (36°F to 46°F) for up to 24 hours.

Mechanism of Action Etoposide phosphate is converted *in vivo* to the active moiety, etoposide, by dephosphorylation. Etoposide inhibits mitotic activity; inhibits cells from entering prophase; inhibits DNA synthesis. Initially thought to be mitotic inhibitors similar to podophyllotoxin, but actually have no effect on microtubule assembly. However, later shown to induce DNA strand breakage and inhibition of topoisomerase II (an enzyme which breaks and repairs DNA); etoposide acts in late S or early G2 phases.

Pharmacodynamics/Kinetics

Distribution: Average V$_d$: 7 to 17 L/m^2; poor penetration across blood-brain barrier; concentrations in CSF being <10% that of plasma

Protein binding: 97%

Metabolism:

Etoposide phosphate: Rapidly and completely converted to etoposide in plasma

Etoposide: Hepatic, via CYP3A4 and 3A5 to various metabolites; in addition, conversion of etoposide to the O-demethylated metabolites (catechol and quinine) via prostaglandin synthases or myeloperoxidase occurs, as well as glutathione and glucuronide conjugation via GSTT1/GSTP1 and UGT1A1 (Yang 2009)

Half-life elimination: Terminal: 4 to 11 hours; Children: Normal renal/hepatic function: 6 to 8 hours

Excretion: Urine (56%; 45% as etoposide) within 120 hours; feces (44%) within 120 hours

Children: Urine (~55% as etoposide) in 24 hours

Dosing

Adult & Geriatric Note: Etoposide phosphate is a prodrug of etoposide; equivalent doses should be used when converting from etoposide to etoposide phosphate. Each 100 mg vial of etoposide phosphate is equivalent to 100 mg of etoposide.

Small cell lung cancer (in combination with other approved chemotherapeutic drugs): IV: Etoposide 35 mg/m^2/day for 4 days up to 50 mg/m^2/day for 5 days. Courses are repeated at 3- to 4-week intervals after adequate recovery from toxicity.

Testicular cancer, refractory (in combination with other approved chemotherapeutic agents): IV: Etoposide 50 to 100 mg/m^2/day on days 1 to 5 to 100 mg/m^2/day on days 1, 3, and 5. Courses are repeated at 3- to 4-week intervals after adequate recovery from toxicity.

Indication-specific off-label dosing: Refer to Etoposide monograph.

Renal Impairment

CrCl >50 mL/minute: No dosage adjustment necessary.

CrCl 15 to 50 mL/minute: Administer 75% of dose.

CrCl <15 mL minute: Data are not available; consider further dose reductions.

Etoposide phosphate is rapidly and completely converted to etoposide in plasma, please refer to Etoposide monograph for additional renal dosing adjustments (for etoposide).

Hepatic Impairment There are no dosage adjustments provided in the manufacturer's labeling. Etoposide phosphate is rapidly and completely converted to etoposide in plasma; please refer to Etoposide monograph for etoposide hepatic dosing adjustments.

Obesity *ASCO Guidelines for appropriate chemotherapy dosing in obese adults with cancer (**Note:** Excludes HSCT dosing):* Utilize patient's actual body weight (full weight) for calculation of body surface area- or weight-based dosing, particularly when the intent of therapy is curative; manage regimen-related toxicities in the same manner as for nonobese patients; if a dose reduction is utilized due to toxicity, consider resumption of full weight-based dosing with subsequent cycles, especially if cause of toxicity (eg, hepatic or renal impairment) is resolved (Griggs 2012).

Adjustment for Toxicity

Hematologic (ANC <500/mm^3 and/or platelets <50,000/mm^3): Interrupt treatment until blood counts have sufficiently recovered.

Severe adverse reactions: Reduce dose, interrupt treatment, or discontinue.

Administration Infuse by slow IV infusion over 5 to 210 minutes; risk of hypotension may increase with rate of infusion. Do not administer as a bolus injection.

Hazardous agent; use appropriate precautions for handling and disposal (NIOSH 2014 [group 1]).

Monitoring Parameters CBC with differential and platelets (prior to initial treatment and each cycle), bilirubin, AST/ALT, renal function, vital signs (blood pressure)

Dosage Forms Excipient information presented when available (limited, particularly for generics); consult specific product labeling.

Solution Reconstituted, Intravenous [strength expressed as base]:

Etopophos: 100 mg (1 ea)

♦ **ETR** *see* Etravirine *on page 719*

Etravirine (et ra VIR een)

Brand Names: US Intelence

Brand Names: Canada Intelence®

Index Terms ETR; TMC125

Pharmacologic Category Antiretroviral, Reverse Transcriptase Inhibitor, Non-nucleoside (Anti-HIV)

Use Treatment of HIV-1 infection in combination with at least two additional antiretroviral agents in treatment-experienced patients exhibiting viral replication with documented non-nucleoside reverse transcriptase inhibitor (NNRTI) resistance

Dosing

Adult Treatment of HIV-1 infection: Oral: 200 mg twice daily

Pediatric Treatment of HIV-1 infection: Oral: Children 6 to <18 years:

≥16 kg to <20 kg: 100 mg twice daily

≥20 kg to <25 kg: 125 mg twice daily

≥25 kg to <30 kg: 150 mg twice daily

≥30 kg: 200 mg twice daily

Renal Impairment No dosage adjustment necessary.

Due to extensive protein binding, significant removal by hemodialysis or peritoneal dialysis is unlikely.

Hepatic Impairment

Mild-to-moderate impairment (Child-Pugh class A or B): No dosage adjustment necessary.

Severe impairment (Child-Pugh class C): There are no dosage adjustments provided in the manufacturer's labeling (has not been studied).

Additional Information Complete prescribing information should be consulted for additional detail.

Dosage Forms Excipient information presented when available (limited, particularly for generics); consult specific product labeling.

Tablet, Oral:

Intelence: 25 mg [scored]

Intelence: 100 mg, 200 mg

♦ **Euflex (Can)** *see* Flutamide *on page 791*

♦ **Euflexxa** *see* Hyaluronate and Derivatives *on page 879*

♦ **Euglucon (Can)** *see* GlyBURIDE *on page 847*

♦ **Eulexin** *see* Flutamide *on page 791*

♦ *Euphorbia peplus* Derivative *see* Ingenol Mebutate *on page 952*

♦ **Eurax** *see* Crotamiton *on page 452*

♦ **Eurax Cream (Can)** *see* Crotamiton *on page 452*

♦ **Euro-Cyproheptadine (Can)** *see* Cyproheptadine *on page 465*

♦ **Euro-Docusate C [OTC] (Can)** *see* Docusate *on page 578*

♦ **Euro-Lac (Can)** *see* Lactulose *on page 1023*

♦ **Eutectic Mixture of Lidocaine and Tetracaine** *see* Lidocaine and Tetracaine *on page 1077*

♦ **Evac [OTC]** *see* Psyllium *on page 1529*

♦ **Evamist** *see* Estradiol (Systemic) *on page 681*

♦ **Evekeo** *see* Amphetamine *on page 115*

Everolimus (e ver OH li mus)

Brand Names: US Afinitor; Afinitor Disperz; Zortress

Brand Names: Canada Afinitor

Index Terms RAD001

Pharmacologic Category Antineoplastic Agent, mTOR Kinase Inhibitor; Immunosuppressant Agent; mTOR Kinase Inhibitor

Use

Breast cancer, advanced (Afinitor only): Treatment of advanced hormone receptor-positive, HER2-negative breast cancer in postmenopausal women (in combination with exemestane and after letrozole or anastrozole failure)

Pancreatic neuroendocrine tumors (Afinitor only): Treatment of locally advanced, metastatic or unresectable progressive pancreatic neuroendocrine tumors (PNET)

Limitations of use: Not indicated for the treatment of functional carcinoid tumors.

Renal angiomyolipoma with tuberous sclerosis complex (Afinitor only): Treatment of renal angiomyolipoma with tuberous sclerosis complex (TSC) not requiring immediate surgery

Renal cell carcinoma, advanced (Afinitor only): Treatment of advanced renal cell cancer (RCC) after sunitinib or sorafenib failure

Subependymal giant cell astrocytoma (Afinitor or Afinitor Disperz only): Treatment of subependymal giant cell astrocytoma (SEGA) associated with TSC which requires intervention, but cannot be curatively resected

Liver transplantation (Zortress only): Prophylaxis of organ rejection in liver transplantation (in combination with corticosteroids and reduced doses of tacrolimus)

Renal transplantation (Zortress only): Prophylaxis of organ rejection in renal transplant patients at low to moderate immunologic risk (in combination with basiliximab induction and concurrent with corticosteroids and reduced doses of cyclosporine)

Pregnancy Considerations Adverse events were observed in animal reproduction studies with exposures lower than expected with human doses. Based on the mechanism of action, may cause fetal harm if administered during pregnancy. Women of reproductive potential should be advised to avoid pregnancy and use highly effective birth control during treatment and for up to 8 weeks after everolimus discontinuation.

The National Transplantation Pregnancy Registry (NTPR) (Temple University) is a registry for pregnant women taking immunosuppressants following any solid organ transplant. The NTPR encourages reporting of all immunosuppressant exposures during pregnancy in transplant recipients at 877-955-6877.

Breast-Feeding Considerations It is not known if everolimus is excreted in breast milk. Due to the potential for serious adverse reactions in the nursing infant, breast-feeding should be avoided.

Medication Guide Available Yes

Contraindications Hypersensitivity to everolimus, sirolimus, other rapamycin derivatives, or any component of the formulation.

Warnings/Precautions Hazardous agent - use appropriate precautions for handling and disposal (NIOSH 2014 [group 1]).

To avoid potential contact with everolimus, caregivers should wear gloves when preparing suspension from tablets for oral suspension. Noninfectious pneumonitis, interstitial lung disease (ILD), and/or noninfectious fibrosis have been observed with mTOR inhibitors including everolimus; some cases were fatal. Symptoms include

dyspnea, cough, hypoxia and/or pleural effusion; promptly evaluate worsening respiratory symptoms. Cases of ILD have been reported with pulmonary hypertension (including pulmonary arterial hypertension) as a secondary event. Consider opportunistic infections such as *Pneumocystis jiroveci* pneumonia (PCP) when evaluating clinical symptoms. May require treatment interruption followed by dose reduction (pneumonitis has developed even with reduced doses) and/or corticosteroid therapy; discontinue for grade 4 pneumonitis. Consider discontinuation for recurrence of grade 3 toxicity after dosage reduction. In patients who require steroid therapy for symptom management, consider PCP prophylaxis. Imaging may overestimate the incidence of clinical pneumonitis. **[US Boxed Warning]: Everolimus has immunosuppressant properties which may result in infection;** the risk of developing bacterial (including mycobacterial), viral, fungal and protozoal infections and for local, opportunistic (including polyomavirus infection), and/or systemic infections is increased; may lead to sepsis, respiratory failure, hepatic failure, or fatality. Polyomavirus infection in transplant patients may be serious and/or fatal. Polyoma virus-associated nephropathy (due to BK virus), which may result in serious cases of deteriorating renal function and renal graft loss, has been observed with use. JC virus-associated progressive multiple leukoencephalopathy (PML) may also be associated with everolimus use in transplantation. Reduced immunosuppression (taking into account the risks of rejection) should be considered with evidence of polyoma virus infection or PML. Reactivation of hepatitis B has been observed in patients receiving everolimus. Resolve preexisting invasive fungal infections prior to treatment initiation. Cases (some fatal) of *Pneumocystis jiroveci* pneumonia (PCP) have been reported with everolimus use. Consider PCP prophylaxis in patients receiving concomitant corticosteroid or other immunosuppressant therapy. In addition, transplant recipient patients should receive prophylactic therapy for PCP and for cytomegalovirus (CMV). Monitor for signs and symptoms of infection during treatment. Discontinue if invasive systemic fungal infection is diagnosed (and manage with appropriate antifungal therapy).

[US Boxed Warning]: Immunosuppressant use may result in the development of malignancy, including lymphoma and skin cancer. The risk is associated with treatment intensity and the duration of therapy. To minimize the risk for skin cancer, limit exposure to sunlight and ultraviolet light; wear protective clothing and use effective sunscreen.

[US Boxed Warning]: Due to the increased risk for nephrotoxicity in renal transplantation, avoid standard doses of cyclosporine in combination with everolimus; reduced cyclosporine doses are recommended when everolimus is used in combination with cyclosporine. Therapeutic monitoring of cyclosporine and everolimus concentrations is recommended. Monitor for proteinuria; the risk of proteinuria is increased when everolimus is used in combination with cyclosporine, and with higher serum everolimus concentrations. Everolimus and cyclosporine combination therapy may increase the risk for thrombotic microangiopathy/thrombotic thrombocytopenic purpura/hemolytic uremic syndrome (TMA/TTP/HUS); monitor blood counts. In liver transplantation, the tacrolimus dose and target range should be reduced to minimize the risk of nephrotoxicity. Eliminating calcineurin inhibitors from the immunosuppressive regimen may result in acute rejection. Elevations in serum creatinine (generally mild), renal failure, and proteinuria have been also observed with everolimus use; monitor renal function (BUN, creatinine, and/or urinary protein). Risk of nephrotoxicity may be increased when administered with calcineurin inhibitors (eg, cyclosporine, tacrolimus); dosage adjustment of calcineurin inhibitor is necessary. An increased incidence of rash, infection and dose interruptions have been reported in patients with renal insufficiency (CrCl ≤60 mL/minute) who received mTOR inhibitors for the treatment of renal cell cancer (Gupta, 2011); serum creatinine elevations and proteinuria have been reported. Monitor renal function (BUN, serum creatinine, urinary protein) at baseline and periodically, especially if risk factors for further impairment exist; pharmacokinetic studies have not been conducted; dosage adjustments are not required based on renal impairment. **[US Boxed Warning]: An increased risk of renal arterial and venous thrombosis has been reported with use in renal transplantation, generally within the first 30 days after transplant; may result in graft loss.** MTOR inhibitors are associated with an increase in hepatic artery thrombosis, most cases have been reported within 30 days after transplant and usually proceeded to graft loss or death; do not use everolimus prior to 30 days post liver transplant.

Potentially significant drug-drug/drug-food interactions may exist, requiring dose or frequency adjustment, additional monitoring, and/or selection of alternative therapy. In transplant patients, avoid the use of certain HMG-CoA reductase inhibitors (eg, simvastatin, lovastatin); may increase the risk for rhabdomyolysis due to the potential interaction with cyclosporine (which may be given in combination with everolimus for transplantation).

Use is associated with mouth ulcers, mucositis and stomatitis; manage with topical therapy; avoid the use of alcohol-, hydrogen peroxide-, iodine-, or thyme-based mouthwashes (due to the high potential for drug interactions, avoid the use of systemic antifungals unless fungal infection has been diagnosed). Everolimus is associated with the development of angioedema; concomitant use with other agents known to cause angioedema (eg, ACE inhibitors) may increase the risk. Everolimus use may delay wound healing and increase the occurrence of wound-related complications (eg, wound dehiscence, infection, incisional hernia, lymphocele, seroma); may require surgical intervention; use with caution in the perisurgical period. Generalized edema, including peripheral edema and lymphedema, and local fluid accumulation (eg, pericardial effusion, pleural effusion, ascites) may also occur.

Everolimus exposure is increased in patients with hepatic impairment. For patients with breast cancer, PNET, RCC, or renal angiomyolipoma with mild and moderate hepatic impairment, reduced doses are recommended; in patients with severe hepatic impairment, use is recommended (at reduced doses) if the potential benefit outweighs risks. Reduced doses are recommended in transplant patients with hepatic impairment; pharmacokinetic information does not exist for renal transplant patients with severe impairment (Child-Pugh class B or C); monitor whole blood trough levels closely for patients with SEGA, reduced doses may be needed for mild and moderate hepatic impairment (based on therapeutic drug monitoring), and are recommended in severe hepatic impairment; monitor whole blood trough levels. The Canadian labeling recommends against the use of everolimus in patients <18 years of age with SEGA and hepatic impairment.

[US Boxed Warning]: Increased mortality (usually associated with infections) within the first 3 months after transplant was noted in a study of patients with *de novo* heart transplant receiving immunosuppressive regimens containing everolimus (with or without induction therapy). Use in heart transplantation is not recommended. Hyperglycemia, hyperlipidemia, and hypertriglyceridemia have been reported. Higher serum everolimus concentrations are associated with an increased risk for hyperlipidemia. Use has not been studied in patients with baseline cholesterol >350 mg/dL. Monitor fasting glucose and lipid profile prior to treatment initiation and periodically thereafter; monitor more frequently in patients with concomitant medications affecting glucose. Manage with appropriate medical therapy (if possible, optimize glucose control and lipids prior to treatment initiation). Antihyperlipidemic therapy may not normalize levels. May alter insulin and/or oral hypoglycemic therapy requirements in patients with diabetes; the risk for new onset diabetes is increased with everolimus use after transplantation. Decreases in hemoglobin, neutrophils, platelets, and lymphocytes have been reported; monitor blood counts at baseline and periodically. Increases in serum glucose are common; may alter insulin and/or oral hypoglycemic therapy requirements in patients with diabetes; the risk for new-onset diabetes is increased with everolimus use after transplantation. Patients should not be immunized with live viral vaccines during or shortly after treatment and should avoid close contact with recently vaccinated (live vaccine) individuals; consider the timing of routine immunizations prior to the start of therapy in pediatric patients treated for SEGA. In pediatric patients treated for SEGA, complete recommended series of live virus childhood vaccinations prior to treatment (if immediate everolimus treatment is not indicated); an accelerated vaccination schedule may be appropriate. Continue treatment with everolimus for renal cell cancer as long as clinical benefit is demonstrated or until occurrence of unacceptable toxicity. Safety and efficacy have not been established for the use of everolimus in the treatment of carcinoid tumors.

Tablets (Afinitor, Zortress) and tablets for oral suspension (Afinitor Disperz) are not interchangeable; Afinitor Disperz is only indicated in conjunction with therapeutic monitoring for the treatment of SEGA. Do not combine formulations to achieve total desired dose. May cause infertility; in females, menstrual irregularities, secondary amenorrhea,

and increases in luteinizing hormone and follicle-stimulating hormone have occurred; azoospermia and oligospermia have been observed in males. Avoid use in patients with hereditary galactose intolerance, Lapp lactase deficiency, or glucose-galactose malabsorption; may result in diarrhea and malabsorption. The safety and efficacy of everolimus in renal transplantation patients with high-immunologic risk or in solid organ transplant other than renal or liver have not been established. **[US Boxed Warning]: In transplantation, everolimus should only be used by physicians experienced in immunosuppressive therapy and management of transplant patients. Adequate laboratory and supportive medical resources must be readily available.** For indications requiring whole blood trough concentrations to determine dosage adjustments, a consistent method should be used; concentration values from different assay methods may not be interchangeable.

Adverse Reactions

Transplantation: Frequency not always defined. Reactions occur in kidney and liver transplantation unless otherwise specified.

>10%:

Cardiovascular: Peripheral edema (kidney transplant: 45%; liver transplant: 18%), hypertension (kidney transplant: 30%; liver transplant: 17%)

Central nervous system: Headache (18% to 19%), insomnia (kidney transplant: 17%), procedural pain (kidney transplant: 15%)

Endocrine & metabolic: Diabetes mellitus (new onset: liver transplant: 32%; kidney transplant: 9%), hypercholesterolemia (15% to 24%), hyperkalemia (renal transplant: 18%), hypomagnesemia (kidney transplant: 14%), hypophosphatemia (kidney transplant: 13%), hyperglycemia (kidney transplant: 12%), hypokalemia (kidney transplant: 12%)

Gastrointestinal: Constipation (kidney transplant: 38%), nausea (kidney transplant: 29%; liver transplant: 14%), diarrhea (19%), vomiting (kidney transplant: 15%), abdominal pain (13%; upper abdominal pain, kidney transplant: 2%)

Genitourinary: Urinary tract infection (kidney transplant: 22%), hematuria (kidney transplant: 12%), dysuria (kidney transplant: 11%)

Hematologic & oncologic: Anemia (kidney transplant: 26%), leukopenia (3% to 12%)

Infection: Infection (kidney transplant: 62%; liver transplant: 50%), viral infection (liver transplant: 17%; kidney transplant: 10%), bacterial infection (liver transplant: 16%), hepatitis C (liver transplant: 11%)

Local: Incisional pain (kidney transplant: 16%)

Neuromuscular & skeletal: Limb pain (kidney transplant: 12%), back pain (kidney transplant: 11%)

Renal: Increased serum creatinine (kidney transplant: 18%)

Respiratory: Upper respiratory tract infection (kidney transplant: 16%)

Miscellaneous: Postoperative wound complication (kidney transplant: 35%; liver transplant: 11%; includes incisional hernia, lymphocele, seroma, wound dehiscence), fever (13% to 19%)

1% to 10%:

Cardiovascular: Hypertensive crisis (1%), angina pectoris, atrial fibrillation, cardiac failure, chest discomfort, chest pain, deep vein thrombosis, edema, hypotension, palpitations, pulmonary embolism, renal artery thrombosis, syncope, tachycardia, venous thromboembolism

Central nervous system: Fatigue (9%), agitation, anxiety, chills, depression, dizziness, drowsiness, hallucination, hemiparesis, hypoesthesia, lethargy, malaise, migraine, myasthenia, neuralgia, pain, paresthesia

Dermatologic: Acneiform eruption, acne vulgaris, alopecia, cellulitis, diaphoresis, folliculitis, hypertrichosis, night sweats, onychomycosis, pruritus, skin rash, tinea pedis

Endocrine & metabolic: Acidosis, amenorrhea, cushingoid appearance, cyanocobalamin deficiency, dehydration, fluid retention, gout, hirsutism, hypercalcemia, hyperparathyroidism, hypertriglyceridemia, hyperuricemia, hypocalcemia, hypoglycemia, hyponatremia, iron deficiency, ovarian cyst

Gastrointestinal: Stomatitis (kidney transplant: 8%), dyspepsia (kidney transplant: 4%), abdominal distention, anorexia, decreased appetite, dysphagia, epigastric distress, flatulence, gastroenteritis, gastroesophageal reflux disease, gingival hyperplasia, hematemesis, hemorrhoids, intestinal obstruction, oral candidiasis, oral herpes, oral mucosa ulcer, peritoneal effusion, peritonitis

Genitourinary: Erectile dysfunction (kidney transplant: 5%), bladder spasm, perinephric abscess, perinephric hematoma, pollakiuria, proteinuria, pyuria, scrotal edema, urethritis, urinary retention, urinary urgency

Hematologic & oncologic: Neoplasm (3% to 4%), leukocytosis, lymphadenopathy, lymphorrhea, neutropenia, pancytopenia, thrombocythemia, thrombocytopenia

Hepatic: Abnormal hepatic function tests (liver transplant: 7%), ascites (liver transplant: 4%), hepatitis (noninfectious), increased liver enzymes, increased serum alkaline phosphatase, increased serum bilirubin

Hypersensitivity: Angioedema (<1%)

Infection: BK virus (kidney transplant: 1%), bacteremia, candidiasis, herpes virus infection, influenza, sepsis, wound infection

Neuromuscular & skeletal: Tremor (8% to 9%), arthralgia, joint swelling, muscle spasm, musculoskeletal pain, myalgia, osteomyelitis, osteonecrosis, osteoporosis, spondylitis, weakness

Ophthalmic: Blurred vision, cataract, conjunctivitis

Renal: Hydronephrosis, increased blood urea nitrogen, interstitial nephritis, polyuria, pyelonephritis, renal failure (acute), renal insufficiency, renal tubular necrosis

Respiratory: Cough (kidney transplant: 7%), atelectasis, bronchitis, dyspnea, epistaxis, lower respiratory tract infection, nasal congestion, nasopharyngitis, oropharyngeal pain, pleural effusion, pneumonia, pulmonary edema, rhinorrhea, sinus congestion, sinusitis, wheezing

Antineoplastic: Antineoplastic indications include advanced hormone receptor-positive, HER2-negative breast cancer (advanced HR + BC), pancreatic neuroendocrine tumors (PNET), renal cell carcinoma (RCC), renal angiomyolipoma and tuberous sclerosis complex (TSC), and subependymal giant cell astrocytoma (SEGA)

>10%:

Cardiovascular: Edema (PNET: ≤39%), peripheral edema (PNET: ≤39%; advanced HR + BC, RCC, TSC: 13% to 25%), hypertension (PNET, RCC: 4% to 13%)

Central nervous system: Malaise (PNET: ≤45%), fatigue (advanced HR + BC, PNET, RCC: 31% to ≤45%; SEGA: 14%), headache (PNET: ≤30%; advanced HR + BC, RCC: 19% to 21%), migraine (PNET: ≤30%), behavioral problems (SEGA: 21%; includes abnormal behavior, aggressive behavior, agitation, anxiety, obsessive compulsive symptoms, panic attack), insomnia (advanced HR + BC, PNET, RCC, SEGA: 6% to 14%), dizziness (PNET, RCC: 7% to 12%)

Dermatologic: Skin rash (PNET: 59%; advanced HR + BC: 39%; RCC, SEGA: 21% to 29%; may include allergic dermatitis, macular eruption, maculopapular rash, papular rash, urticaria), cellulitis (SEGA: 29%), acne vulgaris (TSC: 22%; SEGA: 10%), nail disease (PNET: 22%; RCC: 5%), pruritus (advanced HR + BC, PNET, RCC: 13% to 21%), xeroderma (PNET, RCC: 13%)

Endocrine & metabolic: Hypercholesterolemia (TSC, SEGA: 81% to 85%), decreased serum bicarbonate (PNET: 56%), hypertriglyceridemia (TSC: 52%; SEGA: 27%), hypophosphatemia (TSC: 49%; SEGA: 9%), decreased serum calcium (PNET: 37%), decreased serum albumin (advanced HR + BC: 33%; PNET: 13%), hyperglycemia (SEGA: 25%; advanced HR + BC: 14%), amenorrhea (TSC, SEGA: 15% to 17%)

Gastrointestinal: Stomatitis (advanced HR + BC, PNET, SEGA, TSC: 62% to 78%; grades 3/4: ≤9%; RCC: 44%, grades 3/4: ≤4%), diarrhea (PNET: 50%; advanced HR + BC, RCC: 30% to 33%; TSC, SEGA: 14% to 17%; may include bowel urgency, colitis, enteritis, enterocolitis, steatorrhea), abdominal pain (PNET: 36%; RCC: 9%), decreased appetite (advanced HR + BC, PNET: 30%; TSC: 6%), nausea (advanced HR + BC, RCC: 26% to 29%; SEGA: 8%), vomiting (15% to 29%), weight loss (advanced HR + BC, PNET: 25% to 28%; RCC: 9%), anorexia (RCC: 25%), dysgeusia (advanced HR + BC, PNET: 19% to 22%; RCC: 10%; TSC: 5%), mucositis (RCC: 19%; grades 3/4: ≤1%), constipation (advanced HR + BC, PNET, SEGA: 10% to 14%), xerostomia (advanced HR + BC, PNET, RCC: 8% to 11%)

Genitourinary: Urinary tract infection (PNET: 16%; advanced HR + BC, RCC: 5% to 10%), irregular menses (TSC, PNET: 10% to 11%)

Hematologic & oncologic: Increase in fasting plasma glucose (PNET: 75%, grades 3/4: 17%; TSC: 14%), prolonged partial thromboplastin time (SEGA: 72%), anemia (TSC: 61%; SEGA: 41%), lymphocytopenia (advanced HR + BC, PNET, RCC: 45% to 54%; advanced HR + BC, RCC grade 3: 11% to 16%, RCC grade 4: 2%; PNET grades 3/4: 16%; TSC: 20%, grade 3: 1%), thrombocytopenia (advanced HR + BC, PNET:

45% to 54%; advanced HR + BC grade 3: 3%, PNET grades 3/4: 3%; RCC, TSC: 19% to 23%, RCC grade 3: 1%), neutropenia (SEGA: 46%, grade 3: 9%; advanced HR + BC, PNET: 30% to 31%, PNET grades 3/4: 4%, advanced HR + BC grade 3: 2%; RCC 14%, grade 4: <1%), leukopenia (TSC: 37%)

Hepatic: Increased serum alkaline phosphatase (PNET: 74%; TSC: 32%, grade 3: 1%), increased serum AST (advanced HR + BC: 69%; PNET: 56%; RCC, TSC, SEGA: 23% to 33%; advanced HR + BC, RCC, TSC grade 3: ≤4%; advanced HR + BC, RCC grade 4: <1%), increased serum ALT (advanced HR + BC, PNET: 48% to 51%, advanced HR + BC grade 4: <1%; RCC, TSC, SEGA: 18% to 21%; RCC, TSC grade 3: 1%)

Infection: Infection (advanced HR + BC: 50%; RCC: 37%; advanced HR + BC, RCC grade 3: 4% to 7%; advanced HR + BC, RCC grade 4: 1% to 3%)

Neuromuscular & skeletal: Weakness (RCC: 33%; advanced HR + BC: 13%), arthralgia (advanced HR + BC, PNET, TSC: 13% to 20%), back pain (advanced HR + BC, PNET: 14% to 15%), limb pain (PNET, RCC, SEGA: 8% to 14%)

Renal: Increased serum creatinine (RCC: 50%; advanced HR + BC, PNET: 19% to 24%, advanced HR + BC, RCC grade 3: 1% to 2%, PNET grades 3/4: 2%)

Respiratory: Respiratory tract infection (SEGA: 31%, grade 3: 1%, grade 4: 1%; includes viral respiratory tract infection), cough (advanced HR + BC, PNET, RCC, TSC: 20% to 30%; includes productive cough), nasopharyngitis (PNET: ≤25%; advanced HR + BC, RCC: 6% to 10%), rhinitis (PNET: ≤25%), upper respiratory tract infection (PNET: ≤25%; TSC: 11%; advanced HR + BC: 5%), dyspnea (advanced HR + BC, PNET, RCC: 20% to 24%; includes dyspnea on exertion), epistaxis (advanced HR + BC, PNET, RCC: 17% to 22%; TSC, SEGA: 5% to 9%), pneumonitis (advanced HR + BC, PNET, RCC: 14% to 19%; TSC, SEGA: 1%; advanced HR + BC, PNET, RCC grade 3: 3% to 4%; advanced HR + BC, PNET grade 4: <1%; may include interstitial pulmonary disease, pulmonary alveolar hemorrhage, pulmonary alveolitis, pulmonary fibrosis, pulmonary infiltrates, pulmonary toxicity, restrictive pulmonary disease), oropharyngeal pain (PNET: 11%)

Miscellaneous: Fever (advanced HR + BC, PNET, RCC, SEGA: 15% to 31%)

1% to 10%:

Cardiovascular: Chest pain (RCC: 5%), tachycardia (RCC: 3%), cardiac failure (RCC: 1%), deep vein thrombosis (RCC: <1%)

Central nervous system: Depression (TSC: 5%), paresthesia (RCC: 5%), chills (RCC: 4%)

Dermatologic: Alopecia (advanced HR + BC: 10%), palmar-plantar erythrodysesthesia (RCC: 5%), erythema (RCC: 4%), onychoclasis (RCC: 4%), skin lesion (RCC: 4%), acneiform eruption (RCC: 3%)

Endocrine & metabolic: Diabetes mellitus (PNET: 10%; RCC: exacerbation of diabetes mellitus: 2%, new onset: <1%), hypermenorrhea (TSC, SEGA: 6% to 10%), menstrual disease (TSC, SEGA: 6% to 10%), increased luteinizing hormone (TSC, SEGA: 1% to 4%), increased follicle-stimulating hormone (TSC: 3%), ovarian cyst (TSC: 3%)

Gastrointestinal: Gastroenteritis (SEGA: 10%; includes viral gastroenteritis, gastrointestinal infection), hemorrhoids (RCC: 5%), dysphagia (RCC: 4%)

Genitourinary: Vaginal hemorrhage (TSC: 8%), dysmenorrhea (SEGA: 6%), uterine hemorrhage (SEGA: 6%), cystitis (advanced HR + BC: 3%)

Hematologic & oncologic: Hemorrhage (RCC: 3%)

Hepatic: Increased serum bilirubin (RCC: 3%; grade 3: <1%, grade 4: <1%)

Hypersensitivity: Hypersensitivity (TSC, SEGA: 3%; includes anaphylaxis, chest pain, dyspnea, flushing), angioedema (RCC, TSC: ≤1%)

Infection: Candidiasis (advanced HR + BC, RCC: <1%), hepatitis C (advanced HR + BC: <1%), sepsis (advanced HR + BC, RCC: <1%)

Neuromuscular & skeletal: Muscle spasm (PNET: 10%), jaw pain (RCC: 3%)

Ophthalmic: Eyelid edema (RCC: 4%), conjunctivitis (RCC: 2%)

Otic: Otitis media (TSC: 6%)

Renal: Renal failure (RCC: 3%)

Respiratory: Streptococcal pharyngitis (SEGA: 10%), pleural effusion (RCC: 7%), pneumonia (advanced HR + BC, RCC, SEGA: 4% to 6%), bronchitis (advanced HR + BC, RCC: 4%), pharyngolaryngeal pain (RCC: 4%), rhinorrhea (RCC: 3%), sinusitis (advanced HR + BC, RCC: 3%)

Miscellaneous: Postoperative wound complication (RC: <1%; wound healing impairment)

<1% (Limited to important or life-threatening): Ageusia, arterial thrombosis, aspergillosis, azoospermia, cardiac arrest, cholecystitis, cholelithiasis, complex regional pain syndrome, contact dermatitis, decreased plasma testosterone, eczema, excoriation, gastritis, hemolytic uremic syndrome, hypersensitivity angiitis, male infertility, nephrotoxicity, noninfectious pneumonitis, oligospermia, pancreatitis (including acute pancreatitis), pericardial effusion, pharyngitis, pityriasis rosea, pneumonia due to *Pneumocystis jiroveci*, polyoma virus infection, progressive multifocal leukoencephalopathy, reactivation of HBV, respiratory distress, seizure, thrombosis of vascular graft (kidney), thrombotic thrombocytopenic purpura

Drug Interactions

Metabolism/Transport Effects Substrate of CYP3A4 (major), P-glycoprotein; **Note:** Assignment of Major/Minor substrate status based on clinically relevant drug interaction potential

Avoid Concomitant Use

Avoid concomitant use of Everolimus with any of the following: BCG (Intravesical); Conivaptan; CYP3A4 Inducers (Strong); CYP3A4 Inhibitors (Strong); Deferiprone; Dipyrone; Fusidic Acid (Systemic); Grapefruit Juice; Idelalisib; Natalizumab; Pimecrolimus; St Johns Wort; Tacrolimus (Topical); Tofacitinib; Vaccines (Live); Voriconazole

Increased Effect/Toxicity

Everolimus may increase the levels/effects of: ACE Inhibitors; CloZAPine; Deferiprone; Fingolimod; Leflunomide; Natalizumab; Tofacitinib; Vaccines (Live)

The levels/effects of Everolimus may be increased by: Conivaptan; CycloSPORINE (Systemic); CYP3A4 Inhibitors (Moderate); CYP3A4 Inhibitors (Strong); Dasatinib; Denosumab; Dipyrone; Fosaprepitant; Fusidic Acid (Systemic); Grapefruit Juice; Idelalisib; Luliconazole; Mifepristone; Osimertinib; Palbociclib; P-glycoprotein/ABCB1 Inhibitors; Pimecrolimus; Roflumilast; Stiripentol; Tacrolimus (Topical); Trastuzumab; Voriconazole

Decreased Effect

Everolimus may decrease the levels/effects of: Antidiabetic Agents; BCG (Intravesical); Coccidioides immitis Skin Test; Sipuleucel-T; Vaccines (Inactivated); Vaccines (Live)

The levels/effects of Everolimus may be decreased by: Bosentan; CYP3A4 Inducers (Moderate); CYP3A4 Inducers (Strong); Dabrafenib; Deferasirox; Echinacea; Efavirenz; Osimertinib; P-glycoprotein/ABCB1 Inducers; Siltuximab; St Johns Wort; Tocilizumab

Food Interactions Grapefruit juice may increase levels of everolimus. Absorption with food may be variable. Management: Avoid grapefruit juice. Take with or without food, but be consistent with regard to food.

Storage/Stability Tablets and tablets for suspension: Store at room temperature of 25°C (77°F); excursions permitted to 15°C to 30°C (59°F to 86°F). Protect from light; protect from moisture.

Mechanism of Action Everolimus is a macrolide immunosuppressant and a mechanistic target of rapamycin (mTOR) inhibitor which has antiproliferative and antiangiogenic properties, and also reduces lipoma volume in patients with angiomyolipoma. Reduces protein synthesis and cell proliferation by binding to the FK binding protein-12 (FKBP-12), an intracellular protein, to form a complex that inhibits activation of mTOR (mechanistic target of rapamycin) serine-threonine kinase activity. Also reduces angiogenesis by inhibiting vascular endothelial growth factor (VEGF) and hypoxia-inducible factor (HIF-1) expression. Angiomyolipomas may occur due to unregulated mTOR activity in TSC-associated renal angiomyolipoma (Budde, 2012); everolimus reduces lipoma volume (Bissler, 2012).

Pharmacodynamics/Kinetics

Absorption: Rapid, but moderate

Distribution: Apparent V_d: 128 to 589 L; volume of distribution in children (3 to 16 years) lower than adults (Van Damme-Lombaerts 2002)

Protein binding: ~74%

Metabolism: Extensively metabolized in the liver via CYP3A4; forms 6 weak metabolites

Bioavailability:

Tablets: ~30%; Systemic exposure reduced by 22% with a high-fat meal and by 32% with a light-fat meal

Tablets for suspension: AUC equivalent to tablets although peak concentrations are 20% to 36% lower; steady state concentrations are similar; systemic exposure reduced by 12% with a high-fat meal and by 30% with a low-fat meal

Half-life elimination: ~30 hours; in children (3 to 16 years), half-life similar to adult data (Van Damme-Lombaerts 2002)

Time to peak, plasma: 1 to 2 hours

Excretion: Feces (80%, based on solid organ transplant studies); Urine (~5%, based on solid organ transplant studies); clearance in pediatric patients lower than adults possibly due to distributive differences (Van Damme-Lombaerts 2002)

Dosing

Adult & Geriatric Note: Tablets (Afinitor, Zortress) and tablets for oral suspension (Afinitor Disperz) are not interchangeable; Afinitor Disperz is only indicated for the treatment of subependymal giant cell astrocytoma (SEGA), in conjunction with therapeutic monitoring. Do not combine formulations to achieve total desired dose.

Breast cancer, advanced, hormone receptor-positive, HER2-negative: Oral: 10 mg once daily (in combination with exemestane), continue treatment until disease progression or unacceptable toxicity

Pancreatic neuroendocrine tumors (PNET), advanced: Oral: 10 mg once daily, continue treatment until disease progression or unacceptable toxicity

Renal angiomyolipoma: Oral: 10 mg once daily, continue treatment until disease progression or unacceptable toxicity

Renal cell cancer, advanced (RCC): Oral: 10 mg once daily, continue treatment until disease progression or unacceptable toxicity

Liver transplantation, rejection prophylaxis (begin at least 30 days post-transplant): Oral: Initial: 1 mg twice daily; adjust maintenance dose if needed at a 4- to 5-day interval (from prior dose adjustment) based on serum concentrations, tolerability, and response; goal serum concentration is between 3 and 8 ng/mL (based on an LC/MS/MS assay method). If trough is <3 ng/mL, double total daily dose (using available tablet strengths); if trough >8 ng/mL on 2 consecutive measures, decrease dose by 0.25 mg twice daily. Administer in combination with tacrolimus (reduced dose required) and corticosteroids

Renal transplantation, rejection prophylaxis: Oral: Initial: 0.75 mg twice daily; adjust maintenance dose if needed at a 4- to 5-day interval (from prior dose adjustment) based on serum concentrations, tolerability, and response; goal serum concentration is between 3 and 8 ng/mL (based on an LC/MS/MS assay method). If trough is <3 ng/mL, double total daily dose (using available tablet strengths); if trough >8 ng/mL on 2 consecutive measures, decrease dose by 0.25 mg twice daily. Administer in combination with basiliximab induction and concurrently with cyclosporine (dose adjustment required) and corticosteroids

Subependymal giant cell astrocytoma (SEGA; dosing based on body surface area [BSA]): Oral: **Note:** Continue until disease progression or unacceptable toxicity.

Initial dose: 4.5 mg/m^2 once daily; round to nearest tablet (tablet or tablet for oral suspension) size.

If trough <5 ng/mL: Increase dose by 2.5 mg daily (tablets) or 2 mg daily (tablets for oral suspension).

If trough >15 ng/mL: Reduce dose by 2.5 mg daily (tablets) or 2 mg daily (tablets for oral suspension). If dose reduction necessary in patients receiving the lowest strength available, administer every other day.

Therapeutic drug monitoring: Assess trough concentration ~2 weeks after initiation or with dosage modifications, initiation or changes to concurrent CYP3A4/P-glycoprotein (P-gp) inhibitor/inducer therapy, changes in hepatic impairment, or when changing dosage forms between tablets and tablets for oral suspension; adjust maintenance dose if needed at 2-week intervals to achieve and maintain trough concentrations between 5 and 15 ng/mL; once stable dose is attained and if BSA is stable throughout treatment, monitor trough concentrations every 6 to 12 months (monitor every 3 to 6 months if BSA is changing).

Carcinoid tumors, advanced (off-label use): Oral: 10 mg once daily (in combination with octreotide LAR) until disease progression or toxicity (Pavel, 2010)

Waldenström macroglobulinemia, relapsed or refractory (off-label use): Oral: 10 mg once daily until disease progression or toxicity (Ghobrial, 2010)

Dosage adjustment for concomitant CYP3A4 inhibitors/inducers and/or P-gp inhibitors:

Breast cancer, PNET, RCC, renal angiomyolipoma:

CYP3A4/P-gp inducers: Strong inducers: Avoid coadministration with strong CYP3A4/P-gp inducers (eg, carbamazepine, phenobarbital, phenytoin, rifabutin, rifampin, rifapentine, St John's wort); if concomitant use cannot be avoided, consider doubling the everolimus dose, using increments of 5 mg or less, with careful monitoring (Canadian labeling recommends a maximum daily dose of 20 mg in patients with renal angiomyolipoma). If the strong CYP3A4/P-gp enzyme inducer is discontinued, consider allowing 3 to 5 days to elapse prior to reducing the everolimus to the dose used prior to initiation of the CYP3A4/P-gp inducer.

CYP3A4/P-gp inhibitors:

Strong inhibitors: Avoid concomitant administration with strong CYP3A4/P-gp inhibitors (eg, atazanavir, clarithromycin, indinavir, itraconazole, ketoconazole, nefazodone, nelfinavir, ritonavir, saquinavir, telithromycin, voriconazole).

Moderate CYP3A4/P-gp inhibitors (eg, amprenavir, aprepitant, diltiazem, erythromycin, fluconazole, fosamprenavir, verapamil):

US labeling: Reduce everolimus dose to 2.5 mg once daily; may consider increasing from 2.5 mg to 5 mg once daily based on patient tolerance. When the moderate inhibitor is discontinued, allow ~2 to 3 days to elapse prior to adjusting the everolimus upward to the recommended starting dose or to the dose used prior to initiation of the moderate inhibitor.

Canadian labeling: Reduce everolimus dose by 50%; further reductions may be necessary for adverse reactions. If dose reduction is required for patients receiving the lowest available strength, consider alternate-day dosing. When the moderate inhibitor is discontinued, allow at least 3 days or 4 elimination half-lives to elapse prior to adjusting the everolimus to the dose used prior to initiation of the moderate inhibitor.

Renal transplantation: Dosage adjustments may be necessary based on everolimus serum concentrations

SEGA:

CYP3A4/P-gp inducers: Strong inducers:

US labeling: Avoid concomitant administration with strong CYP3A4/P-gp inducers (eg, carbamazepine, phenobarbital, phenytoin, rifabutin, rifampin, rifapentine, St John's wort); if concomitant use cannot be avoided, an initial starting everolimus dose of 9 mg/m^2 once daily is recommended, or, double the everolimus dose and assess tolerability; assess trough concentration after ~2 weeks; adjust dose as necessary based on therapeutic drug monitoring to maintain target trough concentrations of 5 to 15 ng/mL. If the strong CYP3A4 enzyme inducer is discontinued, reduce the everolimus dose by ~50% or to the dose used prior to initiation of the CYP3A4/P-gp inducer; reassess trough concentration after ~2 weeks.

Canadian labeling: Avoid concomitant administration with strong CYP3A4 inducers (eg, carbamazepine, oxcarbazepine, phenobarbital, phenytoin, rifampin, rifabutin, rifapentine, St John's wort); if concomitant use cannot be avoided and everolimus level <5 ng/mL, may increase daily dose by 2.5 mg every 2 weeks (tablets) or 2 mg every 2 weeks (tablets for oral suspension) until target everolimus trough concentration is 5 to 15 ng/mL. If the strong CYP3A4/P-gp inducer is discontinued, reduce everolimus to the dose used prior to initiation of the CYP3A4/P-gp inducer. Assess trough concentrations ~2 weeks after any change in dose or after any initiation or change in CYP3A4/P-gp inducer therapy.

CYP3A4/P-gp inhibitors:

Strong inhibitors: Avoid concomitant administration with strong CYP3A4/P-gp inhibitors (eg, atazanavir, clarithromycin, indinavir, itraconazole, ketoconazole, nefazodone, nelfinavir, ritonavir, saquinavir, telithromycin, voriconazole).

Moderate CYP3A4/P-gp inhibitors (eg, amprenavir, aprepitant, diltiazem, erythromycin, fluconazole, fosamprenavir, verapamil):

US labeling:

Currently taking a moderate CYP3A4/P-gp inhibitor and starting everolimus: 2.5 mg/m^2 once daily.

Currently taking everolimus and starting a moderate CYP3A4/P-gp inhibitor: Reduce everolimus dose by ~50%; if dose reduction is required for patients receiving the lowest strength available, administer every other day.

Discontinuing a moderate CYP3A4/P-gp inhibitor after concomitant use with everolimus: Discontinue moderate inhibitor and allow 2 to 3 days to elapse prior to resuming the everolimus dose used prior to initiation of the moderate inhibitor.

Therapeutic drug monitoring: Assess trough concentration ~2 weeks after everolimus initiation or dosage modifications, or initiation or changes to concurrent CYP3A4/P-gp inhibitor therapy; adjust maintenance dose if needed at 2-week intervals to achieve and maintain trough concentrations between 5 and 15 ng/mL.

Canadian labeling: Reduce everolimus dose by ~50% (if dose reduction is required for patients receiving the lowest strength available, consider alternate-day dosing). If the moderate inhibitor is discontinued, the everolimus dose should be returned to the dose used prior to initiation of the inhibitor.

Therapeutic drug monitoring: Assess trough concentration ~2 weeks after everolimus initiation or dosage modifications, or initiation or changes to concurrent CYP3A4/P-gp inhibitor therapy. Maintain trough concentrations between 5 and 15 ng/mL; may increase dose within the target range to achieve higher concentrations as tolerated.

Pediatric Note: Tablets (Afinitor, Zortress) and tablets for oral suspension (Afinitor Disperz) are not interchangeable. Do not combine formulations to achieve total desired dose.

Subependymal giant cell astrocytoma (SEGA): Children ≥1 year: Refer to adult dosing.

Renal Impairment No dosage adjustment is necessary.

Hepatic Impairment

Mild impairment (Child-Pugh class A):

Breast cancer, PNET, RCC, renal angiomyolipoma: Reduce dose to 7.5 mg once daily; if not tolerated, may further reduce to 5 mg once daily.

Liver or renal transplantation: Reduce initial dose by ~33%; individualize subsequent dosing based on therapeutic drug monitoring (target trough concentration: 3 to 8 ng/mL).

SEGA:

U.S. labeling: Adjustment to initial dose may not be necessary; subsequent dosing is based on therapeutic drug monitoring (monitor ~2 weeks after initiation, dosage modifications, or after any change in hepatic status; target trough concentration: 5 to 15 ng/mL).

Canadian labeling: Initial:

Patients ≥18 years of age: 75% of usual dose based on calculated BSA (rounded to the nearest strength). Assess trough concentrations ~2 weeks after initiation, dosage modifications, or after any change in hepatic status. Target trough concentration: 5 to 15 ng/mL; may increase dose within the target range to achieve higher concentrations as tolerated.

Patients <18 years of age: Use is not recommended.

Moderate impairment (Child-Pugh class B):

Breast cancer, PNET, RCC, renal angiomyolipoma: Reduce dose to 5 mg once daily; if not tolerated, may further reduce to 2.5 mg once daily.

Liver or renal transplantation: Reduce initial dose by ~50%; individualize subsequent dosing based on therapeutic drug monitoring (target trough concentration: 3 to 8 ng/mL).

SEGA:

US labeling: Adjustment to initial dose may not be necessary; subsequent dosing is based on therapeutic drug monitoring (monitor ~2 weeks after initiation, dosage modifications, or after any change in hepatic status; target trough concentration: 5 to 15 ng/mL).

Canadian labeling: Initial:

Patients ≥18 years of age: 50% of usual dose based on calculated BSA (rounded to the nearest strength). Assess trough concentrations ~2 weeks after initiation, dosage modifications, or after any change in hepatic status. Target trough concentration: 5 to 15 ng/mL; may increase dose within the target range to achieve higher concentrations as tolerated.

Patients <18 years of age: Use is not recommended.

Severe impairment (Child-Pugh class C):

Breast cancer, PNET, RCC, renal angiomyolipoma: If potential benefit outweighs risks, a maximum dose of 2.5 mg once daily may be used.

Liver or renal transplantation: Reduce initial dose by ~50%; individualize subsequent dosing based on therapeutic drug monitoring (target trough concentration: 3 to 8 ng/mL).

SEGA:

US labeling: Reduce initial dose to 2.5 mg/m² once daily (or current dose by ~50%); subsequent dosing is based on therapeutic drug monitoring (monitor ~2 weeks after initiation, dosage modifications, or after any change in hepatic status; target trough concentration: 5 to 15 ng/mL).

Canadian labeling: Use is not recommended.

Adjustment for Toxicity

Breast cancer (adjustments apply to everolimus), PNET, RCC, renal angiomyolipoma, SEGA: Toxicities may require temporary dose interruption (with or without a subsequent dose reduction) or discontinuation; reduce everolimus dose by ~50% if dosage adjustment is necessary:

Noninfectious pneumonitis:

Grade 1 (asymptomatic radiological changes suggestive of pneumonitis): No dosage adjustment is necessary; monitor appropriately.

Grade 2 (symptomatic but not interfering with activities of daily living [ADL]): Consider interrupting treatment, rule out infection, and consider corticosteroids until symptoms improve to ≤ grade 1; reinitiate at a lower dose. Discontinue if recovery does not occur within 4 weeks.

Grade 3 (symptomatic, interferes with ADL; oxygen indicated): Interrupt treatment until symptoms improve to ≤ grade 1; rule out infection and consider corticosteroid treatment; may reinitiate at a lower dose. If grade 3 toxicity recurs, consider discontinuing.

Grade 4 (life-threatening; ventilatory support indicated): Discontinue treatment; rule out infection; consider corticosteroid treatment.

Stomatitis (avoid the use of products containing alcohol, hydrogen peroxide, iodine, or thyme derivatives):

Grade 1 (minimal symptoms, normal diet): No dosage adjustment is necessary; manage with mouth wash (nonalcoholic or isotonic salt water) several times a day

Grade 2 (symptomatic but can eat and swallow modified diet): Interrupt treatment until symptoms improve to ≤ grade 1; reinitiate at same dose; if stomatitis recurs at grade 2, interrupt treatment until symptoms improve to ≤ grade 1 and then reinitiate at a lower dose. Also manage with topical (oral) analgesics (eg, benzocaine, butyl aminobenzoate, tetracaine, menthol, or phenol) ± topical (oral) corticosteroids (eg, triamcinolone).

Grade 3 (symptomatic and unable to orally aliment or hydrate adequately): Interrupt treatment until symptoms improve to ≤ grade 1; then reinitiate at a lower dose. Also manage with topical (oral) analgesics (eg, benzocaine, butyl aminobenzoate, tetracaine, menthol, or phenol) ± topical (oral) corticosteroids (eg, triamcinolone).

Grade 4 (life-threatening symptoms): Discontinue treatment; initiate appropriate medical intervention.

Metabolic toxicity (eg, hyperglycemia, dyslipidemia):

Grade 1: No dosage adjustment is necessary; initiate appropriate medical intervention and monitor.

Grade 2: No dosage adjustment is necessary; manage with appropriate medical intervention and monitor.

Grade 3: Temporarily interrupt treatment; reinitiate at a lower dose; manage with appropriate medical intervention and monitor.

Grade 4: Discontinue treatment; manage with appropriate medical intervention.

Nonhematologic toxicities (excluding pneumonitis, stomatitis, or metabolic toxicity):

Grade 1: If toxicity is tolerable, no dosage adjustment is necessary; initiate appropriate medical intervention and monitor.

Grade 2: If toxicity is tolerable, no dosage adjustment is necessary; initiate appropriate medical intervention and monitor. If toxicity becomes intolerable, temporarily interrupt treatment until improvement to ≤ grade 1 and reinitiate at the same dose; if toxicity recurs at grade 2, temporarily interrupt treatment until improvement to ≤ grade 1 and then reinitiate at a lower dose.

Grade 3: Temporarily interrupt treatment until improvement to ≤ grade 1; initiate appropriate medical intervention and monitor. May reinitiate at a lower dose; if toxicity recurs at grade 3, consider discontinuing.

Grade 4 (life-threatening symptoms): Discontinue treatment; initiate appropriate medical intervention.

Liver or renal transplantation:

Evidence of polyoma virus infection or PML: Consider reduced immunosuppression (taking into account the allograft risks associated with decreased immunosuppression)

Pneumonitis (grade 4 symptoms) or invasive systemic fungal infection: Discontinue

SEGA: Severe/intolerable adverse reactions: Temporarily interrupt or permanently discontinue treatment; if dose reduction is required upon reinitiation, reduce dose by ~50%; if dose reduction is required for patients receiving the lowest available strength, consider alternate-day dosing.

Dietary Considerations Avoid grapefruit juice.

Administration May be taken with or without food; to reduce variability, take consistently with regard to food. Afinitor missed doses may be taken up to 6 hours after regularly scheduled time; if >6 hours, resume at next regularly scheduled time.

Tablets: Swallow whole with a glass of water. Do not break, chew, or crush (do not administer tablets that are crushed or broken). Avoid contact with or exposure to crushed or broken tablets.

Tablets for oral suspension: Administer as a suspension only. Administer immediately after preparation; discard if not administered within 60 minutes after preparation. Prepare suspension in water only. Do not break or crush tablets.

Preparation in an oral syringe: Place dose into 10 mL oral syringe (maximum: 10 mg/syringe; use an additional syringe for doses >10 mg). Draw ~5 mL of water and ~4 mL of air into oral syringe; allow to sit (tip up) in a container until tablets are in suspension (3 minutes). Gently invert syringe 5 times immediately prior to administration; administer contents, then add ~5 mL water and ~4 mL of air to same syringe, swirl to suspend remaining particles and administer entire contents.

Preparation in a small glass: Place dose into a small glass (≤100 mL) containing ~25 mL water (maximum: 10 mg/glass; use and additional glass for doses >10 mg); allow to sit until tablets are in suspension (3 minutes). Stir gently with spoon immediately prior to administration; administer contents, then add ~25 mL water to same glass, swirl with same spoon to suspend remaining particles and administer entire contents.

Breast cancer, pancreatic neuroendocrine tumors, renal cell cancer, renal angiolipoma, SEGA: Administer at the same time each day.

Liver transplantation: Administer consistently ~12 hours apart; administer at the same time as tacrolimus.

Renal transplantation: Administer consistently ~12 hours apart; administer at the same time as cyclosporine.

Hazardous agent; use appropriate precautions for handling and disposal (NIOSH 2014 [group 1]). To avoid potential contact with everolimus, caregivers should wear gloves when preparing suspension from tablets for oral suspension. NIOSH recommends single gloving for administration of intact tablets (NIOSH 2014). Avoid exposure to crushed tablets. When it is necessary to manipulate the tablets (eg, to prepare an oral liquid or suspension), it is recommended to double glove, wear a protective gown, and prepare in a controlled device (NIOSH 2014).

Monitoring Parameters CBC with differential (baseline and periodic), liver function; serum creatinine, urinary protein, and BUN (baseline and periodic); fasting serum glucose and lipid profile (baseline and periodic); monitor for signs and symptoms of infection, noninfectious pneumonitis, or malignancy

For liver or renal transplantation, monitor everolimus whole blood trough concentrations (based on an LC/MS/MS assay method), especially in patients with hepatic impairment, with concomitant CYP3A4 inhibitors and inducers, and when cyclosporine formulations or doses are changed; dosage adjustments should be made on trough concentrations obtained 4 to 5 days after a previous dosage adjustment; monitor cyclosporine concentrations; monitor for proteinuria

For SEGA, monitor everolimus whole blood trough concentrations ~2 weeks after treatment initiation or with dosage modifications, initiation or changes to concurrent CYP3A4/P-glycoprotein (P-gp) inhibitor/inducer therapy, changes in hepatic function and when changing dosage forms between Afinitor tablets and Afinitor Disperz. Maintain trough concentrations between 5 and 15 ng/mL; once stable dose is attained and if BSA is stable throughout treatment, monitor trough concentrations every 6 to 12 months (monitor every 3 to 6 months if BSA is changing).

Reference Range Recommended range for everolimus whole blood trough concentrations:

Liver and renal transplantation: 3-8 ng/mL (based on an LCMSMS assay method)

Subependymal giant cell astrocytoma (SEGA): 5-15 ng/mL (high concentrations may be associated with larger reductions in SEGA volumes, responses have been observed at concentrations as low as 5 ng/mL)

Dosage Forms Excipient information presented when available (limited, particularly for generics); consult specific product labeling.

Tablet, Oral:

Afinitor: 2.5 mg, 5 mg, 7.5 mg, 10 mg

Zortress: 0.25 mg, 0.5 mg, 0.75 mg

Tablet Soluble, Oral:

Afinitor Disperz: 2 mg, 3 mg, 5 mg

Extemporaneous Preparations Hazardous agent: Use appropriate precautions for handling and disposal (NIOSH 2014 [group 1]). When compounding an oral liquid or suspension, NIOSH recommends double gloving, a protective gown, and preparation in a controlled device; if not prepared in a controlled device, respiratory and eye protection as well as ventilated engineering controls are recommended (NIOSH 2014).

Tablets: An oral liquid may be prepared using tablets. Disperse tablet in ~30 mL (1 oz) of water; gently stir. Administer and rinse container with additional 30 mL (1 oz) water and administer to ensure entire dose is administered. Administer immediately after preparation.

Afinitor (everolimus) [prescribing information]. East Hanover, NJ: Novartis Pharmaceuticals Corporation; July 2012.

Tablets for oral suspension: Administer as a suspension only. Administer immediately after preparation; discard if not administered within 60 minutes after preparation. Prepare suspension in water only. Do not break or crush tablets.

Preparation in an oral syringe: Place dose into 10 mL oral syringe (maximum: 10 mg/syringe; use an additional syringe for doses >10 mg). Draw ~5 mL of water and ~4 mL of air into oral syringe; allow to sit (tip up) in a container until tablets are in suspension (3 minutes). Gently invert syringe 5 times immediately prior to administration; administer contents, then add ~5 mL water and ~4 mL of air to same syringe, swirl to suspend remaining particles and administer entire contents.

Preparation in a small glass: Place dose into a small glass (≤100 mL) containing ~25 mL water (maximum 10 mg/glass; use an additional glass for doses >10 mg); allow to sit until tablets are in suspension (3 minutes). Stir gently with spoon immediately prior to administration; administer contents, then add ~25 mL water to same glass, swirl with same spoon to suspend remaining particles and administer entire contents.

Administer immediately after preparation; discard if not administered within 60 minutes after preparation.

Afinitor and Afinitor Disperz (everolimus) [prescribing information]. East Hanover, NJ: Novartis Pharmaceuticals Corporation; August 2012.

◆ EVG/COBI/FTC/TDF *see* Elvitegravir, Cobicistat, Emtricitabine, and Tenofovir Disoproxil Fumarate *on page 632*

◆ Evista *see* Raloxifene *on page 1548*

◆ Evoclin *see* Clindamycin (Topical) *on page 409*

Evolocumab (e voe LOK ue mab)

Brand Names: US Repatha; Repatha SureClick
Brand Names: Canada Repatha
Index Terms AMG145
Pharmacologic Category Antilipemic Agent, PCSK9 Inhibitor; Monoclonal Antibody
Use

Hyperlipidemia, primary: Adjunct to diet and maximally tolerated statin therapy for the treatment of adults with heterozygous familial hypercholesterolemia (HeFH) or clinical atherosclerotic cardiovascular disease (CVD), who require additional lowering of low density lipoprotein cholesterol (LDL-C).

Homozygous familial hypercholesterolemia: Adjunct to diet and other LDL-lowering therapies (eg, statins, ezetimibe, LDL apheresis) for the treatment of patients with homozygous familial hypercholesterolemia (HoFH) who require additional lowering of LDL-C.

Limitation of use: The effect of evolocumab on cardiovascular morbidity and mortality has not been determined.

Dosing
Adult & Geriatric

Hyperlipidemia, primary: SubQ: 140 mg every 2 weeks or 420 mg once monthly

Switching regimens: Administer the first dose of the new regimen on the next scheduled day of the prior regimen.

Homozygous familial hypercholesterolemia: SubQ:

US labeling: 420 mg once monthly

Canadian labeling: Initial: 420 mg once monthly; if clinical response is not achieved after 12 weeks of treatment, dose frequency may be titrated up to 420 mg once every 2 weeks. Patients on apheresis

may initiate treatment with 420 mg every 2 weeks to correspond with their apheresis schedule.

Missed doses: Administer as soon as possible if there are more than 7 days until next scheduled dose, or omit the missed dose and administer next dose according to the original schedule.

Pediatric

Homozygous familial hypercholesterolemia:

US labeling: Adolescents 13 to 17 years: SubQ: Refer to adult dosing

Canadian labeling: Children ≥12 years and Adolescents: SubQ: Refer to adult dosing.

Missed doses: Administer as soon as possible if there are more than 7 days until next scheduled dose, or omit the missed dose and administer next dose according to the original schedule.

Renal Impairment

Mild to moderate impairment: No dosage adjustment necessary.

Severe impairment (estimated GFR <30 mL/minute/1.73 m²):

US labeling: There are no dosage adjustments provided in the manufacturer's labeling (has not been studied); however, dosage adjustment is unlikely to be required as monoclonal antibodies are not known to be renally eliminated.

Canadian labeling: There are no dosage adjustments provided in the manufacturer's labeling (has not been studied); use is not recommended.

Hepatic Impairment

Mild to moderate impairment (Child Pugh class A and B): No dosage adjustment necessary.

Severe impairment (Child Pugh class C): There are no dosage adjustments provided in the manufacturer's labeling (has not been studied).

Additional Information Complete prescribing information should be consulted for additional detail.

Dosage Forms Excipient information presented when available (limited, particularly for generics); consult specific product labeling.

Solution Auto-injector, Subcutaneous [preservative free]:

Repatha SureClick: 140 mg/mL (1 mL) [contains mouse protein (murine) (hamster), polysorbate 80]

Solution Prefilled Syringe, Subcutaneous [preservative free]:

Repatha: 140 mg/mL (1 mL) [contains mouse protein (murine) (hamster), polysorbate 80]

Exemestane (ex e MES tane)

Brand Names: US Aromasin

Brand Names: Canada Aromasin; CO Exemestane

Pharmacologic Category Antineoplastic Agent, Aromatase Inhibitor

Use Breast cancer: Treatment of advanced breast cancer in postmenopausal women whose disease has progressed following tamoxifen therapy; adjuvant treatment of postmenopausal women with estrogen receptor-positive early breast cancer following 2-3 years of tamoxifen (for a total of 5 consecutive years of adjuvant therapy).

Pregnancy Considerations Adverse events were observed in animal reproduction studies. Exemestane is not indicated for use in premenopausal women and use during pregnancy is contraindicated. Based on the mechanism of action, exemestane is expected to cause fetal harm if administered to a pregnant woman.

Breast-Feeding Considerations Exemestane is indicated for use only in postmenopausal women. Due to the potential for serious adverse reactions in the nursing infant, the manufacturer recommends a decision be made whether to discontinue nursing or to discontinue the drug, taking into account the importance of treatment to the mother.

Contraindications Known hypersensitivity to exemestane or any component of the formulation; women who are or may become pregnant; premenopausal women

Warnings/Precautions Hazardous agent - use appropriate precautions for handling and disposal (NIOSH 2014 [group 1]). Due to decreased circulating estrogen levels, exemestane is associated with a reduction in bone mineral density over time; decreases (from baseline) in lumbar spine and femoral neck density have been observed; assess bone mineral density at baseline in patients with, or at risk for osteoporosis; monitor exemestane therapy and initiate osteoporosis treatment if indicated. Due to high prevalence of vitamin D deficiency in women with breast cancer, assess 25-hydroxy vitamin D levels at baseline and supplement accordingly. Grade 3 or 4 lymphopenia has been observed with exemestane, although most patients had preexisting lower grade lymphopenia; some patients improved or recovered while continuing exemestane; lymphopenia did not result in a significant increase in viral infections, and no opportunistic infections were observed. Elevations of AST, ALT, alkaline phosphatase, and gamma glutamyl transferase >5 times ULN have been observed (rarely) in patients with advanced breast cancer; may be attributable to underlying liver and/or bone metastases. In patients with early breast cancer, elevations of bilirubin, alkaline phosphatase, and serum creatinine were more common with exemestane treatment than with tamoxifen or placebo. Potentially significant drug-drug interactions may exist, requiring dose or frequency adjustment, additional monitoring, and/or selection of alternative therapy. Not to be given with estrogen-containing agents. Dose adjustment recommended with concomitant strong CYP3A4 inducers.

Adverse Reactions

>10%:

Cardiovascular: Hypertension (5% to 15%)

Central nervous system: Fatigue (8% to 22%), insomnia (11% to 14%), pain (13%), headache (7% to 13%), depression (6% to 13%)

Dermatological: Hyperhidrosis (4% to 18%), alopecia (15%)

Endocrine & metabolic: Hot flashes (13% to 33%)

Gastrointestinal: Nausea (9% to 18%), abdominal pain (6% to 11%)

Hepatic: Alkaline phosphatase increased (14% to 15%)

Neuromuscular & skeletal: Arthralgia (15% to 29%)

1% to 10%:

Cardiovascular: Edema (6% to 7%); cardiac ischemic events (2%: MI, angina, myocardial ischemia); chest pain

Central nervous system: Dizziness (8% to 10%), anxiety (4% to 10%), fever (5%), confusion, hypoesthesia

Dermatological: Dermatitis (8%), itching, rash

Endocrine & metabolic: Weight gain (8%)

Gastrointestinal: Diarrhea (4% to 10%), vomiting (7%), anorexia (6%), constipation (5%), appetite increased (3%), dyspepsia

Genitourinary: Urinary tract infection (2% to 5%)

Hepatic: Bilirubin increased (5% to 7%)

Neuromuscular & skeletal: Back pain (9%), limb pain (9%), myalgia (6%), osteoarthritis (6%), weakness (6%), osteoporosis (5%), pathological fracture (4%), paresthesia (3%), carpal tunnel syndrome (2%), cramps (2%)

Ocular: Visual disturbances (5%)

Renal: Creatinine increased (6%)

Respiratory: Dyspnea (10%), cough (6%), bronchitis, pharyngitis, rhinitis, sinusitis, upper respiratory infection

Miscellaneous: Flu-like syndrome (6%), lymphedema, infection

<1% (Limited to important or life-threatening): Acute generalized exanthematous pustulosis, cardiac failure, cholestatic hepatitis, endometrial hyperplasia, gastric ulcer, GGT increased, hepatitis, hypersensitivity, neuropathy, osteochondrosis, pruritus, thromboembolism, transaminases increased, trigger finger, urticaria, uterine polyps

A dose-dependent decrease in sex hormone-binding globulin has been observed with daily doses of ≥2.5 mg. Serum luteinizing hormone and follicle-stimulating hormone levels have increased with this medicine.

Drug Interactions

Metabolism/Transport Effects Substrate of CYP3A4 (major); **Note:** Assignment of Major/Minor substrate status based on clinically relevant drug interaction potential

Avoid Concomitant Use

Avoid concomitant use of Exemestane with any of the following: Estrogen Derivatives

Increased Effect/Toxicity

Exemestane may increase the levels/effects of: Methadone

The levels/effects of Exemestane may be increased by: Osimertinib

Decreased Effect

The levels/effects of Exemestane may be decreased by: Bosentan; CYP3A4 Inducers (Moderate); CYP3A4 Inducers (Strong); Dabrafenib; Deferasirox; Enzalutamide; Estrogen Derivatives; Mitotane; Osimertinib; Siltuximab; St Johns Wort; Tocilizumab

Food Interactions Plasma levels increased by 40% when exemestane was taken with a fatty meal. Management: Administer after a meal.

Storage/Stability Store at 25°C (77°F); excursions permitted to 15°C to 30°C (59°F to 86°F).

Mechanism of Action Exemestane is an irreversible, steroidal aromatase inactivator. It is structurally related to androstenedione, and is converted to an intermediate that irreversibly blocks the active site of the aromatase enzyme, leading to inactivation ("suicide inhibition") and thus preventing conversion of androgens to estrogens in peripheral tissues. Significantly lowers circulating estrogens in postmenopausal breast cancers where growth is estrogen-dependent.

Pharmacodynamics/Kinetics

Absorption: Rapid and moderate (~42%) following oral administration; AUC and C_{max} increased by 59% and 39%, respectively, following a high-fat breakfast (compared to fasted state)

Distribution: Extensive into tissues

Protein binding: 90%, primarily to albumin and α_1-acid glycoprotein

Metabolism: Extensively hepatic; oxidation (CYP3A4) of methylene group, reduction of 17-keto group with formation of many secondary metabolites; metabolites are inactive

Half-life elimination: ~24 hours

Time to peak: Women with breast cancer: 1.2 hours

Excretion: Urine (<1% as unchanged drug, 39% to 45% as metabolites); feces (36% to 48%)

Dosing

Adult & Geriatric

Breast cancer, advanced: Postmenopausal females: Oral: 25 mg once daily; continue until tumor progression

Breast cancer, early (adjuvant treatment): Postmenopausal females: Oral: 25 mg once daily (following 2 to 3 years of tamoxifen therapy) for a total duration of 5 years of endocrine therapy (in the absence of recurrence or contralateral breast cancer). **Note:** The American Society of Clinical Oncology (ASCO) guidelines for Adjuvant Endocrine Therapy of Hormone Receptor-Positive Breast Cancer (Focused Update) recommend a maximum duration of 5 years of aromatase inhibitor (AI) therapy for postmenopausal women; AIs may be combined with tamoxifen for a total duration of up to 10 years of endocrine therapy. Refer to the guidelines for specific recommendations based on menopausal status and tolerability (Burstein 2014).

Breast cancer, early (first-line adjuvant treatment; off-label use): Postmenopausal females: Oral: 25 mg once daily for 5 years (Burstein 2010; van de Velde 2011). **Note:** ASCO guidelines for Adjuvant Endocrine Therapy of Hormone Receptor-Positive Breast Cancer (Focused Update) recommend a maximum duration of 5 years of aromatase inhibitor (AI) therapy for postmenopausal women; AIs may be combined with tamoxifen for a total duration of up to 10 years of endocrine therapy. Refer to the guidelines for specific recommendations based on menopausal status and tolerability (Burstein 2014).

Breast cancer, risk reduction (off-label use): Postmenopausal females ≥35 years: Oral: 25 mg once daily for 5 years (Goss 2011; Visvanathan 2013)

Dosage adjustment with strong CYP3A4 inducers: U.S. labeling: 50 mg once daily when used with potent inducers (eg, rifampin, phenytoin)

Renal Impairment No adjustment necessary (although the safety of chronic doses in patients with moderate-to-severe renal impairment has not been studied, dosage adjustment does not appear necessary).

Hepatic Impairment No adjustment necessary (although the safety of chronic doses in patients with moderate-to-severe hepatic impairment has not been studied, dosage adjustment does not appear necessary).

Dietary Considerations Patients on aromatase inhibitor therapy should receive vitamin D and calcium supplements.

Administration Administer after a meal. Hazardous agent; use appropriate precautions for handling and disposal (NIOSH 2014 [group 1]).

Monitoring Parameters 25-hydroxy vitamin D levels (at baseline); bone mineral density

Dosage Forms Excipient information presented when available (limited, particularly for generics); consult specific product labeling.

Tablet, Oral:

Aromasin: 25 mg

Generic: 25 mg

Exenatide (ex EN a tide)

Brand Names: US Bydureon; Byetta 10 MCG Pen; Byetta 5 MCG Pen

Brand Names: Canada Byetta

Index Terms AC 2993; AC002993; Exendin-4; LY2148568

Pharmacologic Category Antidiabetic Agent, Glucagon-Like Peptide-1 (GLP-1) Receptor Agonist

Use

Type 2 diabetes mellitus: Treatment of type 2 diabetes mellitus (noninsulin dependent, NIDDM) to improve glycemic control as an adjunct to diet and exercise.

Limitations of use: Because of the uncertain relevance of the rat thyroid C-cell tumor findings to humans, prescribe exenatide ER only to patients for whom the potential benefits are considered to outweigh the potential risks. Exenatide ER is not recommended as first-line therapy for patients who have inadequate glycemic control on diet and exercise.

Pregnancy Considerations Adverse events were observed in some animal reproduction studies. Based on *in vitro* data, exenatide has a low potential to cross the placenta (Hiles 2003).

In women with diabetes, maternal hyperglycemia can be associated with congenital malformations as well as adverse effects in the fetus, neonate, and the mother (ACOG 2005; ADA 2015; Kitzmiller 2008; Metzger 2007). To prevent adverse outcomes, prior to conception and throughout pregnancy maternal blood glucose and HbA_{1c} should be kept as close to target goals as possible but without causing significant hypoglycemia (ACOG 2013; ADA 2015; Blumer 2013; Kitzmiller 2008). Prior to pregnancy, effective contraception should be used until glycemic control is achieved (Kitzmiller 2008). Other agents are currently recommended to treat diabetes in pregnant women (ACOG 2013; Blumer 2013).

Health care providers are encouraged to enroll women exposed to exenatide during pregnancy in the pregnancy registry (800-633-9081).

Breast-Feeding Considerations It is not known if exenatide is excreted in breast milk. According to the manufacturer, the decision to continue or discontinue breast-feeding during therapy should take into account the risk of exposure to the infant and the benefits of treatment to the mother; use caution if administering exenatide to nursing women.

Medication Guide Available Yes

Contraindications

History of or family history of medullary thyroid carcinoma (exenatide ER only); patients with multiple endocrine neoplasia syndrome type 2 (exenatide ER only); hypersensitivity to exenatide or any component of the formulation.

Byetta: Canadian labeling: Additional contraindications (not in U.S. labeling): End-stage renal disease (ESRD) or severe renal impairment (CrCl <30 mL/minute) including dialysis patients; diabetic ketoacidosis, diabetic coma/precoma or type 1 diabetes mellitus

Warnings/Precautions Bydureon: **[US Boxed Warning] Thyroid C-cell tumors have developed in animal studies with exenatide ER; it is not known if exenatide ER causes thyroid C-cell tumor, including medullary thyroid carcinoma (MTC) in humans. Patients should be counseled on the potential risk of MTC with the use of exenatide and informed of symptoms of thyroid tumors (eg, neck mass, dysphagia, dyspnea, persistent hoarseness). Use is contraindicated in patients with a personal or a family history of medullary thyroid cancer and in patients with multiple endocrine neoplasia syndrome type 2 (MEN2).** Consultation with an endocrinologist is recommended in patients who develop elevated calcitonin concentrations or have thyroid nodules detected during imaging studies or physical exam. Routine monitoring of serum calcitonin or using thyroid ultrasound for early detection of MTC is of unknown value.

Mechanism requires the presence of insulin, therefore use in type 1 diabetes (insulin dependent, IDDM) or diabetic ketoacidosis is not recommended (use is contraindicated in the Canadian labeling); it is not a substitute for insulin in insulin-requiring patients. Bydureon is not recommended for first-line therapy in patients inadequately controlled on diet and exercise alone.

Exenatide is frequently associated with gastrointestinal adverse effects and is not recommended for use in patients with gastroparesis or severe gastrointestinal disease. Gastrointestinal effects may be dose-related and may decrease in frequency/severity with gradual titration and continued use. Cases of acute pancreatitis (including hemorrhagic and necrotizing with some fatalities) have been reported; monitor for signs and symptoms of pancreatitis, (eg, persistent severe abdominal pain which may radiate to the back, and which may or may not be accompanied by vomiting). If pancreatitis is suspected, discontinue use. Do not resume unless an alternative etiology of pancreatitis is confirmed. Consider alternative antidiabetic therapy in patients with a history of pancreatitis. Use may be associated with the development of anti-exenatide antibodies. Low titers are not associated with a loss of efficacy; however, high titers (observed in 6% to 12% of patients in clinical studies) may result in an attenuation of response. May be associated with weight loss (due to reduced intake) independent of the change in hemoglobin A_{1c}. Serious hypersensitivity reactions (eg, anaphylaxis, angioedema) have been reported discontinue therapy in the event of a hypersensitivity reaction. Serious injection-site reactions (eg, abscess, cellulitis, and necrosis), with or without subcutaneous nodules have been reported with use. Isolated cases required surgical intervention. Potentially significant drug-drug interactions may exist, requiring dose or frequency adjustment, additional monitoring, and/or selection of alternative therapy.

Not recommended in severe renal impairment (CrCl <30 mL/minute) or end-stage renal disease (ESRD) (use in these patients and in dialysis patients is contraindicated in the Canadian labeling). Patients with ESRD receiving dialysis may be more susceptible to GI effects (eg, nausea, vomiting) which may result in hypovolemia and further reductions in renal function. Use with caution in patients with renal transplantation or in patients with moderate renal impairment (CrCl 30-50 mL/minute). Cases of acute renal failure and chronic renal failure exacerbation, including severe cases requiring hemodialysis, have been reported, predominately in patients with nausea/vomiting/diarrhea or dehydration; renal dysfunction was usually reversible with appropriate corrective measures, including discontinuation of exenatide. Risk may be increased in patients receiving concomitant medications affecting renal function and/or hydration status.

According to the Centers for Disease Control and Prevention (CDC), pen-shaped injection devices should never be used for more than one person (even when the needle is changed) because of the risk of infection. The injection device should be clearly labeled with individual patient information to ensure that the correct pen is used (CDC, 2012). Serious injection-site reactions (eg, abscess, cellulitis, necrosis), with or without subcutaneous nodules have been reported with Bydureon.

Adverse Reactions Note: Combination therapy may include a sulfonylurea, a thiazolidinedione, insulin glargine, or a combination of oral agents unless otherwise specified.
>10%:
  Central nervous system: Headache (8% to 14%)
  Endocrine & metabolic: Hypoglycemia (combination therapy with a sulfonylurea: Byetta: 14% to 36%, Bydureon 20%; combination therapy without a sulfonylurea ≤11%; monotherapy ≤5%; Bydureon with metformin 1% to 4%), severe hypoglycemia (Byetta combination therapy with metformin and a sulfonylurea <1%)
  Gastrointestinal: Nausea (dose-dependent and usually decreases over time; Byetta combination therapy 40% to 44%, Bydureon combination therapy 13% to 24%, monotherapy 8% to 11%), diarrhea (combination therapy 6% to 20%, Bydureon monotherapy 11%, Byetta monotherapy 1% to <2%), vomiting (combination therapy 11% to 18%, Byetta monotherapy 4%)
  Local: Injection site nodule (Bydureon 6% to 77%), injection site reaction (13% to 17%)
1% to 10%:
  Central nervous system: Jitteriness (Byetta combination therapy 9%), dizziness (Byetta combination therapy 9%, Byetta monotherapy 1% to <2%), fatigue (Bydureon combination therapy 6%)
  Dermatologic: Hyperhidrosis (Byetta combination therapy 3%)

  Gastrointestinal: Constipation (6% to 10%), viral gastroenteritis (6% to 9%), dyspepsia (3% to 7%), decreased appetite (1% to 5%), abdominal distension (Byetta combination therapy 4%), gastroesophageal reflux disease (Byetta combination therapy 2% to 3%), flatulence (Byetta 2%)
  Immunologic: Antibody development to exenatide (2% to 6%, associated with attenuated glycemic response)
  Local: Itching at injection site (Byetta ≥5%)
  Neuromuscular & skeletal: Weakness (Byetta combination therapy 4% to 5%)
<1% (Limited to important or life-threatening): Abscess at injection site (Bydureon), acute pancreatitis (Byetta), acute renal failure (Byetta), alopecia (Byetta), anaphylaxis (Byetta), angioedema (Byetta), cellulitis at injection site (Bydureon), chest pain (Byetta combination therapy), drowsiness (Byetta), exacerbation of renal failure (Byetta), hemorrhagic pancreatitis (Byetta), hypersensitivity pneumonitis (chronic; Byetta combination therapy), influenza, kidney transplant dysfunction (Byetta), necrotizing pancreatitis (Byetta, sometimes resulting in death), pain (stomach, side, or abdominal pain possibly radiating to the back), renal insufficiency (Byetta), severe diarrhea (Byetta), severe nausea (Byetta), severe vomiting (Byetta), tissue necrosis at injection site (Bydureon), upper respiratory tract infection, urticaria (Byetta)

Drug Interactions
Metabolism/Transport Effects None known.
Avoid Concomitant Use There are no known interactions where it is recommended to avoid concomitant use.
Increased Effect/Toxicity
Exenatide may increase the levels/effects of: Hypoglycemia-Associated Agents; Insulin; Sulfonylureas; Vitamin K Antagonists

The levels/effects of Exenatide may be increased by: Alpha-Lipoic Acid; Androgens; MAO Inhibitors; Pegvisomant; Quinolone Antibiotics; Salicylates; Selective Serotonin Reuptake Inhibitors
Decreased Effect
Exenatide may decrease the levels/effects of: Contraceptives (Estrogens); Oral Contraceptive (Progestins)

The levels/effects of Exenatide may be decreased by: Hyperglycemia-Associated Agents; Quinolone Antibiotics; Thiazide Diuretics
Preparation for Administration Bydureon: Reconstitute vial using provided diluent; use immediately.
Storage/Stability
Bydureon: Store under refrigeration at 2°C to 8°C (36°F to 46°F); vials may be stored at ≤25°C (≤77°F) for up to 4 weeks. Do not freeze (discard if freezing occurs). Protect from light.
Byetta: Prior to initial use, store under refrigeration at 2°C to 8°C (36°F to 46°F); after initial use, may store at ≤25°C (≤77°F). Do not freeze (discard if freezing occurs). Protect from light. Pen should be discarded 30 days after initial use.
Mechanism of Action Exenatide is an analog of the hormone incretin (glucagon-like peptide 1 or GLP-1) which increases glucose-dependent insulin secretion, decreases inappropriate glucagon secretion, increases B-cell growth/replication, slows gastric emptying, and decreases food intake. Exenatide administration results in decreases in hemoglobin A_{1c} by approximately 0.5% to 1% (immediate release) or 1.5% to 1.9% (extended release).
Pharmacodynamics/Kinetics
Distribution: V_d: 28.3 L
Metabolism: Minimal systemic metabolism; proteolytic degradation may occur following glomerular filtration
Half-life elimination:
  Immediate release (daily) formulation: 2.4 hours
  Extended release (weekly) formulation: ~2 weeks
Time to peak, plasma: SubQ:
  Immediate release (daily) formulation: 2.1 hours
  Extended release (weekly) formulation: Triphasic: Phase 1: 2-5 hours; Phase 2: ~2 weeks; Phase 3: ~7 weeks
Excretion: Urine (majority of dose)
Dosing
Adult & Geriatric Type 2 diabetes: SubQ:
  Immediate release: Initial: 5 mcg twice daily within 60 minutes prior to a meal; after 1 month, may be increased to 10 mcg twice daily (based on response)
  Extended release: 2 mg once weekly
  Note: May administer a missed dose as soon as noticed if the next regularly scheduled dose is due in ≥3 days; resume normal schedule thereafter. To establish a new day of the week administration schedule, wait ≥3 days after last dose given, then administer next dose on new desired day of the week.

Conversion from immediate release to extended release: Initiate weekly administration of exenatide extended release the day after discontinuing exenatide immediate release. **Note:** May experience increased blood glucose levels for ~2 weeks after conversion. Pretreatment with immediate release exenatide is not required when initiating extended release exenatide.

Renal Impairment

Mild impairment (CrCl ≥50 mL/minute): No dosage adjustment necessary

Moderate impairment (CrCl 30-50 mL/minute): There are no dosage adjustments provided in manufacturer's labeling; use caution.

Severe impairment (CrCl <30 mL/minute) or end-stage renal disease (ESRD):

U.S. labeling: Use is not recommended

Canadian labeling: Use is contraindicated.

Renal transplantation: Use with caution

Hepatic Impairment There are no dosage adjustments provided in manufacturer's labeling (has not been studied); however, hepatic dysfunction is not expected to affect exenatide pharmacokinetics.

Administration SubQ:

Immediate release: Use only if clear, colorless, and free of particulate matter. Administer via injection in the upper arm, thigh, or abdomen. Administer within 60 minutes prior to morning and evening meal (or prior to the 2 main meals of the day, approximately ≥6 hours apart). Set up each new pen before the first use by priming it. See pen user manual for further details. Dial the dose into the dose window before each administration.

Extended release: Administer subcutaneously in the upper arm, thigh, or abdomen; rotate injection sites weekly. Administer immediately after reconstitution in diluent, the mixture should be white to off-white and cloudy. Do not substitute needles or any other components provided with the single-dose tray. May administer without regard to meals or time of day.

Monitoring Parameters Serum glucose, hemoglobin A_{1c}, renal function, signs/symptoms of pancreatitis

Reference Range

Recommendations for glycemic control in nonpregnant adults with diabetes (ADA, 2015):

HbA_{1c}: <7% (a more aggressive [<6.5%] or less aggressive [<8%] HbA_{1c} goal may be targeted based on patient-specific characteristics)

Preprandial capillary plasma glucose: 80 to 130 mg/dL

Peak postprandial capillary blood glucose: <180 mg/dL

Recommendations for glycemic control in pediatric (all age groups) patients with type 1 diabetes (ADA, 2015):

HbA_{1c}: <7.5% (individualization may be appropriate based on patient-specific characteristics; <7% is reasonable if it can be achieved without excessive hypoglycemia)

Preprandial capillary plasma glucose: 90 to 130 mg/dL

Bedtime and overnight capillary blood glucose: 90 to 150 mg/dL

Additional Information A dosing strategy which employs progressive dose escalation of exenatide (initiating at 0.02 mcg/kg 3 times daily and increasing in increments of 0.02 mcg/kg every 3 days) has been described, limiting the frequency and severity of gastrointestinal adverse effects. The complexity of this regimen may limit its clinical application.

In animal models, exenatide has been a useful adjunctive therapy when added to immunotherapy protocols, resulting in recovery of beta cell function and sustained remission.

Dosage Forms Considerations

Bydureon: extended release formulation

Byetta: immediate release formulation

Dosage Forms Excipient information presented when available (limited, particularly for generics); consult specific product labeling.

Pen-injector, Subcutaneous:

Bydureon: 2 mg (1 ea)

Solution Pen-injector, Subcutaneous:

Byetta 10 MCG Pen: 10 mcg/0.04 mL (2.4 mL) [contains metacresol]

Byetta 5 MCG Pen: 5 mcg/0.02 mL (1.2 mL) [contains metacresol]

Suspension Reconstituted, Subcutaneous:

Bydureon: 2 mg (1 ea)

◆ Exendin-4 *see* Exenatide *on page 727*

◆ Exforge® *see* Amlodipine and Valsartan *on page 105*

◆ Exforge HCT® *see* Amlodipine, Valsartan, and Hydrochlorothiazide *on page 105*

◆ Exjade *see* Deferasirox *on page 509*

◆ Ex-Lax Ultra [OTC] *see* Bisacodyl *on page 231*

◆ Exparel *see* Bupivacaine (Liposomal) *on page 263*

◆ Exparel *see* Bupivacaine (Liposomal) *on page 263*

◆ Expecta LIPIL [OTC] [DSC] *see* Omega-3 Fatty Acids *on page 1329*

◆ Extavia *see* Interferon Beta-1b *on page 972*

◆ Extended Release Epidural Morphine *see* Morphine (Liposomal) *on page 1236*

◆ Extina *see* Ketoconazole (Topical) *on page 1014*

◆ Extraneal *see* Icodextrin *on page 910*

◆ Extra Strength Allergy Relief [OTC] (Can) *see* Cetirizine *on page 364*

◆ Exuviance Lightening Complex [OTC] *see* Hydroquinone *on page 893*

◆ EYE001 *see* Pegaptanib *on page 1407*

◆ EyeFlur *see* Fluorescein and Benoxinate *on page 782*

◆ Eye-Sed [OTC] *see* Zinc Sulfate *on page 1929*

◆ Eylea *see* Aflibercept (Ophthalmic) *on page 52*

◆ EZ Char [OTC] *see* Charcoal, Activated *on page 368*

Ezetimibe (ez ET i mibe)

Brand Names: US Zetia

Brand Names: Canada ACH-Ezetimibe; ACT Ezetimibe; Apo-Ezetimibe; Bio-Ezetimibe; Ezetrol; JAMP-Ezetimibe; Mar-Ezetimibe; Mint-Ezetimibe; Mylan-Ezetimibe; PMS-Ezetimibe; Priva-Ezetimibe; RAN-Ezetimibe; Riva-Ezetimibe; Sandoz Ezetimibe; Teva-Ezetimibe

Pharmacologic Category Antilipemic Agent, 2-Azetidinone

Use

Homozygous familial hypercholesterolemia: In combination with atorvastatin or simvastatin for the reduction of elevated total cholesterol (total-C) and low-density lipoprotein cholesterol (LDL-C) levels in patients with homozygous familial hypercholesterolemia as an adjunct to other lipid-lowering treatments (eg, LDL apheresis) or if such treatments are unavailable.

Homozygous sitosterolemia: As adjunctive therapy to diet for the reduction of elevated sitosterol and campesterol levels in patients with homozygous familial sitosterolemia.

Primary hyperlipidemia:

Combination therapy with HMG-CoA reductase inhibitors: In combination with a 3-hydroxy-3-methylglutaryl-coenzyme A (HMG-CoA) reductase inhibitor (statin) as adjunctive therapy to diet for the reduction of elevated total-C, LDL-C, apolipoprotein B (apo B), and non-high-density lipoprotein cholesterol (non-HDL-C) in patients with primary (heterozygous familial and nonfamilial) hyperlipidemia.

Combination therapy with fenofibrate: In combination with fenofibrate as adjunctive therapy to diet for the reduction of elevated total-C, LDL-C, apo B, and non-HDL-C in adult patients with mixed hyperlipidemia.

Monotherapy: As adjunctive therapy to diet for the reduction of elevated total-C, LDL-C, apo B, and non-HDL-C in patients with primary (heterozygous familial and nonfamilial) hyperlipidemia.

Pregnancy Considerations Use is contraindicated in women who are or who may become pregnant.

Breast-Feeding Considerations It is not known if ezetimibe is excreted in breast milk. According to the manufacturer, the decision to continue or discontinue breast-feeding during therapy should take into account the risk of exposure to the infant and the benefits of treatment to the mother. Use is contraindicated in nursing women who require combination therapy with an HMG-CoA reductase inhibitor.

Contraindications Hypersensitivity to ezetimibe or any component of the formulation; concomitant use with an HMG-CoA reductase inhibitor (statin) in patients with active hepatic disease or unexplained persistent elevations in serum transaminases; pregnancy and breast-feeding (when used concomitantly with a statin)

Warnings/Precautions Secondary causes of hyperlipidemia should be ruled out prior to therapy. Use caution with severe renal (CrCl ≤30 mL/minute/1.73 m²); systemic exposure is increased ~1.5-fold. If using concurrent simvastatin in patients with moderate to severe renal impairment (CrCl <60 mL/minute/1.73m²), the manufacturer of ezetimibe recommends that simvastatin doses exceeding 20 mg be used with caution and close monitoring for adverse events (eg, myopathy). Myopathy, including rhabdomyolysis, has been reported (rarely) with ezetimibe monotherapy; risk may be increased with concomitant use of a statin or fibrate. Discontinue ezetimibe and statin or fibrate immediately if myopathy is suspected or confirmed (symptomatic patient with CPK >10 x ULN).

A higher incidence of elevated transaminases (≥3 x ULN) has been observed with concomitant use of ezetimibe and statins compared to statin monotherapy; transaminase changes were generally not associated with symptoms or cholestasis and returned to baseline with or without discontinuation of therapy. Consider discontinuation of ezetimibe and/or the statin for persistently elevated transaminases (ALT or AST ≥3 x ULN). Systemic exposure is increased in hepatic impairment. Use caution with mild hepatic impairment (Child-Pugh class A); use is not recommended in patients with moderate or severe hepatic impairment (Child-Pugh classes B and C). Potentially significant drug-drug interactions may exist, requiring dose or frequency adjustment, additional monitoring, and/or selection of alternative therapy.

Adverse Reactions
1% to 10%:
Central nervous system: Fatigue (2%)
Gastrointestinal: Diarrhea (4%)
Hepatic: Transaminases increased (with HMG-CoA reductase inhibitors) (≥3 x ULN, 1%)
Neuromuscular & skeletal: Arthralgia (3%), pain in extremity (3%)
Respiratory: Upper respiratory tract infection (4%), sinusitis (3%)
Miscellaneous: Influenza (2%)
Postmarketing and/or case reports: Abdominal pain, anaphylaxis, angioedema, autoimmune hepatitis (Stolk, 2006), cholecystitis, cholelithiasis, cholestatic hepatitis (Stolk, 2006), CPK increased, depression, dizziness, erythema multiforme, headache, hepatitis, hypersensitivity reactions, myalgia, myopathy, nausea, pancreatitis, paresthesia, rash, rhabdomyolysis, thrombocytopenia, urticaria

Drug Interactions
Metabolism/Transport Effects Substrate of SLCO1B1
Avoid Concomitant Use
Avoid concomitant use of Ezetimibe with any of the following: Bezafibrate; Gemfibrozil
Increased Effect/Toxicity
Ezetimibe may increase the levels/effects of: CycloSPORINE (Systemic)

The levels/effects of Ezetimibe may be increased by: Bezafibrate; CycloSPORINE (Systemic); Eltrombopag; Fenofibrate and Derivatives; Gemfibrozil; Teriflunomide
Decreased Effect
The levels/effects of Ezetimibe may be decreased by: Bile Acid Sequestrants

Storage/Stability Store at 25°C (77°F); excursions are permitted between 15°C and 30°C (59°F and 86°F). Protect from moisture.

Mechanism of Action Inhibits absorption of cholesterol at the brush border of the small intestine via the sterol transporter, Niemann-Pick C1-Like1 (NPC1L1). This leads to a decreased delivery of cholesterol to the liver, reduction of hepatic cholesterol stores and an increased clearance of cholesterol from the blood; decreases total C, LDL-cholesterol (LDL-C), ApoB, and triglycerides (TG) while increasing HDL-cholesterol (HDL-C).

Pharmacodynamics/Kinetics Note: Pharmacokinetic data in children and adolescents ≥10 years of age are reported to be similar to that in adult patients.
Onset of action: Within 1 week; Maximum effect: 2-4 weeks
Protein binding: >90% to plasma proteins
Metabolism: Undergoes glucuronide conjugation in the small intestine and liver; forms metabolite (active); may undergo enterohepatic recycling
Bioavailability: Variable
Hepatic impairment: Moderate hepatic impairment (Child-Pugh score 7-9): AUC increased 3-4 times; Severe hepatic impairment (Child-Pugh 10-15): AUC increased 5-6 times
Renal impairment: Severe renal dysfunction (CrCl <30 mL/minute/1.73 m²): AUC increased 1.5 times
Half-life elimination: 22 hours (ezetimibe and metabolite)
Time to peak, plasma: 4-12 hours (ezetimibe); 1-2 hours (active metabolite); Effects: ~2 weeks
Excretion: Feces (78%, 69% as ezetimibe); urine (11%, 9% as metabolite)

Dosing
Adult & Geriatric Homozygous familial hypercholesterolemia, primary hyperlipidemia, homozygous sitosterolemia: Oral: 10 mg daily
Pediatric Children ≥10 years and Adolescents: Refer to adult dosing.
Renal Impairment No dosage adjustment necessary.
Hepatic Impairment
Mild impairment (Child-Pugh class A): No dosage adjustment necessary.

Moderate to severe impairment (Child-Pugh class B or C): Use of ezetimibe not recommended.
Dietary Considerations Before initiation of therapy, patients should be placed on a standard cholesterol-lowering diet for 6 weeks and the diet should be continued during drug therapy.
Administration May be administered without regard to meals. May be taken at the same time as a statin or fenofibrate. Administer ≥2 hours before or ≥4 hours after bile acid sequestrants.
Monitoring Parameters Total cholesterol profile prior to therapy, and when clinically indicated and/or periodically thereafter. When used in combination with fenofibrate, monitor LFTs and signs and symptoms of cholelithiasis.

2013 ACC/AHA Blood Cholesterol Guideline recommendations (Stone, 2013): Baseline LFTs (reasonable); when used in combination with statin therapy, monitor LFTs when clinically indicated; discontinue use of ezetimibe if ALT elevations >3 times upper limit of normal persist.
Dosage Forms Excipient information presented when available (limited, particularly for generics); consult specific product labeling.
Tablet, Oral:
Zetia: 10 mg
Dosage Forms: Canada Excipient information presented when available (limited, particularly for generics); consult specific product labeling.
Tablet, Oral:
Ezetrol: 10 mg

Ezetimibe and Atorvastatin
(ez ET i mibe & a TORE va sta tin)

Brand Names: US Liptruzet
Index Terms Atorvastatin and Ezetimibe
Pharmacologic Category Antilipemic Agent, 2-Azetidinone; Antilipemic Agent, HMG-CoA Reductase Inhibitor
Use
Homozygous familial hypercholesterolemia: As an adjunct to diet for the reduction of elevated total cholesterol, and low-density lipoprotein cholesterol (LDL-C) in patients with homozygous familial hypercholesterolemia, as an adjunct to other lipid-lowering treatments (eg, LDL apheresis) or if such treatments are unavailable.
Primary hyperlipidemia: As an adjunct to diet for the reduction of elevated total cholesterol, LDL-C, apolipoprotein B (apo B), triglycerides, and non-high-density lipoprotein cholesterol (non-HDL-C), and to increase HDL-C in patients with primary (heterozygous familial and nonfamilial) hyperlipidemia or mixed hyperlipidemia.
Atorvastatin: Primary and secondary prevention of atherosclerotic cardiovascular disease (ASCVD) according to the American College of Cardiology/ American Heart Association: To reduce the risk of ASCVD in patients with clinical ASCVD (eg, coronary heart disease, stroke/TIA, or peripheral arterial disease presumed to be of atherosclerotic origin); in patients without clinical ASCVD if LDL-C is 190 mg/dL or greater; in patients without clinical ASCVD who have type 1 or type 2 diabetes and are between 40 and 75 years of age; in patients with an estimated 10-year ASCVD risk 7.5% or greater and who are between 40 and 75 years of age (Stone, 2013). Specific recommendations from the Kidney Disease: Improving Global Outcomes (KDIGO) organization have also been released for patients with chronic kidney disease (KDIGO [Tonelli, 2013]).
Dosing
Adult & Geriatric
Homozygous familial hypercholesterolemia: Oral: Ezetimibe 10 mg and atorvastatin 40 or 80 mg once daily
Primary hyperlipidemia: Oral: Initial: Ezetimibe 10 mg and atorvastatin 10 or 20 mg once daily; dosing range: Ezetimibe 10 mg and atorvastatin 10 to 80 mg once daily
Patients requiring >55% reduction in LDL-C: Initial: Ezetimibe 10 mg and atorvastatin 40 mg once daily

Dosage adjustment with concomitant medications:
Clarithromycin, itraconazole, saquinavir plus ritonavir, darunavir plus ritonavir, fosamprenavir, or fosamprenavir plus ritonavir: Use lowest effective dose; atorvastatin dose should not exceed 20 mg once daily.
Lopinavir plus ritonavir: Use lowest effective dose.
Nelfinavir or boceprevir: Use lowest effective dose; atorvastatin dose should not exceed 40 mg once daily.
Renal Impairment No dosage adjustment necessary.
Hepatic Impairment There are no dosage adjustments provided in the manufacturer's labeling; however, use is contraindicated in active liver disease or in patients with unexplained persistent elevations of serum transaminases.

Additional Information Complete prescribing information should be consulted for additional detail.

Dosage Forms Excipient information presented when available (limited, particularly for generics); consult specific product labeling.

Tablet, oral:

Liptruzet 10/10: Ezetimibe 10 mg and atorvastatin 10 mg
Liptruzet 10/20: Ezetimibe 10 mg and atorvastatin 20 mg
Liptruzet 10/40: Ezetimibe 10 mg and atorvastatin 40 mg
Liptruzet 10/80: Ezetimibe 10 mg and atorvastatin 80 mg

Ezetimibe and Simvastatin
(ez ET i mibe & SIM va stat in)

Brand Names: US Vytorin
Index Terms Simvastatin and Ezetimibe
Pharmacologic Category Antilipemic Agent, 2-Azetidinone; Antilipemic Agent, HMG-CoA Reductase Inhibitor

Use
Homozygous familial hypercholesterolemia: As an adjunct to diet for the reduction of elevated total cholesterol (total-C) and low-density lipoprotein cholesterol (LDL-C) in patients with homozygous familial hypercholesterolemia, as an adjunct to other lipid-lowering treatments (eg, LDL apheresis), or if such treatments are unavailable

Primary hyperlipidemia: As an adjunct to diet for the reduction of elevated total-C, LDL-C, apolipoprotein B (apo B), triglycerides, and non-high-density lipoprotein cholesterol (HDL-C), and to increase HDL-C in patients with primary (heterozygous familial and nonfamilial) hyperlipidemia or mixed hyperlipidemia

Simvastatin: Primary and secondary prevention of atherosclerotic cardiovascular disease (ASCVD) according to the American College of Cardiology/ American Heart Association: To reduce the risk of ASCVD in patients with clinical ASCVD (eg, coronary heart disease, stroke/TIA, or peripheral arterial disease presumed to be of atherosclerotic origin) who are greater than 75 years of age or not a candidate for high-intensity statin therapy; in patients without clinical ASCVD if LDL-C is 190 mg/dL or greater and not a candidate for high-intensity statin therapy; in patients without clinical ASCVD who have type 1 or type 2 diabetes and are between 40 and 75 years of age; in patients with an estimated 10-year ASCVD risk 7.5% or greater and who are between 40 and 75 years of age (Stone, 2013). Specific recommendations from the Kidney Disease: Improving Global Outcomes (KDIGO) organization have also been released for patients with chronic kidney disease (KDIGO [Tonelli, 2013]).

Limitations of use: No incremental benefit of ezetimibe/ simvastatin on cardiovascular morbidity and mortality over and above that demonstrated for simvastatin has been established. Ezetimibe/simvastatin has not been studied in Fredrickson type I, III, IV, and V dyslipidemias.

Dosing
Adult & Geriatric Note: Dosing limitation: Simvastatin 80 mg is limited to patients that have been taking this dose for >12 consecutive months without evidence of myopathy and are not currently taking or beginning a simvastatin dose-limiting or contraindicated interacting medication. If patient is unable to achieve low-density lipoprotein-cholesterol (LDL-C) goal using the 40 mg dose of simvastatin, increasing to 80 mg dose is not recommended. Instead, switch patient to an alternative LDL-C-lowering treatment providing greater LDL-C reduction. After initiation or titration, monitor lipid response after ≥2 weeks and adjust dose as necessary.

Homozygous familial hypercholesterolemia: Oral: Ezetimibe 10 mg and simvastatin 40 mg once daily in the evening.

Primary hyperlipidemia: Oral: Initial: Ezetimibe 10 mg and simvastatin 10 to 20 mg once daily in the evening. Start patients who require >55% reduction in LDL-C at ezetimibe 10 mg and simvastatin 40 mg once daily in the evening. Dosing range: Ezetimibe 10 mg and simvastatin 10 to 40 mg once daily.

Dosage adjustment with concomitant medications: Oral: **Note:** Patients currently tolerating and requiring a dose of simvastatin 80 mg who require initiation of an interacting drug with a dose cap for simvastatin should be switched to an alternative statin with less potential for drug-drug interaction.

Amiodarone, amlodipine, or ranolazine: Simvastatin dose should **not** exceed 20 mg once daily.
Diltiazem, dronedarone, or verapamil: Simvastatin dose should **not** exceed 10 mg once daily.

Lomitapide: Reduce simvastatin dose by 50% when initiating lomitapide. Simvastatin dose should **not** exceed 20 mg once daily (or 40 mg once daily for those who previously tolerated simvastatin 80 mg daily for ≥1 year without evidence of muscle toxicity).
Dosage adjustment in Chinese patients on niacin doses ≥1 g daily: Oral: Use caution with simvastatin doses exceeding 20 mg daily; because of an increased risk of myopathy, do not administer simvastatin 80 mg

Pediatric
Primary hyperlipidemia: Heterozygous familial hypercholesterolemia (HeFH) (off-label use): Children and Adolescents 10 to 17 years (males and postmenarchal females): Oral: Initial: Ezetimibe 10 mg and simvastatin 10 to 20 mg once daily in the evening (van der Graaf, 2008). Dosing range: Ezetimibe 10 mg and simvastatin 10 to 40 mg once daily; maximum dose: Ezetimibe 10 mg and simvastatin 40 mg once daily.

Dosage adjustment with concomitant medications: Refer to adult dosing.

Renal Impairment
GFR ≥60 mL/minute/1.73 m^2: No dosage adjustment necessary.
GFR <60 mL/minute/1.73 m^2: Ezetimibe 10 mg and simvastatin 20 mg once daily in the evening (higher doses should be used with caution).

Hepatic Impairment Use is contraindicated in patients with active liver disease or with unexplained transaminase elevations.

Additional Information Complete prescribing information should be consulted for additional detail.

Dosage Forms Excipient information presented when available (limited, particularly for generics); consult specific product labeling.

Tablet:

Vytorin 10/10: Ezetimibe 10 mg and simvastatin 10 mg
Vytorin 10/20: Ezetimibe 10 mg and simvastatin 20 mg
Vytorin 10/40: Ezetimibe 10 mg and simvastatin 40 mg
Vytorin 10/80: Ezetimibe 10 mg and simvastatin 80 mg

◆ **Ezetrol (Can)** *see* Ezetimibe *on page 729*
◆ **EZFE 200 [OTC]** *see* Polysaccharide-Iron Complex *on page 1469*
◆ **EZG** *see* Ezogabine *on page 731*

Ezogabine (e ZOG a been)

Brand Names: US Potiga
Index Terms D-23129; EZG; Retigabine; RTG
Pharmacologic Category Anticonvulsant, Neuronal Potassium Channel Opener
Use Partial-onset seizures: As adjunctive treatment for partial-onset seizures in patients ≥18 years who have responded inadequately to several alternative treatments and for whom the benefits outweigh the risk of retinal abnormalities and potential decline in visual acuity

Pregnancy Considerations Adverse events have been observed in animal reproduction studies. Patients exposed to ezogabine during pregnancy are encouraged to enroll themselves into the North American Antiepileptic Drug (NAAED) Pregnancy Registry by calling 1-888-233-2334. Additional information is available at www.aedpregnancyregistry.org.

Breast-Feeding Considerations It is not known if ezogabine is excreted in breast milk. Due to the potential for serious adverse reactions in the nursing infant, the manufacturer recommends a decision be made to continue nursing or to discontinue the drug, taking into account the importance of treatment to the mother.

Medication Guide Available Yes

Contraindications There are no contraindications listed in the manufacturer's labeling.

Warnings/Precautions [US Boxed Warning]: Retinal abnormalities that may progress to vision loss have been reported and were seen in about one-third of patients after approximately 4 years of treatment. These retinal abnormalities exhibited funduscopic features similar to those of retinal pigment dystrophies. The rate of progression and reversibility of these retinal abnormalities is unknown. Limit use to patients who have responded inadequately to other treatments and in whom the benefits of therapy exceed the risk of vision loss. Visual monitoring (at least visual acuity and dilated fundus photography) by an ophthalmic professional is recommended at baseline and at 6-month intervals. Other visual tests may include fluorescein angiograms, optical coherence tomography, perimetry, and electroretinograms. Discontinue use if there is no substantial benefit after adequate titration or if retinal pigmentary abnormalities or vision changes are detected. If no other treatment options are available and the benefits

of treatment outweigh the potential risk of vision loss, then may cautiously continue treatment with ezogabine.

Skin discoloration has been reported; typically blue in color (but may also be gray-blue or brown) and is predominantly located on or around the lips, nail beds of the fingers or toes, face and legs; discoloration of the palate, sclera, and conjunctiva may also occur. Skin discoloration developed in ~10% of patients, generally after ≥2 years of treatment and at higher doses (≥900 mg). If detected, consider other treatment options or discontinue use.

Urinary retention, including retention requiring catheterization, has been reported, generally within the first 6 months of treatment. All patients should be monitored for urologic symptoms; close monitoring is recommended in patients with other risk factors for urinary retention (eg, benign prostatic hyperplasia), patients unable to communicate clinical symptoms, or patients who use concomitant medications that may affect voiding (eg, anticholinergics). Dose-related neuropsychiatric disorders, including confusion, psychotic symptoms, and hallucinations, have been reported, generally within the first 8 weeks of treatment; some patients required hospitalization. Symptoms resolved in most patients within 7 days of discontinuation of therapy. The risk appears to be greatest with rapid titration at greater than the recommended doses. Dose-related dizziness and somnolence (generally mild-to-moderate) have been reported; effects generally occur during dose titration and appear to diminish with continued use. Patients must be cautioned about performing tasks which require mental alertness (eg, operating machinery or driving). QT prolongation has been observed; monitor ECG in patients with electrolyte abnormalities (eg, hypokalemia, hypomagnesemia), concomitant medications which may augment QT prolongation, or any underlying cardiac abnormality which may also potentiate risk (eg, heart failure, ventricular hypertrophy). Pooled analysis of trials involving various antiepileptics (regardless of indication) showed an increased risk of suicidal thoughts/behavior (incidence rate: 0.43% treated patients compared to 0.24% of patients receiving placebo); risk observed as early as 1 week after initiation and continued through duration of trials (most trials ≤24 weeks). Monitor all patients for notable changes in behavior that might indicate suicidal thoughts or depression; notify healthcare provider immediately if symptoms occur.

Dosage adjustment recommended in hepatic impairment; ezogabine exposure increases in moderate-to-severe impairment. Dosage adjustment recommended in renal impairment; ezogabine undergoes significant renal elimination. Use caution in elderly due to potential for urinary retention, particularly in older men with symptomatic BPH. Systemic exposure is increased in the elderly; dosage adjustment is recommended in patients ≥65 years of age.

Anticonvulsants should not be discontinued abruptly because of the possibility of increasing seizure frequency. Unless safety concerns require a more rapid withdrawal, therapy should be withdrawn gradually over a period of ≥3 weeks to minimize the potential of increased seizure frequency.

Adverse Reactions

>10%: Central nervous system: Dizziness (dose related; 23%), drowsiness (dose related; 22%), fatigue (15%)

2% to 10%:

Central nervous system: Confusion (dose related; 9%), vertigo (8%), coordination impaired (dose related; 7%), lack of concentration (6%), memory impairment (dose related; 6%), abnormal gait (dose related; 4%), aphasia (dose related; 4%), dysarthria (4%), equilibrium disturbance (dose related; 4%), anxiety (3%), paresthesia (3%), amnesia (2%), disorientation (2%), dysphasia (2%), hallucination (2%)

Endocrine & metabolic: Weight gain (dose related; 3%)

Gastrointestinal: Nausea (7%), constipation (dose related; 3%), dysphagia (2%)

Genitourinary: Dysuria (dose related; 2%), hematuria (2%), urinary hesitancy (2%), urinary retention (2%), urine discoloration (dose related; 2%)

Infection: Influenza (3%)

Ophthalmic: Diplopia (7%), blurred vision (dose related; 5%)

Neuromuscular & skeletal: Tremor (dose related; 8%), weakness (5%)

<2% (Limited to important or life-threatening): Alopecia, brain disease, coma, euphoria, hydronephrosis, hyperhidrosis, hypokinesia, increased appetite, increased liver enzymes, leukopenia, muscle spasm, nephrolithiasis, neutropenia, nystagmus, peripheral edema, prolonged Q-T Interval on ECG (mean: 7.7 msec), psychotic symptoms, renal colic, skin rash, syncope, thrombocytopenia

Drug Interactions

Metabolism/Transport Effects Inhibits OAT3, P-glycoprotein

Avoid Concomitant Use

Avoid concomitant use of Ezogabine with any of the following: Azelastine (Nasal); Orphenadrine; Paraldehyde; Thalidomide

Increased Effect/Toxicity

Ezogabine may increase the levels/effects of: Azelastine (Nasal); Buprenorphine; CNS Depressants; Highest Risk QTc-Prolonging Agents; Hydrocodone; Methotrimeprazine; Metyrosine; Mirtazapine; Moderate Risk QTc-Prolonging Agents; Orphenadrine; Paraldehyde; Pramipexole; ROPINIRole; Rotigotine; Selective Serotonin Reuptake Inhibitors; Suvorexant; Thalidomide; Zolpidem

The levels/effects of Ezogabine may be increased by: Alcohol (Ethyl); Brimonidine (Topical); Cannabis; Doxylamine; Dronabinol; Droperidol; HydrOXYzine; Kava Kava; Magnesium Sulfate; Methotrimeprazine; Mifepristone; Minocycline; Nabilone; Perampanel; Rufinamide; Sodium Oxybate; Tapentadol; Tetrahydrocannabinol

Decreased Effect

Ezogabine may decrease the levels/effects of: LamoTRIgine

The levels/effects of Ezogabine may be decreased by: CarBAMazepine; Fosphenytoin-Phenytoin; Mefloquine; Mianserin; Orlistat

Storage/Stability Store at 25°C (77°F); excursions permitted to 15°C to 30°C (59°F to 86°F).

Mechanism of Action Ezogabine binds the KCNQ (Kv7.2-7.5) voltage-gated potassium channels, thereby stabilizing the channels in the open formation and enhancing the M-current. As a result, neuronal excitability is regulated and epileptiform activity is suppressed. In addition, ezogabine may also exert therapeutic effects through augmentation of GABA-mediated currents.

Pharmacodynamics/Kinetics

Absorption: Rapid

Distribution: V_{dss}: 2 to 3 L/kg

Protein binding: Ezogabine: ~80%; N-acetyl active metabolite (NAMR): ~45%

Metabolism: Glucuronidation via UGT1A4, UGT1A1, UGT1A3, and UGT1A9 and acetylation via NAT2 to an N-acetyl active metabolite (NAMR) and other inactive metabolites (eg, N-glucuronides, N-glucoside)

Bioavailability: Oral: ~60%

Half-life elimination: Ezogabine and NAMR: 7 to 11 hours; increased by ~30% in elderly patients

Time to peak, plasma: 0.5 to 2 hours; delayed by 0.75 hours when administered with high-fat food

Excretion: Urine (~85%, 36% of total dose as unchanged drug, 18% of total dose as NAMR); feces (~14%, 3% of total dose as unchanged drug)

Dosing

Adult Partial-onset seizures, adjunct: Oral: Initial: 100 mg 3 times daily; may increase at weekly intervals in increments of ≤150 mg per day to a maintenance dose of 200 to 400 mg 3 times daily based on tolerability (maximum: 400 mg 3 times daily [1,200 mg per day]). In clinical trials, no additional benefit and an increase in adverse effects was observed with doses >900 mg per day. **Note:** If there is no substantial benefit after adequate titration, then discontinue use and consider other treatment options.

Geriatric Partial-onset seizures, adjunct: Oral: Initial: 50 mg 3 times daily; may increase at weekly intervals in increments of ≤150 mg per day to a maximum dose of 250 mg 3 times daily (750 mg per day). **Note:** If there is no substantial benefit after adequate titration, then discontinue use and consider other treatment options.

Renal Impairment

CrCl ≥50 mL/minute: No dosage adjustment necessary.

CrCl <50 mL/minute: Initial: 50 mg 3 times daily; may increase at weekly intervals in increments of ≤150 mg per day to a maximum dose of 200 mg 3 times daily (600 mg per day).

ESRD requiring hemodialysis: Initial: 50 mg 3 times daily; may increase at weekly intervals in increments of ≤150 mg per day to a maximum dose of 200 mg 3 times daily (600 mg per day).

Hepatic Impairment

Mild impairment (Child-Pugh 5 to 6): No dosage adjustment necessary.

Moderate impairment (Child-Pugh 7 to 9): Initial: 50 mg 3 times daily; may increase at weekly intervals in increments of ≤150 mg per day to a maximum dose of 250 mg 3 times daily (750 mg per day).

Severe impairment (Child-Pugh >9): Initial: 50 mg 3 times daily; may increase at weekly intervals in increment of ≤150 mg per day to a maximum dose of 200 mg 3 times daily (600 mg per day).

Administration Administer in 3 equally divided doses daily with or without food. Swallow tablets whole; do not break, crush, dissolve, or chew. If therapy is discontinued, gradually reduce dose over at least 3 weeks unless safety concerns require abrupt withdrawal.

Monitoring Parameters Seizures; electrolytes, bilirubin, QT interval (in patients with risk factors for QT prolongation), renal and hepatic function; urologic symptoms; observe patient for excessive sedation, confusion, psychotic symptoms, and hallucinations; suicidality (eg, suicidal thoughts, depression, behavioral changes); skin discoloration (blue, or gray-blue or brown in color) around the lips, nail beds of fingers or toes, face and legs.

Ophthalmic exams (at least visual acuity testing and dilated fundus photography) at baseline and 6-month intervals; fluorescein angiograms, optical coherence tomography, perimetry, and electroretinograms may also be considered.

Test Interactions May falsely elevate serum and urine bilirubin assays

Dosage Forms Excipient information presented when available (limited, particularly for generics); consult specific product labeling.
Tablet, Oral:
Potiga: 50 mg [contains fd&c blue #2 (indigotine)]
Potiga: 200 mg
Potiga: 300 mg, 400 mg [contains fd&c blue #2 (indigotine)]

Controlled Substance C-V

◆ F₃T see Trifluridine on page 1844

◆ FA-8 [OTC] see Folic Acid on page 804

◆ FaBB see Folic Acid, Cyanocobalamin, and Pyridoxine on page 805

◆ Fabior see Tazarotene on page 1740

◆ Fabrazyme see Agalsidase Beta on page 52

◆ Factive see Gemifloxacin on page 836

◆ Factive® (Can) see Gemifloxacin on page 836

Factor VIIa (Recombinant)
(FAK ter SEV en aye ree KOM be nant)

Brand Names: US NovoSeven RT
Brand Names: Canada Niastase; Niastase RT
Index Terms Coagulation Factor VIIa; Eptacog Alfa (Activated); rFVIIa
Pharmacologic Category Antihemophilic Agent
Use Bleeding episodes and perioperative management: Treatment of bleeding episodes and perioperative management in adults and children with hemophilia A or B with inhibitors, congenital factor VII (FVII) deficiency, and Glanzmann's thrombasthenia with refractoriness to platelet transfusions, with or without antibodies to platelets; treatment of bleeding episodes and perioperative management in adults with acquired hemophilia.
Pregnancy Considerations Adverse events have been observed in animal reproduction studies. Factor VII concentrations may vary significantly in pregnant women with coagulation disorders. Pregnant women with hemophilia should have clotting factors monitored, particularly at 28 and 34 weeks gestation and prior to invasive procedures. Recombinant factor VIIa is recommended for the management of bleeding disorders in pregnant women with factor VII deficiency. Prophylaxis at delivery may be needed if factor VII concentrations are <10 to 20 units /dL or in women with a significant bleeding history and treatment should continue for 3 to 5 days postpartum depending on route of delivery. The neonate may also be at an increased risk of bleeding following delivery and should be tested for the coagulation disorder (Kadir 2009; Lee 2006).
Breast-Feeding Considerations It is not known if factor VIIa (recombinant) is excreted in breast milk. Due to the potential for serious adverse reactions in the nursing infant, the manufacturer recommends that a decision be made whether to discontinue nursing or to discontinue the drug, taking into account the importance of treatment to the mother.
Contraindications There are no contraindications listed in the manufacturer's labeling.
Warnings/Precautions [US Boxed Warning]: Serious arterial and venous thrombotic events following administration of Factor VIIa (recombinant) have been reported. Discuss the risks and explain the signs and symptoms of thrombotic and thromboembolic events to patients who will receive factor VIIa (recombinant). Monitor patients for signs and symptoms of activation

of the coagulation system and for thrombosis. All patients receiving factor VIIa should be monitored for signs and symptoms of activation of the coagulation system or thrombosis; thrombotic events due to circulating tissue factor or predisposing coagulopathy may be increased in patients with disseminated intravascular coagulation (DIC), advanced atherosclerotic disease, septicemia, crush injury, concomitant treatment with activated or nonactivated prothrombin complex concentrates, or uncontrolled postpartum hemorrhage. Use with caution in patients with an increased risk of thromboembolic complications (eg, coronary heart disease, liver disease, DIC, postoperative immobilization, elderly patients, and neonates). Decreased dosage or discontinuation is warranted with confirmed intravascular coagulation or presence of clinical thrombosis.

Hypersensitivity reactions, including anaphylaxis, have been reported with use. Use with caution in patients with known hypersensitivity to mouse, hamster, or bovine proteins, or factor VIIa, or any components of the product. If hypersensitivity reaction occurs, discontinue use and administer appropriate treatment; carefully consider the benefits versus the risk of continued treatment with factor VIIa. Some dosage forms may contain polysorbate 80 (also known as Tweens). Hypersensitivity reactions, usually a delayed reaction, have been reported following exposure to pharmaceutical products containing polysorbate 80 in certain individuals (Isaksson, 2002; Lucente 2000; Shelley, 1995). Thrombocytopenia, ascites, pulmonary deterioration, and renal and hepatic failure have been reported in premature neonates after receiving parenteral products containing polysorbate 80 (Alade, 1986; CDC, 1984). See manufacturer's labeling. A number of factors influence the efficacy of factor VIIa, including hypothermia, thrombocytopenia, acidosis, and the amount of blood products transfused prior to administration (Dunkley, 2008). In patients with factor VII deficiency, if factor VIIa activity does not reach the expected level, prothrombin time is not corrected, or bleeding is uncontrolled (with recommended doses), suspect antibody formation and perform antibody analysis. Prothrombin time and factor VII coagulant activity should be measured before and after administration in patients with factor VII deficiency.

Adverse Reactions
1% to 10%:
Cardiovascular: Thrombosis (4%), hypertension (2%), bradycardia (1%), edema (1%), hypotension (1%)
Central nervous system: Cerebrovascular disease (<2%), headache (1%), pain (1%)
Dermatologic: Pruritus (1%), skin rash (1%)
Endocrine & metabolic: Decreased serum fibrinogen (2%)
Gastrointestinal: Vomiting (1%)
Hematologic & oncologic: Decreased prothrombin time (1%), disseminated intravascular coagulation (1%), increased fibrinolysis (1%), purpura (1%)
Hepatic: Abnormal hepatic function tests (<2%)
Hypersensitivity: Hypersensitivity reaction (1%)
Local: Injection site reaction (1%)
Neuromuscular & skeletal: Osteoarthrosis (1%)
Renal: Renal function abnormality (1%)
Respiratory: Pneumonia (1%)
Miscellaneous: Fever (4%), decreased therapeutic response (<2%)
<1% (Limited to important or life-threatening): Anaphylactic shock, anaphylaxis, angina pectoris, angioedema, antibody development, arterial embolism (retinal), arterial thrombosis, arterial thrombosis (limb, retinal), bowel infarction, cerebral infarction, cerebral ischemia, cerebrovascular accident, deep vein thrombosis, hepatic artery thrombosis, hypersensitivity, immunogenicity, increased fibrin degradation products (including D-dimer elevation), intracardiac thrombus, local phlebitis, myocardial infarction, myocardial ischemia, nausea, occlusion of cerebral arteries, peripheral ischemia, portal vein thrombosis, pulmonary embolism, renal artery thrombosis, thrombophlebitis, venous thrombosis at injection site

Drug Interactions
Metabolism/Transport Effects None known.
Avoid Concomitant Use There are no known interactions where it is recommended to avoid concomitant use.
Increased Effect/Toxicity
The levels/effects of Factor VIIa (Recombinant) may be increased by: Factor XIII A-Subunit (Recombinant)
Decreased Effect There are no known significant interactions involving a decrease in effect.
Preparation for Administration Prior to reconstitution, bring vials to a temperature not above 37°C (98.6°F). Add recommended diluent along wall of vial; do not inject directly onto powder. Gently swirl until dissolved. Do not mix with other infusion solutions.

NovoSeven RT: Reconstitute each vial to a final concentration of 1 mg/mL using the provided histidine diluent as follows:

1 mg vial: 1.1 mL histidine diluent vial or 1 mL prefilled histidine diluent syringe

2 mg vial: 2.1 mL histidine diluent vial or 2 mL prefilled histidine diluent syringe

5 mg vial: 5.2 mL histidine diluent vial or 5 mL prefilled histidine diluent syringe

8 mg vial: 8.1 mL histidine diluent vial or 8 mL prefilled histidine diluent syringe

Storage/Stability NovoSeven RT: Prior to reconstitution, store between 2°C to 25°C (36°F to 77°F); do not freeze. Protect from light. Reconstituted solutions may be stored at room temperature or under refrigeration, but must be infused within 3 hours of reconstitution. Do not freeze reconstituted solutions. Do not store reconstituted solutions in syringes.

Mechanism of Action Recombinant factor VIIa, a vitamin K-dependent glycoprotein, promotes hemostasis by activating the extrinsic pathway of the coagulation cascade. It replaces deficient activated coagulation factor VII, which complexes with tissue factor and may activate coagulation factor X to Xa and factor IX to IXa. When complexed with other factors, coagulation factor Xa converts prothrombin to thrombin, a key step in the formation of a fibrin-platelet hemostatic plug.

Pharmacodynamics/Kinetics

Hemophilia A or B:

Distribution: V_{ss}: Children 2 to 12 years: 164 mL/kg; Adults: 107 to 128 mL/kg

Half-life, terminal: Children 2 to 12 years: 2.6 hours; Adults: 2.9 to 3.1 hours

Excretion: Clearance: Children 2 to 12 years: 58 mL/hour/kg; Adults: 31 to 39 mL/hour/kg

Factor VII deficiency:

Distribution: V_{ss}: 280 to 290 mL/kg

Half-life, terminal: 2.8 to 3.1 hours

Excretion: Clearance: 71 to 79 mL/kg/hour

Dosing

Adult & Geriatric IV:

Congenital hemophilia A or B with inhibitors:

Bleeding episodes: 90 mcg/kg/dose every 2 hours until hemostasis is achieved or until the treatment is judged ineffective. Doses between 35 and 90 mcg/kg/dose have been used successfully in clinical trials. The dose, interval, and duration of therapy may be adjusted based upon the severity of bleeding and the degree of hemostasis achieved. For patients experiencing severe bleeds, dosing should be continued at 3- to 6-hour intervals post-hemostasis. The duration of any post-hemostatic dosing should be minimized.

Perioperative management: 90 mcg/kg/dose immediately before surgery (additional bolus doses may be administered for major surgery if required); repeat at 2-hour intervals for the duration of surgery. For minor surgery, continue 90 mcg/kg/dose postoperatively every 2 hours for 48 hours, then every 2 to 6 hours until healed. For major surgery, continue 90 mcg/kg/dose postoperatively every 2 hours for 5 days, then every 4 hours until healed.

Congenital factor VII deficiency:

Bleeding episodes: 15 to 30 mcg/kg/dose every 4 to 6 hours until hemostasis is achieved. Doses as low as 10 mcg/kg have been effective.

Perioperative management: 15 to 30 mcg/kg/dose immediately before surgery; repeat every 4 to 6 hours for the duration of surgery and until hemostasis achieved. Doses as low as 10 mcg/kg have been effective.

Acquired hemophilia:

Bleeding episodes: 70 to 90 mcg/kg/dose every 2 to 3 hours until hemostasis is achieved.

Perioperative management: 70 to 90 mcg/kg/dose immediately before surgery; repeat every 2 to 3 hours for the duration of surgery and until hemostasis achieved.

Glanzmann's thrombasthenia:

Bleeding episodes (severe, refractory to platelet transfusions): 90 mcg/kg/dose every 2 to 6 hours until hemostasis is achieved.

Perioperative management: 90 mcg/kg/dose immediately before surgery; repeat at 2-hour intervals for the duration of surgery. Continue 90 mcg/kg/dose every 2 to 6 hours to prevent postoperative bleeding.

Note: Higher average infused doses (median 100 mcg/kg) were noted for surgical patients who had clinical refractoriness with or without platelet-specific antibodies compared to those with neither.

Intracerebral hemorrhage (ICH) (warfarin-related) (off-label use; Freeman 2004; Ilyas 2008): 10 to 100 mcg/kg/dose (see **"Note"** below) administered concurrently with IV vitamin K (to correct the nonfactor VII coagulation factors).

Note: Lower doses (10 to 20 mcg/kg) are generally preferred given the higher risk of thromboembolic complications with higher doses; response is highly variable; monitor INR frequently after administration since rebound increases in INR occur quickly given the short half-life of rFVIIa; duration of INR correction is dose dependent. Routine use as a sole agent is not recommended for warfarin-related ICH (Morgenstern 2010).

Treatment of refractory bleeding after cardiac surgery in nonhemophiliac patients: Dosing not established; doses in the range of 35 to 70 mcg/kg/dose have been recommended based on low-quality evidence (case series, observational studies) (Chapman 2011; Ferraris 2011; Karkouti 2007); in patients with a left ventricular assist device, lower doses (ie, 10 to 20 mcg/kg) may be preferred to reduce thromboembolic events (Bruckner 2009).

Pediatric

Congenital factor VII deficiency: Children and Adolescents: Refer to adult dosing.

Glanzmann's thrombasthenia: Children and Adolescents: Refer to adult dosing.

Congenital hemophilia A or B with inhibitors: Children and Adolescents: Refer to adult dosing.

Renal Impairment There are no dosage adjustments provided the in manufacturer's labeling.

Hepatic Impairment There are no dosage adjustments provided in the manufacturer's labeling; use with caution.

Dietary Considerations Some products may contain sodium.

Administration IV: For IV administration only as a bolus over 2 to 5 minutes (depending on the dose administered). Use NS to flush line (if necessary) before and after administration. Administer within 3 hours after reconstitution.

Monitoring Parameters Monitor for evidence of hemostasis and thrombosis (including laboratory confirmation of intravascular coagulation, if appropriate). Although the prothrombin time (PT)/INR, aPTT, and factor VII clotting activity have shown no direct correlation with achieving hemostasis, these parameters may be useful as adjunct tests to evaluate efficacy and guide dose or interval adjustments. In factor VII–deficient patients, monitor PT and factor VII clotting activity before and after administration; if the factor VIIa activity fails to reach the expected level, if PT is not corrected, or if bleeding is not controlled after treatment with recommended doses, monitor for factor VII antibodies.

Additional Information The Hemophilia and Thrombosis Research Society (HTRS) Registry surveillance program is designed to collect data on the treatment of congenital and acquired bleeding disorders. All prescribers can obtain information regarding contribution of patient data to this program by calling 1-877-362-7355 or at www.novosevensurveillance.com.

Dosage Forms Excipient information presented when available (limited, particularly for generics); consult specific product labeling.

Solution Reconstituted, Intravenous [preservative free]:

NovoSeven RT: 1 mg (1 ea); 2 mg (1 ea); 5 mg (1 ea); 8 mg (1 ea) [contains polysorbate 80]

◆ Factor Eight Inhibitor Bypassing Activity *see* Antiinhibitor Coagulant Complex (Human) *on page 134*

◆ Factor VIII Concentrate *see* Antihemophilic Factor/von Willebrand Factor Complex (Human) *on page 133*

◆ Factor VIII (Human) *see* Antihemophilic Factor (Human) *on page 131*

◆ Factor VIII (Human)/von Willebrand Factor *see* Antihemophilic Factor/von Willebrand Factor Complex (Human) *on page 133*

◆ Factor VIII Inhibitor Bypassing Activity *see* Anti-inhibitor Coagulant Complex (Human) *on page 134*

◆ Factor VIII (Recombinant) *see* Antihemophilic Factor (Recombinant) *on page 132*

◆ Factor VIII (Recombinant [Porcine Sequence]) *see* Antihemophilic Factor (Recombinant [Porcine Sequence]) *on page 133*

Factor IX Complex (Human) [(Factors II, IX, X)] (FAK ter nyne KOM pleks HYU man FAKter too nyne ten)

Brand Names: US Bebulin; Bebulin VH; Profilnine; Profilnine SD

Index Terms 3 Factor PCC; 3-Factor PCC; PCC (Caution: Confusion-prone synonym); Prothrombin Complex Concentrate (Caution: Confusion-prone synonym); Three-Factor PCC

Pharmacologic Category Antihemophilic Agent; Blood Product Derivative; Prothrombin Complex Concentrate (PCC)

Additional Appendix Information
Reversal of Oral Anticoagulants *on page 1959*

Use
Factor IX deficiency (hemophilia B [Christmas disease]): Prevention and control of bleeding in patients with factor IX deficiency (hemophilia B or Christmas disease)
Limitations of use: Not indicated for the treatment of other factor deficiencies (eg, factor II, VII, VIII, X), treatment of hemophilia A patients with inhibitors to factor VIII, or treatment of bleeding caused by low levels of liver-dependent coagulation factors.

Pregnancy Considerations Animal reproduction studies have not been conducted. Factor IX concentrations do not change significantly in pregnant women with coagulation disorders and women with factor IX deficiency may be at increased risk of postpartum hemorrhage. Pregnant women should have clotting factors monitored, particularly at 28 and 34 weeks gestation and prior to invasive procedures. Prophylaxis may be needed if factor IX concentrations are <50 units/mL at term and treatment should continue for 3 to 5 days postpartum depending on route of delivery. Because parvovirus infection may cause hydrops fetalis or fetal death, a recombinant product is preferred if prophylaxis or treatment is needed. The neonate may also be at an increased risk of bleeding following delivery and should be tested for the coagulation disorder (Chi 2012; Kadir 2009; Lee 2006).

Contraindications
Profilnine: There are no contraindications listed in the manufacturer's labeling.
Bebulin: Hypersensitivity reactions to factor IX complex or any component of the formulation; known allergy to heparin; history of heparin-induced thrombocytopenia.

Warnings/Precautions Factor IX Complex (Human) [Factors II, IX, X] (Bebulin, Profilnine) contains low or nontherapeutic levels of factor VII component and should not be confused with Prothrombin complex concentrate (Human) [(Factors II, VII, IX, X), Protein C, Protein S] (Kcentra, Octaplex) which contains therapeutic levels of factor VII. Factor IX Complex (Human) [Factors II, IX, X] (Bebulin, Profilnine) should not be used for the treatment of factor VII deficiency. When treating warfarin-associated hemorrhage (off-label use), administration of additional fresh frozen plasma (FFP) or factor VIIa should be considered. Hypersensitivity and anaphylactic/anaphylactoid reactions have been reported with use. Delayed reactions (up to 20 days after infusion) in previously untreated patients may also occur. Due to potential for allergic reactions, the initial ~10 to 20 administrations should be performed under appropriate medical supervision. The development of factor IX antibodies (or inhibitors) has been reported with factor IX therapy (usually occurs within the first 10 to 20 exposure days); the risk of severe hypersensitivity reactions occurring may be greater in these patients. Patients experiencing allergic reactions should be evaluated for factor IX inhibitors. If severe hypersensitivity reactions occur, consider the use of alternative hemostatic measures (WFH [Srivastava 2013]). When clinical response is suboptimal, the patient has reached a specified number of exposure days, or patient is to undergo surgical procedure, screen for inhibitors. Patients with severe hemophilia compared to those with mild or moderate hemophilia are more likely to develop inhibitors (WFH [Srivastava 2013]).

Thrombotic events (eg, deep vein thrombosis, pulmonary embolism, thrombotic strokes) as well as disseminated intravascular coagulation (DIC) have occurred. Monitor closely for signs or symptoms of intravascular coagulation or thrombosis; risk is higher in patients with congenital or acquired coagulation disorders, and with repeated dosing or high doses. Use with caution when administering to patients with liver disease, history of coronary artery disease, pre- or postoperatively, neonates, or patients at risk of thromboembolic phenomena, disseminated intravascular coagulation or patients with signs of fibrinolysis due to the potential risk of thromboembolic complications. Discontinue infusion immediately if signs or symptoms of thrombosis or embolism occur. Use with extreme caution in patients with hepatic dysfunction due to the risk of thromboembolic complications. Product of human plasma; may potentially contain infectious agents that could transmit disease. Screening of donors, as well as testing and/or inactivation or removal of certain viruses, reduces the risk.

Infections thought to be transmitted by this product should be reported to the manufacturer. Some products may contain heparin. Use with caution in patients with a history of heparin-induced thrombocytopenia (use of Bebulin is contraindicated). Some product packaging may contain natural rubber latex.

Response to factor IX administration may vary. If bleeding is not controlled with the recommended dose, determine plasma level of factor IX and follow with a sufficient dose to achieve satisfactory clinical response. If plasma levels of factor IX fail to increase as expected or bleeding continues, suspect the presence of an inhibitor; test as appropriate. Safety and efficacy have not been established in immune tolerance induction with factor IX products. Nephrotic syndrome has occurred following immune tolerance induction in patients with hemophilia B with factor IX inhibitors receiving factor IX products.

Adverse Reactions Frequency not defined.
Cardiovascular: Flushing, thrombosis (sometimes fatal)
Central nervous system: Chills, fever, headache, lethargy, somnolence
Dermatologic: Rash, urticaria
Gastrointestinal: Nausea, vomiting
Hematologic: DIC
Neuromuscular & skeletal: Paresthesia
Respiratory: Dyspnea
Miscellaneous: Anaphylactic shock, clotting factor antibodies (development of), heparin-induced thrombocytopenia (with products containing heparin)

Drug Interactions
Metabolism/Transport Effects None known.
Avoid Concomitant Use
Avoid concomitant use of Factor IX Complex (Human) [(Factors II, IX, X)] with any of the following: Aminocaproic Acid
Increased Effect/Toxicity
The levels/effects of Factor IX Complex (Human) [(Factors II, IX, X)] may be increased by: Aminocaproic Acid
Decreased Effect There are no known significant interactions involving a decrease in effect.

Preparation for Administration Prior to reconstitution, bring diluent (sterile water for injection) and factor IX concentrate to room temperature (but not above 37°C [98.6°F]); gently rotate or agitate to dissolve, do not shake. Following reconstitution, do not refrigerate and use as soon as possible within 3 hours. Do not mix with other drugs or solvents. Vials are intended for single use (does not contain preservative; discard unused portion of the vial.
Bebulin: The reconstituted product should be a colorless to slightly yellowish and clear to slightly turbid solution.
Profilnine: A few particles may remain in solution following reconstitution; the Mix2Vial set will remove the particles and the labeled potency will not be reduced.

Storage/Stability
Bebulin: Store undiluted vials at 2°C to 8°C (35°F to 46°F); do not freeze.
Profilnine: Storage temperature should not exceed 25°C (77°F); do not freeze.

Mechanism of Action Replaces deficient clotting factor including factor X; hemophilia B, or Christmas disease, is an X-linked recessively inherited disorder of blood coagulation characterized by insufficient or abnormal synthesis of the clotting protein factor IX. Factor IX is a vitamin K-dependent coagulation factor which is synthesized in the liver. Factor IX is activated by factor XIa in the intrinsic coagulation pathway. Activated factor IX (IXa), in combination with factor VII:C, activates factor X to Xa, resulting ultimately in the conversion of prothrombin to thrombin and the formation of a fibrin clot. The infusion of exogenous factor IX to replace the deficiency present in hemophilia B temporarily restores hemostasis.

Pharmacodynamics/Kinetics Half-life elimination: IX component: ~19 to 25 hours

Dosing
Adult & Geriatric Note: Factor IX complex (Human) [Factors II, IX, X] (Bebulin, Profilnine) contains low or nontherapeutic levels of factor VII component and should not be confused with Prothrombin Complex Concentrate (Human) [(Factors II, VII, IX, X), Protein C, Protein S] (Kcentra, Octaplex) which contains therapeutic levels of factor VII.

Control or prevention of bleeding in patients with factor IX deficiency (hemophilia B [Christmas disease]): Dosage is expressed in units of factor IX activity and must be individualized based on severity of factor IX deficiency, extent and location of bleeding, and clinical status of patient. Close laboratory monitoring of the factor IX level is required to determine proper dosage, particularly with severe hemorrhage and major surgery. Larger doses than those derived from the

formula below may be required, especially if treatment is delayed. When multiple doses are required, administer at 24-hour intervals unless otherwise specified.

Formula for units required to raise blood level %:

Bebulin: In general, factor IX 1 unit/kg will increase the plasma factor IX level by 0.8%

Number of Factor IX units required = body weight (kg) x desired factor IX increase (as % of normal) x 1.2 units/kg

Profilnine: In general, factor IX 1 unit/kg will increase the plasma factor IX level by 1%:

Number of factor IX units required = bodyweight (kg) x desired factor IX increase (as % of normal) x 1 unit/kg

For example, to increase factor IX level to 25% of normal in a 70 kg patient: Number of factor IX units needed = 70 kg x 25 x 1 unit/kg = 1,750 units

As a general rule, the level of factor IX required for treatment of different conditions is listed below:
Hemorrhage: IV:

Minor bleeding (early hemarthrosis, minor epistaxis, gingival bleeding, mild hematuria):

Bebulin: Raise factor IX level to 20% of normal (typical initial dose: 25 to 35 units/kg); average duration of treatment is 1 day. A single dose is usually sufficient or a second dose may be given after 24 hours.

Profilnine: Raise factor IX level to 20% to 30% of normal (initial dose: 20 to 30 units/kg) every 16 to 24 hours for 1 to 2 days for minor hemorrhage or until hemorrhage stops and healing has been achieved.

Moderate bleeding (severe joint bleeding, early hematoma, major open bleeding, minor trauma, minor hemoptysis, hematemesis, melena, major hematuria):

Bebulin: Raise factor IX level to 40% of normal (typical initial dose: 50 to 65 units/kg); average duration of treatment is 2 days or until adequate wound healing.

Profilnine: Raise factor IX level to 20% to 30% of normal (initial dose: 20 to 30 units/kg) every 16 to 24 hours for 2 to 7 days for moderate hemorrhage or until hemorrhage stops and healing has been achieved.

Major bleeding (severe hematoma, major trauma, severe hemoptysis, hematemesis, melena):

Bebulin: Raise factor IX level to ≥60% of normal (typical initial dose: 75 to 90 units/kg); average duration of treatment is 2 to 3 days or until adequate wound healing.

Profilnine: Raise factor IX level to 30% to 50% of normal (initial dose: 30 to 50 units/kg) every 16 to 24 hours; following this treatment period, maintain factor IX levels at 20% of normal (maintenance dose: 20 units/kg) for 3 to 10 days or until healing has been achieved.

Surgical procedures: IV:

Dental surgery:

Bebulin: Raise factor IX level to 40% to 60% of normal on day of surgery (typical dose: 50 to 75 units/kg). One infusion, administered 1 hour prior to surgery, is generally sufficient for the extraction of one tooth; for the extraction of multiple teeth, replacement therapy may be required for up to 1 week (See dosing guidelines for *Minor Surgery*).

Profilnine: Raise factor IX level to 50% of normal immediately prior to procedure; maintain factor IX levels at 30% to 50% of normal (maintenance dose: 30 to 50 units/kg) every 16 to 24 hours for 7 to 10 days following surgery or until healing has been achieved.

Minor surgery:

Bebulin: Raise factor IX level to 40% to 60% of normal on day of surgery (typical initial dose: 50 to 75 units/kg). Decrease factor IX level from 40% to 60% of normal to 20% to 40% of normal during initial postoperative period (1 to 2 weeks or until adequate wound healing) [typical dose: 26 to 65 units/kg]. The preoperative dose should be given 1 hour prior to surgery. The average dosing interval may be every 12 hours initially, then every 24 hours later in the postoperative period.

Profilnine: Raise factor IX level to 30% to 50% of normal (initial dose: 30 to 50 units/kg) prior to surgery (**Note:** Surgery type not specified by the manufacturer); maintain factor IX levels at 30% to 50% of normal (maintenance dose: 30 to 50 units/kg) every 16 to 24 hours for 7 to 10 days following surgery or until healing is achieved.

Major surgery:

Bebulin: Raise factor IX level to ≥60% of normal on day of surgery (typical initial dose: 75 to 90 units/kg). Decrease factor IX level from ≥60% of normal to 20% to 60% of normal during initial postoperative period (1 to 2 weeks) [typical dose: 25 to 75 units/kg]; further decrease to maintain a factor IX level of 20% of normal during late postoperative period (≥3 weeks) and continuing until adequate wound healing is achieved [typical dose: 25 to 35 units/kg]. The preoperative dose should be given 1 hour prior to surgery. The average dosing interval may be every 12 hours initially, then every 24 hours later in the postoperative period.

Profilnine: Raise factor IX level to 30% to 50% of normal (initial dose: 30 to 50 units/kg) prior to surgery (**Note:** Surgery type not specified by the manufacturer); maintain factor IX levels at 30% to 50% of normal (maintenance dose: 30 to 50 units/kg) every 16 to 24 hours for 7 to 10 days following surgery or until healing is achieved.

Warfarin associated hemorrhage (off-label use): IV: **Note:** Products contain low or nontherapeutic levels of factor VII component; therefore, additional fresh frozen plasma (FFP) or factor VIIa may be considered (Masotti 2011). When immediate INR reversal is required, concomitant use of 1 to 2 units of FFP should be considered to ensure acute INR reversal (Baker 2004; Holland 2009). Coadminister vitamin K (phytonadione) 5 to 10 mg by slow IV infusion (ACCP [Guyatt 2012]); vitamin K may be repeated every 12 hours if INR is persistently elevated. Dosing has not been established; the following regimens have been used with some success.

The following 2 methods have been suggested, but are not product specific:

Adjusted-dose regimen, weight based (Liumbruno 2009):

INR <2: 20 units/kg

INR 2 to 4: 30 units/kg

INR >4: 50 units/kg

Note: If after administration, INR remains >1.5 consider repeating dose appropriate for INR.

May also determine dose based on presenting INR and estimated functional prothrombin complex (PC) expressed as percentage of normal plasma levels (see table; Masotti 2011):

Units needed to be infused = (**target** % of functional PC to be reached − **current** estimated % of functional PC) x kg of body weight

Example:

Patient (weight: 70 kg) presents with INR of 4.5 which corresponds to an **estimated % functional PC** of 10% (see table). Target INR of 1.4 corresponds to an **estimated target % functional PC** of 40%.

Units needed to be infused = (40 - 10) x 70 kg = 2,100 units

Conversion of the INR to Estimated Functional Prothrombin Complex (PC)

INR Value	Estimated Functional PC
≥5	5%
4 to 4.9	10%
2.6 to 3.2	15%
2.2 to 2.5	20%
1.9 to 2.1	25%
1.7 to 1.8	30%
1.4 to 1.6	40%
1 to 1.3	100%

Warfarin associated intracranial hemorrhage (off-label use): IV: **Note:** Products contain low or nontherapeutic levels of factor VII component; therefore, additional FFP or factor VIIa may be considered (Masotti 2011). When immediate INR reversal is required, concomitant use of 1 to 2 units of FFP should be considered to ensure acute INR reversal (Baker 2004; Chong 2010; Holland 2009). Coadminister vitamin K (phytonadione) 5 to 10 mg by slow IV infusion (ACCP [Guyatt 2012]); vitamin K may be repeated every 12 hours if INR is persistently elevated. Dosing has not been established; the following regimens have been used with some success.

Fixed-dose regimen, weight based (Frontera 2014): 50 units/kg irrespective of INR; if after administration INR is not corrected to <1.4, FFP may be administered. **Note:** Bebulin used during study.

Adjusted-dose regimen, weight based (Chong 2010):
INR <5: 30 units/kg
INR >5 (emergent): 50 units/kg
Note: Profilnine used during study. If after administration INR remains >1.2, consider repeating dose and administering more FFP until INR <1.2

Pediatric Control or prevention of bleeding in patients with factor IX deficiency (hemophilia B [Christmas disease]) (off-label use): IV: Refer to adult dosing.

Renal Impairment There are no dosage adjustments provided in the manufacturer's labeling.

Hepatic Impairment There are no dosage adjustments provided in the manufacturer's labeling; monitor factor IX levels. Use with caution due to the risk of thromboembolic complications.

Administration Solution should be infused at room temperature. Rate should not exceed 2 mL/minute for Bebulin or 10 mL/minute for Profilnine. Vasomotor reactions may result from rapid administration; do not exceed the recommended infusion rates. Slowing the rate of infusion, changing the lot of medication, or administering antihistamines may relieve some adverse reactions.

Monitoring Parameters Levels of factor IX; PT, PTT; INR (when used for warfarin reversal); signs and symptoms of hypersensitivity reactions, DIC, thrombosis, especially in patients with liver disease, surgical patients, and patients with known risk factors predisposing to thrombosis

Reference Range Average normal factor IX levels are 50% to 150%; patients with severe hemophilia B will have factor IX levels <1%, often undetectable. Moderate forms of the disease have levels of 1% to 5% while some mild cases may have 5% to 49% of normal factor IX.

Additional Information Vaccination with hepatitis A and hepatitis B vaccines are recommended at diagnosis for patients with hemophilia.

Factor IX concentrate containing only factor IX is also available and preferable for hemophilia B (or Christmas disease). Prothrombin complex concentrates also contain factor II, factor VII, and factor X and are of intermediate purity. Heparin may be present in some products to decrease thrombotic effects.

Dosage Forms Considerations
Strengths expressed as an approximate value. Consult individual vial labels for exact potency within each vial.
Bebulin VH packaged contents may contain natural rubber latex.

Dosage Forms Excipient information presented when available (limited, particularly for generics); consult specific product labeling.
Solution Reconstituted, Intravenous:
Bebulin: 200-1200 units (1 ea)
Bebulin VH: 200-1200 units (1 ea)
Profilnine: 500 units (1 ea); 1000 units (1 ea); 1500 units (1 ea) [contains polysorbate 80]
Profilnine SD: 500 units (1 ea); 1000 units (1 ea); 1500 units (1 ea) [contains polysorbate 80]

◆ Factor IX Concentrate *see* Factor IX (Human) *on page 737*

◆ Factor IX Concentrate *see* Factor IX (Recombinant) *on page 738*

Factor IX (Human) (FAK ter nyne HYU man)

Brand Names: US AlphaNine SD; Mononine
Brand Names: Canada Immunine VH
Index Terms Factor IX Concentrate
Pharmacologic Category Antihemophilic Agent; Blood Product Derivative
Use Prevention and control of bleeding in patients with hemophilia B (congenital factor IX deficiency or Christmas disease)

NOTE: Contains **nondetectable levels of factors II, VII, and X.** Therefore, **NOT INDICATED** for replacement therapy of any other clotting factor besides factor IX or for reversal of anticoagulation due to either vitamin K antagonists or other anticoagulants (eg, dabigatran), for hemophilia A patients with factor VIII inhibitors, or for patients in a hemorrhagic state caused by reduced production of liver-dependent coagulation factors (eg, hepatitis, cirrhosis).

Dosing
Adult & Geriatric NOTE: Contains **nondetectable levels of factors II, VII, and X.** Therefore, **NOT INDICATED** for replacement therapy of any other clotting factor besides factor IX or for reversal of anticoagulation due to either vitamin K antagonists or other anticoagulants

(eg, dabigatran), for hemophilia A patients with factor VIII inhibitors, or for patients in a hemorrhagic state caused by reduced production of liver-dependent coagulation factors (eg, hepatitis, cirrhosis).

Control or prevention of bleeding in patients with factor IX deficiency (hemophilia B or Christmas disease): IV: *AlphaNine SD, Mononine:* Dosage is expressed in units of factor IX activity; dosing must be individualized based on severity of factor IX deficiency, extent and location of bleeding, and clinical status of patient. Refer to product information for specific manufacturer recommended dosing. Alternatively, the World Federation of Hemophilia (WFH) has recommended general dosing for factor IX products.

Formula to determine units required to obtain desired factor IX level: **Note:** If patient has severe hemophilia (ie, baseline factor IX level is or presumed to be <1%), then may just use "desired factor IX level" instead of "desired factor IX level increase".

Number of factor IX units required = patient weight (in kg) x desired factor IX level increase (as % or units/dL) x 1 unit/kg

For example, to attain an 80% level in a 70 kg patient who has a baseline level of 20%: Number of factor IX units needed = 70 kg x 60% x 1 unit/kg = 4200 units

Alternative dosing (off-label): Note: The following recommendations may vary from those found within prescribing information or practitioner preference.

Prophylaxis: 15 to 30 units/kg/dose twice weekly (Utrecht protocol; WFH [Srivastava 2013]) **or** 25 to 40 units/kg/dose twice weekly (Malmö protocol; WFH [Srivastava 2013]) **or** 40 to 100 units/kg/dose 2 to 3 times weekly (National Hemophilia Foundation, MASAC recommendation, 2007); optimum regimen has yet to be defined.

Treatment:

2013 World Federation of Hemophilia Treatment Recommendations (When No Significant Resource Constraint Exists):

Site of Hemorrhage/ Clinical Situation	Desired Factor IX Level to Maintain	Duration
Joint	40 to 60 units/dL	1 to 2 days, may be longer if response is inadequate
Superficial muscle/ no neurovascular compromise	40 to 60 units/dL	2 to 3 days, sometimes longer if response is inadequate
Iliopsoas and deep muscle with neurovascular injury, or substantial blood loss	*Initial:* 60 to 80 units/dL *Maintenance:* 30 to 60 units/dL	*Initial:* 1 to 2 days *Maintenance:* 3 to 5 days, sometimes longer as secondary prophylaxis during physiotherapy
CNS/head	*Initial:* 60 to 80 units/dL *Maintenance:* 30 units/dL	*Initial:* 1 to 7 days *Maintenance:* 8 to 21 days
Throat and neck	*Initial:* 60 to 80 units/dL *Maintenance:* 30 units/dL	*Initial:* 1 to 7 days *Maintenance:* 8 to 14 days
Gastrointestinal	*Initial:* 60 to 80 units/dL *Maintenance:* 30 units/dL	*Initial:* 7 to 14 days *Maintenance:* Not specified
Renal	40 units/dL	3 to 5 days
Deep laceration	40 units/dL	5 to 7 days
Surgery (major)	*Preop:* 60 to 80 units/dL	
	Postop: 40 to 60 units/dL 30 to 50 units/dL 20 to 40 units/dL	*Postop:* 1 to 3 days 4 to 6 days 7 to 14 days
Surgery (minor)	*Preop:* 50to 80 units/dL	
	Postop: 30 to 80 units/dL	*Postop:* 1 to 5 days depending on procedure type

Note: Factor IX level may either be expressed as units/dL or as %. Dosing frequency most commonly corresponds to the half-life of factor IX but should be determined based on an assessment of factor IX levels before the next dose.

Continuous infusion (for patients who require prolonged periods of treatment [eg, intracranial hemorrhage or surgery] to avoid peaks and troughs associated with intermittent infusions) (Batorova, 2002; Poon, 2012; Rickard, 1995; WFH [Srivastava 2013]): Following initial bolus to achieve the desired factor IX level: Initiate 4 to 6 units/kg/hour; adjust dose based on frequent factor assays and calculation of factor IX clearance at steady-state using the following equations:

Factor IX clearance (mL/kg/hour) = (current infusion rate in units/kg/hour) divided by (plasma level in units/mL)

New infusion rate (units/kg/hour) = (factor IX clearance in mL/kg/hour) x (desired plasma level in units/mL)

Pediatric NOTE: Contains **nondetectable levels of factors II, VII, and X.** Therefore, **NOT INDICATED** for replacement therapy of any other clotting factor besides factor IX or for reversal of anticoagulation due to either vitamin K antagonists or other anticoagulants (eg, dabigatran), for hemophilia A patients with factor VIII inhibitors, or for patients in a hemorrhagic state caused by reduced production of liver-dependent coagulation factors (eg, hepatitis, cirrhosis).

Control or prevention of bleeding in patients with factor IX deficiency (hemophilia B or Christmas disease): Infants, Children, and Adolescents: IV: *AlphaNine SD, Mononine:* Dosage is expressed in units of factor IX activity; dosing must be individualized based on severity of factor IX deficiency, extent and location of bleeding, and clinical status of patient. Refer to product information for specific manufacturer recommended dosing. Alternatively, the World Federation of Hemophilia (WFH) has recommended general dosing for factor IX products.

Formula to determine units required to obtain desired factor IX level: **Note:** If patient has severe hemophilia (ie, baseline factor IX level is or presumed to be <1%), then may just use "desired factor IX level" instead of "desired factor IX level increase".

Number of factor IX units required = patient weight (in kg) x desired factor IX level increase (as % or units/dL) x 1 unit/kg

For example, to attain an 80% level in a 70 kg patient who has a baseline factor IX level of 20%: Number of factor IX units needed = 70 kg x 60% x 1 unit/kg = 4200 units

Alternative recommendations (off-label): Infants, Children, and Adolescents:

Prophylaxis, primary: Refer to adult dosing.

Treatment: Refer to adult dosing.

Additional Information Complete prescribing information should be consulted for additional detail.

Dosage Forms Considerations

Strengths expressed with approximate values. Consult individual vial labels for exact potency within each vial.

Dosage Forms Excipient information presented when available (limited, particularly for generics); consult specific product labeling.

Solution Reconstituted, Intravenous [preservative free]:

AlphaNine SD: 500 units (1 ea); 1000 units (1 ea); 1500 units (1 ea) [contains polysorbate 80]

Mononine: 250 units (1 ea); 500 units (1 ea); 1000 units (1 ea) [contains polysorbate 80]

Factor IX (Recombinant)
(FAK ter nyne ree KOM be nant)

Brand Names: US Alprolix; BeneFIX; Ixinity; Rixubis
Brand Names: Canada BeneFix
Index Terms Factor IX Concentrate
Pharmacologic Category Antihemophilic Agent
Use

Factor IX deficiency: Prevention and control of bleeding in patients with factor IX deficiency (hemophilia B [Christmas disease]); perioperative management in patients with hemophilia B.

Alprolix and Rixubis: Routine prophylaxis to prevent or reduce the frequency of bleeding episodes in patients with hemophilia B

Limitations of use: **Not indicated** for the treatment of other factors deficiencies (eg, factors II, VII, VIII, and X), hemophilia A patients with inhibitors to factor VIII, reversal of coumarin-induced anticoagulation, and bleeding due to low levels of liver-dependent clotting factors.

Dosing

Adult & Geriatric Note: Contains **only factor IX**. Therefore, **NOT INDICATED** for the treatment of other factors deficiencies (eg, factors II, VII, VIII, and X), hemophilia A patients with inhibitors to factor VIII, reversal of coumarin-induced anticoagulation, and bleeding due to low levels of liver-dependent clotting factors.

Control or prevention of bleeding in patients with factor IX deficiency (hemophilia B or Christmas disease): IV: Dosage is expressed in units of factor IX activity; dosing must be individualized based on severity of factor IX deficiency, extent and location of bleeding, clinical status of patient, and recovery of factor IX. As compared to Benefix, Ixinity, and Rixubis, Alprolix displays a longer half-life. Therefore, Alprolix dosing and frequency may differ. **Refer to product information for specific manufacturer recommended dosing.** Alternatively, the World Federation of Hemophilia (WFH) has recommended general dosing for factor IX products.

Formula for units required to raise blood level %: **Note:** If patient has severe hemophilia (ie, baseline factor IX level is or presumed to be <1%), then may just use "desired factor IX level" instead of "desired factor IX level *increase*". On average, the observed recovery for BeneFix is 0.8 units/dL per units/kg in adults.

Number of factor IX units required = patient weight (in kg) x desired factor IX level increase (as % or units/dL) x reciprocal of observed recovery (as units/kg per units/dL)

Alternative dosing (off-label): Note: The following recommendations may vary from those found within prescribing information or practitioner preference.

Prophylaxis: 15 to 30 units/kg/dose twice weekly (Utrecht protocol; WFH [Srivastava 2013]) **or** 25 to 40 units/kg/dose twice weekly (Malmö protocol; WFH [Srivastava 2013]) **or** 40 to 100 units/kg/dose 2 to 3 times weekly (National Hemophilia Foundation, MASAC recommendation 2007); optimum regimen has yet to be defined.

Treatment:

2013 World Federation of Hemophilia Treatment Recommendations (When No Significant Resource Constraint Exists):

Site of Hemorrhage/ Clinical Situation	Desired Factor IX Level to Maintain	Duration
Joint	40-60 units/dL	1-2 days, may be longer if response is inadequate
Superficial muscle/ no neurovascular compromise	40-60 units/dL	2-3 days, sometimes longer if response is inadequate
Iliopsoas and deep muscle with neurovascular injury, or substantial blood loss	Initial: 60-80 units/dL Maintenance: 30-60 units/dL	Initial: 1-2 days Maintenance: 3-5 days, sometimes longer as secondary prophylaxis during physiotherapy
CNS/head	Initial: 60-80 units/dL Maintenance: 30 units/dL	Initial: 1-7 days Maintenance: 8-21 days
Throat and neck	Initial: 60-80 units/dL Maintenance: 30 units/dL	Initial: 1-7 days Maintenance: 8-14 days
Gastrointestinal	Initial: 60-80 units/dL Maintenance: 30 units/dL	Initial: 7-14 days Maintenance: Not specified
Renal	40 units/dL	3-5 days
Deep laceration	40 units/dL	5-7 days
Surgery (major)	Preop: 60-80 units/dL	
	Postop: 40-60 units/dL 30-50 units/dL 20-40 units/dL	Postop: 1-3 days 4-6 days 7-14 days
Surgery (minor)	Preop: 50-80 units/dL	
	Postop: 30-80 units/dL	Postop: 1-5 days depending on procedure type

Note: Factor IX level may either be expressed as units/dL or as %. Dosing frequency most commonly corresponds to the half-life of factor IX but should be determined based on an assessment of factor IX levels before the next dose.

Continuous infusion (For patients who require prolonged periods of treatment [eg, intracranial hemorrhage or surgery] to avoid peaks and troughs associated with intermittent infusions) (Batorova 2002; Poon 2012; Rickard, 1995; WFH [Srivastava 2013]): **Note:** Evidence supporting the use of continuous infusion is primarily with BeneFix (Chowdary 2001); however manufacturer's labeling states that safety and efficacy of BeneFIX administration by continuous infusion has not been established: Following initial bolus to achieve the desired factor IX level, initiate 4 to 6 units/kg/hour; adjust dose based on frequent factor assays and calculation of factor IX clearance at steady-state using the following equations:

Factor IX clearance (mL/kg/hour) = (current infusion rate in units/kg/hour)/(plasma level in units/mL)

New infusion rate (units/kg/hour) = (factor IX clearance in mL/kg/hour) x (desired plasma level in units/mL)

Routine prophylaxis to prevent bleeding episodes in patients with factor IX deficiency (hemophilia B or Christmas disease): IV:

Alprolix: 50 units/kg once weekly or 100 units/kg once every 10 days; adjust dose based on individual response

Rixubis: 40 to 60 units/kg twice weekly; may titrate dose depending upon age, bleeding pattern, and physical activity

Pediatric Note: Contains **only factor IX**. Therefore, **NOT INDICATED** for the treatment of other factors deficiencies (eg, factors II, VII, VIII, and X), hemophilia A patients with inhibitors to factor VIII, reversal of coumarin-induced anticoagulation, and bleeding due to low levels of liver-dependent clotting factors.

Control or prevention of bleeding in patients with factor IX deficiency (hemophilia B or Christmas disease): IV: Dosage is expressed in units of factor IX activity; dosing must be individualized based on severity of factor IX deficiency, extent and location of bleeding, clinical status of patient, and recovery of factor IX. As compared to Benefix, Ixinity, and Rixubis, Alprolix displays a longer half-life. Therefore, Alprolix dosing and frequency may differ. **Refer to product information for specific manufacturer recommended dosing.** Alternatively, the World Federation of Hemophilia (WFH) has recommended general dosing for factor IX products.

Formula for units required to raise blood level %:
Note: If patient has severe hemophilia (ie, baseline factor IX level is or presumed to be <1%), then may just use "desired factor IX level" instead of "desired factor IX level *increase*". On average, the observed recovery for BeneFix is 0.7 units/dL per units/kg in children <15 years of age.

Infants, Children, and Adolescents: IV: Number of factor IX units required = patient weight (in kg) x desired factor IX level increase (as % or units/dL) x reciprocal of observed recovery (as units/kg per units/dL)

Alternative recommendations (off label): Infants, Children, and Adolescents:
Prophylaxis: Refer to adult dosing.
Treatment: Refer to adult dosing.

Routine prophylaxis to prevent bleeding episodes in patients with factor IX deficiency (hemophilia B or Christmas disease): IV:
Alprolix: 50 units/kg once weekly or 100 units/kg once every 10 days; adjust dose based on individual response
Rixubis:
Children <12 years: 60 to 80 units/kg twice weekly; may titrate dose depending upon age, bleeding pattern, and physical activity.
Children ≥12 years and Adolescents: 40 to 60 units/kg twice weekly; may titrate dose depending upon age, bleeding pattern, and physical activity.

Renal Impairment
There are no dosage adjustments provided in the manufacturer's labeling; monitor factor IX levels.

Hepatic Impairment
There are no dosage adjustments provided in the manufacturer's labeling; monitor factor IX levels. Use with caution due to the risk of thromboembolic complications.

Additional Information Complete prescribing information should be consulted for additional detail.

Dosage Forms Considerations
Strengths expressed with approximate values. Consult individual vial labels for exact potency within each vial.

Dosage Forms Excipient information presented when available (limited, particularly for generics); consult specific product labeling.
Solution Reconstituted, Intravenous [preservative free]:
Alprolix: 500 units (1 ea); 1000 units (1 ea); 2000 units (1 ea); 3000 units (1 ea)
BeneFIX: 250 units (1 ea); 500 units (1 ea); 1000 units (1 ea); 2000 units (1 ea) [contains polysorbate 80]
Ixinity: 500 units (1 ea); 1000 units (1 ea); 1500 units (1 ea) [contains mouse protein (murine) (hamster), polysorbate 80]
Rixubis: 250 units (1 ea); 500 units (1 ea); 1000 units (1 ea); 2000 units (1 ea); 3000 units (1 ea) [contains polysorbate 80]

◆ 3 Factor PCC *see* Factor IX Complex (Human) [(Factors II, IX, X)] *on page 734*

◆ 4 Factor PCC *see* Prothrombin Complex Concentrate (Human) [(Factors II, VII, IX, X), Protein C, and Protein S] *on page 1525*

◆ Factor 13 *see* Factor XIII Concentrate (Human) *on page 739*

Factor XIII Concentrate (Human)
(FAK ter THIR teen KON cen trate HYU man)

Brand Names: US Corifact
Brand Names: Canada Corifact
Index Terms Activated Factor XIII; Corifact; Factor 13; FXIII
Pharmacologic Category Antihemophilic Agent; Blood Product Derivative
Use Prophylaxis against bleeding episodes and management of perioperative surgical bleeding in patients with congenital factor XIII deficiency

Dosing
Adult & Geriatric Congenital factor XIII deficiency: IV:
Prophylaxis:
Initial: 40 units/kg
Maintenance: Dose adjustment should be based on factor XIII activity trough levels (target level of 5% to 20% using Berichrom activity assay) and clinical response; repeat every 28 days
One trough level of <5%: Increase dosage by 5 units/kg
Trough level of 5% to 20%: No dosage change
Two trough levels of >20%: Decrease dosage by 5 units/kg
One trough level of >25%: Decrease dosage by 5 units/kg
Perioperative management of surgical bleeding: Individualize dosing based on factor XIII activity level, type of surgery, and clinical response; monitor factor XIII activity levels during and after surgery:
If time since last prophylactic dose ≤7 days: Additional dose may not be needed.
If time since last prophylactic dose 8 to 21 days: Additional partial or full dose may be necessary based on factor XIII activity level
If time since last prophylactic dose 21 to 28 days: Administer full prophylactic dose

Pediatric Infants, Children, and Adolescents: Refer to adult dosing.

Renal Impairment There are no dosage adjustments provided in the manufacturer's labeling.

Hepatic Impairment There are no dosage adjustments provided in the manufacturer's labeling.

Additional Information Complete prescribing information should be consulted for additional detail.

Dosage Forms Excipient information presented when available (limited, particularly for generics); consult specific product labeling.
Kit, Intravenous [preservative free]:
Corifact: 1000 - 1600 units

Dosage Forms: Canada Note: Refer also to dosage forms.
Excipient information presented when available (limited, particularly for generics); consult specific product labeling.
Solution Reconstituted, Intravenous [preservative free]
Corifact: 200 - 320 units

◆ FAG-201 *see* Dimethyl Fumarate *on page 557*
◆ FaLessa Kit *see* Ethinyl Estradiol and Levonorgestrel *on page 703*
◆ Falmina *see* Ethinyl Estradiol and Levonorgestrel *on page 703*

Famciclovir (fam SYE kloe veer)

Brand Names: US Famvir
Brand Names: Canada Apo-Famciclovir®; Ava-Famciclovir; CO Famciclovir; Famvir®; PMS-Famciclovir; Sandoz-Famciclovir
Pharmacologic Category Antiviral Agent
Use Treatment of acute herpes zoster (shingles) in immunocompetent patients; treatment and suppression of recurrent episodes of genital herpes in immunocompetent patients; treatment of herpes labialis (cold sores) in immunocompetent patients; treatment of recurrent orolabial/genital (mucocutaneous) herpes simplex in HIV-infected patients
Pregnancy Considerations Adverse events have not been observed in animal reproduction studies. Based on available data, use during pregnancy appears to be well tolerated (CDC [Workowski 2015]; HHS [opportunistic; adult] 2015).

Health care providers are encouraged to enroll women exposed to famciclovir during pregnancy in the Famvir Pregnancy reporting system (888-669-6682).

Breast-Feeding Considerations It is not known if famciclovir is excreted in breast milk. Breast-feeding is not recommended by the manufacturer unless the potential benefits outweigh any possible risk. If herpes lesions are on breast, breast-feeding should be avoided in order to avoid transmission to infant (AAP 2012).

Contraindications Hypersensitivity to famciclovir, penciclovir, or any component of the formulation

Warnings/Precautions Has not been established for use in immunocompromised patients (except HIV-infected patients with orolabial or genital herpes, patients with ophthalmic or disseminated zoster or with relapse of genital herpes, and in Black and African American patients with recurrent episodes of genital herpes. Acute renal failure has been reported with use of inappropriate high doses in patients with underlying renal disease.

Dosage adjustment is required in patients with renal insufficiency. Tablets contain lactose; do not use with galactose intolerance, severe lactase deficiency, or glucose-galactose malabsorption syndromes.

Adverse Reactions Note: Frequencies vary with dose and duration.

>10%:
Central nervous system: Headache (9% to 39%)
Gastrointestinal: Nausea (2% to 13%)
1% to 10%:
Central nervous system: Fatigue (1% to 5%), migraine (1% to 3%)
Dermatologic: Pruritus (≤4%), rash (≤3%)
Endocrine & metabolic: Dysmenorrhea (≤8%)
Gastrointestinal: Diarrhea (2% to 9%), abdominal pain (≤8%), vomiting (1% to 5%), flatulence (≤5%)
Hematologic: Neutropenia (3%)
Hepatic: Transaminases increased (2% to 3%), bilirubin increased (2%)
Neuromuscular & skeletal: Paresthesia (≤3%)
<1% (Limited to important or life-threatening): Anemia, angioedema (eyelid, face, periorbital, pharyngeal edema), cholestatic jaundice, confusion, delirium, disorientation, dizziness, erythema multiforme, hallucinations, leukocytoclastic vasculitis, palpitations, somnolence, Stevens-Johnson syndrome, thrombocytopenia, toxic epidermal necrolysis, urticaria

Drug Interactions
Metabolism/Transport Effects None known.
Avoid Concomitant Use
Avoid concomitant use of Famciclovir with any of the following: Varicella Virus Vaccine; Zoster Vaccine
Increased Effect/Toxicity There are no known significant interactions involving an increase in effect.
Decreased Effect
Famciclovir may decrease the levels/effects of: Talimogene Laherparepvec; Varicella Virus Vaccine; Zoster Vaccine

Food Interactions Rate of absorption and/or conversion to penciclovir and peak concentration are reduced with food, but bioavailability is not affected. Management: Administer without regard to meals.

Storage/Stability Store at 25°C (77°F); excursions permitted to 15°C to 30°C (59°F to 86°F).

Mechanism of Action Famciclovir undergoes rapid biotransformation to the active compound, penciclovir (prodrug), which is phosphorylated by viral thymidine kinase in HSV-1, HSV-2, and VZV-infected cells to a monophosphate form; this is then converted to penciclovir triphosphate and competes with deoxyguanosine triphosphate to inhibit HSV-2 polymerase, therefore, herpes viral DNA synthesis/replication is selectively inhibited.

Pharmacodynamics/Kinetics
Absorption: Food decreases maximum peak penciclovir concentration and delays time to penciclovir peak; AUC remains the same
Distribution: V_d: Healthy adults: Penciclovir: 1.08 ± 0.17 L/kg
Protein binding: Penciclovir: <20%
Metabolism: Famciclovir is rapidly deacetylated and oxidized to penciclovir (active prodrug); *in vitro* data demonstrate that metabolism does not occur via CYP isoenzymes
Bioavailability: Penciclovir: 77% ± 8%
Half-life elimination:
Penciclovir: 2 to 4 hours; Prolonged in renal impairment:
CrCl 40 to 59 mL/minute: ~3.4 hours
CrCl 20 to 39 mL/minute: ~6.2 hours,
CrCl <20 mL/minute: ~13.4 hours
Intracellular penciclovir triphosphate: HSV 1: 10 hours; HSV 2: 20 hours; VZV: 7 hours
Time to peak: Penciclovir: ~1 hour
Excretion: Urine (73% primarily as penciclovir); feces (27%)

Dosing
Adult & Geriatric
Genital herpes simplex virus (HSV) infection: Oral:
Note: Initiate therapy as soon as possible after diagnosis and within 72 hours of rash onset
Immunocompetent patients:
Initial episode: 250 mg 3 times/day for 7 to 10 days (CDC, 2010)
Recurrence: 1,000 mg twice daily for 1 day (**Note:** Initiate therapy as soon as possible and within 6 hours of symptoms/lesions onset)
Alternatively, the following regimens are also recommended: 125 mg twice daily for 5 days or 500 mg as a single dose, followed by 250 mg twice daily for 2 days (CDC, 2010). **Note:** Canadian labeling recommends 125 mg twice daily for 5 days.

Suppressive therapy: 250 mg twice daily for up to 1 year; **Note:** Duration not established, but efficacy/safety have been demonstrated for 1 year (CDC, 2010)
HIV-infected patients:
Manufacturer's labeling: Recurrent episodes: 500 mg twice daily for 7 days
Alternate dosing:
Initial or recurrent episodes: 500 mg twice daily for 5 to 14 days (HHS [OI adult 2015])
Chronic suppressive therapy (off-label use): 500 mg twice daily; continue indefinitely regardless of CD4 count in patients with severe recurrences of genital herpes or in patients who want to minimize frequency of recurrences (HHS [OI adult 2015])
Herpes labialis/orolabial (cold sores): Oral: **Note:** Initiate therapy as soon as possible after diagnosis and within 72 hours of rash onset
Immunocompetent patients:
Recurrent episodes: 1,500 mg as a single dose; initiate therapy at first sign or symptom such as tingling, burning, or itching (initiated within 1 hour in clinical studies)
HIV patients:
Manufacturer's labeling: Recurrent episodes: 500 mg twice daily for 7 days
Alternate dosing: Treatment: 500 mg twice daily for 5 to 10 days (HHS [OI adult 2015])
Herpes zoster (shingles): Oral: **Note:** Initiate therapy as soon as possible after diagnosis and within 72 hours of rash onset
Immunocompetent patients: 500 mg every 8 hours for 7 days
HIV-infected patients (off-label use): 500 mg 3 times daily for 7 to 10 days; consider longer duration if lesions heal slowly (HHS [OI adult 2015])
Varicella infection (chickenpox) in HIV-infected patients (uncomplicated cases) (off-label use): Oral: 500 mg 3 times daily for 5 to 7 days (HHS [OI adult 2015])

Pediatric
Genital herpes simplex virus (HSV) in HIV-infected patients: Adolescents (off-label population): Oral:
Initial or recurrent episodes: 500 mg twice daily for 5 to 14 days (HHS [OI adult 2015])
Chronic suppressive therapy (off-label use): 500 mg twice daily; continue indefinitely regardless of CD4 count in patients with severe recurrences of genital herpes or in patients who want to minimize frequency of recurrences (HHS [OI adult 2015])
Herpes labialis/orolabial (cold sores) in HIV-infected patients: Adolescents (off-label population): Oral: Treatment: 500 mg twice daily for 5 to 10 days (HHS [OI adult 2015])
Herpes zoster (shingles) in HIV-infected patients (off-label use): Adolescents: Oral: 500 mg 3 times daily for 7 to 10 days; consider longer duration if lesions heal slowly (HHS [OI adult 2015])
Varicella infection (chickenpox) in HIV-infected patients (uncomplicated cases) (off-label use): Adolescents: Oral: 500 mg 3 times daily for 5 to 7 days (HHS [OI adult 2015])

Renal Impairment
Herpes zoster:
CrCl ≥60 mL/minute: No dosage adjustment necessary
CrCl 40 to 59 mL/minute: Administer 500 mg every 12 hours
CrCl 20 to 39 mL/minute: Administer 500 mg every 24 hours
CrCl <20 mL/minute: Administer 250 mg every 24 hours
Hemodialysis: Administer 250 mg after each dialysis session.
Recurrent genital herpes: Treatment:
U.S. labeling (single-day regimen):
CrCl ≥60 mL/minute: No dosage adjustment necessary
CrCl 40 to 59 mL/minute: Administer 500 mg every 12 hours for 1 day
CrCl 20 to 39 mL/minute: Administer 500 mg as a single dose
CrCl <20 mL/minute: Administer 250 mg as a single dose
Hemodialysis: Administer 250 mg as a single dose after a dialysis session.
Canadian labeling:
CrCl >20 mL/minute/1.73 m^2: No dosage adjustment necessary
CrCl <20 mL/minute/1.73 m^2: Administer 125 mg every 24 hours
Hemodialysis: Administer 125 mg after each dialysis session.

Recurrent genital herpes: Suppression:
CrCl ≥40 mL/minute: No dosage adjustment necessary
CrCl 20 to 39 mL/minute: Administer 125 mg every 12 hours
CrCl <20 mL/minute: Administer 125 mg every 24 hours
Hemodialysis: Administer 125 mg after each dialysis session.

Recurrent herpes labialis: Treatment (single-dose regimen):
CrCl ≥60 mL/minute: No dosage adjustment necessary
CrCl 40 to 59 mL/minute: Administer 750 mg as a single dose
CrCl 20 to 39 mL/minute: Administer 500 mg as a single dose
CrCl <20 mL/minute: Administer 250 mg as a single dose
Hemodialysis: Administer 250 mg as a single dose after a dialysis session.

Recurrent orolabial/genital (mucocutaneous) herpes in HIV-infected patients:
CrCl ≥40 mL/minute: No dosage adjustment necessary
CrCl 20 to 39 mL/minute: Administer 500 mg every 24 hours
CrCl <20 mL/minute: Administer 250 mg every 24 hours
Hemodialysis: Administer 250 mg after each dialysis session.

Hepatic Impairment
Mild-to-moderate impairment: No dosage adjustment is necessary
Severe impairment: No dosage adjustment provided in manufacturer's labeling; has not been studied. However, a 44% decrease in the C_{max} of penciclovir (active metabolite) was noted in patients with mild-to-moderate impairment; impaired conversion of famciclovir to penciclovir may affect efficacy.

Dietary Considerations May be taken without regard to meals.

Administration May be administered without regard to meals.

Monitoring Parameters Periodic CBC during long-term therapy

Additional Information Most effective for herpes zoster if therapy is initiated within 48 hours of initial lesion. Resistance may occur by alteration of thymidine kinase, resulting in loss of or reduced penciclovir phosphorylation (cross-resistance occurs between acyclovir and famciclovir). When treatment for herpes labialis is initiated within 1 hour of symptom onset, healing time is reduced by ~2 days.

Dosage Forms Excipient information presented when available (limited, particularly for generics); consult specific product labeling.
Tablet, Oral:
Famvir: 125 mg, 250 mg, 500 mg
Generic: 125 mg, 250 mg, 500 mg

Famotidine (fa MOE ti deen)

Brand Names: US Acid Reducer Maximum Strength [OTC]; Acid Reducer [OTC]; Heartburn Relief Max St [OTC]; Heartburn Relief [OTC]; Pepcid
Brand Names: Canada Acid Control; Apo-Famotidine; Famotidine Omega; Maximum Strength Pepcid AC; Mylan-Famotidine; Pepcid AC; Pepcid Complete; Peptic guard; Teva-Famotidine; Ulcidine
Index Terms Pepcid
Pharmacologic Category Histamine H_2 Antagonist
Use Maintenance therapy and treatment of duodenal ulcer; treatment of gastroesophageal reflux disease (GERD), active benign gastric ulcer; pathological hypersecretory conditions
OTC labeling: Relief of heartburn, acid indigestion, and sour stomach
Pregnancy Considerations Adverse events have not been observed in animal reproduction studies; therefore, famotidine is classified as pregnancy category B. Famotidine crosses the placenta. An increased risk of congenital malformations or adverse events in the newborn has generally not been observed following maternal use of famotidine during pregnancy. Histamine H_2 antagonists have been evaluated for the treatment of gastroesophageal reflux disease (GERD), as well as gastric and duodenal ulcers, during pregnancy. Although if needed, famotidine is not the agent of choice. Histamine H_2 antagonists may be used for aspiration prophylaxis prior to cesarean delivery.
Breast-Feeding Considerations Famotidine is excreted into breast milk with peak concentrations occurring ~6 hours after the maternal dose. According to the manufacturer, the decision to continue or discontinue breast-feeding during therapy should take into account the risk of

exposure to the infant and the benefits of treatment to the mother.
Contraindications Hypersensitivity to famotidine, other H_2 antagonists, or any component of the formulation
Warnings/Precautions Modify dose in patients with moderate-to-severe renal impairment. Prolonged QT interval has been reported in patients with renal dysfunction. The FDA has received reports of torsade de pointes occurring with famotidine (Poluzzi, 2009). Relief of symptoms does not preclude the presence of a gastric malignancy. Reversible confusional states, usually clearing within 3-4 days after discontinuation, have been linked to use. Prolonged treatment (≥2 years) may lead to vitamin B_{12} malabsorption and subsequent vitamin B_{12} deficiency. The magnitude of the deficiency is dose-related and the association is stronger in females and those younger in age (<30 years); prevalence is decreased after discontinuation of therapy (Lam, 2013). Increased age (>50 years) and renal or hepatic impairment are thought to be associated.

Benzyl alcohol and derivatives: Some dosage forms may contain benzyl alcohol and/or sodium benzoate/benzoic acid; benzoic acid (benzoate) is a metabolite of benzyl alcohol; large amounts of benzyl alcohol (≥99 mg/kg/day) have been associated with a potentially fatal toxicity ("gasping syndrome") in neonates; the "gasping syndrome" consists of metabolic acidosis, respiratory distress, gasping respirations, CNS dysfunction (including convulsions, intracranial hemorrhage), hypotension, and cardiovascular collapse (AAP ["Inactive" 1997]; CDC, 1982); some data suggests that benzoate displaces bilirubin from protein binding sites (Ahlfors, 2001); avoid or use dosage forms containing benzyl alcohol and/or benzyl alcohol derivative with caution in neonates. See manufacturer's labeling.

OTC labeling: When used for self-medication, patients should be instructed not to use if they have difficulty swallowing, are vomiting blood, or have bloody or black stools. Not for use with other acid reducers.
Adverse Reactions Note: Agitation and vomiting have been reported in up to 14% of pediatric patients <1 year of age.
1% to 10%:
Central nervous system: Headache (5%), dizziness (1%)
Gastrointestinal: Diarrhea (2%), constipation (1%), necrotizing enterocolitis (VLBW neonates; Guillet, 2006)
<1% (Limited to important or life-threatening): Abdominal discomfort, acne, agitation, agranulocytosis, allergic reaction, alopecia, anaphylaxis, angioedema, anorexia, anxiety, arrhythmia, arthralgia, AV block, bronchospasm, cholestatic jaundice, confusion, conjunctival injection, depression, dry skin, facial edema, fatigue, fever, flushing, hallucinations, hepatitis, injection site reactions, insomnia, interstitial pneumonia, leukopenia, libido decreased, liver function tests increased, muscle cramps, nausea, palpitation, pancytopenia, paresthesia, pruritus, QT-interval prolongation, rash, rhabdomyolysis, seizure, somnolence, Stevens-Johnson syndrome, taste disorder, tinnitus, thrombocytopenia, torsade de pointes, toxic epidermal necrolysis, urticaria, vomiting, weakness, xerostomia
Drug Interactions
Metabolism/Transport Effects Substrate of OCT2
Avoid Concomitant Use
Avoid concomitant use of Famotidine with any of the following: Dasatinib; Delavirdine; PAZOPanib; Risedronate
Increased Effect/Toxicity
Famotidine may increase the levels/effects of: Dexmethylphenidate; Highest Risk QTc-Prolonging Agents; Methylphenidate; Moderate Risk QTc-Prolonging Agents; Risedronate; Saquinavir; Varenicline

The levels/effects of Famotidine may be increased by: BuPROPion; Mifepristone
Decreased Effect
Famotidine may decrease the levels/effects of: Atazanavir; Bosutinib; Cefditoren; Cefpodoxime; Cefuroxime; Cysteamine (Systemic); Dabrafenib; Dasatinib; Delavirdine; Erlotinib; Fosamprenavir; Gefitinib; Indinavir; Iron Salts; Itraconazole; Ketoconazole (Systemic); Ledipasvir; Mesalamine; Multivitamins/Minerals (with ADEK, Folate, Iron); Nelfinavir; Nilotinib; PAZOPanib; Posaconazole; Rilpivirine
Food Interactions Prolonged treatment (≥2 years) may lead to malabsorption of dietary vitamin B_{12} and subsequent vitamin B_{12} deficiency (Lam, 2013).
Preparation for Administration Solution for injection:
IV push: Dilute famotidine with NS (or another compatible solution) to a total of 5-10 mL (may also administer undiluted [Lipsy, 1995])

Infusion: Dilute with D_5W 100 mL or another compatible solution.

Storage/Stability

Oral:

Powder for oral suspension: Prior to mixing, dry powder should be stored at controlled room temperature of 25°C (77°F). Reconstituted oral suspension is stable for 30 days at room temperature; do not freeze.

Tablet: Store controlled room temperature. Protect from moisture.

IV:

Solution for injection: Prior to use, store at 2°C to 8°C (36°F to 46°F). If solution freezes, allow to solubilize at controlled room temperature. May be stored at room temperature for up to 3 months (data on file [Bedford Laboratories, 2011]).

IV push: Following preparation, solutions for IV push should be used immediately, or may be stored in refrigerator and used within 48 hours.

Infusion: Following preparation, the manufacturer states may be stored for up to 48 hours under refrigeration; however, solutions for infusion have been found to be physically and chemically stable for 7 days at room temperature.

Solution for injection, premixed bags: Store at controlled room temperature of 25°C (77°F); avoid excessive heat.

Mechanism of Action Competitive inhibition of histamine at H_2 receptors of the gastric parietal cells, which inhibits gastric acid secretion

Pharmacodynamics/Kinetics

Onset of action: Antisecretory effect: Oral: Within 1 hour; IV: Within 30 minutes

Peak effect: Antisecretory effect: Oral: Within 1 to 3 hours (dose-dependent)

Duration: Antisecretory effect: IV, Oral: 10 to 12 hours

Absorption: Oral: Incompletely absorbed

Distribution: V_d:

Infants: 0 to 3 months: 1.4 ± 0.4 L/kg to 1.8 ± 0.3 L/kg; >3 to 12 months: 2.3 ± 0.7 L/kg

Children: 2 ± 1.5 L/kg

Adolescents: 1.5 ± 0.4 L/kg

Adults: 0.94 to 1.33 L/kg

Protein binding: 15% to 20%

Metabolism: 30% to 35%; minimal first-pass metabolism; forms one metabolite (S-oxide)

Bioavailability: Oral: 40% to 45%

Half-life elimination:

Infants: 0 to 3 months: 8.1 ± 3.5 hours to 10.5 ± 5.4 hours; >3 to 12 months: 4.5 ± 1.1 hours

Children: 3.3 ± 2.5 hours

Adolescents: 2.3 ± 0.4 hours

Adults: 2.5 to 3.5 hours; prolonged with renal impairment; Oliguria: >20 hours; Anuria: 24 hours

Time to peak, serum: Oral: ~1 to 3 hours; orally disintegrating tablet: 2.5 hours

Excretion: Urine (25% to 30% [oral], 65% to 70% [IV] as unchanged drug)

Clearance:

Infants: 0 to 3 months: 0.13 to 0.21 ± 0.06 L/hour/kg; >3 to 12 months: 0.49 ± 0.17 L/hour/kg

Children 1 to 11 years: 0.54 ± 0.34 L/hour/kg

Adolescents: 0.48 ± 0.14 L/hour/kg

Adults: 0.39 ± 0.14 L/hour/kg

Dosing

Adult & Geriatric

Duodenal ulcer: Oral: Acute therapy: 40 mg/day at bedtime (or 20 mg twice daily) for 4-8 weeks; maintenance therapy: 20 mg/day at bedtime

Gastric ulcer: Oral: Acute therapy: 40 mg/day at bedtime

GERD: Oral: 20 mg twice daily for 6 weeks

Hypersecretory conditions: Oral: Initial: 20 mg every 6 hours, may increase in increments up to 160 mg every 6 hours

Esophagitis and accompanying symptoms due to GERD: Oral: 20 mg or 40 mg twice daily for up to 12 weeks

Peptic ulcer disease: Eradication of *Helicobacter pylori* (off-label use): Oral: 40 mg once daily; requires combination therapy with antibiotics

Stress ulcer prophylaxis, ICU patients (off-label use): Oral, IV, or nasogastric (NG) tube: 20 mg twice daily (ASHP, 1999; Baghaie, 1995); **Note:** Intended for patients with associated risk factors (eg, coagulopathy, mechanical ventilation for >48 hours, severe sepsis); discontinue use once risk factors have resolved. The Surviving Sepsis Campaign guidelines suggest the use of proton pump inhibitors rather than H_2 antagonist therapy (Dellinger, 2013).

Patients unable to take oral medication: IV: 20 mg every 12 hours

Heartburn, indigestion, sour stomach: OTC labeling: Oral: 10-20 mg every 12 hours; dose may be taken 15-60 minutes before eating foods known to cause heartburn

Pediatric Treatment duration and dose should be individualized

Peptic ulcer: 1-16 years:

Oral: 0.5 mg/kg/day at bedtime or divided twice daily (maximum dose: 40 mg/day); doses of up to 1 mg/kg/day have been used in clinical studies

IV: 0.25 mg/kg every 12 hours (maximum dose: 40 mg/day); doses of up to 0.5 mg/kg have been used in clinical studies

GERD: Oral:

<3 months: 0.5 mg/kg once daily

3-12 months: 0.5 mg/kg twice daily

1-16 years: 1 mg/kg/day divided twice daily (maximum dose: 40 mg twice daily); doses of up to 2 mg/kg/day have been used in clinical studies

Heartburn, indigestion, sour stomach: OTC labeling: Oral: Children ≥12 years: Refer to adult dosing.

Renal Impairment CrCl <50 mL/minute: Manufacturer's labeling: Administer 50% of dose **or** increase the dosing interval to every 36 to 48 hours (to limit potential CNS adverse effects).

Dietary Considerations May be taken without regard to meals.

Administration

Oral: May administer with antacids.

Suspension: Shake vigorously before use. May be taken without regard to meals.

Tablet: May be taken without regard to meals.

IV:

IV push: Inject over at least 2 minutes.

Solution for infusion: Administer over 15-30 minutes.

Dosage Forms Excipient information presented when available (limited, particularly for generics); consult specific product labeling. [DSC] = Discontinued product

Solution, Intravenous:

Generic: 20 mg (50 mL); 20 mg/2 mL (2 mL); 40 mg/4 mL (4 mL); 200 mg/20 mL (20 mL); 500 mg/50 mL (50 mL)

Solution, Intravenous [preservative free]:

Generic: 20 mg/2 mL (2 mL); 40 mg/4 mL (4 mL [DSC])

Suspension Reconstituted, Oral:

Pepcid: 40 mg/5 mL (50 mL) [contains methylparaben sodium, propylparaben sodium, sodium benzoate; cherry banana mint flavor]

Generic: 40 mg/5 mL (50 mL)

Tablet, Oral:

Acid Reducer: 10 mg

Acid Reducer Maximum Strength: 20 mg

Heartburn Relief: 10 mg

Heartburn Relief Max St: 20 mg

Pepcid: 20 mg

Pepcid: 20 mg [DSC] [scored]

Pepcid: 40 mg

Pepcid: 40 mg [DSC] [scored]

Generic: 10 mg, 20 mg, 40 mg

Extemporaneous Preparations An 8 mg/mL oral suspension may be made with tablets. Crush seventy 40 mg tablets in a mortar and reduce to a fine powder. Add small portions of sterile water and mix to a uniform paste. Mix while adding a 1:1 mixture of Ora-Plus® and Ora-Sweet® in incremental proportions to almost 350 mL; transfer to a calibrated bottle, rinse mortar with vehicle, and add quantity of vehicle sufficient to make 350 mL. Label "shake well". Stable for 95 days at room temperature.

Dentinger PJ, Swenson CF, and Anaizi NH, "Stability of Famotidine in an Extemporaneously Compounded Oral Liquid," *Am J Health Syst Pharm,* 2000, 57(14):1340-2.

Fat Emulsion (Plant Based)
(fat e MUL shun plant baste)

Brand Names: US Intralipid; Liposyn II [DSC]; Liposyn III; Nutrilipid

Brand Names: Canada Intralipid

Index Terms Clinolipid; Intravenous Fat Emulsion; Lipid Emulsion (Plant Based)

Pharmacologic Category Caloric Agent

Use Caloric/fatty acid source: Source of calories and essential fatty acids for patients requiring parenteral nutrition for extended periods of time (usually for longer than 5 days) or when oral or enteral nutrition is not possible, insufficient, or contraindicated; to prevent and treat essential fatty acid deficiency (except Clinolipid and Nutrilipid)

Dosing

Adult & Geriatric Note: At the onset of therapy, the patient should be observed for any immediate allergic reactions (eg, dyspnea, cyanosis, and fever).

Caloric source: IV: **Note:** Fat emulsion should not exceed 60% of the total daily calories.

Initial dose: 1-1.5 g/kg/day (not to exceed 500 mL Intralipid 10% or 20% or 330 mL Intralipid 30% [over 4-6 hours] on the first day of therapy); daily dose may be infused over 12-24 hours; maximum daily dose: 2.5 g/kg/day

Essential fatty acid deficiency (EFAD), prevention: IV: Administer at least 2% to 4% of total caloric intake as linoleic acid and 0.25% to 0.5% as alpha linolenic acid (Mirtallo, 2004; Mirtallo, 2010)

Essential fatty acid deficiency (EFAD), treatment: Intralipid, Liposyn III: IV: Administer 8% to 10% of total caloric intake as fat emulsion; may infuse up to once daily (Riella, 1975). If EFAD occurs with stress, the dosage needed to correct EFAD may be increased.

Local anesthetic toxicity (off-label use): 20%: IV: 1.5 **mL**/kg administered over 1 minute, followed immediately by an infusion of 0.25 **mL**/kg/minute. Continue chest compressions (lipid must circulate). Repeat the bolus 1-2 times as needed for persistent asystole, pulseless electrical activity, or re-emergence of hemodynamic instability. Increase the infusion rate to 0.5 **mL**/kg/minute if hemodynamic instability persists or recurs. Continue the infusion for at least 10 minutes after hemodynamic stability is restored; discontinue within 1 hour, if possible (ACMT, 2010; Neal, 2012).

Pediatric Note: At the onset of therapy, the patient should be observed for any immediate allergic reactions (eg, dyspnea, cyanosis, and fever).

Caloric source: IV: **Note:** Fat emulsion should not exceed 60% of the total daily calories.

Infants: Initial dose: 1-2 g/kg/day, increase by 0.5-1 g/kg/day to a maximum of 3 g/kg/day depending on needs/nutritional goals; daily dose may be infused over 24 hours (ASPEN Guidelines, 2002; ASPEN Pediatric Nutrition Support Core Curriculum, 2010)

Children 1-10 years: Initial dose: 1-2 g/kg/day, increase by 0.5-1 g/kg/day to a maximum of 2-3 g/kg/day depending on needs/nutritional goals; daily dose may be infused over 24 hours (ASPEN Guidelines, 2002; ASPEN Pediatric Nutrition Support Core Curriculum, 2010)

Adolescents: Initial dose: 1 g/kg/day (not to exceed 500 mL Intralipid 10% or 20% or 330 mL Intralipid 30% [over 4-6 hours] on the first day of therapy); increase by 1 g/kg/day to a maximum of 2.5 g/kg/day depending upon the needs/nutritional goals; daily dose may be infused over 12-24 hours (ASPEN Guidelines, 2002; ASPEN Pediatric Nutrition Support Core Curriculum, 2010)

Essential fatty acid deficiency (EFAD), prevention: IV: Children and Adolescents: Refer to adult dosing.

Essential fatty acid deficiency (EFAD), treatment: IV: Intralipid, Liposyn III: Children and Adolescents: Refer to adult dosing.

Renal Impairment There are no dosage adjustments provided in manufacturer's labeling; use with caution.

Hepatic Impairment There are no dosage adjustments provided in manufacturer's labeling; use with caution.

Additional Information Complete prescribing information should be consulted for additional detail.

Product Availability Clinolipid: FDA approved October 2013; anticipated availability is currently unknown. Refer to the prescribing information for additional information.

Dosage Forms Considerations Product oil source for Intralipid, Liposyn III, and Nutrilipid: soybean

Dosage Forms Excipient information presented when available (limited, particularly for generics); consult specific product labeling. [DSC] = Discontinued product

Emulsion, Intravenous:

Intralipid: 20% (100 mL, 250 mL, 500 mL, 1000 mL); 30% (500 mL) [contains egg yolk phospholipids, glycerin]

Liposyn II: 10% (500 mL [DSC])

Liposyn II: 20% (200 mL [DSC], 250 mL [DSC]) [contains egg phosphatides]

Liposyn III: 10% (200 mL, 250 mL, 500 mL); 20% (200 mL, 250 mL, 500 mL)

Liposyn III: 30% (500 mL [DSC]) [contains egg phosphatides]

Nutrilipid: 20% (250 mL, 500 mL, 1000 mL) [contains egg yolk phospholipids, glycerin]

◆ **Father John's® Plus [OTC]** *see* Chlorpheniramine, Phenylephrine, and Dextromethorphan *on page* 378

◆ **FazaClo** *see* CloZAPine *on page* 428

◆ **5-FC** *see* Flucytosine *on page* 778

◆ **FC1157a** *see* Toremifene *on page* 1816

◆ **FC1271a** *see* Ospemifene *on page* 1347

◆ **FE200486** *see* Degarelix *on page* 513

Febuxostat (feb UX oh stat)

Brand Names: US Uloric

Brand Names: Canada Uloric

Index Terms TEI-6720; TMX-67

Pharmacologic Category Antigout Agent; Xanthine Oxidase Inhibitor

Use Hyperuricemia: Chronic management of hyperuricemia in patients with gout. **Note:** Not recommended for treatment of asymptomatic hyperuricemia.

Pregnancy Considerations Animal studies have demonstrated increased neonatal mortality and reduction in weight gain, but not teratogenic effects. Use during pregnancy only if potential benefit to the mother outweighs potential risk to the fetus.

Breast-Feeding Considerations It is not known if febuxostat is excreted in breast milk. The U.S. manufacturer labeling recommends that caution be exercised when administering febuxostat to nursing women. Canadian labeling recommends avoiding use in nursing women.

Contraindications

Concurrent use with azathioprine or mercaptopurine

Canadian labeling: Additional contraindications (not in U.S. labeling): Hypersensitivity to febuxostat or any component of the formulation.

Warnings/Precautions Hypersensitivity and serious skin reactions (eg, Stevens-Johnson syndrome) have been reported, particularly in patients with prior skin reactions to allopurinol; use with caution if a patient has a history of hypersensitivity reaction to allopurinol. Administer concurrently with an NSAID or colchicine (up to 6 months) to prevent gout flare which may occur upon initiation of therapy. Do not use to treat asymptomatic or secondary hyperuricemia. Use in secondary hyperuricemia has not been studied; avoid use in patients at increased risk of urate formation (eg, malignancy and its treatment; Lesch-Nyhan syndrome). Postmarketing cases of hepatic failure (both fatal and nonfatal) have been reported (causal relationship has not been established). Significant hepatic transaminase elevations (>3 x ULN), MI, stroke and cardiovascular deaths have been reported in controlled trials (causal relationship not established). Monitor patients for signs/symptoms of MI and stroke. Liver function tests should be evaluated at baseline and periodically thereafter; evaluate liver function tests promptly in patients experiencing signs and symptoms of hepatic injury (eg, fatigue, anorexia, right upper quadrant pain, dark urine, jaundice). Interrupt therapy in patients who develop abnormal liver function tests (eg, ALT >3 x ULN); permanently discontinue use if no other explanation for the abnormalities is elucidated and in patients who develop ALT >3 x ULT **and** serum total bilirubin >2 x ULN. All other patients may be cautiously restarted on febuxostat. Use with caution in patients with severe hepatic impairment (Child-Pugh class C); has not been studied. Canadian labeling recommends avoiding use in severe impairment.

Use with caution in patients with severe renal impairment (CrCl <30 mL/minute); insufficient data. Canadian labeling recommends avoiding use in severe impairment or end-stage renal disease (ESRD) requiring dialysis. Formulation contains lactose; Canadian labeling recommends avoiding use in patients with hereditary conditions of galactose intolerance, Lapp lactase deficiency, or glucose-galactose malabsorption.

Adverse Reactions
1% to 10%:
Dermatologic: Rash (1% to 2%)
Gastrointestinal: Nausea (1%)
Hepatic: Liver function abnormalities (5% to 7%)
Neuromuscular & skeletal: Arthralgia (1%)
<1% (Limited to important or life-threatening): Aggression, agitation, alkaline phosphatase increased, alopecia, amylase increased, anaphylactic reaction, anaphylaxis, anemia, angina, angioedema, anorexia, anxiety, aPTT prolonged, atrial fibrillation/flutter, bicarbonate decreased, blurred vision, bruising, BUN increased, cardiac murmur, cerebrovascular accident, cholecystitis, cholelithiasis, constipation, CPK increased, creatinine increased, deafness, dehydration, depression, dermatitis, dermographism, diabetes mellitus, dyspepsia, dyspnea, ECG abnormal, eczema, edema, EEG abnormal, epistaxis, erectile dysfunction, flushing, gait disturbance, gastritis, gastroesophageal reflux, gingival pain, Guillain-Barré syndrome, gynecomastia, hair color change, hair growth abnormal, hematemesis, hematochezia, hematocrit decreased, hematuria, hemiparesis, hepatic failure (fatal and nonfatal), hepatic steatosis, hepatitis, hepatomegaly, herpes zoster, hot flashes, hyperchlorhydria, hypercholesterolemia, hyperglycemia, hyperhidrosis, hyperkalemia, hyperlipidemia, hypernatremia, hypersensitivity, hyper/hypotension, hypertriglyceridemia, hypokalemia, immune thrombocytopenia (ITP), incontinence, influenza-like syndrome, jaundice, joint swelling, lacunar infarction, LDH increased, lethargy, leukocytosis, leukopenia, libido decreased, lymphocytopenia, MCV increased, MI, migraine, mouth ulceration, muscle spasm/twitching, myalgia, nephrolithiasis, neutropenia, pain, palpitation, pancreatitis, pancytopenia, panic attack, paresthesia, peptic ulcer, personality change, petechiae, pharyngeal edema, photosensitivity, pollakiuria, proteinuria, PSA increased, psychotic behavior, PT prolonged, renal failure, respiratory infection, rhabdomyolysis, sinus bradycardia, skin/pigmentation discoloration, splenomegaly, Stevens-Johnson syndrome, stroke, tachycardia, taste altered, thrombocytopenia, TIA, tinnitus, tremor, TSH increased, tubulointerstitial nephritis, urinary tract infection, urine output decreased/increased, urticaria, vertigo, vomiting, weakness, weight gain/loss

Drug Interactions
Metabolism/Transport Effects None known.
Avoid Concomitant Use
Avoid concomitant use of Febuxostat with any of the following: AzaTHIOprine; Didanosine; Mercaptopurine; Pegloticase
Increased Effect/Toxicity
Febuxostat may increase the levels/effects of: AzaTHIOprine; Didanosine; Mercaptopurine; Pegloticase; Theophylline Derivatives
Decreased Effect There are no known significant interactions involving a decrease in effect.
Storage/Stability Store at 25°C (77°F); excursions permitted to 15°C to 30°C (59°F to 86°F). Protect from light.
Mechanism of Action Selectively inhibits xanthine oxidase, the enzyme responsible for the conversion of hypoxanthine to xanthine to uric acid thereby decreasing uric acid. At therapeutic concentration does not inhibit other enzymes involved in purine and pyrimidine synthesis.
Pharmacodynamics/Kinetics
Absorption: ≥49%
Distribution: V_{ss}: ~50 L
Protein binding: ~99%, primarily to albumin
Metabolism: Extensive conjugation via uridine diphosphate glucuronosyltransferases (UGTs) 1A1, 1A3, 1A9, and 2B7 and oxidation via cytochrome P450 (CYP) 1A2, 2C8, and 2C9 as well as non-P450 enzymes. Oxidation leads to formation of active metabolites (67M-1, 67M-2, 67M-4)
Half-life elimination: ~5 to 8 hours
Time to peak, plasma: 1 to 1.5 hours
Excretion: Urine (~49% mostly as metabolites, 3% as unchanged drug); feces (~45% mostly as metabolites, 12% as unchanged drug)
Dosing
Adult & Geriatric Note: It is recommended to take an NSAID or colchicine with initiation of therapy and may continue for up to 6 months to help prevent gout flares. If a gout flare occurs, febuxostat does not need to be discontinued.
Hyperuricemia: Oral:
U.S. labeling: Initial: 40 mg once daily; may increase to 80 mg once daily in patients who do not achieve a serum uric acid level <6 mg/dL after 2 weeks. The dose may be increased further to 120 mg once daily if clinically indicated (ACR guidelines [Khanna, 2012]).
Canadian labeling: 80 mg once daily

Renal Impairment
Mild-to-moderate impairment (CrCl 30 to 89 mL/minute): No dosage adjustment necessary
Severe impairment (CrCl <30 mL/minute): There are no dosage adjustments provided in the manufacturer's labeling (insufficient data); use caution (use not recommended in the Canadian labeling)
Dialysis: There are no dosage adjustments provided in the manufacturer's labeling; has not been studied (use not recommended in the Canadian labeling)
Hepatic Impairment
Mild-to-moderate impairment (Child-Pugh class A or B): No dosage adjustment necessary
Severe impairment (Child-Pugh class C): There are no dosage adjustments provided in the manufacturer's labeling (has not been studied); use caution (use not recommended in the Canadian labeling)
Dietary Considerations Take with or without meals or antacids.
Administration Administer with or without meals or antacids.
Monitoring Parameters Liver function tests at baseline and then periodically, serum uric acid levels (as early as 2 weeks after initiation); signs/symptoms of MI or stroke, signs/symptoms of hypersensitivity or severe skin reactions
Reference Range Uric acid, serum: An increase occurs during childhood
Adults:
Males: 3.4 to 7 mg/dL or slightly more
Females: 2.4 to 6 mg/dL or slightly more
Target: <6 mg/dL
Values >7 mg/dL are sometimes arbitrarily regarded as hyperuricemia, but there is no sharp line between normals on the one hand, and the serum uric acid of those with clinical gout. Normal ranges cannot be adjusted for purine ingestion, but high purine diet increases uric acid. Uric acid may be increased with body size, exercise, and stress.
Dosage Forms Excipient information presented when available (limited, particularly for generics); consult specific product labeling.
Tablet, Oral:
Uloric: 40 mg, 80 mg

◆ FEIBA *see* Anti-inhibitor Coagulant Complex (Human) on page 134

◆ FEIBA NF *see* Anti-inhibitor Coagulant Complex (Human) on page 134

◆ FEIBA VH *see* Anti-inhibitor Coagulant Complex (Human) on page 134

Felbamate (FEL ba mate)

Brand Names: US Felbatol
Pharmacologic Category Anticonvulsant, Miscellaneous
Use Monotherapy or adjunctive therapy in the treatment of partial seizures (with and without generalization); adjunctive therapy in the treatment of partial and generalized seizures associated with Lennox-Gastaut syndrome; not indicated for use as first-line treatment
Prescribing and Access Restrictions A patient "informed consent" form should be completed and signed by the patient and physician. Copies are available from MEDA Pharmaceuticals by calling 800-526-3840.
Medication Guide Available Yes
Dosing
Adult & Geriatric
Anticonvulsant, monotherapy: Oral:
Initial: 1200 mg/day in divided doses 3 or 4 times/day; titrate previously untreated patients under close clinical supervision, increasing the dosage in 600 mg increments every 2 weeks to 2400 mg/day based on clinical response and thereafter to 3600 mg/day if clinically indicated
Conversion to monotherapy: Initiate at 1200 mg/day in divided doses 3 or 4 times/day, reduce the dosage of the concomitant anticonvulsant(s) by 33% at the initiation of felbamate therapy; at week 2, increase the felbamate dosage to 2400 mg/day while reducing the dosage of the other anticonvulsant(s) up to an additional 33% of their original dosage; at week 3, increase the felbamate dosage up to 3600 mg/day and continue to reduce the dosage of the other anticonvulsant(s) as clinically indicated
Anticonvulsant, adjunctive therapy: Oral: Initial: 1200 mg/day in divided doses 3 or 4 times/day; increase once per week by 1200 mg/day increments up to 3600 mg/day in divided doses 3 or 4 times/day.

Note: Dose of concomitant carbamazepine, phenobarbital, phenytoin, or valproic acid should be decreased by 20% when initiating felbamate therapy. Further dosage reductions may be necessary as dose of felbamate is increased.

Pediatric

Anticonvulsant, monotherapy: Oral: Children >14 years: Refer to adult dosing.

Adjunctive therapy: Oral:

Children 2-14 years with Lennox-Gastaut syndrome: Initial: 15 mg/kg/day in divided doses 3 or 4 times/day; increase once per week by 15 mg/kg/day increments up to 45 mg/kg/day in divided doses 3 or 4 times/day.

Children >14 years: Refer to adult dosing.

Note: Dose of concomitant carbamazepine, phenobarbital, phenytoin, or valproic acid should be decreased by 20% when initiating felbamate therapy. Further dosage reductions may be necessary as dose of felbamate is increased.

Renal Impairment Use caution; reduce initial and maintenance doses by 50%.

Hepatic Impairment Use is contraindicated.

Additional Information Complete prescribing information should be consulted for additional detail.

Dosage Forms Excipient information presented when available (limited, particularly for generics); consult specific product labeling.

Suspension, Oral:

Felbatol: 600 mg/5 mL (237 mL, 946 mL)

Generic: 600 mg/5 mL (237 mL, 240 mL, 473 mL, 946 mL)

Tablet, Oral:

Felbatol: 400 mg, 600 mg [scored]

Generic: 400 mg, 600 mg

◆ **Felbatol** see Felbamate *on page 744*

◆ **Feldene** see Piroxicam *on page 1459*

Felodipine (fe LOE di peen)

Brand Names: Canada Plendil; Sandoz-Felodipine

Index Terms Plendil

Pharmacologic Category Antihypertensive; Calcium Channel Blocker; Calcium Channel Blocker, Dihydropyridine

Use

Hypertension: Treatment of hypertension

The 2014 guideline for the management of high blood pressure in adults (JNC 8) recommends initiation of pharmacologic treatment to lower blood pressure for the following patients (JNC8 [James, 2013]):

• Patients ≥60 years of age, with systolic blood pressure (SBP) ≥150 mm Hg or diastolic blood pressure (DBP) ≥90 mm Hg. Goal of therapy is SBP <150 mm Hg and DBP <90 mm Hg.

• Patients <60 years of age, with SBP ≥140 mm Hg or DBP ≥90 mm Hg. Goal of therapy is SBP <140 mm Hg and DBP <90 mm Hg.

• Patients ≥18 years of age with diabetes, with SBP ≥140 mm Hg or DBP ≥90 mm Hg. Goal of therapy is SBP <140 mm Hg and DBP <90 mm Hg.

• Patients ≥18 years of age with chronic kidney disease (CKD), with SBP ≥140 mm Hg or DBP ≥90 mm Hg. Goal of therapy is SBP <140 mm Hg and DBP <90 mm Hg.

In patients with chronic kidney disease (CKD), regardless of race or diabetes status, the use of an ACE inhibitor (ACEI) or angiotensin receptor blocker (ARB) as initial therapy is recommended to improve kidney outcomes. In the general nonblack population (without CKD) including those with diabetes, initial antihypertensive treatment should consist of a thiazide-type diuretic, calcium channel blocker, ACEI, or ARB. In the general black population (without CKD) including those with diabetes, initial antihypertensive treatment should consist of a thiazide-type diuretic or a calcium channel blocker **instead of** an ACEI or ARB.

Pregnancy Considerations Adverse events were observed in animal reproduction studies. Untreated chronic maternal hypertension is associated with adverse events in the fetus, infant, and mother. If treatment for hypertension during pregnancy is needed, other agents are preferred (ACOG, 2013). The Canadian labeling contraindicates use in women of childbearing potential and during pregnancy.

Breast-Feeding Considerations It is not known if felodipine is excreted in breast milk. Due to the potential for serious adverse reactions in the nursing infant, the U.S. labeling recommends a decision be made whether to discontinue nursing or to discontinue the drug, taking into account the importance of treatment to the mother. The Canadian labeling contraindicates use in nursing women.

Contraindications

Hypersensitivity to felodipine or any component of the formulation.

Canadian labeling: Additional contraindications (not in U.S. labeling): Hypersensitivity to other dihydropyridines; women of childbearing potential, in pregnancy, and during lactation.

Warnings/Precautions Increased angina and/or MI has occurred with initiation or dosage titration of dihydropyridine calcium channel blockers, reflex tachycardia may occur resulting in angina and/or MI in patients with obstructive coronary disease especially in the absence of concurrent beta-blockade. Use with extreme caution in patients with severe aortic stenosis. Use caution in patients with hypertrophic cardiomyopathy with outflow tract obstruction. The ACCF/AHA heart failure guidelines recommend to avoid use in patients with heart failure due to lack of benefit and/or worse outcomes with calcium channel blockers in general (Yancy, 2013). Elderly patients and patients with hepatic impairment should start off with a lower dose. Peripheral edema (dose dependent) is the most common side effect (occurs within 2 to 3 weeks of starting therapy). Symptomatic hypotension with or without syncope can rarely occur; blood pressure must be lowered at a rate appropriate for the patient's clinical condition. Potentially significant drug-drug interactions may exist, requiring dose or frequency adjustment, additional monitoring, and/or selection of alternative therapy. May contain lactose; if necessary, consider alternative agents in patients intolerant of lactose.

Adverse Reactions

>10%: Central nervous system: Headache (11% to 15%)

2% to 10%: Cardiovascular: Peripheral edema (2% to 17%), tachycardia (0.4% to 2.5%), flushing (4% to 7%)

<1% (Limited to important or life-threatening): Angina, angioedema, anxiety, arrhythmia, CHF, CVA, libido decreased, depression, dizziness, gingival hyperplasia, dyspnea, dysuria, gynecomastia, hypotension, impotence, insomnia, irritability, leukocytoclastic vasculitis, MI, nervousness, paresthesia, somnolence, syncope, urticaria, vomiting

Drug Interactions

Metabolism/Transport Effects Substrate of CYP3A4 (major); **Note:** Assignment of Major/Minor substrate status based on clinically relevant drug interaction potential; **Inhibits** CYP2C8 (moderate), CYP2C9 (weak), CYP2D6 (weak)

Avoid Concomitant Use

Avoid concomitant use of Felodipine with any of the following: Amodiaquine; Conivaptan; Fusidic Acid (Systemic); Idelalisib; Itraconazole; Ketoconazole (Systemic)

Increased Effect/Toxicity

Felodipine may increase the levels/effects of: Amifostine; Amodiaquine; Antipsychotic Agents (Second Generation [Atypical]); ARIPiprazole; Atosiban; Calcium Channel Blockers (Nondihydropyridine); CYP2C8 Substrates; DULoxetine; Fosphenytoin; Hypotension-Associated Agents; Levodopa; Magnesium Salts; Neuromuscular-Blocking Agents (Nondepolarizing); Nitroprusside; Phenytoin; Tacrolimus (Systemic)

The levels/effects of Felodipine may be increased by: Alfuzosin; Alpha1-Blockers; Antifungal Agents (Azole Derivatives, Systemic); Aprepitant; Barbiturates; Bitter Orange; Brimonidine (Topical); Calcium Channel Blockers (Nondihydropyridine); Cimetidine; Conivaptan; CycloSPORINE (Systemic); CYP3A4 Inhibitors (Moderate); CYP3A4 Inhibitors (Strong); Dapoxetine; Dasatinib; Diazoxide; Fluconazole; Fosaprepitant; Fusidic Acid (Systemic); Grapefruit Juice; Herbs (Hypotensive Properties); Idelalisib; Itraconazole; Ivacaftor; Ketoconazole (Systemic); Luliconazole; Macrolide Antibiotics; Magnesium Salts; Mifepristone; Molsidomine; Netupitant; Nicorandil; Obinutuzumab; Osimertinib; Palbociclib; Pentoxifylline; Phosphodiesterase 5 Inhibitors; Prostacyclin Analogues; Simeprevir; Stiripentol

Decreased Effect

Felodipine may decrease the levels/effects of: Clopidogrel

The levels/effects of Felodipine may be decreased by: Amphetamines; Barbiturates; Bosentan; Calcium Salts; CarBAMazepine; CYP3A4 Inducers (Moderate); CYP3A4 Inducers (Strong); Dabrafenib; Deferasirox; Efavirenz; Enzalutamide; Herbs (Hypertensive Properties); Melatonin; Methylphenidate; Mitotane; Nafcillin; Osimertinib; Phenytoin; Rifamycin Derivatives; Siltuximab; St Johns Wort; Tocilizumab; Yohimbine

Food Interactions

Ethanol: Ethanol increases felodipine absorption. Management: Monitor for a greater hypotensive effect if ethanol is consumed.

Food: Compared to a fasted state, felodipine peak plasma concentrations are increased up to twofold when taken after a meal high in fat or carbohydrates. Grapefruit juice similarly increases felodipine C_{max} by twofold. Increased therapeutic and vasodilator side effects, including severe hypotension and myocardial ischemia, may occur. Management: May be taken with a small meal that is low in fat and carbohydrates; avoid grapefruit juice during therapy.

Storage/Stability Store below 30°C (86°F); protect from light.

Mechanism of Action Inhibits calcium ions from entering the "slow channels" or select voltage-sensitive areas of vascular smooth muscle and myocardium during depolarization, producing a relaxation of coronary vascular smooth muscle and coronary vasodilation; increases myocardial oxygen delivery in patients with vasospastic angina

Pharmacodynamics/Kinetics

Onset of action: Antihypertensive: 2 to 5 hours

Duration of antihypertensive effect: 24 hours

Absorption: 100%; Absolute: 20% due to first-pass effect

Protein binding: >99%

Metabolism: Hepatic; CYP3A4 substrate (major); extensive first-pass effect

Half-life elimination: Immediate release: 11 to 16 hours

Time to peak: 2.5 to 5 hours

Excretion: Urine (70% as metabolites); feces 10%

Dosing

Adult Hypertension: Oral: Initial: 5 mg once daily; adjust dose as needed at no less than 2-week intervals. Usual dose range: 5 to 10 once daily (ASH/ISH [Weber, 2014]) although some patients may benefit from 2.5 mg once daily. Doses >10 mg daily are associated with greater antihypertensive effects but also a large increase in the incidence of peripheral edema and other vasodilatory adverse effects.

Geriatric Hypertension: Oral: Consider lower initial doses (eg, 2.5 mg once daily) and titrate at no less than 2-week intervals to response (Aronow, 2011). The Canadian labeling recommends a maximum dose of 10 mg daily.

Pediatric Hypertension: Children ≥6 years and Adolescents (off-label use): Oral: Initial: 2.5 mg once daily; may increase as needed at no less than 2-week intervals to a maximum of 10 mg once daily (NHLBI, 2011)

Renal Impairment No dosage adjustment necessary.

Hepatic Impairment Initial: 2.5 mg once daily; monitor blood pressure closely during titration. The Canadian labeling recommends a maximum dose of 10 mg daily.

Dietary Considerations May be taken with a small meal that is low in fat and carbohydrates.

Administration Swallow tablet whole; tablet should not be divided, crushed, or chewed. May be administered without food or with a small meal that is low in fat and carbohydrates.

Dosage Forms Excipient information presented when available (limited, particularly for generics); consult specific product labeling.

Tablet Extended Release 24 Hour, Oral:

Generic: 2.5 mg, 5 mg, 10 mg

Fenofibrate and Derivatives

(fen oh FYE brate & dah RIV ah tives)

Brand Names: US Antara; Fenoglide; Fibricor; Lipofen; Lofibra; Tricor; Triglide; Trilipix

Brand Names: Canada Apo-Feno-Micro; Apo-Feno-Super; Apo-Fenofibrate; Ava-Fenofibrate Micro; Dom-Fenofibrate Micro; Feno-Micro-200; Fenofibrate Micro; Fenofibrate-S; Lipidil EZ; Lipidil Micro; Lipidil Supra; Mylan-Fenofibrate Micro; Novo-Fenofibrate Micronized; PHL-Fenofibrate Micro; PMS-Fenofibrate Micro; PRO-Feno-Super; Q-Fenofibrate Micro; ratio-Fenofibrate MC; Riva-Fenofibrate Micro; Sandoz-Fenofibrate E; Sandoz-Fenofibrate S; Teva-Fenofibrate S

Index Terms ABT-335; Choline Fenofibrate; Fenofibric Acid; Procetofene; Proctofene

Pharmacologic Category Antilipemic Agent, Fibric Acid

Use

Hypercholesterolemia or mixed dyslipidemia: Adjunctive therapy to diet for the reduction of low-density lipoprotein cholesterol (LDL-C), total cholesterol (total-C), triglycerides, and apolipoprotein B (apo B), and to increase high-density lipoprotein cholesterol (HDL-C) in adults with primary hypercholesterolemia or mixed dyslipidemia (Fredrickson types IIa and IIb). Use lipid-altering agents in addition to a diet restricted in saturated fat and cholesterol when response to diet and nonpharmacological interventions alone has been inadequate.

Hypertriglyceridemia: Adjunctive therapy to diet for treatment of adult patients with severe hypertriglyceridemia (Fredrickson types IV and V hyperlipidemia).

Pregnancy Considerations Maternal toxicity was observed in pregnant rats at doses approximately equivalent to the human dose; adverse events have not been observed in animal reproduction studies done in rabbits. Reports of using fenofibrate during pregnancy are limited (Goldberg, 2012; Sunman, 2012; Whitten, 2011). Other agents are generally preferred if treatment for hypertriglyceridemia during pregnancy (Berglund, 2012) or treatment of lipid disorders in women of reproductive age (NCEP, 2001) is required. Use during pregnancy is specifically contraindicated in Canadian product labeling; some products recommend using effective birth control when treating women of reproductive age and discontinuing therapy several months prior to conception if planning a pregnancy.

Breast-Feeding Considerations It is not known if fenofibrate is excreted in breast milk. Use is contraindicated in nursing women. The manufacturer recommends a decision be made whether to discontinue nursing or to discontinue the drug, taking into account the importance of treatment to the mother.

Medication Guide Available Yes

Contraindications

Hypersensitivity to fenofibrate or fenofibric acid or any component of the formulation; active liver disease, including primary biliary cirrhosis and unexplained, persistent liver function abnormality; severe renal dysfunction or end-stage renal disease (ESRD), including those receiving dialysis; preexisting gallbladder disease; breast-feeding

Documentation of allergenic cross-reactivity for fibrates is limited. However, because of similarities in chemical structure and/or pharmacologic actions, the possibility of cross-sensitivity cannot be ruled out with certainty.

Canadian labeling: Additional contraindications (not in US labeling): Pregnancy; known photoallergy or phototoxic reaction during treatment with fibrates or ketoprofen

Lipidil EZ, Lipidil Micro, Lipidil Supra: Additional contraindications: Allergy to soya lecithin or peanut or arachis oil; chronic or acute pancreatitis; patients <18 years of age; coadministration with HMG-CoA reductase inhibitors in patients with a predisposition for myopathy.

Warnings/Precautions Secondary causes of hyperlipidemia should be ruled out prior to therapy. Hepatic transaminases can become significantly elevated (dose-related); hepatocellular, chronic active, and cholestatic hepatitis have been reported after weeks to several years of therapy. Regular monitoring of liver function tests is required; discontinue therapy in patients whose enzyme levels persist above 3 times the upper limit of normal. Use with caution in patients with mild to moderate renal impairment; dosage adjustment may be required. Contraindicated with severe renal impairment including those receiving dialysis. Avoid use of Triglide in patients with mild or moderate renal impairment. Contraindicated active liver disease, including primary biliary cirrhosis and unexplained persistent liver function abnormalities. Increases in serum creatinine (>2 mg/dL) have been observed with use; clinical significance unknown. These elevations tend to return to baseline following discontinuation of fenofibrate. Fenofibrate has been shown to increase creatinine production (unknown mechanism) resulting in an equal increase of creatinuria thereby demonstrating that the increase does not reflect a reduction in creatinine clearance (Hottelart, 2002). Monitor renal function in patients with renal impairment and consider monitoring patients with increased risk for developing renal impairment (eg, elderly and patients with diabetes). May cause cholelithiasis.

Therapy should be discontinued in patients who develop markedly elevated CPK concentrations or if myopathy/myositis is suspected or diagnosed. No incremental benefit of combination therapy on cardiovascular morbidity and mortality over statin monotherapy has been established. In patients with type 2 diabetes mellitus, neither fenofibrate monotherapy nor the addition of fenofibrate to simvastatin compared to placebo has been shown to reduce cardiovascular disease morbidity and mortality in patients with type 2 diabetes. Potentially significant drug-drug interactions may exist, requiring dose or frequency adjustment, additional monitoring, and/or selection of alternative therapy. In combination with HMG-CoA reductase inhibitors, fenofibrate is generally regarded as safer than gemfibrozil due to limited pharmacokinetic interaction with statins. According to the 2013 ACC/AHA Blood Cholesterol Guidelines, fenofibrate may be considered in patients on low- or moderate-intensity statin therapy (ie, statin therapy intended to lower LDL-C by <30% or ~30% to 50%, respectively) only if the benefits from atherosclerotic cardiovascular disease (ASCVD) risk reduction or triglyceride lowering when triglycerides are >500 mg/dL, outweigh the potential risk for adverse effects (Stone, 2013). Therapy should be withdrawn if an adequate response is not obtained after 2 to 3 months of therapy at the maximal daily dose. In patients with severe hypertriglyceridemia, the occurrence of pancreatitis may represent a failure of efficacy, a direct effect of the drug, or obstruction of the common bile duct due to biliary tract stone or sludge formation. A paradoxical, severe, and reversible decrease in HDL-C (as low as 2 mg/dL) with a simultaneous decrease in apolipoprotein A1 has been reported within 2 weeks to years after initiation of fibrate therapy; clinical significance unknown. Monitor HDL-C within a few months of initiation of therapy and discontinue if HDL-C becomes severely depressed; do not restart therapy. The occurrence of pancreatitis may represent a failure of efficacy in patients with severely elevated triglycerides. May cause mild to moderate decreases in hemoglobin, hematocrit, and WBC upon initiation of therapy which usually stabilizes with long-term therapy. Agranulocytosis and thrombocytopenia have been reported. Periodic monitoring of blood counts is recommended during the first year of therapy.

Hypersensitivity reactions have been reported. Use has been associated with pulmonary embolism (PE) and deep vein thrombosis (DVT). Use with caution in patients with risk factors for VTE. Dose adjustment may be required for elderly patients.

Some products may contain soya lecithin or peanut or arachis oil; use is contraindicated in patients with a soya lecithin allergy or a peanut or arachis allergy for applicable formulations.

Adverse Reactions Frequency not always defined.
Cardiovascular: Pulmonary embolism (≤5%), thrombophlebitis (≤5%)
Central nervous system: Pain (1% to 4%), dizziness (≥3%), insomnia (≥3%), fatigue (2% to 3%)
Dermatologic: Skin rash (1%), urticaria (1%), Stevens-Johnson syndrome, toxic epidermal necrolysis
Gastrointestinal: Abdominal pain (5%), diarrhea (≥3%), dyspepsia (≥3%), cholecystitis (requiring surgery: 2%), constipation (2%)
Hematologic & oncologic: Agranulocytosis, decreased hematocrit (acute; levels stabilize with chronic therapy), decreased hemoglobin (acute; levels stabilize with chronic therapy), decreased white blood cell count (acute; levels stabilize with chronic therapy), thrombocytopenia
Hepatic: Increased serum ALT (≤13%; >3 x ULN; dose dependent), increased serum AST (≤13%; >3 x ULN; dose dependent), abnormal hepatic function tests (8%), cholestatic hepatitis, chronic active hepatitis, hepatocellular hepatitis
Neuromuscular & skeletal: Arthralgia (≥3%), limb pain (≥3%), myalgia (≥3%), increased creatine phosphokinase (3%), myopathy, toxic myopathy
Respiratory: Nasopharyngitis (≥3%), sinusitis (≥3%), upper respiratory tract infection (≥3%), rhinitis (2%)
<1% (Limited to important or life-threatening): Acute renal failure, anemia, decreased HDL cholesterol, hepatic cirrhosis, hepatitis, muscle spasm, myalgia, pancreatitis, renal failure, rhabdomyolysis

Drug Interactions
Metabolism/Transport Effects Inhibits CYP2A6 (weak), CYP2C8 (weak), CYP2C9 (weak)
Avoid Concomitant Use
Avoid concomitant use of Fenofibrate and Derivatives with any of the following: Amodiaquine; Ciprofibrate

Increased Effect/Toxicity
Fenofibrate and Derivatives may increase the levels/effects of: Amodiaquine; Colchicine; Ezetimibe; HMG-CoA Reductase Inhibitors; Sulfonylureas; Vitamin K Antagonists; Warfarin

The levels/effects of Fenofibrate and Derivatives may be increased by: Acipimox; Ciprofibrate; CycloSPORINE (Systemic); Raltegravir; Tacrolimus (Systemic)
Decreased Effect
Fenofibrate and Derivatives may decrease the levels/effects of: Chenodiol; CycloSPORINE (Systemic); Ursodiol

The levels/effects of Fenofibrate and Derivatives may be decreased by: Bile Acid Sequestrants
Food Interactions
Antara (micronized): When administered under fasted conditions or with a low-fat meal, the extent of absorption and the time to peak did not change; however peak concentrations were increased in the presence of a low-fat meal. When administered with a high fat meal, a 26% increase in the AUC and 108% increase in the peak concentration were seen in comparison to the fasted state. Management: Administer with or without food.
Fenoglide: When administered with a high-fat meal, the peak concentration was increased by 44% as compared to fasting conditions. Management: Administer with meals.
Fibricor: When administered with a high-fat meal, the peak concentration was decreased by ~35% while AUC remained unchanged as compared to fasting conditions. Management: Administer with or without food.
Lipidil EZ [Canadian product]: Bioavailability was not significantly different when administered under fasting and nonfasting conditions. Management: Administer with or without food.
Lipidil Micro [Canadian product]: In comparison with non-micronized fenofibrate formulations, micronized fenofibrate is better absorbed when administered with a low-fat meal; absorption is less influenced by a higher fat content meal. Management: Administer with meals.
Lipidil Supra [Canadian product]: In general, fenofibrate absorption is low and variable when administered under fasting conditions; absorption is increased when administered with food. Management: Administer with meals.
Lipofen: When administered with a low-fat and high-fat meal, the extent of absorption is increased by ~25% and ~58%, respectively, as compared to fasting conditions. Management: Administer with meals.
Lofibra (micronized) capsules: Absorption is increased by ~35% under fed as compared to fasting conditions. Management: Administer with meals.
Lofibra tablets: Peak concentrations and AUC were not significantly different when a single dose was administered under fasting and nonfasting conditions. Management: Administer with or without food.
TriCor: Peak concentrations and AUC were not significantly different when a single dose was administered under fasting and nonfasting conditions. Management: Administer with or without food.
Triglide: When administered with food, the rate of absorption was increased ~55% as compared to fasting conditions; the AUC remained unchanged. Management: Administer with or without food.
Trilipix: Peak concentrations and AUC were not significantly different when a single dose was administered under fasting and nonfasting conditions. Management: Administer with or without food.
Storage/Stability Store at 25°C (77°F); excursions are permitted between 15°C and 30°C (59°F and 86°F). Protect Fibricor, Lipofen, Lofibra, TriCor, Triglide, and Trilipix from moisture. Protect Fibricor, Lofibra tablets, Lipofen, and Triglide from light.
Canadian products: Lipidil EZ, Lipidil Micro, Lipidil Supra: Store at 15°C to 25°C (59°F to 77°F). Protect Lipidil EZ, Lipidil Micro, and Lipidil Supra from moisture. Protect Lipidil EZ and Lipidil Supra from light.
Mechanism of Action Fenofibric acid, an agonist for the nuclear transcription factor peroxisome proliferator-activated receptor-alpha (PPAR-alpha), downregulates apoprotein C-III (an inhibitor of lipoprotein lipase) and upregulates the synthesis of apolipoprotein A-I, fatty acid transport protein, and lipoprotein lipase resulting in an increase in VLDL catabolism, fatty acid oxidation, and elimination of triglyceride-rich particles; as a result of a decrease in VLDL levels, total plasma triglycerides are reduced by 30% to 60%; modest increase in HDL occurs in some hypertriglyceridemic patients.
Pharmacodynamics/Kinetics
Absorption: Increased when taken with meals
Distribution: Widely to most tissues
Protein binding: ~99%

Metabolism: Fenofibrate is metabolized in the tissue and plasma via esterases to the active form, fenofibric acid; fenofibric acid then undergoes inactivation by glucuronidation hepatically or renally

Bioavailability: Fenofibric acid: ~81%

Half-life elimination: Fenofibric acid: Mean: 20 hours (range: 10 to 35 hours); half-life prolonged in patients with renal impairment

Time to peak: 2 to 8 hours

Excretion: Urine (~60% as metabolites); feces (25%); hemodialysis has no effect on removal of fenofibric acid from plasma

Dosing

Adult Note: At least 2 to 3 months of therapy is required to determine efficacy.

Hypertriglyceridemia: Oral: Initial:

Antara (micronized): 30 to 90 mg once daily; maximum dose: 90 mg once daily

Fenoglide: 40 to 120 mg once daily; maximum dose: 120 mg once daily

Fibricor: 35 to 105 mg once daily; maximum dose: 105 mg once daily

Lipidil EZ [Canadian product]: 145 mg once daily; maximum dose: 145 mg once daily

Lipidil Micro [Canadian product]: 200 mg once daily; maximum dose: 200 mg once daily

Lipidil Supra [Canadian product]: 160 mg once daily; maximum dose: 200 mg once daily

Lipofen: 50 to 150 mg once daily; maximum dose: 150 mg once daily

Lofibra (micronized): 67 to 200 mg once daily; maximum dose: 200 mg once daily

Lofibra (tablets): 54 to 160 mg once daily; maximum dose: 160 mg once daily

TriCor: 48 to 145 mg once daily; maximum dose: 145 mg once daily

Triglide: 160 mg once daily

Trilipix: 45 to 135 mg once daily; maximum dose: 135 mg once daily

Hypercholesterolemia or mixed hyperlipidemia: Oral: Initial:

Antara (micronized): 90 mg once daily; maximum dose: 90 mg once daily

Fenoglide: 120 mg once daily

Fibricor: 105 mg once daily

Lipidil EZ [Canadian product]: 145 mg once daily; maximum dose: 145 mg once daily

Lipidil Micro [Canadian product]: 200 mg once daily; maximum dose: 200 mg once daily

Lipidil Supra [Canadian product]: 160 mg once daily; maximum dose: 200 mg once daily

Lipofen: 150 mg once daily

Lofibra (micronized): 200 mg once daily

Lofibra (tablets): 160 mg once daily

TriCor: 145 mg once daily

Triglide: 160 mg once daily

Trilipix: 135 mg once daily

Geriatric Oral: Initial: Adjust dosage based on renal function; additional product-specific recommendations for initial dose:

Lipidil EZ [Canadian product]: 48 mg once daily

Lofibra (micronized): 67 mg once daily

Lofibra (tablets): 54 mg once daily

Renal Impairment Monitor renal function and lipid panel before adjusting.

Antara (micronized):

CrCl >80 mL/minute or eGFR ≥60 mL/minute/1.73 m^2: No dosage adjustment necessary.

CrCl >30 to 80 mL/minute or eGFR 30 to 59 mL/minute/1.73 m^2: Initiate at 30 mg once daily

CrCl ≤30 mL/minute or eGFR <30 mL/minute/1.73 m^2: Use is contraindicated.

Dialysis: Use is contraindicated.

Fenoglide:

CrCl >80 mL/minute or eGFR ≥60 mL/minute/1.73 m^2: No dosage adjustment necessary.

CrCl >30 to 80 mL/minute or eGFR 30 to 59 mL/minute/1.73 m^2: Initiate at 40 mg once daily

CrCl ≤30 mL/minute or eGFR <30 mL/minute/1.73 m^2: Use is contraindicated.

Dialysis: Use is contraindicated.

Fibricor:

CrCl >80 mL/minute: No dosage adjustment necessary.

CrCl >30 to 80 mL/minute: Initiate at 35 mg once daily

CrCl ≤30 mL/minute: Use is contraindicated.

Dialysis: Use is contraindicated.

Lipidil EZ [Canadian product]: **Note:** Interrupt treatment in patients with an increase in creatinine concentrations >50% the upper limit of normal (ULN).

CrCl >50 mL/minute: No dosage adjustment necessary.

CrCl 20 to 50 mL/minute: Initiate at 48 mg once daily

CrCl <20 mL/minute: Use is contraindicated.

Dialysis: Use is contraindicated.

Lipidil Micro [Canadian product]: **Note:** Interrupt treatment in patients with an increase in creatinine concentrations >50% the upper limit of normal (ULN).

CrCl >85 mL/minute (women) or >95 mL/minute (men): No dosage adjustment necessary.

CrCl 20 to 85 mL/minute (women) or 20 to 95 mL/minute (men): Initiate therapy with Lipidil EZ formulation with a dose of 48 mg once daily.

CrCl <20 mL/minute: Use is contraindicated.

Dialysis: Use is contraindicated.

Lipidil Supra [Canadian product]: **Note:** Interrupt treatment in patients with an increase in creatinine concentrations >50% the upper limit of normal (ULN).

CrCl >100 mL/minute: No dosage adjustment necessary.

CrCl 20 to 100 mL/minute: Initiate at 100 mg once daily

CrCl <20 mL/minute: Use is contraindicated.

Dialysis: Use is contraindicated.

Lipofen:

eGFR ≥90 mL/minute/1.73 m^2: No dosage adjustment necessary.

eGFR 30 to 89 mL/minute/1.73 m^2: Initiate at 50 mg once daily

eGFR <30 mL/minute/1.73 m^2: Use is contraindicated.

Dialysis: Use is contraindicated.

Lofibra (micronized):

CrCl >80 mL/minute: No dosage adjustment necessary.

CrCl >30 to 80 mL/minute: Initiate at 67 mg once daily

CrCl ≤30 mL/minute: Use is contraindicated.

Dialysis: Use is contraindicated.

Lofibra (tablets):

eGFR ≥60 mL/minute/1.73 m^2: No dosage adjustment necessary.

eGFR 30 to 59 mL/minute/1.73 m^2: Initiate at 54 mg once daily

eGFR <30 mL/minute/1.73 m^2: Use is contraindicated.

Dialysis: Use is contraindicated.

TriCor:

eGFR ≥60 mL/minute/1.73 m^2: No dosage adjustment necessary.

eGFR 30 to 59 mL/minute/1.73 m^2: Initiate at 48 mg once daily

eGFR <30 mL/minute/1.73 m^2: Use is contraindicated.

Dialysis: Use is contraindicated.

Triglide:

CrCl >80 mL/minute or eGFR ≥60 mL/minute/1.73 m^2: No dosage adjustment necessary.

CrCl >30 to 80 mL/minute or eGFR 30 to 59 mL/minute/1.73 m^2: Avoid use.

CrCl ≤30 mL/minute or eGFR <30 mL/minute/1.73 m^2: Use is contraindicated.

Dialysis: Use is contraindicated.

Trilipix:

eGFR ≥60 mL/minute/1.73 m^2: No dosage adjustment necessary.

eGFR 30 to 59 mL/minute/1.73 m^2: Initiate at 45 mg once daily.

eGFR <30 mL/minute/1.73 m^2: Use is contraindicated.

Dialysis: Use is contraindicated.

Hepatic Impairment Use is contraindicated. Regular monitoring of liver function tests is required; discontinue therapy in patients whose enzyme levels persist above 3 times the upper limit of normal.

Adjustment for Toxicity

Cholelithiasis: Discontinue if gallstones are found upon gallbladder studies.

CPK elevation, myopathy, and/or myositis: Discontinue therapy if the patient develops markedly elevated CPK concentrations or if myopathy/myositis is suspected or diagnosed.

HDL-C reductions: Permanently discontinue therapy if HDL-C becomes severely depressed; monitor HDL-C concentrations until returned to baseline.

Dietary Considerations

Antara, Fibricor, Lipidil EZ [Canadian product], Lofibra tablets, TriCor, Triglide, Trilipix: May be taken with or without food.

Fenoglide, Lipidil Micro [Canadian product], Lipidil Supra [Canadian product], Lipofen, Lofibra (micronized capsules): Take with meals.

Administration

Antara, Fibricor, Lipidil EZ [Canadian product], Lofibra tablets, TriCor, Triglide, Trilipix: Administer with or without food. Swallow whole; do not open (capsules), crush, dissolve, or chew.

Lipidil Micro [Canadian product]; Lofibra (micronized) capsules: Administer with meals.

Fenoglide, Lipofen, Lipidil Supra [Canadian product]: Administer with meals. Swallow whole; do not open (capsules), crush, dissolve, or chew.

Monitoring Parameters Periodic blood counts during first year of therapy. Monitor lipid profile periodically. Monitor LFTs regularly and discontinue therapy if levels remain >3 times normal limits. Monitor renal function in patients with renal impairment or in those at increased risk for developing renal impairment.

2013 ACC/AHA Blood Cholesterol Guideline recommendations (Stone, 2013): Evaluate renal status at baseline, within 3 months after initiation, and every 6 months thereafter.

Dosage Forms Considerations
Micronized formulations: Antara, Lofibra capsules
Strength of choline fenofibrate products are expressed in terms of fenofibric acid.

Dosage Forms Excipient information presented when available (limited, particularly for generics); consult specific product labeling. [DSC] = Discontinued product
Capsule, Oral, as fenofibrate:
Antara: 30 mg, 43 mg [DSC] [contains fd&c blue #2 (indigotine), fd&c yellow #10 (quinoline yellow)]
Antara: 90 mg [contains brilliant blue fcf (fd&c blue #1), fd&c yellow #10 (quinoline yellow), fd&c yellow #6 (sunset yellow)]
Antara: 130 mg [DSC] [contains fd&c blue #2 (indigotine), fd&c yellow #10 (quinoline yellow)]
Lipofen: 50 mg [contains brilliant blue fcf (fd&c blue #1), fd&c blue #2 (indigotine), fd&c red #40, fd&c yellow #10 (quinoline yellow)]
Lipofen: 150 mg
Lofibra: 67 mg, 134 mg, 200 mg
Generic: 43 mg, 50 mg, 67 mg, 130 mg, 134 mg, 150 mg, 200 mg
Capsule Delayed Release, Oral, as choline fenofibrate:
Trilipix: 45 mg
Trilipix: 135 mg [contains fd&c blue #2 (indigotine)]
Generic: 45 mg, 135 mg
Tablet, Oral, as fenofibrate:
Fenoglide: 40 mg, 120 mg
Lofibra: 54 mg [contains fd&c yellow #10 aluminum lake]
Lofibra: 160 mg
Tricor: 48 mg [contains fd&c blue #2 aluminum lake, fd&c yellow #10 aluminum lake, fd&c yellow #6 aluminum lake, soybean lecithin]
Tricor: 145 mg [contains soybean lecithin]
Triglide: 160 mg
Generic: 40 mg, 48 mg, 54 mg, 120 mg, 145 mg, 160 mg
Tablet, Oral, as fenofibric acid:
Fibricor: 35 mg, 105 mg
Generic: 35 mg, 105 mg

◆ Fenofibrate Micro (Can) *see* Fenofibrate and Derivatives *on page 746*

◆ Fenofibrate-S (Can) *see* Fenofibrate and Derivatives *on page 746*

◆ Fenofibric Acid *see* Fenofibrate and Derivatives *on page 746*

◆ Fenoglide *see* Fenofibrate and Derivatives *on page 746*

Fenoldopam (fe NOL doe pam)

Brand Names: US Corlopam
Index Terms Fenoldopam Mesylate
Pharmacologic Category Antihypertensive; Dopamine Agonist
Additional Appendix Information
Hypertension *on page 1996*
Use Treatment of severe hypertension (up to 48 hours in adults), including in patients with renal compromise; short-term (up to 4 hours) blood pressure reduction in pediatric patients
Pregnancy Considerations Fetal harm was not observed in animal studies; however, safety and efficacy have not been established for use during pregnancy. Use during pregnancy only if clearly needed.
Breast-Feeding Considerations It is not known if fenoldopam is excreted in breast milk. The manufacturer recommends that caution be exercised when administering fenoldopam to nursing women.
Contraindications There are no contraindications listed within the manufacturer's approved labeling.
Warnings/Precautions Use with caution in patients with open-angle glaucoma or intraocular hypertension; fenoldopam causes a dose-dependent increase in intraocular pressure. Dose-related tachycardia can occur, especially at infusion rates >0.1 mcg/kg/minute. Use with extreme caution in patients with obstructive coronary disease or ongoing angina pectoris; can increase myocardial oxygen demand due to tachycardia leading to angina pectoris. Serum potassium concentrations <3 mEq/L were observed

within 6 hours of fenoldopam initiation; monitor potassium concentrations appropriately. Use with caution in patients with increased intracranial pressure; use has not been studied in this population. For continuous infusion only (no bolus doses). Some dosage forms may contain propylene glycol; large amounts are potentially toxic and have been associated hyperosmolality, lactic acidosis, seizures, and respiratory depression; use caution (AAP, 1997; Zar, 2007). Contains sulfites; may cause allergic reaction in susceptible individuals.

Adverse Reactions
≥5%:
Cardiovascular: Cutaneous flushing, hypotension
Central nervous system: Headache
Gastrointestinal: Nausea
<5%:
Cardiovascular: Angina, bradycardia, chest pain, extrasystoles, heart failure, MI, orthostatic hypotension, palpitation, ST-T abnormalities, T-wave inversion, tachycardia
Central nervous system: Anxiety, dizziness, fever, insomnia
Endocrine & metabolic: Hyperglycemia, hypokalemia, LDH increased
Gastrointestinal: Abdominal pain/fullness, constipation, diarrhea, vomiting
Genitourinary: Urinary tract infection
Hematologic: Bleeding, leukocytosis
Hepatic: Transaminases increased
Local: Injection site reactions
Neuromuscular & skeletal: Back pain, limb cramps
Ocular: Intraocular pressure increased
Renal: BUN increased, creatinine increased, oliguria
Respiratory: Dyspnea, nasal congestion
Miscellaneous: Diaphoresis

Drug Interactions
Metabolism/Transport Effects None known.
Avoid Concomitant Use There are no known interactions where it is recommended to avoid concomitant use.
Increased Effect/Toxicity
Fenoldopam may increase the levels/effects of: Amifostine; Antipsychotic Agents (Second Generation [Atypical]); DULoxetine; Hypotension-Associated Agents; Levodopa

The levels/effects of Fenoldopam may be increased by: Alfuzosin; Barbiturates; Brimonidine (Topical); Diazoxide; Herbs (Hypotensive Properties); Molsidomine; Nicorandil; Obinutuzumab; Pentoxifylline; Phosphodiesterase 5 Inhibitors; Prostacyclin Analogues
Decreased Effect
The levels/effects of Fenoldopam may be decreased by: Amphetamines; Herbs (Hypertensive Properties); Methylphenidate; Yohimbine
Storage/Stability Store undiluted product at 2°C to 30°C (35°F to 86°F). Following dilution, store at room temperature and use solution within 24 hours.
Mechanism of Action A selective postsynaptic dopamine agonist (D_1-receptors) which exerts hypotensive effects by decreasing peripheral vasculature resistance with increased renal blood flow, diuresis, and natriuresis; 6 times as potent as dopamine in producing renal vasodilatation; has minimal adrenergic effects
Pharmacodynamics/Kinetics
Onset of action: IV: Children: 5 minutes; Adults: 10 minutes; **Note:** Majority of effect of a given infusion rate is attained within 15 minutes.
Duration: IV: 1 hour
Distribution: V_d: 0.6 L/kg
Half-life elimination: IV: Children: 3-5 minutes; Adults: ~5 minutes
Metabolism: Hepatic via methylation, glucuronidation, and sulfation; the 8-sulfate metabolite may have some activity; extensive first-pass effect
Excretion: Urine (90%); feces (10%)
Clearance: Children: 3 L/hour/kg
Dosing
Adult & Geriatric Hypertension, severe: IV: Initial: 0.03-0.1 mcg/kg/minute (associated with less reflex tachycardia); may be increased in increments of 0.05-0.1 mcg/kg/minute every 15 minutes until target blood pressure is reached; the maximal infusion rate reported in clinical studies was 1.6 mcg/kg/minute
Pediatric Hypertension, severe: IV: Initial: 0.2 mcg/kg/minute; may be increased to dosages of 0.3-0.5 mcg/kg/minute every 20-30 minutes (maximum dose: 0.8 mcg/kg/minute); limited to short-term (4 hours) use
Renal Impairment No dosage adjustment required; the effects of hemodialysis on fenoldopam have not been evaluated.
Hepatic Impairment No dosage adjustment required.

◀ **Usual Infusion Concentrations: Pediatric IV infusion:** 60 **mcg**/mL

Usual Infusion Concentrations: Adult IV infusion: 10 mg in 250 mL (concentration: 40 **mcg**/mL) of D_5W or NS

Administration For continuous IV infusion only.

Monitoring Parameters Blood pressure, heart rate, ECG; serum potassium concentrations (eg, every 6 hours)

Dosage Forms Excipient information presented when available (limited, particularly for generics); consult specific product labeling.

Solution, Intravenous:
Corlopam: 10 mg/mL (1 mL); 20 mg/2 mL (2 mL) [contains propylene glycol, sodium metabisulfite]
Generic: 10 mg/mL (1 mL); 20 mg/2 mL (2 mL)

◆ Fenoldopam Mesylate *see* Fenoldopam *on page 749*

◆ Feno-Micro-200 (Can) *see* Fenofibrate and Derivatives *on page 746*

Fenoprofen (fen oh PROE fen)

Brand Names: US Nalfon
Index Terms Fenoprofen Calcium
Pharmacologic Category Nonsteroidal Anti-inflammatory Drug (NSAID), Oral
Use
Osteoarthritis: Relief of the signs and symptoms of osteoarthritis.
Pain: Relief of mild to moderate pain in adult patients.
Rheumatoid arthritis (RA): Relief of the signs and symptoms of RA.
Medication Guide Available Yes
Dosing
Adult & Geriatric
Rheumatoid arthritis, osteoarthritis: Oral: 400 to 600 mg 3 to 4 times daily; maximum dose: 3.2 g/day
Mild to moderate pain: Oral: 200 mg every 4 to 6 hours as needed; maximum dose: 3.2 g/day
Renal Impairment There are no dosage adjustments provided in the manufacturer's labeling. Contraindicated in patients with significantly impaired renal function; not recommended in patients with advanced renal disease. Not removed by hemodialysis.
Hepatic Impairment There are no dosage adjustments provided in the manufacturer's labeling.
Additional Information Complete prescribing information should be consulted for additional detail.
Dosage Forms Excipient information presented when available (limited, particularly for generics); consult specific product labeling.
Capsule, Oral:
Nalfon: 400 mg [contains brilliant blue fcf (fd&c blue #1), fd&c red #40]
Generic: 400 mg
Tablet, Oral:
Generic: 600 mg

◆ Fenoprofen Calcium *see* Fenoprofen *on page 750*

FentaNYL (FEN ta nil)

Brand Names: US Abstral; Actiq; Duragesic; Fentora; Ionsys; Lazanda; Onsolis [DSC]; Subsys
Brand Names: Canada Abstral; Apo-Fentanyl Matrix; Co-Fentanyl; Duragesic MAT; Fentanyl Citrate Injection, USP; Fentora; Mylan-Fentanyl Matrix Patch; PMS-Fentanyl MTX; RAN-Fentanyl Matrix Patch; Sandoz Fentanyl Patch; Teva-Fentanyl
Index Terms Fentanyl Citrate; Fentanyl Hydrochloride; Fentanyl Patch; Ionsys; OTFC (Oral Transmucosal Fentanyl Citrate)
Pharmacologic Category Analgesic, Opioid; Anilidopiperidine Opioid; General Anesthetic
Additional Appendix Information
Opioid Conversion Table and Morphine Equivalent Dose Table *on page 1955*
Use
Injection:
Pain management: Relief of pain, preoperative medication.
Surgery: Adjunct to general or regional anesthesia.
Transdermal device (eg, Ionsys): **Postoperative pain, acute:** Short-term management of acute postoperative pain in adult patients requiring opioid analgesia in the hospital.
Limitations of use: Only for use in patients who are alert enough and have adequate cognitive ability to understand the directions for use. Not for home use. Transdermal device is for use only in patients in the hospital. Discontinue treatment with the device before patients

leave the hospital. The device is for use after patients have been titrated to an acceptable level of analgesia using alternate opioid analgesics.
Transdermal patch (eg, Duragesic): **Chronic pain:** Management of pain in opioid-tolerant patients, severe enough to require daily, around-the-clock, long-term opioid treatment and for which alternative treatment options are inadequate.
Limitations of use: Because of the risks of addiction, abuse, and misuse with opioids, even at recommended doses, and because of the greater risks of overdose and death with extended-release opioid formulations, reserve fentanyl transdermal patch for use in patients for whom alternative treatment options (eg, nonopioid analgesics, immediate-release opioids) are ineffective, not tolerated, or would be otherwise inadequate to provide sufficient management of pain.
Transmucosal lozenge (eg, Actiq), buccal tablet (Fentora), buccal film (Onsolis), nasal spray (Lazanda), sublingual tablet (Abstral), sublingual spray (Subsys): **Cancer pain:** Management of breakthrough cancer pain in opioid-tolerant patients who are already receiving and who are tolerant to around-the-clock opioid therapy for their underlying persistent cancer pain.
Note: "Opioid-tolerant" patients are defined as patients who are taking at least:
Oral morphine 60 mg/day, **or**
Transdermal fentanyl 25 mcg/hour, **or**
Oral oxycodone 30 mg/day, **or**
Oral hydromorphone 8 mg/day, **or**
Oral oxymorphone 25 mg/day, **or**
Equianalgesic dose of another opioid for at least 1 week
Pregnancy Considerations Adverse events have been observed in some animal reproduction studies. Fentanyl crosses the placenta.

Fentanyl injection may be used for the management of pain during labor (ACOG, 2002). When used for pain relief during labor, opioids may temporarily affect the heart rate of the fetus (ACOG, 2002). Transient muscular rigidity has been observed in the neonate with fentanyl; symptoms of respiratory or neurological depression were not different than those observed in infants of untreated mothers.

[U.S. Boxed Warning]: Prolonged maternal use of opioids during pregnancy can cause neonatal withdrawal syndrome in the newborn which may be life-threatening if not recognized and treated according to protocols developed by neonatology experts. If prolonged opioid therapy is required in a pregnant woman, ensure treatment is available and warn patient of risk to the neonate. If chronic opioid exposure occurs in pregnancy, adverse events in the newborn (including withdrawal) may occur; monitoring of the neonate is recommended. The minimum effective dose should be used if opioids are needed (Chou, 2009). Symptoms characteristic of neonatal abstinence syndrome have been observed following chronic fentanyl use in pregnant women. Neonatal abstinence syndrome following opioid exposure may present with autonomic (eg, fever, temperature instability), gastrointestinal (eg, diarrhea, vomiting, poor feeding/weight gain), or neurologic (eg, high pitched crying, increased muscle tone, irritability, seizure, tremor) symptoms (Dow, 2012; Hudak, 2012).

Long-term opioid use may cause secondary hypogonadism, which may lead to sexual dysfunction or infertility (Brennan, 2013).

Transdermal patch, transmucosal lozenge, nasal spray (Lazanda), sublingual tablet, sublingual spray (Subsys), buccal tablet (Fentora), and buccal film (Onsolis) are not recommended for analgesia during labor and delivery. Transdermal patch Canadian labeling contraindicates use in pregnant women and during labor and delivery.
Breast-Feeding Considerations Fentanyl is excreted in low concentrations in breast milk and breast-feeding is not recommended by the manufacturers.

Parenteral opioids used during labor have the potential to interfere with a newborn's natural reflex to nurse within the first few hours after birth. When needed, a short-acting opioid, such as fentanyl, is preferred for women who is nursing (Montgomery, 2012)

Breast-feeding is considered acceptable following single doses to the mother; however, limited information is available when used long-term (Spigset, 2000). Nursing infants exposed to large doses of opioids should be monitored for apnea and sedation (Montgomery, 2012).

Note: Transdermal patch, transmucosal lozenge, sublingual tablet, sublingual spray (Subsys), buccal tablet (Fentora), and buccal film (Onsolis) are not recommended in nursing women due to potential for sedation and/or

respiratory depression. Transdermal patch Canadian labeling contraindicates use in nursing women. Sublingual tablet Canadian labeling recommends that breast-feeding not be started until 48 hours after the last dose of fentanyl.

Prescribing and Access Restrictions As a requirement of the REMS program, access is restricted.

Transmucosal immediate-release fentanyl products (eg, sublingual tablets and spray, oral lozenges, buccal tablets and soluble film, nasal spray) are only available through the Transmucosal Immediate-Release Fentanyl (TIRF) REMS ACCESS program. Enrollment in the program is required for outpatients, prescribers for outpatient use, pharmacies (inpatient and outpatient), and distributors. Enrollment is not required for inpatient administration (eg, hospitals, hospices, long-term care facilities), inpatients, and prescribers who prescribe to inpatients. Further information is available at 1-866-822-1483 or at www.TIRFREMSaccess.com

Note: Effective December, 2011, individual REMs programs for TIRF products were combined into a single access program (TIRF REMS Access). Prescribers and pharmacies that were enrolled in at least one individual REMS program for these products will automatically be transitioned to the single access program.

Medication Guide Available Yes

Contraindications Hypersensitivity to fentanyl or any component of the formulation

Additional contraindications for transdermal device (eg, Ionsys): Significant respiratory depression; acute or severe bronchial asthma; known or suspected paralytic ileus or GI obstruction; hypersensitivity to cetylpyridinium chloride (eg, Cepacol)

Additional contraindications for transdermal patches (eg, Duragesic): Severe respiratory disease or depression including acute asthma (unless patient is mechanically ventilated); paralytic ileus; patients requiring short-term therapy, management of acute or intermittent pain, postoperative or mild pain, and in patients who are **not** opioid tolerant

Additional contraindications for transmucosal buccal tablets (Fentora), buccal films (Onsolis), lozenges (eg, Actiq), sublingual tablets (Abstral), sublingual spray (Subsys), nasal spray (Lazanda): Contraindicated in the management of acute or postoperative pain (including headache, migraine, or dental pain), and in patients who are **not** opioid tolerant. Abstral and Onsolis also are contraindicated for acute pain management in the emergency room.

Canadian labeling: Additional contraindication (not in US labeling):

Injection: Septicemia; severe hemorrhage or shock; local infection at proposed injection site; disturbances in blood morphology and/or anticoagulant therapy or other concomitant drug therapy or medical conditions which could contraindicate the technique of epidural administration

Sublingual tablets (Abstral): Severe respiratory depression or severe obstructive lung disease.

Transdermal patch: Hypersensitivity to other opioids; suspected surgical abdomen (eg, acute appendicitis, pancreatitis); known or suspected mechanical GI obstruction (eg, bowel obstruction, strictures); acute alcoholism, delirium tremens, and convulsive disorders; severe CNS depression, increased cerebrospinal or intracranial pressure and head injury; concurrent use of monoamine oxidase (MAO) inhibitors or within 14 days of therapy; women who are nursing, pregnant, or during labor and delivery

Warnings/Precautions An opioid-containing analgesic regimen should be tailored to each patient's needs and based upon the type of pain being treated (acute versus chronic), the route of administration, degree of tolerance for opioids (naive versus chronic user), age, weight, and medical condition. The optimal analgesic dose varies widely among patients. Doses should be titrated to pain relief/prevention. May cause CNS depression, which may impair physical or mental abilities; patients must be cautioned about performing tasks which require mental alertness (eg, operating machinery or driving). Effects may be potentiated when used with other sedative drugs or ethanol. Fentanyl shares the toxic potentials of opioid agonists, and precautions of opioid agonist therapy should be observed; use with caution in patients with bradycardia or bradyarrhythmias; rapid IV infusion may result in skeletal muscle and chest wall rigidity leading to respiratory distress and/or apnea, bronchoconstriction, laryngospasm; inject slowly over 3 to 5 minutes. Monitor for respiratory depression in patients with significant chronic obstructive pulmonary disease or cor pulmonale, and patients having a substantially decreased respiratory reserve, hypoxia, hypercarbia, or preexisting respiratory depression,

particularly when initiating therapy and titrating with fentanyl; even therapeutic doses may decrease respiratory drive to the point of apnea. Consider the use of alternative nonopioid analgesics in these patients. **[U.S. Boxed Warning]: Users are exposed to the risks of addiction, abuse, and misuse, potentially leading to overdose and death. Assess each patient's risk prior to prescribing; monitor all patients for development of these behaviors or conditions.** The risk for opioid abuse is increased in patients with a personal or family history of substance abuse (including drug or alcohol abuse or addiction) or mental illness (eg, major depression). Tolerance or drug dependence may result from extended use. The elderly may be particularly susceptible to the CNS depressant and constipating effects of opioids. Use extreme caution in patients with COPD or other chronic respiratory conditions (some products may be contraindicated). Use caution with biliary tract impairment, pancreatitis, head injuries (some products may be contraindicated), morbid obesity, renal impairment, or hepatic dysfunction. **[U.S. Boxed Warning]: Use with strong or moderate CYP3A4 inhibitors may result in increased effects and potentially fatal respiratory depression. In addition, discontinuation of a concomitant CYP 3A4 inducer may result in increased fentanyl concentrations. Monitor patients receiving any CYP 3A4 inhibitor or inducer.** Concurrent use of mixed agonist/antagonist analgesics (eg, pentazocine, nalbuphine, butorphanol) or partial agonist (eg, buprenorphine) analgesics may precipitate withdrawal symptoms and/or reduced analgesic efficacy in patients following prolonged therapy with mu opioid agonists. Abrupt discontinuation following prolonged use may also lead to withdrawal symptoms. May aggravate convulsions in patients with convulsive disorders, and may induce or aggravate seizures in some clinical settings. Monitor patients with a history of seizure disorders for worsened seizure control. May cause severe hypotension including orthostatic hypotension and syncope in ambulatory patients; risk is increased in patients whose ability to maintain blood pressure has already been compromised by a reduced blood volume; monitor these patients for signs of hypotension after initiating therapy. Potentially significant interactions may exist, requiring dose or frequency adjustment, additional monitoring, and/or selection of alternative therapy.

Pediatric patients: **[U.S. Boxed Warning]: Buccal film, buccal tablet, nasal spray, sublingual tablet, sublingual spray, and lozenge preparations contain an amount of medication that can be fatal to children. Keep all used and unused products out of the reach of children at all times and discard products properly.** Patients and caregivers should be counseled on the dangers to children including the risk of exposure to partially-consumed products.

[U.S. Boxed Warning] Abstral, Actiq, Duragesic, Fentora, Ionsys, Lazanda, Onsolis, Subsys: May cause serious, life-threatening, or fatal respiratory depression, even when used as recommended. Monitor closely for respiratory depression, especially during initiation or dose escalation. Abstral, Actiq, Duragesic, Fentora, Lazanda, Onsolis, or Subsys should only be prescribed for opioid-tolerant patients. Risk of respiratory depression increased in elderly patients, debilitated patients, and patients with conditions associated with hypoxia or hypercapnia; usually occurs after administration of initial dose in nontolerant patients or when given with other drugs that depress respiratory function.

Transmucosal (buccal film/tablet, sublingual spray/tablet, lozenge) and nasal spray: **[U.S. Boxed Warning]: Transmucosal and nasal fentanyl formulations are contraindicated in the management of acute or postoperative pain and in opioid nontolerant patients.** Should be used only for the care of opioid-tolerant cancer patients with breakthrough pain and is intended for use by specialists who are knowledgeable in treating cancer pain. **[U.S. Boxed Warning]: Substantial differences exist in the pharmacokinetic profile of fentanyl products. Do not convert patients on a mcg-per-mcg basis from one fentanyl product to another fentanyl product; the substitution of one fentanyl product for another fentanyl product may result in a fatal overdose. [U.S. Boxed Warning]: Available only through the TIRF REMS ACCESS program, a restricted distribution program with outpatients, prescribers who prescribe to outpatients, pharmacies (inpatient and outpatient), and distributor-required enrollment.** Avoid use of topical nasal decongestants (eg, oxymetazoline) during episodes of rhinitis when using fentanyl nasal spray; response to fentanyl may be delayed or reduced. Avoid use of sublingual spray in cancer patients with grade 2 or higher mucositis (fentanyl exposure increased); use with caution

in patients with grade 1 mucositis, and closely monitor for respiratory and CNS depression.

Transdermal device: **[U.S. Boxed Warning]: Available only through a restricted program under a Risk Evaluation and Mitigation Strategy (REMS) called the Ionsys REMS Program. [U.S. Boxed Warning]: For use only in patients in the hospital. Discontinue treatment before patients leave the hospital. Only the patient should activate Ionsys dosing. Accidental exposure to an intact Ionsys device or to the hydrogel component, especially by children, through contact with skin or contact with mucous membranes, can result in a fatal overdose of fentanyl.** Following accidental contact with the device or its components, immediately rinse the affected area thoroughly with water. Do not use soap, alcohol, or other solvent because they may enhance the drug's ability to penetrate the skin; monitor for signs of respiratory or CNS depression. If the device is not handled correctly using gloves, healthcare professionals are at risk of accidental exposure to a fatal overdose of fentanyl. Ionsys device is considered magnetic resonance unsafe. The device contains metal parts and must be removed and properly disposed of before an MRI procedure to avoid injury to the patient and damage to device. It is unknown if exposure to an MRI procedure increases release of fentanyl from the device. Monitor any patients wearing the device with inadvertent exposure to an MRI for signs of CNS and respiratory depression. Use of Ionsys device during cardioversion, defibrillation, X-ray, CT, or diathermy can damage the device from the strong electromagnetic fields set up by these procedures. The device contains radio-opaque components and may interfere with an X-ray image or CT scan. Remove and properly dispose of the device prior to cardioversion, defibrillation, X-ray, CT, or diathermy. Avoid contact with synthetic materials (such as carpeted flooring) to reduce the possibility of electrostatic discharge and damage to the device. Avoid exposing the device to electronic security systems to reduce the possibility of damage. Use near communications equipment (eg, base stations for radio telephones and land mobile radios, amateur radio, AM and FM radio broadcast and TV broadcast Radio) and Radio Frequency Identification (RFID) transmitters can damage the device. Depending on the rated maximum output power and frequency of the transmitter, the recommended separation distance between the device and communications equipment or the RFID transmitter ranges between 0.12 and 23 meters. The low-level electrical current provided by the device does not result in electromagnetic interference with other electromechanical devices like pacemakers or electrical monitoring equipment. If exposure to the procedures listed above, electronic security systems, electrostatic discharge, communications equipment, or RFID transmitters occurs, and if the device does not appear to function normally, remove and replace with a new device. Topical skin reactions (erythema, sweating, vesicles, papules/pustules) may occur with use and are typically limited to the application site area. If a severe skin reaction is observed, remove device and discontinue further use. Ionsys is not for use in patients who are not alert and able to follow directions; avoid use in patients with impaired consciousness or coma. Avoid use in patients with circulatory shock; may cause vasodilation that can further reduce cardiac output and blood pressure.

Transdermal patch (Duragesic): **[U.S. Boxed Warning]: Transdermal patch is contraindicated for use as an as-needed analgesic, in the management of acute or postoperative pain, or in patients who are opioid non-tolerant. Monitor closely for respiratory depression during use, particularly during initiation of therapy or after dose increases.** Should only be prescribed by health care professionals who are knowledgeable in the use of potent opioids in the management of chronic pain. For patients undergoing cordotomy or other pain-relieving procedures, the Canadian labeling recommends withholding transdermal fentanyl within 72 hours prior to the procedure and in the immediate postoperative period; dose adjustment may be necessary upon resuming therapy. **[U.S. Boxed Warning]: Exposure of application site and surrounding area to direct external heat sources (eg, heating pads, electric blankets, heat or tanning lamps, sunbathing, hot tubs) may increase fentanyl absorption and has resulted in fatalities. Patients who experience fever or increase in core body temperature should be monitored closely.** Serum fentanyl concentrations may increase by approximately one-third for patients with a body temperature of 40°C (104°F) secondary to a temperature-dependent increase in fentanyl release from the patch and increased skin permeability. **[U.S. Boxed Warning]: Accidental exposure to fentanyl transdermal patch has resulted in fatal overdose in children and adults. Strict adherence to recommended handling and disposal instructions is necessary to prevent accidental exposures.** Avoid unclothed/unwashed application site exposure, inadvertent person-to-person patch transfer (eg, while hugging), incidental exposure (eg, sharing same bed, sitting on patch), intentional exposure (eg, chewing), or accidental exposure by caregivers when applying/removing patch. **[U.S. Boxed Warning]: Prolonged maternal use of opioids during pregnancy can cause neonatal withdrawal syndrome in the newborn which may be life-threatening if not recognized and treated according to protocols developed by neonatology experts. If prolonged opioid therapy is required in a pregnant woman, patient should be warned of risk to the neonate and ensure treatment is available.** Should be applied only to intact skin. Use of a patch that has been cut, damaged, or altered in any way may result in overdosage. Patients who experience adverse reactions should be monitored for at least 24 hours after removal of the patch. Drug continues to be absorbed from the skin for 24 hours or more following removal of the patch. May contain conducting metal (eg, aluminum); remove patch prior to MRI.

Adverse Reactions

>10%:

Central nervous system: Confusion, dizziness, drowsiness, fatigue, headache, sedation

Endocrine & metabolic: Dehydration

Gastrointestinal: Constipation, nausea, vomiting

Local: Application site erythema (transdermal device)

Neuromuscular & skeletal: Weakness

Respiratory: Dyspnea

1% to 10%:

Cardiovascular: Atrial fibrillation, bigeminy, cardiac arrhythmia, cardiorespiratory arrest, chest pain, deep vein thrombosis, edema, hypertension, hypotension, myocardial infarction, orthostatic hypotension, palpitations, peripheral edema, pulmonary embolism (nasal spray), sinus tachycardia, syncope, tachycardia, vasodilatation

Central nervous system: Abnormal dreams, abnormal gait, abnormality in thinking, agitation, altered sense of smell, amnesia, anxiety, ataxia, chills, depression, disorientation, dysphoria, euphoria, hallucination, hypertonia, hypoesthesia, hypothermia, insomnia, irritability, lack of concentration, lethargy, malaise, mental status changes, migraine, nervousness, neuropathy, paranoia, paresthesia, restlessness, speech disturbance, stupor, vertigo, withdrawal syndrome

Dermatologic: Alopecia, cellulitis, decubitus ulcer, diaphoresis, erythema, exfoliation of skin (application site, transdermal device), hyperhidrosis, local papules (application site, transdermal device), night sweats, pallor, papule, pruritus, pustules (application site, transdermal device), skin rash, vesicobullous rash (application site, transdermal device)

Endocrine & metabolic: Hot flash, hypercalcemia, hyperglycemia, hypoalbuminemia, hypocalcemia, hypokalemia, hypomagnesemia, hyponatremia, weight loss

Gastrointestinal: Abdominal distention, abdominal pain, anorexia, decreased appetite, diarrhea, dysgeusia, dyspepsia, dysphagia (buccal tablet/film/sublingual spray), flatulence, gastritis, gastroenteritis, gastroesophageal reflux disease, gastrointestinal hemorrhage, gastrointestinal ulcer (gingival, lip, mouth; transmucosal use/nasal spray), gingival pain (buccal tablet), gingivitis (lozenge), glossitis (lozenge), hematemesis, intestinal obstruction, periodontal abscess (lozenge/buccal tablet), rectal pain, stomatitis (lozenge/buccal tablet/sublingual tablet/sublingual spray), tongue disease (sublingual tablet), xerostomia

Genitourinary: Urinary retention (3%), difficulty in micturition, dysuria, erectile dysfunction, mastalgia, urinary incontinence, urinary tract infection, urinary urgency, vaginal hemorrhage, vaginitis

Hematologic & oncologic: Anemia (3%), bruise, leukopenia, lymphadenopathy, neutropenia, thrombocytopenia

Hepatic: Ascites, increased serum alkaline phosphatase, increased serum AST, jaundice

Hypersensitivity: Hypersensitivity

Infection: Abscess

Local: Application site burning (transdermal device), application site discharge (transdermal device), application site edema (transdermal device), application site irritation, application site itching (transdermal device), application site pain, application site rash (transdermal device), application site vesicles (transdermal device)

Neuromuscular & skeletal: Arthralgia, back pain, leg cramps, limb pain, myalgia, tremor

Ophthalmic: Blepharoptosis, blurred vision, diplopia, dry eye syndrome, strabismus, swelling of eye, visual disturbance

Renal: Renal failure

Respiratory: Apnea, asthma, atelectasis, bronchitis, cough, dyspnea (exertional), epistaxis, flu-like symptoms, hemoptysis, hyperventilation, hypoventilation, hypoxia, laryngitis, nasal congestion (nasal spray), nasal discomfort (nasal spray), nasopharyngitis, pharyngitis, pharyngolaryngeal pain, pneumonia, postnasal drip (nasal spray), rhinitis, rhinorrhea (nasal spray), sinusitis, upper respiratory tract infection, wheezing

Miscellaneous: Fever, wound healing impairment

<1% (Limited to important or life-threatening): Anaphylaxis, angina pectoris, bradycardia, chest wall rigidity (high dose IV), drug dependence (physical and psychological; with prolonged use), esophageal stenosis, exfoliative dermatitis, fecal impaction, genitourinary tract spasm, gingival hemorrhage (lozenge), gum line erosion (lozenge), hematuria, hostility, hypoglycemia, hypogonadism (Brennan 2013; Debono 2011), local hemorrhage (transdermal device), localized infection (transdermal device), local tissue necrosis (transdermal device), nocturia, oliguria, pancytopenia, pleural effusion, polyuria, seizure, skin erosion (application site, transdermal device), tooth loss (lozenge)

Drug Interactions

Metabolism/Transport Effects Substrate of CYP3A4 (major); **Note:** Assignment of Major/Minor substrate status based on clinically relevant drug interaction potential

Avoid Concomitant Use

Avoid concomitant use of FentaNYL with any of the following: Azelastine (Nasal); Conivaptan; Crizotinib; Dapoxetine; Eluxadoline; Enzalutamide; Fusidic Acid (Systemic); Idelalisib; MAO Inhibitors; Mifepristone; Mixed Agonist / Antagonist Opioids; Orphenadrine; Paraldehyde; Thalidomide

Increased Effect/Toxicity

FentaNYL may increase the levels/effects of: Alcohol (Ethyl); Alvimopan; Antipsychotic Agents; Azelastine (Nasal); Beta-Blockers; Calcium Channel Blockers (Nondihydropyridine); CNS Depressants; Desmopressin; Diuretics; Eluxadoline; Hydrocodone; MAO Inhibitors; Methotrimeprazine; Metoclopramide; Metyrosine; Orphenadrine; Paraldehyde; Pramipexole; Ramosetron; ROPINIRole; Rotigotine; Serotonin Modulators; Suvorexant; Thalidomide; Zolpidem

The levels/effects of FentaNYL may be increased by: Amphetamines; Anticholinergic Agents; Antiemetics (5HT3 Antagonists); Antipsychotic Agents; Antipsychotic Agents (Phenothiazines); Brimonidine (Topical); Cannabis; Conivaptan; Crizotinib; CYP3A4 Inhibitors (Moderate); CYP3A4 Inhibitors (Strong); Dapoxetine; Dasatinib; Doxylamine; Dronabinol; Droperidol; Fosaprepitant; Fusidic Acid (Systemic); HydrOXYzine; Idelalisib; Ivacaftor; Kava Kava; Luliconazole; Magnesium Sulfate; Metaxalone; Methotrimeprazine; Mifepristone; Minocycline; Nabilone; Ombitasvir, Paritaprevir, Ritonavir, and Dasabuvir; Osimertinib; Palbociclib; Perampanel; Rufinamide; Simeprevir; Sodium Oxybate; Stiripentol; Succinylcholine; Tapentadol; Tetrahydrocannabinol

Decreased Effect

FentaNYL may decrease the levels/effects of: Ioflupane I 123; Pegvisomant

The levels/effects of FentaNYL may be decreased by: Alpha-/Beta-Agonists (Indirect-Acting); Alpha1-Agonists; Ammonium Chloride; CYP3A4 Inducers (Moderate); CYP3A4 Inducers (Strong); Enzalutamide; Mixed Agonist / Antagonist Opioids; Naltrexone; Osimertinib; St Johns Wort

Food Interactions Fentanyl concentrations may be increased by grapefruit juice. Management: Avoid concurrent intake of large quantities (>1 quart/day) of grapefruit juice.

Storage/Stability

Injection formulation: Store intact vials/ampules at controlled room temperature of 20°C to 25°C (68°F to 77°F). Protect from light. Canadian labeling (not in U.S. labeling) recommends that when admixing injection formulation in NS for epidural administration, the resulting solution be used within 24 hours.

Nasal spray: Do not store above 25°C (77°F); do not freeze. Protect from light. Bottle should be stored in the provided child-resistant container when not in use and kept out of the reach of children at all times.

Transdermal device: Store at 25°C (77°F); excursions permitted to 15°C to 30°C (59°F to 86°F).

Transdermal patch: Do not store above 25°C (77°F). Keep out of the reach of children.

Transmucosal (buccal film, buccal tablet, lozenge, sublingual spray, sublingual tablet): Store at controlled room temperature of 20°C to 25°C (68°F to 77°F). Protect from freezing and moisture. Keep out of the reach of children.

Mechanism of Action Binds with stereospecific receptors at many sites within the CNS, increases pain threshold, alters pain reception, inhibits ascending pain pathways

Pharmacodynamics/Kinetics

Onset of action:

Children 3-12 years: Intranasal: 5 to 10 minutes (Borland 2002)

Adults: Analgesic: IM: 7 to 8 minutes; IV: Almost immediate (maximal analgesic and respiratory depressant effects may not be seen for several minutes); Transdermal (initial placement): 6 hours; Transmucosal: 5 to 15 minutes

Duration: IM: 1 to 2 hours; IV: 0.5 to 1 hour; Transdermal (removal of patch/no replacement): Related to blood level; some effects may last 72 to 96 hours due to extended half-life and absorption from the skin, fentanyl concentrations decrease by ~50% in 20 to 27 hours; Transmucosal: Related to blood level; respiratory depressant effect may last longer than analgesic effect

Absorption:

Transdermal, patch: Initial application: Drug is released at a nearly constant rate from the transdermal matrix system into the skin, where it accumulates; this results in a depot of fentanyl in the outer layer of skin. Fentanyl is absorbed into systemic circulation from the depot. This results in a gradual increase in serum concentration over the first 12 to 24 hours, followed by fairly constant concentrations for the remainder of the dosing interval. Absorption is decreased in cachectic patients (compared to normal size patients). Exposure to external heat increases drug absorption from patch.

Transdermal, device: At the activation of each dose, an electrical current is activated for 10 minutes, which moves a dose of fentanyl from the drug-containing reservoir through the skin and into the systemic circulation. Fentanyl concentrations increase slowly with device activation and continue to increase for ~5 minutes after the completion of each 10 minute dose. Absorption of fentanyl from the device increases as a function of time and is independent of frequency of dosing.

Transmucosal, buccal tablet and buccal film: Rapid, ~50% from the buccal mucosa; remaining 50% swallowed with saliva and slowly absorbed from GI tract

Transmucosal, lozenge: Rapid, ~25% from the buccal mucosa; 75% swallowed with saliva and slowly absorbed from GI tract

Distribution: Highly lipophilic, redistributes into muscle and fat; **Note:** IV fentanyl exhibits a 3-compartment distribution model. Changes in blood pH may alter ionization of fentanyl and affect its distribution between plasma and CNS

V_{dss}: Children: 0.05 to 14 years of age (after long-term continuous infusion): ~15 L/kg (range: 5 to 30 L/kg)

V_{dss}: Adults: 4 to 6 L/kg

Protein binding: 79% to 87%, primarily to alpha-1 acid glycoprotein; also binds to albumin and erythrocytes; **Note:** Free fraction increases with acidosis

Metabolism: Hepatic, primarily via CYP3A4 by N-dealkylation (to norfentanyl) and hydroxylation to other inactive metabolites

Bioavailability: **Note:** Comparative studies have found the buccal film to have a 40% greater systemic exposure (ie, AUC) than the transmucosal lozenge, and the buccal tablet to have a 30% to 50% greater exposure than the transmucosal lozenge.

Buccal film: 71% (mucositis did not have a clinically significant effect on C_{max} and AUC; however, bioavailability is expected to decrease if film is inappropriately chewed and swallowed)

Buccal tablet: 65%

Lozenge: ~50%

Sublingual spray: 76%

Sublingual tablet: 54%

Half-life elimination:

IV:

Pediatric patients 5 months to 4.5 years: 2.4 hours

Pediatric patients 6 months to 14 years (after long-term continuous infusion): ~21 hours (range: 11-36 hours)

Adults: 2 to 4 hours; when administered as a continuous infusion, the half-life prolongs with infusion duration due to the large volume of distribution (Sessler 2008)

Transdermal device: Terminal: ~16 hours

Transdermal patch: 20 to 27 hours (apparent half-life is influenced by continued fentanyl absorption from skin)

Transmucosal products: 3 to 14 hours (dose dependent)

◀

Nasal spray: 15 to 25 hours (based on a multiple-dose pharmacokinetic study when doses are administered in the same nostril and separated by a 1-, 2-, or 4-hour time lapse)

Buccal film: ~14 hours

Buccal tablet: 100-200 mcg: 3 to 4 hours; 400 to 800 mcg: 11 to 12 hours

Time to peak:

Buccal film: 0.75 to 4 hours (median: 1 hour)

Buccal tablet: 20 to 240 minutes (median: 47 minutes)

Lozenge: 20 to 480 minutes (median: 20 to 40 minutes)

Nasal spray: Median: 15 to 21 minutes

Sublingual spray: 10 to 120 minutes (median: 90 minutes)

Sublingual tablet: 15 to 240 minutes (median: 30 to 60 minutes)

Transdermal patch: 20 to 72 hours; steady state serum concentrations are reached after two sequential 72-hour applications

Excretion: Urine 75% (primarily as metabolites, <7% to 10% as unchanged drug); feces ~9%

Clearance: Newborn infants: Clearance may be significantly correlated to gestational age and birth weight (Saarenmaa 2000)

Dosing

Adult Note: Ranges listed may not represent the maximum doses that may be required in some patients. Doses and dosage intervals should be titrated to pain relief/prevention. Monitor vital signs routinely. Single IM doses have duration of 1-2 hours, single IV doses last 0.5 to 1 hour.

Surgery:

Premedication: IM, slow IV: 50 to 100 mcg administered 30 to 60 minutes prior to surgery **or** slow IV: 25 to 50 mcg given shortly before induction (Barash, 2009)

Adjunct to general anesthesia: Slow IV:

Low dose: 1 to 2 mcg/**kg** depending on the indication (Miller, 2010); additional maintenance doses are generally not needed.

Moderate dose (fentanyl plus a sedative/hypnotic): Initial: 2 to 4 mcg/**kg**; Maintenance (bolus or infusion): 25 to 50 mcg every 15 to 30 minutes or 0.5 to 2 mcg/kg/**hour**. Discontinuing fentanyl infusion 30 to 60 minutes prior to the end of surgery will usually allow adequate ventilation upon emergence from anesthesia.

High dose (opioid anesthesia): 4 to 20 mcg/**kg** bolus then 2 to 10 mcg/kg/**hour** (Miller, 2010); **Note:** High-dose fentanyl (ie, 20 to 50 mcg/kg) is rarely used, but is still described in the manufacturer's label. The concept of fast-tracking and early intubation following cardiac surgery has essentially replaced high-dose fentanyl anesthesia.

Adjunct to regional anesthesia: 50 to 100 mcg IM or slow IV over 1 to 2 minutes. **Note:** An IV should be in place with regional anesthesia so the IM route is rarely used but still maintained as an option in the manufacturer's labeling.

Postoperative recovery: IM, slow IV: 50 to 100 mcg every 1 to 2 hours as needed.

Postoperative pain: Epidural (Canadian labeling; not in U.S. labeling): Initial: 100 mcg (diluted in 8 mL of preservative free NS to final concentration of 10 mcg/mL); may repeat with additional 100 mcg boluses on demand or alternatively may administer by continuous infusion at a rate of 1 mcg/kg/hour.

Pain management:

Postoperative pain, acute: Transdermal device (Ionsys): Apply one device to chest or upper outer arm only. Only the patient may activate the device (40 mcg dose of fentanyl per activation; maximum 6 doses per hour). Only one device may be applied at a time for up to 24 hours or 80 doses, whichever comes first. May be used for a maximum of 72 hours, with each subsequent device applied to a different skin site. If inadequate analgesia is achieved with one device, either provide additional supplemental analgesic medication or replace with an alternate analgesic medication. Refer to manufacturer's labeling for activation instructions.

Note: For hospital use only by patients under medical supervision and direction and only after patients have been titrated to an acceptable level of analgesia using another opioid analgesic.

Severe pain:

Intermittent dosing: IM, IV (off-label dose): Slow IV: 25 to 35 mcg (based on ~70 kg patient) **or** 0.35 to 0.5 mcg/kg every 30 to 60 minutes as needed (SCCM [Barr, 2013]). **Note:** After the first dose, if severe pain persists and adverse effects are minimal at the time of expected peak effect (eg, ~5 minutes after IV administration), may repeat dose (APS, 2008). In addition, since the duration of activity with IV administration is 30 to 60 minutes, more frequent administration may be necessary when administered by this route.

Patient-controlled analgesia (PCA) (off-label use; American Pain Society, 2008; Miller, 2010): Opioid-naive: IV:

Usual concentration: 10 mcg/mL

Demand dose: Usual: 10 to 20 mcg

Lockout interval: 4 to 10 minutes

Usual basal rate: ≤50 mcg/hour. **Note:** Continuous basal infusions are not recommended for initial programming and should rarely be used; consider limiting infusion rate to 10 mcg/hour if used (Grass, 2005).

Critically-ill patients (off-label dose): Slow IV: 25 to 35 mcg (based on ~70 kg patient) **or** 0.35 to 0.5 mcg/kg every 30 to 60 minutes as needed (SCCM [Barr, 2013]). **Note:** More frequent dosing may be needed (eg, mechanically-ventilated patients).

Continuous infusion: 50 to 700 mcg/hour (based on ~70 kg patient) **or** 0.7 to 10 mcg/kg/**hour** (SCCM [Barr, 2013]).

Alternative continuous infusion dosing: 1 to 2 mcg/kg bolus followed by an initial rate of 1 to 2 mcg/**kg**/hour (Peng, 1999) **or** 25 to 100 mcg bolus followed by an initial rate of 25 to 200 mcg/**hour** (Liu, 2003). **Note:** When pain is not controlled, may administer an additional small bolus dose (eg, 25 to 50 mcg) prior to increasing the infusion rate (Loper 1990; Peng, 1999; Salomaki, 1991).

Intrathecal (off-label use; American Pain Society, 2008): **Must be preservative-free.** Doses must be adjusted for age, injection site, and patient's medical condition and degree of opioid tolerance.

Single dose: 5 to 25 mcg; may provide adequate relief for up to 6 hours

Continuous infusion: Not recommended in acute pain management due to risk of excessive accumulation. For chronic cancer pain, infusion of very small doses may be practical (American Pain Society, 2008).

Epidural (off-label use; American Pain Society, 2008): **Must be preservative-free.** Doses must be adjusted for age, injection site, and patient's medical condition and degree of opioid tolerance

Single dose: 25 to 100 mcg; may provide adequate relief for up to 8 hours

Continuous infusion: 25 to 100 mcg/hour (fentanyl alone). When combined with a local anesthetic (eg, bupivacaine or ropivacaine), fentanyl requirement are less (Manion, 2011).

Breakthrough cancer pain: Transmucosal: For patients who are tolerant to and currently receiving opioid therapy for persistent cancer pain; dosing should be individually titrated to provide adequate analgesia with minimal side effects. Dose titration should be done if patient requires more than 1 dose/breakthrough pain episode for several consecutive episodes. Patients experiencing >4 breakthrough pain episodes per day should have the dose of their long-term opioid re-evaluated. **Patients must remain on around-the-clock opioids during use.**

Lozenge (Actiq): **Note: Do not** convert patients from any other fentanyl product to Actiq on a mcg-per-mcg basis. Patients previously using another fentanyl product should be initiated at a dose of 200 mcg; individually titrate to provide adequate analgesia while minimizing adverse effects.

Initial dose: 200 mcg (consumed over 15 minutes) for all patients; if after 30 minutes from the start of the lozenge (ie, 15 minutes following the completion of the lozenge), the pain is unrelieved, a second 200 mcg dose may be given over 15 minutes. A maximum of 1 additional dose can be given per pain episode; **must wait at least 4 hours before treating another episode**. To limit the number of units in the home during titration, only prescribe an initial titration supply of six 200 mcg lozenges.

Dose titration: From the initial dose, closely follow patients and modify the dose until patient reaches a dose providing adequate analgesia using a single dosage unit per breakthrough cancer pain episode. If signs/symptoms of excessive opioid effects (eg, respiratory depression) occur, immediately remove the dosage unit from the patient's mouth, dispose of properly, and reduce subsequent doses. If adequate relief is not achieved 15 minutes after completion of the first dose (ie, 30 minutes after the start of the lozenge), only 1 additional lozenge of the same strength may be given for that episode; **must wait at least 4 hours before treating another episode.**

Maintenance dose: Once titrated to an effective dose, patients should generally use a single dosage unit per breakthrough pain episode. During any pain episode, if adequate relief is not achieved 15 minutes after completion of the first dose (ie, 30 minutes after the start of the lozenge), only 1 additional lozenge of the same strength may be given over 15 minutes for that episode; **must wait at least 4 hours before treating another episode**. Consumption should be limited to ≤4 units per day (once an effective breakthrough dose is found). If adequate analgesia is **not** provided after treating several episodes of breakthrough pain using the same dose, increase dose to next highest lozenge strength (initially dispense no more than 6 units of the new strength). Consider increasing the around-the-clock opioid therapy in patients experiencing >4 breakthrough pain episodes per day. If signs/symptoms of excessive opioid effects (eg, respiratory depression) occur, immediately remove the dosage unit from the patient's mouth, dispose of properly, and reduce subsequent doses.

Buccal film (Onsolis): **Note:** Do **not** convert patients from any other fentanyl product to Onsolis on a mcg-per-mcg basis. Patients previously using another fentanyl product should be initiated at a dose of 200 mcg; individually titrate to provide adequate analgesia while minimizing adverse effects.

Initial dose: 200 mcg for all patients; if after 30 minutes pain is unrelieved, the patient may use an alternative rescue medication as directed by their health care provider. Do **not** redose with Onsolis within an episode; buccal film should only be used once per breakthrough cancer pain episode. **Must wait at least 2 hours before treating another episode with buccal film.**

Dose titration: If titration required, increase dose in 200 mcg increments once per episode using multiples of the 200 mcg film (for doses up to 800 mcg); do not redose within a single episode of breakthrough pain and separate single doses by ≥2 hours. During titration, do not exceed 4 simultaneous applications of the 200 mcg films (800 mcg) (when using multiple films, do not place on top of each other; film may be placed on both sides of mouth); if >800 mcg required, treat next episode with one 1200 mcg film (maximum dose: 1200 mcg). Once maintenance dose is determined, all other unused films should be disposed of and that strength (using a single film) should be used. During any pain episode, if adequate relief is not achieved after 30 minutes following buccal film application, a rescue medication (as determined by health care provider) may be used.

Maintenance dose: Determined dose applied as a single film once per episode and separated by ≥2 hours (dose range: 200 to 1200 mcg); limit to 4 applications per day. Consider increasing the around-the-clock opioid therapy in patients experiencing >4 breakthrough pain episodes per day.

Buccal tablet (Fentora): **Note:** Do **not** convert patients from any other fentanyl product to Fentora on a mcg-per-mcg basis. Patients previously using another fentanyl product should be initiated at a dose of 100 mcg; individually titrate to provide adequate analgesia while minimizing adverse effects. For patients previously using the transmucosal lozenge (Actiq), the initial dose should be selected using the conversions listed; see *Conversion from lozenge (Actiq) to buccal tablet (Fentora)*.

Initial dose: 100 mcg for all patients unless patient already using Actiq; see *Conversion from lozenge (Actiq) to buccal tablet (Fentora)*; if after 30 minutes pain is unrelieved, the U.S. labeling suggests that a second 100 mcg dose may be administered (maximum of 2 doses per breakthrough pain episode). The Canadian labeling recommends only a single dose per breakthrough pain episode; patients experiencing breakthrough pain after administration may take an alternative analgesic as rescue medication after 30 minutes. **Must wait at least 4 hours before treating another episode with Fentora buccal tablet.**

Dose titration: If titration required, 100 mcg dose may be increased to 200 mcg using two 100 mcg tablets (one on each side of mouth) with the next breakthrough pain episode. If 200 mcg dose is not successful, patient can use four 100 mcg tablets (two on each side of mouth) with the next breakthrough pain episode. If titration requires >400 mcg per dose, titrate using 200 mcg tablets; do not use more than

4 tablets simultaneously (maximum single dose: 800 mcg). During any pain episode, if adequate relief is not achieved after 30 minutes following buccal tablet application, a second dose of same strength per breakthrough pain episode may be used. The Canadian labeling recommends only a single dose per breakthrough pain episode; patients experiencing breakthrough pain after administration may take an alternative analgesic as rescue medication after 30 minutes. **Must wait at least 4 hours before treating another episode with Fentora buccal tablet.**

Maintenance dose: Following titration, the effective maintenance dose using 1 tablet of the appropriate strength should be administered once per episode; if after 30 minutes pain is unrelieved, may administer a second dose of the same strength; The Canadian labeling recommends only a single dose per breakthrough pain episode; patients experiencing breakthrough pain after administration may take an alternative analgesic as rescue medication after 30 minutes. **Must wait ≥4 hours before treating another episode with Fentora buccal tablet.** Limit to 4 applications per day. Consider increasing the around-the-clock opioid therapy in patients experiencing >4 breakthrough pain episodes per day. Once an effective maintenance dose has been established, the buccal tablet may be administered sublingually (alternate route). To prevent confusion, patient should only have one strength available at a time. Once maintenance dose is determined, all other unused tablets should be disposed of and that strength (using a single tablet) should be used. Using more than four buccal tablets at a time has not been studied.

Conversion from lozenge (Actiq) to buccal tablet (Fentora):

Lozenge dose 200 to 400 mcg: Initial buccal tablet dose is 100 mcg; may titrate using multiples of 100 mcg

Lozenge dose 600 to 800 mcg: Initial buccal tablet dose is 200 mcg; may titrate using multiples of 200 mcg

Lozenge dose 1200 to 1600 mcg: Initial buccal tablet dose is 400 mcg (using two 200 mcg tablets); may titrate using multiples of 200 mcg

Nasal spray (Lazanda): **Note:** Do **not** convert patients from any other fentanyl product to Lazanda on a mcg-per-mcg basis. Patients previously using another fentanyl product should be initiated at a dose of 100 mcg; individually titrate to provide adequate analgesia while minimizing adverse effects.

Initial dose: 100 mcg (one 100 mcg spray in one nostril) for all patients; if after 30 minutes pain is unrelieved, an alternative rescue medication may be used as directed by their health care provider. **Must wait at least 2 hours before treating another episode with Lazanda nasal spray.** However, for the next pain episode, increase to a higher dose using the recommended dose titration steps.

Dose titration: If titration required, increase to a higher dose for the next pain episode using these titration steps **(Note: Must wait at least 2 hours before treating another episode with Lazanda nasal spray)**: If no relief with 100 mcg dose, increase to 200 mcg dose per episode (one 100 mcg spray in each nostril); if no relief with 200 mcg dose, increase to 400 mcg per episode (one 400 mcg spray in one nostril or two 100 mcg sprays in each nostril); if no relief with 400 mcg dose, increase to 800 mcg dose per episode (one 400 mcg spray in each nostril). **Note:** Single doses >800 mcg have not been evaluated. There are no data supporting the use of a combination of dose strengths.

Maintenance dose: Once maintenance dose for breakthrough pain episode has been determined, use that dose for subsequent episodes. For pain that is not relieved after 30 minutes of Lazanda administration or if a separate breakthrough pain episode occurs within the 2 hour window before the next Lazanda dose is permitted, a rescue medication may be used. Limit Lazanda use to ≤4 episodes of breakthrough pain per day. If patient is experiencing >4 breakthrough pain episodes per day, consider increasing the around-the-clock, long-acting opioid therapy; if long-acting opioid therapy dose is altered, re-evaluate and retitrate Lazanda dose as needed. If response to maintenance dose changes (increase in adverse reactions or alterations in pain relief), dose readjustment may be necessary.

Sublingual spray (Subsys): **Note:** Do **not** convert patients from any other fentanyl product to Subsys on a mcg-per-mcg basis. Patients previously using another fentanyl product should be initiated at a dose of 100 mcg; individually titrate to provide adequate analgesia while minimizing adverse effects. For patients previously using the transmucosal lozenge (Actiq), the initial dose should be selected using the conversions listed; see *Conversion from lozenge (Actiq) to sublingual spray (Subsys)*.

Initial dose: 100 mcg for all patients unless patient already using Actiq; see *Conversion from lozenge (Actiq) to sublingual spray (Subsys)*. If pain is unrelieved, 1 additional 100 mcg dose may be given 30 minutes after administration of the first dose. A maximum of 2 doses can be given per breakthrough pain episode. **Must wait at least 4 hours before treating another episode with sublingual spray.**

Dose titration: If titration required, titrate to a dose that provides adequate analgesia (with tolerable side effects) using the following titration steps: If no relief with 100 mcg dose, increase to 200 mcg dose (using one 200 mcg unit); if no relief with 200 mcg dose, increase to 400 mcg dose (using one 400 mcg unit); if no relief with 400 mcg dose, increase to 600 mcg dose (using one 600 mcg unit); if no relief with 600 mcg dose, increase to 800 mcg dose (using one 800 mcg unit); if no relief with 800 mcg dose, increase to 1200 mcg dose (using two 600 mcg units); if no relief with 1200 mcg dose, increase to 1600 mcg dose (using two 800 mcg units). During dose titration, if breakthrough pain unrelieved 30 minutes after Subsys administration, 1 additional dose using the same strength may be administered (maximum: 2 doses per breakthrough pain episode); **patient must wait 4 hours before treating another breakthrough pain episode with sublingual spray.**

Maintenance dose: Once maintenance dose for breakthrough pain episode has been determined, use that dose for subsequent episodes. If occasional episodes of unrelieved breakthrough pain occur following 30 minutes of Subsys administration, 1 additional dose using the same strength may be administered (maximum: 2 doses per breakthrough pain episode); **patient must wait 4 hours before treating another breakthrough pain episode with Subsys.** Once maintenance dose is determined, limit Subsys use to ≤4 episodes of breakthrough pain per day. If response to maintenance dose changes (increase in adverse reactions or alterations in pain relief), dose readjustment may be necessary. If patient is experiencing >4 breakthrough pain episodes per day, consider increasing the around-the-clock, long-acting opioid therapy.

Conversion from lozenge (Actiq) to sublingual spray (Subsys):

Lozenge dose 200 to 400 mcg: Initial sublingual spray dose is 100 mcg; may titrate using multiples of 100 mcg

Lozenge dose 600 to 800 mcg: Initial sublingual spray dose is 200 mcg; may titrate using multiples of 200 mcg

Lozenge dose 1,200 to 1,600 mcg: Initial sublingual spray dose is 400 mcg; may titrate using multiples of 400 mcg

Sublingual tablet (Abstral): **Note:** Do **not** convert patients from any other fentanyl product to Abstral on a mcg-per-mcg basis. Patients previously using another fentanyl product should be initiated at a dose of 100 mcg (except Actiq); individually titrate to provide adequate analgesia while minimizing adverse effects.

Initial dose:

U.S. labeling: 100 mcg for all patients; if pain is unrelieved, a second 100 mcg dose may be given 30 minutes after administration of the first dose. A maximum of 2 doses can be given per breakthrough pain episode. **Must wait at least 2 hours before treating another episode with sublingual tablet.**

Canadian labeling: 100 mcg for all patients; if pain is unrelieved 30 minutes after administration of Abstral, an alternative rescue medication (other than Abstral) may be given. Administer only 1 dose of Abstral per breakthrough pain episode. **Must wait at least 2 hours before treating another episode with sublingual tablet.**

Dose titration: If titration required, increase in 100 mcg increments (up to 400 mcg) over consecutive breakthrough episodes. If titration requires >400 mcg per dose, increase in increments of 200 mcg, starting with 600 mcg dose and titrating up to 800 mcg.

During titration, patients may use multiples of 100 mcg and/or 200 mcg tablets for any single dose; do not exceed 4 tablets at one time; safety and efficacy of doses >800 mcg have not been evaluated. During dose titration, if breakthrough pain unrelieved 30 minutes after sublingual tablet administration, the U.S. labeling suggests that 1 additional dose using the same strength may be administered (maximum: 2 doses per breakthrough pain episode); the Canadian labeling recommends use of an alternative rescue medication and limits use of Abstral to 1 dose per breakthrough pain episode. **Patient must wait 2 hours before treating another breakthrough pain episode with sublingual tablet.**

Maintenance dose: Once maintenance dose for breakthrough pain episode has been determined, use only 1 tablet in the appropriate strength per episode; if pain is unrelieved with maintenance dose:

U.S. labeling: A second dose may be given after 30 minutes; maximum of 2 doses/episode of breakthrough pain; separate treatment of subsequent episodes by ≥2 hours; limit treatment to ≤4 breakthrough episodes per day.

Canadian labeling: Administer alternative rescue medication after 30 minutes; maximum of 1 Abstral dose/episode of breakthrough pain; separate treatment of subsequent episodes by ≥2 hours; limit treatment to ≤4 breakthrough episodes per day.

Consider increasing the around-the-clock long-acting opioid therapy in patients experiencing >4 breakthrough pain episodes per day; if long-acting opioid therapy dose altered, re-evaluate and retitrate Abstral dose as needed.

Conversion from lozenge (Actiq) to sublingual tablet (Abstral):

Lozenge dose 200 mcg: Initial sublingual tablet dose is 100 mcg; may titrate using multiples of 100 mcg

Lozenge dose 400 to 1,200 mcg: Initial sublingual tablet dose is 200 mcg; may titrate using multiples of 200 mcg

Lozenge dose 1,600 mcg: Initial sublingual tablet dose is 400 mcg; may titrate using multiples of 400 mcg

Chronic pain management (opioid-tolerant patients only): Transdermal patch: Discontinue or taper all other around-the-clock or extended release opioids when initiating therapy with fentanyl transdermal patch.

Initial: To convert patients from oral or parenteral opioids to transdermal patch, a 24-hour analgesic requirement should be calculated (based on prior opioid use). Using the tables, the appropriate initial dose can be determined. The initial fentanyl dosage may be approximated from the 24-hour morphine dosage equivalent and titrated to minimize adverse effects and provide analgesia. Substantial interpatient variability exists in relative potency. Therefore, it is safer to underestimate a patient's daily fentanyl requirement and provide breakthrough pain relief with rescue medication (eg, immediate release opioid) than to overestimate requirements. With the initial application, the absorption of transdermal fentanyl requires several hours to reach plateau; therefore transdermal fentanyl is inappropriate for management of acute pain. Change patch every 72 hours.

Conversion from continuous infusion of fentanyl: In patients who have adequate pain relief with a fentanyl infusion, fentanyl may be converted to transdermal dosing at a rate equivalent to the intravenous rate. A two-step taper of the infusion to be completed over 12 hours has been recommended (Kornick, 2001) after the patch is applied. The infusion is decreased to 50% of the original rate six hours after the application of the first patch, and subsequently discontinued twelve hours after application.

Titration: Short-acting agents may be required until analgesic efficacy is established and/or as supplements for "breakthrough" pain. The amount of supplemental doses should be closely monitored. Appropriate dosage increases may be based on daily supplemental dosage using the ratio of 45 mg/24 hours of oral morphine to a 12.5 mcg/hour increase in fentanyl dosage (U.S. labeling) or using the ratio of 45 to 59 mg/24 hours of oral morphine to a 12 mcg/hour increase in fentanyl dosage (Canadian labeling).

Frequency of adjustment: The dosage should not be titrated more frequently than every 3 days after the initial dose or every 6 days thereafter. Titrate dose based on the daily dose of supplemental opioids required by the patient on the second or third day of the initial application. **Note:** Upon discontinuation, ~17 hours are required for a 50% decrease in fentanyl levels.

Frequency of application: The majority of patients may be controlled on every 72-hour administration; however, a small number of adult patients require every 48-hour administration.

Discontinuation: When discontinuing transdermal fentanyl and not converting to another opioid, use a gradual downward titration, such as decreasing the dose by 50% every 6 days, to reduce the possibility of withdrawal symptoms.

Dose conversion guidelines for transdermal fentanyl (see tables).

Note: U.S. and Canadian dose conversion guidelines differ; consult appropriate table. The conversion factors in these tables are only to be used for the conversion from current opioid therapy to Duragesic. Conversion factors in this table cannot be used to convert from Duragesic to another opioid (doing so may lead to fatal overdose due to overestimation of the new opioid). These are not tables of equianalgesic doses.

U.S. Labeling: Dose Conversion Guidelines: Recommended Initial Duragesic® Dose Based Upon Daily Oral Morphine Dose[1,2]

Oral 24-Hour Morphine (mg/day)	Duragesic Dose[3] (mcg/h)
60 to 134	25
135 to 224	50
225 to 314	75
315 to 404	100
405 to 494	125
495 to 584	150
585 to 674	175
675 to 764	200
765 to 854	225
855 to 944	250
945 to 1034	275
1035 to 1124	300

[1]The table should NOT be used to convert from transdermal fentanyl (Duragesic) to other opioid analgesics. Rather, following removal of the patch, titrate the dose of the new opioid until adequate analgesia is achieved.

[2]Recommendations are based on U.S. product labeling for Duragesic.

[3]Pediatric patients initiating therapy on a 25 mcg/hour Duragesic system should be opioid-tolerant and receiving at least 60 mg oral morphine equivalents per day.

U.S. Labeling: Dose Conversion Guidelines[1,2]

Current Analgesic	Daily Dosage (mg/day)			
Morphine (IM/IV)	10 to 22	23 to 37	38 to 52	53 to 67
Oxycodone (oral)	30 to 67	67.5 to 112	112.5 to 157	157.5 to 202
Codeine (oral)	150 to 447	-	-	-
Hydromorphone (oral)	8 to 17	17.1 to 28	28.1 to 39	39.1 to 51
Hydromorphone (IV)	1.5 to 3.4	3.5 to 5.6	5.7 to 7.9	8 to 10
Meperidine (IM)	75 to 165	166 to 278	279 to 390	391 to 503
Methadone (oral)	20 to 44	45 to 74	75 to 104	105 to 134
Fentanyl transdermal recommended dose (mcg/h)	25 mcg/h	50 mcg/h	75 mcg/h	100 mcg/h

[1]The table should NOT be used to convert from transdermal fentanyl (Duragesic) to other opioid analgesics. Rather, following removal of the patch, titrate the dose of the new opioid until adequate analgesia is achieved.

[2]Recommendations are based on U.S. product labeling for Duragesic.

Transdermal patch (Duragesic MAT [Canadian product]): Adults:

Canadian Labeling: Dose Conversion Guidelines (Adults): Recommended Initial Duragesic MAT Dose Based Upon Daily Oral Morphine Dose[1,2]

Oral 24-Hour Morphine (Current Dose in mg/day)	Duragesic MAT Dose (Initial Dose in mcg/h)
45 to 59	12
60 to 134	25
135 to 179	37
180 to 224	50
225 to 269	62
270 to 314	75
315 to 359	87
360 to 404	100
405 to 494	125
495 to 584	150
585 to 674	175
675 to 764	200
765 to 854	225
855 to 944	250
945 to 1034	275
1035 to 1124	300

[1]The table should NOT be used to convert from transdermal fentanyl (Duragesic MAT) to other opioid analgesics. Rather, following removal of the patch, titrate the dose of the new opioid until adequate analgesia is achieved.

[2]Recommendations are based on Canadian product labeling for Duragesic MAT.

Note: The 12 mcg/hour dose included in this table is to be used for incremental dose adjustment and is generally not recommended for initial dosing, except for patients in whom lower starting doses are deemed clinically appropriate.

Canadian Labeling: Dosing Conversion Guidelines (Adults)[1,2]

Current Analgesic	Daily Dosage (mg/day)						
Morphine[3] (IM/IV)	20 to 44	45 to 60	61 to 75	76 to 90	n/a[4]	n/a[4]	n/a[4]
Oxycodone (oral)	30 to 66	67 to 90	91 to 112	113 to 134	135 to 157	158 to 179	180 to 202
Codeine (oral)	150 to 447	448 to 597	598 to 747	748 to 897	898 to 1047	1048 to 1197	1198 to 1347
Hydromorphone (oral)	8 to 16	17 to 22	23 to 28	29 to 33	34 to 39	40 to 45	46 to 51
Hydromorphone (IV)	4 to 8.4	8.5 to 11.4	11.5 to 14.4	14.5 to 16.5	16.6 to 19.5	19.6 to 22.5	22.6 to 25.5
Fentanyl transdermal recommended dose (mcg/h)	25 mcg/h	37 mcg/h	50 mcg/h	62 mcg/h	75 mcg/h	87 mcg/h	100 mcg/h

[1]The table should NOT be used to convert from transdermal fentanyl (Duragesic MAT) to other opioid analgesics. Rather, following removal of the patch, titrate the dose of the new opioid until adequate analgesia is achieved.

[2]Recommendations are based on Canadian product labeling for Duragesic MAT.

[3]Morphine dose conversion based upon I.M to oral dose ratio of 1:3.

[4]Insufficient data available to provide specific dosing recommendations. Use caution; adjust dose conservatively.

Geriatric Elderly have been found to be twice as sensitive as younger patients to the effects of fentanyl. A wide range of doses may be used. When choosing a dose, take into consideration the following patient factors: age, weight, physical status, underlying disease states, other drugs used, type of anesthesia used, and the surgical procedure to be performed.

Transmucosal lozenge (eg, Actiq): In clinical trials, patients who were >65 years of age were titrated to a mean dose that was 200 mcg less than that of younger patients.

Pediatric Note: Ranges listed may not represent the maximum doses that may be required in some patients. Doses and dosage intervals should be titrated to pain relief/prevention. Monitor vital signs routinely. Single IM doses have duration of 1 to 2 hours, single IV doses last 0.5 to 1 hour.

Surgery adjunct to anesthesia (induction and maintenance): Children ≥2 years and Adolescents: IV: 2 to 3 mcg/**kg**/dose every 1 to 2 hours as needed

◀

Breakthrough cancer pain: Adolescents ≥16 years: Transmucosal lozenge (Actiq): Refer to adult dosing.

Chronic pain management: Children ≥2 years and Adolescents (opioid-tolerant patients): Transdermal patch (U.S. labeling): Refer to adult dosing. **Note:** Canadian labeling does not approve of use in patients <18 years.

Pain management (off-label use): *Patient-controlled analgesia (PCA) (off-label use; American Pain Society, 2008):* Children <50 kg: IV: **Note:** Opioid-naive:
Usual concentration: 10 to 50 mcg/mL (varies by patient weight and institution)
Demand dose: 0.5 to 1 mcg/kg/dose
Lockout interval: 6 to 8 minutes
Usual basal rate (optional): ≤0.5 mcg/kg/**hour. Note:** Due to safety concerns, continuous basal infusions are not recommended for initial programming and should rarely be used (Grass, 2005).

Renal Impairment
Injection: No dosage adjustment provided in manufacturer's labeling; use with caution.
Transdermal (device): There are no dosage adjustments provided in the manufacturer's labeling (has not been studied); fentanyl pharmacokinetics may be altered in renal disease.
Transdermal (patch): Degree of impairment (ie, CrCl) not defined in manufacturer's labeling.
US labeling:
Mild-to-moderate impairment: Initial: Reduce dose by 50%.
Severe impairment: Use not recommended.
Canadian labeling: There are no specific dosage adjustments provided in the manufacturer's labeling; monitor closely for toxicity and reduce dose if necessary.
Transmucosal (buccal film/tablet, sublingual spray/tablet, lozenge) and nasal spray: Although fentanyl pharmacokinetics may be altered in renal disease, fentanyl can be used successfully in the management of breakthrough cancer pain. Doses should be titrated to reach clinical effect with careful monitoring of patients with severe renal disease.

Hepatic Impairment
Injection: No dosage adjustment provided in manufacturer's labeling; use with caution.
Transdermal (device): There are no dosage adjustments provided in the manufacturer's labeling (has not been studied); fentanyl pharmacokinetics may be altered in hepatic disease.
Transdermal (patch):
US labeling:
Mild-to-moderate impairment: Initial: Reduce dose by 50%.
Severe impairment: Use not recommended.
Canadian labeling: There are no specific dosage adjustments provided in the manufacturer's labeling; monitor closely for toxicity and reduce dose if necessary.
Transmucosal (buccal film/tablet, sublingual spray/tablet, lozenge) and nasal spray: Although fentanyl pharmacokinetics may be altered in hepatic disease, fentanyl can be used successfully in the management of breakthrough cancer pain. Doses should be titrated to reach clinical effect with careful monitoring of patients with severe hepatic disease.

Dietary Considerations Transmucosal lozenge contains 2 g sugar per unit.

Usual Infusion Concentrations: Pediatric IV infusion: 10 **mcg**/mL

Usual Infusion Concentrations: Adult IV infusion: 10 mcg/mL

Administration
Epidural (Canadian labeling; not in U.S. labeling): For postoperative pain management may administer as bolus dose (diluted in preservative free NS to a final concentration of 10 mcg/mL) or by continuous infusion at a rate of 1 mcg/kg/hour. Use within 24 hours.
IV: Administer as slow IV infusion over 1 to 2 minutes. May also be administered as continuous infusion or PCA (off-label use) routes. Muscular rigidity may occur with rapid IV administration.
Transdermal device (eg, Ionsys): Always wear gloves when handling the device. Avoid contact with synthetic materials (such as carpeted flooring) while assembling and avoid exposing the device to electronic security systems. Prior to administration, clip excessive hair from application site if necessary (do not shave); clean the site with alcohol and let dry; do not use soaps, lotions, or other agents. Apply one device to healthy, unbroken/intact, non-irritated, and non-irradiated skin on the chest or upper outer arm only. Allow only the patient to self-administer doses; each on-demand dose is delivered over a 10-minute period. Each device operates up to 24 hours or 80 doses, whichever comes first. After 24 hours

have elapsed, or 80 doses have been delivered, the device will not deliver any additional doses; if the patient tries to initiate a dose, the device will ignore the dose request. Ionsys may be used for a maximum of 72 hours, with each subsequent device applied to a different skin site. Refer to manufacturer's labeling for complete activation, administration, and removal instructions.
Transdermal patch (eg, Duragesic): Apply to nonirritated and nonirradiated skin, such as chest, back, flank, or upper arm. Do not shave skin; hair at application site should be clipped. Prior to application, clean site with clear water and allow to dry completely. Do not use damaged, cut or leaking patches; patch may be less effective. Skin exposure from fentanyl gel leaking from patch may lead to serious adverse effects; thoroughly wash affected skin surfaces with water (do not use soap). Firmly press in place and hold for 30 seconds. Change patch every 72 hours. Do **not** use soap, alcohol, or other solvents to remove transdermal gel if it accidentally touches skin; use copious amounts of water. Avoid exposing application site to external heat sources (eg, heating pad, electric blanket, heat lamp, hot tub). If there is difficulty with patch adhesion, the edges of the system may be taped in place with first-aid tape. If there is continued difficulty with adhesion, an adhesive film dressing (eg, Bioclusive, Tegaderm) may be applied over the system. Dispose of any used or unused patches by removing patch from protective pouch and liner, fold adhesive ends together and flush patch down toilet immediately. Do not flush pouch or protective liner as such items can be discarded in the trash.
Lozenge: Foil overwrap should be removed just prior to administration. Place the unit in mouth between the cheek and gum and allow it to dissolve. Do not chew. Lozenge may be moved from one side of the mouth to the other. The unit should be consumed over a period of 15 minutes. Handle should be removed after the lozenge is consumed; early removal should be considered if the patient has achieved an adequate response and/or shows signs of respiratory depression. After consumption of a complete unit, the handle may be disposed of in a trash container that is out of the reach of children. For a partially consumed unit, or a unit that still has any drug matrix remaining on the handle, the handle should be placed under hot running tap water until the drug matrix has dissolved. Special child-resistant containers are available to temporarily store partially consumed units that cannot be disposed of immediately.
Buccal film: Foil overwrap should be removed just prior to administration. Prior to placing film, wet inside of cheek using tongue or by rinsing with water. Place film inside mouth with the pink side of the unit against the inside of the moistened cheek. With finger, press the film against cheek and hold for 5 seconds. The film should stick to the inside of cheek after 5 seconds. The film should be left in place until it dissolves (usually within 15-30 minutes after application). Liquids may be consumed after 5 minutes of application. Food can be eaten after film dissolves. If using more than 1 film simultaneously (during titration period), apply films on either side of mouth (do not apply on top of each other). Do not chew or swallow film. Do not cut or tear the film. All patients must initiate therapy using the 200 mcg film. To dispose of film; remove foil overwrap from any unused, unneeded films and dispose by flushing down the toilet.
Buccal tablet: Patient should not open blister until ready to administer. The blister backing should be peeled back to expose the tablet; tablet should not be pushed out through the blister. Immediately use tablet once removed from blister. Place entire tablet in the buccal cavity (above a rear molar, between the upper cheek and gum) or under the tongue (U.S. labeling recommends for maintenance dosing only; Canadian labeling does not restrict sublingual use to maintenance dosing only); should dissolve in about 14 to 25 minutes. If remnants remain after 30 minutes, they may be swallowed with water. Tablet should not be split, crushed, sucked, chewed, or swallowed whole. When possible, alternate sides of mouth with each dose.
Nasal spray: Prior to initial use, prime device by spraying 4 sprays into the provided pouch (the counting window will show a green bar when the bottle is ready for use). Insert nozzle a short distance into the nose (~1/2 inch or 1 cm) and point towards the bridge of the nose (while closing off the other nostril using 1 finger). Press on finger grips until a "click" sound is heard and the number in the counting window advances by one. The "click" sound and dose counter are the only reliable methods for ensuring a dose has been administered (spray is not always felt on the nasal mucosa). Patient should remain seated for at least 1 minute following administration. Do not blow nose for ≥30 minutes after administration. Wash hands before and

after use. If not used within 5 days, re-prime by spraying once. There are 8 full therapeutic sprays in each bottle; do not continue to use bottle after "8" sprays have been used. Dispose of bottle and contents if it has been ≥60 days since first use. Before disposal, all unopened or partially used bottles must be completely emptied by spraying the contents into the provided pouch. After "8" therapeutic sprays has been reached on the counter, patients should continue to spray an additional four sprays into the pouch to ensure that any residual fentanyl has been expelled (an audible click will no longer be heard and the counter will not advance beyond "8"). The empty bottle and the sealed pouch must be put into the child-resistant container before placing in the trash. Wash hands with soap and water immediately after handling the pouch. If the pouch is lost, another one can be ordered by the patient or caregiver by calling 1-866-458-6389.

Sublingual spray: Open sealed blister unit with scissors immediately prior to administration. Contents of unit should be sprayed into mouth under the tongue. Dispose of each unit dose immediately after use; place used unit into one of the provided white disposal bags. After sealing appropriately, discard in the trash. Dispose of any unused units as soon as no longer needed. Prior to disposal, empty all the medicine into the provided charcoal-lined disposal pouch. The disposal pouch should then be placed into the white disposal bag, sealed appropriately, and discarded in the trash.

Sublingual tablet: Remove from the blister unit immediately prior to administration. Place tablet directly under the tongue on the floor of the mouth and allow to completely dissolve; do not chew, suck, or swallow. Do not eat or drink anything until tablet is completely dissolved. In patients with a dry mouth, water may be used to moisten the buccal mucosa just before administration. All patients must initiate therapy using the 100 mcg tablet. To dispose of sublingual tablets; remove any unused tablets from the blister cards and dispose by flushing down the toilet.

Monitoring Parameters
Respiratory and cardiovascular status, blood pressure, heart rate; signs of misuse, abuse, or addiction; signs or symptoms of hypogonadism or hypoadrenalism (Brennan, 2013)

Transdermal patch: Monitor for 24 hours after application of first dose

Additional Information Fentanyl is 50 to 100 times as potent as morphine; morphine 10 mg IM is equivalent to fentanyl 0.1 to 0.2 mg IM; fentanyl has less hypotensive effects than morphine due to lack of histamine release. However, fentanyl may cause rigidity with high doses. If the patient has required high-dose analgesia or has used for a prolonged period (~7 days), taper dose to prevent withdrawal; monitor for signs and symptoms of withdrawal.

Product Availability
Ionsys (iontophoretic transdermal system): FDA approved May 2015; availability anticipated in the third quarter of 2015. Information pertaining to this product within the monograph is pending revision. Consult prescribing information for additional information.

Onsolis: Reformulated product FDA approved August 2015; availability anticipated in 2016. Consult prescribing information for additional information.

Dosage Forms Excipient information presented when available (limited, particularly for generics); consult specific product labeling. [DSC] = Discontinued product

Film, for buccal application, as citrate [strength expressed as base]:
Onsolis: 200 mcg (30s); 400 mcg (30s); 600 mcg (30s); 800 mcg (30s); 1200 mcg (30s) [DSC]

Injection, solution, as citrate [strength expressed as base, preservative free]:
Generic: 0.05 mg/mL (2 mL, 5 mL, 10 mL, 20 mL, 50 mL)

Liquid, sublingual, as base [spray]:
Subsys: 100 mcg (30s); 200 mcg (30s); 400 mcg (30s); 600 mcg (30s); 800 mcg (30s) [contains dehydrated ethanol 63.6%, propylene glycol]

Lozenge, oral, as citrate [strength expressed as base, transmucosal]:
Actiq: 200 mcg (30s); 400 mcg (30s); 600 mcg (30s); 800 mcg (30s); 1200 mcg (30s); 1600 mcg (30s) [contains sugar 2 g/lozenge; berry flavor]
Generic: 200 mcg (30s); 400 mcg (30s); 600 mcg (30s); 800 mcg (30s); 1200 mcg (30s); 1600 mcg (30s)

Patch, transdermal, as base:
Duragesic: 12 [delivers 12.5 mcg/hr] (5s) [contains ethanol 0.1 mL/10 cm²; 5 cm²]
Duragesic: 25 [delivers 25 mcg/hr] (5s) [contains ethanol 0.1 mL/10 cm²; 10 cm²]
Duragesic: 50 [delivers 50 mcg/hr] (5s) [contains ethanol 0.1 mL/10 cm²; 20 cm²]

Duragesic: 75 [delivers 75 mcg/hr] (5s) [contains ethanol 0.1 mL/10 cm²; 30 cm²]
Duragesic: 100 [delivers 100 mcg/hr] (5s) [contains ethanol 0.1 mL/10 cm²; 40 cm²]
Ionsys: 40 mcg/actuation (6s) [iontophoretic transdermal system]
Generic: 12 [delivers 12.5 mcg/hr] (5s); 25 [delivers 25 mcg/hr] (5s); 50 [delivers 50 mcg/hr] (5s); 75 [delivers 75 mcg/hr] (5s); 87.5 [delivers 87.5 mcg/hr] (5s); 100 [delivers 100 mcg/hr] (5s)

Powder, for prescription compounding, as citrate: USP: 100% (1 g)

Solution, intranasal, as citrate [strength expressed as base, spray]:
Lazanda: 100 mcg/spray (5 mL); 400 mcg/spray (5 mL) [delivers 8 metered sprays]

Tablet, for buccal application, as citrate [strength expressed as base]:
Fentora: 100 mcg (28s); 200 mcg (28s); 400 mcg (28s); 600 mcg (28s); 800 mcg (28s)

Tablet, sublingual, as citrate [strength expressed as base]:
Abstral: 100 mcg (12s, 32s); 200 mcg (12s, 32s); 300 mcg (12s, 32s); 400 mcg (12s, 32s); 600 mcg (32s); 800 mcg (32s)

Dosage Forms: Canada Excipient information presented when available (limited, particularly for generics); consult specific product labeling.

Patch, transdermal, as base: 12 mcg/hr (5s); 25 mcg/hr (5s); 50 mcg/hr (5s); 75 mcg/hr (5s); 100 mcg/hr (5s)
Duragesic MAT: 12 mcg/hr (5s)
Duragesic MAT: 25 mcg/hr (5s)
Duragesic MAT: 50 mcg/hr (5s)
Duragesic MAT: 75 mcg/hr (5s)
Duragesic MAT: 100 mcg/hr (5s)

Controlled Substance C-II

Ferric Carboxymaltose
(FER ik kar box ee MAWL tose)

Brand Names: US Injectafer
Index Terms Ferinject; Iron Carboxymaltose; Iron Dextri-Maltose; VIT 45
Pharmacologic Category Iron Salt
Use Iron-deficiency anemia (IDA): Treatment of IDA in adults with intolerance to oral iron or unsatisfactory response to oral iron; treatment of IDA in adults with nondialysis-dependent chronic kidney disease (ND-CKD)
Pregnancy Considerations Adverse events were observed in some animal reproduction studies.
Breast-Feeding Considerations Ferric carboxymaltose is excreted into breast milk. Iron concentrations are higher than those following oral ferrous sulfate administration.
Contraindications Hypersensitivity to ferric carboxymaltose or any component of the formulation
Warnings/Precautions Serious hypersensitivity reactions, including anaphylactic-type reactions (some life-threatening and fatal) have been reported. Monitor during and for ≥30 minutes after administration and until clinically stable. Signs/symptoms of serious hypersensitivity reaction include shock, hypotension, loss of consciousness, and/or collapse. Equipment for resuscitation, medication, and trained personnel experienced in handling emergencies should be immediately available during infusion. Transient elevations in systolic blood pressure, ▶

◄

(sometimes with facial flushing, dizziness, or nausea) were observed in studies; generally occurred immediately after dosing and resolved within 30 minutes. Monitor blood pressure following infusion. Lab assays may overestimate serum iron and transferrin bound irons for ~24 hours after infusion.

Adverse Reactions

>10%: Endocrine & metabolic: Decreased serum phosphate (27%; <2 mg/dL [0.65 mmol/L]; transient)

1% to 10%:

Cardiovascular: Increased blood pressure (6%; transient, systolic), flushing (4%), hypertension (4%), hypotension

Central nervous system: Dizziness (2%), headache (1%)

Dermatologic: Skin discoloration at injection site (1%)

Endocrine & metabolic: Hypophosphatemia (2%)

Gastrointestinal: Nausea (7%), vomiting (2%), constipation (1%), dysgeusia (1%)

Hepatic Increased serum ALT (1%)

<1% (Limited to important or life-threatening): Anaphylaxis, angioedema, hypersensitivity, syncope, tachycardia

Drug Interactions

Metabolism/Transport Effects None known.

Avoid Concomitant Use

Avoid concomitant use of Ferric Carboxymaltose with any of the following: Dimercaprol

Increased Effect/Toxicity

The levels/effects of Ferric Carboxymaltose may be increased by: Dimercaprol

Decreased Effect There are no known significant interactions involving a decrease in effect.

Preparation for Administration May administer undiluted (for IV push) or diluted (for infusion). When administering as an IV infusion, dilute up to 750 mg in a maximum of 250 mL of 0.9% sodium chloride injection to a concentration of 2-4 mg/mL; concentration should be ≥2 mg/mL. Discard unused portion of vial (single-use).

Storage/Stability Store intact vials at 20°C to 25°C (68°F to 77°F); excursions permitted between 15°C to 30°C (59°F to 86°F); do not freeze. Solutions diluted in 0.9% sodium chloride at concentrations of 2-4 mg/mL are stable for 72 hours at room temperature.

Mechanism of Action Ferric carboxymaltose is a colloidal iron (III) hydroxide in complex with carboxymaltose, a carbohydrate polymer that releases iron necessary to the function of hemoglobin, myoglobin, and specific enzyme systems; allows transport of oxygen via hemoglobin. Ferric carboxymaltose is a non-dextran formulation that allows for iron uptake (into reticuloendothelial system) without the release of free iron (Szczech, 2010).

Pharmacodynamics/Kinetics

Onset of action: Maximum iron levels (37-333 mcg/mL): 0.25-1.2 hours

Distribution: V_d: ~3 L

Half-life elimination: 7-12 hours

Excretion: Urine (negligible)

Dosing

Adult & Geriatric Note: Dose expressed as elemental iron

Iron-deficiency anemia (IDA): IV:

<50 kg: 15 mg/kg elemental iron on day 1; repeat dose after at least 7 days (maximum: 1500 mg elemental iron per course). May repeat course of therapy if anemia reoccurs.

≥50 kg: 750 mg on day 1; repeat dose after at least 7 days (maximum: 1500 mg per course). May repeat course if anemia reoccurs.

Renal Impairment Chronic kidney disease, nondialysis dependent: No dosage adjustment necessary (indicated for use in nondialysis CKD)

Hepatic Impairment No dosage adjustment provided in manufacturer's labeling.

Administration

Administer as slow IV push (undiluted) at a rate of ~100 mg/minute or by IV infusion (diluted to ≥2 mg/mL) over at least 15 minutes.

Avoid extravasation (may cause persistent discoloration). Monitor; if extravasation occurs, discontinue administration at that site.

Monitoring Parameters Hemoglobin and hematocrit, serum ferritin, iron saturation; vital signs (including blood pressure); signs and symptoms of hypersensitivity (monitor for ≥30 minutes following the end of administration and until clinically stable); monitor infusion site for extravasation.

NKF KDOQI guidelines (2006) recommend monitoring iron status every 1-3 months, with more frequent monitoring after course of IV iron therapy.

Reference Range CKD patients should have sufficient iron to achieve and maintain hemoglobin of 11-12 g/dL; to achieve and maintain this target hemoglobin for patients with nondialysis dependent CKD, sufficient iron should be

administered to maintain a transferrin saturation (TSAT) of 20%, and a serum ferritin level ≥100 ng/mL (NKF KDOQI, 2006)

Test Interactions Serum or transferrin bound iron levels may be falsely elevated if assessed within 24 hours of ferric carboxymaltose administration.

Dosage Forms Considerations Each mL of Injectafer contains 50 mg of elemental iron

Dosage Forms Excipient information presented when available (limited, particularly for generics); consult specific product labeling.

Solution, Intravenous:

Injectafer: 750 mg/15 mL (15 mL)

Ferric Citrate (FER ik SIT rate)

Brand Names: US Auryxia

Index Terms Tetraferric Tricitrate Decahydrate

Pharmacologic Category Phosphate Binder

Use Hyperphosphatemia: For the control of serum phosphorus levels in patients with chronic kidney disease (CKD) receiving dialysis

Dosing

Adult & Geriatric Note: Each tablet contains 210 mg of ferric iron equivalent to 1 g ferric citrate.

Hyperphosphatemia: Oral:

Initial: 2 tablets (420 mg ferric iron) 3 times daily

Maintenance: Increase or decrease dose by 1 tablet or 2 tablets (210 mg to 420 mg ferric iron) as needed at 1 week or longer intervals to achieve target serum phosphorus levels (maximum dose: 12 tablets [2,520 mg ferric iron] daily).

Renal Impairment There are no dosage adjustments provided in the manufacturer's labeling.

Hepatic Impairment There are no dosage adjustments provided in the manufacturer's labeling.

Additional Information Complete prescribing information should be consulted for additional detail.

Dosage Forms Excipient information presented when available (limited, particularly for generics); consult specific product labeling.

Tablet, Oral:

Auryxia: Ferric iron 210 mg (ferric citrate 1 g) [contains fd&c blue #2 aluminum lake, fd&c red #40 aluminum lake, fd&c yellow #6 aluminum lake]

◆ **Ferric Ferrocyanide** *see* Ferric Hexacyanoferrate *on page 761*

Ferric Gluconate (FER ik GLOO koe nate)

Brand Names: US Ferrlecit; Nulecit [DSC]

Brand Names: Canada Ferrlecit

Index Terms Sodium Ferric Gluconate; Sodium Ferric Gluconate Complex

Pharmacologic Category Iron Salt

Use Iron deficiency anemia: Treatment of iron-deficiency anemia in patients undergoing hemodialysis in conjunction with erythropoietin therapy

Dosing

Adult & Geriatric

Iron-deficiency anemia, hemodialysis patients: IV: 125 mg elemental iron per dialysis session. Most patients will require a cumulative dose of 1 g elemental iron over approximately 8 sequential dialysis treatments to achieve a favorable response.

Note: A test dose of 2 mL diluted in NS 50 mL administered over 60 minutes was previously recommended (not in current manufacturer labeling). Doses >125 mg are associated with increased adverse events.

Chemotherapy-associated anemia (off-label use): IV infusion: 125 mg once every week for 6 doses (Pedrazzoli, 2008) or for 8 doses (Henry, 2007)

Pediatric Iron-deficiency anemia, hemodialysis patients: Children ≥6 years: IV: 1.5 mg/kg of elemental iron (maximum: 125 mg/dose) per dialysis session. Doses >1.5 mg/kg are associated with increased adverse events.

Renal Impairment No dosage adjustment necessary. The ferric gluconate iron complex is not dialyzable.

Hepatic Impairment No dosage adjustment necessary.

Additional Information Complete prescribing information should be consulted for additional detail.

Dosage Forms Considerations Strength of ferric gluconate injection is expressed as elemental iron.

Dosage Forms Excipient information presented when available (limited, particularly for generics); consult specific product labeling. [DSC] = Discontinued product
Solution, Intravenous:
Ferrlecit: 12.5 mg/mL (5 mL) [contains benzyl alcohol, sucrose]
Nulecit: 12.5 mg/mL (5 mL [DSC]) [contains benzyl alcohol, sucrose]
Generic: 12.5 mg/mL (5 mL)

Ferric Hexacyanoferrate (FER ik hex a SYE an oh fer ate)

Brand Names: US Radiogardase
Index Terms Ferric (III) Hexacyanoferrate (II); Ferric Ferrocyanide; Insoluble Prussian Blue; Prussian Blue
Pharmacologic Category Antidote
Use Internal contamination: Treatment of patients with known or suspected internal contamination with radioactive cesium and/or radioactive or nonradioactive thallium to increase their rates of elimination.
Dosing
Adult & Geriatric
Internal contamination with radioactive cesium and/ or radioactive or nonradioactive thallium: Oral:
Note: Treatment should begin as soon as possible following exposure, but is also effective if therapy is delayed. Treatment typically continues for ≥30 days.
Manufacturer's labeling: 3 g 3 times daily
Alternative recommendations: Cesium exposure: 1 to 3 g 3 times daily (REMM, 2014)
Pediatric
Internal contamination with radioactive cesium and/ or radioactive or nonradioactive thallium: Oral:
Note: treatment should begin as soon as possible following exposure, but is also effective if therapy is delayed. Treatment typically continues for ≥30 days.
Children 2 to 12 years: 1 g 3 times daily
Adolescents: Refer to adult dosing.
Renal Impairment There are no dosage adjustments provided in the manufacturer's labeling; however, ferric hexacyanoferrate is not systemically absorbed.
Hepatic Impairment There are no dosage adjustments provided in the manufacturer's labeling; however, effectiveness may be decreased due to decreased biliary excretion of cesium and thallium.
Additional Information Complete prescribing information should be consulted for additional detail.
Dosage Forms Excipient information presented when available (limited, particularly for generics); consult specific product labeling.
Capsule, Oral:
Radiogardase: 0.5 g

♦ Ferric x-150 [OTC] see Polysaccharide-Iron Complex on page 1469
♦ Ferrimin 150 [OTC] see Ferrous Fumarate on page 761
♦ Ferriprox see Deferiprone on page 512
♦ Ferrlecit see Ferric Gluconate on page 760
♦ Ferro-Bob [OTC] see Ferrous Sulfate on page 762
♦ Ferrocite [OTC] see Ferrous Fumarate on page 761

Ferrous Fumarate (FER us FYOO ma rate)

Brand Names: US Ferretts [OTC]; Ferrimin 150 [OTC]; Ferrocite [OTC]; Hemocyte [OTC]
Brand Names: Canada Palafer®
Index Terms Iron Fumarate
Pharmacologic Category Iron Salt
Use Prevention and treatment of iron-deficiency anemias
Dosing
Adult Note: Doses expressed in terms of elemental iron; ferrous fumarate contains 33% elemental iron.
Dietary Reference Intake: Oral:
19 to 50 years: Males: 8 mg/day; Females: 18 mg/day; Pregnant females: 27 mg/day; Lactating females: 9 mg/day
≥50 years: 8 mg/day

Iron deficiency anemia, prevention: Oral: 60 mg once daily (Stoltzfus 1998; WHO 2001)
Iron deficiency anemia, treatment of iron deficiency: Oral: 100 to 200 mg daily in 2 to 3 divided doses (Liu 2012; Stoltzfus 1998; WHO 2001)
Note: To avoid GI upset, start with a single daily dose and increase by 1 tablet/day each week or as tolerated until desired daily dose is achieved

Geriatric Lower doses (15 to 50 mg elemental iron/day) may have similar efficacy and less GI adverse events (eg, nausea,constipation) as compared to higher doses (eg, 150 mg elemental iron/day) (Rimon 2005).
Pediatric Note: Doses expressed in terms of elemental iron; ferrous fumarate contains 33% elemental iron.
Dietary Reference Intake: Oral:
0 to 6 months: 0.27 mg/day (adequate intake)
7 to 12 months: 11 mg/day
1 to 3 years: 7 mg/day
4 to 8 years: 10 mg/day
9 to 13 years: 8 mg/day
14 to 18 years: Males: 11 mg/day; Females: 15 mg/day; Pregnant females: 27 mg/day; Lactating females: 10 mg/day

Iron deficiency anemia, prevention: Oral:
Children ≥5 years in areas where anemia prevalence is >40%: 30 mg daily with folic acid (WHO 2001)
Adolescents in areas where anemia prevalence is >40%: 60 mg daily with folic acid (WHO 2001)
Iron deficiency anemia, treatment of iron deficiency: Oral: 3 to 6 mg/kg/day in 3 divided doses (Carney 2010, Kliegman 2011)
Additional Information Complete prescribing information should be consulted for additional detail.
Dosage Forms Excipient information presented when available (limited, particularly for generics); consult specific product labeling.
Tablet, Oral:
Ferretts: 325 mg (106 mg elemental iron) [scored]
Ferrimin 150: Elemental iron 150 mg
Ferrocite: 324 mg (106 mg elemental iron) [contains fd&c blue #1 aluminum lake, fd&c yellow #5 aluminum lake]
Hemocyte: 324 mg (106 mg elemental iron)
Generic: 90 mg (29.5 mg elemental iron), 324 mg (106 mg elemental iron), Elemental iron 29 mg

Ferrous Gluconate (FER us GLOO koe nate)

Brand Names: US Ferate [OTC]; Fergon [OTC]
Brand Names: Canada Apo-Ferrous Gluconate®; Novo-Ferrogluc
Index Terms Iron Gluconate
Pharmacologic Category Iron Salt
Use Prevention and treatment of iron-deficiency anemias
Dosing
Adult Note: Dose expressed in terms of elemental iron; ferrous gluconate contains ~12% elemental iron:
Dietary Reference Intake: Oral:
19 to 50 years: Males: 8 mg/day; Females: 18 mg/day; Pregnant females: 27 mg/day; Lactating females: 9 mg/day
≥50 years: 8 mg/day

Iron deficiency anemia, prevention: Oral: 60 mg daily (Stoltzfus 1998; WHO 2001)
Iron deficiency anemia, treatment of iron deficiency: Oral: 100 to 200 mg daily in 2 to 3 divided doses (Liu 2012; Stoltzfus 1998; WHO 2001)
Geriatric Lower doses (15 to 50 mg elemental iron/day) may have similar efficacy and less GI adverse events (eg, nausea, constipation) as compared to higher doses (eg, 150 mg elemental iron/day) (Rimon 2005).
Pediatric Note: Dose expressed in terms of elemental iron; ferrous gluconate contains ~12% elemental iron:
Dietary Reference Intake: Oral:
0 to 6 months: 0.27 mg/day (adequate intake)
7 to 12 months: 11 mg/day
1 to 3 years: 7 mg/day
4 to 8 years: 10 mg/day
9 to 13 years: 8 mg/day
14 to 18 years: Males: 11 mg/day; Females: 15 mg/day; Pregnant females: 27 mg/day; Lactating females: 10 mg/day

Iron deficiency anemia, prevention: Oral:
Children ≥5 years in areas where anemia prevalence is >40%: 30 mg daily with folic acid (WHO 2001)
Adolescents in areas where anemia prevalence is >40%: 60 mg /daily with folic acid (WHO 2001)
Iron deficiency anemia, treatment of iron deficiency: Oral: 3 to 6 mg/kg/day in 3 divided doses (Carney 2010; Kliegman 2011)
Additional Information Complete prescribing information should be consulted for additional detail.
Dosage Forms Excipient information presented when available (limited, particularly for generics); consult specific product labeling. [DSC] = Discontinued product
Tablet, Oral:
Fergon: 240 mg [elemental iron 27 mg] [contains tartrazine (fd&c yellow #5)]

Generic: 240 mg [elemental iron 27 mg], 324 mg [elemental iron 38 mg], 325 mg [elemental iron 36 mg]
Tablet, Oral [preservative free]:
Ferate: 240 mg [elemental iron 27 mg] [corn free, dairy free, egg free, fragrance free, gluten free, no artificial flavor(s), sodium free, soy free, starch free, sugar free, wheat free, yeast free; contains fd&c blue #1 aluminum lake, fd&c yellow #6 aluminum lake]
Ferate: 256 mg [elemental iron 28 mg] [DSC] [gluten free, lactose free, milk free, no artificial color(s), no artificial flavor(s), sodium free, soy free, sugar free, wheat free, yeast free]

Ferrous Sulfate (FER us SUL fate)

Brand Names: US BProtected Pedia Iron [OTC]; Feosol [OTC] [DSC]; Fer-In-Sol [OTC]; Fer-Iron [OTC]; FeroSul [OTC]; Ferro-Bob [OTC]; FerrouSul [OTC]; Iron Supplement Childrens [OTC]; Slow Fe [OTC]; Slow Iron [OTC]; Slow Release Iron [OTC] [DSC]
Brand Names: Canada Apo-Ferrous Sulfate; Fer-In-Sol; Ferodan
Index Terms Feosol Original; FeSO₄; Iron Sulfate; Slow FE
Pharmacologic Category Iron Salt
Use Prevention and treatment of iron-deficiency anemias
Dosing
Adult Note: Multiple concentrations of ferrous sulfate oral liquid exist; close attention must be paid to the concentration when ordering and administering ferrous sulfate; incorrect selection or substitution of one ferrous sulfate liquid for another without proper dosage volume adjustment may result in serious over- or underdosing. Dose expressed in terms of elemental iron; ferrous sulfate contains ~20% elemental iron; ferrous sulfate exsiccated (dried) contains ~30% elemental iron:

Dietary Reference Intake: Oral:
19 to 50 years: Males: 8 mg daily; Females: 18 mg daily; Pregnant females: 27 mg daily; Lactating females: 9 mg daily
≥50 years: 8 mg daily

Iron deficiency anemia, prevention: Oral: 60 mg once daily (Stoltzfus, 1998; WHO, 2001).
Iron deficiency anemia, treatment of iron deficiency: Oral: 100 to 200 mg daily in 2 to 3 divided doses (Liu, 2012; Stoltzfus, 1998; WHO, 2001). **Note:** Extended release tablets are intended for once daily use.
Geriatric Lower doses (15-50 mg elemental iron/day) may have similar efficacy and less GI adverse events (eg, nausea, constipation) as compared to higher doses (eg, 150 mg elemental iron/day) (Rimon 2005).
Pediatric Note: Multiple concentrations of ferrous sulfate oral liquid exist; close attention must be paid to the concentration when ordering and administering ferrous sulfate; incorrect selection or substitution of one ferrous sulfate liquid for another without proper dosage volume adjustment may result in serious over- or underdosing. Dosage expressed in terms of elemental iron; ferrous sulfate contains ~20% elemental iron; ferrous sulfate exsiccated (dried) contains ~30% elemental iron:

Dietary Reference Intake: Oral:
0 to 6 months: 0.27 mg daily (adequate intake)
7 to 12 months: 11 mg daily
1 to 3 years: 7 mg daily
4 to 8 years: 10 mg daily
9 to 13 years: 8 mg daily
14 to 18 years: Males: 11 mg daily; Females: 15 mg daily; Pregnant females: 27 mg daily; Lactating females: 10 mg daily

Iron deficiency anemia, prevention: Oral:
Infants ≥4 months (receiving human milk as only nutritional source or >50% as source of nutrition without iron fortified food): 1 mg/kg/day (Baker, 2010); **Note:** In healthy, term infants, AAP does not recommend routine additional supplementation of iron be considered until at least 4 to 6 months of age if breast-fed (full or partial) (Baker, 2010; Schanler, 2011).
Infants and Children 6 months to <2 years in areas where anemia prevalence is >40% and iron fortified foods not available: 2 mg/kg/day (WHO, 2001).
Children 2 years to <5 years in areas where anemia prevalence is >40%: 2 mg/kg/day (maximum dose: 30 mg/day) (WHO, 2001).
Children ≥5 years in areas where anemia prevalence is >40%: 30 mg daily with folic acid (WHO, 2001).
Adolescents in areas where anemia prevalence is >40%: 60 mg daily with folic acid (WHO, 2001).
Iron deficiency anemia, treatment of iron deficiency: Oral: 3 to 6 mg/kg/day in 3 divided doses (Carney, 2010; Kliegman, 2011).

Additional Information Complete prescribing information should be consulted for additional detail.
Dosage Forms Excipient information presented when available (limited, particularly for generics); consult specific product labeling. [DSC] = Discontinued product
Elixir, Oral:
FeroSul: 220 (44 Fe) mg/5 mL (473 mL) [contains alcohol, usp, fd&c yellow #6 (sunset yellow), propylene glycol, saccharin sodium, sodium benzoate; lemon flavor]
Generic: 220 (44 Fe) mg/5 mL (5 mL [DSC], 473 mL)
Liquid, Oral:
Generic: 220 (44 Fe) mg/5 mL (473 mL)
Solution, Oral:
BProtected Pedia Iron: 75 (15 Fe) mg/mL (50 mL) [alcohol free, gluten free; contains sodium metabisulfite; citrus flavor]
Fer-In-Sol: 75 (15 Fe) mg/mL (50 mL) [contains alcohol, usp, sodium bisulfite]
Fer-Iron: 75 (15 Fe) mg/mL (50 mL) [contains sodium metabisulfite; lemon flavor]
Iron Supplement Childrens: 75 (15 Fe) mg/mL (50 mL) [alcohol free, dye free, gluten free, lactose free; contains sodium bisulfite]
Generic: 75 (15 Fe) mg/mL (50 mL)
Syrup, Oral:
Generic: 300 (60 Fe) mg/5 mL (5 mL)
Tablet, Oral:
Feosol: 200 (65 Fe) mg [DSC] [contains brilliant blue fcf (fd&c blue #1), fd&c yellow #6 (sunset yellow)]
Ferro-Bob: 325 (65 Fe) mg
Generic: 325 (65 Fe) mg
Tablet, Oral [preservative free]:
FerrouSul: 325 (65 Fe) mg [sodium free, starch free]
Generic: 325 (65 Fe) mg
Tablet Delayed Release, Oral:
Generic: 324 (65 Fe) mg, 325 (65 Fe) mg
Tablet Extended Release, Oral:
Slow Fe: 160 (50 Fe) mg
Slow Fe: 142 (45 Fe) mg [contains fd&c blue #1 aluminum lake, fd&c red #40 aluminum lake, fd&c yellow #6 aluminum lake]
Slow Release Iron: 140 (45 Fe) mg [DSC] [contains brilliant blue fcf (fd&c blue #1), fd&c red #40 aluminum lake, fd&c yellow #6 aluminum lake]
Tablet Extended Release, Oral [preservative free]:
Slow Iron: 160 (50 Fe) mg [gluten free]
Generic: 140 (45 Fe) mg

♦ FerrouSul [OTC] see Ferrous Sulfate on page 762

Ferumoxytol (fer ue MOX i tol)

Brand Names: US Feraheme
Brand Names: Canada Feraheme
Pharmacologic Category Iron Salt
Use Iron-deficiency anemia in chronic kidney disease: Treatment of iron-deficiency anemia in adults with chronic kidney disease
Dosing
Adult & Geriatric Doses expressed in mg of **elemental** iron. **Note:** Test dose: Product labeling does not indicate need for a test dose.

Iron-deficiency anemia in chronic kidney disease: IV:
US labeling: 510 mg as an IV infusion, followed by a second 510 mg IV infusion 3 to 8 days after initial dose. Assess response at least 30 days following the second dose. The recommended dose may be readministered in patients with persistent or recurrent iron-deficiency anemia.
Canadian labeling:
Baseline hemoglobin >10 to 12 g/dL:
Body weight ≤50 kg: 510 mg as an IV infusion.
Body weight >50 kg: 510 mg as an IV infusion, followed by a second 510 mg IV infusion 2 to 8 days after initial dose.
Baseline hemoglobin ≤10 g/dL (regardless of weight): 510 mg as an IV infusion, followed by a second 510 mg IV infusion 2 to 8 days after initial dose.
Renal Impairment No dosage adjustment necessary.
Hemodialysis: Not removed by hemodialysis; however, administer dose after at least 1 hour of hemodialysis has been completed and once blood pressure has stabilized.
Hepatic Impairment There are no dosage adjustments provided in the manufacturer's labeling.
Additional Information Complete prescribing information should be consulted for additional detail.
Dosage Forms Considerations Strength of ferumoxytol is expressed as elemental iron

Dosage Forms Excipient information presented when available (limited, particularly for generics); consult specific product labeling.
Solution, Intravenous [preservative free]:
Feraheme: 510 mg/17 mL (17 mL)

◆ FerUS [OTC] [DSC] *see* Polysaccharide-Iron Complex *on page 1469*

◆ FESO *see* Fesoterodine *on page 763*

◆ FeSO₄ *see* Ferrous Sulfate *on page 762*

Fesoterodine (fes oh TER oh deen)

Brand Names: US Toviaz
Brand Names: Canada Toviaz
Index Terms FESO; Fesoterodine Fumarate
Pharmacologic Category Anticholinergic Agent
Use Treatment of patients with an overactive bladder with symptoms of urinary frequency, urgency, or urge incontinence.
Pregnancy Considerations Adverse effects have been observed in some animal reproduction studies.
Breast-Feeding Considerations It is not known if fesoterodine is excreted in breast milk. According to the manufacturer, the decision to continue or discontinue breast-feeding during therapy should take into account the risk of exposure to the infant and the benefits of treatment to the mother.
Contraindications Hypersensitivity to fesoterodine or tolterodine (both are metabolized to 5-hydroxymethyl tolterodine) or any component of the formulation; urinary retention; gastric retention; uncontrolled narrow-angle glaucoma
Warnings/Precautions Cases of angioedema involving the face, lips, tongue, and/or larynx have been reported. Immediately discontinue if tongue, hypopharynx, or larynx are involved. May cause drowsiness and/or blurred vision, which may impair physical or mental abilities; patients must be cautioned about performing tasks which require mental alertness (eg, operating machinery or driving). CNS effects may be potentiated when used with other sedative drugs or ethanol. Consider dose reduction or discontinuation if CNS effects occur. Patients may experience decreased sweating; caution use in hot weather or during exercise. Use is not recommended in patients with severe hepatic impairment (Child-Pugh class C). Doses >4 mg are not recommended for patients with severe renal impairment (CrCl <30 mL/minute) or patients receiving concurrent therapy with strong CYP3A4 inhibitors (no dosing adjustments are recommended in patients receiving moderate CYP3A4 inhibitors). Use caution in patients with bladder flow obstruction, gastrointestinal obstructive disorders, myasthenia gravis, and treated narrow-angle glaucoma. This medication is associated with potent anticholinergic properties which may be inappropriate in older adults depending on comorbidities (eg, dementia, delirium) (Beers Criteria). In addition, risk of adverse effects may be increased in elderly patients.
Adverse Reactions
>10%: Gastrointestinal: Xerostomia (19% to 35%; dose related)
1% to 10%:
Central nervous system: Insomnia (1%)
Dermatological: Rash (1%)
Gastrointestinal: Constipation (4% to 6%), dyspepsia (2%), nausea (1% to 2%), abdominal pain (1%)
Genitourinary: Urinary tract infection (3% to 4%), dysuria (1% to 2%), urinary retention (1%)
Hepatic: ALT increased (1%), GGT increased (1%)
Neuromuscular & skeletal: Back pain (1% to 2%)
Ocular: Dry eyes (1% to 4%)
Respiratory: Upper respiratory tract infection (2% to 3%), cough (1% to 2%), dry throat (1% to 2%)
Miscellaneous: Peripheral edema (1%)
<1% (Limited to important or life-threatening): Angina, angioedema, diverticulitis, gastroenteritis, heat prostration, hypersensitivity reactions, irritable bowel syndrome, QTc prolongation
Drug Interactions
Metabolism/Transport Effects **Substrate** of CYP2D6 (minor), CYP3A4 (major); **Note:** Assignment of Major/Minor substrate status based on clinically relevant drug interaction potential
Avoid Concomitant Use
Avoid concomitant use of Fesoterodine with any of the following: Aclidinium; Cimetropium; Conivaptan; Eluxadoline; Fusidic Acid (Systemic); Glucagon; Glycopyrrolate; Glycopyrrolate (Oral Inhalation); Idelalisib; Ipratropium (Oral Inhalation); Levosulpiride; Potassium Chloride; Tiotropium; Umeclidinium

Increased Effect/Toxicity
Fesoterodine may increase the levels/effects of: AbobotulinumtoxinA; Analgesics (Opioid); Anticholinergic Agents; Cannabinoid-Containing Products; Cimetropium; Eluxadoline; Glucagon; Glycopyrrolate; Glycopyrrolate (Oral Inhalation); Mirabegron; OnabotulinumtoxinA; Potassium Chloride; Ramosetron; RimabotulinumtoxinB; Thiazide Diuretics; Tiotropium; Topiramate

The levels/effects of Fesoterodine may be increased by: Aclidinium; Alcohol (Ethyl); Aprepitant; Conivaptan; CYP2D6 Inhibitors; CYP3A4 Inhibitors (Moderate); CYP3A4 Inhibitors (Strong); Dasatinib; Fosaprepitant; Fusidic Acid (Systemic); Idelalisib; Ipratropium (Oral Inhalation); Ivacaftor; Luliconazole; Mianserin; Mifepristone; Netupitant; Osimertinib; Palbociclib; Pramlintide; Simeprevir; Stiripentol; Umeclidinium
Decreased Effect
Fesoterodine may decrease the levels/effects of: Acetylcholinesterase Inhibitors; Gastrointestinal Agents (Prokinetic); Itopride; Levosulpiride; Secretin

The levels/effects of Fesoterodine may be decreased by: Acetylcholinesterase Inhibitors; Bosentan; CYP3A4 Inducers (Moderate); CYP3A4 Inducers (Strong); Dabrafenib; Deferasirox; Enzalutamide; Mitotane; Osimertinib; Siltuximab; St Johns Wort; Tocilizumab
Storage/Stability Store at 20°C to 25°C (68°F to 77°F); excursions permitted between 15°C to 30°C (59°F to 86°F). Protect from moisture.
Mechanism of Action Fesoterodine acts as a prodrug and is converted to an active metabolite, 5-hydroxymethyl tolterodine (5-HMT); 5-HMT is responsible for fesoterodine's antimuscarinic activity and acts as a competitive antagonist of muscarinic receptors.

Urinary bladder contractions are mediated by muscarinic receptors; fesoterodine inhibits the receptors in the bladder preventing symptoms of urgency and frequency.
Pharmacodynamics/Kinetics
Absorption: Well absorbed
Distribution: IV: 5-HMT: V_d: 169 L
Protein binding: 5-HMT: ~50% (primarily to albumin and alpha₁-acid glycoprotein)
Metabolism: Fesoterodine is rapidly and extensively metabolized to its active metabolite (5-hydroxymethyl tolterodine; 5-HMT) by nonspecific esterases; 5-HMT is further metabolized via CYP2D6 and CYP3A4 to inactive metabolites.
Bioavailability: 5-HMT: 52%
Half-life elimination: ~7 hours
Time to peak, plasma: 5-HMT: ~5 hours; C_{max} higher in poor CYP2D6 metabolizers
Excretion: Urine (~70%; 16% as 5-HMT, ~53% as inactive metabolites); feces (7%)
Dosing
Adult & Geriatric Overactive bladder: Oral: 4 mg once daily; may be increased to 8 mg once daily based on individual response and tolerability
Dosing adjustment for concomitant strong CYP3A4 inhibitors (eg, ketoconazole, itraconazole, clarithromycin): 4 mg once daily; maximum dose: 4 mg once daily
Renal Impairment
CrCl ≥30 mL/minute: No dosage adjustment necessary.
CrCl <30 mL/minute: 4 mg once daily; maximum dose: 4 mg once daily
Hepatic Impairment
Mild-to-moderate impairment (Child-Pugh class A or B): No dosage adjustment necessary.
Severe impairment (Child-Pugh class C): Use is not recommended; has not been studied.
Dietary Considerations May be taken with or without food.
Administration May be administered with or without food. Swallow whole; do not chew, crush, or divide.
Dosage Forms Excipient information presented when available (limited, particularly for generics); consult specific product labeling.
Tablet Extended Release 24 Hour, Oral, as fumarate:
Toviaz: 4 mg, 8 mg [contains fd&c blue #2 aluminum lake, soybean lecithin]

◆ Fesoterodine Fumarate *see* Fesoterodine *on page 763*

◆ FeverAll Adult [OTC] *see* Acetaminophen *on page 25*

◆ FeverAll Childrens [OTC] *see* Acetaminophen *on page 25*

◆ FeverAll Infants [OTC] *see* Acetaminophen *on page 25*

◆ FeverAll Junior Strength [OTC] *see* Acetaminophen *on page 25*

◆ Fexmid *see* Cyclobenzaprine *on page 454*

Fexofenadine (feks oh FEN a deen)

Brand Names: US Allegra Allergy Childrens [OTC]; Allegra Allergy [OTC]; Allergy 24-HR [OTC]; Fexofenadine HCl Childrens [OTC]; Mucinex Allergy [OTC]

Brand Names: Canada Allegra 12 Hour (OTC); Allegra 24 Hour (OTC)

Index Terms Fexofenadine Hydrochloride

Pharmacologic Category Histamine H_1 Antagonist; Histamine H_1 Antagonist, Second Generation; Piperidine Derivative

Use

Chronic idiopathic urticaria: Treatment of chronic idiopathic urticaria

OTC labeling: Relief of symptoms associated with allergic rhinitis

Pregnancy Considerations Adverse events have been observed in animal reproduction studies; therefore, the manufacturer classifies fexofenadine as pregnancy category C. The use of antihistamines for the treatment of rhinitis during pregnancy is generally considered to be safe at recommended doses. Information related to the use of fexofenadine during pregnancy is limited; therefore, other agents are preferred.

Breast-Feeding Considerations Following administration of terfenadine to nursing mothers, fexofenadine (active metabolite of terfenadine) was found to cross into human breast milk (Allegra Canadian product monograph, 2006). The U.S. manufacturer recommends that caution be exercised when administering fexofenadine to nursing women. The Canadian labeling recommends avoiding use in nursing women.

Contraindications Hypersensitivity to fexofenadine or any component of the formulation

Warnings/Precautions Use with caution in patients with renal impairment; dosage adjustment recommended. Orally disintegrating tablet contains phenylalanine. Effects may be potentiated when used with other sedative drugs or ethanol.

Adverse Reactions

>10%:

Central nervous system: Headache (5% to 11%)

Gastrointestinal: Vomiting (children 6 months to 5 years: 4% to 12%)

1% to 10%:

Central nervous system: Fatigue (1% to 3%), somnolence (1% to 3%), dizziness (2%), fever (2%), pain (2%), drowsiness (1%)

Endocrine & metabolic: Dysmenorrhea (2%)

Gastrointestinal: Diarrhea (3% to 4%), nausea (2%), dyspepsia (1% to 2%)

Neuromuscular & skeletal: Myalgia (3%), back pain (2% to 3%), pain in extremities (2%)

Otic: Otitis media (2% to 4%)

Respiratory: Upper respiratory tract infection (3% to 4%), cough (2% to 4%), rhinorrhea (1% to 2%)

Miscellaneous: Viral infection (3%)

<1% (Limited to important or life-threatening): Hypersensitivity reactions (anaphylaxis, angioedema, chest tightness, dyspnea, flushing, pruritus, rash, urticaria); insomnia, nervousness, sleep disorders, paroniria

Drug Interactions

Metabolism/Transport Effects Substrate of CYP3A4 (minor), P-glycoprotein, SLCO1B1; **Note:** Assignment of Major/Minor substrate status based on clinically relevant drug interaction potential; **Inhibits** CYP2D6 (weak)

Avoid Concomitant Use

Avoid concomitant use of Fexofenadine with any of the following: Aclidinium; Azelastine (Nasal); Cimetropium; Eluxadoline; Glucagon; Glycopyrrolate; Glycopyrrolate (Oral Inhalation); Ipratropium (Oral Inhalation); Levosulpiride; Orphenadrine; Paraldehyde; Potassium Chloride; Thalidomide; Tiotropium; Umeclidinium

Increased Effect/Toxicity

Fexofenadine may increase the levels/effects of: AbobotulinumtoxinA; Alcohol (Ethyl); Analgesics (Opioid); Anticholinergic Agents; ARIPiprazole; Azelastine (Nasal); Buprenorphine; Cimetropium; CNS Depressants; Eluxadoline; Glucagon; Glycopyrrolate; Glycopyrrolate (Oral Inhalation); Hydrocodone; Methotrimeprazine; Metyrosine; Mirabegron; Mirtazapine; OnabotulinumtoxinA; Orphenadrine; Paraldehyde; Potassium Chloride; Pramipexole; Ramosetron; RimabotulinumtoxinB; ROPINIRole; Rotigotine; Selective Serotonin Reuptake Inhibitors; Suvorexant; Thalidomide; Thiazide Diuretics; Tiotropium; Topiramate; Zolpidem

The levels/effects of Fexofenadine may be increased by: Aclidinium; Brimonidine (Topical); Cannabis; Doxylamine; Dronabinol; Droperidol; Eltrombopag; Erythromycin (Systemic); HydrOXYzine; Ipratropium (Oral Inhalation); Itraconazole; Kava Kava; Ketoconazole (Systemic); Lumacaftor; Magnesium Sulfate; Methotrimeprazine; Mianserin; Minocycline; Nabilone; Perampanel; P-glycoprotein/ABCB1 Inhibitors; Pramlintide; Ranolazine; Rifampin; Rufinamide; Sodium Oxybate; Tapentadol; Teriflunomide; Tetrahydrocannabinol; Umeclidinium; Verapamil

Decreased Effect

Fexofenadine may decrease the levels/effects of: Acetylcholinesterase Inhibitors; Benzylpenicilloyl Polylysine; Betahistine; Gastrointestinal Agents (Prokinetic); Hyaluronidase; Itopride; Levosulpiride; Secretin

The levels/effects of Fexofenadine may be decreased by: Acetylcholinesterase Inhibitors; Amphetamines; Antacids; Grapefruit Juice; Lumacaftor; P-glycoprotein/ABCB1 Inducers; Rifampin

Food Interactions High-fat meals decrease the bioavailability of fexofenadine by ~50%. Fruit juice (apple, grapefruit, orange) may decrease bioavailability of fexofenadine by ~36%. Management: Administer with water only, avoid fruit juice.

Storage/Stability

U.S. labeling: Store at controlled room temperature of 20°C to 25°C (68°F to 77°F). Protect from excessive moisture.

Canadian labeling: Store at 15°C to 30°C (59°F to 86°F). Protect from moisture.

Mechanism of Action Fexofenadine is an active metabolite of terfenadine and like terfenadine it competes with histamine for H_1-receptor sites on effector cells in the gastrointestinal tract, blood vessels and respiratory tract; it appears that fexofenadine does not cross the blood-brain barrier to any appreciable degree, resulting in a reduced potential for sedation

Pharmacodynamics/Kinetics

Onset of action: 2 hours (Simons 2004)

Duration of action: 24 hours (Simons 2004)

Absorption: Rapid

Distribution: V_d: Children: 5.4 to 5.8 L/kg

Protein binding: 60% to 70% (Brunton 2011); primarily albumin and alpha$_1$-acid glycoprotein

Metabolism: Minimal (Hepatic ~5%); 3.5% transformed into methylester metabolite found only in feces (possibly transformed by gut microflora)

Half-life elimination: 14.4 hours (59% longer in patients with mild to moderate renal impairment [CrCl 41 to 80 mL/minute]; 72% longer in patients with severe impairment [CrCl 11 to 40 mL/minute]) (Simons 2004)

Time to peak, serum: ODT: 2 hours (4 hours with high-fat meal); Tablet: ~2.6 hours (Simons 2004); Suspension: ~1 hour

Excretion: Feces (~80%) and urine (~11%) as unchanged drug (Simons 2004)

Dosing

Adult

Chronic idiopathic urticaria: Oral:

U.S. labeling: 60 mg twice daily **or** 180 mg once daily

Canadian labeling: 60 mg every 12 hours

Allergic rhinitis (OTC labeling): Oral:

U.S. labeling: 60 mg twice daily or 180 mg once daily

Canadian labeling: 60 mg every 12 hours **or** 120 mg once daily

Geriatric Chronic idiopathic urticaria, allergic rhinitis: Oral: Use caution; adjust dose for renal impairment.

Pediatric Note: Canadian labeling does not approve of use in children <12 years.

Chronic idiopathic urticaria: Oral:

Children 6 months to <2 years: 15 mg twice daily

Children 2 to 11 years: 30 mg twice daily

Children ≥12 years and Adolescents: Refer to adult dosing.

Allergic rhinitis (OTC labeling): Oral:

Children 2 to 11 years: Oral: 30 mg twice daily

Children ≥12 years and Adolescents: Refer to adult dosing.

Renal Impairment Note: Canadian labeling does not approve of use in children <12 years

CrCl <80 mL/minute:

Children ≥12 years and Adults: Initial: 60 mg once daily

Children 2 to 11 years: Initial: 30 mg once daily

Children 6 months to <2 years: Initial: 15 mg once daily

Hemodialysis: Not effectively removed by hemodialysis.

Hepatic Impairment There are no dosage adjustment provided in the manufacturer's labeling; however, need for adjustment not likely since undergoes minimal hepatic metabolism.

Dietary Considerations Some products may contain phenylalanine and/or sodium. Take suspension and tablets with water only; do not administer with fruit juices.

Administration

Suspension, tablet: Administer with water only; do not administer with fruit juices. Shake suspension well before use.

Orally disintegrating tablet: Take on an empty stomach. Do not remove from blister pack until administered. Using dry hands, place immediately on tongue. Tablet will dissolve within seconds, and may be swallowed with or without liquid (do not administer with fruit juices). Do not split or chew.

Monitoring Parameters Relief of symptoms

Test Interactions May suppress the wheal and flare reactions to skin test antigens.

Dosage Forms Excipient information presented when available (limited, particularly for generics); consult specific product labeling.

Suspension, Oral, as hydrochloride:
Allegra Allergy Childrens: 30 mg/5 mL (240 mL) [alcohol free, dye free; contains butylparaben, edetate disodium, propylene glycol, propylparaben; berry flavor]
Allegra Allergy Childrens: 30 mg/5 mL (120 mL) [alcohol free, dye free; contains butylparaben, edetate disodium, propylene glycol, propylparaben; raspberry creme flavor]
Fexofenadine HCl Childrens: 30 mg/5 mL (118 mL) [alcohol free, dye free; contains butylparaben, edetate disodium, propylene glycol, propylparaben; berry flavor]
Tablet, Oral:
Allegra Allergy: 60 mg
Allegra Allergy: 180 mg [contains brilliant blue fcf (fd&c blue #1)]
Tablet, Oral, as hydrochloride:
Allegra Allergy: 60 mg, 180 mg
Allegra Allergy Childrens: 30 mg
Allergy 24-HR: 180 mg
Mucinex Allergy: 180 mg [contains fd&c red #40]
Generic: 60 mg, 180 mg
Tablet Dispersible, Oral, as hydrochloride:
Allegra Allergy Childrens: 30 mg [contains aspartame; orange cream flavor]

Dosage Forms: Canada Excipient information presented when available (limited, particularly for generics); consult specific product labeling.

Tablet, Oral, as hydrochloride:
Allegra 12 Hour: 60 mg
Allegra 24 Hour: 120 mg

Fexofenadine and Pseudoephedrine
(feks oh FEN a deen & soo doe e FED rin)

Brand Names: US Allegra-D® 12 Hour; Allegra-D® 24 Hour
Brand Names: Canada Allegra-D®
Index Terms Pseudoephedrine and Fexofenadine
Pharmacologic Category Alpha/Beta Agonist; Decongestant; Histamine H$_1$ Antagonist; Histamine H$_1$ Antagonist, Second Generation; Piperidine Derivative
Use Relief of symptoms associated with seasonal allergic rhinitis in adults and children ≥12 years of age

Dosing
Adult & Geriatric Allergic symptoms and nasal congestion: Oral:
Allegra-D® 12 Hour: One tablet twice daily
Allegra-D® 24 Hour: One tablet once daily
Pediatric Children ≥12 years: Refer to adult dosing.
Renal Impairment
Allegra-D® 12 Hour: CrCl <80 mL/minute (based on fexofenadine component): One tablet once daily.
Allegra-D® 24 Hour: Avoid use.
Hepatic Impairment No dosage adjustment provided in manufacturer's labeling; however, need for adjustment not likely since fexofenadine undergoes minimal hepatic metabolism; impact of hepatic impairment on pseudoephedrine pharmacokinetics are unknown.
Additional Information Complete prescribing information should be consulted for additional detail.
Dosage Forms Excipient information presented when available (limited, particularly for generics); consult specific product labeling.
Tablet, extended release: Fexofenadine hydrochloride 60 mg [immediate release] and pseudoephedrine hydrochloride 120 mg [extended release]; fexofenadine hydrochloride 180 mg [immediate release] and pseudoephedrine hydrochloride 240 mg [extended release]
Allegra-D® 12 Hour: Fexofenadine hydrochloride 60 mg [immediate release] and pseudoephedrine hydrochloride 120 mg [extended release]
Allegra-D® 24 Hour: Fexofenadine hydrochloride 180 mg [immediate release] and pseudoephedrine hydrochloride 240 mg [extended release]

♦ Fexofenadine HCl Childrens [OTC] *see* Fexofenadine *on page 764*
♦ Fexofenadine Hydrochloride *see* Fexofenadine *on page 764*
♦ Fiber Therapy [OTC] *see* Psyllium *on page 1529*
♦ Fibricor *see* Fenofibrate and Derivatives *on page 746*

Fibrinogen Concentrate (Human)
(fi BRIN o gin KON suhn trate HYU man)

Brand Names: US RiaSTAP
Index Terms Coagulation Factor I
Pharmacologic Category Blood Product Derivative
Use Congenital fibrinogen deficiency: Treatment of acute bleeding episodes in patients with congenital fibrinogen deficiency, including afibrinogenemia and hypofibrinogenemia.

Dosing
Adult & Geriatric Congenital fibrinogen deficiency:
IV: **Note:** Adjust dose based on laboratory values and condition of patient. Maintain a target fibrinogen level of 100 mg/dL until hemostasis is achieved.
When baseline fibrinogen level is known:
Dose (mg/kg) = [Target level (mg/dL) - measured level (mg/dL)] **divided by** 1.7 (mg/dL per mg/kg body weight)
When baseline fibrinogen level is not known: 70 mg/kg
Pediatric Congenital fibrinogen deficiency: IV: Refer to adult dosing.
Renal Impairment There are no dosage adjustments provided in the manufacturer's labeling.
Hepatic Impairment There are no dosage adjustments provided in the manufacturer's labeling.
Additional Information Complete prescribing information should be consulted for additional detail.
Dosage Forms Excipient information presented when available (limited, particularly for generics); consult specific product labeling. [DSC] = Discontinued product
Injection, powder for reconstitution:
RiaSTAP: 900-1300 mg [contains albumin (human); exact potency labeled on vial]

♦ Fibristal (Can) *see* Ulipristal *on page 1851*

Fidaxomicin (fye DAX oh mye sin)

Brand Names: US Dificid
Brand Names: Canada Dificid™
Index Terms Difimicin; Lipiarrmycin; OPT-80; PAR-101; Tiacumicin B
Pharmacologic Category Antibiotic, Macrolide
Use Treatment of *Clostridium difficile*-associated diarrhea (CDAD)
Pregnancy Considerations Adverse events were not observed in animal reproduction studies. Due to the limited systemic absorption of fidaxomicin, exposure to the fetus is expected to be low.
Breast-Feeding Considerations It is not known if fidaxomicin is excreted in breast milk. The manufacturer recommends that caution be exercised when administering fidaxomicin to nursing women.
Contraindications Hypersensitivity to fidaxomicin
Warnings/Precautions Do not use for systemic infections; fidaxomicin systemic absorption is negligible. Hypersensitivity reactions (angioedema [mouth, face, throat], dyspnea, pruritus, and rash) to fidaxomicin have been reported. Patients with a history of macrolide allergy may be at increased risk. If a severe reaction occurs, discontinue drug and institute supportive care. Use only in patients with proven or strongly suspected *Clostridium difficile (C. difficile)* infections.

Adverse Reactions
>10%: Gastrointestinal: Nausea (11%)
2% to 10%:
Gastrointestinal: Gastrointestinal hemorrhage (4%), abdominal pain, vomiting
Hematologic & oncologic: Anemia (2%), neutropenia (2%)
<2% (Limited to important or life-threatening): Abdominal distention, abdominal tenderness, angioedema, decreased platelet count, decreased serum bicarbonate, dyspepsia, dysphagia, dyspnea, fixed drug eruption, flatulence, hepatotoxicity (idiosyncratic) (Chalasani, 2014), hyperglycemia, hypersensitivity reaction, increased liver enzymes, increased serum alkaline phosphatase, intestinal obstruction, megacolon, metabolic acidosis, pruritus, skin rash

Drug Interactions
Metabolism/Transport Effects None known.

Avoid Concomitant Use There are no known interactions where it is recommended to avoid concomitant use.

Increased Effect/Toxicity
Fidaxomicin may increase the levels/effects of: Rilpivirine

Decreased Effect
Fidaxomicin may decrease the levels/effects of: Sodium Picosulfate

Storage/Stability Store at 20°C to 25°C (68°F to 77°F); excursions permitted to 15°C to 30°C (59°F to 86°F).

Mechanism of Action Inhibits RNA polymerase sigma subunit resulting in inhibition of protein synthesis and cell death in susceptible organisms including *C. difficile*; bactericidal

Pharmacodynamics/Kinetics
Absorption: Oral: Minimal systemic absorption

Distribution: Largely confined to the gastrointestinal tract; in single- and multiple-dose studies, fecal concentrations of fidaxomicin and its active metabolite (OP-1118) are very high while serum concentrations are minimally detectable to undetectable

Metabolism: Intestinal hydrolysis to less active metabolite (OP-1118)

Excretion: Feces (>92% as unchanged drug and metabolites); urine (<1% as metabolite)

Dosing
Adult & Geriatric Treatment of diarrhea due to *Clostridium difficile* (CDAD): Oral: 200 mg twice daily for 10 days

Renal Impairment No dosage adjustment necessary (minimal systemic absorption).

Hepatic Impairment No dosage adjustment provided in manufacturer's label (has not been studied); However, due to minimal systemic absorption no dosage adjustment predicted.

Administration May be administered with or without food.

Additional Information Fidaxomicin is bactericidal against gram-positive anaerobes (including *C. difficile* NAP1/B1/027 strain) and gram-positive aerobes. Fidaxomicin spectrum does **not** include gram-negative aerobes or gram-negative anaerobes (eg, *Bacteroides spp*). At the approved dose, concentrations in feces substantially exceed the 90% MIC of *C. difficile*. Postantibiotic effects against *C. difficile* in clinical studies range from 6-10 hours. Clinical studies excluded patients with a history of >1 recurrent *C. difficile*-associated diarrhea (CDAD) episode within 3 months.

Dosage Forms Excipient information presented when available (limited, particularly for generics); consult specific product labeling.
Tablet, Oral:
Dificid: 200 mg [contains soybean lecithin]

Filgrastim (fil GRA stim)

Brand Names: US Granix; Neupogen; Zarxio
Brand Names: Canada Neupogen
Index Terms Filgrastim-Sndz; G-CSF; Granulocyte Colony Stimulating Factor; Tbo-Filgrastim; Tevagrastim
Pharmacologic Category Colony Stimulating Factor; Hematopoietic Agent

Use
Myelosuppressive chemotherapy recipients with non-myeloid malignancies:

Neupogen, Zarxio: To decrease the incidence of infection (neutropenic fever) in patients with nonmyeloid malignancies receiving myelosuppressive chemotherapy associated with a significant incidence of severe neutropenia with fever.

Granix: To decrease the duration of severe neutropenia in patients with nonmyeloid malignancies receiving myelosuppressive chemotherapy associated with a clinically significant incidence of neutropenic fever.

Acute myeloid leukemia (AML) patients following induction or consolidation chemotherapy (Neupogen, Zarxio): To reduce the time to neutrophil recovery and the duration of fever following induction or consolidation chemotherapy in adults with AML.

Bone marrow transplantation (Neupogen, Zarxio): To reduce the duration of neutropenia and neutropenia-related events (eg, neutropenic fever) in patients with nonmyeloid malignancies receiving myeloablative chemotherapy followed by marrow transplantation.

Hematopoietic radiation injury syndrome, acute (Neupogen): To increase survival in patients acutely exposed to myelosuppressive doses of radiation.

Peripheral blood progenitor cell collection and therapy (Neupogen, Zarxio): Mobilization of autologous hematopoietic progenitor cells into the peripheral blood for apheresis collection.

Severe chronic neutropenia (Neupogen, Zarxio): Long-term administration to reduce the incidence and duration of neutropenic complications (eg, fever, infections, oropharyngeal ulcers) in symptomatic patients with congenital, cyclic, or idiopathic neutropenia.

Pregnancy Considerations Adverse events have been observed in animal reproduction studies. Filgrastim has been shown to cross the placenta in humans.

Women who become pregnant during Neupogen treatment are encouraged to enroll in the manufacturer's Pregnancy Surveillance Program (1-800-772-6436).

Breast-Feeding Considerations It is not known if filgrastim, filgrastim-sndz, or tbo-filgrastim is excreted in breast milk. The manufacturers recommend that caution be exercised when administering filgrastim products to breast-feeding women.

Women who are nursing during Neupogen treatment are encouraged to enroll in the manufacturer's Lactation Surveillance program (1-800-772-6436).

Contraindications
Neupogen, Zarxio: History of serious allergic reactions to human granulocyte colony-stimulating factors, such as filgrastim or pegfilgrastim, or any component of the formulation

Granix: There are no contraindications listed in the manufacturer's labeling

Warnings/Precautions Serious allergic reactions (including anaphylaxis) have been reported, usually with the initial exposure; may be managed symptomatically with administration of antihistamines, steroids, bronchodilators, and/or epinephrine. Allergic reactions may recur within days after the initial allergy management has been stopped. Do not administer filgrastim products to patients who experienced serious allergic reaction to filgrastim or pegfilgrastim. Permanently discontinue filgrastim products in patients with serious allergic reactions. Rare cases of splenic rupture have been reported (may be fatal); in patients with upper abdominal pain, left upper quadrant pain, or shoulder tip pain, withhold treatment and evaluate for enlarged spleen or splenic rupture. Moderate or severe cutaneous vasculitis has been reported, generally occurring in patients with severe chronic neutropenia on chronic therapy. Withhold treatment if cutaneous vasculitis occurs; may be restarted with a dose reduction once symptoms resolve and the absolute neutrophil count (ANC) has decreased. Capillary leak syndrome (CLS), characterized by hypotension, hypoalbuminemia, edema, and hemoconcentration, may occur in patients receiving human granulocyte colony-stimulating factors (G-CSF). CLS episode may vary in frequency and severity. If CLS develops, monitor closely and manage symptomatically (may require intensive care). CLS may be life-threatening if treatment is delayed.

White blood cell counts of ≥100,000/mm³ have been reported with filgrastim doses >5 mcg/kg/day. When filgrastim products are used as an adjunct to myelosuppressive chemotherapy, discontinue when ANC exceeds 10,000/mm³ after the ANC nadir has occurred (to avoid potential excessive leukocytosis). Doses that increase the ANC beyond 10,000/mm³ may not result in additional clinical benefit. Monitor complete blood cell count (CBC) twice weekly during therapy. In patients receiving myelosuppressive chemotherapy, filgrastim discontinuation generally resulted in a 50% decrease in circulating neutrophils within 1 to 2 days, and a return to pretreatment levels in 1 to 7 days. When used for peripheral blood progenitor cell collection, discontinue filgrastim products if leukocytes >100,000/mm³. Thrombocytopenia has also been reported with filgrastim products; monitor platelet counts. Filgrastim products should not be routinely used in the treatment of established neutropenic fever. Colony-stimulating factors may be considered in cancer patients with febrile neutropenia who are at high risk for infection-associated complications or who have prognostic factors indicative of a poor clinical outcome (eg, prolonged and severe neutropenia, age >65 years, hypotension, pneumonia, sepsis syndrome, presence of invasive fungal infection, uncontrolled primary disease, hospitalization at the time of fever development) (Freifeld, 2011; Smith, 2006). Colony-stimulating factors (CSF) should not be routinely used for patients with neutropenia who are afebrile. Dose-dense regimens that require colony-stimulating factors should only be used within the context of a clinical trial or if supported by convincing evidence (Smith, 2015). Recommendations for the Use of WBC Growth Factors Clinical Practice Guideline Update recommend that prophylactic CSF be used in patients ≥65 years with diffuse aggressive lymphoma treated with curative chemotherapy (eg, rituximab, cyclophosphamide, doxorubicin, vincristine, prednisone), especially if patients have comorbid conditions (Smith, 2015). CSF use in pediatric patients is typically directed

by clinical pediatric protocols. The American Society of Clinical Oncology (ASCO) Recommendations for the Use of WBC Growth Factors Clinical Practice Guideline Update states that CSFs may be reasonable as primary prophylaxis in pediatric patients when chemotherapy regimens with a high likelihood of febrile neutropenia are employed. Likewise, secondary CSF prophylaxis should be limited to high-risk patients. In pediatric cancers in which dose-intense chemotherapy (with a survival benefit) is used, CSFs should be given to facilitate chemotherapy administration. CSFs should not be used in the pediatric population for nonrelapsed acute lymphoblastic or myeloid leukemia when no infection is present (Smith, 2015). Do not use filgrastim products in the period 24 hours before to 24 hours after administration of cytotoxic chemotherapy because of the potential sensitivity of rapidly dividing myeloid cells to cytotoxic chemotherapy. Transient increase in neutrophil count is seen 1 to 2 days after filgrastim initiation; however, for sustained neutrophil response, continue until post-nadir ANC reaches 10,000/mm³. Avoid simultaneous use of filgrastim products with chemotherapy and radiation therapy. Avoid concurrent radiation therapy with filgrastim; safety and efficacy have not been established with patients receiving radiation therapy. The G-CSF receptor through which filgrastim products act has been found on tumor cell lines. May potentially act as a growth factor for any tumor type (including myeloid malignancies and myelodysplasia). When used for stem cell mobilization, may release tumor cells from marrow, which could be collected in leukapheresis product; potential effect of tumor cell reinfusion is unknown.

May precipitate severe sickle cell crises, sometimes resulting in fatalities, in patients with sickle cell disorders (sickle cell trait or sickle cell disease); carefully evaluate potential risks and benefits. Discontinue in patients undergoing sickle cell crisis. Establish diagnosis of severe chronic neutropenia (SCN) prior to initiation; use prior to appropriate diagnosis of SCN may impair or delay proper evaluation and treatment for neutropenia due to conditions other than SCN. Based on findings of azotemia, hematuria (micro- and macro-scopic), proteinuria, and renal biopsy, glomerulonephritis has occurred in patients receiving filgrastim. Glomerulonephritis usually resolved after filgrastim dose reduction or discontinuation. If glomerulonephritis is suspected, evaluate for cause; if likely due to filgrastim, consider dose reduction or treatment interruption. Myelodysplastic syndrome (MDS) and acute myeloid leukemia (AML) have been reported to occur in the natural history of congenital neutropenia (without cytokine therapy). Cytogenetic abnormalities and transformation to MDS and AML have been observed with filgrastim when used to manage SCN, although the risk for MDS and AML appears to be in patients with congenital neutropenia. Abnormal cytogenetics and MDS are associated with the development of AML. The effects of continuing filgrastim products in patients who have developed abnormal cytogenetics or MDS are unknown; consider risk versus benefits of continuing treatment. Acute respiratory distress syndrome (ARDS) has been reported. Evaluate patients who develop fever and lung infiltrates or respiratory distress for ARDS; discontinue in patients with ARDS. Reports of alveolar hemorrhage, manifested as pulmonary infiltrates and hemoptysis (requiring hospitalization), have occurred in healthy donors undergoing PBPC mobilization (off-label for use in healthy donors); hemoptysis resolved upon discontinuation. Increased bone marrow hematopoietic activity due to CSF use has been associated with transient bone-imaging changes; interpret results accordingly.

The packaging of some dosage forms may contain latex.

Some products available internationally may have vial strength and dosing expressed as units (instead of as micrograms). Refer to prescribing information for specific strength and dosing information.

Some dosage forms may contain polysorbate 80 (also known as Tweens). Hypersensitivity reactions, usually a delayed reaction, have been reported following exposure to pharmaceutical products containing polysorbate 80 in certain individuals (Isaksson, 2002; Lucente 2000; Shelley, 1995). Thrombocytopenia, ascites, pulmonary deterioration, and renal and hepatic failure have been reported in premature neonates after receiving parenteral products containing polysorbate 80 (Alade, 1986; CDC, 1984). See manufacturer's labeling.

Adverse Reactions
>10%:
Cardiovascular: Chest pain (5% to 13%)
Central nervous system: Fatigue (20%), dizziness (14%), pain (12%)
Dermatologic: Skin rash (2% to 14%)

Endocrine & metabolic: Increased lactate dehydrogenase (6% to ≤58%; reversible mild to moderate elevations), increased uric acid (≤58%; reversible mild to moderate elevations)
Gastrointestinal: Nausea (10% to 43%)
Hematologic & oncologic: Thrombocytopenia (5% to 38%), splenomegaly (≥5%; severe chronic neutropenia: 30%), petechia (17%)
Hepatic: Increased serum alkaline phosphatase (6% to 11%)
Neuromuscular & skeletal: Ostealgia (5% to 33%; dose and cycle related), back pain (2% to 15%)
Respiratory: Epistaxis (2% to 15%), cough (14%), dyspnea (13%)
Miscellaneous: Fever (12% to 48%; dose and cycle related)
1% to 10%:
Cardiovascular: Peripheral edema (≥5%), hypertension (≥4%), cardiac arrhythmia (≤3%), myocardial infarction (≤3%)
Central nervous system: Headache (7% to 10%), hypoesthesia (≥5%), insomnia (≥5%), malaise (≥5%), mouth pain (≥5%)
Dermatologic: Alopecia (≥5%), erythema (≥2%), maculopapular rash (≥2%)
Gastrointestinal: Vomiting (5% to 7%), constipation (≥2%), diarrhea (≥2%)
Genitourinary: Decreased appetite (≥5%), urinary tract infection (≥5%)
Hematologic & oncologic: Anemia (≥5%), leukocytosis (≤2%)
Hypersensitivity: Transfusion reaction (2% to 10%), hypersensitivity reaction (≥5%)
Immunologic: Antibody development (3%; no evidence of neutralizing response)
Infection: Sepsis (≥5%)
Neuromuscular & skeletal: Arthralgia (5% to 9%), limb pain (2% to 7%), muscle spasm (≥5%), musculoskeletal pain (≥5%) weakness (≥5%)
Respiratory: Bronchitis (≥5%), upper respiratory tract infection (≥5%)
<1% (Limited to important or life-threatening): Capillary leak syndrome, cerebral hemorrhage, decreased bone mineral density, decreased hemoglobin, erythema nodosum, exacerbation of psoriasis, glomerulonephritis, hematuria, hemoptysis, hepatomegaly, hypersensitivity angiitis, proteinuria, pulmonary hemorrhage, pulmonary infiltrates, renal insufficiency, respiratory distress syndrome, severe sickle cell crisis, splenic rupture, Sweet syndrome, tachycardia

Drug Interactions
Metabolism/Transport Effects None known.
Avoid Concomitant Use There are no known interactions where it is recommended to avoid concomitant use.
Increased Effect/Toxicity
Filgrastim may increase the levels/effects of: Bleomycin; Cyclophosphamide; Topotecan
Decreased Effect There are no known significant interactions involving a decrease in effect.
Preparation for Administration Visually inspect prior to use; discard if discolored or if particulates are present.
Neupogen: **Do not dilute with saline at any time; product may precipitate.** Filgrastim (vial only; do not use prefilled syringe for IV preparation) may be diluted with D₅W to a concentration of 5 to 15 mcg/mL for IV infusion administration (minimum concentration: 5 mcg/mL). Concentrations of 5 to 15 mcg/mL require addition of albumin (final albumin concentration of 2 mg/mL) to prevent adsorption to plastics. Dilution to <5 mcg/mL is not recommended. Do not shake. May be prepared in glass bottles, polyvinyl chloride (PVC) or polyolefin bags, and polypropylene syringes. Discard unused portion of vial.
Granix: Remove needle shield and expel extra volume if needed (depending on dose). Prefilled syringe is single use; discard unused portion.
Zarxio: **Do not dilute with saline at any time; product may precipitate.** Filgrastim-sndz may be diluted with D₅W to a concentration of 5 to 15 mcg/mL for IV infusion administration. Concentrations of 5 to 15 mcg/mL require addition of albumin (final albumin concentration of 2 mg/mL) to prevent adsorption to plastics. Do not shake. May be prepared in glass, PVC, polyolefin, and polypropylene. Discard unused portion of syringe.
Storage/Stability
Neupogen: Store at 2°C to 8°C (36°F to 46°F). Store in the original carton. Protect from light. Protect from direct sunlight. Avoid freezing; if frozen, thaw in the refrigerator before administration. Discard if frozen more than once. Do not shake. Transport via a pneumatic tube has not been studied. Prior to injection, allow to reach room temperature for up to 30 minutes and a maximum of 24 hours. Discard any vial or prefilled syringe left at room ▶

temperature for more than 24 hours. Solutions diluted for infusion may be stored at room temperature for up to 24 hours (infusion must be completed within 24 hours of preparation).

Extended storage information may be available for undiluted filgrastim; contact product manufacturer to obtain current recommendations. Sterility has been assessed and maintained for up to 7 days when prepared under strict aseptic conditions (Jacobson, 1996; Singh, 1994). The manufacturer recommends using within 24 hours due to the potential for bacterial contamination.

Granix: Store prefilled syringes at 2°C to 8°C (36°F to 46°F). Protect from light. Do not shake. May be removed from 2°C to 8°C (36°F to 46°F) storage for a single period of up to 5 days between 23°C to 27°C (73°F to 81°F). If not used within 5 days, the product may be returned to 2°C to 8°C (36°F to 46°F) up to the expiration date. Exposure to -1°C to -5°C (23°F to 30°F) for up to 72 hours and temperatures as low as -15°C to -25°C (5°F to -13°F) for up to 24 hours do not adversely affect stability. Discard unused product.

Zarxio: Store at 2°C to 8°C (36°F to 46°F). Store in the original carton. Protect from light. Avoid freezing; if frozen, thaw in the refrigerator before administration. Discard if frozen more than once. Do not shake. Transport via a pneumatic tube has not been studied. Prior to injection, allow to reach room temperature for up to 30 minutes and a maximum of 24 hours. Discard any prefilled syringe left at room temperature for more than 24 hours. Solutions diluted for infusion may be stored at room temperature for up to 24 hours (infusion must be completed within 24 hours of preparation).

Mechanism of Action Filgrastim and tbo-filgrastim are granulocyte colony stimulating factors (G-CSF) produced by recombinant DNA technology. G-CSFs stimulate the production, maturation, and activation of neutrophils to increase both their migration and cytotoxicity.

Pharmacodynamics/Kinetics

Onset of action:
Filgrastim: 1 to 2 days
Tbo-filgrastim: Time to maximum ANC: 3 to 5 days

Duration:
Filgrastim: Neutrophil counts generally return to baseline within 4 days
Tbo-filgrastim: ANC returned to baseline by 21 days after completion of chemotherapy

Distribution: V_d: 150 mL/kg; Continuous infusion: No evidence of drug accumulation over a 11- to 20-day period

Metabolism: Systemically degraded

Bioavailability: Filgrastim: SubQ: 60% to 70%; Tbo-filgrastim: SubQ: 33%

Half-life elimination: Filgrastim: ~3.5 hours; Tbo-filgrastim: 3 to 4 hours

Time to peak, serum: SubQ: Filgrastim: 2 to 8 hours; Tbo-filgrastim: 4 to 6 hours

Dosing

Adult & Geriatric Note: Do not administer in the period 24 hours before to 24 hours after cytotoxic chemotherapy. May round the dose to the nearest vial size for convenience and cost minimization (Ozer, 2000). **International considerations:** Dosages below expressed as micrograms; 1 mcg = 100,000 units (Hoglund, 1998).

Myelosuppressive chemotherapy recipients with nonmyeloid malignancies (Neupogen, Zarxio): SubQ, IV: 5 mcg/kg/day; doses may be increased by 5 mcg/kg (for each chemotherapy cycle) according to the duration and severity of the neutropenia; continue for up to 14 days until the absolute neutrophil count (ANC) reaches 10,000/mm³. Discontinue if the ANC surpasses 10,000/mm³ after the expected chemotherapy-induced neutrophil nadir.

Myelosuppressive chemotherapy recipients with nonmyeloid malignancies (Granix): SubQ: 5 mcg/kg/day; continue until anticipated nadir has passed and neutrophil count has recovered to normal range.

Acute myeloid leukemia (AML) following induction or consolidation chemotherapy (Neupogen, Zarxio): SubQ, IV: 5 mcg/kg/day; doses may be increased by 5 mcg/kg (for each chemotherapy cycle) according to the duration and severity of the neutropenia; continue for up to 14 days until the ANC reaches 10,000/mm³. Discontinue if the ANC surpasses 10,000/mm³ after the expected chemotherapy-induced neutrophil nadir.

Bone marrow transplantation (Neupogen, Zarxio): IV infusion: 10 mcg/kg/day (administer ≥24 hours after chemotherapy and ≥24 hours after bone marrow infusion); adjust the dose according to the duration and severity of neutropenia; recommended steps based on neutrophil response:

When ANC >1,000/mm³ for 3 consecutive days: Reduce dose to 5 mcg/kg/day

If ANC remains >1,000/mm³ for 3 more consecutive days: Discontinue

If ANC decreases to <1,000/mm³: Resume at 5 mcg/kg/day.

If ANC decreases to <1,000/mm³ during the 5 mcg/kg/day dose: Increase dose to 10 mcg/kg/day and follow the above steps.

Hematopoietic radiation injury syndrome, acute (Neupogen): SubQ: 10 mcg/kg once daily; begin as soon as possible after suspected or confirmed radiation doses >2 gray (Gy) and continue filgrastim until ANC remains >1,000/mm³ for 3 consecutive CBCs or ANC exceeds 10,000/mm³ after the radiation-induced nadir. ASCO guidelines recommend initiating within 24 hours of exposure of a dose ≥2 Gy and/or significant decrease in absolute lymphocyte count, or for anticipated neutropenia <500/mm³ for ≥7 days (Smith, 2015).

Peripheral blood progenitor cell collection and therapy (Neupogen, Zarxio): SubQ: 10 mcg/kg daily, usually for 6 to 7 days (with apheresis occurring on days 5, 6, and 7). Begin at least 4 days before the first apheresis and continue until the last apheresis; discontinue for WBC >100,000/mm³

Severe chronic neutropenia (Neupogen, Zarxio): SubQ:

Congenital: Initial: 6 mcg/kg/day in 2 divided doses; adjust the dose based on ANC and clinical response; mean dose: 6 mcg/kg/day

Idiopathic: Initial: 5 mcg/kg once daily; adjust the dose based on ANC and clinical response; mean dose: 1.2 mcg/kg/day

Cyclic: Initial: 5 mcg/kg once daily; adjust the dose based on ANC and clinical response; mean dose: 2.1 mcg/kg/day

Anemia in myelodysplastic syndrome (off-label use; in combination with epoetin): SubQ: 300 mcg weekly in 2 to 3 divided doses (Malcovati, 2013) or 1 mcg/kg once daily (Greenberg, 2009) or 75 mcg, 150 mcg, or 300 mcg per dose 3 times weekly (Hellstrom-Lindberg, 2003)

Hematopoietic stem cell mobilization in autologous transplantation in patients with non-Hodgkin lymphoma or multiple myeloma (in combination with plerixafor; off-label combination): SubQ: 10 mcg/kg once daily; begin 4 days before initiation of plerixafor; continue G-CSF on each day prior to apheresis for up to 8 days (DiPersio, 2009a; DiPersio, 2009b)

Hepatitis C treatment-associated neutropenia (off-label use): SubQ: 150 mcg once weekly to 300 mcg 3 times weekly; titrate to maintain ANC between 750 and 10,000/mm³ (Younossi, 2008)

Pediatric Note: Do not administer in the period 24 hours before to 24 hours after cytotoxic chemotherapy. **International considerations:** Dosages below expressed as micrograms; 1 mcg = 100,000 units (Hoglund, 1998).

Myelosuppressive chemotherapy recipients with nonmyeloid malignancies (Neupogen, Zarxio): SubQ, IV: 5 mcg/kg/day; doses may be increased by 5 mcg/kg (for each chemotherapy cycle) according to the duration and severity of the neutropenia; continue for up to 14 days until the absolute neutrophil count (ANC) reaches 10,000/mm³. Discontinue if the ANC surpasses 10,000/mm³ after the expected chemotherapy-induced neutrophil nadir.

Bone marrow transplantation (Neupogen, Zarxio): IV infusion: 10 mcg/kg/day (administer ≥24 hours after chemotherapy and ≥24 hours after bone marrow infusion); adjust the dose according to the duration and severity of neutropenia; recommended steps based on neutrophil response:

When ANC >1,000/mm³ for 3 consecutive days: Reduce dose to 5 mcg/kg/day

If ANC remains >1,000/mm³ for 3 more consecutive days: Discontinue

If ANC decreases to <1,000/mm³: Resume at 5 mcg/kg/day

If ANC decreases to <1,000/mm³ during the 5 mcg/kg/day dose, increase dose to 10 mcg/kg/day and follow the above steps

Hematopoietic radiation injury syndrome, acute (Neupogen): SubQ: 10 mcg/kg once daily; begin as soon as possible after suspected or confirmed radiation doses >2 gray (Gy) and continue filgrastim until ANC remains >1,000/mm³ for 3 consecutive CBCs or ANC exceeds 10,000/mm³ after the radiation-induced nadir. ASCO guidelines recommend initiating within 24 hours of exposure of a dose ≥2 Gy and/or significant decrease in absolute lymphocyte count, or for anticipated neutropenia <500/mm³ for ≥7 days (Smith, 2015).

Peripheral blood progenitor cell collection and therapy (Neupogen, Zarxio): SubQ: 10 mcg/kg daily, usually for 6 to 7 days (with apheresis occurring on days 5, 6, and 7). Begin at least 4 days before the first apheresis and continue until the last apheresis; discontinue for WBC >100,000/mm^3

Severe chronic neutropenia (Neupogen, Zarxio):
Infants ≥1 month, Children, and Adolescents: SubQ:
Congenital: Initial: 6 mcg/kg/day in 2 divided doses; adjust the dose based on ANC and clinical response; mean dose: 6 mcg/kg/day
Idiopathic: Initial: 5 mcg/kg once daily; adjust the dose based on ANC and clinical response; mean dose: 1.2 mcg/kg/day
Cyclic: Initial: 5 mcg/kg once daily; adjust the dose based on ANC and clinical response; mean dose: 2.1 mcg/kg/day

Renal Impairment
Renal impairment at treatment initiation:
Neupogen, Zarxio: No dosage adjustment necessary.
Granix:
Mild impairment: No dosage adjustment necessary.
Moderate to severe impairment: There are no dosage adjustments provided in the manufacturer's labeling (has not been studied).
Renal toxicity during treatment: Glomerulonephritis due to filgrastim: Consider dose reduction or treatment interruption.

Hepatic Impairment
Neupogen, Zarxio: No dosage adjustment necessary.
Granix: There are no dosage adjustments provided in the manufacturer's labeling (has not been studied).

Dietary Considerations Some products may contain sodium.

Administration Do not administer earlier than 24 hours after or in the 24 hours prior to cytotoxic chemotherapy.
IV (Neupogen, Zarxio): May be administered IV as a short infusion over 15 to 30 minutes (chemotherapy-induced neutropenia) or by continuous infusion (chemotherapy-induced neutropenia) or as an infusion of no longer than 24 hours (bone marrow transplantation).
SubQ: May be administered SubQ (chemotherapy-induced neutropenia, peripheral blood progenitor cell collection, severe chronic neutropenia, hematopoietic radiation injury syndrome). Administer into the outer upper arm, abdomen (except within 2 inches of navel), front middle thigh, or the upper outer buttocks area. Rotate injection site; do not inject into areas that are tender, red, bruised, hardened, or scarred, or sites with stretch marks.
Some patients (or caregivers) may be appropriate candidates for subQ self-administration with proper training; patients/caregivers should follow the manufacturer instructions for preparation and administration. Granix is available in prefilled syringes with and without a needle guard; the prefilled syringe without a safety needle guard is intended for patient/caregiver self-administration.

Monitoring Parameters
Chemotherapy-induced neutropenia: complete blood cell count (CBC) with differential and platelets prior to chemotherapy and twice weekly during growth factor treatment.
Bone marrow transplantation: CBC with differential and platelets frequently.
Hematopoietic radiation injury syndrome (acute): CBC at baseline (do not delay filgrastim for baseline CBC) and approximately every 3 days until ANC remains >1,000/mm^3 for 3 consecutive CBCs. Estimate absorbed radiation dose (radiation exposure) based on information from public health authorities, biodosimetry (if available), or clinical findings (eg, onset of vomiting or lymphocyte depletion kinetics).
Peripheral progenitor cell collection: Neutrophil counts after 4 days of filgrastim treatment.
Severe chronic neutropenia: CBC with differential and platelets twice weekly during the first month of therapy and for 2 weeks following dose adjustments; once clinically stable, monthly for 1 year and quarterly thereafter. Monitor bone marrow and karyotype prior to treatment; and monitor marrow and cytogenetics annually throughout treatment.

Test Interactions May interfere with bone imaging studies; increased hematopoietic activity of the bone marrow may appear as transient positive bone imaging changes

Dosage Forms Considerations Vials: Neupogen: 300 mcg/mL (1 mL); 480 mcg/1.6 mL (1.6 mL)

Dosage Forms Excipient information presented when available (limited, particularly for generics); consult specific product labeling.
Solution, Injection:
Neupogen: 300 mcg/mL (1 mL); 480 mcg/1.6 mL (1.6 mL) [contains polysorbate 80]

Solution Prefilled Syringe, Injection [preservative free]:
Neupogen: 300 mcg/0.5 mL (0.5 mL); 480 mcg/0.8 mL (0.8 mL) [contains polysorbate 80]
Zarxio: 300 mcg/0.5 mL (0.5 mL); 480 mcg/0.8 mL (0.8 mL) [contains polysorbate 80]
Solution Prefilled Syringe, Subcutaneous [preservative free]:
Granix: 300 mcg/0.5 mL (0.5 mL); 480 mcg/0.8 mL (0.8 mL) [contains polysorbate 80]

◆ **Filgrastim-Sndz** *see* Filgrastim *on page 766*

◆ **Finacea** *see* Azelaic Acid *on page 187*

Finasteride (fi NAS teer ide)

Brand Names: US Propecia; Proscar
Brand Names: Canada ACH-Finasteride; ACT-Finasteride; Apo-Finasteride; Auro-Finasteride; Dom-Finasteride; JAMP-Finasteride; Mint-Finasteride; Mylan-Finasteride; Mylan-Finasteride HG; PMS-Finasteride; Propecia; Proscar; RAN-Finasteride; ratio-Finasteride; Sandoz-Finasteride; Sandoz-Finasteride A; Teva-Finasteride; VAN-finasteride

Pharmacologic Category 5 Alpha-Reductase Inhibitor

Use
Androgenetic alopecia (Propecia): Treatment of male pattern hair loss in **men only**.
Limitations of use: Efficacy in bitemporal recession has not been established; not indicated for use in women.
Benign prostatic hyperplasia (Proscar): Treatment (monotherapy) of symptomatic benign prostatic hyperplasia (BPH) to improve symptoms, reduce the risk of acute urinary retention, and to reduce the risk of need for BPH-related surgery); used in combination with an alpha-blocker (doxazosin) to reduce the risk of symptomatic progression.
Limitations of use: Not approved for the prevention of prostate cancer.

Pregnancy Considerations Abnormalities of external male genitalia were reported in animal reproduction studies. Use is not indicated in women. Pregnant women are advised to avoid contact with crushed or broken tablets and the semen from a male partner exposed to finasteride.

Breast-Feeding Considerations It is not known if finasteride is excreted in breast milk. Use is contraindicated in women of childbearing potential.

Contraindications Hypersensitivity to finasteride or any component of the formulation; pregnancy or women of childbearing potential

Warnings/Precautions Hazardous agent - use appropriate precautions for handling and disposal (NIOSH 2014 [group 3]). Other urological diseases (including prostate cancer) should be ruled out before initiating. For BPH, a minimum of 6 months of treatment may be necessary to determine whether an individual will respond to finasteride; for male pattern hair loss, daily use for 3 months or longer may be required before benefit is observed (withdrawal of treatment leads to reversal of hair growth effect within 12 months). Reduces prostate specific antigen (PSA) concentration by ~50% within 6 months of treatment. To interpret serial PSAs, a new PSA baseline should be established ≥6 months after treatment initiation and PSA monitored periodically thereafter. A confirmed PSA increase while on this medication, even if within normal limits, may be associated with an increased risk for prostate cancer and should be evaluated. Finasteride does not interfere with free PSA levels. Use with caution in patients with hepatic dysfunction; finasteride is extensively metabolized in the liver. When compared to placebo, 5-ARIs have been associated with an increase in the incidence of high-grade prostate cancers; 5-ARIs are not approved in the US or Canada for the prevention of prostate cancer. Carefully monitor patients with a large residual urinary volume or severely diminished urinary flow for obstructive uropathy; these patients may not be candidates for finasteride therapy. Active ingredient of crushed or broken tablets can be absorbed through the skin; unbroken tablets are coated which prevents contact with the active ingredient during normal handling. Women should avoid contact with crushed or broken tablets and the semen from a male partner exposed to finasteride; finasteride may negatively impact fetal development.

Adverse Reactions Note: "Combination therapy" refers to finasteride and doxazosin.
>10%:
Cardiovascular: Orthostatic hypotension (combination therapy 18%; monotherapy 9%)
Central nervous system: Dizziness (combination therapy 23%; monotherapy 7%)
Endocrine & metabolic: Decreased libido (combination therapy 12%; monotherapy 2% to 10%)

Genitourinary: Impotence (combination therapy 23%; monotherapy 5% to 19%), ejaculatory disorder (combination therapy 14%; monotherapy <1% to 7%)

Neuromuscular & skeletal: Weakness (combination therapy 17%; monotherapy 5%)

1% to 10%:

Cardiovascular: Edema (combination therapy 3%; monotherapy 1%)

Central nervous system: Drowsiness (combination therapy 3%; monotherapy 2%)

Dermatologic: Skin rash (monotherapy 1%)

Endocrine & metabolic: Gynecomastia (monotherapy 1% to 2%)

Genitourinary: Decreased ejaculate volume (monotherapy 2% to 4%), breast tenderness (monotherapy ≤1%)

Respiratory: Dyspnea (combination therapy 2%; monotherapy 1%), rhinitis (combination therapy 2%; monotherapy 1%)

<1% (Limited to important or life-threatening): Altered mental status, decreased testicular size, depression, disturbed sleep, hypersensitivity (angioedema, facial swelling, pharyngeal edema, pruritus, skin rash, swelling of the lips, swollen tongue, urticaria), male infertility (temporary), malignant neoplasm of the male breast, prostate cancer - high grade, prostatitis, reduction in penile curvature, reduction in penile size, sexual disorder (may not be reversible with discontinuation), testicular pain

Drug Interactions

Metabolism/Transport Effects Substrate of CYP3A4 (minor); **Note:** Assignment of Major/Minor substrate status based on clinically relevant drug interaction potential

Avoid Concomitant Use There are no known interactions where it is recommended to avoid concomitant use.

Increased Effect/Toxicity There are no known significant interactions involving an increase in effect.

Decreased Effect There are no known significant interactions involving a decrease in effect.

Storage/Stability

Propecia: Store at 15°C to 30°C (59°F to 86°F). Keep container tightly closed and protect from moisture.

Proscar: Store below 30°C (86°F). Protect from light. Keep container tightly closed.

Mechanism of Action Finasteride competitively inhibits type II 5-alpha reductase, resulting in inhibition of the conversion of testosterone to dihydrotestosterone and markedly suppresses serum dihydrotestosterone levels

Pharmacodynamics/Kinetics

Duration: Dihydrotestosterone levels return to normal within 14 days of discontinuation of treatment; prostate volume returns to baseline within ~3 months after discontinuation

Distribution: V_{dss}: 76 L

Protein binding: ~90%

Metabolism: Hepatic (extensive) via CYP3A4; two active metabolites (<20% activity of finasteride)

Bioavailability: Mean: 5 mg: ~63%; 1 mg: 65% (not affected by food)

Half-life elimination, serum: 5 to 6 hours (range: 3 to 16 hours); Elderly (≥70 years): 8 hours (range: 6 to 15 hours)

Time to peak, serum: 1 to 2 hours

Excretion: Feces (57%) and urine (39%; as metabolites)

Dosing

Adult & Geriatric

Benign prostatic hyperplasia (Proscar): Males: Oral: 5 mg once daily (either as a single agent or in combination with doxazosin); early responses may occur although 6 months of treatment is usually needed to assess benefit.

Male pattern baldness (Propecia): Males: Oral: 1 mg once daily; may take 3 months or longer of daily use for observed benefit; continued use is recommended to sustain benefit.

Female hirsutism, idiopathic (off-label use): Females: Oral: 5 mg once daily (Beigi, 2004; Lumachi, 2003; Moghetti, 2000) or 2.5 mg once daily (Tartagni 2004).

Female hirsutism, related to polycystic ovary syndrome (off-label use): Females: Oral: 5 mg once daily (Beigi 2004; Moghetti 2000) or 2.5 mg once daily (Tartagni 2004).

Renal Impairment No adjustment is necessary.

Hepatic Impairment Use with caution (finasteride is metabolized extensively in the liver)

Administration May be administered with or without meals. Women of childbearing age should not touch or handle crushed or broken tablets.

Hazardous agent; use appropriate precautions for handling and disposal (NIOSH 2014 [group 3]).

Monitoring Parameters To interpret serial PSAs, establish a new PSA baseline ≥6 months after treatment initiation and monitor PSA periodically thereafter. Objective and subjective signs of relief of benign prostatic hyperplasia, including improvement in urinary flow, reduction in symptoms of urgency, and relief of difficulty in micturition.

Test Interactions PSA levels decrease in treated patients. After 6 months of therapy, PSA levels stabilize to a new baseline that is ~50% of pretreatment values. If following serial PSAs in a patient, re-establish a new baseline after ≥6 months of use.

Dosage Forms Excipient information presented when available (limited, particularly for generics); consult specific product labeling.

Tablet, Oral:

Propecia: 1 mg

Proscar: 5 mg [contains fd&c blue #2 aluminum lake]

Generic: 1 mg, 5 mg

Fingolimod (fin GOL i mod)

Brand Names: US Gilenya

Brand Names: Canada Gilenya

Index Terms FTY720

Pharmacologic Category Sphingosine 1-Phosphate (S1P) Receptor Modulator

Use Multiple sclerosis: Treatment of relapsing forms of multiple sclerosis (MS) to reduce the frequency of clinical exacerbations and to delay the accumulation of physical disability.

Pregnancy Considerations Adverse events have been observed in animal reproduction studies. Elimination of fingolimod takes approximately 2 months; to avoid potential fetal harm, women of childbearing potential should use effective contraception to avoid pregnancy during and for 2 months after discontinuing treatment. Health care providers are encouraged to enroll pregnant women, or pregnant women may enroll themselves, in the Gilenya Pregnancy Registry (1-877-598-7237 or https://www.gilenyapregnancyregistry.com).

Breast-Feeding Considerations It is not known if fingolimod is excreted in breast milk. Due to the potential for serious adverse reactions in the nursing infant, the manufacturer recommends a decision be made whether to discontinue nursing or to discontinue the drug, taking into account the importance of treatment to the mother.

Medication Guide Available Yes

Contraindications

MI, unstable angina, stroke, transient ischemic attack, decompensated heart failure requiring hospitalization, or New York Heart Association (NYHA) class III/IV heart failure in the past 6 months; Mobitz Type II second- or third-degree atrioventricular (AV) block or sick sinus syndrome (unless patient has a functioning pacemaker); baseline QTc interval ≥500 msec; concurrent use of a class Ia or III antiarrhythmic.

Canadian labeling: Additional contraindications (not in U.S. labeling): Hypersensitivity to fingolimod or any component of the formulation; patients at increased risk for opportunistic infections, including those who are immunocompromised; severe active infections; known active malignancy (excluding basal cell carcinoma); severe hepatic impairment (Child-Pugh class C)

Warnings/Precautions Hazardous agent - use appropriate precautions for handling and disposal (NIOSH 2014 [group 2]).

Increased blood pressure may occur ~1 month after initiation of therapy; monitor blood pressure throughout treatment. Therapy may result in transient and asymptomatic atrioventricular (AV) conduction delays; recurrence may be observed following discontinuation (>2 weeks) and subsequent reinitiation of therapy. Third-degree AV block and AV block with junctional escape occurred within the first 6 hours of the initial dose, and transient asystole and unexplained death have occurred within the first 24 hours; syncope has also occurred. Decreased heart rate may occur with initiation of therapy. Initiation must occur in a setting with resources and personnel capable of appropriately managing symptomatic bradycardia. Following the first dose, heart rate may decrease as soon as 1 hour postdose, with the maximal decrease usually occurring ~6 hours postdose with recovery (but not to baseline levels) 8 to 10 hours postdose. A second heart rate decrease occurs within 24 hours after the first dose and may be more pronounced than the first 6-hour rate decrease. Most patients are asymptomatic; however, hypotension, dizziness, fatigue, palpitations and/or chest pain may occur; symptoms usually resolve within 24 hours. With the second dose, heart rate may also decrease, but to a lesser magnitude than observed with the first dose. Heart rate typically returns to baseline after 1 month of chronic therapy.

Heart rate typically returns to baseline after 1 month of therapy. Due to the risk of bradycardia and AV conduction delays, electrocardiogram (ECG) is required prior to initiation of therapy and after the initial observation period (6 hours) in all patients. Patients receiving concomitant therapy with drugs that slow heart rate or AV conduction (eg, beta-blockers, heart rate–lowering calcium channel blockers, digoxin) or with other cardiac risk factors (eg, AV block, sick sinus syndrome, prolonged QT interval, ischemic cardiac disease, history of myocardial infarction [MI], symptomatic bradycardia, and/or cardiac arrest, heart failure, cerebrovascular disease, uncontrolled hypertension, recurrent syncope, severe sleep apnea [untreated]) require continuous overnight ECG monitoring in a medical facility after the first dose. May cause QT prolongation; patients with a prolonged QT interval at baseline (males: >450 msec; females: >470 msec) or during the first 6 hours of treatment initiation, or are at an increased risk of QT prolongation (eg, hypokalemia, hypomagnesemia, concomitant QT-prolonging drugs, congenital long-QT syndrome, concomitant QT-prolonging drugs, congenital long-QT syndrome) require continuous overnight ECG monitoring in a medical facility after the initial dose.

Cases of progressive multifocal leukoencephalopathy (PML) due to the JC virus have been reported. At the first sign or symptom suggestive of PML, perform a diagnostic evaluation (MRI signs may appear before clinical symptoms) and withhold therapy; symptoms progress over days to weeks and may include progressive weakness on one side of the body or clumsiness of limbs; vision disturbances; mental status changes. Posterior reversible encephalopathy syndrome (PRES) has been observed. Monitor for signs/symptoms of PRES (eg, sudden onset of severe headache, altered mental status, visual disturbances, seizure); symptoms are usually reversible, but may evolve into ischemic stroke or cerebral hemorrhage. Delayed diagnosis and treatment may result in permanent neurological sequelae. Discontinue use if PRES is suspected. May increase risk of infection (including serious infections) due to reversible dose-dependent reduction of lymphocytes; lymphocyte counts may be decreased for up to 2 months following discontinuation of therapy. Obtain a complete blood cell count (CBC) (within 6 months or after discontinuation of prior therapy) before starting therapy. Monitor for signs and symptoms of infection; consider therapy interruption in patients who develop serious infection; reassess benefits and risks prior to reinitiation of therapy. Serious, life-threatening herpes infections, including fatalities (eg, disseminated primary herpes zoster and herpes simplex encephalitis) have occurred. Consider disseminated herpes infections as an etiology if an atypical MS relapse or multiorgan failure occur. Consider varicella zoster virus vaccination prior to initiation of treatment in patients without a health care professional-confirmed history of chickenpox, without a documented full course of varicella zoster vaccination, and patients who are VZV antibody negative; postpone fingolimod treatment for 1 month after varicella zoster vaccination. Cryptococcal infections have been reported, including cases of cryptococcal meningitis. Patients with signs and symptoms of cryptococcal meningitis should undergo prompt diagnostic evaluation and treatment.

Use with caution and closely monitor patients with severe hepatic impairment (contraindicated in the Canadian labeling). Elevated liver enzymes may occur; most elevations occurred within 6 to 9 months. Recurrence of liver transaminase elevations may occur with rechallenge. Obtain baseline liver enzymes in all patients prior to therapy initiation (within 6 months); monitor liver enzymes in patients who develop symptoms of hepatic dysfunction (eg, nausea, vomiting, abdominal pain, fatigue, anorexia, jaundice, dark urine). Use caution in patients with preexisting liver disease; may be at increased risk of increased liver enzymes. Discontinue treatment with confirmation of liver injury; transaminases tend to return to normal within 2 months of discontinuation. Macular edema may occur, typically within the first 6 months of treatment. Patients may present with blurred vision, decreased visual acuity, or without symptoms. Signs and symptoms generally improve or resolve with discontinuation of treatment; however, residual decreased visual acuity has occurred in some patients. Patients with a history of diabetes mellitus or uveitis are at increased risk; use with caution. Ophthalmologic exams (including the fundus and macula) should be performed prior to therapy, 3 to 4 months after treatment initiation, and anytime visual disturbances are reported; more frequent examination is warranted in patients with diabetes or a history of uveitis. Reductions of forced expiratory volume in the first second of expiration (FEV_1) and diffusion lung capacity for carbon monoxide (DLCO) are dose dependent and may occur within the first month

of therapy or when switching from other immunosuppressants (consider the duration and mode of action for each substance to avoid additive effects). FEV_1 changes may be reversible with drug discontinuation.

Potentially significant drug-drug interactions may exist, requiring dose or frequency adjustment, additional monitoring, and/or selection of alternative therapy.

Adverse Reactions

>10%:

Central nervous system: Headache (25%)

Endocrine & metabolic: Increased gamma-glutamyl transfer (5% to ≤15%)

Gastrointestinal: Nausea (13%), diarrhea (12% to 13%), abdominal pain (11%)

Hepatic: Increased serum ALT (14% to ≤15%), increased serum AST (14% to ≤15%)

Infection: Influenza (11% to 13%)

Neuromuscular & skeletal: Back pain (10% to 12%)

Respiratory: Cough (10% to 12%), sinusitis (7% to 11%)

1% to 10%:

Cardiovascular: Hypertension (6% to 8%), atrioventricular block (first degree: 5%; second degree: 4%; third degree: ≤1%), bradycardia (≤4%)

Central nervous system: Depression (8%), dizziness (7%), migraine (5% to 6%), paresthesia (5%)

Dermatologic: Alopecia (3% to 4%), tinea (2% to 4%), eczema (3%), pruritus (3%), actinic keratosis (2%)

Endocrine & metabolic: Weight loss (5%), increased serum triglycerides (3%)

Gastrointestinal: Gastroenteritis (5%)

Hematologic & oncologic: Lymphocytopenia (4% to 7%), cutaneous papilloma (3%), leukopenia (2% to 3%), basal cell carcinoma (2%)

Neuromuscular & skeletal: Leg pain (≤10%), upper extremity pain (≤10%), weakness (2% to 3%)

Ophthalmic: Blurred vision (4%), eye pain (3%)

Respiratory: Dyspnea (8% to 9%), bronchitis (8%)

Miscellaneous: Herpes virus infection (9%), herpes zoster (2%)

<1% (Limited to important or life-threatening): Asystole, cerebrovascular accident (ischemic and hemorrhagic), lymphoma, macular edema, multi-organ failure, peripheral arterial disease, pneumonia, progressive multifocal leukoencephalopathy (FDA Safety Alert, Aug 4, 2015), prolonged Q-T interval on ECG, reversible posterior leukoencephalopathy syndrome, syncope

Drug Interactions

Metabolism/Transport Effects Substrate of CYP3A4 (minor), CYP4F2 (major); **Note:** Assignment of Major/Minor substrate status based on clinically relevant drug interaction potential

Avoid Concomitant Use

Avoid concomitant use of Fingolimod with any of the following: Antiarrhythmic Agents (Class Ia); Antiarrhythmic Agents (Class III); BCG (Intravesical); Ceritinib; Natalizumab; Pimecrolimus; Tacrolimus (Topical); Tofacitinib; Vaccines (Live)

Increased Effect/Toxicity

Fingolimod may increase the levels/effects of: Antiarrhythmic Agents (Class Ia); Antiarrhythmic Agents (Class III); Bradycardia-Causing Agents; Ceritinib; Highest Risk QTc-Prolonging Agents; Ivabradine; Lacosamide; Leflunomide; Moderate Risk QTc-Prolonging Agents; Natalizumab; Tofacitinib; Vaccines (Live); Zoster Vaccine

The levels/effects of Fingolimod may be increased by: Beta-Blockers; Bretylium; Denosumab; Diltiazem; Immunosuppressants; Ketoconazole (Systemic); Mifepristone; Pimecrolimus; Roflumilast; Tacrolimus (Topical); Trastuzumab; Verapamil

Decreased Effect

Fingolimod may decrease the levels/effects of: BCG (Intravesical); Coccidioides immitis Skin Test; Sipuleucel-T; Vaccines (Inactivated); Vaccines (Live); Zoster Vaccine

The levels/effects of Fingolimod may be decreased by: CarBAMazepine; Echinacea

Storage/Stability Store at 25°C (77°F); excursions are permitted between 15°C and 30°C (59°F and 86°F). Protect from moisture.

Mechanism of Action Fingolimod-phosphate, active metabolite of fingolimod, binds to sphingosine 1-phosphate receptors 1, 3, 4, and 5. Fingolimod-phosphate blocks the lymphocytes' ability to emerge from lymph nodes; therefore, the amount of lymphocytes available to the central nervous system is decreased, which reduces central inflammation.

Pharmacodynamics/Kinetics

Distribution: V_d: ~1,200 L: distributes into red blood cells (86%)

Protein binding: >99.7% (fingolimod and fingolimod-phosphate)

Metabolism: Hepatic via CYP4F2 to fingolimod-phosphate (active) and other metabolites (inactive); CYP2D6, 2E1, 3A4, and 4F12 also contribute to metabolism

Bioavailability: 93%

Half-life elimination: 6 to 9 days; prolonged by approximately 50% in patients with moderate or severe hepatic impairment

Time to peak, plasma: 12 to 16 hours

Excretion: Urine (~81% as inactive metabolites); feces (fingolimod and fingolimod phosphate: <2.5% of dose)

Dosing

Adult & Geriatric Multiple sclerosis: Oral: 0.5 mg once daily; doses >0.5 mg daily associated with increased adverse events and no additional benefit. **Note:** The first dose and doses following therapy interruption should be administered in a setting in which resources to appropriately manage symptomatic bradycardia are available.

Renal Impairment There are no dosage adjustments provided in the manufacturer's labeling; use with caution in severe renal impairment (exposure is increased).

Hepatic Impairment

Mild to moderate impairment: No dosage adjustment necessary.

Severe impairment: There are no dosage adjustments provided in the manufacturer's labeling; use with caution and closely monitor; exposure is doubled in severe hepatic impairment. Use is contraindicated in the Canadian labeling.

Administration Administer with or without food.

Hazardous agent; use appropriate precautions for handling and disposal (NIOSH 2014 [group 2]).

Monitoring Parameters Complete blood cell count (CBC) (baseline [within 6 months of initiation] and periodically thereafter); monitor for infection during treatment and at least 2 months after discontinuation. ECG (baseline; repeat after initial dose observation period); heart rate, blood pressure, and signs and symptoms of bradycardia (hourly for 6 hours following first dose; continued observation (until resolved) required if 6-hour postdose heart rate is <45 bpm, is lowest postbaseline measurement, or new-onset second degree or higher AV block occurs on repeat ECG); continuous (until symptoms resolved) ECG monitoring if postdose symptomatic bradycardia occurs (overnight continuous ECG in a medical facility and repeat observation period for second dose if pharmacologic intervention for bradycardia necessary)

Initial monitoring procedures (ECG, heart rate, blood pressure) must be repeated for
- treatment interruption of ≥1 day during the first 2 weeks after treatment initiation, or
- treatment interruption of >7 days during weeks 3 to 4 after treatment initiation, or
- treatment interruption of >14 days after ≥1 month of treatment initiation

Ophthalmologic exam at baseline and 3 to 4 months after initiation of treatment (continue periodic examinations for duration of therapy in patients with diabetes, history of uveitis, or visual complaints); baseline liver enzymes in all patients prior to therapy initiation (within 6 months); monitor liver enzymes in patients who develop symptoms of hepatic dysfunction; respiratory function (FEV$_1$, DLCO) if clinically indicated; VZV antibodies (patients with no health care professional–confirmed history of chickenpox or without documented previous full series VZV vaccination); signs and symptoms of infection and/or PRES

Dosage Forms Excipient information presented when available (limited, particularly for generics); consult specific product labeling.

Capsule, Oral:
Gilenya: 0.5 mg

FlavoxATE (fla VOKS ate)

Brand Names: Canada Apo-Flavoxate®; Urispas®

Index Terms Flavoxate Hydrochloride; Urispas

Pharmacologic Category Antispasmodic Agent, Urinary

Use Antispasmodic to provide symptomatic relief of dysuria, nocturia, suprapubic pain, urgency, and incontinence in patients with cystitis, urethritis, urethrocystitis, urethrotrigonitis, and prostatitis

Dosing

Adult & Geriatric Urinary spasms: Oral: 100-200 mg 3-4 times daily; reduce the dose when symptoms improve.

Pediatric Children >12 years: Refer to adult dosing.

Renal Impairment No dosage adjustment provided in manufacturer's labeling.

Hepatic Impairment No dosage adjustment provided in manufacturer's labeling.

Additional Information Complete prescribing information should be consulted for additional detail.

Dosage Forms Excipient information presented when available (limited, particularly for generics); consult specific product labeling.

Tablet, Oral, as hydrochloride:
Generic: 100 mg

Flecainide (fle KAY nide)

Brand Names: US Tambocor [DSC]

Brand Names: Canada Apo-Flecainide; Tambocor

Index Terms Flecainide Acetate; Tambocor

Pharmacologic Category Antiarrhythmic Agent, Class Ic

Use

Paroxysmal atrial fibrillation/flutter and paroxysmal supraventricular tachycardias (prevention): For the prevention of paroxysmal atrial fibrillation/flutter associated with disabling symptoms and paroxysmal supraventricular tachycardias (PSVT), including atrioventricular nodal reentrant tachycardia, atrioventricular reentrant tachycardia, and other supraventricular tachycardias of unspecified mechanism associated with disabling symptoms in patients without structural heart disease.

Ventricular arrhythmias (prevention): Prevention of documented life-threatening ventricular tachyarrhythmias (eg, sustained ventricular tachycardia) in patients without structural heart disease.

Limitations of use: Use of flecainide is not recommended in patients with less severe ventricular arrhythmias, even if symptomatic. Because of the proarrhythmic effects of flecainide, its use should be reserved for patients in whom the benefits of treatment outweigh the risks. Flecainide should not be used in patients with chronic atrial fibrillation (not adequately studied) or recent MI. No evidence from controlled trials have demonstrated favorable effects of flecainide on survival or the incidence of sudden death.

Pregnancy Considerations Adverse events have been observed in some animal reproduction studies.

Breast-Feeding Considerations Flecainide is excreted into breast milk. Concentrations of flecainide in breast milk are as high as 4 times those in the maternal serum. The estimated daily dose of flecainide to a nursing infant would be <3 mg (assuming ~700 mL breast milk over 24 hours).

Contraindications Hypersensitivity to flecainide or any component of the formulation; preexisting second- or third-degree AV block or with right bundle branch block when associated with a left hemiblock (bifascicular block) (except in patients with a functioning artificial pacemaker); cardiogenic shock; concurrent use of ritonavir

According to the American College of Cardiology/American Heart Association/European Society of Cardiology, the use of flecainide is considered contraindicated in patients with structural heart disease (ACC/AHA/ESC [Blomstrom-Lundqvist 2003]).

Warnings/Precautions [US Boxed Warning]: In the Cardiac Arrhythmia Suppression Trial (CAST), recent (>6 days but <2 years ago) myocardial infarction patients with asymptomatic, nonlife-threatening ventricular arrhythmias did not benefit and may have been harmed by attempts to suppress the arrhythmia with flecainide or encainide. An increased mortality or nonfatal cardiac arrest rate (7.7%) was seen in the active treatment group compared with patients in the placebo group (3%). The applicability of the CAST results to other populations is unknown. The risks of class 1C agents and the lack of improved survival make use in patients without life-threatening arrhythmias generally unacceptable. **[US Boxed Warning]: Proarrhythmic effects (including increased premature ventricular contractions, ventricular tachycardia, ventricular fibrillation, and death) have been reported in patients with atrial fibrillation/fibrillation who received flecainide; use is not recommended for patients with chronic atrial fibrillation.** Flecainide can cause new or worsened supraventricular or ventricular arrhythmias in all patients; effect is dose-related. Patients with sustained ventricular tachycardia and serious underlying heart disease are at an increased risk; initiation of therapy should occur in a hospital setting. In the treatment of atrial fibrillation in the elderly, avoid antiarrhythmics as first-line treatment. In older adults, data suggests rate control may provide more benefits than risks compared to rhythm control for most patients (Beers Criteria). **[US Boxed Warning]: When treating atrial flutter, 1:1 atrioventricular conduction may occur; pre-emptive negative chronotropic therapy (eg, digoxin, beta-blockers) may lower the risk.** Dose-related increases in PR and QRS intervals occur. If second- or third-degree AV block, or right bundle branch block associated with a left hemiblock occur, flecainide therapy should be discontinued unless a temporary or implanted ventricular pacemaker is in place to ensure an adequate ventricular rate. Use with extreme caution in patients with sick sinus syndrome; treatment with flecainide may result in sinus bradycardia, sinus pause, or sinus arrest. Use with caution in patients with permanent pacemakers or temporary pacing wires; can increase endocardial pacing thresholds and suppress ventricular escape rhythms. Do not use in patients with existing poor thresholds or nonprogrammable pacemakers unless suitable pacing rescue is available. The pacing threshold in patients with pacemakers should be determined at baseline, 1 week after initiation and at regular intervals thereafter.

Correct electrolyte disturbances, especially hypokalemia or hypomagnesemia, prior to use and throughout therapy. Avoid use in patients with heart failure; may precipitate or exacerbate condition, increase the risk of proarrhythmia, and contribute to an increased risk of mortality (ACCF/AHA [Yancy 2013]). According to the manufacturer, use with extreme caution in patients with structural heart disease as the risk of death and cardiac events may be increased. According to the ACC/AHA/ESC, the use of flecainide is considered relatively contraindicated in patients with coronary artery disease, LV dysfunction, or other significant heart disease (ACC/AHA/ESC [Blomström-Lundqvist 2003]). Use with caution in patients with significant hepatic impairment; benefit should outweigh risk. Consider careful monitoring during initiation of therapy. Dose titration should occur only after steady state has been achieved (≥4 days after initiation) in these patients. Frequent plasma level monitoring is required in patients with severe hepatic impairment; if unavailable, use is not recommended. Use with caution in patients with significant renal impairment. Frequent plasma level monitoring is required in patients with severe renal impairment; if unavailable, use is not recommended. Small changes in dose may lead to disproportionate increases in plasma concentrations in pediatric patients. Following initiation of therapy or changes in dose in pediatric patients, obtain plasma trough concentrations and ECG once steady state has been achieved

(>5 doses after initiation or change); regular monitoring of trough concentrations and ECG is recommended by the manufacturer during the first year of therapy in these patients.

Potentially significant interactions may exist, requiring dose or frequency adjustment, additional monitoring, and/or selection of alternative therapy.

Adverse Reactions

>10%:

Central nervous system: Dizziness (19% to 30%)

Ocular: Visual disturbances (16%)

Respiratory: Dyspnea (~10%)

1% to 10%:

Cardiovascular: Palpitation (6%), chest pain (5%), edema (3.5%), tachycardia (1% to 3%), proarrhythmic (4% to 12%), sinus node dysfunction (1.2%), syncope

Central nervous system: Headache (4% to 10%), fatigue (8%), nervousness (5%) additional symptoms occurring at a frequency between 1% and 3%: fever, malaise, hypoesthesia, paresis, ataxia, vertigo, somnolence, tinnitus, anxiety, insomnia, depression

Dermatologic: Rash (1% to 3%)

Gastrointestinal: Nausea (9%), constipation (1%), abdominal pain (3%), anorexia (1% to 3%), diarrhea (0.7% to 3%)

Neuromuscular & skeletal: Tremor (5%), weakness (5%), paresthesia (1%)

Ocular: Diplopia (1% to 3%), blurred vision

<1% (Limited to important or life-threatening): Alopecia, alters pacing threshold, amnesia, angina, AV block, bradycardia, bronchospasm, CHF, corneal deposits, depersonalization, euphoria, exfoliative dermatitis, granulocytopenia, heart block, increased P-R, leukopenia, metallic taste, neuropathy, paradoxical increase in ventricular rate in atrial fibrillation/flutter, paresthesia, photophobia, pneumonitis, pruritus, QRS duration, swollen lips/tongue/mouth, tardive dyskinesia, thrombocytopenia, urinary retention, urticaria, ventricular arrhythmia

Drug Interactions

Metabolism/Transport Effects Substrate of CYP1A2 (minor), CYP2D6 (major); **Note:** Assignment of Major/Minor substrate status based on clinically relevant drug interaction potential; **Inhibits** CYP2D6 (weak)

Avoid Concomitant Use

Avoid concomitant use of Flecainide with any of the following: Fosamprenavir; Highest Risk QTc-Prolonging Agents; Ivabradine; Mifepristone; Ritonavir; Saquinavir; Tipranavir

Increased Effect/Toxicity

Flecainide may increase the levels/effects of: ARIPiprazole; Digoxin; Highest Risk QTc-Prolonging Agents; Moderate Risk QTc-Prolonging Agents

The levels/effects of Flecainide may be increased by: Abiraterone Acetate; Amiodarone; Antihepaciviral Combination Products; Boceprevir; Carbonic Anhydrase Inhibitors; Cobicistat; CYP2D6 Inhibitors (Moderate); CYP2D6 Inhibitors (Strong); Darunavir; Fosamprenavir; Ivabradine; Mifepristone; Mirabegron; Panobinostat; Peginterferon Alfa-2b; QTc-Prolonging Agents (Indeterminate Risk and Risk Modifying); Ritonavir; Saquinavir; Sodium Bicarbonate; Sodium Lactate; Telaprevir; Tipranavir; Tromethamine; Verapamil

Decreased Effect

The levels/effects of Flecainide may be decreased by: Etravirine; Peginterferon Alfa-2b; Sodium Bicarbonate

Food Interactions Clearance may be decreased in patients following strict vegetarian diets due to urinary pH ≥8. Milk may interfere with the absorption of flecainide (Russell 1989; Thompson 2012). Management: Dose reduction should be considered when milk is removed from the diet (eg, during weaning or bouts of gastroenteritis). Plasma trough flecainide levels should be monitored during major changes in dietary milk intake.

Storage/Stability Store at 20°C to 25°C (68°F to 77°F) in a tight, light-resistant container

Mechanism of Action Class Ic antiarrhythmic; slows conduction in cardiac tissue by altering transport of ions across cell membranes; causes slight prolongation of refractory periods; decreases the rate of rise of the action potential without affecting its duration; increases electrical stimulation threshold of ventricle, His-Purkinje system; possesses local anesthetic and moderate negative inotropic effects

Pharmacodynamics/Kinetics

Absorption: Oral: Nearly complete; decreased when administered with milk

Protein binding: ~40%

Half-life elimination:

Infants: At birth: Up to ≤29 hours; 3 months: 11 to 12 hours; 12 months: 6 hours

Children: ~8 hours

Adolescents: ~11 to 12 hours
Adults: ~20 hours (range: 12 to 27 hours); increased in patients with heart failure or renal dysfunction
Time to peak, serum: ~3 hours (range: 1 to 6 hours)
Excretion: Urine (30% [range: 10% to 50%] as unchanged drug); feces (5%)

Dosing

Adult & Geriatric

Ventricular arrhythmias: (prevention): Oral:
Initial: 100 mg every 12 hours; increase by 50 mg twice daily at 4-day intervals; maximum: 400 mg per day. Some patients inadequately controlled with or intolerant to dosing every 12 hours may require dosing every 8 hours. **Note:** Initiate therapy in a hospital setting in patients with sustained ventricular tachycardia. Use of higher initial doses and more rapid dosage adjustments have resulted in an increased incidence of proarrhythmic events and congestive heart failure, particularly during the first few days. Do not use a loading dose. Use very cautiously in patients with history of congestive heart failure or myocardial infarction.

Paroxysmal atrial fibrillation/flutter and paroxysmal supraventricular tachycardias (prevention): Oral: Initial: 50 mg every 12 hours; increase by 50 mg twice daily at 4-day intervals; maximum total dose: 300 mg. The AHA/ACC/HRS atrial fibrillation guidelines recommend a maximum total daily dose of 400 mg (AHA/ACC/HRS [January 2014]).

Atrial fibrillation or flutter (pharmacological cardioversion) (off-label dose): Oral: Outpatient: "Pill-in-the-pocket" dose: **Note:** May not repeat in ≤24 hours (Alboni 2004; AHA/ACC/HRS [January 2014]). An initial inpatient cardioversion trial should have been successful before sending patient home on this approach. Patient must be taking an AV nodal-blocking agent (eg, beta-blocker, nondihydropyridine calcium channel blocker) prior to initiation of antiarrhythmic.
<70 kg: 200 mg
≥70 kg: 300 mg

Conversion from another antiarrhythmic agent: Allow for 2 to 4 half-lives of the other agent after discontinuation to pass before initiating flecainide therapy.

Dosage adjustment for concomitant therapy: Amiodarone: Reduce the flecainide dose by 50% and monitor the patient closely for adverse effects; monitoring of plasma concentrations is strongly recommended to guide dosage.

Pediatric

Arrhythmias (prevention): Manufacturer's labeling: BSA-directed dosing: Use caution with dose titration, as small change in dose may result in disproportionate increase in plasma concentrations.
Infants ≤6 months: Oral: Initial: 50 mg/m²/day divided every 8 to 12 hours; may titrate dose at 4 day intervals; maximum daily dose: 200 mg/m²/day; higher doses have been associated with an increased risk of proarrhythmic effects
Infants >6 months, Children, and Adolescents: Oral: Initial: 100 mg/m²/day divided every 8 to 12 hours; may titrate dose at 4 day intervals; maximum daily dose: 200 mg/m²/day; higher doses have been associated with an increased risk of proarrhythmic effects

Renal Impairment

CrCl >35 mL/minute/1.73 m²: Adults: Initial: 100 mg every 12 hours; consider obtaining plasma concentrations to guide dosage adjustments. Dose increases should be made very cautiously at intervals >4 days.
CrCl ≤35 mL/minute/1.73 m²: Adults: Initial: 100 mg once daily or 50 mg every 12 hours; obtain plasma concentrations to guide dosage adjustments. Dose increases should be made very cautiously at intervals >4 days and serum trough concentrations monitored frequently. In patients with end stage renal disease, renal clearance is very low as compared to patients with moderate renal impairment and the plasma half-life may extend up to 58 hours (Conard 1984).
Hemodialysis: Removal by hemodialysis is negligible (only ~1% of an oral dose)

Hepatic Impairment

There are no dosage adjustments provided in the manufacturer's labeling; however elimination from the plasma may be slower in patients with hepatic impairment. Use with caution; obtain plasma concentrations to guide dosage adjustments. Dose increases should be made very cautiously at intervals >4 days and serum concentrations monitored frequently. Frequent plasma level monitoring is required in patients with severe hepatic impairment; if unavailable, use is not recommended.

Monitoring Parameters ECG, blood pressure, pulse, periodic serum trough concentrations, especially in patients with renal or hepatic impairment, concomitant administration of amiodarone and pediatric patients.

Reference Range Therapeutic: Trough concentration: 0.2 to 1 mcg/mL. **Note:** Pediatric patients may respond at the lower end of the recommended therapeutic range (0.2 to 0.5 mcg/mL) but up to 0.8 mcg/mL may be required.

Dosage Forms Excipient information presented when available (limited, particularly for generics); consult specific product labeling. [DSC] = Discontinued product
Tablet, Oral, as acetate:
Tambocor: 50 mg [DSC], 100 mg [DSC], 150 mg [DSC]
Generic: 50 mg, 100 mg, 150 mg

Extemporaneous Preparations A 20 mg/mL oral liquid suspension may be made from tablets and one of three different vehicles (cherry syrup, a 1:1 mixture of Ora-Sweet® and Ora-Plus®, or a 1:1 mixture of Ora-Sweet® SF and Ora-Plus®). Crush twenty-four 100 mg tablets in a mortar and reduce to a fine powder. Add 20 mL of the chosen vehicle and mix to a uniform paste; mix while adding the vehicle in incremental proportions to **almost** 120 mL; transfer to a calibrated bottle, rinse mortar with vehicle, and add quantity of vehicle sufficient to make 120 mL. Label "shake well" and "protect from light". Stable for 60 days when stored in amber plastic prescription bottles in the dark at room temperature or refrigerated.
Allen LV and Erickson III MA, "Stability of Baclofen, Captopril, Diltiazem, Hydrochloride, Dipyridamole, and Flecainide Acetate in Extemporaneously Compounded Oral Liquids," *Am J Health Syst Pharm.* 1996, 53:2179-84.

- ◆ Flecainide Acetate *see* Flecainide *on page 772*
- ◆ Fleet Bisacodyl [OTC] *see* Bisacodyl *on page 231*
- ◆ Fleet Enema [OTC] *see* Sodium Phosphates *on page 1677*
- ◆ Fleet Enema (Can) *see* Sodium Phosphates *on page 1677*
- ◆ Fleet Enema Extra [OTC] *see* Sodium Phosphates *on page 1677*
- ◆ Fleet Laxative [OTC] *see* Bisacodyl *on page 231*
- ◆ Fleet Pedia-Lax Enema [OTC] *see* Sodium Phosphates *on page 1677*
- ◆ Flexbumin *see* Albumin *on page 55*
- ◆ Flexeril *see* Cyclobenzaprine *on page 454*
- ◆ Flexeril [DSC] *see* Cyclobenzaprine *on page 454*

Flibanserin (flib AN ser in)

Brand Names: US Addyi
Pharmacologic Category Mixed 5-HT$_{1A}$ Agonist/5-HT$_{2A}$ Antagonist

Use

Hypoactive sexual desire disorder: Treatment of premenopausal women with acquired, generalized hypoactive sexual desire disorder (HSDD), as characterized by low sexual desire that causes marked distress or interpersonal difficulty and **not** due to a coexisting medical or psychiatric condition, problems within the relationship, or the effects of a medication or other drug substance.
Limitations of use: Flibanserin is not indicated for the treatment of HSDD in postmenopausal women or in men, or to enhance sexual performance.

Prescribing and Access Restrictions As a requirement of the REMS program, access to the medication is restricted. Prescribers and pharmacies must be certified with the ADDYI REMS program; certified pharmacies may only dispense to patients pursuant to a prescription from a certified prescriber. More information, including a list of certified pharmacies, is available at www.AddyiREMS.com or 844-746-5745.

Medication Guide Available Yes

Dosing

Adult Hypoactive sexual desire disorder: Females (premenopausal): Oral: 100 mg once daily at bedtime; assess treatment efficacy at 8 weeks and discontinue if symptoms have not improved.
Missed dose: If a dose is missed, skip the missed dose and resume the normal dosing schedule at bedtime on the next day.

Dosage adjustment for the transition to or from treatment with a moderate or strong CYP3A4 inhibitors: The concomitant use of flibanserin and moderate or strong CYP3A4 inhibitors is contraindicated. The following guidelines are recommended by the manufacturer when transitioning to or from treatment with a moderate or strong CYP3A4 inhibitor:
Initiation of a moderate or strong CYP3A4 inhibitor following the use of flibanserin: Initiate the CYP3A4 inhibitor 2 **days** after the last dose of flibanserin. If the

benefit of starting the CYP3A4 inhibitor outweighs the risk of hypotension and syncope, monitor the patient closely.

Initiation of flibanserin following the use of a moderate or strong CYP3A4 inhibitor: Initiate flibanserin therapy 2 **weeks** after the last dose of the CYP3A4 inhibitor.

Renal Impairment There are no dosage adjustments provided in the manufacturer's labeling; however, dosage adjustments are unlikely to be required due to minimal change in AUC in patients with mild to severe renal impairment.

Hepatic Impairment Use is contraindicated.

Additional Information Complete prescribing information should be consulted for additional detail.

Dosage Forms Excipient information presented when available (limited, particularly for generics); consult specific product labeling.
Tablet, Oral:
Addyi: 100 mg

Fluconazole (floo KOE na zole)

Brand Names: US Diflucan
Brand Names: Canada ACT Fluconazole; Apo-Fluconazole; CanesOral; CO Fluconazole; Diflucan; Diflucan injection; Diflucan One; Diflucan PWS; Dom-Fluconazole; Fluconazole Injection; Fluconazole Injection SDZ; Fluconazole Omega; Monicure; Mylan-Fluconazole; Novo-Fluconazole; PHL-Fluconazole; PMS-Fluconazole; PRO-Fluconazole; Riva-Fluconazole; Taro-Fluconazole
Index Terms Diflucan
Pharmacologic Category Antifungal Agent, Oral; Antifungal Agent, Parenteral
Use Treatment of candidiasis (esophageal, oropharyngeal, peritoneal, urinary tract, vaginal); systemic candida infections (eg, candidemia, disseminated candidiasis, and pneumonia); cryptococcal meningitis; antifungal prophylaxis in allogeneic bone marrow transplant recipients
Pregnancy Considerations Adverse events have been observed in some animal reproduction studies. When used in high doses, fluconazole is teratogenic in animal studies. Following exposure during the first trimester, case reports have noted similar malformations in humans when used in higher doses (400 mg/day) over extended periods of time (Aleck 1997). Abnormalities reported include abnormal facies, abnormal calvarial development, arthrogryposis, brachycephaly, cleft palate, congenital heart disease, femoral bowing, thin ribs and long bones. Use of lower doses (150 mg as a single dose) does not suggest an increase risk to the fetus. Most azole antifungals, including fluconazole, are recommended to be avoided during pregnancy (Pappas 2009).
Breast-Feeding Considerations Fluconazole is excreted in breast milk. The manufacturer recommends that caution be exercised when administering fluconazole

to nursing women. Fluconazole is found in breast milk at concentrations similar to maternal plasma.

Contraindications Hypersensitivity to fluconazole or any component of the formulation (cross-reaction with other azole antifungal agents may occur, but has not been established; use caution); coadministration of terfenadine in adult patients receiving multiple doses of 400 mg or higher or with CYP3A4 substrates which may lead to QTc prolongation (eg, astemizole, cisapride, erythromycin, pimozide, or quinidine)

Warnings/Precautions Hazardous agent; use appropriate precautions for handling and disposal (NIOSH 2014 [group 3]). Serious (and sometimes fatal) hepatic toxicity (eg, hepatitis, cholestasis, fulminant hepatic failure) has been observed. Use with caution in patients with renal and hepatic dysfunction or previous hepatotoxicity from other azole derivatives. Patients who develop abnormal liver function tests during fluconazole therapy should be monitored closely and discontinued if symptoms consistent with liver disease develop. Rare exfoliative skin disorders have been observed; fatal outcomes have been reported in patients with serious concomitant diseases. Monitor patients with deep seated fungal infections closely for rash development and discontinue if lesions progress. In patients with superficial fungal infections who develop a rash attributable to fluconazole, treatment should also be discontinued. Cases of QTc prolongation and torsade de pointes associated with fluconazole use have been reported (usually high dose or in combination with agents known to prolong the QT interval); use caution in patients with concomitant medications or conditions which are arrhythmogenic. Potentially significant drug-drug interactions may exist, requiring dose or frequency adjustment, additional monitoring, and/or selection of alternative therapy. May occasionally cause dizziness or seizures; use caution driving or operating machines.

Powder for oral suspension contains sucrose; use caution with fructose intolerance, sucrose-isomaltase deficiency, or glucose-galactose malabsorption.

Benzyl alcohol and derivatives: Some dosage forms may contain sodium benzoate/benzoic acid; benzoate is a metabolite of benzyl alcohol; large amounts of benzyl alcohol (≥99 mg/kg/day) have been associated with a potentially fatal toxicity ("gasping syndrome") in neonates; the "gasping syndrome" consists of metabolic acidosis, respiratory distress, gasping respirations, CNS dysfunction (including convulsions, intracranial hemorrhage), hypotension, and cardiovascular collapse (AAP 1997; CDC 1982); some data suggests that benzoate displaces bilirubin from protein binding sites (Ahlfors 2001); avoid or use dosage forms containing benzyl alcohol derivative with caution in neonates. See manufacturer's labeling.

Adverse Reactions Frequency not always defined.
Cardiovascular: Angioedema (rare)
Central nervous system: Headache (2% to 13%), dizziness (1%)
Dermatologic: Rash (2%)
Gastrointestinal: Nausea (2% to 7%), abdominal pain (2% to 6%), vomiting (2% to 5%), diarrhea (2% to 3%), dysgeusia (1%), dyspepsia (1%)
Hepatic: Alkaline phosphatase increased, ALT increased, AST increased, hepatic failure (rare), hepatitis, jaundice
Miscellaneous: Anaphylactic reactions (rare)
Postmarketing and/or case reports: Agranulocytosis, alopecia, cholestasis, diaphoresis, drug eruption, exanthematous pustulosis, fatigue, fever, hypercholesterolemia, hypertriglyceridemia, hypokalemia, insomnia, leukopenia, malaise, myalgia, neutropenia, paresthesia, QT prolongation, seizure, somnolence, Stevens-Johnson syndrome, thrombocytopenia, torsade de pointes, toxic epidermal necrolysis, tremor, vertigo, weakness, xerostomia

Drug Interactions
Metabolism/Transport Effects Inhibits CYP1A2 (weak), CYP2C19 (strong), CYP2C9 (moderate), CYP3A4 (moderate)
Avoid Concomitant Use
Avoid concomitant use of Fluconazole with any of the following: Aprepitant; Bosutinib; Cisapride; Citalopram; Cobimetinib; Domperidone; Erythromycin (Systemic); Flibanserin; Ibrutinib; Ivabradine; Lomitapide; Naloxegol; Olaparib; Ospemifene; Pimozide; QuiNIDine; Saccharomyces boulardii; Simeprevir; Tolvaptan; Trabectedin; Ulipristal; Voriconazole
Increased Effect/Toxicity
Fluconazole may increase the levels/effects of: Alfentanil; Amitriptyline; Apixaban; Aprepitant; ARIPiprazole; AtorvaSTATin; Avanafil; Bosentan; Bosutinib; Brexpiprazole; Bromocriptine; Budesonide (Systemic); Budesonide (Topical); BusPIRone; Busulfan; Calcium Channel ▶

Blockers; Cannabis; CarBAMazepine; Carvedilol; Cilostazol; Cisapride; Citalopram; Cobimetinib; Colchicine; CycloSPORINE (Systemic); CYP2C19 Substrates; CYP2C9 Substrates; CYP3A4 Substrates; Dapoxetine; Domperidone; DOXOrubicin (Conventional); Dronabinol; Eletriptan; Eliglustat; Eplerenone; Erythromycin (Systemic); Etravirine; Everolimus; FentaNYL; Flibanserin; Fluvastatin; Fosphenytoin; Halofantrine; Highest Risk QTc-Prolonging Agents; Hydrocodone; Ibrutinib; Imatinib; Ivabradine; Ivacaftor; Lomitapide; Lovastatin; Lurasidone; Methadone; Moderate Risk QTc-Prolonging Agents; Naloxegol; Nevirapine; NiMODipine; Olaparib; Ospemifene; OxyCODONE; Parecoxib; Phenytoin; Pimecrolimus; Pimozide; PredniSONE; Propafenone; Proton Pump Inhibitors; QuiNIDine; Ramelteon; Ranolazine; Red Yeast Rice; Rifamycin Derivatives; Ruxolitinib; Salmeterol; Saxagliptin; Sildenafil; Simeprevir; Simvastatin; Sirolimus; Solifenacin; Sonidegib; Sulfonylureas; SUNItinib; Suvorexant; Tacrolimus (Systemic); Tadalafil; Temsirolimus; Tetrahydrocannabinol; Tipranavir; TiZANidine; Tofacitinib; Tolvaptan; Trabectedin; Ulipristal; Vardenafil; Vilazodone; Vindesine; Vitamin K Antagonists; Voriconazole; Zidovudine; Zolpidem; Zopiclone

The levels/effects of Fluconazole may be increased by: Amitriptyline; Etravirine; Mifepristone

Decreased Effect
Fluconazole may decrease the levels/effects of: Amphotericin B; Clopidogrel; Ifosfamide; Losartan; Saccharomyces boulardii

The levels/effects of Fluconazole may be decreased by: Didanosine; Etravirine; Rifamycin Derivatives

Storage/Stability
Tablet: Store at <30°C (86°F).
Powder for oral suspension: Store dry powder at <30°C (86°F). Following reconstitution, store at 5°C to 30°C (41°F to 86°F). Discard unused portion after 2 weeks. Do not freeze.
Injection: Store injection in glass at 5°C to 30°C (41°F to 86°F). Store injection in plastic flexible containers at 5°C to 25°C (41°F to 77°F). Brief exposure of up to 40°C (104°F) does not adversely affect the product. Do not freeze. Do not unwrap unit until ready for use.

Mechanism of Action Interferes with fungal cytochrome P450 activity (lanosterol 14-α-demethylase), decreasing ergosterol synthesis (principal sterol in fungal cell membrane) and inhibiting cell membrane formation

Pharmacodynamics/Kinetics
Absorption: Oral: Well absorbed; food does not affect extent of absorption
Distribution: V_d: ~0.6 L/kg; widely throughout body with good penetration into CSF, eye, peritoneal fluid, sputum, skin, and urine
Relative diffusion blood into CSF: Adequate with or without inflammation (exceeds usual MICs)
CSF:blood level ratio: Normal meninges: 50% to 90%; Inflamed meninges: ~80%
Protein binding, plasma: 11% to 12%
Bioavailability: Oral: >90%
Half-life elimination:
Premature neonates (GA: 26 to 29 weeks): 73.6 hours
PNA: 6 days: 53 hours
PNA: 12 days: 47 hours
Pediatric patients (9 months to 15 years):
9 months to 13 years: Oral: 19.5 to 25 hours
5 to 15 years: IV: 15 to 18 hours
Adults: Normal renal function: ~30 hours (range: 20 to 50 hours); Elderly: ~46 hours
Time to peak, serum: Oral: 1 to 2 hours
Excretion: Urine (80% as unchanged drug)

Dosing
Adult & Geriatric The daily dose of fluconazole is the same for both oral and IV administration
Usual dosage range: Oral, IV: 150 mg once **or** Loading dose: 200 to 800 mg; maintenance: 200 to 800 mg once daily; duration and dosage depend on location and severity of infection

Indication-specific dosing:
Blastomycosis (off-label use): Oral: *CNS disease:* Consolidation: 800 mg daily for ≥12 months and until resolution of CSF abnormalities (Chapman 2008)
Candidiasis: Oral, IV:
Candidemia (neutropenic and non-neutropenic): Loading dose: 800 mg (12 mg/kg) on day 1, then 400 mg daily (6 mg/kg/day) for 14 days after first negative blood culture and resolution of signs/symptoms. **Note:** Not recommended for patients with recent azole exposure, critical illness, or if *C. krusei* or *C. glabrata* are suspected (Pappas 2009).
Chronic, disseminated: 400 mg daily (6 mg/kg/day) until calcification or lesion resolution (Pappas 2009)

CNS candidiasis (alternative therapy): 400 to 800 mg daily (6 to 12 mg/kg/day) until CSF/radiological abnormalities resolved. **Note:** Recommended as alternative therapy in patients intolerant of amphotericin B (Pappas 2009).
Endocarditis, prosthetic valve (off-label use): 400 to 800 mg daily (6 to 12 mg/kg/day) for 6 weeks after valve replacement (as step-down in stable, culture-negative patients); long-term suppression in absence of valve replacement: 400 to 800 mg daily (Pappas 2009)
Endophthalmitis (off-label use): 400 to 800 mg daily (6 to 12 mg/kg/day) for 4 to 6 weeks until examination indicates resolution (Pappas 2009)
Esophageal:
Manufacturer's labeling: Loading dose: 200 mg on day 1, then maintenance dose of 100 to 400 mg daily for 21 days and for at least 2 weeks following resolution of symptoms
Alternative dosing: 200 to 400 mg daily for 14 to 21 days; suppressive therapy of 100 to 200 mg 3 times weekly may be used for recurrent infections (Pappas 2009)
Intertrigo (off-label use): 50 mg daily or 150 mg once weekly (Coldiron 1991; Nozickova 1998; Stengel 1994)
Oropharyngeal:
Manufacturer's labeling: Loading dose: 200 mg on day 1; maintenance dose 100 mg daily for ≥2 weeks. **Note:** Therapy with 100 mg daily is associated with resistance development (Rex 1995).
Alternative dosing: 100 to 200 mg daily for 7 to 14 days for uncomplicated, moderate-to-severe disease; chronic therapy of 100 mg 3 times weekly is recommended in immunocompromised patients with history of oropharyngeal candidiasis (OPC) (Pappas 2009)
Osteoarticular: 400 mg daily for 6 to 12 months (osteomyelitis) or 6 weeks (septic arthritis) (Pappas 2009)
Pacemaker (or ICD, VAD) infection (off-label use): 400 to 800 mg daily (6 to 12 mg/kg/day) for 4 to 6 weeks after device removal (as step-down in stable, culture-negative patients); long-term suppression when VAD cannot be removed: 400 to 800 mg daily (Pappas 2009)
Pericarditis or myocarditis: 400 to 800 mg daily for several months (Pappas 2009)
Peritonitis: 50 to 200 mg daily. **Note:** Some clinicians do not recommend using <200 mg daily (Chen 2004).
Prophylaxis:
Bone marrow transplant: 400 mg once daily. Patients anticipated to have severe granulocytopenia should start therapy several days prior to the anticipated onset of neutropenia and continue for 7 days after the neutrophil count is >1000 mm^3.
High-risk ICU patients in units with high incidence of invasive candidiasis: 400 mg once daily (Pappas 2009)
Neutropenic patients: 400 mg once daily for duration of neutropenia (Pappas 2009)
Peritoneal dialysis associated infection (concurrently treated with antibiotics), prevention of secondary fungal infection: 200 mg every 48 hours (Restrepo 2010)
Solid organ transplant: 200 to 400 mg once daily for at least 7 to 14 days (Pappas 2009)
Surgical (perioperative) prophylaxis in high-risk patients undergoing liver, pancreas, kidney, or pancreas-kidney transplantation (off-label use): IV: 400 mg given in the perioperative period and continued in the postoperative period for ≤28 days. Time of initiation and duration varies with transplant type and operative protocol (Bratzler 2013).
Thrombophlebitis, suppurative (off-label use): 400 to 800 mg daily (6 to 12 mg/kg/day) and as step-down in stable patients for ≥2 weeks (Pappas 2009)
Urinary tract:
Cystitis:
Manufacturer's labeling: UTI: 50 to 200 mg once daily
Asymptomatic, patient undergoing urologic procedure: 200 to 400 mg once daily several days before and after the procedure (Pappas 2009)
Symptomatic: 200 mg once daily for 2 weeks (Pappas 2009)
Fungus balls: 200 to 400 mg once daily (Pappas 2009)
Pyelonephritis: 200 to 400 mg once daily for 2 weeks (Pappas 2009)

Vaginal:
Uncomplicated: Manufacturer's labeling: 150 mg as a single oral dose
Complicated: 150 mg every 72 hours for 3 doses (Pappas 2009)
Recurrent: 150 mg once daily for 10 to 14 days, followed by 150 mg once weekly for 6 months (Pappas 2009), **or** fluconazole (oral) 100 mg, 150 mg, or 200 mg every third day for a total of 3 doses (day 1, 4, and 7), then 100 mg, 150 mg, or 200 mg dose weekly for 6 months (CDC 2010)

Coccidioidomycosis, treatment (off-label use):
HIV-infected (HHS [OI adult 2015]):
Meningeal infections (consultation with specialist is advised): IV, Oral: 400 to 800 mg once daily; patients who complete initial therapy should be considered for lifelong suppressive therapy using fluconazole 400 mg once daily if CD4 counts remain <250 cells/mm^3.
Mild infections (eg, focal pneumonia): Oral: 400 mg once daily; patients who complete initial therapy should be considered for lifelong suppressive therapy using fluconazole 400 mg once daily if CD4 counts remain <250 cells/mm^3.
Non-HIV infected (off-label use): Oral, IV:
Disseminated, extrapulmonary: 400 mg once daily (some experts use 2000 mg daily [Galgiani 2005])
Meningitis: 400 mg once daily (some experts use initial doses of 800 to 1000 mg daily), lifelong duration (Galgiani 2005)
Pneumonia, acute, uncomplicated: 200 to 400 mg daily for 3 to 6 months (Catanzaro 1995; Galgiani 2000)
Pneumonia, chronic progressive, fibrocavitary: 200 to 400 mg daily for 12 months (Catanzaro 1995; Galgiani 2000)
Pneumonia, diffuse: Consolidation after amphotericin B induction: 400 mg daily for 12 months (lifelong in chronically immunosuppressed) (Galgiani 2005)

Coccidioidomycosis, prophylaxis (off-label use):
Oral:
HIV-infected patients (HHS [OI adult 2015]):
Primary prophylaxis in patients with a new positive IgM or IgG serologic test who live in disease-endemic areas and have CD4 counts <250 cells/mm^3: 400 mg once daily
Chronic suppressive therapy (secondary prophylaxis): 400 mg once daily
Solid organ transplant (off-label use): **Note:** Prophylaxis regimens in this setting have not been established; the following regimen has been proposed for transplant recipients who maintain residence in a *Coccidioides* spp endemic area.
Previous history >12 months prior to transplant: 200 mg once daily for 6 to 12 months (Vikram 2009; Vucicevic 2011)
Previous history ≤12 months prior to transplant: 400 mg once daily, lifelong treatment (Vikram 2009; Vucicevic 2011)
Positive serology before or at transplant: 400 mg once daily, lifelong treatment; if serology is negative at 12 months, consider a dose reduction to 200 mg daily (Vikram 2009; Vucicevic 2011)
No history (at risk for *de novo* post-transplant disease): some clinicians treat with 200 mg daily for 6 to 12 months (Vucicevic 2011)

Cryptococcosis:
Meningitis:
Manufacturer's labeling: Oral, IV: 400 mg for 1 dose, then 200 to 400 mg once daily for 10 to 12 weeks following negative CSF culture
Alternate dosing: HIV-infected:
Induction (alternative to preferred therapy): Oral, IV: 800 to 1,200 mg once daily with concomitant flucytosine for 6 weeks (Perfect 2010) **or** 400 to 800 mg once daily with concomitant flucytosine for at least 2 weeks (HHS [OI adult 2015]) **or** 1,200 mg once daily as monotherapy for at least 2 weeks (HHS [OI adult 2015])
Consolidation (preferred therapy): Oral, IV: 400 mg once daily for at least 8 weeks (HHS [OI adult 2015])
Maintenance (suppression) (preferred therapy): Oral: 200 mg once daily for at least 12 months; maintenance therapy may be stopped if the following criteria are fulfilled: induction, consolidation, and at least 12 months of maintenance therapy has been completed, patient remains asymptomatic from cryptococcal infection, and CD4 count ≥100 cells/mm^3 for ≥3 months and

HIV RNA suppressed in response to effective ART (HHS [OI adult 2015])
Pulmonary (immunocompetent) (off-label use):
400 mg once daily for 6 to 12 months (Perfect 2010)
Pediatric The daily dose of fluconazole is the same for oral and IV administration
Usual dosage range: Oral, IV: Loading dose: 6 to 12 mg/kg/dose; maintenance: 3 to 12 mg/kg/dose once daily; duration and dosage depend on location and severity of infection

Indication-specific dosing:
Candidiasis: Oral, IV:
Esophageal:
Manufacturer's recommendation: Loading dose: 6 mg/kg/dose; maintenance: 3-12 mg/kg/dose once daily for 21 days and for at least 2 weeks following resolution of symptoms (maximum: 600 mg/day)
HIV-exposed/-infected: Loading dose: 6 mg/kg/dose once on day 1; maintenance: 3 to 6 mg/kg/dose once daily for 4 to 21 days (maximum: 400 mg/day) (CDC 2009)
Relapse suppression (HIV-exposed/-infected): 3 to 6 mg/kg/dose once daily (maximum: 200 mg/day) (CDC 2009)
Invasive disease (alternative therapy): 5 to 6 mg/kg/dose every 12 hours for ≥28 days (maximum: 600 mg/day) (CDC 2009)
Oropharyngeal:
Manufacturer's recommendation: Loading dose: 6 mg/kg/dose; maintenance: 3 mg/kg/dose once daily for ≥2 weeks (maximum: 600 mg/day)
HIV-exposed/-infected: 3 to 6 mg/kg/dose once daily for 7 to 14 days (maximum: 400 mg/day) (CDC 2009)
Surgical (perioperative) prophylaxis in high-risk patients undergoing liver, pancreas, kidney, or pancreas-kidney transplantation (off-label use): IV: 6 mg/kg given in the perioperative period and continued in the postoperative period for ≤28 days (maximum dose 400 mg). Time of initiation and duration varies with transplant type and operative protocol (Bratzler 2013).
Coccidioidomycosis: Oral, IV:
Children: *Meningeal infection, or in a stable patient with diffuse pulmonary or disseminated disease* (HIV-exposed/-infected):
Treatment: 5 to 6 mg/kg/dose twice daily (maximum daily dose: 800 mg/**day**) (CDC 2009) followed by chronic suppressive therapy (see below)
Relapse suppression: 6 mg/kg/dose once daily (maximum daily dose: 400 mg/**day**) (CDC 2009)
Adolescents: Treatment, primary prophylaxis, or chronic suppressive therapy (secondary prophylaxis): Refer to adult dosing.
Cryptococcosis: Oral, IV:
Meningitis: Manufacturer's labeling: 12 mg/kg/dose for 1 dose, then 6 to 12 mg/kg/day for 10-12 weeks following negative CSF culture
HIV-exposed/-infected:
CNS disease (alternative therapy in patients intolerant of amphotericin B):
Children:
Induction: 12 mg/kg/dose for 1 dose, then 6 to 12 mg/kg/day (maximum: 800 mg/day) for ≥2 weeks (in combination with flucytosine) (CDC 2009)
Consolidation: 10 to 12 mg/kg/day for 8 weeks (Perfect 2010) **or** 12 mg/kg/dose for 1 dose, then 6 to 12 mg/kg/day (maximum: 800 mg/day) for 8 weeks (CDC 2009)
Maintenance (suppression): 6 mg/kg/day (maximum: 200 mg/day) (CDC 2009; Perfect 2010)
Adolescents: Refer to adult dosing.
Non-CNS disease, disseminated (including severe pulmonary disease) (alternative therapy; off-label use): Induction: 12 mg/kg/dose for 1 dose, then 6 to 12 mg/kg/day (maximum: 600 mg/day) (CDC 2009)
Non-CNS disease, localized (including isolated pulmonary disease) (off-label use): 12 mg/kg/dose for 1 dose, then 6 to 12 mg/kg/day (maximum: 600 mg/day). **Note:** Duration depends upon infection site and severity (CDC 2009). For patients with pulmonary disease (not delineated by severity), the IDSA recommends a duration of 6 to 12 months (Perfect 2010).

Primary antifungal prophylaxis in pediatric oncology patients (guideline recommendations; Science 2014): Oral, IV:

Allogeneic hematopoietic stem cell transplant (HSCT): Infants ≥1 month, Children, and Adolescents <19 years: 6 to 12 mg/kg/day (maximum: 400 mg/day), begin at the start of conditioning; continue until engraftment

Allogeneic HSCT with grades 2 to 4 acute graft-versus-host-disease (GVHD) or chronic extensive GVHD: Begin with GVHD diagnosis, continue until GVHD resolves:

Infants ≥1 month and Children <13 years: 6 to 12 mg/kg/day (maximum: 400 mg/day)

Adolescents ≥13 years (where posaconazole is contraindicated): 6 to 12 mg/kg/day (maximum: 400 mg/day)

Autologous HSCT with neutropenia anticipated >7 days: Infants ≥1 month, Children, and Adolescents <19 years: 6 to 12 mg/kg/day (maximum: 400 mg/day), begin at the start of conditioning; continue until engraftment

Acute myeloid leukemia (AML) or myelodysplastic syndromes (MDS): Infants ≥1 month, Children, and Adolescents <19 years: 6 to 12 mg/kg/day (maximum: 400 mg/day) during chemotherapy associated neutropenia; alternative antifungals may be suggested for children ≥13 years in centers with a high local incidence of mold infections or if fluconazole is not available

Renal Impairment

Manufacturer's labeling: **Note:** Renal function estimated using the Cockcroft-Gault formula

No adjustment for vaginal candidiasis single-dose therapy

For multiple dosing in adults, administer loading dose of 50 to 400 mg, then adjust daily doses as follows (dosage reduction in children should parallel adult recommendations):

CrCl >50 mL/minute: No dosage adjustment necessary

CrCl ≤50 mL/minute (no dialysis): Reduce dose by 50%

End-stage renal disease on intermittent hemodialysis (IHD):

Manufacturer's labeling: 100% of daily dose (according to indication) after each dialysis session; on non-dialysis days, patient should receive a reduced dose according to their CrCl.

Alternate recommendations: Doses of 200 to 400 mg every 48 to 72 hours **or** 100 to 200 mg every 24 hours have been recommended. **Note:** Dosing dependent on the assumption of 3 times/week, complete IHD sessions (Heintz 2009).

Continuous renal replacement therapy (CRRT) (Heintz 2009; Trotman 2005): Drug clearance is highly dependent on the method of renal replacement, filter type, and flow rate. Appropriate dosing requires close monitoring of pharmacologic response, signs of adverse reactions due to drug accumulation, as well as drug concentrations in relation to target trough (if appropriate). The following are general recommendations only (based on dialysate flow/ultrafiltration rates of 1 to 2 L/hour and minimal residual renal function) and should not supersede clinical judgment:

CVVH: Loading dose of 400 to 800 mg followed by 200 to 400 mg every 24 hours

CVVHD/CVVHDF: Loading dose of 400 to 800 mg followed by 400 to 800 mg every 24 hours (CVVHD or CVVHDF) **or** 800 mg every 24 hours (CVVHDF)

Note: Higher maintenance doses of 400 mg every 24 hours (CVVH), 800 mg every 24 hours (CVVHD), and 500 to 600 mg every 12 hours (CVVHDF) may be considered when treating resistant organisms and/or when employing combined ultrafiltration and dialysis flow rates of ≥2 L/hour for CVVHD/CVVHDF (Heintz 2009; Trotman 2005).

Hepatic Impairment There are no dosage adjustments provided in the manufacturer's labeling; use with caution.

Administration

IV: Do not use if cloudy or precipitated. Infuse over ~1 to 2 hours; do not exceed 200 mg/hour.

Oral: May be administered without regard to meals.

Hazardous agent; use appropriate precautions for handling and disposal (NIOSH 2014 [group 3]).

Monitoring Parameters Periodic liver function tests (AST, ALT, alkaline phosphatase) and renal function tests, potassium

Dosage Forms Excipient information presented when available (limited, particularly for generics); consult specific product labeling.

Solution, Intravenous:

Generic: 100 mg (50 mL); 200 mg (100 mL); 400 mg (200 mL)

Solution, Intravenous [preservative free]:

Generic: 200 mg (100 mL); 400 mg (200 mL)

Suspension Reconstituted, Oral:

Diflucan: 10 mg/mL (35 mL); 40 mg/mL (35 mL) [orange flavor]

Generic: 10 mg/mL (35 mL); 40 mg/mL (35 mL)

Tablet, Oral:

Diflucan: 50 mg, 100 mg, 150 mg, 200 mg

Generic: 50 mg, 100 mg, 150 mg, 200 mg

◆ Fluconazole Injection (Can) *see* Fluconazole *on page 775*

◆ Fluconazole Injection SDZ (Can) *see* Fluconazole *on page 775*

◆ Fluconazole Omega (Can) *see* Fluconazole *on page 775*

Flucytosine (floo SYE toe seen)

Brand Names: US Ancobon

Index Terms 5-FC; 5-Fluorocytosine; 5-Flurocytosine

Pharmacologic Category Antifungal Agent, Oral

Use Adjunctive treatment of systemic fungal infections (eg, septicemia, endocarditis, UTI, meningitis, or pulmonary) caused by susceptible strains of *Candida* or *Cryptococcus*

Dosing

Adult & Geriatric Usual dosage ranges: Oral: 50 to 150 mg/kg/day in divided doses every 6 hours

Cryptococcal meningitis, treatment: Oral:

Non-HIV-infected: Induction: 25 mg/kg/dose (with amphotericin B) every 6 hours for at least 4 weeks; if clinical improvement, may discontinue both amphotericin and flucytosine and follow with an extended course of fluconazole (Perfect 2010).

HIV-infected: Oral: Induction: 25 mg/kg/dose (with an amphotericin B formulation [liposomal amphotericin B is preferred]) every 6 hours for at least 2 weeks (HHS [OI adult 2015]).

Endocarditis (off-label use): Oral: 100 mg/kg daily in 3 or 4 divided doses (with amphotericin B) for at least 4 to 6 weeks after valve replacement (Gould 2012; Pappas 2009)

Pediatric

Cryptococcal meningitis, treatment:

Non-HIV-infected: Children (off-label population): Oral: Induction: 25 mg/kg/dose (with amphotericin B) every 6 hours for at least 4 weeks; if clinical improvement, may discontinue both amphotericin and flucytosine and follow with an extended course of fluconazole (Perfect 2010).

HIV-infected: Adolescents (off-label population): Refer to adult dosing.

Renal Impairment No dosage adjustment provided in manufacturer's labeling (**Note:** Manufacturer recommends dose reduction); however, the following adjustments have been recommended:

Adults (based upon dosing of 25 mg/kg every 6 hours):

CrCl >40 mL/minute: No dosage adjustment recommended (Perfect 2010)

CrCl 20 to 40 mL/minute: 50% of standard dose every 6 hours (Perfect 2010)

CrCl 10 to 20 mL/minute: 25% of standard dose every 6 hours (Perfect 2010)

ESRD on intermittent hemodialysis (IHD): 25 to 50 mg/kg every 48 to 72 hours; administer dose after hemodialysis (Drew 1999; HHS [OI adult 2015])

Adults and Adolescents (HIV-infected patients) (based upon dosing of 25 mg/kg every 6 hours) (HHS [OI adult 2015]):

CrCl >40 mL/minute: No dosage adjustment recommended

CrCl 20 to 40 mL/minute: 25 mg/kg every 12 hours

CrCl 10 to ≤20 mL/minute: 25 mg/kg every 24 hours

CrCl <10 mL/minute: 25 mg/kg every 48 hours

ESRD on intermittent hemodialysis (IHD): 25 to 50 mg/kg every 48 to 72 hours; administer dose after hemodialysis

Infants, Children, and non-HIV positive Adolescents (based upon dosing of 100 to 150 mg/kg/day divided every 6 hours) (Aronoff 2007): **Note:** Flucytosine should be avoided in children with severe renal impairment (DHHS [pediatric] 2013):

CrCl 30 to 50 mL/minute: 25 to 37.5 mg/kg every 8 hours

CrCl 10 to 29 mL/minute: 25 to 37.5 mg/kg every 12 hours

CrCl <10 mL/minute: 25 to 37.5 mg/kg every 24 hours

Hemodialysis: 25 to 37.5 mg/kg every 24 hours

Peritoneal dialysis: 25 to 37.5 mg/kg every 24 hours

Continuous renal replacement therapy: 25 to 37.5 mg/kg every 8 hours (monitor serum concentrations)

Hepatic Impairment No dosage adjustment provided in manufacturer's labeling; use with caution.

Additional Information Complete prescribing information should be consulted for additional detail.

Dosage Forms Excipient information presented when available (limited, particularly for generics); consult specific product labeling.

Capsule, Oral:

Ancobon: 250 mg, 500 mg

Generic: 250 mg, 500 mg

◆ Fludara *see* Fludarabine *on page 779*

Fludarabine (floo DARE a been)

Brand Names: US Fludara

Brand Names: Canada Fludara; Fludarabine Phosphate for Injection; Fludarabine Phosphate for Injection, USP; Fludarabine Phosphate Injection, PPC STD.

Index Terms 2F-ara-AMP; Fludarabine Phosphate

Pharmacologic Category Antineoplastic Agent, Antimetabolite; Antineoplastic Agent, Antimetabolite (Purine Analog)

Use

Chronic lymphocytic leukemia: Treatment of progressive or refractory B-cell chronic lymphocytic leukemia (CLL)

Canadian labeling: Second-line treatment of chronic lymphocytic leukemia (CLL); second-line treatment of low-grade, refractory non-Hodgkin lymphoma (NHL)

Dosing

Adult & Geriatric

Chronic lymphocytic leukemia (CLL), progressive or refractory:

IV: 25 mg/m^2/day for 5 days every 28 days

Oral (Canadian labeling; not available in U.S.): 40 mg/m^2 once daily for 5 days every 28 days

CLL combination regimens (off-label dosing): IV:

FC: 30 mg/m^2/day for 3 days every 28 days for 6 cycles (in combination with cyclophosphamide) (Eichhorst, 2006) **or** 20 mg/m^2/day for 5 days every 28 days for 6 cycles (in combination with cyclophosphamide) (Flinn, 2007)

FCR: 25 mg/m^2/day for 3 days every 28 days for 6 cycles (in combination with cyclophosphamide and rituximab) (Keating, 2005; Robak, 2010; Wierda, 2005)

FR: 25 mg/m^2/day for 5 days every 28 days for 6 cycles (in combination with rituximab) (Byrd, 2003)

OFAR: 30 mg/m^2/day for 2 days every 28 days for 6 cycles (in combination with oxaliplatin, cytarabine, and rituximab) (Tsimberidou, 2008)

Acute myeloid leukemia (AML), high-risk patients (off-label use): IV: 30 mg/m^2/day for 5 days induction therapy, followed by post remission therapy of 30 mg/m^2/day for 4 days every other cycle (in combination with cytarabine with or without filgrastim) (Borthakur, 2008)

AML, refractory (off-label use): IV: 30 mg/m^2/day for 5 days (in combination with cytarabine and filgrastim), may repeat once for partial remission (Montillo, 1998) **or** 30 mg/m^2/day for 5 days for 1 or 2 cycles (in combination with cytarabine, idarubicin, and filgrastim) (Virchis, 2004)

Non-Hodgkin lymphomas: IV:

Canadian labeling: 25 mg/m^2 for 5 days every 28 days; dosage adjustment may be necessary for hematologic or nonhematologic toxicity.

Follicular lymphoma (off-label use):

FCR: 25 mg/m^2/day for 3 days every 21 days for 4 cycles (in combination with cyclophosphamide and rituximab) (Sacchi, 2007)

FCMR: 25 mg/m^2/day for 3 days every 28 days for 4 cycles (in combination with cyclophosphamide, mitoxantrone, and rituximab) (Forstpointner, 2004; Forstpointner, 2006)

FND: 25 mg/m^2/day for 3 days every 28 days for up to 8 cycles (in combination with mitoxantrone and dexamethasone) (McLaughlin, 1996; Tsimberidou, 2002)

FNDR: 25 mg/m^2/day for 3 days every 28 days for up to 8 cycles (in combination with mitoxantrone, dexamethasone, and rituximab) (McLaughlin, 2000)

FR: 25 mg/m^2/day for 5 days every 28 days for 6 cycles (in combination with rituximab) (Czuczman, 2005)

Mantle cell lymphoma (off-label use):

FC: 20 mg/m^2/day for 4 to 5 days or 25 mg/m^2/day for 3-5 days (in combination with cyclophosphamide) (Cohen, 2001)

FCMR: 25 mg/m^2/day for 3 days every 28 days for 4 cycles (in combination with cyclophosphamide, mitoxantrone, and rituximab) (Forstpointner, 2004; Forstpointner, 2006)

Waldenstron macroglobulinemia (off-label use): IV: 25 mg/m^2/day for 5 days every 28 days (Foran, 1999) **or** 25 mg/m^2/day for 5 days every 28 days for 6 cycles (in combination with rituximab) (Treon, 2009)

Stem cell transplant (allogeneic) conditioning regimen, reduced-intensity, (off-label use): IV: 30 mg/m^2/dose for 6 doses beginning 10 days prior to transplant **or** 30 mg/m^2/dose for 5 days beginning 6 days prior to transplant (in combination with busulfan with or without antithymocyte globulin) (Schetelig, 2003)

Stem cell transplant (allogeneic) nonmyeloablative conditioning regimen (off-label use): IV: 30 mg/m^2/dose for 3 doses beginning 5 days prior to transplant (in combination with cyclophosphamide and rituximab) (Khouri, 2008) **or** 30 mg/m^2/dose for 3 doses beginning 4 days prior to transplant (in combination with total body irradiation) (Rezvani, 2008)

Pediatric

Acute myeloid leukemia (AML) (off-label use): IV: 10.5 mg/m^2 bolus infusion followed by a continuous infusion of 30.5 mg/m^2/day for 48 hours (Lange, 2008)

Acute lymphocytic leukemia (ALL) or AML, relapsed (off-label use): IV: 10.5 mg/m^2 bolus over 15 minutes followed by a continuous infusion of 30.5 mg/m^2/day for 48 hours (Avramis, 1998)

Stem cell transplant (allogeneic) conditioning regimen, reduced-intensity (off-label use): IV: 30 mg/m^2/dose for 6 doses beginning 7-10 days prior to transplant (in combination with busulfan and antithymocyte globulin) (Pulsipher, 2009)

Renal Impairment

U.S. labeling: Adults: CLL: IV:

CrCl 50-79 mL/minute: Decrease dose to 20 mg/m^2.

CrCl 30-49 mL/minute: Decrease dose to 15 mg/m^2.

CrCl <30 mL/minute: Avoid use.

Canadian labeling: CLL (Oral, IV), NHL (IV):

CrCl 30-70 mL/minute: Reduce dose by up to 50%.

CrCl <30 mL/minute: Use is contraindicated.

The following guidelines have been used by some clinicians: Aronoff, 2007: IV:

Adults:

CrCl 10-50 mL/minute: Administer 75% of dose.

CrCl <10 mL/minute: Administer 50% of dose.

Hemodialysis: Administer after dialysis

Continuous ambulatory peritoneal dialysis (CAPD): Administer 50% of dose.

Continuous renal replacement therapy (CRRT): Administer 75% of dose.

Children:

CrCl 30-50 mL/minute: Administer 80% of dose.

CrCl <30 mL/minute: Not recommended.

Hemodialysis: Administer 25% of dose

Continuous ambulatory peritoneal dialysis (CAPD): Not recommended.

Continuous renal replacement therapy (CRRT): Administer 80% of dose.

Hepatic Impairment There are no dosage adjustments provided in the manufacturer's labeling.

Obesity

American Society of Clinical Oncology (ASCO) Guidelines for appropriate chemotherapy dosing in obese adults with cancer (Note: Excludes leukemias and HSCT dosing): Utilize patient's actual body weight (full weight) for calculation of body surface area- or weight-based dosing, particularly when the intent of therapy is curative; manage regimen-related toxicities in the same manner as for nonobese patients; if a dose reduction is utilized due to toxicity, consider resumption of full weight-based dosing with subsequent cycles, especially if cause of toxicity (eg, hepatic or renal impairment) is resolved (Griggs, 2012).

American Society for Blood and Marrow Transplantation (ASBMT) practice guideline committee position statement on chemotherapy dosing in obesity: Utilize actual body weight (full weight) for calculation of body surface area in fludarabine dosing for hematopoietic stem cell transplant conditioning regimens in adults (Bubalo, 2014).

Adjustment for Toxicity

Hematologic or nonhematologic toxicity (other than neurotoxicity): Consider treatment delay or dosage reduction.

Hemolysis: Discontinue treatment.

Neurotoxicity: Consider treatment delay or discontinuation.

Additional Information Complete prescribing information should be consulted for additional detail.

Dosage Forms Excipient information presented when available (limited, particularly for generics); consult specific product labeling. [DSC] = Discontinued product
Solution, Intravenous, as phosphate:
Generic: 50 mg/2 mL (2 mL)
Solution, Intravenous, as phosphate [preservative free]:
Generic: 50 mg/2 mL (2 mL [DSC])
Solution Reconstituted, Intravenous, as phosphate:
Fludara: 50 mg (1 ea)
Generic: 50 mg (1 ea)
Solution Reconstituted, Intravenous, as phosphate [preservative free]:
Generic: 50 mg (1 ea)

Dosage Forms: Canada Excipient information presented when available (limited, particularly for generics); consult specific product labeling.
Tablet, as phosphate:
Fludara: 10 mg

◆ Fludarabine Phosphate see Fludarabine on page 779
◆ Fludarabine Phosphate for Injection (Can) see Fludarabine on page 779
◆ Fludarabine Phosphate for Injection, USP (Can) see Fludarabine on page 779
◆ Fludarabine Phosphate Injection, PPC STD. (Can) see Fludarabine on page 779

Fludrocortisone (floo droe KOR ti sone)

Brand Names: Canada Florinef®
Index Terms 9α-Fluorohydrocortisone Acetate; Florinef; Fludrocortisone Acetate; Fluohydrisone Acetate; Fluohydrocortisone Acetate
Pharmacologic Category Corticosteroid, Systemic
Additional Appendix Information
Corticosteroids Systemic Equivalencies on page 1950
Use Partial replacement therapy for primary and secondary adrenocortical insufficiency in Addison's disease; treatment of salt-losing adrenogenital syndrome (or congenital adrenal hyperplasia)
Dosing
Adult & Geriatric
Addison's disease: Oral: Initial: 0.1 mg daily; if transient hypertension develops, reduce dose to 0.05 mg daily; maintenance dosage range: 0.1 mg 3 times weekly to 0.2 mg daily. Preferred administration with cortisone (10-37.5 mg daily) or hydrocortisone (10-30 mg daily).
Salt-losing adrenogenital syndrome (or congenital adrenal hyperplasia): Oral: 0.1-0.2 mg daily
The Endocrine Society recommends a maintenance dose range of 0.05-0.2 mg once daily (in combination with hydrocortisone) for patients with congenital adrenal hyperplasia due to 21-hydroxylase deficiency (Speiser, 2010).
Orthostatic hypotension (off-label use; Kearney, 2009; Lahrmann, 2006; Lanier, 2011): Oral: Initial: 0.1 mg daily in conjunction with a high-salt diet and adequate fluid intake; may be increased in increments of 0.1 mg per week; maximum dose: 1 mg daily. **Note:** Doses exceeding 0.3 mg daily may not be beneficial and predispose patient to unwanted side effects (eg, hypertension, hypokalemia).
Pediatric Congenital adrenal hyperplasia due to 21-hydroxylase deficiency (Endocrine Society guidelines): Oral: Infants, Children, and Adolescents: 0.05-0.2 mg daily in 1-2 divided doses in combination with sodium chloride supplementation (Speiser, 2010).
Renal Impairment No dosage adjustment provided in manufacturer's labeling; use with caution.
Hepatic Impairment No dosage adjustment provided in manufacturer's labeling.
Additional Information Complete prescribing information should be consulted for additional detail.
Dosage Forms Excipient information presented when available (limited, particularly for generics); consult specific product labeling.
Tablet, Oral, as acetate:
Generic: 0.1 mg

◆ Fludrocortisone Acetate see Fludrocortisone on page 780
◆ Flugerel see Flutamide on page 791
◆ Flulaval Quadrivalent see Influenza Virus Vaccine (Inactivated) on page 945
◆ Flulaval Tetra (Can) see Influenza Virus Vaccine (Inactivated) on page 945
◆ Flumadine see Rimantadine on page 1589
◆ Flumadine® (Can) see Rimantadine on page 1589

Flumazenil (FLOO may ze nil)

Brand Names: US Romazicon [DSC]
Brand Names: Canada Anexate; Flumazenil Injection; Flumazenil Injection, USP; Romazicon
Pharmacologic Category Antidote
Use Benzodiazepine antagonist; reverses sedative effects of benzodiazepines used in conscious sedation and general anesthesia; treatment of benzodiazepine overdose
Dosing
Adult
Reversal of conscious sedation and general anesthesia: IV:
Initial dose: 0.2 mg over 15 seconds
Repeat doses (maximum: 4 doses): If desired level of consciousness is not obtained, 0.2 mg may be repeated at 1-minute intervals.
Maximum total cumulative dose: 1 mg (usual total dose: 0.6-1 mg). In the event of resedation: Repeat doses may be given at 20-minute intervals as needed at 0.2 mg per minute to a maximum of 1 mg total dose and 3 mg in 1 hour.
Suspected benzodiazepine overdose: IV:
Initial dose: 0.2 mg over 30 seconds; if the desired level of consciousness is not obtained 30 seconds after the dose, 0.3 mg can be given over 30 seconds
Repeat doses: 0.5 mg over 30 seconds repeated at 1-minute intervals
Maximum total cumulative dose: 3 mg (usual total dose: 1-3 mg). Patients with a partial response at 3 mg may require (rare) additional titration up to a total dose of 5 mg (although doses >3 mg do not reliably produce additional effects). If a patient has not responded 5 minutes after cumulative dose of 5 mg, the major cause of sedation is not likely due to benzodiazepines. In the event of resedation, repeat doses may be given at 20-minute intervals if needed, at 0.5 mg per minute to a maximum of 1 mg total dose and 3 mg in 1 hour.
Geriatric Refer to adult dosing. No differences in safety or efficacy have been reported; however, increased sensitivity may occur in some elderly patients.
Pediatric Reversal of benzodiazepine when used in conscious sedation: Children ≥1 year: IV:
Initial dose: 0.01 mg/kg over 15 seconds (maximum: 0.2 mg)
Repeat doses (maximum: 4 doses): If desired level of consciousness is not obtained, 0.01 mg/kg (maximum: 0.2 mg) repeated at 1-minute intervals
Maximum total cumulative dose: 1 mg or 0.05 mg/kg (whichever is lower)
Mean total dose: 0.65 mg (range: 0.08-1 mg)
Renal Impairment No dosage adjustment provided in manufacturer's labeling; however, pharmacokinetics are not significantly affected by renal failure (CrCl <10 mL/minute) or hemodialysis.
Hepatic Impairment Initial reversal: No dosage adjustment necessary. Repeat doses: Reduce dose or frequency.
Additional Information Complete prescribing information should be consulted for additional detail.
Dosage Forms Excipient information presented when available (limited, particularly for generics); consult specific product labeling. [DSC] = Discontinued product
Solution, Intravenous:
Romazicon: 1 mg/10 mL (10 mL [DSC])
Generic: 0.5 mg/5 mL (5 mL); 1 mg/10 mL (10 mL)

◆ Flumazenil Injection (Can) see Flumazenil on page 780
◆ Flumazenil Injection, USP (Can) see Flumazenil on page 780
◆ FluMist Quadrivalent see Influenza Virus Vaccine (Live/Attenuated) on page 950

Flunisolide (Nasal) (floo NISS oh lide)

Brand Names: Canada Apo-Flunisolide®; Nasalide®; Rhinalar®
Pharmacologic Category Corticosteroid, Nasal
Use Seasonal or perennial rhinitis
Dosing
Adult & Geriatric Seasonal allergic rhinitis: Intranasal: 2 sprays each nostril twice daily (morning and evening); may increase to 2 sprays 3 times daily; maximum dose: 8 sprays/day in each nostril (400 mcg/day)
Pediatric Seasonal allergic rhinitis: Intranasal:
Children 6-14 years: 1 spray each nostril 3 times daily **or** 2 sprays in each nostril twice daily; not to exceed 4 sprays/day in each nostril
Children ≥15 years: Refer to adult dosing.

Renal Impairment No dosage adjustment provided in manufacturer's labeling.

Hepatic Impairment No dosage adjustment provided in manufacturer's labeling.

Additional Information Complete prescribing information should be consulted for additional detail.

Dosage Forms Excipient information presented when available (limited, particularly for generics); consult specific product labeling. [DSC] = Discontinued product

Solution, Nasal:

Generic: 25 mcg/actuation (0.025%) (25 mL); 29 mcg/actuation (0.025%) (25 mL [DSC])

Fluocinolone (Topical) (floo oh SIN oh lone)

Brand Names: US Capex; Derma-Smoothe/FS Body; Derma-Smoothe/FS Scalp; Fluocinolone Acetonide Body; Fluocinolone Acetonide Scalp; Synalar; Synalar (Cream); Synalar (Ointment); Synalar TS

Brand Names: Canada Capex®; Derma-Smoothe/FS®; Synalar®

Index Terms Fluocinolone Acetonide

Pharmacologic Category Corticosteroid, Topical

Additional Appendix Information

Topical Corticosteroids on page 1952

Use Relief of susceptible inflammatory dermatosis (low, medium corticosteroid); dermatitis or psoriasis of the scalp; atopic dermatitis in adults and children ≥3 months of age

Dosing

Adult & Geriatric

Atopic dermatitis (Derma-Smoothe/FS® body oil): Apply thin film to affected area 3 times/day

Corticosteroid-responsive dermatoses: Topical: Cream, ointment, solution: Apply a thin layer to affected area 2-4 times/day; may use occlusive dressings to manage psoriasis or recalcitrant conditions

Inflammatory and pruritic manifestations (dental use): Topical: Apply to oral lesion 4 times/day, after meals and at bedtime

Scalp psoriasis (Derma-Smoothe/FS® scalp oil): Topical: Massage thoroughly into wet or dampened hair/scalp; cover with shower cap. Leave on overnight (or for at least 4 hours). Remove by washing hair with shampoo and rinsing thoroughly.

Seborrheic dermatitis of the scalp (Capex®): Topical: Apply no more than 1 ounce to scalp once daily; work into lather and allow to remain on scalp for ~5 minutes. Remove from hair and scalp by rinsing thoroughly with water.

Pediatric

Atopic dermatitis: Topical: Children ≥3 months (Derma-Smoothe/FS® body oil): Moisten skin; apply a thin film to affected area twice daily; do not use for longer than 4 weeks

Corticosteroid-responsive dermatoses: Topical: Refer to adult dosing.

Additional Information Complete prescribing information should be consulted for additional detail.

Dosage Forms Excipient information presented when available (limited, particularly for generics); consult specific product labeling.

Cream, External, as acetonide:

Synalar: 0.025% (120 g) [contains cetyl alcohol, edetate disodium, methylparaben, propylene glycol, propylparaben]

Generic: 0.01% (15 g, 60 g); 0.025% (15 g, 60 g)

Kit, External, as acetonide:

Synalar (Cream): 0.025% [contains cetyl alcohol, edetate disodium, methylparaben, propylene glycol, propylparaben]

Synalar (Ointment): 0.025%

Synalar TS: 0.01% [contains propylene glycol]

Oil, External, as acetonide:

Derma-Smoothe/FS Body: 0.01% (118.28 mL) [contains isopropyl alcohol, peanut oil]

Derma-Smoothe/FS Scalp: 0.01% (118.28 mL) [contains isopropyl alcohol, peanut oil]

Fluocinolone Acetonide Body: 0.01% (118.28 mL) [contains isopropyl alcohol, peanut oil]

Fluocinolone Acetonide Scalp: 0.01% (118.28 mL) [contains isopropyl alcohol, peanut oil]

Ointment, External, as acetonide:

Synalar: 0.025% (120 g)

Generic: 0.025% (15 g, 60 g)

Shampoo, External, as acetonide:

Capex: 0.01% (120 mL)

Solution, External, as acetonide:

Synalar: 0.01% (60 mL, 90 mL) [contains propylene glycol]

Generic: 0.01% (60 mL)

◆ Fluocinolone Acetonide see Fluocinolone (Topical) on page 781

◆ Fluocinolone Acetonide Body see Fluocinolone (Topical) on page 781

◆ Fluocinolone Acetonide Scalp see Fluocinolone (Topical) on page 781

Fluocinolone, Hydroquinone, and Tretinoin

(floo oh SIN oh lone, HYE droe kwin one, & TRET i noyn)

Brand Names: US Tri-Luma®

Index Terms Hydroquinone, Fluocinolone Acetonide, and Tretinoin; Tretinoin, Fluocinolone Acetonide, and Hydroquinone

Pharmacologic Category Corticosteroid, Topical; Depigmenting Agent; Retinoic Acid Derivative

Use Short-term treatment of moderate-to-severe melasma of the face

Dosing

Adult & Geriatric Melasma: Topical: Apply a thin film once daily to affected areas; not indicated for use beyond 8 weeks

Additional Information Complete prescribing information should be consulted for additional detail.

Dosage Forms Excipient information presented when available (limited, particularly for generics); consult specific product labeling.

Cream, topical:

Tri-Luma®: Fluocinolone acetonide 0.01%, hydroquinone 4%, and tretinoin 0.05% (30 g) [contains sodium metabisulfite]

Fluocinonide (floo oh SIN oh nide)

Brand Names: US Vanos

Brand Names: Canada Lidemol; Lidex; Lyderm; Tiamol; Topactin; Topsyn

Index Terms Lidex

Pharmacologic Category Corticosteroid, Topical

Additional Appendix Information

Topical Corticosteroids on page 1952

Use Inflammatory and pruritic dermatologic conditions: Relief of the inflammatory and pruritic manifestations of corticosteroid-responsive dermatoses.

Dosing

Adult & Geriatric

Atopic dermatitis: Topical: Cream (0.1%): Apply thin layer to affected areas once daily. Not recommended for use >2 consecutive weeks or >60 g/week total exposure. Therapy should be discontinued when control is achieved; if no improvement is seen within 2 weeks, reassessment of diagnosis may be necessary.

Psoriasis: Topical: Cream (0.1%): Apply a thin layer once or twice daily to affected areas. Not recommended for use >2 consecutive weeks or >60 g/week total exposure. Therapy should be discontinued when control is achieved; if no improvement is seen within 2 weeks, reassess diagnosis.

Other inflammatory and pruritic dermatologic conditions besides atopic dermatitis or psoriasis: Topical: Cream, gel, ointment, solution (0.05%): Apply thin layer to affected area 2 to 4 times daily.

Cream (0.1%): Apply thin layer to affected area once or twice daily. Not recommended for use >2 consecutive weeks or >60 g/week total exposure. Therapy should be discontinued when control is achieved; if no improvement is seen within 2 weeks, reassess diagnosis.

Pediatric

Atopic dermatitis and psoriasis: Children ≥12 years and Adolescents: Topical: Cream (0.1%): Refer to adult dosing.

Other inflammatory and pruritic dermatologic conditions besides atopic dermatitis or psoriasis: Children and Adolescents: Topical: Cream, gel, ointment, solution (0.05%): Refer to adult dosing.

Renal Impairment There are no dosage adjustments provided in the manufacturer's labeling.

Hepatic Impairment There are no dosage adjustments provided in the manufacturer's labeling.

Additional Information Complete prescribing information should be consulted for additional detail.

Dosage Forms Excipient information presented when available (limited, particularly for generics); consult specific product labeling.

Cream, External:

Vanos: 0.1% (30 g, 60 g, 120 g)

Generic: 0.05% (15 g, 30 g, 60 g, 120 g); 0.1% (30 g, 60 g, 120 g)

Gel, External:
Generic: 0.05% (15 g, 30 g, 60 g)
Ointment, External:
Generic: 0.05% (15 g, 30 g, 60 g)
Solution, External:
Generic: 0.05% (20 mL, 60 mL)

◆ Fluohydrisone Acetate see Fludrocortisone on page 780
◆ Fluohydrocortisone Acetate see Fludrocortisone on page 780
◆ Fluor-I-Strips A.T. see Fluorescein on page 782
◆ Fluorabon see Fluoride on page 782
◆ Fluor-A-Day see Fluoride on page 782

Fluorescein (FLURE e seen)

Brand Names: US AK-Fluor; Bio Glo; Fluor-I-Strips A.T.; Fluorescein Lite [DSC]; Fluorescite; Fluorets [DSC]; Ful-Glo
Brand Names: Canada Fluorescite®
Index Terms Fluorescein Sodium; Sodium Fluorescein; Soluble Fluorescein
Pharmacologic Category Diagnostic Agent
Use
Injection: Diagnostic aid in ophthalmic angiography and angioscopy
Ophthalmic: To stain the anterior segment of the eye for procedures (such as fitting contact lenses), disclosing corneal injury, and in applanation tonometry
Dosing
Adult & Geriatric
Diagnostic staining: Ophthalmic: Strips: Moisten strip with sterile water, saline or ophthalmic fluid. Touch conjunctiva or fornix with tip of strip until adequately stained.
Ophthalmic angiography: Solution for injection: **Note:** Prior to use, an intradermal test dose of 0.05 mL may be used if an allergy is suspected. Evaluate 30-60 minutes following intradermal injection. A negative skin test does not exclude the potential for a reaction to occur.
IV: 500 mg as a single dose into antecubital vein; a dose of 200 mg may be appropriate in cases when a highly sensitive imaging system (eg, scanning laser ophthalmoscope) is used.
Oral (off-label route): 1 g of injection solution has been administered orally; clarity of photographs, particularly during early arterial phase, is reportedly poorer than photographs obtained following IV administration (Hara, 1998)
Pediatric
Diagnostic staining: Ophthalmic: Strips: Refer to adult dosing.
Ophthalmic angiography: Solution for injection: **Note:** Prior to use, an intradermal test dose of 0.05 mL may be used if an allergy is suspected. Evaluate 30-60 minutes following intradermal injection. A negative skin test does not exclude the potential for a reaction to occur.
IV: 3.5 mg/lb (7.7 mg/kg) as a single dose into antecubital vein; maximum: 500 mg
Renal Impairment No dosage adjustment provided in manufacturer's labeling.
Hepatic Impairment No dosage adjustment provided in manufacturer's labeling.
Additional Information Complete prescribing information should be consulted for additional detail.
Dosage Forms Excipient information presented when available (limited, particularly for generics); consult specific product labeling. [DSC] = Discontinued product
Solution, Injection, as sodium:
AK-Fluor: 10% (5 mL); 25% (2 mL)
Fluorescein Lite: 10% (5 mL [DSC]); 25% (2 mL [DSC])
Fluorescite: 10% (5 mL)
Generic: 10% (5 mL [DSC]); 25% (2 mL [DSC])
Strip, Ophthalmic, as sodium:
Bio Glo: 1 mg (100 ea, 300 ea)
Fluor-I-Strips A.T.: 1 mg (300 ea)
Fluorets: 1 mg (100 ea [DSC])
Ful-Glo: 0.6 mg (300 ea); 1 mg (100 ea)

Fluorescein and Benoxinate
(FLURE e seen & ben OX i nate)

Brand Names: US EyeFlur; Fluress® [DSC]; Flurox™
Index Terms Benoxinate Hydrochloride and Fluorescein Sodium
Pharmacologic Category Anesthetic, Topical; Diagnostic Agent; Ophthalmic Agent
Use For use in ophthalmic procedures when a topical disclosing agent is needed along with an anesthetic

Dosing
Adult
Removal of foreign bodies, sutures, or tonometry: Ophthalmic: Instill 1 or 2 drops (single instillations) into each eye before operating
Deep ophthalmic anesthesia: Ophthalmic: Instill 2 drops into each eye every 90 seconds up to 3 doses
Renal Impairment No dosage adjustment provided in manufacturer's labeling.
Hepatic Impairment No dosage adjustment provided in manufacturer's labeling.
Additional Information Complete prescribing information should be consulted for additional detail.
Dosage Forms Excipient information presented when available (limited, particularly for generics); consult specific product labeling. [DSC] = Discontinued product
Solution, ophthalmic: Fluorescein sodium 0.25% and benoxinate hydrochloride 0.4% (5 mL)
EyeFlur, Fluress® [DSC], Flurox™: Fluorescein sodium 0.25% and benoxinate hydrochloride 0.4% (5 mL)

◆ Fluorescein and Proparacaine see Proparacaine and Fluorescein on page 1515
◆ Fluorescein Lite [DSC] see Fluorescein on page 782
◆ Fluorescein Sodium see Fluorescein on page 782
◆ Fluorescite see Fluorescein on page 782
◆ Fluorescite® (Can) see Fluorescein on page 782
◆ Fluorets [DSC] see Fluorescein on page 782

Fluoride (FLOR ide)

Brand Names: US Act Kids [OTC]; Act Restoring [OTC]; Act Total Care [OTC]; Act [OTC]; CaviRinse; Clinpro 5000; ControlRx; ControlRx Multi; Denta 5000 Plus; DentaGel; Fluor-A-Day; Fluorabon; Fluorinse; Fluoritab; Flura-Drops; Gel-Kam Rinse; Gel-Kam [OTC]; Just For Kids [OTC]; Lozi-Flur; NeutraCare; NeutraGard Advanced; Omni Gel [OTC]; OrthoWash; PerioMed; Phos-Flur; Phos-Flur Rinse [OTC]; PreviDent; PreviDent 5000 Booster; PreviDent 5000 Booster Plus; PreviDent 5000 Dry Mouth; PreviDent 5000 Plus; Sensodyne Repair & Protect [OTC]; StanGard Perio
Brand Names: Canada Fluor-A-Day
Index Terms Acidulated Phosphate Fluoride; Sodium Fluoride; Stannous Fluoride
Pharmacologic Category Nutritional Supplement
Use Prevention of dental caries
Dosing
Adult & Geriatric
Cream or paste:
Clinpro 5000 paste, Control Rx 1.1%, Denta 5000 Plus: Once daily, in place of conventional toothpaste, brush teeth with a thin ribbon or pea-sized amount of paste for at least 2 minutes. Brush teeth with cream or paste once daily regardless of fluoride content of drinking water
Prevident 5000 Sensitive: Twice daily, brush teeth with a 1 inch strip of toothpaste for at least 1 minute. After brushing, expectorate and rinse mouth thoroughly. Brush teeth twice daily regardless of fluoride content of drinking water
Dental rinse or gel:
ACT Restoring 0.02% rinse, ACT Total Care 0.02% rinse: Twice daily after brushing, rinse 10 mL around and between teeth for 1 minute, then spit. Do not eat, drink, or rinse mouth for at least 30 minutes after treatment; do not swallow
ACT 0.05% rinse, Phos-Flur Rinse: Once daily after brushing, rinse 10 mL around and between teeth for 1 minute, then spit. Do not eat, drink, or rinse mouth for at least 30 minutes after treatment; do not swallow
Cavirinse, PreviDent rinse: Once weekly, rinse 10 mL vigorously around and between teeth for 1 minute, then spit; this should be done preferably at bedtime, after thoroughly brushing teeth; do not swallow. For maximum benefit with PreviDent rinse, do not eat, drink, or rinse mouth for at least 30 minutes after treatment.
Gel-Kam rinse: After diluting solution as directed, rinse with 15 mL for 1 minute at least daily, then spit. Repeat with remaining solution.
Lozenge: Lozi-FlurOne lozenge daily regardless of fluoride content of drinking water

Pediatric Oral: Children 6 months to 16 years: Fluor-A-Day, Fluorabon, Fluoritab drops, Flura-drops, Lozi-flur: The recommended daily dose of oral fluoride supplement (mg), based on fluoride ion content (ppm) in drinking water (2.2 mg of sodium fluoride is equivalent to 1 mg of fluoride ion): See table.

Fluoride Ion

Fluoride Content of Drinking Water	Daily Dose, Oral (mg)
<0.3 ppm	
Birth - 6 mo	None
6 mo - 3 y	0.25
3-6 y	0.5
6-16 y	1
0.3-0.6 ppm	
Birth - 6 mo	None
6 mo - 3 y	None
3-6 y	0.25
6-16 y	0.5

Table from: Recommended dosage schedule of The American Dental Association, The American Academy of Pediatric Dentistry, and The American Academy of Pediatrics

Additional Information Complete prescribing information should be consulted for additional detail.

Dosage Forms Excipient information presented when available (limited, particularly for generics); consult specific product labeling.

Cream, oral, as sodium [toothpaste]: 1.1% (51 g) [equivalent to fluoride 2.5 mg/dose]
   Denta 5000 Plus: 1.1% (51 g) [spearmint flavor; equivalent to fluoride 2.5 mg/dose]
   PreviDent 5000 Plus: 1.1% (51 g) [contains sodium benzoate; fruitastic flavor; equivalent to fluoride 2.5 mg/dose]
   PreviDent 5000 Plus: 1.1% (51 g) [contains sodium benzoate; spearmint flavor; equivalent to fluoride 2.5 mg/dose]

Gel, oral, as sodium [toothpaste]:
   PreviDent 5000 Booster: 1.1% (100 mL, 106 mL) [contains sodium benzoate; fruitastic flavor; equivalent to fluoride 2.5 mg/dose]
   PreviDent 5000 Booster: 1.1% (100 mL, 106 mL) [contains sodium benzoate; spearmint flavor; equivalent to fluoride 2.5 mg/dose]
   PreviDent 5000 Booster Plus: 1.1% (100 mL) [contains sodium benzoate; fruitastic flavor; equivalent to fluoride 2.5 mg/dose]
   PreviDent 5000 Booster Plus: 1.1% (100 mL) [contains sodium benzoate; spearmint flavor; equivalent to fluoride 2.5 mg/dose]
   PreviDent 5000 Dry Mouth: 1.1% (100 mL) [mint flavor; equivalent to fluoride 2.5 mg/dose]

Gel, topical, as sodium: 1.1% (56 g) [equivalent to fluoride 2 mg/dose]
   DentaGel: 1.1% (56 g) [fresh mint flavor; neutral pH; equivalent to fluoride 2 mg/dose]
   NeutraCare: 1.1% (60 g) [grape flavor; neutral pH]
   NeutraCare: 1.1% (60 g) [mint flavor; neutral pH]
   NeutraGard Advanced: 1.1% (60 g) [mint flavor; neutral pH]
   NeutraGard Advanced: 1.1% (60 g) [mixed berry flavor; neutral pH]
   Phos-Flur: 1.1% (51 g) [contains propylene glycol, sodium benzoate; mint flavor; equivalent to fluoride 0.5%]
   PreviDent: 1.1% (56 g) [mint flavor; neutral pH; equivalent to fluoride 2 mg/dose]
   PreviDent: 1.1% (56 g) [very berry flavor; neutral pH; equivalent to fluoride 2 mg/dose]

Gel, topical, as stannous fluoride:
   Gel-Kam: 0.4% (129 g) [cinnamon flavor]
   Gel-Kam: 0.4% (129 g) [fruit & berry flavor]
   Gel-Kam: 0.4% (129 g) [mint flavor]
   Just For Kids: 0.4% (122 g) [bubblegum flavor]
   Just For Kids: 0.4% (122 g) [fruit-punch flavor]
   Just For Kids: 0.4% (122 g) [grapey grape flavor]
   Omni Gel: 0.4% (122 g) [cinnamon flavor]
   Omni Gel: 0.4% (122 g) [grape flavor]
   Omni Gel: 0.4% (122 g) [mint flavor]
   Omni Gel: 0.4% (122 g) [natural flavor]
   Omni Gel: 0.4% (122 g) [raspberry flavor]

Liquid, oral, as base:
   Fluoritab: 0.125 mg/drop [dye free]

Lozenge, oral, as sodium:
   Lozi-Flur: 2.21 mg (90s) [sugar free; cherry flavor; equivalent to fluoride 1 mg]

Paste, oral, as sodium [toothpaste]:
   Clinpro 5000: 1.1% (113 g) [vanilla-mint flavor]
   ControlRx: 1.1% (57 g) [berry flavor]
   ControlRx: 1.1% (57 g) [vanilla-mint flavor]
   ControlRx Multi: 1.1% (57 g) [vanilla-mint flavor]

Paste, oral, as stannous fluoride [toothpaste]:
   Sensodyne Repair & Protect: 0.454% (96.4 g) [mint flavor]

Solution, oral, as fluoride [rinse]:
   Act Total Care: 0.02% (1000 mL) [ethanol free; contains menthol, propylene glycol, sodium benzoate, tartrazine; fresh mint flavor; equivalent to fluoride 0.009%]

Solution, oral, as sodium [drops]: 1.1 mg/mL (50 mL) [equivalent to fluoride 0.5 mg/mL]
   Fluor-A-Day: 0.278 mg/drop (30 mL) [equivalent to fluoride 0.125 mg/drop]
   Fluorabon: 0.55 mg/0.6 mL (60 mL) [dye free, sugar free; equivalent to fluoride 0.25 mg/0.6 mL]
   Flura-Drops: 0.55 mg/drop (24 mL) [dye free, sugar free; contains natural rubber/natural latex in packaging; equivalent to fluoride 0.25 mg/drop]

Solution, oral, as sodium [rinse]: 0.2% (473 mL)
   Act: 0.05% (532 mL) [contains benzyl alcohol, propylene glycol, sodium benzoate, tartrazine; cinnamon flavor; equivalent to fluoride 0.02%]
   Act: 0.05% (532 mL) [contains propylene glycol, sodium benzoate, tartrazine; mint flavor; equivalent to fluoride 0.02%]
   Act Kids: 0.05% (532 mL) [ethanol free; contains benzyl alcohol, propylene glycol, sodium benzoate; bubblegum flavor; equivalent to fluoride 0.02%]
   Act Kids: 0.05% (500 mL) [ethanol free; contains benzyl alcohol, propylene glycol, sodium benzoate; ocean berry flavor; equivalent to fluoride 0.02%]
   Act Restoring: 0.02% (1000 mL) [contains ethanol 11%, propylene glycol, sodium benzoate; Cool Splash mint flavor; equivalent to fluoride 0.009%]
   Act Restoring: 0.02% (1000 mL) [contains ethanol 11%, propylene glycol, sodium benzoate; Cool Splash spearmint flavor; equivalent to fluoride 0.009%]
   Act Restoring: 0.05% (532 mL) [contains ethanol 11%, propylene glycol, sodium benzoate; Cool Splash mint flavor; equivalent to fluoride 0.02%]
   Act Restoring: 0.05% (532 mL) [contains ethanol 11%, propylene glycol, sodium benzoate; Cool Splash spearmint flavor; equivalent to fluoride 0.02%]
   Act Restoring: 0.05% (532 mL) [contains ethanol 11%, propylene glycol, sodium benzoate; Cool Splash vanilla-mint flavor; equivalent to fluoride 0.02%]
   Act Total Care: 0.02% (1000 mL) [contains ethanol 11%, propylene glycol, sodium benzoate; icy clean mint flavor; equivalent to fluoride 0.009%]
   Act Total Care: 0.05% (88 mL, 532 mL) [contains ethanol 11%, propylene glycol, sodium benzoate; icy clean mint flavor; equivalent to fluoride 0.02%]
   Act Total Care: 0.05% (88 mL, 532 mL) [ethanol free; contains menthol, propylene glycol, sodium benzoate, tartrazine; fresh mint flavor; equivalent to fluoride 0.02%]
   CaviRinse: 0.2% (240 mL) [mint flavor]
   Fluorinse: 0.2% (480 mL) [ethanol free; cinnamon flavor]
   Fluorinse: 0.2% (480 mL) [ethanol free; mint flavor]
   OrthoWash: 0.044% (480 mL) [contains sodium benzoate; grape flavor]
   OrthoWash: 0.044% (480 mL) [contains sodium benzoate; strawberry flavor]
   Phos-Flur Rinse: 0.044% (473 mL) [ethanol free, sugar free; bubblegum flavor]
   Phos-Flur Rinse: 0.044% (473 mL) [ethanol free, sugar free; gushing grape flavor]
   Phos-Flur Rinse: 0.044% (500 mL) [sugar free; cool mint flavor]
   PreviDent: 0.2% (473 mL) [contains benzoic acid, ethanol 6%, sodium benzoate; cool mint flavor]

Solution, oral, as stannous fluoride [concentrated rinse]: 0.63% (300 mL) [equivalent to fluoride 7 mg/30 mL dose]
   Gel-Kam Rinse: 0.63% (300 mL) [mint flavor; equivalent to fluoride 7 mg/30 mL dose]
   PerioMed: 0.63% (284 mL) [ethanol free; cinnamon flavor; equivalent to fluoride 7 mg/30 mL dose]
   PerioMed: 0.63% (284 mL) [ethanol free; mint flavor; equivalent to fluoride 7 mg/30 mL dose]
   PerioMed: 0.63% (284 mL) [ethanol free; tropical fruit flavor; equivalent to fluoride 7 mg/30 mL dose]
   StanGard Perio: 0.63% (284 mL) [mint flavor]

Tablet, chewable, oral, as sodium: 0.55 mg [equivalent to fluoride 0.25 mg], 1.1 mg [equivalent to fluoride 0.5 mg], 2.2 mg [equivalent to fluoride 1 mg]

Fluor-A-Day: 0.55 mg [raspberry flavor; equivalent to fluoride 0.25 mg]

Fluor-A-Day: 1.1 mg [raspberry flavor; equivalent to fluoride 0.5 mg]

Fluor-A-Day: 2.2 mg [raspberry flavor; equivalent to fluoride 1 mg]

Fluoritab: 2.2 mg [cherry flavor; equivalent to fluoride 1 mg]

Fluoritab: 1.1 mg [dye free; cherry flavor; equivalent to fluoride 0.5 mg]

◆ Fluorinse see Fluoride on page 782

◆ Fluoritab see Fluoride on page 782

◆ 5-Fluorocytosine see Flucytosine on page 778

◆ 9α-Fluorohydrocortisone Acetate see Fludrocortisone on page 780

Fluorometholone (flure oh METH oh lone)

Brand Names: US Flarex; FML; FML Forte; FML Liquifilm

Brand Names: Canada Flarex®; FML Forte®; FML®; PMS-Fluorometholone

Pharmacologic Category Corticosteroid, Ophthalmic

Use Treatment of steroid-responsive inflammatory conditions of the eye

Dosing

Adult & Geriatric Ocular inflammation: Ophthalmic:

Ointment (FML®): Apply small amount (~1/2 inch ribbon) to conjunctival sac 1-3 times daily; may increase application to every 4 hours during the initial 24-48 hours

Suspension:

Flarex®: Instill 1-2 drops into conjunctival sac 4 times daily; may increase application to 2 drops every 2 hours during initial 24-48 hours

FML®, FML® Forte: Instill 1 drop into conjunctival sac 2-4 times daily; may instill 1 drop every 4 hours during initial 24-48 hours

Note: Re-evaluate therapy if improvement is not seen within 2 days; use care not to discontinue prematurely; in chronic conditions, gradually decrease dosing frequency prior to discontinuing treatment.

Pediatric Children ≥2 years and Adolescents (FML®, FML® Forte): Refer to adult dosing.

Renal Impairment No dosage adjustment provided in manufacturer's labeling.

Hepatic Impairment No dosage adjustment provided in manufacturer's labeling.

Additional Information Complete prescribing information should be consulted for additional detail.

Dosage Forms Excipient information presented when available (limited, particularly for generics); consult specific product labeling. [DSC] = Discontinued product

Ointment, Ophthalmic, as base:

FML: 0.1% (3.5 g) [contains phenylmercuric acetate]

Suspension, Ophthalmic, as acetate:

Flarex: 0.1% (5 mL)

Suspension, Ophthalmic, as base:

FML Forte: 0.25% (5 mL, 10 mL)

FML Liquifilm: 0.1% (5 mL, 10 mL, 15 mL [DSC])

Generic: 0.1% (5 mL, 10 mL, 15 mL)

◆ Fluoroplex see Fluorouracil (Topical) on page 786

◆ Fluoro Uracil see Fluorouracil (Systemic) on page 784

◆ 5-Fluorouracil see Fluorouracil (Systemic) on page 784

◆ 5-Fluorouracil see Fluorouracil (Topical) on page 786

Fluorouracil (Systemic) (flure oh YOOR a sil)

Brand Names: US Adrucil

Brand Names: Canada Fluorouracil Injection

Index Terms 5-Fluorouracil; 5-Fluracil; 5-FU; Fluoro Uracil; Fluouracil; FU

Pharmacologic Category Antineoplastic Agent, Antimetabolite; Antineoplastic Agent, Antimetabolite (Pyrimidine Analog)

Use Treatment of breast cancer, colon cancer, rectal cancer, pancreatic cancer, and stomach (gastric) cancer

Pregnancy Considerations Adverse effects (increased resorptions, embryolethality, and teratogenicity) have been observed in animal reproduction studies. Based on the mechanism of action, fluorouracil may cause fetal harm if administered during pregnancy (according to the manufacturer's labeling). The National Comprehensive Cancer Network (NCCN) breast cancer guidelines (v.3.2012) state that chemotherapy, if indicated, may be administered to pregnant women with breast cancer as part of a combination chemotherapy regimen (common regimens administered during pregnancy include doxorubicin, cyclophosphamide, and fluorouracil); chemotherapy should not be administered during the first trimester, after 35 weeks gestation, or within 3 weeks of planned delivery.

Breast-Feeding Considerations Based on the mechanism of action, the manufacturer's labeling recommends against breast-feeding if receiving fluorouracil.

Contraindications Hypersensitivity to fluorouracil or any component of the formulation; poor nutritional states; depressed bone marrow function; potentially serious infections

Warnings/Precautions Hazardous agent - use appropriate precautions for handling and disposal (NIOSH 2014 [group 1]). Use with caution in patients with impaired kidney or liver function. Discontinue if intractable vomiting or diarrhea, precipitous falls in leukocyte or platelet counts, gastrointestinal ulcer or bleeding, stomatitis, or esophagopharyngitis, hemorrhage, or myocardial ischemia occurs. Use with caution in poor-risk patients who have had high-dose pelvic radiation or previous use of alkylating agents and in patients with widespread metastatic marrow involvement. Palmar-plantar erythrodysesthesia (hand-foot) syndrome has been associated with use (symptoms include a tingling sensation, which may progress to pain, and then to symmetrical swelling and erythema with tenderness; desquamation may occur; with treatment interruption, generally resolves over 5-7 days).

Continuous infusion: Serious errors have occurred when doses administered by continuous ambulatory infusion pumps have inadvertently been given over 1 to 4 hours instead of the intended extended continuous infusion duration. Depending on protocol, infusion duration may range from 46 hours to 7 days for continuous infusions of fluorouracil. Ambulatory pumps utilized for continuous infusions should have safeguards to allow for detection of programming errors. If using an elastomeric device for ambulatory continuous infusion, carefully select and double check the flow rate on the device. Appropriate prescribing (in single daily doses [not course doses] with instructions to infuse over a specific time period), appropriate training/certification/education of staff involved with dispensing and administration processes, and independent double checks should be utilized throughout dispensing and administration procedures (ISMP [Smetzer 2015]).

An investigational uridine prodrug, uridine triacetate (formerly called vistonuridine), has been studied in a limited number of cases of fluorouracil overdose. Of 17 patients receiving uridine triacetate beginning within 8-96 hours after fluorouracil overdose, all patients fully recovered (von Borstel, 2009). Updated data has described a total of 28 patients treated with uridine triacetate for fluorouracil overdose (including overdoses related to continuous infusions delivering fluorouracil at rates faster than prescribed), all of whom recovered fully (Bamat, 2010). Refer to Uridine Triacetate monograph.

Administration to patients with a genetic deficiency of dihydropyrimidine dehydrogenase (DPD) has been associated with prolonged clearance and increased toxicity (diarrhea, neutropenia, and neurotoxicity) following administration; rechallenge has resulted in recurrent toxicity (despite dose reduction). **[U.S. Boxed Warning]: Should be administered under the supervision of an experienced cancer chemotherapy physician; the manufacturer's labeling recommends hospitalizing patients during the first treatment course due to the potential for severe toxicity.** Potentially significant drug-drug interactions may exist, requiring dose or frequency adjustment, additional monitoring, and/or selection of alternative therapy.

Adverse Reactions Toxicity depends on duration of treatment and/or rate of administration

Cardiovascular: Angina, arrhythmia, heart failure, MI, myocardial ischemia, vasospasm, ventricular ectopy

Central nervous system: Acute cerebellar syndrome, confusion, disorientation, euphoria, headache, nystagmus, stroke

Dermatologic: Alopecia, dermatitis, dry skin, fissuring, nail changes (nail loss), palmar-plantar erythrodysesthesia syndrome, pruritic maculopapular rash, photosensitivity, Stevens-Johnson syndrome, toxic epidermal necrolysis, vein pigmentation

Gastrointestinal: Anorexia, bleeding, diarrhea, esophagopharyngitis, mesenteric ischemia (acute), nausea, sloughing, stomatitis, ulceration, vomiting

Hematologic: Agranulocytosis, anemia, leukopenia (nadir: days 9-14; recovery by day 30), pancytopenia, thrombocytopenia

Local: Thrombophlebitis

Ocular: Lacrimation, lacrimal duct stenosis, photophobia, visual changes

Respiratory: Epistaxis

Miscellaneous: Anaphylaxis, generalized allergic reactions

Drug Interactions

Metabolism/Transport Effects Inhibits CYP2C9 (strong)

Avoid Concomitant Use

Avoid concomitant use of Fluorouracil (Systemic) with any of the following: BCG (Intravesical); Deferiprone; Dipyrone; Gimeracil; Natalizumab; Pimecrolimus; Tacrolimus (Topical); Tofacitinib; Vaccines (Live)

Increased Effect/Toxicity

Fluorouracil (Systemic) may increase the levels/effects of: Bosentan; Carvedilol; CloZAPine; CYP2C9 Substrates; Deferiprone; Diclofenac (Systemic); Dronabinol; Fingolimod; Fosphenytoin; Lacosamide; Leflunomide; Natalizumab; Ospemifene; Parecoxib; Phenytoin; Ramelteon; Tetrahydrocannabinol; Tofacitinib; Vaccines (Live); Vitamin K Antagonists

The levels/effects of Fluorouracil (Systemic) may be increased by: Cannabis; Cimetidine; Denosumab; Dipyrone; Gemcitabine; Gimeracil; Leucovorin Calcium-Levoleucovorin; MetroNIDAZOLE (Systemic); Pimecrolimus; Roflumilast; SORAfenib; Tacrolimus (Topical); Trastuzumab

Decreased Effect

Fluorouracil (Systemic) may decrease the levels/effects of: BCG (Intravesical); Coccidioides immitis Skin Test; Sipuleucel-T; Vaccines (Inactivated); Vaccines (Live)

The levels/effects of Fluorouracil (Systemic) may be decreased by: Echinacea; SORAfenib

Preparation for Administration Hazardous agent; use appropriate precautions for handling and disposal (NIOSH 2014 [group 1]). May dispense in a syringe or dilute in 50-1000 mL NS or D$_5$W for infusion.

Storage/Stability Store intact vials at room temperature. Do not refrigerate or freeze. Protect from light. Slight discoloration may occur during storage; does not usually denote decomposition. If exposed to cold, a precipitate may form; **gentle** heating to 60°C (140°F) will dissolve the precipitate without impairing the potency. According to the manufacturer, pharmacy bulk vials should be used within 4 hours of initial entry. Solutions for infusion should be used promptly. Fluorouracil 50 mg/mL in NS was stable in polypropylene infusion syringes for 7 days when stored at 30°C (86°F) (Stiles, 1996). Stability of fluorouracil 1 mg/mL or 10 mg/mL in NS or D$_5$W in PVC bags was demonstrated for up to 14 days at 4°C (39.2°F) and 21°C (69.8°F) (Martel, 1996). Stability of undiluted fluorouracil (50 mg/mL) in ethylene-vinyl acetate ambulatory pump reservoirs was demonstrated for 3 days at 4°C (39.2°F) (precipitate formed after 3 days) and for 14 days at 33°C (91.4°F) (Martel, 1996). Stability of undiluted fluorouracil (50 mg/mL) in PVC ambulatory pump reservoirs was demonstrated for 5 days at 4°C (39.2°F) (precipitate formed after 5 days) and for 14 days at 33°C (91.4°F) (Martel, 1996).

Mechanism of Action A pyrimidine analog antimetabolite that interferes with DNA and RNA synthesis; after activation, F-UMP (an active metabolite) is incorporated into RNA to replace uracil and inhibit cell growth; the active metabolite F-dUMP, inhibits thymidylate synthetase, depleting thymidine triphosphate (a necessary component of DNA synthesis).

Pharmacodynamics/Kinetics

Distribution: Penetrates extracellular fluid, CSF, and third space fluids (eg, pleural effusions and ascitic fluid), marrow, intestinal mucosa, liver and other tissues

Metabolism: Hepatic (90%); via a dehydrogenase enzyme; FU must be metabolized to be active metabolites, 5-fluoroxyuridine monophosphate (F-UMP) and 5-5-fluoro-2'-deoxyuridine-5'-O-monophosphate (F-dUMP)

Half-life elimination: 16 minutes (range: 8-20 minutes); two metabolites, F-dUMP and F-UMP, have prolonged half-lives depending on the type of tissue

Excretion: Primarily metabolized in the liver; excreted in lung (as expired CO$_2$) and urine (7% to 20% as unchanged drug within 6 hours; also as metabolites within 9-10 hours)

Dosing

Adult & Geriatric Details concerning dosing in combination regimens should be consulted:

Breast cancer (off-label dosing): IV:

CEF regimen: 500 mg/m^2 on days 1 and 8 every 28 days (in combination with cyclophosphamide and epirubicin) for 6 cycles (Levine, 1998)

CMF regimen: 600 mg/m^2 on days 1 and 8 every 28 days (in combination with cyclophosphamide and methotrexate) for 6 cycles (Goldhirsch, 1998; Levine, 1998)

FAC regimen: 500 mg/m^2 on days 1 and 8 every 21-28 days (in combination with cyclophosphamide and doxorubicin) for 6 cycles (Assikis, 2003)

Colorectal cancer (off-label dosing): IV:

FLOX regimen: 500 mg/m^2 bolus on days 1, 8, 15, 22, 29, and 36 (1 hour after leucovorin) every 8 weeks (in combination with leucovorin and oxaliplatin) for 3 cycles (Kuebler, 2007)

FOLFOX6 and mFOLFOX6 regimen: 400 mg/m^2 bolus on day 1, followed by 1200 mg/m^2/day continuous infusion for 2 days (over 46 hours) every 2 weeks (in combination with leucovorin and oxaliplatin) until disease progression or unacceptable toxicity (Cheeseman, 2002)

FOLFIRI regimen: 400 mg/m^2 bolus on day 1, followed by 1200 mg/m^2/day continuous infusion for 2 days (over 46 hours) every 2 weeks (in combination with leucovorin and irinotecan) until disease progression or unacceptable toxicity; after 2 cycles, may increase continuous infusion fluorouracil dose to 1500 mg/m^2/day (over 46 hours) (Andre, 1999)

Roswell Park regimen: 500 mg/m^2 (bolus) on days 1, 8, 15, 22, 29, and 36 (1 hour after leucovorin) every 8 weeks (in combination with leucovorin) for 4 cycles (Haller, 2005)

Gastric cancer (off-label dosing): IV:

CF regimen: 750-1000 mg/m^2/day continuous infusion days 1-4 and 29-32 of a 35-day treatment cycle (preoperative chemoradiation; in combination with cisplatin) (Tepper, 2008; NCCN Gastric Cancer Guidelines v2.2012)

ECF regimen (resectable disease): 200 mg/m^2/day continuous infusion days 1-21 every 3 weeks (in combination with epirubicin and cisplatin) for 6 cycles (3 cycles preoperatively and 3 cycles postoperatively) (Cunningham, 2006)

ECF or EOF regimen (advanced disease): 200 mg/m^2/day continuous infusion days 1-21 every 3 weeks (in combination with epirubicin and either cisplatin or oxaliplatin) for a planned duration of 24 weeks (Sumpter, 2005)

TCF or DCF regimen: 750 mg/m^2/day continuous infusion days 1-5 every 3 weeks or 1000 mg/m^2/day continuous infusion days 1-5 every 4 weeks (in combination with docetaxel and cisplatin) until disease progression or unacceptable toxicity (Ajani, 2007; Van Cutsem, 2006; NCCN Gastric Cancer Guidelines v2.2012)

ToGA regimen (HER2-positive): 800 mg/m^2/day continuous infusion days 1-5 every 3 weeks (in combination with cisplatin and trastuzumab) until disease progression or unacceptable toxicity (Bang, 2010)

Pancreatic cancer (off-label dosing): IV:

Chemoradiation therapy: 250 mg/m^2/day continuous infusion for 3 weeks prior to and then throughout radiation therapy (Regine, 2008)

Fluorouracil-Leucovorin: 425 mg/m^2/day (bolus) days 1-5 every 28 days (in combination with leucovorin) for 6 cycles (Neoptolemos, 2010)

FOLFIRINOX regimen: 400 mg/m^2 bolus on day 1, followed by 1200 mg/m^2/day continuous infusion for 2 days (over 46 hours) every 14 days (in combination with leucovorin, irinotecan, and oxaliplatin) until disease progression or unacceptable toxicity for a recommended 12 cycles (Conroy, 2011)

Anal carcinoma (off-label use): IV: 1000 mg/m^2/day continuous infusion days 1-4 and days 29-32 (in combination with mitomycin and radiation therapy) (Ajani, 2008)

Bladder cancer (off-label use): IV: 500 mg/m^2/day continuous infusion days 1-5 and days 16-20 (in combination with mitomycin and radiation therapy) (James, 2012)

Cervical cancer (off-label use): IV: 1000 mg/m^2/day continuous infusion days 1-4 (in combination with cisplatin and radiation therapy) every 3 weeks for 3 cycles (Eifel, 2004)

Esophageal cancer (off-label use): IV:

CF regimen: 750-1000 mg/m^2/day continuous infusion days 1-4 and 29-32 of a 35-day treatment cycle (preoperative chemoradiation; in combination with cisplatin) (Tepper, 2008; NCCN Esophageal and Esophagogastric Junction Cancers Guidelines v2.2012)

ECF regimen (resectable disease): 200 mg/m^2/day continuous infusion days 1-21 every 3 weeks (in combination with epirubicin and cisplatin) for 6 cycles (3 cycles preoperatively and 3 cycles postoperatively) (Cunningham, 2006)

ECF or EOF regimen (advanced disease): 200 mg/m²/day continuous infusion days 1-21 every 3 weeks (in combination with epirubicin and either cisplatin or oxaliplatin) for a planned duration of 24 weeks (Sumpter, 2005)

TCF or DCF regimen: 750 mg/m²/day continuous infusion days 1-5 every 3 weeks or 1000 mg/m²/day continuous infusion days 1-5 every 4 weeks (in combination with docetaxel and cisplatin) until disease progression or unacceptable toxicity (Ajani, 2007; Van Cutsem, 2006; NCCN Esophageal and Esophagogastric Junction Cancers Guidelines v2.2012)

Head and neck cancer, squamous cell (off-label use): IV:

Platinum-Fluorouracil regimen: 1000 mg/m²/day continuous infusion days 1-4 every 3 weeks (in combination with cisplatin) for at least 6 cycles (Gibson, 2005) **or** 600 mg/m²/day continuous infusion days 1-4, 22-25, and 43-46 (in combination with carboplatin and radiation) (Denis, 2004; Bourhis, 2012)

TPF regimen: 1000 mg/m²/day continuous infusion days 1-4 every 3 weeks (in combination with docetaxel and cisplatin) for 3 cycles, and followed by chemoradiotherapy (Posner, 2007) **or** 750 mg/m²/day continuous infusion days 1-5 every 3 weeks (in combination with docetaxel and cisplatin) for up to 4 cycles (Vermorken, 2007)

Platinum, 5-FU, and cetuximab regimen: 1000 mg/m²/day continuous infusion days 1-4 every 3 weeks (in combination with either cisplatin or carboplatin and cetuximab) for a total of up to 6 cycles (Vermorken, 2008)

Hepatobiliary cancer (off-label use): IV: 600 mg/m² (bolus) on days 1, 8, and 15 every 4 weeks (in combination with gemcitabine and leucovorin) (Alberts, 2005)

Renal Impairment No dosage adjustment provided in the manufacturer's labeling; however, extreme caution should be used in patients with renal impairment. The following adjustments have been recommended:

CrCl <50 mL/minute and continuous renal replacement therapy (CRRT): No dosage adjustment necessary (Aronoff, 2007).

Hemodialysis:

Administer standard dose following hemodialysis on dialysis days (Janus, 2010).

Administer 50% of standard dose following hemodialysis (Aronoff, 2007).

Hepatic Impairment No dosage adjustment provided in the manufacturer's labeling; however, extreme caution should be used in patients with hepatic impairment. The following adjustments have been recommended:

Floyd, 2006: Bilirubin >5 mg/dL: Avoid use.

Koren, 1992: Hepatic impairment (degree not specified): Administer <50% of dose, then increase if toxicity does not occur.

Obesity *ASCO Guidelines for appropriate chemotherapy dosing in obese adults with cancer:* Utilize patient's actual body weight (full weight) for calculation of body surface area- or weight-based dosing, particularly when the intent of therapy is curative; manage regimen-related toxicities in the same manner as for nonobese patients; if a dose reduction is utilized due to toxicity, consider resumption of full weight-based dosing with subsequent cycles, especially if cause of toxicity (eg, hepatic or renal impairment) is resolved (Griggs, 2012).

Adjustment for Toxicity *According to the manufacturer, treatment should be discontinued for the following:* Stomatitis or esophagopharyngitis, leukopenia (WBC <3500/mm³), rapidly falling white blood cell count, intractable vomiting, diarrhea, frequent bowel movements, watery stools, gastrointestinal ulcer or bleeding, thrombocytopenia (platelets <100,000/mm³), hemorrhage

Dietary Considerations Increase dietary intake of thiamine.

Administration IV: Administration rate varies by protocol; refer to specific reference for protocol. May be administered by IV push, IV bolus, or as a continuous infusion. Avoid extravasation (may be an irritant).

Hazardous agent; use appropriate precautions for handling and disposal (NIOSH 2014 [group 1]).

Monitoring Parameters CBC with differential and platelet count, renal function tests, liver function tests, signs of palmar-plantar erythrodysesthesia syndrome, stomatitis, diarrhea, hemorrhage, or gastrointestinal ulcers or bleeding

Dosage Forms Excipient information presented when available (limited, particularly for generics); consult specific product labeling.

Solution, Intravenous:

Adrucil: 500 mg/10 mL (10 mL); 2.5 g/50 mL (50 mL); 5 g/100 mL (100 mL)

Generic: 500 mg/10 mL (10 mL); 1 g/20 mL (20 mL); 2.5 g/50 mL (50 mL); 5 g/100 mL (100 mL)

Fluorouracil (Topical) (flure oh YOOR a sil)

Brand Names: US Carac; Efudex; Fluoroplex; Tolak

Brand Names: Canada Efudex; Fluoroplex

Index Terms 5-Fluorouracil; 5-FU; FU; Topical Fluorouracil

Pharmacologic Category Antineoplastic Agent, Antimetabolite; Antineoplastic Agent, Antimetabolite (Pyrimidine Analog); Topical Skin Product

Use

Actinic or solar keratosis: Management of multiple actinic or solar keratoses

Basal cell carcinoma (5%): Treatment of superficial basal cell carcinomas when conventional methods are impractical (eg, due to multiple lesions or difficult treatment sites)

Limitations of use: Establish diagnosis of superficial basal cell carcinoma prior to treatment (use has not been proven effective in other types of basal cell carcinomas); surgery is preferred with isolated, easily accessible basal cell carcinomas because success with such lesions is almost 100% and the success rate with fluorouracil cream and solution is ~93%.

Dosing

Adult & Geriatric

Actinic or solar keratosis: Topical:

Cream (0.5%): Apply thin film to lesions once daily for up to 4 weeks, as tolerated

Cream (1%): Apply to lesions twice daily for 2 to 6 weeks

Cream (4%): Apply to lesions once daily for 4 weeks as tolerated

Cream (5%) or solution (2% and 5%): Apply to lesions twice daily for 2 to 4 weeks; complete healing may not be evident for 1 to 2 months following treatment

Superficial basal cell carcinoma: Topical: Cream (5%) or solution (5%): Apply to affected lesions twice daily for 3 to 6 weeks; treatment may be continued for up to 10 to 12 weeks

Renal Impairment There are no dosage adjustments provided in the manufacturer's labeling.

Hepatic Impairment There are no dosage adjustments provided in the manufacturer's labeling.

Additional Information Complete prescribing information should be consulted for additional detail.

Dosage Forms Excipient information presented when available (limited, particularly for generics); consult specific product labeling.

Cream, External:

Carac: 0.5% (30 g) [contains methylparaben, polysorbate 80, propylene glycol, propylparaben, trolamine (triethanolamine)]

Efudex: 5% (40 g)

Fluoroplex: 1% (30 g) [contains benzyl alcohol]

Tolak: 4% (40 g) [contains cetyl alcohol, methylparaben, peanut oil, propylparaben]

Generic: 0.5% (30 g); 5% (40 g)

Solution, External:

Generic: 2% (10 mL); 5% (10 mL)

◆ Fluorouracil Injection (Can) *see* Fluorouracil (Systemic) on page 784

◆ Fluouracil *see* Fluorouracil (Systemic) on page 784

FLUoxetine (floo OKS e teen)

Brand Names: US PROzac; PROzac Weekly; Sarafem

Brand Names: Canada Apo-Fluoxetine; Ava-Fluoxetine; CO Fluoxetine; Dom-Fluoxetine; Fluoxetine Capsules BP; FXT 40; Gen-Fluoxetine; JAMP-Fluoxetine; Mint-Fluoxetine; Mylan-Fluoxetine; Novo-Fluoxetine; Nu-Fluoxetine; PHL-Fluoxetine; PMS-Fluoxetine; PRO-Fluoxetine; Prozac; Q-Fluoxetine; ratio-Fluoxetine; Riva-Fluoxetine; Sandoz-Fluoxetine; Teva-Fluoxetine; ZYM-Fluoxetine

Index Terms Fluoxetine Hydrochloride

Pharmacologic Category Antidepressant, Selective Serotonin Reuptake Inhibitor

Use Treatment of major depressive disorder (MDD); treatment of binge-eating and vomiting in patients with moderate-to-severe bulimia nervosa; obsessive-compulsive disorder (OCD); premenstrual dysphoric disorder (PMDD); panic disorder with or without agoraphobia; in combination with olanzapine for treatment-resistant or bipolar I depression

Pregnancy Considerations Adverse events have been observed in animal reproduction studies. Fluoxetine and its metabolite cross the human placenta. An increased risk of teratogenic effects, including cardiovascular defects, may be associated with maternal use of fluoxetine or other SSRIs; however, available information is conflicting. Nonteratogenic effects in the newborn following SSRI/SNRI exposure late in the third trimester include respiratory distress, cyanosis, apnea, seizures, temperature instability, feeding difficulty, vomiting, hypoglycemia, hypo- or hypertonia, hyper-reflexia, jitteriness, irritability, constant crying, and tremor. Symptoms may be due to the toxicity of the SSRIs/SNRIs or a discontinuation syndrome and may be consistent with serotonin syndrome associated with SSRI treatment. Persistent pulmonary hypertension of the newborn (PPHN) has also been reported with SSRI exposure. The long-term effects of *in utero* SSRI exposure on infant development and behavior are not known.

Due to pregnancy-induced physiologic changes, women who are pregnant may require dose adjustments of fluoxetine to achieve euthymia. The ACOG recommends that therapy with SSRIs or SNRIs during pregnancy be individualized; treatment of depression during pregnancy should incorporate the clinical expertise of the mental health clinician, obstetrician, primary healthcare provider, and pediatrician. According to the American Psychiatric Association (APA), the risks of medication treatment should be weighed against other treatment options and untreated depression. For women who discontinue antidepressant medications during pregnancy and who may be at high risk for postpartum depression, the medications can be restarted following delivery. Treatment algorithms have been developed by the ACOG and the APA for the management of depression in women prior to conception and during pregnancy.

Breast-Feeding Considerations Fluoxetine and its metabolite are excreted into breast milk and can be detected in the serum of breast-feeding infants. Concentrations in breast milk are variable. In comparison to other SSRIs, fluoxetine concentrations in breast milk are higher and adverse events have been observed in nursing infants. Maternal use of an SSRI during pregnancy may cause delayed milk secretion. Breast-feeding is not recommended by the manufacturer. Long-term effects on development and behavior have not been studied.

Medication Guide Available Yes

Contraindications Hypersensitivity to fluoxetine or any component of the formulation; use of MAO inhibitors intended to treat psychiatric disorders (concurrently, within 5 weeks of discontinuing fluoxetine, or within 2 weeks of discontinuing the MAO inhibitor); initiation of fluoxetine in a patient receiving linezolid or intravenous methylene blue; use with pimozide or thioridazine (**Note:** Thioridazine should not be initiated until 5 weeks after the discontinuation of fluoxetine)

Warnings/Precautions [US Boxed Warning]: Antidepressants increase the risk of suicidal thinking and behavior in children, adolescents, and young adults (18 to 24 years of age) with major depressive disorder (MDD) and other psychiatric disorders; consider risk prior to prescribing. Short-term studies did not show an increased risk in patients >24 years of age and showed a decreased risk in patients ≥65 years. Closely monitor all patients for clinical worsening, suicidality, or unusual changes in behavior, particularly during the initial 1 to 2 months of therapy or during periods of dosage adjustments (increases or decreases); the patient's family or caregiver should be instructed to closely observe the patient and communicate condition with healthcare provider. A medication guide concerning the use of antidepressants should be dispensed with each prescription. **Fluoxetine is FDA approved for the treatment of OCD in children ≥7 years of age and MDD in children ≥8 years of age.**

The possibility of a suicide attempt is inherent in major depression and may persist until remission occurs. Use caution in high-risk patients. Worsening depression and severe abrupt suicidality that are not part of the presenting symptoms may require discontinuation or modification of drug therapy. Prescriptions should be written for the smallest quantity consistent with good patient care. The patient's family or caregiver should be alerted to monitor patients for the emergence of suicidality and associated behaviors (such as agitation, irritability, hostility, impulsivity, and hypomania) and call healthcare provider.

May worsen psychosis in some patients or precipitate a shift to mania or hypomania in patients with bipolar disorder. Patients presenting with depressive symptoms should be screened for bipolar disorder. Monotherapy in patients with bipolar disorder should be avoided. **Fluoxetine monotherapy is not FDA approved for the treatment of bipolar depression.** May cause insomnia, anxiety, nervousness, or anorexia. Use with caution in patients where weight loss is undesirable. May impair cognitive or motor performance; caution operating hazardous machinery or driving.

QT prolongation and ventricular arrhythmia including torsade de pointes has occurred. Use with caution in patients with risk factors for QT prolongation, under conditions that predispose to arrhythmias, or increased fluoxetine exposure. Consider discontinuation of fluoxetine if ventricular arrhythmia suspected and initiate cardiac evaluation. Avoid concurrent use with other medications that increase QT interval.

Potentially life-threatening serotonin syndrome (SS) has occurred with serotonergic agents (eg, SSRIs, SNRIs), particularly when used in combination with other serotonergic agents (eg, triptans, TCAs, fentanyl, lithium, tramadol, buspirone, St John's wort, tryptophan) or agents that impair metabolism of serotonin (eg, MAO inhibitors intended to treat psychiatric disorders, other MAO inhibitors [ie, linezolid and intravenous methylene blue]). Discontinue treatment (and any concomitant serotonergic agent) immediately if signs/symptoms arise. Fluoxetine use has been associated with occurrences of significant rash and allergic events, including vasculitis, lupus-like syndrome, laryngospasm, anaphylactoid reactions, and pulmonary inflammatory disease. Discontinue if underlying cause of rash cannot be identified.

Use caution in patients with a previous seizure disorder or condition predisposing to seizures such as brain damage or alcoholism. Use with caution in patients with hepatic or severe renal dysfunction and in elderly patients. Use caution in elderly patients; may be potentially inappropriate in patients with a history of falls or fractures, and may cause or exacerbate syndrome of inappropriate antidiuretic hormone secretion or hyponatremia; monitor sodium closely with initiation or dosage adjustments in older adults (Beers Criteria). May also cause agitation, sleep disturbances, and excessive CNS stimulation. May cause hyponatremia/SIADH (elderly at increased risk); volume depletion (diuretics may increase risk). May increase the risks associated with electroconvulsive treatment. Use caution with history of MI or unstable heart disease; use in these patients is limited. May alter glycemic control in patients with diabetes. Due to the long half-life of fluoxetine and its metabolites, the effects and interactions noted may persist for prolonged periods following discontinuation. May cause or exacerbate sexual dysfunction. May cause mild pupillary dilation, which in susceptible individuals can lead to an episode of narrow-angle glaucoma. Consider evaluating patients who have not had an iridectomy for narrow-angle glaucoma risk factors. Bone fractures have been associated with antidepressant treatment. Consider the possibility of a fragility fracture if an antidepressant-treated patient presents with unexplained bone pain, point tenderness, swelling, or bruising (Rabenda 2013; Rizzoli 2012). Potentially significant drug-drug interactions may exist, requiring dose or frequency adjustment, additional monitoring, and/or selection of alternative therapy.

Abrupt discontinuation or interruption of antidepressant therapy has been associated with a discontinuation syndrome. Symptoms arising may vary with antidepressant however commonly include nausea, vomiting, diarrhea, headaches, light-headedness, dizziness, diminished appetite, sweating, chills, tremors, paresthesias, fatigue, somnolence, and sleep disturbances (eg, vivid dreams, insomnia). Greater risks for developing a discontinuation syndrome have been associated with antidepressants with shorter half-lives, longer durations of treatment, and abrupt discontinuation. For antidepressants of short or intermediate half-lives, symptoms may emerge within 2 to 5 days after treatment discontinuation and last 7 to 14 days (APA 2010; Fava 2006; Haddad 2001; Shelton 2001; Warner 2006).

Benzyl alcohol and derivatives: Some dosage forms may contain sodium benzoate/benzoic acid; benzoic acid (benzoate) is a metabolite of benzyl alcohol; large amounts of benzyl alcohol (≥99 mg/kg/day) have been associated with a potentially fatal toxicity ("gasping syndrome") in neonates; the "gasping syndrome" consists of metabolic acidosis, respiratory distress, gasping respirations, CNS dysfunction (including convulsions, intracranial hemorrhage), hypotension, and cardiovascular collapse (AAP ["Inactive" 1997]; CDC 1982); some data suggests that

benzoate displaces bilirubin from protein binding sites (Ahlfors 2001); avoid or use dosage forms containing benzyl alcohol derivative with caution in neonates. See manufacturer's labeling.

Adverse Reactions Percentages listed for adverse effects as reported in placebo-controlled trials and were generally similar in adults and children; actual frequency may be dependent upon diagnosis and in some cases the range presented may be lower than or equal to placebo for a particular disorder.

>10%:

Central nervous system: Insomnia (10% to 33%), headache (21%), drowsiness (5% to 17%), anxiety (6% to 15%), nervousness (8% to 14%), yawning (≤11%)

Endocrine & metabolic: Decreased libido (1% to 11%)

Gastrointestinal: Nausea (12% to 29%), diarrhea (8% to 18%), anorexia (4% to 17%), xerostomia (4% to 12%)

Neuromuscular & skeletal: Weakness (9% to 21%), tremor (3% to 13%)

Respiratory: Pharyngitis (10% to 11%)

1% to 10%:

Cardiovascular: Vasodilation (1% to 5%), chest pain, hypertension, palpitations

Central nervous system: Dizziness (9%), abnormal dreams (1% to 5%), abnormality in thinking (2%), agitation, amnesia, chills, confusion, emotional lability, sleep disorder

Dermatologic: Diaphoresis (2% to 8%), skin rash (2% to 6%), pruritus (3%)

Endocrine & metabolic: Weight loss (2%), hypermenorrhea (≥2%), increased thirst (≥2%), weight gain

Gastrointestinal: Dyspepsia (6% to 10%), constipation (5%), flatulence (3%), vomiting (3%), dysgeusia, increased appetite

Genitourinary: Ejaculatory disorder (≤7%), impotence (≤7%), urinary frequency

Neuromuscular & skeletal: Hyperkinesia (≥2%)

Ophthalmic: Visual disturbance (2%)

Otic: Otalgia, tinnitus

Respiratory: Flu-like symptoms (3% to 10%), sinusitis (2% to 6%), epistaxis (≥2%)

<1% (Limited to important or life-threatening): Abnormal hepatic function tests, acne vulgaris, acute abdominal condition, akathisia, albuminuria, alopecia, amenorrhea, anaphylactoid reaction, anemia, angina pectoris, angle-closure glaucoma, aphthous stomatitis, aplastic anemia, arthritis, asthma, ataxia, atrial fibrillation, bruise, bruxism, bursitis, cardiac arrest, cardiac arrhythmia, cataract, cerebrovascular accident, cholelithiasis, cholestatic jaundice, colitis, congestive heart failure, dehydration, delusions, depersonalization, dyskinesia, dysphagia, dysuria, ecchymoses, edema, eosinophilic pneumonitis, equilibrium disturbance, erythema multiforme, erythema nodosum, esophagitis, euphoria, exfoliative dermatitis, extrapyramidal reaction (rare), gastritis, gastroenteritis, gastrointestinal ulcer, glossitis, gout, gynecological bleeding, gynecomastia, hallucination, hemolytic anemia (immune-related), hepatic failure, hepatic necrosis, hepatitis, hiccups, hostility, hypercholesteremia, hyperprolactinemia, hypersensitivity reaction, hypertonia, hyperventilation, hypoglycemia, hypokalemia, hyponatremia (possibly in association with SIADH), hypotension, hypothyroidism, immune thrombocytopenia, laryngeal edema, laryngospasm, leg cramps, lupus-like syndrome, malaise, melena, migraine, mydriasis, myocardial infarction, myoclonus, neuroleptic malignant syndrome (Stevens, 2008), optic neuritis, orthostatic hypotension, ostealgia, pancreatitis, pancytopenia, paranoia, petechia, priapism, prolonged Q-T interval on ECG, pulmonary embolism, pulmonary fibrosis, pulmonary hypertension, purpuric rash, renal failure, serotonin syndrome, skin photosensitivity, Stevens-Johnson syndrome, suicidal ideation, syncope, tachycardia, thrombocytopenia, toxic epidermal necrolysis, vasculitis, ventricular tachycardia (including torsades de pointes), violent behavior

Drug Interactions

Metabolism/Transport Effects Substrate of CYP1A2 (minor), CYP2B6 (minor), CYP2C19 (minor), CYP2C9 (major), CYP2D6 (major), CYP2E1 (minor), CYP3A4 (minor); **Note:** Assignment of Major/Minor substrate status based on clinically relevant drug interaction potential; **Inhibits** CYP1A2 (weak), CYP2B6 (weak), CYP2C19 (moderate), CYP2C9 (weak), CYP2D6 (strong)

Avoid Concomitant Use

Avoid concomitant use of FLUoxetine with any of the following: Clarithromycin; Dapoxetine; Dosulepin; Haloperidol; Highest Risk QTc-Prolonging Agents; Iobenguane I 123; Ivabradine; Linezolid; MAO Inhibitors; Mequitazine; Methylene Blue; Mifepristone; Moderate Risk QTc-Prolonging Agents; Pimozide; Propafenone; Tamoxifen; Thioridazine; Tryptophan; Urokinase; Ziprasidone

Increased Effect/Toxicity

FLUoxetine may increase the levels/effects of: Agents with Antiplatelet Properties; Anticoagulants; Antidepressants (Serotonin Reuptake Inhibitor/Antagonist); Antipsychotic Agents; Apixaban; ARIPiprazole; ARIPiprazole Lauroxil; Aspirin; AtoMOXetine; Beta-Blockers; Blood Glucose Lowering Agents; Brexpiprazole; BusPIRone; CarBAMazepine; Cilostazol; Collagenase (Systemic); CYP2C19 Substrates; CYP2D6 Substrates; Dabigatran Etexilate; Deoxycholic Acid; Desmopressin; Dextromethorphan; Dosulepin; DOXOrubicin (Conventional); Edoxaban; Fesoterodine; Fosphenytoin; Haloperidol; Highest Risk QTc-Prolonging Agents; Ibritumomab; Mequitazine; Methylene Blue; Metoprolol; Mexiletine; Nebivolol; NIFEdipine; NiMODipine; NSAID (COX-2 Inhibitor); NSAID (Nonselective); Obinutuzumab; Phenytoin; Pimozide; Propafenone; Rivaroxaban; Salicylates; Serotonin Modulators; Tamsulosin; Thiazide Diuretics; Thioridazine; Thrombolytic Agents; TiZANidine; Tositumomab and Iodine I 131 Tositumomab; TraMADol; Tricyclic Antidepressants; Urokinase; Vitamin K Antagonists; Vortioxetine; Ziprasidone

The levels/effects of FLUoxetine may be increased by: Abiraterone Acetate; Alcohol (Ethyl); Analgesics (Opioid); Antiemetics (5HT3 Antagonists); Antipsychotic Agents; ARIPiprazole; BuPROPion; BusPIRone; Cimetidine; Clarithromycin; CNS Depressants; Cobicistat; CYP2C9 Inhibitors (Moderate); CYP2C9 Inhibitors (Strong); CYP2D6 Inhibitors (Moderate); CYP2D6 Inhibitors (Strong); Dapoxetine; Darunavir; Fosphenytoin; Glucosamine; Herbs (Anticoagulant/Antiplatelet Properties); Ibrutinib; Ivabradine; Limaprost; Linezolid; Lithium; Lumacaftor; MAO Inhibitors; Metaxalone; Metoclopramide; Metyrosine; Mifepristone; Moderate Risk QTc-Prolonging Agents; Multivitamins/Fluoride (with ADE); Multivitamins/Minerals (with ADEK, Folate, Iron); Multivitamins/Minerals (with AE, No Iron); Omega-3 Fatty Acids; Pentosan Polysulfate Sodium; Pentoxifylline; Propafenone; Prostacyclin Analogues; QTc-Prolonging Agents (Indeterminate Risk and Risk Modifying); Tedizolid; TraMADol; Tryptophan; Vitamin E; Vitamin E (Oral); Ziprasidone

Decreased Effect

FLUoxetine may decrease the levels/effects of: Clopidogrel; Codeine; Hydrocodone; Iobenguane I 123; Ioflupane I 123; Tamoxifen; Thyroid Products

The levels/effects of FLUoxetine may be decreased by: CarBAMazepine; CYP2C9 Inducers (Strong); Cyproheptadine; Dabrafenib; Enzalutamide; Lumacaftor; NSAID (COX-2 Inhibitor); NSAID (Nonselective); Peginterferon Alfa-2b

Storage/Stability All dosage forms should be stored at controlled room temperature. Protect from light.

Mechanism of Action Inhibits CNS neuron serotonin reuptake; minimal or no effect on reuptake of norepinephrine or dopamine; does not significantly bind to alpha-adrenergic, histamine, or cholinergic receptors

Pharmacodynamics/Kinetics

Onset of action: Depression: The onset of action is within a week; however, individual response varies greatly and full response may not be seen until 8 to 12 weeks after initiation of treatment.

Absorption: Well absorbed; delayed 1 to 2 hours with weekly formulation

Distribution: V_d: 12 to 43 L/kg

Protein binding: 95% to albumin and alpha$_1$ glycoprotein

Metabolism: Hepatic, via CYP2C19 and 2D6, to norfluoxetine (activity equal to fluoxetine)

Half-life elimination: Adults:

Parent drug: 1 to 3 days (acute), 4 to 6 days (chronic), 7.6 days (cirrhosis)

Metabolite (norfluoxetine): 9.3 days (range: 4 to 16 days), 12 days (cirrhosis)

Time to peak, serum: 6 to 8 hours

Excretion: Urine (10% as norfluoxetine, 2.5% to 5% as fluoxetine)

Note: Weekly formulation results in greater fluctuations between peak and trough concentrations of fluoxetine and norfluoxetine compared to once-daily dosing (24% daily/164% weekly; 17% daily/43% weekly, respectively). Trough concentrations are 76% lower for fluoxetine and 47% lower for norfluoxetine than the concentrations maintained by 20 mg once-daily dosing. Steady-state fluoxetine concentrations are ~50% lower following the once-weekly regimen compared to 20 mg once daily. Average steady-state concentrations of once-daily dosing were highest in children ages 6 to <13 (fluoxetine 171 ng/mL; norfluoxetine 195 ng/mL), followed by adolescents ages 13 to <18 (fluoxetine 86 ng/mL; norfluoxetine 113 ng/mL); concentrations were considered to be within the ranges reported

in adults (fluoxetine 91 to 302 ng/mL; norfluoxetine 72 to 258 ng/mL).

Dosing

Adult

Depression, obsessive-compulsive disorder: Oral: 20 mg/day in the morning; may increase after several weeks by 20 mg/day increments; maximum: 80 mg/day; doses >20 mg may be given once daily or divided twice daily. **Note:** Lower doses of 5 to 10 mg/day have been used for initial treatment.

Indication-specific dosing:

Bulimia nervosa: Oral: 60 mg/day; may titrate dose to 60 mg over several days

Depression: Oral: Initial: 20 mg/day; may increase after several weeks if inadequate response (maximum: 80 mg/day). Patients maintained on Prozac 20 mg/day may be changed to Prozac Weekly 90 mg/week, starting dose 7 days after the last 20 mg/day dose

Depression associated with bipolar I disorder (in combination with olanzapine): Oral: Initial: 20 mg in the evening; adjust as tolerated to usual range of 20 to 50 mg/day. See **"Note"** below.

Fibromyalgia (off-label use): Oral: Initial: 20 mg daily; may adjust dose based on response and tolerability in 10 to 20 mg increments at 2 week intervals up to 80 mg/day. Mean dose in clinical trials was 45 mg (range: 20 to 80 mg/day) (Arnold 2002)

Obsessive-compulsive disorder: Oral: Initial: 20 mg/day; may increase after several weeks if inadequate response; recommended range: 20 to 60 mg/day (maximum: 80 mg/day)

Panic disorder: Oral: Initial: 10 mg/day; after 1 week, increase to 20 mg/day; may increase after several weeks; doses >60 mg/day have not been evaluated

Post-traumatic stress disorder (PTSD) (off-label use): Oral: 20 to 40 mg/day

Premenstrual dysphoric disorder (Sarafem): Oral: 20 mg/day continuously, **or** 20 mg/day starting 14 days prior to menstruation and through first full day of menses (repeat with each cycle)

Raynaud's phenomena (off-label use): Oral: 20 mg/day (Coleiro 2001)

Social anxiety disorder (off-label use): Oral: Initial: 10 mg/day for 7 days; continue to increase the dose based on response and tolerability in 10 mg increments at intervals of at least 7 days to a target dose of 40 mg/day; typical range in clinical trial was 30 to 60 mg/day (Davidson 2004)

Treatment-resistant depression (in combination with olanzapine): Oral: Initial: 20 mg in the evening; adjust as tolerated to usual range of 20 to 50 mg/day. See **"Note"**

Note: When using individual components of fluoxetine with olanzapine rather than fixed-dose combination product (Symbyax), approximate dosage correspondence is as follows:
Olanzapine 2.5 mg + fluoxetine 20 mg = Symbyax 3/25
Olanzapine 5 mg + fluoxetine 20 mg = Symbyax 6/25
Olanzapine 12.5 mg + fluoxetine 20 mg = Symbyax 12/25
Olanzapine 5 mg + fluoxetine 50 mg = Symbyax 6/50
Olanzapine 12.5 mg + fluoxetine 50 mg = Symbyax 12/50

Discontinuation of therapy: Upon discontinuation of antidepressant therapy, gradually taper the dose to minimize the incidence of withdrawal symptoms and allow for the detection of re-emerging symptoms. Evidence supporting ideal taper rates is limited. APA and NICE guidelines suggest tapering therapy over at least several weeks with consideration to the half-life of the antidepressant; antidepressants with a shorter half-life may need to be tapered more conservatively. In addition for long-term treated patients, WFSBP guidelines recommend tapering over 4 to 6 months. If intolerable withdrawal symptoms occur following a dose reduction, consider resuming the previously prescribed dose and/ or decrease dose at a more gradual rate (APA 2010; Bauer 2002; Haddad 2001; NCCMH 2010; Schatzberg 2006; Shelton 2001; Warner 2006).

MAO inhibitor recommendations:
Switching to or from an MAO inhibitor intended to treat psychiatric disorders:
Allow 14 days to elapse between discontinuing an MAO inhibitor intended to treat psychiatric disorders and initiation of fluoxetine.
Allow 5 weeks to elapse between discontinuing fluoxetine and initiation of an MAO inhibitor intended to treat psychiatric disorders.

Use with other MAO inhibitors (linezolid or IV methylene blue):
Do not initiate fluoxetine in patients receiving linezolid or IV methylene blue; consider other interventions for psychiatric condition.
If urgent treatment with linezolid or IV methylene blue is required in a patient already receiving fluoxetine and potential benefits outweigh potential risks, discontinue fluoxetine promptly and administer linezolid or IV methylene blue. Monitor for serotonin syndrome for 5 weeks or until 24 hours after the last dose of linezolid or IV methylene blue, whichever comes first. May resume fluoxetine 24 hours after the last dose of linezolid or IV methylene blue.

Geriatric Depression: Oral: Some patients may require an initial dose of 10 mg/day with dosage increases of 10 mg and 20 mg every several weeks as tolerated; should not be taken at night unless patient experiences sedation. Refer to adult dosing.

Discontinuation of therapy: Refer to adult dosing.
MAO inhibitor recommendations: Refer to adult dosing.

Pediatric

Depression: Children ≥8 years and Adolescents: Oral: 10 to 20 mg/day; lower-weight children can be started at 10 mg/day, may increase to 20 mg/day after 1 week if needed

Depression associated with bipolar I disorder (in combination with olanzapine): Children ≥10 years and Adolescents: Oral: Initial: 20 mg in the evening; adjust dose, if needed, as tolerated; safety of fluoxetine doses >50 mg in combination with doses >12 mg of olanzapine has not been studied in pediatrics. See **"Note"** below.

Obsessive-compulsive disorder: Children ≥7 years and Adolescents: Oral: Initial: 10 mg/day; may increase after 2 weeks if inadequate clinical response to 20 mg/day; further increases may be considered after several weeks to recommended range of 20 to 30 mg/day (lower weight children) or 20 to 60 mg/day (adolescents and higher weight children)

Selective mutism (off-label use): Children ≥5 years and Adolescents: Oral: Initial: 5 mg once daily for 7 days, then increase to 10 mg once daily for 7 days, and 20 mg once daily thereafter; may further titrate in 20 mg/day increments if needed every 2 weeks; maximum daily dose: 60 mg/day (Dummit 1996). Weight-based dosing: 0.2 mg/kg/day for 1 week, then 0.4 mg/kg/day for 1 week, then 0.6 mg/kg/day for 10 weeks; mean final dose in clinical trials: 21.4 mg/day (Black,1994). To fully assess therapeutic response, a therapeutic trial of at least 9 to 12 weeks or longer has been suggested (Black 1994; Dummit 1996; Kaakeh 2008).

Note: When using individual components of fluoxetine with olanzapine rather than fixed-dose combination product (Symbyax), approximate dosage correspondence is as follows:
Olanzapine 2.5 mg + fluoxetine 20 mg = Symbyax 3/25
Olanzapine 5 mg + fluoxetine 20 mg = Symbyax 6/25
Olanzapine 12.5 mg + fluoxetine 20 mg = Symbyax 12/25
Olanzapine 5 mg + fluoxetine 50 mg = Symbyax 6/50
Olanzapine 12.5 mg + fluoxetine 50 mg = Symbyax 12/50

Discontinuation of therapy: Refer to adult dosing.
MAO inhibitor recommendations: Refer to adult dosing.

Renal Impairment

Single dose studies: Pharmacokinetics of fluoxetine and norfluoxetine were similar among subjects with all levels of impaired renal function, including anephric patients on chronic hemodialysis.

Chronic administration: Additional accumulation of fluoxetine or norfluoxetine may occur in patients with severely impaired renal function.

Not removed by hemodialysis; use of lower dose or less frequent dosing is not usually necessary.

Hepatic Impairment Elimination half-life of fluoxetine is prolonged in patients with hepatic impairment. A lower dose or less frequent dosing of fluoxetine should be used in these patients.

Cirrhosis patient: Administer a lower dose or less frequent dosing interval.

Compensated cirrhosis without ascites: Administer 50% of normal dose.

Dietary Considerations May be taken without regard to meals.

Administration Administer without regard to meals.

Bipolar I disorder and treatment-resistant depression: Take once daily in the evening.

Major depressive disorder and obsessive compulsive disorder: Once daily doses should be taken in the morning, or twice daily (morning and noon).

Bulimia: Take once daily in the morning.

Monitoring Parameters Mental status for depression, suicidal ideation (especially at the beginning of therapy or when doses are increased or decreased), anxiety, social functioning, mania, panic attacks; signs/symptoms of serotonin syndrome; akathisia, sleep status; blood glucose (for diabetic patients), baseline liver function; ECG assessment and periodic monitoring in patients with risk factors for QT prolongation and ventricular arrhythmia

Reference Range Therapeutic levels have not been well established

Therapeutic: Fluoxetine: 100 to 800 ng/mL (SI: 289 to 2314 nmol/L); Norfluoxetine: 100 to 600 ng/mL (SI: 289 to 1735 nmol/L)

Toxic: Fluoxetine plus norfluoxetine: >2000 ng/mL

Additional Information ECG may reveal S-T segment depression. Not shown to be teratogenic in rodents; 15 to 60 mg/day, buspirone and cyproheptadine, may be useful in treatment of sexual dysfunction during treatment with a selective serotonin reuptake inhibitor.

Weekly capsules are a delayed release formulation containing enteric-coated pellets of fluoxetine hydrochloride, equivalent to 90 mg fluoxetine. Therapeutic equivalence of weekly formulation with daily formulation for delaying time to relapse has not been established.

Dosage Forms Excipient information presented when available (limited, particularly for generics); consult specific product labeling.

Capsule, Oral:

PROzac: 10 mg, 20 mg, 40 mg

Generic: 10 mg, 20 mg, 40 mg

Capsule Delayed Release, Oral:

PROzac Weekly: 90 mg

Generic: 90 mg

Solution, Oral:

Generic: 20 mg/5 mL (5 mL, 120 mL)

Tablet, Oral:

Sarafem: 10 mg, 20 mg [contains fd&c yellow #10 aluminum lake, fd&c yellow #6 aluminum lake]

Generic: 10 mg, 20 mg, 60 mg

Dosage Forms: Canada Note: Refer to Dosage Forms. Delayed release capsules and tablets are not available in Canada.

Extemporaneous Preparations Note: Commercial oral solution is available (4 mg/mL)

A 1 mg/mL fluoxetine oral solution may be prepared using the commercially available preparation (4 mg/mL). In separate graduated cylinders, measure 5 mL of the commercially available fluoxetine preparation and 15 mL of Simple Syrup, NF. Mix thoroughly in incremental proportions. For a 2 mg/mL solution, mix equal proportions of both the commercially available fluoxetine preparation and Simple Syrup, NF. Label "refrigerate". Both concentrations are stable for up to 56 days.

Nahata MC, Pai VB, and Hipple TF, *Pediatric Drug Formulations*, 5th ed, Cincinnati, OH: Harvey Whitney Books Co, 2004.

◆ **Fluoxetine Capsules BP (Can)** *see* FLUoxetine *on page* 786

◆ **Fluoxetine Hydrochloride** *see* FLUoxetine *on page* 786

Fluoxymesterone (floo oks i MES te rone)

Brand Names: US Androxy

Index Terms Androxy; Halotestin

Pharmacologic Category Androgen

Use Replacement therapy in the treatment of delayed male puberty; male hypogonadism (primary or hypogonadotropic); inoperable metastatic female breast cancer

Dosing

Adult & Geriatric

Hypogonadism (Males): Oral: 5-20 mg daily

Delayed puberty (Males): Oral: 2.5-20 mg daily for 4-6 months

Inoperable breast carcinoma (Females): Oral: 10-40 mg daily in divided doses for ≥3 months

Renal Impairment No dosage adjustment provided in manufacturer's labeling; use with caution.

Hepatic Impairment No dosage adjustment provided in manufacturer's labeling; use with caution.

Additional Information Complete prescribing information should be consulted for additional detail.

Dosage Forms Excipient information presented when available (limited, particularly for generics); consult specific product labeling.

Tablet, Oral:

Androxy: 10 mg [scored; contains fd&c blue #1 aluminum lake, fd&c yellow #10 aluminum lake, fd&c yellow #6 aluminum lake]

Controlled Substance C-III

FluPHENAZine (floo FEN a zeen)

Brand Names: Canada Apo-Fluphenazine Decanoate®; Apo-Fluphenazine®; Modecate®; Modecate® Concentrate; PMS-Fluphenazine Decanoate

Index Terms Fluphenazine Decanoate; Fluphenazine Hydrochloride; Prolixin

Pharmacologic Category First Generation (Typical) Antipsychotic

Use Management of manifestations of psychotic disorders and schizophrenia; depot formulation may offer improved outcome in individuals with psychosis who are nonadherent with oral antipsychotics

Dosing

Adult

Psychosis:

Oral: Initial: 2.5 to 10 mg/day in divided doses at 6- to 8-hour intervals; Maintenance: 1 to 5 mg/day; **Note:** Some patients may require up to 40 mg/day for symptom control (long-term safety of higher doses not established)

PORT guidelines: Acute therapy: 6 to 20 mg/day for up to 6 weeks; Maintenance: 6 to 12 mg/day (Buchanan, 2009)

IM (hydrochloride): Initial: 1.25 mg as a single dose; depending on severity and duration, may need 2.5 to 10 mg/day in divided doses at 6- to 8-hour intervals (4 mg IM fluphenazine HCl is approximately equivalent to 10 mg oral fluphenazine HCl); use caution with doses >10 mg/day; once symptoms stabilized, transition to oral maintenance therapy

Long-acting maintenance injections (decanoate):

IM, SubQ (decanoate): Initial: 12.5 to 25 mg every 2 to 4 weeks; response may last up to 6 weeks in some patients; titrate dose cautiously, if doses >50 mg are needed, increase in 12.5 mg increments (maximum dose: 100 mg)

Conversion from hydrochloride dosage forms to decanoate IM: 12.5 mg of decanoate every 2 to 4 weeks is approximately equivalent to 10 mg of oral hydrochloride/day; **Note:** Clinically, an every-2-week interval is frequently utilized

PORT guidelines: 6.25 to 25 mg every 2 weeks (Buchanan, 2009)

Note: Decrease the oral fluphenazine (or current antipsychotic) dose by half after the initial injection; consider discontinuation of oral therapy after second injection (McEvoy, 2006).

Geriatric Oral: Initial: 1 to 2.5 mg daily; titrated gradually based on patient response.

Renal Impairment Use with caution; not dialyzable (0% to 5%).

Hepatic Impairment Use with caution.

Additional Information Complete prescribing information should be consulted for additional detail.

Dosage Forms Excipient information presented when available (limited, particularly for generics); consult specific product labeling.

Concentrate, Oral, as hydrochloride:

Generic: 5 mg/mL (120 mL)

Elixir, Oral, as hydrochloride:

Generic: 2.5 mg/5 mL (60 mL, 473 mL)

Solution, Injection, as decanoate:

Generic: 25 mg/mL (5 mL)

Solution, Injection, as hydrochloride:

Generic: 2.5 mg/mL (10 mL)

Tablet, Oral, as hydrochloride:

Generic: 1 mg, 2.5 mg, 5 mg, 10 mg

Dosage Forms: Canada Note: Refer also to Dosage Forms. Oral concentrate, oral elixir, and solution for injection (as hydrochloride) are not available in Canada. Excipient information presented when available (limited, particularly for generics); consult specific product labeling.

Solution, Injection, as decanoate: 100 mg/mL (1 mL)

◆ **Fluphenazine Decanoate** *see* FluPHENAZine *on page* 790

◆ **Fluphenazine Hydrochloride** *see* FluPHENAZine *on page* 790

◆ **5-Fluracil** *see* Fluorouracil (Systemic) *on page* 784

◆ **Flura-Drops** *see* Fluoride *on page* 782

Flurandrenolide (flure an DREN oh lide)

Brand Names: US Cordran
Index Terms Flurandrenolone
Pharmacologic Category Corticosteroid, Topical
Additional Appendix Information
Topical Corticosteroids *on page 1952*
Use Corticosteroid-responsive dermatoses: Relief of inflammatory and pruritic manifestations of corticosteroid-responsive dermatoses
Dosing
Adult & Geriatric
Corticosteroid-responsive dermatoses: Topical: **Note:** Therapy should be discontinued when control is achieved; if no improvement is seen within 2 weeks, reassessment of diagnosis may be necessary.
Cream, lotion, ointment: Apply thin film to affected area 2 to 3 times per day
Tape: Apply 1 to 2 times per day
Pediatric
Corticosteroid-responsive dermatoses: Topical: **Note:** Therapy should be discontinued when control is achieved; if no improvement is seen within 2 weeks, reassessment of diagnosis may be necessary.
Cream, lotion, ointment, tape: Children and Adolescents: Refer to adult dosing.
Renal Impairment There are no dosage adjustments provided in the manufacturer's labeling.
Hepatic Impairment There are no dosage adjustments provided in the manufacturer's labeling.
Additional Information Complete prescribing information should be consulted for additional detail.
Dosage Forms Excipient information presented when available (limited, particularly for generics); consult specific product labeling.
Cream, External:
Cordran: 0.05% (15 g, 30 g, 60 g, 120 g) [contains cetyl alcohol, propylene glycol]
Lotion, External:
Cordran: 0.05% (15 mL, 60 mL, 120 mL) [contains benzyl alcohol, cetyl alcohol, menthol]
Ointment, External:
Cordran: 0.05% (60 g) [contains cetyl alcohol]
Tape, External:
Cordran: 4 mcg/cm^2 (1 ea)

◆ Flurandrenolone *see* Flurandrenolide *on page 791*

Flurazepam (flure AZ e pam)

Brand Names: Canada Apo-Flurazepam; Bio-Flurazepam; Dalmane; PMS-Flurazepam; Som Pam
Index Terms Flurazepam Hydrochloride
Pharmacologic Category Hypnotic, Benzodiazepine
Use Insomnia: For the treatment of insomnia characterized by difficulty in falling asleep, frequent nocturnal awakenings, and/or early-morning awakenings.
Medication Guide Available Yes
Dosing
Adult Insomnia: Adults: Oral: Initial: 15 mg at bedtime for women, and 15 to 30 mg at bedtime for men; may increase dose to 30 mg at bedtime as needed based on response
Geriatric Oral: 15 mg at bedtime
Renal Impairment There are no dosage adjustments provided in the manufacturer's labeling; use with caution.
Hepatic Impairment There are no dosage adjustments provided in the manufacturer's labeling; use with caution.
Additional Information Complete prescribing information should be consulted for additional detail.
Dosage Forms Excipient information presented when available (limited, particularly for generics); consult specific product labeling.
Capsule, Oral, as hydrochloride:
Generic: 15 mg, 30 mg
Controlled Substance C-IV

◆ Flurazepam Hydrochloride *see* Flurazepam *on page 791*

Flurbiprofen (Systemic) (flure BI proe fen)

Brand Names: Canada APO-Flurbiprofen FC; Teva-Flurbiprofen
Index Terms Flurbiprofen Sodium
Pharmacologic Category Nonsteroidal Anti-inflammatory Drug (NSAID), Oral
Use Treatment of rheumatoid arthritis and osteoarthritis
Medication Guide Available Yes

Dosing
Adult & Geriatric
Rheumatoid arthritis and osteoarthritis: Oral: 200-300 mg/day in 2, 3, or 4 divided doses; do not administer more than 100 mg for any single dose; maximum: 300 mg/day
Management of postoperative dental pain (off-label use): Oral: 100 mg every 12 hours
Renal Impairment Not recommended in patients with advanced renal disease.
Hepatic Impairment No dosage adjustment provided in manufacturer's labeling; patients with hepatic insufficiency may require reduced doses due to extensive hepatic metabolism.
Additional Information Complete prescribing information should be consulted for additional detail.
Dosage Forms Excipient information presented when available (limited, particularly for generics); consult specific product labeling.
Tablet, Oral:
Generic: 50 mg, 100 mg

Flurbiprofen (Ophthalmic) (flure BI proe fen)

Brand Names: US Ocufen
Index Terms Flurbiprofen Sodium
Pharmacologic Category Nonsteroidal Anti-inflammatory Drug (NSAID), Ophthalmic
Use Inhibition of intraoperative miosis
Dosing
Adult & Geriatric Ophthalmic anti-inflammatory/surgical aid: Ophthalmic: Instill 1 drop every 30 minutes, beginning 2 hours prior to surgery for a total of 4 drops in each affected eye.
Renal Impairment No dosage adjustment provided in manufacturer's labeling.
Hepatic Impairment No dosage adjustment provided in manufacturer's labeling.
Additional Information Complete prescribing information should be consulted for additional detail.
Dosage Forms Excipient information presented when available (limited, particularly for generics); consult specific product labeling.
Solution, Ophthalmic, as sodium:
Ocufen: 0.03% (2.5 mL) [contains edetate disodium, thimerosal]
Generic: 0.03% (2.5 mL)

◆ Flurbiprofen Sodium *see* Flurbiprofen (Ophthalmic) *on page 791*
◆ Flurbiprofen Sodium *see* Flurbiprofen (Systemic) *on page 791*
◆ Fluress® [DSC] *see* Fluorescein and Benoxinate *on page 782*
◆ 5-Flurocytosine *see* Flucytosine *on page 778*
◆ Flurox™ *see* Fluorescein and Benoxinate *on page 782*

Flutamide (FLOO ta mide)

Brand Names: Canada Apo-Flutamide; Euflex; PMS-Flutamide; Teva-Flutamide
Index Terms Eulexin; Flucinom; Flugerel; Niftolid; SCH 13521
Pharmacologic Category Antineoplastic Agent, Antiandrogen
Use Prostate cancer: Management of locally confined Stage B$_2$ to C and Stage D$_2$ metastatic prostate cancer (in combination with a luteinizing hormone-releasing hormone [LHRH] agonist). For Stage B$_2$ to C prostate cancer, flutamide treatment (and goserelin) should start 8 weeks prior to initiating radiation therapy and continue during radiation therapy. To achieve treatment benefit in Stage D$_2$ metastatic prostate cancer, initiate flutamide with the LHRH agonist and continue until disease progression.
Dosing
Adult & Geriatric Prostate cancer, metastatic: Males: Oral: 250 mg 3 times daily (every 8 hours)
Renal Impairment No dosage adjustment is necessary in patients with chronic renal insufficiency.
Hepatic Impairment
Mild to moderate impairment: There are no dosage adjustments provided in the manufacturer's labeling.
Severe impairment: Use is contraindicated.
Additional Information Complete prescribing information should be consulted for additional detail.
Dosage Forms Excipient information presented when available (limited, particularly for generics); consult specific product labeling.
Capsule, Oral:
Generic: 125 mg

◄ **Dosage Forms: Canada** Excipient information presented when available (limited, particularly for generics); consult specific product labeling.
Tablet, Oral: 250 mg

Fluticasone (Oral Inhalation) (floo TIK a sone)

Brand Names: US Arnuity Ellipta; Flovent Diskus; Flovent HFA
Brand Names: Canada Arnuity Ellipta; Flovent Diskus; Flovent HFA
Index Terms Flovent; Fluticasone Furoate; Fluticasone Propionate
Pharmacologic Category Corticosteroid, Inhalant (Oral)
Additional Appendix Information
Inhaled Corticosteroids *on page 1951*
Use
Asthma:
Arnuity Ellipta: Maintenance treatment of asthma as prophylactic therapy in patients 12 years and older
Flovent Diskus and Flovent HFA: Maintenance treatment of asthma as prophylactic therapy in patients 4 years and older; for patients requiring oral corticosteroid therapy for asthma to assist in total discontinuation or reduction of total oral dose
Limitations of use: Not indicated for relief of acute bronchospasm

Guideline recommendations: A low-dose inhaled corticosteroid (*in addition to an as-needed short acting beta$_2$-agonist*) is the initial preferred long term control medication for children, adolescents, and adult patients with persistent asthma who are candidates for treatment according to a step-wise treatment approach (GINA 2015; NAEPP 2007).

Pregnancy Considerations Adverse events were observed in some animal reproduction studies. Hypoadrenalism may occur in infants born to mothers receiving corticosteroids during pregnancy. Based on available data, an overall increased risk of congenital malformations or a decrease in fetal growth has not been associated with maternal use of inhaled corticosteroids during pregnancy (Bakhireva, 2005; NAEPP, 2005; Namazy, 2004). Uncontrolled asthma is associated with adverse events in pregnancy (increased risk of perinatal mortality, pre-eclampsia, preterm birth, low birth weight infants). Inhaled corticosteroids are recommended for the treatment of asthma during pregnancy (most information available using budesonide) (ACOG, 2008; NAEPP, 2005).

Breast-Feeding Considerations Systemic corticosteroids are excreted in human milk. It is not known if sufficient quantities of fluticasone are absorbed following inhalation to produce detectable amounts in breast milk. The manufacturer recommends that caution be exercised when administering fluticasone to nursing women. The use of inhaled corticosteroids is not considered a contraindication to breast-feeding (NAEPP, 2005).

Contraindications
Hypersensitivity to fluticasone or any component of the formulation; severe hypersensitivity to milk proteins or lactose (Arnuity Ellipta and Flovent Diskus); primary treatment of status asthmaticus or other acute episodes of asthma requiring intensive measures
Documentation of allergenic cross-reactivity for corticosteroids in this class is limited. However, because of similarities in chemical structure and/or pharmacologic actions, the possibility of cross-sensitivity cannot be ruled out with certainty.

Canadian labeling: Additional contraindications (not in US labeling): Flovent HFA and Flovent Diskus: Moderate to severe bronchiectasis; untreated fungal, bacterial or tubercular infections of the respiratory tract

Warnings/Precautions May cause hypercorticism or suppression of hypothalamic-pituitary-adrenal (HPA) axis. HPA axis suppression may lead to adrenal crisis. Withdrawal and discontinuation of a corticosteroid should be done slowly and carefully. Particular care is required when patients are transferred from systemic corticosteroids to inhaled corticosteroids due to possible adrenal insufficiency or withdrawal from steroids, including an increase in allergic symptoms. Patients receiving ≥20 mg per day of prednisone (or equivalent) may be most susceptible. Fatalities have occurred due to adrenal insufficiency in asthmatic patients during and after transfer from systemic corticosteroids to aerosol steroids; aerosol steroids do **not** provide the systemic steroid needed to treat patients having trauma, surgery, or infections. Select surgical patients on long-term, high-dose, inhaled corticosteroid (ICS), should be given stress doses of hydrocortisone intravenously during the surgical period and the dose reduced rapidly within 24 hours after surgery (NAEPP, 2007).

Bronchospasm may occur with wheezing after inhalation; if this occurs, stop steroid and treat with a fast-acting bronchodilator. Hypersensitivity reactions including, allergic dermatitis, anaphylaxis, angioedema, bronchospasm, flushing, hypotension, urticaria, and rash have been reported. Supplemental steroids (oral or parenteral) may be needed during stress or severe asthma attacks. Corticosteroid use may cause psychiatric disturbances, including depression, euphoria, insomnia, mood swings, and personality changes. Preexisting psychiatric conditions may be exacerbated by corticosteroid use. Prolonged use of corticosteroids may also increase the incidence of secondary infection, mask acute infection (including fungal infections), prolong or exacerbate viral infections, or limit response to vaccines. Avoid use if possible in patients with ocular herpes; active or quiescent tuberculosis infections of the respiratory tract; or untreated viral, fungal, parasitic or bacterial systemic infections (Flovent Diskus and Flovent HFA Canadian labeling contraindicates use with untreated respiratory infections). Exposure to chickenpox and measles should be avoided; if the patient is exposed, prophylaxis with varicella zoster immune globulin or pooled intramuscular immunoglobulin, respectively, may be indicated; if chickenpox develops, treatment with antiviral agents may be considered. Rare cases of vasculitis (Churg-Strauss syndrome) or other systemic eosinophilic conditions can occur. Prolonged treatment with corticosteroids has been associated with the development of Kaposi's sarcoma (case reports); if noted, discontinuation of therapy should be considered.

Use with caution in patients with thyroid disease, hepatic impairment, renal impairment, cardiovascular disease, diabetes, glaucoma, cataracts, myasthenia gravis, patients at risk for osteoporosis, patients at risk for seizures, or GI diseases (diverticulitis, peptic ulcer, ulcerative colitis) due to perforation risk. Use caution following acute MI (corticosteroids have been associated with myocardial rupture). When transferring to oral inhaler, previously-suppressed allergic conditions (rhinitis, conjunctivitis, eczema) may be unmasked.

Orally-inhaled corticosteroids may cause a reduction in growth velocity in pediatric patients (~1 centimeter per year [range: 0.3-1.8 cm per year] and related to dose and duration of exposure). To minimize the systemic effects of orally-inhaled corticosteroids, each patient should be titrated to the lowest effective dose. Growth should be routinely monitored in pediatric patients.

Potentially significant drug-drug interactions may exist, requiring dose or frequency adjustment, additional monitoring, and/or selection of alternative therapy. Not to be used in status asthmaticus or for the relief of acute bronchospasm. Flovent Diskus and Arnuity Ellipta contain lactose; very rare anaphylactic reactions have been reported in patients with severe milk protein allergy. Withdraw systemic corticosteroid therapy with gradual tapering of dose; consider reducing the daily prednisone dose by 2.5 to 5 mg on a weekly basis beginning at least 1 week after inhalation therapy. Monitor lung function, beta-agonist use, asthma symptoms, and for signs and symptoms of adrenal insufficiency (fatigue, lassitude, weakness, nausea and vomiting, hypotension) during withdrawal. Local yeast infections (eg, oropharyngeal candidiasis) may occur.

Adverse Reactions
>10%:
Central nervous system: Fatigue (≤16%), malaise (≤16%), headache (2% to 14%)
Gastrointestinal: Oral candidiasis (≤31%)
Neuromuscular & skeletal: Arthralgia (≤17%), arthritis (≤17%), musculoskeletal pain (2% to 12%)
Respiratory: Sinus infection (≤33%), sinusitis (≤33%), upper respiratory tract infection (2% to 31%), throat irritation (<1% to 22%), nasal congestion (≥3% to 16%), nasopharyngitis (8% to 13%), rhinitis (<1% to 13%), bronchitis (≤12%)
1% to 10%:
Cardiovascular: Hypertension (≤1%), subarachnoid hemorrhage (≤1%)
Central nervous system: Pain (10%), voice disorder (≤9%), procedural pain (<1% to 3%), herniated disk (≤1%)
Dermatologic: Skin rash (8%), pruritus (6%)
Gastrointestinal: Nausea and vomiting (1% to 9%), viral gastrointestinal infection (3% to 5%), gastrointestinal distress (≤4%), gastrointestinal pain (≤4%), oropharyngeal candidiasis (3%), toothache (3%), viral gastroenteritis (3%), abdominal pain (≤3%)

Hematologic & oncologic: Malignant neoplasm of breast (≤1%)

Infection: Influenza (4% to 7%), viral infection (≤5%), abscess (≤1%)

Neuromuscular & skeletal: Muscle injury (≤5%), back pain (3%)

Respiratory: Cough (≤9%), hoarseness (≤9%), viral respiratory infection (1% to 9%), pharyngitis (3% to 6%), upper respiratory tract inflammation (≤5%), oropharyngeal pain (3% to 4%), allergic rhinitis (≥3%)

Miscellaneous: Fever (1% to 7%), accidental injury (≤5%), amputation (≤1%)

<1% (Limited to important or life-threatening): Adrenocortical insufficiency, aggressive behavior, agitation, allergic skin reaction, anxiety, aphonia, bacterial infection, bacterial reproductive infection, behavioral changes (very rare: includes hyperactivity and irritability in children), blepharoconjunctivitis, bronchospasm (immediate and delayed), bruise, burn, cataract (long-term use), change in appetite, chest tightness, cholecystitis, Churg-Strauss syndrome, conjunctivitis, cranial nerve palsy, Cushingoid appearance, decreased bone mineral density (long-term use) decreased linear skeletal growth rate (children/adolescents), dental caries, dental discoloration, depression, dermatitis, diarrhea, disturbance in fluid balance, dizziness, drug toxicity, dyspnea, ecchymoses, edema, eosinophilia, epistaxis, esophageal candidiasis, exacerbation of asthma, facial edema, folliculitis, fungal infection, gastrointestinal disease, glaucoma (long-term use), hematoma, HPA-axis suppression, hypercorticoidism, hyperglycemia, hypersensitivity reaction (immediate and delayed; includes ear, nose, and throat allergic disorders, anaphylaxis, angioedema, bronchospasm, hypotension, skin rash, urticaria, increased intraocular pressure (long-term use), inflammation (musculoskeletal), keratitis, laceration, laryngitis, migraine, mobility disorder, mood disorder, mouth disease (and tongue disease), muscle cramps, muscle rigidity (stiffness, tightness), muscle spasm, oral discomfort (and pain), oral mucosa ulcer, oral rash (and erythema), oropharyngeal edema, palpitations, paradoxical bronchospasm, paranasal sinus disease, photodermatitis, pneumonia, polyp (ear, nose, throat), pressure-induced disorder, reduced salivation, restlessness, rhinorrhea, sleep disorder, soft tissue injury, urinary tract infection, vasculitis, viral skin infection, wheezing, wound

Drug Interactions

Metabolism/Transport Effects Substrate of CYP3A4 (major); **Note:** Assignment of Major/Minor substrate status based on clinically relevant drug interaction potential

Avoid Concomitant Use

Avoid concomitant use of Fluticasone (Oral Inhalation) with any of the following: Aldesleukin; BCG (Intravesical); Cobicistat; Conivaptan; Fusidic Acid (Systemic); Idelalisib; Loxapine; Natalizumab; Pimecrolimus; Tacrolimus (Topical); Tipranavir; Tofacitinib

Increased Effect/Toxicity

Fluticasone (Oral Inhalation) may increase the levels/effects of: Amphotericin B; Deferasirox; Fingolimod; Leflunomide; Loop Diuretics; Loxapine; Natalizumab; Thiazide Diuretics; Tofacitinib

The levels/effects of Fluticasone (Oral Inhalation) may be increased by: Aprepitant; Cobicistat; Conivaptan; CYP3A4 Inhibitors (Moderate); CYP3A4 Inhibitors (Strong); Dasatinib; Denosumab; Fosaprepitant; Fusidic Acid (Systemic); Idelalisib; Ivacaftor; Luliconazole; Mifepristone; Netupitant; Osimertinib; Palbociclib; Pimecrolimus; Simeprevir; Stiripentol; Tacrolimus (Topical); Tipranavir; Trastuzumab

Decreased Effect

Fluticasone (Oral Inhalation) may decrease the levels/effects of: Aldesleukin; BCG (Intravesical); Coccidioides immitis Skin Test; Corticorelin; Hyaluronidase; Sipuleucel-T; Vaccines (Inactivated)

The levels/effects of Fluticasone (Oral Inhalation) may be decreased by: Echinacea; Osimertinib

Storage/Stability

Arnuity Ellipta:

US labeling: Store at 20°C to 25°C (68°F to 77°F); excursions are permitted from 15°C to 30°C (59°F to 86°F). Store in a dry place away from direct heat or sunlight. Discard after 6 weeks from removal from protective foil pouch or when the dose counter reads "0" (whichever comes first); device is not reusable.

Canadian labeling: Store at ≤25°C (77°F). If stored in a refrigerator, allow to warm to room temperature for at least 1 hour prior to use. Discard after 6 weeks from removal from protective foil pouch or when the dose counter reads "0" (whichever comes first); device is not reusable.

Flovent Diskus: Store at 20°C to 25°C (68°F to 77°F); excursions are permitted from 15°C to 30°C (59°F to 86°F). Store in a dry place away from direct heat or sunlight. Discard after 6 weeks (50 mcg diskus) or after 2 months (100 mcg and 250 mcg diskus) from removal from protective foil pouch or when the dose counter reads "0" (whichever comes first); device is not reusable.

Flovent HFA: Store between 20°C and 25°C (68°F and 77°F); excursions are permitted from 15°C to 30°C (59°F to 86°F). Discard device when the dose counter reads "000". Store with mouthpiece down. Do not expose to temperatures >120°F. Do not puncture or incinerate.

Mechanism of Action

Fluticasone belongs to a group of corticosteroids which utilizes a fluorocarbothioate ester linkage at the 17 carbon position; extremely potent vasoconstrictive and anti-inflammatory activity. The effectiveness of inhaled fluticasone is due to its direct local effect.

Pharmacodynamics/Kinetics

Onset of action: Maximal benefit may take 1 to 2 weeks or longer

Absorption: Absorbed systemically primarily via lungs, minimal GI absorption (<1%) due to presystemic metabolism

Distribution: 4.2 L/kg

Protein binding: >99%

Metabolism: Hepatic via CYP3A4 to 17β-carboxylic acid (negligible activity)

Bioavailability: Oral inhalation: 13.9%; Flovent Diskus: ~8%

Half-life elimination: IV: ~8 hours; Oral inhalation (plasma elimination phase following repeat dosing): 24 hours

Time to peak, plasma: 0.5 to 1 hour

Excretion: Feces (as parent drug and metabolites); urine (<5% as metabolites)

Dosing

Adult & Geriatric Asthma: Inhalation, oral: **Note:** Titrate to the lowest effective dose once asthma stability is achieved

Arnuity Ellipta (fluticasone furoate): Dosing based on previous asthma therapy: **Note:** May increase dose after 2 weeks of therapy in patients who are not adequately controlled.

No prior treatment with inhaled corticosteroids: Initial: 100 mcg once daily; maximum: 200 mcg once daily

Prior treatment with inhaled corticosteroids: Initial: 100 to 200 mcg once daily; maximum: 200 mcg once daily

Flovent HFA (fluticasone propionate):

US labeling: Dosing based on previous asthma therapy: **Note:** May increase dose after 2 weeks of therapy in patients who are not adequately controlled.

Bronchodilator alone: Initial: 88 mcg twice daily; maximum: 440 mcg twice daily

Inhaled corticosteroids: Initial: 88 to 220 mcg twice daily (initial dose >88 mcg twice daily may be considered in patients previously requiring higher doses of inhaled corticosteroids); maximum: 440 mcg twice daily

Oral corticosteroids (OCS): Initial: 440 mcg twice daily; maximum: 880 mcg twice daily.

Canadian labeling: **Note:** May increase dose after ~1 week of therapy in patients who are not adequately controlled.

Mild asthma: 100 to 250 mcg twice daily

Moderate asthma: 250 to 500 mcg twice daily

Severe asthma: 500 mcg twice daily; may increase up to 1000 mcg twice daily in very severe patients (eg, patients using oral corticosteroids [OCS])

Asthma guidelines:

National Asthma Education and Prevention Program guidelines (NAEPP 2007): HFA inhaler (refers to Flovent HFA 44 mcg, 110 mcg, and 220 mcg strengths available in US): **Note:** Administer in divided doses twice daily.

"Low" dose: 88 to 264 mcg/day

"Medium" dose: >264 to 440 mcg/day

"High" dose: >440 mcg/day

Global Initiative for Asthma guidelines (GINA 2015): HFA inhaler (refers to Flovent HFA 50 mcg, 125 mcg, and 250 mcg strengths available in Canada):

"Low" dose: 100 to 250 mcg daily

"Medium" dose: >250 to 500 mcg daily

"High" dose: >500 mcg daily

Flovent Diskus (fluticasone propionate):

US labeling: **Note:** May increase dose after 2 weeks of therapy in patients who are not adequately controlled.

Dosing based on previous asthma therapy:

Bronchodilator alone: Initial: 100 mcg twice daily; maximum: 500 mcg twice daily

Inhaled corticosteroids: Initial: 100 to 250 mcg twice daily; maximum: 500 mcg twice daily; initial dose >100 mcg twice daily may be considered in patients with poorer asthma control or those previously requiring high ranges of inhaled corticosteroids

Oral corticosteroids (OCS): Initial: 500 to 1000 mcg twice daily; maximum: 1000 mcg twice daily

Canadian labeling: Note: May increase dose after ~1 week of therapy in patients who are not adequately controlled.

Mild asthma: 100 to 250 mcg twice daily

Moderate asthma: 250 to 500 mcg twice daily

Severe asthma: 500 mcg twice daily; may increase up to 1000 mcg twice daily in very severe patients (eg, patients using oral corticosteroids [OCS])

Asthma guidelines:

National Asthma Education and Prevention Program guidelines (NAEPP, 2007): Dry powder inhaler (refers to Flovent Diskus 50 mcg, 100 mcg, and 250 mcg strengths available in the US and Canada, and the 500 mcg strength available in Canada): **Note:** Administer in divided doses twice daily:

"Low" dose: 100 to 300 mcg/day

"Medium" dose: >300 to 500 mcg/day

"High" dose: >500 mcg/day

Global Initiative for Asthma guidelines (GINA 2015): Dry powder inhaler (refers to Flovent Diskus 50 mcg, 100 mcg, and 250 mcg strengths available in the US and Canada, and the 500 mcg strength available in Canada)

"Low" dose: 100 to 250 mcg daily

"Medium" dose: >250 to 500 mcg daily

"High" dose: >500 mcg daily

Conversion: Conversion from oral systemic corticosteroids to orally inhaled corticosteroids: When converting from oral corticosteroids (OCS) to orally inhaled corticosteroids, initiate oral inhalation therapy in patients whose asthma is previously stabilized on OCS. Gradual OCS dose reductions should begin ~7 days after starting inhaled therapy. Flovent Diskus and Flovent HFA US labeling recommend reducing prednisone dose no more rapidly than 2.5 to 5 mg/day (or equivalent of other OCS) weekly. Flovent Diskus and Flovent HFA Canadian labeling recommend decreasing the daily dose of prednisone by 1 mg (or equivalent of other OCS) no more rapidly than weekly in adults who are closely monitored or every 10 days if not closely monitored. Arnuity Ellipta Canadian labeling recommends decreasing the daily prednisone dose by 2.5 mg (or equivalent of other OCS) no more rapidly than weekly. If adrenal insufficiency occurs, resume OCS therapy; initiate a more gradual withdrawal. When transitioning from systemic to inhaled corticosteroids, supplemental systemic corticosteroid therapy may be necessary during periods of stress or during severe asthma attacks.

Chronic obstructive pulmonary disease (stable) (off-label use): 50 to 500 mcg/day in combination with a long-acting bronchodilator (GOLD 2014)

Pediatric

Asthma: Inhalation, oral: **Note:** Titrate to lowest effective dose once asthma stability achieved.

Arnuity Ellipta (fluticasone furoate): Children ≥12 years and Adolescents: Refer to adult dosing.

Flovent HFA (fluticasone propionate):

US labeling:

Children 4 to 11 years: Initial: 88 mcg twice daily; maximum: 88 mcg twice daily

Children ≥12 years and Adolescents: Refer to adult dosing.

Canadian labeling:

Children 1 to 3 years: 100 mcg twice daily

Children 4 to 15 years: 100 mcg twice daily. **Note:** Canadian labeling recommends Flovent HFA be administered as a minimum of 2 inhalations twice daily; therefore, patients requiring lower or higher dosages than 100 mcg twice daily should use Flovent Diskus.

Adolescents ≥16 years and Adults: Refer to adult dosing.

Asthma guidelines:

National Asthma Education and Prevention Program guidelines (NAEPP, 2007): HFA inhaler (refers to Flovent HFA 44 mcg, 110 mcg, and 220 mcg strengths available in US) Note: Administer in divided doses twice daily

"Low" dose:

0 to 4 years: 176 mcg/day

5 to 11 years: 88 to 176 mcg/day

≥12 years: 88 to 264 mcg/day

"Medium" dose:

0 to 4 years: >176 to 352 mcg/day

5 to 11 years: >176 to 352 mcg/day

≥12 years: >264 to 440 mcg/day

"High" dose:

0 to 4 years: >352 mcg/day

5 to 11 years: >352 mcg/day

≥12 years: >440 mcg/day

Global Initiative for Asthma guidelines (GINA, 2015): HFA inhaler (refers to Flovent HFA 50 mcg, 125 mcg, and 250 mcg strengths available in Canada):

Children ≤5 years: "Low" dose: 100 mcg daily

Children 6 to 11 years:

"Low" dose: 100 to 200 mcg daily

"Medium" dose: >200 to 500 mcg daily

"High" dose: >500 mcg daily

Children ≥12 years and Adolescents: Refer to adult dosing.

Flovent Diskus (fluticasone propionate):

US labeling:

Children 4 to 11 years: Initial: 50 mcg twice daily; may increase to maximum dose of 100 mcg twice daily in patients not adequately controlled after 2 weeks of therapy. Initial dose >50 mcg twice daily may be considered in patients with poorer asthma control or those previously requiring high ranges of inhaled corticosteroids.

Adolescents: Refer to adult dosing.

Canadian labeling:

Children 4 to 16 years: Initial: 50 to 100 mcg twice daily; may increase up to 200 mcg twice daily after ~1 week of therapy in patients not adequately controlled

Adolescents ≥16 years: Refer to adult dosing.

Asthma guidelines:

National Asthma Education and Prevention Program guidelines (NAEPP, 2007): (administer in divided doses twice daily): Dry powder inhaler (refers to Flovent Diskus 50 mcg, 100 mcg, and 250 mcg strengths available in the US and Canada, and the 500 mcg strength available in Canada)

"Low" dose:

5 to 11 years: 100 to 200 mcg/day

≥12 years: 100 to 300 mcg/day

"Medium" dose:

5 to 11 years: >200 to 400 mcg/day

≥12 years: >300 to 500 mcg/day

"High" dose:

5 to 11 years: >400 mcg/day

≥12 years: >500 mcg/day

Global Initiative for Asthma guidelines (GINA 2015): Dry powder inhaler (refers to Flovent Diskus 50 mcg, 100 mcg, and 250 mcg strengths available in US and Canada, and the 500 mcg strength available in Canada)

Children 6 to 11 years:

"Low" dose: 100 to 200 mcg daily

"Medium" dose: >200 to 400 mcg daily

"High" dose: >400 mcg daily

Children ≥12 years and Adolescents: Refer to adult dosing.

Conversion: Conversion from oral systemic corticosteroids to orally inhaled corticosteroids: When converting from oral corticosteroids (OCS) to orally inhaled corticosteroids, initiate oral inhalation therapy in patients whose asthma is previously stabilized on OCS. Gradual OCS dose reductions should begin ~7 days after starting inhaled therapy. Flovent Diskus and Flovent HFA US labeling recommend reducing prednisone dose no more rapidly than 2.5 to 5 mg/day (or equivalent of other OCS) weekly in children ≥12 years but does not provide a recommendation for children <12 years. A similar approach to OCS dose reduction would however seem advisable. Flovent Diskus and Flovent HFA Canadian labeling recommend decreasing the daily dose of prednisone by 1 mg (or equivalent of other OCS) every 8 days in children who are closely monitored or every 20 days if not closely monitored. Arnuity Ellipta Canadian labeling recommends decreasing the daily prednisone dose by 2.5 mg (or equivalent of other OCS) no more rapidly than weekly. If adrenal insufficiency occurs, resume OCS therapy; initiate a more gradual withdrawal. When transitioning from systemic to inhaled corticosteroids, supplemental systemic corticosteroid therapy may be necessary during periods of stress or during severe asthma attacks.

Renal Impairment

Arnuity Ellipta: No dosage adjustment necessary.

Flovent Diskus and Flovent HFA:

US labeling: There are no dosage adjustment provided in the manufacturer's labeling (has not been studied).

Canadian labeling: No dosage adjustment necessary.

Hepatic Impairment

US labeling: There are no dosage adjustment provided in the manufacturer's labeling (has not been studied); however, fluticasone is primarily cleared in the liver and plasma levels may be increased in patients with hepatic impairment. Arnuity Ellipta product labeling indicates that systemic exposure is increased up to 3-fold. Use with caution and closely monitor.

Canadian labeling:

Arnuity Ellipta:

Mild impairment (Child-Pugh class A): There are no dosage adjustments provided in the manufacturer's labeling; use with caution.

Moderate or severe impairment (Child-Pugh class B or C): Maximum dose: 100 mcg daily

Flovent HFA and Flovent Diskus: No dosage adjustment necessary.

Dietary Considerations Arnuity Ellipta and Flovent Diskus contains lactose; very rare anaphylactic reactions have been reported in patients with severe milk protein allergy.

Administration

Aerosol inhalation: Flovent HFA: Shake container thoroughly before using. Take 3-5 deep breaths. Use inhaler on inspiration. Allow 1 full minute between inhalations. Rinse mouth with water after use to reduce aftertaste and incidence of candidiasis; do not swallow. Inhaler must be primed before first use, when not used for 7 days, or if dropped. To prime the first time, release 4 sprays into air; shake well before each spray and spray away from face. If dropped or not used for 7 days, prime by releasing a single test spray. Patient should contact pharmacy for refill when the dose counter reads "020". Discard device when the dose counter reads "000". Do not use "float" test to determine contents.

Powder for oral inhalation:

Arnuity Ellipta: Administer the dose at the same time every day. Do not shake inhaler. When ready to use, open and prepare mouthpiece of the inhaler and slide the cover down to activate the first dose. Exhale fully (not into mouthpiece), take one deep breath through mouth without blocking air vents and hold breath for about 3 to 4 seconds. If the cover is opened and closed without inhaling the medicine, the dose will be lost. The lost dose will be held in the inhaler, but it will no longer be available to be inhaled. It is not possible to accidentally take a double dose or an extra dose in one inhalation. Following administration, rinse mouth with water after use (do not swallow). Routine cleaning of the inhaler is not required; may clean the mouthpiece if needed, using a dry tissue, before the cover is closed. Discard inhaler 6 weeks after opening the foil tray or when the counter reads "0" (device is not reusable).

Flovent Diskus: Do not use with a spacer device. Do not exhale into Diskus. Do not wash or take apart. Use in horizontal position. Mouth should be rinsed with water after use (do not swallow). Discard after 6 weeks (50 mcg diskus) or after 2 months (100 mcg and 250 mcg diskus) once removed from protective pouch or when the dose counter reads "0", whichever comes first (device is not reusable).

Monitoring Parameters Growth (adolescents and children via stadiometry); signs/symptoms of HPA axis suppression/adrenal insufficiency; possible eosinophilic conditions (including Churg-Strauss syndrome); FEV$_1$, peak flow, and/or other pulmonary function tests; asthma symptoms; bone mineral density; hepatic impairment

Additional Information Effects of inhaled steroids on growth have been observed in the absence of laboratory evidence of HPA axis suppression, suggesting that growth velocity is a more sensitive indicator of systemic corticosteroid exposure in pediatric patients than some commonly used tests of HPA axis function. The long-term effects of this reduction in growth velocity associated with orally-inhaled corticosteroids, including the impact on final adult height, are unknown. The potential for "catch up" growth following discontinuation of treatment with inhaled corticosteroids has not been adequately studied.

In the United States, dosage for the metered dose inhaler (Flovent HFA) is expressed as the amount of drug which leaves the actuater and is delivered to the patient. This differs from other countries, which express the dosage as the amount of drug which leaves the valve.

Dosage Forms Considerations Flovent HFA 10.6 g and 12 g canisters contain 120 inhalations.

Dosage Forms Excipient information presented when available (limited, particularly for generics); consult specific product labeling.

Aerosol, Inhalation, as propionate:

Flovent HFA: 44 mcg/actuation (10.6 g); 110 mcg/actuation (12 g); 220 mcg/actuation (12 g)

Aerosol Powder Breath Activated, Inhalation, as furoate:

Arnuity Ellipta: 100 mcg/actuation (14 ea, 30 ea); 200 mcg/actuation (14 ea, 30 ea) [contains lactose monohydrate]

Aerosol Powder Breath Activated, Inhalation, as propionate:

Flovent Diskus: 50 mcg/blister (60 ea); 100 mcg/blister (28 ea, 60 ea); 250 mcg/blister (28 ea, 60 ea) [contains lactose]

Dosage Forms: Canada Note: Refer also to Dosage Forms

Excipient information presented when available (limited, particularly for generics); consult specific product labeling.

Aerosol, for oral inhalation, as propionate:

Flovent HFA: 50 mcg/inhalation (120 actuations); 125 mcg/inhalation (60 or 120 actuations); 250 mcg/inhalation (60 or 120 actuations)

Powder, for oral inhalation, as propionate:

Flovent Diskus: 50 mcg (60s) [contains lactose; prefilled blister pack]

Flovent Diskus: 100 mcg (60s) [contains lactose; prefilled blister pack]

Flovent Diskus: 250 mcg (60s) [contains lactose; prefilled blister pack]

Flovent Diskus: 500 mcg (60s) [contains lactose; prefilled blister pack]

Fluticasone (Nasal) (floo TIK a sone)

Brand Names: US Flonase Allergy Relief [OTC]; Flonase [DSC]; Veramyst

Brand Names: Canada Apo-Fluticasone; Avamys; Flonase; ratio-Fluticasone

Index Terms Fluticasone Furoate; Fluticasone Propionate

Pharmacologic Category Corticosteroid, Nasal

Additional Appendix Information

Inhaled Corticosteroids *on page 1951*

Use

Nonallergic rhinitis (Flonase): Management of the nasal symptoms of perennial nonallergic rhinitis in adults and pediatric patients ≥4 years.

Allergic rhinitis (Veramyst, Avamys [Canadian product]): Management of seasonal and perennial allergic rhinitis in adults and pediatric patients ≥2 years

OTC labeling: Relief of hay fever or other upper respiratory allergies (eg, nasal congestion, runny nose, sneezing, itchy nose) in adults and children ≥4 years.

Dosing

Adult & Geriatric Rhinitis: Intranasal:

Flonase (fluticasone propionate):

US labeling: Initial: 2 sprays (50 mcg/spray) per nostril once daily (200 mcg/day); alternatively, the same total daily dosage may be divided and given as 1 spray per nostril twice daily (200 mcg/day). After the first few days, dosage may be reduced to 1 spray per nostril once daily for maintenance therapy (100 mcg/day) (maximum: 2 sprays in each nostril [200 mcg]/day).

Canadian labeling: 2 sprays (50 mcg/spray) per nostril once daily (200 mcg/day); for severe rhinitis may administer 2 sprays in each nostril every 12 hours (maximum: 4 sprays in each nostril [400 mcg]/day).

Flonase OTC (fluticasone propionate): Initial: 2 sprays (50 mcg/spray) per nostril once daily (200 mcg/day); after 1 week, may adjust to 1 or 2 sprays per nostril once daily (100 to 200 mcg/day). Do not use for more than 6 months unless instructed by health care provider.

Veramyst (fluticasone furoate): Initial: 2 sprays (27.5 mcg/spray) per nostril once daily (110 mcg/day); once symptoms are controlled, may reduce dosage to 1 spray per nostril once daily (55 mcg/day) for maintenance therapy.

Avamys (fluticasone furoate) [Canadian product]: 2 sprays (27.5 mcg/spray) in each nostril once daily (110 mcg/day). Total daily dosage should not exceed 2 sprays in each nostril (110 mcg/day).

Pediatric Rhinitis: Intranasal:

Flonase (fluticasone propionate):

US labeling: Children ≥4 years and Adolescents: Initial: 1 spray (50 mcg/spray) per nostril once daily (100 mcg/day); may increase to 2 sprays per nostril once daily (200 mcg/day) if response not adequate; once symptoms are controlled, may reduce to 1 spray per nostril once daily (100 mcg/day) (maximum: 2 sprays in each nostril [200 mcg]/day). Dosing should be at regular intervals.

Canadian labeling:

Children ≥4 years to 11 years: 1 to 2 sprays (50 mcg/spray) per nostril once daily (100 to 200 mcg/day); once symptoms are controlled, reduce to 1 spray per nostril once daily (100 mcg/day) (maximum: 2 sprays in each nostril [200 mcg]/day). Dosing should be at regular intervals.

Children ≥12 years and Adolescents: Refer to adult dosing.

Flonase OTC (fluticasone propionate):

Children 4 to 11 years: 1 spray (50 mcg/spray) per nostril once daily (100 mcg/day). Do not use for more than 2 months per year unless instructed by health care provider.

Children ≥12 years and Adolescents: Initial: 2 sprays (50 mcg/spray) per nostril once daily (200 mcg/day); after 1 week, may adjust to 1 or 2 sprays per nostril once daily (100 to 200 mcg/day). Do not use for more than 6 months unless instructed by health care provider.

Veramyst (fluticasone furoate):

Children 2 to 11 years: Initial: 1 spray (27.5 mcg/spray) per nostril once daily (55 mcg/day); patients not adequately responding may use 2 sprays per nostril once daily (110 mcg/day); once symptoms are controlled, dosage may be reduced to 1 spray per nostril once daily (55 mcg/day). Total daily dosage should not exceed 2 sprays in each nostril (110 mcg/day).

Children ≥12 years and Adolescents: Refer to adult dosing.

Avamys (fluticasone furoate) [Canadian product]:

Children 2 to 11 years: Initial: 1 spray (27.5 mcg/spray) per nostril once daily (55 mcg/day); patients not adequately responding may use 2 sprays per nostril once daily (110 mcg/day); once symptoms are controlled, dosage should be reduced to 1 spray per nostril once daily (55 mcg/day). Total daily dosage should not exceed 2 sprays in each nostril (110 mcg/day).

Children ≥12 years and Adolescents: Refer to adult dosing.

Renal Impairment No dosage adjustment necessary.

Hepatic Impairment

US labeling: There are no dosage adjustments provided in the manufacturer's labeling; use caution in moderate to severe impairment due to extensive hepatic metabolism.

Canadian labeling: No dosage adjustment is necessary; however, increased monitoring is recommended.

Additional Information Complete prescribing information should be consulted for additional detail.

Dosage Forms Considerations Flonase 16 g bottles and Veramyst 10 g bottles contain 120 sprays each.

Dosage Forms Excipient information presented when available (limited, particularly for generics); consult specific product labeling. [DSC] = Discontinued product

Suspension, Nasal, as furoate:

Veramyst: 27.5 mcg/spray (10 g) [contains benzalkonium chloride]

Suspension, Nasal, as propionate:

Flonase: 50 mcg/actuation (16 g [DSC]) [contains benzalkonium chloride, polysorbate 80]

Flonase Allergy Relief: 50 mcg/actuation (9.9 mL, 15.8 mL) [contains benzalkonium chloride, polysorbate 80]

Generic: 50 mcg/actuation (16 g)

Dosage Forms: Canada Excipient information presented when available (limited, particularly for generics); consult specific product labeling.

Suspension, Nasal, as furoate:

Avamys: 27.5 mcg/inhalation (4.5 g) [30 metered actuations; contains benzalkonium chloride]; (10 g) [120 metered actuations; contains benzalkonium chloride]

Suspension, Nasal, as propionate:

Flonase: 50 mcg/actuation (16 g) [120 metered actuations; contains benzalkonium chloride, polysorbate 80]

Fluticasone (Topical) (floo TIK a sone)

Brand Names: US Cutivate
Brand Names: Canada Cutivate
Index Terms Fluticasone Propionate

Pharmacologic Category Corticosteroid, Topical
Additional Appendix Information

Topical Corticosteroids *on page 1952*

Use Dermatoses:

Lotion: For the relief of the inflammatory and pruritic manifestations of atopic dermatoses in patients 3 months of age or older.

Cream and ointment: For the relief of the inflammatory and pruritic manifestations of corticosteroid-responsive dermatoses in patients 3 months of age or older. Ointment is indicated for use in adults only.

Dosing

Adult & Geriatric

Corticosteroid-responsive dermatoses: Topical: Cream, ointment: Apply a thin film to affected area twice daily. If no improvement is seen within 2 weeks, reassessment of diagnosis may be necessary.

Atopic dermatitis: Topical:

Cream: Apply a thin film to affected area 1 to 2 times daily. If no improvement is seen within 2 weeks, reassessment of diagnosis may be necessary.

Lotion: Apply a thin film to affected area once daily. If no improvement is seen within 2 weeks, reassessment of diagnosis may be necessary.

Pediatric

Corticosteroid-responsive dermatoses: Topical: Cream: Infants ≥3 months, Children, and Adolescents: Refer to adult dosing.

Atopic dermatitis: Topical: Cream, lotion: Infants ≥3 months, Children, and Adolescents: Refer to adult dosing.

Renal Impairment There are no dosage adjustments provided in the manufacturer's labeling.

Hepatic Impairment There are no dosage adjustments provided in the manufacturer's labeling.

Additional Information Complete prescribing information should be consulted for additional detail.

Dosage Forms Excipient information presented when available (limited, particularly for generics); consult specific product labeling.

Cream, External, as propionate:

Cutivate: 0.05% (30 g, 60 g) [contains cetyl alcohol, propylene glycol]

Generic: 0.05% (15 g, 30 g, 60 g)

Lotion, External, as propionate:

Cutivate: 0.05% (120 mL) [contains cetostearyl alcohol, methylparaben, propylene glycol, propylparaben]

Generic: 0.05% (60 mL, 120 mL)

Ointment, External, as propionate:

Cutivate: 0.005% (30 g, 60 g)

Generic: 0.005% (15 g, 30 g, 60 g)

Fluticasone and Salmeterol
(floo TIK a sone & sal ME te role)

Brand Names: US Advair Diskus; Advair HFA
Brand Names: Canada Advair; Advair Diskus
Index Terms Fluticasone Propionate and Salmeterol Xinafoate; Salmeterol and Fluticasone
Pharmacologic Category Beta$_2$ Agonist; Beta$_2$-Adrenergic Agonist, Long-Acting; Corticosteroid, Inhalant (Oral)
Use

Asthma: Treatment of asthma in patients 4 years and older (Diskus) and in patients 12 years and older (HFA).

Chronic obstructive pulmonary disease (Diskus only): Twice-daily maintenance treatment of airflow obstruction in patients with chronic obstructive pulmonary disease (COPD), including chronic bronchitis and/or emphysema. Fluticasone 250 mcg/salmeterol 50 mcg Diskus is also indicated to reduce exacerbations of COPD in patients with a history of exacerbations.

Fluticasone 250 mcg/salmeterol 50 mcg Diskus twice daily is the only approved dosage for the treatment of COPD because an efficacy advantage of the higher strength fluticasone 500 mcg/salmeterol 50 mcg Diskus over fluticasone 250 mcg/salmeterol 50 mcg Diskus has not been demonstrated.

General information: Fluticasone/salmeterol is not indicated for the relief of acute bronchospasm.

Pregnancy Considerations Adverse events were observed in animal reproduction studies using this combination. Refer to individual agents.

Breast-Feeding Considerations It is not known if fluticasone or salmeterol are excreted into breast milk. The manufacturer recommends that caution be used if administering this combination to breast-feeding women. Refer to individual agents.

Medication Guide Available Yes

Contraindications

Hypersensitivity to fluticasone, salmeterol, or any component of the formulation; status asthmaticus; acute episodes of asthma or COPD; severe hypersensitivity to milk proteins (Advair Diskus)

Documentation of allergenic cross-reactivity for corticosteroids and sympathomimetics are limited. However, because of similarities in chemical structure and/or pharmacologic actions, the possibility of cross-sensitivity cannot be ruled out with certainty.

Warnings/Precautions See individual agents.

Adverse Reactions

>10%:

Central nervous system: Headache (12% to 21%)

Respiratory: Upper respiratory tract infection (16% to 27%), pharyngitis (9% to 13%)

>3% to 10%:

Central nervous system: Dizziness (1% to 4%), pain (1% to 4%)

Gastrointestinal: Nausea (3% to 6%), vomiting (3% to 6%), gastrointestinal infection (≤4%; including viral), diarrhea (2% to 4%), oral candidiasis (1% to 4%)

Neuromuscular & skeletal: Musculoskeletal pain (2% to 7%), myalgia (≤4%)

Respiratory: Throat irritation (7% to 9%), bronchitis (2% to 8%), upper respiratory tract inflammation (4% to 7%), lower respiratory tract infection (1% to 7%; COPD diagnosis and age >65 years increase risk), cough (3% to 6%), sinusitis (4% to 5%), viral respiratory tract infection (3% to 5%), hoarseness (1% to 5%)

1% to 3%:

Cardiovascular: Cardiac arrhythmia, chest symptoms, edema, myocardial infarction, palpitations, syncope, tachycardia

Central nervous system: Migraine, mouth pain, sleep disorder

Dermatologic: Dermatitis, diaphoresis, eczema, exfoliation of skin, urticaria, viral skin infection

Endocrine & metabolic: Fluid retention, hypothyroidism, weight gain

Gastrointestinal: Constipation, dysgeusia, oral mucosa ulcer

Genitourinary: Urinary tract infection

Hematologic & oncologic: Hematoma

Hepatic: Abnormal hepatic function tests

Hypersensitivity: Hypersensitivity reaction

Infection: Candidiasis (≤3%), bacterial infection, viral infection

Neuromuscular & skeletal: Muscle injury (≤3%), arthralgia, bone disease, bone fracture, muscle cramps, muscle rigidity, muscle spasm, ostealgia, rheumatoid arthritis, tremor

Ophthalmic: Conjunctivitis, eye redness, keratitis, xerophthalmia

Respiratory: Chest congestion, ENT infection, epistaxis, laryngitis, lower respiratory signs and symptoms (hemorrhage), nasal signs and symptoms (irritation), rhinitis, rhinorrhea, sneezing

Miscellaneous: Burn, laceration, wound

<1% (Limited to important or life-threatening): Aggressive behavior, atrial fibrillation, cataract, Churg-Strauss syndrome, Cushing's syndrome, decreased linear skeletal growth rate, depression, dysmenorrhea, ecchymoses, esophageal candidiasis, exacerbation of asthma (serious and some fatal), glaucoma, hyperactivity, hyperglycemia, hypersensitivity reaction (immediate and delayed), hypertension, hypokalemia, hypothyroidism, influenza, irritability, lassitude, myositis, osteoporosis, pallor, paranasal sinus disease, paresthesia, pelvic inflammatory disease, photodermatitis, skin rash, supraventricular tachycardia, syncope, tracheitis, ventricular tachycardia, vulvovaginitis

Drug Interactions

Metabolism/Transport Effects Refer to individual components.

Avoid Concomitant Use

Avoid concomitant use of Fluticasone and Salmeterol with any of the following: Aldesleukin; BCG (Intravesical); Beta-Blockers (Nonselective); Cobicistat; Conivaptan; CYP3A4 Inhibitors (Strong); Fusidic Acid (Systemic); Idelalisib; Iobenguane I 123; Long-Acting Beta2-Agonists; Loxapine; Natalizumab; Pimecrolimus; Tacrolimus (Topical); Telaprevir; Tipranavir; Tofacitinib

Increased Effect/Toxicity

Fluticasone and Salmeterol may increase the levels/ effects of: Amphotericin B; Atosiban; Deferasirox; Doxofylline; Fingolimod; Highest Risk QTc-Prolonging Agents; Leflunomide; Long-Acting Beta2-Agonists; Loop Diuretics; Loxapine; Moderate Risk QTc-Prolonging Agents; Natalizumab; Sympathomimetics; Thiazide Diuretics; Tofacitinib

The levels/effects of Fluticasone and Salmeterol may be increased by: Aprepitant; AtoMOXetine; Cannabinoid-Containing Products; Cobicistat; Conivaptan; CYP3A4 Inhibitors (Moderate); CYP3A4 Inhibitors (Strong); Dasatinib; Denosumab; Fosaprepitant; Fusidic Acid (Systemic); Idelalisib; Ivacaftor; Linezolid; Luliconazole; MAO Inhibitors; Mifepristone; Netupitant; Osimertinib; Palbociclib; Pimecrolimus; Simeprevir; Stiripentol; Tacrolimus (Topical); Tedizolid; Telaprevir; Tipranavir; Trastuzumab; Tricyclic Antidepressants

Decreased Effect

Fluticasone and Salmeterol may decrease the levels/ effects of: Aldesleukin; BCG (Intravesical); Coccidioides immitis Skin Test; Corticorelin; Hyaluronidase; Iobenguane I 123; Sipuleucel-T; Vaccines (Inactivated)

The levels/effects of Fluticasone and Salmeterol may be decreased by: Beta-Blockers (Beta1 Selective); Beta-Blockers (Nonselective); Betahistine; Echinacea; Osimertinib

Storage/Stability

Advair Diskus: Store at 20°C to 25°C (68°F to 77°F). Store in a dry place out of direct heat or sunlight. Diskus device should be discarded 1 month after removal from foil pouch, or when dosing indicator reads "0" (whichever comes first); device is not reusable.

Advair HFA: Store at 20°C to 25°C (68°F to 77°F), excursions permitted from 15°C to 30°C (59°F to 86°F). Store with mouthpiece down. Discard after 120 inhalations. Discard device when the dose counter reads "000". Device is not reusable.

Mechanism of Action Combination of fluticasone (corticosteroid) and salmeterol (long-acting beta$_2$-agonist) designed to improve pulmonary function and control over what is produced by either agent when used alone. Because fluticasone and salmeterol act locally in the lung, plasma levels do not predict therapeutic effect.

Fluticasone: The mechanism of action for all topical corticosteroids is believed to be a combination of three important properties: Anti-inflammatory activity, immunosuppressive properties, and antiproliferative actions. Fluticasone has extremely potent vasoconstrictive and anti-inflammatory activity.

Salmeterol: Relaxes bronchial smooth muscle by selective action on beta$_2$-receptors with little effect on heart rate

Pharmacodynamics/Kinetics See individual agents.

Dosing

Adult & Geriatric Do not use to transfer patients from systemic corticosteroid therapy. Patients receiving fluticasone/salmeterol should not use additional salmeterol or other inhaled, long-acting beta$_2$-agonists (eg, formoterol, arformoterol) for any other reason.

COPD: Oral Inhalation: Advair Diskus:

US labeling: Fluticasone 250 mcg/salmeterol 50 mcg twice daily, 12 hours apart. **Note:** This is the maximum dose.

Canadian labeling: Fluticasone 250 mcg/salmeterol 50 mcg or fluticasone 500 mcg/salmeterol 50 mcg twice daily, 12 hours apart.

Asthma (maintenance): Oral inhalation:

Advair Diskus: One inhalation twice daily, morning and evening, 12 hours apart

Maximum dose: Fluticasone 500 mcg/salmeterol 50 mcg per inhalation (2 inhalations/day)

Advair HFA: Two inhalations twice daily, morning and evening, 12 hours apart

Maximum dose: Fluticasone 230 mcg/salmeterol 21 mcg per inhalation (4 inhalations/day)

Advair 125 or Advair 250 [Canadian products]: Two inhalations twice daily, morning and evening, 12 hours apart

Note: Initial dose prescribed should be based upon asthma severity. Dose should be increased after 2 weeks if adequate response is not achieved. Patients should be titrated to lowest effective dose once stable.

Pediatric Patients receiving fluticasone/salmeterol should not use additional salmeterol or other inhaled, long-acting beta$_2$-agonists (eg, formoterol, arformoterol) for any other reason.

Asthma: Oral inhalation:

Children 4 to 11 years: Advair Diskus: Fluticasone 100 mcg/salmeterol 50 mcg twice daily, 12 hours apart. **Note:** This is the maximum dose.

Children ≥12 years: Refer to adult dosing.

Renal Impairment

US labeling: There are no dosage adjustments provided in the manufacturer's labeling (has not been studied).

Canadian labeling: No dosage adjustment necessary.

Hepatic Impairment No dosage adjustment required; manufacturer suggests close monitoring of patients with hepatic impairment.

◄

Dietary Considerations Advair Diskus powder for oral inhalation contains lactose; very rare anaphylactic reactions have been reported in patients with severe milk protein allergy.

Administration

Advair Diskus: After removing from box and foil pouch, write the "Pouch opened" and "Use by" dates on the label on top of the Diskus. The "Use by" date is 1 month from date of opening the pouch. Every time the lever is pushed back, a dose is ready to be inhaled. Do not close or tilt the Diskus after the lever is pushed back. Do not play with the lever or move the lever more than once. The dose indicator tells you how many doses are left. When the numbers 5 to 0 appear in red, only a few doses remain. Discard device 1 month after you remove it from the foil pouch or when the dose counter reads "0" (whichever comes first). Rinse mouth with water after use and spit to reduce risk of oral candidiasis.

Advair HFA: Shake well for 5 seconds before each spray. Prime with 4 test sprays (into air and away from face) before using for the first time. If canister is dropped or not used for >4 weeks, prime with 2 sprays. Patient should contact pharmacy for refill when the dose counter reads "020". Discard device when the dose counter reads "000". Do not spray in eyes. Rinse mouth with water after use and spit to reduce risk of oral candidiasis.

Monitoring Parameters FEV_1, peak flow, and/or other pulmonary function tests; blood pressure, heart rate; CNS stimulation; glaucoma and cataracts. Monitor for increased use of short-acting beta$_2$-agonist inhalers; may be marker of a deteriorating asthma condition. The growth of pediatric patients receiving inhaled corticosteroids should be monitored routinely (eg, via stadiometry).

Additional Information Effects of inhaled/intranasal steroids on growth have been observed in the absence of laboratory evidence of HPA axis suppression, suggesting that growth velocity is a more sensitive indicator of systemic corticosteroid exposure in pediatric patients than some commonly used tests of HPA axis function. The long-term effects of this reduction in growth velocity associated with orally-inhaled and intranasal corticosteroids, including the impact on final adult height, are unknown. The potential for "catch up" growth following discontinuation of treatment with inhaled corticosteroids has not been adequately studied.

Advair HFA: Salmeterol (base) 21 mcg is equivalent to 30.45 mcg of salmeterol xinafoate.

Dosage Forms Excipient information presented when available (limited, particularly for generics); consult specific product labeling.

Aerosol, for oral inhalation:

Advair HFA:

45/21: Fluticasone propionate 45 mcg and salmeterol 21 mcg per inhalation (8 g) [chlorofluorocarbon free; 60 metered actuations]

45/21: Fluticasone propionate 45 mcg and salmeterol 21 mcg per inhalation (12 g) [chlorofluorocarbon free; 120 metered actuations]

115/21: Fluticasone propionate 115 mcg and salmeterol 21 mcg per inhalation (8 g) [chlorofluorocarbon free; 60 metered actuations]

115/21: Fluticasone propionate 115 mcg and salmeterol 21 mcg per inhalation (12 g) [chlorofluorocarbon free; 120 metered actuations]

230/21: Fluticasone propionate 230 mcg and salmeterol 21 mcg per inhalation (8 g) [chlorofluorocarbon free; 60 metered actuations]

230/21: Fluticasone propionate 230 mcg and salmeterol 21 mcg per inhalation (12 g) [chlorofluorocarbon free; 120 metered actuations]

Powder, for oral inhalation:

Advair Diskus:

100/50: Fluticasone propionate 100 mcg and salmeterol 50 mcg (14s, 60s) [contains lactose]

250/50: Fluticasone propionate 250 mcg and salmeterol 50 mcg (14s, 60s) [contains lactose]

500/50: Fluticasone propionate 500 mcg and salmeterol 50 mcg (14s, 60s) [contains lactose]

Dosage Forms: Canada Excipient information presented when available (limited, particularly for generics); consult specific product labeling.

Aerosol, for oral inhalation:

Advair;

125/25: Fluticasone propionate 125 mcg and salmeterol 25 mcg per inhalation (12 g) [120 metered actuations]

250/25: Fluticasone propionate 250 mcg and salmeterol 25 mcg per inhalation (12 g) [120 metered actuations]

Fluticasone and Vilanterol
(floo TIK a sone & VYE lan ter ol)

Brand Names: US Breo Ellipta

Brand Names: Canada Breo Ellipta

Index Terms Fluticasone Furoate and Vilanterol; Vilanterol and Fluticasone; Vilanterol and Fluticasone Furoate

Pharmacologic Category Beta$_2$ Agonist; Beta$_2$-Adrenergic Agonist, Long-Acting; Corticosteroid, Inhalant (Oral)

Use

Asthma: Treatment of asthma in patients ≥18 years.

Chronic obstructive pulmonary disease: Maintenance treatment of airflow obstruction in patients with chronic obstructive pulmonary disease (COPD), including chronic bronchitis and/or emphysema; to reduce exacerbations of COPD in patients with a history of exacerbations Fluticasone 100 mcg/vilanterol 25 mcg is the only strength indicated for the treatment of COPD.

Limitations of use: Not indicated for the relief of acute bronchospasm.

Pregnancy Considerations Adverse events have not been observed in animal reproduction studies. Hypoadrenalism may occur in infants born to mothers receiving corticosteroids during pregnancy (refer to the Fluticasone [Oral Inhalation] monograph for additional details). Beta-agonists have the potential to affect uterine contractility if administered during labor.

Breast-Feeding Considerations It is not known if sufficient quantities of fluticasone or vilanterol are absorbed following inhalation to produce detectable amounts in breast milk. The manufacturer recommends that caution be exercised when administering fluticasone/vilanterol to breast-feeding women.

Medication Guide Available Yes

Contraindications Hypersensitivity to fluticasone, vilanterol or any component of the formulation; severe hypersensitivity to milk proteins; primary treatment of status asthmaticus or other acute episodes of COPD or asthma where intensive measures are required

Warnings/Precautions [US Boxed Warning]: Long-acting beta$_2$-adrenergic agonists (LABAs) increase the risk of asthma-related death; fluticasone and vilanterol should only be used in patients not adequately controlled on other long-term asthma control medication (ie, inhaled corticosteroid) or whose disease severity requires initiation of treatment with both an inhaled corticosteroid and a LABA. Data from a placebo-controlled trial that compared the safety of another LABA (salmeterol) with placebo added to asthma therapy showed an increase in asthma-related deaths in subjects receiving salmeterol; this finding is considered a class effect of LABAs, including vilanterol. Assess patients at regular intervals once asthma control is maintained on combination therapy to determine if step-down therapy is appropriate (without loss of asthma control), and the patient can be maintained on an inhaled corticosteroid only. LABAs are not appropriate in patients whose asthma is adequately controlled on low- or medium-dose inhaled corticosteroids. Data are not available to determine whether the rate of death in patients with COPD is increased by LABA.

Do **not** use for acute bronchospasm or acute symptomatic COPD. Short-acting beta$_2$-agonist (eg, albuterol) should be used for acute symptoms and symptoms occurring between treatments. Do **not** initiate in patients with significantly worsening or acutely deteriorating COPD. Therapy should not be used more than once daily; do not exceed recommended dose. Do not use with other long-acting beta$_2$-agonists; clinically significant cardiovascular effects and fatalities have been reported in association with excessive use of inhaled sympathomimetic drugs. Patients must be instructed to use short-acting beta$_2$-agonist (eg, albuterol) for acute COPD symptoms and to seek medical attention in cases where acute symptoms are not relieved or a previous level of response is diminished. The need to increase frequency of use of inhaled short-acting beta$_2$-agonist may indicate deterioration of COPD, and medical evaluation must not be delayed.

Severe hypersensitivity, including anaphylaxis, angioedema, rash and urticaria may occur; discontinue fluticasone/vilanterol if a hypersensitivity reaction occurs. Contains lactose; anaphylactic reactions have been reported in patients with severe milk protein allergy using other lactose-containing powder products. Can produce paradoxical bronchospasm, which may be life threatening. If paradoxical bronchospasm occurs following, fluticasone/vilanterol should be discontinued immediately and alternative therapy should be instituted. An increase in the incidence of pneumonia and other lower respiratory tract

infections (some fatal) have been reported in patients with COPD following use; monitor COPD patients closely since pneumonia symptoms may overlap symptoms of exacerbations.

Use caution in patients with cardiovascular disease, especially coronary insufficiency (arrhythmia, hypertension), seizure disorders, diabetes, ocular disease (increased intraocular pressure, cataracts, and/or glaucoma), osteoporosis, hepatic impairment (moderate to severe), thyrotoxicosis, or hypokalemia. Long-term use may affect bone mineral density in adults. Infections with Candida albicans in the mouth and throat (thrush) have been reported with use. Withdraw systemic corticosteroid therapy with gradual tapering of dose (eg, patients on prednisone may decrease dose by 2.5 mg weekly during inhaled corticosteroid therapy). Monitor lung function, beta-agonist use, asthma and COPD symptoms, and for signs and symptoms of adrenal insufficiency (fatigue, lassitude, weakness, nausea and vomiting, hypotension) during withdrawal. Allergic conditions (eg, eosinophilic conditions, rhinitis, eczema, arthritis, conjunctivitis) may be unmasked when transitioning from systemic to inhaled corticosteroid therapy. Potentially significant drug-drug interactions may exist, requiring dose or frequency adjustment, additional monitoring, and/or selection of alternative therapy.

Fluticasone may cause hypercorticism or suppression of hypothalamic-pituitary-adrenal (HPA) axis, including adrenal crisis, in patients sensitive to these effects. Withdrawal and discontinuation of a corticosteroid should be done slowly and carefully. Particular care is required when patients are transferred from systemic corticosteroids to inhaled corticosteroids; deaths due to adrenal insufficiency have occurred in patients with asthma during and after transfer from systemic steroids to a less systemically available inhaled corticosteroid. Patients receiving ≥20 mg per day of prednisone (or equivalent) may be most susceptible. Fluticasone/vilanterol does not provide the systemic steroid dose needed to treat patients having trauma, surgery, or infections. Do not use this product to transfer patients from oral corticosteroid therapy. Observe patients carefully for any evidence of systemic corticosteroid effects; particular care should be taken in observing patients postoperatively or during periods of stress for evidence of inadequate adrenal response. If systemic corticosteroid withdrawal effects occur (eg, fatigue, lassitude, weakness, nausea, vomiting, hypotension), taper fluticasone/vilanterol slowly and other treatments for management of COPD symptoms should be considered.

[US Boxed Warning]: Data from controlled clinical trials suggest LABAs increase the risk of asthma-related hospitalization in pediatric and adolescent patients. Orally-inhaled corticosteroids may cause a reduction in growth velocity in pediatric patients (~1 centimeter per year [range: 0.3 to 1.8 cm per year] and related to dose and duration of exposure). To minimize the systemic effects of orally-inhaled corticosteroids, each patient should be titrated to the lowest effective dose. Growth should be routinely monitored in pediatric patients.

Use increases susceptibility to infections (eg, chickenpox and measles, sometimes more serious or even fatal, in susceptible children or adults using corticosteroids). Avoid exposure in such patients who have not had these diseases or been properly immunized. Use with caution (if at all) in patients with active or quiescent tuberculosis infections of the respiratory tract; systemic fungal, bacterial, viral, or parasitic infections; or ocular herpes simplex.

Adverse Reactions Also see fluticasone (oral inhalation) monograph.

1% to 10%:
Cardiovascular: Hypertension (≥3%), peripheral edema (≥3%), extrasystoles (≥2%), supraventricular extrasystole (≥2%), ventricular premature contractions (≥2%)
Central nervous system: Headache (5% to 8%)
Gastrointestinal: Oropharyngeal candidiasis (2% to 5%), diarrhea (≥3%), upper abdominal pain (≥2%)
Infection: Influenza (≥3%)
Neuromuscular & skeletal: Arthralgia (2% to ≥3%), back pain (2% to ≥3%), bone fracture (2%)
Respiratory: Nasopharyngitis (6% to 10%), upper respiratory tract infection (≥2% to 7%), pneumonia (2% to 7%), oropharyngeal pain (2% to ≥3%), pharyngitis (2% to ≥3%), chronic obstructive pulmonary disease (≥3%), cough (1% to ≥3%), sinusitis (1% to ≥3%), bronchitis (<1% to ≥3%), acute sinusitis (≥2%), allergic rhinitis (≥2%), rhinitis (≥2%), viral respiratory tract infection (≥2%), voice disorder (2%)
Miscellaneous: Fever (2% to ≥3%)
<1% (Limited to important or life-threatening): Anaphylaxis, angioedema, glaucoma, hypersensitivity reaction, palpitations, paradoxical bronchospasm, tachycardia

Drug Interactions
Metabolism/Transport Effects Refer to individual components.

Avoid Concomitant Use
Avoid concomitant use of Fluticasone and Vilanterol with any of the following: Aldesleukin; BCG (Intravesical); Beta-Blockers (Nonselective); Cobicistat; Conivaptan; Fusidic Acid (Systemic); Idelalisib; Iobenguane I 123; Long-Acting Beta2-Agonists; Loxapine; Natalizumab; Pimecrolimus; Tacrolimus (Topical); Tipranavir; Tofacitinib

Increased Effect/Toxicity
Fluticasone and Vilanterol may increase the levels/effects of: Amphotericin B; Atosiban; Deferasirox; Doxofylline; Fingolimod; Highest Risk QTc-Prolonging Agents; Leflunomide; Long-Acting Beta2-Agonists; Loop Diuretics; Loxapine; Moderate Risk QTc-Prolonging Agents; Natalizumab; Sympathomimetics; Thiazide Diuretics; Tofacitinib

The levels/effects of Fluticasone and Vilanterol may be increased by: Aprepitant; AtoMOXetine; Cannabinoid-Containing Products; Cobicistat; Conivaptan; CYP3A4 Inhibitors (Moderate); CYP3A4 Inhibitors (Strong); Dasatinib; Denosumab; Fosaprepitant; Fusidic Acid (Systemic); Idelalisib; Ivacaftor; Linezolid; Luliconazole; MAO Inhibitors; Mifepristone; Netupitant; Osimertinib; Palbociclib; Pimecrolimus; Simeprevir; Stiripentol; Tacrolimus (Topical); Tedizolid; Tipranavir; Trastuzumab; Tricyclic Antidepressants

Decreased Effect
Fluticasone and Vilanterol may decrease the levels/effects of: Aldesleukin; BCG (Intravesical); Coccidioides immitis Skin Test; Corticorelin; Hyaluronidase; Iobenguane I 123; Sipuleucel-T; Vaccines (Inactivated)

The levels/effects of Fluticasone and Vilanterol may be decreased by: Beta-Blockers (Beta1 Selective); Beta-Blockers (Nonselective); Betahistine; Echinacea; Osimertinib

Storage/Stability Store between 20°C and 25°C (68°F and 77°F); excursions permitted from 15°C to 30°C (59°F to 86°F). Store in a dry place away from heat and sunlight. Store inside the unopened foil tray prior to initial use. Discard 6 weeks after opening the foil tray or after the labeled number of inhalations have been used, whichever comes first.

Mechanism of Action
Fluticasone is a corticosteroid with anti-inflammatory activity, immunosuppressive properties, and antiproliferative actions.
Vilanterol, a long-acting beta₂-agonist, relaxes bronchial smooth muscle by selective action on beta₂-receptors with little effect on heart rate.

Pharmacodynamics/Kinetics See individual agents.
Dosing
Adult & Geriatric
Asthma: Oral inhalation: One inhalation (fluticasone 100 mcg/vilanterol 25 mcg or fluticasone 200 mcg/vilanterol 25 mcg) once daily (maximum: 1 inhalation [fluticasone 200 mcg/vilanterol 25 mcg] once daily). Recommended starting dose is determined according to asthma severity. For patients not adequately controlled on the lower combination dose, consider the higher dose combination. Reevaluate treatment regimen if previously effective dose does not provide adequate improvement in asthma control.

Chronic obstructive pulmonary disease (COPD): Oral inhalation: One inhalation (fluticasone 100 mcg/vilanterol 25 mcg) once daily (maximum: 1 inhalation [fluticasone 100 mcg/vilanterol 25 mcg] once daily).

Renal Impairment No dosage adjustment necessary.
Hepatic Impairment
US labeling: No dosage adjustment necessary. Use with caution in moderate or severe impairment; systemic fluticasone exposure may be increased up to threefold.
Canadian labeling:
Mild impairment: No dosage adjustment necessary.
Moderate or severe impairment: Maximum dose: One inhalation (fluticasone 100 mg/vilanterol 25 mcg) once daily.

Administration Oral inhalation: Administer at the same time each day. Do not use more than one inhalation in 24 hours; may cause adverse effects. Discard device 6 weeks after it is removed from the foil tray or when the dose counter reads "0" (whichever comes first). Do not open the cover of the inhaler until ready for use; each time cover is opened, 1 dose of medicine is prepared. Exhale fully before taking one long, steady, deep breath through the mouthpiece (do not breathe through nose); hold breath for 3 to 4 seconds and exhale slowly and gently. Patient should rinse mouth with water after inhalation and expectorate rinse solution.

◀ **Monitoring Parameters** FEV_1, peak flow, and/or other pulmonary function tests; bone mineral density (at baseline and periodically thereafter); blood pressure, heart rate; serum potassium (hypokalemic patients) and glucose (diabetic patients); ocular changes (intraocular pressure, cataracts); signs/symptoms of oral or systemic infection, hypercorticism, or adrenal suppression

Dosage Forms Excipient information presented when available (limited, particularly for generics); consult specific product labeling.

Powder, for oral inhalation:

Breo Ellipta: Fluticasone furoate 100 mcg and vilanterol 25 mcg per actuation (28s, 60s) [contains lactose; blister pack]

♦ Fluticasone Furoate see Fluticasone (Nasal) on page 795

♦ Fluticasone Furoate see Fluticasone (Oral Inhalation) on page 792

♦ Fluticasone Furoate and Vilanterol see Fluticasone and Vilanterol on page 798

♦ Fluticasone Propionate see Fluticasone (Nasal) on page 795

♦ Fluticasone Propionate see Fluticasone (Oral Inhalation) on page 792

♦ Fluticasone Propionate see Fluticasone (Topical) on page 796

♦ Fluticasone Propionate and Azelastine Hydrochloride see Azelastine and Fluticasone on page 188

♦ Fluticasone Propionate and Salmeterol Xinafoate see Fluticasone and Salmeterol on page 796

Fluvastatin (FLOO va sta tin)

Brand Names: US Lescol XL; Lescol [DSC]
Brand Names: Canada Lescol; Lescol XL; Teva-Fluvastatin
Pharmacologic Category Antilipemic Agent, HMG-CoA Reductase Inhibitor
Use
Dyslipidemias:
Heterozygous familial and nonfamilial hypercholesterolemia and mixed dyslipidemia: Adjunct to diet to reduce elevated total cholesterol (total-C), low-density lipoprotein-cholesterol (LDL-C), triglyceride, and apolipoprotein B (apo-B) levels and to increase HDL-C in adults with primary hypercholesterolemia and mixed dyslipidemia (Fredrickson types IIa and IIb)

Heterozygous familial hypercholesterolemia: As an adjunct to diet to reduce total-C, LDL-C, and apo B levels in children ≥10 years and adolescents ≤16 years of age (female patients must be at least 1 year postmenarche) with heterozygous familial hypercholesterolemia and an LDL-C that remains ≥190 mg/dL or ≥160 mg/dL (with ≥2 cardiovascular risk factors or a positive family history of premature cardiovascular disease).

Prevention of cardiovascular disease (CVD):
Secondary prevention of CVD: To slow the progression of coronary atherosclerosis in patients with coronary heart disease; reduce risk of coronary revascularization procedures in patients with coronary heart disease

Primary and secondary prevention of atherosclerotic cardiovascular disease (ASCVD) according to the American College of Cardiology/American Heart Association: To reduce the risk of ASCVD in patients with clinical ASCVD (eg, coronary heart disease, stroke/TIA, or peripheral arterial disease presumed to be of atherosclerotic origin) who are greater than 75 years of age or not a candidate for high-intensity statin therapy; in patients without clinical ASCVD if LDL-C is 190 mg/dL or greater and not a candidate for high-intensity statin therapy; in patients without clinical ASCVD who have type 1 or type 2 diabetes and are between 40 and 75 years of age; in patients with an estimated 10-year ASCVD risk 7.5% or greater and who are between 40 and 75 years of age (Stone 2013). Specific recommendations from the Kidney Disease: Improving Global Outcomes (KDIGO) organization have also been released for patients with chronic kidney disease (KDIGO [Tonelli 2013]).

Limitations of use: Has not been studied in conditions where the major abnormality is elevation of chylomicrons, very low-density lipoprotein (VLDL), or intermediate density lipoprotein (IDL) (ie, hyperlipoproteinemia types I, III, IV, or V).

Dosing
Adult & Geriatric
Heterozygous familial and nonfamilial hypercholesterolemia: Oral:
Immediate release: 40 mg once daily in the evening or 40 mg twice daily
Extended release: 80 mg once daily (anytime)
Mixed dyslipidemia: Oral:
Immediate release: 40 mg once daily in the evening or 40 mg twice daily
Extended release: 80 mg once daily (anytime)
Patients requiring ≥25% decrease in LDL-C: Oral:
Immediate release: Initial: 40 mg once daily in the evening or 40 mg twice daily
Extended release: Initial: 80 mg once daily (anytime)
Patients requiring <25% decrease in LDL-C: Oral:
Initial: Immediate release: 20 mg once daily in the evening; may increase based on tolerability and response to a maximum recommended dose of 80 mg/day, given in 2 divided doses (immediate release) or as a single daily dose (extended release)
Prevention of cardiovascular disease: ACC/AHA Blood Cholesterol Guideline recommendations to reduce the risk of atherosclerotic cardiovascular disease (ASCVD) (Stone 2013): Adults ≥21 years: Oral:
Primary prevention:
LDL-C ≥190 mg/dL: High-intensity therapy necessary; use alternate statin therapy (eg, atorvastatin, rosuvastatin)
Type 1 or 2 diabetes and age 40 to 75 years: Moderate intensity therapy:
Immediate release: 40 mg twice daily.
Extended release: 80 mg once daily.
Type 1 or 2 diabetes, age 40 to 75 years, and an estimated 10-year ASCVD risk ≥7.5%: High-intensity therapy necessary; use alternate statin therapy (eg, atorvastatin, rosuvastatin).
Age 40 to 75 years and an estimated 10-year ASCVD risk ≥7.5%: Moderate- to high-intensity therapy:
Immediate release: 40 mg twice daily or consider using high-intensity statin therapy (eg, atorvastatin, rosuvastatin).
Extended release: 80 mg once daily or consider using high-intensity statin therapy (eg, atorvastatin, rosuvastatin).
Secondary prevention:
Patient has clinical ASCVD (eg, coronary heart disease, stroke/TIA, or peripheral arterial disease presumed to be of atherosclerotic origin) or is post-CABG (AHA [Kulik 2015]) **and:**
Age ≤75 years: High-intensity therapy necessary; use alternate statin therapy (eg, atorvastatin, rosuvastatin).
Age >75 years or not a candidate for high-intensity therapy: Moderate-intensity therapy:
Immediate release: 40 mg twice daily.
Extended release: 80 mg once daily.

Concomitant use with cyclosporine or fluconazole: Immediate release: Do not exceed fluvastatin 20 mg twice daily
Pediatric
Heterozygous familial hypercholesterolemia: Children ≥10 years and Adolescents ≤16 years: Oral: Initial: 20 mg once daily; may increase every 6 weeks based on tolerability and response to a maximum recommended dose of 80 mg/day, given in 2 divided doses (immediate release) or as a single daily dose (extended release)
Concomitant use with cyclosporine or fluconazole: Immediate release: Do not exceed fluvastatin 20 mg twice daily
Renal Impairment
Mild to moderate renal impairment: No dosage adjustment necessary.
Severe renal impairment: There are no dosage adjustments provided in the manufacturer's labeling; use with caution, particularly at doses >40 mg/day (has not been studied).
Hepatic Impairment Use is contraindicated in active liver disease or unexplained transaminase elevations.
Adjustment for Toxicity
Severe muscle symptoms or fatigue: Promptly discontinue use; evaluate CPK, creatinine, and urinalysis for myoglobinuria (Stone 2013).
Mild to moderate muscle symptoms: Discontinue use until symptoms can be evaluated; evaluate patient for conditions that may increase the risk for muscle symptoms (eg, hypothyroidism, reduced renal or hepatic function, rheumatologic disorders such as polymyalgia rheumatica, steroid myopathy, vitamin D deficiency, or primary muscle diseases). Upon resolution, resume the

original or lower dose of fluvastatin. If muscle symptoms recur, discontinue fluvastatin use. After muscle symptom resolution, may then use a low dose of a different statin; gradually increase if tolerated. In the absence of continued statin use, if muscle symptoms or elevated CPK continues after 2 months, consider other causes of muscle symptoms. If determined to be due to another condition aside from statin use, may resume statin therapy at the original dose (Stone 2013).

Additional Information Complete prescribing information should be consulted for additional detail.

Dosage Forms Excipient information presented when available (limited, particularly for generics); consult specific product labeling. [DSC] = Discontinued product
Capsule, Oral:
   Lescol: 20 mg [DSC], 40 mg [DSC]
   Generic: 20 mg, 40 mg
Tablet Extended Release 24 Hour, Oral:
   Lescol XL: 80 mg
   Generic: 80 mg

◆ Fluviral (Can) see Influenza Virus Vaccine (Inactivated) on page 945

◆ Fluvirin see Influenza Virus Vaccine (Inactivated) on page 945

FluvoxaMINE (floo VOKS a meen)

Brand Names: US Luvox CR [DSC]
Brand Names: Canada ACT-Fluvoxamine; Apo-Fluvoxamine; Ava-Fluvoxamine; Dom-Fluvoxamine; Luvox; Novo-Fluvoxamine; PHL-Fluvoxamine; PMS-Fluvoxamine; ratio-Fluvoxamine; Riva-Fluvox; Sandoz-Fluvoxamine
Index Terms Luvox
Pharmacologic Category Antidepressant, Selective Serotonin Reuptake Inhibitor
Use
Obsessive-compulsive disorder: Treatment of obsessive-compulsive disorder (OCD) in pediatric patients 8 to 17 years of age and adults.
Canadian labeling: Additional use (not in US labeling): **Depression:** Treatment of depression in adults
Pregnancy Considerations Adverse events have been observed in animal reproduction studies. Fluvoxamine crosses the human placenta. An increased risk of teratogenic effects, including cardiovascular defects, may be associated with maternal use of fluvoxamine or other SSRIs; however, available information is conflicting. Nonteratogenic effects in the newborn following SSRI/SNRI exposure late in the third trimester include respiratory distress, cyanosis, apnea, seizures, temperature instability, feeding difficulty, vomiting, hypoglycemia, hypo- or hypertonia, hyper-reflexia, jitteriness, irritability, constant crying, and tremor. Symptoms may be due to the toxicity of the SSRIs/SNRIs or a discontinuation syndrome and may be consistent with serotonin syndrome associated with SSRI treatment. Persistent pulmonary hypertension of the newborn (PPHN) has also been reported with SSRI exposure. The long-term effects of *in utero* SSRI exposure on infant development and behavior are not known.

The ACOG recommends that therapy with SSRIs or SNRIs during pregnancy be individualized; treatment of depression during pregnancy should incorporate the clinical expertise of the mental health clinician, obstetrician, primary healthcare provider, and pediatrician. According to the American Psychiatric Association (APA), the risks of medication treatment should be weighed against other treatment options and untreated depression. For women who discontinue antidepressant medications during pregnancy and who may be at high risk for postpartum depression, the medications can be restarted following delivery. Treatment algorithms have been developed by the ACOG and the APA for the management of depression in women prior to conception and during pregnancy.

Breast-Feeding Considerations Fluvoxamine is excreted in breast milk. Based on case reports, the dose the infant receives is relatively small and adverse events have not been observed. Adverse events have been reported in nursing infants exposed to some SSRIs. According to the manufacturer, the decision to continue or discontinue breast-feeding during therapy should take into account the risk of exposure to the infant and the benefits of treatment to the mother.

The long-term effects on development and behavior have not been studied; therefore, fluvoxamine should be prescribed to a mother who is breast-feeding only when the benefits outweigh the potential risks. Maternal use of an SSRI during pregnancy may cause delayed milk secretion.

Medication Guide Available Yes

Contraindications
Concurrent use with alosetron, pimozide, ramelteon, thioridazine, or tizanidine; use of MAO inhibitors intended to treat psychiatric disorders (concurrently or within 14 days of discontinuing either fluvoxamine or the MAO inhibitor); initiation of fluvoxamine in a patient receiving linezolid or intravenous methylene blue.
Canadian labeling: Additional contraindications (not in US labeling): Hypersensitivity to fluvoxamine or any component of the formulation; concurrent use with astemizole, cisapride, mesoridazine, or terfenadine.

Warnings/Precautions [US Boxed Warning]: Antidepressants increase the risk of suicidal thinking and behavior in children, adolescents, and young adults (18 to 24 years of age) with major depressive disorder (MDD) and other psychiatric disorders; consider risk prior to prescribing. Short-term studies did not show an increased risk in patients >24 years of age and showed a decreased risk in patients ≥65 years. Closely monitor patients for clinical worsening, suicidality, or unusual changes in behavior, particularly during the initial 1 to 2 months of therapy or during periods of dosage adjustments (increases or decreases); the patient's family or caregiver should be instructed to closely observe the patient and communicate condition with healthcare provider. A medication guide concerning the use of antidepressants should be dispensed with each prescription. **Fluvoxamine is FDA approved for the treatment of OCD in children ≥8 years of age.**

The possibility of a suicide attempt is inherent in major depression and may persist until remission occurs. Use caution in high-risk patients. Worsening depression and severe abrupt suicidality that are not part of the presenting symptoms may require discontinuation or modification of drug therapy. The patient's family or caregiver should be alerted to monitor patients for the emergence of suicidality and associated behaviors (such as agitation, irritability, hostility, impulsivity, and hypomania) and call healthcare provider.

May worsen psychosis in some patients or precipitate a shift to mania or hypomania in patients with bipolar disorder. Patients presenting with depressive symptoms should be screened for bipolar disorder. Monotherapy in patients with bipolar disorder should be avoided. **Fluvoxamine is not FDA approved for the treatment of bipolar depression.**

Potentially life-threatening serotonin syndrome (SS) has occurred with serotonergic agents (eg, SSRIs, SNRIs), particularly when used in combination with other serotonergic agents (eg, triptans, TCAs, fentanyl, lithium, tramadol, buspirone, St John's wort, tryptophan) or agents that impair metabolism of serotonin (eg, MAO inhibitors intended to treat psychiatric disorders, other MAO inhibitors [ie, linezolid and intravenous methylene blue]). Discontinue treatment (and any concomitant serotonergic agent) immediately if signs/symptoms arise. Fluvoxamine has a low potential to impair cognitive or motor performance; caution operating hazardous machinery or driving. Use caution in patients with a previous seizure disorder rand avoid use with unstable seizure disorder. Discontinue use if seizures occur or if seizure frequency increases. Potentially significant drug-drug interactions may exist, requiring dose or frequency adjustment, additional monitoring, and/or selection of alternative therapy. Fluvoxamine levels may be lower in patients who smoke.

Risk:benefits of combined therapy with electroconvulsive therapy have not been established. Bone fractures have been associated with antidepressant treatment. Consider the possibility of a fragility fracture if an antidepressant-treated patient presents with unexplained bone pain, point tenderness, swelling, or bruising (Rabenda, 2013; Rizzoli, 2012). Use with caution in patients with hepatic dysfunction and in elderly patients. May cause hyponatremia/SIADH (elderly at increased risk); volume depletion (diuretics may increase risk). Use with caution in patients at risk of bleeding or receiving concurrent anticoagulant therapy, although not consistently noted, fluvoxamine may cause impairment in platelet function. May cause or exacerbate sexual dysfunction. Use caution in elderly patients; may be potentially inappropriate in patients with a history of falls or fractures, and may cause or exacerbate SIADH or hyponatremia; monitor sodium closely with initiation or dosage adjustments in older adults (Beers Criteria). May cause mild pupillary dilation which in susceptible individuals can lead to an episode of narrow-angle glaucoma. Consider evaluating patients who have not had an iridectomy for narrow-angle glaucoma risk factors. Impaired glucose control (eg, hyperglycemia, hypoglycemia) has been reported; monitor for signs/symptoms of loss of glucose control particularly in diabetic ▸

patients. Abrupt discontinuation or interruption of antidepressant therapy has been associated with a discontinuation syndrome. Symptoms arising may vary with antidepressant however commonly include nausea, vomiting, diarrhea, headaches, light-headedness, dizziness, diminished appetite, sweating, chills, tremors, paresthesias, fatigue, somnolence, and sleep disturbances (eg, vivid dreams, insomnia). Greater risks for developing a discontinuation syndrome have been associated with antidepressants with shorter half-lives, longer durations of treatment, and abrupt discontinuation. For antidepressants of short or intermediate half-lives, symptoms may emerge within 2 to 5 days after treatment discontinuation and last 7 to 14 days (APA, 2010; Fava, 2006; Haddad, 2001; Shelton, 2001; Warner, 2006).

Adverse Reactions Frequency varies by dosage form and indication. Adverse reactions reported as a composite of all indications.

>10%:

Central nervous system: Headache (22% to 35%), insomnia (21% to 35%), drowsiness (22% to 27%), dizziness (11% to 15%), nervousness (10% to 12%)

Gastrointestinal: Nausea (34% to 40%), diarrhea (11% to 18%), xerostomia (10% to 14%), anorexia (6% to 14%)

Genitourinary: Ejaculatory disorder (8% to 11%)

Neuromuscular & skeletal: Weakness (14% to 26%)

1% to 10%:

Cardiovascular: Chest pain (3%), palpitations (3%), vasodilation (2% to 3%), hypertension (1% to 2%), edema (≥1%), hypotension (≥1%), syncope (≥1%)

Central nervous system: Pain (10%), anxiety (5% to 8%), anorgasmia (2% to 5%), yawning (2% to 5%), abnormal dreams (3%), abnormality in thinking (3%), paresthesia (3%), agitation (2% to 3%), apathy (≥1% to 3%), central nervous system stimulation (2%), chills (2%), depression (2%), hypertonia (2%), psychoneurosis (2%), twitching (2%), amnesia (≥1%), manic reaction (≥1%), myoclonus (≥1%), psychotic reaction (≥1%), malaise (≤1%)

Dermatologic: Diaphoresis (6% to 7%), ecchymoses (4%), acne vulgaris (2%)

Endocrine & metabolic: Decreased libido (2% to 10%; incidence higher in males), hypermenorrhea (3%), weight loss (≥1% to 2%), weight gain (≥1%)

Gastrointestinal: Dyspepsia (8% to 10%), constipation (4% to 10%), vomiting (5% to 6%), abdominal pain (5%), flatulence (4%), dysgeusia (2% to 3%), dysphagia (2%), gingivitis (2%)

Genitourinary: Urinary frequency (3%), sexual disorder (2% to 3%), impotence (2%), urinary tract infection (2%), urinary retention (1%)

Hepatic: Abnormal hepatic function tests (2%)

Infection: Viral infection (2%)

Neuromuscular & skeletal: Tremor (5% to 8%), myalgia (5%), hyperkinesia (≥1%), hypokinesia (≥1%)

Ophthalmic: Amblyopia (2% to 3%)

Renal: Polyuria (2%)

Respiratory: Upper respiratory tract infection (9%), pharyngitis (6%), flu-like symptoms (3%), laryngitis (3%), bronchitis (2%), dyspnea (2%), epistaxis (2%), increased cough (≥1%), sinusitis (≥1%)

<1% (Limited to important or life-threatening): Acute renal failure, agranulocytosis, akinesia, anaphylaxis, anemia, angina, angioedema, angle-closure glaucoma, anuria, aplastic anemia, apnea, asthma, ataxia, bradycardia, bullous skin disease, cardiac conduction delay, cardiac failure, cardiomyopathy, cardiorespiratory arrest, cerebrovascular accident, cholecystitis, cholelithiasis, colitis, coronary artery disease, decreased white blood cell count, dental caries, dental extraction, diplopia, dyskinesia, dystonia, extrapyramidal reaction, first degree atrioventricular block, gastrointestinal hemorrhage, goiter, hallucination, hematemesis, hematuria, hemoptysis, hepatitis, homicidal ideation, hypercholesterolemia, hyperglycemia, hypersensitivity reaction, hypoglycemia, hypokalemia, hyponatremia, hypothyroidism, IgA vasculitis, interstitial pulmonary disease, intestinal obstruction, jaundice, leukocytosis, leukopenia, loss of consciousness, lymphadenopathy, myasthenia, myocardial infarction, myopathy, neuroleptic malignant syndrome (Stevens, 2008), pancreatitis, paralysis, pericarditis, porphyria, prolonged Q-T interval on ECG, purpura, rhabdomyolysis, seizure, serotonin syndrome, ST segment changes on ECG, Stevens-Johnson syndrome, suicidal tendencies, supraventricular extrasystole, tachycardia, tardive dyskinesia, thrombocytopenia, thromboembolism, tooth abscess, toothache, toxic epidermal necrolysis, vasculitis, ventricular arrhythmia, ventricular tachycardia (including torsades de pointes)

Drug Interactions

Metabolism/Transport Effects Substrate of CYP1A2 (major), CYP2D6 (major); **Note:** Assignment of Major/Minor substrate status based on clinically relevant drug interaction potential; **Inhibits** CYP1A2 (strong), CYP2B6 (weak), CYP2C19 (strong), CYP2C9 (weak), CYP2D6 (weak), CYP3A4 (weak)

Avoid Concomitant Use

Avoid concomitant use of FluvoxaMINE with any of the following: Agomelatine; Alosetron; Dapoxetine; Dosulepin; DULoxetine; Iobenguane I 123; Linezolid; MAO Inhibitors; Methylene Blue; Pimozide; Pomalidomide; Ramelteon; Tasimelteon; Thioridazine; TiZANidine; Tryptophan; Urokinase

Increased Effect/Toxicity

FluvoxaMINE may increase the levels/effects of: Agents with Antiplatelet Properties; Agomelatine; Alosetron; ALPRAZolam; Anticoagulants; Antidepressants (Serotonin Reuptake Inhibitor/Antagonist); Antipsychotic Agents; Apixaban; ARIPiprazole; Asenapine; Aspirin; Bendamustine; Blood Glucose Lowering Agents; Bromazepam; BusPIRone; CarBAMazepine; Cilostazol; Citalopram; Clopidogrel; CloZAPine; Collagenase (Systemic); CYP1A2 Substrates; CYP2C19 Substrates; Dabigatran Etexilate; Deoxycholic Acid; Desmopressin; Dofetilide; Dosulepin; DULoxetine; Edoxaban; Erlotinib; Etizolam; Flibanserin; Fosphenytoin; Haloperidol; Hydrocodone; Ibritumomab; Lomitapide; Methadone; Methylene Blue; Mexiletine; NiMODipine; NSAID (COX-2 Inhibitor); NSAID (Nonselective); Obinutuzumab; OLANZapine; Pentoxifylline; Phenytoin; Pimozide; Pirfenidone; Pomalidomide; Propafenone; Propranolol; QuiNIDine; Ramelteon; Rivaroxaban; Roflumilast; Ropivacaine; Salicylates; Serotonin Modulators; Tasimelteon; Theophylline Derivatives; Thiazide Diuretics; Thioridazine; Thrombolytic Agents; TiZANidine; Tositumomab and Iodine I 131 Tositumomab; TraMADol; Tricyclic Antidepressants; Urokinase; Vitamin K Antagonists; Zolpidem

The levels/effects of FluvoxaMINE may be increased by: Abiraterone Acetate; Alcohol (Ethyl); Analgesics (Opioid); Antiemetics (5HT3 Antagonists); Antipsychotic Agents; BuPROPion; BusPIRone; Cimetidine; CNS Depressants; Cobicistat; CYP1A2 Inhibitors (Moderate); CYP1A2 Inhibitors (Strong); CYP2D6 Inhibitors (Moderate); CYP2D6 Inhibitors (Strong); Dapoxetine; Darunavir; Dasatinib; Deferasirox; Glucosamine; Grapefruit Juice; Herbs (Anticoagulant/Antiplatelet Properties); Ibrutinib; Limaprost; Linezolid; Lithium; MAO Inhibitors; Metaxalone; Metoclopramide; Metyrosine; Multivitamins/Fluoride (with ADE); Multivitamins/Minerals (with ADEK, Folate, Iron); Multivitamins/Minerals (with AE, No Iron); Omega-3 Fatty Acids; Panobinostat; Peginterferon Alfa-2b; Pentosan Polysulfate Sodium; Pentoxifylline; Prostacyclin Analogues; QuiNIDine; Tedizolid; TraMADol; Tryptophan; Vemurafenib; Vitamin E; Vitamin E (Oral)

Decreased Effect

FluvoxaMINE may decrease the levels/effects of: Clopidogrel; Iobenguane I 123; Ioflupane I 123; Thyroid Products

The levels/effects of FluvoxaMINE may be decreased by: Cannabis; CarBAMazepine; CYP1A2 Inducers (Strong); Cyproheptadine; Cyproterone; NSAID (COX-2 Inhibitor); NSAID (Nonselective); Osimertinib; Peginterferon Alfa-2b; Teriflunomide

Storage/Stability Protect from high humidity and store at controlled room temperature 25°C (77°F); excursions are permitted between 15°C and 30°C (59°F and 86°F).

Mechanism of Action Inhibits CNS neuron serotonin uptake; minimal or no effect on reuptake of norepinephrine or dopamine; does not significantly bind to alpha-adrenergic, histamine or cholinergic receptors

Pharmacodynamics/Kinetics

Onset of action: Individual responses may vary; however, 8 to 12 weeks of treatment are needed for patients with obsessive-compulsive disorder and 4 to 8 weeks of treatment are needed for patients with depression before determining if a patient is partially or nonresponsive (APA, 2010; APA 2007).

Distribution: V_d: ~25 L/kg

Protein binding: ~80%, primarily to albumin

Metabolism: Extensively hepatic via oxidative demethylation and deamination

Bioavailability: Immediate release: 53%; Extended release: 84%; not significantly affected by food.

Half-life elimination: ~14 to 16 hours; ~17 to 26 hours in the elderly

Time to peak, plasma: 3 to 8 hours

Excretion: Urine (~85% as metabolites; ~2% as unchanged drug)

Dosing

Adult

Obsessive-compulsive disorder: Oral:

Immediate release: Initial: 50 mg once daily at bedtime; may be increased in 50 mg increments at 4- to 7-day intervals, as tolerated; usual dose range: 100 to 300 mg daily; maximum dose: 300 mg daily. **Note:** US labeling recommends that daily doses >100 mg be given in 2 divided doses, with the larger dose administered at bedtime. Canadian labeling recommends that daily doses >150 mg be given in 2 divided doses with the larger dose administered at bedtime (maximum bedtime dose: 150 mg); if no improvement within 10 weeks consider discontinuing fluvoxamine therapy.

Extended release: Initial: 100 mg once daily at bedtime; may be increased in 50 mg increments at intervals of at least 1 week; usual dosage range: 100 to 300 mg daily; maximum dose: 300 mg daily

Depression (Canadian labeling; not an approved use in US labeling): Oral: Immediate release: Initial: 50 mg once daily at bedtime then after a few days may increase to 100 mg daily as tolerated; titrate gradually based on response and tolerability in 50 mg increments; usual dosage range: 100 to 200 mg daily; maximum dose: 300 mg daily. Doses >150 mg daily should be divided with maximum dose of 150 mg given at bedtime.

Panic disorder (off-label use): Oral: Immediate release: Initial: 25 to 50 mg daily; titrate gradually based on response and tolerability; usual dosage range: 100 to 200 mg daily (APA, 2009; Asnis, 2001).

Post-traumatic stress disorder (PTSD) (off-label use): Oral: Immediate release: 75 mg twice daily (Spivak, 2006).

Social anxiety disorder (off-label use): Oral:

Immediate release: Initial: 50 mg once daily; may increase in 50 mg increments at intervals of at least 1 week; usual dosage range: 100 to 300 mg daily (Asakura, 2007).

Extended release: Initial: 100 mg once daily at bedtime; may be increased in 50 mg increments at intervals of at least 1 week; usual dosage range: 100 to 300 mg daily; maximum dose: 300 mg daily (Davidson, 2004; Stein, 2003; Westenberg, 2004)

Discontinuation of therapy: Upon discontinuation of antidepressant therapy, gradually taper the dose to minimize the incidence of withdrawal symptoms and allow for the detection of re-emerging symptoms. Evidence supporting ideal taper rates is limited. APA and NICE guidelines suggest tapering therapy over at least several weeks with consideration to the half-life of the antidepressant; antidepressants with a shorter half-life may need to be tapered more conservatively. In addition for long-term treated patients, WFSBP guidelines recommend tapering over 4 to 6 months. If intolerable withdrawal symptoms occur following a dose reduction, consider resuming the previously prescribed dose and/or decrease dose at a more gradual rate (APA, 2007; APA, 2010; Bauer, 2002; Haddad, 2001; NCCMH, 2010; Schatzberg, 2006; Shelton, 2001; Warner, 2006).

MAO inhibitor recommendations:

Switching to or from an MAO inhibitor intended to treat psychiatric disorders:

Allow 14 days to elapse between discontinuing an MAO inhibitor intended to treat psychiatric disorders and initiation of fluvoxamine.

Allow 14 days to elapse between discontinuing fluvoxamine and initiation of an MAO inhibitor intended to treat psychiatric disorders.

Use with other MAO inhibitors (linezolid or IV methylene blue):

Do not initiate fluvoxamine in patients receiving linezolid or IV methylene blue; consider other interventions for psychiatric condition.

If urgent treatment with linezolid or IV methylene blue is required in a patient already receiving fluvoxamine and potential benefits outweigh potential risks, discontinue fluvoxamine promptly and administer linezolid or IV methylene blue. Monitor for serotonin syndrome for 2 weeks or until 24 hours after the last dose of linezolid or IV methylene blue, whichever comes first. May resume fluvoxamine 24 hours after the last dose of linezolid or IV methylene blue. Risk of administering methylene blue by non-intravenous routes or in IV doses <1 mg/kg concurrently with fluvoxamine is unclear.

Geriatric Refer to adult dosing. Consider a lower initial dose; titrate slowly.

Pediatric Obsessive-compulsive disorder: Oral: **Note:** Not approved for use in patients <18 years of age in Canadian labeling.

Children and Adolescents 8 to 17 years:

Immediate release: Initial: 25 mg once daily at bedtime; may be increased in 25 mg increments at 4- to 7-day intervals, as tolerated, to maximum therapeutic benefit; usual dose range: 50 to 200 mg daily. **Note:** When total daily dose of immediate release exceeds 50 mg, the dose should be given in 2 divided doses with larger portion administered at bedtime.

Maximum dose: Children: 8 to 11 years: 200 mg daily; Adolescents: 300 mg daily; lower doses may be effective in female versus male patients

Extended release: The extended release formulation has not been evaluated in pediatric patients; the lowest available dose of extended release capsules may not be appropriate for pediatric patients naïve to fluvoxamine.

Discontinuation of therapy: Refer to adult dosing.

MAO inhibitor recommendations: Refer to adult dosing.

Renal Impairment There are no dosage adjustments provided in manufacturer's labeling. Limited data suggest fluvoxamine does not accumulate in patients with renal impairment. Canadian labeling recommends initiating therapy at a reduced dosage with close monitoring.

Hepatic Impairment There are no dosage adjustments provided in manufacturer's labeling. Limited data suggest fluvoxamine clearance is reduced in patients with hepatic impairment. Reduced initial dose and slow titration may be required. Monitor closely.

Administration Oral: May be administered with or without food. Do not crush, open, or chew extended release capsules. The Canadian labeling recommends that the immediate release tablet be swallowed whole.

Monitoring Parameters Evaluate mental status, suicide ideation (especially at the beginning of therapy or when doses are increased or decreased), anxiety, social functioning, mania, panic attacks or other unusual changes in behavior; signs/symptoms of serotonin syndrome; akathisia; weight and BMI; hepatic function (baseline and as clinically indicated).

Dosage Forms Excipient information presented when available (limited, particularly for generics); consult specific product labeling. [DSC] = Discontinued product

Capsule Extended Release 24 Hour, Oral, as maleate:

Luvox CR: 100 mg [DSC], 150 mg [DSC] [gluten free; contains fd&c blue #2 (indigotine)]

Generic: 100 mg, 150 mg

Tablet, Oral, as maleate:

Generic: 25 mg, 50 mg, 100 mg

Dosage Forms: Canada Note: Refer to Dosage Forms. Extended release capsules are not available in Canada.

Folic Acid (FOE lik AS id)

Brand Names: US FA-8 [OTC]
Brand Names: Canada Apo-Folic®
Index Terms Folacin; Folate; Pteroylglutamic Acid
Pharmacologic Category Vitamin, Water Soluble
Use Treatment of megaloblastic and macrocytic anemias due to folate deficiency

Pregnancy Considerations Water soluble vitamins cross the placenta. Folate requirements increase during pregnancy. Folate supplementation during the periconceptual period decreases the risk of neural tube defects (ACOG 2003; USPSTF 2009). Folate supplementation (doses larger than the RDA) is recommended for women who may become pregnant (IOM 1998). Folic acid is also indicted for the treatment of anemias due to folate deficiency in pregnant women.

Breast-Feeding Considerations Folate is excreted in breast milk; concentrations are not affected by dietary intake unless the mother has a severe deficiency. Folate requirements increase in breast-feeding women (IOM 1998).

Contraindications Hypersensitivity to folic acid or any component of the formulation

Warnings/Precautions Not appropriate for monotherapy with pernicious, aplastic, or normocytic anemias when anemia is present with vitamin B_{12} deficiency. Doses >0.1 mg/day may obscure pernicious anemia with continuing irreversible nerve damage progression. Resistance to treatment may occur with depressed hematopoiesis, alcoholism, and deficiencies of other vitamins. Injection contains benzyl alcohol (1.5%) as preservative (use care in administration to neonates).

Aluminum: The parenteral product may contain aluminum; toxic aluminum concentrations may be seen with high doses, prolonged use, or renal dysfunction. Premature neonates are at higher risk due to immature renal function and aluminum intake from other parenteral sources. Parenteral aluminum exposure of >4 to 5 mcg/kg/day is associated with CNS and bone toxicity; tissue loading may occur at lower doses (Federal Register, 2002). See manufacturer's labeling.

Benzyl alcohol and derivatives: Some dosage forms may contain benzyl alcohol; large amounts of benzyl alcohol (≥99 mg/kg/day) have been associated with a potentially fatal toxicity ("gasping syndrome") in neonates; the "gasping syndrome" consists of metabolic acidosis, respiratory distress, gasping respirations, CNS dysfunction (including convulsions, intracranial hemorrhage), hypotension and cardiovascular collapse (AAP ["Inactive" 1997]; CDC, 1982); some data suggests that benzoate displaces bilirubin from protein binding sites (Ahlfors, 2001); avoid or use dosage forms containing benzyl alcohol with caution in neonates. See manufacturer's labeling.

Adverse Reactions Frequency not defined.
Cardiovascular: Flushing (slight)
Central nervous system: Malaise (general)
Dermatologic: Erythema, pruritus, rash
Respiratory: Bronchospasm
Miscellaneous: Allergic reaction

Drug Interactions
Metabolism/Transport Effects None known.
Avoid Concomitant Use
Avoid concomitant use of Folic Acid with any of the following: Raltitrexed
Increased Effect/Toxicity There are no known significant interactions involving an increase in effect.
Decreased Effect
Folic Acid may decrease the levels/effects of: Fosphenytoin; PHENobarbital; Phenytoin; Primidone; Raltitrexed

The levels/effects of Folic Acid may be decreased by: Green Tea; SulfaSALAzine

Storage/Stability Store at 20°C to 25°C (68°F to 77°F); protect from light.

Mechanism of Action Folic acid is necessary for formation of a number of coenzymes in many metabolic systems, particularly for purine and pyrimidine synthesis; required for nucleoprotein synthesis and maintenance in erythropoiesis; stimulates WBC and platelet production in folate deficiency anemia. Folic acid enhances the metabolism of formic acid, the toxic metabolite of methanol, to nontoxic metabolites (off-label use).

Pharmacodynamics/Kinetics
Onset of action: Peak effect: Oral: 0.5-1 hour
Absorption: Proximal part of small intestine
Metabolism: Hepatic
Bioavailability: Oral: Folic acid supplement: ~100%; In presence of food: 85%; Dietary folate: 50% (IOM 1998)
Time to peak: Oral: 1 hour
Excretion: Urine

Dosing
Adult
Anemia: Oral, IM, IV, SubQ: 0.4 mg/day
Pregnant and lactating women: 0.8 mg/day
Recommended daily allowance (RDA) (IOM, 1998): Expressed as dietary folate equivalents: Oral: 400 mcg/day
Pregnancy: 600 mcg/day
Lactation: 500 mcg/day
Prevention of neural tube defects (off-label use): Oral:
Females of childbearing potential: 400-800 mcg/day (USPSTF, 2009)
Females at high risk or with family history of neural tube defects: 4 mg/day (ACOG, 2003)
Geriatric Refer to adult dosing. Vitamin B_{12} deficiency must be ruled out before initiating folate therapy due to frequency of combined nutritional deficiencies: RDA requirements (1999): 400 mcg/day (0.4 mg) minimum.
Pediatric
Anemia: Oral, IM, IV, SubQ:
Infants: 0.1 mg/day
Children <4 years: Up to 0.3 mg/day
Children >4 years and Adults: Refer to adult dosing.
Adequate intake (AI) (IOM, 1998): Expressed as folate equivalents: Oral: Infants:
1-6 months: 65 mcg/day
7-12 months: 80 mcg/day
Recommended daily allowance (RDA) (IOM, 1998): Expressed as dietary folate equivalents: Oral: Children:
1-3 years: 150 mcg/day
4-8 years: 200 mcg/day
9-13 years: 300 mcg/day
≥14 years: Refer to adult dosing.

Dietary Considerations As of January 1998, the FDA has required manufacturers of enriched flour, bread, corn meal, pasta, rice, and other grain products to add folic acid to their products. The intent is to help decrease the risk of neural tube defects by increasing folic acid intake. Other foods which contain folic acid include dark green leafy vegetables, citrus fruits and juices, and lentils.

Administration Oral preferred, but may also be administered by deep IM, SubQ, or IV injection.
IV administration: May administer ≤5 mg dose undiluted over ≥1 minute **or** may dilute ≤5 mg in 50 mL of NS or D_5W and infuse over 30 minutes. May also be added to IV maintenance solutions and given as an infusion.

Reference Range Therapeutic: 0.005-0.015 mcg/mL

Test Interactions Falsely low serum concentrations may occur with the *Lactobacillus casei* assay method in patients on anti-infectives (eg, tetracycline)

Additional Information The RDA for folic acid is presented as dietary folate equivalents (DFE). DFE adjusts for the difference in bioavailability of folic acid from food as compared to dietary supplements.

Dosage Forms Excipient information presented when available (limited, particularly for generics); consult specific product labeling.
Capsule, Oral [preservative free]:
FA-8: 0.8 mg [dye free, sugar free, yeast free]
Generic: 5 mg, 20 mg
Solution, Injection, as sodium folate:
Generic: 5 mg/mL (10 mL)
Tablet, Oral:
Generic: 400 mcg, 800 mcg, 1 mg
Tablet, Oral [preservative free]:
FA-8: 800 mcg [dye free]
Generic: 400 mcg, 800 mcg

Extemporaneous Preparations A 1 mg/mL folic acid oral solution may be made with tablets. Heat 90 mL of purified water almost to boiling. Dissolve parabens (methylparaben 200 mg and propylparaben 20 mg) in the heated water; cool to room temperature. Crush one-hundred 1 mg tablets, then dissolve folic acid in the solution. Adjust pH to 8-8.5 with sodium hydroxide 10%; add sufficient quantity of purified water to make 100 mL; mix well. Stable for 30 days at room temperature (Allen, 2007).

A 0.05 mg/mL folic acid oral solution may be prepared using the injectable formulation (5 mg/mL). Mix 1 mL of injectable folic acid with 90 mL of purified water. Adjust pH to 8-8.5 with sodium hydroxide 10%; add sufficient quantity of purified water to make 100 mL; mix well. Stable for 30 days at room temperature (Nahata, 2004).

Allen LV Jr, "Folic Acid 1-mg/mL Oral Liquid," *Int J Pharm Compound,* 2007, 11(3):244.

Nahata MC, Pai VB, and Hipple TF, *Pediatric Drug Formulations,* 5th ed, Cincinnati, OH: Harvey Whitney Books Co, 2004.

Folic Acid, Cyanocobalamin, and Pyridoxine

(FOE lik AS id, sye an oh koe BAL a min, & peer i DOKS een)

Brand Names: US Airavite; Av-VITE FB; CenFol; FaBB; Folastin [DSC]; Folbee; Folbic; Folcaps [DSC]; Folgard Rx; Folplex 2.2; Foltabs 800 [OTC]; Homocysteine Formula [OTC]; Virt-Gard; Virt-Vite; Virt-Vite Forte; Vita-Respa

Index Terms Cyanocobalamin, Folic Acid, and Pyridoxine; Folacin, Vitamin B_{12}, and Vitamin B_6; Pyridoxine, Folic Acid, and Cyanocobalamin

Pharmacologic Category Vitamin

Use Nutritional supplement in end-stage renal failure, dialysis, hyperhomocysteinemia, homocystinuria, malabsorption syndromes, dietary deficiencies

Dosing

Adult & Geriatric Dietary supplement: Oral: One tablet daily

Additional Information Complete prescribing information should be consulted for additional detail.

Dosage Forms Excipient information presented when available (limited, particularly for generics); consult specific product labeling. [DSC] = Discontinued product

Tablet, Oral:

Airavite: Folic acid 2.5 mg, cyanocobalamin 1000 mcg, and pyridoxine hydrochloride 25 mg

Av-VITE FB: Folic acid 2.5 mg, cyanocobalamin 1000 mcg, and pyridoxine hydrochloride 25 mg

CenFol: Folic acid 2.3 mg, cyanocobalamin 2000 mcg, and pyridoxine hydrochloride 24.5 mg

FaBB: Folic acid 2.2 mg, cyanocobalamin 1000 mcg, and pyridoxine hydrochloride 25 mg

Folastin: Folic acid 2.5 mg, cyanocobalamin 2000 mcg, and pyridoxine hydrochloride 25 mg [DSC]

Folbee: Folic acid 2.5 mg, cyanocobalamin 1000 mcg, and pyridoxine hydrochloride 25 mg [dye free, lactose free, and sugar free]

Folbic: Folic acid 2.5 mg, cyanocobalamin 2000 mcg, and pyridoxine hydrochloride 25 mg

Folcaps: Folic acid 2.2 mg, cyanocobalamin 500 mcg, and pyridoxine hydrochloride 25 mg [sugar free] [DSC]

Folgard RX: Folic acid 2.2 mg, cyanocobalamin 1000 mcg, and pyridoxine hydrochloride 25 mg

Folplex 2.2: Folic acid 2.2 mg, cyanocobalamin 500 mcg, and pyridoxine hydrochloride 25 mg

Foltabs 800: Folic acid 0.8 mg, cyanocobalamin 115 mcg, and pyridoxine hydrochloride 10 mg [gluten free]

Homocysteine Formula: Folic acid 0.8 mg, cyanocobalamin 100 mcg, and pyridoxine hydrochloride 50 mg

Niva-Fol: Folic acid 2.5 mg, cyanocobalamin 2000 mcg, and pyridoxine hydrochloride 25 mg

NuFol: Folic acid 2.5 mg, cyanocobalamin 1000 mcg, and pyridoxine hydrochloride 25 mg

Virt-Gard: Folic acid 2.2 mg, cyanocobalamin 1000 mcg, and pyridoxine hydrochloride 25 mg

Virt-Vite: Folic acid 2.5 mg, cyanocobalamin 1000 mcg, and pyridoxine hydrochloride 25 mg

Virt-Vite Forte: Folic acid 2.5 mg, cyanocobalamin 2000 mcg, and pyridoxine hydrochloride 25 mg

Vita-Respa: Folic acid 2.2 mg, cyanocobalamin 1300 mcg, and pyridoxine hydrochloride 25 mg [dye free and sugar free]

Generic: Folic acid 0.5 mg, cyanocobalamin 200 mcg, pyridoxine hydrochloride 5 mg; Folic acid 0.8 mg, cyanocobalamin 100 mcg, and pyridoxine hydrochloride 50 mg; Folic acid 2.2 mg, cyanocobalamin 500 mcg, and pyridoxine hydrochloride 25 mg; Folic acid 2.5 mg, cyanocobalamin 200 mcg, and pyridoxine hydrochloride 25 mg

◆ Folinate Calcium *see* Leucovorin Calcium *on page 1049*

◆ Folinic Acid (error prone synonym) *see* Leucovorin Calcium *on page 1049*

◆ Follicle-Stimulating Hormone, Human *see* Urofollitropin *on page 1855*

◆ Follicle Stimulating Hormone, Recombinant *see* Follitropin Alfa *on page 805*

◆ Follicle Stimulating Hormone, Recombinant *see* Follitropin Beta *on page 805*

◆ Follistim AQ *see* Follitropin Beta *on page 805*

Follitropin Alfa (foe li TRO pin AL fa)

Brand Names: US Gonal-f; Gonal-f RFF; Gonal-f RFF Pen; Gonal-f RFF Rediject

Brand Names: Canada Gonal-f; Gonal-f Pen

Index Terms Follicle Stimulating Hormone, Recombinant; FSH; rFSH-alpha; rhFSH-alpha

Pharmacologic Category Gonadotropin; Ovulation Stimulator

Use

Multifollicular development during Assisted Reproductive Technology (ART): To stimulate the development of multiple follicles with ART

Ovulation induction: Induction of ovulation in oligo-anovulatory infertile patients in whom the cause of infertility is functional and not caused by primary ovarian failure

Spermatogenesis induction (Gonal-f only): Induction of spermatogenesis in men with primary and secondary hypogonadotropic hypogonadism in whom the cause of infertility is not due to primary testicular failure

Dosing

Adult Note: Dose should be individualized. Use the lowest dose consistent with the expectation of good results. Over the course of treatment, doses may vary depending on individual patient response.

Ovulation induction: Females: SubQ: Initial: 75 units daily; incremental dose adjustments of up to 37.5 units may be considered after 14 days; further dose increases of the same magnitude can be made, if necessary, every 7 days (maximum dose: 300 units daily). If response to follitropin is appropriate, hCG is given 1 day following the last dose. Withhold hCG if serum estradiol is >2000 pg/mL; discontinue if the ovaries are abnormally enlarged, or if abdominal pain occurs. In general, therapy should not exceed 35 days.

Multifollicular development during ART: Females: SubQ: Initiate therapy with follitropin alfa in the early follicular phase (cycle day 2 or day 3) at a dose of 150 units daily, until sufficient follicular development is attained. In most cases, therapy should not exceed 10 days. In patients ≥35 years whose endogenous gonadotropin levels are suppressed, initiate follitropin alfa at a dose of 225 units daily. Continue treatment until adequate follicular development is indicated as determined by ultrasound in combination with measurement of serum estradiol levels. Consider adjustments to dose after 5 days based on the patient's response; adjust subsequent dosage every 3-5 days by ≤75-150 units additionally at each adjustment. Doses >450 units daily are not recommended. Once adequate follicular development is evident, administer hCG to induce final follicular maturation in preparation for oocyte retrieval. Withhold hCG if the ovaries are abnormally enlarged.

Spermatogenesis induction: Males: *Gonal-f:* SubQ: Therapy should begin with hCG pretreatment until serum testosterone is in normal range, then initiate Gonal-f at 150 units 3 times weekly with hCG 3 times weekly; continue with lowest dose needed to induce spermatogenesis (maximum dose: 300 units 3 times weekly); may be given for up to 18 months

Geriatric Refer to adult dosing. Clinical studies did not include patients >65 years.

Renal Impairment No dosage adjustment provided in manufacturer's labeling (has not been studied).

Hepatic Impairment No dosage adjustment provided in manufacturer's labeling (has not been studied).

Additional Information Complete prescribing information should be consulted for additional detail.

Dosage Forms Excipient information presented when available (limited, particularly for generics); consult specific product labeling.

Solution, Subcutaneous:

Gonal-f RFF Pen: 300 units/0.5 mL (0.5 mL); 450 units/0.75 mL (0.75 mL); 900 units/1.5 mL (1.5 mL) [contains metacresol]

Gonal-f RFF Rediject: 300 units/0.5 mL (0.5 mL); 450 units/0.75 mL (0.75 mL); 900 units/1.5 mL (1.5 mL) [contains metacresol]

Solution Reconstituted, Injection:

Gonal-f: 450 units (1 ea); 1050 units (1 ea)

Solution Reconstituted, Subcutaneous:

Gonal-f RFF: 75 units (1 ea)

Follitropin Beta (foe li TRO pin BAY ta)

Brand Names: US Follistim AQ

Brand Names: Canada Puregon

Index Terms Follicle Stimulating Hormone, Recombinant; FSH; rFSH-beta; rhFSH-beta

Pharmacologic Category Gonadotropin; Ovulation Stimulator

Use

Females: Induction of ovulation and pregnancy in anovulatory infertile patients in whom the cause of infertility is functional and not caused by primary ovarian failure; induction of pregnancy in normal ovulatory women undergoing Assisted Reproductive Technology (ART) (eg, *in vitro* fertilization [IVF], intracytoplasmic sperm injection [ICSI])

Males: Induction of spermatogenesis in men with primary and secondary hypogonadotropic hypogonadism in whom the cause of infertility is not due to primary testicular failure.

Dosing

Adult Note: Dose should be individualized. Use the lowest dose consistent with the expectation of good results. Over the course of treatment, doses may vary depending on individual patient response.

Ovulation induction: Females:

Follistim® AQ: IM, SubQ: Stepwise approach: Initiate therapy with 75 units/day for at least the first 7 days. Increase by 25 or 50 units at weekly intervals until follicular growth or serum estradiol levels indicate an adequate response. The maximum (individualized) daily dose that has been safely used for ovulation induction in patients during clinical trials is 300 units. If response to follitropin is appropriate, hCG is given 1 day following the last dose. Withhold hCG if the ovaries are abnormally enlarged, or if abdominal pain occurs.

Follistim® AQ Cartridge: SubQ: Stepwise approach: Initiate therapy with 50 units/day for at least the first 7 days. Increase by 25 or 50 units at weekly intervals until follicular growth or serum estradiol levels indicate an adequate response. The maximum (individualized) daily dose that has been safely used for ovulation induction in patients during clinical trials is 250 units. If response to follitropin is appropriate, hCG is given 1 day following the last dose. Withhold hCG if the ovaries are abnormally enlarged, or if abdominal pain occurs. See **"Note"** for dosage adjustment for this product.

ART: Females:

Follistim® AQ: IM, SubQ: Stepwise approach: A starting dose of 150-225 units is recommended for at least the first 4 days of treatment. The dose may be adjusted for the individual patient based upon their ovarian response. The maximum daily dose used in clinical studies is 600 units. When a sufficient number of follicles of adequate size are present, the final maturation of the follicles is induced by administering hCG. Oocyte retrieval is performed 34-36 hours later. Withhold hCG in cases where the ovaries are abnormally enlarged on the last day of follitropin beta therapy.

Follistim® AQ Cartridge: SubQ: Stepwise approach: A starting dose of 200 units is recommended for at least the first 7 days of treatment. The dose may be adjusted for the individual patient based upon their ovarian response. The maximum daily dose used in clinical studies is 500 units. When a sufficient number of follicles of adequate size are present, the final maturation of the follicles is induced by administering hCG. Oocyte retrieval is performed 34-36 hours later. Withhold hCG in cases where the ovaries are abnormally enlarged on the last day of follitropin beta therapy. See **"Note"** for dosage adjustment for this product.

Spermatogenesis induction: Males: *Follistim® AQ, Follistim® AQ Cartridge:* **Note:** Pretreatment with hCG monotherapy is required prior to concomitant therapy with follitropin beta and hCG. Follitropin beta therapy may be initiated after normal serum testosterone levels have been reached. SubQ: 450 units/week (administered as 225 units twice weekly or 150 units 3 times/weekly). A lower dose of Follistim® AQ Cartridge may be considered. See **"Note"** for dosage adjustment for this product.

Note: Dose adjustment for Follistim® AQ Cartridge: When administered using the Follistim Pen®, the Follistim® AQ Cartridge delivers 18% more follitropin beta when compared to dissolved lyophilized follitropin beta administered by a conventional syringe. If the above starting doses were previously used when administering a recombinant lyophilized gonadotropin product via a conventional syringe, lower starting and maintenance doses should be considered when switching to Follistim® AQ Cartridge. The following dose conversion may be used:

Follistim® AQ Dosing Conversion[1]

Dose Administered Using Powder for Solution/Conventional Syringe	Follistim® AQ Dose Administered Using Follistim Pen®
75 units	50 units
150 units	125 units
225 units	175 units
300 units	250 units
375 units	300 units
450 units	375 units

[1]Values listed are rounded to the nearest 25 unit increment.

Renal Impairment No dosage adjustment provided in manufacturer's labeling (has not been studied).

Hepatic Impairment No dosage adjustment provided in manufacturer's labeling (has not been studied).

Additional Information Complete prescribing information should be consulted for additional detail.

Dosage Forms Excipient information presented when available (limited, particularly for generics); consult specific product labeling. [DSC] = Discontinued product

Solution, Injection:
Follistim AQ: 75 units/0.5 mL (0.5 mL); 150 units/0.5 mL (0.5 mL [DSC])

Solution, Subcutaneous:
Follistim AQ: 300 units/0.36 mL (0.42 mL); 600 units/0.72 mL (0.78 mL); 900 units/1.08 mL (1.17 mL) [contains benzyl alcohol]

◆ Folotyn *see* PRALAtrexate *on page 1484*

◆ Folplex 2.2 *see* Folic Acid, Cyanocobalamin, and Pyridoxine *on page 805*

◆ Foltabs 800 [OTC] *see* Folic Acid, Cyanocobalamin, and Pyridoxine *on page 805*

Fomepizole (foe ME pi zole)

Brand Names: US Antizol
Brand Names: Canada Antizol
Index Terms 4-Methylpyrazole; 4-MP
Pharmacologic Category Antidote

Use Treatment of methanol or ethylene glycol poisoning alone or in combination with hemodialysis

Pregnancy Considerations Animal reproduction studies have not been conducted. In general, medications used as antidotes should take into consideration the health and prognosis of the mother; antidotes should be administered to pregnant women if there is a clear indication for use and should not be withheld because of fears of teratogenicity (Bailey, 2003).

Breast-Feeding Considerations It is not known if fomepizole is excreted in breast milk. The manufacturer recommends that caution be exercised when administering fomepizole to nursing women.

Contraindications Hypersensitivity to fomepizole, other pyrazoles, or any component of the formulation

Warnings/Precautions Should not be given undiluted or by bolus injection. Fomepizole is metabolized in the liver and excreted in the urine; use caution with hepatic or renal impairment. Hemodialysis should be considered as an adjunct to fomepizole in patients with renal failure, significant acidosis (pH <7.25-7.3), worsening metabolic acidosis, or ethylene glycol or methanol concentrations ≥50 mg/dL. Pediatric administration is not FDA approved; however, safe and efficacious use in this patient population for ethylene glycol and methanol intoxication has been reported (Baum, 2000; Benitez, 2000; Boyer, 2001; Brown, 2001; De Brabander, 2005; Detaille, 2004; Fisher, 1998); consider consultation with a clinical toxicologist or poison control center.

Adverse Reactions
>10%:
Central nervous system: Headache (14%)
Gastrointestinal: Nausea (11%)

1% to 10% (≤3% unless otherwise noted):

Cardiovascular: Bradycardia, facial flush, hypotension, shock, tachycardia

Central nervous system: Dizziness (6%), drowsiness increased (6%), agitation, anxiety, fever, lightheadedness, seizure, vertigo

Dermatologic: Rash

Endocrine & metabolic: Liver function tests increased

Gastrointestinal: Bad/metallic taste (6%), abdominal pain, appetite decreased, diarrhea, heartburn, vomiting

Hematologic: Anemia, disseminated intravascular coagulation (DIC), eosinophilia, lymphangitis

Local: Application site reaction, injection site inflammation, pain during injection, phlebitis

Neuromuscular & skeletal: Backache

Ocular: Nystagmus, transient blurred vision, visual disturbances

Renal: Anuria

Respiratory: Abnormal smell, hiccups, pharyngitis

Miscellaneous: Multiorgan failure, speech disturbances

<1% (Limited to important or life-threatening): Mild allergic reactions (mild rash, eosinophilia)

Drug Interactions

Metabolism/Transport Effects None known.

Avoid Concomitant Use There are no known interactions where it is recommended to avoid concomitant use.

Increased Effect/Toxicity There are no known significant interactions involving an increase in effect.

Decreased Effect There are no known significant interactions involving a decrease in effect.

Food Interactions Ethanol decreases the rate of fomepizole elimination by ~50%; conversely, fomepizole decreases the rate of elimination of ethanol by ~40%.

Preparation for Administration Prior to administration, dilute in at least 100 mL 0.9% sodium chloride or dextrose 5% water for injection. Although, it is chemically and physically stable when diluted as recommended, sterile precautions should be observed because diluents generally do not contain preservatives.

Storage/Stability Store at controlled room temperature, 20°C to 25°C (68°F to 77°F); fomepizole solidifies at temperatures <25°C (77°F). If solution becomes solid in the vial, it be should be carefully warmed by running the vial under warm water or by holding in the hand. Solidification does not affect the efficacy, safety, or stability of the drug. Diluted solution should be used within 24 hours and may be stored at room temperature or under refrigeration.

Mechanism of Action Fomepizole competitively inhibits alcohol dehydrogenase, an enzyme which catalyzes the metabolism of ethanol, ethylene glycol, and methanol to their toxic metabolites. Ethylene glycol is metabolized to glycoaldehyde, then oxidized to glycolate, glyoxylate, and oxalate. Glycolate and oxalate are responsible for metabolic acidosis and renal damage. Methanol is metabolized to formaldehyde, then oxidized to formic acid. Formic acid is responsible for metabolic acidosis and visual disturbances.

Pharmacodynamics/Kinetics

Onset of effect: Peak effect: Maximum: 1.5-2 hours

Absorption: Oral: Readily absorbed

Distribution: V_d: 0.6-1.02 L/kg; rapidly into total body water

Protein binding: Negligible

Metabolism: Hepatic to 4-carboxypyrazole (80% to 85% of dose), 4-hydroxymethylpyrazole, and their N-glucuronide conjugates; following multiple doses, induces its own metabolism via CYP oxidases after 30-40 hours

Half-life elimination: Has not been calculated; varies with dose

Excretion: Urine (1% to 3.5% as unchanged drug and metabolites)

Dosing

Adult Note: Fomepizole therapy should begin immediately upon suspicion of ethylene glycol or methanol ingestion.

Ethylene glycol and methanol toxicity: IV: Loading dose of 15 mg/kg should be administered, followed by doses of 10 mg/kg every 12 hours for 4 doses, then 15 mg/kg every 12 hours thereafter until ethylene glycol levels have been reduced <20 mg/dL and patient is asymptomatic with normal pH. **Note:** For severe toxicity requiring concomitant hemodialysis, see Dosage Adjustment in Renal Impairment.

Geriatric Specific studies have not been conducted in elderly patients.

Pediatric Ethylene glycol and methanol toxicity (off-label use; Baum, 2000; Benitez, 2000; Boyer, 2001; Brown, 2001; De Brabander, 2005; Detaille, 2004; Fisher, 1998): Refer to adult dosing.

Renal Impairment Note: Hemodialysis should be considered as an adjunct to fomepizole in patients with renal failure, significant or worsening metabolic acidosis, or ethylene glycol or methanol concentrations ≥50 mg/dL. The following dosing adjustments should be used for any patient receiving hemodialysis regardless of renal function.

Prior to the start of hemodialysis:

To determine if the patient requires a dose of fomepizole at the start of hemodialysis, determine when the last dose was administered.

If the last dose of fomepizole was given <6 hours ago, do not administer another dose upon beginning hemodialysis.

If the last dose of fomepizole was given ≥6 hours ago, administer next scheduled dose upon beginning hemodialysis.

During hemodialysis: During hemodialysis, administer fomepizole every 4 hours. Alternatively, a loading dose of 10-20 mg/kg followed by 1-1.5 mg/kg/hour continuous infusion during hemodialysis has been described in case reports (Jobard, 1996).

Upon completion of hemodialysis:

To determine if the patient requires a dose of fomepizole at the time of completion of hemodialysis, determine when the last dose was administered.

If the last dose of fomepizole was given <1 hour ago, do not administer a dose at the end of hemodialysis.

If the last dose of fomepizole was given 1-3 hours ago, administer one-half of the next scheduled dose at the end of hemodialysis.

If the last dose of fomepizole was given >3 hours ago, administer the next scheduled dose at the end of hemodialysis.

Maintenance dose when off hemodialysis: Administer fomepizole every 12 hours (starting 12 hours from last dose administered).

Hepatic Impairment Fomepizole is metabolized in the liver. Specific dosage adjustments have not been determined in patients with hepatic impairment.

Administration The appropriate dose of fomepizole should be drawn from the vial with a syringe and injected into at least 100 mL of sterile 0.9% sodium chloride injection or dextrose 5% injection. All doses should be administered as a slow intravenous infusion (IVPB) over 30 minutes.

Monitoring Parameters Fomepizole plasma levels should be monitored; response to fomepizole; monitor plasma/urinary ethylene glycol or methanol levels, urinary oxalate (ethylene glycol), plasma/urinary osmolality, renal/hepatic function, serum electrolytes, arterial blood gases; anion and osmolar gaps, resolution of clinical signs and symptoms of ethylene glycol or methanol intoxication

Reference Range The manufacturer recommends concentrations 100-300 micromole/L (8.2-24.6 mg/L) to achieve enzyme inhibition of alcohol dehydrogenase; according to practice guidelines, serum fomepizole concentrations of ≥0.8 mg/L provide constant inhibition of alcohol dehydrogenase

Dosage Forms Excipient information presented when available (limited, particularly for generics); consult specific product labeling.

Solution, Intravenous [preservative free]:

Antizol: 1 g/mL (1.5 mL)

Generic: 1 g/mL (1.5 mL); 1.5 g/1.5 mL (1.5 mL)

Fondaparinux (fon da PARE i nuks)

Brand Names: US Arixtra

Brand Names: Canada Arixtra

Index Terms Fondaparinux Sodium

Pharmacologic Category Anticoagulant; Anticoagulant, Factor Xa Inhibitor

Use

Acute deep vein thrombosis: Treatment of acute deep vein thrombosis (DVT) in conjunction with warfarin.

Acute pulmonary embolism: Treatment of acute pulmonary embolism (PE) in conjunction with warfarin.

Deep vein thrombosis prophylaxis: Prophylaxis of DVT in patients undergoing surgery for hip replacement, knee replacement, hip fracture (including extended prophylaxis following hip fracture surgery), or abdominal surgery (in patients at risk for thromboembolic complications).

Canadian labeling: Additional uses; not approved in the US: Management of unstable angina or non-ST segment elevation myocardial infarction (UA/NSTEMI) for the prevention of death and subsequent MI; management of ST segment elevation MI (STEMI) for the prevention of death and myocardial reinfarction

Pregnancy Considerations Adverse events have not been observed in animal reproduction studies. Based on case reports, small amounts of fondaparinux have been detected in the umbilical cord following multiple doses during pregnancy (Dempfle, 2004). Use of fondaparinux in pregnancy should be limited to those women who have severe allergic reactions to heparin, including heparin-induced thrombocytopenia, and who cannot receive danaparoid (Guyatt, 2012).

Breast-Feeding Considerations It is not known if fondaparinux is excreted in breast milk. The manufacturer recommends caution be used if administered to nursing women. The use of alternative anticoagulants is preferred (Guyatt, 2012). The Canadian labeling does not recommend use in breast-feeding women.

Contraindications Serious hypersensitivity (eg, angioedema, anaphylactoid/anaphylactic reactions) to fondaparinux or any component of the formulation; severe renal impairment (CrCl <30 mL/minute); body weight <50 kg (prophylaxis); active major bleeding; bacterial endocarditis; thrombocytopenia associated with a positive *in vitro* test for antiplatelet antibody in the presence of fondaparinux

Warnings/Precautions [U.S. Boxed Warning]: Spinal or epidural hematomas, including subsequent long-term or permanent paralysis, may occur with recent or anticipated neuraxial anesthesia (epidural or spinal anesthesia) or spinal puncture in patients anticoagulated with LMWH, heparinoids, or fondaparinux. Consider risk versus benefit prior to spinal procedures; risk is increased by the use of concomitant agents which may alter hemostasis (such as NSAIDS, platelet inhibitors, or other anticoagulants), the use of indwelling epidural catheters, a history of spinal deformity or spinal surgery, as well as a history of traumatic or repeated epidural or spinal punctures. Patient should be observed closely for bleeding and signs and symptoms of neurological impairment (eg, midline back pain, sensory and motor deficits [numbness, tingling, weakness in lower limbs], bowel or bladder dysfunction) if therapy is administered during or immediately following diagnostic lumbar puncture, epidural anesthesia, or spinal anesthesia. **Optimal timing between administration of fondaparinux and neuraxial procedures is unknown.**

Monitor patient closely for signs or symptoms of bleeding. Certain patients are at increased risk of bleeding. Risk factors include bacterial endocarditis; congenital or acquired bleeding disorders; active ulcerative and angiodysplastic GI disease; uncontrolled arterial hypertension; hemorrhagic stroke; recent intracranial hemorrhage; or use shortly after brain, spinal, or ophthalmology surgery; in patients treated concomitantly with platelet inhibitors; or thrombocytopenia or platelet defects; diabetic retinopathy; patients <50 kg. Risk of major bleeding may be increased if initial dose is administered earlier than recommended (initiation recommended at 6 to 8 hours following surgery). Do not administer with other agents that increase the risk of hemorrhage unless they are essential for the management of the underlying condition (eg, vitamin K antagonists for treatment of VTE). PT and aPTT are insensitive measures of fondaparinux activity. If unexpected changes in coagulation parameters or major bleeding occur, discontinue fondaparinux (elevated aPTT associated with bleeding events have been reported in postmarketing data).

Thrombocytopenia has occurred with administration, including very rare reports of thrombocytopenia with thrombosis similar to heparin-induced thrombocytopenia (HIT); however, has been used in patients with current or history of HIT due to a lack of an immune-mediated effect on platelets (ACCP [Guyatt, 2012]; Savi, 2005). Use is contraindicated in patients with thrombocytopenia associated with a positive in vitro test for antiplatelet antibodies in the presence of fondaparinux. Monitor patients closely and discontinue therapy if platelets fall to <100,000/mm³ (US labeling) or <50,000/ mm³ (Canadian labeling).

The administration of fondaparinux as the sole anticoagulant is **not recommended** during PCI due to an increased risk for guiding-catheter thrombosis. Use of an anticoagulant with antithrombin activity (eg, unfractionated heparin) is recommended as adjunctive therapy to PCI even if prior treatment with fondaparinux (must take into account whether GP IIb/IIIa antagonists have been administered) (ACCF/AHA [Anderson, 2013]; Levine, 2011). Use of fondaparinux during primary PCI is not recommended. In STEMI patients undergoing primary PCI for reperfusion, the use of fondaparinux prior to and during PCI is not recommended (Canadian labeling).

Use with caution in patients with hepatic impairment and in the elderly. Use with caution in patients with CrCl 30 to 50 mL/minute; contraindicated in patients with CrCl <30 mL/ minute. Periodically monitor renal function; discontinue if severe renal dysfunction or labile function develops. Increased risk of bleeding in patients <50 kg; use with caution; dosage reduction recommended. Contraindicated in patients <50 kg when used for prophylactic therapy. Potentially significant interactions may exist, requiring dose or frequency adjustment, additional monitoring, and/ or selection of alternative therapy.

For subcutaneous administration; not for IM administration. The needle guard may contain natural latex rubber. For STEMI patients (Canadian labeling; off-label use in United States) may administer initial dose IV. Do not use interchangeably (unit for unit) with low molecular weight heparins, heparin, or heparinoids. Discontinue use 24 hours prior to CABG and dose with unfractionated heparin per institutional practice (ACCF/AHA [Anderson, 2013]). Following discontinuation, the anticoagulant effects of fondaparinux may persist for 2 to 4 days and even longer in patients with renal impairment.

Adverse Reactions As with all anticoagulants, bleeding is the major adverse effect. Hemorrhage may occur at any site. Risk appears increased by a number of factors including renal dysfunction, age (>75 years), and weight (<50 kg).

>10%: Hematologic & oncologic: Anemia (2% to 20%)

1% to 10%:

Cardiovascular: Hypotension (≤4%)

Central nervous system: Insomnia (≤5%), dizziness (≤4%), confusion (1% to 3%)

Dermatologic: Increased wound secretion (≤5%), skin blister (≤3%)

Endocrine & metabolic: Hypokalemia (≤4%)

Hematologic & oncologic: Purpura (≤4%), thrombocytopenia (50,000 to 100,000/mm³: 3%), hematoma (2% to 3%), minor hemorrhage (2% to 3%), major hemorrhage (1% to 3%; risk of major hemorrhage increased as high as 5% in patients receiving initial dose <6 hours following surgery), postoperative hemorrhage (≤2%)

Hepatic: Increased serum ALT (>3 × ULN: 1% to 3%), increased serum AST (>3 × ULN: <1% to ≤2%)

Infection: Postoperative wound infection (abdominal surgery: 5%)

Respiratory: Epistaxis (VTE: 1%)

<1% (Limited to important or life-threatening): Anaphylactoid reaction, anaphylaxis, angioedema, catheter site thrombosis (during PCI; without heparin), elevated aPTT associated with bleeding, epidural hematoma, hemorrhagic death, injection site reaction (bleeding at injection site, skin rash, pruritus), intracranial hemorrhage, reoperation due to bleeding, severe thrombocytopenia (<50,000/mm³), spinal hematoma, thrombocytopenia (with thrombosis)

Drug Interactions

Metabolism/Transport Effects None known.

Avoid Concomitant Use

Avoid concomitant use of Fondaparinux with any of the following: Apixaban; Dabigatran Etexilate; Edoxaban; Hemin; Omacetaxine; Rivaroxaban; Urokinase; Vorapaxar

Increased Effect/Toxicity

Fondaparinux may increase the levels/effects of: Anticoagulants; Collagenase (Systemic); Deferasirox; Deoxycholic Acid; Ibritumomab; Nintedanib; Obinutuzumab; Omacetaxine; Rivaroxaban; Tositumomab and Iodine I 131 Tositumomab

The levels/effects of Fondaparinux may be increased by: Agents with Antiplatelet Properties; Apixaban; Dabigatran Etexilate; Dasatinib; Edoxaban; Hemin; Herbs (Anticoagulant/Antiplatelet Properties); Ibrutinib; Limaprost; Nonsteroidal Anti-Inflammatory Agents; Omega-3 Fatty Acids; Pentosan Polysulfate Sodium; Prostacyclin Analogues; Salicylates; Sugammadex; Thrombolytic Agents; Tibolone; Tipranavir; Urokinase; Vitamin E; Vitamin E (Oral); Vorapaxar

Decreased Effect

Fondaparinux may decrease the levels/effects of: Factor X (Human)

The levels/effects of Fondaparinux may be decreased by: Estrogen Derivatives; Progestins

Preparation for Administration Canadian labeling: For IV administration: May mix with 25 mL or 50 mL NS

Storage/Stability Store at 25°C (77°F); excursions permitted to 15°C to 30°C (59°F to 86°F).

Canadian labeling: Store <25°C (77°F); do not freeze. For IV infusion, use immediately once diluted in NS; can also be stored for up to 24 hours at 15°C to 30°C (59°F to 86°F).

Mechanism of Action Fondaparinux is a synthetic penta-saccharide that causes an antithrombin III-mediated selective inhibition of factor Xa. Neutralization of factor Xa interrupts the blood coagulation cascade and inhibits thrombin formation and thrombus development.

Pharmacodynamics/Kinetics

Absorption: SubQ: Rapid and complete

Distribution: V_d: 7 to 11 L; mainly in blood

Protein binding: ≥94% to antithrombin III

Bioavailability: SubQ: 100%

Half-life elimination: 17 to 21 hours; prolonged with renal impairment and in the elderly

Time to peak: SubQ: ~2 to 3 hours

Excretion: Urine (up to 77%, unchanged drug)

Dosing

Adult & Geriatric Note: PT and aPTT are insensitive measures of fondaparinux activity. If unexpected changes in coagulation parameters or major bleeding occur, discontinue fondaparinux.

DVT prophylaxis: SubQ: Adults ≥50 kg: 2.5 mg once daily. **Note:** Prophylactic use contraindicated in patients <50 kg. Initiate dose after hemostasis has been established, no earlier than 6 to 8 hours postoperatively.

DVT prophylaxis with history of HIT (off-label use): SubQ: 2.5 mg once daily (Blackmer, 2009; Harenberg, 2004; Parody, 2003)

Usual duration: 5 to 9 days (up to 10 days following abdominal surgery or up to 11 days following hip fracture, hip replacement, or knee replacement was administered in clinical trials). The American College of Chest Physicians recommends a minimum of 10 to 14 days for patients undergoing total hip arthroplasty, total knee arthroplasty, or hip fracture surgery; extended duration of up to 35 days suggested (Guyatt, 2012).

Acute DVT/PE treatment: SubQ: **Note:** Start warfarin on the first or second treatment day and continue fondaparinux until INR is ≥2 for at least 24 hours (usually 5 to 7 days) (Guyatt, 2012).

<50 kg: 5 mg once daily

50 to 100 kg: 7.5 mg once daily

>100 kg: 10 mg once daily

Usual duration: 5 to 9 days (administered up to 26 days in clinical trials)

Acute coronary syndrome (Canadian labeling; off-label use in United States):

UA/NSTEMI: SubQ: 2.5 mg once daily; initiate as soon as possible after presentation; treat for the duration of hospitalization, up to 8 days (ACCF/AHA [Anderson, 2013]; Yusuf 2006a)

STEMI: IV: 2.5 mg once; subsequent doses (starting the following day): SubQ: 2.5 mg once daily; treat for the duration of the hospitalization, up to 8 days, or until revascularization (ACCF/AHA [O'Gara, 2013]; Yusuf, 2006b)

Note: Discontinue fondaparinux 24 hours prior to coronary artery bypass graft (CABG) surgery; instead, administer unfractionated heparin per institutional practice (ACCF/AHA [Anderson, 2013]).

Acute symptomatic superficial vein thrombosis (≥5 cm in length) of the legs (off-label use): SubQ: 2.5 mg once daily for 45 days (Decousus, 2010; Guyatt, 2012)

Acute thrombosis (unrelated to HIT) in patients with a past history of HIT (off-label use; Guyatt, 2012; Warkentin, 2011): SubQ:

<50 kg: 5 mg once daily

50 to 100 kg: 7.5 mg once daily

>100 kg: 10 mg once daily

Renal Impairment

CrCl >50 mL/minute: There are no dosage adjustments provided in the manufacturer's labeling. Total clearance is reduced ~25% compared to patients with normal renal function.

CrCl 30 to 50 mL/minute: Use caution; total clearance ~40% lower compared to patients with normal renal function. When used for thromboprophylaxis, the American College of Chest Physicians suggests a 50% reduction in dose or use of low-dose heparin instead of fondaparinux (Garcia, 2012).

CrCl <30 mL/minute: Use is contraindicated.

Hepatic Impairment

Mild-to-moderate impairment (Child-Pugh class A and B): No dosage adjustment necessary; monitor for signs of bleeding.

Severe impairment (Child-Pugh class A and B): There are no dosage adjustment provided in the manufacturer's labeling (has not been studied). Use with caution; monitor closely for signs of bleeding.

Administration For SubQ administration; do **not** administer IM. Alternate injection sites. Do not expel air bubble from syringe before injection. Administer according to

recommended regimen; when used for DVT prophylaxis, early initiation (before 6 hours after orthopedic surgery) has been associated with increased bleeding. For STEMI patients (Canadian labeling; off-label use in United States) may administer initial dose as IV push or mix in NS and infuse over 1 to 2 minutes; flush tubing with NS after infusion to ensure complete administration for fondaparinux.

To convert from IV unfractionated heparin (UFH) infusion to SubQ fondaparinux (Nutescu, 2007): Calculate specific dose for fondaparinux based on indication, discontinue UFH, and begin fondaparinux within 1 hour

To convert from SubQ fondaparinux to IV UFH infusion (Nutescu, 2007): Discontinue fondaparinux; calculate specific dose for IV UFH infusion based on indication; omit heparin bolus/loading dose

For subQ fondaparinux dosed every 24 hours: Start IV UFH infusion 22 to 23 hours after last dose of fondaparinux

Monitoring Parameters Periodically monitor CBC, platelet count, serum creatinine, and occult blood testing of stools. Anti-Xa activity of fondaparinux can be measured by the assay if fondaparinux is used as the calibrator.

Reference Range Note: Routine monitoring is not recommended; the following fondaparinux-specific anti-Xa concentrations have been reported (Garcia, 2012):

Thromboprophylaxis dose: Anti-Xa activity at 3 hours post dose: ~0.39 to 0.5 mg/L

Therapeutic dosing (eg, 7.5 mg once daily): Anti-Xa activity at 3 hours post dose: 1.2 to 1.26 mg/L

Test Interactions International standards of heparin or LMWH are not the appropriate calibrators for antifactor Xa activity of fondaparinux.

Dosage Forms Excipient information presented when available (limited, particularly for generics); consult specific product labeling.

Solution, Subcutaneous, as sodium:

Generic: 2.5 mg/0.5 mL (0.5 mL); 5 mg/0.4 mL (0.4 mL); 7.5 mg/0.6 mL (0.6 mL); 10 mg/0.8 mL (0.8 mL)

Solution, Subcutaneous, as sodium [preservative free]:

Arixtra: 2.5 mg/0.5 mL (0.5 mL); 5 mg/0.4 mL (0.4 mL); 7.5 mg/0.6 mL (0.6 mL); 10 mg/0.8 mL (0.8 mL)

Generic: 2.5 mg/0.5 mL (0.5 mL); 5 mg/0.4 mL (0.4 mL); 7.5 mg/0.6 mL (0.6 mL); 10 mg/0.8 mL (0.8 mL)

◆ Fondaparinux Sodium see Fondaparinux on page 807

◆ Foradil (Can) see Formoterol on page 809

◆ Foradil Aerolizer see Formoterol on page 809

◆ Forfivo XL see BuPROPion on page 269

Formoterol (for MOH te rol)

Brand Names: US Foradil Aerolizer; Perforomist

Brand Names: Canada Foradil; Oxeze Turbuhaler

Index Terms Eformoterol; Formoterol Fumarate; Formoterol Fumarate Dihydrate

Pharmacologic Category Beta$_2$ Agonist; Beta$_2$-Adrenergic Agonist, Long-Acting

Use

U.S. labeling: Treatment of asthma (only as concomitant therapy with an inhaled corticosteroid) in patients with reversible obstructive airway disease, including patients with symptoms of nocturnal asthma (Foradil Aerolizer); maintenance treatment of bronchoconstriction in patients with COPD (Foradil Aerolizer, Perforomist); prevention of exercise-induced bronchospasm when administered on an as-needed basis (monotherapy may be indicated in patients without persistent asthma) (Foradil Aerolizer)

Canadian labeling: Treatment of asthma (only as concomitant therapy with an inhaled corticosteroid) in patients with reversible obstructive airway disease, including patients with symptoms of nocturnal asthma (Foradil, Oxeze Turbuhaler); maintenance treatment of COPD (Foradil); prevention of exercise-induced bronchospasm when administered on an as-needed basis (monotherapy may be indicated in patients without persistent asthma) (Oxeze Turbuhaler)

Pregnancy Considerations Adverse events were observed in some animal reproduction studies. Formoterol has the potential to affect uterine contractility if administered during labor.

Uncontrolled asthma is associated with adverse events on pregnancy (increased risk of perinatal mortality, pre-eclampsia, preterm birth, low birth weight infants). Although data related to its use in pregnancy is limited, formoterol may be used as an alternative agent when a long-acting beta agonist is needed to treat moderate persistent or severe persistent asthma in pregnant women (NAEPP, 2005).

Breast-Feeding Considerations It is not known if formoterol is excreted into breast milk. The manufacturer recommends that caution be exercised when administering formoterol to nursing women. The use of beta$_2$-receptor agonists are not considered a contraindication to breast-feeding (NAEPP, 2005).

Medication Guide Available Yes

Contraindications

Hypersensitivity to formoterol or any component of the formulation (Foradil Aerolizer only); treatment of status asthmaticus or other acute episodes of asthma or COPD (Foradil Aerolizer only); monotherapy in the treatment of asthma (ie, use without a concomitant long-term asthma control medication, such as an inhaled corticosteroid)

Canadian labeling: Additional contraindications (not in U.S. labeling): Presence of tachyarrhythmias

Warnings/Precautions [U.S. Boxed Warning]: Long-acting beta$_2$-agonists (LABAs) increase the risk of asthma-related deaths. Formoterol should only be used in asthma patients as adjuvant therapy in patients who are currently receiving but are not adequately controlled on a long-term asthma control medication (ie, an inhaled corticosteroid). Monotherapy with an LABA is contraindicated in the treatment of asthma. In a large, randomized, placebo-controlled U.S. clinical trial (SMART, 2006), salmeterol was associated with an increase in asthma-related deaths (when added to usual asthma therapy); risk is considered a class effect among all LABAs. Data are not available to determine if the addition of an inhaled corticosteroid lessens this increased risk of death associated with LABA use. Assess patients at regular intervals once asthma control is maintained on combination therapy to determine if step-down therapy is appropriate and the LABA can be discontinued (without loss of asthma control), and the patient can be maintained on an inhaled corticosteroid. LABAs are not appropriate in patients whose asthma is adequately controlled on low- or medium-dose inhaled corticosteroids. Do **not** use for acute bronchospasm. Short-acting beta$_2$-agonist (eg, albuterol) should be used for acute symptoms and symptoms occurring between treatments. Do **not** initiate in patients with significantly worsening or acutely deteriorating asthma; reports of severe (sometimes fatal) respiratory events have been reported when formoterol has been initiated in this situation. Corticosteroids should not be stopped or reduced when formoterol is initiated. Formoterol is not a substitute for inhaled or systemic corticosteroids and should not be used as monotherapy. During initiation, watch for signs of worsening asthma. **[U.S. Boxed Warning] (Foradil Aerolizer): LABAs may increase the risk of asthma-related hospitalization in pediatric and adolescent patients.** In general, a combination product containing a LABA and an inhaled corticosteroid is preferred in patients <18 years of age to ensure compliance.

Because LABAs may disguise poorly controlled persistent asthma, frequent or chronic use of LABAs for exercise-induced bronchospasm is discouraged by the NIH Asthma Guidelines (NIH, 2007). The safety and efficacy of Performomist in asthma patients have not been established and is not FDA approved for the treatment of asthma.

Do **not** use for acute episodes of COPD. Do **not** initiate in patients with significantly worsening or acutely deteriorating COPD. Data are not available to determine if LABA use increases the risk of death in patients with COPD. Increased use and/or ineffectiveness of short-acting beta$_2$-agonists may indicate rapidly deteriorating disease and should prompt re-evaluation of the patient's condition.

Immediate hypersensitivity reactions (urticaria, angioedema, rash, bronchospasm) have been reported. Do not exceed recommended dose or frequency; serious adverse events (including serious asthma exacerbations and fatalities) have been associated with excessive use of inhaled sympathomimetics. Beta$_2$-agonists may increase risk of arrhythmias, decrease serum potassium, prolong QTc interval, or increase serum glucose. These effects may be exacerbated in hypoxemia. Use caution in patients with cardiovascular disease (arrhythmia, coronary insufficiency, hypertension, HF, or aneurysm), seizures, diabetes, hyperthyroidism, pheochromocytoma, or hypokalemia. Beta-agonists may cause elevation in blood pressure and heart rate, and result in CNS stimulation/excitation. Tolerance to the bronchodilator effect, measured by FEV$_1$, has been observed in studies.

Powder for oral inhalation contains lactose; very rare anaphylactic reactions have been reported in patients with severe milk protein allergy. The contents of the Foradil Aerolizer capsules are for inhalation only via the Aerolizer device. There have been reports of incorrect administration (swallowing of the capsules).

Adverse Reactions

1% to 10%:

Cardiovascular: Chest pain (2% to 3%), palpitation

Central nervous system: Anxiety (2%), dizziness (2%), fever (2%), insomnia (2%), dysphonia (1%), headache

Dermatologic: Pruritus (2%), rash (1%)

Gastrointestinal: Diarrhea (5%), nausea (5%), xerostomia (1% to 3%), vomiting (2%), abdominal pain, dyspepsia, gastroenteritis

Neuromuscular & skeletal: Muscle cramps (2%), tremor

Respiratory: Infection (3% to 7%), asthma exacerbation (age 5-12 years: 5% to 6%; age >12 years: <4%), bronchitis (5%), pharyngitis (3% to 4%), sinusitis (3%), dyspnea (2%), tonsillitis (1%)

<1% (Limited to important or life-threatening): Acute asthma deterioration, anaphylactic reactions (severe hypotension/angioedema), agitation, angina, arrhythmia, atrial fibrillation, bronchospasm (paradoxical), cough, fatigue, hyperglycemia, hypertension, hypokalemia, glucose intolerance, malaise, metabolic acidosis, nervousness, QTc prolongation, tachycardia, ventricular extrasystoles

Drug Interactions

Metabolism/Transport Effects Substrate of CYP2C9 (minor); **Note:** Assignment of Major/Minor substrate status based on clinically relevant drug interaction potential

Avoid Concomitant Use

Avoid concomitant use of Formoterol with any of the following: Beta-Blockers (Nonselective); Iobenguane I 123; Long-Acting Beta2-Agonists; Loxapine

Increased Effect/Toxicity

Formoterol may increase the levels/effects of: Atosiban; Doxofylline; Highest Risk QTc-Prolonging Agents; Long-Acting Beta2-Agonists; Loop Diuretics; Loxapine; Moderate Risk QTc-Prolonging Agents; Sympathomimetics; Thiazide Diuretics

The levels/effects of Formoterol may be increased by: AtoMOXetine; Caffeine and Caffeine Containing Products; Cannabinoid-Containing Products; Inhalational Anesthetics; Linezolid; MAO Inhibitors; Mifepristone; Tedizolid; Theophylline Derivatives; Tricyclic Antidepressants

Decreased Effect

Formoterol may decrease the levels/effects of: Iobenguane I 123

The levels/effects of Formoterol may be decreased by: Beta-Blockers (Beta1 Selective); Beta-Blockers (Nonselective); Betahistine

Storage/Stability

Foradil Aerolizer: Prior to dispensing, store in refrigerator at 2°C to 8°C (36°F to 46°F). After dispensing, store at room temperature at 20°C to 25°C (68°F to 77°F). Protect from heat and moisture. Capsules should always be stored in the blister and only removed immediately before use.

Performomist: Prior to dispensing, store in refrigerator at 2°C to 8°C (36°F to 46°F). After dispensing, store at 2°C to 25°C (36°F to 77°F) for up to 3 months. Protect from heat. Unit-dose vials should always be stored in the foil pouch and only removed immediately before use.

Mechanism of Action Relaxes bronchial smooth muscle by selective action on beta$_2$ receptors with little effect on heart rate. Formoterol has a long-acting effect.

Pharmacodynamics/Kinetics

Onset of action: Powder for inhalation: Within 3 minutes

Peak effect: Powder for inhalation: 80% of peak effect within 15 minutes; Solution for nebulization: 2 hours

Duration: Improvement in FEV$_1$ observed for 12 hours in most patients

Absorption: Rapidly into plasma

Protein binding: 61% to 64% *in vitro* at higher concentrations than achieved with usual dosing

Metabolism: Hepatic via direct glucuronidation and O-demethylation; CYP2D6, CYP2C8/9, CYP2C19, CYP2A6 involved in O-demethylation

Half-life elimination: Powder: ~10-14 hours; Nebulized solution: ~7 hours

Time to peak: Maximum improvement in FEV$_1$ in 1-3 hours

Excretion:

Children 5-12 years: Urine (7% to 9% as direct glucuronide metabolites, 6% as unchanged drug)

Adults: Urine (15% to 18% as direct glucuronide metabolites, 2% to 10% as unchanged drug)

Dosing

Adult & Geriatric

Asthma treatment: Inhalation: **Note:** For asthma control, long-acting beta$_2$-agonists (LABAs) should be used in combination with inhaled corticosteroids and not as monotherapy.

U.S. labeling: Foradil Aerolizer: 12 mcg every 12 hours (maximum: 24 mcg daily)

Canadian labeling:
Foradil: 12 mcg every 12 hours; in severe cases, 24 mcg every 12 hours may be given (maximum: 48 mcg daily)
Oxeze Turbuhaler: 6 mcg or 12 mcg every 12 hours (maximum: 48 mcg daily)

Prevention of exercise-induced bronchospasm: Inhalation: **Note:** If already using for asthma maintenance, then should not use additional doses for exercise-induced bronchospasm. Because LABAs may disguise poorly controlled persistent asthma, frequent or chronic use of LABAs for exercise-induced bronchospasm is discouraged by the Asthma Guidelines (NAEPP, 2007).

U.S. labeling: Foradil Aerolizer: 12 mcg at least 15 minutes before exercise on an occasional "as needed" basis; additional doses should not be used for another 12 hours

Canadian labeling: Oxeze Turbuhaler: 6 mcg or 12 mcg at least 15 minutes before exercise on an occasional "as needed" basis (maximum: 48 mcg/24-hour period)

COPD maintenance treatment: Inhalation:
U.S. labeling:
Foradil Aerolizer: 12 mcg every 12 hours (maximum: 24 mcg daily)
Performomist: 20 mcg twice daily (maximum dose: 40 mcg daily)
Canadian labeling: Foradil: 12 mcg or 24 mcg twice daily (maximum dose: 48 mcg daily)

Pediatric

Asthma treatment: Inhalation: **Note:** For asthma control, long-acting beta$_2$-agonists (LABAs) should be used in combination with inhaled corticosteroids and not as monotherapy.

U.S. labeling: Foradil Aerolizer: Children ≥5 years and Adolescents: Refer to adult dosing.

Canadian labeling:
Foradil:
Children 6 to 16 years: 12 mcg every 12 hours (maximum: 24 mcg daily)
Adolescents ≥17 years: Refer to adult dosing.
Oxeze Turbuhaler:
Children 6 to 16 years: 6 mcg or 12 mcg every 12 hours (maximum: 24 mcg daily)
Adolescents ≥17 years: Refer to adult dosing.

Prevention of exercise-induced bronchospasm: Note: If already using for asthma maintenance, then should not use additional doses for exercise-induced bronchospasm. Because LABAs may disguise poorly controlled persistent asthma, frequent or chronic use of LABAs for exercise-induced bronchospasm is discouraged by the Asthma Guidelines (NAEPP, 2007).

U.S. labeling: Foradil Aerolizer: Children ≥5 years and Adolescents: Refer to adult dosing.

Canadian labeling: Oxeze Turbuhaler: Children ≥6 years and Adolescents: 6 mcg or 12 mcg at least 15 minutes before exercise on an occasional "as needed" basis (maximum: 24 mcg/24-hour period)

Renal Impairment No dosage adjustment provided in manufacturer's labeling (has not been studied).

Hepatic Impairment No dosage adjustment provided in manufacturer's labeling (has not been studied).

Administration

Foradil Aerolizer: Remove capsule from foil blister **immediately** before use. Place capsule in the capsule-chamber in the base of the Aerolizer Inhaler. Capsules must not be swallowed whole; must only use the Aerolizer Inhaler. Press both buttons **once only** and then release. Keep inhaler in a level, horizontal position. Exhale fully. Do not exhale into inhaler. Tilt head slightly back and inhale (rapidly, steadily, and deeply). Hold breath as long as possible. If any powder remains in capsule, exhale and inhale again. Repeat until capsule is empty. Throw away empty capsule; do not leave in inhaler. Do not use a spacer with the Aerolizer Inhaler. Always keep capsules and inhaler dry.

Performomist: Remove unit-dose vial from foil pouch **immediately** before use. Solution does not require dilution prior to administration; do not mix other medications with formoterol solution. Place contents of unit-dose vial into the reservoir of a standard jet nebulizer connected to an air compressor; assemble nebulizer based on the manufacturer's instructions and turn nebulizer on; breathe deeply and evenly until all of the medication has been inhaled. Discard any unused medication immediately; do not ingest contents of vial. Clean nebulizer after use.

Oxeze Turbuhaler (Canadian availability): Hold inhaler upright. Turn colored grip as far as it will go in one direction and then turn back to original position; a clicking sound should be heard which means the inhaler is ready for use. Exhale fully. Do not exhale into mouthpiece of inhaler. Place mouthpiece to lips and inhale forcefully and deeply.

Do not chew or bite on mouthpiece. Clean outside of mouthpiece once weekly with a dry tissue. Avoid getting inhaler wet. If the inhaler is accidently dropped or shaken, or if the patient exhales into the inhaler, the dose will be lost and a new dose should be loaded.

Monitoring Parameters FEV$_1$, peak flow, and/or other pulmonary function tests; blood pressure, heart rate; CNS stimulation; serum glucose, serum potassium

Dosage Forms Excipient information presented when available (limited, particularly for generics); consult specific product labeling.
Capsule, Inhalation, as fumarate:
Foradil Aerolizer: 12 mcg [contains milk protein]
Nebulization Solution, Inhalation, as fumarate dihydrate:
Performomist: 20 mcg/2 mL (2 mL)

Dosage Forms: Canada Excipient information presented when available (limited, particularly for generics); consult specific product labeling.
Powder for oral inhalation, as fumarate:
Oxeze Turbuhaler: 6 mcg/inhalation [delivers 60 metered doses; contains lactose 600 mcg/dose]; 12 mcg/inhalation [delivers 60 metered doses; contains lactose 600 mcg/dose]

◆ Formoterol and Budesonide *see* Budesonide and Formoterol *on page 260*

◆ Formoterol and Mometasone *see* Mometasone and Formoterol *on page 1228*

◆ Formoterol and Mometasone Furoate *see* Mometasone and Formoterol *on page 1228*

◆ Formoterol Fumarate *see* Formoterol *on page 809*

◆ Formoterol Fumarate Dihydrate *see* Formoterol *on page 809*

◆ Formoterol Fumarate Dihydrate and Budesonide *see* Budesonide and Formoterol *on page 260*

◆ Formoterol Fumarate Dihydrate and Mometasone *see* Mometasone and Formoterol *on page 1228*

◆ Formula E 400 [OTC] *see* Vitamin E *on page 1906*

◆ Formulex (Can) *see* Dicyclomine *on page 545*

◆ 5-Formyl Tetrahydrofolate *see* Leucovorin Calcium *on page 1049*

◆ Fortamet *see* MetFORMIN *on page 1156*

◆ Fortaz *see* CefTAZidime *on page 345*

◆ Fortaz in D5W *see* CefTAZidime *on page 345*

◆ Forteo *see* Teriparatide *on page 1765*

◆ Fortesta *see* Testosterone *on page 1766*

◆ Fortical *see* Calcitonin *on page 282*

◆ Fortovase *see* Saquinavir *on page 1636*

◆ Fosamax *see* Alendronate *on page 66*

◆ Fosamax Plus D® *see* Alendronate and Cholecalciferol *on page 68*

Fosamprenavir (FOS am pren a veer)

Brand Names: US Lexiva
Brand Names: Canada Telzir
Index Terms Fosamprenavir Calcium; GW433908G
Pharmacologic Category Antiretroviral, Protease Inhibitor (Anti-HIV)
Use HIV-1 infection: Treatment of HIV-1 infection, in combination with other antiretroviral agents
Dosing

Adult & Geriatric

HIV infection: Oral:
Antiretroviral therapy-naive patients: Oral:
Unboosted regimen (per manufacturer's labeling): 1,400 mg twice daily (without ritonavir); **Note:** This regimen is not recommended due to inferior potency compared to other protease inhibitor-based regimens and the potential for cross-resistance to darunavir (HHS [adults] 2015).
Ritonavir-boosted regimens:
Once-daily regimen: Fosamprenavir 1,400 mg plus ritonavir 100 to 200 mg once daily
Twice-daily regimen: Fosamprenavir 700 mg plus ritonavir 100 mg twice daily

Protease inhibitor (PI)-experienced patients: Fosamprenavir 700 mg plus ritonavir 100 mg twice daily. **Note:** Once-daily administration is not recommended in protease inhibitor-experienced patients.

Dosage adjustments for concomitant therapy: Oral:
Combination therapy with efavirenz (ritonavir-boosted regimen):
Once-daily regimen (PI-naive patients only): Fosamprenavir 1,400 mg plus ritonavir 300 mg plus efavirenz 600 mg once daily

Twice-daily regimen: Fosamprenavir 700 mg plus ritonavir 100 mg twice daily plus efavirenz 600 mg once daily

Combination therapy with maraviroc: Fosamprenavir 700 mg plus ritonavir 100 mg plus maraviroc 150 mg twice daily

Pediatric

HIV infection: Oral:

U.S. labeling: Infants ≥4 weeks, Children, and Adolescents <18 years: **Note:** Twice-daily dosing is recommended; once-daily dosing (without or without ritonavir) is **not** recommended in any pediatric patient.

Protease inhibitor (PI)-naive patients:

Ritonavir-boosted regimen: Infants ≥4 weeks, Children, and Adolescents: **Note:** Should not be administered to infants born <38 weeks' gestation and who have not attained a postnatal age of 28 days.

<11 kg: Fosamprenavir 45 mg/kg/dose twice daily **plus** ritonavir 7 mg/kg/dose twice daily (maximum: Fosamprenavir 700 mg/ritonavir 100 mg twice daily)

11 to <15 kg: Fosamprenavir 30 mg/kg/dose twice daily **plus** ritonavir 3 mg/kg/dose twice daily (maximum: Fosamprenavir 700 mg/ritonavir 100 mg twice daily)

15 to <20 kg: Fosamprenavir 23 mg/kg/dose twice daily **plus** ritonavir 3 mg/kg/dose twice daily (maximum: Fosamprenavir 700 mg/ritonavir 100 mg twice daily)

≥20 kg: Fosamprenavir 18 mg/kg/dose twice daily **plus** ritonavir 3 mg/kg/dose twice daily (maximum: Fosamprenavir 700 mg/ritonavir 100 mg twice daily)

Note: When combined with ritonavir, the adult regimen of fosamprenavir 700 mg plus ritonavir 100 mg twice daily can be used in children who weigh ≥39 kg; ritonavir capsules may be used for children who weigh ≥33 kg.

Unboosted regimen:

Children <2 years: Fosamprenavir without ritonavir is not recommended

Children and Adolescents ≥2 years and <47 kg: Fosamprenavir 30 mg/kg/dose twice daily (maximum: 1,400 mg twice daily)

Children and Adolescents ≥2 years and ≥47 kg: The adult regimen of fosamprenavir 1,400 mg twice daily may be used

Protease inhibitor (PI)-experienced patients:

Ritonavir-boosted regimen:

Infants <6 months: Not recommended in PI-experienced patients

Infants ≥6 months, Children, and Adolescents:

<11 kg: Fosamprenavir 45 mg/kg/dose twice daily **plus** ritonavir 7 mg/kg/dose twice daily (maximum: Fosamprenavir 700 mg/ritonavir 100 mg twice daily)

11 to <15 kg: Fosamprenavir 30 mg/kg/dose twice daily **plus** ritonavir 3 mg/kg/dose twice daily (maximum: Fosamprenavir 700 mg/ritonavir 100 mg twice daily)

15 to <20 kg: Fosamprenavir 23 mg/kg/dose twice daily **plus** ritonavir 3 mg/kg/dose twice daily (maximum: Fosamprenavir 700 mg/ritonavir 100 mg twice daily)

≥20 kg: Fosamprenavir 18 mg/kg/dose twice daily **plus** ritonavir 3 mg/kg/dose twice daily (maximum: Fosamprenavir 700 mg/ritonavir 100 mg twice daily)

Note: When combined with ritonavir, the adult regimen of fosamprenavir 700 mg plus ritonavir 100 mg twice daily can be used in children who weigh ≥39 kg; ritonavir capsules may be used for children who weigh ≥33 kg.

Unboosted regimen: **Note:** No information provided in manufacturer's labeling regarding unboosted fosamprenavir in PI-experienced pediatric patients except that fosamprenavir without ritonavir is not recommended in children <2 years of age and the adult unboosted regimen of 1,400 mg twice daily may be used for pediatric patients who weigh ≥47 kg.

Canadian labeling: **Note:** Use of fosamprenavir without ritonavir (unboosted regimen) is not an approved use in the Canadian labeling.

PI-naive and PI-experienced patients: *Ritonavir boosted regimen:* Children ≥6 years: 18 mg/kg/dose **plus** ritonavir 3 mg/kg/dose twice daily; maximum dose: Fosamprenavir 700 mg/ritonavir 100 mg twice daily; adult regimen of fosamprenavir 700 mg/ritonavir 100 mg twice daily can be used in children who weigh ≥39 kg while ritonavir tablets may be used for children who weigh ≥33 kg and can swallow tablets whole.

Renal Impairment There are no dosage adjustments provided in the manufacturer's labeling (has not been studied); however, dosage adjustment unlikely due to minimal (eg, 1%) renal elimination of unchanged amprenavir.

Hepatic Impairment

Adults:

Mild impairment (Child-Pugh class A): Reduce dosage of fosamprenavir to 700 mg twice daily without concurrent ritonavir (therapy naive) **or** fosamprenavir 700 mg twice daily plus ritonavir 100 mg once daily (therapy naive or PI experienced).

Moderate impairment (Child-Pugh class B): Reduce dosage of fosamprenavir to 700 mg twice daily without concurrent ritonavir (therapy naive) **or** fosamprenavir 450 mg twice daily plus ritonavir 100 mg once daily (therapy naive or PI experienced).

Severe impairment (Child-Pugh class C: Reduce dosage of fosamprenavir to 350 mg twice daily without concurrent ritonavir (therapy naive) **or** fosamprenavir 300 mg twice daily plus ritonavir 100 mg once daily (therapy naive or PI experienced).

Children: There are no dosage adjustments provided in the manufacturer's labeling (has not been studied).

Additional Information Complete prescribing information should be consulted for additional detail.

Dosage Forms Excipient information presented when available (limited, particularly for generics); consult specific product labeling.

Suspension, Oral, as calcium:

Lexiva: 50 mg/mL (225 mL) [contains methylparaben, polysorbate 80, propylene glycol, propylparaben; grape bubblegum peppermint flavor]

Tablet, Oral, as calcium:

Lexiva: 700 mg

Dosage Forms: Canada Excipient information presented when available (limited, particularly for generics); consult specific product labeling.

Tablet, as calcium:

Telzir: 700 mg

Suspension, oral, as calcium:

Telzir: 50 mg/mL (225 mL)

◆ **Fosamprenavir Calcium** *see* Fosamprenavir *on page 811*

Fosaprepitant (fos a PRE pi tant)

Brand Names: US Emend

Brand Names: Canada Emend® IV

Index Terms Aprepitant Injection; Fosaprepitant Dimeglumine; L-758,298; MK 0517

Pharmacologic Category Antiemetic; Substance P/Neurokinin 1 Receptor Antagonist

Use Prevention of acute and delayed nausea and vomiting associated with moderately- and highly-emetogenic chemotherapy (in combination with other antiemetics)

Pregnancy Considerations Adverse events were not observed in animal reproduction studies for aprepitant. Efficacy of hormonal contraceptive may be reduced; alternative or additional methods of contraception should be used both during treatment with fosaprepitant or aprepitant and for at least 1 month following the last fosaprepitant/aprepitant dose.

Breast-Feeding Considerations It is not known if fosaprepitant is excreted in breast milk. Due to the potential for serious adverse reactions in the nursing infant, the manufacturer recommends a decision be made whether to discontinue nursing or to discontinue the drug, taking into account the importance of treatment to the mother.

Contraindications Hypersensitivity to fosaprepitant, aprepitant, polysorbate 80, or any component of the formulation; concurrent use with pimozide or cisapride

Canadian labeling: Additional contraindications (not in U.S. labeling): Concurrent use with astemizole or terfenadine

Warnings/Precautions Fosaprepitant is rapidly converted to aprepitant, which has a high potential for drug interactions. Potentially significant drug-drug interactions may exist, requiring dose or frequency adjustment, additional monitoring, and/or selection of alternative therapy. Immediate hypersensitivity has been reported (rarely) with fosaprepitant; stop infusion with hypersensitivity symptoms (dyspnea, erythema, flushing, or anaphylaxis); do not reinitiate. Some dosage forms may contain polysorbate 80 (also known as Tweens). Hypersensitivity reactions, usually a delayed reaction, have been reported following exposure to pharmaceutical products containing polysorbate 80 in certain individuals (Isaksson, 2002; Lucente 2000; Shelley, 1995). Thrombocytopenia, ascites, pulmonary deterioration, and renal and hepatic failure have been reported in premature neonates after receiving parenteral

products containing polysorbate 80 (Alade, 1986; CDC, 1984). See manufacturer's labeling. Use caution with hepatic impairment; has not been studied in patients with severe hepatic impairment (Child-Pugh class C). Not studied for treatment of existing nausea and vomiting. Chronic continuous administration of fosaprepitant is not recommended.

Adverse Reactions Adverse reactions reported with aprepitant and fosaprepitant (as part of a combination chemotherapy regimen) occurring at a higher frequency than standard antiemetic therapy:

1% to 10%:

Central nervous system: Fatigue (1% to 3%), headache (2%)

Gastrointestinal: Anorexia (2%), constipation (2%), dyspepsia (2%), diarrhea (1%), eructation (1%)

Hepatic: ALT increased (1% to 3%), AST increased (1%)

Local: Injection site reactions (3%; includes erythema, induration, pain, pruritus, or thrombophlebitis)

Neuromuscular & skeletal: Weakness (3%)

Miscellaneous: Hiccups (5%)

<1% (Limited to important or life-threatening): Abdominal pain, alkaline phosphatase increased, anaphylactic reaction, anemia, angioedema, bradycardia, candidiasis, cardiovascular disorder, chest discomfort, chills, cognitive disorder, conjunctivitis, cough, disorientation, dizziness, duodenal ulcer (perforating), dyspnea, edema, erythema, flushing, gait disturbance, hematuria (microscopic), hyperglycemia, hyperhydrosis, hypersensitivity reaction, hypertension, hyponatremia, miosis, nausea, neutropenia, neutropenic colitis, neutropenic fever, palpitation, photosensitivity, pollakiuria, polyuria, pruritus, rash, sensory disturbance, somnolence, staphylococcal infection, Stevens-Johnson syndrome, stomatitis, subileus, tinnitus, toxic epidermal necrolysis, urticaria, visual acuity decreased, vomiting, wheezing

Drug Interactions

Metabolism/Transport Effects Substrate of CYP1A2 (minor), CYP2C19 (minor), CYP3A4 (major); **Note:** Assignment of Major/Minor substrate status based on clinically relevant drug interaction potential; **Inhibits** CYP2C19 (weak), CYP2C9 (weak), CYP3A4 (weak); **Induces** CYP2C9 (weak/moderate)

Avoid Concomitant Use

Avoid concomitant use of Fosaprepitant with any of the following: Astemizole; Cisapride; Conivaptan; Fusidic Acid (Systemic); Idelalisib; Pimozide; Terfenadine

Increased Effect/Toxicity

Fosaprepitant may increase the levels/effects of: ARIPiprazole; Astemizole; Cisapride; Corticosteroids (Systemic); CYP3A4 Substrates; Diltiazem; Dofetilide; Flibanserin; Hydrocodone; Ifosfamide; Lomitapide; NiMODipine; Pimozide; Sirolimus; Terfenadine

The levels/effects of Fosaprepitant may be increased by: Aprepitant; Conivaptan; CYP3A4 Inhibitors (Moderate); CYP3A4 Inhibitors (Strong); Dasatinib; Diltiazem; Fusidic Acid (Systemic); Idelalisib; Ivacaftor; Luliconazole; Mifepristone; Netupitant; Osimertinib; Palbociclib; Simeprevir; Stiripentol

Decreased Effect

Fosaprepitant may decrease the levels/effects of: Contraceptives (Estrogens); Contraceptives (Progestins); PARoxetine; TOLBUTamide; Warfarin

The levels/effects of Fosaprepitant may be decreased by: Bosentan; CYP3A4 Inducers (Moderate); CYP3A4 Inducers (Strong); Dabrafenib; Deferasirox; Enzalutamide; Mitotane; Osimertinib; PARoxetine; Rifampin; Siltuximab; St Johns Wort; Tocilizumab

Food Interactions Aprepitant serum concentration may be increased when taken with grapefruit juice. Management: Avoid concurrent use.

Preparation for Administration Reconstitute vial with 5 mL of sodium chloride 0.9%, directing diluent down side of vial to avoid foaming; swirl gently. Add reconstituted contents of the 150 mg vial to 145 mL sodium chloride 0.9%, resulting in a final concentration of 1 mg/mL; gently invert bag to mix. Solutions may be diluted to a final volume of 250 mL (0.6 mg/mL) (data on file [Merck, 2013]).

Storage/Stability Store intact vials at 2°C to 8°C (36°F to 46°F). Solutions diluted to 1 mg/mL for infusion are stable for 24 hours at room temperature or at ≤25°C (≤77°F). Solutions diluted to a final volume of 250 mL (0.6 mg/mL) should be administered within 24 hours (data on file [Merck, 2013]).

Mechanism of Action Fosaprepitant is a prodrug of aprepitant, a substance P/neurokinin 1 (NK1) receptor antagonist. It is rapidly converted to aprepitant which prevents acute and delayed vomiting by inhibiting the substance P/neurokinin 1 (NK1) receptor; augments the antiemetic activity of the 5-HT$_3$ receptor antagonist and corticosteroid activity and inhibits chemotherapy-induced emesis.

Pharmacodynamics/Kinetics

Distribution: Fosaprepitant: ~5 L; Aprepitant: V_d: ~70 L; crosses the blood-brain barrier

Protein binding: Aprepitant: >95%

Metabolism:

Fosaprepitant: Hepatic and extrahepatic; rapidly (within 30 minutes after the end of infusion) converted to aprepitant (nearly complete conversion)

Aprepitant: Hepatic via CYP3A4 (major); CYP1A2 and CYP2C19 (minor); forms 7 weakly-active metabolites

Half-life elimination: Fosaprepitant: ~2 minutes; Aprepitant: ~9-13 hours

Time to peak, plasma: Fosaprepitant is converted to aprepitant within 30 minutes after the end of infusion

Excretion: Urine (57%); feces (45%)

Clearance: 62 to 90 mL/minute

Dosing

Adult & Geriatric Prevention of chemotherapy-induced nausea/vomiting: IV:

Single-dose regimen for highly-emetogenic chemotherapy: 150 mg ~30 minutes prior to chemotherapy on day 1 only (in combination with a 5-HT$_3$ antagonist on day 1 and dexamethasone on days 1 to 4)

Single-dose regimen for moderately-emetogenic chemotherapy: 150 mg ~30 minutes prior to chemotherapy on day 1 only (in combination with a 5-HT$_3$ antagonist and dexamethasone on day 1, and either a 5-HT$_3$ antagonist or dexamethasone on days 2 and 3) (NCCN Antiemesis guidelines v.1.2013)

Renal Impairment

Mild, moderate, or severe impairment: No dosage adjustment necessary.

Dialysis-dependent end-stage renal disease (ESRD): No dosage adjustment necessary.

Hepatic Impairment

Mild or moderate impairment (Child-Pugh class A or B): No dosage adjustment necessary.

Severe impairment (Child-Pugh class C): Has not been evaluated; use with caution.

Administration 150 mg: Infuse over 20-30 minutes ~30 minutes prior to chemotherapy

Dosage Forms Excipient information presented when available (limited, particularly for generics); consult specific product labeling.

Solution Reconstituted, Intravenous:

Emend: 150 mg (1 ea) [contains disodium edta, polysorbate 80]

◆ Fosaprepitant Dimeglumine see Fosaprepitant on page 812

◆ Fosavance (Can) see Alendronate and Cholecalciferol on page 68

Foscarnet (fos KAR net)

Brand Names: US Foscavir

Brand Names: Canada Foscavir

Index Terms Foscavir; PFA; Phosphonoformate; Phosphonoformic Acid

Pharmacologic Category Antiviral Agent

Use

Cytomegalovirus retinitis: Treatment of cytomegalovirus (CMV) retinitis in persons with AIDS

Herpes simplex virus: Treatment of acyclovir-resistant mucocutaneous herpes simplex virus (HSV) infections in immunocompromised persons (eg, with advanced AIDS)

Dosing

Adult & Geriatric

Cytomegalovirus (CMV) retinitis: IV:

Induction treatment: 60 mg/kg/dose every 8 hours for 14 to 21 days or 90 mg/kg every 12 hours for 14 to 21 days

Maintenance therapy: 90 to 120 mg/kg/day as a single daily infusion; due to lower toxicity, begin with 90 mg/kg once daily, may escalate to 120 mg/kg once daily if lower dose tolerated or for retinitis progression

CMV infection (preemptive therapy) after allogeneic stem cell transplantation (off-label use; second-line therapy): IV:

    <100 days posttransplant: Induction: 60 mg/kg every 12 hours for 7 to 14 days, followed by maintenance therapy: 90 mg/kg once daily if CMV is still detectable and declining, continue until indicator test is negative. Minimum total duration (induction and maintenance) is 2 weeks (Tomblyn 2009)

    >100 days posttransplant: 60 mg/kg every 12 hours for 14 days, continue treatment with 90 mg/kg once daily for 7 to 14 days or until indicator test is negative (Tomblyn 2009)

CMV infection (prophylaxis) after allogeneic stem cell transplantation (off-label use; second-line therapy): IV: 60 mg/kg every 12 hours for 7 days, followed by 90 to 120 mg/kg once daily until day 100 after transplant (Tomblyn 2009)

CMV esophagitis or colitis in HIV-infected patients (alternative to preferred therapy) (off-label use): IV: 60 mg/kg/dose every 8 hours or 90 mg/kg/dose every 12 hours for 21 to 42 days or until symptom resolution (HHS [OI adult 2015])

CMV neurological disease in HIV-infected patients (off-label use): IV: 60 mg/kg/dose every 8 hours or 90 mg/kg/dose every 12 hours plus ganciclovir until symptoms improve followed by chronic maintenance suppression (secondary prophylaxis) (HHS [OI adult 2015])

Herpes simplex infections (acyclovir-resistant): Induction: IV: 40 mg/kg/dose every 8 to 12 hours for 14 to 21 days

Pediatric

Cytomegalovirus (CMV) infection (preemptive therapy) after allogeneic stem cell transplantation (off-label use; second-line therapy): IV:

    <100 days posttransplant: Induction: 60 mg/kg every 12 hours for 7 to 14 days, followed by maintenance therapy: 90 mg/kg once daily if CMV is still detectable and declining, continue until indicator test is negative. Minimum total duration (induction and maintenance) is 2 weeks (Tomblyn 2009)

    >100 days posttransplant: 60 mg/kg every 12 hours for 14 days, continue treatment with 90 mg/kg once daily for 7 to 14 days or until indicator test is negative (Tomblyn 2009)

CMV infection (prophylaxis) after allogeneic stem cell transplantation (off-label use; second-line therapy): IV: 60 mg/kg every 12 hours for 7 days, followed by 90 to 120 mg/kg once daily until day 100 after transplant (Tomblyn 2009)

CMV esophagitis or colitis in HIV-infected patients (alternative to preferred therapy) (off-label use): Adolescents: Refer to adult dosing.

CMV neurological disease in HIV-infected patients (off-label use): Adolescents: Refer to adult dosing

Renal Impairment See tables.

Induction Dosing of Foscarnet in Patients With Abnormal Renal Function

CrCl (mL/min/kg)	HSV Equivalent to 40 mg/kg every 12 hours	HSV Equivalent to 40 mg/kg every 8 hours	CMV Equivalent to 60 mg/kg every 8 hours	CMV Equivalent to 90 mg/kg every 12 hours
<0.4	Not recommended	Not recommended	Not recommended	Not recommended
≥0.4-0.5	20 mg/kg every 24 hours	35 mg/kg every 24 hours	50 mg/kg every 24 hours	50 mg/kg every 24 hours
>0.5-0.6	25 mg/kg every 24 hours	40 mg/kg every 24 hours	60 mg/kg every 24 hours	60 mg/kg every 24 hours
>0.6-0.8	35 mg/kg every 24 hours	25 mg/kg every 12 hours	40 mg/kg every 12 hours	80 mg/kg every 24 hours
>0.8-1	20 mg/kg every 12 hours	35 mg/kg every 12 hours	50 mg/kg every 12 hours	50 mg/kg every 12 hours
>1-1.4	30 mg/kg every 12 hours	30 mg/kg every 8 hours	45 mg/kg every 8 hours	70 mg/kg every 12 hours
>1.4	40 mg/kg every 12 hours	40 mg/kg every 8 hours	60 mg/kg every 8 hours	90 mg/kg every 12 hours

Maintenance Dosing of Foscarnet in Patients With Abnormal Renal Function

CrCl (mL/min/kg)	CMV Equivalent to 90 mg/kg every 24 hours	CMV Equivalent to 120 mg/kg every 24 hours
<0.4	Not recommended	Not recommended
≥0.4-0.5	50 mg/kg every 48 hours	65 mg/kg every 48 hours
>0.5-0.6	60 mg/kg every 48 hours	80 mg/kg every 48 hours
>0.6-0.8	80 mg/kg every 48 hours	105 mg/kg every 48 hours
>0.8-1	50 mg/kg every 24 hours	65 mg/kg every 24 hours
>1-1.4	70 mg/kg every 24 hours	90 mg/kg every 24 hours
>1.4	90 mg/kg every 24 hours	120 mg/kg every 24 hours

Hemodialysis:

    Foscarnet is highly removed by hemodialysis (up to ~38% in 2.5 hours HD with high-flux membrane) (Aweeka 1999)

    Doses of 45 to 60 mg/kg/dose posthemodialysis (3 times/week) with the monitoring of weekly plasma concentrations to maintain peak plasma concentrations in the range of 500 to 800 micromolar for the treatment of CMV infection have been recommended (Aweeka 1999; Jayasekara 1999; MacGregor 1991)

Peritoneal dialysis: HSV infection (localized or disseminated): IV: 60 mg/kg/dose every 48 to 72 hours; higher doses may be necessary for herpes encephalitis or herpes zoster infection (Jayasekara 1999)

Hepatic Impairment There are no dosage adjustments provided in manufacturer's labeling.

Additional Information Complete prescribing information should be consulted for additional detail.

Dosage Forms Excipient information presented when available (limited, particularly for generics); consult specific product labeling. [DSC] = Discontinued product

Solution, Intravenous, as sodium:
    Generic: 24 mg/mL (500 mL [DSC])

Solution, Intravenous, as sodium [preservative free]:
    Foscavir: 24 mg/mL (250 mL)
    Generic: 24 mg/mL (250 mL [DSC])

♦ Foscavir see Foscarnet on page 813

Fosfomycin (fos foe MYE sin)

Brand Names: US Monurol
Brand Names: Canada Monurol
Index Terms Fosfomycin Tromethamine
Pharmacologic Category Antibiotic, Miscellaneous

Use

Uncomplicated urinary tract infections: Treatment of uncomplicated urinary tract infections (acute cystitis) in women due to susceptible strains of *Escherichia coli* and *Enterococcus faecalis*.

Limitations of use: Not indicated for the treatment of pyelonephritis or perinephric abscess. If persistence or reappearance of bacteriuria occurs after treatment with fosfomycin, other therapeutic agents should be selected.

Dosing

Adult & Geriatric

Urinary tract infections, uncomplicated: Oral: Females: Single dose of 3 g in 3 to 4 oz (90 to 120 mL) of water

Complicated UTI (off-label): Males: Oral: 3 g every 2 to 3 days for 3 doses (Neuner 2012; Pullukcu 2007)

Prostatitis (off-label): Males: Oral: 3 g every 3 days for a total of 21 days (Shrestha, 2000)

Renal Impairment There are no dosage adjustments provided in the manufacturer's labeling.

Hepatic Impairment There are no dosage adjustments provided in the manufacturer's labeling.

Additional Information Complete prescribing information should be consulted for additional detail.

Dosage Forms Excipient information presented when available (limited, particularly for generics); consult specific product labeling. [DSC] = Discontinued product

Packet, Oral:
    Monurol: 3 g (1 ea, 3 ea [DSC]) [orange flavor]

♦ Fosfomycin Tromethamine see Fosfomycin on page 814

Fosinopril (foe SIN oh pril)

Brand Names: Canada Apo-Fosinopril; Ava-Fosinopril; Jamp-Fosinopril; Mylan-Fosinopril; PMS-Fosinopril; RAN-Fosinopril; Riva-Fosinopril; Teva-Fosinopril
Index Terms Fosinopril Sodium; Monopril

Pharmacologic Category Angiotensin-Converting Enzyme (ACE) Inhibitor; Antihypertensive

Use

Hypertension: Treatment of hypertension, either alone or in combination with other antihypertensive agents

The 2014 guideline for the management of high blood pressure in adults (Eighth Joint National Committee [JNC 8]) recommends initiation of pharmacologic treatment to lower blood pressure for the following patients:

- Patients ≥60 years of age with systolic blood pressure (SBP) ≥150 mm Hg or diastolic blood pressure (DBP) ≥90 mm Hg. Goal of therapy is SBP <150 mm Hg and DBP <90 mm Hg.
- Patients <60 years of age with SBP ≥140 mm Hg or DBP is ≥90 mm Hg. Goal of therapy is SBP <140 mm Hg and DBP <90 mm Hg.
- Patients ≥18 years of age with diabetes and SBP ≥140 mm Hg or DBP ≥90 mm Hg. Goal of therapy is SBP <140 mm Hg and DBP <90 mm Hg.
- Patients ≥18 years of age with chronic kidney disease (CKD) and SBP ≥140 mm Hg or DBP ≥90 mm Hg. Goal of therapy is SBP <140 mm Hg and DBP <90 mm Hg.

In patients with CKD, regardless of race or diabetes status, the use of an ACE inhibitor (ACEI) or angiotensin receptor blocker (ARB) as initial therapy is recommended to improve kidney outcomes. In the general nonblack population (without CKD) including those with diabetes, initial antihypertensive treatment should consist of a thiazide-type diuretic, calcium channel blocker, ACEI, or ARB. In the general black population (without CKD) including those with diabetes, initial antihypertensive treatment should consist of a thiazide-type diuretic or a calcium channel blocker **instead of** an ACEI or ARB.

Heart failure: Adjunctive treatment of heart failure (HF)

The ACCF/AHA 2013 heart failure guidelines recommend the use of ACE inhibitors, along with other guideline directed medical therapies, to prevent heart failure in patients with a reduced ejection fraction who have a history of MI (Stage B HF), to prevent HF in any patient with a reduced ejection fraction (Stage B HF), or to treat those with HF and reduced ejection fraction (Stage C HFrEF) (ACCF/AHA [Yancy 2013]).

Pregnancy Considerations [U.S. Boxed Warning]: Drugs that act on the renin-angiotensin system can cause injury and death to the developing fetus. Discontinue as soon as possible once pregnancy is detected. Fosinopril crosses the placenta. Drugs that act on the renin-angiotensin system are associated with oligohydramnios. Oligohydramnios, due to decreased fetal renal function, may lead to fetal lung hypoplasia and skeletal malformations. The use of these drugs in pregnancy is also associated with anuria, hypotension, renal failure, skull hypoplasia, and death in the fetus/neonate. Teratogenic effects may occur following maternal use of an ACE inhibitor during the first trimester, although this finding may be confounded by maternal disease. Because adverse fetal events are well documented with exposure later in pregnancy, ACE inhibitor use in pregnant women is not recommended (Seely 2014; Weber 2014). Infants exposed to an ACE inhibitor in utero should be monitored for hyperkalemia, hypotension, and oliguria. Oligohydramnios may not appear until after irreversible fetal injury has occurred. Exchange transfusions or dialysis may be required to reverse hypotension or improve renal function, although data related to the effectiveness in neonates is limited.

Chronic maternal hypertension itself is also associated with adverse events in the fetus/infant and mother. ACE inhibitors are not recommended for the treatment of uncomplicated hypertension in pregnancy (ACOG 2013) and they are specifically contraindicated for the treatment of hypertension and chronic heart failure during pregnancy by some guidelines (Regitz-Zagrosek 2011). In addition, ACE inhibitors should generally be avoided in women of reproductive age (ACOG 2013). If treatment for hypertension or chronic heart failure in pregnancy is needed, other agents should be used (ACOG 2013; Regitz-Zagrosek 2011).

Breast-Feeding Considerations Fosinoprilat is excreted in breast milk. Breast-feeding is not recommended by the manufacturer.

Contraindications Hypersensitivity to fosinopril, any other ACE inhibitor, or any component of the formulation; angioedema related to previous treatment with an ACE inhibitor; concomitant use with aliskiren in patients with diabetes mellitus

Warnings/Precautions Anaphylactic reactions may occur rarely with ACE inhibitors. At any time during treatment (especially following first dose), angioedema may occur rarely with ACE inhibitors; it may involve the head and neck (potentially compromising airway) or the intestine (presenting with abdominal pain). African-Americans may be at an increased risk and patients with idiopathic or hereditary angioedema may be at an increased risk. Risk may also be increased with concomitant use of mTOR inhibitor (eg, everolimus) therapy. Prolonged frequent monitoring may be required especially if tongue, glottis, or larynx are involved as they are associated with airway obstruction. Patients with a history of airway surgery may have a higher risk of airway obstruction. Aggressive early and appropriate management is critical. Use in patients with previous angioedema associated with ACE inhibitor therapy is contraindicated. Severe anaphylactoid reactions may be seen during hemodialysis (eg, CVVHD) with high-flux dialysis membranes (eg, AN69), and rarely, during low density lipoprotein apheresis with dextran sulfate cellulose. Rare cases of anaphylactoid reactions have been reported in patients undergoing sensitization treatment with hymenoptera (bee, wasp) venom while receiving ACE inhibitors.

Symptomatic hypotension with or without syncope can occur with ACE inhibitors (usually with the first several doses); effects are most often observed in volume-depleted patients; correct volume depletion prior to initiation; close monitoring of patient is required especially with initial dosing and dosing increases; blood pressure must be lowered at a rate appropriate for the patient's clinical condition. Initiation of therapy in patients with ischemic heart disease or cerebrovascular disease warrants close observation due to the potential consequences posed by falling blood pressure (eg, MI, stroke). Use with caution in hypertrophic cardiomyopathy with outflow tract obstruction and severe aortic stenosis. In patients on chronic ACE inhibitor therapy, intraoperative hypotension may occur with induction and maintenance of general anesthesia; use with caution before, during, or immediately after major surgery. Cardiopulmonary bypass, intraoperative blood loss, or vasodilating anesthesia increases endogenous renin release. Use of ACE inhibitors perioperatively will blunt angiotensin II formation and may result in hypotension. However, discontinuation of therapy prior to surgery is controversial. If continued preoperatively, avoidance of hypotensive agents during surgery is prudent (Hillis 2011). **[U.S. Boxed Warning]: Drugs that act on the renin-angiotensin system can cause injury and death to the developing fetus. Discontinue as soon as possible once pregnancy is detected.**

Hyperkalemia may occur with ACE inhibitors; risk factors include renal dysfunction, diabetes mellitus, concomitant use of potassium-sparing diuretics, potassium supplements, and/or potassium-containing salts. Use cautiously, if at all, with these agents and monitor potassium closely. Cough may occur with ACE inhibitors. Other causes of cough should be considered (eg, pulmonary congestion in patients with heart failure) and excluded prior to discontinuation. Use with caution in hepatic impairment; fosinopril undergoes hepatic and gut wall metabolism to its active form (fosinoprilat) and may accumulate in hepatic impairment. In patients with alcoholic or biliary cirrhosis, the rate of fosinoprilat formation is slowed, its total body clearance decreased and its AUC ~doubled.

May be associated with deterioration of renal function and/or increases in serum creatinine, particularly in patients with low renal blood flow (eg, renal artery stenosis, heart failure) whose glomerular filtration rate (GFR) is dependent on efferent arteriolar vasoconstriction by angiotensin II; deterioration may result in oliguria, acute renal failure, and progressive azotemia. Small increases in serum creatinine may occur following initiation; consider discontinuation only in patients with progressive and/or significant deterioration in renal function. Use with caution in patients with unstented unilateral/bilateral renal artery stenosis. When unstented bilateral renal artery stenosis is present, use is generally avoided due to the elevated risk of deterioration in renal function unless possible benefits outweigh risks. Potentially significant drug-drug interactions may exist, requiring dose or frequency adjustment, additional monitoring, and/or selection of alternative therapy.

Rare toxicities associated with ACE inhibitors include cholestatic jaundice (which may progress to fulminant hepatic necrosis), agranulocytosis, neutropenia or leukopenia with myeloid hypoplasia. Patients with collagen vascular diseases (especially with concomitant renal impairment) or renal impairment alone may be at increased risk for hematologic toxicity; periodically monitor CBC with differential in these patients.

Adverse Reactions Note: Frequency ranges include data from hypertension and heart failure trials. Higher rates of adverse reactions have generally been noted in patients with CHF. However, the frequency of adverse effects associated with placebo is also increased in this population.

>10%: Central nervous system: Dizziness (1.6% to 11.9%)

1% to 10%:

Cardiovascular: Orthostatic hypotension (1.4% to 1.9%), palpitation (1.4%)

Central nervous system: Dizziness (1% to 2%; up to 12% in CHF patients), headache (3.2%), fatigue (1% to 2%)

Endocrine & metabolic: Hyperkalemia (2.6%)

Gastrointestinal: Diarrhea (2.2%), nausea/vomiting (1.2% to 2.2%)

Hepatic: Transaminases increased

Neuromuscular & skeletal: Musculoskeletal pain (<1% to 3.3%), noncardiac chest pain (<1% to 2.2%), weakness (1.4%)

Renal: Serum creatinine increased, renal function worsening (in patients with bilateral renal artery stenosis or hypovolemia)

Respiratory: Cough (2.2% to 9.7%)

Miscellaneous: Upper respiratory infection (2.2%)

>1% but ≤ frequency in patients receiving placebo: Sexual dysfunction, fever, flu-like syndrome, dyspnea, rash, headache, insomnia

<1% (Limited to important or life-threatening): Anaphylactoid reaction, angina, angioedema, arthralgia, bronchospasm, cerebral infarction, cerebrovascular accident, gout, hepatitis, hepatomegaly, myalgia, MI, pancreatitis, paresthesia, photosensitivity, pleuritic chest pain, pruritus, rash, renal insufficiency, shock, sudden death, syncope, TIA, tinnitus, urticaria, vertigo. In a small number of patients, a symptom complex of cough, bronchospasm, and eosinophilia has been observed with fosinopril.

Other events reported with ACE inhibitors: Acute renal failure, agranulocytosis, anemia, aplastic anemia, bullous pemphigus, cardiac arrest, eosinophilic pneumonitis, exfoliative dermatitis, gynecomastia, hemolytic anemia, hepatic failure, jaundice, neutropenia, pancytopenia, Stevens-Johnson syndrome, symptomatic hyponatremia, thrombocytopenia. In addition, a syndrome which may include fever, myalgia, arthralgia, interstitial nephritis, vasculitis, rash, eosinophilia and positive ANA, and elevated ESR has been reported for other ACE inhibitors.

Drug Interactions

Metabolism/Transport Effects None known.

Avoid Concomitant Use

Avoid concomitant use of Fosinopril with any of the following: Sacubitril

Increased Effect/Toxicity

Fosinopril may increase the levels/effects of: Allopurinol; Amifostine; Antipsychotic Agents (Second Generation [Atypical]); AzaTHIOprine; Ciprofloxacin (Systemic); Drospirenone; DULoxetine; Ferric Gluconate; Gold Sodium Thiomalate; Grass Pollen Allergen Extract (5 Grass Extract); Hypotension-Associated Agents; Iron Dextran Complex; Levodopa; Lithium; Nonsteroidal Anti-Inflammatory Agents; Pregabalin; Sacubitril; Sodium Phosphates

The levels/effects of Fosinopril may be increased by: Alfuzosin; Aliskiren; Angiotensin II Receptor Blockers; Barbiturates; Brimonidine (Topical); Canagliflozin; Dapoxetine; Diazoxide; DPP-IV Inhibitors; Eplerenone; Everolimus; Heparin; Heparin (Low Molecular Weight); Herbs (Hypotensive Properties); Loop Diuretics; Molsidomine; Nicorandil; Obinutuzumab; Pentoxifylline; Phosphodiesterase 5 Inhibitors; Potassium Salts; Potassium-Sparing Diuretics; Prostacyclin Analogues; Salicylates; Sirolimus; Temsirolimus; Thiazide Diuretics; TiZANidine; Tolvaptan; Trimethoprim

Decreased Effect

The levels/effects of Fosinopril may be decreased by: Amphetamines; Antacids; Aprotinin; Herbs (Hypertensive Properties); Icatibant; Lanthanum; Methylphenidate; Nonsteroidal Anti-Inflammatory Agents; Salicylates; Yohimbine

Storage/Stability Store at 25°C (77°F); excursions permitted to 15°C to 30°C (59°F to 86°F). Protect from moisture.

Mechanism of Action Competitive inhibitor of angiotensin-converting enzyme (ACE); prevents conversion of angiotensin I to angiotensin II, a potent vasoconstrictor; results in lower levels of angiotensin II which causes an increase in plasma renin activity and a reduction in aldosterone secretion; a CNS mechanism may also be involved in hypotensive effect as angiotensin II increases adrenergic outflow from CNS; vasoactive kallikreins may be decreased in conversion to active hormones by ACE inhibitors, thus reducing blood pressure

Pharmacodynamics/Kinetics

Onset of action: 1 hour

Duration: 24 hours

Absorption: 36%

Protein binding: >99%

Metabolism: Prodrug, hydrolyzed to its active metabolite fosinoprilat by intestinal wall and hepatic esterases; fosinopril is also metabolized to a glucuronide conjugate and a p-hydroxy metabolite of fosinoprilat

Bioavailability: 36%

Half-life elimination, serum (fosinoprilat):

Children and Adolescents 6-16 years: 11-13 hours

Adults: 12 hours

Adults with CHF: 14 hours

Time to peak, serum: ~3 hours

Excretion: Urine and feces (as fosinoprilat and other metabolites in roughly equal proportions)

Dosing

Adult & Geriatric

Heart failure: Oral: Per the manufacturer: Initial: 10 mg once daily (5 mg once daily if moderate to severe renal dysfunction is present or if aggressively diuresed); increase dose as needed and as tolerated over several weeks. Usual dosage range: 20 to 40 mg once daily (maximum dose: 40 mg once daily). If hypotension, orthostasis, or azotemia occurs during titration, consider decreasing concomitant diuretic dose, if any.

ACCF/AHA 2013 heart failure guidelines: Initial: 5 to 10 mg once daily. Target dose: 40 mg once daily (Yancy 2013).

Hypertension: Oral: Initial: 10 mg once daily; maximum dose: 80 mg once daily. May need to divide the dose into two if trough effect is inadequate. If patient is receiving a diuretic prior to initiation, consider discontinuation of the diuretic to reduce likelihood of hypotension, if possible 2 to 3 days before initiation of therapy. If blood pressure response is inadequate, resume diuretic therapy carefully. Usual dose range (ASH/ISH [Weber 2014]): 10 to 40 mg daily.

HIV-associated nephropathy (HIVAN) (off-label use): Oral: 10 mg once daily (Wei 2003).

Pediatric Hypertension: Children ≥6 years and Adolescents >50 kg: Oral: Initial: 5 to 10 mg once daily (maximum: 40 mg once daily)

Renal Impairment

Moderate-severe impairment: Initial dose reduction to 5 mg once daily recommended for heart failure patients. No other dose adjustments are required; hepatobiliary elimination partially compensates for diminished renal elimination.

Hemodialysis: Poorly dialyzed; supplemental dose not required (Gehr, 1993)

Peritoneal dialysis: Poorly dialyzed; supplemental dose not required (Gehr, 1991)

Hepatic Impairment There are no dosage adjustments provided in the manufacturer's labeling.

Dietary Considerations Should not take a potassium salt supplement without the advice of healthcare provider.

Monitoring Parameters Blood pressure; BUN, serum creatinine and potassium; if patient has collagen vascular disease and/or renal impairment, periodically monitor CBC with differential

2013 ACCF/AHA Heart Failure guideline recommendations: Within 1 to 2 weeks after initiation and periodically thereafter, reassess renal function and serum potassium especially in patients with preexisting hypotension, hyponatremia, diabetes mellitus, azotemia, or those taking potassium supplements (ACCF/AHA [Yancy 2013]).

Test Interactions May cause false low serum digoxin levels with the Digi-Tab RIA kit for digoxin.

Dosage Forms Excipient information presented when available (limited, particularly for generics); consult specific product labeling.

Tablet, Oral, as sodium:

Generic: 10 mg, 20 mg, 40 mg

◆ Fosinopril Sodium *see* Fosinopril *on page 814*

Fosphenytoin (FOS fen i toyn)

Brand Names: US Cerebyx

Brand Names: Canada Cerebyx

Index Terms Cerebyx; Fosphenytoin Sodium

Pharmacologic Category Anticonvulsant, Hydantoin

Use Seizures: Control of generalized tonic-clonic status epilepticus and the prevention and treatment of seizures occurring during neurosurgery; short-term parenteral administration when oral phenytoin is not possible.

Pregnancy Considerations Fosphenytoin is the prodrug of phenytoin. Refer to Phenytoin monograph for additional information.

Breast-Feeding Considerations Fosphenytoin is the prodrug of phenytoin. It is not known if fosphenytoin is excreted in breast milk prior to conversion to phenytoin. Breast-feeding is not recommended by the manufacturer. Refer to Phenytoin monograph for additional information.

Contraindications Hypersensitivity to fosphenytoin, phenytoin, other hydantoins, or any component of the formulation; sinus bradycardia, sinoatrial block, second- and third-degree AV block, or Adams-Stokes syndrome; concurrent use with delavirdine

Warnings/Precautions Hazardous agent - use appropriate precautions for handling and disposal (NIOSH 2014 [group 2]). Administer only when oral phenytoin administration is not possible. If rapid phenytoin loading is a primary goal, IV administration of fosphenytoin is preferred. As non-emergency therapy, fosphenytoin IV should be administered more slowly. Fosphenytoin is NOT indicated for the treatment of absence seizures or seizures due to hypoglycemia or other metabolic causes.

[US Boxed Warning]: The rate of fosphenytoin IV administration should not exceed 150 mg phenytoin equivalents (PE)/minute. Severe hypotension and cardiac arrhythmias (eg, bradycardia, heart block, QT interval prolongation, ventricular tachycardia, ventricular fibrillation) may occur with rapid administration (may be fatal) and are commonly occur in critically ill patients, elderly patients, and patients with hypotension and severe myocardial insufficiency. **Careful cardiac monitoring is necessary during and after administration of fosphenytoin IV; reduction in rate of administration or discontinuation of infusion may be necessary. Although the risk of cardiovascular toxicity increases with infusion rates above the recommended infusion rate, these events have also been reported at or below the recommended infusion rate.**

Doses of fosphenytoin are always expressed as their phenytoin sodium equivalent (PE). 1 mg PE is equivalent to 1 mg phenytoin sodium. Do not change the recommended doses when substituting fosphenytoin for phenytoin or vice versa as they are not equivalent on a mg to mg basis. Dosing errors have also occurred due to misinterpretation of vial concentrations resulting in two- or tenfold overdoses (some fatal); ensure correct volume of fosphenytoin is withdrawn from vial. Severe burning or itching, and/or paresthesias, mostly perineal, may occur upon administration, usually at the maximum administration rate and last from minutes to hours; milder sensory disturbances may persist for as long as 24 hours; occurrence and intensity may be lessened by slowing or temporarily stopping the infusion. Anticonvulsants should not be abruptly discontinued. Lymphadenopathy may occur (local or generalized), including benign lymph node hyperplasia, pseudolymphoma, lymphoma, and Hodgkin disease; discontinue if lymphadenopathy occurs. Cases of acute hepatotoxicity, including infrequent cases of acute hepatic failure, have been reported with phenytoin. Other manifestations include jaundice, hepatomegaly, elevated serum transaminase levels, leukocytosis, and eosinophilia. The clinical course of acute phenytoin hepatotoxicity ranges from prompt recovery to fatal outcomes. Immediately discontinue fosphenytoin in patients who develop acute hepatotoxicity and do not readminister. A spectrum of hematologic effects have been reported with phenytoin (eg, leukopenia, granulocytopenia, agranulocytosis, thrombocytopenia, and pancytopenia with or without bone marrow suppression) and may be fatal. Use with caution in patients with hypotension, severe myocardial insufficiency, diabetes mellitus, porphyria, hypoalbuminemia, hypothyroidism, hepatic dysfunction, the elderly, and in patients who are critically ill or debilitated. Use with caution in patients with renal impairment; also consider the phosphate load of fosphenytoin (0.0037 mmol phosphate/mg PE fosphenytoin). Severe reactions, including toxic epidermal necrolysis (TEN) and Stevens-Johnson syndromes, although rarely reported, have resulted in fatalities; drug should be discontinued if there are any signs of rash and patient should be evaluated for signs and symptoms of drug reaction with eosinophilia and systemic symptoms (DRESS). Patients of Asian descent with the variant *HLA-B*1502* may be at an increased risk of developing Stevens-Johnson syndrome and/or TEN. Consider avoiding fosphenytoin as an alternative for carbamazepine patients positive for HLA-B*1502.

The "purple glove syndrome" (ie, discoloration with edema and pain of distal limb) may occur following peripheral IV administration of fosphenytoin. This syndrome may or may not be associated with drug extravasation. Symptoms may resolve spontaneously; however, skin necrosis and limb ischemia may occur. In general, fosphenytoin has significantly less venous irritation and phlebitis compared with an equimolar dose of phenytoin (Jamerson 1994). Plasma concentrations of phenytoin sustained above the optimal range may produce confusional states referred to as delirium, psychosis, or encephalopathy, or rarely, irreversible cerebellar dysfunction. Measure plasma phenytoin concentrations at the first sign of acute toxicity; dosage reduction is indicated if phenytoin concentrations are excessive; if symptoms persist, discontinue administration. Potentially significant interactions may exist, requiring dose or frequency adjustment, additional monitoring, and/or selection of alternative therapy.

Adverse Reactions The more important adverse clinical events caused by the IV use of fosphenytoin or phenytoin are cardiovascular collapse and/or central nervous system depression. Hypotension can occur when either drug is administered rapidly by the IV route.

The adverse clinical events most commonly observed with the use of fosphenytoin in clinical trials were nystagmus, dizziness, pruritus, paresthesia, headache, somnolence, and ataxia. Paresthesia and pruritus were seen more often following fosphenytoin (versus phenytoin) administration and occurred more often with IV fosphenytoin than with IM administration. These events were dose and rate related (adult doses ≥15 mg/kg at a rate of 150 mg PE/minute) and occurred in up to 64% of patients. These sensations, generally described as itching, burning, or tingling are usually not at the infusion site. The location of the discomfort varied with the groin mentioned most frequently. The paresthesia and pruritus were transient events that occurred within several minutes of the start of infusion and generally resolved within 10 minutes after completion of infusion.

Transient pruritus, tinnitus, nystagmus, somnolence, and ataxia occurred 2-3 times more often at adult doses ≥15 mg/kg and rates ≥150 mg PE/minute.

Also refer to Phenytoin monograph for additional adverse reactions.

IV and IM administration (as reported in clinical trials):
1% to 10%:
Cardiovascular: Facial edema, hypertension
Central nervous system: Chills, fever, intracranial hypertension, nervousness
Endocrine & metabolic: Hypokalemia
Neuromuscular & skeletal: Hyperreflexia, myasthenia

IV administration (maximum dose/rate):
>10%:
Central nervous system: Paresthesia (4% to 64%), nystagmus (44%), dizziness (31%), somnolence (20%), ataxia (11%)
Dermatologic: Pruritus (49% to 64%)
1% to 10%:
Cardiovascular: Hypotension (7%), vasodilation (6%), tachycardia (2%)
Central nervous system: Stupor (7%), extrapyramidal syndrome (4%), incoordination (4%), agitation (3%), tremor (3%), brain edema (2%), headache (2%), hypoesthesia (2%), vertigo (2%)
Gastrointestinal: Nausea (9%), tongue disorder (4%), xerostomia (4%), taste perversion (3%), vomiting (2%)
Neuromuscular & skeletal: Pelvic pain (4%), back pain (2%), dysarthria (2%), weakness (2%)
Ocular: Diplopia (3%), amblyopia (2%)
Otic: Tinnitus (9%), deafness (2%)

IM administration (substitute for oral phenytoin):
>10%: Central nervous system: Nystagmus (15%)
1% to 10%:
Central nervous system: Tremor (10%), headache (9%), ataxia (8%), incoordination (8%), somnolence (7%), dizziness (5%), paresthesia (4%), reflexes decreased (3%)
Dermatologic: Bruising (7%), pruritus (3%)
Gastrointestinal: Nausea (5%), vomiting (3%)
Neuromuscular & skeletal: Weakness (4%)

IV and IM administration: <1% (Limited to important or life-threatening): Acidosis, acute hepatic failure, acute hepatotoxicity, alkalosis, akathisia, amnesia, anemia, anorexia, aphasia, apnea, arthralgia, asthma, atrial flutter, Babinski sign positive, bundle branch block, cachexia, cardiac arrest, cardiomegaly, cerebral hemorrhage, cerebral infarct, CHF, circumoral paresthesia, CNS depression, cyanosis, dehydration, diabetes insipidus, dyskinesia, dysphagia, dyspnea, edema, emotional lability, encephalopathy, epistaxis, extrapyramidal symptoms, GI hemorrhage, hemiplegia, hemoptysis, hostility, hyperacusis, hyperesthesia, hyper-/hypokinesia, hyperkalemia, hyperventilation, hypochromic anemia, hypophosphatemia, hypotonia, hypoxia, ileus, injection site (edema, hemorrhage, inflammation), ketosis, leg cramps, leukocytosis, leukopenia, LFTs abnormal, malaise,

migraine, myalgia, mydriasis, myopathy, neurosis, orthostatic hypotension, palpitation, paralysis, parosmia, petechia, photophobia, photosensitivity reaction, psychosis, pulmonary embolus, QT interval prolongation, rash (maculopapular or pustular), renal failure, sinus bradycardia, shock, subdural hematoma, syncope, Stevens-Johnson syndrome, tenesmus, thrombocytopenia, thrombophlebitis, tongue edema, toxic epidermal necrolysis, urticaria, ventricular extrasystoles, visual field defect

Drug Interactions

Metabolism/Transport Effects Substrate of CYP2C19 (major), CYP2C9 (major), CYP3A4 (minor); **Note:** Assignment of Major/Minor substrate status based on clinically relevant drug interaction potential; **Induces** CYP2B6 (strong), CYP2C19 (strong), CYP2C8 (strong), CYP2C9 (strong), CYP3A4 (strong), P-glycoprotein, UGT1A1

Avoid Concomitant Use

Avoid concomitant use of Fosphenytoin with any of the following: Abiraterone Acetate; Antihepaciviral Combination Products; Apixaban; Apremilast; Aprepitant; Artemether; Axitinib; Azelastine (Nasal); Bedaquiline; Boceprevir; Bortezomib; Bosutinib; Cabozantinib; Cariprazine; Ceritinib; CloZAPine; Cobicistat; Cobimetinib; Crizotinib; Dabigatran Etexilate; Dabrafenib; Daclatasvir; Darunavir; Delavirdine; Dienogest; Dolutegravir; Dronedarone; Eliglustat; Elvitegravir; Enzalutamide; Etravirine; Everolimus; Flibanserin; Ibrutinib; Idelalisib; Irinotecan Products; Isavuconazonium Sulfate; Itraconazole; Ivabradine; Ivacaftor; Ixazomib; Lapatinib; Ledipasvir; Lumefantrine; Lurasidone; Macitentan; Mifepristone; Naloxegol; Netupitant; NIFEdipine; Nilotinib; NiMODipine; Nintedanib; Nisoldipine; Olaparib; Ombitasvir, Paritaprevir, Ritonavir, and Dasabuvir; Orphenadrine; Osimertinib; Palbociclib; Panobinostat; Paraldehyde; PAZOPanib; PONATinib; Praziquantel; Ranolazine; Regorafenib; Rilpivirine; Rivaroxaban; Roflumilast; RomiDEPsin; Simeprevir; Sofosbuvir; Sonidegib; SORAfenib; Suvorexant; Tasimelteon; Telaprevir; Thalidomide; Ticagrelor; Tofacitinib; Tolvaptan; Toremifene; Trabectedin; Ulipristal; Vandetanib; Vemurafenib; VinCRIStine (Liposomal); Vorapaxar

Increased Effect/Toxicity

Fosphenytoin may increase the levels/effects of: Amiodarone; Azelastine (Nasal); Buprenorphine; Chloramphenicol; Ciprofloxacin (Systemic); Clarithromycin; CNS Depressants; Cyclophosphamide; FLUoxetine; Fosamprenavir; Highest Risk QTc-Prolonging Agents; Hydrocodone; Lithium; Methotrexate; Methotrimeprazine; Metyrosine; Moderate Risk QTc-Prolonging Agents; Neuromuscular-Blocking Agents (Nondepolarizing); Orphenadrine; Paraldehyde; PHENobarbital; Pramipexole; QuiNIDine; ROPINIRole; Rotigotine; Selective Serotonin Reuptake Inhibitors; Thalidomide; Vitamin K Antagonists; Zolpidem

The levels/effects of Fosphenytoin may be increased by: Alcohol (Ethyl); Amiodarone; Antifungal Agents (Azole Derivatives, Systemic); Benzodiazepines; Brimonidine (Topical); Calcium Channel Blockers; Cannabis; Capecitabine; CarBAMazepine; Carbonic Anhydrase Inhibitors; CeFAZolin; Chloramphenicol; Chlorpheniramine; Cimetidine; Clarithromycin; CYP2C19 Inhibitors (Moderate); CYP2C19 Inhibitors (Strong); CYP2C9 Inhibitors (Moderate); CYP2C9 Inhibitors (Strong); Delavirdine; Dexamethasone (Systemic); Dexketoprofen; Dexmethylphenidate; Disopyramide; Disulfiram; Doxylamine; Dronabinol; Droperidol; Efavirenz; Eslicarbazepine; Ethosuximide; Felbamate; Floxuridine; Fluconazole; Fluorouracil (Systemic); Fluorouracil (Topical); FLUoxetine; FluvoxaMINE; Halothane; HydrOXYzine; Isoniazid; Kava Kava; Luliconazole; Lumacaftor; Magnesium Sulfate; Methotrimeprazine; Methylphenidate; MetroNIDAZOLE (Systemic); Miconazole (Oral); Minocycline; Nabilone; Omeprazole; OXcarbazepine; Rufinamide; Sertraline; Sodium Oxybate; Tacrolimus (Systemic); Tapentadol; Tegafur; Telaprevir; Tetrahydrocannabinol; Ticlopidine; Topiramate; TraZODone; Trimethoprim; Vitamin K Antagonists

Decreased Effect

Fosphenytoin may decrease the levels/effects of: Abiraterone Acetate; Acetaminophen; Afatinib; Amiodarone; Antifungal Agents (Azole Derivatives, Systemic); Antihepaciviral Combination Products; Apixaban; Apremilast; Aprepitant; ARIPiprazole; ARIPiprazole Lauroxil; Artemether; Axitinib; Bazedoxifene; Bedaquiline; Boceprevir; Bortezomib; Bosutinib; Brentuximab Vedotin; Brexpiprazole; Busulfan; Cabozantinib; Canagliflozin; Cannabidiol; Cannabis; CarBAMazepine; Cariprazine; Ceritinib; Chloramphenicol; Clarithromycin; CloZAPine; Cobicistat; Cobimetinib; Contraceptives (Estrogens); Contraceptives (Progestins); Corticosteroids (Systemic); Crizotinib; CycloSPORINE (Systemic); CYP2B6 Substrates; CYP2C19 Substrates; CYP2C8 Substrates; CYP2C9 Substrates; CYP3A4 Substrates; Dabigatran Etexilate; Dabrafenib; Daclatasvir; Darunavir; Dasatinib; Deferasirox; Delavirdine; Dexamethasone (Systemic); Diclofenac (Systemic); Dienogest; Disopyramide; Dolutegravir; Doxofylline; DOXOrubicin (Conventional); Doxycycline; Dronabinol; Dronedarone; Efavirenz; Eliglustat; Elvitegravir; Enzalutamide; Erlotinib; Eslicarbazepine; Ethosuximide; Etoposide; Etoposide Phosphate; Etravirine; Everolimus; Exemestane; Ezogabine; Felbamate; FentaNYL; Flibanserin; Flunarizine; Gefitinib; GuanFACINE; HMG-CoA Reductase Inhibitors; Hydrocortisone (Systemic); Ibrutinib; Idelalisib; Imatinib; Irinotecan Products; Isavuconazonium Sulfate; Itraconazole; Ivabradine; Ivacaftor; Ixabepilone; Ixazomib; Lacosamide; LamoTRIgine; Lapatinib; Ledipasvir; Levodopa; Linagliptin; Loop Diuretics; Lopinavir; Lumefantrine; Lurasidone; Macitentan; Maraviroc; Mebendazole; Meperidine; Methadone; MethylPREDNISolone; MetroNIDAZOLE (Systemic); Metyrapone; Mexiletine; Mianserin; Mifepristone; Naloxegol; Nelfinavir; Netupitant; Neuromuscular-Blocking Agents (Nondepolarizing); NIFEdipine; Nilotinib; NiMODipine; Nintedanib; Nisoldipine; Olaparib; Ombitasvir, Paritaprevir, Ritonavir, and Dasabuvir; Omeprazole; Osimertinib; OXcarbazepine; Palbociclib; Paliperidone; Panobinostat; PAZOPanib; Perampanel; P-glycoprotein/ABCB1 Substrates; PONATinib; Praziquantel; PredniSOLONE (Systemic); PredniSONE; Primidone; Propacetamol; Propafenone; QUEtiapine; QuiNIDine; QuiNINE; Ranolazine; Regorafenib; Rilpivirine; Ritonavir; Rivaroxaban; Roflumilast; Rolapitant; RomiDEPsin; Rufinamide; Saxagliptin; Sertraline; Simeprevir; Sirolimus; Sofosbuvir; Sonidegib; SORAfenib; SUNItinib; Suvorexant; Tacrolimus (Systemic); Tadalafil; Tasimelteon; Telaprevir; Temsirolimus; Teniposide; Tetrahydrocannabinol; Theophylline Derivatives; Thyroid Products; Ticagrelor; Tipranavir; Tofacitinib; Tolvaptan; Topiramate; Topotecan; Toremifene; Trabectedin; TraZODone; Treprostinil; Trimethoprim; Ulipristal; Valproate Products; Vandetanib; Vemurafenib; Vilazodone; VinCRIStine; VinCRIStine (Liposomal); Vorapaxar; Vortioxetine; Zaleplon; Zonisamide

The levels/effects of Fosphenytoin may be decreased by: Alcohol (Ethyl); CarBAMazepine; Ciprofloxacin (Systemic); CYP2C19 Inducers (Strong); CYP2C9 Inducers (Strong); Dexamethasone (Systemic); Diazoxide; Enzalutamide; Folic Acid; Fosamprenavir; Leucovorin Calcium-Levoleucovorin; Levomefolate; Lopinavir; Lumacaftor; Mefloquine; Methotrexate; Methylfolate; Mianserin; Multivitamins/Minerals (with ADEK, Folate, Iron); Nelfinavir; PHENobarbital; Platinum Derivatives; Pyridoxine; Rifampin; Ritonavir; Theophylline Derivatives; Tipranavir; Valproate Products; Vigabatrin; VinCRIStine

Food Interactions Ethanol:

Acute use: Ethanol inhibits metabolism of phenytoin and may also increase CNS depression. Management: Monitor patients. Caution patients about effects.

Chronic use: Ethanol stimulates metabolism of phenytoin. Management: Monitor patients.

Preparation for Administration Hazardous agent; use appropriate precautions for handling and disposal (NIOSH 2014 [group 2]).

Must be diluted to concentrations of 1.5 to 25 mg PE/mL, in NS or D$_5$W (maximum concentration: 25 mg PE/mL).

Storage/Stability Store refrigerate at 2°C to 8°C (36°F to 46°F). Do not store at room temperature for more than 48 hours. Has been shown to be stable at 1, 8, and 20 mg PE/mL in normal saline or D$_5$W at 25°C (77°F) for 30 days in glass container and at 4°C to 20°C (39°F to 68°F) for 30 days in PVC bag. Undiluted fosphenytoin injection (50 mg PE/mL) is stable in polypropylene syringes for 30 days at 25°C, 4°C, or frozen at -20°C. Fosphenytoin at concentrations of 1, 8, and 20 mg PE/mL prepared in D$_5$¹/$_2$NS, D$_5$¹/$_2$NS with KCl 20 mEq/L, D$_5$¹/$_2$NS with 40 mEq/L, LR, D$_5$LR, D$_{10}$W, amino acid 10%, mannitol 20%, hetastarch 6% in NS or Plasma-Lyte A injection is stable in polyvinyl chloride bags for 7 days when stored at 25°C (room temperature) (Fischer 1997).

Mechanism of Action Diphosphate ester salt of phenytoin that acts as a water soluble prodrug of phenytoin; after administration, plasma esterases convert fosphenytoin to phosphate, formaldehyde (not expected to be clinically consequential [Fierro 1996]), and phenytoin as the active moiety. Phenytoin works by stabilizing neuronal membranes and decreasing seizure activity by increasing efflux or decreasing influx of sodium ions across cell membranes in the motor cortex during generation of nerve impulses

Pharmacodynamics/Kinetics The pharmacokinetics of intravenous fosphenytoin in pediatric patients have been evaluated in two studies (n= 49, age range: 1 day to 16.7 years; n=8, age range: 5-18 years) and found to be similar to the pharmacokinetics observed in young adults; the conversion rate of fosphenytoin to phenytoin was consistent throughout childhood (Fischer 2003; Pellock 1996). Also refer to Phenytoin monograph for additional information.

Distribution: Fosphenytoin: V_d: 4.3 to 10.8 L; V_d of fosphenytoin increases with dose and rate of administration (Fischer 2003)

Protein binding: Fosphenytoin: 95% to 99% (primarily to albumin); binding of fosphenytoin to protein is saturable (the percent bound decreases as total concentration increases); fosphenytoin displaces phenytoin from protein binding sites; can displace phenytoin and increase free fraction (up to 30% unbound) during the period required for conversion of fosphenytoin to phenytoin. **Note:** In patients with renal and/or hepatic impairment or hypoalbuminemia, the fraction of unbound phenytoin may be increased.

Metabolism: Fosphenytoin is rapidly converted via hydrolysis to phenytoin; phenytoin is metabolized in the liver and forms metabolites

Bioavailability: Fosphenytoin: IM: 100%

Half-life elimination:

Pediatric patients (ages: 1 day to 16.7 years): 8.3 minutes (range: 2.5 to 18.5 minutes) (Fischer 2003)

Adults:

Fosphenytoin: IV ~15 minutes; IM: ~30 minutes

Phenytoin: Variable (mean: 12 to 29 hours); pharmacokinetics of phenytoin are saturable

Time to peak: Conversion to phenytoin:

IV: Adults: Following IV administration (maximum rate of administration): ~15 minutes

IM:

Neonates and Infants ≤6 months: 1-3 hours was reported in a case series (n=3; PNA: 15 to 47 days) (Fischer 2003)

Pediatric patients >7 months: Therapeutic concentrations within 30 minutes; time to maximum serum concentration not reported (Fischer 2003)

Adults: ~3 hours; therapeutic phenytoin concentrations may be achieved as early as 5 to 20 minutes following IM (gluteal) administration (Pryor 2001)

Excretion: Phenytoin: Urine (as inactive metabolites)

Dosing

Adult

Note: The dose, concentration, and infusion rates for fosphenytoin are expressed as phenytoin equivalents (PE); fosphenytoin should always be prescribed and dispensed in phenytoin equivalents (PE); fosphenytoin 1.5 mg is equivalent to phenytoin 1 mg and is referred to as 1 mg PE.

Status epilepticus: IV: **Note:** Because the full antiepileptic effect is not immediate, other measures, including concomitant administration of an IV benzodiazepine, will usually be necessary for the control of status epilepticus.

Neurocritical Care Society recommendations: Loading dose: 20 mg PE/kg (maximum rate of administration: 150 mg PE/minute); if necessary, may give an additional 5 mg PE/kg 10 minutes after the loading dose (NCS [Brophy 2012]).

Manufacturer's labeling: Loading dose: 15 to 20 mg PE/kg administered at 100 to 150 mg PE/minute. Follow loading dose with maintenance doses of either fosphenytoin or phenytoin.

Nonemergent loading and maintenance dosing: IV or IM:

Loading dose: 10 to 20 mg PE/kg (IV rate: Infuse more slowly [eg, over 30 minutes]; maximum rate: 150 mg PE/minute)

Initial daily maintenance dose: 4 to 6 mg PE/kg/day in divided doses

Substitution for oral phenytoin therapy: IM or IV: May be substituted for oral phenytoin at the same total daily dose; however, Dilantin capsules are ~90% bioavailable by the oral route; phenytoin, supplied as fosphenytoin, is 100% bioavailable by both the IM and IV routes; for this reason, plasma phenytoin concentrations may modestly increase when IM or IV fosphenytoin is substituted for oral phenytoin; in clinical trials, IM fosphenytoin was administered as a single daily dose utilizing either 1 or 2 injection sites; some patients may require more frequent dosing

Geriatric Phenytoin clearance is decreased in geriatric patients; lower doses may be required. In addition, older adults may have lower serum albumin which may increase the free fraction and, therefore, pharmacologic response including adverse events. Refer to adult dosing.

Pediatric

Note: The dose, concentration, and infusion rates for fosphenytoin are expressed as phenytoin equivalents (PE); fosphenytoin should always be prescribed and dispensed in phenytoin equivalents (PE); fosphenytoin 1.5 mg is equivalent to phenytoin 1 mg and is referred to as 1 mg PE.

Infants, Children, and Adolescents (off-label use): IV: **Note:** A limited number of clinical studies have been conducted in pediatric patients; based on pharmacokinetic studies, experts recommend the following (Fischer 2003): Use the pediatric IV phenytoin dosing guidelines to dose fosphenytoin using doses in **PE** equal to the phenytoin doses (ie, phenytoin 1 mg = fosphenytoin 1 mg **PE**). Further pediatric studies are needed.

Status epilepticus (off-label use): IV: Loading dose: 20 mg PE/kg (maximum rate of administration: 3 mg PE/kg/minute); if necessary, may give an additional 5 mg PE/kg 10 minutes after the loading dose (NCS [Brophy 2012]).

Renal Impairment There are no dosage adjustments provided in the manufacturer's labeling. Free (unbound) phenytoin levels should be monitored closely in patients with renal disease or in those with hypoalbuminemia; furthermore, fosphenytoin clearance to phenytoin may be increased without a similar increase in phenytoin clearance in these patients leading to increase frequency and severity of adverse events.

Hepatic Impairment There are no dosage adjustments provided in the manufacturer's labeling. Free (unbound) phenytoin levels should be monitored closely in patients with hepatic disease or in those with hypoalbuminemia; furthermore, fosphenytoin clearance to phenytoin may be increased without a similar increase in phenytoin clearance in these patients leading to increased frequency and severity of adverse events.

Dietary Considerations Provides phosphate 0.0037 mmol/mg PE fosphenytoin

Administration

IM: May be administered as a single daily dose using 1 to 4 injection sites (up to 20 mL per site well tolerated in adults) (Meek 1999; Pryor 2001).

IV: Rates of infusion:

Children and Adolescents: 1 to 3 mg PE/kg/minute (**maximum rate: 150 mg PE/minute**) (Pellock 1996)

Adults: **Do not exceed 150 mg PE/minute.** Slower administration reduces incidence of cardiovascular events (eg, hypotension, arrhythmia) as well as severity of paresthesias and pruritus. For nonemergent situations, may administer loading dose more slowly (eg, over 30 minutes [~33 mg PE/minute for 1,000 mg PE] **or** 50 to 100 mg PE/minute [Fischer 2003]). Highly sensitive patients (eg, elderly, patients with preexisting cardiovascular conditions) should receive fosphenytoin more slowly (eg, 25 to 50 mg PE/minute) (Meek 1999).

Hazardous agent; use appropriate precautions for handling and disposal (NIOSH 2014 [group 2]).

Monitoring Parameters Continuous blood pressure, ECG, and respiratory function monitoring with loading dose and for 10 to 20 minutes following infusion; vital signs, CBC, hepatic function tests, plasma phenytoin concentration monitoring (plasma concentrations should not be measured until conversion to phenytoin is complete, ~2 hours after an IV infusion or ~4 hours after an IM injection). **Note:** If available, free (unbound) phenytoin concentrations should be obtained in patients with renal impairment and/or hypoalbuminemia; if free phenytoin concentrations are unavailable, the adjusted total concentration may be determined based upon equations in adult patients. Trough concentrations are generally recommended for routine monitoring.

Consult individual institutional policies and procedures.

Reference Range Therapeutic range: Total phenytoin: 10 to 20 mcg/mL (SI: 40 to 79 micromole/L); toxicity is measured clinically, and some patients require levels outside the suggested therapeutic range (refer to Phenytoin monograph for additional information)

Test Interactions Falsely high plasma phenytoin concentrations (due to cross-reactivity with fosphenytoin) when measured by immunoanalytical techniques (eg, TD_X, TD_XFL_X, Emit 2000) prior to complete conversion of fosphenytoin to phenytoin. Phenytoin may produce falsely low results for dexamethasone or metyrapone tests. Phenytoin has the potential to lower serum folate levels.

Additional Information 1.5 mg fosphenytoin is approximately equivalent to 1 mg phenytoin. Equimolar fosphenytoin dose is 375 mg (75 mg/mL solution) to phenytoin 250 mg (50 mg/mL). **However, doses of fosphenytoin are always expressed as their phenytoin sodium equivalent (PE). Thus, 1 mg PE is equivalent to 1 mg phenytoin sodium. Do not change the recommended doses when substituting fosphenytoin for phenytoin or vice versa as they are not equivalent on a mg to mg basis.**

Dosage Forms Excipient information presented when available (limited, particularly for generics); consult specific product labeling.

Solution, Injection, as sodium:

Cerebyx: 100 mg PE/2 mL (2 mL); 500 MG PE/10ML (2 mL, 10 mL); 500 mg PE/10 mL (10 mL)

Generic: 100 mg PE/2 mL (2 mL); 500 mg PE/10 mL (10 mL)

◆ **Fosphenytoin Sodium** see Fosphenytoin on page 816

◆ **Fosrenol** see Lanthanum on page 1035

◆ **Four-Factor PCC** see Prothrombin Complex Concentrate (Human) [(Factors II, VII, IX, X), Protein C, and Protein S] on page 1525

◆ **FR901228** see RomiDEPsin on page 1614

◆ **Fragmin** see Dalteparin on page 483

◆ **Fresenius Propoven** see Propofol on page 1516

◆ **Freya (Can)** see Ethinyl Estradiol and Desogestrel on page 701

◆ **Frisium (Can)** see CloBAZam on page 410

◆ **Frova** see Frovatriptan on page 820

Frovatriptan (froe va TRIP tan)

Brand Names: US Frova
Brand Names: Canada Frova
Index Terms Frovatriptan Succinate
Pharmacologic Category Antimigraine Agent; Serotonin 5-HT$_{1B, 1D}$ Receptor Agonist
Use Migraines: Acute treatment of migraine with or without aura in adults.
Pregnancy Considerations Adverse events were observed in animal reproduction studies. Information related to the use of frovatriptan in pregnancy has not been located. Until additional information is available, other agents are preferred for the initial treatment of migraine in pregnancy (Da Silva, 2012; MacGregor, 2012; Williams, 2012).
Breast-Feeding Considerations It is not known if frovatriptan is excreted in breast milk. Due to the potential for serious adverse reactions in the nursing infant, the manufacturer recommends a decision be made whether to discontinue nursing or to discontinue the drug, taking into account the importance of treatment to the mother.
Contraindications
Ischemic coronary artery disease (eg, angina pectoris, history of MI, documented silent ischemia); coronary artery vasospasm, including Prinzmetal's angina; Wolff-Parkinson-White syndrome or arrhythmias associated with other cardiac accessory conduction pathway disorders; history of stroke, transient ischemic attack, or history of hemiplegic or basilar migraine; peripheral vascular disease; ischemic bowel disease; uncontrolled hypertension; recent use (within 24 hours) of another 5-HT$_1$ agonist, an ergotamine containing or ergot-type medication (eg, dihydroergotamine, methysergide); hypersensitivity to frovatriptan or any component of the formulation.
Canadian labeling: Additional contraindications (not in U.S. labeling): Cardiac arrhythmias, valvular heart disease (especially tachycardia), congenital heart disease, atherosclerotic disease; management of ophthalmoplegic migraine; severe hepatic impairment; Raynaud's syndrome
Documentation of allergenic cross-reactivity for triptans is limited. However, because of similarities in chemical structure and/or pharmacologic actions, the possibility of cross-sensitivity cannot be ruled out with certainty.
Warnings/Precautions Not intended for migraine prophylaxis, or treatment of cluster headaches, hemiplegic or basilar migraines. Rule out underlying neurologic disease in patients with atypical headache, migraine (with no prior history of migraine) or inadequate clinical response to initial dosing. Cardiac events (coronary artery vasospasm, transient ischemia, MI, ventricular tachycardia/fibrillation, cardiac arrest, and death), cerebral/subarachnoid hemorrhage, stroke (some fatal), peripheral vascular ischemia, gastrointestinal vascular ischemia and infarction, splenic infarction, and Raynaud's syndrome have been reported with 5-HT$_1$ agonist administration. Partial vision loss and

blindness (transient and permanent) have been reported with use of 5-HT$_1$ agonists; a causal relationship between these events and 5-HT$_1$ agonist administration has not been clearly determined. Patients who experience sensations of chest pain/pressure/tightness or symptoms suggestive of angina following dosing should be evaluated for coronary artery disease or Prinzmetal's angina before receiving additional doses; if dosing is resumed and similar symptoms recur, monitor with ECG. Do not give to patients with risk factors for CAD until a cardiovascular evaluation has been performed; if evaluation is satisfactory, the healthcare provider should administer the first dose (consider ECG monitoring) and cardiovascular status should be periodically evaluated. Significant elevation in blood pressure, including hypertensive crisis with acute impairment of organ systems, has been reported on rare occasions in patients using other 5-HT$_{1D}$ agonists with and without a history of hypertension; monitor blood pressure. Blood pressure was increased to a greater extent in elderly.

Use with caution in severe hepatic impairment (has not been studied) (Canadian labeling contraindicates use in severe impairment). Potentially significant drug-drug interactions may exist, requiring dose or frequency adjustment, additional monitoring, and/or selection of alternative therapy. Symptoms of agitation, confusion, hallucinations, hyper-reflexia, myoclonus, shivering, and tachycardia (serotonin syndrome) may occur with concomitant proserotonergic drugs (ie, SSRIs/SNRIs or triptans) or agents which reduce frovatriptan's metabolism. Concurrent use of serotonin precursors (eg, tryptophan) is not recommended. If concomitant administration with SSRIs is warranted, monitor closely, especially at initiation and with dose increases. Discontinue frovatriptan if serotonin syndrome is suspected. Anaphylaxis, anaphylactoid, and hypersensitivity reactions (including angioedema) have occurred; may be life-threatening or fatal.

Adverse Reactions

1% to 10%:

Cardiovascular: Flushing (4%), hot or cold flashes (3%), chest pain (2%), palpitations (1%)

Central nervous system: Dizziness (8%), fatigue (5%), headache (4%), paresthesia (4%), drowsiness (≥2%), anxiety (1%), dysesthesia (1%), hypoesthesia (1%), insomnia (1%), pain (1%)

Dermatologic: Diaphoresis (1%)

Gastrointestinal: Xerostomia (3%), nausea (≥2%), dyspepsia (2%), abdominal pain (1%), diarrhea (1%), vomiting (1%)

Neuromuscular & skeletal: Musculoskeletal pain (3%)

Ophthalmic: Visual disturbance (1%)

Otic: Tinnitus (1%)

Respiratory: Rhinitis (1%), sinusitis (1%)

<1% (Limited to important or life-threatening): Abnormal gait, abnormal lacrimation, abnormal reflexes, amnesia, anaphylactoid reactions, anaphylaxis, anorexia, ataxia, bradycardia, bullous rash, cheilitis, chest tightness, confusion, conjunctivitis, dehydration, depersonalization, depression, dysgeusia, ECG changes, emotional lability, epistaxis, esophageal spasm, euphoria, eye pain, gastroesophageal reflux disease, hyperacusis, hyperesthesia, hypersensitivity reaction (including angioedema), hypertonia, hyperventilation, hypocalcemia, hypoglycemia, hypotonia, involuntary muscle movements, jaw tightness, lack of concentration, laryngitis, myocardial infarction, nocturia, osteoarthritis, peptic ulcer, personality disorder, pharyngitis, polyuria, purpura, renal pain, rigors, salivary gland pain, seizure, sialorrhea, significant cardiovascular event, speech disturbance, stomatitis, syncope, tachycardia, tightness in chest and throat, tongue paralysis

Drug Interactions

Metabolism/Transport Effects Substrate of CYP1A2 (minor); **Note:** Assignment of Major/Minor substrate status based on clinically relevant drug interaction potential

Avoid Concomitant Use

Avoid concomitant use of Frovatriptan with any of the following: Dapoxetine; Ergot Derivatives

Increased Effect/Toxicity

Frovatriptan may increase the levels/effects of: Antipsychotic Agents; Droxidopa; Ergot Derivatives; Metoclopramide; Serotonin Modulators

The levels/effects of Frovatriptan may be increased by: Antiemetics (5HT3 Antagonists); Antipsychotic Agents; Dapoxetine; Ergot Derivatives; Metaxalone; Tedizolid

Decreased Effect There are no known significant interactions involving a decrease in effect.

Food Interactions Food does not affect frovatriptan bioavailability.

Storage/Stability Store at 25°C (77°F); excursions are permitted between 15°C and 30°C (59°F and 86°F). Protect from moisture.

Mechanism of Action Selective agonist for serotonin (5-HT$_{1B}$ and 5-HT$_{1D}$ receptors) in cranial arteries; causes vasoconstriction and reduces sterile inflammation associated with antidromic neuronal transmission correlating with relief of migraine.

Pharmacodynamics/Kinetics

Distribution: Male: 4.2 L/kg; Female: 3 L/kg

Protein binding: ~15%

Metabolism: Primarily hepatic via CYP1A2

Bioavailability: Male: ~20%; Female: ~30%

Half-life elimination: ~26 hours

Time to peak: 2-4 hours

Excretion: Feces (62%); urine (32%)

Dosing

Adult & Geriatric Note: If the first dose is ineffective, diagnosis needs to be re-evaluated. The safety of treating >4 migraines/month has not been established.

Migraine: Oral:

U.S. labeling: Initial: 2.5 mg; if headache recurs, a second dose may be administered after 2 hours have elapsed since the first dose (maximum: 7.5 mg daily)

Canadian labeling: Initial: 2.5 mg; if headache recurs, a second dose may be administered after 4 hours have elapsed since the first dose (maximum: 5 mg daily)

Renal Impairment No dosage adjustment necessary.

Hepatic Impairment

Mild-to-moderate impairment: No dosage adjustment necessary.

Severe impairment:

U.S. labeling: Use with caution (has not been studied).

Canadian labeling: Use is contraindicated.

Administration Administer orally with fluids as soon as symptoms appear.

Monitoring Parameters Headache severity, blood pressure, signs/symptoms suggestive of angina; perform a cardiovascular evaluation in triptan-naïve patients who have multiple cardiovascular risk factors (eg, increased age, diabetes, hypertension, smoking, obesity, strong family history of CAD), monitor ECG with first dose in patients with multiple cardiovascular risk factors who have a negative cardiovascular evaluation and consider periodic cardiovascular evaluation in such patients if they are intermittent long-term users; signs/symptoms of serotonin syndrome and hypersensitivity reactions.

Dosage Forms Excipient information presented when available (limited, particularly for generics); consult specific product labeling.

Tablet, Oral:

Frova: 2.5 mg

Fulvestrant (fool VES trant)

Brand Names: US Faslodex

Brand Names: Canada Faslodex

Index Terms ICI-182,780; ZD9238

Pharmacologic Category Antineoplastic Agent, Estrogen Receptor Antagonist

Use Breast cancer, metastatic: Treatment of hormone-receptor-positive metastatic breast cancer in postmenopausal women with disease progression following antiestrogen therapy

Dosing

Adult & Geriatric Breast cancer, metastatic (postmenopausal women): IM: Initial: 500 mg on days 1, 15, and 29; Maintenance: 500 mg once monthly. In studies, the 500 mg once monthly dose was administered at 28 days ± 3 days (Di Leo, 2014).

Breast cancer, advanced, second-line endocrine-based combination therapy (relapsed or progressive on prior endocrine therapy; off-label combination): Adults (females, HER-2 negative): IM: 500 mg every 14 days for 3 doses, then every 28 days (in combination with palbociclib [and goserelin if pre- or peri-menopausal]); continue until disease progression or unacceptable toxicity (Turner 2015).

Renal Impairment There are no dosage adjustments provided in the manufacturer's labeling (has not been studied). However, renal elimination of fulvestrant is negligible.

Hepatic Impairment

Mild impairment (Child-Pugh class A): No dosage adjustment is necessary.

Moderate impairment (Child-Pugh class B): Reduce initial doses and maintenance dose to 250 mg.

Severe impairment (Child-Pugh class C): There are no dosage adjustments provided in the manufacturer's labeling (use has not been evaluated).

Additional Information Complete prescribing information should be consulted for additional detail.

Dosage Forms Excipient information presented when available (limited, particularly for generics); consult specific product labeling.

Solution, Intramuscular:

Faslodex: 250 mg/5 mL (5 mL) [contains alcohol, usp, benzyl alcohol, benzyl benzoate]

Furosemide (fyoor OH se mide)

Brand Names: US Lasix

Brand Names: Canada Apo-Furosemide; AVA-Furosemide; Bio-Furosemide; Dom-Furosemide; Furosemide Injection Sandoz Standard; Furosemide Injection, USP; Furosemide Special; Furosemide Special Injection; Lasix; Lasix Special; Novo-Semide; NTP-Furosemide; Nu-Furosemide; PMS-Furosemide; Teva-Furosemide

Index Terms Frusemide

Pharmacologic Category Antihypertensive; Diuretic, Loop

Use

Management of edema associated with heart failure and hepatic or renal disease; acute pulmonary edema; treatment of hypertension (alone or in combination with other antihypertensives)

Note: According to the Eighth Joint National Committee (JNC 8) guidelines, loop diuretics are **not** recommended for the initial treatment of hypertension (James, 2013). In patients with chronic kidney disease (ie, eGFR <30 mL/minute/1.73 m^2), the American Society of Hypertension/International Society of Hypertension (ASH/ISH) suggests that the use of a loop diuretic may be necessary (Weber, 2014).

Canadian labeling: Additional use: Furosemide Special Injection and Lasix Special (products not available in the U.S.): Adjunctive treatment of oliguria in patients with severe renal impairment

Pregnancy Considerations Adverse events have been observed in animal reproduction studies. Furosemide crosses the placenta (Riva 1978). Furosemide has been used to treat heart failure in pregnant women (ESC 2011; Johnson-Coyle 2012). Monitor fetal growth if used during pregnancy; may increase birth weight.

Breast-Feeding Considerations Furosemide is excreted into breast milk; maternal use may suppress lactation. The U.S. manufacturer recommends that caution be used if administered to a nursing woman. Canadian labeling contraindicates use while breast-feeding.

Contraindications Hypersensitivity to furosemide or any component of the formulation; anuria

Canadian labeling: Additional contraindications (not in U.S. labeling): Hypersensitivity to sulfonamide-derived drugs; complete renal shutdown; hepatic coma and precoma; uncorrected states of electrolyte depletion, hypovolemia, or hypotension; jaundiced newborn infants or infants with disease(s) capable of causing hyperbilirubinemia and possibly kernicterus; breast-feeding. **Note:** Manufacturer labeling for Lasix® Special and Furosemide Special

Injection also includes: GFR <5 mL/minute or GFR >20 mL/minute; hepatic cirrhosis; renal failure accompanied by hepatic coma and precoma; renal failure due to poisoning with nephrotoxic or hepatotoxic substances.

Note: Although the approved product labeling states this medication is contraindicated with other sulfonamide-containing drug classes, the scientific basis of this statement has been challenged. See "Warnings/Precautions" for more detail.

Warnings/Precautions [U.S. Boxed Warning]: If given in excessive amounts, furosemide, similar to other loop diuretics, can lead to profound diuresis, resulting in fluid and electrolyte depletion; close medical supervision and dose evaluation are required. Watch for and correct electrolyte disturbances; adjust dose to avoid dehydration. When electrolyte depletion is present, therapy should not be initiated unless serum electrolytes, especially potassium, are normalized. In cirrhosis, avoid electrolyte and acid/base imbalances that might lead to hepatic encephalopathy; correct electrolyte and acid/base imbalances prior to initiation when hepatic coma is present. In contrast to thiazide diuretics, a loop diuretic can also lower serum calcium concentrations. Electrolyte disturbances can predispose a patient to serious cardiac arrhythmias. Coadministration of antihypertensives may increase the risk of hypotension.

Monitor fluid status and renal function in an attempt to prevent oliguria, azotemia, and reversible increases in BUN and creatinine; close medical supervision of aggressive diuresis is required. May increase risk of contrast-induced nephropathy. Diuretic resistance may occur in some patients, despite higher doses of loop diuretic treatment. Diuretic resistance can usually be overcome by intravenous administration, the use of two diuretics together (eg, furosemide and chlorothiazide), or the use of a diuretic with a positive inotropic agent. Rapid IV administration, renal impairment, excessive doses, hypoproteinemia, and concurrent use of other ototoxins is associated with ototoxicity. Asymptomatic hyperuricemia has been reported with use; rarely, gout may precipitate. Photosensitization may occur.

Use with caution in patients with prediabetes or diabetes mellitus; may see a change in glucose control. Use with caution in patients with systemic lupus erythematosus (SLE); may cause SLE exacerbation or activation. Use with caution in patients with prostatic hyperplasia/urinary stricture; may cause urinary retention. May lead to nephrocalcinosis or nephrolithiasis in premature infants or in children <4 years of age with chronic use. May prevent closure of patent ductus arteriosus in premature infants. Some dosage forms may contain propylene glycol; large amounts are potentially toxic and have been associated hyperosmolality, lactic acidosis, seizures, and respiratory depression; use caution. If given the morning of surgery, furosemide may render the patient volume depleted and blood pressure may be labile during general anesthesia.

Sulfonamide ("sulfa") allergy: The approved product labeling for many medications containing a sulfonamide chemical group includes a broad contraindication in patients with a prior allergic reaction to sulfonamides. There is a potential for cross-reactivity between members of a specific class (eg, two antibiotic sulfonamides). However, concerns for cross-reactivity have previously extended to all compounds containing the sulfonamide structure (SO_2NH_2). An expanded understanding of allergic mechanisms indicates cross-reactivity between antibiotic sulfonamides and nonantibiotic sulfonamides may not occur or at the very least this potential is extremely low (Brackett 2004; Johnson 2005; Slatore 2004; Tornero 2004). In particular, mechanisms of cross-reaction due to antibody production (anaphylaxis) are unlikely to occur with nonantibiotic sulfonamides. T-cell-mediated (type IV) reactions (eg, maculopapular rash) are less well understood and it is not possible to completely exclude this potential based on current insights. In cases where prior reactions were severe (Stevens-Johnson syndrome/TEN), some clinicians choose to avoid exposure to these classes.

Adverse Reactions Frequency not defined.

Cardiovascular: Acute hypotension, chronic aortitis, necrotizing angiitis, orthostatic hypotension, vasculitis

Central nervous system: Dizziness, fever, headache, hepatic encephalopathy, lightheadedness, restlessness, vertigo

Dermatologic: Bullous pemphigoid, cutaneous vasculitis, drug rash with eosinophilia and systemic symptoms (DRESS), erythema multiforme, exanthematous pustulosis (generalized), exfoliative dermatitis, photosensitivity, pruritus, purpura, rash, Stevens-Johnson syndrome, toxic epidermal necrolysis, urticaria

Endocrine & metabolic: Cholesterol and triglycerides increased, glucose tolerance test altered, gout, hyperglycemia, hyperuricemia, hypocalcemia, hypochloremia, hypokalemia, hypomagnesemia, hyponatremia, metabolic alkalosis

Gastrointestinal: Anorexia, constipation, cramping, diarrhea, nausea, oral and gastric irritation, pancreatitis, vomiting

Genitourinary: Urinary bladder spasm, urinary frequency

Hematological: Agranulocytosis (rare), anemia, aplastic anemia (rare), eosinophilia, hemolytic anemia, leukopenia, thrombocytopenia

Hepatic: Intrahepatic cholestatic jaundice, ischemic hepatitis, liver enzymes increased

Local: Injection site pain (following IM injection), thrombophlebitis

Neuromuscular & skeletal: Muscle spasm, paresthesia, weakness

Ocular: Blurred vision, xanthopsia

Otic: Hearing impairment (reversible or permanent with rapid IV or IM administration), tinnitus

Renal: Allergic interstitial nephritis, fall in glomerular filtration rate and renal blood flow (due to overdiuresis), glycosuria, transient rise in BUN

Miscellaneous: Anaphylaxis (rare), exacerbate or activate systemic lupus erythematosus

Drug Interactions

Metabolism/Transport Effects Substrate of OAT3

Avoid Concomitant Use

Avoid concomitant use of Furosemide with any of the following: Chloral Hydrate; Ethacrynic Acid; Levosulpiride; Mecamylamine

Increased Effect/Toxicity

Furosemide may increase the levels/effects of: ACE Inhibitors; Allopurinol; Amifostine; Aminoglycosides; Antipsychotic Agents (Second Generation [Atypical]); Cardiac Glycosides; Cefotiam; Ceftizoxime; Chloral Hydrate; CISplatin; Dofetilide; DULoxetine; Ethacrynic Acid; Foscarnet; Hypotension-Associated Agents; Ivabradine; Levodopa; Levosulpiride; Lithium; Mecamylamine; Methotrexate; Neuromuscular-Blocking Agents; Nonsteroidal Anti-Inflammatory Agents; RisperiDONE; Salicylates; Sodium Phosphates; Tobramycin (Oral Inhalation); Topiramate

The levels/effects of Furosemide may be increased by: Alfuzosin; Analgesics (Opioid); Barbiturates; Beta2-Agonists; Brimonidine (Topical); Canagliflozin; Cefazedone; Cephradine; Corticosteroids (Orally Inhaled); Corticosteroids (Systemic); CycloSPORINE (Systemic); Diazoxide; Empagliflozin; Herbs (Hypotensive Properties); Licorice; Methotrexate; Molsidomine; Nicorandil; Obinutuzumab; Pentoxifylline; Phosphodiesterase 5 Inhibitors; Probenecid; Prostacyclin Analogues; Teriflunomide

Decreased Effect

Furosemide may decrease the levels/effects of: Antidiabetic Agents; Lithium; Neuromuscular-Blocking Agents

The levels/effects of Furosemide may be decreased by: Aliskiren; Amphetamines; Bile Acid Sequestrants; Fosphenytoin; Herbs (Hypertensive Properties); Methotrexate; Methylphenidate; Nonsteroidal Anti-Inflammatory Agents; Phenytoin; Probenecid; Salicylates; Sucralfate; Yohimbine

Food Interactions Furosemide serum levels may be decreased if taken with food. Management: Administer on an empty stomach.

Preparation for Administration IV infusion solution may be mixed in NS or D_5W solution. May also be diluted for infusion to 1-2 mg/mL (maximum: 10 mg/mL).

Storage/Stability

Injection: Store at room temperature of 15°C to 30°C (59°F to 86°F). Protect from light. Exposure to light may cause discoloration; do not use furosemide solutions if they have a yellow color. Furosemide solutions are unstable in acidic media, but very stable in basic media. Refrigeration may result in precipitation or crystallization; however, resolubilization at room temperature or warming may be performed without affecting the drug's stability. Infusion solution is stable for 24 hours at room temperature.

Tablet, solution: Store at 25°C (77°F); excursions permitted to 15°C to 30°C (59°F to 89°F). Protect from light. Discard opened bottle of solution after 90 days (10 mg/mL concentration only).

Mechanism of Action Inhibits reabsorption of sodium and chloride in the ascending loop of Henle and distal renal tubule, interfering with the chloride-binding cotransport system, thus causing increased excretion of water, sodium, chloride, magnesium, and calcium

Pharmacodynamics/Kinetics

Onset of action: Diuresis: Oral, SL: 30-60 minutes; IM: 30 minutes; IV: ~5 minutes

Symptomatic improvement with acute pulmonary edema: Within 15-20 minutes; occurs prior to diuretic effect

Peak effect: Oral, SL: 1-2 hours

Duration: Oral, SL: 6-8 hours; IV: 2 hours

Protein binding: 91% to 99%; primarily to albumin

Metabolism: Minimally hepatic

Bioavailability: Oral tablet: 47% to 64%; Oral solution: 50%; SL administration of oral tablet: ~60%; results of a small comparative study (n=11) showed bioavailability of SL administration of tablet was ~12% higher than oral administration of tablet (Haegeli, 2007)

Half-life elimination: Normal renal function: 0.5-2 hours; End-stage renal disease: 9 hours

Excretion: Urine (Oral: 50%, IV: 80%) within 24 hours; feces (as unchanged drug); nonrenal clearance prolonged in renal impairment

Dosing

Adult Note: Dose equivalency for patients with normal renal function (approximate): Furosemide 40 mg = bumetanide 1 mg = torsemide 20 mg = ethacrynic acid 50 mg

Edema, heart failure:

Oral: Initial: 20-80 mg/dose; if response is not adequate, may repeat the same dose or increase dose in increments of 20-40 mg/dose at intervals of 6-8 hours; may be titrated up to 600 mg daily with severe edematous states; usual maintenance dose interval is once or twice daily. ACCF/AHA 2013 heart failure guidelines recommend initial dosing of 20-40 mg once or twice daily and a maximum total daily dose of 600 mg (Yancy, 2013). **Note:** Dosing frequency may be adjusted based on patient-specific diuretic needs.

IM, IV: Initial: 20-40 mg/dose; if response is not adequate, may repeat the same dose or increase dose in increments of 20 mg/dose and administer 1-2 hours after previous dose (maximum dose: 200 mg/dose). Individually determined dose should then be given once or twice daily although some patients may initially require dosing as frequent as every 6 hours.

Continuous IV infusion (ACCF/AHA [Yancy, 2013]; Brater, 1998; Howard, 2001): Initial: IV bolus dose 40-100 mg over 1-2 minutes, followed by continuous IV infusion rate of 10-40 mg/hour; repeat loading dose before increasing infusion rate. **Note:** With lower baseline CrCl (eg, CrCl <25 mL/minute), the upper end of the initial infusion dosage range should be considered. If urine output is <1 mL/kg/hour, double as necessary to a maximum of 80-160 mg/hour (Howard, 2001; Schuller, 1997). The risk associated with higher infusion rates (80-160 mg/hour) must be weighed against alternative strategies.

Acute pulmonary edema: *IV:* 40 mg over 1-2 minutes. If response not adequate within 1 hour, may increase dose to 80 mg. **Note:** Minimal additional response is gained by single doses over 160-200 mg; maximum dose: 200 mg (Brater, 1998).

Hypertension: *Oral:* Initial: 40 mg twice daily; individualize according to patient response and use minimal dose necessary to maintain therapeutic response. If response inadequate, may add another antihypertensive. Usual dosage (ASH/ISH [Weber, 2014]): 40 mg twice daily.

Geriatric Oral, IM, IV: Initial: 20 mg/day; increase slowly to desired response.

Pediatric Note: Dose equivalency for patients with normal renal function (approximate): Furosemide 40 mg = bumetanide 1 mg = torsemide 20 mg = ethacrynic acid 50 mg

Edema, heart failure: Infants and Children:

Oral: Initial: 2 mg/kg/dose increased in increments of 1-2 mg/kg/dose with each succeeding dose at intervals of 6-8 hours until a satisfactory response is achieved; maximum dose: 6 mg/kg/dose

IM, IV: Initial: 1 mg/kg/dose; if response not adequate, may increase dose in increments of 1 mg/kg/dose and administer not sooner than 2 hours after previous dose, until a satisfactory response is achieved; may administer maintenance dose at intervals of every 6-12 hours; maximum dose: 6 mg/kg/dose

Hypertension, resistant (off-label; AAP, 2004): Children 1-17 years: *Oral:* Initial: 0.5-2 mg/kg/dose once or twice daily; maximum dose: 6 mg/kg/dose

Renal Impairment

Acute renal failure: Doses up to 1-3 g daily may be necessary to initiate desired response; avoid use in oliguric states.

Not removed by hemo- or peritoneal dialysis; supplemental dose is not necessary.

Hepatic Impairment Diminished natriuretic effect with increased sensitivity to hypokalemia and volume depletion in cirrhosis. Monitor effects, particularly with high doses.

Dietary Considerations May cause potassium loss; potassium supplement or dietary changes may be required.

Usual Infusion Concentrations: Pediatric IV infusion: 1 mg/mL **or** 2 mg/mL **or** undiluted as 10 mg/mL

Usual Infusion Concentrations: Adult IV infusion: 1 mg/mL **or** 2 mg/mL **or** undiluted as 10 mg/mL

Administration

IV: IV injections should be given slowly. In adults, undiluted direct IV injections may be administered at a rate of 20-40 mg per minute; maximum rate of administration for short-term intermittent infusion is 4 mg/minute; exceeding this rate increases the risk of ototoxicity. In children, a maximum rate of 0.5 mg/kg/minute has been recommended.

Oral: Administer on an empty stomach (Bard, 2004). May be administered with food or milk if GI distress occurs; however, this may reduce diuretic efficacy.

Note: When IV or oral administration is not possible, the sublingual route may be used. Place 1 tablet under tongue for at least 5 minutes to allow for maximal absorption. Patients should be advised not to swallow during disintegration time (Haegeli, 2007).

Monitoring Parameters Monitor weight and I & O daily; blood pressure, orthostasis; serum electrolytes, renal function; monitor hearing with high doses or rapid IV administration

Dosage Forms Excipient information presented when available (limited, particularly for generics); consult specific product labeling.

Solution, Injection:
Generic: 10 mg/mL (2 mL, 4 mL, 10 mL)
Solution, Injection [preservative free]:
Generic: 10 mg/mL (2 mL, 4 mL, 10 mL)
Solution, Oral:
Generic: 8 mg/mL (5 mL, 500 mL); 10 mg/mL (60 mL, 120 mL)
Tablet, Oral:
Lasix: 20 mg
Lasix: 40 mg, 80 mg [scored]
Generic: 20 mg, 40 mg, 80 mg

Dosage Forms: Canada Excipient information presented when available (limited, particularly for generics); consult specific product labeling.

Injection, solution [preservative free]:
Furosemide Special Injection: 10 mg/mL (25 mL)
Tablet, oral:
Lasix Special: 500 mg [scored]

◆ Furosemide Injection Sandoz Standard (Can) *see* Furosemide *on page 821*

◆ Furosemide Injection, USP (Can) *see* Furosemide *on page 821*

◆ Furosemide Special (Can) *see* Furosemide *on page 821*

◆ Furosemide Special Injection (Can) *see* Furosemide *on page 821*

◆ Fusilev *see* LEVOleucovorin *on page 1063*

◆ Fuzeon *see* Enfuvirtide *on page 639*

◆ FVIII/vWF *see* Antihemophilic Factor/von Willebrand Factor Complex (Human) *on page 133*

◆ FXIII *see* Factor XIII Concentrate (Human) *on page 739*

◆ FXT 40 (Can) *see* FLUoxetine *on page 786*

◆ Fycompa *see* Perampanel *on page 1428*

◆ GA101 *see* Obinutuzumab *on page 1305*

◆ GAA *see* Alglucosidase Alfa *on page 69*

Gabapentin (GA ba pen tin)

Brand Names: US Fanatrex FusePaq; Gralise; Gralise Starter; Neurontin

Brand Names: Canada ACT Gabapentin; Apo-Gabapentin; Auro-Gabapentin; Dom-Gabapentin; GD-Gabapentin; JAMP-Gabapentin; JAMP-Gabapentin Tablets; Mar-Gabapentin; Mylan-Gabapentin; Neurontin; PHL-Gabapentin; PMS-Gabapentin; PRO-Gabapentin; RAN-Gabapentin; Riva-Gabapentin; Teva-Gabapentin; Van-Gabapentin

Pharmacologic Category Anticonvulsant, Miscellaneous; GABA Analog

Use

Postherpetic neuralgia: Management of postherpetic neuralgia (PHN) in adults.

Seizures, partial onset (excluding Gralise): As adjunctive therapy in the treatment of partial seizures with and without secondary generalization in adults and pediatric patients 3 years and older with epilepsy.

Pregnancy Considerations Adverse events have been observed in animal reproduction studies. Gabapentin crosses the placenta. In a small study (n=6), the umbilical/maternal plasma concentration ratio was ~1.74. Neonatal concentrations declined quickly after delivery and at 24 hours of life were ~27% of the cord blood concentrations at birth (gabapentin neonatal half-life ~14 hours) (Ohman 2005). Outcome data following maternal use of gabapentin during pregnancy is limited (Holmes 2012).

Patients exposed to gabapentin during pregnancy are encouraged to enroll in the North American Antiepileptic Drug (NAAED) Pregnancy Registry by calling 1-888-233-2334. Additional information is available at www.aedpregnancyregistry.org.

Breast-Feeding Considerations Gabapentin is excreted in human breast milk. Per the manufacturer, a nursed infant could be exposed to ~1 mg/kg/day of gabapentin; the effect on the child is not known. Use in breast-feeding women only if the benefits to the mother outweigh the potential risk to the infant.

In a small study of breast-feeding women (n=6), the estimated exposure of gabapentin to the nursing infants was ~1% to 4% of the weight-adjusted maternal dose (sampling occurred from 12-97 days after delivery and maternal doses ranged from 600-2100 mg daily). Gabapentin was detected in the serum of 2 nursing infants 2-3 weeks after delivery and in 1 infant after 3 months of breast-feeding. Serum concentrations were <12% of the maternal plasma concentrations and <5% of those measured in the umbilical cord. Adverse events were not reported in the breast-fed infants (Ohman 2005).

Medication Guide Available Yes

Contraindications Hypersensitivity to gabapentin or any component of the formulation

Warnings/Precautions Antiepileptics are associated with an increased risk of suicidal behavior/thoughts with use (regardless of indication); patients should be monitored for signs/symptoms of depression, suicidal tendencies, and other unusual behavior changes during therapy and instructed to inform their healthcare provider immediately if symptoms occur. Avoid abrupt withdrawal, may precipitate seizures; Gralise should be withdrawn over ≥1 week. Use cautiously in patients with severe renal dysfunction; male rat studies demonstrated an association with pancreatic adenocarcinoma (clinical implication unknown). May cause CNS depression including somnolence and dizziness, which may impair physical or mental abilities. Patients must be cautioned about performing tasks which require mental alertness (eg, operating machinery or driving). Pediatric patients have shown increased incidence of CNS-related adverse effects, including emotional lability, hostility, changes in behavior and thinking, and hyperkinesia. Gabapentin immediate release and Gralise products are not interchangeable with each other **or** with gabapentin enacarbil (Horizant). The safety and efficacy of Gralise has not been studied in patients with epilepsy. Potentially serious, sometimes fatal multiorgan hypersensitivity (also known as drug reaction with eosinophilia and systemic symptoms [DRESS]) has been reported with some antiepileptic drugs, including gabapentin; may affect lymphatic, hepatic, renal, cardiac, and/or hematologic systems; fever, rash, and eosinophilia may also be present. Discontinue immediately if suspected. Anaphylaxis and/or angioedema may occur after the first dose or at any time during treatment; discontinue therapy and seek immediate medical care if signs or symptoms of anaphylaxis or angioedema occur. Potentially significant interactions may exist, requiring dose or frequency adjustment, additional monitoring, and/or selection of alternative therapy.

Adverse Reactions As reported for immediate release (IR) formulations in patients >12 years of age, unless otherwise noted in children (3-12 years) or with use of Gralise

>10%:

Central nervous system: Dizziness (IR: 17% to 28%; children 3%; Gralise: 11%), drowsiness (IR: 19% to 21%; children 8%; Gralise: 5%), ataxia (1% to 13%), fatigue (11%; children 3%)

Infection: Viral infection (children 11%)

1% to 10%:

Cardiovascular: Peripheral edema (IR: 2% to 8%; Gralise: 4%), vasodilatation (1%)

Central nervous system: Hostility (children 5% to 8%), tremor (7%), emotional lability (children 4% to 6%), hyperkinesia (children 3% to 5%), headache (children and adolescents 3%), abnormality in thinking (2% to 3%; children 2%), abnormal gait (2%), amnesia (2%), depression (2%), nervousness (2%), pain (Gralise: 1% to 2%), hyperesthesia (1%), lethargy (Gralise: 1%), twitching (1%), vertigo (Gralise: 1%)

Dermatologic: Pruritus (1%), skin rash (1%)

Endocrine & metabolic: Weight gain (IR: Adults and children 2% to 3%; Gralise: 2%), hyperglycemia (1%)

Gastrointestinal: Diarrhea (IR: 6%), nausea and vomiting (3% to 4%; children 8%), xerostomia (IR: 2% to 5%; Gralise: 3%), constipation (IR: 1% to 4%; Gralise: 1%), abdominal pain (3%), dyspepsia (IR: 2%; Gralise: 1%), dry throat (2%), dental disease (2%), flatulence (2%), increased appetite (1%)

Genitourinary: Impotence (2%), urinary tract infection (Gralise: 2%)

Hematologic & oncologic: Decreased white blood cell count (1%), leukopenia (1%)

Infection: Infection (5%)

Neuromuscular & skeletal: Weakness (6%), back pain (IR: 2%; Gralise: 2%), dysarthria (2%), limb pain (Gralise: 2%), myalgia (2%), bone fracture (1%)

Ophthalmic: Nystagmus (8%), diplopia (1% to 6%), blurred vision (3% to 4%), conjunctivitis (1%)

Otic: Otitis media (1%)

Respiratory: Rhinitis (4%), bronchitis (children 3%), nasopharyngitis (Gralise: 3%), respiratory tract infection (children 3%), pharyngitis (1% to 3%), cough (2%)

Miscellaneous: Fever (children 10%)

Postmarketing and case reports (Limited to important or life-threatening): Acute renal failure, altered serum glucose, anaphylaxis, anemia, angina pectoris, angioedema, aphasia, aspiration pneumonia, blindness, blood coagulation disorder, bradycardia, brain disease, breast hypertrophy, cardiac arrhythmia (various), cardiac failure, cerebrovascular accident, CNS neoplasm, colitis, confusion, Cushingoid appearance, DRESS syndrome, drug abuse, drug dependence, erythema multiforme, facial paralysis, fecal incontinence, gastroenteritis, glaucoma, glycosuria, hearing loss, heart block, hematemesis, hematuria, hemiplegia, hemorrhage, hepatitis, hepatomegaly, herpes zoster, hyperlipidemia, hypertension, hyperthyroidism, hyperventilation, hyponatremia, hypotension, hypothyroidism, hypoventilation, increased creatine phosphokinase, increased liver enzymes, increased serum creatinine, jaundice, joint swelling, leukocytosis, lymphadenopathy, lymphocytosis, memory impairment, meningism, migraine, movement disorder, myocardial infarction, myoclonus (local), nephrolithiasis, nephrosis, nerve palsy, non-Hodgkin's lymphoma, ovarian failure, pancreatitis, peptic ulcer, pericardial effusion, pericardial rub, pericarditis, peripheral vascular disease, pneumonia, psychosis, pulmonary thromboembolism, purpura, retinopathy, rhabdomyolysis, seasonal allergy, skin necrosis, status epilepticus, Stevens-Johnson syndrome, subdural hematoma, suicidal ideation, suicidal tendencies, syncope, tachycardia, thrombocytopenia, thrombophlebitis, tumor growth, withdrawal syndrome

Drug Interactions

Metabolism/Transport Effects None known.

Avoid Concomitant Use

Avoid concomitant use of Gabapentin with any of the following: Azelastine (Nasal); Orphenadrine; Paraldehyde; Thalidomide

Increased Effect/Toxicity

Gabapentin may increase the levels/effects of: Alcohol (Ethyl); Azelastine (Nasal); Buprenorphine; CNS Depressants; Hydrocodone; Methotrimeprazine; Metyrosine; Mirtazapine; Morphine (Systemic); Orphenadrine; Paraldehyde; Pramipexole; ROPINIRole; Rotigotine; Selective Serotonin Reuptake Inhibitors; Suvorexant; Thalidomide; Zolpidem

The levels/effects of Gabapentin may be increased by: Brimonidine (Topical); Cannabis; Doxylamine; Dronabinol; Droperidol; HydrOXYzine; Kava Kava; Magnesium Salts; Methotrimeprazine; Minocycline; Morphine (Systemic); Nabilone; Perampanel; Rufinamide; Sodium Oxybate; Tapentadol; Tetrahydrocannabinol

Decreased Effect

The levels/effects of Gabapentin may be decreased by: Antacids; Magnesium Salts; Mefloquine; Mianserin; Orlistat

Food Interactions Tablet, solution (immediate release): No significant effect on rate or extent of absorption; tablet (Gralise): Increases rate and extent of absorption. Management: Administer immediate release products without regard to food. Administer Gralise with food.

Storage/Stability

Capsules and tablets: Store at 25°C (77°F); excursions permitted to 15°C to 30°C (59°F to 86°F). Use scored 600 or 800 mg tablets that are broken in half within 28 days of breaking the tablet.

Oral solution: Store refrigerated at 2°C to 8°C (36°F to 46°F).

Mechanism of Action

Gabapentin is structurally related to GABA. However, it does not bind to GABA$_A$ or GABA$_B$ receptors, and it does not appear to influence synthesis or uptake of GABA. High affinity gabapentin binding sites have been located throughout the brain; these sites correspond to the presence of voltage-gated calcium channels specifically possessing the alpha-2-delta-1 subunit. This channel appears to be located presynaptically, and may modulate the release of excitatory neurotransmitters which participate in epileptogenesis and nociception.

Pharmacodynamics/Kinetics

Absorption: Variable, from proximal small bowel by L-amino transport system; saturable process; dose-dependent

Distribution: V$_d$: 58 ± 6 L; CSF concentrations are ~20% of plasma concentrations

Protein binding: <3%

Metabolism: Not metabolized

Bioavailability: Inversely proportional to dose due to saturable absorption:

Immediate release:
900 mg/day: 60%
1,200 mg/day: 47%
2,400 mg/day: 34%
3,600 mg/day: 33%
4,800 mg/day: 27%

Gralise: Variable; increased with higher fat content meal

Half-life elimination:

Infants 1 month to Children 12 years: 4.7 hours

Adults, normal: 5 to 7 hours; increased half-life with decreased renal function; anuric adult patients: 132 hours; adults during hemodialysis: 3.8 hours

Time to peak: Immediate release: Infants 1 month to Children 12 years: 2 to 3 hours; Adults: 2 to 4 hours; Gralise: 8 hours

Excretion: Proportional to renal function; urine (as unchanged drug)

Clearance: Apparent oral clearance is directly proportional to CrCl: Clearance in infants is highly variable; oral clearance (per kg) in children <5 years of age is higher than in children ≥5 years of age

Dosing

Adult & Geriatric

Postherpetic neuralgia: Oral:

Day 1: 300 mg, Day 2: 300 mg twice daily, Day 3: 300 mg 3 times daily; dose may be titrated as needed for pain relief (range: 1,800 to 3,600 mg/day in divided doses, daily doses >1,800 do not generally show greater benefit)

Gralise only: Day 1: 300 mg, Day 2: 600 mg, Days 3 to 6: 900 mg once daily, Days 7 to 10: 1,200 mg once daily, Days 11 to 14: 1,500 mg once daily, Days ≥15: 1,800 mg once daily

Seizures, partial onset: Oral (excluding Gralise):

Initial: 300 mg 3 times daily; increase dosage based on response and tolerability; usual dosage: 900 to 1,800 mg/day administered in 3 divided doses; doses of up to 2,400 mg/day have been tolerated in long-term clinical studies; up to 3,600 mg/day has been tolerated in short-term studies

Note: If gabapentin is discontinued or if another anticonvulsant is added to therapy, it should be done slowly over a minimum of 1 week.

Diabetic neuropathy (off-label use): Oral: Immediate release: 900 to 3,600 mg/day (Bril 2011)

Hot flashes (off-label use): Oral: Immediate release: Day 1: 300 mg at bedtime, Day 2: 300 mg twice daily, followed by 300 mg 3 times/day for 4 weeks and then tapered off (Butt 2008)

Neuropathic pain (off-label use): Oral: Immediate release: 300 to 3,600 mg/day (Attal 2010; Dworkin 2010)

Neuropathic pain, critically-ill patients (off-label use): Oral: Immediate release: Initial: 100 mg 3 times daily in combination with IV opioids; maintenance: 300 to 1,200 mg 3 times daily; maximum dose: 3,600 mg daily (Barr 2013)

Postoperative pain (adjunct; off-label use): Oral: Immediate release: Usual dose: 300 to 1,200 mg given the night before or 1 to 2 hours prior to surgery (Dauri 2009)

Restless legs syndrome (RLS) (off-label use): Oral: Immediate release: Initial: 300 mg once daily 2 hours before bedtime. Doses ≥600 mg/day have been given in 2 divided doses (late afternoon and 2 hours before bedtime). Dose may be titrated every 2 weeks until symptom relief achieved (range: 300 to 1,800 mg/day). Suggested maintenance dosing schedule: One-third of total daily dose given at 12 pm, remaining two-thirds total daily dose given at 8 pm. (Garcia-Borreguero 2002; Happe 2003; Saletu 2010; Vignatelli 2006)

Social anxiety disorder (off-label use): Oral: Initial: 300 mg twice daily; increase dose based on response and tolerability in increments of no more than 300 mg/day up to a maximum of 3,600 mg/day given in 3 divided doses. Doses for responders ranged from 900 to 3,600 mg/day in the clinical trial (Pande 1999). Additional data may be necessary to further define the role of gabapentin in this condition.

Pediatric

Seizures, partial onset:

Children 3 to 4 years: Oral (excluding Gralise) Initial: 10 to 15 mg/kg/day in 3 divided doses; titrate to effective dose over ~3 days; increase dosage based on response and tolerability; usual dosage: 40 mg/kg/day in 3 divided doses; dosages of up to 50 mg/kg/day have been tolerated in clinical studies:

Children 5 to 11 years: Oral (excluding Gralise): Initial: 10 to 15 mg/kg/day in 3 divided doses; titrate to effective dose over ~3 days; increase dosage based on response and tolerability; usual dosage: 25 to 35 mg/kg/day in 3 divided doses; dosages of up to 50 mg/kg/day have been tolerated in clinical studies

Children ≥12 years: Refer to adult dosing.

Note: If gabapentin is discontinued or if another anticonvulsant is added to therapy, it should be done slowly over a minimum of 1 week

Renal Impairment

Children ≥12 years and Adults:

All products, excluding Gralise:
CrCl ≥60 mL/minute: 300 to 1,200 mg 3 times daily
CrCl >30 to 59 mL/minute: 200 to 700 mg twice daily
CrCl >15 to 29 mL/minute: 200 to 700 mg once daily
CrCl 15 mL/minute: 100 to 300 mg once daily
CrCl <15 mL/minute: Reduce daily dose in proportion to creatinine clearance based on dose for creatinine clearance of 15 mL/minute (eg, reduce dose by one-half [range: 50 to 150 mg/day] for CrCl 7.5 mL/minute)

ESRD requiring hemodialysis: Dose based on CrCl plus a single supplemental dose of 125 to 350 mg (given after each 4 hours of hemodialysis)

Gralise only: **Note:** Follow initial dose titration schedule if treatment-naive.
CrCl ≥60 mL/minute: 1,800 mg once daily
CrCl >30 to 59 mL/minute: 600 to 1,800 mg once daily; dependent on tolerability and clinical response
CrCl <30 mL/minute: Use is not recommended
ESRD requiring hemodialysis: Use is not recommended.

Hepatic Impairment

There are no dosage adjustments provided in the manufacturer's labeling; however, gabapentin is not hepatically metabolized.

Dietary Considerations

Gralise should be taken with food.

Administration

Capsule, tablet (excluding Gralise), solution: May administer without regards to meals. Administer first dose on first day at bedtime to avoid somnolence and dizziness. Dosage must be adjusted for renal function; when given 3 times daily, the maximum time between doses should not exceed 12 hours.

Gralise: Take with evening meal. Swallow whole; do not chew, crush, or split.

Monitoring Parameters

Monitor serum levels of concomitant anticonvulsant therapy; suicidality (eg, suicidal thoughts, depression, behavioral changes)

Test Interactions

False positives have been reported with the Ames N-Multistix SG® dipstick test for urine protein

Dosage Forms Considerations

Fanatrex FusePaq is a compounding kit for the preparation of an oral suspension. Refer to manufacturer's labeling for compounding instructions.

Dosage Forms

Excipient information presented when available (limited, particularly for generics); consult specific product labeling.

Capsule, Oral:
Neurontin: 100 mg, 300 mg, 400 mg
Generic: 100 mg, 300 mg, 400 mg

Miscellaneous, Oral:
Gralise Starter: 300 & 600 mg (78 ea) [contains soybean lecithin]

Solution, Oral:
Neurontin: 250 mg/5 mL (470 mL) [strawberry anise flavor]
Generic: 250 mg/5 mL (5 mL, 6 mL, 470 mL, 473 mL)

Suspension, Oral:
Fanatrex FusePaq: 25 mg/mL (420 mL) [contains saccharin sodium, sodium benzoate]

Tablet, Oral:
Gralise: 300 mg [contains soybean lecithin]
Gralise: 600 mg
Neurontin: 600 mg, 800 mg [scored]
Generic: 600 mg, 800 mg
Extemporaneous Preparations Note: Commercial oral solution is available (50 mg/mL)

A 100 mg/mL suspension may be made with tablets (immediate release) and either a 1:1 mixture of Ora-Sweet® (100 mL) and Ora-Plus® (100 mL) or 1:1 mixture of methylcellulose 1% (100 mL) and Simple Syrup N.F. (100 mL). Crush sixty-seven 300 mg tablets in a mortar and reduce to a fine powder. Add small portions of the chosen vehicle and mix to a uniform paste; mix while adding the vehicle in incremental proportions to **almost** 200 mL; transfer to a calibrated bottle, rinse mortar with vehicle, and add sufficient quantity of vehicle to make 200 mL. Label "shake well" and "refrigerate". Stable for 91 days refrigerated (preferred) or 56 days at room temperature.
Nahata MC, Pai VB, and Hipple TF, *Pediatric Drug Formulations*, 5th ed, Cincinnati, OH: Harvey Whitney Books Co, 2004.

Gabapentin Enacarbil (gab a PEN tin en a KAR bil)

Brand Names: US Horizant
Index Terms GSK 1838262; Solzira; XP13512
Pharmacologic Category Anticonvulsant, Miscellaneous
Use Treatment of moderate-to-severe restless leg syndrome (RLS); management of postherpetic neuralgia (PHN)
Medication Guide Available Yes
Dosing
Adult & Geriatric
Postherpetic neuralgia (PHN): Oral: Initial: 600 mg once daily in the morning for 3 days, then increase to 600 mg twice daily; increasing to >1200 mg daily provided no additional benefit and increased side effects
Restless legs syndrome (RLS): Oral: 600 mg once daily (at ~5:00 pm); increasing to 1200 mg daily provided no additional benefit and increased side effects
Renal Impairment Note: Estimation of renal function for the purpose of drug dosing should be done using the Cockcroft-Gault formula.
PHN:
CrCl 30-59 mL/minute: Initial: 300 mg every morning for 3 days, then increase to 300 mg twice daily. May increase to 600 mg twice daily as needed based on tolerability and efficacy. When discontinuing, reduce current dose to once daily in the morning for 1 week.
CrCl 15-29 mL/minute: Initial: 300 mg in the morning on day 1 and on day 3; then increase to 300 mg once daily. May increase to 300 mg twice daily if needed based on tolerability and efficacy. When discontinuing, if current dose is 300 mg twice daily, reduce to 300 mg once daily for 1 week. If current dose is 300 mg once daily, no taper is needed.
CrCl <15 mL/minute: 300 mg every other day in the morning; may increase dose to 300 mg once daily if needed based on tolerability and efficacy. When discontinuing, no taper is needed.
CrCl <15 mL/minute and on hemodialysis: 300 mg following every dialysis. May increase to 600 mg following every dialysis if needed based on tolerability and efficacy. When discontinuing, no taper is needed.
RLS:
CrCl 30-59 mL/minute: Initial dose: 300 mg daily; increase to 600 mg daily as needed
CrCl 15-29 mL/minute: 300 mg daily
CrCl <15 mL/minute: 300 mg every other day
CrCl <15 mL/minute and on hemodialysis: Use is not recommended.
Hepatic Impairment No dosage adjustment provided in manufacturer's labeling.
Additional Information Complete prescribing information should be consulted for additional detail.
Dosage Forms Excipient information presented when available (limited, particularly for generics); consult specific product labeling.
Tablet Extended Release, Oral:
Horizant: 300 mg, 600 mg

♦ Gabitril see TiaGABine on page 1785
♦ Gablofen see Baclofen on page 197

Galantamine (ga LAN ta meen)

Brand Names: US Razadyne; Razadyne ER
Brand Names: Canada Auro-Galantamine ER; Galantamine ER; Mylan-Galantamine ER; PAT-Galantamine ER; PMS-Galantamine ER; Reminyl ER; Teva-Galantamine ER

Index Terms Galantamine Hydrobromide
Pharmacologic Category Acetylcholinesterase Inhibitor (Central)
Use Treatment of mild-to-moderate dementia of Alzheimer's disease
Pregnancy Considerations Adverse events have been observed in animal reproduction studies.
Breast-Feeding Considerations It is not known if galantamine is excreted in breast milk. The manufacturer recommends that caution be exercised when administering galantamine to nursing women.
Contraindications Hypersensitivity to galantamine or any component of the formulation
Canadian labeling: Additional contraindications (not in U.S. labeling): Hypersensitivity to other tertiary alkaloids
Warnings/Precautions Use caution in patients with supraventricular conduction delays (without a functional pacemaker in place); Alzheimer's treatment guidelines consider bradycardia to be a relative contraindication for use of centrally active cholinesterase inhibitors. Use caution in patients taking medicines that slow conduction through SA or AV node. Use caution in peptic ulcer disease (or in patients at risk); seizure disorder; asthma; COPD; mild to moderate liver dysfunction; moderate renal dysfunction. May cause bladder outflow obstruction. May cause CNS depression, which may impair physical or mental abilities; patients must be cautioned about performing tasks that require mental alertness (eg, operating machinery or driving). Skin reactions including Stevens-Johnson syndrome, acute generalized exanthematous pustulosis and erythema multiforme have been reported. Treatment discontinuation may be necessary if skin reaction occurs; if rash is suspected to be drug related, do not resume galantamine and consider alternative therapy. Weight loss has been observed; monitor body weight. Limited safety data in patients ≥85 years of age. Use with caution particularly in elderly patients with low body weight and/or serious comorbidities; adjust dose with caution. Potentially significant drug-drug interactions may exist, requiring dose or frequency adjustment, additional monitoring, and/or selection of alternative therapy.
Adverse Reactions
>10%: Gastrointestinal: Nausea (25%), vomiting (13%)
1% to 10%:
Cardiovascular: Syncope (2%), bradycardia (1%)
Central nervous system: Dizziness (9%), headache (8%), depression (4%), fatigue (4%), drowsiness (2%), malaise (1%)
Dermatologic: Hyperhidrosis (1%)
Gastrointestinal: Diarrhea (9%), decreased appetite (5%), weight loss (5%), anorexia (4%), abdominal pain (2%), dyspepsia (2%), upper abdominal pain (2%), abdominal distress (1%)
Neuromuscular & skeletal: Tremor (2%)
<1% (Limited to important or life-threatening): Acute generalized exanthematous pustulosis, anemia, aphasia, apraxia, arthritis, ataxia, atrial arrhythmia (includes atrial fibrillation and supraventricular tachycardia), atrioventricular block, attempted suicide, bundle branch block, cardiac failure, cataract, cerebrovascular accident, convulsions, cystitis, dehydration (includes rare, severe cases leading to renal insufficiency and renal failure), delirium, dependent edema, diverticulitis, erythema multiforme, esophageal perforation, exacerbation of depression, falling, gastroenteritis, gastrointestinal bleeding, hematuria, hepatitis, hyperglycemia, hyperkinesia, hypersensitivity reaction, hypersomnia, hypertension, hypertonia, hypokalemia, hypokinesia, hypotension, increased liver enzymes, increased nonprotein nitrogen, increased serum alkaline phosphatase, inversion T wave on ECG, ischemic heart disease, myocardial infarction, nephrolithiasis, orthostatic hypotension, paranoia, peripheral edema, pneumonia, prolonged Q-T interval on ECG, purpura, rectal hemorrhage, seizure, severe bradycardia, sinus bradycardia, Stevens-Johnson syndrome, suicidal ideation, supraventricular extrasystole, thrombocytopenia, transient ischemic attacks, trauma, urinary incontinence, urinary retention, urinary tract infection, ventricular tachycardia
Drug Interactions
Metabolism/Transport Effects Substrate of CYP2D6 (minor), CYP3A4 (minor); **Note:** Assignment of Major/Minor substrate status based on clinically relevant drug interaction potential
Avoid Concomitant Use
Avoid concomitant use of Galantamine with any of the following: Ceritinib

Increased Effect/Toxicity

Galantamine may increase the levels/effects of: Antipsychotic Agents; Beta-Blockers; Bradycardia-Causing Agents; Ceritinib; Cholinergic Agonists; Highest Risk QTc-Prolonging Agents; Ivabradine; Lacosamide; Moderate Risk QTc-Prolonging Agents; Succinylcholine

The levels/effects of Galantamine may be increased by: Bretylium; Corticosteroids (Systemic); Mifepristone; Ruxolitinib; Selective Serotonin Reuptake Inhibitors; Tofacitinib

Decreased Effect

Galantamine may decrease the levels/effects of: Anticholinergic Agents; Neuromuscular-Blocking Agents (Nondepolarizing)

The levels/effects of Galantamine may be decreased by: Anticholinergic Agents; Dipyridamole

Storage/Stability Store at 25°C (77°F); excursions permitted to 15°C to 30°C (59°F to 86°F). Do not freeze oral solution.

Mechanism of Action Centrally-acting cholinesterase inhibitor (competitive and reversible). It elevates acetylcholine in cerebral cortex by slowing the degradation of acetylcholine. Modulates nicotinic acetylcholine receptor to increase acetylcholine from surviving presynaptic nerve terminals. May increase glutamate and serotonin levels.

Pharmacodynamics/Kinetics

Distribution: 175 L

Protein binding: 18%

Metabolism: Hepatic metabolism primarily via CYP2D6 to O-desmethyl-galantamine and 3A4 to galantamine-N-oxide; the activity of galantamine metabolites is not considered to be clinically relevant (Farlow 2003; Scott 2000)

Bioavailability: ~90%

Half-life elimination: ~7 hours

Time to peak: Immediate release: 1 hour (2.5 hours with food); extended release: 4.5-5 hours

Excretion: Urine (20%)

Dosing

Adult

Alzheimer dementia, mild-to-moderate: Oral:

Immediate-release tablet or solution: Initial: 4 mg twice daily for 4 weeks; if tolerated, increase to 8 mg twice daily for ≥4 weeks; if tolerated, increase to 12 mg twice daily. Range: 16 to 24 mg daily in 2 divided doses

Extended-release capsule: Initial: 8 mg once daily for 4 weeks; if tolerated, increase to 16 mg once daily for ≥4 weeks; if tolerated, increase to 24 mg once daily. Range: 16 to 24 mg once daily

Note: If therapy is interrupted for ≥3 days, restart at the lowest dose and increase to current dose.

Alzheimer dementia, severe (off-label use): Immediate-release tablet: Initial: 4 mg twice daily for 4 weeks; if tolerated, increase to 8 mg twice daily for ≥4 weeks; if tolerated, increase to 12 mg twice daily. May decrease to 8 mg twice daily if the target dose is not tolerated. Range: 16 to 24 mg daily in 2 divided doses (Burns 2009)

Dementia associated with Parkinson disease and Lewy body dementia (off-label use): Oral: American Psychiatric Association recommends dosing and titration similar to those for patients with Alzheimer disease (APA [Rabins 2007]).

Conversion from immediate release to extended release formulation: Patients may be switched from the immediate-release formulation to the extended-release formulation by taking the last immediate-release dose in the evening and beginning the extended-release dose the following morning; the same total daily dose should be used.

Conversion to galantamine from other cholinesterase inhibitors: Patients experiencing poor tolerability with donepezil or rivastigmine should wait until side effects subside or allow a 7-day washout period prior to beginning galantamine. Patients not experiencing side effects with donepezil or rivastigmine may begin galantamine therapy the day immediately following discontinuation of previous therapy (Morris 2001).

Geriatric Refer to adult dosing; adjust dose with caution in patients with low body weight and/or serious comorbidities.

Renal Impairment

Mild impairment: There are no dosage adjustments provided in the manufacturer's labeling.

Moderate impairment (CrCl 9 to 59 mL/minute): Maximum dose: 16 mg daily.

Severe impairment (CrCl <9 mL/minute): Use is not recommended

Hepatic Impairment

US labeling:

Mild impairment (Child-Pugh score 5 to 6): There are no dosage adjustments provided in the manufacturer's labeling; however, single-dose galantamine pharmacokinetics were similar to that observed in healthy subjects.

Moderate impairment (Child-Pugh score 7 to 9): Maximum dose: 16 mg daily

Severe impairment (Child-Pugh score 10 to 15): Use is not recommended

Canadian labeling:

Mild impairment: (Child-Pugh score 5 to 6): There are no dosage adjustments provided in the manufacturer's labeling; however, single-dose galantamine pharmacokinetics were similar to that observed in healthy subjects.

Moderate impairment: (Child-Pugh score 7 to 9): Initial: 8 mg every other day for at least 1 week, then increase to 8 mg once daily for at least 4 weeks (maximum dose: 16 mg daily)

Severe impairment (Child-Pugh score 10 to 15): Use is not recommended

Dietary Considerations Administration with food is preferred, but not required; should be taken with breakfast and dinner (tablet or solution) or with breakfast (capsule).

Administration Oral: Administer solution or tablet with breakfast and dinner; administer extended release capsule with breakfast. If therapy is interrupted for ≥3 days, restart at the lowest dose and increase to current dose. If using oral solution, mix dose with 3 to 4 ounces of any nonalcoholic beverage; mix well and drink immediately.

Monitoring Parameters Mental status; body weight

Dosage Forms Excipient information presented when available (limited, particularly for generics); consult specific product labeling. [DSC] = Discontinued product

Capsule Extended Release 24 Hour, Oral, as hydrobromide [strength expressed as base]:

Razadyne ER: 8 mg, 16 mg, 24 mg

Generic: 8 mg, 16 mg, 24 mg

Solution, Oral, as hydrobromide:

Razadyne: 4 mg/mL (100 mL [DSC]) [contains methylparaben, propylparaben, saccharin sodium]

Generic: 4 mg/mL (100 mL)

Tablet, Oral, as hydrobromide [strength expressed as base]:

Razadyne: 4 mg, 8 mg

Razadyne: 12 mg [contains fd&c yellow #6 aluminum lake]

Generic: 4 mg, 8 mg, 12 mg

Dosage Forms: Canada Excipient information presented when available (limited, particularly for generics); consult specific product labeling.

Capsule Extended Release 24 Hour, Oral, as hydrobromide [strength expressed as base]:

Reminyl ER: 8 mg, 16 mg, 24 mg

Ganciclovir (Systemic) (gan SYE kloe veer)

Brand Names: US Cytovene

Brand Names: Canada Cytovene; Ganciclovir for Injection

Index Terms DHPG Sodium; GCV Sodium; Nordeoxyguanosine

Pharmacologic Category Antiviral Agent

Use Treatment of CMV retinitis in immunocompromised individuals, including patients with acquired immunodeficiency syndrome; prophylaxis of CMV infection in transplant patients

Pregnancy Considerations [U.S. Boxed Warning]: Animal studies have demonstrated carcinogenic and teratogenic effects, and inhibition of spermatogenesis. Female patients should use effective contraception during therapy; male patients should use a barrier contraceptive during and for at least 90 days after therapy.

Breast-Feeding Considerations Due to the carcinogenic and teratogenic effects observed in animal studies, the possibility of adverse events in a nursing infant is considered likely. Therefore, nursing should be discontinued during therapy. In addition, the CDC recommends **not** to breast-feed if diagnosed with HIV to avoid postnatal transmission of the virus.

Contraindications Hypersensitivity to ganciclovir, acyclovir, or any component of the formulation

Warnings/Precautions Hazardous agent - use appropriate precautions for handling and disposal (NIOSH 2014 [group 2]).

[US Boxed Warning]: Granulocytopenia (neutropenia), anemia, and thrombocytopenia may occur. Dosage adjustment or interruption of ganciclovir therapy may be necessary in patients with neutropenia and/or thrombocytopenia and patients with impaired renal function. **[U.S. Boxed Warning]: Animal studies have demonstrated carcinogenic and teratogenic effects, and inhibition of spermatogenesis;** contraceptive precautions for female and male patients need to be followed during and for at least 90 days after therapy with the drug; take care to administer only into veins with good blood flow. **[US Boxed Warning]: Indicated only for treatment of CMV retinitis in the immunocompromised patient and CMV prevention in transplant patients at risk.**

Adverse Reactions

>10%:

Central nervous system: Fever (48%)

Gastrointestinal: Diarrhea (44%), anorexia (14%), vomiting (13%)

Hematologic: Thrombocytopenia (57%), leukopenia (41%), anemia (16% to 26%), neutropenia with ANC <500/mm^3 (12% to 14%)

Ocular: Retinal detachment (11%; relationship to ganciclovir not established)

Renal: Serum creatinine increased (2% to 14%)

Miscellaneous: Sepsis (15%), diaphoresis (12%)

1% to 10%:

Central nervous system: Chills (10%), neuropathy (9%)

Dermatologic: Pruritus (5%)

<1% (Limited to important or life-threatening): Allergic reaction (including anaphylaxis), alopecia, arrhythmia, bronchospasm, cardiac arrest, cataracts, cholestasis, coma, dyspnea, edema, encephalopathy, exfoliative dermatitis, extrapyramidal symptoms, hepatitis, hepatic failure, pancreatitis, pancytopenia, pulmonary fibrosis, psychosis, rhabdomyolysis, seizure, alopecia, urticaria, eosinophilia, hemorrhage, Stevens-Johnson syndrome, torsade de pointes, renal failure, SIADH, visual loss

Drug Interactions

Metabolism/Transport Effects None known.

Avoid Concomitant Use There are no known interactions where it is recommended to avoid concomitant use.

Increased Effect/Toxicity

Ganciclovir (Systemic) may increase the levels/effects of: Imipenem; Mycophenolate; Reverse Transcriptase Inhibitors (Nucleoside); Tenofovir Products

The levels/effects of Ganciclovir (Systemic) may be increased by: Mycophenolate; Probenecid; Tenofovir Products

Decreased Effect There are no known significant interactions involving a decrease in effect.

Preparation for Administration Hazardous agent; use appropriate precautions for handling and disposal (NIOSH 2014 [group 2]).

Reconstitute 500 mg vial with 10 mL unpreserved sterile water **not** bacteriostatic water because parabens may cause precipitation. Typically, dilute in 100 mL D$_5$W or NS to a concentration ≤10 mg/mL for infusion.

Storage/Stability Store intact vials at temperatures below 40°C (104°F). Reconstituted solution is stable for 12 hours at room temperature, however, conflicting data indicates that reconstituted solution is stable for 60 days under refrigeration (4°C). Stability of parenteral admixture at room temperature (25°C) and at refrigeration temperature (4°C) for 35 days has been reported. However, the manufacturer recommends use within 24 hours of preparation.

Mechanism of Action Ganciclovir is phosphorylated to a substrate which competitively inhibits the binding of deoxyguanosine triphosphate to DNA polymerase resulting in inhibition of viral DNA synthesis

Pharmacodynamics/Kinetics

Distribution: V$_d$: Children 9 months to 12 years: 0.64 ± 0.22 L/kg; Adults: 0.74 ± 0.15 L/kg; widely to all tissues including CSF and ocular tissue

Protein binding: 1% to 2%

Half-life elimination: Prolonged with renal impairment

Neonates 2-49 days of age: 2.4 hours

Children 9 months to 12 years: 2.4 ± 0.7 hours

Adults: Mean: 2.5-3.6 hours (range: 1.7-5.8 hours); End-stage renal disease (ESRD): 5-28 hours

Excretion: Urine (80% to 99% as unchanged drug)

Dosing

Adult & Geriatric

CMV retinitis:

Manufacturer's labeling:

Induction therapy: IV (slow infusion): 5 mg/kg/dose every 12 hours for 14 to 21 days followed by maintenance therapy

Maintenance therapy: IV (slow infusion): 5 mg/kg/day as a single daily dose for 7 days/week or 6 mg/kg/day for 5 days/week

Alternate dosing (HHS [OI adult 2015]):

Peripheral lesions (alternative to preferred therapy): IV: Induction: 5 mg/kg/dose every 12 hours for 14 to 21 days followed by chronic maintenance (secondary prophylaxis)

Immediate sight-threatening lesions (adjacent to the optic nerve or fovea): Intravitreal injection (off-label route): Induction therapy: 2 mg of an extemporaneously prepared solution administered as intravitreal injections for 1 to 4 doses over a period of 7 to 10 days; administer with a concomitant systemically administered agent (oral valganciclovir preferred).

CMV disease, chronic maintenance (secondary prophylaxis) in HIV-infected patients (off-label use; alternative to preferred therapy): IV: 5 mg/kg/dose 5 to 7 times weekly; continue until sustained CD4 count >100 cells/mm^3 in response to ART for 3 to 6 months; discontinue only after consultation with an ophthalmologist) (HHS [OI adult 2015]).

CMV disease, prophylaxis (secondary) in transplant patients: IV (slow infusion): 5 mg/kg/dose every 12 hours for 7 to 14 days, duration of maintenance therapy is dependent on clinical condition and degree of immunosuppression

CMV esophagitis or colitis in HIV-infected patients (off-label use): IV: 5 mg/kg/dose every 12 hours, then change to oral valganciclovir therapy once oral therapy is tolerated (HHS [OI adult 2015])

CMV neurological disease in HIV-infected patients (off-label use): IV: 5 mg/kg/dose every 12 hours plus foscarnet until symptoms improve (HHS [OI adult 2015])

Varicella-zoster: Acute retinal necrosis (ARN) in HIV-infected patients (off-label use): Intravitreal injection (off-label route): 2 mg of an extemporaneously prepared solution administered as an intravitreal injection twice weekly for 1 to 2 doses in combination with IV acyclovir for 10 to 14 days, followed by valacyclovir for 6 weeks (HHS [OI adult 2015])

Varicella-zoster: Progressive outer retinal necrosis in HIV-infected patients (off-label use): IV: 5 mg/kg/dose every 12 hours (with or without foscarnet IV) **plus** intravitreal ganciclovir and/or intravitreal foscarnet (HHS [OI adult 2015])

Pediatric

CMV retinitis:

Children: IV (slow infusion): Manufacturer's labeling:

Induction therapy: 5 mg/kg/dose every 12 hours for 14 to 21 days followed by maintenance therapy

Maintenance therapy: 5 mg/kg/day as a single daily dose for 7 days/week or 6 mg/kg/day for 5 days/week

Adolescents: Refer to adult dosing.

CMV disease, chronic maintenance (secondary prophylaxis) in HIV-exposed/-infected patients (off-label use):

Infants and Children: IV: 5 mg/kg/dose daily (CDC 2009)

Adolescents (alternative to preferred therapy): Refer to adult dosing.

CMV disease, prophylaxis (secondary) in transplant patients: Children: IV (slow infusion): Refer to adult dosing.

CMV esophagitis or colitis in HIV-infected patients (off-label use): Adolescents: Refer to adult dosing.

CMV neurological disease in HIV-exposed/-infected patients (off-label use): Infants, Children, and Adolescents: IV: Refer to adult dosing.

Varicella-zoster: Acute retinal necrosis (ARN) in HIV-infected patients (off-label use): Adolescents: Refer to adult dosing.

Varicella-zoster: Progressive outer retinal necrosis in HIV-exposed/-infected patients (off-label use):

Infants and Children: IV: 5 mg/kg/dose every 12 hours plus systemic foscarnet and intravitreal ganciclovir or intravitreal foscarnet (CDC 2009)

Adolescents: Refer to adult dosing.

Renal Impairment

IV (Induction):

CrCl 50 to 69 mL/minute: Administer 2.5 mg/kg/dose every 12 hours.

CrCl 25 to 49 mL/minute: Administer 2.5 mg/kg/dose every 24 hours.

CrCl 10 to 24 mL/minute: Administer 1.25 mg/kg/dose every 24 hours.

CrCl <10 mL/minute: Administer 1.25 mg/kg/dose 3 times/week following hemodialysis.

IV (Maintenance):

CrCl 50 to 69 mL/minute: Administer 2.5 mg/kg/dose every 24 hours.

CrCl 25 to 49 mL/minute: Administer 1.25 mg/kg/dose every 24 hours.

CrCl 10 to 24 mL/minute: Administer 0.625 mg/kg/dose every 24 hours

CrCl <10 mL/minute: Administer 0.625 mg/kg/dose 3 times/week following hemodialysis.

Intermittent hemodialysis (IHD) (administer after hemodialysis on dialysis days): Dialyzable (50%): CMV Infection: IV: Induction: 1.25 mg/kg every 48 to 72 hours; Maintenance: 0.625 mg/kg every 48 to 72 hours. **Note:** Dosing dependent on the assumption of 3 times/week, complete IHD sessions.

Peritoneal dialysis (PD): Dose as for CrCl <10 mL/minute.

Continuous renal replacement therapy (CRRT) (Heintz 2009; Trotman 2005): Drug clearance is highly dependent on the method of renal replacement, filter type, and flow rate. Appropriate dosing requires close monitoring of pharmacologic response, signs of adverse reactions due to drug accumulation, as well as drug concentrations in relation to target trough (if appropriate). The following are general recommendations only (based on dialysate flow/ultrafiltration rates of 1 to 2 L/hour and minimal residual renal function) and should not supersede clinical judgment: CMV Infection:

CVVH: IV: Induction: 2.5 mg/kg every 24 hours; Maintenance: 1.25 mg/kg every 24 hours

CVVHD/CVVHDF: IV: Induction: 2.5 mg/kg every 12 hours; Maintenance: 2.5 mg/kg every 24 hours

Hepatic Impairment No dosage adjustment provided in manufacturer's labeling.

Dietary Considerations Some products may contain sodium.

Administration Should not be administered by IM, SubQ, or rapid IVP; administer by slow IV infusion over at least 1 hour. Too rapid infusion can cause increased toxicity and excessive plasma levels. Flush line well with NS before and after administration.

Hazardous agent; use appropriate precautions for handling and disposal (NIOSH 2014 [group 2]).

Monitoring Parameters CBC with differential and platelet count, serum creatinine

Dosage Forms Excipient information presented when available (limited, particularly for generics); consult specific product labeling.

Solution Reconstituted, Intravenous:

Cytovene: 500 mg (1 ea)

Generic: 500 mg (1 ea)

◆ Ganciclovir for Injection (Can) *see* Ganciclovir (Systemic) *on page 828*

Ganirelix (ga ni REL ix)

Brand Names: Canada Orgalutran

Index Terms Antagon; Ganirelix Acetate

Pharmacologic Category Gonadotropin Releasing Hormone Antagonist

Use Adjunct to controlled ovarian hyperstimulation: Inhibits premature luteinizing hormone (LH) surges in women undergoing controlled ovarian hyperstimulation.

Dosing

Adult & Geriatric Adjunct to controlled ovarian hyperstimulation: SubQ: 250 mcg once daily during the mid-to-late phase after initiating follicle-stimulating hormone on day 2 or 3 of cycle. Treatment should be continued daily until the day of chorionic gonadotropin administration.

Renal Impairment There are no dosage adjustments provided in the manufacturer's labeling (has not been studied).

Hepatic Impairment There are no dosage adjustments provided in the manufacturer's labeling (has not been studied).

Additional Information Complete prescribing information should be consulted for additional detail.

Dosage Forms Excipient information presented when available (limited, particularly for generics); consult specific product labeling.

Solution, Subcutaneous, as acetate:

Generic: 250 mcg/0.5 mL (0.5 mL)

◆ Ganirelix Acetate *see* Ganirelix *on page 829*

◆ GAR-936 *see* Tigecycline *on page 1789*

◆ Garamycin *see* Gentamicin (Ophthalmic) *on page 840*

◆ Garamycin® (Can) *see* Gentamicin (Ophthalmic) *on page 840*

◆ Gardasil *see* Papillomavirus (Types 6, 11, 16, 18) Vaccine (Human, Recombinant) *on page 1394*

◆ Gardasil 9 *see* Papillomavirus (9-Valent) Vaccine (Human, Recombinant) *on page 1393*

Gatifloxacin (gat i FLOKS a sin)

Brand Names: US Zymaxid

Brand Names: Canada Zymar

Pharmacologic Category Antibiotic, Fluoroquinolone; Antibiotic, Ophthalmic

Use Treatment of bacterial conjunctivitis

Dosing

Adult & Geriatric Bacterial conjunctivitis: Ophthalmic:

Zymar [Canadian product]:

Days 1 and 2: Instill 1 drop into affected eye(s) every 2 hours while awake (maximum: 8 times/day)

Days 3-7: Instill 1 drop into affected eye(s) 4 times/day while awake

Zymaxid:

Day 1: Instill 1 drop into affected eye(s) every 2 hours while awake (maximum: 8 times/day)

Days 2-7: Instill 1 drop into affected eye(s) 2-4 times/day while awake

Pediatric Bacterial conjunctivitis: Children ≥1 year: Ophthalmic: Refer to adult dosing.

Renal Impairment No dosage adjustment provided in manufacturer's labeling. However, dosage adjustment unlikely due to low systemic absorption.

Hepatic Impairment No dosage adjustment provided in manufacturer's labeling. However, dosage adjustment unlikely due to low systemic absorption.

Additional Information Complete prescribing information should be consulted for additional detail.

Dosage Forms Excipient information presented when available (limited, particularly for generics); consult specific product labeling.

Solution, Ophthalmic:

Zymaxid: 0.5% (2.5 mL) [contains benzalkonium chloride, edetate disodium]

Generic: 0.5% (2.5 mL)

Dosage Forms: Canada Excipient information presented when available (limited, particularly for generics); consult specific product labeling.

Solution, ophthalmic [drops]:

Zymar: 0.3% (1 mL, 2.5 mL, 5 mL) [contains benzalkonium chloride]

◆ Gattex *see* Teduglutide *on page 1742*

◆ GaviLAX [OTC] *see* Polyethylene Glycol 3350 *on page 1465*

◆ GaviLyte-C *see* Polyethylene Glycol-Electrolyte Solution *on page 1466*

◆ GaviLyte-G *see* Polyethylene Glycol-Electrolyte Solution *on page 1466*

◆ GaviLyte-N *see* Polyethylene Glycol-Electrolyte Solution *on page 1466*

◆ Gaviscon Extra Strength [OTC] *see* Aluminum Hydroxide and Magnesium Carbonate *on page 84*

◆ Gaviscon Liquid [OTC] *see* Aluminum Hydroxide and Magnesium Carbonate *on page 84*

◆ Gaviscon Tablet [OTC] *see* Aluminum Hydroxide and Magnesium Trisilicate *on page 85*

Gefitinib (ge FI tye nib)

Brand Names: US Iressa
Brand Names: Canada IRESSA
Index Terms ZD1839
Pharmacologic Category Antineoplastic Agent, Epidermal Growth Factor Receptor (EGFR) Inhibitor; Antineoplastic Agent, Tyrosine Kinase Inhibitor

Use

Non-small cell lung cancer:

US labeling: First-line treatment of metastatic non-small cell lung cancer (NSCLC) in tumors with epidermal growth factor receptor (EGFR) exon 19 deletions or exon 21 (L858R) substitution mutations as detected by an approved test.

Limitation of use: Safety and efficacy have not been established in patients with metastatic NSCLC whose tumors have EGFR mutations other than exon 19 deletions or exon 21 (L858R) substitution mutations

Canadian labeling: First-line treatment of locally advanced (nonresponsive to curative therapy) or metastatic NSCLC with activating mutations of the epidermal growth factor receptor tyrosine kinase (EGFR-TK).

Pregnancy Considerations Adverse events have been observed in animal reproduction studies. Gefitinib may cause fetal harm when administered to a pregnant woman. Women of reproductive potential should use effective contraception during and for at least 2 weeks following gefitinib treatment.

Breast-Feeding Considerations It is not known if gefitinib is excreted in breast milk. Due to the potential for serious adverse reactions in the nursing infant, breast-feeding is not recommended by the manufacturer.

Contraindications

There are no contraindications listed in the manufacturer's US labeling.

Canadian labeling: Hypersensitivity to gefitinib or any component of the formulation.

Warnings/Precautions Hazardous agent - use appropriate precautions for handling and disposal (meets NIOSH 2014 criteria).

Interstitial lung disease (ILD) or ILD-like reactions (eg, acute respiratory distress syndrome, lung infiltration, pneumonitis, or pulmonary fibrosis) have occurred (rarely) with gefitinib; some cases were grade 3 or higher and some were fatal. Withhold gefitinib and promptly assess any patient with worsening respiratory symptoms (dyspnea, cough and fever); discontinue permanently if ILD is confirmed. Increased systemic gefitinib exposure is associated with an increased incidence of ILD. An increase in mortality was observed in patients with the following risk factors: Smoking, CT scan evidence of reduced normal lung (≤50%), preexisting ILD, increased age (≥65 years), and extensive areas adherent to pleura (≥50%).

Increases in ALT, AST, and bilirubin, including grade 3 or higher toxicity have been observed. Fatal hepatotoxicity has occurred rarely. Monitor liver functions tests periodically. Withhold gefitinib in patients with worsening liver function; discontinue for severe hepatic impairment. Gefitinib exposure is increased in patients with mild, moderate, and severe hepatic impairment due to cirrhosis. However, in a study of patients with liver metastases, patients with metastases and moderate impairment had similar systemic exposure as patients with metastases and normal hepatic function. Monitor for adverse reactions if administering to patients with moderate or severe hepatic impairment.

Gastrointestinal perforation has occurred (rarely); discontinue permanently if gastrointestinal perforation develops. Nausea, vomiting, decreased appetite, and stomatitis have also been reported. Diarrhea occurs in approximately one-third of patients; grade 3 or 4 diarrhea has been observed. Diarrhea symptoms should be managed as clinically indicated; avoid dehydration. Withhold gefitinib for severe or persistent (up to 14 days) diarrhea.

Ocular disorders, including keratitis, corneal erosion, abnormal eyelash growth, conjunctivitis, blepharitis, and dry eye have been reported; some events were grade 3. Recent corneal surgery and contact lens wearing may be risk factors for ocular toxicity. Advise patients to promptly report developing eye symptoms and promptly refer for ophthalmic evaluation if signs of keratitis (eg, acute or worsening of eye inflammation, lacrimation, blurred vision, pain, red eye, and/or light sensitivity). Interrupt gefitinib treatment or discontinue for severe or worsening ocular disorders. Skin reactions occurred in nearly one-half of patients taking gefitinib. Bullous skin disorders, including toxic epidermal necrolysis, Stevens Johnson syndrome, erythema multiforme, and dermatitis bullous have been reported. Interrupt gefitinib treatment or discontinue for development of severe bullous, blistering, or exfoliating dermatologic conditions.

Establish EGFR mutation status prior to treatment. Do not use in patients with EGFR mutation-negative tumors. Studies have demonstrated a subset of patients who are more likely to respond to gefitinib treatment. This subset includes patients of Asian origin, never-smokers, women, patients with bronchoalveolar adenocarcinoma, and patients with EGFR-mutated tumors. Deletion in exon 19 and mutation in exon 21 are the two most commonly found EGFR mutations; both mutations correlate with clinical response, resulting in increased response rates in patients with the mutation (Riely, 2006). Studies have compared gefitinib in treatment naïve patients to combination chemotherapy in the subsets of patients described above, resulting in a longer progression free survival in the gefitinib arm (Mok, 2009). Based on these data, the ASCO guidelines state that the first-line use of gefitinib may be recommended in stage IV disease with activating EGFR mutations (Azzoli, 2009; Azzoli, 2011). In patients with a KRAS mutation, however, EGFR-TKI therapy is not recommended.

Systemic exposure of gefitinib may be increased in CYP2D6 poor metabolizers; no dosage adjustment is recommended, although patients should be monitored closely for adverse reactions. Potentially significant drug-drug interactions may exist, requiring dose or frequency adjustment, additional monitoring, and/or selection of alternative therapy. Elevated gastric pH may reduce gefitinib plasma concentrations; if possible, avoid concomitant use with proton pump inhibitors. If proton pump inhibitor therapy is necessary, administer gefitinib 12 hours before or 12 hours after the proton pump inhibitor dose. May administer gefitinib 6 hours before or 6 hours after H$_2$-receptor antagonists or antacids. May contain lactose; consider intolerance risk in patients with galactose intolerance, Lapp lactase deficiency, or glucose-galactose malabsorption.

Adverse Reactions

>10%:

Central nervous system: Insomnia (15%), fatigue (14%)

Dermatologic: Dermatological reaction (58%; including pustular rash, itching, dry skin, skin fissures on an erythematous base), skin rash (52%), xeroderma (24%), pruritus (18%), paronychia (14%), acne vulgaris (11%), alopecia (5% to 11%)

Gastrointestinal: Diarrhea (35% to 47%), anorexia (19% to 20%), nausea (17% to 18%), vomiting (13% to 14%), stomatitis (11% to 13%), constipation (12%)

Hepatic: Increased serum ALT (11%)

Neuromuscular & skeletal: Weakness (18%)

1% to 10%:

Central nervous system: Hypoesthesia (4%), peripheral sensory neuropathy (4%), peripheral neuropathy (2%)

Dermatologic: Nail disease (8%), acneiform eruption (6%)

Endocrine & metabolic: Dehydration (2%; secondary to diarrhea, nausea, vomiting, or anorexia)

Gastrointestinal: Xerostomia (2%)

Genitourinary: Proteinuria (8%), cystitis (1%)

Hematologic & oncologic: Anemia (7%), pulmonary hemorrhage (4% to 5%), hemorrhage (4%; including epistaxis, hematuria), neutropenia (3%), leukopenia (2%), thrombocytopenia (1%)

Hepatic: Increased serum AST (8% to 9%), increased serum bilirubin (3%)

Neuromuscular & skeletal: Myalgia (8%), arthralgia (6%)

Ophthalmic: Eye disease (7%; including conjunctivitis, blepharitis, and dry eye)

Renal: Increased serum creatinine (2%)

Respiratory: Cough (9%), interstitial pulmonary disease (grades 3/4: 1% to 3%)

Miscellaneous: Fever (9%)

<1% (Limited to important or life-threatening): Corneal erosion (reversible; may be associated with aberrant eyelash growth), erythema multiforme, gastrointestinal perforation, hemorrhagic cystitis, hepatic failure, hepatitis, hypersensitivity angiitis, hypersensitivity reaction, keratitis, keratoconjunctivitis sicca, pancreatitis, renal failure, Stevens-Johnson syndrome

Drug Interactions

Metabolism/Transport Effects Substrate of BCRP, CYP2D6 (major), CYP3A4 (major); **Note:** Assignment of Major/Minor substrate status based on clinically relevant drug interaction potential; **Inhibits** BCRP, CYP2C19 (weak), CYP2D6 (weak)

Avoid Concomitant Use

Avoid concomitant use of Gefitinib with any of the following: Conivaptan; Fusidic Acid (Systemic); Idelalisib; PAZOPanib

Increased Effect/Toxicity

Gefitinib may increase the levels/effects of: ARIPiprazole; PAZOPanib; Topotecan; Vinorelbine; Vitamin K Antagonists

The levels/effects of Gefitinib may be increased by: Abiraterone Acetate; Aprepitant; Ceritinib; Cobicistat; Conivaptan; CYP2D6 Inhibitors (Moderate); CYP2D6 Inhibitors (Strong); CYP3A4 Inhibitors (Moderate); CYP3A4 Inhibitors (Strong); Darunavir; Dasatinib; Eltrombopag; Fosaprepitant; Fusidic Acid (Systemic); Idelalisib; Ivacaftor; Luliconazole; Mifepristone; Netupitant; Osimertinib; Palbociclib; Panobinostat; Peginterferon Alfa-2b; Rolapitant; Simeprevir; Stiripentol; Teriflunomide

Decreased Effect

The levels/effects of Gefitinib may be decreased by: Antacids; Bosentan; CYP3A4 Inducers (Moderate); CYP3A4 Inducers (Strong); Dabrafenib; Deferasirox; Enzalutamide; H2-Antagonists; Mitotane; Osimertinib; Peginterferon Alfa-2b; Proton Pump Inhibitors; Siltuximab; St Johns Wort; Tocilizumab

Food Interactions Grapefruit juice may increase serum gefitinib concentrations. Management: Avoid concurrent use.

Storage/Stability Store at 20°C to 25°C (68°F to 77°F).

Mechanism of Action Gefitinib is a tyrosine kinase inhibitor (TKI) which reversibly inhibits kinase activity of wildtype and select activation mutations of epidermal growth factor receptor (EGFR). EGFR is expressed on cell surfaces of normal and cancer cells and has a role in cell growth and proliferation. Gefitinib prevents autophosphorylation of tyrosine residues associated with the EGFR receptor, which blocks downstream signaling and EGFR-dependent proliferation. Gefitinib has a higher binding affinity for EGFR exon 19 deletion and exon 21 (L858R) substitution mutation than for wild-type EGFR.

Pharmacodynamics/Kinetics

Absorption: Oral: Slow

Distribution: 1400 L

Protein binding: 90%, albumin and alpha$_1$-acid glycoprotein

Metabolism: Hepatic (extensive), primarily via CYP3A4, as well as CYP2D6; forms metabolites

Bioavailability: 60%

Half-life elimination: Oral: 41 hours

Time to peak, plasma: Oral: 3 to 7 hours

Excretion: Feces (86%); urine (<4%)

Dosing

Adult & Geriatric

Non-small cell lung cancer (NSCLC), metastatic, with EGFR exon 19 deletions or exon 21 (L858R) substitution mutations: Oral: 250 mg once daily until disease progression or unacceptable toxicity.

NSCLC, locally advanced or metastatic with EGFR mutations (Canadian labeling): Oral: 250 mg once daily.

Missed doses: Do not take a missed dose if it is within 12 hours of the next scheduled dose.

Dosage adjustment for concomitant therapy (US labeling): Strong CYP3A4 inducers (eg, phenytoin, rifampin, or tricyclic antidepressants): Increase gefitinib to 500 mg once daily (in the absence of severe adverse drug reactions); reduce gefitinib dose back to 250 mg once daily 7 days after discontinuing the strong CYP3A4 inducer.

Pediatric Non-small cell lung cancer (NSCLC), locally advanced or metastatic with EGFR mutations (Canadian labeling): Adolescents ≥17 years: Oral: Refer to Canadian adult dosing.

Renal Impairment

US labeling: There are no dosage adjustments provided in the manufacturer's labeling; however, due to minimal renal excretion (<4% of gefitinib and metabolites) the need for dosage adjustment is unlikely. Use has not been studied in patients with CrCl ≤20 mL/minute.

Canadian labeling: No dosage adjustment necessary. Use caution in severe impairment (CrCl ≤20 mL/minute).

Hepatic Impairment

Dosage adjustment for hepatic impairment at treatment initiation:

US labeling: There are no dosage adjustments provided in the manufacturer's labeling; systemic exposure is increased in hepatic impairment.

Canadian labeling: No dosage adjustment necessary. Use caution in moderate to severe impairment (Child-Pugh Class B or C) (systemic exposure may be increased); monitor closely.

Dosage adjustment for hepatotoxicity during treatment:

ALT and/or AST elevations (grade 2 or higher): Withhold treatment for up to 14 days; may resume treatment when fully resolved or improved to grade 1.

Severe hepatic impairment: Permanently discontinue.

Adjustment for Toxicity

Dermatologic toxicity:

Skin reactions (grade 3 or higher): Withhold treatment for up to 14 days; may resume treatment when fully resolved or improved to grade 1. Canadian labeling: Discontinue if unable to tolerate rechallenge following treatment interruption.

Severe bullous, blistering or exfoliating dermatologic conditions: Interrupt or discontinue treatment.

Gastrointestinal toxicity:

Diarrhea (grade 3 or higher): Withhold treatment for up to 14 days; may resume treatment when fully resolved or improved to grade 1. Canadian labeling: Discontinue if unable to tolerate rechallenge following treatment interruption.

Gastrointestinal perforation: Permanently discontinue.

Ocular toxicity:

Signs/symptoms of severe or worsening disorders, including keratitis: Withhold treatment for up to 14 days; may resume treatment when fully resolved or improved to grade 1. Canadian labeling: Discontinue if unable to tolerate rechallenge following treatment interruption.

Persistent ulcerative keratitis: Permanently discontinue.

Pulmonary toxicity:

Acute onset or worsening symptoms (dyspnea, cough, fever): Withhold treatment for up to 14 days; may resume treatment when fully resolved or improved to grade 1.

Interstitial lung disease (ILD), confirmed: Permanently discontinue.

Administration Oral: Administer with or without food.

For patients unable to swallow the tablet whole, place tablet in 120 to 240 mL water and stir for ~15 minutes; immediately drink the liquid or administer through a nasogastric tube. Rinse the container with 120 to 240 mL water and immediately drink or administer through naso-gastric tube.

Hazardous agent; use appropriate precautions for handling and disposal (meets NIOSH 2014 criteria). When administering intact tablets, single gloves should be worn. If it is necessary to manipulate the tablets (eg, preparing an oral solution), it is recommended to double glove, wear a protective gown, and prepare in a controlled device (NIOSH, 2014).

Monitoring Parameters EGFR mutation status (prior to treatment initiation); liver function tests (ALT, AST, bilirubin at baseline and periodically thereafter); BUN, creatinine, and electrolytes (baseline and periodically thereafter); INR or prothrombin time (with concurrent warfarin treatment). Monitor for signs/symptoms of dermatologic toxicity, gastrointestinal perforation, ocular toxicity, and pulmonary toxicity; monitor closely for adverse reactions in CYP2D6 poor metabolizers and patients with hepatic impairment.

Dosage Forms Excipient information presented when available (limited, particularly for generics); consult specific product labeling.
Tablet, Oral:
Iressa: 250 mg
Dosage Forms: Canada Excipient information presented when available (limited, particularly for generics); consult specific product labeling.
Tablet, oral:
Iressa: 250 mg
Extemporaneous Preparations
Hazardous agent: Use appropriate precautions for handling and disposal (meets NIOSH 2014 criteria). When manipulating tablets, NIOSH recommends double gloving, a protective gown, and preparation in a controlled device; if not prepared in a controlled device, respiratory and eye protection as well as ventilated engineering controls are recommended (NIOSH 2014).
For patients unable to swallow the tablet whole, place tablet in 120 to 240 ml water and stir for ~15 minutes; immediately drink the liquid or administer through a nasogastric tube. Rinse the container with 120 to 240 mL water and immediately drink or administer through naso-gastric tube.
Iressa (gefitinib) [prescribing information]. Wilmington, DE: AstraZeneca; July 2015.

♦ Gel-Kam [OTC] see Fluoride on page 782
♦ Gel-Kam Rinse see Fluoride on page 782
♦ Gelnique see Oxybutynin on page 1355
♦ Gel-One see Hyaluronate and Derivatives on page 879
♦ Gelucast® see Zinc Gelatin on page 1929
♦ Gelusil [OTC] see Aluminum Hydroxide, Magnesium Hydroxide, and Simethicone on page 85
♦ Gelusil (Can) see Aluminum Hydroxide, Magnesium Hydroxide, and Simethicone on page 85
♦ Gelusil Extra Strength (Can) see Aluminum Hydroxide and Magnesium Hydroxide on page 85

Gemcitabine (jem SITE a been)

Brand Names: US Gemzar
Brand Names: Canada Gemcitabine For Injection; Gemcitabine For Injection Concentrate; Gemcitabine For Injection, USP; Gemcitabine Hydrochloride For Injection; Gemcitabine Injection; Gemcitabine Sun For Injection; Gemzar
Index Terms dFdC; dFdCyd; Difluorodeoxycytidine Hydrochlorothiazide; Gemcitabine Hydrochloride; LY-188011
Pharmacologic Category Antineoplastic Agent, Antimetabolite; Antineoplastic Agent, Antimetabolite (Pyrimidine Analog)
Use
Breast cancer: First-line treatment of metastatic breast cancer (in combination with paclitaxel) after failure of adjuvant chemotherapy which contained an anthracycline (unless contraindicated)
Non-small cell lung cancer (NSCLC): First-line treatment of inoperable, locally-advanced (stage IIIA or IIIB) or metastatic (stage IV) NSCLC (in combination with cisplatin)
Ovarian cancer: Treatment of advanced ovarian cancer (in combination with carboplatin) that has relapsed at least 6 months following completion of platinum-based chemotherapy
Pancreatic cancer: First-line treatment of locally-advanced (nonresectable stage II or III) or metastatic (stage IV) pancreatic adenocarcinoma
Pregnancy Considerations Adverse events were observed in animal reproduction studies. May cause fetal harm if administered during pregnancy; adverse effects in reproduction are anticipated based on the mechanism of action.
Breast-Feeding Considerations It is not known if gemcitabine is excreted in breast milk. Due to the potential for serious adverse reactions in the nursing infant, the decision to discontinue gemcitabine or to discontinue breast-feeding should take into account the benefits of treatment to the mother.
Contraindications Hypersensitivity to gemcitabine or any component of the formulation
Warnings/Precautions Hazardous agent - use appropriate precautions for handling and disposal (NIOSH 2014 [group 1]). Gemcitabine may suppress bone marrow function (neutropenia, thrombocytopenia, and anemia); myelosuppression is usually the dose-limiting toxicity; toxicity is increased when used in combination with other chemotherapy; monitor blood counts; dosage adjustments are frequently required.

Hemolytic uremic syndrome (HUS) has been reported; may lead to renal failure and dialysis (including fatalities); monitor for evidence of anemia with microangiopathic hemolysis (elevation of bilirubin or LDH, reticulocytosis, severe thrombocytopenia, and/or renal failure) and monitor renal function at baseline and periodically during treatment. Permanently discontinue if HUS or severe renal impairment occurs; renal failure may not be reversible despite discontinuation. Serious hepatotoxicity (including liver failure and death) has been reported (when used alone or in combination with other hepatotoxic medications); use in patients with hepatic impairment (history of cirrhosis, hepatitis, or alcoholism) or in patients with hepatic metastases may lead to exacerbation of hepatic impairment. Monitor hepatic function at baseline and periodically during treatment; consider dose adjustments with elevated bilirubin; discontinue if severe liver injury develops. Capillary leak syndrome (CLS) with serious consequences has been reported, both with single-agent gemcitabine and with combination chemotherapy; discontinue if CLS develops.

Pulmonary toxicity, including adult respiratory distress syndrome, interstitial pneumonitis, pulmonary edema, and pulmonary fibrosis, has been observed; may lead to respiratory failure (some fatal) despite discontinuation. Onset for symptoms of pulmonary toxicity may be delayed up to 2 weeks beyond the last dose. Discontinue for unexplained dyspnea (with or without bronchospasm) or other evidence or pulmonary toxicity. Posterior reversible encephalopathy syndrome (PRES) has been reported, both with single-agent therapy and with combination chemotherapy. PRES may manifest with blindness, confusion, headache, hypertension, lethargy, seizure, and other visual and neurologic disturbances. If PRES diagnosis is confirmed (by MRI), discontinue therapy. Not indicated for use with concurrent radiation therapy; radiation toxicity, including tissue injury, severe mucositis, esophagitis, or pneumonitis, has been reported with concurrent and nonconcurrent administration; may have radiosensitizing activity when gemcitabine and radiation therapy are given ≤7 days apart; radiation recall may occur when gemcitabine and radiation therapy are given >7 days apart. Potentially significant drug-drug interactions may exist, requiring dose or frequency adjustment, additional monitoring, and/or selection of alternative therapy.

Prolongation of the infusion duration >60 minutes or more frequent than weekly dosing have been shown to alter the half-life and increase toxicity (hypotension, flu-like symptoms, myelosuppression, weakness); a fixed-dose rate (FDR) infusion rate of 10 mg/m^2/minute has been studied in adults in order to optimize the pharmacokinetics (off-label); prolonged infusion times increase the intracellular accumulation of the active metabolite, gemcitabine triphosphate (Ko, 2006; Tempero, 2003); patients who receive gemcitabine FDR experience more grade 3/4 hematologic toxicity (Ko, 2006; Poplin, 2009).

Adverse Reactions Frequency of adverse reactions reported for single-agent use of gemcitabine only; bone marrow depression is the dose-limiting toxicity.
>10%:
Cardiovascular: Peripheral edema (20%), edema (13%)
Central nervous system: Drowsiness (11%)
Dermatologic: Skin rash (30%), alopecia (15%)
Gastrointestinal: Nausea and vomiting (69%), diarrhea (19%), stomatitis (11%)
Genitourinary: Proteinuria (45%), hematuria (35%)
Hematologic & oncologic: Anemia (68%; grade 3: 7%; grade 4: 1%), neutropenia (63%; grade 3: 19%; grade 4: 6%), thrombocytopenia (24%; grade 3: 4%; grade 4: 1%), hemorrhage (17%; grade 3: <1%; grade 4: <1%)
Hepatic: Increased serum ALT (68%; grade 3: 8%, grade 4: 2%), increased serum AST (67%; grade 3: 6%; grade 4: 2%), increased serum alkaline phosphatase (55%; grade 3: 7%; grade 4: 2%), increased serum bilirubin (13%; grade 3: 2%, grade 4: <1%)
Infection: Infection (16%)
Renal: Increased blood urea nitrogen (16%)
Respiratory: Dyspnea (23%; grade 3: 3%; grade 4: <1%), flu-like symptoms (19%)
Miscellaneous: Fever (41%)
1% to 10%:
Central nervous system: Paresthesia (10%; grade 3: <1%)
Local: Injection site reaction (4%)
Renal: Increased serum creatinine (8%)
Respiratory: Bronchospasm (<2%)
<1% (Limited to important or life-threatening; reported with single-agent use or with combination therapy): Adult respiratory distress syndrome, anaphylactoid reaction, anorexia, arthralgia, bullous skin disease, capillary leak syndrome, cardiac arrhythmia, cardiac failure, cellulitis,

cerebrovascular accident (Kuenen, 2002), constipation, desquamation, digital vasculitis, gangrene of skin or other tissue, hemolytic-uremic syndrome, hepatic failure, hepatic veno-occlusive disease, hepatotoxicity (rare), hyperglycemia, hypertension, hypocalcemia, hypotension, increased gamma-glutamyl transferase, interstitial pneumonitis, myocardial infarction, neuropathy, petechiae (Zupancic, 2007; Nishijima 2013), pruritus (Curtis, 2014), pulmonary edema, pulmonary fibrosis, radiation recall phenomenon, renal failure, respiratory failure, reversible posterior leukoencephalopathy syndrome, sepsis, supraventricular cardiac arrhythmia, thrombotic thrombocytopenic purpura (Zupancic, 2007; Nishijima, 2013)

Drug Interactions

Metabolism/Transport Effects None known.

Avoid Concomitant Use

Avoid concomitant use of Gemcitabine with any of the following: BCG (Intravesical); Deferiprone; Dipyrone; Natalizumab; Pimecrolimus; Tacrolimus (Topical); Tofacitinib; Vaccines (Live)

Increased Effect/Toxicity

Gemcitabine may increase the levels/effects of: Bleomycin; CloZAPine; Deferiprone; Fingolimod; Fluorouracil (Systemic); Fluorouracil (Topical); Leflunomide; Natalizumab; Tofacitinib; Vaccines (Live); Warfarin

The levels/effects of Gemcitabine may be increased by: Denosumab; Dipyrone; Pimecrolimus; Roflumilast; Tacrolimus (Topical); Trastuzumab

Decreased Effect

Gemcitabine may decrease the levels/effects of: BCG (Intravesical); Coccidioides immitis Skin Test; Sipuleucel-T; Vaccines (Inactivated); Vaccines (Live)

The levels/effects of Gemcitabine may be decreased by: Echinacea

Preparation for Administration

Hazardous agent; use appropriate precautions for handling and disposal (NIOSH 2014 [group 1]).

Reconstitute lyophilized powder with preservative free NS; add 5 mL to the 200 mg vial, add 25 mL to the 1000 mg vial, or add 50 mL to the 2000 mg vial, resulting in a reconstituted concentration of 38 mg/mL (solutions must be reconstituted to ≤40 mg/mL to completely dissolve). Gemcitabine is also supplied as a concentrated solution for injection in different concentrations (40 mg/mL [Canada only] and 38 mg/mL); verify product concentration prior to preparation for administration.

Further dilute reconstituted lyophilized powder or concentrated solution for injection in NS for infusion; to concentrations as low as 0.1 mg/mL.

Storage/Stability

Lyophilized powder: Store intact vials at room temperature of 20°C to 25°C (68°F to 77°F); excursions permitted to 15°C to 30°C (59°F to 86°F). Reconstituted vials are stable for 24 hours at room temperature. Do not refrigerate (may form crystals).

Solution for injection: Store intact vials refrigerated at 2°C to 8°C (36°F to 46°F); do not freeze.

Solutions diluted for infusion in NS are stable for 24 hours at room temperature. Do not refrigerate.

Mechanism of Action A pyrimidine antimetabolite that inhibits DNA synthesis by inhibition of DNA polymerase and ribonucleotide reductase, cell cycle-specific for the S-phase of the cycle (also blocks cellular progression at G1/S-phase). Gemcitabine is phosphorylated intracellularly by deoxycytidine kinase to gemcitabine monophosphate, which is further phosphorylated to active metabolites gemcitabine diphosphate and gemcitabine triphosphate. Gemcitabine diphosphate inhibits DNA synthesis by inhibiting ribonucleotide reductase; gemcitabine triphosphate incorporates into DNA and inhibits DNA polymerase.

Pharmacodynamics/Kinetics

Distribution: Widely distributed into tissues; present in ascitic fluid; V_d: Infusions <70 minutes: 50 L/m^2; Long infusion times (70-285 minutes): 370 L/m^2

Protein binding: Negligible

Metabolism: Metabolized intracellularly by nucleoside kinases to the active diphosphate (dFdCDP) and triphosphate (dFdCTP) nucleoside metabolites

Half-life elimination:

Gemcitabine: Infusion time ≤70 minutes: 42 to 94 minutes; infusion time 3 to 4 hours: 4 to 10.5 hours (affected by age and gender)

Metabolite (gemcitabine triphosphate), terminal phase: 1.7 to 19.4 hours

Time to peak, plasma: 30 minutes after completion of infusion

Excretion: Urine (92% to 98%; primarily as inactive uracil metabolite); feces (<1%)

Dosing

Adult & Geriatric Note: Prolongation of the infusion duration >60 minutes and administration more frequently than once weekly have been shown to increase toxicity.

Breast cancer, metastatic: IV: 1250 mg/m^2 over 30 minutes days 1 and 8; repeat cycle every 21 days (in combination with paclitaxel) **or** (off-label dosing; as a single agent) 800 mg/m^2 over 30 minutes days 1, 8, and 15 of a 28-day treatment cycle (Carmichael, 1995)

Non-small cell lung cancer, locally advanced or metastatic: IV: 1000 mg/m^2 over 30 minutes days 1, 8, and 15; repeat cycle every 28 days (in combination with cisplatin) **or** 1250 mg/m^2 over 30 minutes days 1 and 8; repeat cycle every 21 days (in combination with cisplatin) **or** (off-label dosing/combination) 1000 mg/m^2 over 30 minutes days 1 and 8; repeat cycle every 21 days (in combination with carboplatin) for up to 4 cycles (Grønberg, 2009) **or** (off-label combination) 1000 mg/m^2 over 30 minutes days 1, 8, and 15; repeat cycle every 28 days (in combination with carboplatin) for up to 4 cycles (Danson, 2003) **or** (off-label combination) 1000 mg/m^2 over 30 minutes days 1 and 8; repeat cycle every 21 days (in combination with docetaxel) for 8 cycles (Pujol, 2005) **or** (off-label combination) 1000 mg/m^2 days 1, 8, and 15; repeat cycle every 28 days (in combination with vinorelbine) for 6 cycles (Greco, 2007)

Ovarian cancer, advanced: IV: 1000 mg/m^2 over 30 minutes days 1 and 8; repeat cycle every 21 days (in combination with carboplatin) **or** (off-label dosing; as a single agent) 1000 mg/m^2 over 30-60 minutes days 1 and 8; repeat cycle every 21 days (Mutch, 2007)

Pancreatic cancer, locally advanced or metastatic: IV: Initial: 1000 mg/m^2 over 30 minutes once weekly for 7 weeks followed by 1 week rest; then once weekly for 3 weeks out of every 4 weeks **or** (off-label combinations) 1000 mg/m^2 over 30 minutes weekly for up to 7 weeks followed by 1 week rest; then weekly for 3 weeks out of every 4 weeks (in combination with erlotinib) (Moore, 2007) **or** 1000 mg/m^2 over 30 minutes days 1, 8, and 15 every 28 days (in combination with capecitabine) (Cunningham, 2009) **or** 1000 mg/m^2 over 30 minutes days 1 and 15 every 28 days (in combination with cisplatin) (Heinemann, 2006) **or** 1000 mg/m^2 infused at 10 mg/m^2/minute every 14 days (in combination with oxaliplatin) (Louvet, 2005) **or** 1000 mg/m^2 days 1, 8, and 15 every 28 days (in combination with paclitaxel [protein bound]) (Von Hoff, 2013)

Bladder cancer (off-label use):

Advanced or metastatic: IV: 1000 mg/m^2 over 30-60 minutes days 1, 8, and 15; repeat cycle every 28 days (in combination with cisplatin) (von der Maase, 2000) **or** 1000 mg/m^2 over 30 minutes days 1 and 8; repeat cycle every 21 days (in combination with carboplatin) until disease progression or unacceptable toxicity (De Santis, 2012)

Transitional cell carcinoma: Intravesicular instillation: 2000 mg (in 100 mL NS; retain for 1 hour) twice weekly for 3 weeks; repeat cycle every 4 weeks for at least 2 cycles (Dalbagni, 2006)

Cervical cancer, recurrent or persistent (off-label use): IV: 1000 mg/m^2 days 1 and 8; repeat cycle every 21 days (in combination with cisplatin) (Monk, 2009) **or** 1250 mg/m^2 over 30 minutes days 1 and 8; repeat cycle every 21 days (in combination with cisplatin) (Burnett, 2000) **or** 800 mg/m^2 over 30 minutes days 1, 8, and 15; repeat cycle every 28 days (as a single-agent) (Schilder, 2005) **or** 800 mg/m^2 days 1 and 8; repeat cycle every 28 days (in combination with cisplatin) (Brewer, 2006)

Head and neck cancer, nasopharyngeal (off-label use): IV: 1000 mg/m^2 over 30 minutes days 1, 8, and 15 every 28 days (Zhang, 2008) **or** 1000 mg/m^2 over 30 minutes days 1 and 8 every 21 days (in combination with vinorelbine) (Chen, 2012)

Hepatobiliary cancer, advanced (off-label use): IV: 1000 mg/m^2 over 30 minutes days 1 and 8; repeat cycle every 21 days (in combination with cisplatin) (Valle, 2010) **or** 1000 mg/m^2 over 30 minutes days 1 and 8; repeat cycle every 21 days (in combination with capecitabine) (Knox, 2005) **or** 1000 mg/m^2 infused at 10 mg/m^2/minute every 2 weeks (in combination with oxaliplatin) (Andre, 2004)

Hodgkin lymphoma, relapsed (off-label use): IV: 1000 mg/m^2 (800 mg/m^2 for post-transplant patients) over 30 minutes days 1 and 8; repeat cycle every 21 days (in combination with vinorelbine and doxorubicin liposomal) (Bartlett, 2007) **or** 800 mg/m^2 days 1 and 4; repeat cycle every 21 days (in combination with ifosfamide, mesna, vinorelbine, and prednisolone) (Santoro, 2007)

◄ **Malignant pleural mesothelioma (off-label use; in combination with cisplatin):** IV: 1000 mg/m² over 30 minutes days 1, 8 and 15 every 28 days for up to 6 cycles (Nowak, 2002) **or** 1250 mg/m² over 30 minutes days 1 and 8 every 21 days for up to 6 cycles (van Haarst, 2002)

Non-Hodgkin lymphoma, refractory (off-label use): IV: 1000 mg/m² over 30 minutes days 1 and 8; repeat cycle every 21 days (in combination with cisplatin and dexamethasone) (Crump, 2004) **or** 1000 mg/m² every 15-21 days (in combination with oxaliplatin and rituximab) (Lopez, 2008)

Sarcoma (off-label uses): IV:

Ewing's sarcoma, refractory: 675 mg/m² over 90 minutes days 1 and 8; repeat cycle every 21 days (in combination with docetaxel) (Navid, 2008)

Osteosarcoma, refractory: 675 mg/m² over 90 minutes days 1 and 8; repeat cycle every 21 days (in combination with docetaxel) (Navid, 2008) **or** 1000 mg/m² weekly for 7 weeks followed by 1 week rest; then weekly for 3 weeks out of every 4 weeks (Merimsky, 2000)

Soft tissue sarcoma, advanced: 800 mg/m² over 90 minutes days 1 and 8; repeat cycle every 21 days (in combination with vinorelbine) (Dileo, 2007) **or** 675 mg/m² over 90 minutes days 1 and 8; repeat cycle every 21 days (in combination with docetaxel) (Leu, 2004) **or** 900 mg/m² over 90 minutes days 1 and 8; repeat cycle every 21 days (in combination with docetaxel) (Maki, 2007)

Small cell lung cancer, refractory or relapsed (off-label use): IV: 1000-1250 mg/m² over 30 minutes days 1, 8, and 15 every 28 days (as a single agent) (Masters, 2003)

Testicular cancer, refractory germ cell (off-label use): IV: 1000-1250 mg/m² over 30 minutes days 1 and 8 every 21 days (in combination with oxaliplatin) (DeGiorgi, 2006; Kohllmannsberger, 2004; Pectasides, 2004) **or** 1000 mg/m² over 30 minutes days 1, 8, and 15 every 28 days for up to 6 cycles (in combination with paclitaxel) (Hinton, 2002) **or** 800 mg/m² over 30 minutes days 1 and 8 every 21 days (in combination with oxaliplatin and paclitaxel) (Bokemeyer, 2008)

Unknown-primary, adenocarcinoma (off-label use): IV: 1250 mg/m² days 1 and 8 every 21 days (in combination with cisplatin) (Culine, 2003) **or** 1000 mg/m² over 30 minutes days 1 and 8 every 21 days for up to 6 cycles (in combination with docetaxel) (Pouessel, 2004)

Uterine cancer (off-label use): IV: 900 mg/m² over 90 minutes days 1 and 8 every 21 days (in combination with docetaxel) (Hensley, 2008) **or** 1000 mg/m² over 30 minutes days 1, 8, and 15 every 28 days (Look, 2004)

Pediatric Note: Prolongation of the infusion duration >60 minutes and administration more frequently than once weekly have been shown to increase toxicity. Refer to specific references for ages of populations studied:

Germ cell tumor, refractory (off-label use): IV: 1000 mg/m² over 30 minutes days 1, 8, and 15 every 28 days (in combination with paclitaxel) for up to 6 cycles (Hinton, 2002)

Hodgkin lymphoma, relapsed (off-label use): IV: 1000 mg/m² over 100 minutes days 1 and 8; repeat cycle every 21 days (in combination with vinorelbine) (Cole; 2009) **or** 800 mg/m² days 1 and 4; repeat cycle every 21 days (in combination with ifosfamide, mesna, vinorelbine, and prednisolone) (Santoro, 2007)

Sarcomas (off-label use): IV:

Ewing's sarcoma, refractory: 675 mg/m² over 90 minutes days 1 and 8; repeat cycle every 21 days (in combination with docetaxel) (Navid, 2008)

Osteosarcoma, refractory: 675 mg/m² over 90 minutes days 1 and 8; repeat cycle every 21 days (in combination with docetaxel) (Navid, 2008) **or** 1000 mg/m² weekly for 7 weeks followed by 1 week rest; then weekly for 3 weeks out of every 4 weeks (Merimsky, 2000)

Renal Impairment There are no dosage adjustments provided in the manufacturer's labeling; use with caution in patients with preexisting renal dysfunction. Discontinue if severe renal toxicity or hemolytic uremic syndrome (HUS) occur during gemcitabine treatment.

Mild-to-severe renal impairment: No dosage adjustment necessary (Janus, 2010; Li, 2007).

ESRD (on hemodialysis): Hemodialysis should begin 6-12 hours after gemcitabine infusion (Janus 2010; Li, 2007).

Hepatic Impairment There are no dosage adjustments provided in the manufacturer's labeling; use with caution. Discontinue if severe hepatotoxicity occurs during gemcitabine treatment. The following adjustments have been reported:

Transaminases elevated (with normal bilirubin): No dosage adjustment necessary (Venook, 2000).

Serum bilirubin >1.6 mg/dL: Use initial dose of 800 mg/m²; may escalate if tolerated (Ecklund, 2005; Floyd, 2006; Venook, 2000).

Obesity *ASCO Guidelines for appropriate chemotherapy dosing in obese adults with cancer:* Utilize patient's actual body weight (full weight) for calculation of body surface area- or weight-based dosing, particularly when the intent of therapy is curative; manage regimen-related toxicities in the same manner as for nonobese patients; if a dose reduction is utilized due to toxicity, consider resumption of full weight-based dosing with subsequent cycles, especially if cause of toxicity (eg, hepatic or renal impairment) is resolved (Griggs, 2012).

Adjustment for Toxicity

Nonhematologic toxicity (all indications):

Hold or decrease gemcitabine dose by 50% for the following: Severe (grade 3 or 4) nonhematologic toxicity until resolved (excludes nausea, vomiting, or alopecia [no dose modifications recommended])

Permanently discontinue gemcitabine for any of the following: Unexplained dyspnea (or other evidence of severe pulmonary toxicity), severe hepatotoxicity, hemolytic uremic syndrome (HUS), capillary leak syndrome (CLS), posterior reversible encephalopathy syndrome (PRES)

Hematologic toxicity:

Breast cancer:

Day 1:

Absolute granulocyte count (AGC) ≥1500/mm³ and platelet count ≥100,000/mm³: Administer 100% of full dose

AGC <1500/mm³ or platelet count <100,000/mm³: Hold dose

Day 8:

AGC ≥1200/mm³ and platelet count >75,000/mm³: Administer 100% of full dose

AGC 1000-1199/mm³ or platelet count 50,000-75,000/mm³: Administer 75% of full dose

AGC 700-999/mm³ and platelet count ≥50,000/mm³: Administer 50% of full dose

AGC <700/mm³ or platelet count <50,000/mm³: Hold dose

Non-small cell lung cancer (cisplatin dosage may also require adjustment):

AGC ≥1000/mm³ and platelet count ≥100,000/mm³: Administer 100% of full dose

AGC 500-999/mm³ or platelet count 50,000-99,999/mm³: Administer 75% of full dose

AGC <500/mm³ or platelet count <50,000/mm³: Hold dose

Ovarian cancer:

Day 1:

AGC ≥1500/mm³ and platelet count ≥100,000/mm³: Administer 100% of full dose

AGC <1500/mm³ or platelet count <100,000/mm³: Delay treatment cycle

Day 8:

AGC ≥1500/mm³ and platelet count ≥100,000/mm³: Administer 100% of full dose

AGC 1000-1499/mm³ or platelet count 75,000-99,999/mm³: Administer 50% of full dose

AGC <1000/mm³ or platelet count <75,000/mm³: Hold dose

Hematologic toxicity in previous cycle (dosing adjustment for subsequent cycles):

Initial occurrence: AGC <500/mm³ for >5 days, AGC <100/mm³ for >3 days, febrile neutropenia, platelet count <25,000/mm³, or cycle delay >1 week due to toxicity: Permanently reduce gemcitabine to 800 mg/m² on days 1 and 8.

Subsequent occurrence: AGC <500/mm³ for >5 days, AGC <100/mm³ for >3 days, neutropenic fever, platelet count <25,000/mm³, or cycle delay >1 week due to toxicity: Permanently reduce gemcitabine to 800 mg/m² and administer on day 1 only.

Pancreatic cancer:

AGC ≥1000/mm³ and platelet count ≥100,000/mm³: Administer 100% of full dose

AGC 500-999/mm³ or platelet count 50,000-99,999/mm³: Administer 75% of full dose

AGC <500/mm³ or platelet count <50,000/mm³: Hold dose

Administration Infuse over 30 minutes; for off-label uses, infusion times may vary (refer to specific references). **Note:** Prolongation of the infusion time >60 minutes has been shown to increase toxicity. Gemcitabine has been administered at a fixed-dose rate (FDR) infusion rate of 10 mg/m^2/minute to optimize the pharmacokinetics (off-label); prolonged infusion times increase the intracellular accumulation of the active metabolite, gemcitabine triphosphate (Ko, 2006; Tempero, 2003). Patients who receive gemcitabine FDR experience more grade 3/4 hematologic toxicity (Ko, 2006; Poplin, 2009).

For intravesicular (bladder) instillation (off-label route), gemcitabine was diluted in 50 to 100 mL normal saline; patients were instructed to retain in the bladder for 1 hour (Addeo, 2010; Dalbaghi, 2006)

Hazardous agent; use appropriate precautions for handling and disposal (NIOSH 2014 [group 1]).

Monitoring Parameters CBC with differential and platelet count (prior to each dose); hepatic and renal function (prior to initiation of therapy and periodically, thereafter); monitor electrolytes, including potassium, magnesium, and calcium (when in combination therapy with cisplatin); monitor pulmonary function; signs/symptoms of capillary leak syndrome and posterior reversible encephalopathy syndrome

Dosage Forms Excipient information presented when available (limited, particularly for generics); consult specific product labeling.
Solution, Intravenous:
Generic: 200 mg/5.26 mL (5.26 mL); 1 g/26.3 mL (26.3 mL); 2 g/52.6 mL (52.6 mL)
Solution Reconstituted, Intravenous:
Gemzar: 200 mg (1 ea); 1 g (1 ea)
Generic: 200 mg (1 ea); 1 g (1 ea); 2 g (1 ea)
Solution Reconstituted, Intravenous [preservative free]:
Generic: 200 mg (1 ea); 1 g (1 ea)

Dosage Forms: Canada Excipient information presented when available (limited, particularly for generics); consult specific product labeling.
Solution, Intravenous: 200 mg/5mL, 1 g/25 mL, 2 g/50 mL [40 mg/mL]
Solution, Intravenous: 200 mg/5.3 mL, 1 g/26.3 mL, 2 g/52.6 mL [38 mg/mL]
Solution Reconstituted, Intravenous: 200 mg, 1 g, 2 g

◆ Gemcitabine For Injection (Can) see Gemcitabine on page 832

◆ Gemcitabine For Injection Concentrate (Can) see Gemcitabine on page 832

◆ Gemcitabine For Injection, USP (Can) see Gemcitabine on page 832

◆ Gemcitabine Hydrochloride see Gemcitabine on page 832

◆ Gemcitabine Hydrochloride For Injection (Can) see Gemcitabine on page 832

◆ Gemcitabine Injection (Can) see Gemcitabine on page 832

◆ Gemcitabine Sun For Injection (Can) see Gemcitabine on page 832

Gemfibrozil (jem FI broe zil)

Brand Names: US Lopid
Brand Names: Canada Apo-Gemfibrozil; Dom-Gemfibrozil; Mylan-Gemfibrozil; Novo-Gemfibrozil; PHL-Gemfibrozil; PMS-Gemfibrozil; Teva-Gemfibrozil
Index Terms CI-719
Pharmacologic Category Antilipemic Agent, Fibric Acid
Use Treatment of hypertriglyceridemia in Fredrickson types IV and V hyperlipidemia for patients who are at greater risk for pancreatitis and who have not responded to dietary intervention; to reduce the risk of CHD development in Fredrickson type IIb patients without a history or symptoms of existing CHD who have not responded to dietary and other interventions (including pharmacologic treatment) and who have decreased HDL, increased LDL, and increased triglycerides
Pregnancy Considerations Adverse events have been observed in animal reproduction studies. The Canadian product labeling specifically contraindicates use during pregnancy and recommends gemfibrozil be discontinued several months prior to conception.
Breast-Feeding Considerations It is not known if gemfibrozil is excreted in breast milk. Due to the potential for serious adverse reactions in the nursing infant, a decision should be made whether to discontinue nursing or to discontinue the drug, taking into account the importance of treatment to the mother. The Canadian product labeling specifically contraindicates use during breast-feeding.

Contraindications
Hypersensitivity to gemfibrozil or any component of the formulation; hepatic or severe renal dysfunction; primary biliary cirrhosis; preexisting gallbladder disease; concurrent use with repaglinide or simvastatin.
Documentation of allergenic cross-reactivity for fibrates is limited. However, because of similarities in chemical structure and/or pharmacologic actions, the possibility of cross-sensitivity cannot be ruled out with certainty.
Warnings/Precautions Secondary causes of hyperlipidemia should be ruled out prior to therapy. Possible increased risk of malignancy and cholelithiasis. Anemia, leukopenia, thrombocytopenia, and bone marrow hypoplasia have rarely been reported. Periodic monitoring recommended during the first year of therapy. Elevations in serum transaminases can be seen. Discontinue if lipid response not seen. Be careful in patient selection; this is not a first- or second-line choice. Other agents may be more suitable. Has been associated with rare myositis or rhabdomyolysis; patients should be monitored closely. Patients should be instructed to report unexplained muscle pain, tenderness, weakness, or brown urine. Potentially significant drug-drug interactions may exist, requiring dose or frequency adjustment, additional monitoring, and/or selection of alternative therapy. Use with caution in patients with mild-to-moderate renal impairment; contraindicated in patients with severe impairment. Renal function deterioration has been seen when used in patients with a serum creatinine >2 mg/dL.
Adverse Reactions
>10%: Gastrointestinal: Dyspepsia (20%)
1% to 10%:
Cardiovascular: Atrial fibrillation (1%)
Central nervous system: Fatigue (4%), vertigo (2%)
Dermatologic: Eczema (2%), rash (2%)
Gastrointestinal: Abdominal pain (10%), nausea/vomiting (3%)
<1% or case reports with probable causation (limited to important or life-threatening): Alkaline phosphatase increased, anemia, angioedema, arthralgia, bilirubin increased, blurred vision, bone marrow hypoplasia, cholelithiasis, cholecystitis, cholestatic jaundice, creatine phosphokinase increased, depression, dermatitis, dermatomyositis/polymyositis, dizziness, eosinophilia, exfoliative dermatitis, headache, hypoesthesia, hypokalemia, impotence, laryngeal edema, leukopenia, libido decreased, myalgia, myasthenia, myopathy, nephrotoxicity, painful extremities, paresthesia, peripheral neuritis, pruritus, Raynaud's phenomenon, rhabdomyolysis, somnolence, synovitis, taste perversion, transaminases increased, urticaria
Reports where causal relationship has not been established: Alopecia, anaphylaxis, cataracts, colitis, confusion, decreased fertility (male), drug-induced lupus-like syndrome, extrasystoles, hepatoma, intracranial hemorrhage, pancreatitis, peripheral vascular disease, photosensitivity, positive ANA, renal dysfunction, retinal edema, seizure, syncope, thrombocytopenia, vasculitis, weight loss
Drug Interactions
Metabolism/Transport Effects Substrate of CYP3A4 (minor); **Note:** Assignment of Major/Minor substrate status based on clinically relevant drug interaction potential; **Inhibits** CYP1A2 (moderate), CYP2C19 (strong), CYP2C8 (strong), CYP2C9 (strong), SLCO1B1, UGT1A1
Avoid Concomitant Use
Avoid concomitant use of Gemfibrozil with any of the following: Amodiaquine; AtorvaSTATin; Bexarotene (Systemic); Ciprofibrate; Dabrafenib; Enzalutamide; Ezetimibe; Fluvastatin; Irinotecan Products; Lovastatin; Ombitasvir, Paritaprevir, Ritonavir, and Dasabuvir; Pitavastatin; Pravastatin; Repaglinide; Rosuvastatin; Selexipag; Simvastatin; TiZANidine
Increased Effect/Toxicity
Gemfibrozil may increase the levels/effects of: Agomelatine; Amodiaquine; Antidiabetic Agents (Thiazolidinedione); AtorvaSTATin; Bexarotene (Systemic); Bosentan; Carvedilol; Cilostazol; Citalopram; Colchicine; CYP1A2 Substrates; CYP2C19 Substrates; CYP2C8 Substrates; CYP2C9 Substrates; Dabrafenib; Diclofenac (Systemic); Dronabinol; Eluxadoline; Enzalutamide; Ezetimibe; Flibanserin; Fluvastatin; Irinotecan Products; Lacosamide; Lovastatin; Montelukast; Ombitasvir, Paritaprevir, Ritonavir, and Dasabuvir; Ospemifene; Parecoxib; Pioglitazone; Pirfenidone; Pitavastatin; Pravastatin; Ramelteon; Repaglinide; Rosuvastatin; Selexipag; Simvastatin; Sulfonylureas; Tetrahydrocannabinol; TiZANidine; Treprostinil; Vitamin K Antagonists

The levels/effects of Gemfibrozil may be increased by: Acipimox; Cannabis; Ciprofibrate; CycloSPORINE (Systemic); Raltegravir

Decreased Effect

Gemfibrozil may decrease the levels/effects of: Chenodiol; Clopidogrel; CycloSPORINE (Systemic); Imatinib; Ursodiol

The levels/effects of Gemfibrozil may be decreased by: Bile Acid Sequestrants

Food Interactions When given after meals, the AUC of gemfibrozil is decreased. Management: Administer 30 minutes prior to breakfast and dinner.

Storage/Stability Store at 20°C to 25°C (68°F to 77°F). Protect from light and moisture.

Mechanism of Action The exact mechanism of action of gemfibrozil is unknown, however, several theories exist regarding the VLDL effect; it can inhibit lipolysis and decrease subsequent hepatic fatty acid uptake as well as inhibit hepatic secretion of VLDL; together these actions decrease serum VLDL levels; increases HDL-cholesterol; the mechanism behind HDL elevation is currently unknown

Pharmacodynamics/Kinetics

Onset of action: May require several days

Absorption: Well absorbed

Protein binding: 99%

Metabolism: Hepatic via oxidation to two inactive metabolites; undergoes enterohepatic recycling

Half-life elimination: 1.5 hours

Time to peak, serum: 1 to 2 hours

Excretion: Urine (~70% primarily as conjugated drug); feces (6%)

Dosing

Adult & Geriatric Hyperlipidemia/hypertriglyceridemia: Oral: 600 mg twice daily 30 minutes before breakfast and dinner. **Note:** Discontinue if lipid response is inadequate after 3 months of therapy.

Renal Impairment

Manufacturer's labeling:

Mild-to-moderate impairment: There are no dosage adjustments provided in the manufacturer's labeling; use with caution; deterioration of renal function has been reported in patients with baseline serum creatinine >2 mg/dL

Severe impairment: There are no dosage adjustments provided in the manufacturer's labeling; use is contraindicated

Alternate recommendations (Aronoff, 2007):

GFR >50 mL/minute: No dosage adjustment necessary.

GFR 10 to 50 mL/minute: Administer 75% of dose.

GFR <10 mL/minute: Administer 50% of dose.

Intermittent hemodialysis: Supplemental dose not necessary.

Peritoneal dialysis: Administer 50% of dose as supplement for dialysis.

Hepatic Impairment There are no dosage adjustments provided in the manufacturer's labeling; use is contraindicated.

Dietary Considerations Before initiation of therapy, patients should be placed on a standard cholesterol-lowering diet for 3 to 6 months and the diet should be continued during drug therapy. Administer 30 minutes prior to breakfast and dinner

Administration Administer 30 minutes prior to breakfast and dinner.

Monitoring Parameters Serum cholesterol, LFTs periodically, CBC periodically (first year)

Dosage Forms Excipient information presented when available (limited, particularly for generics); consult specific product labeling.

Tablet, Oral:

Lopid: 600 mg [scored]

Generic: 600 mg

Dosage Forms: Canada Refer also to Dosage Forms. Excipient information presented when available (limited, particularly for generics); consult specific product labeling.

Capsule, Oral: 300 mg

Gemifloxacin (je mi FLOKS a sin)

Brand Names: US Factive

Brand Names: Canada Factive®

Index Terms DW286; Gemifloxacin Mesylate; LA 20304a; SB-265805

Pharmacologic Category Antibiotic, Fluoroquinolone; Antibiotic, Respiratory Fluoroquinolone

Use Treatment of acute exacerbation of chronic bronchitis; treatment of community-acquired pneumonia (CAP), including pneumonia caused by multidrug-resistant strains of *S. pneumoniae* (MDRSP)

Medication Guide Available Yes

Dosing

Adult & Geriatric

Susceptible infections: Oral: 320 mg once daily

Acute exacerbations of chronic bronchitis: Oral: 320 mg once daily for 5 days

Community-acquired pneumonia (mild-to-moderate): Oral: 320 mg once daily for 5 or 7 days (decision to use 5- or 7-day regimen should be guided by initial sputum culture; 7 days are recommended for MDRSP, *Klebsiella*, or *M. catarrhalis* infection)

Acute bacterial rhinosinusitis (off-label use): Oral: 320 mg once daily for 5 to 7 days (Ferguson 2002)

Renal Impairment

CrCl >40 mL/minute: No adjustment required.

CrCl ≤40 mL/minute (or patients on hemodialysis/CAPD): 160 mg once daily (administer dose following hemodialysis).

Hepatic Impairment No adjustment required.

Additional Information Complete prescribing information should be consulted for additional detail.

Dosage Forms Excipient information presented when available (limited, particularly for generics); consult specific product labeling.

Tablet, Oral:

Factive: 320 mg [scored]

◆ **Gemifloxacin Mesylate** *see* Gemifloxacin *on page 836*

Gemtuzumab Ozogamicin
(gem TOO zoo mab oh zog a MY sin)

Index Terms CMA-676; Mylotarg

Pharmacologic Category Antineoplastic Agent, Anti-CD33; Antineoplastic Agent, Antibody Drug Conjugate; Antineoplastic Agent, Monoclonal Antibody

Use Due to safety concerns, as well as lack of clinical benefit demonstrated in a post-approval clinical trial, gemtuzumab was withdrawn from the U.S. commercial market in 2010.

Pregnancy Considerations Teratogenic effects have been observed in animal reproduction studies. May cause fetal harm when administered to a pregnant woman. Women of childbearing potential should avoid becoming pregnant while receiving treatment.

Breast-Feeding Considerations It is not known if gemtuzumab ozogamicin is excreted in breast milk. Because human IgG is secreted in breast milk and the potential for serious adverse reactions in the nursing infant exists, a decision should be made whether to discontinue nursing or to discontinue the drug, taking into account the importance of treatment to the mother.

Prescribing and Access Restrictions As of June 2010, gemtuzumab has been withdrawn from the U.S. market and is no longer commercially available to new patients; gemtuzumab is only available in the U.S. under an Investigational New Drug (IND) protocol.

In Canada, gemtuzumab is available through a special access program (access information is available from Health Canada).

Contraindications Hypersensitivity to gemtuzumab ozogamicin, calicheamicin derivatives, or any component of the formulation; patients with anti-CD33 antibody

Warnings/Precautions Hazardous agent - use appropriate precautions for handling and disposal (NIOSH 2014 [group 1]).

Gemtuzumab has been associated with hepatotoxicity, including severe hepatic sinusoidal obstruction syndrome (SOS; formerly called veno-occlusive disease [VOD]). Symptoms of SOS include right upper quadrant pain, rapid weight gain, ascites, hepatomegaly, and bilirubin/transaminase elevations. Risk may be increased by combination chemotherapy, underlying hepatic disease, or hematopoietic stem cell transplant.

Severe hypersensitivity reactions (including anaphylaxis) and other infusion-related reactions may occur. Infusion-related events are common, generally reported to occur with the first dose after the end of the 2-hour intravenous infusion. These symptoms usually resolved after 2-4 hours with a supportive therapy of acetaminophen, diphenhydramine, and intravenous fluids. Other severe and potentially fatal infusion related pulmonary events (including dyspnea and hypoxia) have been reported infrequently. Symptomatic intrinsic lung disease or high peripheral blast counts may increase the risk of severe reactions. Fewer infusion-related events were observed after the second dose. Postinfusion reactions (may include fever, chills, hypotension, or dyspnea) may occur during the first 24 hours after administration. Consider discontinuation in patients who develop severe infusion-related reactions. In addition to infusion-related pulmonary events,

gemtuzumab therapy is also associated with acute respiratory distress syndrome, pulmonary infiltrates, pleural effusion, noncardiogenic pulmonary edema, and pulmonary insufficiency.

Severe myelosuppression occurs in all patients at recommended dosages. Tumor lysis syndrome may occur as a consequence of leukemia treatment, adequate hydration and prophylactic allopurinol must be instituted prior to use. Other methods to lower WBC <30,000 cells/mm^3 may be considered (hydroxyurea or leukapheresis) to minimize the risk of tumor lysis syndrome, and/or severe infusion reactions. An increased number of deaths have been reported in patients receiving gemtuzumab in combination with chemotherapy, compared to those receiving chemotherapy alone.

Adverse Reactions Frequency not defined.

Cardiovascular: Cerebral hemorrhage, hyper-/hypotension, peripheral edema, tachycardia

Central nervous system: Anxiety, chills, depression, dizziness, fever, headache, insomnia, intracranial hemorrhage, pain

Dermatologic: Bruising, petechiae, pruritus, rash

Endocrine & metabolic: Hyperglycemia, hypocalcemia, hypokalemia, hypomagnesemia, hypophosphatemia

Gastrointestinal: Abdominal pain, anorexia, diarrhea, dyspepsia, gingival hemorrhage, melena, mucositis, nausea, stomatitis, vomiting

Genitourinary: Vaginal bleeding, vaginal hemorrhage

Hematologic: Anemia, disseminated intravascular coagulation (DIC), hemorrhage, leukopenia, lymphopenia, neutropenia (median recovery 40-51 days), neutropenic fever, thrombocytopenia (median recovery 36-51 days)

Hepatic: Alkaline phosphatase increased, ALT increased, ascites, AST increased, hyperbilirubinemia, LDH increased, prothrombin time increased, PTT increased, sinusoidal obstruction syndrome (SOS; veno-occlusive disease; higher frequency in patients with prior history of or subsequent hematopoietic stem cell transplant)

Local: Local reaction

Neuromuscular & skeletal: Arthralgia, back pain, myalgia, weakness

Renal: Creatinine increased, hematuria

Respiratory: Cough, dyspnea, epistaxis, hypoxia, pharyngitis, pneumonia, rhinitis

Miscellaneous: Cutaneous herpes simplex, infection, infusion reaction, sepsis

Infrequent and/or case reports (limited to important or life-threatening): Acute respiratory distress syndrome, anaphylaxis, bradycardia, Budd-Chiari syndrome, gastrointestinal hemorrhage, hepatic failure, hepatosplenomegaly, hypersensitivity reactions, jaundice, neutropenic sepsis, noncardiogenic pulmonary edema, portal vain thrombosis, pulmonary hemorrhage, renal impairment, renal failure (including renal failure secondary to tumor lysis syndrome)

Drug Interactions

Metabolism/Transport Effects None known.

Avoid Concomitant Use

Avoid concomitant use of Gemtuzumab Ozogamicin with any of the following: BCG (Intravesical); Belimumab; Deferiprone; Dipyrone; Natalizumab; Pimecrolimus; Tacrolimus (Topical); Tofacitinib; Vaccines (Live)

Increased Effect/Toxicity

Gemtuzumab Ozogamicin may increase the levels/effects of: Belimumab; CloZAPine; Deferiprone; Fingolimod; Leflunomide; Natalizumab; Tofacitinib; Vaccines (Live)

The levels/effects of Gemtuzumab Ozogamicin may be increased by: Denosumab; Dipyrone; Pimecrolimus; Roflumilast; Tacrolimus (Topical); Trastuzumab

Decreased Effect

Gemtuzumab Ozogamicin may decrease the levels/effects of: BCG (Intravesical); Coccidioides immitis Skin Test; Sipuleucel-T; Vaccines (Inactivated); Vaccines (Live)

The levels/effects of Gemtuzumab Ozogamicin may be decreased by: Echinacea

Preparation for Administration Hazardous agent; use appropriate precautions for handling and disposal (NIOSH 2014 [group 1]). Protect from light during preparation (and administration). Prepare in biologic safety hood with shielded fluorescent light; (some institutions prepare in a darkened room with the lights in the biologic safety cabinet turned off). Allow to warm to room temperature prior to reconstitution. Reconstitute each 5 mg vial with sterile water for injection to a concentration of 1 mg/mL. Dilute in 100 mL of 0.9% sodium chloride injection.

Storage/Stability Light sensitive; protect from light (including direct and indirect sunlight, and unshielded fluorescent light). The infusion container should be placed in a UV protectant bag immediately after preparation. Store intact vials under refrigeration at 2°C to 8°C (36°F to 46°F). Reconstituted solutions may be stored for up to 2 hours at room temperature or under refrigeration. Following dilution for infusion, solutions are stable for up to 16 hours at room temperature. Administration requires 2 hours; therefore, the maximum elapsed time from initial reconstitution to completion of infusion should be 20 hours.

Mechanism of Action Antibody to CD33 antigen, which is expressed on leukemic blasts in 80% of AML patients. Binds to the CD33 antigen, resulting in internalization of the antibody-antigen complex. Following internalization, the calicheamicin derivative is released inside the myeloid cell. The calicheamicin derivative binds to DNA resulting in double strand breaks and cell death. Pluripotent stem cells and nonhematopoietic cells are not affected.

Pharmacodynamics/Kinetics

Distribution: V_{ss}: Adults: Initial dose: 21 L; Repeat dose: 10 L

Half-life elimination: Total calicheamicin: Initial: 41-45 hours, Repeat dose: 60-64 hours; Unconjugated: 100-143 hours (no change noted in repeat dosing)

Dosing

Adult & Geriatric Note: Patients should receive diphenhydramine 50 mg orally and acetaminophen 650-1000 mg orally 1 hour prior to administration of each dose. Acetaminophen dosage should be repeated as needed every 4 hours for 2 additional doses. Pretreatment with methylprednisolone may ameliorate infusion-related symptoms.

Acute myeloid leukemia (off-label/investigational use): IV:

<60 years: 9 mg/m^2 infused over 2 hours. A full treatment course is a total of 2 doses administered with 14-28 days between doses (Larson, 2005).

≥60 years: 9 mg/m^2 infused over 2 hours. A full treatment course is a total of 2 doses administered with 14-28 days between doses (Larson, 2002; Larson, 2005).

Acute promyelocytic leukemia (off-label/investigational use): IV:

Single-agent therapy: 6 mg/m^2 infused over 2 hours on days 1 and 15; for patients testing PCR negative after 2 doses, a third dose was administered (LoCoco, 2004).

Combination therapy (high-risk patients; Ravandi, 2009):

Induction: 9 mg/m^2 as a single dose on day 1 (in combination with arsenic trioxide and tretinoin)

Post remission therapy (if arsenic trioxide or tretinoin discontinued due to toxicity): 9 mg/m^2 once every 4-5 weeks until 28 weeks after complete remission.

Renal Impairment No dosage adjustment provided in manufacturer's labeling (has not been studied).

Hepatic Impairment No dosage adjustment provided in manufacturer's labeling (has not been studied); use with caution.

Adjustment for Toxicity

Dyspnea or significant hypotension: Interrupt infusion; monitor

Anaphylaxis, pulmonary edema, acute respiratory distress syndrome: Strongly consider discontinuing treatment

Administration Do not administer as IV push or bolus. Administer via IV infusion, over at least 2 hours through a low protein-binding (0.2 to 1.2 micron) in-line filter. Protect from light during infusion. Premedicate with acetaminophen and diphenhydramine prior to each infusion.

Hazardous agent; use appropriate precautions for handling and disposal (NIOSH 2014 [group 1]).

Monitoring Parameters Monitor vital signs during the infusion and for 4 hours following the infusion. Monitor for signs/symptoms of postinfusion reaction. Monitor electrolytes, liver function, CBC with differential and platelets frequently. Monitor for signs and symptoms of hepatic sinusoidal obstruction syndrome (SOS; veno-occlusive disease; weight gain, right upper quadrant abdominal pain, hepatomegaly, ascites).

Product Availability No longer commercially available in the US market for new patients. Available in Canada through a special access program.

♦ Gemzar *see* Gemcitabine *on page 832*

♦ Genac *see* Triprolidine and Pseudoephedrine *on page 1847*

♦ Genahist [OTC] *see* DiphenhydrAMINE (Systemic) *on page 561*

♦ Genaphed [OTC] *see* Pseudoephedrine *on page 1527*

Gentamicin (Systemic) (jen ta MYE sin)

Brand Names: Canada Gentamicin Injection, USP

Index Terms Gentamicin Sulfate

Pharmacologic Category Antibiotic, Aminoglycoside

Use Treatment of susceptible bacterial infections, normally gram-negative organisms, including *Pseudomonas, Proteus, Serratia,* and gram-positive *Staphylococcus*; treatment of bone infections, respiratory tract infections, skin and soft tissue infections, as well as abdominal and urinary tract infections, and septicemia; treatment of infective endocarditis

Pregnancy Considerations [US Boxed Warning]: Aminoglycosides may cause fetal harm if administered to a pregnant woman. Gentamicin crosses the placenta. There are several reports of total irreversible bilateral congenital deafness in children whose mothers received another aminoglycoside (streptomycin) during pregnancy. Although serious side effects to the fetus/infant have not been reported following maternal use of all aminoglycosides, a potential for harm exists.

Due to pregnancy-induced physiologic changes, some pharmacokinetic parameters of gentamicin may be altered (Popović 2007). Gentamicin use has been evaluated for various infections in pregnant women including the treatment of acute pyelonephritis (Jolley 2010) and as an alternative antibiotic for prophylactic use prior to cesarean delivery (Bratzler 2013).

Breast-Feeding Considerations Gentamicin is found in breast milk (Celiloglu 1994). As a class, aminoglycosides are expected to be poorly distributed into breast milk, limiting systemic exposure to a nursing infant. In general, modification of bowel flora may occur with any antibiotic exposure (Chung 2002).

Contraindications Hypersensitivity to gentamicin or other aminoglycosides

Warnings/Precautions [U.S. Boxed Warning]: Aminoglycosides may cause neurotoxicity and/or nephrotoxicity; usual risk factors include preexisting renal impairment, concomitant neuro-/nephrotoxic medications, advanced age and dehydration. Ototoxicity may be directly proportional to the amount of drug given and the duration of treatment; tinnitus or vertigo are indications of vestibular injury and impending hearing loss; renal damage is usually reversible. May cause neuromuscular blockade and respiratory paralysis; especially when given soon after anesthesia or muscle relaxants.

Not intended for long-term therapy due to toxic hazards associated with extended administration; use caution in preexisting renal insufficiency, vestibular or cochlear impairment, myasthenia gravis, hypocalcemia, conditions which depress neuromuscular transmission. Dosage modification required in patients with impaired renal function. Prolonged use may result in fungal or bacterial superinfection, including *C. difficile*-associated diarrhea (CDAD) and pseudomembranous colitis; CDAD has been observed >2 months postantibiotic treatment.

Adverse Reactions Frequency not defined.

Cardiovascular: Edema, hyper/hypotension

Central nervous system: Ataxia, confusion, depression, dizziness, drowsiness, encephalopathy, fever, headache, lethargy, pseudomotor cerebri, seizures, vertigo

Dermatologic: Alopecia, erythema, itching, purpura, rash, urticaria

Endocrine & metabolic: Hypocalcemia, hypokalemia, hypomagnesemia, hyponatremia

Gastrointestinal: Anorexia, appetite decreased, *C. difficile*-associated diarrhea, enterocolitis, nausea, salivation increased, splenomegaly, stomatitis, vomiting, weight loss

Hematologic: Agranulocytosis, anemia, eosinophilia, granulocytopenia, leukopenia, reticulocytes increased/decreased, thrombocytopenia

Hepatic: Hepatomegaly, LFTs increased

Local: Injection site reactions, pain at injection site, phlebitis/thrombophlebitis

Neuromuscular & skeletal: Arthralgia, gait instability, muscle cramps, muscle twitching, muscle weakness, myasthenia gravis-like syndrome, numbness, paresthesia, peripheral neuropathy, tremor, weakness

Ocular: Visual disturbances

Otic: Hearing impairment, hearing loss (associated with persistently increased serum concentrations; early toxicity usually affects high-pitched sound), tinnitus

Renal: BUN increased, casts (hyaline, granular) in urine, creatinine clearance decreased, distal tubular dysfunction, Fanconi-like syndrome (high dose, prolonged course) (infants and adults), oliguria, renal failure (high trough serum concentrations), polyuria, proteinuria, serum creatinine increased, tubular necrosis, urine specific gravity decreased

Respiratory: Dyspnea, laryngeal edema, pulmonary fibrosis, respiratory depression

Miscellaneous: Allergic reaction, anaphylaxis, anaphylactoid reactions

Drug Interactions

Metabolism/Transport Effects None known.

Avoid Concomitant Use

Avoid concomitant use of Gentamicin (Systemic) with any of the following: Agalsidase Alfa; Agalsidase Beta; BCG (Intravesical); Foscarnet; Mannitol; Mannitol (Systemic); Mecamylamine

Increased Effect/Toxicity

Gentamicin (Systemic) may increase the levels/effects of: AbobotulinumtoxinA; Bisphosphonate Derivatives; CARBOplatin; Colistimethate; CycloSPORINE (Systemic); Mecamylamine; Neuromuscular-Blocking Agents; OnabotulinumtoxinA; RimabotulinumtoxinB; Tenofovir Products

The levels/effects of Gentamicin (Systemic) may be increased by: Amphotericin B; Capreomycin; Cefazedone; Cephalosporins (2nd Generation); Cephalosporins (3rd Generation); Cephalosporins (4th Generation); Cephradine; CISplatin; Foscarnet; Loop Diuretics; Mannitol; Mannitol (Systemic); Nonsteroidal Anti-Inflammatory Agents; Tenofovir Products; Vancomycin

Decreased Effect

Gentamicin (Systemic) may decrease the levels/effects of: Agalsidase Alfa; Agalsidase Beta; BCG (Intravesical); BCG Vaccine (Immunization); Cardiac Glycosides; Sodium Picosulfate; Typhoid Vaccine

The levels/effects of Gentamicin (Systemic) may be decreased by: Penicillins

Storage/Stability Gentamicin is a colorless to slightly yellow solution which should be stored between 2°C to 30°C, but refrigeration is not recommended. IV infusion solutions mixed in NS or D_5W solution are stable for 48 hours at room temperature and refrigeration (Goodwin, 1991). Premixed bag: Manufacturer expiration date; remove from overwrap stability: 30 days.

Mechanism of Action Interferes with bacterial protein synthesis by binding to 30S and 50S ribosomal subunits resulting in a defective bacterial cell membrane

Pharmacodynamics/Kinetics

Absorption: Intramuscular: Rapid and complete; Oral: Poorly absorbed (<2%)

Distribution: Primarily into extracellular fluid (highly hydrophilic); high concentration in the renal cortex; minimal penetration to CSF and ocular tissues via IV route; small amounts distribute into bile, sputum, saliva, and tears

V_d: Higher in neonates than older pediatric patients; increased by edema, ascites, fluid overload; decreased with dehydration

Neonates: 0.45 ± 0.1 L/kg

Infants: 0.4 ± 0.1 L/kg

Children: 0.35 ± 0.15 L/kg

Adolescents: 0.3 ± 0.1 L/kg

Adults: 0.2-0.3 L/kg

Relative diffusion from blood into CSF: Minimal even with inflammation

CSF:blood level ratio: Normal meninges: Nil; Inflamed meninges: 10% to 30%

Protein binding: <30%

Half-life elimination:

Neonates: <1 week: 3-11.5 hours; 1 week to 1 month: 3 to 6 hours

Infants: 4 ± 1 hour

Children: 2 ± 1 hour

Adolescents: 1.5 ± 1 hour

Adults: 1.5-3 hours; End-stage renal disease (ESRD): 36-70 hours

Time to peak, serum: IM: 30-90 minutes; IV: 30 minutes after 30-minute infusion; **Note:** Distribution may be prolonged after larger doses. One study reported a 1.7-hour distribution period after a 60-minute, high-dose aminoglycoside infusion (Demczar 1997).

Excretion: Urine (as unchanged drug)

Clearance: Directly related to renal function

Neonates: 0.045 ± 0.01 L/hour/kg

Infants: 0.1 ± 0.05 L/hour/kg

Children: 0.1 ± 0.03 L/hour/kg

Adolescents: 0.09 ± 0.03 L/hour/kg

Dosing

Adult & Geriatric Individualization is **critical** because of the low therapeutic index.

In underweight and nonobese patients, use of total body weight (TBW) instead of ideal body weight for determining the initial mg/kg/dose is widely accepted (Nicolau, 1995). Ideal body weight (IBW) also may be used to determine doses for patients who are neither underweight nor obese (Gilbert, 2009).

Initial and periodic plasma drug levels (eg, peak and trough with conventional dosing, post dose level at a prespecified time with extended-interval dosing) should be determined, particularly in critically-ill patients with serious infections or in disease states known to significantly alter aminoglycoside pharmacokinetics (eg, cystic fibrosis, burns, or major surgery).

Usual dosage ranges:

IM, IV:

Conventional: 1-2.5 mg/kg/dose every 8-12 hours; to ensure adequate peak concentrations early in therapy, higher initial dosage may be considered in selected patients when extracellular water is increased (edema, septic shock, postsurgical, or trauma)

Once daily: 4-7 mg/kg/dose once daily; some clinicians recommend this approach for all patients with normal renal function; this dose is at least as efficacious with similar, if not less, toxicity than conventional dosing

Intrathecal: 4-8 mg/day

Indication-specific dosing: IM, IV:

Brucellosis: 240 mg (IM) daily or 5 mg/kg (IV) daily for 7 days; either regimen recommended in combination with doxycycline

Cholangitis: 4-6 mg/kg once daily with ampicillin

Diverticulitis (complicated): 1.5-2 mg/kg every 8 hours (with ampicillin and metronidazole)

Endocarditis: Treatment: 3 mg/kg/day in 1-3 divided doses

Meningitis Enterococcus sp or Pseudomonas aeruginosa: IV: Loading dose 2 mg/kg, then 1.7 mg/kg/dose every 8 hours (administered with another bacteriocidal drug)

Pelvic inflammatory disease: Loading dose: 2 mg/kg, then 1.5 mg/kg every 8 hours

Alternate therapy: 4.5 mg/kg once daily

Plague (Yersinia pestis): Treatment: 5 mg/kg/day, followed by postexposure prophylaxis with doxycycline

Pneumonia, hospital- or ventilator-associated: 7 mg/kg/day (with antipseudomonal beta-lactam or carbapenem)

Surgical (preoperative) prophylaxis (off-label use): IV: 5 mg/kg within 60 minutes prior to surgical incision with or without other antibiotics (procedure dependent). **Note:** Dose is based on actual body weight unless >20% above ideal body weight, then dosage requirement may best be estimated using a dosing weight of IBW + 0.4 (TBW - IBW) (Bratzler, 2013).

Synergy (for gram-positive infections): 3 mg/kg/day in 1-3 divided doses (with ampicillin)

Tularemia: 5 mg/kg/day divided every 8 hours for 1-2 weeks

Urinary tract infection: 1.5 mg/kg/dose every 8 hours

Pediatric Individualization is **critical** because of the low therapeutic index.

Use of ideal body weight (IBW) for determining the mg/kg/dose appears to be more accurate than dosing on the basis of total body weight (TBW).

Initial and periodic plasma drug levels (eg, peak and trough with conventional dosing) should be determined, particularly in critically-ill patients with serious infections or in disease states known to significantly alter aminoglycoside pharmacokinetics (eg, cystic fibrosis, burns, or major surgery).

Usual dosage ranges: IM, IV:

Infants and Children <5 years: 2.5 mg/kg/dose every 8 hours*

Children ≥5 years: 2-2.5 mg/kg/dose every 8 hours*

*Note: Higher individual doses and/or more frequent intervals (eg, every 6 hours) may be required in selected clinical situations (cystic fibrosis) or serum levels document the need.

Surgical (preoperative) prophylaxis (off-label use): Children ≥1 year: IV: 2.5 mg/kg within 60 minutes prior to surgical incision with or without other antibiotics (procedure dependent). **Note:** Dose is based on actual body weight unless >20% above ideal body weight, then dosage requirement may best be estimated using a dosing weight of IBW + 0.4 (TBW - IBW) (Bratzler, 2013).

Renal Impairment

Conventional dosing:

CrCl ≥60 mL/minute: Administer every 8 hours

CrCl 40-60 mL/minute: Administer every 12 hours

CrCl 20-40 mL/minute: Administer every 24 hours

CrCl <20 mL/minute: Loading dose, then monitor levels

High-dose therapy: Interval may be extended (eg, every 48 hours) in patients with moderate renal impairment (CrCl 30-59 mL/minute) and/or adjusted based on serum level determinations.

Intermittent hemodialysis (IHD) (administer after hemodialysis on dialysis days) (Heintz, 2009): Dialyzable (~50%; variable; dependent on filter, duration, and type of IHD):

Loading dose of 2-3 mg/kg loading dose followed by:

Mild UTI or synergy: 1 mg/kg every 48-72 hours; monitor levels

Moderate-to-severe UTI: 1-1.5 mg/kg every 48-72 hours; monitor levels

Systemic gram-negative rod infection: 1.5-2 mg/kg every 48-72 hours; monitor levels

Note: Dosing dependent on the assumption of 3 times/week, complete IHD sessions.

Peritoneal dialysis (PD):

Administration via PD fluid:

Gram-positive infection (eg, synergy): 3-4 mg/L (3-4 mcg/mL) of PD fluid

Gram-negative infection: 4-8 mg/L (4-8 mcg/mL) of PD fluid

Administration via IV, IM route during PD: Dose as for CrCl <10 mL/minute and follow levels

Continuous renal replacement therapy (CRRT) (Heintz, 2009; Trotman, 2005): Drug clearance is highly dependent on the method of renal replacement, filter type, and flow rate. Appropriate dosing requires close monitoring of pharmacologic response, signs of adverse reactions due to drug accumulation, as well as target drug concentrations (if appropriate). The following are general recommendations only (based on dialysate flow/ultrafiltration rates of 1-2 L/hour and minimal residual renal function) and should not supersede clinical judgment:

CVVH/CVVHD/CVVHDF: Loading dose of 2-3 mg/kg followed by:

Mild UTI or synergy: 1 mg/kg every 24-36 hours; monitor levels

Moderate-to-severe UTI: 1-1.5 mg/kg every 24-36 hours; monitor levels

Systemic gram-negative infection: 1.5-2.5 mg/kg every 24-48 hours; monitor levels

Hepatic Impairment Monitor plasma concentrations.

Obesity In moderate obesity (TBW/IBW ≥1.25) or greater (eg, morbid obesity [TBW/IBW >2]), initial dosage requirement may be estimated using a dosing weight of IBW + 0.4 (TBW - IBW) (Traynor, 1995).

Dietary Considerations Calcium, magnesium, potassium: Renal wasting may cause hypocalcemia, hypomagnesemia, and/or hypokalemia.

Administration

IM: Administer by deep IM route if possible. Slower absorption and lower peak concentrations, probably due to poor circulation in the atrophic muscle, may occur following IM injection; in paralyzed patients, suggest IV route.

IV: Infuse over 30-120 minutes.

Some penicillins (eg, carbenicillin, ticarcillin, and piperacillin) have been shown to inactivate aminoglycosides *in vitro*. This has been observed to a greater extent with tobramycin and gentamicin, while amikacin has shown greater stability against inactivation. Concurrent use of these agents may pose a risk of reduced antibacterial efficacy *in vivo*, particularly in the setting of profound renal impairment. However, definitive clinical evidence is lacking. If combination penicillin/aminoglycoside therapy is desired in a patient with renal dysfunction, separation of doses (if feasible), and routine monitoring of aminoglycoside levels, CBC, and clinical response should be considered.

Monitoring Parameters Urinalysis, urine output, BUN, serum creatinine, plasma gentamicin levels (as appropriate to dosing method). Levels are typically obtained after the third dose in conventional dosing. Hearing should be tested before, during, and after treatment; particularly in those at risk for ototoxicity or who will be receiving prolonged therapy (>2 weeks)

Some penicillin derivatives may accelerate the degradation of aminoglycosides *in vitro*. This may be clinically-significant for certain penicillin (ticarcillin, piperacillin, carbenicillin) and aminoglycoside (gentamicin, tobramycin) combination therapy in patients with significant renal impairment. Close monitoring of aminoglycoside levels is warranted.

Reference Range

Timing of serum samples: Draw peak 30 minutes after 30-minute infusion has been completed or 1 hour after IM injection; draw trough immediately before next dose

Therapeutic levels:

Peak:

Serious infections: 6-8 mcg/mL (12-17 micromole/L)

Life-threatening infections: 8-10 mcg/mL (17-21 micromole/L)

Urinary tract infections: 4-6 mcg/mL

Synergy against gram-positive organisms: 3-5 mcg/mL

Trough:

Serious infections: 0.5-1 mcg/mL

Life-threatening infections: 1-2 mcg/mL

The American Thoracic Society (ATS) recommends trough levels of <1 mcg/mL for patients with hospital-acquired pneumonia.

Obtain drug levels after the third dose unless renal dysfunction/toxicity suspected

Test Interactions Some penicillin derivatives may accelerate the degradation of aminoglycosides *in vitro*, leading to a potential underestimation of aminoglycoside serum concentration.

Dosage Forms Excipient information presented when available (limited, particularly for generics); consult specific product labeling.

Solution, Injection:

Generic: 10 mg/mL (2 mL); 40 mg/mL (2 mL, 20 mL)

Solution, Injection [preservative free]:

Generic: 10 mg/mL (2 mL)

Solution, Intravenous:

Generic: 60 mg (50 mL); 70 mg (50 mL); 80 mg (50 mL, 100 mL); 90 mg (100 mL); 100 mg (50 mL, 100 mL); 120 mg (100 mL); 10 mg/mL (6 mL, 8 mL, 10 mL)

Gentamicin (Ophthalmic) (jen ta MYE sin)

Brand Names: US Garamycin; Gentak

Brand Names: Canada Diogent®; Garamycin®; Gentak®; Gentocin; PMS-Gentamicin

Index Terms Gentamicin Sulfate

Pharmacologic Category Antibiotic, Aminoglycoside; Antibiotic, Ophthalmic

Use Treatment of ophthalmic infections caused by susceptible bacteria

Dosing

Adult & Geriatric Ophthalmic infections: Ophthalmic:

Ointment: Instill 1/2" (1.25 cm) 2-3 times/day to every 3-4 hours

Solution: Instill 1-2 drops every 4 hours, up to 2 drops every hour for severe infections

Pediatric Ophthalmic infections: Children: Refer to adult dosing.

Additional Information Complete prescribing information should be consulted for additional detail.

Dosage Forms Excipient information presented when available (limited, particularly for generics); consult specific product labeling. [DSC] = Discontinued product

Ointment, Ophthalmic:

Garamycin: 0.3% (3.5 g [DSC])

Gentak: 0.3% (3.5 g) [contains methylparaben, propylparaben]

Generic: 0.3% (3.5 g)

Solution, Ophthalmic:

Garamycin: 0.3% (5 mL) [contains benzalkonium chloride]

Generic: 0.3% (5 mL, 15 mL)

◆ **Gentamicin and Prednisolone** *see* Prednisolone and Gentamicin *on page 1496*

◆ **Gentamicin Injection, USP (Can)** *see* Gentamicin (Systemic) *on page 838*

◆ **Gentamicin Sulfate** *see* Gentamicin (Ophthalmic) *on page 840*

◆ **Gentamicin Sulfate** *see* Gentamicin (Systemic) *on page 838*

Gentian Violet (JEN shun VYE oh let)

Index Terms Crystal Violet; Methylrosaniline Chloride

Pharmacologic Category Antibiotic, Topical; Antifungal Agent, Topical

Use Topical infection: Treatment of abrasions, minor cuts, surface injuries, and superficial fungus infections of the skin.

Dosing

Adult & Geriatric Topical infection: Topical: Apply to affected area once or twice daily.

Pediatric Topical infection: Infants, Children, and Adolescents: Topical: Refer to adult dosing.

Renal Impairment There are no dosage adjustments provided in the manufacturer's labeling.

Hepatic Impairment There are no dosage adjustments provided in the manufacturer's labeling.

Additional Information Complete prescribing information should be consulted for additional detail.

Dosage Forms Excipient information presented when available (limited, particularly for generics); consult specific product labeling. [DSC] = Discontinued product

Solution, External:

Generic: 1% (30 mL [DSC], 59 mL, 100 mL [DSC], 500 mL [DSC]); 2% (59 mL, 59.14 mL, 100 mL [DSC], 500 mL [DSC])

◆ **Gen-Tizanidine (Can)** *see* TiZANidine *on page 1798*

◆ **Gentle Laxative [OTC]** *see* Bisacodyl *on page 231*

◆ **Gentocin (Can)** *see* Gentamicin (Ophthalmic) *on page 840*

◆ **Genvoya** *see* Elvitegravir, Cobicistat, Emtricitabine, and Tenofovir Alafenamide *on page 632*

◆ **Genz-112638** *see* Eliglustat *on page 624*

◆ **Geodon** *see* Ziprasidone *on page 1930*

◆ **Geri-Dryl [OTC]** *see* DiphenhydrAMINE (Systemic) *on page 561*

◆ **Geri-Lanta Supreme [OTC]** *see* Calcium Carbonate and Magnesium Hydroxide *on page 288*

◆ **Geri-Mox [OTC]** *see* Aluminum Hydroxide, Magnesium Hydroxide, and Simethicone *on page 85*

◆ **Geri-Mucil [OTC]** *see* Psyllium *on page 1529*

◆ **Geri-Pectate [OTC]** *see* Bismuth Subsalicylate *on page 232*

◆ **Geri-Stool [OTC]** *see* Docusate and Senna *on page 579*

◆ **Geri-Tussin [OTC]** *see* GuaiFENesin *on page 860*

◆ **GF196960** *see* Tadalafil *on page 1730*

◆ **GG** *see* GuaiFENesin *on page 860*

◆ **GHB** *see* Sodium Oxybate *on page 1676*

◆ **GI87084B** *see* Remifentanil *on page 1567*

◆ **Gianvi** *see* Ethinyl Estradiol and Drospirenone *on page 702*

◆ **Giazo** *see* Balsalazide *on page 200*

◆ **Gildagia** *see* Ethinyl Estradiol and Norethindrone *on page 708*

◆ **Gildess 24 Fe** *see* Ethinyl Estradiol and Norethindrone *on page 708*

◆ **Gildess FE 1.5/30** *see* Ethinyl Estradiol and Norethindrone *on page 708*

◆ **Gildess FE 1/20** *see* Ethinyl Estradiol and Norethindrone *on page 708*

◆ **Gilenya** *see* Fingolimod *on page 770*

◆ **Gilotrif** *see* Afatinib *on page 50*

◆ **Giotrif (Can)** *see* Afatinib *on page 50*

◆ **Glargine Insulin** *see* Insulin Glargine *on page 956*

Glatiramer Acetate (gla TIR a mer AS e tate)

Brand Names: US Copaxone; Glatopa

Brand Names: Canada Copaxone

Index Terms Copolymer-1; Glatopa
Pharmacologic Category Biological, Miscellaneous
Use

Multiple sclerosis: Treatment of patients with relapsing forms of multiple sclerosis (MS)

Canadian labeling: Additional use (not in US labeling): Treatment of patients who have experienced a single demyelinating event, accompanied by abnormal MRI scans and are considered to be at risk of developing clinically definite MS, after alternative diagnoses are excluded.

Pregnancy Considerations Adverse events were not observed in animal reproduction studies. Limited information is available related to the use of glatiramer acetate in pregnancy (Amato 2015; Fragoso 2014; Ghezzi 2013; Giannini 2012). Until additional information is available, consideration should be given to discontinuing treatment if a woman becomes pregnant, or 1 month prior to becoming pregnant in women with mild disease (Coyle, 2012; Ghezzi 2013; Houtchens, 2013; Lu, 2013).

Breast-Feeding Considerations It is not known if glatiramer acetate is excreted in breast milk. The manufacturer recommends that caution be exercised when administering glatiramer acetate to nursing women. Although glatiramer acetate would not likely be bioavailable if absorbed orally via breast-milk (Amato 2015), it is generally recommended to avoid use if breast-feeding (Amato 2015; Ghezzi 2013; Houtchens, 2013).

Contraindications Hypersensitivity to glatiramer acetate, mannitol, or any component of the formulation

Warnings/Precautions Glatiramer acetate is antigenic and may interfere with recognition of foreign antigens affecting tumor surveillance and infection defense systems. Immediate postinjection systemic reactions occur in a substantial percentage of patients (~16% [20 mg/mL] and ~2% [40 mg/mL] in studies); symptoms (anxiety, chest pain, constriction of the throat, dyspnea, flushing, palpitations, urticaria) are usually self-limited and transient. These symptoms generally occur several months after initiation of treatment. Chest pain may or may not occur with the immediate postinjection reaction; described as a transient pain usually resolving in a few minutes; often unassociated with other symptoms. Episodes usually begin ≥1 month after initiation of treatment. Lipoatrophy may occur locally at injection site at various times after treatment (sometimes after several months) and may not resolve; to possibly minimize occurrence, advise patient to follow proper injection technique and rotate site with each injection. Skin necrosis has also been observed.

Anaphylactoid reactions (rare) have been reported. Potentially significant drug-drug interactions may exist, requiring dose or frequency adjustment, additional monitoring, and/or selection of alternative therapy.

Adverse Reactions

>10%:

Cardiovascular: Vasodilatation (3% to 20%), chest pain (2% to 13%)

Central nervous system: Pain (20%), anxiety (13%)

Dermatologic: Skin rash (2% to 19%), diaphoresis (15%)

Gastrointestinal: Nausea (2% to 15%)

Hypersensitivity: Immediate hypersensitivity (2% to 16%; postinjection, including flushing, chest pain, palpitations, anxiety, dyspnea, throat constriction, and/or urticaria)

Immunologic: Development of IgG antibodies (3 months: ≥3 x baseline: 80%; 12 months: 90%; ≥3 x baseline: 30%)

Infection: Infection (30%)

Local: Inflammation at injection site (2% to 49%), erythema at injection site (22% to 43%), pain at injection site (10% to 40%), itching at injection site (6% to 27%), residual mass at injection site (6% to 27%), swelling (1% to 19%)

Neuromuscular & skeletal: Weakness (22%), back pain (12%)

Respiratory: Dyspnea (3% to 14%), flu-like symptoms (3% to 14%), nasopharyngitis (11%)

1% to 10%:

Cardiovascular: Palpitations (7% to 9%), edema (8%), tachycardia (5%), facial edema (3%), peripheral edema (3%), syncope (3%), hypertension (1%)

Central nervous system: Migraine (4%), chills (2% to 3%), nervousness (2%), speech disturbance (2%), abnormal dreams (1%), emotional lability (1%), stupor (1%)

Dermatologic: Hyperhidrosis (7%), pruritus (5%), erythema (2% to 4%), urticaria (3%), skin atrophy (≥1%), warts (≥1%), eczema (1%), pustular rash (1%)

Endocrine & metabolic: Weight gain (3%), amenorrhea (1%), hypermenorrhea (1%)

Gastrointestinal: Vomiting (7%), gastroenteritis (6%), dysphagia (2%), aphthous stomatitis (≥1%), bowel urgency (≥1%), dental caries (≥1%), enlargement of salivary glands (≥1%), oral candidiasis (≥1%)

Genitourinary: Urinary urgency (5%), vulvovaginal candidiasis (4%), abnormal Pap smear (≥1%), hematuria (≥1%), vaginal hemorrhage (≥1%), impotence (1%)

Hematologic & oncologic: Bruise (8%), lymphadenopathy (7%), benign skin neoplasm (2%)

Hypersensitivity: Hypersensitivity (3%)

Infection: Abscess (≥1%), herpes zoster (≥1%)

Local: Bleeding at injection site (5%), hypersensitivity reaction at injection site (4%), fibrosis at injection site (2%), lipoatrophy at injection site (≤2%), abscess at injection site (1%)

Neuromuscular & skeletal: Neck pain (8%), tremor (4%), laryngospasm (2%)

Ophthalmic: Diplopia (3%), visual field defect (1%)

Respiratory: Rhinitis (7%), bronchitis (6%), cough (6%), laryngismus (5%), viral respiratory tract infection (3%), hyperventilation (1%)

Miscellaneous: Fever (3% to 6%)

<1% (Limited to important or life-threatening): Amyotrophy, anaphylactoid reaction, anemia, angina pectoris, angioedema, aphasia, arthritis, asthma, ataxia, atrial fibrillation, blepharoptosis, blindness, bradycardia, bursitis, carcinoma (breast, bladder, lung, ovarian), cardiac arrhythmia, cardiac failure, cardiomegaly, cardiomyopathy, cataract, cerebral edema, cerebrovascular accident, cholecystitis, cholelithiasis, CNS neoplasm, colitis, coma, corneal ulcer, coronary occlusion, Cushing's syndrome, cyanosis, decreased libido, deep vein thrombophlebitis, depersonalization, dermatitis, dry eye syndrome, duodenal ulcer, eosinophilia, erythema nodosum, esophageal ulcer, esophagitis, facial paralysis, fibrocystic breast disease, fourth heart sound, fungal dermatitis, furunculosis, gastrointestinal carcinoma, gastrointestinal hemorrhage, gastrointestinal ulcer, genitourinary neoplasm, glaucoma, gout, hallucination, hematemesis, hepatic cirrhosis, hepatitis, hepatomegaly, hernia, hydrocephalus, hypercholesterolemia, hyperthyroidism, hypokinesia, hypotension, hypothyroidism, hypoventilation, increased appetite, leukemia, leukopenia, lupus erythematosus, lymphedema, maculopapular rash, malignant neoplasm of cervix, malignant neoplasm of skin, mania, memory impairment, meningitis, mitral valve prolapse syndrome, moon face, muscle spasm, mydriasis, myelitis, myocardial infarction, myoclonus, nephrolithiasis, nephrosis, neuralgia, optic neuritis, oral mucosa ulcer, orthostatic hypotension, osteomyelitis, otitis externa, ovarian cyst, pancreatitis, pancytopenia, paraplegia, pericardial effusion, peripheral vascular disease, photophobia, pneumonia, priapism, pseudolymphoma, psoriasis, psychotic depression, pulmonary embolism, pyelonephritis, rectal hemorrhage, renal failure, seizures, sepsis, serum sickness, skin hypertrophy, skin photosensitivity, skin pigmentation, splenomegaly, stomatitis, suicidal tendencies, systemic lupus erythematosus, systolic heart murmur, tenosynovitis, thrombocytopenia, thrombophlebitis, thrombosis, tissue necrosis at injection site, urethritis, vesicobullous rash, weight loss, xeroderma

Drug Interactions

Metabolism/Transport Effects None known.

Avoid Concomitant Use

Avoid concomitant use of Glatiramer Acetate with any of the following: BCG (Intravesical); Natalizumab; Pimecrolimus; Tacrolimus (Topical); Tofacitinib; Vaccines (Live)

Increased Effect/Toxicity

Glatiramer Acetate may increase the levels/effects of: Fingolimod; Leflunomide; Natalizumab; Tofacitinib; Vaccines (Live)

The levels/effects of Glatiramer Acetate may be increased by: Denosumab; Pimecrolimus; Roflumilast; Tacrolimus (Topical); Trastuzumab

Decreased Effect

Glatiramer Acetate may decrease the levels/effects of: BCG (Intravesical); Coccidioides immitis Skin Test; Sipuleucel-T; Vaccines (Inactivated); Vaccines (Live)

The levels/effects of Glatiramer Acetate may be decreased by: Echinacea

Storage/Stability Store at 2°C to 8°C (36°F to 46°F). If needed, may store at 15°C to 30°C (59°F to 86°F) for up to 1 month (refrigeration is preferred). Avoid exposure to high temperatures; protect from intense light. Do not freeze. Discard if syringe freezes.

Mechanism of Action Glatiramer is a mixture of random polymers of four amino acids; L-alanine, L-glutamic acid, L-lysine, and L-tyrosine, the resulting mixture is antigenically similar to myelin basic protein, which is an important component of the myelin sheath of nerves; glatiramer is thought to induce and activate T-lymphocyte suppressor

◄ cells specific for a myelin antigen, it is also proposed that glatiramer interferes with the antigen-presenting function of certain immune cells opposing pathogenic T-cell function

Pharmacodynamics/Kinetics

Distribution: Small amounts of intact and partial hydrolyzed drug enter lymphatic circulation

Metabolism: SubQ: Large percentage hydrolyzed locally

Dosing

Adult & Geriatric Multiple sclerosis (MS) (relapsing): SubQ:

US labeling: Note: Glatiramer 20 mg/mL and 40 mg/mL formulations are not interchangeable.

MS (relapsing-remitting): 20 mg once daily or 40 mg 3 times per week administered at least 48 hours apart

Canadian labeling: MS (relapsing-remitting or at risk following single demyelinating event): 20 mg once daily

Renal Impairment There are no dosage adjustments provided in the manufacturer's labeling (has not been studied).

Hepatic Impairment There are no dosage adjustments provided in the manufacturer's labeling.

Administration For SubQ administration in the arms, abdomen, hips, or thighs; rotate injection sites to possibly minimize the occurrence of lipoatrophy. Do not administer IV. Administer the 40 mg dose on the same 3 days each week (eg, Monday, Wednesday, Friday) at least 48 hours apart. Allow syringe to stand at room temperature for 20 minutes prior to injection. Discard unused portions.

Dosage Forms Excipient information presented when available (limited, particularly for generics); consult specific product labeling.

Solution Prefilled Syringe, Subcutaneous:

Copaxone: 20 mg/mL (1 mL) [contains mannitol]

Copaxone: 40 mg/mL (1 mL)

Glatopa: 20 mg/mL (1 mL) [contains mannitol]

◆ Glatopa see Glatiramer Acetate on page 840
◆ GlcCerase see Velaglucerase Alfa on page 1883
◆ Gleevec see Imatinib on page 919
◆ Gleostine see Lomustine on page 1096
◆ Gliadel Wafer see Carmustine on page 320
◆ Glibenclamide see GlyBURIDE on page 847

Glimepiride (GLYE me pye ride)

Brand Names: US Amaryl

Brand Names: Canada Amaryl; Apo-Glimepiride; Novo-Glimepiride; PMS-Glimepiride; ratio-Glimepiride; Sandoz-Glimepiride

Pharmacologic Category Antidiabetic Agent, Sulfonylurea

Use Type 2 diabetes mellitus: As an adjunct to diet and exercise to improve glycemic control in adults with type 2 diabetes mellitus

Pregnancy Considerations Adverse events have been observed in some animal reproduction studies. Severe hypoglycemia lasting 4 to 10 days has been noted in infants born to mothers taking a sulfonylurea at the time of delivery.

In women with diabetes, maternal hyperglycemia can be associated with congenital malformations as well as adverse effects in the fetus, neonate, and the mother (ACOG 2005; ADA 2015; Kitzmiller 2008; Metzger 2007). To prevent adverse outcomes, prior to conception and throughout pregnancy maternal blood glucose and HbA$_{1c}$ should be kept as close to target goals as possible but without causing significant hypoglycemia (ACOG 2013; ADA 2015; Blumer 2013; Kitzmiller 2008). Prior to pregnancy, effective contraception should be used until glycemic control is achieved (Kitzmiller 2008). Other agents are currently recommended to treat diabetes in pregnant women (ACOG 2013; Blumer 2013).

Breast-Feeding Considerations It is not known if glimepiride is excreted in breast milk. According to the manufacturer, due to the potential for hypoglycemia in the nursing infant, a decision should be made whether to discontinue nursing or to discontinue the drug, taking into account the importance of treatment to the mother.

Contraindications

Hypersensitivity to glimepiride, any component of the formulation, or sulfonamides; diabetic ketoacidosis (with or without coma)

Note: Although the FDA approved product labeling states this medication is contraindicated with other sulfonamide-containing drug classes, the scientific basis of this statement has been challenged. See "Warnings/Precautions" for more detail.

Documentation of allergenic cross-reactivity for drugs in this class is limited. However, because of similarities in chemical structure and/or pharmacologic actions, the possibility of cross-sensitivity cannot be ruled out with certainty.

Canadian labeling: Additional contraindications (not in U.S. labeling): Pregnancy; breast-feeding; type 1 diabetes; severe renal or hepatic impairment

Warnings/Precautions All sulfonylurea drugs are capable of producing severe hypoglycemia. Hypoglycemia is more likely to occur when caloric intake is deficient, after severe or prolonged exercise, when ethanol is ingested, or when more than one glucose-lowering drug is used. It is also more likely in elderly patients, malnourished patients and in patients with impaired renal or hepatic function; use with caution. Reduce dosage in patients with renal impairment.

Loss of efficacy may be observed following prolonged use as a result of the progression of type 2 diabetes mellitus which results in continued beta cell destruction. In patients who were previously responding to sulfonylurea therapy, consider additional factors which may be contributing to decreased efficacy (eg, inappropriate dose, nonadherence to diet and exercise regimen). If no contributing factors can be identified, consider discontinuing use of the sulfonylurea due to secondary failure of treatment. Additional antidiabetic therapy (eg, insulin) will be required. It may be necessary to discontinue therapy and administer insulin if the patient is exposed to stress (fever, trauma, infection, surgery).

Patients with G6PD deficiency may be at an increased risk of sulfonylurea-induced hemolytic anemia; however, cases have also been described in patients without G6PD deficiency during postmarketing surveillance. Use with caution and consider a nonsulfonylurea alternative in patients with G6PD deficiency. Systemic exposure of glimepiride is increased in patients with CYP2C9*3 allele; dose reductions may be necessary (Niemi, 2002).

Product labeling states oral hypoglycemic drugs may be associated with an increased cardiovascular mortality as compared to treatment with diet alone or diet plus insulin. Data to support this association are limited, and several studies, including a large prospective trial (UKPDS) have not supported an association.

Sulfonamide ("sulfa") allergy: The FDA-approved product labeling for many medications containing a sulfonamide chemical group includes a broad contraindication in patients with a prior allergic reaction to sulfonamides. There is a potential for cross-reactivity between members of a specific class (eg, two antibiotic sulfonamides). However, concerns for cross-reactivity have previously extended to all compounds containing the sulfonamide structure (SO_2NH_2). An expanded understanding of allergic mechanisms indicates cross-reactivity between antibiotic sulfonamides and nonantibiotic sulfonamides may not occur or at the very least this potential is extremely low (Brackett 2004; Johnson 2005; Slatore 2004; Tornero 2004). In particular, mechanisms of cross-reaction due to antibody production (anaphylaxis) are unlikely to occur with nonantibiotic sulfonamides. T-cell-mediated (type IV) reactions (eg, maculopapular rash) are less well understood and it is not possible to completely exclude this potential based on current insights. In cases where prior reactions were severe (Stevens-Johnson syndrome/TEN), some clinicians choose to avoid exposure to these classes.

Adverse Reactions

>10%: Endocrine & metabolic: Hypoglycemia (4% to 20%)

1% to 10%:

Central nervous system: Dizziness (2%), headache

Gastrointestinal: Nausea (5%)

Hepatic: Increased serum ALT (2%)

Respiratory: Flu-like symptoms (5%)

Miscellaneous: Accidental injury (6%)

<1% (Limited to important or life-threatening): Abnormal hepatic function tests, accommodation disturbance (early treatment), agranulocytosis, anaphylaxis, angioedema, anorexia, aplastic anemia, cholestatic jaundice, disulfiram-like reaction, epigastric fullness, hemolytic anemia, hepatic failure, hepatic porphyria, hepatitis, hypersensitivity, hypersensitivity angiitis, hyponatremia, hypotension, leukopenia, maculopapular rash, morbilliform rash, pancytopenia, porphyria cutanea tarda, shock, SIADH, skin photosensitivity, Stevens-Johnson syndrome, thrombocytopenia, weight gain

Drug Interactions

Metabolism/Transport Effects Substrate of CYP2C9 (major); **Note:** Assignment of Major/Minor substrate status based on clinically relevant drug interaction potential

Avoid Concomitant Use

Avoid concomitant use of Glimepiride with any of the following: Mecamylamine

Increased Effect/Toxicity

Glimepiride may increase the levels/effects of: Alcohol (Ethyl); Carbocisteine; Hypoglycemia-Associated Agents; Mecamylamine; Porfimer; Verteporfin; Vitamin K Antagonists

The levels/effects of Glimepiride may be increased by: Alpha-Lipoic Acid; Androgens; Antidiabetic Agents; Antidiabetic Agents (Thiazolidinedione); Beta-Blockers; Ceritinib; Chloramphenicol; Cimetidine; Cyclic Antidepressants; CYP2C9 Inhibitors (Moderate); CYP2C9 Inhibitors (Strong); Dexketoprofen; DPP-IV Inhibitors; Fibric Acid Derivatives; Fluconazole; GLP-1 Agonists; Herbs (Hypoglycemic Properties); Lumacaftor; MAO Inhibitors; Metreleptin; Miconazole (Oral); Mifepristone; Pegvisomant; Probenecid; Quinolone Antibiotics; Ranitidine; Salicylates; Selective Serotonin Reuptake Inhibitors; SGLT2 Inhibitors; Sulfonamide Derivatives; Vitamin K Antagonists; Voriconazole

Decreased Effect

The levels/effects of Glimepiride may be decreased by: Colesevelam; CYP2C9 Inducers (Strong); Dabrafenib; Enzalutamide; Hyperglycemia-Associated Agents; Lumacaftor; Quinolone Antibiotics; Rifampin; Thiazide Diuretics

Food Interactions Ethanol may cause rare disulfiram reactions. Management: Monitor patients.

Storage/Stability Store at 25°C (77°F); excursions permitted between 20°C and 25°C (68°F and 77°F)

Mechanism of Action Stimulates insulin release from the pancreatic beta cells; reduces glucose output from the liver; insulin sensitivity is increased at peripheral target sites

Pharmacodynamics/Kinetics

Onset of action: Peak effect: Blood glucose reductions: 2-3 hours

Duration: 24 hours

Absorption: 100%; delayed when given with food

Distribution: V_d: 8.8 L

Protein binding: >99.5%

Metabolism: Hepatic oxidation via CYP2C9 to M1 metabolite (~33% activity of parent compound); further oxidative metabolism to inactive M2 metabolite

Half-life elimination: 5-9 hours

Time to peak, plasma: 2-3 hours

Excretion: Urine (60%, 80% to 90% as M1 and M2 metabolites); feces (40%, 70% as M1 and M2 metabolites)

Dosing

Adult

Type 2 diabetes: Oral: Initial: 1-2 mg once daily, administered with breakfast or the first main meal; based on response, may increase dose by 1-2 mg every 1-2 weeks up to maximum of 8 mg once daily. If inadequate response to maximal dose, combination therapy with other agents (eg, metformin, insulin) may be considered. Combination therapy is individualized based on glycemic response.

Conversion from therapy with long half-life agents: Observe patient carefully for 1-2 weeks when converting from a longer half-life agent (eg, chlorpropamide) to glimepiride due to overlapping hypoglycemic effects.

Geriatric Type 2 diabetes: Oral: *Initial:* 1 mg once daily; dose titration and maintenance dosing should be conservative to avoid hypoglycemia.

Renal Impairment

U.S. labeling: Initial: 1 mg once daily; titrate carefully based on fasting blood glucose levels

Canadian labeling:

Mild-to-moderate impairment: Initial: 1 mg once daily; titrate carefully based on fasting blood glucose levels

Severe impairment: Use is contraindicated

Hepatic Impairment

U.S. labeling: No dosage adjustment provided in manufacturer's labeling (has not been studied).

Canadian labeling:

Mild-to-moderate impairment: No dosage adjustment provided in manufacturer's labeling (has not been studied).

Severe impairment: Use is contraindicated.

Dietary Considerations Take with breakfast or the first main meal of the day. Individualized medical nutrition therapy (MNT) based on ADA recommendations is an integral part of therapy.

Administration Administer once daily with breakfast or first main meal of the day. Patients that are NPO or require decreased caloric intake may need doses held to avoid hypoglycemia.

Monitoring Parameters Monitor for signs and symptoms of hypoglycemia (fatigue, excessive hunger, profuse sweating, numbness of extremities), fasting blood glucose, hemoglobin A_{1c}

Reference Range

Recommendations for glycemic control in nonpregnant adults with diabetes (ADA, 2015):

HbA_{1c}: <7% (a more aggressive [<6.5%] or less aggressive [<8%] HbA_{1c} goal may be targeted based on patient-specific characteristics)

Preprandial capillary plasma glucose: 80 to 130 mg/dL

Peak postprandial capillary blood glucose: <180 mg/dL

Recommendations for glycemic control in pediatric (all age groups) patients with type 1 diabetes (ADA, 2015):

HbA_{1c}: <7.5% (individualization may be appropriate based on patient-specific characteristics; <7% is reasonable if it can be achieved without excessive hypoglycemia)

Preprandial capillary plasma glucose: 90 to 130 mg/dL

Bedtime and overnight capillary blood glucose: 90 to 150 mg/dL

Dosage Forms Excipient information presented when available (limited, particularly for generics); consult specific product labeling.

Tablet, Oral:

Amaryl: 1 mg [scored]

Amaryl: 2 mg, 4 mg [scored; contains fd&c blue #2 aluminum lake]

Generic: 1 mg, 2 mg, 4 mg

◆ Glimepiride and Pioglitazone *see* Pioglitazone and Glimepiride *on page 1455*

◆ Glimepiride and Pioglitazone Hydrochloride *see* Pioglitazone and Glimepiride *on page 1455*

◆ Glimepiride and Rosiglitazone Maleate *see* Rosiglitazone and Glimepiride *on page 1619*

GlipiZIDE (GLIP i zide)

Brand Names: US GlipiZIDE XL; Glucotrol; Glucotrol XL

Index Terms Glydiazinamide

Pharmacologic Category Antidiabetic Agent, Sulfonylurea

Use

Diabetes mellitus, type 2: Adjunct to diet and exercise to improve glycemic control in adults with type 2 diabetes mellitus (noninsulin dependent, NIDDM).

Limitations of use: Not recommended for the treatment of type 1 diabetes mellitus or diabetic ketoacidosis.

Pregnancy Considerations Adverse events have been observed in some animal reproduction studies. Glipizide was found to cross the placenta in vitro (Elliott 1994). Severe hypoglycemia lasting 4 to 10 days has been noted in infants born to mothers taking a sulfonylurea at the time of delivery.

In women with diabetes, maternal hyperglycemia can be associated with congenital malformations as well as adverse effects in the fetus, neonate, and the mother (ACOG 2005; ADA 2015; Kitzmiller 2008; Metzger 2007). To prevent adverse outcomes, prior to conception and throughout pregnancy maternal blood glucose and HbA_{1c} should be kept as close to target goals as possible but without causing significant hypoglycemia (ACOG 2013; ADA 2015; Blumer 2013; Kitzmiller 2008). Prior to pregnancy, effective contraception should be used until glycemic control is achieved (Kitzmiller 2008). Other agents are currently recommended to treat diabetes in pregnant women (ACOG 2013; Blumer 2013).

The manufacturer recommends if glipizide is used during pregnancy, it should be discontinued at least 1 month before the expected delivery date.

Breast-Feeding Considerations Data from two mother-infant pairs note that glipizide was not detected in breast milk (Feig 2005). According to the manufacturer, due to the potential for hypoglycemia in the nursing infant, a decision should be made whether to discontinue nursing or to discontinue the drug, taking into account the importance of treatment to the mother. Current guidelines note that breast-feeding is encouraged for all women, including those with diabetes (ACOG 2005; Blumer 2013; Metzger 2007). A small snack (such as milk) before nursing may help decrease the risk of hypoglycemia in women with pregestational diabetes (ACOG 2005; ADA 2015; Reader 2004). All types of insulin may be used while breast-feeding and some oral agents, including glipizide, may be acceptable for use as well (Metzger 2007).

Contraindications Hypersensitivity to glipizide, sulfonamide derivatives, or any component of the formulation; type 1 diabetes mellitus (insulin dependent, IDDM); diabetic ketoacidosis (with or without coma)

Warnings/Precautions All sulfonylurea drugs are capable of producing severe hypoglycemia. Hypoglycemia is more likely to occur when caloric intake is deficient, after severe or prolonged exercise, when ethanol is ingested, or when more than one glucose-lowering drug is used. It is also more likely in elderly or debilitated patients, malnourished patients and in patients with impaired renal or hepatic function, adrenal and/or pituitary insufficiency; use with caution. Autonomic neuropathy, advanced age, and concomitant use of beta-blockers or other sympatholytic agents may impair the patient's ability to recognize the signs and symptoms of hypoglycemia; use with caution.

Use with caution in patients with hepatic (hypoglycemia may be prolonged) or renal impairment. It may be necessary to discontinue therapy and administer insulin if the patient is exposed to stress (fever, trauma, infection, surgery). Loss of efficacy may be observed following prolonged use as a result of the progression of type 2 diabetes mellitus which results in continued beta cell destruction. In patients who were previously responding to sulfonylurea therapy, consider additional factors which may be contributing to decreased efficacy (eg, inappropriate dose, nonadherence to diet and exercise regimen). If no contributing factors can be identified, consider discontinuing use of the sulfonylurea due to secondary failure of treatment. Additional antidiabetic therapy (eg, insulin) will be required.

Patients with G6PD deficiency may be at an increased risk of sulfonylurea-induced hemolytic anemia; however, cases have also been described in patients without G6PD deficiency during postmarketing surveillance. Use with caution and consider a nonsulfonylurea alternative in patients with G6PD deficiency.

Product labeling states oral hypoglycemic drugs may be associated with an increased cardiovascular mortality as compared to treatment with diet alone or diet plus insulin. Data to support this association are limited, and several studies, including a large prospective trial (UKPDS) have not supported an association. Avoid use of extended release tablets (Glucotrol XL®) in patients with known stricture/narrowing of the GI tract.

Sulfonamide ("sulfa") allergy: The FDA-approved product labeling for many medications containing a sulfonamide chemical group includes a broad contraindication in patients with a prior allergic reaction to sulfonamides. There is a potential for cross-reactivity between members of a specific class (eg, two antibiotic sulfonamides). However, concerns for cross-reactivity have previously extended to all compounds containing the sulfonamide structure (SO_2NH_2). An expanded understanding of allergic mechanisms indicates cross-reactivity between antibiotic sulfonamides and nonantibiotic sulfonamides may not occur or at the very least this potential is extremely low (Brackett 2004; Johnson 2005; Slatore 2004; Tornero 2004). In particular, mechanisms of cross-reaction due to antibody production (anaphylaxis) are unlikely to occur with nonantibiotic sulfonamides. T-cell-mediated (type IV) reactions (eg, maculopapular rash) are less well understood and it is not possible to completely exclude this potential based on current insights. In cases where prior reactions were severe (Stevens-Johnson syndrome/TEN), some clinicians choose to avoid exposure to these classes. Potentially significant drug-drug interactions may exist, requiring dose or frequency adjustment, additional monitoring and/or selection of alternative therapy.

Adverse Reactions Frequency not always defined.
Cardiovascular: Syncope (<3%)
Central nervous system: Dizziness (2% to 7%), nervousness (4%), anxiety (<3%), depression (<3%), hypoesthesia (<3%), insomnia (<3%), pain (<3%), drowsiness (2%), headache (2%)
Dermatologic: Pruritus (1% to <3%), eczema (1%), erythema (1%), maculopapular eruptions (1%), morbilliform eruptions (1%), rash (1%), urticaria (1%)
Endocrine & metabolic: Hypoglycemia (<3%)
Gastrointestinal: Diarrhea (1% to 5%), flatulence (3%), constipation (1% to <3%), nausea (1% to <3%), dyspepsia (<3%), vomiting (<3%), abdominal pain (1%)
Hepatic: Alkaline phosphatase increased, AST increased, LDH increased
Neuromuscular & skeletal: Tremor (4%), arthralgia (<3%), leg cramps (<3%), myalgia (<3%), paresthesia (<3%)
Ocular: Blurred vision (<3%)
Renal: Blood urea nitrogen increased, creatinine increased
Respiratory: Rhinitis (<3%)
Miscellaneous: Diaphoresis (<3%)

<1% (Limited to important or life-threatening): Agranulocytosis, anorexia, aplastic anemia, arrhythmia, blood in stool, cholestatic jaundice, conjunctivitis, disulfiram-like reaction, edema, gait instability, hemolytic anemia, hypertension, hypertonia, hyponatremia, jaundice, leukopenia, liver injury, migraine, pancytopenia, photosensitivity, porphyria, retinal hemorrhage, SIADH, thrombocytopenia, vertigo

Drug Interactions

Metabolism/Transport Effects Substrate of CYP2C9 (major); **Note:** Assignment of Major/Minor substrate status based on clinically relevant drug interaction potential

Avoid Concomitant Use
Avoid concomitant use of GlipiZIDE with any of the following: Mecamylamine

Increased Effect/Toxicity
GlipiZIDE may increase the levels/effects of: Alcohol (Ethyl); Carbocisteine; Hypoglycemia-Associated Agents; Mecamylamine; Porfimer; Verteporfin; Vitamin K Antagonists

The levels/effects of GlipiZIDE may be increased by: Alpha-Lipoic Acid; Androgens; Antidiabetic Agents; Antidiabetic Agents (Thiazolidinedione); Beta-Blockers; Ceritinib; Chloramphenicol; Cimetidine; Clarithromycin; Cyclic Antidepressants; CYP2C9 Inhibitors (Moderate); CYP2C9 Inhibitors (Strong); Dexketoprofen; DPP-IV Inhibitors; Fibric Acid Derivatives; Fluconazole; GLP-1 Agonists; Herbs (Hypoglycemic Properties); Lumacaftor; MAO Inhibitors; Metreleptin; Miconazole (Oral); Mifepristone; Pegvisomant; Posaconazole; Probenecid; Quinolone Antibiotics; Ranitidine; Salicylates; Selective Serotonin Reuptake Inhibitors; SGLT2 Inhibitors; Sulfonamide Derivatives; Vitamin K Antagonists; Voriconazole

Decreased Effect
The levels/effects of GlipiZIDE may be decreased by: Colesevelam; CYP2C9 Inducers (Strong); Dabrafenib; Enzalutamide; Hyperglycemia-Associated Agents; Lumacaftor; Quinolone Antibiotics; Rifampin; Thiazide Diuretics

Food Interactions
Ethanol: May cause rare disulfiram reactions. Management: Monitor patients.
Food: A delayed release of insulin may occur if glipizide is taken with food. Management: Immediate release tablets should be administered 30 minutes before meals to avoid erratic absorption.

Storage/Stability
Extended release: Store at 68°F to 77°F (20°C to 25°C); excursions permitted between 59°F to 86°F (15°C to 30°C). Protect from moisture and humidity.
Immediate release: Store below 30°C (86°F).

Mechanism of Action Stimulates insulin release from the pancreatic beta cells; reduces glucose output from the liver; insulin sensitivity is increased at peripheral target sites

Pharmacodynamics/Kinetics
Duration: 12 to 24 hours
Absorption: Immediate release: Rapid and complete; delayed with food
Distribution: 10 to 11 L
Protein binding: 98% to 99%; primarily to albumin
Bioavailability: 90% to 100%
Metabolism: Hepatic via CYP2C9; forms metabolites (inactive)
Half-life elimination: 2 to 5 hours
Time to peak: 1 to 3 hours; extended release tablets: 6 to 12 hours
Excretion: Urine (<10% as unchanged drug; 80% as metabolites); feces (10%)

Dosing

Adult

Diabetes mellitus, type 2: Oral:
Immediate release: Initial: 5 mg once daily; titrate in 2.5 to 5 mg increments no more frequently than every few days based on blood glucose response; if once-daily dose is ineffective, may divide the dose; doses >15 mg/day should be administered in divided doses. Maximum recommended once-daily dose: 15 mg; maximum recommended total daily dose: 40 mg (some clinicians recommend a maximum total daily dose of 20 mg [Defronzo 1999]).
Extended release: Initial: 5 mg once daily; start patients at risk for hypoglycemia at 2.5 mg; adjust dose based on glycemic control; maximum: 20 mg/day.

When transferring from immediate release to extended release glipizide: May switch the total daily dose of immediate release to the nearest equivalent daily dose of the extended release tablet and administer once daily.

When transferring from insulin to glipizide immediate release:
Current insulin requirement ≤20 units: Discontinue insulin and initiate glipizide at usual dose
Current insulin requirement >20 units: Decrease insulin by 50% and initiate glipizide at usual dose; gradually decrease insulin dose based on patient response.

Conversion from therapy with long half-life agents: Observe patient carefully for 1 to 2 weeks when converting from a longer half-life agent (eg, chlorpropamide) to glipizide due to overlapping hypoglycemic effects.

Geriatric
Immediate release: Initial: 2.5 mg once daily; consider titrating by 2.5 to 5 mg/day at 1- to 2-week intervals
Extended release: 2.5 mg once daily; maintenance dosing should be conservative to avoid hypoglycemia.

Renal Impairment There are no specific dosage adjustments provided in the manufacturer's labeling. Glipizide is primarily converted to inactive metabolites and may be less likely to cause hypoglycemia in patients with renal impairment compared to other sulfonylureas. A reduced dose may be necessary (Alsahli 2015). Avoidance of sustained release formulation has been suggested. (Snyder 2004)

Hepatic Impairment Initial: 2.5 mg once daily

Dietary Considerations Take immediate release tablets 30 minutes before meals (preferably before breakfast if once-daily dosing); extended release tablets should be taken with breakfast or the first meal of the day. Individualized medical nutrition therapy (MNT) based on ADA recommendations is an integral part of therapy.

Administration
Patients that are NPO or require decreased caloric intake may need doses held to avoid hypoglycemia.
Extended release: Administer with breakfast or the first meal of the day; swallow tablets whole, do not chew, divide or crush.
Immediate release: Administer 30 minutes before a meal (preferably before breakfast if once-daily dosing) to achieve greatest reduction in postprandial hyperglycemia.

Monitoring Parameters Signs and symptoms of hypoglycemia (fatigue, excessive hunger, profuse sweating, numbness of extremities), blood glucose, hemoglobin A_{1c} every 3 months for unstable patients and twice yearly for stable patients

Reference Range
Recommendations for glycemic control in nonpregnant adults with diabetes (ADA 2015):
HbA_{1c}: <7% (a more aggressive [<6.5%] or less aggressive [<8%] HbA_{1c} goal may be targeted based on patient-specific characteristics)
Preprandial capillary plasma glucose: 80 to 130 mg/dL
Peak postprandial capillary blood glucose: <180 mg/dL

Recommendations for glycemic control in pediatric (all age groups) patients with type 1 diabetes (ADA 2015):
HbA_{1c}: <7.5% (individualization may be appropriate based on patient-specific characteristics; <7% is reasonable if it can be achieved without excessive hypoglycemia)
Preprandial capillary plasma glucose: 90 to 130 mg/dL
Bedtime and overnight capillary blood glucose: 90 to 150 mg/dL

Dosage Forms Excipient information presented when available (limited, particularly for generics); consult specific product labeling.
Tablet, Oral:
Glucotrol: 5 mg, 10 mg [scored]
Generic: 5 mg, 10 mg
Tablet Extended Release 24 Hour, Oral:
GlipiZIDE XL: 2.5 mg, 5 mg, 10 mg
Glucotrol XL: 2.5 mg, 5 mg, 10 mg
Generic: 2.5 mg, 5 mg, 10 mg

♦ GlipiZIDE XL see GlipiZIDE on page 843

Glipizide and Metformin
(GLIP i zide & met FOR min)

Index Terms Glipizide and Metformin Hydrochloride; Metaglip; Metformin and Glipizide
Pharmacologic Category Antidiabetic Agent, Biguanide; Antidiabetic Agent, Sulfonylurea
Use Diabetes mellitus, type 2: Indicated as an adjunct to diet and exercise to improve glycemic control in adults with type 2 diabetes mellitus (noninsulin dependent, NIDDM)

Dosing
Adult Diabetes mellitus, type 2:
Patients inadequately controlled on diet and exercise alone: Initial dose: Glipizide 2.5 mg/metformin 250 mg once daily with a meal. In patients with fasting plasma glucose (FPG) 280-320 mg/dL, initiate therapy with glipizide 2.5 mg/metformin 500 mg twice daily.
Note: Increase dose by 1 tablet/day every 2 weeks (maximum daily dose: Glipizide 10 mg/metformin 2000 mg in divided doses)
Patients inadequately controlled on a sulfonylurea and/or metformin: Initial dose: Glipizide 2.5 mg/metformin 500 mg or glipizide 5 mg/metformin 500 mg twice daily with morning and evening meals; starting dose should not exceed current daily dose of glipizide (or sulfonylurea equivalent) and/or metformin.
Note: Increase dose in increments of no more than glipizide 5 mg/metformin 500 mg (maximum daily dose: Glipizide 20 mg/metformin 2000 mg)

Geriatric Conservative doses are recommended in the elderly due to potentially decreased renal function; **do not titrate to maximum dose**; should not be used in patients ≥80 years unless renal function is verified as normal

Renal Impairment
Manufacturer's labeling: Serum creatinine (SCr) ≥1.5 mg/dL (males) or ≥1.4 mg/dL (females) or abnormal CrCl (not defined): Use is contraindicated.
Alternate recommendations: **Note:** The United Kingdom National Institute for Health and Clinical Excellence (NICE) Guidelines recommend prescribing metformin with caution in those patients who are at risk of sudden deterioration in renal function and at risk of an estimated glomerular filtration rate (eGFR) <45 mL/minute/1.73 m^2 (NICE 2008]). Some evidence suggests that use of metformin is unsafe when eGFR <30 mL/minute/1.73 m^2 (calculated using MDRD) (Shaw 2007). A review of the available data by members of the American Diabetes Association proposed the following recommendations based on eGFR (Lipska 2011):
eGFR ≥60 mL/minute/1.73 m^2: No contraindications; monitor renal function annually.
eGFR ≥45 to <60 mL/minute/1.73 m^2: Continue use; monitor renal function every 3 to 6 months.
eGFR ≥30 to <45 mL/minute/1.73 m^2: In patients currently receiving metformin, use with caution, consider dosage reduction (eg, 50% reduction or 50% of maximal dose), monitor renal function every 3 months. Do not initiate therapy in patients with eGFR <45 mL/minute/1.73 m^2.
eGFR <30 mL/minute/1.73 m^2: Discontinue use.

Hepatic Impairment The manufacturer recommends to avoid metformin since liver disease is considered a risk factor for the development of lactic acidosis during metformin therapy. However, continued use of metformin in diabetics with liver dysfunction, including cirrhosis, has been used successfully and may be associated with a survival benefit in carefully selected patients; use cautiously in patients at risk for lactic acidosis (eg, renal impairment, alcohol use) (Brackett 2010; Zhang 2014). Glipizide undergoes hepatic metabolism and use of a lower initial and maintenance dose should be considered.

Additional Information Complete prescribing information should be consulted for additional detail.

Dosage Forms Excipient information presented when available (limited, particularly for generics); consult specific product labeling.
Tablet, oral: 2.5/250: Glipizide 2.5 mg and metformin hydrochloride 250 mg; 2.5/500: Glipizide 2.5 mg and metformin hydrochloride 500 mg; 5/500: Glipizide 5 mg and metformin hydrochloride 500 mg

♦ Glipizide and Metformin Hydrochloride see Glipizide and Metformin on page 845

♦ Glivec see Imatinib on page 919

♦ Gln see Glutamine on page 847

♦ GlucaGen (Can) see Glucagon on page 845

♦ GlucaGen Diagnostic see Glucagon on page 845

♦ GlucaGen HypoKit see Glucagon on page 845

Glucagon (GLOO ka gon)

Brand Names: US GlucaGen Diagnostic; GlucaGen HypoKit; Glucagon Emergency
Brand Names: Canada GlucaGen; GlucaGen HypoKit
Index Terms Glucagon Hydrochloride
Pharmacologic Category Antidote; Antidote, Hypoglycemia; Diagnostic Agent

◄

Use

Diagnostic aid: As a diagnostic aid during radiologic examinations to temporarily inhibit movement of the GI tract in adults.

Hypoglycemia: Treatment of severe hypoglycemia in pediatric and adult patients. **Note:** The American Diabetes Association (ADA) recommends that glucagon be prescribed for all diabetic patients at significant risk of severe hypoglycemia; caregivers or family members of these patients should be trained on how to administer glucagon (ADA 2015).

Limitations of use: Products not packaged with a syringe and diluent necessary for rapid preparation and administration during an emergency outside of a health care facility are not indicated for the emergency treatment of hypoglycemia.

Pregnancy Considerations Adverse events have not been observed in animal reproduction studies.

Breast-Feeding Considerations Glucagon is not absorbed from the GI tract and therefore, it is unlikely adverse effects would occur in a breast-feeding infant.

Contraindications Known hypersensitivity to glucagon, lactose, or any component of the formulation; pheochromocytoma; insulinoma; glucagonoma (excluding GlucaGen)

Warnings/Precautions Use of glucagon is contraindicated in insulinoma; exogenous glucagon may cause an initial rise in blood glucose followed by rebound hypoglycemia. Use of glucagon is contraindicated in pheochromocytoma; exogenous glucagon may cause the release of catecholamines, resulting in an increase in blood pressure. Use caution with prolonged fasting, starvation, adrenal insufficiency, glucagonoma, or chronic hypoglycemia; levels of glucose stores in liver may be decreased. Use of glucagon is contraindicated in patients with glucagonoma (excluding GlucaGen). Allergic reactions including skin rash and anaphylactic shock (with hypotension and respiratory difficulties) have been reported; reactions have generally been associated with endoscopic patients. Use with caution in patients with cardiac disease. Use caution if using as diagnostic aid in patients with diabetes on insulin; may cause hyperglycemia. Supplemental carbohydrates should be given to patients who respond to glucagon for severe hypoglycemia to prevent secondary hypoglycemia.

In patients with hypoglycemia secondary to insulin or sulfonylurea overdose, dextrose should be immediately administered; if IV access cannot be established or if dextrose is not available, glucagon may be considered as alternative acute treatment until dextrose can be administered.

May contain lactose; avoid administration in hereditary galactose intolerance, Lapp lactase deficiency, or glucose-galactose malabsorption. Potentially significant interactions may exist, requiring dose or frequency adjustment, additional monitoring, and/or selection of alternative therapy.

Adverse Reactions Frequency not defined.

Cardiovascular: Hypertension, hypotension (up to 2 hours after GI procedures), increased blood pressure, increased pulse, tachycardia

Gastrointestinal: Nausea, vomiting (high incidence with rapid administration of high doses)

Miscellaneous: Anaphylaxis, hypersensitivity reaction

<1% (Limited to important or life-threatening): Hypoglycemia, hypoglycemic coma, respiratory distress, urticaria

Drug Interactions

Metabolism/Transport Effects None known.

Avoid Concomitant Use

Avoid concomitant use of Glucagon with any of the following: Anticholinergic Agents

Increased Effect/Toxicity

Glucagon may increase the levels/effects of: Vitamin K Antagonists

The levels/effects of Glucagon may be increased by: Anticholinergic Agents

Decreased Effect

Glucagon may decrease the levels/effects of: Antidiabetic Agents

The levels/effects of Glucagon may be decreased by: Indomethacin

Food Interactions Glucagon depletes glycogen stores.

Preparation for Administration Reconstitute powder for injection by adding 1 mL of manufacturer-supplied sterile diluent or sterile water for injection to a vial containing 1 unit of the drug, to provide solutions containing 1 mg of glucagon/mL. Shake vial gently to dissolve. Solution for infusion may be prepared by reconstitution with and further dilution in NS or D_5W (Love, 1998).

Storage/Stability Prior to reconstitution, store at 20°C to 25°C (69°F to 77°F) for up to 24 months. Do not freeze. Protect from light. Use reconstituted solution immediately; discard unused portion.

Mechanism of Action Stimulates adenylate cyclase to produce increased cyclic AMP, which promotes hepatic glycogenolysis and gluconeogenesis, causing a raise in blood glucose levels; antihypoglycemic effect requires preexisting hepatic glycogen stores. Extra hepatic effects of glucagon include relaxation of the smooth muscle of the stomach, duodenum, small bowel, and colon.

Pharmacodynamics/Kinetics

Onset of action:

Blood glucose levels: Peak effect: IV: 5 to 20 minutes; IM: 30 minutes; SubQ: 30 to 45 minutes

GI relaxation: IV: 45 seconds; IM: 4 to 10 minutes

Duration:

Glucose elevation: IV, IM, SubQ: 60 to 90 minutes

GI relaxation: IV: 9 to 25 minutes; IM: 12 to 32 minutes

Distribution: V_d: ~0.25 L/kg

Metabolism: Primarily hepatic; some inactivation occurring renally and in plasma

Half-life elimination, plasma: IV: 8 to 18 minutes; IM (apparent): 26 to 45 minutes

Time to peak: IM: ~10 to 12.5 minutes; SubQ: 20 minutes

Dosing

Adult & Geriatric

Diagnostic aid:

Relaxation of stomach, duodenal bulb, duodenum, and small bowel:

IM: 1 mg

IV: 0.2 to 0.5 mg

Relaxation of colon:

IM: 1 to 2 mg

IV: 0.5 to 0.75 mg

Hypoglycemia: IM, IV, SubQ: 1 mg; may repeat in 15 minutes as needed. **Note:** IV dextrose should be administered as soon as it is available; if patient fails to respond to glucagon, IV dextrose must be given.

Anaphylactic reaction (refractory) in patients on beta-blocker therapy (off-label use): IV: Initial: 1 to 5 mg; followed by an infusion of 5 to 15 mcg/minute; titrate the infusion rate to achieve an adequate clinical response (Lieberman 2010).

Beta-blocker- or calcium channel blocker-induced myocardial depression (with or without hypotension) unresponsive to standard measures (off-label use; AHA [Vanden Hoek 2010]; Bailey 2003): IV: 3 to 10 mg (or 0.05 to 0.15 mg/kg) bolus followed by an infusion of 3 to 5 mg/hour (or 0.05 to 0.1 mg/kg/hour); titrate infusion rate to achieve adequate clinical response (AHA [Vanden Hoek 2010])

Pediatric

Hypoglycemia: Note: IV dextrose should be administered as soon as it is available; if patient fails to respond to glucagon, IV dextrose must be given.

Infants, Children, and Adolescents: IM, IV, SubQ:

Glucagon Emergency Kit:

<20 kg: 0.5 mg or 0.02 to 0.03 mg/kg/dose; may repeat in 15 minutes as needed

≥20 kg: 1 mg; may repeat in 15 minutes as needed

GlucaGen:

Age-based dosing (if weight is unknown):

Infants and Children <6 years: 0.5 mg; may repeat in 15 minutes if needed

Children ≥6 years and Adolescents: 1 mg; may repeat in 15 minutes if needed

Weight-based dosing:

<25 kg: 0.5 mg; may repeat in 15 minutes if needed

≥25 kg: 1 mg; may repeat in 15 minutes if needed

Anaphylactic reaction (refractory) in patients on beta-blocker therapy (off-label use): Children: IV: Initial: 20 to 30 **mcg/kg** (maximum: 1 mg); followed by an infusion of 5 to 15 **mcg/minute**; titrate the infusion rate to achieve an adequate clinical response (Lieberman 2010)

Beta-blocker- or calcium channel blocker-induced myocardial depression (with or without hypotension) unresponsive to standard measures (off-label use): IV:

Children: Initial bolus of 30 to 150 **mcg**/kg followed by an infusion of 70 **mcg**/kg/hour (maximum: 5 mg/hour) (Hegenbarth 2008)

Adolescents: Initial: 5 to 10 mg over several minutes followed by infusion of 1 to 5 mg/hour (Hegenbarth 2008; PALS [Kleinman 2010])

Renal Impairment There are no dosage adjustments provided in the manufacturer's labeling.

Hepatic Impairment There are no dosage adjustments provided in the manufacturer's labeling.

Dietary Considerations Administer oral carbohydrates to patient as soon as possible after response to treatment.

Usual Infusion Concentrations: Adult IV infusion: 4 mg in 50 mL (concentration: 0.08 mg/mL) of D$_5$W

Administration

Diagnostic aid: For IM or IV administration. If given IV, administer over 1 minute. After the diagnostic procedure, administer oral carbohydrates to patients who have been fasting, if this is compatible with the diagnostic procedure applied. Bolus IV doses >1 mg are not recommended.

Hypoglycemia: For SubQ, IM, or IV administration in the upper arms, thighs, or buttocks. Administer fast-acting and long-acting oral carbohydrates to patient as soon as possible after response to treatment.

IV: Rapid injection may be associated with increased nausea and vomiting; place patient in lateral recumbent position to protect airway (Liberman 2010) and to prevent choking when consciousness returns.

Anaphylactic reaction (refractory) in patients on beta-blocker therapy: Administer bolus over 5 minutes (Lieberman 2010).

Beta-blocker/calcium channel blocker toxicity: Administer bolus over 3 to 5 minutes; continuous infusions may be used. Ensure adequate supply available to continue therapy (AHA [Vanden Hoek 2010]).

Monitoring Parameters Blood pressure, blood glucose, ECG, heart rate, mentation; signs or symptoms of a hypersensitivity reaction.

Additional Information 1 unit = 1 mg

Dosage Forms Excipient information presented when available (limited, particularly for generics); consult specific product labeling.

Kit, Injection:
Glucagon Emergency: 1 mg
Solution Reconstituted, Injection, as hydrochloride:
GlucaGen Diagnostic: 1 mg (1 ea)
GlucaGen HypoKit: 1 mg (1 ea)
Generic: 1 mg (1 ea)

◆ Glucagon Emergency see Glucagon on page 845
◆ Glucagon Hydrochloride see Glucagon on page 845

Glucarpidase (gloo KAR pid ase)

Brand Names: US Voraxaze
Index Terms Carboxypeptidase-G2; CPDG2; CPG2; Voraxaze
Pharmacologic Category Antidote; Enzyme
Use Treatment of toxic plasma methotrexate concentrations (>1 micromole/L) in patients with delayed clearance due to renal impairment

Note: Due to the risk of subtherapeutic methotrexate exposure, glucarpidase is **NOT** indicated when methotrexate clearance is within expected range (plasma methotrexate concentration ≤2 standard deviations of mean methotrexate excretion curve specific for dose administered) **or** with normal renal function or mild renal impairment.

Prescribing and Access Restrictions Voraxaze® is distributed through ASD Healthcare; procurement information is available (24 hours a day; 365 days a year) at 1-855-7-VORAXAZE (1-855-786-7292). Voraxaze® is also commercially available in the U.S. through certain pharmacy wholesalers on a drop-ship basis; orders will only be processed during business hours for overnight delivery. For additional information, refer to http://www.btgplc.com/products/specialty-pharmaceuticals/voraxaze.

Dosing

Adult & Geriatric

Methotrexate toxicity: IV: 50 units/kg (Buchen, 2005; Widemann, 1997; Widemann, 2010)

Intrathecal methotrexate overdose (off-label route/use): Intrathecal: 2000 units as soon as possible after accidental methotrexate overdose (Widemann, 2004)

Pediatric

Methotrexate toxicity: IV: Refer to adult dosing.
Intrathecal methotrexate overdose (off-label route/use): Intrathecal: Refer to adult dosing.

Renal Impairment No dosage adjustment necessary.

Hepatic Impairment There are no dosage adjustments provided in the manufacturer's labeling (has not been studied).

Additional Information Complete prescribing information should be consulted for additional detail.

Dosage Forms Excipient information presented when available (limited, particularly for generics); consult specific product labeling.

Solution Reconstituted, Intravenous [preservative free]:
Voraxaze: 1000 units (1 ea)

◆ Glucobay (Can) see Acarbose on page 24
◆ GlucoNorm (Can) see Repaglinide on page 1569
◆ Glucophage see MetFORMIN on page 1156

◆ Glucophage XR see MetFORMIN on page 1156
◆ Glucotrol see GlipiZIDE on page 843
◆ Glucotrol XL see GlipiZIDE on page 843
◆ Glucovance see Glyburide and Metformin on page 849
◆ Glulisine Insulin see Insulin Glulisine on page 957
◆ Glumetza see MetFORMIN on page 1156

Glutamine (GLOO ta meen)

Brand Names: US NutreStore; Sympt-X G.I. [OTC]; Sympt-X [OTC]
Index Terms Gln; L-Glutamine
Pharmacologic Category Amino Acid; Gastrointestinal Agent, Miscellaneous
Use

NutreStore™: Treatment of short bowel syndrome (SBS) when used in combination with specialized nutritional support and growth hormone therapy

OTC products: Medical food used to promote GI tract healing and nutritional supplementation with GI disorders, HIV/AIDS, cancer, and other critical illnesses

Dosing

Adult & Geriatric

Nutritional supplement (Enterex® Glutapak-10®, Resource® GlutaSolve®, Sympt-X, Sympt-X G.I.): Oral: Average dose: 10 g 3 times/day; dosing range: 5-30 g/day

Short bowel syndrome (NutreStore™): Oral: 30 g/day administered as 5 g 6 times/day (every 2-3 hours while awake) for up to 16 weeks; to be used in combination with growth hormone and nutritional support

Renal Impairment No dosage adjustment provided in manufacturer's labeling.

Hepatic Impairment No dosage adjustment provided in manufacturer's labeling; use with caution.

Additional Information Complete prescribing information should be consulted for additional detail.

Dosage Forms Excipient information presented when available (limited, particularly for generics); consult specific product labeling. [DSC] = Discontinued product

Capsule, Oral:
Generic: 500 mg
Packet, Oral:
NutreStore: 5 g (84 ea)
Sympt-X: 10 g (60 ea [DSC])
Sympt-X G.I.: 10 g (60 ea)
Powder, Oral:
Sympt-X: (480 g)
Tablet, Oral:
Generic: 500 mg

◆ Glybenclamide see GlyBURIDE on page 847
◆ Glybenzcyclamide see GlyBURIDE on page 847

GlyBURIDE (GLYE byoor ide)

Brand Names: US Diabeta; Glynase
Brand Names: Canada Apo-Glyburide; Ava-Glyburide; DiaBeta; Dom-Glyburide; Euglucon; Mylan-Glybe; PMS-Glyburide; PRO-Glyburide; ratio-Glyburide; Riva-Glyburide; Sandoz-Glyburide; Teva-Glyburide
Index Terms Diabeta; Glibenclamide; Glybenclamide; Glybenzcyclamide; Micronase
Pharmacologic Category Antidiabetic Agent, Sulfonylurea
Use Type 2 diabetes mellitus: Adjunct to diet and exercise to improve glycemic control in adults with type 2 diabetes mellitus (noninsulin dependent, NIDDM)
Pregnancy Considerations Outcomes of animal reproduction studies differ by manufacturer labeling. Glyburide crosses the placenta. Some pharmacokinetic properties of glyburide may change during pregnancy (Hebert 2009).

Severe hypoglycemia lasting 4 to 10 days has been noted in infants born to mothers taking a sulfonylurea at the time of delivery. Additional adverse maternal and fetal events have been noted in some studies and may be influenced by maternal glycemic control and/or differences in study design (Bertini 2005; Ekpebegh 2007; Joy 2012; Langer 2000; Langer 2005).

In women with diabetes, maternal hyperglycemia can be associated with congenital malformations as well as adverse effects in the fetus, neonate, and the mother (ACOG 2005; ADA 2015; Kitzmiller 2008; Metzger 2007). To prevent adverse outcomes, prior to conception and throughout pregnancy maternal blood glucose and HbA$_{1c}$ should be kept as close to target goals as possible but without causing significant hypoglycemia (ACOG 2013; ADA 2015; Blumer 2013; Kitzmiller 2008). Prior to

pregnancy, effective contraception should be used until glycemic control is achieved (Kitzmiller 2008).

Glyburide may be used to treat GDM when nonpharmacologic therapy is not effective in maintaining glucose control (ACOG 2013; ADA 2015; Blumer 2013). Women with type 2 diabetes are usually treated with insulin prior to and during pregnancy (Blumer 2013). According to the manufacturer, if glyburide is used during pregnancy, it should be discontinued at least 2 weeks before the expected delivery date.

Breast-Feeding Considerations Data from initial studies note that glyburide was not detected in breast milk (Feig 2005). According to the manufacturer, due to the potential for hypoglycemia in the nursing infant, a decision should be made whether to discontinue nursing or to discontinue the drug, taking into account the importance of treatment to the mother. Current guidelines note that breast-feeding is encouraged for all women, including those with diabetes (ACOG 2005; Blumer 2013; Metzger 2007). A small snack (such as milk) before nursing may help decrease the risk of hypoglycemia in women with pregestational diabetes (ACOG 2005; ADA 2015; Reader 2004). Glyburide may be used in breast-feeding women (Blumer 2013; Metzger 2007).

Contraindications

Hypersensitivity to glyburide or any component of the formulation; type 1 diabetes mellitus or diabetic ketoacidosis, with or without coma; concomitant use with bosentan.

Canadian labeling: Additional contraindications (not in U.S. labeling): Diabetic precoma or coma, stress conditions (eg, severe infections, trauma, surgery); liver disease or frank jaundice; renal impairment; pregnancy; breast-feeding.

Documentation of allergenic cross-reactivity for sulfonylureas is limited. However, because of similarities in chemical structure and/or pharmacologic actions, the possibility of cross-sensitivity cannot be ruled out with certainty.

Warnings/Precautions All sulfonylurea drugs are capable of producing severe hypoglycemia. Hypoglycemia is more likely to occur when caloric intake is deficient, after severe or prolonged exercise, when ethanol is ingested, or when more than one glucose-lowering drug is used. It is also more likely in elderly patients, malnourished, or debilitated patients and in patients with severe renal or hepatic impairment; adrenal and/or pituitary insufficiency; use with caution.

It may be necessary to discontinue therapy and administer insulin if the patient is exposed to stress (fever, trauma, infection, surgery). Loss of efficacy may be observed following prolonged use as a result of the progression of type 2 diabetes mellitus which results in continued beta cell destruction. In patients who were previously responding to sulfonylurea therapy, consider additional factors which may be contributing to decreased efficacy (eg, inappropriate dose, nonadherence to diet and exercise regimen). If no contributing factors can be identified, consider discontinuing use of the sulfonylurea due to secondary failure of treatment. Additional antidiabetic therapy (eg, insulin) will be required.

Avoid use in elderly patients due to increased risk of prolonged hypoglycemia (Beers Criteria). If therapy is initiated, dosing should be conservative; monitor closely for hypoglycemia.

Product labeling states oral hypoglycemic drugs may be associated with an increased cardiovascular mortality as compared to treatment with diet alone or diet plus insulin. Data to support this association are limited, and several studies, including a large prospective trial (UKPDS) have not supported an association.

Patients with G6PD deficiency may be at an increased risk of sulfonylurea-induced hemolytic anemia; however, cases have also been described in patients without G6PD deficiency during postmarketing surveillance. Use with caution and consider a nonsulfonylurea alternative in patients with G6PD deficiency. Use caution in advanced renal insufficiency due to accumulation of active metabolites (Snyder 2004).

Micronized glyburide tablets are **not** bioequivalent to *conventional* glyburide tablets; retitration should occur if patients are being transferred to a different glyburide formulation (eg, micronized-to-conventional or vice versa) or from other hypoglycemic agents.

Sulfonamide ("sulfa") allergy: The FDA-approved product labeling for many medications containing a sulfonamide chemical group includes a broad contraindication in patients with a prior allergic reaction to sulfonamides.

There is a potential for cross-reactivity between members of a specific class (eg, two antibiotic sulfonamides). However, concerns for cross-reactivity have previously extended to all compounds containing the sulfonamide structure (SO_2NH_2). An expanded understanding of allergic mechanisms indicates cross-reactivity between antibiotic sulfonamides and nonantibiotic sulfonamides may not occur or at the very least this potential is extremely low (Brackett 2004; Johnson 2005; Slatore 2004; Tornero 2004). In particular, mechanisms of cross-reaction due to antibody production (anaphylaxis) are unlikely to occur with nonantibiotic sulfonamides. T-cell-mediated (type IV) reactions (eg, maculopapular rash) are less well understood and it is not possible to completely exclude this potential based on current insights. In cases where prior reactions were severe (Stevens-Johnson syndrome/TEN), some clinicians choose to avoid exposure to these classes.

Adverse Reactions Frequency not defined.

Cardiovascular: Vasculitis

Central nervous system: Dizziness, headache

Dermatologic: Angioedema, erythema, maculopapular eruptions, morbilliform eruptions, photosensitivity reaction, pruritus, purpura, rash, urticaria

Endocrine & metabolic: Disulfiram-like reaction, hypoglycemia, hyponatremia (SIADH reported with other sulfonylureas)

Gastrointestinal: Anorexia, constipation, diarrhea, epigastric fullness, heartburn, nausea

Genitourinary: Nocturia

Hematologic: Agranulocytosis, aplastic anemia, hemolytic anemia, leukopenia, pancytopenia, porphyria cutanea tarda, thrombocytopenia

Hepatic: Cholestatic jaundice, hepatitis, liver failure, transaminase increased

Neuromuscular & skeletal: Arthralgia, myalgia, paresthesia

Ocular: Blurred vision

Renal: Diuretic effect (minor)

Miscellaneous: Allergic reaction

Drug Interactions

Metabolism/Transport Effects Substrate of CYP2C9 (major); **Note:** Assignment of Major/Minor substrate status based on clinically relevant drug interaction potential; **Inhibits** CYP2C8 (weak)

Avoid Concomitant Use

Avoid concomitant use of GlyBURIDE with any of the following: Amodiaquine; Bosentan; Mecamylamine

Increased Effect/Toxicity

GlyBURIDE may increase the levels/effects of: Alcohol (Ethyl); Amodiaquine; Bosentan; Carbocisteine; CycloSPORINE (Systemic); Hypoglycemia-Associated Agents; Mecamylamine; Porfimer; Verteporfin; Vitamin K Antagonists

The levels/effects of GlyBURIDE may be increased by: Alpha-Lipoic Acid; Androgens; Antidiabetic Agents; Antidiabetic Agents (Thiazolidinedione); Beta-Blockers; Ceritinib; Chloramphenicol; Cimetidine; Clarithromycin; Cyclic Antidepressants; CYP2C9 Inhibitors (Moderate); CYP2C9 Inhibitors (Strong); Dexketoprofen; DPP-IV Inhibitors; Fibric Acid Derivatives; Fluconazole; GLP-1 Agonists; Herbs (Hypoglycemic Properties); Lumacaftor; MAO Inhibitors; Metreleptin; Miconazole (Oral); Mifepristone; Pegvisomant; Probenecid; Quinolone Antibiotics; Ranitidine; Salicylates; Selective Serotonin Reuptake Inhibitors; SGLT2 Inhibitors; Sulfonamide Derivatives; Vitamin K Antagonists; Voriconazole

Decreased Effect

GlyBURIDE may decrease the levels/effects of: Bosentan

The levels/effects of GlyBURIDE may be decreased by: Bosentan; Colesevelam; CycloSPORINE (Systemic); CYP2C9 Inducers (Strong); Dabrafenib; Enzalutamide; Hyperglycemia-Associated Agents; Lumacaftor; Quinolone Antibiotics; Rifampin; Thiazide Diuretics

Food Interactions Ethanol may cause rare disulfiram reactions. Management: Monitor patients.

Storage/Stability

Conventional tablets (Diaβeta): Store at 25°C (77°F); excursions are permitted between 15°C and 30°C (59°F and 86°F).

Micronized tablets (Glynase PresTab): Store at 20°C to 25°C (68°F to 77°F).

Mechanism of Action Stimulates insulin release from the pancreatic beta cells; reduces glucose output from the liver; insulin sensitivity is increased at peripheral target sites

Pharmacodynamics/Kinetics

Onset of action: Serum insulin levels begin to increase 15-60 minutes after a single dose

Duration: ≤24 hours

Absorption: Significant within 1 hour

Protein binding, plasma: Extensive, primarily to albumin

Metabolism: Hepatic; forms metabolites (weakly active)

Bioavailability: Variable among oral dosage forms

Half-life elimination: Diaβeta: 10 hours; Glynase PresTab: ~4 hours; may be prolonged with renal or hepatic impairment

Time to peak, serum: Adults: 2-4 hours

Excretion: Feces (50%) and urine (50%) as metabolites

Dosing

Adult Micronized glyburide tablets are **not** bioequivalent to conventional glyburide tablets; retitration should occur if patients are being transferred to a different glyburide formulation (eg, micronized-to-conventional or vice versa) or from other hypoglycemic agents. When converting to glyburide from other oral hypoglycemic agents with a long half-life (eg, chlorpropamide), observe patient carefully for 2 weeks due to overlapping hypoglycemic effects.

Type 2 diabetes: Oral:

Conventional tablets (Diaβeta):

Initial: 2.5-5 mg daily, administered with breakfast or the first main meal of the day. In patients who are more sensitive to hypoglycemic drugs, start at 1.25 mg daily.

Adjustment: Increase in increments of no more than 2.5 mg daily at weekly intervals based on the patient's blood glucose response

Maintenance: 1.25-20 mg daily given as single or divided doses. Some patients (especially those receiving >10 mg daily) may have a more satisfactory response with twice-daily dosing. Maximum: 20 mg daily

Micronized tablets (Glynase PresTab):

Initial: 1.5-3 mg daily, administered with breakfast or the first main meal of the day. In patients who are more sensitive to hypoglycemic drugs, start at 0.75 mg daily. Increase in increments of no more than 1.5 mg daily in weekly intervals based on the patient's blood glucose response.

Maintenance: 0.75-12 mg daily given as a single dose or in divided doses. Some patients (especially those receiving >6 mg daily) may have a more satisfactory response with twice-daily dosing. Maximum: 12 mg daily

Management of noninsulin-dependent diabetes mellitus in patients previously maintained on insulin: Oral: Initial dosage dependent upon current insulin dosage, see table.

Dose Conversion: Insulin to Glyburide

Current Daily Insulin Dosage (units daily)	Initial Glyburide Dosage Conventional Formulation (mg daily)	Initial Glyburide Dosage Micronized Formulation (mg daily)	Insulin Dosage Change (after glyburide started)
<20	2.5-5	1.5-3	Discontinue
20-40	5	3	Discontinue
>40	5 (increase in increments of 1.25-2.5 mg every 2-10 days)	3 (increase in increments of 0.75-1.5 mg every 2-10 days)	Reduce insulin dosage by 50% (gradually taper off insulin as glyburide dosage increased)

Geriatric

Conventional tablets (Diaβeta): Oral: Initial: 1.25 mg daily. Conservative initial and maintenance doses are recommended to avoid hypoglycemic reactions.

Micronized tablets (Glynase PresTab): Initial: 0.75 mg daily. Conservative initial and maintenance doses are recommended to avoid hypoglycemic reactions.

Renal Impairment There are no specific dosage adjustments provided in the manufacturer's labeling; however, use in patients with eGFR <60 mL/minute is not recommended (Alsahli 2015).

Hepatic Impairment There are no dosage adjustments provided in the manufacturer's labeling; however, use conservative initial and maintenance doses.

Dietary Considerations Should be taken with meals at the same time each day (twice-daily dosing may be beneficial if conventional glyburide doses are >10 mg or micronized glyburide doses are >6 mg). Individualized medical nutrition therapy (MNT) based on ADA recommendations is an integral part of therapy.

Administration Administer with meals at the same time each day (twice-daily dosing may be beneficial if conventional glyburide doses are >10 mg or micronized glyburide doses are >6 mg). Patients that are NPO or require decreased caloric intake may need doses held to avoid hypoglycemia.

Monitoring Parameters Signs and symptoms of hypoglycemia, urine glucose test, fasting blood glucose, hemoglobin A_{1c}

Reference Range

Recommendations for glycemic control in nonpregnant adults with diabetes (ADA, 2015):

HbA_{1c}: <7% (a more aggressive [<6.5%] or less aggressive [<8%] HbA_{1c} goal may be targeted based on patient-specific characteristics)

Preprandial capillary plasma glucose: 80 to 130 mg/dL

Peak postprandial capillary blood glucose: <180 mg/dL

Recommendations for glycemic control in pediatric (all age groups) patients with type 1 diabetes (ADA, 2015):

HbA_{1c}: <7.5% (individualization may be appropriate based on patient-specific characteristics; <7% is reasonable if it can be achieved without excessive hypoglycemia)

Preprandial capillary plasma glucose: 90 to 130 mg/dL

Bedtime and overnight capillary blood glucose: 90 to 150 mg/dL

Dosage Forms Considerations Micronized formulation: Glynase

Dosage Forms Excipient information presented when available (limited, particularly for generics); consult specific product labeling.

Tablet, Oral:

Diabeta: 1.25 mg, 2.5 mg, 5 mg [scored]

Glynase: 1.5 mg, 3 mg, 6 mg [scored]

Generic: 1.25 mg, 1.5 mg, 2.5 mg, 3 mg, 5 mg, 6 mg

Glyburide and Metformin

(GLYE byoor ide & met FOR min)

Brand Names: US Glucovance

Index Terms Glyburide and Metformin Hydrochloride; Metformin and Glyburide

Pharmacologic Category Antidiabetic Agent, Biguanide; Antidiabetic Agent, Sulfonylurea

Use Type 2 diabetes mellitus: As an adjunct to diet and exercise, to improve glycemic control in adults with type 2 diabetes (noninsulin dependent, NIDDM)

Dosing

Adult Note: Dose must be individualized. Dosages expressed as glyburide/metformin components.

Type 2 diabetes: Oral:

Patients with inadequate glycemic control on diet and exercise alone: Initial: 1.25 mg/250 mg once daily with a meal; patients with HbA_{1c} >9% or fasting plasma glucose (FPG) >200 mg/dL may start with 1.25 mg/250 mg twice daily with meals.

Adjustment: Dosage may be increased in increments of 1.25 mg/250 mg per day, at intervals of not less than 2 weeks; maximum daily dose: 10 mg/2000 mg (limited experience with higher doses). **Note:** Doses of 5 mg/500 mg should not be used as initial therapy, due to risk of hypoglycemia.

Patients with inadequate glycemic control on a sulfonylurea and/or metformin: Initial: 2.5 mg/500 mg or 5 mg/500 mg twice daily with meals.

Adjustment: Dosage may be increased in increments no greater than 5 mg/500 mg; maximum daily dose: 20 mg/2000 mg. **Note:** When switching patients previously on a sulfonylurea and metformin together, do not exceed the daily dose of glyburide (or glyburide equivalent) or metformin.

Combination with thiazolidinedione: May be combined with a thiazolidinedione in patients with an inadequate response to glyburide/metformin therapy; however, the risk of hypoglycemia may be increased. When adding a thiazolidinedione, continue glyburide and metformin at current dose and initiate thiazolidinedione at recommended starting dose; may increase based on the thiazolidinedione suggested titration schedule.

Geriatric Refer to adult dosing. Conservative doses are recommended in the elderly due to potentially decreased renal function; adjust carefully to renal function. Should not be used in patients ≥80 years of age unless renal function is verified as normal. Do not titrate to maximum dose.

Renal Impairment

Manufacturer's labeling: Serum creatinine (SCr) ≥1.5 mg/dL (males) or ≥1.4 mg/dL (females) or abnormal CrCl (not defined): Use is contraindicated.

◀ *Alternate recommendations:* **Note:** The United Kingdom National Institute for Health and Clinical Excellence (NICE) Guidelines recommend prescribing metformin with caution in those patients who are at risk of sudden deterioration in renal function and at risk of an estimated glomerular filtration rate (eGFR) <45 mL/minute/1.73 m^2 (NICE, 2008]). Some evidence suggests that use of metformin is unsafe when eGFR <30 mL/minute/1.73 m^2 (calculated using MDRD) (Shaw, 2007). A review of the available data by members of the American Diabetes Association proposed the following recommendations based on eGFR (Lipska, 2011):

eGFR ≥60 mL/minute/1.73 m^2: No contraindications, monitor renal function annually

eGFR ≥45 to <60 mL/minute/1.73 m^2: Continue use; monitor renal function every 3 to 6 months

eGFR ≥30 to <45 mL/minute/1.73 m^2: In patients currently receiving metformin, use with caution, consider dosage reduction (eg, 50% reduction or 50% of maximal dose), monitor renal function every 3 months. Do not initiate therapy in patients with eGFR <45 mL/minute/1.73 m^2

eGFR <30 mL/minute/1.73 m^2: Discontinue use

Hepatic Impairment The manufacturer recommends avoiding metformin since liver disease is considered a risk factor for the development of lactic acidosis during metformin therapy. However, continued use of metformin in diabetics with liver dysfunction, including cirrhosis, has been used successfully and may be associated with a survival benefit in carefully selected patients; use cautiously in patients at risk for lactic acidosis (eg, renal impairment, alcohol use) (Brackett, 2010; Zhang, 2014). Glyburide undergoes hepatic metabolism and use of a lower initial and maintenance dose should be considered.

Additional Information Complete prescribing information should be consulted for additional detail.

Dosage Forms Excipient information presented when available (limited, particularly for generics); consult specific product labeling. [DSC] = Discontinued product

Tablet, oral: 1.25 mg/250 mg: Glyburide 1.25 mg and metformin hydrochloride 250 mg; 2.5 mg/500 mg: Glyburide 2.5 mg and metformin hydrochloride 500 mg; 5 mg/ 500 mg: Glyburide 5 mg and metformin hydrochloride 500 mg

Glucovance: 1.25 mg/250 mg: Glyburide 1.25 mg and metformin hydrochloride 250 mg [DSC]

Glucovance: 2.5 mg/500 mg: Glyburide 2.5 mg and metformin hydrochloride 500 mg

Glucovance: 5 mg/500 mg: Glyburide 5 mg and metformin hydrochloride 500 mg

◆ Glyburide and Metformin Hydrochloride *see* Glyburide and Metformin *on page 849*

◆ Glycate *see* Glycopyrrolate *on page 850*

◆ Glycerol Guaiacolate *see* GuaiFENesin *on page 860*

◆ Glyceryl Trinitrate *see* Nitroglycerin *on page 1289*

◆ GlycoLax [OTC] *see* Polyethylene Glycol 3350 *on page 1465*

◆ Glycon (Can) *see* MetFORMIN *on page 1156*

◆ Glycophos *see* Sodium Glycerophosphate Pentahydrate *on page 1674*

Glycopyrrolate (glye koe PYE roe late)

Brand Names: US Cuvposa; Glycate; Robinul; Robinul-Forte

Brand Names: Canada Glycopyrrolate Injection, USP; Seebri Breezhaler

Index Terms Glycopyrronium Bromide; NVA237; Seebri Neohaler

Pharmacologic Category Anticholinergic Agent

Use Inhibit salivation and excessive secretions of the respiratory tract preoperatively; control of upper airway secretions; intraoperatively to counteract drug-induced or vagal mediated bradyarrhythmias; adjunct in treatment of peptic ulcer (indication listed in product labeling but currently has no place in management of peptic ulcer disease)

Cuvposa: Reduce chronic, severe drooling in those with neurologic conditions (eg, cerebral palsy) associated with drooling

Seebri Breezhaler [Canadian product]: Maintenance treatment of chronic obstructive pulmonary disease (COPD) including chronic bronchitis and emphysema

Pregnancy Considerations Adverse effects were not observed in animal reproduction studies. Small amounts of glycopyrrolate cross the human placenta. Glycopyrrolate in doses of 0.004 mg/kg has not been found to affect fetal heart rate.

Breast-Feeding Considerations It is not known if glycopyrrolate is excreted in breast milk. The manufacturer recommends caution be exercised when administering glycopyrrolate to nursing women. May suppress lactation.

Contraindications Hypersensitivity to glycopyrrolate or any component of the formulation; medical conditions that preclude use of anticholinergic medication; severe ulcerative colitis, toxic megacolon complicating ulcerative colitis, paralytic ileus, obstructive disease of GI tract (eg, pyloric stenosis), intestinal atony in the elderly or debilitated patient; unstable cardiovascular status in acute hemorrhage; narrow-angle glaucoma; acute hemorrhage; tachycardia; obstructive uropathy; myasthenia gravis

Oral solution: Additional contraindication: Concomitant use of potassium chloride in a solid oral dosage form

Seebri Breezhaler [Canadian product]: Hypersensitivity to glycopyrronium bromide or any component of the formulation

Warnings/Precautions Diarrhea may be a sign of incomplete intestinal obstruction, treatment should be discontinued if this occurs. Use caution in elderly and in patients with autonomic neuropathy, narrow-angle glaucoma, renal disease, or ulcerative colitis; may precipitate/aggravate ileus or toxic megacolon, hyperthyroidism, CAD, CHF, arrhythmias, tachycardia, BPH, bladder neck obstruction, or hiatal hernia with reflux. Use of anticholinergics in gastric ulcer treatment may cause a delay in gastric emptying. Caution should be used in individuals demonstrating decreased pigmentation (skin and iris coloration, dark versus light) since there has been some evidence that these individuals have an enhanced sensitivity to the anticholinergic response. May cause drowsiness, eye sensitivity to light, or blurred vision; caution should be used when performing tasks which require mental alertness, such as driving. The risk of heat stroke with this medication may be increased during exercise or hot weather. Seebri® Breezhaler® [Canadian product] is not indicated for the initial (rescue) treatment of acute episodes of bronchospasm or with acutely deteriorating COPD; after initiation of therapy, patients should use short-acting bronchodilators only on an as needed basis for acute symptoms. Rarely, paradoxal bronchospasm may occur with use of inhaled bronchodilating agents; discontinue use of inhaler and consider other therapy if bronchospasm occurs. Patients using Seebri® Breezhaler® should avoid getting the powder into their eyes.

Benzyl alcohol and derivatives: Some dosage forms may contain benzyl alcohol; large amounts of benzyl alcohol (≥99 mg/kg/day) have been associated with a potentially fatal toxicity ("gasping syndrome") in neonates; the "gasping syndrome" consists of metabolic acidosis, respiratory distress, gasping respirations, CNS dysfunction (including convulsions, intracranial hemorrhage), hypotension and cardiovascular collapse (AAP ["Inactive" 1997]; CDC, 1982); some data suggests that benzoate displaces bilirubin from protein binding sites (Ahlfors, 2001); avoid or use dosage forms containing benzyl alcohol with caution in neonates. See manufacturer's labeling. Some dosage forms may contain propylene glycol; large amounts are potentially toxic and have been associated hyperosmolality, lactic acidosis, seizures, and respiratory depression; use caution (AAP, 1997; Zar, 2007).

Adverse Reactions

>10% (as reported with Cuvposa™):

Cardiovascular: Flushing (30%)

Central nervous system: Headache (15%)

Gastrointestinal: Vomiting (40%), xerostomia (40%), constipation (35%)

Genitourinary: Urinary retention (15%)

Respiratory: Nasal congestion (30%), sinusitis (15%), upper respiratory tract infection (15%)

<10% (frequency not always defined):

Cardiovascular: Pallor (≤2%), arrhythmias, cardiac arrest, heart block, hyper-/hypotension, malignant hyperthermia, palpitation, QTc-interval prolongation, tachycardia

Central nervous system: Aggressiveness (≤2%), agitation (≤2%), crying (abnormal; ≤2%), irritability (≤2%), mood changes (≤2%), pain (≤2%), restlessness (≤2%), confusion, dizziness, drowsiness, excitement, insomnia, nervousness, seizure

Dermatologic: Dry skin (≤2%), pruritus (≤2%), rash (≤2%), urticaria

Endocrine & metabolic: Dehydration (≤2%), lactation suppression

Gastrointestinal: Abdominal distention (≤2%), abdominal pain (≤2%), flatulence (≤2%), retching (≤2%), bloated feeling, intestinal obstruction, loss of taste, nausea, pseudo-obstruction

Genitourinary: Urinary tract infection (≤2%), impotence, urinary hesitancy

Local: Injection site reactions (edema, erythema, pain)

Neuromuscular & skeletal: Weakness

Ocular: Nystagmus (≤2%), blurred vision, cycloplegia, mydriasis, ocular tension increased, photophobia, sensitivity to light increased

Respiratory: Bronchial secretion (thickening; ≤2%), nasal dryness (≤2%), pneumonia (≤2%), respiratory depression

Miscellaneous: Anaphylactoid reactions, diaphoresis decreased, hypersensitivity reactions

As reported with Seebri® Breezhaler® [Canadian product]:

1% to 10%:

Central nervous system: Headache (elderly: 2%)

Gastrointestinal: Xerostomia (2% to 3%), gastroenteritis (1% to 3%), dyspepsia (1%), vomiting (1%)

Genitourinary: Urinary tract infection (elderly: 3%), dysuria (1%)

Neuromuscular & skeletal: Musculoskeletal pain (2%)

Respiratory: Nasopharyngitis (9%), rhinitis (2%)

<1% (Limited to important or life-threatening): Cough, cystitis, dental caries, diabetes mellitus, epistaxis, fatigue, hypoesthesia, palpitations, rash, throat irritation, urinary retention, weakness

Drug Interactions

Metabolism/Transport Effects None known.

Avoid Concomitant Use

Avoid concomitant use of Glycopyrrolate with any of the following: Aclidinium; Anticholinergic Agents; Cimetropium; Eluxadoline; Glucagon; Glycopyrrolate (Oral Inhalation); Ipratropium (Oral Inhalation); Levosulpiride; Potassium Chloride; Tiotropium; Umeclidinium

Increased Effect/Toxicity

Glycopyrrolate may increase the levels/effects of: AbobotulinumtoxinA; Analgesics (Opioid); Atenolol; Cannabinoid-Containing Products; Cimetropium; Digoxin; Eluxadoline; Glucagon; Glycopyrrolate (Oral Inhalation); MetFORMIN; Mirabegron; OnabotulinumtoxinA; Potassium Chloride; Ramosetron; RimabotulinumtoxinB; Thiazide Diuretics; Tiotropium; Topiramate

The levels/effects of Glycopyrrolate may be increased by: Aclidinium; Amantadine; Anticholinergic Agents; Ipratropium (Oral Inhalation); Mianserin; Pramlintide; Umeclidinium

Decreased Effect

Glycopyrrolate may decrease the levels/effects of: Acetylcholinesterase Inhibitors; Gastrointestinal Agents (Prokinetic); Haloperidol; Itopride; Levodopa; Levosulpiride; Secretin

The levels/effects of Glycopyrrolate may be decreased by: Acetylcholinesterase Inhibitors

Food Interactions Administration with a high-fat meal significantly reduced absorption. Management: Administer on an empty stomach.

Storage/Stability Store at 20°C to 25°C (68°F to 77°F).

Oral capsules for inhalation [Canadian product]: Store at 15°C to 25°C (59°F to 77°F) in blister. Capsules should be stored in the blister pack and only removed immediately before use. Once protective foil is peeled back and/or removed the capsule should be used immediately; if capsule is not used immediately, it should be discarded. Do not store capsules in Seebri® Breezhaler®. Protect from moisture.

Mechanism of Action Blocks the action of acetylcholine at parasympathetic sites in smooth muscle, secretory glands, and the CNS; indirectly reduces the rate of salivation by preventing the stimulation of acetylcholine receptors

In COPD, competitively and reversibly inhibits the action of acetylcholine at muscarinic receptor subtypes 1-3 (greater affinity for subtypes 1 and 3) in bronchial smooth muscle thereby causing bronchodilation

Pharmacodynamics/Kinetics Note: Oral powder for inhalation is not available in the U.S.

Onset of action: Oral: 50 minutes; IM: 15-30 minutes; IV: ~1 minute

Peak effect: Oral: ~1 hour; IM: 30-45 minutes

Duration: Vagal effect: 2-3 hours; Inhibition of salivation: Up to 7 hours; Anticholinergic: Oral: 8-12 hours; Parenteral: 7 hours

Absorption: Oral tablet: Poor (~3%); variable and erratic; Oral solution: 23% lower compared to tablet; Oral powder for inhalation: Rapid

Distribution: V_d: Children (1 to 14 years): Mean range: 1.3-1.8 L/kg; Adults: 0.2-0.62 L/kg

Metabolism: Hepatic (minimal)

Bioavailability: Tablet: ~1% to 13%; Oral powder for inhalation: ~40%

Half-life elimination: Infants: 22-130 minutes; Children 19-99 minutes; Adults: ~60-75 minutes; Oral solution: Adults: 3 hours; Oral powder for inhalation: 13-22 hours (Sechaud, 2012)

Time to peak, plasma: Oral powder for inhalation: 5 minutes

Excretion: Urine (as unchanged drug, IM: 80%, IV: 85%); bile (as unchanged drug)

Clearance: Children (1 to 14 years): Mean range: 1 to 1.4 L/kg/hour; Adults: Mean range: 0.4 to 0.68 L/kg/hour

Dosing

Adult & Geriatric

Chronic obstructive pulmonary disease (COPD): Oral powder for inhalation: Seebri® Breezhaler® [Canadian product]: 50 mcg (contents of one capsule) once daily

Reduction of secretions:

Preoperative: IM: 4 mcg/kg 30-60 minutes before procedure

Intraoperative: IV: 0.1 mg repeated as needed at 2- to 3-minute intervals

Reversal of neuromuscular blockade: IV: 0.2 mg for each 1 mg of neostigmine or 5 mg of pyridostigmine administered or 5-15 mcg/kg glycopyrrolate with 25-70 mcg/kg of neostigmine or 0.1-0.3 mg/kg of pyridostigmine (agents usually administered simultaneously, but glycopyrrolate may be administered first if bradycardia is present)

Pediatric

Reduction of secretions:

Preoperative: IM:

<2 years: 4-9 mcg/kg 30-60 minutes before procedure

>2 years: 4 mcg/kg 30-60 minutes before procedure

Intraoperative: IV: 4 mcg/kg not to exceed 0.1 mg; repeat at 2- to 3-minute intervals as needed.

Chronic (off-label):

Oral: 40-100 mcg/kg/dose 3-4 times/day

IM, IV: 4-10 mcg/kg/dose every 3-4 hours; maximum: 0.2 mg/dose or 0.8 mg/24 hours

Drooling, chronic: Children 3-16 years: Oral solution (Cuvposa™): 0.02 mg/kg 3 times/day; titrate in increments of 0.02 mg/kg every 5-7 days as tolerated, up to a maximum dose of 0.1 mg/kg 3 times/day, not to exceed 1.5-3 mg/dose

Reversal of neuromuscular blockade: Refer to adult dosing.

Renal Impairment No dosage adjustment provided in manufacturer's labeling. However, data suggest renal impairment reduces glycopyrrolate elimination; use with caution.

Hepatic Impairment No dosage adjustment provided in manufacturer's labeling (has not been studied).

Administration

IV: Administer IV at a rate of 0.2 mg over 1-2 minutes. May be administered IM or IV without dilution. May also be administered via the tubing of a running IV infusion of a compatible solution. May be administered IV in the same syringe with neostigmine or pyridostigmine.

Oral: Administer oral solution on an empty stomach, 1 hour before or 2 hours after meals

Oral inhalation [Canadian product]: Administer once daily preferably at the same time each day using the Seebri® Breezhaler® only. Remove capsule from foil blister immediately before use. Do not swallow capsule. Avoid getting powder into eyes. Place capsule in the capsule-chamber in the base of the Seebri® Breezhaler®. A click is heard as it fully closes. Hold inhaler with mouthpiece in upright position and pierce capsule within chamber by simultaneously pressing piercing buttons on base of inhaler (click is heard as capsule is pierced). Release buttons. Exhale fully. Do not exhale into inhaler. Tilt head slightly back and place mouthpiece in mouth with piercing buttons on base of inhaler in horizontal position and not up and down. Do not press piercing buttons. Inhale (rapidly, steadily and deeply); the capsule vibration should be heard within the device. Hold breath for at least 5-10 seconds or as long as possible. Remove mouthpiece prior to exhalation. Patient should not breathe out through the mouthpiece. If any powder remains in capsule, exhale and inhale again. Repeat until capsule is empty. Throw away empty capsule; do not leave in inhaler. Always keep capsules and inhaler dry. **Note:** If a dose is missed, take as soon as possible on that day; do not take 2 doses on the same day.

Monitoring Parameters Heart rate; anticholinergic effects; bowel sounds; bowel movements; effects on drooling

Oral inhalation: FEV_1, peak flow (or other pulmonary function studies)

Product Availability Seebri Neohaler: FDA approved October 2015; anticipated availability in first quarter of 2016.

◄

Dosage Forms Excipient information presented when available (limited, particularly for generics); consult specific product labeling.

Solution, Injection:

Robinul: 0.2 mg/mL (1 mL); 0.4 mg/2 mL (2 mL); 1 mg/5 mL (5 mL); 4 mg/20 mL (20 mL) [contains benzyl alcohol]

Generic: 0.2 mg/mL (1 mL); 0.4 mg/2 mL (2 mL); 1 mg/5 mL (5 mL); 4 mg/20 mL (20 mL)

Solution, Oral:

Cuvposa: 1 mg/5 mL (473 mL) [contains methylparaben, propylene glycol, propylparaben, saccharin sodium; cherry flavor]

Tablet, Oral:

Glycate: 1.5 mg [dye free]

Robinul: 1 mg [scored]

Robinul-Forte: 2 mg [scored]

Generic: 1 mg, 2 mg

Dosage Forms: Canada Excipient information presented when available (limited, particularly for generics); consult specific product labeling.

Powder, for oral inhalation:

Seebri® Breezhaler®: 50 mcg/capsule (30s) [contains lactose]

Extemporaneous Preparations A 0.5 mg/mL oral suspension may be made with 1 mg tablets and a 1:1 mixture of Ora-Plus® and either Ora-Sweet® or Ora-Sweet® SF. Crush thirty 1 mg tablets in a mortar and reduce to a fine powder. Prepare diluent by mixing 30 mL of Ora-Plus® with 30 mL of either Ora-Sweet® or Ora-Sweet® SF and stir vigorously. Add 30 mL of diluent (via geometric dilution) to powder until smooth suspension is obtained. Transfer suspension to 60 mL amber bottle. Rinse contents of mortar into bottle with sufficient quantity of remaining diluent to obtain 60 mL (final volume). Label "shake well". Stable at room temperature for 90 days. Due to bitter aftertaste, chocolate syrup may be administered prior to or mixed (1:1 v/v) with suspension immediately before administration (Cober, 2011).

A 0.5 mg/mL oral solution can be made from tablets. Crush fifty 1 mg tablets in a mortar and reduce to a fine powder. Add enough distilled water to make about 90 mL, mix well. Transfer to a bottle, rinse mortar with water, and add a quantity of water sufficient to make 100 mL. Label "shake well" and "protect from light". Stable at room temperature for 25 days (Gupta, 2001).

A 0.1 mg/mL oral solution may be made using glycopyrrolate 0.2 mg/mL injection without preservatives. Withdraw 50 mL from vials with a needle and syringe, add to 50 mL of a 1:1 mixture of Ora-Sweet® and Ora-Plus® in a bottle. Label "shake well", "protect from light," and "refrigerate". Stable refrigerated for 35 days (Landry, 2005).

Cober MP, Johnson CE, Sudekum D, et al, "Stability of Extemporaneously Prepared Glycopyrrolate Oral Suspensions," *Am J Health Syst Phar,*. 2011, 68(9):843-5.

Gupta VD, "Stability of an Oral Liquid Dosage Form of Glycopyrrolate Prepared from Tablets," *IJPC* 2001, 5(6):480-1.

Landry C, "Stability and Subjective Taste Acceptability of Four Glycopyrrolate Solutions for Oral Administration," *IJPC*, 2005, 9(5):396-98.

♦ Glycopyrrolate and Indacaterol *see* Indacaterol and Glycopyrrolate *on page 934*

♦ Glycopyrrolate and Indacaterol Maleate *see* Indacaterol and Glycopyrrolate *on page 934*

♦ Glycopyrrolate Injection, USP (Can) *see* Glycopyrrolate *on page 850*

♦ Glycopyrronium and Indacaterol *see* Indacaterol and Glycopyrrolate *on page 934*

♦ Glycopyrronium Bromide *see* Glycopyrrolate *on page 850*

♦ Glycopyrronium Bromide and Indacaterol Maleate *see* Indacaterol and Glycopyrrolate *on page 934*

♦ Glydiazinamide *see* GlipiZIDE *on page 843*

♦ Glydo *see* Lidocaine (Topical) *on page 1074*

♦ Glynase *see* GlyBURIDE *on page 847*

♦ Gly-Oxide [OTC] *see* Carbamide Peroxide *on page 307*

♦ Glyquin® XM (Can) *see* Hydroquinone *on page 893*

♦ Glyset *see* Miglitol *on page 1207*

♦ GM-CSF *see* Sargramostim *on page 1637*

♦ GnRH Agonist *see* Histrelin *on page 878*

Golimumab (goe LIM ue mab)

Brand Names: US Simponi; Simponi Aria
Brand Names: Canada Simponi; Simponi I.V.
Index Terms CNTO-148

Pharmacologic Category Antipsoriatic Agent; Antirheumatic, Disease Modifying; Monoclonal Antibody; Tumor Necrosis Factor (TNF) Blocking Agent

Use

Ankylosing spondylitis (Simponi): Treatment of adults with active ankylosing spondylitis

Psoriatic arthritis (Simponi): Treatment of adults with active psoriatic arthritis (alone or in combination with methotrexate)

Rheumatoid arthritis (Simponi, Simponi Aria): Treatment of adults with moderately-to-severely active rheumatoid arthritis (in combination with methotrexate)

Ulcerative colitis (Simponi): Treatment of adults with moderately-to-severely active ulcerative colitis in patients with corticosteroid dependence or who are refractory or intolerant to oral aminosalicylates, oral corticosteroids, azathioprine, or 6-mercaptopurine (to induce and maintain clinical response, improve mucosal appearance during induction, induce clinical remission, and achieve and sustain remission in induction responders)

Pregnancy Considerations Adverse events have not been observed in animal reproduction studies. Golimumab crosses the placenta. Based on data from other TNF-blockers, antibodies may be present in the newborn serum for up to 6 months and infants exposed to golimumab *in utero* may be at risk of increased infection. Administration of live vaccines to newborns is not recommended until 6 months after the last maternal dose. The Canadian labeling recommends that women of childbearing potential use reliable contraception during and for at least 6 months after discontinuation of golimumab therapy.

Breast-Feeding Considerations It is not known whether golimumab is excreted in breast milk. Because many immunoglobulins are excreted in milk and the potential for serious adverse reactions exists, the US labeling recommends a decision should be made whether to discontinue breast-feeding or discontinue the drug, taking into account the importance of the drug to the mother. The Canadian labeling recommends avoiding breast-feeding during therapy and for at least 6 months after discontinuation of therapy.

Medication Guide Available Yes

Contraindications

There are no contraindications listed in the manufacturer's US labeling.

Canadian labeling: Hypersensitivity to golimumab, latex, or any other component of formulation or packaging; patients with severe infections (eg, sepsis, tuberculosis, opportunistic infections); moderate or severe heart failure (NYHA class III/IV)

Warnings/Precautions [US Boxed Warning]: Patients receiving golimumab are at increased risk for serious infections which may result in hospitalization and/or fatality; infections usually developed in patients receiving concomitant immunosuppressive agents (eg, methotrexate or corticosteroids). Active tuberculosis (or reactivation of latent tuberculosis), invasive fungal (including aspergillosis, blastomycosis, candidiasis, coccidioidomycosis, histoplasmosis, and pneumocystosis) and bacterial, viral or other opportunistic infections (including legionellosis and listeriosis) have been reported in patients receiving TNF-blocking agents, including golimumab. May present as disseminated (rather than local) disease. Histoplasmosis testing (antigen or antibody) may be negative in some patients with active infection. Monitor closely for signs/symptoms of infection. Discontinue for serious infection or sepsis. Consider risks versus benefits prior to use in patients with a history of chronic or recurrent infection. Consider empiric antifungal therapy in patients who are at risk for invasive fungal infection and develop severe systemic illness. Caution should be exercised when considering use in the elderly, patients taking concomitant immunosuppressants, patients with chronic or recurrent infection, patients who have been exposed to tuberculosis, patients with a history of opportunistic infection, patients with comorbid conditions that predispose them to infections (eg, diabetes), or residence/travel from areas of endemic mycoses (blastomycosis, coccidioidomycosis, histoplasmosis). Do not initiate golimumab therapy in patients with with active infection, including localized infection which is clinically important. Patients who develop a new infection while undergoing treatment should be monitored closely.

[US Boxed Warning]: Tuberculosis (disseminated or extrapulmonary) has been reported in patients receiving golimumab; both reactivation of latent infection and new infections have been reported. Patients should be evaluated for tuberculosis risk factors and latent tuberculosis infection (with a tuberculin skin test) prior to and during therapy. Treatment of latent

tuberculosis should be initiated before use. **Patients with initial negative tuberculin skin tests should receive continued monitoring for tuberculosis throughout treatment;** active tuberculosis has developed in this population during treatment with TNF-blocking agents. Use with caution in patients who have resided in regions where tuberculosis is endemic. Consider antituberculosis therapy if an adequate course of treatment cannot be confirmed in patients with a history of latent or active tuberculosis or for patients with risk factors despite negative skin test.

Rare reactivation of hepatitis B virus (HBV), sometimes fatal, has occurred in chronic virus carriers (usually in patients receiving concomitant immunosuppressants); evaluate prior to initiation in all patients. Patients who test positive for HBV surface antigen should be referred for hepatitis B evaluation/treatment prior to golimumab initiation. Monitor during and for several months following discontinuation of treatment in HBV carriers; interrupt therapy if reactivation occurs and treat appropriately with antiviral therapy; if resumption of therapy is deemed necessary, exercise caution and monitor patient closely. Patients should be brought up to date with all immunizations before initiating therapy. Live vaccines should not be given concurrently; there is no data available concerning secondary transmission of infection by live vaccines in patients receiving therapy. In clinical trials, humoral response to pneumococcal vaccine was not suppressed in psoriatic arthritis patients.

[US Boxed Warning]: Lymphoma and other malignancies (some fatal) have been reported in children and adolescent patients receiving TNF-blocking agents. Half of the malignancies reported in children were lymphomas (Hodgkin's and non-Hodgkin's) while other cases varied and included malignancies not typically observed in this population. The onset of malignancy was after a median of 30 months (range: 1 to 84 months) after the initiation of the TNF-blocking agent; most patients were receiving concomitant immunosuppressants. The impact of golimumab on the development and course of malignancy is not fully defined. Compared to the general population, an increased risk of lymphoma has been noted in clinical trials; however, rheumatoid arthritis alone has been previously associated with an increased rate of lymphoma. Lymphomas and other malignancies were also observed (at rates higher than expected for the general population) in adult patients receiving TNF-blocking agents. Hepatosplenic T-cell lymphoma (HSTCL), a rare T-cell lymphoma, has also been associated with TNF-blocking agents, primarily reported in adolescent and young adult males with Crohn disease or ulcerative colitis treated with a TNF-blocking agent and concurrent or prior azathioprine or mercaptopurine. Melanoma and Merkel cell carcinoma have been reported in patients receiving TNF-blocking agents including golimumab. Perform periodic skin examinations in all patients during therapy, particularly those at increased risk for skin cancer. Consider risks versus benefits in patients with a known malignancy (other than a successfully treated nonmelanoma skin cancer) and if considering continuing treatment in a patient who develops a malignancy. Cases of pancytopenia and other significant cytopenias, including aplastic anemia, have been reported with TNF-blocking agents. Pancytopenia, leukopenia, neutropenia and thrombocytopenia have occurred with golimumab; use with caution in patients with underlying hematologic disorders. Consider discontinuing therapy with significant hematologic abnormalities. Treatment may result in the formation of autoimmune antibodies; cases of autoimmune disease have not been described.

Use with caution in patients with preexisting or recent onset central or peripheral nervous system demyelinating disorders; rare cases of new-onset or exacerbation of demyelinating disorders (eg, multiple sclerosis, optic neuritis, Guillain-Barré syndrome, polyneuropathy) have been reported. Consider discontinuing use in patients who develop peripheral or central nervous system demyelinating disorders during treatment. Use with caution in patients with heart failure or decreased left ventricular function; monitor closely and discontinue with new-onset or worsening of symptoms. Canadian labeling contraindicates use in moderate or severe heart failure (NYHA class III/IV). Severe systemic hypersensitivity reactions (including anaphylaxis), have been reported (some have occurred with the first dose) following subcutaneous administration; discontinue immediately if signs develop and initiate appropriate treatment.

Avoid concomitant use with abatacept (increased incidence of serious infections) or anakinra (increased incidence of neutropenia and serious infection). Potentially significant drug-drug interactions may exist, requiring dose or frequency adjustment, additional monitoring, and/or selection of alternative therapy. Use caution when switching between biological disease-modifying antirheumatic drugs (DMARDs); overlapping of biological activity may increase the risk for infection. Use with caution in the elderly (general incidence of infection is higher). Packaging (prefilled syringe and needle cover) contains dry natural rubber (latex). Some dosage forms may contain dry natural rubber (latex). Some dosage forms may contain polysorbate 80 (also known as Tweens). Hypersensitivity reactions, usually a delayed reaction, have been reported following exposure to pharmaceutical products containing polysorbate 80 in certain individuals (Isaksson, 2002; Lucente 2000; Shelley, 1995). Thrombocytopenia, ascites, pulmonary deterioration, and renal and hepatic failure have been reported in premature neonates after receiving parenteral products containing polysorbate 80 (Alade, 1986; CDC, 1984). See manufacturer's labeling. The safety and efficacy of switching between the IV and SubQ formulations and routes have not been studied.

Adverse Reactions

>10%:

Hematologic & oncologic: Positive ANA titer (≥1:160 titer, newly positive; 17% intravenous, 4% subcutaneous)

Infection: Infection (27% to 28%)

Respiratory: Upper respiratory tract infection (includes laryngitis, nasopharyngitis, pharyngitis, and rhinitis; 13% to 16%)

1% to 10%:

Cardiovascular: Hypertension (3%)

Central nervous system: Dizziness (<1% to 2%), paresthesia (<1% to 2%)

Dermatologic: Skin rash (3%)

Gastrointestinal: Constipation (≤1%)

Hematologic & oncologic: Leukopenia (≤1%)

Hepatic: Increased serum ALT (subcutaneous 4%; ≥3 x ULN: 2%; ≥5 x ULN: <1%), increased serum AST (<1% to 3%)

Immunologic: Antibody development (3% to 7%)

Infection: Viral infection (4% to 5%; includes herpes and influenza), fungal infection (superficial; <1% to 2%), bacterial infection (intravenous 1%), serious infection (≤1%)

Local: Injection site reaction (subcutaneous 3% to 6%)

Respiratory: Bronchitis (2% to 3%)

Miscellaneous: Fever (2%), infusion related reaction (intravenous 1%)

<1% (Limited to important or life-threatening): Anaphylaxis, antibody development (anti-dsDNA), aspergillosis, atypical mycobacterial infection (subcutaneous), blastomycosis, bullous skin disease, candidiasis, cardiac failure (worsening or new onset), cellulitis, coccidioidomycosis, demyelinating disease of the central nervous system, hepatotoxicity (idiosyncratic) (Chalasani 2014), histoplasmosis, Hodgkin lymphoma (initiation of therapy ≤18 years old), hypersensitivity angiitis (subcutaneous), hypersensitivity reaction, infective bursitis (subcutaneous), interstitial pulmonary disease (subcutaneous), leukemia, lupus-like syndrome, malignant lymphoma, malignant melanoma, malignant neoplasm (other than nonmelanoma skin cancer), Merkel cell carcinoma, multiple sclerosis, non-Hodgkin lymphoma (initiation of therapy ≤18 years old), neutropenia, optic neuritis, pancytopenia, peripheral demyelinating polyneuropathy, pneumocystosis, pneumonia, psoriasis (subcutaneous) including new onset, palmoplantar, pustular, or exacerbation), pyelonephritis, reactivation of HBV, sarcoidosis, sepsis, septic arthritis (subcutaneous), septic shock (subcutaneous), serious infection, thrombocytopenia, tuberculosis (including reactivation of latent and new infection), vasculitis (subcutaneous)

Drug Interactions

Metabolism/Transport Effects None known.

Avoid Concomitant Use

Avoid concomitant use of Golimumab with any of the following: Abatacept; Anakinra; BCG (Intravesical); Belimumab; Canakinumab; Certolizumab Pegol; InFLIXimab; Natalizumab; Pimecrolimus; Rilonacept; Tacrolimus (Topical); Tocilizumab; Tofacitinib; Vaccines (Live); Vedolizumab

Increased Effect/Toxicity

Golimumab may increase the levels/effects of: Abatacept; Anakinra; Belimumab; Canakinumab; Certolizumab Pegol; Fingolimod; InFLIXimab; Leflunomide; Natalizumab; Rilonacept; Tofacitinib; Vaccines (Live); Vedolizumab

The levels/effects of Golimumab may be increased by: Denosumab; Pimecrolimus; Roflumilast; Tacrolimus (Topical); Tocilizumab; Trastuzumab

◀

Decreased Effect

Golimumab may decrease the levels/effects of: BCG (Intravesical); Coccidioides immitis Skin Test; Sipuleucel-T; Vaccines (Inactivated); Vaccines (Live)

The levels/effects of Golimumab may be decreased by: Echinacea

Preparation for Administration Intact solution should be colorless to light yellow; solution may develop a few fine, translucent particles.

SubQ: Bring to room temperature by allowing syringe/ autoinjector to sit at room temperature outside the carton for 30 minutes prior to administration (do not warm in any other way). Do not use if discolored, cloudy, or if foreign particles are present.

IV: Do not use if solution is discolored, or contains opaque or foreign particles. Dilute for infusion by slowly adding calculated dose/volume to sodium chloride 0.9% to a total volume of 100 mL. Gently mix.

Discard unused portion of vial/syringe/autoinjector.

Storage/Stability Store intact vials and syringes refrigerated at 2°C to 8°C (36°F to 46°F); do not freeze. Do not shake. Protect from light.

IV: Solutions diluted for infusion may be stored at room temperature for 4 hours.

Mechanism of Action Human monoclonal antibody that binds to human tumor necrosis factor alpha (TNFα), thereby interfering with endogenous TNFα activity. Biological activities of TNFα include the induction of proinflammatory cytokines (interleukin [IL]-6, IL-8, Granulocyte-colony stimulating factor, granulocyte-macrophage colony stimulating factor), expression of adhesion molecules (E-selectin, vascular cell adhesion molecule [VCAM]-1, intercellular adhesion molecule [ICAM]-1) necessary for leukocyte infiltration, activation of neutrophils and eosinophils.

Pharmacodynamics/Kinetics

Distribution: V_d: IV: 151 ± 61 mL/kg (distributed primarily to circulatory system with limited extravascular distribution)

Bioavailability: SubQ: ~53%

Metabolism: Pathway unknown

Half-life elimination: ~2 weeks

Time to peak, serum: SubQ: 2-6 days

Dosing

Adult & Geriatric Note: Corticosteroids, *nonbiologic* disease-modifying antirheumatic drugs (DMARDs), and/ or NSAIDs may be continued for the treatment of rheumatoid arthritis, psoriatic arthritis, or ankylosing spondylitis. Golimumab should not be used in combination with *biologic* DMARDs.

Ankylosing spondylitis: SubQ: 50 mg once a month (either alone or in combination with methotrexate or other nonbiologic DMARDs)

Psoriatic arthritis: SubQ: 50 mg once a month (either alone or in combination with methotrexate or other nonbiologic DMARDs)

Rheumatoid arthritis:

IV: 2 mg/kg at weeks 0, 4, and then every 8 weeks thereafter (in combination with methotrexate)

SubQ: 50 mg once a month (in combination with methotrexate)

Ulcerative colitis:

US labeling: SubQ: Induction: 200 mg at week 0, then 100 mg at week 2, followed by maintenance therapy of 100 mg every 4 weeks

Canadian labeling: SubQ: Induction: 200 mg at week 0, then 100 mg at week 2, followed by maintenance therapy of 50 mg every 4 weeks (maintenance dose may be increased to 100 mg every 4 weeks if needed)

Renal Impairment There are no dosage adjustments provided in manufacturer's labeling (has not been studied).

Hepatic Impairment There are no dosage adjustments provided in manufacturer's labeling (has not been studied).

Administration

IV: Dilute prior to use. Infuse over 30 minutes, using an infusion set with an in-line low protein-binding 0.22 micron filter. Do not infuse in the same line with other medications.

Subcutaneous injection: Hold autoinjector firmly against skin and inject subcutaneously into thigh, lower abdomen (below navel), or upper arm. A loud click is heard when injection has begun. Continue to hold autoinjector against skin until second click is heard (may take 3-15 seconds). Following second click, lift autoinjector from injection site. Rotate injection sites and avoid injecting into tender, red, scaly, hard, or bruised skin, or areas with scars or stretch marks. If multiple injections are required for a single dose, administer at different sites on body.

Monitoring Parameters CBC with differential; latent TB screening (prior to initiating and periodically during therapy); HBV screening (prior to initiating [all patients]; during and for several months following therapy [HBV carriers]); monitor improvement of symptoms and physical function assessments; signs/symptoms of infection (prior to, during, and following therapy); signs/symptoms/worsening of heart failure signs and symptoms of hypersensitivity reaction; symptoms of lupus-like syndrome; signs/symptoms of malignancy (eg, splenomegaly, hepatomegaly, abdominal pain, persistent fever, night sweats, weight loss) including periodic skin examination

Dosage Forms Excipient information presented when available (limited, particularly for generics); consult specific product labeling.

Solution, Intravenous [preservative free]:

Simponi Aria: 50 mg/4 mL (4 mL) [latex free; contains polysorbate 80]

Solution Auto-injector, Subcutaneous [preservative free]:

Simponi: 50 mg/0.5 mL (0.5 mL); 100 mg/mL (1 mL) [contains polysorbate 80]

Solution Prefilled Syringe, Subcutaneous [preservative free]:

Simponi: 50 mg/0.5 mL (0.5 mL); 100 mg/mL (1 mL) [contains polysorbate 80]

Goserelin (GOE se rel in)

Brand Names: US Zoladex

Brand Names: Canada Zoladex; Zoladex LA

Index Terms Goserelin Acetate; ICI-118630; ZDX

Pharmacologic Category Antineoplastic Agent, Gonadotropin-Releasing Hormone Agonist; Gonadotropin Releasing Hormone Agonist

Use

US labeling:

Breast cancer, advanced (3.6 mg only): Palliative treatment of advanced breast cancer in pre- and perimenopausal women (estrogen and progesterone receptor values may help to predict if goserelin is likely to be beneficial).

Endometrial thinning (3.6 mg only): Endometrial-thinning agent prior to endometrial ablation for dysfunctional uterine bleeding.

Endometriosis (3.6 mg only): Management of endometriosis, including pain relief and reduction of endometriotic lesions for the duration of therapy (goserelin experience for endometriosis has been limited to women 18 years and older treated for 6 months).

Prostate cancer, advanced (3.6 mg or 10.8 mg): Palliative treatment of advanced carcinoma of the prostate.

Prostate cancer, stage B2 to C (3.6 mg or 10.8 mg):: Management of locally confined stage T2b to T4 (stage B2 to C) prostate cancer (in combination with an antiandrogen [eg, flutamide]); begin goserelin and antiandrogen therapy 8 weeks prior to initiating radiation therapy and continue during radiation therapy.

Canadian labeling:

Breast cancer, advanced (3.6 mg only): Palliative treatment of advanced breast cancer in pre- and perimenopausal women (with estrogen and/or progesterone receptor-positive tumors).

Breast cancer, early (3.6 mg only): Alternative to standard adjuvant chemotherapy in pre- and perimenopausal women with early breast cancer (with estrogen and/or progesterone receptor-positive tumors) who are unsuitable for, intolerant to, or decline chemotherapy.

Endometrial thinning (3.6 mg only): Endometrial-thinning agent prior to endometrial ablation.

Endometriosis (3.6 mg or 10.8 mg): Hormonal management of endometriosis, including pain relief and reduction of endometriotic lesions (goserelin experience for endometriosis has been limited to women 18 years and older treated for 6 months).

Prostate cancer, advanced (3.6 mg or 10.8 mg): Palliative treatment of hormone-dependent advanced carcinoma of the prostate (stage M1 or D2).

Prostate cancer, locally advanced (3.6 mg or 10.8 mg): Management of locally advanced (T3 or T4) or bulky stage T2b to T2c prostate cancer (in combination with a nonsteroidal antiandrogen and radiation therapy); begin goserelin and antiandrogen therapy 8 weeks prior to initiating radiation therapy and continue until completion of radiation therapy.

Prostate cancer, locally advanced (3.6 mg or 10.8 mg): Adjuvant hormone therapy to external beam irradiation in locally advanced prostate cancer (stage T3 to T4).

Pregnancy Considerations Adverse events were observed in animal reproduction studies. Goserelin induces hormonal changes which increase the risk for fetal loss and use is contraindicated in pregnancy unless being used for palliative treatment of advanced breast cancer.

Breast cancer: If used for the palliative treatment of breast cancer during pregnancy, the potential for increased fetal loss should be discussed with the patient.

Endometriosis, endometrial thinning: Use is contraindicated during pregnancy. Women of childbearing potential should not receive therapy until pregnancy has been excluded. Nonhormonal contraception is recommended for premenopausal women during therapy and for 12 weeks after therapy is discontinued. Although ovulation is usually inhibited and menstruation may stop, pregnancy prevention is not ensured during goserelin therapy. Changes in reproductive function may occur following chronic administration.

Breast-Feeding Considerations It is not known if goserelin is excreted in breast milk, although goserelin is inactivated when used orally. Due to the potential for serious adverse reactions in the breast-feeding infant, a decision should be made to discontinue breast-feeding or to discontinue the drug, taking into account the importance of treatment to the mother.

Contraindications

US labeling: Hypersensitivity to goserelin, GnRH, GnRH agonist analogues, or any component of the formulation; pregnancy (except if using for palliative treatment of advanced breast cancer)

Canadian labeling: Hypersensitivity to goserelin or any component of the formulation; undiagnosed vaginal bleeding

Warnings/Precautions Hazardous agent - use appropriate precautions for handling and disposal (NIOSH 2014 [group 1]). Transient increases in serum testosterone (in men with prostate cancer) and estrogen (in women with breast cancer) may result in a worsening of disease signs and symptoms (tumor flare) during the first few weeks of treatment. Some patients experienced a temporary worsening of bone pain, which may be managed symptomatically. Spinal cord compression and urinary tract obstruction have been reported when used for prostate cancer; closely observe patients for symptoms (eg, ureteral obstruction, weakness, paresthesias) in first few weeks of therapy. Manage with standard treatment; consider orchiectomy for extreme cases.

Androgen deprivation therapy may increase the risk for cardiovascular disease (Levine, 2010). An increased risk for MI, sudden cardiac death, and stroke has been observed. Monitor for signs/symptoms of cardiovascular disease; manage according to current clinical practice. Androgen deprivation therapy may cause prolongation of the QT/QTc interval; evaluate risk versus benefit in patients with congenital long QT syndrome, heart failure, frequent electrolyte abnormalities, and in patients taking medication known to prolong the QT interval. Correct electrolytes prior to initiation and consider periodic electrolyte and ECG monitoring. Hyperglycemia has been reported in males and may manifest as diabetes or worsening of preexisting diabetes (worsening glycemic control); monitor blood glucose and HbA$_{1c}$ and manage diabetes appropriately.

Injection site and vascular injury, including pain, hematoma, hemorrhage and hemorrhagic shock (requiring blood transfusions or surgical intervention) have been reported with goserelin. Use extra caution when administering to patients with a low BMI and/or to patients receiving full dose anticoagulation (Canadian labeling does not recommend use of goserelin in these patients due to the risk of vascular injury/bleeding). Use caution while injecting goserelin into the anterior abdominal wall (due to the proximity of underlying inferior epigastric artery and its branches). Monitor for signs/symptoms of abdominal hemorrhage. Inform patient to immediately report abdominal pain, abdominal distention, dyspnea, dizziness, hypotension, and/or altered level of consciousness. Hypersensitivity reactions (including acute anaphylactic reactions) and antibody formation may occur; monitor. Hypercalcemia has been reported in prostate and breast cancer patients with bone metastases; initiate appropriate management if hypercalcemia occurs. Rare cases of pituitary apoplexy (frequently secondary to pituitary adenoma) have been observed with GnRH agonist administration (onset from 1 hour to usually <2 weeks); may present as sudden headache, vomiting, visual or mental status changes, and infrequently cardiovascular collapse; immediate medical attention required. A decreased AUC may be observed when using the 3-month implant in obese patients; monitor testosterone levels if desired clinical response is not observed. Use extra care when administering to patients with a low BMI. If implant removal is necessary, implant may be located by ultrasound.

Decreased bone density has been reported in women and may be irreversible; use caution if other risk factors are present; evaluate and institute preventive treatment if necessary. Cervical resistance may be increased; use caution when dilating the cervix for endometrial ablation. Women of childbearing potential should not receive therapy until pregnancy has been excluded. Nonhormonal contraception is recommended during therapy and for 12 weeks after therapy is discontinued. Chronic administration may result in effects on reproductive function due to antigonadotropic properties. Potentially significant drug-drug interactions may exist, requiring dose or frequency adjustment, additional monitoring, and/or selection of alternative therapy.

Adverse Reactions Some frequencies not defined. Percentages reported with the 1-month implant:

>10%:

Cardiovascular: Vasodilatation (females 57%), peripheral edema (females 21%)

Central nervous system: Headache (females 32% to 75%; males 1% to 5%), emotional lability (females 60%), depression (females 54%; males 1% to 5%), pain (8% to 17%), dyspareunia (females 14%), insomnia (5% to 11%)

Dermatologic: Diaphoresis (females 16% to 45%; males 6%), acne vulgaris (females 42%; usually within 1 month after starting treatment), seborrhea (females 26%)

Endocrine & metabolic: Hot flash (females 57% to 96%; males 64%), decreased libido (females 48% to 61%), increased libido (females 12%)

Gastrointestinal: Abdominal pain (females 7% to 11%), nausea (5% to 11%)

Genitourinary: Vaginitis (75%), breast atrophy (females 33%), sexual disorder (males 21%), breast hypertrophy (females 18%), decrease in erectile frequency (18%), pelvic symptoms (females 18%), genitourinary signs and symptoms (lower; males 13%)

Hematologic & oncologic: Tumor flare (females 23%; males: Incidence not reported)

Infection: Infection (females 13%; males: Incidence not reported)

Neuromuscular & skeletal: Decreased bone mineral density (females 23%; ~4% decrease from baseline in 6 months; male: Incidence not reported), weakness (females 11%)

1% to 10%:

Cardiovascular: Edema (females 5%; male 7%), hypertension (1% to 6%), cardiac failure (males 5%), cardiac arrhythmia (males >1% to <5%), cerebrovascular accident (males >1% to <5%), peripheral vascular disease (males >1% to <5%), varicose veins (males >1% to <5%), chest pain (1% to <5%), myocardial infarction (males <1% to <5%), palpitations, tachycardia (females)

Central nervous system: Lethargy (females ≤8%), migraine (females 1% to 7%), dizziness (females 6%; male 5%), malaise (females ≤5%), chills (males >1% to <5%), anxiety (1% to <5%), nervousness (females 3% to 5%), voice disorder (females 3%), abnormality in thinking, drowsiness, paresthesia

Dermatologic: Skin rash (males 6% to 8%; female frequency not reported), hair disease (females 4%), pruritus (females 2%), alopecia, skin discoloration, xeroderma

Endocrine & metabolic: Gynecomastia (males 8%), hirsutism (7%), gout (males >1% to <5%), hyperglycemia (males >1% to <5%), weight gain (>1% to <5%)

Gastrointestinal: Anorexia (1% to 5%), gastric ulcer (males >1% to <5%), constipation (1% to <5%), diarrhea (1% to <5%), vomiting (1% to <5%), increased appetite (females 2%), dyspepsia, flatulence, xerostomia

Genitourinary: Pelvic pain (females 9%; males 6%), mastalgia (>1% to 7%), uterine hemorrhage (6%), vulvovaginitis (5%), breast swelling (males >1% to <5%), urinary tract obstruction (males: >1% to <5%), urinary tract infection (1% to <5%), urinary frequency, vaginal hemorrhage

Hematologic & oncologic: Anemia (males >1% to <5%), bruise, hemorrhage

Hypersensitivity: Hypersensitivity reaction

Infection: Sepsis (males >1% to <5%)

Local: Application site reaction (females 6%)

Neuromuscular & skeletal: Myalgia (females 3%, males frequency not reported), leg cramps (females 2%, males frequency not reported), hypertonia (females 1%; male frequency not reported), arthralgia, arthropathy

Ophthalmic: Amblyopia, dry eye syndrome

Renal: Renal insufficiency (<1% to >5%)

Respiratory: Upper respiratory tract infection (males 7%), chronic obstructive pulmonary disease (males 5%), flu-like symptoms (females 5%, male frequency not reported), pharyngitis (females 5%), sinusitis (females ≥1%; male frequency not reported), bronchitis, cough, epistaxis, rhinitis

Miscellaneous: Fever

<1% (Limited to important or life-threatening): Anaphylaxis, convulsions, deep vein thrombosis, diabetes mellitus, hypercalcemia, hypercholesterolemia, increased HDL cholesterol, increased serum ALT, increased serum AST, injection site reaction (including vascular injury, pain, hematoma, hemorrhage, hemorrhagic shock), osteoporosis, ovarian cyst, ovarian hyperstimulation syndrome, pituitary apoplexy, pituitary neoplasm (including adenoma), pulmonary embolism, psychotic reaction, transient ischemic attacks

Drug Interactions

Metabolism/Transport Effects None known.

Avoid Concomitant Use

Avoid concomitant use of Goserelin with any of the following: Corifollitropin Alfa; Highest Risk QTc-Prolonging Agents; Indium 111 Capromab Pendetide; Ivabradine; Mifepristone

Increased Effect/Toxicity

Goserelin may increase the levels/effects of: Corifollitropin Alfa; Highest Risk QTc-Prolonging Agents; Moderate Risk QTc-Prolonging Agents

The levels/effects of Goserelin may be increased by: Ivabradine; Mifepristone; QTc-Prolonging Agents (Indeterminate Risk and Risk Modifying)

Decreased Effect

Goserelin may decrease the levels/effects of: Antidiabetic Agents; Choline C 11; Indium 111 Capromab Pendetide

Storage/Stability Store at room temperature not to exceed 25°C (77°F). Keep in foil pouch until ready to use to protect from light and moisture.

Mechanism of Action Goserelin (a gonadotropin-releasing hormone [GnRH] analog) causes an initial increase in luteinizing hormone (LH) and follicle stimulating hormone (FSH), chronic administration of goserelin results in a sustained suppression of pituitary gonadotropins. Serum testosterone falls to levels comparable to surgical castration. The exact mechanism of this effect is unknown, but may be related to changes in the control of LH or down-regulation of LH receptors.

Pharmacodynamics/Kinetics

Onset:

Females: Estradiol suppression reaches postmenopausal levels within 3 weeks and FSH and LH are suppressed to follicular phase levels within 4 weeks of initiation

Males: Testosterone suppression reaches castrate levels within 2 to 4 weeks after initiation

Duration:

Females: Estradiol, LH and FSH generally return to baseline levels within 12 weeks following the last monthly implant.

Males: Testosterone levels maintained at castrate levels throughout the duration of therapy.

Absorption: SubQ: Rapid and can be detected in serum in 30 to 60 minutes; 3.6 mg: released slowly in first 8 days, then rapid and continuous release for 28 days

Distribution: V_d: Male: 44.1 L; Female: 20.3 L

Protein binding: ~27%

Metabolism: Hepatic hydrolysis of the C-terminal amino acids

Time to peak, serum: SubQ: Male: 12 to 15 days, Female: 8 to 22 days

Excretion: Urine (>90%; 20% as unchanged drug)

Dosing

Adult

US labeling:

Prostate cancer, advanced: Males: SubQ:
28-day implant: 3.6 mg every 28 days
12-week implant: 10.8 mg every 12 weeks

Prostate cancer, stage B2 to C (in combination with an antiandrogen and radiotherapy; begin 8 weeks prior to radiotherapy): Males: SubQ:
Combination 28-day/12-week implant: 3.6 mg implant, followed in 28 days by 10.8 mg implant
28-day implant (alternate dosing): 3.6 mg; repeated every 28 days for a total of 4 doses

Breast cancer, advanced: Females: SubQ: 3.6 mg every 28 days

Endometriosis: Females: SubQ: 3.6 mg every 28 days for 6 months

Endometrial thinning: Females: SubQ: 3.6 mg every 28 days for 1 or 2 doses

Canadian labeling:

Prostate cancer, advanced: Males: SubQ:
28-day implant: 3.6 mg every 28 days
3-month implant: 10.8 mg every 13 weeks

Prostate cancer, stage B2 to C (in combination with an antiandrogen and radiotherapy; begin 8 weeks prior to radiotherapy): Males: SubQ:
Combination 28-day/3-month implant: 3.6 mg implant, followed in 28 days by 10.8 mg implant
28-day implant (alternate dosing): 3.6 mg; repeated every 28 days for a total of 4 doses

Breast cancer, advanced: Females: SubQ: 3.6 mg every 28 days

Breast cancer, early: Females: SubQ: 3.6 mg every 28 days

Endometriosis: Females: SubQ:
28-day implant: 3.6 mg every 28 days for 6 months
3-month implant: 10.8 mg every 12 weeks for 6 months

Endometrial thinning: Females: SubQ: 3.6 mg every 28 days for 2 doses

Off-label dosing:

Prevention of early menopause during chemotherapy for early stage hormone receptor negative breast cancer (off-label use): Adult females: SubQ: 3.6 mg every 28 days starting 1 week prior to the first chemotherapy dose; continue until within 2 weeks before or after the final chemotherapy dose (Moore, 2015).

Geriatric Males: Refer to adult dosing.

Renal Impairment No dosage adjustment necessary.

Hepatic Impairment No dosage adjustment necessary.

Administration SubQ: Administer implant by inserting needle at a 30 to 45 degree angle into the anterior abdominal wall below the navel line. Use caution while injecting goserelin into the anterior abdominal wall (due to the proximity of underlying inferior epigastric artery and its branches). Goserelin is an implant; therefore, do not attempt to eliminate air bubbles prior to injection (may displace implant). Do not attempt to aspirate prior to injection; if a large vessel is penetrated, blood will be visualized in the syringe chamber (if vessel is penetrated, withdraw needle and inject elsewhere with a new syringe). Do not penetrate into muscle or peritoneum. Implant may be detected by ultrasound if removal is required. Monitor for signs/symptoms of abdominal hemorrhage. Use extra care when administering goserelin to patients with a low BMI and/or to patients receiving full dose anticoagulation (Canadian labeling does not recommend use in these patients due to the risk of vascular injury/bleeding).

Hazardous agent; use appropriate precautions for handling and disposal (NIOSH 2014 [group 1]).

Monitoring Parameters Monitor blood glucose and HbA_{1c} (periodically), bone mineral density, serum calcium, cholesterol/lipids; monitor for signs/symptoms of abdominal hemorrhage following injection.

Prostate cancer: Consider periodic ECG and electrolyte monitoring. Monitor for weakness, paresthesias, tumor flare, urinary tract obstruction, and spinal cord compression in first few weeks of therapy.

Test Interactions Interferes with pituitary gonadotropic and gonadal function tests during and for up to 12 weeks after discontinued

Dosage Forms Excipient information presented when available (limited, particularly for generics); consult specific product labeling.
Implant, Subcutaneous:
Zoladex: 3.6 mg (1 ea); 10.8 mg (1 ea)
Dosage Forms: Canada Excipient information presented when available (limited, particularly for generics); consult specific product labeling.
Implant, Subcutaneous:
Zoladex: 3.6 mg
Zoladex LA: 10.8 mg

♦ Goserelin Acetate *see* Goserelin *on page 854*

♦ GP 47680 *see* OXcarbazepine *on page 1352*

♦ GR38032R *see* Ondansetron *on page 1335*

♦ Gralise *see* Gabapentin *on page 823*

♦ Gralise Starter *see* Gabapentin *on page 823*

♦ Gramicidin, Neomycin, and Polymyxin B *see* Neomycin, Polymyxin B, and Gramicidin *on page 1267*

Granisetron (gra NI se tron)

Brand Names: US Granisol [DSC]; Sancuso
Brand Names: Canada Granisetron Hydrochloride Injection; Kytril
Index Terms BRL 43694; Granisetron Hydrochloride; Granisol; Kytril
Pharmacologic Category Antiemetic; Selective 5-HT$_3$ Receptor Antagonist
Use
Chemotherapy-associated nausea and vomiting: Prevention of nausea and vomiting associated with initial and repeat courses of emetogenic chemotherapy, including high-dose cisplatin (injection and tablets); prevention of nausea and vomiting associated with moderately and/or highly emetogenic chemotherapy regimens of up to 5 consecutive days of duration (transdermal).
Radiation-associated nausea and vomiting: Prevention of nausea and vomiting associated with radiation therapy, including total body radiation and fractionated abdominal radiation (tablets).
Pregnancy Considerations Adverse events have not been observed in animal reproduction studies. Injection (1 mg/mL strength) may contain benzyl alcohol which may cross the placenta.
Breast-Feeding Considerations It is not known if granisetron is excreted in breast milk. The US manufacturer recommends that caution be exercised when administering granisetron to nursing women. The Canadian manufacturer does not recommend use in nursing women.
Contraindications
Hypersensitivity to granisetron or any component of the formulation
Canadian labeling: Additional contraindications (not in U.S. labeling): Concomitant use with apomorphine
Warnings/Precautions Use with caution in patients with congenital long QT syndrome or other risk factors for QT prolongation (eg, medications known to prolong QT interval, electrolyte abnormalities, and cumulative high-dose anthracycline therapy). 5-HT$_3$ antagonists have been associated with a number of dose-dependent increases in ECG intervals (eg, PR, QRS duration, QT/QTc, JT), usually occurring 1 to 2 hours after IV administration. In general, these changes are not clinically relevant, however, when used in conjunction with other agents that prolong these intervals, arrhythmia may occur. When used with agents that prolong the QT interval (eg, Class I and III antiarrhythmics), clinically relevant QT interval prolongation may occur resulting in torsade de pointes. IV formulations of 5-HT$_3$ antagonists have more association with ECG interval changes, compared to oral formulations.

Antiemetics are most effective when used prophylactically (Roila 2010). If emesis occurs despite optimal antiemetic prophylaxis, re-evaluate emetic risk, disease, concurrent morbidities and medications to assure antiemetic regimen is optimized (Basch 2011).

Serotonin syndrome has been reported with 5-HT$_3$ receptor antagonists, predominantly when used in combination with other serotonergic agents (eg, SSRIs, SNRIs, MAOIs, mirtazapine, fentanyl, lithium, tramadol, and/or methylene blue). Some of the cases have been fatal. The majority of serotonin syndrome reports due to 5-HT$_3$ receptor antagonist have occurred in a postanesthesia setting or in an infusion center. Serotonin syndrome has also been reported following overdose of another 5-HT$_3$ receptor antagonist. Monitor patients for signs of serotonin syndrome, including mental status changes (eg, agitation, hallucinations, delirium, coma); autonomic instability (eg, tachycardia, labile blood pressure, diaphoresis, dizziness, flushing, hyperthermia); neuromuscular changes (eg, tremor, rigidity, myoclonus, hyperreflexia, incoordination); gastrointestinal symptoms (eg, nausea, vomiting, diarrhea); and/or seizures. If serotonin syndrome occurs, discontinue 5-HT$_3$ receptor antagonist treatment and begin supportive management. Use with caution in patients allergic to other 5-HT$_3$ receptor antagonists; cross-reactivity has been reported. Does not stimulate gastric or intestinal peristalsis (should not be used instead of nasogastric suction); may mask progressive ileus and/or gastric distension. Potentially significant drug-drug interactions may exist, requiring dose or frequency adjustment, additional monitoring, and/or selection of alternative therapy.

Transdermal patch: Do not apply patch to red, irritated, or damaged skin. Application-site reactions have occurred with transdermal patch use; local reactions were generally mild and did not require discontinuation. If skin reaction is severe or generalized (allergic rash including erythematous, macular, or papular rash or pruritus), remove patch. Cover patch application site with clothing to protect from natural or artificial sunlight exposure while patch is applied and for 10 days following removal; granisetron may potentially be affected by natural or artificial sunlight. Do not apply heat (eg, heating pad) over or in area of the transdermal patch; avoid prolonged exposure to heat (may increase plasma concentrations).

Benzyl alcohol and derivatives: Some dosage forms may contain benzyl alcohol; large amounts of benzyl alcohol (≥99 mg/kg/day) have been associated with a potentially fatal toxicity ("gasping syndrome") in neonates; the "gasping syndrome" consists of metabolic acidosis, respiratory distress, gasping respirations, CNS dysfunction (including convulsions, intracranial hemorrhage), hypotension and cardiovascular collapse (AAP ["Inactive" 1997]; CDC 1982); some data suggests that benzoate displaces bilirubin from protein binding sites (Ahlfors 2001); avoid or use dosage forms containing benzyl alcohol with caution in neonates. See manufacturer's labeling.

Polysorbate 80: Some dosage forms may contain polysorbate 80 (also known as Tweens). Hypersensitivity reactions, usually a delayed reaction, have been reported following exposure to pharmaceutical products containing polysorbate 80 in certain individuals (Isaksson 2002; Lucente 2000; Shelley 1995). Thrombocytopenia, ascites, pulmonary deterioration, and renal and hepatic failure have been reported in premature neonates after receiving parenteral products containing polysorbate 80 (Alade 1986; CDC 1984). See manufacturer's labeling.

Adverse Reactions
>10%:
Central nervous system: Headache (oral and IV: 3% to 21%; transdermal: <1%)
Gastrointestinal: Nausea (20%), constipation (oral and IV: 3% to 18%; transdermal: 5%), vomiting (12%)
Neuromuscular & skeletal: Weakness (oral: 14% to 18%; IV: 5%)
1% to 10%:
Cardiovascular: Prolonged Q-T interval on ECG (1% to 3%; >450 milliseconds, not associated with any arrhythmias), hypertension (oral and IV: 1% to 2%)
Central nervous system: Dizziness (5%), insomnia (oral and IV: ≤5%), drowsiness (1% to 4%), anxiety (oral and IV: ≤2%), agitation (IV: <2%), central nervous system stimulation (IV: <2%)
Dermatologic: Alopecia (3%), skin rash (IV: 1%)
Gastrointestinal: Diarrhea (oral and IV: 4% to 9%), decreased appetite (6%), dyspepsia (oral: 6%), abdominal pain (4% to 6%), dysgeusia (IV: 2%)
Hematologic & oncologic: Leukopenia (9%), anemia (4%), thrombocytopenia (2%)
Hepatic: Increased serum ALT (>2 x ULN: 3% to 6%), increased serum AST (>2 x ULN: 3% to 5%)
Miscellaneous: Fever (3% to 9%)
<1% (Limited to important or life-threatening): Angina pectoris, application site reaction (transdermal: including allergic rash, burn, discoloration, erythema, erythematous rash, irritation, macular rash, pain, papular rash, pruritus, urticaria, vesicles), atrial fibrillation, atrioventricular block (IV), bradycardia, cardiac arrhythmia, chest pain, ECG abnormality (IV), extrapyramidal reaction (oral), hypersensitivity reaction (includes anaphylaxis, dyspnea, hypotension, urticaria), hypotension, palpitations, serotonin syndrome, sick sinus syndrome, sinus bradycardia (IV), syncope, ventricular ectopy (IV; includes non-sustained tachycardia)

Drug Interactions

Metabolism/Transport Effects Substrate of CYP3A4 (minor); **Note:** Assignment of Major/Minor substrate status based on clinically relevant drug interaction potential

Avoid Concomitant Use

Avoid concomitant use of Granisetron with any of the following: Apomorphine; Highest Risk QTc-Prolonging Agents; Ivabradine; Mifepristone

Increased Effect/Toxicity

Granisetron may increase the levels/effects of: Apomorphine; Highest Risk QTc-Prolonging Agents; Moderate Risk QTc-Prolonging Agents; Panobinostat; Serotonin Modulators

The levels/effects of Granisetron may be increased by: Ivabradine; Mifepristone; QTc-Prolonging Agents (Indeterminate Risk and Risk Modifying)

Decreased Effect

Granisetron may decrease the levels/effects of: Tapentadol; TraMADol

Preparation for Administration IV: May be given undiluted or may be further diluted in NS or D5W.

Storage/Stability

IV: Store at 15°C to 30°C (59°F to 86°F). Protect from light. Do not freeze vials. Stable when mixed in NS or D5W for at least 24 hours at room temperature.

Oral: Store tablet or oral solution at 15°C to 30°C (59°F to 86°F). Protect from light.

Transdermal patch: Store at 20°C to 25°C (68°F to 77°F). Keep patch in original packaging until immediately prior to use.

Mechanism of Action Selective 5-HT$_3$-receptor antagonist, blocking serotonin, both peripherally on vagal nerve terminals and centrally in the chemoreceptor trigger zone

Pharmacodynamics/Kinetics

Onset of action: IV: 1-3 minutes

Duration: Oral, IV: Generally up to 24 hours

Absorption: Oral: Tablets and oral solution are bioequivalent; Transdermal patch: ~66% over 7 days

Distribution: V_d: 2 to 4 L/kg; widely throughout body

Protein binding: ~65%

Metabolism: Hepatic via N-demethylation, oxidation, and conjugation; some metabolites may have 5-HT$_3$ antagonist activity

Half-life elimination: Oral: 6 hours; IV: Mean range: 5 to 9 hours

Time to peak, plasma: Transdermal patch: Maximum systemic concentrations: ~48 hours after application (range: 24 to 168 hours)

Excretion: Urine (11% to 12% as unchanged drug, 48% to 49% as metabolites); feces (34% to 38% as metabolites)

Dosing

Adult & Geriatric

Prevention of chemotherapy-associated nausea and vomiting:

Oral: 2 mg once daily up to 1 hour before chemotherapy or 1 mg twice daily; the first 1 mg dose should be given up to 1 hour before chemotherapy (with the second 1 mg dose 12 hours later). Administer only on the day(s) chemotherapy is given.

IV: 10 mcg/kg 30 minutes prior to chemotherapy; only on the day(s) chemotherapy is given.

Transdermal patch: Prophylaxis of chemotherapy-related emesis: Apply 1 patch at least 24 hours prior to chemotherapy; may be applied up to 48 hours before chemotherapy. Remove patch a minimum of 24 hours after chemotherapy completion. Maximum duration: Patch may be worn up to 7 days, depending on chemotherapy regimen duration.

Adult guideline recommendations:

American Society of Clinical Oncology (ASCO; Basch 2011): High emetic risk:

IV: 1 mg or 10 mcg/kg on the day(s) chemotherapy is administered (antiemetic regimen also includes dexamethasone and aprepitant or fosaprepitant)

Oral: 2 mg on the day(s) chemotherapy is administered (antiemetic regimen also includes dexamethasone and aprepitant or fosaprepitant)

Multinational Association of Supportive Care in Cancer (MASCC) and European Society of Medical Oncology (ESMO) (Roila 2010):

Highly emetic chemotherapy:

IV: 1 mg or 10 mcg/kg (antiemetic regimen includes dexamethasone and aprepitant/fosaprepitant) prior to chemotherapy on day 1

Oral: 2 mg (antiemetic regimen includes dexamethasone and aprepitant/fosaprepitant) prior to chemotherapy on day 1

Moderately emetic chemotherapy:

IV: 1 mg or 10 mcg/kg (antiemetic regimen includes dexamethasone [and aprepitant/fosaprepitant for AC chemotherapy regimen]) prior to chemotherapy on day 1

Oral: 2 mg (antiemetic regimen includes dexamethasone [and aprepitant/fosaprepitant for AC chemotherapy regimen]) prior to chemotherapy on day 1

Low emetic risk:

IV: 1 mg or 10 mcg/kg prior to chemotherapy on day 1

Oral: 2 mg prior to chemotherapy on day 1

Prophylaxis of radiation therapy-associated emesis: Oral: 2 mg once daily within 1 hour of radiation therapy.

Prevention of postoperative nausea and vomiting (off-label use): IV: 0.35 to 3 mg (5 to 20 **mcg/kg**) administered at the end of surgery (Gan 2014).

Pediatric

Prevention of chemotherapy-associated nausea and vomiting: Children ≥2 years and Adolescents: IV: 10 mcg/kg 30 minutes prior to chemotherapy; only on the day(s) chemotherapy is given.

Pediatric guideline recommendations:

Prevention of chemotherapy-induced nausea and vomiting (off-label dosing; Dupuis 2013):

Highly emetogenic chemotherapy: Infants ≥1 month and Children <12 years: IV: 40 mcg/kg as a single daily dose prior to chemotherapy. Antiemetic regimen also includes dexamethasone.

Highly emetogenic chemotherapy: Children ≥12 years and Adolescents: IV: 40 mcg/kg as a single daily dose prior to chemotherapy. Antiemetic regimen includes dexamethasone and (if no known or suspected drug interactions) aprepitant.

Moderately emetogenic chemotherapy: Infants ≥1 month, Children, and Adolescents:

IV: 40 mcg/kg as a single daily dose. Antiemetic regimen also includes dexamethasone

Oral: 40 mcg/kg every 12 hours. Antiemetic regimen also includes dexamethasone

Low emetogenic chemotherapy: Infants ≥1 month, Children, and Adolescents:

IV: 40 mcg/kg as a single daily dose.

Oral: 40 mcg/kg every 12 hours.

Renal Impairment No dosage adjustment necessary.

Hepatic Impairment Kinetic studies in patients with hepatic impairment showed that total clearance was approximately halved; however, standard doses were very well tolerated, and dose adjustments are not necessary.

Administration

Oral: Doses should be given up to 1 hour prior to initiation of chemotherapy/radiation

IV: Administer IV push over 30 seconds or as a 5-minute infusion

Transdermal (Sancuso): Apply patch to clean, dry, intact skin on upper outer arm. Do not use on red, irritated, or damaged skin. Remove patch from pouch immediately before application. Do not cut patch. Cover patch application site with clothing to protect from natural or artificial sunlight exposure while patch is applied and for 10 days following removal; granisetron may potentially be affected by natural or artificial sunlight. Do not apply heat (eg, heating pad) over or in area of the transdermal patch; avoid prolonged exposure to heat (may increase plasma concentrations).

Dosage Forms Excipient information presented when available (limited, particularly for generics); consult specific product labeling. [DSC] = Discontinued product

Patch, Transdermal:

Sancuso: 3.1 mg/24 hr (1 ea)

Solution, Intravenous:

Generic: 0.1 mg/mL (1 mL); 1 mg/mL (1 mL); 4 mg/4 mL (4 mL)

Solution, Intravenous [preservative free]:

Generic: 0.1 mg/mL (1 mL); 1 mg/mL (1 mL)

Solution, Oral:

Granisol: 2 mg/10 mL (30 mL [DSC]) [contains fd&c yellow #6 (sunset yellow), sodium benzoate; orange flavor]

Tablet, Oral:

Generic: 1 mg

Dosage Forms: Canada Refer to Dosage Forms. **Note:** Transdermal patch is not available in Canada

Extemporaneous Preparations Note: Commercial oral solution is available (0.2 mg/mL)

A 0.2 mg/mL oral suspension may be made with tablets. Crush twelve 1 mg tablets in a mortar and reduce to a fine powder. Add 30 mL distilled water, mix well, and transfer to a bottle. Rinse the mortar with 10 mL cherry syrup and add to bottle. Add sufficient quantity of cherry syrup to make a final volume of 60 mL. Label "shake well". Stable 14 days at room temperature or refrigerated (Quercia 1997).

A 50 mcg/mL oral suspension may be made with tablets and one of three different vehicles (Ora-Sweet®, Ora-Plus®, or a mixture of methylcellulose 1% and Simple Syrup, N.F.). Crush one 1 mg tablet in a mortar and reduce to a fine powder. Add 20 mL of the chosen vehicle and mix to a uniform paste; transfer to a calibrated bottle. Label "shake well" and "refrigerate". Stable for 91 days refrigerated (Nahata 1998).

Nahata MC, Morosco RS, and Hipple TF, "Stability of Granisetron Hydrochloride in Two Oral Suspensions," *Am J Health Syst Pharm*, 1998, 55(23):2511-3.

Quercia RA, Zhang J, Fan C, et al, "Stability of Granisetron Hydrochloride in an Extemporaneously Prepared Oral Liquid," *Am J Health Syst Pharm*, 1997, 54(12):1404-6.

◆ **Granisetron Hydrochloride** *see* Granisetron *on page 857*

◆ **Granisetron Hydrochloride Injection (Can)** *see* Granisetron *on page 857*

◆ **Granisol** *see* Granisetron *on page 857*

◆ **Granisol [DSC]** *see* Granisetron *on page 857*

◆ **Granix** *see* Filgrastim *on page 766*

◆ **Granulex®** *see* Trypsin, Balsam Peru, and Castor Oil *on page 1849*

◆ **Granulocyte Colony Stimulating Factor** *see* Filgrastim *on page 766*

◆ **Granulocyte Colony Stimulating Factor (PEG Conjugate)** *see* Pegfilgrastim *on page 1407*

◆ **Granulocyte-Macrophage Colony Stimulating Factor** *see* Sargramostim *on page 1637*

Grass Pollen Allergen Extract (Timothy Grass) (GRAS POL uhn al er juhn EK strakt TIM oh thee GRAS)

Brand Names: US Grastek
Brand Names: Canada Grastek
Index Terms Timothy Grass
Pharmacologic Category Allergen-Specific Immunotherapy
Use
Grass pollen-induced allergic rhinitis: Immunotherapy for the treatment of grass pollen-induced allergic rhinitis with or without conjunctivitis confirmed by positive skin test or *in vitro* testing for pollen-specific IgE antibodies for timothy grass or cross-reactive grass pollens in patients 5 through 65 years of age. Not indicated for the immediate relief of allergy symptoms.
Canadian labeling: Treatment of signs and symptoms of moderate to severe seasonal timothy and related grass pollen induced allergic rhinitis with or without conjunctivitis in patients ≥5 years of age who have a positive skin test and/or positive titer to *Phleum pretense* specific IgE; symptoms for ≥2 pollen seasons; and patients who are not tolerant or responsive to conventional therapy.
Medication Guide Available Yes
Dosing
Adult Dosage strength expressed in Bioequivalent Allergy Units (BAU). **Note:** Initiate treatment ≥12 weeks (U.S. labeling) or ≥8 weeks (Canadian labeling) before expected onset of each pollen season and continue throughout pollen season. May be taken daily for 3 consecutive years (including intervals between grass pollen seasons). Safety and efficacy of initiating treatment during grass pollen season or restarting treatment after missing a dose have not been established. In clinical trials, treatment interruptions ≤7 days were allowed.

Grass pollen-induced allergic rhinitis: Adults ≤65 years: Sublingual: One tablet (2,800 BAU) once daily
Pediatric Dosage strength expressed in Bioequivalent Allergy Units (BAU).
Grass pollen-induced allergic rhinitis: Children ≥5 years and Adolescents: Refer to adult dosing.
Renal Impairment There are no dosage adjustments provided in the manufacturer's labeling.
Hepatic Impairment There are no dosage adjustments provided in the manufacturer's labeling.
Additional Information Complete prescribing information should be consulted for additional detail.

Dosage Forms Excipient information presented when available (limited, particularly for generics); consult specific product labeling.
Tablet Sublingual, Sublingual:
  Grastek: 2800 bau [contains gelatin (fish)]

◆ **Grastek** *see* Grass Pollen Allergen Extract (Timothy Grass) *on page 859*

◆ **Gravol [OTC] (Can)** *see* DimenhyDRINATE *on page 556*

◆ **Gravol IM (Can)** *see* DimenhyDRINATE *on page 556*

◆ **Grifulvin V** *see* Griseofulvin *on page 859*

Griseofulvin (gri see oh FUL vin)

Brand Names: US Grifulvin V; Gris-PEG
Index Terms Griseofulvin Microsize; Griseofulvin Ultramicrosize
Pharmacologic Category Antifungal Agent, Oral
Use Treatment of tinea infections of the skin, hair, and nails caused by susceptible species of *Microsporum, Epidermophyton,* or *Trichophyton*
Dosing
Adult & Geriatric Tinea infections: Oral:
Microsize:
  Tinea corporis, tinea cruris, tinea capitis: 500 mg daily in single or divided doses
  Tinea pedis, tinea unguium: 1000 mg daily in single or divided doses
Ultramicrosize: 375 mg daily in single or divided doses; doses up to 750 mg daily in divided doses have been used for infections more difficult to eradicate such as tinea unguium and tinea pedis

Duration of therapy depends on the site of infection:
  Tinea corporis: 2-4 weeks
  Tinea cruris: 2-6 weeks (*Red Book*, 2012)
  Tinea capitis: 4-6 weeks
  Tinea pedis: 4-8 weeks
  Tinea unguium: 4-6 months or longer
Pediatric Tinea infections: Oral: Children >2 years:
Microsize: 10-20 mg/kg/day in single or 2 divided doses (maximum: 1000 mg daily) (*Red Book*, 2012)
  Tinea capitis: Higher dosages (20-25 mg/kg/day) have been recommended (Ali, 2007; Lipozenic, 2002; Sethi, 2006)
Ultramicrosize: 5-15 mg/kg/day in single dose or 2 divided doses (maximum: 750 mg daily) (*Red Book*, 2012)

Duration of therapy depends on the site of infection:
  Tinea corporis: 2-4 weeks
  Tinea cruris: 2-6 weeks (*Red Book*, 2012)
  Tinea capitis:
    Manufacturer's labeling: 4-6 weeks
    Alternate recommendations: Children: 6-12 weeks; use up to 16 weeks may be required (AAP *Red Book*® recommends continuing treatment for 2 weeks after clinical resolution of symptoms) (Ali, 2007; Lipozenic, 2002; Sethi, 2006)
  Tinea pedis: 4-8 weeks
  Tinea unguium: 4-6 months or longer
Additional Information Complete prescribing information should be consulted for additional detail.
Dosage Forms Considerations
Microsized formulations: Suspensions, Grifulvin V tablets
Ultramicrosize formulation: Gris-PEG tablets
Dosage Forms Excipient information presented when available (limited, particularly for generics); consult specific product labeling.
Suspension, Oral:
  Generic: 125 mg/5 mL (118 mL, 120 mL)
Tablet, Oral:
  Grifulvin V: 500 mg [scored]
  Gris-PEG: 125 mg, 250 mg [scored]
  Generic: 125 mg, 250 mg, 500 mg

◆ **Griseofulvin Microsize** *see* Griseofulvin *on page 859*

◆ **Griseofulvin Ultramicrosize** *see* Griseofulvin *on page 859*

◆ **Gris-PEG** *see* Griseofulvin *on page 859*

◆ **Growth Hormone, Human** *see* Somatropin *on page 1686*

◆ **GRx HiCort 25 [DSC]** *see* Hydrocortisone (Topical) *on page 886*

◆ **GS-1101** *see* Idelalisib *on page 911*

◆ **GS-5885** *see* Ledipasvir and Sofosbuvir *on page 1038*

◆ **GSK-580299** *see* Papillomavirus (Types 16, 18) Vaccine (Human, Recombinant) *on page 1394*

◆ **GSK1120212** *see* Trametinib *on page 1823*

◆ **GSK 1838262** *see* Gabapentin Enacarbil *on page 826*

◆ **GSK2118436** *see* Dabrafenib *on page 476*

◆ **GTN** *see* Nitroglycerin *on page 1289*

◆ **Guaiatussin AC** *see* Guaifenesin and Codeine *on page 861*

◆ **Guaicon DMS [OTC]** *see* Guaifenesin and Dextromethorphan *on page 861*

GuaiFENesin (gwye FEN e sin)

Brand Names: US Altarussin [OTC]; Bidex [OTC]; Buckleys Chest Congestion [OTC]; Cough Syrup [OTC]; Diabetic Siltussin DAS-Na [OTC]; Diabetic Tussin Mucus Relief [OTC]; Diabetic Tussin [OTC]; Fenesin IR [OTC]; Geri-Tussin [OTC]; GoodSense Mucus Relief [OTC]; Iophen-NR [OTC]; Liquibid [OTC]; Liquituss GG [OTC]; Mucinex Chest Congestion Child [OTC]; Mucinex For Kids [OTC]; Mucinex Maximum Strength [OTC]; Mucinex [OTC]; Mucosa [OTC]; Mucus Relief Childrens [OTC]; Mucus Relief [OTC]; Mucus-ER [OTC]; Organ-I NR [OTC]; Q-Tussin [OTC]; Refenesen 400 [OTC]; Refenesen [OTC]; Robafen [OTC]; Robitussin Chest Congestion [OTC]; Robitussin Mucus+Chest Congest [OTC]; Scot-Tussin Expectorant [OTC]; Siltussin DAS [OTC]; Siltussin SA [OTC]; Tussin [OTC]; Xpect [OTC]

Brand Names: Canada Balminil Expectorant; Benylin Chest Congestion Extra Strength; Robitussin Mucus & Phlegm; Vicks DayQuil Mucus Control

Index Terms Cheratussin; GG; Glycerol Guaiacolate; Organidin NR

Pharmacologic Category Expectorant

Use Cough (expectorant): Help loosen phlegm (mucus) and thin bronchial secretions to make coughs more productive

Dosing

Adult & Geriatric

Cough (expectorant): Oral:

Granules: 200 to 400 mg every 4 hours as needed; maximum: 2,400 mg/24 hours

Extended-release tablet: 600 mg to 1,200 mg every 12 hours as needed; maximum: 2,400 mg/24 hours

Immediate-release tablet: 200 to 400 mg every 4 hours as needed; maximum: 2,400 mg/24 hours

Liquid: 200 to 400 mg every 4 hours as needed; maximum: 2,400 mg/24 hours

Pediatric

Cough (expectorant): Oral:

Granules:

Children 4 years to <6 years: 100 mg every 4 hours as needed; maximum: 600 mg/24 hours

Children 6 years to <12 years: 100 to 200 mg every 4 hours as needed; maximum: 1,200 mg/24 hours

Children ≥12 years and Adolescents: 200 to 400 mg every 4 hours as needed; maximum: 2,400 mg/24 hours

Extended-release tablet: Children ≥12 years and Adolescents: 600 mg to 1,200 mg every 12 hours as needed; maximum: 2,400 mg/24 hours

Immediate-release tablet: Children ≥12 years and Adolescents: 200 to 400 mg every 4 hours as needed; maximum: 2,400 mg/24 hours

Liquid:

Children 2 years to <4 years: Limited data available: 50 to 100 mg every 4 hours as needed; maximum: 600 mg/24 hours (Kliegman, 2007)

Children 4 years to <6 years: 50 to 100 mg every 4 hours as needed; maximum: 600 mg/24 hours

Children 6 years to <12 years: 100 to 200 mg every 4 hours as needed; maximum: 1,200 mg/24 hours

Children ≥12 years and Adolescents: 200 to 400 mg every 4 hours as needed; maximum: 2,400 mg/24 hours

Renal Impairment There are no dosage adjustments provided in manufacturer's labeling.

Hepatic Impairment There are no dosage adjustments provided in manufacturer's labeling.

Additional Information Complete prescribing information should be consulted for additional detail.

Dosage Forms Excipient information presented when available (limited, particularly for generics); consult specific product labeling. [DSC] = Discontinued product

Liquid, Oral:

Buckleys Chest Congestion: 100 mg/5 mL (118 mL) [alcohol free, sugar free; contains butylparaben, menthol, propylene glycol, propylparaben]

Diabetic Siltussin DAS-Na: 100 mg/5 mL (118 mL) [alcohol free, color free, fructose free, sodium free, sorbitol free, sugar free; contains aspartame, benzoic acid, methylparaben, propylene glycol; strawberry flavor]

Diabetic Tussin: 100 mg/5 mL (118 mL) [alcohol free, dye free, fructose free, sodium free, sorbitol free, sugar free; contains aspartame, menthol, methylparaben]

Diabetic Tussin Mucus Relief: 200 mg/5 mL (118 mL) [alcohol free, dye free, fructose free, sodium free, sorbitol free, sugar free; contains aspartame, benzoic acid, menthol, polyethylene glycol, propylene glycol]

Iophen-NR: 100 mg/5 mL (473 mL) [contains propylene glycol, saccharin sodium, sodium benzoate; raspberry flavor]

Liquituss GG: 200 mg/5 mL (118 mL, 473 mL) [alcohol free, sugar free; contains methylparaben, propylene glycol, propylparaben, saccharin sodium]

Mucinex Chest Congestion Child: 100 mg/5 mL (118 mL) [alcohol free; contains brilliant blue fcf (fd&c blue #1), edetate disodium, fd&c red #40, propylene glycol, sodium benzoate; grape flavor]

Mucinex Chest Congestion Child: 100 mg/5 mL (118 mL) [alcohol free; contains brilliant blue fcf (fd&c blue #1), fd&c red #40, propylene glycol, saccharin sodium, sodium benzoate; grape flavor]

Mucus Relief Childrens: 100 mg/5 mL (118 mL) [alcohol free; contains brilliant blue fcf (fd&c blue #1), fd&c red #40, propylene glycol, saccharin sodium, sodium benzoate]

Robitussin Mucus+Chest Congest: 100 mg/5 mL (118 mL) [alcohol free; contains fd&c red #40, menthol, propylene glycol, saccharin sodium, sodium benzoate]

Scot-Tussin Expectorant: 100 mg/5 mL (30 mL, 118 mL [DSC], 240 mL, 480 mL, 3780 mL) [alcohol free, dye free, saccharine free, sodium free, sorbitol free, sugar free]

Siltussin DAS: 100 mg/5 mL (118 mL) [alcohol free, dye free, sugar free; strawberry flavor]

Packet, Oral:

Mucinex For Kids: 50 mg (12 ea [DSC]) [contains aspartame; grape flavor]

Mucinex For Kids: 100 mg (12 ea) [contains aspartame; bubble-gum flavor]

Solution, Oral:

Q-Tussin: 100 mg/5 mL (120 mL [DSC], 240 mL [DSC]) [alcohol free; contains fd&c red #40, saccharin sodium, sodium benzoate]

Q-Tussin: 100 mg/5 mL (118 mL, 240 mL, 473 mL) [alcohol free; contains fd&c red #40, saccharin sodium, sodium benzoate; cherry flavor]

Generic: 100 mg/5 mL (5 mL, 10 mL, 15 mL, 118 mL [DSC], 237 mL [DSC], 473 mL [DSC]); 200 mg/10 mL (10 mL); 300 mg/15 mL (15 mL)

Syrup, Oral:

Altarussin: 100 mg/5 mL (120 mL, 236 mL, 473 mL, 3840 mL)

Altarussin: 100 mg/5 mL (120 mL, 240 mL, 480 mL, 3840 mL) [contains alcohol, usp]

Cough Syrup: 100 mg/5 mL (118 mL, 473 mL) [alcohol free; contains fd&c red #40, menthol, propylene glycol, saccharin sodium, sodium benzoate; fruit flavor]

Geri-Tussin: 100 mg/5 mL (473 mL) [alcohol free, sugar free; contains fd&c red #40, menthol, saccharin sodium, sodium benzoate]

Robafen: 100 mg/5 mL (118 mL, 240 mL [DSC], 473 mL) [contains alcohol, usp; cherry flavor]

Robitussin Chest Congestion: 100 mg/5 mL (118 mL, 237 mL) [alcohol free; contains fd&c red #40, saccharin sodium, sodium benzoate; flavored flavor]

Siltussin SA: 100 mg/5 mL (118 mL, 237 mL, 473 mL) [strawberry flavor]

Tussin: 100 mg/5 mL (118 mL, 237 mL) [alcohol free]

Generic: 100 mg/5 mL (480 mL)

Tablet, Oral:

Bidex: 400 mg [DSC] [scored]

Bidex: 400 mg [scored; contains saccharin sodium]

Diabetic Tussin Mucus Relief: 400 mg [scored; dye free, sodium free, sugar free]

Fenesin IR: 400 mg

GoodSense Mucus Relief: 400 mg [scored]

Liquibid: 400 mg

Mucosa: 400 mg [scored]

Mucus Relief: 400 mg

Mucus Relief: 400 mg [scored; dye free]

Organ-I NR: 200 mg [DSC] [scored]

Organ-I NR: 200 mg [scored; contains fd&c red #40 aluminum lake]

Refenesen: 200 mg [scored; contains fd&c red #40 aluminum lake]

Refenesen 400: 400 mg [scored; dye free]

Xpect: 400 mg [scored; contains saccharin sodium]

Generic: 200 mg, 400 mg

Tablet Extended Release 12 Hour, Oral:

Mucinex: 600 mg [contains fd&c blue #1 aluminum lake]

Mucinex Maximum Strength: 1200 mg [contains fd&c blue #1 aluminum lake]

Mucus-ER: 600 mg [gluten free]

Generic: 600 mg

◆ Guaifenesin AC Liquid *see* Guaifenesin and Codeine *on page 861*

Guaifenesin and Codeine
(gwye FEN e sin & KOE deen)

Brand Names: US Allfen CD; Allfen CDX; Codar GF; Dex-Tuss; Guaiatussin AC; Guaifenesin AC Liquid; Iophen C-NR; M-Clear; M-Clear WC; Mar-Cof CG; Ninjacof-XG; Robafen AC; Virtussin A/C

Index Terms Codeine and Guaifenesin; Robitussin AC

Pharmacologic Category Antitussive; Cough Preparation; Expectorant

Use Temporary control of cough due to minor throat and bronchial irritation

Dosing

Adult & Geriatric Cough (antitussive/expectorant): Oral:

Capsule: Guaifenesin 200 mg and codeine 9 mg: Two capsules every 4 hours (maximum: 12 capsules/24 hours)

Liquid:

Guaifenesin 100 mg and codeine 6.33 mg per 5 mL: 15 mL every 4-6 hours (maximum: 45 mL/24 hours)

Guaifenesin 100-200 mg and codeine 8-10 mg per 5 mL: 10 mL every 4 hours (maximum: 60 mL/24 hours)

Guaifenesin 300 mg and codeine 10 mg per 5 mL: 5 mL every 4-6 hours (maximum: 40 mL/24 hours)

Tablet: Guaifenesin 400 mg and codeine 10-20 mg: One tablet every 4-6 hours (maximum: 6 tablets/24 hours)

Pediatric Cough (antitussive/expectorant): Oral:

Children 6-11 years:

Capsule: Guaifenesin 200 mg and codeine 9 mg: One capsule every 4 hours (maximum: 6 capsules/24 hours)

Liquid:

Guaifenesin 100 mg and codeine 6.33 mg per 5 mL: 7.5 mL every 4-6 hours (maximum: 45 mL/24 hours)

Guaifenesin 100-200 mg and codeine 8-10 mg per 5 mL: 5 mL every 4 hours (maximum: 30 mL/24 hours)

Guaifenesin 300 mg and codeine 10 mg per 5 mL: 2.5 mL every 4-6 hours (maximum: 20 mL/24 hours)

Tablet: Guaifenesin 400 mg and codeine 10-20 mg: One-half tablet every 4-6 hours (maximum: 3 tablets/24 hours)

Children ≥12 years: Refer to adult dosing.

Additional Information Complete prescribing information should be consulted for additional detail.

Dosage Forms Excipient information presented when available (limited, particularly for generics); consult specific product labeling.

Capsule, oral:

M-Clear: Guaifenesin 200 mg and codeine phosphate 9 mg [contains tartrazine]

Liquid, oral:

Codar GF: Guaifenesin 200 mg and codeine phosphate 8 mg per 5 mL (473 mL) [contains propylene glycol; cotton candy flavor]

Dex-Tuss: Guaifenesin 300 mg and codeine phosphate 10 mg per 5 mL (473 mL) [ethanol free, gluten free, sugar free; contains propylene glycol; grape flavor]

Iophen C-NR: Guaifenesin 100 mg and codeine phosphate 10 mg per 5 mL (473 mL) [contains propylene glycol, sodium benzoate; raspberry flavor]

M-Clear WC: Guaifenesin 100 mg and codeine phosphate 6.33 mg per 5 mL (473 mL) [contains propylene glycol; cotton candy flavor]

Ninjacof-XG: Guaifenesin 200 mg and codeine phosphate 8 mg per 5 mL (473 mL) [dye free, ethanol free, sugar free; contains propylene glycol; cotton candy flavor]

Solution, oral: Guaifenesin 100 mg and codeine phosphate 10 mg per 5 mL (5 mL, 10 mL, 118 mL, 473 mL)

Mar-Cof CG: Guaifenesin 225 mg and codeine phosphate 7.5 mg per 5 mL (473 mL) [ethanol free, sugar free; contains propylene glycol, sodium benzoate, sodium 6 mg/5 mL]

Virtussin A/C: Guaifenesin 100 mg and codeine phosphate 10 mg per 5 mL (118 mL, 473 mL) [sugar free; contains propylene glycol; cherry flavor]

Syrup, oral: Guaifenesin 100 mg and codeine phosphate 10 mg per 5 mL (473 mL)

Guaiatussin AC: Guaifenesin 100 mg and codeine phosphate 10 mg per 5 mL (5 mL, 10 mL, 118 mL, 473 mL) [sugar free; contains ethanol 3.5%, sodium 1 mg/5 mL, sodium benzoate; cherry flavor]

Robafen AC: Guaifenesin 100 mg and codeine phosphate 10 mg per 5 mL (120 mL, 480 mL) [contains ethanol 3.5%, sodium 4 mg/5 mL, sodium benzoate; cherry flavor]

Tablet, oral:

Allfen CD: Guaifenesin 400 mg and codeine phosphate 10 mg

Allfen CDX: Guaifenesin 400 mg and codeine phosphate 20 mg

Controlled Substance Capsule: C-V; Liquid products: C-V; Tablet: C-III

Guaifenesin and Dextromethorphan
(gwye FEN e sin & deks troe meth OR fan)

Brand Names: US Cheracol D [OTC]; Cheracol Plus [OTC]; Coricidin HBP Chest Congestion and Cough [OTC]; Delsym Cough + Chest Congestion DM [OTC]; Diabetic Siltussin-DM DAS-Na Maximum Strength [OTC]; Diabetic Siltussin-DM DAS-Na [OTC]; Diabetic Tussin DM Maximum Strength [OTC]; Diabetic Tussin DM [OTC]; Double Tussin DM [OTC]; Fenesin DM IR [OTC]; Guaicon DMS [OTC]; Iophen DM-NR [OTC]; Kolephrin GG/DM [OTC]; Mucinex DM Maximum Strength [OTC]; Mucinex DM [OTC]; Mucinex Fast-Max DM Max [OTC]; Mucinex Kid's Cough Mini-Melts [OTC]; Mucinex Kid's Cough [OTC]; Q-Tussin DM [OTC]; Refenesen DM [OTC]; Robafen DM [OTC]; Robitussin Maximum Strength Cough + Congestion DM [OTC]; Robitussin Peak Cold Cough + Chest Congestion DM [OTC]; Robitussin Peak Cold Maximum Strength Cough + Chest Congestion DM [OTC]; Robitussin Peak Cold Sugar-Free Cough + Chest Congestion DM [OTC]; Safe Tussin DM [OTC]; Scot-Tussin Senior [OTC]; Silexin [OTC]; Siltussin DM DAS [OTC]; Siltussin DM [OTC]; Triaminic Cough & Congestion [OTC]; Vicks 44E [OTC]; Vicks DayQuil Mucus Control DM [OTC]; Vicks Nature Fusion Cough & Chest Congestion [OTC]; Vicks Pediatric Formula 44E [OTC]; Zyncof [OTC]

Brand Names: Canada Balminil DM E; Benylin DM-E

Index Terms Dextromethorphan and Guaifenesin

Pharmacologic Category Antitussive; Cough Preparation; Expectorant

Use Temporary control of cough due to minor throat and bronchial irritation

Dosing

Adult & Geriatric Cough (antitussive/expectorant): Oral:

General dosing guidelines: Guaifenesin 200-400 mg and dextromethorphan 10-20 mg every 4 hours (maximum dose: Guaifenesin 2400 mg and dextromethorphan 120 mg per day)

Product-specific labeling:

Mucinex DM: 1-2 tablets every 12 hours (maximum: 4 tablets/24 hours)

Vicks 44E: 15 mL every 4 hours (maximum: 6 doses/24 hours)

Vicks Pediatric Formula 44E: 30 mL every 4 hours (maximum: 6 doses/24 hours)

Pediatric Cough (antitussive/expectorant): Oral: Children:

2-6 years:

General dosing guidelines: Guaifenesin 50-100 mg and dextromethorphan 2.5-5 mg every 4 hours (maximum dose: Guaifenesin 600 mg and dextromethorphan 30 mg per day)

Product-specific labeling: Vicks Pediatric Formula 44E: 7.5 mL every 4 hours (maximum: 6 doses/24 hours)

6-12 years:

General dosing guidelines: Guaifenesin 100-200 mg and dextromethorphan 5-10 mg every 4 hours (maximum dose: Guaifenesin 1200 mg and dextromethorphan 60 mg per day)

Product-specific labeling:

Vicks 44E: 7.5 mL every 4 hours (maximum: 6 doses/24 hours)

Vicks Pediatric Formula 44E: 15 mL every 4 hours (maximum: 6 doses/24 hours)

≥12 years: Refer to adult dosing.

Additional Information Complete prescribing information should be consulted for additional detail.

Dosage Forms Excipient information presented when available (limited, particularly for generics); consult specific product labeling. [DSC] = Discontinued product.

Caplet, oral:

Fenesin DM IR: Guaifenesin 400 mg and dextromethorphan hydrobromide 15 mg [DSC]

Fenesin DM IR: Guaifenesin 400 mg and dextromethorphan hydrobromide 20 mg

Refenesen DM: Guaifenesin 400 mg and dextromethorphan hydrobromide 20 mg

Capsule, oral:

Coricidin HBP Chest Congestion and Cough: Guaifenesin 200 mg and dextromethorphan hydrobromide 10 mg

Robitussin Maximum Strength Cough + Congestion DM: Guaifenesin 200 mg and dextromethorphan hydrobromide 10 mg

Granules, oral:

Mucinex Kid's Cough Mini-Melts: Guaifenesin 100 mg and dextromethorphan hydrobromide 5 mg per packet (12s) [contains magnesium 6 mg/pack, phenylalanine 2 mg/packet, sodium 3 mg/packet; orange crème flavor]

Liquid, oral:

Delsym Cough + Chest Congestion DM: Guaifenesin 100 mg and dextromethorphan hydrobromide 5 mg per 5 mL (180 mL) [contains edetate disodium, proylene glycol, sodium benzoate; cherry flavor]

Diabetic Tussin DM: Guaifenesin 100 mg and dextromethorphan hydrobromide 10 mg per 5 mL (120 mL) [dye free, ethanol free, sugar free; contains phenylalanine 8.4 mg/5 mL]

Diabetic Tussin DM Maximum Strength: Guaifenesin 200 mg and dextromethorphan hydrobromide 10 mg per 5 mL (120 mL) [dye free, ethanol free, sugar free; contains phenylalanine 8.4 mg/5 mL]

Double Tussin DM: Guaifenesin 300 mg and dextromethorphan hydrobromide 20 mg per 5 mL (120 mL, 480 mL) [dye free, ethanol free, sugar free]

Iophen DM-NR: Guaifenesin 100 mg and dextromethorphan hydrobromide 10 mg per 5 mL (480 mL) [contains propylene glycol, sodium benzoate; raspberry flavor]

Kolephrin GG/DM: Guaifenesin 150 mg and dextromethorphan hydrobromide 10 mg per 5 mL (120 mL) [ethanol free; cherry flavor]

Mucinex Fast-Max DM Max: Guaifenesin 400 mg and dextromethorphan hydrobromide 20 mg per 20 mL (180 mL) [contains propylene glycol, potassium 6 mg/20 mL, sodium 13 mg/20 mL]

Mucinex Kid's Cough: Guaifenesin 100 mg and dextromethorphan hydrobromide 5 mg per 5 mL (120 mL) [contains propylene glycol, sodium 3 mg/5 mL; cherry flavor]

Robitussin Peak Cold Cough + Chest Congestion DM: Guaifenesin 100 mg and dextromethorphan hydrobromide 10 mg per 5 mL (120 mL, 240 mL) [contains menthol, propylene glycol, sodium 3.5 mg/5 mL, sodium benzoate]

Robitussin Peak Cold Sugar-Free Cough + Chest Congestion DM: Guaifenesin 100 mg and dextromethorphan hydrobromide 10 mg per 5 mL (120 mL) [sugar free; contains propylene glycol, sodium 3 mg/5 mL, sodium benzoate]

Robitussin Peak Cold Maximum Strength Cough + Chest Congestion DM: Guaifenesin 200 mg and dextromethorphan hydrobromide 10 mg per 5 mL (120 mL, 240 mL) [contains menthol, propylene glycol, sodium 5 mg/5 mL, sodium benzoate]

Safe Tussin DM: Guaifenesin 100 mg and dextromethorphan hydrobromide 15 mg per 5 mL (120 mL) [contains benzoic acid, phenylalanine 4.2 mg/5 mL, and propylene glycol; orange and mint flavors]

Scot-Tussin Senior: Guaifenesin 200 mg and dextromethorphan hydrobromide 15 mg per 5 mL (120 mL) [ethanol free, sodium free, sugar free]

Vicks 44E: Guaifenesin 200 mg and dextromethorphan hydrobromide 20 mg per 15 mL (120 mL, 235 mL) [contains ethanol, sodium 31 mg/15 mL, sodium benzoate]

Vicks DayQuil Mucus Control DM: Guaifenesin 200 mg and dextromethorphan hydrobromide 10 mg per 15 mL (295 mL) [contains propylene glycol, sodium 25 mg/15 mL, sodium benzoate; citrus blend flavor]

Vicks Nature Fusion Cough & Chest Congestion: Guaifenesin 200 mg and dextromethorphan hydrobromide 20 mg per 30 mL (236 mL) [dye free, ethanol free, gluten free; contains propylene glycol, sodium 36 mg/30 mL; honey flavor]

Vicks Pediatric Formula 44E: Guaifenesin 100 mg and dextromethorphan hydrobromide 10 mg per 15 mL (120 mL) [ethanol free; contains sodium 30 mg/15 mL, sodium benzoate; cherry flavor]

Generic: Guaifenesin 100 mg and dextromethorphan hydrobromide 10 mg per 5 mL (480 mL)

Syrup, oral:

Cheracol D: Guaifenesin 100 mg and dextromethorphan hydrobromide 10 mg per 5 mL (120 mL, 180 mL) [contains benzoic acid, ethanol 4.75%]

Cheracol Plus: Guaifenesin 100 mg and dextromethorphan hydrobromide 10 mg per 5 mL (120 mL) [contains benzoic acid, ethanol 4.75%]

Diabetic Siltussin-DM DAS-Na: Guaifenesin 100 mg and dextromethorphan hydrobromide 10 mg per 5 mL (118 mL) [ethanol free, sugar free; contains benzoic acid, phenylalanine 3 mg/5 mL, propylene glycol; strawberry flavor]

Diabetic Siltussin-DM DAS-Na Maximum Strength: Guaifenesin 200 mg and dextromethorphan hydrobromide 10 mg per 5 mL (118 mL) [ethanol free, sugar free; contains benzoic acid, phenylalanine 3 mg/5 mL, propylene glycol; strawberry flavor]

Guaicon DMS: Guaifenesin 100 mg and dextromethorphan hydrobromide 10 mg per 5 mL (10 mL) [ethanol free, sugar free]

Q-Tussin DM: Guaifenesin 100 mg and dextromethorphan hydrobromide 10 mg per 5 mL (118 mL, 237 mL, 473 mL) [ethanol free, contains sodium benzoate; cherry flavor]

Robafen DM: Guaifenesin 100 mg and dextromethorphan hydrobromide 10 mg per 5 mL (120 mL, 240 mL, 480 mL) [cherry flavor]

Silexin: Guaifenesin 100 mg and dextromethorphan hydrobromide 10 mg per 5 mL (45 mL) [ethanol free, sugar free)]

Siltussin DM: Guaifenesin 100 mg and dextromethorphan hydrobromide 10 mg per 5 mL (120 mL, 240 mL, 480 mL) [strawberry flavor]

Siltussin DM DAS: Guaifenesin 100 mg and dextromethorphan hydrobromide 10 mg per 5 mL (120 mL) [dye free, ethanol free, sugar free; strawberry flavor]

Triaminic Cough & Cold: Guaifenesin 100 mg and dextromethorphan hydrobromide 5 mg per 5 mL (118 mL) [contains propylene glycol, sodium benzoate; cherry flavor]

Zyncof: Guaifenesin 400 mg and dextromethorphan hydrobromide 20 mg per 5 mL (120 mL, 480 mL) [dye free, ethanol free, sugar free; contains propylene glycol; grape flavor]

Generic: Guaifenesin 100 mg and dextromethorphan hydrobromide 10 mg per 5 mL (5 mL, 10 mL, 120 mL, 480 mL)

Tablet, oral:

Silexin: Guaifenesin 100 mg and dextromethorphan hydrobromide 10 mg

Generic: Guaifenesin 1000 mg and dextromethorphan hydrobromide 60 mg; guaifenesin 1200 mg and dextromethorphan hydrobromide 60 mg

Tablet, extended release, oral:

Mucinex DM: Guaifenesin 600 mg and dextromethorphan hydrobromide 30 mg

Mucinex DM Maximum Strength: Guaifenesin 1200 mg and dextromethorphan hydrobromide 60 mg

Generic: Guaifenesin 1200 mg and dextromethorphan hydrobromide 60 mg

Guaifenesin and Phenylephrine
(gwye FEN e sin & fen il EF rin)

Brand Names: US Ambi 10PEH/400GFN [OTC]; Ed Bron GP [OTC]; Fenesin PE IR [OTC]; J-Max [OTC]; Liquibid® D-R [OTC]; Liquibid® PD-R [OTC]; Medent®-PEI [OTC]; MucaphEd [OTC]; Mucinex® Cold [OTC]; Mucus Relief Sinus [OTC]; Nu-COPD [OTC]; OneTab™ Congestion & Cold [OTC]; Refenesen™ PE [OTC]; Rescon GG [OTC]; Sudafed PE® Non-Drying Sinus [OTC]; Triaminic® Children's Chest & Nasal Congestion [OTC]

Index Terms Guaifenesin and Phenylephrine Tannate; Phenylephrine Hydrochloride and Guaifenesin

Pharmacologic Category Decongestant; Expectorant

Use Temporary relief of nasal congestion, sinusitis, rhinitis, and hay fever; temporary relief of cough associated with upper respiratory tract conditions, especially when associated with dry, nonproductive cough

Dosing

Adult & Geriatric Expectorant/decongestant: Oral (Rescon GG): 10 mL every 4-6 hours; maximum: 40 mL/24 hours

Pediatric Expectorant/decongestant: Oral:

Children 2-5 years (Rescon GG): 2.5 mL every 4-6 hours; maximum: 10 mL/24 hours

Children 6-11 years (Rescon GG): 5 mL every 4-6 hours; maximum: 20 mL/24 hours

Children ≥12 years (Rescon GG): Refer to adult dosing

Additional Information Complete prescribing information should be consulted for additional detail.

Dosage Forms Excipient information presented when available (limited, particularly for generics); consult specific product labeling. [DSC] = Discontinued product

Caplet, oral:

Fenesin PE IR: Guaifenesin 400 mg and phenylephrine hydrochloride 10 mg

OneTab™ Congestion & Cold: Guaifenesin 400 mg and phenylephrine hydrochloride 10 mg

Refenesen™ PE: Guaifenesin 400 mg and phenylephrine hydrochloride 10 mg

Sudafed PE® Non-Drying Sinus: Guaifenesin 200 mg and phenylephrine hydrochloride 5 mg

Liquid, oral:

Ed Bron GP: Guaifenesin 100 mg and phenylephrine hydrochloride 5 mg per 5 mL (480 mL) [dye free, ethanol free, sugar free; contains propylene glycol; orange flavor]

Mucinex® Cold: Guaifenesin 100 mg and phenylephrine hydrochloride 2.5 mg per 5 mL (480 mL) [contains propylene glycol, sodium 3 mg/5 mL; mixed berry flavor]

Nu-COPD: Guaifenesin 200 mg and phenylephrine hydrochloride 10 mg per 5 mL (480 mL)

Rescon GG: Guaifenesin 100 mg and phenylephrine hydrochloride 5 mg per 5 mL (120 mL, 480 mL) [dye free, ethanol free; contains propylene glycol; wild cherry flavor]

Syrup, oral:

J-Max: Guaifenesin 200 mg and phenylephrine hydrochloride 5 mg per 5 mL (473 mL) [ethanol free, sugar free; contains propylene glycol; strawberry cream flavor]

Triaminic® Children's Chest & Nasal Congestion: Guaifenesin 50 mg and phenylephrine hydrochloride 2.5 mg per 5 mL (118 mL) [contains benzoic acid, propylene glycol, sodium 3 mg/5 mL; tropical flavor]

Tablet, oral:

Ambi 10PEH/400GFN: Guaifenesin 400 mg and phenylephrine hydrochloride 10 mg

Liquibid® D-R: Guaifenesin 400 mg and phenylephrine hydrochloride 10 mg

Liquibid® PD-R: Guaifenesin 200 mg and phenylephrine hydrochloride 5 mg

Medent®-PEI: Guaifenesin 400 mg and phenylephrine hydrochloride 10 mg

MucaphEd: Guaifenesin 400 mg and phenylephrine hydrochloride 10 mg

Mucus Relief Sinus: Guaifenesin 400 mg and phenylephrine hydrochloride 10 mg

Nu-COPD: Guaifenesin 400 mg and phenylephrine hydrochloride 10 mg

◆ Guaifenesin and Phenylephrine Tannate see Guaifenesin and Phenylephrine on page 862

Guaifenesin and Pseudoephedrine
(gwye FEN e sin & soo doe e FED rin)

Brand Names: US Ambifed-G [OTC]; Congestac® [OTC]; ExeFen-IR [DSC]; Maxifed [OTC]; Maxifed-G [OTC] [DSC]; Mucinex® D Maximum Strength [OTC]; Mucinex® D [OTC]; Refenesen Plus [OTC]

Brand Names: Canada Contac® Cold-Chest Congestion, Non Drowsy, Regular Strength; Entex® LA; Novahistex® Expectorant with Decongestant

Index Terms Pseudoephedrine and Guaifenesin

Pharmacologic Category Alpha/Beta Agonist; Expectorant

Use Temporary relief of nasal congestion and to help loosen phlegm and thin bronchial secretions in the treatment of cough

Dosing

Adult Expectorant/decongestant: Oral:

Ambifed-G, Mucinex® D Maximum Strength: One tablet every 12 hours (maximum: 2 tablets/24 hours)

Congestac®: One caplet every 4-6 hours (maximum: 4 caplets in 24 hours)

Maxifed-G®, Mucinex® D: 1-2 tablets every 12 hours (maximum: 4 tablets/24 hours)

Maxifed®: One to 1½ tablets every 12 hours (maximum: 3 tablets/24 hours)

Geriatric Refer to adult dosing; use with caution.

Pediatric Expectorant/decongestant: Oral:

Children 2-6 years (Maxifed-G®): One-third to ½ tablet every 12 hours (maximum: 1 tablet/12 hours)

Children 6-12 years:

Ambifed-G, Maxifed®: One-half caplet or tablet every 12 hours (maximum: 1 tablet/24 hours)

Congestac®: One-half caplet every 4-6 hours (maximum: 2 caplets/24 hours)

Maxifed-G®: One-half to 1 tablet every 12 hours (maximum: 2 tablets/24 hours)

>12 years: Refer to adult dosing.

Additional Information Complete prescribing information should be consulted for additional detail.

Dosage Forms Excipient information presented when available (limited, particularly for generics); consult specific product labeling. [DSC] = Discontinued product

Caplet, oral:

Congestac, Refenesen Plus: Guaifenesin 400 mg and pseudoephedrine hydrochloride 60 mg

Tablet, oral:

Ambifed-G: Guaifenesin 400 mg and pseudoephedrine hydrochloride 20 mg

ExeFen-IR [DSC]: Guaifenesin 400 mg and pseudoephedrine hydrochloride 60 mg

Maxifed: Guaifenesin 400 mg and pseudoephedrine hydrochloride 60 mg

Maxifed-G [DSC]: Guaifenesin 400 mg and pseudoephedrine hydrochloride 40 mg

Tablet, extended release, oral:

Mucinex D: Guaifenesin 600 mg and pseudoephedrine hydrochloride 60 mg

Mucinex D Maximum Strength: Guaifenesin 1200 mg and pseudoephedrine hydrochloride 120 mg

◆ Guaifenesin DAC see Guaifenesin, Pseudoephedrine, and Codeine on page 863

Guaifenesin, Pseudoephedrine, and Codeine (gwye FEN e sin, soo doe e FED rin, & KOE deen)

Brand Names: US Cheratussin DAC; Guaifenesin DAC; Lortuss EX; Mytussin DAC [DSC]; Tricode GF; Virtussin DAC

Brand Names: Canada Balminil Codeine + Decongestant + Expectorant; Benylin 2 Cold and Flu with Codeine; Calmylin PSE with Codeine

Index Terms Codeine, Guaifenesin, and Pseudoephedrine; Pseudoephedrine, Guaifenesin, and Codeine

Pharmacologic Category Antitussive/Decongestant/Expectorant

Use Cough/nasal congestion: Temporarily relieves cough and nasal congestion associated with the common cold, allergic rhinitis, or other upper respiratory allergies

Dosing

Adult

Cough/nasal congestion: Oral: Codeine 10 mg/guaifenesin 100 mg/pseudoephedrine 30 mg per 5 mL: 10 mL every 4 hours (maximum: 40 mL/24 hours)

Note: Calmylin PSE with Codeine [Canadian product] contains codeine 3.33 mg/guaifenesin 100 mg/pseudoephedrine 30 mg per 5 mL

Geriatric Refer to adult dosing. Use with caution.

Pediatric

Cough/nasal congestion: Oral: Codeine 10 mg/guaifenesin 100 mg/pseudoephedrine 30 mg per 5 mL:

Children 6 to <12 years: 5 mL every 4 hours (maximum: 20 mL/24 hours)

Note: Calmylin PSE with Codeine [Canadian product] contains codeine 3.33 mg/guaifenesin 100 mg/pseudoephedrine 30 mg per 5 mL; use of this product is not recommended in children <12 years per the manufacturer labeling:

Children ≥12 years and Adolescents: Refer to adult dosing.

Renal Impairment There are no dosage adjustments provided in the manufacturer's labeling.

Hepatic Impairment There are no dosage adjustments provided in the manufacturer's labeling.

Additional Information Complete prescribing information should be consulted for additional detail.

Dosage Forms Excipient information presented when available (limited, particularly for generics); consult specific product labeling. [DSC] = Discontinued product

Liquid, oral:

Lortuss EX: Guaifenesin 100 mg, pseudoephedrine 30 mg and codeine phosphate 10 mg per 5 mL (473 mL) [dye free, ethanol free, sugar free; contains propylene glycol; apple cinnamon flavor]

Tricode GF: Guaifenesin 200 mg, pseudoephedrine hydrochloride 30 mg, and codeine phosphate 8 mg per 5 mL (473 mL) [ethanol free, dye free, gluten free, sugar free; contains propylene glycol; grape flavor]

Virtussin DAC: Guaifenesin 100 mg, pseudoephedrine hydrochloride 30 mg, and codeine phosphate 10 mg per 5 mL (473 mL) [sugar free; contains ethanol 2.1% v/v, propylene glycol, sodium benzoate]

Syrup, oral: Guaifenesin 100 mg, pseudoephedrine hydrochloride 30 mg, and codeine phosphate 10 mg per 5 mL (473 mL)

Cheratussin DAC: Guaifenesin 100 mg, pseudoephedrine 30 mg and codeine phosphate 10 mg per 5 mL (473 mL) [sugar free; contains ethanol 2.1% v/v, sodium benzoate; cherry flavor]

Mytussin DAC: Guaifenesin 100 mg, pseudoephedrine hydrochloride 30 mg, and codeine phosphate 10 mg per 5 mL (118 mL [DSC], 473 mL [DSC]) [sugar free; contains ethanol 1.7%; strawberry-raspberry flavor]

◄ **Dosage Forms: Canada** Excipient information presented when available (limited, particularly for generics); consult specific product labeling. [DSC] = Discontinued product
Liquid, oral:
Calmylin PSE with Codeine: Guaifenesin 100 mg, pseudoephedrine hydrochloride 30 mg, and codeine phosphate 3.3 mg per 5 mL (100 mL, 250 mL, 350 mL) [gluten free, sugar free; contains propylene glycol; raspberry flavor]
Controlled Substance C-V

Guaifenesin, Pseudoephedrine, and Dextromethorphan

(gwye FEN e sin, soo doe e FED rin, & deks troe meth OR fan)

Brand Names: US Aldex GS DM; AMBI 60PSE/400GFN/20DM; BP 8 Cough [OTC]; Capmist DM [OTC]; Entex PAC [OTC]; Entre-Cough [OTC]; Tusnel Pediatric [OTC]; Tusnel [OTC]; Tusnel-DM Pediatric [OTC]; Z-Cof 1 [OTC] [DSC]; Z-Cof 12 DM [OTC] [DSC]

Brand Names: Canada Balminil DM + Decongestant + Expectorant; Balminil DM + Decongestant + Expectorant Extra Strength; Benylin Cough and Chest Congestion; Benylin Cough Plus Cold Relief; Robitussin Cough & Cold Extra Strength

Index Terms Dextromethorphan, Guaifenesin, and Pseudoephedrine; Pseudoephedrine, Dextromethorphan, and Guaifenesin

Pharmacologic Category Antitussive/Decongestant/Expectorant

Use Cough and upper respiratory tract symptoms: Temporarily relieves nasal congestion and controls cough due to minor throat and bronchial irritation; helps loosen phlegm and thin bronchial secretions to make coughs more productive

Dosing

Adult & Geriatric Cough and upper respiratory tract symptoms: Oral: **Note:** Dosing may vary by product. Consult specific product labeling.
Liquid (dextromethorphan 15 mg/guaifenesin 175 mg/pseudoephedrine 30 mg per 5 mL): 10 mL every 8 hours, up to 30 mL per day.
Liquid (dextromethorphan 15 mg/guaifenesin 200 mg/pseudoephedrine 30 mg per 5 mL): 10 mL every 6 hours, up to 40 mL per day.
Liquid (dextromethorphan 20 mg per 5 mL) and tablets (guaifenesin 375 mg/pseudoephedrine 60 mg):
Liquid: 5 mL every 4 hours, up to 20 mL per day.
Tablets: One tablet every 4 to 6 hours, up to 4 tablets per day.
Suspension (dextromethorphan 15 mg/guaifenesin 211 mg/pseudoephedrine 30 mg per 5 mL): 10 mL every 8 hours, up to 30 mL per day.
Tablets (dextromethorphan 15 mg/guaifenesin 190 mg/pseudoephedrine 30 mg): Two tablets every 6 hours, up to 8 tablets per day.
Tablets (dextromethorphan 15 mg/guaifenesin 400 mg/pseudoephedrine 60 mg): One tablet every 4 hours, up to 4 tablets per day.
Tablets (dextromethorphan 20 mg/guaifenesin 400 mg/pseudoephedrine 60 mg): One tablet every 4 to 6 hours, up to 4 tablets per day.

Pediatric Cough and upper respiratory tract symptoms: Oral:
Note: Dosing may vary by product. Consult specific product labeling.
Drops (dextromethorphan 2.5 mg/guaifenesin 25 mg/pseudoephedrine 7.5 mg per mL):
Children 2 to 5 years: 2 mL every 4 to 6 hours, up to 8 mL per day
Liquid (dextromethorphan 5 mg/guaifenesin 50 mg/pseudoephedrine 15 mg per 5 mL):
Children 2 to 5 years: 5 mL every 4 to 6 hours, up to 20 mL per day
Children 6 to 11 years: 10 mL every 4 to 6 hours, up to 40 mL per day
Liquid (dextromethorphan 15 mg/guaifenesin 175 mg/pseudoephedrine 30 mg per 5 mL):
Children 6 to 11 years: 5 mL every 8 hours, up to 15 mL per day
Children ≥12 years and Adolescents: 10 mL every 8 hours, up to 30 mL per day
Liquid (dextromethorphan 15 mg/guaifenesin 200 mg/pseudoephedrine 30 mg per 5 mL):
Children 6 to <12 years: 5 mL every 6 hours, up to 20 mL per day
Children >12 years and Adolescents: 10 mL every 6 hours, up to 40 mL per day

Liquid (dextromethorphan 20 mg per 5 mL) and tablets (guaifenesin 375 mg/pseudoephedrine 60 mg):
Children 6 to 11 years:
Liquid: 2.5 mL every 4 hours, up to 10 mL per day
Tablets: One-half tablet every 4 to 6 hours, up to 2 tablets per day
Children ≥12 years and Adolescents:
Liquid: 5 mL every 4 hours, up to 20 mL per day
Tablets: One tablet every 4 to 6 hours, up to 4 tablets per day
Suspension (dextromethorphan 15 mg/guaifenesin 211 mg/pseudoephedrine 30 mg per 5 mL):
Children 6 to 11 years: 5 mL every 8 hours, up to 15 mL per day
Children ≥12 years and Adolescents: 10 mL every 8 hours, up to 30 mL per day
Tablets (dextromethorphan 15 mg/guaifenesin 190 mg/pseudoephedrine 30 mg):
Children 6 to 11 years: One tablet every 6 hours, up to 4 tablets per day
Children ≥12 years and Adolescents: Two tablets every 6 hours, up to 8 tablets per day
Tablets (dextromethorphan 15 mg/guaifenesin 400 mg/pseudoephedrine 60 mg):
Children 6 to 11 years: One-half tablet every 4 hours, up to 2 tablets per day
Children ≥12 years and Adolescents: One tablet every 4 hours, up to 4 tablets per day
Tablets (dextromethorphan 20 mg/guaifenesin 400 mg/pseudoephedrine 60 mg):
Children 6 to <12 years: One-half tablet every 4 to 6 hours, up to 2 tablets per day
Children >12 years and Adolescents: One tablet every 4 to 6 hours, up to 4 tablets per day

Renal Impairment There are no dosage adjustments provided in the manufacturer's labeling.
Hepatic Impairment There are no dosage adjustments provided in the manufacturer's labeling.
Additional Information Complete prescribing information should be consulted for additional detail.
Dosage Forms Excipient information presented when available (limited, particularly for generics); consult specific product labeling. DSC = Discontinued product
Combination package, oral:
Entex PAC:
Liquid (Entex S): Dextromethorphan hydrobromide 20 mg per 5 mL [contains benzoic acid, propylene glycol; strawberry flavor]
Tablet (Entex T): Guaifenesin 375 mg, pseudoephedrine hydrochloride 60 mg [alcohol free, contains propylene glycol; grape flavor]
Liquid, Oral:
BP 8 Cough: Guaifenesin 175 mg, pseudoephedrine hydrochloride 30 mg, and dextromethorphan hydrobromide 15 mg per 5 mL (473 mL) [alcohol free, contains propylene glycol; grape flavor]
Entre-Cough: Guaifenesin 175 mg, pseudoephedrine hydrochloride 30 mg, and dextromethorphan hydrobromide 15 mg per 5 mL (473 mL) [contains aspartame, sodium benzoate; cherry flavor]
Tusnel: Guaifenesin 200 mg, pseudoephedrine hydrochloride 30 mg, and dextromethorphan hydrobromide 15 mg per 5 mL (178 mL) [alcohol free, dye free, sugar free; contains aspartame, propylene glycol]
Tusnel-DM Pediatric: Guaifenesin 25 mg, pseudoephedrine hydrochloride 7.5 mg, and dextromethorphan hydrobromide 2.5 mg per 1 mL (60 mL) [contains propylene glycol, sodium benzoate]
Tusnel Pediatric: Guaifenesin 50 mg, pseudoephedrine hydrochloride 15 mg, and dextromethorphan hydrobromide 5 mg per 5 mL (118 mL) [alcohol free; contains aspartame, propylene glycol; grape flavor]
Z-Cof 12 DM: Guaifenesin 175 mg, pseudoephedrine hydrochloride 30 mg, and dextromethorphan hydrobromide 15 mg per 5 mL (473 mL [DSC]) [alcohol free; contains propylene glycol; grape flavor]
Suspension, Oral:
Z-Cof 1: Guaifenesin 211 mg, pseudoephedrine hydrochloride 30 mg, and dextromethorphan hydrobromide 15 mg per 5 mL (473 mL) [contains aspartame, sodium benzoate; grape flavor] [DSC]
Tablet, Oral:
Aldex GS DM: Guaifenesin 190 mg, pseudoephedrine hydrochloride 30 mg, and dextromethorphan hydrobromide 15 mg
AMBI 60PSE/400GFN/20DM: Guaifenesin 400 mg, pseudoephedrine hydrochloride 60 mg, and dextromethorphan hydrobromide 20 mg
Capmist DM: Guaifenesin 400 mg, pseudoephedrine hydrochloride 60 mg, and dextromethorphan hydrobromide 15 mg [contains tartrazine]

GuanFACINE (GWAHN fa seen)

Brand Names: US Intuniv; Tenex
Brand Names: Canada Intuniv XR
Index Terms Guanfacine Hydrochloride
Pharmacologic Category Alpha$_2$-Adrenergic Agonist; Antihypertensive

Use

Attention-deficit/hyperactivity disorder (extended release only): Treatment of attention-deficit/hyperactivity disorder (ADHD) as monotherapy and as adjunctive therapy to stimulant medications.

Hypertension (immediate release only): Management of hypertension.

Dosing

Adult Hypertension: Immediate release: Oral: 1 mg once daily at bedtime, may increase if needed after 3 to 4 weeks of therapy to 2 mg daily at bedtime. **Note:** Adverse reactions increase significantly with doses above 3 mg/day.

Geriatric Immediate release: Refer to adult dosing. In the management of hypertension, consider lower initial doses and titrate to response (Aronow 2011).

Pediatric

ADHD: Extended release: Children ≥6 years and Adolescents ≤17 years: Oral: Initial: 1 mg once daily; may adjust by increments of no more than 1 mg/week. Recommended target dose is 0.05 to 0.12 mg/kg/dose (1 to 7 mg) once daily, depending on clinical response and tolerability.

Maximum daily doses: Doses above the following have not been evaluated.

Monotherapy: Children 6 to 12 years: 4 mg/**day**; Adolescents: 13 to 17 years: 7 mg/**day**

Adjunct therapy (with psychostimulants): 4 mg/**day**

Suggested fixed target dose range for patients weighing ≥25 kg: All doses administered once daily at the same time (either in the morning or evening) not to exceed age-based maximum daily doses.

25 to 33.9 kg: 2 to 3 mg/day
34 to 41.4 kg: 2 to 4 mg/day
41.5 to 49.4 kg: 3 to 5 mg/day
49.5 to 58.4 kg: 3 to 6 mg/day
58.5 to 91 kg: 4 to 7 mg/day
>91 kg: 5 to 7 mg/day

Dosage adjustment for concomitant CYP3A4 inhibitors/inducers:

Strong CYP3A4 inhibitors: If initiating guanfacine while taking a strong CYP3A4 inhibitor or if continuing guanfacine and adding a strong CYP3A4 inhibitor, decrease guanfacine dose by 50%. If continuing guanfacine and discontinuing the strong CYP3A4 inhibitor, increase guanfacine to the recommended dose.

Strong CYP3A4 inducers: If initiating guanfacine while taking a strong CYP3A4 inducer, consider increasing guanfacine to double the recommended dose. If continuing guanfacine and adding a strong CYP3A4 inducer, consider increasing guanfacine gradually over 1 to 2 weeks to double the recommended dose. If continuing guanfacine and discontinuing the strong CYP3A4 inducer, gradually decrease guanfacine dose to the recommended dose over 1 to 2 weeks.

Conversion from immediate release to extended release: Discontinue the immediate release formulation, and titrate according to extended release recommendations.

Missed doses of extended release: If ≥2 consecutive doses are missed, consider repeating dosage titration based on patient tolerability.

Discontinuation of extended release: Gradually discontinue by tapering dose in decrements of ≤1 mg every 3 to 7 days to avoid rebound hypertension.

Hypertension: Children ≥12 years and Adolescents: Immediate release: Oral: Refer to adult dosing.

Tourette syndrome (off-label use): Children ≥6 years and Adolescents ≤16 years: Immediate release: Oral: Initial: 0.5 mg once daily at bedtime for 3 days, then 0.5 mg twice daily for 4 days, then 0.5 mg 3 times daily; may further increase dose after 7 days based on clinical response to maximum daily dose of 4 mg/day in 3 divided doses (Scahill 2001); twice daily dosing may be effective for some patients (Chappell, 1995; Cummings 2002). **Note:** Limited data available; greater efficacy shown in patients with ADHD comorbidity (AACAP [Murphy 2013]; ESSTS [Roessner 2011]; Pringsheim 2012; Weisman 2013).

Renal Impairment

Immediate release: Children ≥12 years, Adolescents, and Adults: There are no specific dosage adjustments provided in the manufacturer's labeling; however, the lower end of the dosing range is recommended in patients with renal impairment.

Extended release: Children ≥6 years and Adolescents ≤17 years: There are no dosage adjustments provided in the manufacturer's labeling (has not been studied); however, dosage adjustments may be necessary in patients with significant renal impairment.

Hemodialysis: Immediate release or extended release: Dialysis clearance is low (~15% of total clearance).

Hepatic Impairment

Immediate release: Children ≥12 years, Adolescents, and Adults: There are no dosage adjustments provided in the manufacturer's labeling; however, use with caution in chronic hepatic impairment.

Extended release: Children ≥6 years and Adolescents ≤17 years: There are no dosage adjustments provided in the manufacturer's labeling (has not been studied); however, dosage adjustments may be necessary in patients with significant hepatic impairment.

Additional Information Complete prescribing information should be consulted for additional detail.

Dosage Forms Excipient information presented when available (limited, particularly for generics); consult specific product labeling.

Tablet, Oral:
Tenex: 1 mg [contains fd&c red #40 aluminum lake]
Tenex: 2 mg [contains fd&c yellow #10 aluminum lake]
Generic: 1 mg, 2 mg
Tablet Extended Release 24 Hour, Oral:
Intuniv: 1 mg, 2 mg, 3 mg, 4 mg
Generic: 1 mg, 2 mg, 3 mg, 4 mg

Dosage Forms: Canada Excipient information presented when available (limited, particularly for generics); consult specific product labeling.

Tablet Extended Release 24 Hour, Oral:
Intuniv XR: 1 mg, 2 mg, 3 mg, 4 mg

Haemophilus b Conjugate and Hepatitis B Vaccine
(he MOF i lus bee KON joo gate & hep a TYE tis bee vak SEEN)

Brand Names: US Comvax
Index Terms *Haemophilus* b (meningococcal protein conjugate) Conjugate Vaccine; Hepatitis B Vaccine (Recombinant); Hib Conjugate Vaccine; Hib-HepB
Pharmacologic Category Vaccine; Vaccine, Inactivated (Bacterial); Vaccine, Inactivated (Viral)
Additional Appendix Information
Immunization Administration Recommendations *on page 1974*
Immunization Schedules *on page 1979*

Use

Haemophilus b and Hepatitis B disease prevention: Active immunization against invasive disease caused by *H. influenzae* type b and against infection caused by all known subtypes of hepatitis B virus in infants 6 weeks to 15 months of age born of hepatitis B surface antigen (HBsAg)-negative mothers

Infants born of HBsAg-positive mothers or mothers of unknown HBsAg status should receive hepatitis B vaccine (recombinant) at birth and should complete the hepatitis B vaccination series given according to a particular schedule (refer to current ACIP recommendations).

◄ **Dosing**
Pediatric
Immunization: Infants: IM: 0.5 mL/dose; one dose at 2, 4, and 12-15 months of age (total of 3 doses). **Note:** If the recommended schedule cannot be followed, the interval between the first two doses should be at least 6 weeks and the interval between the second and third dose should be as close as possible to 8-11 months. Minimum age for first dose is 6 weeks.

Modified Schedule: Children who receive one dose of hepatitis B vaccine at or shortly after birth may receive Comvax® on a schedule of 2, 4, and 12-15 months of age

Renal Impairment There are no dosage adjustments provided in the manufacturer's labeling.

Hepatic Impairment There are no dosage adjustments provided in the manufacturer's labeling.

Additional Information Complete prescribing information should be consulted for additional detail.

Product Availability Production of Comvax has been discontinued by the manufacturer (Merck). As of December 31, 2014, Comvax is no longer available for direct purchase from Merck. Product may still be available from wholesalers and physician distributors. Refer to the following for additional information https://www.merckvaccines.com/is-bin/intershop.static/WFS/Merck-MerckVaccines-Site/Merck-MerckVaccines/en_US/Professional-Resources/Documents/announcements/VACC-1114028-0000.pdf.

Dosage Forms Excipient information presented when available (limited, particularly for generics); consult specific product labeling.

Injection, suspension [preservative free]:
Comvax®: *Haemophilus* b capsular polysaccharide 7.5 mcg (bound to *Neisseria meningitides* OMPC 125 mcg) and hepatitis B surface antigen 5 mcg per 0.5 mL (0.5 mL) [contains aluminum; contains natural rubber/natural latex in packaging]

◆ *Haemophilus* B Conjugate (Hib) *see* Diphtheria and Tetanus Toxoids, Acellular Pertussis, Poliovirus and *Haemophilus* b Conjugate Vaccine *on page 567*

Haemophilus b Conjugate Vaccine
(he MOF fi lus bee KON joo gate vak SEEN)

Brand Names: US ActHIB; Hiberix; PedvaxHIB
Brand Names: Canada ActHIB
Index Terms *Haemophilus influenzae* Type b; Hib; PRP-OMP (PedvaxHIB); PRP-T (ActHIB); PRP-T (Hiberix)
Pharmacologic Category Vaccine; Vaccine, Inactivated (Bacterial)
Additional Appendix Information
Immunization Administration Recommendations *on page 1974*
Immunization Schedules *on page 1979*
Use
Active immunization for the prevention of invasive disease caused by *Haemophilus influenzae* type b (Hib):
ActHIB: Immunization of infants and children 2 months to 5 years of age.
Hiberix: Booster dose in children 15 months to 4 years of age (prior to fifth birthday).
PedvaxHIB: Routine vaccination of infants and children 2 to 71 months of age.

The Advisory Committee on Immunization Practices (ACIP) recommends vaccination for the following (CDC/ACIP [Kim 2015]; CDC/ACIP [Strikas 2015]); CDC/ACIP [Briere 2014]):
- Routine immunization of all infants and children through age 59 months
- Unimmunized (defined as those who have not received a primary series and booster dose or at least 1 dose of a Hib vaccine after 14 months of age) children 12 to 59 months including chemotherapy recipients, anatomic or functional asplenia (including sickle cell disease), HIV infection, immunoglobulin deficiency or early component complement deficiency
Efficacy data are not available for use in older children and adults with chronic conditions associated with an increased risk of Hib disease. However, use may be considered for:
- Unimmunized (defined as those who have not received a primary series and booster dose or at least 1 dose of a Hib vaccine after 14 months of age) children ≥5 years, adolescents and adults with functional or anatomic asplenia, (including sickle cell disease)

- Unimmunized (defined as those who have not received a primary series and booster dose or at least 1 dose of a Hib vaccine after 14 months of age) children ≥5 years and adolescents with HIV infection
- Children <5 years undergoing chemotherapy or radiation treatment
- Successful hematopoietic stem cell transplant recipients
- Children ≥15 months and adolescents undergoing elective splenectomy

Medication Guide Available Yes
Dosing
Adult
Immunization: IM:
Adults who have not received the childhood Hib series **and** are at increased risk for invasive Hib disease due to to sickle cell disease, anatomic/functional asplenia or splenectomy. ACIP recommendations: One dose (0.5 mL); may use any of the Hib conjugate vaccines (CDC/ACIP [Briere 2014])
Adults who are recipients of a successful hematopoietic stem cell transplant: Revaccinate with a 3-dose regimen beginning 6-12 months after the transplant, regardless of vaccination history. Doses should be administered ≥4 weeks apart (CDC/ACIP [Briere 2014]).

Pediatric
Primary immunization (CDC/ACIP [Briere 2014]):
Note: The number of doses for completion of Hib series is dependent upon products including some combination formulations (3 doses: ActHIB; 2 doses: Pedvax-HIB) (see combination product monographs for specific dosing information)
Infants 6 weeks to 6 months: Minimum age for first dose is 6 weeks.
ActHib (PRP-T): IM: 0.5 mL per dose for a total of 3 doses administered as follows: 2, 4, and 6 months of age
PedvaxHIB (PRP-OMP): IM: 0.5 mL per dose for a total of 2 doses administered as follows: 2 and 4 months of age
Booster immunization (CDC/ACIP [Briere 2014]):
ActHIB, PedvaxHIB: Children 12 to 15 months: IM: 0.5 mL as a single dose
Hiberix: Children 12 months to 4 years: IM: 0.5 mL as a single dose
Primary immunization of older patients at risk: Children ≥5 years and Adolescents who have not received the childhood Hib series **and** are at increased risk for invasive Hib disease due to HIV infection, anatomic/functional asplenia or splenectomy, immunoglobulin deficiency, early component complement deficiency, or chemotherapy or radiation therapy. ACIP recommendations: One dose (0.5 mL); may use any of the Hib conjugate vaccines (CDC/ACIP [Briere 2014])
Repeat immunization for high-risk conditions (CDC/ACIP [Briere 2014]):
Invasive Hib disease: Infants and Children <24 months: Revaccinate with a second primary series beginning 4 weeks after onset of disease
Undergoing chemotherapy or radiation therapy: Infants and Children <60 months: If dose administered within 14 days of starting or given during therapy: Repeat the vaccine doses at least 3 months after therapy completion
Hematopoietic stem cell transplant recipient: Children and Adolescents: Revaccinate with a 3-dose regimen beginning 6 to 12 months after successful transplant, regardless of vaccination history. Doses should be administered ≥4 weeks apart.
Renal Impairment There are no dosage adjustments provided in manufacturer's labeling.
Hepatic Impairment There are no dosage adjustments provided in manufacturer's labeling.
Additional Information Complete prescribing information should be consulted for additional detail.
Dosage Forms Excipient information presented when available (limited, particularly for generics); consult specific product labeling.
Injection, powder for reconstitution [preservative free]:
ActHIB *Haemophilus* b capsular polysaccharide 10 mcg [bound to tetanus toxoid 24 mcg] per 0.5 mL [contains sucrose; may be reconstituted with provided diluent (forms solution; contains natural rubber/natural latex in packaging)]
Hiberix: *Haemophilus* b capsular polysaccharide 10 mcg [bound to tetanus toxoid 25 mcg] per 0.5 mL (0.5 mL) [contains lactose 12.6 mg]
Injection, suspension:
PedvaxHIB: *Haemophilus* b capsular polysaccharide 7.5 mcg [bound to *Neisseria meningitidis* OMPC 125 mcg] per 0.5 mL (0.5 mL) [contains aluminum; natural rubber/natural latex in packaging]

Halcinonide (hal SIN oh nide)

Brand Names: US Halog
Pharmacologic Category Corticosteroid, Topical
Additional Appendix Information
Topical Corticosteroids *on page 1952*
Use Relief of inflammatory and pruritic effects of corticosteroid-responsive dermatoses [high potency topical corticosteroid]
Dosing
Adult & Geriatric Steroid-responsive dermatoses: Topical: Apply sparingly 2-3 times daily, occlusive dressing may be used for severe or resistant dermatoses; a thin film is effective; avoid excessive application. Therapy should be discontinued when control is achieved; if no improvement is seen, reassessment of diagnosis may be necessary.
Pediatric Refer to adult dosing.
Additional Information Complete prescribing information should be consulted for additional detail.
Dosage Forms Excipient information presented when available (limited, particularly for generics); consult specific product labeling.
Cream, External:
Halog: 0.1% (30 g, 60 g, 216 g) [contains cetyl alcohol, propylene glycol]
Ointment, External:
Halog: 0.1% (30 g, 60 g)

Halobetasol (hal oh BAY ta sol)

Brand Names: US Halonate; Ultravate; Ultravate PAC [DSC]
Brand Names: Canada Ultravate®
Index Terms Halobetasol Propionate
Pharmacologic Category Corticosteroid, Topical
Additional Appendix Information
Topical Corticosteroids *on page 1952*
Use Relief of inflammatory and pruritic manifestations of corticosteroid-response dermatoses [super high potency topical corticosteroid]
Dosing
Adult & Geriatric Steroid-responsive dermatoses: Topical: Apply sparingly to skin once or twice daily, rub in gently and completely; treatment should not exceed 2 consecutive weeks and total dosage should not exceed 50 g/week. Therapy should be discontinued when control is achieved; if no improvement is seen, reassessment of diagnosis may be necessary.
Pediatric Children ≥12 years: Refer to adult dosing.
Additional Information Complete prescribing information should be consulted for additional detail.
Dosage Forms Excipient information presented when available (limited, particularly for generics); consult specific product labeling. [DSC] = Discontinued product
Cream, External, as propionate:
Ultravate: 0.05% (50 g) [contains cetyl alcohol]
Generic: 0.05% (15 g, 50 g)
Kit, External, as propionate:
Halonate: 0.05 & 12% (Foam) [contains cetyl alcohol, propylene glycol, trolamine (triethanolamine)]
Ultravate PAC: 0.05 & 12% (Cream) [DSC] [contains cetyl alcohol, methylparaben, propylene glycol, propylparaben]

Ointment, External, as propionate:
Ultravate: 0.05% (50 g) [contains propylene glycol]
Generic: 0.05% (15 g, 50 g)

Haloperidol (ha loe PER i dole)

Brand Names: US Haldol; Haldol Decanoate
Brand Names: Canada Apo-Haloperidol; Haloperidol Injection, USP; Haloperidol-LA; Haloperidol-LA Omega; Novo-Peridol; PMS-Haloperidol; PMS-Haloperidol LA
Index Terms Haloperidol Decanoate; Haloperidol Lactate
Pharmacologic Category First Generation (Typical) Antipsychotic
Use
Behavioral disorders (tablet, concentrate): Treatment of severe behavioral problems in children with combative, explosive hyperexcitability that cannot be accounted for by immediate provocation. Reserve for use in these children only after failure to respond to psychotherapy or medications other than antipsychotics.
Hyperactivity (tablet, concentrate): Short-term treatment of hyperactive children who show excessive motor activity with accompanying conduct disorders consisting of some or all of the following symptoms: impulsivity, difficulty sustaining attention, aggression, mood lability, or poor frustration tolerance. Reserve for use in these children only after failure to respond to psychotherapy or medications other than antipsychotics.
Psychotic disorders (tablet, concentrate): Management of manifestations of psychotic disorders.
Schizophrenia:
IM, lactate: Treatment of schizophrenia.
IM, decanoate: Treatment of patients with schizophrenia who require prolonged parenteral antipsychotic therapy.
Tourette disorder (tablet, concentrate, IM lactate): Control of tics and vocal utterances in Tourette syndrome in adults and children.
Pregnancy Considerations Adverse events were observed in animal reproduction studies. Haloperidol crosses the placenta in humans (Newport 2007). Although haloperidol has not been found to be a major human teratogen, an association with limb malformations following first trimester exposure in humans cannot be ruled out (ACOG 2008; Diav-Citrin 2005). Antipsychotic use during the third trimester of pregnancy has a risk for abnormal muscle movements (extrapyramidal symptoms [EPS]) and withdrawal symptoms in newborns following delivery. Symptoms in the newborn may include agitation, feeding disorder, hypertonia, hypotonia, respiratory distress, somnolence, and tremor; these effects may be self-limiting or require hospitalization. If needed, the minimum effective maternal dose should be used in order to decrease the risk of EPS (ACOG 2008).
Breast-Feeding Considerations Haloperidol is found in breast milk and has been detected in the plasma and urine of nursing infants (Whalley 1981; Yoshida 1999). Breast engorgement, gynecomastia, and lactation are known side effects with the use of haloperidol. Breast-feeding is not recommended by the manufacturer.
Contraindications Hypersensitivity to haloperidol or any component of the formulation; Parkinson disease; severe CNS depression; coma
Warnings/Precautions [US Boxed Warning]: Elderly patients with dementia-related psychosis treated with antipsychotics are at an increased risk of death compared to placebo. Most deaths appeared to be either cardiovascular (eg, heart failure, sudden death) or infectious (eg, pneumonia) in nature. Haloperidol is not approved for the treatment of dementia-related psychosis. Hypotension may occur, particularly with parenteral administration. Although the short-acting form (lactate) is used clinically, the IV use of the injection is not an FDA-approved route of administration; the decanoate form should never be administered intravenously.

Cases of sudden death, QT prolongation, and torsades de pointes have been reported with haloperidol use; risk may be increased with doses exceeding recommendations and/or intravenous administration (off-label route) of intramuscular lactate injection. Use with caution or avoid use in patients with electrolyte abnormalities (eg, hypokalemia, hypomagnesemia), hypothyroidism, familial long QT syndrome, concomitant medications that may augment QT prolongation, or any underlying cardiac abnormality that may also potentiate risk. Prior to initiation of intravenous therapy, obtain a baseline ECG. Consider continuous ECG monitoring, especially if the patients has risk factors for QTc prolongation, the baseline ECG reveals a prolonged

QTc, or cumulative doses of ≥2 mg are needed. Monitor electrolyte concentrations throughout therapy. If the baseline QTc interval increases by 20% to 25%, increases >500 msec, or if T-waves flatten or U-waves develop on the ECG, reduce the dosage or consider alternative therapy (Hassballa 2003; Meyer-Massetti 2010).

Leukopenia, neutropenia, and agranulocytosis (sometimes fatal) have been reported in clinical trials and postmarketing reports with antipsychotic use; presence of risk factors (eg, preexisting low WBC or history of drug-induced leuko-/neutropenia) should prompt periodic blood count assessment. Discontinue therapy at first signs of blood dyscrasias or if absolute neutrophil count <1,000/mm³.

May cause CNS depression, which may impair physical or mental abilities; patients must be cautioned about performing tasks that require mental alertness (eg, operating machinery, driving). Use with caution in patients with severe cardiovascular disease because of the possibility of transient hypotension and/or precipitation of anginal pain. Use with caution in patients at risk of seizures, including those with a history of seizures, EEG abnormalities, or concurrent anticonvulsant therapy; haloperidol may lower the seizure threshold. Avoid in thyrotoxicosis; severe neurotoxicity (rigidity, inability to walk or talk) may occur with use. Use is contraindicated in patients with Parkinson disease; these patients may be more sensitive to adverse effects (APA [Lehman 2004]). Use with caution in patients with narrow-angle glaucoma; condition may be exacerbated by cholinergic blockade (APA [Lehman 2004]). Use with caution in patients with bipolar disorder; when used to control mania, there may be a rapid mood swing to depression. Haloperidol does not possess antidepressant effects (Cipriani 2006). Esophageal dysmotility and aspiration have been associated with antipsychotic use - use with caution in patients at risk of pneumonia (eg, Alzheimer disease) (Maddalena 2004). Use associated with increased prolactin levels; clinical significance of hyperprolactinemia in patients with breast cancer or other prolactin-dependent tumors is unknown. May alter temperature regulation or mask toxicity of other drugs due to antiemetic effects (Kwok 2005; Martinez 2002). May cause orthostatic hypotension; use with caution in patients at risk of this effect or those who would tolerate transient hypotensive episodes (cerebrovascular disease, cardiovascular disease, or other medications which would predispose to hypotension/bradycardia). Relative to other neuroleptics, the risk of orthostatic hypotension is low (APA [Lehman 2004]).

May cause anticholinergic effects (confusion, agitation, constipation, xerostomia, blurred vision, urinary retention). Therefore, they should be used with caution in patients with decreased gastrointestinal motility, urinary retention, BPH, xerostomia, visual problems, or narrow-angle glaucoma (screening is recommended). Relative to other neuroleptics, haloperidol has a low potency of cholinergic blockade (APA [Lehman 2004]).

May cause extrapyramidal symptoms, including pseudoparkinsonism, acute dystonic reactions, akathisia, and tardive dyskinesia. Risk of dystonia (and possibly other EPS) may be greater with increased doses, use of conventional antipsychotics, males, and younger patients (APA [Lehman 2004]). Risk of tardive dyskinesia and potential for irreversibility may be increased in elderly patients (particularly women), prolonged therapy, and higher total cumulative dose; antipsychotics may also mask signs/symptoms of tardive dyskinesia. Use may be associated with neuroleptic malignant syndrome (NMS); monitor for mental status changes, fever, muscle rigidity, and/or autonomic instability. Following recovery from NMS, reintroduction of drug therapy should be carefully considered; if an antipsychotic agent is resumed, monitor closely for NMS. Use in elderly patients with dementia is associated with an increased risk of mortality and cerebrovascular accidents; avoid antipsychotic use for behavioral problems associated with dementia unless alternative nonpharmacologic therapies have failed and patient may harm self or others. In addition, use may cause or exacerbate syndrome of inappropriate antidiuretic hormone secretion or hyponatremia; monitor sodium closely with initiation or dosage adjustments in older adults (Beers Criteria). Increased risk for developing tardive dyskinesia, particularly elderly women.

Benzyl alcohol and derivatives: Some dosage forms may contain benzyl alcohol; large amounts of benzyl alcohol (≥99 mg/kg/day) have been associated with a potentially fatal toxicity ("gasping syndrome") in neonates; the "gasping syndrome" consists of metabolic acidosis, respiratory distress, gasping respirations, CNS dysfunction (including convulsions, intracranial hemorrhage), hypotension and cardiovascular collapse (AAP ["Inactive" 1997]; CDC 1982); some data suggests that benzoate displaces bilirubin from protein binding sites (Ahlfors 2001); avoid or use dosage forms containing benzyl alcohol with caution in neonates. See manufacturer's labeling.

Adverse Reactions Frequency not defined.

Cardiovascular: Abnormal T waves with prolonged ventricular repolarization, arrhythmia, hyper-/hypotension, QT prolongation, sudden death, tachycardia, torsade de pointes

Central nervous system: Agitation, akathisia, altered central temperature regulation, anxiety, confusion, depression, drowsiness, dystonic reactions, euphoria, extrapyramidal reactions, headache, insomnia, lethargy, neuroleptic malignant syndrome (NMS), pseudoparkinsonian signs and symptoms, restlessness, seizure, tardive dyskinesia, tardive dystonia, vertigo

Dermatologic: Alopecia, contact dermatitis, hyperpigmentation, photosensitivity (rare), pruritus, rash

Endocrine & metabolic: Amenorrhea, breast engorgement, galactorrhea, gynecomastia, hyper-/hypoglycemia, hyponatremia, lactation, mastalgia, menstrual irregularities, sexual dysfunction

Gastrointestinal: Anorexia, constipation, diarrhea, dyspepsia, hypersalivation, nausea, vomiting, xerostomia

Genitourinary: Priapism, urinary retention

Hematologic: Agranulocytosis (rare), leukopenia, leukocytosis, neutropenia, anemia, lymphomonocytosis

Hepatic: Cholestatic jaundice, obstructive jaundice

Ocular: Blurred vision

Respiratory: Bronchospasm, laryngospasm

Miscellaneous: Diaphoresis, heat stroke

Drug Interactions

Metabolism/Transport Effects Substrate of CYP1A2 (minor), CYP2D6 (major), CYP3A4 (major); **Note:** Assignment of Major/Minor substrate status based on clinically relevant drug interaction potential; **Inhibits** CYP2D6 (moderate)

Avoid Concomitant Use

Avoid concomitant use of Haloperidol with any of the following: Aclidinium; Amisulpride; Azelastine (Nasal); Cimetropium; Conivaptan; Eluxadoline; FLUoxetine; Fusidic Acid (Systemic); Glucagon; Glycopyrrolate (Oral Inhalation); Highest Risk QTc-Prolonging Agents; Idelalisib; Ipratropium (Oral Inhalation); Ivabradine; Levosulpiride; Metoclopramide; Mifepristone; Orphenadrine; Paraldehyde; Potassium Chloride; QuiNIDine; Sulpiride; Thalidomide; Thioridazine; Tiotropium; Umeclidinium

Increased Effect/Toxicity

Haloperidol may increase the levels/effects of: AbobotulinumtoxinA; Alcohol (Ethyl); Amisulpride; Analgesics (Opioid); Anticholinergic Agents; ARIPiprazole; Azelastine (Nasal); Brexpiprazole; ChlorproMAZINE; Cimetropium; CNS Depressants; CYP2D6 Substrates; DOXOrubicin (Conventional); Eluxadoline; Fesoterodine; Glucagon; Glycopyrrolate (Oral Inhalation); Highest Risk QTc-Prolonging Agents; Hydrocodone; Mequitazine; Methotrimeprazine; Methylphenidate; Metoprolol; Metyrosine; Mirabegron; Mirtazapine; Moderate Risk QTc-Prolonging Agents; Nebivolol; OnabotulinumtoxinA; Orphenadrine; Paraldehyde; Potassium Chloride; QuiNIDine; Ramosetron; RimabotulinumtoxinB; Selective Serotonin Reuptake Inhibitors; Serotonin Modulators; Sulpiride; Suvorexant; Thalidomide; Thiazide Diuretics; Thioridazine; Tiotropium; Topiramate; Zolpidem

The levels/effects of Haloperidol may be increased by: Abiraterone Acetate; Acetylcholinesterase Inhibitors (Central); Aclidinium; Aprepitant; ARIPiprazole; Brimonidine (Topical); Cannabis; ChlorproMAZINE; Conivaptan; CYP2D6 Inhibitors (Moderate); CYP2D6 Inhibitors (Strong); CYP3A4 Inhibitors (Moderate); CYP3A4 Inhibitors (Strong); Dasatinib; Doxylamine; Dronabinol; Droperidol; FLUoxetine; FluvoxaMINE; Fosaprepitant; Fusidic Acid (Systemic); HydrOXYzine; Idelalisib; Ipratropium (Oral Inhalation); Ivabradine; Ivacaftor; Kava Kava; Lithium; Luliconazole; Magnesium Sulfate; Methotrimeprazine; Methylphenidate; Metoclopramide; Metyrosine; Mianserin; Mifepristone; Minocycline; Nabilone; Netupitant; Nonsteroidal Anti-Inflammatory Agents; Palbociclib; Panobinostat; Peginterferon Alfa-2b; Perampanel; Pramlintide; QTc-Prolonging Agents (Indeterminate Risk and Risk Modifying); QuiNIDine; Rufinamide; Serotonin Modulators; Simeprevir; Sodium Oxybate; Stiripentol; Tapentadol; Tetrahydrocannabinol; Umeclidinium

Decreased Effect

Haloperidol may decrease the levels/effects of: Acetylcholinesterase Inhibitors; Amphetamines; Anti-Parkinson's Agents (Dopamine Agonist); Codeine; Gastrointestinal Agents (Prokinetic); Itopride; Levosulpiride; Quinagolide; Secretin; Tamoxifen; TraMADol; Urea Cycle Disorder Agents

The levels/effects of Haloperidol may be decreased by: Acetylcholinesterase Inhibitors; Anti-Parkinson's Agents (Dopamine Agonist); ARIPiprazole; Bosentan; CarBAMazepine; CYP3A4 Inducers (Moderate); CYP3A4 Inducers (Strong); Dabrafenib; Deferasirox; Enzalutamide; Glycopyrrolate; Glycopyrrolate (Systemic); Lithium; Mitotane; Peginterferon Alfa-2b; Siltuximab; St Johns Wort; Tocilizumab

Preparation for Administration Haloperidol lactate may be administered IVPB or IV infusion in D_5W solutions. NS solutions should not be used due to reports of decreased stability and incompatibility.

Usual concentration range: 0.5 to 100 mg/50 to 100 mL D_5W.

Storage/Stability
Concentrate, tablets: Store at 20°C to 25°C (68°F to 77°F). Protect from light. Dispense in a tight, light-resistant container. Do not freeze concentrate.
Solution for injection, decanoate: Store at 15°C to 30°C (59°F to 86°F). Protect from light. Do not refrigerate or freeze.
Solution for injection, lactate: Store at 15°C to 30°C (59°F to 86°F). Protect from light. Do not refrigerate or freeze.
Solution for injection, lactate (preservative free): Store at 20°C to 25°C (68°F to 77°F). Protect from light. Do not freeze.

Mechanism of Action Haloperidol is a butyrophenone antipsychotic that nonselectively blocks postsynaptic dopaminergic D_2 receptors in the brain (Richelson 1999; Risch 1996).

Pharmacodynamics/Kinetics
Distribution:
IV: V_z: 9.5 to 21.7 L/kg (Kudo 1999)
Oral: V_z/F: 52.6 ± 14.5 L/kg (Kudo 1999)
Protein binding: 88.4% to 92.5% (Kudo 1999)
Metabolism: Hepatic: 50% to 60% glucuronidation (inactive); 23% CYP3A4-mediated reduction to inactive metabolites (some back-oxidation to haloperidol); and 20% to 30% CYP3A4-mediated N-dealkylation, including minor oxidation pathway to toxic pyridinium derivative (Kudo 1999)
Bioavailability: Oral: 60% to 70% (Kudo 1999)
Half-life elimination:
Decanoate: 21 days
Lactate:
IM: 20 hours (Kudo 1999)
IV: 14 to 26 hours (Kudo 1999)
Oral: 14 to 37 hours (Kudo 1999)
Time to peak, serum:
Decanoate: 6 days
Lactate:
IM: 20 minutes (Kudo 1999)
Oral: 2 to 6 hours (Kudo 1999)
Excretion: Urine (30%, 1% as unchanged drug) (Kudo 1999)

Dosing
Adult
Psychosis:
Manufacturer's labeling: Oral: 0.5 to 5 mg 2 to 3 times daily; adjust dose based on response and tolerability. According to the manufacturer, daily dosages up to 100 mg may be necessary in some cases to achieve an optimal response; infrequently, doses >100 mg have been used in severely treatment resistant patients. Recommended dose range for schizophrenia: 5 to 20 mg/day (APA [Lehman 2004]).
Schizophrenia:
IM (as lactate): 2 to 5 mg; subsequent doses may be administered as often as every 60 minutes, although 4- to 8-hour intervals may be satisfactory.
IM (as decanoate): **Note:** Establish tolerance to oral haloperidol prior to changing to IM decanoate injection.
Initial: 10 to 20 times the daily oral dose. The initial dose should not exceed 100 mg regardless of previous antipsychotic requirements. If the initial dose conversion requires >100 mg, administer the dose in 2 injections (maximum of 100 mg for first injection) separated by 3 to 7 days.
Oral haloperidol ≤10 mg/day, elderly, or debilitated: Initiate dose at 10 to 15 times the daily oral dose
Oral haloperidol >10 mg/day or high risk of relapse: Initiate dose at 20 times the daily oral dose
Maintenance dose: 10 to 15 times the previous daily oral dose or 50 to 200 mg administer doses at 4-week intervals (Buchanan 2009; Hasan 2013).
Oral overlap: Following initial dose, taper the oral dose and discontinue after the first 2 or 3 injections (McEvoy 2006).

Alternative dosing regimen:
Loading dose regimen: Initial: 20 times the previous daily oral dose, divide total dose and give every 3 to 7 days, do not exceed 250 mg per injection; discontinue oral haloperidol prior to first injection. Reduce the dose by 25% each month, depending on clinical response, in months 2 to 4, and establish the maintenance dose.
Usual maintenance dose: 200 mg per month (Ereshefsky 1993)

Tourette syndrome: Oral: 0.5 to 5 mg 2 to 3 times daily; adjust dose based on response and tolerability. Tourette Canada Guidelines recommend a dosing range of 0.5 to 3 mg/day (Pringsheim 2012) and European Society for the Study of Tourette Syndrome recommend a dosing range of 0.25 to 15 mg/day (Roessner 2011). According to the manufacturer, daily dosages up to 100 mg may be necessary in some cases to achieve an optimal response; infrequently doses >100 mg have been used in severely treatment resistant patients.

Chemotherapy-induced nausea and vomiting (off-label use): Breakthrough nausea/vomiting: Oral, IV (off-label route): 0.5 to 1 mg every 6 hours as needed (Lohr 2008)

Delirium in the intensive care unit, treatment (off-label use): Note: The optimal dose and regimen of haloperidol for the treatment of severe agitation and/or delirium has not been established. Currently, there are no studies evaluating the role of haloperidol on duration or severity of delirium. Haloperidol has been used for symptomatic treatment (severe agitation) of delirious patients. Current guidelines do not advocate use of haloperidol for the treatment or prevention of delirium due to insufficient evidence (Barr 2013).
IV (off-label route): Initial: 0.5 to 10 mg depending on degree of agitation; if inadequate response, may repeat bolus dose (with sequential doubling of initial bolus dose) every 15 to 30 minutes until calm achieved, then administer 25% of the last bolus dose every 6 hours; monitor ECG and QTc interval. After the patient is controlled, haloperidol therapy should be tapered over several days. This strategy is based upon expert opinion; efficacy and safety have not been formally evaluated (Tesar 1988).
Note: Continuous infusions have also been used with doses in the range of 0.5 to 2 mg/hour with an optional loading dose of 2.5 mg (Reade 2009).

Delirium in the intensive care unit (patients at high risk of delirium), prevention (off-label use): Note: The optimal dose and regimen of haloperidol for prevention of ICU delirium has not been established. Current guidelines do not advocate use of haloperidol for the treatment or prevention of delirium due to insufficient evidence (Barr 2013). Haloperidol may decrease the incidence of delirium (Van den Boogaard 2013; Wang 2012).
IV (off-label route): 0.5 mg followed by a continuous infusion of 0.1 mg/hour for 12 hours (Wang 2012) **or** 0.5 to 1 mg every 8 hours (Van den Boogaard 2013)

Phencyclidine psychosis (off-label use): IM, IV (off-label route), Oral: 5 mg (Giannini 1984; MacNeal 2012). **Note:** Additional data may be necessary to further define the role of haloperidol in this condition.

Postoperative nausea and vomiting (PONV), prevention (off-label use): IM, IV (off-label route): 0.5 to 2 mg (Gan 2014)

Rapid tranquilization (agitation/aggression/violent behavior) (off-label use): IM (as lactate): 2.5 to 10 mg (Clinton 1987; MacDonald 2012; Powney 2012; Wilson 2012)

Geriatric
Psychosis: Oral: 0.5 to 2 mg 2 to 3 times daily; adjust dose based on response and tolerability. Maximum dosage per manufacturer's labeling: 100 mg/day. Recommended dose range for schizophrenia: 5 to 20 mg/day (APA [Lehman 2004]).

Psychosis/agitation related to Alzheimer disease and other dementias (off-label use): Initial: Oral: 0.25 to 0.5 mg/day (APA [Rabins 2007]; slowly increase dose based on response and tolerability every 4 to 7 days in increments of 0.25 to 1 mg (De Deyn 1999; Devanand 1998); usual maximum dose of 2 mg/day (APA [Rabins 2007]; Doses up to 6 mg/day in 1 to 2 divided doses were evaluated in clinical trials (Lonergan 2002).

Pediatric

Behavior disorders, nonpsychotic:

Children 3 to 12 years weighing 15 to 40 kg: Oral: Initial: 0.5 mg/day in 2 to 3 divided doses; may increase by 0.5 mg every 5 to 7 days to usual maintenance range of 0.05 to 0.075 mg/kg/day in 2 to 3 divided doses; maximum dose not established; children with severe, nonpsychotic disturbance may require higher doses; however, no improvement has been shown with doses >6 mg/day.

Children >40 kg and Adolescents (off-label dose): Oral: 0.5 to 15 mg/day in 2 to 3 divided doses; begin at lower end of the range and may increase as needed (no more frequently than every 5 to 7 days); maximum daily dose: 15 mg/day. **Note:** Higher doses may be necessary in severe or refractory cases (Kliegman 2011).

Psychosis:

Children 3 to 12 years weighing 15 to 40 kg: Oral: Initial: 0.5 mg/day in 2 to 3 divided doses; increase by 0.5 mg every 5 to 7 days to usual maintenance range of 0.05 to 0.15 mg/kg/day in 2 to 3 divided doses; higher doses may be necessary in severe or refractory cases; maximum dose not established; in adolescents, the maximum daily dose is 15 mg/day (Kliegman 2011)

Children >40 kg and Adolescents (off-label dose): Oral: 0.5 to 15 mg/day in 2 to 3 divided doses; begin at lower end of the range and may increase as needed (no more frequently than every 5 to 7 days); maximum daily dose: 15 mg/day (Kliegman 2011; Willner 1969). **Note:** Higher doses may be necessary in severe or refractory cases (Kliegman 2011).

Tourette syndrome:

Children 3 to 12 years weighing 15 to 40 kg: Oral:
Manufacturer's labeling: Initial: 0.5 mg/day in 2 to 3 divided doses; increase by 0.5 mg every 5 to 7 days to usual maintenance of 0.05 to 0.075 mg/kg/day in 2 to 3 divided doses; maximum dose not established; however, no improvement has been shown with doses >6 mg/day in patients with nonpsychotic disturbances

Alternate dosing: Initial: 0.25 to 0.5 mg/day in 2 to 3 divided doses titrated to a usual daily dose range of 1 to 4 mg/day (Roessner 2011; Scahill 2006)

Children >40 kg and Adolescents (off-label dose): Oral: 0.25 to 15 mg/day in 2 to 3 divided doses; begin at lower end of the range and may increase as needed (no more frequently than every 5 to 7 days) (Kleigman 2011; Roessner 2011); usual dose range: 1 to 4 mg/day (Roessner 2011; Scahill 2006); maximum dose not established; however, no improvement has been shown with doses >6 mg/day in patients with nonpsychotic disturbances

Renal Impairment There are no dosage adjustments provided in the manufacturer's labeling.

Hepatic Impairment There are no dosage adjustments provided in the manufacturer's labeling.

Administration

Injection oil (decanoate): The decanoate injectable formulation should be administered IM only, **do not administer decanoate IV.** A 21-gauge needle is recommended. The maximum volume per injection site should not exceed 3 mL. Administer in the gluteal muscle by deep IM injection; Z-track injection techniques are recommended to limit leakage after injections (Baweja 2012; Gillespie 2013; McEvoy 2006).

Injection solution (lactate): The lactate injectable formulation may be administered IM or IV (off-label route). Rate of IV administration not well defined; rates of a maximum of 5 mg/minute (Lerner 1979) and 0.125 mg/kg (in 10 mL NS) over 1 to 2 minutes (Magliozzi 1985) have been reported. **Note:** IV administration has been associated with QT prolongation and the manufacturer recommends ECG monitoring for QT prolongation and arrhythmias. Consult individual institutional policies and procedures prior to administration.

Monitoring Parameters Mental status; vital signs (as clinically indicated); ECG (as clinically indicated and with off-label intravenous administration); weight, height, BMI, waist circumference (baseline; at every visit for the first 6 months; quarterly with stable antipsychotic dose); CBC (as clinically indicated; monitor frequently during the first few months of therapy in patients with preexisting low WBC or history of drug-induced leukopenia/neutropenia); electrolytes and liver function (annually and as clinically indicated); fasting plasma glucose level/ HbA$_{1c}$ (baseline, then yearly; in patients with diabetes risk factors or if gaining weight repeat 4 months after starting antipsychotic, then yearly); lipid panel (baseline; repeat every 2 years if LDL level is normal; repeat every 6 months if LDL level is >130 mg/dL); changes in menstruation, libido,

development of galactorrhea, erectile and ejaculatory function (at each visit for the first 12 weeks after the antipsychotic is initiated or until the dose is stable, then yearly); abnormal involuntary movements or parkinsonian signs (baseline; repeat weekly until dose stabilized for at least 2 weeks after introduction and for 2 weeks after any significant dose increase); tardive dyskinesia (every 6 months; high-risk patients every 3 months); visual changes (inquire yearly); ocular examination (yearly in patients >40 years; every 2 years in younger patients) (ADA 2004; Lehman 2004; Marder 2004).

ICU delirium: Monitor either the Confusion Assessment Method for the ICU (CAM-ICU) or the Intensive Care Delirium Screening Checklist (ICDSC)

Reference Range Schizophrenia: Therapeutic drug monitoring is not routinely warranted; a clear correlation between plasma concentrations and therapeutic response has not been demonstrated. Clinical studies suggest a therapeutic window may range from 5 to 18 ng/mL (SI: 10 to 48 nmol/L) (Boyer 1984; Michel 2001) with concerns for toxicity at levels >50 ng/mL (SI: >133 nmol/L) (Darby 1995)

Dosage Forms Excipient information presented when available (limited, particularly for generics); consult specific product labeling.

Concentrate, Oral, as lactate [strength expressed as base]:
Generic: 2 mg/mL (5 mL, 15 mL, 120 mL)

Solution, Intramuscular, as decanoate [strength expressed as base]:
Haldol Decanoate: 50 mg/mL (1 mL); 100 mg/mL (1 mL) [contains benzyl alcohol, sesame oil]
Generic: 50 mg/mL (1 mL, 5 mL); 100 mg/mL (1 mL, 5 mL)

Solution, Injection, as lactate [strength expressed as base]:
Haldol: 5 mg/mL (1 mL)
Generic: 5 mg/mL (1 mL, 10 mL)

Solution, Injection, as lactate [strength expressed as base, preservative free]:
Generic: 5 mg/mL (1 mL)

Tablet, Oral:
Generic: 0.5 mg, 1 mg, 2 mg, 5 mg, 10 mg, 20 mg

◆ Helixate FS *see* Antihemophilic Factor (Recombinant) *on page 132*

◆ Hemabate *see* Carboprost Tromethamine *on page 314*

◆ Hemangeol *see* Propranolol *on page 1518*

◆ Hemmorex-HC *see* Hydrocortisone (Topical) *on page 886*

◆ Hemocyte [OTC] *see* Ferrous Fumarate *on page 761*

◆ Hemofil M *see* Antihemophilic Factor (Human) *on page 131*

◆ Hemorrhoidal HC *see* Hydrocortisone (Topical) *on page 886*

◆ Hemril-30 [DSC] *see* Hydrocortisone (Topical) *on page 886*

◆ HepA *see* Hepatitis A Vaccine *on page 874*

◆ HepaGam B *see* Hepatitis B Immune Globulin (Human) *on page 875*

◆ HepA-HepB *see* Hepatitis A and Hepatitis B Recombinant Vaccine *on page 874*

Heparin (HEP a rin)

Brand Names: US Hep Flush-10
Brand Names: Canada Heparin Leo; Heparin Lock Flush; Heparin Sodium Injection, USP
Index Terms Heparin Calcium; Heparin Lock Flush; Heparin Sodium; Heparinized Saline
Pharmacologic Category Anticoagulant; Anticoagulant, Heparin
Additional Appendix Information
Reversal of Oral Anticoagulants *on page 1959*
Use Anticoagulation: Prophylaxis and treatment of thromboembolic disorders. As an anticoagulant for extracorporeal and dialysis procedures

Note: Heparin lock flush solution is intended only to maintain patency of IV devices and is **not** to be used for systemic anticoagulant therapy.

Pregnancy Considerations Increased resorptions were observed in some animal reproduction studies. Heparin does not cross the placenta. Heparin may be used for the prevention and treatment of thromboembolism in pregnant women; however the use of low molecular weight heparin (LMWH) is preferred. Twice-daily heparin should be discontinued prior to induction of labor or a planned cesarean delivery. In pregnant women with mechanical heart valves, adjusted-dose LMWH or adjusted-dose heparin may be used throughout pregnancy or until week 13 of gestation when therapy can be changed to warfarin. LMWH or heparin should be resumed close to delivery. In women who are at a very high risk for thromboembolism (older generation prosthesis in mitral position or history of thromboembolism), warfarin can be used throughout pregnancy and replaced with LMWH or heparin near term; the use of low-dose aspirin is also recommended. When choosing therapy, fetal outcomes (ie, pregnancy loss, malformations), maternal outcomes (ie, VTE, hemorrhage), burden of therapy, and maternal preference should be considered (Guyatt, 2012).

Some products contain benzyl alcohol as a preservative; their use in pregnant women is contraindicated by some manufacturers; use of a preservative free formulation is recommended.

Breast-Feeding Considerations Heparin is not excreted into breast milk and can be used in breast-feeding women (Guyatt, 2012). Some products contain benzyl alcohol as a preservative; their use in breast-feeding women is contraindicated by some manufacturers due to the association of gasping syndrome in premature infants.

Contraindications Hypersensitivity to heparin or any component of the formulation (unless a life-threatening situation necessitates use and use of an alternative anticoagulant is not possible); severe thrombocytopenia; uncontrolled active bleeding except when due to disseminated intravascular coagulation (DIC); not for use when appropriate blood coagulation tests cannot be obtained at appropriate intervals (applies to full-dose heparin only)

Note: Some products contain benzyl alcohol as a preservative; their use in neonates, infants, or pregnant or nursing mothers is contraindicated by some manufacturers.

Warnings/Precautions Hypersensitivity reactions can occur. Only in life-threatening situations when use of an alternative anticoagulant is not possible should heparin be cautiously used in patients with a documented hypersensitivity reaction. Hemorrhage is the most common complication. Monitor for signs and symptoms of bleeding. Certain patients are at increased risk of bleeding. Risk factors for bleeding include bacterial endocarditis;

congenital or acquired bleeding disorders; active ulcerative or angiodysplastic GI diseases; continuous GI tube drainage; severe uncontrolled hypertension; history of hemorrhagic stroke; or use shortly after brain, spinal, or ophthalmology surgery; patient treated concomitantly with platelet inhibitors; conditions associated with increased bleeding tendencies (hemophilia, vascular purpura); recent GI bleeding; thrombocytopenia or platelet defects; severe liver disease; hypertensive or diabetic retinopathy; renal failure; or in patients undergoing invasive procedures including spinal tap or spinal anesthesia. Many concentrations of heparin are available ranging from 1 unit/mL to 20,000 units/mL. Clinicians **must** carefully examine each prefilled syringe or vial prior to use ensuring that the correct concentration is chosen; fatal hemorrhages have occurred related to heparin overdose especially in pediatric patients. A higher incidence of bleeding has been reported in patients >60 years of age, particularly women. They are also more sensitive to the dose. Discontinue heparin if hemorrhage occurs; severe hemorrhage or overdosage may require protamine (consult Protamine monograph for dosing recommendations).

May cause thrombocytopenia; monitor platelet count closely. Patients who develop HIT may be at risk of developing a new thrombus (heparin-induced thrombocytopenia and thrombosis [HITT]). Discontinue therapy and consider alternatives if platelets are <100,000/mm^3 and/or thrombosis develops. HIT or HITT may be delayed and can occur up to several weeks after discontinuation of heparin. Use with extreme caution (for a limited duration) or avoid in patients with history of HIT, especially if administered within 100 days of HIT episode (Dager, 2007; Warkentin, 2001); monitor platelet count closely. Osteoporosis may occur with prolonged use (>6 months) due to a reduction in bone mineral density. Monitor for hyperkalemia; can cause hyperkalemia by suppressing aldosterone production. Patients >60 years of age may require lower doses of heparin.

Benzyl alcohol and derivatives: Some dosage forms may contain benzyl alcohol as a preservative. In neonates, large amounts of benzyl alcohol (≥99 mg/kg/day) have been associated with a potentially fatal toxicity ("gasping syndrome"); the "gasping syndrome" consists of metabolic acidosis, respiratory distress, gasping respirations, CNS dysfunction (including convulsions, intracranial hemorrhage), hypotension, and cardiovascular collapse (AAP ["Inactive" 1997]; CDC, 1982); some data suggests that benzoate displaces bilirubin from protein binding sites (Ahlfors, 2001); avoid or use dosage forms containing benzyl alcohol with caution in neonates. See manufacturer's labeling. Use in neonates, infants, or pregnant or nursing mothers is contraindicated by some manufacturers; the use of preservative-free heparin is, therefore, recommended in these populations. Some preparations contain sulfite which may cause allergic reactions.

Heparin resistance may occur in patients with antithrombin deficiency, increased heparin clearance, elevations in heparin-binding proteins, elevations in factor VIII and/or fibrinogen; frequently encountered in patients with fever, thrombosis, thrombophlebitis, infections with thrombosing tendencies, MI, cancer, and in postsurgical patients; measurement of anticoagulant effects using antifactor Xa levels may be of benefit.

Adverse Reactions Note: Thrombocytopenia has been reported to occur at an incidence between 0% and 30%. It is often of no clinical significance. However, immunologically mediated heparin-induced thrombocytopenia (HIT) has been estimated to occur in 1% to 2% of patients, and is marked by a progressive fall in platelet counts and, in some cases, thromboembolic complications (skin necrosis, pulmonary embolism, gangrene of the extremities, stroke, or MI).

Frequency not defined.
Cardiovascular: Allergic vasospastic reaction (possibly related to thrombosis), chest pain, hemorrhagic shock, shock, thrombosis
Central nervous system: Chills, fever, headache
Dermatologic: Alopecia (delayed, transient), bruising (unexplained), cutaneous necrosis, dysesthesia pedis, erythematous plaques (case reports), eczema, urticaria, purpura
Endocrine & metabolic: Adrenal hemorrhage, hyperkalemia (suppression of aldosterone synthesis), ovarian hemorrhage, rebound hyperlipidemia on discontinuation
Gastrointestinal: Constipation, hematemesis, nausea, tarry stools, vomiting
Genitourinary: Frequent or persistent erection

Hematologic: Bleeding from gums, epistaxis, hemorrhage, ovarian hemorrhage, retroperitoneal hemorrhage, thrombocytopenia (see **Note**)

Hepatic: Liver enzymes increased

Local: Irritation, erythema, pain, hematoma, and ulceration have been rarely reported with deep SubQ injections; IM injection (not recommended) is associated with a high incidence of these effects

Neuromuscular & skeletal: Peripheral neuropathy, osteoporosis (chronic therapy effect)

Ocular: Conjunctivitis (allergic reaction), lacrimation

Renal: Hematuria

Respiratory: Asthma, bronchospasm (case reports), hemoptysis, pulmonary hemorrhage, rhinitis

Miscellaneous: Allergic reactions, anaphylactoid reactions, heparin resistance, hypersensitivity (including chills, fever, and urticaria)

Drug Interactions

Metabolism/Transport Effects None known.

Avoid Concomitant Use

Avoid concomitant use of Heparin with any of the following: Apixaban; Corticorelin; Dabigatran Etexilate; Edoxaban; Hemin; Omacetaxine; Oritavancin; Rivaroxaban; Streptokinase; Telavancin; Urokinase; Vorapaxar

Increased Effect/Toxicity

Heparin may increase the levels/effects of: ACE Inhibitors; Aliskiren; Angiotensin II Receptor Blockers; Anticoagulants; Canagliflozin; Collagenase (Systemic); Corticorelin; Deferasirox; Deoxycholic Acid; Eplerenone; Ibritumomab; Nintedanib; Obinutuzumab; Omacetaxine; Palifermin; Potassium Salts; Potassium-Sparing Diuretics; Rivaroxaban; Tositumomab and Iodine I 131 Tositumomab

The levels/effects of Heparin may be increased by: 5-ASA Derivatives; Agents with Antiplatelet Properties; Apixaban; Aspirin; Dabigatran Etexilate; Dasatinib; Edoxaban; Hemin; Herbs (Anticoagulant/Antiplatelet Properties); Ibrutinib; Limaprost; Nonsteroidal Anti-Inflammatory Agents; Omega-3 Fatty Acids; Pentosan Polysulfate Sodium; Pentoxifylline; Prostacyclin Analogues; Salicylates; Streptokinase; Sugammadex; Thrombolytic Agents; Tibolone; Tipranavir; Urokinase; Vitamin E; Vitamin E (Oral); Vorapaxar

Decreased Effect

Heparin may decrease the levels/effects of: Factor X (Human)

The levels/effects of Heparin may be decreased by: Estrogen Derivatives; Nitroglycerin; Oritavancin; Progestins; Telavancin

Storage/Stability Heparin solutions are colorless to slightly yellow. Minor color variations do not affect therapeutic efficacy. Heparin should be stored at controlled room temperature. Protect from freezing and temperatures >40°C.

Stability at room temperature and refrigeration:
Prepared bag: 24-72 hours (specific to solution, concentration, and/or study conditions)
Premixed bag: After seal is broken, 4 days.
Out of overwrap stability: 30 days.

Mechanism of Action Potentiates the action of antithrombin III and thereby inactivates thrombin (as well as activated coagulation factors IX, X, XI, XII, and plasmin) and prevents the conversion of fibrinogen to fibrin; heparin also stimulates release of lipoprotein lipase (lipoprotein lipase hydrolyzes triglycerides to glycerol and free fatty acids)

Pharmacodynamics/Kinetics Note: Increased interpatient variability of pharmacokinetic parameters in pediatric patients compared to adults; however, age-related decreases in volume of distribution and clearance with increasing pediatric patient age have been reported (ACCP [Monagle 2012]; McDonald 1981).

Onset of action: Anticoagulation: IV: Immediate; SubQ: ~20 to 30 minutes

Absorption: Oral, rectal: Erratic at best from these routes of administration; SubQ absorption is also erratic, but considered acceptable for prophylactic use

Distribution:
Premature neonates (data based on single dose of 100 units/kg within 4 hours of birth) (McDonald 1981): Inversely proportional to gestational age
GA 25 to 28 weeks: 81 ± 41 mL/kg
GA 29 to 32 weeks: 73.3 ± 24.8 mL/kg
GA 33 to 36 weeks: 57.8 ± 32.2 mL/kg
Adults: Following a single 75 unit/kg dose: 36.6 ± 7.4 mL/kg (McDonald 1981)

Metabolism: Hepatic; may be partially metabolized in the reticuloendothelial system

Half-life elimination:
Age-related: Shorter half-life reported in premature neonates compared to adult patients
Premature neonates GA 25 to 36 weeks (data based on single dose of 100 units/kg within 4 hours of birth): Mean range: 35.5 to 41.6 minutes (McDonald 1981)
Dose-dependent: IV bolus: 25 units/kg: 30 minutes (Bjornsson 1982); 100 units/kg: 60 minutes (de Swart 1982); 400 units/kg: 150 minutes (Olsson 1963)
Mean: 1.5 hours; Range: 1 to 2 hours; affected by obesity, renal function, malignancy, presence of pulmonary embolism, and infections
Note: At therapeutic doses, elimination occurs rapidly via nonrenal mechanisms. With very high doses, renal elimination may play more of a role; however, dosage adjustment remains unnecessary for patients with renal impairment (Kandrotas 1992).

Excretion: Urine (small amounts as unchanged drug); **Note:** At therapeutic doses, elimination occurs rapidly via nonrenal mechanisms. With very high doses, renal elimination may play more of a role; however, dosage adjustment remains unnecessary for patients with renal impairment (Kandrotas 1992).

Clearance: Age-related changes; within neonatal population, slower clearance with lower GA; however, when compared to adults, the overall clearance in neonatal and pediatric patients is faster than adults (ACCP [Monagle 2012]; McDonald 1981)

Dosing

Adult Note: Many concentrations of heparin are available ranging from 1 unit/mL to 20,000 units/mL. Carefully examine each prefilled syringe or vial prior to use ensuring that the correct concentration is chosen. Heparin lock flush solution is intended only to maintain patency of IV devices and is not to be used for anticoagulant therapy.

Acute coronary syndromes (off-label use): IV infusion (weight-based dosing per institutional nomogram recommended):
STEMI: Adjunct to fibrinolysis (full-dose alteplase, reteplase, or tenecteplase) (Antman, 2008): Initial bolus of 60 units/kg (maximum: 4000 units), then 12 units/kg/hour (maximum: 1000 units/hour) as continuous infusion. Check aPTT every 4 to 6 hours; adjust to target of 1.5 to 2 times the upper limit of control (50 to 70 seconds). Continue for a minimum of 48 hours, and preferably for the duration of hospitalization (up to 8 days) or until revascularization (if performed) (ACCF/AHA [O'Gara, 2013]).
Unstable angina (UA)/non-ST-elevation myocardial infarction (NSTEMI): Initial bolus of 60 units/kg (maximum: 4000 units), followed by an initial infusion of 12 units/kg/hour (maximum: 1000 units/hour). Check aPTT every 4 to 6 hours; adjust to target of 1.5 to 2 times the upper limit of control (50 to 70 seconds). Optimal duration of therapy is unknown; however, most trials continued therapy for 2 to 5 days. Recommended duration is 48 hours or until percutaneous coronary intervention is performed (AHA/ACC [Amsterdam, 2014]).

Anticoagulation (Intermittent administration): IV: Initial: 10,000 units, then 50 to 70 units/kg (5000 to 10,000 units) every 4 to 6 hours

Atrial fibrillation (off-label use): Guidelines pertaining to peri-cardioversion use (ACCP [You, 2012]):
Patients with atrial fibrillation (for more than 48 hours or unknown duration) undergoing cardioversion: IV heparin to maintain an aPTT prolongation that corresponds to plasma heparin levels of 0.3 to 0.7 units/mL anti-Xa activity started at the time of transesophageal echocardiography (TEE) is recommended with cardioversion performed within 24 hours of the TEE if no thrombus is seen.
Patients with atrial fibrillation (for 48 hours or less) undergoing cardioversion: Cardioversion may be performed without prolonged anticoagulation. However, anticoagulation with IV heparin to maintain an aPTT prolongation that corresponds to plasma heparin levels of 0.3 to 0.7 units/mL anti-Xa activity should be started at presentation in patients with no contraindications to anticoagulation.
Emergency cardioversion in hemodynamically unstable patient: Cardioversion may be performed without prolonged anticoagulation. Anticoagulation with IV heparin to maintain an aPTT prolongation that corresponds to plasma heparin levels of 0.3 to 0.7 units/mL anti-Xa activity should be started prior to cardioversion in patients with no contraindications to anticoagulation.

Interstitial cystitis (bladder pain syndrome) (off-label use): Intravesical: **Note:** Various dosage regimens of heparin (20,000 to 50,000 units) alone or with alkalinized lidocaine (1% to 4%) have been used. When lidocaine and heparin are mixed, there is a risk of precipitation if proper alkalinization does not occur. Lidocaine stability and pH should be determined after the components have been mixed, prior to administration.

Single-dose regimen: Instill the combination of 50,000 units of heparin, lidocaine 200 mg, and sodium bicarbonate 420 mg in 15 mL of sterile water into the bladder via catheter and allow to dwell for 30 minutes before draining (Parsons, 2012).

Once-weekly dosing regimen: Instill the combination of 20,000 units of heparin, lidocaine 4% (5 mL), and sodium bicarbonate 7% (25 mL) into an empty bladder via catheter once weekly for 12 weeks and allow to dwell for 30 minutes before draining (Nomiya, 2013).

Twice-weekly dosing regimen: Instill 25,000 units of heparin (diluted with 5 mL of sterile water) into bladder via catheter twice weekly for 3 months (Kuo, 2001).

Maintenance of line patency (line flushing): When using daily flushes of heparin to maintain patency of single and double lumen central catheters, 10 units/mL is commonly used for younger infants (eg, <10 kg) while 100 units/mL is used for older infants, children, and adults. Capped PVC catheters and peripheral heparin locks require flushing more frequently (eg, every 6 to 8 hours). Volume of heparin flush is usually similar to volume of catheter (or slightly greater). Additional flushes should be given when stagnant blood is observed in catheter, after catheter is used for drug or blood administration, and after blood withdrawal from catheter.

Parenteral nutrition: Addition of heparin (0.5 to 3 unit/mL) to peripheral and central parenteral nutrition has not been shown to decrease catheter-related thrombosis. The final concentration of heparin used for TPN solutions may need to be decreased to 0.5 units/mL in small infants receiving larger amounts of volume in order to avoid approaching therapeutic amounts. Arterial lines are heparinized with a final concentration of 1 unit/mL.

Percutaneous coronary intervention (off-label use; Levine, 2011):

No prior anticoagulant therapy:

If no GPIIb/IIIa inhibitor use planned: Initial bolus of 70 to 100 units/kg (target ACT 250 to 300 seconds for HemoTec®, 300 to 350 seconds for Hemochron®)

or

If planning GPIIb/IIIa inhibitor use: Initial bolus of 50 to 70 units/kg (target ACT 200 to 250 seconds regardless of device)

Prior anticoagulant therapy:

If no GPIIb/IIIa inhibitor use planned: Additional heparin as needed (eg, 2000 to 5000 units) (target ACT 250 to 300 seconds for HemoTec®, 300 to 350 seconds for Hemochron®)

or

If planning GPIIb/IIIa inhibitor use: Additional heparin as needed (eg, 2000 to 5000 units) (target ACT 200 to 250 seconds regardless of device)

Thromboprophylaxis (low-dose heparin): SubQ: 5000 units every 8 to 12 hours. **Note:** The American College of Chest Physicians recommends a minimum of 10 to 14 days for patients undergoing total hip arthroplasty, total knee arthroplasty, or hip fracture surgery (Guyatt, 2012).

Venous thromboembolism (treatment): Note: Start warfarin on the first or second treatment day and continue warfarin until INR is ≥2 for at least 24 hours (usually 5 to 7 days) (Guyatt, 2012).

DVT/PE (off-label dosing): IV: 80 units/kg (or alternatively 5000 units) IV push followed by continuous infusion of 18 units/kg/hour (or alternatively 1000 units/hour) (Guyatt, 2012)

or

DVT/PE (off-label dosing): SubQ: *Unmonitored dosing regimen:* Initial: 333 units/kg then 250 units/kg every 12 hours (Guyatt, 2012; Kearon, 2006)

Geriatric Patients >60 years of age may have higher serum levels and clinical response (longer aPTTs) as compared to younger patients receiving similar dosages. Lower dosages may be required.

Pediatric Note: Many concentrations of heparin are available ranging from 1 unit/mL to 20,000 units/mL. Carefully examine each prefilled syringe or vial prior to use ensuring that the correct concentration is chosen. Heparin lock flush solution is intended only to maintain patency of IV devices and is not to be used for anticoagulant therapy.

Prophylaxis for cardiac catheterization (arterial approach): IV: Bolus: 100 units/kg (Freed, 1974; Monagle, 2012)

Systemic heparinization:

Intermittent IV: Initial: 50-100 units/kg, then 50-100 units/kg every 4 hours (**Note:** Continuous IV infusion is preferred)

IV infusion: Initial loading dose: 75 units/kg given over 10 minutes, then initial maintenance dose: 20 units/kg/hour; adjust dose to maintain aPTT of 60-85 seconds (assuming this reflects an antifactor Xa level of 0.35-0.7 units/mL); see table.

Pediatric Protocol For Systemic Heparin Adjustment

To be used after initial loading dose and maintenance IV infusion dose (see usual dosage listed above) to maintain aPTT of 60-85 seconds (assuming this reflects antifactor Xa level of 0.35-0.7 units/mL).

Obtain blood for aPTT 4 hours after heparin loading dose and 4 hours after every infusion rate change.

Obtain daily CBC and aPTT after aPTT is therapeutic.

aPTT (seconds)	Dosage Adjustment	Time to Repeat aPTT
<50	Give 50 units/kg bolus and increase infusion rate by 10%	4 h after rate change
50-59	Increase infusion rate by 10%	4 h after rate change
60-85	Keep rate the same	Next day
86-95	Decrease infusion rate by 10%	4 h after rate change
96-120	Hold infusion for 30 minutes and decrease infusion rate by 10%	4 h after rate change
>120	Hold infusion for 60 minutes and decrease infusion rate by 15%	4 h after rate change

Modified from Andrew M, et al, "Heparin Therapy in Pediatric Patients: A Prospective Cohort Study," *Pediatr Research,* 1994, 35(1):78-83.
Note: The aPTT range of 60-85 seconds corresponds to an anti-Xa level of 0.35-0.7 units/mL.

Note: Refer to adult dosing for notes on line flushing and TPN.

Renal Impairment No dosage adjustment required; adjust therapeutic heparin according to aPTT or anti-Xa activity.

Hepatic Impairment No dosage adjustment required; adjust therapeutic heparin according to aPTT or anti-Xa activity.

Usual Infusion Concentrations: Pediatric Note: Premixed solutions available

IV infusion: 100 units/mL

Usual Infusion Concentrations: Adult Note: Premixed solutions available

IV infusion: 25,000 units in 250 mL (concentration: 100 units/mL) of D$_5$W, ½NS, or NS

Administration

SubQ: Inject in subcutaneous tissue only (not muscle tissue). Injection sites should be rotated (usually left and right portions of the abdomen, above iliac crest).

IM: Do not administer IM due to pain, irritation, and hematoma formation.

Continuous IV infusion: Infuse via infusion pump. If preparing solution, mix thoroughly prior to administration.

Heparin lock: Inject via injection cap using positive pressure flushing technique. Heparin lock flush solution is intended only to maintain patency of IV devices and is **not** to be used for anticoagulant therapy.

Central venous catheters: Must be flushed with heparin solution when newly inserted, daily (at the time of tubing change), after blood withdrawal or transfusion, and after an intermittent infusion through an injectable cap. A volume of at least 10 mL of blood should be removed and discarded from a heparinized line before blood samples are sent for coagulation testing.

Intravesical (off-label use): Various dosage regimens of heparin (20,000 to 50,000 units) alone or with alkalinized lidocaine (1% to 4%) have been instilled into the bladder.

Monitoring Parameters Hemoglobin, hematocrit, signs of bleeding; fecal occult blood test; aPTT (or antifactor Xa activity levels) or ACT depending upon indication

Platelet counts should be routinely monitored (eg, every 2-3 days on days 4-14 of heparin therapy) when the risk of HIT is >1% (eg, receiving therapeutic dose heparin, postoperative antithrombotic prophylaxis), if the patient has received heparin or low molecular weight heparin (eg, enoxaparin) within the past 100 days, if pre-exposure history is uncertain, or if anaphylactoid reaction to heparin occurs. When the risk of HIT is <1% (eg, medical/obstetrical patients receiving heparin flushes), routine platelet count monitoring is not recommended (Guyatt, 2012).

For intermittent IV injections, aPTT is measured 3.5-4 hours after IV injection.

Note: Continuous IV infusion is preferred over IV intermittent injections. For full-dose heparin (ie, nonlow-dose), the dose should be titrated according to aPTT results. For anticoagulation, an aPTT 1.5-2.5 times normal is usually desired. Because of variation among hospitals in the control aPTT values, nomograms should be established at each institution, designed to achieve aPTT values in the target range (eg, for a control aPTT of 30 seconds, the target range [1.5-2.5 times control] would be 45-75 seconds). Measurements should be made prior to heparin therapy, 6 hours (pediatric: 4 hours) after initiation, and 6 hours (pediatric: 4 hours) after any dosage change, and should be used to adjust the heparin infusion until the aPTT exhibits a therapeutic level. When two consecutive aPTT values are therapeutic, subsequent measurements may be made every 24 hours, and if necessary, dose adjustment carried out. In addition, a significant change in the patient's clinical condition (eg, recurrent ischemia, bleeding, hypotension) should prompt an immediate aPTT determination, followed by dose adjustment if necessary. In general, may increase or decrease infusion by 2-4 units/kg/hour dependent upon aPTT.

Heparin infusion dose adjustment: A number of dose-adjustment nomograms have been developed which target an aPTT range of 1.5-2.5 times control (Cruickshank, 1991; Flaker, 1994; Hull, 1992; Raschke, 1993). However, institution-specific and indication-specific nomograms should be consulted for dose adjustment. **Note:** aPTT values vary throughout the day with maximum values occurring during the night (Decousus, 1985).

Reference Range Venous thromboembolism: Heparin: 0.3 to 0.7 unit/mL (children: 0.35 to 0.7 unit/mL) anti-Xa activity (by chromogenic assay) or 0.2 to 0.4 unit/mL (by protamine titration); aPTT: 1.5 to 2.5 times control (usually reflects an aPTT of 60 to 85 seconds) (Garcia, 2012; Monagle, 2012)

When used with thrombolytic therapy in patients with acute MI, a lower therapeutic range corresponding to an aPTT of 1.5 to 2 times control (or approximately an aPTT of 50 to 70 seconds) is recommended (ACCF/AHA [O'Gara, 2013).

Test Interactions Increased thyroxine (competitive protein binding methods); increased PT

Aprotinin significantly increases aPTT and celite Activated Clotting Time (ACT) which may not reflect the actual degree of anticoagulation by heparin. Kaolin-based ACTs are not affected by aprotinin to the same degree as celite ACTs. While institutional protocols may vary, a minimal celite ACT of 750 seconds or kaolin-ACT of 480 seconds is recommended in the presence of aprotinin. Consult the manufacturer's information on specific ACT test interpretation in the presence of aprotinin.

Dosage Forms Excipient information presented when available (limited, particularly for generics); consult specific product labeling. [DSC] = Discontinued product

Solution, Injection, as sodium:
Generic: 1000 units (500 mL); 2000 units (1000 mL); 12,500 units (250 mL); 25,000 units (250 mL, 500 mL); 1000 units/mL (1 mL, 10 mL, 30 mL); 2500 units/mL (10 mL); 5000 units/mL (1 mL, 10 mL); 10,000 units/mL (1 mL, 4 mL, 5 mL); 20,000 units/mL (1 mL)

Solution, Injection, as sodium [preservative free]:
Generic: 1000 units/mL (2 mL); 5000 units/0.5 mL (0.5 mL)

Solution, Intravenous, as sodium:
Hep Flush-10: 10 units/mL (10 mL)
Generic: 10,000 units (250 mL); 12,500 units (250 mL); 20,000 units (500 mL); 25,000 units (250 mL, 500 mL); 1 units/mL (1 mL, 2 mL, 2.5 mL, 3 mL, 5 mL, 10 mL); 2 units/mL (3 mL); 10 units/mL (1 mL, 2 mL, 2.5 mL, 3 mL, 5 mL, 10 mL, 30 mL); 100 units/mL (1 mL, 2 mL, 2.5 mL, 3 mL, 5 mL, 10 mL, 30 mL, 100 mL [DSC], 250 mL); 2000 units/mL (5 mL)

Solution, Intravenous, as sodium [preservative free]:
Generic: 1 units/mL (3 mL); 10 units/mL (1 mL, 3 mL, 5 mL); 100 units/mL (1 mL, 3 mL, 5 mL)

- ♦ Heparin Calcium *see* Heparin *on page 871*
- ♦ Heparinized Saline *see* Heparin *on page 871*
- ♦ Heparin Leo (Can) *see* Heparin *on page 871*
- ♦ Heparin Lock Flush *see* Heparin *on page 871*
- ♦ Heparin Sodium *see* Heparin *on page 871*
- ♦ Heparin Sodium Injection, USP (Can) *see* Heparin *on page 871*

Hepatitis A and Hepatitis B Recombinant Vaccine
(hep a TYE tis aye & hep a TYE tis bee ree KOM be nant vak SEEN)

Brand Names: US Twinrix
Brand Names: Canada Twinrix; Twinrix Junior

Index Terms Engerix-B and Havrix; Havrix and Engerix-B; HepA-HepB; Hepatitis B and Hepatitis A Vaccine
Pharmacologic Category Vaccine; Vaccine, Inactivated (Viral)
Additional Appendix Information
Immunization Administration Recommendations *on page 1974*

Immunization Schedules *on page 1979*
Use
Hepatitis A and B diseases prevention:
Twinrix: Active immunization of persons 18 years and older (US labeling) or 19 years and older (Canadian labeling) against disease caused by hepatitis A virus and hepatitis B virus (all known subtypes)
Canadian labeling: Additional uses (not in US labeling): Approved for active immunization of children and adolescents ages 1 to 15 years.
Twinrix Junior [Canadian product]: Active immunization of children and adolescents ages 1 to 18 years against disease caused by hepatitis A virus and hepatitis B virus (all known subtypes).
Limitations of use: Hepatitis A/hepatitis B vaccine cannot be used for postexposure prophylaxis.
Dosing
Adult & Geriatric
Primary immunization: IM:
US labeling: 1 mL given on a 0-, 1-, and 6-month schedule for a total of 3 doses
Accelerated regimen: 1 mL on day 0, day 7, and days 21 to 30, followed by a booster at 12 months for a total of 4 doses
Canadian labeling: Adults ≥19 years (Twinrix): 1 mL given on a 0-, 1-, and 6-month schedule for a total of 3 doses
Accelerated regimen: 1 mL on day 0, day 7, and day 21, followed by a booster at 12 months for a total of 4 doses
Pediatric
Primary immunization: Canadian labeling: IM:
Children and Adolescents:
Twinrix Junior: Ages 1 to 18 years: 0.5 mL given on a 0-, 1-, and 6-month schedule for a total of 3 doses
Twinrix: Ages 1 to 15 years: 1 mL given on elected date followed by second dose (1 mL) 6 to 12 months later for a total of 2 doses
Renal Impairment There are no dosage adjustments provided in the manufacturer's labeling.
Hepatic Impairment There are no dosage adjustments provided in the manufacturer's labeling.
Additional Information Complete prescribing information should be consulted for additional detail.
Dosage Forms Excipient information presented when available (limited, particularly for generics); consult specific product labeling.
Injection, suspension [preservative free]:
Twinrix: Hepatitis A virus antigen 720 ELISA units and hepatitis B surface antigen 20 mcg per mL (1 mL) [contains aluminum, yeast protein, and trace amounts of neomycin; may contain natural rubber/natural latex in prefilled syringe]
Dosage Forms: Canada Also refer to Dosage Forms. Excipient information presented when available (limited, particularly for generics); consult specific product labeling.
Injection, suspension [preservative free]:
Twinrix Junior: Hepatitis A virus antigen 360 ELISA units and hepatitis B surface antigen 10 mcg per 0.5 mL (0.5 mL) [contains aluminum and trace amounts of neomycin]

Hepatitis A Vaccine (hep a TYE tis aye vak SEEN)

Brand Names: US Havrix; VAQTA
Brand Names: Canada Avaxim; Avaxim-Pediatric; HAVRIX; VAQTA
Index Terms HepA
Pharmacologic Category Vaccine; Vaccine, Inactivated (Viral)
Additional Appendix Information
Immunization Administration Recommendations *on page 1974*

Immunization Schedules *on page 1979*
Use Hepatitis A virus disease prevention:
For active immunization of persons 12 months and older against disease caused by hepatitis A virus (HAV).
The Advisory Committee on Immunization Practices (ACIP) recommends routine vaccination for:
- All children ≥12 months of age (CDC/ACIP [Fiore 2006])
- All unvaccinated adults requesting protection from HAV infection (CDC/ACIP [Fiore 2006])

- Unvaccinated persons with any of the following conditions: Men who have sex with men; injection and non-injection illicit drug users; persons who work with HAV-infected primates or with HAV in a research laboratory setting; persons with chronic liver disease; patients who receive clotting-factor concentrates; persons traveling to or working in countries with high or intermediate levels of endemic HAV infection (CDC/ACIP [Fiore 2006])
- Unvaccinated persons who anticipate close personal contact with international adoptee from a country of intermediate to high endemicity of HAV, during their first 60 days of arrival into the United States (eg, household contacts, babysitters) (CDC/ACIP 58[36] 2009)
- Vaccination can be a component of hepatitis A outbreak response or as postexposure prophylaxis, as determined by local public health authorities (CDC/ACIP 56 [41] 2007; CDC/ACIP [Fiore 2006])

Medication Guide Available Yes

Dosing

Adult & Geriatric

Immunization: Note: Although it is preferred to use the vaccines according to their approved labeling, Havrix and VAQTA are considered to be interchangeable for booster doses (CDC/ACIP [Fiore 2006]).

Primary immunization: Note: When used for primary immunization, the vaccine should be given at least 2 weeks prior to expected HAV exposure. When used prior to an international adoption, the vaccination series should begin when adoption is being planned, but ideally ≥2 weeks prior to expected arrival of adoptee (CDC 58[36] 2009).

Manufacturer's labeling:

Avaxim [Canadian product]: IM: 160 units (0.5 mL) with a booster dose of 160 units (0.5 mL) to be given 6 to 36 months following primary immunization

Havrix: IM: 1440 ELISA units (1 mL) with a booster dose of 1440 ELISA units (1 mL) to be given 6 to 12 months following primary immunization.

VAQTA: IM: 50 units (1 mL) with a booster dose of 50 units (1 mL) to be given 6-18 months after primary immunization (6 to 12 months if initial dose was with Havrix). **Note:** Canadian labeling recommends that adults with HIV receive a booster dose 6 months after primary immunization.

Postexposure prophylaxis (off-label use): Adults without immunity: IM: 0.5 mL once as soon as possible following recent exposure to hepatitis A virus (during last 2 weeks) (CDC 56[41] 2007).

Pediatric Immunization: Note: Although it is preferred to use the vaccines according to their approved labeling, Havrix and VAQTA are considered to be interchangeable for booster doses (CDC/ACIP [Fiore 2006]).

Primary immunization: Advisory Committee on Immunization Practices (ACIP): Children ≥12 months: All children should receive primary immunization with a two-dose series. The series should be initiated at 12 to 23 months; the two doses should be separated by 6 to 18 months (CDC/ACIP [Fiore 2006]). **Note:** When used for primary immunization, the vaccine should be given at least 2 weeks prior to expected HAV exposure. When used prior to an international adoption, the vaccination series should begin when adoption is being planned, but ideally ≥2 weeks prior to expected arrival of adoptee (CDC 58[36] 2009).

Manufacturer's labeling:

Avaxim [Canadian product]: Children ≥12 years and Adolescents: Refer to adult dosing.

Avaxim-Pediatric [Canadian product]: Children ≥12 months and Adolescents ≤15 years: IM: 80 units (0.5 mL) with a booster dose of 80 units (0.5 mL) to be given 6 to 12 months following primary immunization

Havrix: Children ≥12 months and Adolescents: IM: 720 ELISA units (0.5 mL) with a booster dose of 720 ELISA units (0.5 mL) to be given 6 to 12 months following primary immunization

VAQTA: Children ≥12 months and Adolescents: IM: 25 units (0.5 mL) with a booster dose of 25 units (0.5 mL) to be given 6 to 18 months after primary immunization (6 to 12 months if initial dose was with HAVRIX)

Postexposure prophylaxis (off-label use): Children and Adolescents without immunity: IM: 0.5 mL once as soon as possible following recent exposure to hepatitis A virus (during last 2 weeks) (CDC 56[41] 2007).

Renal Impairment There are no dosage adjustments provided in the manufacturer's labeling.

Hepatic Impairment There are no specific recommendations provided in manufacturer's labeling. However, data suggest patients with chronic liver disease have a lower antibody response to HAVRIX than healthy subjects.

Additional Information Complete prescribing information should be consulted for additional detail.

Dosage Forms Excipient information presented when available (limited, particularly for generics); consult specific product labeling.

Injection, suspension [adult, preservative free]:

Havrix: Hepatitis A virus antigen 1440 ELISA units/mL (1 mL) [contains aluminum, neomycin (may have trace amounts); may contain natural rubber/natural latex in prefilled syringe]

VAQTA: Hepatitis A virus antigen 50 units/mL (1 mL) [contains aluminum, natural rubber/natural latex in packaging]

Injection, suspension [pediatric, preservative free]:

Havrix: Hepatitis A virus antigen 720 ELISA units/0.5 mL (0.5 mL) [contains aluminum, neomycin (may have trace amounts); may contain natural rubber/natural latex in prefilled syringe]

Injection, suspension [pediatric/adolescent, preservative free]:

VAQTA: Hepatitis A virus antigen 25 units/0.5 mL (0.5 mL) [contains aluminum, natural rubber/natural latex in packaging]

Dosage Forms: Canada Also refer to Dosage Forms. Excipient information presented when available (limited, particularly for generics); consult specific product labeling.

Injection, suspension [pediatric/adolescent]:

Avaxim-Pediatric: Hepatitis A virus antigen 80 units/0.5 mL [contains aluminum, polysorbate 80, neomycin (may have trace amounts)]

Injection, suspension [adolescent/adult]:

Avaxim: Hepatitis A virus antigen 160 units/0.5 mL [contains aluminum, polysorbate 80, neomycin (may have trace amounts)]

◆ Hepatitis B and Hepatitis A Vaccine *see* Hepatitis A and Hepatitis B Recombinant Vaccine *on page 874*

Hepatitis B Immune Globulin (Human)
(hep a TYE tis bee i MYUN GLOB yoo lin YU man)

Brand Names: US HepaGam B; HyperHEP B S/D; Nabi-HB

Brand Names: Canada HepaGam B; HyperHEP B S/D

Index Terms HBIG

Pharmacologic Category Blood Product Derivative; Immune Globulin

Additional Appendix Information

Immunization Administration Recommendations *on page 1974*

Immunization Schedules *on page 1979*

Use

Passive prophylactic immunity to hepatitis B following: Acute exposure to blood containing hepatitis B surface antigen (HBsAg); perinatal exposure of infants born to HBsAg-positive mothers; sexual exposure to HBsAg-positive persons; household exposure to persons with acute HBV infection

Prevention of hepatitis B virus recurrence after liver transplantation in HBsAg-positive transplant patients

Note: Hepatitis B immune globulin is not indicated for treatment of active hepatitis B infection and is ineffective in the treatment of chronic active hepatitis B infection.

Dosing

Adult & Geriatric

Postexposure prophylaxis: IM: 0.06 mL/kg as soon as possible after exposure (ie, within 24 hours of needle-stick, ocular, or mucosal exposure or within 14 days of sexual exposure); repeat at 28-30 days after exposure in nonresponders to hepatitis B vaccine or in patients who refuse vaccination

Postexposure management of health care personnel (HCP) (CDC 62 [10], 2013): IM: 0.06 mL/kg

If the HCP has prior documentation of ≥3 doses of a hepatitis B vaccine and a postvaccination anti-HBs ≥10 milliunits/mL, then HBIG is not needed, regardless of the patients HBsAg status.

If the HCP is unvaccinated or incompletely vaccinated, and if the source patient is HBsAG positive or their status is unknown, one dose HBIG should be administered. If the source patient is HBsAG negative, then HBIG is not needed.

If the HCP is vaccinated with 3 doses of hepatitis B vaccine but postvaccination anti-HBs status is unknown, test HCP for anti-HBs. If anti-HBs ≥10 milliunits/mL then HBIG is not needed. If anti-HBs <10 milliunits/mL, and if the source patient is HBsAG positive or their status is unknown, 1 dose of HBIG should be administered. If anti-HBs <10 milliunits/mL, and if the source patient is HBsAG negative, then HBIG is not needed.

If the HCP is vaccinated with 6 doses of hepatitis B vaccine but documented as a nonresponder to the vaccine, and if the source patient is HBsAG negative, then HBIG is not needed. If the source patient is HBsAG positive or unknown, administer 2 doses of HBIG separated by 1 month.

Prevention of hepatitis B virus recurrence after liver transplantation (HepaGam B): IV: 20,000 units/dose according to the following schedule:

Anhepatic phase (Initial dose): One dose given with the liver transplant

Week 1 postop: One dose daily for 7 days (days 1-7)

Weeks 2-12 postop: One dose every 2 weeks starting day 14

Month 4 onward: One dose monthly starting on month 4

Dose adjustment: Adjust dose to reach anti-HBs levels of 500 units/L within the first week after transplantation. In patients with surgical bleeding, abdominal fluid drainage >500 mL or those undergoing plasmapheresis, administer 10,000 units/dose every 6 hours until target anti-HBs levels are reached.

Pediatric

Infants born to HBsAg-positive mothers: IM: 0.5 mL as soon after birth as possible (within 12 hours); active vaccination with hepatitis B vaccine may begin at the same time in a different site (if not contraindicated). If first dose of hepatitis B vaccine is delayed for as long as 3 months, dose may be repeated. If hepatitis B vaccine is refused, dose may be repeated at 3 and 6 months.

Infants born to mothers with unknown HBsAg status at birth (CDC, 2005): IM:

Birth weight <2 kg: 0.5 mL within 12 hours of birth (along with hepatitis B vaccine) if unable to determine maternal HBsAg status within that time

Birth weight ≥2 kg: If the mother is determined to be HBsAg positive, administer 0.5 mL as soon as possible, but within 7 days of birth

Household exposure prophylaxis in infants <12 months: IM: 0.5 mL (to be administered if mother or primary caregiver has acute HBV infection).

Postexposure prophylaxis: IM: Children ≥12 months: Refer to adult dosing.

Note: HBIG may be administered at the same time (but at a different site) or up to 1 month preceding hepatitis B vaccination without impairing the active immune response

Renal Impairment No dosage adjustment provided in manufacturer's labeling.

Hepatic Impairment No dosage adjustment provided in manufacturer's labeling.

Additional Information Complete prescribing information should be consulted for additional detail.

Dosage Forms Excipient information presented when available (limited, particularly for generics); consult specific product labeling.

Solution, Injection [preservative free]:

HepaGam B: (1 mL, 5 mL) [contains polysorbate 80]

Solution, Intramuscular:

HyperHEP B S/D: (0.5 mL, 1 mL, 5 mL)

Nabi-HB: (1 mL, 5 mL) [thimerosal free]

◆ **Hepatitis B Inactivated Virus Vaccine (recombinant DNA)** see Hepatitis B Vaccine (Recombinant) on page 876

Hepatitis B Vaccine (Recombinant)

(hep a TYE tis bee vak SEEN ree KOM be nant)

Brand Names: US Engerix-B; Recombivax HB

Brand Names: Canada Engerix-B; Recombivax HB

Index Terms Hepatitis B Inactivated Virus Vaccine (recombinant DNA); HepB

Pharmacologic Category Vaccine; Vaccine, Inactivated (Viral)

Additional Appendix Information

Immunization Administration Recommendations on page 1974

Immunization Schedules on page 1979

Use Hepatitis B disease prevention: Active immunization against infection caused by all known subtypes of hepatitis B virus (HBV)

The Advisory Committee on Immunization Practices (ACIP) recommends routine vaccination for the following:

- All neonates before hospital discharge (CDC/ACIP [Mast 2005])
- All unvaccinated infants and children (CDC/ACIP [Mast 2005])
- All unvaccinated adults requesting protection from HBV infection (CDC/ACIP [Mast 2006])
- All unvaccinated adults at risk for HBV infection such as those with:

Behavioral risks: Sexually-active persons with >1 partner in a 6-month period; persons seeking evaluation or treatment for a sexually-transmitted disease; men who have sex with men; injection drug users (CDC/ACIP [Mast 2006])

Occupational risks: Healthcare personnel (HCP) and public safety workers with reasonably anticipated risk for exposure to blood or blood contaminated body fluids (CDC/ACIP [Mast 2006])

Medical risks: Persons with end-stage renal disease (including predialysis, hemodialysis, peritoneal dialysis, and home dialysis); persons with HIV infection; persons with chronic liver disease (CDC/ACIP [Mast 2006]). Adults (19 through 59 years of age) with diabetes mellitus type 1 or type 2 should be vaccinated as soon as possible following diagnosis. Adults ≥60 years with diabetes mellitus may also be vaccinated at the discretion of their treating clinician based on the likelihood of acquiring HBV infection (CDC/ACIP 60[50] 2011).

Other risks: Household contacts and sex partners of persons with chronic HBV infection; residents and staff of facilities for developmentally disabled persons; international travelers to regions with high or intermediate levels of endemic HBV infection (CDC/ACIP [Mast 2006])

In addition, the ACIP recommends vaccination for any persons who are wounded in bombings or similar mass casualty events who have penetrating injuries or non-intact skin exposure, or who have contact with mucous membranes (exception - superficial contact with intact skin), and who cannot confirm receipt of a hepatitis B vaccination (CDC [Chapman 2008]).

Medication Guide Available Yes

Dosing

Adult & Geriatric

Primary immunization: IM: **Note:** Adult formulations of hepatitis B vaccine products differ by concentration (mcg/mL) but when dosed in terms of volume (mL), the dose of Engerix-B and Recombivax HB are the same (both 1 mL).

Immunocompetent adults: 1 mL/dose (adult formulation) for 3 total doses administered at 0, 1, and 6 months. **Note:** Refer to CDC guideline (Mast 2006) for other options. Manufacturer labeling may include alternate immunization schedules.

Adults with immunocompromising conditions (CDC/ACIP [Kim 2015]):

Engerix-B 20 mcg/mL: Administer 2 mL per dose at 0, 1, 2, and 6 months

Recombivax HB 40 mcg/mL: Administer 1 mL per dose at 0, 1, and 6 months

Bombings or similar mass casualty events: IM: In persons without a reliable history of vaccination against HepB and who have no known contraindications to the vaccine, vaccination should begin within 24 hours (but no later than 7 days) following the event (CDC [Chapman 2008]).

Postexposure management of health care personnel (HCP) (CDC [Schillie 2013]): IM:

Documented vaccine responder: If the HCP has prior documentation of ≥3 doses of a hepatitis B vaccine and a postvaccination anti-HBs ≥10 milliunits/mL, then additional hepatitis B vaccine is not needed, regardless of the patients HBsAg status. HCP is considered seroprotected.

Unvaccinated or incompletely vaccinated: The primary vaccination series should be completed regardless of the source patients HBsAg status. If the source patient is HBsAg positive or their status is unknown, 1 dose of hepatitis B vaccine and 1 dose of hepatitis B immunoglobulin (HBIG) should be administered as soon as possible.

Vaccinated with 3 doses of hepatitis B vaccine but postvaccination anti-HBs status is unknown: Test HCP for anti-HBs. If anti-HBs ≥10 milliunits/mL additional hepatitis B vaccine is not needed. If anti-HBs <10 milliunits/mL, initiate revaccination by administering a single dose of the vaccine and retesting for anti-HBs in 1 to 2 months; if needed 2 additional doses may be given and then retest anti-HBs level.

Alternately, administer 3 consecutive doses of the vaccine and then retest anti-HBs level. Minimum dosing intervals are 4 weeks between doses 1 and 2, and 8 weeks between doses 2 and 3; maximum total 6 doses of hepatitis B vaccine (including the original series). If the source patient is HBsAg positive or their status is unknown, 1 dose of HBIG should also be administered.

Vaccinated with 6 doses of hepatitis B vaccine but documented as a nonresponder to the vaccine: No postexposure vaccination is recommended. If the source patient is HBsAg positive or unknown, administer two doses of HBIG separated by 1 month.

Pediatric

Primary immunization: IM:

Infants: **Note:** Doses are presented using the pediatric/adolescent formulations. Pediatric/adolescent formulations of hepatitis B vaccine products differ by concentration (mcg/mL). However, when dosed in terms of volume (mL), the dose of Engerix-B and Recombivax HB are the same (both 0.5 mL). Combination vaccines should not be used for the "birth" dose but may be used to complete the course beginning after the infant is ≥6 weeks of age (CDC/ACIP [Mast 2005]). Please see combination vaccine monographs for dose and schedule details.

US labeling: 0.5 mL/dose (pediatric/adolescent formulation) for 3 total doses administered at 0, 1 and 6 months. Alternate dosing regimens are also available for children who begin vaccination ≥1 year of age.

Canadian labeling: 0.5 mL/dose (pediatric/adolescent formulation) for 3 total doses administered at 0, 1, and 6 months. For accelerated protection, a 4 dose series can be administered at 0, 1, and 2 months plus a booster at 12 months.

ACIP recommendations (CDC/ACIP [Mast 2005]): IM:

Infants (HBsAg-**negative** mothers):

First dose: 0.5 mL at birth or before discharge (may be delayed in certain cases)

Second dose: 0.5 mL at 1 to 2 months of age

Third dose: 0.5 mL at 6 to 18 months of age, but no sooner than 24 weeks of age

Note: Premature neonates <2 kg should have the initial dose deferred up to 30 days of chronological age or at hospital discharge.

Infants (HBsAg-**positive** mothers):

First dose: 0.5 mL within first 12 hours of life, even if premature and regardless of birth weight (hepatitis immune globulin should also be administered at the same time at a different site)

Second dose: 0.5 mL at 1 to 2 months of age

Third dose: 0.5 mL at 6 months of age but no sooner than 24 weeks of age

Note: Anti-HBs and HBsAg levels should be checked at 9 to 18 months of age (ie, next well-child visit after series completion). If HBsAg negative and anti-HBs levels <10 milliunits/mL, reimmunize with 3 doses and reassess 1 to 2 months after the third dose.

Note: In premature neonates <2 kg, the birth dose should not be counted as part of the 3-dose vaccine series.

Infants (mother's HBsAg status **unknown**):

First dose: 0.5 mL within 12 hours of birth even if premature and regardless of birth weight; if the mother's blood HBsAg test is positive, the infant should receive hepatitis immune globulin as soon as possible (no later than 12 hours of age if <2 kg or age 1 week if ≥2 kg).

Second dose: 0.5 mL at 1 to 2 months of age

Third dose: 0.5 mL at 6 months of age but no sooner than 24 weeks of age

Note: In premature neonates <2 kg, the birth dose should not be counted as part of the 3-dose vaccine series.

Children and Adolescents: 0.5 mL/dose (pediatric/adolescent formulation) administered at 0, 1, and 6 months (for 3 total doses). Alternate dosing regimens are also available for children who begin vaccination ≥1 year of age. **Note:** Refer to CDC guideline (Mast, 2005) for other options. Manufacturer labeling may include alternate immunization schedules, refer to CDC Catch-up Schedules for guidance (CDC/ACIP [Strikas 2015]).

Bombings or similar mass casualty events: Refer to adult dosing.

Renal Impairment Adults ≥20 years:

Predialysis patients: Recombivax HB 40 mcg/mL: Administer 1 mL per dose at 0, 1, and 6 months

Dialysis patients:

Engerix-B 20 mcg/mL: Administer 2 mL per dose at 0, 1, 2, and 6 months

Recombivax HB 40 mcg/mL: Administer 1 mL per dose at 0, 1, and 6 months

Note: Serologic testing is recommended 1 to 2 months after the final dose of the primary vaccine series and annually to determine the need for booster doses. Persons with anti-HBs concentrations of <10 milliunits/mL should be revaccinated with 3 doses of the vaccine (CDC/ACIP [Mast 2006]).

Hepatic Impairment There are no dosage adjustments provided in the manufacturer's labeling.

Additional Information Complete prescribing information should be consulted for additional detail.

Dosage Forms Excipient information presented when available (limited, particularly for generics); consult specific product labeling.

Injection, suspension [adult, preservative free]:

Engerix-B: Hepatitis B surface antigen 20 mcg/mL (1 mL) [contains aluminum, yeast protein, may contain natural rubber/natural latex in prefilled syringe]

Engerix-B: Hepatitis B surface antigen 20 mcg/mL (1 mL) [contains aluminum, yeast protein; vial]

Recombivax HB: Hepatitis B surface antigen 10 mcg/mL (1 mL) [contains aluminum, natural rubber/natural latex in packaging, yeast protein]

Injection, suspension [dialysis formulation, preservative free]:

Recombivax HB: Hepatitis B surface antigen 40 mcg/mL (1 mL) [contains aluminum, natural rubber/natural latex in packaging, yeast protein]

Injection, suspension [pediatric/adolescent, preservative free]:

Engerix-B: Hepatitis B surface antigen 10 mcg/0.5 mL (0.5 mL) [contains aluminum, yeast protein, may contain natural rubber/natural latex in prefilled syringe]

Recombivax HB: Hepatitis B surface antigen 5 mcg/0.5 mL (0.5 mL) [contains aluminum, natural rubber/natural latex in packaging, yeast protein]

Hetastarch (HET a starch)

Brand Names: US Hespan; Hextend

Brand Names: Canada Hextend

Index Terms HES; HES 450/0.7; Hydroxyethyl Starch

Pharmacologic Category Plasma Volume Expander, Colloid

Use

Granulocyte yield increase (Hespan): Used as an adjunct in leukapheresis to improve harvesting and increase the yield of granulocytes by centrifugation

Hypovolemia: Blood volume expander used in treatment of hypovolemia

Dosing

Adult & Geriatric

Plasma volume expansion: IV: 500-1000 mL (up to 1500 mL daily) or 20 mL/kg/day (up to 1500 mL daily). **Note:** With severe dehydration, administer crystalloid first. Daily dose and rate of infusion dependent on amount of blood lost, on maintenance or restoration of hemodynamics, and on amount of hemodilution. Titrate to individual colloid needs, hemodynamics, and hydration status. Do not use in the critically ill, those undergoing open heart surgery and cardiopulmonary bypass, or those with preexisting renal dysfunction.

Leukapheresis (Hespan): 250-700 mL; **Note:** Citrate anticoagulant is added before use and then the mixture is administered to the input line of the centrifuge apparatus.

Renal Impairment Avoid use in patients with preexisting renal dysfunction. Use is contraindicated in renal failure with oliguria or anuria (not related to hypovolemia). Discontinue use at the first sign of renal injury.

Hepatic Impairment No dosage adjustment provided in manufacturer's labeling; use with caution.

Additional Information Complete prescribing information should be consulted for additional detail.

Dosage Forms Excipient information presented when available (limited, particularly for generics); consult specific product labeling.

Solution, Intravenous:
Hespan: 6% (500 mL)
Hextend: 6% (500 mL)
Generic: 6% (500 mL)

Histrelin (his TREL in)

Brand Names: US Supprelin LA; Vantas
Brand Names: Canada Vantas
Index Terms GnRH Agonist; Histrelin Acetate; LH-RH Agonist
Pharmacologic Category Antineoplastic Agent, Gonadotropin-Releasing Hormone Agonist; Gonadotropin Releasing Hormone Agonist
Use
Central precocious puberty: Treatment of central precocious puberty (CPP) in children
Prostate cancer, advanced: Palliative treatment of advanced prostate cancer
Dosing
Adult & Geriatric Prostate cancer, advanced (Vantas):
SubQ: 50 mg implant surgically inserted every 12 months
Pediatric Central precocious puberty (CPP) (Supprelin LA): Children ≥2 years: SubQ: 50 mg implant surgically inserted every 12 months. Discontinue at the appropriate time for the onset of puberty.
Renal Impairment
Vantas: CrCl ≥15 mL/minute: No dosage adjustment necessary.
Supprelin LA: There are no dosage adjustments provided in the manufacturers' labeling.
Hepatic Impairment There are no dosage adjustments provided in the manufacturer's labeling (has not been studied).
Additional Information Complete prescribing information should be consulted for additional detail.
Dosage Forms Excipient information presented when available (limited, particularly for generics); consult specific product labeling.
Kit, Subcutaneous:
Supprelin LA: 50 mg
Vantas: 50 mg

Homatropine (hoe MA troe peen)

Brand Names: US Homatropaire; Isopto Homatropine
Index Terms Homatropine Hydrobromide
Pharmacologic Category Anticholinergic Agent, Ophthalmic; Ophthalmic Agent, Mydriatic
Use
Ciliary spasm: Relief of ciliary spasm.
Iritis/iridocyclitis: Treatment of iritis and iridocyclitis.
Mydriasis and cycloplegia for refraction: Producing cycloplegia and mydriasis for refraction; for pre- and postoperative states when cycloplegic and mydriasis is required.
Optical aid: Use as an optical aid in some cases of axial lens opacities.
Uveitis: Treatment of inflammatory conditions of the uveal tract.
Dosing
Adult & Geriatric Note: Patients with heavily pigmented irides may require increased dose.
Ciliary spasm/iritis/iridocyclitis/uveitis: Ophthalmic: 2% or 5% solution: 1-2 drops 2-3 times daily, up to every 4 hours for severe uveitis (Alexander, 2004)
Refraction: Ophthalmic:
2% solution: 1-2 drops into eye(s); repeat every 10-15 minutes if necessary; maximum: 5 doses
5% solution: 1-2 drops into eye(s); repeat dose in 15 minutes.
Pediatric Note: Children (>3 months of age) should only use the 2% strength solution; patients with heavily pigmented irides may require increased dose.
Ciliary spasm/iritis/iridocyclitis/uveitis: Ophthalmic: 2% solution: 1-2 drops 2-3 times daily, up to every 4 hours for severe uveitis (Alexander, 2004)
Refraction: Ophthalmic: 2% solution: 1-2 drops into eye(s); repeat every 10-15 minutes if necessary; maximum: 5 doses
Renal Impairment No dosage adjustment provided in manufacturer's labeling.
Hepatic Impairment No dosage adjustment provided in manufacturer's labeling.
Additional Information Complete prescribing information should be consulted for additional detail.
Dosage Forms Excipient information presented when available (limited, particularly for generics); consult specific product labeling.
Solution, Ophthalmic, as hydrobromide:
Homatropine: 5% (5 mL)
Isopto Homatropine: 2% (5 mL); 5% (5 mL)
Generic: 5% (5 mL)

◆ HPV Vaccine (Quadrivalent) *see* Papillomavirus (Types 6, 11, 16, 18) Vaccine (Human, Recombinant) *on page 1394*

◆ HRIG *see* Rabies Immune Globulin (Human) *on page 1547*

◆ HU *see* Hydroxyurea *on page 895*

◆ HuLuc63 *see* Elotuzumab *on page 625*

◆ HumaLOG *see* Insulin Lispro *on page 958*

◆ Humalog (Can) *see* Insulin Lispro *on page 958*

◆ HumaLOG KwikPen *see* Insulin Lispro *on page 958*

◆ Humalog Mix 25 (Can) *see* Insulin Lispro Protamine and Insulin Lispro *on page 959*

◆ Humalog Mix 50 (Can) *see* Insulin Lispro Protamine and Insulin Lispro *on page 959*

◆ HumaLOG® Mix 50/50™ *see* Insulin Lispro Protamine and Insulin Lispro *on page 959*

◆ HumaLOG® Mix 50/50™ KwikPen™ *see* Insulin Lispro Protamine and Insulin Lispro *on page 959*

◆ HumaLOG® Mix 75/25™ *see* Insulin Lispro Protamine and Insulin Lispro *on page 959*

◆ HumaLOG® Mix 75/25™ KwikPen™ *see* Insulin Lispro Protamine and Insulin Lispro *on page 959*

◆ Human Albumin Grifols *see* Albumin *on page 55*

◆ Human Antitumor Necrosis Factor Alpha *see* Adalimumab *on page 41*

◆ Human C1 Inhibitor *see* C1 Inhibitor (Human) *on page 276*

◆ Human Corticotrophin-Releasing Hormone, Analogue *see* Corticorelin *on page 448*

◆ Human Diploid Cell Cultures Rabies Vaccine *see* Rabies Vaccine *on page 1547*

◆ Human Growth Hormone *see* Somatropin *on page 1686*

◆ Humanized IgG1 Anti-CD52 Monoclonal Antibody *see* Alemtuzumab *on page 62*

◆ Human Menopausal Gonadotropin *see* Menotropins *on page 1143*

◆ Human Normal Immunoglobulin *see* Immune Globulin *on page 927*

◆ Human Papillomavirus Vaccine (Bivalent) *see* Papillomavirus (Types 16, 18) Vaccine (Human, Recombinant) *on page 1394*

◆ Human Papillomavirus Vaccine (Quadrivalent) *see* Papillomavirus (Types 6, 11, 16, 18) Vaccine (Human, Recombinant) *on page 1394*

◆ Human Rotavirus Vaccine, Attenuated (HRV) *see* Rotavirus Vaccine *on page 1623*

◆ Human Thyroid Stimulating Hormone *see* Thyrotropin Alfa *on page 1784*

◆ Humate-P *see* Antihemophilic Factor/von Willebrand Factor Complex (Human) *on page 133*

◆ Humatin (Can) *see* Paromomycin *on page 1398*

◆ Humatrope *see* Somatropin *on page 1686*

◆ HuMax-CD20 *see* Ofatumumab *on page 1311*

◆ Humira *see* Adalimumab *on page 41*

◆ Humira Pediatric Crohns Start *see* Adalimumab *on page 41*

◆ Humira Pen *see* Adalimumab *on page 41*

◆ Humira Pen-Crohns Starter *see* Adalimumab *on page 41*

◆ Humira Pen-Psoriasis Starter *see* Adalimumab *on page 41*

◆ Humist [OTC] *see* Sodium Chloride *on page 1671*

◆ Humulin 20/80 (Can) *see* Insulin NPH and Insulin Regular *on page 960*

◆ HumuLIN 70/30 *see* Insulin NPH and Insulin Regular *on page 960*

◆ Humulin 70/30 (Can) *see* Insulin NPH and Insulin Regular *on page 960*

◆ HumuLIN 70/30 KwikPen *see* Insulin NPH and Insulin Regular *on page 960*

◆ HumuLIN N [OTC] *see* Insulin NPH *on page 959*

◆ Humulin N (Can) *see* Insulin NPH *on page 959*

◆ HumuLIN N KwikPen [OTC] *see* Insulin NPH *on page 959*

◆ HumuLIN N Pen [OTC] [DSC] *see* Insulin NPH *on page 959*

◆ HumuLIN R [OTC] *see* Insulin Regular *on page 961*

◆ Humulin R (Can) *see* Insulin Regular *on page 961*

◆ HumuLIN R U-500 (CONCENTRATED) *see* Insulin Regular *on page 961*

◆ Hurricaine [OTC] *see* Benzocaine *on page 217*

◆ HurriCaine One [OTC] *see* Benzocaine *on page 217*

◆ Hyalgan *see* Hyaluronate and Derivatives *on page 879*

◆ Hyaluronan *see* Hyaluronate and Derivatives *on page 879*

Hyaluronate and Derivatives

(hye al yoor ON ate & dah RIV ah tives)

Brand Names: US Amvisc; Amvisc Plus; Bionect; Euflexxa; Gel-One; Hyalgan; HyGel; Hylase Wound; Juvederm Ultra; Juvederm Ultra Plus; Juvederm Ultra Plus XC; Juvederm Ultra XC; Juvederm Voluma XC; Monovisc; Orthovisc; Perlane; Perlane-L [DSC]; Provisc; Restylane; Restylane Lyft; Restylane Silk; Restylane-L; Supartz FX; Supartz [DSC]; Synvisc; Synvisc-One

Brand Names: Canada Cystistat; Durolane; OrthoVisc; Suplasyn

Index Terms Hyaluronan; Hyaluronic Acid; Hylan G-F 20; Hylan Polymers; Sodium Hyaluronate

Pharmacologic Category Antirheumatic Miscellaneous; Cosmetic Agent, Implant; Ophthalmic Agent, Viscoelastic; Skin and Mucous Membrane Agent, Miscellaneous

Use

Intra-articular injection: Treatment of pain in osteoarthritis in knee in patients who have failed nonpharmacologic treatment or simple analgesics (Euflexxa, Gel-One, Hyalgan, Monovisc, OrthoVisc, Supartz, Supartz FX, Synvisc, Synvisc-One) or nonsteroidal anti-inflammatory drugs (NSAIDS) (Gel-One)

Intradermal:

Juvederm (all formulations except Voluma XC), Perlane, Restylane, Restylane Lyft, Restylane-L: Correction of moderate to severe facial wrinkles or folds

Restylane Silk: Correction of perioral rhytids in adults >21 years.

Subcutaneous/supraperiosteal: Juvederm Voluma XC, Restylane Lyft: Correction of age-related volume deficit (deep [subcutaneous and/or supraperiosteal] injection) for cheek augmentation in the mid-face in adults >21 years

Ophthalmic: Surgical aid in cataract extraction (Amvisc, Amvisc Plus, Provisc); intraocular lens implantation (Amvisc, Amvisc Plus, Provisc); corneal transplant (Amvisc, Amvisc Plus); glaucoma filtration (Amvisc, Amvisc Plus); and retinal attachment surgery (Amvisc, Amvisc Plus)

Submucosal: Lip augmentation in adults >21 years (Restylane, Restylane-L, Restylane Silk)

Topical cream, gel: Management of skin ulcers and wounds (Bionect, Hylase Wound)

Dosing

Adult & Geriatric

Surgical aid: Ophthalmic (Amvisc, Amvisc Plus, Provisc): Intraocular: Depends upon procedure (slowly introduce a sufficient quantity into eye)

Osteoarthritis of the knee: Intra-articular:

Euflexxa: Inject 20 mg (2 mL) once weekly for 3 weeks (total of 3 injections)

Gel-One: Inject 30 mg (3 mL) once

Hyalgan: Inject 20 mg (2 mL) once weekly for 5 weeks (total of 5 injections); some patients may benefit with a total of 3 injections

Monovisc: Inject 88 mg (4 mL) once

Orthovisc: Inject 30 mg (2 mL) once weekly for 3 to 4 weeks (total of 3 to 4 injections)

Supartz, Supartz FX: Inject 25 mg (2.5 mL) once weekly for 5 weeks (total of 5 injections); some patients may benefit with a total of 3 injections

Synvisc: Inject 16 mg (2 mL) once weekly for 3 weeks (total of 3 injections)

Synvisc-One: Inject 48 mg (6 mL) once

Facial wrinkles/folds: Intradermal:

Note: Formulations differ in terms of recommended injection depth: Juvederm (all formulations except Voluma XC), Restylane, and Restylane-L are intended for mid to deep intradermal injection; Perlane and Restylane Lyft are intended for injection into the deep dermis to superficial subcutis

Juvederm (all formulations except Voluma XC): Inject as required for cosmetic result; typical treatment regimen requires 1.6 mL/treatment site typical volume for repeat treatment is 0.7 mL/treatment site; maximum: 20 mL/60 kg/year

Perlane, Restylane Lyft: Inject as required into deep dermis/superficial subcutis for cosmetic result; median total dose: 3 mL (Perlane); maximum: 6 mL per treatment

Restylane, Restylane-L: Inject as required for cosmetic result; median total dose: 3 mL; maximum: 6 mL per treatment

Cheek augmentation: Subcutaneous/Supraperiosteal: Adults >21 years:

Juvaderm Voluma XC: Inject as required for cosmetic result; typical treatment regimen requires small boluses of 0.1 to 0.2 mL over a large area to volumize and contour the cheek; an additional treatment may be needed to achieve the desired level of correction; maximum: 20 mL/60 kg/year

Restylane Lyft: Maximum: 6 mL per treatment

Lip augmentation: Submucosal (Restylane, Restylane-L, Restylane Silk): Adults ≥21 years: Maximum: 1.5 mL per lip (upper or lower) per treatment session

Perioral rhytids: Intradermal (Restylane Silk): Adults >21 years: Maximum: 1 mL per correction per treatment session

Skin ulcers and wounds: Topical:

Bionect cream, gel: Apply a thin layer to clean and disinfected wound or ulcer 2 to 3 times daily

Hylase Wound gel: Apply liberally to ulcer cavity or wound and to surrounding areas once daily

Interstitial cystitis, refractory (off-label use): Intravesical (off-label route): 40 mg in 50 mL saline intravesically (retain in bladder for at least 30 minutes) once weekly for 4 weeks, then monthly for up to 1 year in patients showing an initial response (Morales 1996)

Additional Information Complete prescribing information should be consulted for additional detail.

Dosage Forms Excipient information presented when available (limited, particularly for generics); consult specific product labeling. [DSC] = Discontinued product

Cream, topical [sodium hyaluronate]:
Bionect: 0.2% (25 g)

Foam, topical [sodium hyaluronate]:
Bionect: 0.2% (113.4 g)

Gel, topical [sodium hyaluronate]:
Bionect: 0.2% (30 g, 60 g)
HyGel: 2.5% (10 g)
Hylase Wound: 2.5% (75 g)

Injection, gel, intra-articular [cross-linked hyaluronate]:
Gel-One: 10 mg/mL (3 mL) [derived from or manufactured using an avian source]

Injection, gel, intradermal [hyaluronic acid]:
Juvederm Ultra: 24 mg/mL (0.4 mL, 0.8 mL) [derived from or manufactured from bacterial source]
Juvederm Ultra Plus: 24 mg/mL (0.4 mL, 0.8 mL) [derived from or manufactured from bacterial source]
Juvederm Ultra Plus XC: Hyaluronic acid 24 mg/mL and lidocaine 0.3% (0.4 mL, 0.8 mL) [derived from or manufactured from bacterial source]
Juvederm Ultra XC: Hyaluronic acid 24 mg/mL and lidocaine 0.3% (0.4 mL, 0.8 mL) [derived from or manufactured from bacterial source]
Perlane-L: Hyaluronic acid 20 mg/mL and lidocaine 0.3% (1 mL [DSC], 2 mL [DSC]) [derived from or manufactured from bacterial source]
Restylane-L: Hyaluronic acid 20 mg/mL and lidocaine 0.3% (0.5 mL, 1 mL, 2 mL) [derived from or manufactured from bacterial source]
Restylane Lyft: Hyaluronic acid 20 mg/mL and lidocaine 0.3% [derived from or manufactured from bacterial source]
Restylane Silk: Hyaluronic acid 20 mg/mL and lidocaine 0.3% [derived from or manufactured from bacterial source]

Injection, gel, intradermal [sodium hyaluronate]:
Perlane: 20 mg/mL (1 mL) [derived from or manufactured from bacterial source]
Restylane: 20 mg/mL (0.4 mL, 1 mL, 2 mL) [derived from or manufactured from bacterial source]

Injection, gel, subcutaneous/supraperiosteal [cross-linked hyaluronic acid]:
Juvederm Voluma XC: Hyaluronic acid 20 mg/mL and lidocaine 0.3% [derived from or manufactured from bacterial source]

Injection, solution, intra-articular [hyaluronan]:
Monovisc: 88 mg/4 mL (4 mL) [derived from or manufactured from bacterial source]

Injection, solution, intra-articular [hylan polymers A and B]:
Synvisc-One: 8 mg/mL (6 mL) [derived from or manufactured using an avian source]
Synvisc: 8 mg/mL (2 mL) [derived from or manufactured using an avian source]

Injection, solution, intra-articular [sodium hyaluronate]:
Euflexxa: 10 mg/mL (2 mL)
Hyalgan: 10 mg/mL (2 mL) [derived from or manufactured using an avian source]
Orthovisc: 15 mg/mL (2 mL) [derived from or manufactured from avian source]
Supartz: 10 mg/mL (2.5 mL [DSC]) [derived from or manufactured using an avian source]
Supartz FX: 25 mg/2.5 mL (2.5 mL) [derived from or manufactured using an avian source]

Injection, solution, intraocular [sodium hyaluronate]:
Amvisc: 12 mg/mL (0.5 mL, 0.8 mL)
Amvisc Plus: 16 mg/mL (0.5 mL, 0.8 mL)
Provisc: 10 mg/mL (0.4 mL, 0.55 mL, 0.85 mL) [contains natural rubber/natural latex in packaging]

♦ **Hyaluronic Acid** see Hyaluronate and Derivatives on page 879

♦ **Hycamptamine** see Topotecan on page 1814

♦ **Hycamtin** see Topotecan on page 1814

♦ **hycet®** see Hydrocodone and Acetaminophen on page 884

♦ **Hycodan** see Hydrocodone and Homatropine on page 885

♦ **Hycort (Can)** see Hydrocortisone (Topical) on page 886

♦ **Hydeltra T.B.A. (Can)** see PrednisoLONE (Systemic) on page 1493

♦ **Hyderm (Can)** see Hydrocortisone (Topical) on page 886

HydrALAZINE (hye DRAL a zeen)

Brand Names: Canada Apo-Hydralazine; Apresoline; Novo-Hylazin; Nu-Hydral

Index Terms Apresoline; Hydralazine Hydrochloride

Pharmacologic Category Antihypertensive; Vasodilator

Additional Appendix Information
Hypertension on page 1996

Use

Hypertension: Management of moderate to severe hypertension

Note: According to the Eighth Joint National Committee (JNC 8) guidelines, hydralazine is **not** recommended for the initial treatment of hypertension (James, 2013).

Pregnancy Considerations Adverse events were observed in some animal reproduction studies. Hydralazine crosses the placenta (Liedholm, 1982). Intravenous hydralazine is recommended for use in the management of acute onset, severe hypertension (systolic BP ≥160 mm Hg or diastolic BP ≥110 mm Hg) with preeclampsia or eclampsia in pregnant and postpartum women. Untreated chronic maternal hypertension is associated with adverse events in the fetus, infant, and mother. If treatment for chronic hypertension in pregnancy is needed, other oral agents are preferred as initial therapy (ACOG, 2013; Magee, 2014).

Breast-Feeding Considerations Hydralazine is excreted into breast milk. In a case report, following a maternal dose of hydralazine 50 mg three times daily, exposure to the infant was calculated to be 0.013 mg per 75 mL breast milk (Liedholm, 1982). The manufacturer recommends that caution be used if administered to a nursing woman.

Contraindications Hypersensitivity to hydralazine or any component of the formulation; coronary artery disease; mitral valve rheumatic heart disease

Warnings/Precautions May cause peripheral neuritis or a drug-induced lupus-like syndrome (more likely on larger doses, longer duration). Discontinue hydralazine in patients who develop SLE-like syndrome or positive ANA. Use with caution in patients with severe renal disease or cerebral vascular accidents or with known or suspected coronary artery disease; monitor blood pressure closely with IV use. Slow acetylators, patients with decreased renal function, and patients receiving >200 mg/day (chronically) are at higher risk for SLE. Titrate dosage cautiously to patient's response. Hypotensive effect after IV administration may be delayed and unpredictable in some patients. Usually administered with diuretic and a beta-blocker to counteract side effects of sodium and water retention and reflex tachycardia.

Adjust dose in severe renal dysfunction. Use is contraindicated in patients with coronary artery disease (CAD); in patients with obstructive CAD, increase in tachycardia may increase myocardial oxygen demand. According to the AHA/ACC/ASH 2015 scientific statement for the treatment of hypertension in patients with CAD, hydralazine (without a concomitant nitrate [eg, isosorbide dinitrate]) should be avoided for the treatment of hypertension in patients with heart failure (with reduced ejection fraction) of ischemic origin (AHA/ACC/ASH [Rosendorff, 2015]). Use with caution in pulmonary hypertension (may cause hypotension). Patients may be poorly compliant because of frequent dosing. Hydralazine-induced fluid and sodium retention may require addition or increased dosage of a diuretic.

Adverse Reactions Frequency not defined.
Cardiovascular: Angina pectoris, flushing, orthostatic hypotension, palpitations, paradoxical hypertension, peripheral edema, tachycardia, vascular collapse

Central nervous system: Anxiety, chills, depression, disorientation, dizziness, fever, headache, increased intracranial pressure (IV; in patient with preexisting increased intracranial pressure), psychotic reaction

Dermatologic: Pruritus, rash, urticaria

Gastrointestinal: Anorexia, constipation, diarrhea, nausea, paralytic ileus, vomiting

Genitourinary: Dysuria, impotence

Hematologic: Agranulocytosis, eosinophilia, erythrocyte count reduced, hemoglobin decreased, hemolytic anemia, leukopenia, thrombocytopenia (rare)

Neuromuscular & skeletal: Muscle cramps, peripheral neuritis, rheumatoid arthritis, tremor, weakness

Ocular: Conjunctivitis, lacrimation

Respiratory: Dyspnea, nasal congestion

Miscellaneous: Diaphoresis, drug-induced lupus-like syndrome (dose related; fever, arthralgia, splenomegaly, lymphadenopathy, asthenia, myalgia, malaise, pleuritic chest pain, edema, positive ANA, positive LE cells, maculopapular facial rash, positive direct Coombs' test, pericarditis, pericardial tamponade)

Drug Interactions

Metabolism/Transport Effects None known.

Avoid Concomitant Use There are no known interactions where it is recommended to avoid concomitant use.

Increased Effect/Toxicity

HydrALAZINE may increase the levels/effects of: Amifostine; Antipsychotic Agents (Second Generation [Atypical]); DULoxetine; Hypotension-Associated Agents; Levodopa

The levels/effects of HydrALAZINE may be increased by: Alfuzosin; Barbiturates; Brimonidine (Topical); Dapoxetine; Diazoxide; Herbs (Hypotensive Properties); Molsidomine; Nicorandil; Obinutuzumab; Pentoxifylline; Phosphodiesterase 5 Inhibitors; Prostacyclin Analogues

Decreased Effect

The levels/effects of HydrALAZINE may be decreased by: Amphetamines; Herbs (Hypertensive Properties); Methylphenidate; Nonsteroidal Anti-Inflammatory Agents; Yohimbine

Food Interactions Food enhances bioavailability of hydralazine. Management: Administer without regard to food, but keep consistent.

Preparation for Administration Hydralazine should be diluted in NS for IVPB administration due to decreased stability in D_5W. Stability of IVPB solution in NS is 4 days at room temperature.

Storage/Stability Intact ampuls/vials of hydralazine should not be stored under refrigeration because of possible precipitation or crystallization.

Mechanism of Action Direct vasodilation of arterioles (with little effect on veins) with decreased systemic resistance

Pharmacodynamics/Kinetics

Onset of action: Oral: 20-30 minutes; IV: 5-20 minutes

Duration: Oral: Up to 8 hours; IV: 1-4 hours; **Note:** Duration may vary depending on acetylator status of patient. Hypotension due to hydralazine may last longer even though the circulating half-life is much shorter (Marik, 2007; O'Malley, 1975).

Protein binding: 85% to 90%

Metabolism: Hepatically acetylated; extensive first-pass effect (oral)

Bioavailability: 30% to 50%; increased with food

Half-life elimination: Normal renal function: 2-8 hours; End-stage renal disease: 7-16 hours

Excretion: Urine (14% as unchanged drug)

Dosing

Adult & Geriatric

Hypertension: Oral: Initial: 10 mg 4 times daily for the first 2 to 4 days; increase to 25 mg 4 times daily for the balance of the first week; further increase by 10 to 25 mg/dose gradually (every 2 to 5 days) to 50 mg 4 times daily (maximum: 300 mg daily in divided doses)

Hypertensive emergency (off-label dose): Note: Use is generally not recommended due to unpredictable and prolonged antihypertensive effects (Marik, 2007): IM, IV: 10 to 20 mg every 4 to 6 hours as needed (Rhoney, 2009)

Hypertensive emergency in pregnancy (systolic BP ≥160 mm Hg or diastolic BP ≥110 mm Hg) (off-label dose): IM, IV: Initial: 5 or 10 mg; may repeat dose in 20 to 40 minutes with 5 to 10 mg if blood pressure continues to exceed thresholds (ACOG, 2015; Magee, 2014; Too, 2013). Also refer to administration protocols developed by the American College of Obstetricians and Gynecologists (ACOG, 2015). A maximum total cumulative dose of 20 mg (IV) or 30 mg (IM) is recommended (Magee, 2014). **Note:** After the initial dose, may initiate a continuous infusion of 0.5 to 10 mg/hour instead of intermittent dosing (Magee, 2014).

Perioperative hypertension (off-label dose): IV: 3 to 20 mg every 20 to 60 minutes as needed (Varon, 2008). **Note:** The lower end of the dosage range is preferred in the immediate perioperative period and in patients with renal failure. The use of hydralazine in this setting especially in patients with ischemic heart disease, aortic dissection, or an intracranial process is best avoided due to unpredictable and prolonged antihypertensive effects (Lien, 2012; Varon, 2008).

Heart failure (off-label use): Oral: Initial dose: 25 to 50 mg 3 or 4 times daily; use in combination with isosorbide dinitrate; maximum dose: 300 mg daily in divided doses (ACCF/AHA [Yancy, 2013])

Pediatric

Hypertension: Oral: Initial: 0.75 to 1 mg/kg/day in 2 to 4 divided doses; increase over 3 to 4 weeks to maximum of 7.5 mg/kg/day in 2 to 4 divided doses; maximum daily dose: 200 mg/day

Acute hypertension: IM, IV: 0.1 to 0.2 mg/kg/dose (not to exceed 20 mg) every 4 to 6 hours as needed, up to 1.7 to 3.5 mg/kg/day in 4 to 6 divided doses

Renal Impairment

CrCl 10 to 50 mL/minute: Administer every 8 hours.

CrCl <10 mL/minute: Administer every 8 to 16 hours in fast acetylators and every 12 to 24 hours in slow acetylators.

Hemodialysis effects: Supplemental dose is not necessary.

Peritoneal dialysis effects: Supplemental dose is not necessary.

Hepatic Impairment No dosage adjustment provided in manufacturer's labeling. However, hydralazine undergoes extensive hepatic metabolism.

Administration

Oral: May be administered without regard to meals. However, food enhances bioavailability, administer consistently with regard to meals.

Solution for injection: Administer as a slow IV push; maximum rate: 5 mg/minute

Monitoring Parameters Blood pressure (monitor closely with IV use), standing and sitting/supine, heart rate, ANA titer

Dosage Forms Excipient information presented when available (limited, particularly for generics); consult specific product labeling.

Solution, Injection, as hydrochloride:
Generic: 20 mg/mL (1 mL)

Tablet, Oral, as hydrochloride:
Generic: 10 mg, 25 mg, 50 mg, 100 mg

Extemporaneous Preparations A 4 mg/mL oral suspension may be made with tablets and a 1:1 mixture of Ora-Sweet SF and Ora-Plus. Crush four 100 mg tablets in a mortar and reduce to a fine powder. Add 15 mL of the vehicle and mix to a uniform paste; mix while adding the vehicle in incremental proportions to almost 100 mL; transfer to a calibrated bottle, rinse mortar with vehicle, and add quantity of vehicle sufficient to make 100 mL. Label "Shake Well", "Protect From Light", "Store in a Refrigerator". Stable for 2 days when stored in amber plastic prescription bottles in the dark and refrigerated (Allen, 1998).

Note: Stability reduced to 24 hours if Ora-Sweet is substituted for Ora-Sweet SF.

Allen LV Jr, Erickson MA 3rd. Stability of alprazolam, chloroquine phosphate, cisapride, enalapril maleate, and hydralazine hydrochloride in extemporaneously compounded oral liquids. *Am J Health-Syst Pharm.* 1998;55(18):1915-1920.

◆ Hydralazine and Isosorbide Dinitrate *see* Isosorbide Dinitrate and Hydralazine *on page 994*

◆ Hydralazine Hydrochloride *see* HydrALAZINE *on page 880*

◆ Hydrea *see* Hydroxyurea *on page 895*

◆ Hydro 35 *see* Urea *on page 1853*

◆ Hydro 40 *see* Urea *on page 1853*

Hydrochlorothiazide (hye droe klor oh THYE a zide)

Brand Names: US Microzide

Brand Names: Canada Apo-Hydro; Ava-Hydrochlorothiazide; Bio-Hydrochlorothiazide; PMS-Hydrochlorothiazide; Teva-Hydrochlorothiazide; Urozide

Index Terms HCTZ (error-prone abbreviation); Hydrodiuril

Pharmacologic Category Antihypertensive; Diuretic, Thiazide

Use

Edema: Treatment of edema due to heart failure, hepatic cirrhosis (see **"Note"**), various forms of renal dysfunction (eg, nephrotic syndrome, acute glomerulosclerosis, chronic renal failure) (see **"Note"**), corticosteroid and estrogen therapy

Note: The use of hydrochlorothiazide in the treatment of edema for hepatic cirrhosis has largely been replaced by spironolactone. The use of hydrochlorothiazide in the management of edema in patients with renal dysfunction has largely been replaced by the use of loop diuretics (eg, furosemide).

Hypertension: Management of mild-to-moderate hypertension

Guideline recommendations:

Hypertension: The 2014 guideline for the management of high blood pressure in adults (Eighth Joint National Committee [JNC 8]) recommends initiation of pharmacologic treatment to lower blood pressure for the following patients:

- Patients ≥60 years of age with systolic blood pressure (SBP) ≥150 mm Hg or diastolic blood pressure (DBP) ≥90 mm Hg. Goal of therapy is SBP <150 mm Hg and DBP <90 mm Hg.
- Patients <60 years of age with SBP ≥140 mm Hg or DBP is ≥90 mm Hg. Goal of therapy is SBP <140 mm Hg and DBP <90 mm Hg.
- Patients ≥18 years of age with diabetes and SBP ≥140 mm Hg or DBP ≥90 mm Hg. Goal of therapy is SBP <140 mm Hg and DBP <90 mm Hg.
- Patients ≥18 years of age with chronic kidney disease (CKD) and SBP ≥140 mm Hg or DBP ≥90 mm Hg. Goal of therapy is SBP <140 mm Hg and DBP <90 mm Hg.

Chronic kidney disease (CKD) and hypertension: Regardless of race or diabetes status, the use of an ACE inhibitor (ACEI) or angiotensin receptor blocker (ARB) as initial therapy is recommended to improve kidney outcomes. In the general nonblack population (without CKD) including those with diabetes, initial antihypertensive treatment should consist of a thiazide-type diuretic, calcium channel blocker, ACEI, or ARB. In the general black population (without CKD), including those with diabetes, initial antihypertensive treatment should consist of a thiazide-type diuretic or a calcium channel blocker **instead of** an ACEI or ARB.

Coronary artery disease (CAD) and hypertension: The American Heart Association, American College of Cardiology and American Society of Hypertension (AHA/ACC/ASH) 2015 scientific statement for the treatment of hypertension in patients with coronary artery disease (CAD) recommends the use of a thiazide (or thiazide-like diuretic) as part of a regimen in patients with hypertension and chronic stable angina. A BP target of <140/90 mm Hg is reasonable for the secondary prevention of cardiovascular events. A lower target BP (<130/80 mm Hg) may be appropriate in some individuals with CAD, previous MI, stroke or transient ischemic attack, or CAD risk equivalents (AHA/ACC/ASH [Rosendorff 2015]).

Canadian labeling: Additional uses (not in U.S. labeling):

Premenstrual tension with edema: Management of premenstrual tension with edema

Toxemia of pregnancy: Management of toxemia of pregnancy (including eclampsia). **Note:** Guidelines recommend alternative agents (Magee, 2008)

Pregnancy Considerations Adverse events were not observed in animal reproduction studies. Thiazide diuretics cross the placenta and are found in cord blood. Maternal use may cause may cause fetal or neonatal jaundice, thrombocytopenia, or other adverse events observed in adults. Use of thiazide diuretics to treat edema during normal pregnancies is not appropriate; use may be considered when edema is due to pathologic causes (as in the nonpregnant patient); monitor. Untreated chronic maternal hypertension is associated with adverse events in the fetus, infant, and mother (ACOG, 2013). Women who required thiazide diuretics for the treatment of hypertension prior to pregnancy may continue their use (ACOG, 2013).

Breast-Feeding Considerations Thiazide diuretics are found in breast milk. Following a single oral maternal dose of hydrochlorothiazide 50 mg, the mean breast milk concentration was 80 ng/mL (samples collected over 24 hours) and hydrochlorothiazide was not detected in the blood of the breast-feeding infant (limit of detection 20 ng/mL) (Miller, 1982). Peak plasma concentrations reported in adults following hydrochlorothiazide 12.5-100 mg are 70-490 ng/mL. Due to the potential for serious adverse reactions in the nursing infant, the manufacturer recommends a decision be made whether to discontinue nursing or to discontinue the drug, taking into account the importance of treatment to the mother (Canadian labeling contraindicates use in nursing women). Diuretics have the potential to decrease milk volume and suppress lactation.

Contraindications

Hypersensitivity to hydrochlorothiazide, any component of the formulation, or sulfonamide-derived drugs; anuria

Note: Although the FDA approved product labeling states this medication is contraindicated with other sulfonamide-containing drug classes, the scientific basis of this statement has been challenged. See "Warnings/Precautions" for more detail.

Canadian labeling: Additional contraindications (not in U.S. labeling): Increasing azotemia and oliguria during treatment of severe progressive renal disease; breast-feeding

Warnings/Precautions Hypersensitivity reactions may occur with hydrochlorothiazide. Risk is increased in patients with a history of allergy or bronchial asthma. Avoid in severe renal disease (ineffective as a diuretic). Electrolyte disturbances (hypokalemia, hypochloremic alkalosis, hypomagnesemia, hyponatremia) can occur. Development of electrolyte disturbances can be minimized when used in combination with other electrolyte sparing antihypertensives (eg, ACE inhibitors or angiotensin receptor blockers). (Sica, 2011) Use with caution in severe hepatic dysfunction; hepatic encephalopathy can be caused by electrolyte disturbances. Gout may be precipitated in certain patients with a history of gout, a familial predisposition to gout, or chronic renal failure. Thiazide diuretics reduce calcium excretion; pathologic changes in the parathyroid glands with hypercalcemia and hypophosphatemia have been observed with prolonged use. Should be discontinued prior to testing for parathyroid function. Use with caution in patients with prediabetes and diabetes; may alter glucose control. May cause SLE exacerbation or activation. Use with caution in patients with moderate or high cholesterol concentrations. Photosensitization may occur. Correct hypokalemia before initiating therapy. Thiazide diuretics may decrease renal calcium excretion; consider avoiding use in patients with hypercalcemia. May cause acute transient myopia and acute angle-closure glaucoma, typically occurring within hours to weeks following initiation; discontinue therapy immediately in patients with acute decreases in visual acuity or ocular pain. Risk factors may include a history of sulfonamide or penicillin allergy. Cumulative effects may develop, including azotemia, in patients with impaired renal function. If given the morning of surgery, hydrochlorothiazide may render the patient volume depleted and blood pressure may be labile during general anesthesia.

Sulfonamide ("sulfa") allergy: The FDA-approved product labeling for many medications containing a sulfonamide chemical group includes a broad contraindication in patients with a prior allergic reaction to sulfonamides. There is a potential for cross-reactivity between members of a specific class (eg, two antibiotic sulfonamides). However, concerns for cross-reactivity have previously extended to all compounds containing the sulfonamide structure (SO_2NH_2). An expanded understanding of allergic mechanisms indicates cross-reactivity between antibiotic sulfonamides and nonantibiotic sulfonamides may not occur or at the very least this potential is extremely low (Brackett 2004; Johnson 2005; Slatore 2004; Tornero 2004). In particular, mechanisms of cross-reaction due to antibody production (anaphylaxis) are unlikely to occur with nonantibiotic sulfonamides. T-cell-mediated (type IV) reactions (eg, maculopapular rash) are less well understood and it is not possible to completely exclude this potential based on current insights. In cases where prior reactions were severe (Stevens-Johnson syndrome/TEN), some clinicians choose to avoid exposure to these classes.

Adverse Reactions Frequency not defined; the occurrence of adverse events are dose related, with the majority occurring with doses ≥25 mg.

Cardiovascular: Hypotension, necrotizing angiitis, orthostatic hypotension

Central nervous system: Dizziness, headache, paresthesia, restlessness, vertigo

Dermatologic: Alopecia, erythema multiforme, exfoliative dermatitis, skin photosensitivity, skin rash, Stevens-Johnson syndrome, toxic epidermal necrolysis, urticaria

Endocrine & metabolic: Glycosuria, hypercalcemia, hyperglycemia, hyperuricemia, hypochloremic alkalosis, hypokalemia, hypomagnesemia, hyponatremia

Gastrointestinal: Abdominal cramps, anorexia, constipation, diarrhea, gastric irritation, nausea, pancreatitis, sialadenitis, vomiting

Genitourinary: Impotence

Hematologic & oncologic: Agranulocytosis, aplastic anemia, hemolytic anemia, leukopenia, purpura, thrombocytopenia

Hepatic: Jaundice

Hypersensitivity: Anaphylaxis

Neuromuscular & skeletal: Muscle spasm, weakness

Ophthalmic: Blurred vision (transient), xanthopsia

Renal: Interstitial nephritis, renal failure, renal insufficiency

Respiratory: Respiratory distress, pneumonitis, pulmonary edema

Miscellaneous: Fever

<1% (Limited to important or life-threatening): Allergic myocarditis, eosinophilic pneumonitis, hepatic insufficiency, lip cancer (Friedman, 2012), systemic lupus erythematosus

Drug Interactions

Metabolism/Transport Effects None known.

Avoid Concomitant Use

Avoid concomitant use of Hydrochlorothiazide with any of the following: Dofetilide; Levosulpiride; Mecamylamine

Increased Effect/Toxicity

Hydrochlorothiazide may increase the levels/effects of: ACE Inhibitors; Allopurinol; Amifostine; Antipsychotic Agents (Second Generation [Atypical]); Benazepril; Calcium Salts; CarBAMazepine; Cardiac Glycosides; Cyclophosphamide; Diazoxide; Dofetilide; DULoxetine; Hypotension-Associated Agents; Ivabradine; Levodopa; Levosulpiride; Lithium; Mecamylamine; Multivitamins/Minerals (with ADEK, Folate, Iron); Multivitamins/Minerals (with AE, No Iron); Nonsteroidal Anti-Inflammatory Agents; OXcarbazepine; Porfimer; Sodium Phosphates; Topiramate; Toremifene; Valsartan; Verteporfin; Vitamin D Analogs

The levels/effects of Hydrochlorothiazide may be increased by: Alcohol (Ethyl); Alfuzosin; Analgesics (Opioid); Anticholinergic Agents; Barbiturates; Beta2-Agonists; Brimonidine (Topical); Corticosteroids (Orally Inhaled); Corticosteroids (Systemic); Dexketoprofen; Diazoxide; Herbs (Hypotensive Properties); Licorice; Molsidomine; Multivitamins/Fluoride (with ADE); Nicorandil; Obinutuzumab; Pentoxifylline; Phosphodiesterase 5 Inhibitors; Prostacyclin Analogues; Selective Serotonin Reuptake Inhibitors; Valsartan

Decreased Effect

Hydrochlorothiazide may decrease the levels/effects of: Antidiabetic Agents

The levels/effects of Hydrochlorothiazide may be decreased by: Amphetamines; Benazepril; Bile Acid Sequestrants; Herbs (Hypertensive Properties); Methylphenidate; Nonsteroidal Anti-Inflammatory Agents; Yohimbine

Storage/Stability Store at 20°C to 25°C (68°F to 77°F) (USP Controlled Room Temperature). Protect from light and moisture.

Mechanism of Action Inhibits sodium reabsorption in the distal tubules causing increased excretion of sodium and water as well as potassium and hydrogen ions

Pharmacodynamics/Kinetics

Onset of action: Diuresis: Infants: 2 to 6 hours (Chemtob 1989); Adults: ~2 hours

Peak effect: 4 to 6 hours

Duration: Infants: 8 hours (Chemtob 1989); Adults: 6 to 12 hours

Absorption: Well absorbed; when administered with food, time to maximum concentration increases from 1.6 to 2.9 hours. Absorption is reduced in patients with CHF.

Distribution: 3.6 to 7.8 L/kg (correlates with dose administered and concentration achieved)

Protein binding: ~40% to 68%

Metabolism: Not metabolized

Bioavailability: 65% to 75% (reduced by 10% when administered with food)

Half-life elimination: 6 to 15 hours

Time to peak: ~1 to 5 hours

Excretion: Urine (as unchanged drug)

Dosing

Adult

Manufacturer's labeling:

Edema: Oral: 25 to 100 mg daily in 1 to 2 divided doses; may administer intermittently on alternate days or on 3 to 5 days each week.

Hypertension: Oral:

U.S. labeling: Initial: 12.5 to 25 mg once daily administered alone or in combination with other antihypertensives; may increase up to 50 mg daily in 1 to 2 divided doses; minimal increase in response and more electrolyte disturbances are seen with doses >50 mg daily.

Canadian labeling: Initial: 12.5 to 100 mg daily as a single dose or in divided doses; titrate for effect. Up to 200 mg daily (in divided doses) may be necessary. If used concomitantly with other antihypertensive agents, reduce the dose of the concomitant antihypertensive by 50%.

Premenstrual tension with edema: Canadian labeling (not in U.S. labeling): Oral: 25 to 50 mg daily once or twice daily (initiate at onset of symptoms and continue through the start of menses).

Toxemia of pregnancy: Canadian labeling (not in U.S. labeling): Oral: 100 mg daily; may temporarily increase to 200 mg daily in divided doses for severe cases. May administer daily or intermittently once every 4 days. **Note:** Guidelines recommend use of alternative agents (Magee, 2008).

Alternate recommendations:

Fluid retention (mild) in heart failure: Oral: Initial: 25 mg once or twice daily; maximum daily dose: 200 mg (ACCF/AHA [Yancy, 2013])

Hypertension: Oral: Initial: 12.5 to 25 mg once daily; may increase dose to a target dose range of 25 to 50 mg once daily in 1 to 2 divided doses (JNC 8 [James, 2014]); usual dosage range (ASH/ISH [Weber, 2013]): 12.5 to 50 mg daily

Off-label use:

Calcium nephrolithiasis: 50 mg daily in 1 or 2 divided doses (AUA Guidelines [Pearle, 2014])

Geriatric Oral: 12.5 to 25 mg once daily; titrate as necessary in increments of 12.5 mg. Minimal increase in response and more electrolyte disturbances are seen with doses >50 mg daily.

Pediatric Edema, hypertension: Infants and Children (in pediatric patients, chlorothiazide may be preferred over hydrochlorothiazide as there are more dosage formulations [eg, suspension] available): Oral (effect of drug may be decreased when used every day):

Manufacturer's labeling: Usual dose:

<6 months: 1 to 3 mg/kg/day in 1 to 2 divided doses; maximum: 37.5 mg daily

6 months to 2 years: 1 to 2 mg/kg/day in a single or 2 divided doses; maximum: 37.5 mg daily

2 to 12 years: 1 to 2 mg/kg/day in a single or 2 divided doses; maximum: 100 mg daily

Alternate recommendations: Children and Adolescents: Initial: 1 mg/kg once daily; maximum 3 mg/kg/day not to exceed 50 mg daily (NHBPEP, 2005)

Renal Impairment There are no dosage adjustments provided in the manufacturer's labeling; however, the following adjustments have been recommended (Aronoff, 2007):

CrCl ≥10 mL/minute: There is no dosage adjustment necessary. Usually ineffective with CrCl <30 mL/minute unless in combination with a loop diuretic.

CrCl <10 mL/minute: Use not recommended; use is contraindicated with anuria.

Hepatic Impairment There are no dosage adjustments provided in the manufacturer's labeling. However, use with caution and monitor for precipitation of hepatic coma.

Administration May be administered with or without food. Take early in day to avoid nocturia. Take the last dose of multiple doses no later than 6 PM unless instructed otherwise.

Monitoring Parameters Assess weight, I & O reports daily to determine fluid loss; blood pressure, serum electrolytes, BUN, creatinine

Test Interactions May interfere with parathyroid function tests and may decrease serum iodine (protein bound) without signs of thyroid disturbance.

Dosage Forms Excipient information presented when available (limited, particularly for generics); consult specific product labeling.

Capsule, Oral:

Microzide: 12.5 mg

Generic: 12.5 mg

Tablet, Oral:

Generic: 12.5 mg, 25 mg, 50 mg

Dosage Forms: Canada

Note: Refer also to Dosage Forms

Excipient information presented when available (limited, particularly for generics); consult specific product labeling.

Tablet, Oral: 100 mg

◆ Hydrochlorothiazide, Aliskiren, and Amlodipine *see* Aliskiren, Amlodipine, and Hydrochlorothiazide *on page 72*

◆ Hydrochlorothiazide, Amlodipine, and Aliskiren *see* Aliskiren, Amlodipine, and Hydrochlorothiazide *on page 72*

◆ Hydrochlorothiazide, Amlodipine, and Valsartan *see* Amlodipine, Valsartan, and Hydrochlorothiazide *on page 105*

◆ Hydrochlorothiazide and Aliskiren *see* Aliskiren and Hydrochlorothiazide *on page 72*

Hydrochlorothiazide and Triamterene
(hye droe klor oh THYE a zide & trye AM ter een)

Brand Names: US Dyazide; Maxzide; Maxzide-25
Brand Names: Canada Apo-Triazide; Pro-Triazide; Teva-Triamterene HCTZ
Index Terms Triamterene and Hydrochlorothiazide
Pharmacologic Category Antihypertensive; Diuretic, Potassium-Sparing; Diuretic, Thiazide
Use Treatment of hypertension or edema (not recommended for initial treatment) when hypokalemia has developed on hydrochlorothiazide alone or when the development of hypokalemia must be avoided
Dosing
Adult & Geriatric Hypertension, edema: Oral:
Hydrochlorothiazide 25 mg and triamterene 37.5 mg: 1-2 tablets/capsules once daily
Hydrochlorothiazide 50 mg and triamterene 75 mg: ¹/₂-1 tablet daily
Renal Impairment Efficacy of hydrochlorothiazide is limited in patients with CrCl <30 mL/minute, contraindicated in patients with anuria, acute and chronic renal insufficiency, or significant renal impairment.
Hepatic Impairment No dosage adjustment provided in manufacturer's labeling; use with caution. Use with caution and monitor for precipitation of hepatic coma.
Additional Information Complete prescribing information should be consulted for additional detail.
Dosage Forms Excipient information presented when available (limited, particularly for generics); consult specific product labeling.
Capsule, oral: Hydrochlorothiazide 25 mg and triamterene 37.5 mg; hydrochlorothiazide 25 mg and triamterene 50 mg
Dyazide: Hydrochlorothiazide 25 mg and triamterene 37.5 mg
Tablet: Hydrochlorothiazide 25 mg and triamterene 37.5 mg; hydrochlorothiazide 50 mg and triamterene 75 mg
Maxzide: Hydrochlorothiazide 50 mg and triamterene 75 mg [scored]
Maxzide-25: Hydrochlorothiazide 25 mg and triamterene 37.5 mg [scored]

Hydrocodone and Acetaminophen
(hye droe KOE done & a seet a MIN oh fen)

Brand Names: US hycet®; Lorcet® 10/650 [DSC]; Lorcet® Plus [DSC]; Lortab®; Maxidone [DSC]; Norco; Stagesic [DSC]; Verdrocet; Vicodin ES; Vicodin HP; Vicodin®; Xodol 10/300; Xodol 5/300; Xodol 7.5/300; Zamicet; Zolvit [DSC]; Zydone [DSC]
Index Terms Acetaminophen and Hydrocodone
Pharmacologic Category Analgesic Combination (Opioid); Analgesic, Opioid
Use Pain: Relief of moderate-to-severe pain

Dosing
Adult Pain management (analgesic): Oral (doses should be titrated to appropriate analgesic effect): Average starting dose in opioid naive patients: Hydrocodone 5-10 mg 4 times/day; the dosage of acetaminophen should be limited to ≤4 g/day (and possibly less in patients with hepatic impairment or ethanol use).

Dosage ranges (based on specific product labeling): Hydrocodone 2.5-10 mg every 4-6 hours (maximum dose of hydrocodone may be limited by the acetaminophen content of specific product)
Geriatric Doses should be titrated to appropriate analgesic effect; 2.5-5 mg of the hydrocodone component every 4-6 hours. Do not exceed 4 g/day of acetaminophen.
Pediatric Pain management (analgesic): Oral (doses should be titrated to appropriate analgesic effect):
Children 2-13 years or <50 kg: Hydrocodone 0.1-0.2 mg/kg/dose every 4-6 hours; do not exceed 6 doses/day or the maximum recommended dose of acetaminophen
Children ≥50 kg: Refer to adult dosing.
Renal Impairment No dosage adjustment provided in manufacturer's labeling; use with caution.
Hepatic Impairment Use with caution. Limited, low-dose therapy usually well tolerated in hepatic disease/cirrhosis; however, cases of hepatotoxicity at daily acetaminophen dosages <4 g/day have been reported. Avoid chronic use in hepatic impairment.
Additional Information Complete prescribing information should be consulted for additional detail.
Dosage Forms Excipient information presented when available (limited, particularly for generics); consult specific product labeling. [DSC] = Discontinued product
Capsule, oral:
Stagesic™: Hydrocodone bitartrate 5 mg and acetaminophen 500 mg [DSC]
Elixir, oral:
Lortab®: Hydrocodone bitartrate 7.5 mg and acetaminophen 500 mg per 15 mL (480 mL) [contains ethanol 7%, propylene glycol; tropical fruit punch flavor] [DSC]
Lortab®: Hydrocodone bitartrate 10 mg and acetaminophen 300 mg per 15 mL (480 mL) [contains ethanol 7%, propylene glycol; tropical fruit punch flavor] [DSC]
Solution, oral: Hydrocodone bitartrate 7.5 mg and acetaminophen 325 mg per 15 mL; hydrocodone bitartrate 7.5 mg and acetaminophen 500 mg per 15 mL (5 mL [DSC], 10 mL [DSC], 15 mL [DSC], 118 mL [DSC], 473 mL [DSC])
hycet®: Hydrocodone bitartrate 7.5 mg and acetaminophen 325 mg per 15 mL (473 mL) [contains ethanol 7%, propylene glycol; tropical fruit punch flavor]
Zamicet™: Hydrocodone bitartrate 10 mg and acetaminophen 325 mg per 15 mL (7.5 mL, 15 mL, 473 mL) [contains ethanol 6.7%, propylene glycol; fruit flavor]
Zolvit®: Hydrocodone bitartrate 10 mg and acetaminophen 300 mg per 15 mL (480 mL) [contains ethanol 7%, propylene glycol; tropical fruit punch flavor] [DSC]
Tablet, oral:
Hydrocodone bitartrate 2.5 mg and acetaminophen 325 mg
Hydrocodone bitartrate 2.5 mg and acetaminophen 500 mg [DSC]
Hydrocodone bitartrate 5 mg and acetaminophen 300 mg
Hydrocodone bitartrate 5 mg and acetaminophen 325 mg
Hydrocodone bitartrate 5 mg and acetaminophen 500 mg [DSC]
Hydrocodone bitartrate 7.5 mg and acetaminophen 300 mg
Hydrocodone bitartrate 7.5 mg and acetaminophen 325 mg
Hydrocodone bitartrate 7.5 mg and acetaminophen 500 mg [DSC]
Hydrocodone bitartrate 7.5 mg and acetaminophen 650 mg [DSC]
Hydrocodone bitartrate 7.5 mg and acetaminophen 750 mg DSC]
Hydrocodone bitartrate 10 mg and acetaminophen 300 mg
Hydrocodone bitartrate 10 mg and acetaminophen 325 mg
Hydrocodone bitartrate 10 mg and acetaminophen 500 mg [DSC]
Hydrocodone bitartrate 10 mg and acetaminophen 650 mg DSC]
Hydrocodone bitartrate 10 mg and acetaminophen 750 mg [DSC]
Lorcet® 10/650: Hydrocodone bitartrate 10 mg and acetaminophen 650 mg [DSC]
Lorcet® Plus: Hydrocodone bitartrate 7.5 mg and acetaminophen 650 mg [DSC]

Lortab®:

5/500: Hydrocodone bitartrate 5 mg and acetaminophen 500 mg [DSC]

7.5/500: Hydrocodone bitartrate 7.5 mg and acetaminophen 500 mg [DSC]

10/500: Hydrocodone bitartrate 10 mg and acetaminophen 500 mg [DSC]

Maxidone®: Hydrocodone bitartrate 10 mg and acetaminophen 750 mg [DSC]

Norco®:

Hydrocodone bitartrate 5 mg and acetaminophen 325 mg

Hydrocodone bitartrate 7.5 mg and acetaminophen 325 mg

Hydrocodone bitartrate 10 mg and acetaminophen 325 mg

Verdrocet: Hydrocodone bitartrate 2.5 mg and acetaminophen 325 mg

Vicodin®: Hydrocodone bitartrate 5 mg and acetaminophen 300 mg

Vicodin ES®: Hydrocodone bitartrate 7.5 mg and acetaminophen 300 mg

Vicodin HP®: Hydrocodone bitartrate 10 mg and acetaminophen 300 mg

Xodol®:

5/300: Hydrocodone bitartrate 5 mg and acetaminophen 300 mg

7.5/300: Hydrocodone bitartrate 7.5 mg and acetaminophen 300 mg

10/300: Hydrocodone bitartrate 10 mg and acetaminophen 300 mg

Zydone®:

Hydrocodone bitartrate 5 mg and acetaminophen 400 mg [DSC]

Hydrocodone bitartrate 7.5 mg and acetaminophen 400 mg [DSC]

Hydrocodone bitartrate 10 mg and acetaminophen 400 mg [DSC]

Controlled Substance C-II

Hydrocodone and Chlorpheniramine
(hye droe KOE done & klor fen IR a meen)

Brand Names: US TussiCaps; Tussionex Pennkinetic; Vituz

Index Terms Chlorpheniramine Maleate and Hydrocodone Bitartrate; Hydrocodone Polistirex and Chlorpheniramine Polistirex; Tussionex

Pharmacologic Category Alkylamine Derivative; Analgesic, Opioid; Antitussive; Histamine H_1 Antagonist; Histamine H_1 Antagonist, First Generation

Use Symptomatic relief of cough and upper respiratory symptoms associated with cold and allergy

Dosing

Adult & Geriatric Antitussive/antihistamine: Oral:

Capsules: Extended release: Hydrocodone 10 mg and chlorpheniramine 8 mg: One capsule every 12 hours (maximum: 2 capsules daily)

Solution: Immediate release: 5 mL every 4-6 hours as needed; do not exceed 20 mL daily

Suspension: Extended release: 5 mL every 12 hours; do not exceed 10 mL daily

Pediatric Antitussive/antihistamine: Oral: **Note:** Solution is not indicated for patients <18 years.

Children 6 to <12 years:

Capsules: Extended release: Hydrocodone 5 mg and chlorpheniramine 4 mg: One capsule every 12 hours (maximum: 2 capsules daily)

Suspension: Extended release: 2.5 mL every 12 hours; do not exceed 5 mL daily

Children ≥12 years and Adolescents: Refer to adult dosing.

Additional Information Complete prescribing information should be consulted for additional detail.

Dosage Forms Excipient information presented when available (limited, particularly for generics); consult specific product labeling.

Capsule, extended release, oral:

TussiCaps® 5/4: Hydrocodone polistirex [equivalent to hydrocodone bitartrate 5 mg] and chlorpheniramine polistirex [equivalent to chlorpheniramine maleate 4 mg]

TussiCaps® 10/8: Hydrocodone polistirex [equivalent to hydrocodone bitartrate 10 mg] and chlorpheniramine polistirex [equivalent to chlorpheniramine maleate 8 mg]

Solution, oral:

Vituz®: Hydrocodone bitartrate 5 mg and chlorpheniramine maleate 4 mg per 5 mL (480 mL) [contains propylene glycol; grape flavor]

Suspension, extended release, oral: Hydrocodone polistirex [equivalent to hydrocodone bitartrate 10 mg] and chlorpheniramine polistirex [equivalent to chlorpheniramine maleate 8 mg] per 5 mL (480 mL)

Tussionex® Pennkinetic®: Hydrocodone polistirex [equivalent to hydrocodone bitartrate 10 mg] and chlorpheniramine polistirex [equivalent to chlorpheniramine maleate 8 mg] per 5 mL (115 mL, 480 mL [DSC]) [contains propylene glycol]

Controlled Substance C-II

Hydrocodone and Homatropine
(hye droe KOE done & hoe MA troe peen)

Brand Names: US Hydromet; Tussigon

Index Terms Homatropine and Hydrocodone; Hycodan; Hydrocodone Bitartrate and Homatropine Methylbromide

Pharmacologic Category Antitussive

Use Cough: Symptomatic relief of cough

Dosing

Adult & Geriatric Antitussive: Oral: One tablet or 5 mL every 4 to 6 hours as needed (maximum: 6 tablets/24 hours or 30 mL/24 hours)

Pediatric Antitussive: Oral:

Children 6 to 12 years: 1/2 tablet or 2.5 mL every 4 to 6 hours as needed (maximum: 3 tablets or 15 mL/24 hours)

Children >12 years and Adolescents: Refer to adult dosing.

Renal Impairment There are no dosage adjustments provided in the manufacturer's labeling; use with caution.

Hepatic Impairment There are no dosage adjustments provided in the manufacturer's labeling; use with caution.

Additional Information Complete prescribing information should be consulted for additional detail.

Dosage Forms Excipient information presented when available (limited, particularly for generics); consult specific product labeling. [DSC] = Discontinued product

Syrup:

Hydromet: Hydrocodone bitartrate 5 mg and homatropine methylbromide 1.5 mg per 5 mL (480 mL) [cherry flavor]

Generic: Hydrocodone bitartrate 5 mg and homatropine methylbromide 1.5 mg per 5 mL (473 mL)

Tablet:

Tussigon: Hydrocodone bitartrate 5 mg and homatropine methylbromide 1.5 mg

Generic: Hydrocodone bitartrate 5 mg and homatropine methylbromide 1.5 mg

Controlled Substance C-II

Hydrocodone and Ibuprofen
(hye droe KOE done & eye byoo PROE fen)

Brand Names: US Ibudone; Reprexain; Vicoprofen; Xylon

Brand Names: Canada Vicoprofen

Index Terms Hydrocodone Bitartrate and Ibuprofen; Ibuprofen and Hydrocodone

Pharmacologic Category Analgesic Combination (Opioid); Nonsteroidal Anti-inflammatory Drug (NSAID), Oral

Use Pain: Short-term (generally less than 10 days) management of acute pain (not indicated for treatment of chronic conditions [eg, osteoarthritis or rheumatoid arthritis]).

Medication Guide Available Yes

Dosing

Adult Pain: Oral: One tablet (hydrocodone 2.5 mg to 10 mg/ibuprofen 200 mg) every 4 to 6 hours as needed; (maximum: 5 tablets/24 hours). **Note:** Short-term use is recommended (<10 days total therapy).

Geriatric Use with caution and at reduced doses. Refer to adult dosing.

Pediatric Pain: Oral: Adolescents ≥16 years: Refer to adult dosing.

Renal Impairment There are no dosage adjustments provided in the manufacturer's labeling (has not been studied). Not recommended in advanced renal disease.

Hepatic Impairment There are no dosage adjustments provided in the manufacturer's labeling (has not been studied); use with caution in severe impairment.

Additional Information Complete prescribing information should be consulted for additional detail.

◀ **Dosage Forms** Excipient information presented when available (limited, particularly for generics); consult specific product labeling. [DSC] = discontinued product

Tablet, oral:

Ibudone:

5/200: Hydrocodone bitartrate 5 mg and ibuprofen 200 mg

10/200: Hydrocodone bitartrate 10 mg and ibuprofen 200 mg

Reprexain:

2.5/200: Hydrocodone bitartrate 2.5 mg and ibuprofen 200 mg [DSC]

5/200: Hydrocodone bitartrate 5 mg and ibuprofen 200 mg

10/200: Hydrocodone bitartrate 10 mg and ibuprofen 200 mg

Vicoprofen: 7.5/200: Hydrocodone bitartrate 7.5 mg and ibuprofen 200 mg

Xylon: 10/200: Hydrocodone bitartrate 10 mg and ibuprofen 200 mg

Generic: Hydrocodone bitartrate 2.5 mg and ibuprofen 200 mg [DSC]; Hydrocodone bitartrate 5 mg and ibuprofen 200 mg; Hydrocodone bitartrate 7.5 mg and ibuprofen 200 mg; Hydrocodone bitartrate 10 mg and ibuprofen 200 mg

Controlled Substance C-II

◆ Hydrocodone Bitartrate and Homatropine Methylbromide *see* Hydrocodone and Homatropine *on page* 885

◆ Hydrocodone Bitartrate and Ibuprofen *see* Hydrocodone and Ibuprofen *on page* 885

◆ Hydrocodone Polistirex and Chlorpheniramine Polistirex *see* Hydrocodone and Chlorpheniramine *on page* 885

Hydrocortisone (Systemic)
(hye droe KOR ti sone)

Brand Names: US A-Hydrocort; Cortef; Solu-CORTEF

Brand Names: Canada Cortef; Solu-Cortef

Index Terms A-hydroCort; Compound F; Cortisol; Hydrocortisone Sodium Succinate

Pharmacologic Category Corticosteroid, Systemic

Additional Appendix Information

Corticosteroids Systemic Equivalencies *on page* 1950

Use Primarily as an anti-inflammatory or immunosuppressant agent in the treatment of a variety of diseases including those of dermatologic, endocrine, GI, hematologic, allergic, inflammatory, neoplastic, neurologic, ophthalmic, renal, respiratory, and autoimmune origin.

Dosing

Adult & Geriatric Dose should be based on severity of disease and patient response.

Adrenal insufficiency (acute) (off-label dosing): IM, IV: 100 mg IV bolus, then 50-75 mg every 6 hours for 24 hours then slowly taper over the next 72 hours administering every 4-6 hours during taper. Alternatively, after the bolus dose, may administer as a continuous infusion at a rate of 10 mg/hour for the first 24 hours followed by a gradual reduction in dose over the next 72 hours. Once patient is stable, may change to an oral maintenance regimen. **Note:** Patients with primary adrenal insufficiency may require mineralocorticoid supplementation (eg, fludrocortisone) when shifting to an oral maintenance regimen (Gardner, 2011).

Adrenal insufficiency (chronic), physiologic replacement (off-label dosing): Oral: 15-25 mg/day in 2-3 divided doses. **Note:** Studies suggest administering one-half to two-thirds of the daily dose in the morning in order to mimic the physiological cortisol secretion pattern. If the twice-daily regimen is utilized, the second dose should be administered 6-8 hours following the first dose (Arlt, 2003).

Anti-inflammatory or immunosuppressive: Oral, IM, IV: 15-240 mg every 12 hours

Congenital adrenal hyperplasia (off-label dosing): Oral: 15-25 mg/day in 2-3 divided doses (Speiser, 2010)

Status asthmaticus: IV: 1-2 mg/kg/dose every 6 hours for 24 hours, then maintenance of 0.5-1 mg/kg every 6 hours

Stress dosing (surgery) in patients known to be adrenally-suppressed or on chronic systemic steroids: IV:

Minor stress (ie, inguinal herniorrhaphy): 25 mg/day for 1 day

Moderate stress (ie, joint replacement, cholecystectomy): 50-75 mg/day (25 mg every 8-12 hours) for 1-2 days

Major stress (pancreatoduodenectomy, esophagogastrectomy, cardiac surgery): 100-150 mg/day (50 mg every 8-12 hours) for 2-3 days

Septic shock (off-label use): IV: 50 mg every 6 hours (Annane, 2002; COIITSS Study Investigators, 2010). Practice guidelines suggest administering 200 mg daily as a continuous infusion over 24 hours to prevent adverse effects (eg, hyperglycemia) (Dellinger, 2013; Weber-Carstens, 2007); however, the impact of continuous infusion on patient outcomes has not been formally evaluated. Taper slowly (over several days) when vasopressors are no longer required; do not stop abruptly. **Note:** Hydrocortisone should be used alone (ie, without fludrocortisone) (Dellinger, 2013).

Thyroid storm (off-label use): IV: 300 mg loading dose, followed by 100 mg every 8 hours (Bahn, 2011)

Pediatric Dose should be based on severity of disease and patient response.

Anti-inflammatory or immunosuppressive:

Infants and Children:

Oral: 2.5-10 mg/kg/day **or** 75-300 mg/m²/day every 6-8 hours

IM, IV: 1-5 mg/kg/day **or** 30-150 mg/m²/day divided every 12-24 hours

Adolescents: Oral, IM, IV: 15-240 mg every 12 hours

Congenital adrenal hyperplasia (off-label dosing): Oral: **Note:** Doses must be individualized by monitoring growth, bone age, and hormonal levels.

Children: 10-15 mg/m²/day in 3 divided doses; higher initial doses may be required to achieve initial target hormone serum concentrations in infancy (Speiser, 2010)

Adolescents: Refer to adult dosing.

Physiologic replacement: Children: Oral: 8-10 mg/m²/day divided every 8 hours; up to 12 mg/m²/day in some patients (Ahmet, 2011; Gupta, 2008; Maguire, 2007)

Status asthmaticus: Children: IV: 1-2 mg/kg/dose every 6 hours for 24 hours, then maintenance of 0.5-1 mg/kg every 6 hours.

Septic shock (off-label use): Children: IV: Initial: 1-2 mg/kg/day (intermittent or as continuous infusion); may titrate up to 50 mg/kg/day for shock reversal (Brierley, 2009); alternative dosing suggests 50 mg/m²/day (Dellinger, 2008). **Note:** Use recommended only in fluid refractory, catecholamine-resistant shock, and suspected or proven absolute (classic) adrenal insufficiency.

Renal Impairment There are no dosage adjustments provided in the manufacturer's labeling; use with caution.

Hepatic Impairment There are no dosage adjustments provided in the manufacturer's labeling.

Additional Information Complete prescribing information should be consulted for additional detail.

Dosage Forms Excipient information presented when available (limited, particularly for generics); consult specific product labeling.

Solution Reconstituted, Injection, as sodium succinate [strength expressed as base]:

A-Hydrocort: 100 mg (1 ea)

Solu-CORTEF: 100 mg (1 ea)

Solution Reconstituted, Injection, as sodium succinate [strength expressed as base, preservative free]:

Solu-CORTEF: 100 mg (1 ea); 250 mg (1 ea); 500 mg (1 ea); 1000 mg (1 ea)

Tablet, Oral, as base:

Cortef: 5 mg, 10 mg, 20 mg [scored]

Generic: 5 mg, 10 mg, 20 mg

Hydrocortisone (Topical) (hye droe KOR ti sone)

Brand Names: US Advanced Allergy Collection; Ala Cort; Ala Scalp; Anti-Itch Maximum Strength [OTC]; Anucort-HC; Anusol-HC; Aqua Glycolic HC Scalp & Body [DSC]; Aquanil HC [OTC]; Beta HC [OTC]; Colocort; Cortaid Maximum Strength [OTC]; CortAlo; Cortenema; Corticool [OTC]; Cortifoam; Dermasorb HC; First-Hydrocortisone; GRx HiCort 25 [DSC]; Hemmorex-HC; Hemril-30 [DSC]; Hydro Skin Maximum Strength [OTC]; Hydrocortisone Max St [OTC]; Hydrocortisone Max St/12 Moist [OTC]; Hydro-SKIN [OTC]; Instacort 10 [OTC]; Instacort 5 [OTC]; Locoid; Locoid Lipocream; Med-Derm Hydrocortisone [OTC]; Medi-First Hydrocortisone [OTC]; NuCort; NuZon [DSC]; Pandel; Pediaderm HC; Preparation H Hydrocortisone [OTC]; Procto-Pak; Proctocort; Proctocream HC [DSC]; Proctosol HC; Proctozone-HC; Recort Plus [OTC]; Rectacort-HC [DSC]; Rederm [OTC]; Sarnol-HC [OTC]; Scalacort; Scalacort DK; Scalpicin Maximum Strength [OTC]; Texacort; TheraCort [OTC]; Westcort

Brand Names: Canada Aquacort; Cortamed; Cortenema; Cortifoam; Emo-Cort; Hycort; Hyderm; HydroVal; Locoid; Prevex HC; Sarna HC; Westcort

Index Terms A-hydroCort; Compound F; Cortisol; Hemorrhoidal HC; Hydrocortisone Acetate; Hydrocortisone Butyrate; Hydrocortisone Probutate; Hydrocortisone Valerate; Nutracort

Pharmacologic Category Antihemorrhoidal Agent; Corticosteroid, Rectal; Corticosteroid, Topical

Use

Anal and genital itching (external): Use in postirradiation (factitial) proctitis, cryptitis, other inflammatory conditions of the anorectum; external genital, feminine, and anal itching.

Dermatoses: Relief of the inflammatory and pruritic manifestations of corticosteroid-responsive dermatoses (eg, eczema; psoriasis; poison ivy, oak, or sumac; insect bites; minor skin irritation; atopic dermatitis [mild to moderate]; seborrheic dermatitis).

Hemorrhoids: Use in inflamed hemorrhoids.

Ulcerative colitis (adjunctive therapy): Adjunctive treatment of ulcerative colitis, especially distal forms including ulcerative proctitis, ulcerative proctosigmoiditis, left-sided ulcerative colitis, and in some cases involving the transverse and ascending colons.

Dosing

Adult & Geriatric

Dermatosis: Topical:

Rx: Apply thin film to affected area 2 to 4 times daily.

Hydrocortisone butyrate (Locoid cream, Lipocream, ointment, solution): Apply thin film to affected area 2 to 3 times daily.

Hydrocortisone probutate (Pandel): Topical: Apply thin film to affected area 1 to 2 times daily.

Hydrocortisone valerate (Westcort): Topical: Apply thin film to affected area 2 to 3 times daily.

OTC: Apply thin film to the affected area up to 3 to 4 times daily.

Anal and genital itching, external: Topical: OTC labeling: Apply to affected area up to 3 to 4 times daily.

Hemorrhoids: Rectal: One suppository (25 or 30 mg) twice daily for 2 weeks. For severe cases of proctitis, 1 suppository 3 times daily or 2 suppositories twice daily may be needed. For factitial proctitis, duration of treatment may be up to 6 to 8 weeks.

Ulcerative colitis: Rectal:

Foam: One applicatorful (90 mg) 1 to 2 times daily for 2 to 3 weeks, and then every other day thereafter; use lowest dose to maintain clinical response; taper dose to discontinue long-term therapy

Suspension: One enema (100 mg) every night for 21 days or until remission (clinical improvement may precede improvement of mucosal integrity); 2 to 3 months of therapy may be required; to discontinue long-term therapy, gradually reduce administration to every other night for 2 or 3 weeks.

Pediatric

Atopic dermatitis: Topical: Infants ≥3 months, Children, and Adolescents: Hydrocortisone butyrate (Locoid Lipocream, Locoid lotion): Apply thin film to affected area twice daily.

Dermatosis: Topical:

Rx: Apply thin film to affected area 2 to 4 times daily.

Hydrocortisone butyrate (Locoid cream, Lipocream, ointment, solution): Apply thin film to affected area 2 to 3 times daily.

OTC: Apply thin film to the affected area up to 3 to 4 times daily. Products labeled for OTC use (self-medication) should not be used in children <2 years of age.

Anal and genital itching, external: Topical: Children ≥12 years and Adolescents: OTC labeling: Refer to adult dosing.

Renal Impairment There are no dosage adjustments provided in the manufacturer's labeling.

Hepatic Impairment There are no dosage adjustments provided in the manufacturer's labeling.

Additional Information Complete prescribing information should be consulted for additional detail.

Dosage Forms Considerations First-Hydrocortisone 10% gel is a compounding kit. Refer to manufacturer's labeling for compounding instructions.

Dosage Forms Excipient information presented when available (limited, particularly for generics); consult specific product labeling. [DSC] = Discontinued product

Cream, External, as acetate:

Hydrocortisone Max St: 1% (28.4 g)

Cream, External, as base:

Ala Cort: 1% (28.4 g, 85.2 g) [contains cetyl alcohol, propylene glycol]

Anti-Itch Maximum Strength: 1% (28 g) [contains cetyl alcohol, methylparaben]

Anti-Itch Maximum Strength: 1% (28 g) [contains cetyl alcohol, methylparaben, propylene glycol, propylparaben]

Cortaid Maximum Strength: 1% (14 g, 28 g) [contains cetyl alcohol, disodium edta, ethylparaben, methylparaben, propylparaben]

Hydrocortisone Max St/12 Moist: 1% (28.4 g) [contains cetearyl alcohol, methylparaben, propylene glycol, propylparaben]

HydroSKIN: 1% (28 g [DSC]) [contains benzyl alcohol]

HydroSKIN: 1% (28 g) [contains methylparaben, propylene glycol, propylparaben]

Instacort 5: 0.5% (28.4 g)

Med-Derm Hydrocortisone: 0.5% (30 g); 1% (30 g)

Medi-First Hydrocortisone: 1% (1 ea) [contains trolamine (triethanolamine)]

Preparation H Hydrocortisone: 1% (26 g)

Recort Plus: 1% (30 g)

Generic: 0.5% (15 g, 28.35 g, 28.4 g, 30 g); 1% (1 g, 1.5 g, 14.2 g, 20 g, 28 g, 28.35 g, 28.4 g, 30 g, 120 g, 453.6 g, 454 g [DSC]); 2.5% (20 g, 28 g, 28.35 g, 30 g, 453.6 g)

Cream, Rectal, as base:

Anusol-HC: 2.5% (30 g)

Procto-Pak: 1% (28.4 g)

Proctocort: 1% (28.35 g) [contains cetyl alcohol, propylene glycol]

Proctocream HC: 2.5% (30 g [DSC]) [contains benzyl alcohol]

Proctosol HC: 2.5% (28.35 g)

Proctozone-HC: 2.5% (30 g)

Proctozone-HC: 2.5% (30 g) [contains cetearyl alcohol, methylparaben, propylene glycol, propylparaben]

Generic: 1% (28.4 g)

Cream, External, as butyrate:

Locoid: 0.1% (15 g [DSC], 45 g [DSC])

Locoid: 0.1% (15 g, 45 g) [contains butylparaben, propylparaben]

Locoid Lipocream: 0.1% (15 g [DSC], 45 g, 60 g) [contains butylparaben, cetostearyl alcohol, propylparaben]

Generic: 0.1% (15 g, 45 g, 60 g)

Cream, External, as probutate:

Pandel: 0.1% (15 g, 45 g, 80 g) [contains butylparaben, methylparaben, propylene glycol]

Cream, External, as valerate:

Generic: 0.2% (15 g, 45 g, 60 g)

Enema, Rectal, as base:

Colocort: 100 mg/60 mL (60 mL)

Cortenema: 100 mg/60 mL (60 mL) [contains methylparaben, polysorbate 80]

Generic: 100 mg/60 mL (60 mL)

Foam, Rectal, as acetate:

Cortifoam: 10% [90 mg/applicatorful] (15 g) [contains cetyl alcohol, methylparaben, propylene glycol, propylparaben, trolamine (triethanolamine)]

Gel, External, as acetate:

CortAlo: 2% (43 g) [contains benzyl alcohol, menthol, trolamine (triethanolamine)]

NuZon: 2% (43 g [DSC]) [contains menthol, trolamine (triethanolamine)]

Generic: 2% (43 g [DSC])

Gel, External, as base:

Corticool: 1% (42.53 g) [contains cremophor el, propylene glycol]

First-Hydrocortisone: 10% (60 g) [contains propylene glycol, simethicone]

Instacort 10: 1% (30 g)

Kit, External, as base:

Advanced Allergy Collection: 2.5% [contains cetyl alcohol, methylparaben, propylene glycol, propylparaben]

Aqua Glycolic HC Scalp & Body: 2% [DSC] [contains benzalkonium chloride, isopropyl alcohol, propylene glycol]

Dermasorb HC: 2% [contains menthol, methylparaben, propylene glycol, propylparaben]

Pediaderm HC: 2% [contains benzalkonium chloride, cetyl alcohol, isopropyl alcohol, methylparaben, propylene glycol, propylparaben]

Scalacort DK: Hydrocortisone lotion 2% and Sal Acid 2% and sulfur 2% [contains benzalkonium chloride, isopropyl alcohol, methylparaben, propylene glycol, propylparaben, soybean lecithin]

Lotion, External, as acetate:

NuCort: 2% (60 g) [contains benzyl alcohol, cetyl alcohol, menthol, trolamine (triethanolamine)]

Lotion, External, as base:

Ala Scalp: 2% (29.6 mL) [contains benzalkonium chloride, isopropyl alcohol, propylene glycol]

Aquanil HC: 1% (120 mL)

Beta HC: 1% (60 mL)

Hydro Skin Maximum Strength: 1% (118 mL) [contains benzyl alcohol]

HydroSKIN: 1% (118 mL) [contains benzyl alcohol, cetyl alcohol, propylene glycol]

Rederm: 1% (120 mL)

Sarnol-HC: 1% (59 mL)

Scalacort: 2% (29.6 mL) [contains benzalkonium chloride, isopropyl alcohol, propylene glycol]

TheraCort: 1% (118 mL) [contains methylparaben, propylene glycol, propylparaben, trolamine (triethanolamine)]

Generic: 1% (114 g, 120 mL [DSC]); 2.5% (59 mL, 118 mL)

Lotion, External, as butyrate:

Locoid: 0.1% (59 mL, 118 mL) [contains butylparaben, cetostearyl alcohol, propylparaben]

Ointment, External, as base:

Generic: 0.5% (28.35 g, 30 g); 1% (25 g, 28 g, 28.35 g, 28.4 g, 30 g, 110 g, 430 g, 453.6 g); 2.5% (20 g, 28.35 g, 453.6 g, 454 g)

Ointment, External, as butyrate:

Locoid: 0.1% (15 g, 45 g)

Generic: 0.1% (15 g, 45 g)

Ointment, External, as valerate:

Westcort: 0.2% (15 g, 45 g, 60 g) [contains propylene glycol]

Generic: 0.2% (15 g, 45 g, 60 g)

Solution, External, as base:

Scalpicin Maximum Strength: 1% (44 mL) [contains disodium edta, menthol, propylene glycol]

Texacort: 2.5% (30 mL) [lipid free, paraben free; contains alcohol, usp]

Solution, External, as butyrate:

Locoid: 0.1% (60 mL) [contains isopropyl alcohol]

Generic: 0.1% (20 mL, 60 mL)

Suppository, Rectal, as acetate:

Anucort-HC: 25 mg (12 ea, 24 ea, 100 ea)

Anusol-HC: 25 mg (12 ea, 24 ea)

GRx HiCort 25: 25 mg (12 ea [DSC])

Hemmorex-HC: 25 mg (12 ea, 24 ea); 30 mg (12 ea)

Hemril-30: 30 mg (12 ea [DSC], 24 ea [DSC])

Proctocort: 30 mg (12 ea)

Rectacort-HC: 25 mg (12 ea [DSC], 24 ea [DSC])

Generic: 25 mg (12 ea, 24 ea); 30 mg (12 ea)

HYDROmorphone (hye droe MOR fone)

Brand Names: US Dilaudid; Dilaudid-HP; Exalgo

Brand Names: Canada Apo-Hydromorphone; Dilaudid; Dilaudid-HP; Hydromorph Contin; Hydromorphone HP; Hydromorphone HP Forte Injection; Hydromorphone Hydrochloride Injection USP HP 10; Hydromorphone Hydrochloride Injection, USP; Jurnista; PMS-Hydromorphone; Teva-Hydromorphone

Index Terms Dihydromorphinone; Hydromorphone Hydrochloride; Palladone

Pharmacologic Category Analgesic, Opioid

Additional Appendix Information

Opioid Conversion Table and Morphine Equivalent Dose Table on page 1955

Use

Pain:

Immediate-release formulations:

Tablet, liquid, injection: Management of pain in patients where an opioid analgesic is appropriate

HP injection: Management of moderate to severe pain in opioid-tolerant patients who require higher doses of opioids

Suppository: Management of moderate to severe pain

Extended-release formulations: Management of pain in opioid-tolerant patients severe enough to require daily, around-the-clock, long-term opioid treatment and for which alternative treatment options are inadequate

Limitations of use: Not indicated as an as-needed analgesic. Because of the risks of addiction, abuse, and misuse with opioids, even at recommended doses, and because of the greater risks of overdose and death with extended-release opioid formulations, reserve for use in patients for whom alternative treatment options (eg, nonopioid analgesics, immediate-release opioids) are ineffective, not tolerated, or would be otherwise inadequate to provide sufficient management of pain

Pregnancy Considerations Adverse events have been observed in some animal reproduction studies. Hydromorphone crosses the placenta. Some dosage forms are specifically contraindicated for use in obstetrical analgesia. The Canadian labeling contraindicates use of some dosage forms during pregnancy and/or labor and delivery.

When used for pain relief during labor, opioids may temporarily affect the heart rate of the fetus (ACOG 2002). Monitor the neonate for respiratory depression if hydromorphone is used during labor.

[US Boxed Warning]: Prolonged maternal use of opioids during pregnancy can cause neonatal withdrawal syndrome in the newborn, which may be life-threatening if not recognized and treated according to protocols developed by neonatology experts. If prolonged opioid therapy is required in a pregnant woman, ensure treatment is available and warn patient of risk to the neonate. If chronic opioid exposure occurs in pregnancy, adverse events in the newborn (including withdrawal) may occur; monitoring of the neonate is recommended. The minimum effective dose should be used if opioids are needed (Chou 2009). Neonatal abstinence syndrome following opioid exposure may present with autonomic (eg, fever, temperature instability), GI (eg, diarrhea, vomiting, poor feeding/weight gain), or neurologic (eg, high-pitched crying, increased muscle tone, irritability, seizure, tremor) symptoms (Dow 2012; Hudak 2012). Long-term opioid use may cause secondary hypogonadism, which may lead to sexual dysfunction or infertility (Brennan 2013).

Breast-Feeding Considerations Low concentrations of hydromorphone can be found in breast milk. Withdrawal symptoms may be observed in breast-feeding infants when opioid analgesics are discontinued. The US labeling does not recommend use in breast-feeding women. The Canadian labeling contraindicates use. Parenteral opioids used during labor have the potential to interfere with a newborn's natural reflex to nurse within the first few hours after birth. Breast-feeding infants exposed to large doses of opioids should be monitored for apnea and sedation (Montgomery, 2012).

Prescribing and Access Restrictions Exalgo: As a requirement of the REMS program, healthcare providers who prescribe Exalgo need to receive training on the proper use and potential risks of Exalgo. For training, please refer to http://www.exalgorems.com. Prescribers will need retraining every 2 years or following any significant changes to the Exalgo REMS program.

Medication Guide Available Yes

Contraindications

US labeling: Hypersensitivity to hydromorphone, or any component of the formulation; acute or severe asthma, respiratory depression (in absence of resuscitative equipment or ventilatory support)

Additional product-specific contraindications:

Dilaudid liquid and tablets: Obstetrical analgesia

Dilaudid injection, Dilaudid-HP injection: Opioid-nontolerant patients (Dilaudid-HP injection only); patients with risk of developing GI obstruction, especially paralytic ileus

Exalgo: Opioid-nontolerant patients, paralytic ileus (known or suspected), preexisting GI surgery and/or diseases resulting in narrowing of GI tract, blind loops in the GI tract, or GI obstruction

Suppository: Intracranial lesion associated with increased intracranial pressure; whenever ventilatory function is depressed (eg, COPD, cor pulmonale, emphysema, kyphoscoliosis, status asthmaticus)

Canadian labeling: Hypersensitivity to hydromorphone or any component of the formulation

Dilaudid, Hydromorph Contin, Jurnista: Known or suspected mechanical GI obstruction (eg, bowel obstruction or strictures) or any disease that affects bowel transit (eg, ileus of any type); suspected surgical abdomen (eg, acute appendicitis or pancreatitis); mild, intermittent, or short-duration pain that can be managed with other pain medications; acute respiratory depression, hypercarbia and cor pulmonale; acute alcoholism, delirium tremens, and convulsive disorders; severe CNS depression, increased cerebrospinal or intracranial pressure, and head injury; coadministration with monoamine oxidase inhibitors (concomitant use or within 14 days); women during pregnancy, labor and delivery, or breast-feeding

Hydromorphone HP, Hydromorphone HP Forte: Patients not already receiving high doses or high concentrations of opioids; respiratory depression in the absence of resuscitative equipment; severe CNS depression; status asthmaticus; obstetrical analgesia; mild or moderate pain

Suppository, syrup: Respiratory depression in the absence of resuscitative equipment; status asthmaticus

Additional product-specific contraindications:

Dilaudid: Hypersensitivity to other opioid analgesics; acute asthma or other obstructive airway and status asthmaticus

Hydromorph Contin: Hypersensitivity to other opioid analgesics; acute asthma or severe bronchial asthma or status asthmaticus; management of acute pain, including use in outpatient or day surgeries; management of perioperative pain (unless GI function is normal)

Jurnista: Prior surgical procedures and/or underlying disease that may result in narrowing of the GI tract, blind loops of the GI tract, or GI obstruction; acute asthma or other obstructive airway and status asthmaticus; management of acute or perioperative pain

Warnings/Precautions Use with caution in patients with hypersensitivity reactions to other phenanthrene derivative opioid agonists (codeine, hydrocodone, levorphanol, oxycodone, oxymorphone). Hydromorphone shares toxic potential of opioid agonists, including CNS depression and respiratory depression. Precautions associated with opioid agonist therapy should be observed. May cause CNS depression, which may impair physical or mental abilities; patients must be cautioned about performing tasks that require mental alertness (eg, operating machinery or driving). Myoclonus and seizures have been reported with high doses; use with caution in patients with a history of seizure disorder (some Canadian labels specifically contraindicate use in patients with seizure disorder, refer to Contraindications). Use with caution in patients with cardiovascular disease, morbid obesity, adrenocortical insufficiency, hypothyroidism, acute alcoholism, delirium tremens, toxic psychoses, prostatic hyperplasia and/or urinary stricture, or severe liver or renal failure. Use with caution and monitor for respiratory depression in patients with significant chronic obstructive pulmonary disease or cor pulmonale, and patients having a substantially decreased respiratory reserve, hypoxia, hypercarbia, or preexisting respiratory depression, particularly when initiating therapy and titrating with hydromorphone; even therapeutic doses may decrease respiratory drive to the point of apnea. Consider the use of alternative nonopioid analgesics in these patients. Avoid use in patients with CNS depression or coma, as these patients are susceptible to intracranial effects of CO_2 retention. Use with caution in patients with biliary tract dysfunction. Hydromorphone may increase biliary tract pressure following spasm in sphincter of Oddi. Use caution in patients with inflammatory or obstructive bowel disorder, acute

pancreatitis secondary to biliary tract disease, and patients undergoing biliary surgery. Use extreme caution in patients with head injury, intracranial lesions, or elevated intracranial pressure (ICP); exaggerated elevation of ICP may occur (in addition, hydromorphone may complicate neurologic evaluation due to pupillary dilation and CNS depressant effects). Use with caution in patients with depleted blood volume or drugs which may exaggerate hypotensive effects (including phenothiazines or general anesthetics). Avoid use in patients with circulatory shock. May obscure diagnosis or clinical course of patients with acute abdominal conditions. Effects may be potentiated when used with other CNS depressants (eg, sedatives, anxiolytics, hypnotics, neuroleptics, other opioids). Potentially significant interactions may exist, requiring dose or frequency adjustment, additional monitoring, and/or selection of alternative therapy.

An opioid-containing analgesic regimen should be tailored to each patient's needs and based upon the type of pain being treated (acute versus chronic), the route of administration, degree of tolerance for opioids (naive versus chronic user), age, weight, and medical condition. The optimal analgesic dose varies widely among patients. Doses should be titrated to pain relief/prevention. IM use may result in variable absorption and a lag time to peak effect. Concurrent use of mixed agonist/antagonist analgesics (eg, pentazocine, nalbuphine, butorphanol) or partial agonist (eg, buprenorphine) analgesics may precipitate withdrawal symptoms and/or reduced analgesic efficacy in patients following prolonged therapy with mu opioid agonists. Abrupt discontinuation following prolonged use may also lead to withdrawal symptoms. May cause constipation. Consider preventive measures to reduce the potential for constipation. Use with extreme caution in patients with chronic constipation. Use immediate-release formulations with caution in the perioperative setting; severe pain may antagonize the respiratory depressant effects of hydromorphone. The Canadian labeling (immediate-release formulations) recommends withholding hydromorphone within 24 hours of procedures that interfere with pain transmission pathways (eg, cordotomy); the Canadian labeling for extended-release formulations contraindicates use in the perioperative setting (Hydromorph Contin may be used in this setting only if GI function is normal).

Dosage form specific warnings:

Some dosage forms may contain trace amounts of sodium metabisulfite, which may cause allergic reactions, including anaphylactic symptoms and life-threatening or less severe asthmatic episodes in susceptible individuals. Some formulations may contain lactose; consider lactose content prior to initiating therapy in patients with hereditary diseases of galactose intolerance (eg, galactosemia, glucose-galactose malabsorption).

Immediate-release formulations: **[US Boxed Warning]: High potential for abuse and risk of producing respiratory depression. Alcohol, other opioids, and CNS depressants potentiate the respiratory depressant effects of hydromorphone, increasing the risk of respiratory depression that might result in death.**

Injection: Vial stoppers of single-dose injectable vials may contain latex. **[US Boxed Warning]: Dilaudid-HP: Extreme caution should be taken to avoid confusing the highly concentrated (Dilaudid-HP) injection with the less-concentrated (Dilaudid) injectable product.** Dilaudid-HP should only be used in patients who are opioid tolerant. Highly concentrated products available in Canada (Hydromorphone HP and Hydromorphone HP Forte) are for use only in opioid-tolerant patients with severe pain.

Extended-release tablets: **[US Boxed Warning]: May cause serious, life-threatening, or fatal respiratory depression. Monitor closely for respiratory depression, especially during initiation or dose escalation. Patients should swallow tablets whole; crushing, chewing, or dissolving can cause rapid release and a potentially fatal dose.** Carbon dioxide retention from opioid-induced respiratory depression can exacerbate the sedating effects of opioids. **[US Boxed Warning]: Users are exposed to the risks of addiction, abuse, and misuse, potentially leading to overdose and death. Assess each patient's risk prior to prescribing; monitor all patients regularly for development of these behaviors or conditions.** Risk of opioid abuse is increased in patients with a history or family history of alcohol or drug abuse or mental illness. Tolerance or drug dependence may result from extended use; however, concerns for abuse should not prevent effective management of pain. In general,

abrupt discontinuation of therapy in dependent patients should be avoided. **[US Boxed Warning]: Prolonged maternal use of opioids during pregnancy can cause neonatal withdrawal syndrome in the newborn, which may be life-threatening if not recognized and treated according to protocols developed by neonatology experts. If prolonged opioid therapy is required in a pregnant woman, ensure treatment is available and warn patient of risk to the neonate.** Signs and symptoms include irritability, hyperactivity and abnormal sleep pattern, high-pitched cry, tremor, vomiting, diarrhea, and failure to gain weight. Onset, duration, and severity depend on the drug used, duration of use, maternal dose, and rate of drug elimination by the newborn. Therapy should only be prescribed by health care professionals familiar with the use of potent opioids for chronic pain. Exalgo and Jurnista [Canadian product] tablets are nondeformable; do not administer to patients with preexisting severe GI narrowing (eg, esophageal motility, small bowel inflammatory disease, short gut syndrome, history of peritonitis, cystic fibrosis, chronic intestinal pseudo-obstruction, Meckel's diverticulum); obstruction may occur. Tablets may be visible on abdominal x-rays, especially when digital enhancing techniques are used. The tablet shell may appear in the excreted stool.

Adverse Reactions Frequency not defined.

Cardiovascular: Bradycardia, extrasystoles, flushing (facial), hypertension, hypotension, palpitations, peripheral edema, peripheral vasodilation, syncope, tachycardia

Central nervous system: Abnormal dreams, abnormal gait, abnormality in thinking, aggressive behavior, agitation, apprehension, ataxia, brain disease, burning sensation of skin (Exalgo), central nervous system depression, chills, cognitive dysfunction, confusion, decreased body temperature (Exalgo), depression, disruption of body temperature regulation (Exalgo), dizziness, drowsiness, drug dependence, dysarthria, dysphoria, equilibrium disturbance, euphoria, fatigue, hallucination, headache, hyperesthesia, hyperreflexia, hypoesthesia, hypothermia, increased intracranial pressure, insomnia, lack of concentration, lethargy, malaise, memory impairment, mood changes, myoclonus, nervousness, painful defecation, panic attack, paranoia, paresthesia, psychomotor agitation, restlessness, sedation, seizure, sleep disorder (Exalgo), suicidal ideation, uncontrolled crying, vertigo

Dermatologic: Diaphoresis, erythema (Exalgo), hyperhidrosis, pruritus, skin rash, urticaria

Endocrine & metabolic: Antidiuretic effect, decreased amylase, decreased libido, decreased plasma testosterone, dehydration, fluid retention, hyperuricemia, hypokalemia, weight loss

Gastrointestinal: Abdominal distention, anal fissure, anorexia, bezoar formation (Exalgo), biliary tract spasm, constipation, decreased appetite, decreased gastrointestinal motility (Exalgo), delayed gastric emptying, diarrhea, diverticulitis, diverticulosis, duodenitis, dysgeusia, dysphagia, eructation, flatulence, gastroenteritis, gastroesophageal reflux disease (aggravated; Exalgo), hematochezia, increased appetite, intestinal perforation (large intestine; Exalgo), nausea, paralytic ileus, stomach cramps, vomiting, xerostomia

Genitourinary: Bladder spasm, decreased urine output, difficulty in micturition, dysuria, erectile dysfunction, hypogonadism, sexual disorder, ureteral spasm, urinary frequency, urinary hesitancy, urinary retention

Hematologic & oncologic: Oxygen desaturation

Hepatic: Increased liver enzymes

Hypersensitivity: Histamine release

Local: Pain at injection site, post-injection flare

Neuromuscular & skeletal: Arthralgia, dyskinesia, laryngospasm, muscle rigidity, muscle spasm, myalgia, tremor, weakness

Ophthalmic: Blurred vision, diplopia, dry eye syndrome, miosis, nystagmus

Otic: Tinnitus

Respiratory: Apnea, bronchospasm, dyspnea, flu-like symptoms (Exalgo), hyperventilation, hypoxia, respiratory depression, respiratory distress, rhinorrhea

Postmarketing and/or case reports (Limited to important or life-threatening): Angioedema, hypersensitivity

Drug Interactions

Metabolism/Transport Effects None known.

Avoid Concomitant Use

Avoid concomitant use of HYDROmorphone with any of the following: Azelastine (Nasal); Eluxadoline; MAO Inhibitors; Mixed Agonist / Antagonist Opioids; Orphenadrine; Paraldehyde; Thalidomide

Increased Effect/Toxicity

HYDROmorphone may increase the levels/effects of: Alcohol (Ethyl); Alvimopan; Azelastine (Nasal); CNS Depressants; Desmopressin; Diuretics; Eluxadoline; Hydrocodone; Methotrimeprazine; Metyrosine; Mirtazapine; Orphenadrine; Paraldehyde; Pramipexole; Ramosetron; ROPINIRole; Rotigotine; Selective Serotonin Reuptake Inhibitors; Suvorexant; Thalidomide; Zolpidem

The levels/effects of HYDROmorphone may be increased by: Amphetamines; Anticholinergic Agents; Antipsychotic Agents (Phenothiazines); Brimonidine (Topical); Cannabis; Doxylamine; Dronabinol; Droperidol; HydrOXYzine; Kava Kava; Magnesium Sulfate; MAO Inhibitors; Methotrimeprazine; Minocycline; Nabilone; Perampanel; Rufinamide; Sodium Oxybate; Succinylcholine; Tapentadol; Tetrahydrocannabinol

Decreased Effect

HYDROmorphone may decrease the levels/effects of: Pegvisomant

The levels/effects of HYDROmorphone may be decreased by: Ammonium Chloride; Mixed Agonist / Antagonist Opioids; Naltrexone

Storage/Stability

Injection: Store at 15°C to 30°C (59°F to 86°F). Protect from light. A slightly yellowish discoloration has not been associated with a loss of potency. Stable for at least 24 hours when protected from light and stored at 25°C in most common large volume parenteral solutions.

Oral dosage forms: Store at 25°C (77°F); excursions permitted from 15°C to 30°C (59°F to 86°F). Protect tablets from light.

Suppository:

US labeling: Store in refrigerator. Protect from light.

Canadian labeling: Store at 15°C to 30°C (59°F to 86°F). Protect from light.

Mechanism of Action Binds to opioid receptors in the CNS, causing inhibition of ascending pain pathways, altering the perception of and response to pain; causes cough suppression by direct central action in the medulla; produces generalized CNS depression

Pharmacodynamics/Kinetics

Onset of action: Analgesic:

Immediate-release formulations:

Oral: 15 to 30 minutes; Peak effect: 30 to 60 minutes

IV: 5 minutes; Peak effect: 10 to 20 minutes

Extended-release tablet: 6 hours; Peak effect: ~9 hours (Angst 2001)

Duration:

Immediate-release formulations: Oral, IV: 3 to 4 hours

Extended-release tablet: ~13 hours (Angst 2001)

Absorption: Extended-release tablet: Delayed; IM: Variable and delayed

Distribution: V_d: 4 L/kg

Protein binding: ~8% to 19%

Metabolism: Hepatic via glucuronidation; to inactive metabolites

Bioavailability: Oral, immediate release: ~24%

Half-life elimination:

Immediate-release formulations: 2 to 3 hours

Extended-release tablets: Apparent half-life: ~11 hours (range: 8 to 15 hours)

Time to peak, plasma:

Immediate-release tablet: ≤1 hour

Extended-release tablet: 12 to 16 hours

Extended-release capsule [Canadian product]: ~5 hours

Excretion: Urine (primarily as glucuronide conjugates)

Dosing

Adult

Acute pain (moderate to severe): Note: These are guidelines and do not represent the maximum doses that may be required in all patients. Doses should be titrated to provide adequate pain relief. When changing routes of administration, oral doses and parenteral doses are **NOT** equivalent; parenteral doses are up to 5 times more potent. Therefore, when administered parenterally, one-fifth of the oral dose will provide similar analgesia.

Oral: Immediate release: Initial: Opioid naive: 2 to 4 mg every 4 to 6 hours as needed (tablets) or 2.5 mg to 10 mg every 3 to 6 hours as needed (liquid); elderly/debilitated patients may require lower doses; patients with prior opioid exposure may require higher initial doses. **Note:** In adults with severe pain, the American Pain Society recommends an initial dose of 4 to 8 mg. Therapy discontinuation (Canadian labeling): Decrease the previous daily dose by 50% (administered every 6 hours) for 2 days then decrease daily dose by 25% every 2 days.

IV: Initial: Opioid naive: 0.2 to 1 mg every 2 to 3 hours as needed; patients with prior opioid exposure may require higher initial doses. Dilaudid HP should **NOT** be used in opioid-naive patients.

Critically ill patients (off-label dosing): 0.2 to 0.6 mg every 1 to 2 hours as needed **or** 0.5 mg every 3 hours as needed (Barr 2013)

Continuous infusion: Usual dosage range: 0.5 to 3 mg/hour (Barr 2013)

Patient-controlled analgesia (PCA) (off-label dosing) (American Pain Society 2008): **Note:** Opioid naive: Consider lower end of dosing range. A continuous (basal) infusion is not recommended in opioid-naive patients (ISMP 2009):

Usual concentration: 0.2 mg/mL

Demand dose: Usual initial dose: 0.2 mg; range: 0.05 to 0.4 mg

Lockout interval: 5 to 10 minutes

Epidural PCA (off-label dosing) (de Leon-Casasola 1996; Liu 2010; Smith 2009):

Usual concentration: 0.01 mg/mL

Bolus dose: 0.4 to 1 mg

Infusion rate: 0.03 to 0.3 mg/**hour**

Demand dose: 0.02 to 0.05 mg

Lockout interval: 10 to 15 minutes

IM, SubQ: **Note:** IM use may result in variable absorption and lag time to peak effect; IM route not recommended for use (American Pain Society 2008). Equianalgesic doses: Morphine 10 mg IM = hydromorphone 1.5 mg IM.

US labeling: Initial: 1 to 2 mg every 2 to 3 hours as needed; lower initial doses may be used in opioid-naive patients. Patients with prior opioid exposure may require higher initial doses.

Canadian labeling: Opioid naive: 2 mg every 4 to 6 hours as needed; for severe pain, may administer 3 to 4 mg every 4 to 6 hours as needed. When discontinuation of therapy is necessary, decrease the previous daily dose by 50% (administered every 6 hours) for 2 days then decrease daily dose by 25% every 2 days. Hydromorphone HP or Hydromorphone HP Forte should **NOT** be used in opioid-naive patients.

Rectal:

US labeling: 3 mg (1 suppository) every 6 to 8 hours as needed

Canadian labeling: 3 mg (1 suppository) at bedtime as needed

Chronic pain: Note: Patients taking opioids chronically may become tolerant and require doses higher than the usual dosage range to maintain the desired effect. Tolerance can be managed by appropriate dose titration. There is no optimal or maximal dose for hydromorphone in chronic pain. The appropriate dose is one that relieves pain throughout its dosing interval without causing unmanageable side effects.

Controlled-release capsule (Hydromorph Contin [Canadian product]): Oral: **Note:** A patient's hydromorphone requirement should be established using prompt release formulations; conversion to long-acting products may be considered when chronic, continuous treatment is required. Higher dosages should be reserved for use only in opioid-tolerant patients. Capsule strengths ≥18 mg or a single dose >12 mg should be reserved for use only in opioid-tolerant patients requiring hydromorphone equivalent dosages ≥36 mg daily.

Opioid naive or receiving low intermittent doses of weak opioids: Initial: 3 mg every 12 hours.

Current therapy with other oral hydromorphone formulations: Initial: Initiate at same total daily hydromorphone dosage divided in 2 equal doses every 12 hours

Current therapy with other opioids: Initial: Determine equivalent oral hydromorphone daily dosage and initiate in 2 equally divided doses every 12 hours. See table below for examples of equivalent dosing (refer to manufacturer labeling for additional equivalency dosing information).

Approximate Opioid Analgesic Equivalent Dosing (Oral)	
Hydromorphone	1 mg
Morphine	8 mg (5 to 7.5 mg with chronic dosing of morphine)
Oxycodone	4 mg
Codeine	~27 mg

Extended-release tablet (Exalgo): **Note:** For use in opioid-tolerant patients only. Patients considered opioid tolerant are those who are receiving, for 1 week or longer, at least 60 mg of oral morphine daily, 25 mcg of transdermal fentanyl per hour, 30 mg of oral oxycodone daily, 8 mg of oral hydromorphone daily, 25 mg of oral oxymorphone daily, or an equianalgesic dose of another opioid.

Opioid-tolerant patients: Discontinue or taper all other extended-release opioids when starting therapy.

Individualization of dose: Suggested recommendations for converting to Exalgo from other analgesics are presented, but when selecting the initial dose, other characteristics (eg, patient status, degree of opioid tolerance, concurrent medications, type of pain, risk factors for addiction, abuse, and misuse) should also be considered. Pain relief and adverse events should be assessed frequently.

Conversion from other oral hydromorphone formulations to Exalgo: Start with the equivalent total daily dose of immediate-release hydromorphone administered once daily.

Conversion from other opioids to Exalgo: Discontinue all other around-the-clock opioids when therapy is initiated. Substantial interpatient variability exists in relative potency. Therefore, it is safer to underestimate a patient's daily oral hydromorphone requirement and provide breakthrough pain relief with rescue medication (eg, immediate release opioid) than to overestimate requirements. In general, start Exalgo at 50% of the calculated total daily dose every 24 hours (see Conversion Factors to Exalgo). The following conversion ratios may be used to convert from oral opioid therapy to Exalgo.

Conversion factors to Exalgo (see table): Select the opioid, sum the current total daily dose, multiply by the conversion factor on the table to calculate the approximate oral hydromorphone daily dose, then calculate the approximate starting dose for Exalgo at 50% of the calculated oral hydromorphone daily does; administer every 24 hours. Round down, if necessary, to the nearest strength available. For patients on a regimen of more than one opioid, calculate the approximate oral hydromorphone dose for each opioid and sum the totals to obtain the approximate total hydromorphone daily dose. For patients on a regimen of fixed-ratio opioid/nonopioid analgesic medications, only the opioid component of these medications should be used in the conversion. **Note:** The conversion factors in this conversion table are only to be used for the conversion from current oral opioid therapy to Exalgo. Conversion factors in this table cannot be used to convert from Exalgo to another oral opioid (doing so may lead to fatal overdose due to overestimation of the new opioid). This is not a table of equianalgesic doses.

Conversion Factors to Exalgo[1]

Previous Oral Opioid	Oral Conversion Factor
Hydromorphone	1
Codeine	0.06
Hydrocodone	0.4
Methadone[2]	0.6
Morphine	0.2
Oxycodone	0.4
Oxymorphone	0.6

[1]The conversion factors are only to be used for the conversion from current oral opioid therapy to Exalgo.

[2]Monitor closely; ratio between methadone and other opioid agonists may vary widely as a function of previous drug exposure. Methadone has a long half-life and may accumulate in the plasma.

Conversion from transdermal fentanyl to Exalgo: Treatment with Exalgo can be started 18 hours after the removal of the transdermal fentanyl patch. For every fentanyl 25 mcg/hour transdermal dose, the equianalgesic dose of Exalgo is 12 mg every 24 hours. An appropriate starting dose is 50% of the calculated total daily dose given every 24 hours. If necessary, round down to the appropriate Exalgo tablet strength available.

Titration and maintenance: Dose adjustments in 4 to 8 mg increments may occur every 3 to 4 days. In patients experiencing breakthrough pain, consider increasing the dose of Exalgo or providing rescue medication of an immediate-release analgesic at an appropriate dose. Do not administer Exalgo more frequently than every 24 hours.

Discontinuing Exalgo: Taper by gradually decreasing the dose by 25% to 50% every 2 to 3 days to a dose of 8 mg every 24 hours before discontinuing therapy.

Extended-release tablet: Jurnista [Canadian product]:
Note: May be used in conjunction with usual doses of nonopioid analgesics and analgesic adjuvants. If appropriate, initiate therapy with an immediate-release opioid formulation to establish a safe and effective dosage, then convert to an equivalent daily dose of extended-release hydromorphone. Tablets ≥16 mg are intended only for opioid-tolerant patients requiring hydromorphone equivalent dosages ≥16 mg daily.

Initial:

Patients who are opioid naive or receiving low intermittent doses of weak opioid analgesics (eg, <40 mg daily oral morphine equivalents): Initial: 4 mg once daily (if clinically indicated, an initial dose of 8 mg may be used; maximum initial dose: 8 mg once daily); titrate dose in increments of 4 or 8 mg as needed but no sooner than every fourth dose (eg, if first dose is administered on Tuesday, increase no sooner than on Friday).

Patients receiving opioids regularly: Discontinue all other around-the-clock opioid analgesics; initial Jurnista dose is based on previous daily opioid dose. For opioids other than morphine, estimate the equivalent daily dose of morphine then determine the equivalent total daily dose of Jurnista by multiplying the equivalent morphine dose by a factor of 0.2. For example, morphine 60 mg daily multiplied by 0.2 is equivalent to hydromorphone 12 mg daily. If necessary, round down to nearest Jurnista dose available and administer once daily.

Maintenance: Dose is individualized based on response. May consider dose increases of 25% to 75% of current daily dose made no sooner than every 4th dose (eg, if first dose is administered on Tuesday, increase no sooner than on Friday). Reassess the need for around-the-clock pain control periodically. Supplemental analgesia for breakthrough pain should typically not exceed 10% to 25% of the equivalent daily Jurnista dose.

Discontinuing Jurnista: Taper by gradually decreasing the dose by 50% every 2 days until lowest possible dose is reached and then discontinue. If signs of withdrawal occur during taper, stop taper and increase dose slightly until signs of withdrawal are no longer present. May then resume taper but with longer periods of time between each dose reduction, or before switching to an equianalgesic dose of another opioid to continue tapering.

Geriatric Doses should be titrated to appropriate analgesic effects. When changing routes of administration, oral doses and parenteral doses are **NOT** equivalent; parenteral doses are up to 5 times more potent. Therefore, when administered parenterally, one-fifth of the oral dose will provide similar analgesia.

Acute pain, opioid-naive:
Oral: Use with caution; initiation at the low end of dosage range is recommended. For patients >70 years, the American Pain Society recommends consideration to lowering initial doses by 25% to 50% followed by upward or downward titration (APS 2008).
IM, SubQ: Refer to adult dosing. Reduce initial doses as necessary.
IV: Reduce initial dose to 0.2 mg

Renal Impairment
Injectable:
US labeling: Initiate with 25% to 50% of the usual starting dose depending on the degree of impairment. Use with caution and monitor closely for respiratory and CNS depression.
Canadian labeling: There are no specific dosage adjustments provided in the manufacturer's labeling; however, a reduced initial dose is recommended for severe renal impairment. Use with caution and monitor closely for respiratory and CNS depression.
Oral (immediate release):
US labeling: There are no specific dosage adjustments provided in the manufacturer's labeling; however, a reduced initial dose is recommended for moderate impairment (CrCl ≤60 mL/minute) and an even lower initial dose is recommended for severe impairment (CrCl <30 mL/minute). Use with caution and monitor closely for respiratory and CNS depression.
Canadian labeling: There are no specific dosage adjustments provided in the manufacturer's labeling; however, a reduced initial dose is recommended for severe renal impairment. Use with caution and monitor closely for respiratory and CNS depression.

Oral (extended-release tablet):
Exalgo:
Mild impairment: There are no dosage adjustments provided in the manufacturer's labeling.
Moderate impairment (CrCl ≤60 mL/minute): Initiate with 50% of the usual starting dose for patients with normal renal function. Use with caution and monitor closely for respiratory and CNS depression.
Severe impairment (CrCl <30 mL/minute): Initiate with 25% of the usual starting dose for patients with normal renal function. Use with caution and monitor closely for respiratory and CNS depression. Consider use of an alternate analgesic with better dosing flexibility.
Jurnista [Canadian product]:
Mild impairment: There are no dosage adjustments provided in the manufacturer's labeling.
Moderate impairment: There are no specific dosage adjustments provided in the manufacturer's labeling; however, an initial dosage reduction is recommended. Use with caution and monitor closely for respiratory and CNS depression.
Severe impairment: There are no specific dosage adjustments provided in the manufacturer's labeling. Reduce initial dose and consider extending the dosing interval. Use with caution and monitor closely for respiratory and CNS depression.
Oral (extended-release capsule): Hydromorph contin [Canadian product]:
Mild impairment: There are no dosage adjustments provided in the manufacturer's labeling; use with caution and monitor closely for respiratory and CNS depression.
Moderate impairment: Initiate at 50% of initial dose for normal renal function; titrate cautiously. Monitor closely for respiratory and CNS depression following initiation of therapy and during titration.
Severe impairment: Initiate at 25% of initial dose for normal renal function; titrate cautiously. Monitor closely for respiratory and CNS depression following initiation of therapy and during titration.
Rectal suppository:
US labeling: There are no dosage adjustments provided in the manufacturer's labeling. Use with caution and monitor closely for respiratory and CNS depression.
Canadian labeling: There are no specific dosage adjustments provided in the manufacturer's labeling; however, an initial dosage reduction is recommended for severe renal impairment. Use with caution and monitor closely for respiratory and CNS depression

Hepatic Impairment
Injectable:
US labeling:
Mild impairment: There are no specific dosage adjustments provided in the manufacturer's labeling.
Moderate impairment: Initiate therapy with 25% to 50% of the usual initial dose. Use with caution and monitor closely for respiratory and CNS depression.
Severe impairment: There are no specific dosage adjustments provided in the manufacturer's labeling (has not been studied); however, further dose reductions (compared with those recommended for moderate impairment) are recommended. Use with caution and monitor closely for respiratory and CNS depression.
Canadian labeling: There are no specific dosage adjustments provided in the manufacturer's labeling; however, a reduced initial dose is recommended in severe hepatic impairment. Use with caution and monitor closely for respiratory and CNS depression.
There are no specific dosage adjustments provided in the manufacturer's labeling; however, an initial dosage reduction is recommended. Use with caution and monitor closely for respiratory and CNS depression.
Oral (immediate release):
US labeling:
Mild impairment: There are no specific dosage adjustments provided in the manufacturer's labeling.
Moderate impairment: There are no specific dosage adjustments provided in the manufacturer's labeling; however, an initial dosage reduction is recommended. Use with caution and monitor closely for respiratory and CNS depression.
Severe impairment: There are no specific dosage adjustments provided in the manufacturer's labeling (has not been studied); initial dose reduction is recommended. Use with caution and monitor closely for respiratory and CNS depression.

Canadian labeling: There are no specific dosage adjustments provided in the manufacturer's labeling; however, a reduced initial dose is recommended in severe hepatic impairment. Use with caution and monitor closely for respiratory and CNS depression.

Oral (extended-release tablet):

Exalgo:

Mild impairment: There are no dosage adjustments provided in the manufacturer's labeling.

Moderate impairment: Initiate with 25% of the usual starting dose for patients with normal hepatic function. Use with caution and monitor closely for respiratory and CNS depression.

Severe impairment: Use alternate analgesic.

Jurnista [Canadian product]:

Mild impairment: There are no dosage adjustments provided in the manufacturer's labeling.

Moderate impairment: There are no specific dosage adjustments provided in the manufacturer's labeling; however, a reduced initial dosage is recommended. Use with caution and monitor closely for respiratory and CNS depression.

Severe impairment: There are no specific dosage adjustments provided in the manufacturer's labeling; reduce initial dose and use with caution. Monitor closely for respiratory and CNS depression.

Oral (extended-release capsule): Hydromorph contin [Canadian product]:

Mild impairment: There are no dosage adjustments provided in the manufacturer's labeling; use with caution and monitor for respiratory and CNS depression.

Moderate impairment: Initiate at 25% of initial dose for normal hepatic function; titrate cautiously. Monitor closely for respiratory and CNS depression following initiation of therapy and during titration.

Severe impairment: Use is not recommended (has not been studied); consider alternative analgesics. If therapy with hydromorphone is initiated, the manufacturer recommends a more conservative dose than that recommended for moderate impairment but does not provide specific dosing recommendations. Monitor closely for respiratory and CNS depression.

Rectal suppository:

US labeling: There are no dosage adjustments provided in the manufacturer's labeling. Use with caution and monitor closely for respiratory and CNS depression.

Canadian labeling: There are no specific dosage adjustments provided in the manufacturer's labeling; however, an initial dosage reduction is recommended for severe hepatic impairment. Use with caution and monitor closely for respiratory and CNS depression.

Administration

Parenteral: Note: Vial stopper may contain latex. May be given SubQ or IM; IM route is not recommended (APS 2008).

IV: For IVP, must be given slowly over 2 to 3 minutes (rapid IVP has been associated with an increase in side effects, especially respiratory depression and hypotension)

Oral: Hydromorphone is available in an 8 mg immediate-release tablet and an 8 mg extended-release tablet. Extreme caution should be taken to avoid confusing dosage forms.

Exalgo, Jurnista [Canadian product]: Tablets should be swallowed whole; do not crush, break, chew, dissolve or inject. May be taken with or without food.

Hydromorph Contin [Canadian product]: For oral use only. Capsule should be swallowed whole; do not crush or chew. Contents may be sprinkled on a tablespoon of applesauce (stored at room temperature or under refrigeration) or custard (stored at room temperature) and swallowed without chewing as soon as possible (discard if not consumed within 30 minutes); patient should then rinse mouth with water to ensure entire contents are swallowed.

Monitoring Parameters Pain relief, respiratory and mental status, blood pressure; signs of misuse, abuse, and addiction; signs or symptoms of hypogonadism or hypoadrenalism (Brennan 2013)

Test Interactions Some quinolones may produce a false-positive urine screening result for opioids using commercially-available immunoassay kits. This has been demonstrated most consistently for levofloxacin and ofloxacin, but other quinolones have shown cross-reactivity in certain assay kits. Confirmation of positive opioid screens by more specific methods should be considered.

Dosage Forms Excipient information presented when available (limited, particularly for generics); consult specific product labeling. [DSC] = Discontinued product

Liquid, Oral, as hydrochloride:

Dilaudid: 1 mg/mL (473 mL) [contains methylparaben, propylparaben, sodium metabisulfite; sweet flavor]

Generic: 1 mg/mL (473 mL)

Solution, Injection, as hydrochloride:

Dilaudid: 1 mg/mL (1 mL [DSC]); 2 mg/mL (1 mL); 4 mg/mL (1 mL)

Dilaudid-HP: 10 mg/mL (1 mL, 5 mL, 50 mL [DSC])

Generic: 1 mg/mL (0.5 mL, 1 mL); 2 mg/mL (1 mL, 20 mL); 4 mg/mL (1 mL); 10 mg/mL (1 mL); 50 mg/5 mL (5 mL); 500 mg/50 mL (50 mL)

Solution, Injection, as hydrochloride [preservative free]:

Generic: 10 mg/mL (1 mL); 50 mg/5 mL (5 mL); 500 mg/ 50 mL (50 mL)

Solution Prefilled Syringe, Intravenous:

Generic: 10 mg/50 mL (50 mL)

Solution Reconstituted, Injection, as hydrochloride:

Dilaudid-HP: 250 mg (1 ea [DSC])

Suppository, Rectal, as hydrochloride:

Generic: 3 mg (6 ea)

Tablet, Oral, as hydrochloride:

Dilaudid: 2 mg, 4 mg [contains fd&c yellow #10 aluminum lake, sodium metabisulfite]

Dilaudid: 8 mg [scored; contains sodium metabisulfite]

Generic: 2 mg, 4 mg, 8 mg

Tablet ER 24 Hour Abuse-Deterrent, Oral, as hydrochloride:

Exalgo: 8 mg, 12 mg, 16 mg, 32 mg [contains sodium metabisulfite]

Generic: 8 mg, 12 mg, 16 mg, 32 mg

Dosage Forms: Canada Excipient information presented when available (limited, particularly for generics); consult specific product labeling.

Capsule, controlled release:

Hydromorph Contin: 3 mg, 4.5 mg, 6 mg, 9 mg, 12 mg, 18 mg, 24 mg, 30 mg

Tablet extended release 24 Hour, Oral, as hydrochloride:

Jurnista: 4 mg, 8 mg, 16 mg, 32 mg (may contain traces of sodium metabisulfite)

Controlled Substance C-II

♦ Hydromorphone HP (Can) *see* HYDROmorphone *on page* 888

♦ Hydromorphone HP Forte Injection (Can) *see* HYDROmorphone *on page* 888

♦ Hydromorphone Hydrochloride *see* HYDROmorphone *on page* 888

♦ Hydromorphone Hydrochloride Injection, USP (Can) *see* HYDROmorphone *on page* 888

♦ Hydromorphone Hydrochloride Injection USP HP 10 (Can) *see* HYDROmorphone *on page* 888

♦ Hydroquinol *see* Hydroquinone *on page* 893

Hydroquinone (HYE droe kwin one)

Brand Names: US Aclaro; Aclaro PD; Alphaquin HP; Blanche; Eldopaque Forte [DSC]; Eldopaque [OTC] [DSC]; Eldoquin Forte [DSC]; Eldoquin [OTC] [DSC]; EpiQuin Micro; EpiQuin Micro/Pump [DSC]; Esoterica Daytime [OTC]; Esoterica Facial [OTC]; Esoterica Fade Nighttime [OTC]; Esoterica Regular [OTC] [DSC]; Esoterica Sensitive Skin [OTC]; Exuviance Lightening Complex [OTC]; Hydroquinone Time Release; Lustra [DSC]; Lustra-AF [DSC]; Lustra-Ultra [DSC]; Melpaque HP; Melquin 3; Melquin HP [DSC]; NAVA-SC; NeoCeuticals Post-Acne Fade [OTC]; NeoStrata HQ Skin Lightening [OTC]; Nuquin HP [DSC]; Remergent HQ; Skin Bleaching; Skin Bleaching-Sunscreen; TL Hydroquinone

Brand Names: Canada Eldopaque®; Eldoquin®; Glyquin® XM; Lustra®; NeoStrata® HQ; Solaquin Forte®; Solaquin®; Ultraquin™

Index Terms Hydroquinol; Quinol

Pharmacologic Category Depigmenting Agent

Use Gradual bleaching of hyperpigmented skin conditions

Dosing

Adult & Geriatric Bleaching: Topical: Apply a thin layer and rub in twice daily.

Pediatric Refer to adult dosing.

Additional Information Complete prescribing information should be consulted for additional detail.

Dosage Forms Excipient information presented when available (limited, particularly for generics); consult specific product labeling. [DSC] = Discontinued product

Cream, External:

Alphaquin HP: 4% (28.4 g, 56.7 g)

Blanche: 4% (30 g) [contains cetearyl alcohol, disodium edta, sodium metabisulfite]

Eldopaque: 2% (28.35 g [DSC])
Eldopaque Forte: 4% (28.35 g [DSC])
Eldoquin: 2% (28.35 g [DSC])
Eldoquin Forte: 4% (28.35 g [DSC]) [contains sodium metabisulfite]
EpiQuin Micro: 4% (30 g) [contains benzyl alcohol, methylparaben, sodium metabisulfite, trolamine (triethanolamine), vitamin a, vitamin e]
EpiQuin Micro/Pump: 4% (40 g [DSC]) [contains benzyl alcohol, cetyl alcohol, edetate disodium, methylparaben, sodium metabisulfite, trolamine (triethanolamine)]
Esoterica Daytime: 2% (70 g) [contains disodium edta, methylparaben, propylene glycol, propylparaben, sodium bisulfite]
Esoterica Daytime: 2% (70 g) [contains disodium edta, methylparaben, propylene glycol, propylparaben, sodium metabisulfite]
Esoterica Facial: 2% (85 g)
Esoterica Fade Nighttime: 2% (70 g) [contains disodium edta, methylparaben, propylene glycol, propylparaben, sodium metabisulfite]
Esoterica Regular: 2% (85 g [DSC])
Esoterica Sensitive Skin: 1.5% (85 g)
Hydroquinone Time Release: 4% (30 g) [contains benzyl alcohol, cetyl alcohol, edetate disodium, sodium metabisulfite, trolamine (triethanolamine)]
Lustra: 4% (56.8 g [DSC]) [contains sodium metabisulfite]
Lustra-AF: 4% (56.8 g [DSC]) [contains sodium metabisulfite, trolamine (triethanolamine)]
Lustra-Ultra: 4% (28.4 g [DSC], 56.8 g [DSC]) [contains methylparaben, octyl methoxycinnamate (octinoxate), propylparaben, sodium metabisulfite, vitamin a]
Melpaque HP: 4% (14.2 g [DSC], 28.4 g)
Melquin HP: 4% (14.2 g [DSC], 28.4 g [DSC])
NAVA-SC: 4% (28.4 g) [contains propylene glycol, sodium metabisulfite]
Nuquin HP: 4% (14.2 g [DSC], 28.4 g [DSC], 56.7 g [DSC]) [contains propylene glycol, sodium metabisulfite]
Remergent HQ: 4% (30 mL) [contains sodium metabisulfite]
Skin Bleaching: 4% (28.35 g)
Skin Bleaching-Sunscreen: 4% (28.35 g) [contains cetostearyl alcohol, glycerin, isopropyl palmitate, propylene glycol, sodium lauryl sulfate, sodium metabisulfite, sorbic acid, water, purified]
TL Hydroquinone: 4% (30 g) [contains benzyl alcohol, cetearyl alcohol, cetyl alcohol, edetate disodium, methylparaben, sodium metabisulfite, trolamine (triethanolamine)]
Generic: 4% (28.35 g, 28.4 g [DSC])
Emulsion, External:
Aclaro: 4% (48.2 g) [contains benzyl alcohol, sodium metabisulfite]
Aclaro PD: 4% (42.5 g)
Generic: 4% (48.2 g [DSC])
Gel, External:
Exuviance Lightening Complex: 2% (30 g) [contains denatured alcohol, propylene glycol, sodium bisulfite, sodium sulfite, tartrazine (fd&c yellow #5)]
NeoCeuticals Post-Acne Fade: 2% (30 g) [contains denatured alcohol, propylene glycol, sodium bisulfite, sodium sulfite, tartrazine (fd&c yellow #5)]
NeoStrata HQ Skin Lightening: 2% (30 g) [fragrance free, oil free; contains propylene glycol, sodium bisulfite, sodium sulfite]
Nuquin HP: 4% (14.2 g [DSC], 28.4 g [DSC])
Generic: 4% (28.35 g [DSC])
Solution, External:
Melquin 3: 3% (29.57 mL)

◆ Hydroquinone, Fluocinolone Acetonide, and Tretinoin see Fluocinolone, Hydroquinone, and Tretinoin on page 781
◆ Hydroquinone Time Release see Hydroquinone on page 893
◆ HydroSKIN [OTC] see Hydrocortisone (Topical) on page 886
◆ Hydro Skin Maximum Strength [OTC] see Hydrocortisone (Topical) on page 886
◆ HydroVal (Can) see Hydrocortisone (Topical) on page 886

Hydroxocobalamin (hye droks oh koe BAL a min)

Brand Names: US Cyanokit
Brand Names: Canada Cyanokit
Index Terms Vitamin B$_{12a}$
Pharmacologic Category Antidote; Vitamin, Water Soluble

Use
IM injection: Treatment of pernicious anemia; treatment of vitamin B$_{12}$ deficiency due to dietary deficiencies or malabsorption diseases, inadequate secretion of intrinsic factor, competition for vitamin B$_{12}$ by intestinal parasites/bacteria, or inadequate utilization of B$_{12}$ (eg, during neoplastic treatment)
IV infusion (Cyanokit®): Treatment of cyanide poisoning (known or suspected)
Dosing
Adult & Geriatric
Cyanide poisoning: IV: **Note:** If cyanide poisoning is suspected, antidotal therapy must be given immediately. Initial: 5 **g** as single infusion; may repeat a second 5 **g** dose depending on the severity of poisoning and clinical response. Maximum cumulative dose: 10 **g**.
Vitamin B$_{12}$ deficiency: IM: Initial: 30 mcg once daily for 5-10 days; maintenance: 100-200 mcg once per month. **Note:** Larger doses may be required in critically-ill patients or if patient has neurologic disease, an infectious disease, or hyperthyroidism.
Pediatric
Vitamin B$_{12}$ deficiency: IM: 100 mcg once daily for ≥2 weeks (total dose: 1-5 **mg**); maintenance: 30-50 mcg once per month
Cyanide poisoning (off-label use): IV: **Note:** If cyanide poisoning is suspected, antidotal therapy must be given immediately; Initial: 70 mg/kg (maximum: 5 **g**) as a single infusion; may repeat a second dose of 35 mg/kg depending on the severity of poisoning and clinical response (Shepherd, 2008).
Renal Impairment No dosage adjustments provided in manufacturer's labeling (has not been studied).
Hepatic Impairment No dosage adjustments provided in manufacturer's labeling (has not been studied).
Additional Information Complete prescribing information should be consulted for additional detail.
Dosage Forms Excipient information presented when available (limited, particularly for generics); consult specific product labeling. [DSC] = Discontinued product
Solution, Intramuscular:
Generic: 1000 mcg/mL (30 mL)
Solution Reconstituted, Intravenous:
Cyanokit: 5 g (1 ea)

◆ 4-Hydroxybutyrate see Sodium Oxybate on page 1676
◆ Hydroxycarbamide see Hydroxyurea on page 895

Hydroxychloroquine (hye droks ee KLOR oh kwin)

Brand Names: US Plaquenil
Brand Names: Canada Apo-Hydroxyquine; Gen-Hydroxychloroquine; Mylan-Hydroxychloroquine; Plaquenil; PRO-Hydroxyquine
Index Terms Hydroxychloroquine Sulfate
Pharmacologic Category Aminoquinoline (Antimalarial); Antimalarial Agent
Use Suppression and treatment of acute attacks of malaria; treatment of systemic lupus erythematosus (SLE) and rheumatoid arthritis
Dosing
Adult & Geriatric Note: Hydroxychloroquine sulfate 200 mg is equivalent to 155 mg hydroxychloroquine base and 250 mg chloroquine phosphate. All doses below expressed as hydroxychloroquine sulfate. Second-line alternative treatment for malaria (chloroquine is preferred).

Malaria, chemoprophylaxis: Oral: 400 mg weekly on same day each week; begin 2 weeks before exposure; continue for 4 weeks (per CDC guidelines) after leaving endemic area; if suppressive therapy is not begun prior to the exposure, double the initial dose and give in 2 doses, 6 hours apart and continue treatment for 8 weeks
Malaria, acute attack: Oral: 800 mg initially, followed by 400 mg at 6, 24, and 48 hours
Rheumatoid arthritis: Oral: Initial: 400 to 600 mg daily taken with food or milk; increase dose gradually until optimum response level is reached; usually after 4 to 12 weeks dose should be reduced by 1/2 to a maintenance dose of 200 to 400 mg daily in 1 to 2 divided doses.
Lupus erythematosus: Oral: 400 mg every day or twice daily for several weeks-months depending on response; 200 to 400 mg daily in 1 to 2 divided doses for prolonged maintenance therapy
Q fever, chronic (off-label use; CDC, 2013): Oral:
Endocarditis or vascular infection: 200 mg every 8 hours in combination with doxycycline for ≥18 months
Noncardiac organ disease: 200 mg every 8 hours in combination with doxycycline (duration based on serologic response; ID consult recommended)

Postpartum with serologic evidence present >12 months after delivery: 200 mg every 8 hours in combination with doxycycline for 12 months

Pediatric Note: Hydroxychloroquine sulfate 200 mg is equivalent to 155 mg hydroxychloroquine base and 250 mg chloroquine phosphate. All doses below expressed as hydroxychloroquine sulfate. Second-line alternative treatment for malaria (chloroquine is preferred).

Malaria, chemoprophylaxis: Oral: 6.5 mg/kg once weekly (not to exceed 400 mg/dose); begin 2 weeks before exposure; continue for 4 weeks (per CDC guidelines) after leaving endemic area; if suppressive therapy is not begun prior to the exposure, double the initial dose and give in 2 doses, 6 hours apart and continue treatment for 8 weeks

Malaria, acute attack: Oral: 13 mg/kg initially (not to exceed 800 mg/dose), followed by 6.5 mg/kg (not to exceed 400 mg/dose) at 6, 24, and 48 hours

Renal Impairment Use with caution; dosage adjustment may be necessary in severe dysfunction (Bernstein, 1992); specific guidelines not available.

Hepatic Impairment Use with caution; dosage adjustment may be necessary.

Additional Information Complete prescribing information should be consulted for additional detail.

Dosage Forms Excipient information presented when available (limited, particularly for generics); consult specific product labeling.
Tablet, Oral, as sulfate:
Plaquenil: 200 mg
Generic: 200 mg

◆ Hydroxychloroquine Sulfate *see* Hydroxychloroquine *on page 894*

◆ Hydroxydaunomycin Hydrochloride *see* DOXOrubicin (Conventional) *on page 593*

◆ Hydroxyethyl Starch *see* Hetastarch *on page 877*

◆ Hydroxyethyl Starch *see* Tetrastarch *on page 1774*

◆ Hydroxyldaunorubicin Hydrochloride *see* DOXOrubicin (Conventional) *on page 593*

Hydroxyprogesterone Caproate
(hye droks ee proe JES te rone CAP ro ate)

Brand Names: US Makena
Index Terms 17OHPC
Pharmacologic Category Progestin
Use
Preterm birth: To reduce the risk of preterm birth in women with a singleton pregnancy who have a history of singleton spontaneous preterm birth.
Limitation of use: Safety and efficacy have been demonstrated only in women with a prior spontaneous singleton preterm birth. Use is not intended for women with multiple gestations or other risk factors for preterm birth.

Prescribing and Access Restrictions The Makena Care Connection™ is a comprehensive program for patients and healthcare providers which provides administrative support (including insurance benefit investigation and prescription fulfillment); financial and co-pay assistance for eligible patients; and treatment support (including educational information, home health care service and scheduled treatment reminders). The Makena Care Connection™ is available by calling 1-800-847-3418, Monday-Friday, 8 AM to 9 PM EST.

Dosing
Adult Preterm birth: Pregnant females ≥16 years: IM: 250 mg once weekly (every 7 days). Treatment may begin between 16 weeks 0 days and 20 weeks 6 days of gestation. Continue weekly administration until 37 weeks gestation or until delivery, whichever comes first.

Renal Impairment No dosage adjustment provided in manufacturer's labeling (has not been studied).

Hepatic Impairment No dosage adjustment provided in manufacturer's labeling (has not been studied). However, hydroxyprogesterone caproate is extensively metabolized and hepatic impairment may reduce its elimination.

Additional Information Complete prescribing information should be consulted for additional detail.

Dosage Forms Excipient information presented when available (limited, particularly for generics); consult specific product labeling.
Oil, Intramuscular:
Makena: 250 mg/mL (5 mL) [contains benzyl alcohol, benzyl benzoate]

◆ 9-hydroxy-risperidone *see* Paliperidone *on page 1374*

Hydroxyurea (hye droks ee yoor EE a)

Brand Names: US Droxia; Hydrea
Brand Names: Canada Apo-Hydroxyurea; Gen-Hydroxyurea; Hydrea; Mylan-Hydroxyurea
Index Terms HU; Hydroxycarbamide; Hydurea
Pharmacologic Category Antineoplastic Agent, Miscellaneous
Use
Chronic myeloid leukemia: Treatment of refractory chronic myeloid leukemia (CML)
Head and neck cancer: Management (with concomitant radiation therapy) of locally advanced squamous cell head and neck cancer (excluding lip cancer)
Sickle cell anemia: Management of sickle cell anemia (to reduce the frequency of painful crises and to reduce the need for blood transfusions in patients with recurrent moderate to severe painful crises)

Pregnancy Considerations Animal reproduction studies have demonstrated teratogenicity and embryotoxicity at doses lower than the usual human dose (based on BSA). Hydroxyurea may cause fetal harm if administered during pregnancy. Women of childbearing potential should be advised to avoid becoming pregnant during treatment and should use effective contraception during and for at least 30 days after completion of therapy. Males of childbearing potential should use effective contraception during and for at least 1 year after therapy.

Breast-Feeding Considerations Hydroxyurea is excreted in breast milk. Due to the potential for serious adverse reactions in the nursing infant, breast-feeding is not recommended by the manufacturer.

Contraindications Hypersensitivity to hydroxyurea or any component of the formulation

Warnings/Precautions Hazardous agent - use appropriate precautions for handling and disposal (NIOSH 2014 [group 1]); to decrease risk of exposure, wear gloves when handling and wash hands before and after contact. **[US Boxed Warning]: Hydroxyurea may cause severe myelosuppression. Monitor blood counts at baseline and throughout treatment. Interrupt treatment and reduce dose as necessary.** Leukopenia and neutropenia commonly occur (thrombocytopenia and anemia are less common); leukopenia/neutropenia occur first. Severe or life-threatening myelosuppression may occur at the recommended dose. Hematologic toxicity reversible (rapid) with treatment interruption. Correct severe anemia prior to initiating treatment. Do not initiate therapy if bone marrow function is markedly reduced. Hydroxyurea should not be used in sickle cell anemia with severe bone marrow suppression (neutrophils <2,000/mm³, platelets <80,000/mm³, hemoglobin <4.5 g/dL, or reticulocytes <80,000/mm³ when hemoglobin <9 g/dL per manufacturer's labeling). Use with caution in patients with a history of prior chemotherapy or radiation therapy; myelosuppression is more common. Patients with a history of radiation therapy are also at risk for exacerbation of post irradiation erythema. Self-limiting macrocytosis/megaloblastic erythropoiesis may be seen early in treatment (may resemble pernicious anemia, but is unrelated to vitamin B_{12} or folic acid deficiency). Prophylactic folic acid supplementation is recommended. Plasma iron clearance may be delayed and iron utilization rate (by erythrocytes) may be reduced. Potentially significant drug-drug interactions may exist, requiring dose or frequency adjustment, additional monitoring, and/or selection of alternative therapy. When treated concurrently with hydroxyurea and antiretroviral agents (including didanosine and stavudine), HIV-infected patients are at higher risk for potentially fatal pancreatitis, hepatotoxicity, hepatic failure, and severe peripheral neuropathy; discontinue immediately if signs of these toxicities develop. Hyperuricemia may occur with antineoplastic treatment; adequate hydration and initiation or dosage adjustment of uricosuric agents (eg, allopurinol) may be necessary.

In patients with sickle cell anemia, Droxia is not recommended if neutrophils <2,000/mm³, platelets <80,000/mm³, hemoglobin <4.5 g/dL, or reticulocytes <80,000/mm³ when hemoglobin <9 g/dL per manufacturer's labeling. May cause macrocytosis, which can mask folic acid deficiency; prophylactic folic acid supplementation is recommended. **[US Boxed Warning]: Hydroxyurea is carcinogenic. Advise sun protection and monitor patients for malignancies.** Treatment of myeloproliferative disorders (eg, polycythemia vera, thrombocythemia) with long-term hydroxyurea is associated with secondary leukemia; it is unknown if this is drug-related or disease-related. Skin cancer has been reported with long-term hydroxyurea use. Monitor for signs/symptoms of secondary malignancies. Cutaneous vasculitic toxicities (vasculitic ulceration and gangrene) have been reported ▶

with hydroxyurea treatment, most often in patients with a history of or receiving concurrent interferon therapy; discontinue hydroxyurea and consider alternate cytoreductive therapy if cutaneous vasculitic toxicity develops. Use caution with renal dysfunction; may require dose reductions. Elderly patients may be more sensitive to the effects of hydroxyurea; may require lower doses.

Adverse Reactions Frequency not always defined.

Cardiovascular: Edema, hypersensitivity angiitis

Central nervous system: Chills, disorientation, dizziness, drowsiness (dose-related), hallucination, headache, malaise, peripheral neuropathy (HIV-infected patients), seizure, vasculitic ulcerations

Dermatologic: Eczema (infants and children 9 to 18 months: 13% [Thornburg 2012]), leg ulcer (7% [Hernández-Boluda 2011]), dermal ulcer (3% [Antonioli 2012]), nail discoloration (2% [Randi 2005]), alopecia (infrequent, [Hernández-Boluda 2011]), changes in nails (infrequent, [Hernández-Boluda 2011]), hyperpigmentation (infrequent, [Hernández-Boluda 2011]), atrophy of nail, dermatomyositis-like skin changes, desquamation, erythema (peripheral), facial erythema, gangrene of skin or other tissue, maculopapular rash, papule (violet), skin atrophy, skin carcinoma

Endocrine & metabolic: Increased uric acid

Gastrointestinal: Acute mucocutaneous toxicity (5% [Hernández-Boluda 2011]), diarrhea (infrequent, [Antonioli 2012]), gastric distress (infrequent, [Antonioli 2012]), nausea (infrequent, [Antonioli 2012]), oral mucosa ulcer (infrequent, [Hernández-Boluda 2011]), anorexia, BSP abnormality (retention), constipation, gastrointestinal irritation (potentiated with radiation therapy), mucositis (potentiated with radiation therapy), pancreatitis (HIV-infected patients), stomatitis, vomiting

Genitourinary: Dysuria

Hematologic & oncologic: Leukemia (4% [Hernández-Boluda 2011]; secondary; long-term use), leukopenia (2% [Hernández-Boluda 2011]), bone marrow depression (neutropenia [common], thrombocytopenia; hematologic recovery: within 2 weeks; abnormal erythropoiesis (megaloblastic; self-limiting), macrocytosis (MCV >97: 42% [Randi 2005]), reticulocytopenia (infants and children 9 to 18 months [Wang 2011])

Hepatic: Hepatic failure (HIV-infected patients), hepatotoxicity, increased liver enzymes

Neuromuscular & skeletal: Panniculitis (Antonioli 2012), weakness

Renal: Increased blood urea nitrogen, increased serum creatinine, renal tubular disease

Respiratory: Asthma (infants and children 9 to 18 months: 9% [Thornburg 2012]), dyspnea, pulmonary fibrosis (rare), pulmonary infiltrates (diffuse, rare)

<1% (Limited to important or life-threatening): Actinic keratosis (Antonioli 2012), basal cell carcinoma (Antonioli 2012), hyperkeratosis (Antonioli 2012), lesion (dyschromic [Antonioli 2012]), malignant neoplasm (Wong 2014), mucous membrane lesion (Antonioli 2012), pneumonitis (Antonioli 2012), squamous cell carcinoma (Antonioli 2012)

Drug Interactions

Metabolism/Transport Effects None known.

Avoid Concomitant Use

Avoid concomitant use of Hydroxyurea with any of the following: BCG (Intravesical); Deferiprone; Didanosine; Dipyrone; Natalizumab; Pimecrolimus; Stavudine; Tacrolimus (Topical); Tofacitinib; Vaccines (Live)

Increased Effect/Toxicity

Hydroxyurea may increase the levels/effects of: CloZAPine; Deferiprone; Didanosine; Fingolimod; Leflunomide; Natalizumab; Stavudine; Tofacitinib; Vaccines (Live)

The levels/effects of Hydroxyurea may be increased by: Denosumab; Didanosine; Dipyrone; Pimecrolimus; Roflumilast; Stavudine; Tacrolimus (Topical); Trastuzumab

Decreased Effect

Hydroxyurea may decrease the levels/effects of: BCG (Intravesical); Coccidioides immitis Skin Test; Sipuleucel-T; Vaccines (Inactivated); Vaccines (Live)

The levels/effects of Hydroxyurea may be decreased by: Echinacea

Storage/Stability Store at 25°C (77°F); excursions permitted between 15°C and 30°C (59°F and 86°F). Keep bottle tightly closed.

Mechanism of Action Antimetabolite which selectively inhibits ribonucleoside diphosphate reductase, preventing the conversion of ribonucleotides to deoxyribonucleotides, halting the cell cycle at the G1/S phase and therefore has radiation sensitizing activity by maintaining cells in the G_1 phase and interfering with DNA repair. In sickle cell anemia, hydroxyurea increases red blood cell (RBC) hemoglobin F levels, RBC water content, deformability of sickled cells, and alters adhesion of RBCs to endothelium.

Pharmacodynamics/Kinetics Note: In pediatric patients, large interpatient variability and phenotypic differences have been reported (Ware 2011).

Onset: Sickle cell anemia: Fetal hemoglobin increase: 4 to 12 weeks

Absorption: Readily absorbed (≥80%); relatively rapid (Rodriguez 1998)

Distribution: Distributes widely into tissues (including into the brain); estimated volume of distribution approximates total body water (Gwilt 1998); concentrates in leukocytes and erythrocytes

V_d: Children: ~12 L (range: 2.5 to 52) (Ware 2011); Adults: ~20 L/m² (Rodriguez 1998)

Metabolism: Up to 60% via hepatic metabolism and urease found in intestinal bacteria

Bioavailability: ~100% (Rodriguez 1998)

Protein binding: 75% to 80% bound to serum proteins (Gwilt 1998)

Half-life elimination: 1.9 to 3.9 hours (Gwilt 1998); Children: Sickle cell anemia: 1.7 hours (range: 0.7 to 3 hours) (Ware 2011)

Time to peak: Children: "Fast" phenotype: 15 to 30 minutes; "Slow" phenotype: 60 to 120 minutes (Ware 2011); Adults: 1 to 4 hours

Excretion: Urine (sickle cell anemia: ~40% of administered dose)

Clearance: Children: ~7 L/hour (range: 1.6 to 22) (Ware 2011); Adults: ~7.5 L/hour (Rodriguez 1998)

Dosing

Adult Note: Doses should be based on ideal or actual body weight, whichever is less (per manufacturer). Prophylactic administration of folic acid is recommended.

Antineoplastic uses (chronic myeloid leukemia [CML], head and neck cancer): Oral: Initial: 15 mg/kg/day; individualize treatment based on tumor type, disease state, response to treatment, patient risk factors, and current clinical practice standards. May be used alone or in combination with other agents or radiation.

Sickle cell anemia: Oral:

Manufacturer's labeling: Initial: 15 mg/kg/day as a single dose; if blood counts are in an acceptable range, may increase by 5 mg/kg/day every 12 weeks until the maximum tolerated dose of 35 mg/kg/day is achieved or the dose that does not produce toxic effects over 24 consecutive weeks (do not increase dose if blood counts are between acceptable and toxic ranges). Monitor for toxicity every 2 weeks; if toxicity occurs, withhold treatment until the bone marrow recovers, then restart with a dose reduction of 2.5 mg/kg/day; if no toxicity occurs over the next 12 weeks, then the subsequent dose may be increased by 2.5 mg/kg/day every 12 weeks to a maximum tolerated dose (dose which does not produce hematologic toxicity for 24 consecutive weeks). If hematologic toxicity recurs a second time at a specific dose, do not retry that dose.

Acceptable hematologic ranges: Neutrophils ≥2,500/mm³; platelets ≥95,000/mm³; hemoglobin >5.3 g/dL, and reticulocytes ≥95,000/mm³ if the hemoglobin concentration is <9 g/dL

Toxic hematologic ranges: Neutrophils <2,000/mm³; platelets <80,000/mm³; hemoglobin <4.5 g/dL; and reticulocytes <80,000/mm³ if the hemoglobin concentration is <9 g/dL

Alternate recommendations (off-label dose): Initial: 15 mg/kg/day; if dosage escalation is warranted based on clinical/laboratory findings, may increase by 5 mg/kg/day increments every 8 weeks. Monitor for toxicity at least every 4 weeks when adjusting dose; aim for a target absolute neutrophils ≥2,000/mm³ (younger patients with lower baseline counts may safely tolerate absolute neutrophils down to 1,250/mm³; maintain platelet count ≥80,000/mm³. Give until mild myelosuppression is achieved (absolute neutrophils: 2,000/mm³ to 4,000/mm³), up to a maximum dose of 35 mg/kg/day. If toxicity occurs (neutropenia or thrombocytopenia), withhold treatment until the bone marrow recovers (monitor weekly), then restart at a dose 5mg/kg/day lower than the dose given prior to onset of cytopenias (NHLBI 2014). **Note:** A clinical response to treatment may take 3 to 6 months; a 6 month trial on the maximum tolerated dose is recommended prior to considering discontinuation due to treatment failure; effectiveness of hydroxyurea depends upon daily dosing adherence. For patients who have a clinical response, long-term hydroxyurea therapy is indicated (NHLBI 2014)

Acute myeloid leukemia (AML), cytoreduction (off-label use): Oral: 50 to 100 mg/kg/day until WBC <100,000/mm³ (Grund 1977) **or** 50 to 60 mg/kg/day until WBC <10,000 to 20,000/mm³ (Dohner 2010)

Essential thrombocythemia, high-risk (off-label use): Oral: 500 to 1000 mg daily; adjust dose to maintain platelets <400,000/mm^3 (Harrison 2005)

Head and neck cancer (off-label dosing; with concurrent radiation therapy and fluorouracil): Oral: 1000 mg every 12 hours for 11 doses per cycle (Garden 2004)

Hypereosinophilic syndrome (off-label use): Oral: 1,000 to 3,000 mg/day (Klion 2006)

Meningioma (off-label use): Oral: 20 mg/kg once daily (Newton 2000; Rosenthal 2002)

Polycythemia vera, high-risk (off-label use): Oral: 15 to 20 mg/kg/day (Finazzi 2007)

Geriatric Refer to adult dosing. May require lower doses.

Pediatric Note: Doses should be based on ideal or actual body weight, whichever is less (per manufacturer). Prophylactic administration of folic acid is recommended.

Sickle cell anemia (off-label use): Infants ≥6 months, Children, and Adolescents: Oral: 20 mg/kg/dose once daily; increase by 5 mg/kg/**day** every 8 weeks until mild myelosuppression (neutrophils 2,000 to 4,000/mm^3) is achieved up to a maximum of 35 mg/kg/**day** (Hankins 2005; NHLBI 2014; Strouse 2012). If myelosuppression occurs (platelets <80,000/mm^3, neutrophils <2,000/mm^3; younger patients with lower baseline counts may safely tolerate ANC down to 1,250/mm^3), hold therapy until counts recover (monitor weekly); reinitiate at a dose 5 mg/kg/**day** lower than the dose given prior to onset of cytopenias (NHLBI 2014); some have recommended reinitiating at a dose 2.5 mg/kg/**day** lower (Hankins 2005; Heeney 2008; Wang 2001; Wang 2011; Zimmerman 2004). **Note:** A clinical response to treatment may take 3 to 6 months; a 6-month trial on the maximum tolerated dose is recommended prior to considering discontinuation due to treatment failure; effectiveness of hydroxyurea depends upon daily dosing adherence. For patients who have a clinical response, long-term hydroxyurea therapy is indicated (NHLBI 2014).

Renal Impairment

The manufacturer's labeling recommends the following adjustments:

Antineoplastic uses (CML, head and neck cancer):
CrCl ≥60 mL/minute: No dosage adjustment (of initial dose) necessary.
CrCl <60 mL/minute: Reduce initial dose by 50% to 7.5 mg/kg/day; titrate to response/avoidance of toxicity
End-stage renal diosorder (ESRD): Reduce initial dose by 50% to 7.5 mg/kg/dose (administer after dialysis on dialysis days); titrate to response/avoidance of toxicity

Sickle cell anemia:
CrCl ≥60 mL/minute: No dosage adjustment (of initial dose) necessary.
CrCl <60 mL/minute: Reduce initial dose to 7.5 mg/kg/day (Yan 2005); titrate to response/avoidance of toxicity (refer to usual dosing).
ESRD: Reduce initial dose to 7.5 mg/kg/dose (administer after dialysis on dialysis days); titrate to response/avoidance of toxicity.

The following adjustments have also been reported:
Aronoff 2007: Adults:
CrCl >50 mL/minute: No dosage adjustment necessary
CrCl 10 to 50 mL/minute: Administer 50% of dose.
CrCl <10 mL/minute: Administer 20% of dose.
Hemodialysis: Administer dose after dialysis on dialysis days.
Continuous renal replacement therapy (CRRT): Administer 50% of dose.
NHLBI 2014: Sickle cell anemia: Adults: Chronic kidney disease: Initial 5 to 10 mg/kg/day
Kintzel 1995:
CrCl 46 to 60 mL/minute: Administer 85% of dose.
CrCl 31 to 45 mL/minute: Administer 80% of dose.
CrCl <30 mL/minute: Administer 75% of dose.

Hepatic Impairment There are no dosage adjustments provided in the manufacturer's labeling; closely monitor for bone marrow toxicity.

Obesity *ASCO Guidelines for appropriate chemotherapy dosing in obese adults with cancer (solid tumors):* Utilize patient's actual body weight (full weight) for calculation of body surface area- or weight-based dosing, particularly when the intent of therapy is curative; manage regimen-related toxicities in the same manner as for nonobese patients; if a dose reduction is utilized due to toxicity, consider resumption of full weight-based dosing with subsequent cycles, especially if cause of toxicity (eg, hepatic or renal impairment) is resolved (Griggs 2012). **Note:** The manufacturer recommends dosing based on ideal or actual body weight, whichever is less.

Adjustment for Toxicity
Cutaneous vasculitic ulcerations: Discontinue
Pancreatitis: Discontinue permanently
Hematologic toxicity:
Antineoplastic uses (CML, head and neck cancer): Do not initiate therapy if bone marrow function is markedly reduced. Monitor blood counts prior to and during treatment; modify dose or discontinue hydroxyurea as needed.
Sickle cell anemia:
Manufacturer's labeling: Neutrophils <2,000/mm^3, platelets <80,000/mm^3, hemoglobin <4.5 g/dL, or reticulocytes <80,000/mm^3 with hemoglobin <9 g/dL: Interrupt treatment; following recovery, may resume with a dose reduction of 2.5 mg/kg/day. If no toxicity occurs over the next 12 weeks, subsequent dose may be increased by 2.5 mg/kg/day every 12 weeks to a dose which does not produce hematologic toxicity for 24 consecutive weeks. If hematologic toxicity recurs a second time at a specific dose, do not retry that dose.
Alternate recommendations (off-label dose): Absolute neutrophils <2,000/mm^3 (younger patients with lower baseline counts may safely tolerate absolute neutrophils down to 1,250/mm^3), platelets <80,000/mm^3; Interrupt treatment; following recovery, may restart at a dose 5mg/kg/day lower than the dose given prior to onset of cytopenias (NHLBI 2014).

Dietary Considerations Supplemental administration of folic acid is recommended; hydroxyurea may mask development of folic acid deficiency.

Administration Administer at the same time each day.

Hazardous agent; use appropriate precautions for handling and disposal (NIOSH 2014 [group 1]). Impervious gloves should be worn when handling bottles containing hydroxyurea or when handling/administering intact capsules (single gloves are recommended). Wash hands with soap and water before and after contact with the bottle or capsules when handling. Avoid exposure to crushed or open capsules. If skin contact with crushed or opened capsules occurs, immediately wash the affected area thoroughly with soap and water. If eye(s) contact with crushed or opened capsules occurs, the affected area should be flushed thoroughly with water or isotonic eyewash designated for that purpose for at least 15 minutes. If the powder from the capsule is spilled, immediately wipe it up with a damp disposable towel and discard (along with the empty capsules) in a closed container, such as a plastic bag. The spill areas should then be cleaned 3 times using a detergent solution followed by clean water.

Although the manufacturer does not recommend opening the capsules, if it is necessary to manipulate the capsules (eg, to prepare an oral suspension or solution), it is recommended to double glove, wear a protective gown, and prepare in a controlled device (NIOSH 2014).

Monitoring Parameters CBC with differential and platelets (once weekly for antineoplastic indications; every 2 weeks initially for sickle cell anemia), renal function and liver function tests, serum uric acid; hemoglobin F levels (sickle cell disease); monitor for cutaneous toxicities

Sickle cell disease: Monitor for toxicity every 2 weeks during dose escalation (neutrophils, platelets, hemoglobin, reticulocytes) (manufacturer's labeling) or at least every 4 weeks when adjusting the dose (CBC with WBC differential, reticulocytes) [NHLBI 2014]). Once on a stable dose, may monitor CBC with differential, reticulocyte count and platelets every 2 to 3 months (NHLBI 2014). Monitor RBC, MCV (mean corpuscular volume) and HbF (fetal hemoglobin) levels for evidence of consistent or progressive laboratory response (NHLBI 2014).

Test Interactions False-negative triglyceride measurement by a glycerol oxidase method. An analytical interference between hydroxyurea and enzymes (lactate dehydrogenase, urease, and uricase) may result in false elevations of lactic acid, urea, and uric acid.

Dosage Forms Excipient information presented when available (limited, particularly for generics; consult specific product labeling.
Capsule, Oral:
Droxia: 200 mg, 300 mg, 400 mg
Hydrea: 500 mg
Generic: 500 mg

Extemporaneous Preparations Hazardous agent: Use appropriate precautions for handling and disposal (NIOSH 2014 [group 1]). When manipulating capsules, NIOSH recommends double gloving, a protective gown, and preparation in a controlled device; if not prepared in a controlled device, respiratory and eye protection as well as ventilated engineering controls are recommended (NIOSH 2014). ▶

A 40 mg/mL oral suspension may be prepared with capsules and either a 1:1 mixture of Ora-Sweet® and Ora-Plus® or a 1:1 mixture of methylcellulose 1% and simple syrup NF. Empty the contents of eight 500 mg capsules into a mortar. Add small portions of chosen vehicle and mix to a uniform paste; mix while incrementally adding the vehicle to **almost** 100 mL; transfer to a calibrated bottle, rinse mortar with vehicle, and add sufficient quantity of vehicle to make 100 mL. Label "shake well" and "refrigerate". Store in plastic prescription bottles. Stable for 14 days at room temperature or refrigerated (preferred) (Nahata 2003).

A 100 mg/mL oral solution may be prepared with capsules. Mix the contents of twenty 500 mg capsules with enough room temperature sterile water (~50 mL) to initially result in a 200 mg/mL concentration. Stir vigorously using a magnetic stirrer for several hours, then filter to remove insoluble contents. Add 50 mL Syrpalta® (flavored syrup, HUMCO) to filtered solution, resulting in 100 mL of a 100 mg/mL hydroxyurea solution. Stable for 1 month at room temperature in amber plastic bottle (Heeney 2004).

Heeney MM, Whorton MR, Howard TA, et al, "Chemical and Functional Analysis of Hydroxyurea Oral Solutions," *J Pediatr Hematol Oncol* 2004, 26(3):179-84.

Nahata MC, Morosco RS, Boster EA, et al, "Stability of Hydroxyurea in Two Extemporaneously Prepared Oral Suspensions Stored at Two Temperatures," 2003, 38:P-161(E) [abstract from 2003 ASHP Midyear Clinical Meeting].

HydrOXYzine (hye DROKS i zeen)

Brand Names: US Vistaril
Brand Names: Canada Apo-Hydroxyzine; Atarax; Hydroxyzine Hydrochloride Injection, USP; Novo-Hydroxyzin; Nu-Hydroxyzine; PMS-Hydroxyzine; Riva-Hydroxyzine
Index Terms Hydroxyzine Hydrochloride; Hydroxyzine Pamoate; Vistaril
Pharmacologic Category Antiemetic; Histamine H$_1$ Antagonist; Histamine H$_1$ Antagonist, First Generation; Piperazine Derivative
Use Treatment of anxiety/agitation (including adjunctive therapy in alcoholism); adjunct to pre- and postoperative analgesia and anesthesia; antipruritic; antiemetic
Pregnancy Considerations Adverse events were observed in animal reproduction studies. Hydroxyzine crosses the placenta. Maternal hydroxyzine use has generally not resulted in an increased risk of birth defects. Use of hydroxyzine early in pregnancy is contraindicated but hydroxyzine is approved for pre- and postpartum adjunctive therapy to reduce opioid dosage, treat anxiety, and control emesis. Antihistamines are recommended for the treatment pruritus with rash in pregnant women (although second generation antihistamines may be preferred). Antihistamines are not recommended for treatment of pruritus associated with intrahepatic cholestasis in pregnancy. Possible withdrawal symptoms have been observed in neonates following chronic maternal use of hydroxyzine during pregnancy.
Breast-Feeding Considerations It is not known if hydroxyzine is excreted in breast milk. Breast-feeding is not recommended by the manufacturer. Antihistamines may decrease maternal serum prolactin concentrations when administered prior to the establishment of nursing.
Contraindications Hypersensitivity to hydroxyzine or any component of the formulation; early pregnancy; SubQ, intra-arterial, or IV injection
Warnings/Precautions Causes sedation, caution must be used in performing tasks which require alertness (eg, operating machinery or driving). Sedative effects of CNS depressants or ethanol are potentiated. Use with caution with narrow-angle glaucoma, prostatic hyperplasia, bladder neck obstruction, asthma, or COPD. In the elderly, avoid use of this potent anticholinergic agent due to increased risk of confusion, dry mouth, constipation, and other anticholinergic effects; clearance decreases in patients of advanced age (Beers Criteria).

For IM use only. Subcutaneous, IV, and intra-arterial routes of administration are contraindicated. Intravascular hemolysis, thrombosis, and digital gangrene have been reported with IV or intra-arterial administration (Baumgartner, 1979); SubQ administration may result in significant tissue damage. If inadvertent IV administration results in extravasation, stop infusion immediately and disconnect (leave cannula/needle in place); gently aspirate extravasated solution (do **NOT** flush the line); remove needle/cannula; elevate extremity.

Benzyl alcohol and derivatives: Some dosage forms may contain benzyl alcohol and/or sodium benzoate/benzoic acid; benzoic acid (benzoate) is a metabolite of benzyl alcohol; large amounts of benzyl alcohol (≥99 mg/kg/day) have been associated with a potentially fatal toxicity ("gasping syndrome") in neonates; the "gasping syndrome" consists of metabolic acidosis, respiratory distress, gasping respirations, CNS dysfunction (including convulsions, intracranial hemorrhage), hypotension and cardiovascular collapse (AAP ["Inactive" 1997]; CDC, 1982); some data suggests that benzoate displaces bilirubin from protein binding sites (Ahlfors, 2001); avoid or use dosage forms containing benzyl alcohol and/or benzyl alcohol derivative with caution in neonates. See manufacturer's labeling.

Adverse Reactions Frequency not defined.
Central nervous system: Dizziness, drowsiness (transient), fatigue, involuntary movements
Gastrointestinal: Xerostomia
Hypersensitivity: Hypersensitivity reaction
Ophthalmic: Blurred vision
Respiratory: Respiratory depression (at higher than recommended doses)
<1% (Limited to important or life-threatening): Fixed drug eruption, hallucination, seizure (at considerably higher than recommended doses), skin rash, tremor (at considerably higher than recommended doses)
Drug Interactions
Metabolism/Transport Effects Inhibits CYP2D6 (weak)
Avoid Concomitant Use
Avoid concomitant use of HydrOXYzine with any of the following: Aclidinium; Azelastine (Nasal); Cimetropium; Eluxadoline; Glucagon; Glycopyrrolate; Glycopyrrolate (Oral Inhalation); Ipratropium (Oral Inhalation); Levosulpiride; Orphenadrine; Paraldehyde; Potassium Chloride; Thalidomide; Tiotropium; Umeclidinium
Increased Effect/Toxicity
HydrOXYzine may increase the levels/effects of: Abobotulinumtoxin A; Alcohol (Ethyl); Anticholinergic Agents; ARIPiprazole; Azelastine (Nasal); Barbiturates; Buprenorphine; Cimetropium; CNS Depressants; Eluxadoline; Glucagon; Glycopyrrolate; Glycopyrrolate (Oral Inhalation); Highest Risk QTc-Prolonging Agents; Hydrocodone; Meperidine; Methotrimeprazine; Metyrosine; Mirabegron; Mirtazapine; Moderate Risk QTc-Prolonging Agents; OnabotulinumtoxinA; Orphenadrine; Paraldehyde; Potassium Chloride; Pramipexole; Ramosetron; RimabotulinumtoxinB; ROPINIRole; Rotigotine; Selective Serotonin Reuptake Inhibitors; Suvorexant; Thalidomide; Thiazide Diuretics; Tiotropium; Topiramate; Zolpidem

The levels/effects of HydrOXYzine may be increased by: Aclidinium; Brimonidine (Topical); Cannabis; Doxylamine; Dronabinol; Droperidol; Ipratropium (Oral Inhalation); Kava Kava; Magnesium Sulfate; Methotrimeprazine; Mianserin; Mifepristone; Minocycline; Nabilone; Perampanel; Pramlintide; Rufinamide; Sodium Oxybate; Tapentadol; Tetrahydrocannabinol; Umeclidinium
Decreased Effect
HydrOXYzine may decrease the levels/effects of: Acetylcholinesterase Inhibitors; Benzylpenicilloyl Polylysine; Betahistine; Gastrointestinal Agents (Prokinetic); Hyaluronidase; Itopride; Levosulpiride; Secretin

The levels/effects of HydrOXYzine may be decreased by: Acetylcholinesterase Inhibitors; Amphetamines
Storage/Stability
Injection: Store at 20°C to 25°C (68°F to 77°F); excursions permitted to 15°C to 30°C (59°F to 86°F). Protect from light.
Capsules: Store below 30°C (86°F); protect from light.
Solution (hydrochloride salt): Store at 15°C to 30°C (59°F to 86°F); protect from light.
Tablets: Store at 20°C to 25°C (68°F to 77°F).
Mechanism of Action Competes with histamine for H$_1$-receptor sites on effector cells in the gastrointestinal tract, blood vessels, and respiratory tract. Possesses skeletal muscle relaxing, bronchodilator, antihistamine, antiemetic, and analgesic properties.
Pharmacodynamics/Kinetics
Onset of action: Oral: 15 to 30 minutes; Injection: Rapid
Duration: Decreased histamine-induced wheal and flare areas: 2 to ≥36 hours; Suppression of pruritus: 1 to 12 hours (Simon F 1984)
Absorption: Oral: Rapid
Distribution: Children and Adolescents 1 to 14 years: 18.5 ± 8.6 L/kg (Simons F 1984a); Adults: V$_d$: 16 ± 3 L/kg (Simons F 1984); Elderly: ~23 L/kg (Simons K 1989); Hepatic dysfunction: ~23 L/kg (Simons F 1989)
Metabolism: Hepatic to multiple metabolites, including cetirizine (active) (Simons F 1989)

Half-life elimination:

Children and Adolescents 1 to 14 years (mean age: 6.1 ± 4.6 years): 7.1 ± 2.3 hours; **Note:** Half-life increased with increasing age and was 4 hours in patients 1-year old and 11 hours in a 14-year old patient (Simons F 1984a)

Adults: ~20 hours (Simons 1984); Elderly: ~29 hours (Simons K 1989); Hepatic dysfunction: ~37 hours (Simons F 1989)

Time to peak: Oral administration: Serum: ~2 hours; Peak suppression of antihistamine-induced wheal and flare: 4 to 12 hours (Simons F 1984)

Excretion: Urine; active metabolite (cetirizine) is renally eliminated (Simons F 1994)

Dosing

Adult Note: Adjust dose based on patient response.

Antiemetic: IM: 25 to 100 mg/dose

Anxiety:

Oral:

Manufacturer's labeling: 50 to100 mg 4 times daily

Alternative recommendations (off-label dosing): 37.5 to 75 mg daily in divided doses (WFSBP [Bandelow, 2008]; WFSBP [Bandelow, 2012])

IM: Initial: 50 to 100 mg, then every 4-6 hours as needed

Preoperative sedation:

Oral: 50 to 100 mg

IM: 25 to 100 mg

Pruritus: Oral: 25 mg 3 to 4 times daily

Geriatric Initiate dosing using the lower end of the recommended dosage range due to an increased potential for anticholinergic side effects. Refer to adult dosing.

Pediatric Note: Adjust dose based on patient response.

Antiemetic: IM: 1.1 mg/kg/dose

Preoperative sedation:

Oral: 0.6 mg/kg/dose

IM: 1.1 mg/kg/dose

Pruritus, anxiety: Oral:

<6 years: 50 mg daily in divided doses

≥6 years: 50-100 mg daily in divided dose

Renal Impairment No dosage adjustment provided in the manufacturer's labeling; however, the following guidelines have been used by some clinicians (Aronoff, 2007): Adults:

GFR >50 mL/minute: No adjustment recommended.

GFR ≤50 mL/minute: Administer 50% of normal dose.

Continuous renal replacement therapy (CRRT), hemodialysis, peritoneal dialysis: Administer 50% of the normal dose.

Hepatic Impairment Change dosing interval to every 24 hours in patients with primary biliary cirrhosis (Simons F, 1989)

Administration

Injection: For IM use only. Do **NOT** administer IV, SubQ, or intra-arterially. Administer IM deep in large muscle. In adults, the preferred site is the upper outer quadrant of the buttock or midlateral thigh. In children, the preferred site is the midlateral thigh. The upper outer quadrant of the gluteal region should be used only when necessary to minimize potential damage to the sciatic nerve.

Oral: Shake suspension vigorously prior to use.

Monitoring Parameters Relief of symptoms, mental status, blood pressure

Test Interactions May cause false-positive serum TCA screen.

Dosage Forms Excipient information presented when available (limited, particularly for generics); consult specific product labeling. [DSC] = Discontinued product

Capsule, Oral, as pamoate:

Vistaril: 25 mg, 50 mg

Generic: 25 mg, 50 mg, 100 mg

Solution, Intramuscular, as hydrochloride:

Generic: 25 mg/mL (1 mL [DSC]); 50 mg/mL (1 mL [DSC], 2 mL [DSC], 10 mL [DSC])

Solution, Oral, as hydrochloride:

Generic: 10 mg/5 mL (473 mL [DSC])

Syrup, Oral, as hydrochloride:

Generic: 10 mg/5 mL (25 mL, 118 mL, 120 mL [DSC], 473 mL)

Tablet, Oral, as hydrochloride:

Generic: 10 mg, 25 mg, 50 mg

◆ Hydroxyzine Hydrochloride *see* HydrOXYzine *on page 898*

◆ Hydroxyzine Hydrochloride Injection, USP (Can) *see* HydrOXYzine *on page 898*

◆ Hydroxyzine Pamoate *see* HydrOXYzine *on page 898*

◆ Hydurea *see* Hydroxyurea *on page 895*

◆ HyGel *see* Hyaluronate and Derivatives *on page 879*

◆ Hygroton *see* Chlorthalidone *on page 380*

◆ Hylan G-F 20 *see* Hyaluronate and Derivatives *on page 879*

◆ Hylan Polymers *see* Hyaluronate and Derivatives *on page 879*

◆ Hylase Wound *see* Hyaluronate and Derivatives *on page 879*

◆ Hyolev MB *see* Methenamine, Sodium Phosphate Monobasic, Phenyl Salicylate, Methylene Blue, and Hyoscyamine *on page 1166*

◆ Hyomax-SL *see* Hyoscyamine *on page 899*

◆ HyoMax-SL *see* Hyoscyamine *on page 899*

◆ Hyophen™ *see* Methenamine, Phenyl Salicylate, Methylene Blue, Benzoic Acid, and Hyoscyamine *on page 1166*

◆ Hyoscine Butylbromide *see* Scopolamine (Systemic) *on page 1640*

Hyoscyamine (hye oh SYE a meen)

Brand Names: US Anaspaz; Colidrops [DSC]; Ed-Spaz; HyoMax-SL; Hyosyne; Levbid; Levsin; Levsin/SL; NuLev; Oscimin; Oscimin SR; Symax Duotab; Symax FasTabs; Symax-SL; Symax-SR

Brand Names: Canada Levsin

Index Terms *l*-Hyoscyamine Sulfate; Cystospaz-M; ED-SPAZ; Hyomax-SL; Hyoscyamine Sulfate

Pharmacologic Category Anticholinergic Agent

Use

Anesthesia:

Preoperative antimuscarinic: Preoperative antimuscarinic to reduce salivary, tracheobronchial, and pharyngeal secretions; to reduce volume and acidity of gastric secretions; to block cardiac vagal inhibitory reflexes during induction of anesthesia and intubation

Reversal of neuromuscular blockade and associated muscarinic effects: Protects against peripheral muscarinic effects (such as bradycardia and excessive secretions produced by halogenated hydrocarbons and cholinergic agents [such as physostigmine, neostigmine, and pyridostigmine]) given to reverse actions of curariform agents

Antidote for anticholinesterase agent poisoning: Antidote for poisoning by anticholinesterase agents

Biliary and renal colic: Adjunctive therapy with morphine or other opioids for the symptomatic relief of biliary and renal colic

Diagnostic procedures: Reduces GI motility to facilitate diagnostic procedures such as endoscopy or hypotonic duodenography; may also improve radiologic visibility of the kidneys

GI disorders:

Aid in the control of acute episodes of gastric secretion, visceral spasm, hypermotility in spastic colitis, pylorospasm, and associated abdominal cramps; relieve symptoms in functional intestinal disorders (eg, mild dysenteries, diverticulitis) and infant colic (elixir and oral solution)

Adjunctive therapy for treatment in peptic ulcer; irritable bowel syndrome (irritable colon, spastic colon, acute enterocolitis, mucous colitis) and other functional GI disorders; neurogenic bowel disturbances (including splenic flexure syndrome and neurogenic colon)

Pancreatitis: Reduce pain and hypersecretion in pancreatitis

Parkinsonism: In parkinsonism, to reduce rigidity and tremors and to control associated sialorrhea and hyperhidrosis

Partial heart block: For use in certain cases of partial heart block associated with vagal activity

Rhinitis: "Drying agent" in the relief of symptoms of acute rhinitis

Urinary system disorder: To control hypermotility in spastic bladder and cystitis; adjunctive therapy in the treatment of neurogenic bladder

Dosing

Adult & Geriatric

Gastrointestinal disorders:

Oral:

Tablet, dispersible:

Anaspaz, ED-SPAZ, NuLev, Symax FasTab: 0.125 to 0.25 mg every 4 hours or as needed; maximum: 1.5 mg daily

Oscimin: 0.125 to 0.25 mg 3 to 4 times daily; may increase to every 4 hours as needed; maximum: 1.5 mg daily

Tablet, extended release:

Levbid: 0.375 to 0.75 mg every 12 hours; maximum: 1.5 mg daily

Oscimin SR, Symax Duotab, Symax SR: 0.375 to 0.75 mg every 12 hours or 0.375 mg every 8 hours; maximum: 1.5 mg daily

Tablet, regular release:

Levsin: 0.125 to 0.25 mg every 4 hours or as needed; maximum: 1.5 mg daily

Oscimin: 0.125 to 0.25 mg 3 to 4 times daily; may increase to every 4 hours as needed; maximum: 1.5 mg daily

Tablet, sublingual (Oscimin, Symax SL): 0.125 to 0.25 mg 3 to 4 times daily; may increase to every 4 hours as needed; maximum: 1.5 mg daily

Drops (Hyosyne [0.125 mg/**mL**]): 0.125 mg (1 mL) to 0.25 mg (2 mL) every 4 hours or as needed; maximum: 1.5 mg (12 mL) daily

Elixir (Hyosyne [0.125 mg/**5 mL**]): 0.125 mg (5 mL) to 0.25 mg (10 mL) every 4 hours or as needed; maximum: 1.5 mg (60 mL) daily

IM, IV, SubQ: 0.25 to 0.5 mg; may repeat as needed up to 4 times daily, at 4-hour intervals

Diagnostic procedures: IV: 0.25 to 0.5 given 5 to 10 minutes prior to procedure

Preanesthesia: IM, IV, SubQ: 5 **mcg**/kg given 30 to 60 minutes prior to induction of anesthesia or at the time preoperative opioids or sedatives are administered

To reduce drug-induced bradycardia during surgery: IV: 0.125 mg; repeat as needed

Reverse neuromuscular blockade: IM, IV, SubQ: 0.2 mg for every 1 mg neostigmine (or the physostigmine/pyridostigmine equivalent)

Pediatric

Gastrointestinal disorders:

Children <2 years: Oral: Drops (Hyosyne [0.125 mg/**mL**]): Dose as listed, based on age and weight (kg); repeat dose every 4 hours or as needed:

3.4 kg: 4 **drops**; maximum: 24 **drops** daily

5 kg: 5 **drops**; maximum: 30 **drops** daily

7 kg: 6 **drops**; maximum: 36 **drops** daily

10 kg: 8 **drops**; maximum: 48 **drops** daily

Children 2 to <12 years: Oral:

Tablets (regular release [Levsin], dispersible [Anaspaz, ED-SPAZ, NuLev, Symax FasTab]): 0.0625 to 0.125 mg every 4 hours or as needed; maximum: 0.75 mg daily

Drops (Hyosyne [0.125 mg/**mL**]): 0.03125 mg (0.25 mL) to 0.125 mg (1 mL) every 4 hours or as needed; maximum: 0.75 mg (6 mL) daily

Elixir (Hyosyne [0.125 mg/**5 mL**]): Dose as listed, based on age and weight (kg); repeat dose every 4 hours or as needed:

10 kg: 0.03125 mg (1.25 mL); maximum: 0.75 mg (30 mL) daily

20 kg: 0.0625 mg (2.5 mL); maximum: 0.75 mg (30 mL) daily

40 kg: 0.09375 mg (3.75 mL); maximum: 0.75 mg (30 mL) daily

50 kg: 0.125 mg (5 mL); maximum: 0.75 mg (30 mL) daily

Children ≥12 years and Adolescents: Oral: Regular release tablets, dispersible tablets, sublingual tablets, elixir/drops, extended release tablets: Refer to adult dosing.

Preanesthesia: Children >2 years and Adolescents: IV: Refer to adult dosing.

Renal Impairment No dosage adjustment provided in manufacturer's labeling, use with caution.

Hepatic Impairment No dosage adjustment provided in manufacturer's labeling.

Additional Information Complete prescribing information should be consulted for additional detail.

Dosage Forms Excipient information presented when available (limited, particularly for generics); consult specific product labeling. [DSC] = Discontinued product

Elixir, Oral, as sulfate:

Hyosyne: 0.125 mg/5 mL (473 mL) [contains alcohol, usp; lemon flavor]

Generic: 0.125 mg/5 mL (473 mL)

Solution, Injection, as sulfate:

Levsin: 0.5 mg/mL (1 mL) [contains benzyl alcohol]

Solution, Oral, as sulfate:

Colidrops: 0.125 mg/mL (30 mL [DSC])

Hyosyne: 0.125 mg/mL (15 mL) [lemon flavor]

Generic: 0.125 mg/mL (15 mL)

Tablet, Oral, as sulfate:

Levsin: 0.125 mg

Oscimin: 0.125 mg [peppermint flavor]

Generic: 0.125 mg

Tablet Dispersible, Oral, as sulfate:

Anaspaz: 0.125 mg [scored]

Ed-Spaz: 0.125 mg [scored]

NuLev: 0.125 mg [peppermint flavor]

Oscimin: 0.125 mg [peppermint flavor]

Symax FasTabs: 0.125 mg [mint flavor]

Generic: 0.125 mg

Tablet Extended Release, Oral, as sulfate:

Symax Duotab: 0.375 mg [contains brilliant blue fcf (fd&c blue #1)]

Tablet Extended Release 12 Hour, Oral, as sulfate:

Levbid: 0.375 mg

Oscimin SR: 0.375 mg

Symax-SR: 0.375 mg [scored]

Generic: 0.375 mg

Tablet Sublingual, Sublingual, as sulfate:

HyoMax-SL: 0.125 mg

Levsin/SL: 0.125 mg

Oscimin: 0.125 mg [peppermint flavor]

Symax-SL: 0.125 mg [mint flavor]

Generic: 0.125 mg

Hyoscyamine, Atropine, Scopolamine, and Phenobarbital

(hye oh SYE a meen, A troe peen, skoe POL a meen, & fee noe BAR bi tal)

Brand Names: US B-Donna; Donnatal Extentabs®; Donnatal®

Index Terms Atropine, Hyoscyamine, Phenobarbital, and Scopolamine; Belladonna Alkaloids With Phenobarbital; Phenobarbital, Hyoscyamine, Atropine, and Scopolamine; Scopolamine, Hyoscyamine, Atropine, and Phenobarbital

Pharmacologic Category Anticholinergic Agent; Antispasmodic Agent, Gastrointestinal

Use Adjunct in treatment of irritable bowel syndrome, acute enterocolitis, duodenal ulcer

Dosing

Adult & Geriatric Spasmolytic: Oral:

Immediate release: 1-2 tablets or 5-10 mL of elixir 3-4 times/day

Extended release: One tablet every 12 hours; may increase to 1 tablet every 8 hours if needed

Pediatric Spasmolytic: Children ≥2 years: Oral: Elixir: To be given every 4-6 hours; initial dose based on weight:

9.1 kg: 1 mL every 4 hours **or** 1.5 mL every 6 hours

13.6 kg: 1.5 mL every 4 hours **or** 2 mL every 6 hours

22.7 kg: 2.5 mL every 4 hours **or** 3.75 mL every 6 hours

34 kg: 3.75 mL every 4 hours **or** 5 mL every 6 hours

45.4 kg: 5 mL every 4 hours **or** 7.5 mL every 6 hours

Additional Information Complete prescribing information should be consulted for additional detail.

Dosage Forms Considerations Elixir contains ethanol (up to 23.8%).

Dosage Forms Excipient information presented when available (limited, particularly for generics); consult specific product labeling.

Elixir, Oral:

Donnatal®: Hyoscyamine sulfate 0.1037 mg, atropine sulfate 0.0194 mg, scopolamine hydrobromide 0.0065 mg, and phenobarbital 16.2 mg per 5 mL (120 mL, 480 mL) [contains ethanol <23.8%; grape flavor]

Donnatal®: Hyoscyamine sulfate 0.1037 mg, atropine sulfate 0.0194 mg, scopolamine hydrobromide 0.0065 mg, and phenobarbital 16.2 mg per 5 mL (120 mL, 480 mL) [contains ethanol <23.8%, tartrazine; mint flavor]

Tablet, Oral:

B-Donna: Hyoscyamine sulfate 0.1037 mg, atropine sulfate 0.0194 mg, scopolamine hydrobromide 0.0065 mg, and phenobarbital 16.2 mg

Donnatal®: Hyoscyamine sulfate 0.1037 mg, atropine sulfate 0.0194 mg, scopolamine hydrobromide 0.0065 mg, and phenobarbital 16.2 mg

Tablet, extended release, Oral:

Donnatal Extentabs®: Hyoscyamine sulfate 0.3111 mg, atropine sulfate 0.0582 mg, scopolamine hydrobromide 0.0195 mg, and phenobarbital 48.6 mg

Controlled Substance C-IV or nonscheduled (DEA exemption status dependent)

◆ Hyoscyamine, Methenamine, Benzoic Acid, Phenyl Salicylate, and Methylene Blue *see* Methenamine, Phenyl Salicylate, Methylene Blue, Benzoic Acid, and Hyoscyamine *on page 1166*

◆ Hyoscyamine, Methenamine, Methylene Blue, Phenyl Salicylate, and Sodium Phosphate Monobasic *see* Methenamine, Sodium Phosphate Monobasic, Phenyl Salicylate, Methylene Blue, and Hyoscyamine *on page 1166*

- **Hyoscyamine, Methenamine, Sodium Phosphate Monobasic, Phenyl Salicylate, and Methylene Blue** *see* Methenamine, Sodium Phosphate Monobasic, Phenyl Salicylate, Methylene Blue, and Hyoscyamine *on page 1166*
- **Hyoscyamine Sulfate** *see* Hyoscyamine *on page 899*
- **Hyosyne** *see* Hyoscyamine *on page 899*
- **Hyperal** *see* Total Parenteral Nutrition *on page 1818*
- **Hyperalimentation** *see* Total Parenteral Nutrition *on page 1818*
- **HyperHEP B S/D** *see* Hepatitis B Immune Globulin (Human) *on page 875*
- **HyperRAB S/D** *see* Rabies Immune Globulin (Human) *on page 1547*
- **HyperRHO S/D** *see* Rh$_o$(D) Immune Globulin *on page 1572*
- **HyperSal** *see* Sodium Chloride *on page 1671*
- **HyperTET S/D** *see* Tetanus Immune Globulin (Human) *on page 1771*
- **Hypertonic Saline** *see* Sodium Chloride *on page 1671*
- **HyQvia** *see* Immune Globulin *on page 927*
- **Hyqvia** *see* Immune Globulin *on page 927*
- **HySept [OTC]** *see* Sodium Hypochlorite *on page 1675*
- **Hytrin** *see* Terazosin *on page 1758*
- **HyVee Advanced Antacid [OTC]** *see* Aluminum Hydroxide, Magnesium Hydroxide, and Simethicone *on page 85*
- **HyVee Ibuprofen Childrens [OTC]** *see* Ibuprofen *on page 905*
- **Hyzaar** *see* Losartan and Hydrochlorothiazide *on page 1109*
- **Hyzaar DS (Can)** *see* Losartan and Hydrochlorothiazide *on page 1109*
- **HZV** *see* Zoster Vaccine *on page 1944*

Ibandronate (eye BAN droh nate)

Brand Names: US Boniva
Index Terms Ibandronate Sodium; Ibandronic Acid
Pharmacologic Category Bisphosphonate Derivative
Use Treatment and prevention of osteoporosis in postmenopausal females
Pregnancy Considerations Adverse effects were observed in animal reproduction studies. It is not known if bisphosphonates cross the placenta, but fetal exposure is expected (Djokanovic, 2008; Stathopoulos, 2011). Bisphosphonates are incorporated into the bone matrix and gradually released over time. The amount available in the systemic circulation varies by dose and duration of therapy. Theoretically, there may be a risk of fetal harm when pregnancy follows the completion of therapy; however, available data have not shown that exposure to bisphosphonates during pregnancy significantly increases the risk of adverse fetal events (Djokanovic, 2008; Levy, 2009; Stathopoulos, 2011). Until additional data is available, most sources recommend discontinuing bisphosphonate therapy in women of reproductive potential as early as possible prior to a planned pregnancy; use in premenopausal women should be reserved for special circumstances when rapid bone loss is occurring (Bhalla, 2010; Pereira, 2012; Stathopoulos, 2011). Because hypocalcemia has been described following *in utero* bisphosphonate exposure, exposed infants should be monitored for hypocalcemia after birth (Djokanovic, 2008; Stathopoulos, 2011).
Breast-Feeding Considerations It is not known if ibandronate is excreted into breast milk. The manufacturer recommends caution be exercised when administering ibandronate to nursing women.
Medication Guide Available Yes
Contraindications Hypersensitivity to ibandronate or any component of the formulation; hypocalcemia; oral tablets are also contraindicated in patients unable to stand or sit upright for at least 60 minutes and in patients with abnormalities of the esophagus which delay esophageal emptying, such as stricture or achalasia
Warnings/Precautions Hypocalcemia must be corrected before therapy initiation. Ensure adequate calcium and vitamin D intake. Osteonecrosis of the jaw (ONJ) has been reported in patients receiving bisphosphonates. Risk factors include invasive dental procedures (eg, tooth extraction, dental implants, boney surgery); a diagnosis of cancer, with concomitant chemotherapy or corticosteroids; poor oral hygiene, ill-fitting dentures; and comorbid disorders (anemia, coagulopathy, infection, preexisting dental disease); risk may increase with duration of bisphosphonate use. Most reported cases occurred after IV

bisphosphonate therapy; however, cases have been reported following oral therapy. A dental exam and preventive dentistry should be performed prior to placing patients with risk factors on chronic bisphosphonate therapy. The manufacturer's labeling states that discontinuing bisphosphonates in patients requiring invasive dental procedures may reduce the risk of ONJ. However, other experts suggest that there is no evidence that discontinuing therapy reduces the risk of developing ONJ (Assael, 2009). The risk:benefit must be assessed by the treating physician and/or dentist/surgeon prior to any invasive dental procedure. Patients developing ONJ while on bisphosphonates should receive care by an oral surgeon.

Atypical femur fractures have been reported in patients receiving bisphosphonates for treatment/prevention of osteoporosis. The fractures include subtrochanteric femur (bone just below the hip joint) and diaphyseal femur (long segment of the thigh bone). Some patients experience prodromal pain weeks or months before the fracture occurs. It is unclear if bisphosphonate therapy is the cause for these fractures, although the majority of cases have been reported in patients taking bisphosphonates. Patients receiving long-term (>3-5 years) therapy may be at an increased risk. Discontinue bisphosphonate therapy in patients who develop a femoral shaft fracture.

Infrequently, severe (and occasionally debilitating) bone, joint, and/or muscle pain have been reported during bisphosphonate treatment. The onset of pain ranged from a single day to several months. Discontinue intravenous ibandronate therapy in patients who experience severe symptoms; symptoms usually resolve upon discontinuation. Some patients experienced recurrence when rechallenged with same drug or another bisphosphonate; avoid use in patients with a history of these symptoms in association with bisphosphonate therapy.

Oral bisphosphonates may cause dysphagia, esophagitis, esophageal or gastric ulcer; risk may increase in patients unable to comply with dosing instructions; discontinue use if new or worsening symptoms develop. Intravenous bisphosphonates may cause transient decreases in serum calcium and have also been associated with renal toxicity.

Use not recommended with severe renal impairment (CrCl <30 mL/minute). In the management of osteoporosis, re-evaluate the need for continued therapy periodically; the optimal duration of treatment has not yet been determined. Consider discontinuing after 3-5 years of use in patients at low-risk for fracture; following discontinuation, re-evaluate fracture risk periodically. Potentially significant drug-drug interactions may exist, requiring dose or frequency adjustment, additional monitoring, and/or selection of alternative therapy.

Adverse Reactions Percentages vary based on frequency of administration (daily vs monthly). Unless specified, percentages are reported with oral use.
>10%:
Gastrointestinal: Dyspepsia (4% to 12%)
Neuromuscular & skeletal: Back pain (4% to 14%)
Respiratory: Upper respiratory tract infection (2% to 34%)
1% to 10%:
Cardiovascular: Hypertension (6% to 7%)
Central nervous system: Headache (3% to 7%), dizziness (1% to 4%), fatigue (3%), insomnia (1% to 2%), depression (2%)
Dermatologic: Skin rash (1% to 2%)
Gastrointestinal: Abdominal pain (5% to 8%), diarrhea (2% to 7%), nausea (4% to 5%), dental disease (4%), constipation (3% to 4%), vomiting (3%), gastritis (2%), gastroenteritis (3%)
Genitourinary: Urinary tract infection (2% to 6%), cystitis (3%)
Hypersensitivity: Acute phase reaction-like symptoms (IV: 10%; oral: 3% to 9%), hypersensitivity reaction (3%)
Infection: Influenza (4% to 8%)
Local: Injection site reaction (<2%)
Neuromuscular & skeletal: Limb pain (1% to 8%), arthralgia (4% to 9%), myalgia (1% to 6%), arthropathy (4%), weakness (4%), localized osteoarthritis (1% to 3%), muscle cramps (2%)
Respiratory: Bronchitis (3% to 10%), pneumonia (6%), nasopharyngitis (3% to 4%), flu-like symptoms (1% to 3%), pharyngitis (3%)
Postmarketing and/or case reports (Limited to important or life-threatening): Acute renal failure, anaphylactic shock, anaphylaxis, angioedema, bullous dermatitis, erythema multiforme, exacerbation of asthma, femur fracture (diaphyseal or subtrochanteric), hypocalcemia, iritis, musculoskeletal pain (bone, joint, or muscle; incapacitating), ophthalmic inflammation, osteonecrosis of the jaw, prolonged Q-T interval on ECG (Bonilla 2014), scleritis, Stevens-Johnson syndrome, uveitis ▶

Drug Interactions

Metabolism/Transport Effects None known.

Avoid Concomitant Use There are no known interactions where it is recommended to avoid concomitant use.

Increased Effect/Toxicity

Ibandronate may increase the levels/effects of: Deferasirox; Highest Risk QTc-Prolonging Agents; Moderate Risk QTc-Prolonging Agents

The levels/effects of Ibandronate may be increased by: Aminoglycosides; Mifepristone; Nonsteroidal Anti-Inflammatory Agents; Systemic Angiogenesis Inhibitors

Decreased Effect

The levels/effects of Ibandronate may be decreased by: Antacids; Calcium Salts; Iron Salts; Magnesium Salts; Multivitamins/Minerals (with ADEK, Folate, Iron); Multivitamins/Minerals (with AE, No Iron); Proton Pump Inhibitors

Food Interactions Food may reduce absorption; mean oral bioavailability is decreased up to 90% when given with food. Management: Take with a full glass (6-8 oz) of plain water, at least 60 minutes prior to any food, beverages, or medications. Mineral water with a high calcium content should be avoided. Wait at least 60 minutes after taking ibandronate before taking anything else.

Storage/Stability Store at controlled room temperature of 25°C (77°F); excursions permitted to 15°C to 30°C (59°F to 86°F).

Mechanism of Action A bisphosphonate which inhibits bone resorption via actions on osteoclasts or on osteoclast precursors; decreases the rate of bone resorption, leading to an indirect increase in bone mineral density.

Pharmacodynamics/Kinetics

Distribution: Terminal V_d: 90 L; 40% to 50% of circulating ibandronate binds to bone

Protein binding: 85.7% to 99.5%

Metabolism: Not metabolized

Bioavailability: Oral: Minimal; reduced ~90% following standard breakfast

Half-life elimination:

Oral: 150 mg dose: Terminal: 37-157 hours

IV: Terminal: ~5-25 hours

Time to peak, plasma: Oral: 0.5-2 hours

Excretion: Urine (50% to 60% of absorbed dose, excreted as unchanged drug); feces (unabsorbed drug)

Dosing

Adult & Geriatric

Postmenopausal osteoporosis (treatment): Note: Consider discontinuing after 3-5 years of use for osteoporosis in patients at low-risk for fracture. Patients should receive supplemental calcium and vitamin D if dietary intake is inadequate.

Oral: 150 mg once monthly

IV: 3 mg every 3 months

Postmenopausal osteoporosis (prevention): Oral: 150 mg once monthly. **Note:** Patients should receive supplemental calcium and vitamin D if dietary intake is inadequate.

Hypercalcemia of malignancy (off-label use): IV: 2-6 mg over 1-2 hours (Pecherstorfer, 2003; Ralston, 1997)

Metastatic bone disease due to breast cancer (off-label use): IV: 6 mg every 3-4 weeks (Diel, 2004)

Missed doses:

Oral: If once-monthly oral dose is missed, it should be given the next morning after remembered if the next month's scheduled dose is >7 days away. If the next month's scheduled dose is within 7 days, wait until the next month's scheduled dose. May then return to the original monthly schedule (original scheduled day of the month). Do not give >150 mg within 7 days.

IV: If an IV dose is missed, it should be administered as soon as it can be rescheduled. Thereafter, it should be given every 3 months from the date of the last injection.

Renal Impairment

Osteoporosis: Oral, IV:

CrCl ≥30 mL/minute: No dosage adjustment necessary.

CrCl <30 mL/minute: Use not recommended.

Oncologic uses (off-label): IV: CrCl <30 mL/minute: 2 mg every 3-4 weeks (von Moos, 2005)

Hepatic Impairment No dosage adjustment necessary (has not been studied); however, ibandronate does not undergo hepatic metabolism.

Dietary Considerations

Ensure adequate calcium and vitamin D intake; if dietary intake is inadequate, dietary supplementation is recommended. Women and men should consume:

Calcium: 1,000 mg/day (men: 50 to 70 years) **or** 1,200 mg/day (women ≥51 years and men ≥71 years) (IOM, 2011; NOF [Cosman 2014])

Vitamin D: 800 to 1,000 int. units daily (men and women ≥50 years) (NOF [Cosman 2014]). Recommended Dietary Allowance (RDA): 600 int. units daily (men and women ≤70 years) **or** 800 int. units daily (men and women ≥71 years) (IOM, 2011).

Ibandronate tablet should be taken with a full glass (6 to 8 oz) of plain water, at least 60 minutes prior to any food, beverages, or medications. Mineral water with a high calcium content should be avoided.

Administration

Oral: Administer 60 minutes before the first food or drink of the day (other than water) and prior to taking any oral medications or supplements (eg, calcium, antacids, vitamins). Ibandronate should be taken in an upright position with a full glass (6-8 oz) of plain water and the patient should avoid lying down for 60 minutes to minimize the possibility of GI side effects. Mineral water with a high calcium content should be avoided. The tablet should be swallowed whole; do not chew or suck. Do not eat or drink anything (except water) for 60 minutes following administration of ibandronate.

IV: Administer as a 15-30 second bolus intravenously; avoid paravenous or intraarterial administration (may cause tissue damage). Do not mix with calcium-containing solutions or other drugs. For osteoporosis, do not administer more frequently than every 3 months. Infuse over 1 hour for metastatic bone disease due to breast cancer (Diel, 2004) and over 1-2 hours for hypercalcemia of malignancy (Pecherstorfer, 2003; Ralston, 1997).

Monitoring Parameters

Osteoporosis: Bone mineral density (BMD) should be evaluated 1 to 2 years after initiating therapy and every 2 years thereafter (NOF [Cosman 2014]); annual measurements of height and weight, assessment of chronic back pain; serum calcium and 25(OH)D; may consider measuring biochemical markers of bone turnover

Serum creatinine prior to each IV dose

Reference Range

Calcium (total): Adults: 9.0 to 11.0 mg/dL (2.05 to 2.54 mmol/L), may slightly decrease with aging

Phosphorus: 2.5 to 4.5 mg/dL (0.81 to 1.45 mmol/L)

Vitamin D: There is no clear consensus on a reference range for total serum 25(OH)D concentrations or the validity of this level as it relates clinically to bone health. In addition, there is significant variability in the reporting of serum 25(OH)D levels as a result of different assay types in use; however, the following ranges have been suggested:

Adults (IOM 2011): Sufficient levels in practically all persons: ≥20 ng/mL (50 nmol/L); concern for risk of toxicity: >50 ng/mL (125 nmol/L)

Osteoporosis patients (NOF [Cosman 2014]): Recommended level to reach and maintain: ~30 ng/mL (75 nmol/L)

Test Interactions Bisphosphonates may interfere with diagnostic imaging agents such as technetium-99m-diphosphonate in bone scans.

Dosage Forms Excipient information presented when available (limited, particularly for generics); consult specific product labeling.

Solution, Intravenous:

Boniva: 3 mg/3 mL (3 mL)

Generic: 3 mg/3 mL (3 mL)

Solution, Intravenous [preservative free]:

Generic: 3 mg/3 mL (3 mL)

Tablet, Oral:

Boniva: 150 mg

Generic: 150 mg

Ibrutinib (eye BROO ti nib)

Brand Names: US Imbruvica

Brand Names: Canada Imbruvica

Index Terms BTK inhibitor PCI-32765; CRA-032765; PCI-32765

Pharmacologic Category Antineoplastic Agent; Antineoplastic Agent, Bruton Tyrosine Kinase Inhibitor; Antineoplastic Agent, Tyrosine Kinase Inhibitor

Use

Chronic lymphocytic leukemia: Treatment of patients with chronic lymphocytic leukemia (CLL) who have received at least 1 prior therapy; treatment of CLL patients with 17p deletion.

Mantle cell lymphoma: Treatment of mantle cell lymphoma (MCL) in patients who have received at least 1 prior therapy

Waldenström macroglobulinemia: Treatment of patients with Waldenström macroglobulinemia

Pregnancy Considerations Adverse events were observed in animal reproduction studies. The US labeling recommends women of reproductive potential avoid pregnancy during therapy. The Canadian labeling recommends women of reproductive potential use highly effective contraception during and for 3 months after completion of treatment; if using a hormonal method of contraception, add a barrier method; male patients should use a condom (during and for 3 months after completion of treatment) when engaging in sexual activity with a pregnant woman.

Breast-Feeding Considerations It is not known if ibrutinib is excreted in breast milk. Due to the potential for serious adverse reactions in the nursing infant, the manufacturer recommends a decision be made whether to discontinue nursing or to discontinue the drug, taking into account the importance of treatment to the mother.

Contraindications

US labeling: There are no contraindications listed in the manufacturer's labeling.

Canadian labeling: Known hypersensitivity to ibrutinib or any component of the formulation.

Warnings/Precautions Hazardous agent – use appropriate precautions for handling and disposal (meets NIOSH 2014 criteria). Grade 3 and 4 neutropenia, thrombocytopenia, and anemia occurred commonly during clinical studies. Monitor blood counts monthly or as clinically necessary. Lymphocytosis (≥50% increase from baseline) may occur upon therapy initiation, generally within the first few weeks of therapy. The increase in lymphocytes is temporary, and resolves by a median of 8 weeks (mantle cell lymphoma) or 23 weeks (chronic lymphocytic leukemia). Some patients who developed lymphocytosis (lymphocytes >400,000/mcL) have developed intracranial hemorrhage, lethargy, headache, and gait instability (some cases may have been associated with disease progression). Monitor for leukostasis, particularly in patients experiencing a rapid increase in lymphocytes to >400,000/mcL. Grade 3 or higher bleeding events (subdural hematoma, gastrointestinal bleeding, hematuria, and post-procedural bleeding) have occurred; some events were fatal. Bleeding events of any grade, including bruising and petechiae have occurred in approximately half of patients receiving ibrutinib. Patients receiving concurrent antiplatelet or anticoagulant treatment may have an increased risk for bleeding. Evaluate the risk-benefit of withholding ibrutinib for 3 to 7 days prior to and after surgery, depending on the procedure type and risk of bleeding. Serious infections (some fatal) have been observed; monitor closely for fever and other signs/symptoms of infection. Evaluate promptly. Progressive multifocal encephalopathy (PML) has been observed; monitor closely and evaluate promptly. Patients treated with ibrutinib have developed second primary malignancies, including skin cancers and other carcinomas. Evaluate for sign/symptoms of malignancy during treatment.

Atrial fibrillation and atrial flutter have occurred, particularly in patients with cardiac risk factors, infections (acute), or with a history of atrial fibrillation. Monitor periodically for clinical symptoms of atrial fibrillation (eg, palpitations, lightheadedness); an ECG should be performed if symptoms or new onset dyspnea develop. For persistent atrial fibrillation, evaluate the risk-benefit of ibrutinib treatment and dose modification. Atrial fibrillation, hypertension, infections (eg, pneumonia, cellulitis, urinary tract infection), and gastrointestinal toxicity (eg, diarrhea and dehydration) were observed more frequently in elderly patients; maintain adequate hydration. Hyperviscosity may require plasmapheresis prior to or during ibrutinib treatment in patients with Waldenström macroglobulinemia; adjustment of ibrutinib dose due to plasmapheresis is not necessary. Use with caution in patients with preexisting renal impairment; has not been studied in those with severe impairment or in patients on dialysis. Renal failure has been reported with use; some cases were fatal. Clinical trials report serum creatinine increases of up to 3 times ULN; monitor renal function periodically and maintain hydration. Tumor lysis syndrome has been reported; increased uric acid levels have been observed, including grade 4 elevations. Monitor for tumor lysis syndrome in patients at risk (eg, high tumor burden). Ibrutinib is hepatically metabolized, and exposure is increased in patients with hepatic dysfunction. Dosage adjustment is recommended in patients with mild (Child-Pugh class A) impairment; avoid use in patients with moderate or severe (Child-Pugh class B or C) impairment. Monitor closely for toxicity. May cause dizziness, fatigue, and/or weakness which may impair physical or mental abilities; patients must be cautioned about performing tasks that require mental alertness (eg, operating machinery or driving). Potentially significant drug-drug/drug-food interactions may exist, requiring dose or frequency adjustment, additional monitoring, and/or selection of alternative therapy.

Adverse Reactions Incidences combined for mantle cell lymphoma (MCL), chronic lymphocytic leukemia (CLL), Waldenström macroglobulinemia (WM) and unless otherwise specified.

>10%:

Cardiovascular: Peripheral edema (MCL: 35%, CLL: 23%; grades 3/4: MCL: 3%), hypertension (CLL: 17%; grades 3/4: CLL: 8%)

Central nervous system: Fatigue (MCL: 41%, CLL, WM: 21% to 31%; grades 3/4: CLL, MCL: 2% to 5%), dizziness (11% to 21%), headache (13% to 19%; grades 3/4: CLL: 1% to 2%), chills (CLL: 13%)

Dermatologic: Skin rash (22% to 27%; grades 3/4: CCL, MCL: 3%), skin infection (14% to 17%; grades 3/4: 2% to 6%), pruritus (WM: 11%)

Endocrine & metabolic: Increased uric acid (MCL: 40%; increased uric acid >10 mg/dL: MCL: 13%), hyperuricemia (MCL: 15%), dehydration (MCL: 12%; grades 3/4: MCL: 4%)

Gastrointestinal: Diarrhea (CLL, MCL: 48% to 63%, WM: 37%; grades 3/4: CCL: 4% to 5%), nausea (21% to 31%; grades 3/4: CLL: 2%), constipation (CLL, MCL: 15% to 25%; grades 3/4: CLL: 2%), abdominal pain (MCL: 24%, CLL: 15%; grades 3/4: MCL: 5%), vomiting (CLL, MCL: 14% to 23%; grades 3/4: CLL: ≤2%), decreased appetite (CLL, MCL: 17% to 21%; grades 3/4: CLL, MCL: 2%), stomatitis (16% to 21%; grades 3/4: CLL, MCL: 1%), gastroesophageal reflux disease (WM: 13%), dyspepsia (CLL, MCL: 11% to 13%)

Genitourinary: Urinary tract infection (CLL, MCL: 10% to 14%; grades 3/4: CLL, MCL: 3% to 4%)

Hematologic & oncologic: Decreased platelet count (CLL, MCL: 52% to 71%, WM: 43%; grades 3/4: 5% to 17%), bruise (11% to 54%; grades 3/4: CLL: 2%), neutropenia (44% to 54%; grades 3/4: 19% to 29%), decreased hemoglobin (CLL, MCL: 36% to 44%, WM: 13%; grades 3/4: MCL, WM: 8% to 9%), petechia (CLL, MCL: 11% to 17%), thrombocytopenia (5% to 17%), malignant neoplasm (secondary; 5% to 14%; includes one death due to histiocytic sarcoma), malignant neoplasm of skin (4% to 11%; nonmelanoma)

Infection: Infection (≥ grade 3: 14% to 26%)

Neuromuscular & skeletal: Musculoskeletal pain (CLL, MCL: 27% to 37%; grades 3/4: CLL: 2% to 6%; grades 3/4: MCL: 1%), arthralgia (CLL: 17% to 23%, MCL: 11%; grades 3/4: CLL: 1%), muscle spasm (14% to 21%; grades 3/4: CLL: 2%), weakness (CLL, MCL: 13% to 14%; grades 3/4: CLL, MCL: 3% to 4%), arthropathy (WM: 13%)

Respiratory: Upper respiratory tract infection (16% to 48%; grades 3/4: CLL: 1% to 2%), dyspnea (MCL: 27%, CLL: 10%; grades 3/4: MCL: 4%), sinusitis (11% to 21%; grades 3/4: CLL, MCL: 1% to 6%), cough (13% to 19%), oropharyngeal pain (CLL: 15%), pneumonia (10% to 15%; grades 3/4: 6% to 10%), epistaxis (MCL, WM: 11% to 19%)

Miscellaneous: Fever (CLL, MCL: 18% to 25%; grades 3/4: CLL, MCL: 1% to 2%)

1% to 10%:

Cardiovascular: Atrial fibrillation (≤6% to 9%), atrial flutter (≤6% to 9%)

Central nervous system: Anxiety (CLL: 10%), insomnia (CLL: 10%), peripheral neuropathy (CLL: 10%)

Hematologic & oncologic: Anemia (grades 3/4: ≤9%), hemorrhage (≤6%; grade 3 or higher bleeding events including gastrointestinal bleeding, hematuria, postprocedural bleeding, subdural hematoma), carcinoma (1% to 3%, other nonskin carcinoma)

Ophthalmic: Blurred vision (CLL: 10%)

Renal: Increased serum creatinine (1.5 to 3 x ULN: 9%)

Miscellaneous: Laceration (CLL: 10%; grades 3/4: CLL: 2%)

<1% (Limited to important or life threatening): Hypersensitivity (includes anaphylactic shock, angioedema, urticaria), progressive multifocal leukoencephalopathy, renal failure, tumor lysis syndrome

Drug Interactions

Metabolism/Transport Effects Substrate of CYP2D6 (minor), CYP3A4 (major); **Note:** Assignment of Major/Minor substrate status based on clinically relevant drug interaction potential; **Inhibits** BCRP, P-glycoprotein

Avoid Concomitant Use

Avoid concomitant use of Ibrutinib with any of the following: BCG (Intravesical); Bitter Orange; Bosutinib; Conivaptan; CYP3A4 Inducers (Strong); CYP3A4 Inhibitors (Moderate); CYP3A4 Inhibitors (Strong); Deferiprone; Dipyrone; Fusidic Acid (Systemic); Idelalisib;

Natalizumab; PAZOPanib; Pimecrolimus; Silodosin; St Johns Wort; Tacrolimus (Topical); Tofacitinib; Topotecan; Vaccines (Live); VinCRIStine (Liposomal)

Increased Effect/Toxicity

Ibrutinib may increase the levels/effects of: Afatinib; Agents with Antiplatelet Properties; Anticoagulants; Bosutinib; Brentuximab Vedotin; CloZAPine; Colchicine; Dabigatran Etexilate; Deferiprone; DOXOrubicin (Conventional); Edoxaban; Everolimus; Fingolimod; Ledipasvir; Leflunomide; Naloxegol; Natalizumab; PAZOPanib; P-glycoprotein/ABCB1 Substrates; Prucalopride; Ranolazine; Rifaximin; Silodosin; Tofacitinib; Topotecan; Vaccines (Live); VinCRIStine (Liposomal)

The levels/effects of Ibrutinib may be increased by: Bitter Orange; Conivaptan; CYP3A4 Inhibitors (Moderate); CYP3A4 Inhibitors (Strong); Dasatinib; Denosumab; Dipyrone; Flaxseed Oil; Fosaprepitant; Fusidic Acid (Systemic); Idelalisib; Ivacaftor; Luliconazole; Omega-3 Fatty Acids; Osimertinib; Palbociclib; Pimecrolimus; Roflumilast; Simeprevir; Stiripentol; Tacrolimus (Topical); Trastuzumab; Vitamin E; Vitamin E (Oral)

Decreased Effect

Ibrutinib may decrease the levels/effects of: BCG (Intravesical); Coccidioides immitis Skin Test; Sipuleucel-T; Vaccines (Inactivated); Vaccines (Live)

The levels/effects of Ibrutinib may be decreased by: CYP3A4 Inducers (Moderate); CYP3A4 Inducers (Strong); Dabrafenib; Deferasirox; Echinacea; Osimertinib; Siltuximab; St Johns Wort; Tocilizumab

Food Interactions Grapefruit and Seville oranges moderately inhibit CYP3A and may increase ibrutinib exposure. Management: Avoid grapefruit and Seville oranges during therapy.

Storage/Stability Store at 20°C to 25°C (68°F to 77°F); excursions are permitted between 15°C and 30°C (59°F and 86°F). Keep in original container until dispensing.

Mechanism of Action Ibrutinib is a potent and irreversible inhibitor of Bruton's tyrosine kinase (BTK), an integral component of the B-cell receptor (BCR) and cytokine receptor pathways. Constitutive activation of B-cell receptor signaling is important for survival of malignant B-cells; BTK inhibition results in decreased malignant B-cell proliferation and survival.

Pharmacodynamics/Kinetics

Distribution: ~10,000 L (Marostica 2015)

Bioavailability: Administration with food increased the C_{max} by ~2- to 4-fold and the AUC 2-fold (compared with overnight fasting). Administration under fasting conditions resulted in exposure of ~60% compared to when administered either 30 minutes before or after a meal, or 2 hours after a high-fat meal (de Jong 2015).

Protein binding: ~97%

Metabolism: Hepatic via CYP3A (major) and CYP2D6 (minor) to active metabolite PCI-45227

Half-life elimination: 4 to 6 hours

Time to peak: 1 to 2 hours (4 hours under fed conditions [de Jong 2015])

Excretion: Feces (80%; ~1% as unchanged drug); urine (<10%, as metabolites)

Dosing

Adult & Geriatric

Chronic lymphocytic leukemia (CLL), previously treated: Oral: 420 mg once daily (Byrd 2014).

CLL with 17p deletion: Oral: 420 mg once daily (Byrd 2014).

Mantle cell lymphoma (MCL), previously treated: Oral: 560 mg once daily (Wang 2013).

Waldenström macroglobulinemia (WM): Oral: 420 mg once daily (Treon 2015)

Missed doses: Administer as soon as the missed dose is remembered on the same day; return to normal scheduling the following day. Do not take extra capsules to make up for the missed dose.

Dosage adjustment for concomitant therapy:

Moderate or strong CYP3A inhibitors:

US labeling: Avoid concurrent use with moderate or strong CYP3A inhibitors which are taken chronically; consider an alternative agent with less CYP3A inhibition. If short term use (≤7 days) of a strong inhibitor is necessary, consider withholding ibrutinib therapy until the strong CYP3A inhibitor is discontinued. If concomitant use of a moderate inhibitor is necessary, reduce ibrutinib dose to 140 mg once daily. Monitor closely for toxicity during concomitant use.

Canadian labeling: Avoid concurrent use with moderate or strong CYP3A inhibitors; consider an alternative agent with less CYP3A inhibition. If use of a strong inhibitor is necessary, withhold ibrutinib temporarily until the strong CYP3A inhibitor is discontinued. If concomitant use of a moderate inhibitor is

necessary, reduce ibrutinib dose to 140 mg once daily until the inhibitor is discontinued. Monitor closely for toxicity during concomitant use.

Strong CYP3A inducers: Avoid concurrent use with strong CYP3A inducers; consider alternative agents with less CYP3A induction.

Renal Impairment

Mild to moderate impairment (CrCl ≥25 mL/minute [US labeling] or CrCl >30 mL/minute [Canadian labeling]): There are no dosage adjustments provided in the manufacturer's labeling; however, renal excretion is minimal and drug exposure is not altered in patients with mild to moderate impairment.

Severe impairment (CrCl <25 mL/minute [US labeling] or CrCl ≤30 mL/minute [Canadian labeling]): There are no dosage adjustments provided in the manufacturer's labeling (has not been studied).

End-stage renal disease (ESRD) requiring dialysis: There are no dosage adjustments provided in the manufacturer's labeling (has not been studied).

Hepatic Impairment

US labeling:

Mild impairment (Child-Pugh class A): Reduce dose to 140 mg once daily.

Moderate and severe impairment (Child-Pugh class B and C): Avoid use.

Canadian labeling:

Mild impairment (Child-Pugh class A): May consider dose reduction to 140 mg once daily (based on preliminary data) only if clinically indicated; monitor closely.

Moderate and severe impairment (Child-Pugh class B and C): Avoid use.

Adjustment for Toxicity

Hematologic toxicity: ≥ grade 3 neutropenia with infection or fever, or grade 4 toxicity: Interrupt therapy; upon improvement to grade 1 toxicity or baseline, resume dosing at the starting dose. If toxicity recurs, reduce daily dose by 140 mg. If toxicity recurs after first dose reduction, reduce daily dose by an additional 140 mg. If toxicity persists following 2 dose reductions, discontinue therapy.

Nonhematologic toxicity: ≥ grade 3 toxicity: Interrupt therapy; upon improvement to grade 1 toxicity or baseline, resume dosing at the starting dose. If toxicity recurs, reduce daily dose by 140 mg. If toxicity recurs after first dose reduction, reduce daily dose by an additional 140 mg. If toxicity persists following 2 dose reductions, discontinue therapy.

Recommend dose reductions for toxicity (following recovery):

Chronic lymphocytic leukemia and Waldenström macroglobulinemia:

First occurrence: Restart at 420 mg once daily

Second occurrence: Restart at 280 mg once daily

Third occurrence: Restart at 140 mg once daily

Fourth occurrence: Discontinue

Mantle cell lymphoma:

First occurrence: Restart at 560 mg once daily

Second occurrence: Restart at 420 mg once daily

Third occurrence: Restart at 280 mg once daily

Fourth occurrence: Discontinue

Dietary Considerations Avoid grapefruit, grapefruit juice, and Seville oranges during therapy.

Administration Administer orally with water at approximately the same time every day. Swallow capsules whole; do not open, break, or chew the capsules. Maintain adequate hydration during treatment. Hazardous agent; use appropriate precautions for handling and disposal (meets NIOSH 2014 criteria).

Based on an analysis of 3 pharmacokinetic studies, it is suggested that ibrutinib may be administered without regard to food (de Jong 2015).

Monitoring Parameters Monitor blood counts monthly or as clinically necessary; renal and hepatic function; uric acid levels as clinically necessary; sign/symptoms of bleeding, infections, progressive multifocal encephalopathy, tumor lysis syndrome, and second primary malignancies; signs/symptoms of atrial fibrillation; ECG prior to initiation (patients with cardiac risk factors or history of atrial fibrillation) and during therapy if clinically indicated.

Dosage Forms Excipient information presented when available (limited, particularly for generics); consult specific product labeling.

Capsule, Oral:

Imbruvica: 140 mg

◆ IBU-200 [OTC] see Ibuprofen *on page 905*

◆ Ibudone see Hydrocodone and Ibuprofen *on page 885*

Ibuprofen (eye byoo PROE fen)

Brand Names: US Addaprin [OTC]; Advil Junior Strength [OTC]; Advil Migraine [OTC]; Advil [OTC]; Caldolor; Childrens Advil [OTC]; Childrens Ibuprofen [OTC]; Childrens Motrin Jr Strength [OTC]; Childrens Motrin [OTC]; Dyspel [OTC]; EnovaRX-Ibuprofen; Genpril [OTC]; HyVee Ibuprofen Childrens [OTC]; I-Prin [OTC]; IBU-200 [OTC]; Ibuprofen Childrens [OTC]; Ibuprofen Comfort Pac; Ibuprofen Junior Strength [OTC]; Infants Advil [OTC]; Infants Ibuprofen [OTC]; KS Ibuprofen [OTC]; Motrin IB [OTC]; Motrin Infants Drops [OTC]; Motrin Junior Strength [OTC]; Motrin [OTC]; NeoProfen; Provil [OTC]

Brand Names: Canada Advil; Advil Pediatric Drops; Apo-Ibuprofen; Caldolor; Children's Advil; Children's Europrofen; Ibuprofen Muscle and Joint; Jamp-Ibuprofen; Motrin; Motrin (Children's); Motrin IB; Novo-Profen; Pamprin Ibuprofen Formula; PMS-Ibuprofen; Super Strength Motrin IB Liquid Gel Capsules

Index Terms *p*-Isobutylhydratropic Acid; Ibuprofen Lysine

Pharmacologic Category Nonsteroidal Anti-inflammatory Drug (NSAID), Oral; Nonsteroidal Anti-inflammatory Drug (NSAID), Parenteral

Use

Oral: Inflammatory diseases and rheumatoid disorders, mild to moderate pain, fever, dysmenorrhea, osteoarthritis

Ibuprofen injection (Caldolor): Management of mild to moderate pain and management of moderate to severe pain as an adjunct to opioid analgesics in adults and children 6 months and older; reduction of fever in adults and children 6 months and older.

Ibuprofen lysine injection (NeoProfen): Patent ductus arteriosus (PDA): To close a clinically significant PDA in premature infants weighing between 500-1500 g who are no more than 32 weeks of gestational age when usual medical management (eg, diuretics, fluid restriction, respiratory support) is ineffective.

OTC labeling: Reduction of fever; management of pain due to headache, sore throat, arthritis, physical or athletic overexertion (eg, sprains/strains), menstrual pain, dental pain, minor muscle/bone/joint pain, backache, pain due to the common cold and flu

Pregnancy Considerations According to the Canadian prescribing information, use is contraindicated during the third trimester and during labor and delivery.

The chronic use of NSAIDs in women of reproductive age may be associated with infertility that is reversible upon discontinuation of the medication. Nonteratogenic effects, including prenatal constriction of the ductus arteriosus, persistent pulmonary hypertension of the newborn, oligohydramnios, necrotizing enterocolitis, renal dysfunction or failure, and intracranial hemorrhage have been observed in the fetus/neonate following in utero NSAID exposure. In addition, non-closure of the ductus arteriosus postnatally may occur and be resistant to medical management (Bermas 2014; Bloor 2013). Because they may cause premature closure of the ductus arteriosus, the use of NSAIDs late in pregnancy should be avoided. Product labeling for Caldolor specifically states use should be avoided starting at 30 weeks gestation.

Breast-Feeding Considerations According to the Canadian prescribing information, ibuprofen is contraindicated in women who are nursing.

Based on limited data, ibuprofen is excreted into breast milk, providing a relative infant dose of 0.06 to 0.6% of the weight adjusted maternal dose. Adverse events have not been reported in nursing infants. Due to the potential for serious adverse reactions in the nursing infant, the US manufacturers recommend that a decision be made whether to discontinue nursing or to discontinue the drug, taking into account the importance of treatment to the mother.

Medication Guide Available Yes

Contraindications

Hypersensitivity to ibuprofen (eg, anaphylactic reactions, serious skin reactions) or any component of the formulation; history of asthma, urticaria, or allergic-type reaction to aspirin or other NSAIDs; aspirin triad (eg, bronchial asthma, aspirin intolerance, rhinitis); in the setting of coronary artery bypass graft (CABG) surgery

Ibuprofen lysine (NeoProfen): Preterm neonates: With proven or suspected infection that is untreated; congenital heart disease in whom patency of the PDA is necessary for satisfactory pulmonary or systemic blood flow (eg, pulmonary atresia, severe coarctation of the aorta, severe tetralogy of Fallot); bleeding (especially those with active intracranial hemorrhage or GI bleeding); thrombocytopenia; coagulation defects; proven or suspected necrotizing enterocolitis; or significant renal function impairment.

Canadian labeling: Additional contraindications (not in US labeling): Cerebrovascular bleeding or other bleeding disorders; active gastric/duodenal/peptic ulcer, active GI bleeding; inflammatory bowel disease; uncontrolled heart failure; moderate [IV formulation only] to severe renal impairment (creatinine clearance [CrCl] <30 mL/minute); deteriorating renal disease; moderate [IV formulation only] to severe hepatic impairment; active hepatic disease; hyperkalemia; third trimester of pregnancy; breast-feeding; patients <18 years of age [IV formulation only]; patients <12 years of age [oral formulation only]; systemic lupus erythematosus [oral formulation only]

OTC labeling: When used for self-medication, do not use if previous allergic reaction to any other pain reliever/fever reducer; prior to or following cardiac surgery.

Warnings/Precautions [US Boxed Warning]: NSAIDs are associated with an increased risk of adverse cardiovascular thrombotic events, including fatal MI and stroke. Risk may be increased with duration of use or preexisting cardiovascular risk factors or disease. Carefully evaluate individual cardiovascular risk profiles prior to prescribing. May cause new-onset hypertension or worsening of existing hypertension. Use caution with fluid retention. Avoid use in heart failure (ACCF/AHA [Yancy 2013]). Avoid Caldolor in patients with a recent MI. Concurrent administration of ibuprofen, and potentially other nonselective NSAIDs, may interfere with aspirin's cardioprotective effect. **[US Boxed Warning]: Use is contraindicated for treatment of perioperative pain in the setting of coronary artery bypass graft (CABG) surgery.** Risk of MI and stroke may be increased with use following CABG surgery.

May increase the risk of aseptic meningitis, especially in patients with systemic lupus erythematosus (SLE) and mixed connective tissue disorders. Platelet adhesion and aggregation may be decreased; may prolong bleeding time; patients with coagulation disorders or who are receiving anticoagulants should be monitored closely. Anemia may occur; patients on long-term NSAID therapy should be monitored for anemia. Rarely, NSAID use may cause severe blood dyscrasias (eg, agranulocytosis, aplastic anemia, thrombocytopenia).

NSAID use may compromise existing renal function; dose-dependent decreases in prostaglandin synthesis may result from NSAID use, reducing renal blood flow which may cause renal decompensation. NSAID use may increase the risk for hyperkalemia. Patients with impaired renal function, dehydration, heart failure, liver dysfunction, those taking diuretics, and ACE inhibitors, and the elderly are at greater risk of renal toxicity and hyperkalemia. Rehydrate patient before starting therapy; monitor renal function closely. The Canadian labeling contraindicates use in moderate (IV only) to severe renal impairment, with deteriorating renal disease and in patients with hyperkalemia. Use of ibuprofen lysine (NeoProfen) is contraindicated in preterm infants with significant renal impairment. Long-term NSAID use may result in renal papillary necrosis.

NSAIDs may increase risk of gastrointestinal irritation, inflammation, ulceration, bleeding, and perforation. These events can be fatal and may occur at any time during therapy and without warning. Elderly patients are at increased risk for serious adverse events. Use caution with a history of GI disease (bleeding or ulcers), concurrent therapy with aspirin, anticoagulants and/or corticosteroids, smoking, use of ethanol, the elderly or debilitated patients. When used concomitantly with aspirin, a substantial increase in the risk of gastrointestinal complications (eg, ulcer) occurs; concomitant gastroprotective therapy (eg, proton pump inhibitors) is recommended (Bhatt 2008). The Canadian labeling contraindicates use in patients with active GI disease (eg, peptic ulcer) or GI bleeding and inflammatory bowel disease.

Use the lowest effective dose for the shortest duration of time, consistent with individual patient goals, to reduce risk of cardiovascular or GI adverse events. Alternate therapies should be considered for patients at high risk.

NSAIDs may cause potentially fatal serious skin adverse events including exfoliative dermatitis, Stevens-Johnson Syndrome (SJS) and toxic epidermal necrolysis (TEN); discontinue use at first sign of skin rash or hypersensitivity. Anaphylactoid reactions may occur, even without prior exposure; patients with "aspirin triad" (bronchial asthma, aspirin intolerance, rhinitis) may be at increased risk. Do not use in patients who experience bronchospasm,

asthma, rhinitis, or urticaria with NSAID or aspirin therapy. Use caution in other forms of asthma.

NSAIDS may cause drowsiness, dizziness, blurred vision and other neurologic effects which may impair physical or mental abilities; patients must be cautioned about performing tasks which require mental alertness (eg, operating machinery or driving). Monitor vision with long-term therapy. Blurred/diminished vision, scotomata, and changes in color vision have been reported. Discontinue use with altered vision and perform ophthalmologic exam.

Use with caution in patients with decreased hepatic function. Closely monitor patients with any abnormal LFT. Severe hepatic reactions (eg, fulminant hepatitis, jaundice, liver necrosis, liver failure) have occurred with NSAID use, rarely; discontinue if signs or symptoms of liver disease develop, or if systemic manifestations occur. The Canadian labeling contraindicates use in moderate (IV only) to severe hepatic impairment and with active hepatic disease.

In the elderly, avoid chronic use (unless alternative agents ineffective and patient can receive concomitant gastroprotective agent); nonselective oral NSAID use is associated with an increased risk of GI bleeding and peptic ulcer disease in older adults in high risk category (eg, >75 years or age or receiving concomitant oral/parenteral corticosteroids, anticoagulants, or antiplatelet agents) (Beers Criteria). Potentially significant drug interactions may exist, requiring dose or frequency adjustment, additional monitoring, and/or selection of alternative therapy.

Withhold for at least 4 to 6 half-lives prior to surgical or dental procedures.

Ibuprofen injection (Caldolor) must be diluted prior to administration; hemolysis can occur if not diluted.

Ibuprofen lysine injection (NeoProfen): Hold second or third doses if urinary output is <0.6 mL/kg/hour. May alter signs of infection. May inhibit platelet aggregation; monitor for signs of bleeding. May displace bilirubin; use caution when total bilirubin is elevated. Long-term evaluations of neurodevelopment, growth, or diseases associated with prematurity following treatment have not been conducted. A second course of treatment, alternative pharmacologic therapy or surgery may be needed if the ductus arteriosus fails to close or reopens following the initial course of therapy.

Benzyl alcohol and derivatives: Some dosage forms may contain sodium benzoate/benzoic acid; benzoic acid (benzoate) is a metabolite of benzyl alcohol; large amounts of benzyl alcohol (≥99 mg/kg/day) have been associated with a potentially fatal toxicity ("gasping syndrome") in neonates; the "gasping syndrome" consists of metabolic acidosis, respiratory distress, gasping respirations, CNS dysfunction (including convulsions, intracranial hemorrhage), hypotension, and cardiovascular collapse (AAP ["Inactive" 1997]; CDC 1982); some data suggests that benzoate displaces bilirubin from protein binding sites (Ahlfors 2001); avoid or use dosage forms containing benzyl alcohol derivative with caution in neonates. See manufacturer's labeling.

Propylene glycol: Some dosage forms may contain propylene glycol; large amounts are potentially toxic and have been associated hyperosmolality, lactic acidosis, seizures and respiratory depression; use caution (AAP ["Inactive" 1997]; Zar 2007).

Polysorbate 80: Some dosage forms may contain polysorbate 80 (also known as Tweens). Hypersensitivity reactions, usually a delayed reaction, have been reported following exposure to pharmaceutical products containing polysorbate 80 in certain individuals (Isaksson 2002; Lucente 2000; Shelley 1995). Thrombocytopenia, ascites, pulmonary deterioration, and renal and hepatic failure have been reported in premature neonates after receiving parenteral products containing polysorbate 80 (Alade 1986; CDC 1984). See manufacturer's labeling.

Phenylalanine: Some products may contain phenylalanine.

Self medication (OTC use): Prior to self-medication, patients should contact healthcare provider if they have had recurring stomach pain or upset, ulcers, bleeding problems, high blood pressure, heart or kidney disease, other serious medical problems, are currently taking a diuretic, aspirin, anticoagulant, or are ≥60 years of age. If patients are using for migraines, they should also contact healthcare provider if they have not had a migraine diagnosis by healthcare provider, a headache that is different from usual migraine, worst headache of life, fever and neck stiffness, headache from head injury or coughing, first headache at ≥50 years of age, daily headache, or migraine requiring bed rest. Recommended dosages should not be

exceeded, due to an increased risk of GI bleeding. Stop use and consult a healthcare provider if symptoms get worse, newly appear, fever lasts for >3 days or pain lasts >3 days (children) and >10 days (adults). Do not give for >10 days unless instructed by healthcare provider. Consuming ≥3 alcoholic beverages/day or taking longer than recommended may increase the risk of GI bleeding.

Adverse Reactions

Oral:

1% to 10%:

Cardiovascular: Edema (1% to 3%)

Central nervous system: Dizziness (3% to 9%), headache (1% to 3%), nervousness (1% to 3%)

Dermatologic: Skin rash (3% to 9%), pruritus (1% to 3%)

Endocrine & metabolic: Fluid retention (1% to 3%)

Gastrointestinal: Epigastric pain (3% to 9%), heartburn (3% to 9%), nausea (3% to 9%), abdominal pain (1% to 3%), constipation (1% to 3%), decreased appetite (1% to 3%), diarrhea (1% to 3%), dyspepsia (1% to 3%), flatulence (1% to 3%), vomiting (1% to 3%)

Otic: Tinnitus (3% to 9%)

<1% (Limited to important or life-threatening): Abnormal liver function tests, acute renal failure, agranulocytosis, anaphylaxis, aplastic anemia, azotemia, blurred vision, bone marrow depression, confusion, decreased creatinine clearance, decreased hematocrit, decreased hemoglobin, decreased platelet aggregation, duodenal ulcer, eosinophilia, epistaxis, erythema multiforme, gastric ulcer, gastrointestinal hemorrhage, gastrointestinal ulcer, hallucination, hearing loss, hematuria, hemolytic anemia, hepatitis, hepatotoxicity (idiosyncratic) (Chalasani, 2014), hypertension, jaundice, leukopenia, melena, neutropenia, pancreatitis, skin photosensitivity, Stevens-Johnson syndrome, thrombocytopenia, toxic amblyopia, toxic epidermal necrolysis, urticaria, vesiculobullous dermatitis, visual disturbance

Injection: Ibuprofen (Caldolor): Frequency not defined.

Cardiovascular: Edema, hypertension

Central nervous system: Dizziness, headache

Dermatologic: Pruritus

Endocrine & metabolic: Hypernatremia, hypokalemia

Gastrointestinal: Abdominal pain, dyspepsia, flatulence, nausea, vomiting

Genitourinary: Urinary retention

Hematologic & oncologic: Anemia, hemorrhage, neutropenia

Renal: Increased blood urea nitrogen

Respiratory: Cough

Postmarketing and/or case reports (Limited to important or life-threatening): Hepatotoxicity (idiosyncratic) (Chalasani, 2014)

Injection: Ibuprofen lysine (NeoProfen): Frequency not always defined.

Cardiovascular: Edema (4%), cardiac failure, hypotension, tachycardia

Central nervous system: Intraventricular hemorrhage (29%; grades 3/4: 15%), seizure

Dermatologic: Skin irritation (16%)

Endocrine & metabolic: Hypocalcemia (12%), hypoglycemia (12%), adrenocortical insufficiency (7%), hypernatremia (7%), hyperglycemia

Gastrointestinal: Gastrointestinal disease (non NEC; 22%), abdominal distension, cholestasis, gastritis, gastroesophageal reflux disease, inguinal hernia, intestinal obstruction

Genitourinary: Urinary tract infection (9%), uremia (7%), decreased urine output (3%; small decrease reported on days 2 to 6 with compensatory increase in output on day 9)

Hematologic & oncologic: Anemia (32%), neutropenia, thrombocytopenia

Hepatic: Jaundice

Infection: Sepsis (43%), infection

Local: Injection site reaction

Renal: Renal insufficiency (6%), increased serum creatinine (3%), renal failure (1%)

Respiratory: Apnea (28%), respiratory tract infection (19%), respiratory failure (10%), atelectasis (4%)

Miscellaneous: Sepsis (43%), Reduced intake of food/fluids

Postmarketing and/or case reports (Limited to important or life-threatening): Gastrointestinal perforation, hepatotoxicity (idiosyncratic) (Chalasani, 2014), necrotizing enterocolitis

Drug Interactions

Metabolism/Transport Effects Substrate of CYP2C19 (minor), CYP2C9 (minor); **Note:** Assignment of Major/Minor substrate status based on clinically relevant drug interaction potential; **Inhibits** CYP2C9 (weak)

Avoid Concomitant Use

Avoid concomitant use of Ibuprofen with any of the following: Dexketoprofen; Floctafenine; Ketorolac (Nasal); Ketorolac (Systemic); Morniflumate; NSAID (COX-2 Inhibitor); Omacetaxine; Talniflumate; Urokinase

Increased Effect/Toxicity

Ibuprofen may increase the levels/effects of: 5-ASA Derivatives; Agents with Antiplatelet Properties; Aliskiren; Aminoglycosides; Anticoagulants; Apixaban; Bisphosphonate Derivatives; Collagenase (Systemic); CycloSPORINE (Systemic); Dabigatran Etexilate; Deferasirox; Deoxycholic Acid; Desmopressin; Digoxin; Drospirenone; Edoxaban; Eplerenone; Haloperidol; Ibritumomab; Lithium; Methotrexate; Nonsteroidal Anti-Inflammatory Agents; NSAID (COX-2 Inhibitor); Obinutuzumab; Omacetaxine; PEMEtrexed; Porfimer; Potassium-Sparing Diuretics; PRALAtrexate; Quinolone Antibiotics; Rivaroxaban; Salicylates; Tacrolimus (Systemic); Tenofovir Products; Thrombolytic Agents; Tositumomab and Iodine I 131 Tositumomab; Urokinase; Vancomycin; Verteporfin; Vitamin K Antagonists

The levels/effects of Ibuprofen may be increased by: ACE Inhibitors; Alcohol (Ethyl); Angiotensin II Receptor Blockers; Antidepressants (Tricyclic, Tertiary Amine); Corticosteroids (Systemic); CycloSPORINE (Systemic); Dasatinib; Dexketoprofen; Diclofenac (Systemic); Floctafenine; Glucosamine; Herbs (Anticoagulant/Antiplatelet Properties); Ibrutinib; Ketorolac (Nasal); Ketorolac (Systemic); Limaprost; Loop Diuretics; Morniflumate; Multivitamins/Fluoride (with ADE); Multivitamins/Minerals (with ADEK, Folate, Iron); Multivitamins/Minerals (with AE, No Iron); Omega-3 Fatty Acids; Pentosan Polysulfate Sodium; Pentoxifylline; Probenecid; Prostacyclin Analogues; Selective Serotonin Reuptake Inhibitors; Serotonin/Norepinephrine Reuptake Inhibitors; Sodium Phosphates; Talniflumate; Thiazide Diuretics; Tipranavir; Treprostinil; Vitamin E; Vitamin E (Oral); Voriconazole

Decreased Effect

Ibuprofen may decrease the levels/effects of: ACE Inhibitors; Aliskiren; Angiotensin II Receptor Blockers; Beta-Blockers; Eplerenone; HydrALAZINE; Imatinib; Loop Diuretics; Potassium-Sparing Diuretics; Prostaglandins (Ophthalmic); Salicylates; Selective Serotonin Reuptake Inhibitors; Thiazide Diuretics

The levels/effects of Ibuprofen may be decreased by: Bile Acid Sequestrants; Salicylates

Food Interactions Ibuprofen peak serum levels may be decreased if taken with food. Management: Administer with food.

Preparation for Administration

Ibuprofen injection (Caldolor): Must be diluted prior to use. Dilute with D$_5$W, NS or LR to a final concentration ≤4 mg/mL.

Ibuprofen lysine injection (NeoProfen): Dilute with dextrose or saline to an appropriate volume.

Storage/Stability

Ibuprofen injection (Caldolor): Store intact vials at 20°C to 25°C (68°F to 77°F); excursions permitted to 15°C to 30°C (59°F to 86°F). Must be diluted prior to use. Diluted solutions stable for 24 hours at 20°C to 25°C (68°F to 77°F).

Ibuprofen lysine injection (NeoProfen): Store at 20°C to 25°C (68°F to 77°F); excursions are permitted between 15°C and 30°C (59°F and 86°F). Protect from light. Store vials in carton until use. After first withdrawal from vial, discard remaining solution (preservative free). Following dilution, use within 30 minutes.

Suspension: Store at 15°C to 30°C (59°F to 86°F).

Tablet: Store at 20°C to 25°C (68°F to 77°F).

Mechanism of Action Reversibly inhibits cyclooxygenase-1 and 2 (COX-1 and 2) enzymes, which results in decreased formation of prostaglandin precursors; has antipyretic, analgesic, and anti-inflammatory properties

Other proposed mechanisms not fully elucidated (and possibly contributing to the anti-inflammatory effect to varying degrees), include inhibiting chemotaxis, altering lymphocyte activity, inhibiting neutrophil aggregation/activation, and decreasing proinflammatory cytokine levels.

Pharmacodynamics/Kinetics

Onset of action: Oral: Analgesic: Within 30 to 60 minutes (Davies, 1998; Mehlisch, 2013); Antipyretic: <1 hour (Sullivan, 2011)

Duration: Oral: Antipyretic: 6 to 8 hours (Sullivan, 2011)

Absorption: Oral: Rapid

Distribution: V$_d$: 6.35 L; Premature infants (highly variable between studies; Van Overmeire, 2001):

Day 3: 160 to 328 mL/kg; Subset with ductal closure: 145 to 349 mL/kg

Day 5: 94 to 248 mL/kg; Subset with ductal closure: 72 to 222 mL/kg

Protein binding: >99%; Premature infants: ~95% (Aranda, 1997)

Bioavailability: 80%

Metabolism: Hepatic via oxidation

Half-life elimination:

Premature infants (highly variable between studies): 23 to 75 hours (Aranda, 2006; Capparelli, 2007)

Children 3 months to 10 years: 1.6 ± 0.7 hours

Adults: ~2 hours; End-stage renal disease: Unchanged (Aronoff, 2007)

Time to peak: Oral: ~1 to 2 hours

Excretion: Urine (primarily as metabolites; 1% as unchanged drug); some feces

Dosing

Adult

Analgesia/pain/dysmenorrhea: Oral: 400 mg every 4 to 6 hours as needed

Analgesic: IV (Caldolor): 400 to 800 mg every 6 hours as needed (maximum: 3,200 mg/day). **Note:** Patients should be well hydrated prior to administration.

Antipyretic: IV (Caldolor): **Note:** Patients should be well hydrated prior to administration.

US labeling: Initial: 400 mg, then every 4 to 6 hours or 100 to 200 mg every 4 hours as needed (maximum: 3,200 mg/day)

Canadian labeling: Initial: 200 to 400 mg, then every 4 to 6 hours as needed up to 24 hours (maximum: 2,400 mg/day)

Osteoarthritis, rheumatoid arthritis: Oral:

US labeling: 400 to 800 mg 3 to 4 times daily (maximum: 3,200 mg/day)

Canadian labeling: Initial: 600 mg 2 times daily; if necessary, may increase to 600 mg 3 times daily (maximum: 1,800 mg/day). Maintenance: 600 mg once or twice daily

OTC labeling:

Analgesic, antipyretic: Oral: 200 mg every 4 to 6 hours as needed; if no relief may increase to 400 mg every 4 to 6 hours as needed (maximum: 1,200 mg/day); Duration: treatment for >10 days as an analgesic or >3 days as an antipyretic is not recommended unless directed by health care provider.

Migraine: Oral: 400 mg at onset of symptoms (maximum: 400 mg/24 hours unless directed by health care provider)

Pericarditis (off-label use): Oral: 400 to 800 mg 3 to 4 times daily (maximum dose: 3,200 mg/day) (Imazio 2009); with pericarditis postmyocardial infarction, the ACCF/AHA prefers the use of aspirin (O'Gara 2013).

Geriatric Refer to adult dosing. Use with caution; consider reduced initial dosage in debilitated or frail patients.

Pediatric

Analgesic:

IV (Caldolor): **Note:** Patients should be well hydrated prior to administration.

Infants 6 months and Children <12 years: 10 mg/kg every 4 to 6 hours as needed; maximum single dose: 400 mg; maximum daily dose: 40 mg/kg/day up to 2,400 mg/day.

Children and Adolescents 12 to 17 years: 400 mg every 4 to 6 hours as needed (maximum: 2,400 mg/day)

Oral: Infants and Children <50 kg: Limited data available in infants <6 months: 4 to 10 mg/kg/dose every 6 to 8 hours; maximum single dose: 400 mg; maximum daily dose: 40 mg/kg/day (American Pain Society 2008; Berde 1990; Berde 2002; Kliegman 2011)

Antipyretic:

IV (Caldolor): **Note:** Patients should be well hydrated prior to administration.

Infants 6 months and Children <12 years: 10 mg/kg every 4 to 6 hours as needed; maximum single dose: 400 mg; maximum daily dose: 40 mg/kg/day up to 2,400 mg/day.

Children and Adolescents 12 to 17 years: 400 mg every 4 to 6 hours as needed (maximum: 2,400 mg/day)

Oral: Infants ≥6 months, Children, and Adolescents: 5 to 10 mg/kg/dose every 6 to 8 hours; maximum single dose: 400 mg; maximum daily dose: 40 mg/kg/day up to 1,200 mg, unless directed by physician (under physician supervision, not to exceed maximum of 2,400 mg daily) (Litalien 2001; Sullivan 2011)

Juvenile idiopathic arthritis (JIA) (off-label use): Oral: Children and Adolescents: 30 to 40 mg/kg/**day** in 3 to 4 divided doses; start at lower end of dosing range and titrate; patients with milder disease may be treated with 20 mg/kg/day; patients with more severe disease may require up to 50 mg/kg/day; maximum single dose: 800 mg; maximum daily dose: 2,400 mg (Giannini 1990; Kliegman 2011; Litalien 2001)

Patent ductus arteriosus: IV (ibuprofen lysine [Neo-Profen]): Infants weighing between 500 to 1,500 g and ≤32 weeks' GA: Initial dose: Ibuprofen 10 mg/kg, followed by two doses of 5 mg/kg at 24 and 48 hours. Dose should be based on birth weight.

OTC labeling (analgesic, antipyretic): Oral: **Note:** Discontinue use and consult health care provider if no improvement within 24 hours after initiating therapy or if symptoms persist >3 days or worsen.

Children 6 months to 11 years: See table; use of weight to select dose is preferred; doses may be repeated every 6 to 8 hours (maximum: 4 doses/day)

Children ≥12 years: Refer to adult dosing.

Ibuprofen Dosing

Weight (lb)	Age	Dosage (mg)
12 to 17	6 to 11 mo	50
18 to 23	12 to 23 mo	75
24 to 35	2 to 3 y	100
36 to 47	4 to 5 y	150
48 to 59	6 to 8 y	200
60 to 71	9 to 10 y	250
72 to 95	11 y	300

Renal Impairment

US labeling: There are no dosage adjustment provided in manufacturer's labeling; avoid use in advanced disease

Canadian labeling:

Mild impairment: There are no dosage adjustments provided in the manufacturer's labeling (has not been studied).

Moderate impairment:

Oral: There are no dosage adjustments provided in the manufacturer's labeling; use with caution.

IV: Use is contraindicated.

Severe impairment (CrCl <30 mL/minute) or deteriorating renal disease: Use is contraindicated.

KDIGO 2012 guidelines provide the following recommendations for NSAIDs:

eGFR 30 to <60 mL/minute/1.73 m^2: Avoid use in patients with intercurrent disease that increases risk of acute kidney injury.

eGFR <30 mL/minute/1.73 m^2: Avoid use.

Neoprofen: If anuria or marked oliguria (urinary output <0.6 mL/kg/hour) evident at the scheduled time of the second or third dose, hold dose until renal function returns to normal. Use is contraindicated in preterm infants with significant renal impairment.

Hepatic Impairment

US labeling: There are no dosage adjustments provided in the manufacturer's labeling; use caution and discontinue if hepatic function worsens

Canadian labeling:

Mild impairment: There are no dosage adjustments provided in the manufacturer's labeling

Moderate impairment:

Oral: There are no dosage adjustments provided in the manufacturer's labeling.

IV: Use is contraindicated

Severe impairment or active hepatic disease: Use is contraindicated.

Dietary Considerations Some products may contain phenylalanine and/or potassium.

Administration

Oral: Administer with food or milk.

IV:

Caldolor: For IV administration only; infuse over at least 30 minutes (adults) or 10 minutes (pediatric)

NeoProfen (ibuprofen lysine): For IV administration only; administration via umbilical arterial line has not been evaluated. Infuse over 15 minutes through port closest to insertion site. Avoid extravasation. Do not administer simultaneously via same line with TPN. If needed, interrupt TPN for 15 minutes prior to and after ibuprofen administration, keeping line open with dextrose or saline.

Monitoring Parameters CBC, chemistry profile, occult blood loss and periodic liver function tests; monitor response (pain, range of motion, grip strength, mobility, ADL function), inflammation; observe for weight gain, edema; monitor renal function (urine output, serum BUN and creatinine); observe for bleeding, bruising; evaluate gastrointestinal effects (abdominal pain, bleeding, dyspepsia); mental confusion, disorientation; blood pressure; periodic ophthalmic exams with long-term therapy; signs of infection (ibuprofen lysine)

Reference Range Plasma concentrations >200 mcg/mL may be associated with severe toxicity

Test Interactions May interfere with urine detection of phencyclidine, cannabinoids, and barbiturates (false-positives) (Marchei 2007; Rollins 1990)

Dosage Forms Considerations

EnovaRX-Ibuprofen cream is compounded from a kit. Refer to manufacturer's labeling for compounding instructions.

Dosage Forms Excipient information presented when available (limited, particularly for generics); consult specific product labeling. [DSC] = Discontinued product

Capsule, Oral:

Advil: 200 mg

Advil Migraine: 200 mg

KS Ibuprofen: 200 mg [contains fd&c blue #2 (indigotine)]

Generic: 200 mg

Cream, External:

EnovaRX-Ibuprofen: 10% (60 g, 120 g) [contains cetearyl alcohol]

Kit, Combination:

Ibuprofen Comfort Pac: 800 mg [contains methylparaben, trolamine (triethanolamine)]

Solution, Intravenous:

Caldolor: 400 mg/4 mL (4 mL); 800 mg/8 mL (8 mL)

Solution, Intravenous, as lysine [preservative free]:

NeoProfen: 10 mg/mL (2 mL)

Suspension, Oral:

Childrens Advil: 100 mg/5 mL (120 mL) [fruit flavor]

Childrens Advil: 100 mg/5 mL (120 mL) [contains edetate disodium, fd&c red #40, polysorbate 80, propylene glycol, sodium benzoate]

Childrens Advil: 100 mg/5 mL (120 mL) [alcohol free; grape flavor]

Childrens Advil: 100 mg/5 mL (120 mL) [alcohol free; contains brilliant blue fcf (fd&c blue #1), edetate disodium, fd&c red #40, polysorbate 80, propylene glycol, sodium benzoate; grape flavor]

Childrens Advil: 100 mg/5 mL (120 mL) [alcohol free; contains brilliant blue fcf (fd&c blue #1), propylene glycol, sodium benzoate; blue raspberry flavor]

Childrens Advil: 100 mg/5 mL (30 mL, 120 mL) [alcohol free, dye free; contains edetate disodium, polysorbate 80, propylene glycol, sodium benzoate; white grape flavor]

Childrens Advil: 100 mg/5 mL (120 mL) [alcohol free, dye free, sugar free; contains edetate disodium, polysorbate 80, propylene glycol, sodium benzoate; berry flavor]

Childrens Ibuprofen: 100 mg/5 mL (118 mL) [alcohol free; contains brilliant blue fcf (fd&c blue #1), fd&c red #40, polysorbate 80, sodium benzoate; grape flavor]

Childrens Ibuprofen: 100 mg/5 mL (120 mL) [alcohol free; contains butylparaben, fd&c red #40, polysorbate 80, propylene glycol, sodium benzoate; bubble-gum flavor]

Childrens Ibuprofen: 100 mg/5 mL (5 mL, 118 mL, 237 mL, 240 mL) [alcohol free; contains fd&c red #40, fd&c yellow #10 (quinoline yellow), polysorbate 80, sodium benzoate; berry flavor]

Childrens Ibuprofen: 100 mg/5 mL (118 mL) [alcohol free; contains fd&c red #40, polysorbate 80, sodium benzoate]

Childrens Ibuprofen: 40 mg/mL (15 mL) [alcohol free; berry flavor]

Childrens Ibuprofen: 100 mg/5 mL (118 mL) [alcohol free, dye free; contains polysorbate 80, sodium benzoate]

Childrens Ibuprofen: 100 mg/5 mL (118 mL) [alcohol free, gluten free; contains brilliant blue fcf (fd&c blue #1), fd&c red #40, polysorbate 80, sodium benzoate; grape flavor]

Childrens Motrin: 40 mg/mL (15 mL) [berry flavor]

Childrens Motrin: 100 mg/5 mL (120 mL) [alcohol free]

Childrens Motrin: 100 mg/5 mL (60 mL, 120 mL) [alcohol free; contains fd&c red #40, fd&c yellow #10 (quinoline yellow), polysorbate 80, sodium benzoate; berry flavor]

Childrens Motrin: 100 mg/5 mL (120 mL [DSC]) [alcohol free; contains fd&c red #40, fd&c yellow #10 (quinoline yellow), sodium benzoate]

Childrens Motrin: 100 mg/5 mL (120 mL) [alcohol free; contains fd&c red #40, fd&c yellow #10 (quinoline yellow), sodium benzoate; berry flavor]

Childrens Motrin: 100 mg/5 mL (120 mL) [alcohol free; contains fd&c red #40, polysorbate 80, sodium benzoate]

Childrens Motrin: 100 mg/5 mL (120 mL) [alcohol free; contains fd&c red #40, sodium benzoate]

Childrens Motrin: 100 mg/5 mL (120 mL) [alcohol free; contains fd&c red #40, sodium benzoate; bubble-gum flavor]

Childrens Motrin: 100 mg/5 mL (120 mL) [alcohol free; contains fd&c red #40, sodium benzoate; tropical punch flavor]

Childrens Motrin: 100 mg/5 mL (120 mL) [alcohol free, dye free; contains polysorbate 80, sodium benzoate]

Childrens Motrin: 100 mg/5 mL (120 mL) [alcohol free, dye free; contains sodium benzoate; berry flavor]

HyVee Ibuprofen Childrens: 100 mg/5 mL (120 mL) [gluten free; contains fd&c red #40, fd&c yellow #10 (quinoline yellow), polysorbate 80, sodium benzoate; berry flavor]

Ibuprofen Childrens: 100 mg/5 mL (120 mL) [alcohol free; contains butylparaben, fd&c red #40, fd&c yellow #6 (sunset yellow), polysorbate 80, propylene glycol, sodium benzoate; fruit flavor]

Ibuprofen Childrens: 100 mg/5 mL (118 mL, 237 mL) [alcohol free; contains fd&c red #40, fd&c yellow #10 (quinoline yellow), polysorbate 80, sodium benzoate; berry flavor]

Ibuprofen Childrens: 100 mg/5 mL (120 mL) [alcohol free, gluten free; contains brilliant blue fcf (fd&c blue #1), fd&c red #40, polysorbate 80, sodium benzoate; grape flavor]

Ibuprofen Childrens: 100 mg/5 mL (120 mL, 240 mL) [alcohol free, gluten free; contains fd&c red #40, fd&c yellow #10 (quinoline yellow), polysorbate 80, sodium benzoate; berry flavor]

Ibuprofen Childrens: 100 mg/5 mL (118 mL) [alcohol free, gluten free; contains fd&c red #40, polysorbate 80, sodium benzoate; bubble-gum flavor]

Infants Advil: 50 mg/1.25 mL (30 mL) [alcohol free, dye free; contains edetate disodium, polysorbate 80, propylene glycol, sodium benzoate]

Infants Advil: 50 mg/1.25 mL (15 mL) [alcohol free, dye free; contains edetate disodium, polysorbate 80, propylene glycol, sodium benzoate; white grape flavor]

Infants Ibuprofen: 50 mg/1.25 mL (15 mL) [alcohol free; contains butylparaben, fd&c red #40, polysorbate 80, propylene glycol, sodium benzoate; berry flavor]

Infants Ibuprofen: 50 mg/1.25 mL (15 mL, 30 mL) [alcohol free, dye free; contains polysorbate 80, sodium benzoate; berry flavor]

Infants Ibuprofen: 50 mg/1.25 mL (15 mL) [alcohol free, gluten free; contains butylparaben, fd&c red #40, polysorbate 80, propylene glycol, sodium benzoate; berry flavor]

Motrin: 40 mg/mL (15 mL) [alcohol free, dye free; berry flavor]

Motrin Infants Drops: 50 mg/1.25 mL (15 mL) [alcohol free; contains fd&c red #40, polysorbate 80, sodium benzoate; berry flavor]

Motrin Infants Drops: 50 mg/1.25 mL (15 mL, 30 mL) [alcohol free, dye free; contains polysorbate 80, sodium benzoate]

Generic: 100 mg/5 mL (5 mL, 10 mL [DSC], 118 mL, 120 mL, 473 mL)

Tablet, Oral:
Addaprin: 200 mg
Advil: 200 mg
Advil Junior Strength: 100 mg
Dyspel: 200 mg
Genpril: 200 mg
I-Prin: 200 mg
IBU-200: 200 mg
Motrin IB: 200 mg
Motrin IB: 200 mg [contains fd&c yellow #6 (sunset yellow)]
Motrin Junior Strength: 100 mg [scored]
Provil: 200 mg
Generic: 200 mg, 400 mg, 600 mg, 800 mg

Tablet Chewable, Oral:
Advil Junior Strength: 100 mg [scored; contains aspartame, fd&c blue #2 aluminum lake; grape flavor]
Childrens Motrin: 50 mg [scored; contains aspartame, fd&c yellow #6 (sunset yellow); orange flavor]
Childrens Motrin Jr Strength: 100 mg [scored; contains aspartame, brilliant blue fcf (fd&c blue #1); grape flavor]
Ibuprofen Junior Strength: 100 mg [contains aspartame, fd&c yellow #6 (sunset yellow), soybean oil, whey protein]
Motrin Junior Strength: 100 mg [contains aspartame, brilliant blue fcf (fd&c blue #1)]
Motrin Junior Strength: 100 mg [scored; contains aspartame, fd&c yellow #6 (sunset yellow); orange flavor]

♦ Ibuprofen and Hydrocodone see Hydrocodone and Ibuprofen on page 885

♦ Ibuprofen and Oxycodone see Oxycodone and Ibuprofen on page 1362

♦ Ibuprofen and Pseudoephedrine see Pseudoephedrine and Ibuprofen on page 1528

♦ Ibuprofen Childrens [OTC] see Ibuprofen on page 905

♦ Ibuprofen Comfort Pac see Ibuprofen on page 905

♦ Ibuprofen Junior Strength [OTC] see Ibuprofen on page 905

♦ Ibuprofen Lysine see Ibuprofen on page 905

♦ Ibuprofen Muscle and Joint (Can) see Ibuprofen on page 905

Ibutilide (i BYOO ti lide)

Brand Names: US Convert
Index Terms Ibutilide Fumarate
Pharmacologic Category Antiarrhythmic Agent, Class III
Use Acute termination of atrial fibrillation or flutter of recent onset; the effectiveness of ibutilide has not been determined in patients with arrhythmias >90 days in duration
Note: According to the American Heart Association/American College of Cardiology/Heart Rhythm Society guidelines for the management of atrial fibrillation, in patients with pre-excited atrial fibrillation and rapid ventricular response who are not hemodynamically compromised, the use of ibutilide to restore sinus rhythm or slow the ventricular rate is recommended (AHA/ACC/HRS [January, 2014]).
Dosing
Adult Atrial fibrillation/flutter: IV:
<60 kg: 0.01 mg/kg over 10 minutes
≥60 kg: 1 mg over 10 minutes
Note: Discontinue infusion if arrhythmia terminates, if sustained or nonsustained ventricular tachycardia occurs, or if marked prolongation of QT/QTc occurs. If the arrhythmia does not terminate within 10 minutes after the end of the initial infusion, a second infusion of equal strength may be infused over a 10-minute period.
Geriatric Refer to adult dosing. Dose selection should be cautious, usually starting at the lower end of the dosing range.
Renal Impairment No dosage adjustment necessary.
Hepatic Impairment No dosage adjustment necessary.
Additional Information Complete prescribing information should be consulted for additional detail.
Dosage Forms Excipient information presented when available (limited, particularly for generics); consult specific product labeling.
Solution, Intravenous, as fumarate:
Convert: 1 mg/10 mL (10 mL)
Generic: 1 mg/10 mL (10 mL)

♦ Ibutilide Fumarate see Ibutilide on page 909

♦ IC51 see Japanese Encephalitis Virus Vaccine (Inactivated) on page 1011

Icatibant (eye KAT i bant)

Brand Names: US Firazyr
Brand Names: Canada Firazyr
Index Terms HOE 140; Icatibant Acetate
Pharmacologic Category Selective Bradykinin B2 Receptor Antagonist
Use Hereditary angioedema: Treatment of acute attacks of hereditary angioedema (HAE)
Dosing
Adult
Hereditary angioedema (HAE): SubQ: 30 mg; may repeat every 6 hours if response is inadequate or symptoms recur (maximum daily dose: 90 mg).
ACE inhibitor-induced angioedema (off-label use): SubQ: 30 mg; if symptoms of angioedema continue to worsen after 6 hours, a second injection may be administered. The authors administered intravenous prednisolone (not available in the US) with the second dose of icatibant (Bas, 2015).
Geriatric Refer to adult dosing. Systemic exposure may be increased; however, no dosage adjustments are recommended.
Renal Impairment No dosage adjustments are recommended (has not been studied); however, icatibant is cleared by nonrenal mechanisms and is not expected to accumulate in patients with renal impairment.
Hepatic Impairment No dosage adjustments necessary.
Additional Information Complete prescribing information should be consulted for additional detail.
Dosage Forms Excipient information presented when available (limited, particularly for generics); consult specific product labeling.
Solution, Subcutaneous [preservative free]:
Firazyr: 30 mg/3 mL (3 mL)

♦ Icatibant Acetate see Icatibant on page 909

♦ ICI-182,780 see Fulvestrant on page 821

♦ ICI-204,219 see Zafirlukast on page 1922

♦ ICI-46474 see Tamoxifen on page 1733

◆ ICI-118630 *see* Goserelin *on page 854*

◆ ICI-176334 *see* Bicalutamide *on page 230*

◆ ICI-D1033 *see* Anastrozole *on page 128*

◆ ICL670 *see* Deferasirox *on page 509*

◆ Iclusig *see* PONATinib *on page 1472*

Icodextrin (eye KOE dex trin)

Brand Names: US Adept; Extraneal

Pharmacologic Category Adhesiolytic; Peritoneal Dialysate, Osmotic

Additional Appendix Information

Peritoneal Dialysis Solutions *on page 1965*

Use

Adept: Adjunct to surgery for the reduction of postsurgical adhesions in gynecologic laparoscopic adhesiolysis

Extraneal: Daily exchange for the long dwell (8- to 16-hour) during continuous ambulatory peritoneal dialysis (CAPD) or automated peritoneal dialysis (APD) for the management of end-stage renal disease (ESRD); improvement of long-dwell ultrafiltration and clearance of creatinine and urea nitrogen (compared to 4.25% dextrose) in patients with high average or greater transport characteristics as measured by peritoneal equilibration test (PET)

Medication Guide Available Yes

Dosing

Adult & Geriatric

CAPD or APD (Extraneal): Intraperitoneal: Given as a single daily exchange in CAPD or APD; dwell time of 8 to 16 hours is suggested

Laparoscopic gynecologic surgery (Adept): Intraperitoneal: Irrigate with at least 100 mL every 30 minutes during surgery; aspirate remaining fluid after surgery is completed, then instill 1 L into the cavity

Additional Information Complete prescribing information should be consulted for additional detail.

Dosage Forms Excipient information presented when available (limited, particularly for generics); consult specific product labeling.

Solution, Intraperitoneal:

Adept: 4% (1000 mL, 1500 mL)

Extraneal: 7.5% (2000 mL, 2500 mL)

◆ Icosapent Ethyl *see* Omega-3 Fatty Acids *on page 1329*

◆ ICRF-187 *see* Dexrazoxane *on page 531*

◆ Icy Hot [OTC] *see* Methyl Salicylate and Menthol *on page 1187*

◆ Idamycin PFS *see* IDArubicin *on page 910*

IDArubicin (eye da ROO bi sin)

Brand Names: US Idamycin PFS

Brand Names: Canada Idamycin PFS; Idarubicin Hydrochloride Injection

Index Terms 4-Demethoxydaunorubicin; 4-DMDR; Idarubicin Hydrochloride; IDR; IMI 30; SC 33428

Pharmacologic Category Antineoplastic Agent, Anthracycline; Antineoplastic Agent, Topoisomerase II Inhibitor

Use Acute myeloid leukemia: Treatment of acute myeloid leukemia (AML) in adults (in combination with other approved chemotherapy agents).

Dosing

Adult & Geriatric Idarubicin is associated with a moderate emetic potential; antiemetics are recommended to prevent nausea and vomiting (Basch, 2011; Roila, 2010).

Acute myeloid leukemia (AML): IV:

Manufacturer labeling: Induction: 12 mg/m^2/day for 3 days (in combination with cytarabine); a second induction cycle may be administered if necessary.

Indication-specific dosing:

AML, relapsed/refractory: FLAG-IDA regimen: 10 mg/m^2/day for 3 days (in combination with fludarabine, cytarabine, and filgrastim); a second course was given for consolidation upon hematologic recovery (Parker, 1997)

Acute promyelocytic leukemia (APL):

LPA 2005 (high-risk patients; Sanz, 2010):

Induction (all patients): 12 mg/m^2/day on days 2, 4, 6, and 8 (dose was omitted in patients >70 years) in combination with ATRA (tretinoin) (Sanz, 2010)

Consolidation (patients ≤60 years): 5 mg/m^2/day for 4 days in consolidation cycle 1 and 12 mg/m^2/day for 1 day in consolidation cycle 3 (in combination with ATRA [tretinoin] and cytarabine) (Sanz, 2010)

APML4 protocol (Iland, 2012): Induction (age-adjusted dosing):

Age <60 years: 12 mg/m^2/day on days 2, 4, 6, and 8 (in combination with ATRA [tretinoin] and arsenic trioxide)

Age 61 to 70 years: 9 mg/m^2/day on days 2, 4, 6, and 8 (in combination with ATRA [tretinoin] and arsenic trioxide)

Age >70 years: 6 mg/m^2/day on days 2, 4, 6, and 8 (in combination with ATRA [tretinoin] and arsenic trioxide)

Pediatric Note: Idarubicin is associated with a moderate emetic potential; antiemetics are recommended to prevent nausea and vomiting (Dupuis, 2011).

Acute myeloid leukemia (AML) (off-label use): IV:

Newly diagnosed (CCG-2961) (Lange, 2008):

Induction: IdaDCTER: Idarubicin 5 mg/m^2/dose daily for 4 days on days 0 to 3 in combination with cytarabine, etoposide, thioguanine, and dexamethasone

Consolidation:

IdaDCTER: Idarubicin 5 mg/m^2/dose daily for 4 days on days 0 to 3 in combination with cytarabine, etoposide, thioguanine, and dexamethasone

or

Idarubicin 12 mg/m^2/dose daily for 3 days on days 0 to 2 in combination with fludarabine and cytarabine

Relapsed/refractory: 12 mg/m^2 once daily for 3 days on days 0 to 2 in combination with fludarabine and cytarabine (Dinndorf, 1997; Leahey, 1997)

Renal Impairment There are no dosage adjustments provided in the manufacturer's labeling; however, it does recommend that dosage reductions be made. Patients with S$_{cr}$ ≥2 mg/dL did not receive treatment in many clinical trials. The following adjustments have been recommended (Aronoff, 2007):

Adults:

CrCl >50 mL/minute: No dosage adjustment is necessary.

CrCl 10 to 50 mL/minute: Administer 75% of dose.

CrCl <10 mL/minute: Administer 50% of dose.

Hemodialysis: Supplemental dose not needed.

Continuous ambulatory peritoneal dialysis (CAPD): Supplemental dose not needed.

Infants, Children, and Adolescents:

GFR >50 mL/minute/1.73 m^2: No dosage adjustment is necessary.

GFR ≤50 mL/minute/1.73 m^2: Administer 75% of dose

Intermittent hemodialysis: Administer 75% of dose

Peritoneal dialysis (PD): Administer 75% of dose

Continuous renal replacement therapy (CRRT): Administer 75% of dose

Hepatic Impairment

Bilirubin 2.6 to 5 mg/dL: Administer 50% of dose (Perry, 2012)

Bilirubin >5 mg/dL: Avoid use

Adjustment for Toxicity Manufacturer labeling: If patients experience severe mucositis during the first induction cycle, delay administration of the second cycle until mucositis has resolved; consider reducing the dose by 25%.

Additional Information Complete prescribing information should be consulted for additional detail.

Dosage Forms Excipient information presented when available (limited, particularly for generics); consult specific product labeling.

Solution, Intravenous, as hydrochloride [preservative free]:

Idamycin PFS: 5 mg/5 mL (5 mL); 10 mg/10 mL (10 mL); 20 mg/20 mL (20 mL)

Generic: 5 mg/5 mL (5 mL); 10 mg/10 mL (10 mL); 20 mg/20 mL (20 mL)

◆ Idarubicin Hydrochloride *see* IDArubicin *on page 910*

◆ Idarubicin Hydrochloride Injection (Can) *see* IDArubicin *on page 910*

IdaruCIZUMAB (eye da roo SIZ uh mab)

Brand Names: US Praxbind

Index Terms aDabi-Fab

Pharmacologic Category Antidote; Monoclonal Antibody

Use Reversal of dabigatran: Reversal of the anticoagulant effects of dabigatran for emergency surgery/urgent procedures or in life-threatening or uncontrolled bleeding

Pregnancy Considerations Animal reproduction studies have not been conducted.

Breast-Feeding Considerations It is not known if idarucizumab is excreted in breast milk. The manufacturer recommends that caution be used if administered to a nursing woman.

Contraindications There are no contraindications listed in the manufacturer's labeling.

Warnings/Precautions Although the duration of effect typically lasts at least 24 hours, in the phase 3 clinical trial, coagulation parameters (eg, aPTT, TT, ecarin clotting time [not routinely available]) re-elevated in a limited number of patients between 12 and 24 hours after administration; some patients experienced re-elevation as early as 1 to 4 hours after administration which may have been due to high initial baseline dabigatran concentrations (Pollack 2015). If clinically relevant bleeding in conjunction with elevated coagulation parameters reoccurs following an idarucizumab 5 g dose, administration of a second dose may be considered.

Although there is insufficient clinical experience with idarucizumab to fully evaluate the risk of hypersensitivity reactions, some reported adverse events possibly indicative of hypersensitivity reactions could not exclude a potential relationship. The risk of using idarucizumab in patients with known hypersensitivity (eg, anaphylactoid reaction) to idarucizumab or any of the components of the formulation should be evaluated cautiously against the potential benefit of emergency dabigatran reversal. Discontinue use if serious allergic reaction occurs (eg, anaphylaxis) and institute appropriate management.

Since patients being treated with dabigatran, have underlying disease states predisposing them to thromboembolic events and reversing the effects of dabigatran will expose the patient to an elevated thrombotic risk; resume anticoagulant therapy as soon as it is appropriate. Dabigatran can be re-initiated 24 hours after idarucizumab administration if appropriate. In the phase 3 clinical trial, not all thromboembolic events that occurred reflected the underlying disease state being treated with dabigatran; adverse thromboembolic events included DVT, PE, atrial thrombus, NSTEMI, and ischemic stroke (Pollack 2015). IV administration of sorbitol in patients with hereditary fructose intolerance has been reported to result in serious reactions (eg, acute hepatic failure, hypoglycemia, hypophosphatemia, metabolic acidosis, uric acid elevations) including fatalities; consider the combined daily metabolic load of sorbitol/fructose from all sources including idarucizumab and other drugs containing sorbitol; minimum amount of sorbitol known to cause serious adverse reactions is unknown.

Adverse Reactions Frequency not always defined.
Central nervous system: Delirium (7%), headache (5%)
Endocrine & metabolic: Hypokalemia (7%)
Gastrointestinal: Constipation (7%)
Hypersensitivity: Hypersensitivity (including bronchospasm, hyperventilation, rash, and pruritus)
Respiratory: Pneumonia (6%)
Miscellaneous: Fever (6%)
<1% (Limited to important or life-threatening) (Pollack 2015): Acute ischemic stroke, cardiac arrest, circulatory shock, deep vein thrombosis, intracardiac thrombus (left atrium), multiorgan failure, non-ST-segment elevation myocardial infarction, pulmonary edema, pulmonary embolism, respiratory failure, right heart failure

Drug Interactions
Metabolism/Transport Effects None known.
Avoid Concomitant Use There are no known interactions where it is recommended to avoid concomitant use.
Increased Effect/Toxicity There are no known significant interactions involving an increase in effect.
Decreased Effect There are no known significant interactions involving a decrease in effect.
Preparation for Administration May withdraw contents of each vial using a 60 mL syringe to be administered as an IV bolus or may hang each vial and administer as an infusion.
Storage/Stability Store intact vials at 2°C to 8°C (36°F to 46°F). Do not freeze. Do not shake. May store intact vial in the original packaging (to protect from light) prior to use at room temperature 25°C (77°F) for up to 48 hours, or up to 6 hours if exposed to light.
Mechanism of Action Idarucizumab, a specific reversal agent for dabigatran, is a humanized monoclonal antibody fragment (Fab) that binds specifically to dabigatran and its acylglucuronide metabolites with an affinity for dabigatran that is ~350 times greater than that of thrombin, and neutralizes the anticoagulant effect within minutes (Das 2015; Schiele 2013).

Pharmacodynamics/Kinetics
Onset: Uncontrolled bleeding: Effects observed within minutes and hemostasis is restored at a median of 11.4 hours (Pollack 2015)
Duration: Usually at least 24 hours
Distribution: V_{dss}: 8.9 L
Metabolism: Biodegradation to small peptides and amino acids
Half-life elimination: 47 minutes (initial); 10.3 hours (terminal)

Excretion: Urine (~32% within the first 6 hours and <1% in the following 18 hours)
Dosing
Adult & Geriatric
Reversal of dabigatran: IV: 5 g (administered as 2 separate 2.5 g doses no more than 15 minutes apart) (Pollack 2015). If coagulation parameters (eg, aPTT) re-elevate and clinically relevant bleeding occurs or if a second emergency surgery/urgent procedure is required and patient has elevated coagulation parameters, may consider administration of an additional 5 g (limited data to support).
Renal Impairment No dosage adjustment necessary; renal impairment does not impact the reversal effect of idarucizumab.
Hepatic Impairment There are no dosage adjustments provided in the manufacturer's labeling (has not been studied).
Administration IV: Prior to administration, flush preexisting IV line with sodium chloride 0.9%. Administer dose undiluted as an IV bolus either via syringe or as an infusion by hanging the vials. Infusion of each vial should take no longer than 5 to 10 minutes with the second vial of 2.5 g administered no later than 15 minutes after the end of the first 2.5 g vial (Pollack 2015 [protocol]). Do not administer any other infusion in the same IV line. Begin administration within 1 hour of removing the solution from the vial.
Monitoring Parameters
Monitor for re-elevation of coagulation parameters (eg, aPTT); signs/symptoms of clinically relevant bleeding and thromboembolic events.
In patients overdosed with dabigatran, consider the following monitoring schedule (Alikhan 2014): Baseline aPTT (at presentation), repeat at 2 hours postexposure (if exposure time is known) or post-presentation (if exposure time is unknown) and every 12 hours thereafter until aPTT returns to normal.
Dosage Forms Excipient information presented when available (limited, particularly for generics); consult specific product labeling.
Solution, Intravenous [preservative free]:
Praxbind: 2.5 g/50 mL (50 mL)

◆ IDEC-C2B8 *see* RiTUXimab *on page 1600*

Idelalisib (eye del a LIS ib)

Brand Names: US Zydelig
Brand Names: Canada Zydelig
Index Terms CAL-101; GS-1101; PI₃K Delta Inhibitor CAL-101
Pharmacologic Category Antineoplastic Agent, Phosphatidylinositol 3-Kinase Inhibitor
Use
Chronic lymphocytic leukemia: Treatment of relapsed chronic lymphocytic leukemia (CLL) (in combination with rituximab) when rituximab alone is appropriate therapy due to other comorbidities
Follicular B-cell non-Hodgkin lymphoma: Treatment of relapsed follicular B-cell non-Hodgkin lymphoma after at least 2 prior systemic therapies
Small lymphocytic lymphoma: Treatment of relapsed small lymphocytic lymphoma (SLL) after at least 2 prior systemic therapies
Pregnancy Considerations Adverse events were observed in animal reproduction studies. Women of reproductive potential should use effective contraception during therapy and for at least 1 month after treatment discontinuation.
Breast-Feeding Considerations It is not known if idelalisib is excreted in breast milk. Due to the potential for serious adverse reactions in the nursing infant, the manufacturer recommends a decision be made whether to discontinue nursing or to discontinue the drug, taking into account the importance of treatment to the mother.
Prescribing and Access Restrictions Available through specialty pharmacies. Further information may be obtained at http://www.zydeligaccessconnect.com/.
Contraindications Serious hypersensitivity reactions, including anaphylaxis and toxic epidermal necrolysis, to idelalisib or any component of the formulation
Warnings/Precautions Hazardous agent - use appropriate precautions for handling and disposal (meets NIOSH 2014 criteria). **[US Boxed Warning]: Serious hepatotoxicity (some fatal) has been observed. Monitor hepatic function at baseline and during therapy. May require treatment interruption and/or dosage reduction.** ALT/AST elevations >5 times ULN have occurred, and were generally observed during the first 12 weeks of therapy; transaminase elevations were reversible upon therapy interruption. Hepatotoxicity may recur upon rechallenge, even at a reduced dose; discontinue for recurrent ▶

hepatotoxicity. Avoid concomitant use with other hepato-toxic agents. Monitor ALT/AST at baseline and every 2 weeks for the first 3 months, every 4 weeks for the next 3 months, then every 1 to 3 months thereafter, or as clinically necessary. Increase monitoring to weekly if ALT or AST >3 times ULN until resolved. Interrupt therapy if ALT/AST >3 times ULN; monitor LFTs weekly until resolved. **[US Boxed Warning]: Serious and/or fatal diarrhea and colitis have been reported. Monitor closely; may require treatment interruption, dosage reduction, and/or discontinuation.** Grade 3 or higher diarrhea or colitis have been reported in clinical trials. Diarrhea may occur at any time during therapy and responds poorly to antidiarrheal (antimotility) medications. The median time to resolution of diarrhea was 1 week to 1 month (following therapy interruption); corticosteroids were used in some cases to manage toxicity. Avoid concomitant use with other promotility agents. **[US Boxed Warning]: Serious and fatal intestinal perforation may occur; discontinue permanently if perforation develops.** In some patients, perforation was preceded by moderate to severe diarrhea. Monitor closely for new or worsening abdominal pain, chills, fever, nausea, or vomiting.

[US Boxed Warning]: Serious and fatal pneumonitis may occur. Monitor for pulmonary symptoms and bilateral interstitial infiltrates. May require therapy interruption or discontinuation. Symptoms such as cough, dyspnea, hypoxia, interstitial infiltrates, or an oxygen saturation decrease of more than 5% should be promptly evaluated. Interrupt therapy for suspected pneumonitis; if diagnosis is confirmed, discontinue idelalisib and administer corticosteroids as appropriate. Serious allergic/hypersensitivity reactions, including anaphylaxis, have been reported. Discontinue permanently for serious reactions and manage appropriately.

Severe and/or life-threatening cutaneous reactions (grade 3 or higher), such as exfoliative dermatitis, rash (generalized, erythematous, macular-papular, pruritic, exfoliative), and skin disorder, have been observed. One case of toxic epidermal necrolysis (TEN) was reported when idelalisib was administered in combination with rituximab and bendamustine. Monitor closely for dermatologic toxicity and discontinue for severe reactions. Grade 3 or 4 neutropenia occurred in close to one-third of patients in clinical trials; thrombocytopenia and anemia (any grade) have also been reported. Monitor blood counts at least every 2 weeks for the first 3 months, and at least weekly in patients with neutropenia. May require treatment interruption and dosage reduction. Potentially significant interactions may exist, requiring dose or frequency adjustment, additional monitoring, and/or selection of alternative therapy. Consult drug interactions database for more detailed information.

Adverse Reactions As reported with monotherapy.

>10%:
- Central nervous system: Fatigue (30%), insomnia (12%), headache (11%)
- Dermatologic: Skin rash (21%; grade ≥3: 3%), night sweats (12%)
- Gastrointestinal: Diarrhea (47%; grade ≥3: 14%), nausea (29%), abdominal pain (26%), decreased appetite (16%), vomiting (15%)
- Hematologic & oncologic: Decreased neutrophils (53%; grade 3: 14%; grade 4: 11%), decreased hemoglobin (28%; grade 3: 2%), decreased platelet count (26%; grade 3: 3%; grade 4: 3%)
- Hepatic: Increased serum ALT (50%; grade 3: 14%; grade 4: 5%), increased serum AST (41%; grade 3: 8%; grade 4: 4%), severe hepatotoxicity (14%)
- Neuromuscular & skeletal: Weakness (12%)
- Respiratory: Cough (29%), pneumonia (25%; grade ≥3: 16%), dyspnea (17%), upper respiratory tract infection (12%)
- Miscellaneous: Fever (28%)

1% to 10%: Cardiovascular: Peripheral edema (10%)

Postmarketing and/or case reports (Limited to important or life-threatening; reported with mono- or combination therapy): Anaphylaxis, hypersensitivity reaction, intestinal perforation, toxic epidermal necrolysis

Drug Interactions

Metabolism/Transport Effects Substrate of CYP3A4 (major), P-glycoprotein, UGT1A4; **Note:** Assignment of Major/Minor substrate status based on clinically relevant drug interaction potential; **Inhibits** CYP2C19 (weak), CYP2C8 (weak), CYP3A4 (strong), UGT1A1

Avoid Concomitant Use

Avoid concomitant use of Idelalisib with any of the following: Ado-Trastuzumab Emtansine; Alfuzosin; Amodiaquine; Aprepitant; Astemizole; Avanafil; Axitinib; Barnidipine; BCG (Intravesical); Bosutinib; Bromocriptine; Cabozantinib; Ceritinib; Cobimetinib; Conivaptan; Crizotinib; CYP3A4 Inducers (Strong); CYP3A4 Substrates; Dabrafenib; Dapoxetine; Domperidone; Dronedarone; Eletriptan; Eplerenone; Everolimus; Flibanserin; Halofantrine; Ibrutinib; Isavuconazonium Sulfate; Ivabradine; Lapatinib; Lercanidipine; Lomitapide; Lovastatin; Lurasidone; Macitentan; Naloxegol; Natalizumab; Nilotinib; NiMODipine; Nisoldipine; Olaparib; Osimertinib; Palbociclib; Pimecrolimus; Pimozide; Ranolazine; Red Yeast Rice; Regorafenib; Salmeterol; Silodosin; Simeprevir; Simvastatin; Sonidegib; St Johns Wort; Suvorexant; Tacrolimus (Topical); Tamsulosin; Terfenadine; Ticagrelor; Tofacitinib; Tolvaptan; Toremifene; Trabectedin; Ulipristal; Vaccines (Live); Vemurafenib; VinCRIStine (Liposomal); Vorapaxar

Increased Effect/Toxicity

Idelalisib may increase the levels/effects of: Ado-Trastuzumab Emtansine; Alfuzosin; Alitretinoin (Systemic); Almotriptan; Alosetron; Amodiaquine; Apixaban; Aprepitant; Astemizole; Avanafil; Axitinib; Barnidipine; Bedaquiline; Bortezomib; Bosentan; Bosutinib; Brentuximab Vedotin; Brinzolamide; Bromocriptine; Budesonide (Nasal); Budesonide (Oral Inhalation); Budesonide (Topical); Cabozantinib; Cannabis; Ceritinib; Cobimetinib; Conivaptan; Corticosteroids (Orally Inhaled); Corticosteroids (Systemic); Crizotinib; CYP3A4 Substrates; Dabrafenib; Dapoxetine; Dienogest; Dofetilide; Domperidone; Dronabinol; Dronedarone; Drospirenone; Dutasteride; Eletriptan; Eplerenone; Estazolam; Everolimus; Fingolimod; Flibanserin; Fluticasone (Nasal); Halofantrine; Ibrutinib; Iloperidone; Imatinib; Imidafenacin; Isavuconazonium Sulfate; Ivabradine; Lacosamide; Lapatinib; Leflunomide; Lercanidipine; Levobupivacaine; Lomitapide; Lovastatin; Lumefantrine; Lurasidone; Macitentan; MedroxyPROGESTERone; MethylPREDNISolone; Naloxegol; Natalizumab; Nilotinib; NiMODipine; Nisoldipine; Olaparib; Osimertinib; Ospemifene; Oxybutynin; Palbociclib; Parecoxib; Paricalcitol; Pimozide; PONATinib; Pranlukast; PrednisoLONE (Systemic); PredniSONE; Propafenone; Ramelteon; Ranolazine; Red Yeast Rice; Regorafenib; Repaglinide; Retapamulin; Rilpivirine; RomiDEPsin; Salmeterol; Silodosin; Simeprevir; Simvastatin; Sonidegib; SORAfenib; Suvorexant; Tamsulosin; Tasimelteon; Terfenadine; Tetrahydrocannabinol; Ticagrelor; Tofacitinib; Tolvaptan; Toremifene; Trabectedin; TraMADol; Ulipristal; Vaccines (Live); Vemurafenib; Vilazodone; VinCRIStine (Liposomal); Vindesine; Vinorelbine; Vorapaxar; Zuclopenthixol

The levels/effects of Idelalisib may be increased by: CYP3A4 Inhibitors (Strong); Denosumab; Pimecrolimus; Roflumilast; Tacrolimus (Topical); Trastuzumab

Decreased Effect

Idelalisib may decrease the levels/effects of: BCG (Intravesical); Coccidioides immitis Skin Test; Ifosfamide; Prasugrel; Sipuleucel-T; Ticagrelor; Vaccines (Inactivated); Vaccines (Live)

The levels/effects of Idelalisib may be decreased by: Bosentan; CYP3A4 Inducers (Moderate); CYP3A4 Inducers (Strong); Deferasirox; Echinacea; Siltuximab; St Johns Wort; Tocilizumab

Storage/Stability Store at 20°C to 30°C (68°F to 86°F); excursions are permitted between 15°C and 30°C (59°F and 86°F). Dispense in the original container.

Mechanism of Action Potent small molecule inhibitor of the delta isoform of phosphatidylinositol 3-kinase (PI3Kδ), which is highly expressed in malignant lymphoid B-cells. PI3Kδ inhibition results in apoptosis of malignant tumor cells. In addition, idelalisib inhibits several signaling pathways, including B-cell receptor, CXCR4 and CXCR5 signaling which may play important roles in CLL pathophysiology (Furman, 2014).

Pharmacodynamics/Kinetics

Distribution: 23 L

Protein binding: >84%

Metabolism: Hepatic; primarily via aldehyde oxidase and CYP3A (to major metabolite GS-563117); minor metabolism via UGT1A4

Half-life elimination: ~8 hours

Time to peak: Median: 1.5 hours

Excretion: Feces (78%; 44% as GS-563117); urine (14%; 49% as GS-563117)

Dosing

Adult & Geriatric Note: The maximum recommended starting dose is 150 mg twice daily. Optimal duration and safety of therapy beyond several months is currently unknown.

Chronic lymphocytic leukemia, relapsed: Oral: 150 mg twice daily (in combination with rituximab); continue until disease progression or unacceptable toxicity (Furman, 2014)

Follicular B-cell non-Hodgkin lymphoma, relapsed:
Oral: 150 mg twice daily; continue until disease progression or unacceptable toxicity (Gopal, 2014)

Small lymphocytic lymphoma, relapsed: Oral: 150 mg twice daily; continue until disease progression or unacceptable toxicity (Gopal, 2014)

Renal Impairment

US labeling:
CrCl ≥15 mL/minute: No dosage adjustment necessary.
CrCl <15 mL/minute: There are no dosage adjustments provided in the manufacturer's labeling (has not been studied).

Canadian labeling: No dosage adjustment necessary.

Hepatic Impairment

Preexisting hepatic impairment: Exposure is increased in patients with ALT/AST or bilirubin >ULN as compared to patients with normal hepatic function; patients with ALT/AST >2.5 times ULN or bilirubin >1.5 times ULN were excluded from some studies. Based on a pharmacokinetic study in patients with moderate and severe hepatic impairment, single oral doses of 150 mg were well tolerated; idelalisib and GS-563117 exposure differences were not considered clinically relevant (Jin, 2014). Monitor closely for toxicity. The Canadian labeling recommends no initial dosage adjustment for mild to moderate hepatic impairment; however, data are insufficient to make a dosing recommendation for severe impairment.

Hepatotoxicity during treatment:

US labeling:
ALT/AST >3 to 5 times ULN or bilirubin >1.5 to 3 times ULN: Continue current dose; monitor LFTs at least weekly until ALT/AST and/or bilirubin ≤1 times ULN.
ALT/AST >5 to 20 times ULN or bilirubin >3 to 10 times ULN: Temporarily interrupt therapy. Monitor LFTs at least weekly until ALT/AST and/or bilirubin ≤1 times ULN, then may reinitiate therapy at 100 mg twice daily.
ALT/AST >20 times ULN or bilirubin >10 times ULN: Discontinue permanently.
Recurrent hepatotoxicity: Discontinue.

Canadian labeling:
Grade 1 (ALT/AST ≤3 times ULN) or Grade 2 (ALT/AST >3 to 5 times ULN): Continue current dose; monitor LFTs at least weekly until ALT/AST ≤1 times ULN.
Grade 3 (ALT/AST >5 to 20 times ULN) or Grade 4 (ALT/AST >20 times ULN): Temporarily interrupt therapy. Monitor LFTs at least weekly until ALT/AST ≤1 times ULN, then may reinitiate therapy at 100 mg twice daily.
Recurrent hepatotoxicity: Discontinue.

Adjustment for Toxicity

Anaphylaxis: Permanently discontinue.

Dermatologic toxicity:
Severe cutaneous reactions: Discontinue.
Rash (Canadian labeling):
Grade 1: Continue current dose
Grade 2: Temporarily interrupt therapy until resolved to ≤ grade 1.
Grade 3 or 4: Temporarily interrupt therapy; monitor at least weekly until resolved to ≤ grade 1 then reinitiate at 100 mg twice daily.

Hematologic toxicity:

Neutropenia:
ANC 1,000 to <1,500 cells/mm^3: Continue current dose.
ANC 500 to <1,000 cells/mm^3: Continue current dose; monitor blood counts at least weekly.
ANC <500 cells/mm^3: Temporarily interrupt therapy; monitor blood counts at least weekly until ANC ≥500 cells/mm^3, then may reinitiate therapy at 100 mg twice daily.

Thrombocytopenia:

US labeling:
Platelets 50,000 to <75,000 cells/mm^3: Continue current dose.
Platelets 25,000 to <50,000 cells/mm^3: Continue current dose; monitor platelet counts at least weekly.
Platelets <25,000 cells/mm^3: Temporarily interrupt therapy; monitor platelet counts at least weekly, may reinitiate therapy at 100 mg twice daily when platelets recover to ≥25,000 cells/mm^3.
Canadian labeling: There are no specific recommendations provided in the manufacturer's labeling.

Gastrointestinal toxicity:

US labeling:
Moderate diarrhea (increase of 4 to 6 stools/day over baseline): Continue current dose; monitor at least weekly until resolved.

Severe diarrhea (increase of ≥7 stools/day over baseline) or hospitalization: Temporarily interrupt therapy; monitor at least weekly until resolved, then may reinitiate therapy at 100 mg twice daily.
Life-threatening diarrhea: Discontinue permanently.

Canadian labeling:
Diarrhea/colitis:
Grade 1: Continue current dose; provide antidiarrheal (eg, loperamide)
Grade 2: Temporarily interrupt therapy; monitor at least weekly until resolved to ≤ grade 1.
Grade 3 or 4: Temporarily interrupt therapy and consider addition of anti-inflammatory drugs (eg, budesonide, sulfasalazine); monitor at least weekly until resolved to ≤ grade 1, then may reinitiate at 100 mg twice daily.
Ongoing inflammatory bowel disease: Use is not recommended.

Pulmonary toxicity: If pneumonitis is suspected, interrupt therapy and evaluate; discontinue for symptomatic pneumonitis of any severity thought to be associated with therapy (may also require corticosteroids). For patients in whom an infectious etiology has been established, the Canadian labeling recommends monitoring until resolved then reinitiate therapy at 100 mg twice daily.

Other toxicity (not listed above): If severe or life-threatening toxicities occur, interrupt therapy until toxicity is resolved. If the decision is made to resume therapy, reduce the dose to 100 mg twice daily. Discontinue permanently if severe or life-threatening toxicities recur upon rechallenge.

Administration Administer orally twice daily with or without food. Swallow tablets whole.

Missed doses: May administer a missed dose if within 6 hours of usual dosing time. If >6 hours, skip the missed dose and resume therapy with the next scheduled dose.

Hazardous agent; use appropriate precautions for handling and disposal (meets NIOSH 2014 criteria).

Monitoring Parameters Liver function tests at baseline and every 2 weeks for the first 3 months, every 4 weeks for the next 3 months, then every 1 to 3 months thereafter, or as clinically necessary; complete blood counts at least every 2 weeks for the first 3 months, and at least weekly in patients with neutropenia, or as clinically necessary; signs/symptoms of diarrhea/colitis, intestinal perforation, pneumonitis, dermatologic toxicity, and hypersensitivity reactions

Dosage Forms Excipient information presented when available (limited, particularly for generics); consult specific product labeling.
Tablet, Oral:
Zydelig: 100 mg, 150 mg

◆ **IDR** *see* IDArubicin *on page 910*

Idursulfase (eye dur SUL fase)

Brand Names: US Elaprase
Brand Names: Canada Elaprase
Pharmacologic Category Enzyme
Use Hunter syndrome: Replacement therapy in Hunter syndrome (mucopolysaccharidosis II; MPS II) for improvement of walking capacity

Dosing

Adult Hunter syndrome (mucopolysaccharidosis II): IV: 0.5 mg/kg once weekly

Pediatric Hunter syndrome (mucopolysaccharidosis II): Children ≥5 years and Adolescents: Refer to adult dosing.

Renal Impairment No dosage adjustment provided in manufacturer's labeling.

Hepatic Impairment No dosage adjustment provided in manufacturer's labeling.

Additional Information Complete prescribing information should be consulted for additional detail.

Dosage Forms Excipient information presented when available (limited, particularly for generics); consult specific product labeling.
Solution, Intravenous [preservative free]:
Elaprase: 6 mg/3 mL (3 mL)

◆ **IDV** *see* Indinavir *on page 937*

◆ **iFerex 150 [OTC]** *see* Polysaccharide-Iron Complex *on page 1469*

◆ **Ifex** *see* Ifosfamide *on page 913*

Ifosfamide (eye FOSS fa mide)

Brand Names: US Ifex
Brand Names: Canada Ifex; Ifosfamide for Injection

◄ **Index Terms** Isophosphamide; Z4942
Pharmacologic Category Antineoplastic Agent, Alkylating Agent; Antineoplastic Agent, Alkylating Agent (Nitrogen Mustard)
Use
US labeling: Treatment (third-line) of germ cell testicular cancer (in combination with other chemotherapy drugs and with concurrent mesna)
Canadian labeling (not approved indications in the US): Treatment of soft tissue sarcoma, pancreatic cancer (relapsed or refractory), cervical cancer (advanced or recurrent; as monotherapy or in combination with cisplatin and bleomycin)
Pregnancy Considerations Embryotoxic and teratogenic effects have been observed in animal reproduction studies. Fetal growth retardation and neonatal anemia have been reported with exposure to ifosfamide-containing regimens during human pregnancy. Male and female fertility may be affected (dose and duration dependent). Ifosfamide interferes with oogenesis and spermatogenesis; amenorrhea, azoospermia, and sterility have been reported and may be irreversible. Avoid pregnancy during treatment; male patients should not father a child for at least 6 months after completion of therapy.
Breast-Feeding Considerations Breast-feeding should be avoided during ifosfamide treatment. According to the manufacturer, due to the potential for serious adverse reactions in the nursing infant, a decision should be made to discontinue ifosfamide or to discontinue breast-feeding, taking into account the benefits of treatment to the mother.
Contraindications Hypersensitivity to ifosfamide or any component of the formulation; urinary outflow obstruction
Canadian labeling: Additional contraindications (not in U.S. labeling): Severe myelosuppression; severe renal or hepatic impairment; active infection (bacterial, fungal, viral); severe immunosuppression; urinary tract disease (eg, cystitis); advanced cerebral arteriosclerosis
Warnings/Precautions Hazardous agent: Use appropriate precautions for handling and disposal (NIOSH 2014 [group 1]). **[US Boxed Warning]: Hemorrhagic cystitis may occur (may be severe); concomitant mesna reduces the risk of hemorrhagic cystitis.** Hydration (at least 2 L/day in adults), dose fractionation, and/or mesna administration will reduce the incidence of hematuria and protect against hemorrhagic cystitis. Obtain urinalysis prior to each dose; if microscopic hematuria is detected, withhold until complete resolution. Exclude or correct urinary tract obstructions prior to treatment. Use with caution (if at all) in patients with active urinary tract infection. Hemorrhagic cystitis is dose-dependent and is increased with high single doses (compared with fractionated doses); past or concomitant bladder radiation or busulfan treatment may increase the risk for hemorrhagic cystitis. **[US Boxed Warning]: May cause severe nephrotoxicity, resulting in renal failure.** Acute and chronic renal failure as well as renal parenchymal and tubular necrosis (including acute) have been reported; tubular damage may be delayed and may persist. Renal manifestations include decreased glomerular rate, increased creatinine, proteinuria, enzymuria, cylindruria, aminoaciduria, phosphaturia, and glycosuria. Syndrome of inappropriate antidiuretic hormone (SIADH), renal rickets, and Fanconi syndrome have been reported. Evaluate renal function prior to and during treatment; monitor urine for erythrocytes and signs of urotoxicity.

[US Boxed Warning]: May cause CNS toxicity which may be severe, resulting in encephalopathy and death; monitor for CNS toxicity; discontinue for encephalopathy. Symptoms of CNS toxicity (somnolence, confusion, dizziness, disorientation, hallucinations, cranial nerve dysfunction, psychotic behavior, extrapyramidal symptoms, seizures, coma blurred vision, and/or incontinence) have been observed within a few hours to a few days after initial dose and generally resolve within 2-3 days of treatment discontinuation (although may persist longer); maintain supportive care until complete resolution. Risk factors may include hypoalbuminemia, renal dysfunction, and prior history of ifosfamide-induced encephalopathy. Concomitant centrally-acting medications may result in additive CNS effects. Peripheral neuropathy has been reported.

[US Boxed Warning]: Severe bone marrow suppression may occur (may be severe and lead to fatal infections); monitor blood counts before and after each cycle. Leukopenia, neutropenia, thrombocytopenia and anemia are associated with ifosfamide. Myelosuppression is dose dependent, increased with single high doses (compared with fractionated doses) and increased with decreased renal function. Severe myelosuppression may occur when administered in combination with other chemotherapy agents or radiation therapy. Use with caution in patients with compromised bone marrow reserve. Unless clinically necessary, avoid administering to patients with WBC <2000/mm^3 and platelets <50,000/mm^3. Antimicrobial prophylaxis may be necessary in some neutropenic patients; Administer antibiotics and/or antifungal agents for neutropenic fever. May cause significant suppression of the immune responses; may lead to serious infection, sepsis or septic shock; reported infections have included bacterial, viral, fungal, and parasitic; latent infections may be reactivated; use with caution with other immunosuppressants or in patients with infection.

Arrhythmias, ST-segment or T-wave changes, cardiomyopathy, pericardial effusion, pericarditis, and epicardial fibrosis have been observed; the risk for cardiotoxicity is dose-dependent; concomitant cardiotoxic agents (eg, anthracyclines), irradiation of the cardiac region, and renal impairment may also increase the risk; use with caution in patients with cardiac risk factors or preexisting cardiac disease. Interstitial pneumonitis, pulmonary fibrosis, and pulmonary toxicity leading to respiratory failure have been reported; monitor for signs and symptoms of pulmonary toxicity.

Anaphylactic/anaphylactoid reactions have been associated with ifosfamide; cross sensitivity with similar agents may occur. Hepatic sinusoidal obstruction syndrome (SOS), formerly called veno-occlusive disease (VOD), has been reported with ifosfamide-containing regimens. Secondary malignancies may occur; the risk for myelodysplastic syndrome (which may progress to acute leukemia) is increased with treatment. May interfere with wound healing. Potentially significant drug-drug interactions may exist, requiring dose or frequency adjustment, additional monitoring, and/or selection of alternative therapy. Use with caution in patients with prior radiation therapy. Ifosfamide is associated with a moderate emetic potential; antiemetics are recommended to prevent nausea and vomiting (Basch 2011; Dupuis 2011; Roila 2010).

Adverse Reactions
>10%:
Central nervous system: CNS toxicity or encephalopathy (12% to 15%)
Dermatologic: Alopecia (83% to 90%; 100% with combination therapy)
Endocrine & metabolic: Metabolic acidosis (31%)
Gastrointestinal: Nausea/vomiting (47% to 58%)
Hematologic: Leukopenia (50% to ≤100%; grade 4: ≤50%; nadir: 8-14 days), anemia (38%), thrombocytopenia (20%; grades 3/4: ≤8%)
Renal: Hematuria (6% to 92%; reduced with mesna; grade 2 [gross hematuria]: 8% to 12%)
1% to 10%:
Central nervous system: Fever (1%)
Gastrointestinal: Anorexia (1%)
Hematologic: Neutropenic fever (1%)
Hepatic: Bilirubin increased (2% to 3%), liver dysfunction (2% to 3%), transaminases increased (2% to 3%)
Local: Phlebitis (2% to 3%)
Renal: Renal impairment (6%)
Miscellaneous: Infection (8% to 10%)
<1% (Limited to important or life-threatening): Acute respiratory distress syndrome, acute tubular necrosis, agranulocytosis, alkaline phosphatase increased, allergic reaction, alveolitis (allergic), amenorrhea, aminoaciduria, amnesia, anaphylactic reaction, angina, angioedema, anuria, arrhythmia, arthralgia, asterixis, atrial ectopy, atrial fibrillation/flutter, azoospermia, bladder irritation, bleeding, blurred vision, bone marrow failure, bradycardia, bradyphrenia, bronchospasm, bundle branch block, BUN increased, capillary leak syndrome, cardiac arrest, cardiogenic shock, cardiomyopathy, cardiotoxicity, catatonia, cecitis, chest pain, cholestasis, coagulopathy, colitis, conjunctivitis, creatinine clearance decreased/increased, creatinine increased, cylindruria, cytolytic hepatitis, delirium, delusion, dermatitis, diarrhea, DIC, DVT, dysesthesia, dyspnea, dysuria, echolalia, edema, ejection fraction decreased, enterocolitis, enuresis, enzymuria, erythema, extrapyramidal disorder, facial swelling, Fanconi syndrome, fatigue, gait disturbance, GGT increased, GI hemorrhage, glycosuria, gonadotropin increased, granulocytopenia, growth retardation (children), hemolytic anemia, hemolytic uremic syndrome, hemorrhagic cystitis, hepatic failure, hepatic sinusoidal obstruction syndrome (SOS; formerly veno-occlusive disease [VOD]), hepatitis fulminant, hepatitis (viral), hepatorenal syndrome, herpes zoster, hyperglycemia, hyper-/hypotension, hypersensitivity reactions, hypocalcemia, hypokalemia, hyponatremia, hypophosphatemia, hypoxia, ileus, immunosuppression, infertility, infusion site reactions (erythema, inflammation, pain, pruritus, swelling, tenderness), interstitial lung disease, jaundice, LDH increased, leukoencephalopathy, lymphopenia, malaise, mania, mental status change, methemoglobinemia, MI,

mucosal inflammation/ulceration, multiorgan failure, mutism, myocardial hemorrhage, myocarditis, nephrogenic diabetes insipidus, neuralgia, neutropenia, oligospermia, oliguria, osteomalacia (adults), ovarian failure, ovulation disorder, palmar-plantar erythrodysesthesia syndrome, pancreatitis, pancytopenia, panic attack, paranoia, paresthesia, pericardial effusion, pericarditis, peripheral neuropathy, petechiae, phosphaturia, pleural effusion, *Pneumocystis jiroveci* pneumonia, pneumonia, pneumonitis, pollakiuria, polydipsia, polyneuropathy, polyuria, portal vein thrombosis, premature atrial contractions, premature menopause, progressive multifocal leukoencephalopathy, proteinuria, pruritus, pulmonary edema, pulmonary embolism, pulmonary fibrosis, pulmonary hypertension, QRS complex abnormal, radiation recall dermatitis, rash (including macular and papular), renal failure, renal parenchymal damage, renal tubular acidosis, respiratory failure, reversible posterior leukoencephalopathy syndrome (RPLS), rhabdomyolysis, rickets, salivation, secondary malignancy, seizure, sepsis, septic shock, SIADH, skin necrosis, spermatogenesis impaired, status epilepticus, sterility, Stevens-Johnson syndrome, stomatitis, ST segment abnormal, supraventricular extrasystoles, tachycardia, tinnitus, toxic epidermal necrolysis, tubulointerstitial nephritis, tumor lysis syndrome, T-wave inversion, uremia, urticaria, vasculitis, ventricular extrasystoles/fibrillation/tachycardia, ventricular failure, vertigo, visual impairment, wound healing impairment

Drug Interactions

Metabolism/Transport Effects Substrate of CYP2B6 (major), CYP2C19 (minor), CYP2C8 (minor), CYP2C9 (minor), CYP3A4 (minor); **Note:** Assignment of Major/Minor substrate status based on clinically relevant drug interaction potential; **Induces** CYP2C9 (weak/moderate)

Avoid Concomitant Use

Avoid concomitant use of Ifosfamide with any of the following: BCG (Intravesical); Deferiprone; Dipyrone; Natalizumab; Pimecrolimus; Tacrolimus (Topical); Tofacitinib; Vaccines (Live)

Increased Effect/Toxicity

Ifosfamide may increase the levels/effects of: CloZAPine; Deferiprone; Fingolimod; Leflunomide; Natalizumab; Tofacitinib; Vaccines (Live); Vitamin K Antagonists

The levels/effects of Ifosfamide may be increased by: Aprepitant; Busulfan; CYP2B6 Inhibitors (Moderate); CYP3A4 Inducers (Moderate); CYP3A4 Inducers (Strong); Denosumab; Dipyrone; Fosaprepitant; Pimecrolimus; Quazepam; Roflumilast; Tacrolimus (Topical); Trastuzumab

Decreased Effect

Ifosfamide may decrease the levels/effects of: BCG (Intravesical); Coccidioides immitis Skin Test; Sipuleucel-T; Vaccines (Inactivated); Vaccines (Live)

The levels/effects of Ifosfamide may be decreased by: CYP2B6 Inducers (Strong); CYP3A4 Inducers (Moderate); CYP3A4 Inducers (Strong); CYP3A4 Inhibitors (Moderate); CYP3A4 Inhibitors (Strong); Dabrafenib; Echinacea; Lumacaftor

Preparation for Administration Hazardous agent; use appropriate precautions for handling and disposal (NIOSH 2014 [group 1]). Reconstitute powder with SWFI or bacteriostatic SWFI (1 g in 20 mL or 3 g in 60 mL) to a concentration of 50 mg/mL. Further dilution in 50-1000 mL D$_5$W, NS, or lactated Ringer's (to a final concentration of 0.6-20 mg/mL) is recommended for IV infusion (may also dilute in D$_{2.5}$W, $\frac{1}{2}$NS, or D$_5$NS).

Storage/Stability Store intact vials of powder for injection at room temperature of 20°C to 25°C (68°F to 77°F); avoid temperatures >30°C (86°F). Store intact vials of solution under refrigeration at 2°C to 8°C (36°F to 46°F). Reconstituted solutions and solutions diluted for administration are stable for 24 hours refrigerated.

Mechanism of Action Causes cross-linking of strands of DNA by binding with nucleic acids and other intracellular structures; inhibits protein synthesis and DNA synthesis

Pharmacodynamics/Kinetics Pharmacokinetics are dose dependent

Distribution: V$_d$: Approximates total body water; penetrates CNS, but not in therapeutic levels

Protein binding: Negligible

Metabolism: Hepatic to active metabolites isofosforamide mustard, 4-hydroxy-ifosfamide, acrolein, and inactive dichloroethylated and carboxy metabolites; acrolein is the agent implicated in development of hemorrhagic cystitis

Half-life elimination (increased in the elderly):

High dose (3,800 to 5,000 mg/m^2): ~15 hours

Lower dose (1,600 to 2,400 mg/m^2): ~7 hours

Excretion:

High dose (5,000 mg/m^2): Urine (70% to 86%; 61% as unchanged drug)

Lower dose (1,600 to 2,400 mg/m^2): Urine (12% to 18% as unchanged drug)

Dosing

Adult & Geriatric Note: To prevent bladder toxicity, ifosfamide should be given with the urinary protector mesna and hydration of at least 2 L of oral or IV fluid per day. Ifosfamide is associated with a moderate emetic potential; antiemetics are recommended to prevent nausea and vomiting (Basch 2011; Roila 2010).

Testicular cancer: IV:

US manufacturer's labeling; as part of combination chemotherapy and with mesna: 1,200 mg/m^2/day for 5 days every 3 weeks or after hematologic recovery

VIP regimen: 1,200 mg/m^2/day for 5 days every 3 weeks for 4 cycles (in combination with etoposide, mesna, and cisplatin) (Nichols 1998)

VeIP regimen: 1,200 mg/m^2/day for 5 days every 3 weeks for 4 cycles (in combination with vinblastine, mesna, and cisplatin) (Loehrer 1998)

Canadian labeling: **Soft tissue sarcoma, cervical cancer (advanced or recurrent), pancreatic cancer (relapsed or refractory):** IV: 2,000- to 2,400 mg/m^2/day for 5 consecutive days (with mesna), may repeat after 3 to 4 weeks (or longer depending on patient status) or if lower daily dosage or total dosage over a longer time period is indicated, administer every other day (eg, days 1, 3, 5, 7, 9) or over 10 consecutive days at reduced doses.

High **single-dose** infusions of up to 5,000 to 8,000 mg/m^2/24 hour with continuous mesna may also be feasible; may repeat after 3 to 4 weeks (or longer depending on patient's condition).

Adult off-label uses and/or dosing:

Testicular cancer: IV:

TIP regimen (off-label dosing): 1,500 mg/m^2/day for 4 days (days 2 to 5) every 3 weeks for 4 cycles (in combination with paclitaxel, mesna, and cisplatin) (Kondagunta 2005)

TICE regimen (off-label dosing): 2,000 mg/m^2/day for 3 days (days 2 to 4) over 4 hours every 2 weeks for 2 cycles (in combination with paclitaxel and mesna; followed by carboplatin and etoposide) (Kondagunta 2007)

Cervical cancer, recurrent or metastatic: IV: 1,500 mg/m^2/day for 5 days every 3 weeks (with mesna) (Coleman 1986; Sutton 1993)

Hodgkin lymphoma, relapsed or refractory: IV:

ICE regimen: 5,000 mg/m^2 (over 24 hours) beginning on day 2 every 2 weeks for 2 cycles (in combination with mesna, carboplatin, and etoposide) (Moskowitz 2001)

IGEV regimen: 2,000 mg/m^2/day for 4 days every 3 weeks for 4 cycles (in combination with mesna, gemcitabine, vinorelbine, and prednisolone) (Santoro 2007)

Non-Hodgkin lymphomas: IV:

CODOX-M/IVAC regimen:

Adults ≤65 years: Cycles 2 and 4 (IVAC): 1,500 mg/m^2/day for 5 days (IVAC is combination with cytarabine, mesna, and etoposide; IVAC alternates with CODOX-M) (Mead 2008)

Adults >65 years: Cycles 2 and 4 (IVAC): 1,000 mg/m^2/day for 5 days (IVAC is combination with cytarabine, mesna, and etoposide; IVAC alternates with CODOX-M) (Mead 2008)

RICE regimen: 5,000 mg/m^2 (over 24 hours) beginning on day 4 every 2 weeks for 3 cycles (in combination with mesna, carboplatin, etoposide, and rituximab) (Kewalramani 2004)

Ewing sarcoma: IV:

VAC/IE regimen: Adults ≤30 years: IE: 1,800 mg/m^2/day for 5 days (in combination with mesna and etoposide) alternate with VAC (vincristine, doxorubicin, and cyclophosphamide) every 3 weeks for a total of 17 courses (Grier 2003)

VAIA regimen: 3,000 mg/m^2 day on days 1, 2, 22, 23, 43, and 44 for 4 courses (in combination with vincristine, doxorubicin, dactinomycin, and mesna) (Paulussen 2001) **or** Adults ≤35 years: 2,000 mg/m^2/day for 3 days every 3 weeks for 14 courses (in combination with vincristine, doxorubicin, dactinomycin, and mesna) (Paulussen 2008)

VIDE regimen: Adults ≤50 years: 3,000 mg/m^2/day over 1 to 3 hours for 3 days every 3 weeks for 6 courses (in combination with vincristine, doxorubicin, etoposide, and mesna) (Juergens 2006)

IE regimen: 1,800 mg/m^2/day over 1 hour for 5 days every 3 weeks for 12 cycles (in combination with etoposide and mesna) (Miser 1987)

ICE regimen: Adults ≤22 years: 1,800 mg/m^2/day for 5 days every 3 weeks for up to 12 cycles (in combination with carboplatin and etoposide [and mesna]) (van Winkle 2005)

Osteosarcoma: IV:

Ifosfamide/cisplatin/doxorubicin/HDMT regimen: Adults <40 years: 3,000 mg/m^2/day continuous infusion for 5 days during weeks 4 and 10 (preop) and during weeks 16, 25, and 34 (postop) (in combination with cisplatin, doxorubicin, methotrexate [high-dose], and mesna) (Bacci 2003)

Ifosfamide/cisplatin/epirubicin regimen: 2,000 mg/m^2/day over 4 hours for 3 days (days 2, 3, and 4) every 3 weeks for 3 cycles (preop) and every 4 weeks for 3 cycles (postop) (in combination with cisplatin, epirubicin, and mesna) (Basaran 2007)

ICE regimen (adults ≤22 years): 1,800 mg/m^2/day for 5 days every 3 weeks for up to 12 cycles (in combination with carboplatin and etoposide [and mesna]) (van Winkle 2005)

Soft tissue sarcoma: IV:

Single-agent ifosfamide: 3,000 mg/m^2/day over 4 hours for 3 days every 3 weeks for at least 2 cycles or until disease progression (van Oosterom 2002)

ICE regimen: 1,500 mg/m^2/day for 4 days every 4 weeks for 4 to 6 cycles (in combination with carboplatin, etoposide, and regional hyperthermia) (Nickenig 2009)

MAID regimen: 2,000 mg/m^2/day continuous infusion for 3 days every 3 weeks (in combination with mesna, doxorubicin, and dacarbazine) (Antman 1993) **or** 2,500 mg/m^2/day continuous infusion for 3 days every 3 weeks (in combination with mesna, doxorubicin, and dacarbazine); reduce ifosfamide to 1,500mg/m^2/day if prior pelvic irradiation (Elias 1989)

Ifosfamide/epirubicin: 1,800 mg/m^2/day over 1 hour for 5 days every 3 weeks for 5 cycles (in combination with mesna and epirubicin) (Frustaci 2001)

AIM regimens: 1,500 mg/m^2/day over 2 hours for 4 days every 3 weeks for 4 to 6 cycles (in combination with mesna and doxorubicin) (Worden 2005) **or** 2,000 to 3,000 mg/m^2/day over 3 hours for 3 days (in combination with mesna and doxorubicin) (Grobmyer 2004)

Pediatric Note: To prevent bladder toxicity, ifosfamide should be given with the urinary protector mesna and hydration of at least 2 L of oral or IV fluid per day. Ifosfamide is associated with a moderate emetic potential; antiemetics are recommended to prevent nausea and vomiting (Dupuis 2011).

Ewing sarcoma (off-label use): IV:

VAC/IE regimen: IE: 1,800 mg/m^2/day for 5 days (in combination with mesna and etoposide) alternate with VAC (vincristine, doxorubicin, and cyclophosphamide) every 3 weeks for a total of 17 courses (Grier 2003)

ICE-CAV regimen: ICE: 1,800 mg/m^2/day for 5 days every 3 to 4 weeks for 2 courses (in combination with carboplatin and etoposide [and mesna]), followed by CAV (cyclophosphamide, doxorubicin, and vincristine) (Milano 2006)

VAIA regimen: 3,000 mg/m^2/day on days 1, 2, 22, 23, 43, and 44 for 4 courses (in combination with vincristine, doxorubicin, dactinomycin, and mesna) (Paulussen 2001) **or** 2,000 mg/m^2/day for 3 days every 3 weeks for 14 courses (in combination with vincristine, doxorubicin, dactinomycin, and mesna) (Paulussen 2008)

VIDE regimen: 3,000 mg/m^2/day over 1 to 3 hours for 3 days every 3 weeks for 6 courses (in combination with vincristine, doxorubicin, etoposide, and mesna) (Juergens 2006)

IE regimen: 1,800 mg/m^2/day over 1 hour for 5 days every 3 weeks for 12 cycles (in combination with etoposide and mesna) (Miser 1987)

ICE regimen: 1,800 mg/m^2/day for 5 days every 3 weeks for up to 12 cycles (in combination with carboplatin and etoposide [and mesna]) (van Winkle 2005)

Osteosarcoma (off-label use): IV:

Ifosfamide/cisplatin/doxorubicin/HDMT regimen: 3,000 mg/m^2/day continuous infusion for 5 days during weeks 4 and 10 (preop) and during weeks 16, 25, and 34 (postop) (in combination with cisplatin, doxorubicin, methotrexate [high-dose], and mesna) (Bacci 2003)

Ifosfamide/cisplatin/epirubicin regimen: Children ≥15 years: 2,000 mg/m^2/day over 4 hours for 3 days (days 2, 3, and 4) every 3 weeks for 3 cycles (preop) and every 4 weeks for 3 cycles (postop) (in combination with cisplatin, epirubicin, and mesna) (Basaran 2007)

IE regimen: 3,000 mg/m^2/day over 3 hours for 4 days every 3 to 4 weeks (in combination with etoposide and mesna) (Gentet 1997)

ICE regimen: Children ≥1 year: 1,800 mg/m^2/day for 5 days every 3 weeks for up to 12 cycles (in combination with carboplatin and etoposide [and mesna]) (van Winkle 2005)

Ifosfamide/HDMT/etoposide regimen: 3,000 mg/m^2/day over 3 hours for 4 days during weeks 4 and 9 (3 additional postop courses were administered in good responders) (in combination with methotrexate [high-dose], etoposide, and mesna) (Le Deley 2007)

Renal Impairment

US labeling: Consider dosage reduction in patients with renal impairment; however, there are no dosage adjustments provided in the manufacturer's labeling; ifosfamide (and metabolites) are excreted renally and may accumulate in patients with renal dysfunction. Ifosfamide and metabolites are dialyzable.

Canadian labeling:

Mild to moderate impairment: There are no dosage adjustments provided in the manufacturer's labeling.

Severe impairment: Use is contraindicated.

The following adjustments have also been recommended:

Aronoff 2007:

CrCl ≥10 mL/minute: Children and Adults: No dosage adjustment necessary.

CrCl <10 mL/minute: Children and Adults: Administer 75% of dose.

Hemodialysis (supplement for dialysis):

Children: 1 g/m^2 followed by hemodialysis 6 to 8 hours later

Adults: No supplemental dose needed

Kintzel 1995:

CrCl 46 to 60 mL/minute: Administer 80% of dose

CrCl 31 to 45 mL/minute: Administer 75% of dose

CrCl <30 mL/minute: Administer 70% of dose

Hepatic Impairment There are no dosage adjustments provided in the manufacturer's labeling; however, ifosfamide is extensively hepatically metabolized to both active and inactive metabolites; use with caution. The following adjustments have been recommended:

Floyd 2006: Bilirubin >3 mg/dL: Administer 25% of dose.

Canadian labeling:

Mild to moderate impairment: There are no dosage adjustments provided in the manufacturer labeling; use with caution.

Severe impairment: Use is contraindicated.

Obesity *ASCO Guidelines for appropriate chemotherapy dosing in obese adults with cancer:* Utilize patient's actual body weight (full weight) for calculation of body surface area- or weight-based dosing, particularly when the intent of therapy is curative; manage regimen-related toxicities in the same manner as for nonobese patients; if a dose reduction is utilized due to toxicity, consider resumption of full weight-based dosing with subsequent cycles, especially if cause of toxicity (eg, hepatic or renal impairment) is resolved (Griggs 2012).

Administration Ifosfamide is associated with a moderate emetic potential; antiemetics are recommended to prevent nausea and vomiting (Basch 2011; Dupuis 2011; Roila 2010).

Administer IV over at least 30 minutes (infusion times may vary by protocol; refer to specific protocol for infusion duration)

Hazardous agent; use appropriate precautions for handling and disposal (NIOSH 2014 [group 1]).

Monitoring Parameters CBC with differential (prior to each dose), urine output, urinalysis (prior to each dose), liver function, and renal function tests; signs and symptoms of neurotoxicity, pulmonary toxicity, and/or hemorrhagic cystitis

Dosage Forms Excipient information presented when available (limited, particularly for generics); consult specific product labeling.

Solution, Intravenous:

Generic: 1 g/20 mL (20 mL); 3 g/60 mL (60 mL)

Solution, Intravenous [preservative free]:

Generic: 1 g/20 mL (20 mL); 3 g/60 mL (60 mL)

Solution Reconstituted, Intravenous:

Ifex: 1 g (1 ea); 3 g (1 ea)

Generic: 1 g (1 ea); 3 g (1 ea)

◆ Ifosfamide for Injection (Can) *see* Ifosfamide *on page 913*

◆ IG *see* Immune Globulin *on page 927*

◆ IgG4-Kappa Monoclonal Antibody *see* Natalizumab *on page 1261*

◆ IGIM *see* Immune Globulin *on page 927*

- IGIV *see* Immune Globulin *on page 927*
- IGIVnex (Can) *see* Immune Globulin *on page 927*
- IGSC *see* Immune Globulin *on page 927*
- IIV *see* Influenza Virus Vaccine (Inactivated) *on page 945*
- IIV3 *see* Influenza Virus Vaccine (Inactivated) *on page 945*
- IIV4 *see* Influenza Virus Vaccine (Inactivated) *on page 945*
- IL-1Ra *see* Anakinra *on page 127*
- IL-2 *see* Aldesleukin *on page 60*
- IL-11 *see* Oprelvekin *on page 1339*
- Ilaris *see* Canakinumab *on page 293*
- Ilevro *see* Nepafenac *on page 1269*

Iloperidone (eye loe PER i done)

Brand Names: US Fanapt; Fanapt Titration Pack
Pharmacologic Category Second Generation (Atypical) Antipsychotic
Use Schizophrenia: Treatment of adults with schizophrenia
Pregnancy Considerations Adverse events were observed in animal reproduction studies. Antipsychotic use during the third trimester of pregnancy has a risk for abnormal muscle movements (extrapyramidal symptoms [EPS]) and/or withdrawal symptoms in newborns following delivery. Symptoms in the newborn may include agitation, feeding disorder, hypertonia, hypotonia, respiratory distress, somnolence, and tremor; these effects may be self-limiting or require hospitalization. Iloperidone may cause hyperprolactinemia, which may decrease reproductive function in both males and females.

The ACOG recommends that therapy during pregnancy be individualized; treatment with psychiatric medications during pregnancy should incorporate the clinical expertise of the mental health clinician, obstetrician, primary healthcare provider, and pediatrician. Safety data related to atypical antipsychotics during pregnancy is limited and routine use is not recommended. However, if a woman is inadvertently exposed to an atypical antipsychotic while pregnant, continuing therapy may be preferable to switching to a typical antipsychotic that the fetus has not yet been exposed to; consider risk:benefit (ACOG, 2008).

Healthcare providers are encouraged to enroll women 18 to 45 years of age exposed to iloperidone during pregnancy in the Atypical Antipsychotics Pregnancy Registry (1-866-961-2388 or http://www.womensmentalhealth.org/pregnancyregistry).
Breast-Feeding Considerations It is not known if iloperidone is excreted into breast milk. Breast-feeding is not recommended by the manufacturer.
Contraindications Hypersensitivity to iloperidone or any component of the formulation
Warnings/Precautions [U.S. Boxed Warning]: Elderly patients with dementia-related psychosis treated with antipsychotics are at an increased risk of death compared to placebo. Most deaths appeared to be either cardiovascular (eg, heart failure, sudden death) or infectious (eg, pneumonia) in nature. In addition, an increased incidence of cerebrovascular effects (eg, transient ischemic attack, cerebrovascular accidents) has been reported in studies of placebo-controlled trials of antipsychotics in elderly patients with dementia-related psychosis. Iloperidone is not approved for the treatment of dementia-related psychosis.

May cause CNS depression, which may impair physical or mental abilities; patients must be cautioned about performing tasks that require mental alertness (eg, operating machinery or driving). Caution in patients with predisposition to seizures. Use is not recommended in patients with hepatic impairment. Esophageal dysmotility and aspiration have been associated with antipsychotic use; use with caution in patients at risk of aspiration pneumonia (ie, Alzheimer's disease). Use is associated with increased prolactin levels; clinical significance of hyperprolactinemia in patients with breast cancer or other prolactin-dependent tumors is unknown. May alter temperature regulation. Leukopenia, neutropenia, and agranulocytosis (sometimes fatal) have been reported in clinical trials and postmarketing reports; presence of risk factors (eg, preexisting low WBC or history of drug-induced leuko-/neutropenia) should prompt periodic blood count assessment and discontinuation at first signs of blood dyscrasias.

May alter cardiac conduction and prolong the QTc interval; life-threatening arrhythmias have occurred with therapeutic doses of antipsychotics. Risks may be increased by conditions or concomitant medications which cause bradycardia, hypokalemia, and/or hypomagnesemia. Avoid use in combination with QTc-prolonging drugs and in patients with congenital long QT syndrome, history of cardiac arrhythmia, recent MI, or uncompensated heart failure. Discontinue treatment in patients found to have persistent QTc intervals >500 msec. Further cardiac evaluation is warranted in patients with symptoms of dizziness, palpitations, or syncope. May cause orthostatic hypotension; use with caution in patients at risk of this effect (eg, concurrent medication use which may predispose to hypotension/bradycardia or presence of hypovolemia) or in those who would not tolerate transient hypotensive episodes. Use with caution in patients with cardiovascular diseases (eg, heart failure, history of myocardial infarction or ischemia, cerebrovascular disease, conduction abnormalities).

May cause anticholinergic effects (confusion, agitation, constipation, xerostomia, blurred vision, urinary retention); therefore, use with caution in patients with decreased gastrointestinal motility, urinary retention, BPH, xerostomia, or visual problems (including narrow-angle glaucoma). May cause extrapyramidal symptoms (EPS), including pseudoparkinsonism, acute dystonic reactions, akathisia, and tardive dyskinesia. Risk of dystonia (and probably other EPS) may be greater with increased doses, use of conventional antipsychotics, males, and younger patients. Risk of neuroleptic malignant syndrome (NMS) may be increased in patients with Parkinson's disease or Lewy body dementia. May cause hyperglycemia; in some cases may be extreme and associated with ketoacidosis, hyperosmolar coma, or death. Use with caution in patients with diabetes or other disorders of glucose regulation; monitor for worsening of glucose control. Dyslipidemia has been reported with atypical antipsychotics; risk profile may differ between agents. In clinical trials, changes in triglyceride and total cholesterol levels observed with iloperidone were similar to those observed with placebo or were clinically insignificant. Small reductions in cholesterol and triglycerides have been observed in longer term iloperidone trials.

Significant weight gain has been observed with antipsychotic therapy; incidence varies with product. Monitor waist circumference and BMI. Rare cases of priapism have been reported.

Use in elderly patients with dementia is associated with an increased risk of mortality and cerebrovascular accidents; avoid antipsychotic use for behavioral problems associated with dementia unless alternative nonpharmacologic therapies have failed and patient may harm self or others. In addition, use may cause or exacerbate syndrome of inappropriate antidiuretic hormone secretion or hyponatremia; monitor sodium closely with initiation or dosage adjustments in older adults (Beers Criteria).

Potentially significant interactions may exist, requiring dose or frequency adjustment, additional monitoring, and/or selection of alternative therapy. The possibility of a suicide attempt is inherent in psychotic illness; use caution in high-risk patients during initiation of therapy. Prescriptions should be written for the smallest quantity consistent with good patient care. Continued use for >6 weeks has not been evaluated.
Adverse Reactions
>10%:
Cardiovascular: Tachycardia (3% to 12%; dose related)
Central nervous system: Dizziness (10% to 20%; dose related), somnolence (9% to 15%)
1% to 10%:
Cardiovascular: Orthostatic hypotension (3% to 5%), hypotension (<1% to 3%; dose related), palpitations (≥1%)
Central nervous system: Fatigue (4% to 6%), extrapyramidal symptoms (4% to 5%), tremor (3%), lethargy (1% to 3%), akathisia (2%), aggression (≥1%), delusion (≥1%), restlessness (≥1%)
Dermatologic: Rash (2% to 3%)
Gastrointestinal: Nausea (≤10%), xerostomia (8% to 10%), weight gain (1% to 9%; dose related), diarrhea (5% to 7%), abdominal discomfort (≤3%; dose related), weight loss (≥1%)
Genitourinary: Ejaculation failure (2%), erectile dysfunction (≥1%), urinary incontinence (≥1%)
Neuromuscular & skeletal: Arthralgia (3%), stiffness (1% to 3%; dose related), dyskinesia (<2%), muscle spasm (≥1%), myalgia (≥1%)
Ocular: Blurred vision (≤3%), conjunctivitis (≥1%)
Respiratory: Nasal congestion (5% to 8%), nasopharyngitis (≤4%), upper respiratory tract infection (2% to 3%), dyspnea (2%)

◀ <1% (Limited to important or life-threatening): Acute renal failure, amenorrhea, amnesia, anemia, anorgasmia, aphthous stomatitis, appetite increased, arrhythmia, asthma, AV block (first degree), blepharitis, bradykinesia, breast pain, bulimia nervosa, cataract, catatonia, cholelithiasis, confusion, dehydration, delirium, difficulty walking, dry eye, duodenal ulcer, dystonia, dysuria, edema, enuresis, epistaxis, esophageal reflux, eyelid edema, eye swelling, fecal incontinence, fluid retention, gastric acid secretion increased, gastritis, gynecomastia, heart failure, hematocrit/hemoglobin decreased, hiatal hernia, hostility, hyperemia, hyperthermia, hypokalemia, hypothyroidism, impulse control disorder, lenticular opacities, leukopenia, libido decreased, major depression, mania, menorrhagia, menstrual irregularities, metrorrhagia, mood swings, mouth ulceration, nasal dryness, nephrolithiasis, neutrophils increased, nystagmus, obsessive compulsive disorder, panic attack, paraesthesia, paranoia, parkinsonism, pollakiuria, polydipsia psychogenic, postmenopausal hemorrhage, prostatitis, pruritus, psychomotor hyperactivity, QTc interval prolongation, restless leg syndrome, retrograde ejaculation, rhinorrhea, salivation, sinus congestion, sleep apnea syndrome, stomatitis, testicular pain, thirst, tinnitus, torticollis, urinary retention, urticaria, vertigo

Drug Interactions
Metabolism/Transport Effects Substrate of CYP2D6 (major), CYP3A4 (minor); **Note:** Assignment of Major/Minor substrate status based on clinically relevant drug interaction potential; **Inhibits** CYP3A4 (weak)

Avoid Concomitant Use
Avoid concomitant use of Iloperidone with any of the following: Amisulpride; Azelastine (Nasal); Highest Risk QTc-Prolonging Agents; Ivabradine; Metoclopramide; Mifepristone; Moderate Risk QTc-Prolonging Agents; Orphenadrine; Paraldehyde; Pimozide; Sulpiride; Thalidomide

Increased Effect/Toxicity
Iloperidone may increase the levels/effects of: Alcohol (Ethyl); Amisulpride; Azelastine (Nasal); CNS Depressants; Flibanserin; Highest Risk QTc-Prolonging Agents; Hydrocodone; Lomitapide; Methotrimeprazine; Methylphenidate; Metyrosine; NiMODipine; Orphenadrine; Paraldehyde; Pimozide; Selective Serotonin Reuptake Inhibitors; Serotonin Modulators; Sulpiride; Suvorexant; Thalidomide; Zolpidem

The levels/effects of Iloperidone may be increased by: Abiraterone Acetate; Acetylcholinesterase Inhibitors (Central); Blood Pressure Lowering Agents; Brimonidine (Topical); Cannabis; CYP2D6 Inhibitors (Moderate); CYP2D6 Inhibitors (Strong); CYP3A4 Inhibitors (Strong); Doxylamine; Dronabinol; Ivabradine; Kava Kava; Magnesium Sulfate; Methotrimeprazine; Methylphenidate; Metoclopramide; Metyrosine; Mifepristone; Minocycline; Moderate Risk QTc-Prolonging Agents; Nabilone; Peginterferon Alfa-2b; Perampanel; QTc-Prolonging Agents (Indeterminate Risk and Risk Modifying); Rufinamide; Serotonin Modulators; Sodium Oxybate; Tapentadol; Tetrahydrocannabinol

Decreased Effect
Iloperidone may decrease the levels/effects of: Amphetamines; Antidiabetic Agents; Anti-Parkinson's Agents (Dopamine Agonist); Quinagolide

The levels/effects of Iloperidone may be decreased by: CYP2D6 Inhibitors (Strong); Peginterferon Alfa-2b

Storage/Stability Store at 25°C (77°F); excursions permitted to 15°C to 30°C (59°F to 86°F). Protect from light and moisture.

Mechanism of Action Iloperidone is a piperidinyl-benzisoxazole atypical antipsychotic with mixed $D_2/5-HT_2$ antagonist activity. It exhibits high affinity for $5-HT_{2A}$, D_2, and D_3 receptors, low to moderate affinity for D_1, D_4, H_1, $5-HT_{1A}$, $5-HT_6$, $5-HT_7$, and $NE_{\alpha1}$ receptors, and no affinity for muscarinic receptors. The addition of serotonin antagonism to dopamine antagonism (classic neuroleptic mechanism) is thought to improve negative symptoms of psychoses and reduce the incidence of extrapyramidal side effects. Iloperidone's low affinity for histamine H_1 receptors may decrease the risk for weight gain and somnolence while its affinity for $NE_{\alpha1/\alpha2C}$ may provide antidepressant and anxiolytic activity and improved cognitive function.

Pharmacodynamics/Kinetics
Absorption: Well absorbed

Distribution: V_d: 1340 to 2800 L

Protein binding: ~97% iloperidone; ~92% active metabolites (P88 and P95)

Metabolism: Hepatic via carbonyl reduction, hydroxylation (CYP2D6) and O-demethylation (CYP3A4); forms active metabolites (P88 and P95)

Bioavailability: Oral: Tablet (relative to solution): 96%

Half-life elimination:
Extensive metabolizers: Iloperidone: 18 hours; P88: 26 hours; P95: 23 hours
Poor metabolizers: Iloperidone: 33 hours; P88: 37 hours; P95: 31 hours

Time to peak, plasma: 2 to 4 hours

Excretion: Urine (58% extensive metabolizers, 45% poor metabolizers); feces (20% extensive metabolizers, 22% poor metabolizers)

Dosing
Adult & Geriatric Schizophrenia: Oral: Initial: 1 mg twice daily; titrate to the recommended dosage range with dosage adjustments not to exceed 2 mg twice daily (4 mg daily) every 24 hours; recommended dosage range: 6 to 12 mg twice daily (maximum: 24 mg daily)
> **Note:** Titrate dose to effect (to avoid orthostatic hypotensive effects); treatment >6 weeks has not been evaluated; when reinitiating treatment after discontinuation (>3 days), the initial titration schedule should be followed.

Dosage adjustment in patients receiving strong CYP2D6 inhibitors (eg, paroxetine, fluoxetine, quinidine): Decrease iloperidone dose by 50%; when the CYP2D6 inhibitor is discontinued, return to previous dose.

Dosage adjustment in patients receiving strong CYP3A4 inhibitors (eg, ketoconazole, clarithromycin): Decrease iloperidone dose by 50%; when the CYP3A4 inhibitor is discontinued, return to previous dose.

Dosage adjustment in poor metabolizers of CYP2D6: Decrease iloperidone dose by 50%.

Renal Impairment There are no dosage adjustments provided in manufacturer's labeling; however, pharmacokinetics of iloperidone do not appear to be altered by renal impairment due to extensive hepatic metabolism.

Hepatic Impairment
Mild impairment: No dosage adjustment necessary.

Moderate impairment: There are no dosage adjustments provided in the manufacturer's labeling; use with caution.

Severe hepatic impairment: Use is not recommended.

Administration Administer with or without food.

Monitoring Parameters Mental status; vital signs (as clinically indicated); blood pressure (baseline; repeat 3 months after antipsychotic initiation, then yearly); ECG (as clinically indicated); weight, height, BMI, waist circumference (baseline; repeat at 4, 8, and 12 weeks after initiating or changing therapy, then quarterly; consider switching to a different antipsychotic for a weight gain ≥5% of initial weight); CBC (as clinically indicated; monitor frequently during the first few months of therapy in patients with preexisting low WBC or history of drug-induced leukopenia/neutropenia); electrolytes (annually and as clinically indicated; perform baseline serum potassium and magnesium with periodic monitoring in patients at risk for significant electrolyte disturbances); liver function (annually and as clinically indicated); personal and family history of obesity, diabetes, dyslipidemia, hypertension, or cardiovascular disease (baseline; repeat annually); fasting plasma glucose level/HbA$_{1c}$ (baseline; repeat 3 months after starting antipsychotic, then yearly); fasting lipid panel (baseline; repeat 3 months after initiation of antipsychotic; if LDL level is normal, repeat at 2- to 5-year intervals or more frequently if clinical indicated); changes in menstruation, libido, development of galactorrhea, erectile and ejaculatory function (at each visit for the first 12 weeks after the antipsychotic is initiated or until the dose is stable, then yearly); abnormal involuntary movements or parkinsonian signs (baseline; repeat weekly until dose stabilized for at least 2 weeks after introduction and for 2 weeks after any significant dose increase); tardive dyskinesia (every 12 months; high-risk patients every 6 months); ocular examination (yearly in patients >40 years; every 2 years in younger patients) (ADA, 2004; Lehman, 2004; Marder, 2004).

Dosage Forms Excipient information presented when available (limited, particularly for generics); consult specific product labeling.
Tablet, Oral:
Fanapt: 1 mg, 2 mg, 4 mg, 6 mg, 8 mg, 10 mg, 12 mg
Fanapt Titration Pack: 1 mg (2s), 2 mg (2s), 4 mg (2s), and 6 mg (2s)

Iloprost (EYE loe prost)

Brand Names: US Ventavis
Index Terms Iloprost Tromethamine; Prostacyclin PGI_2
Pharmacologic Category Prostacyclin; Prostaglandin; Vasodilator

Use Pulmonary arterial hypertension: Treatment of pulmonary arterial hypertension (World Health Organization [WHO] group I) in patients with New York Heart Association (NYHA) class III or IV symptoms to improve exercise tolerance, symptoms, and diminish clinical deterioration.

Dosing

Adult & Geriatric Pulmonary arterial hypertension (PAH): Inhalation: Initial: 2.5 mcg/dose; if tolerated, increase to 5 mcg/dose. Administer 6-9 times daily (dosing at intervals ≥2 hours while awake according to individual need and tolerability). Maintenance dose: 2.5-5 mcg/dose; maximum daily dose: 45 mcg (ie, 5 mcg/dose 9 times daily)

Renal Impairment Inhaled iloprost has not been studied in renal impairment; however, according to the manufacturer, no adjustment is required in patients with renal impairment who are not on dialysis (the effect of dialysis on iloprost is unknown).

Hepatic Impairment Child-Pugh class B or C: Consider increasing dosing interval (eg, every 3-4 hours) based on response at the end of the dose interval.

Additional Information Complete prescribing information should be consulted for additional detail.

Dosage Forms Excipient information presented when available (limited, particularly for generics); consult specific product labeling.

Solution, Inhalation [preservative free]:
Ventavis: 10 mcg/mL (1 mL); 20 mcg/mL (1 mL) [contains alcohol, usp, tromethamine]

◆ **Iloprost Tromethamine** see Iloprost on page 918
◆ **Ilotycin** see Erythromycin (Ophthalmic) on page 672

Imatinib (eye MAT eh nib)

Brand Names: US Gleevec
Brand Names: Canada ACT-Imatinib; Apo-Imatinib; Gleevec; Teva-Imatinib
Index Terms CGP-57148B; Glivec; Imatinib Mesylate; STI-571
Pharmacologic Category Antineoplastic Agent, BCR-ABL Tyrosine Kinase Inhibitor; Antineoplastic Agent, Tyrosine Kinase Inhibitor

Use

Acute lymphoblastic leukemia: Treatment of relapsed or refractory Philadelphia chromosome–positive (Ph+) acute lymphoblastic leukemia (ALL) in adults
Treatment of newly diagnosed Ph+ ALL in children (in combination with chemotherapy)

Aggressive systemic mastocytosis: Treatment of aggressive systemic mastocytosis without D816V c-Kit mutation (or c-Kit mutational status unknown) in adults

Chronic myeloid leukemia: Treatment of Ph+ chronic myeloid leukemia (CML) in chronic phase (newly diagnosed) in adults and children
Treatment of Ph+ CML in blast crisis, accelerated phase, or chronic phase after failure of interferon-alfa therapy

Dermatofibrosarcoma protuberans: Treatment of unresectable, recurrent, and/or metastatic dermatofibrosarcoma protuberans (DFSP) in adults

Gastrointestinal stromal tumors: Treatment of Kit (CD117)-positive unresectable and/or metastatic malignant gastrointestinal stromal tumors (GIST)
Adjuvant treatment of Kit (CD117)-positive GIST following complete gross resection

Hypereosinophilic syndrome and/or chronic eosinophilic leukemia: Treatment of hypereosinophilic syndrome (HES) and/or chronic eosinophilic leukemia (CEL) in adult patients who have the FIP1L1-platelet-derived growth factor (PDGF) receptor alpha fusion kinase (mutational analysis or fluorescent in situ hybridization [FISH] demonstration of CHIC2 allele deletion) and for patients with HES and/or CEL who are FIP1L1-PDGF receptor alpha fusion kinase negative or unknown

Myelodysplastic/Myeloproliferative diseases: Treatment of myelodysplastic syndrome/myeloproliferative diseases (MDS/MPD) associated with PDGF receptor gene rearrangements in adults

Canadian labeling (not an approved indication in the US): Treatment of newly diagnosed Ph+ ALL in adults as a single agent for induction therapy

Pregnancy Considerations Adverse events have been observed in animal reproduction studies. Women of childbearing potential are advised not to become pregnant (female patients and female partners of male patients); highly effective contraception is recommended. The Canadian labeling recommends women of childbearing potential have a negative pregnancy test (urine or serum) with a sensitivity of at least 25 milliunits/mL within 1 week prior to therapy initiation. Case reports of pregnancies while on therapy (both males and females) include reports of spontaneous abortion, minor abnormalities (hypospadias, pyloric stenosis, and small intestine rotation) at or shortly after birth, and other congenital abnormalities including skeletal malformations, hypoplastic lungs, exomphalos, kidney abnormalities, hydrocephalus, cerebellar hypoplasia, and cardiac defects.

Retrospective case reports of women with CML in complete hematologic response (CHR) with cytogenic response (partial or complete) who interrupted imatinib therapy due to pregnancy, demonstrated a loss of response in some patients while off treatment. At 18 months after treatment reinitiation following delivery, CHR was again achieved in all patients and cytogenic response was achieved in some patients. Cytogenetic response rates may not be at as high as compared to patients with 18 months of uninterrupted therapy (Ault, 2006; Pye, 2008).

Breast-Feeding Considerations Imatinib and its active metabolite are found in human breast milk; the milk/plasma ratio is 0.5 for imatinib and 0.9 for the active metabolite. Based on body weight, up to 10% of a therapeutic maternal dose could potentially be received by a breast-fed infant. Due to the potential for serious adverse reactions in the breast-feeding infant, the manufacturer recommends a decision be made to discontinue breast-feeding or to discontinue the drug, taking into account the importance of treatment to the mother.

Contraindications

There are no contraindications listed in the manufacturer's US labeling.
Canadian labeling: Hypersensitivity to imatinib or any component of the formulation

Warnings/Precautions Hazardous agent - use appropriate precautions for handling and disposal (NIOSH 2014 [group 1]). Often associated with fluid retention, weight gain, and edema (risk increases with higher doses and age >65 years); occasionally serious and may lead to significant complications, including pleural effusion, pericardial effusion, pulmonary edema, and ascites. Monitor regularly for rapid weight gain or other signs/symptoms of fluid retention. Use with caution in patients where fluid accumulation may be poorly tolerated, such as in cardiovascular disease (heart failure [HF] or hypertension) and pulmonary disease. Severe HF and left ventricular dysfunction (LVD) have been reported occasionally, usually in patients with comorbidities and/or risk factors; carefully monitor patients with preexisting cardiac disease or risk factors for HF or history of renal failure. With initiation of imatinib treatment, cardiogenic shock and/or LVD have been reported in patients with hypereosinophilic syndrome and cardiac involvement (reversible with systemic steroids, circulatory support and temporary cessation of imatinib). Patients with high eosinophil levels and an abnormal echocardiogram or abnormal serum troponin level may benefit from prophylactic systemic steroids (for 1 to 2 weeks) with the initiation of imatinib.

Severe bullous dermatologic reactions (including erythema multiforme and Stevens-Johnson syndrome) have been reported; recurrence has been described with rechallenge. Case reports of successful resumption at a lower dose (with corticosteroids and/or antihistamine) have been described; however, some patients may experience recurrent reactions. Drug reaction with eosinophilia and systemic symptoms (DRESS) has been reported; if DRESS occurs, interrupt therapy and consider permanent discontinuation.

Hepatotoxicity may occur (may be severe); fatal hepatic failure and severe hepatic injury requiring liver transplantation have been reported with both short- and long-term use; monitor liver function prior to initiation and monthly or as needed thereafter; therapy interruption or dose reduction may be necessary. Transaminase and bilirubin elevations, and acute liver failure have been observed with imatinib in combination with chemotherapy. Use with caution in patients with preexisting hepatic impairment; dosage adjustment recommended in patients with severe impairment. Use with caution in renal impairment; dosage adjustment recommended for moderate and severe impairment. Tumor lysis syndrome (TLS), including fatalities, has been reported in patients with acute lymphoblastic leukemia (ALL), chronic myeloid leukemia (CML) eosinophilic leukemias, and gastrointestinal stromal tumors (GIST); risk for TLS is higher in patients with a high tumor burden or high proliferation rate; monitor closely; correct clinically significant dehydration and treat high uric acid levels prior to initiation of imatinib.

Imatinib is associated with a moderate emetic potential; antiemetics may be recommended to prevent nausea and vomiting (Dupuis, 2011; Roila, 2010). May cause GI irritation, severe hemorrhage (grades 3 and 4; including GI

hemorrhage and/or tumor hemorrhage; hemorrhage incidence is higher in patients with GIST [GI tumors may have been hemorrhage source; gastric antral vascular ectasia has also been reported]), or hematologic toxicity (anemia, neutropenia, and thrombocytopenia; usually occurring within the first several months of treatment). Monitor blood counts weekly for the first month, biweekly for the second month, and as clinically necessary thereafter; median duration of neutropenia is 2 to 3 weeks; median duration of thrombocytopenia is 3 to 4 weeks. In CML, cytopenias are more common in accelerated or blast phase than in chronic phase. Hypothyroidism has been reported in patients who were receiving thyroid hormone replacement therapy prior to the initiation of imatinib; monitor thyroid function; the average onset for imatinib-induced hypothyroidism is 2 weeks; consider doubling levothyroxine doses upon initiation of imatinib (Hamnvik, 2011). Potentially significant drug-drug interactions may exist, requiring dose or frequency adjustment, additional monitoring, and/or selection of alternative therapy. Imatinib exposure may be reduced in patients who have had gastric surgery (eg, bypass, major gastrectomy, or resection); monitor imatinib trough concentrations (Liu, 2011; Pavlovsky, 2009; Yoo, 2010). Growth retardation has been reported in children receiving imatinib for the treatment of CML; generally where treatment was initiated in prepubertal children; growth velocity was usually restored as pubertal age was reached (Shima, 2011); monitor growth closely. The incidence of edema was increased with age older than 65 years in CML and GIST studies. Reports of accidents have been received but it is unclear if imatinib has been the direct cause in any case; advise patients regarding side effects such as dizziness, blurred vision, or somnolence; use caution when driving/operating motor vehicles and heavy machinery.

Adverse Reactions Adverse reactions listed as a composite of data across many trials, except where noted for a specific indication. Frequency not always defined.

>10%:

Cardiovascular: Edema (11% to 86%; grades 3/4: 3% to 13%; includes aggravated edema, anasarca, ascites, pericardial effusion, peripheral edema, pulmonary edema, and superficial edema), facial edema (≤17%), hypotension (Ph+ ALL [pediatric] grades 3/4: 11%), chest pain (7% to 11%)

Central nervous system: Fatigue (20% to 75%), pain (≤47%), headache (8% to 37%), dizziness (5% to 19%), insomnia (9% to 15%), depression (3% to 15%), taste disorder (≤13%), rigors (10% to 12%), anxiety (8% to 12%), paresthesia (≤12%), chills (≤11%)

Dermatologic: Skin rash (9% to 50%; grades 3/4: 1% to 9%), dermatitis (GIST ≤39%), pruritus (7% to 26%), night sweats (CML 13% to 17%), alopecia (7% to 15%), diaphoresis (GIST ≤13%)

Endocrine & metabolic: Increased lactate dehydrogenase (≤60%), hypokalemia (6% to 13%; Ph+ ALL [pediatric] grades 3/4: 34%), weight gain (≤32%), decreased serum albumin (≤21%; grades 3/4: ≤4%)

Gastrointestinal: Nausea (41% to 73%; Ph+ ALL [pediatric] grades 3/4: 16%), diarrhea (25% to 59%; Ph+ ALL [pediatric] grades 3/4: 9%), vomiting (11% to 58%), abdominal pain (3% to 57%), anorexia (≤36%), dyspepsia (11% to 27%), flatulence (≤25%), abdominal distension (≤19%), constipation (8% to 16%), stomatitis (≤16%)

Hematologic & oncologic: Neutropenia (grades 3/4: 8% to 64%), thrombocytopenia (grades 3/4: 1% to 63%), anemia (grades 3/4: 3% to 53%), hemorrhage (3% to 53%; grades 3/4: ≤19%), leukopenia (GIST 5% to 47%; grades 3/4: 2%), hypoproteinemia (≤32%)

Hepatic: Increased serum transaminases (Ph+ ALL [pediatric] grades 3/4: 57%), increased serum AST (≤38%; grades 3/4: ≤6%), increased serum ALT (≤34%; grades 3/4: ≤8%), increased alkaline phosphatase (≤17%; grades 3/4: ≤6%), increased serum bilirubin (≤13%; grades 3/4: ≤4%)

Infection: Infection (Ph+ ALL [pediatric] grades 3/4: 53%; GIST ≤28%), influenza (Ph+ CML ≤14%)

Neuromuscular & skeletal: Muscle cramps (16% to 62%), musculoskeletal pain (children 21%; adults 38% to 49%), arthralgia (11% to 40%), myalgia (9% to 32%), weakness (≤21%), back pain (≤17%), limb pain (≤16%), ostealgia (≤11%)

Ophthalmic: Periorbital edema (15% to 74%), increased lacrimation (DFSP 25%; GIST ≤18%), eyelid edema (Ph+ CML 19%), blurred vision (≤11%)

Renal: Increased serum creatinine (≤44%; grades 3/4: ≤8%)

Respiratory: Nasopharyngitis (1% to 31%), cough (11% to 27%), upper respiratory tract infection (3% to 21%), dyspnea (≤21%), pharyngolaryngeal pain (≤18%), rhinitis (DFSP 17%), pharyngitis (CML 10% to 15%), flu-like symptoms (1% to 14%), pneumonia (CML 4% to 13%), sinusitis (4% to 11%)

Miscellaneous: Fever (6% to 41%)

1% to 10%:

Cardiovascular: Pleural effusion (Ph+ ALL [pediatric] grades 3/4: 7%), palpitations (≤5%), hypertension (≤4%), cardiac failure (Ph+ CML 1%; grades 3/4: <1%), flushing

Central nervous system: Cerebral hemorrhage (≤9%), hypoesthesia, peripheral neuropathy

Dermatologic: Skin photosensitivity (4% to 7%), xeroderma (≤7%), erythema, nail disease

Endocrine & metabolic: Hypophosphatemia (10%), hyperglycemia (≤10%), weight loss (≤10%), hypocalcemia (GIST ≤6%; Ph+ CML grades 3/4: <1%), fluid retention (Ph+ CML 3%; pleural effusion, pericardial effusion, ascites, or pulmonary edema 2%), hyperkalemia (1%)

Gastrointestinal: Decreased appetite (10%), gastroenteritis (≤10%), gastrointestinal hemorrhage (1% to 8%), increased serum lipase (CML grades 3/4: 4%), gastritis, gastroesophageal reflux, xerostomia

Hematologic & oncologic: Lymphocytopenia (≤10%; grades 3/4: 1% to 2%), eosinophilia, febrile neutropenia, pancytopenia, purpura

Neuromuscular & skeletal: Joint swelling

Ophthalmic: Conjunctivitis (5% to 8%), conjunctival hemorrhage, dry eyes

Respiratory: Hypoxia (9%), pneumonitis (Ph+ ALL [pediatric] grades 3/4: 8%), oropharyngeal pain (Ph+ CML ≤6%), epistaxis

<1% (Limited to important or life-threatening): Actinic keratosis, acute generalized exanthematous pustulosis, anaphylactic shock, angina pectoris, angioedema, aplastic anemia, arthritis, ascites, atrial fibrillation, avascular necrosis of bones, bullous rash, cardiac arrest, cardiac arrhythmia, cardiac tamponade, cardiogenic shock, cataract, cellulitis, cerebral edema, decreased linear skeletal growth rate (children), diverticulitis, DRESS syndrome, dyschromia, embolism, erythema multiforme, exfoliative dermatitis, fungal infection, gastric ulcer, gastrointestinal obstruction, gastrointestinal perforation, glaucoma, gout, hearing loss, hematemesis, hematoma, hematuria, hemolytic anemia, hepatic failure, hepatic necrosis, hepatitis, hepatotoxicity, herpes simplex infection, herpes zoster, hypercalcemia, hyperkalemia, hypersensitivity angiitis, hyperuricemia, hypomagnesemia, hyponatremia, hypophosphatemia, hypothyroidism, IgA vasculitis, increased intracranial pressure, inflammatory bowel disease, interstitial pneumonitis, interstitial pulmonary disease, intestinal obstruction, left ventricular dysfunction, lichen planus, lower respiratory tract infection, lymphadenopathy, macular edema, melena, memory impairment, migraine, myocardial infarction, myopathy, optic neuritis, osteonecrosis (hip), ovarian cyst (hemorrhagic), palmar-plantar erythrodysesthesia, pancreatitis, papilledema, pericarditis, psoriasis, pulmonary fibrosis, pulmonary hemorrhage, pulmonary hypertension, Raynaud phenomenon, renal failure, respiratory failure, restless leg syndrome, retinal hemorrhage, rhabdomyolysis, ruptured corpus luteal cyst, sciatica, seizure, sepsis, Stevens-Johnson syndrome, subconjunctival hemorrhage, subdural hematoma, Sweet syndrome, syncope, tachycardia, telangiectasia (gastric antral), thrombocythemia, thrombosis, toxic epidermal necrolysis, tumor hemorrhage (GIST), tumor lysis syndrome, urinary tract infection, vitreous hemorrhage

Drug Interactions

Metabolism/Transport Effects Substrate of CYP1A2 (minor), CYP2C19 (minor), CYP2C8 (minor), CYP2C9 (minor), CYP2D6 (minor), CYP3A4 (major), P-glycoprotein; **Note:** Assignment of Major/Minor substrate status based on clinically relevant drug interaction potential; **Inhibits** BCRP, CYP2C9 (weak), CYP2D6 (weak), CYP3A4 (moderate), P-glycoprotein

Avoid Concomitant Use

Avoid concomitant use of Imatinib with any of the following: Aprepitant; BCG (Intravesical); Bosutinib; Cobimetinib; Deferiprone; Dipyrone; Domperidone; Flibanserin; Ibrutinib; Ivabradine; Lomitapide; Naloxegol; Natalizumab; Olaparib; PAZOPanib; Pimecrolimus; Pimozide; Simeprevir; Tacrolimus (Topical); Tofacitinib; Tolvaptan; Trabectedin; Ulipristal; Vaccines (Live)

Increased Effect/Toxicity

Imatinib may increase the levels/effects of: Apixaban; Aprepitant; ARIPiprazole; Avanafil; Bosentan; Bosutinib; Brexpiprazole; Bromocriptine; Budesonide (Systemic); Budesonide (Topical); Cannabis; Cilostazol; CloZAPine;

Cobimetinib; Colchicine; CycloSPORINE (Systemic); CYP3A4 Substrates; Dapoxetine; Deferiprone; Dofetilide; Domperidone; DOXOrubicin (Conventional); Dronabinol; Eletriptan; Eliglustat; Eplerenone; Everolimus; FentaNYL; Fingolimod; Flibanserin; Halofantrine; Hydrocodone; Ibrutinib; Ivabradine; Ivacaftor; Leflunomide; Lomitapide; Lurasidone; Naloxegol; Natalizumab; NiMODipine; Olaparib; OxyCODONE; PAZOPanib; Pimozide; Propafenone; Ranolazine; Salmeterol; Saxagliptin; Simeprevir; Simvastatin; Sonidegib; Suvorexant; Tetrahydrocannabinol; Tofacitinib; Tolvaptan; Topotecan; Trabectedin; Ulipristal; Vaccines (Live); Vilazodone; Vindesine; Warfarin; Zopiclone; Zuclopenthixol

The levels/effects of Imatinib may be increased by: Acetaminophen; CYP3A4 Inhibitors (Moderate); CYP3A4 Inhibitors (Strong); Denosumab; Dipyrone; Lansoprazole; Osimertinib; P-glycoprotein/ABCB1 Inhibitors; Pimecrolimus; Propacetamol; Roflumilast; Tacrolimus (Topical); Trastuzumab

Decreased Effect

Imatinib may decrease the levels/effects of: BCG (Intravesical); Coccidioides immitis Skin Test; Fludarabine; Ifosfamide; Sipuleucel-T; Vaccines (Inactivated); Vaccines (Live)

The levels/effects of Imatinib may be decreased by: Bosentan; CYP3A4 Inducers (Moderate); CYP3A4 Inducers (Strong); Dabrafenib; Deferasirox; Dexamethasone (Systemic); Echinacea; Enzalutamide; Gemfibrozil; Ibuprofen; Mitotane; Osimertinib; P-glycoprotein/ABCB1 Inducers; Rifamycin Derivatives; Siltuximab; St Johns Wort; Tocilizumab

Food Interactions Food may reduce GI irritation. Grapefruit juice may increase imatinib plasma concentration. Management: Take with a meal and a large glass of water. Avoid grapefruit juice. Maintain adequate hydration, unless instructed to restrict fluid intake.

Storage/Stability Store at 25°C (77°F); excursions permitted between 15°C to 30°C (59°F to 86°F). Protect from moisture.

Mechanism of Action Inhibits Bcr-Abl tyrosine kinase, the constitutive abnormal gene product of the Philadelphia chromosome in chronic myeloid leukemia (CML). Inhibition of this enzyme blocks proliferation and induces apoptosis in Bcr-Abl positive cell lines as well as in fresh leukemic cells in Philadelphia chromosome positive CML. Also inhibits tyrosine kinase for platelet-derived growth factor (PDGF), stem cell factor (SCF), c-Kit, and cellular events mediated by PDGF and SCF.

Pharmacodynamics/Kinetics

Absorption: Rapid

Protein binding: Parent drug and metabolite: ~95% to albumin and alpha$_1$-acid glycoprotein

Metabolism: Hepatic via CYP3A4 (minor metabolism via CYP1A2, CYP2D6, CYP2C9, CYP2C19); primary metabolite (active): N-demethylated piperazine derivative (CGP74588); severe hepatic impairment (bilirubin >3 to 10 times ULN) increases AUC by 45% to 55% for imatinib and its active metabolite, respectively

Bioavailability: 98%; may be decreased in patients who have had gastric surgery (eg, bypass, total or partial resection) (Liu, 2011; Pavlovsky, 2009; Yoo, 2010)

Half-life elimination: Adults: Parent drug: ~18 hours; N-desmethyl metabolite: ~40 hours; Children: Parent drug: ~15 hours

Time to peak: 2 to 4 hours

Excretion: Feces (68% primarily as metabolites, 20% as unchanged drug); urine (13% primarily as metabolites, 5% as unchanged drug)

Dosing

Adult & Geriatric Note: Treatment may be continued until disease progression or unacceptable toxicity. The optimal duration of therapy for chronic myeloid leukemia (CML) in complete remission is not yet determined. Discontinuing CML treatment is not recommended unless part of a clinical trial (Baccarani, 2009). Imatinib is associated with a moderate emetic potential; antiemetics may be recommended to prevent nausea and vomiting (Roila, 2010).

Philadelphia chromosome-positive (Ph+) chronic myeloid leukemia (CML): Oral:

Chronic phase: 400 mg once daily; may be increased to 600 mg daily, if tolerated, for disease progression, lack of hematologic response after 3 months, lack of cytogenetic response after 6-12 months, or loss of previous hematologic or cytogenetic response. An increase to 800 mg daily has been used (Cortes, 2010; Hehlmann, 2014).

Canadian labeling: 400 mg once daily; may be increased to 600-800 mg daily

Accelerated phase or blast crisis: 600 mg once daily; may be increased to 800 mg daily (400 mg twice daily), if tolerated, for disease progression, lack of hematologic response after 3 months, lack of cytogenetic response after 6-12 months, or loss of previous hematologic or cytogenetic response

Ph+ acute lymphoblastic leukemia (ALL) (relapsed or refractory): Oral: 600 mg once daily

Gastrointestinal stromal tumors (GIST) (adjuvant treatment following complete resection): Oral: 400 mg once daily; recommended treatment duration: 3 years

GIST (unresectable and/or metastatic malignant): Oral: 400 mg once daily; may be increased up to 800 mg daily (400 mg twice daily), if tolerated, for disease progression. **Note:** Significant improvement (progression-free survival, objective response rate) was demonstrated in patients with KIT exon 9 mutation with 800 mg (versus 400 mg), although overall survival (OS) was not impacted. The higher dose did not demonstrate a difference in time to progression or OS patients with Kit exon 11 mutation or wild-type status (Debiec-Rychter, 2006; Heinrich, 2009).

Canadian labeling: 400-600 mg daily (depending on disease stage/progression); may be increased to 600-800 mg daily

Aggressive systemic mastocytosis (ASM) with eosinophilia: Oral: Initiate at 100 mg once daily; titrate up to a maximum of 400 mg once daily (if tolerated) for insufficient response to lower dose

ASM without D816V c-Kit mutation or c-Kit mutation status unknown: Oral: 400 mg once daily

Dermatofibrosarcoma protuberans (DFSP): Oral: 400 mg twice daily

Hypereosinophilic syndrome (HES) and/or chronic eosinophilic leukemia (CEL): Oral: 400 mg once daily

HES/CEL with FIP1L1-PDGFRα fusion kinase: Oral: Initiate at 100 mg once daily; titrate up to a maximum of 400 mg once daily (if tolerated) if insufficient response to lower dose

Myelodysplastic/myeloproliferative disease (MDS/MPD): Oral: 400 mg once daily

Ph+ ALL (induction, newly diagnosed): *Canadian labeling (not an approved use in the US):* Oral: 600 mg once daily

Chordoma, progressive, advanced, or metastatic expressing PDGFRB and/or PDGFB (off-label use): Oral: 400 mg twice daily (Stacchiotti, 2012)

Desmoid tumors, unresectable and/or progressive (off-label use): Oral: 300 mg twice daily (BSA ≥1.5 m^2), 200 mg twice daily (BSA 1-1.49 m^2), 100 mg twice daily (BSA <1 m^2) (Chugh, 2010) **or** 400 mg once daily; may increase to 400 mg twice daily if progressive disease on 400 mg daily (Penel, 2011)

Melanoma, advanced or metastatic with C-KIT mutation (off-label use): Oral: 400 mg twice daily (Carvajal, 2011)

Stem cell transplant (SCT, off-label use) for CML (in patients who have not failed imatinib therapy prior to transplant): Oral:

Prophylactic use to prevent relapse post SCT: 400 mg daily starting after engraftment for 1 year post transplant (Carpenter, 2007) **or** 300 mg daily starting on day +35 post SCT (increased to 400 mg within 4 weeks) and continued until 12 months post transplant (Olavarria, 2007)

Relapse post SCT: Initial: 400 mg daily; if inferior response after 3 months, dose may be increased to 600-800 mg daily (Hess, 2005) **or** 400-600 mg daily (chronic phase) **or** 600 mg daily (blast or accelerated phase) (DeAngelo, 2004)

Dosage adjustment with concomitant strong CYP3A4 inducers: Avoid concomitant use of strong CYP3A4 inducers (eg, dexamethasone, carbamazepine, phenobarbital, phenytoin, rifabutin, rifampin); if concomitant use cannot be avoided, increase imatinib dose by at least 50% with careful monitoring.

Pediatric Note: Treatment may be continued until disease progression or unacceptable toxicity. The optimal duration of therapy for CML in complete remission is not yet determined. Imatinib is associated with a moderate emetic potential; antiemetics may be recommended to prevent nausea and vomiting (Dupuis, 2011).

Philadelphia chromosome-positive (Ph+) acute lymphoblastic leukemia (ALL) (newly diagnosed): Children ≥1 year and Adolescents: Oral: 340 mg/m^2/day (in combination with chemotherapy); maximum: 600 mg daily

Ph+ chronic myeloid leukemia (CML), chronic phase, newly diagnosed: Children ≥1 year and Adolescents: Oral: 340 mg/m^2/day; maximum: 600 mg daily

Dosage adjustment with concomitant strong CYP3A4 inducers: Avoid concomitant use of strong CYP3A4 inducers (eg, dexamethasone, carbamazepine, phenobarbital, phenytoin, rifabutin, rifampin); if concomitant use cannot be avoided, increase imatinib dose by at least 50% with careful monitoring.

Dosage adjustment for hepatotoxicity: Refer to Dosing: Hepatic Impairment.

Dosage adjustment for hematologic adverse reactions: Refer to Dosing Adjustment for Toxicity.

Dosage adjustment for nonhematologic adverse reactions: Refer to Dosing Adjustment for Toxicity.

Renal Impairment

US labeling:

Mild impairment (CrCl 40-59 mL/minute): Maximum recommended dose: 600 mg.

Moderate impairment (CrCl 20-39 mL/minute): Decrease recommended starting dose by 50%; dose may be increased as tolerated; maximum recommended dose: 400 mg.

Severe impairment (CrCl <20 mL/minute): Use caution; a dose of 100 mg daily has been tolerated in a limited number of patients with severe impairment (Gibbons, 2008).

Canadian labeling:

Mild impairment (CrCl 40-59 mL/minute): Initial dose: 400 mg once daily (minimum effective dose); titrate to efficacy and tolerability.

Moderate impairment (CrCl 20-39 mL/minute): Initial dose: 400 mg once daily (minimum effective dose); titrate to efficacy and tolerability; the use of 800 mg dose is not recommended.

Severe impairment (CrCl <20 mL/minute): Use is not recommended.

Hepatic Impairment

US labeling:

Mild-to-moderate impairment: No dosage adjustment necessary.

Severe impairment: Reduce dose by 25%.

Canadian labeling:

Mild-to-moderate impairment: Initial dose: 400 mg once daily (minimum effective dose).

Severe impairment: Initial dose: 200 mg once daily; may increase up to 300 mg once daily in the absence of severe toxicity; decrease dose with unacceptable toxicity.

Dosage adjustment for hepatotoxicity (during therapy): If elevations of bilirubin >3 times ULN or transaminases >5 times ULN occur, withhold treatment until bilirubin <1.5 times ULN and transaminases <2.5 times ULN. Resume treatment at a reduced dose as follows (**Note:** The decision to resume treatment should take into consideration the initial severity of hepatotoxicity):

Adults:

If current dose 400 mg daily, reduce dose to 300 mg daily

If current dose 600 mg daily, reduce dose to 400 mg daily

If current dose 800 mg daily, reduce dose to 600 mg daily

Children ≥1 year and Adolescents: If current dose 340 mg/m^2/day, reduce dose to 260 mg/m^2/day

Adjustment for Toxicity

Hematologic toxicity:

Chronic phase CML (initial dose 400 mg daily in adults or 340 mg/m^2/day in children); ASM, MDS/MPD, and HES/CEL (initial dose 400 mg daily); or GIST (initial dose 400 mg daily [US labeling] or 400-600 mg daily [Canadian labeling]): If ANC <1 x 10^9/L and/or platelets <50 x 10^9/L: Withhold until ANC ≥1.5 x 10^9/L and platelets ≥75 x 10^9/L; resume treatment at original starting dose. For recurrent neutropenia and/or thrombocytopenia, withhold until recovery, and reinstitute treatment at a reduced dose as follows:

Children ≥1 year and Adolescents: If initial dose 340 mg/m^2/day, reduce dose to 260 mg/m^2/day.

Adults:

If initial dose 400 mg daily, reduce dose to 300 mg daily.

If initial dose 600 mg daily (Canadian labeling; not in US labeling), reduce dose to 400 mg daily.

CML (accelerated phase or blast crisis): Adults (initial dose 600 mg daily): If ANC <0.5 x 10^9/L and/or platelets <10 x 10^9/L, establish whether cytopenia is related to leukemia (bone marrow aspirate or biopsy). If unrelated to leukemia, reduce dose to 400 mg daily. If cytopenia persists for an additional 2 weeks, further reduce dose to 300 mg daily. If cytopenia persists for 4 weeks and is still unrelated to leukemia, withhold treatment until ANC ≥1 x 10^9/L and platelets ≥20 x 10^9/L, then resume treatment at 300 mg daily.

ASM associated with eosinophilia and HES/CEL with FIP1L1-PDGFRα fusion kinase: Adults (starting dose 100 mg daily): If ANC <1 x 10^9/L and/or platelets <50 x 10^9/L: Withhold until ANC ≥1.5 x 10^9/L and platelets ≥75 x 10^9/L; resume treatment at previous dose.

DFSP: Adults (initial dose 800 mg daily): If ANC <1 x 10^9/L and/or platelets <50 x 10^9/L, withhold until ANC ≥1.5 x 10^9/L and platelets ≥75 x 10^9/L; resume treatment at reduced dose of 600 mg daily. For recurrent neutropenia and/or thrombocytopenia, withhold until recovery, and reinstitute treatment with a further dose reduction to 400 mg daily.

Ph+ ALL:

Pediatrics (Schultz, 2009): Hematologic toxicity requiring dosage adjustments was not observed in the study. No major toxicities were observed with imatinib at 340 mg/m^2/day in combination with intensive chemotherapy.

Adults (initial dose 600 mg daily): If ANC <0.5 x 10^9/L and/or platelets <10 x 10^9/L, establish whether cytopenia is related to leukemia (bone marrow aspirate or biopsy). If unrelated to leukemia, reduce dose to 400 mg daily. If cytopenia persists for an additional 2 weeks, further reduce dose to 300 mg daily. If cytopenia persists for 4 weeks and is still unrelated to leukemia, withhold treatment until ANC ≥1 x 10^9/L and platelets ≥20 x 10^9/L, then resume treatment at 300 mg daily.

Nonhematologic toxicity (eg, severe edema): Withhold treatment until toxicity resolves; may resume if appropriate (depending on initial severity of adverse event).

Dietary Considerations Avoid grapefruit juice.

Administration Imatinib is associated with a moderate emetic potential; antiemetics may be recommended to prevent nausea and vomiting (Dupuis, 2011; Roila, 2010).

Should be administered with a meal and a large glass of water. It is not recommended to crush or chew tablets due to bitter taste. Tablets may be dispersed in water or apple juice (using ~50 mL for 100 mg tablet, ~200 mL for 400 mg tablet); stir until dissolved and administer immediately. In adults, doses ≤600 mg may be given once daily; 800 mg dose should be administered as 400 mg twice daily. Dosing in children may be once or twice daily for chronic myeloid leukemia (CML) and once daily for Philadelphia chromosome–positive (Ph+) acute lymphoblastic leukemia (ALL). For daily dosing ≥800 mg, the 400 mg tablets should be used in order to reduce iron exposure.

Hazardous agent; use appropriate precautions for handling and disposal (NIOSH 2014 [group 1]). Avoid skin or mucous membrane contact with crushed tablets; if contact occurs, wash thoroughly. Avoid exposure to crushed tablets. If it is necessary to manipulate the tablets (eg, to prepare an oral solution), it is recommended to double glove, wear a protective gown, and prepare in a controlled device (NIOSH, 2014).

Monitoring Parameters CBC (weekly for first month, biweekly for second month, then periodically thereafter), liver function tests (at baseline and monthly or as clinically indicated; more frequently [at least weekly] in patients with moderate-to-severe hepatic impairment [Ramanathan, 2008]), renal function, serum electrolytes (including calcium, phosphorus, potassium and sodium levels); bone marrow cytogenetics (in CML; at 6-, 12-, and 18 months), pregnancy test (Canadian labeling recommends women of reproductive potential have a negative test [urine or serum] with a sensitivity of at least 25 milliunits/mL within 1 week prior to therapy initiation); fatigue, weight, and edema/fluid status; consider echocardiogram and serum troponin levels in patients with HES/CEL, and in patients with MDS/MPD or ASM with high eosinophil levels; in pediatric patients, also monitor serum glucose, albumin, and growth

Gastric surgery (eg, bypass, major gastrectomy, or resection) patients: Monitor imatinib trough concentrations (Liu, 2011; Pavlovsky, 2009; Yoo, 2010)

Thyroid function testing (Hamnvik, 2011):

Preexisting levothyroxine therapy: Obtain baseline TSH levels, then monitor every 4 weeks until levels and levothyroxine dose are stable, then monitor every 2 months

Without preexisting thyroid hormone replacement: TSH at baseline, then every 4 weeks for 4 months, then every 2-3 months

Monitor for signs/symptoms of CHF in patients with at risk for cardiac failure or patients with preexisting cardiac disease. In Canada, a baseline evaluation of left ventricular ejection fraction is recommended prior to initiation of imatinib therapy in all patients with known underlying heart disease or in elderly patients. Monitor for signs/symptoms

of gastrointestinal irritation or perforation and dermatologic toxicities.

Dosage Forms Excipient information presented when available (limited, particularly for generics); consult specific product labeling.

Tablet, Oral:

Gleevec: 100 mg, 400 mg [scored]

Extemporaneous Preparations Hazardous agent: Use appropriate precautions for handling and disposal (NIOSH 2014 [group 1]). When manipulating tablets, NIOSH recommends double gloving, a protective gown, and preparation in a controlled device; if not prepared in a controlled device, respiratory and eye protection as well as ventilated engineering controls are recommended (NIOSH, 2014).

An oral suspension may be prepared by placing tablets (whole, do not crush) in a glass of water or apple juice. Use ~50 mL for 100 mg tablet, or ~200 mL for 400 mg tablet. Stir until tablets are disintegrated, then administer immediately. To ensure the full dose is administered, rinse the glass and administer residue.

Gleevec (imatinib) [prescribing information]. East Hanover, NJ: Novartis Pharmaceuticals; January 2015.

◆ Imatinib Mesylate see Imatinib on page 919
◆ Imbruvica see Ibrutinib on page 902
◆ IMC-11F8 see Necitumumab on page 1263
◆ IMC-1121B see Ramucirumab on page 1554
◆ IMC-C225 see Cetuximab on page 366
◆ Imdur see Isosorbide Mononitrate on page 995
◆ Imdur [DSC] see Isosorbide Mononitrate on page 995
◆ Imferon see Iron Dextran Complex on page 986
◆ IMI 30 see IDArubicin on page 910
◆ IMid-1 see Lenalidomide on page 1042
◆ Imidazole Carboxamide see Dacarbazine on page 479
◆ Imidazole Carboxamide Dimethyltriazene see Dacarbazine on page 479
◆ IMIG see Immune Globulin on page 927

Imiglucerase (i mi GLOO ser ace)

Brand Names: US Cerezyme
Brand Names: Canada Cerezyme
Pharmacologic Category Enzyme
Use Gaucher disease:

U.S. labeling: Long-term enzyme replacement therapy for patients with type 1 Gaucher disease that results in at least one of the following: anemia, bone disease, hepatomegaly or splenomegaly, and thrombocytopenia

Canadian labeling: Long-term enzyme replacement therapy for patients with type 1 Gaucher disease or patients with type 3 Gaucher disease who display non-neurological manifestations (anemia, bone disease, hepatomegaly or splenomegaly, and thrombocytopenia) of the disease.

Dosing

Adult & Geriatric

Gaucher disease, type 1: IV (dose is individualized): Initial range: 2.5 units/kg 3 times weekly, up to 60 units/kg every 2 weeks. **Note:** Dosage adjustments are made based on assessment and therapeutic goals. Most benefits observed with doses of 30-60 units/kg every 2 weeks (Charrow, 2004).

Gaucher disease, type 3 (Canadian labeling; not in U.S. labeling): IV (dose is individualized): Initial range: 2.5 units/kg 3 times weekly, up to 60 units/kg every 2 weeks. Doses up to 120 units/kg every 2 weeks have been safely administered.

Pediatric Children ≥2 years and Adolescents: Refer to adult dosing.

Renal Impairment No dosage adjustment provided in the manufacturer's labeling.

Hepatic Impairment No dosage adjustment provided in the manufacturer's labeling.

Additional Information Complete prescribing information should be consulted for additional detail.

Dosage Forms Excipient information presented when available (limited, particularly for generics); consult specific product labeling.

Solution Reconstituted, Intravenous:

Cerezyme: 200 units (1 ea); 400 units (1 ea)

◆ Imipemide see Imipenem and Cilastatin on page 923

Imipenem and Cilastatin
(i mi PEN em & sye la STAT in)

Brand Names: US Primaxin I.V.

Brand Names: Canada Imipenem and Cilastatin for Injection; Imipenem and Cilastatin for Injection, USP; Primaxin; RAN-Imipenem-Cilastatin

Index Terms Cilastatin and Imipenem; Imipemide; Primaxin I.M. [DSC]

Pharmacologic Category Antibiotic, Carbapenem

Use Treatment of lower respiratory tract, urinary tract, intra-abdominal, gynecologic, bone and joint, skin and skin structure, endocarditis (caused by *Staphylococcus aureus*) and polymicrobic infections as well as bacterial septicemia. Antibacterial activity includes gram-positive bacteria (methicillin-sensitive *S. aureus* and *Streptococcus* spp), resistant gram-negative bacilli (including extended spectrum beta-lactamase-producing *Escherichia coli* and *Klebsiella* spp, *Enterobacter* spp, and *Pseudomonas aeruginosa*), and anaerobes.

Pregnancy Considerations Teratogenic events have not been observed in animal reproduction studies. Due to pregnancy induced physiologic changes, some pharmacokinetic parameters of imipenem/cilastatin may be altered. Pregnant women have a larger volume of distribution resulting in lower serum peak levels than for the same dose in nonpregnant women. Clearance is also increased.

Breast-Feeding Considerations Imipenem is excreted in human milk. The low concentrations and low oral bioavailability suggest minimal exposure risk to the infant. The US labeling recommends that caution be exercised when administering imipenem/cilastatin to breast-feeding women. The Canadian labeling recommends discontinuing breast-feeding if therapy is considered necessary. Non-dose-related effects could include modification of bowel flora.

Contraindications Hypersensitivity to imipenem/cilastatin or any component of the formulation

Warnings/Precautions Dosage adjustment required in patients with impaired renal function; elderly patients often require lower doses (adjust to renal function). Prolonged use may result in fungal or bacterial superinfection, including *C. difficile*-associated diarrhea (CDAD) and pseudomembranous colitis; CDAD has been observed >2 months postantibiotic treatment. Carbapenems have been associated with CNS adverse effects, including confusional states and seizures (myoclonic); use caution with CNS disorders (eg, brain lesions and history of seizures) and adjust dose in renal impairment to avoid drug accumulation, which may increase seizure risk. Use with caution in patients with hypersensitivity to beta-lactams (including penicillins or cephalosporins); patients with impaired renal function are at increased risk of seizures if not properly dose adjusted. May decrease divalproex sodium/valproic acid concentrations leading to breakthrough seizures; concomitant use is not recommended. Not recommended in pediatric CNS infections due to seizure risk. Serious hypersensitivity reactions, including anaphylaxis, have been reported (some without a history of previous allergic reactions to beta-lactams).

Adverse Reactions

>10%

Hematologic & oncologic: Decreased hematocrit (infants and children 3 months to 12 years: 18%; neonates and infants <3 months: 2%), decreased hemoglobin (infants and children 3 months to 12 years: 15%), eosinophilia (neonates, infants, and children to 12 years: 9% to 13%), thrombocythemia (infants and children 3 months to 12 years: 13%; neonates and infants <3 months: 4%)

Hepatic: Increased serum AST (infants and children 3 months to 12 years: 18%; neonates and infants <3 months: 6%), increased serum ALT (infants and children 3 months to 12 years: 11%; neonates and infants <3 months: 3%)

1% to 10%:

Cardiovascular: Phlebitis (2% to 3%), tachycardia (neonates and infants ≤3 months: 2%; adults <1%)

Central nervous system: Seizure (neonates and infants ≤3 months: 6%; adults <1%)

Dermatologic: Skin rash (≤2%)

Gastrointestinal: Diarrhea (neonates, infants, and children to 12 years: 3% to 4%; adults 2%), nausea (2%), oral candidiasis (neonates and infants ≤3 months: 2%), vomiting (≤1% to 2%), gastroenteritis (≤1%)

Genitourinary: Proteinuria (infants and children 3 months to 12 years: 8%), urine discoloration (≤1%), oliguria (neonates and infants ≤3 months: 2%; adults <1%)

Hematologic & oncologic: Neutropenia (infants and children 3 months to 12 years: 3%; adults <1%), decreased platelet count (neonates and infants <3 months: 2%), increased hematocrit (neonates and infants <3 months: 1%)

Hepatic: Increased serum alkaline phosphatase (neonates and infants <3 months: 3%), increased serum bilirubin (neonates and infants <3 months: 3%), decreased serum bilirubin (neonates and infants <3 months: 1%)

Local: Irritation at injection site (infants, children, and adolescents 3 months to 16 years: 1%)

Renal: Increased serum creatinine (neonates and infants <3 months: 5%)

<1% (Limited to important or life-threatening): Acute renal failure, agranulocytosis, back pain (thoracic spinal), basophilia, bilirubinuria, bone marrow depression, brain disease, candidiasis, casts in urine, change in prothrombin time, *Clostridium difficile* associated diarrhea, confusion, cyanosis, decreased serum sodium, dental discoloration, drug fever, dyskinesia, erythema multiforme, hallucination, hearing loss, heartburn, hematuria, hemolytic anemia, hemorrhagic colitis, hepatic failure, hepatitis (including fulminant onset), hyperchloremia, hypersensitivity, hyperventilation, hypotension, increased blood urea nitrogen, increased lactate dehydrogenase, increased serum potassium, increased urinary urobilinogen, injection site infection, jaundice, leukocytosis, leukocyturia, leukopenia, lymphocytosis, myoclonus, neutropenia, pancytopenia, positive direct Coombs' test, pseudomembranous colitis, pseudomonas infection (resistant *P. aeruginosa*), psychiatric disturbances, Stevens-Johnson syndrome, thrombocytopenia, toxic epidermal necrolysis

Drug Interactions

Metabolism/Transport Effects None known.

Avoid Concomitant Use

Avoid concomitant use of Imipenem and Cilastatin with any of the following: BCG (Intravesical)

Increased Effect/Toxicity

Imipenem and Cilastatin may increase the levels/effects of: CycloSPORINE (Systemic)

The levels/effects of Imipenem and Cilastatin may be increased by: CycloSPORINE (Systemic); Ganciclovir-Valganciclovir; Probenecid

Decreased Effect

Imipenem and Cilastatin may decrease the levels/effects of: BCG (Intravesical); BCG Vaccine (Immunization); CycloSPORINE (Systemic); Sodium Picosulfate; Typhoid Vaccine; Valproate Products

Preparation for Administration IV: Prior to use, dilute dose into 100-250 mL of an appropriate solution. Imipenem is inactivated at acidic or alkaline pH. Final concentration should not exceed 5 mg/mL.

Storage/Stability Imipenem/cilastatin powder for injection should be stored at <25°C (77°F).

IV: Reconstituted IV solutions are stable for 4 hours at room temperature and 24 hours when refrigerated. Do not freeze.

Mechanism of Action Inhibits bacterial cell wall synthesis by binding to one or more of the penicillin-binding proteins (PBPs); which in turn inhibits the final transpeptidation step of peptidoglycan synthesis in bacterial cell walls, thus inhibiting cell wall biosynthesis. Bacteria eventually lyse due to ongoing activity of cell wall autolytic enzymes (autolysins and murein hydrolases) while cell wall assembly is arrested. Cilastatin prevents renal metabolism of imipenem by competitive inhibition of dehydropeptidase along the brush border of the renal tubules.

Pharmacodynamics/Kinetics

Distribution: Rapidly and widely to most tissues and fluids including sputum, pleural fluid, peritoneal fluid, interstitial fluid, bile, aqueous humor, and bone; highest concentrations in pleural fluid, interstitial fluid, and peritoneal fluid; low concentrations in CSF

Protein binding: Imipenem: 20%; cilastatin: 40%

Metabolism: Imipenem is metabolized in the kidney by dehydropeptidase I; cilastatin prevents imipenem metabolism by this enzyme; cilastatin is partially metabolized renally

Half-life elimination: IV: Both drugs: Prolonged with renal impairment:
Neonates (Freij 1985): Imipenem: 1.7-2.4 hours; Cilastatin: 3.9-6.3 hours
Infants and Children: Imipenem: 1.2 hours (Blumer 1996)
Adults: 60 minutes

Excretion: Both drugs: Urine (~70% as unchanged drug; 70% to 80% of a cilastatin dose is excreted unchanged)

Dosing

Adult & Geriatric Doses based on **imipenem** content.

Usual dosage range: Weight ≥70 kg: 250-1000 mg every 6-8 hours; maximum: 4 g/day. **Note:** For adults weighing <70 kg, refer to Dosing Adjustment in Renal Impairment.

Indication-specific dosing:

Burkholderia pseudomallei (melioidosis) (off-label use): IV: Initial: 20 mg/kg every 8 hours for at least 10 days (White 2003) or 25 mg/kg (up to 1 g) every 6 hours for at least 10 days (Currie 2003); continue parenteral therapy until clinical improvement then switch to oral therapy if tolerated and/or appropriate.

Intra-abdominal infections: IV:
Mild infection: 250-500 mg every 6 hours
Severe infection: 500 mg every 6 hours **or** 1 g every 8 hours for 4-7 days (provided source controlled). **Note:** Not recommended for mild-to-moderate, community-acquired intra-abdominal infections due to risk of toxicity and the development of resistant organisms (Solomkin 2010)

Liver abscess (off-label use): IV: 500 mg every 6 hours for 4-6 weeks (Ulug 2010)

Moderate infections: IV:
Fully-susceptible organisms: 500 mg every 6-8 hours
Moderately-susceptible organisms: 500 mg every 6 hours or 1 g every 8 hours

Neutropenic fever (off-label use): IV: 500 mg every 6 hours (Paul 2006)

Pseudomonas infections: IV: 500 mg every 6 hours; **Note:** Higher doses may be required based on organism sensitivity.

Severe infections: IV:
Fully-susceptible organisms: 500 mg every 6 hours
Moderately-susceptible organisms: 1 g every 6-8 hours
Maximum daily dose should not exceed 50 mg/kg or 4 g/day, whichever is lower

Skin and soft tissue necrotizing infections (off-label use): IV: 1 g every 6 to 8 hours in combination with an agent effective against MRSA (eg, vancomycin, linezolid, daptomycin) for empiric therapy of polymicrobial [mixed] infections. Continue until further debridement is not necessary, patient has clinically improved, and patient is afebrile for 48 to 72 hours (IDSA [Stevens 2014]).

Surgical site infection (intestinal or genitourinary tract surgery) (off-label use): IV: 500 mg every 6 hours (IDSA [Stevens 2014]).

Urinary tract infection, uncomplicated: IV: 250 mg every 6 hours

Urinary tract infection, complicated: IV: 500 mg every 6 hours

Mild infections: Note: Rarely a suitable option in mild infections; normally reserved for moderate-severe cases: IV:
Fully-susceptible organisms: 250 mg every 6 hours
Moderately-susceptible organisms: 500 mg every 6 hours

Pediatric Dosage based on **imipenem** content:

Non-CNS infections: IV: Children: >3 months: 15-25 mg/kg every 6 hours
Maximum dosage: Susceptible infections: 2 g/day; moderately-susceptible organisms: 4 g/day

Burkholderia pseudomallei (melioidosis) (off-label use): IV: Initial: 20 mg/kg every 8 hours for at least 10 days (White 2003) or 25 mg/kg (up to 1 g) every 6 hours for at least 10 days (Currie 2003); continue parenteral therapy until clinical improvement, then switch to oral therapy if tolerated and/or appropriate

Cystic fibrosis: IV: Infants, Children, and Adolescents: Up to 100 mg/kg/day divided every 6 hours; maximum dose: 4 g daily has been used. **Note:** Efficacy in exacerbations may be limited due to rapid development of resistance (Zobell 2013).

Renal Impairment IV:

Patients with a CrCl ≤5 mL/minute/1.73 m² should not receive imipenem/cilastatin unless hemodialysis is instituted within 48 hours.

Patients weighing <30 kg with impaired renal function should not receive imipenem/cilastatin.

Reduced IV dosage regimen based on creatinine clearance and/or body weight: See table.

Intermittent hemodialysis (IHD) (administer after hemodialysis on dialysis days): Use the dosing recommendation for patients with a CrCl 6-20 mL/minute; administer dose after dialysis session and every 12 hours thereafter **or** 250-500 mg every 12 hours (Heintz 2009). **Note:** Dosing dependent on the assumption of 3 times/week, complete IHD sessions.

Peritoneal dialysis (off-label dosing): Dose as for CrCl 6-20 mL/minute (Somani 1988)

Continuous renal replacement therapy (CRRT) (Heintz 2009; Trotman 2005): Drug clearance is highly dependent on the method of renal replacement, filter type, and flow rate. Appropriate dosing requires close monitoring of pharmacologic response, signs of adverse reactions due to drug accumulation, as well as drug concentrations in relation to target trough (if appropriate). The following are general recommendations only (based on dialysate flow/ultrafiltration rates of 1-2 L/hour and minimal residual renal function) and should not supersede clinical judgment:

CVVH: Loading dose of 1 g followed by either 250 mg every 6 hours **or** 500 mg every 8 hours

CVVHD: Loading dose of 1 g followed by either 250 mg every 6 hours **or** 500 mg every 6-8 hours

CVVHDF: Loading dose of 1 g followed by either 250 mg every 6 hours **or** 500 mg every 6 hours

Note: Data suggest that 500 mg every 8-12 hours may provide sufficient time above MIC to cover organisms with MIC values ≤2 mg/L; however, a higher dose of 500 mg every 6 hours is recommended for resistant organisms (particularly *Pseudomonas* spp) with MIC ≥4 mg/L or deep-seated infections (Fish 2005).

Reduced IV dosage regimen based on creatinine clearance and/or body weight:
U.S. labeling: See table.

Imipenem and Cilastatin Dosage in Renal Impairment

Reduced IV Dosage Regimen Based on Creatinine Clearance (mL/minute/1.73 m²) and/or Body Weight <70 kg	Body Weight (kg)				
	≥70	60	50	40	30
Total daily dose for normal renal function: 1 g/day					
CrCl ≥71	250 mg q6h	250 mg q8h	125 mg q6h	125 mg q6h	125 mg q8h
CrCl 41-70	250 mg q8h	125 mg q6h	125 mg q6h	125 mg q8h	125 mg q8h
CrCl 21-40	250 mg q12h	125 mg q12h	125 mg q8h	125 mg q12h	125 mg q12h
CrCl 6-20	250 mg q12h	125 mg q12h	125 mg q12h	125 mg q12h	125 mg q12h
Total daily dose for normal renal function: 1.5 g/day					
CrCl ≥71	500 mg q8h	250 mg q6h	250 mg q6h	250 mg q8h	125 mg q6h
CrCl 41-70	250 mg q6h	250 mg q8h	250 mg q8h	125 mg q6h	125 mg q8h
CrCl 21-40	250 mg q8h	250 mg q8h	250 mg q12h	125 mg q8h	125 mg q8h
CrCl 6-20	250 mg q12h	250 mg q12h	250 mg q12h	125 mg q12h	125 mg q12h
Total daily dose for normal renal function: 2 g/day					
CrCl ≥71	500 mg q6h	500 mg q8h	250 mg q6h	250 mg q6h	250 mg q8h
CrCl 41-70	500 mg q8h	250 mg q6h	250 mg q8h	250 mg q6h	250 mg q6h
CrCl 21-40	250 mg q6h	250 mg q8h	250 mg q8h	250 mg q12h	125 mg q8h
CrCl 6-20	250 mg q12h	250 mg q12h	250 mg q12h	250 mg q12h	125 mg q12h
Total daily dose for normal renal function: 3 g/day					
CrCl ≥71	1000 mg q8h	750 mg q8h	500 mg q6h	500 mg q8h	250 mg q6h
CrCl 41-70	500 mg q6h	500 mg q8h	500 mg q8h	250 mg q6h	250 mg q8h
CrCl 21-40	500 mg q8h	500 mg q8h	250 mg q6h	250 mg q8h	250 mg q8h
CrCl 6-20	500 mg q12h	500 mg q12h	250 mg q12h	250 mg q12h	250 mg q12h
Total daily dose for normal renal function: 4 g/day					
CrCl ≥71	1000 mg q6h	1000 mg q8h	750 mg q8h	500 mg q6h	500 mg q8h
CrCl 41-70	750 mg q8h	750 mg q8h	500 mg q8h	500 mg q8h	250 mg q6h
CrCl 21-40	500 mg q6h	500 mg q8h	500 mg q8h	250 mg q6h	250 mg q8h
CrCl 6-20	500 mg q12h	500 mg q12h	500 mg q12h	250 mg q12h	250 mg q12h

Canadian labeling: Reduced IV dosage regimen based on creatinine clearance (mL/minute/1.73 m²) and body weight ≥70 kg (**Note:** The manufacturer labeling recommends further proportionate dose reductions for patients <70 kg, but does not provide specific dosing recommendations):

Mild renal impairment (CrCl 31-70 mL/minute/1.73 m²):
Fully-susceptible organisms: Maximum dosage: 500 mg every 8 hours
Less susceptible organisms (primarily some *Pseudomonas* strains): Maximum dosage: 500 mg every 6 hours

Moderate renal impairment (CrCl 21-30 mL/minute/1.73 m²):
Fully-susceptible organisms: Maximum dosage: 500 mg every 12 hours
Less susceptible organisms (primarily some *Pseudomonas* strains): Maximum dosage: 500 mg every 8 hours

Severe renal impairment (CrCl 0-20 mL/minute/1.73 m²):
Fully-susceptible organisms: Maximum dosage: 250 mg every 12 hours
Less susceptible organisms (primarily some *Pseudomonas* strains): Maximum dosage: 500 mg every 12 hours

Note: Patients with CrCl 6-20 mL/minute/1.73 m² should receive 250 mg every 12 hours or 3.5 mg/kg (whichever is lower) every 12 hours for most pathogens; seizure risk may increase with higher dosing.

Hepatic Impairment Hepatic dysfunction may further impair cilastatin clearance in patients receiving chronic renal replacement therapy; consider decreasing the dosing frequency.

Dietary Considerations Some products may contain sodium.

Administration IV: Do not administer IV push. Infuse doses ≤500 mg over 20-30 minutes; infuse doses ≥750 mg over 40-60 minutes.

Monitoring Parameters Periodic renal, hepatic, and hematologic function tests; monitor for signs of anaphylaxis during first dose

Test Interactions Interferes with urinary glucose determination using Clinitest®; positive Coombs' [direct]

Dosage Forms Excipient information presented when available (limited, particularly for generics); consult specific product labeling.

Injection, powder for reconstitution: Imipenem 250 mg and cilastatin 250 mg; imipenem 500 mg and cilastatin 500 mg
Primaxin® I.V.: Imipenem 250 mg and cilastatin 250 mg [contains sodium 18.8 mg (0.8 mEq)]; imipenem 500 mg and cilastatin 500 mg [contains sodium 37.5 mg (1.6 mEq)]

◆ Imipenem and Cilastatin for Injection (Can) *see* Imipenem and Cilastatin *on page* 923

◆ Imipenem and Cilastatin for Injection, USP (Can) *see* Imipenem and Cilastatin *on page* 923

Imipramine (im IP ra meen)

Brand Names: US Tofranil; Tofranil-PM
Brand Names: Canada Impril; Novo-Pramine; PMS Imipramine
Index Terms Imipramine Hydrochloride; Imipramine Pamoate
Pharmacologic Category Antidepressant, Tricyclic (Tertiary Amine)
Use
Childhood enuresis: As temporary adjunctive therapy in reducing enuresis in children ≥6 years of age, after possible organic causes have been excluded by appropriate tests
Depression: Treatment of depression
Medication Guide Available Yes
Dosing
Adult
Depression: Oral:
Outpatients: Initial: 75 mg daily; may increase gradually to 150 mg daily. May be given in divided doses or as a single bedtime dose; Maintenance 50-150 mg daily; maximum: 200 mg daily
Inpatients: Initial: 100-150 mg daily; may increase gradually to 200 mg daily; if no response after 2 weeks, may further increase to 250-300 mg daily. May be given in divided doses or as a single bedtime dose; maximum: 300 mg daily.
Neuropathic pain (off-label use): Oral: **Note:** Not the preferred TCA (Bril 2011; Dworkin 2007). Initial: 50 mg once daily or in divided doses twice daily; increase gradually up to 150 mg daily (Kvinesdal 1984; Sindrup 2003) or to a dosage sufficient to achieve an imipramine plus desipramine plasma concentration of 113-170 ng/mL (SI: 400-600 nmol/L) (Sindrup 1989; Sindrup 1990)
Panic disorder (off-label use): Oral: Initial: 10 mg once daily; increase gradually to a usual dose of 75-300 mg daily (APA 2009; Bandelow 2008)
Post-traumatic stress disorder (PTSD) (off-label use): Oral: Initial: 50 mg once daily; increase gradually to 200-300 mg once daily to achieve blood levels in the therapeutic range (>150 ng/mL) (Frank 1988; Kosten 1991)

Discontinuation of therapy: Upon discontinuation of antidepressant therapy, gradually taper the dose to minimize the incidence of withdrawal symptoms and allow for the detection of re-emerging symptoms. Evidence supporting ideal taper rates is limited. APA and NICE guidelines suggest tapering therapy over at least several weeks with consideration to the half-life of the antidepressant; antidepressants with a shorter half-life may need to be tapered more conservatively. In addition for long-term treated patients, WFSBP guidelines recommend tapering over 4 to 6 months. If intolerable withdrawal symptoms occur following a dose reduction, consider resuming the previously prescribed dose and/or decrease dose at a more gradual rate (APA 2010; Bauer 2002; Haddod 2001; NCCMH 2010; Schatzberg 2006; Shelton 2001; Warner 2006).

MAO inhibitor recommendations:
Switching to or from an MAO inhibitor intended to treat psychiatric disorders:

Allow 14 days to elapse between discontinuing an MAO inhibitor intended to treat psychiatric disorders and initiation of imipramine.

Allow 14 days to elapse between discontinuing imipramine and initiation of an MAO inhibitor intended to treat psychiatric disorders.

Use with other MAO inhibitors (linezolid or IV methylene blue):

Do not initiate imipramine in patients receiving linezolid or IV methylene blue; consider other interventions for psychiatric condition.

If urgent treatment with linezolid or IV methylene blue is required in a patient already receiving imipramine and potential benefits outweigh potential risks, discontinue imipramine promptly and administer linezolid or IV methylene blue. Monitor for serotonin syndrome for 2 weeks or until 24 hours after the last dose of linezolid or IV methylene blue, whichever comes first. May resume imipramine 24 hours after the last dose of linezolid or IV methylene blue.

Geriatric
Depression: Initial: 25-50 mg at bedtime; may increase every 3 days for inpatients and weekly for outpatients if tolerated to a recommended maximum of 100 mg daily
Discontinuation of therapy: Refer to adult dosing.
MAO inhibitor recommendations: Refer to adult dosing.

Pediatric Note: Manufacturer labeling warns against use of doses >2.5 mg/kg/**day** in pediatric patients; ECG changes (of unknown significance) have been reported in pediatric patients who received twice this amount.

Depression: Adolescents: Oral: Initial: 25 to 50 mg daily; increase gradually; maximum: 100 mg daily in single or divided doses. **Note:** Controlled clinical trials have not shown tricyclic antidepressants to be superior to placebo for the treatment of depression in children and adolescents; not recommended as first-line medication; may be beneficial for patient with comorbid conditions (ADHD, enuresis) (Birmaher 2007; Dopheide 2006; Wagner 2005)

Enuresis: *Imipramine hydrochloride:* Children ≥6 years and Adolescents: Oral: Initial: 25 mg 1 hour before bedtime, if inadequate response still seen after 1 week of therapy, increase by 25 mg daily; dose should not exceed 2.5 mg/kg/day or 50 mg at bedtime if 6 to 12 years or 75 mg at bedtime if ≥12 years

Attention-deficit/hyperactivity disorder (off-label use): Children ≥6 years and Adolescents: Oral: Initial: 1 mg/kg/day in 1 to 3 divided doses; titrate as needed; maximum daily dose: 4 mg/kg/**day** or 200 mg **daily**; for doses >2 mg/kg/day, monitor serum concentrations (target: ≤200 ng/mL) (Himpel 2005; Pliszka 2007)

Neuropathic pain (off-label use): Children: Oral: Initial: 0.2 to 0.4 mg/kg at bedtime; dose may be increased by 50% every 2 to 3 days up to 1 to 3 mg/kg/dose at bedtime (Berde 1990)

Discontinuation of therapy: Refer to adult dosing.

MAO inhibitor recommendations: Refer to adult dosing.
Renal Impairment No dosage adjustment provided in manufacturer's labeling; use with caution.
Hepatic Impairment No dosage adjustment provided in manufacturer's labeling; use with caution.
Additional Information Complete prescribing information should be consulted for additional detail.
Dosage Forms Excipient information presented when available (limited, particularly for generics); consult specific product labeling.

Capsule, Oral, as pamoate:
Tofranil-PM: 75 mg, 100 mg, 125 mg, 150 mg
Generic: 75 mg, 100 mg, 125 mg, 150 mg

Tablet, Oral, as hydrochloride:
Tofranil: 10 mg, 25 mg, 50 mg
Generic: 10 mg, 25 mg, 50 mg
Dosage Forms: Canada Note: Refer also to Dosage Forms. Excipient information presented when available (limited, particularly for generics); consult specific product labeling.
Tablet, Oral, as hydrochloride: 75 mg

♦ Imiquimod Hydrochloride *see* Imipramine *on page 925*
♦ Imiquimod Pamoate *see* Imipramine *on page 925*

Imiquimod (i mi KWI mod)

Brand Names: US Aldara; Zyclara; Zyclara Pump
Brand Names: Canada Aldara P; Apo-Imiquimod; Vyloma; Zyclara
Pharmacologic Category Skin and Mucous Membrane Agent; Topical Skin Product
Use
Aldara®: Treatment of external genital and perianal warts/condyloma acuminata; nonhyperkeratotic, nonhypertrophic actinic keratosis on face or scalp; superficial basal cell carcinoma (sBCC) with a maximum tumor diameter of 2 cm located on the trunk (excluding anogenital skin), neck, or extremities (excluding hands or feet)
Vyloma™ (Canadian availability; not available in the U.S.): Treatment of external genital and perianal warts/condyloma acuminata
Zyclara®:
U.S. labeling: Treatment of external genital and perianal warts/condyloma acuminata (3.75% formulation); treatment of clinically typical visible or palpable, actinic keratoses on face or scalp (2.5% or 3.75% formulation)
Canadian labeling: Treatment of clinically typical visible or palpable, actinic keratoses on face or scalp
Dosing
Adult & Geriatric Note: Imiquimod treatment should not be prolonged beyond recommended period due to missed doses or rest periods.
U.S. labeling:
Perianal warts/condyloma acuminata: Topical:
Aldara®: Apply a thin layer 3 times/week on alternative days prior to bedtime and leave on skin for 6-10 hours. Remove by washing with mild soap and water. Continue imiquimod treatment until there is total clearance of the genital/perianal warts or a maximum duration of therapy of 16 weeks.
Zyclara® 3.75%: Apply a thin layer using up to 1 packet or 1 full actuation of pump once daily prior to bedtime and leave on skin for ~8 hours. Remove with mild soap and water. Continue treatment until there is total clearance of the warts or a maximum duration of therapy of 8 weeks. Patient should not receive more than 56 packets or 2 x 7.5 g pumps or 1 x 15 g pump per course of treatment.
Actinic keratosis: Topical: **Note:** Prescribed course of therapy should be completed even if all lesions appear to be gone. Safety and efficacy of repeated use in a previously treated area has not been established.
Aldara®: Treatment should be limited to areas ≤25 cm²; apply 2 times/week for 16 weeks to a treatment area on face or scalp (but not both concurrently); no more than 1 packet should be applied at each application and no more than 36 packets applied per 16 weeks; apply prior to bedtime and leave on skin for ~8 hours. Remove with mild soap and water.
Zyclara® 2.5%, 3.75%: Treatment consists of 2 cycles (14 days each) separated by 1 rest period (14 days) with no treatment. Apply up to 2 packets or 2 full actuations of pump once daily at bedtime to affected area on either face or balding scalp (but not both concurrently); leave on skin for ~8 hours. Remove with mild soap and water. Patient should not receive more than 56 packets or 2 x 7.5 g pumps or 1 x 15 g pump per 2 cycles of treatment.
Superficial basal cell carcinoma: Topical: Aldara®: Apply once daily prior to bedtime, 5 days/week for 6 weeks. No more than 36 packets should be used during the 6-week treatment period. Tumor treatment area should not exceed 3 cm (maximum of 2 cm tumor diameter plus a 1 cm margin of skin around the tumor). The diameter of cream droplet applied should range from 4 mm to 7 mm for tumor areas of 0.5 cm to 2 cm, respectively. Leave on skin for ~8 hours. Remove with mild soap and water. Safety and efficacy of repeated use in a previously treated area have not been established.

Canadian labeling:

Actinic keratosis: Topical: **Note:** Prescribed course of therapy should be completed even if all lesions appear to be gone; safety and efficacy of repeated use in a previously treated area have not been established.

Aldara®: Treatment should be limited to areas ≤25 cm^2; apply 2 times/week for 16 weeks to a treatment area on face or scalp (but not both concurrently); no more than 1 packet should be applied at each application; apply prior to bedtime and leave on skin for ~8 hours. Remove with mild soap and water.

Zyclara®: Treatment should be limited to an area <200 cm^2 on the face or scalp and consists of 2 cycles (14 days each) separated by 1 rest period (14 days) with no treatment. Apply up to 2 packets or 2 full actuations of pump once daily at bedtime to affected area on either face or balding scalp (but not both concurrently). Leave on skin for ~8 hours. Remove with mild soap and water. Patient should not receive more than 56 packets or 2 x 7.5 g pumps or 1 x 15 g pump per 2 cycles of treatment.

External genital and/or perianal warts/condyloma acuminata: Topical:

Aldara®: Apply a thin layer 3 times/week prior to bedtime and leave on skin for 6-10 hours. Remove with mild soap and water. Examples of 3 times/week application schedules are: Monday, Wednesday, Friday; or Tuesday, Thursday, Saturday. Continue treatment until there is total clearance of the warts or a maximum duration of therapy of 16 weeks.

Vyloma™: Apply a thin layer once daily prior to bedtime and leave on skin for ~8 hours. Remove with mild soap and water. Continue treatment until there is total clearance of the warts or maximum duration of therapy of 8 weeks.

Superficial basal cell carcinoma: Topical: Aldara®: Apply once daily prior to bedtime, 5 days/week for 6 weeks. Tumor treatment area should not exceed 3 cm (maximum of 2 cm tumor diameter plus a 1 cm margin of skin around the tumor). The diameter of cream droplet applied should range from 4 mm to 7 mm for tumor areas of 0.5 cm to 2 cm, respectively. Leave on skin for ~8 hours. Remove with mild soap and water. Safety and efficacy of repeated use in a previously treated area have not been established.

Common warts (off-label use): Topical (5% cream): Apply once daily prior to bedtime for 5 days/week for up to 16 weeks (Hengge, 2000) or apply twice daily for up to 24 weeks (Grussendorf-Conen, 2002)

Dosing adjustment for toxicity:

Local skin reactions (eg, erythema, edema, scabbing, etc): Temporarily interrupt treatment for up to several days for severe or intolerable reactions; may consider resuming therapy once reaction subsides.

Systemic/flu-like reactions (eg, malaise, fever, rigors, etc): Consider temporary interruption of therapy.

Vulvar swelling: Interrupt or discontinue therapy for severe vulvar swelling.

Pediatric Perianal warts/condyloma acuminata: Topical: Aldara®: Children ≥12 years: Refer to adult dosing.

Renal Impairment No dosage adjustment provided in manufacturer's labeling.

Hepatic Impairment No dosage adjustment provided in manufacturer's labeling.

Additional Information Complete prescribing information should be consulted for additional detail.

Dosage Forms Excipient information presented when available (limited, particularly for generics); consult specific product labeling. [DSC] = Discontinued product

Cream, External:

Aldara®: 5% (12 ea, 24 ea [DSC]) [contains benzyl alcohol, cetyl alcohol, methylparaben, propylparaben, sorbitan monostearate(sorbitan stearate)]

Zyclara®: 3.75% (28 ea) [contains benzyl alcohol, cetyl alcohol, methylparaben, propylparaben]

Zyclara Pump: 2.5% (7.5 g); 3.75% (7.5 g) [contains benzyl alcohol, cetyl alcohol, methylparaben, propylparaben]

Generic: 5% (1 ea, 12 ea, 24 ea)

Dosage Forms: Canada Excipient information presented when available (limited, particularly for generics); consult specific product labeling.

Cream, topical:

Vyloma™: 3.75% (28s) [contains benzyl alcohol; 0.25 g/packet]

◆ Imitrex *see* SUMAtriptan *on page 1717*

◆ Imitrex DF (Can) *see* SUMAtriptan *on page 1717*

◆ Imitrex Injection (Can) *see* SUMAtriptan *on page 1717*

◆ Imitrex Nasal Spray (Can) *see* SUMAtriptan *on page 1717*

◆ Imitrex STATdose Refill *see* SUMAtriptan *on page 1717*

◆ Imitrex STATdose System *see* SUMAtriptan *on page 1717*

◆ ImmuCyst (Can) *see* BCG (Intravesical) *on page 203*

Immune Globulin (i MYUN GLOB yoo lin)

Brand Names: US Bivigam; Carimune NF; Flebogamma DIF; Flebogamma [DSC]; GamaSTAN S/D; Gammagard; Gammagard S/D Less IgA; Gammagard S/D [DSC]; Gammaked; Gammaplex; Gamunex [DSC]; Gamunex-C; Hizentra; Hyqvia; Octagam; Privigen

Brand Names: Canada Gamastan S/D; Gammagard Liquid; Gammagard S/D; Gamunex; Hizentra; IGIVnex; Octagam 10%; Privigen

Index Terms Gamma Globulin; Human Normal Immunoglobulin; HyQvia; IG; IGIM; IGIV; IGSC; IMIG; Immune Globulin Subcutaneous (Human); Immune Serum Globulin; ISG; IV Immune Globulin; IVIG; Normal Immunoglobulin; Octagam 10%; Panglobulin; SCIG

Pharmacologic Category Blood Product Derivative; Immune Globulin

Additional Appendix Information

Immune Globulin Product Comparison *on page 1953*

Immunization Administration Recommendations *on page 1974*

Immunization Schedules *on page 1979*

Use

Treatment of primary humoral immunodeficiency syndromes (congenital agammaglobulinemia, severe combined immunodeficiency syndromes [SCIDS], common variable immunodeficiency, X-linked immunodeficiency, Wiskott-Aldrich syndrome) (Bivigam, Carimune NF, Flebogamma DIF, HyQvia, Gammagard Liquid, Gammagard S/D, Gammaked, Gammaplex, Gamunex-C, Hizentra, Octagam 5%, Privigen)

Treatment of acute and chronic immune thrombocytopenia (ITP) (Carimune NF, Gammagard S/D, Gammaked, Gammaplex [chronic only], Gamunex-C, Octagam 10% [chronic only], Privigen [chronic only])

Treatment of chronic inflammatory demyelinating polyneuropathy (CIDP) (Gammaked, Gamunex-C)

Treatment of multifocal motor neuropathy (MMN) (Gammagard Liquid)

Prevention of coronary artery aneurysms associated with Kawasaki syndrome (in combination with aspirin) (Gammagard S/D)

Prevention of bacterial infection in patients with hypogammaglobulinemia and/or recurrent bacterial infections with B-cell chronic lymphocytic leukemia (CLL) (Gammagard S/D)

Provision of passive immunity in the following susceptible individuals (GamaSTAN S/D):

Hepatitis A: Pre-exposure prophylaxis; postexposure: within 14 days and/or prior to manifestation of disease

Measles: For use within 6 days of exposure in an unvaccinated person, who has not previously had measles

Rubella: Postexposure prophylaxis to reduce the risk of infection and fetal damage in exposed pregnant women who will not consider therapeutic abortion

Varicella: For immunosuppressed patients when varicella zoster immune globulin is not available

Pregnancy Considerations Animal reproduction studies have not been conducted. Immune globulins cross the placenta in increased amounts after 30 weeks gestation. Intravenous immune globulin has been recommended for use in fetal-neonatal alloimmune thrombocytopenia and pregnancy-associated ITP (Anderson, 2007). Intravenous immune globulin is recommended to prevent measles in nonimmune women exposed during pregnancy (CDC, 2013). May also be used in postexposure prophylaxis for rubella to reduce the risk of infection and fetal damage in exposed pregnant women who will not consider therapeutic abortion (per GamaSTAN S/D product labeling; use for postexposure rubella prophylaxis is not currently recommended [CDC, 2013]).

HyQvia: Women who become pregnant during treatment are encouraged to enroll in the HyQvia Pregnancy Registry (1-866-424-6724).

Breast-Feeding Considerations It is not known if immune globulin from these preparations is excreted in breast milk. The manufacturer recommends that caution be exercised when administering immune globulin to nursing women. The manufacturer of HyQvia recommends administration to nursing women only if clearly indicated.

Contraindications Hypersensitivity to immune globulin or any component of the formulation; IgA deficiency (with anti-IgA antibodies and history of hypersensitivity); hyperprolinemia (Hizentra, Privigen); isolated IgA deficiency (GamaSTAN S/D); severe thrombocytopenia or

coagulation disorders where IM injections are contraindicated (GamaSTAN S/D); hypersensitivity to corn (Octagam); hereditary intolerance to fructose (excluding Flebogamma); infants/neonates for whom sucrose or fructose tolerance has not been established (Gammaplex); hypersensitivity to hyaluronidase or recombinant human hyaluronidase (HyQvia)

Warnings/Precautions [U.S. Boxed Warning]: IV administration only: Acute renal dysfunction (increased serum creatinine, oliguria, acute renal failure, osmotic nephrosis) can rarely occur and has been associated with fatalities; usually within 7 days of use (more likely with products stabilized with sucrose). Use with caution in the elderly, patients with renal disease, diabetes mellitus, overweight, hypovolemia, volume depletion, sepsis, paraproteinemia, and nephrotoxic medications due to risk of renal dysfunction. In patients at risk of renal dysfunction, ensure adequate hydration prior to administration; the dose, rate of infusion and concentration of solution should be minimized. Discontinue if renal function deteriorates.

[U.S. Boxed Warning]: Thrombosis may occur with immune globulin products even in the absence of risk factors for thrombosis. For patients at risk for thrombosis (eg, advanced age, history of atherosclerosis, impaired cardiac output, prolonged immobilization, hypercoagulable conditions, history of venous or arterial thrombosis, use of estrogens, indwelling central vascular catheters, hyperviscosity, and cardiovascular risk factors), administer at the minimum dose and infusion rate practicable. Ensure adequate hydration before administration. Monitor for signs and symptoms of thrombosis and assess blood viscosity in patients at risk for hyperviscosity such as those with cryoglobulins, fasting chylomicronemia/severe hypertriglyceridemia, or monoclonal gammopathies.

High-dose regimens (1 g/kg for 1 to 2 days) are not recommended for individuals with fluid overload or where fluid volume may be of concern. Hypersensitivity and anaphylactic reactions can occur (some severe); patients with anti-IgA antibodies are at greater risk; a severe fall in blood pressure may rarely occur with anaphylactic reaction; discontinue therapy and institute immediate treatment (including epinephrine 1:1000) should be available. Product of human plasma; may potentially contain infectious agents which could transmit disease, including unknown or emerging viruses and other pathogens. Screening of donors, as well as testing and/or inactivation or removal of certain viruses, reduces the risk. Infections thought to be transmitted by this product should be reported to the manufacturer. Aseptic meningitis may occur with high doses (≥1 g/kg) and/or rapid infusion; syndrome usually appears within several hours to 2 days following treatment; usually resolves within several days after product is discontinued; patients with a migraine history may be at higher risk for AMS. Increased risk of hypersensitivity, especially in patients with anti-IgA antibodies; use is contraindicated in patients with IgA deficiency (with antibodies against IgA and history of hypersensitivity) or isolated IgA deficiency (GamaSTAN S/D). Increased risk of hematoma formation when administered subcutaneously for the treatment of ITP.

Intravenous immune globulin has been associated with antiglobulin hemolysis (acute or delayed); monitor for signs of hemolytic anemia. Cases of hemolysis-related renal dysfunction/failure or disseminated intravascular coagulation (DIC) have been reported. Risk factors include high doses (≥2 g/kg) and non-O blood type (FDA, 2012). In chronic ITP, assess risk versus benefit of high-dose regimen in patients with increased risk of thrombosis, hemolysis, acute kidney injury, or volume overload.

Patients should be adequately hydrated prior to initiation of therapy. Hyperproteinemia, increased serum viscosity and hyponatremia may occur; distinguish hyponatremia from pseudohyponatremia to prevent volume depletion, a further increase in serum viscosity, and a higher risk of thrombotic events. Patients should be monitored for adverse events during and after the infusion. Stop administration with signs of infusion reaction (fever, chills, nausea, vomiting, and rarely shock). Risk may be increased with initial treatment, when switching brands of immune globulin, and with treatment interruptions of >8 weeks. Monitor for transfusion-related acute lung injury (TRALI); noncardiogenic pulmonary edema has been reported with immune globulin use. TRALI is characterized by severe respiratory distress, pulmonary edema, normal left ventricular function, hypoxemia, and fever (in the presence of normal left ventricular function) and usually occurs within 1 to 6 hours after infusion. Response to live vaccinations may be impaired. Some clinicians may administer intravenous immune globulin products as a subcutaneous infusion based on patient tolerability and clinical judgment. SubQ infusion should begin 1 week after the last IV dose; dose should be individualized based on clinical response and serum IgG trough concentrations; consider premedicating with acetaminophen and diphenhydramine.

Use with caution in the elderly; may be at increased risk for renal dysfunction/failure and thromboembolic events. Some products may contain maltose, which may result in falsely elevated blood glucose readings; maltose-containing products may be contraindicated in patients with an allergy to corn. Some products may contain sodium and/or sucrose. Some dosage forms may contain polysorbate 80 (also known as Tweens). Hypersensitivity reactions, usually a delayed reaction, have been reported following exposure to pharmaceutical products containing polysorbate 80 in certain individuals (Isaksson, 2002; Lucente 2000; Shelley, 1995). Thrombocytopenia, ascites, pulmonary deterioration, and renal and hepatic failure have been reported in premature neonates after receiving parenteral products containing polysorbate 80 (Alade, 1986; CDC, 1984). See manufacturer's labeling. Some products may contain sorbitol; do not use in patients with fructose intolerance. Hizentra and Privigen contain the stabilizer L-proline and are contraindicated in patients with hyperprolinemia. Packaging of some products may contain natural latex/natural rubber; skin testing should not be performed with GamaSTAN S/D as local irritation can occur and be misinterpreted as a positive reaction. Potentially significant interactions may exist, requiring dose or frequency adjustment, additional monitoring, and/or selection of alternative therapy.

Adverse Reactions Frequency not always defined. Adverse effects are reported as class effects rather than for specific products. Adverse effects occur with intravenous administration unless otherwise specified. Some clinical trials were extremely small and skewed the incidence upward ("≤" indicates this trend).

Cardiovascular: Hypotension (≤14%, children 2 to 16 years: 25%), tachycardia (5%, children 2 to 16 years: 25%), decreased diastolic blood pressure (5%, children 2 to 16 years: 21%), decreased heart rate (16%), chest pain (≤9%), hypertension (≤9%), peripheral edema (8%), cardiac arrest (Octagam 5%: ≤8%), heart murmur (7%), chest discomfort (≤7%), flushing (6%), thrombosis (≤2%), facial flushing

Central nervous system: Headache (2% to 75%, children 2 to 16: 42%; subcutaneous: 13% to 21%), fatigue (6% to 29%; subcutaneous: 11%), chills (5% to 19%), pain (5% to 15%), rigors (7% to 13%), dizziness (≤13%), insomnia (9%), migraine (5% to 7%), lethargy (≤6%), fibromyalgia syndrome (exacerbation: 5%), malaise (≤5%), vertigo (≤5%), drowsiness

Dermatologic: Ecchymosis (≤40%), skin rash (5% to 10%), pruritus (6% to 8%), urticaria (5% to 8%, may be transient), cellulitis (≤8%), hyperhidrosis (6%), eczema (≤5%, may be transient), xeroderma (≤5%), localized erythema (subcutaneous)

Endocrine & metabolic: Ketonuria (Octagam 5%: ≤8%), dehydration (≤6%), increased lactate dehydrogenase (5%)

Gastrointestinal: Sore throat (11% to 35%), abdominal pain (6% to ≤33%, children 2 to 16 years: 8%), diarrhea (5% to 28%, children 2 to 16 years: 8%), vomiting (≤26%, children 2 to 16 years: 8%; subcutaneous: 7%), nausea (5% to 22%, children 2 to 16 years: 8%; subcutaneous: 7%), upper abdominal pain (6% to 20%, children 2 to 16 years: ≤15%), dyspepsia (6% to 9%), gastroenteritis (≤8%), pseudomembranous colitis (≤8%), gastritis (6%), stomach discomfort (6%)

Genitourinary: Vulvovaginal candidiasis (9%), urinary tract infection (≤9%), cystitis (≤5%), dysuria (≤5%)

Hematologic & oncologic: Positive direct Coombs test (≤47%), purpura (≤40%), hemorrhage (29%), petechiae (21%), thrombocytopenia (15%), anemia (6% to 11%), decreased hematocrit (5%), hematoma

Hepatic: Increased serum ALT (all elevations were transient and generally mild: ≤18%, children 2 to 16 years, >2.5 x ULN: ≤7%; subcutaneous: ≤3%), increased serum alkaline phosphatase (subcutaneous: ≤13%; mild and transient), hyperbilirubinemia (unconjugated: 11%, conjugated: 9%; total: 5%), increased serum AST (intravenous/subcutaneous: ≤9%), decreased serum alkaline phosphatase (subcutaneous: ≤3%)

Immunologic: Antibody development (subcutaneous: 18%; nonneutralizing antibodies to recombinant human hyaluronidase)

Infection: Fungal infection (7% to 9%), influenza (5%), coxsackievirus (≤2%)

Local: Infusion site reaction (6% to 13%; subcutaneous: 75%), pain at injection site (injection/infusion site: ≤15%), local inflammation (at infusion site: 7%), localized tenderness (intramuscular), local pain (intramuscular/subcutaneous), local swelling (subcutaneous)

Neuromuscular & skeletal: Arthralgia (<5% to 20%; subcutaneous: 6%), limb pain (intravenous/subcutaneous: 6% to 15%), muscle cramps (≤14%), back pain (5% to 11%), weakness (≤10%), myalgia (≤8%), muscle spasm (7%), myasthenia (7%), neck pain (6%), joint effusion (≤6%), joint swelling (≤6%), leg cramps

Ophthalmic: Conjunctivitis (9%), eye discharge (7%), eye irritation (7%), blurred vision

Otic: Otalgia (9% to 18%; subcutaneous: 6%), otitis media (7% to 8%)

Renal: Nephrolithiasis (≤16%), increased serum creatinine (9%), increased blood urea nitrogen

Respiratory: Cough (6% to 54%), nasal congestion (≤52%), rhinitis (5% to 51%), sinusitis (≤50%), pharyngitis (5% to 41%), asthma (9% to 29%; including exacerbation), upper respiratory tract infection (8% to 25%), epistaxis (7% to 23%), bronchitis (5% to 22%), nasopharyngitis (17%), rhinorrhea (7% to 17%), sinus congestion (15%), nasal mucosa swelling (≤13%), wheezing (9% to 11%), exacerbation of asthma (7% to 9%), tonsil disease (children: 8%), dyspnea (7% to 8%), pharyngolaryngeal pain (5% to 8%), pneumonia (≤8%), oropharyngeal pain (7%), post nasal drip (7%), throat irritation (7%), flu-like symptoms (6%)

Miscellaneous: Fever (10% to 33%; subcutaneous: 6% to 7%), accidental injury (13%), positive culture (≤8%)

<1% (Limited to important or life-threatening): Acute renal disease, acute renal failure, acute respiratory distress, agitation, allergic dermatitis, alopecia, anaphylactic shock, anaphylaxis, anxiety, apnea, arterial thrombosis, aseptic meningitis, bradycardia, bronchospasm, bullous dermatitis, burning sensation, cerebrovascular accident, chest tightness, circulatory shock, coma, cyanosis, deep vein thrombosis, disseminated intravascular coagulation (intravenous, subcutaneous, intramuscular; FDA Safety Communication, November 13, 2012), edema, epidermolysis, erythema (may be transient), erythema multiforme, erythematous rash, exacerbation of autoimmune pure red cell aplasia, eye pain, facial edema, hematuria, hemoglobinuria, hemolysis (may be mild), hemolytic anemia (may be delayed), hepatic insufficiency, hepatitis (non-infectious), hypersensitivity, hyperventilation, hypervolemia, hypoxemia, jaundice, leukopenia, loss of consciousness, lymphadenopathy, musculoskeletal pain, myocardial infarction, osmotic nephrosis, oxygen saturation decreased, pallor, palpitations, pancytopenia, paresthesia, peripheral vascular insufficiency, pharyngeal edema, phlebitis, photophobia, proximal tubular nephropathy, pulmonary edema, pulmonary embolism, renal failure, renal insufficiency, renal tubular necrosis, respiratory distress, respiratory failure, restlessness, retinal thrombosis, seizure, Stevens-Johnson syndrome, syncope, thromboembolism, thrombophlebitis, thrombosis, transfusion-related acute lung injury, transient ischemic attacks, tremor, urine discoloration, vena cava thrombosis

Drug Interactions

Metabolism/Transport Effects None known.

Avoid Concomitant Use There are no known interactions where it is recommended to avoid concomitant use.

Increased Effect/Toxicity

The levels/effects of Immune Globulin may be increased by: Estrogen Derivatives

Decreased Effect

Immune Globulin may decrease the levels/effects of: Vaccines (Live)

Preparation for Administration Dilution is dependent upon the manufacturer and brand. Gently swirl; do not shake; avoid foaming. Do not heat. Do not mix products from different manufacturers together. Discard unused portion of vials.

Bivigam: Dilution is not recommended.

Carimune NF: In a sterile laminar air flow environment, reconstitute with NS, D₅W, or SWFI. Complete dissolution may take up to 20 minutes. Begin infusion within 24 hours.

Flebogamma DIF: Dilution is not recommended.

Gammagard Liquid: May dilute in D₅W only.

Gammagard S/D: Reconstitute with SWFI.

Gammaked: May dilute in D₅W only.

Gamunex-C: May dilute in D₅W only.

HyQvia: Bring refrigerated product to room temperature before use. Do **not** mix hyaluronidase and immune globulin prior to administration.

Octagam 10%: Do not dilute. Bottles may be pooled into sterile infusion bags and infused within 8 hours after pooling.

Privigen: If necessary to further dilute, D₅W may be used.

Storage/Stability Stability is dependent upon the manufacturer and brand. Do not freeze (do not use if previously frozen). Do not shake. Do not heat (do not use if previously heated).

Bivigam: Store under refrigeration at 2°C to 8°C (36°F to 46°F). Dilution is not recommended.

Carimune NF: Prior to reconstitution, store at or below 30°C (86°F). Reconstitute with NS, D₅W, or SWFI. Following reconstitution in a sterile laminar air flow environment, store under refrigeration. Begin infusion within 24 hours.

Flebogamma DIF: Store at 2°C to 25°C (36°F to 77°F). Keep in original carton to protect from light. Do not freeze or use if solution has been frozen.

GamaSTAN S/D: Store under refrigeration at 2°C to 8°C (36°F to 46°F). The following stability information has also been reported for GamaSTAN S/D: May be exposed to room temperature for a cumulative 7 days (Cohen, 2007).

Gammagard Liquid: Prior to use, store at 2°C to 8°C (36°F to 46°F). May store at room temperature of 25°C (77°F) within the first 24 months of manufacturing. Storage time at room temperature varies with length of time previously refrigerated; refer to product labeling for details.

Gammagard S/D: Store at ≤25°C (≤77°F). May store diluted solution under refrigeration at 2°C to 8°C (36°F to 46°F) for up to 24 hours if originally prepared in a sterile laminar air flow environment.

Gammaked: Store at 2°C to 8°C (36°F to 46°F); may be stored at ≤25°C (≤77°F) for up to 6 months.

Gammaplex: Store at 2°C to 25°C (36°F to 77°F). Keep in original carton to protect from light. Do not freeze or use if solution has been frozen.

Gamunex-C: Store at 2°C to 8°C (36°F to 46°F); may be stored at ≤25°C (≤77°F) for up to 6 months.

Hizentra: Store at ≤25°C (≤77°F). Keep in original carton to protect from light.

HyQvia: Store at 2°C to 8°C (36°F to 46°F) for up to 36 months; may store at ≤25°C (≤77°F) for up to 3 months during the first 24 months from the date of manufacture (after 3 months at room temperature, discard); do not return vial to refrigerator after it has been stored at room temperature.

Octagam 5%: Store at 2°C to 25°C (36°F to 77°F).

Octagam 10%: Store at 2°C to 8°C (36°F to 46°F) for 24 months from the date of manufacture; within these first 12 months, may store up to 6 months at ≤25°C (77°F); after storage at ≤25°C (77°F), the product must be used or discarded.

Privigen: Store at ≤25°C (≤77°F). Protect from light.

Mechanism of Action Replacement therapy for primary and secondary immunodeficiencies, and IgG antibodies against bacteria, viral, parasitic and mycoplasma antigens; interference with F_c receptors on the cells of the reticuloendothelial system for autoimmune cytopenias and ITP; provides passive immunity by increasing the antibody titer and antigen-antibody reaction potential

Pharmacodynamics/Kinetics

Onset of action: IV: Provides immediate antibody levels

Duration: IM, IV: Immune effect: 3 to 4 weeks (variable)

Distribution: V_d: 0.05 to 0.13 L/kg

Intravascular portion (primarily): Healthy subjects: 41% to 57%; Patients with congenital humoral immunodeficiencies: ~70%

Half-life elimination: IM: ~23 days; SubQ: ~59 days (HyQvia); IV: IgG (variable among patients): Healthy subjects: 14 to 24 days; Patients with congenital humoral immunodeficiencies: 26 to 40 days; hypermetabolism associated with fever and infection have coincided with a shortened half-life

Time to peak:

Plasma: SubQ: Gammagard Liquid: 2.9 days; Hizentra: 2.9 days; HyQvia: ~5 days.

Serum: IM: ~48 hours

Dosing

Adult & Geriatric Note: Some clinicians may administer IGIV formulations FDA approved only for intravenous administration as a subcutaneous infusion based on clinical judgment and patient tolerability.

B-cell chronic lymphocytic leukemia (CLL) with hypogammaglobulinemia, prevention of bacterial infections (Gammagard S/D): IV: 400 mg/kg every 3 to 4 weeks

Chronic inflammatory demyelinating polyneuropathy (CIDP) (Gammaked, Gamunex-C): IV: Loading dose: 2,000 mg/kg (given in divided doses over 2 to 4 consecutive days); Maintenance: 1,000 mg/kg every 3 weeks. Alternatively, administer 500 mg/kg/day for 2 consecutive days every 3 weeks.

Hepatitis A (GamaSTAN S/D): IM:

Preexposure prophylaxis upon travel into endemic areas (hepatitis A vaccine preferred):

0.02 **mL**/kg for anticipated risk of exposure <3 months 0.06 **mL**/kg for anticipated risk of exposure ≥3 months; repeat every 4 to 6 months.

Postexposure prophylaxis: 0.02 **mL**/kg given within 14 days of exposure and/or prior to manifestation of disease; not needed if at least 1 dose of hepatitis A vaccine was given at ≥1 month before exposure (CDC 2006)

Immune thrombocytopenia (ITP):

Carimune NF: IV: Initial: 400 mg/kg/day for 2 to 5 consecutive days (6% solution recommended); Maintenance: 400 mg/kg (no more frequent than daily) as needed to maintain platelet count ≥30,000/mm³ and/or to control significant bleeding; may increase dose if needed (range: 800 to 1,000 mg/kg).

Gammagard S/D: IV: 1,000 mg/kg; up to 3 total doses may be given on alternate days based on patient response and/or platelet count.

Gammaked, Gamunex-C: IV: 1,000 mg/kg/day for 2 consecutive days (second dose may be withheld if adequate platelet response in 24 hours) **or** 400 mg/kg once daily for 5 consecutive days

Gammaplex, Octagam 10%, Privigen: IV: 1,000 mg/kg/day for 2 consecutive days

Measles:

GamaSTAN S/D: IM:

Immunocompetent: 0.25 **mL**/kg given within 6 days of exposure

Immunocompromised children: 0.5 **mL**/kg (maximum dose: 15 **mL**) immediately following exposure

Postexposure prophylaxis, any nonimmune person (off-label population): Patients ≤30 kg: 0.5 **mL**/kg (maximum dose: 15 **mL**) within 6 days of exposure. If patient >30 kg, patient will have lower titers than what is recommended due to the maximum volume that can be administered (CDC 2013)

Gammaked, Gamunex-C, Octagam 5%: IV:

Preexposure prophylaxis in patients with primary humoral immunodeficiency (**ONLY** if routine dose is <400 mg/kg): ≥400 mg/kg immediately before expected exposure followed by resumption of prior dosing in 3 to 4 weeks.

Postexposure prophylaxis in patients with primary humoral immunodeficiency: 400 mg/kg administered as soon as possible after exposure followed by resumption of prior dosing in 3 to 4 weeks.

Postexposure prophylaxis, any nonimmune person (off-label population): 400 mg/kg within 6 days of exposure (CDC 2013)

Hizentra: SubQ infusion:

Preexposure prophylaxis in patients with primary humoral immunodeficiency at risk of measles exposure (eg, during an outbreak; travel to endemic area):

Patients receiving weekly or more frequent dosing: Ensure total weekly dose of ≥200 mg/kg for 2 consecutive weeks followed by resumption of prior dosing schedule

Patients receiving biweekly dosing: Administer ≥400 mg/kg once followed by resumption of prior dosing schedule.

Postexposure prophylaxis in patients with primary humoral immunodeficiency regardless of prior dosing schedule (daily, weekly, or biweekly): 400 mg/kg administered as soon as possible after exposure followed by resumption of prior dosing schedule.

ACIP recommendations: The Advisory Committee on Immunization Practices (ACIP) recommends postexposure prophylaxis with immune globulin (IG) to any nonimmune person exposed to measles. The following patient groups are at risk for severe measles complications and should receive IG therapy: Infants <12 months of age, pregnant women without evidence of immunity; severely compromised persons (eg, persons with severe primary immunodeficiency; some bone marrow transplant patients; some ALL patients; and some patients with AIDS or HIV infection [refer to guidelines for additional details]). IGIM is recommended for infants <12 months of age. IGIV is recommended for pregnant women and immunocompromised persons. Although prophylaxis may be given to any nonimmune person, priority should be given to those at greatest risk for measles complications and also to persons exposed in settings with intense, prolonged, close contact (eg, households, daycare centers, classrooms). Following IG administration, any nonimmune person should then receive the measles mumps and rubella (MMR) vaccine if the person is ≥12 months of age at the time of vaccine administration and the vaccine is not otherwise contraindicated. MMR should not be given until 6 months following IGIM or 8 months following IGIV administration. If a person is already receiving IGIV therapy, a dose of 400 mg/kg IV within 3 weeks prior to exposure (or 200 mg/kg SubQ for 2 consecutive weeks prior to exposure if previously on SubQ therapy) should be sufficient to prevent measles infection. IG therapy is not indicated for any person who already received one dose of a measles-containing vaccine at ≥12 months of age unless they are severely immunocompromised (CDC 2013).

Multifocal motor neuropathy (MMN) (Gammagard Liquid): IV: 500 to 2400 mg/kg/**month** based upon response

Primary humoral immunodeficiency disorders:

IV infusion dosing:

Bivigam, Gammaplex: IV: 300 to 800 mg/kg every 3 to 4 weeks; dose adjusted based on monitored trough serum IgG concentrations and clinical response

Carimune NF: IV: 400 to 800 mg/kg every 3 to 4 weeks. **Note:** In previously untreated agammaglobulinemic or hypogammaglobulinemic patients use a 3% solution; may administer subsequent infusions with a higher concentration if patient tolerates lower concentration.

Flebogamma DIF 5%, Flebogamma DIF 10%, Gammagard Liquid, Gammagard S/D, Gammaked, Gamunex-C, Octagam 5%: IV: 300 to 600 mg/kg every 3 to 4 weeks; dose adjusted based on monitored trough serum IgG concentrations and clinical response

Privigen: IV: 200 to 800 mg/kg every 3 to 4 weeks; dose adjusted based on monitored trough serum IgG concentrations and clinical response

Switching to weekly subcutaneous infusion dosing:

Gammagard Liquid, Gammaked, Gamunex-C: SubQ infusion: Begin 1 week after last IV dose. Use the following equation to calculate initial dose:

Initial weekly dose (g) = [1.37 x IGIV dose (g)] divided by [IV dose interval (weeks)]

Note: For subsequent dose adjustments, refer to product labeling.

Hizentra: SubQ infusion: For weekly or frequent (up to daily) dosing, begin 1 week after last IV infusion or SubQ infusion. For biweekly (every 2 week) dosing, begin 1 or 2 weeks after last IV infusion or 1 week after the last SubQ weekly infusion. **Note:** Patient should have received an IV immune globulin routinely for at least 3 months before switching to SubQ. Use the following equation to calculate initial weekly dose:

Initial weekly dose (g) = [Previous IGIV dose (g)] divided by [IV dose interval (eg, 3 or 4 weeks)] then multiply by 1.37. To convert the dose (in g) to mL, multiply the calculated dose (in g) by 5.

Note: Provided the total weekly dose is maintained, any dosing interval from daily up to biweekly (every 2 weeks) may be used. For patients switching to Hizentra from a different SubQ formulation, the previous weekly SubQ dose should be used initially. Use the following calculations to calculate frequent or biweekly dosing:

Biweekly dosing (g) = multiply the calculated or previous weekly dose by 2.

Frequent (2 to 7 times per week) dosing (g) = divide the calculated or previous weekly dose by the desired number of times per week (eg, for 3 times per week dosing, divide weekly dose by 3)

Note: For subsequent dose adjustments, refer to product labeling.

SubQ infusion dosing:

HyQvia: SubQ: See manufacturer's labeling for initial ramp-up schedule (initiating treatment with a full monthly dose has not been evaluated); dose adjusted based on monitored trough serum IgG concentrations and clinical response after initial ramp-up. **Note:** For patients previously on another IgG treatment, administer the first dose ~1 week after the last infusion of previous treatment.

Patients naive to IgG therapy or switching from IG SubQ therapy: SubQ infusion: 300 to 600 mg/kg every 3 to 4 weeks, after the initial dose ramp-up

Patients switching from IGIV therapy: SubQ infusion: Administer the same dose and frequency as the previous IGIV therapy after the initial dose ramp-up. For subsequent dose adjustments, refer to product labeling.

Rubella (GamaSTAN S/D): IM: Postexposure prophylaxis during pregnancy: 0.55 **mL**/kg

Varicella (GamaSTAN S/D): IM: Prophylaxis: 0.6 to 1.2 **mL**/kg (varicella zoster immune globulin preferred) within 72 hours of exposure (Gershon 1978). **Note:** For patients at risk of thrombosis, administer at the lower end of the recommended dosage range.

Off-label uses: IV:

Acquired hypogammaglobulinemia secondary to malignancy (off-label use): 400 mg/kg/dose every 3 weeks; reevaluate every 4 to 6 months (Anderson 2007)

Dermatomyositis/polymyositis (refractory) (use in combination with other agents in patients with dermatomyositis) (off-label use): 2,000 mg/kg per treatment course administered in divided doses over 2 to 5 consecutive days (eg, 400 mg/kg/day for 5 days); maximum (per treatment course): 2,000 mg/kg (Feasby 2007).

Guillain-Barré syndrome (off-label use): A total dose of 2 g/kg per treatment course, given in divided doses over 2 to 5 consecutive days (eg, 400 mg/kg/day for 5 days) (Feasby 2007; Hughes 2014). European Federation of Neurological Societies (EFNS) guidelines recommend the 5-day treatment regimen (Elovaara, 2008).

Hematopoietic cell transplantation (HCT) with hypogammaglobulinemia (IgG <400 mg/dL), prevention of bacterial infection (off-label use): Note: Increase dose or frequency to maintain IgG concentration >400 mg/dL.
≤100 days post-HCT: 500 mg/kg/dose once weekly (Tomblyn 2009)
>100 days post-HCT: 500 mg/kg/dose every 3 to 4 weeks (Tomblyn 2009)

HIV-associated thrombocytopenia (off-label use): 1,000 mg/kg/day for 2 days (Anderson 2007)

Lambert-Eaton myasthenic syndrome (LEMS) (off-label use): 1,000 mg/kg/day for 2 days (Bain 1996; Patwa 2012)

Myasthenia gravis (acute exacerbation) (off-label use): Adjunctive therapy: 2 g/kg per treatment course, administered in divided doses over 2 to 5 consecutive days (eg, 400 mg/kg/day for 5 days) (Barth 2011; Feasby 2007; Zinman 2007). **Note:** A single dose of 1 g/kg may have similar efficacy to 1 g/kg given on 2 consecutive days (Gajdos 2005)

Relapsing-remitting multiple sclerosis (off-label use): 1,000 mg/kg per month, with or without an induction of 400 mg/kg/day for 5 days (Feasby 2007). Optimal dosing has not been established.

Pediatric Note: Flebogamma DIF 10%, HyQvia, and Octagam 10% are **not** FDA-approved for use in children. Children and Adolescents:

Hepatitis A: Refer to adult dosing.

Immune thrombocytopenia (ITP):
Carimune NF: IV: Initial: 400 mg/kg/day for 2 to 5 consecutive days (6% solution recommended); Maintenance: 400 mg/kg (no more frequent than daily) as needed to maintain platelet count ≥30,000/mm^3 and/or to control significant bleeding; may increase dose if needed (range: 800 to 1,000 mg/kg). For acute ITP, may discontinue after day 2 if platelet response is adequate (30,000 to 50,000/mm^3) after the first 2 doses.
Gammaked, Gamunex-C: IV: 1,000 mg/kg/day for 2 consecutive days (second dose may be withheld if adequate platelet response in 24 hours) **or** 400 mg/kg once daily for 5 consecutive days.
Privigen: IV: 1,000 mg/kg/day for 2 consecutive days (not approved for use in pediatric patients <15 years of age).

Kawasaki syndrome: IV:
Gammagard S/D: 1,000 mg/kg as a single dose **or** 400 mg/kg/day for 4 consecutive days. Begin within 7 days of onset of fever.
AHA guidelines (2004): 2,000 mg/kg as a single dose within 10 days of disease onset
Note: Must be used in combination with aspirin: 80 to 100 mg/kg/day orally, divided every 6 hours for up to 14 days (until fever resolves for at least 48 hours); then decrease dose to 3 to 5 mg/kg/day once daily. In patients without coronary artery abnormalities, give lower dose for 6 to 8 weeks. In patients with coronary artery abnormalities, low-dose aspirin should be continued indefinitely.

Measles: Refer to adult dosing.

Primary humoral immunodeficiency disorders:
IV infusion dosing:
Bivigam: IV: Children ≥6 years and Adolescents: 300 to 800 mg/kg every 3 to 4 weeks; dose adjusted based on monitored trough serum IgG concentrations and clinical response
Carimune NF: IV: Children and Adolescents: 400 to 800 mg/kg every 3 to 4 weeks. **Note:** In previously untreated agammaglobulinemic or hypogammaglobulinemic patients use a 3% solution; may administer subsequent infusions with a higher concentration if patient tolerates lower concentration.
Flebogamma DIF 5%: IV: Children ≥2 years, and Adolescents: 300 to 600 mg/kg every 3 to 4 weeks; dose adjusted based on monitored trough serum IgG concentrations and clinical response
Gammagard Liquid, Gammagard S/D: IV: Children ≥2 years and Adolescents: 300 to 600 mg/kg every 3 to 4 weeks; dose adjusted based on monitored trough serum IgG concentrations and clinical response.
Gammaked, Gamunex-C, Octagam 5%: IV: Children and Adolescents: 300 to 600 mg/kg every 3 to 4 weeks; dose adjusted based on monitored trough serum IgG concentrations and clinical response.
Gammaplex: IV: Children ≥2 years, and Adolescents: 300 to 800 mg/kg every 3 to 4 weeks; dose adjusted based on monitored trough serum IgG concentrations and clinical response.
Privigen: IV: Children ≥3 years and Adolescents: 200 to 800 mg/kg every 3 to 4 weeks; dose adjusted based on monitored trough serum IgG concentrations and clinical response
Switching to weekly subcutaneous infusion dosing:
Gammagard Liquid: Children ≥2 years and Adolescents:
SubQ infusion: Begin 1 week after last IV dose. Use the following equation to calculate initial dose:
Initial weekly dose (g) = [1.37 x IGIV dose (g)] divided by [IV dose interval (weeks)]
Note: For subsequent dose adjustments, refer to product labeling.
Hizentra: SubQ infusion: Children ≥2 years and Adolescents: For weekly or frequent (up to daily) dosing, begin 1 week after last IV infusion or SubQ infusion. For biweekly (every 2 week) dosing, begin 1 or 2 weeks after last IV infusion or 1 week after the last SubQ weekly infusion. **Note:** Patient should have received an IV immune globulin routinely for at least 3 months before switching to SubQ. Use the following equation to calculate initial weekly dose:
Initial weekly dose (g) = [Previous IGIV dose (g)] divided by [IV dose interval (eg, 3 or 4 weeks)] then multiply by 1.37. To convert the dose (in g) to mL, multiply the calculated dose (in g) by 5.
Note: Provided the total weekly dose is maintained, any dosing interval from daily up to biweekly (every 2 weeks) may be used. For patients switching to Hizentra from a different SubQ formulation, the previous weekly SubQ dose should be used initially. Use the following calculations to calculate frequent or biweekly dosing:
Biweekly dosing (g) = multiply the calculated or previous weekly dose by 2.
Frequent (2 to 7 times per week) dosing (g) = divide the calculated or previous weekly dose by the desired number of times per week (eg, for 3 times per week dosing, divide weekly dose by 3).
Note: For subsequent dose adjustments, refer to product labeling.

Varicella: Refer to adult dosing.

Dermatomyositis/polymyositis (refractory) (use in combination with other agents in patients with dermatomyositis) (off-label use): IV: 2,000 mg/kg per treatment course administered in divided doses over 2 consecutive days (eg, 1,000 mg/kg/day for 2 days); maximum (per treatment course): 2,000 mg/kg (Feasby 2007)

Guillain-Barré syndrome (off-label use): Children and Adolescents: IV: 1,000 mg/kg/day for 2 days (Feasby 2007; Korinthenberg 2005) **or** 400 mg/kg/day for 5 days (El-Bayoumi 2011; Korinthenberg 2005).Two-day regimens have been associated with a higher incidence of early relapse (Korinthenberg 2005). American Academy of Neurology guidelines state optimal dosing has not been established (Patwa 2012).

Hematopoietic cell transplantation (HCT) with hypogammaglobulinemia (IgG <400 mg/dL), prevention of bacterial infection (off-label use) (Tomblyn 2009): IV: **Note:** Increase dose or frequency to maintain IgG concentration >400 mg/dL.

≤100 days post-HCT:

Infants and Children (Allogeneic HCT recipients): IV: 400 mg/kg/dose once monthly

Adolescents: IV: 500 mg/kg/dose once weekly

>100 days post-HCT: Infants, Children, and Adolescents: IV: 500 mg/kg/dose every 3 to 4 weeks

Myasthenia gravis (acute exacerbation) (off-label use): Adolescents: Refer to adult dosing.

Renal Impairment

IV: Use with caution due to risk of immune globulin-induced renal dysfunction; the rate of infusion and concentration of solution should be minimized.

IM, SubQ infusion: There are no dosage adjustments provided in the manufacturer's labeling; risk of immune globulin-induced renal dysfunction has not been identified with IM and SubQ infusion administration.

Hepatic Impairment IM, IV, SubQ infusion: There are no dosage adjustments provided in manufacturer's labeling.

Obesity Some clinicians dose IGIV on ideal body weight or an adjusted ideal body weight in morbidly obese patients (Siegel 2010).

Dietary Considerations Some products may contain sodium.

Administration Note: If plasmapheresis employed for treatment of condition, administer immune globulin **after** completion of plasmapheresis session.

IM: Administer IM in the anterolateral aspects of the upper thigh or deltoid muscle of the upper arm. Avoid gluteal region due to risk of injury to sciatic nerve. Divide doses >10 mL and inject in multiple sites.

GamaSTAN S/D is for IM administration only.

IV infusion: Infuse over 2 to 24 hours; administer in separate infusion line from other medications; if using primary line, flush with NS or D$_5$W (product specific; consult product prescribing information) prior to administration. Decrease dose, rate and/or concentration of infusion in patients who may be at risk of renal failure. Decreasing the rate or stopping the infusion may help relieve some adverse effects (flushing, changes in pulse rate, changes in blood pressure). Epinephrine should be available during administration. For initial treatment or in the elderly, a lower concentration and/or a slower rate of infusion should be used. Initial rate of administration and titration is specific to each IGIV product. Refrigerated product should be warmed to room temperature prior to infusion. Some products require filtration; refer to individual product labeling. Antecubital veins should be used, especially with concentrations ≥10% to prevent injection site discomfort.

Bivigam 10%: Primary humoral immunodeficiency: Initial (first 10 minutes): 0.5 mg/kg/minute (0.3 **mL**/kg/**hour**); Maintenance: Increase every 20 minutes (if tolerated) by 0.8 mg/kg/minute (0.48 **mL**/kg/**hour**) up to 6 mg/kg/minute (3.6 **mL**/kg/**hour**)

Carimune NF: Refer to product labeling.

Flebogamma DIF 5%: Primary humoral immunodeficiency: Initial: 0.5 mg/kg/minute (0.6 **mL**/kg/**hour**); Maintenance: Increase slowly (if tolerated) up to 5 mg/kg/minute (6 **mL**/kg/**hour**)

Flebogamma DIF 10%: Primary humoral immunodeficiency: Initial: 1 mg/kg/minute (0.6 **mL**/kg/**hour**); Maintenance: Increase slowly (if tolerated) up to 8 mg/kg/minute (4.8 **mL**/kg/**hour**)

Gammagard Liquid 10%:

Multifocal motor neuropathy (MMN): Initial: 0.8 mg/kg/minute (0.5 **mL**/kg/**hour**); Maintenance: Increase gradually (if tolerated) up to 9 mg/kg/minute (5.4 **mL**/kg/**hour**)

Primary humoral immunodeficiency: Initial (first 30 minutes): 0.8 mg/kg/minute (0.5 **mL**/kg/**hour**); Maintenance: Increase every 30 minutes (if tolerated) up to: 8 mg/kg/minute (5 **mL**/kg/**hour**)

Gammagard S/D: 5% solution: Initial: 0.5 **mL**/kg/**hour**; may increase (if tolerated) to a maximum rate of 4 **mL**/kg/**hour**. If 5% solution is tolerated at maximum rate, may administer 10% solution with an initial rate of 0.5 **mL**/kg/**hour**; may increase (if tolerated) to a maximum rate of 8 **mL**/kg/**hour**

Gammaked 10%:

CIDP: Initial (first 30 minutes): 2 mg/kg/minute (1.2 **mL**/kg/**hour**); Maintenance: Increase gradually (if tolerated) up to 8 mg/kg/minute (4.8 **mL**/kg/**hour**)

Primary humoral immunodeficiency or ITP: Initial (first 30 minutes): 1 mg/kg/minute (0.6 **mL**/kg/**hour**); Maintenance: Increase gradually (if tolerated) up to 8 mg/kg/minute (4.8 **mL**/kg/**hour**)

Gammaplex 5%: Primary humoral immunodeficiency or ITP: Initial (first 15 minutes): 0.5 mg/kg/minute (0.6 **mL**/kg/**hour**); Maintenance: Increase every 15 minutes (if tolerated) up to 4 mg/kg/minute (4.8 **mL**/kg/**hour**)

Gamunex-C 10%:

CIDP: Initial (first 30 minutes): 2 mg/kg/minute (1.2 **mL**/kg/**hour**); Maintenance: Increase gradually (if tolerated) up to 8 mg/kg/minute (4.8 **mL**/kg/**hour**)

Primary humoral immunodeficiency or ITP: Initial (first 30 minutes): 1 mg/kg/minute (0.6 **mL**/kg/**hour**); Maintenance: Increase gradually (if tolerated) up to 8 mg/kg/minute (4.8 **mL**/kg/**hour**)

Octagam 5%: Primary humoral immunodeficiency: Initial (first 30 minutes): 0.5 mg/kg/minute (0.6 **mL**/kg/**hour**); Maintenance: Double infusion rate (if tolerated) every 30 minutes up to a maximum rate of <3.33 mg/kg/minute (4.2 **mL**/kg/**hour**)

Octagam 10%: ITP: Initial (first 30 minutes):1 mg/kg/minute (0.6 **mL**/kg/**hour**); Maintenance: Double infusion rate (if tolerated) every 30 minutes up to a maximum rate of 12 mg/kg/minute (7.2 **mL**/kg/**hour**)

Privigen 10%:

ITP: Initial: 0.5 mg/kg/minute (0.3 **mL**/kg/**hour**); Maintenance: Increase gradually (if tolerated) up to 4 mg/kg/minute (2.4 **mL**/kg/**hour**)

Primary humoral immunodeficiency: Initial: 0.5 mg/kg/minute (0.3 **mL**/kg/**hour**); Maintenance: Increase gradually (if tolerated) up to 8 mg/kg/minute (4.8 **mL**/kg/**hour**)

SubQ infusion: Initial dose should be administered in a healthcare setting capable of providing monitoring and treatment in the event of hypersensitivity. Using aseptic technique, follow the infusion device manufacturer's instructions for filling the reservoir and preparing the pump. Remove air from administration set and needle by priming. For products excluding HyQvia, appropriate injection sites include the abdomen, thigh, upper arm, lower back, and/or lateral hip; dose may be infused into multiple sites (spaced ≥2 inches apart) simultaneously. HyQvia may be injected into the middle to upper abdomen or thigh (avoid bony prominences, or areas that are scarred, inflamed, or infected). If two sites are used simultaneously for HyQvia, the two infusion sites should be on opposite sides of the body. After the sites are clean and dry, insert subcutaneous needle and prime administration set. Attach sterile needle to administration set, gently pull back on the syringe to assure a blood vessel has not been inadvertently accessed (do not use needle and tubing if blood present). Repeat for each injection site; deliver the dose following instructions for the infusion device. Rotate the site(s) between successive infusions. Treatment may be transitioned to the home/home care setting in the absence of adverse reactions.

Gammagard Liquid:

Injection sites: ≤8 simultaneous injection sites

Initial infusion rate:

<40 kg: 15 mL/hour per injection site (maximum volume: 20 mL per injection site)

≥40 kg: 20 mL/hour per injection site (maximum volume: 30 mL per injection site)

Maintenance infusion rate:

<40 kg: 15 to 20 mL/hour per injection site (maximum volume: 20 mL per injection site)

≥40 kg: 20 to 30 mL/hour per injection site (maximum volume: 30 mL per injection site)

Gammaked, Gamunex-C:

Injection sites: ≤8 simultaneous injection sites

Recommended infusion rate: 20 mL/hour per injection site

Hizentra:

Injection sites: ≤4 simultaneous injection sites or ≤12 sites consecutively per infusion

Maximum infusion rate: First infusion: 15 mL/hour per injection site; subsequent infusions: 25 mL/hour per injection site

Maximum infusion volume: First 4 infusions: 15 mL per injection site; subsequent infusions: 20 mL per injection site (maximum: 25 mL per site as tolerated)

HyQvia: Administer components of HyQvia (immune globulin and hyaluronidase) sequentially; do not use either component alone. Infusion pump capable of infusing rates up to 300 mL/hour/site required; must also have the ability to titrate the flow rate. Use a 24 gauge subcutaneous needle set labeled for high flow rates. Infuse the two components of HyQvia sequentially, beginning with the hyaluronidase. Initiate the infusion of the full dose of the immune globulin through the same subcutaneous needle set within ~10 minutes of hyaluronidase infusion. For each full or partial vial of immune globulin used, administer the entire contents of the hyaluronidase vial. A second site can be used based on tolerability and total volume; if a

second site is used, administer half of total volume of the hyaluronidase in each site. Flush the infusion line with NS or D$_5$W if required.

Injection sites:

Volume per site:

<40 kg: ≤300 mL per injection site

≥40 kg: ≤600 mL per injection site

Infusion rate:

Hyaluronidase: ~1 to 2 mL/minute, or as tolerated.

Immune globulin:

First 2 infusions:

<40 kg: 5 mL/hour for 5 to 15 minutes; 10 mL/hour for 5 to 15 minutes; 20 mL/hour for 5 to 15 minutes; 40 mL/hour for 5 to 15 minutes; then 80 mL/hour for remainder of infusion

≥40 kg: 10 mL/hour for 5 to 15 minutes; 30 mL/hour for 5 to 15 minutes; 60 mL/hour for 5 to 15 minutes; 120 mL/hour for 5 to 15 minutes; then 240 mL/hour for remainder of infusion

Next 2 or 3 infusions:

<40 kg: 10 mL/hour for 5 to 15 minutes; 20 mL/hour for 5 to 15 minutes; 40 mL/hour for 5 to 15 minutes; 80 mL/hour for 5 to 15 minutes; then 160 mL/hour for remainder of infusion

≥40 kg: 10 mL/hour for 5 to 15 minutes; 30 mL/hour for 5 to 15 minutes; 120 mL/hour for 5 to 15 minutes; 240 mL/hour for 5 to 15 minutes; then 300 mL/hour for remainder of infusion

Monitoring Parameters Renal function, urine output, IgG concentrations, hemoglobin and hematocrit, platelets (in patients with ITP); infusion- or injection-related adverse reactions, anaphylaxis, signs and symptoms of hemolysis; blood viscosity (in patients at risk for hyperviscosity); presence of antineutrophil antibodies (if TRALI is suspected); volume status; neurologic symptoms (if AMS suspected); pulmonary adverse reactions; clinical response

For patients at high risk of hemolysis (dose ≥2 g/kg, given as a single dose or divided over several days, and non-O blood type): Hemoglobin or hematocrit prior to and 36 to 96 hours postinfusion.

SubQ infusion: Monitor IgG trough levels every 2 to 3 months before/after conversion from IV; subcutaneous infusions provide more constant IgG levels than usual IV immune globulin treatments.

Test Interactions Octagam 5% and Octagam 10% contain maltose. Falsely elevated blood glucose levels may occur when glucose monitoring devices and test strips utilizing the glucose dehydrogenase pyrroloquinolinequinone (GDH-PQQ) based methods are used. Glucose monitoring devices and test strips which utilize the glucose-specific method are recommended. Passively transferred antibodies may yield false-positive serologic testing results; may yield false-positive direct and indirect Coombs' test. Skin testing should not be performed with GamaSTAN S/D because local chemical irritation can occur and be misinterpreted as a positive reaction.

Additional Information IM: When administering immune globulin for hepatitis A prophylaxis, use should be considered for the following close contacts of persons with confirmed hepatitis A: unvaccinated household and sexual contacts, persons who have shared illicit drugs, regular babysitters, staff and attendees of child care centers, food handlers within the same establishment (CDC, 2006).

For travelers, immune globulin is not an alternative to careful selection of foods and water; immune globulin can interfere with the antibody response to parenterally administered live virus vaccines. Frequent travelers should be tested for hepatitis A antibody, immune hemolytic anemia, and neutropenia (with ITP, IV route is usually used).

IgA content:

Bivigam: ≤200 mcg/mL

Carimune NF: 1000 to 2000 mcg/mL

Flebogamma 5% DIF: <50 mcg/mL

Flebogamma 10% DIF: <100 mcg/mL

Gammagard Liquid: 37 mcg/mL

Gammagard S/D 5% solution: <1 mcg/mL or <2.2 mcg/mL (product dependent) (see **Note**)

Gammaked: 46 mcg/mL

Gammaplex: <10 mcg/mL

Gamunex-C: 46 mcg/mL

Hizentra: ≤50 mcg/mL

Octagam 5%: ≤200 mcg/mL

Octagam 10%: 106 mcg/mL

Privigen: ≤25 mcg/mL

Note: Manufacturer has discontinued Gammagard S/D 5% solution; however, the lower IgA product will remain available by special request for patients with known reaction to IgA or IgA deficiency with antibodies.

Dosage Forms Considerations

Carimune NF may contain a significant amount of sodium and also contains sucrose.

Gammagard S/D may contain a significant amount of sodium and also contains glucose.

Octagam contains maltose.

Hyqvia Kit is supplied with a Hyaluronidase (Human Recombinant) component intended for injection prior to Immune Globulin administration to improve dispersion and absorption of the Immune Globulin.

Dosage Forms Excipient information presented when available (limited, particularly for generics); consult specific product labeling. [DSC] = Discontinued product

Injectable, Intramuscular [preservative free]:

GamaSTAN S/D: 15% to 18% [150 to 180 mg/mL] (2 mL, 10 mL)

Kit, Subcutaneous:

Hyqvia: 2.5 g/25 mL, 5 g/50 mL, 10 g/100 mL, 20 g/200 mL, 30 g/300 mL [contains albumin human, edetate disodium dihydrate, mouse protein (murine) (hamster)]

Solution, Injection [preservative free]:

Gammagard: 1 g/10 mL (10 mL); 2.5 g/25 mL (25 mL); 5 g/50 mL (50 mL); 10 g/100 mL (100 mL); 20 g/200 mL (200 mL); 30 g/300 mL (300 mL) [latex free]

Gammaked: 1 g/10 mL (10 mL); 2.5 g/25 mL (25 mL); 5 g/50 mL (50 mL); 10 g/100 mL (100 mL); 20 g/200 mL (200 mL) [latex free]

Gamunex-C: 1 g/10 mL (10 mL); 2.5 g/25 mL (25 mL); 5 g/50 mL (50 mL); 10 g/100 mL (100 mL); 20 g/200 mL (200 mL); 40 g/400 mL (400 mL) [latex free]

Solution, Intravenous:

Gamunex: 10 g/100 mL (100 mL [DSC])

Solution, Intravenous [preservative free]:

Bivigam: 5 g/50 mL (50 mL); 10 g/100 mL (100 mL) [sugar free; contains polysorbate 80]

Flebogamma: 0.5 g/10 mL (10 mL [DSC])

Flebogamma DIF: 0.5 g/10 mL (10 mL); 2.5 g/50 mL (50 mL); 5 g/50 mL (50 mL); 5 g/100 mL (100 mL); 10 g/100 mL (100 mL); 10 g/200 mL (200 mL); 20 g/200 mL (200 mL); 20 g/400 mL (400 mL) [contains polyethylene glycol]

Gammaplex: 2.5 g/50 mL (50 mL); 5 g/100 mL (100 mL); 10 g/200 mL (200 mL); 20 g/400 mL (400 mL) [contains polysorbate 80]

Octagam: 1 g/20 mL (20 mL); 2 g/20 mL (20 mL); 2.5 g/50 mL (50 mL); 5 g/50 mL (50 mL); 5 g/100 mL (100 mL); 10 g/100 mL (100 mL); 10 g/200 mL (200 mL); 20 g/200 mL (200 mL); 25 g/500 mL (500 mL) [sucrose free]

Privigen: 5 g/50 mL (50 mL); 10 g/100 mL (100 mL); 20 g/200 mL (200 mL); 40 g/400 mL (400 mL)

Solution, Subcutaneous [preservative free]:

Hizentra: 1 g/5 mL (5 mL); 2 g/10 mL (10 mL); 4 g/20 mL (20 mL); 10 g/50 mL (50 mL) [contains polysorbate 80]

Solution Reconstituted, Intravenous [preservative free]:

Carimune NF: 3 g (1 ea [DSC]); 6 g (1 ea); 12 g (1 ea)

Gammagard S/D: 2.5 g (1 ea [DSC]); 5 g (1 ea [DSC]); 10 g (1 ea [DSC])

Gammagard S/D Less IgA: 5 g (1 ea); 10 g (1 ea)

- Inapsine *see* Droperidol *on page 607*
- INCB424 *see* Ruxolitinib *on page 1626*
- INCB 18424 *see* Ruxolitinib *on page 1626*
- Incivek [DSC] *see* Telaprevir *on page 1743*

IncobotulinumtoxinA
(in kuh BOT yoo lin num TOKS in aye)

Brand Names: US Xeomin
Brand Names: Canada Xeomin Cosmetic™; Xeomin®
Index Terms Botulinum Toxin Type A
Pharmacologic Category Neuromuscular Blocker Agent, Toxin; Ophthalmic Agent, Toxin
Use
U.S. labeling: Treatment of blepharospasm in patients previously treated with onabotulinumtoxinA (Botox®); treatment of cervical dystonia in botulinum toxin-naïve and previously treated patients; temporary improvement in the appearance of moderate-to-severe glabellar lines associated with corrugator and/or procerus muscle activity

Canadian labeling:
Xeomin®: Treatment of hypertonicity disorders of the seventh nerve (eg, blepharospasm, hemifacial spasm); treatment of poststroke spasticity of upper limb(s); treatment of cervical dystonia (spasmodic torticollis)
Xeomin Cosmetic™: Temporary improvement in the appearance of moderate-to-severe glabellar lines
Medication Guide Available Yes
Dosing
Adult
Blepharospasm: IM:
U.S. labeling: Initial: Total dose should be the same as previously administered onabotulinumtoxinA dose. If prior onabotulinumtoxinA dose is not known: 1.25-2.5 units/injection site (maximum initial dose: 35 units/eye or 70 units/both eyes). Number and location of injection sites based on disease severity and previous dose/response to onabotulinumtoxinA (in clinical trials, a mean number of 6 injections per eye were administered). Cumulative dose should not exceed 35 units/eye or 70 units/both eyes administered no more frequently than every 3 months.
Canadian labeling: Initial: 1.25-2.5 units/injection site (maximum initial dose: 25 units/eye). Dose may be increased up to twice the previous dose if the response from the initial dose lasted ≤2 months; maximum dose per site: 5 units. Cumulative dose should not exceed 35 units/eye or 70 units/both eyes administered no more frequently than every 3 months.
Cervical dystonia: IM:
U.S. labeling: Initial total dose: 120 units (in clinical trials, similar efficacy was noted with initial total doses of 120 and 240 units and between treatment experienced and treatment naïve patients. Dose and number of injection sites should be individualized based on prior treatment, response, duration of effect, adverse events, number/location of muscle(s) to be treated and disease severity. In clinical trials most patients received a total of 2-10 injections into treated muscles. Administer no more frequently than every 3 months
Canadian labeling: Usual total dose: 200 units (maximum: 300 units; maximum dose per injection site: 50 units); administer no more frequently than every 3 months
Reduction of glabellar lines: IM: Inject 4 units into each of the 5 sites (2 injections in each corrugator muscle and 1 injection in the procerus muscle) for a total dose of 20 units per treatment session. Administer no more frequently than every 3 months.
Spasticity of upper limb (poststroke): *Canadian labeling (not in U.S. labeling):* IM: Individualize dose based on patient size, extent, and location of muscle involvement, degree of spasticity, local muscle weakness, and response to prior treatment. In clinical trials, total doses up to 400 units were administered as separate injections typically divided among selected muscles; may repeat therapy at ≥3 months with appropriate dosage based upon the clinical condition of patient at time of retreatment.
Suggested guidelines for the treatment of stroke-related upper limb spasticity: **Note:** The lowest recommended starting dose should be used. Dosage and number of injection sites should be individualized. Multiple injections may minimize adverse effects. Dose listed is total dose administered to site:
Biceps: 80 units
Brachialis: 50 units
Brachioradialis: 60 units
Flexor carpi radialis: 50 units
Flexor carpi ulnaris: 40 units
Flexor digitorum profundus: 40 units
Flexor digitorum superficialis: 40 units
Adductor pollicis: 10 units
Flexor pollicis brevis: 10 units
Flexor pollicis longus: 20 units
Pronator quadratus 25 units
Pronator teres: 40 units
Geriatric Refer to adult dosing. Initiate therapy at lowest recommended dose.
Renal Impairment There are no dosage adjustments provided in manufacturer's labeling.
Hepatic Impairment There are no dosage adjustments provided in manufacturer's labeling.
Additional Information Complete prescribing information should be consulted for additional detail.
Dosage Forms Excipient information presented when available (limited, particularly for generics); consult specific product labeling.
Solution Reconstituted, Intramuscular [preservative free]:
Xeomin: 50 units (1 ea); 100 units (1 ea) [contains albumin human]
Dosage Forms: Canada Excipient information presented when available (limited, particularly for generics); consult specific product labeling.
Injection, powder for reconstitution:
Xeomin Cosmetic™: 100 units [contains albumin (human), sucrose 4.7 mg]

- Incruse Ellipta *see* Umeclidinium *on page 1852*

Indacaterol (in da KA ter ol)

Brand Names: US Arcapta Neohaler
Brand Names: Canada Onbrez Breezhaler
Index Terms Indacaterol Maleate; QAB149
Pharmacologic Category Beta$_2$ Agonist; Beta$_2$-Adrenergic Agonist, Long-Acting
Use
Chronic obstructive pulmonary disease (maintenance): Long-term maintenance treatment of airflow obstruction in chronic obstructive pulmonary disease (COPD) including chronic bronchitis and/or emphysema
Limitations of use: Not indicated for treatment of acute deterioration of COPD or for treatment of asthma.
Medication Guide Available Yes
Dosing
Adult & Geriatric
COPD (maintenance): Inhalation: Contents of 1 capsule (75 mcg) inhaled once daily using Neohaler inhaler (US labeling) or Onbrez Breezhaler inhalation device (Canadian labeling). Maximum dose: 1 capsule (75 mcg)/day.
Note: A dose of 75 to 300 mcg once daily is recommended by the 2015 Updated GOLD Guidelines.
Renal Impairment No dosage adjustment necessary.
Hepatic Impairment
Mild-to-moderate impairment: No dosage adjustment necessary.
Severe impairment: There are no dosage adjustments provided in the manufacturer's labeling (has not been studied).
Additional Information Complete prescribing information should be consulted for additional detail.
Dosage Forms Excipient information presented when available (limited, particularly for generics); consult specific product labeling.
Capsule, Inhalation:
Arcapta Neohaler: 75 mcg [contains lactose monohydrate, milk protein]
Dosage Forms: Canada Excipient information presented when available (limited, particularly for generics); consult specific product labeling.
Capsule, Inhalation:
Onbrez Breezhaler: 75 mcg [contains lactose monohydrate, milk protein]

Indacaterol and Glycopyrrolate
(in da KA ter ol & glye koe PIR oh late)

Brand Names: US Utibron Neohaler [DSC]
Brand Names: Canada Ultibro Breezhaler
Index Terms Glycopyrrolate and Indacaterol; Glycopyrrolate and Indacaterol Maleate; Glycopyrronium and Indacaterol; Glycopyrronium Bromide and Indacaterol Maleate; Indacaterol Maleate and Glycopyrronium Bromide; QVA149
Pharmacologic Category Anticholinergic Agent; Beta$_2$ Agonist; Beta$_2$-Adrenergic Agonist, Long-Acting
Use Chronic obstructive pulmonary disease:
Long-term maintenance treatment of airflow obstruction in chronic obstructive pulmonary disease (COPD) including chronic bronchitis and/or emphysema.

Limitations of use: Not indicated for the relief of acute bronchospasm or for the treatment of asthma.

Pregnancy Considerations Animal reproduction studies have not been conducted with this combination. Refer to individual monographs.

Breast-Feeding Considerations It is not known if indacaterol or glycopyrrolate are excreted in breast milk. The US manufacturer recommends that caution be used if administering this combination to breast-feeding women. The Canadian manufacturer recommends use only if the potential benefits to the mother are expected to be greater than the possible risks to the fetus. Refer to individual monographs.

Contraindications

Hypersensitivity to indacaterol, glycopyrrolate, or any component of the formulation; monotherapy in patients with asthma (ie, without concurrent use of a long-term asthma control medication)

Canadian labeling: Additional contraindications (not in US labeling): Severe hypersensitivity to milk proteins

Warnings/Precautions [US Boxed Warning]: Long-acting beta₂-agonists (LABAs) increase the risk of asthma-related death. The safety and efficacy of indacaterol/glycopyrrolate in patients with asthma have not been established. Indacaterol/glycopyrrolate is not indicated for the treatment of asthma. In a large, randomized, placebo-controlled U.S. clinical trial (SMART, 2006), salmeterol was associated with an increase in asthma-related deaths (when added to usual asthma therapy); risk is considered a class effect among all LABAs. Data are not available to determine if LABA use increases the risk of death in patients with COPD. Rarely, paradoxical, life-threatening bronchospasm may occur with use of inhaled beta₂-agonists; distinguish from inadequate response and discontinue medication immediately if paradoxical bronchospasm occurs.

Do not use for acute episodes of COPD or for acute bronchospasm; always prescribe with an inhaled short-acting beta₂-agonist (eg, albuterol) and educate patient on appropriate use. Upon initiation of the combination inhaler, use of short-acting beta₂-agonists should be limited to treat acute symptoms. Do not initiate in patients with significantly worsening, potentially life-threatening or acutely deteriorating COPD. Do not increase the dose or frequency beyond what is recommended. Hypersensitivity reactions may occur; discontinue immediately if signs and symptoms of an allergic reaction occur; the Canadian labeling does not recommend a rechallenge.

Use with caution in severe hepatic impairment, seizure disorder, diabetes, hyperthyroidism, hypokalemia, narrow angle glaucoma, prostatic hyperplasia/bladder neck obstruction, cardiovascular disease (arrhythmia, coronary insufficiency, hypertension, or HF), and severe renal impairment (GFR <30 mL/minute/1.73 m²) or end-stage renal disease (ESRD) on dialysis. Potentially significant interactions may exist, requiring dose or frequency adjustment, additional monitoring, and/or selection of alternative therapy. Some products may contain lactose; allergic reactions possible in patients with severe milk protein allergy. Use with caution in patients with severe hypersensitivity to milk proteins; use of the Canadian product is contraindicated in patients with severe milk protein allergy. May cause drowsiness, dizziness, and/or blurred vision; patients must be cautioned about performing tasks which require mental alertness (eg, operating machinery or driving).

Adverse Reactions Adverse reactions listed below are reflective of both the US and Canadian product information. Also see Indacaterol monograph. Frequency not always defined. Incidence not specifically defined, but reported in the range of >10%.

Cardiovascular: Chest pain (2%), hypertension (2%), cardiac arrhythmia

Central nervous system: Headache (2% to 3%), dizziness (2%)

Endocrine & metabolic: Hyperglycemia (≥2%)

Gastrointestinal: Gastroenteritis (3%), xerostomia (≤3%), diarrhea (≥2%), gastroesophageal reflux disease (≥2%), dyspepsia (1% to 2%)

Genitourinary: Urinary tract infection (2% to 4%), dysuria (1%)

Neuromuscular & skeletal: Back pain (2%), musculoskeletal pain (1% to 2%)

Respiratory: Nasopharyngitis (4% to >10%), cough (6%), pneumonia (2% to 4%), lower respiratory tract infection (>2%), oropharyngeal pain (2%), sinusitis (2%), rhinitis (1% to 2%), paradoxical bronchospasm, upper respiratory tract infection

Miscellaneous: Fever (2%)

<1% (Limited to important or life-threatening): Atrial fibrillation, bladder outflow obstruction, cystitis, dental caries, diabetes mellitus, glaucoma, hypersensitivity reaction, ischemic heart disease, peripheral edema, tachycardia

Drug Interactions

Metabolism/Transport Effects Refer to individual components.

Avoid Concomitant Use

Avoid concomitant use of Indacaterol and Glycopyrronium with any of the following: Aclidinium; Anticholinergic Agents; Beta-Blockers (Nonselective); Cimetropium; Eluxadoline; Glucagon; Glycopyrrolate; Iobenguane I 123; Ipratropium (Oral Inhalation); Levosulpiride; Long-Acting Beta2-Agonists; Loxapine; Potassium Chloride; Tiotropium; Umeclidinium

Increased Effect/Toxicity

Indacaterol and Glycopyrronium may increase the levels/effects of: AbobotulinumtoxinA; Analgesics (Opioid); Atosiban; Cannabinoid-Containing Products; Cimetropium; Corticosteroids (Systemic); Doxofylline; Eluxadoline; Glucagon; Glycopyrrolate; Highest Risk QTc-Prolonging Agents; Long-Acting Beta2-Agonists; Loop Diuretics; Loxapine; Mirabegron; Moderate Risk QTc-Prolonging Agents; OnabotulinumtoxinA; Potassium Chloride; Ramosetron; RimabotulinumtoxinB; Sympathomimetics; Thiazide Diuretics; Tiotropium; Topiramate

The levels/effects of Indacaterol and Glycopyrronium may be increased by: Aclidinium; Anticholinergic Agents; AtoMOXetine; Caffeine and Caffeine Containing Products; Cannabinoid-Containing Products; Ipratropium (Oral Inhalation); Linezolid; MAO Inhibitors; Mianserin; Mifepristone; Pramlintide; Tedizolid; Theophylline Derivatives; Umeclidinium

Decreased Effect

Indacaterol and Glycopyrronium may decrease the levels/effects of: Acetylcholinesterase Inhibitors; Gastrointestinal Agents (Prokinetic); Iobenguane I 123; Itopride; Levosulpiride; Secretin

The levels/effects of Indacaterol and Glycopyrronium may be decreased by: Acetylcholinesterase Inhibitors; Beta-Blockers (Beta1 Selective); Beta-Blockers (Nonselective); Betahistine

Storage/Stability Store at 15°C to 25°C (59°F to 77°F). Protect from light and moisture. Remove from blister pack immediately before use; discard capsule if not used immediately.

Mechanism of Action

Indacaterol: Relaxes bronchial smooth muscle by selective action on beta2-receptors with little effect on heart rate; acts locally in the lung.

Glycopyrrolate: In COPD, competitively and reversibly inhibits the action of acetylcholine at muscarinic receptor subtypes 1-3 (greater affinity for subtypes 1 and 3) in bronchial smooth muscle thereby causing bronchodilation.

Pharmacodynamics/Kinetics Refer to individual agents

Dosing

Adult & Geriatric

COPD (maintenance): Oral inhalation:
US labeling: 1 capsule (indacaterol 27.5 mcg/glycopyrrolate 15.6 mcg) inhaled twice daily (maximum: 2 capsules/day)
Canadian labeling: 1 capsule (indacaterol 110 mcg/glycopyrrolate 50 mcg) inhaled once daily (maximum: 1 capsule/day)

Renal Impairment

GFR ≥30 mL/minute/1.73 m²: No dosage adjustment necessary.

GFR <30 mL/minute/1.73 m²: There are no dosage adjustments provided in the manufacturer's labeling; use with caution.

ESRD requiring dialysis: There are no dosage adjustments provided in the manufacturer's labeling; use with caution.

Hepatic Impairment

Mild-to-moderate impairment: No dosage adjustment necessary.

Severe impairment: There are no dosage adjustments provided in the manufacturer's labeling (has not been studied); use with caution.

Administration For inhalation using Neohaler (US) or Ultibro Breezhaler (Canada) only; do not swallow capsules. Use the new inhaler included with each prescription. Do not remove capsules from blister until immediately before use. Use at the same time each day. Discard any capsules that are exposed to air and not used immediately. ▶

◄ **Monitoring Parameters** FEV$_1$, FVC, and/or other pulmonary function tests; serum potassium, serum glucose; blood pressure, heart rate; CNS stimulation. Monitor for increased use of short-acting beta$_2$-agonist inhalers; may be marker of a deteriorating condition. Monitor for changes in risk factors (eg, environmental exposure, smoking status).

Product Availability Utibron Neohaler: FDA approved October 2015; availability anticipated in the first quarter of 2016.

Dosage Forms Excipient information presented when available (limited, particularly for generics); consult specific product labeling.

Capsule, Inhalation:
Utibron Neohaler: Indacaterol 27.5 mcg and glycopyrrolate 15.6 mcg [contains milk protein]

Dosage Forms: Canada Excipient information presented when available (limited, particularly for generics); consult specific product labeling.

Capsule, Inhalation:
Ultibro Breezhaler: Indacaterol 110 mcg and glycopyrrolate 50 mcg [contains lactose monohydrate, milk protein, tartrazine]

♦ Indacaterol Maleate *see* Indacaterol *on page 934*

♦ Indacaterol Maleate and Glycopyrronium Bromide *see* Indacaterol and Glycopyrrolate *on page 934*

Indapamide (in DAP a mide)

Brand Names: Canada Apo-Indapamide; Dom-Indapamide; JAMP-Indapamide; Lozide; Mylan-Indapamide; PHL-Indapamide; PMS-Indapamide; PRO-Indapamide; Riva-Indapamide; Teva-Indapamide

Index Terms Lozol

Pharmacologic Category Antihypertensive; Diuretic, Thiazide-Related

Use

Heart failure: Treatment of edema in heart failure

Hypertension: Management of mild-to-moderate hypertension

Guideline recommendations:

Hypertension: The 2014 guideline for the management of high blood pressure in adults (Eighth Joint National Committee [JNC 8]) recommends initiation of pharmacologic treatment to lower blood pressure for the following patients:

• Patients ≥60 years of age with systolic blood pressure (SBP) ≥150 mm Hg or diastolic blood pressure (DBP) ≥90 mm Hg. Goal of therapy is SBP <150 mm Hg and DBP <90 mm Hg.

• Patients <60 years of age with SBP ≥140 mm Hg or DBP is ≥90 mm Hg. Goal of therapy is SBP <140 mm Hg and DBP <90 mm Hg.

• Patients ≥18 years of age with diabetes and SBP ≥140 mm Hg or DBP ≥90 mm Hg. Goal of therapy is SBP <140 mm Hg and DBP <90 mm Hg.

• Patients ≥18 years of age with chronic kidney disease (CKD) and SBP ≥140 mm Hg or DBP ≥90 mm Hg. Goal of therapy is SBP <140 mm Hg and DBP <90 mm Hg.

Chronic kidney disease (CKD) and hypertension: Regardless of race or diabetes status, the use of an ACE inhibitor (ACEI) or angiotensin receptor blocker (ARB) as initial therapy is recommended to improve kidney outcomes. In the general non-black population (without CKD) including those with diabetes, initial antihypertensive treatment should consist of a thiazide-type diuretic, calcium channel blocker, ACEI, or ARB. In the general black population (without CKD), including those with diabetes, initial antihypertensive treatment should consist of a thiazide-type diuretic or a calcium channel blocker **instead of** an ACEI or ARB.

Coronary artery disease (CAD) and hypertension: The American Heart Association, American College of Cardiology and American Society of Hypertension (AHA/ACC/ASH) 2015 scientific statement for the treatment of hypertension in patients with coronary artery disease (CAD) recommends the use of a thiazide (or thiazide-like diuretic) as part of a regimen in patients with hypertension and chronic stable angina. A BP target of <140/90 mm Hg is reasonable for the secondary prevention of cardiovascular events. A lower target BP (<130/80 mm Hg) may be appropriate in some individuals with CAD, previous MI, stroke or transient ischemic attack, or CAD risk equivalents (AHA/ACC/ASH [Rosendorff 2015]).

Pregnancy Considerations Adverse events were not observed in animal reproduction studies. Diuretics cross the placenta and are found in cord blood. Maternal use may cause may cause fetal or neonatal jaundice, thrombocytopenia, or other adverse events observed in adults. Use of diuretics during normal pregnancies is not appropriate; use may be considered when edema is due to pathologic causes (as in the nonpregnant patient); monitor. Canadian labeling contraindicates use in pregnant women.

Breast-Feeding Considerations It is not known if indapamide is excreted in breast milk. If therapy is needed, the manufacturer recommends that nursing be discontinued.

Contraindications

Hypersensitivity to indapamide or any component of the formulation or sulfonamide-derived drugs; anuria

Note: Although the FDA approved product labeling states this medication is contraindicated with other sulfonamide-containing drug classes, the scientific basis of this statement has been challenged. See "Warnings/Precautions" for more detail.

Canadian labeling: Additional contraindications (not in U.S. labeling): Severe renal failure (CrCl <30 mL/minute); hepatic encephalopathy; severe hepatic impairment; hypokalemia; concomitant use with antiarrhythmic agents causing torsade de pointes; pregnancy; breast-feeding; hereditary problems of galactose intolerance, glucose-galactose malabsorption, or Lapp lactase deficiency

Warnings/Precautions Use with caution in severe renal disease; Canadian labeling contraindicates use in severe renal failure (CrCl <30 mL/minute). Electrolyte disturbances including severe hyponatremia (with hypokalemia, hypochloremic alkalosis, hypomagnesemia, or hypercalcemia) can occur; risk may be dose dependent. Correct hypokalemia before initiating therapy (Canadian labeling contraindicates use in hypokalemia). Use in severe hepatic dysfunction; hepatic encephalopathy can be caused by electrolyte disturbances (Canadian labeling contraindicates use in severe hepatic impairment or hepatic encephalopathy). Gout may be precipitated in certain patients with a history of gout, a familial predisposition to gout, or chronic renal failure. Use caution in patients with prediabetes or diabetes; may alter glucose control. May cause SLE exacerbation or activation. Use with caution in patients with moderate or high cholesterol concentrations. Photosensitization may occur.

Formulation may contain lactose; Canadian labeling recommends avoiding use in patients with hereditary conditions of galactose intolerance, glucose-galactose malabsorption, or lactase deficiency.

Sulfonamide ("sulfa") allergy: The FDA-approved product labeling for many medications containing a sulfonamide chemical group includes a broad contraindication in patients with a prior allergic reaction to sulfonamides. There is a potential for cross-reactivity between members of a specific class (eg, two antibiotic sulfonamides). However, concerns for cross-reactivity have previously extended to all compounds containing the sulfonamide structure (SO_2NH_2). An expanded understanding of allergic mechanisms indicates cross-reactivity between antibiotic sulfonamides and nonantibiotic sulfonamides may not occur or at the very least this potential is extremely low (Brackett 2004; Johnson 2005; Slatore 2004; Tornero 2004). In particular, mechanisms of cross-reaction due to antibody production (anaphylaxis) are unlikely to occur with nonantibiotic sulfonamides. T-cell-mediated (type IV) reactions (eg, maculopapular rash) are less well understood and it is not possible to completely exclude this potential based on current insights. In cases where prior reactions were severe (Stevens-Johnson syndrome/TEN), some clinicians choose to avoid exposure to these classes.

Adverse Reactions

≥5%:
Central nervous system: Agitation, anxiety, dizziness, fatigue, headache, irritability, lethargy, malaise, nervousness (dose dependent), pain, tension, tiredness
Endocrine & metabolic: Hypokalemia (<3.5 mEq/L: 20% to 72%, dose dependent)
Neuromuscular & skeletal: Back pain, muscle cramps/spasm, paresthesia, weakness
Respiratory: Rhinitis
Miscellaneous: Infection

≥1% to <5%:
Cardiovascular: Arrhythmia, chest pain, flushing, orthostatic hypotension, palpitation, peripheral edema, PVC, vasculitis
Central nervous system: Depression, drowsiness, insomnia, lightheadedness, vertigo
Dermatologic: Hives, pruritus, rash
Endocrine & metabolic: Hyperglycemia, hyperuricemia, hypochloremia, hyponatremia, libido decreased
Gastrointestinal: Abdominal pain, anorexia, constipation, cramping, diarrhea, dyspepsia, gastric irritation, nausea, vomiting, weight loss, xerostomia
Genitourinary: Nocturia, polyuria

Neuromuscular & skeletal: Hypertonia
Ocular: Blurred vision, conjunctivitis
Renal: BUN increased, creatinine increased, glycosuria
Respiratory: Cough, pharyngitis, rhinorrhea, sinusitis
Miscellaneous: Flu-like syndrome

<1% (Limited to important or life-threatening): Agranulocytosis, anaphylactic reaction, aplastic anemia, bullous eruptions, erythema multiforme, fever, hepatitis, hypercalcemia, jaundice (cholestatic jaundice), leukopenia, liver function test abnormality, pancreatitis, photosensitivity, pneumonitis, purpura, Stevens-Johnson syndrome, thrombocytopenia, torsade de pointes

Drug Interactions

Metabolism/Transport Effects None known.

Avoid Concomitant Use

Avoid concomitant use of Indapamide with any of the following: Dofetilide; Levosulpiride; Mecamylamine

Increased Effect/Toxicity

Indapamide may increase the levels/effects of: ACE Inhibitors; Allopurinol; Amifostine; Antipsychotic Agents (Second Generation [Atypical]); Calcium Salts; CarBAMazepine; Cardiac Glycosides; Cyclophosphamide; Diazoxide; Dofetilide; DULoxetine; Highest Risk QTc-Prolonging Agents; Hypotension-Associated Agents; Ivabradine; Levodopa; Levosulpiride; Lithium; Mecamylamine; Moderate Risk QTc-Prolonging Agents; Multivitamins/Minerals (with ADEK, Folate, Iron); Multivitamins/Minerals (with AE, No Iron); Nonsteroidal Anti-Inflammatory Agents; OXcarbazepine; Porfimer; Sodium Phosphates; Topiramate; Verteporfin; Vitamin D Analogs

The levels/effects of Indapamide may be increased by: Alcohol (Ethyl); Alfuzosin; Analgesics (Opioid); Anticholinergic Agents; Barbiturates; Beta2-Agonists; Brimonidine (Topical); Corticosteroids (Orally Inhaled); Corticosteroids (Systemic); Dexketoprofen; Diazoxide; Herbs (Hypotensive Properties); Licorice; Mifepristone; Molsidomine; Multivitamins/Fluoride (with ADE); Nicorandil; Obinutuzumab; Pentoxifylline; Phosphodiesterase 5 Inhibitors; Prostacyclin Analogues; Selective Serotonin Reuptake Inhibitors

Decreased Effect

Indapamide may decrease the levels/effects of: Antidiabetic Agents

The levels/effects of Indapamide may be decreased by: Amphetamines; Bile Acid Sequestrants; Herbs (Hypertensive Properties); Methylphenidate; Nonsteroidal Anti-Inflammatory Agents; Yohimbine

Storage/Stability Store at 20°C to 25°C (68°F to 77°F).

Mechanism of Action Diuretic effect is localized at the proximal segment of the distal tubule of the nephron; it does not appear to have significant effect on glomerular filtration rate nor renal blood flow; like other diuretics, it enhances sodium, chloride, and water excretion by interfering with the transport of sodium ions across the renal tubular epithelium

Pharmacodynamics/Kinetics

Absorption: Rapid and complete
Distribution: V_d: 25 L (Grebow, 1982)
Protein binding, plasma: 71% to 79%
Metabolism: Extensively hepatic
Bioavailability: 93% (Ernst, 2009)
Half-life elimination: Biphasic: 14 and 25 hours
Time to peak: 2 hours
Excretion: Urine (~70%; 7% as unchanged drug within 48 hours); feces (23%)

Dosing

Adult

Edema: Oral: Initial: 2.5 mg daily; if inadequate response after 1 week, may increase dose to 5 mg daily. **Note:** There is little therapeutic benefit to increasing the dose >5 mg daily; there is, however, an increased risk of electrolyte disturbances

Hypertension: Oral: Initial: 1.25 mg daily; if inadequate response, may increase dose once every 4 weeks to 2.5 mg daily and then to 5 mg daily if needed. Consider adding another antihypertensive and decreasing the dose if response is not adequate. Usual dosage range (ASH/ISH [Weber, 2014]): 1.25 to 2.5 mg daily. **Note:** Canadian labeling recommends a maximum dose of 2.5 mg daily.

Calcium nephrolithiasis (off-label use): Oral: 2.5 mg once daily (AUA [Pearle, 2014])

Geriatric

U.S. labeling: Refer to adult dosing.
Canadian labeling: 1.25 mg daily

Renal Impairment There are no dosage adjustments provided in manufacturer's labeling; use with caution. Canadian labeling contraindicates use in severe impairment (CrCl <30 mL/minute).

Hepatic Impairment There are no dosage adjustments provided in manufacturer's labeling; use with caution. Canadian labeling contraindicates use in severe hepatic impairment or hepatic encephalopathy.

Dietary Considerations May be taken without regard to meals (Caruso, 1983); however, administration with food or milk may to decrease GI adverse effects.

Administration May be administered without regard to meals (Caruso, 1983); however, administration with food or milk may decrease GI adverse effects. Administer early in day to avoid nocturia.

Monitoring Parameters Blood pressure (both standing and sitting/supine); serum electrolytes, hepatic function, renal function, uric acid; assess weight, I & O reports daily to determine fluid loss

Test Interactions May interfere with parathyroid function tests and may decrease serum iodine (protein bound) without signs of thyroid disturbance

Dosage Forms Excipient information presented when available (limited, particularly for generics); consult specific product labeling.
Tablet, Oral:
Generic: 1.25 mg, 2.5 mg

◆ Inderal *see* Propranolol *on page 1518*
◆ Inderal XL *see* Propranolol *on page 1518*
◆ Inderal LA *see* Propranolol *on page 1518*

Indinavir (in DIN a veer)

Brand Names: US Crixivan
Brand Names: Canada Crixivan
Index Terms IDV; Indinavir Sulfate
Pharmacologic Category Antiretroviral, Protease Inhibitor (Anti-HIV)
Use Treatment of HIV infection; should always be used as part of a multidrug regimen (at least three antiretroviral agents)

Dosing

Adult & Geriatric HIV infection: Oral:
Unboosted regimen: 800 mg every 8 hours
Ritonavir-boosted regimen: Ritonavir 100-200 mg twice daily plus indinavir 800 mg twice daily

Dosage adjustments for indinavir when administered in combination therapy:
Delavirdine, itraconazole, or ketoconazole: Reduce indinavir dose to 600 mg every 8 hours
Efavirenz: Increase indinavir dose to 1000 mg every 8 hours
Lopinavir and ritonavir (Kaletra™): Indinavir 600 mg twice daily
Nelfinavir: Increase indinavir dose to 1200 mg twice daily
Nevirapine: Increase indinavir dose to 1000 mg every 8 hours
Rifabutin: Reduce rifabutin to 1/2 the standard dose plus increase indinavir to 1000 mg every 8 hours

Pediatric HIV: Children and Adolescents 4 to 15 years (off-label use): 400 mg/m^2 every 12 hours is currently under study (HHS [pediatric], 2014)

Renal Impairment There are no dosage adjustments provided in the manufacturer's labeling (has not been studied).

Hepatic Impairment
Mild-moderate impairment due to cirrhosis, monotherapy: 600 mg every 8 hours
Severe impairment: There are no dosage adjustments provided in the manufacturer's labeling (has not been studied).

Additional Information Complete prescribing information should be consulted for additional detail.

Dosage Forms Excipient information presented when available (limited, particularly for generics); consult specific product labeling.
Capsule, Oral:
Crixivan: 200 mg, 400 mg

◆ Indinavir Sulfate *see* Indinavir *on page 937*
◆ Indocin *see* Indomethacin *on page 937*

Indomethacin (in doe METH a sin)

Brand Names: US Indocin; Tivorbex
Brand Names: Canada Novo-Methacin; Pro-Indo; ratio-Indomethacin; Sandoz-Indomethacin

Index Terms Indomethacin; Indomethacin Sodium Trihydrate

Pharmacologic Category Nonsteroidal Anti-inflammatory Drug (NSAID), Oral; Nonsteroidal Anti-inflammatory Drug (NSAID), Parenteral

Use

Acute pain, mild to moderate (Tivorbex only): Treatment of mild to moderate acute pain in adults

Arthritis (excluding Tivorbex): Treatment of moderate to severe rheumatoid arthritis (RA), including acute flares of chronic disease; moderate to severe osteoarthritis (OA); acute gouty arthritis (except extended-release [ER] capsules)

Inflammatory conditions (excluding Tivorbex): Treatment of moderate to severe ankylosing spondylitis; acute painful bursitis and/or tendinitis of the shoulder (excluding Canadian products)

Patent ductus arteriosus (IV only): To close a hemodynamically significant patent ductus arteriosus in premature infants weighing between 500 and 1,750 g when 48 hours usual medical management (eg, fluid restriction, diuretics, digitalis, respiratory support) is ineffective.

Pregnancy Considerations Adverse events have been observed in animal reproduction studies; studies in pregnant women have demonstrated risk to the fetus if administered at ≥30 weeks gestation. Indomethacin crosses the placenta and can be detected in fetal plasma and amniotic fluid. Indomethacin exposure during the first trimester is not strongly associated with congenital malformations; however, cardiovascular anomalies and cleft palate have been observed following NSAID exposure in some studies. The use of an NSAID close to conception may be associated with an increased risk of miscarriage. Nonteratogenic effects have been observed following NSAID administration during the third trimester, including myocardial degenerative changes, prenatal constriction of the ductus arteriosus, failure of the ductus arteriosus to close postnatally, and fetal tricuspid regurgitation; renal dysfunction or failure, oligohydramnios; gastrointestinal bleeding or perforation, increased risk of necrotizing enterocolitis; intracranial bleeding (including intraventricular hemorrhage), platelet dysfunction with resultant bleeding; and pulmonary hypertension. The risk of fetal ductal constriction following maternal use of indomethacin is increased with gestational age and duration of therapy. Because they may cause premature closure of the ductus arteriosus, use of NSAIDs late in pregnancy should be avoided (use after 31 or 32 weeks gestation is not recommended by some clinicians). Indomethacin has been used for a short duration (eg, ≤48 hours) in the management of preterm labor. Indomethacin should be used with caution in pregnant women with hypertension. The chronic use of NSAIDs in women of reproductive age may be associated with infertility that is reversible upon discontinuation of the medication. Use during pregnancy (third trimester) is contraindicated in the Canadian labeling.

Breast-Feeding Considerations Indomethacin is excreted into breast milk and low amounts have been measured in the plasma of nursing infants. Seizures in a nursing infant were observed in one case report, although adverse events have not been noted in other cases. Breast-feeding is not recommended by most manufacturers (use is contraindicated in the Canadian labeling); Tivorbex may be used with caution during breast-feeding. (The therapeutic use of indomethacin is contraindicated in neonates with significant renal failure.) Hypertensive crisis and psychiatric side effects have been noted in case reports following use of indomethacin for analgesia in postpartum women. Use with caution in nursing women with hypertensive disorders of pregnancy or preexisting renal disease.

Medication Guide Available Yes

Contraindications

Hypersensitivity (eg, anaphylactic reactions, serious skin reactions) to indomethacin, aspirin, other NSAIDs, or any component of the formulation; perioperative pain in the setting of coronary artery bypass graft (CABG) surgery; history of asthma, urticaria, or allergic-type reactions after taking aspirin or other NSAID agents (severe, even fatal, anaphylactic-like reactions have been reported); patients with a history of proctitis or recent rectal bleeding (suppositories)

Neonates (IV only): Necrotizing enterocolitis (proven or suspected); significant renal impairment; active bleeding (including intracranial hemorrhage and gastrointestinal bleeding), thrombocytopenia, coagulation defects; untreated infection (proven or suspected); congenital heart disease where patency of the ductus arteriosus is necessary for adequate pulmonary or systemic blood flow (eg, pulmonary atresia, severe tetralogy of Fallot, severe coarctation of the aorta)

Canadian labeling: Additional contraindications (not in US labeling): Severe uncontrolled heart failure; known hyperkalemia; active gastric/duodenal/peptic ulcer; active GI bleed; history of recurrent GI ulceration; active GI inflammatory disease; cerebrovascular bleeding or other bleeding disorders; severe hepatic impairment or active liver disease; severe renal impairment (CrCl <30 mL/minute) or deteriorating renal function; concurrent use with other NSAIDs; complete or partial syndrome of nasal polyps; children and adolescents <14 years of age; breast-feeding; pregnancy (third trimester)

Warnings/Precautions [US Boxed Warning]: NSAIDs are associated with an increased risk of adverse cardiovascular thrombotic events, including MI and stroke. Risk may be increased with duration of use or preexisting cardiovascular risk factors or disease. May cause new-onset hypertension or worsening of existing hypertension. Monitor blood pressure closely during initiation of treatment and throughout the course of therapy. Use caution in patients with fluid retention. Avoid use in heart failure (ACCF/AHA [Yancy, 2013]). Concurrent administration of ibuprofen, and potentially other nonselective NSAIDs, may interfere with aspirin's cardioprotective effect. **[US Boxed Warning]: Use is contraindicated for treatment of perioperative pain in the setting of coronary artery bypass graft (CABG) surgery.** Risk of MI and stroke may be increased with use following CABG surgery.

Platelet adhesion and aggregation may be decreased; may prolong bleeding time; patients with coagulation disorders or who are receiving anticoagulants should be monitored closely. Anemia may occur; patients on long-term NSAID therapy should be monitored for anemia. Rarely, NSAID use may cause severe blood dyscrasias (eg, agranulocytosis, aplastic anemia, thrombocytopenia).

NSAID use may compromise existing renal function; dose-dependent decreases in prostaglandin synthesis may result from NSAID use, reducing renal blood flow which may cause renal decompensation. NSAID use may increase the risk for hyperkalemia. Patients with impaired renal function, dehydration, heart failure, liver dysfunction, those taking diuretics, and ACE inhibitors are at greater risk of renal toxicity and hyperkalemia. Rehydrate patient before starting therapy; monitor renal function closely. Long-term NSAID use may result in renal papillary necrosis. Not recommended for use in patients with advanced renal disease; monitor closely if therapy must be initiated. The injection formulation is contraindicated in neonates with significant renal impairment. Canadian labeling contraindicates use in severe renal impairment (CrCl <30 mL/minute) or deteriorating renal function.

[US Boxed Warning]: NSAIDs may increase risk of gastrointestinal irritation, inflammation, ulceration, bleeding, and perforation. Use caution with a history of GI disease (bleeding or ulcers), concurrent therapy with aspirin, anticoagulants and/or corticosteroids, smoking, use of alcohol, the elderly or debilitated patients. When used concomitantly with aspirin, a substantial increase in the risk of gastrointestinal complications (eg, ulcer) occurs; concomitant gastroprotective therapy (eg, proton pump inhibitors) is recommended (Bhatt, 2008).

Use the lowest effective dose for the shortest duration of time, consistent with individual patient goals, to reduce risk of cardiovascular or GI adverse events. Alternate therapies should be considered for patients at high risk.

NSAIDS may cause drowsiness, dizziness, blurred vision and other neurologic effects which may impair physical or mental abilities; patients must be cautioned about performing tasks which require mental alertness (eg, operating machinery or driving). Headache may occur; cessation of therapy required if headache persists after dosage reduction.

NSAIDs may cause potentially fatal serious skin adverse events including exfoliative dermatitis, Stevens-Johnson syndrome (SJS) and toxic epidermal necrolysis (TEN); discontinue use at first sign of skin rash or hypersensitivity. Anaphylactoid reactions may occur, even without prior exposure; patients with "aspirin triad" (bronchial asthma, aspirin intolerance, rhinitis) may be at increased risk. Use is contraindicated in patients who experience bronchospasm, asthma, rhinitis, or urticaria with NSAID or aspirin therapy. Use caution in other forms of asthma.

Use with caution in patients with decreased hepatic function. Canadian labeling contraindicates use in severe hepatic impairment or active liver disease. Closely monitor patients with any abnormal LFT. Notable elevations of ALT or AST (eg, >3 x ULN) have been reported. Severe hepatic reactions (eg, jaundice, fulminant hepatitis, liver necrosis,

liver failure) have occurred with NSAID use, some with fatal outcomes; discontinue immediately if clinical signs or symptoms of liver disease develop, or if systemic manifestations occur (eg, eosinophilia, rash). The elderly are at increased risk for adverse effects (especially peptic ulceration, CNS effects, renal toxicity) from NSAIDs even at low doses. Prolonged therapy may cause corneal deposits and retinal disturbances, including those of the macula. Discontinue use with blurred or diminished vision and perform ophthalmologic exam. Periodically evaluate vision in all patients receiving long-term therapy. Use caution with depression, epilepsy, or Parkinson disease.

Withhold for at least 4 to 6 half-lives prior to surgical or dental procedures. Potentially significant drug-drug interactions may exist, requiring dose or frequency adjustment, additional monitoring, and/or selection of alternative therapy. Tivorbex is not indicated for long-term use.

Elderly: Nonselective oral NSAID use is associated with an increased risk of GI bleeding and peptic ulcer disease in older adults in high risk category (eg, >75 years or age or receiving concomitant oral/parenteral corticosteroids, anticoagulants, or antiplatelet agents). Risk of adverse events may be higher with indomethacin compared to other NSAIDs; avoid use in this age group (Beers Criteria). Indomethacin may cause confusion or, rarely, psychosis; remain alert to the possibility of such adverse reactions in elderly patients.

Oral: There have been cases of hepatotoxicity reported in pediatric patients with juvenile rheumatoid arthritis, including fatalities. Closely monitor if needed in pediatric patients ≥2 years and periodically assess liver function.

Adverse Reactions

>10%:
Central nervous system: Headache (12% to 16%)
Gastrointestinal: Vomiting (≤12%)
Hematologic & oncologic: Postoperative hemorrhage (≤11%)

1% to 10%:
Cardiovascular: Presyncope (≤3%), syncope (≤2%)
Central nervous system: Dizziness (3% to 9%), depression (<3%), drowsiness (<3%), fatigue (<3%), malaise (<3%), vertigo (<3%)
Dermatologic: Pruritus (1% to 4%), hyperhidrosis (2%), skin rash (1% to 2%)
Endocrine & metabolic: Hot flash (2%)
Gastrointestinal: Epigastric pain (3% to 9%), heartburn (3% to 9%), nausea (3% to 9%), dyspepsia (2% to 9%), constipation (≤6%), diarrhea (≤3%), abdominal pain (<3%), decreased appetite (≥2%), rectal irritation (suppository), tenesmus (suppository)
Otic: Tinnitus (<3%)
Miscellaneous: Swelling (3%; postprocedural)

<1% (Limited to important or life-threatening): Acute respiratory distress, agranulocytosis, anaphylaxis, anemia, angioedema, aphthous stomatitis, aplastic anemia, aseptic meningitis, asthma, bone marrow depression, cardiac arrhythmia, cardiac failure, cerebrovascular accident, chest pain, cholestatic jaundice, coma, confusion, convulsions, corneal deposits, depersonalization, depression, diplopia, disseminated intravascular coagulation, dysarthria, edema, erythema multiforme, erythema nodosum, exacerbation of epilepsy, exacerbation of Parkinson's disease, exfoliative dermatitis, fluid retention, gastritis, gastroenteritis, gastrointestinal hemorrhage, gastrointestinal perforation (rare), gastrointestinal ulcer, glycosuria, gynecomastia, hearing loss, hematuria, hemodynamic deterioration (patients with severe heart failure and hyponatremia), hemolytic anemia, hepatic failure, hepatic necrosis, hepatitis (including fatal cases), hepatotoxicity (idiosyncratic) (Chalasani, 2014), hyperglycemia, hyperkalemia, hypersensitivity reaction, hypertension, hypotension, immune thrombocytopenia, interstitial nephritis, intestinal obstruction, intestinal stenosis, involuntary muscle movements, jaundice, leukopenia, maculopathy, myocardial infarction, necrotizing fasciitis, nephrotic syndrome, oliguria, peripheral neuropathy, proctitis, psychosis, pulmonary edema, purpura, rectal hemorrhage, regional ileitis, renal failure, renal insufficiency, retinal disturbance, shock, significant cardiovascular event, Stevens-Johnson syndrome, stomatitis, syncope, thrombocytopenia, thrombophlebitis, toxic amblyopia, toxic epidermal necrolysis, ulcerative colitis, vaginal hemorrhage

Drug Interactions

Metabolism/Transport Effects Substrate of CYP2C19 (minor), CYP2C9 (minor); **Note:** Assignment of Major/Minor substrate status based on clinically relevant drug interaction potential; **Inhibits** CYP2C19 (weak), CYP2C9 (weak)

Avoid Concomitant Use
Avoid concomitant use of Indomethacin with any of the following: Dexketoprofen; Floctafenine; Ketorolac (Nasal); Ketorolac (Systemic); Morniflumate; NSAID (COX-2 Inhibitor); Omacetaxine; Talniflumate; Urokinase

Increased Effect/Toxicity
Indomethacin may increase the levels/effects of: 5-ASA Derivatives; Agents with Antiplatelet Properties; Aliskiren; Aminoglycosides; Anticoagulants; Apixaban; Bisphosphonate Derivatives; Collagenase (Systemic); CycloSPORINE (Systemic); Dabigatran Etexilate; Deferasirox; Deoxycholic Acid; Desmopressin; Digoxin; Drospirenone; Edoxaban; Eplerenone; Haloperidol; Ibritumomab; Lithium; Methotrexate; Nonsteroidal Anti-Inflammatory Agents; NSAID (COX-2 Inhibitor); Obinutuzumab; Omacetaxine; PEMEtrexed; Porfimer; Potassium-Sparing Diuretics; PRALAtrexate; Quinolone Antibiotics; Rivaroxaban; Salicylates; Tacrolimus (Systemic); Tenofovir Products; Thrombolytic Agents; Tiludronate; Tositumomab and Iodine I 131 Tositumomab; Triamterene; Urokinase; Vancomycin; Verteporfin; Vitamin K Antagonists

The levels/effects of Indomethacin may be increased by: ACE Inhibitors; Alcohol (Ethyl); Angiotensin II Receptor Blockers; Antidepressants (Tricyclic, Tertiary Amine); Corticosteroids (Systemic); CycloSPORINE (Systemic); Dasatinib; Dexketoprofen; Diclofenac (Systemic); Floctafenine; Glucosamine; Herbs (Anticoagulant/Antiplatelet Properties); Ibrutinib; Ketorolac (Nasal); Ketorolac (Systemic); Limaprost; Loop Diuretics; Morniflumate; Multivitamins/Fluoride (with ADE); Multivitamins/Minerals (with ADEK, Folate, Iron); Multivitamins/Minerals (with AE, No Iron); Omega-3 Fatty Acids; Pentosan Polysulfate Sodium; Pentoxifylline; Probenecid; Prostacyclin Analogues; Selective Serotonin Reuptake Inhibitors; Serotonin/Norepinephrine Reuptake Inhibitors; Sodium Phosphates; Talniflumate; Thiazide Diuretics; Tipranavir; Treprostinil; Vitamin E; Vitamin E (Oral)

Decreased Effect
Indomethacin may decrease the levels/effects of: ACE Inhibitors; Aliskiren; Angiotensin II Receptor Blockers; Beta-Blockers; Eplerenone; Glucagon; HydrALAZINE; Loop Diuretics; Potassium-Sparing Diuretics; Prostaglandins (Ophthalmic); Salicylates; Selective Serotonin Reuptake Inhibitors; Thiazide Diuretics

The levels/effects of Indomethacin may be decreased by: Bile Acid Sequestrants; Salicylates

Food Interactions Food may decrease the rate but not the extent of absorption. Indomethacin peak serum levels may be delayed if taken with food. Management: Administer with food or milk to minimize GI upset.

Preparation for Administration IV: Reconstitute with 1 mL of preservative-free NS or SWFI to a concentration of 0.1 mg per 0.1 mL, or with 2 mL diluent to a concentration of 0.05 mg per 0.1 mL. Reconstitute solution just prior to each administration; further dilution after reconstitution is not recommended. Discard any unused portion. Do not use preservative-containing diluents for reconstitution.

Storage/Stability
Capsules: Store at 20°C to 25°C (68°F to 77°F). Protect ER capsules from moisture.
Tivorbex: Store at 25°C (77°F); excursions permitted to 15°C to 30°C (59°F to 86°F). Store in the original container; protect from moisture and light.
IV: Store at 25°C (77°F); excursions permitted to 15°C to 30°C (59°F to 86°F). Protect from light. Store vials in original carton until contents used.
Suppositories: Store refrigerated at 2°C to 8°C (36°F to 46°F).
Canadian labeling: Store below 30°C (86°F). Protect from light; elevated humidity; and excessive heat.
Suspension: Store below 30°C (86°F). Avoid temperatures above 50°C (122°F). Protect from freezing.

Mechanism of Action Reversibly inhibits cyclooxygenase-1 and 2 (COX-1 and 2) enzymes, which results in decreased formation of prostaglandin precursors; has antipyretic, analgesic, and anti-inflammatory properties

Other proposed mechanisms not fully elucidated (and possibly contributing to the anti-inflammatory effect to varying degrees), include inhibiting chemotaxis, altering lymphocyte activity, inhibiting neutrophil aggregation/activation, and decreasing proinflammatory cytokine levels.

Pharmacodynamics/Kinetics
Onset of action: ~30 minutes
Duration: 4 to 6 hours
Absorption: Oral: Immediate release: Neonates: Formulation specific; Adults: Prompt and extensive; Extended release: Adults: 90% over 12 hours (**Note:** 75 mg product is designed to initially release 25 mg and then 50 mg over an extended period of time)

Distribution: Crosses blood-brain barrier; Neonates: PDA: 0.36 L/kg; Post-PDA closure: 0.26 L/kg; Adults: 0.34-1.57 L/kg

Protein binding: 99%

Metabolism: Hepatic; significant enterohepatic recirculation; metabolites include desmethyl, desbenzoyl and desmethyl-desbenzoyl (all in unconjugated form)

Bioavailability:

Neonates, premature: Percent bioavailability reported in the literature is highly variable and may be influenced by formulation components and indomethacin physicochemical properties (Scanlon 1982); some have suggested that aqueous formulations are less bioavailable compared to ethanol based formulations (Mrongovious 1982; Scanlon 1982); aqueous suspension (in saline): 13% to 20% (Mrongovious 1982; Sharma 2003); ethanol based (96% v/v) suspension: 98.6% (Al Za'abi 2007)

Adults: Oral: 100%; rectal: 80% to 90% (than that absorbed from capsule form)

Half-life elimination:

Neonates: Postnatal age (PNA) <2 weeks: ~20 hours; PNA >2 weeks: ~11 hours

Adults: 2.6-11.2 hours; 7.6 hours (Tivorbex)

Time to peak: Oral: Immediate release: 2 hours; Tivorbex capsules: 1.67 hours

Excretion: Urine (60%, primarily as glucuronide conjugates); feces (33%, primarily as metabolites; 1.5% as unchanged drug)

Clearance: Preterm neonates: ~19 mL/hour/kg (range: 4.7-45.5 mL/hour/kg) (Al Za'abi 2007)

Dosing

Adult

Inflammatory/rheumatoid disorders: Note: Use lowest effective dose for the shortest duration possible.

Oral (immediate-release [excluding Tivorbex)]], rectal: 25 mg 2 to 3 times daily; if well tolerated, increase daily dosage by 25 or 50 mg at weekly intervals until satisfactory response or a total daily dose of 150 to 200 mg/day (maximum dose: 200 mg/day) is reached. In patients with arthritis and persistent night pain and/or morning stiffness may give the larger portion (up to maximum of 100 mg) of the total daily dose at bedtime.

Oral (extended-release capsules): Initial: 75 mg once daily, may increase to 75 mg twice daily (maximum dose: 150 mg/day).

Bursitis/tendonitis of the shoulder: Oral (excluding Tivorbex and Canadian products), rectal (excluding Canadian products): Initial dose: 75 to 150 mg/day in 3 to 4 divided doses **or** 1 to 2 divided doses for extended release; usual treatment is 7 to 14 days; discontinue after signs/symptoms of inflammation have been controlled for several days.

Acute gouty arthritis: Oral (excluding extended-release capsules and Tivorbex), rectal: 50 mg 3 times daily until pain is tolerable then rapidly reduce dose to complete cessation of drug.

Acute pain (mild to moderate): Oral (Tivorbex only): 20 mg 3 times daily or 40 mg 2 or 3 times daily

Prevention of pancreatitis post-endoscopic retrograde cholangiopancreatography (ERCP) (off-label use): Rectal: 100 mg immediately after ERCP (Elmunzer, 2012)

Geriatric Refer to adult dosing. Use lowest recommended dose and frequency in elderly to initiate therapy for indications listed in adult dosing.

Pediatric

Patent ductus arteriosus:

Neonates weighing between 500 to 1,750 g: IV: Initial: 0.2 mg/kg, followed by 2 doses depending on postnatal age (PNA):

PNA at time of FIRST dose <48 hours: 0.1 mg/kg at 12- to 24-hour intervals

PNA at time of FIRST dose 2 to 7 days: 0.2 mg/kg at 12- to 24-hour intervals

PNA at time of FIRST dose >7 days: 0.25 mg/kg at 12- to 24-hour intervals

Note: In general, may use 12-hour dosing interval if urine output >1 mL/kg/hour after prior dose; use 24-hour dosing interval if urine output is <1 mL/kg/hour but >0.6 mL/kg/hour. Doses should be withheld if patient has oliguria (urine output <0.6 mL/kg/hour) or anuria at the scheduled time of the second or third dose; do not give additional doses until renal function has returned to normal. If the ductus arteriosus closes or is significantly reduced in size after 48 hours or more from completion of first course, no further doses are necessary. If the ductus arteriosus reopens, a second course of 1 to 3 doses may be given; if unresponsive after 2 doses, surgery may be necessary.

Inflammatory/rheumatoid disorders: Note: Use lowest effective dose for the shortest duration possible. Canadian labeling contraindicates use in children and adolescents <14 years.

Children ≥2 years (limited data available): Oral (excluding extended release capsules and Tivorbex): 1 to 2 mg/kg/day in 2 to 4 divided doses; maximum daily dose: 4 mg/kg/day or 200 mg/day, whichever is less

Adolescents >14 years:

Oral (immediate release [excluding Tivorbex]), rectal: Refer to adult dosing.

Oral (extended release capsules): Refer to adult dosing.

Renal Impairment

US labeling:

Oral/rectal: There are no dosage adjustments provided in the manufacturer's labeling; not recommended in patients with advanced renal disease.

Injection: If anuria or marked oliguria (urinary output <0.6 mL/kg/hour) evident at the scheduled time of the second or third dose, hold dose until renal function returns to normal. Use is contraindicated in neonates with significant renal impairment.

Canadian labeling:

Mild to moderate impairment: There are no dosage adjustments provided in the manufacturer's labeling; use with caution and consider lower doses.

Severe impairment (CrCl <30 mL/minute) or deteriorating renal function: Use is contraindicated.

Dosage adjustment in hepatic impairment:

Hepatic Impairment

US labeling: There are no dosage adjustments provided in the manufacturer's labeling; use with caution.

Canadian labeling: There are no dosage adjustments provided in the manufacturer's labeling. Use is contraindicated in severe liver impairment or active liver disease.

Dietary Considerations May cause GI upset; take with food or milk to minimize

Administration

Oral: Administer with food, immediately after meals, or with milk or antacids to decrease GI adverse effects. Extended-release capsules must be swallowed whole; do not crush.

IV: Administer over 20 to 30 minutes. Reconstitute IV formulation just prior to administration; discard any unused portion; avoid IV bolus administration or infusion via an umbilical catheter into vessels near the superior mesenteric artery as these may cause vasoconstriction and can compromise blood flow to the intestines. Do not administer intra-arterially. Avoid extravascular injection or leakage; solution may be irritating to tissue.

Monitoring Parameters Monitor response (pain, range of motion, grip strength, mobility, ADL function), inflammation; observe for weight gain, edema; monitor renal function (serum creatinine, BUN); observe for bleeding, bruising; evaluate gastrointestinal effects (abdominal pain, bleeding, dyspepsia); mental confusion, disorientation, CBC, blood pressure, liver function tests (particularly with pediatric use); ophthalmologic exams with prolonged therapy

Test Interactions False-negative dexamethasone suppression test

Dosage Forms Excipient information presented when available (limited, particularly for generics); consult specific product labeling.

Capsule, Oral:

Tivorbex: 20 mg, 40 mg [contains brilliant blue fcf (fd&c blue #1), fd&c blue #2 (indigotine), fd&c red #40]

Generic: 25 mg, 50 mg

Capsule Extended Release, Oral:

Generic: 75 mg

Solution Reconstituted, Intravenous:

Indocin: 1 mg (1 ea)

Generic: 1 mg (1 ea)

Solution Reconstituted, Intravenous [preservative free]:

Generic: 1 mg (1 ea)

Suppository, Rectal:

Indocin: 50 mg (30 ea)

Suspension, Oral:

Indocin: 25 mg/5 mL (237 mL) [contains alcohol, usp; pineapple-coconut-mint flavor]

Dosage Forms: Canada Note: Refer also to Dosage Forms. Extended release capsule, intravenous solution, and oral suspension are not available in Canada.

Excipient information presented when available (limited, particularly for generics); consult specific product labeling.

Suppository, Rectal: 100 mg

♦ Indomethacin see Indomethacin on page 937

♦ Indomethacin Sodium Trihydrate see Indomethacin on page 937

◆ INF-alpha 2 *see* Interferon Alfa-2b *on page 966*

◆ Infanrix *see* Diphtheria and Tetanus Toxoids, and Acellular Pertussis Vaccine *on page 567*

◆ Infanrix-IPV (Can) *see* Diphtheria and Tetanus Toxoids, Acellular Pertussis, and Poliovirus Vaccine *on page 566*

◆ Infanrix-IPV/HIB (Can) *see* Diphtheria and Tetanus Toxoids, Acellular Pertussis, Poliovirus and *Haemophilus* b Conjugate Vaccine *on page 567*

◆ Infants Advil [OTC] *see* Ibuprofen *on page 905*

◆ Infants Ibuprofen [OTC] *see* Ibuprofen *on page 905*

◆ Infasurf *see* Calfactant *on page 293*

◆ Infed *see* Iron Dextran Complex *on page 986*

◆ Inflectra (Can) *see* InFLIXimab *on page 941*

InFLIXimab (in FLIKS e mab)

Brand Names: US Remicade
Brand Names: Canada Inflectra; Remicade; Remsima
Index Terms Avakine; Infliximab, Recombinant
Pharmacologic Category Antirheumatic, Disease Modifying; Gastrointestinal Agent, Miscellaneous; Immunosuppressant Agent; Monoclonal Antibody; Tumor Necrosis Factor (TNF) Blocking Agent
Use

Ankylosing spondylitis: Treatment of adults with active ankylosing spondylitis (to reduce signs/symptoms)

Crohn disease: Treatment adults and children ≥6 years (US labeling) or ≥9 years (Canadian labeling) with moderately- to severely-active Crohn disease with inadequate response to conventional therapy (to reduce signs/symptoms and induce and maintain clinical remission) or to reduce the number of draining enterocutaneous and rectovaginal fistulas and maintain fistula closure

Plaque psoriasis: Treatment of adults with chronic severe (extensive and/or disabling) plaque psoriasis as an alternative to other systemic therapy

Psoriatic arthritis: Treatment of adults with psoriatic arthritis (to reduce signs/symptoms of active arthritis and inhibit progression of structural damage and improve physical function)

Rheumatoid arthritis: Treatment of adults with moderately- to severely-active rheumatoid arthritis (with methotrexate) (to reduce signs/symptoms of active arthritis and inhibit progression of structural damage and improve physical function)

Ulcerative colitis: Treatment of adults and children ≥6 years with moderately- to severely-active ulcerative colitis with inadequate response to conventional therapy (to reduce signs/symptoms and induce and maintain clinical remission, mucosal healing and eliminate corticosteroid use)

Note: Remsima and Inflectra [Canadian products] are biosimilar agents and are not approved for use in pediatric patients or in patients with Crohn disease or ulcerative colitis.

Pregnancy Considerations Animal reproduction studies have not been conducted. Infliximab crosses the placenta and can be detected in the serum of infants for up to 6 months following in utero exposure. A fatal outcome has been reported in an infant who received a live vaccine (BCG) after in utero exposure to infliximab; it is recommended to wait ≥6 months following birth before administering any live vaccine to infants exposed to infliximab in utero. If a biologic agent such as infliximab is needed to treat inflammatory bowel disease during pregnancy, it is recommended to hold therapy after 30 weeks gestation (Habal, 2012). The Canadian labeling recommends that women of childbearing potential use effective contraception during therapy and for at least 6 months after discontinuation.

Healthcare providers are also encouraged to enroll women exposed to infliximab during pregnancy in the Mother-ToBaby Autoimmune Diseases Study by contacting the Organization of Teratology Information Specialists (OTIS) (877-311-8972).

Breast-Feeding Considerations Small amounts of infliximab have been detected in breast milk. Information is available from three postpartum women who were administered infliximab 5 mg/kg 1-24 weeks after delivery. Infliximab was detected within 12 hours and the highest milk concentrations (0.09-0.105 mcg/mL) were seen 2-3 days after the dose. Corresponding maternal serum concentrations were 18-64 mcg/mL (Ben-Horin, 2011). Due to the potential for serious adverse reactions in the nursing infant, the manufacturer recommends a decision be made whether to discontinue nursing or to discontinue the drug, taking into account the importance of treatment to the mother.

Medication Guide Available Yes
Contraindications

Hypersensitivity to infliximab, murine proteins, or any component of the formulation; doses >5 mg/kg in patients with moderate or severe heart failure (NYHA Class III/IV)

Canadian labeling: Additional contraindications (not in US labeling): Severe infections (eg, sepsis, abscesses, tuberculosis, and opportunistic infections); use in patients with moderate or severe heart failure (NYHA Class III/IV)

Warnings/Precautions [US Boxed Warning]: Patients receiving infliximab are at increased risk for serious infections which may result in hospitalization and/or fatality; infections usually developed in patients receiving concomitant immunosuppressive agents (eg, methotrexate or corticosteroids) and may present as disseminated (rather than local) disease. Active tuberculosis (or reactivation of latent tuberculosis), invasive fungal (including aspergillosis, blastomycosis, candidiasis, coccidioidomycosis, histoplasmosis, and pneumocystosis) and bacterial, viral or other opportunistic infections (including legionellosis and listeriosis) have been reported. Monitor closely for signs/symptoms of infection. Discontinue for serious infection or sepsis. Consider risks versus benefits prior to use in patients with a history of chronic or recurrent infection. Consider empiric antifungal therapy in patients who are at risk for invasive fungal infection and develop severe systemic illness. Caution should be exercised when considering use the elderly or in patients with conditions that predispose them to infections (eg, diabetes) or residence/travel from areas of endemic mycoses (blastomycosis, coccidioidomycosis, histoplasmosis), or with latent or localized infections. Do not initiate infliximab therapy in patients with an active infection, including clinically important localized infection. Patients who develop a new infection while undergoing treatment should be monitored closely. Potentially significant drug interactions may exist, requiring dose or frequency adjustment, additional monitoring, and/or selection of alternative therapy.

[US Boxed Warning]: Infliximab treatment has been associated with active tuberculosis (may be disseminated or extrapulmonary) or reactivation of latent infections; evaluate patients for tuberculosis risk factors and latent tuberculosis infection (with a tuberculin skin test) prior to and during therapy; treatment of latent tuberculosis should be initiated before use. Patients with initial negative tuberculin skin tests should receive continued monitoring for tuberculosis throughout treatment. Most cases of reactivation have been reported within the first couple months of treatment. Caution should be exercised when considering the use of infliximab in patients who have been exposed to tuberculosis.

Patients should be brought up to date with all immunizations before initiating therapy. Live vaccines should not be given concurrently; there is no data available concerning secondary transmission of live vaccines in patients receiving therapy. A fatal outcome has been reported in an infant who received a live vaccine (BCG) after in utero exposure to infliximab; infliximab crosses the placenta and has been detected in infants' serum for up to 6 months. It is recommended to wait ≥6 months following birth before administering any live vaccine to infants exposed to infliximab in utero. Reactivation of hepatitis B virus (HBV) has occurred in chronic virus carriers (may be fatal); use with caution; evaluate prior to initiation and during treatment.

[US Boxed Warning]: Lymphoma and other malignancies (may be fatal) have been reported in children and adolescent patients receiving TNF-blocking agents including infliximab. Half the cases are lymphomas (Hodgkin's and non-Hodgkin's). **[US Boxed Warning]: Postmarketing cases of hepatosplenic T-cell lymphoma have been reported in patients treated with infliximab. Almost all patients had received and concurrent or prior treatment with azathioprine or mercaptopurine at or prior to diagnosis and the majority of reported cases occurred in adolescent and young adult males with Crohn disease or ulcerative colitis.** Malignancies occurred after a median of 30 months (range: 1 to 84 months) after the first dose of TNF blocker therapy; most patients were receiving concomitant immunosuppressants. The impact of infliximab on the development and course of malignancies is not fully defined. As compared to the general population, an increased risk of lymphoma has been noted in clinical trials; however, rheumatoid arthritis alone has been previously associated with an increased rate of lymphoma. Use caution in patients with a history of COPD, higher rates of malignancy were reported in COPD patients treated with infliximab.

Psoriasis patients with a history of phototherapy had a higher incidence of nonmelanoma skin cancers. Melanoma and Merkel cell carcinoma have been reported in patients receiving TNF-blocking agents including infliximab. Perform periodic skin examinations in all patients during therapy, particularly those at increased risk for skin cancer.

Severe hepatic reactions (including hepatitis, jaundice, acute hepatic failure, and cholestasis) have been reported during treatment; reactions occurred between 2 weeks to >1 year after initiation of therapy and some cases were fatal or necessitated liver transplantation; discontinue with jaundice and/or marked increase in liver enzymes (≥5 times ULN). Use caution with heart failure; if a decision is made to use with heart failure, monitor closely and discontinue if exacerbated or new symptoms occur. Doses >5 mg/kg should not be administered in patients with moderate to severe heart failure (HF) (NYHA Class III/IV). The Canadian labeling contraindicates use in moderate or severe HF. Use caution with history of hematologic abnormalities; hematologic toxicities (eg, leukopenia, neutropenia, thrombocytopenia, pancytopenia) have been reported (may be fatal); discontinue if significant abnormalities occur. Positive antinuclear antibody titers have been detected in patients (with negative baselines). Rare cases of autoimmune disorder, including lupus-like syndrome, have been reported; monitor and discontinue if symptoms develop. Rare cases of optic neuritis and demyelinating disease (including multiple sclerosis, systemic vasculitis, and Guillain-Barré syndrome) have been reported; use with caution in patients with preexisting or recent onset CNS demyelinating disorders, or seizures; discontinue if significant CNS adverse reactions develop.

Acute infusion reactions may occur. Hypersensitivity reaction may occur within 2 hours of infusion. Medication and equipment for management of hypersensitivity reaction should be available for immediate use. Interruptions and/or reinstitution at a slower rate may be required (consult protocols). Pretreatment may be considered, and may be warranted in all patients with prior infusion reactions. Serum sickness-like reactions have occurred; may be associated with a decreased response to treatment. The development of antibodies to infliximab may increase the risk of hypersensitivity and/or infusion reactions; concomitant use of immunosuppressants may lessen the development of anti-infliximab antibodies. The risk of infusion reactions may be increased with re-treatment after an interruption or discontinuation of prior maintenance therapy. Re-treatment in psoriasis patients should be resumed as a scheduled maintenance regimen without any induction doses; use of an induction regimen should be used cautiously for re-treatment of all other patients.

Some dosage forms may contain polysorbate 80 (also known as Tweens). Hypersensitivity reactions, usually a delayed reaction, have been reported following exposure to pharmaceutical products containing polysorbate 80 in certain individuals (Isaksson, 2002; Lucente 2000; Shelley, 1995). Thrombocytopenia, ascites, pulmonary deterioration, and renal and hepatic failure have been reported in premature neonates after receiving parenteral products containing polysorbate 80 (Alade, 1986; CDC, 1984). See manufacturer's labeling.

Efficacy was not established in a study to evaluate infliximab use in juvenile idiopathic arthritis (JIA).

Adverse Reactions Although profile is similar, frequency of adverse effects may vary with disease state. Except where noted, percentages reported in adults with rheumatoid arthritis:

>10%:
Central nervous system: Headache (18%)
Gastrointestinal: Nausea (21%), diarrhea (12%), abdominal pain (Crohn's: 26%; other indications: 12%)
Hepatic: Increased serum ALT (risk increased with concomitant methotrexate)
Immunologic: Increased ANA titer (~50%), antibody development (double-stranded DNA, 20%), antibody development (anti-infliximab; variable; ~10% to 15% [range: 6% to 61%]; Mayer, 2006)
Infection: Infection (36%), abscess (Crohn's patients with fistulizing disease: 15%)
Respiratory: Upper respiratory tract infection (32%), sinusitis (14%), cough (12%), pharyngitis (12%)
Miscellaneous: Infusion related reaction (20%; severe <1%)
5% to 10%:
Cardiovascular: Hypertension (7%)
Central nervous system: Fatigue (9%), pain (8%)
Dermatologic: Skin rash (1% to 10%), pruritus (7%)
Gastrointestinal: Dyspepsia (10%)
Genitourinary: Urinary tract infection (8%)

Infection: Candidiasis (5%)
Neuromuscular & skeletal: Arthralgia (1% to 8%), back pain (8%)
Respiratory: Bronchitis (10%), rhinitis (8%), dyspnea (6%)
Miscellaneous: Fever (7%)
<5%: Abscess, adult respiratory distress syndrome, anemia, basal cell carcinoma, biliary colic, bradycardia, cardiac arrest, cardiac arrhythmia, cardiac failure, cellulitis, cerebral infarction, cholecystitis, cholelithiasis, circulatory shock, confusion, constipation, dehydration, delayed hypersensitivity (plaque psoriasis), diaphoresis, dizziness, edema, gastrointestinal hemorrhage, hemolytic anemia, hepatitis, herniated disk, hypersensitivity reaction, hypotension, intestinal obstruction, intestinal perforation, intestinal stenosis, leukopenia, lupus-like syndrome, lymphadenopathy, malignant lymphoma, malignant neoplasm, malignant neoplasm of breast, meningitis, menstrual disease, myalgia, myocardial infarction, nephrolithiasis, neuritis, pancreatitis, pancytopenia, peripheral neuropathy, peritonitis, pleural effusion, pleurisy, pulmonary edema, pulmonary embolism, rectal pain, renal failure, respiratory insufficiency, sarcoidosis, seizure, sepsis, serum sickness, suicidal tendencies, syncope, tachycardia, tendon disease, thrombocytopenia, thrombophlebitis (deep), ulcer

The following adverse events were reported in children with Crohn's disease and were found more frequently in children than adults:
>10%:
Hepatic: Increased liver enzymes (18%; ≥5 times ULN: 1%)
Hematologic & oncologic: Anemia (11%)
Infection: Infection (56%; more common with every 8-week vs every 12-week infusions)
1% to 10%:
Cardiovascular: Flushing (9%)
Gastrointestinal: Bloody stools (10%)
Hematologic & oncologic: Leukopenia (9%), neutropenia (7%)
Hypersensitivity: Hypersensitivity reaction (respiratory, 6%)
Immunologic: Antibody development (anti-infliximab, 3%)
Infection: Viral infection (8%), bacterial infection (6%)
Neuromuscular & skeletal: Bone fracture (7%)

Postmarketing and/or case reports (adults or children; limited to important or life-threatening): Agranulocytosis, anaphylactic shock, anaphylaxis, angina pectoris, angioedema, autoimmune hepatitis, cardiac failure (worsening), cholestasis, demyelinating disease of the central nervous system (eg, multiple sclerosis, optic neuritis), demyelinating disease (peripheral; eg, Guillain-Barré syndrome, chronic inflammatory demyelinating polyneuropathy, multifocal motor neuropathy), dysgeusia, erythema multiforme, hepatic carcinoma, hepatic failure, hepatic injury, hepatitis B (reactivation), hepatotoxicity (idiosyncratic) (Chalasani, 2014), Hodgkin lymphoma, immune thrombocytopenia, interstitial fibrosis, interstitial pneumonitis, jaundice, leukemia, liver function tests increased, lupus-like syndrome (drug-induced), malignant lymphoma (hepatosplenic T-cell [HSTCL]), malignant melanoma, malignant neoplasm (leiomyosarcoma), Merkel cell carcinoma, neuropathy, opportunistic infection, pericardial effusion, pneumonia, psoriasis (including new onset, palmoplantar, pustular, or exacerbation), reactivated tuberculosis, renal cell carcinoma, seizure, Stevens-Johnson syndrome, thrombotic thrombocytopenia purpura, toxic epidermal necrolysis, transverse myelitis, tuberculosis, vasculitis (systemic and cutaneous)

Drug Interactions
Metabolism/Transport Effects None known.
Avoid Concomitant Use
Avoid concomitant use of InFLIXimab with any of the following: Abatacept; Adalimumab; Anakinra; BCG (Intravesical); Belimumab; Canakinumab; Certolizumab Pegol; Etanercept; Golimumab; Natalizumab; Pimecrolimus; Rilonacept; Tacrolimus (Topical); Tocilizumab; Tofacitinib; Ustekinumab; Vaccines (Live); Vedolizumab
Increased Effect/Toxicity
InFLIXimab may increase the levels/effects of: Abatacept; Anakinra; Belimumab; Canakinumab; Certolizumab Pegol; Fingolimod; Leflunomide; Natalizumab; Rilonacept; Tofacitinib; Vaccines (Live); Vedolizumab

The levels/effects of InFLIXimab may be increased by: Adalimumab; Denosumab; Etanercept; Golimumab; Pimecrolimus; Roflumilast; Tacrolimus (Topical); Tocilizumab; Trastuzumab; Ustekinumab
Decreased Effect
InFLIXimab may decrease the levels/effects of: BCG (Intravesical); Coccidioides immitis Skin Test; Sipuleucel-T; Vaccines (Inactivated); Vaccines (Live)

The levels/effects of InFLIXimab may be decreased by: Echinacea

Preparation for Administration Reconstitute vials with 10 mL sterile water for injection (SWFI) with a 21-guage or smaller needle, directing the SWFI towards the wall of the vial. Swirl vial gently to dissolve powder; do not shake. Allow solution to stand for 5 minutes. Total dose of reconstituted product should be further diluted to 250 mL of 0.9% sodium chloride injection (add reconstituted infliximab slowly) to a final concentration of 0.4 to 4 mg/mL. Do not dilute reconstituted infliximab solution with any other diluent. Infusion should begin within 3 hours of preparation (see Storage/Stability for additional information).

Storage/Stability Store intact vials at 2°C to 8°C (36°F to 46°F). The manufacturer recommends that diluted solutions for infusion should be used within 3 hours of preparation. However, a stability study of infliximab 0.4 mg/mL prepared in 0.9% sodium chloride in polyvinyl chloride (PVC) bags found no loss of biological activity when stored refrigerated at 4°C for up to 14 days (Ikeda 2012).

Mechanism of Action Infliximab is a chimeric monoclonal antibody that binds to human tumor necrosis factor alpha (TNFα), thereby interfering with endogenous TNFα activity. Elevated TNFα levels have been found in involved tissues/fluids of patients with rheumatoid arthritis, ankylosing spondylitis, psoriatic arthritis, plaque psoriasis, Crohn disease and ulcerative colitis. Biological activities of TNFα include the induction of proinflammatory cytokines (interleukins), enhancement of leukocyte migration, activation of neutrophils and eosinophils, and the induction of acute phase reactants and tissue degrading enzymes. Animal models have shown TNFα expression causes polyarthritis, and infliximab can prevent disease as well as allow diseased joints to heal.

Pharmacodynamics/Kinetics

Onset of action: Crohn disease: 1-2 weeks; Rheumatoid arthritis: 3-7 days

Duration of action: Crohn disease: 8-48 weeks; Rheumatoid arthritis: 6-12 weeks

Distribution: Within the vascular compartment; V_d: 3-6 L (Klotz 2007)

Half-life elimination: 7-12 days (Klotz 2007)

Dosing

Adult & Geriatric Note: Premedication with antihistamines (H_1-antagonist +/- H_2-antagonist), acetaminophen, and/or corticosteroids may be considered to prevent and/or manage infusion-related reactions. Remsima and Inflectra [Canadian products] are biosimilar agents and are not approved for use in Crohn disease or ulcerative colitis.

Ankylosing spondylitis: IV: 5 mg/kg at 0, 2, and 6 weeks, followed by 5 mg/kg every 6 weeks thereafter (Canadian labeling recommends every 6 to 8 weeks thereafter)

Crohn disease: IV: 5 mg/kg at 0, 2, and 6 weeks, followed by 5 mg/kg every 8 weeks thereafter; dose may be increased to 10 mg/kg in patients who respond but then lose their response. If no response by week 14, consider discontinuing therapy.

Plaque psoriasis: IV: 5 mg/kg at 0, 2, and 6 weeks, followed by 5 mg/kg every 8 weeks thereafter. **Note:** The Canadian labeling recommends discontinuing therapy at 14 weeks if response to therapy is inadequate.

Psoriatic arthritis (with or without methotrexate): IV: 5 mg/kg at 0,2, and 6 weeks, followed by 5 mg/kg every 8 weeks thereafter. **Note:** The Canadian labeling recommends discontinuing therapy at 24 weeks in patients unresponsive to therapy.

Rheumatoid arthritis (in combination with methotrexate therapy): IV 3 mg/kg at 0, 2, and 6 weeks, followed by 3 mg/kg every 8 weeks thereafter; Remicade doses have ranged from 3 to 10 mg/kg repeated at 4- to 8-week intervals

Ulcerative colitis: IV: 5 mg/kg at 0, 2, and 6 weeks, followed by 5 mg/kg every 8 weeks thereafter. The Canadian labeling suggests that after assessment of infliximab trough levels and antibody titers, dose adjustment to 10 mg/kg may be considered in some patients to sustain response/remission.

Pustular psoriasis (off-label use): IV: 5 mg/kg at week 0, 2, and 6, followed by 5 mg/kg every 8 weeks for up to 46 weeks (Suguira 2014; Torii 2011)

Dosage adjustment with heart failure (HF): Weigh risk versus benefits for individual patient:

Mild HF (NYHA Class I/II):

US labeling: No dosage adjustment necessary; use with caution and monitor closely for worsening of HF

Canadian labeling: ≤5 mg/kg

Moderate to severe (NYHA Class III or IV):

US labeling: ≤5 mg/kg

Canadian labeling: Use is contraindicated.

Pediatric Note: Premedication with antihistamines (H_1-antagonist +/- H_2-antagonist), acetaminophen, and/or corticosteroids may be considered to prevent and/or manage infusion-related reactions. Remsima and Inflectra [Canadian products] are biosimilar agents and are not approved for use in pediatric patients.

Crohn disease: Children and Adolescents: US labeling ≥6 years, Canadian labeling ≥9 years: IV: 5 mg/kg at 0, 2, and 6 weeks, followed by 5 mg/kg every 8 weeks thereafter; if no response by week 14, consider discontinuing therapy

Ulcerative colitis: Children ≥6 years and Adolescents: IV: 5 mg/kg at 0, 2, and 6 weeks, followed by 5 mg/kg every 8 weeks thereafter

Juvenile idiopathic arthritis (off-label use): Children ≥4 years and Adolescents: IV: Initial: 3 mg/kg at 0, 2, and 6 weeks; then 3 to 6 mg/kg/dose every 8 weeks thereafter, in combination with methotrexate during induction and maintenance (Ruperto, 2010). Alternatively, some studies used 6 mg/kg starting at week 14 of a methotrexate induction regimen (weeks 0 to 13); repeat dose (6 mg/kg) at week 16 and 20, then every 8 weeks thereafter (Ruperto, 2007; Visvanathan, 2012).

Renal Impairment There are no dosage adjustments provided in the manufacturer's labeling.

Hepatic Impairment There are no dosage adjustments provided in the manufacturer's labeling.

Administration The infusion should begin within 3 hours of reconstitution and dilution. Infuse over at least 2 hours; do not infuse with other agents; use in-line low protein binding filter (≤1.2 micron). Temporarily discontinue or decrease infusion rate with infusion-related reactions. Antihistamines (H_1-antagonist +/- H_2-antagonist), acetaminophen and/or corticosteroids may be used to manage reactions. Infusion may be reinitiated at a lower rate upon resolution of mild to moderate symptoms.

Note: The Canadian labeling suggests that patients with rheumatoid arthritis who have tolerated 3 infusions over 2 hours (doses ≤6 mg/kg) may receive subsequent infusions at the same dose over not less than 1 hour. Safety of shortened infusion has not been studied with doses >6 mg/kg.

Guidelines for the treatment and prophylaxis of infusion reactions: (Note: Limited to adult patients and dosages used in Crohn disease; prospective data for other populations [pediatrics, other indications/dosing] are not available).

A protocol for the treatment of infusion reactions, as well as prophylactic therapy for repeat infusions, has been published (Mayer, 2006).

Treatment of infusion reactions: Medications for the treatment of hypersensitivity reactions should be available for immediate use. For mild reactions, the rate of infusion should be decreased to 10 mL/hour. Initiate a normal saline infusion (500 to 1,000 mL/hour) and appropriate symptomatic treatment (eg, acetaminophen and diphenhydramine); monitor vital signs every 10 minutes until normal. After 20 minutes, the infusion may be increased at 15-minute intervals, as tolerated, to completion (initial increase to 20 mL/hour, then 40 mL/hour, then 80 mL/hour, etc [maximum of 125 mL/hour]). For moderate reactions, the infusion should be stopped or slowed. Initiate a normal saline infusion (500 to 1,000 mL/hour) and appropriate symptomatic treatment. Monitor vital signs every 5 minutes until normal. After 20 minutes, the infusion may be reinstituted at 10 mL/hour; then increased at 15-minute intervals, as tolerated, to completion (initial increase 20 mL/hour, then 40 mL/hour, then 80 mL/hour, etc [maximum of 125 mL/hour]). For severe reactions, the infusion should be stopped with administration of appropriate symptomatic treatment (eg, hydrocortisone/methylprednisolone, diphenhydramine and epinephrine) and frequent monitoring of vitals (consult institutional policies, if available). Re-treatment after a severe reaction should only be done if the benefits outweigh the risks and with appropriate prophylaxis. Delayed infusion reactions typically occur 1 to 7 days after an infusion. Treatment should consist of appropriate symptomatic treatment (eg, acetaminophen, antihistamine, methylprednisolone).

Prophylaxis of infusion reactions: Premedication with acetaminophen and diphenhydramine 90 minutes prior to infusion may be considered in all patients with prior infusion reactions, and in patients with severe repeated corticosteroid administration is recommended. Steroid dosing may be oral (prednisone 50 mg orally every 12 hours for 3 doses prior to infusion) or intravenous (a single dose of hydrocortisone 100 mg or methylprednisolone 20 to 40 mg administered 20 minutes prior to the

infusion). On initiation of the infusion, begin with a test dose at 10 mL/hour for 15 minutes. Thereafter, the infusion may be increased at 15-minute intervals, as tolerated, to completion (initial increase 20 mL/hour, then 40 mL/hour, then 80 mL/hour, etc). A maximum rate of 125 mL/hour is recommended in patients who experienced prior mild to moderate reactions and 100 mL/hour is recommended in patients who experienced prior severe reactions. In patients with cutaneous flushing, aspirin may be considered (Becker, 2004). For delayed infusion reactions, premedicate with acetaminophen and diphenhydramine 90 minutes prior to infusion. On initiation of the infusion, begin with a test dose at 10 mL/hour for 15 minutes. Thereafter, the infusion may be increased to infuse over 3 hours. Postinfusion therapy with acetaminophen for 3 days and an antihistamine for 7 days is recommended.

Monitoring Parameters Monitor improvement of symptoms and physical function assessments. During infusion, if reaction is noted, monitor vital signs every 2-10 minutes, depending on reaction severity, until normal. Latent TB screening prior to initiating and during therapy; signs/symptoms of infection (prior to, during, and following therapy); CBC with differential; signs/symptoms/worsening of heart failure; HBV screening prior to initiating (all patients), HBV carriers (during and for several months following therapy); signs and symptoms of hypersensitivity reaction; symptoms of lupus-like syndrome; LFTs (discontinue if >5 times ULN); signs and symptoms of malignancy (eg, splenomegaly, hepatomegaly, abdominal pain, persistent fever, night sweats, weight loss).

Psoriasis patients with history of phototherapy should be monitored for nonmelanoma skin cancer.

Dosage Forms Considerations Remicade contains sucrose 500 mg per vial

Dosage Forms Excipient information presented when available (limited, particularly for generics); consult specific product labeling.

Solution Reconstituted, Intravenous [preservative free]:
Remicade: 100 mg (1 ea) [contains polysorbate 80]

Dosage Forms: Canada Excipient information presented when available (limited, particularly for generics); consult specific product labeling.

Solution Reconstituted, Intravenous (preservative-free):
Remicade: 100 mg (contains polysorbate 80, sucrose 500 mg)
Inflectra: 100 mg (contains polysorbate 80, sucrose 500 mg; biosimilar agent)
Remsima 100 mg (contains polysorbate 80, sucrose 500 mg; biosimilar agent)

♦ Infliximab, Recombinant see InFLIXimab on page 941

Influenza A Virus Vaccine (H5N1)
(in floo EN za aye VYE rus vak SEEN H5N1)

Index Terms Avian Influenza Virus Vaccine; Bird Flu Vaccine; H5N1 Influenza Vaccine; Highly Pathogenic Avian Influenza (HPAI) A (H5N1) Virus Vaccine; Influenza Virus Vaccine (H5N1); Influenza Virus Vaccine (Monovalent); Q-Pan H5N1 Influenza Vaccine

Pharmacologic Category Vaccine, Inactivated (Viral)

Additional Appendix Information

Immunization Administration Recommendations on page 1974

Immunization Schedules on page 1979

Use Influenza A (H5N1) immunization:

GlaxoSmithKline product (adjuvanted): For active immunization of persons ≥18 years of age at increased risk of exposure to the influenza A (H5N1) virus subtype contained in the vaccine

Sanofi Pasteur product: For active immunization of persons 18-64 years of age at increased risk of exposure to the influenza A (H5N1) virus subtype contained in the vaccine

Pregnancy Considerations Adverse events were not observed in animal reproduction studies using the H5N1 vaccine GlaxoSmithKline adjuvanted product; animal reproduction studies have not been conducted with the Sanofi Pasteur product. Inactivated viral vaccines have not been shown to cause increased risks to the fetus (CDC, 2011).

Breast-Feeding Considerations It is not known if this vaccine is excreted into breast milk. Inactivated virus vaccines do not affect the safety of breast-feeding for the mother or the infant (CDC, 2011).

Prescribing and Access Restrictions Commercial distribution is not planned. The vaccine will be included as part of the U.S. Strategic National Stockpile. It will be distributed by public health officials if needed.

Contraindications

GlaxoSmithKline product (adjuvanted): Known severe allergic reactions (eg, anaphylaxis) to any component of the vaccine, including egg protein, or after a previous dose of an influenza vaccine.

Sanofi Pasteur product: There are no contraindications listed in the manufacturer's labeling.

Warnings/Precautions Immediate treatment (including epinephrine 1:1000) for anaphylactoid and/or hypersensitivity reactions should be available during vaccine use. Use with caution in patients with a history of Guillain-Barré syndrome (GBS); these patients may have a greater likelihood of developing GBS. If recent occurrence of GBS (≤6 weeks), decision to administer vaccine should entail careful consideration of risk:benefit. Recent studies of patients who received the trivalent inactivated influenza vaccine or the monovalent H1N1 influenza vaccine have shown the risk of GBS is lower with vaccination than with influenza infection (Baxter, 2013; Greene, 2013; Kwong, 2013). Vaccination may not result in effective immunity in all patients. Response depends upon multiple factors (eg, type of vaccine, age of patient) and may be improved by administering the vaccine at the recommended dose, route, and interval. Vaccines may not be effective if administered during periods of altered immune competence (CDC, 2011). Use with caution in severely immunocompromised patients (eg, patients receiving chemo/radiation therapy or other immunosuppressive therapy [including high-dose corticosteroids]); may have a reduced response to vaccination (CDC, 2011). In general, household and close contacts of persons with altered immunocompetence may receive all age appropriate vaccines (CDC, 2011); inactivated vaccines should be administered ≥2 weeks prior to planned immunosuppression when feasible (Rubin, 2014). Syncope has been reported with use of injectable vaccines and may be accompanied by transient visual disturbances, weakness, or tonic-clonic movements. Procedures should be in place to avoid injuries from falling and to restore cerebral perfusion if syncope occurs. Sanofi Pasteur product has not been evaluated in patients ≥65 years of age. Some products may be manufactured with chicken egg protein. Some products may contain thimerosal; hypersensitivity reactions may occur

Adverse Reactions All serious adverse reactions must be reported to the U.S. Department of Health and Human Services (DHHS) Vaccine Adverse Event Reporting System (VAERS) 1-800-822-7967 or online at https://vaers.hhs.gov/esub/index.

>10%:
Central nervous system: Headache (3% to 35%), fatigue (34%), shivering (17%)
Dermatologic: Diaphoresis (11%)
Local: Pain at injection site (74% to 83%), tenderness at injection site (70%), erythema at injection site (9% to 20%), swelling at injection site (10% to 15%)
Neuromuscular & skeletal: Myalgia (45%), arthralgia (25%)

1% to 10%:
Gastrointestinal: Nausea (10%), diarrhea (6%)
Local: Itching at injection site (2%), burning sensation at injection site (1%)
Respiratory: Nasal congestion (1%)
Miscellaneous: Fever (5%)

<1% (Limited to important or life-threatening): Celiac disease, cerebrovascular accident, convulsions, cranial nerve palsy (IV), Crohn's disease, erythema nodosum, facial paralysis, giant-cell arteritis, hepatitis, malignant neoplasm of thyroid, organ transplant rejection (corneal), polymyalgia rheumatica, psoriasis, pulmonary embolism, radiculopathy, rheumatoid arthritis, rheumatoid lung

Drug Interactions

Metabolism/Transport Effects None known.

Avoid Concomitant Use There are no known interactions where it is recommended to avoid concomitant use.

Increased Effect/Toxicity There are no known significant interactions involving an increase in effect.

Decreased Effect

The levels/effects of Influenza A Virus Vaccine (H5N1) may be decreased by: Belimumab; Fingolimod; Immunosuppressants

Preparation for Administration GlaxoSmithKline product (adjuvanted): Prior to mixing, bring one vial of H5N1 antigen and one vial of AS03 adjuvant to room temperature (minimum of 15 minutes). Invert each vial to mix; do not use if particulate matter or discoloration are present. Withdraw contents of adjuvant vial and add to the H5N1 antigen vial. Mix thoroughly by inversion and label with the time and date of mixing on vial. After mixing, the final volume provides 10 doses (0.5 mL each). Use within 24 hours of mixing.

Storage/Stability

Sanofi Pasteur product: Store in a refrigerator at 2°C to 8°C (35°F to 46°F). Do not freeze. Discard if frozen. Protect from light.

GlaxoSmithKline product (adjuvanted): Prior to mixing, the H5N1 antigen and AS03 adjuvant vials should be stored in a refrigerator between 2°C and 8°C (36°F and 46°F). Do not freeze. Discard if frozen. Protect from light. After mixing, the vaccine may be stored under refrigeration between 2°C and 8°C (36°F and 46°F) or at room temperature up to 30°C (86°F) for up to 24 hours. Do not freeze. Discard if frozen. Protect from light.

Mechanism of Action

The GlaxoSmithKline product is an adjuvanted monovalent split virus (inactivated) preparation of the type A, subtype H5N1 avian strain of influenza virus (A/Indonesia/05/2005)

The Sanofi Pasteur product is a monovalent, split virus (inactivated) preparation of the type A, subtype H5N1 avian strain of influenza virus (A/Vietnam/1203/2004)

Both promote active immunity to influenza A H5N1 (avian).

Pharmacodynamics/Kinetics Onset of action:

GlaxoSmithKline product (adjuvanted): Fourfold increase in antibody titers (measured by hemagglutination inhibition [HI]) occurred in up to 90% of patients 18-64 years of age and 74% of patients ≥65 years of age 21 days after the second dose

Sanofi Pasteur product: Fourfold increase in antibody titers (measured by HI) occurred in up to 58% of patients 28 days after the second dose (Treanor, 2006).

Dosing

Adult Immunization:

GlaxoSmithKline product (adjuvanted): Adults ≥18 years: IM: 0.5 mL, followed by a second 0.5 mL dose given 21 days later

Sanofi Pasteur product: Adults 18-64 years: IM: 1 mL, followed by second 1 mL dose given 28 days later (acceptable range: 21-35 days)

Renal Impairment No dosage adjustment provided in manufacturer's labeling.

Hepatic Impairment No dosage adjustment provided in manufacturer's labeling.

Administration For IM administration only. Inspect for particulate matter and discoloration prior to administration. Vaccinate in the deltoid muscle using a ≥1 inch needle length. Suspension should be shaken well prior to use.

GlaxoSmithKline product (adjuvanted): If vaccine is stored under refrigeration after mixing, bring to room temperature prior to administration (minimum 15 minutes).

Note: For patients at risk of hemorrhage following intramuscular injection, the ACIP recommends "it should be administered intramuscularly if, in the opinion of the physician familiar with the patient's bleeding risk, the vaccine can be administered by this route with reasonable safety. If the patient receives antihemophilia or other similar therapy, intramuscular vaccination can be scheduled shortly after such therapy is administered. A fine needle (23 gauge or smaller) can be used for the vaccination and firm pressure applied to the site (without rubbing) for at least 2 minutes. The patient should be instructed concerning the risk of hematoma from the injection." Patients on anticoagulant therapy should be considered to have the same bleeding risks and treated as those with clotting factor disorders (CDC, 2011).

Simultaneous administration of vaccines helps ensure the patients will be fully vaccinated by the appropriate age. Simultaneous administration of vaccines is defined as administering >1 vaccine on the same day at different anatomic sites. Separate vaccines should not be combined in the same syringe unless indicated by product specific labeling. Separate needles and syringes should be used for each injection. The ACIP prefers each dose of a specific vaccine in a series come from the same manufacturer when possible. Adolescents and adults should be vaccinated while seated or lying down. In general, preterm infants should be vaccinated at the same chronological age as full-term infants (CDC, 2011).

Antipyretics have not been shown to prevent febrile seizures. Antipyretics may be used to treat fever or discomfort following vaccination (CDC, 2011). One study reported that routine prophylactic administration of acetaminophen to prevent fever prior to vaccination decreased the immune response of some vaccines; the clinical significance of this reduction in immune response has not been established (Prymula, 2009).

Monitoring Parameters Monitor for syncope for 15 minutes following administration. If seizure-like activity associated with syncope occurs, maintain patient in supine or Trendelenburg position to reestablish adequate cerebral perfusion (CDC, 2011).

Additional Information U.S. federal law requires that the name of medication, date of administration, the vaccine manufacturer, lot number of vaccine, and the administering person's name, title, and address be entered into the patient's permanent medical record.

Because there are many strains of the H5N1 virus, multiple vaccines are under development. The antibody level needed for protection is not well established (Abdel-Ghafar, 2008) and a fourfold increase in hemagglutination inhibition antibody titers is generally used to measure immune response in clinical trials. The 2-dose regimen studied using H5N1 vaccine (Sanofi Pasteur product) prompted antibody response consistent with a protective titer in up to 58% of patients (Treanor, 2006). A second study has shown that a third dose of the vaccine further increases the antibody response (Zangwill, 2008). The GlaxoSmithKline product (adjuvant) was shown to increase the immune response while sparing the amount of antigen needed per dose. This would allow for more vaccine to be produced using available antigen; however, the risk of adverse events was also increased (Langley, 2011).

Health care workers involved in the care of patients with known or suspected H5N1 viral subtype influenza infection should be vaccinated with the most recent seasonal human influenza vaccine in order to reduce the risk of coinfection of human influenza A viruses (OSHA, 2006).

Product Availability Products will not be commercially available; distribution will be limited as part of the US Strategic National Stockpile.

GlaxoSmithKline product (adjuvanted) product, (also referred to as Q-Pan H5N1 influenza vaccine): FDA approved November 2013.

Dosage Forms Excipient information presented when available (limited, particularly for generics); consult specific product labeling.

Injection, emulsion [monovalent]: GlaxoSmithKline product: Adjuvanted Hemagglutinin [A/Indonesia/05/2005 (H5N1)] 3.75 mcg/0.5 mL (5 mL) [contains egg protein, polysorbate 80, and thimerosal]

Injection, suspension [monovalent]: Sanofi Pasteur product: Hemagglutinin [A/Vietnam/1203/2004 (H5N1)] 90 mcg/mL (5 mL) [contains chicken and egg protein, porcine gelatin, and thimerosal]

◆ Influenza Vaccine see Influenza Virus Vaccine (Inactivated) on page 945

◆ Influenza Vaccine see Influenza Virus Vaccine (Live/Attenuated) on page 950

◆ Influenza Virus Vaccine (H5N1) see Influenza A Virus Vaccine (H5N1) on page 944

Influenza Virus Vaccine (Inactivated)
(in floo EN za VYE rus vak SEEN, in ak ti VAY ted)

Brand Names: US Afluria; Fluad; Fluarix Quadrivalent; Flucelvax; Flulaval Quadrivalent; Fluvirin; Fluzone; Fluzone High-Dose; Fluzone Intradermal Quadrivalent; Fluzone Quadrivalent

Brand Names: Canada Agriflu; Fluad; Fluad Pediatric; Flulaval Tetra; Fluviral; Fluzone Quadrivalent; Influvac

Index Terms ccIIV3 [Flucelvax]; Cell Culture Inactivated Influenza Vaccine, Trivalent [Flucelvax]; Fluad; H1N1 Influenza Vaccine; IIV; IIV3; IIV4; Inactivated Influenza Vaccine, Quadrivalent; Inactivated Influenza Vaccine, Trivalent; Influenza Vaccine; Influenza Virus Vaccine (Purified Surface Antigen); Influenza Virus Vaccine (Split-Virus); TIV (Trivalent Inactivated Influenza Vaccine)

Pharmacologic Category Vaccine; Vaccine, Inactivated (Viral)

Additional Appendix Information

Immunization Administration Recommendations on page 1974

Immunization Schedules on page 1979

Use Influenza disease prevention: Active immunization against influenza disease caused by influenza virus subtypes A and type B contained in the vaccine in the following persons:

US labeling:
- 6 months and older (Fluzone, Fluzone Quadrivalent)
- 3 years and older (Fluarix Quadrivalent, FluLaval Quadrivalent)
- 4 years and older (Fluvirin)
- 5 years and older (Afluria)
- 18 years and older (Flucelvax)
- 18 through 64 years of age (Fluzone Intradermal Quadrivalent)
- 65 years and older (Fluad, Fluzone High-Dose)

Canadian labeling:
- 6 months to <2 years (Fluad Pediatric)
- 6 months and older (Agriflu, Flulaval Tetra, Fluviral, Fluzone Quadrivalent)
- 18 years and older (Influvac)
- 65 years and older (Fluad)

The Advisory Committee on Immunization Practices (ACIP) recommends routine annual vaccination with the seasonal influenza vaccine for all persons ≥6 months of age who do not otherwise have contraindications to the vaccine (ACIP [Grohskopf 2015]).

The ACIP recommends use of any age and risk factor appropriate product and does not have a preferential recommendation for use of the trivalent inactivated influenza vaccine (IIV_3) or the quadrivalent inactivated influenza vaccine (IIV_4). In addition to the IIV products, other alternative products are available for certain patient populations: Healthy nonpregnant persons aged 2 to 49 years may receive vaccination with the live attenuated influenza vaccine (LAIV). Persons 18 years and older may receive vaccination with the recombinant influenza vaccine (RIV) (ACIP [Grohskopf 2015]).

The Canadian National Advisory Committee on Immunization (NACI) recommends annual vaccination with seasonal influenza vaccine for all persons ≥6 months who do not otherwise have contraindications to the vaccine. Healthy, nonpregnant persons aged 2 to 59 years may receive vaccination with the seasonal live, attenuated influenza vaccine (LAIV) (nasal spray). When readily available, NACI prefers use of LAIV (nasal spray) in healthy persons 2 to 17 years of age. LAIV is not recommended in patients with severe asthma or wheezing requiring medical attention in the 7 days prior to vaccination, adults with chronic health conditions, and children and adults who are immunocompromised. Where LAIV is not recommended, use of quadrivalent inactivated influenza vaccine (QIV) or trivalent inactivated influenza vaccine (TIV) if QIV not available, is recommended.

When vaccine supply is limited, target groups for vaccination (those at higher risk of complications from influenza infection and their close contacts) include the following (CDC/ACIP [Grohskopf 2013]):
- Infants and children 6 to 59 months of age
- Persons ≥50 years of age
- Infants, children, and adolescents (6 months to 18 years of age) who are receiving long-term aspirin therapy, and therefore, may be at risk for developing Reye's syndrome after influenza
- Women who are or will be pregnant during the influenza season
- Patients with chronic pulmonary disorders (including asthma) or cardiovascular systems disorders (except hypertension), renal, hepatic, neurologic, or metabolic disorders (including diabetes mellitus)
- Persons who have immunosuppression (including immunosuppression caused by medications or HIV)
- Residents of nursing homes and other long-term care facilities
- American Indians/Alaska Natives
- Morbidly obese (BMI ≥40)
- Healthcare personnel
- Household contacts (including children) and caregivers of neonates, infants, and children <5 years (particularly children <6 months) and adults ≥50 years
- Household contacts (including children) and caregivers of persons with medical conditions which put them at high risk of complications from influenza infection

Pregnancy Considerations Adverse events were not observed in animal reproduction studies. Inactivated influenza vaccine has not been shown to cause fetal harm when given to pregnant women, although information related to use in the first trimester is limited (CDC/ACIP [Grohskopf 2013]). Following maternal immunization with the inactivated influenza virus vaccine, vaccine specific antibodies are observed in the newborn (Englund 1993; Steinhoff 2010; Zaman 2008; Zuccotti 2010). Vaccination of pregnant women protects infants from influenza infection, including infants <6 months of age who are not able to be vaccinated (CDC/ACIP [Grohskopf 2013]).

Pregnant women are at an increased risk of complications from influenza infection (Rasmussen 2008). Influenza vaccination with the inactivated influenza vaccine (IIV) is recommended for all women who are or will become pregnant during the influenza season and who do not otherwise have contraindications to the vaccine (CDC/ACIP [Grohskopf 2013]). Pregnant women should observe the same precautions as nonpregnant women to reduce the risk of exposure to influenza and other respiratory infections (CDC 2010). When vaccine supply is limited, focus on delivering the vaccine should be given to women who are pregnant or will be pregnant during the flu season, as well as mothers of newborns and contacts or caregivers of children <5 years of age (CDC/ACIP [Grohskopf 2013]).

Health care providers are encouraged to refer women exposed to the influenza vaccine during pregnancy to the Vaccines and Medications in Pregnancy Surveillance System (VAMPSS) by contacting The Organization of Teratology Information Specialists (OTIS) at (877) 311-8972.

Women exposed to Flulaval Quadrivalent or Fluarix Quadrivalent vaccine during pregnancy or their healthcare provider may also contact the GlaxoSmithKline registry at 888-452-9622.

Healthcare providers may enroll women exposed to Fluzone Intradermal Quadrivalent or Fluzone Quadrivalent during pregnancy in the Sanofi Pasteur vaccination registry at 800-822-2463.

Breast-Feeding Considerations It is not known if inactivated influenza vaccine is excreted into breast milk. The manufacturers recommend that caution be used if administered to nursing women. Anti-influenza IgA antibodies can be detected in breast milk following maternal vaccination with the trivalent IIV vaccine (Schlaudecker 2013). Inactivated vaccines do not affect the safety of breastfeeding for the mother or the infant (NCIRD/ACIP 2011). Postpartum women may be vaccinated with either IIV or LAIV (CDC/ACIP [Grohskopf 2013]). When vaccine supply is limited, focus on delivering the vaccine should be given to women who are pregnant or will be pregnant during the flu season, as well as mothers of newborns and contacts or caregivers of children <5 years of age (CDC/ACIP [Grohskopf 2013]). Breast-feeding infants should be vaccinated according to the recommended schedules (NCIRD/ACIP 2011).

Medication Guide Available Yes

Contraindications
Severe allergic reaction (eg, anaphylaxis) to a previous influenza vaccination; hypersensitivity to any component of the formulation

Additional manufacturer contraindications for Afluria, Fluad, Fluarix Quadrivalent, FluLaval Quadrivalent, Flu-virin, Fluzone, Fluzone High-Dose, Fluzone Intradermal Quadrivalent, Fluzone Quadrivalent: History of severe allergic reaction (eg, anaphylaxis) to egg protein

Agriflu, Flulaval Tetra, Fluviral [Canadian products]: Hypersensitivity to egg protein.

Warnings/Precautions Immediate treatment (including epinephrine 1:1,000) for anaphylactoid and/or hypersensitivity reactions should be available during vaccine use (NCIRD/ACIP 2011). Oculorespiratory syndrome (ORS) is an acute, self-limiting reaction to IIV with one or more of the following symptoms appearing within 2 to 24 hours after the dose: Chest tightness, cough, difficulty breathing, facial swelling, red eyes, sore throat, or wheezing. Symptoms resolve within 48 hours of onset. The cause of ORS has not been established, but studies have suggested that it is not IgE-mediated. However, because ORS symptoms may be similar to those of an IgE-mediated hypersensitivity reaction, health care providers unsure of etiology of symptoms should seek advice from an allergist/immunologist when determining whether a patient may be revaccinated in subsequent seasons (CDC/ACIP [Grohskopf 2013]).

Most products are manufactured with chicken egg protein (expressed as ovalbumin content when content is disclosed on prescribing information). The ovalbumin content may vary from season to season and lot to lot of vaccine. Allergy to eggs must be distinguished from allergy to the vaccine. Recommendations are available from the ACIP and NACI regarding influenza vaccination to persons who report egg allergies; however, ACIP states a prior severe allergic reaction to influenza vaccine, regardless of the component suspected, is a contraindication to vaccination. Patients with a history of egg allergy who have experienced only hives following egg exposure should receive influenza vaccine using IIV (egg- or cell-culture based) or RIV, if otherwise appropriate; however, the vaccine should only be administered by a health care provider familiar with the manifestations of egg allergy and patients should be monitored for at least 30 minutes after vaccination (ACIP [Grohskopf 2015]). NACI does not consider an egg allergy as a contraindication to vaccination (NACI, July 2015). Flucelvax (ccIIV3) is an inactivated influenza vaccine manufactured using cell culture technology and provides an alternative to vaccines cultured with chicken egg protein but should not be considered egg free. It may be used in persons with a mild egg allergy if age appropriate and there are no other contraindications; appropriate precautions should be observed (ACIP [Grohskopf 2015]). Some products are manufactured with gentamicin, kanamycin,

neomycin, polymyxin, or thimerosal; some packaging may contain natural latex rubber.

Some dosage forms may contain polysorbate 80 (also known as Tweens). Hypersensitivity reactions, usually a delayed reaction, have been reported following exposure to pharmaceutical products containing polysorbate 80 in certain individuals (Isaksson 2002; Lucente 2000; Shelley 1995). Thrombocytopenia, ascites, pulmonary deterioration, and renal and hepatic failure have been reported in premature neonates after receiving parenteral products containing polysorbate 80 (Alade 1986; CDC 1984). See manufacturer's labeling.

The decision to administer or delay vaccination because of current or recent febrile illness depends on the severity of symptoms and the etiology of the disease. Consider deferring administration in patients with moderate or severe acute illness (with or without fever); vaccination should not be delayed for patients with mild acute illness (with or without fever) (NCIRD/ACIP, 2011). Postmarketing reports of increased incidence of fever and febrile seizures in children <5 years of age has been observed with the use of the 2010 Southern Hemisphere formulation of the Afluria vaccine. Febrile events have also been reported in children 5 to <9 years of age. Based on information from the CDC, an increased rate of febrile seizures has been reported in young children 6 months to 4 years who received vaccination with inactivated influenza vaccine (IIV) and the 13-valent pneumococcal conjugate vaccine (PCV13) simultaneously. However, due to the risks associated with delaying either vaccine, administering them at separate visits or deviating from the recommended vaccine schedule is not currently recommended. The ACIP does not recommend use of Afluria in children <9 years of age (ACIP [Grohskopf 2015]; CDC/ACIP [Grohskopf 2013]). Antipyretics have not been shown to prevent febrile seizures; antipyretics may be used to treat fever or discomfort following vaccination (NCIRD/ACIP, 2011). One study reported that routine prophylactic administration of acetaminophen to prevent fever prior to vaccination decreased the immune response of some vaccines; the clinical significance of this reduction in immune response has not been established (Prymula 2009).

Syncope has been reported with use of injectable vaccines and may result in serious secondary injury (eg, skull fracture, cerebral hemorrhage); typically reported in adolescents and young adults and within 15 minutes after vaccination. Procedures should be in place to avoid injuries from falling and to restore cerebral perfusion if syncope occurs (NCIRD/ACIP 2011).

Use with caution in patients with history of Guillain-Barré syndrome (GBS); patients with history of GBS have a greater likelihood of developing GBS than those without. As a precaution, the ACIP recommends that patients with a history of GBS and who are at low risk for severe influenza complications, and patients known to have experienced GBS within 6 weeks following previous vaccination should generally not be vaccinated (consider influenza antiviral chemoprophylaxis in these patients). The benefits of vaccination may outweigh the potential risks in persons with a history of GBS who are also at high risk for complications of influenza (CDC/ACIP [Grohskopf 2013]). Recent studies of patients who received the trivalent inactivated influenza vaccine or the monovalent H1N1 influenza vaccine have shown the risk of GBS is lower with vaccination than with influenza infection (Baxter 2013; Greene 2013; Kwong 2013). Some Canadian product labeling recommends delaying therapy in patients with active neurologic disorders.

Use with caution in severely immunocompromised patients (eg, patients receiving chemo/radiation therapy or other immunosuppressive therapy [including high-dose corticosteroid]); may have a reduced response to vaccination. Inactivated vaccine (IIV or RIV) is preferred over live virus vaccine for household members, healthcare workers and others coming in close contact with severely-immunosuppressed persons requiring care in a protected environment (ACIP [Grohskopf 2015]; NCIRD/ACIP 2011). In general, inactivated vaccines should be administered ≥2 weeks prior to planned immunosuppression when feasible (IDSA [Rubin 2014]). Antigenic response may not be as great as expected in HIV-infected persons with CD4 cells <100/mm³ and viral copies of HIV type 1 >30,000/mL, and a second dose does not improve immune response in these persons (CDC/ACIP [Grohskopf 2013]). Antibody responses may be lower and decline faster in older adults ≥65 years compared to younger adults, especially by 6 months postvaccination; however, deferral to later in the season may result in missed vaccination opportunities or early season infection (ACIP [Grohskopf 2015]). Use of this vaccine for specific medical and/or other indications

(eg, immunocompromising conditions, hepatic or kidney disease, diabetes) is also addressed in the ACIP Recommended Adult Immunization Schedule (CDC/ACIP [Kim 2015]). Specific recommendations for use of this vaccine in immunocompromised patients with asplenia, cancer, HIV infection, cerebrospinal fluid leaks, cochlear implants, hematopoietic stem cell transplant (prior to or after), sickle cell disease, solid organ transplant (prior to or after), or those receiving immunosuppressive therapy for chronic conditions are available from the IDSA (Rubin 2014).

Seasonal influenza immunization (with inactivated vaccine) is recommended for all patients receiving chemotherapy for malignancy, and for all family and household contacts (Flowers 2013). Life-long seasonal influenza immunization (with inactivated vaccine) is also recommended for hematopoietic cell transplant candidates and recipients; vaccination of family members and close or household contacts is strongly recommended during each flu season and continuing annually as long the recipient is immunocompromised, even if beyond 24 months after transplant (Tomblyn 2009).

Use with caution in patients with a history of bleeding disorders (including thrombocytopenia) and/or patients on anticoagulant therapy; bleeding/hematoma may occur from IM administration; if the patient receives antihemophilia or other similar therapy, IM injection can be scheduled shortly after such therapy is administered (NCIRD/ACIP 2011). In order to maximize vaccination rates, the ACIP, as well as the Canadian National Advisory Committee on Immunization (NACI), recommends simultaneous administration (ie, >1 vaccine on the same day at different anatomic sites) of all age-appropriate vaccines (live or inactivated) for which a person is eligible at a single clinic visit, unless contraindications exist. The ACIP prefers each dose of a specific vaccine in a series come from the same manufacturer when possible (NACI July 2015; NCIRD/ACIP 2011). Vaccination may not result in effective immunity in all patients. Response depends upon multiple factors (eg, type of vaccine, age of patient) and may be improved by administering the vaccine at the recommended dose, route, and interval. Vaccines may not be effective if administered during periods of altered immune competence (NCIRD/ACIP 2011). Influenza vaccines from previous seasons must not be used (CDC/ACIP [Grohskopf 2013]).

Adverse Reactions All serious adverse reactions must be reported to the US Department of Health and Human Services (DHHS) Vaccine Adverse Event Reporting System (VAERS) 1-800-822-7967 or online at https://vaers.hhs.gov/esub/index. In Canada, adverse reactions may be reported to local provincial/territorial health agencies or to the Vaccine Safety Section at Public Health Agency of Canada (1-866-844-0018).

Frequency not defined. Adverse reactions in adults ≥65 years of age may be greater using the high-dose vaccine, but are typically mild and transient.

Cardiovascular: Chest tightness, hypertension

Central nervous system: Chills, drowsiness, fatigue, headache, irritability, malaise, migraine, shivering

Dermatologic: Diaphoresis, ecchymoses

Gastrointestinal: Decreased appetite, diarrhea, gastroenteritis, nausea, sore throat, upper abdominal pain, vomiting

Infection: Infection, varicella

Local: Injection site reactions (including bruising, erythema, induration, inflammation, itching at injection site, pain, soreness, swelling at injection site, tenderness at injection site)

Neuromuscular & skeletal: Arthralgia, back pain, myalgia (may start within 6 to 12 hours and last 1 to 2 days; incidence generally equal to placebo in adults; occurs more frequently than placebo in children)

Ophthalmic: Eye redness

Respiratory: Bronchitis, cough, dyspnea, nasal congestion, nasopharyngitis, oropharyngeal pain, pharyngitis, pharyngolaryngeal pain, respiratory congestion (upper), rhinitis, rhinorrhea, upper respiratory tract infection, wheezing

Miscellaneous: Crying (infants and children 6 to 35 months), fever

Postmarketing and/or case reports (limited to important or life-threatening): Bell's palsy, erythema multiforme, febrile seizures, Guillain-Barre syndrome, hypersensitivity reaction (including oculorespiratory syndrome, an acute, self-limited reaction with ocular and respiratory symptoms) (CDC/ACIP [Grohskopf, 2013]), IgA vasculitis, limb paralysis, lymphadenopathy, maculopapular rash, microscopic polyangiitis (vasculitis), myelitis (including encephalomyelitis), neuralgia, optic neuritis, optic neuropathy, paralysis (including limb), photophobia, seizure, serum sickness, Stevens-Johnson syndrome, syncope,

tachycardia, thrombocytopenia, transverse myelitis, vasculitis, vesicobullous rash

Drug Interactions

Metabolism/Transport Effects None known.

Avoid Concomitant Use There are no known interactions where it is recommended to avoid concomitant use.

Increased Effect/Toxicity

Influenza Virus Vaccine (Inactivated) may increase the levels/effects of: Doxofylline

Decreased Effect

Influenza Virus Vaccine (Inactivated) may decrease the levels/effects of: Pneumococcal Conjugate Vaccine (13-Valent)

The levels/effects of Influenza Virus Vaccine (Inactivated) may be decreased by: Belimumab; Fingolimod; Immunosuppressants; Pneumococcal Conjugate Vaccine (13-Valent)

Storage/Stability Store all products between 2°C to 8°C (36°F to 46°F). Potency is destroyed by freezing; do not use if product has been frozen.

Afluria: Discard multiple dose vials 28 days after initial entry. Between uses, the multiple dose vial should be stored at 2°C to 8°C (36°F to 46°F).

Fluad, Fluarix Quadrivalent, Flucelvax, Influvac: Protect from light.

Agriflu, Fluad, Fluad Pediatric: Protect from light. May be used if exposed to temperatures between 8°C to 25°C for less than 2 hours.

Fluviral: Discard multiple dose vials 28 days after initial entry. Protect from light.

Flulaval Quadrivalent, Flulaval Tetra [Canadian product]: Between uses, the multiple dose vial should be stored at 2°C to 8°C (36°F to 46°F). Do not freeze. Protect from light. Discard multiple dose vials 28 days after initial entry.

Fluvirin: Between uses, the multiple dose vial should be stored at 2°C to 8°C (36°F to 46°F). Protect from light.

Fluzone: Between uses, the multiple dose vial should be stored at 2°C to 8°C (36°F to 46°F).

Mechanism of Action Promotes immunity to seasonal influenza virus by inducing specific antibody production. Each year the formulation is standardized according to the US Public Health Service. Preparations from previous seasons must not be used.

Pharmacodynamics/Kinetics

Onset of action: Most adults have antibody protection within 2 weeks of vaccination (CDC/ACIP [Grohskopf 2013])

Duration: ≥6 to 8 months when vaccine is antigenically similar to circulating virus (CDC/ACIP [Grohskopf 2013]); response may be diminished in persons ≥65 years and limited evidence suggests titers may decline significantly 6 months following vaccination in this population (ACIP [Grohskopf 2015]).

Dosing

Adult It is important to note that influenza seasons vary in their timing and duration from year to year. In general, vaccination should begin soon after the vaccine becomes available (and, if possible, by October) and prior to onset of influenza activity in the community. However, vaccination should continue throughout the influenza season as long as vaccine is available. Unless noted, the ACIP does not have a preference for any given inactivated influenza vaccine (IIV) formulation when used within their specified age indications.

Immunization:

Afluria:

Adults ≤64 years: IM or via PharmaJet Stratis Needle-Free Injection System: 0.5 mL per dose as a single dose (1 dose per season)

Adults >64 years: IM: 0.5 mL per dose as a single dose (1 dose per season)

Fluarix Quadrivalent, Flucelvax, FluLaval Quadrivalent, Fluvirin, Fluzone, Fluzone Quadrivalent: 0.5 mL/dose (1 dose per season)

Fluzone Intradermal Quadrivalent: Adults 18 to 64 years: Intradermal: 0.1 mL/dose (1 dose per season)

Canadian labeling:

Agriflu, Flulaval Tetra, Fluviral, Fluzone Quadrivalent: IM: 0.5 mL/dose (1 dose per season)

Influvac: IM, SubQ: 0.5 mL/dose (1 per season)

Geriatric It is important to note that influenza seasons vary in their timing and duration from year to year. In general, vaccination should begin soon after the vaccine becomes available (and, if possible, by October) and prior to onset of influenza activity in the community. However, vaccination should continue throughout the influenza season as long as vaccine is available. Unless noted, the ACIP does not have a preference for any given inactivated influenza vaccine (IIV) formulation when used within their specified age indications.

Immunization: Adults ≥65 years:

Afluria, Fluad, Fluarix Quadrivalent, Flucelvax, FluLaval Quadrivalent, Fluvirin, Fluzone, Fluzone High-Dose, Fluzone Quadrivalent: IM: 0.5 mL/dose (1 dose per season).

Flulaval Tetra [Canadian product]: IM: 0.5 mL/dose (1 dose per season)

Pediatric It is important to note that influenza seasons vary in their timing and duration from year to year. In general, vaccination should begin soon after the vaccine becomes available (and, if possible, by October) and prior to onset of influenza activity in the community. However, vaccination should continue throughout the influenza season as long as vaccine is available. Unless noted, the ACIP does not have a preference for any given inactivated influenza vaccine (IIV) formulation when used within their specified age indications.

Immunization: IM:

Afluria:

Children 5 to 8 years: 0.5 mL/dose (1 or 2 doses per season; see **"Note"**): Although FDA-approved for use in children ≥5 years of age, the ACIP does not recommend use of Afluria in children <9 years due to an increased incidence of fever and febrile seizures observed with use of the 2010 Southern Hemisphere formulation of Afluria in this age group. However, if other age-appropriate vaccines are not available, children 5 to 8 years of age who are also considered at risk for influenza complications may be given Afluria. The benefits and risks of this vaccine should be discussed with parents or caregivers prior to administration (ACIP [Grohskopf 2015]).

Children ≥9 years and Adolescents: Refer to adult dosing.

Fluarix Quadrivalent, FluLaval Quadrivalent:

Children 3 to 8 years: 0.5 mL/dose (1 or 2 doses per season; see **"Note"**)

Children ≥9 years and Adolescents: Refer to adult dosing.

Fluzone, Fluzone Quadrivalent:

Infants and Children 6 to 35 months: 0.25 mL/dose (1 or 2 doses per season; see **"Note"**)

Children 3 to 8 years: 0.5 mL/dose (1 or 2 doses per season; see **"Note"**)

Children ≥9 years and Adolescents: Refer to adult dosing.

Fluvirin:

Children 4 to 8 years: 0.5 mL/dose (1 or 2 doses per season; see **"Note"**)

Children ≥9 years and Adolescents: Refer to adult dosing.

Note: Infants and children 6 months to <9 years who received at least two doses of trivalent or quadrivalent influenza vaccine prior to July 1, 2015, need only 1 dose of the 2015 to 2016 seasonal influenza vaccine. The 2 doses need not have been received during the same season or consecutive seasons. All other children <9 years (including those whose vaccination status cannot be determined) should receive 2 doses separated by ≥4 weeks, in order to achieve satisfactory antibody response. (ACIP [Grohskopf 2015]).

Canadian labeling:

Agriflu, Fluzone Quadrivalent: IM:

Infants and Children 6 to 35 months: Manufacturer labeling: 0.25 mL/dose; NACI recommendation: 0.5 mL/dose (NACI 2015) (1 dose per season); a second dose should be administered 4 weeks after the first in previously unvaccinated patients

Children 3 to 8 years: 0.5 mL/dose (1 dose per season); a second dose should be administered 4 weeks after the first in previously unvaccinated patients

Children ≥9 years and Adolescents: Refer to adult dosing.

Fluad Pediatric: IM: Infants and Children 6 months to <2 years: 0.25 mL/dose (1 dose per season); a second dose should be administered 4 weeks after the first in previously unvaccinated patients and in patients who were vaccinated for the first time last season and only one dose was received.

Flulaval Tetra: IM:

Infants ≥6 months and Children <9 years: 0.5 mL/dose (1 dose per season); a second dose should be administered 4 weeks after the first in previously unvaccinated patients

Children ≥9 years and Adolescents: Refer to adult dosing.

Fluviral: IM:

Infants and Children 6 months to 8 years: 0.5 mL/dose (1 dose per season); a second dose should be administered 4 weeks after the first in previously unvaccinated patients

Children ≥9 years and Adolescents: Refer to adult dosing.

Renal Impairment There are no dosage adjustments provided in the manufacturer's labeling.

Hepatic Impairment There are no dosage adjustments provided in the manufacturer's labeling.

Administration *Fluzone Intradermal Quadrivalent:* For intradermal administration, preferably into the skin over the deltoid muscle only. Gently shake gently prior to use. Hold system using the thumb and middle finger (do not place fingers on windows). Insert needle perpendicular to the skin; inject using index finger to push on plunger. Do not aspirate.

Afluria, Fluarix Quadrivalent, Flucelvax, FluLaval Quadrivalent, Fluvirin, Fluzone, Fluzone High-Dose, Fluzone Quadrivalent, Agriflu [Canadian product], Fluad, Fluad Pediatric [Canadian product], FluLaval Tetra [Canadian product], Fluviral [Canadian product]: For IM administration only. Suspensions should be shaken well prior to use. Inspect for particulate matter and discoloration prior to administration. Some manufacturers recommend avoiding use if visible particles are present in the suspension after shaking. See manufacturer labeling for specific recommendations. Adults and older children should be vaccinated in the deltoid muscle using a ≥1 inch needle length. Infants and young children should be vaccinated in the anterolateral aspect of the thigh using a 1 inch needle length. Children ≥1 years with adequate deltoid muscle mass should be vaccinated using a 1 inch needle. A ⅝-inch needle may be adequate in younger children (refer to guidelines) (CDC/ACIP [Grohskopf 2013]; NCIRD/ACIP, 2011). Do not inject into the gluteal region or areas where there may be a major nerve trunk.

Afluria via PharmaJet Stratis Needle-free Injection System: For IM administration in adults 18 to 64 years of age only. For detailed instructions on preparation and administration of a dose, refer to the information available online at www.pharmajet.com.

Influvac [Canadian product]: May be administered by IM or deep subcutaneous injection. Shake well prior to use. Allow to warm to room temperature prior to use.

Unless otherwise indicated in product labeling, jet injectors should **not** be used to administer inactivated influenza vaccines. Currently, *Afluria* is the only influenza vaccine licensed in the United States that can be given IM by a jet-injector device.

To prevent syncope related injuries, adolescents and adults should be vaccinated while seated or lying down (NCIRD/ACIP 2011). US law requires that the date of administration, the vaccine manufacturer, lot number of vaccine, and the administering person's name, title, and address be entered into the patient's permanent medical record.

If a pediatric vaccine (0.25 mL) is inadvertently administered to an adult, an additional 0.25 mL should be administered to provide the full adult dose (0.5 mL). If the error is discovered after the patient has left, an adult dose should be given as soon as the patient can return. If an adult vaccine (0.5 mL) is inadvertently given to a child, no action needs to be taken (CDC/ACIP [Grohskopf 2013]). *Agriflu [Canadian product]:* If 0.25 mL dose is to be given, discard half the contained syringe volume prior to administration.

Note: For patients at risk of hemorrhage following intramuscular injection, the vaccine should be administered intramuscularly if, in the opinion of the physician familiar with the patient's bleeding risk, the vaccine can be administered by this route with reasonable safety. If the patient receives antihemophilia or other similar therapy, intramuscular vaccination can be scheduled shortly after such therapy is administered. A fine needle (23 gauge or smaller) can be used for the vaccination and firm pressure applied to the site (without rubbing) for at least 2 minutes. The patient should be instructed concerning the risk of hematoma from the injection. Patients on anticoagulant therapy should be considered to have the same bleeding risks and treated as those with clotting factor disorders (NCIRD/ACIP 2011).

Monitoring Parameters Monitor for syncope for 15 minutes following administration (NCIRD/ACIP 2011). If seizure-like activity associated with syncope occurs, maintain patient in supine or Trendelenburg position to reestablish adequate cerebral perfusion. For those individuals who report a history of egg allergy but it is determined that

the inactivated vaccine can be used, observe vaccine recipient for at least 30 minutes after receipt of vaccine (ACIP [Grohskopf 2015]).

Additional Information Pharmacies will stock the formulation(s) standardized according to the USPHS requirements for the season. Influenza vaccines from previous seasons must not be used.

Seasonal quadrivalent influenza vaccines contain two subtype A strains and two subtype B strains; trivalent influenza vaccines contain two subtype A strains and one subtype B strain.

Product Availability Fluad: FDA approved November 2015; anticipated availability is currently unknown. Information pertaining to this product within the monograph is pending revision.

Dosage Forms Excipient information presented when available (limited, particularly for generics); consult specific product labeling.

Suspension, Intramuscular:

Afluria: (5 mL) [contains egg white (egg protein), neomycin sulfate, polymyxin b, thimerosal]

Flulaval Quadrivalent: (5 mL) [contains egg white (egg protein), formaldehyde solution, polysorbate 80, thimerosal]

Fluvirin: (5 mL) [contains egg white (egg protein), neomycin, polymyxin, thimerosal]

Fluzone: (5 mL) [contains egg white (egg protein), formaldehyde solution, gelatin (pork), thimerosal]

Fluzone Quadrivalent: (5 mL) [contains egg white (egg protein), formaldehyde solution, thimerosal]

Suspension, Intramuscular [preservative free]:

Fluzone Quadrivalent: (0.5 mL) [contains egg white (egg protein), formaldehyde solution]

Suspension Pen-injector, Intradermal [preservative free]:

Fluzone Intradermal Quadrivalent: 9 mcg/strain (0.1 mL) [contains egg white (egg protein), formaldehyde solution]

Suspension Prefilled Syringe, Intramuscular [preservative free]:

Afluria: (0.5 mL) [contains egg white (egg protein), neomycin sulfate, polymyxin b]

Fluarix Quadrivalent: (0.5 mL) [contains egg white (egg protein), formaldehyde solution, gentamicin, polysorbate 80]

Flucelvax: (0.5 mL) [contains polysorbate 80]

Flulaval Quadrivalent: (0.5 mL) [contains egg white (egg protein), polysorbate 80, formaldehyde solution]

Fluvirin: (0.5 mL) [contains egg white (egg protein), neomycin, polymyxin]

Fluzone: (5 mL) [contains egg white (egg protein), formaldehyde solution, gelatin (pork)]

Fluzone High-Dose: (0.5 mL) [contains egg white (egg protein), formaldehyde solution]

Fluzone Quadrivalent: (0.25 mL, 0.5 mL) [contains egg white (egg protein), formaldehyde solution]

Dosage Forms: Canada Excipient information presented when available (limited, particularly for generics); consult specific product labeling.

Injection, suspension:

Agriflu: Hemagglutinin 45 mcg/0.5 mL (0.5 mL) [contains chicken egg protein, neomycin (may have trace amounts), kanamycin (may have trace amounts), formaldehyde, polysorbate 80, thimerosal]

Flulaval Tetra: (5 mL) [contains chicken egg protein, formaldehyde solution, polysorbate 80, thimerosal]

Fluviral: Hemagglutinin 45 mcg/0.5 mL (5 mL) [contains chicken egg protein, formaldehyde, polysorbate 80, thimerosal]

Fluzone Quadrivalent: Hemagglutinin 45 mcg/0.5 mL (5 mL) [contains chicken egg protein, formaldehyde, thimerosal]

Injection, suspension [preservative free]:

Agriflu: Hemagglutinin 45 mcg/0.5 mL (0.5 mL) [contains chicken egg protein, neomycin (may have trace amounts), kanamycin (may have trace amounts), formaldehyde, polysorbate 80]

Fluad: Hemagglutinin 45 mcg/0.5 mL (0.5 mL) [contains chicken egg protein, formaldehyde, neomycin (may have trace amounts), kanamycin (may have trace amounts), polysorbate 80]

Fluad Pediatric: Hemagglutinin 22.5 mcg/0.25 mL (0.25 mL) [contains chicken egg protein, formaldehyde, neomycin (may have trace amounts), kanamycin (may have trace amounts), polysorbate 80]

Fluzone Quadrivalent: Hemagglutinin 45 mcg/0.5 mL (0.25 ml, 0.5 mL) [contains chicken egg protein, formaldehyde]

Influvac: Hemagglutinin 45 mcg/0.5 mL (0.5 mL) [contains chicken egg protein, formaldehyde, gentamicin (may have trace amounts), polysorbate 80]

Influenza Virus Vaccine (Live/Attenuated)

(in floo EN za VYE rus vak SEEN live ah TEN yoo aye ted)

Brand Names: US FluMist Quadrivalent

Brand Names: Canada FluMist Quadrivalent

Index Terms H1N1 Influenza Vaccine; Influenza Vaccine; LAIV; LAIV$_4$; Live Attenuated Influenza Vaccine; Live Attenuated Influenza Vaccine (Quadrivalent)

Pharmacologic Category Vaccine; Vaccine, Live (Viral)

Additional Appendix Information

Immunization Administration Recommendations *on page 1974*

Immunization Schedules *on page 1979*

Use Influenza disease prevention:

US labeling: Active immunization of individuals 2 to 49 years of age against influenza disease caused by influenza virus subtypes A and type B contained in the vaccine.

The Advisory Committee on Immunization Practices (ACIP) recommends routine annual vaccination with seasonal influenza vaccine for all persons ≥6 months who do not otherwise have contraindications to the vaccine. ACIP recommends use of any age and risk factor appropriate product. Healthy, nonpregnant persons aged 2 to 49 years may receive vaccination with the seasonal live, attenuated influenza vaccine (LAIV) (nasal spray). In addition, other alternative products are available for certain patient populations: Persons ≥6 months of age may receive the trivalent inactivated influenza vaccine (IIV$_3$) or the quadrivalent inactivated influenza vaccine (IIV$_4$); persons 18 years and older may receive vaccination with the recombinant influenza vaccine (RIV) (ACIP [Grohskopf 2015]).

Canadian labeling: Active immunization of individuals 2 to 59 years of age against influenza disease caused by influenza virus subtypes A and type B contained in the vaccine.

The National Advisory Committee on Immunization (NACI) recommends annual vaccination with seasonal influenza vaccine for all persons ≥6 months who do not otherwise have contraindications to the vaccine. Healthy, nonpregnant persons aged 2 to 59 years may receive vaccination with the seasonal live, attenuated influenza vaccine (LAIV) (nasal spray). When readily available, NACI prefers use of LAIV (nasal spray) in healthy persons 2 to 17 years of age. LAIV is not recommended in patients with severe asthma or wheezing requiring medical attention in the 7 days prior to vaccination, adults with chronic health conditions, and children and adults who are immunocompromised. Where LAIV is not recommended, use of quadrivalent inactivated influenza vaccine (QIV) or trivalent inactivated influenza vaccine (TIV) if QIV not available, is recommended (NACI 2015).

Pregnancy Considerations Adverse events were not observed in animal reproduction studies. LAIV is not recommended for use during pregnancy. Influenza vaccination with the inactivated influenza vaccine (IIV) is recommended for all women who are or will become pregnant during the influenza season and who do not otherwise have contraindications to the vaccine (CDC/ACIP [Grohskopf 2013]).

Healthy pregnant women do not need to avoid contact with persons vaccinated with LAIV (CDC/ACIP [Grohskopf 2013]). The nasal vaccine contains the same strains of influenza A and B found in the injection. Information specific to the use of LAIV in pregnancy is limited.

Health care providers are encouraged to refer women exposed to the influenza vaccine during pregnancy to the Vaccines and Medications in Pregnancy Surveillance System (VAMPSS) by contacting The Organization of Teratology Information Specialists (OTIS) at (877) 311-8972.

Breast-Feeding Considerations It is not known if the vaccine is excreted into breast milk. LAIV should be used with caution in breast-feeding women (per manufacturer) due to the possibility of virus excretion into breast milk; however, LAIV may be administered to breast-feeding women unless contraindicated due to other reasons (per CDC). Postpartum women may be vaccinated with either IIV or LAIV. When vaccine supply is limited, focus on delivering the vaccine should be given to mothers of newborns and contacts or caregivers of children <5 years of age (CDC/ACIP [Grohskopf 2013]).

Medication Guide Available Yes

Contraindications Severe allergic reaction (eg, anaphylaxis) to any component of the vaccine, including egg protein, or with life-threatening reactions to previous influenza vaccination; children and adolescents (2 to 17 years

of age) receiving aspirin therapy or aspirin-containing therapy because of the association of Reye syndrome with aspirin and wild-type influenza infection.

Warnings/Precautions Immediate treatment (including epinephrine 1:1000) for anaphylactoid and/or hypersensitivity reactions should be available during vaccine use (NCIRD/ACIP 2011). Manufactured with chicken egg protein. Allergy to eggs must be distinguished from allergy to the vaccine. Recommendations are available from the CDC regarding influenza vaccination to persons who report egg allergies; however, a prior severe allergic reaction to influenza vaccine, regardless of the component suspected, is a contraindication to vaccination. ACIP recommends use of IIV or RIV (if RIV is age appropriate) over LAIV when considering vaccination in persons reporting an egg allergy (due to lack of data of LAIV use in this setting) (ACIP [Grohskopf 2015]). Also manufactured with arginine, gelatin, and gentamicin.

Use with caution in patients with history of Guillain-Barré syndrome (GBS); patients with history of GBS have a greater likelihood of developing GBS than those without. As a precaution, the ACIP recommends that patients with a history of GBS and who are at low risk for severe influenza complications, and patients known to have experienced GBS within 6 weeks following previous vaccination should generally not be vaccinated (consider influenza antiviral chemoprophylaxis in these patients). Based on limited data, the benefits of vaccinating persons with a history of GBS who are also at high risk for complications of influenza may outweigh the risks (CDC/ACIP [Grohskopf 2013]). Recent studies of patients who received the trivalent inactivated influenza vaccine or the monovalent H1N1 influenza vaccine have shown the risk of GBS is lower with vaccination than with influenza infection (Baxter 2013; Greene 2013; Kwong 2013).

Data on the use of LAIV in immunocompromised patients is limited. **Avoid contact with severely immunocompromised individuals for at least 7 days following vaccination (at least 14 days per Canadian labeling).** ACIP does not recommend the use of LAIV in immunosuppressed patients (ACIP [Grohskopf 2015]). ACIP does not recommend the use of LAIV for persons who care for severely immunocompromised individuals who require a protective environment due to the theoretical risk of transmitting the live virus from the vaccine. Persons who care for the severely immunocompromised should receive either IIV or RIV (CDC/ACIP [Grohskopf 2013]). In general, live vaccines should be administered ≥4 weeks prior to planned immunosuppression and avoided within 2 weeks of immunosuppression when feasible (IDSA [Rubin 2014]).

Children <24 months of age had increased wheezing and hospitalizations following administration in clinical trials; use of the nasal spray is not approved in this age group. ACIP recommends not using LAIV in patients with chronic pulmonary disorders including asthma and children 2 to 4 years of age who have had asthma or wheezing episodes within the past year (ACIP [Grohskopf 2015]). Risk of wheezing following vaccination is increased in children <5 years of age with a history of recurrent wheezing and in persons of any age with asthma. Patients with severe asthma or active wheezing were not included in clinical trials. The safety of LAIV has not been established in individuals with underlying medical conditions that may predispose them to complications following wild-type influenza infection.

The decision to administer or delay vaccination because of current or recent febrile illness depends on the severity of symptoms and the etiology of the disease. Consider deferring administration in patients with moderate or severe acute illness (with or without fever); vaccination should not be delayed for patients with mild acute illness (with or without fever) (NCIRD/ACIP, 2011). ACIP does not recommend the use of LAIV in patients with chronic disorders of the cardiovascular system (except isolated hypertension), persons with HIV (ACIP [Grohskopf, 2015]). ACIP and NACI do not recommend the use of LAIV in pregnant women (ACIP [Grohskopf, 2015]; NACI, 2015). Use of this vaccine for specific medical and/or other indications (eg, immunocompromising conditions, hepatic or kidney disease, diabetes) is also addressed in the ACIP Recommended Adult Immunization Schedule (CDC/ACIP [Kim, 2015]). Specific recommendations for use of this vaccine in immunocompromised patients with asplenia, cancer, HIV infection, cerebrospinal fluid leaks, cochlear implants, hematopoietic stem cell transplant (prior to or after), sickle cell disease, solid organ transplant (prior to or after), or those receiving immunosuppressive therapy for chronic conditions as well as contacts of immunocompromised patients are available from the IDSA (Rubin, 2014).

Defer immunization if nasal congestion is present which may impede delivery of vaccine (CDC/ACIP [Grohskopf 2013]). In order to maximize vaccination rates, the ACIP recommends simultaneous administration (ie, >1 vaccine on the same day at different anatomic sites) of all age-appropriate vaccines (live or inactivated) for which a person is eligible at a single clinic visit, unless contraindications exist. The ACIP prefers each dose of a specific vaccine in a series come from the same manufacturer when possible (NCIRD/ACIP 2011).

The safety and efficacy of LAIV have not been established in adults ≥50 years of age (US labeling) or ≥60 years of age (Canadian labeling). Vaccination may not result in effective immunity in all patients. Response depends upon multiple factors (eg, type of vaccine, age of patient) and may be improved by administering the vaccine at the recommended dose, route, and interval. Vaccines may not be effective if administered during periods of altered immune competence (NCIRD/ACIP 2011). Influenza vaccines from previous seasons must not be used (CDC/ACIP [Grohskopf 2013]).

Adverse Reactions All serious adverse reactions must be reported to the U.S. Department of Health and Human Services (DHHS) Vaccine Adverse Event Reporting System (VAERS) 1-800-822-7967 or online at https://vaers.hhs.gov/esub/index. In Canada, adverse reactions may be reported to local provincial/territorial health agencies or to the Vaccine Safety Section at Public Health Agency of Canada (1-866-844-0018).

Frequency of events reported within 10 days.
>10%:
Central nervous system: Headache (children 3% to 9%; adults 40%), irritability (children 12% to 21%), lethargy (children 7% to 14%)
Gastrointestinal: Appetite decreased (children 13% to 21%), abdominal pain (children 2% to 12%)
Neuromuscular & skeletal: Tiredness/weakness (adults 26%), muscle aches (children 2% to 6%; adults 17%)
Respiratory: Cough (adults 14%), nasal congestion/runny nose (children 51% to 58%; adults 9% to 44%), sore throat (children 5% to 11%; adults 28%)
1% to 10%:
Central nervous system: Chills (children 2% to 4%, adults 9%), fever (100°F to 101°F: children 6% to 9%; >101°F: children 1% to 4%)
Otic: Otitis media (children 3%)
Respiratory: Sinusitis (adults 4%), sneezing (children 2%), wheezing (children 6-23 months 6%; children 24-59 months 2%)
Postmarketing and/or case reports: Anaphylactic reactions, asthma exacerbations, Bell's palsy, encephalitis (vaccine associated), epistaxis, Guillain-Barré syndrome, hypersensitivity reaction, meningitis (including eosinophilic meningitis), mitochondrial encephalomyopathy (Leigh syndrome) exacerbation, pericarditis

Drug Interactions
Metabolism/Transport Effects None known.
Avoid Concomitant Use
Avoid concomitant use of Influenza Virus Vaccine (Live/Attenuated) with any of the following: Belimumab; Fingolimod; Immunosuppressants; Salicylates
Increased Effect/Toxicity
Influenza Virus Vaccine (Live/Attenuated) may increase the levels/effects of: Salicylates

The levels/effects of Influenza Virus Vaccine (Live/Attenuated) may be increased by: AzaTHIOprine; Belimumab; Corticosteroids (Systemic); Dimethyl Fumarate; Fingolimod; Immunosuppressants; Leflunomide; Mercaptopurine; Methotrexate
Decreased Effect
Influenza Virus Vaccine (Live/Attenuated) may decrease the levels/effects of: Tuberculin Tests

The levels/effects of Influenza Virus Vaccine (Live/Attenuated) may be decreased by: Antiviral Agents (Influenza A and B); AzaTHIOprine; Corticosteroids (Systemic); Dimethyl Fumarate; Fingolimod; Immunosuppressants; Leflunomide; Mercaptopurine; Methotrexate
Storage/Stability Store in refrigerator at 2°C to 8°C (35°F to 46°F). **Do not freeze**; protect from light. The cold chain (2°C to 8°C [35°F to 46°F]) must be maintained when transporting intranasal influenza vaccine. The vaccine may be exposed to temperatures of up to 25°C for up to 12 hours without adverse impact; return to refrigerator as soon as possible; only a single excursion outside of the recommended storage conditions is permitted. Once intranasal influenza vaccine has been administered, the sprayer should be disposed of according to the standard procedures for medical waste (eg, sharps or biohazard container).

Mechanism of Action The vaccine contains live attenuated viruses which infect and replicate within the cells lining the nasopharynx. Promotes immunity to seasonal influenza virus by inducing specific antibody production. Each year the formulation is standardized according to the US Public Health Service. Preparations from previous seasons must not be used.
Pharmacodynamics/Kinetics
Onset of action: Most adults have antibody protection within 2 weeks of vaccination (CDC/ACIP [Grohskopf 2013])
Duration: ≥6 to 8 months when vaccine is antigenically similar to circulating virus (CDC/ACIP [Grohskopf 2013]); response may be diminished in persons ≥65 years and limited evidence suggests titers may decline significantly 6 months following vaccination in this population (ACIP [Grohskopf 2015])
Distribution: Following nasal administration, vaccine is distributed in the nasal cavity (~90%), stomach (~3%), brain (~2%), and lung (0.4%)
Dosing
Adult It is important to note that influenza seasons vary in their timing and duration from year to year. In general, vaccination should begin soon after the vaccine becomes available (and, if possible, by October) and prior to onset of influenza activity in the community. However, vaccination should continue throughout the influenza season as long as vaccine is available (ACIP [Grohskopf 2015]).

Immunization: Intranasal:
US labeling: Adults ≤49 years: 0.2 mL/dose (0.1 mL per nostril) (1 dose per season)
Canadian labeling: Adults ≤59 years: 0.2 mL/dose (0.1 mL per nostril) (1 dose per season)
Not indicated for use in patients ≥50 years (US labeling) or ≥60 years (Canadian labeling).
Geriatric Not indicated for use in patients ≥50 years (US labeling) or ≥60 years (Canadian labeling).
Pediatric It is important to note that influenza seasons vary in their timing and duration from year to year. In general, vaccination should begin soon after the vaccine becomes available (and, if possible, by October) and prior to onset of influenza activity in the community. However, vaccination should continue throughout the influenza season as long as vaccine is available (ACIP [Grohskopf 2015]).

Immunization: Intranasal:

US labeling:
Children 2 to 8 years: 0.2 mL/dose (0.1 mL per nostril) (1 or 2 doses per season; see **"Note"**)
Children ≥9 years and Adolescents: Refer to adult dosing.
Note: Infants and children 6 months to <9 years who received at least 2 doses of trivalent or quadrivalent influenza vaccine prior to July 1, 2015, need only 1 dose of the 2015 to 2016 seasonal influenza vaccine. The two doses need not have been received during the same season or consecutive seasons. All other children <9 years (including those whose vaccination status cannot be determined) should receive 2 doses separated by ≥4 weeks, in order to achieve satisfactory antibody response (ACIP [Grohskopf 2015]).

Canadian labeling:
Children 2 to 8 years: 0.2 mL/dose (0.1 mL per nostril) (1 dose per season); a second dose should be administered 4 weeks after the first in previously unvaccinated patients.
Children ≥9 years and Adolescents: Refer to adult dosing.
Renal Impairment There are no dosage adjustments provided in the manufacturer's labeling.
Hepatic Impairment There are no dosage adjustments provided in the manufacturer's labeling.
Administration For intranasal administration only; do not inject. Half the dose (0.1 mL) is administered to each nostril; patient should be in upright position. A dose divider clip is provided to allow administration of 0.1 mL into each nostril. Place the tip of the sprayer inside the nostril and depress plunger as rapidly as possible to deliver the dose. Remove dose divider clip and repeat into opposite nostril. The patient does not need to inhale during administration (may breath normally). If recipient sneezes following administration, the dose should not be repeated. Defer immunization if nasal congestion is present which may impede delivery of vaccine (CDC/ACIP [Grohskopf 2013]).

US law requires that the date of administration, name of the vaccine manufacturer, lot number of vaccine, and the administering person's name, title, and address and documentation of the vaccine information statement (VIS; date on VIS, and date given to patient) be entered into the patient's permanent medical record.

Test Interactions Administration of the intranasal influenza virus vaccine (live, LAIV) may cause a positive result on the rapid influenza diagnostic test for the 7 days after vaccine administration; for a person with influenza-like illness during this time, the positive test could be caused by either the live attenuated vaccine or wild-type influenza virus (Ali 2004).

Additional Information Seasonal quadrivalent influenza vaccines contain two subtype A strains and two subtype B strains; trivalent influenza vaccines contain two subtype A strains and one subtype B strain.

When vaccine supply is limited, target groups for vaccination (those at higher risk of complications from influenza infection and their close contacts) include the following (CDC/ACIP [Grohskopf 2013]): **Note:** Only use LAIV if appropriate:
• Infants and children 6 to 59 months of age
• Persons ≥50 years of age
• Infants, children, and adolescents (6 months to 18 years of age) who are receiving long-term aspirin therapy, and therefore, may be at risk for developing Reye syndrome after influenza
• Women who are or will be pregnant during the influenza season
• Patients with chronic pulmonary disorders (including asthma) or cardiovascular systems disorders (except hypertension), renal, hepatic, neurologic, or metabolic disorders (including diabetes mellitus)
• Persons who have immunosuppression (including immunosuppression caused by medications or HIV)
• Residents of nursing homes and other long-term care facilities
• American Indians/Alaska Natives
• Morbidly obese (BMI ≥40)
• Health care personnel
• Household contacts (including children) and caregivers of neonates, infants, and children <5 years (particularly children <6 months) and adults ≥50 years
• Household contacts (including children) and caregivers of persons with medical conditions which put them at high risk of complications from influenza infection

Dosage Forms Excipient information presented when available (limited, particularly for generics); consult specific product labeling. [DSC] = Discontinued product
Liquid, Nasal [preservative free]:
  FluMist: (1 ea) [contains egg white (egg protein), gelatin (pork)]
Suspension, Nasal [preservative free]:
  FluMist Quadrivalent: (1 ea [DSC]) [latex free; contains egg white (egg protein), gelatin (pork)]
  FluMist Quadrivalent: (1 ea) [contains egg white (egg protein), gelatin (pork)]

◆ Influenza Virus Vaccine (Monovalent) *see* Influenza A Virus Vaccine (H5N1) *on page* 944
◆ Influenza Virus Vaccine (Purified Surface Antigen) *see* Influenza Virus Vaccine (Inactivated) *on page* 945
◆ Influenza Virus Vaccine (Split-Virus) *see* Influenza Virus Vaccine (Inactivated) *on page* 945
◆ Influvac (Can) *see* Influenza Virus Vaccine (Inactivated) *on page* 945
◆ Infufer (Can) *see* Iron Dextran Complex *on page* 986
◆ Infumorph 200 *see* Morphine (Systemic) *on page* 1230
◆ Infumorph 500 *see* Morphine (Systemic) *on page* 1230

Ingenol Mebutate (IN je nol MEB u tate)

Brand Names: US Picato
Index Terms Euphorbia peplus Derivative; PEP005
Pharmacologic Category Topical Skin Product
Use Actinic keratosis: Topical treatment of actinic keratosis
Dosing
  Adult & Geriatric Actinic keratosis: Topical:
    Face or scalp: Apply 0.015% gel once daily to affected area for 3 consecutive days; patients not achieving clearance or that experience recurrence after achieving clearance ≥8 weeks after initial treatment may benefit from a second treatment course.
    Trunk or extremities: Apply 0.05% gel once daily to affected area for 2 consecutive days
  Renal Impairment There are no dosage adjustments provided in the manufacturer's labeling. However, dosage adjustment unlikely due to low systemic absorption.

Hepatic Impairment There are no dosage adjustments provided in the manufacturer's labeling. However, dosage adjustment unlikely due to low systemic absorption.
Additional Information Complete prescribing information should be consulted for additional detail.
Dosage Forms Excipient information presented when available (limited, particularly for generics); consult specific product labeling.
Gel, External:
  Picato: 0.015% (3 ea); 0.05% (2 ea) [contains benzyl alcohol, isopropyl alcohol]

◆ INH *see* Isoniazid *on page* 990
◆ Injectafer *see* Ferric Carboxymaltose *on page* 759
◆ Inlyta *see* Axitinib *on page* 182
◆ Innohep® (Can) *see* Tinzaparin *on page* 1791
◆ InnoPran XL *see* Propranolol *on page* 1518
◆ Insoluble Prussian Blue *see* Ferric Hexacyanoferrate *on page* 761
◆ Inspra *see* Eplerenone *on page* 651
◆ Instacort 5 [OTC] *see* Hydrocortisone (Topical) *on page* 886
◆ Instacort 10 [OTC] *see* Hydrocortisone (Topical) *on page* 886

Insulin Aspart (IN soo lin AS part)

Brand Names: US NovoLOG; NovoLOG FlexPen; NovoLOG PenFill
Brand Names: Canada NovoRapid®
Index Terms Aspart Insulin
Pharmacologic Category Insulin, Rapid-Acting
Use Treatment of type 1 diabetes mellitus (insulin dependent, IDDM) and type 2 diabetes mellitus (noninsulin dependent, NIDDM) to improve glycemic control
Dosing
  Adult & Geriatric Note: Insulin aspart is a rapid-acting insulin analog which is normally administered SubQ as a premeal component of the insulin regimen or as a continuous SubQ infusion and should be used with intermediate- or long-acting insulin. When compared to insulin regular, insulin aspart has a more rapid onset and shorter duration of activity. In carefully controlled clinical settings with close medical supervision and monitoring of blood glucose and potassium, insulin aspart may also be administered IV. Insulin requirements vary dramatically between patients and dictate frequent monitoring and close medical supervision.
  Diabetes mellitus, type 1:
  General insulin dosing:
    Type 1: SubQ: **Note:** Multiple daily doses or continuous subcutaneous infusions guided by blood glucose monitoring are the standard of diabetes care. Combinations of insulin formulations are commonly used. The daily doses presented below are expressed as the **total units/kg/day of all insulin formulations combined.**
      Initial total insulin dose: 0.2 to 0.6 units/kg/day in divided doses. Conservative initial doses of 0.2 to 0.4 units/kg/day are often recommended to avoid the potential for hypoglycemia. A rapid-acting insulin may be the only insulin formulation used initially.
      Usual maintenance range: 0.5 to 1 units/kg/day in divided doses. An estimate of anticipated needs may be based on body weight and/or activity factors as follows:
        Nonobese: 0.4 to 0.6 units/kg/day
        Obese: 0.8 to 1.2 units/kg/day
        Pubescent Children and Adolescents: During puberty, requirements may substantially increase to >1 unit/kg/day and in some cases up to 2 units/kg/day (IDF-ISPAD 2011).
      Division of daily insulin requirement ("conventional therapy"): Generally, 50% to 75% of the total daily dose (TDD) is given as an intermediate- or long-acting form of insulin (in 1 to 2 daily injections). The remaining portion of the TDD is then divided and administered before or at mealtimes (depending on the formulation) as a rapid-acting (eg, insulin aspart) or short-acting form of insulin. Some patients may benefit from the use of CSII which delivers rapid-acting insulin (insulin aspart) as a continuous infusion throughout the day and as boluses at mealtimes via an external pump device.
      Division of daily insulin requirement ("intensive therapy"): Basal insulin delivery with 1 or 2 doses of intermediate- or long-acting insulin formulations superimposed with doses of short- or rapid-acting insulin (eg, insulin aspart) formulations 3 or more times daily.

Adjustment of dose: Dosage must be titrated to achieve glucose control and avoid hypoglycemia. Adjust dose to maintain premeal and bedtime glucose in target range. Since combinations of agents are frequently used, dosage adjustment must address the individual component of the insulin regimen which most directly influences the blood glucose value in question, based on the known onset and duration of the insulin component. Treatment and monitoring regimens must be individualized.

Continuous SubQ insulin infusion (insulin pump): A combination of a "basal" continuous insulin infusion rate with preprogrammed, premeal bolus doses which are patient controlled. When converting from multiple daily SubQ doses of maintenance insulin, it is advisable to reduce the basal rate to less than the equivalent of the total daily units of the longer acting insulin (eg, NPH); divide the total number of units by 24 to get the basal rate in units/hour. Do not include the total units of regular insulin or other rapid-acting insulin formulations in this calculation. The same premeal regular insulin dosage may be used.

Diabetes mellitus, type 2: SubQ:

General considerations for insulin use in type 2 diabetes:

Timing of initiation: The goal of therapy is to achieve an HbA$_{1c}$ <7%. According to a position statement by the ADA and European Association for the Study of Diabetes (EASD), dual therapy (metformin + a second antihyperglycemic agent) is recommended in patients with type 2 diabetes who fail to achieve glycemic goals after ~3 months with lifestyle interventions and metformin monotherapy (unless contraindications to metformin exist). Preference is not given for adding insulin or a noninsulin agent as the second antihyperglycemic agent (drug choice should be individualized based on patient characteristics). However, insulin should be considered as part of a combination regimen when hyperglycemia is severe, particularly if patient is symptomatic or has catabolic features (eg, weight loss, ketosis). If insulin is selected, the addition of **basal** insulin with a long-acting insulin (ie, glargine or detemir [*not* insulin aspart]) is recommended. If HbA$_{1c}$ target not achieved after ~3 months of dual therapy, may proceed to triple therapy (Inzucchi 2015).

Intensification of therapy: If HbA$_{1c}$ target has not been met, despite titrating **basal** insulin (ie, long-acting insulin) to provide acceptable fasting blood glucose concentrations, intensification of therapy should be considered to cover postprandial glucose excursions. Options include: adding a GLP-1 receptor agonist (eg, exenatide, liraglutide) **or** adding a mealtime insulin (1 injection of a rapid-acting insulin analog [lispro, aspart, glulisine] initiated at a dose of 4 units or 0.1 units/kg or 10% basal dose before largest meal; may progress to "basal-bolus" dosing of 3 injections of a rapid-acting insulin analog [lispro, aspart, glulisine] per meal **or** dose by adding up the total current insulin dose, and provide one-half of this amount as basal and one-half as mealtime insulin (split evenly between 3 meals). Alternatively, although less studied, may transition from basal insulin (ie, long-acting insulin) to a twice daily premixed (or biphasic) insulin analog (70/30 aspart mix, 75/25 or 50/50 lispro mix) (Inzucchi 2015).

Hyperglycemia, critically ill (off-label use): IV continuous infusion: Insulin therapy should be implemented when blood glucose ≥150 mg/dL with a goal to maintain blood glucose <150 mg/dL (with values absolutely <180 mg/dL) using a protocol that achieves a low rate of hypoglycemia (ie, ≤70 mg/dL). Before discontinuation, stable ICU patients should be transitioned to a protocol-driven basal/bolus insulin regimen, based on insulin infusion history and carbohydrate intake, to avoid loss of glycemic control. Subcutaneous insulin therapy may be considered for selected clinically stable ICU patients (Jacobi 2012). **Note:** The Surviving Sepsis Campaign guidelines recommend initiating insulin dosing in patients with severe sepsis when 2 consecutive blood glucose concentrations are >180 mg/dL and to target an upper blood glucose ≤180 mg/dL (Dellinger 2013).

Pediatric

Diabetes mellitus, type 1: Children ≥2 years and Adolescents: Refer to adult dosing.

Diabetic ketoacidosis (DKA), mild-to-moderate (off-label use): Children and Adolescents: Treatment should continue until reversal of acid-base derangement/ketonemia. Serum glucose is not a direct indicator of these abnormalities, and may decrease more rapidly than correction of the metabolic abnormalities. Also refer to institution-specific protocols where appropriate. SubQ (**Note:** Use of IV regular insulin is preferred; only use the SubQ route if IV infusion access is unavailable): 0.3 units/kg followed in 1 hour by 0.1 units/kg given every hour or 0.15 to 0.2 units/kg every 2 hours; continue until acidosis clears, then decrease to 0.05 units/kg given every hour until maintenance SubQ replacement dosing can be initiated (Kitabchi 2004; Wolfsdorf 2007).

Renal Impairment No dosage adjustment provided in manufacturer's labeling; insulin requirements may be reduced due to changes in insulin clearance or metabolism; monitor blood glucose closely.

Hepatic Impairment No dosage adjustment provided in manufacturer's labeling; insulin requirements may be reduced due to changes in insulin clearance or metabolism; monitor blood glucose closely.

Obesity Refer to indication-specific dosing for obesity-related information (may not be available for all indications).

Additional Information Complete prescribing information should be consulted for additional detail.

Dosage Forms Excipient information presented when available (limited, particularly for generics); consult specific product labeling.

Solution, Subcutaneous:
NovoLOG: 100 units/mL (10 mL) [contains metacresol, phenol]

Solution Cartridge, Subcutaneous:
NovoLOG PenFill: 100 units/mL (3 mL) [contains metacresol, phenol]

Solution Pen-injector, Subcutaneous:
NovoLOG FlexPen: 100 units/mL (3 mL) [contains metacresol, phenol]

◆ **Insulin Aspart and Insulin Aspart Protamine** *see* Insulin Aspart Protamine and Insulin Aspart *on page 953*

◆ **Insulin aspart and insulin degludec** *see* Insulin Degludec and Insulin Aspart *on page 954*

Insulin Aspart Protamine and Insulin Aspart (IN soo lin AS part PROE ta meen & IN soo lin AS part)

Brand Names: US NovoLOG® Mix 70/30; NovoLOG® Mix 70/30 FlexPen®

Brand Names: Canada NovoMix® 30

Index Terms Insulin Aspart and Insulin Aspart Protamine; NovoLog 70/30

Pharmacologic Category Insulin, Combination

Use Treatment of type 1 diabetes mellitus (insulin dependent, IDDM) and type 2 diabetes mellitus (noninsulin dependent, NIDDM) to improve glycemic control

Dosing

Adult & Geriatric Note: Insulin aspart protamine is an intermediate-acting insulin and insulin aspart is a rapid-acting insulin administered by SubQ injection. Insulin aspart protamine and insulin aspart combination products are approximately equipotent to insulin NPH and insulin regular combination products with a similar duration of activity, but with a more rapid onset. With combination insulin products, the proportion of rapid-acting to long-acting insulin is fixed; basal vs prandial dose adjustments cannot be made. Fixed ratio insulins (such as insulin aspart protamine and insulin aspart combination) are typically administered as 2 daily doses with each dose intended to cover two meals and a snack. Because of variability in the peak effect and individual patient variability in activities, meals, etc, it may be more difficult to achieve complete glycemic control using fixed combinations of insulins; frequent monitoring and close medical supervision may be necessary.

General insulin dosing:

Diabetes mellitus, type 1: SubQ: **Note:** Multiple daily doses are utilized and guided by blood glucose monitoring. Combinations of different insulin formulations are commonly used. The daily doses presented below are expressed as the **total units/kg/day of all insulin formulations combined.** Insulin aspart protamine and insulin aspart combination product is **not** intended for initial therapy; basal insulin requirements should be established **first** to direct dosing of combination insulin products.

Usual maintenance range: 0.5-1 units/kg/day in divided doses. An estimate of anticipated needs may be based on body weight and/or activity factors as follows:

Nonobese: 0.4-0.6 units/kg/day

Obese: 0.8-1.2 units/kg/day

Pubescent Children and Adolescents: During puberty, requirements may substantially increase to >1 unit/kg/day and in some cases up to 2 units/kg/day (IDF-ISPAD, 2011).

Division of daily insulin requirement ("conventional therapy"): Generally, 50% to 75% of the daily insulin dose is given as an intermediate- or long-acting form of insulin (in 1-2 daily injections). The remaining portion of the 24-hour insulin requirement is divided and administered as either regular insulin or a rapid-acting form of insulin at the same time before breakfast and dinner.

Adjustment of dose: Dosage must be titrated to achieve glucose control and avoid hypoglycemia. Adjust dose to maintain premeal and bedtime glucose in target range. Since combinations of agents are frequently used, dosage adjustment must address the individual component of the insulin regimen which most directly influences the blood glucose value in question, based on the known onset and duration of the insulin component. Treatment and monitoring regimens must be individualized.

Diabetes mellitus, type 2: SubQ: Augmentation therapy (patients for which diet, exercise, weight reduction, and oral hypoglycemic agents have not been adequate): **Note:** Insulin aspart protamine and insulin aspart combination product is **not** intended for initial therapy; basal insulin requirements should be established **first** to direct dosing of combination insulin products. Dosage must be carefully adjusted.

Renal Impairment No dosage adjustment provided in manufacturer's labeling; insulin requirements may be reduced due to changes in insulin clearance or metabolism; monitor blood glucose closely.

Hepatic Impairment No dosage adjustment provided in manufacturer's labeling; insulin requirements may be reduced due to changes in insulin clearance or metabolism; monitor blood glucose closely.

Obesity Refer to indication-specific dosing for obesity-related information (may not be available for all indications).

Additional Information Complete prescribing information should be consulted for additional detail.

Dosage Forms Excipient information presented when available (limited, particularly for generics); consult specific product labeling.

Injection, suspension:

NovoLOG® Mix 70/30: Insulin aspart protamine suspension 70% [intermediate acting] and insulin aspart solution 30% [rapid acting]: 100 units/mL (10 mL)

NovoLOG® Mix 70/30 FlexPen®: Insulin aspart protamine suspension 70% [intermediate acting] and insulin aspart solution 30% [rapid acting]: 100 units/mL (3 mL)

Insulin Degludec (IN su lin de GLOO dek)

Brand Names: US Tresiba FlexTouch

Pharmacologic Category Insulin, Long-Acting

Use Diabetes mellitus: To improve glycemic control in adults with diabetes mellitus

Dosing

Adult & Geriatric

Diabetes mellitus: SubQ:

Note: Do not perform dose conversion when using the FlexTouch pen. The dose window for both U-100 and U-200 FlexTouch pens show the number of insulin units to be delivered and no conversion is needed. Individualize and titrate dose every 3 to 4 days based on patient's metabolic needs, blood glucose monitoring results, and glycemic control goal.

Diabetes mellitus, type 1:

Insulin-naive: Initial: One-third to one-half the total daily insulin dose (general rule for total daily dose, 0.2 to 0.4 units/kg); remainder of total daily dose should be given as a short-acting insulin and divided between each daily meal

Insulin-experienced: Initiate with same unit dose as the total daily long or intermediate-acting insulin unit dose

Diabetes mellitus, type 2:

Insulin-naive: Initial: 10 units once daily

Insulin-experienced: Initiate with same unit dose as the total daily long or intermediate-acting insulin unit dose

Missed dose: Administer as soon as possible, ensure at least 8 hours between consecutive doses.

Renal Impairment There are no dosage adjustments provided in the manufacturer's labeling; insulin requirements may be reduced due to changes in insulin clearance or metabolism; monitor blood glucose closely.

Hepatic Impairment There are no dosage adjustments provided in the manufacturer's labeling; insulin requirements may be reduced due to changes in insulin clearance or metabolism; monitor blood glucose closely.

Additional Information Complete prescribing information should be consulted for additional detail.

Dosage Forms Excipient information presented when available (limited, particularly for generics); consult specific product labeling.

Solution Pen-injector, Subcutaneous:

Tresiba FlexTouch: 100 units/mL (3 mL); 200 units/mL (3 mL) [contains metacresol, phenol]

Insulin Degludec and Insulin Aspart
(IN su lin de GLOO dek & IN soo lin AS part)

Index Terms Insulin aspart and insulin degludec; Ryzodeg 70/30

Pharmacologic Category Insulin, Combination

Use Diabetes mellitus: To improve glycemic control in adults with diabetes mellitus

Dosing

Adult & Geriatric Note: Insulin degludec is a long-acting insulin analog and insulin aspart is a rapid-acting insulin analog administered by SubQ injection. With combination insulin products, the proportion of short-acting to long-acting insulin is fixed; basal versus prandial dose adjustments cannot be made. Fixed-ratio insulins (such as insulin degludec and insulin aspart combination) are typically administered as 2 daily doses with each dose intended to cover two meals and a snack. Because of variability in the peak effect and individual patient variability in activities, meals, etc., it may be more difficult to achieve complete glycemic control using fixed combinations of insulins; frequent monitoring and close medical supervision may be necessary.

Diabetes mellitus, type 1: SubQ:

Insulin degludec and insulin aspart combination-specific dosing: Insulin-naive: Initial: Approximately one-third to one-half of the total daily insulin dose administered as insulin degludec and insulin aspart combination once or twice daily with any main meal; administer remainder of total daily insulin dose as short- or rapid-acting insulin divided between each daily meal. Titrate dose every 3 to 4 days.

Conversion from a once or twice daily premix or self-mix insulin: Initiate insulin degludec and insulin aspart combination at same dose and schedule as the premix or self-mix; short- or rapid-acting mealtime insulins should be continued for meals not covered by insulin degludec and insulin aspart combination.

Conversion from basal insulin: Initiate insulin degludec and insulin aspart combination at same dose as basal insulin and administer once daily with main meal. Short- or rapid-acting mealtime insulins should be continued for meals not covered by insulin degludec and insulin aspart combination.

General insulin dosing:

Type 1: **Note:** Multiple daily doses or continuous subcutaneous infusions guided by blood glucose monitoring are the standard of diabetes care. Combinations of different insulin formulations are commonly used. The daily doses presented below are expressed as the **total units/kg/day of all insulin formulations combined.**

Initial total insulin dose: 0.2 to 0.6 units/kg/day in divided doses. Conservative initial doses of 0.2 to 0.4 units/kg/day are often recommended to avoid the potential for hypoglycemia. A rapid-acting insulin may be the only insulin formulation used initially.

Usual maintenance range: 0.5 to 1 units/kg/day in divided doses. An estimate of anticipated needs may be based on body weight and/or activity factors as follows:

Nonobese: 0.4 to 0.6 units/kg/day

Obese: 0.8 to 1.2 units/kg/day

Pubescent Children and Adolescents: During puberty, requirements may substantially increase to >1 unit/kg/day and in some cases up to 2 units/kg/day (IDF-ISPAD 2011).

Division of daily insulin requirement ("conventional therapy"): Generally, 50% to 75% of the total daily dose (TDD) is given as an intermediate-acting (eg, NPH) or a long-acting form of insulin (in 1 to 2 daily injections). The remaining portion of the TDD is then divided and administered

before or at mealtimes (depending on the formulation) as a rapid-acting or short-acting form of insulin.

Division of daily insulin requirement ("intensive therapy"): Basal insulin delivery with 1 or 2 doses of intermediate- or long-acting insulin formulations superimposed with doses of short- or rapid-acting insulin (eg, insulin aspart) formulations 3 or more times daily.

Adjustment of dose: Dosage must be titrated to achieve glucose control and avoid hypoglycemia. Adjust dose to maintain premeal and bedtime glucose in target range. Because combinations of agents are frequently used, dosage adjustment must address the individual component of the insulin regimen that most directly influences the blood glucose value in question, based on the known onset and duration of the insulin component. Treatment and monitoring regimens must be individualized.

Continuous SubQ insulin infusion (insulin pump): A combination of a "basal" continuous insulin infusion rate with preprogrammed, premeal bolus doses which are patient controlled. When converting from multiple daily SubQ doses of maintenance insulin, it is advisable to reduce the basal rate to less than the equivalent of the total daily units of the longer acting insulin (eg, NPH); divide the total number of units by 24 to get the basal rate in units/hour. Do not include the total units of regular insulin or other rapid-acting insulin formulations in this calculation. The same premeal regular insulin dosage may be used.

Diabetes mellitus, type 2: SubQ:

Insulin degludec and insulin aspart combination-specific dosing: Insulin-naive: Initial: 10 units once daily.

Conversion from a once or twice daily premix or self-mix insulin: Initiate insulin degludec and insulin aspart combination at same dose and schedule as the premix or self-mix. Short- or rapid-acting mealtime insulins should be continued for meals not covered by insulin degludec and insulin aspart combination.

Conversion from basal insulin monotherapy: Initiate insulin degludec and insulin aspart combination at same dose and frequency as the basal insulin.

Conversion from combination basal insulin and short- or rapid-acting insulin therapy: Initiate insulin degludec and insulin aspart combination at same dose and frequency as the basal insulin. Short- or rapid-acting mealtime insulins should be continued for meals not covered by insulin degludec and insulin aspart combination.

General considerations for insulin use in type 2 diabetes:

Timing of initiation: The goal of therapy is to achieve an HbA$_{1c}$ <7%. According to a position statement by the ADA and European Association for the Study of Diabetes (EASD), dual therapy (metformin + a second antihyperglycemic agent) is recommended in patients with type 2 diabetes who fail to achieve glycemic goals after ~3 months with lifestyle interventions and metformin monotherapy (unless contraindications to metformin exist). Preference is not given for adding insulin or a non-insulin agent as the second antihyperglycemic agent (drug choice should be individualized based on patient characteristics). However, insulin should be considered as part of a combination regimen when hyperglycemia is severe, particularly if patient is symptomatic or has catabolic features (eg, weight loss, ketosis). If insulin is selected, the addition of **basal** insulin with a long-acting insulin (ie, glargine or detemir [*not* insulin NPH and insulin regular combination]) is recommended. If HbA$_{1c}$ target not achieved after ~3 months of dual therapy, may proceed to triple therapy (Inzucchi 2015).

Intensification of therapy: If HbA$_{1c}$ target has not been met, despite titrating **basal** insulin (ie, long-acting insulin) to provide acceptable fasting blood glucose concentrations, intensification of therapy should be considered to cover postprandial glucose excursions. Options include adding a mealtime insulin (1 to 3 injections of a rapid-acting insulin analog [lispro, aspart, glulisine]) **or** adding a GLP-1 receptor agonist (eg, exenatide, liraglutide). Alternatively, although less studied, may transition from basal insulin (ie, long-acting insulin) to a twice daily premixed (or biphasic) insulin analog (70/30 aspart mix, 75/25 or 50/50 lispro mix) (Inzucchi 2015).

Renal Impairment There are no dosage adjustments provided in the manufacturer's labeling; insulin requirements may be reduced due to changes in insulin clearance or metabolism; monitor blood glucose closely.

Hepatic Impairment There are no dosage adjustments provided in the manufacturer's labeling; insulin requirements may be reduced due to changes in insulin clearance or metabolism; monitor blood glucose closely.

Additional Information Complete prescribing information should be consulted for additional detail.

Product Availability Ryzodeg 70/30: FDA approved September 2015; anticipated availability is currently undetermined.

Insulin Detemir (IN soo lin DE te mir)

Brand Names: US Levemir; Levemir FlexPen [DSC]; Levemir FlexTouch

Brand Names: Canada Levemir®

Index Terms Detemir Insulin

Pharmacologic Category Insulin, Long-Acting

Use Treatment of type 1 diabetes mellitus (insulin dependent, IDDM) and type 2 diabetes mellitus (noninsulin dependent, NIDDM) to improve glycemic control

Dosing

Adult & Geriatric Note: Insulin detemir is a long-acting insulin administered by SubQ injection. When compared to insulin NPH, insulin detemir has slower, more prolonged absorption; duration of activity is dose-dependent. Insulin detemir may be given once or twice daily when used as the basal insulin component of therapy. Changing the basal insulin component from another insulin to insulin detemir can be done on a unit-to-unit basis. Insulin requirements vary dramatically between patients and dictate frequent monitoring and close medical supervision.

General insulin dosing:

Diabetes mellitus, type 1: SubQ: **Note:** Multiple daily doses are utilized and guided by blood glucose monitoring. Combinations of insulin formulations are commonly used. The daily doses presented below are expressed as the **total units/kg/day of all insulin formulations combined.**

Usual maintenance range: 0.5-1 units/kg/day in divided doses. An estimate of anticipated needs may be based on body weight and/or activity factors as follows:

Nonobese: 0.4-0.6 units/kg/day

Obese: 0.8-1.2 units/kg/day

Pubescent Children and Adolescents: During puberty, requirements may substantially increase to >1 unit/kg/day and in some cases up to 2 units/kg/day (IDF-ISPAD, 2011).

Division of daily insulin requirement ("conventional therapy"): Generally, 50% to 75% of the total daily dose (TDD) is given as an intermediate-acting or a long-acting form of insulin (in 1-2 daily injections). The remaining portion of the TDD is then divided and administered before or at mealtimes (depending on the formulation) as a rapid-acting or short-acting form of insulin.

Division of daily insulin requirement ("intensive therapy"): Basal insulin delivery with 1 or 2 doses of intermediate-acting or long-acting insulin formulations superimposed with doses of short- or rapid-acting insulin formulations 3 or more times daily.

Adjustment of dose: Dosage must be titrated to achieve glucose control and avoid hypoglycemia. Adjust dose to maintain premeal and bedtime glucose in target range. Since combinations of agents are frequently used, dosage adjustment must address the individual component of the insulin regimen which most directly influences the blood glucose value in question, based on the known onset and duration of the insulin component. Treatment and monitoring regimens must be individualized.

Insulin detemir-specific dosing: Manufacturer's labeling:

Diabetes mellitus, type 1: SubQ: Initial dose: Approximately one-third of the total daily insulin requirement administered in 1-2 divided doses. A rapid- or short-acting insulin should be used to complete the balance (~2/3) of the total daily insulin requirement.

Conversion from insulin glargine or NPH insulin: May be substituted on an equivalent unit-per-unit basis; in one Type 2 diabetes clinical trial, higher doses of insulin detemir were required than insulin NPH.

◀

Diabetes mellitus, type 2: SubQ: Initial:

Inadequately controlled on oral antidiabetic agents: 10 units (or 0.1-0.2 units/kg) once daily in the evening; may also administer total daily dose in 2 divided doses.

Inadequately controlled on GLP-1 receptor agonist: 10 units once daily in the evening.

Conversion from insulin glargine or NPH insulin: May be substituted on an equivalent unit-per-unit basis; in one Type 2 diabetes clinical trial, higher doses of insulin detemir were required than insulin NPH.

Pediatric Diabetes mellitus, type 1: Children ≥2 years and Adolescents: Refer to adult dosing.

Renal Impairment No dosage adjustment provided in manufacturer's labeling; insulin requirements may be reduced due to changes in insulin clearance or metabolism; monitor blood glucose closely.

Hepatic Impairment No dosage adjustment provided in manufacturer's labeling; insulin requirements may be reduced due to changes in insulin clearance or metabolism; monitor blood glucose closely.

Obesity Refer to indication-specific dosing for obesity-related information (may not be available for all indications).

Additional Information Complete prescribing information should be consulted for additional detail.

Dosage Forms Excipient information presented when available (limited, particularly for generics); consult specific product labeling. [DSC] = Discontinued product

Solution, Subcutaneous:

Levemir: 100 units/mL (10 mL) [contains metacresol, phenol]

Solution Pen-injector, Subcutaneous:

Levemir FlexPen: 100 units/mL (3 mL [DSC]) [contains metacresol, phenol]

Levemir FlexTouch: 100 units/mL (3 mL) [contains metacresol, phenol]

Insulin Glargine (IN soo lin GLAR jeen)

Brand Names: US Lantus; Lantus SoloStar; Toujeo SoloStar

Brand Names: Canada Lantus; Toujeo SoloStar

Index Terms Basaglar; Glargine Insulin

Pharmacologic Category Insulin, Long-Acting

Use

Diabetes mellitus: To improve glycemic control in adults with type 1 diabetes mellitus (insulin dependent, IDDM) and type 2 diabetes mellitus (noninsulin, NIDDM); to improve glycemic control in children ≥6 years with type 1 diabetes mellitus (Lantus only)

Limitations of use: Not recommended for the treatment of diabetic ketoacidosis.

Dosing

Adult & Geriatric Note: Insulin glargine is a long-acting insulin administered by SubQ injection. Insulin glargine is approximately equipotent to human insulin, but has a slower onset, no pronounced peak, and a longer duration of activity. Insulin requirements vary dramatically between patients and dictates frequent monitoring and close medical supervision.

Diabetes mellitus, type 1: SubQ:

Insulin glargine-specific dosing: Lantus, Toujeo: Initial dose: Approximately one-third to one-half of the total daily insulin requirement administered once daily. A rapid-acting or short-acting insulin should also be used to complete the balance (~1/2 to 2/3) of the total daily insulin requirement. Adjust dosage according to patient response.

Conversion to insulin glargine from other insulin therapies:

Converting from once-daily NPH insulin to insulin glargine: May be substituted on an equivalent unit-per-unit basis

Converting from twice-daily NPH insulin to insulin glargine: Initial dose: Use 80% of the total daily dose of NPH (eg, 20% reduction); administer once daily; adjust dosage according to patient response

Conversion between Toujeo and Lantus:

Conversion from once-daily Toujeo to once-daily Lantus: Initial dose: Use 80% of the dose of Toujeo (eg, 20% reduction); adjust dosage according to patient blood glucose response.

Conversion from once-daily Lantus to once-daily Toujeo: Initial dose: May be substituted on an equivalent unit-per-unit basis; however, generally a higher daily dosage of Toujeo will be required to achieve the same level of glycemic control as with Lantus.

General insulin dosing:

Type 1: SubQ: **Note:** Multiple daily doses are utilized and guided by blood glucose monitoring. Combinations of insulin formulations are commonly used. The daily doses presented below are expressed as the total units/kg/day of all insulin formulations used. Insulin glargine must be used in combination with a rapid- or short-acting insulin.

Usual maintenance range: 0.5 to 1 units/kg/day in divided doses. An estimate of anticipated needs may be based on body weight and/or activity factors as follows:

Nonobese: 0.4 to 0.6 units/kg/day

Obese: 0.8 to 1.2 units/kg/day

Pubescent Children and Adolescents: During puberty, requirements may substantially increase to >1 unit/kg/day and in some cases up to 2 units/kg/day (IDF-ISPAD 2011).

Division of daily insulin requirement ("conventional therapy"): Generally, 50% to 75% of the total daily dose (TDD) is given as an intermediate-acting or a long-acting form of insulin (eg, insulin glargine) (in 1 or 2 daily injections). The remaining portion of the TDD is then divided and administered before or at mealtimes (depending on the formulation) as a rapid-acting or short-acting form of insulin.

Division of daily insulin requirement ("intensive therapy"): Basal insulin delivery with 1 or 2 doses of intermediate-acting or long-acting insulin formulations superimposed with doses of short- or rapid-acting insulin formulations 3 or more times daily.

Adjustment of dose: Dosage must be titrated to achieve glucose control and avoid hypoglycemia. Adjust dose to maintain premeal and bedtime glucose in target range. Since combinations of agents are frequently used, dosage adjustment must address the individual component of the insulin regimen which most directly influences the blood glucose value in question, based on the known onset and duration of the insulin component.

Diabetes mellitus, type 2: SubQ:

Insulin glargine-specific dosing: Initial basal insulin dose: 0.2 units/kg once daily; for Lantus, up to 10 units/day initially is recommended. Adjust dosage according to patient response

Conversion to insulin glargine from other insulin therapies:

Converting from once-daily NPH insulin to insulin glargine: May be substituted on an equivalent unit-per-unit basis

Converting from twice-daily NPH insulin to insulin glargine: Initial dose: Use 80% of the total daily dose of NPH (eg, 20% reduction); administer once daily; adjust dosage according to patient response

Conversion between Toujeo and Lantus:

Conversion from once-daily Toujeo to once-daily Lantus: Initial dose: Use 80% of the dose of Toujeo (eg, 20% reduction); adjust dosage according to patient blood glucose response.

Conversion from once-daily Lantus to once-daily Toujeo: Initial dose: May be substituted on an equivalent unit-per-unit basis; however, generally a higher daily dosage of Toujeo will be required to achieve the same level of glycemic control as with Lantus

General considerations for insulin use in type 2 diabetes:

Timing of initiation: The goal of therapy is to achieve an HbA$_{1c}$ <7%. According to a position statement by the ADA and European Association for the Study of Diabetes (EASD), dual therapy (metformin + a second antihyperglycemic agent) is recommended in patients with type 2 diabetes who fail to achieve glycemic goals after ~3 months with lifestyle interventions and metformin monotherapy (unless contraindications to metformin exist). Preference is not given for adding insulin or a noninsulin agent as the second antihyperglycemic agent (drug choice should be individualized based on patient characteristics). However, insulin should be considered as part of a combination regimen when hyperglycemia is severe, particularly if patient is symptomatic or has catabolic features (eg, weight loss, ketosis). If insulin is selected, the addition of **basal** insulin with a long-acting insulin (ie, glargine or detemir) at 10 units (or 0.1 to 0.2 units/kg) once daily is recommended. If HbA$_{1c}$ target not achieved after ~3 months of dual therapy, may proceed to triple therapy (Inzucchi 2015).

Intensification of therapy: If HbA_{1c} target has not been met, despite titrating **basal** insulin (ie, long-acting insulin) to provide acceptable fasting blood glucose concentrations, intensification of therapy should be considered to cover postprandial glucose excursions. Options include adding a mealtime insulin (1 to 3 injections of a rapid-acting insulin analog [lispro, aspart, glulisine]) **or** adding a GLP-1 receptor agonist (eg, exenatide, liraglutide). Alternatively, although less studied, may transition from basal insulin (ie, long-acting insulin) to a twice daily premixed (or biphasic) insulin analog (70/30 aspart mix, 75/25 or 50/50 lispro mix) (Inzucchi 2015).

Pediatric

Diabetes mellitus, type 1: Lantus: SubQ: Children ≥6 years and Adolescents: Approximately one-third of the total daily insulin requirement administered once daily. A rapid-acting or short-acting insulin should also be used to complete the balance (~2/3) of the total daily insulin requirement. Adjust dosage according to patient response.

Conversion to insulin glargine from other insulin therapies: Refer to adult dosing.

Conversion between Toujeo and Lantus: Refer to adult dosing

Renal Impairment There are no dosage adjustments provided in the manufacturer's labeling; insulin requirements may be reduced due to changes in insulin clearance or metabolism; monitor blood glucose closely.

Hepatic Impairment There are no dosage adjustments provided in the manufacturer's labeling; insulin requirements may be reduced due to changes in insulin clearance or metabolism; monitor blood glucose closely.

Obesity Refer to indication-specific dosing for obesity-related information (may not be available for all indications).

Additional Information Complete prescribing information should be consulted for additional detail.

Product Availability Basaglar: FDA approved December 2015; availability anticipated late 2016. Consult prescribing information for additional detail.

Dosage Forms Excipient information presented when available (limited, particularly for generics); consult specific product labeling.

Solution, Subcutaneous:

Lantus: 100 units/mL (10 mL) [contains metacresol]

Solution Pen-injector, Subcutaneous:

Lantus SoloStar: 100 units/mL (3 mL) [contains metacresol]

Toujeo SoloStar: 300 units/mL (1.5 mL) [contains metacresol]

Insulin Glulisine (IN soo lin gloo LIS een)

Brand Names: US Apidra; Apidra SoloStar

Brand Names: Canada Apidra®

Index Terms Glulisine Insulin

Pharmacologic Category Insulin, Rapid-Acting

Use Treatment of type 1 diabetes mellitus (insulin dependent, IDDM) and type 2 diabetes mellitus (noninsulin dependent, NIDDM) to improve glycemic control

Dosing

Adult & Geriatric Note: Insulin glulisine is a rapid-acting insulin analog which is normally administered SubQ as a premeal component of the insulin regimen or as a continuous SubQ infusion and should be used with an intermediate- or long-acting insulin. When compared to insulin regular, insulin glulisine has a more rapid onset and shorter duration of activity. In carefully controlled clinical settings with close medical supervision and monitoring of blood glucose and potassium, insulin glulisine may be administered IV. Insulin requirements vary dramatically between patients and dictate frequent monitoring and close medical supervision.

Diabetes mellitus, type 1: SubQ:

General insulin dosing:

Type 1: **Note:** Multiple daily doses or continuous subcutaneous infusions guided by blood glucose monitoring are the standard of diabetes care. Combinations of insulin formulations are commonly used. The daily doses presented below are expressed as the **total units/kg/day of all insulin formulations combined.**

Initial total insulin dose: 0.2 to 0.6 units/kg/day in divided doses. Conservative initial doses of 0.2 to 0.4 units/kg/day are often recommended to avoid the potential for hypoglycemia. A rapid-acting insulin may be the only insulin formulation used initially.

Usual maintenance range: 0.5 to 1 units/kg/day in divided doses. An estimate of anticipated needs may be based on body weight and/or activity factors as follows:

Nonobese: 0.4 to 0.6 units/kg/day

Obese: 0.8 to 1.2 units/kg/day

Pubescent Children and Adolescents: During puberty, requirements may substantially increase to >1 unit/kg/day and in some cases up to 2 units/kg/day (IDF-ISPAD, 2011).

Division of daily insulin requirement ("conventional therapy"): Generally, 50% to 75% of the total daily dose (TDD) is given as an intermediate- or long-acting form of insulin (in 1 to 2 daily injections). The remaining portion of the TDD is then divided and administered before or at mealtimes (depending on the formulation) as a rapid-acting insulin (eg, insulin glulisine) or short-acting form of insulin. Some patients may benefit from the use of CSII which delivers rapid-acting insulin (insulin aspart) as a continuous infusion throughout the day and as boluses at mealtimes via an external pump device.

Division of daily insulin requirement ("intensive therapy"): Basal insulin delivery with 1 or 2 doses of intermediate- or long-acting insulin formulations superimposed with doses of short- or rapid-acting insulin (eg, insulin glulisine) formulations 3 or more times daily.

Adjustment of dose: Dosage must be titrated to achieve glucose control and avoid hypoglycemia. Adjust dose to maintain premeal and bedtime glucose in target range. Since combinations of agents are frequently used, dosage adjustment must address the individual component of the insulin regimen which most directly influences the blood glucose value in question, based on the known onset and duration of the insulin component. Treatment and monitoring regimens must be individualized.

Continuous SubQ insulin infusion (insulin pump): A combination of a "basal" continuous insulin infusion rate with preprogrammed, premeal bolus doses which are patient controlled. When converting from multiple daily SubQ doses of maintenance insulin, it is advisable to reduce the basal rate to less than the equivalent of the total daily units of the longer-acting insulin (eg, NPH); divide the total number of units by 24 to get the basal rate in units/hour. Do not include the total units of regular insulin or other rapid-acting insulin formulations in this calculation. The same premeal regular insulin dosage may be used.

Diabetes mellitus, type 2: SubQ:

General considerations for insulin use in type 2 diabetes:

Timing of initiation: The goal of therapy is to achieve an HbA_{1c} <7%. According to a position statement by the ADA and European Association for the Study of Diabetes (EASD), dual therapy (metformin + a second antihyperglycemic agent) is recommended in patients with type 2 diabetes who fail to achieve glycemic goals after ~3 months with lifestyle interventions and metformin monotherapy (unless contraindications to metformin exist). Preference is not given for adding insulin or a noninsulin agent as the second antihyperglycemic agent (drug choice should be individualized based on patient characteristics). However, insulin should be considered as part of a combination regimen when hyperglycemia is severe, particularly if patient is symptomatic or has catabolic features (eg, weight loss, ketosis). If insulin is selected, the addition of **basal** insulin with a long-acting insulin (ie, glargine or detemir [*not* insulin glulisine]) is recommended. If HbA_{1c} target not achieved after ~3 months of dual therapy, may proceed to triple therapy (Inzucchi, 2015).

Intensification of therapy: If HbA_{1c} target has not been met, despite titrating **basal** insulin (ie, long-acting insulin) to provide acceptable fasting blood glucose concentrations, intensification of therapy should be considered to cover postprandial glucose excursions. Options include adding a GLP-1 receptor agonist (eg, exenatide, liraglutide) **or** adding a mealtime insulin (1 injection of a rapid-acting insulin analog [lispro, aspart, glulisine]) initiated at a dose of 4 units or 0.1 units/kg or 10% basal dose before largest meal; may progress to "basal-bolus" dosing of 3 injections of a rapid-acting insulin analog [lispro, aspart, glulisine] per meal **or** dose by adding up the total current insulin dose, and provide one-half of this amount as basal and one-half as mealtime insulin

(split evenly between 3 meals). Alternatively, although less studied, may transition from basal insulin (ie, long-acting insulin) to a twice daily premixed (or biphasic) insulin analog (70/30 aspart mix, 75/25 or 50/50 lispro mix) (Inzucchi, 2015).

Hyperglycemia, critically ill (off-label use): IV continuous infusion: Insulin therapy should be implemented when blood glucose ≥150 mg/dL with a goal to maintain blood glucose <150 mg/dL (with values absolutely <180 mg/dL) using a protocol that achieves a low rate of hypoglycemia (ie, ≤70 mg/dL). Before discontinuation, stable ICU patients should be transitioned to a protocol-driven basal/bolus insulin regimen, based on insulin infusion history and carbohydrate intake, to avoid loss of glycemic control. Subcutaneous insulin therapy may be considered for selected clinically stable ICU patients (Jacobi, 2012). **Note:** The Surviving Sepsis Campaign guidelines recommend initiating insulin dosing in patients with severe sepsis when 2 consecutive blood glucose concentrations are >180 mg/dL and to target an upper blood glucose ≤180 mg/dL (Dellinger, 2013).

Pediatric Diabetes mellitus, type 1: Children ≥4 years and Adolescents: Refer to adult dosing.

Renal Impairment No dosage adjustment provided in manufacturer's labeling; insulin requirements may be reduced due to changes in insulin clearance or metabolism; monitor blood glucose closely.

Hepatic Impairment No dosage adjustment provided in manufacturer's labeling; insulin requirements may be reduced due to changes in insulin clearance or metabolism; monitor blood glucose closely.

Obesity Refer to indication-specific dosing for obesity-related information (may not be available for all indications).

Additional Information Complete prescribing information should be consulted for additional detail.

Dosage Forms Excipient information presented when available (limited, particularly for generics); consult specific product labeling.

Solution, Injection:
Apidra: 100 units/mL (10 mL) [contains metacresol]
Solution Pen-injector, Subcutaneous:
Apidra SoloStar: 100 units/mL (3 mL) [contains metacresol]

Insulin Lispro (IN soo lin LYE sproe)

Brand Names: US HumaLOG; HumaLOG KwikPen
Brand Names: Canada Humalog; HumaLOG KwikPen
Index Terms Lispro Insulin
Pharmacologic Category Insulin, Rapid-Acting
Use
Diabetes mellitus: Treatment of type 1 diabetes mellitus (insulin dependent, IDDM) and type 2 diabetes mellitus (noninsulin dependent, NIDDM) to improve glycemic control

According to the manufacturer's labeling, only the U 100 (eg, 100 units/mL) strength is approved for use in children ≥3 years by continuous subcutaneous insulin infusion (CSII) pumps.

Dosing
Adult & Geriatric Note: Insulin lispro is a rapid-acting insulin analog which is normally administered SubQ as a premeal component of the insulin regimen or as a continuous SubQ infusion and should be used with intermediate- or long-acting insulin. When compared to insulin regular, insulin lispro has a more rapid onset and shorter duration of activity. In carefully controlled clinical settings with close medical supervision and monitoring of blood glucose and potassium, insulin lispro U 100 (100 units/mL) may also be administered IV. Insulin requirements vary dramatically between patients and dictate frequent monitoring and close medical supervision.

Diabetes mellitus, type 1: SubQ:
General insulin dosing:
Type 1: **Note:** Multiple daily doses or continuous subcutaneous infusions guided by blood glucose monitoring are the standard of diabetes care. Combinations of insulin formulations are commonly used. The daily doses presented below are expressed as the **total units/kg/day of all insulin formulations combined.**
Initial total insulin dose: 0.2 to 0.6 units/kg/day in divided doses. Conservative initial doses of 0.2 to 0.4 units/kg/day are often recommended to avoid the potential for hypoglycemia. A rapid-acting insulin may be the only insulin formulation used initially.

Usual maintenance range: 0.5 to 1 units/kg/day in divided doses. An estimate of anticipated needs may be based on body weight and/or activity factors as follows:
Nonobese: 0.4 to 0.6 units/kg/day
Obese: 0.8 to 1.2 units/kg/day
Pubescent Children and Adolescents: During puberty, requirements may substantially increase to >1 unit/kg/day and in some cases up to 2 units/kg/day (IDF-ISPAD, 2011).
Division of daily insulin requirement ("conventional therapy"): Generally, 50% to 75% of the total daily dose (TDD) is given as an intermediate- or long-acting form of insulin (in 1 to 2 daily injections). The remaining portion of the TDD is then divided and administered before or at mealtimes (depending on the formulation) as a rapid-acting (eg, insulin aspart) or short-acting form of insulin. Some patients may benefit from the use of CSII which delivers rapid-acting insulin (insulin aspart) as a continuous infusion throughout the day and as boluses at mealtimes via an external pump device.
Division of daily insulin requirement ("intensive therapy"): Basal insulin delivery with 1 or 2 doses of intermediate- or long-acting insulin formulations superimposed with doses of short- or rapid-acting insulin (eg, insulin aspart) formulations 3 or more times daily.
Adjustment of dose: Dosage must be titrated to achieve glucose control and avoid hypoglycemia. Adjust dose to maintain premeal and bedtime glucose in target range. Since combinations of agents are frequently used, dosage adjustment must address the individual component of the insulin regimen which most directly influences the blood glucose value in question, based on the known onset and duration of the insulin component. Treatment and monitoring regimens must be individualized.
Continuous SubQ insulin infusion (insulin pump): A combination of a "basal" continuous insulin infusion rate with preprogrammed, premeal bolus doses which are patient controlled. When converting from multiple daily SubQ doses of maintenance insulin, it is advisable to reduce the basal rate to less than the equivalent of the total daily units of the longer acting insulin (eg, NPH); divide the total number of units by 24 to get the basal rate in units/hour. Do not include the total units of regular insulin or other rapid-acting insulin formulations in this calculation. The same premeal regular insulin dosage may be used.

Diabetes mellitus, type 2: SubQ:
General considerations for insulin use in type 2 diabetes:
Timing of initiation: The goal of therapy is to achieve an HbA$_{1c}$ <7%. According to a position statement by the ADA and European Association for the Study of Diabetes (EASD), dual therapy (metformin + a second antihyperglycemic agent) is recommended in patients with type 2 diabetes who fail to achieve glycemic goals after ~3 months with lifestyle interventions and metformin monotherapy (unless contraindications to metformin exist). Preference is not given for adding insulin or a noninsulin agent as the second antihyperglycemic agent (drug choice should be individualized based on patient characteristics). However, insulin should be considered as part of a combination regimen when hyperglycemia is severe, particularly if patient is symptomatic or has catabolic features (eg, weight loss, ketosis). If insulin is selected, the addition of **basal** insulin with a long-acting insulin (ie, glargine or detemir [*not* insulin lispro]) is recommended. If HbA$_{1c}$ target not achieved after ~3 months of dual therapy, may proceed to triple therapy (Inzucchi, 2015).
Intensification of therapy: If HbA$_{1c}$ target has not been met, despite titrating **basal** insulin (ie, long-acting insulin) to provide acceptable fasting blood glucose concentrations, intensification of therapy should be considered to cover postprandial glucose excursions. Options include adding a GLP-1 receptor agonist (eg, exenatide, liraglutide) **or** adding a mealtime insulin (1 injection of a rapid-acting insulin analog [lispro, aspart, glulisine]) initiated at a dose of 4 units or 0.1 units/kg or 10% basal dose before largest meal; may progress to "basal-bolus" dosing of 3 injections of a rapid-acting insulin analog [lispro, aspart, glulisine] per meal **or** dose by adding up the total current insulin dose, and provide one-half of this amount as basal and one-half as mealtime insulin

(split evenly between 3 meals). Alternatively, although less studied, may transition from basal insulin (ie, long-acting insulin) to a twice daily pre-mixed (or biphasic) insulin analog (70/30 aspart mix, 75/25 or 50/50 lispro mix) (Inzucchi, 2015).

Pediatric

Diabetes mellitus, type 1: Children ≥3 years and Adolescents: Refer to adult dosing.

Diabetic ketoacidosis (DKA), mild-to-moderate (off-label use): Children and Adolescents: Treatment should continue until reversal of acid-base derangement/ketonemia. Serum glucose is not a direct indicator of these abnormalities, and may decrease more rapidly than correction of the metabolic abnormalities. Also refer to institution-specific protocols where appropriate. SubQ (Note: Use of IV regular insulin is preferred; only use the SubQ route if IV infusion access is unavailable): 0.3 units/kg followed in 1 hour by 0.1 units/kg given every hour or 0.15-0.2 units/kg every 2 hours; continue until acidosis clears, then decrease to 0.05 units/kg given every hour until maintenance SubQ replacement dosing can be initiated (Kitabchi, 2004; Wolfsdorf, 2007).

Renal Impairment Adults: Insulin requirements are reduced due to changes in insulin clearance or metabolism. There are no dosage adjustments provided in the manufacturer's labeling; however, the following adjustments have been recommended (Aronoff, 2007):

CrCl >50 mL/minute: No adjustment necessary

CrCl 10-50 mL/minute: Administer at 75% of recommended dose

CrCl <10 mL/minute: Administer at 50% of recommended dose and monitor glucose closely

Hemodialysis: Because of a large molecular weight (6000 daltons), insulin is not significantly removed by either peritoneal or hemodialysis; supplemental dose is not necessary

Peritoneal dialysis: Supplemental dose is not necessary

Continuous renal replacement therapy: Administer at 75% of recommended dose

Hepatic Impairment There are no dosage adjustments provided in the manufacturer's labeling; dosage requirements may be reduced and patients may require more frequent dose adjustment and glucose monitoring.

Obesity Refer to indication-specific dosing for obesity-related information (may not be available for all indications).

Additional Information Complete prescribing information should be consulted for additional detail.

Dosage Forms Excipient information presented when available (limited, particularly for generics); consult specific product labeling.

Solution, Subcutaneous:

HumaLOG: 100 units/mL (3 mL, 10 mL) [contains metacresol, phenol]

Solution Pen-injector, Subcutaneous:

HumaLOG KwikPen: 100 units/mL (3 mL); 200 units/mL (3 mL) [contains metacresol, phenol]

◆ Insulin Lispro and Insulin Lispro Protamine see Insulin Lispro Protamine and Insulin Lispro on page 959

Insulin Lispro Protamine and Insulin Lispro

(IN soo lin LYE sproe PROE ta meen & IN soo lin LYE sproe)

Brand Names: US HumaLOG® Mix 50/50™; HumaLOG® Mix 50/50™ KwikPen™; HumaLOG® Mix 75/25™; HumaLOG® Mix 75/25™ KwikPen™

Brand Names: Canada Humalog Mix 25; Humalog Mix 50

Index Terms Insulin Lispro and Insulin Lispro Protamine

Pharmacologic Category Insulin, Combination

Use Treatment of type 1 diabetes mellitus (insulin dependent, IDDM) and type 2 diabetes mellitus (noninsulin dependent, NIDDM) to improve glycemic control

Dosing

Adult & Geriatric Note: Lispro protamine is an intermediate-acting insulin and lispro is a rapid-acting insulin administered by SubQ injection. Insulin lispro protamine and insulin lispro combination products are approximately equipotent to insulin NPH and insulin regular combination products with a similar duration of activity but a more rapid onset. With combination insulin products, the proportion of rapid-acting to long-acting insulin is fixed; basal vs prandial dose adjustments cannot be made. Fixed ratio insulins (such as insulin lispro protamine and insulin lispro combination) are typically administered as 2 daily doses with each dose intended to cover two meals and a snack. Because of variability in the peak effect and individual patient variability in activities, meals, etc, it may be more difficult to achieve complete glycemic

control using fixed combinations of insulins; frequent monitoring and close medical supervision may be necessary.

General insulin dosing:

Diabetes mellitus, type 1: SubQ: **Note:** Multiple daily doses are utilized and guided by blood glucose monitoring. Combinations of different insulin formulations are commonly used. The daily doses presented below are expressed as the **total units/kg/day of all insulin formulations combined.** Insulin lispro protamine and insulin lispro combination product is **not** intended for initial therapy; basal insulin requirements should be established **first** to direct dosing of combination insulin products.

Usual maintenance range: SubQ: 0.5-1 units/kg/day in divided doses. An estimate of anticipated needs may be based on body weight and/or activity factors as follows:

Nonobese: 0.4-0.6 units/kg/day

Obese: 0.8-1.2 units/kg/day

Pubescent Children and Adolescents: During puberty, requirements may substantially increase to >1 unit/kg/day and in some cases up to 2 units/kg/day (IDF-ISPAD, 2011).

Division of daily insulin requirement ("conventional therapy"): Generally, 50% to 75% of the daily insulin dose is given as an intermediate- or long-acting form of insulin (in 1-2 daily injections). The remaining portion of the 24-hour insulin requirement is divided and administered as either regular insulin or a rapid-acting form of insulin at the same time before breakfast and dinner.

Adjustment of dose: Dosage must be titrated to achieve glucose control and avoid hypoglycemia. Adjust dose to maintain premeal and bedtime glucose in target range. Since combinations of agents are frequently used, dosage adjustment must address the individual component of the insulin regimen which most directly influences the blood glucose value in question, based on the known onset and duration of the insulin component. Treatment and monitoring regimens must be individualized.

Diabetes mellitus, type 2: SubQ: Augmentation therapy (patients for which diet, exercise, weight reduction, and oral hypoglycemic agents have not been adequate): **Note:** Insulin lispro protamine and insulin lispro combination product is **not** intended for initial therapy; basal insulin requirements should be established **first** to direct dosing of combination insulin products. Dosage must be carefully adjusted.

Renal Impairment No dosage adjustment provided in manufacturer's labeling; insulin requirements may be reduced due to changes in insulin clearance or metabolism; monitor blood glucose closely.

Hepatic Impairment No dosage adjustment provided in manufacturer's labeling; insulin requirements may be reduced due to changes in insulin clearance or metabolism; monitor blood glucose closely.

Obesity Refer to indication-specific dosing for obesity-related information (may not be available for all indications).

Additional Information Complete prescribing information should be consulted for additional detail.

Dosage Forms Excipient information presented when available (limited, particularly for generics); consult specific product labeling.

Injection, suspension:

HumaLOG® Mix 50/50™: Insulin lispro protamine suspension 50% [intermediate acting] and insulin lispro solution 50% [rapid acting]: 100 units/mL (10 mL)

HumaLOG® Mix 50/50™ KwikPen™: Insulin lispro protamine suspension 50% [intermediate acting] and insulin lispro solution 50% [rapid acting]: 100 units/mL (3 mL)

HumaLOG® Mix 75/25™: Insulin lispro protamine suspension 75% [intermediate acting] and insulin lispro solution 25% [rapid acting]: 100 units/mL (10 mL)

HumaLOG® Mix 75/25™ KwikPen™: Insulin lispro protamine suspension 75% [intermediate acting] and insulin lispro solution 25% [rapid acting]: 100 units/mL (3 mL)

Insulin NPH (IN soo lin N P H)

Brand Names: US HumuLIN N KwikPen [OTC]; HumuLIN N Pen [OTC] [DSC]; HumuLIN N [OTC]; NovoLIN N ReliOn [OTC]; NovoLIN N [OTC]

Brand Names: Canada Humulin N; Novolin ge NPH

Index Terms Isophane Insulin; NPH Insulin

Pharmacologic Category Insulin, Intermediate-Acting

Use Treatment of type 1 diabetes mellitus (insulin dependent, IDDM) and type 2 diabetes mellitus (noninsulin dependent, NIDDM) to improve glycemic control

Dosing

Adult & Geriatric Note: Insulin NPH is an intermediate-acting insulin formulation which is usually administered subcutaneously once or twice daily. When compared to insulin regular, insulin NPH has a slower onset and longer duration of activity. Insulin requirements vary dramatically between patients and dictate frequent monitoring and close medical supervision.

General insulin dosing:

Diabetes mellitus, type 1: SubQ: **Note:** Multiple daily doses are utilized and guided by blood glucose monitoring. Combinations of different insulin formulations are commonly used. The daily doses presented below are expressed as the **total units/kg/day of all insulin formulations combined.** Insulin NPH is **not** intended for initial therapy; basal insulin requirements should be established **first** to direct dosing of combination insulin products.

Usual maintenance range: SubQ: 0.5-1 units/kg/day in divided doses. An estimate of anticipated needs may be based on body weight and/or activity factors as follows:

Nonobese: 0.4-0.6 units/kg/day

Obese: 0.8-1.2 units/kg/day

Pubescent Children and Adolescents: During puberty, requirements may substantially increase to >1 unit/kg/day and in some cases up to 2 units/kg/day (IDF-ISPAD, 2011).

Division of daily insulin requirement ("conventional therapy"): Generally, 50% to 75% of the total daily dose (TDD) is given as an intermediate-acting (eg, NPH) or a long-acting form of insulin (in 1-2 daily injections). The remaining portion of the TDD is then divided and administered before or at mealtimes (depending on the formulation) as a rapid-acting or short-acting form of insulin.

Adjustment of dose: Dosage must be titrated to achieve glucose control and avoid hypoglycemia. Adjust dose to maintain premeal and bedtime glucose in target range. Since combinations of agents are frequently used, dosage adjustment must address the individual component of the insulin regimen which most directly influences the blood glucose value in question, based on the known onset and duration of the insulin component. Treatment and monitoring regimens must be individualized.

Diabetes mellitus, type 2: Augmentation therapy (patients for which diet, exercise, weight reduction, and oral hypoglycemic agents have not been adequate): SubQ: Initial dosage of 0.2 units/kg/day or 10 units/day of an intermediate-acting (eg, NPH) or long-acting insulin administered at bedtime has been recommended. As an alternative, regular insulin or rapid-acting insulin formulations administered before meals have also been used. Dosage must be carefully adjusted.

Pediatric

Diabetes mellitus, type 1: SubQ: Children and Adolescents: Refer to adult dosing.

Renal Impairment No dosage adjustment provided in manufacturer's labeling; insulin requirements may be reduced due to changes in insulin clearance or metabolism; monitor blood glucose closely.

Hepatic Impairment No dosage adjustment provided in manufacturer's labeling; insulin requirements may be reduced due to changes in insulin clearance or metabolism; monitor blood glucose closely.

Obesity Refer to indication-specific dosing for obesity-related information (may not be available for all indications).

Additional Information Complete prescribing information should be consulted for additional detail.

Dosage Forms Excipient information presented when available (limited, particularly for generics); consult specific product labeling. [DSC] = Discontinued product

Suspension, Subcutaneous:

HumuLIN N: 100 units/mL (3 mL, 10 mL) [contains metacresol, phenol]

NovoLIN N: 100 units/mL (10 mL) [contains metacresol, phenol]

NovoLIN N ReliOn: 100 units/mL (10 mL) [contains metacresol, phenol]

Suspension Pen-injector, Subcutaneous:

HumuLIN N KwikPen: 100 units/mL (3 mL) [contains metacresol, phenol]

HumuLIN N Pen: 100 units/mL (3 mL [DSC]) [contains metacresol, phenol]

Dosage Forms: Canada Excipient information presented when available (limited, particularly for generics); consult specific product labeling.

Injection, suspension:

Novolin® ge NPH: 100 units/mL (3 mL) [NovolinSet® prefilled syringe or PenFill® prefilled cartridge]; 10 mL [vial]

Insulin NPH and Insulin Regular

(IN soo lin N P H & IN soo lin REG yoo ler)

Brand Names: US HumuLIN 70/30; HumuLIN 70/30 KwikPen; NovoLIN 70/30

Brand Names: Canada Humulin 20/80; Humulin 70/30; Novolin ge 30/70; Novolin ge 40/60; Novolin ge 50/50

Index Terms Insulin Regular and Insulin NPH; Isophane Insulin and Regular Insulin; NPH Insulin and Regular Insulin

Pharmacologic Category Insulin, Combination

Use Treatment of type 1 diabetes mellitus (insulin dependent, IDDM) and type 2 diabetes mellitus (noninsulin dependent, NIDDM) to improve glycemic control

Dosing

Adult & Geriatric Note: Insulin NPH is an intermediate-acting insulin and regular insulin is a short-acting insulin administered by SubQ injection. When compared to insulin NPH, the combination product (insulin NPH and insulin regular) has a shorter onset of action and a similar duration of action. With combination insulin products, the proportion of short-acting to long-acting insulin is fixed; basal vs prandial dose adjustments cannot be made. Fixed-ratio insulins (such as insulin NPH and insulin regular combination) are typically administered as 2 daily doses with each dose intended to cover two meals and a snack. Because of variability in the peak effect and individual patient variability in activities, meals, etc, it may be more difficult to achieve complete glycemic control using fixed combinations of insulins; frequent monitoring and close medical supervision may be necessary.

Diabetes mellitus, type 1:

General insulin dosing:

Type 1: **Note:** Multiple daily doses are utilized and guided by blood glucose monitoring. Combinations of different insulin formulations are commonly used. The daily doses presented below are expressed as the **total units/kg/day of all insulin formulations combined.** Insulin NPH and insulin regular combination product is **not** intended for initial therapy; basal insulin requirements should be established **first** to direct dosing of combination insulin products.

Usual maintenance range: SubQ: 0.5 to 1 units/kg/day in divided doses. An estimate of anticipated needs may be based on body weight and/or activity factors as follows:

Nonobese: 0.4 to 0.6 units/kg/day

Obese: 0.8 to 1.2 units/kg/day

Pubescent Children and Adolescents: During puberty, requirements may substantially increase to >1 unit/kg/day and in some cases up to 2 units/kg/day (IDF-ISPAD 2011).

Division of daily insulin requirement ("conventional therapy"): Generally, 50% to 75% of the total daily dose (TDD) is given as an intermediate-acting (eg, NPH) or a long-acting form of insulin (in 1 to 2 daily injections). The remaining portion of the TDD is then divided and administered before or at mealtimes (depending on the formulation) as a rapid-acting or short-acting form of insulin.

Adjustment of dose: Dosage must be titrated to achieve glucose control and avoid hypoglycemia. Adjust dose to maintain premeal and bedtime glucose in target range. Since combinations of agents are frequently used, dosage adjustment must address the individual component of the insulin regimen which most directly influences the blood glucose value in question, based on the known onset and duration of the insulin component. Treatment and monitoring regimens must be individualized.

Diabetes mellitus, type 2: SubQ:

General considerations for insulin use in type 2 diabetes:

Timing of initiation: The goal of therapy is to achieve an HbA$_{1c}$ <7%. According to a position statement by the ADA and European Association for the Study of Diabetes (EASD), dual therapy (metformin + a second antihyperglycemic agent) is recommended in patients with type 2 diabetes who fail to achieve glycemic goals after ~3 months with lifestyle interventions and metformin monotherapy (unless

contraindications to metformin exist). Preference is not given for adding insulin or a noninsulin agent as the second antihyperglycemic agent (drug choice should be individualized based on patient characteristics). However, insulin should be considered as part of a combination regimen when hyperglycemia is severe, particularly if patient is symptomatic or has catabolic features (eg, weight loss, ketosis). If insulin is selected, the addition of **basal** insulin with a long-acting insulin (ie, glargine or detemir [*not* insulin NPH and insulin regular combination]) is recommended. If HbA$_{1c}$ target not achieved after ~3 months of dual therapy, may proceed to triple therapy (Inzucchi 2015).

Intensification of therapy: If HbA$_{1c}$ target has not been met, despite titrating **basal** insulin (ie, long-acting insulin) to provide acceptable fasting blood glucose concentrations, intensification of therapy should be considered to cover postprandial glucose excursions. Options include adding a mealtime insulin (1 to 3 injections of a rapid-acting insulin analog [lispro, aspart, glulisine] **or** adding a GLP-1 receptor agonist (eg, exenatide, liraglutide). Alternatively, although less studied, may transition from basal insulin (ie, long-acting insulin) to a twice daily premixed (or biphasic) insulin analog (70/30 aspart mix, 75/25 or 50/50 lispro mix) (Inzucchi 2015).

Pediatric

Diabetes mellitus, type 1: SubQ: Children and Adolescents: Refer to adult dosing.

Renal Impairment There are no dosage adjustments provided in manufacturer's labeling; insulin requirements may be reduced due to changes in insulin clearance or metabolism; monitor blood glucose closely.

Hepatic Impairment There are no dosage adjustments provided in manufacturer's labeling; insulin requirements may be reduced due to changes in insulin clearance or metabolism; monitor blood glucose closely.

Obesity Refer to indication-specific dosing for obesity-related information (may not be available for all indications).

Additional Information Complete prescribing information should be consulted for additional detail.

Dosage Forms Excipient information presented when available (limited, particularly for generics); consult specific product labeling.

Injection, suspension:

HumuLIN 70/30: Insulin NPH suspension 70% [intermediate acting] and insulin regular solution 30% [short acting]: 100 units/mL (3 mL, 10 mL) [vial]

HumuLIN 70/30 KwikPen: Insulin NPH suspension 70% [intermediate acting] and insulin regular solution 30% [short acting]: 100 units/mL (3 mL)

NovoLIN 70/30: Insulin NPH suspension 70% [intermediate acting] and insulin regular solution 30% [short acting]: 100 units/mL (10 mL) [vial]

Dosage Forms: Canada Excipient information presented when available (limited, particularly for generics); consult specific product labeling.

Injection, suspension:

Humulin 20/80: Insulin regular solution 20% [short acting] and insulin NPH suspension 80% [intermediate acting]: 100 units/mL (3 mL) [PenFill prefilled cartridge]

Novolin ge 30/70: Insulin regular solution 30% [short acting] and insulin NPH suspension 70% [intermediate acting]: 100 units/mL (3 mL) [prefilled syringe or PenFill prefilled cartridge]; (10 mL) [vial]

Novolin ge 40/60: Insulin regular solution 40% [short acting] and insulin NPH suspension 60% [intermediate acting]: 100 units/mL (3 mL) [PenFill prefilled cartridge]

Novolin ge 50/50: Insulin regular solution 50% [short acting] and insulin NPH suspension 50% [intermediate acting]: 100 units/mL (3 mL) [PenFill prefilled cartridge]

Insulin Regular (IN soo lin REG yoo ler)

Brand Names: US HumuLIN R U-500 (CONCENTRATED); HumuLIN R [OTC]; NovoLIN R ReliOn [OTC]; NovoLIN R [OTC]

Brand Names: Canada Humulin R; Novolin ge Toronto

Index Terms Regular Insulin

Pharmacologic Category Insulin, Short-Acting

Use Diabetes mellitus, type 1 or type 2: Treatment of diabetes mellitus (type 1 or type 2) to improve glycemic control

Pregnancy Considerations Recombinant human insulin for injection is identical to endogenous insulin; therefore, animal reproduction studies have not been conducted. Minimal amounts of endogenous insulin cross the placenta. Exogenous insulin bound to anti-insulin antibodies can be detected in cord blood (Menon 1990)

In women with diabetes, maternal hyperglycemia can be associated with congenital malformations as well as adverse effects in the fetus, neonate, and the mother (ACOG 2005; ADA 2015; Kitzmiller 2008; Metzger 2007). To prevent adverse outcomes, prior to conception and throughout pregnancy maternal blood glucose and HbA$_{1c}$ should be kept as close to target goals as possible but without causing significant hypoglycemia (ACOG 2013; ADA 2015; Blumer 2013; Kitzmiller 2008; Lambert 2013). Prior to pregnancy, effective contraception should be used until glycemic control is achieved (Kitzmiller 2008).

Insulin requirements tend to fall during the first trimester of pregnancy and increase in the later trimesters, peaking at 28 to 32 weeks of gestation. Following delivery, insulin requirements decrease rapidly (ACOG 2005).

Rapid acting insulins, such as insulin aspart or insulin lispro may be preferred over regular human insulin in women trying to conceive (Blumer 2013); however, there is no need to switch a pregnant woman who is well controlled on injectable human insulin to a short acting analogue (Lambert 2013).

Breast-Feeding Considerations Both exogenous and endogenous insulin are excreted into breast milk (study not conducted with this preparation) (Whitmore 2012). Breast-feeding is encouraged for all women, including those with type 1, type 2, or GDM (ACOG 2005; Blumer 2013; Metzger 2007). A small snack (such as milk) before nursing may help decrease the risk of hypoglycemia in women with pregestational diabetes (ACOG 2005; ADA 2015; Reader 2004).

Adverse events have not been reported in nursing infants following use of regular insulin for injection; adjustments of the mothers insulin dose may be needed.

Contraindications

Hypersensitivity to regular insulin or any component of the formulation; during episodes of hypoglycemia.

Documentation of allergenic cross-reactivity for insulin is limited. However, because of similarities in chemical structure and/or pharmacologic actions, the possibility of cross-sensitivity cannot be ruled out with certainty.

Warnings/Precautions Hypoglycemia is the most common adverse effect of insulin. The timing of hypoglycemia differs among various insulin formulations. Hypoglycemia may result from increased work or exercise without eating; use of long-acting insulin preparations (eg, insulin detemir, insulin glargine) may delay recovery from hypoglycemia. Profound and prolonged episodes of hypoglycemia may result in convulsions, unconsciousness, temporary or permanent brain damage or even death. Insulin requirements may be altered during illness, emotional disturbances or other stressors. Instruct patients to use caution with ethanol; may increase risk of hypoglycemia. Insulin may produce hypokalemia which, if left untreated, may result in respiratory paralysis, ventricular arrhythmia and even death. Use with caution in patients at risk for hypokalemia (eg, IV insulin use). Severe, life-threatening, generalized allergic reactions, including anaphylaxis, may occur. If hypersensitivity reactions occur, discontinue therapy, treat the patient with supportive care and monitor until signs and symptoms resolve. Use with caution in renal or hepatic impairment. In the elderly, avoid use of sliding scale injectable insulin in this population due to increased risk of hypoglycemia without benefits in management of hyperglycemia regardless of care setting (Beers Criteria).

Human insulin differs from animal-source insulin. Any change of insulin should be made cautiously; changing manufacturers, type, and/or method of manufacture may result in the need for a change of dosage. U-500 regular insulin is a concentrated insulin formulation which contains 500 units of insulin per mL; for SubQ administration only using a U-100 insulin syringe or tuberculin syringe; **not for IV administration**. To avoid dosing errors when using a U-100 insulin syringe, the prescribed dose should be written in actual insulin units and as unit markings on the U-100 insulin syringe (eg, 50 units [10 units on a U-100 insulin syringe]). To avoid dosing errors when using a tuberculin syringe, the prescribed dose should be written in actual insulin units and as a volume (eg, 50 units [0.1 mL]). Mixing U-500 regular insulin with other insulin formulations is not recommended.

Regular insulin may be administered IV or IM in selected clinical situations; close monitoring of blood glucose and serum potassium, as well as medical supervision, is required.

The general objective of exogenous insulin therapy is to approximate the physiologic pattern of insulin secretion which is characterized by two distinct phases. Phase 1 insulin secretion suppresses hepatic glucose production and phase 2 insulin secretion occurs in response to ▶

carbohydrate ingestion; therefore, exogenous insulin therapy may consist of basal insulin (eg, intermediate- or long-acting insulin or via continuous subcutaneous insulin infusion [CSII]) and/or preprandial insulin (eg, short- or rapid-acting insulin). Patients with type 1 diabetes do not produce endogenous insulin; therefore, these patients require both basal and preprandial insulin administration. Patients with type 2 diabetes retain some beta-cell function in the early stages of their disease; however, as the disease progresses, phase 1 insulin secretion may become completely impaired and phase 2 insulin secretion becomes delayed and/or inadequate in response to meals. Therefore, patients with type 2 diabetes may be treated with oral antidiabetic agents, basal insulin, and/or preprandial insulin depending on the stage of disease and current glycemic control. Since treatment regimens often consist of multiple agents, dosage adjustments must address the specific phase of insulin release that is primarily contributing to the patient's impaired glycemic control. Diabetes self-management education (DSME) is essential to maximize the effectiveness of therapy. Treatment and monitoring regimens must be individualized. Exclusive use of a sliding scale insulin regimen to manage persistent hyperglycemia in the hospital is discouraged. An effective insulin regimen will achieve the goal glucose range without the risk of severe hypoglycemia (ADA 2015).

Potentially significant drug-drug interactions may exist, requiring dose or frequency adjustment, additional monitoring, and/or selection of alternative therapy. In particular, concurrent use with peroxisome proliferator-activated receptor (PPAR)-gamma agonists, including thiazolidinediones (TZDs) may cause dose-related fluid retention and lead to or exacerbate heart failure.

Adverse Reactions Frequency not always defined.

Cardiovascular: Peripheral edema

Dermatologic: Erythema at injection site, injection site pruritus

Endocrine & metabolic: Hypoglycemia, hypokalemia, weight gain

Hypersensitivity: Anaphylaxis, hypersensitivity, hypersensitivity reaction

Local: Hypertrophy at injection site, lipoatrophy at injection site

Drug Interactions

Metabolism/Transport Effects None known.

Avoid Concomitant Use

Avoid concomitant use of Insulin Regular with any of the following: Rosiglitazone

Increased Effect/Toxicity

Insulin Regular may increase the levels/effects of: Hypoglycemia-Associated Agents; Rosiglitazone

The levels/effects of Insulin Regular may be increased by: Alpha-Lipoic Acid; Androgens; Antidiabetic Agents; Beta-Blockers; DPP-IV Inhibitors; Edetate CALCIUM Disodium; Edetate Disodium; GLP-1 Agonists; Herbs (Hypoglycemic Properties); Liraglutide; MAO Inhibitors; Metreleptin; Pegvisomant; Pioglitazone; Pramlintide; Quinolone Antibiotics; Salicylates; Selective Serotonin Reuptake Inhibitors; SGLT2 Inhibitors

Decreased Effect

The levels/effects of Insulin Regular may be decreased by: Hyperglycemia-Associated Agents; Quinolone Antibiotics; Thiazide Diuretics

Preparation for Administration

For SubQ administration:

Humulin R: May be diluted with the universal diluent, Sterile Diluent for Humalog, Humulin N, Humulin R, Humulin 70/30, and Humulin R U-500, to a concentration of 10 units/mL (U-10) or 50 units/mL (U-50).

Novolin R: Insulin Diluting Medium for NovoLog is **not** intended for use with Novolin R or any insulin product other than insulin aspart.

For IV infusion:

Humulin R: May be diluted in NS or D5W to concentrations of 0.1-1 unit/mL.

Novolin R: May be diluted in NS, D5W, or D10W with 40 mEq/L potassium chloride at concentrations of 0.05 to 1 unit/mL.

Storage/Stability

Humulin R: Store unopened vials in refrigerator between 2°C and 8°C (36°F to 46°F); do not freeze; keep away from heat and sunlight. Once punctured (in use), vials may be stored for up to 31 days in the refrigerator between 2°C and 8°C (36°F to 46°F) or at room temperature of ≤30°C (≤86°F).

Humulin R U-500: Store unopened vials (not in use) in a refrigerator (2°C to 8°C [36°F to 46°F]). Do not freeze and do not use if the vial has been frozen. Store vials currently opened (in use) unrefrigerated as long as they are kept as cool as possible (below 30°C [86°F]) and away from heat and light for up to 40 days.

Novolin R: Store unopened vials in refrigerator between 2°C and 8°C (36°F to 46°F) until product expiration date or at room temperature ≤25°C (≤77°F) for up to 42 days; do not freeze; keep away from heat and sunlight. Once punctured (in use), store vials at room temperature ≤25°C (≤77°F) for up to 42 days (this includes any days stored at room temperature prior to opening vial); refrigeration of in-use vials is not recommended.

Canadian labeling (not in U.S. labeling): All products: Unopened vials, cartridges, and pens should be stored under refrigeration between 2°C and 8°C (36°F to 46°F) until the expiration date; do not freeze; keep away from heat and sunlight. Once punctured (in use), Humulin vials, cartridges, and pens should be stored at room temperature <25°C (<77°F) for up to 4 weeks. Once punctured (in use), Novolin ge vials, cartridges, and pens may be stored for up to 1 month at room temperature <25°C (<77°F) for vials or <30°C (<86°F) for pens/cartridges; do not refrigerate.

For SubQ administration:

Humulin R: According to the manufacturer, diluted insulin should be stored at 30°C (86°F) and used within 14 days **or** at 5°C (41°F) and used within 28 days.

For IV infusion:

Humulin R: Stable for 48 hours at room temperature or for 48 hours under refrigeration followed by 48 hours at room temperature.

Novolin R: Stable for 24 hours at room temperature

Mechanism of Action Insulin acts via specific membrane-bound receptors on target tissues to regulate metabolism of carbohydrate, protein, and fats. Target organs for insulin include the liver, skeletal muscle, and adipose tissue.

Within the liver, insulin stimulates hepatic glycogen synthesis. Insulin promotes hepatic synthesis of fatty acids, which are released into the circulation as lipoproteins. Skeletal muscle effects of insulin include increased protein synthesis and increased glycogen synthesis. Within adipose tissue, insulin stimulates the processing of circulating lipoproteins to provide free fatty acids, facilitating triglyceride synthesis and storage by adipocytes; also directly inhibits the hydrolysis of triglycerides. In addition, insulin stimulates the cellular uptake of amino acids and increases cellular permeability to several ions, including potassium, magnesium, and phosphate. By activating sodium-potassium ATPases, insulin promotes the intracellular movement of potassium.

Normally secreted by the pancreas, insulin products are manufactured for pharmacologic use through recombinant DNA technology using either *E. coli* or *Saccharomyces cerevisiae*. Insulins are categorized based on the onset, peak, and duration of effect (eg, rapid-, short-, intermediate-, and long-acting insulin).

Pharmacodynamics/Kinetics Note: Onset and duration of hypoglycemic effects depend upon the route of administration (adsorption and onset of action are more rapid after deeper IM injections than after SubQ), site of injection (onset and duration are progressively slower with SubQ injection into the abdomen, arm, buttock, or thigh respectively), volume and concentration of injection, and the preparation administered. Rate of absorption, onset, and duration of activity may be affected by exercise, presence of lipodystrophy, local blood supply, and/or temperature.

Onset of action: SubQ: 0.5 hours

Peak effect: SubQ: 2.5 to 5 hours

Duration:

IV: U-100: 2 to 6 hours

SubQ: U-100: 4 to 12 hours (may increase with dose); U-500: Up to 24 hours

Distribution: IV, SubQ: V$_d$: 0.26 to 0.36 L/kg

Bioavailability: SubQ: 55% to 77%

Half-life elimination: IV: ~0.5 to 1 hour (dose-dependent); SubQ: 1.5 hours

Time to peak, plasma: SubQ: 0.8 to 2 hours

Excretion: Urine

Dosing

Adult & Geriatric

Diabetes mellitus: SubQ: **Note:** Insulin requirements vary dramatically between patients and therapy requires dosage adjustments with careful medical supervision. Specific formulations may require distinct administration procedures; please see individual agents.

Diabetes mellitus, type 1:

General insulin dosing:

Note: Multiple daily doses or continuous subcutaneous infusions guided by blood glucose monitoring are the standard of diabetes care. Combinations of insulin formulations are commonly used. The daily doses presented below are expressed as the **total units/ kg/day of all insulin formulations combined.**

Initial total insulin dose: 0.2 to 0.6 units/kg/day in divided doses. Conservative initial doses of 0.2 to 0.4 units/kg/day are often recommended to avoid the potential for hypoglycemia. A rapid-acting insulin may be the only insulin formulation used initially.

Usual maintenance range: 0.5 to 1 units/kg/day in divided doses. An estimate of anticipated needs may be based on body weight and/or activity factors as follows:

Nonobese: 0.4 to 0.6 units/kg/day

Obese: 0.8 to 1.2 units/kg/day

Pubescent Children and Adolescents: During puberty, requirements may substantially increase to >1 unit/kg/day and in some cases up to 2 units/kg/day (IDF/ISPAD 2011).

Division of daily insulin requirement ("conventional therapy"): Generally, 50% to 75% of the total daily dose (TDD) is given as an intermediate- or long-acting form of insulin (in 1 to 2 daily injections). The remaining portion of the TDD is then divided and administered before or at mealtimes (depending on the formulation) as a rapid-acting (eg, insulin aspart) or short-acting form of insulin. Some patients may benefit from the use of CSII which delivers rapid-acting insulin (insulin aspart) as a continuous infusion throughout the day and as boluses at mealtimes via an external pump device.

Division of daily insulin requirement ("intensive therapy"): Basal insulin delivery with 1 or 2 doses of intermediate- or long-acting insulin formulations superimposed with doses of short- or rapid-acting insulin (eg, insulin aspart) formulations 3 or more times daily.

Adjustment of dose: Dosage must be titrated to achieve glucose control and avoid hypoglycemia. Adjust dose to maintain premeal and bedtime glucose in target range. Since combinations of agents are frequently used, dosage adjustment must address the individual component of the insulin regimen which most directly influences the blood glucose value in question, based on the known onset and duration of the insulin component. Treatment and monitoring regimens must be individualized. Also see Additional Information.

Continuous SubQ insulin infusion (insulin pump): A combination of a "basal" continuous insulin infusion rate with preprogrammed, premeal bolus doses that are patient controlled. When converting from multiple daily SubQ doses of maintenance insulin, it is advisable to reduce the basal rate to less than the equivalent of the total daily units of the longer acting insulin (eg, NPH); divide the total number of units by 24 to get the basal rate in units/hour. Do not include the total units of regular insulin or other rapid-acting insulin formulations in this calculation. The same premeal regular insulin dosage may be used.

Diabetes mellitus, type 2:

General considerations for insulin use in type 2 diabetes:

Timing of initiation: The goal of therapy is to achieve an HbA$_{1c}$ <7%. According to a position statement by the ADA and European Association for the Study of Diabetes (EASD), dual therapy (metformin + a second antihyperglycemic agent) is recommended in patients with type 2 diabetes who fail to achieve glycemic goals after ~3 months with lifestyle interventions and metformin monotherapy (unless contraindications to metformin exist). Preference is not given for adding insulin or a noninsulin agent as the second antihyperglycemic agent (drug choice should be individualized based on patient characteristics). However, insulin should be considered as part of a combination regimen when hyperglycemia is severe, particularly if patient is symptomatic or has catabolic features (eg, weight loss, ketosis). If insulin is selected, the addition of **basal** insulin with a long-acting insulin (ie, glargine or detemir [*not* insulin regular]) is recommended. If HbA$_{1c}$ target not achieved after ~3 months of dual therapy, may proceed to triple therapy (Inzucchi 2015).

Intensification of therapy: If HbA$_{1c}$ target has not been met, despite titrating basal insulin (ie, long-acting insulin) to provide acceptable fasting blood glucose concentrations, intensification of therapy should be considered to cover postprandial glucose excursions. Options include: adding a mealtime insulin (1 to 3 injections of a rapid-acting insulin analog [lispro, aspart, glulisine]) or adding a GLP-1 receptor agonist (eg, exenatide, liraglutide). Alternatively, although less studied, may transition from basal insulin (ie, long-acting insulin) to a twice daily premixed (or biphasic) insulin analog (70/30 aspart mix, 75/25 or 50/50 lispro mix) (Inzucchi 2015).

In the setting of glucose toxicity (loss of beta-cell sensitivity to glucose concentrations), insulin therapy may be used for short-term management to restore sensitivity of beta-cells; in these cases, the dose may need to be rapidly reduced/withdrawn when sensitivity is re-established.

Cadaveric organ recovery (hormonal resuscitation) (off-label use): IV: Continuous infusion of 1 unit/hour (minimum dose) to maintain blood glucose of 120 to 180 mg/dL **or** 20 units as a bolus dose (after an IV bolus of dextrose 25 g) administered to the brain-dead donor who is hemodynamically unstable requiring significant vasopressor support; give concomitantly with levothyroxine or liothyronine (preferred), vasopressin, and methylprednisolone (Rosendale 2003a; Rosendale 2003b; Rosengard 2002; Salim 2007; Zaroff 2002).

Diabetic ketoacidosis (DKA) (off-label use): Only IV regular insulin should be used for severe DKA (Kitabchi 2009). Treatment should continue until reversal of acid-base derangement/ketonemia. Serum glucose is not a direct indicator of these abnormalities, and may decrease more rapidly than correction of the metabolic abnormalities. Also, refer to institution-specific protocols where appropriate.

Adults <20 years (Kitabchi 2004):

IV infusion: 0.1 units/kg/hour

Adjustment: If serum glucose does not fall by 50 mg/dL in the first hour, check hydration status; if acceptable, double insulin dose hourly until glucose levels fall at rate of 50 to 75 mg/dL per hour. Once serum glucose reaches 250 mg/dL, decrease dose to 0.05 to 0.1 units/kg/hour; dextrose-containing IV fluids should be administered to maintain serum glucose between 150 to 250 mg/dL until the acidosis clears. After resolution of DKA, supplement IV insulin with SubQ insulin as needed until the patient is able to eat and transition fully to a SubQ insulin regimen. An overlap of ~1 to 2 hours between discontinuation of IV insulin and administration of SubQ insulin is recommended to ensure adequate plasma insulin levels.

SubQ, IM (**Note:** Only use the SubQ and IM route if IV infusion access is unavailable): 0.1 to 0.3 units/kg SubQ bolus, followed by 0.1 units/kg given every hour SubQ or IM or 0.15 to 0.2 units/kg every 2 hours SubQ; continue until acidosis clears, then decrease to 0.05 units/kg given every hour until SubQ replacement dosing can be initiated (Kitabchi 2004; Wolfsdorf 2007)

Adults ≥20 years (Kitabchi 2009):

IV:

Bolus: 0.1 units/kg (optional)

Infusion: 0.1 to 0.14 units/kg/hour. **Note:** If no IV bolus was administered, patients should receive a continuous infusion of 0.14 units/kg/hour; lower doses may not achieve adequate insulin concentrations to suppress hepatic ketone body production.

Adjustment: If serum glucose does not fall by at least 10% in the first hour, give an IV bolus of 0.14 units/kg and continue previous regimen. In addition, if serum glucose does not fall by 50 to 70 mg/dL in the first hour, the insulin infusion dose should be increased hourly until a steady glucose decline is achieved Once serum glucose reaches 200 mg/dL, decrease infusion dose to 0.02 to 0.05 units/kg/hour or switch to SubQ rapid-acting insulin (eg, aspart, lispro) at 0.1 units/kg every 2 hours; dextrose-containing IV fluids should be administered to maintain serum glucose between 150 to 250 mg/dL until the acidosis clears. After resolution of DKA, supplement IV insulin with SubQ insulin as needed until the patient is able to eat and transition fully to a SubQ insulin regimen. An overlap of ~1 to 2 hours between discontinuation of IV insulin and administration of SubQ insulin is recommended to ensure adequate plasma insulin levels.

SubQ, IM: The following dosing regimen from the 2004 ADA position statement recommends regular insulin (Kitabchi 2004):

Bolus: 0.4 units/kg; **Note:** Give half of the dose (0.2 units/kg) as an IV bolus and half of the dose (0.2 units/kg) as SubQ or IM

Intermittent: 0.1 units/kg given every hour SubQ or IM

Adjustment: If serum glucose does not fall by 50 to 70 mg/dL in the first hour, administer 10 units hourly by IV bolus until glucose levels fall at a rate of 50 to 70 mg/dL per hour. Once serum glucose reaches 250 mg/dL, decrease dose to 5 to 10 units SubQ every 2 hours; dextrose-containing IV fluids should be administered to maintain serum glucose between 150 to 250 mg/dL until the acidosis clears.

Gestational diabetes mellitus (off-label use): SubQ: Insulin therapy should be considered when medical nutrition therapy has not achieved GDM glycemic goals (fasting plasma glucose: <95 mg/dL; 1-hour postprandial levels: <130 to 140 mg/dL; 2-hour postprandial levels: <120 mg/dL); dose and timing of administration should be based on frequent monitoring of plasma glucose levels (ACOG 2001; ADA 2004). Human insulin may be preferred (ADA 2004); however, rapid-acting insulin analogues may also be considered (ACOG 2001).

Hyperglycemia, critically ill (off-label use): Adults: IV continuous infusion: Insulin therapy should be implemented when blood glucose ≥150 mg/dL with a goal to maintain blood glucose <150 mg/dL (with values absolutely <180 mg/dL) using a protocol that achieves a low rate of hypoglycemia (ie, ≤70 mg/dL). Alternatively, other rapid acting insulin analogues (eg, insulin aspart or insulin glulisine) may also be used as a continuous infusion to maintain glycemic control (in place of regular insulin). Before discontinuation, stable ICU patients should be transitioned to a protocol-driven basal/bolus insulin regimen, based on insulin infusion history and carbohydrate intake, to avoid loss of glycemic control. Subcutaneous insulin therapy may be considered for selected clinically stable ICU patients (Jacobi 2012). **Note:** The Surviving Sepsis Campaign guidelines recommend initiating insulin dosing in patients with severe sepsis when 2 consecutive blood glucose concentrations are >180 mg/dL and to target an upper blood glucose ≤180 mg/dL (Dellinger 2013).

Hyperkalemia, moderate-to-severe (off-label use): IV: 10 units regular insulin mixed with 25 g dextrose (50 mL D$_{50}$W) given over 15 to 30 minutes (ACLS 2010); alternatively, 50 mL D$_{50}$W over 5 minutes followed by 10 units regular insulin IV push over seconds may be administered in the setting of imminent cardiac arrest. In patients with ongoing cardiac arrest (eg, PEA with presumed hyperkalemia), administration of D$_{50}$W over <5 minutes is routine. Effects on potassium are temporary. As appropriate, consider methods of enhancing potassium removal/excretion.

Hyperosmolar hyperglycemic state (HHS) (off-label use): Only regular injectable insulin should be used. Infusion should continue until reversal of mental status changes and hyperosmolality. Serum glucose is not a direct indicator of these abnormalities, and may decrease more rapidly than correction of the metabolic abnormalities. Also, refer to institution-specific protocols where appropriate.

Adults <20 years (Kitabchi 2004):
IV:
Infusion: 0.1 units/kg/hour
Adjustment: If serum glucose does not fall by 50 mg/dL in the first hour, check hydration status; if acceptable, double insulin dose hourly until glucose levels fall at rate of 50 to 75 mg/dL per hour. Once serum glucose reaches 300 mg/dL, decrease dose to 0.05 to 0.1 units/kg/hour; dextrose-containing IV fluids should be administered to maintain serum glucose between 250 to 300 mg/dL until hyperosmolality clears and mental status returns to normal. After resolution of HHS, supplement IV insulin with SubQ insulin as needed until the patient is able to eat and transition fully to a SubQ insulin regimen. An overlap of ~1 to 2 hours between discontinuation of IV insulin and administration of SubQ insulin is recommended to ensure adequate plasma insulin levels.
SubQ, IM (**Note:** Only use the SubQ and IM route if IV infusion access is unavailable): 0.1 to 0.3 units/kg SubQ bolus, followed by 0.1 units/kg given every hour SubQ or IM or 0.15 to 0.2 units/kg every 2 hours SubQ; continue until resolution of hyperosmolality, then decrease to 0.05 units/kg given every hour until SubQ replacement dosing can be initiated (Kitabchi 2004; Wolfsdorf 2007)

Adults ≥20 years (Kitabchi 2009):
IV:
Bolus: 0.1 units/kg bolus (optional)

Infusion: 0.1 to 0.14 units/kg/hour. **Note:** If no IV bolus was administered, patients should receive a continuous infusion of 0.14 units/kg/hour.
Adjustment: If serum glucose does not fall by at least 10% in the first hour, give an IV bolus of 0.14 units/kg and continue previous regimen. In addition, if serum glucose does not fall by 50 to 70 mg/dL in the first hour, the insulin infusion dose should be increased hourly until a steady glucose decline is achieved. Once serum glucose reaches 300 mg/dL, decrease dose to 0.02 to 0.05 units/kg/hour; dextrose-containing IV fluids should be administered to maintain serum glucose between 200 to 300 mg/dL until the patient is mentally alert. After resolution of HHS, supplement IV insulin with SubQ insulin as needed until the patient is able to eat and transition fully to a SubQ insulin regimen. An overlap of ~1 to 2 hours between discontinuation of IV insulin and administration of SubQ insulin is recommended to ensure adequate plasma insulin levels.

Pediatric

Diabetes mellitus: SubQ: Refer to adult dosing.

Diabetic ketoacidosis (DKA) (off-label use): Only IV regular insulin should be used for severe DKA; use of SubQ rapid-acting insulin analogs (eg, aspart, lispro) may be appropriate for mild-moderate DKA (Kitabchi 2009). Treatment should continue until reversal of acid-base derangement/ketonemia. Serum glucose is not a direct indicator of these abnormalities, and may decrease more rapidly than correction of the metabolic abnormalities. Also, refer to institution-specific protocols where appropriate.
IV: (Kitabchi 2004):
Infusion: 0.1 units/kg/hour
Adjustment: If serum glucose does not fall by 50 mg/dL in the first hour, check hydration status; if acceptable, double insulin dose hourly until glucose levels fall at rate of 50 to 75 mg/dL per hour. Once serum glucose reaches 250 mg/dL, decrease dose to 0.05 to 0.1 units/kg/hour; dextrose-containing IV fluids should be administered to maintain serum glucose between 150 to 250 mg/dL until the acidosis clears. After resolution of DKA, supplement IV insulin with SubQ insulin as needed until the patient is able to eat and transition fully to a SubQ insulin regimen. An overlap of ~1 to 2 hours between discontinuation of IV insulin and administration of SubQ insulin is recommended to ensure adequate plasma insulin levels.
SubQ, IM (**Note:** Only use the SubQ and IM route if IV infusion access is unavailable): 0.1 to 0.3 units/kg SubQ bolus, followed by 0.1 units/kg given every hour SubQ or IM or 0.15 to 0.2 units/kg every 2 hours SubQ; continue until acidosis clears, then decrease to 0.05 units/kg given every hour until SubQ replacement dosing can be initiated (Kitabchi 2004; Wolfsdorf 2007)

Hyperkalemia, moderate-to-severe (off-label use): IV: 0.1 units/kg regular insulin with dextrose 400 mg/kg infused over 15 to 30 minutes; ratio of ~1 unit of insulin to every 4 g of dextrose (Hegenbarth 2008). **Note:** Dextrose monotherapy may be sufficient to correct hyperkalemia.

Hyperosmolar hyperglycemic state (HHS) (off-label use): Only regular injectable insulin should be used. Infusion should continue until reversal of mental status changes and hyperosmolality. Serum glucose is not a direct indicator of these abnormalities, and may decrease more rapidly than correction of the metabolic abnormalities. Also, refer to institution-specific protocols where appropriate.
IV (Kitabchi 2004):
Infusion: 0.1 units/kg/hour
Adjustment: If serum glucose does not fall by 50 mg/dL in the first hour, check hydration status; if acceptable, double insulin dose hourly until glucose levels fall at rate of 50 to 75 mg/dL per hour. Once serum glucose reaches 300 mg/dL, decrease dose to 0.05 to 0.1 units/kg/hour; dextrose-containing IV fluids should be administered to maintain serum glucose between 250 to 300 mg/dL until hyperosmolality clears and mental status returns to normal. After resolution of HHS, supplement IV insulin with SubQ insulin as needed until the patient is able to eat and transition fully to a SubQ insulin regimen. An overlap of ~1 to 2 hours between discontinuation of IV insulin and administration of SubQ insulin is recommended to ensure adequate plasma insulin levels.

SubQ, IM (**Note:** Only use the SubQ and IM route if IV infusion access is unavailable): 0.1 to 0.3 units/kg SubQ bolus, followed by 0.1 units/kg given every hour SubQ or IM or 0.15 to 0.2 units/kg every 2 hours SubQ; continue until resolution of hyperosmolality, then decrease to 0.05 units/kg given every hour until SubQ replacement dosing can be initiated (Kitabchi 2004; Wolfsdorf 2007)

Renal Impairment Note: Insulin requirements are reduced due to changes in insulin clearance or metabolism. Close monitoring of blood glucose and adjustment of therapy may be required in renal impairment.

SubQ, IV:

CrCl 10 to 50 mL/minute: Administer at 75% of normal dose and monitor glucose closely

CrCl <10 mL/minute: Administer at 25% to 50% of normal dose and monitor glucose closely

Hemodialysis: Because of a large molecular weight (6000 daltons), insulin is not significantly removed by hemodialysis; supplemental dose is not necessary

Peritoneal dialysis: Because of a large molecular weight (6000 daltons), insulin is not significantly removed by peritoneal dialysis; supplemental dose is not necessary

Continuous renal replacement therapy: Administer 75% of normal dose and monitor glucose closely; supplemental dose is not necessary

Hepatic Impairment Note: Insulin requirements may be reduced. Close monitoring of blood glucose and adjustment of therapy may be required in hepatic impairment.

Dietary Considerations Individualized medical nutrition therapy (MNT) based on ADA recommendations is an integral part of therapy.

Usual Infusion Concentrations: Pediatric IV infusion: 0.1 unit/mL, 0.5 unit/mL, or 1 unit/mL

Usual Infusion Concentrations: Adult IV infusion: 100 units in 100 mL (concentration: 1 unit/mL) of NS

Administration

SubQ administration: Do not use if solution is viscous or cloudy; use only if clear and colorless. Regular insulin should be administered within 30 to 60 minutes before a meal. Cold injections should be avoided. SubQ administration is usually made into the thighs, arms, buttocks, or abdomen; rotate injection sites. When mixing regular insulin with other preparations of insulin, regular insulin should be drawn into syringe first. Regular insulin is not recommended for use in external SubQ insulin infusion pump.

IM administration: Do not use if solution is viscous or cloudy; use only if clear and colorless. May be administered IM in selected clinical situations; close monitoring of blood glucose and serum potassium as well as medical supervision is required.

IV administration: Do not use if solution is viscous or cloudy; use only if clear and colorless. May be administered IV with close monitoring of blood glucose and serum potassium; appropriate medical supervision is required. If possible, avoid IV bolus administration in pediatric patients with DKA; may increase risk of cerebral edema. **Do not administer mixtures of insulin formulations intravenously.** IV administration of U-500 regular insulin is not recommended.

IV infusions: To minimize insulin adsorption to IV tubing: Flush the IV tubing with a priming infusion of 20 mL from the insulin infusion, whenever a new IV tubing set is added to the insulin infusion container (Jacobi 2012; Thompson 2012).

Note: Also refer to institution-specific protocols where appropriate.

If insulin is required prior to the availability of the insulin drip, regular insulin should be administered by IV push injection.

Because of insulin adsorption to IV tubing or infusion bags, the actual amount of insulin being administered via IV infusion could be substantially less than the apparent amount. Therefore, adjustment of the IV infusion rate should be based on effect and not solely on the apparent insulin dose. The apparent dose may be used as a starting point for determining the subsequent SubQ dosing regimen (Moghissi 2009); however, the transition to SubQ administration requires continuous medical supervision, frequent monitoring of blood glucose, and careful adjustment of therapy. In addition, SubQ insulin should be given 1 to 4 hours prior to the discontinuation of IV insulin to prevent hyperglycemia (Moghissi 2009).

Monitoring Parameters

Critically-ill patients receiving insulin infusion: Blood glucose every 1 to 2 hours. **Note:** Every 4 hour blood glucose monitoring is not recommended unless a low hypoglycemia rate is demonstrated with the insulin protocol used. Arterial or venous whole blood sampling is

recommended for patients in shock, on vasopressor therapy, or with severe edema, and when on a prolonged insulin infusion (Jacobi 2012).

Diabetes mellitus: Plasma glucose, electrolytes, HbA$_{1c}$

DKA/HHS: Serum electrolytes, glucose, BUN, creatinine, osmolality, venous pH (repeat arterial blood gases are generally unnecessary), anion gap, urine output, urinalysis, mental status

Hyperkalemia: Serum potassium and glucose must be closely monitored to avoid hypokalemia, rebound hyperkalemia, and hypoglycemia.

Reference Range

Therapeutic, serum insulin (fasting): 5 to 20 microunits/mL (SI: 35 to 145 pmol/L)

Glucose, fasting:

Newborns: 60 to 110 mg/dL

Adults: 60 to 110 mg/dL

Elderly: 100 to 180 mg/dL

Recommendations for glycemic control in nonpregnant adults with diabetes (ADA 2015):

HbA$_{1c}$: <7% (a more aggressive [<6.5%] or less aggressive [<8%] HbA$_{1c}$ goal may be targeted based on patient-specific characteristics)

Preprandial capillary plasma glucose: 80 to 130 mg/dL

Peak postprandial capillary blood glucose: <180 mg/dL

Recommendations for glycemic control in pediatric (all age groups) patients with type 1 diabetes (ADA 2015):

HbA$_{1c}$: <7.5% (individualization may be appropriate based on patient-specific characteristics; <7% is reasonable if it can be achieved without excessive hypoglycemia)

Preprandial capillary plasma glucose: 90 to 130 mg/dL

Bedtime and overnight capillary blood glucose: 90 to 150 mg/dL

Additional Information

Split-mixed or basal-bolus regimens: Combination regimens which optimize differences in the onset and duration of different insulin products are commonly used to approximate physiologic secretion. In split-mixed regimens, an intermediate-acting insulin (eg, NPH insulin) is administered once or twice daily and supplemented by short-acting (regular) or rapid-acting (lispro, aspart, or glulisine) insulin. Blood glucose measurements are completed several times daily. Dosages are adjusted emphasizing the individual component of the regimen which most directly influences the blood sugar in question (either the intermediate-acting component or the shorter-acting component). Fixed-ratio formulations (eg, 70/30 mix) may be used as twice daily injections in this scenario; however, the ability to titrate the dosage of an individual component is limited. An example of a "split-mixed" regimen would be 21 units of NPH plus 9 units of regular insulin in the morning and an evening meal dose consisting of 14 units of NPH plus 6 units of regular insulin.

Basal-bolus regimens are designed to more closely mimic physiologic secretion. These regimens employ a long-acting insulin (eg, glargine) to simulate basal insulin secretion. The basal component is frequently administered at bedtime or in the early morning. This is supplemented by multiple daily injections of rapid-acting products (lispro, aspart, or glulisine) immediately prior to a meal, which provides insulin at the time when nutrients are absorbed. An example of a basal-bolus regimen would be 30 units of glargine at bedtime and 12 units of lispro insulin prior to each meal.

Estimation of the effect per unit: A "Rule of 1500" has been frequently used as a means to estimate the change in blood sugar relative to each unit of insulin administered. In fact, the recommended values used in these calculations may vary from 1500-2200 (a value of 1500 is generally recommended for regular insulin while 1800 is recommended for "rapid-acting insulins"). The higher values lead to more conservative estimates of the effect per unit of insulin, and therefore lead to more cautious adjustments. The effect per unit of insulin is approximated by dividing the selected numerical value (eg, 1500-2200) by the number of units/day received by the patient. This may be used as a crude approximation of the patient's insulin sensitivity as adjustments to individual components of the regimen are made. Each additional unit of insulin added to the corresponding insulin dose may be expected to lower the blood glucose by this amount.

To illustrate, in the "basal-bolus" regimen example presented above, the rule of 1800 would indicate an expected change of 27 mg/dL per unit of lispro insulin (the total daily insulin dose is 66 units; using the formula: 1800/66 = 27). A patient may be instructed to add additional insulin if the preprandial glucose is >125 mg/dL. For a prelunch glucose of 195 mg/dL, this would mean

the patient would administer the scheduled 12 units of lispro along with an additional "correctional" 3 units for a total of 15 units prior to the meal. If correctional doses are required on a consistent basis, an adjustment of the patients diet and/or scheduled insulin dose may be necessary.

Product Availability Humulin R U-500 KwikPen: FDA approved December 2015; anticipated availability is currently unknown. Information pertaining to this product within the monograph is pending revision.

Dosage Forms Excipient information presented when available (limited, particularly for generics); consult specific product labeling.

Solution, Injection:
HumuLIN R: 100 units/mL (3 mL, 10 mL) [contains metacresol, phenol]
NovoLIN R: 100 units/mL (10 mL) [contains metacresol]
NovoLIN R ReliOn: 100 units/mL (10 mL) [contains metacresol]
Solution, Subcutaneous:
HumuLIN R U-500 (CONCENTRATED): 500 units/mL (20 mL) [contains metacresol]

- ◆ **Insulin Regular and Insulin NPH** see Insulin NPH and Insulin Regular *on page 960*
- ◆ **Integrilin** see Eptifibatide *on page 661*
- ◆ **Intelence** see Etravirine *on page 719*
- ◆ **Intelence® (Can)** see Etravirine *on page 719*
- ◆ **α-2-interferon** see Interferon Alfa-2b *on page 966*
- ◆ **Interferon Alfa-2a (PEG Conjugate)** see Peginterferon Alfa-2a *on page 1409*
- ◆ **Interferon Alfa-2b (PEG Conjugate)** see Peginterferon Alfa-2b *on page 1411*

Interferon Alfa-2b (in ter FEER on AL fa too bee)

Brand Names: US Intron A
Brand Names: Canada Intron A
Index Terms INF-alpha 2; Interferon Alpha-2b; rLFN-α2; α-2-interferon
Pharmacologic Category Antineoplastic Agent, Biological Response Modulator; Biological Response Modulator; Immunomodulator, Systemic; Interferon

Use

AIDS-related Kaposi sarcoma: Treatment of patients 18 years and older with AIDS-related Kaposi sarcoma

Chronic hepatitis B: Treatment of chronic hepatitis B in patients 1 year and older with compensated liver disease

Chronic hepatitis C: Treatment of chronic hepatitis C in patients 18 years and older with compensated liver disease who have a history of blood or blood-product exposure and/or are hepatitis C virus (HCV) antibody-positive; in combination with ribavirin for treatment of chronic hepatitis C in patients 3 years and older with compensated liver disease previously untreated with alpha interferon therapy and in patients 18 years and older who have relapsed following alpha interferon therapy

Condylomata acuminata: Treatment of patients 18 years and older with condylomata acuminata involving external surfaces of the genital and perianal areas

Follicular lymphoma: Initial treatment of clinically aggressive follicular non-Hodgkin lymphoma in conjunction with anthracycline-containing combination chemotherapy in patients 18 years and older

Hairy cell leukemia: Treatment of patients 18 years and older with hairy cell leukemia

Malignant melanoma: Adjuvant to surgical treatment in patients 18 years and older with malignant melanoma who are free of disease but at high risk for systemic recurrence, within 56 days of surgery

Pregnancy Considerations Animal reproduction studies have demonstrated abortifacient effects. Disruption of the normal menstrual cycle was also observed in animal studies; therefore, the manufacturer recommends that reliable contraception is used in women of childbearing potential. Alfa interferon is endogenous to normal amniotic fluid. *In vitro* administration studies have reported that when administered to the mother, it does not cross the placenta. Case reports of use in pregnant women are limited. The Perinatal HIV Guidelines Working Group does not recommend that interferon-alfa be used during pregnancy. Interferon alfa-2b monotherapy should only be used in pregnancy when the potential benefit to the mother justifies the possible risk to the fetus. Combination therapy with ribavirin is contraindicated in pregnancy (refer to Ribavirin monograph); two forms of contraception should be used during combination therapy and patients should have monthly pregnancy tests. A pregnancy registry has

been established for women inadvertently exposed to ribavirin while pregnant (800-593-2214).

Breast-Feeding Considerations Breast milk samples obtained from a lactating mother prior to and after administration of interferon alfa-2b showed that interferon alfa is present in breast milk and administration of the medication did not significantly affect endogenous levels. Breast-feeding is not linked to the spread of hepatitis C virus; however, if nipples are cracked or bleeding, breast-feeding is not recommended. Mothers coinfected with HIV are discouraged from breast-feeding to decrease potential transmission of HIV.

Medication Guide Available Yes

Contraindications

Hypersensitivity to interferon alfa or any component of the formulation; decompensated liver disease; autoimmune hepatitis

Combination therapy with interferon alfa-2b and ribavirin is also contraindicated in women who are pregnant, in males with pregnant partners; in patients with hemoglobinopathies (eg, thalassemia major, sickle-cell anemia); creatinine clearance <50 mL/minute; or hypersensitivity to ribavirin or any component of the formulation

Documentation of allergenic cross-reactivity for interferons is limited. However, because of similarities in chemical structure and/or pharmacologic actions, the possibility of cross-sensitivity cannot be ruled out with certainty.

Warnings/Precautions [US Boxed Warning]: May cause or aggravate fatal or life-threatening autoimmune disorders, neuropsychiatric symptoms (including depression and/or suicidal thoughts/behaviors), ischemic, and/or infectious disorders; monitor closely with clinical and laboratory evaluations (periodic); discontinue treatment for severe persistent or worsening symptoms; some cases may resolve with discontinuation.

Neuropsychiatric disorders: May cause neuropsychiatric events, including depression, psychosis, mania, suicidal behavior/ideation, attempts and completed suicides and homicidal ideation; may occur in patients with or without previous psychiatric symptoms. Effects are usually rapidly reversible upon therapy discontinuation, but have persisted up to three weeks. If psychiatric symptoms persist or worsen, or suicidal or homicidal ideation or aggressive behavior towards others is identified, discontinue treatment, and follow the patient closely. Careful neuropsychiatric monitoring is recommended during and for 6 months after treatment in patients who develop psychiatric disorders (including clinical depression). New or exacerbated neuropsychiatric or substance abuse disorders are best managed with early intervention. Use with caution in patients with a history of psychiatric disorders. Drug screening and periodic health evaluation (including monitoring of psychiatric symptoms) is recommended if initiating treatment in patients with coexisting psychiatric condition or substance abuse disorders. Suicidal ideation or attempts may occur more frequently in pediatric patients (eg, adolescents) when compared to adults. Higher doses, usually in elderly patients, may result in increased CNS toxicity (eg, obtundation and coma).

Hepatic disease: May cause hepatotoxicity; monitor closely if abnormal liver function tests develop. A transient increase in ALT (≥2 times baseline) may occur in patients treated with interferon alfa-2b for chronic hepatitis B. Therapy generally may continue; monitor. Worsening and potentially fatal liver disease, including jaundice, hepatic encephalopathy, and hepatic failure have been reported in patients receiving interferon alfa for chronic hepatitis B and C with decompensated liver disease, autoimmune hepatitis, history of autoimmune disease, and immunosuppressed transplant recipients; avoid use in these patients; use is contraindicated in decompensated liver disease. Patients with cirrhosis are at increased risk of hepatic decompensation. Therapy should be discontinued for any patient developing signs and symptoms of liver failure. Permanently discontinue for severe (grade 3) hepatic injury or hepatic decompensation (Child-Pugh class B and C [score >6]). Chronic hepatitis B or C patients with a history of autoimmune disease or who are immunosuppressed transplant recipients should not receive interferon alfa-2b.

Bone marrow suppression: Causes bone marrow suppression, including potentially severe cytopenias, and very rarely, aplastic anemia. Discontinue treatment for severe neutropenia (ANC <500/mm³) or thrombocytopenia (platelets <25,000/mm³). Hemolytic anemia (hemoglobin <10 g/dL) was observed when combined with ribavirin; anemia occurred within 1 to 2 weeks of initiation of therapy. Use caution in patients with preexisting myelosuppression and in patients with concomitant medications which cause myelosuppression.

Autoimmune disorders: Avoid use in patients with history of autoimmune disorders; development of autoimmune disorders (thrombocytopenia, vasculitis, Raynaud's disease, rheumatoid arthritis, lupus erythematosus and rhabdomyolysis) has been associated with use. Monitor closely; consider discontinuing. Worsening of psoriasis and sarcoidosis (and the development of new sarcoidosis) have been reported; use extreme caution.

Cardiovascular disease/coagulation disorders: Use caution and monitor closely in patients with cardiovascular disease (ischemic or thromboembolic), arrhythmias, hypertension, and in patients with a history of MI or prior therapy with cardiotoxic drugs. Patients with preexisting cardiac disease and/or advanced cancer should have baseline and periodic ECGs. May cause hypotension (during administration or delayed up to 2 days), arrhythmia, tachycardia (≥150 bpm), cardiomyopathy (~2% in AIDS-related Kaposi Sarcoma patients), and/or MI. Some experiencing cardiovascular adverse effects had no prior history of cardiac disease. Supraventricular arrhythmias occur rarely, and are associated with preexisting cardiac disease or prior therapy with cardiotoxic agents. Dose modification, discontinuation, and/or additional therapies may be necessary. Hemorrhagic cerebrovascular events have been observed with therapy. Use caution in patients with coagulation disorders.

Endocrine disorders: Thyroid disorders (possibly reversible) have been reported; use caution in patients with preexisting thyroid disease. TSH levels should be within normal limits prior to initiating interferon. Treatment should not be initiated in patients with preexisting thyroid disease who cannot be maintained in normal ranges by medication. Discontinue interferon use in patients who develop thyroid abnormalities during treatment and in patients with thyroid disease who subsequently cannot maintain normal ranges with thyroid medication. Discontinuation of interferon therapy may or may not reverse thyroid dysfunction. Diabetes mellitus has been reported; discontinue if cannot effectively manage with medication. Use with caution in patients with a history of diabetes mellitus, particularly if prone to DKA. Hypertriglyceridemia has been reported; discontinue if persistent and severe, and/or combined with symptoms of pancreatitis.

Pulmonary disease: Dyspnea, pulmonary infiltrates, pulmonary hypertension, interstitial pneumonitis, pneumonia, bronchiolitis obliterans, and sarcoidosis may be induced or aggravated by treatment, sometimes resulting in respiratory failure or fatality. Has been reported more in patients being treated for chronic hepatitis C, although has also occurred with use for oncology indications. Patients with fever, cough, dyspnea or other respiratory symptoms should be evaluated with a chest x-ray; monitor closely and consider discontinuing treatment with evidence of impaired pulmonary function. Use with caution in patients with a history of pulmonary disease.

Ophthalmic disorders: Decreased or loss of vision, macular edema, optic neuritis, retinal hemorrhages, cotton wool spots, papilledema, retinal detachment (serous), and retinal artery or vein thrombosis have occurred (or been aggravated) in patients receiving alpha interferons. Use caution in patients with preexisting eye disorders; monitor closely; a complete eye exam should be done promptly in patients who develop ocular symptoms; discontinue with new or worsening ophthalmic disorders.

Dental and periodontic disorders: In patients receiving combination interferon and ribavirin therapy, dental and periodontal disorders have been reported; additionally, dry mouth can damage teeth and mouth mucous membranes during chronic therapy.

Commonly associated with fever and flu-like symptoms; rule out other causes/infection with persistent fever; use with caution in patients with debilitating conditions. Acute hypersensitivity reactions (eg, urticaria, angioedema, bronchoconstriction, anaphylaxis) have been reported (rarely) with alfa interferons. If an acute reaction develops, discontinue therapy immediately; transient rashes have occurred in some patients following injection, but have not necessitated treatment interruption. Do not treat patients with visceral AIDS-related Kaposi sarcoma associated with rapidly-progressing or life-threatening disease. Some formulations contain albumin, which may carry a remote risk of viral transmission. Due to differences in dosage, patients should not change brands of interferons without the concurrence of their healthcare provider. Combination therapy with ribavirin is associated with birth defects and/or fetal mortality and hemolytic anemia. Do not use combination therapy with ribavirin in patients with CrCl <50 mL/minute. Interferon alfa-2b at doses ≥10 million units/m^2 is associated with a moderate emetic

potential; antiemetics may be recommended to prevent nausea and vomiting. Potentially significant drug-drug interactions may exist, requiring dose or frequency adjustment, additional monitoring, and/or selection of alternative therapy.

Some dosage forms may contain polysorbate 80 (also known as Tweens). Hypersensitivity reactions, usually a delayed reaction, have been reported following exposure to pharmaceutical products containing polysorbate 80 in certain individuals (Isaksson, 2002; Lucente 2000; Shelley 1995). Thrombocytopenia, ascites, pulmonary deterioration, and renal and hepatic failure have been reported in premature neonates after receiving parenteral products containing polysorbate 80 (Alade 1986; CDC 1984). See manufacturer's labeling.

Adverse Reactions Note: In a majority of patients, a flu-like symptom (fever, chills, tachycardia, malaise, myalgia, headache), occurs within 1-2 hours of administration; may last up to 24 hours and may be dose limiting.

>10%:
Cardiovascular: Chest pain (≤28%)
Central nervous system: Fatigue (8% to 96%), headache (21% to 62%), chills (≤54%), rigors (≤42%), depression (3% to 40%; grades 3/4: 2%), drowsiness (≤33%), dizziness (≤24%), irritability (≤22%), paresthesia (1% to 21%), pain (≤18%), right upper quadrant pain (≤15%), amnesia (≤14%), lack of concentration (≤14%), malaise (≤14%), confusion (≤12%), insomnia (≤12%)
Dermatologic: Alopecia (≤38%), skin rash (≤25%), diaphoresis (1% to 21%), pruritus (≤11%)
Endocrine & metabolic: Weight loss (<1% to 13%), amenorrhea (≤12%)
Gastrointestinal: Anorexia (1% to 69%), nausea, (17% to 66%), diarrhea (2% to 45%), vomiting (children 27%; adults 2% to 32%), xerostomia (≤28%), dysgeusia (≤24%), abdominal pain (1% to 23%), constipation (≤14%), gingivitis (≤14%)
Hematologic & oncologic: Neutropenia (≤92%; grade 4: 1% to 4%), leukopenia (≤68%), anemia (≤32%), thrombocytopenia (≤15%)
Hepatic: Increased serum AST (≤63%; grades 3/4: 14%), increased serum ALT (≤15%), increased serum alkaline phosphatase (≤13%)
Infection: Candidiasis (≤17%)
Local: Injection site reaction (≤20%)
Neuromuscular & skeletal: Myalgia (28% to 75%), weakness (≤63%), skeletal pain (≤21%), arthralgia (≤19%), back pain (≤19%)
Renal: Increased blood urea nitrogen (≤12%)
Respiratory: Flu-like symptoms (≤79%), dyspnea (≤34%), cough (≤31%), pharyngitis (≤31%), sinusitis (≤21%)
Miscellaneous: Fever (34% to 94%; more common in children)
5% to 10%:
Cardiovascular: Edema (≤10%), hypertension (≤9%)
Central nervous system: Hypoesthesia (≤10%), anxiety (≤9%), vertigo (≤8%), agitation (≤7%)
Dermatologic: Xeroderma (≤10%), dermatitis (≤8%)
Endocrine & metabolic: Decreased libido (≤5%)
Gastrointestinal: Loose stools (≤10%), dyspepsia (≤8%)
Genitourinary: Urinary tract infection (≤5%)
Hematologic & oncologic: Purpura (≤5%)
Infection: Infection (≤7%), herpes virus infection (≤5%)
Renal: Polyuria (≤10%), increased serum creatinine (≤6%)
Respiratory: Bronchitis (≤10%), nasal congestion (≤10%), epistaxis (≤7%)
<5% (Limited to important or life-threatening): Abnormal hepatic function tests, aggressive behavior, albuminuria, alcohol intolerance, amyotrophy, anaphylaxis, angina pectoris, angioedema, aphasia, aplastic anemia (rarely), ascites, asthma, atrial fibrillation, Bell's palsy, bradycardia, bronchiolitis obliterans, bronchoconstriction, bronchospasm, cardiac arrhythmia, cardiac failure, cardiomegaly, cardiomyopathy, cellulitis, cerebrovascular accident, colitis, coma, conjunctivitis, coronary artery disease, cyanosis, cystitis, dehydration, diabetes mellitus, dysphasia, dysuria, eczema, epidermal cyst, erythema, erythema multiforme, erythematous rash, exacerbation of psoriasis, exacerbation of sarcoidosis, extrapyramidal reaction, extrasystoles, gastrointestinal hemorrhage, granulocytopenia, hallucination, hearing loss, heart valve disease, hematuria, hemolytic anemia, hemoptysis, hepatic encephalopathy, hepatic failure, hepatitis, hepatotoxicity, hot flash, homicidal ideation, hyperbilirubinemia, hypercalcemia, hyperglycemia, hypermenorrhea, hypersensitivity reaction (acute), hypertriglyceridemia, hyperthyroidism, hypochromic anemia, hypotension, hypothermia, hypothyroidism, hypoventilation, immune thrombocytopenia, impotence, increased

lactate dehydrogenase, interstitial pneumonitis, jaundice, leukorrhea, lupus erythematosus, lymphadenitis, lympha-denopathy, lymphocytopenia, lymphocytosis, macular edema, maculopapular rash, migraine, myocardial infarc-tion, myositis, nephrotic syndrome, neuralgia, neuropa-thy, nystagmus, optic neuritis, palpitations, pancreatitis, pancytopenia, papilledema, paranoia, peripheral ische-mia, peripheral neuropathy, photophobia, pituitary insuffi-ciency, pleural effusion, pneumonia, psychoneurosis, pneumothorax, proteinuria, psychosis, pulmonary embo-lism, pulmonary fibrosis, pulmonary hypertension, pulmo-nary infiltrates, pure red cell aplasia, Raynaud's phenomenon, reduced ejection fraction, renal failure, renal insufficiency, respiratory insufficiency, retinal detachment (serous), retinal thrombosis, retinal cotton-wool spot, retinal vein occlusion, rhabdomyolysis, seiz-ure, sepsis, sexual disorder, skin photosensitivity, Ste-vens-Johnson syndrome, stomatitis, suicidal ideation, syncope, systemic lupus erythematosus, tachycardia, tendonitis, tissue necrosis at injection site, thrombotic thrombocytopenic purpura, thrombosis, toxic epidermal necrolysis, upper respiratory tract infection, urinary incon-tinence, urticaria, uterine hemorrhage, vasculitis, Vogt-Koyanagi-Harada syndrome, wheezing

Drug Interactions

Metabolism/Transport Effects Inhibits CYP1A2 (weak)

Avoid Concomitant Use
Avoid concomitant use of Interferon Alfa-2b with any of the following: BCG (Intravesical); Deferiprone; Dipyrone; Telbivudine

Increased Effect/Toxicity
Interferon Alfa-2b may increase the levels/effects of: Aldesleukin; CloZAPine; Deferiprone; Methadone; Riba-virin (Oral Inhalation); Ribavirin (Systemic); Telbivudine; Theophylline Derivatives; TiZANidine; Zidovudine

The levels/effects of Interferon Alfa-2b may be increased by: Dipyrone

Decreased Effect
Interferon Alfa-2b may decrease the levels/effects of: BCG (Intravesical)

Preparation for Administration Powder for injection: The manufacturer recommends reconstituting vial with the diluent provided (SWFI). When reconstituted with SWFI 1 mL, the 10 million unit vial concentration is 10 million units/mL, the 18 million unit vial concentration is 18 million units/mL, and the 50 million unit vial concentration is 50 million units/mL. Swirl gently. To prepare solution for infusion, further dilute appropriate dose in NS 100 mL. Final concentration should be ≥10 million units/100 mL.

Storage/Stability Store intact vials under refrigeration at 2°C to 8°C (36°F to 46°F); do not freeze. After reconstitu-tion of powder for injection, product should be used imme-diately, but may be stored under refrigeration for ≤24 hours.

Mechanism of Action Binds to a specific receptor on the cell wall to initiate intracellular activity; multiple effects can be detected including induction of gene transcription. Inhibits cellular growth, alters the state of cellular differ-entiation, interferes with oncogene expression, alters cell surface antigen expression, increases phagocytic activity of macrophages, and augments cytotoxicity of lympho-cytes for target cells

Pharmacodynamics/Kinetics
Distribution: V_d: 31 L; but has been noted to be much greater (370-720 L) in leukemia patients receiving con-tinuous infusion IFN; IFN does not penetrate the CSF
Metabolism: Primarily renal, filtered and absorbed at the renal tubule
Bioavailability: IM: 83%; SubQ: 90%
Half-life elimination: IV: ~2 hours; IM, SubQ: ~2-3 hours
Time to peak, serum: IM, SubQ: ~3-12 hours; IV: By the end of a 30-minute infusion

Dosing
Adult & Geriatric Consider premedication with acetami-nophen prior to administration to reduce the incidence of some adverse reactions. Not all dosage forms and strengths are appropriate for all indications; refer to product labeling for details. Interferon alfa-2b at doses ≥10 million units/m² is associated with a moderate emetic potential; antiemetics may be recommended to prevent nausea and vomiting.
Hairy cell leukemia: IM, SubQ: 2 million units/m² 3 times weekly for up to 6 months (may continue treatment with sustained treatment response); discontinue for disease progression or failure to respond after 6 months
Lymphoma (follicular): SubQ: 5 million units 3 times weekly for up to 18 months

Malignant melanoma: Induction: 20 million units/m² IV for 5 consecutive days per week for 4 weeks, followed by maintenance dosing of 10 million units/m² SubQ 3 times weekly for 48 weeks
AIDS-related Kaposi sarcoma: IM, SubQ: 30 million units/m² 3 times weekly; continue until disease pro-gression or until maximal response has been achieved after 16 weeks
Chronic hepatitis B: IM, SubQ: 5 million units/ daily or 10 million units 3 times weekly for 16 weeks
Chronic hepatitis C: IM, SubQ: 3 million units 3 times weekly. In patients with normalization of ALT at 16 weeks, continue treatment (if tolerated) for 18-24 months; consider discontinuation if normalization does not occur at 16 weeks. **Note:** May be used in combina-tion therapy with ribavirin in previously untreated patients or in patients who relapse following alpha interferon therapy.
Condyloma acuminata: Intralesionally: 1 million units/ lesion (maximum: 5 lesions per treatment) 3 times weekly (on alternate days) for 3 weeks. May administer a second course at 12-16 weeks.
Pediatric Consider premedication with acetaminophen prior to administration to reduce the incidence of some adverse reactions. Not all dosage forms and strengths are appropriate for all indications; refer to product label-ing for details.

Note: The following dosing may also be used in **infants** in the setting of HIV-exposure/-infection (CDC 2009).
Chronic hepatitis B (including HIV coinfection): SubQ: Children and Adolescents 1 to 17 years: 3 million units/m² 3 times weekly for 1 week, followed by 6 million units/m² 3 times weekly (maximum: 10 million units per dose); total duration of therapy 16 to 24 weeks (treat for 24 weeks in HIV-exposure/-infection)
Chronic hepatitis C with HIV coinfection: IM, SubQ: Children and Adolescents 1 to 17 years: 3 to 5 million units/m² 3 times weekly (maximum: 3 million units per dose) with ribavirin for 48 weeks, regardless of HCV genotype (CDC 2009)
Renal Impairment
Renal impairment at treatment initiation: Combination therapy with ribavirin (hepatitis C) is contraindicated in patients with CrCl <50 mL/minute; use combination therapy with ribavirin (hepatitis C) with caution in patients with impaired renal function and CrCl ≥50 mL/minute.
Renal toxicity during treatment: *Indication-specific adjustments:* Lymphoma (follicular): Serum creatinine >2 mg/dL: Permanently discontinue.
Hepatic Impairment
Hepatic impairment at treatment initiation: There are no dosage adjustments provided in the manufacturer's labeling. Contraindicated in patients with decompen-sated liver disease or autoimmune hepatitis.
Hepatotoxicity during treatment: Permanently discon-tinue for severe (grade 3) hepatic injury or hepatic decompensation (Child-Pugh class B and C [score >6]). *Indication-specific adjustments:*
Lymphoma (follicular): AST >5 times ULN: Perma-nently discontinue.
Malignant melanoma (induction and maintenance):
ALT/AST >5 to 10 times ULN: Temporarily withhold; resume with a 50% dose reduction when adverse reaction abates
ALT/AST >10 times ULN: Permanently discontinue.

Adjustment for Toxicity
Hematologic toxicity (also refer to indication specified adjustments below): ANC <500/mm³ or platelets <25,000/mm³: Discontinue treatment.

Hypersensitivity reaction (acute, serious), ophthalmic dis-orders (new or worsening), thyroid abnormality develop-ment (which cannot be normalized with medication), signs or symptoms of liver failure: Discontinue treatment.

Liver function abnormality, pulmonary infiltrate develop-ment, evidence of pulmonary function impairment, or autoimmune disorder development, triglycerides >1,000 mg/dL: Monitor closely and discontinue if appro-priate. Permanently discontinue for severe (grade 3) hepatic injury or hepatic decompensation (Child-Pugh class B and C [score >6]).

Neuropsychiatric disorders (during treatment):
Clinical depression or other psychiatric problem: Mon-itor closely during and for 6 months after treatment.
Severe depression or other psychiatric disorder: Dis-continue treatment.

Persistent or worsening psychiatric symptoms, suicidal ideation, aggression towards others: Discontinue treatment and follow with appropriate psychiatric intervention.

Manufacturer-recommended adjustments, listed according to indication:

Lymphoma (follicular):

Neutrophils >1000/mm^3 to <1,500/mm^3: Reduce dose by 50%; may re-escalate to starting dose when neutrophils return to >1,500/mm^3

Severe toxicity (neutrophils <1000/mm^3 or platelets <50,000/mm^3): Temporarily withhold.

AST >5 times ULN or serum creatinine >2 mg/dL: Permanently discontinue.

Hairy cell leukemia:

Platelet count <50,000/mm^3: Do not administer intramuscularly (administer SubQ instead).

Severe toxicity: Reduce dose by 50% or temporarily withhold and resume with 50% dose reduction; permanently discontinue if persistent or recurrent severe toxicity is noted.

Chronic hepatitis B:

WBC <1,500/mm^3, granulocytes <750/mm^3, or platelet count <50,000/mm^3, or other laboratory abnormality or severe adverse reaction: Reduce dose by 50%; may re-escalate to starting dose upon resolution of hematologic toxicity. Discontinue for persistent intolerance.

WBC <1,000/mm^3, granulocytes <500/mm^3, or platelet count <25,000/mm^3: Permanently discontinue

Chronic hepatitis C: Severe toxicity: Reduce dose by 50% or temporarily withhold until subsides; permanently discontinue for persistent toxicities after dosage reduction.

AIDS-related Kaposi sarcoma: Severe toxicity: Reduce dose by 50% or temporarily withhold; may resume at reduced dose with toxicity resolution; permanently discontinue for persistent/recurrent toxicities.

Malignant melanoma (induction and maintenance):

Severe toxicity including neutrophils >250/mm^3 to <500/mm^3 or ALT/AST >5 to 10 times ULN: Temporarily withhold; resume with a 50% dose reduction when adverse reaction abates.

Neutrophils <250/mm^3, ALT/AST >10 times ULN, or severe/persistent adverse reactions: Permanently discontinue.

Administration Administer dose in the evening (if possible) to enhance tolerability. Not all dosage forms are recommended for all administration routes; refer to manufacturer's labeling. Interferon alfa-2b at doses ≥10 million units/m^2 is associated with a moderate emetic potential; antiemetics may be recommended to prevent nausea and vomiting.

IM: Rotate injection sites; preferred sites for injection are anterior thigh, deltoid, and superolateral buttock. Some patients may be appropriate for self-administration with appropriate training. Allow to reach room temperature prior to injection. In hairy cell leukemia treatment, if platelets are <50,000/mm^3, do not administer intramuscularly (administer SubQ instead).

IV: Infuse over ~20 minutes

SubQ: Suggested for those who are at risk for bleeding or are thrombocytopenic. Rotate SubQ injection site; preferred sites for injection are abdomen (except around the navel), anterior thigh, and outer upper arm. Patient should be well hydrated. Some patients may be appropriate for self-administration with appropriate training. Allow to reach room temperature prior to injection.

Intralesional: Inject at an angle nearly parallel to the plane of the skin, directing the needle to center of the base of the wart to infiltrate the lesion core and cause a small wheal. Only infiltrate the keratinized layer; avoid administration which is too deep or shallow. Allow to reach room temperature prior to injection.

Monitoring Parameters

General monitoring parameters for *all indications*:

At baseline (repeat during therapy if clinically indicated): Chest x-ray, serum creatinine, albumin, prothrombin time, triglycerides.

At baseline and periodically thereafter: CBC with differential, platelets and hemoglobin, liver function tests, electrolytes and TSH; ophthalmic exam (or with new ocular symptoms); ECG (in patients with preexisting cardiac abnormalities or in advanced stages of cancer). Monitor serum bilirubin, ALT, AST, alkaline phosphatase and LDH at 2, 8 and 12 weeks following initiation, then every 6 months during treatment. Permanently discontinue for severe (grade 3) hepatic injury or hepatic decompensation (Child-Pugh class B and C [score >6]). During therapy: Weight; neuropsychiatric changes during and for 6 months after therapy.

Additional *indication-specific* monitoring parameters:

Chronic hepatitis B: CBC with differential and platelets and liver function tests: Baseline, weeks 1, 2, 4, 8, 12, and 16, at the end of treatment, and then 3 and 6 months post treatment

Chronic hepatitis C:

CBC with differential and platelets: Baseline, weeks 1 and 2, then monthly

Liver function: Every 3 months

TSH: Baseline and periodically during treatment; in patients with preexisting thyroid disorders also repeat at 3 months and 6 months

Condyloma acuminate (intralesional administration): Monitor CBC with differential, liver function tests (elevations have been reported).

Malignant melanoma: CBC with differential and platelets and liver function tests: Weekly during induction phase, then monthly during maintenance

Oncology patients: Thyroid function monitoring (Hamnvik 2011): TSH and anti-TPO antibodies at baseline; if TPO antibody positive, monitor TSH every 2 months; if TPO antibody negative, monitor TSH every 6 months

Dosage Forms Excipient information presented when available (limited, particularly for generics); consult specific product labeling.

Solution, Injection:

Intron A: 6,000,000 units/mL (3.8 mL); 10,000,000 units/mL (3.2 mL) [contains edetate disodium, metacresol, polysorbate 80]

Solution Reconstituted, Injection [preservative free]:

Intron A: 10,000,000 units (1 ea); 18,000,000 units (1 ea); 50,000,000 units (1 ea) [contains albumin human]

Interferon Alfa-n3 (in ter FEER on AL fa en three)

Brand Names: US Alferon N

Brand Names: Canada Alferon N

Pharmacologic Category Interferon

Use Condylomata acuminata: Intralesional treatment of refractory or recurring external condylomata acuminata (venereal or genital warts) in patients 18 years of age or older.

Medication Guide Available Yes

Dosing

Adult & Geriatric

Condylomata acuminata: Intralesional: 250,000 units (0.05 mL) per wart twice weekly for a maximum of 8 weeks; maximum dose per treatment session: 2.5 million units (0.5 mL). Therapy should not be repeated for at least 3 months after the initial 8-week course of therapy (unless existing warts grow or new warts appear).

Renal Impairment There are no dosage adjustments provided in the manufacturer's labeling.

Hepatic Impairment There are no dosage adjustments provided in the manufacturer's labeling.

Additional Information Complete prescribing information should be consulted for additional detail.

Dosage Forms Excipient information presented when available (limited, particularly for generics); consult specific product labeling.

Solution, Injection:

Alferon N: 5,000,000 units/mL (1 mL)

◆ Interferon Alpha-2b *see* Interferon Alfa-2b *on page 966*

Interferon Beta-1a (in ter FEER on BAY ta won aye)

Brand Names: US Avonex; Avonex Pen; Rebif; Rebif Rebidose; Rebif Rebidose Titration Pack; Rebif Titration Pack

Brand Names: Canada Avonex; Rebif

Index Terms rIFN beta-1a

Pharmacologic Category Interferon

Use

US labeling: Treatment of relapsing forms of multiple sclerosis (MS) to decrease the frequency of clinical exacerbations and delay the accumulation of physical disability

Canadian labeling:

Treatment of relapsing forms of multiple sclerosis (MS) to decrease the frequency of clinical exacerbations, delay the accumulation of physical disability, reduce the requirement for steroids, reduce the number of hospitalizations, and reduce disease burden

To decrease the number and volume of active brain lesions, decrease overall disease burden, and delay onset of clinically definite MS in patients who have experienced a single demyelinating event.

Pregnancy Considerations Adverse events have not been observed in animal reproduction studies; however, the possibility of adverse effects cannot be ruled out. Preliminary data from the Avonex pregnancy registry (published in abstract) do not show an increased risk of adverse fetal events when exposure occurs during pregnancy (Richman, 2012; Tomczyk, 2013); however, other studies have reported conflicting results. Until additional information is available, consideration should be given to discontinuing treatment if a woman becomes pregnant, or 1 month prior to becoming pregnant in women with mild disease (Coyle, 2012; Houtchens, 2013; Lu, 2013). Rebif Canadian product monograph contraindicates use in pregnant women.

Breast-Feeding Considerations Small amounts of interferon beta-1a are excreted in breast milk. Milk samples were obtained from six lactating women (6-23 months postpartum) receiving Avonex 30 mcg IM once weekly; sampling occurred at intervals for 72 hours after the dose. The highest reported concentration was 179 pg/mL and the relative infant dose was calculated to be <1% of the maternal dose. Adverse events were not observed in the nursing infants (Hale, 2012). The manufacturer recommends that caution be exercised when administering interferon beta-1a to nursing women. Canadian labeling recommends discontinuing breast-feeding or discontinuing therapy.

Medication Guide Available Yes

Contraindications

Hypersensitivity to natural or recombinant interferon beta, human albumin (albumin-containing formulations only), or any other component of the formulation

Documentation of allergenic cross-reactivity for interferons is limited. However, because of similarities in chemical structure and/or pharmacologic actions, the possibility of cross-sensitivity cannot be ruled out with certainty.

Canadian labeling: Additional contraindications (not in US labeling): Rebif: Pregnancy; decompensated liver disease

Warnings/Precautions Interferons have been associated with psychiatric adverse events (psychosis, depression, suicidal behavior/ideation) in patients with and without previous psychiatric symptoms; use with caution in patients with depression. Patients exhibiting depressive symptoms or other severe psychiatric symptoms should be closely monitored and discontinuation of therapy should be considered.

Autoimmune disorders including idiopathic thrombocytopenia, hyper- and hypothyroidism and rarely autoimmune hepatitis have been reported. Consider discontinuation of treatment if patient develops a new autoimmune disorder. Cases of thrombotic microangiopathy manifesting as thrombotic thrombocytopenic purpura (TTP) or hemolytic uremic syndrome (HUS) (some fatal) have been reported (Hunt 2014; Mahe 2013; Rebif Canadian product monograph 2014). Some cases may occur after several years of therapy. Monitor for new onset hypertension, thrombocytopenia, or impaired renal function; discontinuation of therapy and prompt treatment may be necessary if TTP/HUS are confirmed. Allergic reactions, including anaphylaxis, have been reported; some reactions may occur after prolonged use. Discontinue therapy if anaphylaxis or other allergic reactions occur. Rare cases of severe hepatic injury, including cases of hepatic failure requiring transplantation, have been reported in patients receiving interferon beta-1a; risk may be increased by ethanol use or concurrent therapy with hepatotoxic drugs. Some reports indicate symptoms began after 1-6 months of treatment. Transaminase elevations may be asymptomatic. Use with caution in patients with active or a history of liver disease, alcohol abuse, or increased serum ALT (>2.5 times ULN) at baseline. Obtain liver function tests at 1-, 3-, and 6 months post therapy initiation and periodically thereafter. Treatment should be suspended immediately if jaundice or symptoms of hepatic dysfunction occur. Consider dose reductions or temporary discontinuation if ALT >5 times ULN. Hematologic effects, including pancytopenia (rare), leukopenia, and thrombocytopenia, have been reported. Monitor blood counts at 1-, 3-, and 6 months post therapy initiation and periodically thereafter. Events may recur with rechallenge.

Associated with a high incidence of flu-like adverse effects; use of analgesics and/or antipyretics on treatment days may be helpful. Use caution in patients with preexisting cardiovascular disease. Rare cases of new-onset cardiomyopathy and/or HF have been reported. Use caution in patients with seizure disorders. Thyroid abnormalities may develop with use; may worsen preexisting thyroid conditions. Monitor thyroid function tests every 6 months or as clinically necessary. Safety and efficacy in patients with chronic progressive MS have not been established.

Severe injection site reactions have occurred, including pain, erythema, edema, cellulitis, abscess, and necrosis. Necrosis may occur at single and multiple sites. Some reactions have occurred ≥2 years after initiation; reactions typically resolve with conservative treatment (antibiotics or surgical intervention may be required). Patient and/or caregiver competency in injection technique should be confirmed and periodically re-evaluated. Albumin is a component of some formulations (contraindicated in albumin-sensitive patients); rare risk of CJD or viral transmission. The packaging (prefilled syringe tip cap) may contain latex.

Adverse Reactions Adverse reactions reported as a composite of both commercially-available products. Spectrum and incidence of reactions is generally similar between products, but consult individual product labels for specific incidence.

>10%:

Central nervous system: Headache (58% to 70%), fatigue (33% to 41%), depression (18% to 25%), pain (23%), chills (19%), dizziness (14%)

Gastrointestinal: Nausea (23%), abdominal pain (8% to 22%)

Genitourinary: Urinary tract infection (17%)

Hematologic & oncologic: Leukopenia (28% to 36%), lymphadenopathy (11% to 12%)

Hepatic: Increased serum ALT (20% to 27%), increased serum AST (10% to 17%)

Immunologic: Antibody development (neutralizing; significance not known; Rebif: 24% to 31%; Avonex: 5%)

Local: Injection site reaction (3% to 92%)

Neuromuscular & skeletal: Myalgia (25% to 29%), back pain (23% to 25%), weakness (24%), skeletal pain (10% to 15%), rigors (6% to 13%)

Ophthalmic: Visual disturbance (7% to 13%)

Respiratory: Flu-like symptoms (49% to 59%), sinusitis (14%), upper respiratory tract infection (14%)

Miscellaneous: Fever (20% to 28%)

1% to 10%:

Cardiovascular: Chest pain (5% to 8%), vasodilation (2%)

Central nervous system: Hypertonia (6% to 7%), migraine (5%), ataxia (4% to 5%), drowsiness (4% to 5%), malaise (4% to 5%), seizure (1% to 5%), suicidal tendencies (4%)

Dermatologic: Erythematous rash (5% to 7%), maculopapular rash (4% to 5%), alopecia (4%), hyperhidrosis (4%), urticaria

Endocrine & metabolic: Thyroid disease (4% to 6%)

Gastrointestinal: Xerostomia (1% to 5%), toothache (3%)

Genitourinary: Urinary frequency (2% to 7%), urinary incontinence (2% to 4%), urine abnormality (3%)

Hematologic & oncologic: Thrombocytopenia (2% to 8%), anemia (3% to 5%)

Hepatic: Hyperbilirubinemia (2% to 3%)

Infection: Infection (7%)

Local: Pain at injection site (8%), bruising at injection site (6%), inflammation at injection site (6%), tissue necrosis at injection site (1% to 3%)

Neuromuscular & skeletal: Arthralgia (9%)

Ophthalmic: Eye disease (4%), xerophthalmia (1% to 3%)

Respiratory: Bronchitis (8%)

<1% (Limited to important and life-threatening): Abnormal healing, abscess, abscess at injection site, amnesia, anaphylaxis, arteritis, arthritis, bloody stools, breast fibroadenosis, cardiac arrest, cardiac failure, cellulitis at injection site, conjunctivitis, depersonalization, dermal ulcer, diverticulitis, drug dependence, emphysema, epididymitis, erythema multiforme, facial paralysis, fibrosis at injection site, furunculosis, gallbladder disease, gastritis, gastrointestinal hemorrhage, gingivitis, gynecomastia, hemolytic uremic syndrome, hemorrhage, hepatic failure, hepatic neoplasm, hepatitis, hepatomegaly, hepatotoxicity (idiosyncratic) (Chalasani, 2014), hernia, hypersensitivity reaction at injection site, hyperthyroidism, hypoglycemia, hypokalemia, hypomagnesemia, hypotension, hypothyroidism, immune thrombocytopenia, intestinal obstruction, intestinal perforation, lipoma, lupus erythematosus, menopause, neoplasm, nephrolithiasis, neurological signs and symptoms (transient; may mimic multiple sclerosis exacerbations), nevus, orthostatic hypotension, osteonecrosis, pancytopenia, pelvic inflammatory disease, pericarditis, periodontitis, peripheral vascular disease, Peyronie's disease, pneumonia, postmenopausal bleeding, proctitis, psychiatric disorders (new or worsening; including suicidal ideation), psychoneurosis, pulmonary embolism, pyelonephritis, retinal vascular disease, sepsis, severe weakness (transient), skin photosensitivity, Stevens-Johnson syndrome, synovitis, tachycardia, telangiectasia, testicular disease, thromboembolism, thrombotic thrombocytopenic

purpura, uterine fibroids, vaginal hemorrhage, vascular disease, vesicular eruption

Drug Interactions

Metabolism/Transport Effects None known.

Avoid Concomitant Use There are no known interactions where it is recommended to avoid concomitant use.

Increased Effect/Toxicity

Interferon Beta-1a may increase the levels/effects of: Theophylline Derivatives; Zidovudine

Decreased Effect There are no known significant interactions involving a decrease in effect.

Preparation for Administration Avonex: Reconstitute with 1.1 mL of diluent (SWFI) and swirl gently to dissolve. Do not shake. The reconstituted product contains no preservative and is for single-use only; discard unused portion.

Storage/Stability

Avonex:

Prefilled syringe or pen: Store at 2°C to 8°C (36°F to 46°F); do not freeze. Protect from light. Allow to warm to room temperature prior to use (do not use external heat source). If refrigeration is not available, product may be stored at ≤25°C (77°F) for up to 7 days.

Vial: Store unreconstituted vial at 2°C to 8°C (36°F to 46°F). If refrigeration is not available, may be stored at 25°C (77°F) for up to 30 days; do not freeze. Protect from light. Following reconstitution, use immediately, but may be stored up to 6 hours at 2°C to 8°C (36°F to 46°F); do not freeze.

Rebif: Store at 2°C to 8°C (36°F to 46°F); do not freeze. Protect from heat and light. Allow to warm to room temperature prior to use (do not use external heat source). Refrigeration is preferred; however, if needed, may be stored at 2°C to 25°C (36°F to 77°F) for up to 30 days.

Mechanism of Action Interferon beta differs from naturally occurring human protein by a single amino acid substitution and the lack of carbohydrate side chains; alters the expression and response to surface antigens and can enhance immune cell activities. Properties of interferon beta that modify biologic responses are mediated by cell surface receptor interactions; mechanism in the treatment of MS is unknown.

Pharmacodynamics/Kinetics

Onset of action: Avonex: 12 hours (based on biological response markers)

Duration: Avonex: 4 days (based on biological response markers)

Half-life elimination: Avonex: ~19 hours (range: 8-54 hours); Rebif: 69 hours

Time to peak, serum: Avonex (IM): ~15 hours (range: 6-36 hours); Rebif (SubQ): 16 hours

Dosing

Adult & Geriatric

Multiple sclerosis (MS): Note: Analgesics and/or antipyretics may help decrease flu-like symptoms on treatment days:

IM (Avonex):

US labeling: 30 mcg once weekly; to decrease flu-like symptoms, may initiate once-weekly dosing with 7.5 mcg (week 1) then increase dose in increments of 7.5 mcg once weekly (weeks 2 to 4) up to recommended dose (30 mcg once weekly)

Canadian labeling: 30 mcg once weekly; to decrease flu-like symptoms, may initiate once-weekly dosing with 7.5 mcg (week 1) then increase dose in increments of 7.5 mcg once weekly (weeks 2 to 4) or once every 2 weeks (to week 7) up to recommended dose (30 mcg once weekly). In progressive relapsing MS or secondary progressive MS with recurrent neurologic dysfunction may consider increasing to 60 mcg once weekly.

SubQ (Rebif): Target dose is either 22 or 44 mcg 3 times weekly; doses should be separated by at least 48 hours:

Target dose 44 mcg 3 times weekly:

Initial: 8.8 mcg (20% of target dose) 3 times weekly for 2 weeks

Titration: 22 mcg (50% of target dose) 3 times weekly for 2 weeks

Target dose: 44 mcg 3 times weekly

Target dose 22 mcg 3 times weekly:

Initial: 4.4 mcg (20% of target dose) 3 times weekly for 2 weeks

Titration: 11 mcg (50% of target dose) 3 times weekly for 2 weeks

Target dose: 22 mcg 3 times weekly

Single demyelinating event (Canadian labeling [Rebif]; not in US labeling): SubQ:

Target dose 44 mcg 3 times weekly: Note: Analgesics and/or antipyretics prior to and for 24 hours after dosing may help decrease flu-like symptoms:

Initial: 8.8 mcg (20% of target dose) 3 times weekly for 2 weeks

Titration: 22 mcg (50% of target dose) 3 times weekly for 2 weeks

Target dose: 44 mcg 3 times weekly

Renal Impairment There are no dosage adjustments provided in the manufacturer's labeling (has not been studied).

Hepatic Impairment There are no dosage adjustment provided in the manufacturer's labeling; use with caution in patients with active liver disease, alcohol abuse, ALT >2.5 x ULN, or a history of significant liver disease. Rebif Canadian labeling contraindicates use in decompensated liver disease.

Adjustment for Toxicity

Autoimmune disorder development: Consider discontinuing treatment.

Depression or other severe psychiatric symptoms: Consider discontinuing treatment.

Hepatotoxicity:

ALT >5 x ULN: Temporarily discontinue therapy or consider dose reduction until ALT normalizes, then may consider retitration of dose.

Symptomatic (eg, jaundice): Discontinue immediately.

Leukopenia: May require temporary discontinuation or dose reduction until resolution.

Administration The first injection should be administered under the supervision of a health care professional.

Avonex: Administer IM; rotate injection site; do not inject into area where skin is irritated, red, bruised, scarred, or infected. Two hours after injection, examine site for redness, swelling, or tenderness. Discard any unused portion.

Rebif: Administer SubQ at the same time of day on the same 3 days each week (eg, Mon, Wed, Fri), preferably in the late afternoon or evening; doses should be at least 48 hours apart; rotate injection site; do not inject into area where skin is irritated, red, bruised, or scarred. Discard any unused portion.

Monitoring Parameters Thyroid function tests, CBC with differential, transaminase levels, blood chemistries, symptoms of autoimmune disorders, signs/symptoms of psychiatric disorder (including depression and/or suicidal ideation), signs/symptoms of new onset/worsening cardiovascular disease, signs/symptoms of thrombotic microangiopathy (new-onset hypertension, thrombocytopenia, renal impairment)

Avonex: Frequency of monitoring for patients receiving Avonex® has not been specifically defined; in clinical trials, monitoring was at 6-month intervals. Canadian labeling recommends liver function testing monthly for first 6 months, then every 6 months thereafter or as clinically indicated.

Rebif: CBC and liver function testing at 1-, 3-, and 6 months, then periodically thereafter. Thyroid function every 6 months (in patients with preexisting abnormalities and/or clinical indications). Canadian labeling recommends liver function testing monthly for first 6 months, then every 6 months thereafter or as clinically indicated.

Dosage Forms Excipient information presented when available (limited, particularly for generics); consult specific product labeling.

Injection, powder for reconstitution [preservative free]:

Avonex: 30 mcg [contains albumin (human); derived from or manufactured using Chinese hamster ovary cells; supplied with diluent]

Injection, solution:

Avonex: 30 mcg/0.5 mL (0.5 mL) [albumin free; derived from or manufactured using Chinese hamster ovary cells; prefilled syringe]

Avonex Pen: 30 mcg/0.5 mL (0.5 mL) [albumin free; derived from or manufactured using Chinese hamster ovary cells]

Injection, solution [preservative free]:

Rebif: 22 mcg/0.5 mL (0.5 mL), 44 mcg/0.5 mL (0.5 mL) [contains albumin (human); derived from or manufactured using Chinese hamster ovary cells; prefilled syringe]

Rebif Rebidose: 22 mcg/0.5 mL (0.5 mL), 44 mcg/0.5 mL (0.5 mL) [contains albumin (human); derived from or manufactured using Chinese hamster ovary cells; autoinjector]

Injection, solution [preservative free, combination package]:

Rebif Titration Pack: 8.8 mcg/0.2 mL (6s) and 22 mcg/0.5 mL (6s) [contains albumin (human); derived from or manufactured using Chinese hamster ovary cells; prefilled syringe]

Rebif Rebidose Titration Pack: 8.8 mcg/0.2 mL (6s) and 22 mcg/0.5 mL (6s) [contains albumin (human); derived from or manufactured using Chinese hamster ovary cells; autoinjector]

Interferon Beta-1b (in ter FEER on BAY ta won bee)

Brand Names: US Betaseron; Extavia
Brand Names: Canada Betaseron; Extavia
Index Terms rIFN beta-1b
Pharmacologic Category Interferon
Use

Multiple sclerosis: Treatment of relapsing forms of multiple sclerosis (MS) to reduce the frequency of clinical exacerbations.
Canadian labeling: Additional use (not in US labeling): Treatment of secondary progressive MS

Pregnancy Considerations Adverse events have been observed in animal reproduction studies. Spontaneous abortions were reported in 4 women during a clinical trial. Women with multiple sclerosis are generally recommended to discontinue therapy prior to conception (Lu, 2012). The Canadian labeling contraindicates use in pregnant women.

Breast-Feeding Considerations It is not known if interferon beta-1b is excreted in breast milk. Due to the potential for serious adverse reactions in the nursing infant, the decision to continue or discontinue breastfeeding during therapy should take into account the risk of exposure to the infant and the benefits of treatment to the mother.

Medication Guide Available Yes
Contraindications

History of hypersensitivity to natural or recombinant interferon beta, albumin (human), or any component of the formulation.

Documentation of allergenic cross-reactivity for interferons is limited. However, because of similarities in chemical structure and/or pharmacologic actions, the possibility of cross-sensitivity cannot be ruled out with certainty.

Canadian labeling: Additional contraindication (not in US labeling): Pregnancy, decompensated liver disease (Betaseron, Extavia); current severe depression and/or suicidal ideation (Extavia)

Warnings/Precautions Allergic reactions (eg, bronchospasm, dyspnea, skin rash, tongue edema, urticaria), including anaphylaxis (rare), have been reported with use; discontinue use if anaphylaxis occurs. Associated with a high incidence of flu-like adverse effects; use of analgesics and/or antipyretics on treatment days may be helpful. Improvement in symptoms occurs over time. Hepatotoxicity has been reported with beta interferons, including rare reports of hepatitis (autoimmune) and hepatic failure requiring transplant; use with caution in patients with concurrent exposure to other hepatotoxic drugs. Monitor liver function tests as clinically necessary. Consider discontinuation if serum transaminase levels increase significantly or are associated with clinical symptoms (eg, jaundice). Interferons have been associated with severe psychiatric adverse events (psychosis, mania, depression, suicidal behavior/ideation) in patients with and without previous psychiatric symptoms; avoid use in severe psychiatric disorders and use caution in patients with a history of depression; patients exhibiting symptoms of depression should be closely monitored and discontinuation of therapy should be considered. Use with caution in patients with a history of seizure disorder. Cases of thrombotic microangiopathy manifesting as thrombotic thrombocytopenic purpura (TTP) or hemolytic uremic syndrome (HUS) (some fatal) have been reported with interferon beta products. Some cases may occur after several years of therapy. Monitor for new onset hypertension, thrombocytopenia, or impaired renal function; discontinuation of therapy and prompt treatment may be necessary if TTP/HUS are confirmed.

Use with caution in patients with preexisting cardiovascular disease. Rare cases of new-onset cardiomyopathy and/or HF have been reported. If HF worsens in the absence of another etiology, consider discontinuation of therapy. Use with caution in patients with hepatic impairment or in combination with alcohol. The Canadian labeling contraindicates use in patients with decompensated hepatic disease. Use with caution in patients with bone marrow suppression; may require increased monitoring. Leukopenia has also been observed; routine monitoring of

complete blood counts with differentials is recommended. Dose reduction may be required. Thyroid abnormalities may develop with use; may worsen preexisting thyroid conditions. Monitor thyroid function tests every 6 months or as clinically necessary.

Severe injection site reactions (necrosis) may occur, which may or may not heal with continued therapy. Reactions generally arise within the first 4 months of therapy, but have occurred ≥1 year after initiation. Incidence of reactions tend to improve over time. Patient and/or caregiver competency in injection technique should be confirmed and periodically re-evaluated. Do not inject into affected area until completely healed; if multiple lesions occur, discontinue use until they are fully healed. Contains albumin, which may carry a remote risk of transmitting viral diseases.

Adverse Reactions Note: Flu-like syndrome (including at least two of the following - headache, fever, chills, malaise, diaphoresis, and myalgia) are reported in the majority of patients (60%) and decrease over time (average duration ~1 week).

>10%:
Cardiovascular: Peripheral edema (12% to 15%), chest pain (9% to 11%)
Central nervous system: Headache (50% to 57%), pain (42% to 51%), hypertonia (40% to 50%), myasthenia (46%), chills (21% to 25%), dizziness (24%), insomnia (21% to 24%), ataxia (17% to 21%)
Dermatologic: Skin rash (21% to 24%), dermatological disease (10% to 12%)
Gastrointestinal: Nausea (27%), constipation (20%), diarrhea (19%), abdominal pain (16% to 19%), dyspepsia (14%)
Genitourinary: Urinary urgency (11% to 13%), uterine hemorrhage (9% to 11%)
Hematologic & oncologic: Lymphocytopenia (86% to 88%), leukopenia (13% to 18%), neutropenia (13% to 14%)
Immunologic: Antibody development (≤45%; neutralizing; significance not known)
Local: Injection site reaction (78% to 85%, including inflammation [53%], pain [18%], tissue necrosis [4% to 5%], hypersensitivity reaction [4%], swelling [2% to 3%], residual mass [2%])
Neuromuscular & skeletal: Weakness (53% to 61%), arthralgia (31%), myalgia (23% to 27%)
Respiratory: Flu-like symptoms (decreases over treatment course; 57% to 60%)
Miscellaneous: Fever (31% to 36%)
1% to 10%:
Cardiovascular: Vasodilatation (8%), hypertension (6% to 7%), peripheral vascular disease (6%), palpitations (4%), tachycardia (4%)
Central nervous system: Anxiety (10%), malaise (6% to 8%), nervousness (7%)
Dermatologic: Diaphoresis (8%), alopecia (4%)
Endocrine & metabolic: Hypermenorrhea (8%), dysmenorrhea (7%), weight gain (7%)
Genitourinary: Impotence (8% to 9%), cystitis (8%), urinary frequency (7%), pelvic pain (6%), prostatic disease (3%)
Hematologic & oncologic: Lymphadenopathy (6% to 8%)
Hepatic: Increased serum ALT (>5x baseline: 10% to 12%), increased serum AST (>5x baseline: 3% to 4%)
Hypersensitivity: Hypersensitivity (3%)
Neuromuscular & skeletal: Leg cramps (4%)
Respiratory: Dyspnea (6% to 7%)
<1% (Limited to important or life-threatening): Anaphylaxis, anorexia, apnea, ataxia, autoimmune hepatitis, capillary leak syndrome (in patients with preexisting monoclonal gammopathy), cardiac arrest, cardiac arrhythmia, cardiac failure, cardiomegaly, cardiomyopathy, cerebral hemorrhage, coma, confusion, convulsion, deep vein thrombosis, delirium, depersonalization, depression, emotional lability, erythema nodosum, ethanol sensitization, exfoliative dermatitis, gastrointestinal hemorrhage, hallucinations, hematemesis, hepatic failure, hepatitis, hepatotoxicity (idiosyncratic) (Chalasani, 2014), hyperthyroidism, hyperuricemia, hypocalcemia, increased gamma-glutamyl transferase, increased serum triglycerides maculopapular rash, manic behavior, myocardial infarction, pancreatitis, pericardial effusion, pneumonia, pruritus, psychosis, pulmonary embolism, rash, sepsis, shock, skin discoloration, skin photosensitivity, suicidal ideation, syncope, SIADH, thrombocytopenia, thyroid dysfunction, urinary tract infection, urosepsis, vasculitis, vaginal hemorrhage, vesiculobullous dermatitis, weight loss
Drug Interactions
Metabolism/Transport Effects None known.

Avoid Concomitant Use There are no known interactions where it is recommended to avoid concomitant use.

Increased Effect/Toxicity
Interferon Beta-1b may increase the levels/effects of: Theophylline Derivatives; Zidovudine

Decreased Effect There are no known significant interactions involving a decrease in effect.

Preparation for Administration To reconstitute solution, inject 1.2 mL of diluent (provided); gently swirl to dissolve, do not shake. Reconstituted solution provides 0.25 mg/mL. Use product within 3 hours of reconstitution. Discard unused portion of vial. Foaming may occur if swirled or shaken too vigorously; allow vial to sit until foam settles.

Storage/Stability Store intact vials at 20°C to 25°C (68°F to 77°F); excursions permitted to 15°C to 30°C (59°F to 86°F) for ≤3 months. If not used immediately following reconstitution, refrigerate solution at 2°C to 8°C (35°F to 46°F) and use within 3 hours; do not freeze or shake solution. Discard unused portion of vial.

Mechanism of Action Interferon beta-1b differs from naturally occurring human protein by a single amino acid substitution and the lack of carbohydrate side chains; mechanism in the treatment of MS is unknown; however, immunomodulatory effects attributed to interferon beta-1b include enhancement of suppressor T cell activity, reduction of proinflammatory cytokines, down-regulation of antigen presentation, and reduced trafficking of lymphocytes into the central nervous system. Improves MRI lesions, decreases relapse rate, and disease severity in patients with secondary progressive MS.

Pharmacodynamics/Kinetics Limited data due to small doses used
Half-life elimination: 8 minutes to 4.3 hours
Time to peak, serum: 1-8 hours

Dosing

Adult & Geriatric Note: Analgesics and/or antipyretics may help decrease flu-like symptoms on treatment days:
US labeling:
Multiple sclerosis (relapsing): SubQ: Initial: 0.0625 mg (2 million units [0.25 mL]) every other day; gradually increase dose by 0.0625 mg every 2 weeks to a target dose of 0.25 mg (8 million units [1 mL]) every other day. **Note:** In clinical trials involving patients with a single clinical event suggestive of MS, dose titration occurred at weekly intervals (Kappos 2006).

Canadian labeling:
Multiple sclerosis (relapsing): SubQ: Initial: 0.0625 mg (2 million units [0.25 mL]) every other day; gradually increase dose by 0.0625 mg every week to a target dose of 0.25 mg (8 million units [1 mL]) every other day. May titrate more slowly if significant adverse reactions occur.

Multiple sclerosis (secondary progressive): SubQ: Initial: 0.125 mg (4 million units [0.5 mL]) every other day for 2 weeks; gradually increase to target dose of 0.25 mg (8 million units [1 mL]) every other day

Renal Impairment There are no dosage adjustments provided in the manufacturer's labeling.

Hepatic Impairment There are no dosage adjustments provided in the manufacturer's labeling. The Canadian labeling contraindicates use in decompensated liver disease.

Administration For SubQ administration. The first injection should be administered under the supervision of a health care professional. Withdraw dose of reconstituted solution from the vial into a sterile syringe fitted with a 27-gauge (Extavia) or 30-gauge (Betaseron) needle and inject the solution subcutaneously. The Betaconnect autoinjector may be used with prepared Betaseron syringes after health care provider selects proper depth setting and injection technique (see prescribing information for more detailed use of autoinjector). Sites for self-injection include outer surface of the arms, abdomen (**except** 2-inch area around the navel), buttocks, and thighs. If patient is very thin, only use the thigh or outer surface of arms. Rotate SubQ injection site. Do not inject into area where skin is bruised, infected, or broken. Patient should be well hydrated. If a dose is missed, administer as soon as remembered; do not administer on 2 consecutive days. Time subsequent doses every 48 hours.

Monitoring Parameters Complete blood chemistries (including platelet count) and liver function tests are recommended at 1, 3, and 6 months following initiation of therapy and periodically thereafter. Thyroid function should be assessed every 6 months in patients with history of thyroid dysfunction or as clinically necessary. Monitor for flu-like symptoms, allergic or anaphylactic reactions, injection-site reactions, worsening of cardiac symptoms (in HF patients); and for sign/symptoms of depression.

Canadian labeling: Additional monitoring recommendations (not in US labeling): Baseline pregnancy test, chest X-ray, and electrocardiogram

Additional Information American Academy of Neurology and MS Council guidelines suggest that, based upon published data, 6 million units of Avonex® (interferon beta-1a) (30 mcg) is equivalent to approximately 7-9 million units of Betaseron® (220-280 mcg).

Dosage Forms Excipient information presented when available (limited, particularly for generics); consult specific product labeling.
Kit, Subcutaneous:
Betaseron: 0.3 mg [contains albumin human]
Kit, Subcutaneous [preservative free]:
Extavia: 0.3 mg [contains albumin human]

Interferon Gamma-1b
(in ter FEER on GAM ah won bee)

Brand Names: US Actimmune
Pharmacologic Category Interferon
Use
Chronic granulomatous disease: Reduction in the frequency and severity of serious infections associated with chronic granulomatous disease
Malignant osteopetrosis (severe): To delay time to disease progression in patients with severe, malignant osteopetrosis

Pregnancy Considerations Adverse events have been observed in animal reproduction studies.

Breast-Feeding Considerations It is not known if interferon gamma 1b is excreted in breast milk. Due to the potential for serious adverse reactions in the nursing infant, the manufacturer recommends a decision be made to discontinue nursing or to discontinue the drug, taking into account the importance of treatment to the mother.

Contraindications Hypersensitivity to interferon gamma, *E. coli* derived products, or any component of the formulation

Warnings/Precautions Acute serious hypersensitivity reactions have been reported (case reports); transient cutaneous rashes may occur, although treatment interruption has rarely been necessary. Discontinue therapy immediately if an acute reaction occurs. Dose-related reversible neutropenia and thrombocytopenia (may be severe) have been reported; use caution in patients with myelosuppression. Elevations of AST and/or ALT (up to 25-fold) have been observed and were reversible with dose reduction or interruption of treatment. Incidence may be increased in children <1 year of age; perform monthly liver function assessments in this age group; modify dosage if severe elevations of liver enzyme develop. Neurologic disorders (ie, decreased mental status, gait disturbances, dizziness) have been noted at the higher doses (>250 mcg/m²/day); most of these abnormalities were reversible within a few days after dose reduction or discontinuation. Use with caution in patients with a history of seizure disorder or compromised CNS function. Acute and transient flu-like symptoms (eg, fever, headache, chills, myalgia, fatigue) have been noted at the higher doses (>250 mcg/m²/day) and may exacerbate preexisting cardiovascular disorders; some of the flu-like symptoms may be minimized by bedtime administration. Use with caution in patients with preexisting cardiovascular disease, including ischemia, heart failure, or arrhythmia. Drug accumulation may occur in patients with advanced hepatic disease and severe renal insufficiency; renal toxicity has been reported. The vial stopper may contain dry natural rubber and may cause allergic reactions. Potentially significant drug-drug interactions may exist, requiring dose or frequency adjustment, additional monitoring, and/or selection of alternative therapy.

Adverse Reactions Based on 50 mcg/m² dose administered 3 times weekly for chronic granulomatous disease

>10%:
Central nervous system: Fever (52%), headache (33%), chills (14%), fatigue (14%)
Dermatologic: Rash (17%)
Gastrointestinal: Diarrhea (14%), vomiting (13%)
Local: Injection site erythema or tenderness (14%)
1% to 10%:
Central nervous system: Depression (3%)
Gastrointestinal: Nausea (10%), abdominal pain (8%)
Neuromuscular & skeletal: Myalgia (6%), arthralgia (2%), back pain (2%)
Postmarketing and/or case reports: Alkaline phosphatase elevated, atopic dermatitis, granulomatous colitis, hepatomegaly, hypersensitivity reactions, hypokalemia, neutropenia, Stevens-Johnson syndrome

Additional adverse reactions noted at doses >100 mcg/m^2 administered 3 times weekly: ALT increased, AST increased, autoantibodies increased, bronchospasm, chest discomfort, confusion, dermatomyositis exacerbation, disorientation, DVT, gait disturbance, GI bleeding, hallucinations, heart block, heart failure, hepatic insufficiency, hyperglycemia, hypertriglyceridemia, hyponatremia, hypotension, interstitial pneumonitis, lupus-like syndrome, MI, neutropenia, pancreatitis (may be fatal), Parkinsonian symptoms, PE, proteinuria, renal insufficiency (reversible), seizure, syncope, tachyarrhythmia, tachypnea, thrombocytopenia, TIA

Drug Interactions

Metabolism/Transport Effects Inhibits CYP1A2 (weak), CYP2E1 (weak)

Avoid Concomitant Use There are no known interactions where it is recommended to avoid concomitant use.

Increased Effect/Toxicity

Interferon Gamma-1b may increase the levels/effects of: Theophylline Derivatives; TiZANidine; Zidovudine

Decreased Effect There are no known significant interactions involving a decrease in effect.

Preparation for Administration Do not mix with other drugs in the same syringe. Vials are intended for single use (does not contain preservative); discard unused portion of the vial.

Storage/Stability Store intact vials at 2°C to 8°C (36°F to 46°F); do not freeze. Avoid excessive or vigorous agitation; do not shake. Discard if intact vial is left at room temperature for >12 hours prior to use.

Mechanism of Action Interferon gamma participates in immunoregulation by enhancing the oxidative metabolism of macrophages; it also enhances antibody dependent cellular cytotoxicity, activates natural killer cells and has a role in the expression of Fc receptors and major histocompatibility antigens.

Pharmacodynamics/Kinetics

Absorption: IM, SubQ: >89%

Half-life elimination: IM: ~3 hours, SubQ: ~6 hours

Time to peak, plasma: IM: ~4 hours (1.5 ng/mL); SubQ: ~7 hours (0.6 ng/mL)

Dosing

Adult & Geriatric Note: Dosing expressed in mcg; 50 mcg is equivalent to 1 million units (50 mcg/m^2 is equivalent to 1 million units/m^2).

Chronic granulomatous disease: SubQ: 50 mcg/m^2 (1 million units/m^2) 3 times/week; doses above 50 mcg/m^2 are not recommended.

Malignant osteopetrosis (severe): SubQ: 50 mcg/m^2 (1 million units/m^2) 3 times/week; doses above 50 mcg/m^2 are not recommended.

Pediatric Note: Dosing expressed in mcg; 50 mcg is equivalent to 1 million units (50 mcg/m^2 is equivalent to 1 million units/m^2).

Chronic granulomatous disease: Children and Adolescents: SubQ:

Body surface area (BSA) ≤0.5 m^2: 1.5 mcg/kg/dose 3 times/week

BSA >0.5 m^2: 50 mcg/m^2 (1 million units/m^2) 3 times/week; doses above 50 mcg/m^2 are not recommended.

Malignant osteopetrosis (severe): Infants, Children, and Adolescents: SubQ:

Body surface area (BSA) ≤0.5 m^2: 1.5 mcg/kg/dose 3 times/week

BSA >0.5 m^2: 50 mcg/m^2 (1 million units/m^2) 3 times/week; doses above 50 mcg/m^2 are not recommended.

Renal Impairment There are no dosage adjustments provided in the manufacturer's labeling; drug accumulation may occur in patients with severe renal insufficiency.

Hepatic Impairment There are no dosage adjustments provided in the manufacturer's labeling; drug accumulation may occur in patients with advanced hepatic disease. If severe transaminase elevations occur during treatment, interrupt and reduce the dose upon resolution.

Adjustment for Toxicity If severe reactions occur, reduce dose by 50% or therapy should be interrupted until adverse reaction abates.

Administration Administer by SubQ injection into the right and left deltoid or anterior thigh. Consider premedication with acetaminophen and/or bedtime administration to minimize adverse reactions (eg, flu-like symptoms).

Monitoring Parameters CBC with differential, platelets, LFTs (monthly in children <1 year), electrolytes, BUN, creatinine, and urinalysis prior to therapy and at 3-month intervals

Dosage Forms Considerations Actimmune Injection, solution: 100 mcg (2 million units) per 0.5 mL (50 mcg is equivalent to 1 million units)

Dosage Forms Excipient information presented when available (limited, particularly for generics); consult specific product labeling.

Solution, Subcutaneous:

Actimmune: 2,000,000 units/0.5 mL (0.5 mL)

◆ Interleukin-1 Receptor Antagonist see Anakinra on page 127

◆ Interleukin 2 see Aldesleukin on page 60

◆ Interleukin-11 see Oprelvekin on page 1339

◆ Intermezzo see Zolpidem on page 1940

◆ Intralipid see Fat Emulsion (Plant Based) on page 743

◆ Intrapleural Talc see Talc (Sterile) on page 1732

◆ Intravenous Fat Emulsion see Fat Emulsion (Plant Based) on page 743

◆ Intrifiban see Eptifibatide on page 661

◆ Intron A see Interferon Alfa-2b on page 966

◆ Intropin see DOPamine on page 585

◆ Introvale see Ethinyl Estradiol and Levonorgestrel on page 703

◆ Intuniv see GuanFACINE on page 865

◆ Intuniv XR (Can) see GuanFACINE on page 865

◆ INVanz see Ertapenem on page 668

◆ Invanz (Can) see Ertapenem on page 668

◆ Invega see Paliperidone on page 1374

◆ Invega Sustenna see Paliperidone on page 1374

◆ Invega Trinza see Paliperidone on page 1374

◆ Invirase see Saquinavir on page 1636

◆ Iodine and Potassium Iodide see Potassium Iodide and Iodine on page 1482

Iodoquinol (eye oh doe KWIN ole)

Brand Names: US Aloquin; Yodoxin

Brand Names: Canada Diodoquin

Index Terms Diiodohydroxyquin

Pharmacologic Category Amebicide

Use Treatment of intestinal amebiasis due to trophozoite and cyst forms of *Entamoeba histolytica*

Dosing

Adult Treatment of susceptible infections: Oral: 650 mg 3 times daily after meals for 20 days; not to exceed 1.95 g daily

Geriatric Due to optic nerve damage, use cautiously in the elderly.

Pediatric Treatment of susceptible infections: Oral: Children: 30-40 mg/kg daily (maximum: 650 mg per dose) in 3 divided doses for 20 days; not to exceed 1.95 g daily

Renal Impairment No dosage adjustment provided in manufacturer's labeling.

Hepatic Impairment No dosage adjustment provided in manufacturer's labeling.

Additional Information Complete prescribing information should be consulted for additional detail.

Dosage Forms Excipient information presented when available (limited, particularly for generics); consult specific product labeling.

Gel, External:

Aloquin: 1.25% (60 g) [contains benzyl alcohol, brilliant blue fcf (fd&c blue #1), fd&c yellow #10 (quinoline yellow), propylene glycol, sd alcohol 40b, trolamine (triethanolamine)]

Tablet, Oral:

Yodoxin: 210 mg, 650 mg

Iodoquinol and Hydrocortisone
(eye oh doe KWIN ole & hye droe KOR ti sone)

Brand Names: US Alcortin A; Dermazene; Vytone

Index Terms Hydrocortisone and Iodoquinol

Pharmacologic Category Antifungal Agent, Topical; Corticosteroid, Topical

Use Dermatoses: Treatment of eczema (including impetiginized, nuchal, and nummular); acne urticata; anogenital pruritus (vulvae, scroti, ani); atopic and contact dermatitis, endogenous chronic infectious dermatitis; chronic eczematoid otitis externa; folliculitis, intertrigo; lichen simplex chronicus; moniliasis; dermatoses (mycotic or bacterial); neurodermatitis (localized or systemic); pyoderma, stasis dermatitis

Dosing

Adult & Geriatric Dermatoses: Topical: Apply 3-4 times daily to affected area(s)

Pediatric Dermatoses: Children ≥12 years and Adolescents: Topical: Refer to adult dosing.

Renal Impairment There are no dosage adjustments provided in the manufacturer's labeling.

Hepatic Impairment There are no dosage adjustments provided in the manufacturer's labeling.

Additional Information Complete prescribing information should be consulted for additional detail.

Dosage Forms Excipient information presented when available (limited, particularly for generics); consult specific product labeling.

Cream, topical:

Dermazene: Iodoquinol 1% and hydrocortisone acetate 1% (30 g)

Vytone: Iodoquinol 1% and hydrocortisone 1.9% per 2 g packet (30s) [contains benzyl alcohol]

Generic: Iodoquinol 1% and hydrocortisone acetate 1% (30 g); Iodoquinol 1% and hydrocortisone 1.9% per 2 g packet (30s)

Gel, topical:

Alcortin A: Iodoquinol 1% and hydrocortisone 2% (2 g, 48 g) [contains aloe, benzyl alcohol]

◆ **Ionsys** *see* FentaNYL *on page 750*

◆ **Iophen C-NR** *see* Guaifenesin and Codeine *on page 861*

◆ **Iophen DM-NR [OTC]** *see* Guaifenesin and Dextromethorphan *on page 861*

◆ **Iophen-NR [OTC]** *see* GuaiFENesin *on page 860*

◆ **Iopidine** *see* Apraclonidine *on page 142*

Ipilimumab (ip i LIM u mab)

Brand Names: US Yervoy
Brand Names: Canada Yervoy
Index Terms MDX-010; MDX-CTLA-4; MOAB-CTLA-4
Pharmacologic Category Antineoplastic Agent, Monoclonal Antibody

Use

US labeling:

Melanoma, unresectable or metastatic: Treatment of unresectable or metastatic melanoma

Melanoma, adjuvant treatment: Adjuvant treatment of cutaneous melanoma in patients with pathologic involvement of regional lymph nodes of more than 1 mm who have undergone complete resection, including total lymphadenectomy

Canadian labeling:

Melanoma, unresectable or metastatic: Treatment of unresectable or metastatic melanoma

Pregnancy Considerations Adverse effects were observed in animal reproduction studies. Ipilimumab is an IgG1 immunoglobulin and human IgG1 is known to cross the placenta, therefore, ipilimumab may be expected to reach the fetus. Ipilimumab may cause fetal harm if administered during pregnancy (based on the mechanism of action). Women of reproductive potential should use effective contraception during treatment and for 3 months following the last ipilimumab dose.

Breast-Feeding Considerations It is not known if ipilimumab is excreted in breast milk. The manufacturer recommends to discontinue breast-feeding during treatment and for 3 months following the final dose.

Medication Guide Available Yes

Contraindications

There are no contraindications listed in the manufacturer's US labeling.

Canadian labeling: Hypersensitivity to ipilimumab or any component of the formulation; active life-threatening autoimmune disease, or with organ transplantation graft where further immune activation is potentially imminently life-threatening

Warnings/Precautions [US Boxed Warning]: Severe and fatal immune-mediated adverse effects may occur. While any organ system may be involved, common severe effects include dermatitis (including toxic epidermal necrolysis), endocrinopathy, enterocolitis, hepatitis, and neuropathy. Reactions generally occur during treatment, although some reactions have occurred weeks to months after treatment discontinuation. Discontinue treatment (permanently) and initiate high-dose systemic corticosteroid treatment for severe immune mediated reactions. Evaluate liver function, adrenocorticotropic hormone (ACTH) level, and thyroid function tests at baseline and prior to each dose. Assess for signs and symptoms of enterocolitis, dermatitis, neuropathy, and endocrinopathy at baseline and prior to each dose. Initiate systemic corticosteroids (prednisone 1 to 2 mg/kg/day or equivalent) for severe reactions. Uncommon immune-mediated adverse effects reported include eosinophilia, hemolytic anemia, iritis, meningitis, myocarditis (fatal), nephritis, pancreatitis, pericarditis, pneumonitis, sarcoidosis, and uveitis. Other rare immune-mediated reactions reported in clinical trials

include angiopathy, arthritis, autoimmune central neuropathy (encephalitis), autoimmune thyroiditis, blepharitis, conjunctivitis, episcleritis, erythema multiforme, leukocytoclastic vasculitis, myositis, neurosensory hypoacusis, ocular myositis, polymyalgia rheumatica, polymyositis, psoriasis, scleritis, temporal arteritis, and vasculitis, Administer corticosteroid ophthalmic drops in patients who develop episcleritis, iritis, or uveitis; permanently discontinue ipilimumab if unresponsive to topical ophthalmic immunosuppressive treatments. For severe immune-mediated episcleritis or uveitis, initiate systemic corticosteroids (prednisone 1 to 2 mg/kg/day or equivalent); taper over at least 1 month (Weber, 2012).

Immune-mediated enterocolitis (including fatal cases) may occur. The median time to onset of grade 3 to 5 enterocolitis was 1.1 to 1.7 months. Monitor for signs and symptoms of enterocolitis (abdominal pain, blood in stool, diarrhea, or mucous in stool; with or without fever) and intestinal perforation (peritoneal signs, ileus). If enterocolitis develops, infectious causes should be ruled out; consider endoscopy for persistent or severe symptoms. Withhold ipilimumab treatment and administer antidiarrheals for moderate enterocolitis (diarrhea with ≤6 stools over baseline abdominal pain, mucous or blood in stool); if persists for >1 week, initiate systemic corticosteroids (prednisone at 0.5 mg/kg/day or equivalent). If severe enterocolitis (diarrhea ≥7 stools above baseline, fever, ileus, peritoneal signs) develops, permanently discontinue ipilimumab and initiate systemic corticosteroids (prednisone 1 to 2 mg/kg/day or equivalent); when resolved to ≤ grade 1, taper corticosteroids slowly over ≥1 month (rapid tapering may cause recurrence or worsen symptoms). May consider adding anti-tumor necrosis factor (TNF) or other immunosuppressive therapy for management of immune-mediated enterocolitis unresponsive to 3 to 5 days of systemic corticosteroids or recurring after symptomatic improvement.

Severe, life-threatening or fatal hepatotoxicity and immune-mediated hepatitis have been observed. The median time to onset for grade 3 or 4 immune-mediated hepatitis in patients receiving ipilimumab for adjuvant treatment of melanoma was 2 months. Monitor liver function tests (LFTs) and evaluate for signs of hepatotoxicity prior to each dose; if hepatotoxicity develops, infectious or malignant causes should be ruled out and liver function should be monitored more frequently until resolves. Withhold treatment for grade 2 hepatotoxicity (ALT or AST 2.5 to 5 times ULN or total bilirubin 1.5 to 3 times ULN). If severe or grade 3 or 4 hepatotoxicity develops (ALT or AST >5 times ULN or total bilirubin >3 times ULN), permanently discontinue ipilimumab and initiate systemic corticosteroids (prednisone 1 to 2 mg/kg/day or equivalent). If transaminases do not decrease within 48 hours of steroid initiation, consider adding mycophenolate mofetil (Weber, 2012). May begin tapering corticosteroid (over 1 month) when LFTs show sustained improvement or return to baseline

Severe, life-threatening, or fatal immune-mediated dermatitis has been reported. The median time to onset for dermatologic toxicity is 2 to 3 weeks. Monitor for signs/symptoms of dermatitis, including rash and pruritus; dermatitis should be considered immune-mediated unless identified otherwise. Mild-to-moderate dermatitis (localized rash and pruritus) should be treated symptomatically; topical or systemic corticosteroids should be administered if not resolved within 1 week. Withhold treatment for moderate to severe dermatologic symptoms. Permanently discontinue ipilimumab and initiate systemic corticosteroid (prednisone 1 to 2 mg/kg/day or equivalent) for Stevens-Johnson syndrome, toxic epidermal necrolysis, or rash complicated by dermal ulceration (full thickness) or necrotic, bullous, or hemorrhagic manifestations; when dermatitis is controlled, taper corticosteroid over at least 1 month.

Severe or life-threatening endocrine disorders (hypophysitis, adrenal insufficiency [including adrenal crisis], hyperthyroidism and hypothyroidism) have been reported; may require hospitalization. Endocrine disorders of moderate severity (including hypothyroidism, adrenal insufficiency, hypopituitarism, and less commonly hyperthyroidism and Cushing's syndrome) which have required hormone replacement therapy or medical intervention have also been reported. The median onset for moderate-to-severe endocrine disorders was 2.2 to 2.5 months; long-term hormone replacement therapy has been required in many cases. Monitor thyroid function tests, adrenocorticotropic hormone (ACTH) level, and serum chemistries prior to each dose and as clinically necessary; also monitor for signs of hypophysitis, adrenal insufficiency and thyroid disorders (eg, abdominal pain, fatigue, headache, hypotension, mental status changes, unusual bowel habits);

rule out other potential causes such as underlying disease or brain metastases. Endocrine disorders should be considered immune-mediated unless identified otherwise; consider endocrinology referral for further evaluation. If symptomatic, withhold ipilimumab treatment and initiate systemic corticosteroids (prednisone 1 to 2 mg/kg/day or equivalent) and appropriate hormone replacement therapy.

Immune-mediated neuropathies (some fatal) may occur. Severe peripheral motor neuropathy and fatal Guillain-Barré syndrome have been reported (rare). The median time to onset of grade 2 to 5 immune-mediated neuropathy in patients receiving ipilimumab for adjuvant treatment of melanoma was 1.4 to 27.4 months. Monitor for signs of motor or sensory neuropathy (unilateral or bilateral weakness, sensory changes or paresthesia). Withhold treatment in patients with neuropathy that does not interfere with daily activities (moderate neuropathy). Permanently discontinue for severe neuropathy (interferes with daily activities, including symptoms similar to Guillain-Barré syndrome) and treat accordingly. Consider initiating systemic corticosteroids (prednisone 1 to 2 mg/kg/day or equivalent) for severe neuropathies.

Adverse Reactions
>10%:

Central nervous system: Fatigue (41%), headache (15% [Hodi 2010])

Dermatologic: Pruritus (24% to 31% [Hodi 2010]), skin rash (19% to 29%; grades 3 to 5: 2% [Hodi 2010]), dermatitis (grade 2: 12%; grades 3 to 5: 2% to 3% [includes Stevens-Johnson syndrome, toxic epidermal necrolysis, dermal ulceration, necrotic, bullous or hemorrhagic dermatitis])

Gastrointestinal: Nausea (35% [Hodi 2010]), diarrhea (32%; grades 3 to 5: 5%), decreased appetite (27% [Hodi 2010]), vomiting (24% [Hodi 2010]), constipation (21% [Hodi 2010]), abdominal pain (15% [Hodi 2010])

Hematologic & oncologic: Anemia (12% [Hodi 2010])

Respiratory: Cough (16% [Hodi 2010]), dyspnea (15% [Hodi 2010])

Miscellaneous: Fever (12% [Hodi 2010])

1% to 10%:

Dermatologic: Urticaria (2%), vitiligo (2% [Hodi 2010])

Endocrine & metabolic: Pituitary insufficiency (4%; grade ≥2: ≤2%), hypophysitis (2% [Hodi 2010]), adrenal insufficiency (≤2% [Hodi 2010]), hypothyroidism (≤2% [Hodi 2010])

Gastrointestinal: Colitis (8%; grades 3 to 5: 5%), enterocolitis (grade 2: 5%; grades 3 to 5: 7%), intestinal perforation (1%)

Hematologic & oncologic: Eosinophilia (1%)

Hepatic: Hepatotoxicity (grade 2: 3%; grades 3 to 5: 1% to 2%), ALT increased (≤2% [Hodi 2010])

Immunologic: Antibody development (1%)

Renal: Nephritis (≤1%)

<1% (Limited to important or life-threatening): Acute respiratory distress syndrome, adrenocortical insufficiency (Hodi 2010), arthritis, blepharitis, bronchiolitis obliterans organizing pneumonia (Barjaktarevic 2013), capillary leak syndrome (Hodi 2010), conjunctivitis, Cushing's syndrome, DRESS syndrome, encephalitis, episcleritis, erythema multiforme, esophagitis, gastrointestinal ulcer, giant-cell arteritis, Guillain-Barré syndrome, hemolytic anemia, hepatic failure, hepatitis (immune-mediated), hypersensitivity angiitis, hyperthyroidism, hypoacusis (neurosensory), hypogonadism, increased serum AST, increased serum bilirubin, increased thyroid stimulating hormone level, infusion related reaction, iritis, meningitis, myasthenia gravis, myelofibrosis, myocarditis, myositis, myositis (ocular), neuropathy (sensory and motor), pancreatitis, pericarditis, peritonitis, pneumonitis, polymyalgia rheumatica, polymyositis, psoriasis, renal failure, sarcoidosis, scleritis, sepsis, thyroiditis (autoimmune), uveitis, vascular disease, vasculitis

Drug Interactions

Metabolism/Transport Effects None known.

Avoid Concomitant Use There are no known interactions where it is recommended to avoid concomitant use.

Increased Effect/Toxicity

Ipilimumab may increase the levels/effects of: Vemurafenib

Decreased Effect There are no known significant interactions involving a decrease in effect.

Preparation for Administration Prior to preparation, allow vials to sit at room temperature for ~5 minutes. Inspect vial prior to use; solution may have a pale yellow color or may contain translucent or white amorphous ipilimumab particles; discard if cloudy or discolored. Withdraw appropriate ipilimumab volume and transfer to IV bag, dilute with NS or D5W to a final concentration between 1 to 2 mg/mL. Mix by gently inverting, do not shake.

Storage/Stability Store intact vials refrigerated at 2°C to 8°C (36°F to 46°F); do not freeze. Protect from light. Prior to preparation, allow vials to sit at room temperature for ~5 minutes. Solutions diluted for infusion are stable for up to 24 hours refrigerated or at room temperature.

Mechanism of Action Ipilimumab is a recombinant human IgG1 immunoglobulin monoclonal antibody which binds to the cytotoxic T-lymphocyte associated antigen 4 (CTLA-4). CTLA-4 is a down-regulator of T-cell activation pathways. Blocking CTLA-4 allows for enhanced T-cell activation and proliferation. In melanoma, ipilimumab may indirectly mediate T-cell immune responses against tumors.

Pharmacodynamics/Kinetics Half-life elimination: Terminal: 15.4 days

Dosing

Adult

Melanoma, unresectable or metastatic: IV: 3 mg/kg every 3 weeks for a maximum of 4 doses; doses may be delayed due to toxicity, but all doses must be administered within 16 weeks of the initial dose.

Melanoma, adjuvant treatment: IV: 10 mg/kg every 3 weeks for 4 doses, followed by 10 mg/kg every 12 weeks for up to 3 years; if toxicity occurs, doses are omitted (not delayed).

Melanoma, unresectable or metastatic, first-line combination therapy (off-label use): IV: 3 mg/kg every 3 weeks for 4 doses (in combination with nivolumab; with nivolumab continued until disease progression or unacceptable toxicity) (Larkin 2015)

Renal Impairment No dosage adjustment necessary.

Hepatic Impairment

Impairment at baseline:

Mild impairment (total bilirubin >1 to 1.5 x ULN or AST >ULN): No dosage adjustment necessary.

Moderate or severe impairment (total bilirubin >1.5 x ULN and any AST): There are no dosage adjustments provided in the manufacturer's labeling (has not been studied).

Impairment during treatment:

AST or ALT >2.5 to ≤5 x ULN or bilirubin >1.5 to ≤3 x ULN: Temporarily withhold treatment.

ALT or AST >5 times ULN, or total bilirubin >3 times ULN: Permanently discontinue; also administer systemic corticosteroids (prednisone 1 to 2 mg/kg/day or equivalent). May begin tapering corticosteroid (over 1 month) when LFTs show sustained improvement or return to baseline.

Adjustment for Toxicity

US labeling:

Dermatologic toxicity: Treat symptomatically for mild to moderate dermatitis (eg, localized rash and pruritus); topical or systemic corticosteroids should be administered if not resolved within 1 week. Withhold ipilimumab for moderate to severe dermatologic symptoms. Permanently discontinue for Stevens-Johnson syndrome, toxic epidermal necrolysis, or rash complicated by dermal ulceration (full thickness) or necrotic, bullous, or hemorrhagic manifestations; also initiate systemic corticosteroids (prednisone 1 to 2 mg/kg/day or equivalent). When dermatitis is controlled, taper corticosteroid over at least 1 month.

Endocrinopathy: Temporarily withhold ipilimumab for symptomatic endocrinopathy; initiate systemic corticosteroids (prednisone at 1 to 2 mg/kg/day or equivalent), and begin appropriate hormone replacement therapy. Resume treatment in patients with complete or partial resolution of toxicity (≤ grade 1) and who are receiving prednisone <7.5 mg daily (or equivalent). Permanently discontinue ipilimumab for symptomatic endocrinopathy lasting 6 weeks or longer, or if unable to reduce corticosteroid dose to prednisone ≤7.5 mg daily (or equivalent).

Gastrointestinal toxicity:

Moderate enterocolitis: Withhold ipilimumab and administer antidiarrheal treatment; if moderate enterocolitis persists for >1 week, initiate systemic corticosteroids (prednisone at 0.5 mg/kg/day or equivalent). May resume treatment in patients with complete or partial resolution of toxicity (≤ grade 1) and who are receiving prednisone <7.5 mg daily (or equivalent).

Severe enterocolitis: Permanently discontinue. Initiate systemic corticosteroids (prednisone 1 to 2 mg/kg/day or equivalent). Upon improvement to ≤ grade 1, taper corticosteroids slowly over ≥1 month (rapid tapering may cause recurrence or worsen symptoms). May consider adding anti-tumor necrosis factor (TNF) or other immunosuppressive therapy for management of immune-mediated enterocolitis unresponsive to 3 to 5 days of systemic corticosteroids or recurring after symptomatic improvement.

Neuropathy: Withhold therapy for moderate neuropathy (not interfering with daily activities). Permanently discontinue for severe neuropathy which interferes with daily activities, such as Guillain-Barré-like syndromes. Consider initiating systemic corticosteroids (prednisone 1 to 2 mg/kg/day or equivalent) for severe neuropathies.

Ophthalmologic toxicity: Administer corticosteroid eye drops for uveitis, iritis, or episcleritis. Permanently discontinue for grade 2 through 4 immune-mediated reactions which do not improve to ≤ grade 1 within 2 weeks while receiving topical therapy or which require systemic treatment.

Pancreatitis, immune-mediated: Permanent discontinuation is recommended for grades 3 or 4 amylase or lipase increases (Weber 2012)

Other toxicity: Temporarily withhold ipilimumab for grade 2 adverse reactions. May resume treatment in patients (with grade 2 toxicity) with complete or partial resolution of toxicity (≤ grade 1) and who are receiving prednisone <7.5 mg daily (or equivalent). Initiate systemic corticosteroids (prednisone 1 to 2 mg/kg/day or equivalent) for severe immune-mediated adverse reactions. Permanently discontinue for clinically significant or severe immune-mediated adverse reactions, grade 2 reactions lasting 6 weeks or longer, grade 3 or 4 toxicity, or if unable to reduce corticosteroid dose to prednisone ≤7.5 mg daily (or equivalent).

Canadian labeling:

Temporarily withhold scheduled dose for the following:
Moderate immune-mediated reactions
Symptomatic endocrinopathy
Note: If receiving prednisone <7.5 mg daily (or equivalent), may resume with complete or partial resolution (to ≤ grade 1) of symptoms. Resume ipilimumab treatment at 3 mg/kg every 3 weeks until all 4 planned doses have been administered or until 16 weeks from initial dose, whichever occurs first.

Permanently discontinue for the following:
Failure to complete treatment course within 16 weeks of initial dose
Persistent moderate adverse reactions or unable to reduce corticosteroid dose to prednisone 7.5 mg daily (or equivalent)
Severe or life-threatening adverse reactions including:
Central nervous system or neuromuscular toxicity: Severe motor or sensory neuropathy, Guillain-Barré syndrome, or myasthenia gravis
Dermatologic toxicities: Stevens-Johnson syndrome, toxic epidermal necrolysis, or rash complicated by full thickness dermal ulceration, or necrotic, bullous, or hemorrhagic manifestations
Gastrointestinal toxicities: Colitis with abdominal pain, fever, ileus or peritoneal symptoms, increase in stool frequency (≥7 over baseline), stool incontinence, require IV hydration for >24 hours, or GI hemorrhage or perforation; grades 3/4 amylase or lipase increases (Weber, 2012)
Ophthalmic toxicities: Immune-mediated ocular disease unresponsive to topical immunosuppressive treatment
Severe immune-mediated reactions involving any organ system (eg, myocarditis [noninfectious], nephritis, pancreatitis, pneumonitis)

Administration IV: Infuse over 90 minutes through a non-pyrogenic, low protein-binding in-line filter. Do not administer with other medications. Flush with NS or D5W at the end of infusion

Monitoring Parameters Monitor liver function and evaluate for signs of hepatotoxicity prior to each dose; if hepatotoxicity develops, liver function should be monitored more frequently until resolves. If liver functions tests are >8 times ULN, monitor every other day until begin to fall, then weekly until normal (Weber, 2012). Monitor serum chemistries and adrenocorticotropic hormone (ACTH) prior to each dose. Monitor for signs of hypophysitis, adrenal insufficiency and thyroid disorders (eg, abdominal pain, fatigue, headache, hypotension, mental status changes, unusual bowel habits). Monitor TSH, free T_4 and cortisol levels (morning) at baseline, prior to dose, and as clinically indicated. Monitor for signs and symptoms of enterocolitis (abdominal pain, blood or mucus in stool or diarrhea, and intestinal perforation (peritoneal signs, ileus). Monitor for rash and pruritus. Monitor for signs of motor or sensory neuropathy (unilateral or bilateral weakness, sensory changes or paresthesia). Monitor for ocular toxicity at baseline, then at 4 to 8 weeks with further evaluations as clinically indicated (Renouf, 2012).

Dosage Forms Excipient information presented when available (limited, particularly for generics); consult specific product labeling.

Solution, Intravenous [preservative free]:
Yervoy: 50 mg/10 mL (10 mL); 200 mg/40 mL (40 mL) [contains polysorbate 80]

◆ IPOL see Poliovirus Vaccine (Inactivated) *on page 1465*

Ipratropium (Systemic) (i pra TROE pee um)

Brand Names: US Atrovent HFA
Brand Names: Canada Atrovent HFA; Gen-Ipratropium; Mylan-Ipratropium Sterinebs; Novo-Ipramide; Nu-Ipratropium; PMS-Ipratropium; ratio-Ipratropium UDV; Teva-Ipratropium Sterinebs
Index Terms Ipratropium Bromide
Pharmacologic Category Anticholinergic Agent
Use Chronic obstructive pulmonary disease: Maintenance treatment of bronchospasm associated with chronic obstructive pulmonary disease (COPD), including chronic bronchitis and emphysema
Pregnancy Considerations Teratogenic effects were not observed in animal studies. Inhaled ipratropium is recommended for use as additional therapy for pregnant women with severe asthma exacerbations.
Breast-Feeding Considerations It is not known if ipratropium (oral inhalation) is excreted in breast milk. The manufacturer recommends that caution be exercised when administering ipratropium (oral inhalation) to nursing women.
Contraindications Hypersensitivity to ipratropium, atropine (and its derivatives), or any component of the formulation
Warnings/Precautions Immediate hypersensitivity reactions (urticaria, angioedema, rash, bronchospasm) have been reported. Rarely, paradoxical bronchospasm may occur with use of inhaled bronchodilating agents; this should be distinguished from inadequate response. Not indicated for the initial treatment of acute episodes of bronchospasm where rescue therapy is required for rapid response. Should only be used in acute exacerbations of asthma in conjunction with short-acting beta-adrenergic agonists for acute episodes (NAEPP 2007). Use with caution in patients with myasthenia gravis, narrow-angle glaucoma, benign prostatic hyperplasia (BPH), or bladder neck obstruction

Adverse Reactions
>10%: Respiratory: Bronchitis (10% to 23%), COPD exacerbation (8% to 23%), sinusitis (1% to 11%)
1% to 10%:
Central nervous system: Headache (6% to 7%), dizziness (3%)
Gastrointestinal: Dyspepsia (1% to 5%), nausea (4%), xerostomia (2% to 4%), taste perversion (1%)
Genitourinary: Urinary tract infection (2% to 10%)
Neuromuscular & skeletal: Back pain (2% to 7%)
Respiratory: Dyspnea (7% to 8%), cough (>3%), rhinitis (>3%), upper respiratory infection (>3%)
Miscellaneous: Flu-like syndrome (4% to 8%)
<1% (Limited to important or life-threatening): Accommodation disorder, anaphylactic reaction, angioedema, bronchospasm, corneal edema, eye pain (acute), glaucoma, hypersensitivity reactions, hypotension, intraocular pressure increased, laryngospasm, palpitations, stomatitis, tachycardia, urinary retention

Drug Interactions
Metabolism/Transport Effects None known.
Avoid Concomitant Use
Avoid concomitant use of Ipratropium (Oral Inhalation) with any of the following: Aclidinium; Anticholinergic Agents; Cimetropium; Eluxadoline; Glucagon; Glycopyrrolate; Glycopyrrolate (Oral Inhalation); Levosulpiride; Loxapine; Potassium Chloride; Tiotropium; Umeclidinium

Increased Effect/Toxicity
Ipratropium (Oral Inhalation) may increase the levels/effects of: AbobotulinumtoxinA; Analgesics (Opioid); Anticholinergic Agents; Cannabinoid-Containing Products; Cimetropium; Eluxadoline; Glucagon; Glycopyrrolate; Glycopyrrolate (Oral Inhalation); Loxapine; Mirabegron; OnabotulinumtoxinA; Potassium Chloride; Ramosetron; RimabotulinumtoxinB; Thiazide Diuretics; Tiotropium; Topiramate

The levels/effects of Ipratropium (Oral Inhalation) may be increased by: Aclidinium; Mianserin; Pramlintide; Umeclidinium

Decreased Effect
Ipratropium (Oral Inhalation) may decrease the levels/effects of: Acetylcholinesterase Inhibitors; Gastrointestinal Agents (Prokinetic); Itopride; Levosulpiride; Secretin

The levels/effects of Ipratropium (Oral Inhalation) may be decreased by: Acetylcholinesterase Inhibitors

Storage/Stability

Aerosol: Store at controlled room temperature of 25°C (77°F). Do not store near heat or open flame.

Solution: Store at 15°C to 30°C (59°F to 86°F). Protect from light.

Mechanism of Action Blocks the action of acetylcholine at parasympathetic sites in bronchial smooth muscle causing bronchodilation; local application to nasal mucosa inhibits serous and seromucous gland secretions.

Pharmacodynamics/Kinetics

Onset of action: Bronchodilation: Within 15 minutes
  Peak effect: 1-2 hours

Duration: Oral inhalation: 2-4 hours; Nebulization: 4-5 hours, up to 7-8 hours in some patients

Absorption: Not readily absorbed into the systemic circulation from the surface of the lung or from the GI tract; ~7% absorbed after nebulization of a 2 mg dose

Distribution: 15% of dose reaches lower airways

Protein Binding: ≤9%

Metabolism: Partially metabolized to inactive ester hydrolysis products

Half-life elimination: 2 hours

Excretion: Urine (50%)

Dosing

Adult & Geriatric

COPD: Oral inhalation:

Nebulization: 500 mcg every 6 to 8 hours

Metered-dose inhaler (MDI): 2 inhalations 4 times daily; maximum dose: 12 inhalations in 24 hours

Asthma exacerbation, acute (moderate to severe) (off-label use): Oral inhalation: **Note:** Should be given in combination with a short-acting beta-adrenergic agonist.

Nebulization: 0.5 mg (500 mcg) every 20 minutes for 3 doses, then as needed (NAEPP 2007)

MDI: 8 inhalations every 20 minutes as needed for up to 3 hours (NAEPP 2007)

Pediatric

COPD: Oral inhalation: Nebulization: Children ≥12 years and Adolescents: Refer to adult dosing

Asthma exacerbation, acute (moderate to severe) (off-label use): Oral Inhalation: **Note:** Should be given in combination with a short-acting beta-adrenergic agonist

Children ≤5 years:

Nebulization: 0.25 mg (250 mcg) every 20 minutes for 1 hour (GINA 2015)

MDI: 2 inhalations every 20 minutes for 1 hour (GINA 2015)

Children ≤12 years:

Nebulization: 0.25 to 0.5 mg (250 to 500 mcg) every 20 minutes for 3 doses, then as needed (NAEPP 2007)

MDI: 4 to 8 inhalations every 20 minutes as needed for up to 3 hours (NAEPP 2007)

Adolescents ≥13 years: Refer to adult dosing.

Renal Impairment There are no dosage adjustments provided in the manufacturer's labeling (has not been studied).

Hepatic Impairment There are no dosage adjustments provided in the manufacturer's labeling (has not been studied).

Administration Avoid spraying into the eyes.

Atrovent HFA: Prior to initial use, prime inhaler by releasing 2 test sprays into the air. If the inhaler has not been used for >3 days, reprime.

Dosage Forms Considerations Atrovent HFA 12.9 g canister contains 200 inhalations.

Dosage Forms Excipient information presented when available (limited, particularly for generics); consult specific product labeling.

Aerosol Solution, Inhalation, as bromide:
  Atrovent HFA: 17 mcg/actuation (12.9 g) [contains alcohol, usp]

Solution, Inhalation, as bromide:
  Generic: 0.02% (2.5 mL)

Solution, Inhalation, as bromide [preservative free]:
  Generic: 0.02% (2.5 mL)

Ipratropium (Nasal) (i pra TROE pee um)

Brand Names: US Atrovent

Brand Names: Canada Alti-Ipratropium; Apo-Ipravent®; Atrovent®; Mylan-Ipratropium Solution

Index Terms Ipratropium Bromide

Pharmacologic Category Anticholinergic Agent

Use Symptomatic relief of rhinorrhea associated with the common cold and allergic and nonallergic rhinitis

Dosing

Adult & Geriatric

Colds (symptomatic relief of rhinorrhea): Safety and efficacy of use beyond 4 days not established: *Intranasal:* Nasal spray (0.06%): 2 sprays in each nostril 3-4 times/day

Allergic/nonallergic rhinitis: *Intranasal:* Nasal spray (0.03%): 2 sprays in each nostril 2-3 times/day

Seasonal allergic rhinitis (safety and efficacy of use beyond 3 weeks in patients with seasonal allergic rhinitis has not been established): *Intranasal:* Nasal spray (0.06%): 2 sprays in each nostril 4 times/day

Pediatric

Colds (symptomatic relief of rhinorrhea): Intranasal: Safety and efficacy of use beyond 4 days in patients with the common cold have not been established:

Children 5-11 years: 0.06%: 2 sprays in each nostril 3 times/day

Children ≥12 years and Adults: 0.06%: 2 sprays in each nostril 3-4 times/day

Allergic/nonallergic rhinitis: Intranasal: Children ≥6 years: Refer to adult dosing.

Seasonal allergic rhinitis: Intranasal: Children ≥5 years: Refer to adult dosing.

Renal Impairment No dosage adjustment provided in manufacturer's labeling (has not been studied); use with caution.

Hepatic Impairment No dosage adjustment provided in manufacturer's labeling (has not been studied); use with caution.

Additional Information Complete prescribing information should be consulted for additional detail.

Dosage Forms Considerations Atrovent 0.03% (21 mcg/spray) nasal solution 30 mL bottles contain 345 sprays, and the 0.06% (42 mcg/spray) 15 mL bottles contain 165 sprays.

Dosage Forms Excipient information presented when available (limited, particularly for generics); consult specific product labeling.

Solution, Nasal, as bromide:
  Atrovent: 0.03% (30 mL); 0.06% (15 mL)
  Generic: 0.03% (30 mL); 0.06% (15 mL)

Ipratropium and Albuterol
(i pra TROE pee um & al BYOO ter ole)

Brand Names: US Combivent Respimat; Combivent [DSC]; DuoNeb

Brand Names: Canada Apo-Salvent-Ipravent Sterules; Combivent Respimat; Combivent UDV; ratio-Ipra Sal UDV; Teva-Combo Sterinebs

Index Terms Albuterol and Ipratropium; Salbutamol and Ipratropium

Pharmacologic Category Anticholinergic Agent; Beta$_2$-Adrenergic Agonist

Use Treatment of COPD in those patients who are currently on a regular bronchodilator who continue to have bronchospasms and require a second bronchodilator

Dosing

Adult & Geriatric COPD: Inhalation:

Aerosol for inhalation:

Combivent [DSC]: Two inhalations 4 times daily (maximum: 12 inhalations/24 hours)

Combivent Respimat: One inhalation 4 times daily (maximum: 6 inhalations/24 hours)

Solution for nebulization: Initial: 3 mL every 6 hours (maximum: 3 mL every 4 hours)

Renal Impairment No dosage adjustment provided in manufacturer's labeling (has not been studied); use with caution.

Hepatic Impairment No dosage adjustment provided in manufacturer's labeling (has not been studied); use with caution.

Additional Information Complete prescribing information should be consulted for additional detail.

Dosage Forms Excipient information presented when available (limited, particularly for generics); consult specific product labeling. [DSC] = Discontinued product

Aerosol, for oral inhalation:

Combivent: Ipratropium bromide 18 mcg and albuterol (base) 90 mcg per inhalation (14.7 g) [contains chlorofluorocarbon, soya lecithin; 200 metered actuations] [DSC]

Solution, for nebulization: Ipratropium bromide 0.5 mg and albuterol (base) 2.5 mg per 3 mL (30s, 60s)

DuoNeb: Ipratropium bromide 0.5 mg and albuterol (base) 2.5 mg per 3 mL (30s, 60s)

Solution, for oral inhalation [spray]:

Combivent Respimat: Ipratropium bromide 20 mcg and albuterol (base) 100 mcg per inhalation (4 g) [contains benzalkonium chloride; 120 metered actuations]

Irbesartan (ir be SAR tan)

Brand Names: US Avapro

Brand Names: Canada ACT-Irbesartan; Apo-Irbesartan; Auro-Irbesartan; Ava-Irbesartan; Avapro; Dom-Irbesartan; JAMP-Irbesartan; Mylan-Irbesartan; PMS-Irbesartan; RAN-Irbesartan; ratio-Irbesartan; Sandoz-Irbesartan; Teva-Irbesartan

Pharmacologic Category Angiotensin II Receptor Blocker; Antihypertensive

Use

Diabetic nephropathy: Treatment of diabetic nephropathy with an elevated serum creatinine and proteinuria (>300 mg/day) in patients with type 2 diabetes and hypertension.

Hypertension: Treatment of hypertension alone or in combination with other antihypertensives

Guideline recommendations:

Hypertension: The 2014 guideline for the management of high blood pressure in adults (Eighth Joint National Committee [JNC 8; James, 2013]) recommends initiation of pharmacologic treatment to lower blood pressure for the following patients:

• Patients ≥60 years of age with systolic blood pressure (SBP) ≥150 mm Hg or diastolic blood pressure (DBP) ≥90 mm Hg. Goal of therapy is SBP <150 mm Hg and DBP <90 mm Hg.

• Patients <60 years of age with SBP ≥140 mm Hg or DBP ≥90 mm Hg. Goal of therapy is SBP <140 mm Hg and DBP <90 mm Hg.

• Patients ≥18 years of age with diabetes and SBP ≥140 mm Hg or DBP ≥90 mm Hg. Goal of therapy is SBP <140 mm Hg and DBP <90 mm Hg.

• Patients ≥18 years of age with chronic kidney disease (CKD) and SBP ≥140 mm Hg or DBP ≥90 mm Hg. Goal of therapy is SBP <140 mm Hg and DBP <90 mm Hg.

Chronic kidney disease (CKD) and hypertension: Regardless of race or diabetes status, the use of an ACE inhibitor (ACEI) or angiotensin receptor blocker (ARB) as initial therapy is recommended to improve kidney outcomes. In the general nonblack population (without CKD), including those with diabetes, initial antihypertensive treatment should consist of a thiazide-type diuretic, calcium channel blocker, ACEI, or ARB. In the general black population (without CKD), including those with diabetes, initial antihypertensive treatment should consist of a thiazide-type diuretic or a calcium channel blocker instead of an ACEI or ARB.

Coronary artery disease and hypertension: The American Heart Association, American College of Cardiology and American Society of Hypertension (AHA/ACC/ASH) 2015 scientific statement for the treatment of hypertension in patients with coronary artery disease (CAD) recommends the use of an ARB (or ACE inhibitor) as part of a regimen in patients with hypertension and chronic stable angina if there is prior MI, LV systolic dysfunction, diabetes mellitus, or CKD. A BP target of <140/90 mm Hg is reasonable for the secondary prevention of cardiovascular events. A lower target BP (<130/80 mm Hg) may be appropriate in some individuals with CAD, previous MI, stroke or transient ischemic attack, or CAD risk equivalents (AHA/ACC/ASH [Rosendorff 2015]).

Pregnancy Considerations [U.S. Boxed Warning]: Drugs that act on the renin-angiotensin system can cause injury and death to the developing fetus. Discontinue as soon as possible once pregnancy is detected. The use of drugs which act on the renin-angiotensin system are associated with oligohydramnios. Oligohydramnios, due to decreased fetal renal function, may lead to fetal lung hypoplasia and skeletal malformations. Use is also associated with anuria, hypotension, renal failure, skull hypoplasia, and death in the fetus/neonate. The exposed fetus should be monitored for fetal growth, amniotic fluid volume, and organ formation. Infants exposed *in utero* should be monitored for hyperkalemia, hypotension, and oliguria (exchange transfusions or dialysis may be needed). These adverse events are generally associated with maternal use in the second and third trimesters.

Untreated chronic maternal hypertension is also associated with adverse events in the fetus, infant, and mother. The use of angiotensin II receptor blockers is not recommended to treat chronic uncomplicated hypertension in pregnant women and should generally be avoided in women of reproductive potential (ACOG, 2013).

Breast-Feeding Considerations It is not known if irbesartan is excreted into breast milk. Due to the potential for serious adverse reactions in the nursing infant, the manufacturer recommends a decision be made whether to discontinue nursing or to discontinue the drug, taking into account the importance of treatment to the mother.

Contraindications

Hypersensitivity to irbesartan or any component of the formulation; concomitant use with aliskiren in patients with diabetes mellitus

Documentation of allergenic cross-reactivity for drugs in this class is limited. However, because of similarities in chemical structure and/or pharmacologic actions, the possibility of cross-sensitivity cannot be ruled out with certainty.

Canadian labeling: Additional contraindications (not in U.S. labeling): Concomitant use with aliskiren in patients with moderate to severe renal impairment (GFR <60 mL/minute/1.73 m^2)

Warnings/Precautions [U.S. Boxed Warning]: Drugs that act on the renin-angiotensin system can cause injury and death to the developing fetus. Discontinue as soon as possible once pregnancy is detected. May cause hyperkalemia; avoid potassium supplementation unless specifically required by health care provider. May be associated with deterioration of renal function and/or increases in serum creatinine, particularly in patients with low renal blood flow (eg, renal artery stenosis, heart failure) whose glomerular filtration rate (GFR) is dependent on efferent arteriolar vasoconstriction by angiotensin II. Avoid use or use a much smaller dose in patients who are intravascularly volume-depleted; use caution in patients with unstented unilateral or bilateral renal artery stenosis. When unstented bilateral renal artery stenosis is present, use is generally avoided due to the elevated risk of deterioration in renal function unless possible benefits outweigh risks. AUCs of irbesartan (not the active metabolite) are about 50% greater in patients with CrCl <30 mL/minute and are doubled in hemodialysis patients. In surgical patients on chronic angiotensin receptor blocker (ARB) therapy, intraoperative hypotension may occur with induction and maintenance of general anesthesia.

Potentially significant drug interactions may exist, requiring dose or frequency adjustment, additional monitoring, and/or selection of alternative therapy.

Angioedema has been reported rarely with some angiotensin II receptor antagonists (ARBs) and may occur at any time during treatment (especially following first dose). It may involve the head and neck (potentially compromising airway) or the intestine (presenting with abdominal pain). Patients with idiopathic or hereditary angioedema or previous angioedema associated with ACE-inhibitor therapy may be at an increased risk. Prolonged frequent monitoring may be required, especially if tongue, glottis, or larynx are involved, as they are associated with airway obstruction. Patients with a history of airway surgery may have a higher risk of airway obstruction. Discontinue therapy immediately if angioedema occurs. Aggressive early management is critical. Intramuscular (IM) administration of epinephrine may be necessary. Do not readminister to patients who have had angioedema with ARBs.

Adverse Reactions Unless otherwise indicated, percentage of incidence is reported for patients with hypertension.
>10%: Endocrine & metabolic: Hyperkalemia (19%, diabetic nephropathy; rarely seen in HTN)
1% to 10%:
  Cardiovascular: Orthostatic hypotension (5%, diabetic nephropathy)
  Central nervous system: Fatigue (4%), dizziness (10%, diabetic nephropathy)
  Gastrointestinal: Diarrhea (3%), dyspepsia (2%)
  Respiratory: Upper respiratory infection (9%), cough (2.8% versus 2.7% in placebo)
<1%, postmarketing, and/or case reports (Limited to important or life-threatening): Anemia (case report; Simonetti, 2007), angina, angioedema, arrhythmia, cardiopulmonary arrest, conjunctivitis, depression, dyspnea, ecchymosis, epistaxis, gout, heart failure, hepatitis, hypotension, jaundice, libido decreased, MI, orthostatic hypotension, paresthesia, renal failure, renal function impaired, sexual dysfunction, stroke, thrombocytopenia, transaminases increased, urticaria

Drug Interactions

Metabolism/Transport Effects Substrate of CYP2C9 (minor); **Note:** Assignment of Major/Minor substrate status based on clinically relevant drug interaction potential; **Inhibits** CYP2C8 (moderate), CYP2C9 (moderate), CYP2D6 (weak)

Avoid Concomitant Use

Avoid concomitant use of Irbesartan with any of the following: Amodiaquine

Increased Effect/Toxicity

Irbesartan may increase the levels/effects of: ACE Inhibitors; Amifostine; Amodiaquine; Antipsychotic Agents (Second Generation [Atypical]); ARIPiprazole; Bosentan; Cannabis; Carvedilol; Ciprofloxacin (Systemic); CycloSPORINE (Systemic); CYP2C8 Substrates; CYP2C9 Substrates; Dronabinol; Drospirenone; DULoxetine; Hypotension-Associated Agents; Levodopa; Lithium; Nonsteroidal Anti-Inflammatory Agents; Potassium-Sparing Diuretics; Sodium Phosphates; Tetrahydrocannabinol

The levels/effects of Irbesartan may be increased by: Alfuzosin; Aliskiren; Barbiturates; Brimonidine (Topical); Canagliflozin; Dapoxetine; Diazoxide; Eplerenone; Heparin; Heparin (Low Molecular Weight); Herbs (Hypotensive Properties); Molsidomine; Nicorandil; Obinutuzumab; Pentoxifylline; Phosphodiesterase 5 Inhibitors; Potassium Salts; Prostacyclin Analogues; Tolvaptan; Trimethoprim

Decreased Effect

The levels/effects of Irbesartan may be decreased by: Amphetamines; Herbs (Hypertensive Properties); Methylphenidate; Nonsteroidal Anti-Inflammatory Agents; Yohimbine

Storage/Stability Store at 25°C (77°F); excursions are permitted between 15°C and 30°C (59°F and 86°F).

Mechanism of Action Irbesartan is an angiotensin receptor antagonist. Angiotensin II acts as a vasoconstrictor. In addition to causing direct vasoconstriction, angiotensin II also stimulates the release of aldosterone. Once aldosterone is released, sodium as well as water are reabsorbed. The end result is an elevation in blood pressure. Irbesartan binds to the AT1 angiotensin II receptor. This binding prevents angiotensin II from binding to the receptor thereby blocking the vasoconstriction and the aldosterone secreting effects of angiotensin II.

Pharmacodynamics/Kinetics

Onset of action: Peak effect: 1 to 2 hours

Maximum effect: 3-6 hours postdose; with chronic dosing maximum effect: ~2 weeks

Duration: >24 hours

Absorption: Rapid and almost complete

Distribution: V_d: 53 to 93 L

Protein binding, plasma: 90%, primarily to albumin and alpha1 acid gylcoprotein

Metabolism: Hepatic, via glucuronide conjugation and oxidation; oxidation occurs primarily by cytochrome P450 isoenzyme CYP2C9

Bioavailability: 60% to 80%

Half-life elimination: Terminal: 11 to 15 hours

Time to peak, serum: 1.5 to 2 hours

Excretion: Feces (80%); urine (20%)

Dosing

Adult & Geriatric

Hypertension: Oral: 150 mg once daily; patients may be titrated to 300 mg once daily; usual dosage range (ASH/ISH [Weber, 2014]): 150 to 300 mg daily; target dose (JNC 8 [James, 2013]): 300 mg once daily. **Note:** Starting dose in volume-depleted patients should be 75 mg.

Nephropathy in patients with type 2 diabetes and hypertension: Oral: Target dose: 300 mg once daily

Pediatric

Hypertension: Oral:

Children ≥6 to 12 years (off-label use): Initial: 75 mg once daily; may be titrated to a maximum of 150 mg once daily (NHBPEP, 2004).

Adolescents (off-label use): Initial: 150 mg once daily; may be titrated to a maximum dose of 300 mg once daily (NHBPEP, 2004).

Renal Impairment

Mild to severe renal impairment: No dosage adjustment necessary unless the patient is also volume depleted.

Hemodialysis: Not removed by hemodialysis

Hepatic Impairment No dosage adjustment necessary.

Administration May be administered with or without food.

Monitoring Parameters Electrolytes, serum creatinine, BUN, urinalysis

Dosage Forms Excipient information presented when available (limited, particularly for generics); consult specific product labeling.

Tablet, Oral:

Avapro: 75 mg, 150 mg, 300 mg

Generic: 75 mg, 150 mg, 300 mg

Irbesartan and Hydrochlorothiazide

(ir be SAR tan & hye droe klor oh THYE a zide)

Brand Names: US Avalide

Brand Names: Canada ACT Irbesartan/HCT; Apo-Irbesartan/HCTZ; Avalide; Irbesartan-HCT; Irbesartan-HCTZ; JAMP-Irbesartan and Hydrochlorothiazide; Mint-Irbesartan/HCTZ; PMS-Irbesartan HCTZ; Ran-Irbesartan HCTZ; ratio-Irbesartan HCTZ; Sandoz-Irbesartan HCT; Teva-Irbesartan HCTZ

Index Terms Avapro HCT; Hydrochlorothiazide and Irbesartan

Pharmacologic Category Angiotensin II Receptor Blocker; Antihypertensive; Diuretic, Thiazide

Use Hypertension: Treatment of hypertension

Dosing

Adult & Geriatric Dose must be individualized.

Hypertension: Oral: **Note:** Maximum antihypertensive effects are attained within 2 to 4 weeks after initiation or a change in dose; however, if necessary, may carefully titrate dose as soon as after 1 week of treatment.

Add-on therapy: A patient who is not controlled with either agent alone may be switched to the combination product. The lowest dosage available is irbesartan 150 mg/hydrochlorothiazide 12.5 mg.

Initial therapy: Irbesartan 150 mg/hydrochlorothiazide 12.5 mg once daily. If initial response is inadequate, may titrate dose after 1 to 2 weeks (maximum daily dose: irbesartan 300 mg/hydrochlorothiazide 25 mg).

Renal Impairment

Mild-to-moderate impairment (CrCl >30 mL/minute): No dosage adjustment necessary; use with caution.

Severe impairment (CrCl ≤30 mL/minute): Use not recommended.

Hepatic Impairment No dosage adjustment necessary; use with caution.

Additional Information Complete prescribing information should be consulted for additional detail.

Dosage Forms Excipient information presented when available (limited, particularly for generics); consult specific product labeling. [DSC] = Discontinued product

Tablet, oral: 150/12.5: Irbesartan 150 mg and hydrochlorothiazide 12.5 mg; 300/12.5: Irbesartan 300 mg and hydrochlorothiazide 12.5 mg

Avalide 150/12.5: Irbesartan 150 mg and hydrochlorothiazide 12.5 mg

Avalide 300/12.5: Irbesartan 300 mg and hydrochlorothiazide 12.5 mg

Avalide 300/25: Irbesartan 300 mg and hydrochlorothiazide 25 mg [DSC]

◆ **Irbesartan-HCT (Can)** see Irbesartan and Hydrochlorothiazide *on page 980*

◆ **Irbesartan-HCTZ (Can)** see Irbesartan and Hydrochlorothiazide *on page 980*

◆ **Irenka** see DULoxetine *on page 610*

◆ **Iressa** see Gefitinib *on page 830*

◆ **IRESSA (Can)** see Gefitinib *on page 830*

Irinotecan (Conventional)

(eye rye no TEE kan con VEN sha nal)

Brand Names: US Camptosar

Brand Names: Canada Camptosar; Irinotecan For Injection; Irinotecan Hydrochloride Injection; Irinotecan Hydrochloride Trihydrate For Injection; Irinotecan Hydrochloride Trihydrate Injection

Index Terms Camptothecin-11; Conventional Irinotecan; CPT-11; Irinotecan HCl; Irinotecan Hydrochloride

Pharmacologic Category Antineoplastic Agent, Camptothecin; Antineoplastic Agent, Topoisomerase I Inhibitor

Use Colorectal cancer, metastatic: Treatment of metastatic carcinoma of the colon or rectum

Pregnancy Considerations Adverse events were observed in animal reproduction studies. Information related to the use of irinotecan (conventional) during pregnancy is limited (Cirillo 2012; Taylor 2009). May cause fetal harm if administered during pregnancy. Women of childbearing potential should avoid becoming pregnant while receiving treatment.

Breast-Feeding Considerations It is not known if irinotecan is excreted in breast milk. Due to the potential for serious adverse reactions in the nursing infant, the manufacturer recommends a decision be made to discontinue nursing or to discontinue the drug, taking into account the importance of treatment to the mother.

Contraindications Hypersensitivity to irinotecan or any component of the formulation

Warnings/Precautions Hazardous agent - use appropriate precautions for handling and disposal (NIOSH 2014 [group 1]). Severe hypersensitivity reactions (including anaphylaxis) have occurred. Monitor closely; discontinue therapy if hypersensitivity occurs. Irinotecan is an irritant; avoid extravasation. If extravasation occurs, the manufacturer recommends flushing the external site with sterile water and applying ice.

[US Boxed Warning]: Severe diarrhea may be dose-limiting and potentially fatal; early-onset and late-onset diarrhea may occur. Early diarrhea occurs during or within 24 hours of receiving irinotecan and is characterized by cholinergic symptoms; may be prevented or treated with atropine. Late diarrhea may be life-threatening and should be promptly treated with loperamide. Antibiotics may be necessary if patient develops ileus, fever, or severe neutropenia. Interrupt treatment and reduce subsequent doses for severe diarrhea. Early diarrhea is generally transient and rarely severe; cholinergic symptoms may include increased salivation, rhinitis, miosis, diaphoresis, flushing, abdominal cramping, and lacrimation; bradycardia may also occur. Cholinergic symptoms may occur more frequently with higher irinotecan doses. Late diarrhea occurs more than 24 hours after treatment, which may lead to dehydration, electrolyte imbalance, or sepsis. Late diarrhea may be complicated by colitis, ulceration, bleeding, ileus, obstruction, or infection; cases of megacolon and intestinal perforation have been reported. The median time to onset for late diarrhea is 5 days with every-3-week irinotecan dosing and 11 days with weekly dosing. Advise patients to have loperamide readily available for the treatment of late diarrhea. Patients with diarrhea should be carefully monitored and treated promptly; may require fluid and electrolyte therapy. Bowel function should be returned to baseline for at least 24 hours prior to resumption of weekly irinotecan dosing. Avoid diuretics and laxatives in patients experiencing diarrhea. Patients >65 years of age are at greater risk for early and late diarrhea. A dose reduction is recommended for patients ≥70 years of age receiving the every-3-week regimen. Irinotecan is associated with a moderate emetic potential; antiemetics are recommended to prevent nausea and vomiting (Basch 2011; Dupuis 2011; Roila 2010).

[US Boxed Warning]: May cause severe myelosuppression. Deaths due to sepsis following severe neutropenia have been reported. Complications due to neutropenia should be promptly managed with antibiotics. Therapy should be temporarily withheld if neutropenic fever occurs or if the absolute neutrophil count is <1,000/mm³; reduce the dose upon recovery to an absolute neutrophil count ≥1,000/mm³. Patients who have previously received pelvic/abdominal radiation therapy have an increased risk of severe bone marrow suppression; the incidence of grade 3 or 4 neutropenia was higher in patients receiving weekly irinotecan who have previously received pelvic/abdominal radiation therapy. Concurrent radiation therapy is not recommended with irinotecan (based on limited data). Fatal cases of interstitial pulmonary disease (IPD)-like events have been reported with single-agent and combination therapy. Risk factors for pulmonary toxicity include preexisting lung disease, use of pulmonary toxic medications, radiation therapy, and colony-stimulating factors. Patients with risk factors should be monitored for respiratory symptoms before and during irinotecan treatment. Promptly evaluate progressive changes in baseline pulmonary symptoms or any new-onset pulmonary symptoms (eg, dyspnea, cough, fever). Discontinue all chemotherapy if IPD is diagnosed.

Patients with even modest elevations in total serum bilirubin levels (1 to 2 mg/dL) have a significantly greater likelihood of experiencing first-course grade 3 or 4 neutropenia than those with bilirubin levels that were <1 mg/dL. Patients with abnormal glucuronidation of bilirubin, such as those with Gilbert's syndrome, may also be at greater risk of myelosuppression when receiving therapy with irinotecan. Use caution when treating patients with known hepatic dysfunction or hyperbilirubinemia exposure to the active metabolite (SN-38) is increased; toxicities may be increased. Dosage adjustments should be considered.

Patients homozygous for the UGT1A1*28 allele are at increased risk of neutropenia; initial one-level dose reduction should be considered for both single-agent and combination regimens. Heterozygous carriers of the UGT1A1*28 allele may also be at increased neutropenic risk; however, most patients have tolerated normal starting doses. A test is available for clinical determination of UGT phenotype, although a dose reduction is already recommended in patients who have experienced toxicity.

Renal impairment and acute renal failure have been reported, possibly due to dehydration secondary to diarrhea. Use with caution in patients with renal impairment; not recommended in patients on dialysis. Patients with bowel obstruction should not be treated with irinotecan until resolution of obstruction. Contains sorbitol; do not use in patients with hereditary fructose intolerance. Thromboembolic events have been reported. Higher rates of hospitalization, neutropenic fever, thromboembolism, first-cycle discontinuation, and early mortality were observed in patients with a performance status of 2 than in patients with a performance status of 0 or 1. Except as part of a clinical trial, use in combination with fluorouracil and leucovorin administered for 4 or 5 consecutive days ("Mayo Clinic" regimen) is not recommended due to increased toxicity. Potentially significant interactions may exist, requiring dose or frequency adjustment, additional monitoring, and/or selection of alternative therapy. CYP3A4 enzyme inducers may decrease exposure to irinotecan and SN-38 (active metabolite); enzyme inhibitors may increase exposure; for use in patients with CNS tumors (off-label use), selection of antiseizure medications that are not enzyme inducers is preferred. Irinotecan (conventional) and irinotecan (liposomal) are **NOT** interchangeable. Dosing differs between formulations; verify intended product and dose prior to preparation and administration.

Adverse Reactions Frequency of adverse reactions reported for single-agent use of irinotecan only.
>10%:
   Cardiovascular: Vasodilation (9% to 11%)
   Central nervous system: Cholinergic toxicity (47% - includes rhinitis, increased salivation, miosis, lacrimation, diaphoresis, flushing and intestinal hyperperistalsis); fever (44% to 45%), pain (23% to 24%), dizziness (15% to 21%), insomnia (19%), headache (17%), chills (14%)
   Dermatologic: Alopecia (46% to 72%), rash (13% to 14%)
   Endocrine & metabolic: Dehydration (15%)
   Gastrointestinal: Diarrhea, late (83% to 88%; grade 3/4: 14% to 31%), diarrhea, early (43% to 51%; grade 3/4: 7% to 22%), nausea (70% to 86%), abdominal pain (57% to 68%), vomiting (62% to 67%), cramps (57%), anorexia (44% to 55%), constipation (30% to 32%), mucositis (30%), weight loss (30%), flatulence (12%), stomatitis (12%)
   Hematologic: Anemia (60% to 97%; grades 3/4: 5% to 7%), leukopenia (63% to 96%, grades 3/4: 14% to 28%), thrombocytopenia (96%, grades 3/4: 1% to 4%), neutropenia (30% to 96%; grades 3/4: 14% to 31%)
   Hepatic: Bilirubin increased (84%), alkaline phosphatase increased (13%)
   Neuromuscular & skeletal: Weakness (69% to 76%), back pain (14%)
   Respiratory: Dyspnea (22%), cough (17% to 20%), rhinitis (16%)
   Miscellaneous: Diaphoresis (16%), infection (14%)
1% to 10%:
   Cardiovascular: Edema (10%), hypotension (6%), thromboembolic events (5%)
   Central nervous system: Somnolence (9%), confusion (3%)
   Gastrointestinal: Abdominal fullness (10%), dyspepsia (10%)
   Hematologic: Neutropenic fever (grades 3/4: 2% to 6%), hemorrhage (grades 3/4: 1% to 5%), neutropenic infection (grades 3/4: 1% to 2%)
   Hepatic: AST increased (10%), ascites and/or jaundice (grades 3/4: 9%)
   Respiratory: Pneumonia (4%)
<1%, postmarketing, and/or case reports: ALT increased, amylase increased, anaphylactoid reaction, anaphylaxis, angina, arterial thrombosis, bleeding, bradycardia, cardiac arrest, cerebral infarct, cerebrovascular accident, circulatory failure, colitis, dysrhythmia, embolus, gastrointestinal bleeding, gastrointestinal obstruction, hepatomegaly, hyperglycemia, hypersensitivity, hyponatremia, ileus, interstitial pulmonary disease (IPD), intestinal perforation, ischemic colitis, lipase increased, lymphocytopenia, megacolon, MI, myocardial ischemia, neutropenic typhlitis, pancreatitis, paresthesia, peripheral vascular disorder, pulmonary embolus; pulmonary toxicity

(dyspnea, fever, reticulonodular infiltrates on chest x-ray); renal failure (acute), renal impairment, thrombocytopenia (immune mediated), thrombophlebitis, thrombosis, typhlitis, ulcerative colitis

Note: In limited pediatric experience, dehydration (often associated with severe hypokalemia and hyponatremia) was among the most significant grade 3/4 adverse events, with a frequency up to 29%. In addition, grade 3/4 infection was reported in 24%.

Drug Interactions

Metabolism/Transport Effects Substrate of BCRP, CYP3A4 (major), P-glycoprotein, SLCO1B1, UGT1A1; **Note:** Assignment of Major/Minor substrate status based on clinically relevant drug interaction potential

Avoid Concomitant Use

Avoid concomitant use of Irinotecan (Conventional) with any of the following: BCG (Intravesical); Conivaptan; CYP3A4 Inducers (Strong); CYP3A4 Inhibitors (Strong); Deferiprone; Dipyrone; Fusidic Acid (Systemic); Idelalisib; Natalizumab; Pimecrolimus; St Johns Wort; Tacrolimus (Topical); Tofacitinib; UGT1A1 Inhibitors; Vaccines (Live)

Increased Effect/Toxicity

Irinotecan (Conventional) may increase the levels/effects of: CloZAPine; Deferiprone; Fingolimod; Leflunomide; Natalizumab; Tofacitinib; Vaccines (Live)

The levels/effects of Irinotecan (Conventional) may be increased by: Aprepitant; Conivaptan; CYP3A4 Inhibitors (Moderate); CYP3A4 Inhibitors (Strong); Dasatinib; Denosumab; Dipyrone; Fosaprepitant; Fusidic Acid (Systemic); Idelalisib; Ivacaftor; Luliconazole; Mifepristone; Netupitant; Osimertinib; Palbociclib; P-glycoprotein/ABCB1 Inhibitors; Pimecrolimus; Ranolazine; Roflumilast; Rolapitant; Simeprevir; SORAfenib; Stiripentol; Tacrolimus (Topical); Teriflunomide; Trastuzumab; UGT1A1 Inhibitors

Decreased Effect

Irinotecan (Conventional) may decrease the levels/effects of: BCG (Intravesical); Coccidioides immitis Skin Test; Sipuleucel-T; Vaccines (Inactivated); Vaccines (Live)

The levels/effects of Irinotecan (Conventional) may be decreased by: Bosentan; CYP3A4 Inducers (Moderate); CYP3A4 Inducers (Strong); Dabrafenib; Deferasirox; Echinacea; Osimertinib; P-glycoprotein/ABCB1 Inducers; Siltuximab; St Johns Wort; Tocilizumab

Preparation for Administration Hazardous agent; use appropriate precautions for handling and disposal (NIOSH 2014 [group 1]). Dilute in D_5W (preferred) or NS to a final concentration of 0.12 to 2.8 mg/mL.

Storage/Stability Store intact vials at 15°C to 30°C (59°F to 86°F). Protect from light; retain vials in original carton until use. Solutions diluted in NS may precipitate if refrigerated. Solutions diluted in D_5W are stable for 24 hours at room temperature or 48 hours under refrigeration at 2°C to 8°C (36°F to 46°F), although the manufacturer recommends use within 24 hours if refrigerated, or within 4 to 12 hours (manufacturer dependent; refer to specific prescribing information) at room temperature (including infusion time) only if prepared under strict aseptic conditions (eg, laminar flow hood). Do not freeze. Undiluted commercially available injectable solution prepared in oral syringes is stable for 21 days under refrigeration (Wagner 2010).

Mechanism of Action Irinotecan and its active metabolite (SN-38) bind reversibly to topoisomerase I-DNA complex preventing religation of the cleaved DNA strand. This results in the accumulation of cleavable complexes and double-strand DNA breaks. As mammalian cells cannot efficiently repair these breaks, cell death consistent with S-phase cell cycle specificity occurs, leading to termination of cellular replication.

Pharmacodynamics/Kinetics

Distribution:

Children and Adolescents: ~37 L/m^2 (range: 15.2-77 L/m^2) (Ma, 2000); distributes to pleural fluid, sweat, and saliva

Adults: 33-150 L/m^2

Protein binding, plasma: Predominantly albumin; Irinotecan: 30% to 68%, SN-38 (active metabolite): ~95%

Metabolism: Primarily hepatic to SN-38 (active metabolite) by carboxylesterase enzymes; may also undergo CYP3A4-mediated metabolism to inactive metabolites (one of which may be hydrolyzed to release SN-38). SN-38 undergoes conjugation by UDP-glucuronosyl transferase 1A1 (UGT1A1) to form a glucuronide metabolite. SN-38 is increased by UGT1A1*28 polymorphism (10% of North Americans are homozygous for UGT1A1*28 allele).

Bioavailability: Median: 9%; increased in presence of gefitinib (median: 42%) (Furman 2009)

Half-life elimination:

Children and Adolescents (Ma 2000): Irinotecan: 2.66 hours (range: 1.82-4.47 hours); SN-38 (active metabolite): 1.58 hours (range: 0.29-8.28 hours)

Adults: Irinotecan: 6 to 12 hours; SN-38: ~10 to 20 hours

Time to peak:

Irinotecan: Oral: Children and Adolescents: 3 hours (Wagner 2010a)

SN-38: Following 90-minute infusion: ~1 hour

Excretion: Urine: Irinotecan (11% to 20%), metabolites (SN-38 <1%, SN-38 glucuronide, 3%)

Dosing

Adult

Note: A reduction in the starting dose by one dose level should be considered for prior pelvic/abdominal radiotherapy, performance status of 2, or known homozygosity for UGT1A1*28 allele (subsequent dosing/adjustments should be based on individual tolerance). Irinotecan (conventional) and irinotecan (liposomal) are **NOT** interchangeable. Dosing differs between formulations; verify intended product and dose prior to preparation and administration.

Premedications: Consider premedication of atropine 0.25 to 1 mg IV or SubQ in patients with cholinergic symptoms (eg, increased salivation, rhinitis, miosis, diaphoresis, abdominal cramping) or early-onset diarrhea. Irinotecan is associated with a moderate emetic potential; antiemetics are recommended to prevent nausea and vomiting (Basch 2011; Dupuis 2011; Roila 2010).

Colorectal cancer, metastatic (single-agent therapy): IV:

Weekly regimen: 125 mg/m^2 over 90 minutes on days 1, 8, 15, and 22 of a 6-week treatment cycle (may adjust upward to 150 mg/m^2 if tolerated)

Adjusted dose level -1: 100 mg/m^2

Adjusted dose level -2: 75 mg/m^2

Further adjust to 50 mg/m^2 (in decrements of 25 to 50 mg/m^2) if needed

Once-every-3-week regimen: 350 mg/m^2 over 90 minutes, once every 3 weeks

Adjusted dose level -1: 300 mg/m^2

Adjusted dose level -2: 250 mg/m^2

Further adjust to 200 mg/m^2 (in decrements of 25 to 50 mg/m^2) if needed

Colorectal cancer, metastatic (in combination with fluorouracil and leucovorin): IV: Six-week (42-day) cycle:

Regimen 1: 125 mg/m^2 over 90 minutes on days 1, 8, 15, and 22; to be given in combination with bolus leucovorin and fluorouracil (leucovorin administered immediately following irinotecan; fluorouracil immediately following leucovorin)

Adjusted dose level -1: 100 mg/m^2

Adjusted dose level -2: 75 mg/m^2

Further adjust if needed in decrements of ~20%

Regimen 2: 180 mg/m^2 over 90 minutes on days 1, 15, and 29; to be given in combination with infusional leucovorin and bolus/infusion fluorouracil (leucovorin administered immediately following irinotecan; fluorouracil immediately following leucovorin)

Adjusted dose level -1: 150 mg/m^2

Adjusted dose level -2: 120 mg/m^2

Further adjust if needed in decrements of ~20%

Colorectal cancer, metastatic (off-label dosing): IV: FOLFOXIRI regimen: 165 mg/m^2 over 1 hour once every 2 weeks (in combination with oxaliplatin, leucovorin, and fluorouracil) (Falcone 2007)

Cervical cancer, recurrent or metastatic (off-label use): IV: 125 mg/m^2 over 90 minutes once weekly for 4 consecutive weeks followed by a 2-week rest during each 6 week treatment cycle (Verschraegen 1997)

CNS tumor, recurrent glioblastoma (off-label use): IV: 125 mg/m^2 over 90 minutes once every 2 weeks (in combination with bevacizumab). **NOTE:** In patients taking concurrent antiepileptic enzyme-inducing medications irinotecan dose was increased to 340 mg/m^2 (Friedman 2009; Vredenburgh 2007).

Esophageal cancer, metastatic or locally advanced (off-label use): IV: 65 mg/m^2 over 90 minutes days 1, 8, 15, and 22 of a 6-week treatment cycle (in combination with cisplatin) (Ajani 2002; Ilson 1999) **or** 180 mg/m^2 over 90 minutes every 2 weeks (in combination with leucovorin and fluorouracil) (Guimbaud 2014) **or** 250 mg/m^2 every 3 weeks (in combination with capecitabine) (Leary 2009; Moehler 2010)

Ewing sarcoma, recurrent or progressive (off-label use): IV: 20 mg/m^2 days 1 to 5 and days 8 to 12 every 3 weeks (in combination with temozolomide) (Casey 2009)

Gastric cancer, metastatic or locally advanced (off-label use): IV: 150 mg/m^2 (as a single agent) on days 1 and 15 of a 4-week treatment cycle (Hironaka 2013) **or** 65 mg/m^2 over 90 minutes days 1, 8, 15, and 22 of a 6-week treatment cycle (in combination with cisplatin) (Ajani 2002) **or** 70 mg/m^2 over 90 minutes on days 1 and 15 of a 4-week treatment cycle (in combination with cisplatin) for up to 6 cycles (Park 2005) **or** 180 mg/m^2 over 90 minutes every 2 weeks (in combination with leucovorin and fluorouracil) (Bouche 2004; Guimbaud 2014) **or** 250 mg/m^2 every 3 weeks (in combination with capecitabine) (Moehler 2010)

Non-small cell lung cancer, advanced (off-label use): IV: 60 mg/m^2 days 1, 8, and 15 every 4 weeks (in combination with cisplatin) (Ohe 2007)

Ovarian cancer, recurrent, platinum- and taxane-resistant (off-label use): IV: 100 mg/m^2 days 1, 8, and 15 every 4 weeks (as a single-agent) for up to 6 cycles (Matsumoto 2006)

Pancreatic cancer, advanced (off-label use): IV: FOL-FIRINOX regimen: 180 mg/m^2 over 90 minutes every 2 weeks (in combination with oxaliplatin, leucovorin, and fluorouracil) (Conroy 2005; Conroy 2011)

Small cell lung cancer, extensive stage (off-label use): IV: 60 mg/m^2 days 1, 8, and 15 every 4 weeks (in combination with cisplatin) (Noda 2002) **or** 65 mg/m^2 days 1 and 8 every 3 weeks (in combination with cisplatin) (Hanna 2006) **or** 175 mg/m^2 day 1 every 3 weeks (in combination with carboplatin) (Hermes 2008) **or** 50 mg/m^2 days 1, 8 and 15 every 4 weeks (in combination with carboplatin) (Schmittel 2006)

Geriatric

Weekly dosing schedule: No dosing adjustment is recommended

Every 3-week dosing colorectal cancer schedule: Recommended initial dose is 300 mg/m^2/dose for patients ≥70 years

Pediatric See **"Note"** in adult dosing.

Ewing sarcoma, recurrent or progressive (off-label use): IV: Refer to adult dosing.

Rhabdomyosarcoma, relapsed/refractory (off-label use; Vassal 2007): IV:

Children <10 kg: 20 mg/kg once every 3 weeks

Children ≥10 kg and Adolescents: 600 mg/m^2 once every 3 weeks

Renal Impairment

Renal impairment: There are no dosage adjustments provided in the manufacturer's labeling (has not been studied); use with caution.

Dialysis: Use in patients with dialysis is not recommended by the manufacturer; however, literature suggests reducing weekly dose from 125 mg/m^2 to 50 mg/m^2 and administer after hemodialysis or on non-dialysis days (Janus 2010).

Hepatic Impairment

Manufacturer's labeling:

Liver metastases with normal hepatic function: No dosage adjustment necessary.

Bilirubin >ULN to ≤2 mg/dL: Consider reducing initial dose by one dose level

Bilirubin >2 mg/dL: Use is not recommended

Alternate recommendations: The following adjustments have also been recommended:

Bilirubin 1.5 to 3 mg/dL: Administer 75% of dose (Floyd 2006)

Bilirubin 1.51 to 3 times ULN: Reduce dose from 350 mg/m^2 every 3 weeks to 200 mg/m^2 every 3 weeks (Raymond 2002)

Obesity *ASCO Guidelines for appropriate chemotherapy dosing in obese adults with cancer:* Utilize patient's actual body weight (full weight) for calculation of body surface area- or weight-based dosing, particularly when the intent of therapy is curative; manage regimen-related toxicities in the same manner as for nonobese patients; if a dose reduction is utilized due to toxicity, consider resumption of full weight-based dosing with subsequent cycles, especially if cause of toxicity (eg, hepatic or renal impairment) is resolved (Griggs 2012).

Adjustment for Toxicity It is recommended that new courses begin only after the granulocyte count recovers to ≥1,500/mm^3, the platelet counts recover to ≥100,000/mm^3, and treatment-related diarrhea has fully resolved. Depending on the patient's ability to tolerate therapy, doses should be adjusted in increments of 25 to 50 mg/m^2. Treatment should be delayed 1 to 2 weeks to allow for recovery from treatment-related toxicities. If the patient has not recovered after a 2-week delay, consider discontinuing irinotecan. See tables.

Colorectal Cancer: Single-Agent Schedule: Recommended Dosage Modifications[1]

Toxicity NCI Grade[2] (Value)	During a Cycle of Therapy	At Start of Subsequent Cycles of Therapy (After Adequate Recovery), Compared to Starting Dose in Previous Cycle[1]	
	Weekly	Weekly	Once Every 3 Weeks
No toxicity	Maintain dose level	↑ 25 mg/m^2 up to a maximum dose of 150 mg/m^2	Maintain dose level
Neutropenia			
Grade 1 (1,500 to 1,999/mm^3)	Maintain dose level	Maintain dose level	Maintain dose level
Grade 2 (1,000 to 1,499/mm^3)	↓ 25 mg/m^2	Maintain dose level	Maintain dose level
Grade 3 (500 to 999/mm^3)	Omit dose until resolved to ≤ grade 2, then ↓ 25 mg/m^2	↓ 25 mg/m^2	↓ 50 mg/m^2
Grade 4 (<500/mm^3)	Omit dose until resolved to ≤ grade 2, then ↓ 50 mg/m^2	↓ 50 mg/m^2	↓ 50 mg/m^2
Neutropenic Fever (grade 4 neutropenia and ≥ grade 2 fever)	Omit dose until resolved, then ↓ 50 mg/m^2	↓ 50 mg/m^2	↓ 50 mg/m^2
Other Hematologic Toxicities	Dose modifications for leukopenia, thrombocytopenia, and anemia during a course of therapy and at the start of subsequent courses of therapy are based on NCI toxicity criteria and are the same as recommended for neutropenia above.		
Diarrhea			
Grade 1 (2 to 3 stools/day > pretreatment)	Maintain dose level	Maintain dose level	Maintain dose level
Grade 2 (4 to 6 stools/day > pretreatment)	↓ 25 mg/m^2	Maintain dose level	Maintain dose level
Grade 3 (7 to 9 stools/day > pretreatment)	Omit dose until resolved to ≤ grade 2, then ↓ 25 mg/m^2	↓ 25 mg/m^2	↓ 50 mg/m^2
Grade 4 (≥10 stools/day > pretreatment)	Omit dose until resolved to ≤ grade 2, then ↓ 50 mg/m^2	↓ 50 mg/m^2	↓ 50 mg/m^2
Other Nonhematologic Toxicities[3]			
Grade 1	Maintain dose level	Maintain dose level	Maintain dose level
Grade 2	↓ 25 mg/m^2	↓ 25 mg/m^2	↓ 50 mg/m^2
Grade 3	Omit dose until resolved to ≤ grade 2, then ↓ 25 mg/m^2	↓ 25 mg/m^2	↓ 50 mg/m^2
Grade 4	Omit dose until resolved to ≤ grade 2, then ↓ 50 mg/m^2	↓ 50 mg/m^2	↓ 50 mg/m^2

[1]All dose modifications should be based on the worst preceding toxicity.

[2]National Cancer Institute Common Toxicity Criteria (version 1.0).

[3]Excludes alopecia, anorexia, asthenia.

Colorectal Cancer: Combination Schedules: Recommended Dosage Modifications[1]

Toxicity NCI[2] Grade (Value)	During a Cycle of Therapy	At the Start of Subsequent Cycles of Therapy (After Adequate Recovery), Compared to the Starting Dose in the Previous Cycle[1]
No toxicity	Maintain dose level	Maintain dose level
Neutropenia		
Grade 1 (1,500 to 1,999/mm^3)	Maintain dose level	Maintain dose level
Grade 2 (1,000 to 1,499/mm^3)	↓ 1 dose level	Maintain dose level
Grade 3 (500 to 999/mm^3)	Omit dose until resolved to ≤ grade 2, then ↓ 1 dose level	↓ 1 dose level
Grade 4 (<500/mm^3)	Omit dose until resolved to ≤ grade 2, then ↓ 2 dose levels	↓ 2 dose levels
Neutropenic Fever (grade 4 neutropenia and ≥ grade 2 fever)	Omit dose until resolved, then ↓ 2 dose levels	
Other Hematologic Toxicities	Dose modifications for leukopenia or thrombocytopenia during a course of therapy and at the start of subsequent courses of therapy are also based on NCI toxicity criteria and are the same as recommended for neutropenia above.	
Diarrhea		
Grade 1 (2 to 3 stools/day > pretreatment)	Delay dose until resolved to baseline, then give same dose	Maintain dose level
Grade 2 (4 to 6 stools/day > pretreatment)	Omit dose until resolved to baseline, then ↓ 1 dose level	Maintain dose level
Grade 3 (7 to 9 stools/day > pretreatment)	Omit dose until resolved to baseline, then ↓ by 1 dose level	↓ 1 dose level
Grade 4 (≥10 stools/day > pretreatment)	Omit dose until resolved to baseline, then ↓ 2 dose levels	↓ 2 dose levels

(continued)

983

Colorectal Cancer: Combination Schedules: Recommended Dosage Modifications[1] *(continued)*

Toxicity NCI[2] Grade (Value)	During a Cycle of Therapy	At the Start of Subsequent Cycles of Therapy (After Adequate Recovery), Compared to the Starting Dose in the Previous Cycle[1]
Other Nonhematologic Toxicities[3]		
Grade 1	Maintain dose level	Maintain dose level
Grade 2	Omit dose until resolved to ≤ grade 1, then ↓ 1 dose level	Maintain dose level
Grade 3	Omit dose until resolved to ≤ grade 2, then ↓ 1 dose level	↓ 1 dose level
Grade 4	Omit dose until resolved to ≤ grade 2, then ↓ 2 dose levels	↓ 2 dose levels
Mucositis and/or stomatitis	Decrease only 5-FU, not irinotecan	Decrease only 5-FU, not irinotecan

[1]All dose modifications should be based on the worst preceding toxicity.

[2]National Cancer Institute Common Toxicity Criteria (version 1.0).

[3]Excludes alopecia, anorexia, asthenia.

Dietary Considerations Contains sorbitol; do not use in patients with hereditary fructose intolerance.

Administration Administer by IV infusion, usually over 90 minutes. Irinotecan is associated with a moderate emetic potential (Basch 2011; Dupuis 2011; Roila 2010); premedication with dexamethasone and a 5-HT$_3$ blocker is recommended 30 minutes prior to administration; prochlorperazine may be considered for subsequent use (if needed). Consider atropine 0.25 to 1 mg IV or SubQ as premedication for or treatment of cholinergic symptoms (eg, increased salivation, rhinitis, miosis, diaphoresis, abdominal cramping) or early onset diarrhea.

The recommended regimen to manage late diarrhea is loperamide 4 mg orally at onset of late diarrhea, followed by 2 mg every 2 hours (or 4 mg every 4 hours at night) until 12 hours have passed without a bowel movement. If diarrhea recurs, then repeat administration. Loperamide should not be used for more than 48 consecutive hours.

Hazardous agent; use appropriate precautions for handling and disposal (NIOSH 2014 [group 1]).

Monitoring Parameters CBC with differential, platelet count, and hemoglobin with each dose; bilirubin, electrolytes (with severe diarrhea); bowel movements and hydration status; signs/symptoms of pulmonary toxicity or hypersensitivity reactions; monitor infusion site for signs of inflammation and avoid extravasation

A test is available for genotyping of UGT1A1; however, use of the test is not widely accepted and a dose reduction is already recommended in patients who have experienced toxicity.

Dosage Forms Excipient information presented when available (limited, particularly for generics); consult specific product labeling.

Solution, Intravenous, as hydrochloride:
Camptosar: 40 mg/2 mL (2 mL); 100 mg/5 mL (5 mL); 300 mg/15 mL (15 mL)
Generic: 40 mg/2 mL (2 mL); 100 mg/5 mL (5 mL); 500 mg/25 mL (25 mL)

Solution, Intravenous, as hydrochloride [preservative free]:
Generic: 40 mg/2 mL (2 mL); 100 mg/5 mL (5 mL)

Irinotecan (Liposomal)
(eye rye no TEE kan lye po SO mal)

Brand Names: US Onivyde

Index Terms Irinotecan Liposome; Liposomal Irinotecan; Liposome-Encapsulated Irinotecan Hydrochloride PEP02; MM-398; Onivyde

Pharmacologic Category Antineoplastic Agent, Camptothecin; Antineoplastic Agent, Topoisomerase I Inhibitor

Use

Pancreatic adenocarcinoma, metastatic: Treatment of metastatic adenocarcinoma of the pancreas (in combination with fluorouracil and leucovorin) disease progression following gemcitabine-based therapy.

Limitations of use: Irinotecan (liposomal) is not indicated as a single agent for the treatment of metastatic adenocarcinoma of the pancreas.

Pregnancy Considerations Animal reproduction studies have not been conducted with the liposomal formulation. Based on the mechanism of action as well as animal data using irinotecan (conventional), irinotecan (liposomal) may cause fetal harm if administered during pregnancy. Women of childbearing potential should use effective contraception while receiving treatment and avoid pregnancy for one month following the last dose. Males with female partners of reproductive potential should use condoms during therapy and for four months following the last dose.

Breast-Feeding Considerations It is not known if irinotecan (liposomal) is excreted in breast milk. Due to the potential for serious adverse reactions in the nursing infant, the manufacturer does not recommend breast-feeding during therapy or for one month following the last dose.

Contraindications Severe hypersensitivity to irinotecan (liposomal), irinotecan hydrochloride, or any component of the formulation

Warnings/Precautions Hazardous agent - use appropriate precautions for handling and disposal (NIOSH 2014 [group 1]). **[US Boxed Warning]: Fatal neutropenic sepsis occurred in nearly 1% of patients receiving irinotecan (liposomal). Severe or life-threatening neutropenic fever or sepsis occurred in 3% and severe or life-threatening neutropenia occurred in 20% of patients receiving irinotecan (liposomal) in combination with fluorouracil and leucovorin. Withhold irinotecan (liposomal) for absolute neutrophil count below 1,500/mm^3 or neutropenic fever. Monitor blood cell counts periodically during treatment** (days 1 and 8 of each cycle and more frequently if clinically necessary). May require therapy interruption, dose reduction, and/or discontinuation. Anemia, lymphopenia, and thrombocytopenia also commonly occur. The incidence of neutropenia was higher in Asian patients (compared to white patients).

[US Boxed Warning]: Severe diarrhea (may be life-threatening) occurred in 13% of patients receiving irinotecan (liposomal) in combination with fluorouracil and leucovorin. Do not administer irinotecan (liposomal) to patients with bowel obstruction. Withhold irinotecan (liposomal) for diarrhea of grade 2 to 4 severity. Administer loperamide for late diarrhea of any severity. Administer atropine, if not contraindicated, for early diarrhea of any severity. Early onset diarrhea occurs within 24 hours of chemotherapy, and may cause other symptoms of cholinergic reaction. Late onset diarrhea occurs more than 24 hours following chemotherapy. Diarrhea may require therapy interruption, dosage reduction, and/or discontinuation. Nausea, vomiting and stomatitis commonly occur. The pharmacokinetics of irinotecan (liposomal) have not been studied in patients with hepatic impairment. However, exposure to the active metabolite (SN-38) is increased in patients with hepatic impairment receiving irinotecan (conventional); toxicities may be increased.

Irinotecan (conventional) may cause severe and fatal interstitial lung disease (ILD). Withhold irinotecan (liposomal) during diagnostic evaluation if new or progressive dyspnea, cough, or fever occurs during use. Discontinue therapy if ILD diagnosis is confirmed. Severe hypersensitivity reactions (including anaphylaxis) have occurred with irinotecan (conventional). Monitor closely; permanently discontinue irinotecan (liposomal) therapy if severe hypersensitivity occurs. Irinotecan (liposomal) and irinotecan (conventional) are NOT interchangeable. Dosing differs between formulations; verify intended product and dose prior to preparation and administration. Potentially significant interactions may exist, requiring dose or frequency adjustment, additional monitoring, and/or selection of alternative therapy. CYP3A4 enzyme inducers may decrease exposure to irinotecan and SN-38 (active metabolite); avoid concomitant use (substitute non-enzyme inducing therapies at least 2 weeks prior to irinotecan [liposomal] initiation). Enzyme inhibitors may increase exposure; avoid concomitant use (discontinue strong CYP3A4 inhibitors at least 1 week prior to irinotecan [liposomal] initiation).

Adverse Reactions Frequency not always defined. Percentages reported as part of combination chemotherapy regimens.

Cardiovascular: Septic shock (≥2%)

Central nervous system: Fatigue (≤56%)

Dermatologic: Alopecia (14%)

Endocrine & metabolic: Increased serum alanine aminotransferase (51%), hypoalbuminemia (43%), hypomagnesemia (35%), hypocalcemia (32%), hypokalemia (32%), hypophosphatemia (29%), hyponatremia (27%), weight loss (17%), dehydration (8%)

Gastrointestinal: Diarrhea (59%, grade 3/4: 13%; early onset 30%, grade 3/4: 3%; late onset 43%, grade 3/4: 9%), vomiting (52%), nausea (51%), decreased appetite (44%), stomatitis (32%), gastroenteritis (3%)

Hematologic & oncologic: Anemia (97%, grades 3/4: 6%), lymphopenia (81%, grades 3/4: 27%), neutropenia (52%, grades 3/4: 20%; incidence of neutropenia was higher among Asian patients), thrombocytopenia (41%, grades 3/4: 2%), neutropenic fever (≤3%, grades 3/4: ≤3%)

Hypersensitivity: Severe hypersensitivity

Infection: Sepsis (4%, grades 3/4: 3%), neutropenic sepsis (≤3%, grades 3/4: ≤3%)

Local: Catheter infection (3%)

Neuromuscular & skeletal: Weakness (≤56%)

Renal: Increased creatinine clearance (18%)
Respiratory: Pneumonia (≥2%), interstitial pulmonary disease
Renal: Acute renal failure (≥2%)
Miscellaneous: Fever (23%)

Drug Interactions

Metabolism/Transport Effects Substrate of BCRP, CYP3A4 (major), P-glycoprotein, SLCO1B1, UGT1A1; **Note:** Assignment of Major/Minor substrate status based on clinically relevant drug interaction potential

Avoid Concomitant Use

Avoid concomitant use of Irinotecan (Liposomal) with any of the following: BCG (Intravesical); Conivaptan; CYP3A4 Inducers (Strong); CYP3A4 Inhibitors (Strong); Deferiprone; Dipyrone; Fusidic Acid (Systemic); Idelalisib; Natalizumab; Pimecrolimus; St Johns Wort; Tacrolimus (Topical); Tofacitinib; UGT1A1 Inhibitors; Vaccines (Live)

Increased Effect/Toxicity

Irinotecan (Liposomal) may increase the levels/effects of: CloZAPine; Deferiprone; Fingolimod; Leflunomide; Natalizumab; Tofacitinib; Vaccines (Live)

The levels/effects of Irinotecan (Liposomal) may be increased by: Aprepitant; Conivaptan; CYP3A4 Inhibitors (Moderate); CYP3A4 Inhibitors (Strong); Dasatinib; Denosumab; Dipyrone; Fosaprepitant; Fusidic Acid (Systemic); Idelalisib; Ivacaftor; Luliconazole; Mifepristone; Netupitant; Osimertinib; Palbociclib; P-glycoprotein/ABCB1 Inhibitors; Pimecrolimus; Ranolazine; Roflumilast; Rolapitant; Simeprevir; SORAfenib; Stiripentol; Tacrolimus (Topical); Teriflunomide; Trastuzumab; UGT1A1 Inhibitors

Decreased Effect

Irinotecan (Liposomal) may decrease the levels/effects of: BCG (Intravesical); Coccidioides immitis Skin Test; Sipuleucel-T; Vaccines (Inactivated); Vaccines (Live)

The levels/effects of Irinotecan (Liposomal) may be decreased by: Bosentan; CYP3A4 Inducers (Moderate); CYP3A4 Inducers (Strong); Dabrafenib; Deferasirox; Echinacea; Osimertinib; P-glycoprotein/ABCB1 Inducers; Siltuximab; St Johns Wort; Tocilizumab

Preparation for Administration Hazardous agent; use appropriate precautions for handling and disposal (NIOSH 2014 [group 1]). Withdraw appropriate dose from the vial and dilute in 500 mL D_5W or 0.9% sodium chloride injection. Mix by gentle inversion; protect diluted solution from light.

Storage/Stability Store intact vials at 2°C to 8°C (36°F to 46°F); do not freeze. Protect from light. Solution diluted for administration is stable for up to 4 hours when stored at room temperature, or up to 24 hours when refrigerated (administration should be completed within these time frames). Allow diluted solution to come to room temperature prior to administration.

Mechanism of Action Irinotecan (liposomal) is a topoisomerase 1 inhibitor encapsulated in a lipid bilayer (liposome). Irinotecan and its active metabolite (SN-38) bind reversibly to topoisomerase I-DNA complex preventing re-ligation of the cleaved DNA strand. This results in the accumulation of cleavable complexes and double-strand DNA breaks. As mammalian cells cannot efficiently repair these breaks, cell death consistent with S-phase cell cycle specificity occurs, leading to termination of cellular replication.

Pharmacodynamics/Kinetics

Distribution: 4.1 L; 95% of irinotecan remains liposome-encapsulated

Protein binding: <1%

Metabolism: Irinotecan hydrochloride: Primarily hepatic to SN-38 (active metabolite) by carboxylesterase enzymes; may also undergo CYP3A4-mediated metabolism to inactive metabolites (one of which may be hydrolyzed to release SN-38). SN-38 undergoes conjugation by UDP-glucuronosyl transferase 1A1 (UGT1A1) to form a glucuronide metabolite. SN-38 is increased by UGT1A1*28 polymorphism (10% of North Americans are homozygous for UGT1A1*28 allele).

Half-life elimination: Total irinotecan: ~26 hours; SN-38: ~68 hours

Excretion: Urine: Irinotecan hydrochloride (11% to 20%), metabolites (SN-38 <1%, SN-38 glucuronide, 3%)

Dosing

Adult Note: Premedicate with a corticosteroid and an antiemetic 30 minutes prior to infusion. Irinotecan (liposomal) and irinotecan (conventional) are NOT interchangeable. Dosing differs between formulations; verify intended product and dose prior to preparation and administration.

Pancreatic adenocarcinoma, metastatic: IV: 70 mg/m² once every 2 weeks (in combination with fluorouracil and leucovorin). **Note:** Reduce initial starting dose to 50 mg/m² in patients known to be homozygous for the

UGT1A1*28 allele; the dose may be increased to 70 mg/m² as tolerated in subsequent cycles.

Geriatric Refer to adult dosing

Renal Impairment

CrCl 30 to 89 mL/minute: There are no dosage adjustments provided in the manufacturer's labeling; however, a population pharmacokinetic analysis showed no effect on total SN-38 exposure in patients with mild to moderate renal impairment.

CrCl <30 mL/minute: There are no dosage adjustments provided in the manufacturer's labeling (insufficient data).

Hepatic Impairment Bilirubin >ULN: There are no dosage adjustments provided in the manufacturer's labeling.

Adjustment for Toxicity Note: Fluorouracil and leucovorin may also require dosage adjustment.

Hematologic toxicity: ANC <1,500/mm³ or neutropenic fever: Withhold treatment. Resume therapy when ANC ≥1,500/mm³ with a reduced dose for grade 3 or 4 neutropenia or neutropenic fever in subsequent cycles:

First occurrence: Reduce dose to 50 mg/m² (in patients receiving 70 mg/m²); reduce dose to 43 mg/m² in patients homozygous for UGT1A1*28 without previous increase to 70 mg/m²

Second occurrence: Reduce dose to 43 mg/m² (in patients receiving 50 mg/m²); reduce dose to 35 mg/m² in patients homozygous for UGT1A1*28 previously receiving 43 mg/m²

Third occurrence: Discontinue

Nonhematologic toxicity:

Anaphylactic reaction: Discontinue permanently

Diarrhea: Withhold therapy for grade 2 to 4 diarrhea. Administer IV or SubQ atropine 0.25 to 1 mg (unless clinically contraindicated) for early-onset diarrhea of any severity. Administer loperamide for late-onset diarrhea of any severity. Following recovery to ≤ grade 1 diarrhea, resume treatment at a reduced dose:

First occurrence: Reduce dose to 50 mg/m² (in patients receiving 70 mg/m²); reduce dose to 43 mg/m² in patients homozygous for UGT1A1*28 without previous increase to 70 mg/m²

Second occurrence: Reduce dose to 43 mg/m² (in patients receiving 50 mg/m²); reduce dose to 35 mg/m² in patients homozygous for UGT1A1*28 previously receiving 43 mg/m²

Third occurrence: Discontinue

Interstitial lung disease (ILD): Discontinue

Other grade 3 or 4 adverse reactions: Withhold therapy. Upon recovery to ≤ grade 1 toxicity, resume treatment at a reduced dose:

First occurrence: Reduce dose to 50 mg/m² (in patients receiving 70 mg/m²); reduce dose to 43 mg/m² in patients homozygous for UGT1A1*28 without previous increase to 70 mg/m²

Second occurrence: Reduce dose to 43 mg/m² (in patients receiving 50 mg/m²); reduce dose to 35 mg/m² in patients homozygous for UGT1A1*28 previously receiving 43 mg/m²

Third occurrence: Discontinue

Administration

Administer by IV infusion over 90 minutes. Premedicate with a corticosteroid and an antiemetic 30 minutes prior to infusion. Administer irinotecan (liposomal) prior to fluorouracil and leucovorin. Do not use in-line filters for administration.

Administer IV or SubQ atropine 0.25 to 1 mg (unless clinically contraindicated) for early onset diarrhea of any severity; initiate loperamide for late-onset diarrhea of any severity.

Hazardous agent; use appropriate precautions for handling and disposal (NIOSH 2014 [group 1]).

Monitoring Parameters Complete blood counts on days 1 and 8 of each cycle and as clinically indicated; bilirubin, electrolytes (with severe diarrhea); bowel movements (diarrhea episodes) and hydration status; signs/symptoms of pulmonary toxicity or hypersensitivity reactions

Dosage Forms Excipient information presented when available (limited, particularly for generics); consult specific product labeling.

Injectable, Intravenous:

Onivyde: 43 mg/10 mL (10 mL) [contains mpeg-2000-dspe (methoxy-terminated peg)]

◆ Irinotecan For Injection (Can) *see* Irinotecan (Conventional) *on page 980*

◆ Irinotecan HCl *see* Irinotecan (Conventional) *on page 980*

◆ Irinotecan Hydrochloride *see* Irinotecan (Conventional) *on page 980*

Iron Dextran Complex
(EYE ern DEKS tran KOM pleks)

Brand Names: US Dexferrum [DSC]; Infed
Brand Names: Canada Dexiron; Infufer
Index Terms High-Molecular-Weight Iron Dextran (Dexferrum); Imferon; Iron Dextran; Low-Molecular-Weight Iron Dextran (INFeD)
Pharmacologic Category Iron Salt
Use Iron deficiency: Treatment of iron deficiency in patients in whom oral administration is unsatisfactory or infeasible

Pregnancy Considerations Adverse events have been observed in animal reproduction studies. It is not known if iron dextran (as iron dextran) crosses the placenta. It is recommended that pregnant women meet the dietary requirements of iron with diet and/or supplements in order to prevent adverse events associated with iron deficiency anemia in pregnancy. Treatment of iron deficiency anemia in pregnant women is the same as in nonpregnant women and in most cases, oral iron preparations may be used. Except in severe cases of maternal anemia, the fetus achieves normal iron stores regardless of maternal concentrations.

Breast-Feeding Considerations Trace amounts of iron dextran (as iron dextran) are found in human milk. Iron is normally found in breast milk. Breast milk or iron fortified formulas generally provide enough iron to meet the recommended dietary requirements of infants. The amount of iron in breast milk is generally not influenced by maternal iron status.

Contraindications Hypersensitivity to iron dextran or any component of the formulation; any anemia not associated with iron deficiency

Warnings/Precautions [U.S. Boxed Warning]: Deaths associated with parenteral administration following anaphylactic-type reactions have been reported (use only where resuscitation equipment and personnel are available). A test dose should be administered to all patients prior to the first therapeutic dose. Fatal reactions have occurred in patients who tolerated the test dose. Monitor patients for signs/symptoms of anaphylactic reactions during any iron dextran administration; fatalities have occurred with the test dose. A history of drug allergy (including multiple drug allergies) and/or the concomitant use of an ACE inhibitor may increase the risk of anaphylactic-type reactions. Adverse events (including life-threatening) associated with iron dextran usually occur with the high-molecular-weight formulation (Dexferrum), compared to low-molecular-weight (INFeD) (Chertow, 2006). Delayed (1-2 days) infusion reaction (including arthralgia, back pain, chills, dizziness, and fever) may occur with large doses (eg, total dose infusion) of IV iron dextran; usually subsides within 3-4 days. Delayed reaction may also occur (less commonly) with IM administration; subsiding within 3-7 days. Use with caution in patients with a history of significant allergies, asthma, serious hepatic impairment, preexisting cardiac disease (may exacerbate cardiovascular complications), and rheumatoid arthritis (may exacerbate joint pain and swelling). Avoid use during acute kidney infection.

In patients with chronic kidney disease (CKD) requiring iron supplementation, the IV route is preferred for hemodialysis patients; either oral iron or IV iron may be used for nondialysis and peritoneal dialysis CKD patients. In patients with cancer-related anemia (either due to cancer or chemotherapy-induced) requiring iron supplementation, the IV route is superior to oral therapy; IM administration is not recommended for parenteral iron supplementation.

[U.S. Boxed Warning]: Use only in patients where the iron deficient state is not amenable to oral iron therapy. Discontinue oral iron prior to initiating parenteral iron therapy. Exogenous hemosiderosis may result from excess iron stores; patients with refractory anemias and/or hemoglobinopathies may be prone to iron overload with

unwarranted iron supplementation. Anemia in the elderly is often caused by "anemia of chronic disease" or associated with inflammation rather than blood loss. Iron stores are usually normal or increased, with a serum ferritin >50 ng/mL and a decreased total iron binding capacity. IV administration of iron dextran is often preferred over IM in the elderly secondary to a decreased muscle mass and the need for daily injections. Intramuscular injections of iron-carbohydrate complexes may have a risk of delayed injection site tumor development. Iron dextran products differ in chemical characteristics. The high-molecular-weight formulation (Dexferrum) and the low-molecular-weight formulation (INFeD) are not clinically interchangeable. Intramuscular iron dextran use in neonates may be associated with an increased incidence of gram-negative sepsis.

Adverse Reactions Frequency not defined. **Note:** Adverse event risk is reported to be higher with the high-molecular-weight iron dextran formulation.

Cardiovascular: Arrhythmia, bradycardia, cardiac arrest, chest pain, chest tightness, cyanosis, flushing, hyper-/hypotension, shock, syncope, tachycardia

Central nervous system: Chills, disorientation, dizziness, fever, headache, malaise, seizure, unconsciousness, unresponsiveness

Dermatologic: Pruritus, purpura, rash, urticaria

Gastrointestinal: Abdominal pain, diarrhea, nausea, taste alteration, vomiting

Genitourinary: Discoloration of urine

Hematologic: Leukocytosis, lymphadenopathy

Local: Injection site reactions (cellulitis, inflammation, pain, phlebitis, soreness, swelling), muscle atrophy/fibrosis (with IM injection), skin/tissue staining (at the site of IM injection), sterile abscess

Neuromuscular & skeletal: Arthralgia, arthritis/arthritis exacerbation, back pain, myalgia, paresthesia, weakness

Respiratory: Bronchospasm, dyspnea, respiratory arrest, wheezing

Renal: Hematuria

Miscellaneous: Anaphylactic reactions (sudden respiratory difficulty, cardiovascular collapse), diaphoresis

Postmarketing and/or case reports: Angioedema, tumor formation (at former injection site)

Drug Interactions

Metabolism/Transport Effects None known.

Avoid Concomitant Use

Avoid concomitant use of Iron Dextran Complex with any of the following: Dimercaprol

Increased Effect/Toxicity

The levels/effects of Iron Dextran Complex may be increased by: ACE Inhibitors; Dimercaprol

Decreased Effect There are no known significant interactions involving a decrease in effect.

Preparation for Administration Solutions for infusion should be diluted in 250-1000 mL NS.

Storage/Stability Store at 20°C to 25°C (68°F to 77°F); excursions permitted to 15°C to 30°C (59°F to 86°F).

Mechanism of Action The released iron, from the plasma, eventually replenishes the depleted iron stores in the bone marrow where it is incorporated into hemoglobin

Pharmacodynamics/Kinetics

Onset of action: IV: Serum ferritin peak: 7-9 days after dose

Absorption:

IM: 50% to 90% is promptly absorbed, balance is slowly absorbed over month

IV: Uptake of iron by the reticuloendothelial system appears to be constant at about 10-20 mg/hour

Excretion: Urine and feces via reticuloendothelial system

Dosing

Adult & Geriatric

Note: A 0.5 mL test dose should be given prior to starting iron dextran therapy.

Iron-deficiency anemia: IM (INFeD), IV (Dexferrum, INFeD):

Dose (mL) = 0.0442 (desired hemoglobin - observed hemoglobin) x LBW + (0.26 x LBW)

Desired hemoglobin: Usually 14.8 g/dL

LBW = Lean body weight in kg

Iron replacement therapy for blood loss: (INFeD), IV (Dexferrum, INFeD): Replacement iron (mg) = blood loss (mL) x Hct

Maximum daily dosage: Manufacturer's labeling: **Note:** Replacement of larger estimated iron deficits may be achieved by serial administration of smaller incremental dosages. Daily dosages should be limited to 100 mg iron (2 mL)

Cancer-/chemotherapy-associated anemia: IV: **Note:** Use the iron-deficiency anemia equation for determining a calculated dose, when applicable.

Weekly administration (off-label dosing; INFed):
Weeks 1-3: Test dose of 25 mg (over 1-2 minutes), followed by 75 mg (bolus) once weekly
Weeks 4 and after: 100 mg over 5 minutes once weekly until the calculated dose is reached (Auerbach, 2004)

or

Week 1: Test dose of 25 mg (slow IV push), followed 1 hour later by 75 mg over 5 minutes
Weeks 2-10: 100 mg over 5 minutes once weekly for a total cumulative dose of 1000 mg (NCCN anemia guidelines v.2.2014)

Total dose infusion (off-label dosing; INFeD):
Test dose of 25 mg (over 1-2 minutes), followed 1 hour later by the balance of the calculated total dose mixed in 500 mL NS and infused at 175 mL/hour (Auerbach, 2004)

or

Test dose of 25 mg (slow IV push) followed 1 hour later by the balance of the total dose as a single infusion over several hours; if calculated dose exceeds 1000 mg, administer remaining dose in excess of 1000 mg after 4 weeks if inadequate hemoglobin response (NCCN anemia guidelines v.2.2014)

Pediatric Note: A 0.5 mL test dose (0.25 mL in infants) should be given prior to starting iron dextran therapy.

Iron-deficiency anemia: IM (INFeD), IV (Dexferrum, INFeD):
Children 5-15 kg: Should not normally be given in the first 4 months of life:
Dose (mL) = 0.0442 (desired hemoglobin - observed hemoglobin) x W + (0.26 x W)
Desired hemoglobin: Usually 12 g/dL
W = Total body weight in kg
Children >15 kg: Refer to adult dosing.

Iron replacement therapy for blood loss: Refer to adult dosing.

Maximum daily dose:
Children <5 kg: 25 mg iron (0.5 mL)
Children 5-10 kg: 50 mg iron (1 mL)
Children ≥10 kg: Refer to adult dosing.

Renal Impairment No dosage adjustment provided in manufacturer's labeling.

Hepatic Impairment No dosage adjustment provided in manufacturer's labeling.

Administration Note: A test dose should be given on the first day of therapy; patient should be observed for 1 hour for hypersensitivity reaction, then the remainder of the day's dose (dose minus test dose) should be given. Resuscitation equipment, medication, and trained personnel should be available. An uneventful test dose does not ensure an anaphylactic-type reaction will not occur during administration of the therapeutic dose.

IM (INFeD): Use Z-track technique (displacement of the skin laterally prior to injection); injection should be deep into the upper outer quadrant of buttock; alternate buttocks with subsequent injections. Administer test dose at same recommended site using the same technique.

IV: Test dose should be given gradually over at least 30 seconds (INFeD) or 5 minutes (Dexferrum), or over 1-2 minutes (INFeD) for cancer-/chemotherapy-associated anemia (Auerbach, 2004). Subsequent dose(s) may be administered by IV bolus undiluted at a rate not to exceed 50 mg/minute (maximum 100 mg). For total dose infusion in patients with cancer-/chemotherapy-associated anemia (off-label dose): 1 hour after the test dose, administer the balance of the dose diluted in 500 mL NS and infuse at 175 mL/hour (Auerbach, 2004) or administer over several hours (NCCN Anemia guidelines v.2.2104). Avoid dilutions with dextrose (increased incidence of local pain and phlebitis).

Monitoring Parameters Hemoglobin, hematocrit, reticulocyte count, serum ferritin, serum iron, TIBC; monitor for anaphylaxis/hypersensitivity reaction (during test dose and therapeutic dose)

Reference Range
Hemoglobin: Adults:
Males: 13.5-16.5 g/dL
Females: 12.0-15.0 g/dL
Serum iron: 40-160 mcg/dL
Total iron binding capacity: 230-430 mcg/dL
Transferrin: 204-360 mg/dL
Percent transferrin saturation: 20% to 50%

Test Interactions May cause falsely elevated values of serum bilirubin and falsely decreased values of serum calcium. Residual iron dextran may remain in reticuloendothelial cells; may affect accuracy of examination of bone marrow iron stores. Bone scans with 99m Tc-labeled bone seeking agents may show reduced bony uptake, marked renal activity, and excess blood pooling and soft tissue accumulation following IV iron dextran infusion or with high serum ferritin levels. Following IM iron dextran, bone scans with 99m Tc-diphosphonate may show dense activity in the buttocks.

Dosage Forms Considerations Strength of iron dextran complex is expressed as elemental iron.

Dosage Forms Excipient information presented when available (limited, particularly for generics); consult specific product labeling. [DSC] = Discontinued product
Solution, Injection:
Dexferrum: 50 mg/mL (1 mL [DSC], 2 mL [DSC])
Infed: 50 mg/mL (2 mL)

◆ Iron Dextri-Maltose *see* Ferric Carboxymaltose *on page 759*

◆ Iron Fumarate *see* Ferrous Fumarate *on page 761*

◆ Iron Gluconate *see* Ferrous Gluconate *on page 761*

◆ Iron-Polysaccharide Complex *see* Polysaccharide-Iron Complex *on page 1469*

Iron Sucrose (EYE ern SOO krose)

Brand Names: US Venofer
Brand Names: Canada Venofer
Index Terms Iron (III) Hydroxide Sucrose Complex
Pharmacologic Category Iron Salt
Use Iron deficiency anemia: Treatment of iron-deficiency anemia in chronic kidney disease (CKD)

Pregnancy Considerations Teratogenic effects were not observed in animal studies. There are no adequate and well-controlled studies in pregnant women. Based on limited data, iron sucrose may be effective for the treatment of iron-deficiency anemia in pregnancy. It is recommended that pregnant women meet the dietary requirements of iron with diet and/or supplements in order to prevent adverse events associated with iron deficiency anemia in pregnancy. Treatment of iron deficiency anemia in pregnant women is the same as in nonpregnant women and in most cases, oral iron preparations may be used. Except in severe cases of maternal anemia, the fetus achieves normal iron stores regardless of maternal concentrations.

Breast-Feeding Considerations Iron is normally found in breast milk. Breast milk or iron fortified formulas generally provide enough iron to meet the recommended dietary requirements of infants. The amount of iron in breast milk is generally not influenced by maternal iron status.

Contraindications Known hypersensitivity to iron sucrose or any component of the formulation

Warnings/Precautions Hypersensitivity reactions, including rare postmarketing anaphylactic and anaphylactoid reactions (some fatal), have been reported; monitor patients during and for ≥30 minutes postadministration; discontinue immediately for signs/symptoms of a hypersensitivity reaction (shock, hypotension, loss of consciousness). Equipment for resuscitation and trained personnel experienced in handling medical emergencies should always be immediately available. Significant hypotension has been reported frequently in hemodialysis-dependent patients. Hypotension has also been reported in peritoneal dialysis and nondialysis patients. Hypotension may be related to total dose or rate of administration (avoid rapid IV injection), follow recommended guidelines. Withhold iron in the presence of tissue iron overload; periodic monitoring of hemoglobin, hematocrit, serum ferritin, and transferrin saturation is recommended.

Adverse Reactions Events and incidences are associated with use in adults unless otherwise specified.
>10%:
Cardiovascular: Hypotension (2% to 3%; children 2%; 39% in hemodialysis patients; may be related to total dose or rate of administration)
Central nervous system: Headache (3% to 13%; children 6%)
Gastrointestinal: Nausea (5% to 15%; children 3%)
Neuromuscular & skeletal: Muscle cramps (1% to 3%; 29% in hemodialysis patients)
Respiratory: Nasopharyngitis (2% to 16%), pharyngitis (2% to 16%), sinusitis (2% to 16%), upper respiratory infection (2% to 16%; children 4%)
1% to 10%:
Cardiovascular: Hypertension (7% to 8%; children 2%), peripheral edema (3% to 7%), chest pain (1% to 6%), arteriovenous fistula thrombosis (children 2%), heart failure (>1%)
Central nervous system: Dizziness (1% to 7%; children 4%), fever (1% to 3%; children 4%)
Dermatologic: Pruritus (2% to 4%)
Endocrine & metabolic: Hypoglycemia (≤4%), fluid overload (1% to 3%), gout (≤3%), hyperglycemia (≤3%)

Gastrointestinal: Vomiting (5% to 9%; children 4%), diarrhea (5% to 8%), taste perversion (≤8%), peritonitis (children 4%), abdominal pain (1% to 4%)

Local: Injection site reaction (≤6%)

Neuromuscular & skeletal: Extremity pain (3% to 6%), arthralgia (1% to 4%), myalgia (≤4%), weakness (1% to 3%), back pain (1% to 2%)

Ocular: Conjunctivitis (≤3%)

Otic: Ear pain (≤2%)

Respiratory: Dyspnea (1% to 6%), cough (1% to 3%; children 4%), nasal congestion (≤1%)

Miscellaneous: Graft complication (≤10%), sepsis (>1%)

<1% (Limited to important or life-threatening): Anaphylactic shock, anaphylactoid reactions, angioedema, bradycardia, cardiovascular collapse, hypersensitivity (including wheezing), loss of consciousness, necrotizing enterocolitis (reported in premature infants, no causal relationship established), seizure, shock, urine discoloration

Drug Interactions

Metabolism/Transport Effects None known.

Avoid Concomitant Use

Avoid concomitant use of Iron Sucrose with any of the following: Dimercaprol

Increased Effect/Toxicity

Iron Sucrose may increase the levels/effects of: Amifostine; Antipsychotic Agents (Second Generation [Atypical]); DULoxetine; Hypotension-Associated Agents; Levodopa

The levels/effects of Iron Sucrose may be increased by: Alfuzosin; Barbiturates; Blood Pressure Lowering Agents; Brimonidine (Topical); Diazoxide; Dimercaprol; Herbs (Hypotensive Properties); Molsidomine; Nicorandil; Obinutuzumab; Pentoxifylline; Phosphodiesterase 5 Inhibitors; Prostacyclin Analogues

Decreased Effect There are no known significant interactions involving a decrease in effect.

Preparation for Administration

Children: May administer undiluted or diluted in 25 mL of NS. Do not dilute to concentrations <1 mg/mL.

Adults: Doses ≤200 mg may be administered undiluted or diluted in a maximum of 100 mL NS. Doses >200 mg should be diluted in a maximum of 250 mL NS. Do not dilute to concentrations <1 mg/mL.

Storage/Stability Store intact vials at controlled room temperature of 20°C to 25°C (68°F to 77°F); excursions permitted to 15°C to 30°C (59°F to 86°F); do not freeze. Iron sucrose is stable for 7 days at room temperature (23°C to 27°C [73°F to 81°F]) or under refrigeration (2°C to 6°C [36°F to 43°F]) when undiluted in a plastic syringe or following dilution in normal saline in a plastic syringe (concentration 2-10 mg/mL) or for 7 days at room temperature (23°C to 27°C [73°F to 81°F]) following dilution in normal saline in an IV bag (concentration 1-2 mg/mL).

Mechanism of Action Iron sucrose is dissociated by the reticuloendothelial system into iron and sucrose. The released iron increases serum iron concentrations and is incorporated into hemoglobin.

Pharmacodynamics/Kinetics

Distribution: V_{dss}: Healthy adults: 7.9 L

Metabolism: Dissociated into iron and sucrose by the reticuloendothelial system

Half-life elimination: Healthy adults: 6 hours; Nondialysis-dependent adolescents: 8 hours

Excretion: Healthy adults: Urine (5%) within 24 hours

Dosing

Adult & Geriatric Doses expressed in mg of **elemental** iron. **Note:** Test dose: Product labeling does not indicate need for a test dose in product-naive patients.

Iron-deficiency anemia in chronic kidney disease (CKD): IV:

Hemodialysis-dependent patient: 100 mg administered during consecutive dialysis sessions to a cumulative total dose of 1000 mg (10 doses); may repeat treatment if clinically indicated.

Peritoneal dialysis-dependent patient: Two infusions of 300 mg administered 14 days apart, followed by a single 400 mg infusion 14 days later (total cumulative dose of 1000 mg in 3 divided doses); may repeat treatment if clinically indicated.

Nondialysis-dependent patient: 200 mg administered on 5 different occasions within a 14-day period (total cumulative dose: 1000 mg in 14-day period); may repeat treatment if clinically indicated. **Note:** Dosage has also been administered as 2 infusions of 500 mg on day 1 and day 14 (limited experience).

Chemotherapy-associated anemia (off-label use): IV: 200 mg once every 3 weeks for 5 doses (Bastit, 2008) or 100 mg once weekly during weeks 0 to 6, followed by 100 mg every other week from weeks 8 to 14 (Hedenus, 2007)

Pediatric Doses expressed in mg of **elemental** iron. **Note:** Test dose: Product labeling does not indicate need for a test dose in product-naive patients.

Iron-deficiency anemia in chronic kidney disease (CKD): Children ≥2 years and Adolescents: IV: **Note:** Not indicated for iron replacement treatment in children and adolescents.

Hemodialysis-dependent patient: Maintenance therapy: 0.5 mg/kg/dose (maximum: 100 mg) every 2 weeks for 6 doses; may repeat if clinically indicated.

Nondialysis-dependent patient: Maintenance therapy: 0.5 mg/kg/dose (maximum: 100 mg) every 4 weeks for 3 doses; may repeat if clinically indicated

Peritoneal dialysis-dependent patient: Maintenance therapy: 0.5 mg/kg/dose (maximum: 100 mg) every 4 weeks for 3 doses; may repeat if clinically indicated

Renal Impairment No dosage adjustment provided in manufacturer's labeling.

Hepatic Impairment No dosage adjustment provided in manufacturer's labeling.

Administration Administer intravenously as a slow IV injection (**not** for rapid IV injection) or as an IV infusion. Can be administered through dialysis line.

Children and Adolescents:

Slow IV injection: Administer undiluted over 5 minutes

Infusion: Infuse diluted solution over 5-60 minutes

Adults:

Slow IV injection: May administer doses ≤200 mg undiluted by slow IV injection over 2-5 minutes. When administering to hemodialysis-dependent patients, give iron sucrose early during the dialysis session.

Infusion: Infuse diluted doses ≤200 mg over at least 15 minutes; infuse diluted 300 mg dose over 1.5 hours; infuse diluted 400 mg dose over 2.5 hours; infuse diluted 500 mg dose over 3.5-4 hours (limited experience). When administering to hemodialysis-dependent patients, give iron sucrose early during the dialysis session.

Monitoring Parameters

CKD patients: Hematocrit, hemoglobin, serum ferritin, serum iron, transferrin, percent transferrin saturation, TIBC (takes ~4 weeks of treatment to see increased serum iron and ferritin, and decreased TIBC); iron status should be assessed ≥48 hours after last dose (due to rapid increase in values following administration); signs/symptoms of hypersensitivity reactions (during and ≥30 minutes following infusion); hypotension (following infusion)

Chemotherapy-associated anemia (off-label use): Iron, total iron-binding capacity, transferrin saturation, or ferritin levels at baseline and periodically (Rizzo, 2011)

Reference Range

Hemoglobin: Adults:

Males: 13.5-16.5 g/dL

Females: 12.0-15.0 g/dL

Serum iron: 40-160 mcg/dL

Total iron binding capacity: 230-430 mcg/dL

Transferrin: 204-360 mg/dL

Percent transferrin saturation: 20% to 50%

Dosage Forms Considerations Strength of iron sucrose is expressed as elemental iron.

Dosage Forms Excipient information presented when available (limited, particularly for generics); consult specific product labeling.

Solution, Intravenous [preservative free]:

Venofer: 20 mg/mL (2.5 mL, 5 mL, 10 mL)

◆ **Iron Sulfate** *see* Ferrous Sulfate *on page 762*

◆ **Iron Supplement Childrens [OTC]** *see* Ferrous Sulfate *on page 762*

◆ **Isavuconazole** *see* Isavuconazonium Sulfate *on page 988*

Isavuconazonium Sulfate

(eye sa vue koe na ZOE nee um sul FATE)

Brand Names: US Cresemba

Index Terms BAL8557; Isavuconazole

Pharmacologic Category Antifungal Agent, Azole Derivative; Antifungal Agent, Oral; Antifungal Agent, Parenteral

Use

Aspergillosis: Treatment of invasive aspergillosis in adults

Mucormycosis: Treatment of invasive mucormycosis in adults

Pregnancy Considerations Adverse events were observed in animal reproduction studies. Based on animal data, isavuconazonium sulfate may have the potential to increase the risk of adverse developmental events if used in pregnant women.

Breast-Feeding Considerations It is not known if isavuconazonium sulfate is excreted into breast milk. Breast-feeding is not recommended by the manufacturer.

Contraindications Hypersensitivity to isavuconazonium sulfate (eg, isavuconazole) or any component of the formulation; concurrent use of strong CYP3A4 inhibitors (eg, ketoconazole, high-dose ritonavir [400 mg every 12 hours]); concurrent use of strong CYP3A4 inducers (eg, rifampin, carbamazepine, St. John's wort, long acting barbiturates); familial short QT syndrome

Warnings/Precautions Serious hypersensitivity (eg, anaphylaxis) and severe skin reactions (eg, Stevens-Johnson syndrome) have been reported with other azole antifungal agents. Discontinue if a severe skin reaction occurs. There is no information regarding cross sensitivity between isavuconazonium sulfate and other azoles. Use with caution in patients with hypersensitivity reactions to other azoles. Severe hepatic reactions (hepatic failure [including fatalities], hepatitis, and cholestasis) have been reported in patients with serious underlying medical conditions (eg, hematologic malignancy). Other reactions (elevations in AST, ALT, alkaline phosphatase and total bilirubin) have also been reported; these elevations are generally reversible and do not require discontinuation of therapy. Monitor liver function tests at baseline and periodically during therapy. If abnormal liver function tests develop, monitor closely for development of severe hepatic reactions. Discontinue therapy if clinical signs and symptoms of liver disease develop. Use with caution and monitor for adverse effects in patients with severe hepatic impairment (Child-Pugh class C). Infusion reactions (eg, hypotension, dizziness, chills, dyspnea, paresthesia and hypoesthesia) have been reported during IV administration. Discontinue the infusion if these reactions occur. Following dilution for IV infusion, may form precipitate from the insoluble isavuconazole. Use an infusion set with an in-line filter (pore size 0.2 to 1.2 micron) for IV administration. Potentially significant drug-drug interactions may exist, requiring dose or frequency adjustment, additional monitoring, and/or selection of alternative therapy.

Adverse Reactions Frequency not always defined.
>10%:
Cardiovascular: Peripheral edema (11% to 15%)
Central nervous system: Headache (17%), fatigue (11%), insomnia (11%)
Endocrine & metabolic: Hypokalemia (14% to 19%)
Gastrointestinal: Nausea (26% to 28%), vomiting (25%), diarrhea (22% to 24%), abdominal pain (17%), constipation (13% to 14%)
Hepatic: Increased liver enzymes (16% to 17%)
Respiratory: Dyspnea (12% to 17%), cough (12%)
1% to 10%:
Cardiovascular: Chest pain (9%), hypotension (8%), atrial fibrillation (<5%), atrial flutter (<5%), bradycardia (<5%), cardiac arrest (<5%), catheter site thrombosis (<5%), extrasystoles (<5%), palpitations (<5%), shortened QT interval (<5%), supraventricular extrasystole (<5%), supraventricular tachycardia (<5%), syncope (<5%), thrombophlebitis (<5%), ventricular premature contractions (<5%)
Central nervous system: Delirium (9%), anxiety (8%), brain disease (<5%), chills (<5%), confusion (<5%), convulsions (<5%), depression (<5%), drowsiness (<5%), falling (<5%), hallucination (<5%), hypoesthesia (<5%), malaise (<5%), migraine (<5%), peripheral neuropathy (<5%), stupor (<5%), vertigo (<5%), dizziness, hypoesthesia, paresthesia
Dermatologic: Skin rash (9%), pruritus (8%), alopecia (<5%), dermatitis (<5%), erythema (<5%), exfoliative dermatitis (<5%), urticaria (<5%)
Endocrine & metabolic: Hypomagnesemia (5%), hypoalbuminemia (<5%), hypoglycemia (<5%), hyponatremia (<5%)
Gastrointestinal: Decreased appetite (9%), dyspepsia (6%), abdominal distention (<5%), cholecystitis (<5%), cholelithiasis (<5%), cholestasis (<5%), dysgeusia (<5%), gastritis (<5%), gingivitis (<5%), stomatitis (<5%)
Genitourinary: Hematuria (<5%), proteinuria (<5%)
Hematologic & oncologic: Agranulocytosis (<5%), leukopenia (<5%), pancytopenia (<5%), petechia (<5%)
Hepatic: Hepatitis (<5%), hepatomegaly (<5%), increased serum ALT (>3x ULN ≤4%; >10x ULN ≤1%), increased serum AST (>3x ULN ≤4%; >10x ULN ≤1%), hepatic failure, increased serum transaminases
Hypersensitivity: Hypersensitivity (<5%)
Local: Injection site reaction (6%)
Neuromuscular & Skeletal: Back pain (10%), myositis (<5%), neck pain (<5%), ostealgia (<5%), tremor (<5%)
Ophthalmic: Optic neuropathy (<5%)
Otic: Tinnitus (<5%)

Respiratory: Acute respiratory tract failure (7%), bronchospasm (<5%), tachypnea (<5%)

Drug Interactions
Metabolism/Transport Effects Substrate of CYP3A4 (major); **Note:** Assignment of Major/Minor substrate status based on clinically relevant drug interaction potential; **Inhibits** CYP2C19 (weak), CYP2C8 (weak), CYP2C9 (weak), CYP2D6 (weak), CYP3A4 (moderate), OCT2, P-glycoprotein; **Induces** CYP2B6 (weak/moderate), CYP2C8 (weak/moderate), CYP2C9 (weak/moderate)

Avoid Concomitant Use
Avoid concomitant use of Isavuconazonium Sulfate with any of the following: Amodiaquine; Aprepitant; Bosutinib; Cobimetinib; Conivaptan; CYP3A4 Inducers (Strong); CYP3A4 Inhibitors (Strong); Domperidone; Flibanserin; Fusidic Acid (Systemic); Ibrutinib; Idelalisib; Ivabradine; Lomitapide; Naloxegol; Olaparib; Pimozide; Saccharomyces boulardii; Simeprevir; St Johns Wort; Tolvaptan; Trabectedin; Ulipristal

Increased Effect/Toxicity
Isavuconazonium Sulfate may increase the levels/effects of: Amodiaquine; Apixaban; Aprepitant; ARIPiprazole; Avanafil; Bosentan; Bosutinib; Brexpiprazole; Bromocriptine; Budesonide (Systemic); Budesonide (Topical); Cannabis; Cilostazol; Cobimetinib; Colchicine; CYP3A4 Substrates; Dapoxetine; Digoxin; Dofetilide; Domperidone; DOXOrubicin (Conventional); Dronabinol; Eletriptan; Eliglustat; Eplerenone; Everolimus; FentaNYL; Flibanserin; Halofantrine; Hydrocodone; Ibrutinib; Imatinib; Ivabradine; Ivacaftor; Lomitapide; Lurasidone; Mycophenolate; Naloxegol; NiMODipine; Olaparib; OxyCODONE; Pimecrolimus; Pimozide; Propafenone; Ranolazine; Salmeterol; Saxagliptin; Simeprevir; Sonidegib; Suvorexant; Tetrahydrocannabinol; Tolvaptan; Trabectedin; Ulipristal; Vilazodone; Vindesine; Zopiclone; Zuclopenthixol

The levels/effects of Isavuconazonium Sulfate may be increased by: Conivaptan; CYP3A4 Inhibitors (Moderate); CYP3A4 Inhibitors (Strong); Dasatinib; Fosaprepitant; Fusidic Acid (Systemic); Idelalisib; Luliconazole; Mifepristone; Netupitant; Osimertinib; Palbociclib; Stiripentol

Decreased Effect
Isavuconazonium Sulfate may decrease the levels/effects of: Amphotericin B; BuPROPion; Ifosfamide; Saccharomyces boulardii

The levels/effects of Isavuconazonium Sulfate may be decreased by: Bosentan; CYP3A4 Inducers (Moderate); CYP3A4 Inducers (Strong); Dabrafenib; Deferasirox; Osimertinib; Siltuximab; St Johns Wort; Tocilizumab

Preparation for Administration Reconstitute 1 vial of isavuconazonium with 5 mL SWFI. Shake gently to dissolve. The reconstituted solution may be stored below 25°C for a maximum of 1 hour prior to preparation of the admixed solution. Remove 5 mL of the reconstituted solution from the vial and add it to an infusion bag containing 250 mL (approximately isavuconazonium sulfate 1.5 mg/mL) of NS or D_5W. The diluted solution may show visible translucent to white particulates of isavuconazole (will be removed by in-line filtration). Use gentle mixing or roll bag to minimize the formation of particulates. Avoid unnecessary vibration or vigorous shaking of the solution. Do not use a pneumatic transport system. Apply in-line filter with a microporous membrane pore size of 0.2 to 1.2 micron and in-line filter reminder sticker to the infusion bag. The IV administration should be completed within 6 hours at 20°C to 25°C (68°F to 77°F). If this is not possible, immediately refrigerate (2°C to 8°C [36°F to 46°F]) the admixed solution and complete the infusion within 24 hours.

Storage/Stability
Capsules: Store at 20°C to 25°C (68°F to 77°F) in the original packaging to protect from moisture; excursions are permitted between 15°C and 30°C (59°F and 86°F).
IV: Store intact vials at 2°C to 8°C (36°F to 46°F). Following reconstitution of the vial with SWFI, use the solution immediately, or stored below 25°C for a maximum of 1 hour prior to preparation of the admixed solution. The admixed infusion solution should be kept for not more than 6 hours at (20°C to 25°C [68°F to 77°F]) or 24 hours at 2°C to 8°C (36°F to 46°F) prior to use. Do not freeze.

Mechanism of Action Isavuconazonium sulfate is a pro-drug that is rapidly hydrolyzed in the blood to active isavuconazole. Isavuconazole inhibits the synthesis of ergosterol, a key component of the fungal cell membrane, through the inhibition of cytochrome P-450 dependent enzyme lanosterol 14-alpha-demethylase. This enzyme is responsible for the conversion of lanosterol to ergosterol. An accumulation of methylated sterol precursors and a depletion of ergosterol within the fungal cell membrane weakens the membrane structure and function.

◀ **Pharmacodynamics/Kinetics**

Distribution: V$_{ss}$: IV: ~450 L

Protein binding: >99% (primarily to albumin)

Metabolism: Isavuconazonium sulfate (prodrug) is rapidly hydrolyzed in the blood by esterases to active isavuconazole and an inactive cleavage product. Isavuconazole is metabolized by CYP3A4, CYP 3A5 and UGT.

Bioavailability: Oral: 98%

Half-life elimination: IV: 130 hours

Time to peak: Oral: 2 to 3 hours

Excretion: Oral: 46.1% (feces), 45.5% (urine)

Dosing

Adult & Geriatric Note: Dosage expressed as milligrams of isavuconazonium sulfate; switching between the intravenous (IV) and oral formulations of isavuconazonium sulfate is acceptable; for maintenance dosing, it is not necessary to restart dosing with the initial dose regimen when switching between formulations.

Aspergillosis, invasive:

IV: Initial: 372 mg (isavuconazole 200 mg) every 8 hours for 6 doses; Maintenance: 372 mg (isavuconazole 200 mg) once daily. Start maintenance dose 12 to 24 hours after the last loading dose.

Oral: Initial: 372 mg (200 mg isavuconazole) every 8 hours for 6 doses; Maintenance: 372 mg (isavuconazole 200 mg) once daily. Start maintenance dose 12 to 24 hours after the last loading dose.

Mucormycosis, invasive:

IV: Initial: 372 mg (isavuconazole 200 mg) every 8 hours for 6 doses; Maintenance: 372 mg (isavuconazole 200 mg) once daily. Start maintenance dose 12 to 24 hours after the last loading dose.

Oral: Initial: 372 mg (isavuconazole 200 mg) every 8 hours for 6 doses; Maintenance: 372 mg (isavuconazole 200 mg) once daily. Start maintenance dose 12 to 24 hours after the last loading dose.

Renal Impairment No dosage adjustment necessary.

Hepatic Impairment

Mild or moderate impairment (Child-Pugh class A or B): No dosage adjustment necessary.

Severe impairment (Child-Pugh class C): There are no dosage adjustments provided in the manufacturer's labeling (has not been studied); use with caution.

Administration

IV: Infuse over a minimum of 1 hour; must be administered via an infusion set with an in-line filter (pore size 0.2 to 1.2 micron). Do not administer as an IV bolus injection.

Oral: Swallow capsules whole;. do not chew, crush, dissolve, or open. Administer with or without food.

Monitoring Parameters Hypersensitivity reactions with initial doses, liver function tests (eg, AST, ALT, alkaline phosphatase, total bilirubin) at baseline and periodically during therapy. Infusion-related reactions (eg, hypotension, dyspnea, chills, dizziness, paresthesias, hypoesthesia) during IV infusion.

Dosage Forms Excipient information presented when available (limited, particularly for generics); consult specific product labeling.

Capsule, Oral:

Cresemba: 186 mg [contains disodium edta]

Solution Reconstituted, Intravenous:

Cresemba: 372 mg (1 ea)

Isoniazid (eye soe NYE a zid)

Brand Names: Canada Dom-Isoniazid; Isotamine; PDP-Isoniazid

Index Terms INH; Isonicotinic Acid Hydrazide

Pharmacologic Category Antitubercular Agent

Use

Active tuberculosis infections: Treatment of susceptible active tuberculosis (eg, *Mycobacterium tuberculosis*) infections.

Latent tuberculosis infection (LTBI): Treatment of LTBI caused by *Mycobacterium tuberculosis* (also referred to as prophylaxis or preventive therapy). **Note:** To identify candidates for LTBI treatment, refer to CDC guidelines (http://www.cdc.gov/tb/publications/ltbi/pdf/TargetedLTBI.pdf) for current recommendations.

Pregnancy Considerations Adverse events were observed in some animal reproduction studies. Isoniazid crosses the human placenta. Due to the risk of tuberculosis to the fetus, treatment is recommended when the probability of maternal disease is moderate to high. The CDC recommends isoniazid as part of the initial treatment regimen. Pyridoxine supplementation is recommended (25 mg/day) (CDC 2003). Due to biologic changes during pregnancy and early postpartum, pregnant women may have increased susceptibility to tuberculosis infection or reactivation of latent disease (Mathad 2012).

Breast-Feeding Considerations Small amounts of isoniazid are excreted in breast milk; concentrations are considered nontoxic and not therapeutic to the nursing infant. Women with tuberculosis taking isoniazid should not be discouraged from breast-feeding. Pyridoxine supplementation is recommended for the mother and infant (CDC 2003). Women with tuberculosis mastitis should breast-feed using the unaffected breast (Mathad 2012). In the United States, breast-feeding is not recommended for women with tuberculosis who are also coinfected with HIV (HHS [adult] 2015).

Contraindications Hypersensitivity to isoniazid or any component of the formulation, including drug-induced hepatitis; acute liver disease; previous history of hepatic injury during isoniazid therapy; previous severe adverse reaction (drug fever, chills, arthritis) to isoniazid

Warnings/Precautions Use with caution in patients with severe renal impairment and liver disease. **[U.S. Boxed Warning]: Severe and sometimes fatal hepatitis may occur; usually occurs within the first 3 months of treatment, although may develop even after many months of treatment.** The risk of developing hepatitis is age-related, although isoniazid-induced hepatotoxicity has been reported in children; daily ethanol consumption, chronic liver disease, or injection drug use may also increase the risk. Contraindicated in patients with acute liver disease or previous isoniazid-associated hepatic injury. Fatal hepatitis associated with isoniazid may be increased in women (particularly black and Hispanic and in any woman in the postpartum period). Closer monitoring may be considered in these groups. Patients given isoniazid must be monitored carefully and interviewed at monthly intervals. Patients must report any prodromal symptoms of hepatitis, such as fatigue, paresthesias of hands and feet, weakness, dark urine, rash, anorexia, nausea, fever >3 days' duration, and/or abdominal pain (especially right upper quadrant discomfort), icterus, or vomiting. Patients should be instructed to immediately hold therapy if any of these symptoms occur, and contact their prescriber. If abnormalities of liver function exceed 3 to 5 times the upper limit of normal (ULN), strongly consider discontinuation of isoniazid. If isoniazid must be reinstituted, wait for symptoms and laboratory abnormalities to resolve and use very small and gradual increasing doses, withdrawing therapy immediately if an indication of recurrent hepatic involvement. Treatment with isoniazid for latent tuberculosis infection should be deferred in patients with acute hepatic diseases. Periodic ophthalmic examinations are recommended even when usual symptoms do not occur. Potentially significant drug interactions may exist, requiring dose or frequency adjustment, additional monitoring, and/or selection of alternative therapy. Use should be carefully monitored in the following groups: Daily users of alcohol, active chronic liver disease, severe renal dysfunction, age >35 years, concurrent use of any chronically administered drug, history of previous isoniazid discontinuation, existence of or conditions predisposing to peripheral neuropathy, pregnancy, injection drug use, women in minority groups (particularly postpartum), HIV seropositive patients. AST and ALT should be obtained at baseline and at least monthly during LTBI use. Discontinue temporarily or permanently if liver function tests >3 to 5 times ULN. Pyridoxine (10 to 50 mg/day) is recommended in individuals at risk for development of peripheral neuropathies (eg, HIV infection, nutritional deficiency, diabetes, pregnancy). Children with low milk and low meat intake should receive concomitant pyridoxine therapy. Multidrug regimens should be utilized for the treatment of active tuberculosis to prevent the emergence of drug resistance.

Adverse Reactions Frequency not defined.

Cardiovascular: Flushing, hypertension, palpitation, tachycardia, vasculitis

Central nervous system: Peripheral neuropathy (dose-related incidence, 10% to 20% incidence with 10 mg/kg/day), brain disease (including toxic), depression, dizziness, hyper-reflexia, lethargy, memory impairment, paresthesia, psychosis, seizure, slurred speech

Dermatologic: Skin rash (morbilliform, maculopapular, pruritic, or exfoliative)

Endocrine & metabolic: Gynecomastia, hyperglycemia, metabolic acidosis, pellagra, pyridoxine deficiency

Gastrointestinal: Anorexia, epigastric distress, nausea, stomach pain, vomiting

Hematologic & oncologic: Agranulocytosis, anemia (sideroblastic, hemolytic, or aplastic), eosinophilia, lymphadenopathy, thrombocytopenia

Hepatic: Increased liver enzymes (mild, 10% to 20%), bilirubinuria, jaundice, hepatic insufficiency, hepatitis (may involve progressive liver damage; risk increases with age; 2.3% in patients >50 years), hyperbilirubinemia

Neuromuscular & skeletal: Arthralgia, lupus-like syndrome, rheumatic disease, weakness

Ophthalmic: Blurred vision, optic atrophy, optic neuritis, vision loss

Miscellaneous: Fever

Postmarketing and/or case reports (Limited to important or life-threatening): Hepatotoxicity (idiosyncratic) (Chalasani, 2014)

Drug Interactions

Metabolism/Transport Effects Substrate of CYP2E1 (major); **Note:** Assignment of Major/Minor substrate status based on clinically relevant drug interaction potential; **Inhibits** CYP1A2 (weak), CYP2A6 (moderate), CYP2C19 (moderate), CYP2C9 (weak), CYP2D6 (moderate), CYP2E1 (moderate), CYP3A4 (weak); **Induces** CYP2E1 (weak/moderate)

Avoid Concomitant Use

Avoid concomitant use of Isoniazid with any of the following: Artesunate; Pimozide; Tegafur; Thioridazine

Increased Effect/Toxicity

Isoniazid may increase the levels/effects of: Acetaminophen; ARIPiprazole; Artesunate; Brexpiprazole; CarBAMazepine; Chlorzoxazone; Cilostazol; Citalopram; CycloSERINE; CYP2A6 Substrates; CYP2C19 Substrates; CYP2D6 Substrates; CYP2E1 Substrates; Dofetilide; DOXOrubicin (Conventional); Eliglustat; Fesoterodine; Flibanserin; Fosphenytoin; Hydrocodone; Lomitapide; Metoprolol; Nebivolol; NiMODipine; Phenytoin; Pimozide; Propacetamol; Theophylline Derivatives; Thioridazine; TiZANidine

The levels/effects of Isoniazid may be increased by: Disulfiram; Ethionamide; Propafenone; Rifamycin Derivatives

Decreased Effect

Isoniazid may decrease the levels/effects of: Artesunate; Clopidogrel; Codeine; Itraconazole; Ketoconazole (Systemic); Levodopa; Tamoxifen; Tegafur; TraMADol

The levels/effects of Isoniazid may be decreased by: Antacids; Corticosteroids (Systemic); Cyproterone

Food Interactions

Isoniazid may decrease folic acid absorption and alters pyridoxine metabolism. Management: Increase dietary intake of folate, niacin, and magnesium.

Tyramine-containing food: Isoniazid has weak monoamine oxidase inhibiting activity and may potentially inhibit tyramine metabolism. Several case reports of mild reactions (flushing, palpitations, headache, mild increase in blood pressure, diaphoresis) after ingestion of certain types of cheese or red wine, have been reported (Self, 1999; Toutoungi, 1985). Management: Manufacturer's labeling recommends avoiding tyramine-containing foods (eg, aged or matured cheese, air-dried or cured meats including sausages and salamis; fava or broad bean pods, tap/draft beers, Marmite concentrate, sauerkraut, soy sauce, and other soybean condiments). However, the clinical relevance of the tyramine reaction for the vast majority of patients receiving isoniazid has been questioned due to isoniazid's weak MAO inhibition and the relatively few published case reports of the interaction. Although not fully investigated, it has been proposed that the reaction has a genetic component and may only be significant in poor or intermediate acetylators since isoniazid is primarily inactivated by acetylation (DiMartini, 1995; Toutoungi, 1985).

Histamine-containing food: Isoniazid may also inhibit diamine oxidase resulting in headache, sweating, palpitations, flushing, diarrhea, itching, wheezing, dyspnea or hypotension to histamine-containing foods (eg, skipjack, tuna, saury, other tropical fish). Management: Manufacturer's labeling recommends avoiding histamine-containing foods; corticosteroids and antihistamines may be administered if histamine intoxication occurs (Miki 2005).

Storage/Stability

Tablet: Store at 20°C to 25°C (68°F to 77°F). Protect from light.

Oral solution: Store at 15°C to 30°C (59°F to 86°F). Protect from light.

Injection: Store at 20°C to 25°C (68°F to 77°F). Protect from light. Isoniazid injection may crystallize at low temperatures. If this occurs, warm the vial to room temperature before use to redissolve the crystals.

Mechanism of Action Isoniazid inhibits the synthesis of mycoloic acids, an essential component of the bacterial cell wall. At therapeutic levels isoniazid is bacteriocidal against actively growing intracellular and extracellular *Mycobacterium tuberculosis* organisms.

Pharmacodynamics/Kinetics Note: Isoniazid is primarily metabolized by acetylation and dehydrazination. Rate of acetylation is genetically determined. Approximately 50% of blacks and whites are "slow inactivators" and the rest are "rapid inactivators". The large majority of Eskimo and Asian patients are "rapid inactivators". Acetylation rate does not significantly alter the effectiveness, but slow acetylation may lead to higher blood levels and possibly an increase in adverse effects.

Absorption: Oral, IM: Rapid and complete; food reduces rate and extent of absorption

Distribution: All body tissues and fluids including CSF

Protein binding: 10% to 15%

Metabolism: Hepatic to acetylisoniazid with decay rate determined genetically by acetylation phenotype; undergoes further hydrolysis to isonicotinic acid and acetylhydrazine

Half-life: May be prolonged in patients with impaired hepatic function or severe renal impairment

Fast acetylators: 30-100 minutes

Slow acetylators: 2-5 hours

Time to peak, serum: 1 to 2 hours

Excretion: Urine (75% to 95% as unchanged drug and metabolites); small amounts excreted in feces and saliva

Dosing

Adult & Geriatric Recommendations often change due to resistant strains and newly-developed information; consult CDC for current recommendations. Intramuscular injection is available for patients who are unable to either take or absorb oral therapy.

Tuberculosis, active (drug susceptible; excludes meningitis): Oral, IM: Always given in combination with other antitubercular drugs. **Note:** Concomitant administration of pyridoxine is recommended in malnourished patients or those prone to neuropathy (eg, patients with HIV-infection, diabetes, or chronic alcohol abusers). In the initial dosing phase, ethambutol may be discontinued if drug susceptibility studies demonstrate susceptibility to isoniazid, rifampin and pyrazinamide (CDC 2011).

CDC recommendations (MMWR 2003): Initial: 5 mg/kg/day once daily (usual dose: 300 mg daily) with concomitant rifampin, pyrazinamide and with or without ethambutol for 8 weeks.

Continuation phase: 5 mg/kg/day once daily (usual dose: 300 mg daily) with concomitant rifampin for 18 weeks.

Note: The above is the CDC preferred regimen (CDC 2011)

or

Initial phase: 5 mg/kg/day once daily (usual dose: 300 mg daily) with concomitant rifampin, pyrazinamide and with or without ethambutol for 2 weeks, followed by 15 mg/kg/dose 2 times weekly (maximum: 900 mg per dose) with concomitant rifampin, pyrazinamide and with or without ethambutol for 6 weeks.

Continuation phase: 15 mg/kg/dose 2 times weekly (maximum: 900 mg per dose) with concomitant rifampin for 18 weeks.

or

Initial: 15 mg/kg/dose 3 times weekly (maximum: 900 mg per dose) with concomitant rifampin, pyrazinamide and with or without ethambutol for 8 weeks.

Continuation phase: 15 mg/kg/dose 3 times weekly (maximum: 900 mg per dose) with concomitant rifampin for 18 weeks.

Note: Treatment may be defined by the number of doses administered (eg, CDC preferred regimen involves 182 doses of INH and rifampin, and 56 doses of pyrazinamide [CDC 2011]).

Tuberculosis, active, meningitis (drug susceptible): Oral, IM: Always given in combination with other antitubercular drugs. **Note:** Concomitant administration of pyridoxine is recommended in malnourished patients or those prone to neuropathy (eg, patients with HIV-infection, diabetes or chronic alcohol abusers).

CDC recommendations (MMWR 2003): Initial: 5 mg/kg once daily (usual dose: 300 mg) with concomitant rifampin, pyrazinamide and ethambutol for 8 weeks; dexamethasone is given concomitantly in the first 6 weeks

Continuation phase: 5 mg/kg/day once daily (maximum: 300 mg daily) with concomitant rifampin for 7 to 10 months.

Note: The above is the CDC preferred regimen (MMWR 2003)

Tuberculosis, latent infection (LTBI): Oral, IM:

Note: Concomitant administration of pyridoxine 10 to 50 mg daily is recommended in malnourished patients or those prone to neuropathy (eg, patients with HIV-infection, diabetes or chronic alcohol abusers).

CDC recommendations (CDC 2013):

Non-HIV exposed/infected: 5 mg/kg (maximum: 300 mg per dose) once daily for 6 or 9 months or 15 mg/kg (maximum: 900 mg per dose) twice weekly for 6 or 9 months. **Note:** 9 months is optimal; 6 months may be considered to reduce costs of therapy and improve adherence.

HIV-exposed/-infected patients who are receiving antiretroviral therapy: 5 mg/kg (maximum: 300 mg per dose) once daily for 9 months or 15 mg/kg (maximum: 900 mg per dose) twice weekly for 9 months. **Note:** LTBI treatment is recommended in HIV-infected patients testing positive for LTBI (but have no evidence of TB disease and no history of treatment for active or LTBI) **or** in HIV-infected close contacts of anyone who has infectious TB (regardless of screening tests for LTBI). LTBI treatment is not associated with clinical benefit or recommended in HIV infected patients who are anergic and who have not had recent contact with anyone with infectious TB (HHS [OI adult 2015])

Alternate regimen: 15 mg/kg/dose (maximum 900 mg) once weekly in combination with rifapentine for 12 weeks. **Note:** The rifapentine-containing regimen may only be used in patients who are not pregnant and/or not expecting to become pregnant; if used in HIV-infected patients, it may only be used in otherwise healthy HIV-infected patients **not** receiving antiretroviral therapy (ART) (high risk of drug-drug interactions with rifapentine) (CDC 2013; HHS [adult] 2015).

Nontuberculous mycobacterium *(M. kansasii)* (off-label use): 5 mg/kg/day (maximum: 300 mg daily) for duration to include 12 months of culture-negative sputum; typically used in combination with ethambutol and rifampin (Griffith 2007).

Pediatric Recommendations often change due to resistant strains and newly-developed information; consult CDC for current recommendations. Intramuscular injection is available for patients who are unable to either take or absorb oral therapy.

Tuberculosis, active (drug susceptible; excludes meningitis): Always given in combination with other antitubercular drugs. In the initial dosing phase, ethambutol may be discontinued if drug susceptibility studies demonstrate susceptibility to isoniazid, rifampin and pyrazinamide (CDC 2011).

Infants, Children, and Adolescents: Oral, IM:

CDC recommendations (MMWR 2003): Initial: 10 to 15 mg/kg/day once daily (maximum dose: 300 mg daily) with concomitant rifampin and pyrazinamide, with or without ethambutol for 8 weeks.

Continuation phase: 10 to 15 mg/kg/day once daily (maximum: 300 mg daily) with concomitant rifampin for 18 weeks.

Note: The above is the CDC preferred regimen (CDC 2011)

or

Initial phase 1: 10 to 15 mg/kg/day once daily (maximum dose: 300 mg daily) with concomitant rifampin, pyrazinamide and with or without ethambutol for 2 weeks, followed by:

Initial phase 2: 20 to 30 mg/kg/dose 2 times weekly (maximum: 900 mg per dose) with concomitant rifampin, pyrazinamide and with or without ethambutol for 6 weeks.

Continuation phase: 20 to 30 mg/kg/dose 2 times weekly (maximum: 900 mg per dose) with concomitant rifampin for 18 weeks.

Alternate recommendations (Red Book [AAP 2012]): Initial: 10 to 15 mg/kg once daily (maximum dose: 300 mg) or 20 to 30 mg/kg 2 times weekly (maximum dose: 900 mg) with concomitant rifampin, pyrazinamide and ethambutol for 2 months

Continuation phase: 10 to 15 mg/kg once daily (maximum dose: 300 mg) or 20 to 30 mg/kg 2 times weekly (maximum dose: 900 mg) with concomitant rifampin for 4 months.

Tuberculosis, active, meningitis (drug susceptible): Always given in combination with other antitubercular drugs. **Note:** Concomitant administration of pyridoxine is recommended in malnourished patients or those prone to neuropathy (eg, patients with HIV-infection, diabetes or chronic alcohol abusers).

Infants, Children, and Adolescents: Oral, IM:

CDC recommendations (MMWR 2003): Initial: 10 to 15 mg/kg once daily (maximum dose: 300 mg) with concomitant rifampin, pyrazinamide and ethambutol for 8 weeks; dexamethasone is given concomitantly in the first 6 weeks.

Continuation phase: 10 to 15 mg/kg/day once daily (maximum: 300 mg daily) with concomitant rifampin for 7 to 10 months.

Note: The above is the CDC preferred regimen (MMWR 2003)

Alternate recommendations (Red Book [AAP 2012]): Initial: 10 to 15 mg/kg once daily (maximum dose: 300 mg) with concomitant rifampin, pyrazinamide and an aminoglycoside, ethambutol or ethionamide for 8 weeks.

Continuation phase: 10 to 15 mg/kg once daily (maximum dose: 300 mg) or 20 to 30 mg/kg 2 times weekly (maximum dose: 900 mg) with concomitant rifampin for 7 to 10 months.

Tuberculosis, latent infection (LTBI):

Infants and Children <12 years: Oral, IM:

CDC recommendation (CDC 2013): 10 to 20 mg/kg/day once daily (maximum: 300 mg per dose) (preferred regimen) or 20 to 40 mg/kg (maximum: 900 mg per dose) twice weekly for 9 months.

Note: Once weekly regimen of isoniazid and rifapentine may also be considered in children ≥2 or <12 years if completion of 9 month regimen (preferred) is unlikely and the hazard of tuberculosis is great (CDC 2013). Refer to Children ≥12 years and Adolescents dosing.

Alternate recommendations (Red Book [AAP 2012]): 10 to 15 mg/kg/day once daily (maximum: 300 mg per dose) for 9 months.

Children ≥12 years and Adolescents: Oral, IM:

CDC recommendations (CDC 2013): 10 to 20 mg/kg/day once daily (maximum: 300 mg per dose) (preferred regimen) or 20 to 40 mg/kg (maximum: 900 mg per dose) twice weekly for 9 months (CDC 2013), or 15 mg/kg/dose (maximum: 900 mg per dose) once weekly in combination with rifapentine for 12 weeks (CDC 2013). **Note:** The rifapentine-containing regimen may be used in otherwise healthy HIV-infected patients, but only in patients **not** receiving antiretroviral therapy (ART) (CDC 2013; HHS [adult] 2015).

Alternate recommendation (Red Book [AAP 2012]): 10 to 15 mg/kg/day once daily (maximum: 300 mg per dose) for 9 months

Renal Impairment

No dosage adjustments necessary.

ESRD receiving intermittent hemodialysis (IHD): Administer dose postdialysis (Aronoff 2007); Dialyzable (50% to 100%)

Hepatic Impairment There are no dosage adjustments provided in the manufacturer's labeling; however, use with caution, may accumulate and additional liver damage may occur in patients with preexisting liver disease. Contraindicated in patients with acute liver disease or previous isoniazid-associated hepatic injury. For ALT or AST >3 times the ULN: discontinue or temporarily withhold treatment. Treatment with isoniazid for latent tuberculosis infection should be deferred in patients with acute hepatic diseases.

Dietary Considerations Increase dietary intake of folate, niacin, magnesium.

Administration

Oral: May be administered with or without food.

Intramuscular: IM injection may be used for patients who are unable to either take or absorb oral therapy. Inject deep IM into a large muscle mass.

Monitoring Parameters Baseline and periodic (more frequently in patients with higher risk for hepatitis) liver function tests (ALT and AST); sputum cultures monthly (until 2 consecutive negative cultures reported); monitoring for prodromal signs of hepatitis

LTBI therapy: American Thoracic Society/Centers for Disease Control (ATS/CDC) recommendations: Monthly clinical evaluation, including brief physical exam for adverse events. Use should be carefully monitored in the following groups: daily users of alcohol, active chronic liver disease,

severe renal dysfunction, age >35 years, concurrent use of any chronically administered drug, history of previous isoniazid discontinuation, existence of or conditions predisposing to peripheral neuropathy, pregnancy, injection drug use, women in minority groups (particularly postpartum), HIV seropositive patients. AST and ALT should be obtained at baseline and at least monthly during LTBI use. Discontinue temporarily or permanently if liver function tests >3 to 5 times ULN. Routine, periodic monitoring is recommended for any patient with an abnormal baseline or at increased risk for hepatotoxicity.

Test Interactions False-positive urinary glucose with Clinitest®

Additional Information The AAP recommends that pyridoxine supplementation (1 to 2 mg/kg/day) should be administered to malnourished children or adolescents on meat or milk-deficient diets, breast-feeding infants, and those predisposed to neuritis to prevent peripheral neuropathy; administration of isoniazid syrup has been associated with diarrhea.

Dosage Forms Excipient information presented when available (limited, particularly for generics); consult specific product labeling.
Solution, Injection:
  Generic: 100 mg/mL (10 mL)
Syrup, Oral:
  Generic: 50 mg/5 mL (473 mL)
Tablet, Oral:
  Generic: 100 mg, 300 mg

Extemporaneous Preparations Note: Commercial oral solution is available (50 mg/mL)

A 10 mg/mL oral suspension may be made with tablets, purified water, and sorbitol. Crush ten 100 mg tablets in a mortar and reduce to a fine powder. Add 10 mL of purified water and mix to a uniform paste. Mix while adding sorbitol in incremental proportions to almost 100 mL; transfer to a graduated cylinder, rinse mortar with sorbitol, and add quantity of sorbitol sufficient to make 100 mL (do not use sugar-based solutions). Label "shake well" and "refrigerate". Stable for 21 days refrigerated.
Nahata MC, Pai VB, and Hipple TF, *Pediatric Drug Formulations*, 5th ed, Cincinnati, OH: Harvey Whitney Books Co, 2004.

♦ Isonicotinic Acid Hydrazide *see* Isoniazid *on page* 990
♦ Isonipecaine Hydrochloride *see* Meperidine *on page* 1144
♦ Isophane Insulin *see* Insulin NPH *on page* 959
♦ Isophane Insulin and Regular Insulin *see* Insulin NPH and Insulin Regular *on page* 960
♦ Isophosphamide *see* Ifosfamide *on page* 913
♦ Isoprenaline *see* Isoproterenol *on page* 993

Isoproterenol (eye soe proe TER e nole)

Brand Names: US Isuprel
Index Terms Isoprenaline; Isoproterenol Hydrochloride
Pharmacologic Category Beta$_1$- & Beta$_2$-Adrenergic Agonist Agent
Use Manufacturer's labeled indications (see **"Note"**): Mild or transient episodes of heart block that do not require electric shock or pacemaker therapy; serious episodes of heart block and Adams-Stokes attacks (except when caused by ventricular tachycardia or fibrillation); cardiac arrest until electric shock or pacemaker therapy is available; bronchospasm during anesthesia; adjunct to fluid and electrolyte replacement therapy and other drugs and procedures in the treatment of hypovolemic or septic shock and low cardiac output states (eg, decompensated heart failure, cardiogenic shock)

Note: The use of isoproterenol in advanced cardiac life support (ACLS) has largely been supplanted by the use of other adrenergic agents (eg, epinephrine and dopamine). The use of isoproterenol for bronchospasm during anesthesia and cardiogenic, hypovolemic, or septic shock is no longer recommended.
Dosing
Adult & Geriatric Note: Patients may exhibit dose-dependent vasodilation due to unopposed beta$_2$-agonism elicited by isoproterenol.
  Bradyarrhythmias, AV nodal block, or refractory torsade de pointes: Continuous IV infusion: Usual range: 2-10 mcg/minute; titrate to patient response.
  Brugada syndrome with electrical storm (off-label use): IV bolus: Initial: 1-2 mcg, followed by a continuous infusion of 0.15-0.3 mcg/minute for 1 day; may repeat sequence if ventricular tachycardia/fibrillation recurs (Watanabe, 2006; Zipes, 2006).

Tilt table testing for syncope (Benditt, 1996; Brignole, 2004): Continuous IV infusion: Initial: 1 mcg/minute; increase as necessary based on response; maximum dose: 5 mcg/minute. **Note:** Timing of initiation and dose adjustment during test may be institution-specific.
Pediatric Note: Patients may exhibit dose-dependent vasodilation due to unopposed beta$_2$-agonism elicited by isoproterenol.
  Bradyarrhythmias, AV nodal block, or refractory torsade de pointes: Continuous IV infusion: Usual range: 0.05-2 mcg/**kg**/minute; titrate to patient response.
Renal Impairment No dosage adjustment provided in manufacturer's labeling.
Hepatic Impairment No dosage adjustment provided in manufacturer's labeling.
Additional Information Complete prescribing information should be consulted for additional detail.
Dosage Forms Excipient information presented when available (limited, particularly for generics); consult specific product labeling. [DSC] = Discontinued product
Solution, Injection, as hydrochloride:
  Isuprel: 0.2 mg/mL (1 mL, 5 mL) [contains disodium edta]
  Isuprel: 0.2 mg/mL (1 mL [DSC], 5 mL [DSC]) [contains sodium metabisulfite]

♦ Isoproterenol Hydrochloride *see* Isoproterenol *on page* 993
♦ Isoptin SR *see* Verapamil *on page* 1889
♦ Isopto Atropine [DSC] *see* Atropine (Ophthalmic) *on page* 178
♦ Isopto Atropine (Can) *see* Atropine (Ophthalmic) *on page* 178
♦ Isopto Carbachol *see* Carbachol *on page* 303
♦ Isopto® Carbachol (Can) *see* Carbachol *on page* 303
♦ Isopto Carpine *see* Pilocarpine (Ophthalmic) *on page* 1452
♦ Isopto® Carpine (Can) *see* Pilocarpine (Ophthalmic) *on page* 1452
♦ Isopto Homatropine *see* Homatropine *on page* 878
♦ Isordil Titradose *see* Isosorbide Dinitrate *on page* 993

Isosorbide Dinitrate (eye soe SOR bide dye NYE trate)

Brand Names: US Dilatrate-SR; Isochron [DSC]; IsoDitrate ER; Isordil Titradose
Brand Names: Canada ISDN; PMS-Isosorbide
Index Terms ISD; ISDN
Pharmacologic Category Antianginal Agent; Vasodilator
Use
Angina pectoris, prevention: Prevention of angina pectoris due to coronary artery disease.
Note: Due to slower onset of action, isosorbide dinitrate is not the drug of choice to abort an acute anginal episode.
Pregnancy Considerations Adverse events have been observed in some animal reproduction studies. Nitric oxide donors, such as isosorbide, have been evaluated for preeclampsia and cervical ripening; isosorbide dinitrate use in these conditions is not currently recommended (Kalidindi 2012; Ramirez 2011).
Breast-Feeding Considerations It is not known if isosorbide dinitrate is excreted in breast milk. The manufacturer recommends that caution be exercised when administering isosorbide dinitrate to nursing women.
Contraindications
Hypersensitivity to isosorbide dinitrate or any component of the formulation; concurrent use with phosphodiesterase inhibitors (sildenafil, tadalafil, vardenafil, or avanafil); concurrent use with riociguat
Canadian labeling: Additional contraindications (not in US labeling): Cardiogenic shock or risk of cardiogenic shock developing
Warnings/Precautions Severe hypotension can occur; paradoxical bradycardia and increased angina pectoris can accompany hypotension. Orthostatic hypotension can also occur; ethanol can accentuate this. Use with caution in volume depletion and hypotension and use with extreme caution with inferior wall MI and suspected right ventricular infarctions. Severe hypotension, particularly with upright posture, may occur with even small doses. Avoid use in patients with hypertrophic cardiomyopathy (HCM) with outflow tract obstruction; nitrates may reduce preload, exacerbating obstruction and cause hypotension or syncope and/or worsening of heart failure (ACCF/AHA [Gersh 2011]).

Not recommended in patients with acute MI or HF (cannot easily reverse effects if adverse events develop). Nitrates may precipitate or aggravate increased intracranial pressure and subsequently may worsen clinical outcomes in patients with neurologic injury (eg, intracranial

hemorrhage, traumatic brain injury). Appropriate dosing intervals are needed to minimize tolerance development. Tolerance can only be overcome by short periods of nitrate absence from the body. Dose escalation does not overcome this effect. When used for HF in combination with hydralazine, tolerance is less of a concern (Gogia 1995).

Potentially significant drug-drug interactions may exist, requiring dose or frequency adjustment, additional monitoring, and/or selection of alternative therapy.

Adverse Reactions Frequency not defined.

Cardiovascular: Crescendo angina (uncommon), hypotension, orthostatic hypotension, rebound hypertension (uncommon), syncope (uncommon)

Central nervous system: Headache (most common), lightheadedness (related to blood pressure changes)

Hematologic: Methemoglobinemia (rare, overdose)

Drug Interactions

Metabolism/Transport Effects Substrate of CYP3A4 (major); **Note:** Assignment of Major/Minor substrate status based on clinically relevant drug interaction potential

Avoid Concomitant Use

Avoid concomitant use of Isosorbide Dinitrate with any of the following: Conivaptan; Fusidic Acid (Systemic); Idelalisib; Phosphodiesterase 5 Inhibitors; Riociguat

Increased Effect/Toxicity

Isosorbide Dinitrate may increase the levels/effects of: Amifostine; Antipsychotic Agents (Second Generation [Atypical]); DULoxetine; Hypotension-Associated Agents; Levodopa; Prilocaine; Riociguat; Rosiglitazone; Sodium Nitrite

The levels/effects of Isosorbide Dinitrate may be increased by: Alcohol (Ethyl); Alfuzosin; Aprepitant; Barbiturates; Blood Pressure Lowering Agents; Brimonidine (Topical); Conivaptan; CYP3A4 Inhibitors (Moderate); CYP3A4 Inhibitors (Strong); Dapoxetine; Dapsone (Topical); Dasatinib; Diazoxide; Fosaprepitant; Fusidic Acid (Systemic); Herbs (Hypotensive Properties); Idelalisib; Ivacaftor; Luliconazole; Mifepristone; Molsidomine; Netupitant; Nicorandil; Nitric Oxide; Obinutuzumab; Osimertinib; Palbociclib; Pentoxifylline; Phosphodiesterase 5 Inhibitors; Prostacyclin Analogues; Simeprevir; Stiripentol

Decreased Effect

The levels/effects of Isosorbide Dinitrate may be decreased by: Bosentan; CYP3A4 Inducers (Moderate); CYP3A4 Inducers (Strong); Dabrafenib; Deferasirox; Enzalutamide; Mitotane; Osimertinib; Siltuximab; St Johns Wort; Tocilizumab

Storage/Stability

Extended-release tablets: Store at 20°C to 25°C (68°F to 77°F).

Sustained-release capsules and immediate-release tablets: Store at 20°C to 25°C (68°F to 77°F); excursions permitted to 15°C to 30°C (59°F to 86°F). Protect from light.

Mechanism of Action Isosorbide dinitrate and other nitrates form free radical nitric oxide. In smooth muscle, nitric oxide activates guanylate cyclase which increases guanosine 3'5' monophosphate (cGMP) leading to dephosphorylation of myosin light chains and smooth muscle relaxation. Produces a vasodilator effect on the peripheral veins and arteries with more prominent effects on the veins. Primarily reduces cardiac oxygen demand by decreasing preload (left ventricular end-diastolic pressure); may modestly reduce afterload. Additionally, coronary artery dilation improves collateral flow to ischemic regions.

Pharmacodynamics/Kinetics

Onset of action: Sublingual tablet: ~2 to 5 minutes; Oral tablet and capsule (includes extended-release formulations): ~1 hour

Duration: Sublingual tablet: 1 to 2 hours; Oral tablet and capsule (includes extended-release formulations): Up to 8 hours

Distribution: V_d: 2 to 4 L/kg

Metabolism: Extensively hepatic to conjugated active metabolites isosorbide 5-mononitrate and 2-mononitrate

Bioavailability: Highly variable (10% to 90%); increases with chronic therapy

Half-life elimination: Parent drug: ~1 hour; Metabolites (5-mononitrate: 5 hours; 2-mononitrate: 2 hours)

Dosing

Adult

Angina pectoris (prevention): Note: Due to slower onset of action, isosorbide dinitrate is not the drug of choice to abort an acute anginal episode. Tolerance to nitrate effects develops with chronic exposure; dose escalation does not overcome this effect. Tolerance can only be overcome by short periods of nitrate absence from the body. Nitrate-free intervals of ≥14 hours (immediate release products) or >18 hours (sustained release products) may help minimize tolerance.

Oral:

Immediate release: Initial: 5 to 20 mg 2 to 3 times daily; Maintenance: 10 to 40 mg 2 to 3 times daily **or** 5 to 80 mg 2 to 3 times daily (Anderson 2011)

Sustained release: 40 to 160 mg/day has been used in clinical trials (a nitrate free interval of >18 hours is recommended; however, a clinically efficacious dosage interval has not been clearly established) **or** 40 mg 1 to 2 times daily (Anderson 2011). Maximum dose: 160 mg/day (Dilatrate-SR only).

Sublingual [Canadian product]: 5 to 10 mg every 2 to 4 hours for prophylaxis of acute angina; may supplement with 5 to 10 mg prior to activities which may provoke an anginal episode.

Heart failure (off-label use; ACCF/AHA [Yancy 2013]):

Oral: Immediate release (**Note:** Use in combination with hydralazine):

Initial dose: 20 to 30 mg 3 to 4 times daily

Maximum dose: 120 mg daily in divided doses

Esophageal spastic disorders (off-label use; Goyal, 1998): *Oral, sublingual:* Immediate release: 10 to 30 mg before meals

Geriatric Elderly patients should be given lowest recommended adult daily doses initially and titrate upward. Refer to adult dosing.

Renal Impairment There are no dosage adjustments provided in the manufacturer's labeling.

Hemodialysis: Supplemental dose is not necessary.

Peritoneal dialysis: Supplemental dose is not necessary.

Hepatic Impairment There are no dosage adjustments provided in the manufacturer's labeling.

Administration Do not administer around the clock; allow nitrate-free interval ≥14 hours (immediate release products) and >18 hours (sustained release products). Do not chew or crush sublingual tablets or sustained release formulations.

Immediate release products: For twice daily dosing, consider administering at 8 AM and 1 PM. For 3 times daily dosing, consider 8 AM, 1 PM, and 6 PM.

Sustained release products: Consider once daily in morning or twice-daily dosing at 8 AM and between 1 PM and 2 PM.

Monitoring Parameters Blood pressure, heart rate

Product Availability Sublingual tablets have been discontinued in the US for more than 1 year.

Dosage Forms Excipient information presented when available (limited, particularly for generics); consult specific product labeling. [DSC] = Discontinued product

Capsule Extended Release, Oral:

Dilatrate-SR: 40 mg [DSC]

Dilatrate-SR: 40 mg [contains fd&c yellow #10 (quinoline yellow)]

Tablet, Oral:

Isordil Titradose: 5 mg [scored; contains fd&c red #40]

Isordil Titradose: 40 mg [scored; contains brilliant blue fcf (fd&c blue #1), fd&c yellow #10 (quinoline yellow), fd&c yellow #6 (sunset yellow)]

Generic: 5 mg, 10 mg, 20 mg, 30 mg

Tablet Extended Release, Oral:

Isochron: 40 mg [DSC]

IsoDitrate ER: 40 mg

Generic: 40 mg

Tablet Sublingual, Sublingual:

Generic: 2.5 mg [DSC], 5 mg [DSC]

Dosage Forms: Canada Excipient information presented when available (limited, particularly for generics); consult specific product labeling.

Tablet, Oral: 10 mg, 30 mg

Tablet, Sublingual: 5 mg

Isosorbide Dinitrate and Hydralazine
(eye soe SOR bide dye NYE trate & hye DRAL a zeen)

Brand Names: US BiDil

Index Terms Hydralazine and Isosorbide Dinitrate

Pharmacologic Category Antihypertensive; Vasodilator

Use

Heart failure: Treatment of heart failure as an adjunct to standard therapy in self-identified African American patients

American College of Cardiology/American Heart Association heart failure guidelines recommendations (ACCF/AHA [Yancy, 2013]). Patients who are African-American (self-identified) with heart failure with reduced ejection fraction (HFrEF) NYHA class III-IV remaining symptomatic despite optimal guideline-directed medical therapy; Patients with HFrEF who do not tolerate an ACE inhibitor or an angiotensin receptor blocker (ARB)

Dosing

Adult & Geriatric

Heart failure: Oral:

Initial: One tablet 3 times daily.

Maintenance: May titrate in 3 to 5 days to a maximum dose of 2 tablets 3 times daily.

Renal Impairment There are no dosage adjustments provided in the manufacturer's labeling (has not been studied).

Hepatic Impairment There are no dosage adjustments provided in the manufacturer's labeling (has not been studied).

Adjustment for Toxicity If patient experiences intolerable side effects, dose may be reduced to as little as one-half tablet 3 times daily; dose should be titrated upward as soon as tolerated.

Additional Information Complete prescribing information should be consulted for additional detail.

Dosage Forms

Tablet, oral:

BiDil: Isosorbide dinitrate 20 mg and hydralazine hydrochloride 37.5 mg

---

Isosorbide Mononitrate

(eye soe SOR bide mon oh NYE trate)

Brand Names: US Imdur [DSC]; Monoket [DSC]

Brand Names: Canada Apo-ISMN; Imdur; PMS-ISMN; PRO-ISMN

Index Terms Imdur; ISMN

Pharmacologic Category Antianginal Agent; Vasodilator

Use Prevention of angina pectoris

Pregnancy Considerations Adverse events were observed in some animal reproduction studies. Nitric oxide donors, such as isosorbide, have been evaluated for pre-eclampsia and cervical ripening; isosorbide mononitrate use in these conditions is not currently recommended (Kalidindi, 2012; Ramirez, 2011).

Breast-Feeding Considerations It is not known if isosorbide mononitrate is excreted in breast milk. The manufacturer recommends that caution be exercised when administering isosorbide mononitrate to nursing women.

Contraindications Hypersensitivity to isosorbide mononitrate or any component of the formulation; hypersensitivity to organic nitrates; concurrent use with phosphodiesterase-5 (PDE-5) inhibitors (sildenafil, tadalafil, or vardenafil)

Warnings/Precautions Avoid use in hypertrophic cardiomyopathy with outflow tract obstruction; nitrates may reduce preload, exacerbating obstruction and cause hypotension or syncope and/or worsening of heart failure (Gersh, 2011). Use with caution in volume depletion, moderate hypotension, and extreme caution with inferior wall MI and suspected right ventricular infarctions. Instruct patients to use caution with ethanol; may increase risk of hypotension. Nitrates may precipitate or aggravate increased intracranial pressure and subsequently may worsen clinical outcomes in patients with neurologic injury (eg, intracranial hemorrhage, traumatic brain injury). Postural hypotension, transient episodes of weakness, dizziness, or syncope may occur even with small doses; ethanol accentuates these effects; tolerance and cross-tolerance to nitrate antianginal and hemodynamic effects may occur during prolonged isosorbide mononitrate therapy; (minimized by using the smallest effective dose, by alternating coronary vasodilators or offering drug-free intervals of as little as 12 hours). Excessive doses may result in severe headache, blurred vision, or xerostomia; increased anginal symptoms may be a result of dosage increases. Avoid concurrent use with PDE-5 inhibitors (eg, sildenafil, tadalafil, vardenafil). When nitrate administration becomes medically necessary, may administer nitrates only if 24 hours have elapsed after use of sildenafil or vardenafil (48 hours after tadalafil use) (O'Connor, 2010).

Adverse Reactions

>10%: Central nervous system: Headache (13% to 35%)

1% to 10%:

Cardiovascular: Angina (≤2%), flushing (≤2%)

Central nervous system: Dizziness (≤4%), fatigue (≤4%), pain (≤4%), emotional lability (≤2%)

Dermatologic: Pruritus (≤2%), rash (≤2%)

Gastrointestinal: Nausea (≤3%), abdominal pain (≤2%), diarrhea (≤2%)

Respiratory: Upper respiratory infection (≤4%), cough increased (≤2%)

Miscellaneous: Allergic reaction (≤2%)

<1% (Limited to important or life-threatening): Apoplexy, arrhythmia, bradycardia, dyspnea, edema, hyper-/hypotension, methemoglobinemia (rare, overdose), MI, orthostatic hypotension, pallor, palpitation, paresthesia, tachycardia

Drug Interactions

Metabolism/Transport Effects **Substrate** of CYP3A4 (major); **Note:** Assignment of Major/Minor substrate status based on clinically relevant drug interaction potential

Avoid Concomitant Use

Avoid concomitant use of Isosorbide Mononitrate with any of the following: Conivaptan; Fusidic Acid (Systemic); Idelalisib; Phosphodiesterase 5 Inhibitors; Riociguat

Increased Effect/Toxicity

Isosorbide Mononitrate may increase the levels/effects of: Prilocaine; Riociguat; Rosiglitazone; Sodium Nitrite

The levels/effects of Isosorbide Mononitrate may be increased by: Alcohol (Ethyl); Aprepitant; Conivaptan; CYP3A4 Inhibitors (Moderate); CYP3A4 Inhibitors (Strong); Dapoxetine; Dapsone (Topical); Dasatinib; Fosaprepitant; Fusidic Acid (Systemic); Idelalisib; Ivacaftor; Luliconazole; Mifepristone; Molsidomine; Netupitant; Nitric Oxide; Osimertinib; Palbociclib; Phosphodiesterase 5 Inhibitors; Simeprevir; Stiripentol

Decreased Effect

The levels/effects of Isosorbide Mononitrate may be decreased by: Bosentan; CYP3A4 Inducers (Moderate); CYP3A4 Inducers (Strong); Dabrafenib; Deferasirox; Enzalutamide; Mitotane; Osimertinib; Siltuximab; St Johns Wort; Tocilizumab

Storage/Stability Tablets should be stored in a tight container at room temperature of 15°C to 30°C (59°F to 86°F).

Mechanism of Action Nitroglycerin and other nitrates form free radical nitric oxide. In smooth muscle, nitric oxide activates guanylate cyclase which increases guanosine 3'5' monophosphate (cGMP) leading to dephosphorylation of myosin light chains and smooth muscle relaxation. Produces a vasodilator effect on the peripheral veins and arteries with more prominent effects on the veins. Primarily reduces cardiac oxygen demand by decreasing preload (left ventricular end-diastolic pressure); may modestly reduce afterload; dilates coronary arteries and improves collateral flow to ischemic regions.

Pharmacodynamics/Kinetics

Onset of action: 30 to 60 minutes

Duration: Immediate release: ≥6 hours (Thadani, 1987); Extended release: ≥12 to 24 hours (Anderson, 2007)

Absorption: Nearly complete and low intersubject variability in its pharmacokinetic parameters and plasma concentrations

Distribution: V_d: ~0.6 L/kg

Protein binding: <5%

Metabolism: Hepatic

Bioavailability: ~100%

Half-life elimination: Mononitrate: ~5 to 6 hours

Excretion: Predominantly urine (2% as unchanged drug); feces (1% of dose)

Dosing

Adult

Angina: Oral:

Regular release tablet: Initial: 5 to 20 mg twice daily with the 2 doses given 7 hours apart (eg, 8 AM and 3 PM) to decrease tolerance development; patients initiating therapy with 5 mg twice daily (eg, small stature) should be titrated up to 10 mg twice daily in first 2 to 3 days.

Extended release tablet: Initial: 30 to 60 mg given once daily in the morning; titrate upward as needed, giving at least 3 days between increases; maximum daily single dose: 240 mg

Note: Tolerance to nitrate effects develops with chronic exposure. Dose escalation does not overcome this effect. Tolerance can only be overcome by short periods of nitrate absence from the body. Short periods of nitrate withdrawal may help minimize tolerance. Recommended twice daily dosage regimens incorporate this interval. Administer sustained release tablet once daily in the morning.

Geriatric Start with lowest recommended adult dose.

Renal Impairment Dose adjustment not necessary.

Hemodialysis: Dose supplementation is not necessary.

Peritoneal dialysis: Dose supplementation is not necessary.

Hepatic Impairment Dose adjustment not necessary.

Administration Do not administer around-the-clock. Immediate release tablet should be scheduled twice daily with doses 7 hours apart (8 AM and 3 PM); extended release tablet may be administered once daily in the morning upon rising with a half-glassful of fluid. Do not chew or crush extended release tablets. Due to insoluble matrix embedding, extended release tablets that are scored may be split (Gunasekara, 1999).

Monitoring Parameters Monitor for orthostasis, increased hypotension

◀

Dosage Forms Excipient information presented when available (limited, particularly for generics); consult specific product labeling. [DSC] = Discontinued product
Tablet, Oral:
Monoket: 10 mg [DSC], 20 mg [DSC]
Generic: 10 mg, 20 mg
Tablet Extended Release 24 Hour, Oral:
Imdur: 30 mg [DSC], 60 mg [DSC] [scored]
Imdur: 120 mg [DSC]
Generic: 30 mg, 60 mg, 120 mg

♦ **Isotamine (Can)** *see* Isoniazid *on page 990*

ISOtretinoin (eye soe TRET i noyn)

Brand Names: US Absorica; Amnesteem; Claravis; Myorisan; Zenatane
Brand Names: Canada Accutane; Clarus; Epuris
Index Terms 13-*cis*-Retinoic Acid; 13-*cis*-Vitamin A Acid; 13-CRA; *Cis*-Retinoic Acid; Accutane; Isotretinoinum
Pharmacologic Category Acne Products; Antineoplastic Agent, Retinoic Acid Derivative; Retinoic Acid Derivative
Use Treatment of severe recalcitrant nodular acne unresponsive to conventional therapy
Pregnancy Considerations Isotretinoin and its metabolites can be detected in fetal tissue following maternal use during pregnancy (Benifla, 1995; Kraft, 1989). **[U.S. Boxed Warnings]: Use of isotretinoin is contraindicated in females who are or may become pregnant. Birth defects (facial, eye, ear, skull, central nervous system, cardiovascular, thymus and parathyroid gland abnormalities) have been noted following isotretinoin exposure during pregnancy and the risk for severe birth defects is high, with any dose or even with short treatment duration. Low IQ scores have also been reported. The risk for spontaneous abortion and premature births is increased. Because of the high likelihood of teratogenic effects, all patients (male and female), prescribers, wholesalers, and dispensing pharmacists must register and be active in the iPLEDGE™ risk evaluation and mitigation strategy (REMS) program; do not prescribe isotretinoin for women who are or who are likely to become pregnant while using the drug. If pregnancy occurs during therapy, isotretinoin should be discontinued immediately and the patient referred to an obstetrician-gynecologist specializing in reproductive toxicity.** This medication is contraindicated in females of childbearing potential unless they are able to comply with the guidelines of the iPLEDGE™ pregnancy prevention program. Females of childbearing potential must have two negative pregnancy tests with a sensitivity of at least 25 milliunits/mL prior to beginning therapy and testing should continue monthly during therapy. Females of childbearing potential should not become pregnant during therapy or for 1 month following discontinuation of isotretinoin. Upon discontinuation of treatment, females of childbearing potential should have a pregnancy test after their last dose and again one month after their last dose. Two forms of contraception should be continued during this time. Any pregnancies should be reported to the iPLEDGE™ program (www.ipledgeprogram.com or 866-495-0654) and the FDA through MedWatch (800-FDA-1088).
Breast-Feeding Considerations It is not known if isotretinoin is excreted in breast milk. A case report describes a green discharge from the breast of a nonlactating woman which was determined to be iatrogenic galactorrhea due to isotretinoin (Larsen, 1985). Due to the potential for serious adverse reactions in the nursing infant, the manufacturer recommends a decision be made whether to discontinue nursing or to discontinue the drug, taking into account the importance of treatment to the mother.
Prescribing and Access Restrictions As a requirement of the REMS program, access to this medication is restricted. All patients (male and female), prescribers, wholesalers, and dispensing pharmacists must register and be active in the iPLEDGE™ risk management program, designed to eliminate fetal exposures to isotretinoin. This program covers all isotretinoin products (brand and generic). The iPLEDGE™ program requires that all patients meet qualification criteria and monthly program requirements (eg, pregnancy testing). Healthcare providers can only prescribe a maximum 30-day supply at each monthly visit and must counsel patients on the iPLEDGE™ program requirements and confirm counseling via the iPLEDGE™ automated system. Registration, activation, and additional information are provided at www.ipledgeprogram.com or by calling 866-495-0654.
Medication Guide Available Yes

Contraindications Hypersensitivity to isotretinoin or any component of the formulation; sensitivity to parabens, vitamin A, or other retinoids; pregnant women or those who may become pregnant
Warnings/Precautions Hazardous agent - use appropriate precautions for handling and disposal (meets NIOSH 2014 criteria). This medication should only be prescribed by prescribers competent in treating severe recalcitrant nodular acne and experienced with the use of systemic retinoids. Anaphylaxis and other types of allergic reactions, including cutaneous reactions and allergic vasculitis, have been reported. **[U.S. Boxed Warnings]: Birth defects (facial, eye, ear, skull, central nervous system, cardiovascular, thymus and parathyroid gland abnormalities) have been noted following isotretinoin exposure during pregnancy and the risk for severe birth defects is high, with any dose or even with short treatment duration. Low IQ scores have also been reported. The risk for spontaneous abortion and premature births is increased. Because of the high likelihood of teratogenic effects, all patients (male and female), prescribers, wholesalers, and dispensing pharmacists must register and be active in the iPLEDGE risk evaluation and mitigation strategy (REMS) program; do not prescribe isotretinoin for women who are or who are likely to become pregnant while using the drug. If pregnancy occurs during therapy, isotretinoin should be discontinued immediately and the patient referred to an obstetrician-gynecologist specializing in reproductive toxicity (see Additional Information for details).** Women of childbearing potential must be capable of complying with effective contraceptive measures. Patients must select and commit to two forms of contraception. Therapy is begun after two negative pregnancy tests; effective contraception must be used for at least 1 month before beginning therapy, during therapy, and for 1 month after discontinuation of therapy. Prescriptions should be written for no more than a 30-day supply, and pregnancy testing and counseling should be repeated monthly.

May cause depression, psychosis, aggressive or violent behavior, and changes in mood; use with extreme caution in patients with psychiatric disorders. Rarely, suicidal thoughts and actions have been reported during isotretinoin usage. All patients should be observed closely for symptoms of depression or suicidal thoughts. Discontinuation of treatment alone may not be sufficient, further evaluation may be necessary. Cases of pseudotumor cerebri (benign intracranial hypertension) have been reported, some with concomitant use of tetracycline (avoid using together). Patients with papilledema, headache, nausea, vomiting, and visual disturbances should be referred to a neurologist and treatment with isotretinoin discontinued. Hearing impairment, which can continue after therapy is discontinued, may occur. Clinical hepatitis, elevated liver enzymes, inflammatory bowel disease, skeletal hyperostosis, premature epiphyseal closure, vision impairment, corneal opacities, decreased tolerance to contact lenses (due to dry eyes), and decreased night vision have also been reported with the use of isotretinoin. Rare postmarketing cases of severe skin reactions (eg, Stevens-Johnson syndrome, erythema multiforme) have been reported with use.

Use with caution in patients with diabetes mellitus; impaired glucose control has been reported. Use caution in patients with hypertriglyceridemia; acute pancreatitis and fatal hemorrhagic pancreatitis (rare) have been reported. Instruct patients to avoid or limit ethanol; may increase triglyceride levels if taken in excess. Bone mineral density may decrease; use caution in patients with a genetic predisposition to bone disorders (ie, osteoporosis, osteomalacia) and with disease states or concomitant medications that can induce bone disorders. Patients may be at risk when participating in activities with repetitive impact (such as sports). Patients should be instructed not to donate blood during therapy and for 1 month following discontinuation of therapy due to risk of donated blood being given to a pregnant female. Safety of long-term use is not established and is not recommended. Some products may contain tartrazine (FD&C yellow no. 5), which may cause allergic reactions, including bronchial asthma, in certain individuals. Allergy is frequently seen in patients who also have an aspirin hypersensitivity.

Absorica: Absorption is ~83% greater than Accutane when administered under fasting conditions; they are bioequivalent when taken with a high-fat meal. Absorica is **not** interchangeable with other generic isotretinoin products. Isotretinoin and tretinoin (which is also known as all-*trans* retinoic acid, or ATRA) may be confused, while both products may be used in cancer treatment, they are **not**

interchangeable; verify product prior to dispensing and administration to prevent medication errors.

Adverse Reactions Frequency not always defined.

Cardiovascular: Chest pain, edema, flushing, palpitation, stroke, syncope, tachycardia, vascular thrombotic disease

Central nervous system: Aggressive behavior, depression, dizziness, drowsiness, emotional instability, fatigue, headache, insomnia, lethargy, malaise, nervousness, paresthesia, pseudotumor cerebri, psychosis, seizure, stroke, suicidal ideation, suicide attempts, suicide, violent behavior

Dermatologic: Abnormal wound healing acne fulminans, alopecia, bruising, cheilitis, cutaneous allergic reactions, dry nose, dry skin, eczema, eruptive xanthomas, facial erythema, fragility of skin, hair abnormalities, hirsutism, hyperpigmentation, hypopigmentation, increased sunburn susceptibility, nail dystrophy, paronychia, peeling of palms, peeling of soles, photoallergic reactions, photosensitizing reactions, pruritus, purpura, rash

Endocrine & metabolic: Triglycerides increased (25%), abnormal menses, blood glucose increased, cholesterol increased, HDL decreased, hyperuricemia

Gastrointestinal: Bleeding and inflammation of the gums, colitis, esophagitis, esophageal ulceration, inflammatory bowel disease, nausea, nonspecific gastrointestinal symptoms, pancreatitis, weight loss, xerostomia

Genitourinary: Nonspecific urogenital findings

Hematologic: Agranulocytosis (rare), anemia, neutropenia, pyogenic granuloma, thrombocytopenia

Hepatic: Alkaline phosphatase increased, ALT increased, AST increased, GGTP increased, hepatitis, LDH increased

Neuromuscular & skeletal: Back pain (29% in pediatric patients), arthralgia, arthritis, bone abnormalities, bone mineral density decreased, calcification of tendons and ligaments, CPK increased, myalgia, premature epiphyseal closure, skeletal hyperostosis, tendonitis, weakness

Ocular: Conjunctivitis (4%), blepharitis (1%), chalazion (1%), hordeolum (1%), cataracts, color vision disorder, corneal opacities, eyelid inflammation, keratitis, night vision decreased, optic neuritis, photophobia, visual disturbances

Otic: Hearing impairment, tinnitus

Renal: Glomerulonephritis, hematuria, proteinuria, pyuria, vasculitis

Respiratory: Bronchospasms, epistaxis, respiratory infection, voice alteration, Wegener's granulomatosis

Miscellaneous: Allergic reactions, anaphylactic reactions, disseminated herpes simplex, diaphoresis, infection, lymphadenopathy

<1% (Limited to important or life-threatening): Abnormal meibomian gland secretion, erythema multiforme, meibomian gland atrophy, myopia, pseudotumor cerebri, rhabdomyolysis, Stevens-Johnson syndrome, toxic epidermal necrolysis, visual acuity decreased

Drug Interactions

Metabolism/Transport Effects None known.

Avoid Concomitant Use

Avoid concomitant use of ISOtretinoin with any of the following: Multivitamins/Fluoride (with ADE); Multivitamins/Minerals (with ADEK, Folate, Iron); Multivitamins/Minerals (with AE, No Iron); Tetracycline Derivatives; Vitamin A

Increased Effect/Toxicity

ISOtretinoin may increase the levels/effects of: Mipomersen; Porfimer; Verteporfin

The levels/effects of ISOtretinoin may be increased by: Alcohol (Ethyl); Multivitamins/Fluoride (with ADE); Multivitamins/Minerals (with ADEK, Folate, Iron); Multivitamins/Minerals (with AE, No Iron); Tetracycline Derivatives; Vitamin A

Decreased Effect

ISOtretinoin may decrease the levels/effects of: Contraceptives (Estrogens); Contraceptives (Progestins)

Food Interactions Isotretinoin bioavailability increased if taken with food or milk. Management: Administer orally with a meal (except Absorbica™ which may be taken without regard to meals).

Storage/Stability Store at 20°C to 25°C (68°F to 77°F); excursions permitted between 15°C to 30°C (59°F to 86°F). Protect from light.

Mechanism of Action Reduces sebaceous gland size and reduces sebum production in acne treatment; in neuroblastoma, decreases cell proliferation and induces differentiation

Pharmacodynamics/Kinetics Note: Pharmacokinetic parameters in adolescents (12-15 years) are similar to adults.

Absorption: Enhanced with a high-fat meal; Absorica™ absorption is ~83% greater than Accutane® when administered under fasting conditions; they are bioequivalent when taken with a high-fat meal.

Protein binding: 99% to 100%; primarily albumin

Metabolism: Hepatic via CYP2B6, 2C8, 2C9, 2D6, 3A4; forms metabolites; major metabolite: 4-oxo-isotretinoin (active)

Half-life elimination: Terminal: Parent drug: 21 hours; Metabolite: 21-24 hours

Time to peak, serum: 3-5 hours

Excretion: Urine and feces (equal amounts)

Dosing

Adult & Geriatric

Acne, severe recalcitrant nodular: Oral: 0.5-1 mg/kg/day in 2 divided doses for 15-20 weeks; may discontinue earlier if the total cyst count decreases by 70%. Adults with very severe disease/scarring or primarily involves the trunk may require dosage adjustment up to 2 mg/kg/day. A second course of therapy may be initiated after a period of ≥2 months off therapy. A dose of ≤0.5 mg/kg/day may be used to minimize initial flaring (Strauss, 2007).

Acne, moderate (off-label use): Oral: 20 mg/day (~0.3-0.4 mg/kg/day) for 6 months (Amichai, 2006)

Pediatric

Acne, severe recalcitrant nodular: Children 12-17 years: Oral: 0.5-1 mg/kg/day in 2 divided doses for 15-20 weeks; may discontinue earlier if the total cyst count decreases by 70%. A second course of therapy may be initiated after a period of ≥2 months off therapy. A dose of ≤0.5 mg/kg/day may be used to minimize initial flaring (Strauss, 2007).

Acne, moderate (off-label use): Children 12-17 years: Oral: 20 mg/day (~0.3-0.4 mg/kg/day) for 6 months (Amichai, 2006)

Neuroblastoma, high-risk (off-label use): Children 1-17 years: Oral: 160 mg/m^2/day (in 2 divided doses) days 1 through 14 every 28 days for 6 cycles, beginning after continuation chemotherapy or transplantation (Matthay, 1999)

Renal Impairment No dosage adjustment provided in the manufacturer's labeling.

Hepatic Impairment

Hepatic impairment prior to treatment: No dosage adjustment provided in the manufacturer's labeling.

Hepatotoxicity during treatment: Liver enzymes may normalize with dosage reduction or with continued treatment; discontinue if normalization does not readily occur or if hepatitis is suspected.

Dietary Considerations Should be taken with food, except Absorbica™ which may be taken without regard to meals. Limit intake of vitamin A; avoid use of other vitamin A products. Some formulations may contain soybean oil.

Administration Administer orally with a meal (except Absorica™ which may be taken without regard to meals). According to the manufacturers' labeling, capsules should be swallowed whole with a full glass of liquid. For patients unable to swallow capsule whole, an oral liquid may be prepared; may irritate esophagus if contents are removed from the capsule.

Hazardous agent; use appropriate precautions for handling and disposal (meets NIOSH 2014 criteria).

Monitoring Parameters CBC with differential and platelet count, baseline sedimentation rate, glucose, CPK; signs of depression, mood alteration, psychosis, aggression, severe skin reactions

Pregnancy test (for all female patients of childbearing potential): Two negative tests with a sensitivity of at least 25 milliunits/mL prior to beginning therapy (the second performed at least 19 days after the first test and performed during the first 5 days of the menstrual period immediately preceding the start of therapy); monthly tests to rule out pregnancy prior to refilling prescription.

Lipids: Prior to treatment and at weekly or biweekly intervals until response to treatment is established. Test should not be performed <36 hours after consumption of ethanol.

Liver function tests: Prior to treatment and at weekly or biweekly intervals until response to treatment is established.

Additional Information All patients (male and female), must be registered in the iPLEDGE™ risk management program. Females of childbearing potential must receive oral and written information reviewing the hazards of therapy and the effects that isotretinoin can have on a fetus. Therapy should not begin without two negative

pregnancy tests at least 19 days apart. Two forms of contraception (a primary and secondary form as described in the iPLEDGE™ program materials) must be used simultaneously beginning 1 month prior to treatment, during treatment, and for 1 month after therapy is discontinued; limitations to their use must be explained. Microdosed progesterone products that do not contain an estrogen ("mini-pills") are not an acceptable form of contraception during isotretinoin treatment. Prescriptions should be written for no more than a 30-day supply, and pregnancy testing and counseling should be repeated monthly. During therapy, pregnancy tests must be conducted by a CLIA-certified laboratory. Prescriptions must be filled and picked up from the pharmacy within 7 days of specimen collection for pregnancy test for women of childbearing potential. Prescriptions for males and females of non-childbearing potential must be filled and picked up within 30 days of prescribing.

Any cases of accidental pregnancy should be reported to the iPLEDGE™ program or FDA MedWatch. All patients (male and female) must read and sign the informed consent material provided in the pregnancy prevention program.

Dosage Forms Excipient information presented when available (limited, particularly for generics); consult specific product labeling.
Capsule, Oral:
Absorica: 10 mg, 20 mg [contains soybean oil]
Absorica: 25 mg [contains brilliant blue fcf (fd&c blue #1), fd&c yellow #6 (sunset yellow), soybean oil, tartrazine (fd&c yellow #5)]
Absorica: 30 mg [contains soybean oil]
Absorica: 35 mg [contains fd&c blue #2 (indigotine), soybean oil]
Absorica: 40 mg [contains soybean oil]
Amnesteem: 10 mg, 20 mg, 40 mg [contains soybean oil]
Claravis: 10 mg [contains fd&c yellow #6 (sunset yellow), soybean oil]
Claravis: 20 mg [contains soybean oil]
Claravis: 30 mg
Claravis: 40 mg [contains fd&c yellow #6 (sunset yellow), soybean oil]
Myorisan: 10 mg, 20 mg [contains soybean oil]
Myorisan: 30 mg [contains edetate disodium, soybean oil]
Myorisan: 40 mg [contains fd&c yellow #6 (sunset yellow), soybean oil]
Zenatane: 10 mg [contains brilliant blue fcf (fd&c blue #1), edetate disodium, fd&c yellow #10 (quinoline yellow), methylparaben, propylparaben, soybean oil]
Zenatane: 20 mg [contains edetate disodium, methylparaben, propylparaben, soybean oil]
Zenatane: 30 mg [contains edetate disodium, fd&c blue #2 aluminum lake, fd&c yellow #10 (quinoline yellow), methylparaben, propylparaben, soybean oil]
Zenatane: 40 mg [contains brilliant blue fcf (fd&c blue #1), edetate disodium, fd&c blue #2 (indigotine), fd&c yellow #10 (quinoline yellow), methylparaben, propylparaben, soybean oil]

Extemporaneous Preparations Hazardous agent: Use appropriate precautions for handling and disposal of teratogenic capsule contents (meets NIOSH 2014 criteria).

For patients unable to swallow the capsules whole, an oral liquid may be prepared with softgel capsules (not recommended by the manufacturers) by one of the following methods:
Place capsules (softgel formulations only) in small container and add warm (~37°C [97°F]) water or milk to cover capsule(s); wait 2-3 minutes until capsule is softened and then drink the milk or water with the softened capsule, or swallow softened capsule.
Puncture capsule (softgel formulations only) with needle or cut with scissors; squeeze capsule contents into 5-10 mL of milk or tube feed formula; draw mixture up into oral syringe and administer via feeding tube; flush feeding tube with ≥30 mL additional milk or tube feeding formula.
Puncture capsule (softgel formulations only) with needle or cut with scissors and draw contents into oral syringe; add 1-5 mL of medium chain triglyceride, soybean, or safflower oil to the oral syringe; mix gently and administer via feeding tube; flush feeding tube with ≥30 mL milk or tube feeding formula.

Lam MS, "Extemporaneous Compounding of Oral Liquid Dosage Formulations and Alternative Drug Delivery Methods for Anticancer Drugs," *Pharmacotherapy*, 2011, 31(2):164-92.

◆ Isotretinoinum *see* ISOtretinoin *on page 996*

Isradipine (iz RA di peen)

Brand Names: US DynaCirc CR [DSC]
Pharmacologic Category Antihypertensive; Calcium Channel Blocker; Calcium Channel Blocker, Dihydropyridine
Use Hypertension: Management of hypertension (may be used alone or concurrently with thiazide-type diuretics).

The 2014 guideline for the management of high blood pressure in adults (JNC 8) recommends initiation of pharmacologic treatment to lower blood pressure for the following patients (JNC8 [James, 2013]):
• Patients ≥60 years of age, with systolic blood pressure (SBP) ≥150 mm Hg or diastolic blood pressure (DBP) ≥90 mm Hg. Goal of therapy is SBP <150 mm Hg and DBP <90 mm Hg.
• Patients <60 years of age, with SBP ≥140 mm Hg or DBP ≥90 mm Hg. Goal of therapy is SBP <140 mm Hg and DBP <90 mm Hg.
• Patients ≥18 years of age with diabetes, with SBP ≥140 mm Hg or DBP ≥90 mm Hg. Goal of therapy is SBP <140 mm Hg and DBP <90 mm Hg.
• Patients ≥18 years of age with chronic kidney disease (CKD), with SBP ≥140 mm Hg or DBP ≥90 mm Hg. Goal of therapy is SBP <140 mm Hg and DBP <90 mm Hg.
In patients with chronic kidney disease (CKD), regardless of race or diabetes status, the use of an ACE inhibitor (ACEI) or angiotensin receptor blocker (ARB) as initial therapy is recommended to improve kidney outcomes. In the general nonblack population (without CKD) including those with diabetes, initial antihypertensive treatment should consist of a thiazide-type diuretic, calcium channel blocker, ACEI, or ARB. In the general black population (without CKD) including those with diabetes, initial antihypertensive treatment should consist of a thiazide-type diuretic or a calcium channel blocker **instead of** an ACEI or ARB.

Dosing
Adult & Geriatric Hypertension: Oral: 2.5 mg twice daily; antihypertensive response occurs in 2-3 hours; maximal response in 2-4 weeks; increase dose at 2- to 4-week intervals at 2.5-5 mg increments; usual dose range (ASH/ISH [Weber, 2014]): 5-10 mg twice daily. **Note:** Most patients show no improvement with doses >10 mg daily except adverse reaction rate increases; therefore, maximal dose in older adults should be 10 mg daily.
Pediatric Hypertension (off-label use): Oral: Initial: 0.15-0.2 mg/kg/day in 3-4 divided doses; maximum 0.8 mg/kg/day, up to 20 mg daily (NHBPEP, 2004).
Renal Impairment There are no dosage adjustments provided in manufacturer's labeling; however, bioavailability is increased with mild renal impairment and decreased with severe renal impairment. Other sources recommend that no initial dosage adjustment is required (Aronoff, 2007). Isradipine is not removed by hemodialysis; therefore, supplemental doses after hemodialysis are not necessary (Schonholzer, 1992).
Hepatic Impairment There are no dosage adjustments provided in manufacturer's labeling; however, peak serum concentrations are increased by 32% and bioavailability is increased by 52%.
Additional Information Complete prescribing information should be consulted for additional detail.
Dosage Forms Excipient information presented when available (limited, particularly for generics); consult specific product labeling. [DSC] = Discontinued product
Capsule, Oral:
Generic: 2.5 mg, 5 mg
Tablet Extended Release 24 Hour, Oral:
DynaCirc CR: 5 mg [DSC], 10 mg [DSC]

◆ Istalol *see* Timolol (Ophthalmic) *on page 1790*
◆ Istodax *see* RomiDEPsin *on page 1614*
◆ Isuprel *see* Isoproterenol *on page 993*

Itraconazole (i tra KOE na zole)

Brand Names: US Onmel; Sporanox; Sporanox Pulsepak
Brand Names: Canada Sporanox
Pharmacologic Category Antifungal Agent, Oral
Use
Aspergillosis (capsules): Treatment of pulmonary and extrapulmonary aspergillosis in immunocompromised and nonimmunocompromised patients who are intolerant of or refractory to amphotericin B therapy.
Blastomycosis (capsules): Treatment of pulmonary and extrapulmonary blastomycosis in immunocompromised and nonimmunocompromised patients.

Histoplasmosis (capsules): Treatment of histoplasmosis, including chronic cavitary pulmonary disease and disseminated, nonmeningeal histoplasmosis in immunocompromised and nonimmunocompromised patients.

Onychomycosis:

Capsules: Treatment of onychomycosis of the toenail, with or without fingernail involvement, and onychomycosis of the fingernail caused by dermatophytes (tinea unguium) in nonimmunocompromised patients

Tablets: Treatment of onychomycosis of the toenail caused by *Trichophyton rubrum* or *Trichophyton mentagrophytes* in nonimmunocompromised patients

Oropharyngeal/Esophageal candidiasis (oral solution): Treatment of oropharyngeal and esophageal candidiasis

Canadian labeling: Oral capsules: Additional indications (not in US labeling):

Candidiasis, oral and/or esophageal: Treatment of oral and/or esophageal candidiasis in immunocompromised and immunocompetent patients

Chromomycosis: Treatment of chromomycosis in immunocompromised and immunocompetent patients

Dermatomycoses: Treatment of dermatomycoses due to tinea pedis, tinea cruris, tinea corporis, and of pityriasis versicolor in patients for whom oral therapy is appropriate

Onychomycosis: Treatment of onychomycosis in immunocompetent and immunocompetent patients

Paracoccidioidomycosis: Treatment of paracoccidioidomycosis in immunocompromised and immunocompetent patients

Sporotrichosis: Treatment of cutaneous and lymphatic sporotrichosis in immunocompromised and immunocompetent patients

Pregnancy Considerations Dose related adverse events were observed in animal reproduction studies. Use is contraindicated for the treatment of onychomycosis during pregnancy. If used for the treatment of onychomycosis in women of reproductive potential, effective contraception should be used during treatment and for 2 months following treatment. Therapy should begin on the second or third day following menses. Congenital abnormalities have been reported during postmarketing surveillance, but a causal relationship has not been established. The Canadian labeling contraindicates use in the treatment of onychomycosis or dermatomycoses (tinea corporis, tinea cruris, tinea pedis, pityriasis versicolor) in women who are pregnant or intend to become pregnant.

Breast-Feeding Considerations Itraconazole is excreted in breast milk. According to the manufacturer, the decision to continue or discontinue breast-feeding during therapy should take into account the risk of exposure to the infant and the benefits of treatment to the mother.

Contraindications

Hypersensitivity to itraconazole or any component of the formulation; concurrent administration with cisapride, disopyramide, dofetilide, dronedarone, eplerenone, ergot derivatives, felodipine, irinotecan, lovastatin, lurasidone, methadone, midazolam (oral), nisoldipine, pimozide, quinidine, ranolazine, simvastatin, ticagrelor, or triazolam; concurrent administration with colchicine, fesoterodine, telithromycin, and solifenacin in patients with varying degrees of renal or hepatic impairment; treatment of onychomycosis (or other non-life-threatening indications) in patients with evidence of ventricular dysfunction, such as congestive heart failure (CHF) or a history of CHF; treatment of onychomycosis in women who are pregnant or intend to become pregnant

Canadian labeling: Additional contraindications (not in US labeling): Concurrent administration with domperidone, eletriptan, fesoterodine in patients with moderate to severe renal or hepatic impairment, or solifenacin in patients with severe renal impairment or moderate to severe hepatic impairment (capsule, oral solution); Concurrent administration with the following drugs (none of which are available in Canada): Astemizole, bepridil, halofantrine, ivabradine, lercanidipine, levacetylmethadol, mizolastine, telithromycin (in patients with severe renal or hepatic impairment), sertindole, terfenadine (capsule, oral solution); treatment of dermatomycosis (tinea pedis, tinea cruris, tinea corporis, pityriasis versicolor) in women who are pregnant or intend to become pregnant (capsule)

Warnings/Precautions [US Boxed Warning]: Negative inotropic effects have been observed following intravenous administration. Discontinue or reassess use if signs or symptoms of HF (heart failure) occur during treatment. [US Boxed Warning]: Use is contraindicated for treatment of onychomycosis in patients with ventricular dysfunction or a history of HF. Cases of HF, peripheral edema, and pulmonary edema have occurred in patients treated for onychomycosis. HF has been reported, particularly in patients receiving a total daily oral dose of 400 mg. Use with caution in patients with risk factors for HF (COPD, renal failure, edematous disorders, ischemic or valvular disease). Discontinue if signs or symptoms of HF or neuropathy occur during treatment. Due to potential toxicity, the manufacturer recommends confirmation of diagnosis testing of nail specimens prior to treatment of onychomycosis. The Canadian labeling contraindicates use in the treatment of dermatomycoses (tinea corporis, tinea cruris, tinea pedis, pityriasis versicolor) in patients with evidence of ventricular dysfunction or a history of HF.

[US Boxed Warning]: Coadministration with itraconazole can cause elevated plasma concentrations of certain drugs and can lead to QT prolongation and ventricular tachyarrhythmias, including torsades de pointes. Coadministration with methadone, disopyramide, dofetilide, dronedarone, quinidine, ergot alkaloids, irinotecan, lurasidone, oral midazolam, pimozide, triazolam, felodipine, nisoldipine, ranolazine, eplerenone, cisapride, lovastatin, simvastatin, ticagrelor and, in subjects with vaying degrees of renal or hepatic impairment, colchicine, fesoterodine, telithromycin, and solifencacin is contraindicated. Additional potentially significant interactions may exist, requiring dose or frequency adjustment, additional monitoring, and/or selection of alternative therapy.

May cause CNS depression, which may impair physical or mental abilities; patients must be cautioned about performing tasks that require mental alertness (eg, operating machinery, driving). Use with caution in patients with renal impairment; dosage adjustment may be needed. Use caution in patients with a history of hypersensitivity to other azoles. Rare cases of serious hepatotoxicity (including liver failure and death) have been reported (including some cases occurring within the first week of therapy); hepatotoxicity was reported in some patients without preexisting liver disease or risk factors. Use with caution in patients with preexisting hepatic impairment; monitor liver function closely. Not recommended for use in patients with active liver disease, elevated liver enzymes, or prior hepatotoxic reactions to other drugs unless the expected benefit exceeds the risk of hepatotoxicity. Discontinue treatment if signs or symptoms of hepatotoxicity develop. Transient or permanent hearing loss has been reported. Quinidine (a contraindicated drug) was used concurrently in several of these cases. Hearing loss usually resolves after discontinuation, but may persist in some patients.

Large differences in itraconazole pharmacokinetic parameters have been observed in cystic fibrosis patients receiving the solution; if a patient with cystic fibrosis does not respond to therapy, alternate therapies should be considered. Due to differences in bioavailability, oral capsules and oral solution cannot be used interchangeably. Only the oral solution has proven efficacy for oral and esophageal candidiasis. Initiation of treatment with oral solution is not recommended in patients at immediate risk for systemic candidiasis (eg, patients with severe neutropenia). Absorption of itraconazole capsules is reduced when gastric acidity is reduced; administer capsules or tablets with an acidic beverage (eg, cola) in patients with reduced gastric acidity and separate administration from acid suppressive therapy. Some dosage forms may contain propylene glycol; large amounts are potentially toxic and have been associated hyperosmolality, lactic acidosis, seizures and respiratory depression; use caution (AAP, 1997; Zar, 2007). The Canadian labeling contraindicates use in the treatment of dermatomycoses (tinea corporis, tinea cruris, tinea pedis, pityriasis versicolor) in women who are pregnant or intend to become pregnant.

Adverse Reactions

>10%: Gastrointestinal: Diarrhea (2% to 11%), nausea (2% to 11%)

1% to 10%:

Cardiovascular: Edema (4%), chest pain (3%), hypertension (2% to 3%),

Central nervous system: Headache (1% to 10%), dizziness (1% to 4%), anxiety (3%), depression (2% to 3%), fatigue (2% to 3%), pain (2% to 3%), malaise (1% to 3%), abnormal dreams (2%)

Dermatologic: Skin rash (3% to 9%), pruritus (≤5%), diaphoresis (3%)

Endocrine & metabolic: Hypertriglyceridemia (≤3%), hypokalemia (2%)

Gastrointestinal: Vomiting (5% to 7%), abdominal pain (2% to 6%), dyspepsia (≤4%), flatulence (≤4%), gastrointestinal disease (≤4%), gingivitis (3%), aphthous stomatitis (≤3%), constipation (2% to 3%), gastritis (2%), gastroenteritis (2%), increased appetite (2%)

Genitourinary: Cystitis (3%), urinary tract infection (1% to 3%)

Hepatic: Abnormal hepatic function tests (≤4%), increased liver enzymes (3% to 4%)

Infection: Herpes zoster (2%)

Neuromuscular & skeletal: Bursitis (3%), myalgia (≤3%), tremor (2%), weakness (≤2%)

Respiratory: Rhinitis (5% to 9%), upper respiratory tract infection (6% to 8%), sinusitis (2% to 7%), cough (1% to 4%), dyspnea (2%), increased bronchial secretions (2%), pneumonia (2%), pharyngitis (≤2%)

Miscellaneous: Fever (2% to 7%)

<2% (Limited to important or life-threatening): Abnormal urinalysis, acute generalized exanthematous pustulosis, adrenal insufficiency, albuminuria, anaphylactoid reaction, anaphylaxis, angioedema, cardiac arrhythmia, cardiac failure, confusion, congestive heart failure, dehydration, dysphagia, erythema multiforme, erythematous rash, exfoliative dermatitis, gastrointestinal disease, gynecomastia, hearing loss, hematuria, hepatic failure, hepatitis, hepatotoxicity, hyperbilirubinemia, hyperglycemia, hyperhidrosis, hyperkalemia, hypersensitivity angiitis, hypersensitivity reaction, hypomagnesemia, increased blood urea nitrogen, increased creatine phosphokinase, increased gamma-glutamyl transferase, increased lactate dehydrogenase, increased serum alkaline phosphatase, increased serum ALT, increased serum AST, left heart failure, leukopenia, menstrual disease, mucosal inflammation, neutropenia, orthostatic hypotension, pancreatitis, paresthesia, peripheral edema, pollakiuria, pulmonary edema, renal insufficiency, rigors, serum sickness, sinus bradycardia, Stevens-Johnson syndrome, tachycardia, thrombocytopenia, toxic epidermal necrolysis, vasculitis, voice disorder

Drug Interactions

Metabolism/Transport Effects Substrate of CYP3A4 (major); **Note:** Assignment of Major/Minor substrate status based on clinically relevant drug interaction potential; **Inhibits** CYP3A4 (strong), P-glycoprotein

Avoid Concomitant Use

Avoid concomitant use of Itraconazole with any of the following: Ado-Trastuzumab Emtansine; Alfuzosin; Aliskiren; ALPRAZolam; Aprepitant; Astemizole; Avanafil; Axitinib; Barnidipine; Bosutinib; Bromocriptine; Cabozantinib; Ceritinib; Cisapride; Cobimetinib; Conivaptan; Crizotinib; CYP3A4 Inducers (Strong); Dabrafenib; Dapoxetine; Dihydroergotamine; Disopyramide; Dofetilide; Domperidone; Dronedarone; Efavirenz; Eletriptan; Eplerenone; Ergoloid Mesylates; Ergonovine; Ergotamine; Estazolam; Everolimus; Felodipine; Flibanserin; Fusidic Acid (Systemic); Halofantrine; Ibrutinib; Idelalisib; Irinotecan Products; Isavuconazonium Sulfate; Ivabradine; Lapatinib; Lercanidipine; Lomitapide; Lovastatin; Lumacaftor; Lurasidone; Macitentan; Methadone; Methylergonovine; Midazolam; Naloxegol; Nevirapine; Nilotinib; NiMODipine; Nisoldipine; Olaparib; Osimertinib; Palbociclib; PAZOPanib; Pimozide; QuiNIDine; Ranolazine; Red Yeast Rice; Regorafenib; Rivaroxaban; Saccharomyces boulardii; Salmeterol; Silodosin; Simeprevir; Simvastatin; Sonidegib; Suvorexant; Tamsulosin; Telithromycin; Terfenadine; Ticagrelor; Tolvaptan; Topotecan; Toremifene; Trabectedin; Triazolam; Ulipristal; Vemurafenib; VinCRIStine (Liposomal); Vorapaxar

Increased Effect/Toxicity

Itraconazole may increase the levels/effects of: Ado-Trastuzumab Emtansine; Afatinib; Alfuzosin; Aliskiren; Alitretinoin (Systemic); Almotriptan; Alosetron; ALPRAZolam; Apixaban; Aprepitant; ARIPiprazole; ARIPiprazole Lauroxil; Astemizole; AtorvaSTATin; Avanafil; Axitinib; Barnidipine; Bedaquiline; Boceprevir; Bortezomib; Bosentan; Bosutinib; Brentuximab Vedotin; Brexpiprazole; Brinzolamide; Bromocriptine; Budesonide (Nasal); Budesonide (Oral Inhalation); Budesonide (Systemic); Budesonide (Topical); BusPIRone; Busulfan; Cabazitaxel; Cabozantinib; Calcium Channel Blockers; Cannabis; Cardiac Glycosides; Cariprazine; Ceritinib; Cilostazol; Cisapride; Cobicistat; Cobimetinib; Colchicine; Conivaptan; Corticosteroids (Orally Inhaled); Corticosteroids (Systemic); Crizotinib; CycloSPORINE (Systemic); CYP3A4 Substrates; Dabigatran Etexilate; Dabrafenib; Daclatasvir; Dapoxetine; Darunavir; Dasatinib; Dienogest; Dihydroergotamine; Disopyramide; DOCEtaxel; Dofetilide; Domperidone; DOXOrubicin (Conventional); Dronabinol; Dronedarone; Drospirenone; Dutasteride; Edoxaban; Eletriptan; Eliglustat; Elvitegravir; Eplerenone; Ergoloid Mesylates; Ergonovine; Ergotamine; Erlotinib; Estazolam; Etizolam; Etravirine; Everolimus; Felodipine; FentaNYL; Fesoterodine; Fexofenadine; Flibanserin; Fluticasone (Nasal); Fluticasone (Oral Inhalation); Fosamprenavir; Gefitinib; GuanFACINE; Halofantrine; Highest Risk QTc-Prolonging Agents; Hydrocodone; Ibrutinib; Iloperidone; Imatinib; Imidafenacin; Indinavir; Irinotecan Products; Isavuconazonium Sulfate; Ivabradine; Ivacaftor; Ixabepilone;

Lacosamide; Lapatinib; Ledipasvir; Lercanidipine; Levobupivacaine; Levomilnacipran; Lomitapide; Losartan; Lovastatin; Lurasidone; Macitentan; Maraviroc; MedroxyPROGESTERone; Methadone; Methylergonovine; MethylPREDNISolone; Midazolam; Mifepristone; Moderate Risk QTc-Prolonging Agents; Naloxegol; Nilotinib; NiMODipine; Nintedanib; Nisoldipine; Olaparib; Osimertinib; Ospemifene; Oxybutynin; OxyCODONE; Palbociclib; Paliperidone; Panobinostat; Parecoxib; Paricalcitol; PAZOPanib; P-glycoprotein/ABCB1 Substrates; Pimecrolimus; Pimozide; PONATinib; Pranlukast; Pravastatin; PrednisoLONE (Systemic); PredniSONE; Propafenone; Prucalopride; QUEtiapine; QuiNIDine; Ramelteon; Ranolazine; Red Yeast Rice; Regorafenib; Repaglinide; Retapamulin; Rifaximin; Rilpivirine; Riociguat; Rivaroxaban; RomiDEPsin; Rosuvastatin; Ruxolitinib; Salmeterol; Saquinavir; Saxagliptin; Sildenafil; Silodosin; Simeprevir; Simvastatin; Sirolimus; Solifenacin; Sonidegib; SORAfenib; SUNItinib; Suvorexant; Tacrolimus (Systemic); Tacrolimus (Topical); Tadalafil; Tamsulosin; Tasimelteon; Telaprevir; Telithromycin; Temsirolimus; Terfenadine; Tetrahydrocannabinol; Ticagrelor; Tofacitinib; Tolterodine; Tolvaptan; Topotecan; Toremifene; Trabectedin; TraMADol; Triazolam; Ulipristal; Vardenafil; Vemurafenib; Vilazodone; VinBLAStine; VinCRIStine; VinCRIStine (Liposomal); Vindesine; Vinorelbine; Vitamin K Antagonists; Vorapaxar; Zolpidem; Zopiclone; Zuclopenthixol

The levels/effects of Itraconazole may be increased by: Boceprevir; Cobicistat; Conivaptan; CYP3A4 Inhibitors (Moderate); CYP3A4 Inhibitors (Strong); Darunavir; Etravirine; Fosamprenavir; Fusidic Acid (Systemic); Grapefruit Juice; Idelalisib; Indinavir; Lopinavir; Luliconazole; Mifepristone; Netupitant; Ritonavir; Saquinavir; Stiripentol; Telaprevir; Telithromycin; Tipranavir

Decreased Effect

Itraconazole may decrease the levels/effects of: Amphotericin B; Ifosfamide; Meloxicam; Prasugrel; Saccharomyces boulardii; Ticagrelor

The levels/effects of Itraconazole may be decreased by: Antacids; Bosentan; CYP3A4 Inducers (Moderate); CYP3A4 Inducers (Strong); Deferasirox; Didanosine; Efavirenz; Etravirine; Grapefruit Juice; H2-Antagonists; Isoniazid; Lumacaftor; Nevirapine; Proton Pump Inhibitors; Siltuximab; St Johns Wort; Sucralfate; Tocilizumab

Food Interactions

Capsules: Absorption enhanced by food and possibly by gastric acidity. Cola drinks have been shown to increase the absorption of the capsules in patients with achlorhydria or those taking H_2-receptor antagonists or other gastric acid suppressors. Grapefruit/grapefruit juice may increase serum levels. Management: Take capsules immediately after meals. Avoid grapefruit juice.

Solution: Food decreases the bioavailability and increases the time to peak concentration. Management: Take solution on an empty stomach 1 hour before or 2 hours after meals.

Storage/Stability

Capsule: Store at room temperature of 15°C to 25°C (59°F to 77°F). Protect from light and moisture.

Oral solution: Store at ≤25°C (77°F); do not freeze.

Tablet: Store at room temperature 15°C to 25°C (59°F to 77°F); excursions are permitted between 15°C and 30°C (59°F and 86°F). Protect from light and moisture.

Mechanism of Action Interferes with cytochrome P450 activity, decreasing ergosterol synthesis (principal sterol in fungal cell membrane) and inhibiting cell membrane formation

Pharmacodynamics/Kinetics

Absorption: Requires gastric acidity; capsule or tablet better absorbed with food, solution better absorbed on empty stomach

Distribution: V_d (average): >700 L; highly lipophilic and tissue concentrations are higher than plasma concentrations. The highest concentrations: adipose, omentum, endometrium, cervical and vaginal mucus, and skin/nails. Aqueous fluids (eg, CSF and urine) contain negligible amounts; distributes into bronchial exudate and sputum

Protein binding, plasma: 99.8%; metabolite hydroxy-itraconazole: 99.6%

Metabolism: Extensively hepatic via CYP3A4 into >30 metabolites including hydroxy-itraconazole (major metabolite); appears to have in vitro antifungal activity. Main metabolic pathway is oxidation; may undergo saturation metabolism with multiple dosing.

Bioavailability: Variable, ~55% increases by 30% under fasted conditions (oral solution); **Note:** Oral solution has a higher degree of bioavailability (149% ± 68%) relative to oral capsules; should not be interchanged

Half-life elimination:

Children (6 months to 12 years): Oral solution: ~36 hours; Metabolite hydroxy-itraconazole: ~18 hours

Adults: Oral: Single dose: 16 to 28 hours, Multiple doses: 34 to 42 hours; Cirrhosis (single dose): 37 hours (range: 20 to 54 hours)

Time to peak, plasma: Capsules/tablets: 2 to 5 hours; Oral solution: 2.5 hours

Excretion: Urine (<0.03% active drug, 35% as inactive metabolites); feces (54%; ~3% to 18% as unchanged drug)

Dosing

Adult & Geriatric Note: Doses >200 mg daily should be administered in 2 divided doses.

Aspergillosis: Oral capsule: 200 to 400 mg daily. **Note:** For life-threatening infections, the US labeling recommends administering a loading dose of 200 mg 3 times daily (total: 600 mg daily) for the first 3 days of therapy. Continue treatment for at least 3 months and until clinical and laboratory evidence suggest that infection has resolved.

Aspergillosis, invasive (salvage therapy; voriconazole-susceptible): Duration of therapy should be a minimum of 6 to 12 weeks or throughout period of immunosuppression: Oral capsule: 200 to 400 mg daily; **Note:** 2008 IDSA guidelines recommend 600 mg/day for 3 days, followed by 400 mg daily (Walsh, 2008).

Aspergillosis, allergic (ABPA, sinusitis): Oral: 200 mg daily; may be used in conjunction with corticosteroids (Andes, 2000; Walsh, 2008)

Blastomycosis: *Manufacturer labeling:* Oral capsule: Initial: 200 mg once daily; if no clinical improvement or evidence of progressive infection, may increase dose in increments of 100 mg up to maximum of 400 mg daily. **Note:** For life-threatening infections, the US labeling recommends administering a loading dose of 200 mg 3 times daily (total: 600 mg daily) for the first 3 days of therapy. Continue treatment for at least 3 months and until clinical and laboratory evidence suggest that infection has resolved.

Alternative dosing: 200 mg 3 times daily for 3 days, then 200 mg twice daily for 6 to 12 months; in moderately severe to severe infection, therapy should be initiated with ~2 weeks of amphotericin B (Chapman, 2008).

Candidiasis: Oral:

Esophageal:

US labeling: Oral solution: 100 to 200 mg once daily for a minimum of 3 weeks; continue dosing for 2 weeks after resolution of symptoms

Canadian labeling:

Oral solution: 100 to 200 mg once daily for a minimum of 3 weeks; continue dosing for 2 weeks after resolution of symptoms

Oral capsules: 100 mg once daily for 4 weeks; increase dose to 200 mg once daily in patients with AIDS and neutropenic patients

Alternate dosing: HIV-infected patients: Oral solution: 200 mg once daily for 14 to 21 days (HHS [OI adult 2015])

Oropharyngeal:

US labeling: Oral solution: 200 mg once daily for 1 to 2 weeks; in patients unresponsive or refractory to fluconazole: 100 mg twice daily (clinical response expected in 2 to 4 weeks)

Canadian labeling:

Oral solution: 200 mg once daily or in divided doses daily for 1 to 2 weeks

Oral capsules: 100 mg once daily for 2 weeks; increase dose to 200 mg once daily in patients with AIDS and neutropenic patients

Alternate dosing: HIV-infected patients (alternative to preferred therapy): Oral solution: 200 mg once daily for 7 to 14 days (HHS [OI adult 2015])

Vulvo-vaginal (uncomplicated) in HIV-infected patients (alternative to preferred therapy) (off-label use): Oral solution: 200 mg once daily for 3 to 7 days (HHS [OI adult 2015])

Chromomycosis: Canadian labeling (not in US labeling): Oral: 200 mg once daily for 6 months (when due to *Fonsecaea pedrosoi*) or 100 mg once daily for 3 months (when due to *Cladosporium carrioni*)

Coccidioidomycosis (nonprogressive, nondisseminated disease): 200 mg twice daily or 3 times daily (Galgiani 2005)

Coccidioidal pneumonia: Oral:

Mild to moderate: 200 mg twice daily (Galgiani 2005)

HIV-infected patients (focal pneumonia): 200 mg twice daily (HHS [OI adult 2015])

Coccidioidal meningitis: Oral: 400 to 600 mg daily (Galgiani 2005)

Coccidioidal meningitis in HIV-infected patients (off-label use; HHS [OI adult 2015]) (alternative to preferred therapy): Oral:

Treatment: 200 mg 3 times daily for 3 days, then 200 mg twice daily, followed by chronic suppressive therapy

Chronic suppressive therapy: 200 mg twice daily continued indefinitely, even with increase in CD4 count on ART

Histoplasmosis:

Treatment:

Manufacturer's labeling: Oral capsule: Initial: 200 mg once daily; if no clinical improvement or evidence of progressive infection, may increase dose in increments of 100 mg up to maximum of 400 mg daily. Note: For life-threatening infections, the US labeling recommends administering a loading dose of 200 mg 3 times daily (total: 600 mg daily) for the first 3 days of therapy. Continue treatment for at least 3 months and until clinical and laboratory evidence suggest that infection has resolved.

Alternate dosing: 200 mg 3 times daily for 3 days, then 200 mg twice daily (or once daily in mild-moderate disease) for 6 to 12 weeks in mild-moderate disease or ≥12 months in progressive disseminated or chronic cavitary pulmonary histoplasmosis; in moderately-severe to severe infection, therapy should be initiated with ~2 weeks of a lipid formation of amphotericin B (Wheat, 2007). Duration of twice daily maintenance therapy should be at least 12 months in HIV-infected patients (HHS [OI adult 2015])

Prophylaxis (off-label use):

Primary prophylaxis in HIV-infected patients: 200 mg once daily; primary prophylaxis is indicated when CD4 count <150 cells/mm^3 and at increased risk of exposure (HHS [OI adult 2015])

Long-term suppression therapy (secondary prophylaxis) in HIV-infected patients: 200 mg once daily; long-term suppressive therapy is indicated in patients who relapse despite appropriate therapy or in patients with CNS or severe disseminated infection (HHS [OI adult 2015])

Microsporidiosis, disseminated (caused by *Trachipleistophora* or *Anncaliia*) in HIV-infected patients (off-label use): Oral: 400 mg once daily in combination with albendazole (HHS [OI adult 2015])

Onychomycosis (fingernail involvement only): Oral capsule: 200 mg twice daily for 1 week; repeat 1-week course after 3-week off-time

Onychomycosis (toenails due to *Trichophyton rubrum* or *T. mentagrophytes*): Oral tablet: 200 mg once daily for 12 consecutive weeks.

Onychomycosis (toenails with or without fingernail involvement): Oral capsule: 200 mg once daily for 12 consecutive weeks

Canadian labeling (not in US labeling): "Pulse-dosing": 200 mg twice daily for 1 week; repeat 1-week course twice with 3-week off-time between each course

Paracoccidioidomycosis: Canadian labeling (not in US labeling): Oral capsule: 100 mg once daily for 6 months

Penicilliosis in HIV-infected patients (off-label use; HHS [OI adult 2015]): Oral:

Primary prophylaxis: 200 mg once daily for patients with a CD4 count <100 cells/mm^3 who spend extensive time in northern Thailand, Vietnam, and Southern China, especially rural areas

Treatment: 200 mg twice daily for 8 weeks (mild disease) or 10 weeks (severe infections), then continue with maintenance therapy. In severely-ill patients, initiate therapy with 2 weeks of liposomal amphotericin B.

Chronic maintenance (secondary prophylaxis): 200 mg once daily until CD4 count >100 cells/mm^3 for ≥6 months in response to ART

Pityriasis versicolor: Canadian labeling (not in US labeling): Oral: 200 mg once daily for 7 days

Sporotrichosis: Oral:

Lymphocutaneous: 200 mg daily for 3 to 6 months (Kauffman, 2007)

Canadian labeling (not in US labeling): 100 mg once daily for 3 months

Osteoarticular and pulmonary: 200 mg twice daily for ≥1 years (may use amphotericin B initially for stabilization) (Kauffman, 2007)

Tinea corporis or tinea cruris: Canadian labeling (not in US labeling): Oral capsule: 100 mg once daily for 14 consecutive days or 200 mg once daily for 7 consecutive days. **Note:** Equivalency between regimens not established.

Tinea pedis: Canadian labeling (not in US labeling): Oral capsule: 100 mg once daily for 28 consecutive days or 200 mg twice daily for 7 consecutive days. **Note:** Equivalency between regimens not established. Patients with chronic resistant infection may benefit from lower dose and extended treatment time (100 mg once daily for 28 days).

Pediatric Note: Doses >200 mg daily should be administered in 2 divided doses.

Candidiasis:

Infants and Children (HIV-exposed/-positive; off-label use):

Oropharyngeal: Oral solution: 2.5 mg/kg/dose twice daily (maximum: 200 mg daily [400 mg daily if fluconazole-refractory]) for 7 to 14 days (CDC, 2009)

Esophageal: Oral solution: 5 mg/kg/day once daily or divided twice daily for 4 to 21 days (CDC, 2009)

Adolescents (off-label population): HIV-infected patients:

Esophageal: Oral solution: 200 mg once daily for 14 to 21 days (HHS [OI adult 2015])

Oropharyngeal (alternative to preferred therapy): Oral solution: 200 mg once daily for 7 to 14 days (HHS [OI adult 2015])

Vulvo-vaginal (uncomplicated) (off-label use): Refer to adult dosing.

Coccidioidomycosis: Infants and Children (HIV-exposed/-positive; off-label use):

Treatment: Oral: 5 to 10 mg/kg/dose twice daily for 3 days, followed by 2 to 5 mg/kg/dose orally twice daily (maximum: 400 mg daily) (CDC, 2009)

Relapse prevention: Oral: 2 to 5 mg/kg/dose twice daily (maximum: 400 mg daily) (CDC, 2009)

Coccidioidal meningitis in HIV-infected patients (off-label use) (alternative to preferred therapy): Adolescents: Refer to adult dosing.

Coccidioidal pneumonia (focal pneumonia) in HIV-infected patients (off-label use): Adolescents: Refer to adult dosing.

Cryptococcus: Infants and Children (HIV-exposed/-positive; off-label use):

Treatment, consolidation therapy: Oral solution (preferred): Initial: 2.5 to 5 mg/kg/dose 3 times daily (maximum daily dose: 600 mg daily) for 3 days (9 doses) followed by 5 to 10 mg/kg/day divided once or twice daily (maximum daily dose: 400 mg daily) for a minimum of 8 weeks (CDC, 2009)

Relapse prevention: Oral solution: 5 mg/kg/dose once daily (maximum: 200 mg daily) (CDC, 2009)

Histoplasmosis:

Infants and Children (HIV-exposed/-positive; off-label use):

Treatment of mild disseminated disease: Oral solution: 2 to 5 mg/kg/dose 3 times daily for 3 days (9 doses), followed by twice daily for 12 months (maximum: 200 mg per dose) (CDC, 2009)

Consolidation treatment for moderate-severe to severe disseminated disease, including CNS infection (following appropriate induction therapy): Oral solution: 2 to 5 mg/kg/dose 3 times daily for 3 days, followed by 2 to 5 mg/kg/dose (maximum: 200 mg per dose) twice daily for 12 months for non-CNS-disseminated disease or for ≥12 months for CNS infection (CDC, 2009)

Relapse prevention: Oral solution: 5 mg/kg/dose twice daily (maximum: 400 mg daily) (CDC, 2009)

Adolescents (off-label population): HIV-positive patients:

Treatment (off-label dose): 200 mg 3 times daily for 3 days, then 200 mg twice daily. Duration of twice daily maintenance therapy should be at least 12 months (HHS [OI adult 2015])

Primary prophylaxis in HIV-infected patients (off-label use): Refer to adult dosing.

Long-term suppression therapy (secondary prophylaxis) (off-label use): Refer to adult dosing.

Microsporidiosis, disseminated (caused by *Trachipleistophora* or *Anncaliia*) in HIV-infected patients (off-label use): Adolescents: Refer to adult dosing.

Penicilliosis in HIV-infected patients (off-label use): Adolescents: Refer to adult dosing.

Renal Impairment

The manufacturer's labeling states to use with caution in patients with renal impairment; dosage adjustment may be needed. Limited data suggest that no dosage adjustments are required in renal impairment; wide variations observed in plasma concentrations versus time profiles in patients with uremia, or receiving hemodialysis or continuous ambulatory peritoneal dialysis (Boelaert, 1988).

Hemodialysis: Nondialyzable

Hepatic Impairment There are no dosage adjustments provided in the manufacturer's labeling; however, use caution and monitor closely for signs/symptoms of toxicity.

Dietary Considerations

Capsule, tablet: Take with food.

Solution: Take without food, if possible.

Administration Doses >200 mg/day are given in 2 divided doses; do not administer with antacids. Capsule and oral solution formulations are not bioequivalent and thus are not interchangeable. Capsule and tablet absorption is best if taken with food, therefore, it is best to administer itraconazole after meals at the same time each day; solution should be taken on an empty stomach. When treating oropharyngeal and esophageal candidiasis, solution should be swished vigorously in mouth (10 mL at a time), then swallowed.

Monitoring Parameters Liver function in patients with preexisting hepatic dysfunction, and in all patients being treated for longer than 1 month; serum concentrations particularly for oral therapy (due to erratic bioavailability with capsule formulation); renal function; signs/symptoms of CHF

Reference Range Serum concentrations may be performed to assure therapeutic levels. Itraconazole plus the metabolite hydroxyitraconazole concentrations should be >1 mcg/mL (not to exceed 10 mcg/mL).

Timing of serum samples: Obtain level after ~2 weeks of therapy, level may be drawn anytime during the dosing interval.

Dosage Forms Excipient information presented when available (limited, particularly for generics); consult specific product labeling.

Capsule, Oral:

Sporanox: 100 mg [contains brilliant blue fcf (fd&c blue #1), d&c red #22 (eosine), fd&c blue #2 (indigotine)]

Sporanox Pulsepak: 100 mg [contains brilliant blue fcf (fd&c blue #1), d&c red #22 (eosine), fd&c blue #2 (indigotine)]

Generic: 100 mg

Solution, Oral:

Sporanox: 10 mg/mL (150 mL) [contains propylene glycol, saccharin sodium]

Tablet, Oral:

Onmel: 200 mg

Extemporaneous Preparations Note: Commercial oral solution is available (10 mg/mL)

A 20 mg/mL oral suspension may be made with capsules. Empty the contents of forty 100 mg capsules and add 15 mL of Alcohol, USP. Let stand for 5 minutes. Crush the beads in a mortar and reduce to a fine powder. Mix while adding a 1:1 mixture of Ora-Sweet and Ora-Plus in incremental proportions to **almost** 200 mL; transfer to a calibrated bottle, rinse mortar with vehicle, and add quantity of vehicle sufficient to make 200 mL. Label "shake well" and "refrigerate". Stable for 56 days refrigerated.

Nahata MC, Pai VB, and Hipple TF, *Pediatric Drug Formulations*, 5th ed, Cincinnati, OH: Harvey Whitney Books Co, 2004.

Ivabradine (eye VAB ra deen)

Brand Names: US Corlanor

Index Terms Corlanor; Ivabradine Hydrochloride

Pharmacologic Category Cardiovascular Agent, Miscellaneous

Use Heart failure: Reduce the risk of hospitalization for worsening chronic heart failure in patients with stable, symptomatic chronic heart failure with left ventricular ejection fraction ≤35%, who are in sinus rhythm with resting heart rate ≥70 beats per minute (bpm) and either are on maximally tolerated doses of beta blockers or have a contraindication to beta-blocker use.

Pregnancy Considerations Based on information from animal reproduction studies, fetal harm may occur if ivabradine is administered to pregnant women. Effective contraception is recommended in women of reproductive potential. If treatment is needed during pregnancy, closely monitor for destabilization of heart failure that could potentially result from heart rate slowing caused by ivabradine, especially during the first trimester. Pregnant women with chronic heart failure should also be monitored for preterm birth.

Breast-Feeding Considerations It is not known if ivabradine is excreted into breast milk. Due to the potential risk from exposure in the nursing infant, breast-feeding is not recommended by the manufacturer.

Medication Guide Available Yes

Contraindications Acute decompensated heart failure; blood pressure <90/50 mm Hg; sick sinus syndrome, sinoatrial block, or third-degree AV block (unless a functioning demand pacemaker is present); resting heart rate <60 bpm prior to treatment; severe hepatic impairment; pacemaker dependence (heart rate maintained exclusively by the pacemaker); concomitant use with strong CYP3A4 inhibitors

Warnings/Precautions Ivabradine increases the risk of atrial fibrillation; monitor cardiac rhythm. Discontinue use if atrial fibrillation develops. May cause bradycardia, sinus arrest, and heart block; monitor heart rate prior to initiation and with any dosage adjustment. Risk factors for bradycardia include sinus node dysfunction, conduction defects (eg, first- or second-degree AV block, bundle branch block), ventricular dyssynchrony, and use of other negative chronotropes (eg, digoxin, diltiazem, verapamil, amiodarone). Avoid use with verapamil and diltiazem. Avoid use in patients with second-degree AV block (unless a functioning demand pacemaker is present). Use is contraindicated in patients with sick sinus syndrome, sinoatrial block, third-degree AV block (unless a functioning demand pacemaker is present), or pacemaker dependence. Decrease dose or discontinue use if heart rate <50 bpm persists during therapy. Use is contraindicated in patients with pretreatment heart rate <60 bpm. In patients with history of conduction defects or those in whom bradycardia could lead to hemodynamic compromise, initial dosage reduction is recommended. Heart rate reduction may prolong the uncorrected QT interval while QTc interval remains unchanged (Camm 2003; Murat 2009). At concentrations slightly higher than that achieved with therapeutic dosing, ivabradine prolonged ventricular repolarization in perfused guinea-pig hearts (Melgari 2015). Torsades de pointes has been reported when used with other drugs that produce bradycardia or prolong the QT interval (Cocco 2015; Mittal 2014).

Phosphenes (described as transient enhanced brightness in a limited area of the visual field, halos, image decomposition, colored bright lights, or multiple images) may occur with use; onset is generally within the first 2 months of therapy and is reported to be of mild to moderate intensity; most cases resolve during or after treatment discontinuation. Potentially significant drug-drug interactions may exist, requiring dose or frequency adjustment, additional monitoring, and/or selection of alternative therapy.

Adverse Reactions Frequency not always defined.
Cardiovascular: Bradycardia (6% to 10%), hypertension (9%), atrial fibrillation (5% to 8%), heart block, sinoatrial arrest
Central nervous system: Phosphene (3%)
<1% (Limited to important or life-threatening): Angioedema, diplopia, erythema, hypotension, pruritus, skin rash, syncope, urticaria, vertigo, visual impairment

Drug Interactions
Metabolism/Transport Effects Substrate of CYP3A4 (major); **Note:** Assignment of Major/Minor substrate status based on clinically relevant drug interaction potential
Avoid Concomitant Use
Avoid concomitant use of Ivabradine with any of the following: Calcium Channel Blockers (Nondihydropyridine); Ceritinib; Conivaptan; CYP3A4 Inducers (Strong); CYP3A4 Inhibitors (Moderate); CYP3A4 Inhibitors (Strong); Fusidic Acid (Systemic); Grapefruit Juice; Highest Risk QTc-Prolonging Agents; Idelalisib; Moderate Risk QTc-Prolonging Agents; St Johns Wort
Increased Effect/Toxicity
Ivabradine may increase the levels/effects of: Calcium Channel Blockers (Nondihydropyridine); Ceritinib; Highest Risk QTc-Prolonging Agents; Lacosamide; Moderate Risk QTc-Prolonging Agents

The levels/effects of Ivabradine may be increased by: Bradycardia-Causing Agents; Bretylium; Calcium Channel Blockers (Nondihydropyridine); Conivaptan; CYP3A4 Inhibitors (Moderate); CYP3A4 Inhibitors (Strong); Dasatinib; Fosaprepitant; Fusidic Acid (Systemic); Grapefruit Juice; Idelalisib; Ivacaftor; Loop Diuretics; Luliconazole; Palbociclib; Regorafenib; Ruxolitinib; Simeprevir; Stiripentol; Thiazide Diuretics; Tofacitinib
Decreased Effect
The levels/effects of Ivabradine may be decreased by: Bosentan; CYP3A4 Inducers (Moderate); CYP3A4 Inducers (Strong); Dabrafenib; Deferasirox; Siltuximab; St Johns Wort; Tocilizumab

Food Interactions
Food: Absorption delayed by 1 hour and AUC increased by 20% to 40% when taken with food. Management: Take with food to reduce variability in exposure.

Grapefruit juice: Exposure increased twofold after ingestion of grapefruit juice. Management: Avoid consumption of grapefruit juice (Nawarskas 2015).
Storage/Stability Store at 25°C (77°F); excursions are permitted between 15°C and 30°C (59°F and 86°F).
Mechanism of Action Selective and specific inhibition of the hyperpolarization-activated cyclic nucleotide-gated (HCN) channels (f-channels) within the sinoatrial (SA) node of cardiac tissue resulting in disruption of If ion current flow prolonging diastolic depolarization, slowing firing in the SA node, and ultimately reducing heart rate. Has not demonstrated effects on myocardial contractility or relaxation, ventricular repolarization, or conduction apart from the sinus node effects. Partial inhibition of the retinal I_h current (similar to the cardiac I_f current) may explain visual disturbances (eg, phosphenes) (Nawarskas 2015).
Pharmacodynamics/Kinetics
Distribution: V_d: ~100 L
Protein binding: ~70%
Metabolism: Extensively intestinal and hepatic via CYP3A4; major active metabolite equipotent to ivabradine is the N-desmethylated derivative (S 18982) which is also metabolized by CYP3A4
Bioavailability: ~40% due to first pass elimination in gut and liver; AUC increased 20% to 40% with food
Half-life elimination: Distribution: ~2 hours; Effective: ~6 hours
Time to peak, plasma: ~1 hour (fasting); ~2 hours (with food)
Excretion: Urine (~4% as unchanged drug)
Dosing
Adult
Heart failure: Oral: Initial: 5 mg twice daily **or** 2.5 mg twice daily in patients with a history of conduction defects or who may experience hemodynamic compromise due to bradycardia. After 2 weeks, adjust dose to achieve a resting heart rate between 50 and 60 beats per minute (bpm). Thereafter, adjust dose as needed based on resting heart rate and tolerability. Maximum dose: 7.5 mg twice daily.
Dosage adjustment based on resting heart rate:
If heart rate >60 bpm: Increase dose by 2.5 mg twice daily (maximum dose: 7.5 mg twice daily)
If heart rate 50 to 60 bpm: Maintain dose
If heart rate <50 bpm or signs and symptoms of bradycardia: Decrease dose by 2.5 mg twice daily; if current dose is 2.5 mg twice daily, discontinue therapy

Stable angina (off-label use): Adults <75 years: Oral: Initial: 2.5 to 5 mg twice daily; titrate up in increments of 2.5 mg after 3 to 4 weeks if symptoms persist and heart rate is greater than 60 bpm to a maximum dose of 7.5 mg twice daily. Discontinue therapy if angina symptoms do not improve within 3 months of initiation. Also consider discontinuation if improvement of angina symptoms is limited and no clinically significant heart rate reduction occurs in the first 3 months. If heart rate is lower than 50 bpm at rest or patient experiences symptomatic bradycardia (eg, dizziness, fatigue, hypotension) during therapy, decrease dose by 2.5 mg per dose, or discontinue if already at the minimum dose of 2.5 mg twice daily. Monitor heart rate carefully after dosage reduction. If heart rate continues to be lower than 50 bpm or symptoms of bradycardia persist, discontinue ivabradine (Corlentor 2015).
If symptoms are not controlled on beta-blocker or calcium channel blocker monotherapy, addition of ivabradine can be considered. If combined with a calcium channel blocker, use of a dihydropyridine (such as slow-release nifedipine, amlodipine, or felodipine) is suggested. (Montalescot 2013; NICE 2012).
Geriatric
Heart failure: Refer to adult dosing.
Stable angina (off-label use): Adults ≥75 years: Initial: Oral: Consider 2.5 mg twice daily. Titration and maintenance: Refer to adult dosing.
Renal Impairment
CrCl ≥15 mL/minute: No dosage adjustment necessary.
CrCl <15 mL/minute: There are no dosage adjustments provided in manufacturer's labeling (has not been studied); use with caution.
Hepatic Impairment
Mild or moderate impairment (Child-Pugh class A or B): No dosage adjustment necessary.
Severe impairment (Child-Pugh class C): Use is contraindicated (has not been studied; increase in systemic exposure anticipated).
Administration Oral: Administer with meals.

Monitoring Parameters Heart rate (prior to initiation, prior to increasing dose, or after decreasing dose); monitor heart rate more closely if receiving other negative chronotropes (eg, amiodarone, beta-blockers, digoxin); blood pressure; regularly monitor cardiac rhythm (assessing for atrial fibrillation)

Dosage Forms Excipient information presented when available (limited, particularly for generics); consult specific product labeling.

Tablet, Oral:
Corlanor: 5 mg [scored]
Corlanor: 7.5 mg

◆ Ivabradine Hydrochloride see Ivabradine on page 1002

Ivacaftor (eye va KAF tor)

Brand Names: US Kalydeco
Brand Names: Canada Kalydeco
Index Terms VX-770
Pharmacologic Category Cystic Fibrosis Transmembrane Conductance Regulator Potentiator

Use
Cystic fibrosis:
  US labeling: For the treatment of cystic fibrosis (CF) in patients ≥2 years of age who have one of the following mutations in the cystic fibrosis transmembrane conductance regulator (CFTR) gene: G551D, G1244E, G1349D, G178R, G551S, R117H, S1251N, S1255P, S549N, or S549R.
    If the patient's genotype is unknown, a US Food and Drug Administration-cleared cystic fibrosis mutation test should be used to detect the presence of a CFTR mutation followed by verification with bidirectional sequencing when recommended by the mutation test instructions for use.
  Canadian labeling: For the treatment of cystic fibrosis (CF) in patients ≥6 years of age who have one of the following mutations in the cystic fibrosis transmembrane conductance regulator (CFTR) gene: G551D, G1244E, G1349D, G178R, G551S, S1251N, S1255P, S549N, S549R, or G970R; patients ≥18 years with an R117H mutation in the CFTR gene
  Limitations of use: According to the manufacturer labeling, ivacaftor is not effective in patients with CF who are homozygous for the F508del mutation in the CTFR gene.

Pregnancy Considerations Adverse events have not been observed in animal reproduction studies.

Breast-Feeding Considerations Although unknown, the manufacturer suggests that excretion of ivacaftor in breast milk is probable; caution is recommended when administering ivacaftor to nursing women.

Contraindications There are no contraindications listed in the manufacturer's U.S. labeling.
  Canadian labeling: Hypersensitivity to ivacaftor or any component of the formulation

Warnings/Precautions May increase hepatic transaminases. Monitor liver function; increased monitoring may be necessary in patients with a history of elevated hepatic transaminases.Temporarily discontinue treatment if ALT or AST >5 times ULN. Use with caution in patients with moderate or severe hepatic impairment; dosage adjustment recommended. Use caution in patients with severe renal impairment or ESRD. Noncongenital lens opacities and cataracts have been reported in pediatric patients treated with ivacaftor; other risk factors were present in some cases (eg, corticosteroid use, exposure to radiation), but a possible risk related to ivacaftor cannot be excluded. Baseline and follow-up ophthalmological examinations are recommended in pediatric patients. May cause dizziness, which may impair physical or mental abilities; patients must be cautioned about performing tasks that require mental alertness (eg, operating machinery or driving). Potentially significant drug-drug interactions may exist, requiring dose or frequency adjustment, additional monitoring, and/or selection of alternative therapy.

Adverse Reactions Frequency not always defined.
  >10%:
  Central nervous system: Headache (24%)
  Dermatologic: Skin rash (13%)
  Gastrointestinal: Abdominal pain (16%), diarrhea (13%), nausea (12%)
  Respiratory: Oropharyngeal pain (22%), upper respiratory tract infection (22%), nasal congestion (20%), nasopharyngitis (15%)
  1% to 10%:
  Central nervous system: Dizziness (9%)
  Dermatologic: Acne vulgaris (4% to 7%)
  Endocrine & metabolic: Increased serum glucose (4% to 7%), hypoglycemia
  Hepatic: Increased liver enzymes (4% to 7%), increased serum ALT (4% to 7%)

Neuromuscular & skeletal: Arthralgia (4% to 7%), musculoskeletal chest pain (4% to 7%), myalgia (4% to 7%)
Ophthalmic: Cataract (children ≤12)
Respiratory: Change in bronchial secretions (4% to 7%; bacteria present), pharyngeal erythema (4% to 7%), pleuritic chest pain (4% to 7%), rhinitis (4% to 7%), sinus congestion (4% to 7%), sinus headache (4% to 7%), wheezing (4% to 7%)
Miscellaneous: Bacteria in sputum (4% to 7%)

Drug Interactions
Metabolism/Transport Effects Substrate of CYP3A4 (major); **Note:** Assignment of Major/Minor substrate status based on clinically relevant drug interaction potential; **Inhibits** CYP2C8 (weak), CYP2C9 (weak), CYP3A4 (weak), P-glycoprotein

Avoid Concomitant Use
  Avoid concomitant use of Ivacaftor with any of the following: Amodiaquine; Bitter Orange; Bosutinib; Conivaptan; CYP3A4 Inducers (Strong); Fusidic Acid (Systemic); Grapefruit Juice; Idelalisib; PAZOPanib; Pimozide; Silodosin; St Johns Wort; Topotecan; VinCRIStine (Liposomal)

Increased Effect/Toxicity
  Ivacaftor may increase the levels/effects of: Afatinib; Amodiaquine; ARIPiprazole; Bosutinib; Brentuximab Vedotin; Colchicine; CYP3A4 Substrates; Dabigatran Etexilate; Dofetilide; DOXOrubicin (Conventional); Edoxaban; Everolimus; Flibanserin; Hydrocodone; Ledipasvir; Lomitapide; Naloxegol; NiMODipine; PAZOPanib; P-glycoprotein/ABCB1 Substrates; Pimozide; Prucalopride; Ranolazine; Rifaximin; Silodosin; Topotecan; VinCRIStine (Liposomal)

  The levels/effects of Ivacaftor may be increased by: Bitter Orange; Conivaptan; CYP3A4 Inhibitors (Moderate); CYP3A4 Inhibitors (Strong); Dasatinib; Fosaprepitant; Fusidic Acid (Systemic); Grapefruit Juice; Idelalisib; Luliconazole; Mifepristone; Osimertinib; Palbociclib; Simeprevir; Stiripentol

Decreased Effect
  The levels/effects of Ivacaftor may be decreased by: Bosentan; CYP3A4 Inducers (Moderate); CYP3A4 Inducers (Strong); Dabrafenib; Deferasirox; Osimertinib; Siltuximab; St Johns Wort; Tocilizumab

Food Interactions Ivacaftor serum concentrations may be increased when taken with grapefruit or Seville oranges. Management: Avoid concurrent use.

Storage/Stability Store at 20°C to 25°C (68°F to 77°F); excursions permitted to 15°C to 30°C (59°F to 86°F); after mixing the granules, the product is stable for 1 hour.

Mechanism of Action Potentiates epithelial cell chloride ion transport of defective (G551D mutant) cell-surface CFTR protein thereby improving the regulation of salt and water absorption and secretion in various tissues (eg, lung, gastrointestinal tract).

Pharmacodynamics/Kinetics
Onset of action: FEV_1 increased, sweat chloride decreased within ~2 weeks
Absorption: Variable; increased (by two- to fourfold) with fatty foods
Distribution: V_d: 353 L ± 122 L
Protein binding: ~99%; primarily to alpha$_1$ acid glycoprotein, albumin
Metabolism: Hepatic; extensive via CYP3A; forms 2 major metabolites (M1 [active; 1/6 potency] and M6 [inactive])
Half-life elimination: ~12 hours
Time to peak: ~4 hours
Excretion: Feces (88%, 65% of administered dose as metabolites); urine (minimal, as unchanged drug)

Dosing
Adult Cystic fibrosis: Oral: Tablet: 150 mg every 12 hours
  Dosage adjustment for ivacaftor with concomitant medications:
    CYP3A strong inhibitors (eg, ketoconazole, itraconazole, posaconazole, voriconazole, clarithromycin, telithromycin): 150 mg twice **weekly**
    CYP3A moderate inhibitors (eg, erythromycin, fluconazole): 150 mg once daily
    CYP3A strong inducers (eg, carbamazepine, phenobarbital, phenytoin, rifabutin, rifampin, St John's wort): Use is not recommended
  Missed dose: If dose is missed within 6 hours of the usual time it is taken, take the dose as soon as possible; otherwise, skip the missed dose and resume the normal dosing schedule

Pediatric
Cystic fibrosis: Oral:
  Granules:
    Children 2 to <6 years:
      <14 kg: 50 mg packet every 12 hours
      ≥14 kg: 75 mg packet every 12 hours

Tablet: Children ≥6 years and Adolescents: Refer to adult dosing.

Dosage adjustment for ivacaftor with concomitant medications:

CYP3A strong inhibitors (eg, clarithromycin, itraconazole, ketoconazole, posaconazole, telithromycin, voriconazole):

Children 2 to <6 years:

<14 kg: 50 mg granule packet twice **weekly**

≥14 kg: 75 mg granule packet twice **weekly**

Children ≥6 years and Adolescents: Refer to adult dosing.

CYP3A moderate inhibitors (eg, erythromycin, fluconazole):

Children 2 to <6 years:

<14 kg: 50 mg granule packet once daily

≥14 kg: 75 mg granule packet once daily

Children ≥6 years and Adolescents: Refer to adult dosing.

CYP3A strong inducers (eg, carbamazepine, phenobarbital, phenytoin, rifabutin, rifampin, St John's wort): Refer to adult dosing.

Missed dose: If dose is missed within 6 hours of the usual time it is taken, take the dose as soon as possible; otherwise, skip the missed dose and resume the normal dosing schedule

Renal Impairment

Mild to moderate impairment (CrCl >30 mL/minute): No dosage adjustment necessary (has not been studied).

Severe impairment (CrCl ≤30 mL/minute): There are no dosage adjustments provided in the manufacturer's labeling (has not been studied); use with caution.

End-stage renal disease (ESRD): There are no dosage adjustments provided in the manufacturer's labeling (has not been studied); use with caution.

Hepatic Impairment

Mild impairment (Child-Pugh class A): No dosage adjustment necessary.

Moderate impairment (Child-Pugh class B):

Children ≥6 years, Adolescents, and Adults: 150 mg once daily

Children 2 to <6 years:

<14 kg: 50 mg granule packet once daily

≥14 kg: 75 mg granule packet once daily

Severe impairment (Child-Pugh class C): Has not been studied; use with caution

US labeling:

Children ≥6 years, Adolescents, and Adults: 150 mg once daily or less frequently.

Children 2 to <6 years:

<14 kg: 50 mg granule packet once daily or less frequently

≥14 kg: 75 mg granule packet once daily or less frequently

Canadian labeling: Initial:

Children ≥6 years, Adolescents, and Adults: 150 mg once every other day; adjust for tolerance and/or response.

Children 2 to <6 years:

<14 kg: 50 mg granule packet once every other day; adjust for tolerance and/or response.

≥14 kg: 75 mg granule packet once every other day; adjust for tolerance and/or response.

Adjustment for Toxicity ALT or AST >5 times ULN: Hold ivacaftor; may resume if elevated transaminases resolved and after assessing benefits vs risks of continued treatment.

Dietary Considerations Take with high-fat-containing foods (eg, butter, cheese pizza, eggs, peanut butter, whole milk dairy products [eg, whole milk, cheese, yogurt]). Avoid grapefruit or Seville oranges.

Administration Oral:

Granules: Administer before or after high-fat-containing foods (eg, butter, cheese pizza, eggs, peanut butter, whole-milk dairy products [eg, whole milk, cheese, yogurt]). Mix entire packet of granules with 5 mL of soft food (eg, pureed fruits [excluding grapefruit or Seville oranges] or vegetables, yogurt, applesauce) or liquid (eg, water, milk, juice [excluding grapefruit juice]); food or liquid should be at or below room temperature. Granule mixture should be completely consumed within 1 hour.

Tablets: Administer with high-fat-containing foods (eg, butter, cheese pizza, eggs, peanut butter).

Monitoring Parameters CF mutation test (prior to therapy initiation if G551D mutation status unknown); ALT/AST at baseline, every 3 months for 1 year, then annually thereafter or as clinically indicated (consider more frequent monitoring in patients with a history of elevated hepatic transaminases); FEV$_1$; baseline and follow-up ophthalmological exams in pediatric patients

Additional Information G551D mutation is present in approximately 4% to 5% of patients with CF. When used in addition to standard therapy (eg, dornase alfa, inhaled tobramycin), ivacaftor may provide further improvements in FEV$_1$, a reduction in pulmonary exacerbations, and a beneficial weight gain in CF patients. Long-term benefits on disease progression have not been established.

Dosage Forms Excipient information presented when available (limited, particularly for generics); consult specific product labeling.

Packet, Oral:

Kalydeco: 50 mg (56 ea); 75 mg (56 ea)

Tablet, Oral:

Kalydeco: 150 mg [contains fd&c blue #2 (indigotine)]

◆ Ivacaftor and Lumacaftor *see* Lumacaftor and Ivacaftor *on page 1114*

Ivermectin (Systemic) (eye ver MEK tin)

Brand Names: US Stromectol

Pharmacologic Category Anthelmintic

Use Treatment of the following infections: Strongyloidiasis of the intestinal tract due to the nematode parasite *Strongyloides stercoralis*. Onchocerciasis due to the immature form of the nematode parasite *Onchocerca volvulus*

Pregnancy Considerations Adverse events have been observed in animal reproduction studies. Although use in pregnancy is likely low risk, other agents are currently recommended for the treatment of pediculosis pubis or scabies in pregnant women (CDC [Workowski 2015]).

Breast-Feeding Considerations Ivermectin is measurable in low concentrations in breast milk. The manufacturer does not recommend treating women who intend to breastfeed unless the risk of delayed maternal treatment outweighs the potential risk to the nursing infant. Although use is likely low risk, other agents are currently recommended for the treatment of pediculosis pubis or scabies in breastfeeding women (CDC [Workowski 2015]).

Contraindications Hypersensitivity to ivermectin or any component of the formulation

Warnings/Precautions Data have shown that antihelmintic drugs like ivermectin may cause cutaneous and/or systemic reactions (Mazzoti reaction) of varying severity including ophthalmological reactions in patients with onchocerciasis. These reactions are probably due to allergic and inflammatory responses to the death of microfilariae. Patients with hyper-reactive onchodermatitis may be more likely than others to experience severe adverse reactions, especially edema and aggravation of the onchodermatitis. Repeated treatment may be required in immunocompromised patients (eg, HIV); control of extraintestinal strongyloidiasis may necessitate suppressive (once monthly) therapy. Pretreatment assessment for *Loa loa* infection is recommended in any patient with significant exposure to endemic areas (West and Central Africa); serious and/or fatal encephalopathy has been reported (rarely) during treatment in patients with loiasis. Ivermectin has no activity against adult *Onchocerca volvulus* parasites.

Adverse Reactions

>10%: Miscellaneous: Mazzotti-type reaction (with onchocerciasis): Pruritus (28%), fever (23%), skin involvement (23%; including edema/urticarial rash), lymph node tenderness (1% to 14%), lymph node enlargement (3% to 13%), arthralgia/synovitis (9%)

1% to 10%:

Cardiovascular: Tachycardia (4%), peripheral edema (3%), facial edema (1%), orthostatic hypotension (1%)

Central nervous system: Dizziness (3%)

Dermatologic: Pruritus (3%)

Gastrointestinal: Diarrhea (2%), nausea (2%)

Hematologic: Eosinophilia (3%), leukocytes decreased (3%), hemoglobin increased (1%)

Hepatic: ALT increased (2%), AST increased (2%)

<1% (Limited to important or life-threatening): Abdominal distention, abdominal pain, anemia, anorexia, anterior uveitis, asthma exacerbation, back pain, bilirubin increased, chest discomfort, chorioretinitis, choroiditis, coma, confusion, conjunctival hemorrhage (associated with onchocerciasis), conjunctivitis, constipation, dyspnea, encephalopathy (rare; associated with loiasis), eyelid edema, eye sensation abnormal, fatigue, fecal incontinence, headache, hepatitis, hypotension, INR increased (with concomitant warfarin), keratitis, lethargy, leukopenia, mental status changes, myalgia, neck pain, rash, red eye, seizure, somnolence, standing/walking difficulty, Stevens-Johnson syndrome, stupor, toxic epidermal necrolysis, tremor, urinary incontinence, urticaria, vertigo, vision loss (transient), vomiting, weakness

◀

Drug Interactions

Metabolism/Transport Effects Substrate of CYP3A4 (minor), P-glycoprotein; **Note:** Assignment of Major/Minor substrate status based on clinically relevant drug interaction potential

Avoid Concomitant Use

Avoid concomitant use of Ivermectin (Systemic) with any of the following: BCG (Intravesical)

Increased Effect/Toxicity

Ivermectin (Systemic) may increase the levels/effects of: Vitamin K Antagonists

The levels/effects of Ivermectin (Systemic) may be increased by: Azithromycin (Systemic); Lumacaftor; P-glycoprotein/ABCB1 Inhibitors; Ranolazine

Decreased Effect

Ivermectin (Systemic) may decrease the levels/effects of: BCG (Intravesical); BCG Vaccine (Immunization); Sodium Picosulfate; Typhoid Vaccine

The levels/effects of Ivermectin (Systemic) may be decreased by: Lumacaftor; P-glycoprotein/ABCB1 Inducers

Food Interactions Bioavailability is increased 2.5-fold when administered following a high-fat meal. Management: Administer on an empty stomach.

Storage/Stability Store at <30°C (86°F).

Mechanism of Action Ivermectin is a semisynthetic anthelminthic agent; it binds selectively and with strong affinity to glutamate-gated chloride ion channels which occur in invertebrate nerve and muscle cells. This leads to increased permeability of cell membranes to chloride ions then hyperpolarization of the nerve or muscle cell, and death of the parasite.

Pharmacodynamics/Kinetics

Onset of action:

Peak effect in treatment of onchocerciasis: 3-6 months

Peak effect in treatment of strongyloides: 3 months

Absorption: Well absorbed

Distribution: V_d: 3-3.5 L/kg (healthy males); high concentration in the liver and adipose tissue; does not readily cross the blood-brain barrier in patients >15 kg or >2 years

Protein binding: ~93% primarily to albumin

Metabolism: Hepatic via CYP3A4 (major), CYP2D6 (minor), and CYP2E1 (minor)

Bioavailability: Increased with high-fat meal

Half-life elimination: 18 hours (range: 16-35 hours)

Time to peak, serum: ~4 hours

Excretion: Feces; urine (<1%)

Dosing

Adult & Geriatric

Onchocerciasis: Oral: 150 mcg/kg as a single dose; retreatment may be required every 3-12 months until asymptomatic

Strongyloidiasis: Oral:

Manufacturer's labeling: 200 mcg/kg as a single dose; perform follow-up stool examinations.

Alternative dosing: 200 mcg/kg/day for 2 days (CDC, 2012)

Ascariasis due to *Ascaris lumbricoides* **(off-label use):** Oral: 200 mcg/kg as a single dose (Marti, 1996; Naquira, 1989)

Cutaneous larva migrans (CLM) due to *Ancylostoma braziliense* **(off-label use):** Oral: 200 mcg/kg as a single dose (Vanhaecke, 2013)

Demodicosis due to *Demodex folliculorum* **and** *Demodex brevis* **(off-label use):** Oral: 200 mcg/kg as a single dose, followed by topical permethrin (Eismann, 2010)

Filariasis due to *Mansonella ozzardi* **(off-label use):** Oral: 6 mg as a single dose (Gonzales, 1999)

Filariasis due to *Mansonella streptocerca* **(off-label use):** Oral: 150 mcg/kg as a single dose (Fischer, 1997)

Filariasis due to *Wucheria bancrofti* **(off-label use):** Oral: 200-400 mcg/kg as a single dose in combination with albendazole (Addiss, 1997; Ismail, 2001)

Gnathostomiasis due to *Gnathostoma spinigerum* **(off-label use):** Oral: 200 mcg/kg as a single dose (Nontasut, 2000; Kraivichian, 2004)

Lice due to *Pediculus humanus capitis, Pediculus humanus corporis, Phthirus pubis* **(off-label use):** Oral: 200 mcg/kg/dose; generally requires >1 dose; number of doses and dosage intervals have not been established

Pediculus humanus capitis: Oral: 400 mcg/kg/dose every 7 days for 2 doses (Chosidow, 2010)

Pediculus humanus corporis: Oral: 200 mcg/kg/dose every 7 days for 3 doses (Foucault, 2006)

Phthirus pubis: Oral: 250 mcg/kg/dose every 7 days for 2 doses (Burkhart, 2004)

Scabies due to *Sarcoptes scabiei* **in immunocompromised patients (off-label use):** Oral: 200 mcg/kg as a single dose; may repeat dose in 14 days (Meinking, 1995). **Note:** Preferred drug for immunocompromised patients with crusted scabies.

Trichuriasis due to *Trichuris trichiura* **(off-label use):** Oral: 200 mcg/kg as a single dose on day 1; may repeat dose on day 4 (Naquira, 1989)

Pediatric Parasitic infections: Oral: Children ≥15 kg: Refer to adult dosing.

Renal Impairment No dosage adjustment provided in manufacturer's labeling.

Hepatic Impairment No dosage adjustment provided in manufacturer's labeling.

Dietary Considerations Take on an empty stomach with water.

Administration Administer on an empty stomach with water.

Monitoring Parameters Skin and eye microfilarial counts, periodic ophthalmologic exams; follow up stool examinations

Dosage Forms Excipient information presented when available (limited, particularly for generics); consult specific product labeling.

Tablet, Oral:

Stromectol: 3 mg

Generic: 3 mg

Ivermectin (Topical) (eye ver MEK tin)

Brand Names: US Sklice; Soolantra

Index Terms Ivermectin Cream; Ivermectin Lotion

Pharmacologic Category Antiparasitic Agent, Topical; Pediculocide

Use

Head lice (*Pediculus capitis***)** (Sklice lotion): Treatment of head lice infestations in patients 6 months and older.

Rosacea (Soolantra cream): Treatment of inflammatory lesions of rosacea in adult patients.

Dosing

Adult & Geriatric

Head lice: Topical: Lotion: Apply sufficient amount (up to 1 tube) to completely cover dry scalp and hair; for single-dose use only

Rosacea: Topical: Cream: Apply to each affected area (eg, forehead, chin, nose, each cheek) once daily.

Pediatric Head lice: Children ≥6 months and Adolescents: Topical: Lotion: Refer to adult dosing.

Renal Impairment There are no dosage adjustments provided in the manufacturer's labeling.

Hepatic Impairment There are no dosage adjustments provided in the manufacturer's labeling.

Additional Information Complete prescribing information should be consulted for additional detail.

Dosage Forms Excipient information presented when available (limited, particularly for generics); consult specific product labeling.

Cream, External:

Soolantra: 1% (30 g) [contains cetyl alcohol, edetate disodium, methylparaben, propylene glycol, propylparaben]

Lotion, External:

Sklice: 0.5% (117 g) [contains methylparaben, propylparaben]

♦ Ivermectin Cream *see* Ivermectin (Topical) *on page 1006*

♦ Ivermectin Lotion *see* Ivermectin (Topical) *on page 1006*

♦ IVIG *see* Immune Globulin *on page 927*

♦ IV Immune Globulin *see* Immune Globulin *on page 927*

♦ IV-VIG *see* Vaccinia Immune Globulin (Intravenous) *on page 1857*

♦ Ivy Block [OTC] *see* Bentoquatam *on page 217*

♦ Ivy-Rid [OTC] *see* Benzocaine *on page 217*

Ixabepilone (ix ab EP i lone)

Brand Names: US Ixempra Kit

Index Terms Azaepothilone B; BMS-247550; Epothilone B Lactam

Pharmacologic Category Antineoplastic Agent, Antimicrotubular; Antineoplastic Agent, Epothilone B Analog

Use Breast cancer: Treatment of metastatic or locally-advanced breast cancer resistant to treatment with an anthracycline and a taxane, or if taxane-resistant and further anthracycline therapy is contraindicated (in combination with capecitabine) or as monotherapy in tumors are resistant or refractory to anthracyclines, taxanes, and capecitabine.

Anthracycline resistance is defined as progression during treatment or within 3 months in the metastatic setting (within 6 months in the adjuvant setting). Taxane resistance is defined as progression during treatment within 4 months in the metastatic setting (within 12 months in the adjuvant setting).

Pregnancy Considerations Adverse events were observed in animal reproduction studies. Women of child-bearing potential should be advised to use effective contraception during treatment.

Breast-Feeding Considerations It is not known if ixabepilone is excreted in breast milk. Due to the potential for serious adverse reactions in the nursing infant, a decision should be made to discontinue breast-feeding or to discontinue the drug, taking into account the importance of treatment to the mother.

Contraindications History of severe (grade 3 or 4) hypersensitivity to polyoxyethylated castor oil (Cremophor EL) or its derivatives; neutrophil count <1,500/mm^3 or platelet count <100,000/mm^3; combination therapy with ixabepilone and capecitabine in patients with AST or ALT >2.5 times ULN or bilirubin >1 times ULN

Warnings/Precautions Hazardous agent - use appropriate precautions for handling and disposal (NIOSH 2014 [group 1]). **[U.S. Boxed Warning]: Due to increased risk of toxicity and neutropenia-related mortality, combination therapy with capecitabine is contraindicated in patients with AST or ALT >2.5 times ULN or bilirubin >1 times ULN.** Use (as monotherapy) is not recommended if AST or ALT >10 times ULN or bilirubin >3 times ULN; use caution in patients with AST or ALT >5 times ULN. Toxicities and serious adverse reactions are increased (in mono- and combination therapy) with hepatic dysfunction; dosage reductions are necessary. Diluent contains polyoxyethylated castor oil (Cremophor EL), which is associated with hypersensitivity reactions; use is contraindicated in patients with a history of severe hypersensitivity to polyoxyethylated castor oil (Cremophor EL) or its derivatives. Medications for the treatment of reaction should be available for immediate use; reactions may also be managed with a reduction of infusion rate. Premedicate with an H$_1$- and H$_2$-antagonist 1 hour prior to infusion; patients who experience hypersensitivity (eg, bronchospasm, dyspnea, flushing, rash) should also be premedicated with a corticosteroid for all subsequent cycles if treatment is continued.

Dose-dependent myelosuppression, particularly neutropenia, may occur with mono- or combination therapy. Neutropenic fever and infection have been reported with use. The risk for neutropenia is increased with hepatic dysfunction, especially when used in combination with capecitabine. Severe neutropenia and/or thrombocytopenia may require dosage adjustment and/or treatment delay. Peripheral (sensory and motor) neuropathy occurs commonly; may require dose reductions, treatment delays or discontinuation. Usually occurs during the first 3 cycles. Use with caution in patients with preexisting neuropathy. Patients with diabetes may have an increased risk for severe peripheral neuropathy. Use with caution in patients with a history of cardiovascular disease; the incidence of MI, ventricular dysfunction, and supraventricular arrhythmias is higher when ixabepilone is used in combination with capecitabine (as compared to capecitabine alone). Consider discontinuing ixabepilone in patients who develop cardiac ischemia or impaired cardiac function.

Potentially significant drug-drug interactions may exist, requiring dose or frequency adjustment, additional monitoring, and/or selection of alternative therapy. Due to the ethanol content in the diluent, may cause cognitive impairment; patients must be cautioned about performing tasks which require mental alertness (eg, operating machinery or driving). Toxicities or serious adverse events with combination therapy may be increased in the elderly.

Adverse Reactions

Percentages reported with monotherapy:

>10%:

Central nervous system: Headache (11%)

Dermatologic: Alopecia (48%)

Gastrointestinal: Nausea (42%), vomiting (29%), mucositis/stomatitis (29%), diarrhea (22%), anorexia (19%), constipation (16%), abdominal pain (13%)

Hematologic: Leukopenia (grade 3: 36%; grade 4: 13%), neutropenia (grade 3: 31%; grade 4: 23%)

Neuromuscular & skeletal: Peripheral neuropathy (63%; grades 3/4: 14%; grade 3/4 median onset: cycle 4), sensory neuropathy (62%; grades 3/4: 14%), weakness (56%), myalgia/arthralgia (49%), musculoskeletal pain (20%)

1% to 10%:

Cardiovascular: Edema (9%), chest pain (5%)

Central nervous system: Fever (8%), pain (8%), dizziness (7%), insomnia (5%)

Dermatologic: Nail disorder (9%), rash (9%), palmar-plantar erythrodysesthesia/hand-and-foot syndrome (8%), pruritus (6%), skin exfoliation (2%), hyperpigmentation (2%)

Endocrine & metabolic: Hot flush (6%), dehydration (2%)

Gastrointestinal: Gastroesophageal reflux disease (6%), taste perversion (6%), weight loss (6%)

Hematologic: Anemia (grade 3: 6%; grade 4: 2%), neutropenic fever (3%; grade 3: 3%), thrombocytopenia (grade 3: 5%; grade 4: 2%)

Neuromuscular & skeletal: Motor neuropathy (10%; grade 3: 1%)

Ocular: Lacrimation increased (4%)

Respiratory: Dyspnea (9%), upper respiratory tract infection (6%), cough (2%)

Miscellaneous: Hypersensitivity (5%; grade 3: 1%), infection (5%)

Mono- and combination therapy: <1% (Limited to important or life-threatening): Alkaline phosphatase increased, angina, atrial flutter, autonomic neuropathy, cardiomyopathy, cerebral hemorrhage, coagulopathy, colitis, dysphagia, dysphonia, embolism, enterocolitis, erythema multiforme, gastrointestinal hemorrhage, gastroparesis, GGT increased, hemorrhage, hepatic failure (acute), hypokalemia, hyponatremia, hypotension, hypovolemia, hypovolemic shock, hypoxia, ileus, interstitial pneumonia, jaundice, left ventricular dysfunction, metabolic acidosis, MI, nephrolithiasis, neutropenic infection, orthostatic hypotension, pneumonia, pneumonitis, pulmonary edema (acute), radiation recall, renal failure, respiratory failure, sepsis, septic shock, supraventricular arrhythmia, syncope, thrombosis, transaminases increased, trismus, urinary tract infection, vasculitis

Drug Interactions

Metabolism/Transport Effects Substrate of CYP3A4 (major); **Note:** Assignment of Major/Minor substrate status based on clinically relevant drug interaction potential

Avoid Concomitant Use

Avoid concomitant use of Ixabepilone with any of the following: BCG (Intravesical); Conivaptan; Deferiprone; Dipyrone; Fusidic Acid (Systemic); Idelalisib; St Johns Wort

Increased Effect/Toxicity

Ixabepilone may increase the levels/effects of: CloZAPine; Deferiprone

The levels/effects of Ixabepilone may be increased by: Aprepitant; Conivaptan; CYP3A4 Inhibitors (Moderate); CYP3A4 Inhibitors (Strong); Dasatinib; Dipyrone; Fosaprepitant; Fusidic Acid (Systemic); Idelalisib; Ivacaftor; Luliconazole; Mifepristone; Netupitant; Osimertinib; Palbociclib; Simeprevir; Stiripentol

Decreased Effect

Ixabepilone may decrease the levels/effects of: BCG (Intravesical)

The levels/effects of Ixabepilone may be decreased by: Bosentan; CYP3A4 Inducers (Moderate); CYP3A4 Inducers (Strong); Dabrafenib; Deferasirox; Dexamethasone (Systemic); Enzalutamide; Mitotane; Osimertinib; Siltuximab; St Johns Wort; Tocilizumab

Food Interactions Grapefruit juice may increase plasma concentrations of ixabepilone. Management: Avoid grapefruit juice.

Preparation for Administration Hazardous agent; use appropriate precautions for handling and disposal (NIOSH 2014 [group 1]). Allow to reach room temperature for ~30 minutes prior to reconstitution. Diluent vial may contain a white precipitate which should dissolve upon reaching room temperature. **Reconstitute only with the provided diluent.** Dilute the 15 mg vial with 8 mL and the 45 mg vial with 23.5 mL (using provided diluent) to a concentration of 2 mg/mL (contains overfill). Gently swirl and invert vial until dissolved completely. Prior to administration, further dilute using a non-DEHP container (eg, glass, polypropylene or polyolefin), to a final concentration of 0.2 to 0.6 mg/mL in ~250 mL lactated Ringer's, adjusted sodium chloride 0.9% (pH adjusted prior to ixabepilone addition with 2 mEq sodium bicarbonate per 250 to 500 mL sodium chloride) or PLASMA-LYTE A Injection pH 7.4. Mix thoroughly.

◀ **Storage/Stability** Store intact vials under refrigeration at 2°C to 8°C (36°F to 46°F); protect from light. Reconstituted solution (in the vial) is stable for up to 1 hour at room temperature; infusion solution diluted in appropriate solution for infusion is stable for 6 hours at room temperature if a pH range of 6 to 9 is maintained (infusion must be completed within 6 hours).

Mechanism of Action Epothilone B analog; binds to the beta-tubulin subunit of the microtubule, stabilizing microtubular promoting tubulin polymerization and stabilizing microtubular function, thus arresting the cell cycle (at the G2/M phase) and inducing apoptosis. Activity in taxane-resistant cells has been demonstrated.

Pharmacodynamics/Kinetics

Distribution: >1,000 L

Protein binding: 67% to 77%

Metabolism: Extensively hepatic, via CYP3A4; >30 metabolites (inactive) formed

Half-life elimination: ~52 hours

Time to peak, plasma: At the end of infusion (3 hours)

Excretion: Feces (65%; 2% of the total dose as unchanged drug); urine (21%; 6% of the total dose as unchanged drug)

Dosing

Adult & Geriatric Note: Premedicate with an H_1-antagonist (eg, oral diphenhydramine 50 mg) and H_2-antagonist (eg, oral ranitidine 150 to 300 mg) ~1 hour prior to infusion. Patients with a history of hypersensitivity should also be premedicated with corticosteroids (dexamethasone 20 mg orally 1 hour before or IV 30 minutes before infusion). For dose calculation, body surface area (BSA) is capped at a maximum of 2.2 m^2.

Breast cancer (metastatic or locally advanced): IV: 40 mg/m^2/dose over 3 hours every 3 weeks (maximum dose: 88 mg) either as monotherapy or in combination with capecitabine

Dosage adjustment with concomitant strong CYP3A4 inhibitors/inducers:

CYP3A4 inhibitors: Avoid concomitant administration with strong CYP3A4 inhibitors (eg, itraconazole, ketoconazole, voriconazole, clarithromycin, telithromycin, nefazodone, atazanavir, delavirdine, indinavir, nelfinavir, ritonavir, saquinavir); if concomitant administration with a strong CYP3A4 inhibitor cannot be avoided, consider a dose reduction to 20 mg/m^2. When a strong CYP3A4 inhibitor is discontinued, allow ~1 week to elapse prior to adjusting ixabepilone dose upward to the indicated dose.

CYP3A4 inducers: Avoid concomitant administration with strong CYP3A4 inducers (eg, dexamethasone, phenytoin, carbamazepine, rifampin, phenobarbital); if concomitant administration with a strong CYP3A4 inducer cannot be avoided and after maintenance on the strong CYP3A4 inducer is established, consider adjusting the ixabepilone dose gradually up to 60 mg/m^2 (as a 4-hour infusion), with careful monitoring. If the strong CYP3A4 enzyme inducer is discontinued, reduce ixabepilone dose to the dose used prior to initiation of the CYP3A4 inducer.

Renal Impairment There are no dosage adjustments provided in the manufacturer's labeling, however, renal excretion is minimal. Pharmacokinetics (monotherapy) are not affected in patients with mild-to-moderate renal insufficiency (CrCl >30 mL/minute); monotherapy has not been studied in patients with serum creatinine >1.5 times ULN. Combination therapy with capecitabine has not been studied in patients with CrCl <50 mL/minute.

Hepatic Impairment

Ixabepilone monotherapy (initial cycle; adjust doses for subsequent cycles based on toxicity):

AST and ALT ≤2.5 times ULN and bilirubin ≤1 times ULN: No dosage adjustment necessary

AST and ALT >2.5 to ≤10 times ULN and bilirubin >1 to ≤1.5 times ULN: Reduce dose to 32 mg/m^2

AST and ALT ≤10 times ULN and bilirubin >1.5 to ≤3 times ULN: Reduce dose to 20 to 30 mg/m^2 (initiate treatment at 20 mg/m^2, may escalate up to a maximum of 30 mg/m^2 in subsequent cycles if tolerated)

AST or ALT >10 times ULN or bilirubin >3 times ULN: Use is not recommended

Combination therapy of ixabepilone with capecitabine:

AST and ALT ≤2.5 times ULN and bilirubin ≤1 times ULN: No dosage adjustment necessary

AST or ALT >2.5 times ULN or bilirubin >1 times ULN: Use is contraindicated

Obesity *ASCO Guidelines for appropriate chemotherapy dosing in obese adults with cancer:* In general, utilize patient's actual body weight (full weight) for calculation of body surface area- or weight-based dosing, particularly when the intent of therapy is curative; manage regimen-related toxicities in the same manner as for nonobese

patients; if a dose reduction is utilized due to toxicity, consider resumption of full weight-based dosing with subsequent cycles, especially if cause of toxicity (eg, hepatic or renal impairment) is resolved (Griggs, 2012). **Note:** According to the manufacturer, patients with a body surface area (BSA) >2.2 m^2 should be dosed based upon a maximum BSA of 2.2 m^2

Adjustment for Toxicity

Hematologic:

Neutrophils <500/mm^3 for ≥7 days: Reduce ixabepilone dose by 20%

Neutropenic fever: Reduce ixabepilone dose by 20%

Platelets <25,000/mm^3 (or <50,000/mm^3 with bleeding): Reduce ixabepilone dose by 20%

Nonhematologic:

Neuropathy:

Grade 2 (moderate) for ≥7 days: Reduce ixabepilone dose by 20%

Grade 3 (severe) for <7 days: Reduce ixabepilone dose by 20%

Grade 3 (severe or disabling) for ≥7 days: Discontinue ixabepilone treatment

Grade 3 toxicity (severe; other than neuropathy): Reduce ixabepilone dose by 20%

Grade 3 arthralgia/myalgia or fatigue (transient): Continue ixabepilone at current dose

Grade 3 hand-foot syndrome: Continue ixabepilone at current dose

Grade 4 toxicity (disabling): Discontinue ixabepilone treatment

Note: Adjust dosage at the start of a cycle are based on toxicities (hematologic and nonhematologic) from the previous cycle; delay new cycles until neutrophils have recovered to ≥1,500/mm^3, platelets have recovered to ≥100,000/mm^3 and nonhematologic toxicities have resolved or improved to at least grade 1. If toxicities persist despite initial dose reduction, reduce dose an additional 20%.

Capecitabine dosage adjustments for combination therapy with ixabepilone: Refer to Capecitabine monograph.

Dietary Considerations Avoid grapefruit juice (may increase plasma concentrations of ixabepilone).

Administration IV: Infuse over 3 hours. Use non-DEHP administration set (eg, polyethylene); filter with a 0.2 to 1.2 micron inline filter. Administration should be completed within 6 hours of preparation. If the dose is increased (above 40 mg/m^2) due to concomitant CYP3A4 inducer use, infuse over 4 hours.

Hazardous agent; use appropriate precautions for handling and disposal (NIOSH 2014 [group 1]).

Monitoring Parameters CBC with differential; hepatic function (ALT, AST, bilirubin); monitor for hypersensitivity, signs/symptoms of neuropathy

Dosage Forms Considerations

Diluent supplied in Ixempra Kit contains polyoxyethylated castor oil (Cremophor EL)

Dosage Forms Excipient information presented when available (limited, particularly for generics); consult specific product labeling.

Solution Reconstituted, Intravenous:

Ixempra Kit: 15 mg (1 ea); 45 mg (1 ea) [contains alcohol, usp, cremophor el]

Ixazomib (ix AZ oh mib)

Brand Names: US Ninlaro

Index Terms Ixazomib Citrate; MLN9708; Proteasome Inhibitor MLN9708

Pharmacologic Category Antineoplastic Agent, Proteasome Inhibitor

Use Multiple myeloma: Treatment of multiple myeloma (in combination with lenalidomide and dexamethasone) in patients who have received at least one prior therapy

Pregnancy Considerations Based on animal data and the mechanism of action, ixazomib is expected to cause fetal harm if used during pregnancy. Males and females of reproductive potential should use effective contraception during therapy and for 90 days after the last dose.

When used for the treatment of multiple myeloma, ixazomib is indicated to be used with lenalidomide, which is contraindicated for use during pregnancy (refer to Lenalidomide monograph for details).

Breast-Feeding Considerations It is not known if ixazomib is excreted into breast milk. Due to the potential for adverse events in a nursing infant, the manufacturer recommends that breast-feeding be discontinued during therapy.

Prescribing and Access Restrictions Available through specialty pharmacies and distributors. Further information may be obtained from the manufacturer, Takeda Oncology, at 1-800-390-5663 or at http://www.ninlarohcp.com.

Contraindications There are no contraindications listed in the manufacturer's labeling.

Warnings/Precautions Hazardous agent – use appropriate precautions for handling and disposal (meets NIOSH 2014 criteria).

Neutropenia and thrombocytopenia were reported commonly in clinical trials; grade 3 and 4 toxicity was also observed. Platelet nadirs generally occurred between days 14 to 21 of each cycle with a recovery to baseline by the start of the subsequent cycle. Monitor platelet counts at least monthly during treatment, and consider more frequent monitoring during the initial 3 cycles. May require therapy interruption, dosage reduction and/or platelet transfusions. Monitor complete blood counts (with differential) for neutropenia; therapy interruption or dosage modification may be necessary. Diarrhea, constipation, nausea, and vomiting have been reported. Antidiarrheals, antiemetics, and supportive care may be required to manage toxicity. Dosage adjustment is recommended for grade 3 or 4 symptoms.

Peripheral neuropathy (mostly grade 1 or 2) was observed. Peripheral sensory neuropathy was the most commonly reported symptom, while peripheral motor neuropathy was rarely seen. Monitor closely for signs/symptoms of neuropathy; may require dosage adjustment (of ixazomib and/or lenalidomide) or treatment discontinuation. Peripheral edema was reported in one-quarter of patients receiving ixazomib (generally grade 1 or 2 reactions). If peripheral edema occurs, evaluate for potential underlying causes and provide supportive care. If necessary, grade 3 or 4 symptoms may require dosage adjustment of dexamethasone and/or ixazomib. Rash was reported with ixazomib use; the majority of cases were grade 1 or 2 (grade 3 rash was observed in a small number of patients). Maculopapular and macular rashes were the most commonly reported cutaneous reactions. Monitor for dermatologic toxicity and manage with supportive care or with dosage modification of ixazomib and/or lenalidomide (for grade 2 or higher toxicity).

Drug-induced livery injury, hepatocellular injury, hepatic steatosis, hepatitis cholestatic and hepatotoxicity were reported rarely in clinical trials. Monitor liver enzymes regularly; may require dosage adjustment for grade 3 or 4 toxicity. Reduced initial doses are recommended for patients with moderate and severe hepatic impairment (exposure is increased). In patients with severe renal impairment or end stage renal disease requiring dialysis, reduced initial doses are recommended (exposure is increased). Concomitant lenalidomide may also require dose reduction. Potentially significant drug-drug interactions may exist, requiring dose or frequency adjustment, additional monitoring, and/or selection of alternative therapy.

Adverse Reactions Adverse reaction percentages reported as part of a combination regimen with lenalidomide and dexamethasone. Frequency not always defined.
>10%
Cardiovascular: Peripheral edema (25%)
Central nervous system: Peripheral neuropathy (28%; grade 3: 2%), peripheral sensory neuropathy (19%)
Dermatologic: Skin rash (19%; grade 3: 3%)
Gastrointestinal: Diarrhea (42%; grade 3: 6%), constipation (34%; grade 3: <1%), nausea (26%; grade 3: 2%), vomiting (22%; grade 3: 1%)
Hematologic & oncologic: Thrombocytopenia (78%; grades 3/4: 26%), neutropenia (67%; grades 3/4: 26%)
Neuromuscular & skeletal: Back pain (21%)
Ophthalmic: Eye disease (26%)
Respiratory: Upper respiratory tract infection (19%)
1% to 10%:
Hepatic: Hepatic insufficiency (6%)
Ophthalmic: Blurred vision (6%), conjunctivitis (6%), xerophthalmia (5%)
<1% (Limited to important or life-threatening): Cholestatic hepatitis, hepatocellular hepatitis, hepatotoxicity, liver steatosis, peripheral motor neuropathy, reversible posterior leukoencephalopathy syndrome, Stevens-Johnson syndrome, Sweet's syndrome, thrombotic thrombocytopenic purpura, transverse myelitis, tumor lysis syndrome

Drug Interactions
Metabolism/Transport Effects Substrate of CYP3A4 (major), P-glycoprotein; **Note:** Assignment of Major/Minor substrate status based on clinically relevant drug interaction potential

Avoid Concomitant Use
Avoid concomitant use of Ixazomib with any of the following: BCG (Intravesical); CYP3A4 Inducers (Strong); Deferiprone; Dipyrone; St Johns Wort
Increased Effect/Toxicity
Ixazomib may increase the levels/effects of: CloZAPine; Deferiprone

The levels/effects of Ixazomib may be increased by: Dipyrone; Osimertinib
Decreased Effect
Ixazomib may decrease the levels/effects of: BCG (Intravesical)

The levels/effects of Ixazomib may be decreased by: Bosentan; CYP3A4 Inducers (Moderate); CYP3A4 Inducers (Strong); Dabrafenib; Deferasirox; Osimertinib; Siltuximab; St Johns Wort; Tocilizumab
Storage/Stability Store at ≤30°C (86°F). Do not freeze. Store in original packaging until immediately prior to use.
Mechanism of Action Ixazomib reversibly inhibits proteasomes, enzyme complexes which regulate protein homeostasis within the cell. Specifically, it reversibly inhibits chymotrypsin-like activity of the beta 5 subunit of the 20S proteasome, leading to activation of signaling cascades, cell-cycle arrest, and apoptosis.
Pharmacodynamics/Kinetics
Absorption: High-fat meals decreased AUC by 28% and C_{max} by 69%
Distribution: 543 L
Protein binding: 99% to plasma proteins
Metabolism: Likely hepatic via multiple CYP enzymes and non-CYP proteins. At clinically relevant concentrations, no specific CYP isoform contributes predominantly to metabolism; possible CYP isoforms involved in metabolism include CYP3A4, 1A2, 2B6, 2C8, 2D6, 2C19, and 2C9.
Bioavailability: 58%
Half-life elimination: Terminal: 9.5 days
Time to peak: Median: 1 hour
Excretion: Urine (62%; <3.5% as unchanged drug); Feces (22%)

Dosing
Adult Note: ANC should be ≥1,000/mm³, platelets should be ≥75,000/mm³, and nonhematologic toxicities should be at baseline or ≤ grade 1 (per prescriber discretion) prior to initiating a new cycle of therapy.
Multiple myeloma: Oral: 4 mg once weekly on days 1, 8, and 15 of a 28-day treatment cycle (in combination with lenalidomide and dexamethasone); continue until disease progression or unacceptable toxicity (Moreau 2015).
Missed doses: If a dose is delayed or missed, administer only if the next scheduled dose is ≥72 hours away. Do not take a missed dose within 3 days of the next scheduled dose; do not double up on doses to make up for the missed dose. If vomiting occurs, do not repeat the dose; resume dosing at the next scheduled dose.

Renal Impairment
Preexisting renal impairment:
CrCl <30 mL/min: Reduce initial dose to 3 mg once weekly on days 1, 8, and 15 of a 28-day treatment cycle
ESRD requiring dialysis: Reduce initial dose to 3 mg once weekly on days 1, 8, and 15 of a 28-day treatment cycle; ixazomib is not dialyzable and may be administered without regarding to dialysis timing.
Renal toxicity during treatment: Grade 3 or 4 toxicity: Withhold ixazomib until recovery to baseline or improvement to ≤ grade 1 (at prescriber's discretion). If attributable to ixazomib, resume ixazomib at the next lower dose.

Hepatic Impairment
Preexisting hepatic impairment:
Mild impairment (total bilirubin ≤ ULN and AST > ULN or total bilirubin >1 to 1.5 times ULN and any AST): No dosage adjustment is necessary.
Moderate (total bilirubin >1.5 to 3 times ULN) or severe (total bilirubin >3 times ULN) impairment: Reduce initial dose to 3 mg once weekly on days 1, 8, and 15 of a 28-day treatment cycle
Hepatotoxicity during treatment: Grade 3 or 4 toxicity: Withhold ixazomib until recovery to baseline or improvement to ≤ grade 1 (at prescriber's discretion). If attributable to ixazomib, resume ixazomib at the next lower dose.

Adjustment for Toxicity Also refer to Lenalidomide monograph for dosage modification recommendations. Recommended ixazomib dosage reductions for toxicity:
Initial starting dose: 4 mg
First dose reduction: 3 mg
Second dose reduction: 2.3 mg
If unable to tolerate 2.3 mg, discontinue ixazomib

Hematologic toxicity:

Neutropenia: ANC <500/mm^3: Withhold ixazomib and lenalidomide until ANC is ≥500/mm^3. Consider adding growth-colony stimulating factor (G-CSF). Upon recovery, resume lenalidomide at the next lower dose and resume ixazomib at the dose used prior to therapy interruption. If neutropenia recurs, interrupt ixazomib and lenalidomide until ANC is ≥500/mm^3. Following recovery, resume ixazomib at the next lower dose and resume lenalidomide at the dose used prior to therapy interruption. For additional occurrences, alternate dose modification of lenalidomide and ixazomib.

Thrombocytopenia: Platelet count <30,000/mm^3: Withhold ixazomib and lenalidomide until platelet count is ≥30,000/mm^3. Upon recovery, resume lenalidomide at the next lower dose and resume ixazomib at the dose used prior to therapy interruption. If thrombocytopenia to ≤30,000/mm^3 recurs, interrupt ixazomib and lenalidomide until platelets are ≥30,000/mm^3. Following recovery, resume ixazomib at the next lower dose and resume lenalidomide at the dose used prior to therapy interruption. For additional occurrences, alternate dose modification of lenalidomide and ixazomib.

Nonhematologic toxicity:

Dermatologic toxicity:

Grade 2 or 3 rash: Withhold lenalidomide until rash recovers to ≤ grade 1. Upon recovery, resume lenalidomide at the next lower dose and resume ixazomib at the dose used prior to therapy interruption. If grade 2 or 3 rash recurs, interrupt ixazomib and lenalidomide until rash recovers to ≤ grade 1. Following recovery, resume ixazomib at the next lower dose and resume lenalidomide at the dose used prior to therapy interruption. For additional occurrences, alternate dose modification of lenalidomide and ixazomib.

Grade 4 rash: Discontinue treatment regimen.

Peripheral neuropathy:

Grade 1 (with pain) or grade 2: Interrupt ixazomib until peripheral neuropathy recovers to ≤ grade 1 without pain or to baseline. Upon recovery, resume ixazomib at the dose used prior to therapy interruption.

Grade 2 (with pain) or grade 3: Withhold ixazomib until recovery to baseline or improvement to ≤ grade 1 (at prescriber's discretion). Following recovery, resume ixazomib at the next lower dose.

Grade 4: Discontinue treatment regimen.

Other toxicities (nonhematologic): Grade 3 or 4 toxicity: Withhold ixazomib until recovery to baseline or improvement to ≤ grade 1 (at prescriber's discretion). If attributable to ixazomib, resume ixazomib at the next lower dose.

Administration

Oral: Administer on the same day of the week and at approximately the same time on that day; take at least 1 hour before or at least 2 hours after eating. Swallow capsule whole; do not crush, chew, or open the capsule. Hazardous agent; use appropriate precautions for handling and disposal (meets NIOSH 2014 criteria). NIOSH recommends single gloving for administration of intact capsules (NIOSH 2014). Avoid skin or eye exposure to capsule contents. If skin contact occurs, wash thoroughly with soap and water; if eye contact occurs, flush thoroughly with water.

Monitoring Parameters Platelet counts at least monthly during treatment (consider more frequent monitoring during the first 3 cycles), complete blood count (with differential) as clinically necessary, renal and liver function tests; signs/symptoms of gastrointestinal and dermatologic toxicity; signs/symptoms of peripheral neuropathy and peripheral edema.

Dosage Forms Excipient information presented when available (limited, particularly for generics); consult specific product labeling.

Capsule, Oral:

Ninlaro: 2.3 mg, 3 mg, 4 mg

Japanese Encephalitis Virus Vaccine (Inactivated)

(jap a NEESE en sef a LYE tis VYE rus vak SEEN, in ak ti VAY ted)

Brand Names: US Ixiaro; Je-Vax [DSC]
Brand Names: Canada Ixiaro
Index Terms IC51; JE-VC (Ixiaro)
Pharmacologic Category Vaccine, Inactivated (Viral)
Additional Appendix Information
Immunization Administration Recommendations *on page 1974*

Immunization Schedules *on page 1979*

Use Japanese encephalitis vaccination: For active immunization against Japanese encephalitis (JE) for persons 2 months of age and older

The Advisory Committee on Immunization Practices (ACIP) recommends vaccination for (CDC, 2010; CDC, 2013):
- Persons spending ≥1 month in endemic areas during transmission season
- Research laboratory workers who may be exposed to the Japanese encephalitis virus
Vaccination should also be considered for the following:
• Travelers to areas with an ongoing outbreak
• Travelers spending <30 days in endemic areas during the transmission season and planning to go outside of urban areas and have an increased risk of exposure. For example, high-risk activities include extensive outdoor activity in rural areas especially at night; extensive outdoor activities such as camping, hiking, etc; staying in accommodations without air conditioning, screens or bed nets.
• Travelers to endemic areas who are unsure of specific destination, activities, or duration of travel
Japanese encephalitis vaccine is not recommended for short-term travelers whose visit will be restricted to urban areas or periods outside of the well-defined JE virus transmission season.

Medication Guide Available Yes
Dosing
Adult & Geriatric
U.S. recommended primary immunization schedule:
Adults ≥17 years: IM: 0.5 mL/dose; a total of 2 doses given on days 0 and 28. Series should be completed at least 1 week prior to potential exposure.
Booster dose: Booster dose may be given prior to potential re-exposure if the primary series was completed >1 year previously.
Note: If the second dose is missed, limited data from one clinical trial in adults demonstrate a 99% seroconversion rate when the second dose was administered 11 months after the initial dose.
Pediatric U.S. recommended primary immunization schedule:
Children 2 months to <3 years: IM: 0.25 mL/dose; a total of 2 doses given on days 0 and 28. Series should be completed at least 1 week prior to potential exposure.

Children ≥3 years and Adolescent: Refer to adult dosing.
Note: The safety of booster doses in children and adolescents <17 years has not been established.
Renal Impairment No dosage adjustment provided in manufacturer's labeling.
Hepatic Impairment No dosage adjustment provided in manufacturer's labeling.
Additional Information Complete prescribing information should be consulted for additional detail.
Dosage Forms Excipient information presented when available (limited, particularly for generics); consult specific product labeling. [DSC] = Discontinued product
Solution Reconstituted, Subcutaneous:
Je-Vax: (1 ea [DSC]) [contains polysorbate 80, thimerosal]
Suspension, Intramuscular:
Ixiaro: (0.5 mL) [latex free; contains albumin bovine, protamine sulfate, sodium metabisulfite]

Ketamine (KEET a meen)

Brand Names: US Ketalar

Brand Names: Canada Ketalar; Ketamine Hydrochloride Injection, USP

Index Terms Ketamine Hydrochloride

Pharmacologic Category General Anesthetic

Use Induction and maintenance of general anesthesia

Pregnancy Considerations Adverse events have not been observed in animal reproduction studies. Ketamine crosses the placenta and can be detected in fetal tissue. Ketamine produces dose dependent increases in uterine contractions; effects may vary by trimester. The plasma clearance of ketamine is reduced during pregnancy. Dose related neonatal depression and decreased APGAR scores have been reported with large doses administered at delivery (Ghoneim 1977; Little 1972; White 1982).

Breast-Feeding Considerations It is not known if ketamine is excreted in breast milk.

Contraindications

Hypersensitivity to ketamine or any component of the formulation; conditions in which an increase in blood pressure would be hazardous

Additional absolute contraindications according to the American College of Emergency Physicians (ACEP [Green 2011]): Infants <3 months of age; known or suspected schizophrenia (even if currently stable or controlled with medications)

Warnings/Precautions The American College of Emergency Physicians considers the use of ketamine in patients with known or suspected schizophrenia (even if currently stable or controlled with medications) an absolute contraindication and relatively contraindicated for major procedures involving the posterior pharynx (eg, endoscopy), for patients with an active pulmonary infection or disease (including upper respiratory disease or asthma), history of airway instability, tracheal surgery, or tracheal stenosis, in patients with CNS masses, CNS abnormalities, or hydrocephalus, glaucoma, acute globe injury, porphyria, thyroid disorder, or receiving a thyroid medication (ACEP [Green 2011]). Use with caution in patients with coronary artery disease, catecholamine depletion, hypertension, and tachycardia. Cardiac function should be continuously monitored in patients with increased blood pressure or cardiac decompensation. Ketamine increases blood pressure, heart rate, and cardiac output thereby increasing myocardial oxygen demand. The use of concurrent benzodiazepine, inhaled anesthetics, and propofol or administration of ketamine as a continuous infusion may reduce these cardiovascular effects (Miller 2010). The American College of Emergency Physicians recommends avoidance in patients who are already hypertensive and in older adults with risk factors for coronary artery disease (ACEP [Green 2011]). Rapid IV administration or overdose may cause respiratory depression, apnea, and enhanced pressor response. Resuscitative equipment should be available during use.

Use with caution in patients with increased intraocular pressure and avoid use in patients with an open eye injury or other ophthalmologic disorder where an increase in intraocular pressure would prove to be detrimental; ketamine may further increase intraocular pressure (Cunningham 1986; Miller 2010; Nagdeve 2006). Postanesthetic emergence reactions which can manifest as vivid dreams, hallucinations, and/or frank delirium occur; these reactions are less common in patients <15 years of age and >65 years and when given intramuscularly. Emergence reactions, confusion, or irrational behavior may occur up to 24 hours postoperatively and may be reduced by pretreatment with a benzodiazepine and the use of ketamine at the lower end of the dosing range. Avoid use in patients with schizophrenia (Lahti 1995; Malhotra 1997). Use with caution in patients with CSF pressure elevation, the chronic alcoholic or acutely alcohol-intoxicated. May cause dependence (withdrawal symptoms on discontinuation) and tolerance with prolonged use. May cause CNS depression, which may impair physical or mental abilities; patients must be cautioned about performing tasks which require mental alertness (eg, operating machinery or driving). When used for outpatient surgery, the patient be accompanied by a responsible adult. Should be administered under the supervision of a physician experienced in administering general anesthetics.

Adverse Reactions Frequency not always defined.

Cardiovascular: Bradycardia, cardiac arrhythmia, hypotension, increased blood pressure, increased pulse

Central nervous system: Prolonged emergence from anesthesia (~12%; includes confusion, delirium, dreamlike state, excitement, hallucinations, irrational behavior, vivid imagery), drug dependence, hypertonia (tonic-clonic movements sometimes resembling seizures), increased cerebrospinal fluid pressure

Dermatologic: Erythema (transient), morbilliform rash (transient), rash at injection site

Endocrine & metabolic: Central diabetes insipidus (Hatab 2014)

Gastrointestinal: Anorexia, nausea, sialorrhea (Hatab 2014), vomiting

Genitourinary (adverse reactions can be severe in patients with a history of chronic ketamine use/abuse): Cystitis, irritable bladder, urethritis, urinary tract irritation

Hypersensitivity: Anaphylaxis

Local: Pain at injection site

Neuromuscular & skeletal: Laryngospasm

Ophthalmic: Diplopia, increased intraocular pressure, nystagmus

Respiratory: Airway obstruction, apnea, respiratory depression

Drug Interactions

Metabolism/Transport Effects Substrate of CYP2B6 (major), CYP2C9 (major), CYP3A4 (major); **Note:** Assignment of Major/Minor substrate status based on clinically relevant drug interaction potential

Avoid Concomitant Use

Avoid concomitant use of Ketamine with any of the following: Azelastine (Nasal); Conivaptan; Fusidic Acid (Systemic); Idelalisib; Orphenadrine; Paraldehyde; Thalidomide

Increased Effect/Toxicity

Ketamine may increase the levels/effects of: Alcohol (Ethyl); Azelastine (Nasal); Buprenorphine; CNS Depressants; Hydrocodone; Memantine; Methotrimeprazine; Metyrosine; Mirtazapine; Orphenadrine; Paraldehyde; Pramipexole; ROPINIRole; Rotigotine; Selective Serotonin Reuptake Inhibitors; Suvorexant; Thalidomide; Thiopental; Zolpidem

The levels/effects of Ketamine may be increased by: Brimonidine (Topical); Cannabis; Conivaptan; CYP2B6 Inhibitors (Moderate); CYP2C9 Inhibitors (Moderate); CYP2C9 Inhibitors (Strong); CYP3A4 Inhibitors (Moderate); CYP3A4 Inhibitors (Strong); Dasatinib; Doxylamine; Dronabinol; Droperidol; Fosaprepitant; Fusidic Acid (Systemic); HydrOXYzine; Idelalisib; Ivacaftor; Kava Kava; Luliconazole; Lumacaftor; Magnesium Sulfate; Methotrimeprazine; Mifepristone; Minocycline; Nabilone; Netupitant; Osimertinib; Palbociclib; Perampanel; Quazepam; Rufinamide; Simeprevir; Sodium Oxybate; Stiripentol; Tapentadol; Tetrahydrocannabinol

Decreased Effect

The levels/effects of Ketamine may be decreased by: CYP2C9 Inducers (Strong); Dabrafenib; Enzalutamide; Lumacaftor; Osimertinib

Preparation for Administration The 50 mg/mL and 100 mg/mL vials may be further diluted in D$_5$W or NS to prepare a maintenance infusion with a final concentration of 1 mg/mL (or 2 mg/mL in patients with fluid restrictions). The 10 mg/mL vials are not recommended to be further diluted. Do not mix with barbiturates or diazepam (precipitation may occur). **Note:** The 100 mg/mL concentration should not be administered IV unless properly diluted with an equal volume of SWFI, NS, or D$_5$W.

Storage/Stability Store at 20°C to 25°C (68°F to 77°F). Protect from light.

Mechanism of Action Produces a cataleptic-like state in which the patient is dissociated from the surrounding environment by direct action on the cortex and limbic system. Ketamine is a noncompetitive NMDA receptor antagonist that blocks glutamate. Low (subanesthetic) doses produce analgesia, and modulate central sensitization, hyperalgesia and opioid tolerance. Reduces polysynaptic spinal reflexes.

Pharmacodynamics/Kinetics

Onset of action:
IV: Anesthetic effect: 30 seconds
IM: Anesthetic effect: 3-4 minutes

Duration: Anesthetic effect: IV: 5-10 minutes; IM: 12-25 minutes

Distribution: V$_d$: 3 L/kg

Metabolism: Hepatic via hydroxylation and N-demethylation; the metabolite norketamine is 33% as potent as parent compound; greater conversion to norketamine occurs after oral administration as compared to parenteral administration

Bioavailability: Oral: 16%; Intranasal: 50%

Half-life elimination: Alpha: 10-15 minutes; Beta: 2.5 hours

Excretion: Primarily urine

Dosing

Adult & Geriatric May be used in combination with anticholinergic agents to decrease hypersalivation. **Note:** Titrate dose for desired effect.

Anesthesia:

Induction of anesthesia:

Manufacturer's labeling:
IM: 6.5 to 13 mg/kg
IV: 1 to 4.5 mg/kg

Alternate recommendations (off-label dosing): **Note:** lower doses may be used if adjuvant drugs (eg, midazolam) are administered (Miller 2010)
IM: 4 to 10 mg/kg (Green 1990; Miller 2010; White 1982)
IV: 0.5 to 2 mg/kg (Miller 2010; White 1982)

Maintenance of anesthesia: May administer supplemental doses of one-half to the full induction dose or a continuous infusion of 0.1 to 0.5 mg/minute (per manufacturer). **Note:** To maintain an adequate concentration of ketamine for maintenance of anesthesia, 1 to 2 mg/minute has been recommended (White 1982); doses in the range of 15 to 90 mcg/kg/minute (~1 to 6 mg/minute in a 70-kg patient) have also been suggested (Miller 2010). Concurrent use of nitrous oxide reduces ketamine requirements. Recent laboratory/clinical studies support the use of low-dose ketamine to improve postoperative analgesia/outcome (Adam 2005; Menigaux 2000).

Sedation/analgesia (off-label use):

Procedural (operative or nonoperative):

IM: 2 to 4 mg/kg (Miller 2010; White 1982); may follow with a continuous infusion if necessary. According to the American College of Emergency Physicians, the IV route is preferred; however if IV route unavailable, may administer 4 to 5 mg/kg as a single dose; may give a repeat dose (range: 2 to 4 mg/kg) if sedation inadequate after 5 to 10 minutes or if additional doses are required (ACEP [Green 2011]).

IV: 0.2 to 0.8 mg/kg (Miller 2010; Remérand 2009; White 1982; Zakine 2008); a maximum bolus dose of 50 mg was used in one study (Remérand 2009). May follow with a continuous infusion if necessary.

According to the American College of Emergency Physicians, may administer 1 mg/kg over 30 to 60 seconds for procedural sedation. If initial sedation inadequate or repeated doses are necessary to accomplish a longer procedure, may administer incremental doses of 0.5 mg/kg every 5 to 15 minutes as needed (ACEP [Green 2011])

Continuous IV infusion: 2 to 7 mcg/kg/minute (Hocking 2003; Remérand 2009; Zakine 2008)

Critically ill patients (as an adjunct to an opioid analgesic for non-neuropathic pain): IV: Initial: 0.1 to 0.5 mg/kg bolus; followed by 0.83 to 6.7 mcg/kg/minute (equivalent to 0.05 to 0.4 **mg/kg/hour**) (SCCM [Barr 2013])

Pediatric

Anesthesia: Adolescents ≥16 years: Refer to adult dosing.

Sedation/analgesia (off-label use): Adolescents ≥16 years: Refer to adult dosing.

Sedation (procedural) (off-label use): Children: American College of Emergency Physicians recommendations:

IM: 4 to 5 mg/kg as a single dose; may give a repeat dose (range: 2 to 4 mg/kg) if sedation inadequate after 5 to 10 minutes or if additional doses are required (ACEP [Green 2011]).

IV: 1.5 to 2 mg/kg over 30 to 60 seconds. If initial sedation inadequate or repeated doses are necessary to accomplish a longer procedure, may administer incremental doses of 0.5 to 1 mg/kg every 5 to 10 minutes as needed (ACEP [Green 2011]).

Renal Impairment There are no dosage adjustments provided in the manufacturer's labeling.

Hepatic Impairment There are no dosage adjustments provided in the manufacturer's labeling.

Administration

Oral: Mix the appropriate dose (using the 100 mg/mL injectable solution) in cola or other beverage; administer immediately after preparation.

IV: According to the manufacturer, may administer bolus/induction doses over 1 minute or at a rate of 0.5 mg/kg/minute; more rapid administration may result in respiratory depression and enhanced pressor response. Some experts suggest administration over 2 to 3 minutes (Miller 2010).

Monitoring Parameters Heart rate, blood pressure, respiratory rate, transcutaneous O$_2$ saturation, emergence reactions; cardiac function should be continuously monitored in patients with increased blood pressure or cardiac decompensation

Test Interactions May interfere with urine detection of phencyclidine (false-positive).

Additional Information May produce emergence psychosis including auditory and visual hallucinations, restlessness, disorientation, vivid dreams, and irrational behavior in ~12% of patients; pretreatment with a benzodiazepine reduces incidence of psychosis by >50%. Spontaneous involuntary movements, nystagmus, hypertonus, and vocalizations are also common.

The analgesia outlasts the general anesthetic component. Bronchodilation is beneficial in asthmatic or COPD patients. Laryngeal reflexes may remain intact or may be obtunded. The direct myocardial depressant action of ketamine can be seen in stressed, catecholamine-deficient patients. Ketamine increases cerebral metabolism and cerebral blood flow while producing a noncompetitive block of the glutaminergic postsynaptic NMDA receptor. It lowers seizure threshold and stimulates salivary secretions (atropine/scopolamine treatment is recommended).

Dosage Forms Excipient information presented when available (limited, particularly for generics); consult specific product labeling.

Solution, Injection:
Ketalar: 10 mg/mL (20 mL); 50 mg/mL (10 mL); 100 mg/mL (5 mL)
Generic: 10 mg/mL (20 mL); 50 mg/mL (10 mL); 100 mg/mL (5 mL, 10 mL)

Controlled Substance C-III

◆ Ketamine Hydrochloride *see* Ketamine *on page 1012*
◆ Ketamine Hydrochloride Injection, USP (Can) *see* Ketamine *on page 1012*
◆ Ketek *see* Telithromycin *on page 1746*

Ketoconazole (Systemic) (kee toe KOE na zole)

Brand Names: Canada Apo-Ketoconazole; Teva-Ketoconazole

Index Terms Nizoral

Pharmacologic Category Antifungal Agent, Imidazole Derivative; Antifungal Agent, Oral

Use Fungal infections:

U.S. labeling: Systemic fungal infections: Treatment of susceptible fungal infections, including blastomycosis, histoplasmosis, paracoccidioidomycosis, coccidioidomycosis, and chromomycosis in patients who have failed or who are intolerant to other antifungal therapies

Canadian labeling: Treatment of serious or life-threatening systemic fungal infections (eg, systemic candidiasis, chronic mucocutaneous candidiasis, coccidioidomycosis, paracoccidioidomycosis, histoplasmosis, and chromomycosis) where alternate therapy is inappropriate or ineffective; may be considered for severe dermatophytoses unresponsive to other therapy

Medication Guide Available Yes

Dosing

Adult & Geriatric

Fungal infections: Oral: 200-400 mg once daily

Therapy duration: Continue therapy until active fungal infection has resolved (based on clinical and laboratory parameters); some infections may require at least 6 months of therapy.

Prostate cancer, advanced (off-label use): Oral: 400 mg 3 times daily (in combination with oral hydrocortisone) until disease progression (Ryan, 2007; Small, 2004)

Pediatric Fungal infections: Children ≥2 years: Oral: 3.3-6.6 mg/kg once daily

Therapy duration: Continue therapy until active fungal infection has resolved (based on clinical and laboratory parameters); some infections may require at least 6 months of therapy.

Renal Impairment No dosage adjustment provided in manufacturer's labeling. Some clinicians suggest that no dosage adjustment is necessary in mild-to-severe impairment (Aronoff, 2007).

Hemodialysis: Not dialyzable

Hepatic Impairment No dosage adjustment provided in manufacturer's labeling; use with caution due to risks of hepatotoxicity.

Hepatotoxicity during treatment:

U.S. labeling: If ALT >ULN or 30% above baseline (or if patient is symptomatic), interrupt therapy and obtain full hepatic function panel. Upon normalization of liver function, may consider resuming therapy if benefit outweighs risk (hepatotoxicity has been reported on rechallenge).

Canadian labeling: Discontinue therapy for liver function tests >3 times ULN or if abnormalities persist, worsen, or are associated with hepatotoxicity symptoms.

Additional Information Complete prescribing information should be consulted for additional detail.

Dosage Forms Excipient information presented when available (limited, particularly for generics); consult specific product labeling.

Tablet, Oral:

Generic: 200 mg

Ketoconazole (Topical) (kee toe KOE na zole)

Brand Names: US Extina; Ketodan; Nizoral; Nizoral A-D [OTC]; Xolegel

Brand Names: Canada Ketoderm; Nizoral

Pharmacologic Category Antifungal Agent, Imidazole Derivative; Antifungal Agent, Topical

Use

Cream: Treatment of tinea corporis, tinea cruris, tinea versicolor, cutaneous candidiasis, seborrheic dermatitis

Foam, gel: Treatment of seborrheic dermatitis

Shampoo: Treatment of dandruff, seborrheic dermatitis, tinea versicolor

Dosing

Adult & Geriatric

Fungal infections: *Topical:*

Cream: Tinea infections: Rub gently into the affected area once daily. Duration of treatment: Tinea corporis, cruris: 2 weeks; tinea pedis: 6 weeks

Shampoo (ketoconazole 2%): Tinea versicolor: Apply to damp skin, lather, leave on 5 minutes, and rinse (one application should be sufficient)

Seborrheic dermatitis: *Topical:*

Cream: Rub gently into the affected area twice daily for 4 weeks or until clinical response is noted.

Foam: Apply to affected area twice daily for 4 weeks

Gel: Rub gently into the affected area once daily for 2 weeks.

Shampoo (ketoconazole 1%): Apply twice weekly for up to 8 weeks with at least 3 days between each shampoo

Susceptible fungal infections in the oral cavity (candidiasis, oral thrush, and chronic mucocutaneous candidiasis) (off-label use): *Topical:* Cream: Apply locally as directed with a thin coat to inner surface of denture and affected areas after meals

Pediatric Seborrheic dermatitis: *Topical (cream/foam/gel, shampoo):* Children ≥12 years: Refer to adult dosing.

Additional Information Complete prescribing information should be consulted for additional detail.

Dosage Forms Excipient information presented when available (limited, particularly for generics); consult specific product labeling. [DSC] = Discontinued product

Cream, External:

Generic: 2% (15 g, 30 g, 60 g)

Foam, External:

Extina: 2% (50 g, 100 g) [contains alcohol, usp, cetyl alcohol, propylene glycol]

Ketodan: 2% (100 g) [contains alcohol, usp, cetyl alcohol, propylene glycol]

Generic: 2% (50 g, 100 g [DSC])

Gel, External:

Xolegel: 2% (45 g) [contains alcohol, usp, fd&c yellow #10 (quinoline yellow), fd&c yellow #6 (sunset yellow), propylene glycol]

Kit, External:

Ketodan: 2% [contains cetyl alcohol, edetate disodium, propylene glycol]

Shampoo, External:

Nizoral: 2% (120 mL) [contains fd&c red #40]

Nizoral A-D: 1% (125 mL, 200 mL)

Generic: 2% (120 mL)

◆ Ketodan *see* Ketoconazole (Topical) *on page 1014*

◆ Ketoderm (Can) *see* Ketoconazole (Topical) *on page 1014*

Ketoprofen (kee toe PROE fen)

Brand Names: US Active-Ketoprofen

Brand Names: Canada Ketoprofen SR; Ketoprofen-E; PMS-Ketoprofen; PMS-Ketoprofen-E

Index Terms Orudis KT; Oruvail

Pharmacologic Category Nonsteroidal Anti-inflammatory Drug (NSAID), Oral

Use

Osteoarthritis: Treatment of osteoarthritis

Pain: Treatment of mild to moderate pain (regular release only)

Primary dysmenorrhea: Treatment of primary dysmenorrhea (regular release only)

Rheumatoid arthritis: Treatment of rheumatoid arthritis

Canadian labeling: Additional use (not in U.S. labeling): Treatment of ankylosing spondylitis

Medication Guide Available Yes

Dosing

Adult Note: The enteric coated tablet and extended release formulations are not recommended for the treatment of acute pain. Lower doses should be considered in small or debilitated patients.

Oral:

Rheumatoid arthritis or osteoarthritis:

Regular release: U.S. labeling: 50 mg 4 times daily **or** 75 mg 3 times daily; up to a maximum of 300 mg daily

Regular release or enteric coated: Canadian labeling: 50 mg 3 or 4 times daily; up to 200 mg daily; twice daily regimen (eg, 100 mg twice daily) may be considered after maintenance dose is established although some patients respond more favorably to more frequent dosing. For severe rheumatic activity or an inadequate response to lower dosages, may consider dose increase up to a maximum 300 mg daily.

Extended release: 200 mg once daily

Dysmenorrhea, mild to moderate pain: Regular release: 25-50 mg every 6-8 hours up to a maximum of 300 mg daily

Rectal suppository [Canadian product]: **Ankylosing spondylitis, osteoarthritis, or rheumatoid arthritis:** Insert one suppository rectally in the morning and evening (twice daily) or at bedtime (once daily). May supplement with divided oral dosing up to a combined rectal/oral maximum of 200 mg daily; for severe rheumatic activity or an inadequate response to lower dosages, a combined rectal/oral dose up to 300 mg daily may be considered. Patients should be maintained at the lowest effective dose.

Geriatric

U.S. labeling: Oral: Manufacturer labeling recommends that the initial dose should be decreased in patients >75 years but does not provide specific dosing recommendations; use caution when dosage changes are made.

Canadian labeling: Oral: Reduce initial dose by 33% to 50%; Rectal: Manufacturer labeling recommends that the initial dose should be decreased but does not provide specific dosing recommendation.

Renal Impairment In general, NSAIDs are not recommended for use in patients with advanced renal disease, but the manufacturer of ketoprofen does provide some guidelines for adjustment in renal dysfunction:

U.S. labeling:

Mild impairment: Maximum dose: 150 mg daily

Severe impairment: GFR <25 mL/minute/1.73 m^2: Maximum dose: 100 mg daily

Canadian labeling: Reduce initial dose by 33% to 50%.

Hepatic Impairment Hepatic impairment and serum albumin <3.5 g/dL: Maximum initial dose: 100 mg daily

Additional Information Complete prescribing information should be consulted for additional detail.

Dosage Forms Considerations Active-Ketoprofen cream is compounded from a kit. Refer to manufacturer's labeling for compounding instructions.

Dosage Forms Excipient information presented when available (limited, particularly for generics); consult specific product labeling.

Capsule, Oral:

Generic: 50 mg, 75 mg

Capsule Extended Release 24 Hour, Oral:

Generic: 200 mg

Cream, External:

Active-Ketoprofen: 5% (120 g) [contains chlorocresol (chloro-m-cresol)]

Dosage Forms: Canada Note: Refer also to Dosage Forms. Extended release capsule and external cream are not available in Canada.

Excipient information presented when available (limited, particularly for generics); consult specific product labeling.

Enteric coated tablet, Oral: 50 mg, 100 mg

Extended release tablet, Oral: 200 mg

Suppository, Rectal: 50 mg, 100 mg

◆ Ketoprofen-E (Can) *see* Ketoprofen *on page 1014*
◆ Ketoprofen SR (Can) *see* Ketoprofen *on page 1014*

Ketorolac (Systemic) (KEE toe role ak)

Brand Names: Canada Apo-Ketorolac Injectable®; Apo-Ketorolac®; Ketorolac Tromethamine Injection, USP; Novo-Ketorolac; Toradol®; Toradol® IM

Index Terms Ketorolac Tromethamine; Toradol

Pharmacologic Category Nonsteroidal Anti-inflammatory Drug (NSAID), Oral; Nonsteroidal Anti-inflammatory Drug (NSAID), Parenteral

Use Short-term (≤5 days) management of moderate-to-severe acute pain requiring analgesia at the opioid level

Pregnancy Considerations Adverse events were observed in some animal reproduction studies. Ketorolac crosses the placenta (Walker, 1988). NSAID exposure during the first trimester is not strongly associated with congenital malformations; however, cardiovascular anomalies and cleft palate have been observed following NSAID exposure in some studies (Ericson, 2001). The use of an NSAID close to conception may be associated with an increased risk of miscarriage (Li, 2003; Nielsen, 2001). Nonteratogenic effects have been observed following NSAID administration during the third trimester, including myocardial degenerative changes, prenatal constriction of the ductus arteriosus, fetal tricuspid regurgitation, failure of the ductus arteriosus to close postnatally; renal dysfunction or failure, oligohydramnios; gastrointestinal bleeding or perforation, increased risk of necrotizing enterocolitis; intracranial bleeding (including intraventricular hemorrhage), platelet dysfunction with resultant bleeding; pulmonary hypertension (Van den Veyver, 1993). Because they may cause premature closure of the ductus arteriosus, use of NSAIDs late in pregnancy should be avoided (use after 31 or 32 weeks gestation is not recommended by some clinicians) (Moise, 1993). **[U.S. Boxed Warning]: Ketorolac is contraindicated during labor and delivery (may inhibit uterine contractions and adversely affect fetal circulation).** The chronic use of NSAIDs in women of reproductive age may be associated with infertility that is reversible upon discontinuation of the medication.

Breast-Feeding Considerations Low concentrations of ketorolac are found in breast milk (milk concentrations were <1% of the weight-adjusted maternal dose in one study [Wischnik, 1989]). The manufacturer recommends that caution be used if administered to nursing women.

Medication Guide Available Yes

Contraindications Hypersensitivity to ketorolac, aspirin, other NSAIDs, or any component of the formulation; active or history of peptic ulcer disease; recent or history of GI bleeding or perforation; patients with advanced renal disease or risk of renal failure (due to volume depletion); prophylaxis before major surgery; suspected or confirmed cerebrovascular bleeding; hemorrhagic diathesis, incomplete hemostasis, or high risk of bleeding; concurrent use with ASA, other NSAIDs, probenecid or pentoxifylline; epidural or intrathecal administration; perioperative pain in the setting of coronary artery bypass graft (CABG) surgery; labor and delivery

Warnings/Precautions [U.S. Boxed Warning]: Inhibits platelet function; contraindicated in patients with cerebrovascular bleeding (suspected or confirmed), hemorrhagic diathesis, incomplete hemostasis and patients at high risk for bleeding. Effects on platelet adhesion and aggregation may prolong bleeding time. Anemia may occur; patients on long-term NSAID therapy should be monitored for anemia. Rarely, NSAID use has been associated with potentially severe blood dyscrasias (eg, agranulocytosis, thrombocytopenia, aplastic anemia).

[U.S. Boxed Warning]: NSAIDs are associated with an increased risk of adverse cardiovascular thrombotic events, including MI and stroke. Risk may be increased with duration of use or preexisting cardiovascular risk factors or disease. Carefully evaluate individual cardiovascular risk profiles prior to prescribing. May cause new-onset hypertension or worsening of existing hypertension. Use caution with fluid retention. Avoid use in heart failure (ACCF/AHA [Yancy, 2013]). Concurrent use of aspirin has not been shown to consistently reduce thromboembolic events. **[U.S. Boxed Warning]: Use is contraindicated as prophylactic analgesic before any major surgery and is contraindicated for treatment of perioperative pain in the setting of coronary artery bypass graft (CABG) surgery.** Risk of MI and stroke may be increased with use following CABG surgery. Wound bleeding and postoperative hematomas have been associated with ketorolac use in the perioperative setting.

[U.S. Boxed Warning]: Ketorolac is contraindicated in patients with advanced renal impairment and in patients at risk for renal failure due to volume depletion. NSAID use may compromise existing renal function; dose-dependent decreases in prostaglandin synthesis may result from NSAID use, reducing renal blood flow which may cause renal decompensation. NSAID use may increase the risk for hyperkalemia. Patients with impaired renal function, dehydration, heart failure, liver dysfunction, those taking diuretics and ACE inhibitors, and the elderly are at greater risk of renal toxicity. Use with caution in patients with impaired renal function or history of kidney disease; dosage adjustment is required in patients with moderate elevation in serum creatinine. Monitor renal function closely. Acute renal failure, interstitial nephritis, and nephrotic syndrome have been reported with ketorolac use; papillary necrosis and renal injury have been reported with the use of NSAIDs. Use of NSAIDs can compromise existing renal function. Rehydrate patient before starting therapy.

[U.S. Boxed Warning]: NSAIDs may increase risk of gastrointestinal irritation, inflammation, ulceration, bleeding, and perforation. These events may occur at any time during therapy and without warning. Use is contraindicated in patients with active/history of peptic ulcer disease and recent/history of GI bleeding or perforation. Use caution with a history of inflammatory bowel disease, concurrent therapy with anticoagulants, and/or corticosteroids, smoking, use of alcohol, the elderly, or debilitated patients.

[U.S. Boxed Warning]: Ketorolac injection is contraindicated in patients with prior hypersensitivity reaction to aspirin or NSAIDs. NSAIDs may cause serious skin adverse events including exfoliative dermatitis, Stevens-Johnson syndrome (SJS), and toxic epidermal necrolysis (TEN); discontinue use at first sign of skin rash or hypersensitivity. Hypersensitivity or anaphylactoid reactions may occur, even without prior exposure; patients with "aspirin triad" (bronchial asthma, aspirin intolerance, rhinitis) may be at increased risk. Do not use in patients who experience bronchospasm, asthma, rhinitis, or urticaria with NSAID or aspirin therapy. Use caution in other forms of asthma.

Use with caution in patients with hepatic impairment or a history of liver disease. Closely monitor patients with any abnormal LFT. Rarely, severe hepatic reactions (eg, fulminant hepatitis, hepatic necrosis, liver failure) have occurred with NSAID use; discontinue if signs or symptoms of liver disease develop, or if systemic manifestations occur.

[U.S. Boxed Warning]: Dosage adjustment is required for patients ≥65 years of age. Avoid use in older adults; use is associated with an increased risk of GI bleeding and peptic ulcer disease in older adults in high risk category (eg, >75 years or age or receiving concomitant oral/parenteral corticosteroids, anticoagulants, or antiplatelet agents) (Beers Criteria). **[U.S. Boxed Warning]: Dosage adjustment is required for patients weighing <50 kg (<110 pounds). [U.S. Boxed Warning]: Ketorolac is contraindicated during labor and delivery (may inhibit uterine contractions and adversely affect fetal circulation). [U.S. Boxed Warning]: Concurrent use of ketorolac with aspirin or other NSAIDs is contraindicated due to the increased risk of adverse reactions.**

[U.S. Boxed Warning]: Contraindicated for epidural or intrathecal administration (formulation contains alcohol). [U.S. Boxed Warning]: Systemic ketorolac is indicated for short term (≤5 days) use in adults for treatment of moderately severe acute pain requiring opioid-level analgesia. Low doses of opioids may be needed for breakthrough pain. **[U.S. Boxed Warning]: Oral therapy is only indicated for use as continuation treatment, following parenteral ketorolac and is not indicated for minor or chronic painful conditions. Do not exceed maximum daily recommended doses; does not improve efficacy but may increase the risk of serious adverse effects.** The combined therapy duration (oral and parenteral) should not exceed 5 days. Use the lowest effective dose for the shortest duration of time, consistent with individual patient goals, to reduce risk of cardiovascular or GI adverse events. Alternate therapies should be considered for patients at high risk. **[U.S. Boxed Warning]: Ketorolac is not indicated for use in children.**

Potentially significant drug-drug interactions may exist, requiring dose or frequency adjustment, additional monitoring, and/or selection of alternative therapy.

NSAIDS may cause drowsiness, dizziness, blurred vision and other neurologic effects which may impair physical or mental abilities; patients must be cautioned about performing tasks which require mental alertness (eg, operating machinery or driving). Discontinue use with blurred or diminished vision and perform ophthalmologic exam.

Adverse Reactions Frequencies noted for parenteral administration:
>10%:
Central nervous system: Headache (17%)
Gastrointestinal: Gastrointestinal pain (13%), dyspepsia (12%), nausea (12%)
>1% to 10%:
Cardiovascular: Edema (4%), hypertension
Central nervous system: Dizziness (7%), drowsiness (6%)
Dermatologic: Diaphoresis, pruritus, skin rash
Gastrointestinal: Diarrhea (7%), constipation, flatulence, gastrointestinal fullness, gastrointestinal hemorrhage, gastrointestinal perforation, gastrointestinal ulcer, heartburn, stomatitis, vomiting
Hematologic & oncologic: Anemia, prolonged bleeding time, purpura
Hepatic: Increased liver enzymes
Local: Pain at injection site (2%)
Otic: Tinnitus
Renal: Renal function abnormality
<1% (Limited to important or life-threatening): Abnormality in thinking, acute pancreatitis, acute renal failure, agranulocytosis, alopecia, anaphylactoid reaction, anaphylaxis, angioedema, aplastic anemia, aseptic meningitis, asthma, azotemia, bradycardia, bronchospasm, bruise, cardiac arrhythmia, cholestatic jaundice, coma, confusion, congestive heart failure, conjunctivitis, cough, cystitis, depression, dysuria, eosinophilia, epistaxis, eructation, erythema multiforme, euphoria, exacerbation of urinary frequency, exfoliative dermatitis, extrapyramidal reaction, flank pain, gastritis, glossitis, hallucination, hearing loss, hematemesis, hematuria, hemolytic anemia, hemolytic-uremic syndrome, hepatic failure, hepatitis, hepatotoxicity (idiosyncratic) (Chalasani, 2014), hyperglycemia, hyperkalemia, hyperkinesis, hypersensitivity reaction, hyponatremia, hypotension, increased susceptibility to infection, increased thirst, infertility, inflammatory bowel disease, insomnia, interstitial nephritis, jaundice, lack of concentration, laryngeal edema, leukopenia, lymphadenopathy, maculopapular rash, melena, myocardial infarction, nephritis, oliguria, palpitations, pancytopenia, paresthesia, pneumonia, polyuria, proteinuria, psychosis, pulmonary edema, rectal hemorrhage, renal failure, respiratory depression, rhinitis, seizure, sepsis, skin photosensitivity, Stevens-Johnson syndrome, stomatitis (ulcerative), stupor, syncope, tachycardia, thrombocytopenia, tongue edema, toxic epidermal necrolysis, urinary retention, urticaria, vasculitis, weight gain, wound hemorrhage (postoperative)

Drug Interactions
Metabolism/Transport Effects None known.
Avoid Concomitant Use
Avoid concomitant use of Ketorolac (Systemic) with any of the following: Aspirin; Dexketoprofen; Floctafenine; Ketorolac (Nasal); Morniflumate; Nonsteroidal Anti-Inflammatory Agents; Omacetaxine; Pentoxifylline; Probenecid; Talniflumate; Urokinase

Increased Effect/Toxicity
Ketorolac (Systemic) may increase the levels/effects of: 5-ASA Derivatives; Agents with Antiplatelet Properties; Aliskiren; Aminoglycosides; Anticoagulants; Apixaban; Aspirin; Bisphosphonate Derivatives; Collagenase (Systemic); CycloSPORINE (Systemic); Dabigatran Etexilate; Deferasirox; Deoxycholic Acid; Desmopressin; Digoxin; Drospirenone; Edoxaban; Eplerenone; Haloperidol; Ibritumomab; Lithium; Methotrexate; Neuromuscular-Blocking Agents (Nondepolarizing); Nonsteroidal Anti-Inflammatory Agents; Obinutuzumab; Omacetaxine; PEMEtrexed; Pentoxifylline; Porfimer; Potassium-Sparing Diuretics; PRALAtrexate; Quinolone Antibiotics; Rivaroxaban; Salicylates; Tacrolimus (Systemic); Tenofovir Products; Thrombolytic Agents; Tositumomab and Iodine I 131 Tositumomab; Urokinase; Vancomycin; Verteporfin; Vitamin K Antagonists

The levels/effects of Ketorolac (Systemic) may be increased by: ACE Inhibitors; Alcohol (Ethyl); Angiotensin II Receptor Blockers; Antidepressants (Tricyclic, Tertiary Amine); Corticosteroids (Systemic); CycloSPORINE (Systemic); Dasatinib; Dexketoprofen; Floctafenine; Glucosamine; Herbs (Anticoagulant/Antiplatelet Properties); Ibrutinib; Ketorolac (Nasal); Limaprost; Loop Diuretics; Morniflumate; Multivitamins/Fluoride (with ADE); Multivitamins/Minerals (with ADEK, Folate, Iron); Multivitamins/Minerals (with AE, No Iron); Omega-3 Fatty Acids; Pentosan Polysulfate Sodium; Probenecid; Prostacyclin Analogues; Selective Serotonin Reuptake Inhibitors; Serotonin/Norepinephrine Reuptake Inhibitors; Sodium Phosphates; Talniflumate; Thiazide Diuretics; Tipranavir; Treprostinil; Vitamin E; Vitamin E (Oral)

Decreased Effect
Ketorolac (Systemic) may decrease the levels/effects of: ACE Inhibitors; Aliskiren; Angiotensin II Receptor Blockers; Aspirin; Beta-Blockers; Eplerenone; HydrALAZINE; Loop Diuretics; Potassium-Sparing Diuretics; Prostaglandins (Ophthalmic); Salicylates; Selective Serotonin Reuptake Inhibitors; Thiazide Diuretics

The levels/effects of Ketorolac (Systemic) may be decreased by: Bile Acid Sequestrants; Salicylates

Food Interactions High-fat meals may delay time to peak (by ~1 hour) and decrease peak concentrations. Management: Administer tablet with food or milk to decrease gastrointestinal distress.

Storage/Stability
Injection: Store at room temperature of 15°C to 30°C (59°F to 86°F). Protect from light. Injection is clear and has a slight yellow color. Precipitation may occur at relatively low pH values.
Tablet: Store at room temperature of 15°C to 30°C (59°F to 86°F).

Mechanism of Action Reversibly inhibits cyclooxygenase-1 and 2 (COX-1 and 2) enzymes, which results in decreased formation of prostaglandin precursors; has antipyretic, analgesic, and anti-inflammatory properties

Other proposed mechanisms not fully elucidated (and possibly contributing to the anti-inflammatory effect to varying degrees), include inhibiting chemotaxis, altering lymphocyte activity, inhibiting neutrophil aggregation/activation, and decreasing proinflammatory cytokine levels.

Pharmacodynamics/Kinetics
Onset of action: Analgesic: Oral: 30-60 minutes; IM, IV: ~30 minutes
Peak effect: Analgesic: Oral: 1.5-4 hours; IM, IV: ≤2-3 hours
Duration: Analgesic: 4-6 hours
Absorption: Oral: Well absorbed (100%); IM: Rapid and complete
Distribution: Poor penetration into CSF; V_d beta:
Children 4-8 years: 0.19-0.44 L/kg (mean: 0.26 L/kg)
Adults: 0.11-0.33 L/kg (mean: 0.18 L/kg)

Protein binding: 99%

Metabolism: Hepatic; undergoes hydroxylation and glucuronide conjugation; in children 4-8 years, V_{dss} and plasma clearance were twice as high as adults

Bioavailability: Oral, IM: 100%

Half-life elimination:

Infants 6-18 months of age (n=25): S-enantiomer: 0.83 ± 0.7 hours; R-enantiomer: 4 ± 0.8 hours (Lynn 2007)

Children:

1-16 years (n=36): Mean: 3 ± 1.1 hours (Dsida 2002)

3-18 years (n=24): Mean: 3.8 ± 2.6 hours

4-8 years (n=10): Mean: 6 hours; Range: 3.5-10 hours

Adults:

Mean: ~5 hours; Range: 2-9 hours [S-enantiomer ~2.5 hours (biologically active); R-enantiomer ~5 hours]; Prolonged 30% to 50% in elderly

With renal impairment: S_{cr} 1.9-5 mg/dL: Mean: ~11 hours; Range: 4-19 hours

Renal dialysis patients: Mean: ~14 hours; Range: 8-40 hours

Time to peak, serum: Oral: ~45 minutes; IM: 30-60 minutes; IV: 1-3 minutes

Excretion: Urine (92%, ~60% as unchanged drug); feces ~6%

Dosing

Adult Pain management (acute; moderately severe) in patients ≥50 kg: Note: The maximum combined duration of treatment (for parenteral and oral) is 5 days; do not increase dose or frequency; supplement with low-dose opioids if needed for breakthrough pain.

IM: 60 mg as a single dose or 30 mg every 6 hours (maximum daily dose: 120 mg)

IV: 30 mg as a single dose or 30 mg every 6 hours (maximum daily dose: 120 mg)

IM, IV: Critically-ill patients (off-label dose): 30 mg once, followed by 15-30 mg every 6 hours for up to 5 days (maximum daily dose: 120 mg) (Barr, 2013)

Oral: 20 mg, followed by 10 mg every 4-6 hours as needed; do not exceed 40 mg daily; oral dosing is intended to be a continuation of IM or IV therapy only

Dosage adjustment for low body weight (<50 kg): Refer to geriatric dosing.

Geriatric Pain management (acute; moderately severe): Adults ≥65 years: **Note:** May have an increased incidence of GI bleeding, ulceration, and perforation. The maximum combined duration of treatment (for parenteral and oral) is 5 days.

IM: 30 mg as a single dose or 15 mg every 6 hours (maximum daily dose: 60 mg)

IV: 15 mg as a single dose or 15 mg every 6 hours (maximum daily dose: 60 mg)

Oral: 10 mg, followed by 10 mg every 4-6 hours as needed; do not exceed 40 mg daily; oral dosing is intended to be a continuation of IM or IV therapy only

Pediatric Pain management (acute; moderately severe): Adolescents ≥17 years: Refer to adult dosing.

Renal Impairment Use is contraindicated in patients with advanced renal impairment or patients at risk for renal failure due to volume depletion.

Mild-to-moderate impairment:

IM: 30 mg as a single dose or 15 mg every 6 hours (maximum daily dose: 60 mg)

IV: 15 mg as a single dose or 15 mg every 6 hours (maximum daily dose: 60 mg)

Oral: 10 mg, followed by 10 mg every 4-6 hours as needed; do not exceed 40 mg daily; oral dosing is intended to be a continuation of IM or IV therapy only

Note: The maximum combined duration of treatment (for parenteral and oral) is 5 days.

Advanced impairment or patients at risk for renal failure due to volume depletion: Use is contraindicated.

Hepatic Impairment No dosage adjustment provided in manufacturer's labeling. Use with caution, may cause elevation of liver enzymes; discontinue if clinical signs and symptoms of liver disease develop.

Dietary Considerations Administer tablet with food or milk to decrease gastrointestinal distress.

Administration

Oral: May take with food to reduce GI upset.

IM: Administer slowly and deeply into the muscle.

IV: Administer IV bolus over a minimum of 15 seconds.

Monitoring Parameters Monitor response (pain, range of motion, grip strength, mobility, ADL function), inflammation; observe for weight gain, edema; monitor renal function (serum creatinine, BUN, urine output); CBC and platelets, liver function tests; chemistry profile; blood pressure; observe for bleeding, bruising; evaluate gastrointestinal effects (abdominal pain, bleeding, dyspepsia); mental confusion, disorientation

Reference Range Serum concentration: Therapeutic: 0.3-5 mcg/mL; Toxic: >5 mcg/mL

Additional Information Ketorolac 30 mg IM provides analgesia comparable to morphine ≤12 mg or meperidine ≤100 mg (Buckley, 1990).

Dosage Forms Excipient information presented when available (limited, particularly for generics); consult specific product labeling.

Solution, Injection, as tromethamine:

Generic: 15 mg/mL (1 mL); 30 mg/mL (1 mL); 60 mg/2 mL (2 mL); 300 mg/10 mL (10 mL)

Solution, Injection, as tromethamine [preservative free]:

Generic: 15 mg/mL (1 mL); 30 mg/mL (1 mL)

Solution, Intramuscular, as tromethamine:

Generic: 60 mg/2 mL (2 mL); 30 mg/mL (1 mL)

Solution, Intramuscular, as tromethamine [preservative free]:

Generic: 60 mg/2 mL (2 mL)

Tablet, Oral, as tromethamine:

Generic: 10 mg

Ketorolac (Nasal) (KEE toe role ak)

Brand Names: US Sprix

Index Terms Ketorolac Tromethamine

Pharmacologic Category Nonsteroidal Anti-inflammatory Drug (NSAID), Nasal

Use Moderate to moderately severe pain: Short-term (up to 5 days) management of moderate to moderately severe pain in adults that requires analgesia at the opioid level.

Medication Guide Available Yes

Dosing

Adult Pain management (acute; moderate to moderately severe): Note: The maximum combined duration of treatment (for nasal spray or other ketorolac formulations) is 5 days.

Intranasal: Adults <65 years and ≥50 kg: One spray (15.75 mg) in each nostril (total dose: 31.5 mg) every 6-8 hours; maximum dose: 4 doses (126 mg)/day

Dosage adjustments in adults with low body weight (<50 kg): One spray (15.75 mg) in 1 nostril (total dose: 15.75 mg) every 6-8 hours; maximum dose: 4 doses (63 mg)/day

Geriatric Elderly (≥65 years): Intranasal: One spray (15.75 mg) in 1 nostril (total dose: 15.75 mg) every 6-8 hours; maximum dose: 4 doses (63 mg)/day

Renal Impairment

Renal insufficiency: Intranasal: One spray (15.75 mg) in 1 nostril (total dose: 15.75 mg) every 6-8 hours; maximum dose: 4 doses (63 mg)/day

Advanced renal impairment (or at risk for renal failure due to volume depletion): Use is contraindicated

Hepatic Impairment Use with caution with hepatic impairment or history of hepatic disease; use may cause elevation of liver enzymes; discontinue if clinical signs and symptoms of liver disease develop.

Additional Information Complete prescribing information should be consulted for additional detail.

Dosage Forms Excipient information presented when available (limited, particularly for generics); consult specific product labeling.

Solution, Nasal, as tromethamine [preservative free]:

Sprix: 15.75 mg/spray (1 ea) [contains edetate disodium]

Ketorolac (Ophthalmic) (KEE toe role ak)

Brand Names: US Acular; Acular LS; Acuvail

Brand Names: Canada Acular LS®; Acular®; Apo-Ketorolac® Ophthalmic; ratio-Ketorolac

Index Terms Ketorolac Tromethamine

Pharmacologic Category Nonsteroidal Anti-inflammatory Drug (NSAID), Ophthalmic

Use Temporary relief of ocular itching due to seasonal allergic conjunctivitis; postoperative pain and/or inflammation following cataract extraction; reduction of ocular pain, burning, and stinging following corneal refractive surgery

Dosing

Adult

Seasonal allergic conjunctivitis (relief of ocular itching) (Acular®): Ophthalmic: Instill 1 drop to affected eye(s) 4 times daily

Inflammation following cataract extraction (Acular®): Ophthalmic: Instill 1 drop to affected eye(s) 4 times daily beginning 24 hours after surgery; continue for 2 weeks

Pain, burning/stinging following corneal refractive surgery (Acular LS®): Ophthalmic: Instill 1 drop to affected eye(s) 4 times daily as needed for up to 4 days after surgery

Pain and inflammation associated with cataract surgery (Acuvail®): Instill 1 drop to affected eye(s) 2 times daily 24 hours before surgery and on the day of surgery; continue for 2 weeks

Pediatric Ophthalmic uses: Children ≥2 years and Adolescents: Refer to adult dosing.

Renal Impairment No dosage adjustment provided in manufacturer's labeling.

Hepatic Impairment No dosage adjustment provided in manufacturer's labeling.

Additional Information Complete prescribing information should be consulted for additional detail.

Dosage Forms Excipient information presented when available (limited, particularly for generics); consult specific product labeling.

Solution, Ophthalmic, as tromethamine:

Acular: 0.5% (5 mL) [contains benzalkonium chloride, edetate disodium]

Acular LS: 0.4% (5 mL) [contains benzalkonium chloride, edetate disodium]

Generic: 0.4% (5 mL); 0.5% (3 mL, 5 mL, 10 mL)

Solution, Ophthalmic, as tromethamine [preservative free]:

Acuvail: 0.45% (30 ea)

◆ Ketorolac Tromethamine see Ketorolac (Nasal) on page 1017

◆ Ketorolac Tromethamine see Ketorolac (Ophthalmic) on page 1017

◆ Ketorolac Tromethamine see Ketorolac (Systemic) on page 1015

◆ Ketorolac Tromethamine Injection, USP (Can) see Ketorolac (Systemic) on page 1015

Ketotifen (Ophthalmic) (kee toe TYE fen)

Brand Names: US Alaway Childrens Allergy [OTC]; Alaway [OTC]; Claritin Eye [OTC]; Refresh Eye Itch Relief [OTC] [DSC]; Thera Tears Allergy [OTC]; Zaditor [OTC]; ZyrTEC Itchy Eye [OTC]

Brand Names: Canada Zaditor

Index Terms Ketotifen Fumarate

Pharmacologic Category Histamine H_1 Antagonist; Histamine H_1 Antagonist, Second Generation; Mast Cell Stabilizer; Piperidine Derivative

Use Allergic conjunctivitis: Temporary relief of eye itching due to allergic conjunctivitis

Dosing

Adult & Geriatric

Allergic conjunctivitis:

US labeling (OTC labeling): Ophthalmic: Instill 1 drop into the affected eye(s) twice daily every 8 to 12 hours (maximum: do not exceed 2 applications/day)

Canadian labeling: Ophthalmic: Instill 1 drop into the affected eye(s) every 8 to 12 hours

Pediatric

Allergic conjunctivitis: Children ≥3 years and Adolescents: Ophthalmic: Refer to adult dosing.

Renal Impairment There are no dosage adjustments provided in the manufacturer's labeling. However, dosage adjustment unlikely due to low systemic absorption.

Hepatic Impairment There are no dosage adjustments provided in the manufacturer's labeling. However, dosage adjustment unlikely due to low systemic absorption.

Additional Information Complete prescribing information should be consulted for additional detail.

Dosage Forms Excipient information presented when available (limited, particularly for generics); consult specific product labeling. [DSC] = Discontinued product

Solution, Ophthalmic:

Alaway: 0.025% (10 mL) [contains benzalkonium chloride]

Alaway Childrens Allergy: 0.025% (5 mL) [contains benzalkonium chloride]

Claritin Eye: 0.025% (5 mL) [contains benzalkonium chloride]

Refresh Eye Itch Relief: 0.025% (5 mL [DSC]) [contains benzalkonium chloride]

Thera Tears Allergy: 0.025% (10 mL) [contains benzalkonium chloride]

Zaditor: 0.025% (5 mL) [contains benzalkonium chloride]

ZyrTEC Itchy Eye: 0.025% (5 mL) [contains benzalkonium chloride]

Generic: 0.025% (5 mL)

Dosage Forms: Canada Excipient information presented when available (limited, particularly for generics); consult specific product labeling.

Solution, ophthalmic [drops]:

Zaditor: 0.025% (5 mL) [contains benzalkonium chloride]

◆ Ketotifen Fumarate see Ketotifen (Ophthalmic) on page 1018

◆ Keytruda see Pembrolizumab on page 1414

◆ Khedezla see Desvenlafaxine on page 524

◆ Khloditan see Mitotane on page 1221

◆ KI see Potassium Iodide on page 1481

◆ Kidkare Children's Cough/Cold [OTC] see Chlorpheniramine, Pseudoephedrine, and Dextromethorphan on page 379

◆ Kimidess see Ethinyl Estradiol and Desogestrel on page 701

◆ Kineret see Anakinra on page 127

◆ Kinrix see Diphtheria and Tetanus Toxoids, Acellular Pertussis, and Poliovirus Vaccine on page 566

◆ Kionex see Sodium Polystyrene Sulfonate on page 1680

◆ Kitabis Pak see Tobramycin (Oral Inhalation) on page 1802

◆ Kivexa (Can) see Abacavir and Lamivudine on page 18

◆ Klaron see Sulfacetamide (Topical) on page 1707

◆ Klean-Prep (Can) see Polyethylene Glycol-Electrolyte Solution on page 1466

◆ KlonoPIN see ClonazePAM on page 419

◆ K-Lor [DSC] see Potassium Chloride on page 1479

◆ Klor-Con see Potassium Chloride on page 1479

◆ Klor-Con 10 see Potassium Chloride on page 1479

◆ Klor-Con/EF see Potassium Bicarbonate and Potassium Citrate on page 1479

◆ Klor-Con M10 see Potassium Chloride on page 1479

◆ Klor-Con M15 see Potassium Chloride on page 1479

◆ Klor-Con M20 see Potassium Chloride on page 1479

◆ Klor-Con Sprinkle see Potassium Chloride on page 1479

◆ K-Lyte/Cl see Potassium Bicarbonate and Potassium Chloride on page 1478

◆ KMD 3213 see Silodosin on page 1655

◆ Koate-DVI see Antihemophilic Factor (Human) on page 131

◆ Koffex DM-D (Can) see Pseudoephedrine and Dextromethorphan on page 1528

◆ Kogenate FS see Antihemophilic Factor (Recombinant) on page 132

◆ Kogenate FS Bio-Set see Antihemophilic Factor (Recombinant) on page 132

◆ Kolephrin GG/DM [OTC] see Guaifenesin and Dextromethorphan on page 861

◆ Kombiglyze XR see Saxagliptin and Metformin on page 1640

◆ Komboglyze (Can) see Saxagliptin and Metformin on page 1640

◆ Konakion (Can) see Phytonadione on page 1450

◆ Konsyl [OTC] see Psyllium on page 1529

◆ Konsyl-D [OTC] see Psyllium on page 1529

◆ Korlym see Mifepristone on page 1206

◆ K-Phos see Potassium Acid Phosphate on page 1478

◆ K-Phos Neutral see Potassium Phosphate and Sodium Phosphate on page 1484

◆ K-Phos No. 2 see Potassium Phosphate and Sodium Phosphate on page 1484

◆ K-Prime see Potassium Bicarbonate and Potassium Citrate on page 1479

◆ Kristalose see Lactulose on page 1023

◆ Krystexxa see Pegloticase on page 1413

◆ KS Ibuprofen [OTC] see Ibuprofen on page 905

◆ K-Sol see Potassium Chloride on page 1479

◆ KS Stool Softener [OTC] see Docusate on page 578

◆ K-Tab see Potassium Chloride on page 1479

◆ KU-0059436 see Olaparib on page 1318

◆ Kurvelo see Ethinyl Estradiol and Levonorgestrel on page 703

◆ Kuvan see Sapropterin on page 1636

◆ K-Vescent see Potassium Bicarbonate and Potassium Citrate on page 1479

◆ K-Vescent [DSC] see Potassium Chloride on page 1479

◆ Kwell see Lindane on page 1080

◆ Kwellada-P [OTC] (Can) see Permethrin on page 1432

◆ Kybella see Deoxycholic Acid on page 518

◆ Kynamro see Mipomersen on page 1214

◆ Kynesia (Can) see Benztropine on page 219

◆ Kyprolis see Carfilzomib on page 315

◆ Kytril see Granisetron on page 857

◆ L-749,345 see Ertapenem on page 668

◆ L-758,298 see Fosaprepitant on page 812

◆ L 754030 *see* Aprepitant *on page* 143
◆ LA 20304a *see* Gemifloxacin *on page* 836

Labetalol (la BET a lole)

Brand Names: US Trandate [DSC]
Brand Names: Canada Apo-Labetalol; Labetalol Hydrochloride Injection, USP; Normodyne; Trandate
Index Terms Ibidomide Hydrochloride; Labetalol Hydrochloride; Normodyne; Trandate
Pharmacologic Category Antihypertensive; Beta-Blocker With Alpha-Blocking Activity
Additional Appendix Information
Hypertension *on page* 1996
Use Hypertension: Treatment of mild-to-severe hypertension; IV for severe hypertension (eg, hypertensive emergencies)

The 2014 guideline for the management of high blood pressure in adults (Eighth Joint National Committee [JNC 8]) recommends initiation of pharmacologic treatment to lower blood pressure for the following patients (JNC8 [James, 2013]):

• Patients ≥60 years of age, with systolic blood pressure (SBP) ≥150 mm Hg or diastolic blood pressure (DBP) ≥90 mm Hg. Goal of therapy is SBP <150 mm Hg and DBP <90 mm Hg.

• Patients <60 years of age, with SBP ≥140 mm Hg or DBP ≥90 mm Hg. Goal of therapy is SBP <140 mm Hg and DBP <90 mm Hg.

• Patients ≥18 years of age with diabetes, with SBP ≥140 mm Hg or DBP ≥90 mm Hg. Goal of therapy is SBP <140 mm Hg and DBP <90 mm Hg.

• Patients ≥18 years of age with chronic kidney disease (CKD), with SBP ≥140 mm Hg or DBP ≥90 mm Hg. Goal of therapy is SBP <140 mm Hg and DBP <90 mm Hg.

In patients with CKD, regardless of race or diabetes status, the use of an ACE inhibitor (ACEI) or angiotensin receptor blocker (ARB) as initial therapy is recommended to improve kidney outcomes. In the general nonblack population (without CKD) including those with diabetes, initial antihypertensive treatment should consist of a thiazide-type diuretic, calcium channel blocker, ACEI, or ARB. In the general black population (without CKD) including those with diabetes, initial antihypertensive treatment should consist of a thiazide-type diuretic or a calcium channel blocker **instead of** an ACEI or ARB.

Pregnancy Considerations Adverse events have been observed in some animal reproduction studies. Labetalol crosses the placenta and can be detected in cord blood and infant serum after delivery (Haraldsson, 1989; Rogers, 1990). Fetal/neonatal bradycardia, hypoglycemia, hypotension, and/or respiratory depression have been observed following in utero exposure to labetalol. Adequate facilities for monitoring infants at birth should be available.

Untreated chronic maternal hypertension and preeclampsia are also associated with adverse events in the fetus, infant, and mother. Oral labetalol is considered an appropriate agent for the treatment of chronic hypertension in pregnancy (ACOG, 2013; Magee, 2014). Intravenous labetalol is recommended for use in the management of acute onset, severe hypertension (systolic BP ≥160 mm Hg or diastolic BP ≥110 mm Hg) with preeclampsia or eclampsia in pregnant and postpartum women. In general, avoid use of labetalol in women with asthma or heart failure (ACOG, 2015; Magee, 2014).

Breast-Feeding Considerations Low amounts of labetalol are found in breast milk and can be detected in the serum of nursing infants. The manufacturer recommends that caution be exercised when administering labetalol to nursing women.

Contraindications Hypersensitivity to labetalol or any component of the formulation; severe bradycardia; heart block greater than first degree (except in patients with a functioning artificial pacemaker); cardiogenic shock; bronchial asthma; uncompensated cardiac failure; conditions associated with severe and prolonged hypotension

Warnings/Precautions Consider preexisting conditions such as sick sinus syndrome before initiating. Symptomatic hypotension with or without syncope may occur with labetalol; close monitoring of patient is required especially with initial dosing and dosing increases; blood pressure must be lowered at a rate appropriate for the patient's clinical condition. Initiation with a low dose and gradual up-titration may help to decrease the occurrence of hypotension or syncope. Patients should be advised to avoid driving or other hazardous tasks during initiation of therapy due to the risk of syncope. Orthostatic hypotension may occur with IV administration; patient should remain supine during and for up to 3 hours after IV administration. Use

with caution in impaired hepatic function; bioavailability is increased due to decreased first-pass metabolism. Severe hepatic injury including some fatalities have also been rarely reported with use: periodically monitor LFTs with prolonged use. Use with caution in patients with diabetes mellitus; may potentiate hypoglycemia and/or mask signs and symptoms. Bradycardia may be observed more frequently in elderly patients (>65 years of age); dosage reductions may be necessary. May also reduce release of insulin in response to hyperglycemia; dosage of antidiabetic agents may need to be adjusted. May mask signs of hyperthyroidism (eg, tachycardia); if hyperthyroidism is suspected, carefully manage and monitor; abrupt withdrawal may exacerbate symptoms of hyperthyroidism or precipitate thyroid storm. Elimination of labetalol is reduced in elderly patients; lower maintenance doses may be required.

Use only with extreme caution in compensated heart failure and monitor for a worsening of the condition. Beta-blocker therapy should not be withdrawn abruptly (particularly in patients with CAD), but gradually tapered to avoid acute tachycardia, hypertension, and/or ischemia. Chronic beta-blocker therapy should not be routinely withdrawn prior to major surgery. Use caution with concurrent use of digoxin, verapamil, or diltiazem; bradycardia or heart block can occur. Use with caution in patients receiving inhaled anesthetic agents known to depress myocardial contractility. Patients with bronchospastic disease should not receive beta-blockers; if used at all, should be used cautiously with close monitoring. Use with caution in patients with myasthenia gravis or psychiatric disease (may cause or exacerbate CNS depression). Can precipitate or aggravate symptoms of arterial insufficiency in patients with PVD and Raynaud's disease; use with caution and monitor for progression of arterial obstruction. If possible, obtain diagnostic tests for pheochromocytoma prior to use. May induce or exacerbate psoriasis. Labetalol has been shown to be effective in lowering blood pressure and relieving symptoms in patients with pheochromocytoma. However, some patients have experienced paradoxical hypertensive responses; use with caution in patients with pheochromocytoma. Additional alpha-blockade may be required during use of labetalol. Use caution with history of severe anaphylaxis to allergens; patients taking beta-blockers may become more sensitive to repeated challenges. Treatment of anaphylaxis (eg, epinephrine) in patients taking beta-blockers may be ineffective or promote undesirable effects.

Intraoperative floppy iris syndrome has been observed in cataract surgery patients who were on or were previously treated with alpha$_1$-blockers; causality has not been established and there appears to be no benefit in discontinuing alpha-blocker therapy prior to surgery. Instruct patients to inform ophthalmologist of labetalol use when considering eye surgery.

Benzyl alcohol and derivatives: Some dosage forms may contain sodium benzoate/benzoic acid; benzoic acid (benzoate) is a metabolite of benzyl alcohol; large amounts of benzyl alcohol (≥99 mg/kg/day) have been associated with a potentially fatal toxicity ("gasping syndrome") in neonates; the "gasping syndrome" consists of metabolic acidosis, respiratory distress, gasping respirations, CNS dysfunction (including convulsions, intracranial hemorrhage), hypotension, and cardiovascular collapse (AAP ["Inactive" 1997]; CDC, 1982); some data suggests that benzoate displaces bilirubin from protein binding sites (Ahlfors, 2001); avoid or use dosage forms containing benzyl alcohol derivative with caution in neonates. See manufacturer's labeling.

Adverse Reactions
>10%:
  Cardiovascular: Orthostatic hypotension (IV use; ≤58%)
  Central nervous system: Dizziness (1% to 20%), fatigue (1% to 11%)
  Gastrointestinal: Nausea (≤19%)
1% to 10%:
  Cardiovascular: Hypotension (1% to 5%), edema (≤2%), flushing (1%), ventricular arrhythmia (IV use; 1%)
  Central nervous system: Somnolence (3%), headache (2%), vertigo (1% to 2%)
  Dermatologic: Scalp tingling (≤7%), pruritus (1%), rash (1%)
  Gastrointestinal: Dyspepsia (≤4%), vomiting (≤3%), taste disturbance (1%)
  Genitourinary: Ejaculatory failure (≤5%), impotence (1% to 4%)
  Hepatic: Transaminases increased (4%)
  Neuromuscular & skeletal: Paresthesia (≤5%), weakness (1%)
  Ocular: Vision abnormal (1%)
  Renal: BUN increased (≤8%)

Respiratory: Nasal congestion (1% to 6%), dyspnea (2%)
Miscellaneous: Diaphoresis (≤4%)

<1% (Limited to important or life-threatening): Alopecia (reversible), anaphylactoid reaction, ANA positive, angioedema, bradycardia, bronchospasm, cholestatic jaundice, CHF, diabetes insipidus, heart block, hepatic necrosis, hepatitis, hypersensitivity, Peyronie's disease, psoriaform rash, Raynaud's syndrome, syncope, systemic lupus erythematosus, toxic myopathy, urinary retention, urticaria

Other adverse reactions noted with beta-adrenergic blocking agents include mental depression, catatonia, disorientation, short-term memory loss, emotional lability, clouded sensorium, intensification of preexisting AV block, laryngospasm, respiratory distress, agranulocytosis, thrombocytopenic purpura, nonthrombocytopenic purpura, mesenteric artery thrombosis, and ischemic colitis.

Drug Interactions

Metabolism/Transport Effects None known.

Avoid Concomitant Use

Avoid concomitant use of Labetalol with any of the following: Beta2-Agonists; Ceritinib; Floctafenine; Methacholine; Rivastigmine

Increased Effect/Toxicity

Labetalol may increase the levels/effects of: Alpha-/Beta-Agonists (Direct-Acting); Alpha1-Blockers; Alpha2-Agonists; Amifostine; Antipsychotic Agents (Phenothiazines); Antipsychotic Agents (Second Generation [Atypical]); Bradycardia-Causing Agents; Bupivacaine; Cardiac Glycosides; Ceritinib; Cholinergic Agonists; Disopyramide; DULoxetine; Ergot Derivatives; Fingolimod; Grass Pollen Allergen Extract (5 Grass Extract); Hypotension-Associated Agents; Insulin; Ivabradine; Lacosamide; Levodopa; Lidocaine (Systemic); Lidocaine (Topical); Mepivacaine; Methacholine; Midodrine; Sulfonylureas

The levels/effects of Labetalol may be increased by: Acetylcholinesterase Inhibitors; Alpha2-Agonists; Aminoquinolines (Antimalarial); Amiodarone; Anilidopiperidine Opioids; Antipsychotic Agents (Phenothiazines); Barbiturates; Bretylium; Brimonidine (Topical); Calcium Channel Blockers (Nondihydropyridine); Diazoxide; Dipyridamole; Disopyramide; Dronedarone; Floctafenine; Herbs (Hypotensive Properties); Molsidomine; Nicorandil; NIFEdipine; Obinutuzumab; Pentoxifylline; Phosphodiesterase 5 Inhibitors; Propafenone; Prostacyclin Analogues; Regorafenib; Reserpine; Rivastigmine; Ruxolitinib; Tofacitinib

Decreased Effect

Labetalol may decrease the levels/effects of: Beta2-Agonists; Theophylline Derivatives

The levels/effects of Labetalol may be decreased by: Amphetamines; Barbiturates; Herbs (Hypertensive Properties); Methylphenidate; Nonsteroidal Anti-Inflammatory Agents; Rifamycin Derivatives; Yohimbine

Food Interactions Labetalol serum concentrations may be increased if taken with food. Management: Administer with food.

Storage/Stability

Tablets: Store at room temperature (refer to manufacturer's labeling for detailed storage requirements). Protect from light and excessive moisture.

Injectable: Store at room temperature (refer to manufacturer's labeling for detailed storage requirements); do not freeze. Protect from light. The solution is clear to slightly yellow.

Parenteral admixture: Stability of parenteral admixture at room temperature (25°C) and refrigeration temperature (4°C): 3 days.

Mechanism of Action Blocks alpha-, beta$_1$-, and beta$_2$-adrenergic receptor sites; elevated renins are reduced. The ratios of alpha- to beta-blockade differ depending on the route of administration: 1:3 (oral) and 1:7 (IV).

Pharmacodynamics/Kinetics

Onset of action: Oral: 20 minutes to 2 hours; IV: 2 to 5 minutes

Peak effect: Oral: 1-4 hours; IV: 5 to 15 minutes

Duration: Blood pressure response:

Oral: 8 to 12 hours (dose dependent)

IV: 2 to 18 hours (dose dependent; based on single and multiple sequential doses of 0.25 to 0.5 mg/kg with cumulative dosing up to 3.25 mg/kg)

Absorption: Complete

Distribution: V$_d$: Adults: 3 to 16 L/kg; mean: <9.4 L/kg; moderately lipid soluble, therefore, can enter CNS

Protein binding: 50%

Metabolism: Hepatic, primarily via glucuronide conjugation; extensive first-pass effect

Bioavailability: Oral: 25%; increased with liver disease, elderly, and concurrent cimetidine

Half-life elimination: Oral: 6 to 8 hours; IV: ~5.5 hours

Time to peak, plasma: Oral: 1 to 2 hours

Excretion: Urine (55% to 60% as glucuronide conjugates, <5% as unchanged drug)

Clearance: Possibly decreased in neonates/infants

Dosing

Adult & Geriatric

Hypertension: Oral: Initial: 100 mg twice daily, may increase as needed every 2 to 3 days by 100 mg twice daily (titration increments not to exceed 200 mg twice daily) until desired response is obtained; usual dosage range (ASH/ISH [Weber, 2014]): 100 to 300 mg twice daily; may require up to 2400 mg daily.

Acute hypertension (hypertensive emergency/ urgency):

IV bolus: Per the manufacturer: Initial: 20 mg IV push over 2 minutes; may administer 40 to 80 mg at 10-minute intervals, up to 300 mg total cumulative dose; as appropriate, follow with oral antihypertensive regimen

IV infusion (acute loading): Per the manufacturer: Initial: 2 mg/minute; titrate to response up to 300 mg total cumulative dose (eg, discontinue after 2.5 hours of 2 mg/minute); usual total dose required: 50 to 200 mg; as appropriate, follow with oral antihypertensive regimen

Note: Although loading infusions are well described in the product labeling, the labeling is silent in specific clinical situations, such as in the patient who has an initial response to labetalol infusions but cannot be converted to an oral route for subsequent dosing. There is limited documentation of prolonged continuous infusions (ie, >300 mg/day). In rare clinical situations, higher continuous infusion doses up to 6 mg/minute have been used in the critical care setting (eg, aortic dissection) and up to 8 mg/minute (eg, hypertension with ongoing acute ischemic stroke). At these doses, it may be best to consider an alternative agent if the labetalol infusion is not meeting the goals of therapy. At the other extreme, continuous infusions at relatively low doses (0.03 to 0.1 mg/minute) have been used in some settings (following loading infusion in patients who are unable to be converted to oral regimens or in some cases as a continuation of outpatient oral regimens). These prolonged infusions should not be confused with loading infusions. Because of wide variation in the use of infusions, an awareness of institutional policies and practices is extremely important. Careful clarification of orders and specific infusion rates/units is required to avoid confusion. Due to the prolonged duration of action, careful monitoring should be extended for the duration of the infusion and for several hours after the infusion. Excessive administration may result in prolonged hypotension and/or bradycardia.

Arterial hypertension in acute ischemic stroke (off-label use [Jauch, 2013]): IV:

Patient otherwise eligible for reperfusion treatment (eg, alteplase) except blood pressure (BP) >185/110 mm Hg: 10 to 20 mg over 1 to 2 minutes; may repeat once. If BP does not decline and remains >185/110 mm Hg, alteplase should not be administered.

Management of BP during and after reperfusion treatment (eg, alteplase) to maintain BP ≤180/105 mm Hg: If systolic BP >180 to 230 mm Hg or diastolic >105 to 120 mm Hg, then administer 10 mg over 1 to 2 minutes followed by an infusion of 2 to 8 mg/minute. If hypertension is refractory or diastolic BP >140 mm Hg, consider other IV antihypertensives (eg, nitroprusside).

Hypertensive emergency in pregnancy (systolic BP ≥160 mm Hg or diastolic BP ≥110 mm Hg) (off-label dose): IV: Initial: 20 mg; if blood pressure still exceeds thresholds, may increase dose every 10 minutes in increments of 20 to 40 mg to a maximum single dose of 80 mg (Refer to administration protocols developed by the American College of Obstetricians and Gynecologists; ACOG, 2015). A maximum total cumulative dose of 300 mg is recommended (Magee, 2014). **Note:** After the initial dose, may initiate a continuous infusion of 1 to 2 mg/minute instead of intermittent dosing (Magee, 2014).

IV to oral conversion: Upon discontinuation of IV infusion, may initiate oral dose of 200 mg followed in 6 to 12 hours with an additional dose of 200 to 400 mg. Thereafter, dose patients with 400 to 2400 mg/day in divided doses depending on blood pressure response.

Pediatric Note: Due to limited documentation of its use, labetalol should be initiated cautiously in pediatric patients with careful dosage adjustment and blood pressure monitoring.

Hypertension:
Oral: Hypertension (off-label use): Initial: 1 to 3 mg/kg/day, in 2 divided doses; maximum: 10 to 12 mg/kg/day, up to 1200 mg/day

IV: Intermittent bolus doses of 0.3 to 1 mg/kg/dose have been reported.

Pediatric hypertensive emergencies: Initial continuous infusions of 0.4 to 1 mg/kg/hour with a maximum of 3 mg/kg/hour have been used; administration requires the use of an infusion pump.

Renal Impairment There are no dosage adjustments provided in manufacturer's labeling. Not removed by hemo- or peritoneal dialysis; supplemental dose is not necessary.

Hepatic Impairment There are no dosage adjustments provided in manufacturer's labeling. However, dosage reduction may be necessary in hepatic impairment due to decreased metabolism and increased oral bioavailability, use with caution.

Usual Infusion Concentrations: Pediatric IV infusion: 1 mg/mL

Usual Infusion Concentrations: Adult IV infusion: 500 mg in 250 mL (concentration: 2 mg/mL) of D_5W

Administration Bolus dose may be administered IV push at a rate of 10 mg/minute; may follow with continuous IV infusion

Monitoring Parameters Blood pressure, standing and sitting/supine, pulse, cardiac monitor and blood pressure monitor recommended for IV administration; consult individual institutional policies and procedures

Test Interactions False-positive urine catecholamines, vanillylmandelic acid (VMA) if measured by fluorometric or photometric methods; use HPLC or specific catecholamine radioenzymatic technique; false-positive amphetamine if measured by thin-layer chromatography or radioenzymatic assay (gas chromatographic-mass spectrometer technique should be used)

Dosage Forms Excipient information presented when available (limited, particularly for generics); consult specific product labeling. [DSC] = Discontinued product

Solution, Intravenous, as hydrochloride:
Generic: 5 mg/mL (4 mL, 20 mL, 40 mL)

Tablet, Oral, as hydrochloride:
Trandate: 100 mg [DSC], 200 mg [DSC], 300 mg [DSC] [scored]
Generic: 100 mg, 200 mg, 300 mg

Extemporaneous Preparations A 40 mg/mL labetalol hydrochloride oral suspension may be made with tablets and one of three different vehicles (cherry syrup, a 1:1 mixture of Ora-Sweet® and Ora-Plus®, or a 1:1 mixture of Ora-Sweet® SF and Ora-Plus®). Crush sixteen 300 mg tablets in a mortar and reduce to a fine powder. Add 20 mL of the chosen vehicle and mix to a uniform paste; mix while adding the vehicle in incremental proportions to **almost** 120 mL; transfer to a calibrated bottle, rinse mortar with vehicle, and add quantity of vehicle sufficient to make 120 mL. Label "shake well" and "protect from light". Stable for 60 days when stored in amber plastic prescription bottles in the dark at room temperature or refrigerated (Allen, 1996).

Extemporaneously prepared solutions of labetalol hydrochloride (approximate concentrations 7-10 mg/mL) prepared in distilled water, simple syrup, apple juice, grape juice, and orange juice were stable for 4 weeks when stored in amber glass or plastic prescription bottles at room temperature or refrigerated (Nahata, 1991).

Allen LV Jr and Erickson MA 3rd, "Stability of Labetalol Hydrochloride, Metoprolol Tartrate, Verapamil Hydrochloride, and Spironolactone with Hydrochlorothiazide in Extemporaneously Compounded Oral Liquids," *Am J Health Syst Pharm*, 1996, 53(19):2304-9.

Nahata MC, "Stability of Labetalol Hydrochloride in Distilled Water, Simple Syrup, and Three Fruit Juices," *DICP*, 1991, 25(5):465-9.

◆ Labetalol Hydrochloride *see* Labetalol *on page 1019*

◆ Labetalol Hydrochloride Injection, USP (Can) *see* Labetalol *on page 1019*

Lacosamide (la KOE sa mide)

Brand Names: US Vimpat
Brand Names: Canada Vimpat
Index Terms ADD 234037; Harkoseride; LCM; SPM 927
Pharmacologic Category Anticonvulsant, Miscellaneous
Use Partial-onset seizures:
US labeling: Monotherapy or adjunctive therapy in the treatment of partial-onset seizures in patients ≥17 years.
Canadian labeling: Adjunctive therapy in the treatment of partial-onset seizures in adults who are not satisfactorily controlled with conventional therapy.

Pregnancy Considerations Adverse events were observed in animal reproduction studies. Information related to pregnancy outcomes following maternal use of lacosamide is limited (Hoeltzenbein 2011). In general, maternal polytherapy with antiepileptic drugs may increase the risk of congenital malformations; monotherapy with the lowest effective dose is recommended. Newborns of women taking antiepileptic medications may be at an increased risk of adverse events (Harden and Meader 2009).

Patients exposed to lacosamide during pregnancy are encouraged to enroll themselves into the NAAED Pregnancy Registry by calling 1-888-233-2334. Additional information is available at http://www.aedpregnancy-registry.org.

Breast-Feeding Considerations It is not known if lacosamide is excreted in breast milk. According to the manufacturer, the decision to continue or discontinue breast-feeding during therapy should take into account the risk of exposure to the infant and the benefits of treatment to the mother.

Medication Guide Available Yes
Contraindications
U.S. labeling: There are no contraindications listed in manufacturer's labeling.
Canadian labeling: Hypersensitivity to lacosamide or any component of the formulation; second- or third-degree atrioventricular (AV) block (current or history of).

Warnings/Precautions Antiepileptics are associated with an increased risk of suicidal behavior/thoughts with use (regardless of indication); patients should be monitored for signs/symptoms of depression, suicidal tendencies, and other unusual behavior changes during therapy and instructed to inform their healthcare provider immediately if symptoms occur. CNS effects may occur; patients should be cautioned about performing tasks which require alertness (eg, operating machinery or driving). Lacosamide may prolong PR interval; second degree and complete AV block has also been reported. Use caution in patients with conduction problems (eg, first/second degree atrioventricular block and sick sinus syndrome without pacemaker), sodium channelopathies (eg, Brugada Syndrome), myocardial ischemia, heart failure, structural heart disease, or if concurrent use with other drugs that prolong the PR interval; ECG is recommended prior to initiating therapy and when at the steady state maintenance dose. Monitor closely with IV lacosamide administration; bradycardia and AV block have occurred during infusions. Instruct patients to contact their healthcare provider if signs or symptoms of conduction problems occur (eg, low or irregular pulse, feeling of lightheadedness and fainting). During short-term trials, atrial fibrillation/flutter, or syncope occurred slightly more often in patients with diabetic neuropathy and/or cardiovascular disease. In addition, in open-label studies, syncope has been associated with a history of cardiac disease risk factors and use of drugs that slow AV conduction. Use caution with renal or hepatic impairment and if these patients are taking strong inhibitors of CYP3A4 and CYP2C9; dosage adjustment may be necessary. Multiorgan hypersensitivity reactions can occur (rare); monitor patient and discontinue therapy if necessary. Withdraw therapy gradually (≥1 week) to minimize the potential of increased seizure frequency. Blurred vision and diplopia may occur during therapy. If visual disturbances persist, further assessment may be necessary. Consider increased monitoring in patients with known vision-related issues or ocular conditions. Effects with ethanol may be potentiated. Some products may contain phenylalanine. Some dosage forms may contain propylene glycol; large amounts are potentially toxic and have been associated hyperosmolality, lactic acidosis, seizures and respiratory depression; use caution (AAP, 1997; Zar, 2007).

Adverse Reactions The majority of adverse events are dose-dependent.
>10%:
Central nervous system: Dizziness (16% to 53%), fatigue (7% to 15%), ataxia (4% to 15%), headache (11% to 14%)
Gastrointestinal: Nausea (7% to 17%), vomiting (6% to 16%)
Neuromuscular & skeletal: Tremor (4% to 12%)
Ophthalmic: Diplopia (6% to 16%), blurred vision (2% to 16%)
1% to 10%:
Cardiovascular: Syncope (adults 1%; dose-related: >400 mg/day)
Central nervous system: Drowsiness (5% to 8%), memory impairment (2% to 6%), equilibrium disturbance (1% to 6%), vertigo (3% to 5%), abnormal gait (2% to 4%), depression (2%)
Dermatologic: Pruritus (2% to 3%)

Gastrointestinal: Diarrhea (3% to 5%)
Hematologic & oncologic: Bruise (2% to 4%)
Hepatic: Increased serum ALT (1%)
Local: Pain at injection site (3%), local irritation (1%)
Neuromuscular & skeletal: Weakness (2% to 4%)
Ophthalmic: Nystagmus (2% to 10%)
Miscellaneous: Laceration (2% to 3%)
<1% (Limited to important or life-threatening): Abnormal hepatic function tests, acute psychosis, aggressive behavior, agitation, agranulocytosis, anemia, angioedema, atrial fibrillation, atrial flutter, atrioventricular block, bradycardia, cerebellar syndrome, cognitive dysfunction, disturbance in attention, DRESS syndrome, euphoria, falling, hallucination, hepatitis, insomnia, nephritis, neutropenia, Stevens-Johnson syndrome, toxic epidermal necrolysis, urticaria

Drug Interactions

Metabolism/Transport Effects Substrate of CYP2C19 (minor), CYP2C9 (minor), CYP3A4 (minor); **Note:** Assignment of Major/Minor substrate status based on clinically relevant drug interaction potential; **Inhibits** CYP2C19 (weak)

Avoid Concomitant Use There are no known interactions where it is recommended to avoid concomitant use.

Increased Effect/Toxicity
The levels/effects of Lacosamide may be increased by: Bradycardia-Causing Agents; CarBAMazepine; CYP2C9 Inhibitors (Strong); CYP3A4 Inhibitors (Strong); Delavirdine; NiCARdipine

Decreased Effect
The levels/effects of Lacosamide may be decreased by: CarBAMazepine; Fosphenytoin; Mefloquine; Mianserin; Orlistat; PHENobarbital; Phenytoin

Preparation for Administration Injection: May be mixed with compatible diluents (NS, LR, D5W) in glass or PVC.

Storage/Stability
Injection: Store at 20°C to 25°C (68°F to 77°F); excursions are permitted between 15°C and 30°C (59°F and 86°F). Do not freeze. Stable when mixed with compatible diluents (NS, LR, D5W) for up to 4 hours at room temperature [Canadian labeling indicates the admixture in glass or polyvinyl chloride (PVC) bags is stable for at least 24 hours at 15°C to 30°C]. Discard any unused portion.
Oral solution, tablets: Store at 20°C to 25°C (68°F to 77°F); excursions are permitted between 15°C and 30°C (59°F and 86°F). Do not freeze oral solution. Discard any unused portion of oral solution after 7 weeks.

Mechanism of Action In vitro studies have shown that lacosamide stabilizes hyperexcitable neuronal membranes and inhibits repetitive neuronal firing by enhancing the slow inactivation of sodium channels (with no effects on fast inactivation of sodium channels).

Pharmacodynamics/Kinetics
Absorption: Oral: Completely
Distribution: V_d: ~0.6 L/kg
Protein binding: <15%
Metabolism: Hepatic via CYP3A4, CYP2C9, and CYP2C19; forms metabolite, O-desmethyl-lacosamide (inactive)
Bioavailability: ~100%
Half-life elimination: ~13 hours
Time to peak, plasma: Oral: 1-4 hours
Excretion: Urine (95%; 40% as unchanged drug, 30% as inactive metabolite, 20% as uncharacterized metabolite); feces (<0.5%)

Dosing

Adult & Geriatric
Partial onset seizure:
Monotherapy: Oral, IV:
Initial: 100 mg twice daily; may be increased at weekly intervals by 50 mg twice daily based on response and tolerability.
Alternative initial dosage: Loading dose: 200 mg followed approximately 12 hours later by 100 mg twice daily for 1 week; may be increased at weekly intervals by 50 mg twice daily based on response and tolerability. **Note:** Administer loading doses under medical supervision because of the increased incidence of CNS adverse reactions.
Maintenance: 150 to 200 mg twice daily. **Note:** For patients already on a single antiepileptic and converting to lacosamide monotherapy, maintain the maintenance dose for 3 days before beginning withdrawal of the concomitant antiepileptic drug. Gradually taper the concomitant antiepileptic drug over ≥6 weeks.
Adjunctive therapy: Oral, IV:
Initial: 50 mg twice daily; may be increased at weekly intervals by 50 mg twice daily based on response and tolerability.

Alternative initial dosage: Loading dose of 200 mg followed approximately 12 hours later by 100 mg twice daily for 1 week; may be increased at weekly intervals by 50 mg twice daily based on response and tolerability. **Note:** Administer loading doses under medical supervision because of the increased incidence of CNS adverse reactions.
Maintenance dose: 100 to 200 mg twice daily (maximum: 400 mg daily)

Status epilepticus, refractory (off-label use): IV: 200 to 400 mg followed by a daily maintenance dose of 200 to 600 mg daily in 2 divided doses (Albers, 2011; Goodwin, 2011; Kellinghaus, 2011; NCS [Brophy, 2012]). **Note:** Although the Neurocritical Care Society recommends administration of the initial dose at a rate of 200 mg over 15 minutes, others have administered doses of up to 400 mg IV push over ≤5 minutes without apparent harm (Goodwin, 2011; Kellinghaus, 2011; NCS [Brophy, 2012]).

Switching from oral to IV dosing: When switching from oral to IV formulations, the total daily dose and frequency should be the same; IV therapy should only be used temporarily. Clinical study experience of IV lacosamide is limited to 5 days of consecutive treatment.

Pediatric Partial onset seizure: Adolescents ≥17 years: Refer to adult dosing.

Renal Impairment Use caution when titrating dose.
Mild-to-moderate renal impairment (CrCl >30 mL/minute): No dosage adjustment necessary. However, in patients with renal impairment taking concomitant strong CYP3A4 and/or CYP2C9 inhibitors, dosage reduction may be necessary.
Severe renal impairment (CrCl ≤30 mL/minute): Maximum dose: 300 mg daily. Further dosage reduction/limitation may be necessary with concomitant use of strong CYP3A4 and/or CYP2C9 inhibitors.
End-stage renal disease (ESRD) requiring hemodialysis: Maximum dose: 300 mg daily. Further dosage reduction/limitation may be necessary with concomitant use of strong CYP3A4 and/or CYP2C9 inhibitors. Removed by hemodialysis; after 4-hour hemodialysis treatment, a supplemental dose of up to 50% should be considered.

Hepatic Impairment Use caution when titrating dose.
Mild-to-moderate hepatic impairment: Maximum dose: 300 mg daily. Further dosage reduction/limitation may be necessary in patients taking concomitant strong CYP3A4 and/or CYP2C9 inhibitors.
Severe hepatic impairment: Use is not recommended.

Dietary Considerations Some products may contain phenylalanine.

Administration
Injection: Administer over 15 to 60 minutes (US labeling) or 30 to 60 minutes (Canadian labeling); infusions over 30 to 60 minutes are preferred to minimize adverse effects. IV administration has been used for up to 5 days. Can be administered without further dilution or may be mixed with compatible diluents (NS, LR, D5W).
Oral solution, tablets: May be administered with or without food. Oral solution should be administered with a calibrated measuring device (not a household teaspoon or tablespoon).

Monitoring Parameters Patients with conduction problems, sodium channelopathies, concomitant medications that prolong PR interval or severe cardiac disease should have ECG tracing prior to start of therapy and when at steady-state. Monitor these patients closely during IV infusions (cases of bradycardia and AV block have occurred during infusions). Monitor for suicidality (eg, suicidal thoughts, depression, behavioral changes).

Dosage Forms Excipient information presented when available (limited, particularly for generics); consult specific product labeling.
Solution, Intravenous:
Vimpat: 200 mg/20 mL (20 mL)
Solution, Oral:
Vimpat: 10 mg/mL (200 mL, 465 mL) [contains aspartame, methylparaben, polyethylene glycol, propylene glycol; strawberry flavor]
Tablet, Oral:
Vimpat: 50 mg [contains fd&c blue #2 aluminum lake]
Vimpat: 100 mg, 150 mg
Vimpat: 200 mg [contains fd&c blue #2 aluminum lake]

Controlled Substance C-V

◆ LaCrosse Complete [OTC] see Sodium Phosphates on page 1677

◆ Lactoflavin see Riboflavin on page 1579

Lactulose (LAK tyoo lose)

Brand Names: US Constulose; Enulose; Generlac; Kristalose

Brand Names: Canada Apo-Lactulose; Euro-Lac; Jamp-Lactulose; PMS-Lactulose; Ratio-Lactulose; Teva-Lactulose

Pharmacologic Category Ammonium Detoxicant; Laxative, Osmotic

Use Prevention and treatment of portal-systemic encephalopathy (including hepatic precoma and coma); treatment of constipation

Pregnancy Considerations Adverse events have not been observed in animal reproduction studies. Lactulose is poorly absorbed following oral administration. Use of dietary fiber or bulk-forming laxatives along with increased fluid intake is generally considered first line therapy for treating constipation in pregnant women. Short-term use of lactulose is also considered to be safe/low risk when therapy is needed; however, side effects may limit its use (Cullen, 2007; Mahadevan, 2006; Prather, 2004; Wald, 2003).

Breast-Feeding Considerations It is not known if lactulose is excreted into breast milk; however, lactulose is poorly absorbed following oral administration. The manufacturer recommends that caution be used if administered to a nursing woman.

Contraindications Use in patients requiring a low galactose diet

Warnings/Precautions Use with caution in patients with diabetes mellitus; solution contains galactose and lactose. Monitor periodically for electrolyte imbalance when lactulose is used >6 months or in patients predisposed to electrolyte abnormalities (eg, elderly). Hepatic disease may predispose patients to electrolyte imbalance. Infants receiving lactulose may develop hyponatremia and dehydration. Patients receiving lactulose and an oral anti-infective agent should be monitored for possible inadequate response to lactulose. During proctoscopy or colonoscopy procedures involving electrocautery, a theoretical risk of reaction between H_2 gas accumulation and electrical spark may exist; thorough bowel cleansing with a nonfermentable solution is recommended.

Adverse Reactions Frequency not defined.

Endocrine & metabolic: Dehydration, hypernatremia, hypokalemia

Gastrointestinal: Abdominal discomfort, abdominal distention, belching, cramping, diarrhea (excessive dose), flatulence, nausea, vomiting

Drug Interactions

Metabolism/Transport Effects None known.

Avoid Concomitant Use There are no known interactions where it is recommended to avoid concomitant use.

Increased Effect/Toxicity There are no known significant interactions involving an increase in effect.

Decreased Effect

The levels/effects of Lactulose may be decreased by: Glutamine

Storage/Stability Store at room temperature; do not freeze. Protect from light. Discard solution if cloudy or very dark. Prolonged exposure to cold temperatures will cause thickening which will return to normal upon warming to room temperature.

Mechanism of Action The bacterial degradation of lactulose resulting in an acidic pH inhibits the diffusion of NH_3 into the blood by causing the conversion of NH_3 to NH_4+; also enhances the diffusion of NH_3 from the blood into the gut where conversion to NH_4+ occurs; produces an osmotic effect in the colon with resultant distention promoting peristalsis; reduces blood ammonia concentration to reduce the degree of portal systemic encephalopathy

Pharmacodynamics/Kinetics

Onset:

Constipation: Up to 24 to 48 hours to produce a normal bowel movement

Encephalopathy: At least 24 to 48 hours

Absorption: Not appreciable

Metabolism: Via colonic flora to lactic acid and acetic acid; requires colonic flora for drug activation

Excretion: Primarily feces; urine (≤3%)

Dosing

Adult & Geriatric

Constipation: Oral: 10 to 20 g (15 to 30 mL) daily; may increase to 40 g (60 mL) daily if necessary

Prevention of portal systemic encephalopathy (PSE):

Oral: 20 to 30 g (30 to 45 mL) 3 to 4 times/day; adjust dose every 1 to 2 days to produce 2 to 3 soft stools/day

Treatment of acute PSE:

Oral: 20 to 30 g (30 to 45 mL) every 1 hour to induce rapid laxation; reduce to 20 to 30 g (30 to 45 mL) 3 to 4 times/day after laxation is achieved titrate to produce 2 to 3 soft stools/day

Rectal administration (retention enema): 200 g (300 mL) diluted with 700 mL of water or NS via rectal balloon catheter; retain for 30 to 60 minutes; may repeat every 4 to 6 hours; transition to oral treatment prior to discontinuing rectal administration

Treatment of overt hepatic encephalopathy (OHE) episodes: Route not specified: 16.7 g (25 mL) every 1 to 2 hours until at least 2 soft or loose bowel movements are produced daily; titrate to maintain 2 to 3 bowel movements daily (AASLD [Vilstrup 2014]).

Pediatric

Prevention of portal systemic encephalopathy (PSE):

Oral:

Infants: 1.7 to 6.7 g/day (2.5 to 10 mL/day) in divided doses; adjust dosage to produce 2 to 3 stools/day

Children: 26.7 to 60 g/day (40 to 90 mL/day) in divided doses; adjust dosage to produce 2 to 3 stools/day

Constipation (off-label use): Oral: 0.7 to 2 g/kg/day (1 to 3 mL/kg/day) in divided doses, maximum: 40 g/day (60 mL/day) (NASPGHAN, 2006)

Renal Impairment There are no dosage adjustments provided in the manufacturer's labeling.

Hepatic Impairment There are no dosage adjustments provided in the manufacturer's labeling.

Dietary Considerations Contraindicated in patients on galactose-restricted diet.

Administration

Oral solution: May mix with fruit juice, water or milk.

Crystals for oral solution: Dissolve contents of packet in 120 mL water.

Rectal: Mix with water or normal saline; administer as retention enema using a rectal balloon catheter; retain for 30 to 60 minutes. Transition to oral lactulose when appropriate (able to take oral medication and no longer a risk for aspiration) prior to discontinuing rectal administration

Monitoring Parameters Blood pressure, standing/supine; serum electrolytes, serum ammonia; bowel movement patterns, fluid status

Dosage Forms Excipient information presented when available (limited, particularly for generics); consult specific product labeling. [DSC] = Discontinued product

Packet, Oral:

Kristalose: 10 g (30 ea); 20 g (30 ea)

Solution, Oral:

Constulose: 10 g/15 mL (946 mL [DSC])

Constulose: 10 g/15 mL (237 mL, 946 mL) [unflavored flavor]

Enulose: 10 g/15 mL (473 mL [DSC])

Enulose: 10 g/15 mL (473 mL) [unflavored flavor]

Generlac: 10 g/15 mL (473 mL, 1892 mL) [unflavored flavor]

Generic: 10 g/15 mL (15 mL, 30 mL, 236 mL, 237 mL, 473 mL, 500 mL, 946 mL, 1892 mL); 20 g/30 mL (30 mL)

LamiVUDine (la MI vyoo deen)

Brand Names: US Epivir; Epivir HBV
Brand Names: Canada 3TC; Apo-Lamivudine; Apo-Lamivudine HBV; Heptovir
Index Terms 3TC
Pharmacologic Category Antihepadnaviral, Reverse Transcriptase Inhibitor, Nucleoside (Anti-HBV); Antiretroviral, Reverse Transcriptase Inhibitor, Nucleoside (Anti-HIV)
Use

Chronic hepatitis B (Epivir HBV, Heptovir [Canadian product]): Treatment of chronic hepatitis B associated with evidence of hepatitis B viral replication and active liver inflammation.

Limitations of use: Use only when an alternative antiviral agent with a higher genetic barrier to resistance is not available or appropriate; has not been evaluated in patients with HBV-HIV-1 coinfection, hepatitis C virus or hepatitis delta virus; has also not been evaluated in patients with chronic HBV infection with decompensated liver disease or in liver transplant recipients.

HIV-1 infection (Epivir, 3TC [Canadian product]): Treatment of HIV-1 in combination with other antiretroviral agents

Pregnancy Considerations Adverse events were observed in some animal reproduction studies. Lamivudine has a high level of transfer across the human placenta. No increased risk of overall birth defects has been observed following first trimester exposure according to data collected by the antiretroviral pregnancy registry. The pharmacokinetics of lamivudine during pregnancy are not significantly altered and dosage adjustment is not required. Cases of lactic acidosis/hepatic steatosis syndrome related to mitochondrial toxicity have been reported in pregnant women with prolonged use of nucleoside analogues. It is not known if pregnancy itself potentiates this known side effect; however, women may be at increased risk of lactic acidosis and liver damage. In addition, these adverse events are similar to other rare but life-threatening syndromes which occur during pregnancy (eg, HELLP syndrome). Hepatic enzymes and electrolytes should be monitored in women receiving nucleoside analogues and clinicians should watch for early signs of the syndrome. In addition, mitochondrial dysfunction may develop in infants following in utero exposure. The DHHS Perinatal HIV Guidelines consider lamivudine in combination with either abacavir, tenofovir, or zidovudine to be a preferred NRTI backbone for antiretroviral-naive pregnant women. The DHHS Perinatal HIV Guidelines also consider lamivudine plus tenofovir a recommended dual NRTI/NtRTI backbone for HIV/HBV coinfected pregnant women. Use caution with hepatitis B coinfection; hepatitis B flare may occur if lamivudine is discontinued postpartum.

Regardless of CD4 count or HIV RNA copy number, all HIV-infected pregnant women should receive a combination antiretroviral (ARV) drug regimen. A combination of antepartum, intrapartum, and infant ARV prophylaxis is recommended. ARV therapy should be started as soon as possible in women with symptomatic infection. Although earlier initiation may be more effective in reducing the perinatal transmission of HIV, initiation may be delayed until after 12 weeks gestation in women who do not require immediate treatment after careful consideration of maternal conditions (eg, nausea and vomiting) and the potential risks of first trimester fetal exposure for specific agents. A scheduled cesarean delivery at 38 weeks gestation is recommended for all women with HIV RNA >1000 copies/mL or unknown concentrations near delivery in order to decrease transmission. If ARV therapy must be interrupted for <24 hours during the peripartum period, stop then restart all medications simultaneously in order to decrease the chance of developing resistance. Long-term follow-up is recommended for all infants exposed to ARV medications. In couples who want to conceive, the HIV-infected partner should attain maximum viral suppression prior to conception.

Health care providers are encouraged to enroll pregnant women exposed to antiretroviral medications in the Antiretroviral Pregnancy Registry (1-800-258-4263 or www.APRegistry.com). In Canada, health care providers prescribing Heptovir are encouraged to enroll pregnant women at 800-387-7374. Health care providers caring for HIV-infected women and their infants may contact the National Perinatal HIV Hotline (888-448-8765) for clinical consultation (HHS [perinatal], 2014).

Breast-Feeding Considerations Lamivudine is excreted into breast milk and can be detected in the serum of nursing infants.

Maternal or infant antiretroviral therapy does not completely eliminate the risk of postnatal HIV transmission. In addition, multiclass-resistant virus has been detected in breast-feeding infants despite maternal therapy. Therefore, in the United States, where formula is accessible, affordable, safe, and sustainable, and the risk of infant mortality due to diarrhea and respiratory infections is low, complete avoidance of breast-feeding by HIV-infected women is recommended to decrease potential transmission of HIV (HHS [perinatal], 2014).

Contraindications Hypersensitivity (eg, anaphylaxis) to lamivudine or any component of the formulation

Warnings/Precautions Use caution with renal impairment; dosage reduction recommended. Use with extreme caution in children with history of pancreatitis or risk factors for development of pancreatitis. Pancreatitis has been reported, particularly in HIV-infected children with a history of nucleoside use. Do not use as monotherapy in treatment of HIV. Lamivudine combined with emtricitabine is not recommended as a dual-NRTI combination due to similar resistance patterns and negligible additive antiviral activity; lamivudine and abacavir or tenofovir combination is recommended as the NRTIs in a fully suppressive antiretroviral regimen. Do not use lamivudine/abacavir (plus efavirenz or plus atazanavir/ritonavir) in adolescent and adult HIV-1 patients with a pre-ART HIV RNA >100,000 copies/mL (HHS [adult], 2015). Treatment of HBV in patients with unrecognized/untreated HIV may lead to rapid HIV resistance. In addition, treatment of HIV in patients with unrecognized/untreated HBV may lead to rapid HBV resistance. Use with caution in combination with interferon alfa with or without ribavirin in HIV/HBV coinfected patients; monitor closely for hepatic decompensation, anemia, or neutropenia; dose reduction or discontinuation of interferon and/or ribavirin may be required if toxicity evident. In HIV/HBV coinfection, lamivudine and tenofovir are a recommended NRTI backbone in a fully suppressive antiretroviral regimen to provide activity against both HIV and HBV (DHHS [adult], 2015). **[US Boxed Warning]: Do not use Epivir HBV tablets or Epivir HBV oral solution for the treatment of HIV.** In Canada, Heptovir tablets and oral solution are not approved for treatment of HIV. Potentially significant drug-drug interactions may exist, requiring dose or frequency adjustment, additional monitoring, and/or selection of alternative therapy. Lamivudine oral solution contains 3 g of sucrose/15 mL; advise diabetic patients of sucrose content. Some dosage forms may contain propylene glycol; large amounts are potentially toxic and have been associated hyperosmolality, lactic acidosis, seizures and respiratory depression; use caution (AAP, 1997; Zar, 2007).

[US Boxed Warning]: Lactic acidosis and severe hepatomegaly with steatosis have been reported, including fatal cases. Use caution in hepatic impairment. Pregnancy, obesity, and/or prolonged therapy may increase the risk of lactic acidosis and liver damage.

Immune reconstitution syndrome may develop resulting in the occurrence of an inflammatory response to an indolent or residual opportunistic infection during initial HIV treatment or activation of autoimmune disorders (eg, Graves' disease, polymyositis, Guillain-Barré syndrome) later in therapy. May be associated with fat redistribution. Concomitant use of other lamivudine-containing products should be avoided.

[US Boxed Warning]: Monitor patients closely for several months following discontinuation of therapy for chronic hepatitis B; clinical exacerbations may occur, including fatal cases. **Monitor hepatic function with clinical and laboratory follow up for at least several months after hepatitis B treatment discontinuation. Initiate antihepatitis B (HBV) medications if clinically appropriate. [US Boxed Warning]: HIV-1 resistance may emerge in chronic hepatitis B-infection patients with unrecognized or untreated HIV-1 infection. Counseling and (HIV) testing should be offered to all patients before beginning treatment with lamivudine for hepatitis B and then periodically during treatment. Lamivudine dosing for hepatitis B is subtherapeutic if used for HIV-1 infection treatment. Lamivudine monotherapy is not appropriate for HIV-1 infection treatment.** Lamivudine resistant HIV-1 can develop rapidly and limit treatment options if used in unrecognized or untreated HIV-1 infection or if a patient becomes coinfected during HBV treatment. Lamivudine dosing for hepatitis B is also subtherapeutic if used for HIV-1/HBV coinfection treatment. If lamivudine is chosen as part of a HIV-1 treatment regimen in coinfected patients, the higher lamivudine dosage indicated for HIV-1 therapy should be used, with other drugs, in an appropriate combination regimen. Emergence of lamivudine resistant HBV variants

has also been reported in HIV-1/HBV coinfected patients who have received lamivudine-containing antiretroviral regimens.

Not recommended as first-line therapy of chronic HBV due to high rate of resistance. Consider use only if other anti-HBV antiviral regimens with more favorable resistance patterns cannot be used. May be appropriate for short-term treatment of acute HBV (Lok, 2009). Potential compliance problems, frequency of administration, and adverse effects should be discussed with patients before initiating therapy to help prevent the emergence of resistance.

Adverse Reactions Incidence data include patients on combination therapy with other antiretroviral agents.

>10%:

Central nervous system: Headache (21% to 35%), fatigue (24% to 27%), insomnia (11%)

Gastrointestinal: Nausea (15% to 33%), diarrhea (14% to 18%), pancreatitis (range: 0.3% to 18%; higher percentage in pediatric patients), abdominal pain (9% to 16%), vomiting (13% to 15%)

Hematologic: Neutropenia (7% to 15%)

Hepatic: Transaminases increased (2% to 11%)

Neuromuscular & skeletal: Myalgia (8% to 14%), neuropathy (12%), musculoskeletal pain (12%)

Respiratory: Nasal signs and symptoms (20%), cough (18%), sore throat (13%)

Miscellaneous: Infections (25%; includes ear, nose, and throat)

1% to 10%:

Central nervous system: Dizziness (10%), depression (9%), fever (7% to 10%), chills (7% to 10%)

Dermatologic: Rash (5% to 9%)

Gastrointestinal: Anorexia (10%), lipase increased (10%), abdominal cramps (6%), dyspepsia (5%), amylase increased (<1% to 4%), heartburn

Hematologic: Thrombocytopenia (1% to 4%), hemoglobinemia (2% to 3%)

Neuromuscular & skeletal: Creatine phosphokinase increased (9%), arthralgia (5% to 7%)

<1% (Limited to important or life-threatening): Alopecia, anaphylaxis, anemia, body fat redistribution, hepatitis B exacerbation, hepatomegaly, hyperbilirubinemia, hyperglycemia, immune reconstitution syndrome, lactic acidosis, lymphadenopathy, muscle weakness, paresthesia, peripheral neuropathy, pruritus, red cell aplasia, rhabdomyolysis, splenomegaly, steatosis, stomatitis, urticaria, weakness, wheezing

Drug Interactions

Metabolism/Transport Effects None known.

Avoid Concomitant Use

Avoid concomitant use of LamiVUDine with any of the following: Emtricitabine

Increased Effect/Toxicity

LamiVUDine may increase the levels/effects of: Emtricitabine

The levels/effects of LamiVUDine may be increased by: Ganciclovir-Valganciclovir; Ribavirin (Oral Inhalation); Ribavirin (Systemic); Trimethoprim

Decreased Effect There are no known significant interactions involving a decrease in effect.

Food Interactions Food decreases the rate of absorption and C$_{max}$; however, there is no change in the systemic AUC. Management: Administer with or without food.

Storage/Stability

Oral solution:

Epivir: Store at 25°C (77°F) tightly closed.

Epivir HBV: Store at 20°C to 25°C (68°F to 77°F) tightly closed.

3TC [Canadian product]: Store at 2°C to 25°C (35.6°F to 77°F).

Heptovir [Canadian product]: Store at 15°C and 25°C (59°F and 77°F).

Tablet:

Epivir, Epivir HBV: Store at 25°C (77°F); excursions are permitted between 15°C and 30°C (59°F and 86°F).

3TC, Heptovir [Canadian products]: Store at 2°C to 30°C (35.6°F to 86°F).

Mechanism of Action Lamivudine is a cytosine analog. *In vitro*, lamivudine is triphosphorylated, the principle mode of action is inhibition of HIV reverse transcription via viral DNA chain termination; inhibits RNA- and DNA-dependent DNA polymerase activities of reverse transcriptase. In hepatitis B, the monophosphate form of lamivudine is incorporated into the viral DNA by hepatitis B virus polymerase, resulting in DNA chain termination.

Pharmacodynamics/Kinetics

Absorption: Rapid

Distribution: Into extravascular spaces

Children (n=38): CSF concentrations were 14.2 ± 7.9% of the serum concentration

V$_d$: 1.3 ± 0.4 L/kg

Protein binding: Plasma: <36%

Metabolism: Minor; only known metabolite is trans-sulfoxide metabolite

Bioavailability: Absolute; Cp$_{max}$ decreased with food although AUC not significantly affected

Children: Oral solution: 66% ± 26%

Adolescents and Adults: Oral solution: 87% ± 13%; Tablet 150 mg: 86% ± 16%

Half-life:

Intracellular: 10 to 15 hours

Elimination:

Children 4 months to 14 years: 2 ± 0.6 hours

Adults: 5 to 7 hours; increased with renal impairment

Time to peak, plasma:

Pediatric patients 0.5 to 17 years: Median: 1.5 hours (range: 0.5 to 4 hours) (Lewis 1996)

Adolescents 13 to 17 years: 0.5 to 1 hour

Adults: Fed: 3.2 hours; Fasted: 0.9 hours

Excretion: Primarily urine (majority as unchanged drug); weight-corrected oral clearance is highest at age 2 years, then declines from age 2 to 12 years, where values then remain comparable to adult values

Dosing

Adult & Geriatric Note: The formulation and dosage of Epivir HBV or Heptovir [Canadian product] are not appropriate for patients infected with both HBV and HIV; tenofovir and lamivudine are a preferred NRTI backbone in a fully suppressive antiretroviral regimen and for the treatment of HBV coinfection (HHS [adult] 2015).

HIV-1 infection (Epivir, 3TC [Canadian product]): Oral (use in combination with other antiretroviral agents): 150 mg twice daily or 300 mg once daily.

Note: Lamivudine is a component of recommended initial regimens for any ART-naive patient (when coadministered with tenofovir plus dolutegravir, with tenofovir plus raltegravir, or with tenofovir plus darunavir/ritonavir) or for ART-naive patients who are HLA-B*5701 negative (when coadministered with abacavir plus dolutegravir) (HHS [adult] 2015).

Postexposure prophylaxis for HIV exposure (off-label use [CDC 2005]): Oral: 150 mg twice daily or 300 mg once daily (in combination with zidovudine, tenofovir, stavudine, or didanosine, with or without a protease inhibitor depending on risk)

Treatment of hepatitis B (Epivir HBV, Heptovir [Canadian product]): Note: Not a preferred agent in chronic HBV treatment due to high rates of resistance; consider alternative agents. Oral: 100 mg once daily

Treatment duration (AASLD practice guidelines):

Hepatitis Be antigen (HBeAg) positive chronic hepatitis: Treat ≥1 year until HBeAg seroconversion and undetectable serum HBV DNA; continue therapy for ≥6 months after HBeAg seroconversion

HBeAg negative chronic hepatitis: Treat >1 year until hepatitis B surface antigen (HBsAg) clearance

Note: Patients not achieving <2 log decrease in serum HBV DNA after at least 6 months of therapy should either receive additional treatment or be switched to an alternative therapy (Lok 2009).

Treatment of hepatitis B/HIV coinfection (in patients with both infections requiring treatment): Note: The formulation and dosage of Epivir HBV or Heptovir [Canadian product] are not appropriate for patients infected with both HBV and HIV. Tenofovir and lamivudine are a preferred NRTI backbone in a fully suppressive antiretroviral regimen for the treatment of HIV/HBV coinfection (HHS [adult] 2015).

Oral: 150 mg twice daily or 300 mg/dose once daily, in combination with other antiretrovirals in an antiretroviral (ARV) regimen (HHS [adult] 2015)

Pediatric

HIV-1 infection: (Epivir, 3TC [Canadian product]): Note: Use in combination with other antiretroviral agents when treating HIV.

Infants 1 to 3 months (off-label use; HHS [pediatric] 2014): Oral: 4 mg/kg/dose twice daily

Manufacturer's labeling:

Infants ≥3 months, Children, and Adolescents: **Note:** In clinical studies data regarding efficacy of once-daily dosing are limited to subjects transitioned from twice daily dosing to once daily dosing after 36 weeks of treatment.

Oral solution:
US labeling: 8 mg/kg/day in 1 to 2 divided doses (maximum: 300 mg/day)
Canadian labeling:
<25 kg: 8 mg/kg/day in 1 to 2 divided doses (maximum: 300 mg/day)
≥25 kg: 150 mg twice daily or 300 mg once daily (maximum: 300 mg/day)
Oral tablets:
14 to <20 kg: 75 mg twice daily or 150 mg once daily
≥20 to <25 kg: 75 mg in the morning, 150 mg in the evening or 225 mg once daily
≥25 kg: 150 mg twice daily or 300 mg once daily
Alternate dosing (weight-based dosing) (HHS [pediatric] 2014): **Note:** Use scored 150 mg tablets for dosing.
14 to 21 kg: 75 mg twice daily (150 mg/day)
22 to 29 kg: 75 mg in the morning, 150 mg in the evening (225 mg/day)
≥30 kg: 150 mg twice daily (300 mg/day)

Postexposure prophylaxis for HIV exposure (off-label use [CDC 2005]): Adolescents ≥16 years: Refer to adult dosing.

Treatment of hepatitis B/HIV coinfection (in patients with both infections requiring treatment): Note: The formulation and dosage of Epivir HBV or Heptovir [Canadian product] are not appropriate for patients infected with both HBV and HIV.
Infants and Children: Oral: 4 mg/kg/dose (maximum: 150 mg) twice daily, in combination with other antiretrovirals in an ARV regimen (DHHS [pediatric] 2013)
Adolescents: Refer to adult dosing.

Treatment of hepatitis B (Epivir HBV, Heptovir [Canadian product]): Note: Not a preferred agent in chronic HBV treatment due to high rates of resistance; consider alternative agents: Tablets and oral solution may be used interchangeably; for doses <100 mg, oral solution is recommended.
Epivir HBV: Children and Adolescents 2 to 17 years: Oral: 3 mg/kg/dose once daily (maximum: 100 mg/day)
Treatment duration (AASLD practice guidelines):
Hepatitis Be antigen (HBeAg) positive chronic hepatitis: Treat ≥1 year until HBeAg seroconversion and undetectable serum HBV DNA; continue therapy for ≥6 months after HBeAg seroconversion
HBeAg negative chronic hepatitis: Treat >1 year until hepatitis B surface antigen (HBsAg) clearance
Note: Patients not achieving <2 log decrease in serum HBV DNA after at least 6 months of therapy should either receive additional treatment or be switched to an alternative therapy (Lok 2009).
Heptovir [Canadian product]: Adolescents ≥16 years: Refer to adult dosing.
Renal Impairment
HIV-1 infection:
Adults:
End stage renal disease (ESRD) requiring hemodialysis: Administer 50 mg first dose, then 25 mg once daily (IDSA [Lucas 2014]). Negligible amounts are removed by 4-hour hemodialysis or peritoneal dialysis. Supplemental dosing not needed; however, dosing after dialysis is recommended (HHS [adult] 2015).
Adolescents ≥25 kg and Adults:
Manufacturer's labeling:
CrCl ≥50 mL/minute: No dosage adjustment necessary
CrCl 30 to 49 mL/minute: Administer 150 mg once daily
CrCl 15 to 29 mL/minute: Administer 150 mg first dose, then 100 mg once daily
CrCl 5 to 14 mL/minute: Administer 150 mg first dose, then 50 mg once daily
CrCl <5 mL/minute: Administer 50 mg first dose, then 25 mg once daily
Infants ≥3 months, Children, and Adolescents <25 kg:
US labeling: There are no dosage adjustments provided in the manufacturer's labeling (insufficient data); however, dose reduction should be considered.
Canadian labeling:
CrCl 30 to 50 mL/minute: Administer 4 mg/kg once daily
CrCl 15 to 29 mL/minute: Administer 4 mg/kg first dose, then 2.6 mg/kg once daily
CrCl 5 to 14 mL/minute: Administer 4 mg/kg first dose, then 1.3 mg/kg once daily
CrCl <5 mL/minute: Administer 1.3 mg/kg first dose, then 0.7 mg/kg once daily

Treatment of hepatitis B patients: Adults (US labeling) or Adolescents ≥16 years and Adults (Canadian labeling):
CrCl ≥50 mL/minute: No dosage adjustment necessary.
CrCl 30 to 49 mL/minute: Administer 100 mg first dose, then 50 mg once daily.
CrCl 15 to 29 mL/minute: Administer 100 mg first dose, then 25 mg once daily.
CrCl 5 to 14 mL/minute: Administer 35 mg first dose, then 15 mg once daily.
CrCl <5 mL/minute: Administer 35 mg first dose, then 10 mg once daily.
ESRD requiring hemodialysis: Negligible amounts are removed by 4-hour hemodialysis or peritoneal dialysis. Supplemental dosing not needed; however, dosing after dialysis is recommended (HHS [adult] 2015).
Hepatic Impairment No dosage adjustment necessary. However, has not been studied in the setting of decompensated liver disease.
Dietary Considerations Some products may contain sucrose.
Administration Oral: May be administered without regard to meals.
Monitoring Parameters Amylase, bilirubin, liver enzymes (every 3 months during therapy), hematologic parameters, HIV viral load, and CD4 count; signs/symptoms of pancreatitis or hepatonecroinflammation (Epivir HBV), HBV DNA (regularly during therapy), HBeAg and anti-HBe (after 1 year of therapy and every 3 to 6 months thereafter); signs/symptoms of HBV relapse/exacerbation (for at least several months after stopping treatment)
Dosage Forms Excipient information presented when available (limited, particularly for generics); consult specific product labeling.
Solution, Oral:
Epivir: 10 mg/mL (240 mL) [contains methylparaben, propylene glycol, propylparaben; strawberry-banana flavor]
Epivir HBV: 5 mg/mL (240 mL) [contains methylparaben, propylene glycol, propylparaben; strawberry-banana flavor]
Generic: 10 mg/mL (240 mL)
Tablet, Oral:
Epivir: 150 mg [scored]
Epivir: 300 mg
Epivir HBV: 100 mg
Generic: 100 mg, 150 mg, 300 mg
Dosage Forms: Canada Excipient information presented when available (limited, particularly for generics); consult specific product labeling.
Solution, Oral:
3TC: 10 mg/mL (240 mL) [contains methylparaben, propylene glycol, propylparaben; strawberry-banana flavor]
Heptovir: 5 mg/mL (240 mL) [contains methylparaben, propylene glycol, propylparaben; strawberry-banana flavor]
Tablet, Oral:
3TC: 150 mg [scored]
3TC: 300 mg
Heptovir: 100 mg

◆ Lamivudine, Abacavir, and Dolutegravir see Abacavir, Dolutegravir, and Lamivudine on page 18

◆ Lamivudine, Abacavir, and Zidovudine see Abacavir, Lamivudine, and Zidovudine on page 18

◆ Lamivudine and Abacavir see Abacavir and Lamivudine on page 18

Lamivudine and Zidovudine
(la MI vyoo deen & zye DOE vyoo deen)

Brand Names: US Combivir
Brand Names: Canada Combivir; Teva-Lamivudine/Zidovudine
Index Terms AZT + 3TC (error-prone abbreviation); Zidovudine and Lamivudine
Pharmacologic Category Antiretroviral, Reverse Transcriptase Inhibitor, Nucleoside (Anti-HIV)
Use HIV-1 infection: Treatment of HIV-1 infection in combination with other antiretrovirals.
Dosing
Adult Note: Because this is a fixed-dose combination product, avoid use in patients requiring dosage reduction.
HIV-1 infection: Oral: One tablet twice daily.
Pediatric HIV-1 infection: Children and Adolescents weighing ≥30 kg: Refer to adult dosing.
Renal Impairment
CrCl ≥50 mL/minute: No dosage adjustment necessary.
CrCl <50 mL/minute: Use is not recommended (use dose-adjusted individual components).

Hepatic Impairment Use is not recommended (use dose-adjusted individual components).

Additional Information Complete prescribing information should be consulted for additional detail.

Dosage Forms Excipient information presented when available (limited, particularly for generics); consult specific product labeling.

Tablet, oral: Lamivudine 150 mg and zidovudine 300 mg

Combivir: Lamivudine 150 mg and zidovudine 300 mg [scored]

LamoTRIgine (la MOE tri jeen)

Brand Names: US LaMICtal; LaMICtal ODT; LaMICtal Starter; LaMICtal XR

Brand Names: Canada Apo-Lamotrigine; Auro-Lamotrigine; Lamictal; Mylan-Lamotrigine; PMS-Lamotrigine; ratio-Lamotrigine; Teva-Lamotrigine

Index Terms BW-430C; LTG

Pharmacologic Category Anticonvulsant, Miscellaneous

Use

US labeling:

Bipolar I disorder (immediate release only): Maintenance treatment of bipolar I disorder to delay the time to occurrence of mood episodes (depression, mania, hypomania, mixed episodes) in patients treated for acute mood episodes with standard therapy.

Epilepsy:

Adjunctive therapy:

Immediate release: Adjunctive therapy for partial-onset seizures, generalized seizures of Lennox-Gastaut syndrome, and primary generalized tonic-clonic seizures in adults and children 2 years and older.

Extended release: Adjunctive therapy for primary generalized tonic-clonic seizures and partial-onset seizures with or without secondary generalization in patients 13 years and older.

Monotherapy:

Immediate release: Conversion to monotherapy in adults (16 years and older) with partial-onset seizures who are receiving treatment with carbamazepine, phenytoin, phenobarbital, primidone, or valproate as the single antiepileptic drug (AED).

Extended release: Conversion to monotherapy in patients 13 years and older with partial-onset seizures who are receiving treatment with a single AED.

Canadian labeling: **Epilepsy:** Immediate release:

Adjunctive therapy: Adjunctive therapy for epilepsy uncontrolled by conventional therapy in adults; seizures associated with Lennox-Gastaut syndrome in children ≥9 kg and adults.

Monotherapy: Monotherapy in adults with epilepsy following withdrawal of concurrent AEDs

Pregnancy Considerations Adverse events have been observed in animal reproduction studies. Lamotrigine crosses the human placenta and can be measured in the plasma of exposed newborns (Harden and Pennell, 2009; Ohman, 2000). An overall increase in major congenital malformations has not been observed in available studies; however, an increased risk for cleft lip or cleft palate has not been ruled out (Cunnington, 2011; Hernández-Díaz, 2012; Holmes, 2012). An increased risk of malformations following maternal lamotrigine use may be associated with larger doses (Cunnington, 2007; Tomson, 2011). Polytherapy may increase the risk of congenital malformations; monotherapy with the lowest effective dose is recommended (Harden and Meader, 2009).

Due to pregnancy-induced physiologic changes, women who are pregnant may require dose adjustments of lamotrigine in order to maintain clinical response; monitoring during pregnancy should be considered (Harden and Pennell, 2009). For women with epilepsy who are planning a pregnancy in advance, baseline serum concentrations should be measured once or twice prior to pregnancy during a period when seizure control is optimal. Monitoring can then be continued up to once a month during pregnancy and every second day during the first week postpartum (Patsalos, 2008). In women taking lamotrigine who are trying to avoid pregnancy, potentially significant interactions may exist with hormone-containing contraceptives; consult drug interactions database for more detailed information.

Pregnancy registries are available for women who have been exposed to lamotrigine. Patients may enroll themselves in the North American Antiepileptic Drug (NAAED) Pregnancy Registry by calling (888) 233-2334. Additional information is available at www.aedpregnancyregistry.org.

Breast-Feeding Considerations Lamotrigine is excreted in breast milk and may be as high as 50% of the maternal serum concentration. Adverse events observed in breast-feeding infants include apnea, drowsiness, and poor sucking. The manufacturer recommends that caution be exercised when administering lamotrigine to nursing women and to monitor the nursing infant.

Medication Guide Available Yes

Contraindications Hypersensitivity (eg, rash, angioedema, acute urticaria, extensive pruritus, mucosal ulceration) to lamotrigine or any component of the formulation

Warnings/Precautions [US Boxed Warning]: Serious skin rashes requiring hospitalization and discontinuation of treatment have been reported; incidence of serious rash is higher in pediatric patients than adults; risk may be increased by coadministration with valproic acid, higher than recommended initial doses, exceeding recommended initial dose titration, or exceeding the recommended dose escalation for lamotrigine. One rash-related death was reported in a pediatric patients taking lamotrigine immediate-release as adjunctive therapy. Nearly all cases of life-threatening rashes associated with lamotrigine have occurred within 2 to 8 weeks of treatment initiation; however, isolated cases may occur after prolonged treatment (eg, 6 months) or in patients without these risk factors; discontinue at first sign of rash and do not reinitiate therapy unless rash is clearly not drug related. Rare cases of toxic epidermal necrolysis and/or rash-related death have been reported. Discontinuation of treatment may not prevent a rash from becoming life-threatening or permanently disabling or disfiguring.

Antiepileptics are associated with an increased risk of suicidal behavior/thoughts with use (regardless of indication); patients should be monitored for signs/symptoms of depression, suicidal tendencies, and other unusual behavior changes during therapy and instructed to inform their healthcare provider immediately if symptoms occur.

A spectrum of hematologic effects have been reported with use (eg, neutropenia, leukopenia, thrombocytopenia, pancytopenia, anemias, and rarely, aplastic anemia and pure red cell aplasia); patients with a previous history of adverse hematologic reaction to any drug may be at increased risk. Early detection of hematologic change is important; advise patients of early signs and symptoms including fever, sore throat, mouth ulcers, infections, easy bruising, petechial or purpuric hemorrhage. May be associated with hypersensitivity syndrome (eg, anticonvulsant hypersensitivity syndrome). Multiorgan hypersensitivity reactions (drug reaction with eosinophilia and systemic symptoms [DRESS]) have been reported. Symptoms may include fever, rash, and/or lymphadenopathy; monitor for signs and symptoms of possible disparate manifestations associated with lymphatic, hepatic, renal, and/or hematologic organ systems. Evaluate patient with fever and lymphadenopathy, even if rash is not present; discontinuation and conversion to alternate therapy may be required. Increased risk of developing aseptic meningitis has been reported; symptoms (eg, headache, nuchal rigidity, fever, nausea/vomiting, rash, photophobia) have generally occurred within 1 to 45 days following therapy initiation. Use caution in patients with renal or hepatic impairment. Avoid abrupt cessation, taper over at least 2 weeks if possible.

May cause CNS depression, which may impair physical or mental abilities. Patients must be cautioned about performing tasks which require mental alertness (eg, operating machinery or driving). Effects with other sedative drugs or ethanol may be potentiated. Binds to melanin and may accumulate in the eye and other melanin-rich tissues; the clinical significance of this is not known. Safety and efficacy for the treatment of epilepsy have not been established for use as initial monotherapy, conversion to monotherapy from antiepileptic drugs (AED) other than carbamazepine, phenytoin, phenobarbital, primidone or valproic acid or conversion to monotherapy from two or more AEDs. Patients treated for bipolar disorder should be monitored closely for clinical worsening or suicidality; reassess patients to determine the need for maintenance treatment if on therapy >16 weeks. Prescriptions should be written for the smallest quantity consistent with good patient care. Treatment of acute manic or mixed episodes is not recommended; efficacy has not been established and slow titration limits use. Children are at increased risk for developing serious skin rashes during therapy; lower starting doses and slower dose escalations may decrease the risk of rash. Potentially significant drug-drug interactions may exist, requiring dose or frequency adjustment,

additional monitoring, and/or selection of alternative therapy. There is a potential for medication errors with similar-sounding medications and among different lamotrigine formulations; medication errors have occurred.

Some dosage forms may contain polysorbate 80 (also known as Tweens). Hypersensitivity reactions, usually a delayed reaction, have been reported following exposure to pharmaceutical products containing polysorbate 80 in certain individuals (Isaksson, 2002; Lucente, 2000; Shelley, 1995). Thrombocytopenia, ascites, pulmonary deterioration, and renal and hepatic failure have been reported in premature neonates after receiving parenteral products containing polysorbate 80 (Alade, 1986; CDC, 1984). See manufacturer's labeling.

Adverse Reactions Percentages reported in adults on monotherapy for epilepsy or bipolar disorder.

>10%: Gastrointestinal: Nausea (7% to 14%)

1% to 10%:

Cardiovascular: Chest pain (5%), peripheral edema (2% to 5%), edema (1% to 5%)

Central nervous system: Insomnia (5% to 10%), drowsiness (9%), fatigue (8%), dizziness (7%), ataxia (2% to 7%), anxiety (5%), pain (5%), irritability (2% to 5%), suicidal ideation (2% to 5%), abnormal dreams (1% to 5%), abnormality in thinking (1% to 5%), agitation (1% to 5%), amnesia (1% to 5%), depression (1% to 5%), dyspraxia (1% to 5%), emotional lability (1% to 5%), hypoesthesia (1% to 5%), migraine (1% to 5%), hyperreflexia (>2% to <5%), hyporeflexia (>2% to <5%), confusion (1%), paresthesia (≥1%)

Dermatologic: Skin rash (nonserious 7%; requiring hospitalization ≤1%), dermatitis (2% to 5%), diaphoresis (2% to 5%), xeroderma (2% to 5%)

Endocrine & metabolic: Dysmenorrhea (5% to 7%), weight loss (5%), weight gain (1% to 5%)

Gastrointestinal: Vomiting (5% to 9%), dyspepsia (7%), abdominal pain (6%), xerostomia (2% to 6%), constipation (5%), anorexia (2% to 5%), peptic ulcer (2% to 5%), flatulence (1% to 5%),

Genitourinary: Increased libido (2% to 5%), urinary frequency (1% to 5%)

Hematologic & oncologic: Rectal hemorrhage (2% to 5%)

Infection: Infection (5%)

Neuromuscular & skeletal: Back pain (8%), weakness (2% to 5%), arthralgia (1% to 5%), myalgia (1% to 5%), neck pain (1% to 5%)

Ophthalmic: Nystagmus (2% to 5%), visual disturbance (2% to 5%), amblyopia (≥1%)

Respiratory: Rhinitis (7%), cough (5%), pharyngitis (5%), bronchitis (5%), dyspnea (2% to 5%), epistaxis (2% to 5%), sinusitis (1% to 5%), nasopharyngitis (≥3%), upper respiratory tract infection (≥3%)

Miscellaneous: Fever (1% to 5%)

<1% (Limited to important or life-threatening): Abnormal hepatic function tests, abnormal lacrimation, accommodation disturbance, acne vulgaris, acute renal failure, ageusia, agranulocytosis, akathisia, alcohol intolerance, alopecia, altered sense of smell, amyotrophy, anemia, anorgasmia, apathy, aphasia, apnea, arthritis, aseptic meningitis, blepharoptosis, breast abscess, breast neoplasm, bursitis, central nervous system depression, cerebellar syndrome, conjunctivitis, cystitis, deafness, decreased fibrin, decreased libido, decreased serum fibrinogen, deep vein thrombophlebitis, delirium, delusions, depersonalization, depression, dermatitis (exfoliative, fungal), disseminated intravascular coagulation, DRESS syndrome, dry eye syndrome, dysphagia, dysphoria, dysuria, ecchymosis, ejaculatory disorder, eosinophilia, epididymitis, eructation, erythema multiforme, esophagitis, exacerbation of Parkinson disease, extrapyramidal reaction, gastritis, gastrointestinal hemorrhage, gingival hemorrhage, gingival hyperplasia, gingivitis, glossitis, hallucination, hemiplegia, hemorrhage, hepatitis, hepatotoxicity (idiosyncratic) (Chalasani, 2014); herpes zoster, hirsutism, hostility, hot flash, hyperalgesia, hyperbilirubinemia, hyperesthesia, hyperglycemia, hypermenorrhagia, hypersensitivity reaction, hypertension, hyperventilation, hypokinesia, hypothyroidism, hypotonia, immunosuppression (progressive), impotence, increased appetite, increased gamma glutamyl transpeptidase, increased serum alkaline phosphatase, increased serum ALT, increased serum AST, lactation, leg cramps, leukocytosis, leukoderma, leukopenia, lupus-like syndrome, lymphadenopathy, lymphocytosis, maculopapular rash, malaise, manic depressive reaction, memory impairment, multiorgan failure, muscle spasm, myasthenia, myoclonus, neuralgia, neutropenia, nightmares, oral mucosa ulcer, orthostatic hypotension, oscillopsia, otalgia, palpitations, pancreatitis, pancytopenia, panic attack, paralysis, paranoid reaction, pathological fracture, peripheral neuritis, personality disorder, petechia, photophobia, polyuria, psychosis, pure red cell aplasia, pustular rash, racing mind, renal pain, rhabdomyolysis, sialorrhea, skin discoloration, sleep disorder, status epilepticus, Stevens-Johnson syndrome, strabismus, suicidal tendencies, syncope, tachycardia, tendinous contracture, thrombocytopenia, tics, tinnitus, tonic-clonic seizures (exacerbation), urinary incontinence, urinary retention, urinary urgency, uveitis, vasculitis, vasodilation, vesiculobullous dermatitis, visual field defect, withdrawal seizures

Drug Interactions

Metabolism/Transport Effects Inhibits OCT2

Avoid Concomitant Use

Avoid concomitant use of LamoTRIgine with any of the following: Azelastine (Nasal); Dofetilide; Orphenadrine; Paraldehyde; Thalidomide

Increased Effect/Toxicity

LamoTRIgine may increase the levels/effects of: Alcohol (Ethyl); Azelastine (Nasal); Buprenorphine; CarBAMazepine; CNS Depressants; Desmopressin; Dofetilide; Hydrocodone; MetFORMIN; Methotrimeprazine; Metyrosine; Mirtazapine; OLANZapine; Orphenadrine; Paraldehyde; Pramipexole; Procainamide; ROPINIRole; Rotigotine; Selective Serotonin Reuptake Inhibitors; Suvorexant; Thalidomide; Zolpidem

The levels/effects of LamoTRIgine may be increased by: Brimonidine (Topical); Cannabis; Doxylamine; Dronabinol; Droperidol; HydrOXYzine; Kava Kava; Magnesium Sulfate; Methotrimeprazine; Minocycline; Nabilone; Perampanel; Rufinamide; Sodium Oxybate; Tapentadol; Tetrahydrocannabinol; Valproate Products

Decreased Effect

LamoTRIgine may decrease the levels/effects of: Contraceptives (Progestins)

The levels/effects of LamoTRIgine may be decreased by: Atazanavir; Barbiturates; CarBAMazepine; Contraceptives (Estrogens); Ezogabine; Fosphenytoin; Mefloquine; Mianserin; Orlistat; Phenytoin; Primidone; Rifampin; Ritonavir

Food Interactions Food has no effect on absorption.

Storage/Stability Store at 15°C to 30°C (59°F to 86°F). Protect from light.

Mechanism of Action A triazine derivative which inhibits release of glutamate (an excitatory amino acid) and inhibits voltage-sensitive sodium channels, which stabilizes neuronal membranes. Lamotrigine has weak inhibitory effect on the 5-HT$_3$ receptor; *in vitro* inhibits dihydrofolate reductase.

Pharmacodynamics/Kinetics

Absorption: Immediate release: Rapid and complete

Distribution: V_d: 0.9 to 1.3 L/kg

Protein binding: ~55%

Metabolism: Hepatic and renal; metabolized primarily by glucuronic acid conjugation to inactive metabolites

Bioavailability: Immediate release: 98%; **Note:** AUCs were similar for immediate release and extended release preparations in patients receiving nonenzyme-inducing AEDs. In subjects receiving concomitant enzyme-inducing AEDs, bioavailability of extended release product was ~21% lower than immediate release product; in some of these subjects, a decrease in AUC of up to 70% was observed when switching from immediate release to extended release tablets.

Half-life elimination: Immediate release: Adults: 25 to 33 hours, Elderly: 25 to 43 hours; Extended release: Similar to immediate release

Concomitant valproic acid therapy: Adults: 48 to 70 hours; Children 5 to 11 years: 66 hours; Children 10 months to 5 years: 45 hours

Concomitant phenytoin, phenobarbital, primidone, or carbamazepine therapy: Adults: 13 to 14 hours; Children 10 months to 11 years: 7 to 8 hours

Concomitant phenytoin, phenobarbital, primidone, or carbamazepine plus valproate therapy: Adults: 27 hours; Children 5 to 11 years: 19 hours

Chronic renal failure: 43 hours

Hemodialysis: 13 hours during dialysis; 57 hours between dialysis (~20% of a dose is eliminated in a 4-hour dialysis session)

Hepatic impairment:

Mild: 26 to 66 hours

Moderate: 28 to 116 hours

Severe without ascites: 56 to 78 hours

Severe with ascites: 52 to 148 hours

Time to peak, plasma: Immediate release: ~1 to 5 hours (dependent on adjunct therapy); Extended release: 4 to 11 hours (dependent on adjunct therapy)

Excretion: Urine (94%, ~90% as glucuronide conjugates and ~10% unchanged); feces (2%)

Dosing

Adult & Geriatric Note: Drugs that induce lamotrigine glucuronidation include carbamazepine, phenytoin, phenobarbital, primidone, rifampin, lopinavir/ritonavir, and atazanavir/ritonavir. Valproic acid inhibits lamotrigine glucuronidation. Whole tablets should be used for dosing, round calculated dose down to the nearest whole tablet. Alternatively, a suspension may be prepared using immediate release tablets (see also Extemporaneous Preparations).

US labeling:

Lennox-Gastaut (adjunctive): Oral:

Immediate release formulation:

Regimens **not containing** carbamazepine, phenytoin, phenobarbital, primidone, rifampin, lopinavir/ritonavir, or valproic acid: Initial: Weeks 1 and 2: 25 mg once daily; Weeks 3 and 4: 50 mg once daily; Week 5 and beyond: Increase by 50 mg daily every 1-2 weeks; Usual maintenance: 225-375 mg daily in 2 divided doses

Regimens **containing** valproic acid: Initial: Weeks 1 and 2: 25 mg every other day; Weeks 3 and 4: 25 mg once daily; Week 5 and beyond: Increase by 25-50 mg daily every 1-2 weeks; Usual maintenance: 100-200 mg daily (valproic acid alone) or 100-400 mg daily (valproic acid and other drugs that induce glucuronidation) in 1 or 2 divided doses

Regimens **containing** carbamazepine, phenytoin, phenobarbital, primidone, rifampin, lopinavir/ritonavir, and without valproic acid: Initial: Weeks 1 and 2: 50 mg once daily; Weeks 3 and 4: 100 mg daily in 2 divided doses; Week 5 and beyond: Increase by 100 mg daily every 1-2 weeks; Usual maintenance: 300-500 mg daily in 2 divided doses (doses as high as 700 mg/day have been used)

Partial seizures (adjunctive) and primary generalized tonic-clonic seizures (adjunctive): Oral:

Immediate release formulation:

Regimens **not containing** carbamazepine, phenytoin, phenobarbital, primidone, rifampin, lopinavir/ritonavir, or valproic acid: Initial: Weeks 1 and 2: 25 mg once daily; Weeks 3 and 4: 50 mg once daily; Week 5 and beyond: Increase by 50 mg daily every 1-2 weeks; Usual maintenance: 225-375 mg daily in 2 divided doses

Regimens **containing** valproic acid: Initial: Weeks 1 and 2: 25 mg every other day; Weeks 3 and 4: 25 mg once daily; Week 5 and beyond: Increase by 25-50 mg daily every 1-2 weeks; Usual maintenance: 100-200 mg daily (valproic acid alone) or 100-400 mg daily (valproic acid and other drugs that induce glucuronidation) in 1 or 2 divided doses

Regimens **containing** carbamazepine, phenytoin, phenobarbital, primidone, rifampin, lopinavir/ritonavir, and without valproic acid: Initial: Weeks 1 and 2: 50 mg once daily; Weeks 3 and 4: 100 mg daily in 2 divided doses; Week 5 and beyond: Increase by 100 mg daily every 1-2 weeks; Usual maintenance: 300 to 500 mg daily in 2 divided doses (doses as high as 700 mg/day have been used)

Extended release formulation:

Regimens **not containing** carbamazepine, phenytoin, phenobarbital, primidone, rifampin, lopinavir/ritonavir, or valproic acid: Initial: Weeks 1 and 2: 25 mg once daily; Weeks 3 and 4: 50 mg once daily; Week 5: 100 mg once daily; Week 6: 150 mg once daily; Week 7: 200 mg once daily; Week 8 and beyond: Dose increases should not exceed 100 mg daily at weekly intervals; Usual maintenance: 300-400 mg once daily

Regimens **containing** valproic acid: Initial: Weeks 1 and 2: 25 mg every other day; Weeks 3 and 4: 25 mg once daily; Week 5: 50 mg once daily; Week 6: 100 mg once daily; Week 7: 150 mg once daily; Week 8 and beyond: Dose increases should not exceed 100 mg daily at weekly intervals; Usual maintenance: 200-250 mg once daily

Regimens **containing** carbamazepine, phenytoin, phenobarbital, primidone, rifampin, lopinavir/ritonavir, and without valproic acid: Initial: Weeks 1 and 2: 50 mg once daily; Weeks 3 and 4: 100 mg once daily; Week 5: 200 mg once daily; Week 6: 300 mg once daily; Week 7: 400 mg once daily; Week 8 and beyond: Dose increases should not exceed 100 mg daily at weekly intervals; Usual maintenance: 400-600 mg once daily

Conversion strategy from adjunctive therapy with valproic acid to monotherapy with lamotrigine:

Immediate release formulation:

- Initiate and titrate as per escalation recommendations for adjunctive therapy to a lamotrigine dose of 200 mg daily.

- Then taper valproic acid dose in decrements of not >500 mg/day/week to a valproic acid dosage of 500 mg daily; this dosage should be maintained for 1 week. The lamotrigine dosage should then be increased to 300 mg daily while valproic acid is simultaneously decreased to 250 mg daily; this dosage should be maintained for 1 week.
- Valproic acid may then be discontinued, while the lamotrigine dose is increased by 100 mg daily at weekly intervals to achieve a lamotrigine maintenance dose of 500 mg daily in 2 divided doses.

Extended release formulation:

- Initiate and titrate as per escalation recommendations for adjunctive therapy to a lamotrigine dose of 150 mg daily.
- Then taper valproic acid dose in decrements of not >500 mg/day/week to a valproic acid dose of 500 mg daily; this dosage should be maintained for 1 week. The lamotrigine dosage should then be increased to 200 mg daily while valproic acid is simultaneously decreased to 250 mg daily; this dosage should be maintained for 1 week.
- Valproic acid may then be discontinued, while the lamotrigine dose is increased to achieve a maintenance dosage range of 250-300 mg once daily.

Conversion strategy from adjunctive therapy with drugs that induce lamotrigine glucuronidation (carbamazepine, phenytoin, phenobarbital, primidone) to monotherapy with lamotrigine: *Immediate release formulation and extended release formulation:*

- Initiate and titrate as per escalation recommendations for adjunctive therapy to a lamotrigine dose of 500 mg daily
- Concomitant enzyme-inducing drug should then be withdrawn by 20% decrements each week over a 4-week period.
- Two weeks after withdrawal of the enzyme-inducing drug, the dosage of lamotrigine extended release may be tapered in decrements of not >100 mg/day at intervals of 1 week to achieve a maintenance dosage range of 250-300 mg once daily; no further dosage reduction is required for lamotrigine immediate release.

Conversion strategy from adjunctive therapy with drugs that do **not** inhibit or induce lamotrigine glucuronidation to monotherapy with lamotrigine:

Immediate release formulation: No specific guidelines available

Extended release formulation: Initiate and titrate as per escalation recommendations for adjunctive therapy to a lamotrigine dose of 250-300 mg daily. Concomitant drug should then be withdrawn by 20% decrements each week over a 4-week period.

Conversion from immediate release to extended release (Lamictal XR): Initial dose of the extended release tablet should match the total daily dose of the immediate-release formulation. Adjust dose as needed within the recommended dosing guidelines.

Bipolar I disorder (maintenance): Oral:

Immediate release formulation:

Regimens **not containing** carbamazepine, phenytoin, phenobarbital, primidone, rifampin, lopinavir/ritonavir, or valproic acid: Initial: Weeks 1 and 2: 25 mg once daily; Weeks 3 and 4: 50 mg once daily; Week 5: 100 mg once daily; Week 6 and maintenance: 200 mg once daily

Regimens **containing** valproic acid: Initial: Weeks 1 and 2: 25 mg every other day; Weeks 3 and 4: 25 mg once daily; Week 5: 50 mg once daily; Week 6 and maintenance: 100 mg once daily

Regimens **containing** carbamazepine, phenytoin, phenobarbital, primidone, rifampin, or lopinavir/ritonavir, and without valproic acid: Initial: Weeks 1 and 2: 50 mg once daily; Weeks 3 and 4: 100 mg daily in divided doses; Week 5: 200 mg daily in divided doses; Week 6: 300 mg daily in divided doses; Maintenance: Up to 400 mg daily in divided doses

Adjustment following discontinuation of drugs that inhibit or induce lamotrigine glucuronidation:

Discontinuing valproic acid with current dose of lamotrigine 100 mg daily: 150 mg daily for week 1, then increase to 200 mg daily beginning week 2

Discontinuing carbamazepine, phenytoin, phenobarbital, primidone, rifampin, or lopinavir/ritonavir with current dose of lamotrigine 400 mg daily: 400 mg daily for week 1, then decrease to 300 mg daily for week 2, then decrease to 200 mg daily beginning week 3

Bipolar depression (acute treatment) (off-label use):
Oral: *Immediate release formulation:* Initial: Weeks 1 and 2: 25 mg once daily; Weeks 3 and 4: 50 mg once daily; Week 5: 100 mg once daily; Week 6 and maintenance: 200 mg once daily. Doses up to 400 mg/day have been evaluated in clinical trials; however, guidelines recommend dose ranges of 50 to 200 mg/day (Geddes 2009; van der Loos 2009; WFSBP [Grunze 2010]). **Note:** Concurrent psychoactive drugs were excluded in monotherapy clinical trials (Geddes 2009); this titration reflects product labeling recommendations for regimens not containing carbamazepine, phenytoin, phenobarbital, primidone, rifampin, lopinavir/ritonavir, or valproic acid.

Canadian labeling:
Uncontrolled epilepsy (adjunctive) or Lennox-Gastaut syndrome (adjunctive): Oral:
Regimens **containing** inducers of lamotrigine glucuronidation and valproic acid or regimens not containing agents that induce or inhibit lamotrigine glucuronidation: Initial: Weeks 1 and 2: 25 mg once daily; Weeks 3 and 4: 25 mg twice daily; Week 5 and beyond: Increase dose by 25-50 mg every 1-2 weeks until maintenance dose established (usual maintenance dose: 100-200 mg daily in 2 divided doses)

Alternatively, a more cautious titration schedule for regimens containing valproic acid (regardless of any concomitant medication): Initial: Weeks 1 and 2: 25 mg every other day; Weeks 3 and 4: 25 mg once daily; Week 5 and beyond: Increase dose by 25-50 mg every 1-2 weeks until maintenance dose established (usual maintenance dose: 100-200 mg daily in 2 divided doses).

Regimens **containing** inducers of lamotrigine glucuronidation and without valproic acid: Initial: Weeks 1 and 2: 50 mg once daily; Weeks 3 and 4: 50 mg twice daily; Week 5 and beyond: Increase dose by 100 mg every 1-2 weeks until maintenance dose established (usual maintenance dose: 300-500 mg daily in 2 divided doses)

Conversion from adjunctive therapy with concomitant drugs that inhibit or induce lamotrigine glucuronidation to lamotrigine monotherapy: Decrease dose of concomitant antiepileptic agent by ~20% of original dose every week for 5 weeks (slower taper may be considered if clinically indicated). Lamotrigine dosage adjustments during this period should be determined by changes in lamotrigine pharmacokinetics due to withdrawal of the concomitant drugs that inhibit or induce lamotrigine glucuronidation, and by the clinical response of patient.

Additional considerations:
Discontinuing therapy: Decrease dose by ~50% per week, over at least 2 weeks unless safety concerns require a more rapid withdrawal. Discontinuing carbamazepine, phenytoin, phenobarbital, primidone, rifampin, lopinavir/ritonavir, or atazanavir/ritonavir should prolong the half-life of lamotrigine; discontinuing valproic acid should shorten the half-life of lamotrigine

Restarting therapy after discontinuation: If lamotrigine has been withheld for >5 half-lives, consider restarting according to initial dosing recommendations. **Note:** Concomitant medications may affect the half-life of lamotrigine; consider pharmacokinetic interactions when restarting therapy.

Concomitant therapy:
Dosage adjustment with atazanavir/ritonavir: Follow initial lamotrigine dosing guidelines, maintenance dose should be adjusted as follows:
Patients not taking concomitant carbamazepine, phenytoin, phenobarbital, primidone, rifampin, estrogen-containing contraceptives, or lopinavir/ritonavir: Lamotrigine maintenance dose may need to be increased if atazanavir/ritonavir is added or decreased if atazanavir/ritonavir is discontinued.

Dosage adjustment with estrogen-containing hormonal contraceptives: Follow initial lamotrigine dosing guidelines, maintenance dose should be adjusted as follows, based on concomitant medications:
Patients taking concomitant carbamazepine, phenytoin, phenobarbital, primidone, rifampin, lopinavir/ritonavir, or atazanavir/ritonavir: No dosing adjustment required
Patients **not** taking concomitant carbamazepine, phenytoin, phenobarbital, primidone, rifampin, lopinavir/ritonavir, or atazanavir/ritonavir: Lamotrigine maintenance dose may need increased by twofold over target dose. If already taking a stable dose of lamotrigine and starting contraceptive, maintenance dose may need increased by twofold. Dose increases should start when contraceptive is started and

titrated to clinical response increasing no more rapidly than 50-100 mg daily every week. Gradual increases of lamotrigine plasma levels may occur during the inactive "pill-free" week and will be greater when dose increases are made the week before. If increased adverse events consistently occur during "pill-free" week, overall maintenance dose adjustments may be required. When discontinuing estrogen-containing hormonal contraceptive, dose of lamotrigine may need decreased by as much as 50%; do not decrease by more than 25% of total daily dose over a 2-week period unless clinical response or plasma levels indicate otherwise. Dose adjustments during "pill-free" week are not recommended.

Pediatric Note: Drugs that induce lamotrigine glucuronidation include carbamazepine, phenytoin, phenobarbital, primidone, rifampin, lopinavir/ritonavir, and atazanavir/ritonavir. Valproic acid inhibits lamotrigine glucuronidation. Extended release tablets not FDA approved for use in children ≤12 years of age.

US labeling:
Lennox-Gastaut syndrome (adjunctive), primary generalized tonic-clonic seizures (adjunctive), or partial seizures (adjunctive): Oral: **Note:** Whole tablets should be used for dosing, round calculated dose down to the nearest whole tablet. Alternatively, a suspension may be prepared using immediate release tablets (see also Extemporaneous Preparations). Children <30 kg will likely require maintenance doses to be increased by as much as 50% based on clinical response regardless of regimen below:
Children 2 to 12 years: *Immediate release formulation:*
Regimens **not containing** carbamazepine, phenytoin, phenobarbital, primidone, rifampin, lopinavir/ritonavir, or valproic acid: Initial: Weeks 1 and 2: 0.3 mg/kg/day in 1-2 divided doses; Weeks 3 and 4: 0.6 mg/kg/day in 2 divided doses; Week 5 and beyond: Increase by 0.6 mg/kg/day every 1-2 weeks; Usual maintenance: 4.5-7.5 mg/kg/day (maximum: 300 mg daily) in 2 divided doses
Regimens **containing** valproic acid: Initial: Weeks 1 and 2: 0.15 mg/kg/day in 1-2 divided doses (if calculated dose is equal to or rounds down to 1 mg daily, give 2 mg every other day instead); Weeks 3 and 4: 0.3 mg/kg/day in 1-2 divided doses; Week 5 and beyond: Increase by 0.3 mg/kg/day every 1-2 weeks; Usual maintenance: 1-5 mg/kg/day (maximum: 200 mg daily) in 1 or 2 divided doses or 1-3 mg/kg/day with valproic acid alone (maximum: 200 mg daily)
Regimens **containing** carbamazepine, phenytoin, phenobarbital, primidone, rifampin, or lopinavir/ritonavir, and without valproic acid: Initial: Weeks 1 and 2: 0.6 mg/kg/day in 2 divided doses; Weeks 3 and 4: 1.2 mg/kg/day in 2 divided doses; Week 5 and beyond: Increase by 1.2 mg/kg/day every 1-2 weeks; Usual maintenance: 5-15 mg/kg/day (maximum: 400 mg daily) in 2 divided doses
Adolescents >12 years: Refer to adult dosing.

Conversion from adjunctive therapy with drugs that inhibit or induce lamotrigine glucuronidation to monotherapy with lamotrigine:
Immediate release formulation: Adolescents ≥16 years: Refer to adult dosing.
Extended release formulation: Adolescents ≥13 years: Refer to adult dosing.

Canadian labeling:
Lennox-Gastaut syndrome (adjunctive therapy): Oral: **Note:** Whole tablets should be used for dosing, round calculated dose down to the nearest whole tablet. Alternatively, a suspension may be prepared using immediate release tablets (see also Extemporaneous Preparations). Several weeks to months may be required to achieve individualized maintenance dose. Use is not recommended in children <9 kg.
Children ≤12 years (and ≥9 kg):
Regimens **containing** valproic acid regardless of any other concomitant medication: Initial: Weeks 1 and 2: 0.15 mg/kg once daily (if calculated dose is equal to or rounds down to 1 mg daily, give 2 mg every other day instead); Weeks 3 and 4: 0.3 mg/kg once daily; Week 5 and beyond: Increase dose by 0.3 mg/kg every 1-2 weeks (usual maintenance dose: 1-5 mg/kg daily in 1 or 2 divided doses) up to a maximum dose of 200 mg daily. **Note:** Alternatively, refer to manufacturer's labeling for recommended weight-based rounding regimen.

Regimens **containing** carbamazepine, phenytoin, phenobarbital, primidone, or other drugs that induce glucuronidation and without valproic acid: Initial: Weeks 1 and 2: 0.3 mg/kg twice daily; Weeks 3 and 4: 0.6 mg/kg twice daily; Week 5 and beyond: Increase dose by 1.2 mg/kg every 1-2 weeks (usual maintenance dose: 2.5-7.5 mg/kg twice daily) up to a maximum dose of 400 mg daily. **Note:** When necessary, round doses down to closest 5 mg interval (eg, calculated dose >5 mg and <10 mg would be rounded to 5 mg; calculated dose >10 mg and <15 mg would be rounded to 10 mg). For week 5 and beyond, dose increases made every 1-2 weeks should not exceed previous daily dose administered in week 4 (eg, if week 4 dose was 20 mg daily than dose increase in week 5 or beyond should not exceed 20 mg daily). Manufacturer labeling suggests that insufficient data exists to support weight based dosing in patients >59 kg.

Adolescents >12 years: Refer to adult dosing.

Uncontrolled epilepsy (adjunctive therapy); conversion from adjunctive therapy with concomitant drugs that inhibit or induce lamotrigine glucuronidation to monotherapy with lamotrigine: Adolescents ≥16 years: Refer to adult dosing

Additional considerations:

Discontinuing therapy: Refer to adult dosing.

Restarting therapy after discontinuation: Refer to adult dosing.

Dosage adjustment with estrogen-containing hormonal contraceptives: Refer to adult dosing.

Renal Impairment There are no dosage adjustments provided in the manufacturer's labeling. Decreased maintenance dosage may be effective in patients with significant renal impairment; has not been adequately studied; use with caution.

Hepatic Impairment

US labeling:

Mild impairment: No dosage adjustment necessary.

Moderate-to-severe impairment without ascites: Decrease initial, escalation, and maintenance doses by ~25%; adjust according to clinical response and tolerance.

Moderate-to-severe impairment with ascites: Decrease initial, escalation, and maintenance doses by ~50%; adjust according to clinical response and tolerance.

Canadian labeling:

Mild and moderate impairment (Child-Pugh classes A and B): Reduce initial, escalation, and maintenance dosing by ~50%; adjust according to clinical response and tolerance.

Severe impairment (Child-Pugh class C): Reduce initial, escalation, and maintenance dosing by ~75%; adjust according to clinical response and tolerance.

Administration Doses should be rounded down to the nearest whole tablet.

Lamictal chewable/dispersible tablets: May be chewed, dispersed in water or diluted fruit juice, or swallowed whole. To disperse tablets, add to a small amount of liquid (just enough to cover tablet); let sit ~1 minute until dispersed; swirl solution and consume immediately. Do not administer partial amounts of liquid. If tablets are chewed, a small amount of water or diluted fruit juice should be used to aid in swallowing.

Lamictal ODT: Place tablets on tongue and move around in the mouth. Tablets will dissolve rapidly and can be swallowed with or without food or water.

Lamictal XR: Administer without regard to meals. Swallow whole; do not chew, crush, or cut.

Monitoring Parameters Serum levels of concurrent anticonvulsants, LFTs, renal function, hypersensitivity reactions (especially rash); seizure, frequency and duration; suicidality (eg, suicidal thoughts, depression, behavioral changes); signs/symptoms of aseptic meningitis

Reference Range A therapeutic serum concentration range has not been established for lamotrigine. Dosing should be based on therapeutic response. Lamotrigine plasma concentrations of 0.25-29.1 mcg/mL have been reported in the literature.

Test Interactions May interfere with some rapid urine drug screens, particularly phencyclidine (false-positives).

Dosage Forms Considerations

LaMICtal Kits are available as follows:

Blue - for patients already taking valproate

LaMICtal Starter: 25 mg (35s)

LaMICtal ODT (Titration): 25 mg (21s) and 50 mg (7s)

LaMICtal XR (Titration): 25 mg (21s) and 50 mg (7s)

Green - for patients already taking carbamazepine, phenytoin, phenobarbital, or primidone, and **not** taking valproate

LaMICtal Starter: 25 mg (84s) and 100 mg (14s)

LaMICtal ODT (Titration): 50 mg (42s) and 100 mg (14s)

LaMICtal XR (Titration): 50 mg (14s) and 100 mg (14s) and 200 mg (7s)

Orange - for patients not taking carbamazepine, phenytoin, phenobarbital, primidone, or valproate

LaMICtal Starter: 25 mg (42s) and 100 mg (7s)

LaMICtal ODT (Titration): 25 mg (14s) and 50 mg (14s) and 100 mg (7s)

LaMICtal XR (Titration): 25 mg (14s) and 50 mg (14s) and 100 mg (7s)

Dosage Forms Excipient information presented when available (limited, particularly for generics); consult specific product labeling. [DSC] = Discontinued product

Kit, Oral:

LaMICtal ODT: Blue Kit: 25 mg (21s) & 50 mg (7s), Orange Kit: 25 mg (14s) & 50 mg (14s) & 100 mg (7s), Green Kit: 50 mg (42s) & 100 mg (14s)

LaMICtal Starter: Blue Kit: 25 mg (35s)

LaMICtal Starter: Green Kit: 25 mg (84s) & 100 mg (14s), Orange Kit: 25 mg (42s) & 100 mg (7s) [contains fd&c yellow #6 aluminum lake]

LaMICtal XR: Green Kit: 50 mg (14s) & 100 mg (14s) & 200 mg (7s) [contains fd&c blue #2 aluminum lake, polysorbate 80]

LaMICtal XR: Blue Kit: 25 mg (21s) & 50 mg (7s), Orange Kit: 25 mg (14s) & 50 mg (14s) & 100 mg (7s) [contains polysorbate 80]

Generic: Blue Kit: 25 mg (21s) & 50 mg (7s), Green Kit: 50 mg (42s) & 100 mg (14s), Orange Kit: 25 mg (14s) & 50 mg (14s) & 100 mg (7s)

Tablet, Oral:

LaMICtal: 25 mg, 100 mg, 150 mg, 200 mg [scored]

Generic: 25 mg, 100 mg, 150 mg, 200 mg

Tablet Chewable, Oral:

LaMICtal: 2 mg [DSC] [contains saccharin sodium]

LaMICtal: 5 mg [scored; berry flavor]

LaMICtal: 25 mg [berry flavor]

Generic: 5 mg, 25 mg

Tablet Dispersible, Oral:

LaMICtal ODT: 25 mg, 50 mg, 100 mg, 200 mg

Generic: 25 mg, 50 mg, 100 mg, 200 mg

Tablet Extended Release 24 Hour, Oral:

LaMICtal XR: 25 mg, 50 mg, 100 mg [contains polysorbate 80]

LaMICtal XR: 200 mg [contains fd&c blue #2 aluminum lake, polysorbate 80]

LaMICtal XR: 250 mg [contains fd&c blue #2 aluminum lake]

LaMICtal XR: 300 mg [contains polysorbate 80]

Generic: 25 mg, 50 mg, 100 mg, 200 mg, 250 mg, 300 mg

Extemporaneous Preparations A 1 mg/mL oral suspension may be made with tablets and one of two different vehicles (a 1:1 mixture of Ora-Sweet and Ora-Plus or a 1:1 mixture of Ora-Sweet SF and Ora-Plus). Crush one 100 mg tablet in a mortar and reduce to a fine powder. Add small portions of the chosen vehicle and mix to a uniform paste; mix while adding the vehicle in incremental proportions to **almost** 100 mL; transfer to a graduated cylinder, rinse mortar with vehicle, and add quantity of vehicle sufficient to make 100 mL. Label "shake well" and "protect from light". Stable for 91 days when stored in amber plastic prescription bottles in the dark at room temperature or refrigerated.

Nahata M, Morosco R, Hipple T. "Stability of Lamotrigine in Two Extemporaneously Prepared Oral Suspensions at 4 and 25 Degrees C," *Am J Health Syst Pharm*, 1999, 56(3):240-2.

◆ Lanaphilic/Urea [OTC] *see* Urea *on page 1853*

◆ Lanoxicaps *see* Digoxin *on page 547*

◆ Lanoxin *see* Digoxin *on page 547*

◆ Lanoxin Pediatric *see* Digoxin *on page 547*

Lanreotide (lan REE oh tide)

Brand Names: US Somatuline Depot

Brand Names: Canada Somatuline Autogel

Index Terms Lanreotide (Long-Acting Aqueous); Lanreotide Acetate; Lanreotide Autogel

Pharmacologic Category Somatostatin Analog

Use

US labeling:

Acromegaly: Long-term treatment of acromegalic patients who have had an inadequate response to surgery and/or radiotherapy, or for whom surgery and/or radiotherapy is not an option.

◄

Gastroenteropancreatic neuroendocrine tumors: Treatment (to improve progression-free survival) of unresectable, well- or moderately-differentiated, locally advanced or metastatic gastroenteropancreatic neuroendocrine tumors (GEP-NETs).

Canadian labeling:
Acromegaly: Long-term treatment of patients with acromegaly due to pituitary tumors who have had an inadequate response to surgery and/or radiotherapy, or for whom surgery and/or radiotherapy is not an option; relief of symptoms associated with acromegaly.

Enteropancreatic neuroendocrine tumors: Treatment (to delay progression) of enteropancreatic neuroendocrine tumors in patients with grade 1 or a subset of grade 2 (equivalent to Ki67 <10%) unresectable, locally advanced, or metastatic disease.

Dosing

Adult & Geriatric

US labeling:
Acromegaly: SubQ: Initial dose: 90 mg once every 4 weeks for 3 months; after initial 90 days of therapy, adjust dose based on clinical response of patient, growth hormone (GH) levels, and/or insulin-like growth factor 1 (IGF-1) levels as follows:

GH ≤1 ng/mL, IGF-1 normal, symptoms stable: 60 mg once every 4 weeks; once stabilized on 60 mg once every 4 weeks, may consider regimen of 120 mg once every 6 or 8 weeks (extended-interval dosing)

GH >1 to 2.5 ng/mL, IGF-1 normal, symptoms stable: 90 mg once every 4 weeks; once stabilized on 90 mg once every 4 weeks, may consider regimen of 120 mg once every 6 or 8 weeks (extended-interval dosing)

GH >2.5 ng/mL, IGF-1 elevated and/or uncontrolled symptoms: 120 mg once every 4 weeks

Gastroenteropancreatic neuroendocrine tumors (GEP-NETs): SubQ: 120 mg once every 4 weeks until disease progression or unacceptable toxicity

Canadian labeling:
Acromegaly: SubQ: Initial dose: 90 mg once every 4 weeks for 3 months; after initial 90 days of therapy, adjust dose based on clinical response of patient, growth hormone (GH) levels, and/or insulin-like growth factor 1 (IGF-1) levels as follows:

GH ≤1 ng/mL, IGF-1 normal, symptoms stable: 60 mg once every 4 weeks; once stabilized on 60 mg once every 4 weeks, may consider regimen of 120 mg once every 6 or 8 weeks (extended-interval dosing)

GH >1 to 2.5 ng/mL, IGF-1 normal, symptoms stable: 90 mg once every 4 weeks; once stabilized on 90 mg once every 4 weeks, may consider regimen of 120 mg once every 6 or 8 weeks (extended-interval dosing)

GH >2.5 ng/mL, IGF-1 elevated and/or uncontrolled symptoms: 120 mg once every 4 weeks

Enteropancreatic neuroendocrine tumors (NETs): SubQ: 120 mg once every 4 weeks, continue until disease progression

Pediatric Acromegaly: Adolescents ≥16 years (*Canadian labeling*): Refer to adult dosing.

Renal Impairment

Acromegaly:
Mild impairment (CrCl 60 to 89 mL/minute: No dosage adjustment necessary.

Moderate to severe impairment (CrCl ≤59 mL/minute): Initial dose: 60 mg once every 4 weeks for 3 months; adjust dose based on clinical response of patient, GH levels, and/or IGF-1 levels; use of an extended-interval dose of 120 mg once every 6 or 8 weeks should be done with caution.

Gastroenteropancreatic or enteropancreatic neuroendocrine tumors (GEP-NETs):
Mild to moderate impairment (CrCl ≥30 mL/minute): No dosage adjustment necessary.

Severe impairment (CrCl <30 mL/minute): There are no dosage adjustments provided in the manufacturer's labeling (has not been studied).

Hepatic Impairment

Acromegaly:
Mild impairment: No dosage adjustment necessary.
Moderate to severe impairment: Initial dose: 60 mg once every 4 weeks for 3 months; adjust dose based on clinical response of patient, GH levels, and/or IGF-1 levels; use of an extended-interval dose of 120 mg once every 6 or 8 weeks should be done with caution.

Gastroenteropancreatic or enteropancreatic neuroendocrine tumors (GEP-NETs): There are no dosage adjustments provided in the manufacturer's labeling (has not been studied).

Additional Information Complete prescribing information should be consulted for additional detail.

Dosage Forms Excipient information presented when available (limited, particularly for generics); consult specific product labeling.
Solution, Subcutaneous:
Somatuline Depot: 120 mg/0.5 mL (0.5 mL); 60 mg/0.2 mL (0.2 mL); 90 mg/0.3 mL (0.3 mL)

Dosage Forms: Canada Excipient information presented when available (limited, particularly for generics); consult specific product labeling.
Solution, Subcutaneous:
Somatuline Autogel: 60 mg/0.5 mL (0.5 mL); 90 mg/0.5 mL (0.5 mL); 120 mg/0.5 mL (0.5 mL)

◆ Lanreotide Acetate *see* Lanreotide *on page 1031*
◆ Lanreotide Autogel *see* Lanreotide *on page 1031*
◆ Lanreotide (Long-Acting Aqueous) *see* Lanreotide *on page 1031*

Lansoprazole (lan SOE pra zole)

Brand Names: US First-Lansoprazole; Heartburn Relief 24 Hour [OTC] [DSC]; Heartburn Treatment 24 Hour [OTC]; Prevacid; Prevacid 24HR [OTC]; Prevacid SoluTab

Brand Names: Canada Apo-Lansoprazole; Mylan-Lansoprazole; PMS-Lansoprazole; Prevacid; Prevacid FasTab; Q-Lansoprazole; RAN-Lansoprazole; Riva-Lansoprazole; Sandoz-Lansoprazole; Teva-Lansoprazole

Pharmacologic Category Proton Pump Inhibitor; Substituted Benzimidazole

Use Short-term (4 weeks) treatment of active duodenal ulcers; maintenance treatment of healed duodenal ulcers; as part of a multidrug regimen for *H. pylori* eradication to reduce the risk of duodenal ulcer recurrence; short-term (up to 8 weeks) treatment of active benign gastric ulcer; treatment of NSAID-associated gastric ulcer; to reduce the risk of NSAID-associated gastric ulcer in patients with a history of gastric ulcer who require an NSAID; short-term (up to 8 weeks) treatment of symptomatic GERD; short-term (up to 8 weeks) treatment for all grades of erosive esophagitis; to maintain healing of erosive esophagitis; long-term treatment of pathological hypersecretory conditions, including Zollinger-Ellison syndrome

OTC labeling: Relief of frequent heartburn (≥2 days/week)

Pregnancy Considerations Adverse events have not been observed in animal reproduction studies. An increased risk of hypospadias was reported following maternal use of proton pump inhibitors (PPIs) during pregnancy (Anderka, 2012), but this was based on a small number of exposures and the same association was not found in another study (Erichsen, 2012). Most available studies have not shown an increased risk of major birth defects following maternal use of PPIs during pregnancy (Diav-Citrin, 2005; Matok, 2012; Pasternak, 2010). When treating GERD in pregnancy, PPIs may be used when clinically indicated (Katz, 2013).

Breast-Feeding Considerations It is not known if lansoprazole is excreted in breast milk. Due to the potential for serious adverse reactions in the nursing infant, the manufacturer recommends a decision be made whether to discontinue nursing or to discontinue the drug, taking into account the importance of treatment to the mother.

Medication Guide Available Yes

Contraindications Hypersensitivity (eg, anaphylaxis, angioedema, anaphylactic shock, angioedema, bronchospasm, acute interstitial nephritis, urticaria) to lansoprazole, other substituted benzimidazole proton pump inhibitors, or any component of the formulation

Warnings/Precautions Use of proton pump inhibitors (PPIs) may increase the risk of gastrointestinal infections (eg, *Salmonella, Campylobacter*). Relief of symptoms does not preclude the presence of a gastric malignancy. Atrophic gastritis (by biopsy) has been noted with long-term omeprazole therapy; this may also occur with lansoprazole. No reports of enterochromaffin-like (ECL) cell carcinoids, dysplasia, or neoplasia have occurred. Use of proton pump inhibitors (PPIs) may increase risk of CDAD, especially in hospitalized patients; consider CDAD diagnosis in patients with persistent diarrhea that does not improve. Use the lowest dose and shortest duration of PPI therapy appropriate for the condition being treated. Severe liver dysfunction may require dosage reductions. Decreased *H. pylori* eradication rates have been observed with short-term (≤7 days) combination therapy. The American College of Gastroenterology recommends 10-14 days of therapy (triple or quadruple) for eradication of *H. pylori* (Chey, 2007).

PPIs may diminish the therapeutic effect of clopidogrel thought to be due to reduced formation of the active metabolite of clopidogrel. The manufacturer of clopidogrel recommends either avoidance of both omeprazole (even

when scheduled 12 hours apart) and esomeprazole or use of a PPI with comparatively less effect on the active metabolite of clopidogrel (eg, pantoprazole). Although lansoprazole exhibits the most potent CYP2C19 inhibition *in vitro* (Li, 2004; Ogilvie, 2011), an *in vivo* study of extensive CYP2C19 metabolizers showed less reduction of the active metabolite of clopidogrel by lansoprazole/dexlansoprazole compared to esomeprazole/omeprazole (Frelinger, 2012). The manufacturer of lansoprazole states that no dosage adjustment is necessary for clopidogrel when used concurrently. In contrast to these warnings, others have recommended the continued use of PPIs, regardless of the degree of inhibition, in patients with a history of GI bleeding or multiple risk factors for GI bleeding who are also receiving clopidogrel since no evidence has established clinically meaningful differences in outcome; however, a clinically-significant interaction cannot be excluded in those who are poor metabolizers of clopidogrel (Abraham, 2010; Levine, 2011). Additionally, concomitant use of lansoprazole with some drugs may require cautious use, may not be recommended, or may require dosage adjustments.

Increased incidence of osteoporosis-related bone fractures of the hip, spine, or wrist may occur with PPI therapy. Patients on high-dose or long-term therapy should be monitored. Use the lowest effective dose for the shortest duration of time, use vitamin D and calcium supplementation, and follow appropriate guidelines to reduce risk of fractures in patients at risk. Acute interstitial nephritis has been observed in patients taking PPIs; may occur at any time during therapy and is generally due to an idiopathic hypersensitivity reaction. Discontinue if acute interstitial nephritis develops. Lansoprazole has been shown to be ineffective for the treatment of symptomatic GERD in children 1 month to <1 year.

Hypomagnesemia, reported rarely, usually with prolonged PPI use of >3 months (most cases >1 year of therapy); may be symptomatic or asymptomatic; severe cases may cause tetany, seizures, and cardiac arrhythmias. Consider obtaining serum magnesium concentrations prior to beginning long-term therapy, especially if taking concomitant digoxin, diuretics, or other drugs known to cause hypomagnesemia; and periodically thereafter. Hypomagnesemia may be corrected by magnesium supplementation, although discontinuation of lansoprazole may be necessary; magnesium levels typically return to normal within 1 week of stopping.

Prolonged treatment (≥2 years) may lead to vitamin B_{12} malabsorption and subsequent vitamin B_{12} deficiency. The magnitude of the deficiency is dose-related and the association is stronger in females and those younger in age (<30 years); prevalence is decreased after discontinuation of therapy (Lam, 2013).

Benzyl alcohol and derivatives: Some dosage forms may contain benzyl alcohol; large amounts of benzyl alcohol (≥99 mg/kg/day) have been associated with a potentially fatal toxicity ("gasping syndrome") in neonates; the "gasping syndrome" consists of metabolic acidosis, respiratory distress, gasping respirations, CNS dysfunction (including convulsions, intracranial hemorrhage), hypotension, and cardiovascular collapse (AAP ["Inactive" 1997]; CDC, 1982); some data suggests that benzoate displaces bilirubin from protein binding sites (Ahlfors, 2001); avoid or use dosage forms containing benzyl alcohol with caution in neonates. See manufacturer's labeling.

When used for self-medication, patients should be instructed not to use if they have difficulty swallowing, are vomiting blood, or have bloody or black stools. Prior to use, patients should contact healthcare provider if they have liver disease, heartburn for >3 months, heartburn with dizziness, lightheadedness, or sweating, MI symptoms, frequent chest pain, frequent wheezing (especially with heartburn), unexplained weight loss, nausea/vomiting, stomach pain, or are taking antifungals, atazanavir, digoxin, tacrolimus, theophylline, or warfarin. Patients should stop use and consult a healthcare provider if heartburn continues or worsens, or if they need to take for >14 days or more often than every 4 months. Patients should be informed that it may take 1-4 days for full effect to be seen; should not be used for immediate relief.

Adverse Reactions

1% to 10%:

Central nervous system: Headache (children 1-11 years 3%, 12-17 years 7%), dizziness (children 12-17 years 3%; adults <1%)

Gastrointestinal: Diarrhea (1% to 5%; 60 mg/day: 7%), abdominal pain (children 12-17 years 5%; adults 2%), constipation (children 1-11 years 5%; adults 1%), nausea (children 12-17 years 3%; adults 1%)

<1% (Limited to important or life-threatening): Abdomen enlarged, abnormal dreams, abnormal menses, abnormal stools, abnormal vision, agitation, agranulocytosis, albuminuria, allergic reaction, alkaline phosphatase increased, ALT increased, alopecia, amblyopia, amnesia, anaphylactoid reaction, anemia, angina, anorexia, anxiety, aplastic anemia, appetite increased, arrhythmia, AST increased, arthralgia, arthritis, asthma, avitaminosis, bezoar, bilirubinemia, blepharitis, blurred vision, bradycardia, breast enlargement, breast pain, breast tenderness, bronchitis, candidiasis, carcinoma, cardiospasm, cataract, cerebrovascular accident, cerebral infarction, chest pain, chills, cholelithiasis, cholesterol increased/decreased, *Clostridium difficile*-associated diarrhea (CDAD), colitis, confusion, conjunctivitis, cough increased, creatinine increased, deafness, dehydration, dementia, depersonalization, depression, diabetes mellitus, diaphoresis, diplopia, dry eyes, dry skin, dyspepsia, dysphagia, dyspnea, dysmenorrhea, dysuria, edema, electrolyte imbalance, emotional lability, enteritis, eosinophilia, epistaxis, eructation, erythema multiforme, esophageal stenosis, esophageal ulcer, esophagitis, fecal discoloration, fever, fixed eruption, flatulence, flu-like syndrome, fracture, fundic gland polyps, gastric nodules, gastrin levels increased, gastritis, gastroenteritis, gastrointestinal anomaly, gastrointestinal hemorrhage, GGTP increased/decreased, glaucoma, glucocorticoid levels increased, glossitis, glycosuria, goiter, gout, gum hemorrhage, gynecomastia, halitosis, hallucinations, hematemesis, hematuria, hemiplegia, hemolysis, hemolytic anemia, hemoptysis, hepatotoxicity, hostility aggravated, hyper-/hypoglycemia, hyperkinesia, hyperlipemia, hypertonia, hypoesthesia, hyper-/hypotension, hypomagnesemia, hypothyroidism, impotence, infection, insomnia, interstitial nephritis, kidney calculus, laryngeal neoplasia, LDH increased, leg cramps, leukopenia, leukorrhea, libido decreased/increased, liver function test abnormal, lung fibrosis, lymphadenopathy, maculopapular rash, malaise, melena, menorrhagia, migraine, moniliasis (oral), mouth ulceration, musculoskeletal pain, myalgia, myasthenia, myositis, MI, nervousness, neurosis, neutropenia, pain, palpitation, pancreatitis, pancytopenia, paresthesia, parosmia, pelvic pain, peripheral edema, pharyngitis, photophobia, platelet abnormalities, pneumonia, polyuria, pruritus, ptosis, rash, rectal hemorrhage, retinal degeneration, rhinitis, salivation increased, seizure, shock, sinusitis, skin carcinoma, sleep disorder, somnolence, speech disorder, Stevens-Johnson syndrome, stomatitis, stridor, syncope, synovitis, tachycardia, taste loss, taste perversion, tenesmus, thirst, thrombocytopenia, thrombotic thrombocytopenic purpura, tinnitus, tremor, tongue disorder, toxic epidermal necrolysis, ulcerative colitis, ulcerative stomatitis, upper respiratory inflammation, upper respiratory infection, urethral pain, urinary frequency/urgency, urination impaired, urinary retention, urinary tract infection, urticaria, vaginitis, vasodilation, vertigo, visual field defect, vomiting, weakness, WBC abnormal, weight gain/loss, xerostomia

Drug Interactions

Metabolism/Transport Effects Substrate of CYP2C19 (major), CYP2C9 (minor), CYP3A4 (major); **Note:** Assignment of Major/Minor substrate status based on clinically relevant drug interaction potential; **Inhibits** CYP2C19 (weak), CYP2C9 (weak), CYP2D6 (weak); **Induces** CYP1A2 (weak/moderate)

Avoid Concomitant Use

Avoid concomitant use of Lansoprazole with any of the following: Dasatinib; Delavirdine; Erlotinib; Nelfinavir; PAZOPanib; Rilpivirine; Risedronate

Increased Effect/Toxicity

Lansoprazole may increase the levels/effects of: Amphetamine; ARIPiprazole; Dexmethylphenidate; Dextroamphetamine; Imatinib; Methotrexate; Methylphenidate; Raltegravir; Risedronate; Saquinavir; Tacrolimus (Systemic); Vitamin K Antagonists; Voriconazole

The levels/effects of Lansoprazole may be increased by: Fluconazole; Ketoconazole (Systemic); Osimertinib; Voriconazole

Decreased Effect

Lansoprazole may decrease the levels/effects of: Atazanavir; Bisphosphonate Derivatives; Bosutinib; Cefditoren; Clopidogrel; Cysteamine (Systemic); Dabigatran Etexilate; Dabrafenib; Dasatinib; Delavirdine; Erlotinib; Gefitinib; Indinavir; Iron Salts; Itraconazole; Ketoconazole (Systemic); Ledipasvir; Mesalamine; Multivitamins/Minerals (with ADEK, Folate, Iron); Mycophenolate; Nelfinavir; Nilotinib; PAZOPanib; Posaconazole; Rilpivirine; Riociguat; Risedronate

The levels/effects of Lansoprazole may be decreased by: Bosentan; CYP2C19 Inducers (Strong); CYP3A4 Inducers (Moderate); CYP3A4 Inducers (Strong); Dabrafenib; Deferasirox; Enzalutamide; Mitotane; Osimertinib; Siltuximab; St Johns Wort; Tipranavir; Tocilizumab

Food Interactions Prolonged treatment (≥2 years) may lead to malabsorption of dietary vitamin B_{12} and subsequent vitamin B_{12} deficiency (Lam, 2013).

Storage/Stability

Capsules, orally disintegrating tablets: Store at 25°C (77°F); excursions permitted to 15°C to 30°C (59°F to 86°F). Protect from light and moisture.

Powder for suspension (First® compounding kit): Prior to compounding, store at 15°C to 30°C (59°F to 86°F). Once compounded, the product is stable for 30 days at room temperature and under refrigeration; manufacturer recommendation is for the compounded product to be stored under refrigeration; protect from freezing. Protect from light.

Mechanism of Action Decreases acid secretion in gastric parietal cells through inhibition of (H+, K+)-ATPase enzyme system, blocking the final step in gastric acid production.

Pharmacodynamics/Kinetics

Onset of action: Gastric acid suppression: Oral: 1-3 hours
Duration: Gastric acid suppression: Oral: >1 day
Absorption: Rapid
Distribution: V_d: 14-18 L
Protein binding: 97%
Metabolism: Hepatic via CYP2C19 and 3A4, and in parietal cells to two active metabolites that are not present in systemic circulation
Bioavailability: ≥80%; decreased 50% to 70% if given 30 minutes after food
Half-life elimination: 1.5 ± 1 hours; Elderly: 2-3 hours; Hepatic impairment: 3-7 hours
Time to peak, plasma: 1.7 hours
Excretion: Feces (67%); urine (33%)

Dosing

Adult & Geriatric

Symptomatic GERD: Oral: Short-term treatment: 15 mg once daily for up to 8 weeks

Erosive esophagitis: Oral: Short-term treatment: 30 mg once daily for up to 8 weeks; continued treatment for an additional 8 weeks may be considered for recurrence or for patients who do not heal after the first 8 weeks of therapy; maintenance therapy: 15 mg once daily; controlled studies did not extend past 12 months of therapy

Hypersecretory conditions: Oral: Initial: 60 mg once daily; adjust dose based upon patient response and to reduce acid secretion to <10 mEq/hour (5 mEq/hour in patients with prior gastric surgery); doses of 90 mg twice daily have been used; administer doses >120 mg/day in divided doses

Duodenal ulcer: Oral: Short-term treatment: 15 mg once daily for 4 weeks; maintenance therapy: 15 mg once daily

Helicobacter pylori **eradication:**

Manufacturer labeling: 30 mg 3 times daily administered with amoxicillin 1000 mg 3 times daily for 14 days **or** 30 mg twice daily administered with amoxicillin 1000 mg *and* clarithromycin 500 mg twice daily for 10-14 days

American College of Gastroenterology guidelines (Chey, 2007):

Nonpenicillin allergy: 30 mg twice daily administered with amoxicillin 1000 mg *and* clarithromycin 500 mg twice daily for 10-14 days

Penicillin allergy: 30 mg twice daily administered with clarithromycin 500 mg *and* metronidazole 500 mg twice daily for 10-14 days **or** 30 mg once or twice daily administered with bismuth subsalicylate 525 mg *and* metronidazole 250 mg *plus* tetracycline 500 mg 4 times daily for 10-14 days

Gastric ulcer: Oral: Short-term treatment: 30 mg once daily for up to 8 weeks

NSAID-associated gastric ulcer (healing): Oral: 30 mg once daily for 8 weeks; controlled studies did not extend past 8 weeks

NSAID-associated gastric ulcer (to reduce risk): Oral: 15 mg once daily for up to 12 weeks; controlled studies did not extend past 12 weeks

Heartburn (OTC labeling): Oral: 15 mg once daily for 14 days; may repeat 14 days of therapy every 4 months. Do not take for >14 days or more often than every 4 months, unless instructed by healthcare provider.

Stress ulcer prophylaxis, ICU patients (off-label use): Oral: 30 mg once daily (Brophy, 2010; Olsen, 2008). **Note:** Intended for patients with associated risk factors (eg, coagulopathy, mechanical ventilation for ≥48 hours, severe sepsis); discontinue use once risk factors have resolved (Dellinger, 2013).

Pediatric

GERD, erosive esophagitis: Oral: Children 1-11 years:
≤30 kg: 15 mg once daily for up to 12 weeks
>30 kg: 30 mg once daily for up to 12 weeks
Note: Doses were increased in some pediatric patients if still symptomatic after 2 or more weeks of treatment (maximum dose: 30 mg twice daily)

Erosive esophagitis: Children 12-17 years: Oral: 30 mg once daily for up to 8 weeks

Nonerosive GERD: Children 12-17 years: Oral: 15 mg once daily for up to 8 weeks

Renal Impairment No dosage adjustment necessary.

Hepatic Impairment Bioavailability increased in hepatic impairment. Consider dose reduction in severe impairment.

Dietary Considerations Should be taken before eating; best if taken before breakfast. Some products may contain phenylalanine.

Administration

Oral: Administer before food; best if taken before breakfast. The intact granules should not be chewed or crushed; however, several options are available for those patients unable to swallow capsules:

Capsules may be opened and the intact granules sprinkled on 1 tablespoon of applesauce, Ensure® pudding, cottage cheese, yogurt, or strained pears. The granules should then be swallowed immediately.

Capsules may be opened and emptied into ~60 mL orange juice, apple juice, or tomato juice; mix and swallow immediately. Rinse the glass with additional juice and swallow to assure complete delivery of the dose.

Orally-disintegrating tablets: Should not be swallowed whole, broken, cut, or chewed. Place tablet on tongue; allow to dissolve (with or without water) until particles can be swallowed. Orally-disintegrating tablets may also be administered via an oral syringe: Place the 15 mg tablet in an oral syringe and draw up ~4 mL water, or place the 30 mg tablet in an oral syringe and draw up ~10 mL water. After tablet has dispersed, administer within 15 minutes. Refill the syringe with water (2 mL for the 15 mg tablet; 5 mL for the 30 mg tablet), shake gently, then administer any remaining contents.

Nasogastric tube administration:

Capsule: Capsule can be opened, the granules mixed (not crushed) with 40 mL of apple juice and then administered through the NG tube into the stomach, then flush tube with additional apple juice. Do not mix with other liquids. Thirty milligrams has also been suspended in 10 mL of 8.4% sodium bicarbonate solution (or apple juice) and administered via NG tube (Brophy, 2010).

Orally-disintegrating tablet: Nasogastric tube ≥8 French: Place a 15 mg tablet in a syringe and draw up ~4 mL water, or place the 30 mg tablet in a syringe and draw up ~10 mL water. After tablet has dispersed, administer within 15 minutes. Refill the syringe with ~5 mL water, shake gently, and then flush the nasogastric tube.

Monitoring Parameters Patients with Zollinger-Ellison syndrome should be monitored for gastric acid output, which should be maintained at ≤10 mEq/hour during the last hour before the next lansoprazole dose; lab monitoring should include CBC, liver function, renal function, and serum gastrin levels

Dosage Forms Considerations First-Lansoprazole suspension is a compounding kit. Refer to manufacturer's labeling for compounding instructions.

Dosage Forms Excipient information presented when available (limited, particularly for generics); consult specific product labeling. [DSC] = Discontinued product

Capsule Delayed Release, Oral:
Heartburn Relief 24 Hour: 15 mg [DSC] [sodium free; contains brilliant blue fcf (fd&c blue #1), fd&c red #40, fd&c yellow #10 (quinoline yellow)]
Heartburn Treatment 24 Hour: 15 mg [sodium free; contains brilliant blue fcf (fd&c blue #1), fd&c yellow #10 (quinoline yellow)]
Prevacid: 15 mg, 30 mg [contains brilliant blue fcf (fd&c blue #1), fd&c red #40]
Prevacid 24HR: 15 mg [sodium free; contains brilliant blue fcf (fd&c blue #1), fd&c red #40]
Generic: 15 mg, 30 mg

Suspension, Oral:
First-Lansoprazole: 3 mg/mL (90 mL, 150 mL, 300 mL) [contains benzyl alcohol, fd&c red #40, saccharin sodium; strawberry flavor]

Tablet Dispersible, Oral:
Prevacid SoluTab: 15 mg, 30 mg [contains aspartame]
Generic: 15 mg [DSC], 30 mg [DSC]

Extemporaneous Preparations A 3 mg/mL oral solution (Simplified Lansoprazole Solution [SLS]) may be made with capsules and sodium bicarbonate. Empty the contents of ten lansoprazole 30 mg capsules into a beaker. Add 100 mL sodium bicarbonate 8.4% and gently stir until dissolved (about 15 minutes). Transfer solution to an amber-colored syringe or bottle. A prior study showed that SLS was stable for 8 hours at room temperature or for 14 days refrigerated (DiGiancinto, 2000). However, a more recent study, demonstrated SLS to be stable for 48 hours at room temperature and for only 7 days when refrigerated (Morrison, 2013).

Note: A more palatable lansoprazole (3 mg/mL) suspension is commercially available as a compounding kit (First-Lansoprazole).

DiGiancinto JL, Olsen KM, Bergman KL, et al, "Stability of Suspension Formulations of Lansoprazole and Omeprazole Stored in Amber-Colored Plastic Oral Syringes," *Ann Pharmacother*, 2000, 34(5):600-5

Morrison JT, Lugo RA, Thigpen JC, et al, "Stability of Extemporaneously Prepared Lansoprazole Suspension at Two Temperatures," *J Pediatr Pharmacol Ther*, 2013, 18(2):122-7.

Sharma V, "Comparison of 24-hour Intragastric pH Using Four Liquid Formulations of Lansoprazole and Omeprazole," *Am J Health Syst Pharm*, 1999, 56(Suppl 4):18-21.

Sharma VK, Vasudeva R, and Howden CW, "Simplified Lansoprazole Suspension - Liquid Formulations of Lansoprazole - Effectively Suppresses Intragastric Acidity When Administered Through a Gastrostomy," *Am J Gastroenterol*, 1999, 94(7):1813-7.

Lansoprazole, Amoxicillin, and Clarithromycin
(lan SOE pra zole, a moks i SIL in, & kla RITH roe mye sin)

Brand Names: US Prevpac
Brand Names: Canada Hp-PAC
Index Terms Amoxicillin, Clarithromycin, and Lansoprazole; Clarithromycin, Lansoprazole, and Amoxicillin; Lansoprazole, Amoxicillin, and Clarithromycin
Pharmacologic Category Antibiotic, Macrolide Combination; Antibiotic, Penicillin; Gastrointestinal Agent, Miscellaneous; Proton Pump Inhibitor; Substituted Benzimidazole
Use *Helicobacter pylori* **eradication:** Eradication of *H. pylori* infection to reduce the risk of recurrent duodenal ulcer in patients with active or 1-year history of duodenal ulcer
Dosing
Adult & Geriatric *H. pylori* **eradication:** Oral: Lansoprazole 30 mg, amoxicillin 1 g, and clarithromycin 500 mg administered together twice daily for 10 or 14 days (US labeling) or 7, 10, or 14 days (Canadian labeling)
Renal Impairment
US labeling:
CrCl ≥30 mL/minute: There are no dosage adjustments provided in the manufacturer's labeling.
CrCl <30 mL/minute: Use is not recommended.
Canadian labeling: Use of the triple combination product is not recommended.
Hepatic Impairment
US labeling: There are no dosage adjustments provided in the manufacturer's labeling. Bioavailability of lansoprazole increased in hepatic impairment; consider dose reduction in severe hepatic impairment.
Canadian labeling: There are no dosage adjustments provided in the manufacturer's labeling for the combination product; however, for moderate impairment the manufacturer's labeling recommends limiting lansoprazole to 30 mg/day unless there are compelling clinical indications to increase the dosage; consider dose reduction in severe hepatic impairment.
Additional Information Complete prescribing information should be consulted for additional detail.
Dosage Forms Excipient information presented when available (limited, particularly for generics); consult specific product labeling.
Combination package [each administration card contains]:
Prevpac:
Capsule: Amoxicillin 500 mg (4 capsules/day)
Capsule, delayed release (Prevacid): Lansoprazole 30 mg (2 capsules/day)
Tablet (Biaxin): Clarithromycin 500 mg (2 tablets/day)
Generic:
Capsule: Amoxicillin 500 mg (4 capsules/day)
Capsule, delayed release: Lansoprazole 30 mg (2 capsules/day)
Tablet: Clarithromycin 500 mg (2 tablets/day)

Dosage Forms: Canada Excipient information presented when available (limited, particularly for generics); consult specific product labeling.
Combination package [each administration card contains]:
Hp-Pac:
Capsule: Amoxicillin 500 mg (4 capsules/day)
Capsule, delayed release (Prevacid): Lansoprazole 30 mg (2 capsules/day)
Tablet (Biaxin): Clarithromycin 500 mg (2 tablets/day)

◆ Lansoprazole, Amoxicillin, and Clarithromycin *see* Lansoprazole, Amoxicillin, and Clarithromycin *on page 1035*

Lanthanum (LAN tha num)

Brand Names: US Fosrenol
Brand Names: Canada Fosrenol
Index Terms Lanthanum Carbonate
Pharmacologic Category Phosphate Binder
Use Reduction of serum phosphorous: Reduction of serum phosphate in patients with end-stage renal disease (ESRD)
Medication Guide Available Yes
Dosing
Adult & Geriatric Reduction of serum phosphorous:
Oral: Initial: 1500 mg daily (U.S. labeling) or 750 to 1500 mg daily (Canadian labeling) divided and taken with or immediately after meals; typical increases of 750 mg daily every 2 to 3 weeks are suggested as needed to reduce the serum phosphate level <6 mg/dL (1.92 mmol/L); usual dosage range: 1500 to 3000 mg daily; doses of up to 4500 mg have been evaluated
Renal Impairment No dosage adjustment necessary.
Hepatic Impairment There are no dosage adjustments provided in the manufacturer's labeling.
Additional Information Complete prescribing information should be consulted for additional detail.
Dosage Forms Excipient information presented when available (limited, particularly for generics); consult specific product labeling.
Packet, Oral:
Fosrenol: 750 mg (10 ea, 90 ea); 1000 mg (10 ea, 90 ea)
Tablet Chewable, Oral:
Fosrenol: 500 mg, 750 mg, 1000 mg

◆ Lanthanum Carbonate *see* Lanthanum *on page 1035*
◆ Lantus *see* Insulin Glargine *on page 956*
◆ Lantus SoloStar *see* Insulin Glargine *on page 956*
◆ Lanvis® (Can) *see* Thioguanine *on page 1783*

Lapatinib (la PA ti nib)

Brand Names: US Tykerb
Brand Names: Canada Tykerb
Index Terms GW572016; Lapatinib Ditosylate
Pharmacologic Category Antineoplastic Agent, Anti-HER2; Antineoplastic Agent, Epidermal Growth Factor Receptor (EGFR) Inhibitor; Antineoplastic Agent, Tyrosine Kinase Inhibitor
Use
Breast cancer: Treatment of human epidermal growth receptor type 2 (HER2) overexpressing advanced or metastatic breast cancer (in combination with capecitabine) in patients who have received prior therapy (with an anthracycline, a taxane, and trastuzumab); HER2 overexpressing hormone receptor-positive metastatic breast cancer in postmenopausal women where hormone therapy is indicated (in combination with letrozole)
Limitations of use: Patients should have disease progression on trastuzumab prior to initiation of treatment with lapatinib in combination with capecitabine.
Pregnancy Considerations Adverse events were demonstrated in animal reproduction studies. Lapatinib may cause fetal harm if administered during pregnancy. Women of childbearing potential should be advised to avoid pregnancy during treatment.

European Society for Medical Oncology (ESMO) guidelines for cancer during pregnancy recommend delaying treatment with HER-2 targeted agents until after delivery in pregnant patients with HER-2 positive disease (Peccatori 2013).

Breast-Feeding Considerations It is not known if lapatinib is excreted in breast milk. Due to the potential for serious adverse reactions in the nursing infant, the decision to discontinue lapatinib or discontinue breast-feeding during treatment should take in account the benefits of treatment to the mother.

Prescribing and Access Restrictions Lapatinib is available through specialty pharmacies only. Information is available at www.gskcta.com or 1-866-265-6491.

Contraindications Known severe hypersensitivity to lapatinib or any component of the formulation

Warnings/Precautions Hazardous agent - use appropriate precautions for handling and disposal (meets NIOSH 2014 criteria). Decreases in left ventricular ejection fraction (LVEF) have been reported (usually within the first 3 months of treatment); baseline and periodic LVEF evaluations are recommended; interrupt treatment with decreased LVEF ≥ grade 2 or LVEF <LLN; may reinitiate with a reduced dose after a minimum of 2 weeks if the LVEF recovers and the patient is asymptomatic. QTc prolongation has been observed; use caution in patients with a history of QTc prolongation or with medications known to prolong the QT interval; a baseline and periodic 12-lead ECG should be considered; correct electrolyte (potassium, calcium and magnesium) abnormalities prior to and during treatment. Use with caution in conditions which may impair left ventricular function and in patients with a history of or predisposed to (prior treatment with anthracyclines, chest wall irradiation) left ventricular dysfunction. Interstitial lung disease (ILD) and pneumonitis have been reported (with lapatinib monotherapy and with combination chemotherapy); monitor for pulmonary symptoms which may indicate ILD or pneumonitis; discontinue treatment for grade 3 (or higher) pulmonary symptoms indicative of ILD or pneumonitis (eg, dyspnea, dry cough).

[U.S. Boxed Warning]: Hepatotoxicity (ALT or AST >3 times ULN and total bilirubin >2 times ULN) has been reported with lapatinib; may be severe and/or fatal. Onset of hepatotoxicity may occur within days to several months after treatment initiation. Monitor (at baseline and every 4 to 6 weeks during treatment, and as clinically indicated); discontinue with severe changes in liver function; do not reinitiate. Use caution in patients with hepatic dysfunction; dose reductions should be considered in patients with preexisting severe (Child-Pugh class C) hepatic impairment. Potentially significant drug-drug interactions may exist, requiring dose or frequency adjustment, additional monitoring, and/or selection of alternative therapy. Patients who carry the HLA alleles DQA1*02:01 and DRB1*07:01 may experience a greater incidence of severe liver injury than patients who are noncarriers. These alleles are present in ~15% to 25% of Caucasian, Asian, African, and Hispanic patient populations and 1% in Japanese populations. May cause diarrhea (onset is generally within 6 days and duration is 4 to 5 days); may be severe and/or fatal; instruct patients to immediately report any bowel pattern changes. After first unformed stool, administer antidiarrheal agents; severe diarrhea may require hydration, electrolytes, antibiotics (if duration >24 hours, fever, or grade 3/4 neutropenia), and/or treatment interruption, dose reduction, or discontinuation. Severe cutaneous reactions have been reported with use. Discontinue therapy if life-threatening dermatologic reactions (eg, progressive skin rash with blisters or mucosal lesions) such as erythema multiforme, Stevens-Johnson syndrome, or toxic epidermal necrolysis occur.

Adverse Reactions Percentages reported for combination therapy.

>10%:

Central nervous system: Fatigue (≤20%), headache (14%)

Dermatologic: Palmar-plantar erythrodysesthesia (with capecitabine: 53%; grade 3: 12%), skin rash (28% to 44%), alopecia (13%), xeroderma (10% to 13%), pruritus (12%), nail disease (11%)

Gastrointestinal: Diarrhea (64% to 65%; grade 3: 9% to 13%; grade 4: ≤1%), nausea (31% to 44%), vomiting (17% to 26%), mucositis (15%), abdominal pain (≤15%), stomatitis (14%), anorexia (11%), dyspepsia (11%)

Hematologic: Decreased hemoglobin (with capecitabine: 56%; grade 3: <1%), decreased neutrophils (with capecitabine: 22%; grade 3: 3%; grade 4: <1%), decreased platelet count (with capecitabine: 18%; grade 3: <1%)

Hepatic: Increased serum AST (49% to 53%; grade 3: 2% to 6%; grade 4: <1%), increased serum ALT (37% to 46%; grade 3: 2% to 5%; grade 4: <1%), increased serum bilirubin (22% to 45%; grade 3: ≤4%; grade 4: <1%)

Neuromuscular & skeletal: Limb pain (12%), weakness (12%), back pain (11%)

Respiratory: Dyspnea (12%), epistaxis (11%)

1% to 10%: Central nervous system: Insomnia (10%)

<1% (Limited to important or life-threatening): Anaphylaxis, hepatotoxicity, hypersensitivity, interstitial pulmonary disease, left ventricular ejection fraction, paronychia, pneumonitis, prolonged Q-T interval on ECG, severe dermatological reaction

Drug Interactions

Metabolism/Transport Effects Substrate of CYP3A4 (major), P-glycoprotein; **Note:** Assignment of Major/Minor substrate status based on clinically relevant drug interaction potential; **Inhibits** BCRP, CYP2C8 (moderate), CYP3A4 (weak), P-glycoprotein

Avoid Concomitant Use

Avoid concomitant use of Lapatinib with any of the following: Amodiaquine; Bosutinib; Conivaptan; CYP3A4 Inducers (Strong); CYP3A4 Inhibitors (Strong); Dexamethasone (Systemic); Fusidic Acid (Systemic); Grapefruit Juice; Idelalisib; PAZOPanib; Pimozide; Silodosin; St Johns Wort; Topotecan; VinCRIStine (Liposomal)

Increased Effect/Toxicity

Lapatinib may increase the levels/effects of: Afatinib; Amodiaquine; ARIPiprazole; Bosutinib; Brentuximab Vedotin; Colchicine; CYP2C8 Substrates; Dabigatran Etexilate; DOXOrubicin (Conventional); Edoxaban; Everolimus; Flibanserin; Highest Risk QTc-Prolonging Agents; Hydrocodone; Ledipasvir; Lomitapide; Moderate Risk QTc-Prolonging Agents; Naloxegol; NiMODipine; PAZOPanib; P-glycoprotein/ABCB1 Substrates; Pimozide; Prucalopride; Ranolazine; Rifaximin; Silodosin; Topotecan; VinCRIStine (Liposomal)

The levels/effects of Lapatinib may be increased by: Aprepitant; Conivaptan; CYP3A4 Inhibitors (Moderate); CYP3A4 Inhibitors (Strong); Dasatinib; Fosaprepitant; Fusidic Acid (Systemic); Grapefruit Juice; Idelalisib; Ivacaftor; Luliconazole; Mifepristone; Netupitant; Osimertinib; Palbociclib; P-glycoprotein/ABCB1 Inhibitors; Ranolazine; Simeprevir; Stiripentol

Decreased Effect

The levels/effects of Lapatinib may be decreased by: Bosentan; CYP3A4 Inducers (Moderate); CYP3A4 Inducers (Strong); Dabrafenib; Deferasirox; Dexamethasone (Systemic); Osimertinib; P-glycoprotein/ABCB1 Inducers; Siltuximab; St Johns Wort; Tocilizumab

Food Interactions Systemic exposure of lapatinib is increased when administered with food (AUC three- to fourfold higher). Grapefruit juice may increase the levels/effects of lapatinib. Management: Administer once daily on an empty stomach, 1 hour before or 1 hour after a meal at the same time each day. Avoid grapefruit juice. Maintain adequate hydration, unless instructed to restrict fluid intake.

Storage/Stability Store at room temperature of 25°C (77°F); excursions permitted between 15°C and 30°C (59°F and 86°F).

Mechanism of Action Tyrosine kinase (dual kinase) inhibitor; inhibits EGFR (ErbB1) and HER2 (ErbB2) by reversibly binding to tyrosine kinase, blocking phosphorylation and activation of downstream second messengers (Erk1/2 and Akt), regulating cellular proliferation and survival in ErbB- and ErbB2-expressing tumors. Combination therapy with lapatinib and endocrine therapy may overcome endocrine resistance occurring in HER2+ and hormone receptor positive disease.

Pharmacodynamics/Kinetics

Absorption: Incomplete and variable

Protein binding: >99% to albumin and alpha$_1$-acid glycoprotein

Metabolism: Hepatic; extensive via CYP3A4 and 3A5, and to a lesser extent via CYP2C19 and 2C8 to oxidized metabolites

Half-life elimination: ~24 hours

Time to peak, plasma: ~4 hours (Burris, 2009)

Excretion: Feces (27% as unchanged drug; range 3% to 67%); urine (<2%)

Dosing

Adult & Geriatric

Breast cancer, metastatic, HER2+ (with prior anthracycline, taxane, and trastuzumab therapy): Oral: 1250 mg once daily (in combination with capecitabine) until disease progression or unacceptable toxicity (Geyer, 2006)

Breast cancer, metastatic, HER2+, hormonal therapy indicated: Oral: 1500 mg once daily (in combination with letrozole) until disease progression (Johnston, 2009)

Breast cancer, metastatic, HER2+ with brain metastases, first-line therapy (off-label use): Oral: 1250 mg once daily (in combination with capecitabine) until disease progression or unacceptable toxicity (Bachelot, 2013)

Breast cancer, metastatic, HER2+, with progression on prior trastuzumab therapy (off-label use): Oral: 1000 mg once daily (in combination with trastuzumab) (Blackwell, 2010; Blackwell, 2012)

Missed doses: If a dose is missed, resume with the next scheduled daily dose; do not double the dose the next day.

Dosage adjustment for concomitant CYP3A4 inhibitors/inducers:

CYP3A4 inhibitors: Avoid the use of concomitant strong CYP3A4 inhibitors. If concomitant use cannot be avoided, consider reducing lapatinib to 500 mg once daily with careful monitoring. When a strong CYP3A4 inhibitor is discontinued, allow ~1 week to elapse prior to adjusting the lapatinib dose upward.

CYP3A4 inducers: Avoid the use of concomitant strong CYP3A4 inducers.

U.S. labeling: If concomitant use cannot be avoided, consider gradually titrating lapatinib from 1250 mg once daily up to 4500 mg daily (in combination with capecitabine) **or** from 1500 mg once daily up to 5500 mg daily (in combination with letrozole), based on tolerability and with careful monitoring. If the strong CYP3A4 enzyme inducer is discontinued, reduce the lapatinib dose to the indicated dose.

Canadian labeling: If concomitant use cannot be avoided, titrate lapatinib dose gradually upward based on tolerability. If the strong CYP3A4 enzyme inducer is discontinued, reduce the lapatinib dose over 2 weeks.

Renal Impairment There are no dosage adjustments provided in the manufacturer's labeling (has not been studied); however, due to the minimal renal elimination (<2%), dosage adjustments may not be necessary.

Hepatic Impairment

Mild or moderate preexisting impairment (Child-Pugh class A or B): There are no dosage adjustments provided in the manufacturer's labeling.

Severe preexisting impairment (Child-Pugh class C):

US labeling: The following adjustments should be considered (and are predicted to normalize the AUC), however, there are no clinical data associated with the adjustments.

In combination with capecitabine: Reduce dose from 1250 mg once daily to 750 mg once daily.

In combination with letrozole: Reduce dose from 1500 mg once daily to 1000 mg once daily.

Canadian labeling: There are no specific dosage adjustments provided in the manufacturer's labeling; however, a dosage reduction is recommended based on pharmacokinetic modeling (safety and efficacy of dose reduction has not been demonstrated).

Severe hepatotoxicity during treatment: Discontinue permanently (do not rechallenge).

Adjustment for Toxicity

Cardiac toxicity: Discontinue treatment for at least 2 weeks for LVEF < LLN or decreased LVEF ≥ grade 2 (U.S. labeling) or decreased LVEF ≥ grade 3 (Canadian labeling); may be restarted at 1000 mg once daily (in combination with capecitabine) **or** 1250 mg once daily (in combination with letrozole) if LVEF recovers to normal and patient is asymptomatic.

Dermatologic toxicity: Discontinue treatment for suspected erythema multiforme, Stevens-Johnson syndrome, or toxic epidermal necrolysis.

Diarrhea:

Grade 3 diarrhea or grade 1 or 2 diarrhea with complicating features (moderate-to-severe abdominal cramping, grade 2 or higher nausea/vomiting, decreased performance status, fever, sepsis, neutropenia, frank bleeding, or dehydration):

U.S. labeling: Interrupt treatment; may restart at a reduced dose (from 1500 mg once daily to 1250 mg once daily or from 1250 mg once daily to 1000 mg once daily) when diarrhea resolves to ≤ grade 1.

Canadian labeling: Interrupt treatment; may restart at a reduced dose (from 1500 mg once daily to 1250 mg once daily or from 1250 mg once daily to 1000 mg once daily or from 1000 mg once daily to 750 mg once daily) when diarrhea resolves to ≤ grade 1.

Grade 4 diarrhea: Permanently discontinue.

Pulmonary toxicity: Discontinue treatment with pulmonary symptoms indicative of interstitial lung disease or pneumonitis which are ≥ grade 3

Other toxicities: Withhold for any toxicity (other than cardiac) ≥ grade 2 until toxicity resolves to ≤ grade 1 and reinitiate at the standard dose of 1250 or 1500 mg once daily; for persistent toxicity, reduce dosage to 1000 mg once daily (in combination with capecitabine) **or** 1250 mg once daily (in combination with letrozole)

Dietary Considerations Avoid grapefruit juice.

Administration Administer once daily, on an empty stomach, 1 hour before or 1 hour after a meal. Take full dose at the same time each day; dividing dose throughout the day is not recommended.

Note: For combination treatment with capecitabine, capecitabine should be administered in 2 doses (approximately 12 hours apart) and taken with food or within 30 minutes after a meal.

Hazardous agent; use appropriate precautions for handling and disposal (meets NIOSH 2014 criteria).

Monitoring Parameters LVEF (baseline and periodic), CBC with differential, liver function tests, including transaminases, bilirubin, and alkaline phosphatase (baseline and every 4-6 weeks during treatment); electrolytes including calcium, potassium, magnesium; monitor for fluid retention; ECG monitoring if at risk for QTc prolongation; symptoms of ILD or pneumonitis; monitor for diarrhea and dermatologic toxicity

Dosage Forms Excipient information presented when available (limited, particularly for generics); consult specific product labeling.

Tablet, Oral:

Tykerb: 250 mg [contains fd&c yellow #6 (sunset yellow), fd&c yellow #6 aluminum lake]

◆ Lapatinib Ditosylate *see* Lapatinib *on page 1035*

◆ L-Arginine *see* Arginine *on page 147*

◆ L-Arginine Hydrochloride *see* Arginine *on page 147*

◆ Lariam *see* Mefloquine *on page 1135*

◆ Larin 1.5/30 *see* Ethinyl Estradiol and Norethindrone *on page 708*

◆ Larin 1/20 *see* Ethinyl Estradiol and Norethindrone *on page 708*

◆ Larin 24 Fe *see* Ethinyl Estradiol and Norethindrone *on page 708*

◆ Larin Fe 1.5/30 *see* Ethinyl Estradiol and Norethindrone *on page 708*

◆ Larin Fe 1/20 *see* Ethinyl Estradiol and Norethindrone *on page 708*

Laronidase (lair OH ni days)

Brand Names: US Aldurazyme

Brand Names: Canada Aldurazyme®

Index Terms Recombinant α-L-Iduronidase (Glycosaminoglycan α-L-Iduronohydrolase)

Pharmacologic Category Enzyme

Use Treatment of Hurler and Hurler-Scheie forms of mucopolysaccharidosis I (MPS I); treatment of Scheie form of MPS I in patients with moderate-to-severe symptoms

Dosing

Adult & Geriatric Note: Premedicate with antipyretic and/or antihistamines 1 hour prior to start of infusion.

MPS I (Hurler syndrome, Hurler-Scheie, and Scheie forms): IV: 0.58 mg/kg once weekly; dose should be rounded up to the nearest whole vial

Pediatric Note: Premedicate with antipyretic and/or antihistamines 1 hour prior to start of infusion.

MPS I (Hurler syndrome, Hurler-Scheie, and Scheie forms): Children ≥6 months: IV: 0.58 mg/kg once weekly; dose should be rounded up to the nearest whole vial

Renal Impairment No dosage adjustment provided in manufacturer's labeling.

Hepatic Impairment No dosage adjustment provided in manufacturer's labeling.

Additional Information Complete prescribing information should be consulted for additional detail.

Dosage Forms Excipient information presented when available (limited, particularly for generics); consult specific product labeling.

Solution, Intravenous:

Aldurazyme: 2.9 mg/5 mL (5 mL) [contains mouse protein (murine) (hamster), polysorbate 80]

◆ Lasix *see* Furosemide *on page 821*

◆ Lasix Special (Can) *see* Furosemide *on page 821*

◆ L-asparaginase (*Erwinia*) *see* Asparaginase (*Erwinia*) *on page 156*

◆ L-asparaginase with Polyethylene Glycol *see* Pegaspargase *on page 1407*

◆ Lassar's Zinc Paste *see* Zinc Oxide *on page 1929*

Latanoprost (la TA noe prost)

Brand Names: US Xalatan

Brand Names: Canada ACT Latanoprost; Apo-Latanoprost; GD-Latanoprost; Med-Latanoprost; PMS-Latanoprost; Riva-Latanoprost; Sandoz-Latanoprost; Xalatan

Pharmacologic Category Ophthalmic Agent, Antiglaucoma; Prostaglandin, Ophthalmic

Use Elevated intraocular pressure: Reduction of elevated intraocular pressure (IOP) in patients with open-angle glaucoma and ocular hypertension.

Dosing

Adult & Geriatric Elevated intraocular pressure: Ophthalmic: One drop in the affected eye(s) once daily in the evening; do not exceed the once daily dosage (may decrease the IOP-lowering effect)

Renal Impairment There is no dosage adjustment provided in manufacturer's labeling. However, dosage adjustment unlikely due to low systemic absorption.

Hepatic Impairment There is no dosage adjustment provided in manufacturer's labeling. However, dosage adjustment unlikely due to low systemic absorption.

Additional Information Complete prescribing information should be consulted for additional detail.

Dosage Forms Excipient information presented when available (limited, particularly for generics); consult specific product labeling.

Solution, Ophthalmic:

Xalatan: 0.005% (2.5 mL) [contains benzalkonium chloride]

Generic: 0.005% (2.5 mL)

Ledipasvir and Sofosbuvir
(le DIP as vir & soe FOS bue vir)

Brand Names: US Harvoni

Brand Names: Canada Harvoni

Index Terms GS-5885; Sofosbuvir and Ledipasvir

Pharmacologic Category Antihepaciviral, NS5A Inhibitor; Antihepaciviral, Polymerase Inhibitor (Anti-HCV)

Use

US labeling: Treatment of chronic hepatitis C virus (HCV) genotype 1, 4, 5, or 6 infection.

Canadian labeling: Treatment of chronic HCV genotype 1 infection in adults.

Pregnancy Considerations Adverse events were not observed in animal reproduction studies using the components of this combination.

Breast-Feeding Considerations It is not known if ledipasvir or sofosbuvir are excreted into breast milk. According to the U.S. labeling, the decision to breastfeed during therapy should take into account the risk of exposure to the infant and the benefits of treatment to the mother. The Canadian labeling recommends discontinuing breast-feeding prior to initiating therapy.

Contraindications

If ledipasvir/sofosbuvir is administered with ribavirin, the contraindications to ribavirin also apply. See ribavirin manufacturer's information.

Canadian labeling: Hypersensitivity to any component of the formulation.

Warnings/Precautions Potentially significant drug-drug interactions may exist, requiring dose or frequency adjustment, additional monitoring, and/or selection of alternative therapy. Symptomatic bradycardia (some requiring pacemaker intervention) and fatal cardiac arrest has occurred in patients receiving amiodarone and ledipasvir/sofosbuvir. Bradycardia generally occurred within hours to days following coadministration, however some cases have occurred 2 weeks following the initiation of HCV treatment. The risk of bradycardia may be increased in patients taking beta blockers or patients with underlying cardiac comorbidities and/or advanced liver disease. Bradycardia generally resolves following discontinuation of ledipasvir/sofosbuvir. Coadministration of amiodarone and ledipasvir/sofosbuvir is not recommended. However, if patients have no treatment alternatives, patients should have inpatient cardiac monitoring for the first 48 hours, followed by daily outpatient or self-monitoring of heart rate for at least the first 2 weeks of treatment. Due to the long half-life of amiodarone, cardiac monitoring (as described) is also recommended if amiodarone was discontinued just prior to beginning treatment with ledipasvir/sofosbuvir. Patients should seek medical attention immediately if they experience fainting or near-fainting, dizziness, lightheadedness, malaise, weakness, excessive tiredness, shortness of breath, chest pains, confusion or memory problems. Avoid concurrent use with other sofosbuvir-containing products. Therapy should be initiated by a physician experienced in the treatment of chronic hepatitis C. Tablets may contain lactose; consider lactose content prior to initiating therapy in patients with rare hereditary problems of galactose intolerance.

Adverse Reactions Also see individual agents.

>10%: Central nervous system: Fatigue (13% to 18%), headache (11% to 17%)

1% to 10%:

Central nervous system: Insomnia (3% to 6%)

Gastrointestinal: Nausea (6% to 9%), diarrhea (3% to 7%), increased serum lipase (>3 x ULN; ≤3%)

Hepatic: Hyperbilirubinemia (>1.5 x ULN; ≤3%)

Drug Interactions

Metabolism/Transport Effects Refer to individual components.

Avoid Concomitant Use

Avoid concomitant use of Ledipasvir and Sofosbuvir with any of the following: Amiodarone; Bosutinib; Modafinil; OXcarbazepine; PAZOPanib; P-glycoprotein/ABCB1 Inducers; Rifabutin; Rifapentine; Rosuvastatin; Silodosin; Simeprevir; Topotecan; VinCRIStine (Liposomal)

Increased Effect/Toxicity

Ledipasvir and Sofosbuvir may increase the levels/effects of: Afatinib; Amiodarone; Bosutinib; Brentuximab Vedotin; Colchicine; Dabigatran Etexilate; DOXOrubicin (Conventional); Edoxaban; Everolimus; Naloxegol; PAZOPanib; P-glycoprotein/ABCB1 Substrates; Prucalopride; Ranolazine; Rifaximin; Rosuvastatin; Silodosin; Simeprevir; Tenofovir Disoproxil Fumarate; Topotecan; VinCRIStine (Liposomal)

The levels/effects of Ledipasvir and Sofosbuvir may be increased by: Lumacaftor; P-glycoprotein/ABCB1 Inhibitors; Ranolazine; Simeprevir

Decreased Effect

The levels/effects of Ledipasvir and Sofosbuvir may be decreased by: Antacids; H2-Antagonists; Lumacaftor; Modafinil; OXcarbazepine; P-glycoprotein/ABCB1 Inducers; Proton Pump Inhibitors; Rifabutin; Rifapentine

Storage/Stability Store below 30°C (86°F). Dispense in original container.

Mechanism of Action Ledipasvir inhibits the HCV NS5A protein necessary for viral replication; sofosbuvir is a prodrug converted to its pharmacologically active form (GS-461203), inhibits NS5B RNA-dependent RNA polymerase, also essential for viral replication, and acts as a chain terminator.

Pharmacodynamics/Kinetics

Absorption: Ledipasvir and sofosbuvir are well absorbed

Protein binding: Ledipasvir: >99.8%; Sofosbuvir: 61% to 65%

Metabolism: Ledipasvir: Slow oxidative metabolism via an unknown mechanism; Sofosbuvir: Hepatic; forms pharmacologically active nucleoside (uridine) analog triphosphate GS-461203; Dephosphorylation results in the formation of nucleoside inactive metabolite GS-331007

Half-life elimination: Ledipasvir: 47 hours; Sofosbuvir: ~0.5 hours

Time to peak: Ledipasvir: 4 to 4.5 hours; Sofosbuvir: ~0.8 to 1 hour

Excretion: Ledipasvir: Feces (~86%), urine (1%); Sofosbuvir: Urine (80%), feces (14%)

Dosing

Adult & Geriatric

US labeling:

Chronic hepatitis C (CHC) infection in monoinfected (HCV) or coinfected (HCV/HIV-1) genotype 1 patients: Oral: Treatment regimen and duration based on clinical scenario as noted below; fixed-dose tablet is ledipasvir 90 mg and sofosbuvir 400 mg:

Treatment-naive patients with or without cirrhosis or treatment-experienced patients without cirrhosis: One tablet once daily for 12 weeks.

Treatment-experienced patients with cirrhosis:

Used without concomitant ribavirin: One tablet once daily for 24 weeks.

Used with concomitant ribavirin in eligible patients: One tablet daily with concomitant ribavirin for 12 weeks.

Note: Treatment-naive patients without cirrhosis who have HCV RNA <6 million units/mL may be considered for therapy of 8 weeks duration. Treatment-experienced patients are defined as those in whom treatment has failed with a peginterferon alfa plus ribavirin based regimen with or without an HCV protease inhibitor.

Chronic hepatitis C (CHC) infection in monoinfected (HCV) or coinfected (HCV/HIV-1) genotype 4, 5 or 6 patients: Oral: Treatment regimen and duration based on clinical scenario as noted below; fixed-dose tablet is ledipasvir 90 mg and sofosbuvir 400 mg:

Treatment-naive patients with or without cirrhosis or treatment-experienced patients with or without cirrhosis: One tablet once daily for 12 weeks.

Note: Treatment-experienced patients are defined as those in whom treatment has failed with a peginterferon alfa plus ribavirin based regimen with or without an HCV protease inhibitor.

Canadian labeling:

Chronic hepatitis C (CHC) infection genotype 1 patients: Oral: Treatment regimen and duration based on clinical scenario as noted below; fixed-dose tablet is ledipasvir 90 mg and sofosbuvir 400 mg:

Treatment-naive patients with or without cirrhosis or treatment-experienced patients without cirrhosis: One tablet once daily for 12 weeks.

Treatment-experienced patients with cirrhosis: One tablet once daily for 24 weeks.

Note: Treatment-naive patients without cirrhosis who have HCV RNA <6 million units/mL may be considered for therapy of 8 weeks duration. Treatment experienced patients are defined as those who have failed therapy with an interferon-based regimen, including regimens containing an HCV protease inhibitor.

Missed dose: If missed dose is within 18 hours of regularly scheduled time, administer as soon as possible; if >18 hours from regularly scheduled time, resume at next regularly scheduled dose (do not double dose). If patient vomits <5 hours after administration dose should be repeated; if >5 hours, resume administer at next regularly scheduled dose.

Renal Impairment

CrCl ≥30 mL/minute/1.73 m² : No dosage adjustment necessary.

CrCl <30 mL/minute/1.73 m² : There are no dosage adjustments provided in manufacturer's labeling. However, sofosbuvir and metabolite accumulate in patients with severely impaired renal function.

End-stage renal disease (ESRD), including those requiring intermittent hemodialysis (IHD): There are no dosage adjustments provided in manufacturer's labeling However, sofosbuvir and metabolite accumulate in patients with severely impaired renal function. In a 4-hour dialysis session, 18% of sofosbuvir dose was removed.

Hepatic Impairment

Child-Pugh class A, B, or C: No dosage adjustment necessary.

Decompensated cirrhosis: There are no dosage adjustments provided in manufacturer's labeling (has not been studied).

Administration Oral: Administer with or without food.

Monitoring Parameters

Bilirubin, liver enzymes, and serum creatinine at baseline and periodically when clinically indicated. If used in combination with amiodarone (or in patients who discontinued amiodarone just prior to initiating ledipasvir/sofosbuvir), inpatient cardiac monitoring for the first 48 hours of coadministration, then outpatient or self-monitoring of heart rate daily through at least the first 2 weeks of treatment.

Serum HCV-RNA at baseline, during treatment, at the end of treatment, during treatment follow-up, and when clinically indicated.

Dosage Forms Excipient information presented when available (limited, particularly for generics); consult specific product labeling.

Tablet, Oral:

Harvoni: Ledipasvir 90 mg and sofosbuvir 400 mg [contains fd&c yellow #6 aluminum lake]

◆ Leena *see* Ethinyl Estradiol and Norethindrone on page 708

Leflunomide (le FLOO noh mide)

Brand Names: US Arava

Brand Names: Canada Apo-Leflunomide; Arava; Mylan-Leflunomide; PHL-Leflunomide; PMS-Leflunomide; Sandoz-Leflunomide; Teva-Leflunomide

Pharmacologic Category Antirheumatic, Disease Modifying

Use Rheumatoid arthritis: Treatment of adults with active rheumatoid arthritis (RA).

Pregnancy Considerations [US Boxed Warning]: Leflunomide is contraindicated in pregnant women because of the potential for fetal harm. Adverse events were observed in animal reproduction studies with doses lower than the expected human exposure. Exclude pregnancy before the start of treatment in females of reproductive potential. Advise females of reproductive potential to use effective contraception during treatment and during an accelerated elimination procedure after treatment is discontinued. Discontinue therapy and use an accelerated elimination procedure if pregnancy occurs during treatment. Women of reproductive potential should not receive therapy until pregnancy has been excluded, they have been counseled concerning fetal risk, and reliable contraceptive measures have been confirmed. Following treatment, pregnancy should be avoided until undetectable serum concentrations (<0.02 mg/L) are verified. This may be accomplished by the use of an enhanced drug elimination procedure using cholestyramine. Serum concentrations <0.02 mg/L should be verified by 2 separate tests performed at least 14 days apart. If serum concentrations are >0.02 mg/L, additional cholestyramine treatment should be considered. As an alternative to cholestyramine, the Canadian labeling recommends that activated charcoal may be used to enhance drug elimination.

It is not known if males taking leflunomide may contribute to fetal toxicity. Males taking leflunomide who wish to father a child should consider discontinuing therapy and using the cholestyramine procedure to eliminate the medication. The Canadian labeling recommends avoiding use in males capable of fathering a child and who are not using reliable contraception during and for a total of 2 years after treatment unless an elimination procedure is used; for men receiving treatment and desiring to father a child, serum concentrations of the active metabolite should be verified by 2 separate tests performed at least 14 days apart. If levels <0.02 mg/L are confirmed with the second test, an additional waiting period of 3 months is recommended.

Health care providers are encouraged to enroll women exposed to leflunomide during pregnancy in the Pregnancy Registry (877-311-8972 or http://www.pregnancystudies.org/participate-ina-study/).

Breast-Feeding Considerations It is not known whether leflunomide is secreted in human milk. Because the potential for serious adverse reactions exists in breast-feeding infants, a decision should be made whether to discontinue breast-feeding or discontinue the drug, taking into account the importance of the drug to the mother. Canadian labeling contraindicates use in breast-feeding women.

Contraindications

Hypersensitivity to leflunomide or any component of the formulation; severe hepatic impairment; concomitant treatment with teriflunomide; pregnant women.

Canadian labeling: Additional contraindications (not in US labeling): Hypersensitivity to teriflunomide; moderate to severe renal impairment; immunodeficiency states; impaired bone marrow function or significant anemia, leukopenia, neutropenia, or thrombocytopenia due to causes other than rheumatoid arthritis; serious infections; impaired liver function; severe hypoproteinemia; women of childbearing potential who are not using reliable contraception before, during, and for a period of 2 years after treatment with leflunomide (or as long as plasma levels of the active metabolite are above 0.02 mg/L); breast-feeding; patients younger than 18 years of age

Warnings/Precautions Hazardous agent - use appropriate precautions for handling and disposal (NIOSH 2014 [group 2]).

[US Boxed Warning]: Severe liver injury, including fatal liver failure, has been reported in some patients treated with leflunomide. Leflunomide is contraindicated in patients with severe hepatic impairment. Concomitant use of leflunomide with other potentially hepatotoxic drugs may increase the risk of liver injury. Patients with preexisting acute or chronic liver disease, or those with ALT more than twice the upper limit of normal (ULN) before initiating treatment, are at increased risk and should not be treated with leflunomide. Monitor ALT levels at least monthly for 6 months after starting leflunomide, and thereafter every 6 to 8 weeks. If ALT elevation >3-fold the ULN occurs, interrupt therapy and investigate the cause. **If leflunomide-induced liver injury is suspected, stop leflunomide treatment, start an accelerated drug elimination procedure, and monitor liver tests weekly until normalized.** If leflunomide-induced liver injury is unlikely because another cause has been found, resumption of leflunomide therapy may be considered. If given concomitantly with methotrexate, follow the American College of Rheumatology (ACR) guidelines for monitoring methotrexate liver toxicity with ALT, AST, and serum albumin testing.

Use has been associated (rarely) with interstitial lung disease; the risk is increased in patients with a history of interstitial lung disease. Further investigate etiology in patients who develop new-onset or worsening of pulmonary symptoms (eg, cough and dyspnea, with or without associated fever). Accelerated drug elimination procedures should be considered if interstitial lung disease occurs (with some fatalities reported). Blood pressure elevations have been observed; assess blood pressure at baseline and monitor periodically during therapy. May increase susceptibility to infection, including opportunistic pathogens (especially *Pneumocystis jiroveci* pneumonia, tuberculosis [including extrapulmonary tuberculosis], and aspergillosis). Severe infections, sepsis, and fatalities have been reported. Not recommended in patients with severe immunodeficiency, bone marrow dysplasia, or severe, uncontrolled infections. Caution should be exercised when considering use in patients with a history of new/recurrent infections, with conditions that predispose them to infections, or with chronic, latent, or localized infections. Patients who develop a new infection while undergoing treatment should be monitored closely; consider discontinuation of therapy and accelerated drug elimination procedures if infection is serious.

Use of some immunosuppressive medications may increase risk of malignancies; impact on the development and course of malignancies is not fully defined. Pancytopenia, agranulocytosis, and thrombocytopenia have been reported with leflunomide therapy alone; most frequently hematologic toxicity occurs in patients receiving concomitant therapy with methotrexate or other immunosuppressive agents, or who had recently discontinued these therapies. In some cases, patients had a history of a significant hematologic abnormality. All patients should have platelet, white blood cell count (WBC) and hemoglobin or hematocrit monitored at baseline and monthly for 6 months following therapy initiation and then every 6 to 8 weeks thereafter. If used with concomitant methotrexate or other potential immunosuppressive agents, increase chronic monitoring to monthly. If evidence of bone marrow suppression occurs, stop treatment and initiate an accelerated drug elimination procedure. Use with caution in patients with a history of significant hematologic abnormalities; avoid use with bone marrow dysplasia. The Canadian labeling contraindicates use with impaired bone marrow function or significant anemia, leukopenia, neutropenia, or thrombocytopenia due to causes other than rheumatoid arthritis. Use has been associated with rare pancytopenia, agranulocytosis, and thrombocytopenia, generally when given concurrently or recently with methotrexate or other immunosuppressive agents. Monitoring of hematologic function is required; discontinue if evidence of bone marrow suppression and begin drug elimination procedures (eg, cholestyramine or activated charcoal). Rare cases of dermatologic reactions (including Stevens-Johnson syndrome, toxic epidermal necrolysis, and drug reaction with eosinophilia and systemic symptoms [DRESS]) have been reported; discontinue if evidence of severe dermatologic reaction occurs, and begin drug elimination procedures (eg, cholestyramine or activated charcoal). Cases of peripheral neuropathy have been reported; use with caution in patients >60 years of age, receiving concomitant neurotoxic medications, or patients with diabetes; discontinue if evidence of peripheral neuropathy occurs and begin accelerated drug elimination procedures.

Safety has not been established in patients with latent tuberculosis infection. Patients should be screened for tuberculosis and if necessary, treated prior to initiating therapy. Use with caution in patients with renal impairment. The Canadian labeling contraindicates use in moderate to severe impairment. Use in patients with hepatic impairment is not recommended due to risk of increased hepatotoxicity. **[US Boxed Warning]: Leflunomide is contraindicated in pregnant women because of the potential for fetal harm. Adverse events were observed in animal reproduction studies with doses lower than the expected human exposure. Exclude pregnancy before the start of treatment in females of reproductive potential. Advise females of reproductive potential to use effective contraception during treatment and during an accelerated elimination procedure after treatment is discontinued. Discontinue therapy and use an accelerated elimination procedure if pregnancy occurs during treatment.** The Canadian labeling contraindicates use in women of childbearing potential who are not using reliable contraception before, during, and for a period of 2 years after treatment with leflunomide (or as long as plasma levels of the active metabolite are above 0.02 mg/L). No clinical data are available on the efficacy and safety of vaccinations during leflunomide treatment. Vaccination with live vaccines is not recommended; consider the long elimination half-life of the leflunomide active metabolite (eg, teriflunomide) when considering live vaccine administration after leflunomide discontinuation.

Due to variations in clearance, it may take up to 2 years to reach low levels of leflunomide metabolite serum concentrations. An accelerated drug elimination procedure is recommended when a more rapid elimination is needed. Refer to dosing for detailed accelerated elimination procedure. Verify plasma teriflunomide concentrations are less than 0.02 mg/L by tests at least 14 days apart. If concentrations are greater than 0.02 mg/L, repeat the accelerated elimination procedure. Use of accelerated drug elimination may potentially result in return of disease activity if the patient has been responding to leflunomide treatment.

Potentially significant drug-drug interactions may exist, requiring dose or frequency adjustment, additional monitoring, and/or selection of alternative therapy.

Adverse Reactions

>10%:

Central nervous system: Headache (7% to 13%)

Dermatologic: Alopecia (9% to 17%), skin rash (10% to 12%)

Gastrointestinal: Diarrhea (17% to 27%), nausea (9% to 13%)

Respiratory: Respiratory tract infection (15% to 27%)

1% to 10%:

Cardiovascular: Hypertension (9% to 10%; new onset 1% to 2%), chest pain (1% to 4%), angina pectoris (1% to <3%), palpitations (1% to <3%), peripheral edema (1% to <3%), tachycardia (1% to <3%), varicose veins (1% to <3%), vasculitis (1% to <3%), vasodilatation (1% to <3%)

Central nervous system: Dizziness (4% to 7%), paresthesia (2% to 4%), pain (1% to 4%), anxiety (1% to <3%), depression (1% to <3%), insomnia (1% to <3%), malaise (1% to <3%), migraine (1% to <3%), neuralgia (1% to <3%), neuritis (1% to <3%), sleep disorder (1% to <3%), vertigo (1% to <3%)

Dermatologic: Pruritus (4% to 6%), dry skin (2% to 3%), eczema (2% to 3%), acne vulgaris (1% to <3%), contact dermatitis (1% to <3%), cutaneous nodule (1% to <3%), dermal ulcer (1% to <3%), dermatological disease (1% to <3%), diaphoresis (1% to <3%), fungal dermatitis (1% to <3%), hair discoloration (1% to <3%), maculopapular rash (1% to <3%), nail disease (1% to <3%), skin discoloration (1% to <3%), subcutaneous nodule (1% to <3%)

Endocrine & metabolic: Weight loss (2% to 4%); hypokalemia (1% to 3%), albuminuria (1% to <3%), diabetes mellitus (1% to <3%), hyperglycemia (1% to <3%), hyperlipidemia (1% to <3%), hyperthyroidism (1% to <3%), menstrual disease (1% to <3%)

Gastrointestinal: Gastrointestinal pain (5% to 8%), abdominal pain (5% to 6%), dyspepsia (5% to 6%), oral mucosa ulcer (3% to 5%), vomiting (3% to 5%), anorexia (3%), gastroenteritis (3%), cholelithiasis (1% to <3%), colitis (1% to <3%), constipation (1% to <3%), dysgeusia (1% to <3%), enlargement of salivary glands (1% to <3%), esophagitis (1% to <3%), flatulence (1% to <3%), gastritis (1% to <3%), gingivitis (1% to <3%), hernia (1% to <3%), melena (1% to <3%), oral candidiasis (1% to <3%), stomatitis (1% to <3%), xerostomia (1% to <3%)

Genitourinary: Urinary tract infection (5%), cystitis (1% to <3%), dysuria (1% to <3%), hematuria (1% to <3%), pelvic pain (1% to <3%), prostatic disease (1% to <3%), urinary frequency (1% to <3%), vulvo candidiasis (1% to <3%)

Hematologic & oncologic: Anemia (1% to <3%), ecchymoses (1% to <3%), hematoma (1% to <3%)

Hepatic: Abnormal hepatic function tests (5% to 10%), increased serum ALT (>3 x ULN 2% to 4%; reversible)

Hypersensitivity: Hypersensitivity reaction (1% to 5%)

Infection: Abscess (1% to <3%), herpes simplex infection (1% to <3%), herpes zoster (1% to <3%)

Neuromuscular & skeletal: Back pain (5% to 8%), arthropathy (4% to 8%), weakness (3% to 6%), tenosynovitis (2% to 5%), synovitis (2% to 4%), arthralgia (≤4%), leg cramps (≤4%), bursitis (1% to <3%), increased creatine phosphokinase (1% to <3%), muscle cramps (1% to <3%), myalgia (1% to <3%), neck pain (1% to <3%), ostealgia (1% to <3%), osteoarthritis (1% to <3%), osteonecrosis (1% to <3%), rupture of tendon (1% to <3%)

Ophthalmic: Blurred vision (1% to <3%), cataract (1% to <3%), conjunctivitis (1% to <3%), eye disease (1% to <3%)

Respiratory: Bronchitis (5% to 8%), cough (3% to 5%), rhinitis (2% to 5%), flu-like symptoms (≤4%), upper respiratory tract infection (≤4%), pharyngitis (2% to 3%), pneumonia (2% to 3%), asthma (1% to <3%), dyspnea (1% to <3%), epistaxis (1% to <3%), pulmonary disease (1% to <3%), sinusitis (1% to 2%)

Miscellaneous: Accidental injury (5% to 7%), cyst (1% to <3%), fever (1% to <3%)

<1% (Limited to important or life-threatening): Agranulocytosis, cholestasis, cutaneous lupus erythematosus, DRESS syndrome, eosinophilia, erythema multiforme, exacerbation of psoriasis, hepatitis, hepatotoxicity (rare, including hepatic necrosis and hepatic failure), hypophosphaturia, interstitial pulmonary disease, necrotizing angiitis (cutaneous), opportunistic infection, pancreatitis, pancytopenia, peripheral neuropathy, pustular psoriasis, sepsis, Stevens-Johnson syndrome, thrombocytopenia, toxic epidermal necrolysis, uricosuria

Drug Interactions

Metabolism/Transport Effects Inhibits CYP2C9 (moderate)

Avoid Concomitant Use

Avoid concomitant use of Leflunomide with any of the following: BCG (Intravesical); Natalizumab; Pimecrolimus; Tacrolimus (Topical); Teriflunomide; Tofacitinib

Increased Effect/Toxicity

Leflunomide may increase the levels/effects of: Bosentan; Cannabis; Carvedilol; CYP2C9 Substrates; Dronabinol; Fingolimod; Natalizumab; Teriflunomide; Tetrahydrocannabinol; Tofacitinib; TOLBUTamide; Vaccines (Live); Vitamin K Antagonists

The levels/effects of Leflunomide may be increased by: Denosumab; Immunosuppressants; Methotrexate; Pimecrolimus; Rifampin; Roflumilast; Tacrolimus (Topical); TOLBUTamide; Trastuzumab

Decreased Effect

Leflunomide may decrease the levels/effects of: BCG (Intravesical); Coccidioides immitis Skin Test; Sipuleucel-T; Vaccines (Inactivated); Vaccines (Live); Vitamin K Antagonists

The levels/effects of Leflunomide may be decreased by: Bile Acid Sequestrants; Charcoal, Activated; Echinacea

Food Interactions No interactions with food have been noted.

Storage/Stability Store at 25°C (77°F); excursions permitted to 15°C to 30°C (59°F to 86°F). Protect from light.

Mechanism of Action Leflunomide is an immunomodulatory agent that inhibits pyrimidine synthesis, resulting in antiproliferative and anti-inflammatory effects. Leflunomide is a prodrug; the active metabolite is responsible for activity. For CMV, may interfere with virion assembly.

Pharmacodynamics/Kinetics

Distribution: V_d: Teriflunomide: 11 L

Protein binding: Teriflunomide: >99% to albumin

Metabolism: Hepatic to an active metabolite teriflunomide, which accounts for nearly all pharmacologic activity; further metabolism to multiple inactive metabolites; undergoes enterohepatic recirculation

Half-life elimination: Teriflunomide: Mean: 18 to 19 days; enterohepatic recycling appears to contribute to the long half-life of this agent, since activated charcoal and cholestyramine substantially reduce plasma half-life

Time to peak: Teriflunomide: 6 to 12 hours

Excretion: Feces (37.5%); urine (22.6%)

Dosing

Adult & Geriatric

Rheumatoid arthritis: Oral: Loading dose: 100 mg once daily for 3 days; maintenance dose: 20 mg once daily, may reduce dose to 10 mg once daily if higher dose is not tolerated (maximum dose: 20 mg once daily). **Note:** The loading dose may be omitted in patients at increased risk of hepatic or hematologic toxicity (eg, recent concomitant methotrexate or other immunosuppressive agents). Due to the long half-life of the active metabolite, serum concentrations may require a prolonged period to decline after dosage reduction.

CMV disease, resistant to standard antivirals (off-label use): Oral: Some authors recommend 100 to 200 mg/day for 5 to 7 days, followed by 40 to 60 mg/day (Avery 2004; Avery 2010). Others have utilized the standard rheumatoid arthritis dosing (John 2004). Adjust dose based on serum concentrations of metabolite and adverse events (Avery 2008; Avery 2010; Williams 2002).

Pediatric

Juvenile idiopathic arthritis (off-label use) (Silverman 2005): Children ≥3 years and Adolescents: Oral:

<20 kg: 100 mg as a single dose followed by 10 mg every other day

20 kg to 40 kg: 100 mg once daily for 2 days followed by 10 mg once daily

>40 kg: 100 mg once daily for 3 days followed by 20 mg once daily

Renal Impairment

US labeling: There are no dosage adjustments provided in the manufacturer's labeling (has not been studied); use with caution.

Canadian labeling:

Mild impairment: There are no dosage adjustments provided in the manufacturer's labeling; use with caution.

Moderate to severe impairment: Use is contraindicated.

Hepatic Impairment

US labeling: Not recommended for use in patients with preexisting liver disease or those with baseline ALT >2 times ULN; monitor liver function closely. Use is contraindicated in severe hepatic impairment.

Canadian labeling: Use is contraindicated.

Adjustment for Toxicity

Hepatic toxicity:

US labeling: ALT elevations >3 x ULN: Discontinue drug therapy and investigate probable cause; if leflunomide-induced, initiate accelerated drug elimination process and monitor liver tests weekly until normalized.

Canadian labeling:

ALT elevations 2 to 3 x ULN: May reduce maintenance dose to 10 mg once daily; monitor ALT weekly.

Persistent ALT elevations >2 x ULN or ALT elevations >3 x ULN: Discontinue treatment and initiate drug elimination procedures.

Drug elimination procedure: To achieve nondetectable serum concentrations (<0.02 mg/L) of the active metabolite (teriflunomide) administer the following:

Cholestyramine: 8 g 3 times daily for 11 days. If plasma concentrations are still high, additional cholestyramine treatment may be considered.

Activated charcoal: 50 g (made into suspension) every 12 hours for 11 days. If plasma concentrations are still high, additional activated charcoal treatment may be considered. Note: As an alternative, the Canadian labeling recommends activated charcoal 50 g 4 times daily for 11 days (may modify duration based on clinical response or laboratory results).

Administration Administer without regard to meals.

Hazardous agent; use appropriate precautions for handling and disposal (NIOSH 2014 [group 2]).

Monitoring Parameters Pregnancy test to rule out pregnancy prior to initiating therapy; baseline evaluation for active tuberculosis and screen patients for latent tuberculosis; blood pressure (baseline and periodically thereafter); complete blood count (WBC, platelet count, hemoglobin or hematocrit) at baseline and monthly during the initial 6 months of treatment; if stable, monitoring frequency may be decreased to every 6 to 8 weeks thereafter (continue monthly when used in combination with other immunosuppressive agents [eg, methotrexate]); hepatic function (transaminases) at least monthly for the first 6 months of treatment, then every 6 to 8 weeks thereafter (discontinue if ALT >3 x ULN, treat with accelerated elimination procedure, and monitor liver function at least weekly until normal). If coadministered with methotrexate, monitor transaminases (ALT, AST) and serum albumin levels consistent with the American College of

◀ Rheumatology (ACR) guidelines; signs/symptoms of severe infection or pulmonary symptoms (eg, cough, dyspnea).

When used for CMV disease, monitor serum trough concentrations of active metabolite (also see Reference Range).

Reference Range CMV disease:

Timing of serum samples: Initial: Obtain 24 hours after last dose of loading regimen and periodically thereafter

Therapeutic concentration: Active metabolite (teriflunomide): Trough: 50 to 80 mcg/mL (Avery 2010) or up to 100 mcg/mL (Williams 2002)

Dosage Forms Excipient information presented when available (limited, particularly for generics); consult specific product labeling.

Tablet, Oral:

Arava: 10 mg, 20 mg

Generic: 10 mg, 20 mg

◆ Legatrin PM® [OTC] see Acetaminophen and Diphenhydramine on page 29

◆ Lemtrada see Alemtuzumab on page 62

Lenalidomide (le na LID oh mide)

Brand Names: US Revlimid
Brand Names: Canada Revlimid
Index Terms CC-5013; IMid-1
Pharmacologic Category Angiogenesis Inhibitor; Antineoplastic Agent; Immunomodulator, Systemic
Use

US labeling:

Mantle cell lymphoma: Treatment of patients with mantle cell lymphoma that has relapsed or progressed after 2 prior therapies (one of which included bortezomib).

Multiple myeloma: Treatment of multiple myeloma (in combination with dexamethasone)

Myelodysplastic syndromes: Treatment of patients with transfusion-dependent anemia due to low- or intermediate-1-risk myelodysplastic syndromes (MDS) associated with a deletion 5q (del 5q) cytogenetic abnormality with or without additional cytogenetic abnormalities

Canadian labeling:

Multiple myeloma: Treatment of multiple myeloma (in combination with dexamethasone) in patients who have received at least one prior therapy

Myelodysplastic syndromes: Treatment of patients with transfusion-dependent anemia due to low- or intermediate-1-risk myelodysplastic syndromes (MDS) associated with a deletion 5q (del 5q) cytogenetic abnormality with or without additional cytogenetic abnormalities

Limitations of use: In the US and in Canada, lenalidomide is not indicated and is not recommended for the treatment of chronic lymphocytic leukemia (CLL) outside of controlled clinical trials.

Pregnancy Considerations [US Boxed Warning]: Lenalidomide is an analogue of thalidomide (a human teratogen) and could potentially cause severe birth defects or embryo-fetal death; do not use during pregnancy (contraindication); avoid pregnancy while taking lenalidomide. Obtain 2 negative pregnancy tests prior to initiation of treatment; 2 forms of contraception (or abstain from heterosexual intercourse) must be used at least 4 weeks prior to, during, and for 4 weeks after lenalidomide treatment (and during treatment interruptions). In order to decrease the risk of embryo-fetal exposure, lenalidomide is available only through a restricted distribution program (Revlimid REMS). Animal reproduction studies with lenalidomide in nonhuman primates have demonstrated malformations similar to those observed in humans with thalidomide.

Women of childbearing potential should be treated only if they are able to comply with the conditions of the Revlimid REMS program. Women of reproductive potential must avoid pregnancy 4 weeks prior to therapy, during therapy, during therapy interruptions, and for ≥4 weeks after therapy is discontinued. Two forms of effective contraception (eg, tubal ligation, IUD, hormonal birth control methods, male latex or synthetic condom, diaphragm, or cervical cap) or total abstinence from heterosexual intercourse must be used by females who are not infertile or who have not had a hysterectomy. A negative pregnancy test (sensitivity of at least 50 milliunits/mL) 10 to 14 days prior to therapy, within 24 hours prior to beginning therapy, weekly during the first 4 weeks, and every 4 weeks (every 2 weeks for women with irregular menstrual cycles) thereafter is required for women of childbearing potential. Lenalidomide must be immediately discontinued for a missed period, abnormal pregnancy test or abnormal menstrual bleeding; refer patient to a reproductive toxicity specialist if pregnancy occurs during treatment.

Lenalidomide is also present in the semen of males. Males (including those vasectomized) should use a latex or synthetic condom during any sexual contact with women of childbearing age during treatment, during treatment interruptions, and for 4 weeks after discontinuation. Male patients should not donate sperm during, and for 4 weeks after treatment, and during therapy interruptions.

The parent or legal guardian for patients between 12 and 18 years of age must agree to ensure compliance with the required guidelines. Any suspected fetal exposure should be reported to the FDA via the MedWatch program (1-800-FDA-1088) and to Celgene Corporation (1-888-423-5436).

Breast-Feeding Considerations It is not known if lenalidomide is excreted in breast milk. Due to the potential for serious adverse reactions in the infant, a decision should be made to discontinue nursing or discontinue treatment. Use in breast-feeding women is contraindicated in the Canadian labeling.

Prescribing and Access Restrictions As a requirement of the REMS program, access to this medication is restricted. Lenalidomide is approved for marketing in the US only under a Food and Drug Administration (FDA) approved, restricted distribution program called Revlimid REMS (https://www.celgeneriskmanagement.com or 1-888-423-5436). Prescribers and pharmacies must be certified with the program to prescribe or dispense lenalidomide; patients must comply with the program requirements. No more than a 4-week supply should be dispensed. Prescriptions must be filled within 7 days (for females of reproductive potential) or within 30 days (for all other patients) after authorization number obtained. Subsequent prescriptions may be filled only if fewer than 7 days of therapy remain on the previous prescription. A new prescription is required for further dispensing (a telephone prescription may not be accepted). Pregnancy testing is required for females of childbearing potential. In Canada, distribution is restricted through RevAid (www.RevAid.ca or 1-888-738-2431).

Medication Guide Available Yes
Contraindications

Hypersensitivity (eg, angioedema, Stevens-Johnson syndrome, toxic epidermal necrolysis) to lenalidomide or any component of the formulation; pregnancy

Canadian labeling: Additional contraindications (not in US labeling): Platelet count <50,000/mm³ (in MDS patients); hypersensitivity to thalidomide or pomalidomide; women capable of becoming pregnant; breast-feeding women; male patients unable to follow or comply with required contraceptive measures

Warnings/Precautions Hazardous agent - use appropriate precautions for handling and disposal (NIOSH 2014 [group 2]).

[US Boxed Warning]: Hematologic toxicity (neutropenia and thrombocytopenia) occurs in a majority of patients (grade 3/4: 80% in patients with del 5q myelodysplastic syndrome) and may require dose reductions and/or delays; the use of blood product support and/or growth factors may be needed. CBC should be monitored weekly for the first 8 weeks and at least monthly thereafter in patients being treated for del 5q myelodysplastic syndromes. In patients being treated for multiple myeloma, monitor CBC weekly for the first 2 cycles, every 2 weeks during cycle 3, and monthly thereafter. In patients receiving lenalidomide for mantle cell lymphoma (MCL), monitor CBC weekly for the first cycle, every 2 weeks during cycles 2 to 4, and monthly thereafter. Monitor for signs of infection, bleeding, or bruising; may require dosage adjustment. Lenalidomide use (≥4 cycles) may decrease the number of CD34+ cells collected for autologous stem cell transplant. Transplant eligible patients receiving lenalidomide should be referred to an appropriate transplant center in order to optimize the timing of stem cell collection. Cyclophosphamide in combination with G-CSF or G-CSF in combination with a CXC chemokine receptor 4 inhibitor (eg, plerixafor) may be considered when CD34+ cell collection is impaired. **[US Boxed Warning]: Lenalidomide has been associated with a significant increase in risk for arterial and venous thromboembolic events in multiple myeloma patients treated with lenalidomide and dexamethasone combination therapy. Deep vein thrombosis (DVT), pulmonary embolism (PE), myocardial infarction, and stroke have occurred; monitor for signs and symptoms of thromboembolism (shortness of breath, chest pain, or arm or leg swelling) and seek prompt medical attention with development of these symptoms. Thromboprophylaxis is recommended; the choice of**

regimen should be based on assessment of the patient's underlying risk factors. Erythropoietin-stimulating agents (ESAs) and estrogens may contribute to thromboembolic risk; use with caution. Patients with a prior history of arterial thromboembolic events may be at greater risk; minimize modifiable factors such as hyperlipidemia, hypertension, and smoking. Anticoagulant prophylaxis should be individualized and selected based on the thromboembolism risk of the combination treatment regimen, using the safest and easiest to administer (Palumbo, 2008).

In a clinical trial comparing lenalidomide versus chlorambucil single agent therapy in patients >65 years of age with chronic lymphocytic leukemia patients (not an FDA-approved indication), increased mortality was observed in the lenalidomide treatment arm. Atrial fibrillation, cardiac failure, and MI were observed more frequently in lenalidomide-treated patients; lenalidomide (alone or in combination) is not currently recommended for first-line treatment of CLL. Second primary malignancies (SPMs), including hematologic (AML, MDS, and B-cell malignancies, including Hodgkin lymphoma) and solid tumor malignancies, and skin cancers, have been reported with lenalidomide when used for the treatment of MDS and multiple myeloma; the incidence may be higher when lenalidomide is used in combination with an alkylating agent. Monitor for development of secondary malignancies.

Angioedema, Stevens-Johnson syndrome (SJS), and toxic epidermal necrolysis (TEN) have been reported; may be fatal. Consider interrupting or discontinuing treatment with grade 2 or 3 skin rash; discontinue and do not reinitiate treatment with grade 4 rash, exfoliative or bullous rash, or for suspected SJS or TEN. Patients with a history of grade 4 rash with thalidomide should not receive lenalidomide. Discontinue treatment with angioedema. Use caution in renal impairment; may experience an increased rate of toxicities (due to reduced clearance and increased half-life); initial dosage adjustments are recommended for moderate-to-severe and dialysis-dependent renal impairment. Tumor lysis syndrome (with fatalities) has been reported with lenalidomide; patients with a high tumor burden may be at risk for tumor lysis syndrome; monitor closely; institute appropriate management for hyperuricemia. Tumor flare reaction has been observed in studies of lenalidomide for the treatment of chronic lymphocytic leukemia (CLL) and lymphoma; clinical presentation includes low grade fever, pain, rash, and tender lymph node swelling. In patients with MCL, tumor flare may mimic disease progression; monitor closely. In clinical trials, the majority of tumor flare events occurred in the first cycle of therapy. Treatment with corticosteroids, nonsteroidal anti-inflammatory drugs (NSAIDs), and/or analgesics may be considered; therapy interruption may be necessary as well. Hepatic failure, including fatalities, has occurred in patients treated with combination lenalidomide and dexamethasone therapy; may have hepatocellular, cholestatic, or mixed characteristics. Risk factors may include preexisting viral liver disease, elevated liver enzymes at baseline, and concomitant medications. Monitor closely; interrupt therapy in patients with abnormal hepatic function tests. May consider resuming treatment at a lower dose upon return to baseline. Certain adverse reactions (DVT, pulmonary embolism, atrial fibrillation, renal failure) are more likely in elderly patients. Monitor renal function closely, and select dose accordingly.

[US Boxed Warning]: Lenalidomide is an analogue of thalidomide (a human teratogen) and could potentially cause severe birth defects or embryo-fetal death; do not use during pregnancy (contraindication); avoid pregnancy while taking lenalidomide. Obtain 2 negative pregnancy testes prior to initiation of treatment; 2 forms of contraception (or abstain from heterosexual intercourse) must be used at least 4 weeks prior to, during and for 4 weeks after lenalidomide treatment (and during treatment interruptions). Distribution is restricted; physicians, pharmacies, and patients must be registered with the Revlimid REMS program. In order to decrease the risk of embryo-fetal exposure, lenalidomide is available only through a restricted distribution program (Revlimid REMS). Prescribers and pharmacies must be certified with the program to prescribe or dispense lenalidomide. Males taking lenalidomide (even those vasectomized) must use a latex or synthetic condom during any sexual contact with women of childbearing potential and for up to 28 days following discontinuation of therapy. Males taking lenalidomide must not donate sperm. Patients should be advised not to donate blood during therapy and for 1 month following completion of therapy. May cause dizziness or fatigue; caution patients about performing tasks which require mental alertness (eg, operating machinery or driving).

Potentially significant drug-drug interactions may exist, requiring dose or frequency adjustment, additional monitoring, and/or selection of alternative therapy. Formulation contains lactose; avoid use in patients with Lapp lactase deficiency, glucose-galactose malabsorption, or glucose intolerance. Lenalidomide should only be prescribed to patients (male and female) who can understand and comply with the conditions of the Revlimid REMS program. If used in patients between 12 to 18 years of age, the parent or legal guardian must agree to ensure compliance with the Revlimid REMS program.

Adverse Reactions Frequency not always defined; may vary based on indication and/or concomitant therapy.

Cardiovascular: Peripheral edema (8% to 26%), edema (10%), deep vein thrombosis (4% to 10%; grades 3/4: ≤8%), hypotension (7% to 10%), hypertension (6% to 8%), chest pain (5% to 8%), atrial fibrillation (3% to 7%; grades 3/4: ≤4%), palpitations (5%), myocardial infarction (1% to <5%), pulmonary embolism (2% to 4%; grades 3/4: 1% to 4%), syncope (grades 3/4: 1% to 3%), cerebrovascular tachycardia (grades 3/4: 2%), accident (≤2%), angina pectoris (≥1%), bradycardia (≥1%), cerebral ischemia (≥1%), cardiac failure (1%), cardiac arrest, cardiogenic shock, cardiomyopathy, cardiorespiratory arrest, cerebral infarction, increased cardiac enzymes (troponin I), ischemia, ischemic heart disease, septic shock, subarachnoid hemorrhage, supraventricular cardiac arrhythmia, tachyarrhythmia, thrombophlebitis, thrombosis, transiet ischemic attachs, ventricular dysfunction

Central nervous system: Fatigue (29% to 44%), insomnia (10% to 28%), dizziness (20% to 23%), headache (10% to 20%), depression (5% to 11%), chills (5% to 10%), falling (5% to 8%), hypoesthesia (7%), lethargy (7%), pain (7%), neuropathy (including peripheral, 5% to 7%), rigors (6%), noncardiac chest pain (3% to 6%), emotional lability (≥1%), glossalgia (≥1%), hallucination (≥1%), malaise (≥1%), abnormal gait, aphasia, cerebellar infarction, confusion, dysarthria, impaired consciousness, migraine, spinal cord compression, vertigo

Dermatologic: Pruritus (4% to 42%), skin rash (19% to 36%), xeroderma (9% to 14%), diaphoresis (7% to 10%), night sweats (8%), ecchymoses (5%), erythema (5%), cellulitis (≤5%), hyperpigmentation (≥1%), Sweet's syndrome

Endocrine & metabolic: Weight loss (9% to 20%), hypokalemia (7% to 17%), hyperglycemia (4% to 12%), hypocalcemia (3% to 11%), hypothyroidism (7%), hypomagnesemia (6% to 7%), dehydration (3% to 7%), diabetes mellitus (<5%), gout (<5%), hypophosphatemia (<5%, grades 3/4: ≤3%), hyponatremia (2% to <5%), hirsutism (≥1%), loss of libido (≥1%), Graves' disease, hypernatremia, hypoglycemia

Gastrointestinal: Diarrhea (17% to 49%), constipation (16% to 41%), nausea (24% to 30%), decreased appetite (7% to 23%), abdominal pain (8% to 21%), anorexia (10% to 16%), dysgeusia (4% to 15%), vomiting (10% to 12%), dyspepsia (5% to 11%), xerostomia (7%), loose stools (6%), gastroenteritis (2% to 6%), gastrointestinal hemorrhage (≥1%), biliary obstruction, cholecystitis, colonic polyps, diverticulitis, dysphagia, gastritis, gastroesophageal reflux disease, infection of mouth, inguinal hernia (obstructive), intestinal obstruction, intestinal perforation, irritable bowel syndrome, ischemic colitis, melena

Genitourinary: Urinary tract infection (4% to 14%), dysuria (7%), erectile dysfunction (≥1%), azotemia, hematuria, pelvic pain, perirectal obscess, urolithiasis, urosepsis

Hematologic & oncologic: Thrombocytopenia (19% to 62%; grades 3/4: 8% to 50%; MDS: Onset: 28 days [range: 8 to 290 days]; recovery: 22 days [range: 5 to 224 days]), neutropenia (33% to 61%; grades 3/4: 27% to 53%; MDS: Onset: 42 days [range: 14 to 411 days]; recovery: 17 days [range: 2 to 170 days]), anemia (12% to 44%; grades 3/4: 6% to 19%), leukopenia (8% to 15%; grades 3/4: 4% to 7%), tumor flare (10%), lymphocytopenia (5% to 7%; grades 3/4: 3% to 4%), bruise (3% to 6%), febrile neutropenia (1% to 6%; grades 3/4: 1% to 6%), second primary malignant neoplasms (≤5%, including AML, lymphomas, solid tumors), squamous cell carcinoma of skin (3% to <5%; grades 3/4: ≤3%), pancytopenia (<5%; grades 3/4: ≤2%), basal cell carcinoma (<5%; grades 3/4: <1%), granulocytopenia (grades 3/4: 2%), autoimmune hemolytic anemia (≥1%), acute leukemia, blood coagulation disorder, bone marrow depression, bronchogenic carcinoma, decreased hemoglobin, hemolysis, hemolytic anemia (including warm type), lung carcinoma, malignant lymphoma, myelocytic leukemia, neutropenic infection, pancreatitis, postoperative hemorrhage, prostate carcinoma, rectal hemorrhage, splenic infarction

Hepatic: Increased serum ALT (8%), abnormal hepatic function tests (≥1%), hepatic failure, hyperbilirubinemia

Hypersensitivity: Hypersensitivity reaction, transfusion reaction

Infection: Influenza (3% to 6%), sepsis (including *Enterobacter*, 3% to 6%; grades 3/4: 2% to 5%), bacteremia (1%), bacterial infection, clostridium infection, fungal infection, herpes virus infection, kidney infection, Klebsiella infection, localized infection, pseudomonas infection, staphylococcal infection

Local: Catheter infection

Neuromuscular & skeletal: Muscle cramps (18% to 33%), back pain (13% to 32%), weakness (14% to 28%), arthralgia (8% to 22%), tremor (21%), muscle spasm (11% to 21%), ostealgia (11% to 16%), limb pain (5% to 15%), musculoskeletal pain (7% to 13%), musculoskeletal chest pain (7% to 11%), myalgia (9%), myasthenia (5% to 8%), neck pain (2% to 8%), arthritis, bone fracture (femur, femoral neck, pelvis, hip, rib, spinal compression), calcium pyrophosphate deposition disease

Ophthalmic: Blurred vision (17%), cataract (≤14%; grades 3/4: ≤6%), subcapsular posterior cataract (<5%), blindness (≥1%), ocular hypertension (≥1%)

Otic: Otic infection

Renal: Renal failure (4% to 10%), increased serum creatinine

Respiratory: Cough (13% to 28%), upper respiratory tract infection (6% to 25%), dyspnea (17% to 24%), nasopharyngitis (6% to 23%), pneumonia (9% to 18%), bronchitis (6% to 17%), pharyngitis (14% to 16%), epistaxis (3% to 15%), oropharyngeal pain (3% to 10%), sinusitis (7% to 8%), pleural effusion (7%; grades 3/4: 1%), dyspnea on exertion (≤7%), respiratory tract infection (4% to 7%), rhinitis (3% to 7%), lower respiratory tract infection (2% to 6%), hypoxia (2%; grades 3/4: 1%), hoarseness (≥1%), pneumonitis (grades 3/4: 1%), pulmonary hypertension (grades 3/4: 1%), respiratory distress (1%; grades 3/4: 1% to 2%), chronic obstructive pulmonary disease, interstitial pulmonary disease, pulmonary edema, pulmonary infiltrates, respiratory failure, wheezing

Miscellaneous: Fever (14% to 28%), physical health deterioration (2%), multiorgan failure (grades 3/4: 1%), mass (renal), nodule

<1% (Limited to important or life-threatening): Angioedema, atrial flutter, circulatory shock, desquamation, drug overdose, erythema multiforme, Fanconi's syndrome, hematologic disease (impaired stem cell mobilization), hemorrhage, hepatitis, intracranial hemorrhage, leukoencephalopathy, myopathy, nephrolithiasis, orthostatic hypotension, peripheral ischemia, pseudomembranous colitis, renal tubular necrosis, Stevens-Johnson syndrome, stomatitis, toxic epidermal necrolysis, tumor lysis syndrome, urinary retention

Drug Interactions

Metabolism/Transport Effects Substrate of P-glycoprotein

Avoid Concomitant Use

Avoid concomitant use of Lenalidomide with any of the following: Abatacept; Anakinra; BCG (Intravesical); Canakinumab; Certolizumab Pegol; Deferiprone; Dipyrone; Natalizumab; Pimecrolimus; Rilonacept; Tacrolimus (Topical); Tocilizumab; Tofacitinib; Vaccines (Live); Vedolizumab

Increased Effect/Toxicity

Lenalidomide may increase the levels/effects of: Abatacept; Anakinra; Bisphosphonate Derivatives; Canakinumab; Certolizumab Pegol; CloZAPine; Deferiprone; Digoxin; Fingolimod; Leflunomide; Natalizumab; Rilonacept; Tofacitinib; Vaccines (Live); Vedolizumab

The levels/effects of Lenalidomide may be increased by: Denosumab; Dexamethasone (Systemic); Dipyrone; Erythropoiesis-Stimulating Agents; Estrogen Derivatives; Pimecrolimus; Roflumilast; Tacrolimus (Topical); Tocilizumab; Trastuzumab

Decreased Effect

Lenalidomide may decrease the levels/effects of: BCG (Intravesical); Coccidioides immitis Skin Test; Sipuleucel-T; Vaccines (Inactivated); Vaccines (Live)

The levels/effects of Lenalidomide may be decreased by: Echinacea

Storage/Stability Store at 20°C to 25°C (68°F to 77°F); excursions permitted to 15°C and 30°C (59°F and 86°F).

Mechanism of Action Immunomodulatory, antiangiogenic, and antineoplastic characteristics via multiple mechanisms. Selectively inhibits secretion of proinflammatory cytokines (potent inhibitor of tumor necrosis factor-alpha secretion); enhances cell-mediated immunity by stimulating proliferation of anti-CD3 stimulated T cells (resulting in increased IL-2 and interferon gamma secretion); inhibits trophic signals to angiogenic factors in cells. Inhibits the growth of myeloma cells by inducing cell cycle arrest and cell death.

Pharmacodynamics/Kinetics

Absorption: Rapid

Protein binding: ~30%

Half-life elimination: 3 to 5 hours; Moderate to severe renal impairment: Increased threefold; Hemodialysis patients: Increased ~4.5-fold

Time, to peak, plasma: MDS or myeloma patients: 0.5 to 6 hours

Excretion: Urine (~82%; as unchanged drug)

Hemodialysis effect: ~30% of the drug in body is removed in a 4-hour hemodialysis session

Dosing

Adult

Mantle cell lymphoma (MCL): Oral: 25 mg once daily for 21 days of a 28-day treatment cycle; continue until disease progression or unacceptable toxicity

Multiple myeloma: Oral: 25 mg once daily for 21 days of a 28-day treatment cycle (in combination with dexamethasone). In patients not eligible for autologous stem cell transplantation, continue until disease progression or unacceptable toxicity; in transplant eligible patients, hematopoietic stem cell mobilization should occur within 4 cycles.

Myelodysplastic syndrome (MDS) with deletion 5q: Oral:

US labeling: 10 mg once daily

Canadian labeling: 10 mg once daily for 21 days of 28-day treatment cycle; discontinue therapy if within 4 months of initiation, patient fails to achieve a rise in hemoglobin ≥1 g/dL (if not transfused) or ≥50% reduction in transfusion requirements.

Chronic lymphocytic leukemia (CLL), relapsed/refractory (off-label use): Oral: 10 mg once daily beginning on day 9 of cycle 1; administer continuously in combination with cyclic rituximab (Badoux, 2013)

Diffuse large B-cell lymphoma, relapsed/refractory (off-label use): Oral: 25 mg once daily for 21 days of a 28-day treatment cycle for up to 1 year (Wiernik, 2008)

Multiple myeloma, newly diagnosed (off-label combination): Oral: 25 mg once daily for 14 days of a 21-day cycle (in combination with bortezomib and dexamethasone) for 8 cycles (Kumar, 2012; Richardson, 2010)

Multiple myeloma, relapsed (off-label combination): Adults: Oral: 25 mg once daily for 21 days of 28-day cycle (in combination with carfilzomib and dexamethasone) until disease progression or unacceptable toxicity (Stewart, 2015)

Multiple myeloma, maintenance (following autologous stem cell transplant; off-label use): Oral: 10 mg once daily for 3 months, then increased to 15 mg daily if tolerated; continue until relapse (Attal, 2012; McCarthy, 2012) **or** 10 mg once daily for 21 days of a 28-day treatment cycle until relapse (Palumbo, 2010)

Myelodysplastic syndrome (MDS), lower risk, without deletion 5q (off-label use): Oral: 10 mg once daily (Raza, 2008)

Systemic light chain amyloidosis (off-label use): Oral: 15 mg once daily for 21 days of a 28-day cycle (in combination with dexamethasone) (Nair, 2012; Sanchorawala, 2007)

Geriatric Refer to adult dosing. Due to the potential for decreased renal function in the elderly, select dose carefully and closely monitor renal function.

Renal Impairment

Recommended initial dose adjustment in the FDA-approved labeling; further individualize based on tolerance:

MCL:

CrCl >60 mL/minute: No adjustment required

CrCl 30 to 60 mL/minute: 10 mg once daily

CrCl <30 mL/minute (nondialysis dependent): 15 mg every 48 hours

ESRD: CrCl <30 mL/minute and dialysis dependent: 5 mg once daily (administer after dialysis on dialysis days)

MDS:

CrCl >60 mL/minute: No adjustment required

CrCl 30 to 60 mL/minute: 5 mg once daily

CrCl <30 mL/minute (nondialysis dependent): 2.5 mg once daily

ESRD: CrCl <30 mL/minute and dialysis dependent: 2.5 mg once daily (administer after dialysis on dialysis days)

Multiple myeloma:

CrCl >50 mL/minute: No adjustment required

CrCl 30 to 50 mL/minute: 10 mg once daily (may increase to 15 mg once daily after 2 cycles if nonresponsive but tolerating treatment; Chen, 2007)

CrCl <30 mL/minute (nondialysis dependent): 15 mg every 48 hours

ESRD: CrCl <30 mL/minute and dialysis dependent: 5 mg once daily (administer after dialysis on dialysis days)

Recommended adjustment in Canadian labeling:

MDS:

CrCl ≥60 mL/minute: No adjustment required

CrCl 30 to 59 mL/minute: 5 mg once daily

CrCl <30 mL/minute (nondialysis dependent): 5 mg every 48 hours

ESRD: CrCl <30 mL/minute and dialysis dependent: 5 mg 3 times weekly (administer after each dialysis)

Multiple myeloma:

CrCl ≥60 mL/minute: No adjustment required

CrCl 30 to 59 mL/minute: 10 mg once daily (may increase to 15 mg once daily after 2 cycles if nonresponsive but tolerating treatment; Chen, 2007)

CrCl <30 mL/minute (nondialysis dependent): 15 mg every 48 hours

ESRD: CrCl <30 mL/minute and dialysis dependent: 5 mg once daily (administer after dialysis on dialysis days)

Hepatic Impairment There are no dosage adjustments provided in the manufacturer's labeling (has not been studied). However, lenalidomide undergoes minimal hepatic metabolism.

Adjustment for Toxicity

NONHEMATOLOGIC toxicities:

Dermatologic toxicities:

Skin rash, grade 2 or 3: Consider interrupting or discontinuing treatment

Angioedema, grade 4 rash, exfoliative or bullous rash, or suspected Stevens-Johnson syndrome or toxic epidermal necrolysis: Discontinue treatment; do not rechallenge

Tumor flare reaction:

Grade 1 or 2: Continue therapy at physician's discretion; may consider symptom management with corticosteroids, nonsteroidal anti-inflammatory drugs (NSAIDs) and/or analgesic therapy.

Grade 3 or 4: Interrupt therapy until resolved to ≤ grade 1; consider symptom management with corticosteroids, nonsteroidal anti-inflammatory drugs (NSAIDs) and/or analgesic therapy.

Other toxicities: For additional treatment-related grade 3/4 toxicities, hold treatment and restart at next lower dose level when toxicity has resolved to ≤ grade 2.

HEMATOLOGIC toxicities:

Adjustment for thrombocytopenia in MCL:

Platelets <50,000/mm³: Hold treatment, check CBC weekly

When platelets return to ≥50,000/mm³: Resume treatment at 5 mg below previous dose; do not dose below 5 mg daily

Adjustment for neutropenia in MCL:

ANC <1000/mm³ for at least 7 days or associated with fever (≥38.5°C [101°F]): Hold treatment, check CBC weekly

ANC <500/mm³: Hold treatment, check CBC weekly

When ANC returns to ≥1000/mm³: Resume treatment at 5 mg below previous dose; do not dose below 5 mg daily

Adjustment for thrombocytopenia in MDS:

Thrombocytopenia developing within 4 weeks of beginning treatment at 10 mg daily:

Baseline platelets ≥100,000/mm³:

If platelets <50,000/mm³: Hold treatment

When platelets return to ≥50,000/mm³: Resume treatment at 5 mg daily

Baseline platelets <100,000/mm³:

If platelets fall to 50% of baseline: Hold treatment

If baseline ≥60,000/mm³ and platelet level returns to ≥50,000/mm³: Resume at 5 mg daily

If baseline <60,000/mm³ and platelet level returns to ≥30,000/mm³: Resume at 5 mg daily

Thrombocytopenia developing after 4 weeks of beginning treatment at 10 mg daily:

Platelets <30,000/mm³ **or** <50,000/mm³ with platelet transfusions: Hold treatment

When platelets return to ≥30,000/mm³ (without hemostatic failure): Resume at 5 mg daily

Thrombocytopenia developing with treatment at 5 mg daily:

Platelets <30,000/mm³ **or** <50,000/mm³ with platelet transfusions: Hold treatment

When platelets return to ≥30,000/mm³ (without hemostatic failure):

US labeling: Resume at 2.5 mg once daily

Canadian labeling: Resume at 5 mg every other day

Adjustment for neutropenia in MDS:

Neutropenia developing within 4 weeks of beginning treatment at 10 mg daily:

For baseline absolute neutrophil count (ANC) ≥1000/mm³:

ANC <750/mm³: Hold treatment

When ANC returns to ≥1000/mm³: Resume at 5 mg daily

For baseline absolute neutrophil count (ANC) <1000/mm³:

ANC <500/mm³: Hold treatment

When ANC returns to ≥500/mm³: Resume at 5 mg daily

Neutropenia developing after 4 weeks of beginning treatment at 10 mg daily:

ANC <500/mm³ for ≥7 days or associated with fever (≥38.5°C [101°F]): Hold treatment

When ANC returns to ≥500/mm³: Resume at 5 mg daily

Neutropenia developing with treatment at 5 mg daily:

ANC <500/mm³ for ≥7 days or associated with fever (≥38.5°C [101°F]): Hold treatment

When ANC returns to ≥500/mm³:

US labeling: Resume at 2.5 mg once daily

Canadian labeling: Resume at 5 mg every other day

Adjustment for thrombocytopenia in multiple myeloma:

US labeling:

Platelets <30,000/mm³: Hold treatment, check CBC weekly

When platelets return to ≥30,000/mm³: Resume at next lower dose; do not dose below 2.5 mg daily

Additional occurrence of platelets <30,000/mm³: Hold treatment

When platelets return to ≥30,000/mm³: Resume treatment at next lower dose; do not dose below 2.5 mg daily

Canadian labeling:

Platelets <30,000/mm³: Hold treatment, check CBC weekly

When platelets return to ≥30,000/mm³: Resume at 15 mg daily

Additional occurrence of platelets <30,000/mm³: Hold treatment

When platelets return to ≥30,000/mm³: Resume treatment at 5 mg less than previous dose; do not dose below 5 mg daily

Adjustment for neutropenia in multiple myeloma:

US labeling:

ANC <1000/mm³: Hold treatment, check CBC weekly

When ANC returns to ≥1000/mm³ (with neutropenia as only toxicity): Resume at 25 mg daily or initial starting dose

When ANC returns to ≥1000/mm³ (with additional toxicities): Resume at next lower dose; do not dose below 2.5 mg daily

Additional occurrence of ANC <1000/mm³: Hold treatment

When ANC returns to ≥1000/mm³: Resume treatment at next lower dose; do not dose below 2.5 mg daily

Canadian labeling:

ANC <1,000/mm³: Hold treatment, initiate granulocyte-colony stimulating factor (G-CSF), check CBC weekly

When ANC returns to ≥1,000/mm³ (with neutropenia as only toxicity): Resume at 25 mg daily

When ANC returns to ≥1,000/mm³ (with additional toxicities): Resume at 15 mg daily

Additional occurrence of ANC <1,000/mm³: Hold treatment

When ANC returns to ≥1,000/mm³: Resume treatment at 5 mg less than previous dose; do not dose below 5 mg daily

Administration Administer at about the same time each day with water; administer with or without food. Swallow capsule whole; do not break, open, or chew.

Missed doses: May administer a missed dose if within 12 hours of usual dosing time. If greater than 12 hours, patient should skip dose for that day and resume usual dosing the following day. Patient should **not** take 2 doses to make up for a missed dose.

Hazardous agent; use appropriate precautions for handling and disposal (NIOSH 2014 [group 2]).

Monitoring Parameters

CBC with differential (MCL - weekly for the first cycle, every 2 weeks during cycles 2 to 4; MDS - weekly for first 8 weeks; Multiple myeloma - weekly for the first 2 cycles, every 2 weeks during the third cycle), then monthly thereafter; serum creatinine, liver function tests, thyroid function tests (TSH at baseline then every 2 to 3 months during lenalidomide treatment [Hamnvik, 2011]); ECG when clinically indicated; monitor for signs and symptoms of infection (if neutropenic), secondary malignancies, thromboembolism, tumor lysis syndrome, or tumor flare reaction

Women of childbearing potential: Pregnancy test 10 to 14 days **and** 24 hours prior to initiating therapy, weekly during the first 4 weeks of treatment, then every 2 to 4 weeks through 4 weeks after therapy discontinued

Dosage Forms Excipient information presented when available (limited, particularly for generics); consult specific product labeling.

Capsule, Oral:

Revlimid: 2.5 mg [contains fd&c blue #2 (indigotine)]

Revlimid: 5 mg

Revlimid: 10 mg, 15 mg, 20 mg [contains fd&c blue #2 (indigotine)]

Revlimid: 25 mg

Lenvatinib (len VA ti nib)

Brand Names: US Lenvima 10 MG Daily Dose; Lenvima 14 MG Daily Dose; Lenvima 20 MG Daily Dose; Lenvima 24 MG Daily Dose

Index Terms E7080; Lenvatinib Mesylate

Pharmacologic Category Antineoplastic Agent, Tyrosine Kinase Inhibitor; Antineoplastic Agent, Vascular Endothelial Growth Factor (VEGF) Inhibitor

Use Thyroid cancer, differentiated: Treatment of locally recurrent or metastatic, progressive, radioactive iodine-refractory differentiated thyroid cancer (DTC)

Pregnancy Considerations Adverse events were observed in animal reproduction studies. Based on the mechanism of action, lenvatinib may cause fetal harm if administered in pregnancy. Females of reproductive potential should use effective contraception during lenvatinib treatment and for at least 2 weeks after completion of therapy.

Breast-Feeding Considerations It is not known if lenvatinib is excreted into breast milk. The manufacturer recommends that breast-feeding be discontinued during therapy.

Prescribing and Access Restrictions Lenvatinib is available only through specialty pharmacies. For further information on patient assistance, product availability, and prescribing instructions, please refer to the following website: http://www.lenvima.com/hcp/pharmacy-financial-options

Contraindications There are no contraindications listed in the manufacturer's labeling.

Warnings/Precautions Hazardous agent - use appropriate precautions for handling and disposal (meets NIOSH 2014 criteria). Hypertension, including grade 3 and 4 toxicity, occurred in ~75% of patients treated with lenvatinib in a clinical trial; the median time to onset of new or worsening hypertension was 16 days. Blood pressure should be controlled prior to initiating therapy; monitor frequently throughout treatment. Other cardiac events such as decreased left or right ventricular function, cardiac failure, or pulmonary edema were also reported. Decreased ejection fraction (EF) was the most commonly reported of these events; some patients experienced greater than 20% EF reduction. Monitor for signs/symptoms of cardiac decompensation. QT/QTc prolongation was also observed in lenvatinib-treated patients. Monitor and correct electrolyte abnormalities in all patients; obtain electrocardiograms in patients with congenital long QT syndrome, heart failure, bradyarrhythmias, or in those on concomitant medications known to prolong the QT interval. Cardiac effects may require therapy interruption, dosage reduction, or discontinuation. An increased incidence of hypocalcemia (including grade 3 events) was observed in lenvatinib-treated patients compared to the placebo group in a clinical trial. Calcium replacement therapy and dosage interruption or reduction generally corrected hypocalcemia. Monitor serum calcium levels at least monthly; replace calcium as necessary. May require therapy interruption or dosage reduction. Arterial thromboembolic events, including grade 3 events, have been reported. Discontinue treatment if arterial thrombosis occurs; the safety of resuming therapy after such an event has not been established. Lenvatinib has not been studied in patients who have had an arterial thromboembolic event within the preceding 6 months. Hemorrhagic events (most frequently epistaxis) occurred in over one-third of lenvatinib-treated patients.

Monitor; may require therapy interruption, dosage reduction, or discontinuation.

Lenvatinib impairs exogenous thyroid suppression. In patients with a normal thyroid stimulating hormone (TSH) level at baseline, TSH elevations were observed in over half of lenvatinib-treated patients. Monitor TSH levels monthly; adjust thyroid hormone therapy as clinically necessary. Gastrointestinal perforation or fistula formation were reported in a small percentage of patients in a clinical trial. Discontinue use in patients who develop perforation or life-threatening fistula. Lenvatinib is associated with a moderate emetic potential; antiemetics are recommended to prevent nausea and vomiting. Nausea, vomiting, and diarrhea were commonly observed. Initiate appropriate management prior to therapy interruption or dosage reduction. Monitor closely; dehydration or hypovolemia due to diarrhea and vomiting are risk factors for renal toxicity. Reversible posterior leukoencephalopathy syndrome (RPLS) has occurred (rarely). If RPLS diagnosis is confirmed through MRI, interrupt treatment until fully resolved. Therapy may resume at a reduced dose or be discontinued, depending on the severity and persistence of neurologic symptoms. Palmar-plantar erythrodysesthesia (usually grades 1 to 2) was observed in nearly one-third of patients receiving lenvatinib.

Elevations in transaminases (including grade 3 or greater events) were observed. Hepatic failure (some fatal), as well as acute hepatitis have occurred rarely. Monitor liver function tests at baseline and throughout therapy. May require therapy interruption, dosage reduction, or discontinuation. If hepatic failure occurs, discontinue treatment. Proteinuria (including grade 3 toxicity) was commonly observed. Monitor for proteinuria at baseline and throughout therapy. If urine dipstick for proteinuria is 2+, obtain a 24-hour urine protein. If proteinuria ≥2 g/24 hours develops, withhold therapy and resume at a reduced dose when proteinuria is <2 g/24 hours. Discontinue for nephrotic syndrome. Renal impairment may also occur (may be grade 3 or higher); a primary risk factor for severe renal impairment is dehydration or hypovolemia due to diarrhea and vomiting. Monitor renal function throughout treatment; may require therapy interruption, dosage reduction, or discontinuation. Potentially significant drug-drug interactions may exist, requiring dose or frequency adjustment, additional monitoring, and/or selection of alternative therapy.

Adverse Reactions

>10%:

Cardiovascular: Hypertension (73%; grades 3/4: ≤44%), peripheral edema (21%; grades 3/4: <1%)

Central nervous system: Fatigue (67%; grades 3/4: 11%), headache (38%; grades 3/4: 3%), voice disorder (31%; grades 3/4: 1%), mouth pain (25%; grades 3/4: 1%), dizziness (15%; grades 3/4: <1%), insomnia (12%)

Dermatologic: Palmar-plantar erythrodysesthesia (32%; grades 3/4: 3%), skin rash (21%; grades 3/4: <1%), alopecia (12%)

Endocrine & metabolic: Increased thyroid stimulating hormone level (57%), weight loss (51%; grades 3/4: 13%)

Hematologic & oncologic: Hemorrhage (35%)

Gastrointestinal: Diarrhea (67%; grades 3/4: 9%), decreased appetite (54%; grades 3/4: 7%), nausea (47%; grades 3/4: 2%), stomatitis (41%; grades 3/4: 5%), vomiting (36%; grades 3/4: 2%), abdominal pain (31%; grades 3/4: 2%), constipation (29%), dysgeusia (18%), xerostomia (17%; grades 3/4: <1%), dyspepsia (13%; grades 3/4: <1%), infection of mouth (10%; grades 3/4: 1%)

Genitourinary: Proteinuria (34%; grade 3: 11%), urinary tract infection (11%; grades 3/4: 1%)

Neuromuscular & skeletal: Arthralgia (≤62%; grades 3/4: ≤5%), myalgia (≤62%; grades 3/4: ≤5%)

Renal: Renal insufficiency (14%; grade 3 or higher: 3%)

Respiratory: Cough (24%), epistaxis (12%)

1% to 10%:

Cardiovascular: Hypotension (9%; grades 3/4: 2%), prolonged Q-T interval on ECG (9%; grades 3/4: 2%), thromboembolic complications (5%; grade 3 or higher: 3%; arterial events), pulmonary embolism (3%), reduced ejection fraction (2%; ejection fraction reduced by >20%)

Dermatologic: Hyperkeratosis (7%)

Endocrine & metabolic: Dehydration (9%; grades 3/4: 2%), hypocalcemia (grades 3/4: 9%), hypokalemia (grades 3/4: 6%), hypercalcemia (>5%), hypercholesterolemia (>5%), hyperkalemia (>5%), hypoalbuminemia (>5%), hypoglycemia (>5%), hypomagnesemia (>5%)

Gastrointestinal: Increased serum amylase (>5%), increased serum lipase (grades 3/4: 4%), gastrointestinal fistula (2%)

Hematologic & oncologic: Decreased platelet count (grades 3/4: 2%)

Hepatic: Hyperbilirubinemia (>5%), increased serum alkaline phosphatase (>5%), increased serum AST (grades 3 or higher: 5%), increased serum ALT (grades 3 or higher: 4%)

Renal: Increased serum creatinine (grades 3/4: 3%)

Respiratory: Pulmonary edema (7%; grade 3 or higher: 2%)

<1% (Limited to important or life-threatening): Reversible posterior leukoencephalopathy syndrome

Drug Interactions

Metabolism/Transport Effects Substrate of BCRP, CYP3A4 (minor), P-glycoprotein; **Note:** Assignment of Major/Minor substrate status based on clinically relevant drug interaction potential; **Inhibits** BSEP, OAT1, OAT3, OCT1, OCT2, SLCO1B1, UGT1A1, UGT1A4

Avoid Concomitant Use

Avoid concomitant use of Lenvatinib with any of the following: Highest Risk QTc-Prolonging Agents; Irinotecan Products; Ivabradine; Mifepristone

Increased Effect/Toxicity

Lenvatinib may increase the levels/effects of: Highest Risk QTc-Prolonging Agents; Irinotecan Products; Moderate Risk QTc-Prolonging Agents

The levels/effects of Lenvatinib may be increased by: Ivabradine; Mifepristone; QTc-Prolonging Agents (Indeterminate Risk and Risk Modifying)

Decreased Effect There are no known significant interactions involving a decrease in effect.

Storage/Stability Store at 25°C (77°F); excursions are permitted between 15°C and 30°C (59°F and 86°F).

Mechanism of Action Lenvatinib is a multitargeted tyrosine kinase inhibitor of vascular endothelial growth factor (VEGF) receptors VEGFR1 (FLT1), VEGFR2 (KDR), VEGFR3 (FLT4), fibroblast growth factor (FGF) receptors FGFR1, 2, 3, and 4, platelet derived growth factor receptor alpha (PDGFRα), KIT, and RET. Inhibition of these receptor tyrosine kinases leads to decreased tumor growth and slowing of cancer progression.

Pharmacodynamics/Kinetics

Protein binding: 98% to 99%

Metabolism: Primarily enzymatic through CYP3A and aldehyde oxidase; nonenzymatic metabolism also occurs

Half-life elimination: ~28 hours

Time to peak: 1 to 4 hours

Excretion: Feces (~64%); urine (~25%)

Dosing

Adult & Geriatric Note: Lenvatinib is associated with a moderate emetic potential; antiemetics are recommended to prevent nausea and vomiting.

Thyroid cancer, differentiated: Oral: 24 mg once daily until disease progression or unacceptable toxicity (Schlumberger, 2015)

Missed doses: Do not take a missed dose within 12 hours of the next dose (if within 12 hours, skip the missed dose and return to regular administration time).

Renal Impairment

Preexisting renal impairment:

Mild or moderate impairment (CrCl ≥30 mL/minute): No dosage adjustment necessary.

Severe impairment (CrCl <30 mL/minute): 14 mg once daily

End-stage renal disease (ESRD): There are no dosage adjustments provided in the manufacturer's labeling (has not been studied).

Renal toxicity during treatment: Interrupt therapy if grade 3 or 4 renal failure or impairment develops. When improved to ≤ grade 1 or baseline, may either resume at a reduced dose or discontinue, depending on severity and persistence of toxicity.

Hepatic Impairment

Preexisting hepatic impairment:

Mild or moderate impairment (Child-Pugh class A or B): No dosage adjustment necessary.

Severe impairment (Child-Pugh class C): 14 mg once daily

Hepatotoxicity during treatment: Interrupt therapy if grade 3 or 4 hepatotoxicity develops. When improved to ≤ grade 1 or baseline, may either resume at a reduced dose or discontinue, depending on severity and persistence of toxicity. Discontinue for hepatic failure.

Adjustment for Toxicity

Recommended dose modifications for persistent and intolerable grade 2 or grade 3 adverse reactions or grade 4 laboratory abnormalities:

First occurrence: Interrupt therapy until resolved to ≤ grade 1 or baseline, then resume dosing at 20 mg once daily

Second occurrence (same or different toxicity): Interrupt therapy until resolved to ≤ grade 1 or baseline, then resume dosing at 14 mg once daily

Third occurrence (same or different toxicity): Interrupt therapy until resolved to ≤ grade 1 or baseline, then resume dosing at 10 mg once daily

Note: There are currently no recommendations for resuming therapy in patients who experience grade 4 clinical adverse reactions that resolve.

Arterial thrombotic event: Discontinue therapy.

Cardiac:

Cardiac dysfunction: Temporarily interrupt therapy for a grade 3 event until improved to ≤ grade 1 or baseline; depending on severity and persistence of toxicity, may either resume therapy at a reduced dose or discontinue treatment. Discontinue for a grade 4 event.

Hypertension: Monitor blood pressure prior to and throughout therapy; initiate or adjust antihypertensive medication to control blood pressure. Temporarily interrupt therapy for grade 3 hypertension that persists despite optimal medical management. When hypertension is ≤ grade 2, resume therapy at a reduced dose. Discontinue therapy for life-threatening hypertension.

QT prolongation: Temporarily interrupt therapy for ≥ grade 3 QT prolongation. When improved to ≤ grade 1 or baseline, resume therapy at a reduced dose.

Gastrointestinal toxicity:

Nausea, vomiting, or diarrhea: Initiate medical management prior to interrupting dose or reducing therapy.

Perforation or fistula formation: Discontinue in patients who develop gastrointestinal perforation or life-threatening fistula.

Hemorrhage: Temporarily interrupt therapy for a grade 3 event until improved to ≤ grade 1 or baseline; depending on severity and persistence of toxicity, may either resume therapy at a reduced dose or discontinue treatment. Discontinue for a grade 4 event.

Hypocalcemia: Administer calcium replacement therapy as necessary; may require treatment interruption or dose reduction depending on the severity, presence of ECG changes, and persistence of hypocalcemia.

Nephrotic syndrome: Discontinue therapy.

Proteinuria: Temporarily interrupt therapy for ≥2 g proteinuria/24 hours; resume therapy at a reduced dose when improved to <2 g proteinuria/24 hours.

Reversible posterior leukoencephalopathy syndrome (RPLS): Interrupt therapy until fully resolved; depending on severity and persistence of neurologic symptoms, may either resume therapy at a reduced dose when resolved or discontinue treatment.

Administration

Lenvatinib is associated with a moderate emetic potential; antiemetics are recommended to prevent nausea and vomiting.

Administer orally at the same time each day; may be taken without regards to meals. Hazardous agent; use appropriate precautions for handling and disposal (meets NIOSH 2014 criteria).

Monitoring Parameters Liver function tests (at baseline, every 2 weeks for 2 months, and at least monthly thereafter); renal function; electrolytes; serum calcium at least monthly; TSH levels at baseline and monthly or as clinically indicated; monitor for proteinuria at baseline and periodically during treatment (urine dipstick; if 2+ then 24-hour urine protein); monitor blood pressure after 1 week, then every 2 weeks for 2 months, and at least monthly thereafter; electrocardiogram in select patients; monitor for signs/symptoms of cardiac decompensation, arterial thrombosis, reversible posterior leukoencephalopathy syndrome, signs/symptoms of gastrointestinal perforation/fistula, and hemorrhagic events

Dosage Forms Considerations Each Lenvima Therapy Pack contains a 30 day supply of dosage units

Dosage Forms Excipient information presented when available (limited, particularly for generics); consult specific product labeling.

Capsule Therapy Pack, Oral:

Lenvima 10 MG Daily Dose: 10 mg (5 ea, 30 ea)

Lenvima 14 MG Daily Dose: 10 mg & 4 mg (10 ea, 60 ea)

Lenvima 20 MG Daily Dose: 2x10 mg (10 ea, 60 ea)

Lenvima 24 MG Daily Dose: 2x10 mg & 4 mg (15 ea, 90 ea)

◆ Lenvatinib Mesylate *see* Lenvatinib *on page 1046*

Letrozole (LET roe zole)

Brand Names: US Femara
Brand Names: Canada ACH-Letrozole; Apo-Letrozole; Auro-Letrozole; Bio-Letrozole; Femara; JAMP-Letrozole; Mar-Letrozole; MED-Letrozole; Myl-Letrozole; Nat-Letrozole; PMS-Letrozole; RAN-Letrozole; Riva-Letrozole; Sandoz-Letrozole; Teva-Letrozole; Van-Letrozole; Zinda-Letrozole
Index Terms CGS-20267
Pharmacologic Category Antineoplastic Agent, Aromatase Inhibitor
Use Breast cancer in postmenopausal women: Adjuvant treatment of hormone receptor-positive early breast cancer, extended adjuvant treatment of early breast cancer after 5 years of tamoxifen; treatment of advanced breast cancer with disease progression following antiestrogen therapy; first-line treatment of hormone receptor–positive or hormone receptor-unknown, locally-advanced, or metastatic breast cancer
Pregnancy Considerations Adverse events were observed in animal reproduction studies. Letrozole is FDA approved for postmenopausal women only (no clinical benefit for breast cancer has been demonstrated in premenopausal women). Use in women who are or who may become pregnant is contraindicated. Women who are perimenopausal or recently postmenopausal should use adequate contraception until postmenopausal status is fully established.
Breast-Feeding Considerations It is not known if letrozole is excreted in breast milk. Due to the potential for serious adverse reactions in the nursing infant, a decision should be made whether to discontinue nursing or to discontinue the drug, taking into account the importance of treatment to the mother. Use in nursing women is contraindicated in the Canadian labeling.
Contraindications Use in women who are or may become pregnant

Canadian labeling: Additional contraindications (not in U.S. labeling): Hypersensitivity to letrozole, other aromatase inhibitors, or any component of the formulation; use in patients <18 years of age; breast-feeding
Warnings/Precautions Hazardous agent - use appropriate precautions for handling and disposal (NIOSH 2014 [group 1]). Not generally indicated for known hormone-receptor negative disease. Use caution with hepatic impairment; dose adjustment recommended in patients with cirrhosis or severe hepatic dysfunction. May cause dizziness, fatigue, and somnolence; patients should be cautioned before performing tasks which require mental alertness (eg, operating machinery or driving). May increase total serum cholesterol; in patients treated with adjuvant therapy and cholesterol levels within normal limits, an increase of ≥1.5 x ULN in total cholesterol has been demonstrated in 8.2% of letrozole-treated patients (25% requiring lipid-lowering medications) vs 3.2% of tamoxifen-treated patients (16% requiring medications); monitor cholesterol panel; may require antihyperlipidemics. May cause decreases in bone mineral density (BMD); a decrease in hip BMD by 3.8% from baseline in letrozole-treated patients vs 2% in placebo at 2 years has been demonstrated; however, there was no statistical difference in changes to the lumbar spine BMD scores; monitor BMD. Potentially significant drug-drug interactions may exist, requiring dose or frequency adjustment, additional monitoring, and/or selection of alternative therapy.
Adverse Reactions
>10%:
Cardiovascular: Edema (7% to 18%)
Central nervous system: Headache (4% to 20%), dizziness (3% to 14%), fatigue (8% to 13%)

Endocrine & metabolic: Hypercholesterolemia (3% to 52%), hot flashes (6% to 50%)
Gastrointestinal: Nausea (9% to 17%), weight gain (2% to 13%), constipation (2% to 11%)
Neuromuscular & skeletal: Weakness (4% to 34%), arthralgia (8% to 25%), arthritis (7% to 25%), bone pain (5% to 22%), back pain (5% to 18%), bone mineral density decreased/osteoporosis (5% to 15%), bone fracture (10% to 14%)
Respiratory: Dyspnea (6% to 18%), cough (6% to 13%)
Miscellaneous: Diaphoresis (≤24%), night sweats (15%)
1% to 10%:
Cardiovascular: Chest pain (6% to 8%), hypertension (5% to 8%), chest wall pain (6%), peripheral edema (5%); cerebrovascular accident including hemorrhagic stroke, thrombotic stroke (2% to 3%); thromboembolic event including venous thrombosis, thrombophlebitis, portal vein thrombosis, pulmonary embolism (2% to 3%); MI (1% to 2%), angina (1% to 2%), transient ischemic attack
Central nervous system: Insomnia (6% to 7%), pain (5%), anxiety (<5%), depression (<5%), vertigo (<5%), somnolence (3%)
Dermatologic: Rash (5%), alopecia (3% to 5%), pruritus (1%)
Endocrine & metabolic: Breast pain (2% to 7%), hypercalcemia (<5%)
Gastrointestinal: Diarrhea (5% to 8%), vomiting (3% to 7%), weight loss (6% to 7%), abdominal pain (6%), anorexia (1% to 5%), dyspepsia (3%)
Genitourinary: Urinary tract infection (6%), vaginal bleeding (5%), vaginal dryness (5%), vaginal hemorrhage (5%), vaginal irritation (5%)
Neuromuscular & skeletal: Limb pain (4% to 10%), myalgia (7% to 9%)
Ocular: Cataract (2%)
Renal: Renal disorder (5%)
Respiratory: Pleural effusion (<5%)
Miscellaneous: Infection (7%), influenza (6%), viral infection (6%), secondary malignancy (2% to 4%)
<1%, postmarketing, and/or case reports (Limited to important or life-threatening): Anaphylactic reaction, angioedema, arterial thrombosis, cardiac failure, carpal tunnel syndrome, endometrial cancer, endometrial hyperplasia, endometrial proliferation, erythema multiforme, hepatitis, leukopenia, memory impairment, stomatitis, tachycardia, thrombocytopenia, toxic epidermal necrolysis, trigger finger
Drug Interactions
Metabolism/Transport Effects Substrate of CYP2A6 (minor), CYP3A4 (minor); **Note:** Assignment of Major/Minor substrate status based on clinically relevant drug interaction potential; **Inhibits** CYP2A6 (strong), CYP2C19 (weak)
Avoid Concomitant Use
Avoid concomitant use of Letrozole with any of the following: Artesunate; Tegafur
Increased Effect/Toxicity
Letrozole may increase the levels/effects of: Artesunate; CYP2A6 Substrates; Methadone
Decreased Effect
Letrozole may decrease the levels/effects of: Artesunate; Tegafur

The levels/effects of Letrozole may be decreased by: Tamoxifen
Storage/Stability Store at room temperature of 25°C (77°F); excursions permitted to 15°C to 30°C (59°F to 86°F).
Mechanism of Action Nonsteroidal competitive inhibitor of the aromatase enzyme system which binds to the heme group of aromatase, a cytochrome P450 enzyme which catalyzes conversion of androgens to estrogens (specifically, androstenedione to estrone and testosterone to estradiol). This leads to inhibition of the enzyme and a significant reduction in plasma estrogen (estrone, estradiol and estrone sulfate) levels. Does not affect synthesis of adrenal or thyroid hormones, aldosterone, or androgens.
Pharmacodynamics/Kinetics
Absorption: Rapid and well absorbed; not affected by food
Distribution: V_d: ~1.9 L/kg
Protein binding, plasma: Weak
Metabolism: Hepatic via CYP3A4 and 2A6 to an inactive carbinol metabolite
Half-life elimination: Terminal: ~2 days
Time to steady state, plasma: 2 to 6 weeks
Excretion: Urine (90%; 6% as unchanged drug, 75% as glucuronide carbinol metabolite, 9% as unidentified metabolites)

Dosing

Adult & Geriatric

Breast cancer, advanced (first- or second-line treatment): Females: Postmenopausal: Oral: 2.5 mg once daily; continue until tumor progression

Breast cancer, early (adjuvant treatment): Females: Postmenopausal: Oral: 2.5 mg once daily for a planned duration of 5 years; discontinue at relapse. **Note:** American Society of Clinical Oncology (ASCO) guidelines for Adjuvant Endocrine Therapy of Hormone Receptor-Positive Breast Cancer (Focused Update) recommend a maximum duration of 5 years of aromatase inhibitor therapy for postmenopausal women; aromatase inhibitors may be combined with tamoxifen for a total duration of up to 10 years of endocrine therapy. Refer to the guidelines for specific recommendations based on menopausal status and tolerability (Burstein 2014).

Breast cancer, early (extended adjuvant treatment): Females: Postmenopausal: Oral: 2.5 mg once daily for a planned duration of 5 years (after 5 years of tamoxifen); discontinue at relapse. In clinical trials, letrozole was initiated within 3 months of discontinuing tamoxifen (Goss 2003; Jin 2012). **Note:** ASCO guidelines for Adjuvant Endocrine Therapy of Hormone Receptor-Positive Breast Cancer (Focused Update) recommend a maximum duration of 5 years of aromatase inhibitor therapy for postmenopausal women; aromatase inhibitors may be combined with tamoxifen for a total duration of up to 10 years of endocrine therapy. Refer to the guidelines for specific recommendations based on menopausal status and tolerability (Burstein 2014).

Off-label combinations:

Breast cancer, advanced, estrogen receptor-positive, HER2-negative: Females: Oral: 2.5 mg once daily (in combination with palbociclib) until disease progression or unacceptable toxicity (Finn 2015)

Breast cancer, metastatic, hormone receptor-positive, HER2-positive: Females: Oral: 2.5 mg once daily (in combination with lapatinib) until disease progression or unacceptable toxicity (Johnston 2009)

Infertility/ovulation stimulation in anovulatory women with polycystic ovarian syndrome (PCOS; off-label use): Oral: 2.5 to 7.5 mg daily on cycle days 3 to 7 (Franik 2014; Legro 2013; Legro 2014; Misso 2012). Up to 5 treatment cycles may be administered with the dose increased in subsequent cycles for nonresponse or poor ovulatory response as determined by progesterone levels; maximum dose 7.5 mg daily (Legro 2014). Additional trials may be necessary to further define the routine use of letrozole in infertile women with PCOS.

Ovarian (epithelial) cancer (off-label use): Oral: 2.5 mg once daily; continue until disease progression (Ramirez 2008)

Renal Impairment

CrCl ≥10 mL/minute: No dosage adjustment necessary.

CrCl <10 mL/minute: There are no dosage adjustments provided in the manufacturer's labeling.

Hepatic Impairment

U.S. labeling:

Mild to moderate impairment (Child-Pugh class A or B): No dosage adjustment necessary.

Severe impairment (Child-Pugh class C) and cirrhosis: 2.5 mg every other day

Noncirrhotic patients with elevated bilirubin: There are no dosage adjustments provided in the manufacturer's labeling (effect has not been determined).

Canadian labeling:

Mild to moderate impairment (Child-Pugh class A or B): No dosage adjustment necessary.

Severe impairment (Child-Pugh class C): There are no dosage adjustments provided in the manufacturer's labeling (insufficient data). Monitor closely.

Dietary Considerations Calcium and vitamin D supplementation are recommended.

Administration Administer orally with or without food. Hazardous agent; use appropriate precautions for handling and disposal (NIOSH 2014 [group 1]).

Monitoring Parameters

Monitor periodically during therapy: Complete blood counts, thyroid function tests; serum electrolytes, cholesterol, transaminases, and creatinine; blood pressure; bone density

Canadian labeling recommends monitoring LH, FSH, and/or estradiol prior to initiating therapy and regularly for the first 6 months in women whose menopausal status is unclear or who become amenorrheic following chemotherapy. For infertility/ovarian stimulation (off-label use), a pregnancy test is recommended prior to initiation. Midluteal progestin concentrations (in a clinical study, nonresponse to treatment was defined as a progesterone concentration <3 ng/mL during the midluteal phase; poor ovulatory response was defined as progesterone concentrations indicating ovulation but just above the cutoff point) (Legro 2014).

Dosage Forms Excipient information presented when available (limited, particularly for generics); consult specific product labeling.

Tablet, Oral:

Femara: 2.5 mg

Generic: 2.5 mg

◆ Leucovorin *see* Leucovorin Calcium *on page 1049*

Leucovorin Calcium (loo koe VOR in KAL see um)

Brand Names: Canada Lederle Leucovorin; Leucovorin Calcium Injection; Leucovorin Calcium Injection USP

Index Terms 5-Formyl Tetrahydrofolate; Calcium Folinate; Calcium Leucovorin; Citrovorum Factor; Folinate Calcium; Folinic Acid (error prone synonym); Leucovorin

Pharmacologic Category Antidote; Chemotherapy Modulating Agent; Rescue Agent (Chemotherapy); Vitamin, Water Soluble

Use

Colorectal cancer, advanced: Injection: Palliative treatment of advanced colorectal cancer to prolong survival (in combination with 5-fluorouracil).

Methotrexate toxicity:

Injection: Rescue agent after high-dose methotrexate treatment in osteosarcoma and to diminish the toxicity and counteract the effects of impaired methotrexate elimination and of inadvertent overdosage of folic acid antagonists.

Oral: Rescue agent to diminish toxicity and counteract effects of impaired methotrexate elimination and inadvertent overdoses of folic acid antagonists.

Megaloblastic anemia: Injection: Treatment of megaloblastic anemias due to folic acid deficiency (when oral therapy is not feasible).

Pregnancy Considerations Animal reproduction studies have not been conducted. Leucovorin is a biologically active form of folic acid. Adequate amounts of folic acid are recommended during pregnancy. Refer to Folic Acid monograph.

Breast-Feeding Considerations Leucovorin is a biologically active form of folic acid. Adequate amounts of folic acid are recommended in breast-feeding women. Refer to Folic Acid monograph.

Contraindications Pernicious anemia and other megaloblastic anemias secondary to vitamin B_{12}-deficiency

Warnings/Precautions When used for the treatment of accidental folic acid antagonist overdose, administer as soon as possible. When used for the treatment of a methotrexate overdose, administer IV leucovorin as soon as possible. Monitoring of the serum methotrexate concentration is essential to determine the optimal dose/duration of leucovorin; however, do not wait for the results of a methotrexate level before initiating therapy. It is important to adjust the leucovorin dose once a methotrexate level is known. When used for methotrexate rescue therapy, methotrexate serum concentrations should be monitored to determine dose and duration of leucovorin therapy. The dose may need to be increased or administration prolonged in situations where methotrexate excretion may be delayed (eg, ascites, pleural effusion, renal insufficiency, inadequate hydration); **never administer leucovorin intrathecally**. Parenteral administration may be preferred to oral if vomiting or malabsorption is likely. Potentially significant drug-drug interactions may exist, requiring dose or frequency adjustment, additional monitoring, and/or selection of alternative therapy. Combination of leucovorin and sulfamethoxazole-trimethoprim for the acute treatment of PCP in patients with HIV infection has been reported to cause increased rates of treatment failure. Leucovorin may increase the toxicity of 5-fluorouracil; deaths from severe enterocolitis, diarrhea, and dehydration have been reported (in elderly patients); granulocytopenia and fever have also been reported.

Hypersensitivity, including allergic reactions, anaphylactoid reactions, and urticaria have been reported with leucovorin. Because leucovorin is typically administered in combination with other chemotherapy agents, it may be difficult to determine the causative agent for hypersensitivity reactions. In a series of 44 patients with hypersensitivity to leucovorin-containing regimens, hypersensitivity/infusion reaction to leucovorin was confirmed in 5 patients; reactions also occurred with subsequent rechallenge with LEVOleucovorin (Ureña-Tavera, 2015).

Leucovorin is inappropriate treatment for pernicious anemia and other megaloblastic anemias secondary to a lack of vitamin B_{12}; a hematologic remission may occur while neurologic manifestations progress. Leucovorin is

excreted renally; the risk for toxicities may be increased in patients with renal impairment.

Benzyl alcohol and derivatives: When doses >10 mg/m^2 are required using the powder for injection, reconstitute using sterile water for injection, not a solution containing benzyl alcohol; large amounts of benzyl alcohol (≥99 mg/kg/day) have been associated with a potentially fatal toxicity ("gasping syndrome") in neonates; the "gasping syndrome" consists of metabolic acidosis, respiratory distress, gasping respirations, CNS dysfunction (including convulsions, intracranial hemorrhage), hypotension, and cardiovascular collapse (AAP ["Inactive" 1997]; CDC, 1982); some data suggests that benzoate displaces bilirubin from protein binding sites (Ahlfors, 2001); avoid or use dosage forms containing benzyl alcohol with caution in neonates. See manufacturer's labeling.

Injection: Due to calcium content, do not administer IV solutions at a rate >160 mg/minute. Not intended for intrathecal use.

Adverse Reactions Frequency not defined. Toxicities (especially gastrointestinal toxicity) of fluorouracil is higher when used in combination with leucovorin.

Dermatologic: Rash, pruritus, erythema, urticaria

Hematologic: Thrombocytosis

Respiratory: Wheezing

Miscellaneous: Allergic reactions, anaphylactoid reactions

Drug Interactions

Metabolism/Transport Effects None known.

Avoid Concomitant Use

Avoid concomitant use of Leucovorin Calcium with any of the following: Raltitrexed; Trimethoprim

Increased Effect/Toxicity

Leucovorin Calcium may increase the levels/effects of: Capecitabine; Fluorouracil (Systemic); Fluorouracil (Topical); Tegafur

Decreased Effect

Leucovorin Calcium may decrease the levels/effects of: Fosphenytoin; PHENobarbital; Phenytoin; Primidone; Raltitrexed; Trimethoprim

The levels/effects of Leucovorin Calcium may be decreased by: Glucarpidase

Preparation for Administration

Powder for injection: Reconstitute with SWFI or BWFI; dilute in D$_5$W or NS for infusion. When doses >10 mg/m^2 are required, reconstitute using sterile water for injection, not a solution containing benzyl alcohol. For methanol toxicity, dilute in D$_5$W (Barceloux, 2002).

Storage/Stability

Powder for injection: Store at room temperature of 25°C (77°F). Protect from light. Solutions reconstituted with bacteriostatic water for injection U.S.P. must be used within 7 days. Solutions reconstituted with SWFI must be used immediately. Parenteral admixture is stable for 24 hours stored at room temperature (25°C) and for 4 days when stored under refrigeration (4°C).

Solution for injection: Prior to dilution, store vials under refrigeration at 2°C to 8°C (36°F to 46°F). Protect from light.

Tablet: Store at room temperature of 15°C to 30°C (59°F to 86°F).

Mechanism of Action A reduced form of folic acid, leucovorin supplies the necessary cofactor blocked by methotrexate. Leucovorin actively competes with methotrexate for transport sites, displaces methotrexate from intracellular binding sites, and restores active folate stores required for DNA/RNA synthesis. Stabilizes the binding of 5-dUMP and thymidylate synthetase, enhancing the activity of fluorouracil. When administered with pyrimethamine for the treatment of opportunistic infections, leucovorin reduces the risk for hematologic toxicity (HHS [OI adult 2015]).

Methanol toxicity treatment: Formic acid (methanol's toxic metabolite) is normally metabolized to carbon dioxide and water by 10-formyltetrahydrofolate dehydrogenase after being bound to tetrahydrofolate. Administering a source of tetrahydrofolate may aid the body in eliminating formic acid (Barceloux, 2002).

Pharmacodynamics/Kinetics

Absorption: Oral, IM: Well absorbed

Metabolism: Intestinal mucosa and hepatically to 5-methyltetrahydrofolate (5MTHF; active)

Bioavailability: Saturable at oral doses >25 mg; 25 mg (97%), 50 mg (75%), 100 mg (37%)

Half-life elimination: ~4 to 8 hours

Time to peak: Oral: ~2 hours; IV: Total folates: 10 minutes; 5MTHF: ~1 hour

Excretion: Urine (primarily); feces

Dosing

Adult & Geriatric

Colorectal cancer, advanced: IV: 200 mg/m^2/day over at least 3 minutes for 5 days every 4 weeks for 2 cycles, then every 4 to 5 weeks (in combination with fluorouracil) **or** 20 mg/m^2/day for 5 days every 4 weeks for 2 cycles, then every 4 to 5 weeks (in combination with fluorouracil). **Note:** Multiple leucovorin-containing regimens are available for the treatment of colorectal cancer. Refer to appropriate literature/guidelines for additional details.

Folic acid antagonist (eg, trimethoprim, pyrimethamine) overdose: Oral: 5 to 15 mg once daily

Folate-deficient megaloblastic anemia: IM, IV: ≤1 mg once daily

High-dose methotrexate-rescue: Initial: Oral, IM, IV: 15 mg (~10 mg/m^2); start 24 hours after beginning methotrexate infusion; continue every 6 hours for 10 doses, until methotrexate level is <0.05 micromolar. Adjust dose as follows:

Normal methotrexate elimination (serum methotrexate level ~10 micromolar at 24 hours after administration, 1 micromolar at 48 hours, and <0.2 micromolar at 72 hours): Oral, IM, IV: 15 mg every 6 hours for 60 hours (10 doses) beginning 24 hours after the start of methotrexate infusion

Delayed late methotrexate elimination (serum methotrexate level remaining >0.2 micromolar at 72 hours and >0.05 micromolar at 96 hours after administration): Continue leucovorin calcium 15 mg (oral, IM or IV) every 6 hours until methotrexate level is <0.05 micromolar

Delayed early methotrexate elimination and/or acute renal injury (serum methotrexate level ≥50 micromolar at 24 hours, or ≥5 micromolar at 48 hours, or a doubling of serum creatinine level at 24 hours after methotrexate administration): IV: 150 mg every 3 hours until methotrexate level is <1 micromolar, then 15 mg every 3 hours until methotrexate level is <0.05 micromolar

High-dose methotrexate overexposure: Leucovorin nomogram dosing for high-dose methotrexate overexposure (off-label dosing; generalized dosing derived from reference nomogram figures, refer to each reference [Bleyer, 1978; Bleyer, 1981; Widemann, 2006] or institution-specific nomogram for details):

At 24 hours:

For methotrexate levels of ≥100 micromolar at ~24 hours, leucovorin is initially dosed at 1,000 mg/m^2 every 6 hours

For methotrexate levels of ≥10 to <100 micromolar at 24 hours, leucovorin is initially dosed at 100 mg/m^2 every 3 or 6 hours

For methotrexate levels of ~1 to 10 micromolar at 24 hours, leucovorin is initially dosed at 10 mg/m^2 every 3 or 6 hours

At 48 hours:

For methotrexate levels of ≥100 micromolar at 48 hours, leucovorin is dosed at 1,000 mg/m^2 every 6 hours

For methotrexate levels of ≥10 to <100 micromolar at 48 hours, leucovorin is dosed at 100 mg/m^2 every 3 hours

For methotrexate levels of ~1 to 10 micromolar at 48 hours, leucovorin is dosed at 100 mg/m^2 every 6 hours **or** 10 to 100 mg/m^2 every 3 hours

At 72 hours:

For methotrexate levels of ≥10 micromolar at 72 hours, leucovorin is dosed at 100 to 1,000 mg/m^2 every 3 to 6 hours

For methotrexate levels of ~1 to 10 micromolar at 72 hours, leucovorin is dosed at 10 to 100 mg/m^2 every 3 hours

For methotrexate levels of ~0.1 to 1 micromolar at 72 hours, leucovorin is dosed at 10 mg/m^2 every 3 to 6 hours

If serum creatinine is increased more than 50% above baseline, increase the standard leucovorin dose to 100 mg/m^2 every 3 hours, then adjust according to methotrexate levels above.

Follow methotrexate levels daily, leucovorin may be discontinued when methotrexate level is <0.1 micromolar

Methotrexate overdose (inadvertent) (begin as soon as possible after overdose): Oral, IM, IV: 10 mg/m^2 every 6 hours until the methotrexate level is <0.01 micromolar. If serum creatinine is increased more than 50% above baseline 24 hours after methotrexate administration, if 24 hour methotrexate level is >5 micromolar, or if 48 hour methotrexate level is >0.9 micromolar, increase leucovorin dose to 100 mg/m^2 IV every 3 hours until the methotrexate level is <0.01 micromolar.

Do not administer leucovorin intrathecally; the use of intrathecal leucovorin is not advised (Jardine, 1996; Smith, 2008).

Bladder cancer, neoadjuvant treatment (off-label use): IV, Oral: 15 mg every 6 hours for 4 doses on days 2 and 9, starting 24 hours after each methotrexate dose (in combination with methotrexate, vinblastine, and cisplatin) (Griffiths, 2011).

Cofactor therapy in methanol toxicity (off-label use): IV: 1 mg/kg (maximum dose: 50 mg) over 30 to 60 minutes every 4 to 6 hours. Therapy should continue until methanol and formic acid have been completely eliminated (Barceloux, 2002).

Esophageal cancer, advanced or metastatic (off-label use): IV: 400 mg/m^2 over 2 hours once every 2 weeks (in combination with fluorouracil and irinotecan [FOL-FIRI]) until disease progression or unacceptable toxicity (Guimbaud, 2014) **or** 200 mg/m^2 over 2 hours once every 2 weeks (in combination with fluorouracil and oxaliplatin) until disease progression or unacceptable toxicity (Al-Batran, 2008).

Gastric cancer, advanced or metastatic (off-label use): IV: 400 mg/m^2 over 2 hours once every 2 weeks (in combination with fluorouracil and irinotecan [FOL-FIRI]) until disease progression or unacceptable toxicity (Guimbaud, 2014) **or** 200 mg/m^2 over 2 hours once every 2 weeks (in combination with fluorouracil and oxaliplatin) until disease progression or unacceptable toxicity (Al-Batran, 2008).

Pancreatic cancer, metastatic (off-label use): IV: 400 mg/m^2 over 2 hours once every 2 weeks (in combination with fluorouracil, oxaliplatin, and irinotecan [FOLFIRINOX]) for at least 6 months (Conroy, 2011).

Pemetrexed toxicity (off-label dose): IV: 100 mg/m^2 once, followed by 50 mg/m^2 every 6 hours for 8 days (used in clinical trial for CTC grade 4 leukopenia ≥3 days; CTC grade 4 neutropenia ≥3 days; immediately for CTC grade 4 thrombocytopenia, bleeding associated with grade 3 thrombocytopenia, or grade 3 or 4 mucositis) (Alimta [prescribing information], 2013).

Prevention of pyrimethamine hematologic toxicity in HIV-infected patients (off-label use; HHS [OI adult 2015]): Oral:

Isosporiasis (*Isospora belli*):

Treatment: 10 to 25 mg once daily (in combination with pyrimethamine)

Chronic maintenance (secondary prophylaxis): 5 to 10 mg once daily (in combination with pyrimethamine)

Pneumocystis pneumonia (PCP): Prophylaxis (primary and secondary): 25 mg once weekly (in combination with pyrimethamine [with dapsone] **or** 10 mg once daily (in combination with pyrimethamine [with atovaquone])

Toxoplasma gondii encephalitis:

Primary prophylaxis: 25 mg once weekly (in combination with pyrimethamine [with dapsone]) **or** 10 mg once daily (in combination with pyrimethamine [with atovaquone])

Treatment: 10 to 25 mg once daily (in combination with pyrimethamine [with either sulfadiazine, clindamycin, atovaquone, or azithromycin]). **Note:** May increase leucovorin to 50 to 100 mg/day in divided doses in cases of pyrimethamine toxicity (rash, nausea, bone marrow suppression).

Chronic maintenance (secondary prophylaxis): 10 to 25 mg once daily (in combination with pyrimethamine [with either sulfadiazine or clindamycin]) **or** 10 mg once daily (in combination with pyrimethamine [with atovaquone])

Pediatric

Folic acid antagonist (eg, trimethoprim, pyrimethamine) overdose: Refer to adult dosing.

Folate-deficient megaloblastic anemia: Refer to adult dosing.

High-dose methotrexate-rescue: Refer to adult dosing.

Cofactor therapy in methanol toxicity (off-label use): Refer to adult dosing.

Prevention of pyrimethamine hematologic toxicity in HIV-exposed/-positive patients (off-label uses; CDC, 2009):

Infants and Children >1 month of age: **Note:** Leucovorin should continue for 1 week after pyrimethamine is discontinued.

Toxoplasmosis (*Toxoplasma gondii*):

Primary prophylaxis: Oral: 5 mg once every 3 days (in combination with pyrimethamine [with either dapsone or atovaquone])

Secondary prophylaxis: Oral: 5 mg once every 3 days (in combination with pyrimethamine [with either sulfadiazine, atovaquone, or clindamycin])

Treatment (congenital): Oral or IM: 10 mg with every pyrimethamine dose (in combination with either sulfadiazine or clindamycin); treatment duration: 12 months

Treatment (acquired): Oral: Acute induction: 10-25 mg once daily (in combination with pyrimethamine [with either sulfadiazine, clindamycin, or atovaquone]) for ≥6 weeks

Adolescents: Refer to adult dosing

Renal Impairment There are no dosage adjustments provided in the manufacturer's labeling.

Hepatic Impairment There are no dosage adjustments provided in the manufacturer's labeling.

Dietary Considerations Solutions for injection contain calcium 0.004 mEq per leucovorin 1 mg

Administration Due to calcium content, do not administer IV solutions at a rate >160 mg/minute; not intended for intrathecal use.

Refer to individual protocols. Should be administered IM, IV push, or IV infusion (15 minutes to 2 hours). Leucovorin should not be administered concurrently with methotrexate. It is commonly initiated 24 hours after the start of methotrexate. Toxicity to normal tissues may be irreversible if leucovorin is not initiated by ~40 hours after the start of methotrexate.

As a rescue after folate antagonists: Administer by IV bolus, IM, or orally.

Do not administer orally in the presence of nausea or vomiting. Doses >25 mg should not be administered orally (should be converted to parenteral therapy).

Combination therapy with fluorouracil: Fluorouracil is usually given after, or at the midpoint, of the leucovorin infusion. Leucovorin is usually administered by IV bolus injection or short (10 to 120 minutes) IV infusion. Other administration schedules have been used; refer to individual protocols.

For the treatment of methanol toxicity, infuse over 30 to 60 minutes (Barceloux, 2002)

Monitoring Parameters

High-dose methotrexate therapy: Plasma methotrexate concentration; leucovorin is continued until the plasma methotrexate level <0.05 micromolar. With 4- to 6-hour high-dose methotrexate infusions, plasma drug values in excess of 50 and 1 micromolar at 24 and 48 hours after starting the infusion, respectively, are often predictive of delayed methotrexate clearance.

Fluorouracil therapy: CBC with differential and platelets, liver function tests, electrolytes

Dosage Forms Excipient information presented when available (limited, particularly for generics); consult specific product labeling. [DSC] = Discontinued product

Solution, Injection [strength expressed as base]:

Generic: 100 mg/10 mL (10 mL [DSC]); 300 mg/30 mL (30 mL)

Solution Reconstituted, Injection [strength expressed as base]:

Generic: 100 mg (1 ea); 200 mg (1 ea); 350 mg (1 ea); 500 mg (1 ea)

Solution Reconstituted, Injection [strength expressed as base, preservative free]:

Generic: 50 mg (1 ea); 100 mg (1 ea); 200 mg (1 ea); 350 mg (1 ea)

Tablet, Oral [strength expressed as base]:

Generic: 5 mg, 10 mg, 15 mg, 25 mg

Extemporaneous Preparations A 5 mg/mL oral suspension may be prepared with tablets, Cologel, and a 2:1 mixture of simple syrup and wild cherry syrup. Crush twenty-four 25 mg tablets in a glass mortar and reduce to a fine powder; transfer powder to amber bottle. Add 30 mL Cologel and shake mixture thoroughly. Add a quantity of syrup mixture sufficient to make 120 mL. Label "shake well" and "refrigerate". Stable for 28 days refrigerated.

Lam MS. Extemporaneous Compounding of Oral Liquid Dosage Formulations and Alternative Drug Delivery Methods for Anticancer Drugs. *Pharmacotherapy.* 2011;31(2):164-192.

◆ Leucovorin Calcium Injection (Can) *see* Leucovorin Calcium *on page 1049*

◆ Leucovorin Calcium Injection USP (Can) *see* Leucovorin Calcium *on page 1049*

◆ Leukeran *see* Chlorambucil *on page 370*

◆ Leukeran® (Can) *see* Chlorambucil *on page 370*

◆ Leukine *see* Sargramostim *on page 1637*

Leuprolide (loo PROE lide)

Brand Names: US Eligard; Lupron Depot; Lupron Depot-Ped

Brand Names: Canada Eligard; Lupron; Lupron Depot

Index Terms Abbott-43818; Leuprolide Acetate; Leuprorelin Acetate; TAP-144

Pharmacologic Category Antineoplastic Agent, Gonado-tropin-Releasing Hormone Agonist; Gonadotropin Releasing Hormone Agonist

Use

Central precocious puberty: Treatment of children with central precocious puberty

Endometriosis: Management of endometriosis, including pain relief and reduction of endometriotic lesions

Prostate cancer: Palliative treatment of advanced prostate cancer

Uterine leiomyomata (fibroids): Treatment of anemia caused by uterine leiomyomata (fibroids)

Pregnancy Considerations Adverse events were observed in animal reproduction studies. Pregnancy must be excluded prior to the start of treatment. Although leuprolide usually inhibits ovulation and stops menstruation, contraception is not ensured and a nonhormonal contraceptive should be used. Use is contraindicated in pregnant women.

Breast-Feeding Considerations It is not known if leuprolide is excreted into breast milk; use is contraindicated in nursing women.

Contraindications

Hypersensitivity to leuprolide, GnRH, GnRH-agonist analogs, or any component of the formulation; undiagnosed abnormal vaginal bleeding (Lupron Depot 3.75 mg [monthly] and Lupron Depot 11.25 mg [3-month]); pregnancy; breast-feeding (Lupron Depot 3.75 mg [monthly] and Lupron Depot 11.25 mg [3-month])

Lupron Depot 22.5 mg, 30 mg, and 45 mg are also not indicated for use in women

Warnings/Precautions Hazardous agent - use appropriate precautions for handling and disposal (NIOSH 2014 [group 1]). Transient increases in testosterone serum levels (~50% above baseline) occur at the start of treatment. Androgen-deprivation therapy (ADT) may increase the risk for cardiovascular disease (Levine, 2010); sudden cardiac death and stroke have been reported in men receiving GnRH agonists; ADT may prolong the QT/QTc interval; consider the benefits of ADT versus the risk for QT prolongation in patients with a history of QTc prolongation, congenital long QT syndrome, heart failure, frequent electrolyte abnormalities, and in patients with medications known to prolong the QT interval, or with preexisting cardiac disease. Consider periodic monitoring of electrocardiograms and electrolytes in at-risk patients. Tumor flare, bone pain, neuropathy, urinary tract obstruction, and spinal cord compression have been reported when used for prostate cancer; closely observe patients for weakness, paresthesias, hematuria, and urinary tract obstruction in first few weeks of therapy. Observe patients with metastatic vertebral lesions or urinary obstruction closely. Exacerbation of endometriosis or uterine leiomyomata may occur initially. Decreased bone density has been reported when used for ≥6 months; use caution in patients with additional risk factors for bone loss (eg, chronic alcohol use, corticosteroid therapy). In patients with prostate cancer, androgen deprivation therapy may increase the risk for cardiovascular disease, diabetes, insulin resistance, obesity, alterations in lipids, and fractures; monitor as clinically necessary. Use caution in patients with a history of psychiatric illness; alteration in mood, memory impairment, and depression have been associated with use. Rare cases of pituitary apoplexy (frequently secondary to pituitary adenoma) have been observed with GnRH agonist administration (onset from 1 hour to usually <2 weeks); may present as sudden headache, vomiting, visual or mental status changes, and infrequently cardiovascular collapse; immediate medical attention required. Convulsions have been observed in postmarketing reports; patients affected included both those with and without a history of cerebrovascular disorders, central nervous system anomalies or tumors, epilepsy, seizures, and those on concomitant medications which may lower the seizure threshold. If seizures occur, manage accordingly. Females treated for precocious puberty may experience menses or spotting during the first 2 months of treatment; notify healthcare provider if bleeding continues after the second month.

Benzyl alcohol and derivatives: Some dosage forms may contain benzyl alcohol; large amounts of benzyl alcohol (≥99 mg/kg/day) have been associated with a potentially fatal toxicity ("gasping syndrome") in neonates; the "gasping syndrome" consists of metabolic acidosis, respiratory distress, gasping respirations, CNS dysfunction (including convulsions, intracranial hemorrhage), hypotension, and cardiovascular collapse (AAP ["Inactive" 1997]; CDC, 1982); some data suggests that benzoate displaces bilirubin from protein binding sites (Ahlfors, 2001); avoid or use dosage forms containing benzyl alcohol with caution in neonates.

Some dosage forms may contain polysorbate 80 (also known as Tweens). Hypersensitivity reactions, usually a delayed reaction, have been reported following exposure to pharmaceutical products containing polysorbate 80 in certain individuals (Isaksson, 2002; Lucente 2000; Shelley, 1995). Thrombocytopenia, ascites, pulmonary deterioration, and renal and hepatic failure have been reported in premature neonates after receiving parenteral products containing polysorbate 80 (Alade, 1986; CDC, 1984). See manufacturer's labeling.

Vehicle used in depot injectable formulations (polylactide-co-glycolide microspheres) has rarely been associated with retinal artery occlusion in patients with abnormal arteriovenous anastomosis. Due to different release properties, combinations of dosage forms or fractions of dosage forms should not be interchanged.

Adverse Reactions

Children (percentages based on 1-month and 3-month pediatric formulations combined):

>10%: Local: Pain at injection site (≤20%)

2% to 10%:

Cardiovascular: Vasodilatation (2%)

Central nervous system: Emotional lability (5%), mood changes (5%), headache (3% to 5%), pain (3%)

Dermatologic: Acne vulgaris (3%), seborrhea (3%), skin rash (3% including erythema multiforme)

Endocrine & metabolic: Weight gain (≤7%)

Genitourinary: Vaginal discharge (3%), vaginal hemorrhage (3%), vaginitis (3%)

Local: Injection site reaction (≤9%)

<2%: Abnormal gait, alopecia, arthralgia, asthma, body odor, bradycardia, cervix disease, constipation, cough, decreased appetite, decreased visual acuity, depression, dizziness, drowsiness, dysmenorrhea, dyspepsia, dysphagia, epistaxis, excessive crying, feminization, fever, flu-like symptoms, gingivitis, goiter, growth suppression, gynecomastia, hirsutism, hyperhidrosis, hyperkinesia, hypersensitivity reaction, hypertension, increased appetite, infection, lacrimation, leukoderma, limb pain, musculoskeletal pain, myalgia, myopathy, nausea, nervousness, obesity, pallor, peripheral edema, personality disorder, pharyngitis, precocious puberty, purpura, rhinitis, sinusitis, skin striae, syncope, urinary incontinence, vomiting, weakness

Adults: Note: For prostate cancer treatment, an initial rise in serum testosterone concentrations may cause "tumor flare" or worsening of symptoms, including bone pain, neuropathy, hematuria, or ureteral or bladder outlet obstruction during the first 2 weeks. Similarly, an initial increase in estradiol levels, with a temporary worsening of symptoms, may occur in women treated with leuprolide.

Delayed release formulations:

>10%:

Cardiovascular: Edema (≤14%)

Central nervous system: Headache (≤65%), pain (<2% to 33%), depression (≤31%), insomnia (≤31%), fatigue (≤17%), dizziness (≤16%)

Dermatologic: Allergic skin reaction (≤12%)

Endocrine & metabolic: Hot flash (25% to 98%), weight changes (≤13%), hyperlipidemia (≤12%), decreased libido (≤11%)

Gastrointestinal: Nausea and vomiting (≤25%), gastrointestinal disease (14%), change in bowel habits (≤14%)

Genitourinary: Vaginitis (11% to 28%), testicular atrophy (≤20%), genitourinary complaint (13% to 15%)

Local: Burning sensation at injection site burning (transient: ≤35%)

Neuromuscular & skeletal: Weakness (≤18%), arthropathy (≤12%)

Respiratory: Flu-like symptoms (≤12%), respiratory tract disease (11%)

1% to 10% (limited to important or life-threatening):

Cardiovascular: Angina pectoris (<5%), atrial fibrillation (<5%), bradycardia (<5%), cardiac arrhythmia (<5%), cardiac failure (<5%), deep thrombophlebitis (<5%), hyper-/hypotension (<5%), palpitations (<5%), syncope (<5%), tachycardia (<5%)

Central nervous system: Nervousness (≤8%), paresthesia (≤8%), anxiety (≤6%), agitation (<5%), confusion (<5%), delusions (<5%), dementia (<5%), neuropathy (<5%), paralysis (<5%), seizure (<5%), ostealgia (<2%)

Dermatologic: Acne vulgaris (≤10%), alopecia (≤5%), diaphoresis (≤5%), cellulitis (<5%), hair disease (<5%), pruritus (≤3%), skin rash (≤2%)

Endocrine & metabolic: Dehydration (≤8%), gynecomastia (≤7%), decreased serum bicarbonate (≥5%), hypercholesterolemia (≥5%), hyperglycemia (≥5%), hyperphosphatemia (≥5%), hyperuricemia (≥5%), hypoalbuminemia (≥5%), hypocholesterolemia (≥5%), hypoproteinemia (≥5%), increased lactate dehydrogenase (≥5%), increased prostatic acid phosphatase (≥5%), menstrual disorder (≤2%), hirsutism (<2%)

Gastrointestinal: Anorexia (<5%), dysphagia (<5%), eructation (<5%), gastric ulcer (<5%), gastrointestinal hemorrhage (<5%), intestinal obstruction (<5%), peptic ulcer (<5%), constipation (≤3%), gastroenteritis (≤3%), diarrhea (≤2%)

Genitourinary: Mastalgia (≤6%), impotence (≤5%), balanitis (<5%), breast hypertrophy (<5%), lactation (<5%), penile disease (<5%), testicular disease (<5%), urinary incontinence (<5%), urinary tract infection (<5%), nocturia (≤4%), testicular pain (≤4%), dysuria (≤2%), bladder spasm (<2%), erectile dysfunction (<2%), hematuria (<2%), urinary retention (<2%), urinary urgency (<2%)

Hematologic & oncologic: Change in platelet count (increased; ≥5%), decreased prostatic acid phosphatase (≥5%), eosinophilia (≥5%), leukopenia (≥5%), bruise (≤5%), ecchymoses (<5%), lymphadenopathy (<5%), neoplasm (<5%), anemia, decreased hematocrit, decreased hemoglobin

Hepatic: Abnormal hepatic function tests (≥5%), increased serum AST (≥5%), prolonged partial thromboplastin time (≥5%), prolonged prothrombin time (≥5%), hepatomegaly (<5%)

Hypersensitivity: Hypersensitivity reaction (<5%)

Infection: Infection (5%)

Local: Pain at injection site (2% to 5%), injection site reaction (<5%), erythema at injection site (1% to 3%)

Neuromuscular & skeletal: Myalgia (≤8%), neuromuscular disease (<5%), pathological fracture (<5%), arthralgia (≤1%)

Renal: Decreased urine specific gravity (≥5%), increased blood urea nitrogen (≥5%), increased serum creatinine (≥5%), increased urine specific gravity (≥5%), polyuria (2% to 4%)

Respiratory: Emphysema (<5%), epistaxis (<5%), hemoptysis (<5%), increased bronchial secretions (<5%), pleural effusion (<5%), pulmonary edema (<5%), dyspnea (≤2%), cough (≤1%)

Miscellaneous: Fever (<5%)

Immediate release formulation:

>10%:

Cardiovascular: ECG changes (19%), peripheral edema (12%)

Central nervous system: Pain (13%)

Endocrine & metabolic: Hot flash (55%)

1% to 10% (limited to important or life-threatening):

Cardiovascular: Hypertension (8%), heart murmur (3%), thrombophlebitis (2%), cardiac failure (1%), angina pectoris, cardiac arrhythmia, myocardial infarction, pulmonary embolism, syncope

Central nervous system: Headache (7%), insomnia (7%), dizziness (5%), ostealgia (5%), anxiety, depression, fatigue, fever, nervousness, peripheral neuropathy

Dermatologic: Dermatitis (5%), alopecia, hyperpigmentation, pruritus, skin lesion

Endocrine & metabolic: Decreased libido, diabetes mellitus, goiter, gynecomastia, hypercalcemia, hypoglycemia

Gastrointestinal: Constipation (7%), anorexia (6%), nausea and vomiting (5%), diarrhea, dysphagia, gastrointestinal hemorrhage, peptic ulcer, rectal polyps

Genitourinary: Decreased testicular size (7%), hematuria (6%), urinary frequency (6%), impotence (4%), urinary tract infection (3%), bladder spasm, dysuria, incontinence, mastalgia, testicular pain, urinary tract obstruction

Hematologic & oncologic: Anemia (5%), bruise

Infection: Infection

Local: Injection site reaction

Neuromuscular & skeletal: Weakness (10%)

Ophthalmic: Blurred vision

Renal: Increased blood urea nitrogen, increased serum creatinine

Respiratory: Dyspnea (2%), cough, pneumonia, pulmonary fibrosis

Miscellaneous: Fever, inflammation

Children and Adults: *Any formulations:* Postmarketing and/or case reports (Limited to important or life-threatening): Abscess at injection site, anaphylaxis, anaphylactoid reaction, asthma, bone fracture (spine), cerebrovascular accident, convulsions, coronary artery disease, decreased white blood cell count, diabetes mellitus, fibromyalgia syndrome (arthralgia/myalgia), headaches, GI distress), hemoptysis, hepatic injury, hepatic insufficiency, hepatotoxicity, hyperuricemia, hypokalemia, hypoproteinemia, induration at injection site, interstitial pulmonary disease, leukocytosis, myocardial infarction, osteopenia, paralysis, penile swelling, peripheral neuropathy, pituitary apoplexy (cardiovascular collapse, mental status altered, ophthalmoplegia, sudden headache, visual changes, vomiting), prolonged QT interval on ECG, prostate pain, pulmonary embolism, pulmonary infiltrates, retroperitoneal fibrosis (pelvic), seizure, skin photosensitivity, suicidal ideation (rare), tenosynovitis (symptoms), thrombocytopenia, transient ischemic attacks

Drug Interactions

Metabolism/Transport Effects None known.

Avoid Concomitant Use

Avoid concomitant use of Leuprolide with any of the following: Corifollitropin Alfa; Highest Risk QTc-Prolonging Agents; Indium 111 Capromab Pendetide; Ivabradine; Mifepristone

Increased Effect/Toxicity

Leuprolide may increase the levels/effects of: Corifollitropin Alfa; Highest Risk QTc-Prolonging Agents; Moderate Risk QTc-Prolonging Agents

The levels/effects of Leuprolide may be increased by: Ivabradine; Mifepristone; QTc-Prolonging Agents (Indeterminate Risk and Risk Modifying)

Decreased Effect

Leuprolide may decrease the levels/effects of: Antidiabetic Agents; Choline C 11; Indium 111 Capromab Pendetide

Preparation for Administration Hazardous agent; use appropriate precautions for handling and disposal (NIOSH 2014 [group 1]).

Eligard: Packaged in two syringes; one contains the Atrigel polymer system and the second contains leuprolide acetate powder; follow package instructions for mixing

Lupron Depot, Lupron Depot-Ped: Reconstitute only with diluent provided

Storage/Stability

Eligard: Store at 2°C to 8°C (36°F to 46°F). Allow to reach room temperature prior to using; once mixed, must be administered within 30 minutes.

Lupron Depot, Lupron Depot-Ped: Store at room temperature of 25°C (77°F); excursions permitted to 15°C to 30°C (59°F to 86°F). Upon reconstitution, the suspension does not contain a preservative and should be used immediately; discard if not used within 2 hours.

Leuprolide acetate 5 mg/mL solution: Store at 20°C to 25°C (68°F to 77°F); excursions permitted to 15°C to 30°C (59°F to 86°F). Protect from light and store vial in carton until use. Do not freeze.

Mechanism of Action Leuprolide, is an agonist of gonadotropin releasing hormone (GnRH). Acting as a potent inhibitor of gonadotropin secretion; continuous administration results in suppression of ovarian and testicular steroidogenesis due to decreased levels of LH and FSH with subsequent decrease in testosterone (male) and estrogen (female) levels. In males, testosterone levels are reduced to below castrate levels. Leuprolide may also have a direct inhibitory effect on the testes, and act by a different mechanism not directly related to reduction in serum testosterone.

Pharmacodynamics/Kinetics

Onset of action: Following transient increase, testosterone suppression occurs in ~2-4 weeks of continued therapy

Distribution: Males: V_d: 27 L

Protein binding: 43% to 49%

Metabolism: Major metabolite, pentapeptide (M-1)

Bioavailability: SubQ: 94%

Excretion: Urine (<5% as parent and major metabolite)

Dosing

Adult & Geriatric

Prostate cancer, advanced:

IM:

Lupron Depot 7.5 mg (monthly): 7.5 mg every month **or**

Lupron Depot 22.5 mg (3 month): 22.5 mg every 12 weeks **or**

Lupron Depot 30 mg (4 month): 30 mg every 16 weeks **or**

Lupron Depot 45 mg (6 month): 45 mg every 24 weeks

SubQ:

Eligard: 7.5 mg monthly **or** 22.5 mg every 3 months **or** 30 mg every 4 months **or** 45 mg every 6 months

Leuprolide acetate 5 mg/mL solution: 1 mg daily

Endometriosis: IM: Initial therapy may be with leuprolide alone or in combination with norethindrone; if re-treatment for an additional 6 months is necessary, concomitant norethindrone should be used. Re-treatment is not recommended for longer than one additional 6-month course.

◀

Lupron Depot: 3.75 mg every month for up to 6 months **or**

Lupron Depot-3 month: 11.25 mg every 3 months for up to 2 doses (6 months total duration of treatment)

Uterine leiomyomata (fibroids): IM (in combination with iron):

Lupron Depot: 3.75 mg every month for up to 3 months **or**

Lupron Depot-3 month: 11.25 mg as a single injection

Breast cancer, premenopausal ovarian ablation (off-label use):

Lupron Depot: 3.75 mg every 28 days for up to 24 months (Boccardo, 1999) **or**

Lupron Depot-3 month: 11.25 mg every 3 months for up to 24 months (Boccardo, 1999; Schmid, 2007)

Treatment of paraphilia/hypersexuality (off-label use; Guay, 2009; Reilly, 2000): Males: IM:

Note: May cause an initial increase in androgen concentrations which may be treated with an antiandrogen (eg, flutamide, cyproterone) for 1-2 months (Guay, 2009). Avoid use in patients with osteoporosis or active pituitary pathology.

SubQ: Test dose: 1 mg (observe for hypersensitivity)

Depot IM: 3.75-7.5 mg monthly

Pediatric

Precocious puberty (consider discontinuing by age 11 for females and by age 12 for males):

IM:

Lupron Depot-Ped (monthly):

≤25 kg: 7.5 mg every month

>25-37.5 kg: 11.25 mg every month

>37.5 kg: 15 mg every month

Titrate dose upward in increments of 3.75 mg every 4 weeks if down-regulation is not achieved.

Lupron Depot-Ped (3 month): 11.25 mg or 30 mg every 12 weeks

SubQ (leuprolide acetate 5 mg/mL solution): Initial: 50 mcg/kg/day; titrate dose upward by 10 mcg/kg/day if down-regulation is not achieved. **Note:** Higher mg/kg doses may be required in younger children.

Renal Impairment There are no dosage adjustments provided in the manufacturer's labeling (has not been studied).

Hepatic Impairment There are no dosage adjustments provided in the manufacturer's labeling (has not been studied).

Administration

Do not use concurrently a fractional dose of the 3-, 4-, or 6-month depot formulation, or a combination of doses of the monthly depot formulation or any depot formulation due to different release characteristics. Do not use a combination of syringes to achieve a particular dose.

IM: Lupron Depot, Lupron Depot-Ped: Administer as a single injection into the gluteal area, anterior thigh, or deltoid. Vary injection site periodically

SubQ:

Eligard: Vary injection site; choose site with adequate subcutaneous tissue (eg, upper or mid-abdomen, upper buttocks); avoid areas that may be compressed or rubbed (eg, belt or waistband)

Leuprolide acetate 5 mg/mL solution: Vary injection site; if an alternate syringe from the syringe provided is required, insulin syringes should be used

Hazardous agent; use appropriate precautions for handling and disposal (NIOSH 2014 [group 1]).

Monitoring Parameters Bone mineral density

Precocious puberty: GnRH testing (blood LH and FSH levels), measurement of height and bone age every 6-12 months, testosterone in males and estradiol in females (IM [monthly] and SubQ formulations): 1-2 months after initiation of therapy or with dosage change; IM [3 month] formulation: 2-3 months after initiation of therapy, month 6, and as clinically indicated thereafter); Tanner staging

Prostatic cancer: LH and FSH levels, serum testosterone (~4 weeks after initiation of therapy), PSA; weakness, paresthesias, and urinary tract obstruction in first few weeks of therapy. Screen for diabetes (blood glucose and HbA_{1c}) and cardiovascular risk prior to initiating and periodically during treatment. Consider periodic monitoring of electrocardiograms and electrolytes.

Treatment of paraphilia/hypersexuality (off-label use; Reilly, 2000): CBC (baseline, monthly for 4 months then every 6 months); serum testosterone (baseline, monthly for 4 months then every 6 months); serum LH (baseline and every 6 months), FSH (baseline), serum BUN and creatinine (baseline and every 6 months); bone density (baseline and yearly); ECG (baseline)

Test Interactions Interferes with pituitary gonadotropic and gonadal function tests during and up to 3 months after monthly administration of leuprolide therapy.

Additional Information

Eligard Atrigel: A nongelatin-based, biodegradable, polymer matrix

Oncology Comment: Guidelines from the American Society of Clinical Oncology (ASCO) for hormonal management of advanced prostate cancer which is androgen-sensitive (Loblaw, 2007) recommend either orchiectomy or luteinizing hormone-releasing hormone (LHRH) agonists as initial treatment for androgen deprivation.

Dosage Forms Excipient information presented when available (limited, particularly for generics); consult specific product labeling.

Kit, Injection, as acetate:

Generic: 1 mg/0.2 mL

Kit, Intramuscular, as acetate:

Lupron Depot: 7.5 mg, 45 mg [latex free; contains polysorbate 80]

Kit, Intramuscular, as acetate [preservative free]:

Lupron Depot: 3.75 mg, 11.25 mg, 22.5 mg, 30 mg [latex free; contains polysorbate 80]

Lupron Depot-Ped: 7.5 mg, 11.25 mg, 15 mg, 30 mg (Ped), 11.25 mg (Ped) [latex free; contains polysorbate 80]

Kit, Subcutaneous, as acetate:

Eligard: 7.5 mg, 22.5 mg, 30 mg, 45 mg

◆ **Leuprolide Acetate** *see* Leuprolide *on page 1051*

◆ **Leuprolide Acetate and Norethindrone Acetate** *see* Leuprolide and Norethindrone *on page 1054*

Leuprolide and Norethindrone
(loo PROE lide & nor eth IN drone)

Brand Names: US Lupaneta Pack

Index Terms Leuprolide Acetate and Norethindrone Acetate; Norethindrone and Leuprolide

Pharmacologic Category Gonadotropin Releasing Hormone Agonist; Progestin

Use Endometriosis: Management of initial and recurrent painful symptoms of endometriosis

Dosing

Adult Endometriosis: Females: **Note:** Treatment consists of an oral norethindrone tablet used in conjunction with an IM leuprolide injection. The initial therapy should be limited to 6 months duration; a single re-treatment of not more than 6 additional months may be administered if symptoms recur. Maximum total duration of therapy is 12 months.

1 month:

Injection: IM: Leuprolide 3.75 mg as a single dose administered by healthcare provider once every month for up to 6 doses (maximum initial therapy: 6 months; maximum cumulative therapy: 12 months)

Tablet: Oral: Norethindrone 5 mg once daily for up to 6 months (maximum initial therapy: 6 months; maximum cumulative therapy: 12 months)

3 month:

Injection: IM: Leuprolide 11.25 mg as a single dose administered by healthcare provider once every 3 months for up to 2 doses (maximum initial therapy: 6 months; maximum cumulative therapy: 12 months)

Tablet: Oral: Norethindrone 5 mg once daily for up to 6 months (maximum initial therapy: 6 months; maximum cumulative therapy: 12 months)

Geriatric Not for use in postmenopausal women

Pediatric Not for use prior to menarche

Renal Impairment No dosage adjustment provided in manufacturer's labeling (has not been studied).

Hepatic Impairment No dosage adjustment provided in manufacturer's labeling (has not been studied). Use is contraindicated with hepatic tumors or disease.

Additional Information Complete prescribing information should be consulted for additional detail.

Dosage Forms Excipient information presented when available (limited, particularly for generics); consult specific product labeling.

Kit, Combination:

Lupaneta Pack: 1-month kit: leuprolide acetate 3.75 mg depot suspension for injection (1) and norethindrone acetate 5 mg oral tablets (30), 3-month kit: leuprolide acetate 11.25 mg depot suspension for injection (1) and norethindrone acetate 5 mg oral tablets (90) [contains polysorbate 80]

◆ **Leuprorelin Acetate** *see* Leuprolide *on page 1051*

◆ **Leurocristine Sulfate** *see* VinCRIStine *on page 1897*

◆ **Leustatin** *see* Cladribine *on page 401*

◆ **Leustatin [DSC]** *see* Cladribine *on page 401*

Levalbuterol (leve al BYOO ter ole)

Brand Names: US Xopenex; Xopenex Concentrate; Xopenex HFA

Index Terms Levalbuterol Hydrochloride; Levalbuterol Tartrate; Levosalbutamol; R-albuterol

Pharmacologic Category Beta$_2$ Agonist

Use Bronchospasm: Treatment or prevention of bronchospasm in patients with reversible obstructive airway disease

Pregnancy Considerations Adverse events were not observed in animal reproduction studies. Congenital anomalies (cleft palate, limb defects) have rarely been reported following maternal use of racemic albuterol during pregnancy. Multiple medications were used in most cases, no specific pattern of defects has been reported, and no relationship to racemic albuterol has been established. Beta-agonists may interfere with uterine contractility if administered during labor.

Uncontrolled asthma is associated with adverse events on pregnancy (increased risk of perinatal mortality, preeclampsia, preterm birth, low birth weight infants). Other beta$_2$-receptor agonists are currently preferred for the treatment of asthma during pregnancy (NAEPP, 2005).

Breast-Feeding Considerations It is not known whether levalbuterol is excreted in human milk. According to the manufacturer, the decision to continue or discontinue breast-feeding during therapy should take into account the risk of exposure to the infant and the benefits of treatment to the mother. The use of beta$_2$-receptor agonists are not considered a contraindication to breast-feeding (NAEPP, 2005).

Contraindications Hypersensitivity to levalbuterol, albuterol, or any component of the formulation

Warnings/Precautions Optimize anti-inflammatory treatment before initiating maintenance treatment with levalbuterol. Do not use as a component of chronic therapy without an anti-inflammatory agent. Only the mildest form of asthma (Step 1 and/or exercise-induced) would not require concurrent use based upon asthma guidelines (NAEPP, 2007). If patients need more doses than usual, this may be a sign of asthma destabilization; patient should be reevaluated. Patient must be instructed to seek medical attention in cases where acute symptoms are not relieved or a previous level of response is diminished. The need to increase frequency of use may indicate deterioration of asthma, and treatment must not be delayed.

Use caution in patients with cardiovascular disease (arrhythmia or hypertension or HF), convulsive disorders, diabetes, glaucoma, hyperthyroidism, or hypokalemia. Beta-agonists may cause elevation in blood pressure, heart rate, and result in CNS stimulation/excitation. Beta$_2$-agonists may increase risk of arrhythmia, increase serum glucose, or decrease serum potassium.

Immediate hypersensitivity reactions (urticaria, angioedema, rash, bronchospasm, anaphylaxis, oropharyngeal edema) have been reported. Do not exceed recommended dose; serious adverse events including fatalities, have been associated with excessive use of inhaled sympathomimetics. Rarely, paradoxical bronchospasm may occur with use of inhaled bronchodilating agents; this should be distinguished from inadequate response. Potentially significant interactions may exist, requiring dose or frequency adjustment, additional monitoring, and/or selection of alternative therapy.

Adverse Reactions

>10%:
Endocrine & metabolic: Serum glucose increased, serum potassium decreased
Neuromuscular & skeletal: Tremor (≤7%)
Respiratory: Rhinitis (3% to 11%)
Miscellaneous: Viral infection (7% to 12%)

>2% to 10%:
Central nervous system: Headache (8% to 12%), nervousness (3% to 10%), dizziness (1% to 3%), anxiety (≤3%), migraine (≤3%), weakness (3%)
Cardiovascular: Tachycardia (~3%)
Dermatologic: Rash (≤8%)
Gastrointestinal: Diarrhea (2% to 6%), dyspepsia (1% to 3%)
Neuromuscular & skeletal: Leg cramps (≤3%)
Respiratory: Asthma (9%), pharyngitis (3% to 10%), cough (1% to 4%), sinusitis (1% to 4%), nasal edema (1% to 3%)
Miscellaneous: Flu-like syndrome (1% to 4%), accidental injury (≤3%)

<2% (Limited to important or life-threatening): Abnormal ECG, acne, anaphylaxis, angina, angioedema, arrhythmia, atrial fibrillation, chest pain, dysmenorrhea, epistaxis, extrasystole, gastroenteritis, gastroesophageal reflux disease, hematuria, hypertension, hypoesthesia (hand), hypokalemia, lymphadenopathy, metabolic acidosis, myalgia, nausea, oropharyngeal dryness, paresthesia, supraventricular arrhythmia, syncope, vaginal moniliasis

Note: Immediate hypersensitivity reactions have occurred (including angioedema, oropharyngeal edema, urticaria, and anaphylaxis).

Drug Interactions

Metabolism/Transport Effects None known.

Avoid Concomitant Use
Avoid concomitant use of Levalbuterol with any of the following: Beta-Blockers (Nonselective); Iobenguane I 123; Loxapine

Increased Effect/Toxicity
Levalbuterol may increase the levels/effects of: Atosiban; Doxofylline; Highest Risk QTc-Prolonging Agents; Loop Diuretics; Loxapine; Moderate Risk QTc-Prolonging Agents; Sympathomimetics; Thiazide Diuretics

The levels/effects of Levalbuterol may be increased by: AtoMOXetine; Cannabinoid-Containing Products; Linezolid; MAO Inhibitors; Mifepristone; Tedizolid; Tricyclic Antidepressants

Decreased Effect
Levalbuterol may decrease the levels/effects of: Iobenguane I 123

The levels/effects of Levalbuterol may be decreased by: Beta-Blockers (Beta1 Selective); Beta-Blockers (Nonselective); Betahistine

Preparation for Administration Concentrated solution should be diluted with 2.5 mL NS prior to use.

Storage/Stability

Aerosol: Store at 20°C to 25°C (68°F to 77°F); protect from freezing and direct sunlight. Store with mouthpiece down. Discard after 200 actuations (15 g canister) or 80 actuations (8.4 g canister). Do not puncture or incinerate.

Solution for nebulization: Store in protective foil pouch at 20°C to 25°C (68°F to 77°F). Protect from light and excessive heat. Vials should be used within 2 weeks after opening protective pouch. Use within 1 week and protect from light if removed from pouch. Vials of concentrated solution should be used immediately after removing from protective pouch.

Mechanism of Action Relaxes bronchial smooth muscle by action on beta$_2$-receptors with little effect on heart rate

Pharmacodynamics/Kinetics

Onset of action (as measured by a 15% increase in FEV$_1$):
Aerosol: 5.5 to 10.2 minutes
Peak effect: ~77 minutes
Nebulization: 10 to 17 minutes
Peak effect: 1.5 hours

Duration (as measured by a 15% increase in FEV$_1$):
Aerosol: 3 to 4 hours (up to 6 hours in some patients)
Nebulization: 5 to 6 hours (up to 8 hours in some patients)

Absorption: A portion of inhaled dose is absorbed to systemic circulation

Half-life elimination: 3.3 to 4 hours

Time to peak, serum:
Aerosol: Children: 0.8 hours, Adults: 0.5 hours
Nebulization: Children: 0.3 to 0.6 hours, Adults: 0.2 hours

Dosing

Adult

Bronchospasm:
Metered-dose inhaler: 2 inhalations (90 mcg) every 4 to 6 hours as needed; in some patients, 1 inhalation (45 mcg) every 4 hours may be sufficient (maximum: 2 inhalations every 4 hours)

Solution for nebulization: Initial: 0.63 mg 3 times daily at intervals of 6 to 8 hours; dosage may be increased to 1.25 mg 3 times daily with close monitoring for adverse effects (maximum: 1.25 mg 3 times daily)

Exacerbation of asthma (acute, severe) *(off-label; NAEPP, 2007):*
Metered-dose inhaler: 4 to 8 inhalations every 20 minutes for up to 4 hours, then every 1 to 4 hours as needed

Solution for nebulization: 1.25 to 2.5 mg every 20 minutes for 3 doses, then 1.25 to 5 mg every 1 to 4 hours as needed

Geriatric Refer to adult dosing, starting with lowest dose; titrate cautiously.

Pediatric

Bronchospasm:
Metered-dose inhaler: Children ≥4 years and Adolescents: 2 inhalations (90 mcg) every 4 to 6 hours as needed; in some patients, 1 inhalation (45 mcg) every 4 hours may be sufficient (maximum: 2 inhalations every 4 hours)

◄

Solution for nebulization:
Asthma Guidelines (off-label; NAEPP, 2007):
Children ≤4 years: 0.31 to 1.25 mg every 4 to 6 hours as needed
Children 5 to 11 years: 0.31 to 0.63 mg every 8 hours as needed
Manufacturer's labeling:
Children 6 to 11 years: 0.31 mg 3 times daily (maximum: 0.63 mg 3 times daily)
Children ≥12 years and Adolescents: Refer to adult dosing.

Exacerbation of asthma (acute, severe) *(off-label; NAEPP, 2007):*
Metered-dose inhaler:
Children <12 years: 4 to 8 inhalations every 20 minutes for 3 doses, then every 1 to 4 hours as needed
Children ≥12 years and Adolescents: Refer to adult dosing.
Solution for nebulization:
Children <12 years: 0.075 mg/kg (minimum: 1.25 mg) every 20 minutes for 3 doses, then 0.075 to 0.15 mg/kg (maximum: 5 mg) every 1 to 4 hours as needed
Children ≥12 years and Adolescents: Refer to adult dosing.

Renal Impairment There are no dosage adjustments provided in the manufacturer's labeling. Use with caution.

Hepatic Impairment There are no dosage adjustments provided in the manufacturer's labeling (has not been studied).

Administration Inhalation:
Metered-dose inhaler: Shake well before use, avoid spraying in the eyes; prime with 4 test sprays prior to first use or if inhaler has not been used for more than 3 days. Clean actuator (mouthpiece) weekly. A spacer device or valved holding chamber is recommended when using a metered-dose inhaler.
Solution for nebulization: Safety and efficacy were established when administered with the following nebulizers: PARI LC Jet, PARI LC Plus, as well as the following compressors: PARI Master, Dura-Neb 2000, and Dura-Neb 3000. Concentrated solution should be diluted prior to use. Blow-by administration is not recommended, use a mask device if patient unable to hold mouthpiece in mouth for administration.

Monitoring Parameters Asthma symptoms; FEV₁, peak flow, and/or other pulmonary function tests; heart rate, blood pressure, CNS stimulation; arterial blood gases (if condition warrants); serum potassium, serum glucose (in selected patients)

Dosage Forms Considerations Xopenex HFA 15 g canisters contain 200 inhalations and 8.4 g canisters contain 80 inhalations.

Dosage Forms Excipient information presented when available (limited, particularly for generics); consult specific product labeling. [DSC] = Discontinued product
Aerosol, Inhalation, as tartrate [strength expressed as base]:
Xopenex HFA: 45 mcg/actuation (15 g)
Nebulization Solution, Inhalation, as hydrochloride [strength expressed as base]:
Xopenex: 0.63 mg/3 mL (3 mL [DSC]); 1.25 mg/3 mL (3 mL [DSC])
Generic: 0.63 mg/3 mL (3 mL)
Nebulization Solution, Inhalation, as hydrochloride [strength expressed as base, preservative free]:
Xopenex: 0.31 mg/3 mL (3 mL); 0.63 mg/3 mL (3 mL); 1.25 mg/3 mL (3 mL)
Xopenex Concentrate: 1.25 mg/0.5 mL (1 ea, 30 ea)
Generic: 0.31 mg/3 mL (3 mL); 0.63 mg/3 mL (3 mL); 1.25 mg/3 mL (3 mL); 1.25 mg/0.5 mL (1 ea, 30 ea)

LevETIRAcetam (lee va tye RA se tam)

Brand Names: US Keppra; Keppra XR

Brand Names: Canada Abbott-Levetiracetam; ACT Levetiracetam; Apo-Levetiracetam; Auro-Levetiracetam; Dom-Levetiracetam; JAMP-Levetiracetam; Keppra; PHL-Levetiracetam; PMS-Levetiracetam; PRO-Levetiracetam; RAN-Levetiracetam

Index Terms Elepsia XR; Spritam

Pharmacologic Category Anticonvulsant, Miscellaneous

Use

Myoclonic seizures:
Immediate-release tablets/oral solution/orally disintegrating tablets: Adjunctive therapy in the treatment of myoclonic seizures in adults and adolescents 12 years and older with juvenile myoclonic epilepsy.
IV: Adjunctive therapy in the treatment of myoclonic seizures in adults and adolescents 12 years and older with juvenile myoclonic epilepsy.

Partial-onset seizures:
Immediate-release tablets/oral solution/orally disintegrating tablets: Adjunctive therapy in the treatment of partial-onset seizures in adults and children 1 month and older (Keppra) or 4 years and older and more than 20 kg (Spritam) with epilepsy.
Extended-release tablets: Adjunctive therapy in the treatment of partial-onset seizures in adults and adolescents 12 years and older with epilepsy.
IV: Adjunctive therapy in the treatment of partial-onset seizures in adults and children 1 month and older with epilepsy.

Primary generalized tonic-clonic seizures:
Immediate-release tablets/oral solution/orally disintegrating tablets: Adjunctive therapy in the treatment of primary generalized tonic-clonic seizures in adults and children 6 years and older with idiopathic generalized epilepsy.
IV: Adjunctive therapy in the treatment of primary generalized tonic-clonic seizures in adults and children 6 years and older with idiopathic generalized epilepsy.

Pregnancy Considerations Adverse effects were observed in animal reproduction studies. Levetiracetam crosses the placenta and can be detected in the newborn following delivery (Johannessen 2005; Lopez-Fraile 2009; Tomson 2007). An increase in the overall rate of major congenital malformations has not been observed following maternal use of levetiracetam. Available studies have not been large enough to determine if there is an increased risk of specific birth defects (Hernandez-Diaz 2012; Mawhinney 2013; Mølgaard-Nielsen 2011; Vajda 2012). In general, maternal polytherapy with antiepileptic drugs may increase the risk of congenital malformations; monotherapy with the lowest effective dose is recommended. Newborns of women taking antiepileptic medications may be at an increased risk of SGA and a 1 minute APGAR score <7 (Harden and Meader 2009). Plasma concentrations of levetiracetam gradually decrease during pregnancy, especially during the third trimester, due to physiologic changes which occur; patients should be monitored during pregnancy and postpartum.

A registry is available for women exposed to levetiracetam during pregnancy: Pregnant women may enroll themselves into the North American Antiepileptic Drug (AED) Pregnancy Registry (888-233-2334 or http://www.aedpregnancyregistry.org/).

Breast-Feeding Considerations Levetiracetam is excreted into breast milk in concentrations similar to those in the maternal plasma and can be detected in the plasma of a nursing infant (Johannessen 2005; Tomson 2007). Due to the potential for serious adverse reactions in the nursing infant, the manufacturer recommends a decision be made whether to discontinue nursing or to discontinue the drug, taking into account the importance of treatment to the mother.

Medication Guide Available Yes

Contraindications
There are no contraindications listed in the U.S. manufacturer's labeling.
Canadian labeling: Hypersensitivity to levetiracetam or any component of the formulation

Warnings/Precautions Antiepileptics are associated with an increased risk of suicidal behavior/thoughts with use (regardless of indication); patients should be monitored for signs/symptoms of depression, suicidal tendencies, and other unusual behavior changes during therapy and instructed to inform their health care provider immediately if symptoms occur.

Severe reactions, including toxic epidermal necrolysis (TEN) and Stevens-Johnson syndrome (SJS), have been reported in adults and children. Onset is usually within ~2 weeks of treatment initiation, but may be delayed (>4 months); recurrence following rechallenge has been reported. Levetiracetam should be discontinued if there are any signs of a hypersensitivity reaction or unspecified rash; if signs or symptoms suggest SJS or TEN, do not resume therapy and consider alternative treatment.

Psychosis, paranoia, hallucinations, and behavioral symptoms (including aggression, agitation, anger, anxiety, apathy, confusion, depersonalization, depression, emotional lability, hostility, hyperkinesias, irritability, nervousness, neurosis, and personality disorder) may occur; incidence may be increased in children. Dose reduction or discontinuation may be required. Levetiracetam should be withdrawn gradually, when possible, to minimize the potential of increased seizure frequency. Use caution with renal impairment; dosage adjustment may be necessary. In patients with ESRD requiring hemodialysis, it is recommended that immediate-release formulations be used instead of ER formulations. Elepsia XR is not recommended in patients with moderate or severe renal impairment (CrCl <50 mL/minute/1.73 m^2). May cause CNS depression (impaired coordination, ataxia, abnormal gait, fatigue, weakness, dizziness, and somnolence), which may impair physical or mental abilities. Symptoms occur most commonly during the first month of therapy. Patients must be cautioned about performing tasks that require mental alertness (eg, operating machinery or driving). Decreases in red blood cell counts, hemoglobin, hematocrit, white blood cell counts and neutrophils have been observed. Cases of eosinophilia, agranulocytosis, and lymphocytosis have also been reported. Isolated elevations in diastolic blood pressure measurements have been reported in children <4 years of age; however, no observable differences were noted in mean diastolic measurements of children receiving levetiracetam vs placebo. Similar effects have not been observed in older children and adults. Potentially significant drug-drug interactions may exist, requiring dose or frequency adjustment, additional monitoring, and/or selection of alternative therapy.

Adverse Reactions Incidences are for all indications and populations (adults and children) unless otherwise specified.

>10%:

Cardiovascular: Increased blood pressure (diastolic; infants and children: 17%)

Central nervous system: Behavioral problems (includes aggression, agitation, anger, anxiety, apathy, depersonalization, emotional lability, irritability, neurosis: children and adolescents: 7% to 38%; adults: 7% to 13%), headache (14% to 19%), drowsiness (8% to 15%; immediate release 4,000 mg/day, no titration: 45%; serious [patients hospitalized]: <1%), psychotic symptoms (infants and children: 17%; adults: 1%), irritability (infants, children and adolescents: 6% to12%), fatigue (10% to 11%)

Gastrointestinal: Vomiting (children and adolescents: 15%)

Infection: Infection (13%)

Neuromuscular & skeletal: Weakness (15%)

Respiratory: Nasopharyngitis (7% to 15%)

1% to 10%:

Central nervous system: Aggressive behavior (children and adolescents: 10%; adults: 1%), dizziness (5% to 9%), pain (7%), lethargy (children and adolescents: 6%), insomnia (children and adolescents: 5%), depression (3% to 5%), vertigo (3% to 5%), emotional lability (2% to 5%), agitation (children and adolescents: 4%), nervousness (4%), ataxia (partial-onset seizures: 3%; includes abnormal gait, incoordination, falling (children and adolescents: 3%), mood changes (children and adolescents: 3%), confusion (2% to 3%), amnesia (2%), anxiety (2%), hostility (children and adolescents: 2%), paresthesia (2%), sedation (children and adolescents: 2%)

Gastrointestinal: Upper abdominal pain (children and adolescents: 9%), decreased appetite (children and adolescents: 8%), diarrhea (6% to 8%), nausea (5%), anorexia (3% to 4%), constipation (children and adolescents: 3%), gastroenteritis (children and adolescents: 2%)

Hematologic & oncologic: Eosinophilia (children and adolescents: 9%), bruise (children and adolescents: 3%), decreased white blood cell count (3%), decreased neutrophils (2%)

Infection: Influenza (3% to 8%)

Neuromuscular & skeletal: Neck pain (2% to 8%), arthralgia (children and adolescents: 2%), joint sprain (children and adolescents: 2%)

Ophthalmic: Conjunctivitis (children and adolescents: 2%), diplopia (2%)

Otic: Otalgia (children and adolescents: 2%)

Respiratory: Nasal congestion (children and adolescents: 9%), cough (2% to 9%), pharyngolaryngeal pain (children and adolescents: 7%), pharyngitis (6% to 7%), rhinitis (2% to 4%), sinusitis (2%)

Miscellaneous: Head trauma (children and adolescents: 4%)

<1% (Limited to important or life-threatening): Agranulocytosis, decreased red blood cells, dyskinesia, DRESS syndrome, eczema, equilibrium disturbance, erythema multiforme, hepatic failure, hepatitis, hyperkinesia, hyponatremia, memory impairment, myalgia, myasthenia, pancreatitis, pancytopenia (with bone marrow suppression in some cases), panic attack, personality disorder, psychosis, Stevens-Johnson syndrome, suicidal tendencies, thrombocytopenia, toxic epidermal necrolysis

Drug Interactions

Metabolism/Transport Effects None known.

Avoid Concomitant Use

Avoid concomitant use of LevETIRAcetam with any of the following: Azelastine (Nasal); Orphenadrine; Paraldehyde; Thalidomide

Increased Effect/Toxicity

LevETIRAcetam may increase the levels/effects of: Alcohol (Ethyl); Azelastine (Nasal); Buprenorphine; CNS Depressants; Hydrocodone; Methotrimeprazine; Metyrosine; Mirtazapine; Orphenadrine; Paraldehyde; Pramipexole; ROPINIRole; Rotigotine; Selective Serotonin Reuptake Inhibitors; Suvorexant; Thalidomide; Zolpidem

The levels/effects of LevETIRAcetam may be increased by: Brimonidine (Topical); Cannabis; Doxylamine; Dronabinol; Droperidol; HydrOXYzine; Kava Kava; Magnesium Sulfate; Methotrimeprazine; Minocycline; Nabilone; Perampanel; Rufinamide; Sodium Oxybate; Tapentadol; Tetrahydrocannabinol

Decreased Effect

The levels/effects of LevETIRAcetam may be decreased by: Mefloquine; Mianserin; Orlistat

Food Interactions Food may delay, but does not affect the extent of absorption. Management: Administer without regard to meals.

Preparation for Administration Vials for injection: Must dilute dose in 100 mL of NS, LR, or D$_5$W. If a smaller volume is required (eg, pediatric patients) the amount of diluent should be calculated to not exceed a maximum levetiracetam concentration of 15 mg/mL of diluted solution.

Storage/Stability

Oral solution, tablets, orally disintegrating tablets: Store at 25°C (77°F); excursions permitted to 15°C to 30°C (59°F to 86°F).

Premixed solution for infusion: Store at 20°C to 25°C (68°F to 77°F).

Vials for injection: Store at 25°C (77°F); excursions permitted to 15°C to 30°C (59°F to 86°F). Admixed solution is stable for 24 hours in PVC bags kept at room temperature.

Mechanism of Action The precise mechanism by which levetiracetam exerts its antiepileptic effect is unknown. However, several studies have suggested the mechanism may involve one or more of the following central pharmacologic effects: inhibition of voltage-dependent N-type calcium channels; facilitation of GABA-ergic inhibitory transmission through displacement of negative modulators; reduction of delayed rectifier potassium current; and/or binding to synaptic proteins which modulate neurotransmitter release.

Pharmacodynamics/Kinetics

Absorption: Oral: Rapid and almost complete

Immediate release: Food decreases C$_{max}$ by 20% and delays time to C$_{max}$ (T$_{max}$) by 1.5 hours

Extended release: Intake of a high-fat, high-calorie breakfast before the administration results in a higher C$_{max}$ and longer median T$_{max}$; the median T$_{max}$ is 2 hours longer in the fed state (Elepsia XR: 3 to 4.5 hours longer in the fed state)

Distribution: V$_d$: Similar to total body water

Protein binding: <10%

Metabolism: Not extensive; primarily by enzymatic hydrolysis; forms metabolites (inactive)

Bioavailability: 100%

Half-life elimination: ~6 to 8 hours; extended release tablet: ~7 hours

Time to peak, plasma: Oral: Immediate release: ~1 hour; Extended release: ~4 hours

Excretion: Urine (66% as unchanged drug)

Dosing

Adult & Geriatric Note: When switching from oral to IV formulations, the total daily dose should be the same.

Myoclonic seizures:

Oral: Immediate release (tablets, oral solution, orally disintegrating tablets): Initial: 500 mg twice daily; may increase every 2 weeks by 500 mg/dose to the recommended dose of 1,500 mg twice daily. Efficacy of doses other than 3,000 mg/day has not been established.

IV: Initial: 500 mg twice daily; may increase every 2 weeks by 500 mg/dose to the recommended dose of 1,500 mg twice daily. Efficacy of doses other than 3,000 mg/day has not been established.

Partial onset seizures:

Oral:

Immediate release (tablets, oral solution, orally disintegrating tablets): Initial: 500 mg twice daily; may increase every 2 weeks by 500 mg/dose to the maximum recommended dose of 1,500 mg twice daily. Efficacy of doses >3,000 mg/day has not been established.

Extended release: Initial: 1,000 mg once daily; may increase every 2 weeks by 1,000 mg/day to a maximum of 3,000 mg once daily.

IV: Initial: 500 mg twice daily; may increase every 2 weeks by 500 mg/dose to a maximum of 1,500 mg twice daily. Doses >3,000 mg/day have been used in trials; however, there is no evidence of increased benefit.

Tonic-clonic seizures:

Oral: Immediate release (tablets, oral solution, orally disintegrating tablets): Initial: 500 mg twice daily; may increase every 2 weeks by 500 mg/dose to the recommended dose of 1,500 mg twice daily. Efficacy of doses <3,000 mg/day has not been established.

IV: Initial: 500 mg twice daily; may increase every 2 weeks by 500 mg/dose to the recommended dose of 1,500 mg twice daily. Efficacy of doses other than 3,000 mg/day has not been established.

Loading dose (off-label): Oral: Immediate release: Initial doses of 1,500 to 2,000 mg have been well-tolerated (Betts 2000; Koubeissi 2008), although the necessity of a loading dose has not been established

Status epilepticus (off-label use): IV: 1,000 to 3,000 mg administered at a rate of 2 to 5 mg/kg/minute (NCS [Brophy 2012])

Status epilepticus, refractory (off-label use): IV: 1,000 to 3,000 mg administered over 15 minutes (EFNS [Meierkord 2010]); 2,500 mg has been safely administered over 5 minutes in one report (Uges 2009). **Note:** Levetiracetam has not been well studied in comparison to other agents routinely used in this setting. EFNS recommends levetiracetam only for use in refractory *complex partial* status epilepticus; however, data suggests that levetiracetam may be beneficial in other forms of status epilepticus (EFNS [Meierkord 2010]; Knake 2008).

Pediatric Note: Use oral solution in children ≤20 kg; oral solution and immediate release or orally disintegrating tablets may be used in children >20 kg. When switching from oral to IV formulations, the total daily dose should be the same.

Myoclonic seizures:

Oral: Immediate release (tablets, oral solution, orally disintegrating tablets): Children ≥12 years and Adolescents: Refer to adult dosing.

IV: Children ≥12 years and Adolescents: Refer to adult dosing.

Partial onset seizures:

Oral:

Immediate release (tablets, oral solution):

Children 1 month to <6 months: Initial: 7 mg/kg/dose twice daily; may increase every 2 weeks by 7 mg/kg/dose to a recommended dose of 21 mg/kg/dose twice daily

Children 6 months to <4 years: Initial: 10 mg/kg/dose twice daily; may increase every 2 weeks by 10 mg/kg/dose to a recommended dose of 25 mg/kg/dose twice daily

Children and Adolescents 4 to <16 years: Initial: 10 mg/kg/dose twice daily; may increase every 2 weeks by 10 mg/kg/dose to a recommended dose of 30 mg/kg/dose twice daily (maximum daily dose: 3,000 mg/day)

Adolescents ≥16 years: Refer to adult dosing.

Alternate immediate-release fixed tablet dosing for partial onset seizures:

20 to 40 kg: Initial: 250 mg twice daily, increase every 2 weeks by 250 mg twice daily to the maximum recommended dose of 750 mg twice daily

>40 kg: Initial: 500 mg twice daily, increase every 2 weeks by 500 mg twice daily to the maximum recommended dose of 1,500 mg twice daily

Immediate release (orally disintegrating tablets):

Children ≥4 years and weighing 20 kg to 40 kg: Initial: 250 mg twice daily; may increase every 2 weeks by 250 mg/dose to the maximum recommended dose of 750 mg twice daily.

Children ≥4 years (weighing >40 kg) and Adolescents: Initial: 500 mg twice daily; may increase every 2 weeks by 500 mg/dose to the maximum recommended dose of 1,500 mg twice daily. Efficacy of doses >3,000 mg/day has not been established.

Extended release: Children ≥12 years and Adolescents: Refer to adult dosing.

IV:

Children 1 month to <6 months: Initial: 7 mg/kg twice daily; increase every 2 weeks by 7 mg/kg/dose to a recommended dose of 21 mg/kg twice daily. In clinical trials the average daily dose was 35 mg/kg/day. Efficacy of lower doses has not been established.

Children 6 months to <4 years: Initial: 10 mg/kg twice daily; increase every 2 weeks by 10 mg/kg/dose to a recommended dose of 25 mg/kg twice daily. If the patient cannot tolerate 50 mg/kg/day, reduce the daily dose. In clinical trials the average daily dose was 47 mg/kg/day.

Children and Adolescents 4 to <16 years: Initial: 10 mg/kg twice daily; increase every 2 weeks by 10 mg/kg/dose to the recommended dose of 30 mg/kg twice daily. If the patient cannot tolerate 60 mg/kg/day, reduce the daily dose. In clinical trials the average daily dose was 44 mg/kg/day and the maximum daily dose was 3,000 mg/day.

Adolescents ≥16 years: Refer to adult dosing.

Tonic-clonic seizures:

Oral:

Immediate release (tablets, oral solution):

Children and Adolescents 6 to <16 years: Initial: 10 mg/dose twice daily; may increase every 2 weeks by 10 mg/kg/dose to the recommended dose of 30 mg/kg twice daily. Efficacy of doses other than 60 mg/kg/day has not been established.

Adolescents ≥16 years: Refer to adult dosing.

Immediate release (orally disintegrating tablets):

Children ≥6 years and weighing 20 kg to 40 kg: Initial: 250 mg twice daily; may increase every 2 weeks by 250 mg/dose to the maximum recommended dose of 750 mg twice daily.

Children ≥6 years (weighing >40 kg) and Adolescents: Initial: 500 mg twice daily; may increase every 2 weeks by 500 mg/dose to the recommended dose of 1,500 mg twice daily. Efficacy of doses <3,000 mg/day has not been established.

IV:

Children and Adolescents 6 to <16 years: Initial: 10 mg/kg twice daily; increase every 2 weeks by 10 mg/kg/dose to the recommended dose of 30 mg/kg twice daily. Efficacy of doses lower than 60 mg/kg/day has not been established.

Adolescents ≥16 years: Refer to adult dosing.

Status epilepticus (off-label use): Infants, Children, and Adolescents: IV: 20 to 60 mg/kg administered at a rate of 2 to 5 mg/kg/minute (NCS [Brophy 2012])

Renal Impairment Adults:

Immediate release and IV formulations:

CrCl >80 mL/minute/1.73 m^2: 500 to 1,500 mg every 12 hours

CrCl 50 to 80 mL/minute/1.73 m^2: 500 to 1,000 mg every 12 hours

CrCl 30 to 50 mL/minute/1.73 m^2: 250 to 750 mg every 12 hours

CrCl <30 mL/minute/1.73 m^2: 250 to 500 mg every 12 hours

End-stage renal disease (ESRD) requiring hemodialysis: 500 to 1,000 mg every 24 hours; supplemental dose of 250 to 500 mg is recommended posthemodialysis

Peritoneal dialysis (PD): 500 to 1,000 mg every 24 hours (Aronoff 2007)

Continuous renal replacement therapy (CRRT): 250 to 750 mg every 12 hours (Aronoff 2007)

Extended release tablets:

Elepsia XR:

CrCl >80 mL/minute/1.73 m^2: 1,000 to 3,000 mg every 24 hours

CrCl 50 to 80 mL/minute/1.73 m^2: 1,000 to 2,000 mg every 24 hours

CrCl <50 mL/minute/1.73 m^2: Use not recommended.

Keppra XR and generic:
CrCl >80 mL/minute/1.73 m^2: 1,000 to 3,000 mg every 24 hours
CrCl 50 to 80 mL/minute/1.73 m^2: 1,000 to 2,000 mg every 24 hours
CrCl 30 to 50 mL/minute/1.73 m^2: 500 to 1,500 mg every 24 hours
CrCl <30 mL/minute/1.73 m^2: 500 to 1,000 mg every 24 hours
ESRD requiring hemodialysis: Use of immediate release formulation is recommended.

Hepatic Impairment
US labeling: No dosage adjustment necessary
Canadian labeling:
Mild-to-moderate impairment: No dosage adjustment necessary
Severe impairment: Reduce maintenance dose by 50% in patients who **also** have CrCl <60 mL/minute/1.73 m^2

Dietary Considerations May be taken without regard to meals.

Administration
IV: For IV use only; infuse over 15 minutes
Oral: Administer without regard to meals.
Orally disintegrating tablet: Remove from blister by peeling back the foil (do not push tablet through the foil). Place whole tablet on the tongue with dry hand (do not split), follow with a sip of liquid and allow to disintegrate (do not swallow intact tablet); tablet dissolves rapidly in saliva.
Oral solution: Administer with a calibrated measuring device (not a household teaspoon or tablespoon)
Tablet (immediate release and extended release): Only administer as whole tablet; do not crush, break or chew.

Monitoring Parameters CNS depression (impaired coordination, ataxia, abnormal gait, weakness, fatigue, dizziness, and somnolence); psychiatric and behavioral symptoms (aggression, agitation, anger, anxiety, apathy, confusion, depersonalization, depression, emotional lability, hostility, hyperkinesias, irritability, nervousness, neurosis, suicidal thoughts and personality disorder); diastolic blood pressure in children 1 month to <4 years of age

Product Availability
Elepsia XR: FDA approved March 2015; anticipated availability is currently unknown.
Spritam: FDA approved August 2015; availability anticipated in the first quarter of 2016. Spritam tablets are designed using ZipDose technology that allows rapid disintegration with a sip of liquid. Refer to the prescribing information for additional information.

Dosage Forms Excipient information presented when available (limited, particularly for generics); consult specific product labeling. [DSC] = Discontinued product
Solution, Intravenous:
Keppra: 500 mg/5 mL (5 mL)
Generic: 500 mg/100 mL (100 mL); 1000 mg/100 mL (100 mL); 1500 mg/100 mL (100 mL); 500 mg/5 mL (5 mL)
Solution, Intravenous [preservative free]:
Generic: 500 mg/5 mL (5 mL)
Solution, Oral:
Keppra: 100 mg/mL (473 mL) [gluten free, lactose free; contains acesulfame potassium, methylparaben, propylparaben; grape flavor]
Generic: 100 mg/mL (5 mL, 118 mL [DSC], 473 mL, 500 mL)
Tablet, Oral:
Keppra: 250 mg [scored; contains fd&c blue #2 (indigotine)]
Keppra: 500 mg [scored]
Keppra: 750 mg [scored; contains fd&c yellow #6 (sunset yellow)]
Keppra: 1000 mg [scored]
Generic: 250 mg, 500 mg, 750 mg, 1000 mg
Tablet Extended Release 24 Hour, Oral:
Keppra XR: 500 mg, 750 mg
Generic: 500 mg, 750 mg

◆ Levitra *see* Vardenafil *on page 1875*

Levobunolol (lee voe BYOO noe lole)

Brand Names: US Betagan
Brand Names: Canada Apo-Levobunolol®; Betagan®; Novo-Levobunolol; PMS-Levobunolol; Ratio-Levobunolol; Sandoz-Levobunolol
Index Terms *l*-Bunolol Hydrochloride; Levobunolol Hydrochloride
Pharmacologic Category Beta-Adrenergic Blocker, Nonselective; Ophthalmic Agent, Antiglaucoma
Use To lower intraocular pressure in chronic open-angle glaucoma or ocular hypertension

Dosing
Adult & Geriatric Glaucoma (open-angle, chronic), intraocular hypertension: Ophthalmic:
0.25% solution: Instill 1-2 drops into affected eye(s) twice daily
0.5% solution: Instill 1-2 drops into affected eye(s) once daily; may increase to 1 drop twice daily in patients with severe or uncontrolled glaucoma; Maximum dose: Doses >1 drop twice daily (0.5%) are generally not more effective.
Renal Impairment No dosage adjustment provided in manufacturer's labeling.
Hepatic Impairment No dosage adjustment provided in manufacturer's labeling.
Additional Information Complete prescribing information should be consulted for additional detail.
Dosage Forms Excipient information presented when available (limited, particularly for generics); consult specific product labeling.
Solution, Ophthalmic, as hydrochloride:
Betagan: 0.5% (5 mL, 10 mL, 15 mL)
Generic: 0.25% (5 mL, 10 mL); 0.5% (5 mL, 10 mL, 15 mL)

◆ Levobunolol Hydrochloride *see* Levobunolol *on page 1059*

◆ Levocarb CR (Can) *see* Carbidopa and Levodopa *on page 307*

Levocetirizine (LEE vo se TI ra zeen)

Brand Names: US Xyzal
Index Terms Levocetirizine Dihydrochloride
Pharmacologic Category Histamine H$_1$ Antagonist; Histamine H$_1$ Antagonist, Second Generation; Piperazine Derivative
Use Relief of symptoms of perennial and seasonal allergic rhinitis; treatment of skin manifestations (uncomplicated) of chronic idiopathic urticaria

Dosing
Adult
Allergic rhinitis, seasonal allergic rhinitis: Oral: 5 mg once daily (in the evening); some patients may experience relief of symptoms with 2.5 mg once daily.
Chronic idiopathic urticaria: Oral: 5 mg once daily (in the evening); some patients may experience relief of symptoms with 2.5 mg once daily. In one clinical trial, the titrated use of higher doses (up to 10 mg twice daily) in adults demonstrated clinical improvement (Staevska, 2010).
Geriatric Refer to adult dosing; dosing should begin at the lower end of the dosing range.
Pediatric
Perennial allergic rhinitis, chronic urticaria: Oral:
Children 6 months to 5 years: 1.25 mg once daily (in the evening); maximum: 1.25 mg
Children 6-11 years: 2.5 mg once daily (in the evening); maximum: 2.5 mg/day
Children ≥12 years: Refer to adult dosing.
Seasonal allergic rhinitis: Oral:
Children 2-5 years: 1.25 mg once daily (in the evening); maximum: 1.25 mg
Children 6-11 years: 2.5 mg once daily (in the evening); maximum: 2.5 mg/day
Children ≥12 years: Refer to adult dosing.
Renal Impairment
Children ≥12 and Adults:
CrCl 50-80 mL/minute: 2.5 mg once daily
CrCl 30-50 mL/minute: 2.5 mg once every other day
CrCl 10-30 mL/minute: 2.5 mg twice weekly (every 3 or 4 days)
CrCl <10 mL/minute, hemodialysis patients: Contraindicated
Children 6 months to 11 years with renal impairment: Contraindicated
Hepatic Impairment No adjustment required.
Additional Information Complete prescribing information should be consulted for additional detail.
Dosage Forms Excipient information presented when available (limited, particularly for generics); consult specific product labeling.
Solution, Oral, as dihydrochloride:
Xyzal: 2.5 mg/5 mL (148 mL) [contains methylparaben, propylparaben, saccharin]
Generic: 2.5 mg/5 mL (118 mL, 148 mL)
Tablet, Oral, as dihydrochloride:
Xyzal: 5 mg [scored]
Generic: 5 mg

◆ Levocetirizine Dihydrochloride *see* Levocetirizine *on page 1059*

◆ Levodopa and Carbidopa see Carbidopa and Levodopa on page 307

Levodopa, Carbidopa, and Entacapone
(lee voe DOE pa, kar bi DOE pa, & en TA ka pone)

Brand Names: US Stalevo
Brand Names: Canada Stalevo
Index Terms Carbidopa, Entacapone, and Levodopa; Carbidopa, Levodopa, and Entacapone; Entacapone, Carbidopa, and Levodopa
Pharmacologic Category Anti-Parkinson's Agent, COMT Inhibitor; Anti-Parkinson's Agent, Decarboxylase Inhibitor; Anti-Parkinson's Agent, Dopamine Precursor
Additional Appendix Information
Oral Dosages That Should Not Be Crushed on page 2003
Use Parkinson disease: Treatment of Parkinson disease.
Dosing
Adult & Geriatric Note: All strengths of Stalevo contain a carbidopa/levodopa ratio of 1:4 plus entacapone 200 mg.
Parkinson disease: Oral: Dose should be individualized based on therapeutic response; doses may be adjusted by changing strength or adjusting interval. Fractionated doses are not recommended and only 1 tablet should be given at each dosing interval; maximum daily dose: 8 tablets of Stalevo 50, 75, 100, 125, or 150, **or** 6 tablets of Stalevo 200. Patients receiving <70 to 100 mg of the carbidopa component may experience nausea and vomiting.
Patients previously treated with carbidopa/levodopa immediate release tablets (ratio of 1:4):
With current entacapone therapy: May switch directly to corresponding strength of combination tablet. No data available on transferring patients from controlled release preparations or products with a 1:10 ratio of carbidopa/levodopa.
Without entacapone therapy:
If current levodopa dose is >600 mg daily or history of moderate or severe dyskinesias: Levodopa dose reduction may be required when adding entacapone to therapy; therefore, titrate dose using individual products first (carbidopa/levodopa immediate release with a ratio of 1:4 plus entacapone 200 mg); then transfer to combination product once stabilized.
If current levodopa dose is <600 mg and without a history of dyskinesias: May transfer to corresponding dose of combination product; monitor, dose reduction of levodopa may be required.
Patients previously treated with benserazide/levodopa immediate release tablets [Canadian product]:
With current entacapone therapy: Prior to switching to combination product (carbidopa/levodopa/entacapone), withhold treatment for 1 night, then initiate (carbidopa/levodopa/entacapone) therapy the following morning at a dose that provides either an equivalent amount or ~5% to 10% more levodopa.
Renal Impairment
U.S. labeling: There are no dosage adjustments provided in manufacturer's labeling. Use of levodopa and carbidopa has not been studied in patients with renal impairment. Use with caution.
Canadian labeling: There are no dosage adjustments provided in the manufacturer's labeling; titrate dose cautiously in severe impairment. Use is contraindicated in uncompensated renal disease.
Hepatic Impairment
U.S. labeling: There are no dosage adjustments provided in manufacturer's labeling (has not been studied); use with caution in biliary obstruction or hepatic disease.
Canadian labeling: Use is contraindicated. There are no dosage adjustments provided in the manufacturer's labeling; titrate dose cautiously in severe impairment. Use is contraindicated in uncompensated hepatic disease.
Additional Information Complete prescribing information should be consulted for additional detail.
Dosage Forms Excipient information presented when available (limited, particularly for generics); consult specific product labeling.
Tablet:
Stalevo 50: Levodopa 50 mg, carbidopa 12.5 mg, and entacapone 200 mg
Stalevo 75: Levodopa 75 mg, carbidopa 18.75 mg, and entacapone 200 mg
Stalevo 100: Levodopa 100 mg, carbidopa 25 mg, and entacapone 200 mg
Stalevo 125: Levodopa 125 mg, carbidopa 31.25 mg, and entacapone 200 mg
Stalevo 150: Levodopa 150 mg, carbidopa 37.5 mg, and entacapone 200 mg

Stalevo 200: Levodopa 200 mg, carbidopa 50 mg, and entacapone 200 mg
Generic: Levodopa 50 mg, carbidopa 12.5 mg, and entacapone 200 mg; Levodopa 75 mg, carbidopa 18.75 mg, and entacapone 200 mg; Levodopa 100 mg, carbidopa 25 mg, and entacapone 200 mg; Levodopa 125 mg, carbidopa 31.25 mg, and entacapone 200 mg; Levodopa 150 mg, carbidopa 37.5 mg, and entacapone 200 mg; Levodopa 200 mg, carbidopa 50 mg, and entacapone 200 mg

◆ Levo-Dromoran see Levorphanol on page 1067

Levofloxacin (Systemic) (lee voe FLOKS a sin)

Brand Names: US Levaquin
Brand Names: Canada ACT Levofloxacin; APO-Levofloxacin; Levaquin; Levaquin in 5% Dextrose Injection; Mylan-Levofloxacin; PMS-Levofloxacin; Sandoz-Levofloxacin; Teva-Levofloxacin
Pharmacologic Category Antibiotic, Fluoroquinolone; Antibiotic, Respiratory Fluoroquinolone
Use Treatment of community-acquired pneumonia, including multidrug resistant strains of *S. pneumoniae* (MDRSP); nosocomial pneumonia; chronic bronchitis (acute bacterial exacerbation); acute bacterial rhinosinusitis (ABRS); prostatitis (chronic bacterial), urinary tract infection (uncomplicated or complicated); acute pyelonephritis; skin or skin structure infections (uncomplicated or complicated); reduce incidence or disease progression of inhalational anthrax (postexposure); prophylaxis and treatment of plague (pneumonic and septicemic) due to *Y. pestis*
Pregnancy Considerations Adverse events have been observed in some animal reproduction studies. Levofloxacin crosses the placenta and can be detected in the amniotic fluid and cord blood (Ozyüncü and Beksac 2010; Ozyüncü and Nemutl, 2010). Information specific to levofloxacin use during pregnancy is limited (Padberg 2014).
Breast-Feeding Considerations Based on data from a case report, small amounts of levofloxacin are excreted in breast milk (Cahill 2005). Due to the potential for serious adverse reactions in the nursing infant, the manufacturer recommends a decision be made whether to discontinue nursing or to discontinue the drug, taking into account the importance of treatment to the mother.
Medication Guide Available Yes
Contraindications Hypersensitivity to levofloxacin, any component of the formulation, or other quinolones

Canadian labeling: Additional contraindications (not in U.S. labeling): History of tendonitis or tendon rupture associated with use of any quinolone antimicrobial agent
Warnings/Precautions [U.S. Boxed Warning]: There have been reports of tendon inflammation and/or rupture with quinolone antibiotics; risk may be increased with concurrent corticosteroids, organ transplant recipients, and in patients >60 years of age. Rupture of the Achilles tendon sometimes requiring surgical repair has been reported most frequently; but other tendon sites (eg, rotator cuff, biceps) have also been reported. Strenuous physical activity, rheumatoid arthritis, and renal impairment may be an independent risk factor for tendonitis. Discontinue at first sign of tendon inflammation or pain. May occur even after discontinuation of therapy. Use with caution in patients with rheumatoid arthritis; may increase risk of tendon rupture. Safety of use in pediatric patients for >14 days of therapy has not been studied; increased incidence of musculoskeletal disorders (eg, arthralgia, tendon rupture) has been observed in children. CNS effects may occur (toxic psychoses, tremor, restlessness, anxiety, lightheadedness, paranoia, depression, nightmares, confusion, and very rarely hallucinations increased intracranial pressure (including pseudotumor cerebri, seizures, or toxic psychosis). Potential for seizures, although very rare, may be increased with concomitant NSAID therapy. Use with caution in individuals at risk of seizures, with known or suspected CNS disorders or renal dysfunction. Avoid excessive sunlight and take precautions to limit exposure (eg, loose fitting clothing, sunscreen); may cause moderate-to-severe phototoxicity reactions. Discontinue use if photosensitivity occurs.

Rare cases of torsade de pointes have been reported in patients receiving levofloxacin. Use caution in patients with known prolongation of QT interval, bradycardia, hypokalemia, hyponagesemia, or in those receiving concurrent therapy with Class Ia or Class III antiarrhythmics.

Severe hypersensitivity reactions, including anaphylaxis, have occurred with quinolone therapy. Reactions may present as typical allergic symptoms after a single dose, or may manifest as severe idiosyncratic dermatologic,

vascular, pulmonary, renal, hepatic, and/or hematologic events, usually after multiple doses. Prompt discontinuation of drug should occur if skin rash or other symptoms arise. Prolonged use may result in fungal or bacterial superinfection, including *C. difficile*-associated diarrhea (CDAD) and pseudomembranous colitis; CDAD has been observed >2 months postantibiotic treatment. Peripheral neuropathy has been reported (rare); may occur soon after initiation of therapy and may be irreversible; discontinue if symptoms of sensory or sensorimotor neuropathy occur. **[U.S. Boxed Warning]: Quinolones may exacerbate myasthenia gravis; avoid use (rare, potentially life-threatening weakness of respiratory muscles may occur).** Unrelated to hypersensitivity, severe hepatotoxicity (including acute hepatitis and fatalities) has been reported. Elderly patients may be at greater risk. Discontinue therapy immediately if signs and symptoms of hepatitis occur. Hemolytic reactions may (rarely) occur with quinolone use in patients with latent or actual G6PD deficiency.

Fluoroquinolones have been associated with the development of serious, and sometimes fatal, hypoglycemia, most often in elderly diabetics, but also in patients without diabetes. This occurred most frequently with gatifloxacin (no longer available systemically) but may occur at a lower frequency with other quinolones.

Benzyl alcohol and derivatives: Some dosage forms may contain benzyl alcohol; large amounts of benzyl alcohol (≥99 mg/kg/day) have been associated with a potentially fatal toxicity ("gasping syndrome") in neonates; the "gasping syndrome" consists of metabolic acidosis, respiratory distress, gasping respirations, CNS dysfunction (including convulsions, intracranial hemorrhage), hypotension, and cardiovascular collapse (AAP ["Inactive" 1997]; CDC, 1982); some data suggests that benzoate displaces bilirubin from protein binding sites (Ahlfors, 2001); avoid or use dosage forms containing benzyl alcohol with caution in neonates. See manufacturer's labeling.

Adverse Reactions
1% to 10%:
Cardiovascular: Chest pain (1%), edema (1%)
Central nervous system: Headache (6%), insomnia (4%), dizziness (3%)
Dermatologic: Skin rash (2%), pruritus (1%)
Gastrointestinal: Nausea (7%), diarrhea (5%), constipation (3%), abdominal pain (2%), dyspepsia (2%), vomiting (2%)
Genitourinary: Vaginitis (1%)
Infection: Candidiasis (1%)
Local: Injection site reaction (1%)
Respiratory: Dyspnea (1%)
<1% (Limited to important or life-threatening): Abnormal electroencephalogram, abnormal gait, acute renal failure, ageusia, agranulocytosis, anaphylactoid reaction, anemia (including aplastic and hemolytic), anorexia, anosmia, brain disease (rare), cardiac arrest, cardiac arrhythmia (including ventricular tachycardia/fibrillation and torsade de pointes), casts in urine, *Clostridium difficile*-associated diarrhea, confusion, convulsions, crystalluria, depression, elevation in serum levels of skeletal-muscle enzymes, eosinophilia, epistaxis, erythema multiforme, esophagitis, exacerbation of myasthenia gravis, gastritis (including gastroenteritis), glossitis, granulocytopenia, hallucination, hepatic failure (some fatal), hepatic insufficiency, hepatitis, hepatotoxicity (idiosyncratic) (Chalasani, 2014), hyperglycemia, hyperkalemia, hyperkinesias, hypersensitivity reaction (including anaphylaxis, angioedema, rash, pneumonitis, and serum sickness), hypertension, hypertonia, hypoacusis, hypoglycemia, hypotension, increased INR, increased intracranial pressure, increased serum alkaline phosphatase, increased serum transaminases, interstitial nephritis, intestinal obstruction, jaundice, leukocytosis, leukopenia, leukorrhea, lymphadenopathy, multiorgan failure, muscle injury, muscle spasm, pancreatitis, pancytopenia, paralysis, paranoia, peripheral neuropathy (may be irreversible), phlebitis, phototoxicity, prolonged prothrombin time, prolonged Q-T interval on ECG, pseudotumor cerebri, psychosis, renal function abnormality, rhabdomyolysis, rupture of tendon, scotoma, seizure, skeletal pain, skin photosensitivity, sleep disorder (including abnormal dreams and nightmares), Stevens-Johnson syndrome, stomatitis, suicidal ideation, syncope, tachycardia, tendonitis, toxic epidermal necrolysis, toxic psychosis, thrombocytopenia (including thrombotic thrombocytopenic purpura), uveitis, vasculitis (leukocytoclastic), vasodilatation, visual disturbances(including diplopia), voice disorder

Drug Interactions
Metabolism/Transport Effects None known.
Avoid Concomitant Use
Avoid concomitant use of Levofloxacin (Systemic) with any of the following: BCG (Intravesical); Highest Risk QTc-Prolonging Agents; Ivabradine; Mifepristone; Strontium Ranelate
Increased Effect/Toxicity
Levofloxacin (Systemic) may increase the levels/effects of: Blood Glucose Lowering Agents; Highest Risk QTc-Prolonging Agents; Moderate Risk QTc-Prolonging Agents; Porfimer; Tacrolimus (Systemic); Varenicline; Verteporfin; Vitamin K Antagonists

The levels/effects of Levofloxacin (Systemic) may be increased by: Corticosteroids (Systemic); Ivabradine; Mifepristone; Nonsteroidal Anti-Inflammatory Agents; Probenecid; QTc-Prolonging Agents (Indeterminate Risk and Risk Modifying)
Decreased Effect
Levofloxacin (Systemic) may decrease the levels/effects of: BCG (Intravesical); BCG Vaccine (Immunization); Blood Glucose Lowering Agents; Didanosine; Mycophenolate; Sodium Picosulfate; Typhoid Vaccine

The levels/effects of Levofloxacin (Systemic) may be decreased by: Antacids; Calcium Salts; Didanosine; Iron Salts; Lanthanum; Magnesium Salts; Multivitamins/Minerals (with ADEK, Folate, Iron); Multivitamins/Minerals (with AE, No Iron); Quinapril; Sevelamer; Strontium Ranelate; Sucralfate; Zinc Salts
Preparation for Administration Solution for injection: Single-use vials must be further diluted in compatible solution to a final concentration of 5 mg/mL prior to infusion.
Storage/Stability
Solution for injection:
Vial: Store at room temperature. Protect from light. Diluted solution (5 mg/mL) is stable for 72 hours when stored at room temperature; stable for 14 days when stored under refrigeration. When frozen, stable for 6 months; do not refreeze. Do not thaw in microwave or by bath immersion.
Premixed: Store at ≤25°C (77°F); do not freeze. Brief exposure to 40°C (104°F) does not affect product. Protect from light.
Tablet, oral solution: Store at 25°C (77°F); excursions permitted to 15°C to 30°C (59°F to 86°F).
Mechanism of Action As the S(-) enantiomer of the fluoroquinolone, ofloxacin, levofloxacin, inhibits DNA-gyrase in susceptible organisms thereby inhibits relaxation of supercoiled DNA and promotes breakage of DNA strands. DNA gyrase (topoisomerase II), is an essential bacterial enzyme that maintains the superhelical structure of DNA and is required for DNA replication and transcription, DNA repair, recombination, and transposition.
Pharmacodynamics/Kinetics
Absorption: Rapid and complete
Distribution: V_d: 74-112 L; CSF concentrations ~15% of serum levels; high concentrations are achieved in prostate, lung, and gynecological tissues, sinus, saliva
Protein binding: ~24% to 38%; primarily to albumin
Metabolism: Minimally hepatic
Bioavailability: ~99%
Half-life elimination: ~6-8 hours
Time to peak, serum: Oral: 1-2 hours
Excretion: Urine (~87% as unchanged drug, <5% as metabolites); feces (<4%)
Dosing
Adult & Geriatric Note: Sequential therapy (intravenous to oral) may be instituted based on prescriber's discretion.
Acute bacterial rhinosinusitis: Oral, IV:
Manufacturer's labeling: 750 mg every 24 hours for 5 days or 500 mg every 24 hours for 10-14 days
Alternate recommendations: 500 mg every 24 hours for 5-7 days (Chow 2012)
Anthrax (inhalational): Oral, IV: 500 mg every 24 hours for 60 days, beginning as soon as possible after exposure
Bite wounds (animal/human) (off-label use): Oral, IV:
Note: Recommended as an alternative therapy for human bite wound in patients hypersensitive to beta-lactams: 750 mg once daily; in combination with metronidazole or clindamycin (IDSA [Stevens 2014])
Chlamydia trachomatis **sexually transmitted infections (off-label use) (CDC 2010):** Oral: 500 mg every 24 hours for 7 days
Chronic bronchitis (acute bacterial exacerbation): Oral: 500 mg every 24 hours for 7 days; Canadian labeling (not in U.S. labeling) also includes a dosage regimen of 750 mg every 24 hours for 5 days

Diverticulitis, peritonitis (off-label use) (Solomkin, [IDSA] 2010): Oral, IV: 750 mg every 24 hours for 7-10 days; use adjunctive metronidazole therapy

Epididymitis, nongonococcal (off-label use) (CDC 2010): Oral: 500 mg once daily for 10 days

Gonococcal infection (off-label use) (CDC 2010): As of April 2007, the CDC no longer recommends the use of fluoroquinolones for the treatment of uncomplicated or more serious gonococcal disease, unless no other options exist and susceptibility can be confirmed via culture.

Intra-abdominal infection, complicated, community-acquired (in combination with metronidazole) (off-label use) (Solomkin, [IDSA] 2010): IV: 750 mg once daily for 4-7 days (provided source controlled). **Note:** Avoid using in settings where *E. coli* susceptibility to fluoroquinolones is <90%.

Pelvic inflammatory disease (off-label use) (CDC 2010): Oral: 500 mg once daily for 14 days with or without concomitant metronidazole; **Note:** The CDC recommends use as an alternative therapy only if standard parenteral cephalosporin therapy is not feasible and community prevalence of quinolone-resistant gonococcal organisms is low. Culture sensitivity must be confirmed.

Plague (prophylaxis and treatment): Oral, IV: 500 mg every 24 hours for 10-14 days, beginning as soon as possible after exposure. **Note:** Dose of 750 mg once daily may be considered if clinically warranted.

Pneumonia: Oral, IV:
Community-acquired (CAP): 500 mg every 24 hours for 7-14 days or 750 mg every 24 hours for 5 days (efficacy of 5-day regimen for MDRSP not established)
Healthcare-associated (HAP): 750 mg every 24 hours for 7-14 days

Prostatitis (chronic bacterial): Oral, IV: 500 mg every 24 hours for 28 days

Skin and skin structure infections: Oral, IV:
Uncomplicated: 500 mg every 24 hours for 7-10 days
Complicated: 750 mg every 24 hours for 7-14 days

Surgical (preoperative) prophylaxis (off-label use): IV: 500 mg within 120 minutes prior to surgical incision (Bratzler 2013)

Surgical site infections (intestinal or genitourinary tract; perineum or axilla) (off-label use): IV: 750 mg every 24 hours, in combination with metronidazole (IDSA [Stevens 2014])

Traveler's diarrhea (off-label use): Oral: 500 mg for one dose (Sanders 2007)

Tuberculosis, drug-resistant tuberculosis, or intolerance to first-line agents (off-label use): Oral: 500-1000 mg every 24 hours (CDC 2003)

Urethritis, nongonococcal (off-label use) (CDC 2010): Oral: 500 mg every 24 hours for 7 days

Urinary tract infections: Oral, IV:
Uncomplicated: 250 mg once daily for 3 days
Complicated, including pyelonephritis: 250 mg once daily for 10 days **or** 750 mg once daily for 5 days

Pediatric

Acute bacterial rhinosinusitis (off-label use): Oral, IV: 10-20 mg/kg/day divided every 12-24 hours for 10-14 days (maximum: 500 mg daily). **Note:** Recommended in patients with a type I penicillin allergy, after failure of initial therapy or in patients at risk for antibiotic resistance (eg, daycare attendance, age <2 years, recent hospitalization, antibiotic use within the past month) (Chow 2012).

Anthrax (inhalational, postexposure): Oral, IV
Infants ≥6 months and Children ≤50 kg: 8 mg/kg every 12 hours for 60 days (do not exceed 250 mg/dose), beginning as soon as possible after exposure
Children >50 kg: 500 mg every 24 hours for 60 days, beginning as soon as possible after exposure

Community-acquired pneumonia (CAP) (IDSA/PIDS 2011): Note: May consider addition of vancomycin or clindamycin to empiric therapy if community-acquired MRSA suspected; alternative to ceftriaxone or cefotaxime in patients not fully immunized for *H. influenzae* type b and *S. pneumoniae*, or significant local resistance to penicillin in invasive pneumococcal strains.
Infants ≥6 months and Children ≤4 years:
S. pneumoniae (MICs to penicillin ≤2.0 mcg/mL), mild infection or step-down therapy (alternative to amoxicillin): Oral: 8-10 mg/kg/dose every 12 hours (maximum: 750 mg daily)
S. pneumoniae (MICs to penicillin ≥4.0 mcg/mL):
Moderate-to-severe infection (alternative to ceftriaxone): IV: 8-10 mg/kg/dose every 12 hours (maximum: 750 mg daily)
Mild infection, step-down therapy (preferred): Oral: 8-10 mg/kg/dose every 12 hours (maximum: 750 mg daily)

H. influenzae, moderate-to-severe infection (alternative to ampicillin, ceftriaxone, or cefotaxime): IV: 8-10 mg/kg/dose every 12 hours (maximum: 750 mg daily)
Atypical pathogens, moderate-to-severe infection (alternative to azithromycin) or empiric treatment (alternative to azithromycin +/- beta-lactam; should be limited to macrolide allergic/intolerant patients): Oral, IV: 8-10 mg/kg/dose every 12 hours (maximum: 750 mg daily)
Children 5-16 years:
S. pneumoniae (MICs to penicillin ≤2.0 mcg/mL), mild infection or step-down therapy (alternative to amoxicillin): Oral: 8-10 mg/kg/dose once daily (maximum: 750 mg daily)
S. pneumoniae (MICs to penicillin ≥4.0 mcg/mL):
Moderate-to-severe infection (alternative to ceftriaxone): IV: 8-10 mg/kg/dose once daily (maximum: 750 mg daily)
Mild infection, step-down therapy (preferred): Oral: 8-10 mg/kg/dose once daily (maximum: 750 mg daily)
H. influenzae, moderate-to-severe infection (alternative to ampicillin, ceftriaxone, or cefotaxime): IV: 8-10 mg/kg/dose once daily (maximum: 750 mg daily)
Atypical pathogens:
Moderate-to-severe infection (alternative to azithromycin): Oral, IV: 8-10 mg/kg/dose once daily (maximum: 750 mg daily)
Mild infection, step-down therapy (alternative to azithromycin in adolescents with skeletal maturity): Oral: 500 mg once daily

Plague (prophylaxis and treatment): Infants ≥6 months and Children: Oral, IV:
≤50 kg: 8 mg/kg every 12 hours for 10-14 days (do not exceed 250 mg/dose), beginning as soon as possible after exposure
>50 kg: 500 mg every 24 hours for 10-14 days, beginning as soon as possible after exposure. **Note:** Dose of 750 mg once daily may be considered if clinically warranted.

Surgical (preoperative) prophylaxis (off-label use): Children ≥1 year: IV: 10 mg/kg within 120 minutes prior to surgical incision (maximum: 500 mg) (Bratzler 2013)

Renal Impairment IV, Oral:
Normal renal function dosing of 250 mg daily:
CrCl 20-49 mL/minute: No dosage adjustment required.
CrCl 10-19 mL/minute: Administer 250 mg every 48 hours (except in uncomplicated UTI, where no dosage adjustment is required).
Hemodialysis/chronic ambulatory peritoneal dialysis (CAPD): No information available.
Normal renal function dosing of 500 mg daily:
CrCl 20-49 mL/minute: Administer 500 mg initial dose, followed by 250 mg every 24 hours.
CrCl 10-19 mL/minute: Administer 500 mg initial dose, followed by 250 mg every 48 hours.
Hemodialysis/chronic ambulatory peritoneal dialysis (CAPD): Administer 500 mg initial dose, followed by 250 mg every 48 hours; supplemental doses are not required following either hemodialysis or CAPD
Normal renal function dosing of 750 mg daily:
CrCl 20-49 mL/minute: Administer 750 mg every 48 hours.
CrCl 10-19 mL/minute: Administer 750 mg initial dose, followed by 500 mg every 48 hours.
Hemodialysis/chronic ambulatory peritoneal dialysis (CAPD): Administer 750 mg initial dose, followed by 500 mg every 48 hours; supplemental doses are not required following either hemodialysis or CAPD.
Normal renal function dosing of 750 or 1000 mg daily (treatment of tuberculosis **only**) (CDC 2003): CrCl <30 mL/minute: Administer 750 or 1000 mg 3 times per week (in hemodialysis patients administer after dialysis on dialysis days).
Continuous renal replacement therapy (CRRT) (Heintz 2009; Trotman 2005): Drug clearance is highly dependent on the method of renal replacement, filter type, and flow rate. Appropriate dosing requires close monitoring of pharmacologic response, signs of adverse reactions due to drug accumulation, as well as drug concentrations in relation to target trough (if appropriate). The following are general recommendations only (based on dialysate flow/ultrafiltration rates of 1-2 L/hour and minimal residual renal function) and should not supersede clinical judgment:
CVVH: Loading dose of 500-750 mg followed by 250 mg every 24 hours.
CVVHD: Loading dose of 500-750 mg followed by 250-500 mg every 24 hours.

CVVHDF: Loading dose of 500-750 mg followed by 250-750 mg every 24 hours.

Hepatic Impairment IV, Oral: No dosage adjustment provided in manufacturer's labeling (has not been studied). However, dosage adjustment unlikely due to limited hepatic metabolism.

Dietary Considerations Tablets may be taken without regard to meals. Oral solution should be administered on an empty stomach (1 hour before or 2 hours after a meal). Take 2 hours before or 2 hours after multiple vitamins, antacids, or other products containing magnesium, aluminum, iron, or zinc.

Administration

Oral: Tablets may be administered without regard to meals. Oral solution should be administered 1 hour before or 2 hours after meals. Maintain adequate hydration of patient to prevent crystalluria.

IV: Infuse 250-500 mg IV solution over 60 minutes; infuse 750 mg IV solution over 90 minutes. Too rapid of infusion can lead to hypotension. Avoid administration through an intravenous line with a solution containing multivalent cations (eg, magnesium, calcium). Maintain adequate hydration of patient to prevent crystalluria or cylindruria.

Monitoring Parameters Evaluation of organ system functions (renal, hepatic, and hematopoietic) is recommended periodically during therapy; the possibility of crystalluria should be assessed; WBC and signs of infection

Test Interactions Some quinolones may produce a false-positive urine screening result for opioids using commercially-available immunoassay kits. This has been demonstrated most consistently for levofloxacin and ofloxacin, but other quinolones have shown cross-reactivity in certain assay kits. Confirmation of positive opioid screens by more specific methods should be considered.

Dosage Forms Excipient information presented when available (limited, particularly for generics); consult specific product labeling. [DSC] = Discontinued product

Solution, Intravenous [preservative free]:
Levaquin: 250 mg/50 mL (50 mL [DSC]); 500 mg/100 mL (100 mL [DSC]); 750 mg/150 mL (150 mL [DSC])
Generic: 250 mg/50 mL (50 mL); 500 mg/100 mL (100 mL); 750 mg/150 mL (150 mL); 25 mg/mL (20 mL, 30 mL)

Solution, Oral:
Levaquin: 25 mg/mL (480 mL [DSC]) [contains propylene glycol]
Generic: 25 mg/mL (10 mL, 20 mL, 100 mL, 200 mL, 480 mL)

Tablet, Oral:
Levaquin: 250 mg, 500 mg, 750 mg
Generic: 250 mg, 500 mg, 750 mg

Extemporaneous Preparations Note: Commercial oral solution is available (25 mg/mL)

A 50 mg/mL oral suspension may be made with tablets and a 1:1 mixture of Ora-Plus® and strawberry syrup NF. Crush six 500 mg levofloxacin tablets in a mortar and reduce to a fine powder. Add small portions of the vehicle and mix to a uniform paste; mix while adding the vehicle in incremental proportions to almost 60 mL; transfer to a graduated cylinder, rinse mortar with vehicle, and add quantity of vehicle sufficient to make 60 mL. Label "shake well". Stable for 57 days when stored in amber plastic prescription bottles at room temperature or refrigerated.

VandenBussche HL, Johnson CE, and Fontana EM, et al, "Stability of Levofloxacin in an Extemporaneously Compounded Oral Liquid," *Am J Health Syst Pharm*, 1999, 56(22):2316-8.

Levofloxacin (Ophthalmic) (lee voe FLOKS a sin)

Brand Names: US Quixin [DSC]
Index Terms Iquix; Quixin
Pharmacologic Category Antibiotic, Fluoroquinolone; Antibiotic, Ophthalmic
Use Bacterial conjunctivitis: Treatment of bacterial conjunctivitis caused by susceptible strains of *Corynebacterium* species, *Staphylococcus aureus*, *Staphylococcus epidermidis*, *Streptococcus pneumoniae*, *Streptococcus* groups C/F, *Streptococcus* group G, viridans group streptococci, *Acinetobacter lwoffii*, *Haemophilus influenzae*, and *Serratia marcescens*.

Dosing

Adult & Geriatric

Bacterial conjunctivitis: Ophthalmic:
Treatment day 1 and day 2: Instill 1 to 2 drops into affected eye(s) every 2 hours while awake, up to 8 times daily
Treatment day 3 through day 7: Instill 1 to 2 drops into affected eye(s) every 4 hours while awake, up to 4 times daily

Pediatric Bacterial conjunctivitis: Children ≥6 years and Adolescents: Refer to adult dosing.

Renal Impairment There are no dosage adjustments provided in the manufacturer's labeling. However, dosage adjustment unlikely due to low systemic absorption.

Hepatic Impairment There are no dosage adjustments provided in the manufacturer's labeling. However, dosage adjustment unlikely due to low systemic absorption.

Additional Information Complete prescribing information should be consulted for additional detail.

Dosage Forms Excipient information presented when available (limited, particularly for generics); consult specific product labeling. [DSC] = Discontinued product

Solution, Ophthalmic:
Quixin: 0.5% (5 mL [DSC]) [contains benzalkonium chloride]
Generic: 0.5% (5 mL)

◆ **Levo-folinic Acid** see LEVOleucovorin *on page 1063*

LEVOleucovorin (lee voe loo koe VOR in)

Brand Names: US Fusilev
Index Terms 6S-leucovorin; Calcium Levoleucovorin; L-leucovorin; Levo-folinic Acid; Levo-leucovorin; Levoleucovorin Calcium Pentahydrate; S-leucovorin
Pharmacologic Category Antidote; Chemotherapy Modulating Agent; Rescue Agent (Chemotherapy)

Use

Colorectal cancer, metastatic: Palliative treatment of advanced, metastatic colorectal cancer (in combination with fluorouracil)

High-dose methotrexate rescue: Rescue agent after high-dose methotrexate therapy in osteosarcoma treatment

Folic acid antagonist overdose: Antidote for impaired methotrexate elimination and for inadvertent overdosage of folic acid antagonists

Limitations of use: Levoleucovorin is not approved for pernicious anemia and megaloblastic anemias secondary to the lack of vitamin B_{12} (improper use may result in hematologic remission with progressive neurologic manifestations)

Dosing

Adult & Geriatric Note: Levoleucovorin, when substituted in place of leucovorin calcium (the racemic form), is dosed at **one-half** the usual dose of leucovorin calcium:

Colorectal cancer, metastatic: IV: The following regimens have been used (in combination with fluorouracil; fluorouracil doses may need to be adjusted for toxicity; no adjustment is required for the levoleucovorin dose): 100 mg/m²/day over at least 3 minutes (followed by fluorouracil 370 mg/m²/day) for 5 days every 4 weeks for 2 cycles, then every 4 to 5 weeks depending on recovery from toxicities, **or**
10 mg/m²/day (followed by fluorouracil 425 mg/m²/day) for 5 days every 4 weeks for 2 cycles, then every 4 to 5 weeks depending on recovery from toxicities, **or**
Alternative dosing: Levoleucovorin, when substituted in place of leucovorin calcium within a chemotherapy regimen, is dosed at **one-half** the usual dose of leucovorin calcium (Goldberg 1997; Kovoor 2009)

High-dose methotrexate rescue: IV: Usual dose: 7.5 mg (~5 mg/m²) every 6 hours for 10 doses, beginning 24 hours after the start of the methotrexate infusion (based on a methotrexate dose of 12 g/m² IV over 4 hours). Levoleucovorin (and hydration and urinary alkalinization) should be continued and/or adjusted until the methotrexate level is <0.05 micromolar (5 x 10⁻⁸ M) as follows:
Normal methotrexate elimination (serum methotrexate levels ~10 micromolar at 24 hours post administration, 1 micromolar at 48 hours and <0.2 micromolar at 72 hours post infusion): 7.5 mg IV every 6 hours for 10 doses
Delayed late methotrexate elimination (serum methotrexate levels >0.2 micromolar at 72 hours and >0.05 micromolar at 96 hours post methotrexate infusion): Continue 7.5 mg IV every 6 hours until methotrexate level is <0.05 micromolar
Delayed early methotrexate elimination and/or evidence of acute renal injury (serum methotrexate level ≥50 micromolar at 24 hours, ≥5 micromolar at 48 hours or a doubling or more of the serum creatinine level at 24 hours post methotrexate infusion): 75 mg IV every 3 hours until methotrexate level is <1 micromolar, followed by 7.5 mg IV every 3 hours until methotrexate level is <0.05 micromolar
Significant clinical toxicity in the presence of less severe abnormalities in methotrexate elimination or renal function (as described above): Extend levoleucovorin treatment for an additional 24 hours (total of 14 doses) in subsequent treatment cycles.

Delayed methotrexate elimination due to third space fluid accumulation, renal insufficiency, or inadequate hydration: May require higher levoleucovorin doses or prolonged administration.

Folic acid antagonist overdose: IV: 7.5 mg (~5 mg/m^2) every 6 hours; continue until the methotrexate level is <0.01 micromolar (10^{-8} M). Initiate treatment as soon as possible after methotrexate overdose. Increase the levoleucovorin dose to 50 mg/m^2 IV every 3 hours if the 24-hour serum creatinine has increased 50% over baseline, or if the 24 hour methotrexate level is >5 micromolar (5 x 10^{-6} M), or if the 48-hour methotrexate level is >0.9 micromolar (9 x 10^{-7} M); continue levoleucovorin until the methotrexate level is <0.01 micromolar (10^{-8} M). Hydration (aggressive) and urinary alkalinization (with sodium bicarbonate) should also be maintained.

Pediatric Note: Levoleucovorin, when substituted in place of leucovorin calcium (the racemic form), is dosed at **one-half** the usual dose of leucovorin calcium:
High-dose methotrexate rescue: Refer to adult dosing.
Folic acid antagonist overdose: Refer to adult dosing.

Renal Impairment There are no dosage adjustments provided in the manufacturer's labeling.

Hepatic Impairment There are no dosage adjustments provided in the manufacturer's labeling.

Additional Information Complete prescribing information should be consulted for additional detail.

Dosage Forms Excipient information presented when available (limited, particularly for generics); consult specific product labeling.
Solution, Intravenous:
Generic: 175 mg/17.5 mL (17.5 mL)
Solution, Intravenous [preservative free]:
Generic: 175 mg/17.5 mL (17.5 mL); 250 mg/25 mL (25 mL)
Solution Reconstituted, Intravenous:
Fusilev: 50 mg (1 ea)

Levonorgestrel (Systemic) (LEE voe nor jes trel)

Brand Names: US Aftera [OTC]; EContra EZ [OTC]; My Way [DSC]; My Way [OTC]; Next Choice One Dose [DSC]; Next Choice One Dose [OTC]; Opcicon One-Step [OTC]; Plan B; Plan B One-Step; Plan B One-Step [OTC]; Take Action [OTC]
Brand Names: Canada Next Choice; NorLevo; Option 2; Plan B
Index Terms LNg 20; Plan B
Pharmacologic Category Contraceptive; Progestin
Use Emergency contraception: Emergency contraception following unprotected intercourse or possible contraceptive failure

Pregnancy Considerations Use during pregnancy is contraindicated. When pregnancies have continued following levonorgestrel exposure, congenital anomalies have been infrequent. Significant adverse effects on infant growth and development have not been observed (limited data).

Levonorgestrel may be used as an emergency contraceptive in women with contraindications to conventional oral contraceptive agents (eg, cardiovascular disease, migraines, liver disease) (CDC 2010). A rapid return of fertility is expected following use for emergency contraception; routine contraceptive measures should be initiated or continued following use to ensure ongoing prevention of pregnancy. Any regular contraceptive method can be started immediately after levonorgestrel; however, a barrier method (or abstinence from sexual intercourse) is also needed for 7 days (ACOG 2015; CDC 2013).

Breast-Feeding Considerations Following maternal use of the oral tablets or intrauterine device, levonorgestrel is found in breast milk and can be detected in the serum of nursing infants (Shikary 1987). In general, no adverse effects on the growth or development if the infant have been observed. Isolated cases of decreased milk production have been reported. Women who are breast-feeding

may use levonorgestrel for emergency contraception (ACOG 2010).

Contraindications Known or suspected pregnancy
It is not known if the same contraindications associated with long-term progestin-only contraceptives apply to the levonorgestrel emergency contraception dose regimens. A history of ectopic pregnancy is not a contraindication to use in emergency contraception. Canadian labeling contraindicates use in patients with undiagnosed vaginal bleeding.
OTC labeling: When used for self-medication, do not use if you are already pregnant; do not use for regular birth control

Warnings/Precautions Hazardous agent: Use appropriate precautions for handling and disposal (NIOSH 2014 [group 2]).

Potentially significant drug-drug interactions may exist, requiring dose or frequency adjustment, additional monitoring, and/or selection of alternative therapy. Not for use prior to menarche or in postmenopausal women. Hormonal contraceptives do not protect against HIV infection or other sexually-transmitted diseases (CDC, 2013). The use of estrogens and/or progestins may change the results of some laboratory tests (eg, coagulation factors, lipids, glucose tolerance, binding proteins). The dose, route, and the specific estrogen/progestin influence these changes. In addition, personal risk factors (eg, cardiovascular disease, smoking, diabetes, age) also contribute to adverse events; use of specific products may be contraindicated in women with certain risk factors.

Spotting may occur following use; the possibility of pregnancy should be considered if menstruation is delayed for >7 days of the expected menstrual period. When used for emergency contraception, reduced efficacy has been reported in women ≥75 kg to 80 kg and lack of efficacy has been reported in women >80 kg; the Canadian labeling recommends that alternative emergency contraceptive methods be considered (Plan B Canadian product monograph 2014). The CDC recommends that obese women can generally use any type of contraceptive but suggests that levonorgestrel may be less efficacious in obese women compared to ulipristal acetate (CDC, 2013). Not intended to be used for routine contraception and is not effective in terminating an existing pregnancy. Barrier contraception is recommended immediately following emergency contraception and throughout the same menstrual cycle; efficacy of hormonal contraception may be decreased (ACOG, 2010; CDC, 2013).

A history of ectopic pregnancy is not a contraindication for use as an emergency contraceptive. The possibility of ectopic pregnancy should be considered in patients with lower abdominal pain, especially in association with missed periods or vaginal bleeding in women with prior amenorrhea. Ectopic pregnancy may result in loss of fertility.

Adverse Reactions Frequency not always defined.
>10%:
Central nervous system: Fatigue (13%)
Endocrine & metabolic: Hypermenorrhea (31%)
Gastrointestinal: Nausea (14%), abdominal pain (13%)
1% to 10%:
Central nervous system: Dizziness (10%), headache (10%)
Endocrine & metabolic: Suppressed menstruation (5%)
Genitourinary: Breast tenderness (8%)
Postmarketing and/or case reports: Dysmenorrhea

Drug Interactions
Metabolism/Transport Effects Substrate of CYP3A4 (major); **Note:** Assignment of Major/Minor substrate status based on clinically relevant drug interaction potential
Avoid Concomitant Use
Avoid concomitant use of Levonorgestrel (Systemic) with any of the following: Griseofulvin; Tranexamic Acid; Ulipristal
Increased Effect/Toxicity
Levonorgestrel (Systemic) may increase the levels/effects of: C1 inhibitors; Flibanserin; Selegiline; Thalidomide; Tranexamic Acid; Voriconazole

The levels/effects of Levonorgestrel (Systemic) may be increased by: Atazanavir; Boceprevir; Cobicistat; Herbs (Progestogenic Properties); Lopinavir; Metreleptin; Mifepristone; Osimertinib; Tipranavir; Voriconazole
Decreased Effect
Levonorgestrel (Systemic) may decrease the levels/effects of: Anticoagulants; Antidiabetic Agents; Fosamprenavir; Ulipristal; Vitamin K Antagonists

The levels/effects of Levonorgestrel (Systemic) may be decreased by: Acitretin; Aprepitant; Artemether; Barbiturates; Bexarotene (Systemic); Bile Acid Sequestrants;

Bosentan; CarBAMazepine; CloBAZam; CYP3A4 Inducers (Moderate); CYP3A4 Inducers (Strong); Dabrafenib; Darunavir; Deferasirox; Efavirenz; Enzalutamide; Eslicarbazepine; Exenatide; Felbamate; Fosamprenavir; Fosaprepitant; Fosphenytoin; Griseofulvin; LamoTRIgine; Lesinurad; Lopinavir; Lumacaftor; Metreleptin; Mifepristone; Mitotane; Mycophenolate; Nelfinavir; Nevirapine; Osimertinib; OXcarbazepine; Perampanel; Phenytoin; Primidone; Prucalopride; Retinoic Acid Derivatives; Rifamycin Derivatives; Saquinavir; Siltuximab; St Johns Wort; Sugammadex; Telaprevir; Tocilizumab; Topiramate; Ulipristal

Storage/Stability Store at 20°C to 25°C (68°F to 77°F).

Mechanism of Action Pregnancy may be prevented through several mechanisms: Thickening of cervical mucus, which inhibits sperm passage through the uterus and sperm survival; inhibition of ovulation, from a negative feedback mechanism on the hypothalamus, leading to reduced secretion of follicle stimulating hormone (FSH) and luteinizing hormone (LH); altering the endometrium, which may affect implantation. Levonorgestrel is not effective once the implantation process has begun.

Pharmacodynamics/Kinetics

Absorption: Oral: Rapid and complete

Distribution: V_d: ~1.8 L/kg

Protein binding: Highly bound to albumin (~50%) and sex hormone-binding globulin (~47%) (Fotherby, 1995)

Metabolism: Hepatic via CYP3A4; forms inactive metabolites

Half-life elimination: Oral: ~27 hours

Time to peak: Oral: ~2 hours

Excretion: Urine (45%); feces (32%)

Dosing

Adult

Emergency contraception: Females: Oral: May be used at any time during menstrual cycle:

Two-dose regimen: One 0.75 mg tablet as soon as possible within 72 hours of unprotected sexual intercourse; a second 0.75 mg tablet should be taken 12 hours after the first dose.

Single-dose regimen: One 1.5 mg tablet as soon as possible within 72 hours of unprotected sexual intercourse.

Note: Treatment for emergency contraception should begin as soon as possible; however, treatment is still moderately effective if used within 5 days and should be made available to women up to 5 days after unprotected or inadequately protected intercourse. When using the two-dose emergency contraceptive regimen, the second dose is equally effective if taken 12 to 24 hours after the first (ACOG, 2015).

Geriatric Not indicated for use in postmenopausal women.

Pediatric Emergency contraception: Females: Refer to adult dosing. Not for use prior to menarche.

Renal Impairment There are no dosage adjustments provided in the manufacturer's labeling (has not been studied).

Hepatic Impairment There are no dosage adjustments provided in the manufacturer's labeling (has not been studied).

Administration Oral: Consider repeating the dose if vomiting occurs within 2 hours. Hazardous agent; use appropriate precautions for handling and disposal (NIOSH 2014 [group 2]).

Monitoring Parameters Evaluate for pregnancy, spontaneous abortion or ectopic pregnancy if menses is delayed for ≥1 week following emergency contraception, or if lower abdominal pain or persistent irregular bleeding develops.

Dosage Forms Excipient information presented when available (limited, particularly for generics); consult specific product labeling. [DSC] = Discontinued product

Tablet, Oral:

Aftera: 1.5 mg

EContra EZ: 1.5 mg

My Way: 1.5 mg

Next Choice One Dose: 1.5 mg [contains fd&c yellow #6 (sunset yellow)]

Opcicon One-Step: 1.5 mg

Plan B: 0.75 mg

Plan B One-Step: 1.5 mg

Take Action: 1.5 mg

Generic: 0.75 mg [DSC], 1.5 mg

Levonorgestrel (IUD) (LEE voe nor jes trel)

Brand Names: US Liletta; Mirena; Skyla

Brand Names: Canada Jaydess; Mirena

Index Terms LNg 20

Pharmacologic Category Contraceptive; Progestin

Use

Contraception: Prevention of pregnancy

Heavy menstrual bleeding: Mirena: Treatment of heavy menstrual bleeding in women who also choose to use an IUD for contraception

Pregnancy Considerations Use during pregnancy is contraindicated. Pregnancy should be ruled out prior to insertion. Women who become pregnant with an IUD in place risk septic abortion; septicemia, septic shock and death may occur. Hysterectomy may be required in cases of severe infection. Removal of the device is recommended, however, removal or manipulation of IUD may result in pregnancy loss. In addition, miscarriage, sepsis, premature labor, and premature delivery may occur if pregnancy is continued with IUD in place. Following pregnancy, the manufacturer recommends that insertion of the device should not take place until at least 6 weeks postpartum or until involution of the uterus is complete. The device may be inserted immediately following a first trimester abortion. Following removal of the device, ~77% to 87% of women who wished to conceive became pregnant within 12 months.

Breast-Feeding Considerations Following maternal use of the oral tablets or intrauterine device, levonorgestrel is found in breast milk and can be detected in the serum of nursing infants (Shikary 1987). In general, no adverse effects on the growth or development if the infant have been observed. Isolated cases of decreased milk production have been reported. Risk of perforation with IUD is increased in lactating women. Following pregnancy, the manufacturer recommends that insertion of the device should not take place until 6 weeks postpartum or until involution of the uterus is complete.

Contraindications Hypersensitivity to levonorgestrel or any component of the formulation; pregnancy; postcoital contraception, congenital or acquired uterine anomaly including fibroids that distort the uterine cavity, acute pelvic inflammatory disease, history of pelvic inflammatory disease (unless there has been a subsequent intrauterine pregnancy), postpartum endometritis or infected abortion within past 3 months, known or suspected uterine or cervical neoplasia, untreated acute cervicitis or vaginitis (including bacterial vaginosis, known chlamydial or gonococcal cervical infection) or other lower genital tract infections until infection is controlled, conditions which increase susceptibility to pelvic infections, unremoved IUD, undiagnosed uterine bleeding, acute hepatic disease or hepatic tumors, current or history of known or suspected carcinoma of the breast or other progestin-sensitive cancer

Canadian labeling: Additional contraindications (not in US labeling): Bacterial endocarditis, known immunodeficiency, hematologic malignancy, recent trophoblastic disease while human chorionic gonadotropin (hCG) hormone levels are elevated; cervical dysplasia

Warnings/Precautions Hazardous agent: Use appropriate precautions for handling and disposal (NIOSH 2014 [group 2]).

Potentially significant drug-drug interactions may exist, requiring dose or frequency adjustment, additional monitoring, and/or selection of alternative therapy. Not for use prior to menarche or in postmenopausal women. Hormonal contraceptives do not protect against HIV infection or other sexually-transmitted diseases (CDC 2013). The use of estrogens and/or progestins may change the results of some laboratory tests (eg, coagulation factors, lipids, glucose tolerance, binding proteins). The dose, route, and the specific estrogen/progestin influences these changes. In addition, personal risk factors (eg, cardiovascular disease, smoking, diabetes, age) also contribute to adverse events; use of specific products may be contraindicated in women with certain risk factors.

Use of the IUD is contraindicated with acute hepatic disease or hepatic tumors. Use is not effective for emergency contraception. An increased incidence of group A streptococcal sepsis, pelvic inflammatory disease or endometritis (may be asymptomatic), and actinomycosis have been reported with use. Using aseptic technique during insertion is essential to minimizing the risk of serious infections. Pelvic inflammatory disease (PID) occurs more frequently within the first year and most often within the first month after insertion; risk is increased with multiple sexual partners. Women with a history of PID or endometritis are at increased risk. If PID is diagnosed, treat according to current guidelines and reassess in 24 to 48 hours. Remove IUD 24 to 48 hours after beginning antibiotics if there is no clinical improvement or if the woman wishes to discontinue use (CDC 2013). Women with symptomatic actinomycosis should have the device removed and be treated with the appropriate antibiotics. Use caution in patients with previous ectopic pregnancy.

Women with history of ectopic pregnancy were excluded from clinical trials; women with previous ectopic pregnancy, tubal surgery or pelvic infection may be at increased risk for ectopic pregnancy. The possibility of ectopic pregnancy should be considered in patients with lower abdominal pain, especially in association with missed periods or vaginal bleeding in women with prior amenorrhea. Ectopic pregnancy may result in loss of fertility. Menstrual bleeding patterns may be altered with use of the intrauterine device; the possibility of pregnancy should be considered if menstruation does not occur within 6 weeks of the previous menstrual period. If bleeding irregularities continue with prolonged use, appropriate diagnostic measures should be taken to rule out endometrial pathology. Partial or complete expulsion may occur. An increase in menstrual bleeding may indicate a partial or complete expulsion of the IUD. The risk of expulsion may be increased when the uterus is not completely involuted. If expulsion occurs, device may be replaced within 7 days of a menstrual period once pregnancy is ruled out.

Ovarian cysts may occur during IUD use; most are asymptomatic and disappear spontaneously within 2 to 3 months. Evaluate if persistent. Insertion should be done by a trained health care provider. Insertion may be associated with pain bleeding, vasovagal reactions (eg, diaphoresis, syncope, bradycardia); especially in patient's predisposed to these conditions, or seizure in an epileptic patients. Removal of the device may be necessary for the following reasons: pelvic infection, symptomatic genital actinomycosis, endometrial or cervical cancer, uterine or cervical perforation, and pregnancy. Use the intrauterine system with caution if any of the following conditions exist and consider removal if any of them arise during use: Coagulopathy or are receiving anticoagulants; marked increase of blood pressure; severe arterial disease, such as stroke or MI; exceptionally severe headache; and migraine, focal migraine with asymmetrical visual loss, or other symptoms indicating transient cerebral ischemia. In addition, consider removal if uterine or cervical malignancy or jaundice occurs during use. Bradycardia or syncope may occur during insertion or removal of the intrauterine device. Total or partial perforation may occur, most often during insertion, and may include penetration/embedment in the uterus or cervix; risk of perforation is increased in lactating women and when the uterus is fixed retroverted or not completely involuted during the postpartum period. Pregnancy may result if perforation occurs; delayed detection of perforation may result in migration of IUD outside of uterine cavity, adhesions, peritonitis, intestinal perforations, intestinal obstruction, abscesses, and erosion of adjacent viscera. Perforation may decrease effectiveness and lead to difficult removal. BMI had no effect on contraceptive efficacy in clinical trials using the Liletta intrauterine device for the long term prevention of pregnancy. Only under specific conditions may Skyla or Jaydess [Canadian product] be scanned safely by MRI. Image quality may also be impaired if area of interest is relatively close to the device. Liletta is MRI safe. Some products provide a consent form; a copy of the form and lot number should be kept with the woman's medical record.

The use of combination hormonal contraceptives has been associated with a slight increase in the frequency of breast cancer, however, studies are not consistent. Data is insufficient to determine if progestin only contraceptives also increase this risk. Use of the intrauterine device is contraindicated in patients who have or who have had breast cancer. Use with caution in patients with depression; may be more susceptible to recurrence of depressive episodes; consider removal of IUD for serious recurrence. Depression is not a contraindication to use of the intrauterine device (CDC 2010). The risk of cardiovascular side effects increases in women using estrogen containing combined hormonal contraceptives and who smoke cigarettes, especially those who are >35 years of age. This risk relative to progestin-only contraceptives has not been established. Women who take contraceptives should be advised not to smoke. Smoking is not a contraindication to use of the intrauterine device (CDC 2010). IUD may need removed (temporarily or permanently) if ophthalmic problems or discomfort occur, including issues related to contact lenses.

Adverse Reactions Frequency not always defined.
Cardiovascular: Edema (<5%), hypertension (<5%)
Central nervous system: Headache (≤12%), migraine (≤10%), depression (4% to 6%), mood changes (≤6%), nervousness (<5%), bipolar mood disorder (exacerbation), suicidal tendencies
Dermatologic: Acne vulgaris (6% to 15%), seborrhea (1% to 15%), alopecia (<5%), eczema (<5%), pruritus (<5%), skin rash (<5%), urticaria (<5%)

Endocrine & metabolic: Amenorrhea (≤38%, increases with duration of treatment), intermenstrual bleeding (23%), ovarian cyst (3% to 13%; includes symptomatic and asymptomatic cysts), hypermenorrhea (6% to 8%), decreased libido (<5%), hirsutism (<5%), weight gain (<5%), ectopic pregnancy
Gastrointestinal: Abdominal pain (≤23%), nausea (≤8%), vomiting (≤8%), abdominal distension (<5%)
Genitourinary: Abnormal uterine bleeding (52%), vulvovaginitis (≤20%), vaginal infection (14%), pelvic pain (≤23%), mastalgia (3% to 9%), dysmenorrhea (≤9%), breast tenderness (≤7%), dyspareunia (≤7%), vaginal discharge (4% to 5%), cervicitis (<5%; Papanicolaou smear normal/class II), endometritis (≤2%), uterine spasm (≤2%), genitourinary tract infection (upper, 1%), pelvic inflammatory disease
Hematologic & oncologic: Anemia (<5%)
Infection: Vulvovaginal infection (13%)
Neuromuscular & skeletal: Back pain (<5%)
Miscellaneous: Device expulsion (3% to 5%), ovarian follicle stimulation
<1% (Limited to important or life-threatening): Arterial thromboembolism, breakage of IUD, cerebrovascular accident, cervical perforation, hypersensitivity reaction, jaundice, malignant neoplasm of breast, myocardial infarction, sepsis (including Group A streptococcal sepsis), uterine hemorrhage, uterine perforation, venous thromboembolism

Drug Interactions
Metabolism/Transport Effects Substrate of CYP3A4 (minor); **Note:** Assignment of Major/Minor substrate status based on clinically relevant drug interaction potential

Avoid Concomitant Use
Avoid concomitant use of Levonorgestrel (IUD) with any of the following: Griseofulvin; Tranexamic Acid; Ulipristal

Increased Effect/Toxicity
Levonorgestrel (IUD) may increase the levels/effects of: C1 inhibitors; Flibanserin; Selegiline; Thalidomide; Tranexamic Acid; Voriconazole

The levels/effects of Levonorgestrel (IUD) may be increased by: Atazanavir; Boceprevir; Cobicistat; Herbs (Progestogenic Properties); Lopinavir; Metreleptin; Mifepristone; Tipranavir; Voriconazole

Decreased Effect
Levonorgestrel (IUD) may decrease the levels/effects of: Anticoagulants; Antidiabetic Agents; Fosamprenavir; Ulipristal; Vitamin K Antagonists

The levels/effects of Levonorgestrel (IUD) may be decreased by: Acitretin; Aprepitant; Artemether; Barbiturates; Bexarotene (Systemic); Bile Acid Sequestrants; Bosentan; CarBAMazepine; CloBAZam; Dabrafenib; Darunavir; Efavirenz; Eslicarbazepine; Felbamate; Fosamprenavir; Fosaprepitant; Fosphenytoin; Griseofulvin; LamoTRIgine; Lesinurad; Lopinavir; Lumacaftor; Metreleptin; Mifepristone; Mycophenolate; Nelfinavir; Nevirapine; OXcarbazepine; Perampanel; Phenytoin; Primidone; Prucalopride; Retinoic Acid Derivatives; Rifamycin Derivatives; Saquinavir; St Johns Wort; Sugammadex; Telaprevir; Topiramate; Ulipristal

Storage/Stability
Liletta: Store at 20°C to 25°C (68°F to 77°F); excursions permitted between 15°C to 30°C (59°F to 86°F). Protect from light.
Mirena, Skyla: Store at 25°C (77°F); excursions permitted between 15°C to 30°C (59°F to 86°F).

Mechanism of Action Pregnancy may be prevented through several mechanisms: Thickening of cervical mucus, which inhibits sperm passage through the uterus and sperm survival; inhibition of ovulation, from a negative feedback mechanism on the hypothalamus, leading to reduced secretion of follicle stimulating hormone (FSH) and luteinizing hormone (LH); altering the endometrium, which may affect implantation. Levonorgestrel is not effective once the implantation process has begun.

Pharmacodynamics/Kinetics
Duration: Mirena: Up to 5 years; Liletta, Skyla, Jaydess [Canadian product]: Up to 3 years
Distribution: V_d: ~1.8 L/kg
Protein binding: Highly bound to albumin (~50%) and sex hormone-binding globulin (~47%) (Fotherby 1995)
Metabolism: Hepatic via CYP3A4; forms inactive metabolites
Excretion: Urine (45%); feces (32%)

Dosing
Adult
Contraception: Females: Intrauterine device: To be inserted into uterine cavity.
Liletta: Releases levonorgestrel ~15.6 mcg per day over 3 years. Do not leave device in place for >3 years.

Skyla, Jaydess [Canadian product]: Releases levonorgestrel ~6 mcg per day over 3 years. Do not leave device in place for >3 years.

Mirena: Initially releases levonorgestrel 20 mcg per day, then rate subsequently decreases; mean release rate over 5 years is levonorgestrel ~14 mcg per day. Do not leave device in place for >5 years.

Initiation of therapy: The device may be inserted at any time in the menstrual cycle once it is determined that the woman is not pregnant. Back-up contraception is not needed if insertion is within 7 days of onset of menstruation or immediately after first trimester abortion or miscarriage. Following pregnancy or a second trimester abortion or miscarriage, insertion of the device should not take place until 6 weeks postpartum or until involution of the uterus is complete. Do not administer immediately following a septic abortion. If insertion occurs >7 days after menstrual bleeding started, an additional form of contraception must be used for 7 days unless the woman abstains from sexual intercourse (CDC 2013).

Continuation of contraception: When it is time to replace, device may be removed and replaced with a new device immediately, and at any time during menstrual cycle as long as the woman is not pregnant.

Switching from a different contraceptive to levonorgestrel IUD: The device may be inserted immediately if it is determined that the woman is not pregnant. Unless the woman abstains from sexual intercourse, a backup method of contraception is needed if it has been >7 days since menstrual bleeding has begun. When an additional method of contraception is needed, consider continuing the woman's previous method for 7 days after insertion (CDC 2013).

Switching from a copper IUD: If sexual intercourse occurred after the start of the current cycle, and it has been >5 days since bleeding began, consider administering an emergency contraceptive (CDC 2013).

Switching to Liletta from an injectable progestin contraceptive: May be inserted at any time. If inserted >13 weeks after the last injection, a barrier method of contraception should be used for 7 days.

Switching to Liletta from a contraceptive implant or another intrauterine system: May insert on the same day the implant or device is removed, any time during the menstrual cycle.

Switching to Liletta from a hormonal contraceptive (oral, transdermal, vaginal): May be inserted anytime, including hormone free interval. Continue previous method for 7 days or until the end of the current cycle.

Switching from levonorgestrel IUD to a different contraceptive: If the patient wishes to change to a different method of birth control, may remove the device during the first 7 days of menstrual cycle and begin the new therapy. If the device is not removed during the first 7 days of menstruation (or if the patient has irregular menstrual cycles or amenorrhea) and wants to start a different method of birth control, start the new method at least 7 days prior to device removal, otherwise, a back-up barrier contraceptive should be used for 7 days after the device is removed unless the woman abstains from vaginal intercourse.

Treatment of heavy menstrual bleeding: Females: Intrauterine device (Mirena): Refer to dosing for long-term prevention of pregnancy

Geriatric Not indicated for use in postmenopausal women.

Pediatric Long-term prevention of pregnancy, or treatment of heavy menstrual bleeding: Females: Refer to adult dosing. Not for use prior to menarche.

Renal Impairment There are no dosage adjustments provided in the manufacturer's labeling (has not been studied).

Hepatic Impairment There are no dosage adjustments provided in the manufacturer's labeling (has not been studied); use of the intrauterine device is contraindicated with active hepatic disease or hepatic tumor.

Administration Intrauterine device: Consider administering analgesics or cervical anesthetic prior to insertion. Insert into the uterine cavity to the recommended depth with the provided insertion device; should not be forced into the uterus. If necessary, dilate the cervical canal and consider using a paracervical block. Transvaginal ultrasound may be used to check proper placement. Remove if not positioned properly and insert a new IUD; do not reinsert removed IUD. Exclude perforation if exceptional pain or bleeding occurs after insertion.

Hazardous agent; use appropriate precautions for handling and disposal (NIOSH 2014 [group 2]).

Monitoring Parameters
Prior to insertion: Assessment of pregnancy status; cervical examination; weight (optional; BMI at baseline may be helpful to monitor changes during therapy); STD screen (unless already screened according to CDC STD Treatment guidelines) (CDC, 2013). Complete medical and social history which may determine conditions influencing an IUD use for contraception.

Following insertion: Transvaginal ultrasound may be used to check placement. Changes in health status (including medications) should be assessed at routine follow-up visits (CDC, 2013). Re-examine following insertion (4 to 6 weeks Liletta, Mirena, Skyla; 4 to 12 weeks Jaydess [Canadian product]) and then yearly or more frequently if necessary. Threads should be visible; if length of thread has changed device may have become displaced, broken, perforated the uterus, or expelled. Monitor for significant changes in menstrual bleeding during prolonged use, Pap smear, blood pressure, serum glucose in patients with diabetes. Patients presenting with lower abdominal pain should be evaluated for ovarian cysts and ectopic pregnancy. Signs of infection. Monitor for signs/symptoms of thromboembolism in women who require surgery with prolonged immobilization.

Reference Range
Liletta: Plasma concentrations range from a peak of 252 pg/mL (7 days following insertion) to 135 pg/mL (after 3 years)

Mirena: Plasma concentrations range from 150 to 200 pg/mL

Skyla, Jaydess [Canadian product]: Plasma concentrations range from a peak of 192 pg/mL (2 days following insertion) to 59 to 61 pg/mL (after 3 years)

Dosage Forms Considerations
Liletta 52 mg intrauterine device initially releases 18.6 mcg/day of levonorgestrel, then decreases to approximately 16.3 mcg/day at 1 year, 14.3 mcg/day at 2 years, and 12.6 mcg/day at 3 years.

Mirena 52 mg intrauterine device initially releases approximately 20 mcg/day of levonorgestrel, then decreases progressively to half that value after 5 years.

Skyla 13.5 mg intrauterine device initially releases approximately 14 mcg/day of levonorgestrel, then decreases to 10 mcg/day after 60 days, then further declines to 5 mcg/day after 3 years.

Dosage Forms Excipient information presented when available (limited, particularly for generics); consult specific product labeling.
Intrauterine Device, Intrauterine:
Liletta: 18.6 mcg/day
Mirena: 20 mcg/24 hr
Skyla: 13.5 mg

Dosage Forms: Canada
Note: Also refer to Dosage Forms.
Excipient information presented when available (limited, particularly for generics); consult specific product labeling.
Intrauterine Device, Intrauterine: Jaydess: 13.5 mg

◆ **Levonorgestrel and Estradiol** *see* Estradiol and Levonorgestrel *on page 686*

◆ **Levonorgestrel and Ethinyl Estradiol** *see* Ethinyl Estradiol and Levonorgestrel *on page 703*

◆ **Levophed** *see* Norepinephrine *on page 1297*

◆ **Levophed® (Can)** *see* Norepinephrine *on page 1297*

◆ **Levora** *see* Ethinyl Estradiol and Levonorgestrel *on page 703*

Levorphanol (lee VOR fa nole)

Index Terms Levo-Dromoran; Levorphan Tartrate; Levorphanol Tartrate
Pharmacologic Category Analgesic, Opioid
Additional Appendix Information
Opioid Conversion Table and Morphine Equivalent Dose Table *on page 1955*
Use Pain: Management of moderate to severe pain where an opioid analgesic is appropriate
Dosing
Adult Note: These are guidelines and do not represent the maximum doses that may be required in all patients. Doses should be titrated to pain relief/prevention.

Acute pain (moderate to severe): Oral: Initial: Opioid-naive: 2 mg every 6 to 8 hours as needed; may increase to 3 mg every 6 to 8 hours if needed (maximum: 12 mg per 24 hours); higher doses may be appropriate in opioid tolerant patients. Reduce initial dose by ≥50% in patients with conditions affecting respiratory reserve or with coadministration with other drugs affecting the respiratory center.

Note: The American Pain Society recommends an initial dose of 2 to 4 mg for severe pain in adults (APS 2008)

Chronic pain: Patients taking opioids chronically may become tolerant and require doses higher than the usual dosage range to maintain the desired effect. Tolerance can be managed by appropriate dose titration. **There is no optimal or maximal dose for levorphanol in chronic pain. The appropriate dose is one that relieves pain throughout its dosing interval without causing unmanageable side effects.**

Geriatric Reduce initial doses by 50% or more. Refer to adult dosing.

Renal Impairment There are no specific dosage adjustments provided in the manufacturer's labeling; use with caution; reduce initial dose in patients with severe renal impairment.

Hepatic Impairment There are no specific dosage adjustments provided in the manufacturer's labeling; use with caution; reduce initial dose in patients with severe hepatic impairment.

Additional Information Complete prescribing information should be consulted for additional detail.

Dosage Forms Excipient information presented when available (limited, particularly for generics); consult specific product labeling.
Tablet, Oral, as tartrate:
Generic: 2 mg

Controlled Substance C-II

- ◆ Levorphanol Tartrate *see* Levorphanol *on page 1067*
- ◆ Levorphan Tartrate *see* Levorphanol *on page 1067*
- ◆ Levosalbutamol *see* Levalbuterol *on page 1055*
- ◆ Levothroid *see* Levothyroxine *on page 1068*
- ◆ Levothroid [DSC] *see* Levothyroxine *on page 1068*

Levothyroxine (lee voe thye ROKS een)

Brand Names: US Levothroid [DSC]; Levoxyl; Synthroid; Tirosint; Unithroid; Unithroid Direct
Brand Names: Canada Eltroxin; Levothyroxine Sodium; Levothyroxine Sodium for Injection; Synthroid
Index Terms *L*-Thyroxine Sodium; Levothroid; Levothyroxine Sodium; T_4
Pharmacologic Category Thyroid Product
Use

Oral:
Hypothyroidism: Replacement or supplemental therapy in congenital or acquired hypothyroidism of any etiology, except transient hypothyroidism during the recovery phase of subacute thyroiditis. Specific indications include primary (thyroidal), secondary (pituitary), and tertiary (hypothalamic) hypothyroidism and subclinical hypothyroidism. Primary hypothyroidism may result from functional deficiency, primary atrophy, partial or total congenital absence of the thyroid gland, or from the effects of surgery, radiation, or drugs, with or without the presence of goiter. **Note:** ATA/AACE guidelines recommend levothyroxine monotherapy as the preferred thyroid preparation for the treatment of hypothyroidism (ATA/AACE [Garber 2012]).
Pituitary thyrotropin-stimulating hormone suppression: Prevention or treatment of various types of euthyroid goiters, including thyroid nodules, subacute or chronic lymphocytic thyroiditis (Hashimoto thyroiditis), multinodular goiter and as an adjunct to surgery and radioiodine therapy in the management of thyrotropin-dependent well-differentiated thyroid cancer.

Injectable:
US labeling: Treatment of myxedema coma
Canadian labeling: Refer to oral indications; IV may be substituted for oral when rapid repletion is required; IV or IM may be used when oral administration is not possible.

Pregnancy Considerations Endogenous thyroid hormones minimally cross the placenta; the fetal thyroid becomes active around the end of the first trimester. Levothyroxine has not been shown to increase the risk of congenital abnormalities.

Uncontrolled maternal hypothyroidism may result in adverse neonatal outcomes (eg, premature birth, low birth weight, and respiratory distress) and adverse maternal outcomes (eg, spontaneous abortion, pre-eclampsia, stillbirth, and premature delivery). To prevent adverse events, normal maternal thyroid function should be maintained prior to conception and throughout pregnancy. TSH concentrations should be monitored every 4 weeks during the first half of pregnancy, at least once between weeks 26 and 32, and ~6 weeks postpartum. Levothyroxine is considered the treatment of choice for the control of hypothyroidism during pregnancy. Due to alterations of endogenous maternal thyroid hormones, the levothyroxine dose may need to be increased during pregnancy and the dose usually needs to be decreased after delivery (Stagnaro-Green 2011).

Breast-Feeding Considerations Endogenous thyroid hormones are minimally found in breast milk. The manufacturer recommends that caution be used if administered to a nursing woman.

The amount of endogenous thyroxine found in breast milk does not influence infant plasma thyroid values (van Wassenaer 2002). Levothyroxine was not found to cause adverse events to the infant or mother during breastfeeding (Ito 1993). Adequate thyroid hormone concentrations are required to maintain normal lactation. Appropriate levothyroxine doses should be continued during breastfeeding.

Contraindications
Hypersensitivity to levothyroxine sodium or any component of the formulation; acute MI; untreated subclinical (suppressed serum TSH level with normal T3 and T4 levels) or overt thyrotoxicosis of any etiology; uncorrected adrenal insufficiency.
Capsule: Additional contraindication: Inability to swallow capsules (eg, infants, small children)
Injection:
US labeling: There are no contraindications listed in the manufacturer's labeling when used for labeled indication (treatment of myxedema coma); consider contraindications for oral therapy if using as a temporary substitute for oral treatment (off-label use) in patients with chronic hypothyroidism.
Canadian labeling: Hypersensitivity to levothyroxine sodium or any component of the formulation; acute MI; thyrotoxicosis of any etiology; uncorrected adrenal insufficiency.

Warnings/Precautions [US Boxed Warning]: Thyroid supplements are ineffective and potentially toxic when used for the treatment of obesity or for weight reduction, especially in euthyroid patients. High doses may produce serious or even life-threatening toxic effects particularly when used with anorectic drugs (eg, sympathomimetic amines). Levothyroxine, either alone or with other concomitant therapeutic agents, should not be used for the treatment of obesity or for weight loss. Routine use of T_4 for TSH suppression is not recommended in patients with benign thyroid nodules. In patients deemed appropriate candidates, treatment should never be fully suppressive (TSH <0.1 milliunits/L). Use with caution and reduce dosage in patients with cardiovascular disease, including heart failure; patients with developing or worsening cardiac symptoms should have their dose reduced or therapy withheld for 7 days then resumed at a reduced dose. Use cautiously in the elderly; suppressed TSH levels may increase risk of atrial fibrillation and mortality secondary to cardiovascular disease (Gharib 2010; Parle 2001). Increase dose slowly in the elderly and monitor for signs/symptoms of angina (ATA/AACE [Garber 2012]). Patients with adrenal insufficiency, myxedema, diabetes mellitus and insipidus may have symptoms exaggerated or aggravated. Use is contraindicated in patients with uncorrected adrenal insufficiency. Treatment with glucocorticoids should precede levothyroxine therapy in patients with adrenal insufficiency (ATA/AACE [Garber 2012]). Chronic hypothyroidism predisposes patients to coronary artery disease. Long-term therapy can decrease bone mineral density. Levoxyl may rapidly swell and disintegrate causing choking or gagging (should be administered with a full glass of water); use caution in patients with dysphagia or other swallowing disorders. Potentially significant drug-drug interactions may exist, requiring dose or frequency adjustment, additional monitoring, and/or selection of alternative therapy.

Adverse Reactions Frequency not defined.
Cardiovascular: Angina pectoris, cardiac arrest, cardiac arrhythmia, congestive heart failure, flushing, hypertension, increased pulse, myocardial infarction, palpitations, tachycardia
Central nervous system: Anxiety, choking sensation (Levoxyl), emotional lability, fatigue, headache, heat intolerance, hyperactivity, insomnia, irritability, myasthenia, nervousness, pseudotumor cerebri (children), seizure (rare)
Dermatologic: Alopecia, diaphoresis
Endocrine & metabolic: Menstrual disease, weight loss
Gastrointestinal: Abdominal cramps, diarrhea, dysphagia (Levoxyl), gag reflex (Levoxyl), increased appetite, vomiting
Genitourinary: Infertility
Hepatic: Increased liver enzymes

Hypersensitivity: Hypersensitivity (to inactive ingredients; symptoms include urticaria, pruritus, rash, flushing, angioedema, GI symptoms, fever, arthralgia, serum sickness, wheezing)

Neuromuscular & skeletal: Decreased bone mineral density, slipped capital femoral epiphysis (children), tremor

Respiratory: Dyspnea

Miscellaneous: Fever

Drug Interactions

Metabolism/Transport Effects None known.

Avoid Concomitant Use

Avoid concomitant use of Levothyroxine with any of the following: Sodium Iodide I131; Sucroferric Oxyhydroxide

Increased Effect/Toxicity

Levothyroxine may increase the levels/effects of: Tricyclic Antidepressants; Vitamin K Antagonists

The levels/effects of Levothyroxine may be increased by: Piracetam

Decreased Effect

Levothyroxine may decrease the levels/effects of: Sodium Iodide I131; Theophylline Derivatives

The levels/effects of Levothyroxine may be decreased by: Aluminum Hydroxide; Bile Acid Sequestrants; Calcium Polystyrene Sulfonate; Calcium Salts; CarBAMazepine; Ciprofloxacin (Systemic); Estrogen Derivatives; Fosphenytoin; Iron Salts; Lanthanum; Magnesium Salts; Multivitamins/Minerals (with ADEK, Folate, Iron); Orlistat; Phenytoin; Polaprezinc; Raloxifene; Rifampin; Selective Serotonin Reuptake Inhibitors; Sevelamer; Sodium Polystyrene Sulfonate; Sucralfate; Sucroferric Oxyhydroxide

Food Interactions Taking levothyroxine with enteral nutrition may cause reduced bioavailability and may lower serum thyroxine levels leading to signs or symptoms of hypothyroidism. Soybean flour (infant formula), soy, grapefruit juice, espresso coffee, cottonseed meal, walnuts, and dietary fiber may interfere with absorption of levothyroxine from the GI tract. Management: Take in the morning on an empty stomach at least 30 minutes before food. Consider an increase in dose if taken with enteral tube feed.

Preparation for Administration Dilute vial for injection with 5 mL normal saline. Reconstituted concentrations for the 100 mcg, 200 mcg and 500 mcg vials are 20 mcg/mL, 40 mcg/mL, and 100 mcg/mL, respectively. Shake well and use immediately after reconstitution (manufacturer labeling suggests reconstituted vial is stable for 4 hours); discard any unused portions.

Storage/Stability

Capsules and tablets: Store at 25°C (77°F); excursions are permitted between 15°C and 30°C (59°F and 86°F). Protect from light and moisture.

Injection: Store at 20°C to 25°C (68°F to 77°F). Protect from light.

Additional stability data:

Stability in polypropylene syringes (100 mcg/mL in NS) at 5°C ± 1°C is 7 days (Gupta 2000).

Stability in latex-free, PVC minibags protected from light and stored at 15°C to 30°C (59°F to 86°F) was 12 hours for a 2 mcg/mL concentration or 18 hours for a 0.4 mcg/mL concentration in NS. May be exposed to light; however, stability time is significantly reduced, especially for the 2 mcg/mL concentration (Strong 2010).

Mechanism of Action Levothyroxine (T_4) is a synthetic form of thyroxine, an endogenous hormone secreted by the thyroid gland. T_4 is converted to its active metabolite, L-triiodothyronine (T_3). Thyroid hormones (T_4 and T_3) then bind to thyroid receptor proteins in the cell nucleus and exert metabolic effects through control of DNA transcription and protein synthesis; involved in normal metabolism, growth, and development; promotes gluconeogenesis, increases utilization and mobilization of glycogen stores, and stimulates protein synthesis, increases basal metabolic rate

Pharmacodynamics/Kinetics

Absorption: Oral: Erratic (40% to 80% [per manufacturer]); may be decreased by age and specific foods and drugs

Protein binding: >99% bound to plasma proteins including thyroxine-binding globulin, thyroxine-binding prealbumin, and albumin

Metabolism: Hepatic to triiodothyronine (T_3; active); ~80% thyroxine (T_4) deiodinated in kidney and periphery; glucuronidation/conjugation also occurs; undergoes enterohepatic recirculation

Bioavailability: Oral tablets: 64% (nonfasting state) to 79% to 81% (fasting state)

Time to peak, serum: 2 hours

Half-life elimination: Euthyroid: 6 to 8 days; Hypothyroid: 9 to 10 days; Hyperthyroid: 3 to 4 days

Excretion: Urine (major route of elimination; decreases with age); feces (~20%)

Dosing

Adult Doses should be adjusted based on clinical response and laboratory parameters.

Hypothyroidism: Oral:

Adults, healthy adults <50 years of age, children in whom growth and puberty are complete, and older adults who have been recently treated for hyperthyroidism or who have been hypothyroid for only a few months:

~1.7 mcg/kg/day; usual doses are ≤200 mcg daily (range: 100 to 125 mcg daily [70 kg adult]); doses ≥300 mcg daily are rare (consider poor compliance, malabsorption, and/or drug interactions). Titrate dose every 6 weeks. The Canadian labeling includes detailed dosage titration information. Refer to manufacturer labeling for specific recommendations.

Alternate recommendations (off-label dose): Adults (healthy adults <50 years of age): ~1.6 mcg/kg/day. Full replacement doses should be considered when initiating therapy in young healthy adults with overt hypothyroidism and after planned (eg, in preparation for thyroid cancer imaging and therapy) or short-term inadvertent lapses in therapy. Patients presenting with subclinical hypothyroidism do not require full replacement doses (ATA/AACE [Garber 2012]).

Adults <50 years with cardiac disease: Initial: 25 to 50 mcg daily; adjust dose by 12.5 to 25 mcg increments at 6- to 8-week intervals as needed

Adults >50 years: Refer to geriatric dosing.

IM, IV: (Canadian labeling; off-label use [IM] and off-label use in US): 50% of the oral dose; alternatively, some clinicians administer up to 80% of the oral dose. **Note:** Bioavailability of the oral formulation is highly variable, but absorption has been measured to be ~80%, when the oral tablet formulation was administered in the recommended fasting state (Dickerson 2010; Fish 1987).

Severe hypothyroidism: Oral: Initial: 12.5 to 25 mcg daily; adjust dose by 25 mcg daily every 2 to 4 weeks as appropriate

Subclinical hypothyroidism (if treated): Oral: Manufacturer's labeling: 1 mcg/kg/day. Alternate recommendations (off-label dose): 25 to 75 mcg daily, with higher doses usually required for those presenting with higher TSH values (ATA/AACE [Garber 2012])

TSH suppression: Oral:

Well-differentiated thyroid cancer (papillary and follicular): Highly individualized; Doses >2 mcg/kg/day may be needed to suppress TSH to <0.1 milliunits/L in intermediate- to high-risk tumors. Low-risk tumors may be maintained at or slightly below the lower limit of normal (0.1 to 0.5 milliunits/L) (Cooper 2009).

Benign nodules and nontoxic multinodular goiter: Routine use of T_4 for TSH suppression is not recommended in patients with benign thyroid nodules. In patients deemed appropriate candidates, treatment should never be fully suppressive (TSH <0.1 milliunits/L) (Cooper 2009; Gharib 2010). The Canadian labeling recommends an initial dose of 1.7 to 2 mcg/kg/day (target TSH: 0.1 to 0.3 milliunits/L). Avoid use if TSH is already suppressed.

Myxedema coma or stupor: IV: 300 to 500 mcg initially, followed by 50 to 100 mcg once daily until patient is able to tolerate oral administration; smaller doses should be considered in patients with cardiovascular disease

Alternate recommendations (off-label dose): Initial loading dose: 200 to 400 mcg; followed by a daily replacement dose of 1.2 mcg/kg/day (which is 75% of the 1.6 mcg/kg oral daily replacement dose reduced for IV administration); smaller doses should be considered for smaller or older patients and those with a history of coronary disease or arrhythmia; institute oral therapy after the patient improves clinically (ATA [Jonklaas 2014])

Cadaveric organ recovery (hormonal resuscitation) (off-label use): IV: Initial: 20 mcg bolus followed by a continuous infusion of 10 mcg/hour administered to the brain-dead donor who is hemodynamically unstable requiring significant vasopressor support; give concomitantly with methylprednisolone, dextrose, and regular insulin (Salim 2007).

Geriatric Doses should be adjusted based on clinical response and laboratory parameters.

Hypothyroidism:

Adults >50 years without cardiac disease: Initial: 25 to 50 mcg daily; adjust dose by 12.5 to 25 mcg increments at 6- to 8-week intervals as needed

Adults >50 years with cardiac disease: Initial: 12.5 to 25 mcg daily; adjust dose by 12.5 to 25 mcg increments at 4- to 6-week intervals (many clinicians prefer to adjust at 6- to 8-week intervals)

◄

Elderly patients may require <1 mcg/kg/day. Elderly patients often require 20% to 25% less per kilogram than younger patients due to decreased body mass (ATA/AACE [Garber 2012]): Refer to adult dosing.

Myxedema coma: Refer to adult dosing; lower doses may be needed.

Pediatric Hypothyroidism: Infants and Children: Doses should be adjusted based on clinical response and laboratory parameters.

Oral: Daily dosage based on body weight and age as listed below:

1 to 3 months: 10 to 15 mcg/kg/day; if the infant is at risk for development of cardiac failure, use a lower starting dose of 25 mcg daily; if the initial serum T_4 is very low (<5 mcg/dL) begin treatment at a higher dosage of approximately 50 mcg daily (12 to 17 mcg/kg/day) (AAP 2006; Selva 2002)

3 to 6 months: 8 to 10 mcg/kg/day

6 to 12 months: 6 to 8 mcg/kg/day

1 to 5 years: 5 to 6 mcg/kg/day

6 to 12 years: 4 to 5 mcg/kg/day

>12 years: 2 to 3 mcg/kg/day

Growth and puberty complete: 1.7 mcg/kg/day; refer to adult dosing (US labeling) or 1.6 to 1.7 mcg/kg/day (Canadian labeling).

Note: Hyperactivity in older children may be minimized by starting at 1/4 of the recommended dose and increasing each week by that amount until the full dose is achieved (4 weeks).

Children with severe or chronic hypothyroidism should be started at 25 mcg daily; adjust dose by 25 mcg every 2 to 4 weeks.

IM (off-label route in US), IV: Refer to adult dosing.

Renal Impairment There are no dosage adjustments provided in the manufacturer's labeling.

Hepatic Impairment There are no dosage adjustments provided in the manufacturer's labeling.

Adjustment for Toxicity Cardiac symptoms (onset or worsening): Manufacturer labeling recommends reducing dosage or withholding therapy for 7 days and then resuming therapy at reduced dosage. Specific dosing recommendations are not provided.

Administration

Oral: Administer in the morning on an empty stomach, at least 30 to 60 minutes before food.

Capsule: Must be swallowed whole; do not cut, crush, or attempt to dissolve capsules in water to prepare a suspension.

Tablet: May be crushed and suspended in 5 to 10 mL of water; suspension should be used immediately. Levoxyl should be administered with a full glass of water to prevent gagging (due to tablet swelling). **Note:** The Canadian labeling suggests that crushed tablets may also be suspended in breast milk or non-soybean based formula or sprinkled over a small amount of food (eg, apple sauce); avoid the use of foods with high content of iron, fiber, or soybean.

Nasogastric tube: Bioavailability of levothyroxine is reduced if administered with enteral tube feeds. Since holding feedings for at least 1 hour before and after levothyroxine administration may not completely resolve the interaction, an increase in dose (eg, additional 25 mcg) may be necessary (Dickerson 2010).

Parenteral: May be administered by IV injection; may also be administered IM when oral administration is not feasible (Canadian labeling; off-label route in US).

Cadaveric organ recovery (hormonal resuscitation) (off-label use): After IV bolus administration, may administer as a continuous infusion (Salim 2007).

Monitoring Parameters Thyroid function test (serum thyroxine, thyrotropin concentrations), resin triiodothyronine uptake (rT$_3$U), free thyroxine index (FTI), T$_4$, TSH, heart rate, blood pressure, clinical signs of hypo- and hyperthyroidism; TSH is the most reliable guide for evaluating adequacy of thyroid replacement dosage. TSH may be elevated during the first few months of thyroid replacement despite patients being clinically euthyroid. In cases where T$_4$ remains low and TSH is within normal limits, an evaluation of "free" (unbound) T$_4$ is needed to evaluate further increase in dosage

Infants: Monitor closely for cardiac overload, arrhythmias, and aspiration from avid suckling

Infants/children: Monitor closely for under/overtreatment. Undertreatment may decrease intellectual development and linear growth, and lead to poor school performance due to impaired concentration and slowed mentation. Overtreatment may adversely affect brain maturation, accelerate bone age (leading to premature closure of the epiphyses and reduced adult height); craniosynostosis has been reported in infants. Treated children may experience a period of catch-up growth. Monitor TSH and total or free

T$_4$ at 2 and 4 weeks after starting treatment; every 1 to 2 months for first year of life; every 2 to 3 months during years 1 to 3; every 3 to 12 months until growth completed. Perform routine clinical examinations at regular intervals (to assess mental and physical growth and development).

Adults:

Manufacturer's labeling: Monitor TSH every 6 to 8 weeks until normalized; 8 to 12 weeks after dosage changes; every 6 to 12 months throughout therapy

Alternate recommendations: Monitor TSH 4 to 8 weeks after treatment initiation or dose changes, 6 months after adequate replacement dose determined, followed by every 12 months thereafter (or more frequently depending on clinical situation) (ATA/AACE [Garber 2012]).

Reference Range

T$_4$ (thyroxine) serum concentrations: Adults: ~4 to 12 mcg/dL (SI: 51 to 154 nmol/L). **Note:** Normal range is increased in women on birth control pills (5.5 to 12 mcg/dL); normal range in pregnancy: ~5.5 to 16 mcg/dL (SI: ~71 to 206 nmol/L)

T$_4$ free (free thyroxine; free T$_4$) serum concentrations: Adults: 0.7 to 1.8 ng/dL (SI: 9 to 23 pmol/L).

T$_3$ total (triiodothyronine; total T$_3$) serum concentrations: Adults: 80 to 230 ng/dL (SI: 1.2 to 3.5 nmol/L)

Thyroid-stimulating hormone (TSH) serum concentrations: Adults: Varies by laboratory and assay used; refer to laboratory provided reference range. If an upper and lower limit of normal for a third generation TSH assay is not available, a reference range of 0.45 to 4.12 milliunits/L should be considered (ATA/AACE [Garber 2012])

Overt hypothyroidism: Adults: TSH >10 milliunits/L, in combination with a subnormal free T$_4$. These patients are at increased risk for heart failure and cardiovascular mortality and should be considered for treatment with L-thyroxine (ATA/AACE [Garber 2012])

Subclinical hypothyroidism: Adults: TSH: <10 milliunits/L; decision for when to treat should be tailored to individual patient (ATA/AACE [Garber 2012])

Test Interactions

T$_4$-binding globulin (TBG): Factors that alter binding in serum (ATA/AACE [Garber 2012]):

Note: T$_4$ is ~99.97% protein bound. Factors that alter protein binding will affect serum total T$_4$ levels; however, measurement of serum free T$_4$ (the metabolically active moiety) has largely replaced serum total T$_4$ for thyroid status assessment.

Conditions/states that increase TBG binding: Pregnancy, hepatitis, porphyria, neonatal state

Medications that increase TBG binding: Estrogens, 5-fluorouracil, heroin, methadone, mitotane, perphenazine, selective estrogen receptor modulators (eg, tamoxifen, raloxifene)

Conditions/states that decrease TBG binding: Hepatic failure, nephrosis, severe illness

Medications that decrease TBG binding: Androgens, anabolic steroids, glucocorticoids, L-asparaginase, nicotinic acid

Thyroxine (T$_4$) and triiodothyronine (T3): Serum binding inhibitors (ATA/AACE [Garber 2012]):

Medications that inhibit T$_4$ and T$_3$ binding: Carbamazepine, furosemide, free fatty acids, heparin, NSAIDS (variable, transient), phenytoin, salicylates

Thyroid gland hormone: Interference with production and secretion (ATA/AACE [Garber 2012]):

Medications affecting iodine uptake: Amiodarone, iodinated contrast agents, iodine, ethionamide

Medications affecting hormone production: Amiodarone, ethionamide, iodinated contrast agents, iodine, sulfonylureas, sulfonamides, thionamides (carbimazole, methimazole, propylthiouracil),

Medications affecting secretion: Amiodarone, iodinated contrast agents, iodine, lithium

Medications inducing thyroiditis: Alemtuzumab, amiodarone, antiangiogenic agents (lenalidomide, thalidomide), denileukin diftitoxin, interferon alpha, interleukins, lithium, tyrosine kinase inhibitors (sunitinib, sorafenib)

Medications potentially causing the development of Graves': Alemtuzumab, interferon alpha, highly active antiretroviral therapy

Medications potentially ameliorating thyroiditis (if autoimmune) or Graves': Glucocorticoids

Hypothalamic-pituitary axis and TSH: Interference with secretion (ATA/AACE [Garber 2012]):

Medications decreasing TSH secretion: Bexarotene, dopamine, dopaminergic agonists (bromocriptine, cabergoline), glucocorticoids, interleukin-6, metformin, opiates, somatostatin analogues (octreotide, lanreotide), thyroid hormone analogues

Mediations increasing TSH secretion: Amphetamine, interleukin 2, metoclopramide, ritonavir, St John's wort

Medications potentially causing hypophysitis: Ipilimumab

Additional Information Equivalent doses: The following statement on relative potency of thyroid products is included in a joint statement by American Thyroid Association (ATA), American Association of Clinical Endocrinologists (AACE) and The Endocrine Society (TES): For purposes of conversion, levothyroxine sodium (T_4) 100 mcg is usually considered equivalent to desiccated thyroid 60 to 65 mg (1 grain), liothyronine sodium (T_3) 25 mcg, or liotrix 12.5 mcg T_3/50 mcg T_4. However, these are rough guidelines only and do not obviate the careful re-evaluation of a patient when switching thyroid hormone preparations, including a change from one brand of levothyroxine to another. Joint position statement is available at http://www.thyroid.org/thyroxine-products-joint-position-statement/.

Dosage Forms Excipient information presented when available (limited, particularly for generics); consult specific product labeling. [DSC] = Discontinued product
Capsule, Oral, as sodium:
Tirosint: 13 mcg, 25 mcg, 50 mcg, 75 mcg, 88 mcg, 100 mcg, 112 mcg, 125 mcg, 137 mcg, 150 mcg
Solution Reconstituted, Intravenous, as sodium [preservative free]:
Generic: 100 mcg (1 ea); 200 mcg (1 ea); 500 mcg (1 ea)
Tablet, Oral, as sodium:
Levothroid: 25 mcg [DSC] [scored; contains fd&c yellow #6 aluminum lake]
Levothroid: 50 mcg [DSC] [scored]
Levothroid: 75 mcg [DSC] [scored; contains fd&c blue #2 aluminum lake, fd&c red #40 aluminum lake]
Levothroid: 88 mcg [DSC] [scored; contains fd&c blue #1 aluminum lake, fd&c yellow #10 aluminum lake, fd&c yellow #6 aluminum lake]
Levothroid: 100 mcg [DSC] [scored; contains fd&c yellow #10 aluminum lake, fd&c yellow #6 aluminum lake]
Levothroid: 112 mcg [DSC] [scored]
Levothroid: 125 mcg [DSC] [scored; contains fd&c blue #1 aluminum lake, fd&c red #40 aluminum lake, fd&c yellow #6 aluminum lake]
Levothroid: 137 mcg [DSC] [scored; contains fd&c blue #1 aluminum lake]
Levothroid: 150 mcg [DSC] [scored; contains fd&c blue #2 aluminum lake]
Levothroid: 175 mcg [DSC] [scored; contains fd&c blue #1 aluminum lake]
Levothroid: 200 mcg [DSC] [scored; contains fd&c red #40 aluminum lake]
Levothroid: 300 mcg [DSC] [scored; contains fd&c blue #1 aluminum lake, fd&c yellow #10 (quinoline yellow), fd&c yellow #6 aluminum lake]
Levoxyl: 25 mcg [scored; contains fd&c yellow #6 aluminum lake]
Levoxyl: 50 mcg [scored]
Levoxyl: 75 mcg [scored; contains fd&c blue #1 aluminum lake]
Levoxyl: 88 mcg [scored; contains fd&c blue #1 aluminum lake, fd&c yellow #10 aluminum lake, fd&c yellow #6 aluminum lake]
Levoxyl: 100 mcg [scored; contains fd&c yellow #10 aluminum lake, fd&c yellow #6 aluminum lake]
Levoxyl: 112 mcg [scored; contains fd&c red #40 aluminum lake, fd&c yellow #6 aluminum lake]
Levoxyl: 125 mcg [scored; contains fd&c red #40 aluminum lake, fd&c yellow #10 aluminum lake]
Levoxyl: 137 mcg, 150 mcg [scored; contains fd&c blue #1 aluminum lake]
Levoxyl: 175 mcg [scored; contains fd&c blue #1 aluminum lake, fd&c yellow #10 aluminum lake]
Levoxyl: 200 mcg [scored; contains fd&c yellow #10 aluminum lake]
Synthroid: 25 mcg [scored; contains fd&c yellow #6 aluminum lake]
Synthroid: 50 mcg [scored]
Synthroid: 75 mcg [scored; contains fd&c blue #2 aluminum lake, fd&c red #40 aluminum lake]
Synthroid: 88 mcg [scored; contains fd&c blue #1 aluminum lake, fd&c yellow #10 aluminum lake, fd&c yellow #6 aluminum lake]
Synthroid: 100 mcg [scored; contains fd&c yellow #10 aluminum lake, fd&c yellow #6 aluminum lake]
Synthroid: 112 mcg [scored]
Synthroid: 125 mcg [scored; contains fd&c blue #1 aluminum lake, fd&c red #40 aluminum lake, fd&c yellow #6 aluminum lake]
Synthroid: 137 mcg [scored; contains fd&c blue #1 aluminum lake]
Synthroid: 150 mcg [scored; contains fd&c blue #2 aluminum lake]
Synthroid: 175 mcg [scored; contains fd&c blue #1 aluminum lake]
Synthroid: 200 mcg [scored; contains fd&c red #40 aluminum lake]
Synthroid: 300 mcg [scored; contains fd&c blue #1 aluminum lake, fd&c yellow #10 aluminum lake, fd&c yellow #6 aluminum lake]
Unithroid: 25 mcg [contains fd&c yellow #6 aluminum lake]
Unithroid: 25 mcg [DSC] [scored; contains fd&c yellow #6 aluminum lake]
Unithroid: 50 mcg
Unithroid: 50 mcg [DSC], 75 mcg [DSC] [scored]
Unithroid: 75 mcg [contains fd&c blue #2 aluminum lake, fd&c red #40 aluminum lake]
Unithroid: 88 mcg [DSC] [scored]
Unithroid: 88 mcg [contains fd&c blue #1 aluminum lake, fd&c yellow #10 aluminum lake, fd&c yellow #6 aluminum lake]
Unithroid: 100 mcg [contains fd&c yellow #10 aluminum lake, fd&c yellow #6 aluminum lake]
Unithroid: 100 mcg [DSC] [scored; contains fd&c yellow #10 aluminum lake, fd&c yellow #6 aluminum lake]
Unithroid: 112 mcg
Unithroid: 112 mcg [DSC] [scored]
Unithroid: 125 mcg [contains fd&c blue #1 aluminum lake, fd&c red #40 aluminum lake, fd&c yellow #6 aluminum lake]
Unithroid: 125 mcg [DSC] [scored; contains fd&c blue #1 aluminum lake, fd&c red #40 aluminum lake, fd&c yellow #6 aluminum lake]
Unithroid: 137 mcg [contains fd&c blue #1 aluminum lake]
Unithroid: 150 mcg [contains fd&c blue #2 aluminum lake]
Unithroid: 150 mcg [DSC] [scored; contains fd&c blue #2 aluminum lake]
Unithroid: 175 mcg [DSC] [scored]
Unithroid: 175 mcg [contains fd&c blue #1 aluminum lake]
Unithroid: 200 mcg [DSC] [scored]
Unithroid: 200 mcg [contains fd&c red #40 aluminum lake]
Unithroid: 300 mcg [contains fd&c blue #1 aluminum lake, fd&c yellow #10 (quinoline yellow), fd&c yellow #6 aluminum lake]
Unithroid: 300 mcg [DSC] [scored; contains fd&c blue #1 aluminum lake, fd&c yellow #10 aluminum lake, fd&c yellow #6 aluminum lake]
Unithroid Direct: 25 mcg [scored; contains fd&c yellow #6 aluminum lake]
Unithroid Direct: 50 mcg [scored]
Unithroid Direct: 75 mcg, 88 mcg [scored; contains fd&c blue #1 aluminum lake, fd&c blue #2 aluminum lake, fd&c red #40 aluminum lake, fd&c yellow #10 aluminum lake, fd&c yellow #6 aluminum lake]
Unithroid Direct: 100 mcg [scored; contains fd&c yellow #10 aluminum lake, fd&c yellow #6 aluminum lake]
Unithroid Direct: 112 mcg [scored]
Unithroid Direct: 125 mcg [scored; contains fd&c blue #1 aluminum lake, fd&c red #40 aluminum lake, fd&c yellow #6 aluminum lake]
Unithroid Direct: 150 mcg [scored; contains fd&c blue #2 aluminum lake]
Unithroid Direct: 175 mcg [scored; contains fd&c blue #1 aluminum lake]
Unithroid Direct: 200 mcg [scored; contains fd&c red #40 aluminum lake]
Unithroid Direct: 300 mcg [scored; contains fd&c blue #1 aluminum lake, fd&c yellow #10 aluminum lake, fd&c yellow #6 aluminum lake]
Generic: 25 mcg, 50 mcg, 75 mcg, 88 mcg, 100 mcg, 112 mcg, 125 mcg, 137 mcg, 150 mcg, 175 mcg, 200 mcg, 300 mcg

Dosage Forms: Canada Refer also to Dosage Forms.
Note: Capsules are not available in Canada. Excipient information presented when available (limited, particularly for generics); consult specific product labeling
Tablet, Oral, as sodium:
Eltroxin: 50 mcg, 100 mcg, 150 mcg, 200 mcg, 300 mcg
Extemporaneous Preparations A 25 mcg/mL oral suspension may be made with tablets and 40 mL glycerol. Crush twenty-five 0.1 mg levothyroxine tablets in a mortar and reduce to a fine powder. Add small portions of glycerol and mix to a uniform suspension. Transfer to a calibrated 100 mL amber bottle; rinse the mortar with about 10 mL of glycerol and pour into the bottle; repeat until all 40 mL of glycerol is used. Add quantity of water sufficient to make 100 mL. Label "shake well" and "refrigerate". Stable for 8 days refrigerated.
Boulton DW, Fawcett JP, and Woods DJ, "Stability of an Extemporaneously Compounded Levothyroxine Sodium Oral Liquid," *Am J Health Syst Pharm*, 1996, 53(10):1157-61.

♦ **Levothyroxine and Liothyronine** see Liotrix
on page 1084

Lidocaine (Systemic) (LYE doe kane)

Brand Names: US Xylocaine; Xylocaine (Cardiac); Xylocaine-MPF

Brand Names: Canada Lidocaine Hydrochloride Injection USP; Xylocard

Index Terms Lidocaine Hydrochloride; Lignocaine Hydrochloride

Pharmacologic Category Antiarrhythmic Agent, Class Ib; Local Anesthetic

Use Local and regional anesthesia by infiltration, nerve block, epidural, or spinal techniques; acute treatment of ventricular arrhythmias from myocardial infarction or cardiac manipulation (eg, cardiac surgery)

Note: The routine prophylactic use of lidocaine to prevent arrhythmia associated with fibrinolytic administration or to suppress isolated ventricular premature beats, couplets, runs of accelerated idioventricular rhythm, and nonsustained ventricular tachycardia (VT) is not recommended (ACCF/AHA [O'Gara, 2013]).

Pregnancy Considerations Adverse events were not observed in animal reproduction studies. Lidocaine and its metabolites cross the placenta and can be detected in the fetal circulation following injection (Cavalli, 2004; Mitani, 1987). Adverse reactions in the fetus/neonate may affect the CNS, heart, or peripheral vascular tone. Fetal heart monitoring is recommended. Lidocaine injection is approved for obstetric analgesia. Lidocaine administered by local infiltration is used to provide analgesia prior to episiotomy and during repair of obstetric lacerations (ACOG, 2002). Administration by the perineal route may result in greater absorption than administration by the epidural route (Cavalli, 2004). Cumulative exposure from all routes of administration should be considered. When used as an antiarrhythmic, ACLS guidelines recommend using the same dose that would be used in a nonpregnant woman (Vanden Hoek, 2010).

Breast-Feeding Considerations Lidocaine is excreted into breast milk. The manufacturer recommends that caution be used when administered to a nursing woman. When administered by injection for dental or obstetric analgesia, small amounts are detected in breast milk; oral bioavailability to the nursing infant is expected to be low and the amount of lidocaine available to the nursing infant would not be expected to cause adverse events (Lebedevs, 1993; Ortega, 1999). Cumulative exposure from all routes of administration should be considered.

Contraindications Hypersensitivity to lidocaine or any component of the formulation; hypersensitivity to another local anesthetic of the amide type; Adam-Stokes syndrome; Wolff-Parkinson-White syndrome; severe degrees of SA, AV, or intraventricular heart block (except in patients with a functioning artificial pacemaker); premixed injection may contain corn-derived dextrose and its use is contraindicated in patients with allergy to corn or corn-related products

Warnings/Precautions Use caution in patients with severe hepatic dysfunction or pseudocholinesterase deficiency; may have increased risk of lidocaine toxicity.

Intravenous: Constant ECG monitoring is necessary during IV administration. Use cautiously in hepatic impairment, HF, marked hypoxia, severe respiratory depression, hypovolemia, history of malignant hyperthermia, or shock. Increased ventricular rate may be seen when administered to a patient with atrial fibrillation. Correct electrolyte disturbances, especially hypokalemia or hypomagnesemia, prior to use and throughout therapy. Use is contraindicated in patients with Wolff-Parkinson-White syndrome and severe degrees of SA, AV, or intraventricular heart block (except in patients with a functioning artificial pacemaker). Correct any underlying causes of ventricular arrhythmias. Monitor closely for signs and symptoms of CNS toxicity. The elderly may be prone to increased CNS and cardiovascular side effects. Reduce dose in hepatic dysfunction and CHF.

Benzyl alcohol and derivatives: Some dosage forms may contain benzyl alcohol; large amounts of benzyl alcohol (≥99 mg/kg/day) have been associated with a potentially fatal toxicity ("gasping syndrome") in neonates; the "gasping syndrome" consists of metabolic acidosis, respiratory distress, gasping respirations, CNS dysfunction (including convulsions, intracranial hemorrhage), hypotension, and cardiovascular collapse (AAP ["Inactive" 1997]; CDC, 1982); some data suggests that benzoate displaces bilirubin from protein binding sites (Ahlfors, 2001); avoid or use dosage forms containing benzyl alcohol with caution in neonates. See manufacturer's labeling.

Injectable anesthetic: Follow appropriate administration techniques so as not to administer any intravascularly. Continuous intra-articular infusion of local anesthetics after arthroscopic or other surgical procedures is **not** an approved use; chondrolysis (primarily in the shoulder joint) has occurred following infusion, with some cases requiring arthroplasty or shoulder replacement. Solutions containing antimicrobial preservatives should not be used for epidural or spinal anesthesia. Some solutions contain a bisulfite; avoid in patients who are allergic to bisulfite. Resuscitative equipment, medicine and oxygen should be available in case of emergency. Use products containing epinephrine cautiously in patients with significant vascular disease, compromised blood flow, or during or following general anesthesia (increased risk of arrhythmias). Adjust the dose for the elderly, pediatric, acutely ill, and debilitated patients.

Adverse Reactions Effects vary with route of administration. Many effects are dose related.

Frequency not defined.

Cardiovascular: Arrhythmia, bradycardia, arterial spasms, cardiovascular collapse, defibrillator threshold increased, edema, flushing, heart block, hypotension, sinus node supression, vascular insufficiency (periarticular injections)

Central nervous system: Agitation, anxiety, apprehension, coma, confusion, disorientation, dizziness, drowsiness, euphoria, hallucinations, headache, hyperesthesia, hypoesthesia, lethargy, lightheadedness, nervousness, psychosis, seizure, slurred speech, somnolence, unconsciousness

Gastrointestinal: Metallic taste, nausea, vomiting

Local: Thrombophlebitis

Neuromuscular & skeletal: Paresthesia, transient radicular pain (subarachnoid administration; up to 1.9%), tremor, twitching, weakness

Otic: Tinnitus

Respiratory: Bronchospasm, dyspnea, respiratory depression or arrest

Miscellaneous: Allergic reactions, anaphylactic reaction, anaphylactoid reaction, sensitivity to temperature extremes

Following spinal anesthesia: Positional headache (3%), shivering (2%), double vision (<1%), cauda equina syndrome, hypotension, nausea, peripheral nerve symptoms, respiratory inadequacy

Postmarketing and/or case reports: Asystole, disorientation, methemoglobinemia, skin reaction

Drug Interactions

Metabolism/Transport Effects Substrate of CYP1A2 (major), CYP2A6 (minor), CYP2B6 (minor), CYP2C9 (minor), CYP3A4 (major); **Note:** Assignment of Major/Minor substrate status based on clinically relevant drug interaction potential; **Inhibits** CYP1A2 (weak)

Avoid Concomitant Use

Avoid concomitant use of Lidocaine (Systemic) with any of the following: Conivaptan; Fusidic Acid (Systemic); Idelalisib; Saquinavir

Increased Effect/Toxicity

Lidocaine (Systemic) may increase the levels/effects of: Prilocaine; Sodium Nitrite; TiZANidine

The levels/effects of Lidocaine (Systemic) may be increased by: Abiraterone Acetate; Amiodarone; Aprepitant; Beta-Blockers; Conivaptan; CYP1A2 Inhibitors (Moderate); CYP1A2 Inhibitors (Strong); CYP3A4 Inhibitors (Moderate); CYP3A4 Inhibitors (Strong); Dapsone (Topical); Dasatinib; Deferasirox; Disopyramide; Fosaprepitant; Fusidic Acid (Systemic); Hyaluronidase; Idelalisib; Ivacaftor; Luliconazole; Mifepristone; Netupitant; Nitric Oxide; Osimertinib; Palbociclib; Peginterferon Alfa-2b; Saquinavir; Simeprevir; Stiripentol; Telaprevir; Vemurafenib

Decreased Effect

Lidocaine (Systemic) may decrease the levels/effects of: Technetium Tc 99m Tilmanocept

The levels/effects of Lidocaine (Systemic) may be decreased by: Bosentan; Cannabis; CYP1A2 Inducers (Strong); CYP1A2 Inducers (Moderate); CYP3A4 Inducers (Strong); Cyproterone; Dabrafenib; Deferasirox; Enzalutamide; Etravirine; Mitotane; Osimertinib; Siltuximab; St Johns Wort; Teriflunomide; Tocilizumab

Preparation for Administration Local infiltration: Buffered lidocaine for injectable local anesthetic may be prepared: Add 2 mL of sodium bicarbonate 8.4% to 18 mL of lidocaine 1% (Christoph, 1988).

Storage/Stability Injection: Stable at room temperature. Stability of parenteral admixture at room temperature (25°C) is the expiration date on premixed bag; out of overwrap stability is 30 days.

Mechanism of Action Class Ib antiarrhythmic; suppresses automaticity of conduction tissue, by increasing electrical stimulation threshold of ventricle, His-Purkinje system, and spontaneous depolarization of the ventricles during diastole by a direct action on the tissues; blocks both the initiation and conduction of nerve impulses by decreasing the neuronal membrane's permeability to sodium ions, which results in inhibition of depolarization with resultant blockade of conduction

Pharmacodynamics/Kinetics

Onset of action: Single bolus dose: 45 to 90 seconds

Duration: 10 to 20 minutes

Distribution: V_d: 1.1 to 2.1 L/kg; alterable by many patient factors; decreased in CHF and liver disease; crosses blood-brain barrier

Protein binding: 60% to 80% to alpha$_1$ acid glycoprotein

Metabolism: 90% hepatic; active metabolites monoethylglycinexylidide (MEGX) and glycinexylidide (GX) can accumulate and may cause CNS toxicity

Half-life elimination: Biphasic: Prolonged with congestive heart failure, liver disease, shock, severe renal disease; Initial: 7 to 30 minutes; Terminal: Infants, premature: 3.2 hours, Adults: 1.5 to 2 hours

Excretion: Urine (<10% as unchanged drug, ~90% as metabolites)

Dosing

Adult & Geriatric

Antiarrhythmic (ACLS 2010; ACLS 2015):

VF or pulseless VT (after defibrillation attempts, CPR, and vasopressor administration), alternative to amiodarone: IV, intraosseous (I.O.): Initial: 1 to 1.5 mg/kg. If refractory VF or pulseless VT, repeat 0.5 to 0.75 mg/kg bolus every 5 to 10 minutes (maximum cumulative dose: 3 mg/kg). Follow with continuous infusion (1 to 4 mg/minute) after return of perfusion. Reappearance of arrhythmia during constant infusion: 0.5 mg/kg bolus and reassessment of infusion (Zipes, 2000)

Endotracheal (loading dose only): 2 to 3.75 mg/kg (2 to 2.5 times the recommended IV dose); dilute in 5 to 10 mL NS or sterile water. **Note:** Absorption is greater with sterile water and results in less impairment of PaO$_2$.

Hemodynamically stable monomorphic VT: IV: 1 to 1.5 mg/kg; repeat with 0.5 to 0.75 mg/kg every 5 to 10 minutes as necessary (maximum cumulative dose: 3 mg/kg). Follow with continuous infusion of 1 to 4 mg/minute (or 14 to 57 mcg/kg/minute).

Note: Reduce maintenance infusion in patients with CHF, shock, or hepatic disease; initiate infusion at 10 mcg/kg/minute (maximum dose: 1.5 mg/minute or 20 mcg/kg/minute).

Anesthesia, local injectable: Varies with procedure, degree of anesthesia needed, vascularity of tissue, duration of anesthesia required, and physical condition of patient; maximum: 4.5 mg/kg/dose not to exceed 300 mg; do not repeat within 2 hours.

Interstitial cystitis (bladder pain syndrome) (off-label use): Adults: Intravesical:

Various dosage regimens of alkalinized lidocaine alone or with heparin (20,000 to 50,000 units) have been used. There is a risk of precipitation if proper

alkalinization does not occur. Lidocaine stability and pH should be determined after the components have been mixed, prior to administration (Parsons, 2012)

Single instillation: Single intravesical administration of lidocaine (200 mg)/heparin (50,000 units)/sodium bicarbonate (420 mg) in 15 mL of sterile water, instilled into the bladder via catheter and allowed to dwell for 30 minutes before drainage (Parsons, 2012).

Weekly instillation: Weekly bladder instillations for 12 consecutive weeks with lidocaine 4% (5 mL)/heparin (20,000 units)/sodium bicarbonate 7% (25 mL), instilled into an empty bladder via catheter and allowed to dwell for 30 minutes before drainage (Nomiya, 2013).

Daily instillation: Daily bladder instillations for 5 days with lidocaine (200 mg)/sodium bicarbonate 8.4% solution (final volume of 10 mL), instilled into an empty bladder and allowed to dwell for 1 hour before drainage (Nickel, 2009).

Pediatric

Antiarrhythmic:

IV, intraosseous (I.O.): **Note:** For use in VF or pulseless VT if amiodarone is not available; give after defibrillation attempts, CPR, and epinephrine:

Loading dose: 1 mg/kg (maximum: 100 mg); follow with continuous infusion; may administer second bolus of 0.5 to 1 mg/kg if delay between bolus and start of infusion is >15 minutes (PALS, 2000; PALS, 2010)

Continuous infusion: 20 to 50 mcg/kg/minute (PALS, 2010). Per the manufacturer, do not exceed 20 mcg/kg/minute in patients with shock, hepatic disease, cardiac arrest, or CHF.

Endotracheal: 2 to 3 mg/kg; flush with 5 mL of NS and follow with 5 assisted manual ventilations (PALS, 2010)

Anesthesia, local injectable: Refer to adult dosing.

Renal Impairment No dosage adjustment provided in manufacturer's labeling. However, accumulation of metabolites may be increased in renal dysfunction. Not dialyzable (0% to 5%) by hemo- or peritoneal dialysis; supplemental dose is not necessary.

Hepatic Impairment Use with caution; reduce maintenance infusion. Initial: 0.75 mg/minute or 10 mcg/kg/minute; maximum dose: 1.5 mg/minute or 20 mcg/kg/minute. Monitor lidocaine concentrations closely and adjust infusion rate as necessary; consider alternative therapy.

Dietary Considerations Premixed injection may contain corn-derived dextrose and its use is contraindicated in patients with allergy to corn-related products.

Usual Infusion Concentrations: Pediatric Note: Premixed solutions available

IV infusion: 8000 mcg/mL

Usual Infusion Concentrations: Adult Note: Premixed solutions available

IV infusion: 1000 mg in 250 mL (concentration: 4 mg/mL) or 2000 mg in 250 mL (concentration: 8 mg/mL) of D$_5$W

Administration

IV:

Bolus: According to the manufacturer, may administer at 25 to 50 mg/minute. In the setting of cardiac arrest (eg, ventricular fibrillation or pulseless ventricular tachycardia), may be infused rapidly into a peripheral vein (Dorian, 2002).

Continuous infusion: After initial bolus dosing, may administer as a continuous infusion; refer to indication-specific infusion rates in dosing for detailed recommendations. In the setting of cardiac arrest, infusion may be initiated once patient has return of spontaneous circulation resulting from lidocaine administration; however, there is no evidence to support subsequent continuous infusion to prevent recurrence (ACLS [Peberdy, 2010]). Local thrombophlebitis may occur in patients receiving prolonged IV infusions.

Endotracheal (off-label administration route): Dilute in NS or sterile water. Absorption is greater with sterile water and results in less impairment of PaO$_2$ (Hahnel, 1990). Stop compressions, spray drug quickly down tube. Flush with 5 mL of NS and follow immediately with several quick insufflations and continue chest compressions.

Intraosseous (IO; off-label administration route): Intraosseous administration is a safe and effective alternative to venous access in children with cardiac arrest; the onset for most medications is similar to that of IV administration (PALS, 2010). In adults, IO administration is a reasonable alternative when quick IV access is not feasible (ACLS, 2010).

Intravesical (off-label use): Various regimens of alkalinized lidocaine (with or without heparin) have been instilled into the bladder

The On-Q® infusion pump is used to slowly administer local anesthetics (eg, bupivacaine, lidocaine, ropivacaine) to or around surgical wound sites and/or in close proximity to nerves for pre- or postoperative regional anesthesia. When infused directly into the shoulder, destruction of articular cartilage (chondrolysis) has occurred. On-Q® pumps should never be placed directly into any joint (see https://www.ismp.org/Newsletters/acutecare/archives/May09.asp).

Monitoring Parameters Liver function tests, lidocaine concentrations, ECG; in patients requiring drug >24 hrs, blood level monitoring recommended; consult individual institutional policies and procedures

Reference Range

Therapeutic: 1.5 to 5.0 mcg/mL (SI: 6 to 21 micromole/L)
Potentially toxic: >6 mcg/mL (SI: >26 micromole/L)
Toxic: >9 mcg/mL (SI: >38 micromole/L)

Dosage Forms Excipient information presented when available (limited, particularly for generics); consult specific product labeling.

Solution, Injection, as hydrochloride:
Xylocaine: 0.5% (50 mL); 1% (20 mL, 50 mL); 2% (10 mL, 20 mL, 50 mL) [contains methylparaben]
Xylocaine-MPF: 0.5% (50 mL); 1% (2 mL, 5 mL, 10 mL, 30 mL); 1.5% (10 mL, 20 mL); 2% (2 mL, 5 mL, 10 mL); 4% (5 mL) [methylparaben free]
Generic: 0.5% (50 mL); 1% (2 mL, 5 mL, 10 mL, 20 mL, 30 mL, 50 mL); 1.5% (20 mL); 2% (2 mL, 5 mL, 20 mL, 50 mL)
Solution, Injection, as hydrochloride [preservative free]:
Generic: 0.5% (50 mL); 1% (2 mL, 5 mL, 30 mL); 1.5% (20 mL); 2% (2 mL, 5 mL, 10 mL); 4% (5 mL)
Solution, Intravenous, as hydrochloride:
Xylocaine (Cardiac): 20 mg/mL (5 mL)
Generic: 10 mg/mL (5 mL); 20 mg/mL (5 mL); 0.4% [4 mg/mL] (250 mL, 500 mL); 0.8% [8 mg/mL] (250 mL); 2% (5 mL); 5% [50 mg/mL] (2 mL)
Solution, Intravenous, as hydrochloride [preservative free]:
Generic: 10 mg/mL (5 mL); 20 mg/mL (5 mL)

Lidocaine (Topical) (LYE doe kane)

Brand Names: US AneCream [OTC]; AneCream5 [OTC]; CidalEaze; EnovaRX-Lidocaine HCl; Glydo; LC-4 Lidocaine [OTC]; LC-5 Lidocaine [OTC]; Lidocin; Lidoderm; Lidopin; LidoRx; Lidotral; Lidovex; Lidovin; Lidozol; LMX 4 Plus [OTC]; LMX 4 [OTC]; LMX 5 [OTC]; LTA 360 Kit; Predator [OTC]; Premium Lidocaine; Prozena [DSC]; Prozena [OTC] [DSC]; RectiCare [OTC]; Tecnu First Aid [OTC]; Topicaine 5 [OTC]; Topicaine [OTC]; Xolido XP [OTC]; Xolido [OTC]; Xylocaine; Xylocaine Jelly [DSC]; Zingo

Brand Names: Canada Betacaine; Lidodan; Lidoderm; Maxilene; Xylocaine

Index Terms Lidocaine Hydrochloride; Lidocaine Patch; Lignocaine Hydrochloride; Viscous Lidocaine; Xylocaine Viscous

Pharmacologic Category Analgesic, Topical; Local Anesthetic

Use

Intradermal injection (Zingo): Topical local analgesia prior to venipuncture or peripheral intravenous (IV) cannulation in children ≥3 years; topical local analgesia prior to venipuncture in adults.

Jelly: Prevention and control of pain in procedures involving the male and female urethra; for topical treatment of painful urethritis

Oral topical solution (2% viscous): Topical anesthesia of irritated or inflamed oral mucous membranes and pharyngeal tissue; reducing gagging during the taking of x-ray. **Note:** Not approved for relief of teething pain and discomfort in infants and children; serious adverse (toxic) effects have been reported (AAP 2011; AAPD 2012; ISMP 2014).

Oral topical solution (4%): Topical anesthesia of accessible mucous membranes of the oral and nasal cavities and proximal portions of the digestive tract. **Note:** Not approved for relief of teething pain and discomfort in infants and children; serious adverse (toxic) effects have been reported (AAP 2011; AAPD 2012; ISMP 2014).

Oral topical solution (metered-dose spray) [Canadian product]: Topical anesthesia of accessible mucous membranes of the oral and nasal cavities and proximal portions of the digestive tract.

Patch (Lidoderm): Relief of pain associated with postherpetic neuralgia

Patch (LidoPatch): Temporary relief of localized pain

Rectal: Temporary relief of pain and itching due to anorectal disorders

Topical: Local anesthetic for mucous membrane of the oropharynx; lubricant for intubation; use in laser/cosmetic surgeries; pruritus, pruritic eczemas, insect bites, pain, soreness, minor burns (including sunburns), cuts, and abrasions of the skin; discomfort due to pruritus ani, pruritus vulvae, hemorrhoids, anal fissures, and similar conditions of the skin and mucous membranes.

Dosing

Adult Anesthesia, topical:

Cream:
LidaMantle, Lidovex: Skin irritation: Apply a thin film to affected area 2 to 3 times daily as needed
LMX 4: Skin irritation: Apply up to 3 to 4 times daily to intact skin
LMX 5: Relief of anorectal pain and itching: Apply to affected area up to 6 times daily

Gel: Apply to affected area ≤4 times daily as needed (maximum dose: 4.5 mg/kg, not to exceed 300 mg)

Intradermal injection: Apply one intradermal lidocaine (0.5 mg) device to the site planned for venipuncture, 1 to 3 minutes prior to needle insertion.

Topical solution: Apply 1 to 5 mL (40 to 200 mg) to affected area

Jelly: Maximum dose: 30 mL (600 mg) in any 12-hour period:
Anesthesia of male urethra: 5 to 30 mL (100 to 600 mg)
Anesthesia of female urethra: 3 to 5 mL (60 to 100 mg)

Lotion: Apply a thin film to affected area 2 or 3 times daily.

Ointment: Apply as a single application not exceeding 5 g of ointment (equivalent to lidocaine base 250 mg); maximum: 20 g of ointment/day (equivalent to lidocaine base 1,000 mg/day).

Oral topical solution (2% viscous):
Anesthesia of the mouth: 15 mL swished in the mouth and spit out no more frequently than every 3 hours (maximum: 4.5 mg/kg [or 300 mg per dose]; 8 doses per 24-hour period)
Anesthesia of the pharynx: 15 mL gargled no more frequently than every 3 hours (maximum: 4.5 mg/kg [or 300 mg per dose]; 8 doses per 24-hour period); may be swallowed

Oral topical solution (4%): **Note:** For use in mucous membranes of oral and nasal cavities and proximal GI tract. Apply 1 to 5 mL (40 to 200 mg) to affected area (maximum dose: 4.5 mg/kg, not to exceed 300 mg per dose)

Oral topical endotracheal solution, metered-dose spray (10 mg/actuation) [Canadian product]:
Nasal: 20 to 60 mg (maximum dose: 500 mg for procedure <1 minute or 600 mg for procedure >5 minutes)
Oropharyngeal: 20 to 200 mg (maximum dose: 500 mg for procedure <1 minute or 600 mg for procedure >5 minutes)
Respiratory tract: 50 to 400 mg (maximum dose: 400 mg for procedure <1 minute or 600 mg for procedure >5 minutes)
Trachea, larynx, bronchi: 50 to 200 mg (maximum dose: 200 mg for procedure <1 minute or 400 mg for procedure >5 minutes)

Patch:
Lidoderm: Postherpetic neuralgia: Apply patch to most painful area. Up to 3 patches may be applied in a single application. Patch(es) may remain in place for up to 12 hours in any 24-hour period.
LidoPatch: Pain (localized): Apply patch to painful area. Patch may remain in place for up to 12 hours in any 24-hour period. No more than 1 patch should be used in a 24-hour period.

Geriatric Refer to adult dosing. Administer reduced doses commensurate with age and physical status.

Pediatric Anesthesia, topical: Note: Smaller areas of treatment recommended in younger or smaller patients (<12 months or <10 kg) or those with impaired elimination (Fein 2012); use lowest effective dose

Cream:
LidaMantle, Lidovex: Skin irritation: Children and Adolescents: Refer to adult dosing.
LMX 4 (liposomal lidocaine 4%):
Skin irritation: Children ≥2 years and Adolescents: Refer to adult dosing.
Minor dermal procedures (eg, IV access, venipuncture, lumbar puncture, abscess drainage, joint aspiration); anesthetic (off-label):
Infants and Children <4 years: 1 g applied to site (6.25 cm² of skin) 30 minutes prior to procedure (Fein 2012; Taddio 2004)

Children ≥4 years and Adolescents ≤17 years: 1 g to 2.5 g applied to site (6.25 cm^2 of skin) 30 minutes prior to procedure (Eichenfeld 2002; Fein 2012; Koh 2004; Luhman 2004; Taddio 2004).

LMX 5: Relief of anorectal pain and itching: Children ≥12 years and Adolescents: Refer to adult dosing.

Jelly: Children and Adolescents: Dose varies with age and weight (maximum dose: 4.5 mg/kg)

Intradermal injection: Children ≥3 years and Adolescents: Apply one intradermal lidocaine (0.5 mg) device to the site planned for venipuncture or IV cannulation, 1 to 3 minutes prior to needle insertion.

Lotion: Children and Adolescents: Refer to adult dosing.

Ointment: Children and Adolescents: Dose varies with age and weight, apply single application not exceeding 5 g of ointment (equivalent to lidocaine base 250 mg); maximum dose: lidocaine base 4.5 mg/kg.

Oral topical solution (2% viscous): **Note:** Not approved for relief of teething pain and discomfort in infants and children; serious adverse (toxic) effects have been reported; AAP, AAPD, and ISMP strongly discourage use (AAP 2011; AAPD 2012; ISMP 2014).

Infants and Children <3 years: ≤1.2 mL applied to area with a cotton-tipped applicator no more frequently than every 3 hours (maximum: 4 doses per 12-hour period; use only if the underlying condition requires treatment with product volume of ≤1.2 mL)

Children ≥3 years and Adolescents: Do not exceed 4.5 mg/kg/dose (or 300 mg per dose); swished in the mouth and spit out no more frequently than every 3 hours (maximum: 4 doses per 12-hour period)

Oral topical solution (4%): **Note:** For use in mucous membranes of oral and nasal cavities and proximal GI tract. Children and Adolescents: Dose varies with age and weight (maximum dose: 4.5 mg/kg)

Oral topical endotracheal solution, metered-dose spray (10 mg/actuation) [Canadian product]: Children ≥2 years and Adolescents: Dose varies with age and weight (maximum dose [children ≥2 to <12 years]: Laryngotracheal: 3 mg/kg; nasal/oropharyngeal: 4 to 5 mg/kg)

Renal Impairment There are no dosage adjustments provided in the manufacturer's labeling.

Hepatic Impairment There are no dosage adjustments provided in the manufacturer's labeling; use caution in patients with severe hepatic disease.

Additional Information Complete prescribing information should be consulted for additional detail.

Dosage Forms Considerations EnovaRX-Lidocaine cream is compounded from a kit. Refer to manufacturer's package insert for compounding instructions.

Dosage Forms Excipient information presented when available (limited, particularly for generics); consult specific product labeling. [DSC] = Discontinued product

Cream, External:
AneCream: 4% (5 g, 15 g, 30 g) [contains benzyl alcohol, polysorbate 80, propylene glycol, trolamine (triethanolamine)]
AneCream5: 5% (15 g, 30 g) [contains benzyl alcohol, polysorbate 80, propylene glycol, trolamine (triethanolamine)]
LC-4 Lidocaine: 4% (45 g) [contains cetyl alcohol]
LC-5 Lidocaine: 5% (45 g) [contains cetyl alcohol]
Lidotral: 3.88% (85 g) [contains cetearyl alcohol, methylparaben, propylene glycol, propylparaben]
Lidovex: 3.75% (60 g) [contains cetyl alcohol, methylparaben, propylparaben]
Lidovin: 3.95% (60 g) [contains peg-40 castor oil]
Lidozol: 3.75% (60 g) [contains peg-40 castor oil]
LMX 4: 4% (5 g, 15 g, 30 g) [contains benzyl alcohol]
LMX 5: 5% (15 g, 30 g) [contains benzyl alcohol]
RectiCare: 5% (15 g, 30 g) [contains benzyl alcohol, polysorbate 80, propylene glycol, trolamine (triethanolamine)]
Generic: 4% (5 g, 15 g, 30 g); 5% (15 g, 30 g)

Cream, External, as hydrochloride:
CidalEaze: 3% (453.6 g) [contains aluminum sulfate, calcium acetate, cetyl alcohol, methylparaben, propylparaben]
EnovaRX-Lidocaine HCl: 5% (60 g, 120 g); 10% (60 g, 120 g) [contains cetyl alcohol]
Lidopin: 3% (28 g, 85 g); 3.25% (28 g, 85 g) [contains cetyl alcohol, methylparaben, propylparaben]
Predator: 4% (63 g) [contains propylene glycol, trolamine (triethanolamine)]
Xolido: 2% (118 mL) [contains methylisothiazolinone]
Xolido XP: 4% (118 mL) [contains methylisothiazolinone]
Generic: 3% (28.3 g, 28.35 g, 85 g)

Device, Intradermal, as hydrochloride:
Zingo: 0.5 mg (1 ea)

Gel, External:
Topicaine: 4% (10 g, 30 g, 113 g) [contains benzyl alcohol, disodium edta]
Topicaine 5: 5% (10 g, 30 g, 113 g) [contains benzyl alcohol, disodium edta]

Gel, External, as hydrochloride:
Lidocin: 3% (30 g, 120 g, 240 g) [contains brilliant blue fcf (fd&c blue #1), polysorbate 80, tartrazine (fd&c yellow #5), trolamine (triethanolamine)]
LidoRx: 3% (10 mL, 30 mL, 90 mL) [contains isopropyl alcohol, trolamine (triethanolamine)]
Tecnu First Aid: 0.2-2.5% (56.7 g) [contains disodium edta]
Xylocaine Jelly: 2% (5 mL [DSC], 30 mL [DSC]) [contains methylparaben, propylparaben]
Generic: 2% (5 mL, 10 mL [DSC], 20 mL, 30 mL)

Gel, External, as hydrochloride [preservative free]:
Glydo: 2% (6 mL, 11 mL) [pvc free]
Generic: 2% (5 mL, 10 mL)

Kit, External:
AneCream: 4% [contains benzyl alcohol, polysorbate 80, propylene glycol, trolamine (triethanolamine)]
LMX 4 Plus: 4% [contains benzyl alcohol]
Generic: 4%

Lotion, External, as hydrochloride:
Generic: 3% (118 mL, 177 mL)

Ointment, External:
Premium Lidocaine: 5% (50 g)
Generic: 5% (30 g, 35.44 g, 50 g)

Patch, External:
Lidoderm: 5% (1 ea, 30 ea) [contains disodium edta, methylparaben, propylene glycol, propylparaben]
Prozena: 4% (5 ea [DSC], 15 ea [DSC], 30 ea [DSC])
Generic: 5% (1 ea, 30 ea); 5% (30 ea)

Solution, External, as hydrochloride:
Xylocaine: 4% (50 mL) [contains methylparaben]
Generic: 4% (50 mL)

Solution, Mouth/Throat, as hydrochloride:
Generic: 2% (15 mL, 100 mL); 4% (4 mL [DSC])

Solution, Mouth/Throat, as hydrochloride [preservative free]:
LTA 360 Kit: 4% (4 mL)
Generic: 4% (4 mL)

Dosage Forms: Canada Note: Refer also to Dosage Forms

Excipient information presented when available (limited, particularly for generics); consult specific product labeling

Solution, Mouth/Throat:
Xylocaine Endotracheal: 10 mg/actuation (50 mL) [contains ethanol]

Lidocaine and Epinephrine
(LYE doe kane & ep i NEF rin)

Brand Names: US Lignospan® Forte; Lignospan® Standard; Xylocaine® MPF With Epinephrine; Xylocaine® With Epinephrine

Brand Names: Canada Xylocaine® With Epinephrine

Index Terms Epinephrine and Lidocaine

Pharmacologic Category Local Anesthetic

Use Local infiltration anesthesia; AVS for nerve block

Dosing

Adult & Geriatric Dosage varies with the anesthetic procedure, degree of anesthesia needed, vascularity of tissue, duration of anesthesia required, and physical condition of patient.

Dental anesthesia, infiltration, or conduction block:
Children <12 years: 20-30 mg (1-1.5 mL) of lidocaine hydrochloride as a 2% solution with epinephrine 1:100,000; maximum: 4.5 mg of lidocaine hydrochloride/kg of body weight or 100-150 mg as a single dose

Children ≥12 years and Adults: Do not exceed 7 mg/kg body weight up to a maximum range of 300 mg (usual dental practice) to 500 mg (approved product labeling) of lidocaine hydrochloride and 3 mcg (0.003 mg) of epinephrine/kg of body weight or 0.2 mg epinephrine per dental appointment. The effective anesthetic dose varies with procedure, intensity of anesthesia needed, duration of anesthesia required, and physical condition of the patient. Always use the lowest effective dose along with careful aspiration.

Note: For most routine dental procedures, lidocaine hydrochloride 2% with epinephrine 1:100,000 is preferred. When a more pronounced hemostasis is required, a 1:50,000 epinephrine concentration should be used.

Pediatric Dosage varies with the anesthetic procedure, degree of anesthesia needed, vascularity of tissue, duration of anesthesia required, and physical condition of patient.

Dental anesthesia, infiltration, or conduction block:

Children <12 years: 20-30 mg (1-1.5 mL) of lidocaine hydrochloride as a 2% solution with epinephrine 1:100,000; maximum: 4.5 mg of lidocaine hydrochloride/kg of body weight or 100-150 mg as a single dose

Children ≥12 years: Refer to adult dosing.

Note: For most routine dental procedures, lidocaine hydrochloride 2% with epinephrine 1:100,000 is preferred. When a more pronounced hemostasis is required, a 1:50,000 epinephrine concentration should be used.

Renal Impairment No dosage adjustment provided in manufacturer's labeling. However, accumulation of metabolites may be increased in renal dysfunction.

Hepatic Impairment No dosage adjustment provided in manufacturer's labeling; use with caution.

Additional Information Complete prescribing information should be consulted for additional detail.

Dosage Forms Excipient information presented when available (limited, particularly for generics); consult specific product labeling. [DSC] = Discontinued product

Injection, solution:

Xylocaine® with Epinephrine:

0.5% / 1:200,000: Lidocaine hydrochloride 0.5% [5 mg/mL] and epinephrine 1:200,000 (50 mL) [contains methylparaben]

1% / 1:100,000: Lidocaine hydrochloride 1% [10 mg/mL] and epinephrine 1:100,000 (10 mL, 20 mL, 50 mL) [contains methylparaben]

2% / 1:100,000: Lidocaine hydrochloride 2% [20 mg/mL] and epinephrine 1:100,000 (10 mL, 20 mL, 50 mL) [contains methylparaben]

Generic:

0.5% / 1:200,000: Lidocaine hydrochloride 0.5% [5 mg/mL] and epinephrine 1:200,000 (50 mL)

1% / 1:100,000: Lidocaine hydrochloride 1% [10 mg/mL] and epinephrine 1:100,000 (20 mL, 30 mL, 50 mL)

2% / 1:100,000: Lidocaine hydrochloride 2% [20 mg/mL] and epinephrine 1:100,000 (30 mL, 50 mL)

Injection, solution [preservative free]:

Xylocaine®-MPF with Epinephrine:

1% / 1:200,000: Lidocaine hydrochloride 1% [10 mg/mL] and epinephrine 1:200,000 (5 mL, 10 mL, 30 mL) [contains sodium metabisulfite]

1.5% / 1:200,000: Lidocaine hydrochloride 1.5% [15 mg/mL] and epinephrine 1:200,000 (5 mL, 10 mL, 30 mL) [contains sodium metabisulfite]

2% / 1:200,000: Lidocaine hydrochloride 2% [20 mg/mL] and epinephrine 1:200,000 (5 mL, 10 mL, 20 mL) [contains sodium metabisulfite]

Generic:

1.5% / 1:200,000: Lidocaine hydrochloride 1.5% [15 mg/mL] and epinephrine 1:200,000 (5 mL, 30 mL)

2% / 1:200,000: Lidocaine hydrochloride 2% [20 mg/mL] and epinephrine 1:200,000 (20 mL)

Injection, solution [for dental use]:

Lignospan® Forte: 2% / 1:50,000: Lidocaine hydrochloride 2% [20 mg/mL] and epinephrine 1:50,000 (1.7 mL) [contains edetate disodium, potassium metabisulfite]

Lignospan® Standard: 2% / 1:100,000: Lidocaine hydrochloride 2% [20 mg/mL] and epinephrine 1:100,000 (1.7 mL) [contains edetate disodium, potassium metabisulfite]

Xylocaine® Dental with Epinephrine:

2% / 1:50,000: Lidocaine hydrochloride 2% [20 mg/mL] and epinephrine 1:50,000 (1.7 mL; 1.8 mL [DSC]) [contains sodium metabisulfite]

2% / 1:100,000: Lidocaine hydrochloride 2% [20 mg/mL] and epinephrine 1:100,000 (1.7 mL; 1.8 mL [DSC]) [contains sodium metabisulfite]

Generic:

2% / 1:50,000: Lidocaine hydrochloride 2% [20 mg/mL] and epinephrine 1:50,000 (1.7 mL, 1.8 mL)

2% / 1:100,000: Lidocaine hydrochloride 2% [20 mg/mL] and epinephrine 1:100,000 (1.7 mL, 1.8 mL)

Lidocaine and Prilocaine
(LYE doe kane & PRIL oh kane)

Brand Names: US EMLA; Livixil Pak; LP Lite Pak; Oraqix; Relador Pak

Brand Names: Canada EMLA; Oraqix

Index Terms Prilocaine and Lidocaine

Pharmacologic Category Local Anesthetic

Use

US labeling:

Cream: Topical anesthetic for use on normal intact skin to provide local analgesia; for use on genital mucous membranes for superficial minor surgery; and as pretreatment for infiltration anesthesia.

Periodontal gel: Topical anesthetic for use in periodontal pockets during scaling and/or root planing procedures

Canadian labeling:

Cream: Topical anesthetic for use on intact skin in connection with: IV cannulation or venipuncture; superficial surgical procedures (eg, split skin grafting, electrolysis, removal of molluscum contagiosum); laser treatment for superficial skin surgery (eg, telangiectasia, port wine stains, warts, moles, skin nodules, scar tissue); surgical procedures of genital mucosa (≤10 minutes) on small superficial localized lesions (eg, removal of condylomata by laser or cautery, biopsies); local infiltration anesthesia in genital mucous membranes; mechanical cleansing/debridement of leg ulcers; vaccination with measles-mumps-rubella (MMR), diphtheria-pertussis-tetanus-poliovirus (DPTP), *Haemophilus influenzae* b, and hepatitis B.

Patch: Topical anesthetic for use on intact skin in connection with IV cannulation or venipuncture; vaccination with measles-mumps-rubella (MMR), diphtheria-pertussis-tetanus-poliovirus (DPTP), *Haemophilus influenzae* b, and hepatitis B.

Periodontal gel: Topical anesthetic for use in periodontal pockets during scaling and/or root planing procedures

Dosing

Adult Anesthetic: Topical:

Cream (intact skin): **Note:** Apply a thick layer to intact skin and cover with an occlusive dressing. Dermal analgesia can be expected to increase for up to 3 hours under occlusive dressing and persist for 1 to 2 hours after removal of the cream.

US labeling:

Minor dermal procedures (eg, IV cannulation or venipuncture): Apply 2.5 g (1/2 of the 5 g tube) over 20 to 25 cm^2 of skin surface area) for at least 1 hour

Major dermal procedures (eg, more painful dermatological procedures involving a larger skin area such as split thickness skin graft harvesting): Apply 2 g per 10 cm^2 of skin and allow to remain in contact with the skin for at least 2 hours.

Adult male genital skin (eg, pretreatment prior to local anesthetic infiltration): Apply 1 g per 10 cm^2 to the skin surface for 15 minutes. Local anesthetic infiltration should be performed immediately after removal of cream.

Adult female genital mucous membranes: Minor procedures (eg, removal of condylomata acuminata, pretreatment for local anesthetic infiltration): Apply 5 to 10 g for 5 to 10 minutes. The local anesthetic infiltration or procedure should be performed immediately after removal of cream.

Canadian labeling:

Minor dermal procedures (eg, IV cannulation, venipuncture, surgical or laser treatment): Apply 2 g (~1/2 of the 5 g tube) over ~13.5 cm^2 for at least 1 hour but no longer than 5 hours

Major dermal procedures (eg, split-skin grafting): 1.5 to 2 g per 10 cm^2 (maximum: 60 g per 400 cm^2) for at least 2 hours but no longer than 5 hours

Genital mucosa (eg, surgical procedures ≤10 minutes such as localized wart removal, and prior to local anesthetic infiltration): Apply 2 g (~1/2 of 5 g tube) per lesion (maximum: 10 g) for 5 to 10 minutes. Initiate procedure immediately after removing cream.

Leg ulcers (eg, mechanical cleansing/surgical debridement): Apply ~1 to 2 g per 10 cm^2 (maximum: 10 g) for at least 30 minutes and up to 60 minutes for necrotic tissue that is more difficult to penetrate. Initiate procedure immediately after removing cream.

Periodontal gel (Oraqix): Apply on gingival margin around selected teeth using the blunt-tipped applicator included in package. Wait 30 seconds, then fill the periodontal pockets using the blunt-tipped applicator until gel becomes visible at the gingival margin. Wait another 30 seconds before starting treatment. May reapply; maximum recommended dose: One treatment session: 5 cartridges (8.5 g)

Transdermal patch [Canadian product]: Minor procedures (eg, needle insertion): Apply 1 or more patches to intact skin surface area <10 cm^2 for at least 1 hour (maximum application time: 5 hours)

Geriatric Smaller areas of treatment may be necessary depending on status of patient (eg, debilitated, impaired hepatic function). Refer to adult dosing.

Pediatric Although the incidence of systemic adverse effects is very low, caution should be exercised, particularly when applying over large areas and leaving on for >2 hours

Local anesthetic (procedures): Infants and Children (intact skin): Topical: **Note:** If a patient >3 months of age does not meet the minimum weight requirement, the maximum total dose should be restricted to the corresponding maximum based on patient weight.

Cream: Should **not** be used in neonates with a gestation age <37 weeks nor in infants <12 months of age who are receiving treatment with methemoglobin-inducing agents

Dosing is based on child's age and weight:

Age 0 to 3 months or <5 kg: Apply a maximum of 1 g over no more than 10 cm^2 of skin; leave on for no longer than 1 hour

Age 3 months to 12 months and >5 kg: Apply no more than a maximum 2 g total over no more than 20 cm^2 of skin; leave on for no longer than 4 hours

Age 1 to 6 years and >10 kg: Apply no more than a maximum of 10 g total over no more than 100 cm^2 of skin. US labeling recommends leaving on for no longer than 4 hours. Canadian labeling recommends leaving on for no longer than 5 hours.

Age 7 to 12 years and >20 kg: Apply no more than a maximum 20 g total over no more than 200 cm^2 of skin. US labeling recommends leaving on for no longer than 4 hours. Canadian labeling recommends leaving on for no longer than 5 hours.

Transdermal patch [Canadian product]: **Note:** Should not be used in neonates with a gestation age <37 weeks nor in infants <12 months of age who are receiving treatment with methemoglobin-inducing agents

Dosing is based on child's age and weight: Apply patch(es) to skin area(s) <10 cm^2:

Age 0 to 3 months or <5 kg: Apply 1 patch and leave on for ~1 hour (do not exceed 1-hour application time); do not apply more than 1 patch at same time; safety of repeated dosing not established

Age 3 months to 12 months and >5 kg: Apply 1 to 2 patches for ~1 hour (maximum application time: 4 hours); do not apply more than 2 patches at the same time

Age 1 to 6 years and >10 kg: Apply 1 or more patches for minimum of 1 hour (maximum application time: 5 hours); maximum dose: 10 patches

Age 7 to 12 years and >20 kg: Apply 1 or more patches for a minimum of 1 hour (maximum application time: 5 hours); maximum dose: 20 patches

Renal Impairment There are no dosage adjustments provided in the manufacturer's labeling. Lidocaine and prilocaine primarily undergo hepatic metabolism and their pharmacokinetics are not expected to be changed significantly in renal impairment.

Hepatic Impairment Smaller areas of treatment are recommended for patients with severe hepatic impairment.

Additional Information Complete prescribing information should be consulted for additional detail.

Dosage Forms Excipient information presented when available (limited, particularly for generics); consult specific product labeling.

Cream, topical:

EMLA: Lidocaine 2.5% and prilocaine 2.5% (5 g, 30 g)

Livixil Pak: Lidocaine 2.5% and prilocaine 2.5% (3 x 30 g) [packaged with occlusive dressing]

LP Lite Pak: Lidocaine 2.5% and prilocaine 2.5% (2 x 30 g) [packaged with occlusive dressing]

Relador Pak: Lidocaine 2.5% and prilocaine 2.5% (3 x 30 g) [packaged with occlusive dressing]

Generic: Lidocaine 2.5% and prilocaine 2.5% (5 g, 30 g)

Gel, periodontal:

Oraqix: Lidocaine 2.5% and prilocaine 2.5% (1.7 g)

Dosage Forms: Canada Excipient information presented when available (limited, particularly for generics); consult specific product labeling.

Patch, transdermal:

EMLA Patch: Lidocaine 2.5% and prilocaine 2.5% per patch (2s, 20s) [active contact surface area of each 1 g patch: 10 cm^2; surface area of entire patch: 40 cm^2]

Lidocaine and Tetracaine
(LYE doe kane & TET ra kane)

Brand Names: US Pliaglis; Synera

Index Terms Eutectic Mixture of Lidocaine and Tetracaine; Tetracaine and Lidocaine

Pharmacologic Category Analgesic, Topical; Local Anesthetic

Use

Cream: For use on intact skin in adults to provide topical local analgesia for superficial dermatological procedures.

Patch: For use on intact skin in patients ≥3 years to provide local analgesia for superficial venous access and superficial dermatological procedures.

Dosing

Adult & Geriatric Anesthesia, topical:

Cream: Superficial dermatological procedures: Prior to procedure, apply to intact skin for 20 to 60 minutes. Amount of cream varies depending on size of the surface area to be treated; see manufacturer's labeling for detailed information.

Patch:

Venipuncture or intravenous cannulation: Prior to procedure, apply to intact skin for 20 to 30 minutes; **Note:** May use another patch at a new location to facilitate venous access after a failed attempt; remove previous patch.

Superficial dermatological procedures: Prior to procedure, apply to intact skin for 30 minutes

Pediatric Anesthesia, topical: Children ≥3 years and Adolescents: Patch: Refer to adult dosing.

Renal Impairment There are no dosage adjustments provided in the manufacturer's labeling. Lidocaine primarily undergoes hepatic metabolism and its pharmacokinetics are not expected to be changed significantly following topical administration of recommended doses in renal impairment.

Hepatic Impairment There are no dosage adjustments provided in the manufacturer's labeling (has not been studied). Use caution in patients with severe hepatic dysfunction.

Additional Information Complete prescribing information should be consulted for additional detail.

Dosage Forms Excipient information presented when available (limited, particularly for generics); consult specific product labeling.

Cream, external:

Pliaglis: Lidocaine 7% and tetracaine 7% (30 g, 100 g) [contains methylparaben, propylparaben]

Generic: Lidocaine 7% and tetracaine 7% (30 g)

Patch, transdermal:

Synera: Lidocaine 70 mg and tetracaine 70 mg (10s) [contains heating component, metal; each patch is ~50 cm^2]

Linaclotide (lin AK loe tide)

Brand Names: US Linzess

Brand Names: Canada Constella

Index Terms Linaclotide Acetate

Pharmacologic Category Gastrointestinal Agent, Miscellaneous

Use

Chronic idiopathic constipation: Treatment of chronic idiopathic constipation (CIC) in adults

◄

Irritable bowel syndrome with constipation: Treatment of irritable bowel syndrome with constipation (IBS-C) in adults

Pregnancy Considerations Adverse events were observed in some animal reproduction studies. Linaclotide and its metabolite are not measurable in plasma when used at recommended doses.

Breast-Feeding Considerations It is not known if linaclotide is excreted in breast milk; linaclotide and its metabolite are not measurable in plasma when used at recommended doses. The manufacturer recommends to use caution if administered to breast-feeding women.

Medication Guide Available Yes

Contraindications

Use in pediatric patients <6 years of age; known or suspected mechanical gastrointestinal obstruction

Canadian labeling: Additional contraindications (not in U.S. labeling): Hypersensitivity to linaclotide or any component of the formulation

Warnings/Precautions [US Boxed Warning]: Use is contraindicated in pediatric patients <6 years of age. Use in pediatric patients 6 to 17 years of age should be avoided. Deaths due to dehydration were observed in young juvenile animals during nonclinical studies; deaths were not observed in older juvenile animals. There are not sufficient safety and efficacy data to support use in pediatric patients. May cause diarrhea. Patients should be instructed to discontinue use and contact their health care provider if severe diarrhea occurs. Administration with a high-fat meal may worsen diarrhea.

Adverse Reactions Adverse reactions reported with use in IBS-C and CIC.

>10%: Gastrointestinal: Diarrhea (16% to 20%; severe diarrhea: 2%)

1% to 10%:

Central nervous system: Headache (4%), fatigue (<2%)

Endocrine & metabolic: Dehydration (≤1%)

Gastrointestinal: Abdominal pain (7%), flatulence (4% to 6%), abdominal distension (2% to 3%), viral gastroenteritis (≤3%), dyspepsia (<2%), fecal incontinence (<2%), gastroesophageal reflux disease (<2%), vomiting (<2%)

Respiratory: Upper respiratory tract infection (5%), sinusitis (3%)

<1% (Limited to important or life-threatening): Hematochezia, hypersensitivity reaction, rectal hemorrhage

Drug Interactions

Metabolism/Transport Effects None known.

Avoid Concomitant Use There are no known interactions where it is recommended to avoid concomitant use.

Increased Effect/Toxicity There are no known significant interactions involving an increase in effect.

Decreased Effect There are no known significant interactions involving a decrease in effect.

Storage/Stability Store at 25°C (77°F) in tightly closed, original container with included desiccant packet; excursions permitted between 15°C and 30°C (59°F and 86°F). Do not subdivide or repackage; protect from moisture.

Mechanism of Action Linaclotide and its active metabolite bind and agonize guanylate cyclase-C on the luminal surface of intestinal epithelium. Intracellular and extracellular cyclic guanosine monophosphate (cGMP) concentrations are subsequently increased resulting in chloride and bicarbonate secretion into the intestinal lumen. Intestinal fluid increases and GI transit time is decreased. Increased extracellular cGMP may decrease visceral pain by reducing pain-sensing nerve activity.

Pharmacodynamics/Kinetics

Absorption: Minimal systemic availability; plasma concentrations are not measurable when used at recommended doses.

Distribution: Minimal tissue distribution is expected given immeasurable plasma concentrations when used at recommended doses.

Metabolism: Metabolized within GI tract to active metabolite; parent drug and metabolite undergo proteolytic degradation within the intestinal lumen to smaller peptides and amino acids

Excretion: Primarily feces (3% to 5%; as the active metabolite)

Dosing

Adult

Chronic idiopathic constipation (CIC): Oral: 145 mcg once daily

Irritable bowel syndrome with constipation (IBS-C): Oral: 290 mcg once daily

Geriatric Not adequately studied in the elderly. Refer to adult dosing.

Renal Impairment No dosage adjustment necessary.

Hepatic Impairment No dosage adjustment necessary.

Dietary Considerations Administer at least 30 minutes before the first meal of the day on an empty stomach. Loose stools and greater stool frequency may occur after administration with a high-fat breakfast.

Administration

Oral:

Administer at least 30 minutes before the first meal of the day on an empty stomach; loose stools and greater stool frequency may occur after administration with a high-fat breakfast. Swallow capsule whole; do not break, crush, or chew capsules or capsule contents.

For patients with swallowing difficulties, the capsule may be opened and the entire contents (beads) sprinkled on 1 teaspoonful of room temperature applesauce or into 30 mL of room temperature bottled water. For administration on applesauce, consume the entire contents immediately; do not chew the beads. For administration in water, gently swirl beads and water for at least 10 seconds and swallow immediately; add another 30 mL of water to any remaining beads in cup, swirl for 10 seconds, and swallow immediately. Do not store the applesauce or water-bead mixture for future use. **Note:** The drug is coated on surface of beads and will dissolve off the beads in water; beads will remain visible and will not dissolve; therefore not necessary to consume all the beads to deliver complete dose.

Gastric/nasogastric feeding tube: Open capsule and empty entire contents (beads) into 30 mL of room temperature bottled water; gently mix by swirling beads for at least 10 seconds; draw up bead and water mixture with catheter syringe and apply rapid and steady pressure (10 mL per 10 seconds) to dispense the bead-water mixture into the tube. Flush nasogastric/gastric tube with a minimum of 10 mL of water after administration. Note: Not necessary to flush all the beads through tube to deliver complete dose.

After administration of linaclotide in applesauce or water, the first meal of the day may be consumed 30 minutes later.

Monitoring Parameters

IBS-C: Abdominal pain, spontaneous bowel movement quality and frequency

CIC: Frequency of straining during bowel movements; spontaneous bowel movement quality and frequency

Dosage Forms Excipient information presented when available (limited, particularly for generics); consult specific product labeling.

Capsule, Oral:

Linzess: 145 mcg, 290 mcg

◆ Linaclotide Acetate *see* Linaclotide *on page* 1077

Linagliptin (lin a GLIP tin)

Brand Names: US Tradjenta

Brand Names: Canada Trajenta

Index Terms BI-1356; Trajenta

Pharmacologic Category Antidiabetic Agent, Dipeptidyl Peptidase IV (DPP-IV) Inhibitor

Use Type 2 diabetes mellitus: As an adjunct to diet and exercise to improve glycemic control in adults with type 2 diabetes (noninsulin dependent, NIDDM) as monotherapy or in combination with other antidiabetic agents

Pregnancy Considerations Adverse events were not observed in animal reproduction studies, except with doses that were also maternally toxic.

In women with diabetes, maternal hyperglycemia can be associated with congenital malformations as well as adverse effects in the fetus, neonate, and the mother (ACOG 2005; ADA 2015; Kitzmiller 2008; Metzger 2007). To prevent adverse outcomes, prior to conception and throughout pregnancy maternal blood glucose and HbA$_{1c}$ should be kept as close to target goals as possible but without causing significant hypoglycemia (ACOG 2013; ADA 2015; Blumer 2013; Kitzmiller 2008). Prior to pregnancy, effective contraception should be used until glycemic control is achieved (Kitzmiller 2008). Other agents are currently recommended to treat diabetes in pregnant women (ACOG 2013; Blumer 2013).

Breast-Feeding Considerations It is not known if linagliptin is excreted in breast milk. The manufacturer recommends that caution be used if administered to breast-feeding women.

Medication Guide Available Yes

Contraindications

Hypersensitivity (eg, anaphylaxis, angioedema, exfoliative skin conditions, urticaria, or bronchial hyperreactivity) to linagliptin or any component of the formulation

Canadian labeling: Additional contraindications: Use in type 1 diabetes mellitus or diabetic ketoacidosis

Warnings/Precautions Severe and disabling arthralgia has been reported with DPP-IV inhibitor use; onset may occur within one day to years after treatment initiation and may resolve with discontinuation of therapy. Some patients may experience a recurrence of symptoms if DPP-IV inhibitor therapy resumed. Avoid use in type 1 diabetes mellitus (insulin dependent, IDDM) and diabetic ketoacidosis (DKA) due to lack of efficacy in these populations. Diabetes self-management education (DSME) is essential to maximize the effectiveness of therapy. Cases of acute pancreatitis, including fatalities, have been reported with use. Monitor for signs/symptoms of pancreatitis; discontinue use immediately if pancreatitis is suspected and initiate appropriate management. Use with caution in patients with a history of pancreatitis as it is not known if this population is at greater risk. Clinical trials included only a limited number of patients with heart failure (HF). No specific recommendations regarding this population are provided in the approved U.S. labeling (Canadian labeling recommends against use in this population). Potentially significant drug-drug interactions may exist, requiring dose or frequency adjustment, additional monitoring, and/or selection of alternative therapy. Rare hypersensitivity reactions including anaphylaxis, angioedema, and exfoliative skin conditions have been reported in patients treated with linagliptin; discontinue if signs/symptoms of hypersensitivity reactions occur. Events have generally been noted within the first 3 months of therapy, and may occur with the initial dose. Use with caution if patient has experienced angioedema with other DPP-IV inhibitor use.

Adverse Reactions Incidences reported for patients on monotherapy unless otherwise specified

>10%:

Endocrine & metabolic: Hypoglycemia (combination therapy in renal function impairment 63%, combined with metformin and sulfonylurea 23%, monotherapy 4% to 7%), severe hypoglycemia (combination therapy in renal function impairment [life-threatening or requiring hospitalization] 3%, with insulin 2%, with insulin [life-threatening] 1%)

1% to 10%:

Central nervous system: Headache (combination therapy 6%)

Endocrine & metabolic: Increased uric acid (3%), hypertriglyceridemia (combination therapy 2%), weight gain (combination therapy 2%)

Gastrointestinal: Constipation (combination therapy 2%)

Genitourinary: Urinary tract infection (combination therapy 3%)

Neuromuscular & skeletal: Back pain (combination therapy 9%), arthralgia (combination therapy 8%), limb pain (combination therapy 5%)

Respiratory: Nasopharyngitis (7%), cough (monotherapy and combination therapy 2% to 6%)

<1% (Limited to important or life-threatening): Acute pancreatitis, severe arthralgia (FDA Safety Alert, Aug 28, 2015), severe hypersensitivity, stomatitis

Drug Interactions

Metabolism/Transport Effects Substrate of CYP3A4 (major), P-glycoprotein; **Note:** Assignment of Major/Minor substrate status based on clinically relevant drug interaction potential

Avoid Concomitant Use There are no known interactions where it is recommended to avoid concomitant use.

Increased Effect/Toxicity

Linagliptin may increase the levels/effects of: ACE Inhibitors; Hypoglycemia-Associated Agents; Insulin; Sulfonylureas

The levels/effects of Linagliptin may be increased by: Alpha-Lipoic Acid; Androgens; Antihepaciviral Combination Products; MAO Inhibitors; Osimertinib; Pegvisomant; P-glycoprotein/ABCB1 Inhibitors; Quinolone Antibiotics; Ranolazine; Ritonavir; Salicylates; Selective Serotonin Reuptake Inhibitors

Decreased Effect

The levels/effects of Linagliptin may be decreased by: Bosentan; CYP3A4 Inducers (Moderate); CYP3A4 Inducers (Strong); Dabrafenib; Deferasirox; Enzalutamide; Hyperglycemia-Associated Agents; Mitotane; Osimertinib; P-glycoprotein/ABCB1 Inducers; Quinolone Antibiotics; Siltuximab; St Johns Wort; Thiazide Diuretics; Tocilizumab

Storage/Stability Store at 25°C (77°F); excursions permitted between 15°C to 30°C (59°F to 86°F).

Mechanism of Action Linagliptin inhibits dipeptidyl peptidase IV (DPP-IV) enzyme resulting in prolonged active incretin levels. Incretin hormones (eg, glucagon-like peptide-1 [GLP-1] and glucose-dependent insulinotropic polypeptide [GIP]) regulate glucose homeostasis by increasing insulin synthesis and release from pancreatic beta cells and decreasing glucagon secretion from pancreatic alpha cells. Decreased glucagon secretion results in decreased hepatic glucose production. Under normal physiologic circumstances, incretin hormones are released by the intestine throughout the day and levels are increased in response to a meal; incretin hormones are rapidly inactivated by the DPP-IV enzyme.

Pharmacodynamics/Kinetics

Absorption: Rapid

Distribution: Extensive

Protein binding: 70% to 80%; concentration dependent

Metabolism: Not extensively metabolized

Bioavailability: ~30%

Half-life elimination: Effective (therapeutic): ~12 hours; Terminal (DPP-IV saturable binding): >100 hours

Time to peak: 1.5 hours

Excretion: 80% feces unchanged; 5% urine unchanged

Dosing

Adult & Geriatric Type 2 diabetes: Oral: 5 mg once daily

Concomitant use with insulin and/or insulin secretagogues (eg, sulfonylureas): Reduced dose of insulin and/or insulin secretagogues may be needed.

Renal Impairment No dosage adjustment necessary.

Hepatic Impairment No dosage adjustment necessary. **Note:** Canadian labeling does not recommend use in severe hepatic impairment.

Dietary Considerations Individualized medical nutrition therapy (MNT) based on ADA recommendations is an integral part of therapy.

Administration May be administered with or without food.

Monitoring Parameters HbA$_{1c}$, serum glucose; signs/symptoms of pancreatitis

Reference Range

Recommendations for glycemic control in nonpregnant adults with diabetes (ADA, 2015):

HbA$_{1c}$: <7% (a more aggressive [<6.5%] or less aggressive [<8%] HbA$_{1c}$ goal may be targeted based on patient-specific characteristics)

Preprandial capillary plasma glucose: 80 to 130 mg/dL

Peak postprandial capillary blood glucose: <180 mg/dL

Recommendations for glycemic control in pediatric (all age groups) patients with type 1 diabetes (ADA, 2015):

HbA$_{1c}$: <7.5% (individualization may be appropriate based on patient-specific characteristics; <7% is reasonable if it can be achieved without excessive hypoglycemia)

Preprandial capillary plasma glucose: 90 to 130 mg/dL

Bedtime and overnight capillary blood glucose: 90 to 150 mg/dL

Dosage Forms Excipient information presented when available (limited, particularly for generics); consult specific product labeling.

Tablet, Oral:

Tradjenta: 5 mg

Linagliptin and Metformin
(lin a GLIP tin & met FOR min)

Brand Names: US Jentadueto

Brand Names: Canada Jentadueto

Index Terms Linagliptin and Metformin Hydrochloride; Metformin and Linagliptin; Metformin Hydrochloride and Linagliptin

Pharmacologic Category Antidiabetic Agent, Biguanide; Antidiabetic Agent, Dipeptidyl Peptidase IV (DPP-IV) Inhibitor

Use Diabetes mellitus type 2: As an adjunct to diet and exercise to improve glycemic control in adults with type 2 diabetes mellitus (noninsulin dependent, NIDDM) when treatment with both linagliptin and metformin is appropriate.

Medication Guide Available Yes

Dosing

Adult

Type 2 diabetes mellitus: Oral: Initial doses should be based on current dose of linagliptin and metformin.

Patients currently on metformin: Initial dose: Linagliptin 5 mg daily plus current daily dose of metformin given in 2 equally divided doses; maximum: linagliptin 5 mg/metformin 2000 mg daily.

Patients not on metformin: Initial dose: Linagliptin 5 mg daily plus metformin 1000 mg daily given in 2 equally divided doses; maximum: linagliptin 5 mg/metformin 2000 mg daily.

Concomitant use with insulin and/or insulin secretagogues (eg, sulfonylureas): Reduced dose of insulin and/or insulin secretagogues may be needed.

Dosing adjustment: Metformin component may be gradually increased up to the maximum dose. Maximum dose: Linagliptin 5 mg/metformin 2000 mg daily

Geriatric Refer to adult dosing. The initial and maintenance dosing should be conservative, due to the potential for decreased renal function (monitor). Do not use in patients ≥80 years of age unless normal renal function has been established.

Renal Impairment

Manufacturer's labeling:

Serum creatinine (SCr) ≥1.5 mg/dL (males) or ≥1.4 mg/dL (females): Use is contraindicated.

Abnormal CrCl (US labeling: Not defined; Canadian labeling: <60 mL/minute): Use is contraindicated.

Alternate recommendations: **Note:** The United Kingdom National Institute for Health and Clinical Excellence (NICE) Guidelines recommend prescribing metformin with caution in those patients who are at risk of sudden deterioration in renal function and at risk of an estimated glomerular filtration rate (eGFR) <45 mL/minute/1.73 m^2 (NICE, 2008]). Some evidence suggests that use of metformin is unsafe when eGFR <30 mL/minute/1.73 m^2 (calculated using MDRD) (Shaw, 2007). A review of the available data by members of the American Diabetes Association proposed the following recommendations based on eGFR (Lipska, 2011):

eGFR ≥60 mL/minute/1.73 m^2: No contraindications, monitor renal function annually

eGFR ≥45 to <60 mL/minute/1.73 m^2: Continue use; monitor renal function every 3 to 6 months

eGFR ≥30 to <45 mL/minute/1.73 m^2: In patients currently receiving metformin, use with caution, consider dosage reduction (eg, 50% reduction or 50% of maximal dose), monitor renal function every 3 months. Do not initiate therapy in patients with eGFR <45 mL/minute/1.73 m^2

eGFR <30 mL/minute/1.73 m^2: Discontinue use

Hepatic Impairment The manufacturer recommends avoiding metformin since liver disease is considered a risk factor for the development of lactic acidosis during metformin therapy. However, continued use of metformin in diabetics with liver dysfunction, including cirrhosis, has been used successfully and may be associated with a survival benefit in carefully selected patients; use cautiously in patients at risk for lactic acidosis (eg, renal impairment, alcohol use) (Brackett, 2010; Zhang, 2014).

Additional Information Complete prescribing information should be consulted for additional detail.

Dosage Forms Excipient information presented when available (limited, particularly for generics); consult specific product labeling.

Tablet, oral:

Jentadueto 2.5/500: Linagliptin 2.5 mg and metformin hydrochloride 500 mg

Jentadueto 2.5/850: Linagliptin 2.5 mg and metformin hydrochloride 850 mg

Jentadueto 2.5/1000: Linagliptin 2.5 mg and metformin hydrochloride 1000 mg

◆ Linagliptin and Metformin Hydrochloride *see* Linagliptin and Metformin *on page 1079*

Lindane (LIN dane)

Index Terms Benzene Hexachloride; Gamma Benzene Hexachloride; Hexachlorocyclohexane; Kwell

Pharmacologic Category Antiparasitic Agent, Topical; Pediculocide; Scabicidal Agent

Use

Lotion: Treatment of *Sarcoptes scabiei* (scabies)

Shampoo: Treatment of *Pediculus capitis* (head lice) and *Phthirus pubis* (crab lice)

Note: Not recommended for first line-treatment; use should be reserved for patients who are intolerant to or have failed first-line agents.

Medication Guide Available Yes

Dosing

Adult & Geriatric

Scabies: Topical: Apply a thin layer of lotion and massage it on skin from the neck to the toes; after 8-12 hours, bathe and remove the drug; most patients will require 30 mL; larger adults may require up to 60 mL. Do not re-treat. Do not leave on for more than 12 hours.

Head lice, crab lice: Topical: Apply shampoo to dry hair and massage into hair for 4 minutes; add small quantities of water to hair until lather forms, then rinse hair thoroughly and comb with a fine tooth comb to remove nits. Amount of shampoo needed is based on length and density of hair; most patients will require 30 mL (maximum: 60 mL). Do not re-treat.

Pediatric Infants, Children, and Adolescents: Refer to adult dosing.

Additional Information Complete prescribing information should be consulted for additional detail.

Dosage Forms Excipient information presented when available (limited, particularly for generics); consult specific product labeling.

Lotion, External:

Generic: 1% (60 mL)

Shampoo, External:

Generic: 1% (60 mL)

◆ Linessa (Can) *see* Ethinyl Estradiol and Desogestrel *on page 701*

Linezolid (li NE zoh lid)

Brand Names: US Zyvox

Brand Names: Canada Apo-Linezolid; Linezolid Injection; Sandoz-Linezolid; Zyvoxam

Pharmacologic Category Antibiotic, Oxazolidinone

Use

Enterococcal infections, vancomycin-resistant: Treatment of vancomycin-resistant *Enterococcus faecium* infections, including cases with concurrent bacteremia.

Pneumonia:

Community-acquired: Treatment of community-acquired pneumonia caused by *Streptococcus pneumoniae*, including cases with concurrent bacteremia, or *Staphylococcus aureus* (methicillin-susceptible isolates only).

Hospital-acquired or healthcare-associated: Treatment of hospital-acquired or healthcare-associated pneumonia caused by *S. aureus* (methicillin-susceptible and -resistant isolates), or *S. pneumoniae.*

Skin and skin structure infections:

Complicated: Treatment of complicated skin and skin structure infections, including diabetic foot infections, without concomitant osteomyelitis, caused by *S. aureus* (methicillin-susceptible and -resistant isolates), *Streptococcus pyogenes*, or *Streptococcus agalactiae.*

Uncomplicated: Treatment of uncomplicated skin and skin structure infections caused by *S. aureus* (methicillin-susceptible isolates) or *S. pyogenes.*

Limitations of use: Linezolid has not been studied in the treatment of decubitus ulcers. Linezolid is not indicated for treatment of gram-negative infections; if a concomitant gram-negative pathogen is documented or suspected, initiate specific therapy immediately.

Pregnancy Considerations Adverse effects were observed in some animal reproduction studies at doses that were also maternally toxic. Information related to linezolid use during pregnancy is limited.

Breast-Feeding Considerations Linezolid is excreted into breast milk. The manufacturer advises caution if administering linezolid to a breast-feeding woman. Non-dose-related effects could include modification of bowel flora.

Contraindications Hypersensitivity to linezolid or any component of the formulation; concurrent use or within 2 weeks of MAO inhibitors

Warnings/Precautions Myelosuppression has been reported and may be dependent on duration of therapy (generally >2 weeks of treatment); use with caution in patients with preexisting myelosuppression, in patients receiving other drugs which may cause bone marrow suppression, or in chronic infection (previous or concurrent antibiotic therapy). Weekly CBC monitoring is recommended. Consider discontinuation in patients developing myelosuppression (or in whom myelosuppression worsens during treatment).

Lactic acidosis has been reported with use. Use with caution and monitor closely in patients with uncontrolled hypertension, pheochromocytoma, carcinoid syndrome, or untreated hyperthyroidism; do not use in the absence of close monitoring. Hypoglycemic episodes have been reported; use with caution and closely monitor glucose in diabetic patients. Dose reductions/discontinuation of concurrent hypoglycemic agents or discontinuation of linezolid may be required. Potentially significant interactions may exist, requiring dose or frequency adjustment, additional monitoring, and/or selection of alternative therapy. Symptoms of agitation, confusion, hallucinations, hyper-reflexia, myoclonus, shivering, and tachycardia may occur with concomitant proserotonergic drugs, agents which reduce linezolid's metabolism, or in patients with carcinoid syndrome. Avoid use in such patients unless clinically appropriate and under close monitoring for signs/symptoms of serotonin syndrome or neuroleptic malignant syndrome-like reactions. Unnecessary use may lead to the development of resistance to linezolid; consider alternatives before initiating outpatient treatment.

Peripheral and optic neuropathy (with vision loss) has been reported in adults and children and may occur primarily with extended courses of therapy >28 days; any

symptoms of visual change or impairment warrant immediate ophthalmic evaluation and possible discontinuation of therapy. Seizures have been reported; use with caution in patients with a history of seizures. Prolonged use may result in fungal or bacterial superinfection, including *C. difficile*-associated diarrhea (CDAD) and pseudomembranous colitis; CDAD has been observed >2 months post-antibiotic treatment.

The manufacturer does not recommend the use of linezolid for empiric treatment of pediatric CNS infections since therapeutic linezolid concentrations are not consistently achieved or maintained in the CSF of patients with ventriculoperitoneal shunts. However, limited data in the form of case reports in pediatric and adult patients suggest that linezolid may be useful in treating gram-positive CNS infections that have failed to respond to other treatment options describing successful treatment of documented VRE and *Staphylococcus aureus* CNS and shunt infections in the literature (Cook 2005; da Silva 2007; Milstone 2007; Shaikh 2001; Villani 2002). Linezolid should not be used in the empiric treatment of catheter-related bloodstream infection (CRBSI), but may be appropriate for targeted therapy (Mermel 2009).

Benzyl alcohol and derivatives: Some dosage forms may contain sodium benzoate/benzoic acid; benzoic acid (benzoate) is a metabolite of benzyl alcohol; large amounts of benzyl alcohol (≥99 mg/kg/day) have been associated with a potentially fatal toxicity ("gasping syndrome") in neonates; the "gasping syndrome" consists of metabolic acidosis, respiratory distress, gasping respirations, CNS dysfunction (including convulsions, intracranial hemorrhage), hypotension, and cardiovascular collapse (AAP ["Inactive" 1997]; CDC, 1982); some data suggests that benzoate displaces bilirubin from protein binding sites (Ahlfors 2001); avoid or use dosage forms containing benzyl alcohol derivative with caution in neonates. See manufacturer's labeling.

Some products may contain phenylalanine.

Adverse Reactions Percentages as reported in adults; frequency similar in pediatric patients unless otherwise noted.

>10%:
Central nervous system: Headache (<1% to 11%)
Gastrointestinal: Diarrhea (3% to 11%)
Hematologic & oncologic: Decreased hemoglobin (1% to 16%), thrombocytopenia (<1% to 13%), leukopenia (children 1% to 12%; adults <1% to 2%)

1% to 10%:
Central nervous system: Insomnia (3%), dizziness (≤3%), vertigo (children 1%)
Dermatologic: Skin rash (1% to 2%), pruritus (children 1%)
Endocrine & metabolic: Increased amylase (<1% to 2%), increased lactate dehydrogenase (<1% to 2%)
Gastrointestinal: Nausea (1% to 10%), vomiting (1% to 9%), increased serum lipase (3% to 4%), constipation (2%), dysgeusia (1% to 2%), loose stools (children 1% to 2%), oral candidiasis (1% to 2%), abdominal pain (≤2%), tongue discoloration (≤1%), pancreatitis
Genitourinary: Vulvovaginal candidiasis (1% to 2%)
Hematologic & oncologic: Neutropenia (children 1% to 6%; adults ≤1%), anemia (children ≤6%; adults ≤2%), eosinophilia (children ≤2%)
Hepatic: Increased serum ALT (≤10%), increased serum bilirubin (children ≤6%; adults ≤1%), increased serum AST (adults 2% to 5%), increased serum alkaline phosphatase (<1% to 4%), abnormal hepatic function tests (≤2%)
Infection: Fungal infection (≤1% to 2%)
Renal: Increased blood urea nitrogen (≤2%), increased serum creatinine (<1% to 2%)
Miscellaneous: Fever (2%)

<1% (Limited to important or life-threatening): Anaphylaxis, angioedema, bullous skin disease, *Clostridium difficile*-associated diarrhea, convulsions, hypertension, hypoglycemia, lactic acidosis, optic neuropathy, pancytopenia, peripheral neuropathy, rhabdomyolysis, seizures, serotonin syndrome (with concurrent use of other serotonergic agents), Stevens-Johnson syndrome, vision loss

Drug Interactions

Metabolism/Transport Effects Inhibits Monoamine Oxidase

Avoid Concomitant Use

Avoid concomitant use of Linezolid with any of the following: Alcohol (Ethyl); Anilidopiperidine Opioids; Apraclonidine; AtoMOXetine; Atropine (Ophthalmic); BCG (Intravesical); Bezafibrate; Buprenorphine; BuPROPion; BusPIRone; CarBAMazepine; Cyclobenzaprine; Cyproheptadine; Dapoxetine; Deferiprone; Dexmethylphenidate; Dextromethorphan; Diethylpropion; Dipyrone; EPINEPHrine (Oral Inhalation); HYDROmorphone;

Isometheptene; Levonordefrin; MAO Inhibitors; Maprotiline; Meperidine; Mequitazine; Methyldopa; Methylene Blue; Methylphenidate; Mianserin; Mirtazapine; Moclobemide; Morphine (Liposomal); Morphine (Systemic); Nefazodone; Oxymorphone; Pholcodine; Pizotifen; Selective Serotonin Reuptake Inhibitors; Serotonin 5-HT1D Receptor Agonists; Serotonin/Norepinephrine Reuptake Inhibitors; Tapentadol; Tetrabenazine; Tetrahydrozoline (Nasal); Tianeptine; TraZODone; Tricyclic Antidepressants; Tryptophan

Increased Effect/Toxicity

Linezolid may increase the levels/effects of: Antipsychotic Agents; Apraclonidine; AtoMOXetine; Atropine (Ophthalmic); Betahistine; Bezafibrate; Blood Glucose Lowering Agents; Brimonidine (Ophthalmic); Brimonidine (Topical); BuPROPion; CloZAPine; Cyproheptadine; Deferiprone; Dexmethylphenidate; Dextromethorphan; Diethylpropion; Domperidone; EPINEPHrine (Oral Inhalation); Epinephrine (Racemic); Hydrocodone; HYDROmorphone; Isometheptene; Levonordefrin; Lithium; Meperidine; Mequitazine; Methadone; Methyldopa; Methylene Blue; Methylphenidate; Metoclopramide; Mianserin; Mirtazapine; Moclobemide; Morphine (Liposomal); Morphine (Systemic); Nefazodone; OxyCODONE; Pizotifen; Reserpine; Selective Serotonin Reuptake Inhibitors; Serotonin 5-HT1D Receptor Agonists; Serotonin Modulators; Serotonin/Norepinephrine Reuptake Inhibitors; Sympathomimetics; Tetrahydrozoline (Nasal); TraZODone; Tricyclic Antidepressants

The levels/effects of Linezolid may be increased by: Alcohol (Ethyl); Anilidopiperidine Opioids; Antiemetics (5HT3 Antagonists); Antipsychotic Agents; Buprenorphine; BusPIRone; CarBAMazepine; COMT Inhibitors; Cyclobenzaprine; Dapoxetine; Dipyrone; Levodopa; MAO Inhibitors; Maprotiline; Metaxalone; Oxymorphone; Pholcodine; Tapentadol; Tetrabenazine; Tianeptine; TraMADol; Tryptophan

Decreased Effect

Linezolid may decrease the levels/effects of: BCG (Intravesical); BCG Vaccine (Immunization); Domperidone; Sodium Picosulfate; Typhoid Vaccine

The levels/effects of Linezolid may be decreased by: Cyproheptadine; Domperidone

Food Interactions Concurrent ingestion of foods rich in tyramine, dopamine, tyrosine, phenylalanine, tryptophan, or caffeine may cause sudden and severe high blood pressure (hypertensive crisis or serotonin syndrome). Beverages containing tyramine (eg, hearty red wine and beer) may increase toxic effects. Management: Avoid tyramine-containing foods (aged or matured cheese, air-dried or cured meats including sausages and salamis; fava or broad bean pods, tap/draft beers, Marmite concentrate, sauerkraut, soy sauce, and other soybean condiments). Food's freshness is also an important concern; improperly stored or spoiled food can create an environment in which tyramine concentrations may increase. Avoid foods containing dopamine, tyrosine, phenylalanine, tryptophan, or caffeine. Avoid beverages containing tyramine.

Preparation for Administration Oral suspension: Refer to manufacturer's product labeling for reconstitution instructions. Prior to administration mix gently by inverting bottle; do not shake.

Storage/Stability

Infusion: Store at 25°C (77°F). Protect from light and freezing. Keep infusion bags in overwrap until ready for use.

Oral suspension: Store at 25°C (77°F); following reconstitution store at room temperature and use suspension within 21 days. Protect from light.

Tablet: Store at 25°C (77°F). Protect from light and moisture.

Mechanism of Action Inhibits bacterial protein synthesis by binding to bacterial 23S ribosomal RNA of the 50S subunit. This prevents the formation of a functional 70S initiation complex that is essential for the bacterial translation process. Linezolid is bacteriostatic against enterococci and staphylococci and bactericidal against most strains of streptococci.

Pharmacodynamics/Kinetics

Absorption: Rapid and extensive

Distribution: V_{dss}: Adults: 40 to 50 L

Protein binding: Adults: 31%

Metabolism: Hepatic via oxidation of the morpholine ring, resulting in two inactive metabolites (aminoethoxyacetic acid, hydroxyethyl glycine); minimally metabolized, may be mediated by cytochrome P450

Bioavailability: Oral: ~100%

Half-life elimination: Children ≥1 week (full-term) to 11 years: 1.5 to 3 hours; Adults: 4 to 5 hours

Time to peak: Adults: Oral: 1 to 2 hours

Excretion: Urine (~30% of total dose as parent drug, ~50% of total dose as metabolites); feces (~9% of total dose as metabolites)

Nonrenal clearance: Adults: ~65%

Dosing

Adult & Geriatric

Usual dosage: Oral, IV: 600 mg every 12 hours

Indication-specific dosing:

Enterococcal infections, vancomycin-resistant, including concurrent bacteremia: Oral, IV: 600 mg every 12 hours for 14 to 28 days

Pneumonia:

Community-acquired (CAP):

Manufacturer's labeling (includes concurrent bacteremia): Oral, IV: 600 mg every 12 hours for 10 to 14 days.

Alternate dosing (Liu 2011): Oral, IV: S. aureus (methicillin-resistant): 600 mg every 12 hours for 7 to 21 days

Hospital-acquired or healthcare-associated:

Manufacturer's labeling: Oral, IV: 600 mg every 12 hours for 10 to 14 days.

Note: May consider 7-day treatment course (versus manufacturer recommended 10 to 14 days) in patients with healthcare-, hospital-, and ventilator-associated pneumonia who have demonstrated good clinical response (ATS/IDSA 2005).

Alternate dosing (Liu 2011): Oral, IV: S. aureus (methicillin-resistant): 600 mg every 12 hours for 7 to 21 days

Skin and skin structure infections, complicated: Oral, IV: 600 mg every 12 hours for 10 to 14 days. **Note:** For diabetic foot infections, initial treatment duration is up to 4 weeks depending on severity of infection and response to therapy (Lipsky 2012).

Skin and skin structure infections, uncomplicated: Oral: 400 mg every 12 hours for 10 to 14 days. **Note:** 400 mg dose is recommended in the product labeling; however, 600 mg dose is commonly employed clinically; consider 5- to 10-day treatment course as opposed to the manufacturer recommended 10 to 14 days (Liu 2011; Stevens 2014). For diabetic foot infections, may extend treatment duration up to 4 weeks if slow to resolve (Lipsky 2012).

Brain abscess, subdural empyema, spinal epidural abscess (*S. aureus* [methicillin-resistant]) (off-label use) (Liu 2011): Oral, IV: 600 mg every 12 hours for 4 to 6 weeks

Meningitis (*S. aureus* [methicillin-resistant]) (off-label use) (Liu 2011): Oral, IV: 600 mg every 12 hours for 2 weeks

Osteomyelitis (*S. aureus* [methicillin-resistant]) (off-label use) (Liu 2011): Oral, IV: 600 mg every 12 hours for a minimum of 8 weeks (some experts combine with rifampin)

Prosthetic joint infection (off-label use):

Enterococcus spp (penicillin-susceptible or -resistant) (alternative treatment): Oral, IV: 600 mg every 12 hours for 4 to 6 weeks (consider adding an aminoglycoside) followed by an oral antibiotic suppressive regimen (Osmon 2013)

Staphylococci (oxacillin-sensitive or -resistant) (alternative treatment): Oral, IV: 600 mg every 12 hours for 2 to 6 weeks used in combination with rifampin followed by oral antibiotic treatment and suppressive regimens (Osmon 2013)

Septic arthritis (*S. aureus* [methicillin-resistant]) (off-label use) (Liu 2011): Oral, IV: 600 mg every 12 hours for 3 to 4 weeks

Septic thrombosis of cavernous or dural venous sinus (*S. aureus* [methicillin-resistant]) (off-label use) (Liu 2011): Oral, IV: 600 mg every 12 hours for 4 to 6 weeks

Pediatric

Usual dosage: Oral, IV:

Children ≤11 years: 10 mg/kg (maximum: 600 mg/dose) every 8 hours

Children ≥12 years and Adolescents: Refer to adult dosing.

Indication-specific dosing:

Enterococcal infections, vancomycin-resistant, including concurrent bacteremia: Oral, IV:

Infants and Children ≤11 years: 10 mg/kg every 8 hours for 14 to 28 days

Children ≥12 years and Adolescents: Refer to adult dosing.

Pneumonia:

Community-acquired (CAP):

Manufacturer's labeling (includes concurrent bacteremia): Oral, IV:

Infants and Children ≤11 years: 10 mg/kg/dose every 8 hours for 10 to 14 days

Children ≥12 years and Adolescents: Refer to adult dosing.

Alternate dosing:

Infants >3 months and Children ≤11 years (IDSA/PIDS 2011):

S. pneumoniae (MICs to penicillin ≤2.0 mcg/mL), mild infection or step-down therapy (alternative to amoxicillin): Oral: 10 mg/kg/dose every 8 hours

S. pneumoniae (MICs to penicillin ≥4.0 mcg/mL):

Severe infection (alternative to ceftriaxone): IV: 10 mg/kg/dose every 8 hours

Mild infection, step-down therapy (preferred): Oral: 10 mg/kg/dose every 8 hours

S. aureus (methicillin-resistant/clindamycin-susceptible):

Severe infection (alternative to vancomycin or clindamycin): IV: 10 mg/kg/dose every 8 hours

Mild infection, step-down therapy (alternative to clindamycin): Oral: 10 mg/kg/dose every 8 hours

S. aureus (methicillin- and clindamycin-resistant):

Severe infection (alternative to vancomycin): IV: 10 mg/kg/dose every 8 hours

Mild infection, step-down therapy (preferred): Oral: 10 mg/kg/dose every 8 hours

Children ≤11 years (Liu 2011): Oral, IV: S. aureus (methicillin-resistant): 10 mg/kg/dose every 8 hours for 7 to 21 days (maximum: 600 mg/dose)

Children ≥12 years and Adolescents (IDSA/PIDS 2011):

S. pneumoniae (MICs to penicillin ≤2.0 mcg/mL), mild infection or step-down therapy (alternative to amoxicillin): Oral: 10 mg/kg/dose every 12 hours

S. pneumoniae (MICs to penicillin ≥4.0 mcg/mL)

Severe infection (alternative to ceftriaxone): IV: 10 mg/kg/dose every 12 hours

Mild infection, step-down therapy (preferred): Oral: 10 mg/kg/dose every 12 hours

S. aureus (methicillin-resistant/clindamycin-susceptible):

Severe infection (alternative to vancomycin/clindamycin): IV: 10 mg/kg/dose every 12 hours

Mild infection, step-down therapy (alternative to clindamycin): Oral: 10 mg/kg/dose every 12 hours

S. aureus (methicillin- and clindamycin-resistant):

Severe infection (alternative to vancomycin): IV: 10 mg/kg/dose every 12 hours

Mild infection, step-down therapy (preferred): Oral: 10 mg/kg/dose every 12 hours

Children ≥12 years and Adolescents (Liu 2011): S. aureus (methicillin-resistant): Refer to adult dosing.

Hospital-acquired or healthcare-associated: Oral, IV:

Manufacturer's labeling:

Infants and Children ≤11 years: 10 mg/kg every 8 hours for 10 to 14 days

Children ≥12 years and Adolescents: Refer to adult dosing.

Note: May consider 7-day treatment course (versus manufacturer recommended 10 to 14 days) in patients with healthcare-, hospital-, and ventilator-associated pneumonia who have demonstrated good clinical response (ATS/IDSA 2005).

Alternate dosing (Liu 2011): S. aureus (methicillin-resistant):

Infants and Children ≤11 years: 10 mg/kg/dose every 8 hours for 7 to 21 days (maximum: 600 mg/dose)

Children ≥12 years and Adolescents: Refer to adult dosing.

Skin and skin structure infections, complicated: Oral, IV:

Infants and Children ≤11 years: 10 mg/kg every 8 hours for 10 to 14 days

Children ≥12 years and Adolescents: Refer to adult dosing.

Skin and skin structure infections, uncomplicated: Oral:

Infants and Children <5 years: 10 mg/kg every 8 hours for 10 to 14 days

Children 5 to 11 years: 10 mg/kg every 12 hours for 10 to 14 days

Children ≥12 years and Adolescents: 600 mg every 12 hours for 10 to 14 days

Brain abscess, subdural empyema, spinal epidural abscess (S. aureus [methicillin-resistant]) (off-label use) (Liu 2011): Oral, IV: **Note:** The manufacturer does not recommend the use of linezolid for empiric treatment of pediatric CNS infections since therapeutic linezolid concentrations are not consistently achieved or maintained in the CSF of patients with ventriculoperitoneal shunts.

Children ≤11 years: 10 mg/kg every 8 hours for 4 to 6 weeks (maximum: 600 mg/dose)

Children ≥12 years and Adolescents: Refer to adult dosing.

Meningitis (S. aureus [methicillin-resistant]) (off-label use) (Liu 2011): Oral, IV:

Infants and Children ≤11 years: 10 mg/kg every 8 hours for 2 weeks (maximum: 600 mg/dose)

Children ≥12 years and Adolescents: Refer to adult dosing.

Osteomyelitis (S. aureus [methicillin-resistant]) (off-label use) (Liu 2011): Oral, IV:

Infants and Children ≤11 years: 10 mg/kg every 8 hours for a minimum of 4 to 6 weeks (maximum: 600 mg/dose)

Children ≥12 years and Adolescents: Refer to adult dosing.

Septic arthritis (S. aureus [methicillin-resistant]) (off-label use) (Liu 2011): Oral, IV:

Infants and Children ≤11 years: 10 mg/kg every 8 hours for 3 to 4 weeks (maximum: 600 mg/dose)

Children ≥12 years and Adolescents: Refer to adult dosing.

Septic thrombosis of cavernous or dural venous sinus (S. aureus [methicillin-resistant]) (off-label use) (Liu 2011): Oral, IV:

Children ≤11 years: 10 mg/kg every 8 hours for 4 to 6 weeks (maximum: 600 mg/dose)

Children ≥12 years and Adolescents: Refer to adult dosing.

Renal Impairment

Mild to severe impairment: No dosage adjustment necessary. The two primary metabolites may accumulate in patients with renal impairment but the clinical significance is unknown; use with caution.

End-stage renal disease (ESRD) on intermittent hemodialysis (IHD):

Manufacturer's labeling: Dialyzable (~30% removed during 3-hour dialysis session): Administer after hemodialysis on dialysis days.

Alternate dosing: If administration time is not immediately after dialysis session, may consider administration of a supplemental dose especially early in the treatment course to maintain levels above the MIC (Brier 2003). However, others have recommended no supplemental dose or dosage adjustment for patients on IHD (Heintz 2009; Trotman 2005)

Peritoneal dialysis: No supplemental dose or dosage adjustment needed (Heintz 2009; Trotman 2005)

Continuous renal replacement therapy (eg, CVVHD): No supplemental dose or dosage adjustment needed (Heintz 2009; Trotman 2005)

Hepatic Impairment

Mild to moderate impairment (Child-Pugh class A or B): No dosage adjustment necessary.

Severe impairment (Child-Pugh class C): There are no dosage adjustments provided in the manufacturer's labeling (has not been studied).

Dietary Considerations Some products may contain sodium and/or phenylalanine. Avoid consuming large amounts of tyramine-containing foods/beverages. Some examples include aged or matured cheese, air-dried or cured meats (including sausages and salamis), fava or broad bean pods, tap/draft beers, Marmite concentrate, sauerkraut, soy sauce, and other soybean condiments.

Administration

IV: Administer intravenous infusion over 30 to 120 minutes. Do not mix or infuse with other medications. When the same intravenous line is used for sequential infusion of other medications, flush line with D_5W, NS, or LR before and after infusing linezolid. The yellow color of the injection may intensify over time without affecting potency.

Oral: Administer without regard to meals.

Oral suspension: Invert gently to mix prior to administration, do not shake.

Monitoring Parameters Weekly CBC, particularly in patients at increased risk of bleeding, with preexisting myelosuppression, on concomitant medications that cause bone marrow suppression, in those who require >2 weeks of therapy, or in those with chronic infection who have received previous or concomitant antibiotic therapy; visual function with extended therapy (≥3 months) or in patients with new onset visual symptoms, regardless of therapy

length; in patients with renal impairment, monitor for hematopoietic (eg, anemia, leukopenia, thrombocytopenia) and neuropathic (eg, peripheral neuropathy) adverse events when administering for extended periods.

Dosage Forms Excipient information presented when available (limited, particularly for generics); consult specific product labeling.

Solution, Intravenous:

Zyvox: 2 mg/mL (100 mL, 300 mL)

Generic: 2 mg/mL (300 mL)

Suspension Reconstituted, Oral:

Zyvox: 100 mg/5 mL (150 mL) [orange flavor]

Generic: 100 mg/5 mL (150 mL)

Tablet, Oral:

Zyvox: 600 mg

Generic: 600 mg

◆ Linezolid Injection (Can) *see* Linezolid *on page 1080*

◆ Linzess *see* Linaclotide *on page 1077*

◆ Lioresal *see* Baclofen *on page 197*

◆ Lioresal D.S. (Can) *see* Baclofen *on page 197*

◆ Lioresal Intrathecal (Can) *see* Baclofen *on page 197*

Liothyronine (lye oh THYE roe neen)

Brand Names: US Cytomel; Triostat

Brand Names: Canada Cytomel

Index Terms Liothyronine Sodium; Sodium *L*-Triiodothyronine; T_3 Sodium (error-prone abbreviation)

Pharmacologic Category Thyroid Product

Use

Oral: Replacement or supplemental therapy in hypothyroidism; management of nontoxic goiter; a diagnostic aid

IV: Treatment of myxedema coma/precoma

Dosing

Adult

Hypothyroidism: Oral: 25 mcg/day increase by 12.5 to 25 mcg/day every 1 to 2 weeks to a maximum of 100 mcg/day; usual maintenance dose: 25 to 75 mcg/day Patients with cardiovascular disease: Refer to geriatric dosing.

Suppression test: (T_3): Oral: 75 to 100 mcg/day for 7 days; use lowest dose for elderly

Myxedema: Oral: Initial: 5 mcg/day; increase in increments of 5 to 10 mcg/day every 1 to 2 weeks. When 25 mcg/day is reached, dosage may be increased at intervals of 5 to 25 mcg/day every 1 to 2 weeks. Usual maintenance dose: 50 to 100 mcg/day.

Myxedema coma: IV: 25 to 50 mcg

Patients with known or suspected cardiovascular disease: 10 to 20 mcg

Note: Normally, at least 4 hours should be allowed between doses to adequately assess therapeutic response and no more than 12 hours should elapse between doses to avoid fluctuations in hormone levels. Oral therapy should be resumed as soon as the clinical situation has been stabilized and the patient is able to take oral medication. If levothyroxine rather than liothyronine sodium is used in initiating oral therapy, the prescriber should bear in mind that there is a delay of several days in the onset of levothyroxine activity and that IV therapy should be discontinued gradually.

Simple (nontoxic) goiter: Oral: Initial: 5 mcg/day; increase by 5 to 10 mcg every 1 to 2 weeks; after 25 mcg/day is reached, may increase dose by 12.5 to 25 mcg. Usual maintenance dose: 75 mcg/day.

Antidepressant augmentation (off-label use): Oral: Initial: 25 mcg/day; may be increased to 50 mcg/day after ~1 week based on response and tolerability (APA 2010). Dose ranges of 20 to 62.5 mcg/day have been studied in clinical trials (Altshuler 2001; Aronson, 1996; Nierenberg 2006). **Note:** The duration of treatment has not been well studied (APA 2010; Cooper-Kazaz 2008). If the patient has a history of multiple episodes or significant treatment resistance, long-term maintenance treatment is reasonable if there are no symptoms of hyperthyroidism and no known cardiac disease (Rosenthal 2011).

Cadaveric organ recovery (hormonal resuscitation) (off-label use): IV: Initial: 4 mcg bolus followed by a continuous infusion of 3 mcg/hour administered to the brain-dead donor who is hemodynamically unstable requiring significant vasopressor support; give concomitantly with vasopressin, methylprednisolone, and continuous regular insulin infusion (maintain blood glucose 120 to 180 mg/dL) (Rosendale 2003a; Rosendale 2003b; Rosengard 2002; Zaroff 2002).

Geriatric Oral: 5 mcg/day; increase by 5 mcg/day every 2 weeks

Pediatric Congenital hypothyroidism: Oral: 5 mcg/day increase by 5 mcg every 3 to 4 days until the desired response is achieved. Usual maintenance dose: 20 mcg/day for infants, 50 mcg/day for children 1 to 3 years of age, and adult dose for children >3 years.

Renal Impairment No dosage adjustment provided in manufacturer's labeling.

Hepatic Impairment No dosage adjustment provided in manufacturer's labeling.

Additional Information Complete prescribing information should be consulted for additional detail.

Dosage Forms Excipient information presented when available (limited, particularly for generics); consult specific product labeling.
Solution, Intravenous:
Triostat: 10 mcg/mL (1 mL) [contains alcohol, usp]
Generic: 10 mcg/mL (1 mL)
Tablet, Oral:
Cytomel: 5 mcg
Cytomel: 25 mcg, 50 mcg [scored]
Generic: 5 mcg, 25 mcg, 50 mcg

◆ **Liothyronine and Levothyroxine** see Liotrix on page 1084
◆ **Liothyronine Sodium** see Liothyronine on page 1083

Liotrix (LYE oh triks)

Brand Names: US Thyrolar
Brand Names: Canada Thyrolar
Index Terms Levothyroxine and Liothyronine; Liothyronine and Levothyroxine; T_3/T_4 Liotrix
Pharmacologic Category Thyroid Product
Use
Replacement or supplemental therapy in hypothyroidism (uniform mixture of T_4:T_3 in 4:1 ratio by weight)
Thyroid-stimulating hormone (TSH) suppressant therapy used in the management of thyroid cancer (levothyroxine is generally recommended for this indication); prevention or treatment of euthyroid goiters (eg, thyroid nodules, subacute or chronic lymphocytic thyroiditis [Hashimoto's], multinodular goiters)
Diagnostic agent in suppression tests to diagnose suspected mild hyperthyroidism or to demonstrate thyroid gland autonomy

Dosing
Adult Hypothyroidism: Oral: Initial: Levothyroxine 25 mcg/Liothyronine 6.25 mcg once daily; may increase by levothyroxine 12.5 mcg/Liothyronine 3.1 mcg every 2-3 weeks. A lower initial dose (levothyroxine 12.5 mcg/Liothyronine 3.1 mcg) is recommended in patients with long-standing myxedema, especially if cardiovascular impairment coexists. If angina occurs, reduce dose (usual maintenance dose: levothyroxine 50-100 mcg/Liothyronine 12.5-25 mcg)

Geriatric Initial: Levothyroxine 12.5-25 mcg/Liothyronine 3.1-6.25 mcg once daily; may increase by levothyroxine 12.5 mcg/Liothyronine 3.1 mcg every 2-3 weeks

Pediatric Congenital hypothyroidism: Oral: **Note:** In newly diagnosed infants, begin therapy with full dose.
Children 0-6 months: Levothyroxine 12.5-25 mcg/Liothyronine 3.1-6.25 mcg once daily
Children 6-12 months: Levothyroxine 25-37.5 mcg/Liothyronine 6.25-9.35 mcg once daily
Children 1-5 years: Levothyroxine 37.5-50 mcg/Liothyronine 9.35-12.5 mcg once daily
Children 6-12 years: Levothyroxine 50-75 mcg/Liothyronine 12.5-18.75 mcg once daily
Children >12 years: Levothyroxine 75 mcg/Liothyronine 18.75 mcg once daily
Also see individual agents.

Additional Information Complete prescribing information should be consulted for additional detail.

Dosage Forms Excipient information presented when available (limited, particularly for generics); consult specific product labeling.
Tablet, oral:
Thyrolar: 1/4 [levothyroxine sodium 12.5 mcg and liothyronine sodium 3.1 mcg]
Thyrolar: 1/2 [levothyroxine sodium 25 mcg and liothyronine sodium 6.25 mcg]
Thyrolar: 1 [levothyroxine sodium 50 mcg and liothyronine sodium 12.5 mcg]
Thyrolar: 2 [levothyroxine sodium 100 mcg and liothyronine sodium 25 mcg]
Thyrolar: 3 [levothyroxine sodium 150 mcg and liothyronine sodium 37.5 mcg]

◆ **Lipancreatin** see Pancrelipase on page 1384
◆ **Lipase, Protease, and Amylase** see Pancrelipase on page 1384

◆ **Lipiarrmycin** see Fidaxomicin on page 765
◆ **Lipid Emulsion (Plant Based)** see Fat Emulsion (Plant Based) on page 743
◆ **Lipidil EZ (Can)** see Fenofibrate and Derivatives on page 746
◆ **Lipidil Micro (Can)** see Fenofibrate and Derivatives on page 746
◆ **Lipidil Supra (Can)** see Fenofibrate and Derivatives on page 746
◆ **Lipitor** see AtorvaSTATin on page 169
◆ **Lipodox** see DOXOrubicin (Liposomal) on page 597
◆ **Lipodox 50** see DOXOrubicin (Liposomal) on page 597
◆ **Lipofen** see Fenofibrate and Derivatives on page 746
◆ **Liposomal Amphotericin** see Amphotericin B (Liposomal) on page 119
◆ **Liposomal Amphotericin B** see Amphotericin B (Liposomal) on page 119
◆ **Liposomal Bupivacaine** see Bupivacaine (Liposomal) on page 263
◆ **Liposomal Cytarabine** see Cytarabine (Liposomal) on page 471
◆ **Liposomal DAUNOrubicin** see DAUNOrubicin (Liposomal) on page 506
◆ **Liposomal DOXOrubicin** see DOXOrubicin (Liposomal) on page 597
◆ **Liposomal Irinotecan** see Irinotecan (Liposomal) on page 984
◆ **Liposomal Morphine** see Morphine (Liposomal) on page 1236
◆ **Liposomal Vincristine** see VinCRIStine (Liposomal) on page 1900
◆ **Liposome-Encapsulated Irinotecan Hydrochloride PEP02** see Irinotecan (Liposomal) on page 984
◆ **Liposome Vincristine** see VinCRIStine (Liposomal) on page 1900
◆ **Liposyn II [DSC]** see Fat Emulsion (Plant Based) on page 743
◆ **Liposyn III** see Fat Emulsion (Plant Based) on page 743
◆ **Liptruzet** see Ezetimibe and Atorvastatin on page 730
◆ **Liquibid [OTC]** see GuaiFENesin on page 860
◆ **Liquibid® D-R [OTC]** see Guaifenesin and Phenylephrine on page 862
◆ **Liquibid® PD-R [OTC]** see Guaifenesin and Phenylephrine on page 862
◆ **Liquid Antidote** see Charcoal, Activated on page 368
◆ **Liquituss GG [OTC]** see GuaiFENesin on page 860

Liraglutide (lir a GLOO tide)

Brand Names: US Saxenda; Victoza
Brand Names: Canada Victoza
Index Terms NN2211
Pharmacologic Category Antidiabetic Agent, Glucagon-Like Peptide-1 (GLP-1) Receptor Agonist
Use
Chronic weight management (Saxenda): As an adjunct to a reduced-calorie diet and increased physical activity for chronic weight management in adult patients with an initial body mass index of 30 kg/m² or greater (obese) or 27 kg/m² or greater (overweight) in the presence of at least one weight-related comorbid condition (eg, hypertension, type 2 diabetes mellitus, dyslipidemia)
Diabetes mellitus, type 2 (Victoza): As an adjunct to diet and exercise to improve glycemic control in adults with type 2 diabetes mellitus.

Pregnancy Considerations Use for chronic weight management is contraindicated in pregnant women (lack of potential benefit and possible fetal harm). Weight loss therapy is generally not recommended for pregnant women. Obese and overweight women should be encouraged to participate in weight reduction programs prior to attempting pregnancy; weight gain during pregnancy should be determined by prepregnancy BMI and current guidelines (ACOG 549 2013; IOM 2009; NHLBI 1998).

In women with diabetes, maternal hyperglycemia can be associated with congenital malformations as well as adverse effects in the fetus, neonate, and the mother (ACOG 2005; ADA 2015; Kitzmiller 2008; Metzger 2007). To prevent adverse outcomes, prior to conception and throughout pregnancy maternal blood glucose and HbA1c should be kept as close to target goals as possible but without causing significant hypoglycemia (ACOG 137 2013; ADA 2015; Blumer 2013; Kitzmiller 2008). Prior to pregnancy, effective contraception should be used until

glycemic control is achieved (Kitzmiller 2008). Other agents are currently recommended to treat diabetes in pregnant women (ACOG 137 2013; Blumer 2013).

Breast-Feeding Considerations It is not known if liraglutide is excreted in breast milk. Because tumors were observed in animal studies, the manufacturer recommends that a decision be made whether to discontinue nursing or the drug, taking into account the importance of treatment to the mother.

Weight loss therapy is generally not recommended for lactating women (NHLBI 1998). Weight loss programs that include physical activity and nutrition components should be discussed at the 6-week postpartum visit (ADA 2009).

Medication Guide Available Yes

Contraindications Hypersensitivity to liraglutide or any component of the formulation; history of or family history of MTC; patients with multiple endocrine neoplasia syndrome type 2 (MEN2); pregnancy (Saxenda).

Canadian labeling: Additional contraindications (not in US labeling): Pregnancy; breast-feeding

Warnings/Precautions Hazardous agent - use appropriate precautions for handling and disposal (NIOSH 2014 [group 2]).

[US Boxed Warning] Dose-dependent and treatment duration–dependent thyroid C-cell tumors have developed in animal studies with liraglutide therapy; it is unknown whether liraglutide will cause thyroid C-cell tumors, including MTC, in humans, because the human relevance of liraglutide-induced rodent thyroid C-cell tumors has not been determined. Patients should be counseled on the potential risk of MTC with the use of liraglutide and informed of symptoms of thyroid tumors (eg, neck mass, dysphagia, dyspnea, persistent hoarseness). Use is contraindicated in patients with a personal or a family history of MTC and in patients with multiple endocrine neoplasia syndrome type 2 (MEN2). Consultation with an endocrinologist is recommended in patients who develop elevated calcitonin concentrations or have thyroid nodules detected during imaging studies or physical exam; **routine monitoring of serum calcitonin or using thyroid ultrasound monitoring is of uncertain value for early detection of MTC in patients treated with liraglutide.**

Serious hypersensitivity reactions, including anaphylactic reactions and angioedema, have been reported with use; discontinue therapy in the event of a hypersensitivity reaction. Use with caution in patients with a history of angioedema to other GLP-1 receptor agonists (angioedema has been reported with other GLP-1 receptor agonists); potential for cross-sensitivity is unknown. Cases of acute and chronic pancreatitis (including fatal and nonfatal, hemorrhagic or necrotizing pancreatitis) have been reported; monitor for signs and symptoms of pancreatitis (eg, persistent severe abdominal pain which may radiate to the back and which may or may not be accompanied by vomiting. If pancreatitis is suspected, discontinue use. Do not resume unless an alternative etiology of pancreatitis is confirmed. Use with caution in patients with a history of pancreatitis or consider antidiabetic therapies other than liraglutide. Use with caution in patients with cholelithiasis and/or alcohol abuse. Cholelithiasis and cholecystitis have been reported in patients treated with liraglutide for obesity. Most common reactions are gastrointestinal related; these symptoms may be dose-related and may decrease in frequency/severity with gradual titration and continued use. Slows gastric emptying; has not been studied in patients with preexisting gastroparesis. Use may be associated with weight loss (likely due to reduced intake) independent of the change in hemoglobin A$_{1c}$. Use with caution in patients with hepatic impairment. Use with caution in renal impairment, particularly during initiation of therapy and dose escalation; cases of acute renal failure and chronic renal failure exacerbation have been reported; some cases have been reported in patients with no known preexisting renal disease.

Suicidal behavior, with one case of attempted suicide, has been reported in patients treated for obesity; monitor for new or worsening depression, suicidal thoughts or behavior, or unusual changes in mood or behavior. Discontinue use if suicidal thoughts or behaviors occur. Avoid use in patients with history of suicidal attempts or active suicidal ideation. Increased resting heart rate has been reported in patients treated for obesity; monitoring is recommended. Discontinue use in patients who experience a sustained increase in resting heart rate.

Victoza is not recommended for first-line therapy; use as adjunct to diet and exercise. Do not use in patients with type 1 diabetes mellitus or for the treatment of diabetic ketoacidosis; not a substitute for insulin. Saxenda is not indicated for the treatment of type 2 diabetes and concomitant use with insulin is not recommended. Diabetes self-management education (DSME) is essential to maximize the effectiveness of therapy. According to the Centers for Disease Control and Prevention (CDC), pen-shaped injection devices should never be used for more than one person (even when the needle is changed) because of the risk of infection. The injection device should be clearly labeled with individual patient information to ensure that the correct pen is used (CDC, 2012). Potentially significant interactions may exist, requiring dose or frequency adjustment, additional monitoring, and/or selection of alternative therapy.

Adverse Reactions

Obesity:

>10%:

Cardiovascular: Increased heart rate (>10 bpm from baseline: 34%; >20 bpm from baseline: 5%)

Central nervous system: Headache (14%)

Endocrine & metabolic: Hypoglycemia (Type 2 diabetics: combination therapy with sulfonylurea: 44%; monotherapy: 16%; nondiabetic patients 2% to 3%)

Gastrointestinal: Nausea (39%), diarrhea (21%), constipation (19%), vomiting (16%)

1% to 10%:

Cardiovascular: Tachycardia (6%; one resting heart rate >100 bpm)

Central nervous system: Fatigue (8%), dizziness (7%)

Gastrointestinal: Decreased appetite (10%), dyspepsia (10%), abdominal distension (5%), abdominal pain (5%), eructation (5%), gastroenteritis (5%), gastroesophageal reflux disease (5%), increased serum lipase (5%; >3 x ULN: 2%), upper abdominal pain (5%), flatulence (4%), viral gastroenteritis (3%), cholelithiasis (2%), xerostomia (2%)

Genitourinary: Urinary tract infection (4%)

Immunologic: Antibody development (3%; neutralizing: 1%)

Local: Injection site reactions (3% to 14%; including erythema [1% to 3%], itching [1% to 3%], rash [1% to 3%])

Neuromuscular & skeletal: Weakness (2%)

Type 2 diabetes mellitus: Incidence reported in monotherapy trials unless otherwise specified.

>10%: Gastrointestinal: Nausea (28%), diarrhea (17%), vomiting (11%)

1% to 10%:

Central nervous system: Headache (9%)

Gastrointestinal: Constipation (10%), dyspepsia (combination trials: 9%)

Hepatic: Hyperbilirubinemia (monotherapy and combination trials: 4%)

Immunologic: Antibody development: Antiliraglutide antibodies (low titers [concentrations not requiring dilution of serum]; monotherapy and combination trials: 9%), cross-reacting antiliraglutide antibodies to native GLP-1 (monotherapy: 7%; combination trials: 5%)

Local: Injection site reactions (monotherapy and combination trials: 2% [includes rash, erythema])

<1% (Limited to important or life-threatening; any indication): Acute renal failure, asthma, benign gastrointestinal neoplasm (colorectal), carcinoma (papillary thyroid), cholecystitis, cholestasis, chronic renal failure (exacerbation), first degree atrioventricular block, hepatitis, hypersensitivity reaction, increased susceptibility to infection, left bundle branch block, malignant neoplasm (including colorectal carcinoma), malignant neoplasm of breast, medullary thyroid carcinoma, pancreatitis (including acute, chronic, hemorrhagic, and necrotizing), papillary thyroid carcinoma, right bundle branch block, suicidal ideation, systolic hypotension, thyroid disease (C-cell hyperplasia), upper respiratory tract infection

Drug Interactions

Metabolism/Transport Effects None known.

Avoid Concomitant Use There are no known interactions where it is recommended to avoid concomitant use.

Increased Effect/Toxicity

Liraglutide may increase the levels/effects of: Hypoglycemia-Associated Agents; Insulin; Sulfonylureas

The levels/effects of Liraglutide may be increased by: Alpha-Lipoic Acid; Androgens; MAO Inhibitors; Pegvisomant; Quinolone Antibiotics; Salicylates; Selective Serotonin Reuptake Inhibitors

Decreased Effect

The levels/effects of Liraglutide may be decreased by: Hyperglycemia-Associated Agents; Quinolone Antibiotics; Thiazide Diuretics

Storage/Stability Prior to initial use, store at 2°C to 8°C (36°F to 46°F); after initial use, may be stored at 2°C to 8°C (36°F to 46°F) or at 15°C to 30°C (59°F to 86°F). Do not freeze (discard if freezing occurs) or store directly adjacent to the refrigerator cooling element. Protect from heat and light. Pen should be discarded 30 days after initial use.

Mechanism of Action Liraglutide is a long acting analog of human glucagon-like peptide-1 (GLP-1) (an incretin hormone) which increases glucose-dependent insulin secretion, decreases inappropriate glucagon secretion, increases B-cell growth/replication, slows gastric emptying, and decreases food intake. Liraglutide administration results in decreases in hemoglobin A_{1c} by approximately 1%.

Pharmacodynamics/Kinetics
Distribution: V_d: SubQ: ~13 to 25 L; IV: 0.07 L/kg
Protein binding: >98%
Metabolism: Endogenously metabolized by dipeptidyl peptidase IV (DPP-IV) and endogenous endopeptidases (Croom, 2009); metabolism occurs slower than that seen with native GLP-1
Bioavailability: SubQ: ~55%
Half-life, elimination: ~13 hours
Time to peak, plasma: 8 to 12 hours
Excretion: Urine (6%, as metabolites); feces (5%, as metabolites)

Dosing
Adult & Geriatric
Chronic weight management: SubQ: Initial: 0.6 mg once daily for one week; increase by 0.6 mg daily at weekly intervals to a target dose of 3 mg once daily. If the patient cannot tolerate an increased dose during dose escalation, consider delaying dose escalation for one week. If the 3 mg daily dose is not tolerated, discontinue use as efficacy has not been established at lower doses.
Note: Evaluate change in body weight 16 weeks after initiation of therapy; discontinue if at least 4% of baseline body weight loss has not been achieved.
Diabetes mellitus, type 2: SubQ: Initial: 0.6 mg once daily for 1 week; then increase to 1.2 mg once daily; may increase further to 1.8 mg once daily if optimal glycemic response not achieved with 1.2 mg daily.
Note: Initial dose is intended to reduce GI symptoms; does not provide effective glycemic control.

Missed doses: In the event of a missed dose, the once daily regimen can be resumed with the next scheduled dose (an extra dose or an increase in the next dose should **not** be attempted); if >3 days have passed since the last liraglutide dose, reinitiate therapy at 0.6 mg/day to avoid GI symptoms and titrate according to prescriber discretion.

Renal Impairment
US labeling: Mild-to-severe impairment: There are no dosage adjustments provided in the manufacturer's labeling; however, use with caution, due to limited experience and reports of acute renal failure and exacerbation of chronic renal failure.
Canadian labeling:
Mild impairment: No dosage adjustment necessary.
Moderate-to-severe impairment: Use is not recommended.

Hepatic Impairment
US labeling: Mild-to-severe impairment: There are no dosage adjustments provided in the manufacturer's labeling; use with caution, due to limited experience.
Canadian labeling: Mild-to-severe impairment: Use is not recommended.

Dietary Considerations Individualized medical nutrition therapy (MNT) based on ADA recommendations is an integral part of therapy.

Administration Do not inject intravenously or intramuscularly. Inject subcutaneously in the upper arm, thigh, or abdomen. Administer without regard to meals or time of day. Change needle with each administration. Use only if clear, colorless, and free of particulate matter. Do not share pens between patients even if needle is changed. If using concomitantly with insulin, administer as separate injections (do **not** mix); may inject in the same body region as insulin, but not adjacent to one another.

Hazardous agent; use appropriate precautions for handling and disposal (NIOSH 2014 [group 2]).

Monitoring Parameters Plasma glucose, HbA_{1c}; renal function; signs/symptoms of pancreatitis; emergence of worsening depression, suicidal thoughts/behavior, changes in behavior; heart rate

Reference Range Recommendations for glycemic control in nonpregnant adults with diabetes (ADA, 2013):
HbA_{1c}: <7% (a more aggressive [<6.5%] or less aggressive [<8%] HbA_{1c} goal may be targeted based on patient-specific characteristics)

Preprandial capillary plasma glucose: 70-130 mg/dL
Peak postprandial capillary blood glucose: <180 mg/dL
Dosage Forms Excipient information presented when available (limited, particularly for generics); consult specific product labeling.
Solution Pen-injector, Subcutaneous:
Saxenda: 18 mg/3 mL (3 mL) [contains phenol, propylene glycol]
Victoza: 18 mg/3 mL (3 mL) [contains phenol, propylene glycol]

Lisdexamfetamine (lis dex am FET a meen)

Brand Names: US Vyvanse
Brand Names: Canada Vyvanse
Index Terms Lisdexamfetamine Dimesylate; Lisdexamphetamine; NRP104
Pharmacologic Category Central Nervous System Stimulant
Use
Attention-deficit/hyperactivity disorder: Treatment of attention-deficit/hyperactivity disorder (ADHD)
Binge eating disorder: Treatment of moderate to severe binge eating disorder
Pregnancy Considerations Adverse effects have not been observed in animal reproduction studies. Lisdexamfetamine is converted to dextroamphetamine. The majority of human data is based on illicit amphetamine/methamphetamine exposure and not from therapeutic maternal use (Golub 2005). Use of amphetamines during pregnancy may lead to an increased risk of premature birth and low birth weight; newborns may experience symptoms of withdrawal. Behavioral problems may also occur later in childhood (LaGasse 2012).
Breast-Feeding Considerations The majority of human data is based on illicit amphetamine/methamphetamine exposure and not from therapeutic maternal use (Golub 2005). Amphetamines are excreted into breast milk and use may decrease milk production. Increased irritability, agitation, and crying have been reported in nursing infants (ACOG 2011). According to the manufacturer, the decision to continue or discontinue breast-feeding during therapy should take into account the risk of exposure to the infant and the benefits of treatment to the mother.
Medication Guide Available Yes
Contraindications
Hypersensitivity to amphetamine products or any component of the formulation; concurrent use of MAO inhibitor, or within 14 days of the last MAO inhibitor dose.
Canadian labeling: Additional contraindications (not in U.S. labeling): Known hypersensitivity or idiosyncrasy to sympathomimetic amines; advanced arteriosclerosis; symptomatic cardiovascular disease; moderate-to-severe hypertension; hyperthyroidism; glaucoma; agitated states; history of drug abuse
Warnings/Precautions Sudden death, stroke, and myocardial infarction have been reported in adults receiving the recommended doses of CNS stimulants. In children and adolescents with preexisting structural cardiac abnormalities or other serious heart problems, sudden death has been reported while receiving the recommended doses of CNS stimulants for ADHD. These products should be avoided in the patients with known serious structural cardiac abnormalities, cardiomyopathy, serious heart rhythm abnormalities, coronary artery disease (adults), or other serious cardiac problems that could increase the risk of sudden death. Patients should be carefully evaluated for these cardiac disorders prior to initiation of therapy. Patients who develop exertional chest pain, unexplained syncope, or arrhythmias during therapy should be evaluated promptly. CNS stimulants may increase heart rate (mean increase: 3 to 6 bpm) and blood pressure (mean increase: 2 to 4 mm Hg); monitor for adverse events related to tachycardia or hypertension. Stimulants are associated with peripheral vasculopathy, including Raynaud phenomenon; signs/symptoms are usually mild and intermittent, and generally improve with dose reduction or discontinuation. Digital ulceration and/or soft tissue breakdown have been observed rarely; monitor for digital changes during therapy and seek further evaluation (eg, rheumatology) if necessary.

Suicidal ideation and/or behavior (including rare completed suicide) have been reported with ADHD drugs; monitor for signs of suicide-related behavior. Patients with suicidal thoughts/behavior should be evaluated immediately; alternative ADHD therapy may be necessary. Use with caution in patients with preexisting psychosis or bipolar disorder (may induce mixed/manic episode). May exacerbate symptoms of behavior and thought disorder in psychotic patients; new onset psychosis or mania may occur in children or adolescents with stimulant use. Patients should

be screened for bipolar disorder prior to treatment; consider discontinuation if such symptoms (eg, delusional thinking, hallucinations, or mania) occur. May be associated with aggressive behavior or hostility (causal relationship not established); monitor for development or worsening of these behaviors. Use with caution in patients with Tourette syndrome; stimulants may exacerbate tics (motor and phonic) and Tourette syndrome. Evaluate for tics and Tourette syndrome prior to therapy initiation. **[US Boxed Warning]: CNS stimulants (including lisdexamfetamine) have a high potential for abuse and dependence; assess for abuse potential prior to use and monitor for signs of abuse and dependence while on therapy.** Use with caution in patients with history of ethanol or drug abuse (Canadian labeling contraindicates use if history of drug abuse). Prescriptions should be written for the smallest quantity consistent with good patient care to minimize possibility of overdose. Abrupt discontinuation following high doses or for prolonged periods may result in symptoms for withdrawal (eg, depression, extreme fatigue). Canadian labeling recommends discontinuing therapy if improvement is not observed after 1 month of dosage titration. Lisdexamfetamine is not recommended for weight loss; safety and efficacy not established for treatment of obesity.

Elderly patients may have decreased renal, hepatic or cardiac function or other concomitant disease or drug therapy; initiate dose at the low end of the dosing range. Appetite suppression may occur; particularly in children. Use of stimulants has been associated with weight loss and slowing of growth rate; monitor growth rate and weight during treatment. Treatment interruption may be necessary in patients who are not increasing in height or gaining weight as expected. Hypersensitivity, including anaphylaxis, Stevens-Johnson syndrome, angioedema, and urticaria have been observed. Potentially significant drug-drug interactions may exist, requiring dose or frequency adjustment, additional monitoring, and/or selection of alternative therapy.

Adverse Reactions
>10%:
Central nervous system: Insomnia (13% to 27%)
Gastrointestinal: Decreased appetite (children and adolescents: 34% to 39%; adults: 8% to 27%), xerostomia (adults: 26% to 36%; children and adolescents: 4% to 5%), upper abdominal pain (children: 12%; adults: 2%)
1% to 10%:
Cardiovascular: Increased heart rate (adults: 2% to 7%), increased blood pressure (adults: 3%)
Central nervous system: Irritability (children: 10%), anxiety (adults: 5% to 6%), jitteriness (adults: 4% to 6%), dizziness (children: 5%), agitation (adults: 3%), emotional lability (children: 3%), restlessness (adults: 2% to 3%), drowsiness (children: 2%), increased energy (adults: 2%), nightmares (adults: 2%), paresthesia (adults: 2%), tics (children: 2%)
Dermatologic: Hyperhidrosis (adults: 3% to 4%), skin rash (children: 3%), pruritus (adults: 2%)
Endocrine & metabolic: Weight loss (children and adolescents: 9%; adults: 3% to 4%), decreased libido (adults: <2%)
Gastrointestinal: Vomiting (children: 9%; adults: 2%), diarrhea (adults: 7%), nausea (6% to 7%), constipation (adults: 6%), anorexia (adults: 5%), gastroenteritis (adults: 2%)
Genitourinary: Erectile dysfunction (adults: 3%)
Neuromuscular & skeletal: Tremor (adults: 2%)
Respiratory: Dyspnea (adults: 2%), oropharyngeal pain (2%)
Miscellaneous: Fever (children: 2%)
<1% (Limited to important or life-threatening): Accommodation disturbance, bruxism, cardiomyopathy, cerebrovascular accident, decreased linear skeletal growth rate, depression, dermatillomania, diplopia, exacerbation of tics, excoriation, frequent erections, hallucination, headache, hepatitis (eosinophilic), hypersensitivity, hypertension, incoherent speech, mania, mydriasis, myocardial infarction, overstimulation, peripheral vascular insufficiency, prolonged erection, psychotic reaction, Raynaud's phenomenon, seizure, Stevens-Johnson syndrome, suicidal tendencies, tachycardia

Drug Interactions
Metabolism/Transport Effects None known.
Avoid Concomitant Use
Avoid concomitant use of Lisdexamfetamine with any of the following: Iobenguane I 123; MAO Inhibitors
Increased Effect/Toxicity
Lisdexamfetamine may increase the levels/effects of: Analgesics (Opioid); Doxofylline; Sympathomimetics

The levels/effects of Lisdexamfetamine may be increased by: Alkalinizing Agents; Antacids; AtoMOXetine; Cannabinoid-Containing Products; Carbonic Anhydrase Inhibitors; Linezolid; MAO Inhibitors; Tedizolid; Tricyclic Antidepressants
Decreased Effect
Lisdexamfetamine may decrease the levels/effects of: Antihistamines; Antihypertensive Agents; Ethosuximide; Iobenguane I 123; Ioflupane I 123; PHENobarbital; Phenytoin

The levels/effects of Lisdexamfetamine may be decreased by: Ammonium Chloride; Antipsychotic Agents; Ascorbic Acid; Gastrointestinal Acidifying Agents; Lithium; Methenamine; Multivitamins/Fluoride (with ADE); Multivitamins/Minerals (with ADEK, Folate, Iron); Multivitamins/Minerals (with AE, No Iron); Urinary Acidifying Agents
Food Interactions High-fat meal prolongs T_{max} by ~1 hour. Management: Administer without regard to meals.
Storage/Stability Store at 20°C to 25°C (68°F to 77°F); excursions are permitted between 15°C and 30°C (59°F and 86°F). Protect from light.
Mechanism of Action Lisdexamfetamine dimesylate is a prodrug that is converted to the active component dextroamphetamine (a noncatecholamine, sympathomimetic amine). Amphetamines are noncatecholamine, sympathomimetic amines that cause release of catecholamines (primarily dopamine and norepinephrine) from their storage sites in the presynaptic nerve terminals. A less significant mechanism may include their ability to block the reuptake of catecholamines by competitive inhibition.
Pharmacodynamics/Kinetics
Absorption: Rapid
Distribution: Dextroamphetamine: V_d: Adults: 3.5 to 4.6 L/kg; distributes into CNS; mean CSF concentrations are 80% of plasma
Metabolism: Metabolized in the blood by hydrolytic activity of red blood cells to dextroamphetamine and l-lysine; does not undergo CYP mediated metabolism
Half-life elimination: Lisdexamfetamine: <1 hour; Dextroamphetamine: 10 to 13 hours
Time to peak, serum: T_{max}: Lisdexamfetamine: ~1 hour; Dextroamphetamine: ~3.5 hours
Excretion: Urine (96%, 42% as amphetamine-related compounds, 2% as lisdexamfetamine, 25% hippuric acid); feces (minimal)
Dosing
Adult Note: Prior to treatment, assess for presence of cardiac disease and assess for risk of abuse.
Attention-deficit/hyperactivity disorder (ADHD): Oral:
Note: Individualize dosage based on patient need and response to therapy. Administer at the lowest effective dose.
U.S. labeling: Initial: 30 mg once daily in the morning; may increase in increments of 10 mg or 20 mg daily at weekly intervals until optimal response is obtained; maximum: 70 mg daily
Canadian labeling: Initial: 20 to 30 mg once daily in the morning; per clinical discretion, may increase in increments of 10 or 20 mg daily at weekly intervals up to a maximum dose of 60 mg daily. Discontinue therapy if improvement is not observed after 1 month of dosage titration. **Note:** Canadian ADHD Resource Alliance (CADDRA) 2011 practice guidelines recommend a maximum dose of 70 mg daily.
Binge eating disorder: Oral: Initial: 30 mg once daily in the morning; may titrate in increments of 20 mg at weekly intervals to target dose of 50 to 70 mg once daily (maximum: 70 mg daily); discontinue use if binge eating does not improve.
Pediatric
Attention-deficit/hyperactivity disorder (ADHD):
Note: Prior to treatment, assess for presence of cardiac disease and assess for risk of abuse. Individualize dosage based on patient need and response to therapy. Administer at the lowest effective dose.
U.S. labeling: Children ≥6 years and Adolescents: Oral: Refer to adult dosing.
Canadian labeling:
Children ≥6 years and Adolescents: Oral: Initial: 20 to 30 mg once daily in the morning; per clinical discretion, may increase in increments of 10 or 20 mg daily at weekly intervals up to a maximum dose of 60 mg daily. Discontinue therapy if improvement is not observed after 1 month of dosage titration. **Note:** For patients requiring dose titration, the Canadian ADHD Resource Alliance (CADDRA) 2011 practice guidelines recommend weekly increases of 10 mg daily up to a maximum of 60 mg daily.
Adolescents: Refer to adult dosing.

Renal Impairment

U.S. labeling:

GFR ≥30 mL/minute/1.73 m²: There are no dosage adjustments provided in the manufacturer's labeling.

GFR 15 to <30 mL/minute/1.73 m²: Maximum dose: 50 mg daily.

GFR <15 mL/minute/1.73 m²: Maximum dose: 30 mg daily.

ESRD requiring hemodialysis: Maximum dose: 30 mg daily; lisdexamfetamine and dextroamphetamine are not dialyzable.

Canadian labeling:

Mild to moderate impairment (GFR ≥30 mL/minute/1.73 m²): There are no dosage adjustments provided in the manufacturer's labeling.

Severe impairment:

GFR 15 to <30 mL/minute/1.73 m²: Maximum dose: 50 mg daily.

GFR <15 mL/minute/1.73 m²: There are no specific dosage adjustments provided in the manufacturer's labeling.

Dialysis: There are no specific dosage adjustments provided in the manufacturer's labeling; however, the manufacturer recommends considering further maximum dosage reductions (compared to that recommended for severe impairment).

Hepatic Impairment
There are no dosage adjustments provided in the manufacturer's labeling.

Administration
Administer in the morning without regard to meals; swallow capsule whole, do not chew. Capsule may be opened and the entire contents dissolved in glass of water, yogurt, or orange juice; stir until dispersed completely and consume the entire mixture immediately; do not store mixture. The active ingredient dissolves completely once dispersed; however, a film containing the inactive ingredients may remain in the glass or container once the mixture is consumed. Do not take less than one capsule daily; a single capsule should not be divided.

Monitoring Parameters
Cardiac evaluation should be completed on any patient who develops exertional chest pain, unexplained syncope, and any symptom of cardiac disease during treatment with stimulants; growth (height and weight) in children; CNS activity in all patients; signs of peripheral vasculopathy (eg, digital changes); behavioral changes; signs of misuse, abuse, or addiction

When used for the treatment of ADHD, thoroughly evaluate for cardiovascular risk. Monitor heart rate, blood pressure, and consider obtaining ECG prior to initiation (Vetter 2008).

Test Interactions
Amphetamines may elevate plasma corticosteroid levels; may interfere with urinary steroid determinations.

Dosage Forms
Excipient information presented when available (limited, particularly for generics); consult specific product labeling.

Capsule, Oral, as dimesylate:

Vyvanse: 10 mg [contains brilliant blue fcf (fd&c blue #1), fd&c yellow #6 (sunset yellow)]

Vyvanse: 20 mg, 30 mg, 40 mg, 50 mg, 60 mg, 70 mg [contains brilliant blue fcf (fd&c blue #1), fd&c red #40, fd&c yellow #10 (quinoline yellow)]

Dosage Forms: Canada
Refer to Dosage Forms. **Note:** Vyvanse 70 mg capsule is not available in Canada.

Controlled Substance
C-II

◆ Lisdexamfetamine Dimesylate *see* Lisdexamfetamine *on page 1086*

◆ Lisdexamphetamine *see* Lisdexamfetamine *on page 1086*

Lisinopril (lyse IN oh pril)

Brand Names: US
Prinivil; Zestril

Brand Names: Canada
ACT Lisinopril; Apo-Lisinopril; Auro-Lisinopril; Dom-Lisinopril; JAMP-Lisinopril; Mylan-Lisinopril; PMS-Lisinopril; Prinivil; PRO-Lisinopril; RAN-Lisinopril; Riva-Lisinopril; Sandoz-Lisinopril; Teva-Lisinopril (Type P); Teva-Lisinopril (Type Z); Zestril

Pharmacologic Category
Angiotensin-Converting Enzyme (ACE) Inhibitor; Antihypertensive

Use

Acute myocardial infarction: Treatment of acute myocardial infarction (MI) within 24 hours in hemodynamically-stable patients to improve survival

Heart failure: Adjunctive therapy in treatment systolic of heart failure (HF)

Hypertension: Treatment of hypertension, either alone or in combination with other antihypertensive agents in adult and pediatric patients 6 years and older

Guideline recommendations:

Heart failure: The ACCF/AHA 2013 heart failure guidelines recommend the use of ACE inhibitors, along with other guideline directed medical therapies, to prevent HF in patients with a reduced ejection fraction who have a history of MI (stage B HF), to prevent HF in any patient with a reduced ejection fraction (stage B HF), or to treat those with HF and reduced ejection fraction (stage C HFrEF) (Yancy, 2013).

Hypertension: The 2014 guideline for the management of high blood pressure in adults (Eighth Joint National Committee [JNC 8]) recommends initiation of pharmacologic treatment to lower blood pressure for the following patients:

• Patients ≥60 years of age with systolic blood pressure (SBP) ≥150 mm Hg or diastolic blood pressure (DBP) ≥90 mm Hg. Goal of therapy is SBP <150 mm Hg and DBP <90 mm Hg.

• Patients <60 years of age with SBP ≥140 mm Hg or DBP is ≥90 mm Hg. Goal of therapy is SBP <140 mm Hg and DBP <90 mm Hg.

• Patients ≥18 years of age with diabetes and SBP ≥140 mm Hg or DBP ≥90 mm Hg. Goal of therapy is SBP <140 mm Hg and DBP <90 mm Hg.

• Patients ≥18 years of age with chronic kidney disease (CKD) and SBP ≥140 mm Hg or DBP ≥90 mm Hg. Goal of therapy is SBP <140 mm Hg and DBP <90 mm Hg.

Chronic kidney disease (CKD) and hypertension: Regardless of race or diabetes status, the use of an ACE inhibitor (ACEI) or angiotensin receptor blocker (ARB) as initial therapy is recommended to improve kidney outcomes. In the general nonblack population (without CKD) including those with diabetes, initial antihypertensive treatment should consist of a thiazide-type diuretic, calcium channel blocker, ACEI, or ARB. In the general black population (without CKD) including those with diabetes, initial antihypertensive treatment should consist of a thiazide-type diuretic or a calcium channel blocker **instead of** an ACEI or ARB.

Coronary artery disease (CAD) and hypertension: The American Heart Association, American College of Cardiology and American Society of Hypertension (AHA/ACC/ASH) 2015 scientific statement for the treatment of hypertension in patients with CAD recommends the use of an ACE inhibitor (or an ARB) as part of a regimen in patients with hypertension and chronic stable angina if there is prior MI, LV systolic dysfunction, diabetes mellitus, or CKD. A BP target of <140/90 mm Hg is reasonable for the secondary prevention of cardiovascular events. A lower target BP (<130/80 mm Hg) may be appropriate in some individuals with CAD, previous MI, stroke or transient ischemic attack, or CAD risk equivalents (AHA/ACC/ASH [Rosendorff 2015]).

STEMI: The 2013 American College of Cardiology Foundation/American Heart Association (ACCF/AHA) guidelines for the management of patients with ST-elevation myocardial infarction (STEMI) states that an ACE inhibitor should be initiated within the first 24 hours after STEMI in patients with anterior MI, heart failure, or left ventricular ejection fraction (LVEF) of 0.4 or less. It is also reasonable to initiate an ACE inhibitor in all patients with STEMI (O'Gara, 2013).

Pregnancy Considerations [US Boxed Warning]:
Drugs that act on the renin-angiotensin system can cause injury and death to the developing fetus. Discontinue as soon as possible once pregnancy is detected. Lisinopril crosses the placenta.

Drugs that act on the renin-angiotensin system are associated with oligohydramnios. Oligohydramnios, due to decreased fetal renal function, may lead to fetal lung hypoplasia and skeletal malformations. The use of these drugs in pregnancy is also associated with anuria, hypotension, renal failure, skull hypoplasia, and death in the fetus/neonate. Teratogenic effects may occur following maternal use of an ACE inhibitor during the first trimester, although this finding may be confounded by maternal disease. Because adverse fetal events are well documented with exposure later in pregnancy, ACE inhibitor use in pregnant women is not recommended (Seely 2014; Weber 2014). Infants exposed to an ACE inhibitor in utero should be monitored for hyperkalemia, hypotension, and oliguria. Oligohydramnios may not appear until after irreversible fetal injury has occurred. Exchange transfusions or dialysis may be required to reverse hypotension or improve renal function, although data related to the effectiveness in neonates is limited.

Chronic maternal hypertension itself is also associated with adverse events in the fetus/infant and mother. ACE inhibitors are not recommended for the treatment of uncomplicated hypertension in pregnancy (ACOG 2013) and they are specifically contraindicated for the treatment of hypertension and chronic heart failure during pregnancy by some guidelines (Regitz-Zagrosek 2011). In addition, ACE inhibitors should generally be avoided in women of reproductive age (ACOG 2013). If treatment for hypertension or chronic heart failure in pregnancy is needed, other agents should be used (ACOG 2013; Regitz-Zagrosek 2011).

Breast-Feeding Considerations It is not known if lisinopril is excreted in breast milk. Due to the potential for serious adverse reactions in the nursing infant, the manufacturer recommends a decision be made whether to discontinue nursing or to discontinue the drug, taking into account the importance of treatment to the mother.

Contraindications

Hypersensitivity to lisinopril, other ACE inhibitors, or any component of the formulation; angioedema related to previous treatment with an ACE inhibitor; idiopathic or hereditary angioedema; concomitant use with aliskiren in patients with diabetes mellitus

Documentation of allergenic cross-reactivity for ACE inhibitors is limited. However, because of similarities in chemical structure and/or pharmacologic actions, the possibility of cross-sensitivity cannot be ruled out with certainty.

Canadian labeling: Additional contraindications (not in US labeling): Concomitant use with aliskiren-containing drugs in patients with moderate-to-severe renal impairment (GFR <60 mL/minute/1.73 m²)

Warnings/Precautions Anaphylactic reactions may occur rarely with ACE inhibitors. At any time during treatment (especially following first dose), angioedema may occur rarely with ACE inhibitors; it may involve the head and neck (potentially compromising airway) or the intestine (presenting with abdominal pain). African-Americans may be at an increased risk. Risk may also be increased with concomitant use of mTOR inhibitor (eg, everolimus) therapy. Prolonged frequent monitoring may be required especially if tongue, glottis, or larynx are involved as they are associated with airway obstruction. Patients with a history of airway surgery may have a higher risk of airway obstruction. Aggressive early and appropriate management is critical. Use in patients with idiopathic or hereditary angioedema or previous angioedema associated with ACE inhibitor therapy is contraindicated. Severe anaphylactoid reactions may be seen during hemodialysis (eg, CVVHD) with high-flux dialysis membranes (eg, AN69), and rarely, during low density lipoprotein apheresis with dextran sulfate cellulose. Rare cases of anaphylactoid reactions have been reported in patients undergoing sensitization treatment with hymenoptera (bee, wasp) venom while receiving ACE inhibitors.

Symptomatic hypotension with or without syncope can occur with ACE inhibitors (usually with the first several doses). Effects are most often observed in volume depleted patients; correct volume depletion prior to initiation. Other patients at risk include those with heart failure and systolic blood pressure <100 mm Hg, ischemic heart disease, cerebrovascular disease, renal dialysis, hyponatremia, high-dose diuretic therapy, severe aortic stenosis, or hypertrophic cardiomyopathy. Close monitoring of patient is required especially within the first few weeks of initial dosing and with dosing increases; blood pressure must be lowered at a rate appropriate for the patient's clinical condition. Initiation of therapy in patients with ischemic heart disease or cerebrovascular disease warrants close observation due to the potential consequences posed by falling blood pressure (eg, MI, stroke). Avoid use in hemodynamically unstable patients after acute MI. Use with caution in hypertrophic cardiomyopathy with outflow tract obstruction and severe aortic stenosis. In patients on chronic ACE inhibitor therapy, intraoperative hypotension may occur with induction and maintenance of general anesthesia; use with caution before, during, or immediately after major surgery. Cardiopulmonary bypass, intraoperative blood loss, or vasodilating anesthesia increases endogenous renin release. Use of ACE inhibitors perioperatively will blunt angiotensin II formation and may result in hypotension. However, discontinuation of therapy prior to surgery is controversial. If continued preoperatively, avoidance of hypotensive agents during surgery is prudent (Hillis, 2011). **[US Boxed Warning]: Drugs that act on the renin-angiotensin system can cause injury and death to the developing fetus. Discontinue as soon as possible once pregnancy is detected.**

Hyperkalemia may occur with ACE inhibitors; risk factors include renal dysfunction, diabetes mellitus, concomitant use of potassium-sparing diuretics, potassium supplements, and/or potassium-containing salts. Use cautiously, if at all, with these agents and monitor potassium closely. Cough may occur with ACE inhibitors. Other causes of cough should be considered (eg, pulmonary congestion in patients with heart failure) and excluded prior to discontinuation.

May be associated with deterioration of renal function and/or increases in serum creatinine, particularly in patients with low renal blood flow (eg, renal artery stenosis, heart failure) whose glomerular filtration rate (GFR) is dependent on efferent arteriolar vasoconstriction by angiotensin II; deterioration may result in oliguria, acute renal failure, and progressive azotemia. Small increases in serum creatinine may occur following initiation; consider discontinuation only in patients with progressive and/or significant deterioration in renal function. Use with caution in patients with unstented unilateral/bilateral renal artery stenosis. When unstented bilateral renal artery stenosis is present, use is generally avoided due to the elevated risk of deterioration in renal function unless possible benefits outweigh risks. In acute myocardial infarction, the Canadian labeling does not recommend initiating therapy if serum creatinine >177 micromol/L and/or proteinuria >500 mg/24 hour and recommends considering discontinuing therapy if serum creatinine >265 micromol/L or doubles from baseline during therapy. In a retrospective cohort study of elderly patients (≥65 years) with myocardial infarction and impaired left ventricular function, administration of an ACE inhibitor was associated with a survival benefit, including patients with serum creatinine concentrations >3 mg/dL (265 micromol/L) (Frances, 2000).

Potentially significant drug-drug interactions may exist, requiring dose or frequency adjustment, additional monitoring, and/or selection of alternative therapy. Use with caution in patients with preexisting hepatic impairment; consider baseline hepatic function tests prior to initiating therapy. Rare toxicities associated with ACE inhibitors include cholestatic jaundice or hepatitis (which may progress to fulminant hepatic necrosis), agranulocytosis, neutropenia, or leukopenia with myeloid hypoplasia. Patients with collagen vascular diseases (especially with concomitant renal impairment) or renal impairment alone may be at increased risk for hematologic toxicity; periodically monitor CBC with differential in these patients.

Adverse Reactions Note: Frequency not always defined. Frequency ranges include data from hypertension and heart failure trials. Higher rates of adverse reactions have generally been noted in patients with heart failure. However, the frequency of adverse effects associated with placebo is also increased in this population.

>10%:

Cardiovascular: Hypotension (7% to 11%)

Central nervous system: Dizziness (12% to 19%)

Renal: Increased blood urea nitrogen (2% to ≤11%), increased serum creatinine (≤2% to ≤11%; often transient)

1% to 10%:

Cardiovascular: Syncope (5% to 7%), flushing (≥1%), orthostatic effect (≥1%), chest pain

Central nervous system: Altered sense of smell (≥1%), fatigue (≥1%), headache

Dermatologic: Alopecia (≥1%), diaphoresis (≥1%), erythema (≥1%), pruritus (≥1%), skin photosensitivity (≥1%), Stevens-Johnson syndrome (≥1%), toxic epidermal necrolysis (≥1%), urticaria (≥1%)

Endocrine & metabolic: Increased nonprotein nitrogen (7%), hyperkalemia (2% to 6%), diabetes mellitus (≥1%), gout (≥1%), SIADH (≥1%)

Gastrointestinal: Constipation (≥1%), diarrhea (≥1%), dysgeusia (≥1%), flatulence (≥1%), pancreatitis (≥1%), xerostomia (≥1%)

Genitourinary: Impotence (≥1%)

Hematologic & oncologic: Bone marrow depression (≥1%), hemolytic anemia (≥1%), leukopenia (≥1%), neutropenia (≥1%), thrombocytopenia (≥1%), decreased hematocrit (small), decreased hemoglobin (small)

Infection: Common cold (1%)

Neuromuscular & skeletal: Weakness (≥1%)

Ophthalmic: Blurred vision (≥1%), diplopia (≥1%), photophobia (≥1%), vision loss (≥1%)

Otic: Tinnitus (≥1%)

Renal: Renal insufficiency (in patients with acute myocardial infarction: 2%)

Respiratory: Cough

<1% (Limited to important or life-threatening): Acute renal failure, anaphylactoid reactions, angioedema, anuria, arthralgia, arthritis, asthma, ataxia, azotemia, bronchitis, bronchospasm, cardiac arrest, cardiac arrhythmia, cerebrovascular acciden (possibly secondary to excessive hypotension in high risk patients), chills, confusion, cutaneous pseudolymphoma, dehydration, drowsiness, dyspepsia, dyspnea, dysuria, eosinophilia, eosinophilic pneumonitis, epistaxis, facial edema, fever, gastritis, hallucination, heartburn, hemoptysis, hepatic necrosis, hepatitis (hepatocellular jaundice or cholestatic jaundice), herpes zoster, hypersomnia, hypervolemia, hypoglycemia (diabetic patients on oral antidiabetic agents or insulin), hyponatremia, increased erythrocyte sedimentation rate, insomnia, intestinal angioedema, irritability, laryngitis, leukocytosis, malaise, malignant neoplasm of lung, mastalgia, memory impairment, mood changes (including depressive symptoms), muscle spasm, musculoskeletal pain, myalgia, myocardial infarction (possibly secondary to excessive hypotension in high risk patients), oliguria, orthopnea, orthostatic hypotension, palpitations, paresthesia, paroxysmal nocturnal dyspnea, pemphigus, peripheral edema, peripheral neuropathy, pharyngitis, pleural effusion, pneumonia, positive ANA titer, psoriasis, pulmonary embolism, pulmonary infarct, pulmonary infiltrates, pyelonephritis, rhinitis, rhinorrhea, sinusitis, skin infection, skin lesion, skin rash, sore throat, systemic lupus erythematosus, transient ischemic attacks, tremor, uremia, urinary tract infection, vasculitis, vertigo, viral infection, visual hallucination (Doane, 2013), weight gain, weight loss, wheezing

Drug Interactions

Metabolism/Transport Effects None known.

Avoid Concomitant Use

Avoid concomitant use of Lisinopril with any of the following: Sacubitril

Increased Effect/Toxicity

Lisinopril may increase the levels/effects of: Allopurinol; Amifostine; Antipsychotic Agents (Second Generation [Atypical]); AzaTHIOprine; Ciprofloxacin (Systemic); Drospirenone; DULoxetine; Ferric Gluconate; Gold Sodium Thiomalate; Grass Pollen Allergen Extract (5 Grass Extract); Hypotension-Associated Agents; Iron Dextran Complex; Levodopa; Lithium; Nonsteroidal Anti-Inflammatory Agents; Pregabalin; Sacubitril; Sodium Phosphates

The levels/effects of Lisinopril may be increased by: Alfuzosin; Aliskiren; Angiotensin II Receptor Blockers; Barbiturates; Brimonidine (Topical); Canagliflozin; Dapoxetine; Diazoxide; DPP-IV Inhibitors; Eplerenone; Everolimus; Heparin; Heparin (Low Molecular Weight); Herbs (Hypotensive Properties); Loop Diuretics; Molsidomine; Nicorandil; Obinutuzumab; Pentoxifylline; Phosphodiesterase 5 Inhibitors; Potassium Salts; Potassium-Sparing Diuretics; Prostacyclin Analogues; Salicylates; Sirolimus; Temsirolimus; Thiazide Diuretics; TiZANidine; Tolvaptan; Trimethoprim

Decreased Effect

The levels/effects of Lisinopril may be decreased by: Amphetamines; Aprotinin; Herbs (Hypertensive Properties); Icatibant; Lanthanum; Methylphenidate; Nonsteroidal Anti-Inflammatory Agents; Salicylates; Yohimbine

Storage/Stability Store at room temperature. Protect from moisture, freezing, and excessive heat.

Mechanism of Action Competitive inhibitor of angiotensin-converting enzyme (ACE); prevents conversion of angiotensin I to angiotensin II, a potent vasoconstrictor; results in lower levels of angiotensin II which causes an increase in plasma renin activity and a reduction in aldosterone secretion; a CNS mechanism may also be involved in hypotensive effect as angiotensin II increases adrenergic outflow from CNS; vasoactive kallikreins may be decreased in conversion to active hormones by ACE inhibitors, thus reducing blood pressure

Pharmacodynamics/Kinetics

Onset of action: 1 hour

Peak effect: Hypotensive: Oral: ~6 hours

Duration: 24 hours

Absorption: Unaffected by food

Metabolism: Not metabolized

Bioavailability: Adults: ~25% (range: 6% to 60%); decreased to 16% with NYHA Class II-IV heart failure; Children: ~28%

Half-life elimination: 12 hours

Time to peak: ~7 hours

Excretion: Primarily urine (as unchanged drug)

Dosing

Adult

Acute myocardial infarction (within 24 hours in hemodynamically stable patients): Oral: 5 mg immediately, then 5 mg at 24 hours, 10 mg at 48 hours, and 10 mg every day thereafter for 6 weeks. Patients should continue to receive standard treatments such as thrombolytics, aspirin, and beta-blockers.

According to the 2013 ACCF/AHA guidelines for STEMI: Initial: 2.5 to 5 mg once daily; titrate to 10 mg daily or higher as tolerated (O'Gara, 2013).

Note: For patients with SBP 100 to 120 mm Hg following infarct, initiate therapy with 2.5 mg once daily for 3 days; if SBP falls to <100 mm Hg give maintenance dose of 5 mg once daily (may temporarily reduce to 2.5 mg once daily if necessary). Discontinue if SBP <90 mm Hg for >1 hour.

Heart failure:

US labeling: Initial: 2.5 to 5 mg once daily; then increase by no more than 10 mg increments at intervals no less than 2 weeks to a daily dose of 40 mg daily. Usual maintenance: 5 to 40 mg daily as a single dose. Target dose: 20 to 40 mg once daily (ACCF/AHA [Yancy, 2013])

Note: If patient has hyponatremia (serum sodium <130 mEq/L) or renal impairment (CrCl <30 mL/minute or creatinine >3 mg/dL), then initial dose should be 2.5 mg once daily

Canadian labeling: 2.5 mg once daily; then increase by no more than 10 mg increments at intervals no less than 2 weeks to a maximum dose of 35 mg daily

Hypertension: Oral: Initial: 10 mg once daily (not maintained on a diuretic) or 5 mg once daily (maintained on a diuretic). Target dose (JNC 8 [James, 2013]): 40 mg once daily; usual dosage range (ASH/ISH [Weber, 2014]): 10 to 40 mg daily

Note: Antihypertensive effect may diminish toward the end of the dosing interval especially with doses of 10 mg daily. An increased dose may aid in extending the duration of antihypertensive effect. Doses up to 80 mg daily have been used, but do not appear to give greater effect.

Patients taking diuretics should have them discontinued 2 to 3 days prior to initiating lisinopril if possible. Restart diuretic after blood pressure is stable if needed.

Patients with renovascular hypertension (particularly those with unilateral/bilateral renal artery stenosis): Canadian labeling: Initial: 2.5 to 5 mg once daily with close monitoring; titrate dose carefully based on response.

Geriatric Refer to adult dosing. In the management of hypertension, consider lower initial doses (eg, 2.5 to 5 mg once daily) and titrate to response (Aronow, 2011).

Pediatric

Hypertension:

US labeling: Children ≥6 years and Adolescents: Oral: Initial: 0.07 mg/kg once daily (up to 5 mg); increase dose at 1- to 2-week intervals up to a maximum dose of 0.61 mg/kg or 40 mg once daily; doses >0.61 mg/kg or >40 mg have not been evaluated.

Canadian labeling:

20 kg to <50 kg: Initial: 2.5 mg once daily; titrate per response up to a maximum dose of 20 mg daily

≥50 kg: Initial: 5 mg once daily; titrate per response up to a maximum dose of 40 mg daily

Renal Impairment

Acute myocardial infarction (within 24 hours in hemodynamically stable patients): Adults:

US labeling:

CrCl >30 mL/minute: No dosage adjustment necessary.

CrCl 10 to 30 mL/minute: Initial: 2.5 mg once daily

CrCl <10 mL/minute: Initial: 2.5 mg once daily

Hemodialysis: Initial: 2.5 mg once daily (dialyzable)

Canadian labeling: There are no dosage adjustments provided in the manufacturer's labeling; not recommended if serum creatinine >177 micromol/L and/or proteinuria >500 mg/24 hour; consider discontinuing therapy if serum creatinine >265 micromol/L or doubles from baseline during therapy.

Heart failure: Adults: Initial doses should be modified and upward titration should be cautious, based on response (maximum: 40 mg daily)

US labeling:

CrCl >30 mL/minute: No dosage adjustment necessary.

CrCl 10 to 30 mL/minute or creatinine >3 mg/dL: Initial: 2.5 mg once daily

CrCl <10 mL/minute: Initial: 2.5 mg once daily
Hemodialysis: Initial: 2.5 mg once daily (dialyzable)
Canadian labeling: There are no dosage adjustments provided in the manufacturer's labeling.
Hypertension:
Adults: Initial doses should be modified and upward titration should be cautious, based on response (maximum: 40 mg/day)
CrCl >30 mL/minute: No dosage adjustment necessary.
CrCl 10 to 30 mL/minute: Initial: 5 mg once daily (US labeling) or 2.5 to 5 mg once daily (Canadian labeling)
CrCl <10 mL/minute: Initial: 2.5 mg once daily
Hemodialysis: Initial: 2.5 mg once daily (dialyzable)
Children ≥6 years and Adolescents:
GFR >30 mL/minute/1.73 m^2: No dosage adjustment necessary.
GFR <30 mL/minute/1.73 m^2: Use is not recommended.
Hepatic Impairment There are no dosage adjustments provided in the manufacturer's labeling.
Dietary Considerations Use potassium-containing salt substitutes cautiously in patients with diabetes, patients with renal dysfunction, or those maintained on potassium supplements or potassium-sparing diuretics.
Administration Administer as a single daily dose and without regard to meals.
Monitoring Parameters BUN, serum creatinine, renal function, WBC, and potassium; if patient has collagen vascular disease and/or renal impairment, periodically monitor CBC with differential; hypotensive effects within 1 to 3 hours of initial dose or with increased dosages; consider baseline hepatic function tests (if preexisting hepatic impairment)

2013 ACCF/AHA Heart Failure guideline recommendations: Within 1-2 weeks after initiation and periodically thereafter, reassess renal function and serum potassium especially in patients with preexisting hypotension, hyponatremia, diabetes mellitus, azotemia, or those taking potassium supplements (ACCF/AHA [Yancy, 2013]).
Dosage Forms Excipient information presented when available (limited, particularly for generics); consult specific product labeling.
Tablet, Oral:
Prinivil: 5 mg, 10 mg, 20 mg [scored]
Zestril: 2.5 mg
Zestril: 5 mg [scored]
Zestril: 10 mg, 20 mg, 30 mg, 40 mg
Generic: 2.5 mg, 5 mg, 10 mg, 20 mg, 30 mg, 40 mg
Extemporaneous Preparations A 1 mg/mL lisinopril oral suspension may be made with tablets and a mixture of Bicitra and Ora-Sweet SF. Place ten 20 mg tablets into an 8 ounce amber polyethylene terephthalate (PET) bottle and then add 10 mL purified water and shake for at least 1 minute. Gradually add 30 mL of Bicitra and 160 mL of Ora-Sweet SF to the bottle and gently shake after each addition to disperse the contents. Store resulting suspension at ≤25°C (77°F) for up to 4 weeks. Label bottle "shake well" (Prinivil prescribing information, 2013; Thompson, 2003).

A 1 mg/mL lisinopril oral suspension may be made with tablets and a 1:1 mixture of Ora-Plus® and Ora-Sweet®. Crush ten 10 mg tablets in a mortar and reduce to a fine powder. Add small portions of the vehicle and mix to a uniform paste; mix while adding the vehicle in incremental proportions to **almost** 100 mL; transfer to a graduated cylinder; rinse mortar with vehicle, and add quantity of vehicle sufficient to make 100 mL. Store in amber plastic prescription bottles; label "shake well". Stable for 13 weeks at room temperature or refrigerated (Nahata, 2004).

A 1 mg/mL lisinopril oral suspension also be made with tablets, methylcellulose 1% with parabens, and simple syrup NF. Crush ten 10 mg tablets in a mortar and reduce to a fine powder. Add 7.7 mL of methylcellulose gel and mix to a uniform paste; mix while adding the simple syrup in incremental proportions to **almost** 100 mL; transfer to a graduated cylinder; rinse mortar with vehicle, and add quantity of vehicle sufficient to make 100 mL. Store in amber plastic prescription bottles; label "shake well". Stable for 13 weeks refrigerated or 8 weeks at room temperature (Nahata, 2004).

A 2 mg/mL lisinopril syrup may be made with powder (Sigma Chemical Company, St. Louis, MO) and simple syrup. Dissolve 1 g of lisinopril powder in 30 mL of distilled water. Mix while adding simple syrup in incremental proportions in a quantity sufficient to make 500 mL. Label "shake well" and "refrigerate". Stable for 30 days when stored in amber plastic prescription bottles at room temperature or refrigerated. **Note:** Although no visual evidence of

microbial growth was observed, the authors recommend refrigeration to inhibit microbial growth (Webster, 1997).

Nahata MC and Morosco RS, "Stability of Lisinopril in Two Liquid Dosage Forms," *Ann Pharmacother*, 2004, 38(3):396-9.
Prinivil (lisinopril) [prescribing information]. Whitehouse Station, NJ: Merck & Co., Inc; February 2013.
Thompson KC, Zhao Z, Mazakas JM, et al, "Characterization of an Extemporaneous Liquid Formulation of Lisinopril," *Am J Health Syst Pharm*, 2003, 60(1):69-74.
Webster AA, English BA, and Rose DJ, "The Stability of Lisinopril as an Extemporaneous Syrup," *Intr J Pharmaceut Compound*, 1997, 1:352-3.

Lisinopril and Hydrochlorothiazide
(lyse IN oh pril & hye droe klor oh THYE a zide)

Brand Names: US Prinzide [DSC]; Zestoretic
Brand Names: Canada Apo-Lisinopril/Hctz; Mylan-Lisinopril/Hctz; Sandoz-Lisinopril/Hctz; Teva-Lisinopril/Hctz (Type P); Teva-Lisinopril/Hctz (Type Z); Zestoretic
Index Terms Hydrochlorothiazide and Lisinopril
Pharmacologic Category Angiotensin-Converting Enzyme (ACE) Inhibitor; Antihypertensive; Diuretic, Thiazide
Use Hypertension: Treatment of hypertension
Dosing
Adult & Geriatric Note: Not for initial therapy. Dose is individualized; may be substituted for individual components in patients currently maintained on both agents separately or in patients not controlled with monotherapy.
Hypertension: Oral: Initial: Lisinopril 10 mg/hydrochlorothiazide 12.5 mg or lisinopril 20 mg/hydrochlorothiazide 12.5 mg once daily in patients not adequately controlled on monotherapy; titrate dosage based on clinical response; doses >80 mg/day lisinopril or >50 mg/day hydrochlorothiazide are not recommended.
Renal Impairment
CrCl >30 mL/minute/1.7 m^2: No dosage adjustment necessary; use with caution. Avoid rapid dosage escalation, which may lead to further renal impairment.
CrCl ≤30 mL/minute/1.7 m^2: Use is not recommended.
Hepatic Impairment There are no dosage adjustments provided in the manufacturer's labeling; use with caution.
Additional Information Complete prescribing information should be consulted for additional detail.
Dosage Forms Excipient information presented when available (limited, particularly for generics); consult specific product labeling. [DSC] = Discontinued product
Tablet, oral: 10/12.5: Lisinopril 10 mg and hydrochlorothiazide 12.5 mg; 20/12.5: Lisinopril 20 mg and hydrochlorothiazide 12.5 mg; 20/25: Lisinopril 20 mg and hydrochlorothiazide 25 mg
Prinzide:
10/12.5: Lisinopril 10 mg and hydrochlorothiazide 12.5 mg [DSC]
20/12.5: Lisinopril 20 mg and hydrochlorothiazide 12.5 mg [DSC]
Zestoretic:
10/12.5: Lisinopril 10 mg and hydrochlorothiazide 12.5 mg
20/12.5: Lisinopril 20 mg and hydrochlorothiazide 12.5 mg
20/25: Lisinopril 20 mg and hydrochlorothiazide 25 mg

♦ Lispro Insulin *see* Insulin Lispro *on page 958*
♦ Lithane (Can) *see* Lithium *on page 1091*

Lithium (LITH ee um)

Brand Names: US Lithobid
Brand Names: Canada Apo-Lithium Carbonate; Carbolith; Lithane; Lithmax; PMS-Lithium Carbonate; PMS-Lithium Citrate
Index Terms Eskalith; Lithium Carbonate; Lithium Citrate
Pharmacologic Category Antimanic Agent
Use Bipolar disorder: Acute treatment of manic episodes and maintenance therapy for patients with a diagnosis of bipolar disorder.
Pregnancy Considerations Adverse events have been observed in animal reproduction studies. Lithium crosses the placenta in concentrations similar to those in the maternal plasma (Newport, 2005). Cardiac malformations in the infant, including Ebstein's anomaly, are associated with use of lithium during the first trimester of pregnancy. Other adverse events including polyhydramnios, fetal/neonatal cardiac arrhythmias, hypoglycemia, diabetes insipidus, changes in thyroid function, premature delivery, floppy infant syndrome, or neonatal lithium toxicity are associated with lithium exposure when used later in pregnancy (ACOG, 2008). The incidence of adverse events may be associated with higher maternal doses (Newport, 2005).

Due to pregnancy-induced physiologic changes, women who are pregnant may require dose adjustments of lithium to achieve euthymia and avoid toxicity (ACOG, 2008; Grandjean, 2009; Yonkers, 2011).

For planned pregnancies, use of lithium during the first trimester should be avoided if possible (Grandjean, 2009). If lithium is needed during pregnancy, the minimum effective dose should be used, maternal serum concentrations should be monitored, and consideration should be given to start therapy after the period of organogenesis; lithium should be suspended 24 to 48 hours prior to delivery or at the onset of labor when delivery is spontaneous, then restarted when the patient is medically stable after delivery (ACOG, 2008; Grandjean, 2009; Newport, 2005). Fetal echocardiography should be considered if first trimester exposure occurs (ACOG, 2008).

Breast-Feeding Considerations Lithium is excreted into breast milk and serum concentrations of nursing infants may be 10% to 50% of the maternal serum concentration (Grandjean, 2009). Hypotonia, hypothermia, cyanosis, electrocardiogram changes, and lethargy have been reported in nursing infants (ACOG, 2008). It is generally recommended that breast-feeding be avoided during maternal use of lithium; however, treatment may be continued in appropriately selected patients (Grandjean, 2009; Sharma, 2009; Viguera, 2007). The hydration status of the nursing infant and maternal serum concentrations of lithium should be monitored (ACOG, 2008). In addition, monitor the infant for lethargy, growth, and feeding problems; obtain infant serum concentrations only if clinical concerns arise (Bogen, 2012; Yonkers, 2011). Long-term effects on development and behavior have not been studied (ACOG, 2008; Grandjean, 2009).

Contraindications Hypersensitivity to lithium or any component of the formulation; avoid use in patients with severe cardiovascular or renal disease, or with severe debilitation, dehydration, or sodium depletion

Warnings/Precautions [US Boxed Warning]: Lithium toxicity is closely related to serum levels and can occur at therapeutic doses; serum lithium determinations are required to monitor therapy. Use with caution in patients with mild-moderate renal impairment mild-moderate cardiovascular disease, debilitated patients, and elderly patients due to an increased risk of lithium toxicity. Likewise, use caution in patients in patients with significant fluid loss (protracted sweating, diarrhea, or prolonged fever); temporary reduction or cessation of therapy may be warranted. Lithium may unmask Brugada syndrome; avoid use in patients with or suspected of having Brugada Syndrome. Consult with a cardiologist if a patient is suspected of having Brugada syndrome or has risk factors for Brugada syndrome (eg, unexplained syncope, a family history of Brugada syndrome, a family history of sudden death before the age of 45 years), or if unexplained syncope or palpitations develop after starting therapy. Use with caution in patients with thyroid disease; hypothyroidism may occur with treatment. Hypercalcemia with or without hyperparathyroidism has been reported. Risks are greater in women and possibly in older patients; symptom onset does not appear to be related therapy duration (Lehman, 2013). Serum calcium levels typically range from slightly above normal to over 15 mg/dL and PTH levels may range from high normal to several times the upper limit of normal (Lehman, 2013); magnesium levels are often elevated; serum phosphate levels may be either normal or low (Grandjean, 2009). Monitor calcium and PTH levels as clinically indicated. Consider discontinuation if clinical manifestations of hypercalcemia are present (fatigue, weakness, abdominal pain, constipation, nephrolithiasis,bone pain) or if calcium levels are >11.4 mg/dL. Following discontinuation check serum calcium levels weekly for one month for return to baseline. Changes are usually reversible if lithium is discontinued; however, sustained hypercalcemia and parathyroid gland enlargement has been reported (Lehman, 2013). Chronic therapy results in diminished renal concentrating ability (nephrogenic diabetes insipidus); this is usually reversible when lithium is discontinued. Changes in renal function should be monitored, and re-evaluation of treatment may be necessary. Use caution in patients at risk of suicide (suicidal thoughts or behavior) by drug overdose; lithium has a narrow therapeutic index. Lithium may impair the patient's alertness, affecting the ability to operate machinery or driving a vehicle. Neuromuscular-blocking agents should be administered with caution; the response may be prolonged. Higher serum concentrations may be required and tolerated during an acute manic phase; however, the tolerance decreases when symptoms subside. Normal fluid and salt intake must be maintained during therapy.

Benzyl alcohol and derivatives: Some dosage forms may contain benzyl alcohol; large amounts of benzyl alcohol (≥99 mg/kg/day) have been associated with a potentially fatal toxicity ("gasping syndrome") in neonates; the "gasping syndrome" consists of metabolic acidosis, respiratory distress, gasping respirations, CNS dysfunction (including convulsions, intracranial hemorrhage), hypotension, and cardiovascular collapse (AAP ["Inactive" 1997]; CDC, 1982); some data suggests that benzoate displaces bilirubin from protein binding sites (Ahlfors, 2001); avoid or use dosage forms containing benzyl alcohol with caution in neonates. See manufacturer's labeling.

Adverse Reactions Frequency not always defined.

Cardiovascular: Abnormal T waves on ECG, bradycardia, cardiac arrhythmia, chest tightness, circulatory shock, cold extremities, edema, hypotension, myxedema, sinus node dysfunction, startled response, syncope

Central nervous system: Ataxia, blackout spells, cogwheel rigidity, coma, confusion, dizziness, drowsiness, dystonia, EEG pattern changes, extrapyramidal reaction, fatigue, hallucination, headache, hyperactive deep tendon reflex, hypertonia, involuntary choreoathetoid movements, lethargy, local anesthesia, memory impairment, loss of consciousness, metallic taste, myasthenia gravis (rare), pseudotumor cerebri, psychomotor retardation, reduced intellectual ability, restlessness, salty taste, sedation, seizure, slowed intellectual functioning, slurred speech, stupor, tics, vertigo, worsening of organic brain syndromes

Dermatologic: Acne vulgaris, alopecia, blue-gray skin pigmentation, dermal ulcer, dry or thinning of hair, exacerbation of psoriasis, folliculitis, pruritus, psoriasis, skin rash, xerosis

Endocrine & metabolic: Hypothyroidism (females 14%; males 5% [Johnston 1999]), albuminuria, dehydration, diabetes insipidus, euthyroid goiter, glycosuria, hypercalcemia (secondary to hyperparathyroidism [McKnight 2012]), hyperglycemia, hyperparathyroidism, hyperthyroidism, increased radioactive iodine uptake, increased thirst, polydipsia, weight gain, weight loss

Gastrointestinal: Abdominal pain, anorexia, dental caries, diarrhea, dysgeusia, dyspepsia, excessive salivation, flatulence, gastritis, nausea, vomiting, sialadenitis, sialorrhea, swelling of lips, xerostomia

Genitourinary: Impotence, incontinence, oliguria

Hematologic & oncologic: Leukocytosis

Hypersensitivity: Angioedema

Neuromuscular & skeletal: Joint swelling, muscle hyperirritability, neuromuscular excitability, polyarthralgia, tremor

Ophthalmic: Blurred vision, exophthalmos, nystagmus, transient scotoma

Otic: Tinnitus

Renal: Decreased creatinine clearance, polyuria

Miscellaneous: Fever

Drug Interactions

Metabolism/Transport Effects None known.

Avoid Concomitant Use

Avoid concomitant use of Lithium with any of the following: Dapoxetine

Increased Effect/Toxicity

Lithium may increase the levels/effects of: Antipsychotic Agents; Highest Risk QTc-Prolonging Agents; Metoclopramide; Moderate Risk QTc-Prolonging Agents; Neuromuscular-Blocking Agents; Selective Serotonin Reuptake Inhibitors; Serotonin Modulators; Tricyclic Antidepressants

The levels/effects of Lithium may be increased by: ACE Inhibitors; Angiotensin II Receptor Blockers; Antiemetics (5HT3 Antagonists); Calcium Channel Blockers (Nondihydropyridine); CarBAMazepine; Dapoxetine; Desmopressin; Eplerenone; Fosphenytoin; Loop Diuretics; MAO Inhibitors; Metaxalone; Methyldopa; Mifepristone; Nonsteroidal Anti-Inflammatory Agents; Phenytoin; Potassium Iodide; Thiazide Diuretics; Topiramate

Decreased Effect

Lithium may decrease the levels/effects of: Amphetamines; Antipsychotic Agents; Desmopressin

The levels/effects of Lithium may be decreased by: Caffeine and Caffeine Containing Products; Calcitonin; Calcium Polystyrene Sulfonate; Carbonic Anhydrase Inhibitors; Loop Diuretics; Sodium Bicarbonate; Sodium Chloride; Sodium Polystyrene Sulfonate; Theophylline Derivatives

Storage/Stability Store between 15°C and 30°C (59°F to 86°F). Protect tablets and capsules from moisture.

Mechanism of Action The precise mechanism of action in mood disorders is unknown. Traditionally thought to alter cation transport across cell membranes in nerve and muscle cells, influence the reuptake of serotonin and/or norepinephrine, and inhibit second messenger systems involving the phosphatidylinositol cycle (Ward, 1994). May also provide neuroprotective effects by increasing glutamate clearance, inhibiting apoptoctic glycogen synthase kinase activity, increasing the levels of antiapoptotic protein Bcl-2 and, enhancing the expression of neurotropic factors, including brain-derived neurotrophic factor (Sanacora, 2008).

Pharmacodynamics/Kinetics
Absorption: Rapid and complete
Distribution: V_d: Initial: 0.307 L/kg; V_{dss}: 0.7 to 1 L/kg
Protein binding: Not protein bound
Metabolism: Not metabolized
Bioavailability: 80% to 100%
Half-life elimination: 18 to 36 hours
Time to peak, serum: Immediate release: ~0.5 to 3 hours; Extended release: 2 to 6 hours; Solution: 15 to 60 minutes
Excretion: Urine (primarily; unchanged drug); sweat, saliva, and feces (negligible amounts)
Clearance: 80% of filtered lithium is reabsorbed in the proximal convoluted tubules (Ward, 1994)

Dosing
Adult Note: Monitor serum concentrations and clinical response (efficacy and toxicity) to determine proper dose. Each 5 mL of lithium citrate oral solution contains 8 mEq of lithium ion, equivalent to the amount of lithium in 300 mg of lithium carbonate immediate release capsules/tablets.

Bipolar disorder (acute mania, acute depression [off-label use], and maintenance): Oral:
Immediate release: Initial: Initiate at low dose (eg, 300 mg 3 times daily or less); increase gradually based on response and tolerability (APA, 2002); usual dosage: 900 to 1,800 mg daily in 3 to 4 divided doses
Extended release: Initiate at low dose (eg, 450 mg 2 times daily or less); increase gradually based on response and tolerability (APA, 2002); usual dosage: 900 to 1,800 mg daily in 2 divided doses

Depression, augmentation of antidepressant (off-label use): Oral: Initial: Initiate at a low dose (eg, 300 mg once daily or 300 mg twice daily); increase gradually based on response and tolerability; usual dosage: 600 to1200 mg daily in divided doses (Bauer, 2003a; Bauer 2003b; Nelson, 2014)

Geriatric Bipolar disorder (acute mania, acute depression [off-label use], and maintenance): Initiate therapy with lower doses; refer to adult dosing.

Pediatric Note: Monitor serum concentrations and clinical response (efficacy and toxicity) to determine proper dose. Each 5 mL of lithium citrate oral solution contains 8 mEq of lithium ion, equivalent to the amount of lithium in 300 mg of lithium carbonate immediate release capsules/tablets.

Bipolar disorder:
Children 6 to 12 years (off-label use): Oral: 15 to 60 mg/kg/day in 3 to 4 divided doses; dose not to exceed usual adult dosage. Monitor serum concentrations and clinical response (efficacy and toxicity) to determine proper dose (Nelson, 1996).
Children >12 years and Adolescents: Refer to adult dosing.

Renal Impairment
CrCl 10 to 50 mL/minute: Administer 50% to 75% of normal dose.
CrCl <10 mL/minute: Administer 25% to 50% of normal dose.
End stage renal disease (ESRD) with hemodialysis: Dose after dialysis (Aronoff, 2007).

Hepatic Impairment There are no dosage adjustments provided in manufacturer's labeling.

Dietary Considerations May be taken with meals to avoid GI upset; maintain adequate fluid intake.

Administration Administer with meals to decrease GI upset. Extended release tablets must be swallowed whole; do not crush or chew.

Monitoring Parameters Renal function including BUN and SrCr (baseline, every 2 to 3 months during the first 6 months of treatment, then once a year in stable patients or as clinically indicated); serum electrolytes (baseline, then periodically), serum calcium (baseline, 2 to 6 weeks after initiation, then every 6 to 12 months; repeat as clinically indicated) (Broome, 2011); thyroid (baseline, 1 to 2 times with in the first 6 months of treatment, then once a year in stable patients or as clinically indicated); beta-hCG pregnancy test for all females not known to be sterile (baseline); ECG with rhythm strip (baseline for all patients over 40 years, repeat as clinical indicated), CBC with differential (baseline, repeat as clinically indicated); serum lithium levels (twice weekly until both patient's clinical status and levels are stable, then repeat levels every 1 to 3 months or as clinically indicated); weight (baseline, then periodically) (APA, 2002).

Reference Range Levels should be obtained twice weekly until both patient's clinical status and levels are stable then levels may be obtained no less than every 6 months (APA, 2002).
Timing of serum samples: Draw trough just before next dose (8-12 hours after previous dose)
Therapeutic levels:
Acute mania: 0.5 to 1.2 mEq/L (SI: 0.5 to 1.2 mmol/L)
Maintenance: 0.6 to 1 mEq/L (SI: 0.6 to 1.0 mmol/L); a higher rate of relapse is described in subjects who are maintained at <0.4 mEq/L (SI: 0.4 mmol/L) (APA, 2002)
Toxic concentrations
>1.5 mEq/L (SI: >1.5 mmol/L): Early signs and symptoms of intoxication may include marked tremor, nausea, diarrhea, blurred vision, vertigo, confusion, and decreased deep tendon reflexes.
>2.5 mEq/L (SI: >2.5 mmol/L): Intoxication symptoms may progress to include severe neurological complications, seizures, coma, cardiac dysrhythmia, and permanent neurological impairment.
>3.5 mEq/L (SI: >3.5 mmol/L): Potentially lethal toxicity (APA, 2002; Mitchell, 2001).
Note: A 10% to 26% increase in levels can be expected if there is a change to once daily (usually night-time) dosing (Mitchell, 2001; Singh 2011).

Dosage Forms Excipient information presented when available (limited, particularly for generics); consult specific product labeling.
Capsule, Oral, as carbonate:
Generic: 150 mg, 300 mg, 600 mg
Solution, Oral, as citrate:
Generic: 8 mEq/5 mL (5 mL, 500 mL)
Tablet, Oral, as carbonate:
Generic: 300 mg
Tablet Extended Release, Oral, as carbonate:
Lithobid: 300 mg [contains fd&c blue #2 aluminum lake, fd&c red #40 aluminum lake, fd&c yellow #6 aluminum lake]
Generic: 300 mg, 450 mg

Lodoxamide (loe DOKS a mide)

Brand Names: US Alomide
Brand Names: Canada Alomide®
Index Terms Lodoxamide Tromethamine
Pharmacologic Category Mast Cell Stabilizer
Use Treatment of vernal keratoconjunctivitis, vernal conjunctivitis, and vernal keratitis
Dosing

Adult & Geriatric Vernal conjunctivitis, keratitis: Ophthalmic: Instill 1-2 drops in eye(s) 4 times/day for up to 3 months

Pediatric Children >2 years: Refer to adult dosing.

Renal Impairment No dosage adjustment provided in manufacturer's labeling. However, dosage adjustment unlikely due to low systemic absorption.

Hepatic Impairment No dosage adjustment provided in manufacturer's labeling. However, dosage adjustment unlikely due to low systemic absorption.

Additional Information Complete prescribing information should be consulted for additional detail.

Dosage Forms Excipient information presented when available (limited, particularly for generics); consult specific product labeling.

Solution, Ophthalmic:
Alomide: 0.1% (10 mL)

Lomitapide (loe MI ta pide)

Brand Names: US Juxtapid
Brand Names: Canada Juxtapid
Index Terms AEGR-733; BMS 201038; Lomitapide Mesylate
Pharmacologic Category Antilipemic Agent, Microsomal Triglyceride Transfer Protein (MTP) Inhibitor
Use Homozygous familial hypercholesterolemia: Adjunct to a low-fat diet and other lipid-lowering treatments, including low-density lipoprotein (LDL) apheresis where available, to reduce LDL cholesterol, total cholesterol, apolipoprotein B (apo B), and non-high-density lipoprotein cholesterol (non-HDL-C) in patients with homozygous familial hypercholesterolemia.

Pregnancy Considerations Teratogenic effects have been observed in animal reproduction studies using doses lower than equivalent human doses. Use is contraindicated in pregnant women. Discontinue immediately if pregnancy occurs during treatment. Women of reproductive potential should have a negative pregnancy test prior to therapy and effective contraception must be used during treatment. Dose adjustment may be required for women using oral contraceptives.

Health care providers are encouraged to enroll women exposed to lomitapide during pregnancy in the Global Lomitapide Pregnancy Exposure Registry by calling 1-877-902-4099.

Breast-Feeding Considerations It is not known if lomitapide is excreted into breast milk. Due to the potential for serious adverse reactions in the nursing infant, a decision should be made whether to discontinue nursing or to discontinue the drug, taking into account the importance of treatment to the mother.

Prescribing and Access Restrictions As a requirement of the REMS program, access to this medication is restricted. Prescribers must enroll in the Juxtapid REMS program and complete the Prescriber Training Module and complete, sign, and submit the Prescriber Enrollment Form to the Juxtapid REMS program. Pharmacies must educate all pharmacy staff involved in the dispensing of Juxtapid on the REMS program requirements, put processes in place to verify (prior to dispensing Juxtapid) that the prescriber is certified and the Prescription Authorization Form is received with each new prescription. Pharmacies must also agree to be audited to ensure that all processes and procedures in place are being followed in accordance with the program and be able to provide prescription data to the REMS program. Additional information is available at www.JUXTAPIDREMSProgram.com or at 1-855-898-2743.

Medication Guide Available Yes
Contraindications

Pregnancy; coadministration with moderate or strong CYP3A4 inhibitors; moderate or severe hepatic impairment (Child-Pugh class B or C) and patients with active liver disease, including unexplained persistent elevations of serum transaminases.

Canadian labeling: Additional contraindications (not in U.S. labeling): Hypersensitivity to lomitapide or any component of the formulation; known significant, chronic bowel disease (eg, inflammatory bowel disease, malabsorption); concomitant administration of simvastatin >20 mg daily (concomitant use with simvastatin 40 mg daily is permitted in patients previously tolerant of simvastatin 80 mg daily for ≥1 year without evidence of myotoxicity); galactose intolerance, Lapp-lactase deficiency, or glucose-galactose malabsorption

Warnings/Precautions [U.S. Boxed Warning]: May cause transaminase elevations; elevations in ALT or AST ≥3 times upper limit of normal occurred during clinical trials (no clinically meaningful concomitant bilirubin, INR, or alkaline phosphatase elevation was observed). Lomitapide also increases hepatic fat, with or without concomitant transaminase elevations. Hepatic steatosis associated with lomitapide (reversible upon discontinuation) may be a risk factor for progressive liver disease including steatohepatitis and cirrhosis. Monitor hepatic function (ALT, AST, alkaline phosphatase and total bilirubin) prior to treatment; monitor ALT and AST regularly as recommended during treatment; dosage adjustment or discontinuation may be necessary; transaminases typically reduce within 1-4 weeks after discontinuation. Alcohol ingestion may increase the risk of hepatic steatosis; alcohol consumption should be limited to ≤1 drink/day. Use caution when administered concomitantly with other hepatotoxic medications (eg, acetaminophen (>4 g/day for ≥3 days/week), amiodarone, isotretinoin, methotrexate, tetracyclines, and tamoxifen); may require more frequent monitoring of liver function tests. Concomitant administration with other LDL-lowering agents that also have the potential to increase hepatic fat is not recommended (has not been studied). Use with caution in patients with mild (Child-Pugh class A) hepatic impairment due to increased drug exposure; a reduced maximum dose is recommended. Use is contraindicated in patients with moderate to severe (Child-Pugh class B or C) impairment or active liver disease including unexplained persistent elevations of serum transaminases. Monitor liver function as recommended. Use with caution in patients with mild-to-severe renal impairment including end-stage renal disease (ESRD) not receiving dialysis (has not been evaluated); drug exposure may significantly increase. Use with caution in patients with ESRD receiving dialysis; a reduced maximum dose of 40 mg daily is recommended.

Safety and effectiveness have not been established in patients with hypercholesterolemia who do not have homozygous familial hypercholesterolemia. The effect of lomitapide on cardiovascular morbidity and mortality has not been determined.

Significant gastrointestinal events (eg, diarrhea, nausea, dyspepsia, vomiting) occurred during treatment with lomitapide; absorption of other oral medications may be affected; adherence to a low-fat diet (<20% of energy from fat) and gradual titration of dosage will reduce the risk of gastrointestinal adverse events. Lomitapide may reduce the absorption of fat-soluble nutrients (eg, vitamin E, linoleic acid, alpha-linolenic acid, eicosapentaenoic acid,

and docosahexaenoic acid); supplementation is recommended; patients with chronic bowel or pancreatic diseases predisposed to malabsorption are at increased risk for deficiency. Canadian labeling contraindicates use in patients with known significant, chronic bowel disease (eg, inflammatory bowel disease, malabsorption).

Potentially significant drug-drug interactions may exist, requiring dose or frequency adjustment, additional monitoring, and/or selection of alternative therapy. Contains lactose; avoid use in patients with hereditary galactose intolerance, Lapp lactase deficiency, or glucose-galactose malabsorption; may result in diarrhea and malabsorption. **[U.S. Boxed Warning]: Due to the risk for hepatotoxicity, access is restricted through a REMS program (Juxtapid REMS program).** Only certified health care providers and pharmacies may prescribe and dispense lomitapide.

Adverse Reactions

>10%:

Cardiovascular: Chest pain (24%)

Central nervous system: Fatigue (17%)

Gastrointestinal: Diarrhea (79%; severe: 14%), nausea (65%), dyspepsia (38%), vomiting (34%; severe: 10%), abdominal pain (34%; severe: 7%), weight loss (24%), abdominal discomfort (21%; severe: 7%), abdominal distension (21%; severe: 7%), constipation (21%), flatulence (21%), gastroenteritis (14%)

Hepatic: Liver steatosis (increase in hepatic fat >5%: 78%; >20% fat increase: 13%), increased serum transaminases ≥3 times upper limit of normal (34%), increased serum transaminases (17%; severe: 10%)

Neuromuscular & skeletal: Back pain (14%)

Respiratory: Nasopharyngitis (17%), pharyngolaryngeal pain (14%)

Miscellaneous: Influenza (21%)

1% to 10%:

Cardiovascular: Angina pectoris (10%), palpitation (10%)

Central nervous system: Dizziness (10%), fever (10%), headache (10%)

Gastrointestinal: Frequent bowel movement (10%), gastroesophageal reflux disease (10%), rectal tenesmus (10%)

Hepatic: Hepatotoxicity (severe: 10%)

Respiratory: Nasal congestion (10%)

<1% (Limited to important or life-threatening): Abnormal pulmonary function test, anemia, cough, decreased appetite, dehydration, early satiety, eructation, eye swelling, gait disturbance, gastroenteritis, hematemesis, hematuria, hepatomegaly, hyperhidrosis, hypersensitivity, increase neutrophil, increased appetite, increased gamma-glutamyl transferase, increased serum bilirubin, increased white blood cell count, joint swelling, lower gastrointestinal hemorrhage, myalgia, myocardial infarction, pain in extremity, paresthesia, pharyngeal lesion, prolonged prothrombin time, proteinuria, pyrexia, rsinusitis, skin rash, somnolence, transiet ischemic attack, xeroderma

Drug Interactions

Metabolism/Transport Effects Substrate of CYP1A2 (minor), CYP2B6 (minor), CYP2C19 (minor), CYP2C8 (minor), CYP3A4 (major); **Note:** Assignment of Major/Minor substrate status based on clinically relevant drug interaction potential; **Inhibits** CYP3A4 (weak), P-glycoprotein

Avoid Concomitant Use

Avoid concomitant use of Lomitapide with any of the following: Bosutinib; Conivaptan; CYP3A4 Inhibitors (Moderate); CYP3A4 Inhibitors (Strong); Fusidic Acid (Systemic); Idelalisib; Lovastatin; Mipomersen; PAZOPanib; Pimozide; Silodosin; Tipranavir; Topotecan; VinCRIStine (Liposomal)

Increased Effect/Toxicity

Lomitapide may increase the levels/effects of: Afatinib; ARIPiprazole; Bosutinib; Brentuximab Vedotin; Colchicine; Dabigatran Etexilate; Dofetilide; DOXOrubicin (Conventional); Edoxaban; Everolimus; Flibanserin; Hydrocodone; Ledipasvir; Lovastatin; Mipomersen; Naloxegol; NiMODipine; PAZOPanib; P-glycoprotein/ABCB1 Substrates; Pimozide; Prucalopride; Rifaximin; Silodosin; Simvastatin; Topotecan; VinCRIStine (Liposomal); Warfarin

The levels/effects of Lomitapide may be increased by: Alcohol (Ethyl); Conivaptan; CYP3A4 Inhibitors (Moderate); CYP3A4 Inhibitors (Strong); CYP3A4 Inhibitors (Weak); Fusidic Acid (Systemic); Idelalisib; Luliconazole; Osimertinib; Simeprevir; Stiripentol; Tipranavir

Decreased Effect

The levels/effects of Lomitapide may be decreased by: Bile Acid Sequestrants; Bosentan; CYP3A4 Inducers (Moderate); CYP3A4 Inducers (Strong); Dabrafenib; Deferasirox; Enzalutamide; Mitotane; Osimertinib; Siltuximab; St Johns Wort; Tocilizumab

Food Interactions High-fat diets containing ≥20% of total calories from fat may increase the risk of gastrointestinal adverse reactions (eg, abdominal pain/discomfort, constipation, diarrhea, flatulence, and nausea/vomiting). Grapefruit juice may increase lomitapide plasma concentration. Absorption of fat-soluble nutrients may be reduced. Management: Avoid administering with high fat diets. Avoid grapefruit juice. Take recommended daily supplements of vitamin E, alpha-linolenic acid (ALA), linoleic acid, eicosapentaenoic acid (EPA), and docosahexaenoic acid (DHA).

Storage/Stability Store at 20°C to 25°C (68°F to 77°F); excursions permitted between 15°C to 30°C (59°F to 86°F). Brief exposure up to 40°C (104°F) may be tolerated provided the mean temperature does not exceed 25°C (77°F); minimize this type of exposure. Protect from moisture.

Mechanism of Action Lomitapide directly binds to and inhibits microsomal triglyceride transfer protein (MTP) which is located in the lumen of the endoplasmic reticulum. MTP inhibition prevents the assembly of apo-B containing lipoproteins in enterocytes and hepatocytes resulting in reduced production of chylomicrons and VLDL and subsequently reduces plasma LDL-C concentrations.

Pharmacodynamics/Kinetics

Distribution: Mean V_d: 985-1292 L

Protein binding: 99.8% to plasma proteins

Metabolism: Primarily hepatic (extensive) through CYP3A4 to M1 and M3 (major [inactive in vitro] metabolites); CYP1A2, CYP2B6, CYP2C8, and CYP2C19 are also involved in metabolism to a minor degree.

Bioavailability: ~7%

Half-life elimination: 39.7 hours

Time to peak: ~6 hours

Excretion: Urine (53% to 60%; major component: M1 metabolite); feces (33% to 35%; major component: parent drug)

Dosing

Adult & Geriatric Homozygous familial hypercholesterolemia (HoFH):

Note: Transaminases should be measured prior to initiation and any dose increase; obtain a negative pregnancy test in female patients of reproductive potential prior to beginning treatment. Maintenance dose should be individualized, taking into account patient characteristics such as goal of therapy and response to treatment. To reduce development of fat-soluble nutrient deficiency, administer daily supplements containing vitamin E 400 units, linoleic acid ≥200 mg, alpha-linolenic acid (ALA) ≥210 mg, eicosapentaenoic acid (EPA) ≥110 mg, and docosahexaenoic acid (DHA) ≥80 mg. Initiate and maintain a low-fat diet supplying <20% of energy from fat.

Oral: Initial: 5 mg once daily; after 2 weeks of therapy, may increase dose to 10 mg once daily, as tolerated; then at 4-week intervals, the dose may be increased to 20 mg once daily, then to 40 mg once daily, and finally to a maximum dose of 60 mg once daily.

Dosage adjustment for lomitapide with **weak** CYP3A inhibitors (eg, amiodarone, amlodipine, atorvastatin, cyclosporine, fluoxetine, oral contraceptives): Maximum dose: 30 mg once daily

Renal Impairment

Mild-to-severe impairment (not receiving dialysis): There are no dosage adjustments provided in the manufacturer's labeling (has not been studied); however, it is possible that patients with renal impairment not receiving dialysis may experience increases in lomitapide exposure exceeding 50%.

End stage renal disease (ESRD; receiving dialysis): Maximum dose: 40 mg once daily

Hepatic Impairment

Mild impairment (Child-Pugh class A): Maximum dose: 40 mg once daily

Moderate-to-severe impairment (Child-Pugh class B or C), active liver disease (including unexplained persistent transaminase elevations): Use is contraindicated.

Adjustment for Toxicity Hepatotoxicity: Note: If patient experiences clinical symptoms of liver injury (eg, nausea, vomiting, abdominal pain, fever, jaundice, lethargy, flu-like symptoms) with transaminase elevation, increases in bilirubin ≥2 times ULN, or active liver disease, discontinue use and investigate for probable cause.

AST or ALT ≥3 to <5 times ULN: Confirm measurement (within 1 week); once confirmed, reduce dose and obtain additional liver function tests (LFTs) (eg, alkaline phosphatase, total bilirubin, and INR); repeat tests weekly and withhold subsequent doses if signs of abnormal liver function (eg, increased bilirubin or INR), if transaminases rise to >5 times ULN, or if they do not fall to <3 times ULN within ~4 weeks; investigate for probable cause. If resuming after transaminase resolution to <3 times ULN, consider reducing dose and monitor LFTs more frequently.

AST or ALT ≥5 times ULN: Withhold doses, obtain additional LFTs (eg, alkaline phosphatase, total bilirubin, and INR); investigate for probable cause. If resuming after transaminase resolution to <3 times ULN, reduce dose and monitor LFTs more frequently.

Administration Oral: Administer with a glass of water and without food; administer at least 2 hours after the evening meal since administration with food may increase risk of gastrointestinal adverse effects. Swallow capsules whole (do not open, crush, dissolve, or chew).

Monitoring Parameters Baseline: ALT, AST, alkaline phosphatase, total bilirubin; pregnancy test in females of reproductive potential; measure transaminases prior to any increase in dose or monthly (whichever occurs first) during the first year, and then at least every 3 months and prior to dosage increases (also see Dosage Adjustment for Toxicity)

Dosage Forms Excipient information presented when available (limited, particularly for generics); consult specific product labeling.

Capsule, Oral:

Juxtapid: 5 mg, 10 mg, 20 mg, 30 mg, 40 mg, 60 mg

◆ Lomitapide Mesylate see Lomitapide on page 1094
◆ Lomotil see Diphenoxylate and Atropine on page 564

Lomustine (loe MUS teen)

Brand Names: US CeeNU [DSC]; Gleostine
Brand Names: Canada CeeNU
Index Terms CCNU; CeeNU; Lomustinum
Pharmacologic Category Antineoplastic Agent, Alkylating Agent; Antineoplastic Agent, Alkylating Agent (Nitrosourea)

Use

Brain tumors: Treatment of primary and metastatic brain tumors (after appropriate surgical and/or radiotherapeutic procedures).

Hodgkin lymphoma: Treatment of relapsed or refractory Hodgkin lymphoma (secondary therapy) in combination with other chemotherapy agents; however, its use is limited in the management of Hodgkin lymphoma due to efficacy of other chemotherapy agents/regimens.

Dosing

Adult & Geriatric Note: Dispense only enough capsules for a single dose; do not dispense more than one dose at a time (ISMP, 2014). Repeat courses should only be administered after adequate recovery of leukocytes to >4,000/mm³ and platelets to >100,000/mm³. Doses should be rounded to the nearest 10 mg. Lomustine is associated with a moderate emetic potential; antiemetics are recommended to prevent nausea and vomiting.

Brain tumors: *Manufacturer's labeling:* Oral: 130 mg/m² as a single dose once every 6 weeks; reduce dose to 100 mg/m² as a single dose once every 6 weeks in patients with compromised bone marrow function (dosage reductions may be recommended for combination chemotherapy regimens).

Anaplastic oligodendroglioma: PCV regimen (off-label combination): Oral: 130 mg/m² on day 1 every 6 weeks for up to 4 cycles prior to radiation therapy (in combination with procarbazine and vincristine) (Cairncross, 2013; Cairncross, 2006).

Astrocytoma, high grade: POC regimen (off-label dosing): Adults ≤21 years: Oral: 100 mg/m² on day 1 every 6 weeks for 8 cycles (in combination with vincristine and prednisone) (Finlay, 1995).

Glioblastoma, recurrent:

PCV regimen (off-label dosing): Oral: 110 mg/m² on day 1 every 6 weeks for 7 cycles (in combination with procarbazine and vincristine) (Levin, 2000).

Single-agent therapy: Oral: 100 to 130 mg/m² every 6 weeks until disease progression or unacceptable toxicity (Wick, 2010).

Medulloblastoma (off-label dosing): Adults ≤21 years: Oral: 75 mg/m² once every 6 weeks for 8 cycles (in combination with cisplatin and vincristine) (Packer, 2006; Packer, 1999).

Hodgkin lymphoma: *Manufacturer's labeling:* Oral: 130 mg/m² as a single dose once every 6 weeks; reduce dose to 100 mg/m² as a single dose once every 6 weeks in patients with compromised bone marrow function (dosage reductions may be recommended for combination chemotherapy regimens).

Dosing adjustment (based on nadir) for subsequent cycles:

Leukocytes ≥3,000/mm³, platelets ≥75,000/mm³: No dosage adjustment required

Leukocytes 2,000 to 2,999/mm³, platelets 25,000 to 74,999/mm³: Administer 70% of prior dose

Leukocytes <2,000/mm³, platelets <25,000/mm³: Administer 50% of prior dose

Pediatric Note: Dispense only enough capsules for a single dose; do not dispense more than one dose at a time (ISMP, 2014). Repeat courses should only be administered after adequate recovery of leukocytes to >4,000/mm³ and platelets to >100,000/mm³. Doses should be rounded to the nearest 10 mg. Lomustine is associated with a moderate emetic potential; antiemetics are recommended to prevent nausea and vomiting (Dupuis, 2011).

Brain tumors: *Manufacturer's labeling:* Oral: 130 mg/m² as a single dose once every 6 weeks; reduce dose to 100 mg/m² as a single dose once every 6 weeks in patients with compromised bone marrow function (dosage reductions may be recommended for combination chemotherapy regimens).

Astrocytoma, high grade: POC regimen (off-label dosing): Children ≥18 months and Adolescents: Oral: 100 mg/m² on day 1 every 6 weeks for 8 cycles (in combination with vincristine and prednisone) (Finlay, 1995)

Medulloblastoma (off-label dosing): Children ≥3 years and Adolescents: Oral: 75 mg/m² once every 6 weeks for 8 cycles (in combination with cisplatin and vincristine) (Packer, 2006; Packer, 1999)

Hodgkin lymphoma: *Manufacturer's labeling:* Oral: 130 mg/m² as a single dose once every 6 weeks; reduce dose to 100 mg/m² as a single dose once every 6 weeks in patients with compromised bone marrow function (dosage reductions may be recommended for combination chemotherapy regimens)

Dosing adjustment (based on nadir) for subsequent cycles: Refer to adult dosing.

Renal Impairment There are no dosage adjustments provided in the manufacturer's labeling. The following adjustments have been recommended:

Aronoff, 2007: Adults:

CrCl 10 to 50 mL/minute: Administer 75% of dose

CrCl <10 mL/minute: Administer 25% to 50% of dose

Hemodialysis: Supplemental dose is not necessary

Continuous ambulatory peritoneal dialysis (CAPD): Administer 25% to 50% of dose

Kintzel, 1995:

CrCl 46 to 60 mL/minute: Administer 75% of normal dose

CrCl 31 to 45 mL/minute: Administer 70% of normal dose

CrCl ≤30 mL/minute: Avoid use

Hepatic Impairment There are no dosage adjustments provided in the manufacturer's labeling. However, lomustine is hepatically metabolized and caution should be used in patients with hepatic dysfunction.

Obesity *ASCO Guidelines for appropriate chemotherapy dosing in obese adults with cancer:* Utilize patient's actual body weight (full weight) for calculation of body surface area- or weight-based dosing, particularly when the intent of therapy is curative; manage regimen-related toxicities in the same manner as for nonobese patients; if a dose reduction is utilized due to toxicity, consider resumption of full weight-based dosing with subsequent cycles, especially if cause of toxicity (eg, hepatic or renal impairment) is resolved (Griggs, 2012).

Additional Information Complete prescribing information should be consulted for additional detail.

Dosage Forms Excipient information presented when available (limited, particularly for generics); consult specific product labeling. [DSC] = Discontinued product

Capsule, Oral:

CeeNU: 10 mg [DSC], 40 mg [DSC], 100 mg [DSC]

Gleostine: 5 mg, 10 mg, 40 mg, 100 mg

Generic: 10 mg, 40 mg, 100 mg

◆ Lomustinum see Lomustine on page 1096
◆ Longastatin see Octreotide on page 1308
◆ Loniten (Can) see Minoxidil (Systemic) on page 1213
◆ Lonsurf see Trifluridine and Tipiracil on page 1845

♦ Lo Ovral *see* Ethinyl Estradiol and Norgestrel
  on page 711

♦ Loperacap (Can) *see* Loperamide *on page 1097*

Loperamide (loe PER a mide)

Brand Names: US Anti-Diarrheal [OTC]; Diamode [OTC]; Imodium A-D [OTC]; Loperamide A-D [OTC]

Brand Names: Canada Apo-Loperamide®; Diarr-Eze; Dom-Loperamide; Imodium®; Loperacap; Novo-Lopera-mide; PMS-Loperamide; Rhoxal-loperamide; Rho®-Loper-amine; Riva-Loperamide; Sandoz-Loperamide

Index Terms Loperamide Hydrochloride

Pharmacologic Category Antidiarrheal

Use Control and symptomatic relief of chronic diarrhea associated with inflammatory bowel disease and of acute nonspecific diarrhea; to reduce volume of ileostomy discharge

OTC labeling: Control of symptoms of diarrhea, including Traveler's diarrhea

Pregnancy Considerations Teratogenic effects were not observed in animal reproduction studies. Information related to loperamide use in pregnancy is limited and data is conflicting (Einarson, 2000; Källén, 2008). For acute diarrhea in pregnant women, some clinicians recommend oral rehydration and dietary changes; loperamide in small amounts may be used only if symptoms are disabling (Wald, 2003).

Breast-Feeding Considerations Small amounts of loperamide are excreted in human breast milk (information is based on studies using loperamide oxide, the prodrug of loperamide [Nikodem, 1992]). The manufacturer does not recommend use in nursing women.

Contraindications Hypersensitivity to loperamide or any component of the formulation; abdominal pain without diarrhea; children <2 years of age

Avoid use as primary therapy in patients with acute dysentery (bloody stools and high fever), acute ulcerative colitis, bacterial enterocolitis (caused by *Salmonella, Shigella,* and *Campylobacter*), pseudomembranous colitis associated with broad-spectrum antibiotic use

Warnings/Precautions Loperamide is a symptom-directed treatment; if an underlying diagnosis is made, other disease-specific treatment may be indicated. Rare cases of anaphylaxis and anaphylactic shock have been reported. Use is contraindicated if diarrhea is accompanied by high fever or blood in stool. Use caution in young children as response may be variable because of dehydration; contraindicated in children <2 years of age. Concurrent fluid and electrolyte replacement is often necessary in all age groups depending upon severity of diarrhea. Should not be used when inhibition of peristalsis is undesirable or dangerous. Discontinue promptly if constipation, abdominal pain, abdominal distension, blood in stool, or ileus develop. Do not use when peristalsis inhibition should be avoided due to potential for ileus, megacolon, and/or toxic megacolon. Stop therapy in AIDS patients at the first sign of abdominal distention; cases of toxic megacolon have occurred in AIDS patients with infectious colitis (due to viral or bacterial pathogens). Use caution in patients with hepatic impairment due to reduced first-pass metabolism; monitor for signs of CNS toxicity. May cause drowsiness or dizziness, which may impair physical or mental abilities; patients must be cautioned about performing tasks which require mental alertness (eg, operating machinery or driving). Discontinue use and consult health care provider if diarrhea lasts longer than 2 days, symptoms worsen, or abdominal swelling or bulging develops.

Benzyl alcohol and derivatives: Some dosage forms may contain sodium benzoate/benzoic acid; benzoic acid (benzoate) is a metabolite of benzyl alcohol; large amounts of benzyl alcohol (≥99 mg/kg/day) have been associated with a potentially fatal toxicity ("gasping syndrome") in neonates; the "gasping syndrome" consists of metabolic acidosis, respiratory distress, gasping respirations, CNS dysfunction (including convulsions, intracranial hemorrhage), hypotension, and cardiovascular collapse (AAP ["Inactive" 1997]; CDC, 1982); some data suggests that benzoate displaces bilirubin from protein binding sites (Ahlfors, 2001); avoid or use dosage forms containing benzyl alcohol derivative with caution in neonates. See manufacturer's labeling.

Adverse Reactions 1% to 10%:

Central nervous system: Dizziness (1%)

Gastrointestinal: Constipation (2% to 5%), abdominal cramping (≤3%), nausea (≤3%)

Postmarketing and/or case reports: Abdominal distention, abdominal pain, allergic reactions, anaphylactic shock, anaphylactoid reactions, angioedema, bullous eruption (rare), drowsiness, dyspepsia, erythema multiforme (rare), fatigue, flatulence, hypersensitivity, paralytic ileus, megacolon, pruritus, rash, Stevens-Johnson syndrome (rare), toxic epidermal necrolysis (rare), toxic megacolon, urinary retention, urticaria, vomiting, xerostomia

Drug Interactions

Metabolism/Transport Effects Substrate of P-glycoprotein

Avoid Concomitant Use There are no known interactions where it is recommended to avoid concomitant use.

Increased Effect/Toxicity

Loperamide may increase the levels/effects of: Ramosetron

The levels/effects of Loperamide may be increased by: Lumacaftor; P-glycoprotein/ABCB1 Inhibitors; Ranolazine

Decreased Effect

The levels/effects of Loperamide may be decreased by: Lumacaftor; P-glycoprotein/ABCB1 Inducers

Storage/Stability Store at 20°C to 25°C (68°F to 77°F).

Mechanism of Action Acts directly on circular and longitudinal intestinal muscles, through the opioid receptor, to inhibit peristalsis and prolong transit time; reduces fecal volume, increases viscosity, and diminishes fluid and electrolyte loss; demonstrates antisecretory activity. Loperamide increases tone on the anal sphincter

Pharmacodynamics/Kinetics

Absorption: Poor

Distribution: Poor penetration into brain

Metabolism: Hepatic via oxidative N-demethylation

Half-life elimination: 9-14 hours

Time to peak, plasma: Liquid: 2.5 hours; Capsule: 5 hours

Dosing

Adult & Geriatric

Acute diarrhea: Oral: Initial: 4 mg, followed by 2 mg after each loose stool, up to 16 mg/day

Chronic diarrhea: Oral: Initial: Follow acute diarrhea; maintenance dose should be slowly titrated downward to minimum required to control symptoms (typically, 4-8 mg/day in divided doses)

Traveler's diarrhea: Oral: Initial: 4 mg after first loose stool, followed by 2 mg after each subsequent stool (maximum dose: 8 mg/day)

Cancer treatment-induced diarrhea (off-label use): Oral: 4 mg followed by 2 mg every 4 hours or after each unformed stool; Maximum: 16 mg/day (Benson, 2004) **or** 4 mg followed by 2 mg every 2 hours (4 mg every 4 hours at night) until 12 hours have passed without a loose bowel movement (Sharma, 2005)

Irinotecan-induced delayed diarrhea (off-label use): Oral: 4 mg after first loose or frequent bowel movement, then 2 mg every 2 hours (4 mg every 4 hours at night) until 12 hours have passed without a bowel movement (Rothenberg, 1996)

Pediatric

Acute diarrhea: Initial doses (in first 24 hours):

2-5 years (13-20 kg): 1 mg 3 times/day

6-8 years (20-30 kg): 2 mg twice daily

8-12 years (>30 kg): 2 mg 3 times/day

Maintenance: After initial dosing, 0.1 mg/kg doses after each loose stool, daily dose should not exceed the recommended dose for the initial 24 hours

Traveler's diarrhea:

6-8 years: 2 mg after first loose stool, followed by 1 mg after each subsequent stool (maximum dose: 4 mg/day)

9-11 years: 2 mg after first loose stool, followed by 1 mg after each subsequent stool (maximum dose: 6 mg/day)

≥12 years: Refer to adult dosing.

Renal Impairment No dosage adjustment necessary.

Hepatic Impairment No dosage adjustment provided in manufacturer's labeling; use with caution.

Dietary Considerations Some products may contain sodium.

Dosage Forms Excipient information presented when available (limited, particularly for generics); consult specific product labeling. [DSC] = Discontinued product

Capsule, Oral, as hydrochloride:

Generic: 2 mg

Liquid, Oral, as hydrochloride:

Anti-Diarrheal: 1 mg/5 mL (120 mL [DSC]) [contains alcohol, usp, benzoic acid, propylene glycol, sodium benzoate]

Anti-Diarrheal: 1 mg/5 mL (120 mL [DSC]) [contains alcohol, usp, methylparaben, propylparaben]

Imodium A-D: 1 mg/7.5 mL (120 mL, 240 mL) [contains brilliant blue fcf (fd&c blue #1), fd&c yellow #10 (quinoline yellow), propylene glycol, sodium benzoate]

Imodium A-D: 1 mg/7.5 mL (30 mL, 120 mL, 240 mL, 360 mL) [contains brilliant blue fcf (fd&c blue #1), fd&c yellow #10 (quinoline yellow), propylene glycol, sodium benzoate; mint flavor]

Generic: 1 mg/5 mL (5 mL, 10 mL, 118 mL)

Suspension, Oral, as hydrochloride:

Generic: 1 mg/7.5 mL (120 mL)

Tablet, Oral, as hydrochloride:

Anti-Diarrheal: 2 mg

Anti-Diarrheal: 2 mg [scored]

Anti-Diarrheal: 2 mg [contains brilliant blue fcf (fd&c blue #1), fd&c yellow #10 (quinoline yellow)]

Anti-Diarrheal: 2 mg [scored; contains brilliant blue fcf (fd&c blue #1), fd&c yellow #10 (quinoline yellow)]

Anti-Diarrheal: 2 mg [contains fd&c blue #1 aluminum lake, fd&c yellow #10 (quinoline yellow)]

Diamode: 2 mg [scored]

Imodium A-D: 2 mg [scored; contains brilliant blue fcf (fd&c blue #1), fd&c yellow #10 (quinoline yellow)]

Imodium A-D: 2 mg [scored; contains fd&c blue #1 aluminum lake, fd&c yellow #10 aluminum lake]

Loperamide A-D: 2 mg

Tablet Chewable, Oral, as hydrochloride:

Imodium A-D: 2 mg [contains fd&c blue #1 aluminum lake, fd&c yellow #10 aluminum lake; cool mint flavor]

♦ Loperamide A-D [OTC] *see* Loperamide *on page 1097*

Loperamide and Simethicone
(loe PER a mide & sye METH i kone)

Brand Names: US Imodium Multi-Symptom Relief [OTC]
Brand Names: Canada Imodium Advanced Multi-Symptom
Index Terms Simethicone and Loperamide Hydrochloride
Pharmacologic Category Antidiarrheal; Antiflatulent
Use
Acute diarrhea and gas: Control of symptoms of diarrhea and gas (bloating, pressure, and cramps)
Dosing
Adult & Geriatric Acute diarrhea and gas: Oral: Two tablets after first loose stool, followed by 1 tablet with each subsequent loose stool (maximum dose: 4 tablets/24 hours)
Pediatric Acute diarrhea and gas: Note: Weight-based dosing is preferred
Children 6 to 8 years (22 to 26 kg): Oral: One tablet after first loose stool, followed by one-half tablet with each subsequent loose stool (maximum dose: 2 tablets/24 hours)
Children 9 to 11 years (27 to 43 kg): Oral: One tablet after first loose stool, followed by one-half tablet with each subsequent loose stool (maximum dose: 3 tablets/24 hours)
Children ≥12 years and Adolescents: Refer to adult dosing.
Renal Impairment There are no dosage adjustments provided in the manufacturer's labeling.
Hepatic Impairment There are no dosage adjustments provided in the manufacturer's labeling.
Additional Information Complete prescribing information should be consulted for additional detail.
Dosage Forms Excipient information presented when available (limited, particularly for generics); consult specific product labeling.
Caplet:
Imodium Multi-Symptom Relief: Loperamide hydrochloride 2 mg and simethicone 125 mg [contains calcium 65 mg/caplet, sodium 4 mg/caplet]
Tablet, chewable:
Imodium Multi-Symptom Relief: Loperamide hydrochloride 2 mg and simethicone 125 mg [contains calcium 50 mg/tablet; mint flavor]

♦ Loperamide Hydrochloride *see* Loperamide *on page 1097*

♦ Lopid *see* Gemfibrozil *on page 835*

Lopinavir and Ritonavir
(loe PIN a veer & ri TOE na vir)

Brand Names: US Kaletra
Brand Names: Canada Kaletra
Index Terms Ritonavir and Lopinavir
Pharmacologic Category Antiretroviral, Protease Inhibitor (Anti-HIV)

Use Treatment of HIV-1 infection: Treatment of HIV-1 infection in combination with other antiretroviral agents

Pregnancy Considerations Adverse events were not seen in animal reproduction studies, except at doses which were also maternally toxic. Lopinavir/ritonavir has a low level of transfer across the human placenta. Based on information collected by the Antiretroviral Pregnancy Registry, an increased risk of teratogenic effects has not been observed in humans. A small increased risk of preterm birth has been associated with maternal use of protease inhibitor-based combination antiretroviral (ARV) therapy during pregnancy; however, the benefits of use generally outweigh this risk and protease inhibitors (PIs) should not be withheld if otherwise recommended. Hyperglycemia, new onset of diabetes mellitus, or diabetic ketoacidosis have been reported with PIs; it is not clear if pregnancy increases this risk.

The HHS Perinatal HIV Guidelines consider lopinavir/ritonavir to be a preferred protease inhibitor for use in antiretroviral-naive pregnant women. Lopinavir/ritonavir is not recommended for use in pregnant women with lopinavir-resistance-associated amino acid substitutions. In addition, once-daily dosing is not recommended during pregnancy and use of the oral solution should be avoided (due to alcohol and propylene glycol content).

Regardless of CD4 count or HIV RNA copy number, all HIV-infected pregnant women should receive a combination antiretroviral ARV drug regimen. A combination of antepartum, intrapartum, and infant ARV prophylaxis is recommended. ARV therapy should be started as soon as possible in women with symptomatic infection. Although earlier initiation may be more effective in reducing the perinatal transmission of HIV, initiation may be delayed until after 12 weeks gestation in women who do not require immediate treatment after careful consideration of maternal conditions (eg, nausea and vomiting) and the potential risks of first trimester fetal exposure for specific agents. A scheduled cesarean delivery at 38 weeks gestation is recommended for all women with HIV RNA >1000 copies/mL or unknown concentrations near delivery in order to decrease transmission. If ARV therapy must be interrupted for <24 hours during the peripartum period, stop then restart all medications simultaneously in order to decrease the chance of developing resistance. Long-term follow-up is recommended for all infants exposed to ARV medications. In couples who want to conceive, the HIV-infected partner should attain maximum viral suppression prior to conception.

Health care providers are encouraged to enroll pregnant women exposed to antiretroviral medications in the Antiretroviral Pregnancy Registry (1-800-258-4263 or www.APRegistry.com). Health care providers caring for HIV-infected women and their infants may contact the National Perinatal HIV Hotline (888-448-8765) for clinical consultation (HHS [perinatal], 2014).

Breast-Feeding Considerations Lopinavir/ritonavir concentrations are very low to undetectable in breast milk and undetectable in the serum of nursing infants. Maternal or infant antiretroviral therapy does not completely eliminate the risk of postnatal HIV transmission. In addition, multi-class-resistant virus has been detected in breast-feeding infants despite maternal therapy. Therefore, in the United States, where formula is accessible, affordable, safe, and sustainable, and the risk of infant mortality due to diarrhea and respiratory infections is low, complete avoidance of breast-feeding by HIV-infected women is recommended to decrease potential transmission of HIV (HHS [perinatal], 2014).

Medication Guide Available Yes
Contraindications
Hypersensitivity (eg, toxic epidermal necrolysis, Stevens-Johnson syndrome, erythema multiforme, urticaria, angioedema) to lopinavir, ritonavir, or any component of the formulation; coadministration with drugs that are highly dependent on CYP3A for clearance and for which elevated plasma concentrations are associated with serious and/or life-threatening reactions; coadministration with the potent CYP3A inducers (where significantly decreased lopinavir levels may be associated with a potential for loss of virologic response and resistance and cross-resistance to develop): Alfuzosin, cisapride, ergot derivatives (eg, dihydroergotamine, ergotamine, methylergonovine), lovastatin, oral midazolam, pimozide, rifampin, sildenafil (when used to treat pulmonary arterial hypertension), simvastatin, St John's wort, and triazolam.
Canadian labeling: Additional contraindications (not in US labeling): Coadministration with fusidic acid, midazolam, salmeterol, vardenafil, astemizole (not available in Canada), terfenadine (not available in Canada)

Warnings/Precautions Potentially significant drug-drug interactions may exist, requiring dose or frequency adjustment, additional monitoring, and/or selection of alternative therapy. Cases of pancreatitis, some fatal, have been associated with lopinavir/ritonavir; use caution in patients with a history of pancreatitis or advanced HIV-1 disease (may be at increased risk). Patients with signs or symptoms of pancreatitis should be evaluated and therapy suspended as clinically appropriate. May alter cardiac conduction and prolong the QTc and/or PR interval; second and third degree AV block and torsade de pointes have been observed. Possible higher risk of myocardial infarction associated with the cumulative use of lopinavir/ritonavir; consider avoiding lopinavir/ritonavir-based regimens in patients with high cardiac risk (Bavinger, 2013; HHS [adult], 2015). Use with caution in patients with underlying structural heart disease, preexisting conduction system abnormalities, ischemic heart disease or cardiomyopathies. Avoid use in combination with QTc- or PR-interval prolonging drugs or in patients with hypokalemia or congenital long QT syndrome.

Changes in glucose tolerance, hyperglycemia, exacerbation of diabetes, DKA, and new-onset diabetes mellitus have been reported in patients receiving protease inhibitors. May cause hepatitis or exacerbate preexisting hepatic dysfunction; use with caution in patients with hepatitis B or C and in hepatic disease; patients with hepatitis or elevations in transaminases prior to the start of therapy may be at increased risk for further increases in transaminases or hepatic dysfunction (rare fatalities reported postmarketing). Consider more frequent liver function test monitoring during therapy initiation in patients with preexisting hepatic dysfunction. Large increases in total cholesterol and triglycerides have been reported; screening should be done prior to therapy and periodically throughout treatment. Increased bleeding may be seen in patients with hemophilia A or B who are taking protease inhibitors. Redistribution or accumulation of body fat has been observed in patients using antiretroviral therapy. Patients may develop immune reconstitution syndrome resulting in the occurrence of an inflammatory response to an indolent or residual opportunistic infection during initial HIV treatment or activation of autoimmune disorders (eg, Graves' disease, polymyositis, Guillain-Barré syndrome) later in therapy; further evaluation and treatment may be required.

The oral solution is highly concentrated and contains large amounts of alcohol. Monitor patients with renal impairment or with decreased ability to metabolize propylene glycol (eg, patients of Asian origin) for propylene glycol toxicity. Health care providers should pay special attention to accurate calculation, measurement, and administration of dose. Overdose in a child may lead to lethal ethanol or propylene glycol toxicity. Oral solution also contains fructose; consider fructose content in patients with fructose intolerance. Once-daily dosing is not recommended in patients with ≥3 lopinavir-resistance-associated substitutions; those receiving efavirenz, nevirapine, or nelfinavir; carbamazepine, phenobarbital, phenytoin, or in children <18 years of age. Safety, efficacy, and pharmacokinetic profiles of lopinavir and ritonavir have not been established for neonates <14 days of age. Neonates <14 days of age, particularly preterm neonates, are at risk for developing propylene glycol toxicity with use of the lopinavir/ritonavir oral solution. Oral solution contains ethanol and propylene glycol; ethanol competitively inhibits propylene glycol metabolism. Postmarketing reports in preterm neonates following use of the oral solution include cardiotoxicity (complete AV block, bradycardia, cardiomyopathy), lactic acidosis, CNS depression, respiratory complications, acute renal failure, and death. The oral solution should not be used in the immediate postnatal period, including full term neonates age <14 days or preterm neonates until 14 days after their due date, unless the infant is closely monitored and benefits clearly outweigh risk.

Adverse Reactions Data presented for short- and long-term combination antiretroviral therapy in both protease inhibitor experienced and naïve patients.

>10%:
Dermatologic: Skin rash (children 12%; adults ≤5%)
Endocrine & metabolic: Hypercholesterolemia (3% to 39%), increased serum triglycerides (3% to 36%), increased gamma-glutamyl transferase (10% to 29%)
Gastrointestinal: Diarrhea (7% to 28%; greater with once-daily dosing), dysgeusia (children 22%; adults <2%), vomiting (children 21%; adults 2% to 7%), nausea (5% to 16%), abdominal pain (1% to 11%)
Hepatic: Increased serum ALT (grade 3/4: 1% to 11%)
Respiratory: Upper respiratory tract infection (14%)
>2% to 10%:
Cardiovascular: Vasodilation (≤3%)

Central nervous system: Fatigue (8%, including weakness), headache (2% to 6%), anxiety (4%), insomnia (≤4%)
Dermatologic: Skin infection (3%, including cellulitis, folliculitis, furuncle)
Endocrine & metabolic: Hypertriglyceridemia (6%), hyperglycemia (≤5%), hyperuricemia (≤5%), alteration in sodium (children 3%), weight loss (≤3%)
Gastrointestinal: Increased serum amylase (3% to 8%), dyspepsia (≤6%), increased serum lipase (3% to 5%), flatulence (1% to 4%), gastroenteritis (3%)
Hematologic & oncologic: Thrombocytopenia (grade 3/4: 4% children), neutropenia (grade 3/4: 1% to 5%)
Hepatic: Increased serum AST (grade 3/4: 2% to 10%), hepatitis (4%, including increased AST, ALT, and gamma-glutamyl transferase), increased serum bilirubin (children 3%; adults 1%)
Hypersensitivity: Hypersensitivity (3%, including urticaria and angioedema)
Neuromuscular & skeletal: Weakness (≤9%), musculoskeletal pain (6%)
Respiratory: Lower respiratory tract infection (8%)
≤2% (Limited to important or life-threatening): Acne vulgaris, alopecia, amenorrhea, amnesia, anemia, anorexia, asthma, atherosclerotic disease, atrial fibrillation, atrioventricular block (second and third degree), atrophic striae, bacterial infection, benign neoplasm, bradycardia, brain disease, breast hypertrophy, bronchitis, cerebral infarction, cerebrovascular accident, cholangitis, cholecystitis, confusion, Cushing's syndrome, cyst, decreased creatine clearance, decreased glucose tolerance, deep vein thrombosis, dehydration, depression, dermal ulcer, diabetes mellitus, duodenitis, dyskinesia, eczema, edema, enteritis, enterocolitis, erythema multiforme, exfoliative dermatitis, extrapyramidal reaction, facial paralysis, fecal incontinence, first degree atrioventricular block, gastritis, gastroesophageal reflux disease, gastrointestinal hemorrhage, gastrointestinal ulcer, gynecomastia, hematuria, hemorrhagic colitis, hemorrhoids, hepatic insufficiency, hepatomegaly, hyperacusis, hyperhidrosis, hypermenorrhea, hypersensitivity reaction, hypertension, hypertonia, hypogonadism (males), hypophosphatemia, hypothyroidism, immune reconstitution syndrome, impotence, jaundice, lactic acidosis, leukopenia, lipoma, liver steatosis, liver tenderness, lymphadenopathy, maculopapular rash, migraine, myocardial infarction, neoplasm, nephritis, neuropathy, obesity, oral mucosa ulcer, orthostatic hypotension, osteonecrosis, otitis media, pancreatitis, periodontitis, peripheral edema, peripheral neuropathy, prolonged Q-T interval on ECG, propylene glycol toxicity (preterm neonates [includes cardiomyopathy, lactic acidosis, acute renal failure, respiratory complications]), pulmonary edema, rectal hemorrhage, redistribution of body fat (including facial wasting), renal failure, rhabdomyolysis, seborrhea, seizure, sialadenitis, skin discoloration, splenomegaly, Stevens-Johnson syndrome, stomatitis, thrombophlebitis, torsades de pointes, tricuspid regurgitation, vasculitis, viral infection, vitamin deficiency, weight gain

Drug Interactions
Metabolism/Transport Effects Refer to individual components.
Avoid Concomitant Use
Avoid concomitant use of Lopinavir and Ritonavir with any of the following: Ado-Trastuzumab Emtansine; Alfuzosin; Amiodarone; Amodiaquine; Antihepaciviral Combination Products; Aprepitant; Astemizole; Atovaquone; Avanafil; Axitinib; Barnidipine; Bosutinib; Bromocriptine; Cabozantinib; Ceritinib; Cisapride; Clarithromycin; Cobimetinib; Conivaptan; Crizotinib; Dabrafenib; Dapoxetine; Darunavir; Disulfiram; Domperidone; Dronedarone; Eletriptan; Enzalutamide; Eplerenone; Ergot Derivatives; Everolimus; Flecainide; Flibanserin; Fluticasone (Nasal); Fosamprenavir; Fusidic Acid (Systemic); Halofantrine; Highest Risk QTc-Prolonging Agents; Ibrutinib; Irinotecan Products; Isavuconazonium Sulfate; Ivabradine; Lapatinib; Lercanidipine; Lomitapide; Lovastatin; Lurasidone; Macitentan; Mequitazine; Methadone; MetroNIDAZOLE (Systemic); Midazolam; Mifepristone; Moderate Risk QTc-Prolonging Agents; Naloxegol; Nilotinib; NiMODipine; Nisoldipine; Olaparib; Ombitasvir, Paritaprevir, Ritonavir, and Dasabuvir; Osimertinib; Palbociclib; PAZOPanib; Pimozide; Propafenone; QuiNIDine; QuiNINE; Ranolazine; Red Yeast Rice; Regorafenib; Rifampin; Rivaroxaban; Salmeterol; Saquinavir; Silodosin; Simeprevir; Simvastatin; Sonidegib; St Johns Wort; Suvorexant; Tamoxifen; Tamsulosin; Telaprevir; Terfenadine; Thioridazine; Ticagrelor; Tipranavir; Tolvaptan; Topotecan; Toremifene; Trabectedin; TraZODone; Triazolam; Ulipristal; Vemurafenib; VinCRIStine (Liposomal); Vorapaxar; Voriconazole

◀ **Increased Effect/Toxicity**

Lopinavir and Ritonavir may increase the levels/effects of: Ado-Trastuzumab Emtansine; Afatinib; Alfuzosin; Alitretinoin (Systemic); Almotriptan; Alosetron; ALPRAZolam; Amiodarone; Amodiaquine; Antihepaciviral Combination Products; Apixaban; Aprepitant; ARIPiprazole; ARIPiprazole Lauroxil; Astemizole; AtoMOXetine; AtorvaSTATin; Avanafil; Axitinib; Barnidipine; Bedaquiline; Bosentan; Bosutinib; Brentuximab Vedotin; Brexpiprazole; Brinzolamide; Bromocriptine; Budesonide (Nasal); Budesonide (Oral Inhalation); Budesonide (Systemic); Budesonide (Topical); Cabazitaxel; Cabozantinib; Calcium Channel Blockers (Nondihydropyridine); Cannabis; Cariprazine; Ceritinib; Cilostazol; Cisapride; Clarithromycin; Cobimetinib; Colchicine; Conivaptan; Contraceptives (Progestins); Corticosteroids (Orally Inhaled); Corticosteroids (Systemic); Crizotinib; Cyclophosphamide; CycloSPORINE (Systemic); CYP2C8 Substrates; CYP2D6 Substrates; CYP3A4 Substrates; Dabigatran Etexilate; Dabrafenib; Daclatasvir; Dapoxetine; Dasatinib; Digoxin; Disulfiram; Domperidone; DOXOrubicin (Conventional); Dronabinol; Dronedarone; DULoxetine; Dutasteride; Edoxaban; Eletriptan; Eluxadoline; Elvitegravir; Enfuvirtide; Enzalutamide; Eplerenone; Ergot Derivatives; Erlotinib; Estazolam; Etizolam; Everolimus; FentaNYL; Fesoterodine; Flecainide; Flibanserin; Fluticasone (Nasal); Fluticasone (Oral Inhalation); Fusidic Acid (Systemic); GuanFACINE; Halofantrine; Highest Risk QTc-Prolonging Agents; Hydrocodone; Ibrutinib; Idelalisib; Imatinib; Imidafenacin; Irinotecan Products; Isavuconazonium Sulfate; Itraconazole; Ivabradine; Ivacaftor; Ixabepilone; Ketoconazole (Systemic); Lacosamide; Lapatinib; Ledipasvir; Lercanidipine; Levobupivacaine; Levomilnacipran; Linagliptin; Lomitapide; Lovastatin; Lurasidone; Macitentan; Maraviroc; Meperidine; Mequitazine; MethylPREDNISolone; Metoprolol; MetroNIDAZOLE (Systemic); Midazolam; Naloxegol; Nebivolol; Nefazodone; Nelfinavir; Nilotinib; NiMODipine; Nintedanib; Nisoldipine; Olaparib; Ombitasvir, Paritaprevir, Ritonavir, and Dasabuvir; Osimertinib; Ospemifene; Oxybutynin; OxyCODONE; Palbociclib; Parecoxib; Paricalcitol; PAZOPanib; P-glycoprotein/ABCB1 Substrates; Pimecrolimus; Pimozide; Pioglitazone; PONATinib; Pranlukast; PrednisoLONE (Systemic); PredniSONE; Propafenone; Protease Inhibitors; Prucalopride; QuiNIDine; QuiNINE; Ramelteon; Ranolazine; Red Yeast Rice; Regorafenib; Retapamulin; Rifabutin; Rifaximin; Rilpivirine; Riociguat; Rivaroxaban; Rosuvastatin; Ruxolitinib; Salmeterol; Saxagliptin; Sildenafil; Silodosin; Simeprevir; Simvastatin; Sonidegib; Suvorexant; Tacrolimus (Systemic); Tacrolimus (Topical); Tadalafil; Tamsulosin; Tasimelteon; Temsirolimus; Tenofovir Disoproxil Fumarate; Terfenadine; Tetrahydrocannabinol; Thioridazine; Ticagrelor; Tofacitinib; Tolterodine; Tolvaptan; Topotecan; Toremifene; Trabectedin; TraMADol; TraZODone; Treprostinil; Triamcinolone (Systemic); Triazolam; Ulipristal; Vardenafil; Vemurafenib; Vilazodone; VinBLAStine; VinCRIStine; VinCRIStine (Liposomal); Vindesine; Vinorelbine; Vorapaxar; Vortioxetine; Zolpidem; Zopiclone

The levels/effects of Lopinavir and Ritonavir may be increased by: ARIPiprazole; Clarithromycin; Delavirdine; Enfuvirtide; Fusidic Acid (Systemic); Ivabradine; Ketoconazole (Systemic); Methadone; MetroNIDAZOLE (Topical); Mifepristone; Moderate Risk QTc-Prolonging Agents; P-glycoprotein/ABCB1 Inhibitors; QTc-Prolonging Agents (Indeterminate Risk and Risk Modifying); QuiNINE; Rifabutin; Rifampin; Saquinavir; Simeprevir

Decreased Effect

Lopinavir and Ritonavir may decrease the levels/effects of: Abacavir; Antidiabetic Agents; Atovaquone; Boceprevir; BuPROPion; Canagliflozin; Clarithromycin; Codeine; Contraceptives (Estrogens); Contraceptives (Progestins); CYP2C19 Substrates; Darunavir; Deferasirox; Delavirdine; Didanosine; Etravirine; Fosamprenavir; Fosphenytoin; Hydrocodone; Ifosfamide; LamoTRIgine; Meperidine; Methadone; Phenytoin; Prasugrel; Proguanil; QuiNINE; Tamoxifen; Telaprevir; Ticagrelor; TraMADol; Valproate Products; Voriconazole; Warfarin; Zidovudine

The levels/effects of Lopinavir and Ritonavir may be decreased by: Boceprevir; Bosentan; CarBAMazepine; CYP3A4 Inducers (Moderate); CYP3A4 Inducers (Strong); Efavirenz; Fosamprenavir; Fosphenytoin; Garlic; Mitotane; Nelfinavir; Nevirapine; PHENobarbital; Phenytoin; Rifampin; Siltuximab; St Johns Wort; Tipranavir; Tocilizumab

Food Interactions Moderate- to high-fat meals increase the C_{max} and AUC of lopinavir/ritonavir oral solution; no significant changes observed with oral tablets. Management: Take oral solution with food; take tablet with or without food.

Storage/Stability

Oral solution: Store at 2°C to 8°C (36°F to 46°F). Avoid exposure to excessive heat. If stored at room temperature (25°C or 77°F), use within 2 months.

Tablet: Store at USP controlled room temperature of 20°C to 25°C (68°F to 77°F). Exposure to high humidity outside of the original container for >2 weeks is not recommended.

Mechanism of Action A coformulation of lopinavir and ritonavir. The lopinavir component binds to the site of HIV-1 protease activity and inhibits the cleavage of viral Gag-Pol polyprotein precursors into individual functional proteins required for infectious HIV. This results in the formation of immature, noninfectious viral particles. The ritonavir component inhibits the CYP3A metabolism of lopinavir, allowing increased plasma levels of lopinavir.

Pharmacodynamics/Kinetics

Ritonavir: See Ritonavir monograph.

Lopinavir:

Protein binding: 98% to 99%; decreased with mild-to-moderate hepatic dysfunction

Metabolism: Hepatic via CYP3A4; 13 metabolites identified

Half-life elimination: 5-6 hours

Time to peak, plasma: ~4 hours

Excretion: Feces (83%, 20% as unchanged drug); urine (10%; <3% as unchanged drug)

Dosing

Adult

HIV infection (as a component of combination therapy): Oral:

Twice-daily dosing:

Therapy-naive or therapy-experienced: Lopinavir 400 mg/ritonavir 100 mg twice daily.

Therapy-naive or therapy-experienced patients receiving efavirenz, fosamprenavir, nelfinavir, nevirapine: See dosage adjustment for combination therapy.

Once-daily dosing: Therapy-naive or experienced patients with <3 lopinavir resistance-associated substitutions: Lopinavir 800 mg/ritonavir 200 mg once daily. Once-daily dosing is not recommended in those receiving efavirenz, fosamprenavir, nevirapine, nelfinavir, carbamazepine, phenobarbital, or phenytoin.

Pregnant women (with no lopinavir-resistance-associated amino acid substitutions): Lopinavir 400 mg/ritonavir 100 mg twice daily. Once-daily dosing is not recommended. Tablets are recommended; avoid use of the oral solution.

Dosage adjustment for combination therapy with efavirenz, nelfinavir, or nevirapine (US labeling) or efavirenz, fosamprenavir, nelfinavir, or nevirapine (Canadian labeling): Oral:

Twice-daily dosing: Therapy-naive and therapy-experienced patients:

Solution: Lopinavir 533 mg/ritonavir 133 mg (6.5 mL) twice daily

Tablet: Lopinavir 500 mg/ritonavir 125 mg twice daily

Once-daily dosing: Once-daily dosing not recommended.

Dosage adjustment for combination therapy with carbamazepine, phenobarbital, phenytoin: Once-daily dosing not recommended

Geriatric Initial studies did not include enough elderly patients to determine effects based on age. Use with caution due to possible decreased hepatic, renal, and cardiac function.

Pediatric

HIV infection (component of combination therapy): Oral: Dosage based on weight or body surface area (BSA), **presented based on lopinavir component** (maximum dose: Lopinavir 400 mg/ritonavir 100 mg). **Note:** Once daily dosing is not recommended in Infants, Children, or Adolescents <18 years of age. Use in infants <6 months of age is not approved in the Canadian labeling.

14 days to 6 months: 16 mg/kg or 300 mg/m^2 twice daily; **Note:** Should not be administered to neonates age <14 days (defined as postmenstrual age of 42 weeks [first day of mother's last menstrual period to birth plus postnatal age]) and a postnatal age of at least 14 days

6 months to 18 years: **Note:** FDA-approved dose and Health Canada-approved dose are approximately equivalent to lopinavir 230 mg/m^2 per dose.

Oral solution:
<15 kg: 12 mg/kg twice daily
15 to 40 kg: 10 mg/kg twice daily
>40 kg: Lopinavir 400 mg/ritonavir 100 mg twice daily

Tablets:
<15 kg: Tablets are not recommended.
15 to 25 kg: Lopinavir 200 mg/ritonavir 50 mg twice daily
>25 kg to 35 kg: Lopinavir 300 mg/ritonavir 75 mg twice daily
>35 kg: Lopinavir 400 mg/ritonavir 100 mg twice daily

Dosage adjustment for combination therapy with efavirenz, nelfinavir, or nevirapine (US labeling) or efavirenz, fosamprenavir, nelfinavir, or nevirapine (Canadian labeling): Oral:

Twice-daily dosing:
Infants 14 days to 6 months: Combination therapy with these agents is not recommended due to lack of data.
Infants, Children, and Adolescents 6 months to 18 years: Solution or tablet **(based on mg of lopinavir component)**: FDA-approved dose and Health Canada-approved dose are approximately equivalent to lopinavir 300 mg/m^2 per dose:

Oral solution:
<15 kg: 13 mg/kg twice daily
15 to 45 kg: 11 mg/kg twice daily
>45 kg: Refer to adult dosing.

Tablets:
<15 kg: Tablets are not recommended.
15 kg to 20 kg: Lopinavir 200 mg/ritonavir 50 mg twice daily
>20 kg to 30 kg: Lopinavir 300 mg/ritonavir 75 mg twice daily
>30 kg to 45 kg: Lopinavir 400 mg/ritonavir 100 mg twice daily
>45 kg: Refer to adult dosing.

Once-daily dosing: Not recommended in children.

Renal Impairment Has not been studied in patients with renal impairment; however, a decrease in clearance is not expected.

Hemodialysis: Avoid once-daily dosing in hemodialysis patients (HHS [adult], 2015)

Hepatic Impairment Use caution in hepatic impairment (metabolized primarily by the liver).

Mild-to-moderate impairment: Mild-to-moderate impairment: There are no dosage adjustments provided in the manufacturer's labeling; however, lopinavir is primarily metabolized by the liver and its AUC may be increased ~30%; use with caution.

Severe impairment: There are no dosage adjustments provided in the manufacturer's labeling (has not been studied).

Dietary Considerations Solution must be taken with food. Tablet may be taken with or without food

Administration

Solution: Must be administered with food; if using didanosine, take didanosine 1 hour before or 2 hours after lopinavir/ritonavir. Administer using calibrated dosing syringe.

Tablet: May be taken with or without food. Swallow whole, do not break, crush, or chew. May be taken with didanosine when taken without food. Tablets are not recommended in patients <15 kg.

Monitoring Parameters Prior to therapy, consider genotypic or phenotypic testing for lopinavir resistance-associated substitutions.

Triglycerides and cholesterol (prior to initiation then periodically thereafter), LFTs, electrolytes, basic HIV monitoring, viral load and CD4 count, glucose

Dosage Forms Excipient information presented when available (limited, particularly for generics); consult specific product labeling.

Solution, oral:
Kaletra: Lopinavir 80 mg and ritonavir 20 mg per 1 mL (160 mL) [contains ethanol 42.4%, menthol, propylene glycol; cotton candy flavor]]

Tablet:
Kaletra:
Lopinavir 100 mg and ritonavir 25 mg
Lopinavir 200 mg and ritonavir 50 mg

◆ Lopreeza *see* Estradiol and Norethindrone *on page 687*
◆ Lopresor (Can) *see* Metoprolol *on page 1193*
◆ Lopresor SR (Can) *see* Metoprolol *on page 1193*
◆ Lopressor *see* Metoprolol *on page 1193*

◆ Loprox *see* Ciclopirox *on page 384*
◆ Loradamed [OTC] *see* Loratadine *on page 1101*

Loratadine (lor AT a deen)

Brand Names: US Alavert [OTC]; Allergy Relief For Kids [OTC]; Allergy Relief [OTC]; Allergy [OTC]; Childrens Loratadine [OTC]; Claritin Reditabs [OTC]; Claritin [OTC]; Loradamed [OTC]; Loratadine Childrens [OTC]; Loratadine Hives Relief [OTC]; QlearQuil 24 Hour Relief [OTC]; Tri-aminic Allerchews [OTC]

Brand Names: Canada Apo-Loratadine; Claritin®; Claritin® Kids

Index Terms Tavist ND

Pharmacologic Category Histamine H$_1$ Antagonist; Histamine H$_1$ Antagonist, Second Generation; Piperidine Derivative

Use

Allergic rhinitis: Relief of nasal and non-nasal symptoms of seasonal allergic rhinitis

Urticaria: Treatment of itching due to hives (urticarial)

Pregnancy Considerations Maternal use of loratadine has not been associated with an increased risk of major malformations. The use of antihistamines for the treatment of rhinitis during pregnancy is generally considered to be safe at recommended doses. Although safety data is limited, loratadine may be the preferred second generation antihistamine for the treatment of rhinitis or urticaria during pregnancy.

Breast-Feeding Considerations Small amounts of loratadine and its active metabolite, desloratadine, are excreted into breast milk.

Contraindications Hypersensitivity to loratadine or any component of the formulation

Warnings/Precautions Use with caution in patients with liver or renal impairment. Hepatic impairment increases systemic exposure. Some products may contain phenylalanine. May be inappropriate in older adults depending on comorbidities (eg, dementia, delirium) due to its potent anticholinergic effects (Beers Criteria). Effects may be potentiated when used with other sedative drugs or ethanol.

Benzyl alcohol and derivatives: Some dosage forms may contain sodium benzoate/benzoic acid; benzoic acid (benzoate) is a metabolite of benzyl alcohol; large amounts of benzyl alcohol (≥99 mg/kg/day) have been associated with a potentially fatal toxicity ("gasping syndrome") in neonates; the "gasping syndrome" consists of metabolic acidosis, respiratory distress, gasping respirations, CNS dysfunction (including convulsions, intracranial hemorrhage), hypotension, and cardiovascular collapse (AAP ["Inactive" 1997]; CDC, 1982); some data suggests that benzoate displaces bilirubin from protein binding sites (Ahlfors, 2001); avoid or use dosage forms containing benzyl alcohol derivative with caution in neonates. See manufacturer's labeling.

Adverse Reactions

Central nervous system: Headache (12% adults), somnolence (8% adults), nervousness (4% ages 6-12 years), fatigue (4% adults; 3% ages 6-12 years, 2% to 3% ages 2-5 years), malaise (2% ages 6-12 years)

Dermatologic: Rash (2% to 3% ages 2-5 years)

Gastrointestinal: Xerostomia (3% adults), stomatitis (2% to 3% ages 2-5 years), abdominal pain (2% ages 6-12 years)

Neuromuscular & skeletal: Hyperkinesia (3% ages 6-12 years)

Ocular: Conjunctivitis (2% ages 6-12 years)

Respiratory: Wheezing (4% ages 6-12 years), epistaxis (2% to 3% ages 2-5 years), pharyngitis (2% to 3% ages 2-5 years), dysphonia (2% ages 6-12 years), upper respiratory infection (2% ages 6-12 years)

Miscellaneous: Flu-like syndrome (2% to 3% ages 2-5 years), viral infection (2% to 3% ages 2-5 years)

<2% (Limited to important or life-threatening): Abnormal hepatic function, agitation, alopecia, altered lacrimation, altered micturition, altered salivation, altered taste, amnesia, anaphylaxis, angioneurotic edema, anorexia, arthralgia, back pain, blepharospasm, blurred vision, breast enlargement, breast pain, bronchospasm, chest pain, confusion, depression, dizziness, dysmenorrhea, dyspnea, erythema multiforme, hemoptysis, hepatic necrosis, hepatitis, hypotension, impaired concentration, impotence, insomnia, irritability, jaundice, menorrhagia, migraine, nausea, palpitation, paresthesia, paroniria, peripheral edema, photosensitivity, pruritus, purpura, rigors, seizure, supraventricular tachyarrhythmia, syncope, tachycardia, tremor, urinary discoloration, urticaria, thrombocytopenia, vaginitis, vertigo, vomiting, weight gain

Drug Interactions

Metabolism/Transport Effects Substrate of CYP2D6 (minor), CYP3A4 (minor), P-glycoprotein; **Note:** Assignment of Major/Minor substrate status based on clinically relevant drug interaction potential; **Inhibits** CYP2C19 (weak), CYP2C8 (weak), CYP2D6 (weak)

Avoid Concomitant Use

Avoid concomitant use of Loratadine with any of the following: Aclidinium; Amodiaquine; Azelastine (Nasal); Cimetropium; Eluxadoline; Glucagon; Glycopyrrolate; Glycopyrrolate (Oral Inhalation); Ipratropium (Oral Inhalation); Levosulpiride; Orphenadrine; Paraldehyde; Potassium Chloride; Thalidomide; Tiotropium; Umeclidinium

Increased Effect/Toxicity

Loratadine may increase the levels/effects of: AbobotulinumtoxinA; Alcohol (Ethyl); Amodiaquine; Analgesics (Opioid); Anticholinergic Agents; ARIPiprazole; Azelastine (Nasal); Buprenorphine; Cimetropium; CNS Depressants; Eluxadoline; Glucagon; Glycopyrrolate; Glycopyrrolate (Oral Inhalation); Hydrocodone; Methotrimeprazine; Metyrosine; Mirabegron; Mirtazapine; OnabotulinumtoxinA; Orphenadrine; Paraldehyde; Potassium Chloride; Pramipexole; Ramosetron; RimabotulinumtoxinB; ROPINIRole; Rotigotine; Selective Serotonin Reuptake Inhibitors; Suvorexant; Thalidomide; Thiazide Diuretics; Tiotropium; Topiramate; Zolpidem

The levels/effects of Loratadine may be increased by: Aclidinium; Amiodarone; Brimonidine (Topical); Cannabis; Doxylamine; Dronabinol; Droperidol; HydrOXYzine; Ipratropium (Oral Inhalation); Kava Kava; Lumacaftor; Magnesium Sulfate; Methotrimeprazine; Mianserin; Minocycline; Nabilone; Perampanel; P-glycoprotein/ABCB1 Inhibitors; Pramlintide; Ranolazine; Rufinamide; Sodium Oxybate; Tapentadol; Tetrahydrocannabinol; Umeclidinium

Decreased Effect

Loratadine may decrease the levels/effects of: Acetylcholinesterase Inhibitors; Benzylpenicilloyl Polylysine; Betahistine; Gastrointestinal Agents (Prokinetic); Hyaluronidase; Itopride; Levosulpiride; Secretin

The levels/effects of Loratadine may be decreased by: Acetylcholinesterase Inhibitors; Amphetamines; Lumacaftor; P-glycoprotein/ABCB1 Inducers

Food Interactions Food increases bioavailability and delays peak. Management: Administer without regard to meals.

Storage/Stability Store at 20°C to 25°C (68°F to 77°F). Rapidly-disintegrating tablets: Use within 6 months of opening foil pouch, and immediately after opening individual tablet blister. Store in a dry place.

Mechanism of Action Long-acting tricyclic antihistamine with selective peripheral histamine H_1-receptor antagonistic properties

Pharmacodynamics/Kinetics

Onset of action: 1-3 hours
Peak effect: 8-12 hours
Duration: >24 hours
Absorption: Rapid
Metabolism: Extensively hepatic via CYP2D6 and 3A4 to active metabolite (descarboethoxyloratadine)
Half-life elimination: Mean: 8.4 hours (range: 3-20 hours)
Excretion: Urine (40%) and feces (40%) as metabolites

Dosing

Adult & Geriatric Seasonal allergic rhinitis, urticaria: Oral: 10 mg daily once daily or 5 mg twice daily (RediTabs)

Pediatric

Children 2-5 years: Seasonal allergic rhinitis, urticaria: Oral: 5 mg once daily
Children ≥6 years: Refer to adult dosing.

Renal Impairment No dosage adjustment provided in manufacturer's labeling; however, the following recommendations have been recommended (Aronoff, 2007):

Adults:
CrCl 10-50 mL/minute: Recommended dose every 24 to 48 hours.
CrCl <10 mL/minute: Recommended dose every 48 hours.
Dialysis: Recommended dose every 48 hours.
Continuous renal replacement therapy (CRRT): No dosage adjustment necessary if clearance is 2000 mL/minute.
Children ≥2 years: No dosage adjustment necessary for any degree of renal impairment.

Hepatic Impairment No dosage adjustment provided in manufacturer's labeling; however, hepatic impairment increases systemic exposure to loratadine.

Dietary Considerations May be taken without regard to meals. Some products may contain phenylalanine and/or sodium.

Administration May be administered without regard to meals.
Dispersible tablet: Place in mouth and allow to dissolve. Swallow with or without water.

Test Interactions May suppress the wheal and flare reactions to skin test antigens

Dosage Forms Excipient information presented when available (limited, particularly for generics); consult specific product labeling.

Capsule, Oral:
Claritin: 10 mg [contains brilliant blue fcf (fd&c blue #1)]
Solution, Oral:
Childrens Loratadine: 5 mg/5 mL (120 mL) [alcohol free, dye free, sugar free; contains propylene glycol, sodium benzoate; grape flavor]
Loratadine Childrens: 5 mg/5 mL (120 mL) [alcohol free, dye free, sugar free; contains propylene glycol, sodium benzoate; fruit flavor]
Loratadine Hives Relief: 5 mg/5 mL (120 mL) [alcohol free, dye free, sugar free; contains propylene glycol, sodium benzoate; grape flavor]
Syrup, Oral:
Allergy Relief: 5 mg/5 mL (236 mL) [alcohol free; contains propylene glycol, sodium benzoate]
Allergy Relief For Kids: 5 mg/5 mL (120 mL) [contains propylene glycol, sodium benzoate; fruit flavor]
Childrens Loratadine: 5 mg/5 mL (120 mL) [fruit flavor]
Childrens Loratadine: 5 mg/5 mL (120 mL) [alcohol free, dye free; contains propylene glycol, sodium benzoate, sodium metabisulfite; grape flavor]
Claritin: 5 mg/5 mL (60 mL, 120 mL, 150 mL) [alcohol free, color free, dye free, sugar free; contains edetate disodium, propylene glycol, sodium benzoate; grape flavor]
Loratadine Childrens: 5 mg/5 mL (120 mL) [sugar free; contains polyethylene glycol, propylene glycol, sodium benzoate, sodium metabisulfite; grape flavor]
Tablet, Oral:
Alavert: 10 mg
Allergy: 10 mg
Allergy Relief: 10 mg
Claritin: 10 mg
Loradamed: 10 mg
QlearQuil 24 Hour Relief: 10 mg
Generic: 10 mg
Tablet Chewable, Oral:
Claritin: 5 mg [contains aspartame, fd&c blue #2 aluminum lake; grape flavor]
Tablet Dispersible, Oral:
Alavert: 10 mg [contains aspartame]
Alavert: 10 mg [contains aspartame; bubble-gum flavor]
Alavert: 10 mg [contains aspartame; citrus flavor]
Allergy: 10 mg [contains aspartame; fruit flavor]
Allergy Relief: 10 mg [contains aspartame]
Allergy Relief: 10 mg [contains aspartame; fruit flavor]
Claritin Reditabs: 5 mg, 10 mg
Triaminic Allerchews: 10 mg

◆ Loratadine-D 12 Hour [OTC] *see* Loratadine and Pseudoephedrine *on page 1102*

Loratadine and Pseudoephedrine

(lor AT a deen & soo doe e FED rin)

Brand Names: US Alavert™ Allergy and Sinus [OTC]; Claritin-D® 12 Hour Allergy & Congestion [OTC]; Claritin-D® 24 Hour Allergy & Congestion [OTC]; Loratadine-D 12 Hour [OTC]

Brand Names: Canada Chlor-Tripolon ND®; Claritin® Extra; Claritin® Liberator

Index Terms Pseudoephedrine and Loratadine

Pharmacologic Category Alpha/Beta Agonist; Decongestant; Histamine H_1 Antagonist; Histamine H_1 Antagonist, Second Generation; Piperidine Derivative

Use Temporary relief of symptoms of seasonal allergic rhinitis, other upper respiratory allergies, or the common cold

Dosing

Adult & Geriatric Seasonal allergic rhinitis/nasal congestion:
Oral: 1 tablet every 12 hours
Extended release: 1 tablet daily

Pediatric Seasonal allergic rhinitis/nasal congestion: Children ≥12 years: Refer to adult dosing.

Renal Impairment CrCl <30 mL/minute:
Claritin-D® 12-Hour: 1 tablet daily
Claritin-D® 24-Hour: 1 tablet every other day

Hepatic Impairment Should be avoided.

Additional Information Complete prescribing information should be consulted for additional detail.

Dosage Forms Excipient information presented when available (limited, particularly for generics); consult specific product labeling.

Tablet, extended release: Loratadine 10 mg and pseudoephedrine sulfate 240 mg

Alavert™ Allergy and Sinus: Loratadine 5 mg and pseudoephedrine sulfate 120 mg

Claritin-D® 12 Hour Allergy & Congestion: Loratadine 5 mg and pseudoephedrine sulfate 120 mg [contains calcium 30 mg/tablet]

Claritin-D® 24 Hour Allergy & Congestion: Loratadine 10 mg and pseudoephedrine sulfate 240 mg [contains calcium 25 mg/tablet]

Loratadine-D 12 Hour: Loratadine 5 mg and pseudoephedrine sulfate 120 mg

◆ Loratadine Childrens [OTC] see Loratadine on page 1101

◆ Loratadine Hives Relief [OTC] see Loratadine on page 1101

LORazepam (lor A ze pam)

Brand Names: US Ativan; LORazepam Intensol

Brand Names: Canada Apo-Lorazepam; Ativan; Dom-Lorazepam; Lorazepam Injection, USP; PHL-Lorazepam; PMS-Lorazepam; PRO-Lorazepam; Teva-Lorazepam

Pharmacologic Category Benzodiazepine

Use

Anxiety (oral): Management of anxiety disorders, short-term (≤4 months) relief of anxiety symptoms, or anxiety associated with depressive symptoms, or anxiety/stress-associated insomnia

Anesthesia premedication (parenteral): Anesthesia premedication to relieve anxiety or to produce amnesia (diminish recall) or sedation

Anesthesia premedication (sublingual): *Canadian labeling:* Anesthesia premedication to relieve anxiety prior to surgical procedures

Status epilepticus (parenteral): Treatment of status epilepticus

Pregnancy Considerations Teratogenic effects have been observed in some animal reproduction studies. Lorazepam and its metabolite cross the human placenta. Teratogenic effects in humans have been observed with some benzodiazepines (including lorazepam); however, additional studies are needed. The incidence of premature birth and low birth weights may be increased following maternal use of benzodiazepines; hypoglycemia and respiratory problems in the neonate may occur following exposure late in pregnancy. Neonatal withdrawal symptoms may occur within days to weeks after birth and "floppy infant syndrome" (which also includes withdrawal symptoms) have been reported with some benzodiazepines (including lorazepam). Elimination of lorazepam in the newborn infant is slow; following *in utero* exposure, term infants may excrete lorazepam for up to 8 days (Bergman 1992; Iqbal 2002; Wikner 2007).

Breast-Feeding Considerations Lorazepam can be detected in breast milk. Drowsiness, lethargy, or weight loss in nursing infants have been observed in case reports following maternal use of some benzodiazepines (Iqbal 2002). Breast-feeding is not recommended by the manufacturer.

Contraindications

Hypersensitivity to lorazepam, any component of the formulation, or other benzodiazepines (cross-sensitivity with other benzodiazepines may exist); acute narrow-angle glaucoma; sleep apnea (parenteral); intra-arterial injection of parenteral formulation; severe respiratory insufficiency (except during mechanical ventilation)

Canadian labeling: Additional contraindications (not in U.S. labeling): Myasthenia gravis

Warnings/Precautions Use with caution in elderly or debilitated patients, patients with hepatic disease (including alcoholics) or renal impairment. In older adults, benzodiazepines increase the risk of impaired cognition, delirium, falls, fractures, and motor vehicle accidents. Due to increased sensitivity in this age group, avoid use for treatment of insomnia, agitation, or delirium. (Beers Criteria). Use with caution in patients with respiratory disease (COPD or sleep apnea) or limited pulmonary reserve, or impaired gag reflex. Initial doses in elderly or debilitated patients should be at the lower end of the dosing range. May worsen hepatic encephalopathy.

Causes CNS depression (dose-related) resulting in sedation, dizziness, confusion, or ataxia which may impair physical and mental capabilities. Patients must be cautioned about performing tasks which require mental alertness (eg, operating machinery or driving). Effects may be potentiated when used with other sedative drugs or ethanol. Potentially significant drug-drug interactions may exist, requiring dose or frequency adjustment, additional monitoring, and/or selection of alternative therapy. Benzodiazepines have been associated with falls and traumatic injury and should be used with extreme caution in patients who are at risk of these events.

Lorazepam may cause anterograde amnesia. Paradoxical reactions, including hyperactive or aggressive behavior have been reported with benzodiazepines, particularly in adolescent/pediatric or psychiatric patients. Does not have analgesic, antidepressant, or antipsychotic properties.

Preexisting depression may worsen or emerge during therapy. Not recommended for use in primary depressive or psychotic disorders. Should not be used in patients at risk for suicide without adequate antidepressant treatment. Risk of dependence increases in patients with a history of alcohol or drug abuse and those with significant personality disorders; use with caution in these patients. Tolerance, psychological and physical dependence may also occur with higher dosages and prolonged use. The risk of dependence is decreased with short-term treatment (2 to 4 weeks); evaluate the need for continued treatment prior to extending therapy duration. Benzodiazepines have been associated with dependence and acute withdrawal symptoms on discontinuation or reduction in dose. Acute withdrawal, including seizures, may be precipitated after administration of flumazenil to patients receiving long-term benzodiazepine therapy. Lorazepam is a short half-life benzodiazepine. Tolerance develops to the sedative, hypnotic, and anticonvulsant effects. It does not develop to the anxiolytic effects (Vinkers 2012). Chronic use of this agent may increase the perioperative benzodiazepine dose needed to achieve desired effect.

As a hypnotic agent, should be used only after evaluation of potential causes of sleep disturbance. Failure of sleep disturbance to resolve after 7 to 10 days may indicate psychiatric or medical illness. A worsening of insomnia or the emergence of new abnormalities of thought or behavior may represent unrecognized psychiatric or medical illness and requires immediate and careful evaluation.

Status epilepticus should not be treated with injectable benzodiazepines alone; requires close observation and management and possibly ventilatory support. When used as a component of preanesthesia, monitor for heavy sedation and airway obstruction; equipment necessary to maintain airway and ventilatory support should be available. Parenteral formulation of lorazepam contains polyethylene glycol which has resulted in toxicity during high-dose and/or longer-term infusions. Parenteral formulation also contains propylene glycol (PG); may be associated with dose-related toxicity and can occur ≥48 hours after initiation of lorazepam. Limited data suggest increased risk of PG accumulation at doses of ≥6 mg/hour for 48 hours or more (Nelson 2008). Monitor for signs of toxicity which may include acute renal failure, lactic acidosis, and/or osmol gap. May consider using enteral delivery of lorazepam tablets to decrease the risk of PG toxicity (Lugo 1999).

Benzyl alcohol and derivatives: Some dosage forms may contain benzyl alcohol; large amounts of benzyl alcohol (≥99 mg/kg/day) have been associated with a potentially fatal toxicity ("gasping syndrome") in neonates; the "gasping syndrome" consists of metabolic acidosis, respiratory distress, gasping respirations, CNS dysfunction (including convulsions, intracranial hemorrhage), hypotension, and cardiovascular collapse (AAP ["Inactive" 1997]; CDC 1982); some data suggests that benzoate displaces bilirubin from protein binding sites (Ahlfors 2001); avoid or use dosage forms containing benzyl alcohol with caution in neonates. See manufacturer's labeling.

Adverse Reactions Frequency not always defined.

Cardiovascular: Hypotension (≤2%)

Central nervous system: Sedation (≤16%), dizziness (≤7%), drowsiness (2% to 4%), unsteadiness (3%), headache (1%), coma (≤1%), stupor (≤1%), aggressive behavior, agitation, akathisia, amnesia, anxiety, central nervous system stimulation, disinhibition, disorientation, dysarthria, euphoria, excitement, extrapyramidal reaction, fatigue, hostility, hypothermia, irritability, mania, memory impairment, outbursts of anger, psychosis, seizures, sleep apnea (exacerbation), sleep disturbances, slurred speech, suicidal behavior, suicidal ideation, vertigo

Dermatologic: Alopecia, skin rash

Gastrointestinal: Changes in appetite, constipation

Endocrine & metabolic: Change in libido, hyponatremia, SIADH

Genitourinary: Impotence, orgasm disturbance

Hematologic & oncologic: Agranulocytosis, pancytopenia, thrombocytopenia

Hepatic: Increased serum alkaline phosphatase, increased serum bilirubin, increased serum transaminases, jaundice

Hypersensitivity: Anaphylaxis, anaphylactoid reaction, hypersensitivity reaction

Local: Pain at injection site (IM: 1% to 17%; IV: ≤2%), erythema at injection site (≤2%)

Neuromuscular & skeletal: Weakness (≤4%)

Ophthalmic: Visual disturbances (including diplopia and blurred vision)

Respiratory: Respiratory failure (1% to 2%), apnea (1%), hypoventilation (≤1%), exacerbation of obstructive pulmonary disease, nasal congestion, respiratory depression, worsening of sleep apnea

<1% (Limited to important or life-threatening): Abnormal gait, abnormal hepatic function tests, abnormality in thinking, acidosis, cardiac arrhythmia, ataxia, blood coagulation disorder, bradycardia, cardiac arrest, cardiac failure, cerebral edema, confusion, convulsions, cystitis, decreased mental acuity, delirium, depression, drug dependence (with prolonged use), drug toxicity (polyethylene glycol or propylene glycol poisoning [prolonged IV infusion]), excessive crying, gastrointestinal hemorrhage, hallucinations, hearing loss, heart block, hematologic abnormality, hepatotoxicity, hypertension, hyperventilation, hyporeflexia, infection, injection site reaction, myoclonus, neuroleptic malignant syndrome, paralysis, pericardial effusion, pheochromocytoma (aggravation), pneumothorax, pulmonary edema, pulmonary hemorrhage, pulmonary hypertension, seizure, tachycardia, urinary incontinence, ventricular arrhythmia, withdrawal syndrome

Drug Interactions

Metabolism/Transport Effects None known.

Avoid Concomitant Use

Avoid concomitant use of LORazepam with any of the following: Azelastine (Nasal); Methadone; OLANZapine; Orphenadrine; Paraldehyde; Sodium Oxybate; Thalidomide

Increased Effect/Toxicity

LORazepam may increase the levels/effects of: Alcohol (Ethyl); Azelastine (Nasal); Buprenorphine; CloZAPine; CNS Depressants; Fosphenytoin; Hydrocodone; Methadone; Methotrimeprazine; Metyrosine; Mirtazapine; Orphenadrine; Paraldehyde; Phenytoin; Pramipexole; ROPINIRole; Rotigotine; Selective Serotonin Reuptake Inhibitors; Sodium Oxybate; Suvorexant; Thalidomide; Zolpidem

The levels/effects of LORazepam may be increased by: Brimonidine (Topical); Cannabis; Doxylamine; Dronabinol; Droperidol; HydrOXYzine; Kava Kava; Loxapine; Magnesium Sulfate; Methotrimeprazine; Minocycline; Nabilone; OLANZapine; Perampanel; Probenecid; Rufinamide; Tapentadol; Teduglutide; Tetrahydrocannabinol; Valproate Products

Decreased Effect

The levels/effects of LORazepam may be decreased by: Theophylline Derivatives; Yohimbine

Preparation for Administration

IV injection: According to the manufacturer, dilute IV dose prior to use with an equal volume of compatible diluent (D5W, NS, SWFI).

Infusion: Precipitation may occur upon dilution when preparing an infusion. Use 2 mg/mL injectable vial to prepare; there may be decreased stability when using 4 mg/mL vial. Dilute to ≤1 mg/mL with a compatible diluent in a non-PVC (eg, polyolefin, glass) container (consult parenteral admixture resource for additional detailed recommendations). Can also be administered undiluted (up to 4 mg/mL) via infusion into a central vein or into a peripheral vein with a running compatible maintenance IV solution (Johnson 2002).

IM: Administer undiluted.

Storage/Stability

Parenteral: Intact vials should be refrigerated (room temperature storage information may be available; contact product manufacturer to obtain current recommendations). Protect from light. Do not use discolored or precipitate-containing solutions. Parenteral admixture is stable at room temperature (25°C) for 24 hours.

Oral concentrate: Store at colder room temperature or refrigerate at 2°C to 8°C (36°F to 46°F). Discard open bottle after 90 days.

Oral tablet: Store at 25°C (77°F); excursions are permitted between 15°C and 30°C (59°F and 86°F).

Sublingual tablet [Canadian product]: Store at 15°C to 25°C (59°F to 77°F). Protect from light.

Mechanism of Action Binds to stereospecific benzodiazepine receptors on the postsynaptic GABA neuron at several sites within the central nervous system, including the limbic system, reticular formation. Enhancement of the inhibitory effect of GABA on neuronal excitability results by increased neuronal membrane permeability to chloride ions. This shift in chloride ions results in hyperpolarization (a less excitable state) and stabilization. Benzodiazepine receptors and effects appear to be linked to the GABA-A receptors. Benzodiazepines do not bind to GABA-B receptors.

Pharmacodynamics/Kinetics

Duration: Anesthesia premedication: Adults: IM, IV: ~6 to 8 hours

Absorption: IM: Rapid and complete absorption; Oral: Readily absorbed

Distribution: IV: V_d: Neonates: 0.78 L/kg; Children and Adolescents: 1.9 L/kg; Adults: ~1.3 L/kg

Protein binding: ~85% to 93%; free fraction may be significantly higher in elderly (Greenblatt, 1981)

Metabolism: Hepatic; rapidly conjugated to lorazepam glucuronide (inactive)

Bioavailability: Oral: 90%

Half-life elimination:

IM: ~13 to 18 hours (Greenblatt, 1981)

IV: Neonates: ~42 hours; Children 2 to12 years: ~18 hours; Adolescents: ~28 hours; Adults: ~14 hours; End-stage renal disease (ESRD): ~18 hours

Oral: ~12 hours

Time to peak: IM: ≤3 hours; Oral: ~2 hours; Sublingual tablet [Canadian product]: 1 hour

Excretion: Urine (~88%; predominantly as inactive metabolites); feces (~7%)

Dosing

Adult

Anxiety disorder: Oral: Initial: 2 to 3 mg daily in 2 to 3 divided doses; usual dose: 2 to 6 mg daily in divided doses; however, daily dose may vary from 1 to 10 mg/day

Insomnia due to anxiety or stress: Oral: 2 to 4 mg at bedtime

Premedication for anesthesia:

IM: 0.05 mg/kg administered 2 hours before surgery (maximum dose: 4 mg)

IV: 0.044 mg/kg administered 15 to 20 minutes before surgery (usual dose: 2 mg; maximum dose: 4 mg). **Note:** Doses >2 mg should generally not be exceeded in patients >50 years.

Sublingual tablet [Canadian product]: 0.05 mg/kg 1 to 2 hours before surgery (maximum dose: 4 mg)

Status epilepticus: IV:

Neurocritical Care Society recommendation: 0.1 mg/kg (maximum dose: 4 mg) given at a maximum rate of 2 mg/minute; may repeat in 5 to 10 minutes (NCS [Brophy 2012]). **Note:** Dilute dose 1:1 with saline.

Manufacturer's labeling: 4 mg given slowly (2 mg/minute); may repeat in 10 to 15 minutes. May be given IM, but IV preferred.

Agitation in the ICU patient (off-label use): IV: Loading dose: 0.02 to 0.04 mg/kg (maximum single dose: 2 mg); Maintenance: 0.02 to 0.06 mg/kg every 2 to 6 hours as needed **or** 0.01 to 0.1 mg/kg/hour; maximum dose: ≤10 mg/hour (Barr 2013)

Alcohol withdrawal delirium (off-label use) (Mayo-Smith 2004):

IV: 1 to 4 mg every 5 to 15 minutes until calm, then every hour as needed to maintain light somnolence

IM: 1 to 4 mg every 30 to 60 minutes until calm, then every hour as needed to maintain light somnolence

Alcohol withdrawal syndrome (off-label use) (Mayo-Smith, 1997):

Oral, IM, IV (fixed-dose regimen): 2 mg every 6 hours for 4 doses, then 1 mg every 6 hours for 8 additional doses

Oral, IM, IV (symptom-triggered regimen): 2 to 4 mg every 1 hour as needed; dose determined by a validated severity assessment scale

Chemotherapy-associated nausea and vomiting (off-label use): Breakthrough nausea/vomiting or as adjunct to standard antiemetics: Oral, IV, Sublingual (off-label route): 0.5 to 2 mg every 6 hours as needed (Lohr 2008)

Partial complex seizures, refractory (off-label use): Oral: 1 mg twice daily; increase biweekly in increments of 1 mg twice daily until seizures stop or side effects occur (Walker, 1984); however, additional data may be necessary to further define the role of lorazepam in this condition

Psychogenic catatonia (off-label use):
IM, Sublingual (off-label route): 1 to 2 mg; repeat dose in 3 hours then again in another 3 hours if initial and subsequent doses, respectively, are ineffective (Rosebush, 1990; Rosebush 2010); however, additional data may be necessary to further define the role of lorazepam in this condition
or
Oral, IM, IV: Initial: 1 mg; may repeat in 5 minutes if necessary. If initial challenge is unsuccessful, may increase dose up to 4 to 8 mg per day; may continue treatment for up to 5 days (Bush, 1996); however, additional data may be necessary to further define the role of lorazepam in this condition
Rapid tranquilization of the agitated patient (off-label use): Oral, IM: 1 to 3 mg administered every 30 to 60 minutes; may be administered with an antipsychotic (eg, haloperidol) (Allen 2005; Battaglia 2005; De Fruyt 2004). **Note:** When administering IM, may consider a lower initial dose (eg, 0.5 mg) (Allen 2005).

Dosage adjustment for lorazepam with concomitant medications: *Probenecid or valproic acid:* Reduce lorazepam dose by 50%
Geriatric Refer also to adult dosing. Dose selection should generally be on the low end of the dosage range (initial dose not to exceed 2 mg).
Anxiety disorder: Oral:
US labeling: Initial: 1 to 2 mg daily in divided doses; Beers Criteria: Avoid maintenance doses >3 mg daily
Canadian labeling: Initial: 0.5 mg daily; titrate cautiously as tolerated
Premedication for anesthesia: IM, IV: *Canadian labeling:* Reduce the initial dose by approximately 50% and adjust as needed and tolerated; IV dose should generally not exceed 2 mg in patients >50 years.
Pediatric
Chemotherapy-associated nausea and vomiting (off-label use):
Anticipatory nausea/vomiting (prevention and treatment): Infants ≥1 month, Children, and Adolescents: Oral: 0.04 to 0.08 mg/kg/dose (maximum dose: 2 mg) once at bedtime the evening prior to chemotherapy and once the next day before chemotherapy (Dupuis 2014)
Breakthrough nausea/vomiting: Children ≥2 years and Adolescents: IV: 0.025 to 0.05 mg/kg/dose (maximum dose: 2 mg) every 6 hours as needed (Dupuis 2003); however, additional data may be necessary to further define the role of lorazepam in children for chemotherapy-associated nausea and vomiting
Status epilepticus: Infants, Children, and Adolescents (off-label use):
Neurocritical Care Society recommendation: IV: 0.1 mg/kg (maximum dose: 4 mg) given at a maximum rate of 2 mg/minute; may repeat in 5 to 10 minutes (NCS [Brophy 2012]). **Note:** Dilute dose 1:1 with saline.
American Academy of Pediatrics recommendation: IV, IM: 0.05 to 0.1 mg/kg (maximum dose: 4 mg); may repeat dose every 10 to 15 minutes if seizure continues (AAP [Hegenbarth 2008])

Dosage adjustment for lorazepam with concomitant medications: *Probenecid or valproic acid:* Reduce lorazepam dose by 50%
Renal Impairment
Oral: No dosage adjustment necessary (Aronoff 2007).
IM, IV: Risk of propylene glycol toxicity. Monitor closely if using for prolonged periods of time or at high doses.
Mild-to-moderate disease: Use with caution.
Severe disease or failure: Use is not recommended.
Hepatic Impairment
Oral:
Mild-to-moderate disease: No dose adjustment necessary.
Severe insufficiency and/or encephalopathy: Use with caution; may require lower doses.
IM, IV:
Mild-to-moderate disease: Use with caution.
Severe disease or failure: Use is not recommended.
Administration
IM: Should be administered (undiluted) deep into the muscle mass.
IV injection: Dilute prior to use (according to the manufacturer). Do not exceed 2 mg/minute or 0.05 mg/kg over 2 to 5 minutes. Monitor IV site during administration. Avoid intra-arterial administration. Avoid extravasation.
Continuous IV infusion (off-label administration mode; Barr 2013) solutions should have an in-line filter and the solution should be checked frequently for possible precipitation (Grillo 1996).

Oral: Lorazepam oral concentrate: Use only the provided calibrated dropper to withdraw the prescribed dose. Mix the dose with liquid (eg, water, juice, soda, soda-like beverage) or semisolid food (eg, applesauce, pudding), and stir for a few seconds to blend completely. The prepared mixture should be administered immediately.
Sublingual tablet [Canadian product]: Place under tongue; patient should not swallow for at least 2 minutes.
Monitoring Parameters Respiratory and cardiovascular status, blood pressure, heart rate, symptoms of anxiety
CBC, liver function tests; clinical signs of propylene glycol toxicity (for continuous high-dose and/or long duration intravenous use) including serum creatinine, BUN, serum lactate, osmol gap
Critically-ill patients: Monitor depth of sedation with either the Richmond Agitation-Sedation Scale (RASS) or Sedation-Agitation Scale (SAS) (Barr 2013)
Reference Range Therapeutic: 50 to 240 ng/mL (SI: 156 to 746 nmol/L)
Dosage Forms Excipient information presented when available (limited, particularly for generics); consult specific product labeling.
Concentrate, Oral:
LORazepam Intensol: 2 mg/mL (30 mL) [alcohol free, dye free, sugar free; unflavored flavor]
Generic: 2 mg/mL (30 mL)
Solution, Injection:
Ativan: 2 mg/mL (1 mL, 10 mL); 4 mg/mL (1 mL, 10 mL) [contains benzyl alcohol, polyethylene glycol, propylene glycol]
Generic: 2 mg/mL (1 mL, 10 mL); 4 mg/mL (1 mL, 10 mL)
Tablet, Oral:
Ativan: 0.5 mg
Ativan: 1 mg, 2 mg [scored]
Generic: 0.5 mg, 1 mg, 2 mg
Dosage Forms: Canada Excipient information presented when available (limited, particularly for generics); consult specific product labeling
Tablet, Sublingual: 0.5 mg, 1 mg, 2 mg
Controlled Substance C-IV
Extemporaneous Preparations Note: Commercial oral solution is available (2 mg/mL)

Two different 1 mg/mL oral suspensions may be made from different generic lorazepam tablets (Mylan Pharmaceuticals or Watson Laboratories), sterile water, Ora-Sweet, and Ora-Plus.

Mylan tablets: Place one-hundred-eighty 2 mg tablets in a 12-ounce amber glass bottle; add 144 mL of sterile water to disperse the tablets; shake until slurry is formed. Add 108 mL Ora-Plus in incremental proportions; then add a quantity of Ora-Sweet sufficient to make 360 mL. Label "shake well" and "refrigerate". Stable for 91 days when stored in amber glass prescription bottles at room temperature or refrigerated (preferred).

Watson tablets: Place one-hundred-eighty 2 mg tablets in a 12-ounce amber glass bottle; add 48 mL sterile water to disperse the tablets; shake until slurry is formed. Add 156 mL of Ora-Plus in incremental proportions; then add a quantity of Ora-Sweet sufficient to make 360 mL. Label "shake well" and "refrigerate". Store in amber glass prescription bottles. Stable for 63 days at room temperature or 91 days refrigerated.

Lee ME, Lugo RA, Rusho WJ, et al, "Chemical Stability of Extemporaneously Prepared Lorazepam Suspension at Two Temperatures," *J Pediatr Pharmacol Ther,* 2004, 9(4):254-58.

◆ Lorazepam Injection, USP (Can) *see* LORazepam *on page 1103*

◆ LORazepam Intensol *see* LORazepam *on page 1103*

Lorcaserin (lor KA ser in)

Brand Names: US Belviq
Index Terms Lorcaserin Hydrochloride
Pharmacologic Category Anorexiant; Serotonin 5-HT$_{2C}$ Receptor Agonist
Use Chronic weight management, as an adjunct to a reduced-calorie diet and increased physical activity, in patients with either an initial body mass index (BMI) of ≥30 kg/m^2 **or** an initial BMI of ≥27 kg/m^2 and at least one weight-related comorbid condition (eg, hypertension, dyslipidemia, type 2 diabetes)
Pregnancy Considerations Adverse fetal effects were observed in some animal reproduction studies. Due to the fact that weight loss during pregnancy offers no clinical benefit, lorcaserin is contraindicated in pregnancy. Obese and overweight women should be encouraged to participate in weight reduction programs prior to attempting pregnancy; weight gain during pregnancy should be

determined by their prepregnancy BMI and current guidelines (ADA, 2009; IOM, 2009).

Breast-Feeding Considerations Lorcaserin may alter maternal serum prolactin concentrations. It is not known if lorcaserin is excreted into breast milk. According to the manufacturer, the decision to continue or discontinue breast-feeding during therapy should take into account the risk of exposure to the infant and the benefits of treatment to the mother. Weight-loss therapy is generally not recommended for lactating women. Weight-loss programs which include physical activity and nutrition components should be discussed at the 6-week postpartum visit (ADA, 2009; IOM, 2009).

Contraindications Pregnancy

Warnings/Precautions Use may cause confusion, somnolence, fatigue, and cognitive impairment (difficulty with concentration/attention/memory); patients must be cautioned about performing tasks which require mental alertness (eg, operating machinery or driving). Agents affecting the CNS have been associated with depression and suicidal ideation; monitor patients closely during use; discontinue for suicidal thoughts or behaviors. Priapism may occur with use; men with erections >4 hours should immediately discontinue lorcaserin and seek emergency medical attention to avoid irreversible damage to erectile tissue. Use with caution in men with conditions that increase the risk for priapism (eg, sickle cell anemia, multiple myeloma, leukemia) or men with anatomical penis deformities (eg, angulation, cavernosal fibrosis, Peyronie's disease). Rare WBC and RBC count decreases (including leukopenia, lymphopenia, neutropenia, anemia, decreases in hematocrit and hemoglobin) have been observed; consider monitoring CBC periodically during use. Increased prolactin levels may occur; obtain prolactin levels if signs or symptoms of hyperprolactinemia occur (eg, galactorrhea, gynecomastia).

Primary pulmonary hypertension (PPH) is a rare and frequently fatal pulmonary disease, which has been reported in patients receiving other centrally acting, serotonergic weight loss agents. Available data from clinical trials are inadequate to determine if lorcaserin increases the risk for pulmonary hypertension (due to the low incidence of PPH occurring in the general population); however, a theoretical risk cannot be excluded. Cardiac valvular disease has been associated with the use of agents exhibiting potent $5-HT_{2B}$ agonist activity (eg, cabergoline, fenfluramine [not currently on the U.S. market], dexfenfluramine [not currently on the U.S. market]). Cardiac valvular disease is believed to result from activation of $5-HT_{2B}$ receptors in interstitial cardiac cells. Lorcaserin has greater affinity for $5-HT_{2C}$ receptors compared to $5-HT_{2B}$ receptors (at therapeutic doses). However, a slight increase in incidence of regurgitant cardiac valve disease (mitral and/or aortic) has been observed with lorcaserin compared to placebo in some clinical trials (pooled RR: 1.16; 95% CI: 0.81-1.67). The incidence observed in both groups was low, making it difficult to ascertain the risk of valvular disease with lorcaserin therapy based on available data. Evaluate patients if signs/symptoms of valvular heart disease (eg, dyspnea, dependent edema, heart failure, new onset cardiac murmur) arise during therapy; consider discontinuing therapy if present. Use has not been studied in patients with hemodynamically-significant valvular heart disease. Do not use lorcaserin in combination with potent serotonergic and dopaminergic agents that are potent $5-HT_{2B}$ receptor agonists (eg, cabergoline) due to the risk for cardiac valvulopathy.

Serotonin syndrome (SS)/neuroleptic malignant syndrome (NMS)-like reactions have occurred with serotonergic agents such as lorcaserin, particularly when used in combination with other serotonergic agents (eg, triptans, SNRIs, SSRIs, TCAs, bupropion, St John's wort, tryptophan), agents that impair metabolism of serotonin (eg, MAO inhibitors, dextromethorphan, tramadol, lithium), or antidopaminergic agents (eg, antipsychotics). Concurrent use with these agents should be avoided. If concomitant use cannot be avoided, coadminister with extreme caution, and closely monitor patients, particularly during treatment initiation. Discontinue treatment (and any concomitant serotonergic and/or antidopaminergic agents) immediately if signs/symptoms of SS or NMS-like reactions arise.

Use with caution in patients with bradycardia or heart block (second or third degree); bradycardia has been observed rarely with use. Use with caution in patients with heart failure (has not been studied). Effect of lorcaserin on cardiovascular morbidity and mortality has not been established. Use with caution in patients with type 2 diabetes mellitus; weight loss from therapy may result in decreased requirements of antidiabetic agents and an increased risk of hypoglycemia; monitor blood glucose. Use with caution in patients with severe hepatic impairment (not studied);

lorcaserin undergoes extensive hepatic metabolism. Use is not recommended in patients with severe renal impairment or end stage renal disease. Use with caution in patients with moderate renal impairment. Serum concentrations and principal metabolite (M1 and M5) half-lives are increased in renal impairment.

In short-term studies, euphoria, hallucinations, and dissociation have been observed with lorcaserin at supratherapeutic doses. Data suggest lorcaserin may produce psychic dependence. Physical dependence or a withdrawal syndrome has not been observed. Pharmacotherapy for weight loss should be used in conjunction with a comprehensive weight management program including diet and exercise. Discontinue if significant weight loss has not occurred (ie, <5% within the first 12 weeks of treatment). Concomitant use of lorcaserin with other agents intended for weight loss (eg, phentermine, orlistat, OTC, or herbal preparations) has not been evaluated; safety and efficacy of coadministration with other weight loss agents are unknown.

Adverse Reactions

>10%:
Central nervous system: Headache (15% to 17%)
Endocrine & metabolic: Hypoglycemia (diabetic patients 29%; severe: 2%)
Hematologic: Lymphocytes decreased (12%)
Neuromuscular & skeletal: Back pain (6% to 12%)
Respiratory: Upper respiratory tract infection (14%), nasopharyngitis (11% to 13%)

1% to 10%:
Cardiovascular: Peripheral edema (5%), hypertension (5%), valvulopathy (at 1 year: 2.4%; placebo: 2.0%)
Central nervous system: Dizziness (7% to 9%), fatigue (7%), anxiety (4%), insomnia (4%), depression (2% to 3%; placebo: 2%), cognitive impairment (2%), psychiatric disorders (2%)
Dermatologic: Rash (2%)
Endocrine & metabolic: Diabetes mellitus exacerbation (3%), prolactin increased (<2 x ULN: 7%; 2 x ULN: 2%; 5 x ULN: <1%)
Gastrointestinal: Nausea (8% to 9%), diarrhea (7%), constipation (6%), xerostomia (5%), vomiting (4%), gastroenteritis (3%), toothache (3%), appetite decreased (2%)
Genitourinary: Urinary tract infection (7% to 9%)
Hematologic: Hemoglobin decreased (10%), neutrophils decreased (6%)
Neuromuscular & skeletal: Muscle spasms (5%), musculoskeletal pain (2%)
Ocular: Eye disorders (5%; diabetic patients 6%)
Respiratory: Cough (4% to 8%), oropharyngeal pain (4%), sinus congestion (3%)
Miscellaneous: Seasonal allergy (3%), stress (3%)

<1% (Limited to important or life-threatening): Bradycardia, dissociation, euphoria, serotonin syndrome, suicidal ideation

Drug Interactions

Metabolism/Transport Effects Inhibits CYP2D6 (moderate)

Avoid Concomitant Use
Avoid concomitant use of Lorcaserin with any of the following: Dapoxetine; Ergot Derivatives; Thioridazine

Increased Effect/Toxicity
Lorcaserin may increase the levels/effects of: Antipsychotic Agents; ARIPiprazole; Brexpiprazole; CYP2D6 Substrates; DOXOrubicin (Conventional); Eliglustat; Ergot Derivatives; Fesoterodine; Metoclopramide; Metoprolol; Nebivolol; Phosphodiesterase 5 Inhibitors; Serotonin Modulators; Thioridazine

The levels/effects of Lorcaserin may be increased by: Antiemetics (5HT3 Antagonists); Antipsychotic Agents; BuPROPion; Dapoxetine; Metaxalone; Propafenone; Tedizolid

Decreased Effect
Lorcaserin may decrease the levels/effects of: Codeine; Tamoxifen

Storage/Stability Store at 25°C (77°F); excursions permitted to 15°C to 30°C (59°F to 86°F).

Mechanism of Action Lorcaserin is believed to activate serotonin $5-HT_{2C}$ receptors, which stimulate pro-opiomelanocortin (POMC) neurons in the arcuate nucleus of the hypothalamus, leading to increased alpha-melanocortin stimulating hormone release at melanocortin-4 receptors and resulting in satiety and decreased food intake. At recommended doses, lorcaserin has greater affinity for $5-HT_{2C}$ receptors compared to other 5-HT receptor subtypes (including $5-HT_{2A}$ and $5-HT_{2B}$), the 5-HT receptor transporter, and 5-HT reuptake sites (Hurren, 2011).

Pharmacodynamics/Kinetics
Distribution: Distributes to the CNS and cerebrospinal fluid
Protein binding: ~70% to plasma proteins

Metabolism: Extensive hepatic metabolism, via multiple enzymatic pathways, producing two major metabolites (inactive), lorcaserin sulfamate (M1) and N-carbamoyl glucuronide lorcaserin (M5), as well as minor metabolites (glucuronide and sulfate conjugates)

Half-life elimination: ~11 hours

Time to peak: 1.5-2 hours

Excretion: Urine (92%, as metabolites); feces (2%, as metabolites)

Dosing

Adult & Geriatric Weight management: Oral: 10 mg twice daily (maximum: 10 mg twice daily); evaluate response by week 12; if patient has not lost ≥5% of baseline body weight, discontinue therapy

Renal Impairment Note: Renal function was estimated in studies using ideal body weight (IBW) with the Cock-croft-Gault formula.

Mild impairment (CrCl >50 mL/minute): No dosage adjustment necessary.

Moderate impairment (CrCl 30-50 mL/minute): Use with caution; serum concentrations and half-life of major metabolites are increased.

Severe impairment (CrCl <30 mL/minute): Use is not recommended.

ESRD: Use is not recommended; hemodialysis does not remove lorcaserin or M1 metabolite

Hepatic Impairment

Mild-to-moderate impairment (Child-Pugh score 5-9): No dosage adjustment necessary.

Severe impairment: Use with caution (has not been studied); undergoes extensive hepatic metabolism.

Administration Administer orally with or without food.

Monitoring Parameters Weight, waist circumference; CBC (periodically during use); blood glucose (in diabetics); prolactin levels (if galactorrhea, gynecomastia or other signs/symptoms of hyperprolactinemia arise); monitor for depression or suicidal thoughts/behavior; signs/symptoms of SS/NMS-like reaction; signs/symptoms of valvular heart disease (dyspnea, dependent edema)

Additional Information *In vitro*, lorcaserin has an 18-fold and 104-fold greater affinity for $5HT_{2C}$ receptors compared to $5-HT_{2A}$ and $5HT_{2B}$ receptors, respectively (Hurren, 2011).

Dosage Forms Excipient information presented when available (limited, particularly for generics); consult specific product labeling.

Tablet, Oral:

Belviq: 10 mg [contains fd&c blue #2 aluminum lake]

Controlled Substance C-IV

Losartan (loe SAR tan)

Brand Names: US Cozaar

Brand Names: Canada ACT Losartan; Apo-Losartan; Auro-Losartan; Cozaar; JAMP-Losartan; Mint-Losartan; Mylan-Losartan; PMS-Losartan; RAN-Losartan; Sandoz Losartan; Septa Losartan; Teva-Losartan

Index Terms DuP 753; Losartan Potassium; MK594

Pharmacologic Category Angiotensin II Receptor Blocker; Antihypertensive

Use

Diabetic nephropathy: Treatment of diabetic nephropathy with an elevated serum creatinine and proteinuria (urinary albumin to creatinine ratio ≥300 mg/g) in patients with type 2 diabetes and a history of hypertension.

Hypertension: Treatment of hypertension, alone or in combination with other antihypertensive agents.

Hypertension with left ventricular hypertrophy: To reduce the risk of stroke in patients with hypertension and left ventricular hypertrophy (LVH). Evidence suggests that this benefit does not apply to black patients.

Guideline recommendations:

Hypertension: The 2014 guideline for the management of high blood pressure in adults (Eighth Joint National Committee [JNC 8]) recommends initiation of pharmacologic treatment to lower blood pressure for the following patients:

• Patients ≥60 years of age with systolic blood pressure (SBP) ≥150 mm Hg or diastolic blood pressure (DBP) ≥90 mm Hg. Goal of therapy is SBP <150 mm Hg and DBP <90 mm Hg.

• Patients <60 years of age with SBP ≥140 mm Hg or DBP is ≥90 mm Hg. Goal of therapy is SBP <140 mm Hg and DBP <90 mm Hg.

• Patients ≥18 years of age with diabetes and SBP ≥140 mm Hg or DBP ≥90 mm Hg. Goal of therapy is SBP <140 mm Hg and DBP <90 mm Hg.

• Patients ≥18 years of age with chronic kidney disease (CKD) and SBP ≥140 mm Hg or DBP ≥90 mm Hg. Goal of therapy is SBP <140 mm Hg and DBP <90 mm Hg.

Chronic kidney disease (CKD) and hypertension: Regardless of race or diabetes status, the use of an ACE inhibitor (ACEI) or angiotensin receptor blocker (ARB) as initial therapy is recommended to improve kidney outcomes. In the general nonblack population (without CKD) including those with diabetes, initial antihypertensive treatment should consist of a thiazide-type diuretic, calcium channel blocker, ACEI, or ARB. In the general black population (without CKD) including those with diabetes, initial antihypertensive treatment should consist of a thiazide-type diuretic or a calcium channel blocker instead of an ACEI or ARB.

Coronary artery disease and hypertension: The American Heart Association, American College of Cardiology and American Society of Hypertension (AHA/ACC/ASH) 2015 scientific statement for the treatment of hypertension in patients with coronary artery disease (CAD) recommends the use of an ARB (or ACE inhibitor) as part of a regimen in patients with hypertension and chronic stable angina if there is prior MI, LV systolic dysfunction, diabetes mellitus, or CKD. A BP target of <140/90 mm Hg is reasonable for the secondary prevention of cardiovascular events. A lower target BP (<130/80 mm Hg) may be appropriate in some individuals with CAD, previous MI, stroke, or transient ischemic attack, or CAD risk equivalents (AHA/ACC/ASH [Rosendorff 2015]).

Pregnancy Considerations [U.S. Boxed Warning]: Drugs that act on the renin-angiotensin system can cause injury and death to the developing fetus. Discontinue as soon as possible once pregnancy is detected. The use of drugs which act on the renin-angiotensin system are associated with oligohydramnios. Oligohydramnios, due to decreased fetal renal function, may lead to fetal lung hypoplasia and skeletal malformations. Use is also associated with anuria, hypotension, renal failure, skull hypoplasia, and death in the fetus/neonate. The exposed fetus should be monitored for fetal growth, amniotic fluid volume, and organ formation. Infants exposed *in utero* should be monitored for hyperkalemia, hypotension, and oliguria (exchange transfusions or dialysis may be needed). These adverse events are generally associated with maternal use in the second and third trimesters.

Untreated chronic maternal hypertension is also associated with adverse events in the fetus, infant, and mother. The use of angiotensin II receptor blockers is not recommended to treat chronic uncomplicated hypertension in pregnant women and should generally be avoided in women of reproductive potential (ACOG, 2013).

Breast-Feeding Considerations It is not known if losartan is found in breast milk. Due to the potential for serious adverse reactions in the nursing infant, the manufacturer recommends a decision be made whether to discontinue nursing or to discontinue the drug, taking into account the importance of treatment to the mother.

Contraindications

Hypersensitivity to losartan or any component of the formulation; concomitant use with aliskiren in patients with diabetes mellitus

Documentation of allergenic cross-reactivity for angiotensin receptor blockers is limited. However, because of similarities in chemical structure and/or pharmacologic actions, the possibility of cross-sensitivity cannot be ruled out with certainty.

Canadian labeling: Additional contraindications (not in U.S. labeling): Concomitant use with aliskiren in patients with moderate-to-severe renal impairment (GFR <60 mL/minute/1.73 m²)

◄ **Warnings/Precautions [U.S. Boxed Warning]: Drugs that act on the renin-angiotensin system can cause injury and death to the developing fetus. Discontinue as soon as possible once pregnancy is detected.** Avoid use or use a much smaller dose in patients who are volume-depleted; correct depletion first. Use with caution in patients with significant aortic/mitral stenosis. May cause hyperkalemia; avoid potassium supplementation unless specifically required by healthcare provider. May be associated with deterioration of renal function and/or increases in serum creatinine, particularly in patients with low renal blood flow (eg, renal artery stenosis, heart failure) whose glomerular filtration rate (GFR) is dependent on efferent arteriolar vasoconstriction by angiotensin II. Use caution in patients with unstented unilateral/bilateral renal artery stenosis. When unstented bilateral renal artery stenosis is present, use is generally avoided due to the elevated risk of deterioration in renal function unless possible benefits outweigh risks. Use with caution with preexisting renal insufficiency. AUCs of losartan (not the active metabolite) are about 50% greater in patients with CrCl <30 mL/minute and are doubled in hemodialysis patients. Potentially significant drug interactions may exist, requiring dose or frequency adjustment, additional monitoring, and/or selection of alternative therapy. In surgical patients on chronic angiotensin receptor blocker (ARB) therapy, intraoperative hypotension may occur with induction and maintenance of general anesthesia.

Angioedema has been reported rarely with some angiotensin II receptor antagonists (ARBs) and may occur at any time during treatment (especially following first dose). It may involve the head and neck (potentially compromising airway) or the intestine (presenting with abdominal pain). Patients with idiopathic or hereditary angioedema or previous angioedema associated with ACE-inhibitor therapy may be at an increased risk. Prolonged frequent monitoring may be required, especially if tongue, glottis, or larynx are involved, as they are associated with airway obstruction. Patients with a history of airway surgery may have a higher risk of airway obstruction. Discontinue therapy immediately if angioedema occurs. Aggressive early management is critical. Intramuscular (IM) administration of epinephrine may be necessary. Do not readminister to patients who have had angioedema with ARBs.

When used to reduce the risk of stroke in patients with HTN and LVH, may not be effective in the black population. Use caution with hepatic dysfunction, dose adjustment may be needed.

Adverse Reactions Note: The incidence of some adverse reactions varied based on the underlying disease state. Notations are made, where applicable, for data derived from trials conducted in diabetic nephropathy and hypertensive patients, respectively.

>10%:

Cardiovascular: Chest pain (12% diabetic nephropathy)

Central nervous system: Fatigue (14% diabetic nephropathy)

Endocrine: Hypoglycemia (14% diabetic nephropathy)

Gastrointestinal: Diarrhea (2% hypertension to 15% diabetic nephropathy)

Genitourinary: Urinary tract infection (13% diabetic nephropathy)

Hematologic: Anemia (14% diabetic nephropathy)

Neuromuscular & skeletal: Weakness (14% diabetic nephropathy), back pain (2% hypertension to 12% diabetic nephropathy)

Respiratory: Cough (≤3% to 11%; similar to placebo; incidence higher in patients with previous cough related to ACE inhibitor therapy)

1% to 10%:

Cardiovascular: Hypotension (7% diabetic nephropathy), orthostatic hypotension (4% hypertension to 4% diabetic nephropathy), first-dose hypotension (dose related: <1% with 50 mg, 2% with 100 mg)

Central nervous system: Dizziness (4%), hypoesthesia (5% diabetic nephropathy), fever (4% diabetic nephropathy), insomnia (1%)

Dermatology: Cellulitis (7% diabetic nephropathy)

Endocrine: Hyperkalemia (<1% hypertension to 7% diabetic nephropathy)

Gastrointestinal: Gastritis (5% diabetic nephropathy), weight gain (4% diabetic nephropathy), dyspepsia (1% to 4%), abdominal pain (2%), nausea (2%)

Neuromuscular & skeletal: Muscular weakness (7% diabetic nephropathy), knee pain (5% diabetic nephropathy), leg pain (1% to 5%), muscle cramps (1%), myalgia (1%)

Respiratory: Bronchitis (10% diabetic nephropathy), upper respiratory infection (8%), nasal congestion (2%), sinusitis (1% hypertension to 6% diabetic nephropathy)

Miscellaneous: Infection (5% diabetic nephropathy), flu-like syndrome (10% diabetic nephropathy)

<1% (Limited to important or life-threatening): Acute psychosis with paranoid delusions, ageusia, allergic reaction, alopecia, anaphylactic reactions, anemia, angina, angioedema, anorexia, anxiety, arrhythmia, arthralgia, arthritis, ataxia, AV block (second degree), bilirubin increased, blurred vision, bradycardia, bronchitis, BUN increased, confusion, conjunctivitis, constipation, CVA, depression, dermatitis, dysgeusia, dyspnea, ecchymosis, epistaxis, erythroderma, erythema, facial edema, fever, flatulence, flushing, gastritis, gout, hematocrit decreased, hemoglobin decreased, Henoch-Schönlein purpura (IgA vasculitis), hepatitis, hyponatremia, hypotension, impotence, joint swelling, maculopapular rash, malaise, memory impairment, MI, migraine, muscle weakness, myositis, neoplasm, nervousness, orthostatic effects, pancreatitis, paresthesia, peripheral neuropathy, pharyngitis, photosensitivity, pruritus, rash, rhabdomyolysis, rhinitis, serum creatinine increased, sleep disorder, somnolence, syncope, tachycardia, taste perversion, thrombocytopenia, tinnitus, transaminases increased, tremor, urinary frequency, urticaria, vasculitis, ventricular arrhythmia, vertigo, visual acuity decreased, vomiting, xerostomia

Drug Interactions

Metabolism/Transport Effects Substrate of CYP2C9 (major), CYP3A4 (major); **Note:** Assignment of Major/Minor substrate status based on clinically relevant drug interaction potential; **Inhibits** CYP1A2 (weak), CYP2C19 (weak), CYP2C8 (moderate), CYP2C9 (moderate)

Avoid Concomitant Use

Avoid concomitant use of Losartan with any of the following: Amodiaquine

Increased Effect/Toxicity

Losartan may increase the levels/effects of: ACE Inhibitors; Amifostine; Amodiaquine; Antipsychotic Agents (Second Generation [Atypical]); Bosentan; Cannabis; Carvedilol; Ciprofloxacin (Systemic); CycloSPORINE (Systemic); CYP2C8 Substrates; CYP2C9 Substrates; Dronabinol; Drospirenone; DULoxetine; Hypotension-Associated Agents; Levodopa; Lithium; Nonsteroidal Anti-Inflammatory Agents; Potassium-Sparing Diuretics; Sodium Phosphates; Tetrahydrocannabinol; TiZANidine

The levels/effects of Losartan may be increased by: Alfuzosin; Aliskiren; Antifungal Agents (Azole Derivatives, Systemic); Barbiturates; Brimonidine (Topical); Canagliflozin; Ceritinib; CYP2C9 Inhibitors (Moderate); CYP2C9 Inhibitors (Strong); Dapoxetine; Diazoxide; Eplerenone; Heparin; Heparin (Low Molecular Weight); Herbs (Hypotensive Properties); Mifepristone; Molsidomine; Nicorandil; Obinutuzumab; Osimertinib; Pentoxifylline; Phosphodiesterase 5 Inhibitors; Potassium Salts; Prostacyclin Analogues; Tolvaptan; Trimethoprim

Decreased Effect

The levels/effects of Losartan may be decreased by: Amphetamines; Bosentan; CYP2C9 Inducers (Strong); CYP3A4 Inducers (Moderate); CYP3A4 Inducers (Strong); Dabrafenib; Deferasirox; Enzalutamide; Fluconazole; Herbs (Hypertensive Properties); Methylphenidate; Mitotane; Nonsteroidal Anti-Inflammatory Agents; Osimertinib; Rifampin; Siltuximab; St Johns Wort; Tocilizumab; Yohimbine

Storage/Stability Store at 25°C (77°F); excursions are permitted to 15°C to 30°C (59°F to 86°F). Protect from light.

Mechanism of Action As a selective and competitive, nonpeptide angiotensin II receptor antagonist, losartan blocks the vasoconstrictor and aldosterone-secreting effects of angiotensin II; losartan interacts reversibly at the AT1 and AT2 receptors of many tissues and has slow dissociation kinetics; its affinity for the AT1 receptor is 1000 times greater than the AT2 receptor. Angiotensin II receptor antagonists may induce a more complete inhibition of the renin-angiotensin system than ACE inhibitors, they do not affect the response to bradykinin, and are less likely to be associated with nonrenin-angiotensin effects (eg, cough and angioedema). Losartan increases urinary flow rate and in addition to being natriuretic and kaliuretic, increases excretion of chloride, magnesium, uric acid, calcium, and phosphate.

Pharmacodynamics/Kinetics

Onset of action: 6 hours

Distribution: V_d: Losartan: 34 L; E-3174: 12 L; animal studies suggest that losartan does not cross the blood-brain barrier

Protein binding, plasma: High

Metabolism: Hepatic (14%) via CYP2C9 and 3A4 to active metabolite, E-3174 (10 to 40 times more potent than losartan); extensive first-pass effect

Bioavailability: ~33%; AUC of E-3174 is four times greater than that of losartan

Half-life elimination: Losartan: 2 hours; E-3174: 6 to 9 hours

Time to peak, serum: Losartan: 1 to 2 hours; E-3174: 3.5 to 4 hours

Excretion: Urine (4% as unchanged drug, 6% as active metabolite); feces

Dosing

Adult & Geriatric

Hypertension: Oral: Initial: 50 mg once daily; can be administered once or twice daily with total daily doses ranging from 25 to 100 mg; usual dosage range (ASH/ISH [Weber, 2014]): 50 to 100 mg daily; target dose (JNC 8 [James, 2013]): 100 mg daily in 1 or 2 divided doses

Usual initial doses in patients receiving diuretics or those with intravascular volume depletion: 25 mg once daily

Diabetic nephropathy: Oral: Initial: 50 mg once daily; can be increased to 100 mg once daily based on blood pressure response

Hypertension with left ventricular hypertrophy: Oral: Initial: 50 mg once daily; can be increased to 100 mg once daily based on blood pressure response. May be used in combination with a thiazide diuretic

Heart failure (off-label use): Initial: 12.5 to 25 mg once daily; target dose: 150 mg once daily (HFSA, 2010; Konstam, 2009). The ACCF/AHA 2013 heart failure guidelines recommend an initial dose of 25 to 50 mg once daily; target dose: 150 mg once daily (Yancy, 2013).

Pediatric Hypertension: Oral: Children 6 to 16 years:

U.S. labeling: Initial: 0.7 mg/kg once daily (maximum: 50 mg daily); doses >1.4 mg/kg (>100 mg daily) have not been studied

Canadian labeling:

≥20 kg to <50 kg: 25 mg once daily (maximum: 50 mg once daily)

≥50 kg: 50 mg once daily (maximum: 100 mg once daily)

Aortic-root dilation with Marfan's syndrome (off-label use): Children 14 months to 16 years: Initial: 0.6 mg/kg/day; can be increased to a maximum of 1.4 mg/kg/day (not to exceed adult maximum of 100 mg daily) (Brooke, 2008)

Renal Impairment

Adults: Initial: No dosage adjustment necessary.

Children: Use is not recommended if GFR <30 mL/minute/1.73 m^2

Hepatic Impairment

Adults: Reduce the initial dose to 25 mg/day

Children 6 to 16 years:

U.S. labeling: No specific dosing recommendations are provided in the manufacturer's labeling, however it may be advisable to initiate therapy at a reduced dosage.

Canadian labeling: Use is not recommended.

Dietary Considerations May be taken without regard to meals. Some products may contain potassium.

Administration May be administered without regard to meals.

Monitoring Parameters

Supine blood pressure, electrolytes, serum creatinine, BUN, urinalysis, symptomatic hypotension and tachycardia, CBC

Neonates exposed *in utero* should be monitored for oliguria and hypotension.

2013 ACCF/AHA Heart Failure guideline recommendations:

Within 1 to 2 weeks after initiation, reassess blood pressure (including postural blood pressure changes), renal function, and serum potassium; follow closely after dose changes. Patients with systolic blood pressure <80 mm Hg, low serum sodium, diabetes mellitus, and impaired renal function should be closely monitored (ACCF/AHA [Yancy, 2013]).

Dosage Forms Excipient information presented when available (limited, particularly for generics); consult specific product labeling. [DSC] = Discontinued product

Tablet, Oral, as potassium:

Cozaar: 25 mg, 50 mg [DSC]

Cozaar: 50 mg [scored]

Cozaar: 100 mg

Generic: 25 mg, 50 mg, 100 mg

Extemporaneous Preparations A 2.5 mg/mL losartan oral suspension may be made with tablets and a 1:1 mixture of Ora-Plus® and Ora-Sweet® SF. Combine 10 mL of purified water and ten losartan 50 mg tablets in an 8-ounce amber polyethylene terephthalate bottle. Shake well for at least 2 minutes. Allow concentrate to stand for 1 hour, then shake for 1 minute. Separately, prepare 190 mL of a 1:1 mixture of Ora-Plus® and Ora-Sweet® SF; add to tablet and water mixture in the bottle and shake for 1 minute. Label "shake well" and "refrigerate". Return promptly to refrigerator after each use. Stable for 4 weeks when stored in amber polyethylene terephthalate prescription bottles and refrigerated (Cozaar prescribing information, 2014).

Cozaar prescribing information, Merck & Co, Inc, Whitehouse Station, NJ, 2014.

Losartan and Hydrochlorothiazide
(loe SAR tan & hye droe klor oh THYE a zide)

Brand Names: US Hyzaar

Brand Names: Canada ACT Losartan/HCT; Apo-Losartan/HCTZ; Auro-Losartan HCT; Hyzaar; Hyzaar DS; JAMP-Losartan HCTZ; Losartan-HCT; Losartan-HCTZ; Mint-Losartan/HCTZ; Mint-Losartan/HCTZ DS; Mylan-Losartan/HCTZ; PMS-Losartan/HCTZ; Sandoz-Losartan HCT; Sandoz-Losartan HCT DS; Teva-Losartan/HCTZ

Index Terms Hydrochlorothiazide and Losartan

Pharmacologic Category Angiotensin II Receptor Blocker; Antihypertensive; Diuretic, Thiazide

Use

Hypertension: Treatment of hypertension.

Hypertension with left ventricular hypertrophy: To reduce the risk of stroke in patients with hypertension and left ventricular hypertrophy (LVH). Evidence suggests that this benefit does not apply to black patients.

Dosing

Adult & Geriatric

Hypertension: Oral: **Note:** Dose must be individualized; combination product may be substituted for individual components in patients currently maintained on both agents separately or in patients not adequately controlled with monotherapy.

Replacement therapy: Losartan 50 to 100 mg/hydrochlorothiazide 12.5 to 25 mg once daily; as appropriate, dose may be titrated after ~3 weeks of therapy as necessary until maximum daily dose is reached. Maximum daily dose: Losartan 100 mg/hydrochlorothiazide 25 mg once daily.

Severe hypertension: Initial: Losartan 50 mg/hydrochlorothiazide 12.5 mg once daily; dose may be titrated after 2 to 4 weeks of therapy as necessary until maximum daily dose is reached. Maximum daily dose: Losartan 100 mg/hydrochlorothiazide 25 mg once daily.

Hypertension with left ventricular hypertrophy: Oral: **Note:** Initiate treatment with losartan monotherapy. If blood pressure reduction inadequate, then may initiate losartan/hydrochlorothiazide combination.

Losartan 50 mg/hydrochlorothiazide 12.5 mg once daily; may increase to losartan 100 mg/hydrochlorothiazide 12.5 mg once daily, followed by losartan 100 mg/hydrochlorothiazide 25 mg once daily if needed to control blood pressure.

Renal Impairment

Mild to moderate impairment (CrCl >30 mL/minute): No dosage adjustment necessary.

Severe impairment (CrCl ≤30 mL/minute): Use is not recommended.

Hepatic Impairment Use is not recommended as initial therapy.

Additional Information Complete prescribing information should be consulted for additional detail.

Dosage Forms Excipient information presented when available (limited, particularly for generics); consult specific product labeling.

Tablet, oral: 50/12.5: Losartan potassium 50 mg and hydrochlorothiazide 12.5 mg; 100/12.5: Losartan potassium 100 mg and hydrochlorothiazide 12.5 mg; 100/25: Losartan potassium 100 mg and hydrochlorothiazide 25 mg

Hyzaar 50/12.5: Losartan potassium 50 mg and hydrochlorothiazide 12.5 mg [contains potassium 4.24 mg (0.108 mEq)]

Hyzaar 100/12.5: Losartan potassium 100 mg and hydrochlorothiazide 12.5 mg [contains potassium 8.48 mg (0.216 mEq)]

Hyzaar 100/25: Losartan potassium 100 mg and hydrochlorothiazide 25 mg [contains potassium 8.48 mg (0.216 mEq)]

Loteprednol (loe te PRED nol)

Brand Names: US Alrex; Lotemax
Brand Names: Canada Alrex; Lotemax
Index Terms Loteprednol Etabonate
Pharmacologic Category Corticosteroid, Ophthalmic
Use

Seasonal allergic conjunctivitis (0.2% suspension): Temporary relief of signs and symptoms of seasonal allergic conjunctivitis

Postoperative inflammation/pain (0.5% suspension/ointment/gel): Treatment of postoperative inflammation and pain following ocular surgery

Ophthalmic inflammatory conditions (0.5% suspension): Treatment of steroid-responsive inflammatory conditions of the palpebral and bulbar conjunctiva, cornea, and anterior segment of the globe (eg, allergic conjunctivitis, acne rosacea, superficial punctate keratitis, herpes zoster keratitis, iritis, cyclitis, selected infective conjunctivitis, when the inherent hazard of steroid use is accepted to obtain an advisable diminution in edema and inflammation)

Dosing

Adult & Geriatric

Seasonal allergic conjunctivitis: Ophthalmic: 0.2% suspension: Instill 1 drop into affected eye(s) 4 times daily.

Steroid-responsive inflammatory conditions: Ophthalmic: 0.5% suspension: Instill 1 to 2 drops into the conjunctival sac of the affected eye(s) 4 times daily. During the initial treatment within the first week, the dosing may be increased up to 1 drop every hour. Advise patients not to discontinue therapy prematurely. If signs and symptoms fail to improve after 2 days, re-evaluate the patient.

Postoperative inflammation/pain: Ophthalmic:

0.5% ointment: Apply ~1/2 inch ribbon into the conjunctival sac of the affected eye(s) 4 times daily beginning 24 hours after surgery and continuing throughout the first 2 weeks of the postoperative period.

0.5% gel, 0.5% suspension: Instill 1 to 2 drops into the conjunctival sac of the affected eye(s) 4 times daily beginning 24 hours after surgery and continuing throughout the first 2 weeks of the postoperative period.

Renal Impairment There are no dosage adjustments provided in the manufacturer's labeling. However, dosage adjustment unlikely due to low systemic absorption.

Hepatic Impairment There are no dosage adjustments provided in the manufacturer's labeling. However, dosage adjustment unlikely due to low systemic absorption.

Additional Information Complete prescribing information should be consulted for additional detail.

Dosage Forms Excipient information presented when available (limited, particularly for generics); consult specific product labeling.

Gel, Ophthalmic, as etabonate:
Lotemax: 0.5% (5 g) [contains benzalkonium chloride, edetate disodium dihydrate, propylene glycol]
Ointment, Ophthalmic, as etabonate:
Lotemax: 0.5% (3.5 g)
Suspension, Ophthalmic, as etabonate:
Alrex: 0.2% (5 mL, 10 mL)
Lotemax: 0.5% (5 mL, 10 mL, 15 mL)

Loteprednol and Tobramycin
(loe te PRED nol & toe bra MYE sin)

Brand Names: US Zylet
Index Terms Loteprednol Etabonate and Tobramycin; Tobramycin and Loteprednol Etabonate
Pharmacologic Category Antibiotic/Corticosteroid, Ophthalmic

Use Ocular inflammatory conditions: Treatment of steroid-responsive ocular inflammatory conditions (where either a superficial bacterial ocular infection or the risk of a superficial bacterial ocular infection exists) of the palpebral and bulbar conjunctiva, cornea and anterior segment of the globe (eg, allergic conjunctivitis, acne rosacea, superficial punctate keratitis, herpes zoster keratitis, iritis, cyclitis, and where the inherent risk of steroid use in certain infective conjunctivitides is accepted to obtain a diminution in edema and inflammation); chronic anterior uveitis; corneal injury from chemical, radiation or thermal burns; penetration of foreign bodies.

Dosing

Adult & Geriatric Ocular inflammatory conditions: Ophthalmic: Instill 1 to 2 drops into the affected eye(s) every 4 to 6 hours; may increase frequency during the first 24 to 48 hours to every 1 to 2 hours. Frequency should decrease as signs and symptoms improve. Further evaluation should occur for use of greater than 20 mL.

Pediatric Refer to adult dosing.

Renal Impairment There are no dosage adjustments provided in the manufacturer's labeling. However, dosage adjustment unlikely due to low systemic absorption.

Hepatic Impairment There are no dosage adjustments provided in the manufacturer's labeling. However, dosage adjustment unlikely due to low systemic absorption.

Additional Information Complete prescribing information should be consulted for additional detail.

Dosage Forms Excipient information presented when available (limited, particularly for generics); consult specific product labeling.

Suspension, ophthalmic [drops]:
Zylet: Loteprednol etabonate 0.5% and tobramycin 0.3% (2.5 mL, 5 mL, 10 mL) [contains benzalkonium chloride]

Lovastatin (LOE va sta tin)

Brand Names: US Altoprev; Mevacor
Brand Names: Canada ACT Lovastatin; Apo-Lovastatin; CO Lovastatin; Dom-Lovastatin; Mylan-Lovastatin; PHL-Lovastatin; PMS-Lovastatin; PRO-Lovastatin; Riva-Lovastatin; Sandoz-Lovastatin; Teva-Lovastatin
Index Terms Mevinolin; Monacolin K
Pharmacologic Category Antilipemic Agent, HMG-CoA Reductase Inhibitor
Use

Adjunct to dietary therapy to decrease elevated serum total and LDL-cholesterol concentrations in primary hypercholesterolemia

Primary prevention of coronary artery disease (patients without symptomatic disease with average to moderately elevated total and LDL-cholesterol and below average HDL-cholesterol); slow progression of coronary atherosclerosis in patients with coronary heart disease and reduce the risk of myocardial infarction, unstable angina, and coronary revascularization procedures.

Adjunct to dietary therapy in adolescent patients (10-17 years of age, females >1 year postmenarche) with heterozygous familial hypercholesterolemia having LDL >189 mg/dL, **or** LDL >160 mg/dL with positive family history of premature cardiovascular disease (CVD), **or** LDL >160 mg/dL with the presence of at least two other CVD risk factors

Primary and secondary prevention of atherosclerotic cardiovascular disease (ASCVD) according to the American College of Cardiology/American Heart Association: To reduce the risk of ASCVD in patients with clinical ASCVD (eg, coronary heart disease, stroke/TIA, or peripheral arterial disease presumed to be of atherosclerotic origin) who are greater than 75 years of age or not a candidate for high-intensity statin therapy; in patients without clinical ASCVD if LDL-C is 190 mg/dL or greater and not a candidate for high-intensity statin therapy; in patients without clinical ASCVD who have type 1 or type 2 diabetes and are between 40 and 75 years of age; in patients with an estimated 10-year ASCVD risk 7.5% or greater and who are between 40 and 75 years of age (Stone 2013). The American Heart Association (AHA) recommends statin therapy (unless contraindicated) for all coronary artery bypass graft (CABG) surgery patients to help maintain long-term graft patency and help obtain the highest level of physical health and quality of life (AHA [Kulik 2015]). Specific recommendations from the Kidney Disease: Improving Global Outcomes (KDIGO) organization have also been released for patients with chronic kidney disease (KDIGO [Tonelli 2013]).

Pregnancy Considerations Adverse events were observed in animal reproduction studies. There are reports of congenital anomalies following maternal use of HMG-CoA reductase inhibitors in pregnancy; however, maternal disease, differences in specific agents used, and the low rates of exposure limit the interpretation of the available data (Godfrey 2012; Lecarpentier 2012). Cholesterol biosynthesis may be important in fetal development; serum cholesterol and triglycerides increase normally during pregnancy. The discontinuation of lipid lowering medications temporarily during pregnancy is not expected to have significant impact on the long term outcomes of primary hypercholesterolemia treatment.

Use of lovastatin is contraindicated in pregnancy. HMG-CoA reductase inhibitors should be discontinued prior to pregnancy (ADA 2013). If treatment of dyslipidemias is needed in pregnant women or in women of reproductive age, other agents are preferred (Berglund 2012; Stone 2013). The manufacturer recommends administration to women of childbearing potential only when conception is highly unlikely and patients have been informed of potential hazards.

Breast-Feeding Considerations It is not known if lovastatin is excreted into breast milk. Due to the potential for serious adverse reactions in a nursing infant, use while breast-feeding is contraindicated by the manufacturer.

Contraindications

Hypersensitivity to lovastatin or any component of the formulation; active liver disease; unexplained persistent elevations of serum transaminases; concomitant use of strong CYP3A4 inhibitors (eg, clarithromycin, erythromycin, itraconazole, ketoconazole, nefazodone, posaconazole, voriconazole, protease inhibitors [including boceprevir and telaprevir], telithromycin, cobicistat-containing products); pregnancy; breast-feeding

Canadian labeling: Additional contraindications (not in US labeling): Concomitant use of cyclosporine

Warnings/Precautions Secondary causes of hyperlipidemia should be ruled out prior to therapy. Liver enzyme tests should be obtained at baseline and as clinically indicated; routine periodic monitoring of liver enzymes is not necessary. Use with caution in patients who consume large amounts of ethanol or have a history of liver disease; use is contraindicated with active liver disease and with unexplained transaminase elevations. Rhabdomyolysis with or without acute renal failure has occurred. Risk of rhabdomyolysis is dose-related and increased with concurrent use of lipid-lowering agents which may also cause rhabdomyolysis (fibric acid derivatives or niacin at doses ≥1 g/day) or during concurrent use with potent CYP3A4 inhibitors. Use is contraindicated in patients taking strong CYP3A4 inhibitors. Concomitant use of lovastatin with some drugs may require cautious use, may not be recommended, may require dosage adjustments, or may be contraindicated. Increases in HbA$_{1c}$ and fasting blood glucose have been reported with HMG-CoA reductase inhibitors; however, the benefits of statin therapy far outweigh the risk of dysglycemia. Monitor closely if used with other drugs associated with myopathy (eg, colchicine). Patients should be instructed to report unexplained muscle pain or weakness; lovastatin should be discontinued if myopathy is suspected/confirmed. Immune-mediated necrotizing myopathy (IMNM), an autoimmune-mediated myopathy, has been reported (rarely) with HMG-CoA reductase inhibitor therapy. IMNM presents as proximal muscle weakness with elevated CPK levels, which persists despite discontinuation of HMG-CoA reductase inhibitor therapy; additionally, muscle biopsy may show necrotizing myopathy with limited inflammation; immunosuppressive therapy (eg, corticosteroids, azathioprine) may be used for treatment. The manufacturer recommends temporary discontinuation for elective major surgery, acute medical or surgical conditions, or in any patient experiencing an acute or serious condition predisposing to renal failure (eg, sepsis, hypotension, trauma, uncontrolled seizures). Based on current research and clinical guidelines (Fleisher 2009), HMG-CoA reductase inhibitors should be continued in the perioperative period. Use with caution in patients with advanced age; these patients are predisposed to myopathy.

Adverse Reactions Frequency not always defined. Percentages as reported with immediate release tablets; similar adverse reactions seen with extended release tablets.

Central nervous system: Headache (2% to 3%), dizziness (≤1%)

Dermatologic: Rash (≤1%)

Gastrointestinal: Flatulence (4% to 5%), constipation (2% to 4%), abdominal pain (2% to 3%), diarrhea (2% to 3%), nausea (2% to 3%), dyspepsia (1% to 2%)

Genitourinary: Cystitis (interstitial; Huang 2015)

Neuromuscular & skeletal: Increased CPK (>2x normal) (11%), myalgia (2% to 3%), weakness (1% to 2%), muscle cramps (≤1%)

Ocular: Blurred vision (≤1%)

<1% (Limited to important or life-threatening): Acid regurgitation, alopecia, amnesia (reversible), arthralgia, chest pain, cognitive impairment (reversible), confusion (reversible), dermatomyositis, diabetes mellitus (new onset), eye irritation, increased blood glucose, increased glycosylated hemoglobin (HbA$_{1c}$), insomnia, leg pain, memory disturbance (reversible), memory impairment (reversible), paresthesia, pruritus, vomiting, xerostomia

Additional class-related events or case reports (not necessarily reported with lovastatin therapy): Alteration in taste, anaphylaxis, angioedema, anorexia, anxiety, arthritis, cataracts, chills, cholestatic jaundice, cirrhosis, depression, dryness of skin/mucous membranes, dyspnea, eosinophilia, erectile dysfunction, erythema multiforme, facial paresis, fatty liver, fever, flushing, fulminant hepatic necrosis, gynecomastia, hemolytic anemia, hepatic failure (fatal and nonfatal), hepatitis, hepatoma, hyperbilirubinemia, hypersensitivity reaction, immune-mediated necrotizing myopathy (IMNM), impaired extraocular muscle movement, impotence, increased alkaline phosphatase, increased ESR, increased GGT, increased transaminases, interstitial lung disease, leukopenia, libido decreased, malaise, myopathy, nail changes, nodules, ophthalmoplegia, pancreatitis, peripheral nerve palsy, peripheral neuropathy, photosensitivity, polymyalgia rheumatica, positive ANA, psychic disturbance, purpura, renal failure (secondary to rhabdomyolysis), rhabdomyolysis, skin discoloration, Stevens-Johnson syndrome, systemic lupus erythematosus-like syndrome, thrombocytopenia, thyroid dysfunction, toxic epidermal necrolysis, tremor, urticaria, vasculitis, vertigo

Drug Interactions

Metabolism/Transport Effects Substrate of CYP3A4 (major), P-glycoprotein; **Note:** Assignment of Major/Minor substrate status based on clinically relevant drug interaction potential; **Inhibits** CYP2C9 (weak)

Avoid Concomitant Use

Avoid concomitant use of Lovastatin with any of the following: Boceprevir; Clarithromycin; Conivaptan; CycloSPORINE (Systemic); CYP3A4 Inhibitors (Strong); Erythromycin (Systemic); Fusidic Acid (Systemic); Gemfibrozil; Idelalisib; Lomitapide; Mifepristone; Protease Inhibitors; Red Yeast Rice; Telaprevir; Telithromycin

Increased Effect/Toxicity

Lovastatin may increase the levels/effects of: DAPTOmycin; Diltiazem; PAZOPanib; Trabectedin; Vitamin K Antagonists

The levels/effects of Lovastatin may be increased by: Acipimox; Amiodarone; Aprepitant; Azithromycin (Systemic); Bezafibrate; Boceprevir; Ciprofibrate; Clarithromycin; Colchicine; Conivaptan; CycloSPORINE (Systemic); CYP3A4 Inhibitors (Moderate); CYP3A4 Inhibitors (Strong); Cyproterone; Daclatasvir; Danazol; Dasatinib; Diltiazem; Dronedarone; Erythromycin (Systemic); Fenofibrate and Derivatives; Fluconazole; Fosaprepitant; Fusidic Acid (Systemic); Gemfibrozil; Grapefruit Juice; Idelalisib; Ivacaftor; Lomitapide; Luliconazole; Mifepristone; Netupitant; Niacin; Niacinamide; Osimertinib; Palbociclib; P-glycoprotein/ABCB1 Inhibitors; Protease Inhibitors; QuiNINE; Raltegravir; Ranolazine; Red Yeast Rice; Sacubitril; Simeprevir; Stiripentol; Telaprevir; Telithromycin; Ticagrelor; Verapamil

Decreased Effect

Lovastatin may decrease the levels/effects of: Lanthanum

The levels/effects of Lovastatin may be decreased by: Antacids; Bosentan; CYP3A4 Inducers (Moderate); CYP3A4 Inducers (Strong); Dabrafenib; Deferasirox; Efavirenz; Enzalutamide; Etravirine; Fosphenytoin; Mitotane; Osimertinib; P-glycoprotein/ABCB1 Inducers; Phenytoin; Rifamycin Derivatives; Siltuximab; St Johns Wort; Tocilizumab

Food Interactions Food decreases the bioavailability of lovastatin extended release tablets and increases the bioavailability of lovastatin immediate release tablets. Lovastatin serum concentrations may be increased if taken with grapefruit juice. Management: Avoid concurrent intake of large quantities (>1 quart/day) of grapefruit juice.

Storage/Stability
Tablet, immediate release: Store at 20°C to 25°C (68°F to 77°F). Protect from light
Tablet, extended release: Store at 20°C to 25°C (68°F to 77°F); excursions permitted between 15°C to 30°C (59°F to 86°F). Avoid excessive heat and humidity.

Mechanism of Action Lovastatin acts by competitively inhibiting 3-hydroxyl-3-methylglutaryl-coenzyme A (HMG-CoA) reductase, the enzyme that catalyzes the rate-limiting step in cholesterol biosynthesis. In addition to the ability of HMG-CoA reductase inhibitors to decrease levels of high-sensitivity C-reactive protein (hsCRP), they also possess pleiotropic properties including improved endothelial function, reduced inflammation at the site of the coronary plaque, inhibition of platelet aggregation, and anticoagulant effects (de Denus 2002; Ray 2005).

Pharmacodynamics/Kinetics
Onset of action: LDL-cholesterol reductions: 3 days
Absorption: 30%; increased with extended release tablets when taken in the fasting state
Protein binding: >95%
Metabolism: Hepatic; extensive first-pass effect; hydrolyzed to β-hydroxyacid (active)
Bioavailability: Increased with extended release tablets
Half-life elimination: 1.1-1.7 hours
Time to peak, serum: Immediate release: 2-4 hours; extended release: 12-14 hours
Excretion: Feces (~80% to 85%); urine (10%)

Dosing
Adult
Dyslipidemia and primary prevention of CAD: Oral:
Immediate release: Initial: 20 mg once daily with evening meal, then adjust at 4-week intervals; maximum dose: 80 mg daily
Extended release: Initial: 20, 40, or 60 mg once daily at bedtime, then adjust at 4-week intervals; maximum dose: 60 mg daily
Note: Doses should be individualized according to the baseline LDL-cholesterol levels, the recommended goal of therapy, and patient response. For patients requiring smaller reductions in cholesterol, the use of the extended release tablet is not recommended; consider use of immediate release formulation.

Prevention of cardiovascular disease: ACC/AHA Blood Cholesterol Guideline recommendations to reduce the risk of atherosclerotic cardiovascular disease (ASCVD) (Stone 2013): Adults ≥21 years: Oral:
Primary prevention:
LDL-C ≥190 mg/dL: High intensity therapy necessary; use alternate statin therapy (eg, atorvastatin or rosuvastatin)
Type 1 or 2 diabetes and age 40-75 years: Moderate intensity therapy: Immediate release: 40 mg once daily
Type 1 or 2 diabetes, age 40-75 years, and an estimated 10-year ASCVD risk ≥7.5%: High intensity therapy necessary; use alternate statin therapy (eg, atorvastatin or rosuvastatin)
Age 40-75 years and an estimated 10-year ASCVD risk ≥7.5%: Moderate to high intensity therapy: Immediate release: 40 mg once daily or consider using high intensity statin therapy (eg, atorvastatin or rosuvastatin)
Secondary prevention:
Patient has clinical ASCVD (eg, coronary heart disease, stroke/TIA, or peripheral arterial disease presumed to be of atherosclerotic origin) or is post-CABG (AHA [Kulik 2015]) **and:**
Age ≤75 years: High intensity therapy necessary; use alternate statin therapy (eg, atorvastatin or rosuvastatin)
Age >75 years or not a candidate for high intensity therapy: Moderate intensity therapy: Immediate release: 40 mg once daily

Dosage adjustment for lovastatin with concomitant medications:
Amiodarone: Maximum recommended lovastatin dose (extended release and immediate release): 40 mg daily
Danazol, diltiazem, dronedarone, or verapamil: Initial lovastatin (immediate release) dose: 10 mg daily; Maximum recommended lovastatin (extended release and immediate release) dose: 20 mg daily
Lomitapide: Consider lovastatin dose reduction (per lomitapide manufacturer).

Geriatric Immediate release: Refer to adult dosing; Extended release: Initial: 20 mg once daily at bedtime

Pediatric
Heterozygous familial hypercholesterolemia: Oral (immediate release tablet): Adolescents 10-17 years:
LDL reduction <20%: Initial: 10 mg daily with evening meal
LDL reduction ≥20%: Initial: 20 mg daily with evening meal
Usual range: 10-40 mg once daily with evening meal, then adjust dose at 4-week intervals; maximum dose per manufacturer: 40 mg daily
Dosage adjustment for lovastatin with concomitant medications (amiodarone, danazol, diltiazem, dronedarone, lomitapide, or verapamil): Refer to adult dosing.

Renal Impairment CrCl <30 mL/minute: Use with caution and carefully consider doses >20 mg/day.

Hepatic Impairment No dosage adjustment provided in manufacturer's labeling (has not been studied).

Adjustment for Toxicity
Severe muscle symptoms or fatigue: Promptly discontinue use; evaluate CPK, creatinine, and urinalysis for myoglobinuria (Stone 2013).
Mild to moderate muscle symptoms: Discontinue use until symptoms can be evaluated; evaluate patient for conditions that may increase the risk for muscle symptoms (eg, hypothyroidism, reduced renal or hepatic function, rheumatologic disorders such as polymyalgia rheumatica, steroid myopathy, vitamin D deficiency, or primary muscle diseases). Upon resolution, resume the original or lower dose of lovastatin. If muscle symptoms recur, discontinue lovastatin use. After muscle symptom resolution, may then use a low dose of a different statin; gradually increase if tolerated. In the absence of continued statin use, if muscle symptoms or elevated CPK continues after 2 months, consider other causes of muscle symptoms. If determined to be due to another condition aside from statin use, may resume statin therapy at the original dose (Stone 2013).

Dietary Considerations Before initiation of therapy, patients should be placed on a standard cholesterol-lowering diet for 6 weeks and the diet should be continued during drug therapy. Avoid intake of large quantities of grapefruit juice (≥1 quart/day); may increase toxicity. Immediate release tablet should be taken with the evening meal.

Red yeast rice contains variable amounts of several compounds that are structurally similar to HMG-CoA reductase inhibitors, primarily monacolin K (or mevinolin) which is structurally identical to lovastatin; concurrent use of red yeast rice with HMG-CoA reductase inhibitors may increase the incidence of adverse and toxic effects (Lapi 2008; Smith 2003).

Administration Administer immediate release tablet with the evening meal. Administer extended release tablet at bedtime; do not crush or chew.

Monitoring Parameters
2013 ACC/AHA Blood Cholesterol Guideline recommendations (Stone 2013):
Lipid panel (total cholesterol, HDL, LDL, triglycerides): Baseline lipid panel; fasting lipid profile within 4-12 weeks after initiation or dose adjustment and every 3-12 months (as clinically indicated) thereafter. If 2 consecutive LDL levels are <40 mg/dL, consider decreasing the dose.
Hepatic transaminase levels: Baseline measurement of hepatic transaminase levels (ie, ALT); measure hepatic function if symptoms suggest hepatotoxicity (eg, unusual fatigue or weakness, loss of appetite, abdominal pain, dark-colored urine or yellowing of skin or sclera) during therapy.
CPK: CPK should not be routinely measured. Baseline CPK measurement is reasonable for some individuals (eg, family history of statin intolerance or muscle disease, clinical presentation, concomitant drug therapy that may increase risk of myopathy). May measure CPK in any patient with symptoms suggestive of myopathy (pain, tenderness, stiffness, cramping, weakness, or generalized fatigue).

Evaluate for new-onset diabetes mellitus during therapy; if diabetes develops, continue statin therapy and encourage adherence to a heart-healthy diet, physical activity, a healthy body weight, and tobacco cessation. If patient develops a confusional state or memory impairment, may evaluate patient for nonstatin causes (eg, exposure to other drugs), systemic and neuropsychiatric causes, and the possibility of adverse effects associated with statin therapy.

Manufacturer's labeling: Liver enzyme tests at baseline and repeated when clinically indicated. Measure CPK when myopathy is being considered or may measure CPK periodically in patients starting therapy or when dosage increase is necessary. Analyze lipid panel at intervals of 4 weeks or more.

Dosage Forms Excipient information presented when available (limited, particularly for generics); consult specific product labeling.

Tablet, Oral:

Mevacor: 20 mg, 40 mg

Generic: 10 mg, 20 mg, 40 mg

Tablet Extended Release 24 Hour, Oral:

Altoprev: 20 mg, 40 mg, 60 mg [contains fd&c yellow #6 (sunset yellow)]

Dosage Forms: Canada

Refer to Dosage Forms. **Note:** Extended release tablet is not available in Canada.

Loxapine (LOKS a peen)

Brand Names: US Adasuve; Loxitane [DSC]

Brand Names: Canada Apo-Loxapine; Dom-Loxapine; Loxapac; PHL-Loxapine; Xylac

Index Terms Loxapine Succinate; Loxitane; Oxilapine Succinate

Pharmacologic Category First Generation (Typical) Antipsychotic

Use

Schizophrenia: IM, Oral: Treatment of schizophrenia.

Agitation associated with schizophrenia or bipolar I disorder: Inhalation: Acute treatment of agitation associated with schizophrenia or bipolar I disorder in adults.

Prescribing and Access Restrictions Adasuve is only available through a restricted program called Adasuve REMS. In order to distribute, dispense and administer Adasuve, healthcare facilities must be enrolled and comply with REMS requirements (including on-site access to equipment and personnel to provide advance airway management including intubation and mechanical ventilation). Information is available at www.adasuverems.com or 855-755-0492.

Medication Guide Available Yes

Dosing

Adult

Schizophrenia:

Oral: Initial: 10 mg twice daily (up to 50 mg daily may be considered in severely disturbed patients), increase dose until psychotic symptoms are controlled; usual maintenance: 60-100 mg daily in divided doses 2-4 times daily; satisfactory response often observed with doses of 20-60 mg daily (maximum: 250 mg daily). Therapy should be maintained at lowest effective dose.

IM [Canadian product]: 12.5-50 mg every 4-6 hours or longer; individualize dose early in therapy; some patients respond satisfactorily to twice-daily dosing

Acute treatment of agitation associated with schizophrenia or bipolar I disorder: Inhalation: 10 mg once daily; maximum dose 10 mg per 24-hour period

Geriatric Reduced dosing may be indicated due to risks of adverse events associated with high-dose therapy. Refer to adult dosing.

Renal Impairment No dosage adjustment provided in manufacturer's labeling.

Hepatic Impairment No dosage adjustment provided in manufacturer's labeling. Canadian labeling does not recommend use in severe hepatic disease.

Additional Information Complete prescribing information should be consulted for additional detail.

Dosage Forms Excipient information presented when available (limited, particularly for generics); consult specific product labeling. [DSC] = Discontinued product

Aerosol Powder Breath Activated, Inhalation [preservative free]:

Adasuve: 10 mg (1 ea)

Capsule, Oral:

Loxitane: 5 mg [DSC], 10 mg [DSC], 25 mg [DSC], 50 mg [DSC]

Generic: 5 mg, 10 mg, 25 mg, 50 mg

Dosage Forms: Canada Excipient information presented when available (limited, particularly for generics); consult specific product labeling.

Injection, solution, as hydrochloride [strength expressed as base]:

Loxapac: 50 mg/mL (1 mL) [contains polysorbate 80, propylene glycol]

Solution, oral, as hydrochloride [strength expressed as base; concentrate]:

Xylac: 25 mg/mL (100 mL) [contains propylene glycol]

Tablet, oral, as succinate [strength expressed as base]:

Xylac: 2.5 mg, 5 mg, 10 mg, 25 mg, 50 mg

Lubiprostone (loo bi PROS tone)

Brand Names: US Amitiza

Index Terms RU 0211; SPI 0211

Pharmacologic Category Chloride Channel Activator; Gastrointestinal Agent, Miscellaneous

Use Treatment of chronic idiopathic constipation; treatment of opioid-induced constipation with chronic non-cancer pain; treatment of irritable bowel syndrome with constipation in adult women

Dosing

Adult & Geriatric

Chronic idiopathic constipation: Oral: 24 mcg twice daily

Irritable bowel syndrome with constipation: Females ≥18 years: Oral: 8 mcg twice daily

Opioid-induced constipation: Oral: 24 mcg twice daily

Renal Impairment No dosage adjustment necessary.

Hepatic Impairment

Mild hepatic impairment (Child-Pugh class A): No dosage adjustment necessary.

Moderate hepatic impairment (Child-Pugh class B):

Chronic idiopathic constipation: Initial: 16 mcg twice daily; may increase to 24 mcg twice daily if tolerated and an adequate response has not been obtained with lower dosage.

Irritable bowel syndrome with constipation: No dosage adjustment necessary.

Opioid-induced constipation: Initial: 16 mcg twice daily; may increase to 24 mcg twice daily if tolerated and an adequate response has not been obtained with lower dosage.

Severe hepatic impairment (Child-Pugh class C):

Chronic idiopathic constipation: Initial: 8 mcg twice daily; may increase to 16-24 mcg twice daily if tolerated and an adequate response has not been obtained with lower dosage.

Irritable bowel syndrome with constipation: Initial: 8 mcg once daily; may increase to 8 mcg twice daily if tolerated and an adequate response has not been obtained at lower dosage.

Opioid-induced constipation: Initial: 8 mcg twice daily; may increase to 16-24 mcg twice daily if tolerated and an adequate response has not been obtained with lower dosage.

Additional Information Complete prescribing information should be consulted for additional detail.

◄ **Dosage Forms** Excipient information presented when available (limited, particularly for generics); consult specific product labeling.
Capsule, Oral:
Amitiza: 8 mcg
Amitiza: 24 mcg [contains fd&c red #40, fd&c yellow #10 (quinoline yellow)]

◆ Lucentis *see* Ranibizumab *on page 1556*

Lucinactant (loo sin AK tant)

Brand Names: US Surfaxin
Pharmacologic Category Lung Surfactant
Use Prevention of respiratory distress syndrome (RDS) in premature infants at high risk for RDS
Dosing
Pediatric Respiratory distress prophylaxis: Premature infants: Endotracheal: 5.8 mL/kg birth weight; up to 3 subsequent doses (total of 4 doses) may be administered at ≥6-hour intervals within the first 48 hours of life.
Renal Impairment No dosage adjustment provided in manufacturer's labeling.
Hepatic Impairment No dosage adjustment provided in manufacturer's labeling.
Additional Information Complete prescribing information should be consulted for additional detail.
Dosage Forms Excipient information presented when available (limited, particularly for generics); consult specific product labeling.
Suspension, Inhalation:
Surfaxin: 30 mg/mL (8.5 mL)

◆ Ludiomil *see* Maprotiline *on page 1126*
◆ Lugol's Solution *see* Potassium Iodide and Iodine *on page 1482*

Luliconazole (loo li KON a zole)

Brand Names: US Luzu
Pharmacologic Category Antifungal Agent, Topical
Use Fungal infections: Topical treatment of tinea pedis, tinea cruris, and tinea corporis caused by the organisms *Trichophyton rubrum* and *Epidermophyton floccosum*
Dosing
Adult & Geriatric
Fungal Infection: Topical:
Tinea pedis: Apply to affected area and ~1 inch of immediate surrounding area(s) once daily for 2 weeks
Tinea cruris or tinea corporis: Apply to affected area and ~1 inch of immediate surrounding area(s) once daily for 1 week
Renal Impairment No dosage adjustment provided in the manufacturer's labeling.
Hepatic Impairment No dosage adjustment provided in the manufacturer's labeling.
Additional Information Complete prescribing information should be consulted for additional detail.
Dosage Forms Excipient information presented when available (limited, particularly for generics); consult specific product labeling.
Cream, External:
Luzu: 1% (60 g) [contains benzyl alcohol, methylparaben, propylene glycol]

Lumacaftor and Ivacaftor
(loo ma KAF tor & eye va KAF tor)

Brand Names: US Orkambi
Index Terms Ivacaftor and Lumacaftor
Pharmacologic Category Cystic Fibrosis Transmembrane Conductance Regulator Potentiator
Use
Cystic fibrosis: Treatment of cystic fibrosis (CF) in patients age 12 years and older who are homozygous for the F508del mutation in the CFTR gene. If the patient's genotype is unknown, an FDA-cleared CF mutation test should be used to detect the presence of the F508del mutation on both alleles of the CFTR gene.
Limitations of use: Efficacy and safety have not been established in patients with CF other than those homozygous for the F508del mutation.
Pregnancy Considerations Adverse events were not observed in animal reproduction studies when testing the individual agents.
Breast-Feeding Considerations It is not known if lumacaftor or ivacaftor are excreted into breast milk; however excretion is expected. The manufacturer recommends that caution be used if administered to a nursing woman.
Contraindications There are no contraindications listed in the manufacturer's labeling.

Warnings/Precautions May increase hepatic transaminases with or without concomitant elevations in total serum bilirubin. Monitor ALT, AST, and bilirubin at baseline, every 3 months for the first year of therapy, and annually thereafter. Increased monitoring may be necessary in patients with a history of elevated hepatic transaminases or bilirubin. Temporarily discontinue treatment if ALT or AST >5 times ULN without concomitant elevated bilirubin or if ALT or AST >3 times ULN with concomitant bilirubin >2 times ULN. Use with caution in patients with severe renal impairment (CrCl ≤30 mL/minute), end-stage renal disease (ESRD), or hepatic impairment; worsening of liver function (including hepatic encephalopathy) has been reported in patients with advanced liver disease. Dosage adjustment is recommended in patients with moderate to severe (Child-Pugh class B or C) impairment.

Noncongenital lens opacities and cataracts have been reported in pediatric patients treated with ivacaftor; other risk factors were present in some cases (eg, corticosteroid use, exposure to radiation), but a possible risk related to ivacaftor cannot be excluded. Baseline and follow-up ophthalmological examinations are recommended in pediatric patients. Use was associated with an increased incidence of respiratory events (eg, chest discomfort, dyspnea, and abnormal respirations). Careful monitoring during initiation of therapy is recommended in patients with a percent predicted FEV$_1$ <40.

Potentially significant drug-drug interactions may exist, requiring dose or frequency adjustment, additional monitoring, and/or selection of alternative therapy.
Adverse Reactions
>10%:
Gastrointestinal: Nausea (13%), diarrhea (12%)
Respiratory: Changes in respiration (9% to ≤22%), chest discomfort (≤22%), dyspnea (13% to ≤22%), nasopharyngitis (13%)
1% to 10%:
Central nervous system: Fatigue (9%)
Dermatologic: Skin rash (7%)
Endocrine & metabolic: Menstrual disease (10%; including amenorrhea, dysmenorrhea, menorrhagia, menstrual irregular; more common in patients using hormonal contraceptives)
Gastrointestinal: Flatulence (7%)
Infection: Influenza (5%)
Neuromuscular & skeletal: Increased creatine phosphokinase (≤7%)
Respiratory: Upper respiratory tract infection (10%), rhinorrhea (6%)
<1% (Limited to important or life-threatening): Hepatic encephalopathy, increased serum bilirubin, increased serum transaminases
Drug Interactions
Metabolism/Transport Effects Refer to individual components.
Avoid Concomitant Use
Avoid concomitant use of Lumacaftor and Ivacaftor with any of the following: Abiraterone Acetate; Amodiaquine; Antihepaciviral Combination Products; Apixaban; Apremilast; Aprepitant; Artemether; Axitinib; Bedaquiline; Bitter Orange; Boceprevir; Bortezomib; Bosutinib; Cabozantinib; Cariprazine; Ceritinib; CloZAPine; Cobimetinib; Conivaptan; Crizotinib; CYP3A4 Inducers (Strong); Dabrafenib; Daclatasvir; Dienogest; Dronedarone; Eliglustat; Enzalutamide; Everolimus; Flibanserin; Fusidic Acid (Systemic); Grapefruit Juice; Ibrutinib; Idelalisib; Irinotecan Products; Isavuconazonium Sulfate; Itraconazole; Ivabradine; Ivacaftor; Ixazomib; Ketoconazole (Systemic); Lapatinib; Lumefantrine; Lurasidone; Macitentan; Mifepristone; Naloxegol; Netupitant; NIFEdipine; Nilotinib; NiMODipine; Nisoldipine; Olaparib; Osimertinib; Palbociclib; Panobinostat; PAZOPanib; Perampanel; Pimozide; PONATinib; Posaconazole; Praziquantel; Ranolazine; Regorafenib; Rivaroxaban; Roflumilast; RomiDEPsin; Silodosin; Simeprevir; Sonidegib; SORAfenib; St Johns Wort; Suvorexant; Tasimelteon; Telaprevir; Ticagrelor; Tofacitinib; Tolvaptan; Topotecan; Toremifene; Trabectedin; Ulipristal; Vandetanib; Vemurafenib; VinCRIStine (Liposomal); Vorapaxar; Voriconazole

Increased Effect/Toxicity
Lumacaftor and Ivacaftor may increase the levels/effects of: Afatinib; Amodiaquine; Bosutinib; Brentuximab Vedotin; Clarithromycin; Colchicine; CYP2C8 Substrates; CYP2C9 Substrates; CYP3A4 Substrates; Dabigatran Etexilate; Dofetilide; DOXOrubicin (Conventional); Edoxaban; Hydrocodone; Ifosfamide; Ledipasvir; Lomitapide; PAZOPanib; P-glycoprotein/ABCB1 Substrates; Pimozide; Prucalopride; Rifaximin; Silodosin; Topotecan; VinCRIStine (Liposomal)

The levels/effects of Lumacaftor and Ivacaftor may be increased by: Bitter Orange; Clarithromycin; Conivaptan; CYP3A4 Inhibitors (Moderate); CYP3A4 Inhibitors (Strong); Fusidic Acid (Systemic); Grapefruit Juice; Idelalisib; Luliconazole; Stiripentol

Decreased Effect

Lumacaftor and Ivacaftor may decrease the levels/effects of: Abiraterone Acetate; Antihepaciviral Combination Products; Apixaban; Apremilast; Aprepitant; ARIPiprazole; ARIPiprazole Lauroxil; Artemether; Axitinib; Bedaquiline; Boceprevir; Bortezomib; Bosutinib; Brentuximab Vedotin; Brexpiprazole; Buprenorphine; Cabozantinib; Cannabidiol; Cannabis; Cariprazine; Ceritinib; Clarithromycin; CloZAPine; Cobimetinib; Contraceptives (Estrogens); Contraceptives (Progestins); Corticosteroids (Systemic); Crizotinib; CYP2B6 Substrates; CYP2C19 Substrates; CYP2C8 Substrates; CYP2C9 Substrates; CYP3A4 Substrates; Dabrafenib; Daclatasvir; Dasatinib; Dexamethasone (Systemic); Dienogest; DOXOrubicin (Conventional); Dronabinol; Dronedarone; Eliglustat; Enzalutamide; Erlotinib; Etizolam; Etoposide; Etoposide Phosphate; Everolimus; Exemestane; FentaNYL; Flibanserin; Gefitinib; GuanFACINE; Hydrocodone; Hydrocortisone (Systemic); Ibrutinib; Idelalisib; Ifosfamide; Imatinib; Irinotecan Products; Isavuconazonium Sulfate; Itraconazole; Ivabradine; Ivacaftor; Ixabepilone; Ixazomib; Ketoconazole (Systemic); Lapatinib; Linagliptin; Lumefantrine; Lurasidone; Macitentan; Maraviroc; MethylPREDNISolone; Mifepristone; Montelukast; Naloxegol; Netupitant; NIFEdipine; Nilotinib; NiMODipine; Nisoldipine; Olaparib; Osimertinib; Palbociclib; Panobinostat; PAZOPanib; Perampanel; P-glycoprotein/ABCB1 Substrates; PONATinib; Posaconazole; Praziquantel; PrednisoLONE (Systemic); PredniSONE; Propafenone; QUEtiapine; Ranolazine; Regorafenib; Rivaroxaban; Roflumilast; Rolapitant; RomiDEPsin; Saxagliptin; Simeprevir; Sonidegib; SORAfenib; SUNItinib; Suvorexant; Tadalafil; Tasimelteon; Telaprevir; Tetrahydrocannabinol; Ticagrelor; Tofacitinib; Tolvaptan; Toremifene; Trabectedin; Ulipristal; Vandetanib; Vemurafenib; Vilazodone; VinCRIStine (Liposomal); Vorapaxar; Voriconazole; Vortioxetine; Zaleplon; Zuclopenthixol

The levels/effects of Lumacaftor and Ivacaftor may be decreased by: Bosentan; CYP3A4 Inducers (Moderate); CYP3A4 Inducers (Strong); Deferasirox; Siltuximab; St Johns Wort; Tocilizumab

Food Interactions Food increases exposure to lumacaftor and ivacaftor. Ivacaftor serum concentrations may be increased when taken with grapefruit or Seville oranges (Kalydeco prescribing information, 2015). Management: Administer with fat-containing food; avoid grapefruit and Seville oranges during therapy.

Storage/Stability Store at 20°C to 25°C (68°F to 77°F); excursions permitted between 15°C and 30°C (59°F and 86°F)

Mechanism of Action Lumacaftor improves the conformational stability of F508del-CFTR, resulting in increased processing and trafficking of mature protein to the cell surface. Ivacaftor is a CFTR potentiator that facilitates increased chloride transport by potentiating the channel-open probability (or gating) of the CFTR protein at the cell surface.

Pharmacodynamics/Kinetics

Absorption:
Ivacaftor: Variable; increased (by ~3-fold) when administered with fatty foods as compared with fasting
Lumacaftor: Variable; increased (by ~2-fold) when administered with fatty foods as compared with fasting

Distribution: V_d:
Ivacaftor: 353 L
Lumacaftor: 86 ± 69.8 L

Protein binding:
Ivacaftor: ~99%; primarily to alpha$_1$-acid glycoprotein and albumin
Lumacaftor: ~99%; primarily to albumin

Metabolism:
Ivacaftor: Hepatic; extensive via CYP3A; forms 2 major metabolites (M1 [active; 1/6 potency] and M6 [inactive])
Lumacaftor: Not extensively metabolized; undergoes oxidation and glucuronidation

Half-life elimination:
Ivacaftor: ~9 hours (when administered with lumacaftor in healthy subjects)
Lumacaftor: ~26 hours

Time to peak:
Ivacaftor: Median: ~4 hours (fed state)
Lumacaftor: Median: ~4 hours (fed state)

Excretion:
Ivacaftor: Feces (88%; 65% of administered dose as metabolites); urine (6.6% as unchanged drug)
Lumacaftor: Feces (51% as unchanged drug); urine (8.6%; 0.18% of administered dose as unchanged drug)

Dosing

Adult & Geriatric

Cystic fibrosis: Oral: Lumacaftor 400 mg/ivacaftor 250 mg every 12 hours
Missed dose: If a dose is missed ≤6 hours of the usual time it is taken, take the dose as soon as possible; otherwise, skip the missed dose and resume the normal dosing schedule.

Dosage adjustment with concomitant medications:
Coadministration of strong CYP3A inhibitors (eg, itraconazole): When initiating lumacaftor/ivacaftor in patients already maintained on a strong CYP3A inhibitor, reduce the initial dose to lumacaftor 200 mg/ivacaftor 125 mg once daily. Following 1 week of therapy, increase to lumacaftor 400 mg/ivacaftor 250 mg every 12 hours. If lumacaftor/ivacaftor therapy is interrupted for >1 week while taking strong CYP3A inhibitors, re-titration must occur. No dosage adjustment is required for patients already maintained on lumacaftor/ivacaftor who begin therapy with a CYP3A inhibitor.

Pediatric Cystic fibrosis: Children ≥12 years and Adolescents: Oral: Refer to adult dosing

Renal Impairment Children ≥12 years, Adolescents, and Adults:
CrCl >30 mL/minute: No dosage adjustment necessary.
CrCl ≤30 mL/minute: There are no dosage adjustments provided in the manufacturer's labeling; use with caution.
End-stage renal disease (ESRD): There are no dosage adjustments provided in the manufacturer's labeling; use with caution.

Hepatic Impairment Children ≥12 years, Adolescents, and Adults:
Mild impairment (Child-Pugh class A): No dosage adjustment necessary.
Moderate impairment (Child-Pugh class B): Reduce the dose to lumacaftor 400 mg /ivacaftor 250 mg in the morning and lumacaftor 200 mg/ivacaftor 125 mg in the evening.
Severe impairment (Child-Pugh class C): Use with caution, weighing the risks and benefits of treatment. If therapy is appropriate, administer a maximum dose of lumacaftor 200 mg/ivacaftor 125 mg every 12 hours.

Adjustment for Toxicity Children ≥12 years, Adolescents, and Adults:
ALT or AST >5 times ULN without concomitant elevated bilirubin: Temporarily discontinue lumacaftor/ivacaftor; may resume if elevated transaminases resolved and after assessing benefits vs risks of continued treatment
ALT or AST >3 times ULN with concomitant bilirubin >2 times ULN: Temporarily discontinue lumacaftor/ivacaftor; may resume if elevated transaminases resolved and after assessing benefits vs risks of continued treatment

Dietary Considerations Take with fat-containing food (eg, eggs, avocados, nuts, peanut butter, cheese pizza, whole-milk dairy products); avoid grapefruit and Seville oranges (Kalydeco prescribing information, 2015).

Administration Oral: Administer with fat-containing food (eg, eggs, avocados, nuts, butter, peanut butter, cheese pizza, whole-milk dairy products [eg, whole milk, cheese, and yogurt]).

Monitoring Parameters CF mutation test (prior to therapy if genotype is unknown); ophthalmological examinations (baseline and follow-up in pediatric patients); ALT, AST, and bilirubin (baseline, every 3 months for the first year of therapy, and annually thereafter; increased monitoring may be necessary in patients with a history of elevated hepatic transaminases or bilirubin); signs and symptoms of respiratory effects (in patients with a percent predicted FEV$_1$ <40)

Dosage Forms Excipient information presented when available (limited, particularly for generics); consult specific product labeling.
Tablet, Oral:
Orkambi: Lumacaftor 200 mg and ivacaftor 125 mg [contains brilliant blue fcf (fd&c blue #1), fd&c blue #2 (indigotine)]

◆ Lupron Depot *see* Leuprolide *on page 1051*
◆ Lupron Depot-Ped *see* Leuprolide *on page 1051*

Lurasidone (loo RAS i done)

Brand Names: US Latuda
Brand Names: Canada Latuda
Index Terms Lurasidone Hydrochloride; SM-13496
Pharmacologic Category Second Generation (Atypical) Antipsychotic
Use Psychiatric issues: Treatment of schizophrenia; monotherapy or adjunctive therapy of depressive episodes associated with bipolar I disorder
Pregnancy Considerations Adverse events were not observed in animal reproduction studies. Antipsychotic use during the third trimester of pregnancy has a risk for abnormal muscle movements (extrapyramidal symptoms [EPS]) and/or withdrawal symptoms in newborns following delivery. Symptoms in the newborn may include agitation, feeding disorder, hypertonia, hypotonia, respiratory distress, somnolence, and tremor; these effects may be self-limiting or require hospitalization. Lurasidone may cause hyperprolactinemia, which may decrease reproductive function in both males and females.

The ACOG recommends that therapy during pregnancy be individualized; treatment with psychiatric medications during pregnancy should incorporate the clinical expertise of the mental health clinician, obstetrician, primary healthcare provider, and pediatrician. Safety data related to atypical antipsychotics during pregnancy is limited and routine use is not recommended. However, if a woman is inadvertently exposed to an atypical antipsychotic while pregnant, continuing therapy may be preferable to switching to a typical antipsychotic that the fetus has not yet been exposed to; consider risk:benefit (ACOG, 2008).

Healthcare providers are encouraged to enroll women 18-45 years of age exposed to lurasidone during pregnancy in the Atypical Antipsychotics Pregnancy Registry (866-961-2388 or http://www.womensmentalhealth.org/ pregnancyregistry).

Breast-Feeding Considerations It is not known if lurasidone is excreted in breast milk. Due to the potential for serious adverse reactions in the nursing infant, the manufacturer recommends a decision be made whether to discontinue nursing or to discontinue the drug, taking into account the importance of the treatment to the mother.
Contraindications Hypersensitivity to lurasidone or any component of the formulation; concomitant use with strong CYP3A4 inhibitors (eg, ketoconazole) and inducers (eg, rifampin)
Warnings/Precautions [U.S. Boxed Warning]: Antidepressants increase the risk of suicidal thinking and behavior in children, adolescents, and young adults (18-24 years of age) with major depressive disorder and other psychiatric disorders; consider risk prior to prescribing. Lurasidone is not approved in the U.S. for use in children. Short-term studies did not show an increased risk in patients >24 years of age and showed a decreased risk in patients ≥65 years. **[U.S. Boxed Warning]: Closely monitor all patients for clinical worsening, suicidality, or unusual changes in behavior,** particularly during the initial 1-2 months of therapy or during periods of dosage adjustments (increases or decreases); the patient's family or caregiver should be instructed to closely observe the patient and communicate condition with healthcare provider. A medication guide concerning the use of antidepressants should be dispensed with each prescription.

The possibility of a suicide attempt is inherent in major depression and may persist until remission occurs. Patients treated with antidepressants (for any indication) should be observed for clinical worsening and suicidality, especially during the initial few months of a course of drug therapy, or at times of dose changes (increases or decreases). Worsening depression and severe abrupt suicidality that are not part of the presenting symptoms may require discontinuation or modification of drug therapy. Use caution in high-risk patients during initiation of therapy.

Prescriptions should be written for the smallest quantity consistent with good patient care. The patient's family or caregiver should be alerted to monitor patients for the emergence of suicidality and associated behaviors such as anxiety, agitation, panic attacks, insomnia, irritability, hostility, impulsivity, akathisia, hypomania, and mania; patients should be instructed to notify their healthcare provider if any of these symptoms or worsening depression or psychosis occur.

[U.S. Boxed Warning]: Elderly patients with dementia-related psychosis treated with antipsychotics are at an increased risk of death compared to placebo. Most deaths appeared to be either cardiovascular (eg, heart failure, sudden death) or infectious (eg, pneumonia) in nature. **Lurasidone is not approved for the treatment of dementia-related psychosis.** An increased incidence of cerebrovascular effects (eg, transient ischemic attack, stroke), including fatalities, has been reported in placebo-controlled trials of antipsychotics for the unapproved use in elderly patients with dementia-related psychosis.

Leukopenia, neutropenia, and agranulocytosis (sometimes fatal) have been reported in clinical trials and postmarketing reports with antipsychotic use; presence of risk factors (eg, preexisting low WBC or history of drug-induced leuko-/ neutropenia) should prompt periodic blood count assessment. Discontinue therapy at first signs of blood dyscrasias or if absolute neutrophil count <1000/mm^3.

Low to moderately sedating, use with caution in disorders where CNS depression is a feature; patients must be cautioned about performing tasks which require mental alertness (eg, operating machinery or driving). Effects may be potentiated when used with other sedative drugs or ethanol. Use with caution in Parkinson's disease. Caution in patients with predisposition to seizures, including those with a history of seizures, head trauma, brain damage, alcoholism, or concurrent therapy with medications which may lower seizure threshold. Elderly patients may be at increased risk of seizures due to an increased prevalence of predisposing factors. Use with caution in renal or hepatic dysfunction; dose reduction recommended in moderate-to-severe impairment. Esophageal dysmotility and aspiration have been associated with antipsychotic use; use with caution in patients at risk of aspiration pneumonia (ie, Alzheimer's disease). Use is associated with increased prolactin levels; clinical significance of hyperprolactinemia in patients with breast cancer or other prolactin-dependent tumors is unknown. May alter temperature regulation.

Use with caution in patients with severe cardiac disease, hemodynamic instability, prior myocardial infarction or ischemic heart disease. May cause orthostatic hypotension; use with caution in patients at risk of this effect (eg, concurrent medication use which may predispose to hypotension/bradycardia or presence of hypovolemia) or in those who would not tolerate transient hypotensive episodes. Antipsychotics may alter cardiac conduction; life-threatening arrhythmias have occurred with therapeutic doses of antipsychotics. Relative to other antipsychotics, lurasidone has minimal effects on the QTc interval and therefore, risk for arrhythmias is low. However, Canadian labeling recommends avoiding use of lurasidone in patients with a history of cardiac arrhythmias, situations that may increase the risk of torsade de pointes and/or sudden death due to QT prolongation including bradycardia, congenital QT prolongation, electrolyte disturbances (ie, hypokalemia or hypomagnesemia), or in combination with other QTc-prolonging agents. Increases in total cholesterol and triglyceride concentrations have been observed with atypical antipsychotic use; during clinical trials of lurasidone, there were no significant changes in total cholesterol or triglycerides observed. Potentially significant drug-drug interactions may exist, requiring dose or frequency adjustment, additional monitoring, and/or selection of alternative therapy. Consult drug interactions database for more detailed information.

May cause extrapyramidal symptoms (EPS), including pseudoparkinsonism, acute dystonic reactions, akathisia, and tardive dyskinesia (potentially irreversible). Risk of tardive dyskinesia may be increased in elderly patients, particularly elderly women. Risk of dystonia (and probably other EPS) may be greater with increased doses, use of conventional antipsychotics, males, and younger patients. Use may be associated with neuroleptic malignant syndrome (NMS); monitor for mental status changes, fever, muscle rigidity and/or autonomic instability (risk may be increased in patients with Parkinson's disease or Lewy body dementia). May cause hyperglycemia; in some cases may be extreme and associated with ketoacidosis, hyperosmolar coma, or death. Use with caution in patients with diabetes or other disorders of glucose regulation; monitor for worsening of glucose control. Significant weight gain has been observed with antipsychotic therapy; incidence varies with product. Monitor waist circumference and BMI.

Use in elderly patients with dementia is associated with an increased risk of mortality and cerebrovascular accidents; avoid antipsychotic use for behavioral problems associated with dementia unless alternative nonpharmacologic therapies have failed and patient may harm self or others. In addition, use may cause or exacerbate syndrome of

inappropriate antidiuretic hormone secretion or hyponatremia; monitor sodium closely with initiation or dosage adjustments in older adults (Beers Criteria).

Adverse Reactions Frequencies reported for schizophrenia unless otherwise noted.

10%:

Central nervous system: Drowsiness (dose-related: 8% to 27%; depressive episodes, monotherapy: 11%), extrapyramidal reaction (dose-related: 14% to 26%; depressive episodes, monotherapy: 7%), akathisia (dose-related: 6% to 22%; depressive episodes, monotherapy: 8% to 11%), parkinsonian-like syndrome (6% to 17%; depressive episodes, monotherapy: 8%)

Endocrine & metabolic: Increased serum triglycerides (10% to 14%), increased serum glucose (fasting, 10% to 14%), increased serum cholesterol (6% to 14%)

Gastrointestinal: Nausea (dose-related; 10%; depressive episodes, monotherapy: 14%)

1% to 10%:

Cardiovascular: Orthostatic hypotension (1% to 2%), tachycardia

Central nervous system: Insomnia (10%), agitation (5%), anxiety (5%; depressive episodes, monotherapy: 4%), dizziness (4%), dystonia (≤7%; depressive episodes, monotherapy: ≤2%), restlessness (1% to 3%)

Dermatologic: Pruritus, skin rash

Endocrine & metabolic: Increased serum prolactin (≥5 x ULN: females: 8%; males: ≤2%), weight gain (≥7% increase in baseline body weight: 2% to 6%)

Gastrointestinal: Vomiting (8%; depressive episodes, monotherapy: 4%), dyspepsia (6%), xerostomia (depressive episodes, monotherapy: 5%), diarrhea (≥1%; depressive episodes, monotherapy: 4%), sialorrhea (2%), abdominal pain, decreased appetite

Genitourinary: Urinary tract infection (depressive episodes, monotherapy: 2%)

Infection: Influenza (depressive episodes, monotherapy: 2%)

Neuromuscular & skeletal: Back pain (3%; depressive episodes, monotherapy: 2%), increased creatine phosphokinase

Ophthalmic: Blurred vision

Renal: Increased serum creatinine (3% to 7%; depressive episodes, monotherapy: 2% to 4%)

Respiratory: Nasopharyngitis (depressive episodes, monotherapy: 4%)

<1% (Limited to important or life-threatening): Amenorrhea, anemia, angina pectoris, angioedema, atrioventricular block, breast hypertrophy, cerebrovascular accident, gastritis, dysmenorrhea, erectile dysfunction, galactorrhea, hypomania, leukopenia, mania, neuroleptic malignant syndrome, panic attack, renal failure, rhabdomyolysis, seizure, suicidal ideation, tardive dyskinesia, venous thromboembolism

Drug Interactions

Metabolism/Transport Effects Substrate of CYP3A4 (major); **Note:** Assignment of Major/Minor substrate status based on clinically relevant drug interaction potential; **Inhibits** CYP3A4 (weak)

Avoid Concomitant Use

Avoid concomitant use of Lurasidone with any of the following: Amisulpride; Azelastine (Nasal); Conivaptan; CYP3A4 Inducers (Strong); CYP3A4 Inhibitors (Strong); DOPamine; EPINEPHrine (Systemic); Fusidic Acid (Systemic); Grapefruit Juice; Idelalisib; Metoclopramide; Orphenadrine; Paraldehyde; Pimozide; St Johns Wort; Sulpiride; Thalidomide

Increased Effect/Toxicity

Lurasidone may increase the levels/effects of: Alcohol (Ethyl); Amisulpride; ARIPiprazole; Azelastine (Nasal); Buprenorphine; CNS Depressants; Disopyramide; Dofetilide; Flibanserin; Hydrocodone; Lomitapide; Mequitazine; Methotrimeprazine; Methylphenidate; Metyrosine; Mirtazapine; NiMODipine; Orphenadrine; Paraldehyde; Pimozide; Procainamide; QuiNIDine; Selective Serotonin Reuptake Inhibitors; Serotonin Modulators; Sulpiride; Suvorexant; Thalidomide; Zolpidem

The levels/effects of Lurasidone may be increased by: Acetylcholinesterase Inhibitors (Central); Blood Pressure Lowering Agents; Brimonidine (Topical); Cannabis; Conivaptan; CYP3A4 Inhibitors (Moderate); CYP3A4 Inhibitors (Strong); Dasatinib; DOPamine; Doxylamine; Dronabinol; Droperidol; EPINEPHrine (Systemic); Fosaprepitant; Fusidic Acid (Systemic); Grapefruit Juice; HydrOXYzine; Idelalisib; Ivacaftor; Kava Kava; Lithium; Luliconazole; Magnesium Sulfate; Methotrimeprazine; Methylphenidate; Metoclopramide; Metyrosine; Mifepristone; Minocycline; Nabilone; Osimertinib; Palbociclib; Perampanel; Rufinamide; Serotonin Modulators; Simeprevir; Sodium Oxybate; Stiripentol; Tapentadol; Tetrabenazine; Tetrahydrocannabinol

Decreased Effect

Lurasidone may decrease the levels/effects of: Amphetamines; Antidiabetic Agents; Anti-Parkinson's Agents (Dopamine Agonist); Quinagolide

The levels/effects of Lurasidone may be decreased by: Bosentan; CYP3A4 Inducers (Moderate); CYP3A4 Inducers (Strong); Dabrafenib; Deferasirox; Lithium; Osimertinib; Siltuximab; St Johns Wort; Tocilizumab

Food Interactions Administration with food (≥350 calories) increased C_{max} and AUC of lurasidone ~3 times and 2 times, respectively, compared to administration under fasting conditions. Lurasidone exposure was not affected by the fat content of the meal. Management: Administer with food (≥350 calories).

Storage/Stability Store at controlled room temperature of 25°C (77°F); excursions permitted to 15°C to 30°C (59°F to 86°F).

Mechanism of Action Lurasidone is a benzoisothiazol-derivative atypical antipsychotic with mixed serotonin-dopamine antagonist activity. It exhibits high affinity for D_2, 5-HT_{2A}, and 5-HT_7 receptors; moderate affinity for $alpha_{2C}$-adrenergic receptors; and is a partial agonist for 5-HT_{1A} receptors. Lurasidone has no significant affinity for muscarinic M_1 and histamine H_1 receptors. The addition of serotonin antagonism to dopamine antagonism (classic neuroleptic mechanism) is thought to improve negative symptoms of psychoses and reduce the incidence of extrapyramidal side effects as compared to typical antipsychotics.

Pharmacodynamics/Kinetics

Distribution: V_d: 6173 L

Protein binding: ~99%

Metabolism: Primarily via CYP3A4; two active metabolites (ID-14283 and ID-14326) and two major nonactive metabolites (ID-20219 and ID-20220) produced

Bioavailability: 9% to 19%

Half-life elimination: 18 hours; Main active metabolite, ID-14283 (exo-hydroxy metabolite), exhibits a half-life of 7.5-10 hours

Time to peak: 1-3 hours; steady state concentrations achieved within 7 days

Excretion: Urine (~9%); feces (~80%)

Dosing

Adult & Geriatric

Depressive episodes associated with bipolar I disorder (monotherapy or as an adjunct to lithium or valproic acid): Oral: Initial: 20 mg once daily; titration is not required; maximum recommended dose: 120 mg daily. **Note:** Doses ≥80 mg daily during monotherapy studies did not provide additional efficacy compared to lower doses (eg, 20-60 mg daily).

Schizophrenia: Oral: Initial: 40 mg once daily; titration is not required; maximum recommended dose: 160 mg daily

Concomitant CYP3A4 inhibitors/inducers:

CYP3A4 inhibitors:

Concomitant administration with a **strong** CYP3A4 inhibitor (eg, ketoconazole) is contraindicated.

Concomitant administration with a **moderate** CYP3A4 inhibitor (eg, diltiazem):

US labeling: Initial dose: 20 mg once daily; do not exceed 80 mg daily of lurasidone

Canadian labeling: Do not exceed 40 mg daily of lurasidone

CYP3A4 inducers:

Concomitant administration with a **strong** CYP3A4 inducer (eg, rifampin) is contraindicated.

Concomitant administration with a **moderate** CYP3A4 inducer: Lurasidone dose may need to be increased when combined with a moderate CYP3A4 inducer for ≥7 days.

Renal Impairment

US labeling:

CrCl ≥50 mL/minute: No dosage adjustment necessary.

CrCl <50 mL/minute: Initial: 20 mg daily; maximum: 80 mg daily

Canadian labeling:

CrCl ≥50 mL/minute: No dosage adjustment necessary.

CrCl <50 mL/minute: Maximum: 40 mg daily

Hepatic Impairment

US labeling:

Mild impairment (Child-Pugh class A): No dosage adjustment necessary.

Moderate impairment (Child-Pugh class B): Initial: 20 mg daily; maximum: 80 mg daily

Severe impairment (Child-Pugh class C): Initial: 20 mg daily; maximum: 40 mg daily

◀ *Canadian labeling:*
Mild impairment (Child-Pugh class A): No dosage adjustment necessary.
Moderate and severe impairment (Child-Pugh class B and C): Maximum: 40 mg daily

Dietary Considerations Should be taken with food (≥350 calories).

Administration Administer with food (≥350 calories).

Monitoring Parameters Mental status; vital signs (as clinically indicated); blood pressure (baseline; repeat 3 months after antipsychotic initiation, then yearly); weight, height, BMI, waist circumference (baseline; repeat at 4, 8, and 12 weeks after initiating or changing therapy, then quarterly; consider switching to a different antipsychotic for a weight gain ≥5% of initial weight); CBC (as clinically indicated); monitor frequently during the first few months of therapy in patients with preexisting low WBC or history of drug-induced leukopenia/neutropenia); electrolytes, renal and liver function (annually and as clinically indicated); personal and family history of obesity, diabetes, dyslipidemia, hypertension, or cardiovascular disease (baseline; repeat annually); fasting plasma glucose level/HbA$_{1c}$ (baseline; repeat 3 months after starting antipsychotic, then yearly); fasting lipid panel (baseline; repeat 3 months after initiation of antipsychotic; if LDL level is normal repeat at 2- to 5-year intervals or more frequently if clinically indicated); changes in menstruation, libido, development of galactorrhea, erectile and ejaculatory function (at each visit for the first 12 weeks after the antipsychotic is initiated or until the dose is stable, then yearly); abnormal involuntary movements or parkinsonian signs (baseline; repeat weekly until dose stabilized for at least 2 weeks after introduction and for 2 weeks after any significant dose increase); tardive dyskinesia (every 12 months; high-risk patients every 6 months); ocular examination (yearly in patients >40 years; every 2 years in younger patients) (ADA, 2004; Lehman, 2004; Marder, 2004).

Dosage Forms Excipient information presented when available (limited, particularly for generics); consult specific product labeling.
Tablet, Oral, as hydrochloride:
Latuda: 20 mg, 40 mg, 60 mg
Latuda: 80 mg [contains fd&c blue #2 aluminum lake]
Latuda: 120 mg

Mafenide (MA fe nide)

Brand Names: US Sulfamylon
Index Terms Mafenide Acetate
Pharmacologic Category Antibiotic, Topical
Use Burn treatment: For adjunctive therapy of patients with second- and third-degree burns (cream); for use as an adjunctive topical antimicrobial agent to control bacterial infection when used under moist dressings over meshed autografts on excised burn wounds (powder for solution)
Dosing
Adult & Geriatric Burn treatment: Topical:
Cream: Apply once or twice daily with a sterile-gloved hand; apply to a thickness of approximately 1/16 inch (thicker application is not recommended). The burned area should be covered with cream at all times. Continue treatment until healing is progressing well or the burn site is ready for grafting.
Powder for solution: Wet an 8-ply burn dressing with solution and cover graft area. Keep dressing wet using syringe or irrigation tubing every 4 hours (or as necessary) or by moistening dressing every 6 to 8 hours (or as necessary). Continue treatment until autograft vascularization occurs and healing is progressing; may leave dressings in place for ≤5 days.
Pediatric Burn treatment: Topical:
Cream: Children and Adolescents: Refer to adult dosing.
Powder for solution: Infants ≥3 months, Children, and Adolescents: Refer to adult dosing.
Renal Impairment There are no dosage adjustments provided in the manufacturer's labeling; use caution, accumulation of parent drug and metabolite may enhance carbonic anhydrase inhibition.
Hepatic Impairment There are no dosage adjustments provided in the manufacturer's labeling.
Adjustment for Toxicity Acidosis: When acidosis becomes difficult to control, discontinuing treatment for 24 to 48 hours may aid in restoring acid-base balance
Additional Information Complete prescribing information should be consulted for additional detail.
Dosage Forms Excipient information presented when available (limited, particularly for generics); consult specific product labeling. [DSC] = Discontinued product
Cream, External, as acetate [strength expressed as base]:
Sulfamylon: 85 mg/g (56.7 g, 113.4 g, 453.6 g) [contains methylparaben, propylparaben, sodium metabisulfite]
Packet, External, as acetate:
Sulfamylon: 50 g (1 ea, 5 ea)
Generic: 50 g (1 ea [DSC], 5 ea [DSC])

Magaldrate and Simethicone
(MAG al drate & sye METH i kone)

Index Terms Riopan Plus; Simethicone and Magaldrate
Pharmacologic Category Antacid; Antiflatulent
Use Relief of hyperacidity associated with peptic ulcer, gastritis, peptic esophagitis, and hiatal hernia which are accompanied by symptoms of gas
Dosing
Adult & Geriatric Hyperacidity/gas: Oral: 5-10 mL (540-1080 mg magaldrate) between meals and at bedtime
Additional Information Complete prescribing information should be consulted for additional detail.
Dosage Forms Excipient information presented when available (limited, particularly for generics); consult specific product labeling.
Suspension, oral: Magaldrate 540 mg and simethicone 20 mg per 5 mL (360 mL)

Magnesium Chloride (mag NEE zhum KLOR ide)

Brand Names: US Chloromag; Mag-Delay [OTC]; Mag-SR Plus Calcium [OTC]; Mag-SR [OTC] [DSC]; Slow Magnesium/Calcium [OTC]; Slow-Mag [OTC]

Pharmacologic Category Electrolyte Supplement, Oral; Electrolyte Supplement, Parenteral; Magnesium Salt

Use Correction or prevention of hypomagnesemia; dietary supplement

Dosing

Adult & Geriatric Note: Serum magnesium is poor reflection of repletional status as the majority of magnesium is intracellular; serum levels may be transiently normal for a few hours after a dose is given; therefore, aim for consistently high normal serum levels in patients with normal renal function for most efficient repletion.

Dietary supplement: Oral (Mag 64®, Mag Delay™, Slow-Mag®): 2 tablets once daily

Hypomagnesemia, prevention (parenteral nutrition supplementation) (ASPEN [Mirtallo, 2004]): IV (elemental magnesium): 8-20 mEq/day

RDA (elemental magnesium) (IOM, 1997): Oral:
19 to 30 years:
Females: 310 mg/day
Pregnancy: 350 mg/day
Lactation: 310 mg/day
Males: 400 mg/day
≥31 years:
Females: 320 mg/day
Pregnancy: 360 mg/day
Lactation: 320 mg/day
Males: 420 mg/day

Pediatric Note: Serum magnesium is poor reflection of repletional status as the majority of magnesium is intracellular; serum levels may be transiently normal for a few hours after a dose is given; therefore, aim for consistently high normal serum levels in patients with normal renal function for most efficient repletion.

Infants, Children, and Adolescents:
Hypomagnesemia, prevention (parenteral nutrition supplementation) (ASPEN [Mirtallo, 2004]): IV (elemental magnesium):
≤50 kg: 0.3 to 0.5 mEq/kg/day
>50 kg: 10 to 30 mEq/day

RDA (elemental magnesium) (IOM, 1997): Oral:
1 to 3 years: 80 mg/day
4 to 8 years: 130 mg/day
9 to 13 years: 240 mg/day
14 to 18 years:
Females: 360 mg/day
Pregnancy: 400 mg/day
Lactation: 360 mg/day
Males: 410 mg/day

Renal Impairment According to the manufacturer's labeling, use is contraindicated in patients with renal impairment

Hepatic Impairment No dosage adjustment provided in manufacturer's labeling.

Additional Information Complete prescribing information should be consulted for additional detail.

Dosage Forms Considerations
1 g magnesium chloride = elemental magnesium 120 mg = magnesium 9.85 mEq = magnesium 4.93 mmol
Elemental magnesium 64 mg = magnesium 5.26 mEq = magnesium 2.62 mmol

Dosage Forms Excipient information presented when available (limited, particularly for generics); consult specific product labeling. [DSC] = Discontinued product
Solution, Injection, as hexahydrate:
Chloromag: 200 mg/mL (50 mL) [contains benzyl alcohol]
Generic: 200 mg/mL (50 mL)

Tablet Delayed Release, Oral:
Mag-SR Plus Calcium: 535 mg (elemental magnesium 64 mg, plus calcium 106 mg) [starch free, sugar free]
Slow Magnesium/Calcium: 535 mg (elemental magnesium 64 mg, plus calcium 106 mg)
Slow-Mag: Elemental magnesium 71.5 mg (plus calcium 119 mg) [contains fd&c blue #2 aluminum lake]
Tablet Extended Release, Oral:
Mag-Delay: 535 mg (elemental magnesium 64 mg)
Mag-SR: 535 mg (elemental magnesium 64 mg) [DSC] [starch free, sugar free]

Magnesium Citrate (mag NEE zhum SIT rate)

Brand Names: US Citroma [OTC]
Brand Names: Canada Citro-Mag
Index Terms Citrate of Magnesia; Mag Citrate
Pharmacologic Category Laxative, Saline; Magnesium Salt
Use Relieves occasional constipation
Dosing
Adult & Geriatric Laxative: Oral: Solution: 195-300 mL given once or in divided doses
Pediatric Laxative: Oral: Solution:
Children 2-6 years: 60-90 mL given once or in divided doses (maximum: 90 mL/24 hours)
Children 6-12 years: 90-210 mL given once or in divided doses
Children ≥12 years and Adolescents: Refer to adult dosing.
Renal Impairment No dosage adjustment provided in manufacturer's labeling; however, magnesium is renally excreted. Use caution; accumulation of magnesium in renal impairment may lead to magnesium toxicity.
Additional Information Complete prescribing information should be consulted for additional detail.
Dosage Forms Considerations
1 g magnesium citrate ≈ elemental magnesium 160 mg = magnesium 13 mEq = magnesium 6.5 mmol
Dosage Forms Excipient information presented when available (limited, particularly for generics); consult specific product labeling. [DSC] = Discontinued product
Solution, Oral:
Citroma: 1.745 g/30 mL (296 mL) [contains polyethylene glycol, saccharin sodium; lemon flavor]
Citroma: 1.745 g/30 mL (296 mL) [low sodium; lemon flavor]
Citroma: 1.745 g/30 mL (296 mL) [low sodium; contains fd&c red #40, saccharin sodium; cherry flavor]
Generic: 1.745 g/30 mL (296 mL); (300 mL [DSC])
Tablet, Oral:
Generic: 100 mg

Magnesium Gluconate
(mag NEE zhum GLOO koe nate)

Brand Names: US Mag-G [OTC]; Magonate [OTC]
Pharmacologic Category Electrolyte Supplement, Oral; Magnesium Salt
Use Dietary supplement
Dosing
Adult & Geriatric RDA (elemental magnesium): Oral:
19-30 years:
Females: 310 mg/day
Pregnant females: 350 mg/day
Males: 400 mg/day
≥31 years:
Females: 320 mg/day
Pregnant females: 360 mg/day
Males: 420 mg/day
Pediatric RDA (elemental magnesium): Oral:
1-3 years: 80 mg/day
4-8 years: 130 mg/day
9-13 years: 240 mg/day
14-18 years:
Females: 360 mg/day
Pregnant females: 400 mg/day
Males: 410 mg/day
Renal Impairment CrCl <30 mL/minute: Use with caution; monitor for hypermagnesemia
Additional Information Complete prescribing information should be consulted for additional detail.
Dosage Forms Considerations 1 g magnesium gluconate = elemental magnesium 54 mg = magnesium 4.5 mEq = magnesium 2.25 mmol
Dosage Forms Excipient information presented when available (limited, particularly for generics); consult specific product labeling. [DSC] = Discontinued product
Liquid, Oral:
Magonate: 1000 mg (54 mg elemental magnesium) per 5 mL (355 mL [DSC]) [contains sodium benzoate]

Magonate: Magnesium carbonate equivalent to magnesium gluconate 1000 mg (54 mg elemental magnesium) per 5 mL (355 mL) [contains sodium benzoate; mixed melon flavor]

Tablet, Oral:

Mag-G: 500 mg (27 mg elemental magnesium)

Magonate: 500 mg (27 mg elemental magnesium) [scored]

Magonate: 500 mg (27 mg elemental magnesium) [scored; contains fd&c yellow #6 aluminum lake]

Generic: Elemental magnesium 27.5 mg

Tablet, Oral [preservative free]:

Generic: 500 mg (27 mg elemental magnesium)

Magnesium Hydroxide
(mag NEE zhum hye DROKS ide)

Brand Names: US Dulcolax Milk of Magnesia [OTC]; Milk of Magnesia Concentrate [OTC]; Milk of Magnesia [OTC]; Pedia-Lax [OTC]

Index Terms Magnesia Magma; Milk of Magnesia; MOM

Pharmacologic Category Antacid; Laxative; Magnesium Salt

Use Short-term treatment of occasional constipation and symptoms of hyperacidity, laxative

Dosing

Adult & Geriatric

Antacid: OTC labeling: Oral:

Liquid: Magnesium hydroxide 400 mg/5 mL: 5-15 mL as needed up to 4 times/day

Tablet: Magnesium hydroxide 311 mg/tablet: 2-4 tablets every 4 hours up to 4 times/day

Laxative: OTC labeling: Oral:

Liquid:

Magnesium hydroxide 400 mg/5 mL: 30-60 mL/day once daily at bedtime or in divided doses

Magnesium hydroxide 800 mg/5 mL: 15-30 mL/day once daily at bedtime or in divided doses

Tablet: Magnesium hydroxide 311 mg/tablet: 8 tablets/day once daily at bedtime or in divided doses

Pediatric

Antacid: OTC labeling: Oral:

Liquid: Children ≥12 years: Refer to adult dosing.

Tablet:

Children <12 years: Use not recommended.

Children ≥12 years: Refer to adult dosing.

Laxative: Oral:

Liquid: Magnesium hydroxide 400 mg/5 mL: 1-3 mL/kg/day; adjust dose to induce daily bowel movement

OTC labeling:

Children <2 years: Use not recommended.

Children 2-5 years: Magnesium hydroxide 400 mg/5 mL: 5-15 mL/day once daily at bedtime or in divided doses

Children 6-11 years:

Magnesium hydroxide 400 mg/5 mL: 15-30 mL/day once daily at bedtime or in divided doses

Magnesium hydroxide 800 mg/5 mL: 7.5-15 mL/day once daily at bedtime or in divided doses

Children ≥12 years: Refer to adult dosing.

Tablet: OTC labeling:

Children <3 years: Use not recommended.

Children 3-5 years: Magnesium hydroxide 311 mg/tablet: 2 tablets/day once daily at bedtime or in divided doses

Children 6-11 years: Magnesium hydroxide 311 mg/tablet: 4 tablets/day once daily at bedtime or in divided doses

Children ≥12 years: Refer to adult dosing.

Renal Impairment Patients in severe renal failure should not receive magnesium due to toxicity from accumulation. Patients with a CrCl <30 mL/minute should be monitored by serum magnesium levels.

Additional Information Complete prescribing information should be consulted for additional detail.

Dosage Forms Excipient information presented when available (limited, particularly for generics); consult specific product labeling. [DSC] = Discontinued product

Suspension, Oral:

Dulcolax Milk of Magnesia: 400 mg/5 mL (355 mL) [sugar free; unflavored flavor]

Dulcolax Milk of Magnesia: 400 mg/5 mL (355 mL) [sugar free; contains saccharin sodium; mint flavor]

Milk of Magnesia: 400 mg/5 mL (355 mL, 480 mL); 1200 mg/15 mL (355 mL)

Milk of Magnesia: 1200 mg/15 mL (355 mL) [mint flavor]

Milk of Magnesia: 7.75% (360 mL, 480 mL)

Milk of Magnesia: 7.75% (355 mL, 473 mL) [mint flavor]

Milk of Magnesia: 7.75% (30 mL) [spearmint flavor]

Milk of Magnesia: 400 mg/5mL (473 mL [DSC])

Milk of Magnesia: 1200 mg/15 mL (355 mL) [gluten free, stimulant free, sugar free; contains saccharin sodium]

Milk of Magnesia: 400 mg/5 mL (355 mL, 473 mL) [low sodium, sugar free]

Milk of Magnesia: 400 mg/5 mL (473 mL, 769 mL); 1200 mg/15 mL (355 mL) [stimulant free, sugar free]

Milk of Magnesia: 1200 mg/15 mL (355 mL) [stimulant free, sugar free; contains saccharin sodium]

Milk of Magnesia: 400 mg/5 mL (473 mL); 1200 mg/15 mL (355 mL) [sugar free]

Milk of Magnesia Concentrate: 2400 mg/10 mL (100 mL, 400 mL) [lemon flavor]

Milk of Magnesia Concentrate: 2400 mg/10 mL (10 mL) [contains methylparaben, propylene glycol, propylparaben, saccharin sodium; lemon flavor]

Tablet Chewable, Oral:

Pedia-Lax: 400 mg [scored; stimulant free; contains fd&c red #40 aluminum lake; watermelon flavor]

◆ Magnesium Hydroxide, Aluminum Hydroxide, and Simethicone see Aluminum Hydroxide, Magnesium Hydroxide, and Simethicone *on page 85*

◆ Magnesium Hydroxide and Aluminum Hydroxide see Aluminum Hydroxide and Magnesium Hydroxide *on page 85*

◆ Magnesium Hydroxide and Calcium Carbonate see Calcium Carbonate and Magnesium Hydroxide *on page 288*

Magnesium Hydroxide and Mineral Oil
(mag NEE zhum hye DROKS ide & MIN er al oyl)

Brand Names: US Phillips'® M-O [OTC]

Index Terms Haley's M-O; MOM/Mineral Oil Emulsion

Pharmacologic Category Laxative

Use Short-term treatment of occasional constipation

Dosing

Adult & Geriatric Laxative: OTC labeling: Oral: 45-60 mL at bedtime

Pediatric Laxative: OTC labeling: Oral:

Children <6 years: Use not recommended

Children 6-11 years: 20-30 mL at bedtime

Children ≥12 years: Refer to adult dosing.

Renal Impairment Patients in severe renal failure should not receive magnesium due to toxicity from accumulation. Patients with a CrCl <30 mL/minute should be monitored by serum magnesium levels.

Additional Information Complete prescribing information should be consulted for additional detail.

Dosage Forms Excipient information presented when available (limited, particularly for generics); consult specific product labeling.

Suspension, oral:

Phillips'® M-O: Magnesium hydroxide 300 mg and mineral oil 1.25 mL per 5 mL (360 mL, 780 mL) [contains magnesium 125 mg and sodium 1.5 mg per 5 mL mint flavors]

Magnesium L-aspartate Hydrochloride
(mag NEE zhum el as PAR tate hye droe KLOR ide)

Brand Names: US Maginex™ DS [OTC]; Maginex™ [OTC]

Index Terms MAH

Pharmacologic Category Electrolyte Supplement, Oral; Magnesium Salt

Use Dietary supplement

Dosing

Adult & Geriatric

Dietary Reference Intake for Magnesium: Dosage is in terms of elemental magnesium (IOM, 1997): Oral:

RDA:

19-30 years:

Females: 310 mg daily

Pregnant females: 350 mg daily

Lactation: 310 mg daily

Males: 400 mg daily

≥31 years:

Females: 320 mg daily

Pregnant females: 360 mg daily

Lactation: 320 mg daily

Males: 420 mg daily

OTC labeling:

Dietary supplement (dosage in terms of magnesium-L-aspartate hydrochloride salt): Adults: Oral: One packet or 2 tablets (1230 mg) up to 3 times daily

Pediatric

Dietary Reference Intake for Magnesium: Dosage is in terms of elemental magnesium (IOM, 1997): Oral: Children:

1-6 months: Adequate intake: 30 mg daily

7-12 months: Adequate intake: 75 mg daily

1-3 years: RDA: 80 mg daily

4-8 years: RDA: 130 mg daily

9-13 years: RDA: 240 mg daily

14-18 years: RDA:

Females: 360 mg daily

Pregnant females: 400 mg daily

Lactation: 360 mg daily

Males: 410 mg daily

Renal Impairment No dosage adjustment provided in manufacturer's labeling; however, magnesium is renally excreted. Use caution; accumulation of magnesium in renal impairment may lead to magnesium toxicity.

Additional Information Complete prescribing information should be consulted for additional detail.

Dosage Forms Considerations 1 g magnesium L-aspartate Hydrochloride ≈ elemental magnesium 100 mg = magnesium 8.1 mEq = magnesium 4.05 mmol

Dosage Forms Excipient information presented when available (limited, particularly for generics); consult specific product labeling.

Granules for solution, oral [preservative free]:

Maginex™ DS: 1230 mg/packet (30s) [sugar free; lemon flavor; equivalent to elemental magnesium 122 mg]

Tablet, enteric coated, oral [preservative free]:

Maginex™: 615 mg [sugar free; equivalent to elemental magnesium 61 mg]

Magnesium L-lactate (mag NEE zhum el LAK tate)

Brand Names: US Mag-Tab SR [OTC]

Index Terms Magnesium L-lactate Dihydrate

Pharmacologic Category Electrolyte Supplement; Magnesium Salt

Use Dietary supplement

Dosing

Adult & Geriatric

Dietary supplement: Oral: 1-2 caplets every 12 hours

RDA (elemental magnesium):

19-30 years:

Females: 310 mg/day

Pregnant females: 350 mg/day

Males: 400 mg/day

≥31 years:

Females: 320 mg/day

Pregnant females: 360 mg/day

Males: 420 mg/day

Pediatric RDA (elemental magnesium):

Children:

1-3 years: 80 mg/day

4-8 years: 130 mg/day

9-13 years: 240 mg/day

14-18 years:

Females: 360 mg/day

Pregnant females: 400 mg/day

Males: 410 mg/day

Renal Impairment CrCl <30 mL/minute: Use with caution; monitor for hypermagnesemia

Additional Information Complete prescribing information should be consulted for additional detail.

Dosage Forms Considerations 1 g Magnesium L-lactate ≈ elemental magnesium 120 mg = magnesium 9.8 mEq = magnesium 4.9 mmol

Dosage Forms Excipient information presented when available (limited, particularly for generics); consult specific product labeling.

Tablet Extended Release, Oral:

Mag-Tab SR: Elemental magnesium 84 mg [7 mEq]

Magnesium Oxide (mag NEE zhum OKS ide)

Brand Names: US Mag-200 [OTC]; Maox [OTC]; Uro-Mag [OTC]

Index Terms Mag Oxide

Pharmacologic Category Electrolyte Supplement, Oral; Magnesium Salt

Use Dietary supplement; relief of acid indigestion and upset stomach; short-term treatment of occasional constipation

Dosing

Adult & Geriatric

Dietary Reference Intake for Magnesium: Dosage is in terms of elemental magnesium (IOM, 1997): Oral: RDA:

19-30 years:

Females: 310 mg daily

Pregnant females: 350 mg daily

Lactation: 310 mg daily

Males: 400 mg daily

≥31 years:

Females: 320 mg daily

Pregnant females: 360 mg daily

Lactation: 320 mg daily

Males: 420 mg daily

OTC labeling:

Antacid (dosage in terms of magnesium oxide salt): Adults: Oral: Tablet: 1-2 tablets (400-800 mg) daily or in divided doses; maximum: 2 tablets daily

Dietary supplement (dosage in terms of magnesium oxide salt): Adults: Oral:

Mag-Ox 400®: Two tablets (800 mg) daily with food (maximum: 2 tablets/24 hours)

Uro-Mag®: 3-4 capsules (420-560 mg) daily with food

Laxative (dosage in terms of elemental magnesium): Children ≥12 years, Adolescents, and Adults: Oral: Caplet: 2-4 caplets (1000-2000 mg) at bedtime or in divided doses

Pediatric

Dietary Reference Intake for Magnesium: Dosage is in terms of elemental magnesium (IOM, 1997): Oral: Children:

1-6 months: Adequate intake: 30 mg daily

7-12 months: Adequate intake: 75 mg daily

1-3 years: RDA: 80 mg daily

4-8 years: RDA: 130 mg daily

9-13 years: RDA: 240 mg daily

14-18 years: RDA:

Females: 360 mg daily

Pregnant females: 400 mg daily

Lactation: 360 mg daily

Males: 410 mg daily

OTC labeling:

Laxative (dosage in terms of elemental magnesium): Children ≥12 years and Adolescents: Oral: Refer to adult dosing.

Renal Impairment No dosage adjustment provided in manufacturer's labeling; however, magnesium is renally excreted. Use with caution; accumulation in renal impairment may lead to magnesium toxicity.

Additional Information Complete prescribing information should be consulted for additional detail.

Dosage Forms Considerations 400 mg magnesium oxide = elemental magnesium 240 mg = magnesium 19.9 mEq = magnesium 9.85 mmol

Dosage Forms Excipient information presented when available (limited, particularly for generics); consult specific product labeling.

Capsule, Oral:

Uro-Mag: 140 mg

Tablet, Oral:

Mag-200: 200 mg [contains para-aminobenzoic acid]

Maox: 420 mg [contains tartrazine (fd&c yellow #5)]

Generic: 250 mg, 400 mg, 420 mg, 400 mg

Tablet, Oral [preservative free]:

Generic: 400 mg, 500 mg

◆ **Magnesium Oxide, Sodium Picosulfate, and Citric Acid** see Sodium Picosulfate, Magnesium Oxide, and Citric Acid *on page 1680*

Magnesium Salicylate (mag NEE zhum sa LIS i late)

Brand Names: US Doans Extra Strength [OTC]; Doans Pills [OTC]; MST 600 [DSC]

Pharmacologic Category Salicylate

Use Mild-to-moderate pain, fever, various inflammatory conditions; relief of pain and inflammation of rheumatoid arthritis and osteoarthritis

Dosing

Adult Relief of mild-to-moderate pain:

Doan's® Extra Strength, Momentum®: Two caplets every 6 hours as needed (maximum: 8 caplets/24 hours)

Keygesic: One tablet every 4 hours as needed (maximum: 4 tablets/24 hours)

Pediatric Relief of mild-to-moderate pain: Children ≥12 years: Refer to adult dosing.

Additional Information Complete prescribing information should be consulted for additional detail.

Dosage Forms Excipient information presented when available (limited, particularly for generics); consult specific product labeling. [DSC] = Discontinued product

Tablet, Oral:

Doans Pills: 325 mg

Tablet, Oral, as tetrahydrate:

Doans Extra Strength: 580 mg

Doans Extra Strength: 580 mg [contains methylparaben]

MST 600: 600 mg [DSC] [contains fd&c yellow #10 (quinoline yellow)]

Magnesium Sulfate (mag NEE zhum SUL fate)

Brand Names: US Epsom Salt [OTC]

Index Terms Epsom Salts; $MgSO_4$ (error-prone abbreviation)

Pharmacologic Category Anticonvulsant, Miscellaneous; Electrolyte Supplement, Parenteral; Magnesium Salt

Use

Oral: Laxative for the relief of occasional constipation (OTC labeling)

Parenteral: Treatment and prevention of hypomagnesemia; prevention and treatment of seizures in severe pre-eclampsia or eclampsia, pediatric acute nephritis; treatment of cardiac arrhythmias (VT/VF) caused by hypomagnesemia

Topical: Soaking aid for minor cuts and bruises (OTC labeling)

Pregnancy Considerations Magnesium crosses the placenta; serum concentrations in the fetus are similar to those in the mother (Idama, 1998; Osada, 2002). Continuous maternal use for >5-7 days (in doses such as those used for preterm labor, an off-label use) may cause fetal hypocalcemia and bone abnormalities, as well as fractures in the neonate. Magnesium sulfate injection is used for the prevention and treatment of seizures in pregnant or postpartum women with severe pre-eclampsia or eclampsia (ACOG, 2013). Magnesium sulfate may also be used prior to early preterm delivery to reduce the risk of cerebral palsy (ACOG, 2010; Reeves, 2011). Tocolytics may be used for the short-term (48 hour) prolongation of pregnancy to allow for the administration of antenatal steroids and should not be used prior to fetal viability or when the risks of use to the fetus or mother are greater than the risk of preterm birth; maintenance therapy with tocolytics is ineffective and not recommended. Magnesium sulfate injection may be used in conjunction with tocolytics for neuroprotection (it is not preferred for use as a tocolytic); however, an increased risk of maternal complications may be observed when used in combination with some tocolytic agents (ACOG, 2012).

Breast-Feeding Considerations Magnesium is found in breast milk; concentrations remain constant during the first year of lactation and are not influenced by dietary intake under normal conditions. Magnesium requirements are the same in lactating and nonlactating females (IOM, 1997). When magnesium sulfate is used in the intrapartum management of eclampsia, breast milk concentrations are generally increased for only ~24 hours after the end of treatment (Idama, 1998). The manufacturer recommends that caution be used if administered to nursing women.

Contraindications Hypersensitivity to any component of the formulation; heart block; myocardial damage; IV use for pre-eclampsia/eclampsia during the 2 hours prior to delivery

Warnings/Precautions Use magnesium with caution in patients with impaired renal function (accumulation of magnesium may lead to magnesium intoxication). Use with extreme caution in patients with myasthenia gravis or other neuromuscular disease. Magnesium toxicity can lead to fatal cardiovascular arrest and/or respiratory paralysis. The parenteral product may contain aluminum; toxic aluminum concentrations may be seen with high doses, prolonged use, or renal dysfunction. Premature neonates are at higher risk due to immature renal function and aluminum intake from other parenteral sources. Parenteral aluminum exposure of >4 to 5 mcg/kg/day is associated with CNS and bone toxicity; tissue loading may occur at lower doses (Federal Register, 2002). See manufacturer's labeling. Concurrent hypokalemia or hypocalcemia can accompany a magnesium deficit. Unlikely to effectively terminate irregular/polymorphic VT (with normal baseline QT interval) (AHA [Neumar 2010]).

Obstetric use: Vigilant monitoring and safe administration techniques (ISMP, 2005) recommended to avoid potential for errors resulting in toxicity. Monitor mother and fetus closely. Use longer than to -7 days may cause adverse fetal events.

Self-medication (OTC Use): When used as a soaking aid, patients should not use if there is evidence of infection or prompt relief is not obtained. When used as a laxative, patients should consult a healthcare provider prior to use if they have: kidney disease; are on a magnesium-restricted diet; have abdominal pain, nausea, or vomiting; change in bowel habits lasting >2 weeks; have already used a laxative for >1 week

Adverse Reactions Adverse effects on neuromuscular function may occur at lower concentrations in patients with neuromuscular disease (eg, myasthenia gravis).

Frequency not defined:
Cardiovascular: Flushing (IV; dose related), hypotension (IV; rate related), vasodilation (IV; rate related)
Endocrine & metabolic: Hypermagnesemia

Drug Interactions

Metabolism/Transport Effects None known.

Avoid Concomitant Use

Avoid concomitant use of Magnesium Sulfate with any of the following: Calcium Polystyrene Sulfonate; Raltegravir; Sodium Polystyrene Sulfonate

Increased Effect/Toxicity

Magnesium Sulfate may increase the levels/effects of: Calcium Channel Blockers; Calcium Polystyrene Sulfonate; CNS Depressants; Gabapentin; Neuromuscular-Blocking Agents; Sodium Polystyrene Sulfonate

The levels/effects of Magnesium Sulfate may be increased by: Alfacalcidol; Calcitriol (Systemic); Calcium Channel Blockers

Decreased Effect

Magnesium Sulfate may decrease the levels/effects of: Alpha-Lipoic Acid; Bisphosphonate Derivatives; Deferiprone; Dolutegravir; Eltrombopag; Gabapentin; Levothyroxine; Multivitamins/Fluoride (with ADE); Mycophenolate; Phosphate Supplements; Quinolone Antibiotics; Raltegravir; Tetracycline Derivatives; Trientine

The levels/effects of Magnesium Sulfate may be decreased by: Alpha-Lipoic Acid; Trientine

Food Interactions Increased alcohol intake can deplete magnesium stores (IOM, 1997).

Preparation for Administration

IV: Dilute to a ≤20% solution for IV infusion.

IM: A 25% or 50% concentration may be used for adults and dilution to a ≤20% solution is recommended for children.

Oral: Dissolve granules in 8 ounces of water prior to administration. May add lemon juice to improve taste.

Topical: Dissolve 2 cups of granules per gallon of warm water to use as a soaking aid.

Storage/Stability Prior to use, store at room temperature of 20°C to 25°C (68°F to 77°F). Do not freeze. Refrigeration of solution may result in precipitation or crystallization.

Mechanism of Action When taken orally, magnesium promotes bowel evacuation by causing osmotic retention of fluid which distends the colon with increased peristaltic activity; parenterally, magnesium decreases acetylcholine in motor nerve terminals and acts on myocardium by slowing rate of S-A node impulse formation and prolonging conduction time. Magnesium is necessary for the movement of calcium, sodium, and potassium in and out of cells, as well as stabilizing excitable membranes.

Intravenous magnesium may improve pulmonary function in patients with asthma; causes relaxation of bronchial smooth muscle independent of serum magnesium concentration.

Pharmacodynamics/Kinetics

Onset of action: Anticonvulsant: IM: 1 hour; IV: Immediate

Duration of anticonvulsant activity: IM: 3-4 hours; IV: 30 minutes

Distribution: Bone (50% to 60%); extracellular fluid (1% to 2%) (IOM, 1997)

Protein binding: 30%, to albumin

Excretion: Urine (as magnesium)

Dosing

Adult & Geriatric Dose represented as magnesium sulfate unless stated otherwise. **Note:** Serum magnesium is poor reflection of repletional status as the majority of magnesium is intracellular; serum concentrations may be transiently normal for a few hours after a dose is given, therefore, aim for consistently high normal serum concentrations in patients with normal renal function for most efficient repletion.

Note: 1 g of magnesium sulfate = 98.6 mg elemental magnesium = 8.12 mEq elemental magnesium = magnesium 4.06 mmol

Constipation (occasional): Oral: 2 to 4 level teaspoons of granules dissolved in 8 ounces of water; may repeat in 6 hours. Do not exceed 2 doses per day.

Eclampsia/pre-eclampsia (severe):

Manufacturer's labeling: IV: An initial total dose of 10 to 14 g administered as follows: 4 g infusion with simultaneous IM injections of 4 to 5 g in each buttock. After the initial IV/IM doses, may administer a 1 to 2 g/hour continuous infusion or may follow with IM doses of 4 to 5 g into alternate buttocks every 4 hours as necessary. Maximum: 40 g/24 hours. IV use for pre-eclampsia/eclampsia is contraindicated during the 2 hours prior to delivery.

Alternate dosing (off-label): IV: 4 to 6 g loading dose followed by 1 to 2 g/hour continuous infusion for at least 24 hours (ACOG, 2013)

Hypomagnesemia, treatment: Note: Treatment depends on severity and clinical status. In asymptomatic patients (when oral route is available), oral replacement therapy is a better replacement method than IV administration.

Mild deficiency: IM: Manufacturer's labeling: 1 g every 6 hours for 4 doses, or as indicated by serum magnesium concentrations

Mild-to-moderate (serum concentration 1 to 1.5 mg/dL): IV: 1 to 4 g (up to 0.125 g/kg), administer at ≤1 g/hour if asymptomatic; do not exceed 12 g over 12 hours (Kraft, 2005). **Note:** Additional supplementation may be required after the initial dose with replenishment occurring over several days.

Severe deficiency:
IM: Manufacturer's labeling: Up to 250 mg/kg within a 4-hour period
IV:
Severe (<1 mg/dL): 4 to 8 g (up to 0.1875 g/kg), administer at ≤1 g/hour if asymptomatic; in symptomatic patients, may administer ≤4 g over 4-5 minutes (Kraft, 2005)
With polymorphic VT (including torsade de pointes): IV push: 1 to 2 g (ACLS, 2010)
Obesity: Weight >130% of ideal body weight (IBW) or body mass index (BMI) ≥30 kg/m^2: When determining maximum per kg dose for replacement, some clinicians suggest using adjusted body weight (AdjBW) (Kraft, 2005).
AdjBW (men) = ([wt (kg) -IBW (kg)] x 0.3) + IBW
AdjBW (women) = ([wt (kg) -IBW (kg)] x 0.25) + IBW

Hypomagnesemia, prevention (parenteral nutrition supplementation): IV: 8 to 20 mEq elemental magnesium daily (ASPEN [Mirtallo, 2004])

Soaking aid: Topical: Dissolve 2 cupfuls of granules per gallon of warm water; may also soak a towel with the solution to apply as a wet dressing.

Asthma (acute severe exacerbations) (off-label use): IV: 2 g as a single dose over 20 minutes (NAEPP, 2007; GINA, 2015); recommended as adjunctive therapy for severe life-threatening exacerbations and for exacerbations that remain severe after 1 hour of intensive conventional therapy (NAEPP, 2007)

Torsade de pointes or VF/pulseless VT associated with torsade de pointes (off-label use): IV, I.O.: 1 to 2 g over 15 minutes (ACLS, 2010)

RDA (IOM, 1997):
Adults 19 to 30 years:
Females: 310 mg elemental magnesium daily
Pregnant females: 350 mg elemental magnesium daily
Breast-feeding females: 310 mg elemental magnesium daily
Males: 400 mg elemental magnesium daily
Adults ≥31 years:
Females: 320 mg elemental magnesium daily
Pregnant females: 360 mg elemental magnesium daily
Breast-feeding females: 320 mg elemental magnesium daily
Males: 420 mg elemental magnesium daily

Pediatric Dose represented as magnesium sulfate unless stated otherwise. **Note:** Serum magnesium is poor reflection of repletional status as the majority of magnesium is intracellular; serum concentrations may be transiently normal for a few hours after a dose is given, therefore, aim for consistently high normal serum concentrations in patients with normal renal function for most efficient repletion.

Note: 1 g of magnesium sulfate = 98.6 mg elemental magnesium = 8.12 mEq elemental magnesium = magnesium 4.06 mmol

Constipation (occasional): Oral:
Children 6 to <12 years: 1 to 2 level teaspoons of granules dissolved in water; may repeat in 4 to 6 hours (maximum: 2 doses/24 hours)
Children ≥12 years and Adolescents: Refer to adult dosing.

Hypomagnesemia, treatment: Note: Treatment depends on severity and clinical status: IV, I.O.: 25 to 50 mg/kg/dose over 10 to 20 minutes (over several minutes for torsade de pointes); maximum single dose: 2000 mg (PALS, 2010)

Hypomagnesemia, prevention (parenteral nutrition supplementation) (ASPEN [Mirtallo, 2004]): IV:
≤50 kg: 0.3 to 0.5 mEq elemental magnesium/kg/day
>50 kg: 10 to 30 mEq elemental magnesium daily

Asthma (acute severe exacerbations) (off-label use): IV: Children and Adolescents: 25 to 75 mg/kg (maximum: 2000 mg) as a single dose over 20 to 60 minutes (GINA 2015; NAEPP, 2007); recommended as adjunctive therapy for severe life-threatening exacerbations and for exacerbations that remain severe after 1 hour of intensive conventional therapy (NAEPP, 2007)

RDA (IOM, 1997): Children
1 to 3 years: 80 mg elemental magnesium daily
4 to 8 years: 130 mg elemental magnesium daily
9 to 13 years: 240 mg elemental magnesium daily
14 to 18 years:
Females: 360 mg elemental magnesium daily
Pregnant females: 400 mg elemental magnesium daily
Breast-feeding females: 360 mg elemental magnesium daily
Males: 410 mg elemental magnesium daily

Renal Impairment
Hypomagnesemia: Renal dysfunction: Reduce dose by 50% (Kraft, 2005). Use with caution; monitor for hypermagnesemia; Close monitoring is required.
Pre-eclampsia/eclampsia: Severe renal impairment: Per the manufacturer, do not exceed 20 grams during a 48 hour period.

Hepatic Impairment No dosage adjustment necessary.

Obesity Refer to indication-specific dosing for obesity-related information (may not be available for all indications).

Dietary Considerations Whole grains, legumes and dark-green leafy vegetables are dietary sources of magnesium (IOM, 1997).

Administration
Injection: May be administered IM or IV
IM: Must be diluted prior to administration for children (Adults: 25% or 50% concentration; Children: ≤20% diluted solution)
IV: Must be diluted to a ≤20% solution for IV infusion and may be administered IV push, IVPB, or continuous IV infusion. When giving IV push, must dilute first and should generally not be given any faster than 150 mg/minute; may administer over 1 to 2 minutes in patients with persistent pulseless VT or VF with known hypomagnesemia (Dager, 2006). ACLS guidelines recommend administration over 15 minutes in patients with torsade de pointes (ACLS, 2010). In patients not in cardiac arrest, hypotension and asystole may occur with rapid administration. In patients with asthma (acute severe exacerbation) (off-label use), may administer single dose over 20 minutes to 60 minutes (GINA 2015; NAEPP 2007).
Maximal rate of infusion: Up to 50% of an IV dose may be eliminated in the urine, therefore, slower administration may improve retention (maximum rate: 1 g/hour in asymptomatic patients). For doses <6 g, infuse over 8 to 12 hours and for larger doses infuse over 24 hours if patient is asymptomatic. If patient is severely symptomatic (or has conditions such as preeclampsia or eclampsia) more aggressive therapy (≤4 g over 4 to 5 minutes) may be required; patients should be closely monitored (Kraft, 2005).
Oral: When used as a laxative, dissolve dose in 8 ounces of water prior to ingesting. Lemon juice may be added to the solution to improve the taste.
Topical: May dissolve granules to prepare a solution for use as a soaking aid or as a compress. To make a compress, use a towel to apply as a wet dressing.

Monitoring Parameters
IV: Rapid administration: ECG monitoring, vital signs, deep tendon reflexes; magnesium concentrations if frequent or prolonged dosing required particularly in patients with renal dysfunction, calcium, and potassium concentrations; renal function
Obstetrics: Patient status including vital signs, oxygen saturation, deep tendon reflexes, level of consciousness, fetal heart rate, maternal uterine activity.

Reference Range Serum magnesium: 1.5-2.5 mg/dL; slightly different ranges are reported by different laboratories

Dosage Forms Considerations
1 g of magnesium sulfate = elemental magnesium 98.6 mg = magnesium 8.12 mEq = magnesium 4.06 mmol

Magnesium sulfate 1% [10 mg/mL] in Dextrose 5% injection is equivalent to elemental magnesium 0.081 mEq/mL.

Magnesium sulfate 2% [20 mg/mL] in Dextrose 5% injection is equivalent to elemental magnesium 0.162 mEq/mL.

Magnesium sulfate 4% [40 mg/mL] in Water injection is equivalent to elemental magnesium 0.325 mEq/mL.

Magnesium sulfate 8% [80 mg/mL] in Water injection is equivalent to elemental magnesium 0.65 mEq/mL.

Magnesium sulfate 50% injection is equivalent to elemental magnesium 4 mEq/mL.

Dosage Forms Excipient information presented when available (limited, particularly for generics); consult specific product labeling.

Capsule, Oral:
Generic: 70 mg
Granules, Oral:
Epsom Salt: (454 g, 1810 g, 1816 g)
Solution, Injection:
Generic: 50% (2 mL, 10 mL, 20 mL, 50 mL); 40 mg/mL (50 mL, 100 mL, 500 mL, 1000 mL); 80 mg/mL (50 mL)
Solution, Intravenous:
Generic: 10 mg/mL (100 mL); 20 mg/mL (500 mL)

◆ Magnesium Sulfate, Potassium Sulfate, and Sodium Sulfate *see* Sodium Sulfate, Potassium Sulfate, and Magnesium Sulfate *on page 1681*

◆ Magnesium Sulfate, Sodium Sulfate, and Potassium Sulfate *see* Sodium Sulfate, Potassium Sulfate, and Magnesium Sulfate *on page 1681*

◆ Magnesium Trisilicate and Aluminum Hydroxide *see* Aluminum Hydroxide and Magnesium Trisilicate *on page 85*

◆ Magonate [OTC] *see* Magnesium Gluconate *on page 1119*

◆ Mag Oxide *see* Magnesium Oxide *on page 1121*

◆ Mag-SR [OTC] [DSC] *see* Magnesium Chloride *on page 1119*

◆ Mag-SR Plus Calcium [OTC] *see* Magnesium Chloride *on page 1119*

◆ Mag-Tab SR [OTC] *see* Magnesium L-lactate *on page 1121*

◆ MAH *see* Magnesium L-aspartate Hydrochloride *on page 1120*

◆ Makena *see* Hydroxyprogesterone Caproate *on page 895*

◆ Malarone® *see* Atovaquone and Proguanil *on page 173*

◆ Malarone® Pediatric (Can) *see* Atovaquone and Proguanil *on page 173*

Malathion (mal a THYE on)

Brand Names: US Ovide
Pharmacologic Category Antiparasitic Agent, Topical; Pediculocide; Scabicidal Agent
Use Head lice infection: Topical treatment of *Pediculus humanus capitis* (head lice and their ova) of the scalp hair
Dosing
Adult & Geriatric Head lice (*Pediculus humanus capitis*): Topical: Apply sufficient amount to cover and thoroughly moisten dry hair and scalp; allow hair to dry naturally and shampoo after 8 to 12 hours. If required, repeat with second application in 7 to 9 days. Further treatment is generally not necessary.
Pediatric Head lice (*Pediculus humanus capitis*): Children ≥6 years and Adolescents: Topical: Refer to adult dosing. **Note:** Use is contraindicated in neonates and infants.
Renal Impairment There are no dosage adjustments provided in the manufacturer's labeling.
Hepatic Impairment There are no dosage adjustments provided in the manufacturer's labeling.
Additional Information Complete prescribing information should be consulted for additional detail.
Dosage Forms Excipient information presented when available (limited, particularly for generics); consult specific product labeling.
Lotion, External:
Ovide: 0.5% (59 mL) [contains isopropyl alcohol]
Generic: 0.5% (59 mL)

◆ Mandelamine (Can) *see* Methenamine *on page 1165*

◆ Mandrake *see* Podophyllum Resin *on page 1464*

Manganese (MAN ga nees)

Brand Names: US Mangimin [OTC]; MN-50 [OTC]
Index Terms Manganese Chloride; Manganese Sulfate
Pharmacologic Category Dietary Supplement; Trace Element, Parenteral

Use Trace element added to total parenteral nutrition (TPN) solution to prevent manganese deficiency; orally as a dietary supplement
Dosing
Adult & Geriatric
Adequate intake: Oral:
Males: 2.3 mg/day; Females: 1.8 mg/day
Pregnancy: 2 mg/day
Lactation: 2.6 mg/day
Deficiency prevention: IV: 150-800 **mcg**/day usually administered in TPN solutions
Pediatric
Adequate intake: Oral:
0-6 months: 0.003 mg/day
7-12 months: 0.6 mg/day
1-3 years: 1.2 mg/day
4-8 years: 1.5 mg/day
9-13 years: Males: 1.9 mg/day; Females: 1.6 mg/day
14-18 years: Males: 2.2 mg/day; Females: 1.6 mg/day
Deficiency prevention: IV: 2-10 **mcg**/kg/day usually administered in TPN solutions
Note: Use caution in premature neonates; manganese chloride solution for injection contains aluminum.
Renal Impairment Use caution; manganese chloride solution for injection contains aluminum.
Hepatic Impairment Use caution; dose may need to be decreased or withheld.
Additional Information Complete prescribing information should be consulted for additional detail.
Dosage Forms Excipient information presented when available (limited, particularly for generics); consult specific product labeling.
Capsule, Oral, as chelated:
MN-50: Elemental manganese 16.67 mg
Solution, Intravenous, as chloride:
Generic: Elemental manganese 0.1 mg/mL (10 mL)
Solution, Intravenous, as sulfate [preservative free]:
Generic: Elemental manganese 0.1 mg/mL (10 mL)
Tablet, Oral, as aspartate:
Generic: 93 mg [elemental manganese 25 mg]
Tablet, Oral, as chelated:
Mangimin: Elemental manganese 10 mg [corn free, rye free, wheat free]
Generic: Elemental manganese 15 mg, Elemental manganese 50 mg
Tablet, Oral, as gluconate:
Generic: 50 mg [elemental manganese 5.7 mg]

◆ Manganese Chloride *see* Manganese *on page 1124*

◆ Manganese Sulfate *see* Manganese *on page 1124*

◆ Mangimin [OTC] *see* Manganese *on page 1124*

Mannitol (MAN i tole)

Brand Names: US Aridol; Osmitrol; Resectisol
Brand Names: Canada Osmitrol®
Index Terms D-Mannitol
Pharmacologic Category Diagnostic Agent; Diuretic, Osmotic; Genitourinary Irrigant
Use
Injection: Reduction of increased intracranial pressure associated with cerebral edema; reduction of increased intraocular pressure; promoting urinary excretion of toxic substances; genitourinary irrigant in transurethral prostatic resection or other transurethral surgical procedures
Note: Although FDA-labeled indications, the use of mannitol for the prevention of acute renal failure and/or promotion of diuresis is not routinely recommended (Kellum, 2008).
Genitourinary irrigation solution: Irrigation in transurethral prostatic resection or other transurethral surgical procedures
Powder for inhalation: Assessment of bronchial hyperresponsiveness
Pregnancy Considerations Reproduction studies have not been conducted.
Breast-Feeding Considerations It is not known if mannitol is excreted in breast milk. The manufacturer recommends that caution be exercised when administering mannitol to nursing women.
Contraindications
Injection: Hypersensitivity to mannitol or any component of the formulation; severe renal disease (anuria); severe dehydration; active intracranial bleeding except during craniotomy; progressive heart failure, pulmonary congestion, or renal dysfunction after mannitol administration; severe pulmonary edema or congestion
Genitourinary irrigation solution: Anuria

Powder for inhalation: Hypersensitivity to mannitol, gelatin, or any component of the formulation; conditions that may be compromised by induced bronchospasm or repeated spirometry (eg, aortic or cerebral aneurysm, uncontrolled hypertension, recent MI or cerebral vascular accident)

Warnings/Precautions Should not be administered until adequacy of renal function and urine flow is established; use 1-2 test doses to assess renal response. Excess amounts can lead to profound diuresis with fluid and electrolyte loss; close medical supervision and dose evaluation are required. Watch for and correct electrolyte disturbances; adjust dose to avoid dehydration. May cause renal dysfunction especially with high doses; use caution in patients taking other nephrotoxic agents, with sepsis or preexisting renal disease. To minimize adverse renal effects, adjust to keep serum osmolality less than 320 mOsm/L. Discontinue if evidence of acute tubular necrosis.

In patients being treated for cerebral edema, mannitol may accumulate in the brain (causing rebound increases in intracranial pressure) if circulating for long periods of time as with continuous infusion; intermittent boluses preferred. Cardiovascular status should also be evaluated; do not administer electrolyte-free mannitol solutions with blood. If hypotension occurs monitor cerebral perfusion pressure to ensure adequate. Vesicant (at concentrations >5%); ensure proper catheter or needle position prior to and during IV infusion; avoid extravasation of IV infusions.

Powder for inhalation (Aridol): **[U.S. Boxed Warning] Use may result in severe bronchospasm; use only for bronchial challenge testing. Testing should only be done by trained professionals. Not for use in patients with asthma or very low baseline pulmonary function. Medications (eg, short-acting inhaled beta-agonist) and equipment for the treatment of severe bronchospasm should be readily available.** Use with caution in patients with conditions that may increase sensitivity to bronchoconstriction (eg, severe cough, ventilatory impairment, spirometry-induced bronchoconstriction, hemoptysis of unknown origin, pneumothorax, recent abdominal, thoracic, or intraocular surgery, unstable angina, active upper or lower respiratory tract infection). Patients who have ≥10% reduction in FEV_1 on administration of the 0 mg capsule, patients with a positive response to bronchial challenge testing, or patients who develop significant respiratory symptoms should receive short acting inhaled beta-agonist; monitor until full recovery to baseline. Bronchial challenge testing should not be performed in children <6 years of age as these patients are unable to provide reliable spirometric results.

Adverse Reactions

Inhalation:

1% to 10%:

Cardiovascular: Chest discomfort (1%)

Central nervous system: Headache (adults 6%; children 3%), dizziness (1%)

Gastrointestinal: Nausea (adults 2%; children 3%), throat irritation (2%), retching (1%)

Respiratory: Cough (2%), pharyngolaryngeal pain (adults 2%; children 4%), rhinorrhea (2%), dyspnea (1%), wheezing (1%)

<1% (Limited to important or life-threatening): FEV_1 decreased, gagging

Injection: Frequency not defined:

Cardiovascular: Chest pain, CHF, circulatory overload, hyper-/hypotension, peripheral edema, tachycardia

Central nervous system: Chills, convulsions, dizziness, fever, headache

Dermatologic: Bullous eruption, urticaria

Endocrine & metabolic: Fluid and electrolyte imbalance, dehydration and hypovolemia secondary to rapid diuresis, hyperglycemia, hypernatremia, hyponatremia (dilutional), hyperosmolality-induced hyperkalemia, metabolic acidosis (dilutional), osmolar gap increased, water intoxication

Gastrointestinal: Nausea, vomiting, xerostomia

Genitourinary: Dysuria, polyuria

Local: Pain, thrombophlebitis, tissue necrosis

Ocular: Blurred vision

Renal: Acute renal failure, acute tubular necrosis (adult dose >200 g/day; serum osmolality >320 mOsm/L)

Respiratory: Pulmonary edema, rhinitis

Miscellaneous: Allergic reactions

Drug Interactions

Metabolism/Transport Effects None known.

Avoid Concomitant Use

Avoid concomitant use of Mannitol with any of the following: Aminoglycosides; Tobramycin (Oral Inhalation)

Increased Effect/Toxicity

Mannitol may increase the levels/effects of: Aminoglycosides; Sodium Phosphates; Tobramycin (Oral Inhalation)

The levels/effects of Mannitol may be increased by: Analgesics (Opioid)

Decreased Effect There are no known significant interactions involving a decrease in effect.

Storage/Stability

Injection: Should be stored at room temperature of 15°C to 30°C (59°F to 86°F); do not freeze. In concentrations ≥15%, crystallization may occur at low temperatures; do not use solutions that contain crystals. Heating in a hot water bath and vigorous shaking may be utilized for resolubilization. Cool solutions to body temperature before using.

Irrigation: Store at room temperature of 25°C (77°F); excursions permitted up to 40°C. Avoid excessive heat; do not warm above 150°F (66°C). Do not freeze.

Powder for inhalation: Store at <25°C (<77°F); excursions permitted between 15°C to 30°C (59°F to 86°F). Do not freeze.

Mechanism of Action Produces an osmotic diuresis by increasing the osmotic pressure of glomerular filtrate, which inhibits tubular reabsorption of water and electrolytes and increases urinary output. Mechanism of action in reduction of intracranial pressure (ICP) is controversial. However, it is thought that mannitol reduces ICP by reducing blood viscosity which transiently increases cerebral blood flow and oxygen transport. This in turn reduces cerebral blood volume and ICP. Furthermore, mannitol reduces ICP by withdrawing water from the brain parenchyma and excretes water in the urine (Allen, 1998; Bratton, 2007; Miller, 2010).

Pharmacodynamics/Kinetics

Onset of action: Diuresis: Injection: 1-3 hours; Reduction in intracranial pressure: ~15-30 minutes

Duration: Reduction in intracranial pressure: 1.5-6 hours

Distribution: 34.3 L; remains confined to extracellular space (except in extreme concentrations); does not penetrate the blood-brain barrier (generally, penetration is low)

Metabolism: Minimally hepatic to glycogen

Bioavailability: Inhaled: 59% (relative to oral administration: 96%)

Half-life elimination: Terminal: 4.7 hours

Time to peak, plasma: Inhaled: 1.5 hours

Excretion: Urine (~55% to 87% as unchanged drug)

Dosing

Adult

Assessment of bronchial hyper-responsiveness: Inhalation: Administer in a stepwise fashion (measuring FEV_1 in duplicate after each administration) until the patient has a positive response or 635 mg of mannitol has been administered (whichever comes first).

Positive test: 15% reduction in FEV_1 from baseline or 10% incremental reduction in FEV_1 between consecutive doses

Negative test: Administration of full dose (635 mg) without reduction in FEV_1 sufficient to meet criteria for a positive test

Administration should be as follows:

Stepwise Administration Schedule

Dose #	Dose (mg)	Cumulative Dose (mg)	Capsules/Dose
1	0	0	1
2	5	5	1
3	10	15	1
4	20	35	1
5	40	75	1
6	80	155	2 x 40 mg caps
7	160	315	4 x 40 mg caps
8	160	475	4 x 40 mg caps
9	160	635	4 x 40 mg caps

Increased intracranial pressure, cerebral edema (off-label dosing): IV: 0.25 to 1 g/kg/dose; may repeat every 6 to 8 hours as needed (Adelson, 2003; Bratton, 2007); maintain serum osmolality <300 to 320 mOsm/kg (Adelson, 2003; Rabinstein, 2006)

Reduction of intraocular pressure: IV: 0.25 to 2 g/kg administered over 30 to 60 minutes 1 to 1.5 hours prior to surgery

Reduction of intraocular pressure (traumatic hyphema): IV: 1.5 g/kg administered over 45 minutes twice daily for IOP >35 mm Hg; may administer every 8 hours in patients with extremely high pressure (Crouch, 1999)

Kidney transplant:

Donor: 12.5 g (with adequate hydration) prior to nephrectomy; may repeat (Morris, 2008)

Recipient: 50 g before kidney revascularization (Sprung, 2000; Tiggeler, 1984; van Valenberg, 1987; Weimar, 1983)

Transurethral irrigation: Topical: Use 5% urogenital solution as required for irrigation.

Geriatric Refer to adult dosing. Consider initiation at lower end of dosing range.

Pediatric

Assessment of bronchial hyper-responsiveness: Inhalation: Children ≥6 years: Refer to adult dosing.

Increased intracranial pressure (off-label dosing): IV: 0.25 to 1 g/kg/dose; repeat as needed to maintain serum osmolality <300 to 320 mOsm/kg (Adelson, 2003; Broderick, 2007; Hegenbarth, 2008)

Reduction of intraocular pressure: 1 to 2 g/kg or 30 to 60 g/m^2 administered over 30 to 60 minutes 1 to 1.5 hours prior to surgery

Reduction of intraocular pressure (traumatic hyphema): 1.5 g/kg administered over 45 minutes twice daily for IOP >35 mm Hg; may administer every 8 hours in patients with extremely high pressure (Crouch, 1999)

Additional indications: IV: Children ≥12 years: Refer to adult dosing.

Renal Impairment Contraindicated in severe renal impairment. Use caution in patients with underlying renal disease. May be used to reduce the incidence of acute tubular necrosis when administered prior to revascularization during kidney transplantation.

Hepatic Impairment No adjustment required.

Administration

IV: Concentration and rate of administration depends on indication/severity, or may be adjusted to urine flow. For cerebral edema or elevated ICP, administer over 30-60 minutes. Inspect for crystals prior to administration. If crystals are present, redissolve by warming solution. Use filter-type administration set for infusion solutions containing mannitol ≥20%. Do not administer with blood. Crenation and agglutination of red blood cells may occur if administered with whole blood.

Vesicant (at concentrations >5%); ensure proper catheter or needle position prior to and during IV infusion. Avoid extravasation of IV infusions.

Extravasation management: If extravasation occurs, stop infusion immediately and disconnect (leave needle/cannula in place); gently aspirate extravasated solution (do **NOT** flush the line); initiate hyaluronidase antidote; remove needle/cannula; apply dry cold compresses (Hurst, 2004); elevate extremity.

Hyaluronidase: SubQ: Administer multiple 0.5-1 mL injections of a 15 units/mL solution around the periphery of the extravasation (Kumar, 2003).

Inhalation (Aridol): Administer using supplied single patient use inhaler; do not puncture capsule more than once; do not swallow capsules. A nose clip may be used if preferred. The patient should exhale completely, followed by a controlled rapid deep inspiration from the device; hold breath for 5 seconds and exhale through the mouth. Measure FEV$_1$ in duplicate 60 seconds after inhalation; repeat process until positive response or full dose (635 mg) has been administered.

Irrigation: Administer using only the appropriate transurethral urologic instrumentation.

Monitoring Parameters Renal function, daily fluid I & O, serum electrolytes, serum and urine osmolality; for treatment of elevated intracranial pressure, maintain serum osmolality in the range of 300-320 mOsm/kg (serum osmolality >320 mOsm/kg may increase the risk of acute renal tubular damage).

Bronchial challenge test: Standard spirometry prior to bronchial challenge test; FEV$_1$ in duplicate 60 seconds after administration of each step of test

Additional Information May autoclave or heat to redissolve crystals; mannitol 20% has an approximate osmolarity of 1100 mOsm/L and mannitol 25% has an approximate osmolarity of 1375 mOsm/L

Bronchial challenge testing: The dose of inhaled mannitol which causes a 15% reduction in FEV$_1$ is expressed as PD$_{15}$

Dosage Forms Excipient information presented when available (limited, particularly for generics); consult specific product labeling.

Kit, Inhalation:
Aridol:
Solution, Intravenous:
Osmitrol: 5% (1000 mL); 10% (500 mL); 15% (500 mL); 20% (250 mL, 500 mL)
Generic: 5% (1000 mL); 10% (1000 mL); 15% (500 mL); 20% (250 mL, 500 mL); 25% (50 mL)
Solution, Intravenous [preservative free]:
Generic: 25% (50 mL)
Solution, Irrigation:
Resectisol: 5% (2000 mL)

◆ Mantoux *see* Tuberculin Tests *on page 1850*

◆ Maox [OTC] *see* Magnesium Oxide *on page 1121*

◆ Mapap [OTC] *see* Acetaminophen *on page 25*

◆ Mapap Arthritis Pain [OTC] *see* Acetaminophen *on page 25*

◆ Mapap Children's [OTC] *see* Acetaminophen *on page 25*

◆ Mapap Extra Strength [OTC] *see* Acetaminophen *on page 25*

◆ Mapap Infant's [OTC] *see* Acetaminophen *on page 25*

◆ Mapap PM [OTC] *see* Acetaminophen and Diphenhydramine *on page 29*

◆ Mapezine (Can) *see* CarBAMazepine *on page 303*

Maprotiline (ma PROE ti leen)

Brand Names: Canada Teva-Maprotiline
Index Terms Ludiomil; Maprotiline Hydrochloride
Pharmacologic Category Antidepressant, Tetracyclic
Use

Anxiety: Relief of anxiety associated with depression

Depression: Treatment of major depressive disorder (MDD)

Medication Guide Available Yes
Dosing

Adult Depression or anxiety: Oral: Initial: 25 to 75 mg once daily or in divided doses; increase gradually in 25 mg increments after 2 weeks based on response and tolerability. Usual dosage: 100 to 225 mg once daily or in divided doses; maximum dose: 225 mg daily. **Note:** Initial doses of 100 to 150 mg daily may be considered in severely depressed, hospitalized patients (APA, 2010; Bauer, 2013).

Discontinuation of therapy: Upon discontinuation of antidepressant therapy, gradually taper the dose to minimize the incidence of withdrawal symptoms and allow for the detection of re-emerging symptoms. Evidence supporting ideal taper rates is limited. APA and NICE guidelines suggest tapering therapy over at least several weeks with consideration to the half-life of the antidepressant; antidepressants with a shorter half-life may need to be tapered more conservatively. In addition for long-term treated patients, WFSBP guidelines recommend tapering over 4-6 months. If intolerable withdrawal symptoms occur following a dose reduction, consider resuming the previously prescribed dose and/or decrease dose at a more gradual rate (APA, 2010; Bauer, 2002; Haddad, 2001; NCCMH, 2010; Schatzberg, 2006; Shelton, 2001; Warner, 2006).

MAO inhibitor recommendations:

Switching to or from an MAO inhibitor intended to treat psychiatric disorders:

Allow 14 days to elapse between discontinuing an MAO inhibitor intended to treat psychiatric disorders and initiation of maprotiline.

Allow 14 days to elapse between discontinuing maprotiline and initiation of an MAO inhibitor intended to treat psychiatric disorders.

Use with other MAO inhibitors (such as linezolid or IV methylene blue):

Do not initiate maprotiline in patients receiving linezolid or IV methylene blue; consider other interventions for psychiatric condition.

If urgent treatment with linezolid or IV methylene blue is required in a patient already receiving maprotiline and potential benefits outweigh potential risks, discontinue maprotiline promptly and administer linezolid or IV methylene blue. Monitor for serotonin syndrome for 2 weeks or until 24 hours after the last dose of linezolid or IV methylene blue, whichever comes first. May resume maprotiline 24 hours after the last dose of linezolid or IV methylene blue.

Geriatric Depression or anxiety: Oral: Initial: 25 mg once daily; increase gradually in 25 mg increments after 2 weeks based on response and tolerability. Usual dose: 50 to 75 mg once daily or in divided doses

Discontinuation of therapy: Refer to adult dosing.

MAO inhibitor recommendations: Refer to adult dosing.

Renal Impairment There are no dosage adjustments provided in the manufacturer's labeling.

Hepatic Impairment There are no dosage adjustments provided in the manufacturer's labeling.

Additional Information Complete prescribing information should be consulted for additional detail.

Dosage Forms Excipient information presented when available (limited, particularly for generics); consult specific product labeling.

Tablet, Oral, as hydrochloride:
Generic: 25 mg, 50 mg, 75 mg

◆ Maprotiline Hydrochloride see Maprotiline on page 1126

◆ Mar-Allopurinol (Can) see Allopurinol on page 73

◆ Mar-Amlodipine (Can) see AmLODIPine on page 101

◆ Mar-Anastrozole (Can) see Anastrozole on page 128

Maraviroc (mah RAV er rock)

Brand Names: US Selzentry
Brand Names: Canada Celsentri
Index Terms UK-427,857
Pharmacologic Category Antiretroviral, CCR5 Antagonist (Anti-HIV)
Use HIV infection: Treatment of only CCR5-tropic HIV-1 infection, in combination with other antiretroviral agents
Medication Guide Available Yes
Dosing

Adult HIV infection: Oral: 300 mg twice daily; dose recommended when maraviroc administered concomitantly with other medications, including tipranavir/ritonavir, nevirapine, raltegravir, all NRTIs and enfuvirtide.

Dosage adjustment for concomitant CYP3A inhibitors/inducers:
CYP3A inhibitors (with or without a potent CYP3A inducer): 150 mg twice daily; dose recommended when maraviroc administered concomitantly with potent CYP3A inhibitors including (but not limited to) protease inhibitors (excluding tipranavir/ritonavir), delavirdine, elvitegravir/ritonavir, ketoconazole, itraconazole, clarithromycin, nefazodone, telithromycin, and boceprevir.
CYP3A inducers (without a potent CYP3A inhibitor): 600 mg twice daily; dose recommended when maraviroc administered concomitantly with potent CYP3A inducers including (but not limited to) efavirenz, etravirine, rifampin, carbamazepine, phenobarbital, and phenytoin

Pediatric HIV infection: Oral:
Alternate dosing: Adolescents ≥16 years: Refer to adult dosing (HHS [pediatric], 2014).

Renal Impairment
CrCl ≥30 mL/minute:
CrCl ≥30 mL/minute and concomitant potent CYP3A inhibitors (with or without a potent CYP3A inducer): 150 mg twice daily
CrCl ≥30 mL/minute and concomitant potent CYP3A inducer (without a potent CYP3A inhibitor): 600 mg twice daily
CrCl ≥30 mL/minute and other concomitant medications (eg, tipranavir/ritonavir, nevirapine, raltegravir, all NRTIs, and enfuvirtide): 300 mg twice daily
CrCl <30 mL/minute:
CrCl <30 mL/minute and concomitant potent CYP3A inhibitors (with or without a potent CYP3A inducer) **or** concomitant potent CYP3A inducer (without a potent CYP3A inhibitor): Use is contraindicated
CrCl <30 mL/minute and other concomitant medications (eg, tipranavir/ritonavir, nevirapine, raltegravir, all NRTIs, and enfuvirtide): 300 mg twice daily. If postural hypotension occurs, reduce dose to 150 mg twice daily
CrCl <30 mL/minute and experiencing postural hypotension: Reduce dose to 150 mg twice daily
ESRD requiring intermittent hemodialysis (IHD):
Note: Hemodialysis has minimal effect on clearance
With concomitant potent CYP3A inhibitors (with or without a potent CYP3A inducer) or concomitant potent CYP3A inducer (without a potent CYP3A inhibitor): Use is contraindicated

With other concomitant medications (eg, tipranavir/ritonavir, nevirapine, raltegravir, all NRTIs, and enfuvirtide): 300 mg twice daily. If postural hypotension occurs, reduce dose to 150 mg twice daily.

Hepatic Impairment
Mild to moderate impairment: There are no dosage adjustments provided in the manufacturer's labeling; however, maraviroc concentrations are increased in mild to moderate impairment; use caution.
Moderate impairment (with concomitant potent CYP3A inhibitor): There are no dosage adjustments provided in the manufacturer's labeling; however, maraviroc concentrations are increased moderate impairment; use caution and monitor closely for adverse events.
Severe impairment: There are no dosage adjustments provided in the manufacturer's labeling (has not been studied).

Additional Information Complete prescribing information should be consulted for additional detail.

Dosage Forms Excipient information presented when available (limited, particularly for generics); consult specific product labeling.
Tablet, Oral:
Selzentry: 150 mg, 300 mg [contains fd&c blue #2 aluminum lake, soybean lecithin]

◆ Marcaine see Bupivacaine on page 262

◆ Marcaine® (Can) see Bupivacaine on page 262

◆ Marcaine Preservative Free see Bupivacaine on page 262

◆ Marcaine Spinal see Bupivacaine on page 262

◆ Mar-Celecoxib (Can) see Celecoxib on page 355

◆ Mar-Ciprofloxacin (Can) see Ciprofloxacin (Systemic) on page 388

◆ Mar-Citalopram (Can) see Citalopram on page 398

◆ Mar-Clopidogrel (Can) see Clopidogrel on page 424

◆ Mar-Cof CG see Guaifenesin and Codeine on page 861

◆ Mar-Donepezil (Can) see Donepezil on page 583

◆ MarEPA [OTC] [DSC] see Omega-3 Fatty Acids on page 1329

◆ Mar-Escitalopram (Can) see Escitalopram on page 673

◆ Mar-Ezetimibe (Can) see Ezetimibe on page 729

◆ Mar-Gabapentin (Can) see Gabapentin on page 823

◆ Margesic see Butalbital, Acetaminophen, and Caffeine on page 275

◆ Marine Lipid Concentrate [OTC] see Omega-3 Fatty Acids on page 1329

◆ Marinol see Dronabinol on page 606

◆ Mark 1 see Atropine and Pralidoxime on page 179

◆ Mar-Letrozole (Can) see Letrozole on page 1048

◆ Marlissa see Ethinyl Estradiol and Levonorgestrel on page 703

◆ Mar-Metformin (Can) see MetFORMIN on page 1156

◆ Mar-Modafinil (Can) see Modafinil on page 1222

◆ Mar-Montelukast (Can) see Montelukast on page 1229

◆ Mar-Olanzapine (Can) see OLANZapine on page 1314

◆ Mar-Olanzapine ODT (Can) see OLANZapine on page 1314

◆ Mar-Ondansetron (Can) see Ondansetron on page 1335

◆ Mar-Pantoprazole (Can) see Pantoprazole on page 1390

◆ Mar-Pregabalin (Can) see Pregabalin on page 1500

◆ Marqibo see VinCRIStine (Liposomal) on page 1900

◆ Mar-Quetiapine (Can) see QUEtiapine on page 1536

◆ Mar-Ramipril (Can) see Ramipril on page 1552

◆ Mar-Risperidone (Can) see RisperiDONE on page 1593

◆ Mar-Rizatriptan (Can) see Rizatriptan on page 1609

◆ Mar-Rosuvastatin (Can) see Rosuvastatin on page 1620

◆ Mar-Sertraline (Can) see Sertraline on page 1649

◆ Mar-Simvastatin (Can) see Simvastatin on page 1659

◆ Mar-Tramadol/Acet (Can) see Acetaminophen and Tramadol on page 29

◆ Marvelon (Can) see Ethinyl Estradiol and Desogestrel on page 701

◆ Mar-Zolmitriptan (Can) see ZOLMitriptan on page 1938

◆ Matulane see Procarbazine on page 1506

◆ Matzim LA see Diltiazem on page 553

◆ 3M Avagard [OTC] see Chlorhexidine Gluconate on page 373

Measles, Mumps, and Rubella Virus Vaccine (MEE zels, mumpz & roo BEL a VYE rus vak SEEN)

Brand Names: US M-M-R II

Brand Names: Canada M-M-R II; Priorix

Index Terms MMR; Mumps, Measles and Rubella Vaccines; Rubella, Measles and Mumps Vaccines

Pharmacologic Category Vaccine; Vaccine, Live (Viral)

Additional Appendix Information

Immunization Administration Recommendations *on page 1974*

Immunization Schedules *on page 1979*

Use Measles, mumps, and rubella prophylaxis: Active immunization for simultaneous vaccination against measles, mumps, and rubella in patients ≥12 months of age

The Advisory Committee on Immunization Practices (ACIP) recommends routine vaccination for the following (CDC/ACIP [McLean 2013]):

• All children (first dose given at 12 to 15 months of age)

• Adults born 1957 or later (without evidence of immunity or documentation of vaccination). Vaccine may be given to adults born prior to 1957 if they do not have contraindications to the MMR vaccine.

• Adults at higher risk for exposure to and transmission of measles mumps and rubella should receive special consideration for vaccination, unless an acceptable evidence of immunity exists. This includes international travelers, persons attending colleges and other post high school education, persons working in healthcare facilities.

Medication Guide Available Yes

Dosing

Adult Note: The minimum interval between 2 doses of MMR vaccine is 28 days (CDC/ACIP [McLean 2013]).

Immunization: SubQ: 0.5 mL per dose; 1 or 2 doses administered at least 28 days apart based upon the following criteria (CDC/ACIP [McLean 2013]):

Adults born in or after 1957 should be vaccinated unless they have acceptable evidence of immunity.

Adults born prior to 1957 are considered immune to measles, mumps, and rubella but may be vaccinated if they do not have contraindications to the vaccine. Pregnant adults born prior to 1957 are not considered immune to rubella.

Healthcare personnel: Persons born in or after 1957 should have 2 doses of vaccine unless they have acceptable evidence of immunity. Unvaccinated persons born prior to 1957 should also consider vaccination with 2 doses unless they have laboratory evidence or laboratory confirmation of disease.

HIV infection (without severe immunosuppression): Two doses of MMR unless there is acceptable evidence of immunity.

Household/close contacts of immunocompromised persons: Two doses of MMR unless there is acceptable evidence of immunity.

International travelers: Two doses of MMR prior to travel unless there is acceptable evidence of immunity.

Measles, mumps, or rubella outbreak (community): Adults who received 1 dose of MMR should be considered for a second dose if the outbreak involves measles or mumps in adults. Vaccination should also be considered for persons born prior to 1957 without evidence of immunity who may be exposed to mumps. A single dose of a rubella-containing vaccine is considered adequate vaccination during a rubella outbreak.

Measles, mumps, or rubella outbreak (healthcare facility): Unvaccinated health care personnel without evidence of immunity regardless of birth year should receive 2 doses during a measles or mumps outbreak and one dose during a rubella outbreak.

Students: Persons entering post high school educational facilities should receive 2 doses of MMR unless they have acceptable evidence of immunity prior to enrollment.

Women of childbearing potential: One dose of MMR unless they have acceptable evidence of immunity. Vaccination should not be given during pregnancy and pregnancy should be avoided for 28 days after vaccine administration.

Pediatric Note: The minimum interval between 2 doses of MMR vaccine is 28 days (CDC/ACIP [McLean 2013]).

Primary immunization: Children ≥12 months: SubQ: 0.5 mL per dose. One dose is recommended at 12 to 15 months of age and repeated at 4 to 6 years of age; the second dose is recommended prior to entering kindergarten or first grade. The second dose may be administered at any time provided at least 28 days have elapsed since the first dose (CDC/ACIP [McLean 2013]).

HIV infection without evidence of MMR immunity: Children ≥12 months: SubQ: 0.5 mL per dose. Children with HIV infection and without evidence of severe immunosuppression should have 2 doses of MMR. Those with perinatal HIV infection who were vaccinated prior to effective ART should have 2 additional doses of MMR once ART is established (CDC/ACIP [McLean 2013]).

Household/close contacts of immunocompromised persons: Children ≥12 months: SubQ: 0.5 mL per dose; 2 doses of MMR administered at least 28 days apart unless they have acceptable evidence of immunity (CDC/ACIP [McLean 2013]).

International travel:

Infants 6 to 11 months: SubQ: 0.5 mL per dose. Infants without evidence of immunity traveling internationally should receive 1 dose of MMR before departure from the United States; these infants should be revaccinated with 2 doses of MMR with the first dose between 12 to 15 months of age (and at least 28 days after the previous dose; target 12 months of age if child remains in area where disease risk is high) and the second dose at least 28 days later (CDC/ACIP [McLean 2013]; CDC/ACIP [Strikas 2015]).

Children ≥12 months and Adolescents: SubQ: 0.5 mL per dose. Children without evidence of immunity traveling internationally should receive 2 doses of MMR before departure from the United States. The second dose 28 days later (CDC/ACIP [McLean 2013]).

Measles outbreak:
Infants 6 to 11 months: SubQ: 0.5 mL per dose. If there is risk of exposure to measles involving infants, 1 dose of MMR vaccine may be administered (CDC/ACIP [McLean 2013]).

Children ages 1 to 4 years: SubQ: 0.5 mL per dose. Children who received one dose of MMR should be considered for a second dose if the outbreak involves preschool-aged children (CDC/ACIP [McLean 2013]).

Mumps outbreak: Children ages 1 to 4 years: SubQ: 0.5 mL per dose. Children who received 1 dose of MMR should be considered for a second dose if the outbreak involves preschool-aged children (CDC/ACIP [McLean 2013]).

Renal Impairment There are no dosage adjustments provided in manufacturer's labeling.

Hepatic Impairment There are no dosage adjustments provided in manufacturer's labeling.

Additional Information Complete prescribing information should be consulted for additional detail.

Dosage Forms Excipient information presented when available (limited, particularly for generics); consult specific product labeling.

Injection, powder for reconstitution [preservative free]:
M-M-R II: Measles virus ≥1000 $TCID_{50}$, mumps virus ≥20,000 $TCID_{50}$, and rubella virus ≥1000 $TCID_{50}$ [contains albumin (human), bovine serum, chicken egg protein, gelatin, neomycin, sorbitol, and sucrose 1.9 mg/vial; supplied with diluent]

Measles, Mumps, Rubella, and Varicella Virus Vaccine
(MEE zels, mumpz, roo BEL a, & var i SEL a VYE rus vak SEEN)

Brand Names: US ProQuad
Brand Names: Canada Priorix-Tetra; ProQuad
Index Terms MMRV; Mumps, Rubella, Varicella, and Measles Vaccine; Rubella, Varicella, Measles, and Mumps Vaccine; Varicella, Measles, Mumps, and Rubella Vaccine
Pharmacologic Category Vaccine; Vaccine, Live (Viral)
Additional Appendix Information
Immunization Administration Recommendations *on page 1974*
Immunization Schedules *on page 1979*
Use
Measles, mumps, rubella, and varicella vaccination: To provide active immunization for the prevention of measles, mumps, rubella, and varicella in children 12 months to 12 years of age.

The Advisory Committee on Immunization Practices (ACIP) recommends routine vaccination against measles, mumps, rubella, and varicella in healthy children; the first dose should be given at 12 to 15 months of age and the second dose at 4 to 6 years of age. For children receiving their first dose at 12 to 47 months of age, either the MMRV combination vaccine or separate MMR and varicella vaccines can be used. The ACIP prefers administration of separate MMR and varicella vaccines as the first dose in this age group unless the parent or caregiver expresses preference for the MMRV combination. For children receiving the first dose at ≥48 months or their second dose at any age, use of MMRV is preferred. For children with a personal or family history of seizures, the ACIP recommends vaccination with separate MMR and varicella vaccines, as opposed to the MMRV combination vaccine (CDC/ACIP [Marin 2010]).

Canadian labeling (not in US labeling): MMRV combination vaccine is approved for use in healthy children (Priorix-Tetra: 9 months to 6 years; ProQuad: 12 months to 6 years); may consider use in healthy children ≤12 years of age based upon prior experience with the separate component (live-attenuated MMR or live-attenuated varicella [OKA-strain]) vaccines.

Medication Guide Available Yes
Dosing
Pediatric Immunization:
US labeling: Children 12 months to 12 years: SubQ: One dose (0.5 mL). The first dose is usually administered at 12 to 15 months of age. If a second dose of measles, mumps, rubella, and varicella vaccine is needed, ProQuad can be used with the second dose usually administered at 4 to 6 years of age.

At least 1 month should elapse between a previous dose of a measles-containing vaccine (eg, MMR) and at least 3 months should elapse between a dose of varicella-containing vaccine.

ACIP recommendations: Administer the first dose at 12 to 15 months of age and the second dose at 4 to 6 years of age. The second dose may be administered before age 4 years, provided at least 3 months have

elapsed since the first dose. For children receiving their first dose at 12 to 47 months of age, either the MMRV combination vaccine or separate MMR and varicella vaccines can be used. (The ACIP prefers administration of separate MMR and varicella vaccines as the first dose in this age group unless the parent or caregiver expresses preference for the MMRV combination.) For children receiving the first dose at ≥48 months or their second dose at any age, use of MMRV is preferred. The ACIP recommends that children with a personal or family history of seizures be vaccinated with separate MMR and varicella vaccines, as opposed to the MMRV combination vaccine (CDC/ACIP [Marin 2010]).

Canadian labeling:
Priorix-Tetra: SubQ or IM: Infants ≥9 months and Children ≤6 years: Two doses (0.5 mL each dose) administered at least 4 to 6 weeks apart (minimum interval between doses: 4 weeks)
ProQuad: SubQ: Children 12 months to 6 years: Two doses (0.5 mL each dose) administered at least 4 weeks apart

Renal Impairment There are no dosage adjustments provided in the manufacturer's labeling.

Hepatic Impairment There are no dosage adjustments provided in the manufacturer's labeling.

Additional Information Complete prescribing information should be consulted for additional detail.

Dosage Forms Excipient information presented when available (limited, particularly for generics); consult specific product labeling.

Injection, powder for reconstitution [preservative free]:
ProQuad: Measles virus ≥3.00 log_{10} $TCID_{50}$, mumps virus ≥4.3 log_{10} $TCID_{50}$, rubella virus ≥3.00 log_{10} $TCID_{50}$, and varicella virus ≥3.99 log_{10} PFU [contains albumin (human), bovine serum, chicken egg protein, gelatin, neomycin, sorbitol, and sucrose (≤21 mg/vial)]
ProQuad: Measles virus ≥3.00 log_{10} $TCID_{50}$, mumps virus ≥4.3 log_{10} $TCID_{50}$, rubella virus ≥3.00 log_{10} $TCID_{50}$, and varicella virus ≥3.99 log_{10} PFU [contains recombinant albumin (human), bovine serum, chicken egg protein, gelatin, neomycin, sorbitol, and sucrose (≤21 mg/vial)]

Dosage Forms: Canada Excipient information presented when available (limited, particularly for generics); consult specific product labeling.

Injection, powder for reconstitution [preservative free]:
Priorix-Tetra (CAN): Measles virus ≥3.00 log_{10} $CCID_{50}$, mumps virus ≥4.4 log_{10} $CCID_{50}$, rubella virus ≥3.00 log_{10} $CCID_{50}$, and varicella virus ≥3.3 log_{10} PFU [contains chicken egg protein, neomycin, sorbitol, and lactose]
ProQuad (CAN): Measles virus ≥3.00 log_{10} $TCID_{50}$, mumps virus ≥4.3 log_{10} $TCID_{50}$, rubella virus ≥3.00 log_{10} $TCID_{50}$, and varicella virus ≥3.99 log_{10} PFU [contains hydrolyzed gelatin, urea, sorbitol, monosodium L-glutamate, recombinant human albumin, neomycin, bovine serum albumin, and MRC-5 cell residuals]

Mecamylamine (mek a MIL a meen)

Brand Names: US Vecamyl
Index Terms Mecamylamine Hydrochloride
Pharmacologic Category Ganglionic Blocking Agent
Use Hypertension: Management of moderately severe to severe essential hypertension and in uncomplicated malignant hypertension.

Pregnancy Considerations Animal reproduction studies have not been conducted. Mecamylamine crosses the placenta.

Breast-Feeding Considerations
Due to the potential for serious adverse reactions in the nursing infant, the manufacturer recommends a decision be made whether to discontinue nursing or to discontinue the drug, taking into account the importance of treatment to the mother.

Contraindications Hypersensitivity to mecamylamine or any component of the formulation; mild, moderate, labile hypertension (may not be suitable for uncooperative patients); coronary insufficiency or recent myocardial infarction; uremia; glaucoma; organic pyloric stenosis; coadministration with antibiotics or sulfonamides

Warnings/Precautions Do not abruptly discontinue. CNS effects, including tremor, choreiform movements, mental aberrations, and convulsions may occur (rarely), especially with large doses or in patients with cerebral or renal insufficiency. In addition, dizziness, lightheadedness, or fainting may also occur.

Discontinue if signs of paralytic ileus occur (eg, frequent loose bowel movements with abdominal distention, decreased borborygmi). Use with caution in patients with marked cerebral and coronary arteriosclerosis or after a recent cerebral accident. Use with caution in patients with prostatic hyperplasia, bladder obstruction, or urethral stricture; may cause urinary retention. Use with caution in patients with renal impairment. When renal impairment is manifested by a rising or elevated BUN, use with extreme caution, if at all. Since mecamylamine is excreted unchanged in the urine, renal impairment may reduce elimination and increase the risk of adverse effects including hypotension; the risk for neurological adverse effects is increased especially when large doses are administered to patients with renal impairment.

Adverse Reactions Frequency not defined.

Cardiovascular: Orthostatic hypotension, syncope

Central nervous system: Altered mental status, choreiform movements, convulsions, fatigue, orthostatic dizziness, paresthesia, sedation

Endocrine & metabolic: Decreased libido

Gastrointestinal: Anorexia, constipation (sometimes preceded by small, frequent stools), glossitis, intestinal obstruction, nausea, vomiting, xerostomia

Genitourinary: Impotence, urinary retention

Neuromuscular & skeletal: Tremor, weakness

Ophthalmic: Blurred vision, mydriasis

Respiratory: Pulmonary fibrosis, pulmonary interstitial edema

Drug Interactions

Metabolism/Transport Effects None known.

Avoid Concomitant Use

Avoid concomitant use of Mecamylamine with any of the following: Aminoglycosides; Capreomycin; Colistimethate; Lincosamide Antibiotics; Polymyxin B; Sulfonamides; Tetracycline Derivatives

Increased Effect/Toxicity

Mecamylamine may increase the levels/effects of: Amifostine; Antipsychotic Agents (Second Generation [Atypical]); DULoxetine; Hypotension-Associated Agents; Levodopa

The levels/effects of Mecamylamine may be increased by: Alcohol (Ethyl); Alfuzosin; Alkalinizing Agents; Aminoglycosides; Barbiturates; Brimonidine (Topical); Capreomycin; Colistimethate; Diazoxide; Herbs (Hypotensive Properties); Lincosamide Antibiotics; Molsidomine; Nicorandil; Obinutuzumab; Pentoxifylline; Phosphodiesterase 5 Inhibitors; Polymyxin B; Prostacyclin Analogues; Sulfonamides; Tetracycline Derivatives

Decreased Effect

The levels/effects of Mecamylamine may be decreased by: Amphetamines; Herbs (Hypertensive Properties); Methylphenidate; Urinary Acidifying Agents; Yohimbine

Storage/Stability Store at 20°C to 25°C (68°F to 77°F); excursions are permitted between 15°C and 30°C (59°F and 86°F)

Mechanism of Action Mecamylamine inhibits acetylcholine at the autonomic ganglia, causing a decrease in blood pressure. The blood pressure lowering effect is predominantly orthostatic; the supine blood pressure is also significantly decreased.

Pharmacodynamics/Kinetics

Onset: 0.5 to 2 hours

Duration: 6 to ≥12 hours

Absorption: Almost complete

Excretion: Urine (unchanged); rate of elimination is significantly affected by the pH of the urine. Acidic urine promotes excretion; alkalinization reduces excretion

Dosing

Adult & Geriatric

Hypertension: Oral: Initial: 2.5 mg twice daily; may increase by increments of 2.5 mg at intervals ≥2 days until desired blood pressure response is achieved; average dose: 25 mg/day (usually in 3 divided doses; range of 2 to 4 divided doses or more may be required). **Note:** A small dose and sometimes no dose at all, should be administered in the morning as the blood pressure response is heightened early in the day. The larger dose should be given at noontime or the evening. Concomitant therapy: When coadministered with thiazide diuretics, decrease the dose of mecamylamine by ≥50%

Renal Impairment There are no dosage adjustments provided in the manufacturer's labeling; use with caution; use with extreme caution, if at all, if renal impairment is manifested by a rising or elevated BUN. Use is contraindicated in uremia.

Hepatic Impairment There are no dosage adjustments provided in the manufacturer's labeling

Dietary Considerations Take after meals. Concomitant use of alcohol may potentiate the effects of mecamylamine.

Administration Administration after meals may cause a more gradual absorption and smoother control of excessively high blood pressure. Timing of relationship to meals should be consistent.

Monitoring Parameters Monitor blood pressure (assess in the erect position before initiation and with dose increases), orthostatic vital signs, and heart rate

Dosage Forms Excipient information presented when available (limited, particularly for generics); consult specific product labeling. [DSC] = Discontinued product

Tablet, Oral, as hydrochloride:

Vecamyl: 2.5 mg

◆ *Mecamylamine Hydrochloride see* Mecamylamine *on page 1129*

Mechlorethamine (Systemic)
(me klor ETH a meen)

Brand Names: US Mustargen

Index Terms Chlorethazine; Chlorethazine Mustard; HN$_2$; Mechlorethamine Hydrochloride; Mustine; Nitrogen Mustard

Pharmacologic Category Antineoplastic Agent, Alkylating Agent; Antineoplastic Agent, Alkylating Agent (Nitrogen Mustard)

Use

Hodgkin lymphoma: Palliative treatment of Hodgkin lymphoma

Malignant effusion: Palliative treatment of effusions from metastatic carcinomas

Additional approved uses (manufacturer labeling): Treatment of lymphosarcoma, chronic myelocytic or chronic lymphocytic leukemia, polycythemia vera, mycosis fungoides, and bronchogenic carcinoma

Dosing

Adult & Geriatric Dosage should be based on ideal dry weight (evaluate the presence of edema or ascites so that dosage is based on actual weight unaugmented by edema/ascites). Mechlorethamine is associated with a high emetic potential (Basch, 2011; Roila, 2010); antiemetics are recommended to prevent nausea and vomiting

Hodgkin lymphoma (off-label dosing): IV:

MOPP regimen: 6 mg/m^2 on days 1 and 8 of a 28-day treatment cycle for 6 to 8 cycles (Canelos, 1992; DeVita, 1970)

Stanford V regimen: 6 mg/m^2 as a single dose on day 1 in weeks 1, 5, and 9 (Horning, 2000; Horning, 2002)

Malignant effusion: Intracavitary: 0.4 mg/kg as a single dose; although 0.2 mg/kg (10-20 mg) as a single dose has been used by the *intrapericardial* route

Renal Impairment No dosage adjustment provided in manufacturer's labeling.

Hepatic Impairment No dosage adjustment provided in manufacturer's labeling.

The following have also been reported:

Mild-to-moderate impairment: No dosage adjustment necessary (Ecklund, 2005).

Severe liver impairment: No dosage adjustment necessary; concomitant chemotherapy may require alteration until improvement in hepatic function (Ecklund, 2005)

Obesity *ASCO Guidelines for appropriate chemotherapy dosing in obese adults with cancer:* In general, utilize patient's actual body weight (full weight) for calculation of body surface area- or weight-based dosing, particularly when the intent of therapy is curative; manage regimen-related toxicities in the same manner as for nonobese patients; if a dose reduction is utilized due to toxicity, consider resumption of full weight-based dosing with subsequent cycles, especially if cause of toxicity (eg, hepatic or renal impairment) is resolved (Griggs, 2012). **Note:** The manufacturer recommends dosing be based on ideal dry body weight and the presence of edema or ascites should be considered so the dose will be based on unaugmented weight.

Additional Information Complete prescribing information should be consulted for additional detail.

Product Availability Mustargen: Mustargen was acquired by Recordati Rare Diseases in 2013; availability information is currently unknown.

Dosage Forms Excipient information presented when available (limited, particularly for generics); consult specific product labeling.

Solution Reconstituted, Injection, as hydrochloride:

Mustargen: 10 mg (1 ea)

Mechlorethamine (Topical) (me klor ETH a meen)

Brand Names: US Valchlor

Index Terms Mechlorethamine HCl (Topical); Mechlorethamine Topical Gel

Pharmacologic Category Antineoplastic Agent, Alkylating Agent; Antineoplastic Agent, Alkylating Agent (Nitrogen Mustard)

Use Cutaneous T-cell lymphoma: Topical treatment of stage IA and IB mycosis fungoides-type cutaneous T-cell lymphoma in patients who have received prior skin-directed therapy

Prescribing and Access Restrictions Valchlor is only available through a specialty pharmacy; information regarding prescribing and access may be found at www.-valchlor.com.

Medication Guide Available Yes

Dosing

Adult & Geriatric

Cutaneous T-cell lymphoma (mycosis fungoides-type): Topical: Apply a thin film once daily to affected areas of skin

Note: Concurrent use of topical or systemic corticosteroids was not allowed in the clinical study (Lessin, 2013).

Renal Impairment No dosage adjustment provided in the manufacturer's labeling; however, based on the lack of systemic exposure, dosage adjustment is likely not necessary.

Hepatic Impairment No dosage adjustment provided in the manufacturer's labeling; however, based on the lack of systemic exposure, dosage adjustment is likely not necessary.

Adjustment for Toxicity Skin ulceration (any grade), blistering, or dermatitis (moderately severe-to-severe): Withhold treatment; upon improvement, may reinitiate treatment with a reduced frequency of once every 3 days; if every 3-day application is tolerated for at least 1 week, may increase to every other day for at least 1 week, then (if tolerated) may increase to once daily.

Additional Information Complete prescribing information should be consulted for additional detail.

Dosage Forms Considerations Valchlor 0.016% is equivalent to 0.02% mechlorethamine hydrochloride

Dosage Forms Excipient information presented when available (limited, particularly for generics); consult specific product labeling.

Gel, External:

Valchlor: 0.016% (60 g) [contains edetate disodium, isopropyl alcohol, menthol, propylene glycol]

◆ Mechlorethamine HCl (Topical) see Mechlorethamine (Topical) on page 1130

◆ Mechlorethamine Hydrochloride see Mechlorethamine (Systemic) on page 1130

◆ Mechlorethamine Topical Gel see Mechlorethamine (Topical) on page 1130

Meclizine (MEK li zeen)

Brand Names: US Antivert [DSC]; Dramamine Less Drowsy [OTC]; Medi-Meclizine [OTC]; Motion-Time [OTC]; Travel Sickness [OTC]; UniVert; Vertin-32 [OTC] [DSC]

Index Terms Antivert; Meclizine Hydrochloride; Meclozine Hydrochloride

Pharmacologic Category Antiemetic; Histamine H₁ Antagonist; Histamine H₁ Antagonist, First Generation; Piperazine Derivative

Use Prevention and treatment of symptoms of motion sickness; management of vertigo with diseases affecting the vestibular system

Dosing

Adult & Geriatric

Motion sickness: Oral: 25-50 mg 1 hour before travel, repeat dose every 24 hours if needed

Vertigo: Oral: 25-100 mg daily in divided doses

Pediatric Children ≥12 years: Refer to adult dosing.

Renal Impairment No dosage adjustment provided in manufacturer's labeling.

Hepatic Impairment No dosage adjustment provided in manufacturer's labeling.

Additional Information Complete prescribing information should be consulted for additional detail.

Dosage Forms Excipient information presented when available (limited, particularly for generics); consult specific product labeling. [DSC] = Discontinued product

Tablet, Oral, as hydrochloride:

Antivert: 12.5 mg [DSC], 25 mg [DSC], 50 mg [DSC]

Dramamine Less Drowsy: 25 mg [contains fd&c yellow #10 (quinoline yellow)]

Dramamine Less Drowsy: 25 mg [contains fd&c yellow #10 aluminum lake]

Medi-Meclizine: 25 mg

UniVert: 32 mg [scored; contains brilliant blue fcf (fd&c blue #1), fd&c yellow #10 (quinoline yellow)]

Vertin-32: 32 mg [DSC] [contains brilliant blue fcf (fd&c blue #1), fd&c yellow #10 (quinoline yellow)]

Generic: 12.5 mg, 25 mg

Tablet Chewable, Oral, as hydrochloride:

Motion-Time: 25 mg [scored; contains fd&c red #40 aluminum lake, saccharin sodium; raspberry flavor]

Travel Sickness: 25 mg [contains aspartame, fd&c red #40 aluminum lake]

Travel Sickness: 25 mg [DSC] [scored; contains aspartame, fd&c red #40 aluminum lake; raspberry flavor]

Generic: 25 mg

◆ Meclizine Hydrochloride see Meclizine on page 1131

◆ Meclozine Hydrochloride see Meclizine on page 1131

◆ Med-Anastrozole (Can) see Anastrozole on page 128

◆ Med-Derm Hydrocortisone [OTC] see Hydrocortisone (Topical) on page 886

◆ Med-Dutasteride (Can) see Dutasteride on page 613

◆ Medent®-PEI [OTC] see Guaifenesin and Phenylephrine on page 862

◆ Medicinal Carbon see Charcoal, Activated on page 368

◆ Medicinal Charcoal see Charcoal, Activated on page 368

◆ Medi-First Anti-Fungal [OTC] see Tolnaftate on page 1807

◆ Medi-First Hydrocortisone [OTC] see Hydrocortisone (Topical) on page 886

◆ Medi-First Triple Antibiotic [OTC] see Bacitracin, Neomycin, and Polymyxin B (Topical) on page 197

◆ Medi-Meclizine [OTC] see Meclizine on page 1131

◆ Medi-Phenyl [OTC] see Phenylephrine (Systemic) on page 1442

◆ Mediproxen [OTC] see Naproxen on page 1256

◆ Med-Latanoprost (Can) see Latanoprost on page 1037

◆ MED-Letrozole (Can) see Letrozole on page 1048

◆ Med-Memantine (Can) see Memantine on page 1139

◆ Med-Rivastigmine (Can) see Rivastigmine on page 1607

◆ Medrol see MethylPREDNISolone on page 1184

◆ Medrol Dose Pack see MethylPREDNISolone on page 1184

◆ Medrol (Pak) see MethylPREDNISolone on page 1184

◆ Med-Rosuvastatin (Can) see Rosuvastatin on page 1620

◆ Medroxy (Can) see MedroxyPROGESTERone on page 1131

MedroxyPROGESTERone
(me DROKS ee proe JES te rone)

Brand Names: US Depo-Provera; Depo-SubQ Provera 104; Provera

Brand Names: Canada Alti-MPA; Apo-Medroxy; Depo-Prevera; Depo-Provera; Dom-Medroxyprogesterone; Gen-Medroxy; Medroxy; Medroxyprogesterone Acetate Injectable Suspension USP; Novo-Medrone; PMS-Medroxyprogesterone; Provera; Provera-Pak; Teva-Medroxyprogesterone

Index Terms Acetoxymethylprogesterone; Medroxyprogesterone Acetate; Methylacetoxyprogesterone; MPA

Pharmacologic Category Contraceptive; Progestin

Use

Abnormal uterine bleeding (tablet): Treatment of abnormal uterine bleeding due to hormonal imbalance in the absence of organic pathology, such as fibroids or uterine cancer.

Amenorrhea, secondary (tablet): Treatment of secondary amenorrhea due to hormonal imbalance in the absence of organic pathology, such as fibroids or uterine cancer.

Contraception (104 mg/0.65 mL and 150 mg/mL injection): Prevention of pregnancy in women of childbearing potential.

Endometrial hyperplasia (tablet): Prevention of endometrial hyperplasia in nonhysterectomized postmenopausal women receiving daily oral conjugated estrogens 0.625 mg.

Endometrial carcinoma (400 mg/mL injection): Adjunctive therapy and palliative treatment of inoperable, recurrent, and metastatic endometrial carcinoma.

Endometriosis (104 mg/0.65 mL injection): Management of endometriosis-associated pain.

Pregnancy Considerations Most products are contra-indicated in women who are pregnant, suspected to be pregnant or as a diagnostic test for pregnancy. In general, there is not an increased risk of birth defects following inadvertent use of the injectable medroxyprogesterone acetate (MPA) contraceptives early in pregnancy. Hypospadias has been reported in male babies and clitoral enlargement and labial fusion have been reported in female babies exposed to MPA during the first trimester of pregnancy. High doses impair fertility. Ectopic pregnancies have been reported with use of the MPA contraceptive injection. Median time to conception/return to ovulation following discontinuation of MPA contraceptive injection is 10 months following the last injection and is unrelated to the duration of use.

Breast-Feeding Considerations Medroxyprogesterone acetate (MPA) is excreted in breast milk. Composition, quality, and quantity of breast milk are not affected; adverse developmental and behavioral effects have not been noted following exposure of infant to MPA while breast-feeding. The manufacturer does not recommend the use of MPA tablets in breast-feeding mothers; however, guidelines note that the injectable MPA contraceptives can be initiated immediately postpartum in women who are nursing (CDC, 2010; CDC, 2011; CDC, 2013). The manufacturer recommends medroxyprogesterone 400 mg/mL be used with caution in women who are nursing.

Contraindications

Angioedema, anaphylactic reaction, or hypersensitivity to medroxyprogesterone or any component of the formulation

Additional contraindications:

Injection (104 mg/0.65 mL): Active thrombophlebitis; venous thromboembolic disorders or cerebral vascular disease (current or history of); undiagnosed genital bleeding; breast cancer (known, suspected or history of); significant hepatic impairment or disease; pregnancy

Injection (150 mg/mL): Active thrombophlebitis; venous thromboembolic disorders or cerebral vascular disease (current or history of); undiagnosed genital bleeding; breast cancer (known, suspected or history of); significant hepatic impairment or disease; pregnancy; diagnostic test for pregnancy

Injection (400 mg/mL): Active thrombophlebitis; venous thromboembolic disorders or cerebral vascular disease (current or history of)

Tablet: DVT or PE (current or history of); active or history of arterial thromboembolic disease (eg, stroke, MI); estrogen or progesterone dependent tumor (known or suspected); undiagnosed abnormal genital bleeding; breast cancer (known, suspected or history of); hepatic impairment or disease; pregnancy

Warnings/Precautions Hazardous agent - use appropriate precautions for handling and disposal (NIOSH 2014 [group 2]).

Anaphylaxis or anaphylactoid reactions have been reported with use of the injection; medication for the treatment of hypersensitivity reactions should be available for immediate use.

[US Boxed Warning]: Prolonged use of medroxyprogesterone contraceptive injection may result in a loss of bone mineral density (BMD). It is not known if use during adolescence or early adulthood will decrease peak bone mass accretion or increase the risk for osteoporotic fractures later in life. Loss is related to the duration of use, may not be completely reversible on discontinuation of the drug, and incidence is not significantly different between the SubQ and IM dosage forms. The impact on peak bone mass in adolescents should be weighed against the potential for unintended pregnancies in treatment decision. Consider alternative contraceptive methods in patients at risk for osteoporosis (eg, metabolic bone disease, chronic alcohol and/or tobacco use, anorexia nervosa, strong family history of osteoporosis, chronic use of medications associated with osteoporosis such as anticonvulsants or corticosteroids). All patients should have adequate calcium and Vitamin D intake. Consider evaluating bone mineral density in patients receiving high doses of medroxyprogesterone for long term endometrial cancer. **[US Boxed Warning]: Long-term use (ie, >2 years) should be limited to situations where other birth control methods are inadequate.** When used for endometrial carcinoma, the effects of long term use on adrenal, hepatic, ovarian, pituitary, and uterine function is not known. **[US Boxed Warning]: Inform patients that injectable contraceptives do not protect against HIV infection or other sexually-transmitted diseases.**

[US Boxed Warning]: Based on data from the Women's Health Initiative (WHI) studies, an increased risk of invasive breast cancer was observed in postmenopausal women using conjugated estrogens (CE) in combination with medroxyprogesterone acetate (MPA). This risk may be associated with duration of use and declines once combined therapy is discontinued (Chlebowski, 2009). The risk of invasive breast cancer was decreased in postmenopausal women with a hysterectomy using CE only, regardless of weight. However, the risk was not significantly decreased in women at high risk for breast cancer (family history of breast cancer, personal history of benign breast disease) (Anderson, 2012). Women who used depo-medroxyprogesterone within the previous 5 years and for a duration of 12 months or longer were found to have an increased risk of breast cancer. An increase in abnormal mammogram findings has also been reported with estrogen alone or in combination with progestin therapy. Most products are contraindicated in patients with known or suspected breast cancer. Use of medroxyprogesterone for the treatment of endometrial carcinoma is not recommended in women with known or suspected breast cancer and women with a strong family history of breast cancer should be carefully monitored.

[US Boxed Warning]: Estrogens with or without progestin should not be used to prevent dementia. In the Women's Health Initiative Memory Study (WHIMS), an increased incidence of probable dementia was observed in women ≥65 years of age taking CE alone or in combination with MPA.

[US Boxed Warning]: Estrogens with progestin should not be used to prevent cardiovascular disease. Using data from the Women's Health Initiative (WHI) studies, an increased risk of deep vein thrombosis (DVT), and stroke, has been reported with CE and an increased risk of DVT, stroke, pulmonary emboli (PE) and myocardial infarction (MI) has been reported with CE with MPA in postmenopausal women 50 to 79 years of age. Additional risk factors include diabetes mellitus, hypercholesterolemia, hypertension, SLE, obesity, tobacco use, and/or history of venous thromboembolism (VTE). Risk factors should be managed appropriately; discontinue use if adverse cardiovascular events occur or are suspected. Use is contraindicated in women with active DVT, PE, active arterial thromboembolic disease or a history of these conditions. If thrombosis develops with contraceptive treatment, discontinue treatment (unless no other acceptable contraceptive alternative).

[US Boxed Warning]: Estrogens with progestin should be used for the shortest duration possible at the lowest effective dose consistent with treatment goals and risks for the individual woman. Patients should be reevaluated as clinically appropriate to determine if treatment is still necessary. Available data related to treatment risks are from Women's Health Initiative (WHI) studies, which evaluated oral CE 0.625 mg with or without MPA 2.5 mg relative to placebo in postmenopausal women. Other combinations and dosage forms of estrogens and progestins were not studied. **Outcomes reported from clinical trials using CE with or without MPA should be assumed to be similar for other doses and other dosage forms of estrogens and progestins until comparable data becomes available.** Women who are early in menopause, who are in good cardiovascular health, and who are at low risk for adverse cardiovascular events can be considered candidates for estrogen with or without progestin therapy for the relief of menopausal symptoms (ACOG 565 2013). MPA is used to reduce the risk of endometrial hyperplasia in nonhysterectomized postmenopausal women receiving conjugated estrogens. The use of unopposed estrogen in women with a uterus is associated with an increased risk of endometrial cancer. The addition of a progestin to estrogen therapy may decrease the risk of endometrial hyperplasia, a precursor to endometrial cancer. Adequate diagnostic measures, including endometrial sampling if indicated, should be performed to rule out malignancy in postmenopausal women with undiagnosed abnormal vaginal bleeding. There is no evidence that the use of natural estrogens results in a different endometrial risk profile than synthetic estrogens at equivalent estrogen doses. The risk of endometrial cancer is dose and duration dependent; risk appears to be greatest with use ≥5 years and may persist following discontinuation of therapy.

Use with caution in patients with migraine, or a history of depression. Use with caution in patients with diseases which may be exacerbated by fluid retention, including cardiac, or renal dysfunction. Discontinue pending examination in cases of sudden partial or complete vision loss, sudden onset of proptosis, diplopia, or migraine; discontinue permanently if papilledema or retinal vascular lesions

are observed on examination. Unscheduled bleeding/spotting may occur. Presentation of irregular, unresolving vaginal bleeding following previously regular cycles warrants further evaluation including endometrial sampling, if indicated, to rule out malignancy. Potentially significant interactions may exist, requiring dose or frequency adjustment, additional monitoring, and/or selection of alternative therapy. Not for use prior to menarche. Whenever possible, progestins in combination with estrogens should be discontinued at least 4-6 weeks prior to surgery associated with an increased risk of thromboembolism or during periods of prolonged immobilization.

Postmenopausal estrogen therapy and combined estrogen/progesterone therapy may increase the risk of ovarian cancer; however, the absolute risk to an individual woman is small. Although results from various studies are not consistent, risk does not appear to be significantly associated with the duration, route, or dose of therapy. In one study, the risk decreased after 2 years following discontinuation of therapy (Mørch, 2009). Although the risk of ovarian cancer is rare, women who are at an increased risk (eg, family history) should be counseled about the association (NAMS, 2012). In women using estrogen plus progesterone therapy, triglycerides may be increased in women with preexisting hypertriglyceridemia; discontinue if pancreatitis occurs. Estrogen plus progestin therapy may have adverse effects on glucose tolerance; use caution in women with diabetes. Use estrogen plus progestin therapy with caution in patients with asthma, epilepsy, hepatic hemangiomas, porphyria, or SLE; may exacerbate disease. Use estrogen plus progestin therapy with caution in patients with hypoparathyroidism; estrogen-induced hypocalcemia may occur.

Estrogens plus progestins are poorly metabolized in patients with hepatic dysfunction. Use caution with a history of cholestatic jaundice associated with prior estrogen use or pregnancy. Discontinue if jaundice develops or if acute or chronic hepatic disturbances occur. Most products are contraindicated with hepatic impairment or disease. Use of medroxyprogesterone for the treatment of endometrial carcinoma is not recommended in women with significant hepatic dysfunction and should be discontinued if liver dysfunction occurs. The use of estrogens and/or progestins may change the results of some laboratory tests (eg, coagulation factors, lipids, glucose tolerance, binding proteins). The dose, route, and the specific estrogen/progestin influences these changes. In addition, personal risk factors (eg, cardiovascular disease, smoking, diabetes, age) also contribute to adverse events; use of specific products may be contraindicated in women with certain risk factors.

When used for contraception, the possibility of ectopic pregnancy should be considered in patients with severe abdominal pain. Contraceptive therapy with medroxyprogesterone commonly results in an average weight gain of ~3.7 kg after 2 years of treatment.

May cause suppression of hypothalamic-pituitary-adrenal (HPA) axis, resulting in decreased plasma cortisol concentrations, decreased cortisol secretion, and low plasma ACTH concentrations. Cushingoid symptoms may occur.

Use may mask the onset of menopause in women treated for endometrial cancer.

Some dosage forms may contain polysorbate 80 (also known as Tweens). Hypersensitivity reactions, usually a delayed reaction, have been reported following exposure to pharmaceutical products containing polysorbate 80 in certain individuals (Isaksson, 2002; Lucente 2000; Shelley, 1995). Thrombocytopenia, ascites, pulmonary deterioration, and renal and hepatic failure have been reported in premature neonates after receiving parenteral products containing polysorbate 80 (Alade, 1986; CDC, 1984). See manufacturer's labeling.

Adverse Reactions Adverse effects as reported with any dosage form.

>10%:

Central nervous system: Headache (9% to 17%), nervousness (11%)

Endocrine & metabolic: Amenorrhea (IM: 55% at 12 months; 68% at 24 months; SubQ: 6%), weight gain (IM: >10 lbs at 24 months: 38%; SubQ: 6%), menstrual disease (IM: 57% at 12 months; 32% at 24 months; SubQ: 1% to 7%)

Gastrointestinal: Abdominal pain (1% to 11%)

1% to 10%:

Cardiovascular: Edema (2%)

Central nervous system: Dizziness (1% to 6%), anxiety (1% to <5%), depression (1% to <5%), insomnia (1% to <5%), irritability (1% to <5%), fatigue (<5%)

Dermatologic: Acne vulgaris (1% to <5%), alopecia (1%), skin rash (1%)

Endocrine & metabolic: Decreased libido (1% to 6%), change in menstrual flow (menometrorrhagia; 1% to <5%), hypermenorrhea (1% to <5%), hot flash (1% to <5%)

Gastrointestinal: Abdominal distension (1% to <5%), diarrhea (1% to <5%), nausea (1% to <5%), bloating (2%)

Genitourinary: Abnormal Pap smear (1% to <5%), bacterial vaginosis (1% to <5%), breast tenderness (1% to <5%), dysmenorrhea (1% to <5%), mastalgia (1% to <5%), urinary tract infection (1% to <5%), uterine hemorrhage (1% to <5%), vaginal hemorrhage (1% to <5%), vaginitis (1% to <5%), vulvovaginal candidiasis (1% to <5%), leukorrhea (3%)

Infection: Influenza (1% to <5%)

Local: Pain at injection site (SubQ: 1% to <5%), atrophy at injection site (SubQ: ≤1%), induration at injection site (SubQ: ≤1%)

Neuromuscular & skeletal: Arthralgia (1% to <5%), back pain (1% to <5%), limb pain (1% to <5%), leg cramps (4%), weakness (≤4%)

Respiratory: Bronchitis (1% to <5%), nasopharyngitis (1% to <5%), pharyngitis (1% to <5%), sinusitis (1% to <5%), upper respiratory tract infection (1% to <5%)

<1% (Limited to important or life-threatening): Anaphylaxis, anaphylactoid reaction, angioedema, asthma, Bell's palsy, breast changes, cervical cancer, chest pain, chloasma, cholestatic jaundice, decreased bone mineral density, decreased glucose tolerance, decreased lactation, deep vein thrombosis, delayed return to fertility, diaphoresis, dyspnea, galactorrhea, hematologic abnormality, hirsutism, hoarseness, jaundice, malignant neoplasm of breast, nipple bleeding, optic neuritis, osteoporosis, paralysis, paresthesia, pathological fracture due to osteoporosis, pulmonary embolus, rectal hemorrhage, residual mass at injection site (aqueous suspension), retinal thrombosis, scleroderma, seizure, skin discoloration at injection site (aqueous suspension), sterile abscess at injection site (aqueous suspension), syncope, tachycardia, thrombophlebitis, weight loss

Drug Interactions

Metabolism/Transport Effects Substrate of CYP3A4 (major); **Note:** Assignment of Major/Minor substrate status based on clinically relevant drug interaction potential

Avoid Concomitant Use

Avoid concomitant use of MedroxyPROGESTERone with any of the following: Griseofulvin; Indium 111 Capromab Pendetide; Tranexamic Acid; Ulipristal

Increased Effect/Toxicity

MedroxyPROGESTERone may increase the levels/effects of: C1 inhibitors; Flibanserin; Selegiline; Thalidomide; Tranexamic Acid; Voriconazole

The levels/effects of MedroxyPROGESTERone may be increased by: Atazanavir; Boceprevir; Cobicistat; CYP3A4 Inhibitors (Strong); Herbs (Progestogenic Properties); Lopinavir; Metreleptin; Mifepristone; Osimertinib; Tipranavir; Voriconazole

Decreased Effect

MedroxyPROGESTERone may decrease the levels/effects of: Anticoagulants; Antidiabetic Agents; Choline C 11; Fosamprenavir; Indium 111 Capromab Pendetide; Ulipristal; Vitamin K Antagonists

The levels/effects of MedroxyPROGESTERone may be decreased by: Acitretin; Aprepitant; Artemether; Barbiturates; Bexarotene (Systemic); Bile Acid Sequestrants; Bosentan; CarBAMazepine; CloBAZam; CYP3A4 Inducers (Moderate); CYP3A4 Inducers (Strong); Dabrafenib; Darunavir; Deferasirox; Efavirenz; Enzalutamide; Eslicarbazepine; Felbamate; Fosamprenavir; Fosaprepitant; Fosphenytoin; Griseofulvin; LamoTRIgine; Lesinurad; Lopinavir; Lumacaftor; Metreleptin; Mifepristone; Mitotane; Mycophenolate; Nelfinavir; Nevirapine; Osimertinib; OXcarbazepine; Perampanel; Phenytoin; Primidone; Prucalopride; Retinoic Acid Derivatives; Rifamycin Derivatives; Saquinavir; Siltuximab; St Johns Wort; Sugammadex; Telaprevir; Tocilizumab; Topiramate; Ulipristal

Food Interactions Bioavailability of the oral tablet is increased when taken with food; half-life is unchanged. Management: Administer without regard to food.

Storage/Stability Store at 20°C to 25°C (68°F to 77°F).

Mechanism of Action Medroxyprogesterone acetate (MPA) transforms a proliferative endometrium into a secretory endometrium. When administered with conjugated estrogens, MPA reduces the incidence of endometrial hyperplasia and risk of adenocarcinoma. When used as an injection for contraception (doses of 150 mg IM or 104 mg SubQ), MPA inhibits secretion of pituitary gonadotropins, which prevents follicular maturation and ovulation ▶

and causes endometrial thinning. Progestogens, such as medroxyprogesterone when used for endometriosis, lead to atrophy of the endometrial tissue. They may also suppress new growth and implantation. Pain associated with endometriosis is decreased (ASRM, 2014).

Pharmacodynamics/Kinetics

Absorption: Oral: Rapid; IM: Slow

Protein binding: 86% to 90% primarily to albumin; does not bind to sex hormone–binding globulin

Metabolism: Extensively hepatic via hydroxylation and conjugation; forms metabolites

Half-life elimination: Oral: 12 to 17 hours; IM (Depo-Provera Contraceptive): ~50 days; SubQ: ~43 days

Time to peak: Oral: 2 to 4 hours; IM (Depo-Provera Contraceptive): ~3 weeks; SubQ: ~1 week

Excretion: Urine

Dosing

Adult & Geriatric

Abnormal uterine bleeding: Oral: 5 or 10 mg daily for 5 to 10 days starting on day 16 or 21 of menstrual cycle. Secretory transformation of the endometrium will occur when adequately primed with endogenous or exogenous estrogen. Withdrawal bleeding may be expected within 3 to 7 days after discontinuing medroxyprogesterone.

Amenorrhea, secondary: Oral: 5 or 10 mg daily for 5 to 10 days. Therapy may be started at any time. Secretory transformation of the endometrium will occur when adequately primed with endogenous or exogenous estrogen. Withdrawal bleeding may be expected within 3 to 7 days after discontinuing medroxyprogesterone.

Contraception:

Depo-Provera Contraceptive: IM: 150 mg every 3 months (every 13 weeks)

depo-subQ provera 104: SubQ: 104 mg every 3 months (every 12 to 14 weeks)

Endometrial carcinoma, recurrent or metastatic (adjunctive/palliative treatment) (Depo-Provera): IM: Initial: 400 to 1,000 mg/week

Endometrial hyperplasia reduction: Oral: 5 or 10 mg daily for 12 to 14 consecutive days each month, starting on day 1 or day 16 of the cycle. When treating postmenopausal women, use for the shortest duration possible at the lowest effective dose consistent with treatment goals. Reevaluate patients as clinically appropriate to determine if treatment is still necessary. Consider use of an estrogen with a progestin in postmenopausal women with a uterus. Women who have had a hysterectomy generally do not need a progestin. Adjust dose based on patient response. Attempt to taper or discontinue at 3- to 6-month intervals.

Endometriosis (depo-subQ provera 104): SubQ: 104 mg every 3 months (every 12 to 14 weeks)

Paraphilia/hypersexuality (off-label use) (Reilly 2000): Males (**Note:** Avoid use if active pituitary pathology, hepatic failure, or thromboembolic disease):

IM (Depo-Provera): 100 to 600 mg weekly

Oral: 100 to 500 mg daily

Pediatric Adolescents:

Abnormal uterine bleeding: Refer to adult dosing.

Amenorrhea, secondary: Refer to adult dosing.

Contraception: Refer to adult dosing.

Endometriosis: Refer to adult dosing.

Renal Impairment There are no dosage adjustments provided in the manufacturer's labeling (has not been studied).

Hepatic Impairment Medroxyprogesterone is extensively metabolized in the liver. Most products are contraindicated in patients with hepatic impairment. If needed for the palliative treatment metastatic endometrial carcinoma, monitor closely; withhold or discontinue treatment if liver dysfunction develops and do not resume until hepatic function has returned to normal.

Dietary Considerations Ensure adequate calcium and vitamin D intake

Administration

IM: Depo-Provera Contraceptive: Administer first dose during the first 5 days of menstrual period, or within the first 5 days postpartum if not breast-feeding, or at the sixth week postpartum if breast-feeding exclusively. Shake vigorously prior to administration. Administer by deep IM injection in the gluteal or deltoid muscle.

When switching from combined hormonal contraceptives (estrogen plus progestin), the first injection should be on the day after the last active tablet or (at the latest) the day after the final inactive tablet. When switching from other contraceptive methods, ensure continuous contraceptive coverage.

SubQ: depo-subQ provera 104: Administer first dose during the first 5 days of menstrual period, or at the sixth week postpartum if breast-feeding. Shake vigorously for at least 1 minute prior to administration. Administer by

SubQ injection in the anterior thigh or abdomen; avoid boney areas and the umbilicus. Administer slowly over 5 to 7 seconds. Do not rub the injection area.

When switching from combined hormonal contraceptives (estrogen plus progestin), the first injection should be within 7 days after the last active pill, or removal of patch or ring. If switching from the IM to SubQ formulation, the next dose should be given within the prescribed dosing period for the IM injection to ensure continuous coverage.

Hazardous agent; use appropriate precautions for handling and disposal (NIOSH 2014 [group 2]).

Monitoring Parameters Monitor patient closely for loss of vision; sudden onset of proptosis, diplopia, or migraine; signs and symptoms of thromboembolic disorders; signs or symptoms of depression; glucose in patients with diabetes; or blood pressure. Adequate diagnostic measures, including endometrial sampling, if indicated, should be performed to rule out malignancy in all cases of undiagnosed abnormal vaginal bleeding. Monitor blood pressure at regular intervals with estrogen plus progestin therapy.

Contraception: Assessment of pregnancy status (prior to therapy); weight (optional; BMI at baseline may be helpful to monitor changes during therapy); assess potential health status changes at routine visits (CDC, 2013). BMD with long-term use (per manufacturer).

Endometrial cancer: Consider BMD with long term use; breast cancer (in women with a strong family history of breast cancer).

Treatment of paraphilia/hypersexuality (Guay, 2009; Reilly, 2000): Hepatic function test (baseline and during treatment if suspected hepatotoxicity); CBC (baseline); serum testosterone (baseline then monthly for 4 months then every 6 months); serum LH and prolactin (baseline and every 6 months); FSH (baseline); glucose; bone scan (baseline then annually) if serum testosterone significantly suppressed; gallbladder function; blood pressure; weight gain

Dosage Forms Excipient information presented when available (limited, particularly for generics); consult specific product labeling.

Suspension, Intramuscular, as acetate:

Depo-Provera: 150 mg/mL (1 mL)

Depo-Provera: 150 mg/mL (1 mL) [contains methylparaben, polyethylene glycol, polysorbate 80, propylparaben]

Depo-Provera: 400 mg/mL (2.5 mL)

Generic: 150 mg/mL (1 mL)

Suspension, Subcutaneous, as acetate:

Depo-SubQ Provera 104: 104 mg/0.65 mL (0.65 mL) [contains methylparaben, propylparaben]

Tablet, Oral, as acetate:

Provera: 2.5 mg, 5 mg, 10 mg [scored]

Generic: 2.5 mg, 5 mg, 10 mg

◆ Medroxyprogesterone Acetate see MedroxyPROGESTERone on page 1131

◆ Medroxyprogesterone Acetate Injectable Suspension USP (Can) see MedroxyPROGESTERone on page 1131

◆ Med-Sotalol (Can) see Sotalol on page 1694

◆ Mefenamic (Can) see Mefenamic Acid on page 1134

Mefenamic Acid (me fe NAM ik AS id)

Brand Names: US Ponstel

Brand Names: Canada Dom-Mefenamic Acid; Mefenamic; PMS-Mefenamic Acid; Ponstan

Pharmacologic Category Nonsteroidal Anti-inflammatory Drug (NSAID), Oral

Use

Mild to moderate pain: Relief of mild to moderate pain in patients ≥14 years and older, when therapy will not exceed 1 week (7 days)

Primary dysmenorrhea: Treatment of primary dysmenorrhea.

Medication Guide Available Yes

Dosing

Adult & Geriatric Note: Use the lowest effective dose for the shortest possible duration.

Mild to moderate pain: Oral: Initial: 500 mg, then 250 mg every 6 hours as needed; usually not to exceed 1 week

Primary dysmenorrhea: Oral: Initial: 500 mg beginning at the onset of symptoms, followed by 250 mg every 6 hours; continue for 2 to 3 days

Pediatric Adolescents ≥14 years: Refer to adult dosing.

Renal Impairment

US labeling: Use is contraindicated in preexisting renal disease.

Canadian labeling:

CrCl ≥30 mL/minute: There are no dosage adjustments provided in the manufacturer's labeling; use with caution,consider lower doses, and monitor renal function.

CrCl <30 mL/minute or deteriorating renal function: Use is contraindicated.

Hepatic Impairment

US labeling: There are no dosage adjustments provided in the manufacturer's labeling (has not been studied); however, adjustment may be necessary due to extensive hepatic metabolism.

Canadian labeling: There are no dosage adjustments provided in the manufacturer's labeling. Use is contraindicated in severe liver impairment or active liver disease.

Additional Information Complete prescribing information should be consulted for additional detail.

Dosage Forms Excipient information presented when available (limited, particularly for generics); consult specific product labeling.

Capsule, Oral:

Ponstel: 250 mg

Generic: 250 mg

Mefloquine (ME floe kwin)

Index Terms Lariam; Mefloquine Hydrochloride

Pharmacologic Category Antimalarial Agent

Use Treatment of mild-to-moderate acute malarial infections and prevention of malaria caused by *Plasmodium falciparum* (including chloroquine-resistant strains) or *P. vivax*

Note: Due to geographical resistance and cross-resistance, consult current CDC guidelines.

Medication Guide Available Yes

Dosing

Adult & Geriatric Malaria: Oral (dose expressed as mg of mefloquine hydrochloride):

Mild-to-moderate, treatment: 1250 mg (5 tablets) as a single dose. **Note:** If clinical improvement is not seen within 48-72 hours, an alternative therapy should be used for re-treatment.

Uncomplicated, treatment (off-label dose): 750 mg (3 tablets) as initial dose, followed 6-12 hours later by 500 mg (2 tablets) (CDC, 2013b)

Uncomplicated, chloroquine-resistant P. vivax malaria treatment (off-label use): 750 mg (3 tablets) as initial dose, followed 6-12 hours later by 500 mg (2 tablets) with concomitant primaquine (CDC, 2013b)

Chemoprophylaxis: 250 mg weekly starting 1 week (CDC, 2014: ≥2 weeks) before arrival in endemic area, continuing weekly during travel and for 4 weeks after leaving endemic area. **Note:** Prophylaxis may begin 2-3 weeks prior to travel to ensure tolerance.

Pediatric Malaria: Children ≥6 months: Oral (dose expressed as mg of mefloquine hydrochloride):

Mild-to-moderate, treatment: 20-25 mg/kg/day in 2 divided doses, taken 6-8 hours apart (maximum total dose: 1250 mg). **Note:** If clinical improvement is not seen within 48-72 hours, an alternative therapy should be used for re-treatment.

Uncomplicated, treatment (off-label dose): 15 mg/kg, followed 6-12 hours later by 10 mg/kg/dose (maximum total dose: 1250 mg) (CDC, 2013b)

Uncomplicated, chloroquine-resistant P. vivax malaria treatment (off-label use): 15 mg/kg, followed 6-12 hours later by 10 mg/kg/dose (maximum total dose: 1250 mg) with concomitant primaquine (CDC, 2013b)

Chemoprophylaxis: 5 mg/kg/dose once weekly (maximum dose: 250 mg) starting 1 week (CDC, 2014: ≥2 weeks) before arrival in endemic area, continuing weekly during travel and for 4 weeks after leaving endemic area. **Note:** Prophylaxis may begin 2-3 weeks prior to travel to ensure tolerance.

Manufacturer's labeling:

20-30 kg: $^1/_2$ of 250 mg tablet (125 mg) once weekly

30-45 kg: $^3/_4$ of 250 mg tablet (187.5 mg) once weekly

>45 kg: One tablet (250 mg) once weekly

Off-label dosing (CDC, 2014):

≤9 kg: 5 mg/kg/dose once weekly

>9-19 kg: $^1/_4$ of 250 mg tablet (62.5 mg) once weekly

>19-30 kg: $^1/_2$ of 250 mg tablet (125 mg) once weekly

>30-45 kg: $^3/_4$ of 250 mg tablet (187.5 mg) once weekly

>45 kg: One tablet (250 mg) once weekly

Renal Impairment No dosage adjustment necessary; only a small amount of mefloquine is renally eliminated.

Hepatic Impairment No dosage adjustment provided in manufacturer's labeling; however, half-life may be prolonged and plasma levels may be higher in patients with hepatic impairment.

Additional Information Complete prescribing information should be consulted for additional detail.

Dosage Forms Excipient information presented when available (limited, particularly for generics); consult specific product labeling.

Tablet, Oral, as hydrochloride:

Generic: 250 mg

♦ Mefloquine Hydrochloride *see* Mefloquine *on page 1135*

♦ Mefoxin *see* CefOXitin *on page 340*

♦ Mega-C/A Plus *see* Ascorbic Acid *on page 155*

♦ Megace ES *see* Megestrol *on page 1135*

♦ Megace Oral *see* Megestrol *on page 1135*

♦ Megace OS (Can) *see* Megestrol *on page 1135*

Megestrol (me JES trole)

Brand Names: US Megace ES; Megace Oral

Brand Names: Canada Megace OS; Megestrol

Index Terms 5071-1DL(6); Megestrol Acetate

Pharmacologic Category Antineoplastic Agent, Hormone; Appetite Stimulant; Progestin

Use

Anorexia or cachexia: *Suspension:* Treatment of anorexia, cachexia, or unexplained significant weight loss in patients with AIDS

Limitations of use: Treatment of AIDS-related weight loss should only be initiated after addressing the treatable causes (eg, malignancy, infection, malabsorption, endocrine disease, renal disease, psychiatric disorder) for weight loss. Megestrol is not intended to prevent weight loss.

Breast cancer: *Tablet:* Treatment (palliative) of advanced breast cancer

Endometrial cancer: *Tablet:* Treatment (palliative) of advanced endometrial carcinoma

Additional Canadian use (not an approved use in the U.S.): Tablet: Treatment of anorexia, cachexia, or weight loss secondary to metastatic cancer

Pregnancy Considerations Adverse events were demonstrated in animal reproduction studies. May cause fetal harm if administered to a pregnant woman. Use during pregnancy is contraindicated (suspension) and appropriate contraception is recommended in women who may become pregnant. In clinical studies, megestrol was shown to cause breakthrough vaginal bleeding in women.

Breast-Feeding Considerations Megestrol is excreted into breast milk. Information is available from five nursing women, ~8 weeks postpartum, who were administered megestrol 4 mg in combination with ethinyl estradiol 50 mcg daily for contraception. Maternal serum and milk samples were obtained over 5 days, beginning 10 days after therapy began. The highest concentrations of megestrol were found at the samples taken 3 hours after the maternal dose. Mean concentrations of megestrol were 6.5 ng/mL (maternal serum; range: 3.7 to 10.8 ng/mL), 4.6 ng/mL (foremilk; range: 1.1 to 12.7 ng/mL), and 5.6 ng/mL (hindmilk; range: 1.2 to 18.5 ng/mL) (Nilsson, 1977). Due to the potential for adverse reaction in the newborn, the manufacturer recommends discontinuing breast-feeding while receiving megestrol. In addition, in the United States, where formula is accessible, affordable, safe, and sustainable, and the risk of infant mortality due to diarrhea and respiratory infections is low, complete avoidance of breast-feeding by HIV-infected women is recommended to decrease potential transmission of HIV (DHHS [perinatal], 2012).

Contraindications

Hypersensitivity to megestrol or any component of the formulation; known or suspected pregnancy (suspension).

Documentation of allergenic cross-reactivity for progestins is limited. However, because of similarities in chemical structure and/or pharmacologic actions, the possibility of cross-sensitivity cannot be ruled out with certainty.

Warnings/Precautions Hazardous agent - use appropriate precautions for handling and disposal (NIOSH 2014 [group 1]). May suppress hypothalamic-pituitary-adrenal (HPA) axis during chronic administration; consider the possibility of adrenal suppression in any patient receiving or being withdrawn from chronic therapy when signs/symptoms suggestive of hypoadrenalism are noted (during stress or in unstressed state). Laboratory evaluation and replacement/stress doses of rapid-acting glucocorticoid should be considered. Cushing syndrome has been

reported with long-term use. New-onset diabetes and exacerbation of preexisting diabetes have been reported with long-term use. Use with caution in patients with a history of thromboembolic disease. Avoid use in older adults due to minimal effect on weight, and an increased risk of thrombosis and possibly death (Beers Criteria). Vaginal bleeding or discharge may occur in females. The effects on HIV viral replications are unknown in patients with AIDS-related cachexia. Potentially significant drug-drug interactions may exist, requiring dose or frequency adjustment, additional monitoring, and/or selection of alternative therapy.

Megace ES suspension is not equivalent to other formulations on a mg per mg basis; Megace ES suspension 625 mg/5 mL is equivalent to megestrol acetate suspension 800 mg/20 mL.

Benzyl alcohol and derivatives: Some dosage forms may contain sodium benzoate/benzoic acid; benzoic acid (benzoate) is a metabolite of benzyl alcohol; large amounts of benzyl alcohol (≥99 mg/kg/day) have been associated with a potentially fatal toxicity ("gasping syndrome") in neonates; the "gasping syndrome" consists of metabolic acidosis, respiratory distress, gasping respirations, CNS dysfunction (including convulsions, intracranial hemorrhage), hypotension, and cardiovascular collapse (AAP ["Inactive" 1997]; CDC, 1982); some data suggests that benzoate displaces bilirubin from protein binding sites (Ahlfors, 2001); avoid or use dosage forms containing benzyl alcohol derivative with caution in neonates. See manufacturer's labeling.

Adverse Reactions

Frequency not always defined.

Cardiovascular: Hypertension (4% to 8%), cardiomyopathy (1% to 3%), chest pain (1% to 3%), edema (1% to 3%), palpitations (1% to 3%), peripheral edema (1% to 3%), cardiac failure

Central nervous system: Headache (3% to 10%), pain (4% to 6%, similar to placebo), insomnia (1% to 6%), abnormality in thinking (1% to 3%), confusion (1% to 3%), convulsions (1% to 3%), depression (1% to 3%), hypoesthesia (1% to 3%), neuropathy (1% to 3%), paresthesia (1% to 3%), carpal tunnel syndrome, lethargy, malaise, mood changes

Dermatologic: Skin rash (6% to 12%), alopecia (1% to 3%), dermatological disease (1% to 3%), diaphoresis (1% to 3%), pruritus (1% to 3%), vesicobullous dermatitis (1% to 3%)

Endocrine & metabolic: Hyperglycemia (6%), decreased libido (1% to 5%), albuminuria (1% to 3%), gynecomastia (1% to 3%), increased lactate dehydrogenase (1% to 3%), adrenocortical insufficiency, amenorrhea, Cushing's syndrome, diabetes mellitus, hot flash, HPA-axis suppression, hypercalcemia, weight gain (not attributed to edema or fluid retention)

Gastrointestinal: Diarrhea (10%, similar to placebo), flatulence (6% to 10%), vomiting (4% to 6%), nausea (4% to 5%), dyspepsia (2% to 3%), abdominal pain (1% to 3%), constipation (1% to 3%), oral moniliasis (1% to 3%), sialorrhea (1% to 3%), xerostomia (1% to 3%)

Genitourinary: Impotence (4% to 14%), urinary incontinence (1% to 3%), urinary tract infection (1% to 3%), urinary frequency (1% to 2%), breakthrough bleeding

Hematologic & oncologic: Leukopenia (1% to 3%), sarcoma (1% to 3%), tumor flare

Hepatic: Hepatomegaly (1% to 3%)

Infection: Candidiasis (1% to 3%), herpes virus infection (1% to 3%), infection (1% to 3%)

Neuromuscular & skeletal: Weakness (5% to 6%)

Ophthalmic: Amblyopia (1% to 3%)

Respiratory: Cough (1% to 3%), dyspnea (1% to 3%), pharyngitis (1% to 3%), pulmonary disorder (1% to 3%), pneumonia (1%), hyperventilation

Miscellaneous: Fever (1% to 6%)

Postmarketing and/or case reports (Limited to important or life-threatening): Decreased glucose tolerance, thromboembolic phenomena (including deep vein thrombosis, pulmonary embolism, thrombophlebitis)

Drug Interactions

Metabolism/Transport Effects None known.

Avoid Concomitant Use

Avoid concomitant use of Megestrol with any of the following: Dofetilide; Indium 111 Capromab Pendetide; Ulipristal

Increased Effect/Toxicity

Megestrol may increase the levels/effects of: C1 inhibitors; Dofetilide

The levels/effects of Megestrol may be increased by: Herbs (Progestogenic Properties)

Decreased Effect

Megestrol may decrease the levels/effects of: Anticoagulants; Antidiabetic Agents; Choline C 11; Indium 111 Capromab Pendetide; Ulipristal

The levels/effects of Megestrol may be decreased by: Ulipristal

Storage/Stability

Suspension: Store at 15°C to 25°C (59°F to 77°F); protect from heat. Store/dispense in a tight container.

Tablet: Store at 15°C to 30°C (59°F to 86°F); protect from light. Protect from temperatures above 40°C (104°F).

Mechanism of Action A synthetic progestin with antiestrogenic properties which disrupt the estrogen receptor cycle. Megestrol interferes with the normal estrogen cycle and results in a lower LH titer. May also have a direct effect on the endometrium. Megestrol is an antineoplastic progestin thought to act through an antileutenizing effect mediated via the pituitary. May stimulate appetite by antagonizing the metabolic effects of catabolic cytokines.

Pharmacodynamics/Kinetics

Metabolism: Hepatic (to free steroids and glucuronide conjugates)

Half-life elimination: Suspension: 20 to 50 hours; Tablet: 13 to 105 hours

Time to peak, serum: 1 to 3 hours

Excretion: Urine (57% to 78%; 5% to 8% as metabolites); feces (8% to 30%)

Dosing

Adult Note: Megace ES suspension is not equivalent to other formulations on a mg-per-mg basis.

Anorexia or cachexia associated with AIDS: Oral: Suspension:

U.S. labeling: Initial: 625 mg daily (of the 125 mg/mL suspension) or 800 mg daily (of the 40 mg/mL suspension); daily doses of 400 mg to 800 mg have been found to be effective

Canadian labeling: Usual dose: 400 to 800 mg once daily for at least 2 months

Breast cancer, advanced: Oral: Tablet:

U.S. labeling: 160 mg per day in divided doses of 40 mg 4 times daily for at least 2 months

Canadian labeling: 160 mg or 125 mg/m² daily (40 mg 4 times daily or 160 mg once daily) for at least 2 months

Endometrial cancer, advanced: Oral: Tablet:

U.S. labeling: 40 to 320 mg daily in divided doses for at least 2 months

Canadian labeling: 80 to 320 mg or 62.5 to 250 mg/m² daily in divided doses (40 to 80 mg 1 to 4 times daily or 160 to 320mg daily) for at least 2 months

Cancer-related cachexia: *Canadian labeling:* Oral: Tablet: 400 to 800 mg once daily for at least 2 months

Cancer-related cachexia (off-label use/dosing in U.S.): Oral: Doses ranging from 160 to 800 mg per day were effective in achieving weight gain, higher doses (>160 mg) were associated with more weight gain (Beller, 1997; Loprinzi, 1990; Loprinzi, 1993; Vadell, 1998); based on a meta-analysis, an optimal dose has not been determined (Ruiz Garcia, 2013)

Geriatric Use with caution; refer to adult dosing.

Renal Impairment There are no dosage adjustments provided in the manufacturer's labeling; however, the urinary excretion of megestrol acetate is substantial, use caution.

Hepatic Impairment There are no dosage adjustments provided in the manufacturer's labeling.

Administration Oral: Shake suspension well before use. Hazardous agent; use appropriate precautions for handling and disposal (NIOSH 2014 [group 1]).

Monitoring Parameters Observe for signs of thromboembolic events; blood pressure; weight; serum glucose

Dosage Forms Excipient information presented when available (limited, particularly for generics); consult specific product labeling. [DSC] = Discontinued product

Suspension, Oral, as acetate:

Megace ES: 625 mg/5 mL (150 mL) [contains alcohol, usp, sodium benzoate; lemon-lime flavor]

Megace Oral: 40 mg/mL (240 mL) [lemon-lime flavor]

Generic: 40 mg/mL (10 mL, 240 mL, 480 mL); 400 mg/10 mL (10 mL, 20 mL [DSC]); 625 mg/5 mL (150 mL)

Tablet, Oral, as acetate:

Generic: 20 mg, 40 mg

Dosage Forms: Canada Refer also to Dosage Forms. **Note:** Megace ES not available in Canada.

Excipient information presented when available (limited, particularly for generics); consult specific product labeling.

Tablet, Oral, as acetate: 160 mg

◆ Megestrol Acetate *see* Megestrol *on page 1135*

◆ Mekinist *see* Trametinib *on page 1823*

◆ Mellaril *see* Thioridazine *on page 1783*

Meloxicam (mel OKS i kam)

Brand Names: US Meloxicam Comfort Pac; Mobic; Vivlodex

Brand Names: Canada ACT Meloxicam; Apo-Meloxicam; Auro-Meloxicam; Dom-Meloxicam; Mobicox; Mylan-Meloxicam; PHL-Meloxicam; PMS-Meloxicam; Teva-Meloxicam

Index Terms Vivlodex

Pharmacologic Category Nonsteroidal Anti-inflammatory Drug (NSAID), Oral

Use

Osteoarthritis: Relief of the signs and symptoms of osteoarthritis (OA); management of OA pain.

Rheumatoid arthritis (tablet and suspension only): Relief of signs and symptoms of rheumatoid arthritis (RA); relief of the signs and symptoms of pauciarticular or polyarticular course juvenile RA in patients ≥2 years.

Medication Guide Available Yes

Dosing

Adult & Geriatric Note: Capsules are not interchangeable with other formulations of oral meloxicam even if the total mg strength is the same. Do not substitute similar dose strengths of other meloxicam products.

Osteoarthritis: Capsule: Oral: Initial: 5 mg once daily; some patients may receive additional benefit from increasing dose to 10 mg once daily; maximum dose: 10 mg/day

Osteoarthritis, rheumatoid arthritis: Tablet/Suspension: Oral: Initial: 7.5 mg once daily; some patients may receive additional benefit from increasing dose to 15 mg once daily; maximum dose: 15 mg/day

Pediatric Juvenile rheumatoid arthritis: Oral: Tablet/Suspension: Children ≥2 years and Adolescents: 0.125 mg/kg once daily; maximum dose: 7.5 mg/day. **Note:** Capsules are not interchangeable with other formulations of oral meloxicam even if the total mg strength is the same. Do not substitute similar dose strengths of other meloxicam products.

Renal Impairment

US labeling:

Mild to moderate impairment: No dosage adjustment necessary.

Severe impairment: Not recommended.

Hemodialysis: Maximum dose: 7.5 mg/day (tablet/suspension); 5 mg/day (capsule). **Note:** Additional dose not necessary after hemodialysis.

Canadian labeling:

CrCl ≥30 mL/minute: No dosage adjustment necessary.

CrCl <30 mL/minute or deteriorating renal function; Use is contraindicated.

Hemodialysis: Maximum dose: 7.5 mg/day. **Note:** Additional dose not necessary after hemodialysis.

Hepatic Impairment

US labeling:

Mild to moderate impairment: No dosage adjustment necessary.

Severe impairment: There are no dosage adjustments provided in the manufacturer's labeling (has not been studied); use with caution.

Canadian labeling:

Mild to moderate impairment: No dosage adjustment necessary.

Severe impairment or active liver disease: Use is contraindicated.

Additional Information Complete prescribing information should be consulted for additional detail.

Product Availability Vivlodex: FDA approved October 2015; availability anticipated in the first quarter of 2016. Vivlodex is indicated for the management of osteoarthritis pain.

Dosage Forms Considerations Meloxicam Comfort Pac is a kit containing meloxicam oral tablets 15 mg, and Duraflex topical gel.

Dosage Forms Excipient information presented when available (limited, particularly for generics); consult specific product labeling.

Capsule, Oral:

Vivlodex: 5 mg, 10 mg [contains fd&c blue #2 (indigotine), fd&c red #40, fd&c yellow #6 (sunset yellow)]

Kit, Combination:

Meloxicam Comfort Pac: 15 mg [contains methylparaben, trolamine (triethanolamine)]

Suspension, Oral:

Mobic: 7.5 mg/5 mL (100 mL) [contains saccharin sodium, sodium benzoate; raspberry flavor]

Generic: 7.5 mg/5 mL (100 mL)

Tablet, Oral:

Mobic: 7.5 mg, 15 mg

Generic: 7.5 mg, 15 mg

Dosage Forms: Canada Note: Refer also to Dosage Forms. Combination kit and oral suspension are not available in Canada. Excipient information presented when available (limited, particularly for generics); consult specific product labeling.

Tablet, Oral:

Mobicox: 7.5 mg, 15 mg

◆ Meloxicam Comfort Pac *see* Meloxicam *on page* 1137

◆ Melpaque HP *see* Hydroquinone *on page* 893

Melphalan (MEL fa lan)

Brand Names: US Alkeran

Brand Names: Canada Alkeran

Index Terms L-PAM; L-Phenylalanine Mustard; L-Sarcolysin; Phenylalanine Mustard

Pharmacologic Category Antineoplastic Agent, Alkylating Agent; Antineoplastic Agent, Alkylating Agent (Nitrogen Mustard)

Use

Multiple myeloma: Palliative treatment of multiple myeloma (injection and tablets).

Ovarian carcinoma: Palliative treatment of nonresectable epithelial ovarian carcinoma (tablets)

Pregnancy Considerations Animal studies have demonstrated embryotoxicity and teratogenicity. Therapy may suppress ovarian function leading to amenorrhea. There are no adequate and well-controlled studies in pregnant women. May cause fetal harm if administered during pregnancy. Women of childbearing potential should be advised to avoid pregnancy while on melphalan therapy.

Breast-Feeding Considerations According to the manufacturer, melphalan should not be administered if breast-feeding.

Contraindications Hypersensitivity to melphalan or any component of the formulation; patients whose disease was resistant to prior melphalan therapy

Warnings/Precautions Hazardous agent; use appropriate precautions for handling and disposal (NIOSH 2014 [group 1]).

[U.S. Boxed Warning]: Bone marrow suppression is common; may be severe and result in infection or bleeding; has been demonstrated more with the IV formulation (compared to oral); myelosuppression is dose-related. Monitor blood counts; may require treatment delay or dose modification for thrombocytopenia or neutropenia. Use with caution in patients with prior bone marrow suppression, impaired renal function (consider dose reduction), or who have received prior (or concurrent) chemotherapy or irradiation. Myelotoxicity is generally reversible, although irreversible bone marrow failure has been reported. In patients who are candidates for autologous transplantation, avoid melphalan-containing regimens prior to transplant (due to the effects on stem cell reserve). Signs of infection, such as fever and WBC rise, may not occur; lethargy and confusion may be more prominent signs of infection.

[U.S. Boxed Warning]: Hypersensitivity reactions (including anaphylaxis) have occurred in ~2% of patients receiving IV melphalan, usually after multiple treatment cycles. Discontinue infusion and treat symptomatically. Hypersensitivity may also occur (rarely) with oral melphalan. Do not readminister (oral or IV) in patients who experience hypersensitivity to melphalan.

Gastrointestinal toxicities, including nausea, vomiting, diarrhea and mucositis, are common. When administering high-dose melphalan in autologous transplantation, cryotherapy is recommended to prevent oral mucositis (Lalla, 2014). Melphalan is associated with a moderate emetic potential (depending on dose and/or administration route); antiemetics may be recommended to prevent nausea and vomiting (Dupuis, 2011). Abnormal liver function tests may occur; hepatitis and jaundice have also been reported; hepatic sinusoidal obstruction syndrome (SOS; formerly called veno-occlusive disease) has been reported with IV melphalan. Pulmonary fibrosis (some fatal) and interstitial pneumonitis have been observed with treatment. Dosage reduction is recommended with IV melphalan in patients with renal impairment; reduced initial doses may also be recommended with oral melphalan. Closely monitor patients with azotemia.

◄ **[U.S. Boxed Warning]: Produces chromosomal changes and is leukemogenic and potentially mutagenic;** secondary malignancies (including acute myeloid leukemia, myeloproliferative disease, and carcinoma) have been reported reported (some patients were receiving combination chemotherapy or radiation therapy); the risk is increased with increased treatment duration and cumulative doses. Suppresses ovarian function and produces amenorrhea; may also cause testicular suppression.

Extravasation may cause local tissue damage; administration by slow injection into a fast running IV solution into an injection port or via a central line is recommended; do not administer directly into a peripheral vein. Some dosage forms may contain propylene glycol; large amounts are potentially toxic and have been associated hyperosmolality, lactic acidosis, seizures and respiratory depression; use caution (AAP, 1997; Zar, 2007). **[U.S. Boxed Warning]: Should be administered under the supervision of an experienced cancer chemotherapy physician.** Avoid vaccination with live vaccines during treatment if immunocompromised. Toxicity may be increased in elderly; start with lowest recommended adult doses. Potentially significant drug-drug interactions may exist, requiring dose or frequency adjustment, additional monitoring, and/or selection of alternative therapy.

Adverse Reactions

>10%:

Gastrointestinal: Nausea/vomiting, diarrhea, oral ulceration

Hematologic: Myelosuppression, leukopenia (nadir: 14-21 days; recovery: 28-35 days), thrombocytopenia (nadir: 14-21 days; recovery: 28-35 days), anemia

Miscellaneous: Secondary malignancy (<2% to 20%; cumulative dose and duration dependent, includes acute myeloid leukemia, myeloproliferative syndrome, carcinoma)

1% to 10%: Miscellaneous: Hypersensitivity (IV: 2%; includes bronchospasm, dyspnea, edema, hypotension, pruritus, rash, tachycardia, urticaria)

Infrequent, frequency undefined, postmarketing, and/or case reports: Agranulocytosis, allergic reactions, alopecia, amenorrhea, anaphylaxis (rare), bleeding (with high-dose therapy),, bone marrow failure (irreversible), BUN increased, cardiac arrest, cardiotoxicity (angina, arrhythmia, hypertension, MI; with high-dose therapy), encephalopathy, hemolytic anemia, hemorrhagic cystitis, hepatic sinusoidal obstruction syndrome (SOS; veno-occlusive disease; high-dose IV melphalan), hepatitis, infection, injection site reactions (ulceration, necrosis), interstitial pneumonitis, jaundice, mucositis (with high-dose therapy), ovarian suppression, paralytic ileus (with high-dose therapy), pruritus, pulmonary fibrosis, radiation myelopathy, rash (maculopapular), renal toxicity (with high-dose therapy), seizure (with high-dose therapy), sepsis, SIADH, skin hypersensitivity, sterility, stomatitis, testicular suppression, tingling sensation, transaminases increased, vasculitis, warmth sensation

Drug Interactions

Metabolism/Transport Effects None known.

Avoid Concomitant Use

Avoid concomitant use of Melphalan with any of the following: BCG (Intravesical); Deferiprone; Dipyrone; Nalidixic Acid; Natalizumab; Pimecrolimus; Tacrolimus (Topical); Tofacitinib; Vaccines (Live)

Increased Effect/Toxicity

Melphalan may increase the levels/effects of: Carmustine; CloZAPine; CycloSPORINE (Systemic); Deferiprone; Fingolimod; Leflunomide; Natalizumab; Tofacitinib; Vaccines (Live)

The levels/effects of Melphalan may be increased by: Denosumab; Dipyrone; Nalidixic Acid; Pimecrolimus; Roflumilast; Tacrolimus (Topical); Trastuzumab

Decreased Effect

Melphalan may decrease the levels/effects of: BCG (Intravesical); Coccidioides immitis Skin Test; Sipuleucel-T; Vaccines (Inactivated); Vaccines (Live)

The levels/effects of Melphalan may be decreased by: Echinacea

Food Interactions Food interferes with oral absorption. Management: Administer on an empty stomach.

Preparation for Administration Hazardous agent; use appropriate precautions for handling and disposal (NIOSH 2014 [group 1]).

Injection: Stability is limited; must be prepared fresh. **The time between reconstitution/dilution and administration of parenteral melphalan must be kept to a minimum (manufacturer recommends <60 minutes) because reconstituted and diluted solutions are unstable.** Dissolve powder initially with 10 mL of supplied diluent to a concentration of 5 mg/mL; shake immediately and vigorously to dissolve. **Immediately** dilute dose in NS to a concentration of ≤0.45 mg/mL (manufacturer recommended concentration). Do not refrigerate solution; precipitation occurs if stored at 5°C. The manufacturer recommends administration within 60 minutes of reconstitution.

Storage/Stability

Tablet: Store in refrigerator at 2°C to 8°C (36°F to 46°F). Protect from light.

Injection: Store intact vials at 20°C to 25°C (68°F to 77°F). Protect from light. The manufacturer recommends administration be completed within 60 minutes of reconstitution; **immediately** dilute dose in NS. Do not refrigerate solution; precipitation occurs.

Mechanism of Action Alkylating agent which is a derivative of mechlorethamine that inhibits DNA and RNA synthesis via formation of carbonium ions; cross-links strands of DNA; acts on both resting and rapidly dividing tumor cells.

Pharmacodynamics/Kinetics Note: Pharmacokinetics listed are for FDA-approved doses.

Absorption: Oral: Variable and incomplete

Distribution: V_d: 0.5 L/kg; low penetration into CSF

Protein binding: 53% to 92%; primarily to albumin (40% to 60%), ~20% to alpha$_1$-acid glycoprotein

Metabolism: Hepatic; chemical hydrolysis to monohydroxymelphalan and dihydroxymelphalan

Bioavailability: Oral: Variable; 56% to 93%; exposure is reduced with a high-fat meal

Half-life elimination: Terminal: IV: 75 minutes; Oral: 1 to 2 hours

Time to peak, serum: Oral: ~1 to 2 hours

Excretion: Oral: Feces (20% to 50%); urine (~10% as unchanged drug)

Dosing

Adult Note: Melphalan is associated with a moderate emetic potential (depending on dose and/or administration route); antiemetics may be recommended to prevent nausea and vomiting. Adjust dose based on patient response and weekly blood counts.

Multiple myeloma (palliative treatment): Note: Response is gradual; may require repeated courses to realize benefit:

Oral: Usual dose (as described in the manufacturer's labeling):

6 mg once daily for 2 to 3 weeks initially, followed by up to 4 weeks rest, then a maintenance dose of 2 mg daily as hematologic recovery begins **or**

10 mg daily for 7 to 10 days; institute 2 mg daily maintenance dose after WBC >4,000 cells/mm^3 and platelets >100,000 cells/mm^3 (~4 to 8 weeks); titrate maintenance dose to hematologic response **or**

0.15 mg/kg/day for 7 days, with a 2 to 6 week rest, followed by a maintenance dose of ≤0.05 mg/kg/day as hematologic recovery begins **or**

0.25 mg/kg/day for 4 days (or 0.2 mg/kg/day for 5 days); repeat at 4- to 6-week intervals as ANC and platelet counts return to normal

Other dosing regimens in combination therapy (off-label doses):

4 mg/m^2/day for 7 days every 4 weeks (in combination with prednisone **or** with prednisone and thalidomide) (Palumbo, 2006; Palumbo, 2008) **or**

6 mg/m^2/day for 7 days every 4 weeks (in combination with prednisone) (Palumbo, 2004) **or**

0.25 mg/kg/day for 4 days every 6 weeks (in combination with prednisone [Facon, 2006; Facon, 2007] **or** with prednisone and thalidomide [Facon, 2007]) **or**

9 mg/m^2/day for 4 days every 6 weeks (in combination with prednisone **or** with prednisone and bortezomib) (Dimopoulos, 2009; San Miguel, 2008)

IV: 16 mg/m^2 administered at 2-week intervals for 4 doses, then administer at 4-week intervals after adequate hematologic recovery.

Ovarian carcinoma: Oral: 0.2 mg/kg/day for 5 days, repeat every 4 to 5 weeks **or**

Off-label dosing: 7 mg/m^2/day in 2 divided doses for 5 days, repeat every 28 days (Wadler, 1996)

Amyloidosis, light chain (off-label use): Oral: 0.22 mg/kg/day for 4 days every 28 days (in combination with oral dexamethasone) (Palladini, 2004) **or** 10 mg/m^2/day for 4 days every month (in combination with oral dexamethasone) for 12 to 18 treatment cycles (Jaccard, 2007)

Hodgkin lymphoma, relapsed/refractory (off-label use): IV: 30 mg/m^2 on day 6 of combination chemotherapy (mini-BEAM) regimen (Colwill, 1995; Martin, 2001)

Conditioning regimen for autologous hematopoietic stem cell transplantation (off-label use): IV:

200 mg/m² alone 2 days prior to transplantation (Fermand, 2005; Moreau, 2002) **or**

140 mg/m² 2 days prior to transplantation (combined with busulfan) (Fermand, 2005) **or**

140 mg/m² 2 days prior to transplantation (combined with total body irradiation [TBI]) (Moreau, 2002) **or**

140 mg/m² 5 days prior to transplantation (combined with TBI) (Barlogie, 2006)

Geriatric Refer to adult dosing. Use caution and begin at the lower end of dosing range.

Pediatric Note: Melphalan is associated with a moderate emetic potential (depending on dose and/or administration route); antiemetics may be recommended to prevent nausea and vomiting (Dupuis, 2011).

Conditioning regimen for autologous hematopoietic stem cell transplantation (off-label use): IV:

140 mg/m² 2 days prior to transplantation (combined with busulfan) (Canete, 2009; Oberlin, 2006) **or**

180 mg/m² (with pre- and posthydration) 12-30 hours prior to transplantation (Pritchard, 2005) **or**

45 mg/m²/day for 4 days starting 8 days prior to transplantation (combined with busulfan or etoposide and carboplatin) (Berthold, 2005)

Renal Impairment

The manufacturer's labeling contains the following adjustment recommendations (for approved dosing levels) based on route of administration:

Oral: Moderate-to-severe renal impairment: Consider a reduced dose initially.

IV: BUN ≥30 mg/dL: Reduce dose by up to 50%.

The following adjustments have also been recommended:

Aronoff, 2007: Adults: Oral (based on a 6 mg once-daily dose):

CrCl 10 to 50 mL/minute: Administer 75% of dose.

CrCl <10 mL/minute: Administer 50% of dose.

Hemodialysis: Administer dose after hemodialysis.

Continuous ambulatory peritoneal dialysis (CAPD): Administer 50% of dose.

Continuous renal replacement therapy (CRRT): Administer 75% of dose.

Carlson, 2005: Oral (for melphalan-prednisone combination therapy; based on a study evaluating toxicity with melphalan dosed at 0.25 mg/kg/day for 4 days/cycle):

CrCl >10 to <30 mL/minute: Administer 75% of dose

CrCl ≤10 mL/minute: Data is insufficient for a recommendation

Kintzel, 1995:

Oral: Adjust dose in the presence of hematologic toxicity

IV:

CrCl 46 to 60 mL/minute: Administer 85% of normal dose.

CrCl 31 to 45 mL/minute: Administer 75% of normal dose.

CrCl <30 mL/minute: Administer 70% of normal dose.

Badros, 2001: IV: Autologous stem cell transplant (single-agent conditioning regimen; no busulfan or irradiation): Serum creatinine >2 mg/dL: Reduce dose from 200 mg/m² over 2 days (as 100 mg/m²/day for 2 days) to 140 mg/m² given as a single-dose infusion

Hepatic Impairment Melphalan is hepatically metabolized; however, dosage adjustment does not appear to be necessary (King, 2001).

Obesity

American Society of Clinical Oncology (ASCO) Guidelines for appropriate chemotherapy dosing in obese adults with cancer (Note: Excludes HSCT dosing): Utilize patient's actual body weight (full weight) for calculation of body surface area- or weight-based dosing, particularly when the intent of therapy is curative; manage regimen-related toxicities in the same manner as for nonobese patients; if a dose reduction is utilized due to toxicity, consider resumption of full weight-based dosing with subsequent cycles, especially if cause of toxicity (eg, hepatic or renal impairment) is resolved (Griggs, 2012).

American Society for Blood and Marrow Transplantation (ASBMT) practice guideline committee position statement on chemotherapy dosing in obesity: Utilize actual body weight (full weight) for calculation of body surface area in melphalan dosing for hematopoietic stem cell transplant conditioning regimens in adults (Bubalo, 2014).

Adjustment for Toxicity

Oral:

WBC <3000/mm³: Withhold treatment until recovery

Platelets <100,000/mm³: Withhold treatment until recovery

IV: Adjust dose based blood cell count at the nadir and day of treatment

Administration Melphalan is associated with a moderate emetic potential (depending on dose and/or administration route); antiemetics may be recommended to prevent nausea and vomiting (Dupuis, 2011).

Oral: Administer on an empty stomach (Schmidt, 2002)

Parenteral: Due to limited stability, complete administration of IV dose should occur within 60 minutes of reconstitution

IV: Infuse over 15 to 20 minutes. Extravasation may cause local tissue damage; administration by slow injection into a fast running IV solution into an injection port or via a central line is recommended; do not administer by direct injection into a peripheral vein.

Hazardous agent; use appropriate precautions for handling and disposal (NIOSH 2014 [group 1]).

Monitoring Parameters CBC with differential and platelet count, serum electrolytes, serum uric acid

Test Interactions False-positive Coombs' test [direct]

Dosage Forms Excipient information presented when available (limited, particularly for generics); consult specific product labeling.

Solution Reconstituted, Intravenous:

Alkeran: 50 mg (1 ea) [contains alcohol, usp, propylene glycol]

Generic: 50 mg (1 ea)

Tablet, Oral:

Alkeran: 2 mg

◆ Melquin 3 *see* Hydroquinone *on page 893*

◆ Melquin HP [DSC] *see* Hydroquinone *on page 893*

Memantine (me MAN teen)

Brand Names: US Namenda; Namenda Titration Pak; Namenda XR; Namenda XR Titration Pack

Brand Names: Canada ACT Memantine; Apo-Memantine; Ebixa; Med-Memantine; Mylan-Memantine; PMS-Memantine; RAN-Memantine; ratio-Memantine; Riva-Memantine; Sandoz-Memantine

Index Terms Memantine Hydrochloride

Pharmacologic Category N-Methyl-D-Aspartate Receptor Antagonist

Use Alzheimer disease: Treatment of moderate to severe dementia of the Alzheimer type.

Pregnancy Considerations Adverse events have been observed in animal reproduction studies.

Breast-Feeding Considerations It is not known if memantine is excreted in breast milk. The US labeling recommends that caution be exercised when administering memantine to nursing women. The Canadian labeling recommends avoiding use in nursing women.

Contraindications Hypersensitivity to memantine or any component of the formulation

Warnings/Precautions Rare skin hypersensitivity reactions (eg, Stevens Johnson syndrome, erythema multiforme) have been reported; advise patients to report skin reactions immediately. Discontinue use with signs of hypersensitivity reaction. Use with caution in patients with cardiovascular disease; an increased incidence of cardiac failure, angina, bradycardia, and hypertension (compared with placebo) was observed in clinical trials. Use caution with seizure disorders or severe hepatic impairment. The Canadian labeling recommends avoiding use in severe hepatic impairment. Use with caution in severe renal impairment; dose adjustments may be required. Worsening of corneal condition has been observed in a clinical trial; periodic ophthalmic exams during use have been recommended (Canadian labeling). Clearance is significantly reduced by alkaline urine; use caution with medications, dietary changes, or patient conditions which may alter urine pH.

Adverse Reactions Adverse reactions similar in immediate and extended release formulations except as noted.

1% to 10%:

Cardiovascular: Hypertension (4%), hypotension (extended release: 2%)

Central nervous system: Dizziness (5% to 7%), confusion (6%), headache (6%), anxiety (extended release: 4%), depression (extended release: 3%), drowsiness (3%), hallucination (3%), pain (3%), aggressive behavior (2%), fatigue (2%)

Endocrine & metabolic: Weight gain (extended release: 3%)

Gastrointestinal: Diarrhea (5%), constipation (3% to 5%), vomiting (2% to 3%), abdominal pain (2%)

Genitourinary: Urinary incontinence (2%)

Infection: Influenza (4%)

Neuromuscular & skeletal: Back pain (3%)

Respiratory: Cough (4%), dyspnea (2%)

<1% (Limited to important or life-threatening): Anorexia, aspiration pneumonia, atrioventricular block, bone fracture, bradycardia, brain disease, bronchitis, cardiac failure, carpal tunnel syndrome, cerebral infarction, cerebrovascular accident, cholelithiasis, colitis, complete atrioventricular block, deep vein thrombosis, drug-induced Parkinson disease, fecal incontinence, gastritis, gastroesophageal reflux disease, hepatic failure, hepatitis (including cytolytic and cholestatic), hyperglycemia, hypoglycemia, increased INR, increased serum alkaline phosphatase, neuroleptic malignant syndrome, otitis media, pancreatitis, pancytopenia, peripheral edema, prolonged Q-T interval on ECG, psychotic reaction, renal failure, second-degree atrioventricular block, sepsis, SIADH, Stevens-Johnson syndrome, suicidal tendencies, supraventricular tachycardia, thrombotic thrombocytopenic purpura, tonic-clonic seizures, torsades de pointes, upper respiratory tract infection, urinary tract infection

Drug Interactions

Metabolism/Transport Effects Substrate of OCT2

Avoid Concomitant Use There are no known interactions where it is recommended to avoid concomitant use.

Increased Effect/Toxicity

Memantine may increase the levels/effects of: Trimethoprim

The levels/effects of Memantine may be increased by: Alkalinizing Agents; BuPROPion; Carbonic Anhydrase Inhibitors; NMDA Receptor Antagonists; Trimethoprim

Decreased Effect There are no known significant interactions involving a decrease in effect.

Storage/Stability

Capsule (extended release): Store between 20°C to 25°C (68°F to 77°F).

Tablet, oral solution: Store at 25°C (77°C); excursions are permitted between 15°C and 30°C (59°F and 86°F).

Mechanism of Action Glutamate, the primary excitatory amino acid in the CNS, may contribute to the pathogenesis of Alzheimer's disease (AD) by overstimulating various glutamate receptors leading to excitotoxicity and neuronal cell death. Memantine is an uncompetitive antagonist of the N-methyl-D-aspartate (NMDA) type of glutamate receptors, located ubiquitously throughout the brain. Under normal physiologic conditions, the (unstimulated) NMDA receptor ion channel is blocked by magnesium ions, which are displaced after agonist-induced depolarization. Pathologic or excessive receptor activation, as postulated to occur during AD, prevents magnesium from reentering and blocking the channel pore resulting in a chronically open state and excessive calcium influx. Memantine binds to the intra-pore magnesium site, but with longer dwell time, and thus functions as an effective receptor blocker only under conditions of excessive stimulation; memantine does not affect normal neurotransmission.

Pharmacodynamics/Kinetics

Absorption: Well absorbed

Distribution: 9 to 11 L/kg

Protein binding: 45%

Metabolism: Partially hepatic, primarily independent of the CYP enzyme system; forms 3 metabolites (minimal activity)

Half-life elimination: Terminal: ~60 to 80 hours

Time to peak, serum: Immediate release: 3 to 7 hours; Extended release: 9 to 12 hours

Excretion: Urine (74%; ~48% of the total dose as unchanged drug; undergoes active tubular secretion moderated by pH-dependent tubular reabsorption; excretion reduced by alkaline urine pH)

Dosing

Adult & Geriatric

Alzheimer disease, moderate to severe: Oral:

Immediate release: Initial: 5 mg daily; increase dose by 5 mg daily to a target dose of 20 mg daily; wait ≥1 week between dosage changes. Doses >5 mg daily should be given in 2 divided doses. **Note:** If treatment is interrupted for longer than several days, the treatment may need to be restarted at a lower dose and retitrated.

Suggested titration: 5 mg daily for ≥1 week; 5 mg twice daily for ≥1 week; 15 mg daily given in 5 mg and 10 mg separate doses for ≥1 week; then 10 mg twice daily

Extended release: Initial: 7 mg once daily, increase dose by 7 mg daily to a target maximum dose of 28 mg once daily; wait ≥1 week between dosage changes (if previous dose well tolerated)

Note: When switching from immediate release product to the extended release product, begin the extended release product the day after the last dose of the immediate release product. Patients on immediate release 10 mg twice daily should be switched to extended release 28 mg once daily.

Missed dose: If a single dose is missed, do not double up on the next dose; take the next dose as scheduled. If several days of dosing are missed, dosing may need to be resumed at lower doses and retitrated.

Vascular dementia, mild to moderate (off-label use): Oral: Immediate release: Initial: 5 mg once daily; titrate in increments of 5 mg daily each week to a target dose of 10 mg twice daily (Orgogozo, 2002; Wilcock 2002). Additional data may be necessary to further define the role of memantine in this condition.

Renal Impairment Note: Renal function may be estimated using the Cockcroft-Gault formula for dosage adjustment purposes.

Mild impairment: No dosage adjustment necessary.

Moderate impairment:

U.S. labeling: No dosage adjustment necessary.

Canadian labeling: (CrCl 30-49 mL/minute): Initial: 5 mg once daily; after at least 1 week of therapy and if tolerated, titrate up to 5 mg twice daily; based on clinical response and tolerability, may further titrate dosage upward in weekly increments to 20 mg daily according to suggested titration schedule.

Severe impairment:

U.S. labeling: CrCl 5-29 mL/minute: Immediate release: Initial: 5 mg once daily; after at least 1 week of therapy and if tolerated, may titrate up to a target dose of 5 mg twice daily; Extended release: Target dose of 14 mg once daily.

Note: When switching from immediate release product to the extended release product, begin the extended release product the day after the last dose of the immediate release product. Patients on immediate release 5 mg twice daily should be switched to extended release 14 mg once daily.

Canadian labeling: CrCl 15-29 mL/minute: Initial: 5 mg once daily; after at least 1 week of therapy and if tolerated, may titrate up to a target dose of 5 mg twice daily

Hepatic Impairment

Mild-to-moderate impairment: No dosage adjustment necessary.

Severe impairment:

U.S. labeling: There are no dosage adjustments provided in the manufacturer's labeling (has not been studied); use with caution.

Canadian labeling: There are no dosage adjustments provided in the manufacturer's labeling (has not been studied); use is not recommended.

Administration Administer without regard to meals. Extended release capsules may be swallowed whole or entire contents of capsule may be sprinkled on applesauce and swallowed immediately; do not chew, crush, or divide. Withdraw and administer oral solution with provided dosing device; dose should be slowly squirted into the corner of the patient's mouth. Do not mix oral solution with any other liquid. The Canadian labeling recommends tablets to be swallowed whole with water.

Monitoring Parameters Cognitive function; periodic ophthalmic exam (Canadian labeling)

Dosage Forms Excipient information presented when available (limited, particularly for generics); consult specific product labeling.

Capsule Extended Release 24 Hour, Oral, as hydrochloride:

Namenda XR: 7 mg, 14 mg, 21 mg, 28 mg

Namenda XR Titration Pack: 7 mg (7s) and 14 mg (7s) and 21 mg (7s) and 28 mg (7s)

Solution, Oral, as hydrochloride:

Namenda: 10 mg/5 mL (360 mL) [peppermint flavor]

Generic: 2 mg/mL (360 mL)

Tablet, Oral, as hydrochloride:

Namenda: 5 mg [contains fd&c blue #2 (indigotine), fd&c yellow #6 (sunset yellow)]

Namenda: 10 mg

Namenda Titration Pak: 5 mg (28s) and 10 mg (21s) [contains fd&c blue #2 (indigotine), fd&c yellow #6 (sunset yellow)]

Generic: 5 mg, 10 mg, 5 mg (28s) and 10 mg (21s)

◆ Memantine Hydrochloride *see* Memantine *on page 1139*

◆ Menactra *see* Meningococcal (Groups A / C / Y and W-135) Diphtheria Conjugate Vaccine *on page 1141*

◆ MenACWY *see* Meningococcal (Groups A / C / Y and W-135) Diphtheria Conjugate Vaccine *on page 1141*

- ◆ MenACWY-D (Menactra) *see* Meningococcal (Groups A / C / Y and W-135) Diphtheria Conjugate Vaccine *on page 1141*
- ◆ MenACWY-CRM (Menveo) *see* Meningococcal (Groups A / C / Y and W-135) Diphtheria Conjugate Vaccine *on page 1141*
- ◆ M-END DM [OTC] [DSC] *see* Chlorpheniramine, Pseudoephedrine, and Dextromethorphan *on page 379*
- ◆ Menest *see* Estrogens (Esterified) *on page 693*
- ◆ Menest® (Can) *see* Estrogens (Esterified) *on page 693*
- ◆ Menhibrix *see* Meningococcal Polysaccharide (Groups C and Y) and *Haemophilus* b Tetanus Toxoid Conjugate Vaccine *on page 1142*
- ◆ Meningococcal Conjugate Vaccine *see* Meningococcal (Groups A / C / Y and W-135) Diphtheria Conjugate Vaccine *on page 1141*

Meningococcal (Groups A / C / Y and W-135) Diphtheria Conjugate Vaccine

(me NIN joe kok al groops aye, see, why & dubl yoo won thur tee fyve dif THEER ee a KON joo gate vak SEEN)

Brand Names: US Menactra; Menveo
Brand Names: Canada Menactra; Menveo
Index Terms MCV; MCV4; MenACWY; MenACWY-CRM (Menveo); MenACWY-D (Menactra); Meningococcal Conjugate Vaccine
Pharmacologic Category Vaccine; Vaccine, Inactivated (Bacterial)
Additional Appendix Information
Immunization Administration Recommendations *on page 1974*
Immunization Schedules *on page 1979*
Use
Meningococcal disease prevention: Provide active immunization of children and adults against invasive meningococcal disease caused by *N. meningitidis* serogroups A, C, Y, and W-135.

The Advisory Committee on Immunization Practices (ACIP) (CDC/ACIP [Cohn 2013]; CDC/ACIP [MacNeil 2014]):
ACIP recommends routine vaccination of the following:
- Children and adolescents 11 to 18 years of age
- Persons ≥2 months of age who are at increased risk of meningococcal disease
- Persons (in all recommended age groups) at increased risk who are part of outbreaks caused by vaccine preventable serogroups
Those at increased risk of meningococcal disease include the following:
- Persons ≥2 months of age with medical conditions such as anatomic or functional asplenia (including sickle cell disease) or persistent compliment component deficiencies (eg, C₅-C₉, properdin, factor H, or factor D)
- Persons ≥2 months of age that travel to or reside in countries where meningococcal disease is hyperendemic or epidemic, especially if contact with the local population will be prolonged
- Unvaccinated or incompletely vaccinated first year college students living in residence halls
- Military recruits
- Microbiologists with occupational exposure

The Canadian National Advisory Committee on Immunization (NACI): NACI recommends a routine vaccination at ~12 years of age but no booster unless at a continued high risk of exposure. Either quadrivalent vaccine may be used; NACI does not have a preference. NACI recommends use of Menveo (off-label use) for high risk persons 2 months to 2 years of age if vaccination with a quadrivalent vaccine is needed; may also be considered for use in persons ≥56 years of age (NACI, 39[1] 2013). Additional recommendations may be found at www.phac-aspc.gc.ca/publicat/ccdr-rmtc/13vol39/acs-dcc-1/index-eng.php
Medication Guide Available Yes
Dosing
Adult Immunization: IM:
Manufacturer's labeling: Menactra, Menveo: Adults ≤55 years: 0.5 mL/dose given as single dose

ACIP recommendations (CDC/ACIP [Cohn 2013]; CDC/ACIP [Kim 2015]) Use of the abbreviation, MenACWY, refers to either meningococcal quadrivalent conjugate vaccine. MenACWY-CRM refers specifically to Menveo; MenACWY-D refers specifically to Menactra.

Primary vaccination:
Adults 19 to 21 years: Not routinely recommended; may receive one 0.5 mL dose as a catch-up vaccination if no dose was received after the sixteenth birthday. **Note:** Patients who are HIV positive should receive 2 doses 2 months apart.
Adults ≥22 years: Not routinely recommended; see dosing for persons at increased risk
Primary vaccination: Persons at increased risk for meningococcal disease:
Adults ≤55 years not previously vaccinated and who have persistent complement deficiencies, functional or anatomic asplenia, or who have HIV infection plus another indication for vaccination: Two 0.5 mL doses, given ≥2 months apart. If using MenACWY-D (Menactra), administer ≥4 weeks after completion of all PCV doses
Adults ≤55 years not previously vaccinated and who are either: First year college students ≤21 years of age living in residential housing, traveling to or residents of areas where meningococcal disease is endemic/hyperendemic, at risk during a community outbreak, military recruits, or microbiologists routinely exposed to *Neisseria meningitidis*: One 0.5 mL dose. If using MenACWY-D (Menactra), administer ≥4 weeks after completion of all PCV doses. College students ≤21 years should have documentation of a vaccination not more than 5 years before enrollment (preferably a dose on their sixteenth birthday). **Note:** Patients who are HIV positive should receive 2 doses 2 months apart.
Adults ≥56 years: Meningococcal polysaccharide vaccine (MPSV4, Menomune) is preferred for meningococcal vaccine-naïve persons in this age group who require a single dose. If multiple doses are anticipated, see booster dosing for persons at increased risk.
Booster dose: Persons NOT at increased risk for meningococcal disease: Adults ≤21 years: One 0.5 mL dose if the first dose was given prior to the sixteenth birthday. A booster dose is not needed if the primary dose was given after the sixteenth birthday unless the person becomes at increased risk for meningococcal disease.
Booster vaccination: Persons at increased risk for meningococcal disease:
Manufacturer labeling: Menactra: Repeat a single dose ≥4 years after prior dose.
ACIP recommendations (CDC/ACIP [Cohn 2013]; CDC/ACIP [Kim 2015]):
Adults ≤55 years: Repeat dose every 5 years if the person remains at increased risk.
Adults ≥56 years: Persons previously vaccinated with MenACWY and who require revaccination or for whom multiple doses are anticipated, MenACWY (Menactra or Menveo) is preferred. Otherwise, meningococcal polysaccharide vaccine (MPSV4, Menomune) is preferred for meningococcal vaccine naïve persons in this age group who require a single dose.
Pediatric Immunization: IM:
Manufacturer's labeling:
Menactra:
Infants ≥9 months and Children <2 years: 0.5 mL/dose given as a 2-dose series, 3 months apart
Children ≥2 years and Adolescents: Refer to adult dosing.
Menveo: Age at initial vaccination:
Infants 2 months to <7 months: 0.5 mL/dose given as a 4-dose series at 2, 4, 6, and 12 months of age
Infants ≥7 months and Children <2 years: 0.5 mL/dose given as a 2-dose series, with the second dose given during the second year of life and at least 3 months after the first dose
Children 2 to <6 years: 0.5 mL/dose given as a single dose; for children at continued high risk of meningococcal disease, may consider an additional dose given 2 months after the first dose
Children ≥6 years and Adolescents: Refer to adult dosing.

ACIP recommendations (CDC/ACIP [Cohn 2013]; CDC/ACIP [MacNeil 2014; CDC/ACIP [Strikas 2015]): **Note:** Use of the abbreviation, MenACWY, refers to either meningococcal quadrivalent conjugate vaccine. MenACWY-CRM refers specifically to Menveo; MenACWY-D refers specifically to Menactra.

Primary vaccination:

Infants, Children, and Adolescents:

<11 years: Not routinely recommended; see dosing for persons at increased risk

11 to 12 years: One 0.5 mL dose. Children not at increased risk for meningococcal disease who may have been previously vaccinated with Hib-MenCY-TT (MenHibrix) or MenACWY prior to their tenth birthday, should receive the routinely recommended doses of MenACWY at 11 to 12 years. **Note:** Patients who are HIV positive should receive 2 doses 2 months apart.

13 to 18 years: One 0.5 mL dose if not previously vaccinated. **Note:** Patients who are HIV positive should receive 2 doses 2 months apart.

Primary vaccination: Persons at increased risk for meningococcal disease:

Infants ≥2 months and Children <2 years with anatomic or functional asplenia, including sickle-cell disease: Dosing based on age at initial dose:

Infants and Children 8 weeks to 6 months: MenACWY-CRM (Menveo): IM: 0.5 mL per dose for a total of 4 doses given as follows: 2, 4, 6, and 12 months

Children 7 to 23 months (incomplete vaccination): MenACWY-CRM (Menveo): IM: 0.5 mL per dose for a total of 2 doses; the second dose should be given at age ≥12 months and at least 12 weeks after the first dose.

Infants ≥2 months and Children <2 years with persistent complement component deficiency: Dosing based on age at first dose:

Infants 8 weeks to 6 months: MenACWY-CRM (Menveo): IM: 0.5 mL per dose for a total of 4 doses given as follows: 2, 4, 6, and 12 months

Infants and Children 7 to 23 months:

MenACWY-CRM (Menveo): Infants and Children 7 to 23 months: IM: 0.5 mL per dose for a total of 2 doses; the second dose should be given at age ≥12 months and at least 12 weeks after the first dose.

MenACWY-D (Menactra): Infants and Children 9 to 23 months: IM: 0.5 mL per dose for a total of 2 doses; the second dose should be given at least three months after the first dose. May be given as early as 8 weeks apart if needed prior to travel.

Infants and Children 2 months to 2 years for community outbreak (due to vaccine serogroup): Initiate or complete an age appropriate series of MenACWY-CRM (Menveo) or MenACWY-D (Menactra); see Primary vaccination above for dosing.

Infants and Children 2 months to <2 years with travel to or residence in countries with hyperendemic or epidemic meningococcal disease: Initiate or complete an age appropriate series of MenACWY-CRM (Menveo) or MenACWY-D (Menactra); see Primary vaccination above for dosing.

Children ≥2 years and Adolescents not previously vaccinated and who have persistent complement deficiencies, functional or anatomic asplenia, or who have HIV infection plus another indication for vaccination: Two 0.5 mL doses, given ≥2 months apart apart. If using MenACWY-D (Menactra), administer ≥4 weeks after completion of all PCV doses

Children ≥2 years and Adolescents not previously vaccinated and who are either: First year college students ≤21 years of age living in residential housing, traveling to or residents of areas where meningococcal disease is endemic/hyperendemic, at risk during a community outbreak, military recruits, or microbiologists routinely exposed to Neisseria meningitidis: One 0.5 mL dose. If using MenACWY-D (Menactra), administer ≥4 weeks after completion of all PCV doses. College students ≤21 years should have documentation of a vaccination not more than 5 years before enrollment (preferably a dose on their sixteenth birthday). **Note:** Patients who are HIV positive should receive 2 doses 2 months apart.

Booster dose: Persons NOT at increased risk for meningococcal disease: Children ≥11 years and Adolescents: If primary vaccination was at 11 to 12 years, the booster dose should be given at age 16. If the primary vaccination was given at 13 to 15 years, the booster dose should be given at age 16 to 18. Minimum interval between MenACWY (Menveo or Menactra) doses is 8 weeks. A booster dose is not needed if the primary dose was given after the sixteenth birthday unless the person becomes at increased risk for meningococcal disease. (CDC/ACIP [Cohn 2013])

Booster vaccination: Persons at increased risk for meningococcal disease:

Manufacturer labeling: Menactra: Adolescents ≥15 years: Repeat a single dose ≥4 years after prior dose.

ACIP recommendations (CDC/ACIP [Cohn 2013]):

If first dose received at 2 months to 6 years of age: Repeat dose 3 years after primary vaccination, and every 5 years thereafter if the person remains at increased risk.

If first dose received at ≥7 years of age: Repeat dose 5 years after primary vaccination, and every 5 years thereafter if the person remains at increased risk.

Renal Impairment There are no dosage adjustments provided in the manufacturer's labeling.

Hepatic Impairment There are no dosage adjustments provided in the manufacturer's labeling.

Additional Information Complete prescribing information should be consulted for additional detail.

Dosage Forms Excipient information presented when available (limited, particularly for generics); consult specific product labeling.

Injection, solution [preservative free]:

Menactra: 4 mcg each of polysaccharide antigen groups A, C, Y, and W-135 [bound to diphtheria toxoid 48 mcg] per 0.5 mL [MCV4 or MenACWY-D]

Menveo: MenA oligosaccharide 10 mcg, MenC oligosaccharide 5 mcg, MenY oligosaccharide 5 mcg, and MenW-135 oligosaccharide 5 mcg [bound to CRM$_{197}$ protein 32.7-64.1 mcg] per 0.5 mL (0.5 mL) [MenACWY-CRM; supplied in two vials, one containing MenA powder and one containing MenCYW-135 liquid]

Meningococcal Polysaccharide (Groups C and Y) and *Haemophilus* b Tetanus Toxoid Conjugate Vaccine

(me NIN joe kok al pol i SAK a ride groops see & why & he MOF i lus bee TET a nus TOKS oyd KON joo gate vak SEEN)

Brand Names: US Menhibrix

Index Terms Hib-MenCY-TT

Pharmacologic Category Vaccine; Vaccine, Inactivated (Bacterial)

Additional Appendix Information

Immunization Administration Recommendations *on page 1974*

Immunization Schedules *on page 1979*

Use Meningococcal and *Haemophilus influenza* type b disease prevention: To provide active immunity to prevent invasive disease caused by meningococcal serogroups C and Y and *Haemophilus influenzae* type b

The Advisory Committee on Immunization Practices (ACIP) (CDC/ACIP [Cohn 2013]) recommends vaccination only for infants 2-18 months of age who are at increased risk for meningococcal disease, including:

- Infants with persistent complement pathway deficiencies
- Infants with anatomic or functional asplenia, including sickle cell disease
- Infants in communities with serogroups C and Y meningococcal disease outbreaks

The ACIP does not recommend routine vaccination for infants not at increased risk for meningococcal disease. In addition, infants traveling to certain areas (eg, meningitis belt of sub-Saharan Africa) will require a meningococcal vaccine with serogroups A and W$_{135}$; vaccination with Hib-MenCY-TT will not be adequate (CDC/ACIP [Cohn 2013])

Dosing

Pediatric Primary immunization: Infants ≥6 weeks and Children ≤18 months: IM: 0.5 mL/dose given as a four-dose series at 2, 4, 6, and 12 to 15 months of age. The first dose may be given as early as 6 weeks of age and the fourth dose may be given as late as 18 months of age.

Note: If an infant at increased risk is behind on Hib vaccine doses, Hib-MenCY-TT may be used to catch up using the current Hib schedule. If the first dose of Hib-MenCY-TT is given ≥12 months of age, two doses should be given 8 weeks apart. If infants have/will receive a different Hib vaccine, a two-dose series of a quadrivalent meningococcal vaccine is recommended (Menactra for ages 9 to 23 months; Menactra or Menveo for ages >23 months) (CDC/ACIP [Cohn 2013]).

Renal Impairment There are no dosage adjustments provided in manufacturer's labeling.

Hepatic Impairment There are no dosage adjustments provided in manufacturer's labeling.

Additional Information Complete prescribing information should be consulted for additional detail.

Dosage Forms Excipient information presented when available (limited, particularly for generics); consult specific product labeling.

Solution Reconstituted, Intramuscular [preservative free]:
  Menhibrix: 5 mcg each of polysaccharide antigen groups C and Y, and 2.5 mcg Haemophilus b capsular polysaccharide per 0.5 mL dose (1 ea) [contains tetanus toxoid]

♦ Meningococcal Polysaccharide Vaccine *see* Meningococcal Polysaccharide Vaccine (Groups A / C / Y and W-135) *on page 1143*

Meningococcal Polysaccharide Vaccine (Groups A / C / Y and W-135)
(me NIN joe kok al pol i SAK a ride vak SEEN groops aye, see, why & dubl yoo won thur tee fyve)

Brand Names: US Menomune-A/C/Y/W-135
Brand Names: Canada Menomune-A/C/Y/W-135
Index Terms Meningococcal Polysaccharide Vaccine; MPSV; MPSV4
Pharmacologic Category Vaccine; Vaccine, Inactivated (Bacterial)
Additional Appendix Information
  Immunization Administration Recommendations *on page 1974*
  Immunization Schedules *on page 1979*
Use
  Meningococcal disease prevention: Active immunization of patients 2 years and older to prevent invasive meningococcal disease caused by *Neisseria meningitidis* serogroups A, C, Y, and W-135.
  The Advisory Committee on Immunization Practices (ACIP) recommends routine vaccination for persons at increased risk for meningococcal disease. Meningococcal quadrivalent conjugate vaccine (MenACWY; Menactra, Menveo) is preferred; meningococcal polysaccharide vaccine (MPSV4; Menomune) is preferred in meningococcal vaccine-naive adults ≥56 years of age requiring only a single vaccination (CDC/ACIP [Cohn 2013]).
  Those at increased risk of meningococcal disease include the following:
  - Persons ≥2 months of age with medical conditions such as anatomical or functional asplenia or persistent compliment component deficiencies (eg, C_5-C_9, properdin, factor H, or factor D)
  - Persons ≥9 months of age that travel to or reside in countries where meningococcal disease is hyperendemic or epidemic, especially if contact with the local population will be prolonged
  - Unvaccinated or incompletely vaccinated first year college students living in residence halls
  - Military recruits
  - Microbiologists with occupational exposure
  - Persons (in all recommended age groups) at risk who are part of outbreaks caused by vaccine preventable serogroups
Dosing
  Adult & Geriatric
    Immunization: SubQ: 0.5 mL/dose
    ACIP recommendations (CDC/ACIP [Cohn 2013]):
      Adults <56 years: Not routinely recommended.
      Adults ≥56 years: Meningococcal polysaccharide vaccine (MPSV4,Menomune) is preferred for meningococcal vaccine-naive persons in this age group who are at increased risk of meningococcal infection and require a single dose (eg, travelers or during a community outbreak). Persons previously vaccinated with a quadrivalent meningococcal conjugate vaccine (MenACWY, Menveo, or Menactra) and who require revaccination or for whom multiple doses are anticipated, MenACWY-D (Menactra) is preferred (eg, persons with asplenia or microbiologists).
  Pediatric
    Immunization: Children ≥2 years and Adolescents: SubQ: 0.5 mL/dose
    ACIP recommendations (CDC/ACIP [Cohn 2013]):
      Children and Adolescents: Not routinely recommended.
  Renal Impairment There are no dosage adjustments provided in manufacturer's labeling.
  Hepatic Impairment There are no dosage adjustments provided in manufacturer's labeling.
  Additional Information Complete prescribing information should be consulted for additional detail.

Dosage Forms Excipient information presented when available (limited, particularly for generics); consult specific product labeling.
Injection, powder for reconstitution [MPSV4]:
  Menomune-A/C/Y/W-135: 50 mcg each of polysaccharide antigen groups A, C, Y, and W-135 per 0.5 mL dose [contains lactose 2.5-5 mg/0.5 mL, natural rubber/natural latex in packaging, thimerosal in diluent for multidose vial]

♦ Menomune-A/C/Y/W-135 *see* Meningococcal Polysaccharide Vaccine (Groups A / C / Y and W-135) *on page 1143*

♦ Menopur *see* Menotropins *on page 1143*

♦ Menostar *see* Estradiol (Systemic) *on page 681*

Menotropins (men oh TROE pins)

Brand Names: US Menopur; Repronex
Brand Names: Canada Menopur; Repronex
Index Terms hMG; Human Menopausal Gonadotropin
Pharmacologic Category Gonadotropin; Ovulation Stimulator
Use
  Menopur: For multiple follicle development and pregnancy in ovulatory women as part of an assisted reproductive technology (ART) cycle
  Repronex: In conjunction with hCG to for multiple follicular development (controlled ovarian stimulation) and ovulation induction in women who have previously received GnRH agonist or antagonist for pituitary suppression
  Limitations of use: Prior to therapy, preform a complete gynecologic exam and endocrinologic evaluation to diagnose the cause of infertility; exclude the possibility of pregnancy; evaluate the fertility status of the male partner; exclude a diagnosis of primary ovarian failure.
Dosing
  Adult
    Ovulation induction (females): *Repronex:* IM, SubQ: Initial: 150 units once daily for the first 5 days of treatment. Adjustments should not be made more frequently than once every 2 days and should not exceed 75-150 units per adjustment based on ultrasound monitoring of ovarian response and/or measurement of serum estradiol levels. Maximum daily dose: 450 units; treatment >12 days is not recommended. If patient's response is appropriate, administer hCG one day following the last dose of Repronex. Hold dose if serum estradiol is >2000 pg/mL, if the ovaries are abnormally enlarged, or if abdominal pain occurs; the patient should also be advised to refrain from intercourse. May repeat process if follicular development is inadequate or if pregnancy does not occur.
    Assisted reproductive technologies (ART) (females): *Menopur:* SubQ: Initial: 225 units once daily beginning on cycle day 2 or 3; Menotropins may be administered together with urofollitropin and the total initial dose of both products combined should not exceed 225 units (menotropins 150 units and urofollitropin 75 units; or menotropins 75 units and urofollitropin 150 units). Dose should be adjusted after 5 days based on ultrasound monitoring of ovarian response and/or measurement of serum estradiol levels. Do not make additional adjustments more frequently than once every 2 days or by >150 units. Maximum daily dose: 450 units (of menotropins, or menotropins plus urofollitrop); treatment >20 days is not recommended. Once adequate follicular development is evident, hCG should be administered. Withhold the hCG dose if ovarian monitoring suggests an increased risk of ovarian hyperstimulation syndrome (OHSS).
    Repronex: IM, SubQ: Initial: 225 units once daily; adjustments in dose based on ultrasound monitoring of ovarian response and/or measurement of serum estradiol levels should not be made more frequently than once every 2 days and should not exceed more than 75-150 units per adjustment. Maximum daily dose: 450 units; treatment >12 days is not recommended. Once adequate follicular development is evident, hCG should be administered to induce final follicular maturation in preparation for oocyte retrieval. Withhold the hCG dose if ovarian monitoring suggests an increased risk of OHSS.
    Spermatogenesis (males) (off-label use): IM: Following pretreatment with hCG: 75 units 3 times per week with hCG twice weekly until sperm is detected in the ejaculate (4-6 months); if response is inadequate after 6 months, may increase menotropins dosage to 150 units 3 times per week for another 6 months (AACE, 2002)

Renal Impairment There are no dosage adjustments provided in manufacturer's labeling (has not been studied).

Hepatic Impairment There are no dosage adjustments provided in manufacturer's labeling (has not been studied).

Additional Information Complete prescribing information should be consulted for additional detail.

Dosage Forms Considerations 75 units of menotropins represents 75 units each of FSH activity and LH activity

Dosage Forms Excipient information presented when available (limited, particularly for generics); consult specific product labeling.

Injection, powder for reconstitution:
Menopur: 75 units [supplied with diluent]
Repronex: 75 units [supplied with diluent]

◆ Mentax see Butenafine on page 275

◆ Menthol and Methyl Salicylate see Methyl Salicylate and Menthol on page 1187

◆ Menveo see Meningococcal (Groups A / C / Y and W-135) Diphtheria Conjugate Vaccine on page 1141

Meperidine (me PER i deen)

Brand Names: US Demerol; Meperitab
Brand Names: Canada Demerol
Index Terms Isonipecaine Hydrochloride; Meperidine Hydrochloride; Pethidine Hydrochloride
Pharmacologic Category Analgesic, Opioid
Additional Appendix Information
Opioid Conversion Table and Morphine Equivalent Dose Table on page 1955
Use Management of moderate to severe pain; preoperative sedation, and obstetrical analgesia
Pregnancy Considerations Animal reproduction studies have not been conducted by the manufacturer. Meperidine crosses the placenta; meperidine and its active metabolite accumulate in the fetus. Respiratory or CNS depression should be expected to occur in the newborn if maternal IM administration occurs within a few hours of delivery (Mattingly 2003). When used for pain relief during labor, opioids may temporarily affect the heart rate of the fetus. Due to the prolonged half-life of the active metabolite, dose-dependent sedation in the neonate may be observed for 2-3 days following delivery. Meperidine has been used for the management of pain during labor; however, due to adverse maternal and fetal effects, other opioids may be preferred. Meperidine should also be avoided following delivery when postoperative analgesia is needed (ACOG 2002).

If chronic opioid exposure occurs in pregnancy, adverse events in the newborn (including withdrawal) may occur; monitoring of the neonate is recommended. The minimum effective dose should be used if opioids are needed (Chou 2009). Neonatal abstinence syndrome following opioid exposure may present with autonomic (eg, fever, temperature instability), gastrointestinal (eg, diarrhea, vomiting, poor feeding/weight gain), or neurologic (eg, high-pitched crying, increased muscle tone, irritability, seizure, tremor) symptoms (Dow 2012; Hudak 2012).

Breast-Feeding Considerations Meperidine is excreted in breast milk and may cause CNS and/or respiratory depression in the nursing infant. Due to the potential for serious adverse reactions in the nursing infant, the manufacturer recommends a decision be made whether to discontinue nursing or to discontinue the drug, taking into account the importance of treatment to the mother.

Small concentrations of meperidine are excreted into breast milk following single doses. With multiple doses, concentrations of meperidine and the active metabolite may increase and both are slowly eliminated by a nursing infant (Spigset 2000). Parenteral opioids used during labor have the potential to interfere with a newborns natural reflex to nurse within the first few hours after birth. Nursing infants exposed to large doses of opioids should be monitored for apnea and sedation. If treatment for pain in nursing women is needed, other agents are preferred (Montgomery 2012)

Contraindications Hypersensitivity to meperidine or any component of the formulation; use with or within 14 days of MAO inhibitors; severe respiratory insufficiency

Warnings/Precautions Oral meperidine is not recommended for acute/chronic pain management. Meperidine should not be used for acute/cancer pain because of the risk of neurotoxicity. Normeperidine (an active metabolite and CNS stimulant) may accumulate and precipitate anxiety, tremors, or seizures; risk increases with CNS or renal dysfunction, prolonged use (>48 hours), and cumulative dose (>600 mg/24 hours in adults). The Institute for Safe Medication Practice recommends avoiding the use of meperidine for pain control, especially in the elderly and renally impaired (ISMP 2007). In the elderly; meperidine is not an effective oral analgesic at commonly used doses; may cause neurotoxicity; other agents are preferred in the elderly (Beers Criteria).

May cause CNS depression, which may impair physical or mental abilities; patients must be cautioned about performing tasks which require mental alertness (eg, operating machinery or driving). Potentially significant drug interactions may exist, requiring dose or frequency adjustment, additional monitoring, and/or selection of alternative therapy. Use only with extreme caution (if at all) in patients with head injury or increased intracranial pressure (ICP). Avoid use in patients with CNS depression or coma as these patients are susceptible to intracranial effects of CO_2 retention. Use caution with pulmonary, hepatic, or renal disorders, supraventricular tachycardias (including atrial flutter), acute abdominal conditions, biliary tract dysfunction, pancreatitis, delirium tremens, hypothyroidism, myxedema, kyphoscoliosis, morbid obesity, adrenal insufficiency, Addison's disease, seizure disorders, pheochromocytoma, BPH, or urethral stricture. May cause hypotension (including orthostatic hypotension); use with caution in patients with depleted blood volume or drugs which may exaggerate hypotensive effects (including phenothiazines or general anesthetics).

In patients with sickle cell anemia, use with caution and decrease initial dose; normeperidine (active metabolite) may accumulate and induce seizures in these patients; **Note:** Meperidine recommended for use in sickle cell patients by the American Pain Society (APS 2008) and should only be used in sickle cell patients with a vaso-occlusive crisis (VOC) if it is the only effective opioid for an individual patient (NHLBI 2014).

An opioid-containing analgesic regimen should be tailored to each patient's needs and based upon the type of pain being treated (acute versus chronic), the route of administration, degree of tolerance for opioids (naive versus chronic user), age, weight, and medical condition. The optimal analgesic dose varies widely among patients. Some preparations contain sulfites which may cause allergic reaction. Tolerance or drug dependence may result from extended use. Healthcare provider should be alert to problems of abuse, misuse, and diversion. Concurrent use of agonist/antagonist analgesics may precipitate withdrawal symptoms and/or reduced analgesic efficacy in patients following prolonged therapy with mu opioid agonists. Abrupt discontinuation following prolonged use may also lead to withdrawal symptoms. Avoid use in the elderly.

After chronic maternal exposure to opioids, neonatal withdrawal syndrome may occur in the newborn; monitor neonate closely. Signs and symptoms include irritability, hyperactivity and abnormal sleep pattern, high-pitched cry, tremor, vomiting, diarrhea, and failure to gain weight. Onset, duration and severity depend on the drug used, duration of use, maternal dose, and rate of drug elimination by the newborn. Opioid withdrawal syndrome in the neonate, unlike in adults, may be life-threatening and should be treated according to protocols developed by neonatology experts.

Benzyl alcohol and derivatives: Some dosage forms may contain sodium benzoate/benzoic acid; benzoic acid (benzoate) is a metabolite of benzyl alcohol; large amounts of benzyl alcohol (≥99 mg/kg/day) have been associated with a potentially fatal toxicity ("gasping syndrome") in neonates; the "gasping syndrome" consists of metabolic acidosis, respiratory distress, gasping respirations, CNS dysfunction (including convulsions, intracranial hemorrhage), hypotension, and cardiovascular collapse (AAP ["Inactive" 1997]; CDC, 1982); some data suggests that benzoate displaces bilirubin from protein binding sites (Ahlfors 2001); avoid or use dosage forms containing benzyl alcohol derivative with caution in neonates. See manufacturer's labeling.

Use with extreme caution in patients having an acute asthma attack, with chronic obstructive pulmonary disease or cor pulmonale, kyphoscoliosis or other skeletal disorder which may alter respiratory function, and patients having a substantially decreased respiratory reserve, hypoxia, hypercarbia, or preexisting respiratory depression; even therapeutic doses may decrease respiratory drive to the point of apnea.

Adverse Reactions Frequency not defined.
Cardiovascular: Bradycardia, cardiac arrest, circulatory depression, flushing, hypotension, palpitations, shock, syncope, tachycardia

Central nervous system: Agitation, confusion, delirium, disorientation, dizziness, drug dependence (physical dependence), habituation, hallucination, headache, increased intracranial pressure, involuntary muscle movements (including muscle twitching, myoclonus), mood changes (including euphoria, dysphoria), sedation, seizure (associated with metabolite accumulation), serotonin syndrome

Dermatologic: Diaphoresis, pruritus, skin rash, urticaria

Gastrointestinal: Biliary colic, constipation, nausea, spasm of sphincter of Oddi, vomiting, xerostomia

Genitourinary: Urinary retention

Hypersensitivity: Anaphylaxis, histamine release, hypersensitivity reaction

Local: Injection site reaction (including pain, wheal, and flare)

Neuromuscular & skeletal: Tremor, weakness

Ophthalmic: Visual disturbance

Respiratory: Dyspnea, respiratory arrest, respiratory depression

<1% (Limited to important or life-threatening): Hypogonadism (Brennan 2013; Debono 2011)

Drug Interactions

Metabolism/Transport Effects None known.

Avoid Concomitant Use

Avoid concomitant use of Meperidine with any of the following: Azelastine (Nasal); Dapoxetine; Eluxadoline; MAO Inhibitors; Mixed Agonist / Antagonist Opioids; Orphenadrine; Paraldehyde; Thalidomide

Increased Effect/Toxicity

Meperidine may increase the levels/effects of: Alcohol (Ethyl); Alvimopan; Antipsychotic Agents; Azelastine (Nasal); CNS Depressants; Desmopressin; Diuretics; Eluxadoline; Hydrocodone; Methotrimeprazine; Metoclopramide; Metyrosine; Orphenadrine; Paraldehyde; Pramipexole; Ramosetron; ROPINIRole; Rotigotine; Serotonin Modulators; Suvorexant; Thalidomide; Zolpidem

The levels/effects of Meperidine may be increased by: Amphetamines; Anticholinergic Agents; Antiemetics (5HT3 Antagonists); Antipsychotic Agents; Antipsychotic Agents (Phenothiazines); Barbiturates; Brimonidine (Topical); Cannabis; Cimetidine; Dapoxetine; Doxylamine; Dronabinol; Droperidol; HydrOXYzine; Kava Kava; Magnesium Sulfate; MAO Inhibitors; Metaxalone; Methotrimeprazine; Minocycline; Nabilone; Perampanel; Protease Inhibitors; Rufinamide; Sodium Oxybate; Succinylcholine; Tapentadol; Tetrahydrocannabinol

Decreased Effect

Meperidine may decrease the levels/effects of: Pegvisomant

The levels/effects of Meperidine may be decreased by: Ammonium Chloride; Fosphenytoin; Mixed Agonist / Antagonist Opioids; Naltrexone; Phenytoin; Protease Inhibitors

Storage/Stability

Injection solution: Store at 20°C to 25°C (68°F to 77°F); excursions permitted to 15°C to 30°C (59°F to 86°F).

Tablets: Store at 25°C (77°F); excursions permitted to 15°C to 30°C (59°F to 86°F).

Mechanism of Action Binds to opioid receptors in the CNS, causing inhibition of ascending pain pathways, altering the perception of and response to pain; produces generalized CNS depression

Pharmacodynamics/Kinetics

Onset of action: Analgesic: Oral, SubQ: 10-15 minutes; IV: ~5 minutes

Peak effect: SubQ: ~1 hour; Oral: 2 hours

Duration: Oral, SubQ: 2-4 hours

Absorption: IM: Erratic and highly variable

Protein binding: 65% to 75%

Metabolism: Hepatic; hydrolyzed to meperidinic acid (inactive) or undergoes N-demethylation to normeperidine (active; has 1/2 the analgesic effect and 2-3 times the CNS effects of meperidine)

Bioavailability: ~50% to 60%; increased with liver disease

Half-life elimination:

Parent drug: Terminal phase: Adults: 2.5-4 hours, Liver disease: 7-11 hours

Normeperidine (active metabolite): 15-30 hours; can accumulate with high doses (>600 mg/day) or with decreased renal function

Excretion: Urine (as metabolites)

Dosing

Adult Note: The American Pain Society (2008) and ISMP (2007) do not recommend meperidine's use as an analgesic. If use in acute pain (in patients without renal or CNS disease) cannot be avoided, treatment should be limited to ≤48 hours and doses should not exceed 600 mg/24 hours. Oral route is not recommended for treatment of acute or chronic pain. If IV route is required, consider a reduced dose. Patients with prior opioid exposure may require higher initial doses.

Pain, moderate to severe (analgesic): Oral, IM, SubQ: 50 to 150 mg every 3 to 4 hours as needed

Preoperatively: IM, SubQ: 50 to 100 mg given 30 to 90 minutes before the beginning of anesthesia

Obstetrical analgesia: IM, SubQ: 50 to 100 mg when pain becomes regular; may repeat at every 1- to 3-hour intervals

Postoperative shivering (off-label use): IV: 25 to 50 mg once (Crowley 2008; Kranke 2002; Mercandante 1994; Wang 1999)

Geriatric Avoid use (American Pain Society 2008; ISMP 2007).

Pediatric Note: The American Pain Society (2008) and ISMP (2007) do not recommend meperidine's use as an analgesic. If use in acute pain (in patients without renal or CNS disease) cannot be avoided, treatment should be limited to ≤48 hours and doses should not exceed 600 mg/24 hours. Oral route is not recommended for treatment of acute or chronic pain. If IV route is required, consider a reduced dose. Patients with prior opioid exposure may require higher initial doses.

Pain, moderate to severe (analgesic): Oral, IM, SubQ: 1.1 to 1.8 mg/kg/dose every 3 to 4 hours as needed (maximum: 50 to 150 mg/dose)

Preoperatively: IM, SubQ: 1.1 to 2.2 mg/kg given 30 to 90 minutes before the beginning of anesthesia (maximum: 50 to 100 mg/dose)

Renal Impairment Avoid use in renal impairment (American Pain Society 2008; ISMP 2007).

Hepatic Impairment Use with caution in severe hepatic impairment; consider a lower initial dose when initiating therapy. An increased opioid effect may be seen in patients with cirrhosis; dose reduction is more important for the oral than IV route.

Administration

Solution for injection: Meperidine may be administered IM, SubQ, or IV; IV push should be administered slowly using a diluted solution, use of a 10 mg/mL concentration has been recommended.

Oral solution: Administer solution in 1/2 glass of water; undiluted solution may exert topical anesthetic effect on mucous membranes

Monitoring Parameters Pain relief, respiratory and mental status, blood pressure; observe patient for excessive sedation, CNS depression, seizures, respiratory depression; signs or symptoms of hypogonadism or hypoadrenalism (Brennan 2013)

Test Interactions Increased amylase (S), increased BSP retention, increased CPK (IM injections)

Dosage Forms Excipient information presented when available (limited, particularly for generics); consult specific product labeling.

Solution, Injection, as hydrochloride:

Demerol: 25 mg/mL (1 mL); 25 mg/0.5 mL (0.5 mL); 50 mg/mL (1 mL, 30 mL); 75 mg/1.5 mL (1.5 mL); 100 mg/2 mL (2 mL); 75 mg/mL (1 mL); 100 mg/mL (1 mL, 20 mL)

Generic: 10 mg/mL (30 mL); 25 mg/mL (1 mL); 50 mg/mL (1 mL); 100 mg/mL (1 mL)

Solution, Oral, as hydrochloride:

Generic: 50 mg/5 mL (500 mL)

Tablet, Oral, as hydrochloride:

Demerol: 50 mg [scored]

Demerol: 100 mg

Meperitab: 50 mg [scored]

Meperitab: 100 mg

Generic: 50 mg, 100 mg

Controlled Substance C-II

◆ Meperidine Hydrochloride *see* Meperidine *on page 1144*

◆ Meperitab *see* Meperidine *on page 1144*

◆ Mephyton *see* Phytonadione *on page 1450*

Mepivacaine (me PIV a kane)

Brand Names: US Carbocaine; Carbocaine Preservative-Free; Polocaine; Polocaine-MPF

Brand Names: Canada Carbocaine®; Polocaine®

Index Terms Mepivacaine Hydrochloride

Pharmacologic Category Local Anesthetic

Use Local or regional analgesia; anesthesia by local infiltration, peripheral and central neural techniques (epidural and caudal); **not** for use in spinal anesthesia

Dosing
Adult

Injectable local anesthetic: Dose varies with procedure, degree of anesthesia needed, vascularity of tissue, duration of anesthesia required, and physical condition of patient. The smallest dose and concentration required to produce the desired effect should be used.

Maximum single or total dose given for one procedure: 400 mg; 500 mg if epinephrine has been added (Barash, 2009)

Cervical, brachial, intercostal, pudendal nerve block: 5-40 mL of a 1% solution (maximum: 400 mg) **or** 5-20 mL of a 2% solution (maximum: 400 mg). For pudendal block, inject one-half the total dose each side.

Transvaginal block (paracervical plus pudendal): Up to 30 mL (total for both sides) of a 1% solution (maximum: 300 mg). Inject one-half the total dose each side.

Paracervical block: Up to 20 mL (total for both sides) of a 1% solution (maximum: 200 mg). Inject one-half the total dose to each side. This is the maximum recommended dose per 90-minute procedure; inject slowly with 5 minutes between sides.

Caudal and epidural block (preservative free solutions only): 15-30 mL of a 1% solution (maximum: 300 mg) **or** 10-25 mL of a 1.5% solution (maximum: 375 mg) **or** 10-20 mL of a 2% solution (maximum: 400 mg)

Infiltration: Up to 40 mL of a 1% solution (maximum: 400 mg); up to 50 mL if epinephrine has been added (maximum: 500 mg) (Barash, 2009); an equivalent amount of a 0.5% solution (prepared by diluting the 1% solution with NS) may be used for large areas

Peripheral nerve block to provide a surgical level of anesthesia (Miller, 2010):

Major nerve block (blockade of two or more distinct nerves, a nerve plexus, or very large nerves at more proximal sites: 30-50 mL of a 1% or 1.5% solution (maximum: 500 mg)

Minor nerve block (blockade of a single nerve [eg, ulnar or radial]): 5-20 mL of a 1% solution (maximum: 200 mg)

Therapeutic block: 1-5 mL of 1% solution (maximum: 50 mg) **or** 1-5 mL of 2% solution (maximum: 100 mg)

Geriatric Decreased doses suggested by manufacturer's labeling; however, no dosing adjustments provided. Refer to adult dosing.

Pediatric Injectable local anesthetic: Dose varies with procedure, degree of anesthesia needed, vascularity of tissue, duration of anesthesia required, and physical condition of patient. The smallest dose and concentration required to produce the desired effect should be used.

Maximum single or total dose given for one procedure: 5-6 mg/kg; only concentrations <2% should be used in children <3 years or <14 kg (30 lbs)

Renal Impairment No dosage adjustment provided in manufacturer's labeling; use with caution.

Hepatic Impairment No dosage adjustment provided in manufacturer's labeling; use with caution.

Additional Information Complete prescribing information should be consulted for additional detail.

Dosage Forms Excipient information presented when available (limited, particularly for generics); consult specific product labeling.

Solution, Injection, as hydrochloride:
Carbocaine: 1% (50 mL); 2% (50 mL) [contains methylparaben]
Polocaine: 1% (50 mL); 2% (50 mL) [contains methylparaben]
Generic: 3% (1.8 mL)

Solution, Injection, as hydrochloride [preservative free]:
Carbocaine Preservative-Free: 1% (30 mL); 1.5% (30 mL); 2% (20 mL)
Polocaine-MPF: 1% (30 mL); 1.5% (30 mL); 2% (20 mL) [methylparaben free]

◆ Mepivacaine Hydrochloride *see* Mepivacaine *on page 1145*

Mepolizumab (me poe LIZ ue mab)

Brand Names: US Nucala
Pharmacologic Category Interleukin-5 Receptor Antagonist; Monoclonal Antibody, Anti-Asthmatic
Use

Asthma: Add-on maintenance treatment of severe asthma in adults and children 12 years and older with an eosinophilic phenotype
Limitations of use: Not indicated for the relief of acute bronchospasm or status asthmaticus
Dosing
Adult & Geriatric Asthma: SubQ: 100 mg once every 4 weeks

Pediatric Asthma: Children ≥12 years and Adolescents: SubQ: Refer to adult dosing.

Renal Impairment There are no dosage adjustments provided in the manufacturer's labeling (has not been studied); however, adjustment based on renal function is unlikely to be necessary as mepolizumab is not renally eliminated.

Hepatic Impairment There are no dosage adjustments provided in the manufacturer's labeling (has not been studied); however, adjustment based on hepatic function is unlikely to be necessary as mepolizumab is degraded by widely distributed proteolytic enzymes which are not restricted to hepatic tissue.

Additional Information Complete prescribing information should be consulted for additional detail.

Dosage Forms Excipient information presented when available (limited, particularly for generics); consult specific product labeling.
Solution Reconstituted, Subcutaneous [preservative free]:
Nucala: 100 mg (1 ea) [contains mouse protein (murine) (hamster), polysorbate 80]

Meprobamate (me proe BA mate)

Index Terms Equanil
Pharmacologic Category Antianxiety Agent, Miscellaneous
Use Management of anxiety disorders
Dosing
Adult Anxiety: Oral: 1200-1600 mg/day in 3-4 divided doses, up to 2400 mg/day
Pediatric Anxiety: Oral: 6-12 years: 200-600 mg/day in 2-3 divided doses
Renal Impairment No dosage adjustment provided in manufacturer's labeling; however, the following adjustments have been recommended (Aronoff, 2007): Adults:
CrCl 10-50 mL/minute: Administer every 9-12 hours.
CrCl <10 mL/minute: Administer every 12-18 hours.
Hemodialysis: No dosage adjustment necessary.
Peritoneal dialysis: Administer every 12-18 hours.
Continuous renal replacement therapy (CRRT): Administer every 9-12 hours.
Hepatic Impairment No dosage adjustment provided in manufacturer's labeling; use with caution.
Additional Information Complete prescribing information should be consulted for additional detail.
Dosage Forms Excipient information presented when available (limited, particularly for generics); consult specific product labeling.
Tablet, Oral:
Generic: 200 mg, 400 mg
Controlled Substance C-IV

◆ Mepron *see* Atovaquone *on page 172*
◆ Mercaptamine *see* Cysteamine (Systemic) *on page 466*
◆ Mercaptoethane Sulfonate *see* Mesna *on page 1154*

Mercaptopurine (mer kap toe PURE een)

Brand Names: US Purinethol [DSC]; Purixan
Brand Names: Canada Purinethol
Index Terms 6-Mercaptopurine (error-prone abbreviation); 6-MP (error-prone abbreviation); Purinethol
Pharmacologic Category Antineoplastic Agent, Antimetabolite; Antineoplastic Agent, Antimetabolite (Purine Analog); Immunosuppressant Agent
Use Acute lymphoblastic leukemia: Treatment of acute lymphoblastic leukemia (ALL), as part of a combination chemotherapy regimen
Pregnancy Considerations May cause fetal harm if administered during pregnancy. Case reports of fetal loss have been noted with mercaptopurine administration during the first trimester; adverse effects have also been noted with second and third trimester use. Women of child bearing potential should avoid becoming pregnant during treatment.
Breast-Feeding Considerations Mercaptopurine is the active metabolite of azathioprine. Following administration of azathioprine, mercaptopurine can be detected in breast milk (Gardiner 2006). It is not known if/how much mercaptopurine is found in breast milk following oral administration. According to the manufacturer, the decision to discontinue mercaptopurine or discontinue breast-feeding during therapy should take into account the benefits of treatment to the mother.
Prescribing and Access Restrictions Distribution of Purixan is provided by the specialty pharmacy, AnovoRx. For ordering information, call 888-470-0904.

Contraindications Hypersensitivity to mercaptopurine or any component of the formulation; patients whose disease showed prior resistance to mercaptopurine

Warnings/Precautions Hazardous agent - use appropriate precautions for handling and disposal (NIOSH 2014 [group 1]).

Hepatotoxicity has been reported, including jaundice, ascites, hepatic necrosis (may be fatal), intrahepatic cholestasis, parenchymal cell necrosis, and/or hepatic encephalopathy; may be due to direct hepatic cell damage or hypersensitivity. While hepatotoxicity or hepatic injury may occur at any dose, dosages exceeding the recommended dose are associated with a higher incidence. Signs of jaundice generally appear early in treatment, after ~1 to 2 months (range: 1 week to 8 years) and may resolve following discontinuation; recurrence with rechallenge has been noted. Monitor liver function tests, including transaminases, alkaline phosphatase, and bilirubin weekly with treatment initiation, then monthly thereafter (monitor more frequently if used in combination with other hepatotoxic drugs or in patients with preexisting hepatic impairment). Consider a reduced dose in patients with baseline hepatic impairment; monitor closely for toxicity. Withhold treatment for clinical signs of jaundice (hepatomegaly, anorexia, tenderness), deterioration in liver function tests, toxic hepatitis, or biliary stasis until hepatotoxicity is ruled out.

Dose-related leukopenia, thrombocytopenia, and anemia are common; however, may be indicative of disease progression. Hematologic toxicity may be delayed. Bone marrow may appear hypoplastic (could also appear normal). Monitor blood counts; dose may require adjusting for severe neutropenia or thrombocytopenia. Monitor for bleeding (due to thrombocytopenia) or infection (due to neutropenia). Profound severe or repeated hematologic toxicity may be indicative of TPMT deficiency. Patients with homozygous genetic defect of thiopurine methyltransferase (TPMT) are more sensitive to myelosuppressive effects; generally associated with rapid myelosuppression. Significant mercaptopurine dose reductions will be necessary (possibly with continued concomitant chemotherapy at normal doses). Patients who are heterozygous for TPMT defects will have intermediate activity; may have increased toxicity (primarily myelosuppression) although will generally tolerate normal mercaptopurine doses. Consider TPMT testing for severe toxicities/excessive myelosuppression. A germline variant in nucleoside diphophate-linked moiety X-type motif 15 (*NUDT15*) is strongly correlated with mercaptopurine intolerance in children receiving treatment for acute lymphoblastic leukemia (ALL). A genome-wide association study was performed in two prospective clinical childhood ALL trials, and showed that patients homozygous for the TT genotype were extremely sensitive to mercaptopurine, and achieved an average dose intensity of only 8.3%. The *NUDT15* genetic variant is most common in East Asian and Hispanic patients. In patients homozygous for either TPMT or *NUDT15* (or heterozygous for both), mercaptopurine dose reductions of ≥50% were required in 100% of patients (Yang 2015). Potentially significant drug-drug interactions may exist, requiring dose or frequency adjustment, additional monitoring, and/or selection of alternative therapy. Because azathioprine is metabolized to mercaptopurine, concomitant use with azathioprine may result in a significant increase in hematologic toxicity and profound myelosuppression; avoid concurrent use. Hematologic toxicity may be exacerbated by other medications which inhibit TPMT (eg, mesalamine, olsalazine, sulfasalazine) or by other myelosuppressive drugs.

Immunosuppressive agents, including mercaptopurine, are associated with the development of lymphoma and other malignancies including hepatosplenic T-cell lymphoma (HSTCL). Mercaptopurine is immunosuppressive; immune responses to infections may be impaired and the risk for infection is increased; common signs of infection, such as fever and leukocytosis may not occur; lethargy and confusion may be more prominent signs of infection. Immune response to vaccines may be diminished; live virus vaccines impose a risk for infection. Consider adjusting dosage in patients with renal impairment. Some renal adverse effects may be minimized with hydration and prophylactic antihyperuricemic therapy. To avoid potentially serious dosage errors, the terms "6-mercaptopurine" or "6-MP" should be avoided; use of these terms has been associated with six-fold overdosages.

Adverse Reactions Frequency not always defined.
Central nervous system: Malaise (5% to 20%), drug fever
Dermatologic: Skin rash (5% to 20%), hyperpigmentation (<5%), urticaria (<5%), alopecia
Endocrine & metabolic: Hyperuricemia (<5%)

Gastrointestinal: Anorexia (5% to 20%), diarrhea (5% to 20%), nausea (5% to 20%; minimal), vomiting (5% to 20%; minimal), oral lesion (<5%), pancreatitis (<5%), cholestasis, mucositis, sprue-like symptoms, stomach pain, ulcerative bowel lesion

Genitourinary: Oligospermia, renal toxicity, uricosuria

Hematologic & oncologic: Bone marrow depression (>20%; onset 7-10 days; nadir 14 days; recovery: 21 days), anemia, granulocytopenia, hemorrhage, hepatosplenic T-cell lymphomas, leukopenia, lymphocytopenia, metastases, neutropenia, thrombocytopenia

Hepatic: Hyperbilirubinemia (<5%), increased serum transaminases (<5%), ascites, hepatic encephalopathy, hepatic fibrosis, hepatic injury, hepatic necrosis, hepatomegaly, hepatotoxicity, intrahepatic cholestasis, jaundice, toxic hepatitis

Immunologic: Immunosuppression

Infection: Infection

Respiratory: Pulmonary fibrosis

Drug Interactions

Metabolism/Transport Effects None known.

Avoid Concomitant Use

Avoid concomitant use of Mercaptopurine with any of the following: AzaTHIOprine; BCG (Intravesical); Deferiprone; Dipyrone; Febuxostat; Natalizumab; Pimecrolimus; Tacrolimus (Topical); Tofacitinib

Increased Effect/Toxicity

Mercaptopurine may increase the levels/effects of: CloZAPine; Deferiprone; Fingolimod; Leflunomide; Natalizumab; Tofacitinib; Vaccines (Live)

The levels/effects of Mercaptopurine may be increased by: 5-ASA Derivatives; Allopurinol; AzaTHIOprine; Denosumab; Dipyrone; DOXOrubicin (Conventional); Febuxostat; Pimecrolimus; Roflumilast; Sulfamethoxazole; Tacrolimus (Topical); Trastuzumab; Trimethoprim

Decreased Effect

Mercaptopurine may decrease the levels/effects of: BCG (Intravesical); Coccidioides immitis Skin Test; Sipuleucel-T; Vaccines (Inactivated); Vaccines (Live); Vitamin K Antagonists

The levels/effects of Mercaptopurine may be decreased by: Echinacea

Food Interactions Absorption is variable with food. Management: Take on an empty stomach at the same time each day 1 hour before or 2 hours after a meal. Maintain adequate hydration, unless instructed to restrict fluid intake.

Preparation for Administration Hazardous agent; use appropriate precautions for handling and disposal (NIOSH 2014 [group 1]).

Suspension: Wear disposable gloves when handling. Measure dose with an oral dosing syringe to assure proper dose is administered. Oral syringe provided by the manufacturer is intended to be reused, wash with warm soapy water and rinse well (hold syringe under water and move plunger several times to ensure inside of syringe is clean); allow to dry completely.

Storage/Stability

Tablets: Store at 15°C to 25°C (59°F to 77°F). Store in a dry place.

Suspension: Store at 15°C to 25°C (59°F to 77°F). Do not store above 25°C (77°F). Store in a dry place. Use within 6 weeks after opening.

Mechanism of Action Mercaptopurine is a purine antagonist which inhibits DNA and RNA synthesis; acts as false metabolite and is incorporated into DNA and RNA, eventually inhibiting their synthesis; specific for the S phase of the cell cycle

Pharmacodynamics/Kinetics

Absorption: Variable and incomplete (~50% of a dose is absorbed); C_{max} of suspension is 34% higher than the tablet

Distribution: V_d: > total body water; CNS penetration is poor

Protein binding: ~19%

Metabolism: Hepatic and in GI mucosa; hepatically via xanthine oxidase and methylation via TPMT to sulfate conjugates, 6-thiouric acid, and other inactive compounds; first-pass effect

Half-life elimination (age dependent): ~2 hours

Excretion: Urine (46% as mercaptopurine and metabolites)

Dosing

Adult Note: Patients with minimal or no thiopurine S-methyltransferase (TPMT) activity are at increased risk for severe toxicity at conventional mercaptopurine doses and generally require dose reduction; consider TPMT gene polymorphism testing in patients who experience severe bone marrow suppression (homozygous deficient patients may require up to a 90% dosage reduction; ►

heterozygous patients usually tolerate recommended doses, although some may require dosage reduction).

Acute lymphoblastic leukemia (ALL): Maintenance: Oral: 1.5 to 2.5 mg/kg once daily (50 to 75 mg/m^2 once daily); continue based on blood counts **or**

Off-label ALL dosing (combination chemotherapy; refer to specific reference for combinations):

Early intensification (two 4-week courses): 60 mg/m^2/day days 1 to 14 (Larson 1995; Larson 1998)

Interim maintenance (12-week course): 60 mg/m^2/day days 1 to 70 (Larson 1995; Larson 1998)

Maintenance (prolonged): 50 mg 3 times/day for 2 years (Kantarjian 2000) **or** 60 mg/m^2/day for 2 years from diagnosis (Larson 1995; Larson 1998)

Acute promyelocytic leukemia (APL) maintenance (off-label use): 60 mg/m^2/day for 1 year (in combination with tretinoin and methotrexate) (Powell 2010)

Crohn disease, remission maintenance or reduction of steroid use (off-label use): Oral: 1 to 1.5 mg/kg/day (Lichtenstein 2009)

Lymphoblastic lymphoma (off-label use): Maintenance (prolonged): 50 mg 3 times daily for 2 years (Kantarjian 2000; Thomas 2004)

Ulcerative colitis (off-label use): Oral:

Initial: 50 mg once daily; titrate dose up if clinical remission not achieved or down if leukopenia occurs (Lobel 2004) **or**

Initial: 50 mg (25 mg if heterozygous for TPMT activity) once daily; titrate up to goal of 1.5 mg/kg (0.75 mg/kg if heterozygous for TPMT activity) if WBC >4,000/mm^3 (and at least 50% of baseline) and LFTs and amylase are stable (Siegel 2005) **or**

Maintenance: 1 to 1.5 mg/kg/day (Carter 2004) **or**

Remission maintenance: 1.5 mg/kg/day (Danese 2011)

Dosage adjustment with concurrent allopurinol: Reduce mercaptopurine dosage to 25% to 33% of the usual dose.

Geriatric Due to renal decline with age, initiate treatment at the low end of recommended dose range.

Pediatric Note: Patients with minimal or no thiopurine S-methyltransferase (TPMT) activity are at increased risk for severe toxicity at conventional mercaptopurine doses and generally require dose reduction; consider TPMT gene polymorphism testing in patients who experience severe bone marrow suppression (homozygous deficient patients may require up to a 90% dosage reduction; heterozygous patients usually tolerate recommended doses, although some may require dosage reduction).

Acute lymphoblastic leukemia (ALL): Maintenance: Oral: 1.5 to 2.5 mg/kg once daily (50 to 75 mg/m^2 once daily); continue based on blood counts **or**

Off-label ALL dosing (combination chemotherapy; refer to specific reference for combinations): Adolescents ≥15 years:

Consolidation phase: 60 mg/m^2/day days 0 to 27 days (5-week course) (Stock 2008) **or** 60 mg/m^2/day days 0 to 13 and days 28 to 41 (9-week course) (Stock 2008)

Early intensification (two 4-week courses): 60 mg/m^2/day days 1 to 14 (Larson 1995; Larson 1998; Stock 2008)

Interim maintenance: 60 mg/m^2/day days 0-41 (8-week course) (Stock 2008) **or** 60 mg/m^2/day days 1 to 70 (12-week course) (Larson 1995; Larson 1998; Stock 2008)

Maintenance (prolonged): 50 mg 3 times/day for 2 years (Kantarjian 2000) **or** 60 mg/m^2/day for 2 years from diagnosis (Larson 1995; Larson 1998; Stock 2008) **or** 75 mg/m^2/day for 2 years (girls) or 3 years (boys) from first interim maintenance (Stock 2008)

Acute promyelocytic leukemia (APL) maintenance (off-label use): Oral: Adolescents ≥15 years: 60 mg/m^2/day for 1 year (in combination with tretinoin and methotrexate) (Powell 2010)

Autoimmune hepatitis (off-label use): Oral: 1.5 mg/kg/day (in combination with prednisone) (Manns 2010)

Crohn disease, remission maintenance (off-label use): Doses range from 1 to 1.5 mg/kg/day (Grossman 2008; Markowitz 2000); children ≤6 years may require higher doses to achieve clinical improvement (Grossman 2008).

Lymphoblastic lymphoma (off-label use): Adolescents ≥15 years: Maintenance (prolonged): 50 mg 3 times daily for 2 years (Kantarjian 2000; Thomas 2004) **or** 60 mg/m^2/day for 2 years from diagnosis (Stock 2008) **or** 75 mg/m^2/day for 2 years (girls) or 3 years (boys) from first interim maintenance (Stock 2008)

Ulcerative colitis, remission maintenance (off-label use): Doses range from 1 to 1.5 mg/kg/day (Grossman 2008; Sandhu 2010); children ≤6 years may require higher doses to achieve clinical improvement (Grossman 2008); additional trials may be necessary to further define the role of mercaptopurine in pediatric patients with this condition.

Dosage adjustment with concurrent allopurinol: Reduce mercaptopurine dosage to 25% to 33% of the usual dose.

Renal Impairment The manufacturer's labeling recommends starting with reduced doses (starting at the low end of the dosing range) or increasing the dosing interval to every 36 to 48 hours in patients with renal impairment to avoid accumulation; however, no specific dosage adjustment is provided. The following adjustments have also been recommended (Aronoff 2007): Children:

CrCl ≤50 mL/minute/1.73 m^2: Administer every 48 hours

Hemodialysis: Administer every 48 hours

Continuous ambulatory peritoneal dialysis (CAPD): Administer every 48 hours

Continuous renal replacement therapy (CRRT): Administer every 48 hours

Hepatic Impairment The manufacturer's labeling recommends considering a reduced dose (starting at the low end of the dosing range) with close monitoring for toxicity dose in patients with baseline hepatic impairment; however, no specific dosage adjustment is provided.

Adjustment for Toxicity Adjust dosage for excessive hematologic toxicity.

Administration Administer preferably on an empty stomach (1 hour before or 2 hours after meals)

ALL treatment in children (Schmiegelow 1997): Administration in the evening has demonstration superior outcome; administration with food did not significantly affect outcome.

Suspension: Shake well for at least 30 seconds to ensure suspension is mixed thoroughly (suspension is viscous). Measure dose with an oral dosing syringe (a 1 mL and a 5 mL oral dosing syringe are supplied by the manufacturer) to assure proper dose is administered. Patients and caregivers should be trained on appropriate measuring and administration, handling, storage, disposal, cleanup of accidental spills, and proper cleaning of oral dosing syringe. Use within 6 weeks after opening.

Hazardous agent; use appropriate precautions for handling and disposal (NIOSH 2014 [group 1]). Avoid exposure to crushed or broken tablets; if it is necessary to manipulate the tablets (eg, to prepare an oral solution), it is recommended to double glove, wear a protective gown, and prepare in a controlled device. Disposable gloves should be worn when handling tablets or suspension for administration; health care providers should also wear a protective gown (NIOSH 2014).

Monitoring Parameters CBC with differential (weekly initially, although clinical status may require increased frequency), bone marrow exam (to evaluate marrow status), liver function tests (transaminases, alkaline phosphatase, and bilirubin; weekly initially, then monthly; monitor more frequently if on concomitant hepatotoxic agents or in patients with preexisting hepatic impairment), renal function, urinalysis; consider TPMT genotyping to identify TPMT defect (if severe hematologic toxicity occurs)

For use as immunomodulatory therapy in CD or UC, monitor CBC with differential weekly for 1 month, then biweekly for 1 month, followed by monitoring every 1 to 2 months throughout the course of therapy. LFTs should be assessed every 3 months. Monitor for signs/symptoms of malignancy (eg, splenomegaly, hepatomegaly, abdominal pain, persistent fever, night sweats, weight loss).

Test Interactions TPMT testing: Recent transfusions may result in a misinterpretation of the actual TPMT activity. Concomitant drugs may influence TPMT activity in the blood.

Dosage Forms Excipient information presented when available (limited, particularly for generics); consult specific product labeling. [DSC] = Discontinued product

Suspension, Oral:

Purixan: 2000 mg/100 mL (100 mL) [contains aspartame, methylparaben, propylparaben]

Tablet, Oral:

Purinethol: 50 mg [DSC] [scored]

Generic: 50 mg

Extemporaneous Preparations Hazardous agent: Use appropriate precautions for handling and disposal (NIOSH 2014 [group 1]). When manipulating tablets, NIOSH recommends double gloving, a protective gown, and preparation in a controlled device; if not prepared in a controlled device, respiratory and eye protection as well as ventilated engineering controls are recommended (NIOSH 2014).

A 50 mg/mL oral suspension may be prepared in a vertical flow hood with tablets and a mixture of sterile water for injection (SWFI), simple syrup, and cherry syrup. Crush thirty 50 mg tablets in a mortar and reduce to a fine powder. Add ~5 mL SWFI and mix to a uniform paste; then add ~10 mL simple syrup; mix while continuing to add cherry syrup to make a final volume of 30 mL; transfer to a calibrated bottle. Label "shake well" and "caution chemotherapy". Stable for 35 days at room temperature.
Aliabadi HM, Romanick M, Desai, S, et al, "Effect of Buffer and Antioxidant on Stability of a Mercaptopurine Suspension," *Am J Health Syst Pharm* 2008, 65(5):441-7.

◆ **6-Mercaptopurine (error-prone abbreviation)** *see* Mercaptopurine *on page 1146*

◆ **Mercapturic Acid** *see* Acetylcysteine *on page 31*

Meropenem (mer oh PEN em)

Brand Names: US Merrem
Brand Names: Canada Meropenem For Injection; Merrem
Pharmacologic Category Antibiotic, Carbapenem
Use
Bacterial meningitis: Treatment of bacterial meningitis in pediatric patients 3 months and older caused by *Streptococcus pneumoniae*, *Haemophilus influenzae*, and *Neisseria meningitidis*
Complicated skin and skin structure infections: Treatment of complicated skin and skin structure infections in adults and pediatric patients 3 months and older caused by *Staphylococcus aureus* (methicillin-susceptible isolates only), *Streptococcus pyogenes*, *S. agalactiae*, viridans group streptococci, *Enterococcus faecalis* (vancomycin-susceptible isolates only), *Pseudomonas aeruginosa*, *Escherichia coli*, *Proteus mirabilis*, *Bacteroides fragilis*, and *Peptostreptococcus* species
Intra-abdominal infections: Treatment of complicated appendicitis and peritonitis in adult and pediatric patients caused by viridans group streptococci, *E. coli*, *Klebsiella pneumoniae*, *P. aeruginosa*, *B. fragilis*, *B. thetaiotaomicron*, and *Peptostreptococcus* species

Canadian labeling: Additional indications (not in U.S. labeling): Treatment of lower respiratory tract infections (community-acquired and nosocomial pneumonias), uncomplicated skin and skin structure infections, complicated urinary tract infections, gynecologic infections (excluding chlamydia), and septicemia; treatment of bacterial meningitis in adults caused by *S. pneumoniae*, *H. influenzae*, and *N. meningitidis* (use in adult meningitis based on pediatric data)

Pregnancy Considerations Adverse events were not observed in animal reproduction studies. Incomplete transplacental transfer of meropenem was found using an *ex vivo* human perfusion model.

Breast-Feeding Considerations Small amounts of meropenem are excreted into breast milk (case report). The manufacturer recommends that caution be exercised when administering meropenem to breast-feeding women. Non-dose-related effects could include modification of bowel flora.

Contraindications Hypersensitivity to meropenem, other drugs in the same class, or any component of the formulation; patients who have experienced anaphylactic reactions to beta-lactams

Warnings/Precautions Serious hypersensitivity reactions, including anaphylaxis, have been reported (some without a history of previous allergic reactions to beta-lactams). Carbapenems have been associated with CNS adverse effects, including confusional states and seizures (myoclonic); use caution with CNS disorders (eg, brain lesions and history of seizures) and adjust dose in renal impairment to avoid drug accumulation, which may increase seizure risk. Outpatient use may result in paresthesias, seizures, or headaches that can impair neuromotor function and alertness; patients should not operate machinery or drive until it is established that meropenem is well tolerated. Prolonged use may result in fungal or bacterial superinfection, including *C. difficile*-associated diarrhea (CDAD) and pseudomembranous colitis; CDAD has been observed >2 months postantibiotic treatment. Use with caution in patients with renal impairment; dosage adjustment required in patients with moderate-to-severe renal dysfunction. Thrombocytopenia has been reported in patients with renal dysfunction. Lower doses (based upon renal function) are often required in the elderly. Potentially significant drug-drug interactions may exist, requiring dose or frequency adjustment, additional monitoring, and/or selection of alternative therapy.

Adverse Reactions
1% to 10%:
Cardiovascular: Peripheral vascular disease (>1%), shock (1%), bradycardia (≤1%), cardiac arrest (≤1%), cardiac failure (≤1%), chest pain (≤1%), hypertension (≤1%), hypotension (≤1%), myocardial infarction (≤1%), peripheral edema (≤1%), pulmonary embolism (≤1%), syncope (≤1%), tachycardia (≤1%)
Central nervous system: Headache (2% to 8%), convulsions (neonates and infants <3 months: 5%), pain (≤5%), agitation (≤1%), anxiety (≤1%), chills (≤1%), confusion (≤1%), delirium (≤1%), depression (≤1%), dizziness (≤1%), drowsiness (≤1%), hallucination (≤1%), insomnia (≤1%), nervousness (≤1%), paresthesia (≤1%), seizure (≤1%)
Dermatologic: Skin rash (2% to 3%, includes diaper-area moniliasis in infants), pruritus (1%), dermal ulcer (≤1%), diaphoresis (≤1%), urticaria (≤1%)
Endocrine & metabolic: Hypoglycemia (>1%), hypervolemia (≤1%)
Gastrointestinal: Nausea (≤8%), diarrhea (4% to 7%), constipation (1% to 7%), vomiting (≤4%), oral candidiasis (≤2%), gastrointestinal disease (>1%), glossitis (1%), abdominal pain (≤1%), anorexia (≤1%), dyspepsia (≤1%), enlargement of abdomen (≤1%), flatulence (≤1%), intestinal obstruction (≤1%)
Genitourinary: Dysuria (≤1%), pelvic pain (≤1%), urinary incontinence (≤1%), vulvovaginal candidiasis (≤1%)
Hematologic & oncologic: Anemia (≤6%), hypochromic anemia (≤1%)
Hepatic: Hyperbilirubinemia (conjugated; neonates and infants <3 months: 5%), cholestatic jaundice (≤1%), hepatic failure (≤1%), jaundice (≤1%)
Infection: Sepsis (2%)
Local: Inflammation at injection site (2%)
Neuromuscular & skeletal: Back pain (≤1%), weakness (≤1%)
Renal: Renal failure (≤1%)
Respiratory: Pharyngitis (>1%), pneumonia (>1%), apnea (1%), asthma (≤1%), cough (≤1%), dyspnea (≤1%), hypoxia (≤1%), pleural effusion (≤1%), pulmonary edema (≤1%), respiratory tract disease (≤1%)
Miscellaneous: Accidental injury (>1%), fever (≤1%)
<1% (Limited to important or life-threatening): Agranulocytosis, angioedema, anorexia, asthma, bradycardia, cardiac arrest, cardiac failure, change in platelet count, cholestatic jaundice, *Clostridium difficile* associated diarrhea, confusion, decreased hematocrit, decreased hemoglobin, decreased partial thromboplastin time, decreased prothrombin time, decreased white blood cell count, delirium, depression, dermal ulcer, eosinophilia, erythema multiforme, gastrointestinal hemorrhage, hallucination, hematuria, hemolytic anemia, hemoperitoneum, hepatic failure, hypertension, hypervolemia, hypochromic anemia, hypokalemia, hypotension, hypoxia, increased blood urea nitrogen, increased lactate dehydrogenase, increased serum alkaline phosphatase, increased serum ALT, increased serum AST, increased serum bilirubin, increased serum creatinine, ileus, intestinal obstruction, jaundice, leukocytosis, leukopenia, myocardial infarction, neutropenia, peripheral edema, pleural effusion, positive direct Coombs test, pulmonary edema, pulmonary embolism, renal failure, seizure, Stevens-Johnson syndrome, tachycardia, toxic epidermal necrolysis, urinary incontinence, vulvovaginal candidiasis

Drug Interactions
Metabolism/Transport Effects None known.
Avoid Concomitant Use
Avoid concomitant use of Meropenem with any of the following: BCG (Intravesical); Probenecid
Increased Effect/Toxicity
The levels/effects of Meropenem may be increased by: Probenecid
Decreased Effect
Meropenem may decrease the levels/effects of: BCG (Intravesical); BCG Vaccine (Immunization); Sodium Picosulfate; Typhoid Vaccine; Valproate Products

Preparation for Administration Meropenem infusion vials may be reconstituted with SWFI. The 500 mg vials should be reconstituted with 10 mL, and 1 g vials with 20 mL. May be further diluted with compatible solutions for infusion. Consult detailed reference/product labeling for compatibility.
Duplex: Unlatch side tab, unfold, remove foil strip from drug chamber. Point set port in downward direction, fold container just below the diluent meniscus, and squeeze the diluent chamber until the seal between the diluent and drug powder opens. Agitate until dissolved.

Storage/Stability Freshly prepared solutions should be used. However, constituted solutions maintain satisfactory potency under the conditions described below. Solutions should not be frozen.

Store intact vials and unactivated Duplex containers at 20°C to 25°C (68°F to 77°F). Unactivated duplex units with foil strip removed from the drug chamber must be protected from light and used within 7 days at room temperature. Once activated, must be used within 1 hour if stored at room temperature or within 15 hours if stored under refrigeration. Do not freeze.

Dry powder should be stored at controlled room temperature 20°C to 25°C (68°F to 77°F).

Injection reconstitution: Stability in vial when constituted (up to 50 mg/mL) with:

SWFI:

U.S. labeling: Stable for up to 3 hours at up to 25°C (77°F) or for up to 13 hours at up to 5°C (41°F).

Canadian labeling: Stable for up to 3 hours at 15°C to 25°C (59°F to 77°F) or for up to 16 hours at 2°C to 8°C (36°F to 46°F).

Infusion admixture (1 to 20 mg/mL): Solution is stable when diluted in NS for 1 hour at up to 25°C (77°F) or 15 hours at up to 5°C (41°F). Solutions constituted with dextrose injection 5% should be used immediately. **Note:** Meropenem stability (admixed with NS at a concentration of 20 mg/mL) at room temperature for >1 hour or under refrigeration for >15 hours is not supported by the manufacturer. Data exist supporting stability (admixed with NS at a concentration of 20 mg/mL) at room temperature for ≤4 hours and under refrigeration ≤24 hours (Patel, 1997).

Mechanism of Action Inhibits bacterial cell wall synthesis by binding to several of the penicillin-binding proteins, which in turn inhibit the final transpeptidation step of peptidoglycan synthesis in bacterial cell walls, thus inhibiting cell wall biosynthesis; bacteria eventually lyse due to ongoing activity of cell wall autolytic enzymes (autolysins and murein hydrolases) while cell wall assembly is arrested

Pharmacodynamics/Kinetics Note: In the elderly, reduction in plasma clearance correlates with age-associated reduction in creatinine clearance (Craig, 1997). Clearance correlates with creatinine clearance in patients with renal impairment.

Distribution: V_d: Adults: 15 to 20 L, Children: 0.37 to 0.49 L/kg; penetrates well into most body fluids and tissues (Craig, 1997)

Protein binding: ~2%

Metabolism: Hepatic; hydrolysis of beta-lactam bond to open beta-lactam form (inactive) (Craig, 1997)

Half-life elimination: Infants <3 months: ~2.5 hours (mean); Infants ≥3 months, Children, Adolescents, and Adults: Normal renal function: 1 to 1.5 hours

Time to peak: Tissue: ~1 hour following infusion; CSF: 2 to 3 hours with inflamed meninges

Excretion: Urine (~70% as unchanged drug; ~28% inactive metabolite); feces (2%)

Dosing

Adult & Geriatric

Usual dosage range: IV: 1.5 to 6 g daily divided every 8 hours

Extended infusion method (off-label dosing): IV: 0.5 to 2 g over 3 hours every 8 hours (Crandon, 2011; Dandekar, 2003). **Note:** Dosing used at some centers and is based on pharmacokinetic/pharmacodynamic modeling and not clinical efficacy data. Meropenem stability (admixed with NS at a concentration of 20 mg/mL) at room temperature for >1 hour or under refrigeration for >15 hours is not supported by the manufacturer. Data exist supporting stability (admixed with NS at a concentration of 20 mg/mL) at room temperature for ≤4 hours and under refrigeration ≤24 hours (Patel, 1997).

Indication-specific dosing:

Catheter-related bloodstream infections (off-label use): IV: 1 g every 8 hours (Mermel, 2009)

Cholangitis, intra-abdominal infections, complicated: IV: 1 g every 8 hours. **Note:** 2010 IDSA guidelines recommend treatment duration of 4-7 days (provided source controlled). Not recommended for mild-to-moderate, community-acquired intra-abdominal infections due to risk of toxicity and the development of resistant organisms (Solomkin, 2010).

Cystic fibrosis, pulmonary exacerbation (off-label use): IV: 40 mg/kg every 8 hours; maximum single dose: 2 g (Zobell, 2012)

Febrile neutropenia (off-label use): IV: 1 g every 8 hours (Ohata, 2011; Paul, 2010)

Gynecologic and pelvic inflammatory disease: Canadian labeling (not in U.S. labeling): IV: 500 mg every 8 hours

Melioidosis *(Burkholderia pseudomallei)* **(off-label use):** IV: Initial treatment (intensive-phase): 1 g every 8 hours (Cheng 2004; Inglis 2006; Lipsitz 2012). **Note:** Meropenem is an alternative treatment to ceftazidime

for melioidosis; continued treatment with oral antibiotics is recommended after intensive-phase is completed (Lipsitz 2012).

Meningitis: IV:

Off-label use [U.S.]: 2 g every 8 hours; duration of therapy dependent upon pathogen: *N. meningitides*, *H. influenza*: 7 days; *S. pneumoniae*: 10 to 14 days; aerobic gram-negative bacilli: 21 days (Tunkel, 2004)

Canadian labeling (not in U.S. labeling): 2 g every 8 hours

Pneumonia (community-acquired): Canadian labeling (not in U.S. labeling): IV: 500 mg every 8 hours

Pneumonia (hospital-acquired, healthcare-associated, or ventilator-associated) (off-label use): IV: 1 g every 8 hours (ATS/IDSA, 2005)

Pneumonia (nosocomial): Canadian labeling (not in U.S. labeling): IV: 1 g every 8 hours

Prosthetic joint infection, *Pseudomonas aeruginosa* **(off-label use):** IV: 1 g every 8 hours for 4 to 6 weeks (consider addition of aminoglycoside) (Osmon, 2013)

Septicemia: Canadian labeling (not in U.S. labeling): IV: 1 g every 8 hours

Skin and skin structure infections:

Complicated: U.S. labeling: IV:

Pseudomonas aeruginosa-suspected or confirmed: 1 g every 8 hours

Pseudomonas aeruginosa not suspected: 500 mg every 8 hours

Uncomplicated: Canadian labeling (not in U.S. labeling): 500 mg every 8 hours

Skin and soft tissue necrotizing infections (off-label use): IV: 1 g every 8 hours in combination with an agent effective against MRSA (eg, vancomycin, linezolid, daptomycin) for empiric therapy of polymicrobial (mixed) infections. Continue until further debridement is not necessary, patient has clinically improved, and patient is afebrile for 48 to 72 hours (IDSA [Stevens, 2014]).

Surgical site infection (intestinal or genitourinary tract surgery) (off-label use): IV: 1 g every 8 hours (IDSA [Stevens, 2014])

Urinary tract infections (complicated): Canadian labeling (not in U.S. labeling): IV: 500 mg every 8 hours. **Note:** Up to 1 g every 8 hours may be administered (Pallett, 2010).

Pediatric

Usual dosage range:

Infants <3 months: IV:

Gestational age <32 weeks:

Postnatal age <14 days: 20 mg/kg/dose every 12 hours

Postnatal age ≥14 days: 20 mg/kg/dose every 8 hours

Gestational age ≥32 weeks:

Postnatal age <14 days: 20 mg/kg/dose every 8 hours

Postnatal age ≥14 days: 30 mg/kg/dose every 8 hours

Infants ≥3 months, Children, and Adolescents (≤50 kg): IV: 30 to 120 mg/kg/day divided every 8 hours (maximum dose: 6 **g** daily)

Children and Adolescents (>50 kg): IV: 1.5 to 6 g daily divided every 8 hours

Indication-specific dosing:

Catheter-related blood stream infections (off-label use): IV:

Infants ≥3 months, Children, and Adolescents (≤50 kg): IV: 20 mg/kg every 8 hours; maximum single dose: 1,000 mg (Mermel, 2009)

Children and Adolescents (>50 kg): Refer to adult dosing.

Cholangitis, intra-abdominal infections, complicated: IV: Children and Adolescents (>50 kg): Refer to adult dosing.

Cystic fibrosis, pulmonary exacerbation (off-label use): IV:

Infants ≥3 months, Children, and Adolescents (≤50 kg): 40 mg/kg every 8 hours; maximum single dose: 2,000 mg (Zobell, 2012)

Children and Adolescents (>50 kg): Refer to adult dosing.

Febrile neutropenia (off-label use): IV:

Infants ≥3 months, Children, and Adolescents (≤50 kg): 20 mg/kg every 8 hours (maximum dose: 1,000 mg every 8 hours) (Lehrnbecher, 2012; Yildirim, 2008)

Children and Adolescents (>50 kg): Refer to adult dosing.

Intra-abdominal infections (complicated): IV:

Infants <3 months: IV: **Note:** Administer as an IV infusion over 30 minutes; do not administer as an IV bolus

Gestational age <32 weeks:
Postnatal age <14 days: 20 mg/kg/dose every 12 hours
Postnatal age ≥14 days: 20 mg/kg/dose every 8 hours
Gestational age ≥32 weeks:
Postnatal age <14 days: 20 mg/kg/dose every 8 hours
Postnatal age ≥14 days: 30 mg/kg/dose every 8 hours
Infants ≥3 months, Children, and Adolescents: 20 mg/kg every 8 hours (maximum dose: 1,000 mg every 8 hours) (Solomkin, 2010)

Melioidosis (Burkholderia pseudomallei) (off-label use): IV:
Infants ≥6 months, Children, and Adolescents (≤40 kg): Initial treatment (intensive-phase): 25 mg/kg (up to 1 g) every 8 hours (Cheng 2004). **Note:** Meropenem is an alternative treatment to ceftazidime for melioidosis; continued treatment with oral antibiotics is recommended after intensive-phase is completed (Lipitz 2012).
Children and Adolescents (>50 kg): Refer to adult dosing.

Meningitis: IV:
Infants ≥3 months, Children, and Adolescents (≤50 kg): 40 mg/kg every 8 hours (maximum dose: 2,000 mg every 8 hours)
Children and Adolescents (>50 kg): 2 g every 8 hours

Pneumonia (community-acquired): IV:
Infants ≥3 months, Children, and Adolescents (≤50 kg): Canadian labeling (not in U.S. labeling): 10 to 20 mg/kg every 8 hours (maximum dose: 1,000 mg every 8 hours)
Children and Adolescents (>50 kg): Refer to adult dosing.

Pneumonia (hospital-acquired, health care-associated, or ventilator-associated) (off-label use): IV: Children and Adolescents (>50 kg): Refer to adult dosing.

Prosthetic joint infection, Pseudomonas aeruginosa (off-label use): Children and Adolescents (>50 kg): Refer to adult dosing.

Skin and skin structure infections: IV:
Infants ≥3 months, Children, and Adolescents (≤50 kg):
Complicated: U.S. labeling:
Pseudomonas aeruginosa-suspected or confirmed: 20 mg/kg every 8 hours
Pseudomonas aeruginosa not suspected: 10 mg/kg every 8 hours (maximum dose: 500 mg every 8 hours)
Uncomplicated: Canadian labeling (not in U.S. labeling): 10 to 20 mg/kg every 8 hours (maximum dose: 1,000 mg every 8 hours)
Children and Adolescents (>50 kg): Refer to adult dosing.

Skin and soft tissue necrotizing infections (off-label use): IV: 20 mg/kg every 8 hours in combination with an agent effective against MRSA (eg, vancomycin, linezolid, daptomycin) for empiric therapy of polymicrobial (mixed) infections. Continue until further debridement is not necessary, patient has clinically improved, and patient is afebrile for 48 to 72 hours (IDSA [Stevens, 2014])

Urinary tract infection (complicated): IV:
Infants ≥3 months, Children, and Adolescents (≤50 kg): Canadian labeling (not in U.S. labeling): 10 mg/kg every 8 hours (maximum dose: 500 mg every 8 hours)
Children and Adolescents (>50 kg): Refer to adult dosing

Renal Impairment
Adults:
Manufacturer's labeling:
CrCl >50 mL/minute: No dosage adjustment necessary.
CrCl 26 to 50 mL/minute: Administer recommended dose based on indication every 12 hours
CrCl 10 to 25 mL/minute: Administer one-half recommended dose based on indication every 12 hours
CrCl <10 mL/minute: Administer one-half recommended dose based on indication every 24 hours
Alternative recommendations (off-label dosing):
GFR 10 to 50 mL/minute: Administer recommended dose (based on indication) every 12 hours (Aronoff, 2007)
GFR <10 mL/minute: Administer recommended dose (based on indication) every 24 hours (Aronoff, 2007)

Intermittent hemodialysis (IHD) (administer after hemodialysis on dialysis days): Meropenem and its metabolite are readily dialyzable: 500 mg every 24 hours (Heintz, 2009). **Note:** Dosing dependent on the assumption of 3 times weekly, complete IHD sessions.
Peritoneal dialysis (off-label dose): Administer recommended dose (based on indication) every 24 hours (Aronoff, 2007).
Continuous renal replacement therapy (CRRT) (Heintz, 2009; Trotman, 2005): Drug clearance is highly dependent on the method of renal replacement, filter type, and flow rate. Appropriate dosing requires close monitoring of pharmacologic response, signs of adverse reactions due to drug accumulation, as well as drug concentrations in relation to target trough (if appropriate). The following are general recommendations only (based on dialysate flow/ultrafiltration rates of 1 to 2 L/hour and minimal residual renal function) and should not supersede clinical judgment:
CVVH: Loading dose of 1 **g** followed by either 500 mg every 8 hours **or** 1,000 mg every 12 hours
CVVHD/CVVHDF: Loading dose of 1 **g** followed by either 500 mg every 6 to 8 hours **or** 1 **g** every 8 to 12 hours
Note: Consider giving patients receiving CVVHDF dosages of 750 mg every 8 hours **or** 1.5 **g** every 12 hours (Heintz, 2009). Substantial variability exists in various published recommendations, ranging from 1 to 3 **g** daily in 2 to 3 divided doses. One gram every 12 hours achieves a target trough of ~4 mg/L.

Children:
Manufacturer's labeling: There are no dosage adjustments provided in the manufacturer's labeling (has not been studied)
Alternate recommendations (off-label dosing; Aronoff, 2007):
GFR 30 to 50 mL/minute: Administer 20 to 40 mg/kg every 12 hours
GFR 10 to 29 mL/minute: Administer 10 to 20 mg/kg every 12 hours
GFR <10 mL/minute: Administer 10 to 20 mg/kg every 24 hours
Intermittent hemodialysis (IHD): 10 to 20 mg/kg every 24 hours administer after hemodialysis on dialysis days)
Peritoneal dialysis (PD): 10 to 20 mg/kg every 24 hours
Continuous renal replacement therapy (CRRT): 20 to 40 mg/kg every 12 hours

Hepatic Impairment No dosage adjustment necessary.
Dietary Considerations Some products may contain sodium.
Administration IV:
Infants <3 months: Administer as an IV infusion over 30 minutes
Infants ≥3 months, Children, Adolescents, and Adults: Administer IV infusion over 15 to 30 minutes; IV bolus injection (5 to 20 mL) over 3 to 5 minutes
Extended infusion administration (off-label dosing): Adults: Administer over 3 hours (Crandon 2011; Dandekar, 2003). **Note:** Must consider meropenem's limited room temperature stability if using extended infusions
Monitoring Parameters Perform culture and sensitivity testing prior to initiating therapy. Monitor for signs of anaphylaxis during first dose. During prolonged therapy, monitor renal function, liver function, CBC.
Test Interactions Positive Coombs' [direct]
Dosage Forms Excipient information presented when available (limited, particularly for generics); consult specific product labeling.
Solution Reconstituted, Intravenous:
Merrem: 500 mg (1 ea); 1 g (1 ea)
Generic: 500 mg (1 ea); 1 g (1 ea)

◆ Meropenem For Injection (Can) see Meropenem on page 1149
◆ Merrem see Meropenem on page 1149

Mesalamine (me SAL a meen)

Brand Names: US Apriso; Asacol HD; Asacol [DSC]; Canasa; Delzicol; Lialda; Pentasa; Rowasa; SfRowasa
Brand Names: Canada Asacol; Asacol 800; Mesasal; Mezavant; Pentasa; Salofalk; Teva-5 ASA
Index Terms 5-Aminosalicylic Acid; 5-ASA; Asacol; Fisalamine; Mesalazine
Pharmacologic Category 5-Aminosalicylic Acid Derivative

◀ **Use**

US labeling:

Oral:

Apriso: Maintenance of remission of ulcerative colitis in patients ≥18 years

Asacol HD: Treatment of moderately active ulcerative colitis in adults

Delzicol: Treatment of mildly to moderately active ulcerative colitis in patients ≥5 years; maintenance of remission of ulcerative colitis in adults

Lialda, Pentasa: Treatment and maintenance of remission of mildly to moderately active ulcerative colitis

Rectal: Treatment of active mild to moderate distal ulcerative colitis (suspension only), proctosigmoiditis (suspension only), or proctitis (suspension and suppository)

Canadian labeling:

Oral:

Asacol, Mezavant: Treatment and maintenance of remission of mildly- to moderately-active ulcerative colitis

Asacol 800: Treatment of moderately active ulcerative colitis

Mesasal: Treatment and maintenance of remission of ulcerative colitis

Pentasa: Treatment and maintenance of remission of mildly to moderately active ulcerative colitis; treatment and maintenance of remission of mild to moderate Crohn disease

Rectal: Treatment and maintenance of remission of distal ulcerative colitis (extending to splenic flexure) and as adjunctive therapy in more extensive disease (suspension only); treatment and maintenance of ulcerative proctitis (suppository only)

Pregnancy Considerations Adverse events have not been observed in animal reproduction studies. Dibutyl phthalate (DBP) is an inactive ingredient in the enteric coating of Asacol and Asacol HD; adverse effects in male rats were noted at doses greater than the recommended human dose. Mesalamine is known to cross the placenta. An increased rate of congenital malformations has not been observed in human studies. Preterm birth, still birth and decreased birth weight have been observed; however, these events may also be due to maternal disease. When treatment for inflammatory bowel disease is needed during pregnancy, mesalamine may be used, although products with DBP should be avoided (Habal, 2012; Mottet, 2009).

Breast-Feeding Considerations Low concentrations of the parent drug (undetectable to 0.11 mg/L) and higher concentrations of the N-acetyl metabolite of the parent drug (5 to 18 mg/L) have been detected in human breast milk. Adverse effects (diarrhea) in a breast-feeding infant have been reported while the mother received rectal administration of mesalamine within 12 hours after the first dose (Nelis, 1989). The manufacturer recommends that caution be exercised when administering mesalamine to breast-feeding women. Other sources consider use of mesalamine to be safe while breast-feeding (Habal, 2012; Mottet, 2009).

Contraindications

U.S. labeling: Hypersensitivity to mesalamine, aminosalicylates, salicylates, or any component of the formulation (including suppository vehicle of vegetable fatty acid esters)

Canadian labeling: Hypersensitivity to mesalamine, salicylates, or any component of the formulation; severe renal impairment (GFR <30 mL/minute/1.73 m^2); severe hepatic impairment

Additional contraindications per specific Canadian product labeling: Existing gastric or duodenal ulcer, urinary tract obstruction, use in children <2 years of age (Asacol, Asacol 800, Mesasal, Pentasa, Salofalk); hemorrhagic diathesis (Mesasal); patients unable to swallow intact tablet (Asacol, Asacol 800); renal parenchymal disease (Pentasa)

Warnings/Precautions May cause an acute intolerance syndrome (cramping, abdominal pain, bloody diarrhea; sometimes fever, headache, malaise, pruritus, rash, conjunctivitis); may be hard to discern from an exacerbation; discontinue immediately if syndrome occurs or is suspected. Symptoms usually abate if drug is discontinued. If rechallenge is performed to validate the hypersensitivity, use a reduced dose and only if clearly needed. Patients with pyloric stenosis or other organic or functional upper gastrointestinal obstructive disorders may have prolonged gastric retention of tablets, delaying the release of mesalamine in the colon. Mesalamine-induced hypersensitivity reactions have been reported and may include internal organ involvement, such as hepatitis, hematologic abnormalities, and/or pneumonitis. Discontinue treatment for mesalamine-induced hypersensitivity reactions. Pericarditis or myocarditis (mesalamine-induced cardiac hypersensitivity reactions) have been reported. Use with caution in patients predisposed to these conditions. Oligospermia (rare, reversible) has been reported in males. Patients with hypersensitivity to sulfasalazine may react to mesalamine; although usually well-tolerated in this population, use with caution. Use caution in patients with hepatic dysfunction; hepatic failure has been reported. Canadian labeling contraindicates use in severe hepatic impairment. Renal impairment (including minimal change nephropathy, acute/chronic interstitial nephritis, nephrotic syndrome, and rarely renal failure) has been reported; a renal function evaluation is recommended prior to initiation of therapy and periodically during treatment. Mesalamine-induced nephrotoxicity should be suspected in patients developing renal dysfunction during treatment. Use with caution in patients with renal impairment or a history of renal disease. Patients with preexisting renal disease, increased BUN or serum creatinine, or proteinuria should be carefully monitored, especially during the initial phase of treatment. Canadian labeling contraindicates use in severe renal impairment GFR <30 mL/minute/1.73 m^2; urinary tract obstruction and renal parenchymal disease are also included as contraindications in specific Canadian labels (refer to Contraindications). Use with caution in the elderly; postmarketing reports suggest an increased incidence of blood dyscrasias in patients >65 years; consider monitoring CBC periodically during therapy.

Apriso contains phenylalanine. The Asacol HD 800 mg tablet has not been shown to be bioequivalent to two Asacol 400 mg tablets [Canadian product] or two Delzicol 400 mg capsules. Canasa suppositories contain saturated vegetable fatty acid esters (contraindicated in patients with allergy to these components). Rowasa, Salofalk [Canadian product] and Pentasa [Canadian product] enema contain metabisulfite salts that may cause severe hypersensitivity reactions (ie, anaphylaxis) in patients with sulfite allergies. Rowasa, sfRowasa and Canasa Suppositories may stain surfaces including clothing, other fabrics, flooring, painted surfaces, enamel, granite, marble and vinyl; choose a suitable location for product administration and keep away from these surfaces. Potentially significant interactions may exist, requiring dose or frequency adjustment, additional monitoring, and/or selection of alternative therapy.

Delzicol: Intact, partially intact, and/or tablet shells have been reported in the stool. Two Delzicol 400 mg capsules have not been shown to be interchangeable or substitutable with 1 mesalamine 800 mg delayed-release tablet.

Adverse Reactions Adverse effects vary depending upon dosage form; frequency similar in adult and pediatric patients unless otherwise noted. Incidence usually on lower end with enema and suppository dosage forms.

>10%:

Central nervous system: Headache (adults: 2% to 14%; children and adolescents: 10%), pain (≤14%)

Gastrointestinal: Eructation (≤26%), abdominal pain (2% to 21%), exacerbation of ulcerative colitis (children and adolescents: 12%; adults: 2% to 3%), constipation (≤11%)

Respiratory: Nasopharyngitis (children and adolescents: 15%; adults: 1% to 4%), pharyngitis (11%)

1% to 10%:

Cardiovascular: Chest pain (3%), peripheral edema (3%), vasodilation (≥2%), syncope (children and adolescents: 2%), hypertension (1%)

Central nervous system: Dizziness (≤9%), hypertonia (5%), chills (3%), fatigue (<3%), vertigo (<3%), anxiety (≥2%), migraine (≥2%), nervousness (≥2%), paresthesia (≥2%), insomnia (≤2%), malaise (≤2%)

Dermatologic: Skin rash (1% to 6%), diaphoresis (≤3%), pruritus (≤3%), alopecia (<3%), acne vulgaris (≤2%)

Endocrine & metabolic: Increased serum triglycerides (<3%), weight loss (children and adolescents: 2%)

Gastrointestinal: Diarrhea (2% to 8%), flatulence (≤6%), vomiting (≤5%), dyspepsia (≤4%), nausea (≤4%), abnormal stools (≥2%), gastroenteritis (≥2%), gastrointestinal hemorrhage (<1% to ≥2%), tenesmus (≥2%), hemorrhoids (≥2%), bloody diarrhea (children and adolescents: 2%), pancreatitis (children and adolescents: 2%), rectal pain (2%), sclerosing cholangitis (children and adolescents: 2%), abdominal distention (≥1%), anorectal pain (1%; on insertion of enema tip), nausea and vomiting (1%)

Genitourinary: Hematuria (<3%), urinary frequency (<1% to ≥2%)

Hematologic & oncologic: Decreased hemoglobin (<3%), decreased hematocrit (<3%), rectal hemorrhage (<1% to ≥2%), anemia (children and adolescents: 2%)

Hepatic: Cholestatic hepatitis (<3%), increased serum transaminases (<3%), abnormal hepatic function tests (2%), increased serum ALT (1%)

Hypersensitivity: Anaphylaxis (2%)

Infection: Infection (≥2%), viral infection (children and adolescents: 2%; adenovirus)

Neuromuscular & skeletal: Back pain (6%), arthralgia (≤5%), myalgia (≤3%), weakness (<1% to ≥2%), arthritis (2%), musculoskeletal pain (2%; leg/joint)

Ophthalmic: Visual disturbance (≥2%), conjunctivitis (≤2%)

Otic: Tinnitus (<3%), otalgia (≥2%)

Renal: Decreased creatinine clearance (<3%), polyuria (≥2%)

Respiratory: Rhinitis (8%), sinusitis (children and adolescents: 7%; adults: ≥2%), flu-like symptoms (1% to ≥5%), cough (≤5%), dyspnea (<3%), bronchitis (≥2%)

Miscellaneous: Fever (≤1% to ≥5%), intolerance syndrome (3%)

<1% (Limited to important or life-threatening): Abdominal distention, abnormal T waves on ECG, abnormal uterine bleeding, agranulocytosis, albuminuria, alopecia, aplastic anemia, cholecystitis, cholestatic jaundice, DRESS syndrome, drug fever, duodenal ulcer, dysuria, ecchymoses, eczema, edema, eosinophilia, eosinophilic pneumonitis, erythema nodosum, esophageal ulcer, fecal discoloration, granulocytopenia, Guillain-Barré syndrome, hepatic cirrhosis, hepatic failure, hepatic injury, hepatic necrosis, hepatitis, hepatotoxicity, hypersensitivity pneumonitis, hypersensitivity reaction, hypomenorrhea, idiopathic nephrotic syndrome, increased blood urea nitrogen, increased serum amylase, increased serum bilirubin, increased serum creatinine, increased serum lipase, increased thirst, interstitial nephritis, interstitial pneumonitis, jaundice, Kawasaki-like syndrome, leg cramps, leukopenia, lupus-like syndrome, lymphadenopathy, mastalgia, mucus stools, myocarditis, nail disease, nephrotoxicity, neutropenia, oligospermia, palpitations, pancytopenia, paresthesia, perforated peptic ulcer, perianal skin irritation, pericardial effusion, pericarditis, peripheral neuropathy, pharyngolaryngeal pain, pleurisy, pneumonitis, pruritus, pulmonary infiltrates, pulmonary interstitial fibrosis, pyoderma gangrenosum, rectal discharge, rectal polyp, renal failure, skin photosensitivity, Stevens-Johnson syndrome, systemic lupus erythematosus, tachycardia, tenesmus, thrombocythemia, thrombocytopenia, transverse myelitis, vasodilation

Drug Interactions

Metabolism/Transport Effects None known.

Avoid Concomitant Use There are no known interactions where it is recommended to avoid concomitant use.

Increased Effect/Toxicity

Mesalamine may increase the levels/effects of: Heparin; Heparin (Low Molecular Weight); Thiopurine Analogs; Varicella Virus-Containing Vaccines

The levels/effects of Mesalamine may be increased by: Nonsteroidal Anti-Inflammatory Agents

Decreased Effect

Mesalamine may decrease the levels/effects of: Cardiac Glycosides

The levels/effects of Mesalamine may be decreased by: Antacids; H2-Antagonists; Proton Pump Inhibitors

Storage/Stability

Capsule, tablet: Store between 15°C and 30°C (59°F and 86°F). Protect capsules from moisture.

Enema: Store at 20°C to 25°C (68°F to 77°F). Use Rowasa promptly once foil wrap is removed; once the foil wrap is removed from a unit of seven sfRowasa bottles, discard any bottles remaining after 14 days. Contents may darken with time (do not use if dark brown).

Suppository: Store below 25°C (below 77°F). May store under refrigeration; do not freeze. Protect from direct heat, light, and humidity.

Mechanism of Action

Mesalamine (5-aminosalicylic acid) is the active component of sulfasalazine; the specific mechanism of action is unknown; however, it is thought that mesalamine modulates local chemical mediators of the inflammatory response, especially leukotrienes, and is also postulated to be a free radical scavenger or an inhibitor of tumor necrosis factor (TNF); action appears topical rather than systemic

Pharmacodynamics/Kinetics

Absorption: Rectal: Variable and dependent upon retention time, underlying GI disease, and colonic pH; Oral: Tablet: ~20% to 28%, Capsule: ~20% to 43%

Protein binding: Mesalamine (5-ASA): ~43%; N-acetyl-5-ASA: ~78%

Metabolism: Hepatic and via GI tract to N-acetyl-5-aminosalicylic acid

Half-life elimination: 5-ASA and N-acetyl-5-ASA: Variable; ~25 hours (range: 2 to 296 hours)

Time to peak, serum:

Capsule: Apriso: ~4 hours; Delzicol: ~10 hours; Pentasa: ~3 hours

Rectal: Pentasa, Salofalk [Canadian products]: 2 to 6 hours

Tablet: Asacol HD: 10 to 16 hours; Lialda: 9 to 12 hours

Canadian products: Asacol: 7 hours; Asacol 800: 10 hours; Mesasal: ~7 hours; Mezavant: 8 hours (range: 4 to 34 hours)

Excretion:

Oral, suppository: Urine (primarily as N-acetyl-5-ASA, ≤12% as unchanged drug); feces (unabsorbed mesalamine)

Enema: Feces (primarily); urine (10% to 30%)

Dosing

Adult

Crohn disease, mild to moderate (treatment): Pentasa (Canadian labeling; not in US labeling): Initial: 1 g 4 times daily

Crohn disease, mild to moderate (maintenance of remission): Pentasa (Canadian labeling; not in US labeling): 1 g 3 times daily

Distal ulcerative colitis or proctosigmoiditis, active mild to moderate (treatment): Rectal: Retention enema: **Note:** Duration of rectal therapy is 3 to 6 weeks; some patients may require rectal and oral therapy concurrently.

US labeling: 4 g at bedtime, retained overnight, approximately 8 hours

Canadian labeling: Salofalk 4 g or Pentasa 1 to 4 g at bedtime; retained overnight, approximately 8 hours

Distal ulcerative colitis (maintenance of remission): Rectal: Retention enema: Salofalk [Canadian product]: 2 g at bedtime daily or 4 g at bedtime every 2 to 3 days

Ulcerative colitis (treatment): Oral: Usual course of therapy is 6 to 8 weeks:

US labeling:

Asacol HD: 1.6 g 3 times daily for 6 weeks (**Note:** Approved for treatment only)

Delzicol: 800 mg 3 times daily for 6 weeks

Lialda: 2.4 or 4.8 g once daily

Pentasa: 1 g 4 times daily

Canadian labeling:

Asacol: 800 mg to 3.2 g in divided doses daily; for severe active disease may increase to 4.8 g daily

Asacol 800: 1.6 g 3 times daily for 6 weeks (**Note:** Approved for treatment only)

Mesasal: 1.5 to 3 g daily in 3 divided doses

Mezavant: 2.4 to 4.8 g once daily for up to 8 weeks

Pentasa: 500 mg 4 times daily; may increase to 1 g 4 times daily if needed

Ulcerative colitis (maintenance of remission): Oral:

US labeling:

Apriso: 1.5 once daily in the morning

Delzicol: 1.6 g in 2 to 4 divided doses

Lialda: 2.4 g once daily

Pentasa: 1 g 4 times daily

Canadian labeling:

Asacol: 1.6 g daily in divided doses

Mesasal: 1.5 g daily in 3 divided doses

Mezavant: 2.4 g once daily

Pentasa: 500 mg 4 times daily; may increase to 1 g 4 times daily if needed

Ulcerative proctitis, active:

US labeling:

Retention enema: 4 g at bedtime, retained overnight, approximately 8 hours

Rectal suppository: One 1,000 mg suppository rectally at bedtime; retain for at least 1 to 3 hours

Canadian labeling: Rectal suppository:

Pentasa: One 1,000 mg suppository in rectum daily at bedtime; retained for at least 1 to 3 hours to achieve maximum benefit

Salofalk: One 500 mg suppository in rectum 2 to 3 times daily or one 1,000 mg suppository in rectum once daily at bedtime; retained for at least 1 to 3 hours to achieve maximum benefit. Usual dose: 1 to 1.5 g daily until significant clinical response or remission. Taper off gradually; avoid abrupt discontinuation.

Geriatric Refer to adult dosing. Use with caution.

Pediatric

Ulcerative colitis (treatment): Children ≥5 years and Adolescents: Oral: Delzicol:

17 to 32 kg: 36 to 71 mg/kg/day in divided doses twice daily for 6 weeks; maximum dose: 1,200 mg/day

33 to 53 kg: 37 to 61 mg/kg/day in divided doses twice daily for 6 weeks; maximum dose: 2,000 mg/day

54 to 90 kg: 27 to 44 mg/kg/day in divided doses twice daily for 6 weeks; maximum dose: 2,400 mg/day

Renal Impairment

US labeling: There are no dosage adjustments provided in the manufacturer's labeling; however, dosage adjustment may be necessary since mesalamine is renally eliminated. Use with caution.

Canadian labeling:

GFR ≥30 mL/minute/1.73 m²: There are no dosage adjustments provided in the manufacturer's labeling; use with caution.

GFR <30 mL/minute/1.73 m²: Use is contraindicated; urinary tract obstruction and renal parenchymal disease are also contraindicated in specific Canadian labels (refer to Contraindications).

Hepatic Impairment

US labeling: There are no dosage adjustments provided in the manufacturer's labeling; use with caution.

Canadian labeling:

Mild to moderate impairment: There are no dosage adjustments provided in the manufacturer's labeling; use with caution.

Severe impairment: Use is contraindicated.

Dietary Considerations Some products may contain phenylalanine.

Apriso: Do not administer with antacids.

Administration Oral:

Capsules: Administer with or without food.

Apriso: Do not administer with antacids. Opening the capsule and placing the contents (delayed-release granules) on food with a pH <6 is not expected to affect the release of mesalamine once ingested (data on file, Salix Pharmaceuticals Medical Information). There is no safety/efficacy information regarding this practice.

Delzicol: Swallow capsule whole with water; do not break, chew, crush, or cut. If a patient is unable to swallow the capsule, may open capsule and swallow capsule contents whole (do not cut, chew, break, or crush, or cut the contents).

Pentasa: Swallow capsule whole; do not crush or chew; if a patient is unable to swallow the capsule, may open capsule and sprinkle the entire contents (controlled-release beads) onto yogurt or applesauce.

Tablets: Swallow whole; do not break, chew, or crush.

Asacol [Canadian product]: Administer with or without food.

Asacol HD, Asacol 800 [Canadian product]: Administer with or without food.

Lialda: Administer with a meal.

Mesasal [Canadian product]: Administer before meals.

Mezavant [Canadian product]: Administer once daily with a meal.

Pentasa [Canadian product]: Administer with meals.

Rectal enema: Shake bottle well. Instruct patient to lie on left side with left leg extended and right leg flexed forward for balance, or in "knee-chest" position. Insert lubricated applicator tip into the rectum and point slightly toward the navel. Grasp bottle firmly and tilt so nozzle is aimed toward the back; squeeze slowly to instill medication. After administration, withdraw and discard bottle. Retain enemas for 8 hours or as long as practical.

Suppository: Remove foil wrapper; avoid excessive handling. Insert into rectum. Retain suppository for 1 to 3 hours or longer.

Monitoring Parameters Renal function (prior to and periodically during therapy); CBC (particularly in elderly patients); hepatic function

Test Interactions May cause falsely-elevated urinary normetanephrine levels when measured by liquid chromatography with electrochemical detection (due to similarity in the chromatograms of normetanephrine and mesalamine's main metabolite, N-acetylaminosalicylic acid).

Dosage Forms Excipient information presented when available (limited, particularly for generics); consult specific product labeling. [DSC] = Discontinued product

Capsule Delayed Release, Oral:

Delzicol: 400 mg

Capsule Extended Release, Oral:

Pentasa: 250 mg [contains brilliant blue fcf (fd&c blue #1), fd&c yellow #10 (quinoline yellow)]

Pentasa: 500 mg [contains brilliant blue fcf (fd&c blue #1)]

Capsule Extended Release 24 Hour, Oral:

Apriso: 0.375 g [contains aspartame]

Enema, Rectal:

SfRowasa: 4 g/60 mL (60 mL) [sulfite free; contains edetate disodium, sodium benzoate]

Generic: 4 g (60 mL)

Kit, Rectal:

Rowasa: 4 g [contains edetate disodium, potassium metabisulfite, sodium benzoate]

Generic: 4 g

Suppository, Rectal:

Canasa: 1000 mg (30 ea, 42 ea)

Tablet Delayed Release, Oral:

Asacol: 400 mg [DSC]

Asacol HD: 800 mg

Lialda: 1.2 g

Dosage Forms: Canada Excipient information presented when available (limited, particularly for generics); consult specific product labeling.

Enema, Rectal:

Pentasa: 1 g/100 mL, 4 g/100 mL [contains sodium acetate, sodium edetate, sodium metabisulfite]

Salofalk: 2 g/60 mL, 4 g/60 mL [contains edetate disodium, potassium metabisulfite, sodium benzoate]

Suppository, Rectal:

Pentasa: 1000 mg

Salofalk: 500 mg, 1000 mg

Tablet Delayed Release, Oral:

Asacol: 400 mg

Asacol 800: 800 mg

Mesasal: 500 mg

Pentasa: 500 mg, 1 g

Tablet, delayed and extended release: Mezavant: 1.2 g

◆ Mesalazine *see* Mesalamine *on page 1151*

◆ Mesasal (Can) *see* Mesalamine *on page 1151*

◆ M-Eslon (Can) *see* Morphine (Systemic) *on page 1230*

Mesna (MES na)

Brand Names: US Mesnex

Brand Names: Canada Mesna for injection; Uromitexan

Index Terms Mercaptoethane Sulfonate; Sodium 2-Mercaptoethane Sulfonate

Pharmacologic Category Antidote; Chemoprotective Agent

Use

Prevention of ifosfamide-induced hemorrhagic cystitis: Preventive agent to reduce the incidence of ifosfamide-induced hemorrhagic cystitis

Limitations of use: Mesna is not indicted to reduce the risk of hematuria due to other conditions such as thrombocytopenia

Pregnancy Considerations Adverse effects were not observed in animal reproduction studies. Use during pregnancy only if clearly needed.

Breast-Feeding Considerations It is not known if mesna is excreted in breast milk. Benzyl alcohol, a component in some formulations, does enter breast milk and may be absorbed by a nursing infant. Due to the potential for adverse reactions in the nursing infant, a decision should be made to discontinue breast-feeding or to discontinue mesna, taking into account the importance of treatment to the mother.

Contraindications Hypersensitivity to mesna or any component of the formulation

Warnings/Precautions Monitor urine for hematuria. Severe hematuria despite utilization of mesna may require ifosfamide dose reduction or discontinuation. Examine morning urine specimen for hematuria prior to ifosfamide or cyclophosphamide treatment; if hematuria (>50 RBC/HPF) develops, reduce the ifosfamide/cyclophosphamide dose or discontinue the drug; will not prevent hemorrhagic cystitis in all patients. Mesna will not reduce the risk of hematuria related to thrombocytopenia. Patients should receive adequate hydration during treatment. Mesna is intended for the prevention of hemorrhagic cystitis and will not prevent or alleviate other toxicities associated with ifosfamide or cyclophosphamide.

Hypersensitivity reactions have been reported; symptoms ranged from mild hypersensitivity to systemic anaphylactic reactions and may include fever, hypotension, tachycardia, acute renal impairment, hypoxia, respiratory distress, urticaria, angioedema, signs of disseminated intravascular coagulation, hematologic abnormalities, increased liver enzymes, nausea, vomiting, arthralgia, and myalgia. Reactions may occur with the first exposure, or after several months of treatment. Monitor for signs/symptoms of reactions. May require discontinuation. Patients with autoimmune disorders receiving cyclophosphamide and mesna may be at increased risk. Mesna is a thiol compound; it is unknown if the risk for reaction is increased in patients who have had a reaction to other thiol compounds (eg, amifostine). Drug rash with eosinophilia and systemic symptoms and bullous/ulcerative skin and mucosal reactions consistent with Stevens-Johnson syndrome (SJS) or toxic epidermal necrolysis (TEN) have been reported. The skin and mucosal reactions may be characterized by rash, pruritus, urticaria, erythema, burning sensation, angioedema, periorbital edema, flushing, and stomatitis. Reactions may occur with the first exposure, or after several months of treatment. May require discontinuation.

Benzyl alcohol and derivatives: Some dosage forms may contain benzyl alcohol; large amounts of benzyl alcohol (≥99 mg/kg/day) have been associated with a potentially fatal toxicity ("gasping syndrome") in neonates; the

"gasping syndrome" consists of metabolic acidosis, respiratory distress, gasping respirations, CNS dysfunction (including convulsions, intracranial hemorrhage), hypotension, and cardiovascular collapse (AAP ["Inactive" 1997]; CDC, 1982); some data suggests that benzoate displaces bilirubin from protein binding sites (Ahlfors, 2001); avoid or use dosage forms containing benzyl alcohol with caution in neonates. See manufacturer's labeling.

Adverse Reactions

Mesna alone (frequency not defined):

Cardiovascular: Flushing

Central nervous system: Dizziness, fever, headache, hyperesthesia, somnolence

Dermatologic: Rash

Gastrointestinal: Anorexia, constipation, diarrhea, flatulence, nausea, taste alteration/bad taste (with oral administration), vomiting

Local: Injection site reactions

Neuromuscular: Arthralgia, back pain, rigors

Ocular: Conjunctivitis

Respiratory: Cough, pharyngitis, rhinitis

Miscellaneous: Flu-like syndrome

Mesna alone or in combination: Postmarketing and/or case reports: Allergic reaction, anaphylactic reaction, hypersensitivity, hyper-/hypotension, injection site erythema, injection site pain, limb pain, malaise, myalgia, platelets decreased, ST-segment increased, tachycardia, tachypnea, transaminases increased

Drug Interactions

Metabolism/Transport Effects None known.

Avoid Concomitant Use There are no known interactions where it is recommended to avoid concomitant use.

Increased Effect/Toxicity There are no known significant interactions involving an increase in effect.

Decreased Effect There are no known significant interactions involving a decrease in effect.

Preparation for Administration IV: Dilute in D_5W, NS, $D_5^{1/4}NS$, $D_5^{1/3}NS$, $D_5^{1/2}NS$, or lactated Ringer's to a final concentration of 20 mg/mL.

Storage/Stability Store intact vials and tablets at room temperature of 20°C to 25°C (68°F to 77°F); excursions are permitted between 15°C and 30°C (59°F and 86°F). Opened multidose vials may be stored and used for use up to 8 days after initial puncture. Solutions diluted for infusion stored at room temperature should be used within 24 hours. According to the manufacturer, mesna and ifosfamide may be mixed in the same bag if the final ifosfamide concentration is ≤50 mg/mL. Solutions of mesna and ifosfamide (1:1) in NS at a concentration of up to 20 mg/mL are stable for 14 days in PVC bags (Zhang, 2014). Solutions of mesna (0.5 to 3.2 mg/mL) and cyclophosphamide (1.8 to 10.8 mg/mL) in D_5W are stable for 48 hours refrigerated or 6 hours at room temperature (Menard, 2003). Mesna injection prepared for oral administration is stable for at least 9 days undiluted in polypropylene syringes and stored at 5°C, 24°C, 35°C; for 7 days when diluted 1:2 or 1:5 with syrups and stored at 24°C in capped tubes; or for 24 hours at 5°C when diluted to 1:2, 1:10, and 1:100 in orange or apple juice, milk, or carbonated beverages (Goren, 1991).

Mechanism of Action In blood, mesna is oxidized to dimesna which in turn is reduced in the kidney back to mesna, supplying a free thiol group which binds to and inactivates acrolein, the urotoxic metabolite of ifosfamide and cyclophosphamide

Pharmacodynamics/Kinetics

Distribution: 0.65 ± 0.24 L/kg; distributed to total body water

Metabolism: Rapidly oxidized to mesna disulfide (dimesna)

Bioavailability: Oral: Free mesna: 58% (range: 45% to 71%); not affected by food

Half-life elimination: Mesna: ~22 minutes; Dimesna: ~70 minutes

Time to peak, plasma: Oral: Free mesna: 1.5 to 4 hours

Excretion: Urine (32% as mesna; 33% as dimesna)

Dosing

Adult & Geriatric Note: Mesna dosing schedule should be repeated each day ifosfamide is received. If ifosfamide dose is adjusted (decreased or increased), the mesna dose should also be modified to maintain the mesna-to-ifosfamide ratio.

Prevention of ifosfamide-induced hemorrhagic cystitis:

Standard-dose ifosfamide (manufacturer's labeling): IV: Mesna dose is equal to 20% of the ifosfamide dose given for 3 doses: With the ifosfamide dose, hour 4, and at hour 8 after the ifosfamide dose (total daily mesna dose is 60% of the ifosfamide dose)

Oral mesna (following IV mesna; for ifosfamide doses ≤2 g/m²/day): Mesna dose (IV) is equal to 20% of the ifosfamide dose at hour 0, followed by mesna dose (orally) equal to 40% of the ifosfamide dose given 2 and 6 hours after the ifosfamide dose (total daily mesna dose is 100% of the ifosfamide dose). **Note:** If the oral mesna dose is vomited within 2 hours of administration, repeat the dose or administer IV mesna.

Short infusion standard-dose ifosfamide (<2.5 g/m²/day): ASCO guidelines: IV: Total mesna dose is equal to 60% of the ifosfamide dose, in 3 divided doses (each mesna dose as 20% of ifosfamide dose), given 15 minutes before the ifosfamide dose, and 4 and 8 hours after each dose of ifosfamide (Hensley, 2009)

Continuous infusion standard-dose ifosfamide (<2.5 g/m²/day): ASCO guidelines: IV: Mesna dose (as a bolus) is equal to 20% of the ifosfamide dose, followed by a continuous infusion of mesna at 40% of the ifosfamide dose; continue mesna infusion for 12-24 hours after completion of ifosfamide infusion (Hensley, 2009)

High-dose ifosfamide (>2.5 g/m²/day): ASCO guidelines: Evidence for use is inadequate; more frequent and prolonged mesna administration regimens may be required (Hensley, 2009)

Other dosing strategies used in combination with ifosfamide (off-label dosing):

Mesna continuous infusion: IV: 1.8 g/m²/day to 5 g/m²/day as a continuous infusion (100% of the ifosfamide dose), repeated each day ifosfamide is received; see protocols for specific details (Bacci, 2003; Kolb, 2003; Moskowitz, 2011)

Mesna bolus followed by continuous infusion: IV: 1000 mg/m² 1 hour prior to ifosfamide on day 1, followed by 3000 mg/m²/day continuous infusion (continuous infusion is 100% of the ifosfamide dose) on days 1, 2, and 3 (with sufficient hydration) every 3 weeks for 6 courses (Juergens, 2006)

Prevention of cyclophosphamide-induced hemorrhagic cystitis (off-label use):

HDCAV/IE regimen for Ewing sarcoma: Children ≥4 years and Adults <40 years: IV: 2100 mg/m²/day continuous infusion (mesna dose is equivalent to the cyclophosphamide dose) for 2 days with cyclophosphamide infusion during cycles 1, 2, 3, and 6 (Kolb, 2003)

Hyper-CVAD regimen for ALL: Adults: IV: 600 mg/m²/day continuous infusion (mesna continuous infusion is same total dose as cyclophosphamide) on days 1, 2, and 3, beginning with cyclophosphamide and ending 6 hours after the last cyclophosphamide dose during odd-numbered cycles (cycles 1, 3, 5, 7) of an 8-cycle phase (Kantarjian, 2000)

Pediatric

Prevention of ifosfamide-induced hemorrhagic cystitis (off-label use):

Short infusion standard-dose ifosfamide (<2.5 g/m²/day): ASCO guidelines: Refer to adult dosing.

Continuous infusion standard-dose ifosfamide (<2.5 g/m²/day): ASCO guidelines: Refer to adult dosing.

Other dosing strategies used in combination with ifosfamide (off-label dosing):

Mesna continuous infusion: IV: 1.8 g/m²/day to 5 g/m²/day as a continuous infusion (100% of the ifosfamide dose), repeated each day ifosfamide is received; see protocols for specific details (Bacci, 2003; Kolb, 2003; Moskowitz, 2011)

Mesna bolus followed by continuous infusion: IV: 1000 mg/m² 1 hour prior to ifosfamide on day 1, followed by 3000 mg/m²/day continuous infusion (continuous infusion is 100% of the ifosfamide dose) on days 1, 2, and 3 (with sufficient hydration) every 3 weeks for 6 courses (Juergens, 2006)

Mesna (20% higher than ifosfamide) continuous infusion: IV: 3600 mg/m²/day continuous infusion for 4 days (mesna dose is 20% higher than ifosfamide), with hydration, during weeks 4 and 9 (3 additional postop courses were administered in good responders) (Le Deley, 2007)

Prevention of cyclophosphamide-induced hemorrhagic cystitis (off-label use): HDCAV/IE regimen for Ewing sarcoma: Children ≥4 years and Adults <40 years: IV: 2100 mg/m²/day continuous infusion (mesna dose is equivalent to the cyclophosphamide dose) for 2 days with cyclophosphamide infusion during cycles 1, 2, 3, and 6 (Kolb, 2003)

Renal Impairment There are no dosage adjustments provided in the manufacturer's labeling (has not been studied)

◄ **Hepatic Impairment** There are no dosage adjustments provided in the manufacturer's labeling (has not been studied)

Administration Maintain adequate hydration and urinary output during ifosfamide treatment

IV: Administer as an IV bolus (per manufacturer); may also be administered by short infusion or continuous infusion (maintain continuous infusion for 12-24 hours after completion of ifosfamide infusion) (Hensley, 2009); refer to specific protocol for administration rate/details

Oral: Administer orally in tablet formulation; patients who vomit within 2 hours after taking oral mesna should repeat the dose or receive IV mesna. A solution may be prepared from solution for injection by dilution in syrup, juice, carbonate beverages, or milk (Goren, 1991); see Extemporaneous Preparations.

Monitoring Parameters Monitor urine for hematuria; urine output and hydration status; monitor for signs/symptoms of hypersensitivity or dermatologic toxicity

Test Interactions

Urinary ketones: False-positive tests for urinary ketones may occur in patients receiving mesna with the use of nitroprusside-based urine tests, including dipstick tests.

CPK activity: Mesna may interfere with enzymatic creatine kinase (CPK) activity tests which use a thiol compound (eg, N-acetylcysteine) for CPK reactivation; may result in a falsely low CPK level.

Ascorbic acid: Mesna may result in false-positive reactions in Tillman's reagent-based urine screening tests for ascorbic acid.

Additional Information Oncology Comment: Guidelines from the American Society of Clinical Oncology (ASCO) for the use of chemotherapy and radiotherapy protectants (Hensley, 2009 [update]; Schuchter, 2002) recommend mesna to decrease the incidence of ifosfamide-induced urotoxicity associated with short infusion and continuous infusion standard-dose ifosfamide (<2.5 g/m²/day). Although evidence is inadequate regarding mesna's uroprotective effects in high-dose ifosfamide (>2.5 g/m²/day), the guidelines suggest more frequent and prolonged mesna administration times may be required. For prevention of high-dose cyclophosphamide-induced urotoxicity (associated with stem cell transplantation), the guidelines recommend mesna in conjunction with saline diuresis (or forced saline diuresis alone).

Dosage Forms Excipient information presented when available (limited, particularly for generics); consult specific product labeling.

Solution, Intravenous:

Mesnex: 100 mg/mL (10 mL) [contains benzyl alcohol, edetate disodium]

Generic: 100 mg/mL (10 mL)

Tablet, Oral:

Mesnex: 400 mg [scored]

Dosage Forms: Canada Refer also to Dosage Forms.

Note: Tablets are not available in Canada.

Excipient information presented when available (limited, particularly for generics); consult specific product labeling.

Solution, Intravenous:

Mesna for injection: 100 mg/mL (10 mL) [contains benzyl alcohol, edetate disodium]

Uromitexan: 100 mg/mL (4 mL, 10 mL) [contains edetate disodium]

Uromitexan: 100 mg/mL (10 mL, 50 mL) [contains benzyl alcohol, edetate disodium]

Extemporaneous Preparations An oral solution may be prepared from mesna solution for injection. Dilute solution for injection to 20 mg/mL or 50 mg/mL with orange or grape syrup. Prior to administration, syrup-diluted solutions may be diluted to a final concentration of 1, 10, or 50 mg/mL with any of the following: carbonated beverages, apple juice, orange juice, or milk. Mesna injection prepared for oral administration is stable for at least 9 days undiluted in polypropylene syringes and stored at 5°C, 24°C, 35°C; for 7 days when diluted 1:2 or 1:5 with syrups and stored at 24°C in capped tubes; or for 24 hours at 5°C when diluted to 1:2, 1:10, and 1:100 in orange or apple juice, milk, or carbonated beverages. Dilution of mesna with diet or sugar-free preparations has not been evaluated.

Goren MP, Lyman BA, Li JT. The stability of mesna in beverages and syrup for oral administration. *Cancer Chemother Pharmacol.* 1991;28 (4):298-301.

◆ **Mesna for injection (Can)** see Mesna on page 1154

◆ **Mesnex** see Mesna on page 1154

◆ **Mestinon** see Pyridostigmine on page 1531

◆ **Mestinon-SR (Can)** see Pyridostigmine on page 1531

◆ **Mestranol and Norethindrone** see Norethindrone and Mestranol on page 1300

◆ **Metadate CD** see Methylphenidate on page 1180

◆ **Metadate ER** see Methylphenidate on page 1180

◆ **Metadol (Can)** see Methadone on page 1160

◆ **Metadol-D (Can)** see Methadone on page 1160

◆ **MetaFiber [OTC] [DSC]** see Psyllium on page 1529

◆ **Metafolbic Plus** see Methylfolate, Methylcobalamin, and Acetylcysteine on page 1179

◆ **Metafolbic Plus RF** see Methylfolate, Methylcobalamin, and Acetylcysteine on page 1179

◆ **Metaglip** see Glipizide and Metformin on page 845

◆ **Metamucil® (Can)** see Psyllium on page 1529

◆ **Metamucil MultiHealth Fiber [OTC]** see Psyllium on page 1529

Metaproterenol (met a proe TER e nol)

Brand Names: Canada Apo-Orciprenaline®; ratio-Orciprenaline®; Tanta-Orciprenaline®

Index Terms Alupent; Metaproterenol Sulfate; Orciprenaline Sulfate

Pharmacologic Category Beta₂ Agonist

Use Bronchodilator in reversible airway obstruction due to asthma or COPD

Dosing

Adult & Geriatric Bronchoconstriction: Oral: 20 mg 3-4 times/day

Pediatric Bronchoconstriction: Oral:

<6 years (limited experience): 1.3-2.6 mg/kg/day divided every 6-8 hours

6-9 years (or <27 kg): 10 mg/dose 3-4 times/day

>9 years (or ≥27 kg); Refer to adult dosing.

Renal Impairment No dosage adjustment provided in manufacturer's labeling.

Hepatic Impairment No dosage adjustment provided in manufacturer's labeling.

Additional Information Complete prescribing information should be consulted for additional detail.

Dosage Forms Excipient information presented when available (limited, particularly for generics); consult specific product labeling.

Syrup, Oral, as sulfate:

Generic: 10 mg/5 mL (473 mL)

Tablet, Oral, as sulfate:

Generic: 10 mg, 20 mg

◆ **Metaproterenol Sulfate** see Metaproterenol on page 1156

◆ **Metaxall** see Metaxalone on page 1156

Metaxalone (me TAKS a lone)

Brand Names: US Metaxall; Skelaxin

Brand Names: Canada Skelaxin®

Pharmacologic Category Skeletal Muscle Relaxant

Use *Musculoskeletal conditions:* Relief of discomforts associated with acute, painful musculoskeletal conditions.

Dosing

Adult & Geriatric Musculoskeletal conditions: Oral: 800 mg 3 to 4 times daily

Pediatric Musculoskeletal conditions: Adolescents ≥13 years: Refer to adult dosing.

Renal Impairment There are no dosage adjustments provided in the manufacturer's labeling; use with caution; contraindicated with significant renal impairment.

Hepatic Impairment There are no dosage adjustments provided in the manufacturer's labeling; use with caution; contraindicated with significant hepatic impairment.

Additional Information Complete prescribing information should be consulted for additional detail.

Dosage Forms Excipient information presented when available (limited, particularly for generics); consult specific product labeling.

Tablet, Oral:

Metaxall: 800 mg [scored; contains fd&c red #40]

Skelaxin: 800 mg [scored]

Generic: 400 mg, 800 mg

MetFORMIN (met FOR min)

Brand Names: US Fortamet; Glucophage; Glucophage XR; Glumetza; Riomet

Brand Names: Canada ACT-Metformin; Apo-Metformin; Auro-Metformin; Dom-Metformin; ECL-Metformin; Glucophage; Glumetza; Glycon; JAMP-Metformin; JAMP-Metformin Blackberry; Mar-Metformin; Metformin FC; Mint-Metformin; Mylan-Metformin; PHL-Metformin; PMS-Metformin; PRO-Metformin; RAN-Metformin; ratio-Metformin; Riva-Metformin; Sandoz-Metformin FC; Septa-Metformin; Teva-Metformin

Index Terms Metformin Hydrochloride

Pharmacologic Category Antidiabetic Agent, Biguanide

Use

Diabetes mellitus, type 2: Management of type 2 diabetes mellitus (noninsulin dependent, NIDDM) when hyperglycemia cannot be managed with diet and exercise alone.

Note: If not contraindicated and if tolerated, metformin is the preferred initial pharmacologic agent for type 2 diabetes management (ADA 2015).

Pregnancy Considerations Adverse events have not been observed in animal reproduction studies. Metformin has been found to cross the placenta in concentrations which may be comparable to those found in the maternal plasma. Pharmacokinetic studies suggest that clearance of metformin may increase during pregnancy and dosing may need adjusted in some women when used during the third trimester (Charles 2006; de Oliveira Baraldi 2011; Eyal 2010; Gardiner 2003; Hughes 2006; Vanky 2005).

An increased risk of birth defects or adverse fetal/neonatal outcomes has not been observed following maternal use of metformin for GDM or type 2 diabetes when glycemic control is maintained (Balani 2009; Coetzee 1979; Coetzee 1984; Ekpebegh 2007; Niromanesh 2012; Rowan 2008; Rowan 2010; Tertti 2008). In women with diabetes, maternal hyperglycemia can be associated with congenital malformations as well as adverse effects in the fetus, neonate, and the mother (ACOG 2005; ADA 2015; Kitzmiller 2008; Metzger 2007). To prevent adverse outcomes, prior to conception and throughout pregnancy maternal blood glucose and HbA$_{1c}$ should be kept as close to target goals as possible but without causing significant hypoglycemia (ACOG 2013; ADA 2015; Blumer 2013; Kitzmiller 2008). Prior to pregnancy, effective contraception should be used until glycemic control is achieved (Kitzmiller 2008).

Metformin may be used to treat GDM when nonpharmacologic therapy is not effective in maintaining glucose control (ACOG 2013). Metformin or lifestyle intervention may also be used in women with a history of GDM who later develop prediabetes in order to prevent or delay type 2 diabetes (ADA 2015).

Metformin is recommended to treat insulin resistance associated with PCOS; however, its use may also restore spontaneous ovulation. Women with PCOS who do not desire to become pregnant should use effective contraception. Although studied for use in women with anovulatory PCOS, there is no evidence that it improves live birth rates or decreases pregnancy complications. Routine use to treat infertility related to PCOS is not currently recommended (ACOG 2009; Fauser 2012).

Breast-Feeding Considerations Low amounts of metformin (generally ≤1% of the weight-adjusted maternal dose) are excreted into breast milk. Small amounts of metformin have been detected in the serum of nursing infants. Because breast milk concentrations of metformin stay relatively constant, avoiding nursing around peak plasma concentrations in the mother would not be helpful in reducing metformin exposure to the infant (Briggs 2005; Eyal 2010; Gardiner 2003; Hale 2002).

According to the manufacturer, due to the potential for hypoglycemia in the nursing infant, a decision should be made whether to discontinue nursing or to discontinue the drug, taking into account the importance of treatment to the mother. Breast-feeding is encouraged for all women, including those with diabetes (ACOG 2005; Blumer 2013; Metzger 2007). Small snacks before feeds may help decrease the risk of hypoglycemia in women with pregestational diabetes (ACOG 2005; Reader 2004); metformin may be used in breast-feeding women (Blumer 2013).

Contraindications

US labeling: Hypersensitivity to metformin or any component of the formulation; renal disease or renal dysfunction (serum creatinine ≥1.5 mg/dL in males or ≥1.4 mg/dL in females) or abnormal creatinine clearance from any cause, including shock, acute myocardial infarction, or septicemia; acute or chronic metabolic acidosis with or without coma (including diabetic ketoacidosis)

Canadian labeling: Hypersensitivity to metformin or any component of the formulation; renal function unknown, renal impairment, and serum creatinine levels above the upper limit of normal range; renal disease or renal dysfunction (serum creatinine ≥136 micromol/L in males or ≥124 micromol/L in females or abnormal creatinine clearance <60 mL/minute) which may result from conditions such as cardiovascular collapse (shock), acute myocardial infarction, and septicemia; unstable and/or insulin-dependent (type I) diabetes mellitus; acute or chronic metabolic acidosis, including diabetic ketoacidosis, with or without

coma, history of ketoacidosis with or without coma; history of lactic acidosis (regardless of precipitating factors); excessive alcohol intake (acute or chronic); severe hepatic dysfunction or clinical or laboratory evidence of hepatic disease; cardiovascular collapse and disease states associated with hypoxemia including cardiorespiratory insufficiency, which are often associated with hyperlactacidemia; stress conditions (eg, severe infection, trauma, surgery and postoperative recovery phase); severe dehydration; pregnancy; breast-feeding

Note: The manufacturer recommends to temporarily discontinue metformin in patients undergoing radiologic studies in which intravascular iodinated contrast media are utilized.

Warnings/Precautions [US Boxed Warning]: Lactic acidosis is a rare, but potentially severe consequence of therapy with metformin that requires urgent care and hospitalization. The risk is increased in patients with acute congestive heart failure, dehydration, excessive alcohol intake, hepatic or renal impairment, or sepsis. Symptoms may be nonspecific (eg, abdominal distress, malaise, myalgia, respiratory distress, somnolence); low pH, increased anion gap and elevated blood lactate may be observed. Discontinue immediately if acidosis is suspected. Lactic acidosis should be suspected in any patient with diabetes receiving metformin with evidence of acidosis but without evidence of ketoacidosis. Discontinue metformin in patients with conditions associated with dehydration, sepsis, or hypoxemia. The risk of accumulation and lactic acidosis increases with the degree of impairment of renal function. Use caution in patients with congestive heart failure requiring pharmacologic management, particularly in patients with unstable or acute CHF; risk of lactic acidosis may be increased secondary to hypoperfusion.

Metformin is substantially excreted by the kidney. The risk of accumulation and lactic acidosis increases with the degree of impairment of renal function. Patients with renal function below the limit of normal for their age should not receive metformin. Metformin should be withheld in patients with prerenal azotemia. In elderly patients, renal function should be monitored regularly; do not initiate in patients ≥80 years of age unless normal renal function is confirmed; risk of lactic acidosis may be increased. Use of concomitant medications that may affect renal function (ie, affect tubular secretion) may also affect metformin disposition. Therapy should be suspended for any surgical procedures (Canadian labeling recommends discontinuing use 48 hours prior to surgical procedures excluding minor procedures not associated with restricted food and fluid intake). Restart only after normal oral intake resumed and normal renal function is verified. Due to the risk of acute alteration in renal function, the manufacturer's labeling states to temporarily discontinue metformin prior to or at the time of intravascular administration of iodinated contrast media, withhold for 48 hours after the radiologic study, and restart only after renal function has been confirmed as normal. The American College of Radiology (ACR) guidelines also recommend to temporarily discontinue metformin at the time of contrast injection but only for certain patients: Patients with known renal dysfunction (and withhold until renal function monitoring assures safe reinstitution) and patients with normal renal function, but with multiple comorbidities (liver dysfunction, alcohol abuse, cardiac failure, myocardial/peripheral muscle ischemia, sepsis, severe infection) (and withhold for 48 hours). In patients with normal renal function and no known comorbidities, ACR states that discontinuation of metformin is not necessary (ACR 2013). It may be necessary to discontinue metformin and administer insulin if the patient is exposed to stress (fever, trauma, infection, surgery).

Use with caution in patients with impaired liver function. Patient must be instructed to avoid excessive acute or chronic ethanol use; ethanol may potentiate metformin's effect on lactate metabolism. May impair vitamin B$_{12}$ absorption, particularly in those with inadequate vitamin B$_{12}$ or calcium intake/absorption; very rarely associated with anemia. Rapid reversal of vitamin B12 deficiency may be observed with discontinuation of therapy or supplementation. Monitor vitamin B$_{12}$ serum concentrations periodically with long-term therapy. Administration of oral antidiabetic drugs has been reported to be associated with increased cardiovascular mortality; metformin does not appear to share this risk. Potentially significant interactions may exist, requiring dose or frequency adjustment, additional monitoring, and/or selection of alternative therapy. Insoluble tablet shell of Glumetza 1,000 mg extended release tablet may remain intact and be visible in the stool. Other extended released tablets (Fortamet, Glucophage XR, Glumetza 500 mg) may appear in the stool as a soft mass resembling the tablet. Diabetes self-management ▶

education (DSME) is essential to maximize the effectiveness of therapy. Not indicated for use in patients with insulin-dependent diabetes mellitus (IDDM) (type 1) or for the treatment of diabetic ketoacidosis.

Adverse Reactions

>10%: Gastrointestinal: Diarrhea (IR tablet: 53%; ER tablet: 10%), nausea and vomiting (IR tablet: 26%; ER tablet: 7%), flatulence (12%)

1% to 10%:

Cardiovascular: Chest discomfort (1% to 5%), flushing (1% to 5%), palpitations (1% to 5%)

Central nervous system: Headache (6%), chills (1% to 5%), dizziness (1% to 5%), taste disorder (1% to 5%)

Dermatologic: Diaphoresis (1% to 5%), nail disease (1% to 5%), skin rash (1% to 5%)

Endocrine & metabolic: Decreased vitamin B_{12} serum concentrate (7%), hypoglycemia (1% to 5%)

Gastrointestinal: Dyspepsia (≤1% to 7%), abdominal distress (6%), abdominal distention (1% to 5%), abdominal pain (1% to 5%), abnormal stools (1% to 5%), constipation (1% to 5%), heartburn (≤1% to 5%)

Neuromuscular & skeletal: Weakness (9%), myalgia (1% to 5%)

Respiratory: Dyspnea (1% to 5%), flu-like symptoms (1% to 5%), upper respiratory tract infection (1% to 5%)

<1% (Limited to important or life-threatening): Lactic acidosis, megaloblastic anemia

Drug Interactions

Metabolism/Transport Effects Substrate of OCT2

Avoid Concomitant Use

Avoid concomitant use of MetFORMIN with any of the following: Alcohol (Ethyl)

Increased Effect/Toxicity

MetFORMIN may increase the levels/effects of: Dalfampridine; Dofetilide; Hypoglycemia-Associated Agents

The levels/effects of MetFORMIN may be increased by: Alcohol (Ethyl); Alpha-Lipoic Acid; Androgens; BuPROPion; Carbonic Anhydrase Inhibitors; Cephalexin; Cimetidine; Dalfampridine; Dolutegravir; Glycopyrrolate; Glycopyrrolate (Systemic); Iodinated Contrast Agents; LamoTRIgine; MAO Inhibitors; Pegvisomant; Quinolone Antibiotics; Ranolazine; Salicylates; Selective Serotonin Reuptake Inhibitors; Topiramate; Trimethoprim; Vandetanib

Decreased Effect

MetFORMIN may decrease the levels/effects of: Trospium

The levels/effects of MetFORMIN may be decreased by: Hyperglycemia-Associated Agents; Quinolone Antibiotics; Thiazide Diuretics; Verapamil

Food Interactions Food decreases the extent and slightly delays the absorption. Management: Administer with a meal.

Storage/Stability

Oral solution: Store at 15°C to 30°C (59°F to 86°F).

Tablets: Store at 20°C to 25°C (68°F to 77°F); excursion permitted to 15°C to 30°C (59°F to 86°F). Protect from light and moisture.

Mechanism of Action Decreases hepatic glucose production, decreasing intestinal absorption of glucose and improves insulin sensitivity (increases peripheral glucose uptake and utilization)

Pharmacodynamics/Kinetics

Onset of action: Within days; maximum effects up to 2 weeks

Distribution: V_d: 654 ± 358 L; partitions into erythrocytes; concentrates in liver, kidney, and GI tract

Protein binding: Negligible

Metabolism: Not metabolized by the liver

Bioavailability: Absolute: Fasting: 50% to 60%

Half-life elimination: Plasma: 4 to 9 hours

Time to peak, serum: Immediate release: 2 to 3 hours; Extended release: 7 hours (range: 4 to 8 hours)

Excretion: Urine (90% as unchanged drug; active secretion)

Dosing

Adult

Diabetes mellitus, type 2: Oral: **Note:** Allow 1 to 2 weeks between dose titrations: Generally, clinically significant responses are not seen at doses <1,500 mg daily; however, a lower recommended starting dose and gradual increased dosage is recommended to minimize gastrointestinal symptoms.

Immediate-release tablet or solution: Adults ≥17 years: Initial: 500 mg twice daily **or** 850 mg once daily; titrate in increments of 500 mg weekly or 850 mg every other week; may also titrate from 500 mg twice a day to 850 mg twice a day after 2 weeks

If a dose >2,000 mg daily is required, it may be better tolerated in 3 divided doses. Maximum recommended dose: 2,550 mg daily.

Extended-release tablet: **Note:** If glycemic control is not achieved at maximum dose, may divide dose and administer twice daily.

Fortamet: Initial: 500 to 1,000 mg once daily; dosage may be increased by 500 mg weekly; maximum dose: 2,500 mg once daily

Glucophage XR: Initial: 500 mg once daily; dosage may be increased by 500 mg weekly; maximum dose: 2,000 mg once daily

Glumetza: Initial: 500 mg once daily; dosage may be increased by 500 mg weekly; maximum dose: 2,000 mg once daily

Transfer from other antidiabetic agents: No transition period is generally necessary except when transferring from chlorpropamide. When transferring from chlorpropamide, care should be exercised during the first 2 weeks because of the prolonged retention of chlorpropamide in the body, leading to overlapping drug effects and possible hypoglycemia.

Concomitant metformin and oral sulfonylurea therapy: If patients have not responded to 4 weeks of the maximum dose of metformin monotherapy, consider a gradual addition of an oral sulfonylurea, even if prior primary or secondary failure to a sulfonylurea has occurred. Continue metformin at the maximum dose. If adequate response has not occurred following 1 to 3 months of metformin and sulfonylurea combination therapy, consider switching to insulin with or without metformin.

Failed sulfonylurea therapy: Patients with prior failure on glyburide may be treated by gradual addition of metformin. Initiate with glyburide 20 mg and metformin 500 mg daily. Metformin dosage may be increased by 500 mg/day at weekly intervals, up to a maximum metformin dose (dosage of glyburide maintained at 20 mg daily).

Concomitant metformin and insulin therapy: Initial: Metformin 500 mg once daily; continue current insulin dose; may increase by metformin 500 mg after ~1 week and by 500 mg every week thereafter until adequate glycemic control is achieved

Maximum daily dose: Immediate release and solution: 2,550 mg metformin; Extended release: 2,000 to 2,500 mg (varies by product)

Decrease insulin dose 10% to 25% when FPG <120 mg/dL; monitor and make further adjustments as needed

Diabetes mellitus, type 2, prevention (off-label use): *Immediate-release tablet or solution:* Oral: Initial: 850 mg once daily; Target: 850 mg twice daily (Knowler 2002)

Polycystic ovary syndrome with anovulatory infertility (off-label use): Females: Oral:

Immediate release: 1,500 to 2,000 mg/day in 2 or 3 divided doses (Johnson 2010; Moll 2006; Morin-Papunen 2012)

Extended release: 1,000 mg twice daily (Legro 2007)

Note: Metformin should be initiated at lower doses (500 mg daily) and increased gradually over 1 to 2 weeks to the target dose to minimize adverse effects (eg, GI intolerance) (Johnson 2010; Legro 2007; Moll 2006; Morin-Papunen 2012)

Polycystic ovary syndrome with menstrual irregularities (off-label use): Females: Oral: *Immediate release:* 500 mg 2 or 3 times daily, up to 1,000 mg twice daily (Costello 2007; Morin-Papunen 2003; Meyer 2007; Moghetti 2000). The dose of metformin should be increased gradually to minimize GI adverse effects (Meyer 2007)

Note: When metformin is used, cyclic progestin therapy may be added for the first 6 months of metformin treatment, until regular cycles are established.

Prevention of ovarian hyperstimulation syndrome with polycystic ovary syndrome (off-label use): Females: Oral: *Immediate release:* 1,000 mg to 2,550 mg per day as 500 mg 2 or 3 times per day **or** 850 mg 2 or 3 times per day (Palomba 2013; Palomba 2011; Tang 2006; Tso 2014). The dose of metformin should be increased gradually to minimize GI adverse effects.

Note: Pretreatment with metformin may be started as early as 16 weeks prior (but typically 4 to 5 weeks prior) to as late as the first day of gonadotropin-releasing hormone (GnRH) agonist administration; some studies continued metformin therapy during gonadotropin ovarian stimulation (Tso 2014).

Geriatric The initial and maintenance dosing should be conservative, due to the potential for decreased renal function. Generally, elderly patients should **not** be titrated to the maximum dose of metformin.

Pediatric Diabetes mellitus, type 2: Oral: **Note:** Allow 1 to 2 weeks between dose titrations: Generally, clinically significant responses are not seen at doses <1,500 mg daily; however, a lower recommended starting dose and gradual increased dosage is recommended to minimize gastrointestinal symptoms.

Immediate-release tablet or solution:

Children ≥10 years and Adolescents ≤16 years: Initial: 500 mg twice daily; increases in daily dosage should be made in increments of 500 mg at weekly intervals, given in divided doses, up to a maximum of 2,000 mg daily

Adolescents ≥17 years: Refer to adult dosing.

Extended-release tablet: Adolescents ≥17 years: **Note:** If glycemic control is not achieved at maximum dose, may divide dose and administer twice daily.

Fortamet: Initial: 500 to 1,000 mg once daily; dosage may be increased by 500 mg weekly; maximum dose: 2,500 mg once daily

Glucophage XR: Initial: 500 mg once daily; dosage may be increased by 500 mg weekly; maximum dose: 2,000 mg once daily

Renal Impairment

Manufacturer's labeling:

Serum creatinine (SCr) ≥1.5 mg/dL (males) or ≥1.4 mg/dL (females): Use is contraindicated.

Abnormal CrCl (U.S. labeling: Not defined; Canadian labeling: <60 mL/minute): Use is contraindicated.

Alternate recommendations: **Note:** The United Kingdom National Institute for Health and Clinical Excellence (NICE) Guidelines recommends prescribing metformin with caution in those patients who are at risk of sudden deterioration in renal function and at risk of an estimated glomerular filtration rate (eGFR) <45 mL/minute/1.73 m^2 (NICE 2008]). Some evidence suggests that use of metformin is unsafe when eGFR <30 mL/minute/1.73 m^2 (calculated using MDRD) (Shaw 2007). A review of the available data by members of the American Diabetes Association proposed the following recommendations based on eGFR (Lipska 2011):

eGFR ≥60 mL/minute/1.73 m^2: No contraindications, monitor renal function annually

eGFR ≥45 to <60 mL/minute/1.73 m^2: Continue use; monitor renal function every 3 to 6 months

eGFR ≥30 to <45 mL/minute/1.73 m^2: In patients currently receiving metformin, use with caution, consider dosage reduction (eg, 50% reduction or 50% of maximal dose), monitor renal function every 3 months. Do not initiate therapy in patients with eGFR <45 mL/minute/1.73 m^2

eGFR <30 mL/minute/1.73 m^2: Discontinue use.

Hepatic Impairment The manufacturer recommends avoiding metformin since liver disease is considered a risk factor for the development of lactic acidosis during metformin therapy. However, continued use of metformin in diabetics with liver dysfunction, including cirrhosis, has been used successfully and may be associated with a survival benefit in carefully selected patients; use cautiously in patients at risk for lactic acidosis (eg, renal impairment, alcohol use) (Brackett 2010; Zhang 2014).

Dietary Considerations Drug may cause GI upset; take with food (to decrease GI upset). Take at the same time(s) each day. Dietary modification based on ADA recommendations is a part of therapy. Monitor for signs and symptoms of vitamin B_{12} and/or folic acid deficiency; supplementation may be required.

Administration Administer with a meal (to decrease GI upset).

Extended release: Swallow whole; do not crush, break, or chew. Administer once daily doses with the evening meal. Fortamet should also be administered with a full glass of water.

Monitoring Parameters Urine for glucose and ketones, fasting blood glucose, hemoglobin A_{1c}, and fructosamine. Initial and periodic monitoring of hematologic parameters (eg, hemoglobin/hematocrit and red blood cell indices) and renal function should be performed, at least annually (Canadian labeling recommends monitoring renal function every 6 months or more frequently if necessary). Monitor vitamin B_{12} serum concentrations periodically with long-term therapy.

Reference Range

Recommendations for glycemic control in nonpregnant adults with diabetes (ADA 2015):

HbA$_{1c}$: <7% (a more aggressive [<6.5%] or less aggressive [<8%] HbA$_{1c}$ goal may be targeted based on patient-specific characteristics)

Preprandial capillary plasma glucose: 80 to 130 mg/dL

Peak postprandial capillary blood glucose: <180 mg/dL

Recommendations for glycemic control in pediatric (all age groups) patients with type 1 diabetes (ADA 2015):

HbA$_{1c}$: <7.5% (individualization may be appropriate based on patient-specific characteristics; <7% is reasonable if it can be achieved without excessive hypoglycemia)

Preprandial capillary plasma glucose: 90 to 130 mg/dL

Bedtime and overnight capillary blood glucose: 90 to 150 mg/dL

Dosage Forms Considerations Extended release tablets utilize differing release mechanisms: Glucophage XR uses dual hydrophilic polymer matrix systems, Fortamet uses single-composition osmotic technology, and Glumetza uses gastric retention technology.

Dosage Forms Excipient information presented when available (limited, particularly for generics); consult specific product labeling.

Solution, Oral, as hydrochloride:

Riomet: 500 mg/5 mL (118 mL, 473 mL) [contains propylene glycol; strawberry flavor]

Riomet: 500 mg/5 mL (118 mL, 473 mL) [contains saccharin calcium; cherry flavor]

Tablet, Oral, as hydrochloride:

Glucophage: 500 mg, 850 mg

Glucophage: 1000 mg [scored]

Generic: 500 mg, 850 mg, 1000 mg

Tablet Extended Release 24 Hour, Oral, as hydrochloride:

Fortamet: 500 mg, 1000 mg

Glucophage XR: 500 mg, 750 mg

Glumetza: 500 mg, 1000 mg

Generic: 500 mg, 750 mg, 1000 mg

Dosage Forms: Canada Excipient information presented when available (limited, particularly for generics); consult specific product labeling.

Tablet, oral, as hydrochloride:

Glycon: 500 mg, 850 mg

◆ Metformin and Dapagliflozin *see* Dapagliflozin and Metformin *on page 488*

◆ Metformin and Glipizide *see* Glipizide and Metformin *on page 845*

◆ Metformin and Glyburide *see* Glyburide and Metformin *on page 849*

◆ Metformin and Linagliptin *see* Linagliptin and Metformin *on page 1079*

◆ Metformin and Repaglinide *see* Repaglinide and Metformin *on page 1570*

◆ Metformin and Rosiglitazone *see* Rosiglitazone and Metformin *on page 1619*

◆ Metformin and Saxagliptin *see* Saxagliptin and Metformin *on page 1640*

◆ Metformin and Sitagliptin *see* Sitagliptin and Metformin *on page 1666*

◆ Metformin FC (Can) *see* MetFORMIN *on page 1156*

◆ Metformin Hydrochloride *see* MetFORMIN *on page 1156*

◆ Metformin Hydrochloride and Dapagliflozin *see* Dapagliflozin and Metformin *on page 488*

◆ Metformin Hydrochloride and Linagliptin *see* Linagliptin and Metformin *on page 1079*

◆ Metformin Hydrochloride and Pioglitazone Hydrochloride *see* Pioglitazone and Metformin *on page 1455*

◆ Metformin Hydrochloride and Rosiglitazone Maleate *see* Rosiglitazone and Metformin *on page 1619*

◆ Metformin Hydrochloride and Saxagliptin *see* Saxagliptin and Metformin *on page 1640*

Methacholine (meth a KOLE leen)

Brand Names: US Provocholine

Brand Names: Canada Methacholine Omega; Provocholine

Index Terms Methacholine Chloride

Pharmacologic Category Diagnostic Agent

Use Bronchial airway hyperreactivity (diagnosis): Diagnosis of bronchial airway hyperreactivity in patients who do not have clinically apparent asthma

Dosing

Adult & Geriatric Note: For inhalation only mixed in solution; do not inhale powder.

Bronchial airway hyperreactivity (diagnosis): Inhalation: Before inhalation challenge, perform baseline pulmonary function tests; the patient must have an FEV_1 of at least 70% of the predicted value. Patients are given ascending serial concentrations (designated Vials E through A below) of methacholine starting with Vial E and ending with Vial A. At each concentration, 5 breaths are administered via nebulizer (with dosimeter). The following is a suggested schedule for administration of methacholine challenge. Calculate cumulative units by multiplying number of breaths by concentration given. Total cumulative units is the sum of cumulative units for each concentration given. See following breakdown:

Methacholine

Vial	Serial Concentration (mg/mL)	No. of Breaths	Cumulative Units per Concentration	Total Cumulative Units
E	0.025	5	0.125	0.125
D	0.25	5	1.25	1.375
C	2.5	5	12.5	13.88
B	10	5	50	63.88
A	25	5	125	188.88

Determine FEV_1 within 5 minutes of challenge, a positive challenge is a 20% reduction in FEV_1. After challenge completion, an inhaled beta-agonist may be administered to expedite FEV_1 return to baseline and relieve patient discomfort.

Pediatric Children ≥5 years and Adolescents: Refer to adult dosing.

Renal Impairment There are no dosage adjustments provided in the manufacturer's labeling.

Hepatic Impairment There are no dosage adjustments provided in the manufacturer's labeling.

Additional Information Complete prescribing information should be consulted for additional detail.

Dosage Forms Excipient information presented when available (limited, particularly for generics); consult specific product labeling.
Solution Reconstituted, Inhalation, as chloride:
Provocholine: 100 mg (1 ea)

◆ Methacholine Chloride see Methacholine on page 1159
◆ Methacholine Omega (Can) see Methacholine on page 1159

Methadone (METH a done)

Brand Names: US Dolophine; Methadone HCl Intensol; Methadose; Methadose Sugar-Free
Brand Names: Canada Metadol; Metadol-D; Methadose
Index Terms Methadone Hydrochloride
Pharmacologic Category Analgesic, Opioid
Additional Appendix Information
Opioid Conversion Table and Morphine Equivalent Dose Table on page 1955

Use
Chronic pain (except for oral soluble tablets for suspension): Management of pain severe enough to require daily, around-the-clock, long-term opioid treatment and for which alternative treatment options are inadequate.
Limitations of use: Because of the risks of addiction, abuse, and misuse with opioids, even at recommended doses, and because of the greater risks of overdose and death with long-acting opioids, reserve methadone for use in patients for whom alternative analgesic treatment options (eg, nonopioid analgesics, immediate-release opioid analgesics) are ineffective, not tolerated, or would be otherwise inadequate to provide sufficient management of pain. Methadone is not for use as an as-needed analgesic.

Detoxification: Detoxification and maintenance treatment of opioid addiction (heroin or other morphine-like drugs), in conjunction with appropriate social and medical services.

Pregnancy Considerations Adverse events were observed in animal reproduction studies. Methadone crosses the placenta and can be detected in cord blood, amniotic fluid, and newborn urine.

Methadone is considered the standard of care when treating opioid addiction in pregnant women. Women receiving methadone for the treatment of addiction should be maintained on their daily dose of methadone in addition to receiving the same pain management options during labor and delivery as opioid-naïve women; maintenance doses of methadone will not provide adequate pain relief. Narcotic agonist-antagonists should be avoided for the treatment of labor pain in women maintained on methadone due to the risk of precipitating acute withdrawal (ACOG, 2012; Dow, 2012).

Data is available related to fetal/neonatal outcomes following maternal use of methadone during pregnancy. Information collected by the Teratogen Information System is complicated by maternal use of illicit drugs, nutrition, infection, and psychosocial circumstances. However, pregnant women in methadone treatment programs are reported to have improved fetal outcomes compared to pregnant women using illicit drugs. Fetal growth, birth weight, length, and/or head circumference may be decreased in infants born to opioid-addicted mothers treated with methadone during pregnancy. Growth deficits do not appear to persist; however, decreased performance on psychometric and behavioral tests has been found to continue into childhood. Abnormal fetal nonstress tests have also been reported.

[U.S. Boxed Warning]: Prolonged maternal use of opioids during pregnancy can cause neonatal withdrawal syndrome in the newborn, which may be life-threatening if not recognized and treated according to protocols developed by neonatology experts. If prolonged opioid therapy is required in a pregnant woman, ensure treatment is available and warn patient of risk to the neonate. Withdrawal symptoms in the neonate may be observed up to 2 to 4 weeks after delivery and should be expected (ACOG, 2012). Neonatal abstinence syndrome following opioid exposure may present with autonomic (eg, fever, temperature instability), gastrointestinal (eg, diarrhea, vomiting, poor feeding/weight gain), or neurologic (eg, high-pitched crying, increased muscle tone, irritability, seizure, tremor) symptoms (Dow, 2012; Hudak, 2012). Monitoring is recommended for neonates born to mothers receiving methadone for neonatal abstinence syndrome (Chou, 2014).

Methadone clearance in pregnant women is increased and half-life is decreased during the 2nd and 3rd trimesters of pregnancy; the dosage of methadone may need increased or dosing interval decreased during pregnancy to avoid withdrawal symptoms in the mother. Dosage may need decreased following delivery (ACOG, 2012).

Long-term opioid use may cause secondary hypogonadism, which may lead to sexual dysfunction or infertility (Brennan, 2013). Amenorrhea may also develop secondary to substance abuse; pregnancy may occur following the initiation of buprenorphine or methadone maintenance treatment. Contraception counseling is recommended to prevent unplanned pregnancies (Dow, 2012).

Breast-Feeding Considerations Methadone is excreted into breast milk; the dose to a nursing infant has been calculated to be 2% to 3% of the maternal dose (following oral doses of 10 to 80 mg/day). Peak methadone levels appear in breast milk 4 to 5 hours after an oral dose. Methadone has been detected in the plasma of some breast-fed infants whose mothers are taking methadone. Sedation and respiratory depression have been reported in nursing infants. The manufacturer recommends that women monitor their nursing infants for sedation and that they should be instructed as to when to contact their healthcare provider for emergency care. In addition, the manufacturer recommends slowly weaning to prevent withdrawal symptoms in the nursing infant.

When methadone is used to treat opioid addiction in nursing women, guidelines do not contraindicate breast-feeding as long as the infant is tolerant to the dose and other contraindications do not exist (ACOG, 2012). If additional illicit substances are being abused, women treated with methadone should pump and discard breast milk until sobriety is established (ACOG, 2012; Dow, 2012).

Prescribing and Access Restrictions When used for treatment of opioid addiction: May only be dispensed in accordance to guidelines established by the Substance Abuse and Mental Health Services Administration's (SAMHSA) Center for Substance Abuse Treatment (CSAT). Regulations regarding methadone use may vary by state and/or country. Obtain advice from appropriate regulatory agencies and/or consult with pain management/palliative care specialists.

Note: Regulatory Exceptions to the General Requirement to Provide Opioid Agonist Treatment (per manufacturer's labeling):
1. During inpatient care, when the patient was admitted for any condition other than concurrent opioid addiction, to facilitate the treatment of the primary admitting diagnosis.
2. During an emergency period of no longer than 3 days while definitive care for the addiction is being sought in an appropriately licensed facility.

Medication Guide Available Yes

Contraindications

Hypersensitivity to methadone or any component of the formulation; significant respiratory depression; acute or severe bronchial asthma (in the absence of resuscitative equipment or in an unmonitored setting) or hypercarbia; known or suspected paralytic ileus; concurrent use of selegiline (Emsam product labeling)

Methadone is not to be used on an as-needed basis; it is not for pain that is mild or not expected to persist; it is not for acute pain or postoperative pain.

Canadian labeling: Additional contraindications (not in U.S. labeling): Diarrhea associated with pseudomembranous colitis or caused by poisoning until toxic material has been eliminated from the gastrointestinal tract

Warnings/Precautions

The optimal analgesic dose varies widely among patients. Doses should be titrated to pain relief/prevention. Patients maintained on stable doses of methadone may need rescue doses of a immediate release analgesic in case of acute pain (eg, postoperative pain, physical trauma). Methadone is ineffective for the relief of anxiety. May cause CNS depression, which may impair physical or mental abilities. Patients must be cautioned about performing tasks which require mental alertness (eg, operating machinery or driving). Effects may be potentiated when used with other CNS depressants (eg, sedatives, anxiolytics, hypnotics, neuroleptics, other opioids). Contraindicated in patients with respiratory depression and in those with conditions that increase the risk of life-threatening respiratory depression. Use with caution and monitor for respiratory depression in patients with significant chronic obstructive pulmonary disease or cor pulmonale, and patients having a substantially decreased respiratory reserve, hypoxia, hypercarbia, or preexisting respiratory depression, particularly when initiating therapy and titrating with methadone; even therapeutic doses may decrease respiratory drive to the point of apnea. Consider the use of alternative nonopioid analgesics in these patients. Use with caution in patients with depression or suicidal tendencies, or in patients with a history of drug or ethanol abuse. Avoid use of methadone in patients with CNS depression or coma as these patients are susceptible to intracranial effects of CO_2 retention. Use with caution in patients with head injury or increased intracranial pressure; reduced respiratory drive and resultant CO_2 retention may increase intracranial pressure. Elderly may be more susceptible to adverse effects (eg, CNS, respiratory, gastrointestinal). Decrease initial dose and use caution in the elderly, debilitated or cachectic; with hyper/hypothyroidism, morbid obesity, adrenal insufficiency, prostatic hyperplasia, or urethral stricture; or with severe renal or hepatic failure. Should only be prescribed by healthcare professionals who are knowledgeable in the use of potent opioids for chronic pain management.

[U.S. Boxed Warning]: QTc interval prolongation and serious arrhythmias (eg, torsades de pointes) have occurred during treatment. Closely monitor patients during initiation and titration for changes in cardiac rhythm. Patients should be informed of the potential arrhythmia risk, evaluated for any history of structural heart disease, arrhythmia, syncope, and for existence of potential drug interactions including drugs that possess QTc interval-prolonging properties, promote hypokalemia, hypomagnesemia, or hypocalcemia, or reduce elimination of methadone (eg, CYP3A4 inhibitors). Obtain baseline ECG for all patients and risk stratify according to QTc interval; QTc interval prolongation and torsades de pointes may be associated with doses >200 mg/day, but have also been observed with lower doses. Other agents should be used in patients with a baseline QTc interval ≥500 msecs (Chou, 2014).

Potentially significant drug-drug interactions may exist, requiring dose or frequency adjustment, additional monitoring, and/or selection of alternative therapy. May cause severe hypotension; use caution with severe volume depletion or other conditions which may compromise maintenance of normal blood pressure. Use caution with cardiovascular disease or patients predisposed to dysrhythmias. Concurrent use of mixed agonist/antagonist analgesics (eg, pentazocine, nalbuphine, butorphanol) or partial agonist (eg, buprenorphine) analgesics may precipitate withdrawal symptoms and/or reduced analgesic efficacy in patients following prolonged therapy with mu opioid agonists. Abrupt discontinuation following prolonged use may also lead to withdrawal symptoms. Abrupt cessation may precipitate withdrawal symptoms. Gradually taper dose. **[U.S. Boxed Warning]: When used for treatment of opioid addiction:** May only be dispensed by certified opioid treatment programs. Exceptions include inpatient treatment of other conditions and emergency period (not >3 days) while definitive substance abuse treatment is being sought.

Benzyl alcohol and derivatives: Some dosage forms may contain sodium benzoate/benzoic acid; benzoic acid (benzoate) is a metabolite of benzyl alcohol; large amounts of benzyl alcohol (≥99 mg/kg/day) have been associated with a potentially fatal toxicity ("gasping syndrome") in neonates; the "gasping syndrome" consists of metabolic acidosis, respiratory distress, gasping respirations, CNS dysfunction (including convulsions, intracranial hemorrhage), hypotension, and cardiovascular collapse (**AAP, 1997;** CDC, 1982); some data suggests that benzoate displaces bilirubin from protein binding sites (Ahlfors, 2001); avoid or use dosage forms containing benzyl alcohol derivative with caution in neonates. See manufacturer's labeling.

Oral formulations:

[U.S. Boxed Warning]: May cause serious, life-threatening, or fatal respiratory depression. Monitor closely for respiratory depression, especially during initiation or dose escalation. Carbon dioxide retention from opioid-induced respiratory depression can exacerbate the sedating effects of opioids. Peak respiratory depressant effect of methadone occurs later and persists longer than the peak analgesic effect, particularly during the initial dosing phase. Misuse or abuse (chewing, swallowing, snorting, or injecting the dissolved product) causes uncontrolled medication delivery resulting in a significant risk of overdose and death. Incomplete cross tolerance may occur; patients tolerant to other mu opioid agonists may not be tolerant to methadone.

[U.S. Boxed Warning]: Prolonged maternal use of opioids during pregnancy can cause neonatal withdrawal syndrome in the newborn which may be life-threatening if not recognized and treated according to protocols developed by neonatology experts. If prolonged opioid therapy is required in a pregnant woman, ensure treatment is available and warn patient of risk to the neonate. Signs and symptoms include irritability, hyperactivity and abnormal sleep pattern, high pitched cry, tremor, vomiting, diarrhea, and failure to gain weight. Onset, duration, and severity depend on the drug used, duration of use, maternal dose, and rate of drug elimination by the newborn. **[U.S. Boxed Warning]: Users are exposed to the risks of addiction, abuse, and misuse, potentially leading to overdose and death. Assess each patient's risk prior to prescribing; monitor all patients regularly for development of these behaviors or conditions.** Risk of opioid abuse is increased in patients with a history or family history of alcohol or drug abuse or mental illness. **[U.S. Boxed Warning]: Accidental ingestion of even one dose, especially in children, can result in a fatal overdose of methadone.** Use with caution in patients with biliary tract dysfunction including acute pancreatitis; may cause constriction of sphincter of Oddi. May obscure diagnosis or clinical course of patients with acute abdominal conditions. Avoid use in gastrointestinal obstruction.

Soluble tablets (diskets): **[U.S. Boxed Warning]: For oral administration only;** excipients to deter use by injection are contained in tablets.

Adverse Reactions

Frequency not defined. During prolonged administration, adverse effects may decrease over several weeks; however, constipation and sweating may persist.

Cardiovascular: Bigeminy, bradycardia, cardiac arrest, cardiac arrhythmia, cardiac failure, cardiomyopathy, ECG changes, edema, extrasystoles, flushing, hypotension, inversion T wave on ECG, orthostatic hypotension, palpitations, peripheral vasodilation, phlebitis, prolonged Q-T interval on ECG, shock, syncope, tachycardia, torsades de pointes, ventricular fibrillation, ventricular tachycardia

Central nervous system: Agitation, confusion, disorientation, dizziness, drowsiness, drug dependence (physical dependence), dysphoria, euphoria, habituation, hallucination, headache, insomnia, sedation, seizure

Dermatologic: Diaphoresis, hemorrhagic urticaria (can occur locally with intravenous administration [rare]), localized erythema (intravenous/subcutaneous), pruritus, rash at injection site (intravenous), skin rash, urticaria, urticaria at injection site (intravenous)

Endocrine & metabolic: Amenorrhea, antidiuretic effect, decreased libido, hypokalemia, hypomagnesemia, weight gain

Gastrointestinal: Abdominal pain, anorexia, biliary tract spasm, constipation, glossitis, nausea, stomach cramps, vomiting, xerostomia

Genitourinary: Impotence, urinary hesitancy, urinary retention

Hematologic: Thrombocytopenia (reversible, reported in patients with chronic hepatitis)

Local: Local pruritus (intravenous), local pain (intravenous/subcutaneous), local swelling (intravenous/subcutaneous)

Neuromuscular & skeletal: Weakness

Ophthalmic: Miosis, visual disturbance

Respiratory: Pulmonary edema, respiratory arrest, respiratory depression

<1% (Limited to important or life-threatening): Hypogonadism (Brennan, 2013; Debono, 2011)

Drug Interactions

Metabolism/Transport Effects Substrate of CYP2B6 (major), CYP2C19 (minor), CYP2C9 (minor), CYP2D6 (minor), CYP3A4 (major). **Note:** Assignment of Major/Minor substrate status based on clinically relevant drug interaction potential; **Inhibits** CYP2D6 (moderate)

Avoid Concomitant Use

Avoid concomitant use of Methadone with any of the following: Alcohol (Ethyl); Azelastine (Nasal); Benzodiazepines; Conivaptan; Dapoxetine; Eluxadoline; Fusidic Acid (Systemic); Highest Risk QTc-Prolonging Agents; Idelalisib; Itraconazole; Ivabradine; Ketoconazole (Systemic); Lopinavir; Mifepristone; Mixed Agonist / Antagonist Opioids; Orphenadrine; Paraldehyde; Posaconazole; QUEtiapine; Thalidomide; Thioridazine

Increased Effect/Toxicity

Methadone may increase the levels/effects of: Alvimopan; Antipsychotic Agents; ARIPiprazole; Azelastine (Nasal); Brexpiprazole; CNS Depressants; CYP2D6 Substrates; Desmopressin; Diuretics; DOXOrubicin (Conventional); Eluxadoline; Fesoterodine; Highest Risk QTc-Prolonging Agents; Hydrocodone; Lopinavir; Mequitazine; Methotrimeprazine; Metoclopramide; Metoprolol; Metyrosine; Moderate Risk QTc-Prolonging Agents; Nebivolol; Orphenadrine; Paraldehyde; Pramipexole; QUEtiapine; Ramosetron; ROPINIRole; Rotigotine; Saquinavir; Serotonin Modulators; Suvorexant; Thalidomide; Thioridazine; Zidovudine; Zolpidem

The levels/effects of Methadone may be increased by: Alcohol (Ethyl); Amphetamines; Anticholinergic Agents; Antiemetics (5HT3 Antagonists); Antipsychotic Agents; Antipsychotic Agents (Phenothiazines); Aprepitant; ARIPiprazole; Aromatase Inhibitors; Benzodiazepines; Boceprevir; Brimonidine (Topical); Cannabis; Cobicistat; Conivaptan; CYP2B6 Inhibitors (Moderate); CYP3A4 Inhibitors (Moderate); CYP3A4 Inhibitors (Strong); Dapoxetine; Dasatinib; Doxylamine; Dronabinol; Droperidol; Fluconazole; Fosaprepitant; Fusidic Acid (Systemic); HydrOXYzine; Idelalisib; Interferons (Alfa); Itraconazole; Ivabradine; Ivacaftor; Kava Kava; Ketoconazole (Systemic); Luliconazole; Magnesium Sulfate; MAO Inhibitors; Metaxalone; Methotrimeprazine; Mifepristone; Minocycline; Nabilone; Netupitant; Palbociclib; Perampanel; Posaconazole; QTc-Prolonging Agents (Indeterminate Risk and Risk Modifying); QUEtiapine; Rufinamide; Selective Serotonin Reuptake Inhibitors; Sodium Oxybate; Stiripentol; Succinylcholine; Tapentadol; Tetrahydrocannabinol; Voriconazole

Decreased Effect

Methadone may decrease the levels/effects of: Abacavir; Codeine; Didanosine; Fosamprenavir; Lubiprostone; Pegvisomant; Tamoxifen

The levels/effects of Methadone may be decreased by: Abacavir; Ammonium Chloride; Boceprevir; Bosentan; CarBAMazepine; CYP3A4 Inducers (Moderate); CYP3A4 Inducers (Strong); Dabrafenib; Darunavir; Deferasirox; Enzalutamide; Etravirine; Fosamprenavir; Fosphenytoin; Lopinavir; Mitotane; Mixed Agonist / Antagonist Opioids; Naltrexone; Nelfinavir; PHENobarbital; Phenytoin; Primidone; Reverse Transcriptase Inhibitors (Non-Nucleoside); Rifamycin Derivatives; Ritonavir; Saquinavir; Siltuximab; St Johns Wort; Telaprevir; Tipranavir; Tocilizumab

Food Interactions Grapefruit/grapefruit juice may increase levels of methadone. Management: Avoid concurrent use of grapefruit juice.

Storage/Stability

Injection: Store at 15°C to 30°C (59°F to 86°F). Protect from light.

Oral concentrate, oral solution, tablet: Store at 25°C (77°F); excursions are permitted between 15°C and 30°C (59°F and 86°F).

Mechanism of Action Binds to opiate receptors in the CNS, causing inhibition of ascending pain pathways, altering the perception of and response to pain; produces generalized CNS depression. Methadone has also been shown to have weak N-methyl-D-aspartate (NMDA) receptor antagonism (Callahan, 2004).

Pharmacodynamics/Kinetics

Onset of action: Oral: Analgesic: 0.5 to 1 hour; Parenteral: 10 to 20 minutes

Peak effect: Parenteral: 1 to 2 hours; Oral: Continuous dosing: 3 to 5 days

Duration of analgesia: Oral: 4 to 8 hours (single-dose studies), increases to 22 to 48 hours with repeated doses; slow release from the liver and other tissues may prolong duration of action

Distribution: Lipophilic; V_{dss}: 1 to 8 L/kg

Protein binding: 85% to 90% primarily to alpha-1 acid glycoprotein

Metabolism: Hepatic; N-demethylation primarily via CYP3A4, CYP2B6, and CYP2C19 to inactive metabolites

Bioavailability: Oral: 36% to 100%

Half-life elimination: Terminal: 8 to 59 hours; may be prolonged with alkaline pH

Time to peak, plasma: 1 to 7.5 hours

Excretion: Urine (<10% as unchanged drug); increased with urine pH <6

Dosing

Adult Regulations regarding methadone use may vary by state and/or country. Obtain advice from appropriate regulatory agencies and/or consult with pain management/palliative care specialists. **Note:** These are guidelines and do not represent the maximum doses that may be required. Consider total daily dose, potency, prior opioid use, degree of opioid experience and tolerance, conversion from previous opioid, patient's general condition, concurrent medications, and type and severity of pain during prescribing process. Other factors to consider:

- Interpatient variability in absorption, metabolism, and relative analgesic potency.
- Population-based equianalgesic conversion ratios between methadone and other opioids are not accurate when applied to individuals.
- Duration of analgesic action is much shorter than plasma elimination half-life.
- Steady-state plasma concentrations and full analgesic effects are not attained until at least 3 to 5 days after initiation, and may take longer in some patients.
- Methadone has a narrow therapeutic index, particularly when used concomitantly with other medications.

Chronic pain:

Manufacturer's labeling: Opioid-naive: Use as the first opioid analgesic:

Oral: Initial: 2.5 mg every 8 to 12 hours

IV: Initial: 2.5 to 10 mg every 8 to 12 hours; titrate slowly to effect; may also be administered by SubQ or IM injection (manufacturer's labeling)

Alternative recommendations: Opioid-naive: Oral:

Gradual titration (for chronic noncancer pain and situations where frequent monitoring is unnecessary): Initial: 2.5 mg every 8 hours; may increase dose by 2.5 mg per dose (Va/DoD, 2010) or 5 mg per day (Chou, 2014) every 5 to 7 days. Once a stable dose is reached, the dosing interval may be extended to every 8 to 12 hours, or longer (Va/DOD, 2010).

Faster titration (for cancer pain and situations where frequent monitoring is possible): Initial: 2.5 mg every 6 to 8 hours; may increase dose by 2.5 mg per dose as often as every day over about 4 days. Once a stable dose is reached, the dosing interval may be extended to every 8 to 12 hours, or longer (Va/DoD, 2010).

Conversion recommendations:

Manufacturer's labeling:

Conversion from oral opioids to oral methadone: Discontinue all other around-the-clock opioids when methadone therapy is initiated; fatalities have occurred in opioid-tolerant patients during conversion to methadone. Substantial interpatient variability exists in relative potency. Therefore, it is safer to underestimate a patient's daily oral methadone requirement and provide breakthrough pain relief with rescue medication (eg, immediate release opioid) than to overestimate requirements. Patient response to methadone needs to be monitored closely throughout the process of the conversion. Sum the current total daily dose of oral opioid, convert it to a morphine equivalent dose according to conversion factor for that specific opioid, then multiply the morphine equivalent dose by the corresponding percentage in the table to calculate the approximate oral methadone daily dose. Divide total daily methadone dose by intended dosing schedule (ie, divide by 3 for administration every 8 hours). Round down, if necessary, to the nearest strength available. For patients on a regimen of more than one opioid, calculate the approximate oral methadone dose for each opioid and sum the

totals to obtain the approximate total methadone daily dose, and divide the total daily methadone dose by the intended dosing schedule (ie, divide by 3 for administration every 8 hours). For patients on a regimen of fixed-ratio opioid/nonopioid analgesic medications, only the opioid component of these medications should be used in the conversion. **Note:** Conversion factors in table are only for the conversion from another oral opioid analgesic to methadone. Table cannot be used to convert from methadone to another opioid (doing so may lead to fatal overdose due to overestimation of the new opioid). This is not a table of equianalgesic doses.

Daily oral morphine dose <100 mg: Estimated daily oral methadone dose: 20% to 30% of total daily morphine dose

Daily oral morphine dose 100 to 300 mg: Estimated daily oral methadone dose: 10% to 20% of total daily morphine dose

Daily oral morphine dose 300 to 600 mg: Estimated daily oral methadone dose: 8% to 12% of total daily morphine dose

Daily oral morphine dose 600 to 1000 mg: Estimated daily oral methadone dose: 5% to 10% of total daily morphine dose.

Daily oral morphine dose >1000 mg: Estimated daily oral methadone dose: <5% of total daily morphine dose.

Conversion from parenteral methadone to oral methadone: Initial dose: Parenteral: Oral ratio: 1:2 (eg, 5 mg parenteral methadone equals 10 mg oral methadone)

Alternative recommendations: Opioid-tolerant:

Conversion from oral morphine to oral methadone: 1) There is not a linear relationship when converting to methadone from oral morphine. The higher the daily morphine equivalent dose the more potent methadone is, and 2) conversion to methadone is more of a process than a calculation. In general, the starting methadone dose should not exceed 30 to 40 mg/day, even in patients on high doses of other opioids. Patient response to methadone needs to be monitored closely throughout the process of the conversion. There are several proposed ratios for converting from oral morphine to oral methadone (Ayonrinde, 2000; Mercadente, 2001; Ripamonti, 1998). The estimated total daily methadone dose should then be divided to reflect the intended dosing schedule (eg, divide by 3 and administer every 8 hours). Patients who have not taken an opioid for 1 to 2 weeks should be considered opioid naïve (Chou, 2014).

Titration and maintenance: Manufacturer's labeling: May adjust dosage every 3 to 5 days to a dose providing adequate analgesia and minimal adverse reactions. However, because of high interpatient variability, substantially longer periods between dose adjustments may be necessary in some patients (up to 12 days). Breakthrough pain may require a dose increase or rescue medication with an immediate-release analgesic. Some guidelines note that dose increases should not be more than 10 mg per day every 5 to 7 days (Chou, 2014).

Discontinuation: Manufacturer's labeling: When pain management is no longer required, do not abruptly discontinue. Reduce dose every 2 to 4 days to prevent signs or symptoms of withdrawal.

Critically-ill patients (off-label use; Barr, 2013):
Note: May be used to slow development of tolerance when escalation with other opioids is required. Enteral methadone has also been used to wean prolonged continuous opioid infusions (Al Qadheeb, 2012)
Oral: 10 to 40 mg every 6 to 12 hours
IV: 2.5 to 10 mg every 8 to 12 hours

Detoxification: Oral:
Initial: A single dose of 20 to 30 mg is usually sufficient to suppress symptoms. Should not exceed 30 mg; lower doses should be considered in patients with low tolerance at initiation (eg, absence of opioids ≥5 days); an additional 5 to 10 mg of methadone may be provided if withdrawal symptoms have not been suppressed or if symptoms reappear after 2 to 4 hours; total daily dose on the first day should not exceed 40 mg. Do not increase dose without waiting for steady-state to be achieved. Levels will accumulate over the first few days; deaths have occurred in early treatment due to cumulative effects. Reassure the patient that duration of effect will increase as methadone accumulates.

Maintenance: Titrate to a dosage which prevents opioid withdrawal symptoms for 24 hours, prevents craving, attenuates euphoric effect of self-administered opioids, and tolerance to sedative effects of methadone. Usual range: 80 to 120 mg/day (titration should occur cautiously)
Withdrawal: Dose reductions should be <10% of the maintenance dose, every 10 to 14 days

Detoxification (short-term): Oral:
Initial: Titrate to ~40 mg/day in divided doses to achieve stabilization.
Maintenance: May continue 40 mg dose for 2 to 3 days.
Withdrawal: After 2 to 3 days of stabilization at 40 mg, gradually decrease the dose on a daily basis or at 2-day intervals. Keep dose at a level sufficient to keep withdrawal symptoms at a tolerable level. Hospitalized patients may tolerate a total daily dose decrease of 20%; ambulatory patients may require a slower reduction.

Dosage adjustment during pregnancy: Methadone dose may need to be increased or the dosing interval decreased when chronic doses are used during the second or third trimesters. Use is not appropriate for short term analgesia during labor and delivery.

Geriatric Oral, IM: 2.5 mg every 8 to 12 hours; refer to adult dosing.

Renal Impairment Off-label dosing (Aronoff, 2007):
Adults:
CrCl ≥10 mL/minute: No dosage adjustment necessary
CrCl <10 mL/minute: Administer 50% to 75% of normal dose

Hepatic Impairment There are no dosage adjustments provided in the manufacturer's labeling; however, undergoes hepatic metabolism and systemic exposure may be increased after repeated dosing. Avoid in severe liver disease.

Adjustment for Toxicity
Excessive opioid-related adverse events: Reduce next dose. Assess and reduce both the maintenance dose and dosing interval if necessary. Some guidelines recommend holding the dose if there is evidence of sedation (Chou, 2014).
QTc prolongation (Chou, 2014):
QTc >450 to 499 msecs: Discuss potential risks and benefits. Evaluate and correct potential causes of QTc interval prolongation prior to initiating therapy. Consider alternative therapies or reduced methadone dose if QTc interval becomes ≥450 to 499 msecs during treatment.
QTc ≥500 msecs: Alternative therapies for opioid addiction or chronic pain are recommended. If QTc ≥500 msecs occurs during therapy, switch to an alternative therapy or immediately decrease the dose of methadone; correct any reversible causes of QTc interval prolongation and repeat ECG.

Administration Oral dose for detoxification and maintenance may be administered in fruit juice or water. Dispersible tablet should not be chewed or swallowed; add to liquid and allow to dissolve before administering. May rinse if residual remains. Injectable solution can be administered IM, SubQ, or IV; rate of IV administration not defined.

Monitoring Parameters
Assess efficacy of pain control; vital signs and mental status; signs of drug abuse, addiction, or diversion; signs or symptoms of hypogonadism or hypoadrenalism (Brennan, 2013). Also evaluate constipation, nausea, pruritus, respiratory depression, and sedation (Chou, 2014).
Obtain baseline ECG (evaluate QTc interval) prior to therapy in patients with risk factors for QTc interval prolongation, a prior ECG with a QTc >450 msecs, or a history suggesting prior ventricular arrhythmia. If an ECG was obtained within the previous 3 months and it showed a QTc interval <450 msecs, it can be used as a baseline for patients without new risk factors. Repeat ECG 2 to 4 weeks after initiating therapy and after significant dose increases; follow-up ECG should also be done if new risk factors present or signs/symptoms of arrhythmia occur. Repeat ECG when the methadone dose reaches 30 to 40 mg per day (when started at lower doses) and again at 100 mg per day (Chou, 2014).

Reference Range Prevention of opioid withdrawal: Therapeutic: 100 to 400 ng/mL (SI: 0.32 to 1.29 micromole/L); Toxic: >2 mcg/mL (SI: >6.46 micromole/L)

Test Interactions Some quinolones may produce a false-positive urine screening result for opioids using commercially-available immunoassay kits. This has been demonstrated most consistently for levofloxacin and ofloxacin, but other quinolones have shown cross-reactivity in certain assay kits. Confirmation of positive opioid screens by more specific methods should be considered.

◄ **Dosage Forms** Excipient information presented when available (limited, particularly for generics); consult specific product labeling.

Concentrate, Oral, as hydrochloride:
Methadone HCl Intensol: 10 mg/mL (30 mL) [unflavored flavor]
Methadose: 10 mg/mL (1000 mL) [cherry flavor]
Methadose Sugar-Free: 10 mg/mL (1000 mL) [dye free, sugar free; unflavored flavor]
Generic: 10 mg/mL (30 mL, 1000 mL)

Solution, Injection, as hydrochloride:
Generic: 10 mg/mL (20 mL)

Solution, Oral, as hydrochloride:
Generic: 5 mg/5 mL (500 mL); 10 mg/5 mL (500 mL)

Tablet, Oral, as hydrochloride:
Dolophine: 5 mg, 10 mg [scored]
Methadose: 10 mg [scored]
Generic: 5 mg, 10 mg

Tablet Soluble, Oral, as hydrochloride:
Methadose: 40 mg [scored]
Generic: 40 mg

Dosage Forms: Canada Excipient information presented when available (limited, particularly for generics); consult specific product labeling.

Concentrate, Oral, as hydrochloride:
Metadol: 10 mg/mL [unflavored]
Methadose: 10 mg/mL [cherry flavor]
Methadose Sugar-Free: 10 mg/mL [dye free, sugar free; unflavored]

Solution, Oral, as hydrochloride:
Metadol: 1 mg/mL [unflavored]

Tablet, Oral, as hydrochloride:
Metadol: 1 mg, 5 mg, 10 mg, 25 mg [scored]

Controlled Substance C-II

◆ Methadone HCl Intensol see Methadone on page 1160
◆ Methadone Hydrochloride see Methadone on page 1160
◆ Methadose see Methadone on page 1160
◆ Methadose Sugar-Free see Methadone on page 1160
◆ Methaminodiazepoxide Hydrochloride see ChlordiazePOXIDE on page 372

Methamphetamine (meth am FET a meen)

Brand Names: US Desoxyn
Brand Names: Canada Desoxyn
Index Terms Desoxyephedrine Hydrochloride; Methamphetamine Hydrochloride
Pharmacologic Category Anorexiant; Central Nervous System Stimulant; Sympathomimetic

Use

Attention-deficit/hyperactivity disorder (ADHD): For a stabilizing effect in children >6 years with a behavioral syndrome characterized by the following group of developmentally inappropriate symptoms: Moderate to severe distractibility, short attention span, hyperactivity, emotional lability, and impulsivity

Exogenous obesity: Short-term (ie, a few weeks) adjunct in a regimen of weight reduction based on caloric restriction, for patients in whom obesity is refractory to alternative therapy (eg, repeated diets, group programs, other drugs)

Pregnancy Considerations Adverse effects have been observed in animal reproduction studies. Methamphetamine and amphetamine were detected in newborn tissues following intermittent maternal use of Desoxyn during pregnancy (Garriott, 1973). The majority of human data is based on illicit amphetamine/methamphetamine exposure and not from therapeutic maternal use (Golub, 2005). Use of amphetamines during pregnancy may lead to an increased risk of premature birth and low birth weight; newborns may experience symptoms of withdrawal. Behavioral problems may also occur later in childhood (LaGasse, 2012).

Breast-Feeding Considerations Methamphetamine is excreted in breast milk. The majority of human data is based on illicit amphetamine/methamphetamine exposure and not from therapeutic maternal use (Golub, 2005). Amphetamines may decrease milk production. Increased irritability, agitation, and crying have been reported in nursing infants (ACOG, 2011). Due to the potential for serious adverse reactions in the nursing infant, breast-feeding is not recommended by the manufacturer.

Medication Guide Available Yes

Contraindications
During or within 14 days following MAO inhibitors; glaucoma; advanced arteriosclerosis; symptomatic cardiovascular disease; moderate to severe hypertension; hyperthyroidism; hypersensitivity or idiosyncrasy to sympathomimetic amines; agitated state; patients with a history of drug abuse

Documentation of allergic cross-reactivity for amphetamines is limited. However, because of similarities in chemical structure and/or pharmacologic actions, the possibility of cross-sensitivity cannot be ruled out with certainty.

Warnings/Precautions CNS stimulant use has been associated with serious cardiovascular events including sudden death in patients with preexisting structural cardiac abnormalities or other serious heart problems (sudden death in children and adolescents; sudden death, stroke and MI in adults). These products should be avoided in the patients with known serious structural cardiac abnormalities, cardiomyopathy, serious heart rhythm abnormalities, or other serious cardiac problems that could increase the risk of sudden death that these conditions alone carry. Patients should be carefully evaluated for cardiac disease prior to initiation of therapy. Patients who develop angina, unexplained syncope, or other symptoms of cardiac disease during therapy should be evaluated immediately. Use with caution in patients with hypertension and other cardiovascular conditions (heart failure, recent MI, ventricular arrhythmia) that might be exacerbated by increases in blood pressure or heart rate. Use is contraindicated in patients with moderate-to-severe hypertension. Amphetamines may impair the ability to engage in potentially hazardous activities; patients must be cautioned about performing tasks which require mental alertness (eg, operating machinery or driving). Stimulants are associated with peripheral vasculopathy, including Raynaud's phenomenon; signs/symptoms are usually mild and intermittent, and generally improve with dose reduction or discontinuation. Digital ulceration and/or soft tissue breakdown have been observed rarely; monitor for digital changes during therapy and seek further evaluation (eg, rheumatology) if necessary. Difficulty in accommodation and blurred vision has been reported with the use of stimulants.

Use with caution in patients with psychiatric disorders, diabetes, or seizure disorders. May exacerbate symptoms of behavior and thought disorder in psychotic patients; new onset psychosis or mania may occur with stimulant use. Patients should be screened for bipolar disorder prior to treatment; consider discontinuation if such symptoms (eg, delusional thinking, hallucinations, or mania) occur. May be associated with aggressive behavior or hostility (causal relationship not established); monitor for development or worsening of these behaviors. May exacerbate motor and phonic tics and Tourette's syndrome. **[U.S. Boxed Warning]: Potential for drug dependency and abuse exists.** Use is contraindicated in patients with history of drug abuse. Prescriptions should be written for the smallest quantity consistent with good patient care to minimize possibility of overdose. Recommended to be used as part of a comprehensive treatment program for attention deficit disorders. Aggression and hostility has been reported with use of medications for ADHD treatment; no evidence suggests that stimulants cause aggressive behavior, but patient should be monitored for the onset or exacerbation of these behaviors. **[U.S. Boxed Warning]: Use in weight reduction programs only when alternative therapy has been ineffective.** Avoid prolonged treatment durations due to potential for drug dependence. Abrupt discontinuation following high doses or for prolonged periods may result in symptoms for withdrawal. Discontinue if satisfactory weight loss has not occurred within the first 4 weeks of treatment, or if tolerance develops.

Therapy is not appropriate for the treatment of fatigue in normal patients. Use caution in the elderly due to the risk for causing dependence, hypertension, angina, and myocardial infarction. Use of stimulants in pediatric patients has been associated with suppression of growth; monitor growth rate during treatment.

Adverse Reactions Frequency not defined.

Cardiovascular: Hypertension, increased blood pressure, palpitations, tachycardia

Central nervous system: Dizziness, drug dependence (prolonged use), dysphoria, euphoria, exacerbation of tics (motor, phonic, and Tourette's syndrome), headache, insomnia, overstimulation, psychotic symptoms, restlessness

Dermatologic: Urticaria

Endocrine & metabolic: Change in libido, growth suppression (children)

Gastrointestinal: Constipation, diarrhea, gastrointestinal distress, unpleasant taste, xerostomia

Genitourinary: Frequent erections, impotence, prolonged erection

Neuromuscular & skeletal: Rhabdomyolysis, tremor

Drug Interactions

Metabolism/Transport Effects Substrate of CYP2D6 (major); **Note:** Assignment of Major/Minor substrate status based on clinically relevant drug interaction potential

Avoid Concomitant Use

Avoid concomitant use of Methamphetamine with any of the following: Iobenguane I 123; MAO Inhibitors

Increased Effect/Toxicity

Methamphetamine may increase the levels/effects of: Analgesics (Opioid); Doxofylline; Sympathomimetics

The levels/effects of Methamphetamine may be increased by: Abiraterone Acetate; Alkalinizing Agents; Antacids; AtoMOXetine; Cannabinoid-Containing Products; Carbonic Anhydrase Inhibitors; Cobicistat; CYP2D6 Inhibitors (Moderate); CYP2D6 Inhibitors (Strong); Darunavir; Linezolid; MAO Inhibitors; Panobinostat; Peginterferon Alfa-2b; Tedizolid; Tricyclic Antidepressants

Decreased Effect

Methamphetamine may decrease the levels/effects of: Antihistamines; Antihypertensive Agents; Ethosuximide; Iobenguane I 123; Ioflupane I 123; PHENobarbital; Phenytoin

The levels/effects of Methamphetamine may be decreased by: Ammonium Chloride; Antipsychotic Agents; Ascorbic Acid; Gastrointestinal Acidifying Agents; Lithium; Methenamine; Multivitamins/Fluoride (with ADE); Multivitamins/Minerals (with ADEK, Folate, Iron); Multivitamins/Minerals (with AE, No Iron); Peginterferon Alfa-2b; Urinary Acidifying Agents

Food Interactions Amphetamine serum levels may be altered if taken with acidic food, juices, or vitamin C. Management: Administer 30 minutes before a meal.

Storage/Stability Store below 30°C (86°F).

Mechanism of Action A sympathomimetic amine related to ephedrine and amphetamine with CNS stimulant activity; causes release of catecholamines (primarily dopamine and other catecholamines) from their storage sites in the presynaptic nerve terminals. Inhibits reuptake and metabolism of catecholamines through inhibition of monoamine transporters and oxidase.

Pharmacodynamics/Kinetics

Absorption: Rapid from GI tract

Metabolism: Predominately hepatic via aromatic hydroxylation, N-dealkylation and deamination; forms ≥7 metabolites

Half-life elimination: 4-5 hours

Excretion: Urine primarily (dependent on urine pH; alkaline urine increases the half-life); 62% of dose eliminated within first 24 hours as ~33% unchanged drug with remainder as metabolites

Dosing

Adult & Geriatric Exogenous obesity: Oral: 5 mg given 30 minutes before each meal; treatment duration should not exceed a few weeks

Pediatric

ADHD: Oral: Children ≥6 years: Initial: 5 mg 1-2 times daily; may increase by 5 mg increments at weekly intervals until optimum response is achieved; usual effective dose range: 20-25 mg daily in 1 or 2 divided doses

Exogenous obesity: Oral: Children ≥12 years: Refer to adult dosing.

Renal Impairment No dosage adjustment provided in manufacturer's labeling.

Hepatic Impairment No dosage adjustment provided in manufacturer's labeling.

Dietary Considerations Most effective when combined with a low calorie diet and behavior modification counseling.

Administration For obesity, administer 30 minutes before each meal. Late evening doses should be avoided due to potential for insomnia.

Monitoring Parameters Heart rate, respiratory rate, blood pressure, CNS activity, body weight (BMI), signs of peripheral vasculopathy (eg, digital changes); growth rate in children

When used for the treatment of ADHD, thoroughly evaluate for cardiovascular risk. Monitor heart rate, blood pressure, and consider obtaining ECG prior to initiation (Vetter, 2008). Monitor for aggression and hostility.

Reference Range

Adult classification of weight by BMI (kg/m²):

Underweight: <18.5

Normal: 18.5-24.9

Overweight: 25-29.9

Obese, class I: 30-34.9

Obese, class II: 35-39.9

Extreme obesity (class III): ≥40

Waist circumference: In adults with a BMI of 25-34.9 kg/m², high-risk waist circumference is defined as:

Men >102 cm (>40 in)

Women >88 cm (>35 in)

Test Interactions Amphetamines may elevate plasma corticosteroid levels; may interfere with urinary steroid determinations.

Additional Information Illicit methamphetamine may contain lead; alkalinizing urine can result in longer methamphetamine half-life and elevated blood level; ephedrine is a precursor in the illicit manufacture of methamphetamine; ephedrine is extracted by dissolving ephedrine tablets in water or alcohol (50,000 tablets can result in 1 kg of ephedrine); conversion to methamphetamine occurs at a rate of 50% to 70% of the weight of ephedrine. 3,4-methylene dioxymethamphetamine (slang: XTC, Ecstasy, Adam) affects the serotonergic, dopaminergic, and noradrenergic pathways. As such, it can cause the serotonin syndrome associated with malignant hyperthermia and rhabdomyolysis.

Dosage Forms Excipient information presented when available (limited, particularly for generics); consult specific product labeling.

Tablet, Oral, as hydrochloride:

Desoxyn: 5 mg [contains sodium aminobenzoate]

Generic: 5 mg

Controlled Substance C-II

◆ **Methamphetamine Hydrochloride** *see* Methamphetamine *on page 1164*

Methazolamide (meth a ZOE la mide)

Brand Names: US Neptazane

Brand Names: Canada Apo-Methazolamide®

Pharmacologic Category Carbonic Anhydrase Inhibitor; Diuretic, Carbonic Anhydrase Inhibitor; Ophthalmic Agent, Antiglaucoma

Use Treatment of chronic open-angle or secondary glaucoma; short-term therapy of acute angle-closure glaucoma prior to surgery

Dosing

Adult & Geriatric Glaucoma: Oral: 50-100 mg 2-3 times/day

Renal Impairment Contraindicated in marked renal dysfunction.

Hepatic Impairment Contraindicated in marked hepatic dysfunction.

Additional Information Complete prescribing information should be consulted for additional detail.

Dosage Forms Excipient information presented when available (limited, particularly for generics); consult specific product labeling.

Tablet, Oral:

Neptazane: 25 mg

Neptazane: 50 mg [scored]

Generic: 25 mg, 50 mg

Methenamine (meth EN a meen)

Brand Names: US Hiprex; Urex [DSC]

Brand Names: Canada Mandelamine

Index Terms Hexamethylenetetramine; Methenamine Hippurate; Methenamine Mandelate; Urex

Pharmacologic Category Antibiotic, Miscellaneous

Use Urinary tract infection, prophylaxis/suppression: Prophylaxis or suppression of recurrent urinary tract infections when long-term therapy is indicated and infection has been eradicated by appropriate antimicrobial treatment

Dosing

Adult & Geriatric Urinary tract infection, prophylaxis/suppression: Oral:

Hippurate: 1,000 mg twice daily

Mandelate: 1,000 mg 4 times daily

Pediatric Urinary tract infection, prophylaxis/suppression: Oral:

US labeling:

Children <6 years: Mandelate: 250 mg per 14 kg body weight 4 times daily

Children 6 to 12 years:

Hippurate: 500 to 1,000 mg twice daily

Mandelate: 500 mg 4 times daily

Adolescents: Refer to adult dosing.

Canadian labeling: Mandelate:

Children <5 years: 250 mg per 14 kg body weight 4 times daily

Children ≥5 years and Adolescents: 500 mg 4 times daily

Renal Impairment Use is contraindicated.

Hepatic Impairment

Mild to moderate impairment: There are no dosage adjustments provided in the manufacturer's labeling; use with caution.

Severe impairment: Use is contraindicated.

Additional Information Complete prescribing information should be consulted for additional detail.

Dosage Forms Excipient information presented when available (limited, particularly for generics); consult specific product labeling. [DSC] = Discontinued product

Tablet, Oral, as hippurate:

Hiprex: 1 g [scored; contains tartrazine (fd&c yellow #5)]

Urex: 1 g [DSC] [scored]

Generic: 1 g

Tablet, Oral, as mandelate:

Generic: 0.5 g, 1 g

Methenamine and Sodium Acid Phosphate

(meth EN a meen & SOW dee um AS id FOS fate)

Brand Names: US Uroqid-Acid® No. 2

Index Terms Methenamine Mandelate and Sodium Acid Phosphate; Sodium Acid Phosphate and Methenamine

Pharmacologic Category Antibiotic, Miscellaneous

Use Prophylaxis or suppression of bacteriuria associated with recurrent urinary tract infections

Dosing

Adult & Geriatric Prophylaxis or suppression of bacteriuria: Oral: Initial: 2 tablets 4 times daily; maintenance: 2-4 tablets daily in divided doses

Additional Information Complete prescribing information should be consulted for additional detail.

Dosage Forms Excipient information presented when available (limited, particularly for generics); consult specific product labeling.

Tablet: Methenamine mandelate 500 mg and sodium acid phosphate 500 mg [contains 83 mg sodium]

♦ Methenamine Hippurate *see* Methenamine on page 1165

♦ Methenamine Mandelate *see* Methenamine on page 1165

♦ Methenamine Mandelate and Sodium Acid Phosphate *see* Methenamine and Sodium Acid Phosphate on page 1166

Methenamine, Phenyl Salicylate, Methylene Blue, Benzoic Acid, and Hyoscyamine

(meth EN a meen, fen nil sa LIS i late, METH i leen bloo, ben ZOE ik AS id & hye oh SYE a meen)

Brand Names: US Hyophen™; Prosed®/DS; Urophen MB

Index Terms Benzoic Acid, Hyoscyamine, Methenamine, Methylene Blue, and Phenyl Salicylate; Benzoic Acid, Methenamine, Methylene Blue, Phenyl Salicylate, and Hyoscyamine; Hyoscyamine, Methenamine, Benzoic Acid, Phenyl Salicylate, and Methylene Blue; Methylene Blue, Methenamine, Benzoic Acid, Phenyl Salicylate, and Hyoscyamine; Phenyl Salicylate, Methenamine, Methylene Blue, Benzoic Acid, and Hyoscyamine

Pharmacologic Category Antibiotic, Miscellaneous

Use Urinary tract discomfort secondary to hypermotility resulting from infection or diagnostic procedures

Dosing

Adult & Geriatric Urinary tract symptoms: Oral: One tablet 4 times/day

Pediatric Urinary tract symptoms: Children >6 years: Oral: Dosage must be individualized

Renal Impairment No dosage adjustment provided in manufacturer's labeling.

Hepatic Impairment No dosage adjustment provided in manufacturer's labeling.

Additional Information Complete prescribing information should be consulted for additional detail.

Dosage Forms Excipient information presented when available (limited, particularly for generics); consult specific product labeling.

Tablet, oral:

Hyophen™: Methenamine 81.6 mg, phenyl salicylate 36.2 mg, methylene blue 10.8 mg, benzoic acid 9 mg, hyoscyamine sulfate 0.12 mg

Prosed®/DS: Methenamine 81.6 mg, phenyl salicylate 36.2 mg, methylene blue 10.8 mg, benzoic acid 9 mg, hyoscyamine sulfate 0.12 mg

Urophen MB: Methenamine 81.6 mg, phenyl salicylate 36.2 mg, methylene blue 10.8 mg, benzoic acid 9 mg, hyoscyamine sulfate 0.12 mg

Methenamine, Sodium Phosphate Monobasic, Phenyl Salicylate, Methylene Blue, and Hyoscyamine

(meth EN a meen, SOW dee um FOS fate mon oh BAY sik, fen nil sa LIS i late, METH i leen bloo, & hye oh SYE a meen)

Brand Names: US Azuphen MB; Hyolev MB; Phosphasal; Ur N-C; Uramit MB; Urelle; Uribel; Urimar-T; Uro-L; Uro-MP; Ustell; Uticap; Utira-C; Utrona-C

Index Terms Hyoscyamine, Methenamine, Methylene Blue, Phenyl Salicylate, and Sodium Phosphate Monobasic; Hyoscyamine, Methenamine, Sodium Phosphate Monobasic, Phenyl Salicylate, and Methylene Blue; Methylene Blue, Methenamine, Sodium Phosphate Monobasic, Phenyl Salicylate, and Hyoscyamine; Phenyl Salicylate, Methenamine, Methylene Blue, Sodium Biphosphate, and Hyoscyamine; Sodium Phosphate Monobasic, Methenamine, Methylene Blue, Phenyl Salicylate, and Hyoscyamine

Pharmacologic Category Antibiotic, Miscellaneous

Use Treatment of symptoms of irritative voiding; relief of local symptoms associated with urinary tract infections; relief of urinary tract symptoms caused by diagnostic procedures

Dosing

Adult & Geriatric Urinary tract symptoms: Oral: One tablet 4 times daily (follow by liberal fluid intake)

Pediatric Urinary tract symptoms: Children >6 years: Oral: Dosage must be individualized

Renal Impairment No dosage adjustment provided in manufacturer's labeling.

Hepatic Impairment No dosage adjustment provided in manufacturer's labeling.

Additional Information Complete prescribing information should be consulted for additional detail.

Dosage Forms Excipient information presented when available (limited, particularly for generics); consult specific product labeling.

Capsule, oral:

Azuphen MB: Methenamine 120 mg, sodium phosphate monobasic 40.8 mg, phenyl salicylate 36 mg, methylene blue 10 mg, hyoscyamine sulfate 0.12 mg

Uramit MB: Methenamine 118 mg, sodium phosphate monobasic 40.8 mg, phenyl salicylate 36 mg, methylene blue 10 mg, hyoscyamine sulfate 0.12 mg

Uribel: Methenamine 118 mg, sodium phosphate monobasic 40.8 mg, phenyl salicylate 36 mg, methylene blue 10 mg, hyoscyamine sulfate 0.12 mg

Uro-MP: Methenamine 118 mg, sodium phosphate monobasic 40.8 mg, phenyl salicylate 36 mg, methylene blue 10 mg, hyoscyamine sulfate 0.12 mg

Ustell: Methenamine 120 mg, sodium phosphate monobasic 40.8 mg, phenyl salicylate 36 mg, methylene blue 10 mg, hyoscyamine sulfate 0.12 mg

Uticap: Methenamine 120 mg, sodium phosphate monobasic 40.8 mg, phenyl salicylate 36 mg, methylene blue 10 mg, hyoscyamine sulfate 0.12 mg

Tablet, oral:

Hyolev MB: Methenamine 81 mg, sodium phosphate monobasic 40.8 mg, phenyl salicylate 32.4 mg, methylene blue 10.8 mg, hyoscyamine sulfate 0.12 mg

Phosphasal: Methenamine 81.6 mg, sodium phosphate monobasic 40.8 mg, phenyl salicylate 36.2 mg, methylene blue 10.8 mg, hyoscyamine sulfate 0.12 mg

Ur N-C: Methenamine 81.6 mg, sodium phosphate monobasic 40.8 mg, phenyl salicylate 36.2 mg, methylene blue 10.8 mg, hyoscyamine sulfate 0.12 mg

Urelle: Methenamine 81 mg, sodium phosphate monobasic 40.8 mg, phenyl salicylate 32.4 mg, methylene blue 10.8 mg, hyoscyamine sulfate 0.12 mg

Urimar-T: Methenamine 120 mg, sodium phosphate monobasic 40.8 mg, phenyl salicylate 36.2 mg, methylene blue 10.8 mg, hyoscyamine sulfate 0.12 mg

Uro-L: Methenamine 81 mg, sodium phosphate monobasic 40.8 mg, phenyl salicylate 32.4 mg, methylene blue 10.8 mg, hyoscyamine sulfate 0.12 mg

Utira-C: Methenamine 81.6 mg, sodium phosphate monobasic 40.8 mg, phenyl salicylate 36.2 mg, methylene blue 10.8 mg, hyoscyamine sulfate 0.12 mg

Utrona-C: Methenamine 81.6 mg, sodium phosphate monobasic 40.8 mg, phenyl salicylate 36.2 mg, methylene blue 10.8 mg, hyoscyamine sulfate 0.12 mg

♦ Methergine [DSC] *see* Methylergonovine on page 1178

♦ Methergine® (Can) *see* Methylergonovine on page 1178

Methimazole (meth IM a zole)

Brand Names: US Tapazole

Brand Names: Canada Dom-Methimazole; PHL-Methimazole; Tapazole

Index Terms MMI; Thiamazole

Pharmacologic Category Antithyroid Agent; Thioamide

Use Hyperthyroidism: Treatment of hyperthyroidism in patients with Graves' disease or toxic multinodular goiter (surgery or radioactive iodine therapy is not appropriate); amelioration of hyperthyroid symptoms in preparation for thyroidectomy or radioactive iodine therapy.

Pregnancy Considerations Methimazole has been found to readily cross the placenta. Congenital anomalies, including esophageal atresia, choanal atresia, aplasia cutis, and dysmorphic facies, have been observed in neonates born to mothers taking methimazole during pregnancy (Stangaro-Green, 2011). Nonteratogenic adverse events, including fetal and neonatal hypothyroidism, have been observed following maternal methimazole use. The transfer of thyroid-stimulating immunoglobulins can stimulate the fetal thyroid *in utero* and transiently after delivery and may increase the risk of fetal or neonatal hyperthyroidism (De Groot, 2012; Stangaro-Green, 2011).

Uncontrolled maternal hyperthyroidism may result in adverse neonatal outcomes (eg, prematurity, low birth weight, infants born small for gestational age) and adverse maternal outcomes (eg, pre-eclampsia, congestive heart failure) (ACOG, 2002; Stangaro-Green, 2011). To prevent adverse fetal and maternal events, normal maternal thyroid function should be maintained prior to conception and throughout pregnancy. Antithyroid treatment is recommended for the control of hyperthyroidism during pregnancy. Due to an increased risk of congenital anomalies with methimazole, propylthiouracil is preferred during the first trimester of pregnancy and methimazole is preferred during the second and third trimesters of pregnancy (ACOG, 2002; De Groot, 2012; Stangaro-Green, 2011). If drug therapy is changed, maternal thyroid function should be monitored after 2 weeks and then every 2 to 4 weeks (De Groot, 2012).

The severity of hyperthyroidism may fluctuate throughout pregnancy and may result in decreased dose requirements or discontinuation of methimazole 2 to 3 weeks prior to delivery.

Breast-Feeding Considerations Methimazole is excreted into human breast milk. The thyroid function and intellectual development of breast-fed infants are not affected by exposure to maternal methimazole during breast-feeding. The American Thyroid Association considers doses of methimazole <30 mg/day to be safe during breast-feeding. Methimazole should be administered after nursing and in divided doses (Stagnaro-Green, 2011).

Contraindications Hypersensitivity to methimazole or any component of the formulation

Warnings/Precautions May cause significant bone marrow depression; the most severe manifestation is agranulocytosis. Aplastic anemia, thrombocytopenia, and leukopenia may also occur. and with concomitant use of other drugs known to cause myelosuppression (particularly agranulocytosis). Monitor patients closely; discontinue if significant bone marrow suppression occurs, particularly agranulocytosis or aplastic anemia.

May cause hypoprothrombinemia and bleeding. Monitoring is recommended, especially before surgical procedures. Antithyroid agents have been associated with rare but severe dermatologic reactions. Discontinue in the presence of exfoliative dermatitis. Hepatotoxicity (including acute liver failure) may occur. Symptoms suggestive of hepatic dysfunction (eg, anorexia, pruritus, right upper quadrant pain) should prompt evaluation. Discontinue in the presence of hepatitis and clinically significant hepatic abnormality, including transaminase >3 times upper limit of normal. May cause hypothyroidism; routinely monitor TSH and free T_4 levels, adjust dose to maintain euthyroid state. ANCA-positive vasculitis may develop during therapy discontinue use in the presence of vasculitis use. Discontinue in the presence of unexplained fever. A lupus-like syndrome may occur. Potentially significant drug-drug interactions may exist, requiring dose or frequency adjustment, additional monitoring, and/or selection of alternative therapy.

Adverse Reactions Frequency not defined.

Cardiovascular: ANCA-positive vasculitis, edema, leukocytoclastic vasculitis, periarteritis

Central nervous system: Drowsiness, fever, headache, neuritis, vertigo

Dermatologic: Alopecia, exfoliative dermatitis, pruritus, skin pigmentation, skin rash, urticaria

Endocrine & metabolic: Goiter, hypoglycemic coma

Gastrointestinal: Constipation, epigastric distress, loss of taste perception, nausea, salivary gland swelling, vomiting, weight gain

Hematologic: Agranulocytosis, aplastic anemia, granulocytopenia, hypoprothrombinemia, leukopenia, thrombocytopenia

Hepatic: Hepatic necrosis, hepatitis, jaundice

Neuromuscular & skeletal: Arthralgia, myalgia, paresthesia

Renal: Nephritis

Miscellaneous: Insulin autoimmune syndrome, lymphadenopathy, SLE-like syndrome

Drug Interactions

Metabolism/Transport Effects Inhibits CYP1A2 (weak), CYP2A6 (weak), CYP2B6 (weak), CYP2C19 (weak), CYP2C9 (weak), CYP2D6 (weak), CYP2E1 (weak)

Avoid Concomitant Use

Avoid concomitant use of Methimazole with any of the following: BCG (Intravesical); Deferiprone; Dipyrone; Sodium Iodide I131

Increased Effect/Toxicity

Methimazole may increase the levels/effects of: ARIPiprazole; Cardiac Glycosides; CloZAPine; Deferiprone; Theophylline Derivatives; TiZANidine

The levels/effects of Methimazole may be increased by: Dipyrone

Decreased Effect

Methimazole may decrease the levels/effects of: BCG (Intravesical); PredniSOLONE (Systemic); Sodium Iodide I131; Vitamin K Antagonists

Storage/Stability Store at 15°C to 30°C (59°F to 86°F).

Mechanism of Action Inhibits the synthesis of thyroid hormones by blocking the oxidation of iodine in the thyroid gland; blocks synthesis of thyroxine and triiodothyronine (T_3); does not inactivate circulating T_4 and T_3

Pharmacodynamics/Kinetics

Onset of action: Antithyroid: Oral: 12 to 18 hours (Clark, 2006)

Duration: 36 to 72 hours (Clark, 2006)

Distribution: Concentrated in thyroid gland

Protein binding, plasma: None (Cooper, 2005)

Metabolism: Hepatic

Excretion: Urine

Dosing

Adult & Geriatric Note: Administer in 3 equally divided doses at approximately 8-hour intervals.

Hyperthyroidism: Oral: Initial: 15 mg daily in 3 divided doses for mild hyperthyroidism; 30 to 40 mg daily in 3 divided doses for moderately severe hyperthyroidism; 60 mg daily in 3 divided doses for severe hyperthyroidism; maintenance: 5 to 15 mg daily (may be given as a single daily dose in many cases) (Mandana, 2004)

Adjust dosage as required to achieve and maintain serum T_3, T_4, and TSH levels in the normal range. An elevated T_3 may be the sole indicator of inadequate treatment. An elevated TSH indicates excessive antithyroid treatment.

Hyperthyroidism associated with Graves' disease: Oral:

Manufacturer's labeling: Initial: 15 mg daily in 3 divided doses for mild hyperthyroidism; 30 to 40 mg daily in 3 divided doses for moderately severe hyperthyroidism; 60 mg daily in 3 divided doses for severe hyperthyroidism; maintenance: 5 to 15 mg daily.

Alternate dosing: Initial: 10 to 20 mg once daily to restore euthyroidism; maintenance: 5 to 10 mg once daily for a total of 12 to 18 months, then taper or discontinue if TSH is normal at that time (Bahn, 2011).

Iodine-induced thyrotoxicosis (off-label use): Oral: 20 to 40 mg daily given either once or twice daily (Bahn, 2011)

Thyrotoxic crisis (off-label use): Oral: **Note:** Recommendations vary; use in combination with other specific agents. Dosages of 20 to 25 mg every 6 hours have been used; once stable, dosing frequency may be reduced to once or twice daily (Nayak, 2006). The American Thyroid Association and the American Association of Clinical Endocrinologists recommend 60 to 80 mg daily (Bahn, 2011). Rectal administration has also been described (Nabil, 1982).

Thyrotoxicosis (type I amiodarone-induced; off-label use): Oral: 40 mg once daily to restore euthyroidism (generally 3 to 6 months). **Note:** If high doses continue to be required, dividing the dose may be more effective (Bahn, 2011).

Pediatric Note: Administer in 3 equally divided doses at approximately 8-hour intervals.

Hyperthyroidism: Oral: Initial: 0.4 mg/kg/day in 3 divided doses; maintenance: 0.2 mg/kg/day in 3 divided doses

Hyperthyroidism associated with Graves' disease:
Oral:
Manufacturer's labeling: Initial: 0.4 mg/kg/day in 3 divided doses; maintenance: 0.2 mg/kg/day in 3 divided doses
Alternate dosing: Initial: 0.2 to 0.5 mg/kg once daily (range: 0.1 to 1 mg/kg/day) to restore euthyroidism, then reduce dose by 50% or more and continue for a total of 1 to 2 years; may then discontinue or reduce dose to assess if patient is in remission. **Note:** In severe cases, initial doses that are 50% to 100% higher may be used (Bahn, 2011).
The following dosing approach may also be used (Bahn, 2011):
Infants: 1.25 mg daily
Children 1 to 5 years: 2.5 to 5 mg daily
Children 5 to 10 years: 5 to 10 mg daily
Children and Adolescents 10 to 18 years: 10 to 20 mg daily

Renal Impairment There are no dosage adjustments provided in the manufacturer's labeling.

Hepatic Impairment There are no dosage adjustments provided in the manufacturer's labeling.

Administration In thyrotoxic crisis, rectal administration has been described (Nabil, 1982).

Monitoring Parameters Monitor for signs of hypothyroidism, hyperthyroidism, free T_4, T_3; CBC with differential, liver function (baseline and as needed), serum thyroxine, free thyroxine index; prothrombin time (especially before surgical procedures)

Additional Information A potency ratio of methimazole to propylthiouracil of at least 20-30:1 is recommended when changing from one drug to another (eg, 300 mg of propylthiouracil would be roughly equivalent to 10-15 mg of methimazole) (Bahn, 2011).

Dosage Forms Excipient information presented when available (limited, particularly for generics); consult specific product labeling.
Tablet, Oral:
Tapazole: 5 mg, 10 mg [scored]
Generic: 5 mg, 10 mg

Extemporaneous Preparations Suppositories can be made from methimazole tablets; dissolve 1200 mg methimazole in 12 mL of water and add to 52 mL cocoa butter containing 2 drops of Span 80. Stir the resulting mixture to form a water-oil emulsion and pour into 2.6 mL suppository molds to cool.

Nabil N, Miner DJ, and Amatruda JM, "Methimazole: An Alternative Route of Administration," *J Clin Endo Metab*, 1982, 54(1):180-1.

◆ Methitest *see* MethylTESTOSTERone *on page 1188*

Methocarbamol (meth oh KAR ba mole)

Brand Names: US Robaxin; Robaxin-750
Brand Names: Canada Robaxin®
Pharmacologic Category Skeletal Muscle Relaxant
Use Adjunctive treatment of muscle spasm associated with acute painful musculoskeletal conditions (eg, tetanus)

Pregnancy Considerations Animal reproduction studies have not been conducted. The manufacturer notes that fetal and congenital abnormalities have been rarely reported following *in utero* exposure. Use during pregnancy only if clearly needed.

Breast-Feeding Considerations It is not known if methocarbamol is excreted in breast milk. The manufacturer recommends that caution be exercised when administering methocarbamol to nursing women.

Contraindications Hypersensitivity to methocarbamol or any component of the formulation; renal impairment (injection formulation)

Warnings/Precautions May cause CNS depression, which may impair physical or mental abilities; patients must be cautioned about performing tasks which require mental alertness (eg, operating machinery or driving). Effects may be potentiated when used with other sedative drugs or ethanol. Plasma protein binding and clearance are decreased and the half-life is increased in patients with hepatic impairment. Muscle relaxants are poorly tolerated by the elderly due to potent anticholinergic effects, sedation, and risk of fracture. Efficacy is questionable at dosages tolerated by elderly patients; avoid use (Beers Criteria).

Injection: Contraindicated in renal impairment. Contains polyethylene glycol. Rate of injection should not exceed 3 mL/minute; solution is hypertonic; avoid extravasation. Use with caution in patients with a history of seizures. Use caution with hepatic impairment. Vial stopper contains latex. Recommended only for the treatment of tetanus in pediatric patients.

Adverse Reactions Frequency not defined.
Cardiovascular: Bradycardia, flushing, hypotension, syncope
Central nervous system: Amnesia, confusion, coordination impaired (mild), dizziness, drowsiness, fever, headache, insomnia, lightheadedness, sedation, seizures, vertigo
Dermatologic: Angioneurotic edema, pruritus, rash, urticaria
Gastrointestinal: Dyspepsia, metallic taste, nausea, vomiting
Hematologic: Leukopenia
Hepatic: Jaundice
Local: Pain at injection site, thrombophlebitis
Ocular: Blurred vision, conjunctivitis, diplopia, nystagmus
Respiratory: Nasal congestion
Miscellaneous: Hypersensitivity reactions including anaphylaxis

Drug Interactions
Metabolism/Transport Effects None known.
Avoid Concomitant Use
Avoid concomitant use of Methocarbamol with any of the following: Azelastine (Nasal); Orphenadrine; Paraldehyde; Thalidomide

Increased Effect/Toxicity
Methocarbamol may increase the levels/effects of: Alcohol (Ethyl); Azelastine (Nasal); Buprenorphine; CNS Depressants; Hydrocodone; Methotrimeprazine; Metyrosine; Mirtazapine; Orphenadrine; Paraldehyde; Pramipexole; ROPINIRole; Rotigotine; Selective Serotonin Reuptake Inhibitors; Suvorexant; Thalidomide; Zolpidem

The levels/effects of Methocarbamol may be increased by: Brimonidine (Topical); Cannabis; Doxylamine; Dronabinol; Droperidol; Eperisone; HydrOXYzine; Kava Kava; Magnesium Sulfate; Methotrimeprazine; Minocycline; Nabilone; Perampanel; Rufinamide; Sodium Oxybate; Tapentadol; Tetrahydrocannabinol

Decreased Effect
Methocarbamol may decrease the levels/effects of: Pyridostigmine

Preparation for Administration Solution for injection: May administer undiluted or diluted in D_5W or NS (1 vial/≤250 mL diluent).

Storage/Stability
Solution for injection: Prior to dilution, store at controlled room temperature of 20°C to 25°C (68°F to 77°F); excursions permitted to 15°C to 30°C (59°F to 86°F).
Tablet: Store at controlled room temperature of 20°C to 25°C (68°F to 77°F).

Mechanism of Action Causes skeletal muscle relaxation by general CNS depression

Pharmacodynamics/Kinetics
Onset of action: Muscle relaxation: Oral: ~30 minutes
Protein binding: 46% to 50%
Metabolism: Hepatic via dealkylation and hydroxylation
Half-life elimination: 1-2 hours
Time to peak, serum: Oral: 1-2 hours
Excretion: Urine (primarily as metabolites)

Dosing
Adult
Muscle spasm:
Oral: 1.5 g 4 times/day for 2-3 days (up to 8 g/day may be given in severe conditions), then decrease to 4-4.5 g/day in 3-6 divided doses
IM, IV: Initial: 1 g; may repeat every 8 hours if oral administration not possible; maximum dose: 3 g/day for no more than 3 consecutive days. If condition persists, may repeat course of therapy after a drug-free interval of 48 hours.
Tetanus: IV: Initial dose: 1-2 g by direct IV injection, which may be followed by an additional 1-2 g by infusion (maximum initial dose: 3 g total); may repeat initial dose every 6 hours until NG tube or oral therapy possible; total oral daily dose of up to 24 g may be needed; injection should not be used for more than 3 consecutive days

Pediatric
Tetanus (recommended **only** for use in tetanus): IV: 15 mg/kg/dose or 500 mg/m²/dose, may repeat every 6 hours if needed; maximum dose: 1.8 g/m²/day for 3 days only
Muscle spasm: Oral: Children ≥16 years: Refer to adult dosing.

Renal Impairment No dosage adjustment provided in manufacturer's labeling. However, administration of the parenteral formulation is contraindicated in patients with renal dysfunction due to the presence of polyethylene glycol.

Hepatic Impairment No dosage adjustment provided in manufacturer's labeling. However, elimination may be reduced in patients with cirrhosis.

Administration
Solution for injection:
IM: A maximum of 5 mL can be administered into each gluteal region.
IV: Maximum rate: 3 mL/minute; may be administered undiluted or diluted. Monitor closely for extravasation. Administer IV while in recumbent position. Maintain position for at least 10-15 minutes following infusion.
Tablet: May be crushed and mixed with food or liquid if needed.

Monitoring Parameters Monitor closely for extravasation (IV administration).

Test Interactions May cause color interference in certain screening tests for 5-HIAA using nitrosonaphthol reagent and in screening tests for urinary VMA using the Gitlow method.

Dosage Forms Excipient information presented when available (limited, particularly for generics); consult specific product labeling.
Solution, Injection:
Robaxin: 1000 mg/10 mL (10 mL) [contains polyethylene glycol 300]
Solution, Injection [preservative free]:
Generic: 1000 mg/10 mL (10 mL)
Tablet, Oral:
Robaxin: 500 mg [scored; contains fd&c yellow #6 (sunset yellow), saccharin sodium]
Robaxin-750: 750 mg [contains fd&c yellow #10 (quinoline yellow), fd&c yellow #6 (sunset yellow), saccharin sodium]
Generic: 500 mg, 750 mg

Methohexital (meth oh HEKS i tal)

Brand Names: US Brevital Sodium
Brand Names: Canada Brevital
Index Terms Methohexital Sodium
Pharmacologic Category Barbiturate; General Anesthetic
Use Induction of anesthesia; procedural sedation
Dosing
Adult
Anesthesia (doses must be titrated to effect): IV: Induction: 1-1.5 mg/kg
Procedural sedation (off-label dose): IV: 0.75-1 mg/kg; can redose 0.5 mg/kg every 2-5 minutes as needed (Bahn, 2005)
Wada test (off-label use): IV: 3-4 mg over 3 seconds; following signs of recovery, administer a second dose of 2 mg over 2 seconds (Buchtel, 2002)
Geriatric IV: Refer to adult dosing. Reduce dose or administer at the low end of the dosage range.
Pediatric
Anesthesia: Doses must be titrated to effect.
Infants <1 month: Safety and efficacy not established
Infants ≥1 month and Children: Induction:
IM: 6.6-10 mg/kg of a 5% solution
Rectal: Usual: 25 mg/kg of a 1% solution
IV (off-label dose): 1-2 mg/kg/dose of a 1% solution
Procedural sedation (off-label dose): Infants ≥1 month and Children:
IV: Initial: 0.5 mg/kg; may repeat 0.5 mg/kg to a maximum total dose of 2 mg/kg
Rectal: 25 mg/kg of a 10% (100 mg/mL) solution given 5-15 minutes prior to procedure; maximum dose 500 mg
Renal Impairment No dosage adjustment provided in manufacturer's labeling; use with caution.
Hepatic Impairment No dosage adjustment provided in manufacturer's labeling. However, adjustment may be necessary due to hepatic metabolism. Use with caution.
Additional Information Complete prescribing information should be consulted for additional detail.
Dosage Forms Excipient information presented when available (limited, particularly for generics); consult specific product labeling. [DSC] = Discontinued product
Solution Reconstituted, Injection, as sodium:
Brevital Sodium: 200 mg (1 ea [DSC]); 500 mg (1 ea); 2.5 g (1 ea)
Controlled Substance C-IV

◆ Methohexital Sodium see Methohexital on page 1169

Methotrexate (meth oh TREKS ate)

Brand Names: US Otrexup; Rasuvo; Rheumatrex; Trexall
Brand Names: Canada Apo-Methotrexate; JAMP-Methotrexate; Methotrexate Injection USP; Methotrexate Injection, BP; Methotrexate Sodium Injection; Metoject; ratio-Methotrexate Sodium

Index Terms Amethopterin; Methotrexate Sodium; Methotrexatum; MTX (error-prone abbreviation)
Pharmacologic Category Antineoplastic Agent, Antimetabolite (Antifolate); Antirheumatic, Disease Modifying; Immunosuppressant Agent
Use
Oncology uses: Acute lymphoblastic leukemia (ALL) maintenance treatment, ALL meningeal leukemia (prophylaxis and treatment); treatment of trophoblastic neoplasms (gestational choriocarcinoma, chorioadenoma destruens and hydatidiform mole), breast cancer, head and neck cancer (epidermoid), cutaneous T-Cell lymphoma (advanced mycosis fungoides), lung cancer (squamous cell and small cell), advanced non-Hodgkin lymphomas (NHL), osteosarcoma
Nononcology uses: Treatment of psoriasis (severe, recalcitrant, disabling) that is unresponsive to other therapies; severe, active rheumatoid arthritis (RA) that is unresponsive to or intolerant of first-line therapy including full dose non-steroidal anti-inflammatory agents (NSAIDs); active polyarticular-course juvenile idiopathic arthritis (pJIA) that is unresponsive to or intolerant of first-line therapy including full dose non-steroidal anti-inflammatory agents (NSAIDs).
Limitations of use: Otrexup and Rasuvo are not indicated for the treatment of neoplastic diseases.
Pregnancy Considerations [U.S. Boxed Warning]: Methotrexate may cause fetal death and/or congenital abnormalities. Studies in animals and pregnant women have shown evidence of fetal abnormalities; therefore, the manufacturer classifies methotrexate as pregnancy category X (for psoriasis or RA). A pattern of congenital malformations associated with maternal methotrexate use is referred to as the aminopterin/methotrexate syndrome. Features of the syndrome include CNS, skeletal, and cardiac abnormalities. Low birth weight and developmental delay have also been reported. The use of methotrexate may impair fertility and cause menstrual irregularities or oligospermia during treatment and following therapy. Methotrexate is approved for the treatment of trophoblastic neoplasms (gestational choriocarcinoma, chorioadenoma destruens, and hydatidiform mole) and has been used for the medical management of ectopic pregnancy and the medical management of abortion. **[U.S. Boxed Warning]: Use is contraindicated for the treatment of psoriasis or RA in pregnant women.** Pregnancy should be excluded prior to therapy in women of child-bearing potential. Use for the treatment of neoplastic diseases only when the potential benefit to the mother outweighs the possible risk to the fetus. Pregnancy should be avoided for ≥3 months following treatment in male patients and ≥1 ovulatory cycle in female patients. A registry is available for pregnant women exposed to autoimmune medications including methotrexate. For additional information contact the Organization of Teratology Information Specialists, OTIS Autoimmune Diseases Study, at 877-311-8972.
Breast-Feeding Considerations Low amounts of methotrexate are excreted into breast milk. Due to the potential for serious adverse reactions in a breast-feeding infant, use is contraindicated in nursing mothers.
Contraindications Known hypersensitivity to methotrexate or any component of the formulation; breast-feeding

Additional contraindications for patients with psoriasis or rheumatoid arthritis: Pregnancy, alcoholism, alcoholic liver disease or other chronic liver disease, immunodeficiency syndrome (overt or laboratory evidence); preexisting blood dyscrasias (eg, bone marrow hypoplasia, leukopenia, thrombocytopenia, significant anemia)
Warnings/Precautions Hazardous agent - use appropriate precautions for handling and disposal (NIOSH 2014 [group 1]).

[US Boxed Warning]: Methotrexate has been associated with acute (elevated transaminases) and potentially fatal chronic (fibrosis, cirrhosis) hepatotoxicity. Risk is related to cumulative dose (≥1.5 g) and prolonged exposure. Monitor closely (with liver function tests, including serum albumin) for liver toxicities. Liver enzyme elevations may be noted, but may not be predictive of hepatic disease in long term treatment for psoriasis (but generally is predictive in rheumatoid arthritis [RA] treatment). With long-term use, liver biopsy may show histologic changes, fibrosis, or cirrhosis; periodic liver biopsy is recommended with long-term use for psoriasis patients with risk factors for hepatotoxicity and for persistent abnormal liver function tests in psoriasis patients without risk factors for hepatotoxicity and in RA patients; discontinue methotrexate with moderate-to-severe change in liver biopsy. Risk factors for hepatotoxicity include history of above moderate ethanol consumption, persistent abnormal liver chemistries, history of chronic liver disease (including hepatitis B or C), family

history of inheritable liver disease, diabetes, obesity, hyperlipidemia, lack of folate supplementation during methotrexate therapy, cumulative methotrexate dose exceeding 1.5 g, continuous daily methotrexate dosing and history of significant exposure to hepatotoxic drugs. Use caution with preexisting liver impairment; may require dosage reduction. Use caution when used with other hepatotoxic agents (azathioprine, retinoids, sulfasalazine). **[US Boxed Warning]: Methotrexate elimination is reduced in patients with ascites and pleural effusions;** resulting in prolonged half-life and toxicity; may require dose reduction or discontinuation. Monitor closely for toxicity.

[US Boxed Warning]: May cause renal damage leading to acute renal failure, especially with high-dose methotrexate; monitor renal function and methotrexate levels closely, maintain adequate hydration and urinary alkalinization. Use caution in osteosarcoma patients treated with high-dose methotrexate in combination with nephrotoxic chemotherapy (eg, cisplatin). **[US Boxed Warning]: Methotrexate elimination is reduced in patients with renal impairment;** may require dose reduction or discontinuation; monitor closely for toxicity. **[US Boxed Warning]: Tumor lysis syndrome may occur in patients with high tumor burden;** use appropriate prevention and treatment.

[US Boxed Warning]: May cause potentially life-threatening pneumonitis (acute or chronic); may require treatment interruption; may be irreversible. Pulmonary symptoms may occur at any time during therapy and at any dosage; monitor closely for pulmonary symptoms, particularly dry, nonproductive cough. Other potential symptoms include fever, dyspnea, hypoxemia, or pulmonary infiltrate. **[US Boxed Warning]: Methotrexate elimination is reduced in patients with pleural effusions;** may require dose reduction or discontinuation. Monitor closely for toxicity.

[US Boxed Warning]: Bone marrow suppression may occur (sometimes fatal); aplastic anemia has been reported; anemia, pancytopenia, leukopenia, neutropenia, and/or thrombocytopenia may occur. Use caution in patients with preexisting bone marrow suppression. Discontinue treatment (immediately) in RA or psoriasis if a significant decrease in hematologic components is noted. **[US Boxed Warning]: Use of low-dose methotrexate has been associated with the development of malignant lymphomas;** may regress upon treatment discontinuation; treat lymphoma appropriately if regression is not induced by cessation of methotrexate. Discontinue methotrexate if lymphoma does not regress. Other secondary tumors have been reported.

[US Boxed Warning]: Gastrointestinal toxicity may occur; diarrhea and ulcerative stomatitis may require treatment interruption; hemorrhagic enteritis or intestinal perforation (with fatality) may occur. Use with caution in patients with peptic ulcer disease, ulcerative colitis. In children, doses ≥12 g/m^2 (IV) are associated with a high emetic potential; doses ≥250 mg/m^2 (IV) in adults and children are associated with moderate emetic potential (Dupuis, 2011). Antiemetics may be recommended to prevent nausea and vomiting.

May cause neurotoxicity including seizures (usually in pediatric ALL patients receiving intermediate-dose (1 g/m^2 methotrexate), leukoencephalopathy (usually in patients who have received cranial irradiation) and stroke-like encephalopathy (usually with high-dose regimens). Chemical arachnoiditis (headache, back pain, nuchal rigidity, fever) and myelopathy may result from intrathecal administration. Chronic leukoencephalopathy has been reported with high-dose and with intrathecal methotrexate; may be progressive and fatal. May cause dizziness and fatigue; may affect the ability to drive or operate heavy machinery.

[US Boxed Warning]: Any dose level, route of administration, or duration of therapy may cause severe and potentially fatal dermatologic reactions, including toxic epidermal necrolysis, Stevens-Johnson syndrome, exfoliative dermatitis, skin necrosis, and erythema multiforme. Recovery has been reported with treatment discontinuation. Radiation dermatitis and sunburn may be precipitated by methotrexate administration. Psoriatic lesions may be worsened by concomitant exposure to ultraviolet radiation.

Potentially significant drug-drug interactions may exist, requiring dose or frequency adjustment, additional monitoring, and/or selection of alternative therapy. **[US Boxed Warning]: Concomitant administration with NSAIDs may cause severe bone marrow suppression, aplastic anemia, and GI toxicity.** Do not administer NSAIDs prior to or during high-dose methotrexate therapy; may increase and prolong serum methotrexate levels. Doses used for psoriasis may still lead to unexpected toxicities; use caution when administering NSAIDs or salicylates with lower doses of methotrexate for RA. Methotrexate may increase the levels and effects of mercaptopurine; may require dosage adjustments. Vitamins containing folate may decrease response to systemic methotrexate; folate deficiency may increase methotrexate toxicity. Concomitant use of proton pump inhibitors with methotrexate (primarily high-dose methotrexate) may elevate and prolong serum methotrexate and metabolite (hydroxymethotrexate) levels; may lead to toxicities; use with caution. Immunization may be ineffective during methotrexate treatment. Immunization with live vaccines is not recommended; cases of disseminated vaccinia infections due to live vaccines have been reported. **[US Boxed Warning]: Concomitant methotrexate administration with radiotherapy may increase the risk of soft tissue necrosis and osteonecrosis.**

[US Boxed Warnings]: Should be administered under the supervision of a physician experienced in the use of antimetabolite therapy; serious and fatal toxicities have occurred at all dose levels. Immune suppression may lead to potentially fatal opportunistic infections, including *Pneumocystis jirovecii* pneumonia (PCP). Use methotrexate with extreme caution in patients with an active infection (contraindicated in patients with immunodeficiency syndrome). **[US Boxed Warnings]: For rheumatoid arthritis and psoriasis, immunosuppressive therapy should only be used when disease is active, severe, recalcitrant, and disabling; and where less toxic, traditional therapy is ineffective. Methotrexate formulations and/or diluents containing preservatives should not be used for intrathecal or high-dose methotrexate therapy. May cause fetal death or congenital abnormalities; do not use for psoriasis or RA treatment in pregnant women.** May cause impairment of fertility, oligospermia, and menstrual dysfunction. Toxicity from methotrexate or any immunosuppressive is increased in the elderly. Methotrexate injection may contain benzyl alcohol and should not be used in neonates. Errors have occurred (some resulting in death) when methotrexate was administered as a "daily" dose instead of a "weekly" dose intended for some indications. The ISMP Targeted Medication Safety Best Practices for Hospitals recommends hospitals use a weekly dosage regimen default for oral methotrexate orders, with a hard stop override requiring verification of appropriate oncology indication; manual systems should require verification of an oncology indication prior to dispensing oral methotrexate for daily administration. Pharmacists should provide patient education for patients discharged on weekly oral methotrexate; education should include written leaflets that contain clear instructions about the weekly dosing schedule and explain the danger of taking extra doses (ISMP, 2014).

When used for intrathecal administration, should not be prepared during the preparation of any other agents; after preparation, store intrathecal medications in an isolated location or container clearly marked with a label identifying as "intrathecal" use only; delivery of intrathecal medications to the patient should only be with other medications intended for administration into the central nervous system (Jacobson, 2009).

Benzyl alcohol and derivatives: Some dosage forms may contain benzyl alcohol; large amounts of benzyl alcohol (≥99 mg/kg/day) have been associated with a potentially fatal toxicity ("gasping syndrome") in neonates; the "gasping syndrome" consists of metabolic acidosis, respiratory distress, gasping respirations, CNS dysfunction (including convulsions, intracranial hemorrhage), hypotension, and cardiovascular collapse (AAP ["Inactive" 1997]; CDC, 1982); some data suggests that benzoate displaces bilirubin from protein binding sites (Ahlfors, 2001); avoid or use dosage forms containing benzyl alcohol with caution in neonates. See manufacturer's labeling.

Glucarpidase is an enzyme that rapidly hydrolyzes extracellular methotrexate into inactive metabolites, allowing for a rapid reduction of methotrexate concentrations. Glucarpidase may be used for methotrexate overexposure; it is approved for the treatment of toxic plasma methotrexate concentrations (>1 micromole/L) in patients with delayed clearance due to renal impairment.

Adverse Reactions Note: Adverse reactions vary by route and dosage. Frequency not always defined.

Cardiovascular: Arterial thrombosis, cerebral thrombosis, chest pain, deep vein thrombosis, hypotension, pericardial effusion, pericarditis, plaque erosion (psoriasis), pulmonary embolism, retinal thrombosis, thrombophlebitis, vasculitis

Central nervous system: Dizziness (≤3%), headache (pJIA 1%), abnormal cranial sensation, brain disease, chemical arachnoiditis (intrathecal; acute), chills, cognitive dysfunction (has been reported at low dosage), drowsiness, fatigue, leukoencephalopathy (intravenous administration after craniospinal irradiation or repeated high-dose therapy; may be chronic), malaise, mood changes (has been reported at low dosage), neurological signs and symptoms (at high dosages; including confusion, hemiparesis, transient blindness, seizures, and coma), severe neurotoxicity (reported with unexpectedly increased frequency among pediatric patients with acute lymphoblastic leukemia who were treated with intermediate-dose intravenous methotrexate), speech disturbance

Dermatologic: Alopecia (≤10%), burning sensation of skin (psoriasis 3% to 10%), skin photosensitivity (3% to 10%), skin rash (≤3%), dermatitis (rheumatoid arthritis 1% to 3%), pruritus (rheumatoid arthritis 1% to 3%), acne vulgaris, dermal ulcer, diaphoresis, ecchymoses, erythema multiforme, erythematous rash, exfoliative dermatitis, furunculosis, hyperpigmentation, hypopigmentation, skin abnormalities related to radiation recall, skin necrosis, Stevens-Johnson syndrome, telangiectasia, toxic epidermal necrolysis, urticaria

Endocrine & metabolic: Decreased libido, decreased serum albumin, diabetes mellitus, gynecomastia, menstrual disease

Gastrointestinal: Diarrhea (≤11%), nausea and vomiting (≤11%), stomatitis (2% to 10%), abdominal distress, anorexia, aphthous stomatitis, enteritis, gastrointestinal hemorrhage, gingivitis, hematemesis, intestinal perforation, melena

Genitourinary: Azotemia, cystitis, defective oogenesis, defective spermatogenesis, dysuria, hematuria, impotence, infertility, oligospermia, pancreatitis, proteinuria, severe renal disease, vaginal discharge

Hematologic & oncologic: Thrombocytopenia (rheumatoid arthritis 3% to 10%; platelet count <100,000/mm³), leukopenia (1% to 3%; WBC <3000/mm³), pancytopenia (rheumatoid arthritis 1% to 3%), agranulocytosis, anemia, aplastic anemia, bone marrow depression (nadir: 7-10 days), decreased hematocrit, eosinophilia, gastric ulcer, hypogammaglobulinemia, lymphadenopathy, lymphoma, lymphoproliferative disorder, neutropenia, non-Hodgkin's lymphoma (in patients receiving low-dose oral methotrexate), tumor lysis syndrome

Hepatic: Increased liver enzymes (14% to 15%), cirrhosis (chronic therapy), hepatic failure, hepatic fibrosis (chronic therapy), hepatitis (acute), hepatotoxicity

Hypersensitivity: Anaphylactoid reaction

Infection: Cryptococcosis, cytomegalovirus disease (including cytomegaloviral pneumonia, sepsis, nocardiosis), herpes simplex infection, herpes zoster, histoplasmosis, infection, pneumonia due to *pneumocystis jiroveci*, vaccinia (disseminated; following smallpox immunization)

Neuromuscular & skeletal: Arthralgia, myalgia, myelopathy (subacute), osteonecrosis (with radiotherapy), osteoporosis, stress fracture

Ophthalmic: Blurred vision, conjunctivitis, eye pain, visual disturbance

Otic: Tinnitus

Renal: Renal failure

Respiratory: Interstitial pneumonitis (rheumatoid arthritis 1%), chronic obstructive pulmonary disease, cough, epistaxis, pharyngitis, pneumonia, pulmonary alveolitis, pulmonary disease, pulmonary fibrosis, respiratory failure, upper respiratory tract infection

Miscellaneous: Fever, nodule, tissue necrosis

Drug Interactions

Metabolism/Transport Effects Substrate of BCRP, OAT3, P-glycoprotein, SLCO1B1

Avoid Concomitant Use

Avoid concomitant use of Methotrexate with any of the following: Acitretin; BCG (Intravesical); Deferiprone; Dipyrone; Foscarnet; Natalizumab; Pimecrolimus; Tacrolimus (Topical)

Increased Effect/Toxicity

Methotrexate may increase the levels/effects of: CloZAPine; CycloSPORINE (Systemic); Deferiprone; Dipyrone; Fingolimod; Leflunomide; Loop Diuretics; Natalizumab; Tegafur; Theophylline Derivatives; Tofacitinib; Vaccines (Live)

The levels/effects of Methotrexate may be increased by: Acitretin; Alitretinoin (Systemic); Ciprofloxacin (Systemic); CycloSPORINE (Systemic); Denosumab; Dexketoprofen; Dipyrone; Eltrombopag; Foscarnet; Fosphenytoin-Phenytoin; Loop Diuretics; Lumacaftor; Mipomersen; Nonsteroidal Anti-Inflammatory Agents; Penicillins; P-glycoprotein/ABCB1 Inhibitors; Pimecrolimus; Probenecid; Proton Pump Inhibitors; Ranolazine; Roflumilast; Rolapitant; Salicylates; SulfaSALAzine;

Sulfonamide Derivatives; Tacrolimus (Topical); Teriflunomide; Trastuzumab; Trimethoprim

Decreased Effect

Methotrexate may decrease the levels/effects of: BCG (Intravesical); Coccidioides immitis Skin Test; Fosphenytoin-Phenytoin; Loop Diuretics; Sapropterin; Sipuleucel-T; Vaccines (Inactivated); Vaccines (Live)

The levels/effects of Methotrexate may be decreased by: Bile Acid Sequestrants; Echinacea; Lumacaftor; P-glycoprotein/ABCB1 Inducers

Food Interactions Methotrexate peak serum levels may be decreased if taken with food. Milk-rich foods may decrease methotrexate absorption. Management: Administer without regard to food.

Preparation for Administration Hazardous agent; use appropriate precautions for handling and disposal (NIOSH 2014 [group 1]). **Use preservative-free preparations for intrathecal or high-dose methotrexate administration.**

IV: Dilute powder with D₅W or NS to a concentration of ≤25 mg/mL (20 mg and 50 mg vials) and 50 mg/mL (1 g vial). May further dilute in D₅W or NS.

Intrathecal: Prepare intrathecal solutions with preservative-free NS, lactated Ringer's, or Elliot's B solution to a final volume of up to 12 mL (volume generally based on institution or practitioner preference). Intrathecal methotrexate concentrations may be institution specific or based on practitioner preference, generally ranging from a final concentration of 1 mg/mL (per prescribing information; Grossman, 1993; Lin, 2008) up to ~2 to 4 mg/mL (de Lemos, 2009; Glantz, 1999). For triple intrathecal therapy (methotrexate 12 mg/hydrocortisone 24 mg/cytarabine 36 mg), preparation to final volume of 12 mL is reported (Lin, 2008). Intrathecal medications should **NOT** be prepared during the preparation of any other agents.

Storage/Stability

Tablets: Store between 20°C and 25°C (68°F and 77°F); excursions are permitted between 15°C and 30°C (59°F and 86°F). Protect from light.

Injection: Store intact vials and autoinjectors between 20°C and 25°C (68°F and 77°F); excursions may be permitted between 15°C and 30°C (59°F and 86°F). Protect from light.

IV: Solution diluted in D₅W or NS is stable for 24 hours at room temperature (21°C to 25°C).

Intrathecal: Intrathecal dilutions are preservative free and should be used as soon as possible after preparation. After preparation, store intrathecal medications (until use) in an isolated location or container clearly marked with a label identifying as "intrathecal" use only.

Mechanism of Action Methotrexate is a folate antimetabolite that inhibits DNA synthesis, repair, and cellular replication. Methotrexate irreversibly binds to and inhibits dihydrofolate reductase, inhibiting the formation of reduced folates, and thymidylate synthetase, resulting in inhibition of purine and thymidylic acid synthesis, thus interfering with DNA synthesis, repair, and cellular replication. Methotrexate is cell cycle specific for the S phase of the cycle. Actively proliferative tissues are more susceptible to the effects of methotrexate.

The MOA in the treatment of rheumatoid arthritis is unknown, but may affect immune function. In psoriasis, methotrexate is thought to target rapidly proliferating epithelial cells in the skin.

In Crohn disease, it may have immune modulator and antiinflammatory activity.

Pharmacodynamics/Kinetics

Onset of action: Antirheumatic: 3 to 6 weeks; additional improvement may continue longer than 12 weeks

Absorption:
Oral: Highly variable; dose dependent
IM injection: Complete

Distribution: Penetrates slowly into 3rd space fluids (eg, pleural effusions, ascites), exits slowly from these compartments (slower than from plasma); sustained concentrations retained in kidney and liver

V_d: IV: 0.18 L/kg (initial); 0.4 to 0.8 L/kg (steady state)

Protein binding: ~50%

Metabolism: Partially metabolized by intestinal flora (after oral administration) to DAMPA by carboxypeptidase; hepatic aldehyde oxidase converts methotrexate to 7-hydroxy methotrexate; polyglutamates are produced intracellularly and are just as potent as methotrexate; their production is dose- and duration-dependent and they are slowly eliminated by the cell once formed. Polyglutamated forms can be converted back to methotrexate.

Bioavailability: Oral: ~20% to 95%; in general, bioavailability is dose dependent and decreases as the dose increases (especially at doses >80 mg/m²)

Half-life elimination: Low dose: 3 to 10 hours; High dose: 8 to 15 hours; Children: 1 to 6 hours

Time to peak, serum: Oral: 1 to 2 hours; IM: 30 to 60 minutes

Excretion: Dose and route dependent; IV: Urine (80% to 90% as unchanged drug; 5% to 7% as 7-hydroxy methotrexate); feces (<10%)

Dosing

Adult Note: Methotrexate doses between 100 to 500 mg/m^2 **may require** leucovorin calcium rescue. Doses >500 mg/m^2 **require** leucovorin calcium rescue (refer to Dosing: Adjustment for Toxicity for leucovorin calcium dosing). Doses ≥250 mg/m^2 (IV) are associated with moderate emetic potential. Antiemetics may be recommended to prevent nausea and vomiting.

Acute lymphoblastic leukemia (ALL):

Meningeal leukemia prophylaxis or treatment: Intrathecal: Manufacturer's labeling: 12 mg (maximum 15 mg/dose) every 2 to 7 days; continue for 1 dose beyond CSF cell count normalization. **Note:** Optimal intrathecal chemotherapy dosing should be based on age rather than on body surface area (BSA); CSF volume correlates with age and not to BSA (Bleyer, 1983; Kerr, 2001).

CALGB 8811 regimen (Larson, 1995; combination therapy):

Early intensification: Intrathecal: 15 mg day 1 of early intensification phase, repeat in 4 weeks

CNS prophylaxis/interim maintenance phase:
Intrathecal: 15 mg day 1, 8, 15, 22, and 29
Oral: 20 mg/m^2 days 36, 43, 50, 57, and 64

Prolonged maintenance: Oral: 20 mg/m^2 days 1, 8, 15, and 22 every 4 weeks for 24 months from diagnosis

Dose-intensive regimen (Kantarjian, 2000; combination therapy):

IV: 200 mg/m^2 over 2 hours, followed by 800 mg/m^2 over 24 hours beginning day 1, (followed by leucovorin rescue) of even numbered cycles (in combination with cytarabine; alternates with Hyper-CVAD)

CNS prophylaxis: Intrathecal: 12 mg on day 2 of each cycle; duration depends on risk

Maintenance: IV: 10 mg/m^2/day for 5 days every month for 2 years (in combination with prednisone, vincristine, and mercaptopurine)

Breast cancer: IV: CMF regimen: 40 mg/m^2 days 1 and 8 every 4 weeks (in combination with cyclophosphamide and fluorouracil) for 6 to 12 cycles (Bonadonna, 1995; Levine, 1998)

Choriocarcinoma, chorioadenoma, gestational trophoblastic diseases: 15 to 30 mg oral or IM daily for a 5 day course; may repeat for 3 to 5 courses (manufacturer's labeling) **or** 100 mg/m^2 IV over 30 minutes followed by 200 mg/m^2 IV over 12 hours (with leucovorin 24 hours after the start of methotrexate), administer a second course if hCG levels plateau for 3 consecutive weeks (Garrett, 2002)

Head and neck cancer, advanced: IV: 40 mg/m^2 once weekly until disease progression or unacceptable toxicity (Forastiere, 1992; Guardiola, 2004; Stewart, 2009)

Lymphoma, non-Hodgkin: IV:

CODOX-M/IVAC regimen (Mead, 2008): Cycles 1 and 3 of CODOX-M (CODOX-M alternates with IVAC)

Adults ≤65 years: IV: 300 mg/m^2 over 1 hour (on day 10) followed by 2700 mg/m^2 over 23 hours (with leucovorin rescue)

Adults >65 years: IV: 100 mg/m^2 over 1 hour (on day 10) followed by 900 mg/m^2 over 23 hours (with leucovorin rescue)

Hyper-CVAD alternating with high-dose methotrexate/cytarabine regimen: IV: 1000 mg/m^2 over 24 hours on day 1 during even courses (2, 4, 6, and 8) of 21-day treatment cycles (Thomas, 2006) **or** 200 mg/m^2 bolus day 1 followed by 800 mg/m^2 over 24 hours during even courses (2, 4, 6, and 8) of 21-day treatment cycles (Khouri, 1998) with leucovorin rescue

Mycosis fungoides (cutaneous T-cell lymphoma): 5 to 50 mg once weekly or 15 to 37.5 mg twice weekly orally or IM for early stages (manufacturer's labeling) **or** 25 mg orally once weekly, may increase to 50 mg once weekly (Zackheim, 2003)

Osteosarcoma: Adults ≤30 years: IV: MAP regimen: 12 g/m^2 (maximum dose: 20 g) over 4 hours (followed by leucovorin rescue) for 4 doses during induction (before surgery) at weeks 4, 5, 9, and 10, and for 8 doses during maintenance (after surgery) at weeks 15, 16, 20, 21, 25, 26, 30, and 31 (in combination with doxorubicin and cisplatin) (Meyers, 2005); other combinations, intervals, age ranges, and doses (8 to 14 g/m^2/dose) have been described (with leucovorin rescue), refer to specific reference for details (Bacci, 2000;

Bacci, 2003; Goorin, 2003; Le Deley, 2007; Meyers, 1992; Weiner, 1986; Winkler, 1988)

Psoriasis: Note: Some experts recommend concomitant folic acid 1 to 5 mg daily (except the day of methotrexate) to reduce hematologic, gastrointestinal, and hepatic adverse events related to methotrexate.

Oral: Initial: 2.5 to 5 mg/dose every 12 hours for 3 doses per week **or**

Oral, IM, IV, SubQ: Initial: 10 to 25 mg given once weekly; adjust dose gradually to optimal response (doses above 20 mg once weekly are associated with an increased incidence of toxicity); doses >30 mg per week should not be exceeded.

Note: An initial test dose of 2.5 to 5 mg is recommended in patients with risk factors for hematologic toxicity or renal impairment. (Kalb, 2009).

Rheumatoid arthritis: Note: Some experts recommend concomitant folic acid at a dose of at least 5 mg per week (except the day of methotrexate) to reduce hematologic, gastrointestinal, and hepatic adverse events related to methotrexate.

Oral (manufacturer labeling): Initial: 7.5 mg once weekly or 2.5 mg every 12 hours for 3 doses per week; adjust dose gradually to optimal response (dosage exceeding 20 mg once weekly are associated with an increased incidence of toxicity; *alternatively*, 10 to 15 mg once weekly, increased by 5 mg every 2 to 4 weeks to a maximum of 20 to 30 mg once weekly has been recommended by some experts. Consider parenteral therapy with inadequate response or intolerance to oral therapy (Visser, 2009).

SubQ: Initial: 7.5 mg once weekly; adjust dose gradually to optimal response (doses above 20 mg once weekly are associated with an increased incidence of toxicity)

IM: 7.5 mg once weekly; adjust dose gradually to optimal response (doses above 20 mg once weekly are associated with an increased incidence of toxicity)

Off-label uses:

Acute promyelocytic leukemia (APL) maintenance phase:

Oral: 15 mg/m^2 once weekly for 2 years (Ades 2008) or 20 mg/m^2 once weekly for 1 year (Powell 2010)

IM: 15 mg/m^2 once weekly for 2 years (Sanz 2004)

Bladder cancer (off-label use): IV:

Dose-dense MVAC regimen: 30 mg/m^2 day 1 every 2 weeks (in combination with vinblastine, doxorubicin, and cisplatin) (Sternberg, 2001)

CMV regimen: 30 mg/m^2 days 1 and 8 every 3 weeks for 3 cycles (in combination with cisplatin, vinblastine and leucovorin rescue) (Griffiths, 2011)

CNS Lymphoma (off-label use): IV: 8000 mg/m^2 over 4 hours (followed by leucovorin rescue) every 14 days until complete response or a maximum of 8 cycles; if complete response, follow with 2 consolidation cycles at the same dose every 14 days (with leucovorin rescue), followed by 11 maintenance cycles of 8000 mg/m^2 every 28 days with leucovorin rescue (Batchelor, 2003) **or** 2500 mg/m^2 over 2 to 3 hours every 14 days for 5 doses (in combination with vincristine, procarbazine, intrathecal methotrexate, leucovorin, dexamethasone, and cytarabine) (De Angelis, 2002) **or** 3500 mg/m^2 over 2 hours on day 2 every 2 weeks (in combination with rituximab, vincristine, procarbazine, and leucovorin [with intra-omaya methotrexate 12 mg between days 5 and 12 of each cycle if positive CSF cytology]) for 5 to 7 induction cycles (Shah, 2007)

Crohn disease, moderate/severe, corticosteroid-dependent or refractory (off-label use):

Remission induction or reduction of steroid use: IM, SubQ: 25 mg once weekly (Lichtenstein, 2009)

Remission maintenance: IM: 15 mg once weekly (Feagan, 2000; Lichtenstein, 2009)

Dermatomyositis/polymyositis (off-label uses):

Oral: Initial: 7.5 to 15 mg per week, often adjunctively with high-dose corticosteroid therapy; may increase in weekly 2.5 mg increments to target dose of 10 to 25 mg per week (**Note:** Administration of folate 5 to 7 mg per week has been used to reduce side effects) (Briemberg, 2003; Newman, 1995; Wiendl, 2008).

IV, IM: Doses of 20 to 60 mg/week have been employed if failure with oral therapy (doses >50 mg/week may require leucovorin calcium rescue) (Briemberg, 2003)

Ectopic pregnancy (off-label use): IM:

Single-dose regimen: Methotrexate 50 mg/m^2 on day 1; Measure serum hCG levels on days 4 and 7; if needed, repeat dose on day 7 (Barnhart, 2009)

Two-dose regimen: Methotrexate 50 mg/m^2 on day 1; Measure serum hCG levels on day 4 and administer a second dose of methotrexate 50 mg/m^2; Measure serum hCG levels on day 7 and if needed, administer a third dose of 50 mg/m^2 (Barnhart, 2009)

Multidose regimen: Methotrexate 1 mg/kg on day 1; leucovorin calcium 0.1 mg/kg IM on day 2; measure serum hCG on day 2; methotrexate 1 mg/kg on day 3; leucovorin calcium 0.1 mg/kg on day 4; measure serum hCG on day 4; continue up to a total of 4 courses based on hCG concentrations (Barnhart, 2009)

Graft-versus-host disease, acute (aGVHD), prophylaxis: IV: 15 mg/m^2/dose on day 1 and 10 mg/m^2/dose on days 3 and 6 after allogeneic transplant (in combination with cyclosporine and prednisone) (Chao, 1993; Chao, 2000; Ross, 1999) **or** 15 mg/m^2/dose on day 1 and 10 mg/m^2/dose on days 3, 6, and 11 after allogeneic transplant (in combination with cyclosporine) (Chao, 2000) **or** 15 mg/m^2/dose on day 1 and 10 mg/m^2/dose on days 3, 6, and 11 after allogeneic transplant (in combination with cyclosporine, followed by leucovorin); may omit day 11 methotrexate for grade 2 or higher toxicity (Ruutu, 2013)

Nonleukemic meningeal cancer (off-label uses): Intrathecal: 12 mg/dose twice weekly for 4 weeks, then weekly for 4 doses, then monthly for 4 doses (Glantz, 1998) **or** 10 mg twice weekly for 4 weeks, then weekly for 1 month, then every 2 weeks for 2 months (Glantz, 1999) **or** 10 to 15 mg twice weekly for 4 weeks, then once weekly for 4 weeks, then a maintenance regimen of once a month (Chamberlain, 2010)

Soft tissue sarcoma (desmoid tumors, aggressive fibromatosis), advanced (off-label use): IV: 30 mg/m^2 every 7 to 10 days (dose usually rounded to 50 mg) in combination with vinblastine for 1 year (Azzarelli, 2001)

Systemic lupus erythematosus, moderate-to-severe (off-label use): Oral: Initial: 7.5 mg once weekly; may increase by 2.5 mg increments weekly (maximum: 20 mg once weekly), in combination with prednisone (Fortin, 2008)

Takayasu arteritis, refractory or relapsing disease (off-label use): Oral: Initial dose: 0.3 mg/kg/week (maximum: 15 mg per week), titrated by 2.5 mg increments every 1 to 2 weeks until reaching a maximum tolerated weekly dose of 25 mg (use in combination with a corticosteroid; Hoffman, 1994)

Geriatric Refer to adult dosing; adjust for renal impairment.

Breast cancer: Patients >60 years: IV: CMF regimen: 30 mg/m^2 days 1 and 8 every 4 weeks (in combination with cyclophosphamide and fluorouracil) for up to 12 cycles (Bonadonna, 1995)

Meningeal leukemia: Intrathecal: Consider a dose reduction (CSF volume and turnover may decrease with age)

Non-Hodgkin lymphoma: CODOX-M/IVAC regimen (Mead, 2008): Cycles 1 and 3 of CODOX-M (CODOX-M alternates with IVAC): IV: 100 mg over 1 hour (on day 10) followed by 900 mg over 23 hours (with leucovorin rescue)

Rheumatoid arthritis/psoriasis: Oral: Initial: 5 to 7.5 mg per week, not to exceed 20 mg per week

Pediatric Note: Methotrexate doses between 100 to 500 mg/m^2 **may require** leucovorin calcium rescue. Doses >500 mg/m^2 **require** leucovorin calcium rescue (refer to Dosing: Adjustment for Toxicity for leucovorin calcium dosing). In children, doses ≥12 g/m^2 (IV) are associated with a high emetic potential; doses ≥250 mg/m^2 (IV) are associated with moderate emetic potential (Dupuis, 2011). Antiemetics may be recommended to prevent nausea and vomiting.

Polyarticular juvenile idiopathic arthritis (pJIA): Oral, IM, SubQ: Initial: 10 mg/m^2 once weekly, adjust gradually to optimum response; doses up to 20 to 30 mg/m^2 once weekly have been used (doses above 20 mg/m^2 once weekly may be associated with an increased risk of toxicity)

Acute lymphoblastic leukemia (ALL; intrathecal therapy is also administered [refer to specific reference]):

Consolidation/intensification phases (as part of a combination regimen): 1,000 mg/m^2 IV over 24 hours in week 1 of intensification and 20 mg/m^2 IM (use 50% dose reduction if on same day as intrathecal methotrexate) on day 1 of week 2 of intensification phase; Intensification repeats every 2 weeks for a total of 12 courses (Mahoney, 2000) **or** 5000 mg/m^2 IV over 24 hours days 8, 22, 36, and 50 of consolidation phase (Schrappe, 2000) with leucovorin rescue

Interim maintenance (as part of a combination regimen): 15 mg/m^2 orally days 0, 7, 14, 21, 28, and 35 of interim maintenance phase (Seibel, 2008) **or** 100 mg/m^2 (escalate dose by 50 mg/m^2 each dose) IV days 0, 10, 20, 30, and 40 of increased intensity interim maintenance phase (Seibel, 2008)

Maintenance (as part of a combination regimen): 20 mg/m^2 IM weekly in weeks 25 to 130 (Mahoney, 2000) **or** 20 mg/m^2 orally days 7, 14, 21, 28, 35, 42, 49, 56, 63, 70, and 77 (Seibel, 2008)

T-cell acute lymphoblastic leukemia (Asselin, 2011; triple intrathecal therapy is also administered [refer to specific reference]):

Induction (weeks 1 to 6; as part of a combination regimen): IV:

Low dose: 40 mg/m^2 day 2

High dose: 500 mg/m^2 over 30 minutes followed by 4500 mg/m^2 over 23.5 hours (with leucovorin rescue) day 22

Consolidation (weeks 7 to 33; combination chemotherapy): IV: High dose: 500 mg/m^2 over 30 minutes followed by 4500 mg/m^2 over 23.5 hours (with leucovorin rescue) in weeks 7, 10, and 13 with leucovorin rescue

Continuation (weeks 34 to 108; combination chemotherapy): IV, IM: 30 mg/m^2 weekly until 2 years after documented complete remission

ALL, CNS prophylaxis triple intrathecal therapy (off-label dosing): Intrathecal: Age-based dosing (in combination with cytarabine and hydrocortisone): Days of administration vary based on risk status and protocol; refer to institutional protocols or reference for details (Matloub, 2006):

<2 years: 8 mg

2 to <3 years: 10 mg

3 to ≤8 years: 12 mg

>8 years: 15 mg

Meningeal leukemia, prophylaxis or treatment: Intrathecal: 6 to 12 mg/dose (based on age) every 2 to 7 days; continue for 1 dose beyond CSF cell count normalization. **Note:** Optimal intrathecal chemotherapy dosing should be based on age rather than on body surface area (BSA); CSF volume correlates with age and not to BSA (Bleyer, 1983; Kerr, 2001):

<1 year: 6 mg/dose

1 year: 8 mg/dose

2 years: 10 mg/dose

≥3 years: 12 mg/dose

Osteosarcoma: IV: MAP regimen: 12 g/m^2 (maximum dose: 20 g) over 4 hours (followed by leucovorin rescue) for 4 doses during induction (before surgery) at weeks 3, 4, 8, and 9, and for 8 doses during maintenance (after surgery) at weeks 15, 16, 20, 21, 25, 26, 30, and 31 (in combination with doxorubicin and cisplatin) (Meyers, 2005); other combinations, intervals, and doses (8 to 14 g/m^2/dose) have been described (with leucovorin rescue), refer to specific reference for details (Bacci, 2000; Bacci, 2003; Goorin, 2003; Le Deley, 2007; Meyers, 1992; Weiner, 1986; Winkler, 1988)

Crohn disease, induction and maintenance (off-label use): SubQ: 15 mg/m^2 once weekly; maximum dose: 25 mg (Rufo, 2012)

Dermatomyositis (off-label use): Oral, SubQ (preferred): The lesser of 15 mg/m^2 or 1 mg/kg once weekly (maximum dose: 40 mg/week) in combination with corticosteroids (Huber, 2010) **or** 15 mg/m^2 once weekly (range: 10 to 20 mg/m^2 once weekly; maximum dose: 25 mg/week) in combination with prednisone (Ramanan, 2005)

Graft-versus-host disease, acute (aGVHD) prophylaxis (off-label use): IV: Refer to adult dosing.

Renal Impairment There are no dosage adjustments provided in the manufacturer's labeling. The following adjustments have been recommended:

Aronoff, 2007:

Adults:

CrCl 10 to 50 mL/minute: Administer 50% of dose

CrCl <10 mL/minute: Avoid use

Intermittent hemodialysis: Administer 50% of dose (post dialysis)

Continuous renal replacement therapy (CRRT): Administer 50% of dose

Children:

CrCl 10 to 50 mL/minute/1.73 m^2: Administer 50% of dose

CrCl <10 mL/minute/1.73 m^2: Administer 30% of dose

Intermittent hemodialysis: Administer 30% of dose (post dialysis)

Continuous ambulatory peritoneal dialysis (CAPD): Administer 30% of dose

Continuous renal replacement therapy (CRRT): Administer 50% of dose

Kintzel, 1995:

CrCl 46 to 60 mL/minute: Administer 65% of normal dose

CrCl 31 to 45 mL/minute: Administer 50% of normal dose

CrCl <30 mL/minute: Avoid use

Hemodialysis patients with cancer (Janus, 2010): Administer 25% of dose after hemodialysis; monitor closely for toxicity

High-dose methotrexate, dose-intensive regimen for ALL (200 mg/m^2 over 2 hours, followed by 800 mg/m^2 over 24 hours with leucovorin rescue [Kantarjian, 2000]):

Serum creatinine <1.5 mg/dL: No dosage adjustment necessary

Serum creatinine 1.5 to 2 mg/dL: Administer 75% of dose

Serum creatinine >2 mg/dL: Administer 50% of dose

Hepatic Impairment There are no dosage adjustments provided in the manufacturer's labeling; use with caution in patients with impaired hepatic function or preexisting hepatic damage. The following adjustments have been recommended (Floyd, 2006):

Bilirubin 3.1 to 5 mg/dL **or** transaminases >3 times ULN: Administer 75% of dose

Bilirubin >5 mg/dL: Avoid use

Obesity *ASCO Guidelines for appropriate chemotherapy dosing in obese adults with cancer (excludes leukemias):* Utilize patient's actual body weight (full weight) for calculation of body surface area- or weight-based dosing, particularly when the intent of therapy is curative; manage regimen-related toxicities in the same manner as for nonobese patients; if a dose reduction is utilized due to toxicity, consider resumption of full weight-based dosing with subsequent cycles, especially if cause of toxicity (eg, hepatic or renal impairment) is resolved (Griggs, 2012).

Adjustment for Toxicity

Methotrexate toxicities:

Nonhematologic toxicity: Diarrhea, stomatitis, or vomiting which may lead to dehydration: Discontinue until recovery

Hematologic toxicity:

Psoriasis, rheumatoid arthritis: Significant blood count decrease: Discontinue immediately.

Oncologic uses: Profound granulocytopenia and fever: Evaluate immediately; consider broad-spectrum parenteral antimicrobial coverage

Leucovorin calcium dosing (from methotrexate injection prescribing information; other leucovorin dosing/schedules may be specific to chemotherapy protocols):

Normal methotrexate elimination (serum methotrexate level ~10 micromolar at 24 hours after administration, 1 micromolar at 48 hours, and <0.2 micromolar at 72 hours): Leucovorin calcium 15 mg (oral, IM, or IV) every 6 hours for 60 hours (10 doses) beginning 24 hours after the start of methotrexate infusion

Delayed late methotrexate elimination (serum methotrexate level remaining >0.2 micromolar at 72 hours and >0.05 micromolar at 96 hours after administration): Continue leucovorin calcium 15 mg (oral, IM or IV) every 6 hours until methotrexate level is <0.05 micromolar

Delayed early methotrexate elimination and/or acute renal injury (serum methotrexate level ≥50 micromolar at 24 hours, or ≥5 micromolar at 48 hours, or a doubling of serum creatinine level at 24 hours after methotrexate administration): Leucovorin calcium 150 mg IV every 3 hours until methotrexate level is <1 micromolar, then 15 mg IV every 3 hours until methotrexate level <0.05 micromolar

Leucovorin nomogram dosing for high-dose methotrexate overexposure (**generalized dosing** derived from reference nomogram figures, refer to each reference [Bleyer, 1978; Bleyer, 1981; Widemann, 2006] or institution-specific nomogram for details):

At 24 hours:

For methotrexate levels of ≥100 micromolar at ~24 hours, leucovorin is initially dosed at 1000 mg/m^2 every 6 hours

For methotrexate levels of ≥10 to <100 micromolar at 24 hours, leucovorin is initially dosed at 100 mg/m^2 every 3 or 6 hours

For methotrexate levels of ~1 to 10 micromolar at 24 hours, leucovorin is initially dosed at 10 mg/m^2 every 3 or 6 hours

At 48 hours:

For methotrexate levels of ≥100 micromolar at 48 hours, leucovorin is dosed at 1000 mg/m^2 every 6 hours

For methotrexate levels of ≥10 to <100 micromolar at 48 hours, leucovorin is dosed at 100 mg/m^2 every 3 hours

For methotrexate levels of ~1 to 10 micromolar at 48 hours, leucovorin is dosed at 100 mg/m^2 every 6 hours **or** 10 to 100 mg/m^2 every 3 hours

At 72 hours:

For methotrexate levels of ≥10 micromolar at 72 hours, leucovorin is dosed at 100 to 1000 mg/m^2 every 3 to 6 hours

For methotrexate levels of ~1 to 10 micromolar at 72 hours, leucovorin is dosed at 10 to 100 mg/m^2 every 3 hours

For methotrexate levels of ~0.1 to 1 micromolar at 72 hours, leucovorin is dosed at 10 mg/m^2 every 3 to 6 hours

If serum creatinine is increased more than 50% above baseline, increase the standard leucovorin dose to 100 mg/m^2 every 3 hours, then adjust according to methotrexate levels above.

Follow methotrexate levels daily, leucovorin may be discontinued when methotrexate level is <0.1 micromolar

Dietary Considerations Some products may contain sodium.

Administration In children, doses ≥12 g/m^2 are associated with a high emetic potential; doses ≥250 mg/m^2 (IV) in adults and children are associated with moderate emetic potential (Dupuis, 2011). Antiemetics may be recommended to prevent nausea and vomiting.

Methotrexate may be administered orally, IM, IV, intrathecally, or SubQ; IV administration may be as slow push (10 mg/minute), bolus infusion, or 24-hour continuous infusion (route and rate of administration depend on indication and/or protocol; refer to specific references). Must use preservative-free formulation for intrathecal or high-dose methotrexate administration.

Specific dosing schemes vary, but high doses should be followed by leucovorin calcium rescue to prevent toxicity.

Otrexup and Rasuvo are autoinjectors for once weekly subcutaneous use in the abdomen or thigh; patient may self-administer after appropriate training. All schedules should be continually tailored to the individual patient. An initial test dose may be given prior to the regular dosing schedule to detect any extreme sensitivity to adverse effects.

Hazardous agent; use appropriate precautions for handling and disposal (NIOSH 2014 [group 1]). NIOSH recommends single gloving for administration of intact oral tablets (NIOSH 2014).

Monitoring Parameters

Oncologic uses: Baseline and frequently during treatment: CBC with differential and platelets, serum creatinine, BUN, liver function tests (LFTs); methotrexate levels and urine pH (with high-dose methotrexate); closely monitor fluid and electrolyte status in patients with impaired methotrexate elimination; chest x-ray (baseline); pulmonary function test (if methotrexate-induced lung disease suspected); monitor carefully for toxicities (due to impaired elimination) in patients with ascites, pleural effusion, decreased folate stores, renal impairment, and/or hepatic impairment

Psoriasis (Kalb, 2009; Menter, 2009):

CBC with differential and platelets (baseline, 7 to 14 days after initiating therapy or dosage increase, every 2 to 4 weeks for first few months, then every 1 to 3 months depending on leukocyte count and stability of patient) monitor more closely in patients with risk factors for hematologic toxicity (eg, renal insufficiency, advanced age, hypoalbuminemia); BUN and serum creatinine (baseline and every 2 to 3 months) calculate glomerular filtration rate if at risk for renal dysfunction; consider PPD for latent TB screening (baseline); LFTs (baseline, monthly for first 6 months, then every 1 to 2 months; more frequently if at risk for hepatotoxicity or if clinically indicated; liver function tests should be performed at least 5 days after the last dose; pregnancy test (if female of reproductive potential); chest x-ray (baseline if underlying lung disease); pulmonary function test (if methotrexate-induced lung disease suspected)

Liver biopsy for patients **with** risk factors for hepatotoxicity: Baseline or after 2 to 6 months of therapy and with each 1 to 1.5 g cumulative dose interval

Liver biopsy for patients **without** risk factors for hepatotoxicity: If persistent elevations in 5 of 9 AST levels during a 12-month period, or decline of serum albumin below the normal range with normal nutritional status. Consider biopsy after cumulative dose of 3.5 to 4 g and after each additional 1.5 g.

Rheumatoid arthritis (American College of Rheumatology Subcommittee, 2002; Kremer, 1994; Saag, 2008; Singh, 2012):

CBC with differential and platelets serum creatinine, and LFTs at baseline and every 2 to 4 weeks for 3 months after initiation or following dose increases, then every 8 to 12 weeks for 3 to 6 months, then every 12 weeks for 6 months; monitor more frequently if clinically indicated.

Chest x-ray (within 1 year prior to initiation), Hepatitis B and C serology (if at high risk); tuberculosis testing annually for patients who live, travel or work in areas with likely TB exposure

Liver biopsy: Baseline (if persistent abnormal baseline LFTs, history of alcoholism, or chronic hepatitis B or C) or during treatment if persistent LFT elevations (6 of 12 tests abnormal over 1 year or 5 of 9 results when LFTs performed at 6-week intervals)

Crohn disease (off-label use; Lichtenstein, 2009): CBC with differential and platelets (baseline and periodic) and liver function tests (baseline and every 1 to 2 months); baseline liver biopsy (in patients with abnormal baseline LFTs or with chronic liver disease); liver biopsy at 1 year if (over a 1-year span) AST consistently elevated or serum albumin consistently decreased; chest x-ray (baseline)

Ectopic pregnancy (off-label use; Barnhart, 2009): Prior to therapy, measure serum hCG, CBC with differential and platelets, liver function tests, serum creatinine. Serum hCG concentrations should decrease between treatment days 4 and 7. If hCG decreases by >15%, additional courses are not needed however, continue to measure hCG weekly until no longer detectable. If <15% decrease is observed, repeat dose per regimen.

Reference Range Therapeutic levels: Variable; Toxic concentration: Variable; therapeutic range is dependent upon therapeutic approach.

High-dose regimens produce drug levels that are between 0.1 to 1 micromole/L 24 to 72 hours after drug infusion

Toxic: Low-dose therapy: >0.2 micromole/L; high-dose therapy: >1 micromole/L

Dosage Forms Excipient information presented when available (limited, particularly for generics); consult specific product labeling. [DSC] = Discontinued product

Solution, Injection:
Generic: 25 mg/mL (2 mL, 10 mL)
Solution, Injection [preservative free]:
Generic: 25 mg/mL (2 mL, 4 mL, 8 mL, 10 mL, 40 mL); 50 mg/2 mL (2 mL); 100 mg/4 mL (4 mL); 200 mg/8 mL (8 mL [DSC]); 250 mg/10 mL (10 mL); 1 g/40 mL (40 mL)

Solution Auto-injector, Subcutaneous [preservative free]:
Otrexup: 7.5 mg/0.4 mL (0.4 mL); 10 mg/0.4 mL (0.4 mL); 15 mg/0.4 mL (0.4 mL); 20 mg/0.4 mL (0.4 mL); 25 mg/0.4 mL (0.4 mL)

Rasuvo: 7.5 mg/0.15 mL (0.15 mL); 10 mg/0.2 mL (0.2 mL); 12.5 mg/0.25 mL (0.25 mL); 15 mg/0.3 mL (0.3 mL); 17.5 mg/0.35 mL (0.35 mL); 20 mg/0.4 mL (0.4 mL); 22.5 mg/0.45 mL (0.45 mL); 25 mg/0.5 mL (0.5 mL); 27.5 mg/0.55 mL (0.55 mL); 30 mg/0.6 mL (0.6 mL)

Solution Reconstituted, Injection [preservative free]:
Generic: 1 g (1 ea)

Tablet, Oral:
Rheumatrex: 2.5 mg [scored]
Trexall: 5 mg, 7.5 mg, 10 mg, 15 mg [scored]
Generic: 2.5 mg

Methoxsalen (Systemic) (meth OKS a len)

Brand Names: US 8-Mop; Oxsoralen Ultra; Uvadex
Brand Names: Canada Uvadex
Index Terms 8-Methoxypsoralen; 8-MOP; Methoxypsoralen
Pharmacologic Category Psoralen
Use

Oral: Symptomatic control of severe, recalcitrant disabling psoriasis; repigmentation of idiopathic vitiligo; palliative treatment of skin manifestations of cutaneous T-cell lymphoma (CTCL)

Extracorporeal: Palliative treatment of skin manifestations of CTCL that is unresponsive to other forms of treatment

Dosing
Adult & Geriatric Note: Refer to treatment protocols for UVA exposure guidelines.
Psoriasis: Oral:
Initial: 10 to 70 mg 1.5 to 2 hours (Oxsoralen Ultra) or 2 hours (8-MOP) before exposure to UVA light; dose may be repeated 2-3 times per week, based on UVA exposure; doses must be given at least 48 hours apart; dosage is based upon patient's body weight and skin type:
<30 kg: 10 mg
30 to 50 kg: 20 mg
51 to 65 kg: 30 mg
66 to 80 kg: 40 mg
81 to 90 kg: 50 mg
91 to 115 kg: 60 mg
>115 kg: 70 mg
Note: Dosage may be increased (one time) by 10 mg after 15th treatment if minimal or no response.
Maintenance: When 95% psoriasis clearing achieved, may begin 1 treatment every week for at least 2 treatments; followed by 1 treatment every 2 weeks for at least 2 treatments; then every 3 weeks for at least 2 treatments then as needed to maintain response while minimizing UVA exposure.
Vitiligo: Oral (8-MOP): 20 mg 2 to 4 hours before exposure to UVA light; dose may be repeated based on erythema and tenderness of skin; do not give on 2 consecutive days
Cutaneous T-cell lymphoma (CTCL): Extracorporeal (Uvadex): Dose is determined by treatment volume; amount of Uvadex needed for each treatment may be calculated using the following equation: Treatment volume x 0.017 = mL of Uvadex needed. Inject this amount into the recirculation bag prior to the photoactivation phase using the UVAR XTS or CELLEX photopheresis system (consult user's guide).
Treatment schedule: Two consecutive days every 4 weeks for a minimum of 7 treatment cycles, may accelerate to 2 consecutive days every 2 weeks if skin score worsens (eg, increases from baseline) after assessment during the fourth treatment cycle. If skin score improves by 25% after 4 consecutive weeks of accelerated therapy, may resume regular treatment schedule. Patients maintained on accelerated therapy may receive a maximum of 20 accelerated therapy cycles. There is no clinical evidence to show that treatment with methoxsalen for more than 6 months or using a different schedule provides additional benefit.
Renal Impairment There are no dosage adjustments provided in manufacturer's labeling.
Hepatic Impairment There are no dosage adjustments provided in manufacturer's labeling; use with caution.
Additional Information Complete prescribing information should be consulted for additional detail.
Dosage Forms Excipient information presented when available (limited, particularly for generics); consult specific product labeling.
Capsule, Oral:
8-Mop: 10 mg
Oxsoralen Ultra: 10 mg [contains brilliant blue fcf (fd&c blue #1), fd&c yellow #10 (quinoline yellow), fd&c yellow #6 (sunset yellow), methylparaben, propylparaben]
Generic: 10 mg
Solution, Injection:
Uvadex: 20 mcg/mL (10 mL) [contains alcohol, usp, propylene glycol]

Methoxsalen (Topical) (meth OKS a len)

Brand Names: US Oxsoralen
Index Terms Methoxypsoralen
Pharmacologic Category Psoralen
Use Repigmentation of idiopathic vitiligo
Dosing
Adult & Geriatric Note: Refer to treatment protocols for UVA exposure guidelines.
Vitiligo: Topical: Lotion is applied by healthcare provider prior to UVA light exposure, usually no more than once weekly; frequency is determined by erythema response
Pediatric Vitiligo: Topical: Children ≥12 years: Refer to adult dosing.
Additional Information Complete prescribing information should be consulted for additional detail.
Dosage Forms Excipient information presented when available (limited, particularly for generics); consult specific product labeling.
Lotion, External:
Oxsoralen: 1% (29.57 mL)

◆ **Methoxy Peg-Epoetin Beta** *see* Methoxy Polyethylene Glycol-Epoetin Beta *on page 1176*

Methoxy Polyethylene Glycol-Epoetin Beta (meth OX ee pol i ETH i leen GLY kol e POE e tin BAY ta)

Brand Names: US Mircera

Index Terms rHuEPO-Beta; CERA; Continuous Erythropoietin Receptor Activator; Erythropoiesis-Stimulating Agent (ESA); Methoxy Peg-Epoetin Beta; Mircera; MPG-EPO

Pharmacologic Category Colony Stimulating Factor; Erythropoiesis-Stimulating Agent (ESA); Hematopoietic Agent

Use

Anemia: Treatment of anemia associated with chronic kidney disease (CKD) in adult patients on dialysis and patients not on dialysis.

Limitations of use: Not indicated and is not recommended in the treatment of anemia due to cancer chemotherapy or as a substitute for red blood cell (RBC) transfusions in patients who require immediate correction of anemia; has not been shown to improve symptoms, physical functioning or health-related quality of life.

Prescribing and Access Restrictions Distribution is restricted to certain dialysis centers.

Medication Guide Available Yes

Dosing

Adult Note: Evaluate iron status before and during treatment and maintain iron repletion.

Anemia associated with chronic kidney disease (CKD): Individualize dosing and use the lowest dose necessary to reduce the need for RBC transfusions:

Patients not currently taking an ESA:

Chronic kidney disease patients on dialysis (IV route is preferred for hemodialysis patients; initiate treatment when hemoglobin <10 g/dL): Initial: IV, SubQ: 0.6 mcg/kg once every 2 weeks. Reduce dose or interrupt treatment if hemoglobin approaches or exceeds 11 g/dL. After hemoglobin stabilizes, may administer once monthly with a dose that is double the dose administered every 2 weeks; titrate as necessary.

Chronic kidney disease patients NOT on dialysis (consider initiating treatment when hemoglobin <10 g/dL and the rate of hemoglobin decline would likely result in RBC transfusion and goal is to reduce risk of alloimmunization or other RBC transfusion-related risks): Initial: IV, SubQ: 0.6 mcg/kg once every 2 weeks. Reduce dose or interrupt treatment if hemoglobin exceeds 10 g/dL. After hemoglobin stabilizes, may administer once monthly with a dose that is double the dose administered every 2 weeks; titrate as necessary.

Patients converting from epoetin alfa or darbepoetin alfa: IV, SubQ: Based on total weekly ESA dose at the time of conversion (if hemoglobin is stabilized):

For epoetin alfa dose <8,000 units/week or darbepoetin alfa dose <40 mcg/week: Administer methoxy polyethylene glycol-epoetin beta 120 mcg once monthly or 60 mcg every 2 weeks.

For epoetin alfa dose 8,000 to 16,000 units/week or darbepoetin alfa dose 40 to 80 mcg/week: Administer methoxy polyethylene glycol-epoetin beta 200 mcg once monthly or 100 mcg every 2 weeks.

For epoetin alfa dose >16,000 units/week or darbepoetin alfa dose >80 mcg/week: Administer methoxy polyethylene glycol-epoetin beta 360 mcg once monthly or 180 mcg every 2 weeks.

Dosage adjustments for all CKD patients: Do not increase dose more frequently than every 4 weeks (dose decreases may occur more often); avoid frequent dosage adjustments.

If hemoglobin increases >1 g/dL in any 2-week period: Decrease dose by ≥25% as needed to reduce rapid responses.

If hemoglobin does not increase by >1 g/dL after 4 weeks of therapy: Increase dose by 25%.

Inadequate or lack of response over 12 weeks of therapy: If adequate response is not achieved after 12 weeks of therapy, further increases are unlikely to be of benefit and may increase the risk for adverse events; use the minimum effective dose that will maintain a hemoglobin level sufficient to avoid red blood cell transfusions **and** evaluate patient for other causes of anemia. Discontinue treatment if responsiveness does not improve.

Geriatric Refer to adult dosing; initiate at the lower end of dosing ranges.

Renal Impairment There are no dosage adjustments provided in the manufacturer's labeling; however, methoxy polyethylene glycol-epoetin beta is indicated for use in patients with chronic kidney disease.

Hepatic Impairment No dosage adjustment necessary.

Adjustment for Toxicity

Serious allergic/anaphylactic reactions: Discontinue immediately (and permanently).

Hypertension (difficult to control): Reduce dose or withhold treatment (use is contraindicated in uncontrolled hypertension).

Pure red cell aplasia (PRCA): Permanently discontinue treatment.

Additional Information Complete prescribing information should be consulted for additional detail.

Dosage Forms Excipient information presented when available (limited, particularly for generics); consult specific product labeling.

Solution, Injection [preservative free]:

Mircera: 50 mcg/0.3 mL (0.3 mL); 75 mcg/0.3 mL (0.3 mL); 100 mcg/0.3 mL (0.3 mL); 200 mcg/0.3 mL (0.3 mL)

◆ **Methoxypsoralen** *see* Methoxsalen (Systemic) *on page 1175*

◆ **Methoxypsoralen** *see* Methoxsalen (Topical) *on page 1175*

◆ **8-Methoxypsoralen** *see* Methoxsalen (Systemic) *on page 1175*

Methsuximide (meth SUKS i mide)

Brand Names: US Celontin

Brand Names: Canada Celontin®

Pharmacologic Category Anticonvulsant, Succinimide

Use Control of absence (petit mal) seizures that are refractory to other drugs

Medication Guide Available Yes

Dosing

Adult & Geriatric Anticonvulsant: Oral: 300 mg/day for the first week; may increase by 300 mg/day at weekly intervals up to 1.2 g/day in 2-4 divided doses/day

Renal Impairment No dosage adjustment provided in manufacturer's labeling; use with caution.

Hepatic Impairment No dosage adjustment provided in manufacturer's labeling; use with caution.

Additional Information Complete prescribing information should be consulted for additional detail.

Dosage Forms Excipient information presented when available (limited, particularly for generics); consult specific product labeling.

Capsule, Oral:

Celontin: 300 mg

Methyclothiazide (meth i kloe THYE a zide)

Index Terms Enduron

Pharmacologic Category Antihypertensive; Diuretic, Thiazide

Use Management of hypertension; adjunctive therapy of edema

Guideline recommendations:

Hypertension: The 2014 guideline for the management of high blood pressure in adults (Eighth Joint National Committee [JNC 8]) recommends initiation of pharmacologic treatment to lower blood pressure for the following patients:

• Patients ≥60 years of age with systolic blood pressure (SBP) ≥150 mm Hg or diastolic blood pressure (DBP) ≥90 mm Hg. Goal of therapy is SBP <150 mm Hg and DBP <90 mm Hg.

• Patients <60 years of age with SBP ≥140 mm Hg or DBP is ≥90 mm Hg. Goal of therapy is SBP <140 mm Hg and DBP <90 mm Hg.

• Patients ≥18 years of age with diabetes and SBP ≥140 mm Hg or DBP ≥90 mm Hg. Goal of therapy is SBP <140 mm Hg and DBP <90 mm Hg.

• Patients ≥18 years of age with chronic kidney disease (CKD) and SBP ≥140 mm Hg or DBP ≥90 mm Hg. Goal of therapy is SBP <140 mm Hg and DBP <90 mm Hg.

Chronic kidney disease (CKD) and hypertension: Regardless of race or diabetes status, the use of an ACE inhibitor (ACEI) or angiotensin receptor blocker (ARB) as initial therapy is recommended to improve kidney outcomes. In the general nonblack population (without CKD) including those with diabetes, initial antihypertensive treatment should consist of a thiazide-type diuretic, calcium channel blocker, ACEI, or ARB. In the general black population (without CKD), including those with diabetes, initial antihypertensive

treatment should consist of a thiazide-type diuretic or a calcium channel blocker **instead of** an ACEI or ARB.

Coronary artery disease (CAD) and hypertension: The American Heart Association, American College of Cardiology and American Society of Hypertension (AHA/ACC/ASH) 2015 scientific statement for the treatment of hypertension in patients with coronary artery disease (CAD) recommends the use of a thiazide (or thiazide-like diuretic) as part of a regimen in patients with hypertension and chronic stable angina. A BP target of <140/90 mm Hg is reasonable for the secondary prevention of cardiovascular events. A lower target BP (<130/80 mm Hg) may be appropriate in some individuals with CAD, previous MI, stroke or transient ischemic attack, or CAD risk equivalents (AHA/ACC/ASH [Rosendorff 2015]).

Dosing

Adult & Geriatric

Edema: Oral: 2.5 to 10 mg/day

Hypertension: Oral: 2.5 to 5 mg/day; may add another antihypertensive if 5 mg is not adequate after a trial of 8 to 12 weeks of therapy

Renal Impairment There are no dosage adjustments provided in manufacturer's labeling. However, thiazides are usually ineffective with CrCl <30 mL/minute; use with caution.

Hepatic Impairment There are no dosage adjustments provided in manufacturer's labeling; use with caution.

Additional Information Complete prescribing information should be consulted for additional detail.

Dosage Forms Excipient information presented when available (limited, particularly for generics); consult specific product labeling.

Tablet, Oral:

Generic: 5 mg

♦ **Methylacetoxyprogesterone** see MedroxyPROGES-TERone on page 1131

Methyl Aminolevulinate (METH il a mee noe LEV ue lin ate)

Brand Names: US Metvixia

Brand Names: Canada Metvix

Index Terms Methyl Aminolevulinate Hydrochloride; P-1202

Pharmacologic Category Photosensitizing Agent, Topical; Topical Skin Product

Use

Actinic keratosis: Treatment of thin and moderately thick, nonhyperkeratotic, nonpigmented actinic keratoses of the face and scalp in immunocompetent patients (photodynamic therapy [PDT] to be used in conjunction with red light illumination.

Limitations of use: Safety and efficacy have not been established for treatment of cutaneous malignancies or for skin lesions other than nonhyperkeratotic face and scalp actinic keratoses using PDT with methyl aminolevulinate cream; safety and efficacy of methyl aminolevulinate cream have not been established in patients with immunosuppression, porphyria, or pigmented actinic keratosis; has not been tested on patients with inherited or acquired coagulation defects; use without subsequent red light illumination is not recommended.

Dosing

Adult & Geriatric Actinic keratoses: Topical: Apply up to 1 g to prepared actinic keratoses, occlude for 3 hours, followed by red light illumination; repeat in 1 week. **Note:** If multiple lesions being treated, 1 g should not be exceeded for all lesions combined per treatment session.

Additional Information Complete prescribing information should be consulted for additional detail.

Dosage Forms Excipient information presented when available (limited, particularly for generics); consult specific product labeling.

Cream, External:

Metvixia: 16.8% (2 g) [contains cetostearyl alcohol, edetate disodium, methylparaben, peanut oil, propylparaben]

♦ **Methyl Aminolevulinate Hydrochloride** see Methyl Aminolevulinate on page 1177

♦ **Methylcobalamin, Acetylcysteine, and Methylfolate** see Methylfolate, Methylcobalamin, and Acetylcysteine on page 1179

Methyldopa (meth il DOE pa)

Brand Names: Canada Methyldopa; Novo-Medopa

Index Terms Aldomet; Methyldopate Hydrochloride

Pharmacologic Category Alpha$_2$-Adrenergic Agonist; Antihypertensive

Additional Appendix Information

Hypertension on page 1996

Use

Hypertension: Management of moderate to severe hypertension

Note: According to the Eighth Joint National Committee (JNC 8) guidelines, methyldopa is **not** recommended for the initial treatment of hypertension (James, 2013).

Dosing

Adult Hypertension:

Oral: Initial: 250 mg 2 to 3 times daily; increase every 2 days as needed (maximum dose: 3 g daily); usual dose range (ASH/ISH [Weber, 2014]): 250 to 500 mg twice daily. **Note:** When administered with other antihypertensives other than thiazide diuretics, limit initial daily dose of methyldopa to 500 mg daily.

IV: 250 to 1000 mg every 6 to 8 hours; maximum: 1 g every 6 hours

Geriatric Refer to adult dosing. Initiate at the lower end of the dosage range.

Pediatric Hypertension:

Oral: Initial: 10 mg/kg/day in 2 to 4 divided doses; increase every 2 days as needed to maximum dose of 65 mg/kg/day. Do not exceed 3 g daily.

IV: 5 to 10 mg/kg/dose every 6 to 8 hours up to a total maximum daily dose of 65 mg/kg/day or 3 g daily

Renal Impairment

There are no dosage adjustments provided in manufacturer's labeling; however, the following adjustments have been recommended (Aronoff, 2007):

CrCl >50 mL/minute: Administer every 8 hours.

CrCl 10 to 50 mL/minute: Administer every 8 to 12 hours.

CrCl <10 mL/minute: Administer every 12 to 24 hours.

Intermittent hemodialysis (administer after hemodialysis on dialysis days): Moderately dialyzable (up to 60% with a 6-hour session) (Yeh, 1970).

Peritoneal dialysis (PD): Administer every 12 to 24 hours.

Continuous renal replacement therapy (CRRT): Administer every 8 to 12 hours. **Note:** Use of antihypertensives in patients requiring CRRT is generally not recommended since CRRT is typically employed when patient cannot tolerate intermittent hemodialysis due to hypotension.

Hepatic Impairment Use is contraindicated in patients with active hepatic disease.

Additional Information Complete prescribing information should be consulted for additional detail.

Dosage Forms Excipient information presented when available (limited, particularly for generics); consult specific product labeling.

Solution, Intravenous, as hydrochloride:

Generic: 250 mg/5 mL (5 mL)

Tablet, Oral:

Generic: 250 mg, 500 mg

Dosage Forms: Canada Note: Also refer to Dosage Forms. Intravenous solution is not available in Canada. Excipient information presented when available (limited, particularly for generics); consult specific product labeling.

Tablet, Oral: 125 mg

♦ **Methyldopate Hydrochloride** see Methyldopa on page 1177

Methylene Blue (METH i leen bloo)

Index Terms Methylthionine Chloride; Methylthioninium Chloride

Pharmacologic Category Antidote

Use Methemoglobinemia: Treatment of drug-induced methemoglobinemia

Dosing

Adult & Geriatric

Methemoglobinemia: IV: 1 to 2 mg/kg or 25 to 50 mg/m^2 over 5 to 10 minutes; may be repeated in 1 hour if necessary

Chromoendoscopy (off label use): Topical: 0.1% to 1% solution sprayed via catheter or directly applied onto gastrointestinal mucosa during procedure (Areia 2008; Ichimasa 2014; Kaminski 2014; Ngamruengphong 2009)

Ifosfamide-induced encephalopathy (off-label use): Oral, IV: **Note:** Treatment may not be necessary; encephalopathy may improve spontaneously (Patel 2006):

Prevention: 50 mg every 6 to 8 hours (Turner 2003)

Treatment: 50 mg as a single dose or every 4 to 8 hours until symptoms resolve (Patel 2006; Turner 2003)

◄

Onychomycosis (toenail; off-label use): Topical: 2% solution applied to affected area(s) at 15 day intervals for 6 months; used in conjunction with photodynamic therapy (Figueiredo Souza 2014)

Sentinel node mapping in breast cancer surgery (off label use): Intraparenchymal: 5 mg in 3 to 5 mL NS administered once during procedure (Simmons 2001; Simmons 2003; Thevarajah 2005)

Vasoplegia syndrome associated with cardiac surgery (off-label use): IV: 1.5 to 2 mg/kg over 20 to 60 minutes administered once (Levin 2004; Leyh 2003). **Note:** Improvement of vasoplegia (eg, increased systemic vascular resistance, reduced vasopressor dosage) has been observed within 1 to 2 hours following methylene blue administration. Some have employed the use of continuous infusion (0.5 to 1 mg/kg/hour) after administration of the bolus dose; however, prospective clinical trials are necessary to validate this dosing schema (Grayling 2003; Omar 2014; Weiner 2013).

Pediatric Methemoglobinemia: Children and Adolescents: Refer to adult dosing.

Renal Impairment No dosage adjustment provided in manufacturer's labeling. However, use with caution in severe renal impairment.

Hepatic Impairment No dosage adjustment provided in manufacturer's labeling.

Additional Information Complete prescribing information should be consulted for additional detail.

Dosage Forms Excipient information presented when available (limited, particularly for generics); consult specific product labeling.
Solution, Injection:
Generic: 1% (1 mL, 10 mL)

◆ Methylene Blue, Methenamine, Benzoic Acid, Phenyl Salicylate, and Hyoscyamine *see* Methenamine, Phenyl Salicylate, Methylene Blue, Benzoic Acid, and Hyoscyamine *on page 1166*

◆ Methylene Blue, Methenamine, Sodium Phosphate Monobasic, Phenyl Salicylate, and Hyoscyamine *see* Methenamine, Sodium Phosphate Monobasic, Phenyl Salicylate, Methylene Blue, and Hyoscyamine *on page 1166*

◆ Methylergometrine Maleate *see* Methylergonovine *on page 1178*

Methylergonovine (meth il er goe NOE veen)

Brand Names: US Methergine [DSC]
Brand Names: Canada Methergine®
Index Terms Methylergometrine Maleate; Methylergonovine Maleate
Pharmacologic Category Ergot Derivative
Use Management of uterine atony, hemorrhage and subinvolution of the uterus following delivery of the placenta; control of uterine hemorrhage following delivery of the anterior shoulder in the second stage of labor

Pregnancy Considerations Animal reproduction studies have not been conducted. Methylergonovine is intended for use after delivery of the infant; use is contraindicated during pregnancy.

Breast-Feeding Considerations At normal doses used to control postpartum uterine bleeding, small amounts are excreted in breast milk. In one study, ten women were given a single dose of methylergonovine 0.5 mg once lactation was established. Simultaneous maternal milk and plasma samples were taken 1 and 2 hours later. Maximum milk concentrations were 410-830 pg/mL, 2-3 hours after the dose and declined to 0.2 pg/mL (median) at 5 hours. The mean M/P ratios were 0.18 (at 1 hour) and 0.17 (at 2 hours) (Vogel, 2004). Methylergonovine may decrease breast milk production. Some manufacturers do not recommend breast-feeding during therapy or for 12 hours after the last dose due to adverse reactions reported in breast-feeding infants.

Contraindications Hypersensitivity to methylergonovine or any component of the formulation; hypertension; toxemia; pregnancy

Warnings/Precautions Hazardous agent - use appropriate precautions for handling and disposal (NIOSH 2014 [group 3]).

Use caution in patients with sepsis, obliterative vascular disease, cardiovascular disease, hepatic or renal involvement, or second stage of labor; administer with extreme caution if using intravenously. Patients with coronary artery disease (CAD) or risk factors for CAD may be more likely to develop myocardial ischemia and infarction following methylergonovine-induced vasospasm. Pleural and peritoneal fibrosis have been reported with prolonged daily use of other ergot alkaloids. Ergot alkaloid use may result in ergotism (intense vasoconstriction) resulting in peripheral vascular ischemia and possible gangrene. Concomitant use with potent inhibitors of CYP3A4 (includes protease inhibitors, azole antifungals, and some macrolide antibiotics) and ergot alkaloids has been associated with acute ergot toxicity (ergotism); concurrent use of certain ergot alkaloids (eg, ergotamine and dihydroergotamine) are not recommended by the manufacturer. Not for routine IV administration due to risk of inducing sudden hypertensive and cerebrovascular accidents. IV administration should only be considered during life-threatening situations. Inadvertent administration to newborns has been reported.

Adverse Reactions Frequency not defined.

Cardiovascular: Acute MI, angina pectoris, arterial spasm, atrioventricular block, bradycardia, cerebrovascular accident, chest pain, hyper-/hypotension, palpitation, tachycardia, vasospasm, ventricular fibrillation

Central nervous system: Dizziness, hallucinations, headache, seizure

Dermatologic: Rash

Endocrine & metabolic: Water intoxication

Gastrointestinal: Abdominal pain, diarrhea, foul taste, nausea, vomiting

Local: Thrombophlebitis

Neuromuscular & skeletal: Leg cramps, paresthesia

Otic: Tinnitus

Renal: Hematuria

Respiratory: Dyspnea, nasal congestion

Miscellaneous: Anaphylaxis, diaphoresis

Drug Interactions

Metabolism/Transport Effects Substrate of CYP3A4 (major); **Note:** Assignment of Major/Minor substrate status based on clinically relevant drug interaction potential

Avoid Concomitant Use

Avoid concomitant use of Methylergonovine with any of the following: Alpha-/Beta-Agonists; Alpha1-Agonists; Antihepaciviral Combination Products; Boceprevir; Cobicistat; Conivaptan; Dapoxetine; Fusidic Acid (Systemic); Idelalisib; Itraconazole; Ketoconazole (Systemic); Lorcaserin; Nitroglycerin; Posaconazole; Protease Inhibitors; Serotonin 5-HT1D Receptor Agonists; Telaprevir; Voriconazole

Increased Effect/Toxicity

Methylergonovine may increase the levels/effects of: Alpha-/Beta-Agonists; Alpha1-Agonists; Antipsychotic Agents; Metoclopramide; Serotonin 5-HT1D Receptor Agonists; Serotonin Modulators

The levels/effects of Methylergonovine may be increased by: Antiemetics (5HT3 Antagonists); Antihepaciviral Combination Products; Antipsychotic Agents; Aprepitant; Beta-Blockers; Boceprevir; Cobicistat; Conivaptan; CYP3A4 Inhibitors (Moderate); CYP3A4 Inhibitors (Strong); Dapoxetine; Dasatinib; Fosaprepitant; Fusidic Acid (Systemic); Idelalisib; Itraconazole; Ivacaftor; Ketoconazole (Systemic); Lorcaserin; Luliconazole; Macrolide Antibiotics; Metaxalone; Mifepristone; Netupitant; Nitroglycerin; Osimertinib; Palbociclib; Posaconazole; Protease Inhibitors; Serotonin 5-HT1D Receptor Agonists; Simeprevir; Stiripentol; Tedizolid; Telaprevir; Voriconazole

Decreased Effect

Methylergonovine may decrease the levels/effects of: Nitroglycerin

The levels/effects of Methylergonovine may be decreased by: Osimertinib

Storage/Stability

Injection: Store under refrigeration at 2°C to 8°C (36°F to 46°F). Protect from light. The following stability information has also been reported: May be stored at room temperature for up to 14 days (Cohen, 2007).
Tablet: Store below 25°C (77°F).

Mechanism of Action Increases the tone, rate and amplitude of contractions on the smooth muscles of the uterus, producing sustained contractions which shortens the third stage of labor and reduces blood loss.

Pharmacodynamics/Kinetics

Onset of action: Oxytocic: Oral: 5-10 minutes; IM: 2-5 minutes; IV: Immediately

Duration: Oral: ~3 hours; IM: ~3 hours; IV: 45 minutes

Absorption: Rapid

Distribution: V_d: 39-73 L

Metabolism: Hepatic

Bioavailability: Oral: 60%; IM: 78%

Half-life elimination: ~3 hours (range: 1.5-12.7 hours)

Time to peak, serum: Oral: 0.3-2 hours; IM: 0.2-0.6 hours

Excretion: Urine and feces

Dosing

Adult Prevention of hemorrhage:

Oral: 0.2 mg 3-4 times daily in the puerperium for up to 7 days (maximum duration: 1 week)

IM, IV: 0.2 mg after delivery of anterior shoulder, after delivery of placenta, or during puerperium; may be repeated every 2-4 hours as needed. **Note:** IV administration should only be considered during life-threatening situations.

Renal Impairment No dosage adjustment provided in manufacturer's labeling; use with caution.

Hepatic Impairment No dosage adjustment provided in manufacturer's labeling; use with caution.

Administration

IV: Administer over ≥60 seconds. Should not be routinely administered IV because of possibility of inducing sudden hypertension and cerebrovascular accident. IV administration should only be considered during life-threatening situations.

IM: May be administered intramuscularly.

Oral: Available in tablets for oral administration.

Hazardous agent; use appropriate precautions for handling and disposal (NIOSH 2014 [group 3]).

Monitoring Parameters Blood pressure

Dosage Forms Excipient information presented when available (limited, particularly for generics); consult specific product labeling. [DSC] = Discontinued product

Solution, Injection, as maleate:
Methergine: 0.2 mg/mL (1 mL [DSC])
Generic: 0.2 mg/mL (1 mL)

Solution, Injection, as maleate [preservative free]:
Generic: 0.2 mg/mL (1 mL)

Tablet, Oral, as maleate:
Methergine: 0.2 mg [DSC]
Generic: 0.2 mg

◆ **Methylergonovine Maleate** see Methylergonovine on page 1178

Methylfolate, Methylcobalamin, and Acetylcysteine
(meth il FO late meth il koe BAL a min & a se teel SIS teen)

Brand Names: US Cerefolin® NAC; Metafolbic Plus; Metafolbic Plus RF

Index Terms Acetylcysteine, Methylcobalamin, and Methylfolate; Acetylcysteine, Methylfolate, and Methylcobalamin; L-methylfolate, Methylcobalamin, and N-acetylcysteine; Methylcobalamin, Acetylcysteine, and Methylfolate

Pharmacologic Category Dietary Supplement

Use Medicinal food for use in patients with neurovascular oxidative stress and/or hyperhomocysteinemia

Dosing

Adult Medicinal food: Oral: One tablet daily

Pediatric Medicinal food: Oral: Children ≥12 years: Refer to adult dosing.

Additional Information Complete prescribing information should be consulted for additional detail.

Dosage Forms Excipient information presented when available (limited, particularly for generics); consult specific product labeling.

Tablet, oral:
Cerefolin® NAC: L-methylfolate 6 mg, methylcobalamin 2 mg, N-acetylcysteine 600 mg, and Schizochytrium algae [contains soy; gluten free, lactose free, yeast free]
Metafolbic Plus: L-methylfolate 6 mg, methylcobalamin 2 mg, and N-acetylcysteine 600 mg [gluten free, lactose free, sugar free, yeast free]
Metafolbic Plus RF: L-methylfolate 6 mg, methylcobalamin 2 mg, N-acetylcysteine 600 mg, and Schizochytrium algae [contains soy; gluten free, yeast free]

◆ **Methylin** see Methylphenidate on page 1180

◆ **Methylmorphine** see Codeine on page 437

Methylnaltrexone (meth il nal TREKS one)

Brand Names: US Relistor

Brand Names: Canada Relistor

Index Terms Methylnaltrexone Bromide; N-methylnaltrexone Bromide

Pharmacologic Category Gastrointestinal Agent, Miscellaneous; Opioid Antagonist, Peripherally-Acting

Use

Opioid-induced constipation with advanced illness: Treatment of opioid-induced constipation in adult patients with advanced illness (receiving palliative care) who have an inadequate response to conventional laxative regimens.

Opioid-induced constipation with chronic non-cancer pain: Treatment of opioid-induced constipation in adult patients with chronic non-cancer pain.

Pregnancy Considerations Adverse effects were not observed in animal reproduction studies. Maternal use of methylnaltrexone during pregnancy may precipitate opioid withdrawal effects in newborn.

Breast-Feeding Considerations It is not known if methylnaltrexone is excreted in breast milk. Due to the potential for serious adverse reactions in the nursing infant, the manufacturer recommends a decision be made whether to discontinue nursing or to discontinue the drug, taking into account the importance of treatment to the mother.

Medication Guide Available Yes

Contraindications

Known or suspected gastrointestinal obstruction; patients at increased risk of recurrent obstruction due to the potential for gastrointestinal perforation.

Canadian labeling: Additional contraindications (not in U.S. labeling): Hypersensitivity to methylnaltrexone or any component of the formulation

Warnings/Precautions Discontinue treatment for severe or persistent diarrhea. Gastrointestinal perforations have been reported in patients with advanced illnesses associated with impaired structural integrity of the GI wall (eg, Ogilvie's syndrome, peptic ulcer disease, diverticular disease, infiltrative GI tract malignancies, or peritoneal metastases). Use with caution in patients or in patients with other conditions that may result in impaired integrity of the GI wall (eg, Crohn disease); Monitor for development of severe, persistent or worsening abdominal pain; discontinue therapy if this occurs. Use is contraindicated in patients with known or suspected GI obstruction or at increased risk of recurrent obstruction. Use with caution in patients with renal impairment; dosage adjustment recommended for severe renal impairment (CrCl <30 mL/minute). Has not been studied in patients with end-stage renal impairment requiring dialysis. May precipitate symptoms of opioid withdrawal (eg, abdominal pain, anxiety, chills, diarrhea, hyperhidrosis, and yawning). Use with caution in patients with disruptions to the blood-brain barrier; may increase the risk for withdrawal and/or reduced analgesia. Monitor for symptoms of opioid withdrawal in such patients. Discontinue methylnaltrexone if opioids are discontinued. Use beyond 4 months has not been studied.

Appropriate use for patients with opioid-induced constipation with chronic non-cancer pain: Efficacy has been established in patients who have taken opioids for ≥4 weeks; sustained exposure to opioids prior to initiation of methylnaltrexone may increase sensitivity to effects. All laxative maintenance therapy should be discontinued prior to initiation of therapy; laxative therapy may be added if a suboptimal response to therapy is noted after 3 days. When the opioid regimen has been changed, the patient should be re-evaluated for the need to continue methylnaltrexone therapy.

Adverse Reactions

>10%: Gastrointestinal: Abdominal pain (21% to 29%), flatulence (13%), nausea (9% to 12%)

1% to 10%:
Central nervous system: Dizziness (7%), chills (1%)
Dermatologic: Hyperhidrosis (6%)
Endocrine & metabolic: Hot flash (3%)
Gastrointestinal: Diarrhea (6%)
Neuromuscular & skeletal: Tremor (1%)

<1% (Limited to important or life-threatening): Abdominal cramps, gastrointestinal perforation, increased body temperature, muscle spasm, opioid withdrawal syndrome, piloerection, syncope

Drug Interactions

Metabolism/Transport Effects Substrate of CYP2D6 (minor); **Note:** Assignment of Major/Minor substrate status based on clinically relevant drug interaction potential

Avoid Concomitant Use

Avoid concomitant use of Methylnaltrexone with any of the following: Naloxegol; Opioid Antagonists

Increased Effect/Toxicity

Methylnaltrexone may increase the levels/effects of: Naloxegol; Opioid Antagonists

Decreased Effect There are no known significant interactions involving a decrease in effect.

Storage/Stability Store intact vials and prefilled syringes between 20°C and 25°C (68°F and 77°F); excursions are permitted between 15°C and 30°C (59°F and 86°F). Do not freeze. Protect from light. Solution withdrawn from the single use vial is stable in a syringe for 24 hours at room temperature. Do not remove the prefilled syringe from the tray until ready to administer.

Mechanism of Action An opioid receptor antagonist which blocks opioid binding at the mu receptor, methylnaltrexone is a quaternary derivative of naltrexone with restricted ability to cross the blood-brain barrier. It therefore functions as a peripheral acting opioid antagonist,

including actions on the gastrointestinal tract to inhibit opioid-induced decreased gastrointestinal motility and delay in gastrointestinal transit time, thereby decreasing opioid-induced constipation. Does not affect opioid analgesic effects.

Pharmacodynamics/Kinetics
Onset of action: Usually within 30-60 minutes (in responding patients)
Absorption: SubQ: Rapid
Distribution: V_{dss}: ~1.1 L/kg
Protein binding: 11% to 15%
Metabolism: Metabolized to methyl-6-naltrexol isomers, methylnaltrexone sulfate, and other minor metabolites
Half-life elimination: Terminal: ~8 hours
Time to peak, plasma: SubQ: 30 minutes
Excretion: Urine (~54%, primarily as unchanged drug); feces (~17%, primarily as unchanged drug)

Dosing
Adult & Geriatric
Opioid-induced constipation with chronic non-cancer pain: SubQ: 12 mg once daily. **Note:** Discontinue all laxatives prior to use; if response is not optimal after 3 days, laxative therapy may be reinitiated.

Opioid-induced constipation with advanced illness: SubQ: Dosing is according to body weight: Administer 1 dose every other day as needed; maximum: 1 dose/24 hours
<38 kg: 0.15 mg/kg (round dose up to nearest 0.1 mL of volume)
38 to <62 kg: 8 mg
62 to 114 kg: 12 mg
>114 kg: 0.15 mg/kg (round dose up to nearest 0.1 mL of volume)

Renal Impairment
Mild-to-moderate impairment: No dosage adjustment necessary.
Severe impairment (CrCl <30 mL/minute): Administer 50% of normal dose.
End-stage renal impairment (dialysis-dependent): There are no dosing adjustments provided in the manufacturer's labeling (has not been studied).

Hepatic Impairment
Mild-to-moderate impairment (Child-Pugh class A or B): No dosage adjustment necessary.
Severe impairment: There are no dosing adjustments provided in the manufacturer's labeling (has not been studied).

Administration Administer by subcutaneous injection into the upper arm, abdomen, or thigh. Rotate injection sites at each dose. Toilet facilities should be nearby immediately following administration. Discard any unused medication that remains in the vial.

Monitoring Parameters Severe, persistent, or worsening abdominal pain; symptoms of opioid withdrawal; adequate analgesia; signs or symptoms of orthostatic hypotension.

Additional Information In some clinical trials, patients who received methylnaltrexone were on a palliative opioid therapy equivalent to a mean daily oral morphine dose of 172 mg, at a stable dose for ≥3 days. Constipation was defined as <3 bowel movements/week or no bowel movement for >2 days. Patients maintained their regular laxative regimen for at least 3 days prior to treatment and throughout the study.

Dosage Forms Excipient information presented when available (limited, particularly for generics); consult specific product labeling.
Kit, Subcutaneous:
Relistor: 12 mg/0.6 mL [contains edetate calcium disodium]
Solution, Subcutaneous:
Relistor: 8 mg/0.4 mL (0.4 mL); 12 mg/0.6 mL (0.6 mL) [contains edetate calcium disodium]

◆ **Methylnaltrexone Bromide** *see* Methylnaltrexone on page 1179

Methylphenidate (meth il FEN i date)

Brand Names: US Aptensio XR; Concerta; Daytrana; Metadate CD; Metadate ER; Methylin; Quillivant XR; Ritalin; Ritalin LA; Ritalin SR [DSC]
Brand Names: Canada Apo-Methylphenidate; Apo-Methylphenidate SR; Biphentin; Concerta; PHL-Methylphenidate; PMS-Methylphenidate; ratio-Methylphenidate; Ritalin; Ritalin SR; Sandoz-Methylphenidate SR; Teva-Methylphenidate ER-C
Index Terms Methylphenidate Hydrochloride; Quillichew ER
Pharmacologic Category Central Nervous System Stimulant

Use
US labeling: Treatment of attention-deficit/hyperactivity disorder (ADHD); symptomatic management of narcolepsy (except Aptensio XR, Concerta, Daytrana, Metadate CD, Ritalin LA, and Quillivant XR)
Canadian labeling: Treatment of attention-deficit/hyperactivity disorder (ADHD); symptomatic management of narcolepsy (except Biphentin, Concerta)

Pregnancy Considerations Adverse events have been observed in animal reproduction studies. Information related to the use of methylphenidate in pregnant women with attention-deficit/hyperactivity disorder (Bolea-Akmanac, 2013; Dideriksen, 2013) or narcolepsy (Maurovich-Horvat, 2013; Thorpy, 2013) is limited.

Breast-Feeding Considerations Methylphenidate excretion in breast milk has been noted in case reports. In both cases, the authors calculated the relative infant dose to be ≤0.2% of the weight adjusted maternal dose. Adverse events were not noted in either infant, however, both were older (6 months of age and 11 months of age) and exposure was limited (Hackett, 2006; Spigset, 2007). The manufacturer recommends that caution be used if administered to a nursing woman.

Medication Guide Available Yes

Contraindications
US labeling: Hypersensitivity to methylphenidate or any component of the formulation; use during or within 14 days following MAO inhibitor therapy; marked anxiety, tension, and agitation (excluding Aptensio XR and Quillivant XR); glaucoma (excluding Aptensio XR and Quillivant XR); family history or diagnosis of Tourette syndrome or tics (excluding Aptensio XR and Quillivant XR)
Additional contraindications: Metadate CD and Metadate ER: Severe hypertension, heart failure, arrhythmia, hyperthyroidism, recent MI or angina; concomitant use of halogenated anesthetics
Canadian labeling: Hypersensitivity to methylphenidate or any component of the formulation; marked anxiety, tension, and agitation; glaucoma; use during or within 14 days following MAO inhibitor therapy; family history or diagnosis of Tourette's syndrome or tics, thyrotoxicosis, advanced arteriosclerosis, symptomatic cardiovascular disease, or moderate-to-severe hypertension
Additional contraindications: Ritalin and Ritalin SR: Pheochromocytoma

Warnings/Precautions CNS stimulant use has been associated with serious cardiovascular events (eg, sudden death in children and adolescents; sudden death, stroke, and MI in adults) in patients with preexisting structural cardiac abnormalities or other serious heart problems. These products should be avoided in patients with known serious structural cardiac abnormalities, cardiomyopathy, serious heart rhythm abnormalities, or other serious cardiac problems that could further increase their risk of sudden death. Patients should be carefully evaluated for cardiac disease prior to initiation of therapy. Use of stimulants can cause an increase in blood pressure (average 2 to 4 mm Hg) and increases in heart rate (average 3 to 6 bpm), although some patients may have larger than average increases. Use caution with hypertension, hyperthyroidism, or other cardiovascular conditions that might be exacerbated by increases in blood pressure or heart rate. Some products are contraindicated in patients with heart failure, arrhythmias, severe hypertension, hyperthyroidism, angina, or recent MI. Stimulants are associated with peripheral vasculopathy, including Raynaud's phenomenon; signs/symptoms are usually mild and intermittent, and generally improve with dose reduction or discontinuation. Digital ulceration and/or soft tissue breakdown have been observed rarely; monitor for digital changes during therapy and seek further evaluation (eg, rheumatology) if necessary. Prolonged and painful erections (priapism), sometimes requiring surgical intervention, have been reported (rarely) with methylphenidate and atomoxetine use in pediatric and adult patients. Priapism has been reported to develop after some time on the drug, often subsequent to an increase in dose but also during a period of drug withdrawal (drug holidays or discontinuation). Patients with certain hematological dyscrasias (eg, sickle cell disease), malignancies, perineal trauma, or concomitant use of alcohol, illicit drugs, or other medications associated with priapism may be at increased risk. Patients who develop abnormally sustained or frequent and painful erections should discontinue therapy and seek immediate medical attention. An emergent urological consultation should be obtained in severe cases. Priapism has been associated with different dosage forms and products; it is not known if rechallenge with a different formulation will risk recurrence. Avoidance of stimulants and atomoxetine may be preferred in patients with severe cases that were

slow to resolve and/or required detumescence (Eiland, 2014).

Has demonstrated value as part of a comprehensive treatment program for ADHD. Use with caution in patients with bipolar disorder (may induce mixed/manic episode). May exacerbate symptoms of behavior and thought disorder in psychotic patients; new-onset psychosis or mania may occur with stimulant use. Patients should be screened for bipolar disorder prior to treatment; consider discontinuation if such symptoms occur (eg, delusional thinking, hallucinations, mania) occur. May be associated with aggressive behavior or hostility (causal relationship not established); monitor for development or worsening of these behaviors. Use caution with seizure disorders (may reduce seizure threshold). Use caution in patients with history of ethanol or drug abuse. May exacerbate symptoms of behavior and thought disorder in psychotic patients. **[US Boxed Warning]: Potential for drug dependency exists - avoid abrupt discontinuation in patients who have received for prolonged periods.** Visual disturbances have been reported (rare). Not labeled for use in children <6 years of age. Use of stimulants has been associated with suppression of growth in children; monitor growth rate during treatment. Hypersensitivity reactions, such as angioedema and anaphylactic reactions have been reported.

Concerta should not be used in patients with esophageal motility disorders or preexisting severe gastrointestinal narrowing (small bowel disease, short gut syndrome, history of peritonitis, cystic fibrosis, chronic intestinal pseudo-obstruction, Meckel's diverticulum). Concomitant use of Metadate CD and Metadate ER with halogenated anesthetics is contraindicated; may cause sudden elevations in blood pressure; if surgery is planned, do not administer Metadate CD or Metadate ER on the day of surgery. Transdermal system may cause allergic contact sensitization, characterized by intense local reactions (edema, papules) that may spread beyond the patch site; sensitization may subsequently manifest systemically with other routes of methylphenidate administration; monitor closely. Avoid exposure of application site to any direct external heat sources (eg, hair dryers, heating pads, electric blankets); may increase the rate and extent of absorption and risk of overdose. Efficacy of transdermal methylphenidate therapy for >7 weeks has not been established. Transdermal system may cause a persistent loss of skin pigmentation at and around the application site, as well as at distant sites from the application site; loss of skin pigmentation may continue after discontinuation of transdermal system. May resemble vitiligo especially if loss of skin pigmentation occurs at areas distant from application site; use with caution in patients with a history and/or family history of vitiligo. Monitor for signs of skin depigmentation; immediately discontinue use if patient experiences chemical leukoderma. Potentially significant drug-drug interactions may exist, requiring dosage or frequency adjustment, additional monitoring, and/or selection of alternative therapy. Biphentin [Canadian product] controlled release capsules are not interchangeable with other controlled release formulations. Some dosage forms may contain lactose or sucrose; use with caution in patients intolerant to either component (some manufacturer labels recommend avoiding use in such patients).

Some dosage forms may contain sodium benzoate/benzoic acid; benzoic acid (benzoate) is a metabolite of benzyl alcohol; large amounts of benzyl alcohol (≥99 mg/kg/day) have been associated with a potentially fatal toxicity ("gasping syndrome") in neonates; the "gasping syndrome" consists of metabolic acidosis, respiratory distress, gasping respirations, CNS dysfunction (including convulsions, intracranial hemorrhage), hypotension, and cardiovascular collapse (AAP ["Inactive" 1997]; CDC, 1982); some data suggests that benzoate displaces bilirubin from protein binding sites (Ahlfors, 2001); avoid or use dosage forms containing benzyl alcohol derivative with caution in neonates. See manufacturer's labeling.

Adverse Reactions All dosage forms: Frequency not always defined:

Cardiovascular: Tachycardia (5%; children and adolescents: ≤1%, transdermal), palpitations (3%), angina pectoris, cardiac arrhythmia, cerebrovascular accident, decreased pulse, hypertension, increased pulse, myocardial infarction, necrotizing angiitis, Raynaud phenomenon

Central nervous system: Headache (adults: 22%; transdermal), insomnia (adults: 12%; children and adolescents: 3% to 5%), irritability (6% to 11%), emotional lability (children: 6% to 9%; adults: 1%), anxiety (8%), tics (oral: adolescents: 7%, transdermal; children: 2%), dizziness (adolescents: 2% to 7%), depressed mood (4%), initial insomnia (≤4%), nervousness (3%), restlessness (3%), aggressive behavior (2%), agitation (2%),

depression (2%), hypertonia (2%), vertigo (2%), confusion (1%), paresthesia (1%), sedation (1%), tension (1%), tension headache (1%), drowsiness, fatigue, Gilles de la Tourette syndrome (rare), hypervigilance, lethargy, outbursts of anger, toxic psychosis

Dermatologic: Hyperhidrosis (5%), excoriation (children: 4%), skin rash (children: 2%), alopecia, erythema multiforme, exfoliative dermatitis, urticaria

Endocrine & metabolic: Weight loss (6% to 9%), decreased libido (2%), growth suppression

Gastrointestinal: Decreased appetite (≤26%), xerostomia (14%), nausea (10% to 13%), vomiting (2% to 10%), anorexia (2% to 9%; transdermal), abdominal pain (children and adolescents: 5% to 7%), bruxism (2%), dyspepsia (2%), motion sickness (children: 2%), constipation (1%), diarrhea

Genitourinary: Erectile dysfunction

Hematologic & oncologic: Immune thrombocytopenia, leukopenia, pancytopenia, thrombocytopenia

Hepatic: Increased serum bilirubin

Hypersensitivity: Hypersensitivity reaction

Local: Application site reaction

Neuromuscular & skeletal: Tremor (3%), arthralgia, dyskinesia

Ophthalmic: Blurred vision (2%), eye pain (children: 2%), accommodation disturbance, dry eye syndrome, mydriasis

Respiratory: Nasopharyngitis (children and adolescents: 3%), cough (children and adolescents: 2%), upper respiratory tract infection (2%), oropharyngeal pain (1% to 2%), dyspnea, pharyngitis, pharyngolaryngeal pain, rhinitis, sinusitis

Miscellaneous: Fever (children and adolescents: 2%), accidental injury

<1% (Limited to important or life-threatening): Abnormal behavior, abdominal distress, anaphylaxis (transdermal), angioedema (transdermal), bradycardia, cardiac arrest, chest discomfort, decreased platelet count, decreased therapeutic response, disorientation, dyskinesia, extrasystoles, hallucination, heart murmur, hot flash, hyperpyrexia, increased blood pressure, increased heart rate, increased liver enzymes, increased thirst, jitteriness, lack of effectiveness of drug, leukoderma (transdermal, chemical; FDA Safety Alert 2015), macular eruption, mania, migraine, mood changes, muscle spasm, obsessive-compulsive disorder, panic attack, peripheral vascular insufficiency, priapism, psychomotor agitation, rhabdomyolysis, seizure, sleep disorder, supraventricular tachycardia, ventricular premature contractions, visual disturbance, weakness

Drug Interactions

Metabolism/Transport Effects Inhibits CYP2D6 (weak)

Avoid Concomitant Use

Avoid concomitant use of Methylphenidate with any of the following: Alcohol (Ethyl); Inhalational Anesthetics; Iobenguane I 123; MAO Inhibitors

Increased Effect/Toxicity

Methylphenidate may increase the levels/effects of: Anti-Parkinson's Agents (Dopamine Agonist); Antipsychotic Agents; ARIPiprazole; CloNIDine; Doxofylline; Fosphenytoin; Inhalational Anesthetics; PHENobarbital; Phenytoin; Primidone; Sympathomimetics; Tricyclic Antidepressants; Vitamin K Antagonists

The levels/effects of Methylphenidate may be increased by: Alcohol (Ethyl); Antacids; Antipsychotic Agents; AtoMOXetine; Cannabinoid-Containing Products; H2-Antagonists; MAO Inhibitors; Proton Pump Inhibitors

Decreased Effect

Methylphenidate may decrease the levels/effects of: Antihypertensive Agents; Iobenguane I 123; Ioflupane I 123

Food Interactions

Ethanol: Alcohol consumption increases the rate of methylphenidate release from Metadate CD and Ritalin LA (extended-release capsules), but not from Concerta (extended-release tablet); an *in vitro* study involving Metadate CD and Ritalin LA showed that an alcohol concentration of 40% resulted in 84% and 98% of the methylphenidate being released in the first hour, respectively. Management: Avoid consuming alcohol during therapy.

Food: Food may increase oral absorption of immediate release tablet/solution and chewable tablet. Management: Administer 30-45 minutes before meals.

Preparation for Administration

Suspension: *Extended release (Quillivant XR):* Prior to dispensing, reconstitute with an appropriate amount of water (refer to bottle).

Storage/Stability

Capsule:

Extended release:

Aptensio XR: Store at 20°C to 25°C (68°F to 77°F). Protect from moisture.

Metadate CD, Ritalin LA: Store at 25°C (77°F); excursions permitted to 15°C to 30°C (59°F to 86°F). Protect from light.

Controlled release (Biphentin [Canadian product]): Store at 15°C to 30°C (59°F to 86°F).

Solution: *Immediate release (Methylin):* Store at 20°C to 25°C (68°F to 77°F).

Suspension: *Extended release (Quillivant XR):* Store at 25°C (77°F); excursions permitted to 15°C to 30°C (59°F to 86°F), before and after reconstitution. Reconstituted bottle must be used within 4 months.

Tablet:

Chewable (Methylin): Store at 20°C to 25°C (68°F to 77°F). Protect from light and moisture.

Extended release:

Metadate ER: Store at 20°C to 25°C (68°F to 77°F); excursions permitted to 15°C to 30°C (59°F to 86°F). Protect from light and moisture.

Concerta: Store at 25°C (77°F); excursions permitted to 15°C to 30°C (59°F to 86°F). Protect from humidity.

Immediate release (Ritalin): Store at 25°C (77°F); excursions permitted to 15°C to 30°C (59°F to 86°F). Protect from light and moisture.

Sustained release (Ritalin-SR): Store at 25°C (77°F); excursions permitted to 15°C to 30°C (59°F to 86°F). Protect from light and moisture.

Transdermal system: *Daytrana:* Store at 25°C (77°F); excursions permitted to 15°C to 30°C (59°F to 86°F). Keep patches stored in protective pouch. Once tray is opened, use patches within 2 months; once an individual patch has been removed from the pouch and the protective liner removed, use immediately. Do not refrigerate or freeze.

Mechanism of Action Mild CNS stimulant; blocks the reuptake of norepinephrine and dopamine into presynaptic neurons; appears to stimulate the cerebral cortex and subcortical structures similar to amphetamines

Pharmacodynamics/Kinetics

Absorption:

Oral: Readily absorbed

Chewable tablet: Methylin: A high-fat meal delayed peak time (~1 hour) and increased AUC (~20%).

Controlled release capsule: Biphentin [Canadian product]: Food delayed initial peak slightly (~18 minutes); relative to immediate release tablets, AUC is similar in fed or fasted state (~100%)

Extended release capsule:

Aptensio XR: A high-fat meal increased C_{max} (~28%) and AUC (~19%). At an alcohol concentration up to 40% there was 96% release of methylphenidate within 2 hours.

Metadate CD: A high-fat meal delayed the early peak (~1 hour), and increased C_{max} (~30%) and AUC (~17%). At an alcohol concentration of 40%, there was an increase in the release rate of methylphenidate in the first hour, resulting in 84% of the methylphenidate being released.

Ritalin LA: A high-fat meal delayed absorption and peak times, but not the amount absorbed nor initial peak concentration (second peak lowered by ~25%). At an alcohol concentration of 40%, there was a 98% release of methylphenidate in the first hour.

Extended release suspension: Quillivant XR: A high-fat meal led to an earlier peak (~1 hour), and increased C_{max} (~28%) and AUC (~19%).

Extended release tablet: Metadate ER: Food resulted in greater C_{max} and AUC compared to fasting.

Immediate release solution: Methylin: A high-fat meal delayed peak time (~1 hour), and increased C_{max} (~13%) and AUC (~25%).

Transdermal: Absorption increased when applied to inflamed skin or exposed to heat. Absorption is continuous for 9 hours after application.

Distribution: V_d: d-methylphenidate: 2.65 ± 1.11 L/kg, l-methylphenidate: 1.80 ± 0.91 L/kg

Protein binding: 10% to 33%

Metabolism: Extensive metabolism, predominately via de-esterification by carboxylesterase CES1A1 to alpha-phenyl-piperidine acetic acid (PPAA; ritalinic acid) which has little to no pharmacologic activity.

Bioavailability:

Extended release capsule: Aptensio XR: 102% (relative to immediate release oral product)

Extended release suspension: Quillivant XR: 95% (relative to immediate release oral solution)

Half-life elimination:

Chewable tablet: Methylin: Adults: 3 hours

Controlled release capsule: Biphentin [Canadian product]: Children: 2.4 hours; Adults: 2.1 hours

Extended release capsule:

Aptensio XR: Adults: ~5 hours

Metadate CD: Adults: 6.8 hours

Ritalin LA: Children: ~2.45 hours (range: 1.5 to 4 hours); Adults: ~3.3 hours (range: 3 to 4.2 hours)

Extended release suspension: Quillivant XR: Children, Adolescents, and Adults: ~5 hours

Extended release tablet: Concerta: Adolescents and Adults: ~3.5 hours

Immediate release solution: Methylin: Adults: 2.7 hours

Immediate release tablet: Adults: 2.9 hours

Sustained release tablet: Adults: 3.4 hours

Transdermal: Children and Adolescents: d-methylphenidate ~4 to 5 hours, l-methylphenidate 1.4 to 2.9 hours

Time to peak:

Chewable tablet: Methylin: ~1 to 2 hours

Controlled release capsule: Biphentin [Canadian product]: Children: Initial: ~2.5 hours; Adults: Initial: ~2 hours

Extended release capsule:

Aptensio XR: Adults: Initial: ~2 hours; Second peak: ~8 hours

Metadate CD: Children: Initial: ~1.5 hours; Second peak: ~4.5 hours

Ritalin LA:

Children: Initial: 1 to 3 hours; Second peak: 5 to 11 hour

Adults: Initial: 1.3 to 4 hours; Second peak: 4.3 to 6.5 hours

Extended release suspension: Quillivant XR: Children: 4.05 hours (range: 3.98 to 6 hours); Adolescents: 2 hours (range: 1.98 to 4 hours); Adults: 4 hours (range: 1.3 to 7.3 hours)

Extended release tablet: Concerta: Initial: ~1 hours, followed by gradually ascending concentrations over 5 to 9 hours; Mean peak: 6 to 10 hours

Immediate release solution: Methylin: 1 to 2 hours

Immediate release tablet: Children: 1.9 hours (range: 0.3 to 4.4 hours)

Sustained release tablet: Children: 4.7 hours (range: 1.3 to 8.2 hours)

Transdermal: ~8 to 10 hours

Excretion: Urine (90% as metabolites and unchanged drug)

Dosing

Adult & Geriatric

ADHD:

Oral, immediate release (IR) products (tablets, chewable tablets, and solution): Initial: 5 mg twice daily, before breakfast and lunch; increase by 5 to 10 mg daily at weekly intervals; maximum dose: 60 mg daily (in 2 to 3 divided doses).

Oral, extended release (ER), sustained release (SR) products (capsules, tablets, and oral suspension):

Concerta: (Adults <65 years):

Patients not currently taking methylphenidate: Initial: US labeling: 18 to 36 mg once every morning

Canadian labeling: 18 mg once every morning

Patients currently taking immediate release (IR) methylphenidate: Initial: **Note:** Dosing based on current regimen and clinical judgment; suggested dosing listed below:

- Patients taking IR methylphenidate 5 mg 2 to 3 times daily **or** (Canadian labeling; not in US labeling) methylphenidate SR 20 mg daily: 18 mg once every morning

- Patients taking IR methylphenidate 10 mg 2 to 3 times daily **or** (Canadian labeling; not in US labeling) methylphenidate SR 40 mg daily: 36 mg once every morning

- Patients taking IR methylphenidate 15 mg 2 to 3 times daily **or** (Canadian labeling; not in US labeling) methylphenidate SR 60 mg daily: 54 mg once every morning

- Patients taking IR methylphenidate 20 mg 2 to 3 times daily: 72 mg once every morning

Dose adjustment: May increase dose in increments of 18 mg at weekly intervals. A dosage strength of 27 mg is available for situations in which a dosage between 18 to 36 mg is desired. Maximum dose: 72 mg daily.

Aptensio XR: Initial: 10 mg once daily; may be titrated in 10 mg increments at weekly intervals; maximum: 60 mg once daily

Biphentin [Canadian product]: Patients not currently taking methylphenidate: Initial: 10 to 20 mg once daily; may be adjusted in 10 mg increments at weekly intervals to a maximum dose of 80 mg daily.

Conversion from immediate release methylphenidate formulations to Biphentin: Use equivalent total daily dose administered once daily.

Metadate ER, Ritalin-SR: May be given in place of immediate release products (duration of action ~8 hours), once the immediate release formulation daily dose is titrated and the titrated 8-hour dosage corresponds to sustained or extended release tablet size; maximum: 60 mg daily

Metadate CD, Quillivant XR: Initial: 20 mg once daily; may be adjusted in 10 to 20 mg increments at weekly intervals; maximum: 60 mg daily

Ritalin LA: Initial: 20 mg once daily (10 mg once daily may be considered for some patients); may be adjusted in 10 mg increments at weekly intervals; maximum: 60 mg daily

Conversion from immediate release or sustained release methylphenidate formulation to Ritalin LA: Use equivalent total daily dose administered once daily.

Narcolepsy: Oral:

***Immediate release tablets and solution** (Methylin, Ritalin):* Initial: 5 mg twice daily before breakfast and lunch; increase by 5 to 10 mg daily at weekly intervals; maximum dose: 60 mg daily (in 2 to 3 divided doses).

***Extended and sustained release tablets** (Metadate ER, Ritalin-SR):* May be given in place of immediate release products (duration of action ~8 hours), once the immediate release formulation daily dose is titrated and the titrated 8-hour dosage corresponds to sustained or extended release tablet size; maximum: 60 mg daily.

Depression in medically-ill older adults or adult patients with terminal illness and/or receiving palliative care (off-label use): Oral: Initial: *Immediate release:* 2.5 to 5 mg once daily before breakfast or twice daily before breakfast and lunch; increase by 2.5 to 5 mg daily every 1 to 3 days in divided doses before breakfast and lunch as tolerated; maximum dose: 20 to 40 mg daily (Hardy, 2009; Kerr 2012). *Do not use sustained release product.*

Pediatric

ADHD:

Oral, immediate release (IR) products (tablets, chewable tablets, and solution): Children ≥6 years and Adolescents: Initial: 5 mg twice daily, before breakfast and lunch; increase by 5 to 10 mg daily at weekly intervals; maximum dose: 60 mg daily (in 2 to 3 divided doses).

Oral, extended release (ER), sustained release (SR) products (capsules, tablets, and oral suspension): Children ≥6 years and Adolescents <18 years: *Concerta:* **Note:** For adolescents ≥18 years, refer to adult dosing.

Patients not currently taking methylphenidate: Initial: 18 mg once daily in the morning

Patients currently taking immediate release (IR) methylphenidate: Initial: **Note:** Dosing based on current regimen and clinical judgment; suggested dosing listed below:

- Patients taking IR methylphenidate 5 mg 2 to 3 times daily **or** (Canadian labeling; not in US labeling) methylphenidate SR 20 mg daily: 18 mg once every morning

- Patients taking IR methylphenidate 10 mg 2 to 3 times daily **or** (Canadian labeling; not in US labeling) methylphenidate SR 40 mg daily: 36 mg once every morning

- Patients taking IR methylphenidate 15 mg 2 to 3 times daily **or** (Canadian labeling; not in US labeling) methylphenidate SR 60 mg daily: 54 mg once every morning

- Patients taking IR methylphenidate 20 mg 2 to 3 times daily: 72 mg once every morning

Dose adjustment: May increase dose in increments of 18 mg at weekly intervals. A dosage strength of 27 mg is available for situations in which a dosage between 18 to 36 mg is desired.

Maximum dose:

US labeling: 54 mg daily in children 6 to 12 years **or** 2 mg/kg/day (up to 72 mg daily) in adolescents <18 years

Canadian labeling: 54 mg daily in children and adolescents 6 to 18 years

Children ≥6 years and Adolescents:

Aptensio XR: Initial: 10 mg once daily; may be titrated in 10 mg increments at weekly intervals; maximum: 60 mg once daily

Biphentin [Canadian product]: Patients not currently taking methylphenidate: Initial: 10 to 20 mg once daily; may be adjusted in 10 mg increments at weekly intervals. Maximum: 60 mg daily. **Note:** In some children >60 kg, a maximum dose of 1 mg/kg/daily (not to exceed 80 mg daily) may be

necessary; however, close monitoring for adverse events is required. Reduce dose or discontinue if adverse events arise.

Conversion from immediate release methylphenidate formulations to Biphentin: Use equivalent total daily dose administered once daily.

Metadate ER, Ritalin-SR: May be given in place of immediate release products (duration of action ~8 hours), once the immediate release formulation daily dose is titrated and the titrated 8-hour dosage corresponds to sustained or extended release tablet size; maximum: 60 mg daily

Metadate CD, Quillivant XR: Initial: 20 mg once daily; may be adjusted in 10 to 20 mg increments at weekly intervals; maximum: 60 mg daily

Ritalin LA: Initial: 20 mg once daily (10 mg once daily may be considered for some patients); may be adjusted in 10 mg increments at weekly intervals; maximum: 60 mg daily

Conversion from immediate release or sustained release methylphenidate formulation to Ritalin LA: Use equivalent total daily dose administered once daily.

Transdermal: (Daytrana): Children ≥6 years and Adolescents <18 years: Initial: 10 mg patch once daily; remove up to 9 hours after application. Titrate based on response and tolerability; may increase to next transdermal dose no more frequently than every week. **Note:** Application should occur 2 hours prior to desired effect. Drug absorption may continue for a period of time after patch removal. The prescribing information recommends patients converting from another formulation of methylphenidate should be initiated at 10 mg regardless of their previous dose and titrated as needed due to the differences in bioavailability of the transdermal formulation. However, some clinicians have supported higher starting patch doses for patients converting from oral methylphenidate doses of >20 mg daily; for example, the 15 mg (18.75 cm^2) patch has been investigated to have the same effect as 22.5 mg daily of the immediate release preparation, 27 mg/day of the osmotic release preparation, or 20 mg daily of the encapsulated bead preparation (Arnold, 2007).

Narcolepsy: Oral: Children ≥6 years and Adolescents: Refer to adult dosing.

Renal Impairment

Oral: There are no dosage adjustments provided in the manufacturer's labeling (has not been studied); undergoes extensive metabolism to a renally eliminated metabolite with little or no pharmacologic activity.

Transdermal: There are no dosage adjustments provided in the manufacturer's labeling (has not been studied).

Hepatic Impairment

Oral: There are no dosage adjustments provided in the manufacturer's labeling (has not been studied).

Transdermal: There are no dosage adjustments provided in the manufacturer's labeling (has not been studied).

Dietary Considerations Administer immediate release (IR) tablet (Ritalin), IR solution (Methylin), chewable tablet (Methylin), and sustained released tablet (Ritalin-SR) 30-45 minutes before meals. Some products may contain phenylalanine.

Administration

Oral:

Controlled release capsule (Biphentin; Canadian product): Administer in the morning with breakfast. Swallow whole; do not crush or chew capsule. Alternatively, capsules may be opened and the contents sprinkled onto applesauce, ice cream, or yogurt, but the beads must not be crushed or chewed.

Immediate release (IR) tablet (Ritalin), IR solution (Methylin), chewable tablet (Methylin): Administer each dose 30-45 minutes before a meal. Ensure last daily dose is administered before 6 pm if difficulty sleeping occurs. Administer chewable tablet with at least 8 ounces of water or other fluid.

Extended release capsule (Aptensio XR, Metadate CD, Ritalin LA): Administer in the morning with or without food. Alternatively, capsules may be opened and the contents sprinkled onto a small amount (equal to 1 tablespoon) of cold applesauce. Swallow applesauce mixture immediately without chewing. Do not crush or chew capsule contents.

Extended release suspension (Quillivant XR): Administer in the morning with or without food. Shake bottle ≥10 seconds prior to administration. Use the oral dosing dispenser provided; wash after each use.

Extended release tablet:

Metadate ER: May be taken with or without food. Swallow whole with water or other fluid; do not crush or chew tablet.

Concerta: Administer in the morning. May be taken with or without food, but must be taken with water or other fluid. Do not crush, chew, or divide tablet.

Sustained release tablet (Ritalin-SR): Administer 30-45 minutes before a meal. Swallow whole; do not crush or chew tablet.

Topical: Transdermal (Daytrana): Apply to clean, dry, non-oily, intact skin to the hip area, avoiding the waistline; do not premedicate the patch site with hydrocortisone or other solutions, creams, ointments, or emollients. Apply at the same time each day to alternating hips. Press firmly for 30 seconds to ensure proper adherence. Avoid exposure of application site to external heat source, which may increase the amount of drug absorbed. If difficulty is experienced when separating the patch from the liner or if any medication (sticky substance) remains on the liner after separation; discard that patch and apply a new patch. Do not use a patch that has been damaged or torn; do not cut patch. If patch should dislodge, may replace with new patch (to different site) but total wear time should not exceed 9 hours; do not reapply with dressings, tape, or common adhesives. Patch may be removed early if a shorter duration of effect is desired or if late day side effects occur. Wash hands with soap and water after handling. Avoid touching the sticky side of the patch. If patch removal is difficult, an oil-based product (eg, petroleum jelly, olive oil) may be applied to the patch edges to aid removal; never apply acetone-based products (eg, nail polish remover) to patch. Dispose of used patch by folding adhesive side onto itself, and discard in toilet or appropriate lidded container.

Monitoring Parameters Periodic CBC, differential, and platelet counts with prolonged use; blood pressure, heart rate; signs and symptoms of depression, aggression, or hostility; growth rate in children; signs of central nervous system stimulation; signs of peripheral vasculopathy (eg, digital changes)

Transdermal: Signs of worsening erythema, blistering or edema which does not improve within 48 hours of patch removal, or spreads beyond patch site.

When used for the treatment of ADHD, thoroughly evaluate for cardiovascular risk. Monitor heart rate, blood pressure, and consider obtaining ECG prior to initiation (Vetter, 2008).

Test Interactions May interfere with urine detection of amphetamines/methamphetamines (false-positive).

Additional Information Treatment with methylphenidate may include "drug holidays" or periodic discontinuation in order to assess the patient's requirements and to decrease tolerance and limit suppression of linear growth and weight. Specific patients may require 3 doses/day for treatment of ADHD (ie, additional dose at 4 PM).

Concerta is an osmotic controlled release formulation (OROS) of methylphenidate. The tablet has an immediate-release overcoat that provides an initial dose of methylphenidate within 1 hour. The overcoat covers a trilayer core. The trilayer core is composed of two layers containing the drug and excipients, and one layer of osmotic components. As water from the gastrointestinal tract enters the core, the osmotic components expand and methylphenidate is released.

Metadate CD capsules contain a mixture of immediate release and extended release beads, designed to release 30% of the dose immediately and 70% over an extended period.

Ritalin LA uses a combination of immediate release and enteric coated, delayed release beads.

Product Availability Quillichew ER chewable tablet: FDA approved December 2015; availability anticipated in the first quarter of 2016. Information pertaining to this product within the monograph is pending revision.

Dosage Forms Excipient information presented when available (limited, particularly for generics); consult specific product labeling. [DSC] = Discontinued product

Capsule Extended Release, Oral, as hydrochloride:
Metadate CD: 10 mg, 20 mg, 30 mg [contains fd&c blue #2 (indigotine)]
Metadate CD: 40 mg
Metadate CD: 50 mg [contains fd&c blue #2 (indigotine)]
Metadate CD: 60 mg
Generic: 10 mg, 20 mg, 30 mg, 40 mg, 50 mg, 60 mg

Capsule Extended Release 24 Hour, Oral, as hydrochloride:
Aptensio XR: 10 mg [contains brilliant blue fcf (fd&c blue #1)]
Aptensio XR: 15 mg [contains fd&c red #40, fd&c yellow #10 (quinoline yellow)]
Aptensio XR: 20 mg [contains fd&c yellow #10 (quinoline yellow)]

Aptensio XR: 30 mg [contains brilliant blue fcf (fd&c blue #1)]
Aptensio XR: 40 mg [contains brilliant blue fcf (fd&c blue #1), fd&c red #40]
Aptensio XR: 50 mg [contains fd&c yellow #10 (quinoline yellow)]
Aptensio XR: 60 mg
Ritalin LA: 10 mg, 20 mg, 30 mg, 40 mg, 60 mg
Generic: 20 mg, 30 mg, 40 mg

Patch, Transdermal:
Daytrana: 10 mg/9 hr (30 ea); 15 mg/9 hr (30 ea); 20 mg/9 hr (30 ea); 30 mg/9 hr (30 ea)

Solution, Oral, as hydrochloride:
Methylin: 5 mg/5 mL (500 mL); 10 mg/5 mL (500 mL) [contains polyethylene glycol]
Generic: 5 mg/5 mL (500 mL); 10 mg/5 mL (500 mL)

Suspension Reconstituted, Oral, as hydrochloride:
Quillivant XR: 25 mg/5 mL (60 mL, 120 mL, 150 mL, 180 mL) [contains sodium benzoate; banana flavor]

Tablet, Oral, as hydrochloride:
Ritalin: 5 mg
Ritalin: 10 mg, 20 mg [scored]
Generic: 5 mg, 10 mg, 20 mg

Tablet Chewable, Oral, as hydrochloride:
Methylin: 2.5 mg, 5 mg [contains aspartame; grape flavor]
Methylin: 10 mg [scored; contains aspartame; grape flavor]
Generic: 2.5 mg, 5 mg, 10 mg

Tablet Extended Release, Oral, as hydrochloride:
Concerta: 18 mg, 27 mg, 36 mg, 54 mg
Metadate ER: 20 mg [DSC]
Metadate ER: 20 mg [additive free, color free]
Ritalin SR: 20 mg [DSC]
Generic: 10 mg, 18 mg, 20 mg, 27 mg, 36 mg, 54 mg

Dosage Forms: Canada Also refer to Dosage Forms Excipient information presented when available (limited, particularly for generics); consult specific product labeling.

Capsule, Controlled Release, Oral, as hydrochloride:
Biphentin: 10 mg, 15 mg, 20 mg, 30 mg, 40 mg, 50 mg, 60 mg, 80 mg

Controlled Substance C-II

♦ **Methylphenidate Hydrochloride** see Methylphenidate on page 1180

♦ **Methylphenoxy-Benzene Propanamine** see AtoMOXetine on page 167

♦ **Methylphenyl Isoxazolyl Penicillin** see Oxacillin on page 1348

♦ **Methylphytyl Napthoquinone** see Phytonadione on page 1450

MethylPREDNISolone (meth il pred NIS oh lone)

Brand Names: US A-Methapred; Depo-Medrol; Medrol; Medrol (Pak); Solu-MEDROL

Brand Names: Canada Depo-Medrol; Medrol; Methylprednisolone Acetate; Methylprednisolone Sodium Succinate For Injection; Methylprednisolone Sodium Succinate For Injection USP; Solu-Medrol

Index Terms 6-α-Methylprednisolone; A-Methapred; Medrol Dose Pack; Methylprednisolone Acetate; Methylprednisolone Sodium Succinate; Solumedrol

Pharmacologic Category Corticosteroid, Systemic

Additional Appendix Information
Corticosteroids Systemic Equivalencies on page 1950

Use Primarily as an anti-inflammatory or immunosuppressant agent in the treatment of a variety of diseases including those of dermatologic, endocrine, GI, hematologic, allergic, inflammatory, neoplastic, neurologic, ophthalmic, renal, respiratory, and autoimmune origin. Prevention and treatment of graft-versus-host disease following allogeneic bone marrow transplantation.

Pregnancy Considerations Adverse events have been observed with corticosteroids in animal reproduction studies. Methylprednisolone crosses the placenta (Anderson 1981). Some studies have shown an association between first trimester systemic corticosteroid use and oral clefts (Park-Wyllie 2000; Pradat 2003). Systemic corticosteroids may also influence fetal growth (decreased birth weight); however, information is conflicting (Lunghi 2010). Hypoadrenalism may occur in newborns following maternal use of corticosteroids in pregnancy; monitor.

When systemic corticosteroids are needed in pregnancy, it is generally recommended to use the lowest effective dose for the shortest duration of time, avoiding high doses during the first trimester (Leachman 2006; Lunghi 2010; Makol 2011; Østensen 2009). Inhaled corticosteroids are preferred for the treatment of asthma during pregnancy. Systemic corticosteroids such as methylprednisolone may

be used for the treatment of severe persistent asthma if needed; the lowest dose administered on alternate days (if possible) should be used (NAEPP 2005).

Pregnant women exposed to methylprednisolone for antirejection therapy following a transplant may contact the National Transplantation Pregnancy Registry (NTPR) at 215-955-4820. Women exposed to methylprednisolone during pregnancy for the treatment of an autoimmune disease may contact the OTIS Autoimmune Diseases Study at 877-311-8972.

Breast-Feeding Considerations Corticosteroids are excreted in human milk. The manufacturer notes that when used systemically, maternal use of corticosteroids have the potential to cause adverse events in a nursing infant (eg, growth suppression, interfere with endogenous corticosteroid production) and therefore recommends a decision be made whether to discontinue nursing or to discontinue the drug, taking into account the importance of treatment to the mother. If there is concern about exposure to the infant, some guidelines recommend waiting 4 hours after the maternal dose of an oral systemic corticosteroid before breast-feeding in order to decrease potential exposure to the nursing infant (based on a study using prednisolone) (Bae 2011; Leachman 2006; Makol 2011; Ost 1985). Other guidelines note that maternal use of systemic corticosteroids is not a contraindication to breast-feeding (NAEPP 2005).

Contraindications Hypersensitivity to methylprednisolone or any component of the formulation; systemic fungal infection; administration of live virus vaccines; methylprednisolone formulations containing benzyl alcohol preservative are contraindicated in premature infants; IM administration in idiopathic thrombocytopenic purpura; intrathecal administration

Warnings/Precautions Corticosteroids are not approved for epidural injection. Serious neurologic events (eg, spinal cord infarction, paraplegia, quadriplegia, cortical blindness, stroke), some resulting in death, have been reported with epidural injection of corticosteroids, with and without use of fluoroscopy.

Use with caution in patients with thyroid disease, hepatic impairment, renal impairment, cardiovascular disease, diabetes, glaucoma, cataracts, myasthenia gravis, multiple sclerosis, osteoporosis, seizures, or GI diseases (diverticulitis, intestinal anastomoses, peptic ulcer, ulcerative colitis) due to perforation risk. Avoid ethanol may enhance gastric mucosal irritation. Not recommended for the treatment of optic neuritis; may increase frequency of new episodes. Use with caution in patients with a history of ocular herpes simplex; corneal perforation has occurred; do not use in active ocular herpes simplex, Use caution following acute MI (corticosteroids have been associated with myocardial rupture). Cardiomegaly and congestive heart failure have been reported following concurrent use of amphotericin B and hydrocortisone for the management of fungal infections.

Because of the risk of adverse effects, systemic corticosteroids should be used cautiously in the elderly in the smallest possible effective dose for the shortest duration. May affect growth velocity; growth should be routinely monitored in pediatric patients. Withdraw therapy with gradual tapering of dose. Patients may require higher doses when subject to stress (ie, trauma, surgery, severe infection).

May cause hypercorticism or suppression of hypothalamic-pituitary-adrenal (HPA) axis, particularly in younger children or in patients receiving high doses for prolonged periods. HPA axis suppression may lead to adrenal crisis. Withdrawal and discontinuation of a corticosteroid should be done slowly and carefully. Particular care is required when patients are transferred from systemic corticosteroids to inhaled products due to possible adrenal insufficiency or withdrawal from steroids, including an increase in allergic symptoms. Adult patients receiving >20 mg per day of prednisone (or equivalent) may be most susceptible. Fatalities have occurred due to adrenal insufficiency in asthmatic patients during and after transfer from systemic corticosteroids to aerosol steroids; aerosol steroids do not provide the systemic steroid needed to treat patients having trauma, surgery, or infections. Use in septic shock or sepsis syndrome may increase mortality in some populations (eg, patients with elevated serum creatinine, patients who develop secondary infections after use).

Acute myopathy has been reported with high dose corticosteroids, usually in patients with neuromuscular transmission disorders; may involve ocular and/or respiratory muscles; monitor creatine kinase; recovery may be delayed. Corticosteroid use may cause psychiatric disturbances, including depression, euphoria, insomnia, mood swings, and personality changes. Preexisting psychiatric conditions may be exacerbated by corticosteroid use. Prolonged use of corticosteroids may increase the incidence of secondary infection, cause activation of latent infections, mask acute infection (including fungal infections), prolong or exacerbate viral or parasitic infections, or limit response to vaccines. Exposure to chickenpox or measles should be avoided; corticosteroids should not be used to treat ocular herpes simplex. Corticosteroids should not be used for cerebral malaria, fungal infections, or viral hepatitis. Close observation is required in patients with latent tuberculosis and/or TB reactivity; restrict use in active TB (only fulminating or disseminated TB in conjunction with antituberculosis treatment). Amebiasis should be ruled out in any patient with recent travel to tropic climates or unexplained diarrhea prior to initiation of corticosteroids. Use with extreme caution in patients with *Strongyloides* infections; hyperinfection, dissemination and fatalities have occurred. Prolonged treatment with corticosteroids has been associated with the development of Kaposi's sarcoma (case reports); discontinuation may result in clinical improvement.

High-dose corticosteroids should not be used to manage acute head injury. Rare cases of anaphylactoid reactions have been observed in patients receiving corticosteroids. Avoid injection or leakage into the dermis; dermal and/or subdermal skin depression may occur at the site of injection. Avoid deltoid muscle injection; subcutaneous atrophy may occur. Potentially significant drug-drug interactions may exist, requiring dose or frequency adjustment, additional monitoring, and/or selection of alternative therapy.

Benzyl alcohol and derivatives: Methylprednisolone **acetate** IM injection (multiple-dose vial) and the diluent for methylprednisolone **sodium succinate** injection may contain benzyl alcohol; large amounts of benzyl alcohol (≥99 mg/kg/day) have been associated with a potentially fatal toxicity ("gasping syndrome") in neonates; the "gasping syndrome" consists of metabolic acidosis, respiratory distress, gasping respirations, CNS dysfunction (including convulsions, intracranial hemorrhage), hypotension, and cardiovascular collapse (AAP ["Inactive" 1997]; CDC 1982); some data suggests that benzoate displaces bilirubin from protein binding sites (Ahlfors 2001); avoid or use dosage forms containing benzyl alcohol with caution in neonates.

Some dosage forms may contain polysorbate 80 (also known as Tweens). Hypersensitivity reactions, usually a delayed reaction, have been reported following exposure to pharmaceutical products containing polysorbate 80 in certain individuals (Isaksson 2002; Lucente 2000; Shelley 1995). Thrombocytopenia, ascites, pulmonary deterioration, and renal and hepatic failure have been reported in premature neonates after receiving parenteral products containing polysorbate 80 (Alade 1986; CDC 1984). See manufacturer's labeling.

Adverse Reactions Frequency not defined.

Cardiovascular: Arrhythmias, bradycardia, cardiac arrest, cardiomegaly, circulatory collapse, congestive heart failure, edema, fat embolism, hypertension, hypertrophic cardiomyopathy in premature infants, myocardial rupture (post MI), syncope, tachycardia, thromboembolism, vasculitis

Central nervous system: Delirium, depression, emotional instability, euphoria, hallucinations, headache, intracranial pressure increased, insomnia, malaise, mood swings, nervousness, neuritis, personality changes, psychic disorders, pseudotumor cerebri (usually following discontinuation), seizure, vertigo

Dermatologic: Acne, allergic dermatitis, alopecia, dry scaly skin, ecchymoses, edema, erythema, hirsutism, hyper-/hypopigmentation, hypertrichosis, impaired wound healing, petechiae, rash, skin atrophy, sterile abscess, skin test reaction impaired, striae, urticaria

Endocrine & metabolic: Adrenal suppression, amenorrhea, carbohydrate intolerance increased, Cushing's syndrome, diabetes mellitus, fluid retention, glucose intolerance, growth suppression (children), hyperglycemia, hyperlipidemia, hypokalemia, hypokalemic alkalosis, menstrual irregularities, negative nitrogen balance, pituitary-adrenal axis suppression, protein catabolism, sodium and water retention

Gastrointestinal: Abdominal distention, appetite increased, bowel/bladder dysfunction (after intrathecal administration), gastrointestinal hemorrhage, gastrointestinal perforation, nausea, pancreatitis, peptic ulcer, perforation of the small and large intestine, ulcerative esophagitis, vomiting, weight gain

Hematologic: Leukocytosis (transient)

Hepatic: Hepatomegaly, transaminases increased

◄ Local: Postinjection flare (intra-articular use), thrombophlebitis

Neuromuscular & skeletal: Arthralgia, arthropathy, aseptic necrosis (femoral and humoral heads), fractures, muscle mass loss, muscle weakness, myopathy (particularly in conjunction with neuromuscular disease or neuromuscular-blocking agents), neuropathy, osteoporosis, parasthesia, tendon rupture, vertebral compression fractures, weakness

Ocular: Cataracts, exophthalmoses, glaucoma, intraocular pressure increased

Renal: Glycosuria

Respiratory: Pulmonary edema

Miscellaneous: Abnormal fat disposition, anaphylactoid reaction, anaphylaxis, angioedema, avascular necrosis, diaphoresis, hiccups, hypersensitivity reactions, infections, secondary malignancy

<1% (Limited to important or life-threatening): Venous thrombosis (Johannesdottir, 2013)

Drug Interactions

Metabolism/Transport Effects Substrate of CYP3A4 (minor); **Note:** Assignment of Major/Minor substrate status based on clinically relevant drug interaction potential; **Inhibits** CYP2C8 (weak)

Avoid Concomitant Use

Avoid concomitant use of MethylPREDNISolone with any of the following: Aldesleukin; Amodiaquine; BCG (Intravesical); Indium 111 Capromab Pendetide; Mifepristone; Natalizumab; Pimecrolimus; Tacrolimus (Topical); Tofacitinib

Increased Effect/Toxicity

MethylPREDNISolone may increase the levels/effects of: Acetylcholinesterase Inhibitors; Amodiaquine; Amphotericin B; Androgens; CycloSPORINE (Systemic); Deferasirox; Fingolimod; Leflunomide; Loop Diuretics; Natalizumab; Nicorandil; NSAID (COX-2 Inhibitor); NSAID (Nonselective); Quinolone Antibiotics; Thiazide Diuretics; Tofacitinib; Vaccines (Live); Warfarin

The levels/effects of MethylPREDNISolone may be increased by: Aprepitant; CycloSPORINE (Systemic); CYP3A4 Inhibitors (Strong); Denosumab; Estrogen Derivatives; Fosaprepitant; Indacaterol; Mifepristone; Neuromuscular-Blocking Agents (Nondepolarizing); Pimecrolimus; Roflumilast; Salicylates; Tacrolimus (Topical); Telaprevir; Trastuzumab

Decreased Effect

MethylPREDNISolone may decrease the levels/effects of: Aldesleukin; Antidiabetic Agents; BCG (Intravesical); Calcitriol (Systemic); Coccidioides immitis Skin Test; Corticorelin; CycloSPORINE (Systemic); Hyaluronidase; Indium 111 Capromab Pendetide; Isoniazid; Salicylates; Sipuleucel-T; Telaprevir; Urea Cycle Disorder Agents; Vaccines (Inactivated); Vaccines (Live)

The levels/effects of MethylPREDNISolone may be decreased by: Antacids; Bile Acid Sequestrants; CYP3A4 Inducers (Strong); Echinacea; Mifepristone; Mitotane

Preparation for Administration

Standard diluent (Solu-Medrol): 40 mg/50 mL D_5W; 125 mg/50 mL D_5W.

Minimum volume (Solu-Medrol): 50 mL D_5W.

Storage/Stability

Methylprednisolone acetate; tablets: Store at 20°C to 25°C (68°F to 77°F).

Methylprednisolone sodium succinate: Store intact vials at controlled room temperature of 20°C to 25°C (68°F to 77°F). Protect from light. Reconstituted solutions of methylprednisolone sodium succinate should be stored at room temperature of 20°C to 25°C (68°F to 77°F) and used within 48 hours. Stability of parenteral admixture at room temperature (25°C) and at refrigeration temperature (4°C) is 48 hours.

Mechanism of Action In a tissue-specific manner, corticosteroids regulate gene expression subsequent to binding specific intracellular receptors and translocation into the nucleus. Corticosteroids exert a wide array of physiologic effects including modulation of carbohydrate, protein, and lipid metabolism and maintenance of fluid and electrolyte homeostasis. Moreover cardiovascular, immunologic, musculoskeletal, endocrine, and neurologic physiology are influenced by corticosteroids. Decreases inflammation by suppression of migration of polymorphonuclear leukocytes and reversal of increased capillary permeability.

Pharmacodynamics/Kinetics

Onset of action: Peak effect (route dependent): Oral: 1 to 2 hours; IM: 4 to 8 days; Intra-articular: 1 week; methylprednisolone sodium succinate is highly soluble and has a rapid effect by IM and IV routes

Duration (route dependent): Oral: 30 to 36 hours; IM: 1 to 4 weeks; Intra-articular: 1 to 5 weeks; methylprednisolone acetate has a low solubility and has a sustained IM effect

Distribution: V_d: 0.7 to 1.5 L/kg

Half-life elimination: 3 to 3.5 hours; reduced in obese

Excretion: Clearance: Reduced in obese

Dosing

Adult & Geriatric Only sodium succinate may be given IV; methylprednisolone sodium succinate is highly soluble and has a rapid effect by IM and IV routes. Methylprednisolone acetate has a low solubility and has a sustained IM effect.

Acute spinal cord injury (off-label use): IV (sodium succinate): 30 mg/kg over 15 minutes, followed in 45 minutes by a continuous infusion of 5.4 mg/kg/hour for 23 hours. **Note:** Due to insufficient evidence of clinical efficacy (ie, preserving or improving spinal cord function), the routine use of methylprednisolone in the treatment of acute spinal cord injury is no longer recommended. If used in this setting, methylprednisolone should not be initiated >8 hours after the injury; not effective in penetrating trauma (eg, gunshot) (Consortium for Spinal Cord Medicine 2008).

Allergic conditions: Oral: Tapered-dosage schedule (eg, dose-pack containing 21 x 4 mg tablets):

Day 1: 24 mg on day 1 administered as 8 mg (2 tablets) before breakfast, 4 mg (1 tablet) after lunch, 4 mg (1 tablet) after supper, and 8 mg (2 tablets) at bedtime OR 24 mg (6 tablets) as a single dose or divided into 2 or 3 doses upon initiation (regardless of time of day)

Day 2: 20 mg on day 2 administered as 4 mg (1 tablet) before breakfast, 4 mg (1 tablet) after lunch, 4 mg (1 tablet) after supper, and 8 mg (2 tablets) at bedtime

Day 3: 16 mg on day 3 administered as 4 mg (1 tablet) before breakfast, 4 mg (1 tablet) after lunch, 4 mg (1 tablet) after supper, and 4 mg (1 tablet) at bedtime

Day 4: 12 mg on day 4 administered as 4 mg (1 tablet) before breakfast, 4 mg (1 tablet) after lunch, and 4 mg (1 tablet) at bedtime

Day 5: 8 mg on day 5 administered as 4 mg (1 tablet) before breakfast and 4 mg (1 tablet) at bedtime

Day 6: 4 mg on day 6 administered as 4 mg (1 tablet) before breakfast

Anti-inflammatory or immunosuppressive:

Oral: 2 to 60 mg/day in 1 to 4 divided doses to start, followed by gradual reduction in dosage to the lowest possible level consistent with maintaining an adequate clinical response.

IM (sodium succinate): 10 to 80 mg/day once daily

IM (acetate): 10 to 80 mg every 1 to 2 weeks

IV (sodium succinate): 10 to 40 mg over a period of several minutes and repeated IV or IM at intervals depending on clinical response; when high dosages are needed, give 30 mg/kg over a period ≥30 minutes and may be repeated every 4 to 6 hours for 48 hours.

Arthritis: Intra-articular (acetate): Administer every 1 to 5 weeks.

Large joints (eg, knee, ankle): 20 to 80 mg

Medium joints (eg, elbow, wrist): 10 to 40 mg

Small joints: 4 to 10 mg

Asthma exacerbations, including status asthmaticus (emergency medical care or hospital doses): Oral, IV: 40 to 80 mg/day in 1 to 2 divided doses until peak expiratory flow is 70% of predicted or personal best (NAEPP 2007)

Asthma, severe persistent, long-term control: Oral: 7.5 to 60 mg/day (or on alternate days) (NAEPP 2007)

Bronchiolitis obliterans syndrome, prevention (off-label use): IV: 1000 mg daily for 3 days. **Note:** Many centers use 10 to 15 mg/kg/day for smaller patients (Meyer 2014).

Cadaveric organ recovery (hormonal resuscitation) (off-label use): IV: 15 mg/kg **or** 2,000 mg bolus administered to the brain-dead donor who is hemodynamically unstable requiring significant vasopressor support; give concomitantly with vasopressin, levothyroxine or liothyronine (preferred), dextrose (if bolus dose insulin used), and regular insulin (bolus dose or continuous infusion). If continuous infusion insulin is employed, maintain blood glucose 120 to 180 mg/dL (Rosendale 2003a; Rosendale 2003b; Rosengard 2002; Salim 2007; Zaroff 2002).

COPD exacerbation (off-label use): Note: Dose, frequency, and duration of therapy not established. GOLD guidelines recommend the use of oral prednisone; however, methylprednisolone may be used as an alternative (GOLD [Decramer 2014]). No comparative studies exist to examine safety and efficacy between low-, medium-, or high-dose regimens. While several clinical trials have examined the use of methylprednisolone in this setting, these trials included low numbers of patients, employed vastly different regimens, and/or

examined different clinical outcomes (Albert 1980; Alía 2011; Niewoehner 1999; Sayiner 2001; Shortall 2002; Vrondracek 2006; Willaert 2002). Current dosing strategies are empiric and have not been established by clinical trials. Based on expert opinion, commonly used regimens ranging from 60 to 125 mg IV administered 1 to 4 times daily followed by oral therapy (eg, prednisone 40 mg once daily) for a total of 5 to 14 days of therapy may be employed; the shorter duration (ie, 5 days) may be preferred (Leuppi 2013); however, comparative prospective data does not exist. IV administration with a higher dose (eg, ≥60 mg) may be preferred for those patients with impending or actual acute respiratory failure; outcome trials not available for this approach.

Dermatitis, acute severe: IM (acetate): 80 to 120 mg as a single dose

Dermatitis, chronic: IM (acetate): 40 to 120 mg every 5 to 10 days

Dermatologic conditions (eg, keloids, lichen planus): Intralesional (acetate): 20 to 60 mg

Dermatomyositis/polymyositis: IV (sodium succinate): 1 g/day for 3 to 5 days for severe muscle weakness, followed by conversion to oral prednisone (Drake 1996)

Gout, acute: IV, IM: Initial: 0.5 to 2 mg/kg; may be repeated as clinically indicated (ACR guidelines [Khanna 2012])

Lupus nephritis: High-dose "pulse" therapy: IV (sodium succinate): 0.5 to 1 g/day for 3 days (Ponticelli 2010)

***Pneumocystis* pneumonia in AIDS patients:** IV: 30 mg twice daily for 5 days, then 30 mg once daily for 5 days, then 15 mg once daily for 11 days

Pediatric Dosing should be based on the lesser of ideal body weight or actual body weight. **Only sodium succinate may be given IV;** methylprednisolone sodium succinate is highly soluble and has a rapid effect by IM and IV routes. Methylprednisolone acetate has a low solubility and has a sustained IM effect.

Acute spinal cord injury (off-label use): IV (sodium succinate): 30 mg/kg over 15 minutes, followed in 45 minutes by a continuous infusion of 5.4 mg/kg/hour for 23 hours. **Note:** Due to insufficient evidence of clinical efficacy (ie, preserving or improving spinal cord function), the routine use of methylprednisolone in the treatment of acute spinal cord injury is no longer recommended. If used in this setting, methylprednisolone should not be initiated >8 hours after the injury; not effective in penetrating trauma (eg, gunshot) (Consortium for Spinal Cord Medicine 2008).

Anti-inflammatory or immunosuppressive: Oral, IM, IV (sodium succinate): 0.5 to 1.7 mg/kg/day **or** 5 to 25 mg/m²/day in divided doses every 6 to 12 hours; "Pulse" therapy: 15 to 30 mg/kg/dose over ≥30 minutes given once daily for 3 days

Asthma exacerbations, including status asthmaticus (emergency medical care or hospital doses) (NAEPP 2007): Children <12 years: Oral, IV: 1 to 2 mg/kg/day in 2 divided doses (maximum: 60 mg/day) until peak expiratory flow is 70% of predicted or personal best

Lupus nephritis: IV (sodium succinate): 30 mg/kg over ≥30 minutes every other day for 6 doses

Renal Impairment There are no dosage adjustments provided in the manufacturer's labeling; use with caution.

Hepatic Impairment There are no dosage adjustments provided in the manufacturer's labeling.

Dietary Considerations Take with meals to decrease GI upset; need diet rich in pyridoxine, vitamin C, vitamin D, folate, calcium, phosphorus, and protein.

Administration
Administer with meals to decrease GI upset.

Parenteral: Methylprednisolone sodium succinate may be administered IM or IV; IV administration may be IVP over one to several minutes or IVPB or continuous IV infusion.

Acetate salt should not be given IV. Avoid injection into the deltoid muscle due to a high incidence of subcutaneous atrophy. Avoid injection or leakage into the dermis; dermal and/or subdermal skin depression may occur at the site of injection.

IV: Succinate:

Low dose: ≤1.8 mg/kg or ≤125 mg/dose: IV push over 3 to 15 minutes

Moderate dose: ≥2 mg/kg or 250 mg/dose: IV over 15 to 30 minutes

High dose: 15 mg/kg or ≥500 mg/dose: IV over ≥30 minutes

Doses >15 mg/kg or ≥1 g: Administer over 1 hour

Do **not** administer high-dose IV push; hypotension, cardiac arrhythmia, and sudden death have been reported in patients given high-dose methylprednisolone IV push (>0.5 g over <10 minutes); intermittent infusion over 15 to 60 minutes; maximum concentration: IV push 125 mg/mL

IM: Avoid injection into the deltoid muscle due to a high incidence of subcutaneous atrophy. Avoid injection or leakage into the dermis; dermal and/or subdermal skin depression may occur at the site of injection. Do not inject into areas that have evidence of acute local infection.

Monitoring Parameters Blood pressure, blood glucose, electrolytes, growth in children

Test Interactions Interferes with skin tests

Additional Information Sodium content of 1 g sodium succinate injection: 2.01 mEq; 53 mg of sodium succinate salt is equivalent to 40 mg of methylprednisolone base

Methylprednisolone acetate: Depo-Medrol

Methylprednisolone sodium succinate: Solu-Medrol

Dosage Forms Excipient information presented when available (limited, particularly for generics); consult specific product labeling. [DSC] = Discontinued product

Solution Reconstituted, Injection, as sodium succinate [strength expressed as base]:

A-Methapred: 40 mg (1 ea); 125 mg (1 ea) [contains benzyl alcohol]

Solu-MEDROL: 500 mg (1 ea); 1000 mg (1 ea)

Solu-MEDROL: 2 g (1 ea) [contains benzyl alcohol]

Generic: 40 mg (1 ea); 125 mg (1 ea); 500 mg (1 ea [DSC]); 1000 mg (1 ea); 1 g (1 ea [DSC])

Solution Reconstituted, Injection, as sodium succinate [strength expressed as base, preservative free]:

Solu-MEDROL: 40 mg (1 ea); 125 mg (1 ea); 500 mg (1 ea); 1000 mg (1 ea)

Suspension, Injection, as acetate:

Depo-Medrol: 20 mg/mL (5 mL); 40 mg/mL (5 mL, 10 mL) [contains benzyl alcohol, polyethylene glycol, polysorbate 80]

Depo-Medrol: 40 mg/mL (1 mL) [contains polyethylene glycol]

Depo-Medrol: 80 mg/mL (1 mL)

Depo-Medrol: 80 mg/mL (5 mL) [contains benzyl alcohol, polyethylene glycol, polysorbate 80]

Depo-Medrol: 80 mg/mL (1 mL) [contains polyethylene glycol]

Generic: 40 mg/mL (1 mL, 5 mL, 10 mL); 80 mg/mL (1 mL, 5 mL)

Suspension, Injection, as acetate [preservative free]:

Generic: 80 mg/mL (1 mL [DSC])

Tablet, Oral:

Medrol: 2 mg, 4 mg, 8 mg, 16 mg, 32 mg [scored]

Medrol (Pak): 4 mg [scored]

Generic: 4 mg, 8 mg, 16 mg, 32 mg

◆ **6-α-Methylprednisolone** *see* MethylPREDNISolone *on page 1184*

◆ **Methylprednisolone Acetate** *see* MethylPREDNISolone *on page 1184*

◆ **Methylprednisolone Sodium Succinate** *see* Methyl-PREDNISolone *on page 1184*

◆ **Methylprednisolone Sodium Succinate For Injection (Can)** *see* MethylPREDNISolone *on page 1184*

◆ **Methylprednisolone Sodium Succinate For Injection USP (Can)** *see* MethylPREDNISolone *on page 1184*

◆ **4-Methylpyrazole** *see* Fomepizole *on page 806*

◆ **Methylrosaniline Chloride** *see* Gentian Violet *on page 840*

Methyl Salicylate and Menthol
(METH il sa LIS i late & MEN thol)

Brand Names: US BenGay [OTC]; Icy Hot [OTC]; Precise [OTC]; Salonpas Arthritis Pain [OTC]; Salonpas Jet Spray [OTC]; Salonpas Massage Foam [OTC]; Salonpas Pain Relief Patch [OTC]; Thera-Gesic Plus [OTC]; Thera-Gesic [OTC]

Index Terms Menthol and Methyl Salicylate

Pharmacologic Category Analgesic, Topical; Salicylate; Topical Skin Product

Use Temporary relief of minor aches and pains of muscle and joints associated with arthritis, bruises, simple backache, sprains, and strains

Dosing

Adult Pain relief: Topical:

Balm, cream, foam, spray, stick: Apply to affected area; may repeat up to 3-4 times/day

Patch:

Methyl salicylate 10% and menthol 1.5%: Apply 1 patch to affected area not more than 3-4 times daily; leave in place for no more than 8 hours

Methyl salicylate 10% and menthol 3%: Apply 1 patch to affected area and leave in place for up to 8-12 hours; do not exceed 1 patch/application. If pain still present, a second patch may be applied for up to 8-12 hours (maximum: 2 patches/24 hours; 3 days of consecutive use)

Pediatric Pain relief: Topical:

Balm, cream, foam, spray, stick: Children ≥12 years: Refer to adult dosing.

Patch: Methyl salicylate 10% and menthol 1.5%: Children ≥12 years: Refer to adult dosing.

Additional Information Complete prescribing information should be consulted for additional detail.

Dosage Forms Excipient information presented when available (limited, particularly for generics); consult specific product labeling.

Aerosol, foam, topical:

Salonpas Massage Foam: Methyl salicylate 10% and menthol 3% (118 mL)

Aerosol, spray, topical:

Salonpas Jet Spray: Methyl salicylate 10% and menthol 3% (118 mL) [contains ethanol]

Balm, topical:

Icy Hot Balm: Methyl salicylate 29% and menthol 7.6% (99.2 g)

Cream, topical:

BenGay Arthritis Formula: Methyl salicylate 30% and menthol 8% (57 g, 113 g)

BenGay Greaseless: Methyl salicylate 15% and menthol 10% (57 g, 113 g)

Icy Hot: Methyl salicylate 30% and menthol 10% (35.4 g, 85 g)

Precise: Methyl salicylate 30% and menthol 10% (75 g)

Thera-Gesic: Methyl salicylate 15% and menthol 1% (85 g, 142 g)

Thera-Gesic Plus: Methyl salicylate 15% and menthol 4% (85 g) [contains aloe]

Patch, topical:

Salonpas Arthritis Pain®: Methyl salicylate 10% and menthol 3% (5s)

Salonpas Pain Relief Patch®: Methyl salicylate 10% and menthol 1.5% (3s)

Salonpas Pain Relief Patch®: Methyl salicylate 10% and menthol 3% (5s)

Stick, topical:

Icy Hot: Methyl salicylate 30% and menthol 10% (49 g)

MethylTESTOSTERone (meth il tes TOS te rone)

Brand Names: US Android; Methitest; Testred

Pharmacologic Category Androgen

Use

Males:

Delayed puberty: To stimulate puberty in carefully selected males with clearly delayed puberty.

Hypogonadotropic hypogonadism (congenital or acquired): Treatment of idiopathic gonadotropin or luteinizing hormone-releasing hormone (LHRH) deficiency, or pituitary hypothalamic injury from tumors, trauma, or radiation.

Primary hypogonadism (congenital or acquired): Treatment of testicular failure caused by cryptorchidism, bilateral torsion, orchitis, vanishing testis syndrome; or orchidectomy.

Females:

Breast cancer, metastatic: Secondarily in women with advancing inoperable (skeletal) mammary cancer who are 1 to 5 years postmenopausal; has also been used in premenopausal women with breast cancer who have benefited from oophorectomy and are considered to have a hormone-responsive tumor.

Dosing

Adult & Geriatric

Breast cancer, metastatic (females): Oral: 50 to 200 mg daily

Delayed puberty (males): Oral: 10 to 50 mg daily; limit treatment duration to 4 to 6 months; use lower range of dosing and individualize dose based on response and tolerability.

Hypogonadotropic hypogonadism (congenital or acquired) and primary hypogonadism (congenital or acquired) (males): Oral: Initial: 10 to 50 mg daily; individualize dose based on response and tolerability.

Pediatric

Delayed puberty: Adolescent males: Oral: Refer to adult dosing.

Hypogonadotropic hypogonadism (congenital or acquired) and primary hypogonadism (congenital or acquired): Adolescent males: Oral: Refer to adult dosing.

Renal Impairment There are no dosage adjustments provided in the manufacturer's labeling. However, patients with renal disease may be at an increased risk of fluid retention.

Hepatic Impairment There are no dosage adjustments provided in the manufacturer's labeling. However, patients with hepatic disease may be at an increased risk of fluid retention.

Additional Information Complete prescribing information should be consulted for additional detail.

Dosage Forms Excipient information presented when available (limited, particularly for generics); consult specific product labeling.

Capsule, Oral:

Android: 10 mg [contains brilliant blue fcf (fd&c blue #1), fd&c red #40]

Testred: 10 mg [contains brilliant blue fcf (fd&c blue #1), fd&c red #40]

Generic: 10 mg

Tablet, Oral:

Methitest: 10 mg [scored]

Controlled Substance C-III

◆ **Methylthionine Chloride** *see* Methylene Blue *on page 1177*

◆ **Methylthioninium Chloride** *see* Methylene Blue *on page 1177*

◆ **3-methyl TTNEB** *see* Bexarotene (Systemic) *on page 229*

Metipranolol (met i PRAN oh lol)

Brand Names: US Optipranolol [DSC]

Index Terms Metipranolol Hydrochloride

Pharmacologic Category Beta-Blocker, Nonselective; Ophthalmic Agent, Antiglaucoma

Use Treatment of chronic open-angle glaucoma or ocular hypertension

Dosing

Adult & Geriatric Glaucoma: Ophthalmic: Instill 1 drop in the affected eye(s) twice daily

Renal Impairment No dosage adjustment provided in manufacturer's labeling. However, dosage adjustment unlikely due to low systemic absorption.

Hepatic Impairment No dosage adjustment provided in manufacturer's labeling. However, dosage adjustment unlikely due to low systemic absorption.

Additional Information Complete prescribing information should be consulted for additional detail.

Dosage Forms Excipient information presented when available (limited, particularly for generics); consult specific product labeling. [DSC] = Discontinued product

Solution, Ophthalmic:

Optipranolol: 0.3% (5 mL [DSC], 10 mL [DSC])

Generic: 0.3% (5 mL, 10 mL)

◆ **Metipranolol Hydrochloride** *see* Metipranolol *on page 1188*

Metoclopramide (met oh KLOE pra mide)

Brand Names: US Metozolv ODT; Reglan

Brand Names: Canada Apo-Metoclop; Metoclopramide Hydrochloride Injection; Metoclopramide Omega; Metonia; Nu-Metoclopramide; PMS-Metoclopramide

Index Terms Reglan

Pharmacologic Category Antiemetic; Gastrointestinal Agent, Prokinetic

Use

US labeling:

Injection:

Diabetic gastroparesis (diabetic gastric stasis): Relief of symptoms associated with acute and recurrent diabetic gastric stasis.

Prevention of nausea and vomiting associated with emetogenic cancer chemotherapy: Prophylaxis of vomiting associated with emetogenic cancer chemotherapy.

Prevention of postoperative nausea and vomiting: Prophylaxis of postoperative nausea and vomiting in circumstances where nasogastric suction is undesirable.

Radiological examination: To stimulate gastric emptying and intestinal transit of barium when delayed emptying interferes with radiological examination of the stomach and/or small intestine.

Small bowel intubation: To facilitate small bowel intubation in adults and pediatrics in whom the tube does not pass the pylorus with conventional maneuvers.

Oral:

Diabetic gastroparesis (diabetic gastric stasis): Relief of symptoms associated with acute and recurrent diabetic gastroparesis (gastric stasis) in adults.

Gastroesophageal reflux: Short-term (4 to 12 weeks) therapy for adults with documented symptomatic gastroesophageal reflux disease (GERD) who fail to respond to conventional therapy.

Limitations of use: Oral metoclopramide is indicated for adults only. Treatment should not exceed 12-week duration.

Canadian labeling:
Injection:

Gastroparesis: Adjunctive therapy in the management of gastroparesis associated with subacute and chronic gastritis and sequelae of surgical procedures (eg, vagotomy, pyloroplasty).

Prevention of vomiting associated with cancer chemotherapy regimens that include cisplatin: Prophylaxis of vomiting associated with cancer chemotherapy regimens that include cisplatin.

Prevention of postoperative nausea and vomiting: Prophylaxis of postoperative nausea and vomiting.

Small bowel intubation: To facilitate small bowel intubation.

Oral:

Gastroparesis: Adjunctive therapy in the management of gastroparesis associated with subacute and chronic gastritis and sequelae of surgical procedures (eg, vagotomy, pyloroplasty).

Prevention of postoperative vomiting: Prophylaxis of postoperative vomiting induced by narcotics.

Radiological examination: To stimulate gastric emptying and intestinal transit of barium when delayed emptying interferes with radiological examination of the stomach and/or small intestine.

Small bowel intubation: To facilitate small bowel intubation.

Limitations of use: Treatment should not exceed 12-week duration.

Pregnancy Considerations Adverse events were not observed in animal reproduction studies. Metoclopramide crosses the placenta and can be detected in cord blood and amniotic fluid (Arvela, 1983; Bylsma-Howell, 1983). Available evidence suggests safe use during pregnancy (Berkovitch, 2002; Matok, 2009; Sørensen, 2000). Metoclopramide may be used for the treatment of nausea and vomiting of pregnancy (ACOG, 2004; Levichek, 2002) and prophylaxis for nausea and vomiting associated with cesarean delivery (ASA, 2007; Mahadevan, 2006; Smith, 2011). Other agents are preferred for gastroesophageal reflux (Mahadevan, 2006).

Breast-Feeding Considerations Metoclopramide is excreted in breast milk. Information is available from studies conducted in mothers nursing preterm infants (n=14; delivered at 23-34 weeks gestation) or term infants (n=18) and taking metoclopramide 10 mg 3 times daily. The median concentration of metoclopramide in breast milk was ~45 ng/mL in the preterm infants and the mean concentration was ~48 ng/mL in the full term infants. The authors of both studies calculated the relative infant dose to be 3% to 5%, based on a therapeutic infant dose of 0.5 mg/kg/day. Metoclopramide was also detected in the serum of one nursing full term infant (Hansen, 2005; Kauppila, 1983). Metoclopramide may increase prolactin concentrations and cause galactorrhea and gynecomastia, but studies which evaluated its use to increase milk production for women who want to nurse have had mixed results. In addition, due to the potential for adverse events, nonpharmacologic measure should be considered prior to the use of medications as galactagogues (ABM, 2011). The manufacturer recommends that caution be used if administered to a nursing woman.

Medication Guide Available Yes

Contraindications Known sensitivity or intolerance to metoclopramide or any component of the formulation; situations where gastrointestinal (GI) motility may be dangerous, including mechanical GI obstruction, perforation, or hemorrhage; pheochromocytoma; history of seizure disorder (eg, epilepsy), concomitant use with other agents likely to increase extrapyramidal reactions

Canadian labeling: Additional contraindications (not in US labeling): Infants <1 year of age.

Warnings/Precautions [US Boxed Warning]: May cause tardive dyskinesia, a serious movement disorder which is often irreversible; the risk of developing tardive dyskinesia increases with duration of treatment and total cumulative dose. Discontinue metoclopramide in patients who develop signs/symptoms of tardive dyskinesia. There is no known treatment for tardive dyskinesia. In some patients, symptoms lessen or resolve after metoclopramide treatment is stopped. Avoid metoclopramide treatment longer than 12 weeks in all but rare cases in which therapeutic benefit is thought to outweigh the risk of developing tardive dyskinesia. Tardive dyskinesia is characterized by involuntary movements of the face, tongue, or extremities and may be disfiguring. An analysis of utilization patterns showed that ~20% of patients who used metoclopramide took it for longer than 12 weeks. Metoclopramide may mask underlying tardive disease by suppressing or partially suppressing tardive dyskinesia signs (metoclopramide should not be used to control tardive dyskinesia symptoms as the long-term course is unknown). The risk for tardive dyskinesia appears to be increased in the elderly, women, and diabetics, although it is not possible to predict which patients will develop tardive dyskinesia. There is no known effective treatment for established cases of tardive dyskinesia, although in some patients, tardive dyskinesia may remit (partially or completely) within several weeks to months after metoclopramide is withdrawn.

May cause extrapyramidal symptoms (EPS), generally manifested as acute dystonic reactions within the initial 24 to 48 hours of use at the usual adult dose (30 to 40 mg/day). Risk of these reactions is increased at higher doses, and in pediatric patients and adults <30 years of age. Symptoms may include involuntary limb movements, facial grimacing, torticollis, oculogyric crisis, rhythmic tongue protrusion, bulbar type speech, trismus, or dystonic reactions resembling tetanus. May also rarely present as stridor and dyspnea (may be due to laryngospasm). Dystonic symptoms may be managed with IM diphenhydramine or benztropine. Pseudoparkinsonism (eg, bradykinesia, tremor, rigidity, mask-like facies) may also occur (usually within first 6 months of therapy) and is generally reversible within 2 to 3 months following discontinuation. Symptoms of Parkinson disease may be exacerbated by metoclopramide; use with extreme caution (or avoid use) in patients with Parkinson disease.

Metoclopramide has been known to cause sinus arrest (usually with rapid IV administration or higher doses) (Bentsen, 2002; Malkoff 1995). The torsadogenic potential for metoclopramide is considered to be low (Claassen, 2005). Based on case reports, however, metoclopramide may cause QT prolongation and torsades de pointes in certain individuals (eg, heart failure patients with renal impairment); use with caution in these patients (Siddiquie, 2009). There is data in healthy male volunteers to show that metoclopramide actually shortens the QT interval while at the same time increasing QT variance (Ellidokuz, 2003). No human data other than case reports; however, has demonstrated a consistent QT prolonging effect with metoclopramide nor is there any substantiated evidence to show a direct association with the development of torsades de pointes.

Metoclopramide use may be associated (rarely) with neuroleptic malignant syndrome (NMS); may be fatal. Monitor for manifestations of NMS, which include hyperthermia, muscle rigidity, altered consciousness, and autonomic instability (irregular pulse or blood pressure, tachycardia, diaphoresis, and cardiac arrhythmias). Discontinue immediately if signs/symptoms of NMS appear and begin intensive symptomatic management and monitoring. Bromocriptine and dantrolene have been used to manage NMS, although effectiveness have not been established.

Mental depression has occurred (in patients with and without a history of depression), and symptoms range from mild to severe (suicidal ideation and suicide); use in patients with a history of depression only if anticipated benefits outweigh potential risks.

In a study in hypertensive patients, IV metoclopramide was associated with catecholamine release. Use with caution in patients with hypertension. There are reports of hypertensive crises in some patients with undiagnosed pheochromocytoma. Immediately discontinue with any rapid rise in blood pressure that is associated with metoclopramide. Hypertensive crises may be managed with phentolamine. Use with caution in patients who are at risk of fluid overload (HF, cirrhosis); metoclopramide causes a transient increase in serum aldosterone and increases the risk for fluid retention/overload; discontinue if adverse events or signs/symptoms appear.

Patients with NADH-cytochrome b5 reductase deficiency are at increased risk of methemoglobinemia and/or sulfhemoglobinemia. Use with caution in patients with renal impairment; dosage adjustment may be needed. Use with caution following surgical anastomosis/closure; promotility agents may theoretically increase pressure in suture lines.

For patients with diabetic gastroparesis, the usual manifestations of delayed gastric emptying (eg, nausea, vomiting, heartburn, persistent fullness after meals, anorexia) appear to respond to metoclopramide within different time intervals. Significant relief of nausea occurs early and continues to improve over a 3-week period; relief of vomiting and anorexia may precede the relief of abdominal fullness by a week or more. If gastroesophageal reflux symptoms are confined to particular situations, such as following the evening meal, consider use of metoclopramide as a single dose prior to the provocative situation, ▶

◄ rather than using the drug throughout the day. Symptoms of postprandial and daytime heartburn respond better to metoclopramide, with less observed effect on nocturnal symptoms. Because there is no documented correlation between symptoms and healing of esophageal lesions, patients with documented lesions should be monitored endoscopically. Healing of esophageal ulcers and erosions has been endoscopically demonstrated at the end of a 12-week trial using a dosage of 15 mg 4 times daily.

Avoid use in older adults (except for diabetic gastroparesis) due to risk of extrapyramidal effects, including tardive dyskinesia; risk is potentially even greater in frail older adults (Beers Criteria). In addition, risk of tardive dyskinesia may be increased in older women. EPS are increased in pediatric patients. In neonates, prolonged clearance of metoclopramide may lead to increased serum concentrations. Neonates may also have decreased levels of NADH-cytochrome b5 reductase which increases the risk of methemoglobinemia. The Canadian labeling contraindicates use in infants <1 year of age and recommends avoiding use in children >1 year unless clearly necessary. Potentially significant drug-drug interactions may exist, requiring dose or frequency adjustment, additional monitoring, and/or selection of alternative therapy. CNS effects may be potentiated when used with other sedative drugs or ethanol. Abrupt discontinuation may (rarely) result in withdrawal symptoms (dizziness, headache, nervousness).

Benzyl alcohol and derivatives: Some dosage forms may contain sodium benzoate/benzoic acid; benzoic acid (benzoate) is a metabolite of benzyl alcohol; large amounts of benzyl alcohol (≥99 mg/kg/day) have been associated with a potentially fatal toxicity ("gasping syndrome") in neonates; the "gasping syndrome" consists of metabolic acidosis, respiratory distress, gasping respirations, CNS dysfunction (including convulsions, intracranial hemorrhage), hypotension, and cardiovascular collapse (AAP ["Inactive" 1997]; CDC, 1982); some data suggest that benzoate displaces bilirubin from protein binding sites (Ahlfors, 2001); avoid or use dosage forms containing benzyl alcohol derivative with caution in neonates. See manufacturer's labeling.

Adverse Reactions Frequency not always defined.

Cardiovascular: Atrioventricular block, bradycardia, congestive heart failure, flushing (following high IV doses), hypertension, hypotension, supraventricular tachycardia

Central nervous system: Drowsiness (~10% to 70%; dose related), dystonic reaction (<1% to 25%; dose and age related), lassitude (~10%), restlessness (~10%), fatigue (2% to 10%), headache (4% to 5%), dizziness (1% to 4%), somnolence (2% to 3%), akathisia, confusion, depression, drug-induced Parkinson's disease, hallucination (rare), insomnia, neuroleptic malignant syndrome (rare), seizure, suicidal ideation, tardive dyskinesia

Dermatologic: Skin rash, urticaria

Endocrine & metabolic: Amenorrhea, fluid retention, galactorrhea, gynecomastia, hyperprolactinemia, porphyria

Gastrointestinal: Nausea (4% to 6%), vomiting (1% to 2%), diarrhea

Genitourinary: Impotence, urinary frequency, urinary incontinence

Hematologic & oncologic: Agranulocytosis, leukopenia, methemoglobinemia, neutropenia, sulfhemoglobinemia

Hepatic: Hepatotoxicity (rare)

Hypersensitivity: Angioedema (rare), hypersensitivity reaction

Neuromuscular & skeletal: Laryngospasm (rare)

Ophthalmic: Visual disturbance

Respiratory: Bronchospasm, laryngeal edema (rare)

Drug Interactions

Metabolism/Transport Effects Substrate of CYP1A2 (minor), CYP2D6 (minor); **Note:** Assignment of Major/Minor substrate status based on clinically relevant drug interaction potential; **Inhibits** CYP2D6 (weak)

Avoid Concomitant Use

Avoid concomitant use of Metoclopramide with any of the following: Antipsychotic Agents; Droperidol; Promethazine; Rivastigmine; Tetrabenazine; Trimetazidine

Increased Effect/Toxicity

Metoclopramide may increase the levels/effects of: Antipsychotic Agents; CycloSPORINE (Systemic); Highest Risk QTc-Prolonging Agents; Levosulpiride; Moderate Risk QTc-Prolonging Agents; Prilocaine; Promethazine; Selective Serotonin Reuptake Inhibitors; Serotonin/Norepinephrine Reuptake Inhibitors; Sodium Nitrite; Tetrabenazine; Tricyclic Antidepressants; Trimetazidine

The levels/effects of Metoclopramide may be increased by: Dapsone (Topical); Droperidol; Metyrosine; Mifepristone; Nitric Oxide; Rivastigmine; Serotonin Modulators

Decreased Effect

Metoclopramide may decrease the levels/effects of: Anti-Parkinson's Agents (Dopamine Agonist); Atovaquone; Posaconazole; Quinagolide

The levels/effects of Metoclopramide may be decreased by: Anticholinergic Agents

Preparation for Administration Injection: Lower doses (≤10 mg): No dilution required; Higher doses (>10 mg): Dilute in 50 mL of compatible solution (preferably NS).

Storage/Stability

Injection: Store intact vials at 20°C to 25°C (68°F to 77°F); injection is photosensitive and should be protected from light during storage; parenteral admixtures in D_5W, $D_5\frac{1}{2}NS$, NS, LR, or Ringer's injection are stable for up to 24 hours after preparation at normal light conditions or up to 48 hours if protected from light. When mixed with NS, can be stored frozen for up to 4 weeks; metoclopramide is degraded when admixed and frozen with D_5W.

Oral solution: Store at 20°C to 25°C (68°F to 77°F). Do not freeze. Dispense in tight, light-resistant container.

Tablet: Store at 20°C to 25°C (68°F to 77°F). Dispense in tight, light-resistant container.

Tablet, orally disintegrating: Store at 20°C to 25°C (68°F to 77°F). Keep in original packaging until just prior to use.

Mechanism of Action Blocks dopamine receptors and (when given in higher doses) also blocks serotonin receptors in chemoreceptor trigger zone of the CNS; enhances the response to acetylcholine of tissue in upper GI tract causing enhanced motility and accelerated gastric emptying without stimulating gastric, biliary, or pancreatic secretions; increases lower esophageal sphincter tone

Pharmacodynamics/Kinetics

Onset of action: Oral: 30 to 60 minutes; IV: 1 to 3 minutes; IM: 10 to 15 minutes

Duration: Therapeutic: 1 to 2 hours, regardless of route

Absorption: Oral: Rapid, well absorbed

Distribution: V_d: ~3.5 L/kg

Protein binding: ~30%

Bioavailability: Oral: Range: 65% to 95%

Half-life elimination: Normal renal function: Pediatric: ~4 hours; Adults: 5 to 6 hours (may be dose dependent)

Time to peak, serum: Oral: 1 to 2 hours

Excretion: Urine (~85%)

Dosing

Adult

US labeling:

Diabetic gastroparesis:

Oral: 10 mg up to 4 times daily 30 minutes before meals or food and at bedtime for 2 to 8 weeks. Treatment >12 weeks is not recommended.

IM, IV (for severe symptoms): 10 mg over 1 to 2 minutes; 10 days of IV therapy may be necessary before symptoms are controlled to allow transition to oral administration.

Gastroparesis management, regardless of etiology (off-label use): American College of Gastroenterology Guidelines: Oral: Initial: 5 mg 3 times daily before meals. Dosage range: 5 to 10 mg 2 to 3 times daily before meals (maximum: 40 mg daily). Liquid formulation is preferred (to increase absorption) and the use of drug holidays or dose reductions (eg, 5 mg before the two main meals of the day) is also recommended when clinically possible (Camilleri, 2013).

Gastroesophageal reflux: Oral: 10 to 15 mg up to 4 times daily 30 minutes before meals and at bedtime; alternatively, single doses of up to 20 mg (rather than continuous treatment) may be administered prior to provoking situation if symptoms are intermittent. Treatment >12 weeks is not recommended.

Prevention of nausea and vomiting associated with emetogenic chemotherapy: IV: **Note:** Pretreatment with diphenhydramine will decrease risk of extrapyramidal reactions.

Highly emetogenic: Initial dose: 2 mg/kg over 15 minutes 30 minutes before chemotherapy; repeat every 2 hours for 2 doses, then every 3 hours for 3 doses

Less emetogenic: Initial dose: 1 mg/kg over 15 minutes 30 minutes before chemotherapy; repeat every 2 hours for 2 doses, then every 3 hours for 3 doses

Delayed-emesis prophylaxis (off-label): Oral: 20 to 40 mg (or 0.5 mg/kg/dose) 2 to 4 times daily for 3 to 4 days in combination with dexamethasone (ASCO guidelines (Kris, 2006])

Refractory or intolerant to antiemetics with a higher therapeutic index (off-label; Hesketh, 2008):

IV: 1 to 2 mg/kg/dose before chemotherapy and repeat 2 hours after chemotherapy

Oral: 0.5 mg/kg every 6 hours on days 2 to 4

Prevention of postoperative nausea and vomiting: IM, IV (off-label route): Usual dose: 10 mg near end of surgery; some patients may require 20 mg. **Note:** Guidelines discourage use of 10 mg metoclopramide due to lack of effectiveness (Gan, 2007); comparative study indicates higher dose (20 mg) may be efficacious (Quaynor, 2002).

Radiological exam: IV: 10 mg as a single dose

Small bowel intubation (postpyloric feeding tube placement): IV: 10 mg as a single dose

Prevention of radiation therapy-induced nausea and vomiting (minimal emetic risk) (off-label use): Oral: 20 mg as rescue therapy; if rescue therapy is used, then administer prior to each fraction until the end of radiation therapy (Basch, 2011).

Canadian labeling:

Gastroparesis management (adjunctive therapy): Note: Total daily dose should not exceed 0.5 mg/kg.
IM, IV: 10 mg 2 to 3 times daily as needed by IM injection or by slow IV injection
Oral: 5 to 10 mg 3 to 4 times daily before meals based on response and weight

Prevention of vomiting associated with cancer chemotherapy regimens that include cisplatin: IV:
Cisplatin dose ≤100 mg/m^2: Metoclopramide 1 mg/kg over 15 minutes every 2 hours for 2 doses, then every 3 hours for 3 doses
Cisplatin dose >100 mg/m^2: Metoclopramide 2 mg/kg over 15 minutes every 2 hours for 2 doses, then every 3 hours for 2 doses

Prevention of postoperative vomiting: Note: Total daily dose should not exceed 0.5 mg/kg.
IM: 10 mg prior to end of surgical procedure and then every 4 to 6 hours as needed; dose may be increased to 20 mg for high-risk groups (eg, general anesthesia ≥2 hours, abdominal or pelvic surgery with visceral manipulation, absence of gastric suction)
Oral: 20 mg 2 hours prior to anesthesia

Radiological exam: Oral: 20 mg 5 to 10 minutes prior to barium swallow (total daily dose should not exceed 0.5 mg/kg)

Small bowel intubation (postpyloric feeding tube placement):
IV: 10 mg as a single dose by slow injection
Oral: 10 mg as single dose; may not be preferred route due to delayed onset of action when compared to IV route

Geriatric Initial: Dose at the lower end of the recommended range (may require only 5 mg/dose) and use the lowest effective dose. Refer to adult dosing.

Pediatric

US labeling: Children and Adolescents:

Small bowel intubation (postpyloric feeding tube placement): IV:
<6 years: 0.1 mg/kg as a single dose
6 to 14 years: 2.5 to 5 mg as a single dose
>14 years: Refer to adult dosing.

Canadian labeling: Children and Adolescents: **Note:** Total daily dose should not exceed 0.5 mg/kg.

Gastroparesis: Oral:
5 to 14 years: 2.5 mg to 5 mg 3 times daily before meals (based on body weight and response)
>14 years: Refer to adult dosing.

Small bowel intubation: IV:
5 to 14 years: 0.1 mg/kg as single dose by slow IV injection
>14 years: Refer to adult dosing.

Prevention of chemotherapy-associated nausea and vomiting (off-label use): IV: Moderately emetogenic chemotherapy (patients who cannot receive corticosteroids): IV: 1 mg/kg prior to chemotherapy, followed by Oral: 0.0375 mg/kg every 6 hours; regimen also includes ondansetron or granisetron; coadministration of diphenhydramine or benztropine is recommended to prevent metoclopramide-induced adverse effects (Dupuis, 2013).

Renal Impairment
CrCl <40 mL/minute: Administer 50% of normal dose.
Not dialyzable (0% to 5%); supplemental dose is not necessary (Aronoff, 2007).

Hepatic Impairment There are no dosage adjustments provided in the manufacturer's labeling. However, metoclopramide has been used safely in patients with advanced liver disease with normal renal function.

Administration
Injection: May be given IM, direct IV push, short infusion (at least 15 minutes), or continuous infusion; lower doses (≤10 mg) of metoclopramide can be given IV push undiluted over 1 to 2 minutes; higher doses (>10 mg) to be diluted in 50 mL of compatible solution (preferably NS) and given IVPB over at least 15 minutes. **Note:** Rapid IV

administration may be associated with a transient (but intense) feeling of anxiety and restlessness, followed by drowsiness.

Tablets: When used for gastroparesis/reflux, administer 30 minutes prior to meals and at bedtime.

Orally disintegrating tablets: When used for gastroparesis/reflux, administer on an empty stomach at least 30 minutes prior to food and at bedtime (do not repeat if inadvertently taken with food). Do not remove from packaging until time of administration. If tablet breaks or crumbles while handling, discard and remove new tablet. Using dry hands, place tablet on tongue and allow to dissolve (disintegrates within ~1 minute [range: 10 seconds to 14 minutes]). Swallow with saliva.

Oral solution: When used for gastroparesis/reflux, administer 30 minutes prior to meals and at bedtime.

Monitoring Parameters Signs of tardive dyskinesias, extrapyramidal symptoms; signs/symptoms of neuroleptic malignant syndrome

Dosage Forms Excipient information presented when available (limited, particularly for generics); consult specific product labeling. [DSC] = Discontinued product
Solution, Injection:
Generic: 5 mg/mL (2 mL)
Solution, Injection [preservative free]:
Generic: 5 mg/mL (2 mL)
Solution, Oral:
Generic: 5 mg/5 mL (10 mL, 473 mL); 10 mg/10 mL (10 mL)
Tablet, Oral:
Reglan: 5 mg [contains fd&c blue #1 aluminum lake, fd&c yellow #10 aluminum lake]
Reglan: 10 mg [dye free]
Generic: 5 mg, 10 mg
Tablet Dispersible, Oral:
Metozolv ODT: 5 mg, 10 mg [DSC]
Generic: 5 mg, 10 mg

◆ **Metoclopramide Hydrochloride Injection (Can)** *see* Metoclopramide *on page 1188*

◆ **Metoclopramide Omega (Can)** *see* Metoclopramide *on page 1188*

◆ **Metoject (Can)** *see* Methotrexate *on page 1169*

Metolazone (me TOLE a zone)

Brand Names: US Zaroxolyn [DSC]
Brand Names: Canada Zaroxolyn
Index Terms Zaroxolyn
Pharmacologic Category Diuretic, Thiazide-Related
Use

Edema: Treatment of edema in congestive heart failure and edema accompanying renal diseases, including the nephrotic syndrome and states of diminished renal function.

Hypertension: Treatment of hypertension.

Guideline recommendations:

Coronary artery disease (CAD) and hypertension: The American Heart Association, American College of Cardiology and American Society of Hypertension (AHA/ACC/ASH) 2015 scientific statement for the treatment of hypertension in patients with coronary artery disease (CAD) recommends the use of a thiazide (or thiazide-like diuretic) as part of a regimen in patients with hypertension and chronic stable angina. A BP target of <140/90 mm Hg is reasonable for the secondary prevention of cardiovascular events. A lower target BP (<130/80 mm Hg) may be appropriate in some individuals with CAD, previous MI, stroke or transient ischemic attack, or CAD risk equivalents (AHA/ACC/ASH [Rosendorff 2015]).

Pregnancy Considerations Adverse events have not been observed in animal reproduction studies. Metolazone crosses the placenta and appears in cord blood. Hypoglycemia, hypokalemia, hyponatremia, jaundice, and thrombocytopenia are reported as complications to the fetus or newborn following maternal use of thiazide diuretics.

Breast-Feeding Considerations Metolazone is excreted in breast milk. Due to the potential for serious adverse reactions in the nursing infant, the manufacturer recommends a decision be made whether to discontinue nursing or to discontinue the drug, taking into account the importance of treatment to the mother.

Contraindications
Hypersensitivity to metolazone or any component of the formulation; anuria; hepatic coma or precoma.
Documentation of allergic cross-reactivity for diuretics is limited. However, because of similarities in chemical structure and/or pharmacologic actions, the possibility of cross-sensitivity cannot be ruled out with certainty.

Warnings/Precautions Severe hypokalemia and/or hypo-natremia can occur rapidly following initial doses. Hypercalcemia, hypochloremic alkalosis, and/or hypomagnesemia can also occur. Correct hypokalemia before initiating therapy. Sensitivity reactions, including angioedema and bronchospasm, may occur. Orthostatic hypotension may also occur. Ethanol may potentiate orthostatic hypotensive effect of metolazone. Instruct patients to avoid ethanol during therapy. If taken concurrently, monitor for hypotensive effects. Use with caution in severe hepatic dysfunction. Hyperuricemia can occur and gout can be precipitated. Cautious use in patients with prediabetes or diabetes; may see a change in glucose control. Can cause SLE exacerbation or activation. Azotemia and oliguria may occur. Use caution in severe renal impairment. If azotemia and oliguria worsen during treatment in these patients, discontinue therapy. Photosensitization may occur. If given the morning of surgery, metolazone may render the patient volume depleted and blood pressure may be labile during general anesthesia.

Potentially significant drug-drug interactions may exist, requiring dose or frequency adjustment, additional monitoring, and/or selection of alternative therapy. Do not interchange Zaroxolyn with other formulations of metolazone that are not therapeutically equivalent at the same doses (eg, Mykrox, no longer available in the US).

Sulfonamide ("sulfa") allergy: The FDA-approved product labeling for many medications containing a sulfonamide chemical group includes a broad contraindication in patients with a prior allergic reaction to sulfonamides. There is a potential for cross-reactivity between members of a specific class (eg, two antibiotic sulfonamides). However, concerns for cross-reactivity have previously extended to all compounds containing the sulfonamide structure (SO_2NH_2). An expanded understanding of allergic mechanisms indicates cross-reactivity between antibiotic sulfonamides and nonantibiotic sulfonamides may not occur or at the very least this potential is extremely low (Brackett 2004; Johnson 2005; Slatore 2004; Tornero 2004). In particular, mechanisms of cross-reaction due to antibody production (anaphylaxis) are unlikely to occur with nonantibiotic sulfonamides. T-cell-mediated (type IV) reactions (eg, maculopapular rash) are less well understood and it is not possible to completely exclude this potential based on current insights. In cases where prior reactions were severe (Stevens-Johnson syndrome/TEN), some clinicians choose to avoid exposure to these classes.

Adverse Reactions Frequency not defined.

Cardiovascular: Chest pain/discomfort, necrotizing angiitis, orthostatic hypotension, palpitation, syncope, venous thrombosis, vertigo, volume depletion

Central nervous system: Chills, depression, dizziness, drowsiness, fatigue, headache, lightheadedness, restlessness

Dermatologic: Petechiae, photosensitivity, pruritus, purpura, rash, skin necrosis, Stevens-Johnson syndrome, toxic epidermal necrolysis, urticaria

Endocrine & metabolic: Gout attacks, hypercalcemia, hyperglycemia, hyperuricemia, hypochloremia, hypochloremic alkalosis, hypokalemia, hypomagnesemia, hyponatremia, hypophosphatemia

Gastrointestinal: Abdominal bloating, abdominal pain, anorexia, constipation, diarrhea, epigastric distress, nausea, pancreatitis, vomiting, xerostomia

Genitourinary: Impotence

Hematologic: Agranulocytosis, aplastic/hypoplastic anemia, hemoconcentration, leukopenia, thrombocytopenia

Hepatic: Cholestatic jaundice, hepatitis

Neuromuscular & skeletal: Joint pain, muscle cramps/spasm, neuropathy, paresthesia, weakness

Ocular: Blurred vision (transient)

Renal: BUN increased, glucosuria

Drug Interactions

Metabolism/Transport Effects None known.

Avoid Concomitant Use

Avoid concomitant use of Metolazone with any of the following: Dofetilide; Levosulpiride; Mecamylamine

Increased Effect/Toxicity

Metolazone may increase the levels/effects of: ACE Inhibitors; Allopurinol; Amifostine; Antipsychotic Agents (Second Generation [Atypical]); Calcium Salts; CarBAMazepine; Cardiac Glycosides; Cyclophosphamide; Diazoxide; Dofetilide; DULoxetine; Hypotension-Associated Agents; Ivabradine; Levodopa; Levosulpiride; Lithium; Mecamylamine; Multivitamins/Minerals (with ADEK, Folate, Iron); Multivitamins/Minerals (with AE, No Iron); Nonsteroidal Anti-Inflammatory Agents; OXcarbazepine; Porfimer; Sodium Phosphates; Topiramate; Toremifene; Verteporfin; Vitamin D Analogs

The levels/effects of Metolazone may be increased by: Alcohol (Ethyl); Alfuzosin; Analgesics (Opioid); Anticholinergic Agents; Barbiturates; Beta2-Agonists; Brimonidine (Topical); Corticosteroids (Orally Inhaled); Corticosteroids (Systemic); Dexketoprofen; Diazoxide; Herbs (Hypotensive Properties); Licorice; Molsidomine; Multivitamins/Fluoride (with ADE); Nicorandil; Obinutuzumab; Pentoxifylline; Phosphodiesterase 5 Inhibitors; Prostacyclin Analogues; Selective Serotonin Reuptake Inhibitors

Decreased Effect

Metolazone may decrease the levels/effects of: Antidiabetic Agents

The levels/effects of Metolazone may be decreased by: Amphetamines; Bile Acid Sequestrants; Herbs (Hypertensive Properties); Methylphenidate; Nonsteroidal Anti-Inflammatory Agents; Yohimbine

Storage/Stability Store at 25°C (77°F); excursions are permitted between 15°C and 30°C (59°F and 86°F). Protect from light.

Mechanism of Action Inhibits sodium reabsorption in the distal tubules causing increased excretion of sodium and water, as well as, potassium and hydrogen ions

Pharmacodynamics/Kinetics

Onset of action: Diuresis: ~60 minutes

Duration: ≥24 hours

Absorption: Incomplete

Distribution: Crosses placenta; enters breast milk

Protein binding: 90% to 95%

Time to peak, serum: ~8 hours

Excretion: Urine (unchanged)

Dosing

Adult & Geriatric

Edema (renal disease): Oral: Initial: 5-20 mg once daily.

Edema (heart failure) (off-label dose): Oral: Initial: 2.5 mg once daily; maximum daily dose: 20 mg (ACCF/AHA [Yancy, 2013]); Note: Dosing frequency may be adjusted based on patient-specific diuretic needs (eg, administration every other day or weekly) (HFSA [Lindenfeld, 2010]).

Hypertension: Oral: Initial: 2.5-5 mg once daily; adjust dose as necessary to achieve maximum therapeutic effect.

Renal Impairment There are no dosage adjustments provided in the manufacturer's labeling; use caution in patients with severe renal impairment, as most of the drug is excreted by the renal route and accumulation may occur.

Hepatic Impairment There are no dosage adjustments provided in manufacturer's labeling; contraindicated in hepatic coma or precoma.

Dietary Considerations May require potassium supplementation

Administration Administer orally as a single daily dose with or without food. Take early in day to avoid nocturia.

Monitoring Parameters Serum electrolytes, uric acid, fluid balance, renal function, blood pressure (standing, sitting/supine)

Additional Information Metolazone 5 mg is approximately equivalent to hydrochlorothiazide 50 mg.

Dosage Forms Excipient information presented when available (limited, particularly for generics); consult specific product labeling. [DSC] = Discontinued product

Tablet, Oral:

Zaroxolyn: 2.5 mg [DSC], 5 mg [DSC]

Generic: 2.5 mg, 5 mg, 10 mg

Extemporaneous Preparations A 1 mg/mL oral suspension may be made by with tablets and one of three different vehicles (cherry syrup diluted 1:4 with simple syrup; a 1:1 mixture of Ora-Sweet and Ora-Plus; or a 1:1 mixture of Ora-Sweet SF and Ora-Plus). Crush twelve 10 mg tablets in a mortar and reduce to a fine powder. Add small portions of the chosen vehicle and mix to a uniform paste; mix while adding the vehicle in incremental proportions to **almost** 120 mL; transfer to a calibrated bottle, rinse mortar with vehicle, and add quantity of vehicle sufficient to make 120 mL. Label "shake well" and "refrigerate". Stable for 60 days.

A 0.25 mg/mL oral suspension may be made with tablets and a 1:1 mixture of methylcellulose 1% and simple syrup. Crush one 2.5 mg tablet in a mortar and reduce to a fine powder. Add small portions of the vehicle and mix to a uniform paste; mix while adding the vehicle in incremental proportions to **almost** 10 mL; transfer to a calibrated bottle, rinse mortar with vehicle, and add quantity of vehicle sufficient to make 10 mL. Label "shake well" and "refrigerate". Stable for 91 days refrigerated (preferred), 28 days at room temperature in plastic, and 14 days at room temperature in glass.

Nahata, MC, Pai VB, and Hipple TF, *Pediatric Drug Formulations*, 5th ed, Cincinnati, OH: Harvey Whitney Books Co, 2004.

◆ Metonia (Can) *see* Metoclopramide *on page 1188*

Metoprolol (me toe PROE lole)

Brand Names: US Lopressor; Toprol XL
Brand Names: Canada Apo-Metoprolol; Apo-Metoprolol (Type L); Apo-Metoprolol SR; Ava-Metoprolol; Ava-Metoprolol (Type L); Betaloc; Dom-Metoprolol-B; Dom-Metoprolol-L; JAMP-Metoprolol-L; Lopresor; Lopresor SR; Metoprolol Tartrate Injection, USP; Metoprolol-25; Metoprolol-L; Mylan-Metoprolol (Type L); Nu-Metop; PMS-Metoprolol-B; PMS-Metoprolol-L; Riva-Metoprolol-L; Sandoz-Metoprolol (Type L); Sandoz-Metoprolol SR; Teva-Metoprolol
Index Terms Metoprolol Succinate; Metoprolol Tartrate
Pharmacologic Category Antianginal Agent; Antihypertensive; Beta-Blocker, Beta-1 Selective
Use
Immediate-release tablets (metoprolol tartrate): Treatment of angina pectoris, hypertension, or hemodynamically-stable acute myocardial infarction
Extended-release tablets (metoprolol succinate): Treatment of angina pectoris or hypertension; to reduce mortality/hospitalization in patients with heart failure (HF) (stable NYHA Class II or III) already receiving ACE inhibitors, diuretics, and/or digoxin
Injectable (metoprolol tartrate): Treatment of hemodynamically-stable acute myocardial infarction when used in conjunction with metoprolol oral maintenance therapy

Guideline recommendations:
Acute coronary syndromes (eg, myocardial infarction, unstable angina): According to the ACCF/AHA 2013 guidelines for the management of ST-elevation myocardial infarction (STEMI) and the guidelines for the management of unstable angina/non-STEMI, oral beta-blockers should be initiated within the first 24 hours unless the patient has signs of heart failure, evidence of a low-output state, an increased risk for cardiogenic shock, or other contraindications. Intravenous use should be reserved for those patients who have refractory hypertension or ongoing ischemia (ACCF/AHA [Anderson 2013]; ACCF/AHA [O'Gara 2013]).
Heart failure: The ACCF/AHA 2013 heart failure guidelines recommend the use of 1 of 3 beta blockers (ie, bisoprolol, carvedilol, or extended-release metoprolol succinate) for all patients with recent or remote history of MI or ACS and reduced ejection fraction (rEF) to reduce mortality, for all patients with rEF to prevent symptomatic HF (even if no history of MI), and for all patients with current or prior symptoms of HF with reduced ejection fraction (HFrEF), unless contraindicated, to reduce morbidity and mortality (ACCF/AHA [Yancy 2013]).
Hypertension: The 2014 guideline for the management of high blood pressure in adults (Eighth Joint National Committee [JNC 8]) recommends initiation of pharmacologic treatment to lower blood pressure for the following patients (JNC8 [James 2013]):
• Patients ≥60 years of age, with systolic blood pressure (SBP) ≥150 mm Hg or diastolic blood pressure (DBP) ≥90 mm Hg. Goal of therapy is SBP <150 mm Hg and DBP <90 mm Hg.
• Patients <60 years of age, with SBP ≥140 mm Hg or DBP ≥90 mm Hg. Goal of therapy is SBP <140 mm Hg and DBP <90 mm Hg.
• Patients ≥18 years of age with diabetes, with SBP ≥140 mm Hg or DBP ≥90 mm Hg. Goal of therapy is SBP <140 mm Hg and DBP <90 mm Hg.
• Patients ≥18 years of age with chronic kidney disease (CKD), with SBP ≥140 mm Hg or DBP ≥90 mm Hg. Goal of therapy is SBP <140 mm Hg and DBP <90 mm Hg.
Chronic kidney disease (CKD) and hypertension: Regardless of race or diabetes status, the use of an ACE inhibitor (ACEI) or angiotensin receptor blocker (ARB) as initial therapy is recommended to improve kidney outcomes. In the general nonblack population (without CKD) including those with diabetes, initial antihypertensive treatment should consist of a thiazide-type diuretic, calcium channel blocker, ACEI, or ARB. In the general black population (without CKD) including those with diabetes, initial antihypertensive treatment should consist of a thiazide-type diuretic or a calcium channel blocker **instead of** an ACEI or ARB.
Coronary artery disease (CAD) and hypertension: The American Heart Association, American College of Cardiology and American Society of Hypertension (AHA/ACC/ASH) 2015 scientific statement for the treatment of hypertension in patients with coronary artery disease (CAD) recommends the use of a beta blocker as part of a regimen in patients with hypertension and chronic stable angina with a history of prior MI. A BP target of <140/90 mm Hg is reasonable for the secondary prevention of cardiovascular events. A lower target BP (<130/80 mm Hg) may be appropriate in some individuals with CAD, previous MI, stroke or transient ischemic attack, or CAD risk equivalents (AHA/ACC/ASH [Rosendorff 2015]).

Pregnancy Considerations Adverse events were observed in animal studies; therefore, the manufacturer classifies metoprolol as pregnancy category C. Metoprolol crosses the placenta and can be detected in cord blood, amniotic fluid, and the serum of newborn infants. In a cohort study, an increased risk of cardiovascular defects was observed following maternal use of beta-blockers during pregnancy. Intrauterine growth restriction (IUGR), small placentas, as well as fetal/neonatal bradycardia, hypoglycemia, and/or respiratory depression have been observed following *in utero* exposure to beta-blockers as a class. Adequate facilities for monitoring infants at birth should be available. Untreated chronic maternal hypertension and pre-eclampsia are also associated with adverse events in the fetus, infant, and mother. The clearance of metoprolol is increased and serum concentrations and AUC of metoprolol are decreased during pregnancy. Metoprolol has been evaluated for the treatment of hypertension in pregnancy, but other agents may be more appropriate for use.

Breast-Feeding Considerations Small amounts of metoprolol can be detected in breast milk. The manufacturer recommends that caution be exercised when administering metoprolol to nursing women.

Contraindications
Hypersensitivity to metoprolol, any component of the formulation, or other beta-blockers
Note: Additional contraindications are formulation and/or indication specific.
Immediate release tablets/injectable formulation:
Hypertension and angina: Sinus bradycardia; second- and third-degree heart block; cardiogenic shock; overt heart failure; sick sinus syndrome (except in patients with a functioning artificial pacemaker); severe peripheral arterial disease; pheochromocytoma (without alpha blockade)
Myocardial infarction: Severe sinus bradycardia (heart rate <45 beats/minute); significant first-degree heart block (P-R interval ≥0.24 seconds); second- and third-degree heart block; systolic blood pressure <100 mm Hg; moderate-to-severe cardiac failure
Extended release tablet: Severe bradycardia, second- and third degree heart block; cardiogenic shock; decompensated heart failure; sick sinus syndrome (except in patients with a functioning artificial pacemaker)

Warnings/Precautions [U.S. Boxed Warning]: Beta-blocker therapy should not be withdrawn abruptly (particularly in patients with CAD), but gradually tapered over 1 to 2 weeks to avoid acute tachycardia, hypertension, and/or ischemia. Consider preexisting conditions such as sick sinus syndrome before initiating. Metoprolol commonly produces mild first-degree heart block. May also produce severe first-, second-, or third-degree heart block. Patients with acute MI (especially right ventricular MI) have a high risk of developing heart block of varying degrees. If severe heart block occurs, metoprolol should be discontinued and measures to increase heart rate should be employed. Symptomatic hypotension may occur with use. May precipitate or aggravate symptoms of arterial insufficiency in patients with PVD and Raynaud disease; use with caution and monitor for progression of arterial obstruction. Potentially significant interactions may exist, requiring dose or frequency adjustment, additional monitoring, and/or selection of alternative therapy. Consult drug interactions database for more detailed information.

In general, beta-blockers should be avoided in patients with bronchospastic disease. Metoprolol, with B$_1$ selectivity, should be used cautiously in bronchospastic disease with close monitoring. Use cautiously in patients with diabetes because it can mask prominent hypoglycemic symptoms. May mask signs of hyperthyroidism (eg, tachycardia); if hyperthyroidism is suspected, carefully manage and monitor; abrupt withdrawal may exacerbate symptoms of hyperthyroidism or precipitate thyroid storm. Alterations in thyroid function tests may be observed. Use caution with hepatic dysfunction. Use with caution in patients with myasthenia gravis or psychiatric disease (may cause CNS depression). Although perioperative beta-blocker therapy is recommended prior to elective surgery in selected patients, use of high-dose extended release metoprolol in patients naïve to beta-blocker therapy undergoing noncardiac surgery has been associated with ▶

bradycardia, hypotension, stroke, and death. Chronic beta-blocker therapy should not be routinely withdrawn prior to major surgery. Use of beta-blockers may unmask cardiac failure in patients without a history of dysfunction. Adequate alpha-blockade is required prior to use of any beta-blocker for patients with untreated pheochromocytoma. May induce or exacerbate psoriasis. Use caution with history of severe anaphylaxis to allergens; patients taking beta-blockers may become more sensitive to repeated allergen challenges. Treatment of anaphylaxis (eg, epinephrine) in patients taking beta-blockers may be ineffective or promote undesirable effects. Bradycardia may be observed more frequently in elderly patients (>65 years of age); dosage reductions may be necessary.

Extended release: Use with caution in patients with compensated heart failure; monitor for a worsening of heart failure.

Adverse Reactions Frequency not always defined.

Cardiovascular: Hypotension (1% to 27%), bradycardia (2% to 16%), first degree atrioventricular block (5%), arterial insufficiency (usually Raynaud type: 1%), cardiac failure (1%), cerebrovascular accident (1%), cold extremities (1%), palpitations (1%), peripheral edema (1%), claudication

Central nervous system: Dizziness (2% to 10%), fatigue (1% to 10%), depression (>2% to 5%), vertigo (≤2%), confusion, disturbed sleep, hallucination, headache, insomnia, nightmares, temporary amnesia

Dermatology: Pruritus (5%), rash (>2% to 5%), exacerbation of psoriasis, skin photosensitivity

Endocrine & metabolic: Decreased libido, unstable diabetes

Gastrointestinal: Diarrhea (>2% to 5%), constipation (1%), flatulence (1%), heartburn (1%), stomach pain (1%), xerostomia (1%), nausea (≤1%), vomiting

Neuromuscular & skeletal: Musculoskeletal pain

Ophthalmic: Blurred vision, visual disturbance

Otic: Tinnitus

Respiratory: Dyspnea (≤3%), bronchospasm (1%), wheezing (1%), rhinitis

Miscellaneous: Accidental injury (1%)

<1% (Limited to important or life-threatening): Abdominal pain, agranulocytosis, alopecia (reversible), anxiety, arthralgia, arthritis, chest pain, decreased HDL cholesterol, diaphoresis, drowsiness, dry eye syndrome, gangrene, hepatic insufficiency, hepatitis, impotence, increased lactate dehydrogenase, increased serum alkaline phosphatase, increased serum transaminases, increased serum triglycerides, jaundice, nervousness, paresthesia, Peyronie's disease, retroperitoneal fibrosis, syncope, taste disorder, weight gain

Drug Interactions

Metabolism/Transport Effects Substrate of CYP2C19 (minor), CYP2D6 (major); **Note:** Assignment of Major/Minor substrate status based on clinically relevant drug interaction potential; **Inhibits** CYP2D6 (weak)

Avoid Concomitant Use

Avoid concomitant use of Metoprolol with any of the following: Ceritinib; Floctafenine; Methacholine; Rivastigmine

Increased Effect/Toxicity

Metoprolol may increase the levels/effects of: Alpha-/Beta-Agonists (Direct-Acting); Alpha1-Blockers; Alpha2-Agonists; Amifostine; Antipsychotic Agents (Phenothiazines); Antipsychotic Agents (Second Generation [Atypical]); ARIPiprazole; Bradycardia-Causing Agents; Bupivacaine; Cardiac Glycosides; Ceritinib; Cholinergic Agonists; Disopyramide; Ergot Derivatives; Fingolimod; Grass Pollen Allergen Extract (5 Grass Extract); Hypotension-Associated Agents; Insulin; Ivabradine; Lacosamide; Levodopa; Lidocaine (Systemic); Lidocaine (Topical); Mepivacaine; Methacholine; Midodrine; Sulfonylureas

The levels/effects of Metoprolol may be increased by: Abiraterone Acetate; Acetylcholinesterase Inhibitors; Alpha2-Agonists; Aminoquinolines (Antimalarial); Anilidopiperidine Opioids; Antipsychotic Agents (Phenothiazines); Barbiturates; Bretylium; Brimonidine (Topical); Calcium Channel Blockers (Nondihydropyridine); Cobicistat; CYP2D6 Inhibitors; Darunavir; Diazoxide; Dipyridamole; Disopyramide; Dronedarone; Floctafenine; Herbs (Hypotensive Properties); Lercanidipine; Mirabegron; Molsidomine; Nicorandil; NIFEdipine; Obinutuzumab; Panobinostat; Peginterferon Alfa-2b; Pentoxifylline; Phosphodiesterase 5 Inhibitors; Propafenone; Prostacyclin Analogues; Regorafenib; Reserpine; Rivastigmine; Ruxolitinib; Selective Serotonin Reuptake Inhibitors; Tofacitinib

Decreased Effect

Metoprolol may decrease the levels/effects of: Beta2-Agonists; Lercanidipine; Theophylline Derivatives

The levels/effects of Metoprolol may be decreased by: Amphetamines; Barbiturates; Herbs (Hypertensive Properties); Methylphenidate; Mirabegron; Nonsteroidal Anti-Inflammatory Agents; Peginterferon Alfa-2b; Rifamycin Derivatives; Yohimbine

Food Interactions Food increases absorption. Metoprolol serum levels may be increased if taken with food. Management: Take immediate release tartrate tablets with food; succinate can be taken with or without food.

Storage/Stability

Injection: Store at 25°C (77°F); excursions permitted to 15°C to 30°C (59°F to 86°F). Protect from light and heat.

Tablet: Store at 25°C (77°F); excursions permitted to 15°C to 30°C (59°F to 86°F). Protect from moisture and heat.

Mechanism of Action Selective inhibitor of beta$_1$-adrenergic receptors; competitively blocks beta$_1$-receptors, with little or no effect on beta$_2$-receptors at oral doses <100 mg (in adults); does not exhibit any membrane stabilizing or intrinsic sympathomimetic activity

Pharmacodynamics/Kinetics

Onset of action: Peak effect: Oral: 1 to 2 hours (Regàrdh, 1980); IV: 20 minutes (when infused over 10 minutes)

Duration: Oral: Immediate release: Variable (dose-related; 50% reduction in maximum heart rate after single doses of 20, 50, and 100 mg occurred at 3.3, 5, and 6.4 hours, respectively), Extended release: ~24 hours; IV: 5 to 8 hours

Absorption: Rapid and complete

Distribution: V_d: 3.2 to 5.6 L/kg

Protein binding: ~10% to albumin

Metabolism: Extensively hepatic via CYP2D6; significant first-pass effect (~50%)

Bioavailability: Oral: Immediate release: ~40% to 50% (Johnsson, 1975); Extended release: 77% relative to immediate release

Half-life elimination: 3 to 4 hours (7 to 9 hours in poor CYP2D6 metabolizers or hepatic impairment)

Excretion: Urine (<10% as unchanged drug; increased to 30% to 40% in poor CYP2D6 metabolizers)

Dosing

Adult

Angina: Oral:

Immediate release (metoprolol tartrate): Initial: 50 mg twice daily; usual dosage range: 50 to 200 mg twice daily; maximum: 400 mg daily; increase dose at weekly intervals to desired effect

Extended release (metoprolol succinate): Initial: 100 mg daily (maximum: 400 mg daily)

Atrial fibrillation/flutter (ventricular rate control), supraventricular tachycardia (SVT) (acute treatment; off-label use; AHA/ACC/HRS [January 2014]; AHA [Neumar 2010]): IV: 2.5 to 5 mg every 2 to 5 minutes (maximum total dose: 15 mg over a 10- to 15-minute period). **Note:** Initiate cautiously in patients with concomitant heart failure. Avoid in patients with decompensated heart failure; electrical cardioversion preferred.

Maintenance: Oral (immediate release [metoprolol tartrate]): 25 to 100 mg twice daily; Oral (extended release [metoprolol succinate]): 50 to 400 mg once daily

Heart failure: Note: Initiate only in stable patients or hospitalized patients after volume status has been optimized and IV diuretics, vasodilators, and inotropic agents have all been successfully discontinued. Caution should be used when initiating in patients who required inotropes during their hospital course. Increase dose gradually and monitor for congestive signs and symptoms of HF making every effort to achieve target dose shown to be effective (ACCF/AHA [Yancy 2013]; HFSA [Lindenfeld 2010]; MERIT-HF Study Group, 1999).

Oral: *Extended release (metoprolol succinate):* Initial: 25 mg once daily (reduce to 12.5 mg once daily in NYHA class higher than class II); may double dosage every 2 weeks as tolerated (target dose: 200 mg daily).

ACCF/AHA 2013 Heart Failure Guidelines: Oral (extended release [metoprolol succinate]): Initial: 12.5 to 25 mg once daily; maximum daily dose: 200 mg (Yancy 2013).

Hypertension: Oral:

Immediate release (metoprolol tartrate): Initial: 50 mg twice daily; effective dosage range: 100 to 450 mg daily in 2 to 3 divided doses; increase dose at weekly intervals to desired effect; maximum total daily dose: 450 mg; usual dosage range (ASH/ISH [Weber 2014]): 50 to 100 mg twice daily; target dose (JNC 8 [James 2013]): 100 to 200 mg daily

Extended release (metoprolol succinate): Initial: 25 to 100 mg once daily; increase doses at weekly (or longer) intervals to desired effect; maximum: 400 mg daily

Hypertension/ventricular rate control: IV (in patients having nonfunctioning GI tract): Initial: 1.25 to 5 mg every 6 to 12 hours; titrate initial dose to response. Initially, low doses may be appropriate to establish response; however, although not routine, up to 15 mg administered as frequently as every 3 hours has been employed in patients with refractory tachycardia.

Myocardial infarction:

Early treatment:

IV: 5 mg every 5 minutes as tolerated for up to 3 doses in the early treatment of ST elevation myocardial infarction; titrate to heart rate and blood pressure; then begin oral therapy. Note: The ACCF/AHA guidelines for the management of STEMI recommend the use of IV metoprolol at the time of presentation in patients with STEMI who are hypertensive or have ongoing ischemia without contraindications. Do not initiate this regimen in those with signs of heart failure, a low output state, increased risk of cardiogenic shock, or other contraindications (eg, second- or third-degree heart block) (ACCF/AHA [O'Gara 2013]).

Oral: 25 to 50 mg (metoprolol tartrate [immediate release]) orally every 6 to 12 hours; transition over the next 2 to 3 days to twice daily dosing of metoprolol tartrate (immediate release) or to daily metoprolol succinate (extended release) and increase as tolerated to a maximum daily dose of 200 mg. **Note:** The ACCF/AHA guidelines for the management of STEMI recommend initiation within the first 24 hours. Do not initiate this regimen in those with signs of heart failure, a low output state, increased risk of cardiogenic shock, or other contraindications (eg, second- or third-degree heart block) (ACCF/AHA [O'Gara 2013]).

Secondary prevention (off-label use): Oral: Immediate release (metoprolol tartrate): 25 to 100 mg twice daily; optimize dose based on heart rate and blood pressure; continue indefinitely (Olsson, 1992).

Thyrotoxicosis (off-label use): Oral: Immediate release (metoprolol tartrate): 25 to 50 mg every 6 hours; may also consider administering extended release formulation (metoprolol succinate) (Bahn 2011)

Note: Switching dosage forms:

When switching from immediate release (metoprolol tartrate) to extended release (metoprolol succinate), the same total daily dose of metoprolol should be used.

When switching between oral and intravenous dosage forms, in most cases, equivalent beta-blocking effect is achieved when doses in a 2.5:1 (Oral:IV) ratio is used. However, in one bioavailability study including healthy volunteers, a range of Oral:IV conversion ratios was found to be approximately 2:1 to 5:1 (Regardh, 1974). Therefore, patient variability may exist and a specific ratio may not apply to all patients, especially if comorbid conditions are present. For example, based on a range of 2.5:1 to 5:1 ratios, if the patient is receiving a chronic oral dose of 25 mg twice daily (50 mg daily), this would translate to 2.5 to 5 mg IV every 6 hours. Recognizing that patients receiving larger chronic oral doses should not automatically be converted to a large IV dose, consideration should be given to further reducing the initial IV dose and basing subsequent doses on the clinical response (Huckleberry 2003).

Geriatric Refer to adult dosing. In the management of hypertension, consider lower initial doses and titrate to response (Aronow 2011).

Pediatric

Hypertension: Oral:

Immediate release tablet (metoprolol tartrate): Children: 1 to 17 years (National High Blood Pressure Education Program Working Group on High Blood Pressure in Children and Adolescents 2004): Initial: 1 to 2 mg/kg/day; maximum 6 mg/kg/day (≤200 mg daily); administer in 2 divided doses

Extended release tablet (metoprolol succinate): Children ≥6 years: Initial: 1 mg/kg once daily (maximum initial dose: 50 mg daily). Adjust dose based on patient response (maximum: 2 mg/kg/day or 200 mg daily)

Renal Impairment No dosage adjustment necessary.

Hepatic Impairment There are no dosage adjustments provided in manufacturer's labeling. However, reduced dose may be necessary due to extensive hepatic metabolism.

Dietary Considerations Immediate-release tablets should be taken with or immediately following food (Melander, 1977). Extended-release tablets may be taken without regard to meals (Tangeman 2003; van den Berg 1990; Wikstrand 2003).

Administration

Oral: Administer immediate-release tablets (metoprolol tartrate) with or immediately following food (Melander 1977). Extended-release tablets may be taken without regard to meals (Tangeman 2003; van den Berg 1990; Wikstrand 2003). Extended-release tablets (metoprolol succinate) may also be divided in half; do not crush or chew.

IV: IV dose is much smaller than oral dose. When administered acutely for cardiac treatment, monitor ECG and blood pressure; may administer by rapid infusion (IV push) over 1 minute. May also be administered by slow infusion (ie, 5 to 10 mg of metoprolol in 50 mL of fluid) over ~30 to 60 minutes during less urgent situations (eg, substitution for oral metoprolol).

Monitoring Parameters Acute cardiac treatment: Monitor ECG and blood pressure with IV administration; heart rate and blood pressure with oral administration. IV use in a nonemergency situation: Necessary monitoring for surgical patients who are unable to take oral beta-blockers (because of prolonged ileus) has not been defined. Some institutions require monitoring of baseline and postinfusion heart rate and blood pressure when a patient's response to beta-blockade has not been characterized (ie, the patient's initial dose or following a change in dose). Consult individual institutional policies and procedures.

Dosage Forms Excipient information presented when available (limited, particularly for generics); consult specific product labeling. [DSC] = Discontinued product

Solution, Intravenous, as tartrate:

Lopressor: 1 mg/mL (5 mL [DSC])

Generic: 1 mg/mL (5 mL); 5 mg/5 mL (5 mL)

Tablet, Oral, as tartrate:

Lopressor: 50 mg, 100 mg [scored]

Lopressor: 100 mg [scored; contains fd&c blue #2 aluminum lake]

Generic: 25 mg, 50 mg, 100 mg

Tablet Extended Release 24 Hour, Oral, as succinate:

Toprol XL: 25 mg, 50 mg, 100 mg, 200 mg [scored]

Generic: 25 mg, 50 mg, 100 mg, 200 mg

Extemporaneous Preparations A 10 mg/mL oral suspension may be made with metoprolol tartrate tablets and one of three different vehicles (cherry syrup; a 1:1 mixture of Ora-Sweet® and Ora-Plus®; or a 1:1 mixture of Ora-Sweet® SF and Ora-Plus®). Crush twelve 100 mg tablets in a mortar and reduce to a fine powder. Add 20 mL of the chosen vehicle and mix to a uniform paste; mix while adding the vehicle in incremental proportions to **almost** 120 mL; transfer to a calibrated bottle, rinse mortar with vehicle, and add quantity of vehicle sufficient to make 120 mL. Label "shake well" and "protect from light". Stable for 60 days.

Allen LV Jr and Erickson MA 3rd, "Stability of Labetalol Hydrochloride, Metoprolol Tartrate, Verapamil Hydrochloride, and Spironolactone With Hydrochlorothiazide in Extemporaneously Compounded Oral Liquids," *Am J Health Syst Pharm,* 1996, 53(19):2304-9.

◆ Metoprolol-25 (Can) *see* Metoprolol *on page 1193*

◆ Metoprolol-L (Can) *see* Metoprolol *on page 1193*

◆ Metoprolol Succinate *see* Metoprolol *on page 1193*

◆ Metoprolol Tartrate *see* Metoprolol *on page 1193*

◆ Metoprolol Tartrate Injection, USP (Can) *see* Metoprolol *on page 1193*

◆ Metozolv ODT *see* Metoclopramide *on page 1188*

Metreleptin (met re LEP tin)

Brand Names: US Myalept

Index Terms Recombinant Methionyl-Human Leptin

Pharmacologic Category Leptin Analog

Use

Lipodystrophy: Replacement therapy to treat the complications of leptin deficiency, in addition to diet, in patients with congenital or acquired generalized lipodystrophy.

Limitations of use: Not indicated for use in patients with HIV-related lipodystrophy or for use in patients with metabolic disease (eg, diabetes mellitus, hypertriglyceridemia) without concurrent evidence of congenital or acquired generalized lipodystrophy.

Prescribing and Access Restrictions As a requirement of the REMS program, access to this medication is restricted. Prescribers must be certified with the program by enrolling and completing training. Pharmacies must be certified with the program and only dispense metreleptin after the receipt of the prescription authorization form for

each new prescription. Additional information is available at 1-855-669-2537 or www.MYALEPTREMS.com.

Medication Guide Available Yes

Dosing

Adult & Geriatric

Lipodystrophy: SubQ: **Note:** Increase or decrease dose based on clinical response (eg, inadequate metabolic control) or other considerations (eg, tolerability issues, excessive weight loss [especially in pediatric patients]). Baseline weight ≤40 kg: Initial dose: 0.06 mg/kg once daily; increase or decrease by 0.02 mg/kg daily based on response or adverse effects. Maximum dose: 0.13 mg/kg once daily.

Baseline weight >40 kg: Initial dose: 2.5 mg (males) or 5 mg (females) once daily; increase or decrease by 1.25-2.5 mg daily based on response or adverse effects. Maximum dose: 10 mg once daily.

Discontinuation: When discontinuing therapy in patients with risk factors for pancreatitis (eg, history of pancreatitis, severe hypertriglyceridemia), taper the dose over a 1-week period and monitor triglyceride levels; consider initiating or adjusting the dose of lipid-lowering medications as needed.

Pediatric Refer to adult dosing.

Renal Impairment There are no dosage adjustments provided in the manufacturer's labeling (has not been studied).

Hepatic Impairment There are no dosage adjustments provided in the manufacturer's labeling (has not been studied).

Additional Information Complete prescribing information should be consulted for additional detail.

Dosage Forms Excipient information presented when available (limited, particularly for generics); consult specific product labeling.

Solution Reconstituted, Subcutaneous:
Myalept: 11.3 mg (1 ea)

◆ **Metro** see MetroNIDAZOLE (Systemic) *on page 1196*

◆ **MetroCream** see MetroNIDAZOLE (Topical) *on page 1199*

◆ **Metrogel** see MetroNIDAZOLE (Topical) *on page 1199*

◆ **MetroGel-Vaginal** see MetroNIDAZOLE (Topical) *on page 1199*

◆ **MetroLotion** see MetroNIDAZOLE (Topical) *on page 1199*

MetroNIDAZOLE (Systemic)

(met roe NYE da zole)

Brand Names: US Flagyl; Flagyl ER; Metro

Brand Names: Canada Flagyl; Metronidazole Injection USP; Novo-Nidazol; PMS-Metronidazole

Index Terms Flagyl; Metronidazole Hydrochloride

Pharmacologic Category Amebicide; Antibiotic, Miscellaneous; Antiprotozoal, Nitroimidazole

Use

Amebiasis: Oral immediate release tablet and capsule: Treatment of acute intestinal amebiasis (amebic dysentery) and amebic liver abscess

Limitations of use (oral immediate-release tablet, capsule and injection): When used for amebic liver abscess, may be used concurrently with percutaneous needle aspiration when it is clinically indicated

Anaerobic bacterial infections (caused by *Bacteroides spp*, including the *B. fragilis* group): Oral immediate-release tablet, capsule, and injection:

Bacterial septicemia: Treatment of bacterial septicemia (also caused by *Clostridium spp*)

Bone and joint infections: Treatment (adjunctive therapy) of bone and joint infections

CNS Infections: Treatment of CNS infections, including meningitis and brain abscess

Endocarditis: Treatment of endocarditis

Gynecologic infections: Treatment of gynecologic infections including endometritis, endomyometritis, tubo-ovarian abscess, or postsurgical vaginal cuff infection (also caused by *Clostridium spp, Peptococcus spp, Peptostreptococcus spp,* and *Fusobacterium spp*)

Intra-abdominal infections: Treatment of intra-abdominal infections, including peritonitis, intra-abdominal abscess and liver abscess (also caused by *Clostridium spp, Eubacterium spp, Peptococcus spp,* and *Peptostreptococcus spp*)

Lower respiratory tract infections: Treatment of lower respiratory tract infections, including pneumonia, empyema and lung abscess

Skin and skin structure infections: Treatment of skin and skin structure infections (also caused by *Clostridium spp, Peptococcus spp, Peptostreptococcus spp,* and *Fusobacterium spp*)

Bacterial vaginosis: Oral extended-release tablet: Treatment of bacterial vaginosis in nonpregnant women

Surgical prophylaxis (colorectal surgery): Injection: Preoperative, intraoperative, and postoperative prophylaxis to reduce the incidence of postoperative infection in patients undergoing elective colorectal surgery classified as contaminated or potentially contaminated.

Trichomoniasis: Oral immediate-release tablet, capsule, and injection: Treatment of infections caused by *Trichomonas vaginalis,* including treatment of asymptomatic sexual partners

Pregnancy Considerations Adverse events were not observed in animal reproduction studies. Metronidazole crosses the placenta. Cleft lip with or without cleft palate has been reported following first trimester exposure to metronidazole; however, most studies have not shown an increased risk of congenital anomalies or other adverse events to the fetus following maternal use during pregnancy. Because metronidazole was carcinogenic in some animal species, concern has been raised whether metronidazole should be used during pregnancy. Available studies have not shown an increased risk of infant cancer following metronidazole exposure during pregnancy; however, the ability to detect a signal for this may have been limited. Use of metronidazole during the first trimester of pregnancy is contraindicated by the manufacturer.

Metronidazole pharmacokinetics are similar between pregnant and nonpregnant patients (Amon, 1981; Visser, 1984; Wang, 2011). Bacterial vaginosis has been associated with adverse pregnancy outcomes (including preterm labor); metronidazole is recommended for the treatment of symptomatic bacterial vaginosis in pregnant patients (CDC, 2010). Vaginal trichomoniasis has been also associated with adverse pregnancy outcomes (including preterm labor). Treatment may relieve symptoms and prevent sexual transmission; however, metronidazole use has not resulted in reduced perinatal morbidity and should not be used solely to prevent preterm delivery. Some clinicians consider deferring therapy in asymptomatic women until >37 weeks gestation (CDC, 2010). Metronidazole may also be used for the treatment of giardiasis in pregnant women (some sources recommend second and third trimester administration only) (DHHS, 2013; Gardner, 2001) and symptomatic amebiasis during pregnancy (DHHS, 2013; Li, 1996). The use of other agents is preferred when treatment is needed during pregnancy for *Clostridium difficile* (Surawicz, 2013), *Helicobacter pylori* (Mahadevan, 2006), or Crohn disease (Mottet, 2009). Consult current guidelines for appropriate use in pregnant women.

Breast-Feeding Considerations Metronidazole can be detected in breast milk in concentrations similar to the maternal serum. Infant serum concentrations may be near maternal therapeutic concentrations. Due to the potential for tumorigenicity observed in animal studies, the manufacturer recommends a decision be made whether to discontinue nursing or to discontinue the drug, taking into account the importance of treatment to the mother. Alternately, the mother may pump and discard breast milk for 24 hours after the last dose. Some guidelines note if metronidazole is given, breast-feeding should be withheld for 12 to 24 hours after the dose (CDC, 2010). Use of other agents is preferred in some cases, such as when treating breast-feeding women for Crohn disease (Mottet, 2009) or *Clostridium difficile* infection (Surawicz, 2013).

Contraindications Hypersensitivity to metronidazole, nitroimidazole derivatives, or any component of the formulation; pregnant patients (first trimester) with trichomoniasis; use of disulfiram within the past 2 weeks; use of alcohol or propylene glycol-containing products during therapy or within 3 days of therapy discontinuation

Warnings/Precautions [U.S. Boxed Warning]: Possibly carcinogenic based on animal data. Reserve use for conditions described in Use; unnecessary use should be avoided. Use with caution in patients with severe liver impairment and ESRD due to potential accumulation; reduce dosage in patients with severe liver impairment and consider dosage reduction in patients with severe renal impairment (CrCl <10 mL/minute) who are receiving prolonged therapy. Dose should not specifically be reduced in anuric patients (accumulated metabolites may be rapidly removed by dialysis). Hemodialysis patients may need supplemental dosing. Use with caution in patients with blood dyscrasias (monitor CBC with differential at baseline, during and after treatment) or history of seizures.

Aseptic meningitis (symptoms may occur within hours of a dose); encephalopathy (cerebellar toxicity with ataxia, dizziness, dysarthria and/or CNS lesions); seizures; and peripheral and optic neuropathies have been reported especially with increased doses and chronic treatment; monitor and consider discontinuation of therapy if

symptoms occur. Prolonged use may result in fungal or bacterial superinfection, including *C. difficile*-associated diarrhea (CDAD) and pseudomembranous colitis; CDAD has been observed >2 months postantibiotic treatment. Guidelines recommend the use of oral metronidazole for initial treatment of mild to moderate *C. difficile* infection and the use of oral vancomycin for initial treatment of severe *C. difficile* infection (with or without IV metronidazole depending on the presence of complications). May treat recurrent mild to moderate infection once with oral metronidazole; avoid use beyond first reoccurrence (Cohen, 2010, Surawicz, 2013). Candidiasis infection (known or unknown) maybe more prominent during metronidazole treatment, antifungal treatment required.

Abdominal cramps, nausea, vomiting, headaches, and flushing have been reported with oral and injectable metronidazole and concomitant alcohol consumption; avoid alcoholic beverages or products containing propylene glycol during oral and injectable therapy and for at least 3 days after oral therapy. Use with caution in the elderly; dosage adjustment may be required based on renal and/or hepatic function. Do not use extended-release tablets in patients with severe hepatic impairment (Child-Pugh class C) unless benefit outweighs risk. Use injection with caution in patients with heart failure, edema or other sodium retaining states, including corticosteroid treatment. In patients receiving continuous nasogastric secretion aspiration, sufficient metronidazole may be removed in the aspirate to cause a reduction in serum levels. Potentially significant drug-drug interactions may exist, requiring dose or frequency adjustment, additional monitoring, and/or selection of alternative therapy.

Adverse Reactions Frequency not always defined.
Cardiovascular: Flattened T-wave on ECG, flushing, local thrombophlebitis (IV), syncope
Central nervous system: Headache (18%), metallic taste (9%), dizziness (4%), aseptic meningitis, ataxia, brain disease, confusion, depression, disulfiram-like reaction (with alcohol), dysarthria, dyspareunia, insomnia, irritability, peripheral neuropathy, seizure, vertigo
Dermatologic: Erythematous rash, pruritus, Stevens-Johnson syndrome, toxic epidermal necrolysis, urticaria
Gastrointestinal: Nausea (10% to ~12%), abdominal pain (4%), diarrhea (4%), xerostomia (2%), abdominal cramps, anorexia, constipation, epigastric distress, glossitis, hairy tongue, pancreatitis (rare), proctitis, stomatitis, vomiting
Genitourinary: Vaginitis (15%), genital pruritus (5%), dysmenorrhea (3%), urine abnormality (3%), urinary tract infection (2%), cystitis, dark urine (rare), decreased libido, dysuria, sensation of pelvic pressure, urinary incontinence, vaginal dryness, vulvovaginal candidiasis
Hematologic & oncologic: Leukopenia (reversible), thrombocytopenia (reversible, rare)
Immunologic: Serum sickness-like reaction (joint pains)
Infection: Bacterial infection (7%), candidiasis (3%)
Neuromuscular & skeletal: Weakness
Ophthalmic: Optic neuropathy
Renal: Polyuria
Respiratory: Flu-like symptoms (6%), upper respiratory tract infection (4%), pharyngitis (3%), nasal congestion, rhinitis, sinusitis
Miscellaneous: Fever, lesion (central nervous system, reversible)

Drug Interactions
Metabolism/Transport Effects Substrate of CYP2A6 (minor); **Note:** Assignment of Major/Minor substrate status based on clinically relevant drug interaction potential; **Inhibits** CYP2C9 (weak)

Avoid Concomitant Use
Avoid concomitant use of MetroNIDAZOLE (Systemic) with any of the following: Alcohol (Ethyl); BCG (Intravesical); Carbocisteine; Disulfiram; Mebendazole; Ritonavir

Increased Effect/Toxicity
MetroNIDAZOLE (Systemic) may increase the levels/effects of: Alcohol (Ethyl); Busulfan; Capecitabine; Carbocisteine; Fluorouracil (Systemic); Fosphenytoin; Highest Risk QTc-Prolonging Agents; Lopinavir; Moderate Risk QTc-Prolonging Agents; Phenytoin; Tegafur; Tipranavir; Vitamin K Antagonists

The levels/effects of MetroNIDAZOLE (Systemic) may be increased by: Disulfiram; Mebendazole; Mifepristone; Ritonavir

Decreased Effect
MetroNIDAZOLE (Systemic) may decrease the levels/effects of: BCG (Intravesical); BCG Vaccine (Immunization); Mycophenolate; Sodium Picosulfate; Typhoid Vaccine

The levels/effects of MetroNIDAZOLE (Systemic) may be decreased by: Fosphenytoin; PHENobarbital; Phenytoin; Primidone

Food Interactions Peak antibiotic serum concentration lowered and delayed, but total drug absorbed not affected.

Storage/Stability
Oral:
Extended release: Store at 25°C (77°F); excursions are permitted between 15°C and 30°C (59°F and 86°F).
Immediate release: Store at 15°C to 25°C (59°F to 77°F). Protect the tablets from light.
Injection: Store at 20°C to 25°C (68°F to 77°F). Protect from light. Avoid excessive heat. Do not refrigerate. Do not remove unit from overwrap until ready for use. Discard unused solution.

Mechanism of Action After diffusing into the organism, interacts with DNA to cause a loss of helical DNA structure and strand breakage resulting in inhibition of protein synthesis and cell death in susceptible organisms

Pharmacodynamics/Kinetics
Absorption: Oral: Well absorbed
Distribution: To bile, seminal fluid, bone, liver, and liver abscesses, lung and vaginal secretions; crosses blood-brain barrier; saliva and CSF concentrations similar to those in plasma
Protein binding: <20%
Metabolism: Hepatic (30% to 60%) to several metabolites including an active hydroxyl metabolite
Half-life elimination: ~8 hours
Time to peak, serum: Oral: Immediate release: 1 to 2 hours; Extended release: ~5 hours
Excretion: Urine (unchanged drug and metabolites: 60% to 80%; ~20% of total as unchanged drug); feces (6% to 15%)

Dosing
Adult
Amebiasis (acute dysentery): Oral: Immediate-release tablets and capsules: 750 mg every 8 hours for 5 to 10 days
Amebic liver abscess: Oral:
Immediate-release tablets: 500 to 750 mg every 8 hours for 5 to 10 days
Capsules: 750 mg every 8 hours for 5 to 10 days
Anaerobic infections (diverticulitis, peritonitis, cholangitis, or abscess): Oral (immediate release), IV: 500 mg every 6 hours (maximum: 4 g/day); **Note:** Initial: 1 g IV loading dose may be administered
Bacterial vaginosis or vaginitis due to *Gardnerella, Mobiluncus*: Oral: Tablet:
Immediate release: 500 mg twice daily for 7 days (off-label use) (CDC 2010)
Extended release: 750 mg once daily for 7 days
Intra-abdominal infection:
Manufacturer's labeling: Oral (immediate release), IV: 500 mg every 6 hours (maximum: 4 g/day); **Note:** Initial: 1 g IV loading dose may be administered
Alternate dosing: Complicated, community-acquired, mild to moderate (in combination with cephalosporin or fluoroquinolone; off-label dosing): IV: 500 mg every 8 to 12 hours **or** 1.5 g every 24 hours for 4 to 7 days (provided source controlled) (Solomkin 2010)
Pelvic inflammatory disease (off-label dosing): Oral (immediate release): 500 mg twice daily for 14 days (in combination with a third generation parenteral cephalosporin and doxycycline) (CDC 2010)
Trichomoniasis (index case and sex partner): Oral: Immediate-release tablets:
Manufacturer's labeling: 250 mg every 8 hours for 7 days **or** 1 g twice daily for 2 doses (on same day) **or** 2 g as a single dose
Alternate dosing: 500 mg twice daily for 7 days (CDC 2010)
Capsules: 375 mg twice daily for 7 days
Trichomoniasis (failure of nitroimidazole [eg metronidazole] therapy in index case; treatment of sex partner; off-label dosing): Oral (immediate release): 500 mg twice daily for 7 days (CDC 2010)
Balantidiasis (off-label use): IV, Oral (immediate release): 750 mg 3 times daily for ≥5 days (Anagyrou 2003; Schuster 2008)
Bite wounds (animal/human) (off-label use) (IDSA [Stevens 2014]): Note: Use in combination with a second- or third-generation cephalosporin, levofloxacin, or sulfamethoxazole/trimethoprim for animal bites, or in combination with ciprofloxacin or levofloxacin for human bites.
Oral: 250 to 500 mg 3 times daily
IV: 500 mg every 8 hours

Clostridium difficile -associated diarrhea (CDAD) (off-label use):

Mild to moderate infection: Oral (immediate release): 500 mg 3 times daily for 10 to 14 days (Cohen 2010; Surawicz 2013)

Severe complicated infection (no abdominal distention): IV: 500 mg 3 times daily with oral vancomycin for 10 to 14 days (Surawicz 2013)

Severe complicated infection (with ileus, toxic colitis, and/or abdominal distention): IV: 500 mg 3 times daily with oral and rectal vancomycin for 10 to 14 days (Surawicz 2013)

Note: Recent guideline recommends converting to oral vancomycin therapy if the patient does not show a clear clinical response after 5 to 7 days of metronidazole therapy (Surawicz 2013)

Crohn disease (off-label use): Oral (immediate release): 10 to 20 mg/kg/day; long-term (eg, several months) safety has not been established (Lichtenstein 2009). **Note:** Reserved for mild to moderate disease in patients not responsive to sulfasalazine and/or who have colonic involvement (eg, ileocolitis and colitis) (Lichtenstein 2009; Sutherland, 1991).

Dientamoeba fragilis infections (off-label use): Oral (immediate release): 500 to 750 mg 3 times daily for 10 days (CDC 2012)

Giardiasis (off-label use): Oral (immediate release): 250 to 500 mg 3 times daily for 5 to 10 days (Granados 2012)

Helicobacter pylori eradication (off-label use): Oral (immediate release):

Triple therapy: Metronidazole 500 mg twice daily for 10 to 14 days, in combination with clarithromycin and a proton pump inhibitor (Chey 2007)

Quadruple therapy: Metronidazole 250 mg 4 times daily for 10 to 14 days, in combination with bismuth subsalicylate, a tetracycline, and either ranitidine or a proton pump inhibitor (Chey 2007)

Periodontitis (associated with aggressive disease; off-label use): Oral (immediate release): 250 mg every 8 hours in combination with amoxicillin for 10 days; used in addition to scaling, root planing and pocket irrigation (Silva-Senem 2013)

Pouchitis (post ileal pouch-anal anastomosis, acute treatment; off-label use): Oral (immediate release): 400 to 500 mg three times daily for 7 days (Holubar 2010; Wall 2011)

Sexual assault (prophylaxis; off-label use): Oral (immediate release): 2 g as a single dose in combination with ceftriaxone and azithromycin or doxycycline (CDC 2010; CDC 2012)

Skin and soft tissue necrotizing infections (off-label use): IV: 500 mg every 6 hours, in combination with cefotaxime for empiric therapy of polymicrobial infections. Continue until further debridement is not necessary, patient has clinically improved, and patient is afebrile for 48 to 72 hours (IDSA [Stevens 2014]).

Surgical prophylaxis:

Manufacturer's labeling: IV: 15 mg/kg 1 hour prior to surgical incision; followed by 7.5 mg/kg 6 and 12 hours after initial dose

Alternate dosing:

IV: 500 mg within 60 minutes prior to surgical incision in combination with other antibiotics (Bratzler 2013). **Note:** Considered a recommended agent for select procedures other than colorectal surgery (off-label use) (Bratzler 2013).

Oral (for colorectal surgical prophylaxis only; immediate release; off-label use): 1 g every 3 to 4 hours for 3 doses, starting after mechanical bowel preparation the afternoon and evening before the procedure with or without additional oral antibiotics and with an appropriate IV antibiotic prophylaxis regimen (Bratzler 2013).

Surgical site infections (intestinal or GU tract; axilla or perineum) (off-label use): IV: 500 mg every 8 hours; in combination with ceftriaxone, ciprofloxacin, or levofloxacin (IDSA [Stevens 2014]).

Tetanus (Clostridium tetani infection; off-label use): Oral (immediate release): 500 mg every 6 hours for 7 to 10 days in combination with supportive therapy (Ahmadsyah, 1985)

Urethritis (for recurrent or persistent urethritis; off-label use): Oral: 2 g as a single dose with azithromycin. **Note:** Compliance with initial regimen and lack of re-exposure to an untreated sex partner should be excluded prior to use (CDC 2010)

Geriatric Refer to adult dosing.

Pediatric

Infants, Children, and Adolescents:

Amebiasis: Oral: 35 to 50 mg/kg/day in divided doses every 8 hours for 7 to 10 days (Red Book [AAP 2012])

Trichomoniasis: Oral: 15 mg/kg/day in divided doses every 8 hours for 7 days (Red Book [AAP 2012])

Anaerobic infections (off-label dosing):

Oral: 30 to 50 mg/kg/day in divided doses every 8 hours (maximum: 2,250 mg/day) (Red Book [AAP 2012])

IV: 22.5 to 40 mg/kg/day in divided doses every 8 hours (maximum: 1,500 mg/day) (Red Book [AAP 2012])

Balantidiasis (off-label use): Oral: 35 to 50 mg/kg/day in 3 divided doses for 5 days (Red Book [AAP 2012]; Schuster 2008)

Clostridium difficile-associated diarrhea (CDAD; off-label use): Oral: 30 mg/kg/day divided every 6 hours for ≥10 days (maximum: 2 g/day) (Red Book [AAP 2012]; Schutze 2013). **Note:** Recommended agent for the initial treatment of mild to moderate disease and for first relapse (Red Book [AAP 2012]; Schutze 2013).

Giardiasis (off-label use): Oral: 15 mg/kg/day in divided doses every 8 hours for 5 to 10 days (Granados 2012; Red Book [AAP 2012])

Helicobacter pylori eradication (off-label use): Oral: 20 mg/kg/day in 2 divided doses for 10 to 14 days in combination therapy with amoxicillin and either a proton pump inhibitor or bismuth subsalicylate daily or 20 mg/kg/day in 2 divided doses on days 6 through 10 in combination therapy with a proton pump inhibitor and clarithromycin (after treatment with amoxicillin and a proton pump inhibitor for days 1 through 5) (maximum: 1 g/day) (Koletzko 2011)

Skin and soft tissue necrotizing infections (off-label use): IV: 7.5 mg/kg every 6 hours, in combination with cefotaxime for empiric therapy of polymicrobial infections. Continue until further debridement is not necessary, patient has clinically improved, and patient is afebrile for 48 to 72 hours (IDSA [Stevens 2014]).

Surgical (preoperative) prophylaxis (off-label use):

Infants <1,200 g: IV: 7.5 mg/kg within 60 minutes prior to surgical incision in combination with other antibiotics (Bratzler 2013).

Infants ≥1,200 g and Children ≥1 year:

IV: 15 mg/kg within 60 minutes prior to surgical incision in combination with other antibiotics (maximum: 500 mg per dose) (Bratzler 2013).

Oral (for colorectal surgical prophylaxis only): 15 mg/kg (maximum: 1,000 mg) every 3 to 4 hours for 3 doses, starting after mechanical bowel preparation the afternoon and evening before the procedure, with or without additional oral antibiotics and with an appropriate IV antibiotic prophylaxis regimen (Bratzler 2013).

Tetanus (Clostridium tetani infection, off-label use): Oral, IV: 30 mg/kg per day in divided doses every 6 hours for 10 to 14 days in combination with tetanus immune globulin and supportive therapy (maximum: 4 g/day) (Red Book [AAP 2012])

Adolescents: Oral:

Pelvic inflammatory disease (off-label dosing): Refer to adult dosing.

Sexual assault (prophylaxis; off-label use): Refer to adult dosing

Vaginal infections:

Vaginitis: (Trichomonas vaginalis; off-label use): 2 g as a single dose (Red Book [AAP 2012])

Vaginosis (bacterial; off-label use): 500 mg twice daily for 7 days (Red Book [AAP 2012])

Renal Impairment

Manufacturer's labeling:

Mild, moderate, or severe impairment: There are no dosage adjustments provided in the manufacturer's labeling; however, decreased renal function does not alter the single-dose pharmacokinetics

End-stage renal disease (ESRD) requiring dialysis: Metronidazole metabolites may accumulate; monitor for adverse events. Accumulated metabolites may be rapidly removed by dialysis:

Intermittent hemodialysis (IHD): If administration cannot be separated from hemodialysis, consider supplemental dose following hemodialysis.

Peritoneal dialysis (PD): No dosage adjustment necessary.

Alternate dosing:

Intermittent hemodialysis (IHD) (administer after hemodialysis on dialysis days): Dialyzable (50% to 100%): 500 mg every 8 to 12 hours. **Note:** Dosing regimen highly dependent on clinical indication (trichomoniasis vs *C. difficile* colitis) (Heintz 2009). **Note:** Dosing dependent on the assumption of thrice weekly, complete IHD sessions.

Continuous renal replacement therapy (CRRT) (Heintz 2009; Trotman 2005): Drug clearance is highly dependent on the method of renal replacement, filter type, and flow rate. Appropriate dosing requires close monitoring of pharmacologic response, signs of adverse reactions due to drug accumulation, as well as drug concentrations in relation to target trough (if appropriate). The following are general recommendations only (based on dialysate flow/ultrafiltration rates of 1 to 2 L/hour and minimal residual renal function) and should not supersede clinical judgment:

CVVH/CVVHD/CVVHDF: 500 mg every 6 to 12 hours (or per clinical indication; dosage reduction generally not necessary)

Hepatic Impairment

Manufacturer's labeling:

Mild or moderate impairment (Child-Pugh class A or B): No dosage adjustment necessary; use with caution and monitor for adverse events

Severe impairment (Child-Pugh class C):

Extended-release tablets: Use is not recommended.

Immediate-release capsules:

Amebiasis: 375 mg 3 times daily

Trichomoniasis: 375 mg once daily

Immediate-release tablets, injection: Reduce dose by 50%

Alternate dosing: The pharmacokinetics of a single oral 500 mg dose were not altered in patients with cirrhosis; initial dose reduction is therefore not necessary (Daneshmend, 1982). In one study of IV metronidazole, patients with alcoholic liver disease (with or without cirrhosis), demonstrated a prolonged elimination half-life (eg, ~18 hours). The authors recommended the dose be reduced accordingly (clearance was reduced by ~62%) and the frequency may be prolonged (eg, every 12 hours instead of every 6 hours) (Lau, 1987). In another single IV dose study using metronidazole metabolism to predict hepatic function, patients classified as Child-Pugh class C demonstrated a half-life of ~21.5 hours (Muscara, 1995).

Dietary Considerations

Immediate-release tablets and capsules may be administered with food to minimize stomach upset. Extended-release tablets should be taken on an empty stomach (1 hour before or 2 hours after meals).

Sodium: Injectable dosage form may contain sodium.

Ethanol: Use of ethanol is contraindicated during therapy and for 3 days after therapy discontinuation.

Administration

IV: Infuse intravenously over 30 to 60 minutes. Avoid contact of drug solution with equipment containing aluminum.

Oral: Immediate-release tablets and capsules may be administered with food to minimize stomach upset. Extended-release tablets should be administered on an empty stomach (1 hour before or 2 hours after meals); do not split, crush, or chew.

Monitoring Parameters Monitor CBC with differential at baseline and after prolonged or repeated courses of therapy. Closely monitor elderly patients and patients with severe hepatic impairment or ESRD for adverse reactions. Observe patients carefully if neurologic symptoms occur and consider discontinuation of therapy.

Test Interactions May interfere with AST, ALT, triglycerides, glucose, and LDH testing

Dosage Forms Considerations Parenteral solution contains 28 mEq of sodium/gram of metronidazole.

Dosage Forms Excipient information presented when available (limited, particularly for generics); consult specific product labeling.

Capsule, Oral:

Flagyl: 375 mg

Generic: 375 mg

Solution, Intravenous:

Metro: 500 mg (100 mL)

Generic: 500 mg (100 mL)

Solution, Intravenous [preservative free]:

Generic: 500 mg (100 mL)

Tablet, Oral:

Flagyl: 250 mg, 500 mg

Generic: 250 mg, 500 mg

Tablet Extended Release 24 Hour, Oral:

Flagyl ER: 750 mg

Extemporaneous Preparations A 50 mg/mL oral suspension may be made with tablets and a 1:1 mixture of Ora-Sweet and Ora-Plus. Crush twenty-four 250 mg tablets in a mortar and reduce to a fine powder. Add small portions of the vehicle and mix to a uniform paste; mix while adding the vehicle in incremental portions to **almost** 120 mL; transfer to a calibrated bottle, rinse mortar with vehicle, and add quantity of vehicle sufficient to make 120 mL. Label "shake well". Stable for 60 days at room temperature or refrigerated (Allen, 1996).

MetroNIDAZOLE (Topical) (met roe NYE da zole)

Brand Names: US MetroCream; Metrogel; MetroGel-Vaginal; MetroLotion; Noritate; Nuvessa; Rosadan; Vandazole; Vitazol [DSC]

Brand Names: Canada MetroCream; Metrogel; MetroLotion; Nidagel; Noritate; Rosasol

Index Terms Metronidazole Hydrochloride

Pharmacologic Category Antibiotic, Topical

Use

Bacterial vaginosis: Vaginal gel: Treatment of bacterial vaginosis

Rosacea: Topical: Treatment of inflammatory lesions and erythema of rosacea

Dosing

Adult & Geriatric

Bacterial vaginosis: Vaginal:

0.75% (Vandazole): One applicatorful (~37.5 mg metronidazole) intravaginally once daily for 5 days

0.75% (MetroGel-vaginal, other products): One applicatorful (~37.5 mg metronidazole) intravaginally once or twice daily for 5 days

1.3%: One applicatorful (~65 mg metronidazole) intravaginally as a single dose

Rosacea: Topical:

0.75%: Apply and rub a thin film twice daily, morning and evening, to entire affected areas after washing.

1%: Apply thin film to affected area once daily

Renal Impairment There are no dosage adjustments provided in the manufacturer's labeling.

Hepatic Impairment There are no dosage adjustments provided in the manufacturer's labeling; use with caution in severe hepatic impairment.

Additional Information Complete prescribing information should be consulted for additional detail.

Dosage Forms Excipient information presented when available (limited, particularly for generics); consult specific product labeling. [DSC] = Discontinued product

Cream, External:

MetroCream: 0.75% (45 g) [contains benzyl alcohol]

Noritate: 1% (60 g) [contains methylparaben, propylparaben, trolamine (triethanolamine)]

Rosadan: 0.75% (45 g) [contains benzyl alcohol]

Vitazol: 0.75% (60 g [DSC]) [contains benzyl alcohol]

Generic: 0.75% (45 g)

Gel, External:

Metrogel: 1% (55 g, 60 g) [contains methylparaben, propylparaben]

Rosadan: 0.75% (45 g) [contains edetate disodium, methylparaben, propylene glycol, propylparaben]

Generic: 0.75% (45 g); 1% (55 g, 60 g)

Gel, Vaginal:

MetroGel-Vaginal: 0.75% (70 g) [contains edetate disodium, methylparaben, propylene glycol, propylparaben]

Nuvessa: 1.3% (5 g) [contains benzyl alcohol, methylparaben, polyethylene glycol, propylene glycol, propylparaben]

Vandazole: 0.75% (70 g) [contains methylparaben, propylparaben]

Generic: 0.75% (70 g)

Kit, External:

Rosadan: 0.75% [contains benzyl alcohol]

Rosadan: 0.75% [contains edetate disodium, methylparaben, propylene glycol, propylparaben]

Lotion, External:

MetroLotion: 0.75% (59 mL) [contains benzyl alcohol]

Generic: 0.75% (59 mL)

◆ **Metronidazole Hydrochloride** *see* MetroNIDAZOLE (Systemic) *on page 1196*

◆ **Metronidazole Hydrochloride** *see* MetroNIDAZOLE (Topical) *on page 1199*

◆ **Metronidazole Injection USP (Can)** *see* MetroNIDAZOLE (Systemic) *on page 1196*

◆ **MET Tyrosine Kinase Inhibitor PF-02341066** *see* Crizotinib *on page 450*

◆ **Metvix (Can)** *see* Methyl Aminolevulinate *on page 1177*

◆ **Metvixia** *see* Methyl Aminolevulinate *on page 1177*

Metyrosine (me TYE roe seen)

Brand Names: US Demser
Index Terms AMPT; OGMT
Pharmacologic Category Tyrosine Hydroxylase Inhibitor
Use Short-term management of pheochromocytoma before surgery, long-term management when surgery is contraindicated or when chronic malignant pheochromocytoma exists

Dosing

Adult & Geriatric Pheochromocytoma: Oral: Initial: 250 mg 4 times/day, increased by 250-500 mg/day up to 4 g/day in 4 divided doses; titrate hypertensive patients to achieve normal blood pressure and symptom control and titrate normotensive patients to reduce catecholamines by ≥50%. Usual maintenance: 2-3 g/day in 4 divided doses; for preoperative preparation, administer optimum effective dosage for 5-7 days.

Pediatric Children ≥12 years: Refer to adult dosing.

Renal Impairment No dosage adjustment provided in manufacturer's labeling.

Hepatic Impairment No dosage adjustment provided in manufacturer's labeling.

Additional Information Complete prescribing information should be consulted for additional detail.

Dosage Forms Excipient information presented when available (limited, particularly for generics); consult specific product labeling.
Capsule, Oral:
Demser: 250 mg [contains fd&c blue #2 (indigotine)]

◆ Mevacor *see* Lovastatin *on page 1110*

◆ Mevinolin *see* Lovastatin *on page 1110*

◆ Mexar Wash [DSC] *see* Sulfacetamide (Topical) *on page 1707*

Mexiletine (meks IL e teen)

Brand Names: Canada Novo-Mexiletine
Pharmacologic Category Antiarrhythmic Agent, Class Ib
Use

Ventricular arrhythmias: Management of life-threatening ventricular arrhythmias

Note: The American College of Cardiology/American Heart Association/European Society of Cardiology (ACC/AHA/ESC) states that mexiletine may be considered for those with long QT syndrome who present with torsades de pointes (ACC/AHA/ESC [Zipes 2006])

Dosing

Adult & Geriatric

Ventricular arrhythmias (life-threatening): Oral: Initial: 200 mg every 8 hours (may load with 400 mg if necessary); adjust dose in 50 or 100 mg increments no more frequently than every 2 to 3 days; usual dose: 200 to 300 mg every 8 hours; maximum dose: 1.2 g/day. **Note:** Once controlled, patients may be transferred to an every 12-hour dosing schedule; do not exceed 450 mg every 12 hours with this regimen.

Conversion:

Switching from other oral antiarrhythmics (eg, disopyramide, quinidine sulfate): Initiate 200 mg dose of mexiletine 6 to 12 hours after the last dose of the former agent.

Switching from IV lidocaine: Initiate 200 mg dose of mexiletine when lidocaine infusion is stopped.

Switching from oral procainamide: Initiate a 200 mg dose of mexiletine 3 to 6 hours after the last dose of procainamide.

Premature ventricular complex (symptomatic) suppression (off-label use): Oral: 100 or 150 mg 3 times daily; if not controlled, may increase to 200 mg 3 times daily (Saikawa 1992; Tanabe 1991) **or** 100 or 200 mg 2 to 3 times daily; may progressively increase to a maximum dose of 500 mg 3 times daily (Rutledge 1985)

Renal Impairment No dosage adjustment necessary.

Hepatic Impairment There are no dosage adjustments provided in the manufacturer's labeling. Patients with hepatic impairment or hepatic congestion secondary to heart failure may require dose reduction; half-life is approximately doubled in patients with hepatic impairment.

Additional Information Complete prescribing information should be consulted for additional detail.

Dosage Forms Excipient information presented when available (limited, particularly for generics); consult specific product labeling.
Capsule, Oral, as hydrochloride:
Generic: 150 mg, 200 mg, 250 mg

◆ Mezavant (Can) *see* Mesalamine *on page 1151*

◆ MgSO₄ (error-prone abbreviation) *see* Magnesium Sulfate *on page 1122*

◆ Miacalcin *see* Calcitonin *on page 282*

◆ Mi-Acid [OTC] *see* Aluminum Hydroxide, Magnesium Hydroxide, and Simethicone *on page 85*

◆ Mi-Acid Double Strength [OTC] *see* Calcium Carbonate and Magnesium Hydroxide *on page 288*

◆ Mi-Acid Maximum Strength [OTC] [DSC] *see* Aluminum Hydroxide, Magnesium Hydroxide, and Simethicone *on page 85*

◆ Micaderm [OTC] *see* Miconazole (Topical) *on page 1201*

Micafungin (mi ka FUN gin)

Brand Names: US Mycamine
Brand Names: Canada Mycamine
Index Terms Micafungin Sodium
Pharmacologic Category Antifungal Agent, Parenteral; Echinocandin
Use

Candidemia, acute disseminated candidiasis, *Candida* peritonitis and abscesses: Treatment of candidemia, acute disseminated candidiasis, *Candida* peritonitis and abscesses

Esophageal candidiasis: Treatment of esophageal candidiasis

Prophylaxis of *Candida* infections: Prophylaxis of *Candida* infections in patients undergoing hematopoietic stem cell transplantation (HSCT)

Pregnancy Considerations Adverse events have been observed in animal reproduction studies. There are no adequate and well-controlled studies in pregnant women. Use only if benefit outweighs risk.

Breast-Feeding Considerations It is not known if micafungin is excreted in breast milk. The manufacturer recommends that caution be exercised when administering micafungin to nursing women.

Contraindications Hypersensitivity to micafungin, other echinocandins, or any component of the formulation

Warnings/Precautions Severe anaphylactic reactions, including shock, have been reported. New-onset or worsening hepatic impairment, including hepatitis and hepatic failure, has been reported. Monitor closely and evaluate appropriateness of continued use in patients who develop abnormal liver function tests during treatment. Hemolytic anemia and hemoglobinuria have been reported. Increased BUN, serum creatinine, renal dysfunction, and/or acute renal failure has been reported; use with caution in patients that develop worsening renal function during treatment; monitor closely.

Adverse Reactions Frequency of adverse events generally higher following prophylaxis of *Candida* infections in hematopoietic stem cell transplant recipients.

>10%:

Cardiovascular: Tachycardia (3% to 26%), localized phlebitis (with peripheral administration; 5% to 19%)

Central nervous system: Headache (2% to 44%), insomnia (4% to 37%), anxiety (≤23%), dizziness (13%)

Dermatologic: Pruritus (pediatric patients ages 3 days through 16 years: ≤33%; adults 6%), skin rash (2% to 30%), urticaria (pediatric patients ages 3 days through 16 years: ≤19%; adults <5%)

Endocrine & metabolic: Hypokalemia (14% to 18%), hypomagnesemia (6% to 13%)

Gastrointestinal: Diarrhea (7% to 77%), nausea (7% to 71%), vomiting (7% to 66%), abdominal pain (2% to 35%), abdominal distension (pediatric patients ages 3 days through 16 years: 2% to 19%), mucositis (14%), constipation (11%)

Genitourinary: Decreased urine output (pediatric patients ages 3 days through 16 years: ≤23%), hematuria (pediatric patients ages 3 days through 16 years: ≤23%)

Hematologic & oncologic: Neutropenia (5% to 75%), thrombocytopenia (4% to 75%), anemia (pediatric patients ages 3 days through 16 years: 13% to 51%; adults 3% to 10%), febrile neutropenia (≤16%)

Hepatic: Increased serum ALT (pediatric patients ages 3 days through 16 years: ≤16%; adults 5%), abnormal hepatic function tests (pediatric patients ages 3 days through 16 years: <15%; adults 4%), hyperbilirubinemia (pediatric patients ages 3 days through 16 years: <15%; adults <1%)

Renal: Renal failure (pediatric patients ages 3 days through 16 years: <15%)

Miscellaneous: Fever (pediatric patients ages 3 days through 16 years: 9% to 61%; adults 7% to 20%), infusion related reaction (pediatric patients ages 3 days through 16 years: ≤16%; adults <5%)

1% to 10%:
Cardiovascular: Hypotension (6% to 10%), peripheral edema (7%), edema (5%), atrial fibrillation (3% to 5%), bradycardia (3% to 5%), hypertension (3% to 5%), cardiac arrest (<5%), myocardial infarction (<5%), pericardial effusion (<5%)

Central nervous system: Rigors (9%), fatigue (6%), brain disease (<5%), convulsions (<5%), delirium (<5%), intracranial hemorrhage (<5%)

Endocrine & metabolic: Hypocalcemia (7%), hypoglycemia (6% to 7%), hyperglycemia (6%), hypernatremia (4% to 6%), hypervolemia (5%), hyperkalemia (4% to 5%)

Gastrointestinal: Anorexia (6%), dyspepsia (6%)

Hematologic & oncologic: Blood coagulation disorder (<5%), pancytopenia (<5%), thrombotic thrombocytopenic purpura (<5%)

Hepatic: Increased serum alkaline phosphatase (3% to 8%), increased serum AST (3% to 6%), hepatic failure (<5%), hepatic injury (<5%), hepatomegaly (<5%), jaundice (<5%)

Hypersensitivity: Anaphylaxis (<5%), hypersensitivity reaction (<5%)

Infection: Bacteremia (5% to 9%), sepsis (5% to 6%)

Local: Venous thrombosis at injection site (<5%)

Neuromuscular & skeletal: Back pain (5%)

Respiratory: Epistaxis (≤9%), cough (8%), dyspnea (6%)

<1% (Limited to important or life-threatening) or frequency not defined: Acidosis, acute renal failure, anaphylactoid reaction, anuria, apnea, cardiac arrhythmia, cyanosis, decreased white blood cell count, deep vein thrombosis, disseminated intravascular coagulation, erythema multiforme, hemoglobinuria, hemolysis, hemolytic anemia, hepatic insufficiency, hepatitis, hiccups, hyponatremia, hypoxia, increased blood urea nitrogen, increased serum creatinine, infection, injection site reaction, oliguria, pneumonia, pulmonary embolism, renal insufficiency, renal tubular necrosis, seizure, shock, skin necrosis, Stevens-Johnson syndrome, thrombophlebitis, tissue necrosis at injection site, toxic epidermal necrolysis, vasodilatation

Drug Interactions

Metabolism/Transport Effects Substrate of CYP3A4 (minor); **Note:** Assignment of Major/Minor substrate status based on clinically relevant drug interaction potential

Avoid Concomitant Use

Avoid concomitant use of Micafungin with any of the following: Saccharomyces boulardii

Increased Effect/Toxicity There are no known significant interactions involving an increase in effect.

Decreased Effect

Micafungin may decrease the levels/effects of: Saccharomyces boulardii

Preparation for Administration Aseptically add 5 mL of NS (preservative free) or D₅W to each 50 or 100 mg vial. To minimize foaming, gently swirl to dissolve; do not shake. Further dilute 50-150 mg in 100 mL NS or D₅W (when used in children the final concentration should be between 0.5-4 mg/mL; concentrations >1.5 mg/mL should be administered via central catheter). Protect infusion solution from light (it is not necessary to protect the drip chamber or tubing from light).

Storage/Stability Store at 25°C (77°F); excursions permitted to 15°C to 30°C (59°F to 86°F). Reconstituted and diluted solutions are stable for 24 hours at room temperature. Protect infusion solution from light (it is not necessary to protect the drip chamber or tubing from light).

Mechanism of Action Concentration-dependent inhibition of 1,3-beta-D-glucan synthase resulting in reduced formation of 1,3-beta-D-glucan, an essential polysaccharide comprising 30% to 60% of Candida cell walls (absent in mammalian cells); decreased glucan content leads to osmotic instability and cellular lysis

Pharmacodynamics/Kinetics

Distribution: 0.28-0.5 L/kg

Protein binding: >99%; primarily to albumin

Metabolism: Hepatic; forms M-1 (catechol), M-2 (methoxy), and M-5 metabolites (activity unknown)

Half-life elimination: Children: 5-22 hours; Adults: 11-21 hours

Excretion: Primarily feces (71%); urine (<15%)

Dosing

Adult & Geriatric

Aspergillosis (invasive) in HIV-infected patients (off-label use): IV: 100 to 150 mg once daily until infection resolution and CD4 count >200 cells/mm³ (HHS [OI adult 2015])

Candidemia, acute disseminated candidiasis, and Candida peritonitis and abscesses: IV: 100 mg once daily; mean duration of therapy (from clinical trials) was 15 days (range: 10 to 47 days)

Esophageal candidiasis: IV: 150 mg once daily; mean duration of therapy (from clinical trials) was 15 days (range: 10 to 30 days)

Prophylaxis of Candida infection in hematopoietic stem cell transplantation: IV: 50 mg once daily; mean duration of therapy (from clinical trials) was 19 days (range: 6 to 51 days)

Pediatric

Aspergillosis (invasive) in HIV-infected patients (off-label use): IV: Adolescents: Refer to adult dosing.

Candidemia, acute disseminated candidiasis, and Candida peritonitis and abscesses: Infants ≥4 months, Children, and Adolescents: IV: 2 mg/kg once daily; maximum: 100 mg once daily

Esophageal candidiasis: Infants ≥4 months, Children, and Adolescents: IV:
≤30 kg: 3 mg/kg once daily
>30 kg: 2.5 mg/kg once daily; maximum: 150 mg once daily

Prophylaxis of Candida infection in hematopoietic stem cell transplantation: IV: Infants ≥4 months, Children, and Adolescents: IV: 1 mg/kg once daily; maximum: 50 mg once daily

Primary antifungal prophylaxis in allogeneic HSCT (when fluconazole is contraindicated; off-label dosing/population; guideline recommendation): Infants ≥1 month, Children, and Adolescents <19 years: IV: 1 mg/kg once daily; maximum: 50 mg once daily (Science, 2014)

Renal Impairment

No dosage adjustment necessary.

Poorly dialyzed; no supplemental dose or dosage adjustment necessary, including patients on intermittent hemodialysis.

Hepatic Impairment No dosage adjustment necessary.

Administration For intravenous use only; infuse over 1 hour. When used in children, administer infusions >1.5 mg/mL via central catheter to minimize risk of infusion reactions. Flush line with NS prior to administration.

Monitoring Parameters Liver function tests

Dosage Forms Excipient information presented when available (limited, particularly for generics); consult specific product labeling.

Solution Reconstituted, Intravenous, as sodium:
Mycamine: 50 mg (1 ea); 100 mg (1 ea)

Solution Reconstituted, Intravenous, as sodium [preservative free]:
Mycamine: 50 mg (1 ea); 100 mg (1 ea)

◆ Micafungin Sodium see Micafungin on page 1200

◆ Micanol (Can) see Anthralin on page 129

◆ Micardis see Telmisartan on page 1747

◆ Micardis HCT see Telmisartan and Hydrochlorothiazide on page 1748

◆ Micardis Plus (Can) see Telmisartan and Hydrochlorothiazide on page 1748

◆ Micatin [OTC] see Miconazole (Topical) on page 1201

◆ Micatin® (Can) see Miconazole (Topical) on page 1201

◆ Miconazole 3 see Miconazole (Topical) on page 1201

◆ Miconazole 3 Combo Pack [OTC] see Miconazole (Topical) on page 1201

◆ Miconazole 7 [OTC] see Miconazole (Topical) on page 1201

Miconazole (Topical) (mi KON a zole)

Brand Names: US Aloe Vesta Antifungal [OTC]; Antifungal [OTC]; Azolen Tincture [OTC]; Baza Antifungal [OTC]; Carrington Antifungal [OTC]; Critic-Aid Clear AF [OTC]; Cruex Prescription Strength [OTC]; DermaFungal [OTC]; Desenex Jock Itch [OTC]; Desenex Spray [OTC]; Desenex [OTC]; Fungoid Tincture [OTC]; Lotrimin AF Deodorant Powder [OTC]; Lotrimin AF Jock Itch Powder [OTC]; Lotrimin AF Powder [OTC]; Lotrimin AF [OTC]; Micaderm [OTC]; Micatin [OTC]; Miconazole 3; Miconazole 3 Combo Pack [OTC]; Miconazole 7 [OTC]; Micro Guard [OTC]; Miranel AF [OTC]; Mitrazol [OTC] [DSC]; NuZole [DSC]; Podactin [OTC]; Remedy Antifungal Clear [OTC]; Remedy Antifungal [OTC]; Remedy Phytoplex Antifungal [OTC]; Secura Antifungal Extra Thick [OTC]; Secura Antifungal [OTC]; Soothe & Cool INZO Antifungal [OTC]; Triple Paste AF [OTC]; Vagistat-3 [OTC]; Zeasorb-AF [OTC]

Brand Names: Canada Dermazole; Micatin®; Micozole; Monistat®; Monistat® 3

Index Terms Miconazole Nitrate

Pharmacologic Category Antifungal Agent, Imidazole Derivative; Antifungal Agent, Topical; Antifungal Agent, Vaginal

◀ **Use** Treatment of vulvovaginal candidiasis and a variety of skin and mucous membrane fungal infections

Dosing

Adult & Geriatric

Tinea corporis: Topical: Apply twice daily for 4 weeks

Tinea pedis: Topical: Apply twice daily for 4 weeks

Effervescent tablet: Dissolve 1 tablet in ~1 gallon of water; soak feet for 15-30 minutes; pat dry

Tinea cruris: Topical: Apply twice daily for 2 weeks

Vulvovaginal candidiasis: Vaginal:

Cream, 2%: Insert 1 applicatorful at bedtime for 7 days

Cream, 4%: Insert 1 applicatorful at bedtime for 3 days

Suppository, 100 mg: Insert 1 suppository at bedtime for 7 days

Suppository, 200 mg: Insert 1 suppository at bedtime for 3 days

Suppository, 1200 mg: Insert 1 suppository (a one-time dose); may be used at bedtime or during the day

Note: Many products are available as a combination pack, with a suppository for vaginal instillation and cream to relieve external symptoms. External cream may be used twice daily, as needed, for up to 7 days.

Pediatric

Tinea corporis, tinea pedis, tinea cruris: Topical: **Note:** Not for OTC use in children <2 years: Refer to adult dosing.

Vulvovaginal candidiasis: Vaginal: Children ≥12 years: Refer to adult dosing.

Additional Information Complete prescribing information should be consulted for additional detail.

Dosage Forms Excipient information presented when available (limited, particularly for generics); consult specific product labeling. [DSC] = Discontinued product

Aerosol, External, as nitrate:
Desenex Spray: 2% (133 g)
Lotrimin AF: 2% (150 g)

Aerosol Powder, External, as nitrate:
Cruex Prescription Strength: 2% (85 g)
Desenex Jock Itch: 2% (113 g)
Desenex Spray: 2% (113 g)
Lotrimin AF Deodorant Powder: 2% (133 g)
Lotrimin AF Jock Itch Powder: 2% (133 g)
Lotrimin AF Powder: 2% (133 g)

Cream, External, as nitrate:
Antifungal: 2% (14 g, 28 g, 42.5 g) [contains benzoic acid]
Antifungal: 2% (113 g, 198 g) [contains cetyl alcohol, methylparaben, propylene glycol, propylparaben]
Baza Antifungal: 2% (4 g, 57 g, 142 g)
Carrington Antifungal: 2% (141 g) [contains disodium edta, methylparaben, propylene glycol, propylparaben]
Micaderm: 2% (30 g)
Micatin: 2% (14 g) [contains benzoic acid]
Micro Guard: 2% (57 g)
NuZole: 2% (45 g [DSC]) [contains cetyl alcohol, methylparaben, polysorbate 80, propylene glycol, propylparaben]
Podactin: 2% (28.35 g) [contains benzoic acid]
Remedy Antifungal: 2% (118 mL) [contains methylparaben, propylparaben, trolamine (triethanolamine)]
Secura Antifungal: 2% (57 g) [contains cetearyl alcohol, methylparaben, propylparaben]
Secura Antifungal Extra Thick: 2% (92 g) [contains cetearyl alcohol, methylparaben, propylparaben]
Soothe & Cool INZO Antifungal: 2% (56.7 g, 141.7 g)
Generic: 2% (15 g, 28.4 g, 30 g)

Cream, Vaginal, as nitrate:
Miconazole 7: 2% (45 g) [contains benzoic acid]
Generic: 2% (45 g)

Kit, External, as nitrate:
Fungoid Tincture: 2% [contains benzyl alcohol]

Kit, Vaginal, as nitrate:
Miconazole 3 Combo Pack: Cream, topical: 2% (9 g) and Suppository, vaginal: 200 mg (3s)
Miconazole 3 Combo Pack: Cream, topical: 2% (9 g) and Suppository, vaginal: 200 mg (3s) [contains benzoic acid]
Vagistat-3: Cream, topical: 2% (9 g) and Suppository, vaginal: 200 mg (3s) [contains benzoic acid]

Lotion, External, as nitrate:
Zeasorb-AF: 2% (56 g) [contains alcohol, usp]

Ointment, External, as nitrate:
Aloe Vesta Antifungal: 2% (56 g, 141 g)
Critic-Aid Clear AF: 2% (4 g, 57 g, 142 g)
DermaFungal: 2% (113 g)
Remedy Antifungal Clear: 2% (71 g) [contains soybean oil]
Triple Paste AF: 2% (56.7 g) [contains polysorbate 80]

Powder, External, as nitrate:
Desenex: 2% (43 g, 85 g)
Lotrimin AF: 2% (90 g)
Micro Guard: 2% (85 g)
Mitrazol: 2% (30 g [DSC])
Remedy Antifungal: 2% (85 g)
Remedy Antifungal: 2% (85 g) [talc free; contains methylparaben]
Remedy Phytoplex Antifungal: 2% (85 g) [paraben free; contains sodium benzoate, soy protein]
Zeasorb-AF: 2% (71 g)
Zeasorb-AF: 2% (71 g) [starch free]

Solution, External, as nitrate:
Azolen Tincture: 2% (29.57 mL) [contains benzyl alcohol, isopropyl alcohol]
Fungoid Tincture: 2% (29.57 mL) [contains benzyl alcohol]
Miranel AF: 2% (28 g) [contains disodium edta, menthol, propylene glycol, sd alcohol 40b]

Suppository, Vaginal, as nitrate:
Miconazole 7: 100 mg (7 ea)
Miconazole 3: 200 mg (3 ea)
Generic: 100 mg (7 ea)

Midazolam (MID aye zoe lam)

Brand Names: Canada Midazolam Injection

Index Terms Midazolam Hydrochloride; Versed

Pharmacologic Category Benzodiazepine

Use

Anesthesia: IV: Induction of general anesthesia before administration of other anesthetic agents and maintenance of anesthesia as a component of balanced anesthesia

Sedation/anxiolysis/amnesia (preoperative/procedural):

IM: Preoperative sedation, anxiolysis, and amnesia.

IV: Sedation, anxiolysis, and amnesia prior to or during diagnostic, therapeutic, or endoscopic procedures, or prior to surgery.

Oral: Sedation, anxiolysis, and amnesia in children prior to diagnostic, therapeutic or endoscopic procedures or before induction of anesthesia.

Sedation for mechanically-ventilated patients: IV: Sedation of intubated and mechanically-ventilated patients as a component of anesthesia or during treatment in a critical care setting by continuous IV infusion.

Pregnancy Considerations Adverse events were not observed in animal reproduction studies. Midazolam has been found to cross the human placenta and can be detected in the serum of the umbilical vein and artery, as well as the amniotic fluid. Teratogenic effects have been observed with some benzodiazepines; however, additional studies are needed. The incidence of premature birth and low birth weights may be increased following maternal use of benzodiazepines; hypoglycemia and respiratory

problems in the neonate may occur following exposure late in pregnancy. Neonatal withdrawal symptoms may occur within days to weeks after birth and "floppy infant syndrome" (which also includes withdrawal symptoms) have been reported with some benzodiazepines (Bergman, 1992; Iqbal 2002; Wikner 2007).

Breast-Feeding Considerations Midazolam and hydroxymidazolam can be detected in breast milk. Based on information from two women, 2-3 months postpartum, the half-life of midazolam in breast milk is ~1 hour. Milk concentrations were below the limit of detection (<5 nmol/L) 4 hours after a single maternal dose of midazolam 15 mg. Drowsiness, lethargy, or weight loss in nursing infants have been observed in case reports following maternal use of some benzodiazepines (Iqbal 2002; Matheson, 1990). The manufacturer recommends that caution be exercised when administering midazolam to nursing women.

Contraindications Hypersensitivity to midazolam or any component of the formulation; intrathecal or epidural injection of parenteral forms containing preservatives (ie, benzyl alcohol); acute narrow-angle glaucoma; concurrent use of potent inhibitors of CYP3A4 (amprenavir, atazanavir, or ritonavir)

Per respective protease inhibitor manufacturer's labeling: Concurrent use of oral midazolam with amprenavir, atazanavir, darunavir, indinavir, lopinavir-ritonavir, nelfinavir, ritonavir, saquinavir, tipranavir and concurrent use of oral or injectable midazolam with fosamprenavir

Warnings/Precautions [US Boxed Warning]: May cause severe respiratory depression, respiratory arrest, or apnea. Use with extreme caution, particularly in noncritical care settings. Appropriate resuscitative equipment and qualified personnel must be available for administration and monitoring. Initial dosing must be cautiously titrated and individualized, particularly in elderly or debilitated patients, patients with hepatic impairment (including alcoholics), or in renal impairment, particularly if other CNS depressants (including opioids) are used concurrently. **[US Boxed Warning]: Initial doses in elderly or debilitated patients should be conservative; as little as 1 mg, but not to exceed 2.5 mg.** Use with caution in patients with respiratory disease or impaired gag reflex. Use during upper airway procedures may increase risk of hypoventilation. Prolonged responses have been noted following extended administration by continuous infusion (possibly due to metabolite accumulation) or in the presence of drugs which inhibit midazolam metabolism.

Causes CNS depression (dose-related) resulting in sedation, dizziness, confusion, or ataxia which may impair physical and mental capabilities. Patients must be cautioned about performing tasks which require mental alertness (eg, operating machinery or driving). A minimum of 1 day should elapse after midazolam administration before attempting these tasks. Use with caution in patients receiving other CNS depressants or psychoactive agents. Effects with other sedative drugs or ethanol may be potentiated. Benzodiazepines have been associated with falls and traumatic injury and should be used with extreme caution in patients who are at risk of these events (especially the elderly).

Use with caution in patients receiving CYP3A4 inhibitors; may result in more intense and prolonged sedation; consider reducing midazolam dose and anticipate potential for prolongation and intensity of effect. The concurrent use of all protease inhibitors is contraindicated with oral midazolam per their respective manufacturer's labeling. The concurrent use of fosamprenavir is contraindicated with both oral and parenteral forms of midazolam.

May cause hypotension - hemodynamic events are more common in pediatric patients or patients with hemodynamic instability. Hypotension and/or respiratory depression may occur more frequently in patients who have received opioid analgesics. Use with caution in obese patients, chronic renal failure, and HF. Does not protect against increases in heart rate or blood pressure during intubation. Should not be used in shock, coma, or acute alcohol intoxication. **[US Boxed Warning]: Do not administer by rapid IV injection in neonates; severe hypotension and seizures have been reported; risk may be increased with concomitant fentanyl use.**

Avoid intra-arterial administration or extravasation of parenteral formulation. Some formulations may contain cherry flavoring.

Midazolam causes anterograde amnesia. Paradoxical reactions, including hyperactive or aggressive behavior have been reported with benzodiazepines, particularly in adolescent/pediatric or psychiatric patients; may consider

treatment with flumazenil (Massanari, 1997). Does not have analgesic, antidepressant, or antipsychotic properties.

Benzodiazepines have been associated with dependence and acute withdrawal symptoms on discontinuation or reduction in dose. Acute withdrawal, including seizures, may be precipitated after administration of flumazenil to patients receiving long-term benzodiazepine therapy. Midazolam is a short half-life benzodiazepine and may be of benefit in patients where a rapidly and short-acting agent is desired (acute agitation). Tolerance develops to the sedative and anticonvulsant effects. It does not develop to the anxiolytic effects (Vinkers 2012).

Benzyl alcohol and derivatives: Some dosage forms may contain benzyl alcohol; large amounts of benzyl alcohol (≥99 mg/kg/day) have been associated with a potentially fatal toxicity ("gasping syndrome") in neonates; the "gasping syndrome" consists of metabolic acidosis, respiratory distress, gasping respirations, CNS dysfunction (including convulsions, intracranial hemorrhage), hypotension, and cardiovascular collapse (AAP ["Inactive" 1997]; CDC, 1982); some data suggests that benzoate displaces bilirubin from protein binding sites (Ahlfors 2001); avoid or use dosage forms containing benzyl alcohol with caution in neonates. See manufacturer's labeling.

Adverse Reactions As reported in adults unless otherwise noted:

>10%: Respiratory: Decreased tidal volume and/or respiratory rate decrease, apnea (3% children)

1% to 10%:
Cardiovascular: Hypotension (3% children)
Central nervous system: Drowsiness (1%), oversedation, headache (1%), seizure-like activity (1% children)
Gastrointestinal: Nausea (3%), vomiting (3%)
Local: Pain and local reactions at injection site (4% IM, 5% IV; severity less than diazepam)
Neuromuscular & skeletal: Myoclonic jerks (preterm infants)
Ocular: Nystagmus (1% children)
Respiratory: Cough (1%)
Miscellaneous: Physical and psychological dependence with prolonged use, hiccups (4%, 1% children), paradoxical reaction (2% children)

<1% (Limited to important or life-threatening): Agitation, amnesia, bigeminy, bronchospasm, emergence delirium, euphoria, hallucinations, laryngospasm, rash

Drug Interactions

Metabolism/Transport Effects Substrate of CYP2B6 (minor), CYP3A4 (major); **Note:** Assignment of Major/Minor substrate status based on clinically relevant drug interaction potential; **Inhibits** CYP2C8 (weak), CYP2C9 (weak)

Avoid Concomitant Use

Avoid concomitant use of Midazolam with any of the following: Amodiaquine; Antihepaciviral Combination Products; Azelastine (Nasal); Boceprevir; Cobicistat; Conivaptan; Fusidic Acid (Systemic); Idelalisib; Itraconazole; Ketoconazole (Systemic); Methadone; OLANZapine; Orphenadrine; Paraldehyde; Protease Inhibitors; Sodium Oxybate; Telaprevir; Thalidomide

Increased Effect/Toxicity

Midazolam may increase the levels/effects of: Alcohol (Ethyl); Amodiaquine; Azelastine (Nasal); Buprenorphine; CloZAPine; CNS Depressants; Hydrocodone; Methadone; Methotrimeprazine; Metyrosine; Mirtazapine; Orphenadrine; Paraldehyde; Pramipexole; Propofol; ROPINIRole; Rotigotine; Selective Serotonin Reuptake Inhibitors; Sodium Oxybate; Suvorexant; Thalidomide; Zolpidem

The levels/effects of Midazolam may be increased by: Antihepaciviral Combination Products; Aprepitant; AtorvaSTATin; Boceprevir; Brimonidine (Topical); Cannabis; Cobicistat; Conivaptan; CYP3A4 Inhibitors (Moderate); CYP3A4 Inhibitors (Strong); Dasatinib; Doxylamine; Dronabinol; Droperidol; Fosaprepitant; Fusidic Acid (Systemic); HydrOXYzine; Idelalisib; Itraconazole; Ivacaftor; Kava Kava; Ketoconazole (Systemic); Luliconazole; Macrolide Antibiotics; Magnesium Sulfate; Methotrimeprazine; Mifepristone; Minocycline; Nabilone; Netupitant; OLANZapine; Osimertinib; Palbociclib; Perampanel; Propofol; Protease Inhibitors; Rufinamide; Simeprevir; Stiripentol; Tapentadol; Teduglutide; Telaprevir; Tetrahydrocannabinol

Decreased Effect

The levels/effects of Midazolam may be decreased by: Bosentan; CYP3A4 Inducers (Moderate); CYP3A4 Inducers (Strong); Dabrafenib; Deferasirox; Enzalutamide; Ginkgo Biloba; Mitotane; Osimertinib; Siltuximab; St Johns Wort; Theophylline Derivatives; Tocilizumab; Yohimbine

◄ **Food Interactions** Grapefruit juice may increase serum concentrations of midazolam. Management: Avoid concurrent use of grapefruit juice with oral midazolam.

Storage/Stability

Oral: Store at 25°C (77°F); excursions permitted to 15°C to 30°C (59°F to 86°F).

Injection: Store at 20°C to 25°C (68°F to 77°F), excursions permitted to 15°C to 30°C (59°F to 86°F). The manufacturer states that midazolam, at a final concentration of 0.5 mg/mL, is stable for up to 24 hours when diluted with D₅W or NS. A final concentration of 1 mg/mL in NS has been documented to be stable for up to 10 days (McMullin, 1995). Admixtures do not require protection from light for short-term storage.

Mechanism of Action Binds to stereospecific benzodiazepine receptors on the postsynaptic GABA neuron at several sites within the central nervous system, including the limbic system, reticular formation. Enhancement of the inhibitory effect of GABA on neuronal excitability results by increased neuronal membrane permeability to chloride ions. This shift in chloride ions results in hyperpolarization (a less excitable state) and stabilization. Benzodiazepine receptors and effects appear to be linked to the GABA-A receptors. Benzodiazepines do not bind to GABA-B receptors.

Pharmacodynamics/Kinetics

Onset of action: IM: Sedation: ~15 minutes; IV: 3 to 5 minutes; Oral: 10 to 20 minutes; Intranasal: Children: 4 to 8 minutes (Lee-Kim 2004)

Duration: IM: Up to 6 hours; Mean: 2 hours; Intranasal: Children: 18 to 41 minutes (Lee-Kim 2004); IV: Single dose: <2 hours (dose-dependent) (Fragen, 1997); Cirrhosis: Up to 6 hours (MacGilcrhist, 1986)

Absorption: IM: Rapid, complete; Oral: Rapid

Distribution: V$_d$: 1 to 3.1 L/kg; increased in females, elderly, and obesity

Protein binding: ~97%; in patients with cirrhosis, protein binding is reduced with a free fraction of ~5% (Trouvin, 1988)

Metabolism: Extensively hepatic CYP3A4; 60% to 70% of biotransformed midazolam is the active metabolite 1-hydroxy-midazolam (or alpha-hydroxymidazolam)

Bioavailability: Oral: 40% to 50% (Kanto, 1985), ~36% (children); IM: >90%

Half-life elimination: 2 to 7 hours; prolonged in cirrhosis, congestive heart failure, obesity, renal failure, and elderly. **Note:** In patients with renal failure, reduced elimination of active hydroxylated metabolites leads to drug accumulation and prolonged sedation.

Time to peak, serum: IM: 0.5 to 1 hour; Oral: 0.2 to 3 hours

Excretion: IV: Urine (primarily as glucuronide conjugates of the hydroxylated metabolites); Oral: Urine (~90% within 24 hours; primarily [60% to 70%] as glucuronide conjugates of the hydroxylated metabolites; <0.03% as unchanged drug); feces (~2% to 10% over 5 days) (Kanto, 1985; Smith, 1981)

Dosing

Adult Note: The dose of midazolam needs to be individualized based on the patient's age, underlying diseases, and concurrent medications. Consider reducing dose by 20% to 50% in elderly, chronically ill, or debilitated patients and those receiving opioids or other CNS depressants.

Anesthesia: IV:

Induction: Adults <55 years:

Unpremedicated patients: 0.3 to 0.35 mg/kg over 20 to 30 seconds; after 2 minutes, may repeat if necessary at 25% of initial dose every 2 minutes, up to a total dose of 0.6 mg/kg in resistant cases

Premedicated patients: Usual dosage range: 0.05 to 0.2 mg/kg (Barash 2009; Miller 2010). Use of 0.2 mg/kg administered over 5 to 10 seconds has been shown to safely produce anesthesia within 30 seconds (Samuelson, 1981) and is recommended for ASA physical status P1 and P2 patients. When used with other anesthetic drugs (ie, co-induction), the dose is <0.1 mg/kg (Miller 2010).

ASA physical status >P3 or debilitation: Reduce dose by at least 20% (Miller 2010).

Maintenance: 0.05 mg/kg as needed (Miller 2010), or continuous infusion 0.015 to 0.06 mg/kg/**hour** (0.25 to 1 **mcg**/kg/minute) (Barash 2009; Miller 2010)

Sedation/anxiolysis/amnesia (preoperative/procedural):

Manufacturer's labeling:

Healthy adults <60 years:

IM: 0.07 to 0.08 mg/kg 30 to 60 minutes prior to surgery/procedure; usual dose: 5 mg

IV:

Initial: Some patients respond to doses as low as 1 mg; no more than 2.5 mg should be administered over a period of 2 minutes. Additional doses

of midazolam may be administered after a 2-minute waiting period and evaluation of sedation after each dose increment. A total dose >5 mg is generally not needed.

Maintenance: 25% of dose used to reach sedative effect

Adults ≥60 years, debilitated, or chronically ill: Refer to geriatric dosing.

Alternate recommendations:

Intranasal (off-label route): 0.1 mg/kg; administer 15 minutes prior to surgery/procedure (Uygur-Bayramiçli 2002). **Note:** Use 5 mg/mL injectable solution to deliver dose. Due to the low pH of the solution, burning upon administration is likely to occur.

IV: American Society for Gastrointestinal Endoscopy (off-label dosing): Initial: 0.5 to 2 mg administered over at least 2 minutes; slowly titrate to effect by repeating doses every 2 to 3 minutes if needed; usual total dose: 2.5 to 5 mg (ASGE [Waring 2003])

Sedation in mechanically-ventilated patients (off-label dosing): IV: Initial dose: 0.01 to 0.05 mg/kg (~0.5 to 4 mg); may repeat at 5- to 15-minute intervals until adequate sedation achieved; maintenance infusion: 0.02 to 0.1 mg/kg/**hour** (0.3 to 1.7 **mcg**/kg/minute). Titrate to reach desired level of sedation. Titration to maintain a light rather than a deep level of sedation is recommended unless clinically contraindicated (Barr 2013). May consider a trial of daily awakening; if agitated after discontinuation of drip, then restart at 50% of the previous dose (Kress 2000).

Status epilepticus (off-label use): Note: Administered when convulsions last >5 minutes **or** if convulsions are occurring after having intermittent seizures without regaining consciousness for >5 minutes. IM: 10 mg once (Silbergleit 2012) **or** 0.2 mg/kg once (maximum dose: 10 mg) (NCS [Brophy 2012])

Status epilepticus, refractory (off-label use): IV: **Note:** Mechanical ventilation and cardiovascular monitoring required; titrate dose to cessation of electrographic seizures or burst suppression (NCS [Brophy 2012]).

Neurocritical Care Society recommendations (NCS [Brophy 2012]):

Loading dose: 0.2 mg/kg followed by a continuous infusion.

Continuous infusion: 0.05 to 2 mg/kg/**hour** (0.83 to 33.2 **mcg**/kg/minute) titrated to cessation of electrographic seizures or burst suppression. If patient experiences breakthrough status epilepticus while on the continuous infusion, administer a bolus of 0.1 to 0.2 mg/kg and increase infusion rate by 0.05 to 0.1 mg/kg/**hour** (0.83 to 1.66 **mcg**/kg/minute) every 3 to 4 hours. **Note:** A period of at least 24 to 48 hours of electrographic control is recommended prior to withdrawing the continuous infusion; withdraw gradually to prevent recurrent status epilepticus.

Geriatric The dose of midazolam needs to be individualized based on the patient's age, underlying diseases, and concurrent medications. Consider reducing dose by 20% to 50% in elderly, chronically ill, or debilitated patients and those receiving opioids or other CNS depressants.

Anesthesia: IV:

Induction: Adults ≥55 years:

Unpremedicated patients: Initial dose: 0.3 mg/kg

Premedicated patients: Reduce dose by at least 20% (Miller 2010).

Maintenance: Refer to adult dosing.

Sedation/Anxiolysis/Amnesia (preoperative/procedural):

Manufacturer's labeling:

IM: 2 to 3 mg (or 0.02 to 0.05 mg/kg) 30 to 60 minutes prior to surgery/procedure; some may only require 1 mg if anticipated intensity and duration of sedation is less critical.

IV:

Initial: Some patients respond to doses as low as 1 mg; give no more than 1.5 mg in a 2-minute period; if additional titration is needed, give no more than 1 mg over 2 minutes, waiting another 2 or more minutes to evaluate sedative effect; a total dose of >3.5 mg is rarely necessary

Maintenance: 25% of dose used to reach sedative effect

Alternate recommendations: IV: American Society for Gastrointestinal Endoscopy (off-label dosing): Initial: 0.5 to 2 mg administered over at least 2 minutes (smaller doses may be used in the elderly); slowly titrate to effect by repeating doses every 2 to 3 minutes if needed; usual total dose: 2.5 to 5 mg (ASGE [Waring 2003])

Pediatric Note: The dose of midazolam needs to be individualized based on the patient's age, underlying diseases, and concurrent medications. Decrease dose (by ~30%) if opioids or other CNS depressants are administered concomitantly. Children <6 years may require higher doses and closer monitoring than older children; in children with obesity, calculate dose based on ideal body weight.

Sedation/Anxiolysis/Amnesia (preoperative/procedural): Infants ≥6 months, Children, and Adolescents ≤16 years:

Oral: 0.25 to 0.5 mg/kg (maximum: 20 mg) as a single dose 20 to 30 minutes prior to procedure. Children <6 years or less cooperative patients may require as much as 1 mg/kg as a single dose; 0.25 mg/kg may suffice for children 6 to 16 years of age or for cooperative patients. Doses of 0.5 to 0.75 mg/kg administered 20 to 30 minutes prior to procedure have also been suggested; however, doses above 0.5 mg/kg typically do not improve the sedative and anxiolytic effects but increase side effects during recovery (Bozkurt 2007).

IM: 0.1 to 0.15 mg/kg 30 to 60 minutes before surgery or procedure; range: 0.05 to 0.15 mg/kg; doses up to 0.5 mg/kg have been used in more anxious patients; maximum total dose: 10 mg

Intranasal (off-label route): 0.2 to 0.5 mg/kg (maximum total dose: 10 mg or 5 mg per nare); may be administered 10 to 20 minutes prior to procedure (Bozkurt 2007; Chiaretti 2011). **Note:** Use 5 mg/mL injectable concentrated solution to deliver dose. Due to the low pH of the solution, burning upon administration is likely to occur.

IV:

Infants <6 months: Limited information is available in nonintubated infants; dosing recommendations not clear; infants <6 months are at higher risk for airway obstruction and hypoventilation; titrate dose in small increments to desired effect

Infants 6 months to Children 5 years: Initial: 0.05 to 0.1 mg/kg; total dose of 0.6 mg/kg may be required; maximum total dose: 6 mg

Children 6 to 12 years: Initial: 0.025 to 0.05 mg/kg; total doses of 0.4 mg/kg may be required; maximum total dose: 10 mg

Children 12 to 16 years: Dose as adults; maximum total dose: 10 mg

Rectal (off-label route): 0.5 to 0.75 mg/kg (maximum: 20 mg) as a single dose 20 to 30 minutes prior to procedure (Bozkurt 2007).

Sedation in mechanically-ventilated patients (off-label dosing): Infants, Children and Adolescents: IV: Loading dose: 0.05 to 0.2 mg/kg, followed by initial continuous infusion: 0.06 to 0.12 mg/kg/**hour** (1 to 2 **mcg**/kg/minute); range in clinical trials: 0.024 to 0.564 mg/kg/**hour** (0.4 to 9.4 **mcg**/kg/minute) (Hartman 2009)

Seizures (off-label use): Children and Adolescents: IM: 0.2 mg/kg (maximum dose: 6 mg); may repeat every 10 to 15 minutes (AAP [Hegenbarth 2008]; Chamberlain, 1997)

Status epilepticus (off-label use): Children and Adolescents: **Note:** Administered when convulsions last >5 minutes **or** if convulsions are occurring after having intermittent seizures without regaining consciousness for >5 minutes (Silbergleit 2012).

IM (NCS [Brophy 2012]; Silbergleit 2012):
<13 kg: Not evaluated
13 to 40 kg: 5 mg once
>40 kg: 10 mg once

Intranasal: 0.2 mg/kg (NCS [Brophy 2012]) **Note:** Use 5 mg/mL injectable concentrated solution to deliver dose (Ljungman 2000). Due to the low pH of the solution, burning upon administration is likely to occur (Bozkurt 2007).

Buccal: 0.5 mg/kg (NCS [Brophy 2012])

Status epilepticus, refractory (off-label use): Infants, Children, and Adolescents: IV: **Note:** Mechanical ventilation and cardiovascular monitoring required; titrate dose to cessation of electrographic seizures or burst suppression (NCS [Brophy 2012])

Neurocritical Care Society recommendations (NCS [Brophy 2012]):

Loading dose: 0.2 mg/kg followed by a continuous infusion.

Continuous infusion: 0.05 to 2 mg/kg/**hour** (0.83 to 33.2 **mcg**/kg/minute) titrated to cessation of electrographic seizures or burst suppression. If patient experiences breakthrough status epilepticus while on the continuous infusion, administer a bolus of

0.1 to 0.2 mg/kg and increase infusion rate by 0.05 to 0.1 mg/kg/**hour** (0.83 to 1.66 **mcg**/kg/minute) every 3 to 4 hours. **Note:** A period of at least 24 to 48 hours of electrographic control is recommended prior to withdrawing the continuous infusion; withdraw gradually to prevent recurrent status epilepticus.

American Academy of Pediatrics recommendations (AAP [Hegenbarth 2008]):

Loading dose: 0.15 to 0.2 mg/kg followed by a continuous infusion.

Continuous infusion: 1 mcg/kg/minute titrated every 15 minutes by increments of 1 mcg/kg/minute until the cessation of seizures (maximum: 5 mcg/kg/minute)

Renal Impairment There are no dosage adjustments provided in manufacturer's labeling; however, patients with renal failure receiving a continuous infusion cannot adequately eliminate the active hydroxylated metabolites (eg, 1-hydroxymidazolam) contributing to prolonged sedation sometimes for days after discontinuation (Spina 2007).

Intermittent hemodialysis: Supplemental dose is not necessary.

Continuous venovenous hemofiltration (CVVH): Unconjugated 1-hydroxymidazolam not effectively removed; 1-hydroxymidazolamglucuronide effectively removed; sieving coefficient = 0.45 (Swart 2005).

Peritoneal dialysis: Significant drug removal is unlikely based on physiochemical characteristics.

Hepatic Impairment

Severe hepatic impairment (eg, cirrhosis): **Note:** Use with caution in patients with any degree of hepatic impairment; patients with hepatic encephalopathy likely to be more sensitive to midazolam.

Single dose (eg, induction): No dosage adjustment recommended; patients with hepatic impairment may be more sensitive compared to patients without hepatic impairment; anticipate longer duration of action (MacGilchrist, 1986; Trouvin, 1988).

Multiple dosing or continuous infusion: Expect longer duration of action and accumulation; based on patient response, dosage reduction likely to be necessary (Trouvin, 1988).

Dietary Considerations Avoid grapefruit juice with oral syrup.

Usual Infusion Concentrations: Pediatric IV infusion: 0.5 mg/mL **or** 1 mg/mL

Usual Infusion Concentrations: Adult IV infusion: 100 mg in 100 mL (concentration: 1 mg/mL) of D_5W or NS

Administration

Intranasal (off-label route): **Note:** Due to the low pH of the solution, burning upon administration is likely to occur. Use of an atomizer, such as the MAD 300 Mucosal Atomizer which attaches to a tuberculin syringe, can reduce irritation. If possible, based upon dose to be administered, use higher concentration injectable solution to minimize volume administered intranasal. Smaller volume will reduce irritation and swallowing of administered dose. The maximum recommended dose volume per nare is 1 mL.

Using the 5 mg/mL injectable solution, draw up desired dose with a 1 to 3 mL needleless syringe; may attach a nasal mucosal atomization device prior to delivering dose. Deliver half of the total dose volume (of the 5 mg/mL concentration) into the first nare using the atomizer device or by dripping slowly into nostril, then deliver the other half of the dose into the second nare.

Oral: Do not mix with any liquid (such as grapefruit juice) prior to administration

Parenteral:

IM: Administer deep IM into large muscle.

IV: Administer by slow IV injection over at least 2 to 5 minutes at a concentration of 1 to 5 mg/mL or by IV infusion. For induction of anesthesia, administer IV bolus over 5 to 30 seconds. Continuous infusions should be administered via an infusion pump.

Monitoring Parameters

Respiratory and cardiovascular status, blood pressure, blood pressure monitor required during IV administration

Critically-ill patients: Monitor depth of sedation with either the Richmond Agitation-Sedation Scale (RASS) or Sedation-Agitation Scale (SAS) (Barr 2013)

Additional Information Abrupt discontinuation after sustained use (generally >10 days) may cause withdrawal symptoms. For neonates, since both concentrations of the injection contain 1% benzyl alcohol, use the 5 mg/mL injection and dilute to 0.5 mg/mL with SWI without preservatives to decrease the amount of benzyl alcohol delivered to the neonate; with continuous infusion, midazolam may accumulate in peripheral tissues; use lowest effective infusion rate to reduce accumulation effects; midazolam is 3-4 times as potent as diazepam; paradoxical reactions ▶

associated with midazolam use in children (eg, agitation, restlessness, combativeness) have been successfully treated with flumazenil (Massanari, 1997).

Dosage Forms Excipient information presented when available (limited, particularly for generics); consult specific product labeling.

Solution, Injection:

Generic: 2 mg/2 mL (2 mL); 5 mg/5 mL (5 mL); 10 mg/10 mL (10 mL); 5 mg/mL (1 mL, 2 mL, 5 mL, 10 mL); 10 mg/2 mL (2 mL); 25 mg/5 mL (5 mL); 50 mg/10 mL (10 mL)

Solution, Injection [preservative free]:

Generic: 2 mg/2 mL (2 mL); 5 mg/5 mL (5 mL); 5 mg/mL (1 mL); 10 mg/2 mL (2 mL)

Syrup, Oral:

Generic: 2 mg/mL (118 mL)

Controlled Substance C-IV

◆ Midazolam Hydrochloride see Midazolam on page 1202

◆ Midazolam Injection (Can) see Midazolam on page 1202

Midodrine (MI doe dreen)

Brand Names: Canada Amatine; Apo-Midodrine

Index Terms Midodrine Hydrochloride; ProAmatine

Pharmacologic Category Alpha$_1$ Agonist

Use Orthostatic hypotension: Treatment of symptomatic orthostatic hypotension

Pregnancy Considerations Adverse events were observed in animal reproduction studies. Information related to the use of midodrine in pregnancy is limited (Glatter, 2005).

Breast-Feeding Considerations It is not known if midodrine is excreted in breast milk. The manufacturer recommends that caution be exercised when administering midodrine to nursing women.

Contraindications Severe organic heart disease, acute renal disease, urinary retention, pheochromocytoma, thyrotoxicosis, persistent and excessive supine hypertension

Warnings/Precautions [U.S. Boxed Warning]: Indicated for patients for whom orthostatic hypotension significantly impairs their daily life despite standard clinical care. May cause hypertension. Use is not recommended with supine hypertension. Continue therapy only in patients who appear to attain symptomatic improvement during initial treatment. May cause supine hypertension; discontinue use immediately if supine hypertension persists. Use with caution when administered concurrently with vasoconstrictors (eg, phenylephrine, ephedrine, dihydroergotamine, phenylpropanolamine, pseudoephedrine). Use is not recommended in patients with initial supine systolic pressure >180 mm Hg. Due to marked elevation of supine blood pressure (BP greater than 200 mm Hg systolic), use in patients whose lives are considerably impaired despite standard clinical care, including nonpharmacologic treatment (such as support stockings), fluid expansion, and lifestyle alterations. Supine and sitting blood pressure should be monitored. May slow heart rate primarily due to vagal reflex. Use caution when administered concurrently with negative chronotropes (eg, digoxin, beta blockers). Discontinue use if signs or symptoms of bradycardia occur. Desglymidodrine, the active metabolite, is primarily renally excreted; assess renal function prior to initial dose; use with caution in patients with renal impairment (has not been studied) and initiate with a reduced dose; contraindicated in patients with acute renal failure. Caution should be exercised in patients with diabetes, visual problems (especially if receiving fludrocortisone), or hepatic dysfunction.

Adverse Reactions

>10%:

Cardiovascular: Supine hypertension (7% to 13%)

Dermatologic: Piloerection (13%), pruritus (12%)

Genitourinary: Urinary urgency, retention, or polyuria, dysuria (up to 13%)

Neuromuscular & skeletal: Paresthesia (18%)

1% to 10%:

Central nervous system: Chills (5%), pain (5%)

Dermatologic: Rash (2%)

Gastrointestinal: Abdominal pain

<1% (Limited to important or life-threatening): Anxiety, backache, canker sore, confusion, dizziness, dry skin, erythema multiforme, facial flushing, flatulence, flushing, GI distress, headache, heartburn, hyperesthesia, insomnia, ICP increased, leg cramps, nausea, somnolence, visual field defect, weakness, xerostomia

Drug Interactions

Metabolism/Transport Effects None known.

Avoid Concomitant Use

Avoid concomitant use of Midodrine with any of the following: Ergot Derivatives; Iobenguane I 123; MAO Inhibitors

Increased Effect/Toxicity

Midodrine may increase the levels/effects of: Doxofylline; Droxidopa; Sympathomimetics

The levels/effects of Midodrine may be increased by: AtoMOXetine; Beta-Blockers; Calcium Channel Blockers (Nondihydropyridine); Cannabinoid-Containing Products; Cardiac Glycosides; Ergot Derivatives; Linezolid; MAO Inhibitors; Tedizolid; Tricyclic Antidepressants

Decreased Effect

Midodrine may decrease the levels/effects of: Benzylpenicilloyl Polylysine; Iobenguane I 123

The levels/effects of Midodrine may be decreased by: Alpha1-Blockers; Tricyclic Antidepressants

Storage/Stability Store at 20°C to 25°C (68°F to 77°F). Protect from light and moisture.

Mechanism of Action Midodrine forms an active metabolite, desglymidodrine, which is an alpha$_1$-agonist. This agent increases arteriolar and venous tone resulting in a rise in standing, sitting, and supine systolic and diastolic blood pressure in patients with orthostatic hypotension.

Pharmacodynamics/Kinetics

Onset of action: ~1 hour

Duration: 2 to 3 hours

Absorption: Rapid

Distribution: Poorly crosses blood-brain barrier

Protein binding: Minimal

Metabolism: Hepatic and many other tissues; midodrine is a prodrug which undergoes rapid deglycination to desglymidodrine (active metabolite)

Bioavailability: Desglymidodrine: 93%

Half-life elimination: Desglymidodrine: ~3 to 4 hours; Midodrine: 25 minutes

Time to peak, serum: Desglymidodrine: 1 to 2 hours; Midodrine: 30 minutes

Excretion: Urine (Midodrine: Insignificant; Desglymidodrine: 80% by active renal secretion)

Dosing

Adult & Geriatric

Orthostatic hypotension: Oral: 10 mg 3 times daily during daytime hours (every 3 to 4 hours) when patient is upright

Prevention of hemodialysis-induced hypotension (off-label use): Oral: 2.5 to 10 mg given 15 to 30 minutes prior to dialysis session (Cruz, 1998; KDOQI, 2005; Prakash, 2004)

Vasovagal syncope (off-label use): Oral: Initial: 5 mg 3 times/day during daytime hours (every 6 hours) increased up to 15 mg/dose if necessary (Perez-Lugones, 2001; Ward, 1998)

Renal Impairment Orthostatic hypotension: 2.5 mg 3 times daily; gradually increase as tolerated.

Hemodialysis: Dialyzable

Hepatic Impairment No dosage adjustment provided in manufacturer's labeling (has not been studied); use with caution.

Administration Doses may be given in approximately 3- to 4-hour intervals (eg, shortly before or upon rising in the morning, at midday, in the late afternoon not later than 6 PM). Avoid dosing after the evening meal or within 4 hours of bedtime. Continue therapy only in patients who appear to attain symptomatic improvement during initial treatment. Standing systolic blood pressure may be elevated 15-30 mm Hg at 1 hour after a 10 mg dose. Some effect may persist for 2-3 hours.

Monitoring Parameters Blood pressure; renal and hepatic function

Additional Information Single doses as high as 20 mg have been given to patients, but severe and persistent systolic supine hypertension occurs at a high rate (approximately 45%) at this dose. Total daily doses greater than 30 mg have been tolerated by some patients, but their safety and usefulness have not been studied systematically or established.

Dosage Forms Excipient information presented when available (limited, particularly for generics); consult specific product labeling.

Tablet, Oral, as hydrochloride:

Generic: 2.5 mg, 5 mg, 10 mg

◆ Midodrine Hydrochloride see Midodrine on page 1206

◆ Mifeprex see Mifepristone on page 1206

Mifepristone (mi FE pris tone)

Brand Names: US Korlym; Mifeprex

Index Terms RU-38486; RU-486

Pharmacologic Category Abortifacient; Antineoplastic Agent, Hormone Antagonist; Antiprogestin; Cortisol Receptor Blocker

Use

Korlym: To control hyperglycemia occurring secondary to hypercortisolism in patients with endogenous Cushing's syndrome who have type 2 diabetes mellitus or glucose intolerance and who failed surgery or who are not surgical candidates

Mifeprex: Medical termination of intrauterine pregnancy, through day 49 of pregnancy. Patients may need treatment with misoprostol and possibly surgery to complete therapy.

Prescribing and Access Restrictions

Korlym is only available through a restricted access program. For prescriber registration and patient enrollment forms, please refer to http://www.korlym.com/hcp/how-to-prescribe-korlym.php or call 1-855-4Korlym (1-855-456-7596).

Mifeprex: As a requirement of the REMS program, a medication guide must be given to the patient prior to receiving the medication. In addition, the manufacturer recommends distributing a patient agreement form which must be signed by the patient and prescriber confirming the patient's agreement to terminate her pregnancy. A signed copy of the patient agreement should be kept in the patient's medical record.

Mifeprex is only available direct from Danco Laboratories' distributor. To obtain the product, please refer to http://www.earlyoptionpill.com, or call 1-877-432-7596.

Investigators wishing to obtain the agent for use in oncology patients must apply for a patient-specific IND from the FDA.

Medication Guide Available Yes

Dosing

Adult

Hyperglycemia in patients with Cushing syndrome (Korlym): Oral: Initial dose: 300 mg once daily. Dose may be increased in 300 mg increments at intervals of ≥2-4 weeks based on tolerability and symptom control. Maximum dose: 1200 mg once daily, not to exceed 20 mg/kg/day. If treatment is interrupted, reinitiate at 300 mg daily or a dose lower than the dose that caused the treatment to be stopped if interruption due to adverse reactions

Dosage adjustment with concurrent use of strong CYP450 inhibitor therapy (eg, ketoconazole): Maximum dose 300 mg/day

Termination of pregnancy (Mifeprex): Oral: Treatment consists of 3 office visits by the patient; the patient must read medication guide and sign patient agreement prior to treatment:

Day 1 (mifepristone administration): 600 mg (three 200 mg tablets) taken as a single dose under physician supervision

Day 3 (misoprostol administration): Patient must return to the health care provider 2 days following administration of mifepristone; unless abortion has occurred (confirmed using ultrasound or clinical examination): Misoprostol 400 mcg (two 200 mcg tablets); **Note:** Patient may need treatment for cramps or gastrointestinal symptoms at this time

Day 14 (post-treatment exam): Patient must return to the health care provider ~14 days after administration of mifepristone; confirm complete termination of pregnancy by ultrasound or clinical exam. Surgical termination is recommended to manage treatment failures.

Termination of pregnancy (off-label dosing): Mifepristone 200 mg orally followed by misoprostol 800 mcg vaginally 24 to 48 hours later (ACOG, 2014; FIGO, 2011).

Geriatric Hyperglycemia in patients with Cushing syndrome: Refer to adult dosing.

Renal Impairment

Hyperglycemia in patients with Cushing syndrome: Maximum dose 600 mg daily; **Note:** Following doses of 1200 mg daily for 7 days in patients with severe renal impairment (CrCl <30 mL/minute), exposure to mifepristone and its metabolites was increased and a large variability in exposure was observed.

Termination of pregnancy: There are no dosage adjustments provided in the manufacturer's labeling (has not been studied)

Hepatic Impairment

Hyperglycemia in patients with Cushing syndrome:

Mild-to-moderate impairment: Maximum dose 600 mg daily

Severe impairment: Use is not recommended

Note: Following single and multiple doses of 600 mg/day in patients with moderate hepatic impairment (Child-Pugh class B), a large variability in exposure to mifepristone and its metabolites was observed.

Termination of pregnancy: There are no dosage adjustments provided in the manufacturer's labeling (has not been studied); use with caution due to CYP3A4 metabolism.

Additional Information Complete prescribing information should be consulted for additional detail.

Dosage Forms Excipient information presented when available (limited, particularly for generics); consult specific product labeling.

Tablet, Oral:

Korlym: 300 mg [contains fd&c yellow #10 aluminum lake, fd&c yellow #6 aluminum lake]

Mifeprex: 200 mg

Miglitol (MIG li tol)

Brand Names: US Glyset

Pharmacologic Category Antidiabetic Agent, Alpha-Glucosidase Inhibitor

Use Type 2 diabetes mellitus (noninsulin-dependent, NIDDM):

Monotherapy as an adjunct to diet to improve glycemic control in patients with type 2 diabetes mellitus (non-insulin-dependent, NIDDM) whose hyperglycemia cannot be managed with diet alone

Combination therapy with a sulfonylurea when diet plus either miglitol or a sulfonylurea alone do not result in adequate glycemic control. The effect of miglitol to enhance glycemic control is additive to that of sulfonylureas when used in combination.

Dosing

Adult & Geriatric Type 2 diabetes (noninsulin dependent, NIDDM): Oral: Initial: 25 mg 3 times daily at the start of each meal; the dose may be increased to 50 mg 3 times daily after 4-8 weeks and continued for ~3 months; if glycosylated hemoglobin is not satisfactory, may further increase to maximum recommended dose: 100 mg 3 times daily

Renal Impairment

CrCl ≥25 mL/minute: No dosage adjustment necessary. Although miglitol is primarily excreted unchanged, the increased plasma levels in renal impairment are not expected to affect efficacy (clinical response is localized to the GI tract); however, the effects on adverse effects are unknown.

CrCl <25 mL/minute or SCr >2 mg/dL: Use not recommended (not adequately studied).

Hepatic Impairment No dosage adjustment necessary.

Additional Information Complete prescribing information should be consulted for additional detail.

Dosage Forms Excipient information presented when available (limited, particularly for generics); consult specific product labeling.

Tablet, Oral:

Glyset: 25 mg, 50 mg, 100 mg

Miglustat (MIG loo stat)

Brand Names: US Zavesca

Brand Names: Canada Zavesca

Index Terms OGT-918

Pharmacologic Category Enzyme Inhibitor; Glucosylceramide Synthase Inhibitor

Use

Gaucher disease: Treatment of adult patients with mild-to-moderate type 1 Gaucher disease for whom enzyme replacement therapy is not a therapeutic option (eg, due to allergy, hypersensitivity, or poor venous access)

Canadian labeling: Additional use (not in U.S. labeling): Treatment to delay the progression of neurological manifestations in Niemann-Pick type C disease

Dosing

Adult & Geriatric

Type 1 Gaucher disease: Oral: 100 mg 3 times daily; dose may be reduced to 100 mg 1-2 times daily in patients with adverse effects (ie, tremor, GI distress)

Niemann-Pick Type C disease *(Canadian labeling; not in U.S. labeling):* Oral: 200 mg 3 times daily

Pediatric Niemann-Pick Type C disease *(Canadian labeling (not in U.S. labeling):* Oral:

Children <12 years: **Note:** Children <4 years of age were not included in clinical trials; dose based on body surface area (BSA):

BSA >1.25 m^2: Miglustat 200 mg 3 times daily

BSA >0.88-1.25 m^2: Miglustat 200 mg 2 times daily

BSA >0.73-0.88 m^2: Miglustat 100 mg 3 times daily

BSA >0.47-0.73 m^2: Miglustat 100 mg 2 times daily

BSA ≤0.47 m^2: Miglustat 100 mg once daily
Children ≥12 years: Refer to adult dosing.

Renal Impairment
Gaucher disease: Adults:
CrCl 50-70 mL/minute/1.73 m^2: 100 mg twice daily
CrCl 30-50 mL/minute/1.73 m^2: 100 mg once daily
CrCl <30 mL/minute/1.73 m^2: Not recommended
Niemann-Pick Type C disease: Canadian labeling (not in U.S. labeling):
Children ≥12 years and Adults:
CrCl 50-70 mL/minute/1.73 m^2: 200 mg twice daily
CrCl 30-50 mL/minute/1.73 m^2: 100 mg twice daily
CrCl <30 mL/minute/1.73 m^2: Not recommended
Children <12 years:
CrCl 50-70 mL/minute/1.73 m^2: Administer two-thirds of regular dose in 2 equal doses (adjusted for BSA)
CrCl 30-50 mL/minute/1.73 m^2: Administer one-third of regular dose in 2 equal doses (adjusted for BSA)
CrCl <30 mL/minute/1.73 m^2: Not recommended

Hepatic Impairment No dosage adjustment provided in manufacturer's labeling (has not been studied). However, dosage adjustment unlikely because miglustat is not metabolized by the liver.

Additional Information Complete prescribing information should be consulted for additional detail.

Dosage Forms Excipient information presented when available (limited, particularly for generics); consult specific product labeling.
Capsule, Oral:
Zavesca: 100 mg [contains soybean lecithin]

◆ **Migranal** *see* Dihydroergotamine *on page 552*

◆ **Migranal® (Can)** *see* Dihydroergotamine *on page 552*

◆ **Milk of Magnesia** *see* Magnesium Hydroxide *on page 1120*

◆ **Milk of Magnesia [OTC]** *see* Magnesium Hydroxide *on page 1120*

◆ **Milk of Magnesia Concentrate [OTC]** *see* Magnesium Hydroxide *on page 1120*

◆ **Millipred** *see* PrednisoLONE (Systemic) *on page 1493*

◆ **Millipred DP** *see* PrednisoLONE (Systemic) *on page 1493*

◆ **Millipred DP 12-Day** *see* PrednisoLONE (Systemic) *on page 1493*

Milnacipran (mil NAY ci pran)

Brand Names: US Savella; Savella Titration Pack
Pharmacologic Category Antidepressant, Serotonin/Norepinephrine Reuptake Inhibitor
Use Management of fibromyalgia
Pregnancy Considerations Adverse events were observed in some animal reproduction studies. Nonteratogenic effects in the newborn following SSRI/SNRI exposure late in the third trimester include respiratory distress, cyanosis, apnea, seizures, temperature instability, feeding difficulty, vomiting, hypoglycemia, hyper- or hypotonia, hyper-reflexia, jitteriness, irritability, constant crying, and tremor. Symptoms may be due to the toxicity of the SNRIs/SSRIs or a discontinuation syndrome and may be consistent with serotonin syndrome associated with SSRI treatment. The long-term effects of *in utero* SNRI/SSRI exposure on infant development and behavior are not known.

Women inadvertently exposed to milnacipran during pregnancy may be enrolled in the Savella Pregnancy Registry (877-643-3010 or http://www.savellapregnancyregistry.com).

Breast-Feeding Considerations Milnacipran is excreted into breast milk. The manufacturer recommends that caution be exercised when administering milnacipran to nursing women.

Medication Guide Available Yes

Contraindications Use of MAOIs intended to treat psychiatric disorders (concurrently or within 5 days of discontinuing milnacipran, or within 2 weeks of discontinuing the MAOI); initiation of milnacipran in a patient receiving linezolid or methylene blue IV

Warnings/Precautions [U.S. Boxed Warning]: Milnacipran is a serotonin/norepinephrine reuptake inhibitor (SNRI) similar to SNRIs used to treat depression and other psychiatric disorders. Antidepressants increase the risk of suicidal thinking and behavior in children, adolescents, and young adults (18-24 years of age) with major depressive disorder (MDD) and other psychiatric disorders; consider risk prior to prescribing. Short-term studies did not show an increased risk in patients >24 years of age and showed a decreased risk in patients ≥65 years. Closely monitor for clinical worsening, suicidality, or unusual changes in behavior; the patient's family or caregiver should be instructed to closely observe the patient and communicate condition with healthcare provider. A medication guide concerning the use of antidepressants in children and teenagers should be dispensed with each prescription. **Milnacipran is not FDA approved for the treatment of major depressive disorder or for use in children.**

Suicide risks should be monitored in patients treated with SNRIs regardless of the indication. The possibility of a suicide attempt is inherent in major depression and may persist until remission occurs. Patients treated with antidepressants should be observed for clinical worsening and suicidality, especially during initial few months of a course of drug therapy, or at times of dose changes, either increases or decreases. Use caution in high-risk patients. Worsening depression and severe abrupt suicidality that are not part of the presenting symptoms may require discontinuation or modification of drug therapy. Prescriptions should be written for the smallest quantity consistent with good patient care. The patient's family or caregiver should be alerted to monitor patients for the emergence of suicidality and associated behaviors (such as anxiety, agitation, panic attacks, insomnia, irritability, hostility, impulsivity, akathisia, mania, and hypomania); patients should be instructed to notify their health care provider if any of these symptoms or worsening depression or psychosis occur.

Patients with major depressive disorder were excluded from clinical trials evaluating milnacipran for fibromyalgia; however, mania has been reported in patients with mood disorders taking similar medications. May worsen psychosis in some patients or precipitate a shift to mania or hypomania in patients with bipolar disorder. Patients presenting with depressive symptoms should be screened for bipolar disorder. Monotherapy in patients with bipolar disorder should be avoided. **Milnacipran is not FDA approved for the treatment of bipolar depression.**

Potentially life-threatening serotonin syndrome (SS) has occurred with serotonergic agents (eg, SSRIs, SNRIs), particularly when used in combination with other serotonergic agents (eg, triptans, TCAs, fentanyl, lithium, tramadol, buspirone, St John's wort, tryptophan) or agents that impair metabolism of serotonin (eg, MAO inhibitors intended to treat psychiatric disorders, other MAO inhibitors [ie, linezolid and intravenous methylene blue]). Monitor patients closely for signs of SS such as mental status changes (eg, agitation, hallucinations, delirium, coma); autonomic instability (eg, tachycardia, labile blood pressure, dizziness, diaphoresis, flushing, hyperthermia, incoordination); neuromuscular changes (eg, tremor, rigidity, myoclonus, hyperreflexia, incoordination); GI symptoms (eg, nausea, vomiting, diarrhea); and/or seizures. Discontinue treatment (and any concomitant serotonergic agent) immediately if signs/symptoms arise. Potential for severe reaction when used with MAO inhibitors; autonomic instability, coma, death, delirium, diaphoresis, hyperthermia, mental status changes/agitation, muscular rigidity, myoclonus, neuroleptic malignant syndrome features, and seizures may occur; concurrent use with MAO inhibitors is contraindicated. Do not use milnacipran in combination with an MAO inhibitor or within 14 days of discontinuing an MAO inhibitor; do not start an MAO inhibitor until ≥5 days after discontinuing milnacipran. Symptoms of serotonin syndrome may occur with concomitant proserotonergic drugs (ie, SSRIs/SNRIs or triptans), agents which reduce milnacipran's metabolism, or antidopaminergic agents (including antipsychotics). Concurrent use of serotonin precursors (eg, tryptophan) is not recommended. Effects may be potentiated when used with other sedative drugs or ethanol.

May increase blood pressure and heart rate. Preexisting cardiovascular disease (including hypertension and tachyarrhythmias) should be treated prior to initiating therapy. Blood pressure and heart rate should be evaluated prior to initiating therapy and periodically thereafter; consider dose reduction or gradual discontinuation of therapy in individuals with sustained hypertension or tachycardia during therapy. Use with caution in patients with preexisting hypertension, tachyarrhythmias (eg, atrial fibrillation), or other cardiovascular disease; and with concomitant medications known to increase blood pressure or heart rate. May impair platelet aggregation resulting in increased risk of bleeding events, particularly if used concomitantly with aspirin or NSAIDs due to ulcerogenic potential. Data are inconclusive regarding extent of bleeding risk of SNRIs in combination with warfarin or other anticoagulants. Bleeding related to SNRI use has been reported to range from relatively minor bruising and epistaxis to life-threatening hemorrhage. Avoid use in patients with substantial

ethanol intake, evidence of chronic liver disease or hepatic impairment. Cases of increased liver enzymes and severe liver injury (including fulminant hepatitis) have been reported. Discontinue therapy with the presentation of jaundice or other signs of hepatic dysfunction and do not reinitiate therapy unless another source or cause is identified. Use caution in patients with a history of seizures. Use caution in patients with a history of dysuria, especially males with prostatic hypertrophy, prostatitis, or other lower urinary tract disorders. May cause mild pupillary dilation which in susceptible individuals can lead to an episode of narrow-angle glaucoma. Consider evaluating patients who have not had an iridectomy for narrow-angle glaucoma risk factors. SSRIs and SNRIs have been associated with the development of SIADH; hyponatremia has been reported rarely (including severe cases with serum sodium <110 mmol/L), predominately in the elderly. Volume depletion and/or concurrent use of diuretics likely increases risk. Bone fractures have been associated with antidepressant treatment. Use caution in elderly patients; may cause or exacerbate syndrome of inappropriate antidiuretic hormone secretion or hyponatremia. Consider the possibility of a fragility fracture if an antidepressant-treated patient presents with unexplained bone pain, point tenderness, swelling, or bruising (Rabenda, 2013; Rizzoli, 2012).

Abrupt discontinuation or interruption of antidepressant therapy has been associated with a discontinuation syndrome. Symptoms arising may vary with antidepressant however commonly include nausea, vomiting, diarrhea, headaches, light-headedness, dizziness, diminished appetite, sweating, chills, tremors, paresthesias, fatigue, somnolence, and sleep disturbances (eg, vivid dreams, insomnia). Greater risks for developing a discontinuation syndrome have been associated with antidepressants with shorter half-lives, longer durations of treatment, and abrupt discontinuation. For antidepressants of short or intermediate half-lives, symptoms may emerge within 2-5 days after treatment discontinuation and last 7-14 days (APA, 2010; Fava, 2006; Haddad, 2001; Shelton, 2001; Warner, 2006).

Adverse Reactions

>10%:

Central nervous system: Headache (18%), insomnia (12%)

Endocrine & metabolic: Hot flash (12%)

Gastrointestinal: Nausea (37%), constipation (16%)

1% to 10%:

Cardiovascular: Palpitations (7%), increased heart rate (6%), hypertension (5%), increased blood pressure (3%), flushing (3%), tachycardia (2%), peripheral edema (≥1%)

Central nervous system: Dizziness (10%), migraine (5%), chills (2%), depression (≥1%), drowsiness (≥1%), falling (≥1%), fatigue (≥1%), irritability (≥1%)

Dermatologic: Hyperhidrosis (9%), skin rash (3%), night sweats (≥1%)

Endocrine & metabolic: Decreased libido (≥2%), hypercholesterolemia (≥1%), weight changes (≥1%)

Gastrointestinal: Vomiting (7%), xerostomia (5%), abdominal pain (3%), decreased appetite (2%), abdominal distension (≥1%), dysgeusia (≥1%), diarrhea (≥1%), dyspepsia (≥1%), flatulence (≥1%), gastroesophageal reflux disease (≥1%)

Genitourinary: Dysuria (≥2%), ejaculatory disorder (≥2%), ejaculation failure (≥2%), erectile dysfunction (≥2%), prostatitis (≥2%), scrotal pain (≥2%), testicular pain (≥2%), testicular swelling (≥2%), urethral pain (≥2%), urinary hesitancy (≥2%), urinary retention (≥2%), decreased urine output (≥2%), cystitis (≥1%), urinary tract infection (≥1%)

Neuromuscular & skeletal: Tremor (2%)

Ophthalmic: Blurred vision (2%)

Respiratory: Dyspnea (2%)

Miscellaneous: Fever (≥1%)

<1% (Limited to important or life-threatening): Accommodation disturbance, acute renal failure, aggressive behavior, angle-closure glaucoma, anorexia, delirium, erythema multiforme, galactorrhea, hallucination, hepatitis, homicidal ideation, hyperprolactinemia, hypertensive crisis, hyponatremia, leukopenia, loss of consciousness, neuroleptic malignant syndrome (Stevens, 2008), neutropenia, outbursts of anger, parkinsonian-like syndrome, rhabdomyolysis, seizure, serotonin syndrome, Stevens-Johnson syndrome, supraventricular tachycardia, thrombocytopenia

Drug Interactions

Metabolism/Transport Effects None known.

Avoid Concomitant Use

Avoid concomitant use of Milnacipran with any of the following: Dapoxetine; Iobenguane I 123; Linezolid; MAO Inhibitors; Methylene Blue; Urokinase

Increased Effect/Toxicity

Milnacipran may increase the levels/effects of: Agents with Antiplatelet Properties; Alpha-/Beta-Agonists; Anticoagulants; Antipsychotic Agents; Apixaban; Aspirin; Collagenase (Systemic); Dabigatran Etexilate; Deoxycholic Acid; Digoxin; Edoxaban; Ibritumomab; Methylene Blue; NSAID (Nonselective); Obinutuzumab; Rivaroxaban; Salicylates; Serotonin Modulators; Thrombolytic Agents; Tositumomab and Iodine I 131 Tositumomab; Urokinase; Vitamin K Antagonists

The levels/effects of Milnacipran may be increased by: Alcohol (Ethyl); Antiemetics (5HT3 Antagonists); Antipsychotic Agents; ClomiPRAMINE; Dapoxetine; Dasatinib; Glucosamine; Herbs (Anticoagulant/Antiplatelet Properties); Ibrutinib; Limaprost; Linezolid; MAO Inhibitors; Metaxalone; Metoclopramide; Multivitamins/Fluoride (with ADE); Multivitamins/Minerals (with ADEK, Folate, Iron); Multivitamins/Minerals (with AE, No Iron); Omega-3 Fatty Acids; Pentosan Polysulfate Sodium; Pentoxifylline; Prostacyclin Analogues; Tedizolid; Tipranavir; Vitamin E; Vitamin E (Oral)

Decreased Effect

Milnacipran may decrease the levels/effects of: Alpha2-Agonists; Iobenguane I 123; Ioflupane I 123

Storage/Stability Store at 25°C (77°F); excursions permitted between 15°C to 30°C (59°F to 86°F).

Mechanism of Action Potent inhibitor of norepinephrine and serotonin reuptake (3:1). Milnacipran has no significant activity for serotonergic, alpha- and beta-adrenergic, muscarinic, histaminergic, dopaminergic, opiate, benzodiazepine, and GABA receptors. It does not possess MAO-inhibitory activity.

Pharmacodynamics/Kinetics

Absorption: Well absorbed

Distribution: IV: V_d: ~400 L

Protein binding: 13%

Metabolism: Hepatic to inactive metabolites

Bioavailability: 85% to 90%

Half-life elimination: 6-8 hours

Time to peak, plasma: Oral: 2-4 hours

Excretion: Urine (55% as unchanged drug)

Dosing

Adult & Geriatric

Fibromyalgia: Oral: 50 mg twice daily.

Titration schedule: 12.5 mg once on day 1, then 12.5 mg twice daily on days 2-3, 25 mg twice daily on days 4-7, then 50 mg twice daily thereafter. Dose may be increased to 100 mg twice daily, based on individual response. Doses >200 mg daily have not been studied.

Discontinuation of therapy: Upon discontinuation of antidepressant therapy, gradually taper the dose to minimize the incidence of withdrawal symptoms and allow for the detection of re-emerging symptoms. Evidence supporting ideal taper rates is limited. APA and NICE guidelines suggest tapering therapy over at least several weeks with consideration to the half-life of the antidepressant; antidepressants with a shorter half-life may need to be tapered more conservatively. In addition for long-term treated patients, WFSBP guidelines recommend tapering over 4-6 months. If intolerable withdrawal symptoms occur following a dose reduction, consider resuming the previously prescribed dose and/or decrease dose at a more gradual rate (APA, 2010; Bauer, 2002; Haddad, 2001; NCCMH, 2010; Schatzberg, 2006; Shelton, 2001; Warner, 2006).

MAO inhibitor recommendations:

Switching to or from an MAO inhibitor intended to treat psychiatric disorders:

Allow ≥14 days to elapse between discontinuing an MAO inhibitor intended to treat psychiatric disorders and initiation of milnacipran.

Allow ≥5 days to elapse between discontinuing milnacipran and initiation of MAO inhibitor intended to treat psychiatric disorders.

Use with other MAO inhibitors (linezolid or IV methylene blue):

Do not initiate milnacipran in patients receiving linezolid or IV methylene blue; consider other interventions for psychiatric condition.

If urgent treatment with linezolid or IV methylene blue is required in a patient already receiving milnacipran and potential benefits outweigh potential risks, discontinue milnacipran promptly and administer linezolid or IV methylene blue. Monitor for serotonin syndrome for 5 days or until 24 hours after the last dose of linezolid or IV methylene blue, whichever comes first. May resume milnacipran 24 hours after the last dose of linezolid or IV methylene blue.

Renal Impairment

Mild renal impairment: No dosage adjustment necessary.

Moderate renal impairment: Use with caution.

Severe renal impairment (CrCl ≤29 mL/minute): Reduce maintenance dose to 25 mg twice daily; dose may be increased to 50 mg twice daily, based on individual tolerance.

End-stage renal disease (ESRD): Use not recommended.

Hepatic Impairment

Mild-to-moderate hepatic impairment: No dosage adjustment necessary.

Severe hepatic impairment: No dosage adjustment necessary; use with caution

Administration Oral: Administer with or without food; food may improve tolerability.

Monitoring Parameters Blood pressure and heart rate should be regularly monitored; renal function should be monitored for dosing purposes; mental status for suicidal ideation (especially at the beginning of therapy or when doses are increased or decreased); intraocular pressure should be monitored in those with baseline elevations or a history of glaucoma

Dosage Forms Excipient information presented when available (limited, particularly for generics); consult specific product labeling.

Miscellaneous, Oral:

Savella Titration Pack: 12.5 & 25 & 50 mg (55 ea) [contains fd&c blue #2 aluminum lake]

Tablet, Oral:

Savella: 12.5 mg [contains fd&c blue #2 aluminum lake]

Savella: 25 mg, 50 mg

Savella: 100 mg [contains fd&c red #40 aluminum lake]

Milrinone (MIL ri none)

Brand Names: Canada Milrinone Injection; Milrinone Lactate Injection

Index Terms Milrinone Lactate

Pharmacologic Category Inotrope; Phosphodiesterase-3 Enzyme Inhibitor

Use Inotropic support in heart failure: Short-term IV therapy of acutely-decompensated heart failure

American College of Cardiology/American Heart Association heart failure (HF) guideline recommendations (ACCF/AHA [Yancy 2013]): To maintain systemic perfusion and preserve end-organ performance in patients with cardiogenic shock; bridge therapy in stage D HF unresponsive to guideline-directed medical therapy and device therapy in patients awaiting heart transplant or mechanical circulatory support; short-term management of hospitalized patients with severe systolic dysfunction presenting with low blood pressure and significantly depressed cardiac output; long-term management (palliative therapy) in select patients with stage D HF unresponsive to guideline-directed medical therapy and device therapy who are not candidates for heart transplant or mechanical circulatory support.

Pregnancy Considerations Adverse events have not been observed in animal reproduction studies; however, increased resorption was reported in some studies.

Breast-Feeding Considerations It is not known if milrinone is excreted in breast milk. The manufacturer recommends that caution be exercised when administering milrinone to nursing women.

Contraindications Hypersensitivity to milrinone or any component of the formulation

Warnings/Precautions Monitor closely for hypotension. Avoid in severe obstructive aortic or pulmonic valvular disease. Milrinone may aggravate outflow tract obstruction in hypertrophic cardiomyopathy. Ventricular arrhythmias, including nonsustained ventricular tachycardia and supraventricular arrhythmias, have been reported. Observe closely for arrhythmias in this very high-risk patient population; sudden cardiac death has been observed. Due to the prolonged half-life as compared to other inotropic agents, ventricular or atrial arrhythmias may persist even after discontinuation of milrinone especially in patients with renal dysfunction (Cox 2013; Leier 1998). Ensure that ventricular rate is controlled in atrial fibrillation/flutter before initiating; may increase ventricular response rate. In heart transplant candidates, institute appropriate measures to protect patient against risks of sudden cardiac death (Brozena 2004). Monitor and correct fluid and electrolyte problems to minimize the risk of arrhythmias.

Use with caution in patients with renal impairment; reduction in infusion rate recommended. Hypotension may be prolonged in patients with renal dysfunction (Cox 2013; Leier 1998). According to the ACCF/AHA 2013 heart failure guidelines, long-term use of intravenous inotropic therapy without a specific indication or for reasons other than palliation is potentially harmful (ACCF/AHA [Yancy 2013]).

A facility for immediate treatment of potential cardiac events, including life-threatening ventricular arrhythmias, must be available. Safe and effective use beyond 48 hours (prolonged use) has not been demonstrated. An increased risk of death and hospitalization has been observed with prolonged use in NYHA Class III/IV heart failure patients. Sudden cardiac death has been reported with prolonged use. Continuous electrocardiographic monitoring is recommended.

Adverse Reactions

>10%: Cardiovascular: Ventricular arrhythmia (ectopy 9%, NSVT 3%, sustained ventricular tachycardia 1%, ventricular fibrillation <1%)

1% to 10%:

Cardiovascular: Supraventricular arrhythmia (4%), hypotension (3%), angina/chest pain (1%)

Central nervous system: Headache (3%)

<1% (Limited to important or life-threatening): Anaphylaxis, atrial fibrillation, bronchospasm, hypokalemia, injection site reaction, liver function abnormalities, MI, rash, thrombocytopenia, torsade de pointes, tremor, ventricular fibrillation

Drug Interactions

Metabolism/Transport Effects None known.

Avoid Concomitant Use There are no known interactions where it is recommended to avoid concomitant use.

Increased Effect/Toxicity

Milrinone may increase the levels/effects of: Riociguat

Decreased Effect There are no known significant interactions involving a decrease in effect.

Preparation for Administration

Loading dose (optional): May administer undiluted; diluting to a rounded total volume of 10 or 20 mL may simplify the visualization of the injection rate.

Maintenance dose: For a final concentration of 0.2 mg/mL: Dilute 1 mg/mL (20 mL) with 80 mL diluent (final volume: 100 mL) of 1/2NS, NS or D5W. May also dilute 1 mg/mL (10 mL) with 40 mL diluent (final volume: 50 mL).

Storage/Stability

Injection: Store at 20°C to 25°C (68°F to 77°F); excursions permitted between 15°C and 30°C (59°F and 86°F); avoid freezing. Stable at 0.2 mg/mL in 1/2NS, NS, or D5W for 72 hours at room temperature in normal light.

Premixed infusion: Store at room temperature at 25°C (77°F); brief exposure up to 40°C (104°F) will not adversely affect drug; minimize exposure to heat; avoid excessive heat; protect from freezing.

Mechanism of Action A selective phosphodiesterase inhibitor in cardiac and vascular tissue, resulting in vasodilation and inotropic effects with little chronotropic activity.

Pharmacodynamics/Kinetics

Onset of action: IV: 5 to 15 minutes

Distribution: V_d: 0.38 to 0.45 L/kg

Protein binding, plasma: ~70%

Metabolism: Hepatic (minor); majority is not metabolized (Rocci 1987)

Half-life elimination: Normal renal function: ~2.5 hours; Patients with severe heart failure undergoing continuous venovenous hemofiltration (CVVH): 20.1 hours (Taniguchi 2000)

Excretion: Urine (83% as unchanged drug); active tubular secretion is a major elimination pathway for milrinone

Dosing

Adult & Geriatric

Inotropic support in heart failure: IV: Loading dose (optional, not recommended by ACCF/AHA 2013 heart failure guidelines; also see **"Note"**): 50 mcg/kg administered over 10 minutes followed by a maintenance dose titrated according to hemodynamic and clinical response; Maintenance dose: IV infusion: 0.375 to 0.75 mcg/kg/minute; lower initial doses of 0.1 mcg/kg/minute (with final maintenance doses of 0.2 to 0.3 mcg/kg/minute) have also been recommended (HFSA [Lindenfeld 2010]). The ACCF/AHA 2013 heart failure guidelines recommend a maintenance dose of 0.125 to 0.75 mcg/kg/minute (ACCF/AHA [Yancy 2013]).

Note: When initiating an infusion of 0.5 mcg/kg/minute without a loading dose, significant hemodynamic changes seen at 30 minutes with similar effects on pulmonary capillary wedge pressure and cardiac index seen at 2 and 3 hours, respectively, compared to loading dose regimen (Baruch 2011).

Postoperative inotropic support in heart transplant recipients (off-label use): IV: 0.375 to 0.75 mcg/kg/minute; use the lowest effective dose and wean as tolerated over the first 3 to 5 days (ISHLT [Costanzo 2010]).

Renal Impairment Manufacturer recommended adjustment:
CrCl 50 mL/minute/1.73 m²: Administer 0.43 mcg/kg/minute
CrCl 40 mL/minute/1.73 m²: Administer 0.38 mcg/kg/minute
CrCl 30 mL/minute/1.73 m²: Administer 0.33 mcg/kg/minute
CrCl 20 mL/minute/ 1.73 m²: Administer 0.28 mcg/kg/minute
CrCl 10 mL/minute/1.73 m²: Administer 0.23 mcg/kg/minute
CrCl 5 mL/minute/1.73 m²: Administer 0.2 mcg/kg/minute

Alternative Dosing Adjustments in Patients with Renal Impairment[1]

CrCl (mL/min)	Starting dose (mcg/kg/min)		
	0.375	0.5	0.75
50	0.25	0.375	0.5
40	0.125	0.25	0.375
30	0.0625	0.125	0.25
20	Consider alternative therapy	0.0625	0.125
10	Consider alternative therapy		0.0625
5	Consider alternative therapy		

[1]Based on expert opinion

Hepatic Impairment There are no dosage adjustments provided in manufacturer's labeling.
Usual Infusion Concentrations: Pediatric Note: Premixed solutions available
IV infusion: 200 mcg/mL
Usual Infusion Concentrations: Adult Note: Premixed solutions available
IV infusion: 20 mg in 100 mL (total volume) (concentration: 200 mcg/mL) of D₅W
Administration For IV use only. Administer loading dose (optional) undiluted slowly over 10 minutes. Infuse maintenance dose via continuous infusion pump.
Monitoring Parameters Platelet count, electrolytes (especially potassium and magnesium) and fluid status, renal function; ECG, blood pressure, heart rate; infusion site

If pulmonary artery catheter is in place, monitor cardiac index, stroke volume, systemic vascular resistance, pulmonary capillary wedge pressure and pulmonary vascular resistance.

Consult individual institutional policies and procedures.
Dosage Forms Excipient information presented when available (limited, particularly for generics); consult specific product labeling.
Solution, Intravenous:
Generic: 200 mcg/mL (100 mL, 200 mL); 10 mg/10 mL (10 mL); 20 mg/20 mL (20 mL); 50 mg/50 mL (50 mL)
Solution, Intravenous [preservative free]:
Generic: 200 mcg/mL (100 mL, 200 mL)

Minocycline (mi noe SYE kleen)

Brand Names: US Dynacin [DSC]; Minocin; Solodyn
Brand Names: Canada Apo-Minocycline; Dom-Minocycline; Mylan-Minocycline; PHL-Minocycline; PMS-Minocycline; Sandoz-Minocycline; Teva-Minocycline

Index Terms Dynacin; Minocycline Hydrochloride; Ximino
Pharmacologic Category Antibiotic, Tetracycline Derivative
Use
Acute intestinal amebiasis: Adjunctive therapy to amebicides in the treatment of acute intestinal amebiasis
Acne:
Oral (immediate release) and IV: Adjunctive therapy for the treatment of severe acne
Oral (extended-release): Treatment of only inflammatory lesions of non-nodular moderate to severe acne vulgaris in patients 12 years and older
Actinomycosis: Treatment of actinomycosis caused by Actinomyces israelii when penicillin is contraindicated
Anthrax: Treatment of anthrax caused by Bacillus anthracis when penicillin is contraindicated
Asymptomatic carriers of Neisseria meningitides: Oral (immediate-release): To eliminate the meningococci from the nasopharynx of asymptomatic carriers of N. meningitidis
Campylobacter: Treatment of infections caused by Campylobacter fetus
Cholera: Treatment of cholera caused by Vibrio cholerae
Clostridium: Treatment of infections caused by Clostridium spp when penicillin is contraindicated
Gram-negative infections: Treatment of infections caused by susceptible Acinetobacter spp, Escherichia coli, Enterobacter aerogenes, Shigella spp
Listeriosis: Treatment of listeriosis due to Listeria monocytogenes when penicillin is contraindicated
Meningitis: Treatment of meningitis due to Neisseria meningitidis
Ophthalmic infections: Treatment of inclusion conjunctivitis or trachoma caused by Chlamydia trachomatis
Relapsing fever: Treatment of relapsing fever caused by Borrelia recurrentis
Respiratory tract infections: Treatment of respiratory tract infections caused by Haemophilus influenzae, Klebsiella spp, or Mycoplasma pneumonia. For the treatment of upper respiratory tract infections caused by Streptococcus pneumoniae.
Rickettsial infections: Treatment of Rocky Mountain spotted fever, typhus fever and the typhus group, Q fever, rickettsialpox, and tick fevers caused by Rickettsiae
Sexually transmitted infections: Treatment of lymphogranuloma venereum caused by C. trachomatis; nongonococcal urethritis, endocervical, or rectal infections in adults caused by Ureaplasma urealyticum or C. trachomatis; donovanosis (granuloma inguinale) caused by Klebsiella granulomatis; syphilis caused by Treponema pallidum subspecies pallidum, when penicillin is contraindicated
Skin and skin structure infections: Treatment of skin and skin structure infections caused by Staphylococcus aureus
Limitations of use: Not considered a first line agent for any staphylococcal infection
Urinary tract infections: Treatment of urinary tract infections caused by Klebsiella species
Vincent infection: Treatment of Vincent infection caused by Fusobacterium fusiforme when penicillin is contraindicated
Yaws: Treatment of yaws caused by T. pallidum subspecies pertenue when penicillin is contraindicated
Zoonotic infections: Treatment of psittacosis (ornithosis) due to Chlamydia psittaci; plague due to Yersinia pestis; tularemia due to Francisella tularensis; brucellosis due to Brucella spp (in conjunction with streptomycin); bartonellosis due to Bartonella bacilliformis
Pregnancy Considerations Tetracyclines cross the placenta and accumulate in developing teeth and long tubular bones. Rare spontaneous reports of congenital anomalies, including limb reduction, have been reported following maternal minocycline use. Due to limited information, a causal association cannot be established. Tetracyclines may discolor fetal teeth following maternal use during pregnancy; the specific teeth involved and the portion of the tooth affected depends on the timing and duration of exposure relative to tooth calcification. As a class, tetracyclines are generally considered second-line antibiotics in pregnant women and their use should be avoided (Mylonas, 2011). Minocycline should not be used for the treatment of acne in pregnant women, or in males or females attempting to conceive a child.
Breast-Feeding Considerations Minocycline is excreted in breast milk (Brogden, 1975). According to the manufacturer, the decision to continue or discontinue breast-feeding during therapy should take into account the risk of exposure to the infant and the benefits of treatment to the mother. Oral absorption is not affected by dairy products; therefore, oral absorption of minocycline by the breast-feeding infant would not be expected to be ▶

diminished by the calcium in the maternal milk. Nondose-related effects could include modification of bowel flora. There have been case reports of black discoloration of breast milk in women taking minocycline (Basler, 1985; Hunt, 1996).

Contraindications

Hypersensitivity to minocycline, other tetracyclines, or any component of the formulation

Documentation of allergenic cross-reactivity for tetracyclines is limited. However, because of similarities in chemical structure and/or pharmacologic actions, the possibility of cross-sensitivity cannot be ruled out with certainty.

Warnings/Precautions Anaphylaxis has been reported; discontinue drug immediately and institute supportive measures. May be associated with increases in BUN secondary to antianabolic effects; use caution in patients with renal impairment as this may lead to azotemia, hyperphosphatemia, acidosis, and possibly to drug accumulation and potential hepatotoxicity. Serious liver injury, including irreversible drug induced hepatitis and fulminant hepatic failure (sometimes fatal) have been reported with use for acne treatment; use caution in patients with hepatic insufficiency or in conjunction with other hepatotoxic drugs. Autoimmune syndromes (including serum sickness [eg fever, arthralgia and malaise]) have been reported; discontinue if symptoms occur and assess liver function tests, ANA, and CBC. CNS effects (lightheadedness, dizziness, vertigo) may occur; patients must be cautioned about performing tasks which require mental alertness (eg, operating machinery or driving); symptoms usually disappear with continued therapy and when the drug is discontinued. Benign intracranial hypertension (pseudotumor cerebri [PTC]) (including headache, blurred vision, diplopia, vision loss, and/or papilledema) has been associated with use. Women of childbearing age who are overweight or have a history of intracranial hypertension are at greater risk. Concomitant use of isotretinoin (known to cause PTC) and minocycline should be avoided. Benign intracranial hypertension typically resolves after discontinuation of treatment; however, permanent visual loss is possible. If visual symptoms develop during treatment, prompt ophthalmologic evaluation is warranted. Intracranial pressure can remain elevated for weeks after drug discontinuation; monitor patients until they stabilize.

May cause photosensitivity; discontinue if skin erythema occurs. Use skin protection and avoid prolonged exposure to sunlight; avoid use of use tanning equipment or UVA/B treatment. Hyperpigmentation may occur in nails, bone, skin (including scar and injury sites), eyes, sclerae, thyroid, oral cavity, visceral tissue, and heart valves; skin and oral hyperpigmentation are independent of dose or administration duration. Prolonged use may result in fungal or bacterial superinfection, including *C. difficile*-associated diarrhea (CDAD) and pseudomembranous colitis; CDAD has been observed >2 months postantibiotic treatment. May cause tooth enamel hypoplasia, or permanent tooth discoloration; more common with long-term use, but observed with repeated, short courses; use of tetracyclines should be avoided during tooth development (infancy and children <8 years of age) unless other drugs are not likely to be effective or are contraindicated. Do not use during pregnancy. In addition to affecting tooth development, tetracycline use has been associated with retardation of skeletal development and reduced bone growth. Erythema multiforme, Stevens Johnson syndrome, or rash, along with eosinophilia, fever, and organ failure (Drug Rash with Eosinophilia and Systemic Symptoms [DRESS] syndrome) has been reported; discontinue treatment immediately if DRESS syndrome is suspected. Parenteral (IV) formulation contains magnesium; monitor serum magnesium in patients with renal impairment and signs of magnesium intoxication (eg, flushing, sweating, hypotension, depressed reflexes, flaccid paralysis, hypothermia, circulatory collapse, cardiac and CNS depression leading to respiratory paralysis). Also use with caution and closely monitor patients with heart block or myocardial damage. Potentially significant drug-drug interactions may exist, requiring dose or frequency adjustment, additional monitoring, and/or selection of alternative therapy.

Adverse Reactions

1% to 10%:

Central nervous system: Dizziness (9%), fatigue (9%), malaise (4%), drowsiness (2%)

Dermatologic: Pruritus (5%), urticaria (2%)

Neuromuscular & skeletal: Arthralgia (1%)

Otic: Tinnitus (2%)

Postmarketing and/or case reports (Limited to important or life-threatening): Acute renal failure (reversible), autoimmune hepatitis, balanitis, bulging fontanel, *Clostridium difficile* associated diarrhea, DRESS syndrome, enterocolitis, eosinophilia, erythema multiforme, exacerbation of systemic lupus erythematosus, exfoliative dermatitis, fixed drug eruption, glossitis, hearing loss, hemolytic anemia, hepatic failure, hepatitis, hepatotoxicity (idiosyncratic) (Chalasani 2014), hypersensitivity, IgA vasculitis, lupus-like syndrome, malignant neoplasm of thyroid, microscopic thyroid discoloration (brown-black), mucous membrane pigmentation, myocarditis, pancreatitis, pericarditis, pneumonitis, polyarthralgia, pseudomembranous colitis, pseudotumor cerebri, pulmonary infiltrates (with eosinophilia), serum sickness, skin photosensitivity, skin pigmentation, Stevens-Johnson syndrome, thrombocytopenia, thyroid dysfunction, tooth discoloration, vasculitis

Drug Interactions

Metabolism/Transport Effects None known.

Avoid Concomitant Use

Avoid concomitant use of Minocycline with any of the following: BCG (Intravesical); Mecamylamine; Retinoic Acid Derivatives; Strontium Ranelate

Increased Effect/Toxicity

Minocycline may increase the levels/effects of: CNS Depressants; Mecamylamine; Mipomersen; Neuromuscular-Blocking Agents; Porfimer; Retinoic Acid Derivatives; Verteporfin; Vitamin K Antagonists

Decreased Effect

Minocycline may decrease the levels/effects of: Atazanavir; BCG (Intravesical); BCG Vaccine (Immunization); Iron Salts; Penicillins; Sodium Picosulfate; Typhoid Vaccine

The levels/effects of Minocycline may be decreased by: Antacids; Bile Acid Sequestrants; Bismuth Subcitrate; Bismuth Subsalicylate; Calcium Salts; Iron Salts; Lanthanum; Magnesium Salts; Multivitamins/Minerals (with ADEK, Folate, Iron); Multivitamins/Minerals (with AE, No Iron); Quinapril; Strontium Ranelate; Sucralfate; Sucroferric Oxyhydroxide; Zinc Salts

Food Interactions Minocycline serum concentrations are not significantly altered if taken with food or dairy products. Management: Administer without regard to food.

Preparation for Administration Injection: Reconstitute with 5 mL of sterile water for injection. Further dilute in 100 to 1,000 mL of NS, D$_5$W, D$_5$NS, or 250 mL to 1,000 mL of LR. **Note:** Preparation instructions are for the reformulated product (containing magnesium) available as of July 2015.

Storage/Stability

Capsule (including pellet-filled), tablet: Store at 20°C to 25°C (68°F to 77°F); protect from heat. Protect from light and moisture.

Extended-release capsule: Store at 20°C to 25°C (68°F to 77°F); excursions are permitted to 15°C to 30°C (59°F to 86°F). Protect from light, moisture, and excessive heat.

Extended-release tablet: Store at 15°C to 30°C (59°F to 86°F); protect from heat. Protect from light and moisture.

Injection: Store intact vials at 20°C to 25°C (68°F to 77°F). Reconstituted solution is stable at room temperature for up to 4 hours or at 2°C to 8°C (36°F to 46°F) for up to 24 hours.

Mechanism of Action Inhibits bacterial protein synthesis by binding with the 30S and possibly the 50S ribosomal subunit(s) of susceptible bacteria; cell wall synthesis is not affected

Rheumatoid arthritis: The mechanism of action of minocycline in rheumatoid arthritis is not completely understood. It is thought to have antimicrobial, anti-inflammatory, immunomodulatory, and chondroprotective effects. More specifically, it is thought to be a potent inhibitor of metalloproteinases, which are active in rheumatoid arthritis joint destruction.

Pharmacodynamics/Kinetics

Absorption: Oral: Well absorbed

Protein binding: 70% to 75%

Metabolism: Hepatic to inactive metabolites

Half-life elimination: IV: 15 to 23 hours; 18 to 69 hours (renal impairment); Oral: 16 hours (range: 11 to 17 hours)

Time to peak: Capsule, pellet filled: 1 to 4 hours; Extended release tablet: 3.5 to 4 hours

Excretion: Urine, feces

Dosing

Adult & Geriatric

Usual dosage range:

IV: Initial: 200 mg for 1 dose; Maintenance: 100 mg every 12 hours (maximum: 400 mg daily)

Oral: Initial: 200 mg for 1 dose; Maintenance: 100 mg every 12 hours; more frequent dosing intervals may be used (100 to 200 mg initially, followed by 50 mg 4 times daily)

Acne: Oral: Capsule or immediate-release tablet: 50 to 100 mg twice daily

Acne (inflammatory, non-nodular, moderate to severe): Note: Therapy should be continued for 12 weeks. Safety of use beyond 12 weeks has not been established.

Extended-release capsule (Ximino): Oral: 1 mg/kg (rounded to the nearest capsule) once daily
Extended-release tablet (Solodyn): Oral:
45 to 49 kg: 45 mg once daily
50 to 59 kg: 55 mg once daily
60 to 71 kg: 65 mg once daily
72 to 84 kg: 80 mg once daily
85 to 96 kg: 90 mg once daily
97 to 110 kg: 105 mg once daily
111 to 125 kg: 115 mg once daily
126 to 136 kg: 135 mg once daily

Cellulitis (purulent) due to community-acquired MRSA (off-label use): Oral: Initial: 200 mg; Maintenance: 100 mg twice daily for 5-10 days (Liu, 2011)

Chlamydial or *Ureaplasma urealyticum* infection, uncomplicated: Oral, IV: Urethral, endocervical, or rectal: 100 mg every 12 hours for at least 7 days

Gonococcal infection, uncomplicated (males): Oral, IV:
Without urethritis or anorectal infection: Initial: 200 mg for 1 dose; Maintenance: 100 mg every 12 hours for at least 4 days (cultures 2 to 3 days post-therapy)
Urethritis: 100 mg every 12 hours for 5 days

Meningococcal carrier state (manufacturer's labeling): Oral: 100 mg every 12 hours for 5 days. **Note:** CDC recommendations do not mention use of minocycline for eradicating nasopharyngeal carriage of meningococcal

Mycobacterium marinum: Oral: 100 mg every 12 hours for 6 to 8 weeks

Nocardiosis, cutaneous (non-CNS) (off-label use): Oral: 100 to 200 mg every 12 hours

Prosthetic joint infection:
Staphylococci (oxacillin-sensitive or -resistant) oral phase treatment (after completion of pathogen-specific IV therapy) following 1-stage exchange:
Total ankle, elbow, hip, or shoulder arthroplasty: 100 mg twice daily for 3 months; **Note:** Must be used in combination with rifampin (Osmon, 2013)
Total knee arthroplasty: 100 mg twice daily for 6 months; **Note:** Must be used in combination with rifampin (Osmon, 2013)
Chronic oral antimicrobial suppression (off-label use): Oral:
Propionibacterium spp (alternative to penicillin or amoxicillin): 100 mg twice daily (Osmon, 2013)
Staphylococci (oxacillin-resistant): 100 mg twice daily (Osmon, 2013)

Rheumatoid arthritis (off-label use): Oral: 100 mg twice daily (O'Dell, 2001)

Syphilis: Oral, IV: Initial: 200 mg for 1 dose; Maintenance: 100 mg every 12 hours for 10 to 15 days

Pediatric
Usual dosage range: Children >8 years and Adolescents: Oral, IV: Initial: 4 mg/kg/dose for 1 dose; Maintenance: 2 mg/kg/dose every 12 hours (maximum: 400 mg daily)

Acne (inflammatory, non-nodular, moderate to severe): Children ≥12 years and Adolescents: Oral: Refer to adult dosing.

Cellulitis (purulent) infection due to community-acquired MRSA (off-label use): Oral: Children >8 years: Initial: 4 mg/kg (maximum: 200 mg); Maintenance: 2 mg/kg/dose (maximum: 100 mg) every 12 hours for 5 to 10 days (Liu, 2011)

Renal Impairment Use with caution. Consider decreasing dose or increasing dosing interval (extended release).
CrCl ≥80 mL/minute: No dosage adjustment necessary
CrCl <80 mL/minute: Do not exceed 200 mg daily

Hepatic Impairment There are no dosage adjustments provided in the manufacturer's labeling; however, hepatotoxicity has been reported. Use with caution.

Administration
Note: IV administration instructions are for the reformulated product (containing magnesium) available as of July 2015. Refer to the following for additional information: http://links.mkt1283.com/servlet/MailView?ms=MjMwNTcwMzIS1&r=MTI2NjgzODE5NjE3S0&j=N-jAxNDY4MzkzS0&mt=1&rt=0
IV: Infuse over 60 minutes; avoid rapid administration. The injectable route should be used only if the oral route is not feasible or adequate. Prolonged intravenous therapy may be associated with thrombophlebitis.
Oral: May be administered with or without food. Administer with adequate fluid to decrease the risk of esophageal irritation and ulceration. Swallow pellet-filled capsule and extended-release tablet or capsule whole; do not chew, crush, or split.

Monitoring Parameters LFTs, BUN, renal function with long-term treatment, serum magnesium in patients with renal impairment; if symptomatic for autoimmune disorder, include ANA, CBC; ophthalmologic evaluation if visual disturbances occur. If used for syphilis, obtain follow up serologic tests 3 months after treatment.

Test Interactions May cause interference with fluorescence test for urinary catecholamines (false elevations)

Product Availability Ximino: FDA approved August 2015; availability anticipated in fourth quarter of 2015. Ximino is indicated to treat inflammatory lesions of non-nodular moderate to severe acne vulgaris in patients 12 years of age and older. Consult prescribing information for additional information.

Dosage Forms Considerations
Minocin Kit contains minocycline oral capsules packaged with T3 Calming Wipes
Minocin for injection contains magnesium 2.2 mEq per vial

Dosage Forms Excipient information presented when available (limited, particularly for generics); consult specific product labeling. [DSC] = Discontinued product
Capsule, Oral:
Minocin: 50 mg, 75 mg, 100 mg [contains brilliant blue fcf (fd&c blue #1), fd&c yellow #10 (quinoline yellow)]
Generic: 50 mg, 75 mg, 100 mg
Kit, Combination:
Minocin: 50 mg, 100 mg [contains brilliant blue fcf (fd&c blue #1), disodium edta, fd&c yellow #10 (quinoline yellow), sodium benzoate]
Solution Reconstituted, Intravenous:
Minocin: 100 mg (1 ea)
Tablet, Oral:
Dynacin: 50 mg [DSC], 75 mg [DSC], 100 mg [DSC]
Generic: 50 mg, 75 mg, 100 mg
Tablet Extended Release 24 Hour, Oral:
Solodyn: 55 mg [contains fd&c red #40]
Solodyn: 65 mg [contains brilliant blue fcf (fd&c blue #1), fd&c blue #2 (indigotine), fd&c yellow #10 (quinoline yellow)]
Solodyn: 80 mg [contains fd&c blue #2 (indigotine), fd&c red #40, fd&c yellow #6 (sunset yellow)]
Solodyn: 105 mg [contains brilliant blue fcf (fd&c blue #1)]
Solodyn: 115 mg [contains brilliant blue fcf (fd&c blue #1), fd&c blue #2 (indigotine), fd&c yellow #10 (quinoline yellow)]
Generic: 45 mg, 90 mg, 135 mg

♦ Minocycline Hydrochloride *see* Minocycline *on page 1211*

♦ Min-Ovral (Can) *see* Ethinyl Estradiol and Levonorgestrel *on page 703*

♦ Minox (Can) *see* Minoxidil (Topical) *on page 1214*

Minoxidil (Systemic) (mi NOKS i dil)

Brand Names: Canada Loniten
Pharmacologic Category Antihypertensive; Vasodilator, Direct-Acting
Use
Hypertension: Treatment of hypertension that is symptomatic or associated with target organ damage, and is not manageable with maximum therapeutic doses of a diuretic plus 2 other antihypertensives. Use in milder degrees of hypertension is not recommended because the benefit-risk ratio in such patients has not been defined.
Note: According to the Eighth Joint National Committee (JNC 8) guidelines, minoxidil is **not** recommended for the initial treatment of hypertension (James, 2013).

Dosing
Adult
Hypertension: Oral: Initial: 5 mg once daily, increase dose gradually in single or divided doses every 3 days or more (or every 6 hours with careful monitoring if rapid management required) (maximum: 100 mg daily); usual dosage range: 10 to 40 mg (manufacturer's labeling); others have recommended 5 to 10 mg daily (ASH/ISH [Weber, 2014])
Note: Dosage adjustment is needed when added to concomitant therapy. If supine diastolic pressure reduced <30 mm Hg, administer dose once daily; if supine diastolic pressure reduced >30 mm Hg, administer dose in 2 divided equal parts

Dosage adjustment with concomitant therapy: Canadian labeling: Consider initiating minoxidil at a reduced dose in patients receiving strong UGT inhibitors (eg, valproic acid, atazanavir, probenecid)
Geriatric Hypertension: Initial: 2.5 mg once daily; increase gradually (ASH/ISH [Weber, 2014])

◄ **Pediatric**

Hypertension:

Children <12 years: Oral: Initial: 0.2 mg/kg once daily; maximum daily initial dose: 5 mg daily; titrate gradually to effect every 3 days; usual dosage: 0.25 to 1 mg/kg/day in 1 to 3 divided doses (NHLBI, 2005); maximum daily dose: 50 mg daily

Children ≥12 years and Adolescents: Refer to adult dosing

Renal Impairment There are no specific dosage recommendations provided in the manufacturer's labeling; however, the manufacturer suggests that patients with renal failure and/or receiving dialysis may require a dosage reduction.

Hepatic Impairment

US labeling: There are no dosage adjustments provided in the manufacturer's labeling.

Canadian labeling:

Mild or moderate impairment: There are no specific dosage adjustments provided in the manufacturer's labeling; however, a reduced dosage should be considered.

Severe impairment: Use is contraindicated.

Additional Information Complete prescribing information should be consulted for additional detail.

Dosage Forms Excipient information presented when available (limited, particularly for generics); consult specific product labeling.

Tablet, Oral:

Generic: 2.5 mg, 10 mg

Dosage Forms: Canada Excipient information presented when available (limited, particularly for generics); consult specific product labeling.

Tablet, Oral:

Loniten: 2.5 mg, 10 mg

Minoxidil (Topical) (mi NOKS i dil)

Brand Names: US Hair Regrowth Treatment Men [OTC]; Minoxidil for Men [OTC]; Rogaine Mens Extra Strength [OTC]

Brand Names: Canada Apo-Gain; Hair Regrowth Formula; Minox; Rogaine

Pharmacologic Category Topical Skin Product

Use Alopecia: Treatment of alopecia androgenetica of the scalp

Dosing

Adult Alopecia: Topical: **Note:** Continuous therapy for 4 months may be necessary for hair growth.

Females:

Foam, aerosol 5%: Apply 1/2 capful once daily

Solution 2%: Apply 1 mL twice daily

Males:

Foam, aerosol 5%: Apply 1/2 capful twice daily

Solution 2% or 5%: Apply 1 mL twice daily

Renal Impairment There are no dosage adjustments provided in the manufacturer's labeling

Hepatic Impairment There are no dosage adjustments provided in the manufacturer's labeling

Additional Information Complete prescribing information should be consulted for additional detail.

Dosage Forms Excipient information presented when available (limited, particularly for generics); consult specific product labeling. [DSC] = Discontinued product

Foam, External:

Rogaine Mens Extra Strength: 5% (60 g) [contains sd alcohol 40b]

Solution, External:

Hair Regrowth Treatment Men: 5% (60 mL) [contains alcohol, usp, propylene glycol]

Minoxidil for Men: 2% (60 mL)

Minoxidil for Men: 2% (60 mL) [contains alcohol, usp]

Minoxidil for Men: 5% (60 mL, 120 mL) [contains alcohol, usp, propylene glycol, water, purified]

Generic: 5% (60 mL [DSC])

Mipomersen (mi poe MER sen)

Brand Names: US Kynamro

Index Terms ISIS 301012; Mipomersen Sodium

Pharmacologic Category Antihyperlipidemic Agent, Apolipoprotein B Antisense Oligonucleotide

Use Adjunct to dietary therapy and other lipid-lowering treatments to reduce low-density lipoprotein cholesterol (LDL-C), total cholesterol, apolipoprotein B, and non-high-density lipoprotein cholesterol (non-HDL-C) in patients with homozygous familial hypercholesterolemia (HoFH)

Prescribing and Access Restrictions As a requirement of the REMS program, access to this medication is restricted. Prescribers must enroll in the Kynamro™ REMS program and complete the prescriber training and complete, sign, and submit the Prescriber Enrollment Form to the Kynamro™ REMS program. The prescriber must then complete the Prescriber Training before activation within the Kynamro™ REMS program. Pharmacies must educate all pharmacy staff involved in the dispensing of Kynamro™ on the REMS program requirements, put processes in place to verify (prior to dispensing Kynamro™) that the prescriber is certified and the Prescription Authorization Form is received with each new prescription. Pharmacies must also agree to be audited to ensure that all processes and procedures in place are being followed in accordance with the program and be able to provide prescription data to the REMS program.

Medication Guide Available Yes

Dosing

Adult & Geriatric Homozygous familial hypercholesterolemia (HoFH): SubQ: 200 mg once weekly. **Note:** Maximal LDL-C reduction seen after ~6 months.

Renal Impairment No dosage adjustment provided in manufacturer's labeling (has not been studied); use is not recommended in patients with severe renal impairment, clinically significant proteinuria, or receiving hemodialysis.

Hepatic Impairment No dosage adjustment provided in manufacturer's labeling (has not been studied); use is contraindicated in patients with moderate or severe hepatic impairment (Child-Pugh class B or C), active liver disease, or unexplained persistent elevations of hepatic transaminases.

Adjustment for Toxicity

ALT or AST ≥3 x and <5 x ULN: First, repeat measurement within 1 week to confirm elevation. Once confirmed, withhold mipomersen and obtain additional liver function tests (eg, total bilirubin, alkaline phosphatase, and INR); investigate for probable cause. If resumed when AST or ALT <3 x ULN, monitor liver function tests more frequently.

ALT or AST ≥5 x ULN: Withhold mipomersen and obtain additional liver function tests (eg, total bilirubin, alkaline phosphatase, and INR); investigate for probable cause. If resumed when AST or ALT <3 x ULN, monitor liver function tests more frequently.

Clinical symptoms of liver injury (eg, nausea, vomiting, abdominal pain, fever, jaundice, lethargy, flu-like symptoms), bilirubin increase ≥2 x ULN, or active liver disease: Discontinue mipomersen; investigate for probable cause.

Additional Information Complete prescribing information should be consulted for additional detail.

Dosage Forms Excipient information presented when available (limited, particularly for generics); consult specific product labeling.
Solution Prefilled Syringe, Subcutaneous, as sodium [preservative free]:
Kynamro: 200 mg/mL (1 mL)

◆ Mipomersen Sodium *see* Mipomersen *on page 1214*

Mirabegron (mir a BEG ron)

Brand Names: US Myrbetriq
Brand Names: Canada Myrbetriq
Index Terms YM-178
Pharmacologic Category Beta₃ Agonist
Use Overactive bladder: Treatment of overactive bladder (OAB) with symptoms of urinary frequency, urgency, or urge urinary incontinence

Pregnancy Considerations Adverse effects have been observed in some animal reproduction studies. The Canadian labeling contraindicates use in pregnancy.

Breast-Feeding Considerations Mirabegron is expected to be excreted in breast milk. Because of the potential for serious adverse reactions in the nursing infant, the manufacturer recommends a decision be made whether to discontinue nursing or the drug, taking into account the importance of treatment to the mother.

Contraindications

Hypersensitivity to mirabegron or any component of the formulation

Canadian labeling: Additional contraindications (not in U.S. labeling): Severe uncontrolled hypertension (systolic blood pressure ≥180 mm Hg and/or diastolic blood pressure ≥110 mm Hg); pregnancy

Warnings/Precautions Dose-related increases in blood pressure have been reported. Not recommended in patients with severe uncontrolled hypertension (SBP ≥180 and/or DBP ≥110 mm Hg); if used in patients with controlled and less severe hypertension, use with caution and monitor blood pressure closely; exacerbation of pre-existing hypertension has been reported. Use with caution in patients with bladder outlet obstruction (BOO) or in patients taking concomitant antimuscarinic medications; the risk of urinary retention may be increased. Use with caution in patients with a history of QT interval prolongation or those receiving medications known to prolong the QT interval. In one thorough QT study, supratherapeutic doses prolonged the QTc interval based on the individual subject-specific correction method (QTcI) in females but not in males (Malik 2012). In general, mirabegron at the recommended dose has a low risk of QT interval prolongation (Sanford 2013).

Mirabegron is a moderate CYP2D6 inhibitor; potentially significant drug-drug interactions may exist, requiring dose or frequency adjustment, additional monitoring, and/or selection of alternative therapy. Use with caution in patients with mild to moderate hepatic impairment; dosage adjustment is required in patients with moderate hepatic impairment. Use is not recommended in severe hepatic impairment. Use with caution in patients with renal

impairment; dosage adjustment is required in patients with severe renal impairment. Use is not recommended in ESRD. Angioedema of the face, lips, tongue, and/or larynx has been reported; some cases have occurred after the first dose. May be life-threatening. Immediately discontinue and institute supportive care if involvement of the tongue, hypopharynx, or larynx is involved.

Adverse Reactions

>10%: Cardiovascular: Hypertension (9% to 11%)

1% to 10%:
Cardiovascular: Tachycardia (2%)
Central nervous system: Headache (4%), dizziness (3%)
Gastrointestinal: Constipation (2% to 3%), xerostomia (3%), diarrhea (2%), abdominal pain (1%)
Genitourinary: Urinary tract infection (3% to 6%), cystitis (2%)
Infection: Influenza (3%)
Neuromuscular & skeletal: Back pain (3%), arthralgia (2%)
Respiratory: Nasopharyngitis (4%), sinusitis (3%)

<1% (Limited to important or life-threatening): Abdominal distension, angioedema (angioedema of the face, angioedema of the lips, angioedema of the throat, angioedema of the tongue with or without respiratory symptoms), atrial fibrillation, bladder pain, blurred vision, breast cancer, cerebrovascular accident, dry eye syndrome, dyspepsia, gastritis, elevated gamma-glutamyl transferase, glaucoma, increased lactate dehydrogenase, increased serum ALT, increased serum AST, leukocytoclastic vasculitis, lip edema, malignant neoplasm of lung, malignant neoplasm of prostate, nausea, nephrolithiasis, osteoarthritis, palpitations, pruritus, purpura, rhinitis, skin rash, Stevens-Johnson syndrome, urinary retention, urticaria, vaginal infection, vulvovaginal pruritus

Drug Interactions

Metabolism/Transport Effects Substrate of CYP2D6 (minor), CYP3A4 (minor), P-glycoprotein; **Note:** Assignment of Major/Minor substrate status based on clinically relevant drug interaction potential; **Inhibits** CYP2D6 (moderate), P-glycoprotein

Avoid Concomitant Use

Avoid concomitant use of Mirabegron with any of the following: Bosutinib; PAZOPanib; Silodosin; Thioridazine; Topotecan; VinCRIStine (Liposomal)

Increased Effect/Toxicity

Mirabegron may increase the levels/effects of: Afatinib; ARIPiprazole; Bosutinib; Brentuximab Vedotin; Brexpiprazole; Colchicine; CYP2D6 Substrates; Dabigatran Etexilate; Desipramine; Digoxin; DOXOrubicin (Conventional); Edoxaban; Eliglustat; Everolimus; Fesoterodine; Flecainide; Highest Risk QTc-Prolonging Agents; Ledipasvir; Metoprolol; Moderate Risk QTc-Prolonging Agents; Naloxegol; Nebivolol; PAZOPanib; P-glycoprotein/ABCB1 Substrates; Propafenone; Prucalopride; Ranolazine; Rifaximin; Silodosin; Solifenacin; Thioridazine; Topotecan; VinCRIStine (Liposomal)

The levels/effects of Mirabegron may be increased by: Anticholinergic Agents; Ketoconazole (Systemic); Mifepristone

Decreased Effect

Mirabegron may decrease the levels/effects of: Codeine; Metoprolol; Tamoxifen; TraMADol

The levels/effects of Mirabegron may be decreased by: Rifampin

Food Interactions Coadministration with a high-fat meal decreased C_{max} and AUC by 45% and 17%, respectively. Coadministration with a low-fat meal decreased C_{max} and AUC by 75% and 51%, respectively. However, safety and efficacy were unaffected by food intake. Management: Mirabegron may be administered without regard to food.

Storage/Stability Store at 25°C (77°F); excursions permitted to 15°C to 30°C (59°F to 86°F).

Mechanism of Action Mirabegron, a beta-3 adrenergic receptor agonist, activates beta-3 adrenergic receptors in the bladder resulting in relaxation of the detrusor smooth muscle during the urine storage phase, thus increasing bladder capacity. At usual doses, mirabegron is believed to display selectivity for the beta-3 adrenergic receptor subtype compared to its affinity for the beta-1 and -2 adrenoceptor subtypes. Data have shown that beta-adrenoceptors, predominately the beta-3 subtype, mediate detrusor smooth muscle tone and promote the storage function of the human bladder.

Pharmacodynamics/Kinetics

Onset of action: Efficacy is seen within 8 weeks; steady state achieved within 7 days

Distribution: V_{ss}: ~1670 L (following IV administration)

Protein binding: ~71%; binds mainly to albumin and alpha₁-acid glycoprotein

◀

Metabolism: Extensive metabolism via multiple pathways (eg, dealkylation, oxidation, glucuronidation, amide hydrolysis) via multiple enzymes (eg, UGT, esterase, CYP3A4, CYP2D6); two major pharmacologically inactive metabolites produced

Bioavailability: 29% to 35% (following 25 mg and 50 mg oral dosing, respectively); bioavailability is dose-dependent; C_{max} and AUC are higher in females compared to males

Half-life elimination: ~50 hours

Time to peak: ~3.5 hours

Excretion: Urine (radiolabeled drug: 55%; unchanged drug: ~25%); feces (radiolabeled drug: 34%; unchanged drug: 0%)

Dosing

Adult & Geriatric Overactive bladder (OAB): Oral: Initial: 25 mg once daily; efficacy is observed within 8 weeks for 25 mg dose. May increase to 50 mg once daily based on individual patient efficacy and tolerability.

Dosing with concomitant therapy: CYP2D6 substrates: Appropriate monitoring and possible dose adjustment of the CYP2D6 substrate (especially those with a narrow therapeutic index) may be necessary. The Canadian labeling specifically recommends limiting mirabegron to 25 mg once daily in patients receiving concomitant CYP2D6 substrates with a narrow therapeutic index (eg, flecainide, propafenone, thioridazine).

Renal Impairment

CrCl 30 to 89 mL/minute or eGFR 30 to 89 mL/minute/ 1.73 m²: No dosage adjustment necessary.

CrCl 15 to 29 mL/minute or eGFR 15 to 29 mL/minute/ 1.73 m²: Do not exceed 25 mg once daily.

CrCl <15 mL/minute or eGFR <15 mL/minute/1.73 m²: Not recommended (has not been studied).

Hemodialysis: Not recommended (has not been studied).

Hepatic Impairment

Mild impairment (Child-Pugh class A): No dosage adjustment necessary.

Moderate impairment (Child-Pugh class B): Do not exceed 25 mg once daily.

Severe impairment (Child-Pugh class C): Not recommended (has not been studied).

Administration Administer without regard to food. Swallow the tablet whole with water; do not chew, divide, or crush.

Monitoring Parameters Monitor blood pressure at baseline and then periodically during therapy

Dosage Forms Excipient information presented when available (limited, particularly for generics); consult specific product labeling.

Tablet Extended Release 24 Hour, Oral:

Myrbetriq: 25 mg, 50 mg

Mirtazapine (mir TAZ a peen)

Brand Names: US Remeron; Remeron SolTab

Brand Names: Canada Apo-Mirtazapine; Auro-Mirtazapine; Auro-Mirtazapine OD; Ava-Mirtazapine; Dom-Mirtazapine; GD-Mirtazapine OD; Jamp-Mirtazapine; Mylan-Mirtazapine; PMS-Mirtazapine; PRO-Mirtazapine; ratio-Mirtazapine; Remeron; Remeron RD; Riva-Mirtazapine; Sandoz-Mirtazapine; Teva-Mirtazapine; Teva-Mirtazapine OD; ZYM-Mirtazapine

Pharmacologic Category Antidepressant, Alpha-2 Antagonist

Use Major depressive disorder: Treatment of major depressive disorder (MDD)

Pregnancy Considerations Adverse events were observed in some animal reproduction studies. A significant increase in major teratogenic effects has not been observed in humans following exposure to mirtazapine during pregnancy; however, some nonteratogenic adverse events (similar to those observed with SSRI agents) have been reported (Djulus, 2006; Einarson, 2009; Lennestål,

2007). Mirtazapine was found to cross the placenta following a maternal overdose (Hatzidaki, 2008).

The ACOG recommends that therapy with antidepressants during pregnancy be individualized; treatment of depression during pregnancy should incorporate the clinical expertise of the mental health clinician, obstetrician, primary healthcare provider, and pediatrician. According to the American Psychiatric Association (APA), the risks of medication treatment should be weighed against other treatment options and untreated depression. Consideration should be given to using agents with safety data in pregnancy. For women who discontinue antidepressant medications during pregnancy and who may be at high risk for postpartum depression, the medications can be restarted following delivery. Treatment algorithms have been developed by the ACOG and the APA for the management of depression in women prior to conception and during pregnancy (ACOG, 2008; APA, 2010; Yonkers, 2009).

Breast-Feeding Considerations Mirtazapine and its active metabolite are found in breast milk, with higher levels in the hindmilk than foremilk. Mirtazapine can also be detected in the serum of nursing infants; adverse events have generally not been observed, although possible sedation and weight gain was noted in one case report (Kristensen, 2007; Tonn, 2009). The manufacturer recommends that caution be used if administered to a breast-feeding woman.

Medication Guide Available Yes

Contraindications Hypersensitivity to mirtazapine or any component of the formulation; use of MAO inhibitors intended to treat psychiatric disorders (concurrently or within 14 days of discontinuing either mirtazapine or the MAO inhibitor); initiation of mirtazapine in a patient receiving linezolid or intravenous methylene blue

Warnings/Precautions [U.S. Boxed Warning]: Antidepressants increase the risk of suicidal thinking and behavior in children, adolescents, and young adults (18-24 years of age) with major depressive disorder (MDD) and other psychiatric disorders; consider risk prior to prescribing. Short-term studies did not show an increased risk in patients >24 years of age and showed a decreased risk in patients ≥65 years. Closely monitor for clinical worsening, suicidality, or unusual changes in behavior, particularly during the initial 1 to 2 months of therapy or during periods of dosage adjustments (increases or decreases); the patient's family or caregiver should be instructed to closely observe the patient and communicate condition with healthcare provider. A medication guide should be dispensed with each prescription. **Mirtazapine is not FDA approved for use in children.**

The possibility of a suicide attempt is inherent in major depression and may persist until remission occurs. Worsening depression and severe abrupt suicidality that are not part of the presenting symptoms may require discontinuation or modification of drug therapy. The patient's family or caregiver should be alerted to monitor patients for the emergence of suicidality and associated behaviors (such as agitation, irritability, hostility, impulsivity, and hypomania) and call health care provider.

May precipitate a shift to mania or hypomania in patients with bipolar disorder. Patients presenting with depressive symptoms should be screened for bipolar disorder. Monotherapy in patients with bipolar disorder should be avoided. **Mirtazapine is not FDA approved for the treatment of bipolar depression.**

Potentially life-threatening serotonin syndrome (SS) has occurred with serotonergic agents (eg, SSRIs, SNRIs), particularly when used in combination with other serotonergic agents (eg, triptans, TCAs, fentanyl, lithium, tramadol, buspirone, St John's wort, tryptophan) or agents that impair metabolism of serotonin (eg, MAO inhibitors intended to treat psychiatric disorders, other MAO inhibitors such as linezolid and intravenous methylene blue). Discontinue treatment (and any concomitant serotonergic agent) immediately if signs/symptoms arise. Discontinue immediately if signs and symptoms of neutropenia/agranulocytosis occur. May cause CNS depression, which may impair physical or mental abilities; patients must be cautioned about performing tasks that require mental alertness (eg, operating machinery or driving). The degree of sedation is moderate-high relative to other antidepressants. Conversely, may increase psychomotor restlessness within first few weeks of therapy. Dizziness may occur; it is unclear whether or not tolerance may develop to dizziness. The risks of orthostatic hypotension or anticholinergic effects are low relative to other antidepressants. The incidence of sexual dysfunction with mirtazapine is generally lower than with selective serotonin reuptake inhibitors (SSRIs) (Bauer, 2013). May increase appetite and

stimulate weight gain. May increase serum cholesterol and triglyceride levels. Potentially significant interactions may exist, requiring dose or frequency adjustment, additional monitoring, and/or selection of alternative therapy.

QT prolongation, torsade de pointes, and ventricular fibrillation have been reported (rarely) (Remeron Canadian product monograph, 2014); case reports are mostly associated with mirtazapine overdose (although one case series of single-agent mirtazapine overdose in 84 patients did not identify any cases of QT prolongation [Berling, 2014]) or patients with risk factors for QT prolongation or receiving concomitant QT-prolonging agents. Use caution in patients with cardiovascular disease, history of QT prolongation, or receiving concomitant QT-prolonging agents.

Use caution in patients with a previous seizure disorder or condition predisposing to seizures such as brain damage, alcoholism, or concurrent therapy with other drugs which lower the seizure threshold. May cause mild pupillary dilation which in susceptible individuals can lead to an episode of narrow-angle glaucoma. Consider evaluating patients who have not had an iridectomy for narrow-angle glaucoma risk factors. Bone fractures have been associated with antidepressant treatment. Consider the possibility of a fragility fracture if an antidepressant-treated patient presents with unexplained bone pain, point tenderness, swelling, or bruising (Rabenda, 2013; Rizzoli, 2012). Use with caution in patients with hepatic or renal dysfunction. Use caution in elderly patients; may cause or exacerbate syndrome of inappropriate antidiuretic hormone secretion or hyponatremia; monitor sodium closely with initiation or dosage adjustments in older adults (Beers Criteria). Clinically significant transaminase elevations have been observed. SolTab formulation contains phenylalanine.

Abrupt discontinuation or interruption of antidepressant therapy has been associated with a discontinuation syndrome. Symptoms arising may vary with antidepressant however commonly include nausea, vomiting, diarrhea, headaches, lightheadedness, dizziness, diminished appetite, sweating, chills, tremors, paresthesias, fatigue, somnolence, and sleep disturbances (eg, vivid dreams, insomnia). Greater risks for developing a discontinuation syndrome have been associated with antidepressants with shorter half-lives, longer durations of treatment, and abrupt discontinuation. For antidepressants of short or intermediate half-lives, symptoms may emerge within 2 to 5 days after treatment discontinuation and last 7 to 14 days (APA, 2010; Fava, 2006; Haddad, 2001; Shelton, 2001; Warner, 2006).

Adverse Reactions

>10%:

Central nervous system: Drowsiness (54%)

Endocrine & metabolic: Increased serum cholesterol (15%), weight gain (12%; weight gain of >7% reported in 8% of adults, 49% of pediatric patients)

Gastrointestinal: Xerostomia (25%), increased appetite (17%), constipation (13%)

1% to 10%:

Cardiovascular: Peripheral edema (2%), edema (1%), hypertension, vasodilatation

Central nervous system: Dizziness (7%), abnormal dreams (4%), abnormality in thinking (3%), confusion (2%), agitation, amnesia, anxiety, apathy, depression, hypoesthesia, malaise, myasthenia, paresthesia, twitching, vertigo

Dermatologic: Pruritus, skin rash

Endocrine & metabolic: Increased serum triglycerides (6%), increased thirst

Gastrointestinal: Abdominal pain, anorexia, vomiting

Genitourinary: Urinary frequency (2%), urinary tract infection

Hepatic: Increased serum ALT (≥3 times ULN: 2%)

Neuromuscular & skeletal: Weakness (8%), back pain (2%), myalgia (2%), tremor (2%), arthralgia, hyperkinesia, hypokinesia

Respiratory: Flu-like symptoms (5%), dyspnea (1%), increased cough, sinusitis

<1% (Limited to important or life-threatening): Abnormal accommodation, abnormal healing, abnormal hepatic function tests, abnormal lacrimation, alopecia, altered sense of smell, amenorrhea, aphasia, arthritis, asphyxia, asthma, atrial arrhythmia, bigeminy, blepharitis, bradycardia, breast engorgement, breast hypertrophy, bursitis, cellulitis, cerebral ischemia, cholecystitis, colitis, conjunctivitis, cystitis, deafness, dehydration, delirium, dementia, depersonalization, diabetes mellitus, diarrhea, diplopia, drug dependence, dysmenorrhea, ejaculatory disorder, emotional lability, enlargement of abdomen, eosinophilia, erythema multiforme, exfoliative dermatitis, extrapyramidal reaction, facial edema, gastroenteritis, gingival hemorrhage, glaucoma, glossitis, gout, hepatic cirrhosis, herpes simplex infection, herpes zoster, hyperacusis,

hyper-reflexia, hypotension, hypothyroidism, hypotonia, impotence, increased acid phosphatase, increased libido, insomnia, intestinal obstruction, laryngitis, left heart failure, leukorrhea, lymphadenopathy, lymphocytosis, migraine, myocardial infarction, myoclonus, myositis, neck pain, nephrolithiasis, nystagmus, oral candidiasis, ostealgia, osteoporosis, otalgia, pancreatitis, pancytopenia, paralysis, phlebitis, pneumonia, pneumothorax, prolonged Q-T interval on ECG, psychomotor agitation, psychoneurosis, psychotic depression, pulmonary embolism, restless leg syndrome, seborrhea, sedation, seizure, serotonin syndrome, skin hypertrophy, skin photosensitivity, stomatitis, suicidal behavior, syncope, tenosynovitis, torsade de pointes (rare), urethritis, urinary incontinence, urinary retention, urinary urgency, uterine hemorrhage, vaginitis, vascular headache, ventricular fibrillation, ventricular premature contractions, ventricular tachycardia

Drug Interactions

Metabolism/Transport Effects Substrate of CYP1A2 (major), CYP2C9 (minor), CYP2D6 (major), CYP3A4 (major); **Note:** Assignment of Major/Minor substrate status based on clinically relevant drug interaction potential; **Inhibits** CYP1A2 (weak)

Avoid Concomitant Use

Avoid concomitant use of Mirtazapine with any of the following: Alcohol (Ethyl); Azelastine (Nasal); Conivaptan; Dapoxetine; Fusidic Acid (Systemic); Idelalisib; Linezolid; MAO Inhibitors; Methylene Blue; Orphenadrine; Paraldehyde; Thalidomide; Tryptophan

Increased Effect/Toxicity

Mirtazapine may increase the levels/effects of: Azelastine (Nasal); Buprenorphine; Highest Risk QTc-Prolonging Agents; Hydrocodone; Methotrimeprazine; Methylene Blue; Metoclopramide; Metyrosine; Moderate Risk QTc-Prolonging Agents; Orphenadrine; Paraldehyde; Pramipexole; ROPINIRole; Rotigotine; Serotonin Modulators; Suvorexant; Thalidomide; TiZANidine; Warfarin; Zolpidem

The levels/effects of Mirtazapine may be increased by: Abiraterone Acetate; Alcohol (Ethyl); Antiemetics (5HT3 Antagonists); Aprepitant; Brimonidine (Topical); Cannabis; CNS Depressants; Conivaptan; CYP1A2 Inhibitors (Moderate); CYP1A2 Inhibitors (Strong); CYP2D6 Inhibitors (Moderate); CYP2D6 Inhibitors (Strong); CYP3A4 Inhibitors (Moderate); CYP3A4 Inhibitors (Strong); Dapoxetine; Dasatinib; Deferasirox; Doxylamine; Dronabinol; Droperidol; Fosaprepitant; Fusidic Acid (Systemic); HydrOXYzine; Idelalisib; Ivacaftor; Kava Kava; Linezolid; Luliconazole; Magnesium Sulfate; MAO Inhibitors; Metaxalone; Methotrimeprazine; Mifepristone; Minocycline; Nabilone; Netupitant; Osimertinib; Palbociclib; Panobinostat; Peginterferon Alfa-2b; Perampanel; Rufinamide; Simeprevir; Sodium Oxybate; Stiripentol; Tapentadol; Tedizolid; Tetrahydrocannabinol; Tryptophan; Vemurafenib

Decreased Effect

Mirtazapine may decrease the levels/effects of: Alpha2-Agonists

The levels/effects of Mirtazapine may be decreased by: Bosentan; Cannabis; CYP1A2 Inducers (Strong); CYP3A4 Inducers (Moderate); CYP3A4 Inducers (Strong); Cyproterone; Dabrafenib; Deferasirox; Enzalutamide; Mitotane; Osimertinib; Peginterferon Alfa-2b; Siltuximab; St Johns Wort; Teriflunomide; Tocilizumab

Storage/Stability Store at 25°C (77°F); excursions are permitted between 15°C and 30°C (59°F and 86°F). Protect from light and moisture. Use orally disintegrating tablets immediately upon opening individual tablet blister; once removed it cannot be stored.

Mechanism of Action Mirtazapine is a tetracyclic antidepressant that works by its central presynaptic alpha$_2$-adrenergic antagonist effects, which results in increased release of norepinephrine and serotonin. It is also a potent antagonist of 5-HT$_2$ and 5-HT$_3$ serotonin receptors and H$_1$ histamine receptors and a moderate peripheral alpha$_1$-adrenergic and muscarinic antagonist; it does not inhibit the reuptake of norepinephrine or serotonin.

Pharmacodynamics/Kinetics

Absorption: Rapid and complete

Protein binding: ~85%

Metabolism: Extensively hepatic via CYP1A2, 2D6, 3A4 and via demethylation and hydroxylation

Bioavailability: ~50%

Half-life elimination: 20 to 40 hours; increased with renal or hepatic impairment

Time to peak, serum: ~2 hours

Excretion: Urine (75%) and feces (15%) as metabolites

◄ **Dosing**
Adult

Major depressive disorder (MDD): Oral: Initial: 15 mg nightly, may titrate dose up no more frequently than every 1 to 2 weeks to a maximum of 45 mg daily; dosage range: 15 to 45 mg daily

Discontinuation of therapy: Upon discontinuation of antidepressant therapy, gradually taper the dose to minimize the incidence of withdrawal symptoms and allow for the detection of re-emerging symptoms. Evidence supporting ideal taper rates is limited. APA and NICE guidelines suggest tapering therapy over at least several weeks with consideration to the half-life of the antidepressant; antidepressants with a shorter half-life may need to be tapered more conservatively. In addition for long-term treated patients, WFSBP guidelines recommend tapering over 4-6 months. If intolerable withdrawal symptoms occur following a dose reduction, consider resuming the previously prescribed dose and/or decrease dose at a more gradual rate (APA, 2010; Bauer, 2002; Haddad, 2001; NCCMH, 2010; Schatzberg, 2006; Shelton, 2001; Warner, 2006).

MAO inhibitor recommendations:
Switching to or from an MAO inhibitor intended to treat psychiatric disorders:
Allow 14 days to elapse between discontinuing an MAO inhibitor intended to treat psychiatric disorders and initiation of mirtazapine.
Allow 14 days to elapse between discontinuing mirtazapine and initiation of an MAO inhibitor intended to treat psychiatric disorders.
Use with other MAO inhibitors (linezolid or IV methylene blue):
Do not initiate mirtazapine in patients receiving linezolid or IV methylene blue; consider other interventions for psychiatric condition.
If urgent treatment with linezolid or IV methylene blue is required in a patient already receiving mirtazapine and potential benefits outweigh potential risks, discontinue mirtazapine promptly and administer linezolid or IV methylene blue. Monitor for serotonin syndrome for 2 weeks or until 24 hours after the last dose of linezolid or IV methylene blue, whichever comes first. May resume mirtazapine 24 hours after the last dose of linezolid or IV methylene blue.

Geriatric There are no dosage adjustments provided in the manufacturer's labeling; however, clearance may be decreased in the elderly. Use with caution.

Discontinuation of therapy: Refer to adult dosing.
MAO inhibitor recommendations: Refer to adult dosing.

Renal Impairment There are no dosage adjustments provided in the manufacturer's labeling; however, clearance is decreased with moderate and severe renal impairment. Use with caution.

Hepatic Impairment There are no dosage adjustments provided in the manufacturer's labeling; however, clearance may be decreased with hepatic impairment. Use with caution.

Dietary Considerations Some products may contain phenylalanine.

Administration

Orally disintegrating tablet: Administer without regard to meals. Open blister pack and place tablet on the tongue; tablet is formulated to dissolve on the tongue without water; do not split tablet.

Tablet: Administer without regard to meals. The Canadian labeling recommends the tablet be swallowed with water and not be chewed.

Monitoring Parameters Patients should be monitored for signs of agranulocytosis or severe neutropenia such as sore throat, stomatitis or other signs of infection or a low WBC; renal and hepatic function; mental status for depression, suicide ideation (especially at the beginning of therapy or when doses are increased or decreased), anxiety, social functioning, mania, panic attacks; signs/symptoms of serotonin syndrome; lipid profile; weight gain

Dosage Forms Excipient information presented when available (limited, particularly for generics); consult specific product labeling.
Tablet, Oral:
Remeron: 15 mg, 30 mg [scored]
Remeron: 45 mg
Generic: 7.5 mg, 15 mg, 30 mg, 45 mg
Tablet Dispersible, Oral:
Remeron SolTab: 15 mg, 30 mg, 45 mg [contains aspartame]
Generic: 15 mg, 30 mg, 45 mg

◆ Mirvaso *see* Brimonidine (Topical) *on page 254*

Brand Names: US Cytotec
Brand Names: Canada Novo-Misoprostol; PMS-Misoprostol
Pharmacologic Category Prostaglandin
Use
Prevention of NSAID-induced gastric ulcers
Medical termination of pregnancy of ≤49 days in conjunction with mifepristone (refer to Mifepristone monograph for details)
Pregnancy Considerations Use for the prevention of NSAID-induced gastric ulcers is contraindicated in pregnant women.

[US Boxed Warning]: Use of misoprostol during pregnancy may cause abortion, birth defects, or premature birth. Uterine rupture has been reported when used to induce labor after the eighth week of pregnancy. Misoprostol is not to be used to reduce NSAID-induced ulcers in a woman of childbearing potential unless she is capable of complying with effective contraceptive measures and is at high risk of developing gastric ulcers and/or their complications. If needed, the patient must have a negative pregnancy test within 2 weeks of starting therapy, she must use effective contraception during treatment, and therapy should begin on the second or third day of next normal menstrual period. Written and verbal warnings concerning the hazards of misoprostol should be provided. Due to the abortifacient property of this medication, patients must be warned not to give this drug to others.

Congenital anomalies following first trimester exposure have been reported, including skull defects, cranial nerve palsies, facial malformations, and limb defects. Misoprostol may produce uterine contractions; fetal death, uterine perforation, and abortion may occur.

Misoprostol is FDA approved for the medical termination of pregnancy of ≤49 days in conjunction with mifepristone.

Because misoprostol may induce or augment uterine contractions, it has been used off-label as a cervical-ripening agent for induction of labor. Misoprostol should not be used for this purpose during the third trimester in women who have had a prior cesarean delivery or major uterine surgery because the risk of uterine rupture is increased (ACOG 107, 2009; ACOG 115, 2010). It has also been used for the treatment of incomplete or missed abortion (ACOG 427, 2009), early pregnancy loss (ACOG 150, 2015), or severe postpartum hemorrhage (ACOG 76, 2006; FIGO, 2012a; FIGO, 2012b). Some guidelines recommend misoprostol for postpartum hemorrhage only secondary to oxytocin in situations where oxytocin is not available (Leduc, 2000; FIGO, 2012a; FIGO, 2012b). Various routes of administration have been used for postpartum hemorrhage. Sublingual administration has the most rapid onset, the oral route produces the most pronounced initial increase in tonus, and rectal and vaginal routes exhibit longer durations of action as compared to oral and sublingual routes (Leduc, 2009). Adverse events associated with off-label obstetric uses include uterine tachysystole (may impair placental blood flow), uterine rupture, amniotic fluid embolism, or adverse fetal heart changes.

Breast-Feeding Considerations Misoprostol acid (the active metabolite of misoprostol) has been detected in breast milk. Concentrations following a single oral dose were 7.6 to 20.9 pg/mL after 1 hour and decreased to <1 pg/mL by 5 hours. Adverse events have not been reported in nursing infants (FIGO, 2012a; FIGO, 2012b). The manufacturer recommends that caution be used if administered to a nursing woman.

Contraindications Hypersensitivity to prostaglandins; pregnancy (when used to reduce NSAID-induced ulcers)

Warnings/Precautions Hazardous agent; use appropriate precautions for handling and disposal (NIOSH 2014 [group 3]).

[US Boxed Warning]: Use of misoprostol during pregnancy may cause abortion, birth defects, or premature birth. Uterine rupture has been reported when used to induce labor after the eighth week of pregnancy. Misoprostol is not to be used to reduce NSAID-induced ulcers in a woman of childbearing potential unless she is capable of complying with effective contraceptive measures and is at high risk of developing gastric ulcers and/or their complications. If needed, the patient must have a negative pregnancy test within 2 weeks of starting therapy, she must use effective contraception during treatment, and therapy should

begin on the second or third day of next normal menstrual period. Written and verbal warnings concerning the hazards of misoprostol should be provided. Due to the abortifacient property of this medication, patients must be warned not to give this drug to others. Adverse events have been reported when used outside of current product labeling (cervical ripening, induction of labor, postpartum hemorrhage). Uterine tachysystole may occur and progress to uterine tetany; uteroplacental blood flow may be impaired and uterine rupture or amniotic fluid embolism may occur. The risk of uterine rupture may be increased with advanced gestational age, grand multiparity, or prior uterine surgery. Uterine activity and fetal status should be monitored in a hospital setting. Misoprostol should not be used in situations where uterotonic drugs are otherwise contraindicated or inappropriate.

When used for ulcers, use only in patients at high risk of complications from gastric ulcers (eg, the elderly or patients with concomitant diseases) or patients at high risk for developing gastric ulcers (eg, those with a history of ulcers) taking NSAIDs. Misoprostol must be taken during the duration of NSAID therapy. It is not effective in preventing duodenal ulcers in patients taking NSAIDs.

Use with caution in patients with cardiovascular disease, renal impairment, and the elderly.

Adverse Reactions
>10%: Gastrointestinal: Diarrhea, abdominal pain
1% to 10%:
Central nervous system: Headache
Gastrointestinal: Constipation, dyspepsia, flatulence, nausea, vomiting
<1% (Limited to important or life-threatening): Abnormal taste, abnormal vision, alkaline phosphatase increased, alopecia, anaphylaxis, anemia, amylase increase, anxiety, arrhythmia, arterial thrombosis, arthralgia, cardiac enzymes increased, chest pain, chills, confusion, CVA, deafness, depression, diaphoresis, dizziness, drowsiness, dysphagia, dyspnea, dysuria, edema, epistaxis, ESR increased, fatigue, fever, GI bleeding, GI inflammation, gingivitis, glycosuria, gout; gynecological disorders, hematuria, hepatobiliary function abnormal, hyper-/hypotension, impotence, loss of libido, MI, muscle cramps, myalgia, neuropathy, neurosis, nitrogen increased, pallor, phlebitis, polyuria, pulmonary embolism, purpura, rash, reflux, rigors, stiffness, syncope, thirst, thrombocytopenia, tinnitus, uterine rupture, weakness, weight changes

Drug Interactions
Metabolism/Transport Effects None known.
Avoid Concomitant Use
Avoid concomitant use of Misoprostol with any of the following: Antacids; Carbetocin
Increased Effect/Toxicity
Misoprostol may increase the levels/effects of: Carbetocin; Oxytocin

The levels/effects of Misoprostol may be increased by: Antacids
Decreased Effect There are no known significant interactions involving a decrease in effect.
Food Interactions Misoprostol peak serum concentrations may be decreased if taken with food (not clinically significant).
Storage/Stability Store at or below 25°C (77°F).
Mechanism of Action Misoprostol is a synthetic prostaglandin E_1 analog that replaces the protective prostaglandins consumed with prostaglandin-inhibiting therapies (eg, NSAIDs); has been shown to induce uterine contractions
Pharmacodynamics/Kinetics
Absorption: Rapid and extensive
Metabolism: Hepatic; rapidly de-esterified to misoprostol acid (active)
Protein binding: Misoprostol acid: <90%
Half-life elimination: Misoprostol acid: 20-40 minutes
Time to peak, serum: Misoprostol acid: Fasting: 6-22 minutes
Excretion: Urine (80%)
Dosing
Adult
Prevention of NSAID-induced gastric ulcers: Oral: 200 mcg 4 times daily with food; if not tolerated, may decrease dose to 100 mcg 4 times daily with food; last dose of the day should be taken at bedtime
Medical termination of pregnancy: Oral: Refer to Mifepristone monograph.
Early pregnancy loss (off-label use): Intravaginal (off-label route): Initial dose: 800 mcg. May repeat with one dose if needed, ≥3 hours after the first dose and typically within 7 days if no response to the initial dose is observed (ACOG 150, 2015).
Incomplete abortion (treatment) (off-label use): Oral: 600 mcg as a single dose (ACOG 427, 2009)

Labor induction or cervical ripening (off-label uses):
Intravaginal (off-label route): 25 mcg (¼ of 100 mcg tablet); may repeat at intervals no more frequent than every 3 to 6 hours (ACOG 107, 2009).
Missed abortion (treatment) (off-label use):
Intravaginal (off-label route): 800 mcg; may repeat every 3 hours for 2 additional doses if needed (ACOG 427, 2009).
Sublingual (off-label route): 600 mcg; may repeat every 3 hours for 2 additional doses if needed (ACOG 427, 2009).
Postpartum hemorrhage (prevention) (off-label use):
Oral: 600 mcg as a single dose administered immediately after delivery (FIGO, 2012a).
Postpartum hemorrhage (treatment) (off-label use):
Rectal (off-label route): 800 to 1000 mcg (ACOG 76, 2006).
Sublingual (off-label route): 800 mcg as a single dose. Use caution if a prophylactic dose was already given, especially if adverse events were observed (FIGO, 2012b).
Geriatric Prevention of NSAID-induced gastric ulcers: Refer to adult dosing.
Renal Impairment Dose adjustment is not routinely needed; however, the dose may be reduced if the recommended dose is not tolerated. It is not known if misoprostol is removed by dialysis.
Hepatic Impairment No dosage adjustment provided in manufacturer's labeling.
Dietary Considerations When used for the prevention of NSAID-induced ulcers, take with food.
Administration Incidence of diarrhea may be lessened by having patient take dose right after meals and avoiding magnesium-containing antacids. When used for the prevention of NSAID-induced ulcers, therapy is usually begun on the second or third day of the next normal menstrual period in women of childbearing potential.

Hazardous agent; use appropriate precautions for handling and disposal (NIOSH 2014 [group 3]).
Monitoring Parameters
Prevention of NSAID-induced gastric ulcers: Pregnancy test in women of reproductive potential prior to therapy; adequate diagnostic measures in all cases of undiagnosed abnormal vaginal bleeding
Off-label pregnancy-related uses: Uterine activity and fetal status. When used for incomplete or missed abortion, reevaluate 1 to 2 weeks after dosing (ACOG 427, 2009)
Dosage Forms Excipient information presented when available (limited, particularly for generics); consult specific product labeling.
Tablet, Oral:
Cytotec: 100 mcg
Cytotec: 200 mcg [scored]
Generic: 100 mcg, 200 mcg

◆ Misoprostol and Diclofenac see Diclofenac and Misoprostol on page 544

◆ MITC see MitoMYcin (Systemic) on page 1219

◆ Mitigare see Colchicine on page 440

◆ MITO see MitoMYcin (Systemic) on page 1219

◆ MITO-C see MitoMYcin (Systemic) on page 1219

◆ Mitomycin-X see MitoMYcin (Systemic) on page 1219

◆ Mitomycin-C see MitoMYcin (Ophthalmic) on page 1221

◆ Mitomycin-C see MitoMYcin (Systemic) on page 1219

MitoMYcin (Systemic) (mye toe MYE sin)

Brand Names: Canada Mitomycin For Injection; Mitomycin For Injection USP; Mutamycin®
Index Terms MITC; MITO; MITO-C; Mitomycin-C; Mitomycin-X; MMC; MTC; Mutamycin
Pharmacologic Category Antineoplastic Agent, Antibiotic
Use Treatment of adenocarcinoma of stomach or pancreas
Pregnancy Considerations Teratogenic effects have been observed in animal reproduction studies.
Breast-Feeding Considerations It is not known if mitomycin is excreted in human milk; the manufacturer recommends against breast-feeding during treatment.
Contraindications Hypersensitivity to mitomycin or any component of the formulation; thrombocytopenia; coagulation disorders, or other increased bleeding tendency
Warnings/Precautions Hazardous agent - use appropriate precautions for handling and disposal (NIOSH 2014 [group 1]). **[U.S. Boxed Warning]: Bone marrow suppression (thrombocytopenia and leukopenia) is common and may be severe and/or contribute to infections.** Fatalities due to sepsis have been reported; monitor for infections. Myelosuppression is dose-limiting, ▶

delayed in onset, and cumulative; therefore, monitor blood counts closely during and for ≥8 weeks following treatment; treatment delay or dosage adjustment may be required for significant thrombocytopenia (platelets <100,000/mm³) or leukopenia (WBC<4000/mm³) or a progressive decline in either value. Use with caution in patients who have received radiation therapy or in the presence of hepatobiliary dysfunction; reduce dosage in patients who are receiving radiation therapy simultaneously. Monitor for renal toxicity; do not administer if serum creatinine is >1.7 mg/dL. **[U.S. Boxed Warning]: Hemolytic-uremic syndrome (HUS) has been reported (incidence not defined); condition usually involves microangiopathic hemolytic anemia (hematocrit ≤5%), thrombocytopenia (≤100,000/mm³), and irreversible renal failure (serum creatinine ≥1.6 mg/dL). HUS may occur at any time, is generally associated with single doses ≥60 mg, and HUS symptoms may be exacerbated by blood transfusion.** Other less common effects may include pulmonary edema, neurologic abnormalities, and hypertension. High mortality from HUS development has been reported, and is largely the result of renal failure. HUS may also be associated with cumulative doses ≥50 mg/m². Bladder fibrosis/contraction has been reported with intravesical administration (unapproved administration route). Mitomycin is a potent vesicant; ensure proper needle or catheter placement prior to and during infusion. Avoid extravasation. May cause necrosis and tissue sloughing; delayed erythema and/or ulceration have been reported.

Cases of acute respiratory distress syndrome (ARDS) have been reported in patients receiving mitomycin in combination with other chemotherapy who were maintained at FIO_2 concentrations >50% perioperatively; use caution to provide only enough oxygen to maintain adequate arterial saturation and avoid overhydration. Pulmonary toxicity has also been reported as dyspnea with nonproductive cough and appearance of pulmonary infiltrates on radiograph; discontinue therapy if pulmonary toxicity occurs and other potential etiologies have been ruled out. Shortness of breath and bronchospasm have been reported in patients receiving vinca alkaloids in combination with mitomycin or who received mitomycin previously; this acute respiratory distress has occurred within minutes to hours following the vinca alkaloid; may be managed with bronchodilators, steroids and/or oxygen. **[U.S. Boxed Warning]: Should be administered under the supervision of an experienced cancer chemotherapy physician.**

Adverse Reactions
>10%:
Central nervous system: Fever (14%)
Gastrointestinal: Nausea, vomiting, and anorexia (14%)
Hematologic: Myelosuppression (64%; onset: 4 weeks; recovery: 8-10 weeks)
Miscellaneous: Thrombotic thrombocytopenic purpura (TTP)/hemolytic uremic syndrome (HUS) (≤15%)
1% to 10%:
Dermatologic: Alopecia, mucous membrane toxicity (4%)
Gastrointestinal: Stomatitis (4%)
Renal: Serum creatinine increased (2%)
<1% (Limited to important or life-threatening): Adult respiratory distress syndrome (ARDS), bladder fibrosis/contraction (intravesical administration), dyspnea, extravasation reactions, heart failure, hepatic sinusoidal obstruction syndrome (SOS, veno-occlusive liver disease), interstitial fibrosis, nonproductive cough, pulmonary infiltrates, rash, renal failure (irreversible)

Drug Interactions
Metabolism/Transport Effects Substrate of P-glycoprotein

Avoid Concomitant Use
Avoid concomitant use of MitoMYcin (Systemic) with any of the following: BCG (Intravesical); Deferiprone; Dipyrone; Natalizumab; Pimecrolimus; Tacrolimus (Topical); Tofacitinib; Vaccines (Live)

Increased Effect/Toxicity
MitoMYcin (Systemic) may increase the levels/effects of: CloZAPine; Deferiprone; Fingolimod; Leflunomide; Natalizumab; Tofacitinib; Vaccines (Live)

The levels/effects of MitoMYcin (Systemic) may be increased by: Antineoplastic Agents (Vinca Alkaloids); Denosumab; Dipyrone; Lumacaftor; P-glycoprotein/ABCB1 Inhibitors; Pimecrolimus; Ranolazine; Roflumilast; Tacrolimus (Topical); Trastuzumab

Decreased Effect
MitoMYcin (Systemic) may decrease the levels/effects of: BCG (Intravesical); Coccidioides immitis Skin Test; Sipuleucel-T; Vaccines (Inactivated); Vaccines (Live)

The levels/effects of MitoMYcin (Systemic) may be decreased by: Echinacea; Lumacaftor; P-glycoprotein/ABCB1 Inducers

Preparation for Administration Hazardous agent; use appropriate precautions for handling and disposal (NIOSH 2014 [group 1]). Dilute powder with SWFI to a concentration of 0.5 mg/mL. May further dilute in NS or sodium lactate to 20-40 mcg/mL.

Storage/Stability Store intact vials at controlled room temperature; avoid exposure to temperatures >40°C (104°F). Reconstituted solution is stable for 7 days at room temperature and 14 days when refrigerated. Protect reconstituted solution from light. Solution of 0.5 mg/mL in a syringe is stable for 7 days at room temperature and 28 days when refrigerated and protected from light.

Further dilution to 20-40 mcg/mL:
In normal saline: Stable for 12 hours at room temperature.
In sodium lactate: Stable for 24 hours at room temperature.

Mechanism of Action Acts like an alkylating agent and produces DNA cross-linking (primarily with guanine and cytosine pairs); cell-cycle nonspecific; inhibits DNA and RNA synthesis; degrades preformed DNA, causes nuclear lysis and formation of giant cells. While not phase-specific *per se*, mitomycin has its maximum effect against cells in late G and early S phases.

Pharmacodynamics/Kinetics
Metabolism: Hepatic
Half-life elimination: 17-78 minutes; Terminal: 50 minutes
Excretion: Urine (~10% as unchanged drug)

Dosing
Adult & Geriatric Details concerning dosing in combination regimens should also be consulted.
Stomach or pancreas adenocarcinoma (manufacturer's labeling): IV: 20 mg/m² every 6-8 weeks
Anal carcinoma (off-label use): IV: 10 mg/m² as an IV bolus on days 1 and 29 (maximum: 20 mg/dose) in combination with fluorouracil and radiation therapy (Ajani, 2008)
Bladder cancer, nonmuscle invasive (off-label use/route): Intravesical instillation:
Low risk of recurrence (uncomplicated): 40 mg as a single dose postoperatively; retain in bladder for 2 hours (Hall, 2007)
Increased risk of recurrence: 20 mg weekly for 6 weeks, followed by 20 mg monthly for 3 years; retain in bladder for 1-2 hours (Friedrich, 2007)

Renal Impairment The manufacturer's labeling states to avoid use in patients with serum creatine >1.7 mg/dL, but no dosage adjustments are provided. The following adjustments have been used by some clinicians (Aronoff, 2007): Adults:
CrCl <10 mL/minute: Administer 75% of dose.
Continuous ambulatory peritoneal dialysis (CAPD): Administer 75% of dose.

Hepatic Impairment No dosage adjustment provided in manufacturer's labeling (has not been studied).

Obesity *ASCO Guidelines for appropriate chemotherapy dosing in obese adults with cancer:* Utilize patient's actual body weight (full weight) for calculation of body surface area- or weight-based dosing, particularly when the intent of therapy is curative; manage regimen-related toxicities in the same manner as for nonobese patients; if a dose reduction is utilized due to toxicity, consider resumption of full weight-based dosing with subsequent cycles, especially if cause of toxicity (eg, hepatic or renal impairment) is resolved (Griggs, 2012).

Adjustment for Toxicity
Leukocytes 2000 to <3000/mm³: Hold therapy until leukocyte count ≥4000/mm³; reduce to 70% of dose in subsequent cycles
Leukocytes <2000/mm³: Hold therapy until leukocyte count ≥4000/mm³; reduce to 50% of dose in subsequent cycles
Platelets 25,000 to <75,000/mm³: Hold therapy until platelets ≥100,000/mm³; reduce to 70% of dose in subsequent cycles
Platelets <25,000/mm³: Hold therapy until platelets ≥100,000 mm³; reduce to 50% of dose in subsequent cycles

Administration
IV: Administer slow IV push or by slow (15-30 minute) infusion via a freely-running saline infusion. Consider using a central venous catheter.
Vesicant; ensure proper needle or catheter placement prior to and during infusion; avoid extravasation.

Extravasation management: If extravasation occurs, stop infusion immediately and disconnect (leave cannula/needle in place); gently aspirate extravasated solution (do **NOT** flush the line); remove needle/cannula; elevate extremity. Initiate dimethyl sulfate (DMSO) antidote. Apply dry cold compress for 20 minutes 4 times/day for 1-2 days (Pérez Fidalgo, 2012).

DMSO: Apply topically to a region covering twice the affected area every 8 hours for 7 days; begin within 10 minutes of extravasation; do not cover with a dressing (Perez Fidalgo, 2012).

Intravesicular (off-label route): Instill into bladder and retain for up to 2 hours (Friedrich, 2007; Hall, 2007); rotate patient every 15-30 minutes

Hazardous agent; use appropriate precautions for handling and disposal (NIOSH 2014 [group 1]).

Monitoring Parameters Monitor CBC with differential (repeatedly during therapy and for ≥8 weeks following therapy); serum creatinine; pulmonary function tests; monitor for signs/symptoms of HUS

Dosage Forms Excipient information presented when available (limited, particularly for generics); consult specific product labeling.

Solution Reconstituted, Intravenous:

Generic: 5 mg (1 ea); 20 mg (1 ea); 40 mg (1 ea)

MitoMYcin (Ophthalmic) (mye toe MYE sin)

Brand Names: US Mitosol

Index Terms Mitomycin-C; MMC

Pharmacologic Category Antineoplastic Agent, Antibiotic; Ophthalmic Agent, Miscellaneous

Use Adjunct to *ab externo* glaucoma surgery

Dosing

Adult & Geriatric Glaucoma surgery, adjunctive therapy: Topical ophthalmic: 0.2 mg solution is aseptically applied via saturated sponges to surgical site of glaucoma filtration surgery for 2 minutes

Additional Information Complete prescribing information should be consulted for additional detail.

Dosage Forms Excipient information presented when available (limited, particularly for generics); consult specific product labeling.

Kit, Ophthalmic:

Mitosol: 0.2 mg

◆ Mitomycin For Injection (Can) *see* MitoMYcin (Systemic) *on page 1219*

◆ Mitomycin For Injection USP (Can) *see* MitoMYcin (Systemic) *on page 1219*

◆ Mitosol *see* MitoMYcin (Ophthalmic) *on page 1221*

Mitotane (MYE toe tane)

Brand Names: US Lysodren

Brand Names: Canada Lysodren

Index Terms Chlodithan; Chlodithane; Khloditan; Mytotan; o,p'-DDD; Ortho,para-DDD

Pharmacologic Category Antineoplastic Agent, Miscellaneous

Use Adrenocortical carcinoma: Treatment of inoperable adrenocortical carcinoma (both functional and non-functional types)

Dosing

Adult & Geriatric Note: Mitotane is associated with a moderate emetic potential; antiemetics may be needed to prevent nausea and vomiting.

Adrenocortical carcinoma: Oral: Initial: 2 to 6 g daily in 3 to 4 divided doses, then increase incrementally to 9 to 10 g daily in 3 to 4 divided doses (maximum tolerated range: 2 to 16 g daily, usually 9 to 10 g daily; maximum dose studied: 18 to 19 g daily); continue as long as clinical benefit is demonstrated

Off-label dosing: Initial 1 to 2 g daily; increase by 1 to 2 g daily at 1 to 2 week intervals as tolerated to a maximum of 6 to 10 g daily; usual dose 4 to 5 g daily (Veytsman, 2009)

Cushing syndrome (off-label use): Oral: Initial dose: 500 mg 3 times daily; maximum dose: 3 g 3 times daily (Biller, 2008)

Renal Impairment No dosage adjustment provided in manufacturer's labeling.

Hepatic Impairment No dosage adjustment provided in manufacturer's labeling. However, drug accumulation may occur in patients with liver disease; use with caution.

Adjustment for Toxicity

Severe side effects: Reduce dose until a maximum tolerated dose is achieved.

Significant neuropsychiatric adverse effects: Withhold treatment for at least 1 week and restart at a lower dose (Allolio, 2006).

Additional Information Complete prescribing information should be consulted for additional detail.

Dosage Forms Excipient information presented when available (limited, particularly for generics); consult specific product labeling.

Tablet, Oral:

Lysodren: 500 mg [scored]

MitoXANtrone (mye toe ZAN trone)

Brand Names: Canada Mitoxantrone Injection; Mitoxantrone Injection USP

Index Terms CL-232315; DHAD; DHAQ; Dihydroxyanthracenedione; Dihydroxyanthracenedione Dihydrochloride; Mitoxantrone Dihydrochloride; Mitoxantrone HCl; Mitoxantrone Hydrochloride; Mitozantrone; Novantrone

Pharmacologic Category Antineoplastic Agent, Anthracenedione; Antineoplastic Agent, Topoisomerase II Inhibitor

Use Initial treatment of acute nonlymphocytic leukemias (ANLL [includes myelogenous, promyelocytic, monocytic and erythroid leukemias]); treatment of advanced hormone-refractory prostate cancer; secondary progressive or relapsing-remitting multiple sclerosis (MS)

Canadian labeling: Additional uses (not in U.S. labeling): Treatment of metastatic breast cancer, relapsed leukemia (adults), lymphoma, and hepatocellular carcinoma

Medication Guide Available Yes

Dosing

Adult & Geriatric Details concerning dosing in combination regimens should also be consulted.

U.S. labeling:

Acute nonlymphocytic leukemias (ANLL):

Acute myeloid leukemia (AML) induction: 12 mg/m^2 once daily for 3 days (in combination with cytarabine); for incomplete response, may repeat (7-10 days later) at 12 mg/m^2 once daily for 2 days (in combination with cytarabine) (Arlin, 1990)

AML consolidation (beginning ~6 weeks after initiation of the final induction course): 12 mg/m^2 once daily for 2 days (in combination with cytarabine), repeat in 4 weeks (Arlin, 1990)

Multiple sclerosis: 12 mg/m^2 every 3 months (maximum lifetime cumulative dose: 140 mg/m^2; discontinue use with LVEF <50% or clinically significant reduction in LVEF)

Prostate cancer (advanced, hormone-refractory): 12-14 mg/m^2 every 3 weeks (in combination with corticosteroids)

Canadian labeling:

Acute nonlymphocytic leukemias (ANLL):

AML induction: 10-12 mg/m^2 once daily for 3 days (in combination with cytarabine); for incomplete response, may repeat at 10-12 mg/m^2 once daily for 2 days (in combination with cytarabine)

AML consolidation (beginning ~6 weeks after initiation of the final induction course): 12 mg/m^2 once daily for 2 days (in combination with cytarabine), repeat in 4 weeks

Acute leukemias (relapsed): Induction: 12 mg/m^2 once daily for 5 consecutive days; may repeat once if needed (at the same dose and duration)

Breast cancer (metastatic), lymphoma: Initial: Single agent: 14 mg/m^2 every 21 days; reduce initial dose to ≤12 mg/m^2 for myelosuppression due to previous treatment or for poor general health. When used in combination with other agents, reduce initial dose to 10-12 mg/m^2.

Hepatocellular cancer: Initial: Single agent: 14 mg/m^2 every 21 days; reduce initial dose to ≤12 mg/m^2 for myelosuppression due to previous treatment or for poor general health

Adult off-label uses and/or dosing:

AML, refractory:

CLAG-M regimen: 10 mg/m^2 once daily for 3 days (in combination with cladribine, cytarabine, and filgrastim), may repeat once if needed (Wierzbowska, 2008)

MEC or EMA regimen: 6 mg/m^2 once daily for 6 days (in combination with cytarabine and etoposide) (Amadori, 1991)

Mitoxantrone/Etoposide: 10 mg/m^2 once daily for 5 days (in combination with etoposide) (Ho, 1988)

APL consolidation phase (second course): 10 mg/m^2 once daily for 5 days (Sanz, 2004)

Hodgkin lymphoma, refractory:

MINE-ESHAP regimen: 10 mg/m^2 on day 1 every 28 days for up to 2 cycles (MINE is combination with mesna, ifosfamide, mitoxantrone, and etoposide; MINE alternates with ESHAP for up to 2 cycles of each) (Fernandez, 2010)

VIM-D regimen: 10 mg/m^2 on day 1 every 28 days (in combination with etoposide, ifosfamide, mesna, and dexamethasone) (Phillips, 1990)

Non-Hodgkin lymphoma (as part of combination chemotherapy regimens):

CNOP regimen: 10 mg/m^2 every 21 days (Bessell, 2003)

FCMR regimen: 8 mg/m^2 every 28 days (Forstpointner, 2004)

FMR regimen: 10 mg/m^2 every 21 days (Zinzani, 2004)

FND regimen: 10 mg/m^2 every 28 days (Tsimberidou, 2002)

MINE-ESHAP regimen: 8 mg/m^2 every 21 days for 6 cycles (MINE is combination with mesna, ifosfamide, mitoxantrone, and etoposide; followed by ESHAP) (Rodriguez, 1995)

Stem cell transplantation, autologous: 60 mg/m^2 administered 4-5 days prior to autografting (as 3 divided doses over 1 hour each at 1-2 hour intervals on the same day; in combination with other chemotherapeutic agent[s]) (Oyan, 2006; Tarella, 2001)

Pediatric Details concerning dosing in combination regimens should also be consulted.

Acute nonlymphocytic leukemias: IV:

Acute myeloid leukemia (AML) consolidation phase (second course; off-label use): 10 mg/m^2 once daily for 5 days (in combination with cytarabine) (Stevens, 1998)

Acute promyelocytic leukemia (APL) consolidation phase (second course; off-label use): 10 mg/m^2 once daily for 5 days (Ortega, 2005; Sanz, 2004)

Renal Impairment No dosage adjustment provided in manufacturer's labeling (has not been studied).

Hemodialysis: Supplemental dose is not necessary

Peritoneal dialysis: Supplemental dose is not necessary

Elderly: Clearance is decreased in elderly patients; use with caution

Hepatic Impairment

U.S. labeling: No dosage adjustment provided in the manufacturer's labeling; however, clearance is reduced in hepatic dysfunction. Patients with severe hepatic dysfunction (bilirubin >3.4 mg/dL) have an AUC of 3 times greater than patients with normal hepatic function; consider dose adjustments. **Note:** MS patients with hepatic impairment should not receive mitoxantrone.

Canadian labeling:

Mild-to-moderate impairment: No specific dosage adjustment provided; consider dose adjustments and monitor closely.

Severe impairment: Use is contraindicated.

Obesity *ASCO Guidelines for appropriate chemotherapy dosing in obese adults with cancer:* Utilize patient's actual body weight (full weight) for calculation of body surface area- or weight-based dosing, particularly when the intent of therapy is curative; manage regimen-related toxicities in the same manner as for nonobese patients; if a dose reduction is utilized due to toxicity, consider resumption of full weight-based dosing with subsequent cycles, especially if cause of toxicity (eg, hepatic or renal impairment) is resolved (Griggs, 2012).

Adjustment for Toxicity

ANLL patients: Severe or life-threatening nonhematologic toxicity: Withhold treatment until toxicity resolves

MS patients:

Neutrophils <1500/mm^3: Use is not recommended.

Signs/symptoms of HF: Evaluate for cardiac signs/symptoms and LVEF.

LVEF <50% or baseline LVEF below the lower limit of normal (LLN): Use is not recommended.

Canadian labeling (not in U.S. labeling): **Hepatocellular cancer, lymphoma, or breast cancer (metastatic):**

WBC nadir >1500/mm^3 **and** platelet nadir >50,000/mm^3 and recovery ≤21 days: Repeat previous dose or increase dose by 2 mg/m^2 if myelosuppression is inadequate.

WBC nadir >1500/mm^3 **and** platelet nadir >50,000/mm^3 and recovery >21 days: Withhold treatment until recovery then resume at previous dose.

WBC nadir <1500/mm^3 **or** platelet nadir <50,000/mm^3 (regardless of recovery time): Withhold treatment until recovery then decrease previous dose by 2 mg/m^2.

WBC nadir <1000/mm^3 **or** platelet nadir <25,000/mm^3 (regardless of recovery time): Withhold treatment until recovery then decrease previous dose by 4 mg/m^2.

Additional Information Complete prescribing information should be consulted for additional detail.

Dosage Forms Excipient information presented when available (limited, particularly for generics); consult specific product labeling.

Concentrate, Intravenous:

Generic: 20 mg/10 mL (10 mL); 25 mg/12.5 mL (12.5 mL); 30 mg/15 mL (15 mL)

◆ Mitoxantrone Dihydrochloride *see* MitoXANtrone *on page 1221*

◆ Mitoxantrone HCl *see* MitoXANtrone *on page 1221*

◆ Mitoxantrone Hydrochloride *see* MitoXANtrone *on page 1221*

◆ Mitoxantrone Injection (Can) *see* MitoXANtrone *on page 1221*

◆ Mitoxantrone Injection USP (Can) *see* MitoXANtrone *on page 1221*

◆ Mitozantrone *see* MitoXANtrone *on page 1221*

◆ Mitrazol [OTC] [DSC] *see* Miconazole (Topical) *on page 1201*

◆ MK-217 *see* Alendronate *on page 66*

◆ MK383 *see* Tirofiban *on page 1797*

◆ MK-0431 *see* SitaGLIPtin *on page 1665*

◆ MK462 *see* Rizatriptan *on page 1609*

◆ MK 0517 *see* Fosaprepitant *on page 812*

◆ MK-0518 *see* Raltegravir *on page 1549*

◆ MK594 *see* Losartan *on page 1107*

◆ MK0826 *see* Ertapenem *on page 668*

◆ MK 869 *see* Aprepitant *on page 143*

◆ MK-3475 *see* Pembrolizumab *on page 1414*

◆ MK4305 *see* Suvorexant *on page 1723*

◆ MLN341 *see* Bortezomib *on page 243*

◆ MLN9708 *see* Ixazomib *on page 1008*

◆ MM-398 *see* Irinotecan (Liposomal) *on page 984*

◆ MMC *see* MitoMYcin (Ophthalmic) *on page 1221*

◆ MMC *see* MitoMYcin (Systemic) *on page 1219*

◆ MMF *see* Mycophenolate *on page 1240*

◆ MMI *see* Methimazole *on page 1166*

◆ MMR *see* Measles, Mumps, and Rubella Virus Vaccine *on page 1128*

◆ M-M-R II *see* Measles, Mumps, and Rubella Virus Vaccine *on page 1128*

◆ MMRV *see* Measles, Mumps, Rubella, and Varicella Virus Vaccine *on page 1129*

◆ MN-50 [OTC] *see* Manganese *on page 1124*

◆ MOAB 2C4 *see* Pertuzumab *on page 1433*

◆ MOAB ABX-EGF *see* Panitumumab *on page 1386*

◆ MOAB C225 *see* Cetuximab *on page 366*

◆ MoAb CD52 *see* Alemtuzumab *on page 62*

◆ MOAB Ch14.18 *see* Dinutuximab *on page 559*

◆ MOAB-CTLA-4 *see* Ipilimumab *on page 975*

◆ MOAB HER2 *see* Trastuzumab *on page 1831*

◆ Mobic *see* Meloxicam *on page 1137*

◆ Mobicox (Can) *see* Meloxicam *on page 1137*

Modafinil (moe DAF i nil)

Brand Names: US Provigil

Brand Names: Canada Alertec; Apo-Modafinil; Auro-Modafinil; Bio-Modafinil; Mar-Modafinil; Teva-Modafinil

Pharmacologic Category Central Nervous System Stimulant

Use

Narcolepsy: To improve wakefulness in adult patients with excessive sleepiness associated with narcolepsy.

Obstructive sleep apnea: To improve wakefulness in adult patients with obstructive sleep apnea (OSA)

Shift work sleep disorder: To improve wakefulness in adult patients with shift work sleep disorder (SWSD)

Pregnancy Considerations Adverse events have been observed in some animal reproduction studies. An increased risk of spontaneous abortion and intrauterine growth restriction has been reported with modafinil. Efficacy of steroidal contraceptives (including depot and implantable contraceptives) may be decreased; alternate means of contraception should be considered during therapy and for 1 month after modafinil is discontinued.

Health care providers are encouraged to register pregnant patients exposed to modafinil, or pregnant women may enroll themselves, by calling (866-404-4106).

Breast-Feeding Considerations It is not known if modafinil is excreted in breast milk. The manufacturer recommends that caution be exercised when administering modafinil to nursing women.

Medication Guide Available Yes

Contraindications

Hypersensitivity to modafinil, armodafinil, or any component of the formulation

Canadian labeling: Additional contraindications (not in US labeling): Patients in agitated states or with severe anxiety

Warnings/Precautions The degree of sleepiness should be reassessed frequently; some patients may not return to a normal level of wakefulness. In obstructive sleep apnea, modafinil is indicated as treatment for excessive sleepiness and not for the underlying obstruction. If continuous positive airway pressure (CPAP) is the treatment of choice for a patient, a maximal effort to treat with CPAP for an adequate period of time should be made prior to initiating and during treatment with modafinil for excessive sleepiness. Use with caution in patients with cardiovascular disease; increased blood pressure and heart rate monitoring may be required. Use is not recommended in patients with a history of left ventricular hypertrophy or patients with mitral valve prolapse who have developed mitral valve prolapse syndrome with previous CNS stimulant use. Increased monitoring should be considered in patients with a recent history of myocardial infarction or unstable angina.

Serious and life-threatening rashes, including Stevens-Johnson syndrome, toxic epidermal necrolysis and drug rash with eosinophilia and systemic symptoms (DRESS) have been reported. Although initially reported in children during clinical trials, postmarketing cases have occurred in both children and adults. Most cases have occurred within the first 5 weeks of therapy; however, rare cases have occurred after long-term use (eg, 3 months). No risk factors have been identified to predict occurrence or severity. Patients should be advised to discontinue at first sign of rash (unless the rash is clearly not drug-related). As a result of these serious dermatologic adverse events, approval for the use of modafinil in children for ADHD was denied by the FDA. The serious nature of these dermatologic adverse effects, as well reports of psychiatric events, resulted in the FDA's Pediatric Advisory Committee unanimously recommending that a specific warning against the use of modafinil in children be added to the manufacturer's labeling. Modafinil is not FDA-approved for use in pediatrics for any indication.

Rare cases of multiorgan hypersensitivity reactions (with fatality) in association with modafinil use; lone cases of angioedema and anaphylactoid reactions with armodafinil have been reported (angioedema has been noted in postmarketing reports with modafinil). Signs and symptoms are diverse, reflecting the involvement of specific organs; patients typically present with fever and rash associated with organ-system dysfunction. No risk factors have been identified to predict occurrence or severity of multiorgan hypersensitivity reactions. Patients should be advised to report any signs and symptoms related to these effects; discontinuation of therapy is recommended.

Use with caution in patients with a history of psychosis, depression, or mania. Use may result in emergence of or exacerbation of psychiatric symptoms. Observe for symptoms of aggression, hallucinations, mania, delusions, or suicidal ideation. Consider discontinuing therapy if psychiatric symptoms develop. May impair the ability to engage in potentially hazardous activities; patients must be cautioned about performing tasks which require mental alertness (eg, operating machinery or driving). Use with caution in patients with Tourette syndrome; limited evidence suggests stimulants may exacerbate tics and Tourette syndrome (AACAP [Murphy 2013]; Pringsheim 2012; Rossner 2011). Use caution with renal or hepatic impairment (dosage adjustment in severe hepatic impairment is recommended). Instruct patients to avoid concomitant ethanol consumption.

Adverse Reactions

Frequency not always defined.

Cardiovascular: Chest pain (3%), hypertension (3%), palpitations (2%), tachycardia (2%), vasodilatation (2%), edema (1%)

Central nervous system: Headache (adults 34%; children 20% [Biederman 2005]; dose related), nervousness (7%), anxiety (5%; dose related), dizziness (5%), insomnia (5%), depression (2%), drowsiness (2%), paresthesia (2%), agitation (1%), chills (1%), confusion (1%), emotional lability (1%), hypertonia (1%), vertigo (1%)

Dermatologic: Diaphoresis (1%)

Endocrine & metabolic: Weight loss (children 5% [Greenhill 2006]), increased thirst (1%), increased gamma-glutamyl transferase

Gastrointestinal: Decreased appetite (children 16% [Biederman 2005]), abdominal pain (children 12% [Greenhill 2006]), nausea (11%), diarrhea (6%), dyspepsia (5%), xerostomia (4%), anorexia (4%), constipation (2%), dysgeusia (1%), flatulence (1%), oral mucosa ulcer (1%)

Genitourinary: Urine abnormality (1%)

Hematologic & oncologic: Eosinophilia (1%)

Hepatic: Abnormal hepatic function tests (2%), increased serum alkaline phosphatase

Neuromuscular & skeletal: Back pain (6%), dyskinesia (1%), hyperkinesia (1%), tremor (1%)

Ocular: Abnormal vision (1%)

Respiratory: Rhinitis (7%), pharyngitis (4%), asthma (1%), epistaxis (1%)

<1% (Limited to important or life-threatening): Agranulocytosis, DRESS syndrome, erythema multiforme (pediatric patients), hallucination, hypersensitivity, mania, multiorgan hypersensitivity, psychomotor agitation, psychosis, Stevens-Johnson syndrome, suicidal ideation, toxic epidermal necrolysis

Drug Interactions

Metabolism/Transport Effects Substrate of CYP3A4 (major); **Note:** Assignment of Major/Minor substrate status based on clinically relevant drug interaction potential; **Inhibits** CYP2A6 (weak), CYP2C19 (moderate), CYP2C9 (weak), CYP2E1 (weak); **Induces** CYP1A2 (weak/moderate), CYP2B6 (weak/moderate), CYP3A4 (moderate)

Avoid Concomitant Use

Avoid concomitant use of Modafinil with any of the following: Antihepaciviral Combination Products; Axitinib; Bedaquiline; Bosutinib; Cobimetinib; Conivaptan; Flibanserin; Fusidic Acid (Systemic); Idelalisib; Iobenguane I 123; Nisoldipine; Olaparib; Palbociclib; Ranolazine; Simeprevir; Sofosbuvir; Sonidegib

Increased Effect/Toxicity

Modafinil may increase the levels/effects of: Cilostazol; Citalopram; Clarithromycin; CYP2C19 Substrates; Doxofylline; Ifosfamide; Sympathomimetics

The levels/effects of Modafinil may be increased by: Aprepitant; AtoMOXetine; Cannabinoid-Containing Products; Conivaptan; CYP3A4 Inhibitors (Moderate); CYP3A4 Inhibitors (Strong); Dasatinib; Fosaprepitant; Fusidic Acid (Systemic); Idelalisib; Ivacaftor; Linezolid; Luliconazole; Mifepristone; Netupitant; Osimertinib; Stiripentol; Tedizolid

Decreased Effect

Modafinil may decrease the levels/effects of: Antihepaciviral Combination Products; ARIPiprazole; Axitinib; Bedaquiline; Bosutinib; Clarithromycin; Clopidogrel; Cobimetinib; Contraceptives (Estrogens); CycloSPORINE (Systemic); CYP3A4 Substrates; Daclatasvir; FentaNYL; Flibanserin; Hydrocodone; Ibrutinib; Ifosfamide; Iobenguane I 123; NiMODipine; Nisoldipine; Olaparib; Palbociclib; Ranolazine; Rolapitant; Saxagliptin; Simeprevir; Sofosbuvir; Sonidegib

The levels/effects of Modafinil may be decreased by: Bosentan; CYP3A4 Inducers (Moderate); CYP3A4 Inducers (Strong); Dabrafenib; Deferasirox; Enzalutamide; Mitotane; Osimertinib; Siltuximab; St Johns Wort; Tocilizumab

Food Interactions Food delays absorption, but does not affect bioavailability. Management: Administer without regard to meals.

Storage/Stability

Provigil: Store at 20°C to 25°C (68°F to 77°F).

Alertec (Canadian availability; not available in US): Store at 15°C to 30°C (59°F to 86°F).

Mechanism of Action The exact mechanism of action is unclear; it does not appear to alter the release of dopamine or norepinephrine, it may exert its stimulant effects by decreasing GABA-mediated neurotransmission, although this theory has not yet been fully evaluated; several studies also suggest that an intact central alpha-adrenergic system is required for modafinil's activity; the drug increases high-frequency alpha waves while decreasing both delta and theta wave activity, and these effects are consistent with generalized increases in mental alertness

Pharmacodynamics/Kinetics Modafinil is a racemic compound (10% S-isomer and 90% R-isomer at steady state) whose enantiomers have different pharmacokinetics

Distribution: V_d: 0.9 L/kg

Protein binding: ~60%, primarily to albumin

Metabolism: Hepatic; multiple pathways including CYP3A4

Half-life elimination: Effective half-life: 15 hours

Time to peak, serum: 2 to 4 hours; may be delayed ~1 hour with food.

Excretion: Urine (80% as metabolites, <10% as unchanged drug); feces (1%)

Dosing

Adult

US labeling:

Narcolepsy, obstructive sleep apnea (OSA): Oral: Initial: 200 mg as a single daily dose in the morning. **Note:** Doses up to 400 mg once daily have been well tolerated, but there is no consistent evidence that this dose confers additional benefit.

Shift work sleep disorder (SWSD): Oral: Initial: 200 mg as a single dose ~1 hour prior to start of work shift

Canadian labeling:

Narcolepsy: Oral: Initial: 200 mg daily in 2 divided doses (first dose in the morning and second dose at noon [or no later than early afternoon]); may titrate dose upward in 100 mg increments as needed and tolerated (maximum single dose: <300 mg; maximum daily dose: 400 mg). Single doses ≥300 mg and daily doses >400 mg are associated with increased side effects and are not recommended.

Obstructive sleep apnea: Oral: 200 mg once daily in the morning.

Shift work sleep disorder (SWSD): Oral: 200 mg as a single dose taken ~1 hour prior to start of work shift

Off-label uses:

Attention-deficit/hyperactivity disorder (ADHD) (off-label use): Oral: 100 to 400 mg daily (Taylor 2000)

Fatigue, cancer-related, severe (in patients receiving active treatment; off-label use): Oral: 100 mg once daily for 3 days (beginning on day 5 of second chemotherapy cycle), followed by 200 mg once daily during active treatment (Jean-Pierre 2010).

Multiple sclerosis-related fatigue (off-label use): Oral: 100 mg once daily initially, increased as tolerated to 200 mg once daily **or** if patient experiences post-noon fatigue, 100 mg twice daily (ie, morning and noon). Higher daily doses (greater than 200 mg) do not appear to be effective (Brown, 2010; Moller 2011; Rammohan, 2002; Stankoff 2005; Zifko 2002).

Geriatric Consider initiating at lower doses.

Renal Impairment There are no dosage adjustments provided in the manufacturer's labeling.

Hepatic Impairment

Mild to moderate hepatic impairment: There are no dosage adjustments provided in the manufacturer's labeling.

Severe hepatic impairment: Dose should be reduced to one-half of that recommended for patients with normal liver function.

Administration

US labeling: For the treatment of narcolepsy and obstructive sleep apnea/hypopnea syndrome, administer dose in the morning. For the treatment of shift work sleep disorder, administer dose ~1 hour prior to start of work shift.

Canadian labeling: For the treatment of narcolepsy, administer in 2 divided doses with first dose given in the morning and the second dose given at noon (or no later than early afternoon) to avoid potential for insomnia. For treatment of obstructive sleep apnea, administer as a single dose in the morning. For the treatment of shift work sleep disorder, administer dose ~1 hour prior to start of work shift.

Monitoring Parameters Levels of sleepiness; blood pressure; heart rate; increased monitoring in patients with recent MI or unstable angina; development of severe skin reactions; development or exacerbation of psychiatric symptoms (eg, agitation, anxiety, depression)

When used for the treatment of ADHD, thoroughly evaluate for cardiovascular risk. Monitor heart rate, blood pressure, and consider obtaining ECG prior to initiation (Vetter 2008).

Dosage Forms Excipient information presented when available (limited, particularly for generics); consult specific product labeling.

Tablet, Oral:

Provigil: 100 mg

Provigil: 200 mg [scored]

Generic: 100 mg, 200 mg

Dosage Forms: Canada Excipient information presented when available (limited, particularly for generics); consult specific product labeling.

Tablet, oral: 100 mg

Alertec: 100 mg

Controlled Substance C-IV

◆ Modecate® (Can) see FluPHENAZine on page 790

◆ Modecate® Concentrate (Can) see FluPHENAZine on page 790

◆ Modicon see Ethinyl Estradiol and Norethindrone on page 708

◆ Modified Dakin's Solution see Sodium Hypochlorite on page 1675

◆ Modified Shohl's Solution see Sodium Citrate and Citric Acid on page 1673

Moexipril (mo EKS i pril)

Brand Names: US Univasc [DSC]

Index Terms Moexipril Hydrochloride; Univasc

Pharmacologic Category Angiotensin-Converting Enzyme (ACE) Inhibitor; Antihypertensive

Use

Hypertension: Management of hypertension

Guideline recommendations:

Hypertension: The 2014 guideline for the management of high blood pressure in adults (Eighth Joint National Committee [JNC 8]) recommends initiation of pharmacologic treatment to lower blood pressure for the following patients:

• Patients ≥60 years of age with systolic blood pressure (SBP) ≥150 mm Hg or diastolic blood pressure (DBP) ≥90 mm Hg. Goal of therapy is SBP <150 mm Hg and DBP <90 mm Hg.

• Patients <60 years of age with SBP ≥140 mm Hg or DBP is ≥90 mm Hg. Goal of therapy is SBP <140 mm Hg and DBP <90 mm Hg.

• Patients ≥18 years of age with diabetes and SBP ≥140 mm Hg or DBP ≥90 mm Hg. Goal of therapy is SBP <140 mm Hg and DBP <90 mm Hg.

• Patients ≥18 years of age with chronic kidney disease (CKD) and SBP ≥140 mm Hg or DBP ≥90 mm Hg. Goal of therapy is SBP <140 mm Hg and DBP <90 mm Hg.

Chronic kidney disease (CKD) and hypertension: Regardless of race or diabetes status, the use of an ACE inhibitor (ACEI) or angiotensin receptor blocker (ARB) as initial therapy is recommended to improve kidney outcomes. In the general nonblack population (without CKD) including those with diabetes, initial antihypertensive treatment should consist of a thiazide-type diuretic, calcium channel blocker, ACEI, or ARB. In the general black population (without CKD) including those with diabetes, initial antihypertensive treatment should consist of a thiazide-type diuretic or a calcium channel blocker **instead of** an ACEI or ARB.

Coronary artery disease (CAD) and hypertension: The American Heart Association, American College of Cardiology and American Society of Hypertension (AHA/ACC/ASH) 2015 scientific statement for the treatment of hypertension in patients with CAD recommends the use of an ACE inhibitor (or an ARB) as part of a regimen in patients with hypertension and chronic stable angina if there is prior MI, LV systolic dysfunction, diabetes mellitus, or CKD. A BP target of <140/90 mm Hg is reasonable for the secondary prevention of cardiovascular events. A lower target BP (<130/80 mm Hg) may be appropriate in some individuals with CAD, previous MI, stroke or transient ischemic attack, or CAD risk equivalents (AHA/ACC/ASH [Rosendorff 2015]).

Dosing

Adult & Geriatric Hypertension: Oral: Initial: 7.5 mg once daily (in patients **not** receiving a diuretic) **or** 3.75 mg once daily (when combined with a diuretic); adjust dose to blood pressure response; maintenance dose: 7.5 to 30 mg/day in 1 or 2 divided doses

Renal Impairment

CrCl >40 mL/minute/1.73 m^2: There are no dosage adjustments provided in the manufacturer's labeling; use with caution.

CrCl ≤40 mL/minute/1.73 m^2: Initial: 3.75 mg once daily; maximum dose: 15 mg/day

Hepatic Impairment There are no dosage adjustments provided in the manufacturer's labeling. However, hepatic impairment increases systemic exposure.

Additional Information Complete prescribing information should be consulted for additional detail.

Dosage Forms Excipient information presented when available (limited, particularly for generics); consult specific product labeling. [DSC] = Discontinued product

Tablet, Oral, as hydrochloride:

Univasc: 7.5 mg [DSC], 15 mg [DSC] [scored]

Generic: 7.5 mg, 15 mg

Moexipril and Hydrochlorothiazide
(mo EKS i pril & hye droe klor oh THYE a zide)

Brand Names: US Uniretic

Index Terms Hydrochlorothiazide and Moexipril; Uniretic

Pharmacologic Category Angiotensin-Converting Enzyme (ACE) Inhibitor; Antihypertensive; Diuretic, Thiazide

Use Hypertension: Management of hypertension

Dosing

Adult & Geriatric Note: Not for initial therapy. Dose is individualized; may be substituted for individual components in patients currently maintained on both agents separately or in patients not controlled with monotherapy.

Hypertension: Oral: Initial: Moexipril 7.5 mg/hydrochlorothiazide 12.5 mg or moexipril 15 mg/hydrochlorothiazide 12.5 mg or moexipril 15 mg/hydrochlorothiazide 25 mg once daily in patients not adequately controlled on monotherapy; titrate dosage based on clinical response; dose range: moexipril 3.75 to 30 mg/hydrochlorothiazide 6.25 to 50 mg once daily

Renal Impairment
CrCl >40 mL/minute/1.73 m^2: No dosage adjustment necessary.
CrCl ≤40 mL/minute/1.73 m^2: Use not recommended. Also see individual agents.

Hepatic Impairment There are no dosage adjustments provided in the manufacturer's labeling; use with caution; hepatic impairment increases systemic exposure.

Additional Information Complete prescribing information should be consulted for additional detail.

Dosage Forms Excipient information presented when available (limited, particularly for generics); consult specific product labeling.

Tablet, oral:
7.5/12.5: Moexipril hydrochloride 7.5 mg and hydrochlorothiazide 12.5 mg
15/12.5: Moexipril hydrochloride 15 mg and hydrochlorothiazide 12.5 mg
15/25: Moexipril hydrochloride 15 mg and hydrochlorothiazide 25 mg

Uniretic:
7.5/12.5: Moexipril hydrochloride 7.5 mg and hydrochlorothiazide 12.5 mg [scored]
15/12.5: Moexipril hydrochloride 15 mg and hydrochlorothiazide 12.5 mg [scored]
15/25: Moexipril hydrochloride 15 mg and hydrochlorothiazide 25 mg [scored]

♦ Moexipril Hydrochloride see Moexipril on page 1224
♦ MOM see Magnesium Hydroxide on page 1120

Mometasone (Oral Inhalation)
(moe MET a sone)

Brand Names: US Asmanex 120 Metered Doses; Asmanex 14 Metered Doses; Asmanex 30 Metered Doses; Asmanex 60 Metered Doses; Asmanex 7 Metered Doses; Asmanex HFA

Brand Names: Canada Asmanex Twisthaler

Index Terms Mometasone Furoate

Pharmacologic Category Corticosteroid, Inhalant (Oral)

Additional Appendix Information
Inhaled Corticosteroids on page 1951

Use

Asthma: Maintenance treatment of asthma as prophylactic therapy in patients 4 years and older (Asmanex Twisthaler) and 12 years and older (Asmanex HFA)
Limitations of use: Not indicated for the relief of acute bronchospasm.

Guideline recommendations: A low-dose inhaled corticosteroid (in addition to an as-needed short-acting beta-2 agonist) is the initial preferred long-term control medication for children, adolescents, and adult patients with persistent asthma who are candidates for treatment according to a step-wise treatment approach (GINA 2015; NAEPP 2007).

Pregnancy Considerations Adverse events have been observed in some animal reproduction studies. Hypoadrenalism may occur in infants born to mothers receiving corticosteroids during pregnancy. Based on available data, an overall increased risk of congenital malformations or a decrease in fetal growth has not been associated with maternal use of inhaled corticosteroids during pregnancy (Bakhireva, 2005; NAEPP, 2005; Namazy, 2004). Uncontrolled asthma is associated with adverse events in pregnancy (increased risk of perinatal mortality, preeclampsia, preterm birth, low birth weight infants). Inhaled corticosteroids are recommended for the treatment of asthma during pregnancy (most information available using budesonide) (ACOG, 2008; NAEPP, 2005).

Breast-Feeding Considerations Systemic corticosteroids are excreted in human milk. It is not known if sufficient quantities of mometasone are absorbed following oral inhalation to produce detectable amounts in breast milk; however, oral absorption is limited (<1%). The manufacturer recommends that caution be exercised when administering mometasone to nursing women. The use of inhaled corticosteroids is not considered a contraindication to breast-feeding (NAEPP, 2005).

Contraindications

Hypersensitivity to mometasone or any component of the formulation; hypersensitivity to milk proteins (Asmanex Twisthaler only); primary treatment of status asthmaticus or other acute episodes of asthma for which intensive measures are required

Documentation of allergenic cross-reactivity for corticosteroids is limited. However, because of similarities in chemical structure and/or pharmacologic actions, the possibility of cross-sensitivity cannot be ruled out with certainty.

Canadian labeling: Additional contraindications (not in US labeling): Untreated systemic fungal, bacterial, viral, or parasitic infections; active or quiet tuberculosis infection of the respiratory tract; ocular herpes simplex

Warnings/Precautions May cause hypercorticism or suppression of hypothalamic-pituitary-adrenal (HPA) axis, particularly in younger children or in patients receiving high doses for prolonged periods. HPA axis suppression may lead to adrenal crisis. Withdrawal and discontinuation of a corticosteroid should be done slowly and carefully. Particular care is required when patients are transferred from systemic corticosteroids to inhaled products due to possible adrenal insufficiency or withdrawal from steroids, including an increase in allergic symptoms. Adult patients receiving >20 mg per day of prednisone (or equivalent) may be most susceptible. Fatalities have occurred due to adrenal insufficiency in asthmatic patients during and after transfer from systemic corticosteroids to aerosol steroids; aerosol steroids do not provide the systemic steroid needed to treat patients having trauma, surgery, or infections. Select surgical patients on long-term, high-dose, inhaled corticosteroids should be given stress doses of hydrocortisone intravenously during the surgical period and the dose reduced rapidly within 24 hours after surgery (NAEPP, 2007). When transferring to oral inhaler, previously suppressed allergic conditions (rhinitis, conjunctivitis, eczema) may be unmasked.

Paradoxical bronchospasm may occur with wheezing after inhalation; if this occurs, stop steroid and treat with a fast-acting bronchodilator. Supplemental steroids (oral or parenteral) may be needed during stress or severe asthma attacks. Not to be used in status asthmaticus or for the relief of acute bronchospasm. Corticosteroid use may cause psychiatric disturbances, including depression, euphoria, insomnia, mood swings, and personality changes. Preexisting psychiatric conditions may be exacerbated by corticosteroid use. Prolonged use of corticosteroids may increase the incidence of secondary infection, mask acute infection (including fungal infections), prolong or exacerbate viral infections, or limit response to vaccines. Avoid use if possible in patients with ocular herpes; active or quiescent tuberculosis infections of the respiratory tract; or untreated viral, fungal, or bacterial or parasitic systemic infections. Exposure to chickenpox or measles should be avoided; if the patient is exposed to chickenpox, prophylaxis with varicella zoster immune globulin or pooled intravenous immunoglobulin may be indicated; if chickenpox develops, treatment with antiviral agents may be considered. If exposure to measles, prophylaxis with pooled intramuscular immunoglobulin may be indicated. Canadian labeling contraindicates use in patients with untreated systemic fungal, bacterial, viral, or parasitic infections, active or quiet tuberculosis infection of the respiratory tract, and ocular herpes simplex.

Prolonged treatment with corticosteroids has been associated with the development of Kaposi sarcoma (case reports); if noted, discontinuation of therapy should be considered (Goedert, 2002). Rare cases of vasculitis (Churg-Strauss syndrome) or other systemic eosinophilic conditions can occur; often associated with decrease and/or withdrawal of oral corticosteroid therapy following initiation of inhaled corticosteroid. Local oropharyngeal *Candida* infections have been reported; if occurs, treat appropriately while continuing mometasone therapy. Patients should be instructed to rinse mouth after each use.

Hypersensitivity reactions including allergic dermatitis, anaphylaxis, angioedema, bronchospasm, flushing, pruritus, rash, and urticaria have been reported; if these symptoms occur discontinue use. Use with caution in patients with thyroid disease, hepatic impairment, renal impairment, cardiovascular disease, diabetes, glaucoma, cataracts, myasthenia gravis, patients at risk for seizures, or GI diseases (diverticulitis, peptic ulcer, ulcerative colitis) due to perforation risk. Use caution following acute MI (corticosteroids have been associated with myocardial rupture). Use with caution in patients with major risk factors for decreased bone mineral count such as prolonged immobilization, family history of osteoporosis, or chronic use of drugs that can reduce bone mass (eg, anticonvulsants, oral corticosteroids); long-term use of inhaled corticosteroids have been associated with decreases in bone mineral density. Because of the risk of adverse effects, systemic corticosteroids should be used cautiously in the elderly in the smallest possible effective dose for the shortest duration.

Orally inhaled corticosteroids may cause a reduction in growth velocity in pediatric patients (~1 cm per year [range, 0.3 to 1.8 cm per year] and related to dose and duration of exposure). To minimize the systemic effects of orally inhaled corticosteroids, each patient should be titrated to the lowest effective dose. Growth should be routinely monitored in pediatric patients. Prior to use, the dose and duration of treatment should be based on the risk versus benefit for each individual patient. In general, use the smallest effective dose for the shortest duration of time to minimize adverse events. Short-acting beta-2 agonist (eg, albuterol) should be used for acute symptoms and symptoms occurring between treatments. Withdraw systemic corticosteroid therapy with gradual tapering of dose; consider reducing the daily prednisone dose by 2.5 mg on a weekly basis beginning after at least 1 week of inhalation therapy. Monitor lung function, beta-agonist use, asthma symptoms, and for signs and symptoms of adrenal insufficiency (fatigue, lassitude, weakness, nausea and vomiting, hypotension) during withdrawal. Asmanex Twisthaler may contain lactose; very rare anaphylactic reactions have been reported in patients with severe milk protein allergy. Potentially significant interactions may exist, requiring dose or frequency adjustment, additional monitoring, and/or selection of alternative therapy.

Adverse Reactions

>10%:

Central nervous system: Headache (3% to 22%), fatigue (1% to 13%), depression (11%)

Gastrointestinal: Oral candidiasis (≤22%)

Neuromuscular & skeletal: Musculoskeletal pain (8% to 22%), arthralgia (13%)

Respiratory: Sinusitis (3% to 22%), allergic rhinitis (adolescents & adults 14% to 20%; children 4%), upper respiratory tract infection (8% to 15%), pharyngitis (8% to 13%)

1% to 10%:

Central nervous system: Pain (1% to <3%)

Gastrointestinal: Abdominal pain (3% to 6%), dyspepsia (5%), nausea (3%), vomiting (1% to ≤3%), anorexia (1% to <3%), gastroenteritis (1% to <3%)

Genitourinary: Dysmenorrhea (9%), urinary tract infection (children 2%)

Hematologic & oncologic: Bruise (children 2%)

Infection: Influenza (4%), infection (1% to <3%)

Neuromuscular & skeletal: Back pain (6%), myalgia (3%)

Ophthalmic: Increased intraocular pressure (3%)

Otic: Otalgia (1% to <3%)

Respiratory: Sinus congestion (9%), nasopharyngitis (5% to 8%), bronchitis (3%), dry throat (1% to <3%), epistaxis (1% to <3%), flu-like symptoms (1% to <3%), nasal discomfort (1% to <3%), voice disorder (1% to <3%)

Miscellaneous: Fever (children 7%)

<1% (Limited to important or life-threatening): Cataract, exacerbation of asthma, glaucoma, growth suppression, hypersensitivity

Drug Interactions

Metabolism/Transport Effects Substrate of CYP3A4 (minor); **Note:** Assignment of Major/Minor substrate status based on clinically relevant drug interaction potential

Avoid Concomitant Use

Avoid concomitant use of Mometasone (Oral Inhalation) with any of the following: Aldesleukin; Loxapine

Increased Effect/Toxicity

Mometasone (Oral Inhalation) may increase the levels/effects of: Amphotericin B; Ceritinib; Deferasirox; Loop Diuretics; Loxapine; Thiazide Diuretics

The levels/effects of Mometasone (Oral Inhalation) may be increased by: CYP3A4 Inhibitors (Strong)

Decreased Effect

Mometasone (Oral Inhalation) may decrease the levels/effects of: Aldesleukin; Corticorelin; Hyaluronidase

Storage/Stability

Asmanex HFA: Store at 20°C to 25°C (68°F to 77°F); excursions permitted to 15°C to 30°C (59°F to 86°F). Do not puncture. Do not use or store near heat or open flame. Exposure to temperatures above 120°F may cause bursting. Discard when the dose counter reads "0".

Asmanex Twisthaler: Store at 25°C (77°F); excursions permitted to 15°C to 30°C (59°F to 86°F). Discard when oral dose counter reads "00" (or 45 days [U.S. labeling] or 60 days [Canadian labeling] after opening the foil pouch).

Mechanism of Action May depress the formation, release, and activity of endogenous chemical mediators of inflammation (kinins, histamine, liposomal enzymes, prostaglandins). Leukocytes and macrophages may have to be present for the initiation of responses mediated by the above substances. Inhibits the margination and subsequent cell migration to the area of injury, and also reverses the dilatation and increased vessel permeability in the area resulting in decreased access of cells to the sites of injury.

Pharmacodynamics/Kinetics

Onset of action: Maximum effects may not be evident for ≥1 to 2 weeks

Absorption: <1%

Distribution: V_d: 152 L

Protein binding: 98% to 99%

Metabolism: Hepatic via CYP3A4; forms metabolite

Half-life elimination: ~5 hours

Time to peak, plasma: 0.5 to 2.5 hours

Excretion: Feces (~74%), urine (~8%)

Dosing

Adult & Geriatric Asthma: Oral inhalation: **Note:** Dosage forms of Asmanex Twisthaler available in the United States (110 mcg and 220 mcg Twisthaler) deliver 100 and 200 mcg mometasone furoate per actuation respectively. Maximum effects may not be evident for 1 to 2 weeks or longer; higher doses may provide additional asthma control in patients who do not respond adequately after 2 weeks of therapy. Doses should be titrated to the lowest effective dose.

US labeling:

Previous therapy:

Bronchodilators: Asmanex Twisthaler: Initial: 220 mcg daily (maximum: 440 mcg daily); may be given in the evening or in divided doses twice daily

Inhaled corticosteroids:

Asmanex HFA: Maximum: 400 mcg twice daily (800 mcg daily)

Inhaled medium-dose corticosteroids: Asmanex HFA 100 mcg inhaler: 200 mcg twice daily

Inhaled high-dose corticosteroids: Asmanex HFA 200 mcg inhaler: 400 mcg twice daily

Asmanex Twisthaler: Initial: 220 mcg daily (maximum: 440 mcg daily); may be given in the evening or in divided doses twice daily

Oral corticosteroids: **Note:** Prednisone should be reduced slowly (ie, no faster than 2.5 mg daily on a weekly basis), beginning after at least 1 week of mometasone use

Asmanex HFA: Initial: 400 mcg twice daily (maximum: 800 mcg daily)

Asmanex Twisthaler: Initial: 440 mcg twice daily (maximum: 880 mcg daily)

Canadian labeling:

Usual dose: 200 to 400 mcg once daily in the evening or 200 mcg twice daily administered in the morning and evening. **Note:** Manufacturer suggests that there is a greater chance of achieving asthma control if oncedaily dosing is administered in the evening. Some patients (eg, previously receiving high-dose inhaled corticosteroids) may respond more favorably to 400 mcg daily administered in 2 divided doses. Titrate to the lowest effective dose.

Severe asthma and requiring oral corticosteroids: Initial: 400 mcg twice daily administered in the morning and evening (maximum: 800 mcg daily). Taper off oral corticosteroid gradually by decreasing daily prednisone dose by 1 mg daily (or equivalent of other corticosteroid) no sooner than on a weekly basis, beginning after at least 1 week of mometasone use; upon successful taper off of oral steroids, titrate mometasone to lowest effective dose.

Asthma Guidelines: National Asthma Education and Prevention Program guidelines (NAEPP, 2007): Dry powder inhaler (refers to Asmanex 200 mcg strength available in U.S.) **Note:** 220 mcg inhaler delivers 200 mcg mometasone furoate per actuation; NAEPP uses doses based on delivery, while manufacturer recommended doses are based on inhaler amount

"Low" dose: 200 mcg daily
"Medium" dose: 400 mcg daily
"High" dose: >400 mcg daily

Pediatric

Asthma: Oral inhalation: **Note:** Dosage forms of Asmanex Twisthaler available in the United States (110 mcg and 220 mcg Twisthaler) deliver 100 and 200 mcg mometasone furoate per actuation respectively. Maximum effects may not be evident for 1 to 2 weeks or longer; higher doses may provide additional asthma control in patients who do not respond adequately after 2 weeks of therapy. Doses should be titrated to the lowest effective dose.

Children 4 to 11 years: Asmanex Twisthaler: 110 mcg once daily in the evening (maximum: 110 mcg daily)

Children ≥12 years and Adolescents: Asmanex HFA and Asmanex Twisthaler: Refer to adult dosing.

Asthma Guidelines: National Asthma Education and Prevention Program guidelines (NAEPP, 2007): Dry powder inhaler (refers to Asmanex 200 mcg strength available in United States) **Note:** 220 mcg inhaler delivers 200 mcg mometasone furoate per actuation; NAEPP uses doses based on delivery, while manufacturer recommended doses are based on inhaler amount.

Children ≥12 years and Adolescents: Refer to adult dosing.

Renal Impairment There are no dosage adjustments provided in the manufacturer's labeling (has not been studied).

Hepatic Impairment There are no dosage adjustments provided in the manufacturer's labeling (has not been studied). However, mometasone exposure may increase with hepatic impairment.

Dietary Considerations Asmanex Twisthaler contains lactose.

Administration

Asmanex HFA: Shake well prior to each inhalation. Administer as 2 inhalations twice daily (morning and evening). Prime before first use by releasing 4 test sprays into the air, away from the face, shaking well before each spray. If the inhaler has not been used for more than 5 days, prime the inhaler again with 4 test sprays. Rinse mouth with water without swallowing.

Asmanex Twisthaler: Exhale fully prior to bringing the Twisthaler up to the mouth. Place between lips and inhale quickly and deeply. Do not breathe out through the inhaler. Remove inhaler and hold breath for 10 seconds if possible. Rinse mouth after use.

Monitoring Parameters

Growth (adolescents and children via stadiometry); HPA axis suppression; signs/symptoms of oral candidiasis; ocular effects (eg, cataracts, increased intraocular pressure, glaucoma); hepatic impairment; bone mineral density; FEV_1, peak flow, and/or other pulmonary function tests

Dosage Forms Excipient information presented when available (limited, particularly for generics); consult specific product labeling.

Aerosol, Inhalation, as furoate:
Asmanex HFA: 100 mcg/actuation (13 g); 200 mcg/actuation (13 g)

Aerosol Powder Breath Activated, Inhalation, as furoate:
Asmanex 120 Metered Doses: 220 mcg/INH (1 ea) [contains milk protein]
Asmanex 14 Metered Doses: 220 mcg/INH (1 ea) [contains milk protein]
Asmanex 30 Metered Doses: 110 mcg/INH (1 ea); 220 mcg/INH (1 ea) [contains milk protein]
Asmanex 60 Metered Doses: 220 mcg/INH (1 ea) [contains milk protein]
Asmanex 7 Metered Doses: 110 mcg/INH (1 ea) [contains milk protein]

Dosage Forms: Canada Excipient information presented when available (limited, particularly for generics); consult specific product labeling.

Powder, for oral inhalation, as furoate:
Asmanex Twisthaler: 200 mcg (30 doses, 60 doses) [contains lactose; delivers 200 mcg/actuation]
Asmanex Twisthaler: 400 mcg (30 doses, 60 doses) [contains lactose; delivers 400 mcg/actuation]

Mometasone (Nasal) (moe MET a sone)

Brand Names: US Nasonex
Brand Names: Canada Apo-Mometasone; Nasonex
Index Terms Mometasone Furoate
Pharmacologic Category Corticosteroid, Nasal

Additional Appendix Information
Inhaled Corticosteroids *on page 1951*

Use

Allergic rhinitis (seasonal and perennial): Treatment of nasal symptoms of seasonal allergic and perennial allergic rhinitis in adults and pediatric patients ≥2 years (US labeling) and ≥3 years (Canadian labeling).

Nasal congestion associated with seasonal rhinitis: Relief of nasal congestion associated with seasonal allergic rhinitis in adults and pediatric patients ≥2 years.

Nasal polyps: Treatment of nasal polyps in adults.

Seasonal allergic rhinitis (prophylaxis): Prophylaxis of nasal symptoms of seasonal allergic rhinitis in adults and pediatric patients ≥12 years.

Canadian labeling: Additional use (not in US labeling): Treatment of mild-to-moderate uncomplicated rhinosinusitis or as adjunctive treatment (with antimicrobials) in acute rhinosinusitis in adults and pediatric patients ≥12 years

Dosing

Adult & Geriatric

US labeling:

Allergic rhinitis (seasonal and perennial): Intranasal: 2 sprays (100 mcg) in each nostril once daily (total daily dose: 200 mcg)

Nasal congestion associated with seasonal rhinitis: Intranasal: 2 sprays (100 mcg) in each nostril once daily (total daily dose: 200 mcg)

Nasal polyps: Intranasal: 2 sprays (100 mcg) in each nostril twice daily (total daily dose: 400 mcg); 2 sprays (100 mcg) in each nostril once daily may be effective in some patients

Seasonal allergic rhinitis (prophylaxis): Intranasal: 2 sprays (100 mcg) in each nostril once daily (total daily dose: 200 mcg); treatment should begin 2 to 4 weeks prior to the anticipated start of pollen season

Canadian labeling:

Allergic rhinitis (seasonal and perennial): Intranasal: Initial: 2 sprays (100 mcg) in each nostril once daily (total daily dose: 200 mcg); upon symptom control, may consider dose reduction to 1 spray (50 mcg) in each nostril once daily as maintenance therapy. **Note:** If adequate symptom control is not achieved with initial dosing, may increase dose to 4 sprays (200 mcg) in each nostril once daily (total daily dose: 400 mcg). Dose reduction is recommended upon symptom control.

Nasal polyps: Intranasal: 2 sprays (100 mcg) in each nostril twice daily (total daily dose: 400 mcg); upon symptom control, may consider dose reduction to 2 sprays (100 mcg) once daily which may be effective for continued treatment; treatment duration for 4 months has been studied

Rhinosinusitis, adjunctive treatment (acute): Intranasal: 2 sprays (100 mcg) in each nostril twice daily (total daily dose: 400 mcg); if inadequate symptom control, may increase to 4 sprays (200 mcg) in each nostril twice daily (total daily dose: 800 mcg)

Rhinosinusitis treatment (acute, mild to moderate, uncomplicated): Intranasal: 2 sprays (100 mcg) in each nostril twice daily (total daily dose: 400 mcg); use beyond 15 days has not been studied.

Pediatric

US labeling:

Allergic rhinitis (seasonal and perennial): Intranasal:
Children 2 to 11 years: 1 spray (50 mcg) in each nostril once daily (total daily dose: 100 mcg)
Children ≥12 years and Adolescents: Refer to adult dosing.

Nasal congestion associated with seasonal rhinitis: Intranasal:
Children 2 to 11 years: 1 spray (50 mcg) in each nostril once daily (total daily dose: 100 mcg)
Children ≥12 years and Adolescents: Refer to adult dosing

Seasonal allergic rhinitis (prophylaxis): Intranasal: Children ≥12 years and Adolescents: Refer to adult dosing.

Canadian labeling:

Allergic rhinitis (seasonal and perennial): Intranasal:
Children 3 to 11 years: 1 spray (50 mcg) in each nostril once daily (total daily dose: 100 mcg)
Children ≥12 years and Adolescents: Refer to adult dosing.

Rhinosinusitis, adjunctive treatment (acute): Intranasal: Children ≥12 years and Adolescents: Refer to adult dosing.

Rhinosinusitis treatment (acute, mild to moderate, uncomplicated): Intranasal: Children ≥12 years and Adolescents: Refer to adult dosing.

◀ **Renal Impairment** There are no dosage adjustments provided in the manufacturer's labeling (has not been studied)

Hepatic Impairment There are no dosage adjustments provided in the manufacturer's labeling; drug accumulation may increase with severity of hepatic impairment.

Additional Information Complete prescribing information should be consulted for additional detail.

Dosage Forms Considerations Nasonex 17 g bottles contain 120 sprays.

Dosage Forms Excipient information presented when available (limited, particularly for generics); consult specific product labeling.

Suspension, Nasal, as furoate:

Nasonex: 50 mcg/actuation (17 g) [contains benzalkonium chloride]

Dosage Forms: Canada Excipient information presented when available (limited, particularly for generics); consult specific product labeling.

Suspension, intranasal, as furoate [spray]:

Nasonex: 50 mcg/spray [contains benzalkonium chloride; delivers 140 sprays]

Mometasone (Topical) (moe MET a sone)

Brand Names: US Elocon

Brand Names: Canada Elocom; PMS-Mometasone; ratio-Mometasone; Taro-Mometasone

Index Terms Mometasone Furoate

Pharmacologic Category Corticosteroid, Topical

Additional Appendix Information

Topical Corticosteroids *on page 1952*

Use Corticosteroid-responsive dermatoses: Relief of the inflammatory and pruritic manifestations of corticosteroid-responsive dermatoses (medium potency topical corticosteroid)

Dosing

Adult Corticosteroid-responsive dermatoses: Topical: Apply sparingly, do not use occlusive dressings. Therapy should be discontinued when control is achieved; consider reassessment of diagnosis if no improvement is seen within 2 weeks.

U.S. labeling:

Cream, ointment: Apply a thin film to affected area once daily

Lotion: Apply a few drops to affected area once daily

Canadian labeling:

Cream, ointment: Apply a thin film to affected area once daily; do not use on face, axillae or scrotum for more than 5 days and on the body for more than 3 weeks

Lotion: Apply a few drops to the affected area once daily; do not use on the face, scalp, axillae or scrotum for more than 5 days and on the body for more than 3 weeks

Geriatric Refer to adult dosing. Use with caution as elderly patients may be more susceptible to systemic effects.

Pediatric Corticosteroid-responsive dermatoses: Topical: Apply sparingly, do not use occlusive dressings. Therapy should be discontinued when control is achieved; consider reassessment of diagnosis if no improvement is seen within 2 weeks.

Cream, ointment: Children ≥2 years and Adolescents: Refer to adult dosing. Do not use in pediatric patients for longer than 3 weeks. Canadian labeling does not approve for use in patients <18 years.

Lotion: Children ≥12 years and Adolescents: Refer to adult dosing. Canadian labeling does not approve for use in patients <18 years.

Renal Impairment

U.S. labeling: There are no dosage adjustments provided in the manufacturer's labeling.

Canadian labeling: There are no specific dosage adjustments provided in the manufacturer's labeling; however, the manufacturer recommends applying a minimum quantity for the shortest duration

Hepatic Impairment

U.S. labeling: There are no dosage adjustments provided in the manufacturer's labeling.

Canadian labeling: There are no specific dosage adjustments provided in the manufacturer's labeling; however, the manufacturer recommends applying a minimum quantity for the shortest duration

Additional Information Complete prescribing information should be consulted for additional detail.

Dosage Forms Excipient information presented when available (limited, particularly for generics); consult specific product labeling.

Cream, External, as furoate:

Elocon: 0.1% (15 g, 45 g, 50 g) [contains soybean lecithin]

Generic: 0.1% (15 g, 45 g)

Lotion, External, as furoate:

Elocon: 0.1% (30 mL, 60 mL) [contains isopropyl alcohol, propylene glycol]

Ointment, External, as furoate:

Elocon: 0.1% (15 g, 45 g) [contains propylene glycol stearate]

Generic: 0.1% (15 g, 45 g)

Solution, External, as furoate:

Generic: 0.1% (30 mL, 60 mL)

◆ Mometasone and Eformoterol *see* Mometasone and Formoterol *on page 1228*

Mometasone and Formoterol
(moe MET a sone & for MOH te rol)

Brand Names: US Dulera

Brand Names: Canada Zenhale

Index Terms Eformoterol and Mometasone; Formoterol and Mometasone; Formoterol and Mometasone Furoate; Formoterol Fumarate Dihydrate and Mometasone; Mometasone and Eformoterol

Pharmacologic Category Beta$_2$ Agonist, Long-Acting; Beta$_2$-Adrenergic Agonist, Long-Acting; Corticosteroid, Inhalant (Oral)

Use Asthma: Treatment of asthma in patients 12 years and older.

Limitations of use: Mometasone/formoterol is not indicated for the relief of acute bronchospasm.

Medication Guide Available Yes

Dosing

Adult & Geriatric

Asthma: Oral inhalation:

Previous therapy included inhaled low-dose corticosteroids: Canadian labeling (not in US labeling): Mometasone 50 mcg/formoterol 5 mcg: Two inhalations twice daily. Maximum daily dose: Mometasone 200 mcg/formoterol 20 mcg (4 inhalations).

Previous therapy included inhaled medium-dose corticosteroids: Mometasone 100 mcg/formoterol 5 mcg: Two inhalations twice daily. Consider the higher dose combination for patients not adequately controlled on the lower combination following 2 weeks of therapy. Maximum daily dose: Mometasone 400 mcg/formoterol 20 mcg (4 inhalations).

Previous therapy included inhaled high-dose corticosteroids: Mometasone 200 mcg/formoterol 5 mcg: Two inhalations twice daily. Maximum daily dose: Mometasone 800 mcg/formoterol 20 mcg (4 inhalations).

Chronic obstructive pulmonary disease (stable) (off-label use): Oral inhalation: Mometasone 200 mcg/formoterol 10 mcg to mometasone 400 mcg/formoterol 10 mcg twice daily (Doherty, 2012; GOLD, 2014).

Pediatric Asthma: Oral inhalation: Children ≥12 years and Adolescents: Refer to adult dosing.

Renal Impairment There are no dosage adjustments provided in the manufacturer's labeling (has not been studied).

Hepatic Impairment There are no dosage adjustments provided in the manufacturer's labeling (has not been studied) However, mometasone exposure is increased with hepatic impairment.

Additional Information Complete prescribing information should be consulted for additional detail.

Dosage Forms Excipient information presented when available (limited, particularly for generics); consult specific product labeling.

Aerosol, for oral inhalation:

Dulera: Mometasone furoate 100 mcg and formoterol fumarate dihydrate 5 mcg per inhalation (8.8 g) [60 metered actuations]

Dulera: Mometasone furoate 100 mcg and formoterol fumarate dihydrate 5 mcg per inhalation (13 g) [120 metered actuations]

Dulera: Mometasone furoate 200 mcg and formoterol fumarate dihydrate 5 mcg per inhalation (8.8 g) [60 metered actuations]

Dulera: Mometasone furoate 200 mcg and formoterol fumarate dihydrate 5 mcg per inhalation (13 g) [120 metered actuations]

Dosage Forms: Canada Excipient information presented when available (limited, particularly for generics); consult specific product labeling.

Aerosol, for oral inhalation:

Zenhale: Mometasone furoate 50 mcg and formoterol fumarate dihydrate 5 mcg per inhalation [120 metered actuations]

Montelukast (mon te LOO kast)

Brand Names: US Singulair

Brand Names: Canada ACH-Montelukast; Apo-Montelukast; Auro-Montelukast; Auro-Montelukast Chewable Tablets; Dom-Montelukast; Dom-Montelukast FC; Jamp-Montelukast; Mar-Montelukast; Mint-Montelukast; Montelukast Sodium Tablets; Mylan-Montelukast; PMS-Montelukast; PMS-Montelukast FC; RAN-Montelukast; Riva-Montelukast FC; Sandoz-Montelukast; Sandoz-Montelukast Granules; Singulair; Teva-Montelukast

Index Terms Montelukast Sodium

Pharmacologic Category Leukotriene-Receptor Antagonist

Use

Prophylaxis and chronic treatment of asthma; relief of symptoms of seasonal allergic rhinitis and perennial allergic rhinitis; prevention of exercise-induced bronchoconstriction.

Note: American Academy of Otolaryngology, Head and Neck Surgery (AAO-HNS) guidelines recommend *against* montelukast use as first-line therapy for allergic rhinitis (except in patients with concurrent asthma) (Seidman, 2015 [AAO-HNS, 2015]).

Pregnancy Considerations Adverse events have not been observed in animal reproduction studies. Structural defects have been reported in neonates exposed to montelukast *in utero*; however, a specific pattern and relationship to montelukast has not been established. Based on available data, an increased risk of teratogenic effects has not been observed with montelukast use in pregnancy (Bakhireva 2007; Nelsen 2012; Sarkar 2009). Uncontrolled asthma is associated with adverse events on pregnancy (increased risk of perinatal mortality, pre-eclampsia, preterm birth, low birth weight infants). Montelukast may be considered for use in women who had a favorable response prior to becoming pregnant; however, initiating a leukotriene receptor antagonist during pregnancy is an alternative (but not preferred) treatment option for mild persistent asthma (NAEPP 2005).

Breast-Feeding Considerations It is not known if montelukast is excreted into breast milk. The manufacturer recommends that caution be exercised when administering montelukast to nursing women.

Contraindications Hypersensitivity to montelukast or any component of the formulation

Warnings/Precautions Montelukast is not FDA approved for use in the reversal of bronchospasm in acute asthma attacks, including status asthmaticus; some studies, however, support its use as adjunctive therapy (Cylly, 2003; Ferreira, 2001; Harmancik, 2006). Appropriate rescue medication should be available. Montelukast treatment should continue during acute asthma exacerbation. When inhaled or systemic corticosteroid reduction is considered in patients initiating or receiving montelukast, appropriate clinical monitoring and a gradual dose reduction of the steroid are recommended.

Postmarketing reports of behavioral changes (eg, agitation, aggression, anxiety, attention deficit, depression, hallucinations, hostility, insomnia, irritability, restlessness, sleep disturbance, suicide ideation/behavior) have been noted in pediatric, adolescent, and adult patients. In a retrospective analysis performed by Merck, serious behavior-related events were rare (Philip, 2009a); assess patients for behavioral changes. Patients should be instructed to notify the prescriber if behavioral changes occur.

Potentially significant drug-drug interactions may exist, requiring dose or frequency adjustment, additional monitoring, and/or selection of alternative therapy. In rare cases, patients on therapy with montelukast may present with systemic eosinophilia, sometimes presenting with clinical features of vasculitis consistent with Churg-Strauss syndrome, a condition which is often treated with systemic corticosteroid therapy. Healthcare providers should be alert to eosinophilia, vasculitic rash, worsening pulmonary symptoms, cardiac complications, and/or neuropathy presenting in their patients. A causal association between montelukast and these underlying conditions has not been established. Montelukast will not interrupt bronchoconstrictor response to aspirin or other NSAIDs; aspirin sensitive asthmatics should continue to avoid these agents. The chewable tablet contains phenylalanine.

Adverse Reactions

Children ≥15 years and Adults:

>10%: Central nervous system: Headache (18%)

1% to 10%:

Central nervous system: Dizziness (2%), fatigue (2%), fever (2%)

Dermatologic: Skin rash (2%)

Gastrointestinal: Dyspepsia (2%), gastroenteritis (2%), toothache (2%)

Hepatic: Increased serum AST (2%), increased serum ALT (≥1%)

Neuromuscular & skeletal: Weakness (2%)

Respiratory: Nasal congestion (2%), cough (≥1%), epistaxis (≥1%), sinusitis (≥1%), upper respiratory tract infection (≥1%)

Children 2 to ≤14 years: ≥2%:

Central nervous system: Fever, headache

Dermatologic: Dermatitis, eczema, skin rash, urticaria

Gastrointestinal: Abdominal pain, dyspepsia, gastroenteritis, nausea

Infection: Influenza, varicella, viral infection

Ophthalmic: Conjunctivitis

Otic: Otalgia, otitis

Respiratory: Laryngitis, pharyngitis, pneumonia, rhinorrhea, sinusitis, upper respiratory tract infection

Children 6 to 23 months: ≥2%:

Respiratory: Cough, otitis media, pharyngitis, rhinitis, tonsillitis, upper respiratory tract infection, wheezing

Postmarketing and/or case reports (Limited to important or life-threatening): Churg-Strauss syndrome, depression, disorientation, eosinophilia (systemic), eosinophilic pneumonitis, erythema multiforme, erythema nodosum, hallucination, hepatic eosinophilic infiltration, hepatitis (mixed pattern, hepatocellular, and cholestatic), hypersensitivity, insomnia, memory impairment, pancreatitis, paresthesia, seizure, somnambulism, Stevens-Johnson syndrome, suicidal ideation, suicidal tendencies, thrombocytopenia, toxic epidermal necrolysis, urinary incontinence (children)

Drug Interactions

Metabolism/Transport Effects Substrate of CYP2C8 (minor), CYP2C9 (minor), CYP3A4 (minor); **Note:** Assignment of Major/Minor substrate status based on clinically relevant drug interaction potential; **Inhibits** CYP2C8 (weak), CYP2C9 (weak)

Avoid Concomitant Use

Avoid concomitant use of Montelukast with any of the following: Amodiaquine; Loxapine

Increased Effect/Toxicity

Montelukast may increase the levels/effects of: Amodiaquine; Loxapine

The levels/effects of Montelukast may be increased by: Gemfibrozil

Decreased Effect

The levels/effects of Montelukast may be decreased by: Lumacaftor

Storage/Stability Store at room temperature of 25°C (77°F); excursions permitted to 15°C to 30°C (59°F to 86°F). Store in original package. Protect from moisture and light. Granules must be used within 15 minutes of opening packet.

Mechanism of Action Selective leukotriene receptor antagonist that inhibits the cysteinyl leukotriene receptor. Cysteinyl leukotrienes and leukotriene receptor occupation have been correlated with the pathophysiology of asthma, including airway edema, smooth muscle contraction, and altered cellular activity associated with the inflammatory process, which contribute to the signs and symptoms of asthma. Cysteinyl leukotrienes are also released from the nasal mucosa following allergen exposure leading to symptoms associated with allergic rhinitis (Jarvis, 2000).

Pharmacodynamics/Kinetics

Duration: >24 hours

Absorption: Rapid

Distribution: V_d: 8-11 L

Protein binding, plasma: >99%

Metabolism: Extensively hepatic via CYP3A4, 2C8, and 2C9

Bioavailability: Tablet: 10 mg, Mean: 64%; Chewable tablet: 5 mg: 73% (63% when administered with a standard meal)

Half-life elimination: 2.7-5.5 hours; Mild-to-moderate hepatic impairment: 7.4 hours

Time to peak: Tablet: 10 mg: 3-4 hours; Chewable tablet: 2-2.5 hours; granules: 1-3 hours (fasting) and 3.5 to ~9 hours (with high-fat meal)

Excretion: Feces (86%); urine (<0.2%)

Dosing

Adult & Geriatric Note: Patients with **both** asthma and allergic rhinitis should take only one dose in the evening.

Allergic rhinitis (perennial or seasonal): Oral: 10 mg once daily

Asthma: Oral: 10 mg once daily (in the evening)

Bronchoconstriction, exercise-induced (prevention): Oral: 10 mg at least 2 hours prior to exercise. **Note:** Additional doses should not be administered within 24 hours. Daily administration to prevent exercise-induced bronchoconstriction has not been evaluated. Patients receiving montelukast for another indication should not take an additional dose to prevent exercise-induced bronchoconstriction.

Chronic urticaria (off-label use): Oral: 10 mg once daily (DiLorenzo 2004; Nettis 2004)

Urticaria (nonsteroidal anti-inflammatory drug-induced) (off-label use): Oral: 10 mg once daily (Pacor 2001)

Pediatric Note: Patients with **both** asthma and allergic rhinitis should take only one dose in the evening.

Asthma: Oral:

Children ≥1 to <2 years: 4 mg (oral granules) once daily (in the evening)

Children ≥2 to <6 years: 4 mg (chewable tablet or oral granules) once daily (in the evening)

Children ≥6 years and Adolescents <15 years: 5 mg (chewable tablet) once daily (in the evening)

Adolescents ≥15 years: 10 mg once daily (in the evening)

Bronchoconstriction, exercise-induced (prevention): Note: Additional doses should not be administered within 24 hours. Daily administration to prevent exercise-induced bronchoconstriction has not been evaluated. Patients receiving montelukast for another indication should not take an additional dose to prevent exercise-induced bronchoconstriction. Oral:

Children ≥6 years and Adolescents <15 years: 5 mg (chewable tablet) at least 2 hours prior to exercise

Adolescents ≥15 years: 10 mg once daily at least 2 hours prior to exercise

Perennial allergic rhinitis: Oral:

Children 6 months to <2 years: 4 mg (oral granules) once daily

Children ≥2 to <6 years: 4 mg (chewable tablet or oral granules) once daily

Children ≥6 years and Adolescents <15 years: 5 mg (chewable tablet) once daily

Adolescents ≥15 years: 10 mg once daily

Seasonal allergic rhinitis: Oral:

Children ≥2 to <6 years: 4 mg (chewable tablet or oral granules) once daily

Children ≥6 years and Adolescents <15 years: 5 mg (chewable tablet) once daily

Adolescents ≥15 years: 10 mg once daily

Urticaria (nonsteroidal anti-inflammatory drug-induced) (off-label use): Oral: Adolescents ≥15 years: 10 mg once daily (Pacor 2001)

Renal Impairment No dosage adjustment necessary.

Hepatic Impairment

Mild-to-moderate impairment: No dosage adjustment necessary.

Severe impairment: No dosage adjustment provided in manufacturer's labeling; has not been studied.

Dietary Considerations Some products may contain phenylalanine.

Administration When treating asthma, administer dose in the evening. Patients with allergic rhinitis may individualize administration time (morning or evening). Patients with **both** asthma and allergic rhinitis should take a single dose in the evening. May administer without regard to food or meals.

Granules: May be administered directly in the mouth, dissolved in 5 mL of baby formula or breast milk, or mixed with a spoonful of applesauce, carrots, rice, or ice cream; do not add to any other liquids or foods. Administer within 15 minutes of opening packet.

Monitoring Parameters Mood or behavior changes, including suicidal thinking/behavior

Dosage Forms Excipient information presented when available (limited, particularly for generics); consult specific product labeling.

Packet, Oral:

Singulair: 4 mg (30 ea)

Generic: 4 mg (1 ea, 30 ea)

Tablet, Oral:

Singulair: 10 mg

Generic: 10 mg

Tablet Chewable, Oral:

Singulair: 4 mg [contains aspartame]

Singulair: 4 mg [contains aspartame; cherry flavor]

Singulair: 5 mg [contains aspartame]

Singulair: 5 mg [contains aspartame; cherry flavor]

Generic: 4 mg, 5 mg

Morphine (Systemic) (MOR feen)

Brand Names: US Astramorph; AVINza [DSC]; Duramorph; Infumorph 200; Infumorph 500; Kadian; MS Contin

Brand Names: Canada Doloral; Kadian; M-Eslon; M.O.S. 10; M.O.S. 20; M.O.S. 30; M.O.S.-SR; M.O.S.-Sulfate; Morphine Extra Forte Injection; Morphine Forte Injection; Morphine HP; Morphine LP Epidural; Morphine SR; Morphine-EPD; MS Contin; MS Contin SRT; MS-IR; Novo-Morphine SR; PMS-Morphine Sulfate SR; ratio-Morphine; ratio-Morphine SR; Sandoz-Morphine SR; Statex; Teva-Morphine SR

Index Terms MorphaBond; MS (error-prone abbreviation and should not be used); MSO_4 (error-prone abbreviation and should not be used); Oramorph SR; Roxanol

Pharmacologic Category Analgesic, Opioid

Additional Appendix Information

Opioid Conversion Table and Morphine Equivalent Dose Table *on page 1955*

Use

Immediate-release oral products: Relief of moderate to severe acute and chronic pain for which use of an opioid analgesic is appropriate.

Injection: Relief of severe pain, such as myocardial infarction and severe injuries; relief of dyspnea of acute left ventricular failure and pulmonary edema; preanesthetic medication

Preservative-free injectable solution:

Infumorph: Used in continuous microinfusion devices for intrathecal or epidural administration in treatment of intractable chronic pain

Duramorph: For intravenous, epidural, or intrathecal administration in the management of pain for extended periods without attendant loss of motor, sensory, or sympathetic function. **Note:** Not for use in continuous microinfusion devices.

Extended-release oral products: Management of pain severe enough to require daily, around-the-clock, long-term opioid treatment and for which alternative treatment options are inadequate

Limitations of use: Because of the risks of addiction, abuse, and misuse with opioids, even at recommended doses, and because of the greater risks of overdose and death with extended-release formulations, reserve extended-release formulations for use in patients for whom alternative treatment options (eg, nonopioid analgesics, immediate-release opioids) are ineffective, not tolerated, or would be otherwise inadequate to provide sufficient management of pain. MS Contin, Kadian, and Avinza are not indicated as as-needed analgesics.

Pregnancy Considerations Adverse events have been observed in some animal reproduction studies. Morphine crosses the human placenta. The frequency of congenital malformations has not been reported to be greater than expected in children from mothers treated with morphine during pregnancy. However, following *in utero* exposure, infants may exhibit withdrawal, decreased brain volume (reversible), small size, decreased ventilatory response to CO_2, and increased risk of sudden infant death syndrome.

Morphine sulfate injection may be used for the management of pain during labor (ACOG, 2002); however, some manufacturers specifically contraindicate use of the injection during labor when a premature birth is anticipated. When used for pain relief during labor, opioids may temporarily affect the heart rate of the fetus. Morphine injection may also be used to treat pain following delivery (ACOG, 2002).

[U.S. Boxed Warning]: Prolonged maternal use of opioids during pregnancy can cause neonatal withdrawal syndrome in the newborn, which may be life-threatening if not recognized and treated according to protocols developed by neonatology experts. If prolonged opioid therapy is required in a pregnant woman, ensure treatment is available and warn patient of risk to the neonate. If chronic opioid exposure occurs in pregnancy, adverse events in the newborn (including withdrawal) may occur; monitoring of the neonate is recommended. The minimum effective dose should be used if opioids are needed (Chou, 2009). Neonatal abstinence syndrome following opioid exposure may present with autonomic (eg, fever, temperature instability), gastrointestinal (eg, diarrhea, vomiting, poor feeding/weight gain), or neurologic (eg, high-pitched crying, increased muscle tone, irritability, seizure, tremor) symptoms (Dow, 2012; Hudak, 2012).

Long-term opioid use may cause secondary hypogonadism, which may lead to sexual dysfunction or infertility (Brennan, 2013).

Breast-Feeding Considerations Morphine concentrates in breast milk, with a milk to plasma AUC ratio of 2.5:1. Detectable serum levels of morphine can be found in infants following morphine administration to nursing mothers.

Parenteral opioids used during labor have the potential to interfere with a newborn's natural reflex to nurse within the first few hours after birth. Morphine is recommended as an analgesic in nursing women due to the limited amounts found in breast milk and poor oral bioavailability in nursing infants. Nursing infants exposed to large doses of opioids should be monitored for apnea and sedation (Montgomery, 2012).

Treatment of the mother with single doses of morphine is not expected to cause detrimental effects in nursing infants. Breast-feeding following chronic use or in neonates with hepatic or renal dysfunction may lead to higher levels of morphine in the infant and a risk of adverse effects (Spigset, 2000).

The manufacturers of extended release products note that due to the potential for serious adverse reactions in the nursing infant, a decision should be made whether to discontinue nursing or to discontinue the drug, taking into account the importance of treatment to the mother.

Medication Guide Available Yes

Contraindications Note: Some contraindications are product specific. For details, please see detailed product prescribing information.

Hypersensitivity to morphine sulfate or any component of the formulation; severe respiratory depression, acute or severe asthma (in an unmonitored setting or without resuscitative equipment); known or suspected paralytic ileus

Additional contraindication information (based on formulation):

Epidural/intrathecal:

Astramorph/PF, Duramorph: Upper airway obstruction

Astramorph/PF, Duramorph, Infumorph: Usual contraindications related to neuraxial analgesia apply (eg, presence of infection at infusion site, concomitant anticoagulant therapy, uncontrolled bleeding diathesis)

Extended release: GI obstruction

Immediate release tablets/solution: Hypercarbia

Injectable formulation: Heart failure due to chronic lung disease, cardiac arrhythmias; increased intracranial pressure, head injuries, brain tumors; acute alcoholism, deliriums tremens; seizure disorders; use during labor when a premature birth is anticipated

Suppository: Severe CNS depression; cardiac arrhythmias, heart failure due to chronic lung disease; increased intracranial or cerebrospinal pressure, head injuries, brain tumor; acute alcoholism, delirium tremens; seizure disorder; use after biliary tract surgery, suspected surgical abdomen, surgical anastomosis; concurrent use or within 2 weeks of MAO inhibitors

Warnings/Precautions An opioid-containing analgesic regimen should be tailored to each patient's needs and based upon the type of pain being treated (acute versus chronic), the route of administration, degree of tolerance for opioids (naive versus chronic user), age, weight, and medical condition. The optimal analgesic dose varies widely among patients. Doses should be titrated to pain relief/prevention. When used as an epidural injection, monitor for delayed sedation.

All morphine sulfate formulations are capable of causing respiratory depression; risk increased in elderly patients, debilitated patients, and patients with conditions associated with hypoxia or hypercapnia. Monitor for respiratory depression, especially during initiation and titration. Extended-release formulations: **[U.S. Boxed Warning]: May cause serious, life-threatening, or fatal respiratory depression. Monitor closely for respiratory depression, especially during initiation or dose escalation. Instruct patients to swallow extended-release morphine formulations whole (or may sprinkle the contents of the Avinza capsule on applesauce and swallow without chewing); crushing, chewing, or dissolving the extended-release formulations can cause rapid release and absorption of a potentially fatal dose of morphine.** Carbon dioxide retention from opioid-induced respiratory depression can exacerbate the sedating effects of opioids. Use with caution and monitor for respiratory depression in patients with significant chronic obstructive pulmonary disease or cor pulmonale, and patients having a substantially decreased respiratory reserve, hypoxia, hypercarbia, or preexisting respiratory depression, particularly when initiating therapy and titrating with morphine; even therapeutic doses may decrease respiratory drive to the point of apnea. Consider the use of alternative nonopioid analgesics in these patients. Some dosage forms may be contraindicated in patients with severe respiratory disorders. Infants <3 months of age are more susceptible to respiratory depression, use with caution and generally in reduced doses in this age group.

Use caution in morbid obesity, adrenal insufficiency, prostatic hyperplasia, thyroid dysfunction, urinary stricture, renal impairment, or severe hepatic dysfunction and in patients with hypersensitivity reactions to other phenanthrene derivative opioid agonists (codeine, hydrocodone, hydromorphone, levorphanol, oxycodone, oxymorphone). Avoid use in patients with CNS depression or coma as these patients are susceptible to intracranial effects of CO_2 retention. Use with caution in patients with biliary tract dysfunction including acute pancreatitis as may cause constriction of sphincter of Oddi. May obscure diagnosis or clinical course of patients with acute abdominal conditions. May cause constipation which may be problematic in patients with unstable angina and patients post-myocardial infarction. Some preparations contain sulfites which may cause allergic reactions.

May cause CNS depression, which may impair physical or mental abilities; patients must be cautioned about performing tasks which require mental alertness (eg, operating machinery or driving). Potentially significant drug interactions may exist, requiring dose or frequency adjustment, additional monitoring, and/or selection of alternative therapy. Effects may be potentiated when used with other CNS ▶

depressants (eg, sedatives, anxiolytics, hypnotics, neuro-leptics, other opioids). **[U.S. Boxed Warning]: Patients should not consume alcoholic beverages or medication containing ethanol while taking Avinza or Kadian; ethanol may increase morphine plasma levels resulting in a potentially fatal overdose.**

May cause hypotension; use with caution in patients with hypovolemia, cardiovascular disease (including acute MI), circulatory shock, or drugs which may exaggerate hypotensive effects (including phenothiazines or general anesthetics). May cause orthostatic hypotension and syncope in ambulatory patients. Use with extreme caution in patients with head injury, intracranial lesions, or elevated intracranial pressure; exaggerated elevation of ICP may occur if respiratory drive is depressed and CO_2 retention occurs. Use with caution in patients with seizure disorders, may exacerbate preexisting seizures. Tolerance or drug dependence may result from extended use. Concurrent use of mixed agonist/antagonist analgesics (eg, pentazocine, nalbuphine, butorphanol) or partial agonist (eg, buprenorphine) analgesics may precipitate withdrawal symptoms and/or reduced analgesic efficacy in patients following prolonged therapy with mu opioid agonists. Abrupt discontinuation following prolonged use may also lead to withdrawal symptoms; taper dose gradually when discontinuing.

Use epidural/intrathecal formulations with extreme caution in elderly patients.

Extended-release formulations: **[U.S. Boxed Warning]: Users are exposed to the risks of addiction, abuse, and misuse, potentially leading to overdose and death. Assess each patient's risk prior to prescribing; monitor all patients regularly for development of these behaviors or conditions.** Risk of opioid abuse is increased in patients with a history or family history of alcohol or drug abuse or mental illness. Avinza capsules contain fumaric acid; dangerous quantities of fumaric acid may be ingested when >1600 mg/day is used; serious renal toxicity may occur above the maximum dose. **Extended-release products are not interchangeable;** when determining a generic equivalent or switching from one extended-release product to another, review pharmacokinetic properties. **[U.S. Boxed Warning]: Prolonged maternal use of opioids during pregnancy can cause neonatal withdrawal syndrome in the newborn which may be life-threatening if not recognized and treated according to protocols developed by neonatology experts. If prolonged opioid therapy is required in a pregnant woman, ensure treatment is available and warn patient of risk to the neonate.** Signs and symptoms include irritability, hyperactivity, abnormal sleep pattern, high-pitched cry, tremor, vomiting, diarrhea, and failure to gain weight. Onset, duration, and severity depend on the drug used, duration of use, maternal dose, and rate of drug elimination by the newborn. **[U.S. Boxed Warning]: Accidental ingestion of even one dose, especially in children, can result in a fatal overdose of morphine.**

Highly concentrated oral solutions: **[U.S. Boxed Warning]: Check doses carefully when using highly concentrated oral solutions. The 100 mg/5 mL (20 mg/mL) concentration is indicated for use in opioid-tolerant patients only.**

Injections: Products are designed for administration by specific routes (ie, IV, intrathecal, epidural). Use caution when prescribing, dispensing, or administering to use formulations only by intended route(s).

Astramorph/PF, Duramorph, Infumorph: **[U.S. Boxed Warning]: Due to the risk of severe and/or sustained cardiopulmonary depressant effects, must be administered in a fully equipped room for resuscitation and staffed environment.** Naloxone injection should be immediately available. Patient should remain in this environment for at least 24 hours following the initial dose. **[U.S. Boxed Warning]: Accidental dermal exposure to Astramorph/ PF, Duramorph, Infumorph should be rinsed with water. Contaminated clothing should be removed.** For patients receiving Infumorph via microinfusion device, patient may be observed, as appropriate, for the first several days after catheter implantation. Thoracic epidural administration has been shown to dramatically increase the risk of early and late respiratory depression.

[U.S. Boxed Warning]: Improper or erroneous substitution of Infumorph for regular Duramorph is likely to result in serious overdosage, leading to seizures, respiratory depression and possibly a fatal outcome. Infumorph should only be used in microinfusion devices; not for IV, IM, or SubQ administration or for single-dose administration. Monitor closely, especially in the first 24 hours. Inflammatory masses (eg, granulomas), some

resulting in severe neurologic impairment have occurred when receiving Infumorph via indwelling intrathecal catheter; monitor carefully for new neurologic signs/symptoms. **[U.S. Boxed Warning]: Intrathecal dosage is usually ¹/₁₀ (one-tenth) that of epidural dosage.**

Benzyl alcohol and derivatives: Some dosage forms may contain sodium benzoate/benzoic acid; benzoic acid (benzoate) is a metabolite of benzyl alcohol; large amounts of benzyl alcohol (≥99 mg/kg/day) have been associated with a potentially fatal toxicity ("gasping syndrome") in neonates; the "gasping syndrome" consists of metabolic acidosis, respiratory distress, gasping respirations, CNS dysfunction (including convulsions, intracranial hemorrhage), hypotension, and cardiovascular collapse (AAP ["Inactive" 1997]; CDC, 1982); some data suggests that benzoate displaces bilirubin from protein binding sites (Ahlfors, 2001); avoid or use dosage forms containing benzyl alcohol derivative with caution in neonates. See manufacturer's labeling.

Adverse Reactions Note: Individual patient differences are unpredictable, and percentage may differ in acute pain (surgical) treatment. Reactions may be dose, formulation, and/or route dependent.

Frequency not defined:
 Cardiovascular: Circulatory depression, flushing, shock
 Central nervous system: Dysphonia, physical and psychological dependence, sedation
 Endocrine & metabolic: Antidiuretic hormone release, hypogonadism
 Neuromuscular & skeletal: Bone mineral density decreased
>10%:
 Cardiovascular: Bradycardia, hypotension
 Central nervous system: Drowsiness (9% to 48%; tolerance usually develops to drowsiness with regular dosing for 1-2 weeks), dizziness (6% to 20%), fever (<3% to >10%), confusion, headache (following epidural or intrathecal use)
 Dermatologic: Pruritus (may be dose related)
 Gastrointestinal: Xerostomia (78%), constipation (9% to 40%; tolerance develops very slowly if at all), nausea (7% to 28%; tolerance usually develops to nausea and vomiting with chronic use), vomiting
 Genitourinary: Urinary retention (16%; may be prolonged, up to 20 hours, following epidural or intrathecal use)
 Hematologic: Anemia (following intrathecal use)
 Local: Pain at injection site
 Neuromuscular & skeletal: Weakness
 Respiratory: Oxygen saturation decreased
 Miscellaneous: Histamine release
1% to 10%:
 Cardiovascular: Atrial fibrillation (<3%), chest pain (<3%), edema, hypertension, palpitation, peripheral edema, syncope, tachycardia, vasodilation
 Central nervous system: Amnesia, agitation, anxiety, apathy, apprehension, ataxia, chills, coma, delirium, depression, dream abnormalities, euphoria, false sense of well being, hallucination, hypoesthesia, insomnia, lethargy, malaise, nervousness, restlessness, seizure, slurred speech, somnolence, vertigo
 Dermatologic: Dry skin, rash, urticaria
 Endocrine & metabolic: Gynecomastia (<3%), hypokalemia, hyponatremia, libido decreased
 Gastrointestinal: Abdominal distension, abdominal pain, anorexia, biliary colic, diarrhea, dyspepsia, dysphagia, flatulence, gastroenteritis, GERD, GI irritation, paralytic ileus, rectal disorder, taste perversion, weight loss
 Genitourinary: Bladder spasm, dysuria, ejaculation abnormal, impotence, urination decreased
 Hematologic: Leukopenia (<3%), thrombocytopenia (<3%), hematocrit decreased
 Hepatic: Liver function tests increased
 Neuromuscular & skeletal: Arthralgia, back pain, bone pain, foot drop, gait abnormalities, paresthesia, rigors, skeletal muscle rigidity, tremor
 Ocular: Amblyopia, conjunctivitis, eye pain, vision problems/disturbance
 Renal: Oliguria
 Respiratory: Asthma, atelectasis, dyspnea, hiccups, hypercapnia, hypoxia, pulmonary edema (noncardiogenic), respiratory depression, rhinitis
 Miscellaneous: Diaphoresis, flu-like syndrome, infection, thirst, voice alteration, withdrawal syndrome
<1% (Limited to important or life-threatening): Amenorrhea, anaphylaxis, apnea, biliary tract spasm, blurred vision, bronchospasm, cardiac arrest, cough reflex decreased, dehydration, diplopia, disorientation, hemorrhagic urticaria, intestinal obstruction, intracranial pressure increased, laryngospasm, menstrual irregularities, miosis, myoclonus, nystagmus, paradoxical CNS

stimulation, respiratory arrest, sepsis, urinary tract spasm, thermal dysregulation, toxic psychoses

Drug Interactions

Metabolism/Transport Effects Substrate of CYP2D6 (minor), P-glycoprotein, UGT1A1; **Note:** Assignment of Major/Minor substrate status based on clinically relevant drug interaction potential

Avoid Concomitant Use

Avoid concomitant use of Morphine (Systemic) with any of the following: Azelastine (Nasal); Eluxadoline; MAO Inhibitors; Mixed Agonist / Antagonist Opioids; Orphenadrine; Paraldehyde; Thalidomide

Increased Effect/Toxicity

Morphine (Systemic) may increase the levels/effects of: Alcohol (Ethyl); Alvimopan; Amifostine; Antipsychotic Agents (Second Generation [Atypical]); Azelastine (Nasal); CNS Depressants; Desmopressin; Diuretics; DULoxetine; Eluxadoline; Gabapentin; Hydrocodone; Hypotension-Associated Agents; Levodopa; Methotrimeprazine; Metyrosine; Mirtazapine; Orphenadrine; Paraldehyde; Pramipexole; Ramosetron; ROPINIRole; Rotigotine; Selective Serotonin Reuptake Inhibitors; Suvorexant; Thalidomide; Zolpidem

The levels/effects of Morphine (Systemic) may be increased by: Alfuzosin; Amphetamines; Anticholinergic Agents; Antipsychotic Agents (Phenothiazines); Barbiturates; Blood Pressure Lowering Agents; Brimonidine (Topical); Cannabis; Diazoxide; Doxylamine; Dronabinol; Droperidol; Gabapentin; Herbs (Hypotensive Properties); HydrOXYzine; Kava Kava; Lumacaftor; Magnesium Sulfate; MAO Inhibitors; Methotrimeprazine; Minocycline; Molsidomine; Nabilone; Nicorandil; Obinutuzumab; Pentoxifylline; Perampanel; P-glycoprotein/ABCB1 Inhibitors; Phosphodiesterase 5 Inhibitors; Prostacyclin Analogues; Ranolazine; Rufinamide; Sodium Oxybate; Succinylcholine; Tapentadol; Tetrahydrocannabinol

Decreased Effect

Morphine (Systemic) may decrease the levels/effects of: Clopidogrel; Pegvisomant

The levels/effects of Morphine (Systemic) may be decreased by: Ammonium Chloride; Lumacaftor; Mixed Agonist / Antagonist Opioids; Naltrexone; P-glycoprotein/ABCB1 Inducers; Rifamycin Derivatives

Food Interactions

Ethanol: Alcoholic beverages or ethanol-containing products may disrupt extended release formulation resulting in rapid release of entire morphine dose. Management: Avoid alcohol. **Do not administer Avinza with alcoholic beverages or ethanol-containing prescription or nonprescription products.**

Food: Administration of oral morphine solution with food may increase bioavailability (ie, a report of 34% increase in morphine AUC when morphine oral solution followed a high-fat meal). The bioavailability of Avinza, MS Contin, or Kadian does not appear to be affected by food. Management: Take consistently with or without meals.

Storage/Stability

Capsule, extended release: Store at 25°C (77°F); excursions permitted to 15°C to 30°C (59°F to 86°F). Protect from light and moisture.

Injection: Store at controlled room temperature of 20°C to 25°C (68°F to 77°F); do not freeze. Protect from light. Degradation depends on pH and presence of oxygen; relatively stable in pH ≤4; darkening of solutions indicate degradation.

Astramorph/PF, Duramorph, Infumorph: Store in carton until use at controlled room temperature of 20°C to 25°C (68°F to 77°F); excursions permitted to 15°C to 30°C (59°F to 86°F); do not freeze; do not heat-sterilize. Contains no preservative or antioxidant. Protect from light.

Oral solution: Store at controlled room temperature of 15°C to 30°C (59°F to 86°F); do not freeze. Protect from moisture.

Suppositories: Store below controlled room temperature 25°C (77°F).

Tablet, extended release: Store at controlled room temperature of 25°C (77°F); excursions permitted to 15°C to 30°C (59°F to 86°F).

Tablet, immediate release: Store at 15°C to 30°C (59°F to 86°F). Protect from moisture.

Mechanism of Action Binds to opioid receptors in the CNS, causing inhibition of ascending pain pathways, altering the perception of and response to pain; produces generalized CNS depression

Pharmacodynamics/Kinetics

Onset of action (patient dependent; dosing must be individualized): Oral (immediate release): ~30 minutes; IV: 5 to 10 minutes

Duration (patient dependent; dosing must be individualized): Pain relief:

Immediate-release formulations: 4 hours

Extended-release capsule and tablet: 8 to 24 hours (formulation dependent)

Absorption: Variable

Distribution: V_d: 1 to 6 L/kg; binds to opioid receptors in the CNS and periphery (eg, GI tract)

Protein binding: 20% to 35%

Metabolism: Hepatic via conjugation with glucuronic acid primarily to morphine-6-glucuronide (active analgesic) morphine-3-glucuronide (inactive as analgesic); minor metabolites include morphine-3-6-diglucuronide; other minor metabolites include normorphine (active) and morphine 3-ethereal sulfate

Bioavailability: Oral: 17% to 33% (first-pass effect limits oral bioavailability; oral:parenteral effectiveness reportedly varies from 1:6 in opioid-naive patients to 1:3 with chronic use)

Half-life elimination: Adults: Immediate-release forms: 2 to 4 hours; Avinza: ~24 hours; Kadian: 11 to 13 hours

Time to peak, plasma: Avinza: 30 minutes (maintained for 24 hours); Kadian: ~10 hours

Excretion: Urine (primarily as morphine-3-glucuronide, ~2% to 12% excreted unchanged); feces (~7% to 10%). It has been suggested that accumulation of morphine-6-glucuronide might cause toxicity with renal insufficiency. All of the metabolites (ie, morphine-3-glucuronide, morphine-6-glucuronide, and normorphine) have been suggested as possible causes of neurotoxicity (eg, myoclonus).

Dosing

Adult These are guidelines and do not represent the doses that may be required in all patients. Doses and dosage intervals should be titrated to pain relief/prevention.

Acute pain (moderate to severe):

Oral (immediate-release formulations): Opioid naive: Initial: **Note:** Usual dosage range: 10 to 30 mg every 4 hours as needed. Patients with prior opioid exposure may require higher initial doses.

Solution: 10 to 20 mg every 4 hours as needed

Tablet: 15 to 30 mg every 4 hours as needed

IM, SubQ: **Note:** Repeated SubQ administration causes local tissue irritation, pain, and induration. The use of IM injections is no longer recommended especially for repeated administration due to painful administration, variable absorption and lag time to peak effect; other routes are more reliable and less painful (APS, 2008).

Initial: Opioid naive: 5 to 10 mg every 4 hours as needed; usual dosage range: 5 to 15 mg every 4 hours as needed. Patients with prior opioid exposure may require higher initial doses.

IV: Initial: Opioid naive: 2.5 to 5 mg every 3 to 4 hours; patients with prior opioid exposure may require higher initial doses. **Note:** Administration of 2 to 3 mg every 5 minutes until pain relief or if associated sedation, oxygen saturation <95%, or serious adverse event occurs may be appropriate in treating acute moderate to severe pain in settings such as the immediate postoperative period or the emergency department (Aubrun, 2012; Lvovschi, 2008); dose reduction in the immediate postoperative period (postanesthesia care unit) in the elderly is usually not necessary (Aubrun, 2002). A maximum cumulative dose (eg, 10 mg) prompting reevaluation of continued morphine use and/or dose should be included as part of any medication order intended for short-term use (eg, PACU orders). Refer to institution-specific protocols as appropriate.

Acute myocardial infarction, analgesia (off-label use): Initial management: 4 to 8 mg (lower doses in elderly patients); subsequently may give 2 to 8 mg every 5 to 15 minutes as needed (O'Gara, 2012)

Critically ill patients, analgesia (off-label dose): 2 to 4 mg every 1 to 2 hours **or** 4 to 8 mg every 3 to 4 hours as needed (Barr, 2013)

IV, SubQ continuous infusion: 0.8 to 10 mg/hour; usual range: Up to 80 mg/hour. **Note:** May administer a loading dose (amount administered should depend on severity of pain) prior to initiating the infusion. A continuous (basal) infusion is not recommended in an opioid-naive patient (ISMP, 2009)

Continuous infusion for critically ill patients: Usual dosage range: 2 to 30 mg/hour (Barr, 2013)

Patient-controlled analgesia (PCA) (APS, 2008): **Note:** In opioid-naive patients, consider lower end of dosing range:

Usual concentration: 1 mg/mL

Demand dose: Usual: 1 mg; range: 0.5 to 2.5 mg

Lockout interval: 5 to 10 minutes

Epidural: Pain management: **Note: Must be preservative free.** Administer with extreme caution and in reduced dosage to geriatric or debilitated patients. Vigilant monitoring is particularly important in these patients.

Single dose: **Lumbar region:** Astramorph/PF, Duramorph: 30 to 100 mcg/kg (optimal range: 2.5 to 3.75 mg; may depend upon patient comorbidities; Bujedo, 2012; Sultan, 2011)

Continuous infusion (may be combined with bupivacaine): 0.2 to 0.4 mg/hour (Bujedo, 2012)

Continuous microinfusion (Infumorph):

Opioid naive: Initial: 3.5 to 7.5 mg over 24 hours

Opioid tolerant: Initial: 4.5 to 10 mg over 24 hours, titrate to effect; usual maximum is ~30 mg per 24 hours

Intrathecal: **Note: Must be preservative free.** Administer with extreme caution and in reduced dosage to geriatric or debilitated patients. Intrathecal dose is usually 1/10 (one-tenth) that of epidural dosage.

Opioid naive: Single dose: Lumbar region: Astramorph/PF, Duramorph: 0.1 to 0.3 mg (may provide adequate relief for up to 24 hours; APS, 2008); repeat doses are **not** recommended. If pain recurs within 24 hours of administration, use of an alternate route of administration is recommended. **Note:** Although product labeling recommends doses up to 1 mg, an analgesic ceiling exists with doses >0.3 mg and the risk of respiratory depression is higher with doses >0.3 mg (Rathmell, 2005).

Continuous microinfusion (Infumorph): Lumbar region: After initial in-hospital evaluation of response to single-dose injections (Astramorph/PF, Duramorph) the initial dose of Infumorph is 0.2 to 1 mg over 24 hours

Opioid tolerant: Continuous microinfusion (Infumorph): Lumbar region: Dosage range: 1 to 10 mg over 24 hours, titrate to effect; usual maximum is ~20 mg over 24 hours

Rectal: 10 to 20 mg every 3 to 4 hours

Chronic pain: Note: Patients taking opioids chronically may become tolerant and require doses higher than the usual dosage range to maintain the desired effect. Tolerance can be managed by appropriate dose titration. There is no optimal or maximal dose for morphine in chronic pain. The appropriate dose is one that relieves pain throughout its dosing interval without causing unmanageable side effects. Consider total daily dose, potency, prior opioid use, degree of opioid experience and tolerance, conversion from previous opioid (including opioid formulation), patient's general condition, concurrent medications, and type and severity of pain during prescribing process. Opioid tolerance is defined as: Patients already taking at least 60 mg of oral morphine daily, 25 mcg transdermal fentanyl per hour, 30 mg of oral oxycodone daily, 8 mg oral hydromorphone daily, 25 mg of oral oxymorphone daily, or an equivalent dose of another opioid for at least 1 week.

Oral (extended-release formulations): A patient's morphine requirement should be established using immediate-release formulations. Conversion to long-acting products may be considered when chronic, continuous treatment is required. Higher dosages should be reserved for use only in opioid-tolerant patients.

Capsules, extended release (Avinza): Daily dose administered once daily (for best results, administer at same time each day). **Note:** Avinza 90 mg and 120 mg are only indicated for use in opioid-tolerant patents.

Use as the first opioid analgesic or use in patients who are **not** opioid tolerant: Initial: 30 mg once daily

Conversion from other oral morphine formulations to Avinza: Total daily morphine dose given as once daily. The first dose of Avinza may be taken with the last dose of the immediate-release morphine. Maximum: 1600 mg daily due to fumaric acid content.

Conversion from other opioids to Avinza: Discontinue all other around-the-clock opioids when Avinza is initiated. Initial dose: 30 mg once daily; there are no established conversion ratios from other opioids to Avinza. Substantial interpatient variability exists in relative potency. Therefore, it is safer to underestimate a patient's daily oral morphine requirement and provide rescue medication (eg, immediate-release morphine) than to overestimate requirements. The first dose of Avinza may be taken with the last dose of the immediate-release opioid.

Titration and maintenance: Adjust in increments ≤30 mg daily every 3 to 4 days. Maximum: 1600 mg daily due to fumaric acid content.

Discontinuation of Avinza: Gradually titrate dose downward every 2 to 4 days. Do not discontinue abruptly.

Capsules, extended release (Kadian): **Note:** Kadian 100 mg, 130 mg, 150 mg, and 200 mg are only indicated for use in opioid-tolerant patients.

Use as the first opioid analgesic: Has not been evaluated. Use an immediate-release morphine formulation and then convert patients to Kadian in the same fashion as initiating therapy in a non-opioid-tolerant patient.

Use in patients who are **not** opioid tolerant: Initial: 30 mg once daily.

Conversion from other oral morphine formulations to Kadian: Total daily oral morphine dose may be either administered once daily or in 2 divided doses daily (every 12 hours).

Conversion from other opioids to Kadian: Discontinue all other around-the-clock opioids when Kadian is initiated. Initial dose: 30 mg once daily; there are no established conversion ratios from other opioids to Kadian. Substantial interpatient variability exists in relative potency. Therefore, it is safer to underestimate a patient's daily oral morphine requirement and provide rescue medication (eg, immediate-release morphine) than to overestimate requirements.

Titration and maintenance: Dose adjustments may be done every 1 to 2 days.

Discontinuation of Kadian: Gradually titrate dose downward every 2 to 4 days. Do not discontinue abruptly.

Tablets, extended release (MS Contin): **Note:** MS Contin 100 mg and 200 mg tablets are only indicated for use in opioid-tolerant patients.

Use as the first opioid analgesic: Initial: 15 mg every 8 to 12 hours

Use in patients who are **not** opioid tolerant: Initial: 15 mg every 12 hours.

Conversion from other oral morphine formulations to MS Contin: Total daily oral morphine dose may be either administered in 2 divided doses daily (every 12 hours) **or** in 3 divided doses (every 8 hours).

Conversion from other opioids to MS Contin: Discontinue all other around-the-clock opioids when MS Contin is initiated. Initial: 15 mg every 8 to 12 hours; there are no established conversion ratios from other opioids to MS Contin. Substantial interpatient variability exists in relative potency. Therefore, it is safer to underestimate a patient's daily oral morphine requirement and provide rescue medication (eg, immediate-release morphine) than to overestimate requirements.

Titration and maintenance: Dose adjustments may be done every 1 to 2 days.

Discontinuation of MS Contin: Gradually titrate dose downward. Do not discontinue abruptly.

Conversion from parenteral morphine or other opioids to extended-release formulations: Substantial interpatient variability exists in relative potency. Therefore, it is safer to underestimate a patient's daily oral morphine requirement and provide breakthrough pain relief with immediate-release morphine than to overestimate requirements. Consider the parenteral to oral morphine ratio or other oral or parenteral opioids to oral morphine conversions.

Parenteral to oral morphine ratio: Between 2 to 6 mg of oral morphine may be required for analgesia equivalent to 1 mg of parenteral morphine. An oral dose 3 times the daily parenteral dose may be sufficient in chronic pain settings.

Other parenteral or oral nonmorphine opioids to oral morphine: Specific recommendations are not available; refer to published relative potency data realizing that such ratios are only approximations. In general, it is safest to administer half of the estimated daily morphine requirement as the initial dose, and to manage inadequate analgesia by supplementation with immediate-release morphine.

Conversion from methadone to extended-release formulations: Close monitoring is required when converting methadone to another opioid. Ratio between methadone and other opioid agonists varies widely according to previous dose exposure. Methadone has a long half-life and can accumulate in the plasma.

Geriatric Refer to adult dosing. Use with caution; may require reduced dosage in the elderly and debilitated patients.

Pediatric These are guidelines and do not represent the doses that may be required in all patients. Doses and dosage intervals should be titrated to pain relief/prevention.

Acute pain (moderate to severe): Children >6 months and <50 kg:

Oral (immediate release formulations): 0.15 to 0.3 mg/kg every 3 or 4 hours as needed. **Note:** The American Pain Society recommends an initial dose of 0.3 mg/kg for children with severe pain (American Pain Society [APS], 2008)

IM, SubQ: 0.1 or 0.2 mg/kg; **Note:** Repeated SubQ administration causes local tissue irritation, pain, and induration. The use of IM injections is no longer recommended especially for repeated administration due to painful administration, variable absorption and lag time to peak effect.

IV: 0.05 to 0.3 mg/kg every 3 to 4 hours as needed, not to exceed 10 mg per dose

Continuous infusion: Initial: 10 to 30 **mcg/kg/hour**; titrate as needed to control pain

Patient-controlled analgesia (PCA) (APS, 2008): **Note:** Opioid-naive: Consider lower end of dosing range:

Usual concentration: 1 mg/mL

Demand dose: Usual: 0.02 mg/kg/dose; range: 0.01 to 0.03 mg/kg/dose

Lockout interval: 8 to 10 minutes

Usual basal rate: 0 to 0.03 mg/kg/hour

Renal Impairment

CrCl 10 to 50 mL/minute: Children and Adults: Administer at 75% of normal dose.

CrCl <10 mL/minute: Children and Adults: Administer at 50% of normal dose.

Intermittent HD:

Adults: Administer 50% of normal dose. No supplemental dose necessary.

Children: Administer 50% of normal dose.

Peritoneal dialysis: Children: Administer 50% of normal dose.

CRRT: Children and Adults: Administer 75% of normal dose, titrate.

Hepatic Impairment No dosage adjustment provided in manufacturer's labeling. Pharmacokinetics unchanged in mild liver disease; substantial extrahepatic metabolism may occur. In cirrhosis, increases in half-life and AUC suggest dosage adjustment required.

Dietary Considerations Morphine may cause GI upset; take with food if GI upset occurs. Be consistent when taking morphine with or without meals.

Usual Infusion Concentrations: Pediatric IV infusion: 0.1 mg/mL, 0.5 mg/mL, **or** 1 mg/mL

Usual Infusion Concentrations: Adult IV infusion: 1 mg/mL

Administration

Oral: Do not crush, chew, or dissolve extended release drug product; swallow whole. Kadian and Avinza can be opened and sprinkled on applesauce and eaten immediately without chewing; do not crush, dissolve, or chew the beads as it can result in a rapid release of a potentially fatal dose of morphine. Ensure all pellets have been swallowed by rinsing mouth. Contents of Kadian capsules may be opened and sprinkled over 10 mL water and flushed through prewetted 16F gastrostomy tube; do not administer Kadian through gastric/nasogastric tubes.

IV: When giving morphine IV push, it is best to first dilute with sterile water or NS for a final concentration of 1 to 2 mg/mL and then administer slowly over 4 to 5 minutes.

Epidural, intrathecal: Use preservative-free solutions for intrathecal or epidural use. Infumorph may **only** be used as a continuous microinfusion via catheter.

Monitoring Parameters Assess efficacy of pain control, vital signs, and mental status; signs of drug abuse, addiction, or diversion; signs or symptoms of hypogonadism or hypoadrenalism (Brennan, 2013)

Astramorph/PF, Duramorph, Infumorph: Patients should be observed in a fully-equipped and staffed environment for at least 24 hours following initiation, and as appropriate for the first several days after catheter implantation. Naloxone injection should be immediately available. Patient should remain in this environment for at least 24 hours following the initial dose. For patients receiving Infumorph via microinfusion device, patient may be observed, as appropriate, for the first several days after catheter implantation.

Note: Also refer to institution specific protocols as appropriate.

Test Interactions Some quinolones may produce a false-positive urine screening result for opioids using commercially-available immunoassay kits. This has been demonstrated most consistently for levofloxacin and ofloxacin, but other quinolones have shown cross-reactivity in certain assay kits. Confirmation of positive opioid screens by more specific methods should be considered.

Product Availability MorphaBond (morphine sulfate extended-release tablets): FDA approved October 2015; anticipated availability is currently unknown. Information

pertaining to this product within the monograph is pending revision. Consult prescribing information for additional information.

Dosage Forms Excipient information presented when available (limited, particularly for generics); consult specific product labeling. [DSC] = Discontinued product

Capsule Extended Release 24 Hour, Oral, as sulfate:

AVINza: 30 mg [DSC] [contains fd&c yellow #10 (quinoline yellow), fumaric acid]

AVINza: 45 mg [DSC] [contains fd&c blue #2 (indigotine)]

AVINza: 60 mg [DSC] [contains fumaric acid]

AVINza: 75 mg [DSC]

AVINza: 90 mg [DSC] [contains fd&c red #40, fumaric acid]

AVINza: 120 mg [DSC] [contains brilliant blue fcf (fd&c blue #1), fumaric acid]

Kadian: 10 mg [contains brilliant blue fcf (fd&c blue #1)]

Kadian: 20 mg [contains fd&c yellow #10 (quinoline yellow)]

Kadian: 30 mg [contains brilliant blue fcf (fd&c blue #1)]

Kadian: 40 mg [contains brilliant blue fcf (fd&c blue #1), fd&c yellow #10 (quinoline yellow)]

Kadian: 50 mg, 60 mg [contains brilliant blue fcf (fd&c blue #1), fd&c red #40]

Kadian: 70 mg [DSC] [contains brilliant blue fcf (fd&c blue #1)]

Kadian: 80 mg [contains brilliant blue fcf (fd&c blue #1), fd&c red #40, fd&c yellow #6 (sunset yellow)]

Kadian: 100 mg [contains brilliant blue fcf (fd&c blue #1), fd&c yellow #10 (quinoline yellow)]

Kadian: 130 mg [DSC] [contains brilliant blue fcf (fd&c blue #1), fd&c red #40, fd&c yellow #6 (sunset yellow)]

Kadian: 150 mg [DSC] [contains brilliant blue fcf (fd&c blue #1), fd&c yellow #10 (quinoline yellow)]

Kadian: 200 mg

Generic: 10 mg, 20 mg, 30 mg, 45 mg, 50 mg, 60 mg, 75 mg, 80 mg, 90 mg, 100 mg, 120 mg

Device, Intramuscular, as sulfate:

Generic: 10 mg/0.7 mL (0.7 mL)

Solution, Injection, as sulfate:

Astramorph: 1 mg/mL (10 mL [DSC])

Generic: 2 mg/mL (1 mL); 4 mg/mL (1 mL); 5 mg/mL (1 mL); 8 mg/mL (1 mL); 10 mg/mL (1 mL, 10 mL [DSC]); 15 mg/mL (1 mL, 20 mL [DSC])

Solution, Injection, as sulfate [preservative free]:

Astramorph: 0.5 mg/mL (2 mL, 10 mL [DSC]); 1 mg/mL (2 mL)

Duramorph: 0.5 mg/mL (10 mL); 1 mg/mL (10 mL)

Infumorph 200: 200 mg/20 mL (10 mg/mL) (20 mL) [antioxidant free]

Infumorph 500: 500 mg/20 mL (25 mg/mL) (20 mL) [antioxidant free]

Generic: 0.5 mg/mL (10 mL); 1 mg/mL (10 mL)

Solution, Intravenous, as sulfate:

Generic: 1 mg/mL (10 mL, 30 mL, 250 mL [DSC]); 5 mg/mL (30 mL [DSC]); 25 mg/mL (4 mL, 10 mL); 50 mg/mL (20 mL, 50 mL)

Solution, Intravenous, as sulfate [preservative free]:

Generic: 1 mg/mL (30 mL); 2 mg/mL (1 mL); 4 mg/mL (1 mL); 150 mg/30 mL (30 mL); 8 mg/mL (1 mL); 10 mg/mL (1 mL); 15 mg/mL (1 mL); 25 mg/mL (10 mL)

Solution, Oral, as sulfate:

Generic: 10 mg/5 mL (5 mL, 15 mL, 100 mL, 500 mL); 20 mg/5 mL (5 mL, 100 mL, 500 mL); 100 mg/5 mL (15 mL, 30 mL, 120 mL, 240 mL)

Suppository, Rectal, as sulfate:

Generic: 5 mg (12 ea); 10 mg (12 ea); 20 mg (12 ea); 30 mg (12 ea)

Tablet, Oral, as sulfate:

Generic: 15 mg, 30 mg

Tablet Extended Release, Oral, as sulfate:

MS Contin: 15 mg, 30 mg, 60 mg, 100 mg, 200 mg

Generic: 15 mg, 30 mg, 60 mg, 100 mg, 200 mg

Dosage Forms: Canada Excipient information presented when available (limited, particularly for generics); consult specific product labeling.

Solution, oral, as hydrochloride:

Doloral: 1 mg/mL (10 mL, 250 mL, 500 mL); 5 mg/mL (10 mL, 250 mL, 500 mL)

Controlled Substance C-II

Extemporaneous Preparations A 0.4 mg/mL oral solution may be made using the **2 mg/mL** oral morphine solution. Measure 10 mL (20 mg) of the 2 mg/mL oral morphine solution and transfer to a plastic amber bottle. Measure 40 mL of sterile water for irrigation and add to bottle containing the morphine. Shake to mix. Store at room temperature. Stable for 60 days.

Sauberan J, Rossi S, Kim JH. Stability of dilute oral morphine solution for neonatal abstinence syndrome. *J Addict Med.* 2013;7(2):113-115.

Morphine (Liposomal) (MOR feen)

Brand Names: US DepoDur
Index Terms Extended Release Epidural Morphine; Liposomal Morphine; MS (error-prone abbreviation and should not be used); MSO$_4$ (error-prone abbreviation and should not be used)
Pharmacologic Category Analgesic, Opioid
Additional Appendix Information
Opioid Conversion Table and Morphine Equivalent Dose Table *on page 1955*
Use Epidural (lumbar) single-dose management of surgical pain
Dosing
Adult Surgical anesthesia: Epidural: Single-dose (extended release, DepoDur®): Lumbar epidural only; not recommended in patients <18 years of age:
Cesarean section: 10 mg (after clamping umbilical cord)
Lower abdominal/pelvic surgery: 10-15 mg
Major orthopedic surgery of lower extremity: 15 mg;
Note: Some patients may benefit from a 20 mg dose; however, the incidence of adverse effects may be increased.
To minimize the pharmacokinetic interaction resulting in higher peak serum concentrations of morphine, administer the test dose of the local anesthetic at least 15 minutes prior to administration. Use with epidural local anesthetics has not been studied. Other medications should not be administered into the epidural space for at least 48 hours after administration.
Geriatric Refer to adult dosing. Use with caution; may require reduced dosage in the elderly and debilitated patients.
Renal Impairment No dosage adjustment necessary.
Hepatic Impairment No dosage adjustment necessary.
Additional Information Complete prescribing information should be consulted for additional detail.
Dosage Forms Excipient information presented when available (limited, particularly for generics); consult specific product labeling.
Suspension, Epidural, as sulfate:
DepoDur: 10 mg/mL (1 mL); 15 mg/1.5 mL (1.5 mL)
Controlled Substance C-II

Morrhuate Sodium (MOR yoo ate SOW dee um)

Brand Names: US Scleromate
Pharmacologic Category Sclerosing Agent
Use Treatment of small, uncomplicated varicose veins of the lower extremities
Dosing
Adult & Geriatric Varicose veins: IV:
Note: A test dose of 0.25-1 mL of a 5% injection may be given (into a varicosity) 24 hours before full-dose treatment.
Full-dose treatment: 50-250 mg, depending on the size and degree of varicosity (50-100 mg for small or medium veins, 150-250 mg for large veins); may be given as multiple injections at one time or in single doses.
Renal Impairment No dosage adjustment provided in manufacturer's labeling.
Hepatic Impairment No dosage adjustment provided in manufacturer's labeling.
Additional Information Complete prescribing information should be consulted for additional detail.
Dosage Forms Excipient information presented when available (limited, particularly for generics); consult specific product labeling. [DSC] = Discontinued product
Solution, Intravenous:
Scleromate: 5% (30 mL)
Generic: 5% (30 mL [DSC])

Moxifloxacin (Systemic) (moxs i FLOKS a sin)

Brand Names: US Avelox; Avelox ABC Pack
Brand Names: Canada Avelox; Avelox I.V.
Index Terms Moxifloxacin Hydrochloride
Pharmacologic Category Antibiotic, Fluoroquinolone; Antibiotic, Respiratory Fluoroquinolone
Use Treatment of mild to moderate community-acquired pneumonia, including multidrug-resistant *Streptococcus pneumoniae* (MDRSP); acute bacterial exacerbation of chronic bronchitis; acute bacterial sinusitis; complicated and uncomplicated skin and skin structure infections; complicated intra-abdominal infections; prophylaxis and treatment of plague, including pneumonic and septicemic plague, due to *Yersinia pestis*.
Pregnancy Considerations Adverse events have been observed in some animal reproduction studies. Moxifloxacin crosses the placenta and can be detected in the amniotic fluid and cord blood (Ozyüncü and Beksac 2010; Ozyüncü and Nemutlu, 2010). Information specific to moxifloxacin use in pregnant women is limited (Padberg, 2014).
Breast-Feeding Considerations It is not known if moxifloxacin is excreted into breast milk. Due to the potential for serious adverse reactions in the nursing infant, the manufacturer recommends a decision be made whether to discontinue nursing or to discontinue the drug, taking into account the importance of treatment to the mother.
Medication Guide Available Yes
Contraindications Hypersensitivity to moxifloxacin, other quinolone antibiotics, or any component of the formulation
Warnings/Precautions [U.S. Boxed Warning]: There have been reports of tendon inflammation and/or rupture with quinolone antibiotics in all ages; risk may be increased with concurrent corticosteroids, solid organ transplant recipients, and in patients >60 years of age. Rupture of the Achilles tendon sometimes requiring surgical repair has been reported most frequently; but other tendon sites (eg, rotator cuff, biceps) have also been reported. Strenuous physical activity, rheumatoid arthritis, and renal impairment may be an independent risk factor for tendonitis. Inflammation and rupture may occur bilaterally. Cases have been reported within the first 48 hours, during, and up to several months after discontinuation of therapy. Discontinue at first sign of tendon inflammation or pain. Use with caution in patients with rheumatoid arthritis; may increase risk of tendon rupture. Use with caution in patients with a history of tendon disorders.

Fluoroquinolones may prolong QTc interval; avoid use in patients with known QTc prolongation, ventricular arrhythmias including torsades de pointes, proarrhythmic conditions (eg, clinically significant bradycardia, acute myocardial ischemia), uncorrected hypokalemia, hypomagnesemia, or concurrent administration of other medications known to prolong the QT interval (including Class Ia and Class III antiarrhythmics, cisapride, erythromycin, antipsychotics, and tricyclic antidepressants). CNS effects may occur (tremor, restlessness, confusion, and very rarely hallucinations, increased intracranial pressure [including pseudotumor cerebri] or seizures). Use with caution in patients with known or suspected CNS disorder. Potential for seizures, although very rare, may be increased with concomitant NSAID therapy. Use with caution in individuals at risk of seizures. Use with caution in patients with mild, moderate, or severe hepatic impairment or liver cirrhosis; may increase the risk of QT

prolongation. Fulminant hepatitis potentially leading to liver failure (including fatalities) has been reported with use. Use with caution in diabetes; glucose regulation may be altered.

Fluoroquinolones have been associated with the development of serious, and sometimes fatal, hypoglycemia, most often in elderly diabetics, but also in patients without diabetes. This occurred most frequently with gatifloxacin (no longer available systemically) but may occur at a lower frequency with other quinolones.

Severe hypersensitivity reactions, including anaphylaxis, have occurred with quinolone therapy. Reactions may present as typical allergic symptoms after a single dose, or may manifest as severe idiosyncratic dermatologic, vascular, pulmonary, renal, hepatic, and/or hematologic events, usually after multiple doses. Prompt discontinuation of drug should occur if skin rash or other symptoms arise. Avoid excessive sunlight and take precautions to limit exposure (eg, loose fitting clothing, sunscreen); may cause moderate to severe phototoxicity reactions. Discontinue use if photosensitivity occurs. Prolonged use may result in fungal or bacterial superinfection, including *C. difficile*-associated diarrhea (CDAD) and pseudomembranous colitis; CDAD has been observed >2 months post-antibiotic treatment.

[U.S. Boxed Warning]: Quinolones may exacerbate myasthenia gravis; avoid use (rare, potentially life-threatening weakness of respiratory muscles may occur). Peripheral neuropathy has been reported (rare); may occur soon after initiation of therapy and may be irreversible; discontinue if symptoms of sensory or sensorimotor neuropathy occur. Hemolytic reactions may (rarely) occur with quinolone use in patients with latent or actual G6PD deficiency. Adverse effects (eg, tendon rupture, QT changes) may be increased in elderly patients. Some quinolones may exacerbate myasthenia gravis, use with caution (rare, potentially life-threatening weakness of respiratory muscles may occur). Safety and efficacy of systemically administered moxifloxacin (oral, intravenous) in patients <18 years of age have not been established. Potentially significant interactions may exist, requiring dose or frequency adjustment, additional monitoring, and/or selection of alternative therapy.

Adverse Reactions

2% to 10%:
Central nervous system: Headache (≤4%), dizziness (3%), insomnia (2%)
Endocrine & metabolic: Decreased serum glucose (≥2%), hyperchloremia (≥2%), increased serum albumin (≥2%)
Gastrointestinal: Nausea (7%), diarrhea (6%), decreased amylase (≥2%), constipation (2%), vomiting (2%), abdominal pain (1% to 2%)
Hematologic & oncologic: Decreased basophils (≥2%), decreased hemoglobin (≥2%), decreased neutrophils (≥2%), decreased prothrombin time (≥2%), decreased red blood cells (≥2%), eosinopenia (≥2%), increased MCH (≥2%), increased neutrophils (≥2%), leukocytosis (≥2%), prolonged prothrombin time (≥2%)
Hepatic: Decreased serum bilirubin (≥2%), increased serum bilirubin (≥2%)
Immunologic: Increased serum globulins (≥2%)
Renal: Increased ionized serum calcium (≥2%)
Respiratory: Hypoxia (≥2%)
0.1% to <2%:
Cardiovascular: Angina pectoris, atrial fibrillation, bradycardia, cardiac arrest, cardiac failure, chest discomfort, chest pain, edema, hypertension, hypotension, increased blood pressure, palpitations, peripheral edema, phlebitis, prolonged Q-T interval on ECG, syncope, tachycardia
Central nervous system: Agitation, anxiety, chills, confusion, depression, disorientation, drowsiness, facial pain, fatigue, hallucination, hypoesthesia, lethargy, malaise, nervousness, noncardiac chest pain, pain, paresthesia, restlessness, vertigo
Dermatologic: Allergic dermatitis, erythema, hyperhidrosis, night sweats, pruritus, skin rash, urticaria
Endocrine & metabolic: Hypokalemia (1%), dehydration, hyperglycemia, hyperlipidemia, increased gamma-glutamyl transferase, increased lactate dehydrogenase, increased serum glucose, increased serum triglycerides, increased uric acid
Gastrointestinal: Dyspepsia (1%), abdominal discomfort, abdominal distension, anorexia, decreased appetite, dysgeusia, flatulence, gastritis, gastroenteritis, gastroesophageal reflux disease, increased amylase, increased serum lipase, oral candidiasis, xerostomia
Genitourinary: Dysuria, fungal vaginosis, vaginal infection, vulvovaginal candidiasis, vulvovaginal pruritus

Hematologic & oncologic: Anemia (1%), decreased hematocrit, eosinophilia, leukopenia, prolonged partial thromboplastin time, thrombocythemia, thrombocytopenia
Hepatic: Increased serum ALT (1%), abnormal hepatic function tests, increased liver enzymes, increased serum alkaline phosphatase, increased serum AST, increased serum transaminases
Hypersensitivity: Hypersensitivity reaction
Infection: Candidiasis, fungal infection (including oral)
Local: Extravasation
Neuromuscular & skeletal: Arthralgia, back pain, limb pain, muscle spasms, musculoskeletal pain, myalgia, tremor, weakness
Ophthalmic: Blurred vision
Otic: Tinnitus
Renal: Increased blood urea nitrogen, increased serum creatinine, renal failure
Respiratory: Asthma, bronchospasm, dyspnea, wheezing
Miscellaneous: Fever (1%)
<0.1% (Limited to important or life-threatening): Agranulocytosis, anaphylactic shock, anaphylaxis, aplastic anemia, ataxia, auditory impairment, cholestatic jaundice, *Clostridium difficile* associated diarrhea, deafness (reversible), decreased INR, ECG abnormality, exacerbation of myasthenia gravis, hemolytic anemia, hepatic failure, hepatic necrosis, hepatitis (predominantly cholestatic), hepatotoxicity (idiosyncratic) (Chalasani 2014), hypoglycemia, increased intracranial pressure, interstitial nephritis, jaundice, pancytopenia, peripheral neuropathy (may be irreversible), phototoxicity, pneumonitis (allergic), polyneuropathy, pseudomembranous colitis, pseudotumor cerebri, psychotic reaction, renal insufficiency, rupture of tendon, seizure, skin photosensitivity, Stevens-Johnson syndrome, suicidal ideation, suicidal tendencies, tendonitis, thrombotic thrombocytopenic purpura, toxic epidermal necrolysis, ventricular tachyarrhythmias (including torsade de pointes and cardiac arrest [usually in patients with concurrent, severe proarrhythmic conditions]), vasculitis, vision loss (transient)

Drug Interactions

Metabolism/Transport Effects None known.

Avoid Concomitant Use
Avoid concomitant use of Moxifloxacin (Systemic) with any of the following: BCG (Intravesical); Highest Risk QTc-Prolonging Agents; Ivabradine; Mequitazine; Mifepristone; Strontium Ranelate

Increased Effect/Toxicity
Moxifloxacin (Systemic) may increase the levels/effects of: Blood Glucose Lowering Agents; Highest Risk QTc-Prolonging Agents; Mequitazine; Moderate Risk QTc-Prolonging Agents; Porfimer; Varenicline; Verteporfin; Vitamin K Antagonists

The levels/effects of Moxifloxacin (Systemic) may be increased by: Corticosteroids (Systemic); Ivabradine; Mifepristone; Nonsteroidal Anti-Inflammatory Agents; Probenecid; QTc-Prolonging Agents (Indeterminate Risk and Risk Modifying)

Decreased Effect
Moxifloxacin (Systemic) may decrease the levels/effects of: BCG (Intravesical); BCG Vaccine (Immunization); Blood Glucose Lowering Agents; Didanosine; Mycophenolate; Sodium Picosulfate; Typhoid Vaccine

The levels/effects of Moxifloxacin (Systemic) may be decreased by: Antacids; Didanosine; Iron Salts; Lanthanum; Magnesium Salts; Multivitamins/Minerals (with ADEK, Folate, Iron); Multivitamins/Minerals (with AE, No Iron); Quinapril; Sevelamer; Strontium Ranelate; Sucralfate; Zinc Salts

Food Interactions Absorption is not affected by administration with a high-fat meal or yogurt.

Storage/Stability Store at 25°C (77°F); excursions are permitted between 15°C and 30°C (59°F and 86°F). Avoid high humidity. Do not refrigerate infusion solution.

Mechanism of Action Moxifloxacin is a DNA gyrase inhibitor, and also inhibits topoisomerase IV. DNA gyrase (topoisomerase II) is an essential bacterial enzyme that maintains the superhelical structure of DNA. DNA gyrase is required for DNA replication and transcription, DNA repair, recombination, and transposition; inhibition is bactericidal.

Pharmacodynamics/Kinetics
Absorption: Well absorbed; not affected by high-fat meal or yogurt
Distribution: V_d: 1.7 to 2.7 L/kg; tissue concentrations often exceed plasma concentrations in respiratory tissues, alveolar macrophages, abdominal tissues/fluids, uterine tissue (endometrium, myometrium), and sinus tissues
Protein binding: ~30% to 50%
Metabolism: Hepatic (~52% of dose) via glucuronide (~14%) and sulfate (~38%) conjugation

◄ Bioavailability: ~90%

Half-life elimination: Single dose: Oral: 12-16 hours; IV: 8-15 hours

Excretion: Urine (as unchanged drug [20%] and glucuronide conjugates); feces (as unchanged drug [25%] and sulfate conjugates)

Dosing

Adult & Geriatric

Acute bacterial rhinosinusitis: Oral, IV: 400 mg every 24 hours for 10 days or 5 to 7 days (Chow 2012). **Note:** Recommended in patients with beta-lactam allergy; may also be used if initial therapy fails, in areas with high endemic rates of penicillin nonsusceptible *S. pneumoniae*, those with severe infections, age >65 years, recent hospitalization, antibiotic use within the past month, or who are immunocompromised.

Bite wounds (animal/human) (off-label use): Oral, IV: **Note:** Recommended as an alternative therapy for human bite wound in patients hypersensitive to beta-lactams: 400 mg once daily (IDSA [Stevens 2014])

Chronic bronchitis, acute bacterial exacerbation: Oral, IV: 400 mg every 24 hours for 5 days

Community-acquired pneumonia (CAP) (including MDRSP): Oral, IV: 400 mg every 24 hours for 7 to 14 days

Intra-abdominal infections, complicated: 400 mg every 24 hours for 5 to 14 days (initiate with IV); **Note:** 2010 IDSA guidelines recommend a treatment duration of 4 to 7 days (provided source controlled) for community-acquired, mild to moderate IAI

***M. genitalium* infections** (including confirmed cases or clinically significant persistent cervicitis, pelvic inflammatory disease or urethritis in patients who previously received azithromycin or doxycycline; off-label use): Oral, IV: 400 mg every 24 hours for 7 to 10 days (Manhart 2011)

Plague: Oral, IV: 400 mg every 24 hours for 10 to 14 days

Skin and skin structure infections: Oral, IV:
Complicated: 400 mg every 24 hours for 7 to 21 days
Uncomplicated: 400 mg every 24 hours for 7 days

Surgical (perioperative) prophylaxis (off-label use): IV: 400 mg within 120 minutes prior to surgical incision (Bratzler 2013).

Tuberculosis, drug-resistant tuberculosis, or intolerance to first-line agents (off-label use): Oral: 400 mg every 24 hours (*MMWR* 2003)

Pediatric

Community-acquired pneumonia (CAP) due to atypical pathogens (*M. pneumoniae, Chlamydophila* [also known as *Chlamydia*] *pneumoniae, C. trachomatis*), mild infection or step-down therapy in adolescents with skeletal maturity, (alternative to azithromycin) (IDSA/PIDS 2011): Adolescents (off-label): Oral: 400 mg once daily

Surgical (perioperative) prophylaxis (off-label use): Children ≥1 year: IV: 10 mg/kg within 120 minutes prior to surgical incision (maximum dose: 400 mg) (Bratzler 2013)

Renal Impairment No dosage adjustment required in renal impairment.

Poorly dialyzed; no supplemental dose or dosage adjustment necessary, including patients on intermittent hemodialysis, peritoneal dialysis, or continuous renal replacement therapy (eg, CVVHD).

Hepatic Impairment No dosage adjustment is required in mild, moderate, or severe hepatic insufficiency (Child-Pugh class A, B, or C); however, use with caution in this patient population secondary to the risk of QT prolongation.

Dietary Considerations Take 4 hours before or 8 hours after multiple vitamins, antacids, or other products containing magnesium, aluminum, iron, or zinc.

Avelox IV infusion (premixed in sodium chloride 0.8%) contains sodium 34.2 mEq (~787 mg)/250 mL.

Administration Administer without regard to meals.

IV: Infuse over 60 minutes; do not infuse by rapid or bolus intravenous infusion

Monitoring Parameters WBC, signs of infection, signs/symptoms of disordered glucose regulation, blood glucose in diabetic patients, ECG in patients with liver cirrhosis

Test Interactions Some quinolones may produce a false-positive urine screening result for opioids using commercially-available immunoassay kits. This has been demonstrated most consistently for levofloxacin and ofloxacin, but other quinolones have shown cross-reactivity in certain assay kits. Confirmation of positive opioid screens by more specific methods should be considered.

Dosage Forms Excipient information presented when available (limited, particularly for generics); consult specific product labeling.

Solution, Intravenous:
Generic: 400 mg/250 mL (250 mL)

Solution, Intravenous [preservative free]:
Avelox: 400 mg/250 mL (250 mL) [latex free]

Tablet, Oral:
Avelox: 400 mg
Avelox ABC Pack: 400 mg
Generic: 400 mg

Extemporaneous Preparations A 20 mg/mL oral suspension may be made using tablets. Crush three 400 mg tablets and reduce to a fine powder. Carefully sieve powder from enteric-coating remnants to improve pharmaceutical elegance. Add a small amount of a 1:1 mixture of Ora-Plus® and Ora-Sweet® or Ora-Sweet® SF and mix to a uniform paste; mix while adding the vehicle in geometric proportions to **almost** 60 mL; transfer to a calibrated bottle, rinse mortar with vehicle, and add quantity of vehicle sufficient to make 60 mL. Label "shake well". Stable 90 days at room temperature.

Hutchinson DJ, Johnson CE, and Klein KC, "Stability of Extemporaneously Prepared Moxifloxacin Oral Suspensions," *Am J Health Syst Pharm*, 2009, 66(7):665-7.

Moxifloxacin (Ophthalmic) (moxs i FLOKS a sin)

Brand Names: US Moxeza; Vigamox

Brand Names: Canada ACT-Moxifloxacin; Sandoz -Moxifloxacin; Vigamox

Index Terms Moxifloxacin Hydrochloride

Pharmacologic Category Antibiotic, Fluoroquinolone; Antibiotic, Ophthalmic

Use Bacterial conjunctivitis: Treatment of bacterial conjunctivitis caused by susceptible organisms: *Acinetobacter lwoffii, Aerococcus viridams, Corynebacterium spp, Enterococcus faecalis, Micrococcus luteus, Staphylococcus arlettae, S. aureus, S. capitis, S. epidermidis, S. haemolyticus, S. hominis, S. saprophyticus, S. warneri, Streptococcus viridans spp., S. pneumoniae, Escherichia coli, Haemophilus influenzae, H. parainfluenzae, Klebsiella pneumoniae, Propionibacterium acnes, Chlamydia trachomatis*

Dosing

Adult & Geriatric

Bacterial conjunctivitis: Ophthalmic:
Moxeza: Instill 1 drop into affected eye(s) 2 times daily for 7 days
Vigamox: Instill 1 drop into affected eye(s) 3 times daily for 7 days

Surgical prophylaxis (off-label use): Vigamox: Instill 1 drop into operative eye every 5 to 15 minutes for five doses within the hour prior to the start of the procedure (ASHP/IDSA/SIS/SHEA [Bratzler 2013]). **Note:** Prophylactic administration has ranged from preoperatively (including day of surgery only to 1 to 3 days preoperatively), intraoperatively, at end of procedure, and postoperatively. However, no specific recommendations beyond immediate preoperative use, including duration of prophylaxis, can be made due to insufficient evidence. A total duration (pre- and postoperatively) of up to 15 days has been reported (ASHP/IDSA/SIS/SHEA [Bratzler 2013]; Freitas 2007; Speaker 2009).

Pediatric Bacterial conjunctivitis: Ophthalmic:
Children ≥4 months and Adolescents (Moxeza): Refer to adult dosing.
Children ≥1 year and Adolescents (Vigamox): Refer to adult dosing.

Renal Impairment There are no dosage adjustments provided in the manufacturer's labeling. However, dosage adjustment unlikely due to low systemic absorption.

Hepatic Impairment There are no dosage adjustments provided in the manufacturer's labeling. However, dosage adjustment unlikely due to low systemic absorption.

Additional Information Complete prescribing information should be consulted for additional detail.

Dosage Forms Excipient information presented when available (limited, particularly for generics); consult specific product labeling.

Solution, Ophthalmic:
Moxeza: 0.5% (3 mL)
Vigamox: 0.5% (3 mL)

◆ Moxifloxacin Hydrochloride *see* Moxifloxacin (Ophthalmic) *on page 1238*

◆ Moxifloxacin Hydrochloride *see* Moxifloxacin (Systemic) *on page 1236*

◆ Mozobil *see* Plerixafor *on page 1460*

◆ 4-MP *see* Fomepizole *on page 806*

◆ MP-424 *see* Telaprevir *on page 1743*

- MPA *see* MedroxyPROGESTERone *on page 1131*
- MPA *see* Mycophenolate *on page 1240*
- 6-MP (error-prone abbreviation) *see* Mercaptopurine *on page 1146*
- MPG-EPO *see* Methoxy Polyethylene Glycol-Epoetin Beta *on page 1176*
- MPSV *see* Meningococcal Polysaccharide Vaccine (Groups A / C / Y and W-135) *on page 1143*
- MPSV4 *see* Meningococcal Polysaccharide Vaccine (Groups A / C / Y and W-135) *on page 1143*
- MRA *see* Tocilizumab *on page 1802*
- MS Contin *see* Morphine (Systemic) *on page 1230*
- MS Contin SRT (Can) *see* Morphine (Systemic) *on page 1230*
- MS (error-prone abbreviation and should not be used) *see* Morphine (Liposomal) *on page 1236*
- MS (error-prone abbreviation and should not be used) *see* Morphine (Systemic) *on page 1230*
- M-Sildenafil (Can) *see* Sildenafil *on page 1653*
- MS-IR (Can) *see* Morphine (Systemic) *on page 1230*
- MSO$_4$ (error-prone abbreviation and should not be used) *see* Morphine (Liposomal) *on page 1236*
- MSO$_4$ (error-prone abbreviation and should not be used) *see* Morphine (Systemic) *on page 1230*
- MST 600 [DSC] *see* Magnesium Salicylate *on page 1121*
- MT103 *see* Blinatumomab *on page 238*
- MTC *see* MitoMYcin (Systemic) *on page 1219*
- MTX (error-prone abbreviation) *see* Methotrexate *on page 1169*
- MucaphEd [OTC] *see* Guaifenesin and Phenylephrine *on page 862*
- Mucinex [OTC] *see* GuaiFENesin *on page 860*
- Mucinex® D [OTC] *see* Guaifenesin and Pseudoephedrine *on page 863*
- Mucinex® D Maximum Strength [OTC] *see* Guaifenesin and Pseudoephedrine *on page 863*
- Mucinex Allergy [OTC] *see* Fexofenadine *on page 764*
- Mucinex Chest Congestion Child [OTC] *see* GuaiFENesin *on page 860*
- Mucinex® Cold [OTC] *see* Guaifenesin and Phenylephrine *on page 862*
- Mucinex DM [OTC] *see* Guaifenesin and Dextromethorphan *on page 861*
- Mucinex DM Maximum Strength [OTC] *see* Guaifenesin and Dextromethorphan *on page 861*
- Mucinex Fast-Max DM Max [OTC] *see* Guaifenesin and Dextromethorphan *on page 861*
- Mucinex For Kids [OTC] *see* GuaiFENesin *on page 860*
- Mucinex Kid's Cough [OTC] *see* Guaifenesin and Dextromethorphan *on page 861*
- Mucinex Kid's Cough Mini-Melts [OTC] *see* Guaifenesin and Dextromethorphan *on page 861*
- Mucinex Maximum Strength [OTC] *see* GuaiFENesin *on page 860*
- Mucomyst *see* Acetylcysteine *on page 31*
- Mucosa [OTC] *see* GuaiFENesin *on page 860*
- Mucus-ER [OTC] *see* GuaiFENesin *on page 860*
- Mucus Relief [OTC] *see* GuaiFENesin *on page 860*
- Mucus Relief Childrens [OTC] *see* GuaiFENesin *on page 860*
- Mucus Relief Sinus [OTC] *see* Guaifenesin and Phenylephrine *on page 862*
- Multaq *see* Dronedarone *on page 607*
- Mumps, Measles and Rubella Vaccines *see* Measles, Mumps, and Rubella Virus Vaccine *on page 1128*
- Mumps, Rubella, Varicella, and Measles Vaccine *see* Measles, Mumps, Rubella, and Varicella Virus Vaccine *on page 1129*

Mupirocin (myoo PEER oh sin)

Brand Names: US Bactroban; Bactroban Nasal; Centany; Centany AT
Brand Names: Canada Bactroban
Index Terms Mupirocin Calcium; Pseudomonic Acid A
Pharmacologic Category Antibiotic, Topical
Use Topical infection:
Intranasal: Eradication of nasal colonization with methicillin-resistant *S. aureus* (MRSA) in adult and pediatric patients ≥12 years of age and health care workers as part of a comprehensive infection control program to reduce the risk of infection among patients at high risk of MRSA infection during institutional outbreaks of infections with this microorganism

Limitations of use: Insufficient data for use as part of an intervention program to prevent autoinfection of high-risk patients from their own *S. aureus* nasal colonization or for general prophylaxis of any infection in any patient population.

Topical cream: Treatment of secondary infected traumatic skin lesions (up to 10 cm in length or 100 cm^2 in area) due to susceptible strains of *S. aureus* and *S. pyogenes*

Topical ointment: Treatment of impetigo due to *S. aureus* and *S. pyogenes*

Dosing
Adult & Geriatric
Impetigo: Topical: Ointment: Apply to affected area 3 times daily; re-evaluate after 3 to 5 days if no clinical response

Secondary skin infections: Topical: Cream: Apply to affected area 3 times daily for 10 days; re-evaluate after 3 to 5 days if no clinical response

Elimination of MRSA colonization: Intranasal: Approximately one-half of the ointment from the single-use tube should be applied into one nostril and the other half into the other nostril twice daily (morning and evening) for 5 days

Surgical prophylaxis in methicillin-resistant *S. aureus* (MRSA) carriers (off-label use): Intranasal: Approximately one-half of the ointment from the single-use tube should be applied into one nostril and the other half into the other nostril twice daily for 5 days (Bode, 2010; Lee, 2013)

Pediatric
Eradication of nasal MRSA: Intranasal: Children ≥12 years and Adolescents: Refer to adult dosing.

Impetigo: Topical: Ointment: Infants ≥2 months, Children, and Adolescents: Refer to adult dosing.

Secondary skin infections: Topical: Cream: Infants ≥3 months, Children, and Adolescents: Refer to adult dosing.

Renal Impairment There are no dosage adjustments provided in the manufacturer's labeling (has not been studied).

Hepatic Impairment There are no dosage adjustments provided in the manufacturer's labeling.

Additional Information Complete prescribing information should be consulted for additional detail.

Dosage Forms Excipient information presented when available (limited, particularly for generics); consult specific product labeling.
Cream, External, as calcium [strength expressed as base]:
Bactroban: 2% (15 g, 30 g)
Generic: 2% (15 g, 30 g)
Kit, External:
Centany AT: 2% [contains propylene glycol monostearate]
Ointment, External:
Bactroban: 2% (22 g)
Centany: 2% (30 g) [contains propylene glycol monostearate]
Generic: 2% (22 g)
Ointment, Nasal, as calcium [strength expressed as base]:
Bactroban Nasal: 2% (1 g)

- Mupirocin Calcium *see* Mupirocin *on page 1239*
- Muro 128 [OTC] *see* Sodium Chloride *on page 1671*
- Muse *see* Alprostadil *on page 78*
- Muse Pellet (Can) *see* Alprostadil *on page 78*
- Mustargen *see* Mechlorethamine (Systemic) *on page 1130*
- Mustine *see* Mechlorethamine (Systemic) *on page 1130*
- Mutamycin *see* MitoMYcin (Systemic) *on page 1219*
- Mutamycin® (Can) *see* MitoMYcin (Systemic) *on page 1219*
- Mya (Can) *see* Ethinyl Estradiol and Drospirenone *on page 702*
- Myalept *see* Metreleptin *on page 1195*
- Myambutol *see* Ethambutol *on page 699*
- Mycamine *see* Micafungin *on page 1200*
- Mycelex *see* Clotrimazole (Oral) *on page 427*
- Mycobutin *see* Rifabutin *on page 1579*
- Mycocide CX Callus Exfoliator [OTC] *see* Urea *on page 1853*
- Mycocide Clinical NS [OTC] *see* Tolnaftate *on page 1807*
- Mycolog-II *see* Nystatin and Triamcinolone *on page 1305*

Mycophenolate (mye koe FEN oh late)

Brand Names: US CellCept; CellCept Intravenous; Myfortic

Brand Names: Canada Ach-Mycophenolate; Apo-Mycophenolate; CellCept; CellCept I.V.; CO Mycophenolate; JAMP-Mycophenolate; Myfortic; Mylan-Mycophenolate; Novo-Mycophenolate; Sandoz-Mycophenolate Mofetil

Index Terms MMF; MPA; Mycophenolate Mofetil; Mycophenolate Sodium; Mycophenolic Acid

Pharmacologic Category Immunosuppressant Agent

Use Prophylaxis of organ rejection concomitantly with cyclosporine and corticosteroids in patients receiving allogeneic renal (CellCept, Myfortic), cardiac (CellCept), or hepatic (CellCept) transplants

Pregnancy Considerations [US Boxed Warning]: Mycophenolate is associated with an increased risk of congenital malformations and first trimester pregnancy loss when used by pregnant women. Females of reproductive potential must be counseled about pregnancy prevention and planning. Alternative agents should be considered for women planning a pregnancy. Adverse events have been reported in animal reproduction studies. In humans, the following congenital malformations have been reported: external ear abnormalities, cleft lip and palate, anomalies of the distal limbs, heart, esophagus, kidney, and nervous system. Spontaneous abortions have also been noted. Females of reproductive potential (girls who have entered puberty, women with a uterus who have not passed through clinically confirmed menopause) should have a negative pregnancy test with a sensitivity of ≥25 milliunits/mL immediately before therapy and the test should be repeated 8 to 10 days later. Pregnancy tests should be repeated during routine follow-up visits. Acceptable forms of contraception should be used during treatment and for 6 weeks after therapy is discontinued. The effectiveness of hormonal contraceptive agents may be affected by mycophenolate. For women with lupus nephritis taking mycophenolate and who are planning a pregnancy, mycophenolate should be discontinued at least 6 weeks prior to trying to conceive (Hahn, 2012).

Healthcare providers should report female exposures to mycophenolate during pregnancy or within 6 weeks of discontinuing therapy to the Mycophenolate Pregnancy Registry (800-617-8191). The National Transplantation Pregnancy Registry (NTPR, Temple University) is a registry for pregnant women taking immunosuppressants following any solid organ transplant. The NTPR encourages reporting of all immunosuppressant exposures during pregnancy in transplant recipients at 877-955-6877.

Breast-Feeding Considerations It is unknown if mycophenolate is excreted in human milk. Due to potentially serious adverse reactions, the decision to discontinue the drug or discontinue breast-feeding should be considered. Breast-feeding is not recommended during therapy or for 6 weeks after treatment is complete.

Medication Guide Available Yes

Contraindications Hypersensitivity to mycophenolate mofetil, mycophenolic acid, mycophenolate sodium, or any component of the formulation

Cellcept: Intravenous formulation is also contraindicated in patients who are allergic to polysorbate 80

Warnings/Precautions Hazardous agent - use appropriate precautions for handling and disposal (NIOSH 2014 [group 2]).

[US Boxed Warning]: Risk for bacterial, viral, fungal, and protozoal infections, including opportunistic infections, is increased with immunosuppressant therapy; infections may be serious and potentially fatal. Due to the risk of oversuppression of the immune system, which may increase susceptibility to infection, combination immunosuppressant therapy should be used with caution. Polyomavirus associated nephropathy (PVAN), JC virus-associated progressive multifocal leukoencephalopathy (PML), cytomegalovirus (CMV) infections, reactivation of hepatitis B (HBV) or hepatitis C (HCV), have been reported with use. A reduction in immunosuppression should be considered for patients with new or reactivated viral infections; however, in transplant recipients, the risk that reduced immunosuppression presents to the functioning graft should also be considered. PVAN, primarily from activation of BK virus, may lead to the deterioration of renal function and/or renal graft loss. PML, a potentially fatal condition, commonly presents with hemiparesis, apathy, ataxia, cognitive deficiencies, confusion, and hemiparesis. Risk factors for development of PML include treatment with immunosuppressants and immune function impairment; consultation with a neurologist should be considered in any patient with neurological symptoms receiving immunosuppressants. Risk of CMV viremia or

disease is increased in transplant recipients CMV seronegative at the time of transplant who receive a graft from a CMV seropositive donor. In patients infected with HBV or HCV, viral reactivation may occur; these patients should be monitored for signs of active HBV or HCV. **[US Boxed Warning]: Risk of development of lymphoma and skin malignancy is increased.** The risk for malignancies is related to intensity/duration of therapy. Patients should be monitored appropriately, instructed to limit exposure to sunlight/UV light to decrease the risk of skin cancer, and given supportive treatment should these conditions occur. Post-transplant lymphoproliferative disorder related to EBV infection has been reported in immunosuppressed organ transplant patients; risk is highest in EBV seronegative patients (including many young children). Neutropenia (including severe neutropenia) may occur, requiring dose reduction or interruption of treatment (risk greater from day 31-180 post-transplant). Use may rarely be associated with gastric or duodenal ulcers, GI bleeding and/or perforation. Use caution in patients with active serious digestive system disease; patients with active peptic ulcers were not included in clinical studies. Use caution in renal impairment as toxicity may be increased; may require dosage adjustment in severe impairment.

[US Boxed Warning]: Mycophenolate is associated with an increased risk of congenital malformations and first trimester pregnancy loss when used by pregnant women. Females of reproductive potential must be counseled about pregnancy prevention and planning. Alternative agents should be considered for women planning a pregnancy. Females of reproductive potential should have a negative pregnancy test with a sensitivity of ≥25 milliunits/mL immediately before therapy and the test should be repeated 8-10 days later. Pregnancy tests should be repeated during routine follow-up visits. Acceptable forms of contraception should be used during treatment and for 6 weeks after therapy is discontinued. Females of childbearing potential should have a negative pregnancy test within 1 week prior to beginning therapy. Two reliable forms of contraception should be used beginning 4 weeks prior to, during, and for 6 weeks after therapy. Because mycophenolate mofetil has demonstrated teratogenic effects in rats and rabbits, tablets should not be crushed, and capsules should not be opened or crushed. Avoid inhalation or direct contact with skin or mucous membranes of the powder contained in the capsules and the powder for oral suspension. Caution should be exercised in the handling and preparation of solutions of intravenous mycophenolate. Avoid skin contact with the intravenous solution and reconstituted suspension. If such contact occurs, wash thoroughly with soap and water, rinse eyes with plain water.

Theoretically, use should be avoided in patients with the rare hereditary deficiency of hypoxanthine-guanine phosphoribosyltransferase (such as Lesch-Nyhan or Kelley-Seegmiller syndrome). Intravenous solutions should be given over at least 2 hours; never administer intravenous solution by rapid or bolus injection. Live attenuated vaccines should be avoided during use; vaccinations may be less effective during therapy. **[US Boxed Warning]: Should be administered under the supervision of a physician experienced in immunosuppressive therapy.**

Note: CellCept and Myfortic dosage forms should not be used interchangeably due to differences in absorption. Some dosage forms may contain phenylalanine. Some dosage forms may contain polysorbate 80 (also known as Tweens). Hypersensitivity reactions, usually a delayed reaction, have been reported following exposure to pharmaceutical products containing polysorbate 80 in certain individuals (Isaksson, 2002; Lucente 2000; Shelley, 1995). Thrombocytopenia, ascites, pulmonary deterioration, and renal and hepatic failure have been reported in premature neonates after receiving parenteral products containing polysorbate 80 (Alade, 1986; CDC, 1984). See manufacturer's labeling.

Adverse Reactions Data for incidence >20% as reported in adults following oral dosing of CellCept alone in renal, cardiac, and hepatic allograft rejection studies. Profile in 3% to <20% range reflects use in combination with cyclosporine and corticosteroids. In general, lower doses used in renal rejection patients had less adverse effects than higher doses. Rates of adverse effects were similar for each indication, except for those unique to the specific organ involved. The type of adverse effects observed in pediatric patients was similar to those seen in adults, with the exception of abdominal pain, anemia, diarrhea, fever, hypertension, infection, pharyngitis, respiratory tract infection, sepsis, and vomiting; lymphoproliferative disorder was the only type of malignancy observed. Percentages of adverse reactions were similar in studies comparing CellCept to Myfortic in patients following renal transplant.

>20%:
Cardiovascular: Hypertension (28% to 78%), hypotension (33%), peripheral edema (27% to 64%), edema (27% to 28%), chest pain (26%), tachycardia (20% to 22%)
Central nervous system: Pain (31% to 76%), headache (16% to 54%), insomnia (41% to 52%), fever (21% to 52%), dizziness (29%), anxiety (28%)
Dermatologic: Rash (22%)
Endocrine & metabolic: Hyperglycemia (44% to 47%), hypercholesterolemia (41%), hypomagnesemia (39%), hypokalemia (32% to 37%), hypocalcemia (30%), hyperkalemia (22%)
Gastrointestinal: Abdominal pain (25% to 63%), nausea (20% to 55%), diarrhea (31% to 51%), constipation (19% to 41%), vomiting (33% to 34%), anorexia (25%), dyspepsia (22%)
Genitourinary: Urinary tract infection (37%)
Hematologic: Leukopenia (23% to 46%), anemia (26% to 43%; hypochromic 25%), leukocytosis (22% to 41%), thrombocytopenia (24% to 38%)
Hepatic: Liver function tests abnormal (25%), ascites (24%)
Neuromuscular & skeletal: Back pain (35% to 47%), weakness (35% to 43%), tremor (24% to 34%), paresthesia (21%)
Renal: Creatinine increased (39%), BUN increased (35%), kidney function abnormal (22% to 26%)
Respiratory: Dyspnea (31% to 37%), respiratory tract infection (22% to 37%), pleural effusion (34%), cough (31%), lung disorder (22% to 30%), sinusitis (26%)
Miscellaneous: Infection (18% to 27%), sepsis (27%), lactate dehydrogenase increased (23%), Candida (17% to 22%), herpes simplex (10% to 21%)
3% to <20%:
Cardiovascular: Angina, arrhythmia, arterial thrombosis, atrial fibrillation, atrial flutter, bradycardia, cardiac arrest, cardiac failure, CHF, extrasystole, facial edema, hyper-/hypovolemia, orthostatic hypotension, pallor, palpitation, pericardial effusion, peripheral vascular disorder, supraventricular extrasystoles, supraventricular tachycardia, syncope, thrombosis, vasodilation, vasospasm, venous pressure increased, ventricular extrasystole, ventricular tachycardia
Central nervous system: Agitation, chills with fever, confusion, delirium, depression, emotional lability, hallucinations, hypoesthesia, malaise, nervousness, psychosis, seizure, somnolence, thinking abnormal, vertigo
Dermatologic: Acne, alopecia, bruising, cellulitis, fungal dermatitis, hirsutism, petechia, pruritus, skin carcinoma, skin hypertrophy, skin ulcer, vesiculobullous rash
Endocrine & metabolic: Acidosis, alkalosis, Cushing's syndrome, dehydration, diabetes mellitus, gout, hypercalcemia, hyper-hypophosphatemia, hyperlipemia, hyperuricemia, hypochloremia, hypoglycemia, hyponatremia, hypoproteinemia, hypothyroidism, parathyroid disorder
Gastrointestinal: Abdomen enlarged, dysphagia, esophagitis, flatulence, gastritis, gastroenteritis, gastrointestinal hemorrhage, gastrointestinal moniliasis, gingivitis, gum hyperplasia, ileus, melena, mouth ulceration, oral moniliasis, stomach disorder, stomach ulcer, stomatitis, xerostomia, weight gain/loss
Genitourinary: Impotence, nocturia, pelvic pain, prostatic disorder, scrotal edema, urinary frequency, urinary incontinence, urinary retention, urinary tract disorder
Hematologic: Coagulation disorder, hemorrhage, neutropenia, pancytopenia, polycythemia, prothrombin time increased, thromboplastin time increased
Hepatic: Alkaline phosphatase increased, bilirubinemia, cholangitis, cholestatic jaundice, GGT increased, hepatitis, jaundice, liver damage, transaminases increased
Local: Abscess
Neuromuscular & skeletal: Arthralgia, hypertonia, joint disorder, leg cramps, myalgia, myasthenia, neck pain, neuropathy, osteoporosis
Ocular: Amblyopia, cataract, conjunctivitis, eye hemorrhage, lacrimation disorder, vision abnormal
Otic: Deafness, ear disorder, ear pain, tinnitus
Renal: Albuminuria, creatinine increased, dysuria, hematuria, hydronephrosis, oliguria, pyelonephritis, renal failure, renal tubular necrosis
Respiratory: Apnea, asthma, atelectasis, bronchitis, epistaxis, hemoptysis, hiccup, hyperventilation, hypoxia, respiratory acidosis, pharyngitis, pneumonia, pneumothorax, pulmonary edema, pulmonary hypertension, respiratory moniliasis, rhinitis, sputum increased, voice alteration

Miscellaneous: Candida (mucocutaneous 16% to 18%), CMV viremia/syndrome (12% to 14%), CMV tissue invasive disease (6% to 12%), herpes zoster cutaneous disease (4% to 10%), cyst, diaphoresis, flu-like syndrome, healing abnormal, hernia, ileus infection, neoplasm, peritonitis, thirst
<1% (Limited to important or life-threatening): Atypical mycobacterial infection, BK virus-associated nephropathy, bronchiectasis (Boddana 2011, Rook 2006), colitis, gastrointestinal perforation, hypogammaglobulinemia (Boddana 2011; Keven 2003; Robertson 2009), infectious endocarditis, interstitial lung disorder, intestinal villous atrophy, lymphoma, lymphoproliferative disease, malignancy, meningitis, pancreatitis, progressive multifocal leukoencephalopathy (sometimes fatal), pulmonary fibrosis (fatal), pure red cell aplasia, tuberculosis

Drug Interactions

Metabolism/Transport Effects Substrate of OAT3, SLCO1B1, SLCO1B3, UGT1A10, UGT1A8, UGT1A9, UGT2B7

Avoid Concomitant Use
Avoid concomitant use of Mycophenolate with any of the following: BCG (Intravesical); Bile Acid Sequestrants; Cholestyramine Resin; Natalizumab; Pimecrolimus; Rifamycin Derivatives; Tacrolimus (Topical); Tofacitinib; Vaccines (Live)

Increased Effect/Toxicity
Mycophenolate may increase the levels/effects of: Acyclovir-Valacyclovir; Fingolimod; Ganciclovir-Valganciclovir; Leflunomide; Natalizumab; Tofacitinib; Vaccines (Live)

The levels/effects of Mycophenolate may be increased by: Acyclovir-Valacyclovir; Denosumab; Ganciclovir-Valganciclovir; Isavuconazonium Sulfate; Pimecrolimus; Probenecid; Roflumilast; Tacrolimus (Topical); Teriflunomide; Trastuzumab

Decreased Effect
Mycophenolate may decrease the levels/effects of: BCG (Intravesical); Coccidioides immitis Skin Test; Contraceptives (Estrogens); Contraceptives (Progestins); Sipuleucel-T; Vaccines (Inactivated); Vaccines (Live)

The levels/effects of Mycophenolate may be decreased by: Antacids; Bile Acid Sequestrants; Cholestyramine Resin; CycloSPORINE (Systemic); Echinacea; Magnesium Salts; MetroNIDAZOLE (Systemic); Penicillins; Proton Pump Inhibitors; Quinolone Antibiotics; Rifamycin Derivatives; Sevelamer

Food Interactions Food decreases C_{max} of MPA by 40% following CellCept administration and 33% following Myfortic use; the extent of absorption is not changed. Management: Take CellCept or Myfortic on an empty stomach to decrease variability; however, Cellcept may be taken with food if necessary in stable renal transplant patients.

Preparation for Administration Hazardous agent; use appropriate precautions for handling and disposal (NIOSH 2014 [group 2]).

Oral suspension: Should be constituted prior to dispensing to the patient and **not** mixed with any other medication. Add 47 mL of water to the bottle and shake well for ~1 minute. Add another 47 mL of water to the bottle and shake well for an additional minute. Final concentration is 200 mg/mL of mycophenolate mofetil.
IV: Reconstitute the contents of each vial with 14 mL of 5% dextrose injection; dilute the contents of a vial with 5% dextrose in water to a final concentration of 6 mg mycophenolate mofetil per mL. **Note:** Vial is vacuum-sealed; if a lack of vacuum is noted during preparation, the vial should not be used.

Storage/Stability

Capsules: Store at 25°C (77°F); excursions permitted to 15°C to 30°C (59°F to 86°F).
Tablets: Store at 25°C (77°F); excursions permitted to 15°C to 30°C (59°F to 86°F). Protect from moisture and light.
Oral suspension: Store powder for oral suspension at 25°C (77°F); excursions permitted to 15°C to 30°C (59°F to 86°F). Once reconstituted, the oral solution may be stored at room temperature or under refrigeration. Do not freeze. The mixed suspension is stable for 60 days.
Injection: Store intact vials and diluted solutions at 25°C (77°F); excursions permitted to 15°C to 30°C (59°F to 86°F). Begin infusion within 4 hours of reconstitution.

Mechanism of Action MPA exhibits a cytostatic effect on T and B lymphocytes. It is an inhibitor of inosine monophosphate dehydrogenase (IMPDH) which inhibits *de novo* guanosine nucleotide synthesis. T and B lymphocytes are dependent on this pathway for proliferation.

Pharmacodynamics/Kinetics

Onset of action: Peak effect: Correlation of toxicity or efficacy is still being developed, however, one study indicated that 12-hour AUCs >40 mcg/mL/hour were correlated with efficacy and decreased episodes of rejection

Absorption: AUC values for MPA are lower in the early post-transplant period versus later (>3 months) post-transplant period. The extent of absorption in pediatrics is similar to that seen in adults, although there was wide variability reported.

Oral: Myfortic: 93%

Distribution:

CellCept: MPA: Oral: 4 L/kg; IV: 3.6 L/kg

Myfortic: MPA: Oral: 54 L (at steady state); 112 L (elimination phase)

Protein binding: MPA: >97%, MPAG 82%

Metabolism: Hepatic and via GI tract; CellCept is completely hydrolyzed in the liver to mycophenolic acid (MPA; active metabolite); enterohepatic recirculation of MPA may occur; MPA is glucuronidated to MPAG (inactive metabolite)

Bioavailability: Oral: CellCept: 94%; Myfortic: 72%

Half-life elimination:

CellCept: MPA: Oral: 18 hours; IV: 17 hours

Myfortic: MPA: Oral: 8-16 hours; MPAG: 13-17 hours

Time to peak, plasma: Oral: MPA:

CellCept: 1-1.5 hours

Myfortic: 1.5-2.75 hours

Excretion:

CellCept: MPA: Urine (<1%), feces (6%); MPAG: Urine (87%)

Myfortic: MPA: Urine (3%), feces; MPAG: Urine (>60%)

Dosing

Adult Note: May be used IV for up to 14 days; transition to oral therapy as soon as tolerated.

Renal transplant:

CellCept:

Oral: 1 g twice daily. Doses >2 g daily are not recommended.

IV: 1 g twice daily

Myfortic: Oral: 720 mg twice daily (total daily dose: 1440 mg)

Cardiac transplantation: *CellCept:*

Oral: 1.5 g twice daily

IV: 1.5 g twice daily

Hepatic transplantation: *CellCept:*

Oral: 1.5 g twice daily

IV: 1 g twice daily

Autoimmune hepatitis, refractory (off-label use): *CellCept:* Oral: 2 g daily (Manns, 2010)

Lupus nephritis (off-label use): CellCept: Oral:

Induction: 1 g twice daily for 6 months in combination with a glucocorticoid (Ong, 2005) **or** 2-3 g daily for 6 months in combination with glucocorticoids (Hahn, 2012)

Maintenance: 0.5-3 g daily (Contreras, 2004) **or** 1 g twice daily (Dooley, 2011) **or** 1-2 g daily (Hahn, 2012)

Myasthenia gravis (off-label use): *CellCept:* Oral: 1 g twice daily (range: 1-3 g daily) (Cahoon, 2006; Ciafaloni, 2001; Merriggioli, 2003)

Psoriasis, moderate-to-severe (off-label use): *CellCept:* Oral: 2-3 g daily (Menter, 2009)

Geriatric Dosage is the same as younger patients, however, dosing should be cautious due to possibility of increased hepatic, renal, or cardiac dysfunction. Elderly patients may be at an increased risk of certain infections, gastrointestinal hemorrhage, and pulmonary edema, as compared to younger patients.

Pediatric

Renal transplant: Oral:

CellCept: Infants ≥3 months, Children, and Adolescents: *Cellcept suspension:* 600 mg/m^2/dose twice daily; maximum dose: 1 g twice daily

Alternatively, may use Cellcept solid dosage forms according to BSA as follows:

BSA 1.25-1.5 m^2: 750 mg capsule twice daily

BSA >1.5 m^2: 1 g capsule or tablet twice daily

Myfortic: Children ≥5 years and Adolescents: Usual dosage: 400 mg/m^2/dose twice daily; maximum dose: 720 mg twice daily

BSA <1.19 m^2: Use of this formulation is not recommended

BSA 1.19-1.58 m^2: 540 mg twice daily (maximum: 1080 mg daily)

BSA >1.58 m^2: 720 mg twice daily (maximum: 1440 mg daily)

Renal Impairment

Renal transplant: GFR <25 mL/minute/1.73 m^2 in patients outside the immediate post-transplant period:

CellCept: Doses of >1 g administered twice daily should be avoided; patients should also be carefully observed; no dose adjustments are needed in renal transplant patients experiencing delayed graft function postoperatively

Myfortic: No dose adjustments are needed in renal transplant patients experiencing delayed graft function postoperatively; however, monitor carefully for potential concentration dependent adverse events

Cardiac or liver transplant: No data available; mycophenolate may be used in cardiac or hepatic transplant patients with severe chronic renal impairment if the potential benefit outweighs the potential risk.

Autoimmune disease (off-label use): There have been no specific dosage adjustments identified, although use of lower doses may be required. MPA exposure appears to be inversely related to renal function (Abd Rahman, 2013); monitor closely for efficacy and adverse effects, especially in patients with end-stage renal disease (Haubitz, 2002; MacPhee, 2000).

Hemodialysis: Not removed; supplemental dose is not necessary.

Peritoneal dialysis: Supplemental dose is not necessary.

Hepatic Impairment No dosage adjustment is recommended for renal patients with severe hepatic parenchymal disease; however, it is not currently known whether dosage adjustments are necessary for hepatic disease with other etiologies.

Adjustment for Toxicity Neutropenia (ANC <1.3 x 10^3/μL): Dosing should be interrupted or the dose reduced, appropriate diagnostic tests performed and patients managed appropriately

Dietary Considerations Oral dosage formulations should be taken on an empty stomach to avoid variability in MPA absorption. However, in stable renal transplant patients, Cellcept may be administered with food if necessary. Some products may contain phenylalanine.

Administration

Oral dosage formulations (tablet, capsule, suspension) should be administered on an empty stomach (1 hour before or 2 hours after meals) to avoid variability in MPA absorption. The oral solution may be administered via a nasogastric tube (minimum 8 French, 1.7 mm interior diameter); oral suspension should not be mixed with other medications. Delayed release tablets should not be crushed, cut, or chewed. Cellcept may be administered with food in stable renal transplant patients when necessary. If a dose is missed, administer as soon as it is remembered. If it is close to the next scheduled dose, skip the missed dose and resume at next regularly scheduled time; do not double a dose to make up for a missed dose.

Intravenous solutions should be administered over at least 2 hours (either peripheral or central vein); do **not** administer intravenous solution by rapid or bolus injection.

Hazardous agent; use appropriate precautions for handling and disposal (NIOSH 2014 [group 2]).

Monitoring Parameters Complete blood count (weekly for first month, twice monthly during months 2 and 3, then monthly thereafter through the first year); renal and liver function; signs and symptoms of organ rejection; signs and symptoms of bacterial, fungal, protozoal, new or reactivated viral, or opportunistic infections; neurological symptoms (eg, hemiparesis, confusion, cognitive deficiencies, ataxia) suggestive of PML, pregnancy test (immediately prior to initiation and 8-10 days later in females of childbearing potential, followed by repeat tests during therapy); monitor skin (for lesions suspicious of skin cancer); monitor for signs of lymphoma

Additional Information Females of reproductive potential are required to have contraceptive counseling and use acceptable birth control unless heterosexual intercourse is completely avoided. Use of an intrauterine device (IUD), tubal sterilization, or vasectomy of the female patient's partner are acceptable contraceptive methods that can be used alone. If a hormonal contraceptive is used (eg, combination oral contraceptive pills, transdermal patches, vaginal rings, or progestin only products), then one barrier method must also be used (eg, diaphragm or cervical cap with spermicide, contraceptive sponge, male or female condom). Alternatively, the use of two barrier methods is also acceptable (eg, diaphragm or cervical cap with spermicide, or contraceptive sponge **PLUS** male or female condom). Refer to manufacturer's labeling for full details.

Dosage Forms Considerations Single dose pharmacokinetic studies in adult renal transplant patients suggest that bioavailability is similar between oral mycophenolate mofetil (1000 mg) and delayed release mycophenolic acid (720 mg) (Arns, 2005). In clinical trials, comparative efficacy and safety profiles have been observed in adult renal transplant patients randomized to either oral mycophenolate mofetil (1000 mg twice daily) or delayed release mycophenolic acid (720 mg twice daily) (Budde, 2004; Salvadori, 2003).

Dosage Forms Excipient information presented when available (limited, particularly for generics); consult specific product labeling.

Capsule, Oral, as mofetil:
CellCept: 250 mg [contains fd&c blue #2 (indigotine)]
Generic: 250 mg [imprints], 250 mg
Solution Reconstituted, Intravenous, as mofetil hydrochloride:
CellCept Intravenous: 500 mg (1 ea)
Suspension Reconstituted, Oral, as mofetil:
CellCept: 200 mg/mL (160 mL) [contains aspartame, methylparaben, soybean lecithin; mixed fruit flavor]
Generic: 200 mg/mL (160 mL)
Tablet, Oral, as mofetil:
CellCept: 500 mg [contains fd&c blue #2 aluminum lake]
Generic: 500 mg
Tablet Delayed Release, Oral, as mycophenolic acid:
Myfortic: 180 mg [contains fd&c blue #2 (indigotine)]
Myfortic: 360 mg
Generic: 180 mg, 360 mg

Extemporaneous Preparations Hazardous agent; use appropriate precautions for handling and disposal (NIOSH 2014 [group 2]).

A 50 mg/mL oral suspension may be made with mycophenolate mofetil capsules, Ora-Plus, and cherry syrup. In a vertical flow hood, empty six 250 mg capsules into a mortar; add 7.5 mL Ora-Plus and mix to a uniform paste. Mix while adding 15 mL of cherry syrup in incremental proportions; transfer to a calibrated bottle, rinse mortar with cherry syrup, and add sufficient quantity of cherry syrup to make 30 mL. Label "shake well". Stable for 210 days at 5°C, for 28 days at 25°C to 37°C, and for 11 days at 45°C.

Venkataramanan R, McCombs JR, Zuckerman S, et al, "Stability of Mycophenolate Mofetil as an Extemporaneous Suspension," *Ann Pharmacother*, 1998, 32(7-8):755-7.

Nabumetone (na BYOO me tone)

Brand Names: Canada Apo-Nabumetone; Mylan-Nabumetone; Teva-Nabumetone

Index Terms Relafen

Pharmacologic Category Nonsteroidal Anti-inflammatory Drug (NSAID), Oral

Use Arthritis: Relief of signs and symptoms of osteoarthritis and rheumatoid arthritis.

Medication Guide Available Yes

Dosing

Adult & Geriatric

Arthritis: Oral: 1,000 mg as a single dose; adjust dose based on patient response up to 2,000 mg/day in 1 to 2 divided doses; doses >2,000 mg/day have not been studied. Canadian labeling recommends not to adjust dose more frequently than 1-week intervals.

Note: Patients <50 kg are less likely to require doses >1,000 mg/day.

Renal Impairment

US labeling: In general, NSAIDs are not recommended for use in patients with advanced renal disease, but the manufacturer of nabumetone does provide some guidelines for adjustment in renal dysfunction:

CrCl ≥50 mL/minute: No dosage adjustment necessary.

CrCl 30 to 49 mL/minute: Initial maximum dose: 750 mg once daily; maximum daily dose: 1,500 mg/day

CrCl <30 mL/minute: Initial maxim dose: 500 mg once daily; maximum daily dose: 1,000 mg/day

Hemodialysis: Not removed

Canadian labeling:

CrCl ≥50 mL/minute: There are no dosage adjustments provided in the manufacturer's labeling

CrCl 30 to 49 mL/minute: There are no specific dosage adjustments provided in the manufacturer's labeling; however, dose reduction may warranted. Use with caution.

CrCl <30 mL/minute: There are no specific dosage adjustments provided in the manufacturer's labeling; however, lower doses are recommended and should be made on an individual basis; monitor closely. Contraindicated in patients with severely impaired or deteriorating renal function.

Hepatic Impairment There are no dosage adjustments provided in the manufacturer's labeling (data limited). The Canadian labeling contraindicates use in patients with significant hepatic impairment or active hepatic disease. Prodrug activation and metabolism are hepatic function dependent and may be reduced in severe hepatic impairment.

Additional Information Complete prescribing information should be consulted for additional detail.

Dosage Forms Excipient information presented when available (limited, particularly for generics); consult specific product labeling.

Tablet, Oral:

Generic: 500 mg, 750 mg

◆ NAC see Acetylcysteine on page 31

◆ N-Acetyl-L-cysteine see Acetylcysteine on page 31

◆ N Acetylcysteine see Acetylcysteine on page 31

◆ N-acetylgalactosamine-6-sulfatase see Elosulfase Alfa on page 625

◆ N-Acetyl-P-Aminophenol see Acetaminophen on page 25

◆ NaCl see Sodium Chloride on page 1671

Nadolol (NAY doe lol)

Brand Names: US Corgard

Brand Names: Canada Apo-Nadol; Teva-Nadolol

Pharmacologic Category Antianginal Agent; Antihypertensive; Beta-Blocker, Nonselective

Use Treatment of hypertension and angina pectoris

Guideline recommendations:

Hypertension: The 2014 guideline for the management of high blood pressure in adults (Eighth Joint National Committee [JNC 8]) recommends initiation of pharmacologic treatment to lower blood pressure for the following patients (JNC8 [James 2013]):

• Patients ≥60 years of age, with systolic blood pressure (SBP) ≥150 mm Hg or diastolic blood pressure (DBP) ≥90 mm Hg. Goal of therapy is SBP <150 mm Hg and DBP <90 mm Hg.

• Patients <60 years of age, with SBP ≥140 mm Hg or DBP ≥90 mm Hg. Goal of therapy is SBP <140 mm Hg and DBP <90 mm Hg.

• Patients ≥18 years of age with diabetes, with SBP ≥140 mm Hg or DBP ≥90 mm Hg. Goal of therapy is SBP <140 mm Hg and DBP <90 mm Hg.

• Patients ≥18 years of age with chronic kidney disease (CKD), with SBP ≥140 mm Hg or DBP ≥90 mm Hg. Goal of therapy is SBP <140 mm Hg and DBP <90 mm Hg.

Chronic kidney disease (CKD) and hypertension: Regardless of race or diabetes status, the use of an ACE inhibitor (ACEI) or angiotensin receptor blocker (ARB) as initial therapy is recommended to improve kidney outcomes. In the general nonblack population (without CKD) including those with diabetes, initial antihypertensive treatment should consist of a thiazide-type diuretic, calcium channel blocker, ACEI, or ARB. In the general black population (without CKD) including those with diabetes, initial antihypertensive treatment should consist of a thiazide-type diuretic or a calcium channel blocker instead of an ACEI or ARB.

Coronary artery disease (CAD) and hypertension: The American Heart Association, American College of Cardiology, and American Society of Hypertension (AHA/ACC/ASH) 2015 scientific statement for the treatment of

hypertension in patients with CAD recommends the use of a beta blocker as part of a regimen in patients with hypertension and chronic stable angina with a history of prior MI. A BP target of <140/90 mm Hg is reasonable for the secondary prevention of cardiovascular events. A lower target BP (<130/80 mm Hg) may be appropriate in some individuals with CAD, previous MI, stroke or transient ischemic attack, or CAD risk equivalents (AHA/ACC/ASH [Rosendorff 2015]).

Dosing

Adult

U.S. labeling:

Angina: Oral: Initial: 40 mg once daily, increase dosage gradually by 40 to 80 mg increments at 3- to 7-day intervals until optimum clinical response is obtained usual dose: 40 to 80 mg daily; maximum dose: 240 mg daily

Hypertension: Oral: Initial: 40 mg once daily, increase dosage gradually by 40 to 80 mg increments until optimum blood pressure reduction achieved. Usual dosage range (ASH/ISH [Weber, 2014]): 40 to 80 mg once daily. Doses up to 240 to 320 mg once daily in hypertension may be necessary

Canadian labeling:

Angina: Oral: Initial: 80 mg once daily, increase dosage gradually by 80 mg increments at 7-day intervals until optimum clinical response is obtained; may consider dose reduction to 40 mg once daily for patients stable on 80 mg daily; maximum dose: 240 mg daily

Hypertension: Oral: Initial: 80 mg once daily; increase dosage gradually by 80 mg increments at 7-day intervals until optimum blood pressure reduction achieved. Doses ≤240 mg daily are typically effective; maximum dose: 320 mg once daily

Off-label uses:

Atrial fibrillation (rate control): Oral: Usual maintenance dose: 10 to 240 mg once daily (AHA/ACC/HRS [January, 2014])

Variceal hemorrhage prophylaxis (Garcia-Tsao, 2007): Oral:

Primary prophylaxis: Initial: 40 mg once daily; adjust to maximal tolerated dose. **Note:** Risk factors for hemorrhage include Child-Pugh class B/C or variceal red wale markings on endoscopy.

Secondary prophylaxis: Initial: 40 mg once daily; adjust to maximal tolerated dose

Thyrotoxicosis: Oral: 40 to 160 mg once daily (Bahn, 2011)

Geriatric Refer to adult dosing. In the management of hypertension, consider lower initial doses (eg, 20 mg daily) and titrate to response (Aronow, 2011).

Renal Impairment

CrCl >50 mL/minute/1.73 m^2: Administer every 24 hours

CrCl 31 to 50 mL/minute/1.73 m^2: Administer every 24 to 36 hours

CrCl 10 to 30 mL/minute/1.73 m^2: Administer every 24 to 48 hours

CrCl <10 mL/minute/1.73 m^2: Administer every 40 to 60 hours

Dosage adjustments for dialysis are not provided in the manufacturer's labeling; however, the following guidelines have been used by some clinicians (Aronoff, 2007):

ESRD requiring hemodialysis: Administer dose post-dialysis.

Peritoneal dialysis: Administer every 40 to 60 hours

Hepatic Impairment There are no dosage adjustments provided in the manufacturer's labeling.

Additional Information Complete prescribing information should be consulted for additional detail.

Dosage Forms Excipient information presented when available (limited, particularly for generics); consult specific product labeling.

Tablet, Oral:

Corgard: 20 mg, 40 mg, 80 mg [scored]

Generic: 20 mg, 40 mg, 80 mg

Nafarelin (naf a REL in)

Brand Names: US Synarel

Brand Names: Canada Synarel

Index Terms Nafarelin Acetate

Pharmacologic Category Gonadotropin Releasing Hormone Agonist

Use

Central precocious puberty: Treatment of central precocious puberty (CPP) (gonadotropin-dependent precocious puberty) in children of both sexes.

Endometriosis: Management of endometriosis, including pain relief and reduction of endometriotic lesions.

◄ **Dosing**

Adult & Geriatric

Endometriosis: Intranasal: Females: One spray (200 mcg) into 1 nostril each morning and 1 spray (200 mcg) into the other nostril each evening starting between days 2 and 4 of menstrual cycle (total: 2 sprays [400 mcg] daily). If regular menstruation persists after 2 months of therapy, may increase dose to 2 sprays (400 mcg; 1 spray in each nostril) in the morning and evening (total: 4 sprays [800 mcg] daily). Total duration of therapy should not exceed 6 months due to decreases in bone mineral density; re-treatment is not recommended by the manufacturer.

Pediatric Central precocious puberty: Intranasal: Males/Females: Two sprays (400 mcg) into each nostril in the morning and 2 sprays (400 mcg) into each nostril in the evening (total: 8 sprays [1600 mcg] daily). If inadequate suppression, may increase dose to 3 sprays (600 mcg) into alternating nostrils 3 times daily (total: 9 sprays [1800 mcg] daily). Continue therapy until resumption of puberty is desired.

Renal Impairment There are no dosage adjustments provided in the manufacturer's labeling (has not been studied).

Hepatic Impairment There are no dosage adjustments provided in the manufacturer's labeling (has not been studied).

Additional Information Complete prescribing information should be consulted for additional detail.

Dosage Forms Excipient information presented when available (limited, particularly for generics); consult specific product labeling.

Solution, Nasal:
Synarel: 2 mg/mL (8 mL)

◆ Nafarelin Acetate see Nafarelin on page 1245

Nafcillin (naf SIL in)

Brand Names: US Nallpen in Dextrose

Index Terms Ethoxynaphthamido Penicillin Sodium; Nafcillin Sodium; Nallpen; Sodium Nafcillin

Pharmacologic Category Antibiotic, Penicillin

Use Treatment of infections such as osteomyelitis, bacteremia, septicemia, endocarditis, and CNS infections caused by susceptible strains of *Staphylococcus* species

Pregnancy Considerations Adverse events have not been observed in animal reproduction studies. Information specific to nafcillin use in pregnancy is limited. Maternal use of penicillins has generally not resulted in an increased risk of birth defects.

Breast-Feeding Considerations Penicillins are excreted into breast milk. The manufacturer recommends that caution be exercised when administering nafcillin to nursing women. Nondose-related effects could include modification of bowel flora.

Contraindications Hypersensitivity to nafcillin, or any component of the formulation, or penicillins

Warnings/Precautions Serious and occasionally severe or fatal hypersensitivity (anaphylactoid) reactions have been reported in patients on penicillin therapy, especially with a history of beta-lactam hypersensitivity, history of sensitivity to multiple allergens, or previous IgE-mediated reactions (eg, anaphylaxis, angioedema, urticaria). Use with caution in asthmatic patients. Contains sodium; use with caution in patients with heart failure. Vesicant; ensure proper catheter or needle position prior to and during IV infusion; avoid extravasation of IV infusions. Large IV or intraventricular doses have been associated with neurotoxicity. Modification of dosage is necessary in patients with both severe renal and hepatic impairment. Elimination may be decreased in pediatric patients. Prolonged use may result in fungal or bacterial superinfection, including C. difficile-associated diarrhea (CDAD) and pseudomembranous colitis; CDAD has been observed >2 months postantibiotic treatment. Potentially significant drug-drug interactions may exist, requiring dose or frequency adjustment, additional monitoring, and/or selection of alternative therapy.

Adverse Reactions Frequency not always defined.

Central nervous system: Neurotoxicity (high doses)

Gastrointestinal: *C. difficile*-associated diarrhea

Hematologic: Agranulocytosis, bone marrow depression, neutropenia

Local: Inflammation, pain, phlebitis, skin sloughing, swelling, and thrombophlebitis at the injection site; tissue necrosis with sloughing (SubQ extravasation)

Renal: Interstitial nephritis (rare), renal tubular damage (rare)

Miscellaneous: Anaphylaxis, hypersensitivity reactions (immediate and delayed; general incidence of 1% to 10% for penicillins), serum sickness

<1% (Limited to important or life-threatening): ALT increased, AST increased, bilirubin increased, cholestatic hepatitis, diarrhea, drug-induced lupus erythematosus, fever, hypokalemia, itching, nausea, rash (including bullous skin eruptions), vomiting

Drug Interactions

Metabolism/Transport Effects Induces CYP3A4 (moderate)

Avoid Concomitant Use

Avoid concomitant use of Nafcillin with any of the following: Antihepaciviral Combination Products; Axitinib; BCG (Intravesical); Bedaquiline; Bosutinib; Cobimetinib; Flibanserin; Nisoldipine; Olaparib; Palbociclib; Probenecid; Ranolazine; Simeprevir; Sonidegib

Increased Effect/Toxicity

Nafcillin may increase the levels/effects of: Clarithromycin; Ifosfamide; Methotrexate

The levels/effects of Nafcillin may be increased by: Probenecid

Decreased Effect

Nafcillin may decrease the levels/effects of: Antihepaciviral Combination Products; ARIPiprazole; Axitinib; BCG (Intravesical); BCG Vaccine (Immunization); Bedaquiline; Bosutinib; Calcium Channel Blockers; Clarithromycin; Cobimetinib; Contraceptives (Estrogens); CycloSPORINE (Systemic); CYP3A4 Substrates; Daclatasvir; FentaNYL; Flibanserin; Hydrocodone; Ibrutinib; Ifosfamide; Mycophenolate; Nisoldipine; Olaparib; Palbociclib; Ranolazine; Rolapitant; Saxagliptin; Simeprevir; Sodium Picosulfate; Sonidegib; Typhoid Vaccine; Vitamin K Antagonists

The levels/effects of Nafcillin may be decreased by: Tetracycline Derivatives

Storage/Stability

Premixed infusions: Store in a freezer at -20°C (-4°F). Thaw at room temperature or under refrigeration only. Thawed bags are stable for 21 days under refrigeration or 72 hours at room temperature. Do not refreeze.

Vials: Reconstituted parenteral solution is stable for 3 days at room temperature and 7 days when refrigerated. For IV infusion in NS or D₅W, solution is stable for 24 hours at room temperature and 7 days when refrigerated.

Solutions for ambulatory IV infusion reservoirs (eg, >24-hour supply) may be subject to inadvertent exposure to temperatures higher than recommended due to heat radiation from patient's skin; lower concentrations of preparation may be needed to prevent precipitation of solution in some circumstances (Chan 2005).

Mechanism of Action Interferes with bacterial cell wall synthesis during active multiplication, causing cell wall destruction and resultant bactericidal activity against susceptible bacteria; resistant to inactivation by staphylococcal penicillinase

Pharmacodynamics/Kinetics

Distribution: Widely distributed; CSF penetration is poor but enhanced by meningeal inflammation

Protein binding: ~90%; primarily to albumin

Metabolism: Primarily hepatic; undergoes enterohepatic recirculation

Half-life elimination:

Neonates: <3 weeks: 2.2-5.5 hours; 4-9 weeks: 1.2-2.3 hours

Children 1 month to 14 years: 0.75-1.9 hours

Adults: Normal renal/hepatic function: 30-60 minutes

Time to peak, serum: IM: 30-60 minutes

Excretion: Primarily feces; urine (~30% as unchanged drug)

Dosing

Adult & Geriatric

Endocarditis: Methicillin-susceptible *Staphylococcus aureus* (MSSA): IV:

Native valve: 12 g/24 hours in 4-6 divided doses (ie, 2 g every 4 hours or 3 g every 6 hours) for 6 weeks. **Note:** Dosing intended for **complicated** right-sided infective endocarditis (IE) or left-sided IE. For **uncomplicated** right-sided IE, 2 weeks of therapy may be adequate (Baddour 2005). The British Society for Antimicrobial Chemotherapy (BSAC) recommends 4 weeks of therapy with a penicillinase-resistant penicillin for all patients with native valve IE due to MSSA unless patient has intracardiac prostheses, secondary lung abscesses, or osteomyelitis, then extend treatment to ≥6 weeks (Gould 2012).

Prosthetic valve: 12 g/24 hours in 6 divided doses (ie, 2 g every 4 hours) for ≥6 weeks (use with rifampin for entire course and gentamicin for first 2 weeks) (Baddour 2005)

Skin and soft tissue infections(IDSA [Stevens 2014]):

Due to methicillin-susceptible Staphylococcus aureus (MSSA): IV: 1 to 2 g every 4 hours for 7 to 14 days

Necrotizing infection due to MSSA (off-label use): IV: 1 to 2 g every 4 hours; continue until further debridement is not necessary, patient has clinically improved, and patient is afebrile for 48 to 72 hours

Streptococcal skin infections (off-label use): IV: 1 to 2 g every 4 to 6 hours (IDSA [Stevens 2014])

Surgical site infections (trunk or extremity [away from axilla or perineum]) (off-label use): IV: 2 g every 6 hours (IDSA [Stevens 2014])

Pediatric

Mild-to-moderate infections: IM, IV: 100-150 mg/kg/day in divided doses every 6 hours (maximum dose: 4000 mg daily)

Severe infections: IM, IV: 150-200 mg/kg/day in divided doses every 4-6 hours; for life-threatening infection (eg, meningitis) daily doses up to 200 mg/kg are used (maximum dose: 12 g daily)

Skin and soft tissue infections (IDSA [Stevens 2014]):

Due to methicillin-susceptible Staphylococcus aureus (MSSA): IV: 100 to 150 mg/kg/day in divided doses every 6 hours for 7 to 14 days

Necrotizing infection due to MSSA (off-label use): IV: 200 mg/kg/day in divided doses every 6 hours; continue until further debridement is not necessary, patient has clinically improved, and patient is afebrile for 48 to 72 hours

Streptococcal skin infections (off-label use): IV: 200 mg/kg/day in divided doses every 6 hours (IDSA [Stevens 2014])

Renal Impairment No dosage adjustment is necessary unless in the setting of concomitant hepatic impairment; however, manufacturer labeling does not provide specific dosage adjustments.

Poorly dialyzed. No supplemental dose or dosage adjustment necessary, including patients on intermittent hemodialysis, peritoneal dialysis, or continuous renal replacement therapy (eg, CVVHD) (Aronoff 2007; Heintz 2009).

Hepatic Impairment No specific dosage adjustments provided in manufacturer's labeling; however, dosage adjustment may be necessary particularly in the setting of concomitant renal impairment; nafcillin primarily undergoes hepatic metabolism. In patients with both hepatic and renal impairment, monitoring of serum drug levels and modification of dosage may be necessary.

Dietary Considerations Some products may contain sodium.

Administration

IM: Administer as a deep intragluteal injection; rotate injection sites.

IV: Infuse over 30-60 minutes. Vesicant; ensure proper needle or catheter placement prior to and during IV infusion. Avoid extravasation.

Extravasation management: If extravasation occurs, stop infusion immediately and disconnect (leave needle/cannula in place); gently aspirate extravasated solution (do **NOT** flush the line); initiate hyaluronidase antidote; remove needle/cannula (if not using IV hyaluronidase antidote), apply dry cold compresses (Hurst 2004); elevate extremity.

Hyaluronidase: Intradermal or SubQ: Inject a total of 1 mL (15 units/mL) as five separate 0.2 mL injections (using a 25-gauge needle) into area of extravasation at the leading edge in a clockwise manner (MacCara, 1983; Zenk, 1981).

Monitoring Parameters Baseline and periodic CBC with differential; periodic urinalysis, BUN, serum creatinine, AST and ALT; observe for signs and symptoms of anaphylaxis during first dose

Test Interactions Positive Coombs' test (direct), false-positive urinary and serum proteins; may inactivate aminoglycosides *in vitro*

Dosage Forms Excipient information presented when available (limited, particularly for generics); consult specific product labeling.

Solution, Intravenous:

Nallpen in Dextrose: 1 g/50 mL (50 mL); 2 g/100 mL (100 mL)

Solution Reconstituted, Injection:

Generic: 1 g (1 ea); 2 g (1 ea); 10 g (1 ea)

Solution Reconstituted, Injection [preservative free]:

Generic: 1 g (1 ea); 2 g (1 ea); 10 g (1 ea)

Solution Reconstituted, Intravenous:

Generic: 1 g (1 ea); 2 g (1 ea)

◆ Nafcillin Sodium *see* Nafcillin *on page 1246*

Naftifine (NAF ti feen)

Brand Names: US Naftin
Index Terms Naftifine Hydrochloride
Pharmacologic Category Antifungal Agent, Topical

Use

Tinea infections: Cream 1% and 2%, Gel 1%: Topical treatment of tinea cruris (jock itch), tinea corporis (ringworm), and tinea pedis (athlete's foot).

Tinea pedis: Gel 2%: Topical treatment of tinea pedis (athlete's foot).

Dosing

Adult & Geriatric

Tinea corporis, tinea cruris: Topical:

Cream 1% and gel 1%: Apply once daily (cream) or twice daily (gel; morning and evening) to affected area and surrounding skin for up to 4 weeks

Cream 2%: Apply a thin layer once daily to affected area and healthy surrounding skin (1/2 inch margin) for 2 weeks

Tinea pedis: Topical:

Cream 1% and gel 1%: Apply once daily (cream) or twice daily (gel; morning and evening) to affected area and surrounding skin for up to 4 weeks

Cream 2% and gel 2%: Apply a thin layer once daily to affected area and surrounding skin (1/2 inch margin) for 2 weeks

Pediatric

Tinea corporis, tinea cruris: Children ≥12 years and Adolescents: Topical: Cream 2%: Refer to adult dosing.

Tinea pedis: Children ≥12 years and Adolescents:Topical: Cream 2% and gel 2%: Refer to adult dosing.

Additional Information Complete prescribing information should be consulted for additional detail.

Dosage Forms Excipient information presented when available (limited, particularly for generics); consult specific product labeling. [DSC] = Discontinued product

Cream, External, as hydrochloride:

Naftin: 1% (30 g [DSC], 60 g [DSC], 90 g [DSC]); 2% (45 g, 60 g) [contains benzyl alcohol, cetyl alcohol]

Generic: 1% (60 g, 90 g)

Gel, External, as hydrochloride:

Naftin: 1% (40 g, 60 g, 90 g) [contains alcohol, usp, edetate disodium, polysorbate 80]

Naftin: 2% (45 g, 60 g) [contains alcohol, usp, benzyl alcohol, edetate disodium, propylene glycol, trolamine (triethanolamine)]

◆ Naftifine Hydrochloride *see* Naftifine *on page 1247*

◆ Naftin *see* Naftifine *on page 1247*

◆ NaHCO$_3$ *see* Sodium Bicarbonate *on page 1669*

Nalbuphine (NAL byoo feen)

Brand Names: Canada Nubain
Index Terms Nalbuphine Hydrochloride; Nubain
Pharmacologic Category Analgesic, Opioid; Analgesic, Opioid Partial Agonist

Additional Appendix Information

Opioid Conversion Table and Morphine Equivalent Dose Table *on page 1955*

Use

Pain, moderate to severe: Relief of moderate to severe pain

Surgical anesthesia supplement: Supplement to balanced anesthesia, for preoperative and postoperative analgesia, and for obstetrical analgesia during labor and delivery

Pregnancy Considerations Adverse events were observed in some animal reproduction studies. Nalbuphine crosses the placenta. Nalbuphine is approved for use in obstetrical analgesia during labor and delivery. When used for pain relief during labor, opioids may temporarily affect the heart rate of the fetus (ACOG 2002) and severe fetal bradycardia has been reported following use of nalbuphine in labor/delivery. Fetal bradycardia may occur when administered earlier in pregnancy (not documented). Use only if clearly needed, with monitoring to detect and manage possible adverse fetal effects. Naloxone has been reported to reverse bradycardia. Newborn should be monitored for respiratory depression or bradycardia following nalbuphine use in labor.

If chronic opioid exposure occurs in pregnancy, adverse events in the newborn (including withdrawal) may occur; monitoring of the neonate is recommended. The minimum effective dose should be used if opioids are needed (Chou 2009). Neonatal abstinence syndrome following opioid exposure may present with autonomic (eg, fever, temperature instability), gastrointestinal (eg, diarrhea, vomiting, poor feeding/weight gain), or neurologic (eg, high-pitched crying, increased muscle tone, irritability, seizure, tremor) symptoms (Dow 2012; Hudak 2012).

Breast-Feeding Considerations Small amounts (<1% of maternal dose) of nalbuphine are excreted in breast milk. The manufacturer recommends that caution be exercised when administering nalbuphine to nursing women.

Parenteral opioids used during labor have the potential to interfere with a newborns natural reflex to nurse within the first few hours after birth. If nalbuphine is administered to a nursing woman, it is recommended to monitor both the mother and baby for psychotomimetic reactions. Nursing infants exposed to large doses of opioids should also be monitored for apnea and sedation (Montgomery 2012).

Contraindications

Hypersensitivity to nalbuphine or any component of the formulation

Documentation of allergenic cross-reactivity for morphine and related drugs is limited. However, because of similarities in chemical structure and/or pharmacologic actions, the possibility of cross-sensitivity cannot be ruled out with certainty.

Warnings/Precautions Use caution in CNS depression. Sedation and psychomotor impairment are likely, and are additive with other CNS depressants or ethanol. May cause respiratory depression. Ambulatory patients must be cautioned about performing tasks which require mental alertness (eg, operating machinery or driving). Potentially significant drug interactions may exist, requiring dose or frequency adjustment, additional monitoring, and/or selection of alternative therapy. Use with caution in patients with recent myocardial infarction, biliary tract impairment, pancreatitis, morbid obesity, thyroid dysfunction, head trauma, or increased intracranial pressure. Avoid use in patients with CNS depression or coma as these patients are susceptible to intracranial effects of CO_2 retention. Use caution in patients with prostatic hyperplasia and/or urinary stricture, adrenal insufficiency, decreased hepatic or renal function. Use with caution and at low doses in patients with preexisting respiratory compromise (eg, hypoxia and/or hypercapnia, uremia, severe infection, concomitant medications, cyanosis, bronchial asthma), COPD or other obstructive pulmonary disease, and kyphoscoliosis or other skeletal disorder which may alter respiratory function; critical respiratory depression may occur, even at therapeutic dosages. Bradycardia has been reported in patients who did not receive atropine preoperatively. May cause hypotension; use with caution in patients with hypovolemia, or drugs which may exaggerate hypotensive effects (including phenothiazines or general anesthetics). Use with caution in patients with cardiovascular disease, including myocardial infarction patients who have nausea or vomiting. May obscure diagnosis or clinical course of patients with acute abdominal conditions. Use with caution in patients with a history of drug abuse, emotionally unstable patients, or acute alcoholism; potential for drug dependency exists. Tolerance, psychological, and physical dependence may occur with prolonged use. Abrupt discontinuation following prolonged use may lead to withdrawal symptoms. May precipitate withdrawal symptoms in patients following prolonged therapy with mu opioid agonists.

After chronic maternal exposure to opioids, neonatal withdrawal syndrome may occur in the newborn; monitor neonate closely. Signs and symptoms include irritability, hyperactivity and abnormal sleep pattern, high pitched cry, tremor, vomiting, diarrhea and failure to gain weight. Onset, duration and severity depend on the drug used, duration of use, maternal dose, and rate of drug elimination by the newborn. Opioid withdrawal syndrome in the neonate, unlike in adults, may be life-threatening and should be treated according to protocols developed by neonatology experts. Use with caution in the elderly and debilitated patients; may be more sensitive to adverse effects.

Adverse Reactions

>10%: Central nervous system: Sedation (36%)

1% to 10%:
Central nervous system: Dizziness (5%), headache (3%)
Dermatologic: Cold and clammy skin (9%)
Gastrointestinal: Nausea and vomiting (6%), xerostomia (4%)

<1% (Limited to important or life-threatening): Abdominal pain, abnormal dreams, agitation, anaphylactoid reaction, anaphylaxis, anxiety, asthma, bitter taste, blurred vision, bradycardia, burning sensation, cardiac arrest, confusion, crying, delusions, depersonalization, depression, derealization, diaphoresis, drowsiness, dyspepsia, dysphoria, euphoria, fever, floating feeling, flushing, hallucination, hostility, hypersensitivity reaction, hypertension, hypogonadism (Brennan, 2013; Debono, 2011), hypotension, injection site reaction (pain, swelling, redness, burning), intestinal cramps, laryngeal edema, loss of consciousness, nervousness, numbness, pruritus, pulmonary edema, respiratory depression, respiratory distress, restlessness, seizure, skin rash, speech disturbance, stridor, tachycardia, tingling sensation, tremor, urinary urgency, urticaria

Drug Interactions

Metabolism/Transport Effects None known.

Avoid Concomitant Use

Avoid concomitant use of Nalbuphine with any of the following: Analgesics (Opioid); Azelastine (Nasal); Buprenorphine; Eluxadoline; Orphenadrine; Paraldehyde; Thalidomide

Increased Effect/Toxicity

Nalbuphine may increase the levels/effects of: Alcohol (Ethyl); Alvimopan; Azelastine (Nasal); CNS Depressants; Desmopressin; Diuretics; Eluxadoline; Methotrimeprazine; Metyrosine; Mirtazapine; Orphenadrine; Paraldehyde; Pramipexole; Ramosetron; ROPINIRole; Rotigotine; Selective Serotonin Reuptake Inhibitors; Suvorexant; Thalidomide; Zolpidem

The levels/effects of Nalbuphine may be increased by: Amphetamines; Anticholinergic Agents; Antipsychotic Agents (Phenothiazines); Brimonidine (Topical); Cannabis; Doxylamine; Dronabinol; Droperidol; HydrOXYzine; Kava Kava; Magnesium Sulfate; Methotrimeprazine; Minocycline; Nabilone; Perampanel; Rufinamide; Sodium Oxybate; Succinylcholine; Tetrahydrocannabinol

Decreased Effect

Nalbuphine may decrease the levels/effects of: Analgesics (Opioid); Buprenorphine; Pegvisomant

The levels/effects of Nalbuphine may be decreased by: Ammonium Chloride; Naltrexone

Storage/Stability Store at 20°C to 25°C (68°F to 77°F). Store in original carton; protect from light.

Mechanism of Action Agonist of kappa opiate receptors and partial antagonist of mu opiate receptors in the CNS, causing inhibition of ascending pain pathways, altering the perception of and response to pain; produces generalized CNS depression

Pharmacodynamics/Kinetics

Onset of action: Peak effect: SubQ, IM: <15 minutes; IV: 2 to 3 minutes

Duration of action: 3 to 6 hours

Protein binding: ~50% (Jaillon 1989)

Metabolism: Hepatic; extensive first-pass metabolism (Errick 1983)

Half-life elimination:
Children: 0.9 to 3.5 hours; however, overall trend observed is longer half-life as age increases (Bressolle 2011; Jaillon 1989)
Adults: 5 hours

Excretion: Feces; urine (~7% eliminated as unchanged drug and metabolites) (Errick 1983)

Dosing

Adult

Pain, moderate to severe: IM, IV, SubQ: Based on a 70 kg individual, administer 10 mg every 3 to 6 hours as needed; Maximum dose in nonopioid dependent patients: Single dose: 20 mg; Daily dose: 160 mg

Surgical anesthesia supplement: IV:
US labeling: Induction: 0.3 to 3 mg/kg over 10 to 15 minutes; maintenance doses of 0.25 to 0.5 mg/kg may be given as required
Canadian labeling: Induction: 0.3 mg/kg to 5 mg/kg over 10 to 15 minutes; maintenance doses of 0.25 to 0.5 mg/kg may be given as required
Adjunctive therapy in regional anesthesia: 0.2 to 0.5 mg/kg/dose

Opioid-induced pruritus (off-label use): IV: 2.5 to 5 mg; may repeat dose (Cohen 1992; Charuluxananan 1999; Charuluxananan 2001; Charuluxananan 2003; Ganesh 2007)

Geriatric Refer to adult dosing; use with caution.

Pediatric Pain, moderate to severe (off-label use): Children ≥1 year and Adolescents: IM, IV, SubQ: 0.1 to 0.2 mg/kg every 3 to 4 hours as needed; higher single doses of 0.3 mg/kg have also been used; maximum single dose: 20 mg; maximum daily dose: 160 mg (Bhatt-Mehta 1991; Kliegman 2007)

Renal Impairment There are no specific dosage adjustments provided in the manufacturer's labeling; however, a reduced dose is recommended. Use with caution.

Hepatic Impairment There are no specific dosage adjustments provided in the manufacturer's labeling; however, a reduced dose is recommended. Use with caution.

Administration

IM, SubQ: Administer undiluted.

IV: Administer undiluted over at least 2 to 3 minutes; larger induction doses should be administered over 10 to 15 minutes (Nursing 2016)

Monitoring Parameters Relief of pain, respiratory and mental status, blood pressure; signs or symptoms of hypogonadism or hypoadrenalism (Brennan 2013)

Test Interactions May interfere with certain enzymatic methods used to detect opioids, depending on sensitivity and specificity of the test (refer to test manufacturer for details)

Dosage Forms Excipient information presented when available (limited, particularly for generics); consult specific product labeling.
Solution, Injection, as hydrochloride:
Generic: 10 mg/mL (1 mL, 10 mL); 20 mg/mL (1 mL, 10 mL)
Dosage Forms: Canada Excipient information presented when available (limited, particularly for generics); consult specific product labeling.
Solution, Injection, as hydrochloride:
Nubain: 10 mg/mL (1 mL); 20 mg/mL (1 mL)

♦ **Nalbuphine Hydrochloride** see Nalbuphine on page 1247

♦ **Nalfon** see Fenoprofen on page 750

♦ **Nallpen** see Nafcillin on page 1246

♦ **Nallpen in Dextrose** see Nafcillin on page 1246

♦ *N*-allylnoroxymorphine Hydrochloride see Naloxone on page 1250

Naloxegol (nal OX ee gol)

Brand Names: US Movantik
Index Terms Naloxegol Oxalate; NKTR-118
Pharmacologic Category Gastrointestinal Agent, Miscellaneous; Opioid Antagonist, Peripherally-Acting
Use Opioid-induced constipation: Treatment of opioid-induced constipation (OIC) in adult patients with chronic noncancer pain.
Pregnancy Considerations Adverse events were not observed in animal reproduction studies. However, exposure during pregnancy may potentiate opioid withdrawal in the fetus.
Breast-Feeding Considerations It is not known if naloxegol is excreted into breast milk. Due to the potential for serious adverse reactions (which could include opioid withdrawal in the nursing infant), the manufacturer recommends a decision be made whether to discontinue nursing or to discontinue the drug, taking into account the importance of treatment to the mother.
Contraindications Serious or severe hypersensitivity reaction to naloxegol or any component of the formulation; known or suspected GI obstruction or at increased risk of recurrent obstruction; concomitant use with strong CYP3A4 inhibitors (eg, clarithromycin, ketoconazole)
Warnings/Precautions GI perforation has been reported with use of another peripherally acting opioid antagonist (ie, methylnaltrexone) in patients with reduced wall integrity of the GI tract (eg, peptic ulcer disease, Ogilvie syndrome, diverticular disease, infiltrative gastrointestinal tract malignancies, peritoneal metastases). Consider the overall risk-benefit profile when using naloxegol in patients with these conditions or other conditions which might result in impaired integrity of the GI tract wall (eg, Crohn disease). Monitor for development of severe, persistent or worsening abdominal pain; discontinue naloxegol if this occurs. Use is contraindicated in patients with known or suspected GI obstruction or at increased risk of recurrent obstruction.

Symptoms consistent with opioid withdrawal (eg, hyperhidrosis, chills, abdominal pain, anxiety, irritability) have occurred. In clinical trials, patients receiving methadone for pain management were observed to have a higher frequency of GI adverse reactions that may have been related to opioid withdrawal than patients receiving other opioids. Patients having disruptions to the blood-brain barrier may be at increased risk for opioid withdrawal or reduced analgesia. Consider the overall risk-benefit profile when using naloxegol in such patients. Monitor for symptoms of opioid withdrawal in such patients.

Avoid use of naloxegol in patients with severe hepatic impairment (dosage has not been determined). No dosage adjustment is necessary for patients with mild or moderate hepatic impairment. Dosage reduction recommended for patients with CrCl <60 mL/minute (ie, moderate, severe, or end-stage renal disease). No dosage adjustment is necessary for patients with mild renal impairment. Potentially significant interactions may exist, requiring dose or frequency adjustment, additional monitoring, and/or selection of alternative therapy. Discontinue naloxegol if opioids are discontinued.

Adverse Reactions
>10%: Gastrointestinal: Abdominal pain (12% to 21%)
1% to 10%:
Central nervous system: Headache (4%)
Dermatologic: Hyperhidrosis (≤3%)
Gastrointestinal: Diarrhea (6% to 9%), nausea (7% to 8%), flatulence (3% to 6%), vomiting (5%)

<1% (Limited to important or life-threatening):Anxiety, arthritis, back pain, chills, gastrointestinal perforation, irritability, joint pain, yawning
Drug Interactions
Metabolism/Transport Effects Substrate of CYP3A4 (major), P-glycoprotein; **Note:** Assignment of Major/Minor substrate status based on clinically relevant drug interaction potential
Avoid Concomitant Use
Avoid concomitant use of Naloxegol with any of the following: Conivaptan; CYP3A4 Inducers (Strong); CYP3A4 Inhibitors (Moderate); CYP3A4 Inhibitors (Strong); Fusidic Acid (Systemic); Grapefruit Juice; Idelalisib; Methylnaltrexone; Opioid Antagonists; St Johns Wort
Increased Effect/Toxicity
The levels/effects of Naloxegol may be increased by: Conivaptan; CYP3A4 Inhibitors (Moderate); CYP3A4 Inhibitors (Strong); Dasatinib; Fosaprepitant; Fusidic Acid (Systemic); Grapefruit Juice; Idelalisib; Ivacaftor; Luliconazole; Methylnaltrexone; Opioid Antagonists; Osimertinib; Palbociclib; P-glycoprotein/ABCB1 Inhibitors; Ranolazine; Simeprevir; Stiripentol
Decreased Effect
The levels/effects of Naloxegol may be decreased by: Bosentan; CYP3A4 Inducers (Moderate); CYP3A4 Inducers (Strong); Dabrafenib; Deferasirox; Osimertinib; P-glycoprotein/ABCB1 Inducers; Siltuximab; St Johns Wort; Tocilizumab
Storage/Stability Store at 20°C to 25°C (68°F to 77°F); excursions are permitted between 15°C and 30°C (59°F and 86°F).
Mechanism of Action Naloxegol is a mu-opioid receptor antagonist. It is composed of naloxone conjugated with a polyethylene glycol polymer, which limits its ability to cross the blood-brain barrier. When administered at the recommended dose, naloxegol functions peripherally in tissues such as the GI tract, thereby decreasing the constipation associated with opioids (Webster, 2013).
Pharmacodynamics/Kinetics
Absorption: Rapid. With a high-fat meal, C_{max} and AUC increased by 30% and 45%, respectively.
Distribution: V_d: 968 to 2,140 L
Protein binding: ~4.2%
Metabolism: Hepatic via CYP3A (primarily). Data suggests no major metabolites. Minor metabolites formed via N-dealkylation, O-demethylation, oxidation and partial loss of the PEG chain.
Half-life elimination: 6 to 11 hours
Time to peak: <2 hours; in majority of subjects, a secondary C_{max} occurs ~0.4 to 3 hours after the first C_{max}
Excretion: Feces (68%; ~16% as unchanged drug); Urine (16%; <6% as unchanged drug)
Dosing
Adult Note: Discontinue all maintenance laxative therapy prior to use; may reintroduce laxatives as needed if suboptimal response to naloxegol after 3 days. Alteration in analgesic dosing regimen prior to initiating naloxegol is not required.

Opioid-induced constipation: Oral: 25 mg once daily in the morning on an empty stomach. If not tolerated, reduce dose to 12.5 mg once daily. Discontinue treatment if opioid pain medication is discontinued.

Dosing adjustment with concomitant medications:
Moderate CYP3A4 Inhibitors (eg, diltiazem, erythromycin, verapamil): Avoid concomitant use. If concurrent use is unavoidable, reduce dose of naloxegol to 12.5 mg once daily and monitor for adverse reactions.
Strong CYP3A4 inhibitors (eg, clarithromycin, ketoconazole): Concomitant use is contraindicated.
Renal Impairment
CrCl ≥60 mL/minute: No dosage adjustment necessary.
CrCl <60 mL/minute: Initial dose 12.5 mg once daily; if well tolerated but opioid-induced constipation symptoms continue, may increase to 25 mg once daily, taking into consideration the potential for markedly increased exposures in some patients with renal impairment and the increased risk of adverse reactions with higher exposures.
Hepatic Impairment
Mild to moderate impairment: No dosage adjustment necessary.
Severe impairment: Avoid use (has not been studied).
Dietary Considerations Take on an empty stomach. Avoid grapefruit or grapefruit juice.
Administration Oral: Administer naloxegol on an empty stomach at least 1 hour prior to or 2 hours after the first meal of the day. Swallow tablets whole, do not crush or chew. Avoid consumption of grapefruit or grapefruit juice during treatment.

◄ **Monitoring Parameters** Symptoms of GI obstruction (eg, severe, persistent, or worsening abdominal pain); symptoms of opioid withdrawal (eg, chills, diaphoresis, anxiety, irritability, changes in blood pressure or heart rate).

Dosage Forms Excipient information presented when available (limited, particularly for generics); consult specific product labeling.

Tablet, Oral:

Movantik: 12.5 mg, 25 mg

◆ **Naloxegol Oxalate** see Naloxegol on page 1249

Naloxone (nal OKS one)

Brand Names: US Evzio; Narcan

Brand Names: Canada Naloxone Hydrochloride Injection; Naloxone Hydrochloride Injection USP

Index Terms *N*-allylnoroxymorphine Hydrochloride; Naloxone Hydrochloride; Narcan

Pharmacologic Category Antidote; Opioid Antagonist

Use

Opioid overdose: For the complete or partial reversal of opioid depression (including respiratory depression) induced by natural and synthetic opioids (eg, propoxyphene, methadone, nalbuphine, butorphanol, pentazocine). Naloxone is also indicated for the diagnosis of suspected or known acute opioid overdosage.

Evzio (IM, SubQ), Narcan Nasal Spray (intranasal): For the emergency treatment of known or suspected opioid overdose as manifested by respiratory and/or CNS depression. Intended for immediate administration as emergency therapy in settings where opioids may be present. Not a substitute for emergency medical care.

Septic shock: For use as an adjunctive agent to increase blood pressure in the management of septic shock. **Note:** Naloxone is no longer a recommended adjunctive agent for the treatment of septic shock (SCCM [Dellinger 2013]).

Pregnancy Considerations Adverse events were not observed in animal reproduction studies. Naloxone crosses the placenta. Consider the benefit to the mother and the risk to the fetus before administering to a pregnant woman who is known or suspected to be opioid dependent; may precipitate withdrawal in both the mother and fetus. In general, medications used as antidotes should take into consideration the health and prognosis of the mother; antidotes should be administered to pregnant women if there is a clear indication for use and should not be withheld because of fears of teratogenicity (Bailey 2003). Use caution in pregnant women with mild-to-moderate hypertension during labor; severe hypertension may occur.

Breast-Feeding Considerations It is not known if naloxone is excreted into breast milk, however, systemic absorption following oral administration is low (Smith 2012) and any exposure of naloxone to a nursing infant would therefore be limited. Since naloxone is used for opioid reversal, the opioid concentrations in the milk of a breast-feeding mother and potential transfer of the opioid to the infant should be considered.

Contraindications Hypersensitivity to naloxone or any component of the formulation

Warnings/Precautions Use with caution in patients with cardiovascular disease or in patients receiving medications with potential adverse cardiovascular effects (eg, hypotension, pulmonary edema, or arrhythmias); pulmonary edema and cardiovascular instability, including ventricular fibrillation, have been reported in association with abrupt reversal when using opioid antagonists. Administration of naloxone causes the release of catecholamines, which may precipitate acute withdrawal or unmask pain in those who regularly take opioids. Symptoms of acute withdrawal in opioid-dependent patients may include pain, tachycardia, hypertension, fever, sweating, abdominal cramps, diarrhea, nausea, vomiting, agitation, and irritability. In neonates born to mothers with narcotic dependence, opioid withdrawal may be life-threatening and symptoms may include shrill cry, failure to feed, seizures, and hyperactive reflexes. In settings other than acute opioid overdose (eg, postoperative patients), carefully titrate the dose to reverse hypoventilation; do not fully awaken patient or reverse analgesic effect (postoperative patient). Excessive dosages should be avoided after use of opioids in surgery. Abrupt postoperative reversal may result in nausea, vomiting, sweating, tachycardia, hypertension, seizures, and other cardiovascular events (including pulmonary edema and arrhythmias). Reversal of partial opioid agonists or mixed opioid agonist/antagonists (eg, buprenorphine, pentazocine) may be incomplete and larger or repeat doses of naloxone may be required. Recurrence of respiratory and/or CNS depression is possible if the opioid involved is long-acting; continuously observe patients until there is no further risk of recurrent respiratory or CNS depression.

To prevent overdose deaths, there are initiatives to dispense naloxone for self- or buddy-administration to patients at risk of opioid overdose (eg, recipients of high-dose opioids, suspected or confirmed history of illicit opioid use) and individuals likely to be present in an overdose situation (eg, family members of illicit drug users) (Albert 2011; Bennett 2011); Evzio and Narcan Nasal Spray are approved for out-of-hospital emergency treatment. Needleless administration via nebulization and the intranasal route using the injectable solution (with a mucosal atomization device) by first responders and bystanders has also been described (Doe-Simkins 2009; Weber 2012). Needleless administration provides an alternative route of administration in patients with venous scarring due to illicit drug use (eg, heroin). There is a low incidence of death following naloxone reversal of opioid toxicity in patients who refuse transport to a healthcare facility (Wampler 2011). Nevertheless, patients who received naloxone in the out-of-hospital setting should seek immediate emergency medical assistance after the first dose due to the likelihood that respiratory and/or central nervous system depression will return.

When the auto-injector (Evzio) is administered to infants <1 year of age, monitor the injection site for residual needle parts and signs of infection.

Adverse Reactions Adverse reactions are related to reversing dependency and precipitating withdrawal. Withdrawal symptoms are the result of sympathetic excess. Adverse events occur secondarily to reversal (withdrawal) of opioid analgesia and sedation.

Cardiovascular: Cardiac arrest, fever, flushing, hypertension, hypotension, tachycardia, ventricular fibrillation ventricular tachycardia

Central nervous system: Agitation, coma, crying (excessive [neonates]), encephalopathy, hallucination, irritability, nervousness, restlessness, seizure (neonates), tremulousness

Gastrointestinal: Abdominal cramps, diarrhea, nausea, vomiting

Local: Injection site reaction

Neuromuscular & skeletal: Ache, hyperreflexia (neonates), paresthesia, piloerection, tremor, weakness

Respiratory: Dyspnea, hypoxia, pulmonary edema, respiratory depression, rhinorrhea, sneezing

Miscellaneous: Diaphoresis, hot flashes, shivering, yawning

Drug Interactions

Metabolism/Transport Effects None known.

Avoid Concomitant Use

Avoid concomitant use of Naloxone with any of the following: Methylnaltrexone; Naloxegol

Increased Effect/Toxicity

Naloxone may increase the levels/effects of: Naloxegol

The levels/effects of Naloxone may be increased by: Methylnaltrexone

Decreased Effect There are no known significant interactions involving a decrease in effect.

Preparation for Administration

IV push: Dilute naloxone 0.4 mg (1 mL ampul) with 9 mL of NS for a total volume of 10 mL to achieve a concentration of 0.04 mg/mL (APS 2008)

IV infusion: Dilute naloxone 2 mg in 500 mL of NS or D$_5$W to make a final concentration of 4 **mcg**/mL

Inhalation via nebulization (off-label route): Dilute 2 mg of naloxone with 3 mL of normal saline (Mycyk 2003; Weber 2012)

Storage/Stability

Solution, injection: Store at 20°C to 25°C (68°F to 77°F). Protect from light. Use IV infusion within 24 hours of preparation.

Solution, auto-injector (Evzio): Store at 15°C to 25°C (59°F to 77°F); excursions are permitted between 4°C and 40°C (39°F and 104°F). Store in the outer case provided.

Solution, nasal spray (Narcan Nasal Spray): Store at 15°C to 25°C (59°F to 77°F); excursions are permitted between 4°C and 40°C (39°F and 104°F). Do not freeze. Protect from light.

Mechanism of Action Pure opioid antagonist that competes and displaces opioids at opioid receptor sites

Pharmacodynamics/Kinetics

Onset of action: Endotracheal, IM, SubQ: 2 to 5 minutes; Inhalation via nebulization: ~5 minutes (Mycyk 2003); Intranasal: ~8 to 13 minutes (Kelley 2005; Robertson 2009); IV: ~2 minutes

Duration: ~30 to 120 minutes depending on route of administration; IV has a shorter duration of action than IM administration; since naloxone's action is shorter than that of most opioids, repeated doses are usually needed

Protein binding: Relatively weak (to albumin [major] and other plasma constituents)

Metabolism: Primarily hepatic via glucuronidation

Bioavailability: Intranasal: 44% to 47% (compared to 0.4 mg IM dose)

Time to peak: IM, SubQ (Evzio): 15 minutes; Intranasal (Narcan Nasal Spray): 19.8 to 30 minutes

Half-life elimination: Neonates: Mean 3.1 ± 0.5 hours; Adults: IM, IV, or SubQ: 0.5 to 1.5 hours; Intranasal: ~2 hours

Excretion: Urine (as metabolites)

Dosing

Adult & Geriatric Note: Available routes of administration include IV (preferred), IM, SubQ, and intranasal; other available routes (off-label) include inhalation via nebulization (adults only), and intraosseous (IO). Endotracheal administration is the least desirable and is supported by only anecdotal evidence (case report) (AHA [Neumar 2010]):

Opioid overdose:

Note: For the initial treatment of an opioid-associated life-threatening emergency, the American Heart Association recommends, after initiation of CPR, the use of intranasal or IM naloxone with a repeat dose as needed. If there is an initial patient response (ie, purposeful movement, regular breathing, moan or other response) but the patient then stops responding, begin CPR and repeat naloxone dose. If no initial response, continue CPR and use AED as appropriate (AHA [Lavonas 2015]).

IV, IM, SubQ: Initial: 0.4 to 2 mg; may need to repeat doses every 2 to 3 minutes; after reversal, may need to readminister dose(s) at a later interval (ie, 20 to 60 minutes) depending on type/duration of opioid. If no response is observed after 10 mg total, consider other causes of respiratory depression. **Note:** May be given endotracheally (off-label route) as 2 to 2.5 times the initial IV dose (ie, 0.8 to 5 mg) (AHA [Neumar 2010]).

Continuous infusion (off-label dosing): IV: **Note:** For use with exposures to long-acting opioids (eg, methadone), sustained release product, and symptomatic body packers after initial naloxone response. Calculate dosage/hour based on effective intermittent dose used and duration of adequate response seen (Tenenbein 1984) **or** use two-thirds (2/3) of the initial effective naloxone bolus on an hourly basis (typically 0.25 to 6.25 mg/hour); one-half (1/2) of the initial bolus dose should be readministered 15 minutes after initiation of the continuous infusion to prevent a drop in naloxone levels; adjust infusion rate as needed to assure adequate ventilation and prevent withdrawal symptoms (Goldfrank 1986).

IM, SubQ: Evzio: 0.4 mg (contents of 1 auto-injector) as a single dose; may repeat every 2 to 3 minutes until emergency medical assistance becomes available.

Inhalation via nebulization (off-label route): 2 mg; may repeat. Switch to IV or IM administration when possible (Weber 2012). **Note:** This administration method is not included in the AHA recommendations for initial management of opioid-associated life-threatening emergency (AHA [Lavonas 2015]).

Intranasal: **Note:** Onset of action is slightly delayed compared to IM or IV routes (Kelly 2005; Robertson 2009)

Narcan Nasal Spray: 4 mg (contents of 1 nasal spray) as a single dose; may repeat every 2 to 3 minutes in alternating nostrils until medical assistance becomes available.

Off label dosing: 2 mg (1 mg per nostril) using generic injectable solution (with a mucosal atomization device); may repeat in 3 to 5 minutes if respiratory depression persists (AHA [Lavonas 2015]; AHA [Vanden Hoek 2010]; Kelly 2005; Robertson 2009; Walley 2013).

Reversal of respiratory depression with therapeutic opioid doses: IV, IM, SubQ.: Initial: 0.04 to 0.4 mg; may repeat until desired response achieved. If desired response is not observed after 0.8 mg total, consider other causes of respiratory depression. **Note:** May be given endotracheally (off-label route) as 2 to 2.5 times the initial IV dose (ie, 0.08 to 1 mg) (AHA [Neumar 2010]).

Continuous infusion (off-label dosing): IV: **Note:** For use with exposures to long-acting opioids (eg, methadone) or sustained release products. Calculate dosage/hour based on effective intermittent dose used and duration of adequate response seen (Tenenbein 1984) **or** use two-thirds (2/3) of the initial effective naloxone bolus on an hourly basis (typically 0.2 to 0.6 mg/hour); one-half (1/2) of the initial bolus dose should be readministered 15 minutes after initiation of the continuous infusion to prevent a drop in naloxone levels; adjust infusion rate

as needed to assure adequate ventilation and prevent withdrawal symptoms (Goldfrank 1986).

Opioid-dependent patients being treated for cancer pain (NCCN guidelines, v.2.2011): IV: 0.04 to 0.08 mg (40 to 80 **mcg**) slow IV push; administer every 30 to 60 seconds until improvement in symptoms; if no response is observed after total naloxone dose 1 mg, consider other causes of respiratory depression. **Note:** May dilute 0.4 mg/mL (1 mL) ampul into 9 mL of normal saline for a total volume of 10 mL to achieve a 0.04 mg/mL (40 **mcg**/mL) concentration.

Postoperative reversal: IV: 0.1 to 0.2 mg every 2 to 3 minutes until desired response (adequate ventilation and alertness without significant pain). **Note:** Repeat doses may be needed within 1 to 2 hour intervals depending on type, dose, and timing of the last dose of opioid administered.

Opioid-induced pruritus (off-label use): IV infusion: 0.25 **mcg/kg/hour**; **Note:** Monitor pain control; verify that the naloxone is not reversing analgesia (Gan 1997).

Pediatric Note: IV (preferred), IM, SubQ, intranasal, intraosseous (IO) (off-label), and endotracheal (off-label) routes may be used. Endotracheal administration is the least desirable and is supported by only anecdotal evidence (case report) (AHA [Neumar 2010]).

Opioid overdose:

Neonates, Infants, Children, and Adolescents: IV, IM, SubQ, IO (off-label route), endotracheal (off-label route): **Note:** IV administration is preferred; IO and endotracheal routes are alternative routes recommended by the PALS guidelines (AHA [Kleinman 2010]): The use of naloxone is **not** recommended as part of initial resuscitative efforts in the delivery room for neonates with respiratory depression; support ventilation to improve oxygenation and heart rate (AHA [Kattwinkel 2010]):

<5 years or ≤20 kg (off-label dose): 0.1 mg/kg/dose (maximum dose: 2 mg); repeat every 2 to 3 minutes if needed (AHA [Kleinman 2010]; Hegenbarth 2008)

≥5 years or >20 kg: 2 mg; if no response, repeat every 2 to 3 minutes. If no response is observed after 10 mg total, consider other causes of respiratory depression (AHA [Kleinman 2010]; Hegenbarth 2008).

Manufacturer's labeling: IV (preferred), IM, SubQ: Initial: 0.01 mg/kg/dose; if no response, a subsequent dose of 0.1 mg/kg may be given; **Note:** if using IM or SubQ route, dose should be given in divided doses.

Continuous infusion (off-label dosing): IV: If continuous infusion is required, calculate dosage/hour based on effective intermittent dose used and duration of adequate response seen (Tenenbein 1984) **or** use two-thirds (2/3) of the initial effective naloxone bolus on an hourly basis; titrate dose (typically 0.04 to 0.16 mg/hour for 2 to 5 days in children); one-half (1/2) of the initial bolus dose should be readministered 15 minutes after initiation of the continuous infusion to prevent a drop in naloxone levels; increase infusion rate as needed to assure adequate ventilation and prevent withdrawal symptoms (Goldfrank 1986). **Note:** The infusion should be discontinued by reducing the infusion in decrements of 25%; closely monitor the patient (eg, pulse oximetry) after each adjustment and after discontinuation of the infusion for recurrence of opioid-induced respiratory depression (Perry 1996).

IM, SubQ: Evzio: 0.4 mg (contents of 1 auto-injector) as a single dose; may repeat every 2 to 3 minutes until emergency medical assistance becomes available.

Infants, Children, and Adolescents: Intranasal: Narcan Nasal Spray: 4 mg (contents of 1 nasal spray) as a single dose; may repeat every 2 to 3 minutes in alternating nostrils until medical assistance becomes available. **Note:** Onset of action is slightly delayed compared to IM or IV routes (Kelly 2005; Robertson 2009). In neonates with known or suspected exposure to maternal opioid use, consider using another form of naloxone to allow dosing according to weight and titration to effect.

Reversal of respiratory depression with therapeutic opioid dosing: Infants, Children, and Adolescents: IV: 0.001 to 0.015 mg/kg/dose; dose may be repeated as needed (AHA [Kleinman 2010]; Hegenbarth 2008)

Postoperative reversal: IV: 0.005 to 0.01 mg/kg (Fischer 1974); may repeat every 2 to 3 minutes as needed based on response (adequate ventilation without significant pain)

Renal Impairment There are no dosage adjustments provided in the manufacturer's labeling.

Hepatic Impairment There are no dosage adjustments provided in the manufacturer's labeling.

Administration

IV push: Administer over 30 seconds as undiluted preparation **or** administer as diluted preparation slow IV push by diluting 0.4 mg (1 mL) ampul with 9 mL of normal saline for a total volume of 10 mL to achieve a concentration of 0.04 mg/mL (APS 2008)

IV continuous infusion: Dilute to 4 **mcg**/mL in D$_5$W or normal saline

IM, SubQ: May administer IM or SubQ if unable to obtain IV access

Auto-injector: Evzio: For IM or SubQ use only. Intended for buddy administration; the person administering the medication should follow the printed instructions on the device or the electronic voice instructions coming from the speaker on the device. If the voice instruction system does not operate properly, the device will still deliver the intended dose of naloxone when properly administered. Administer IM or SubQ into the anterolateral aspect of the thigh; may be injected through clothing. When being administered to infants <1 year of age, the thigh muscle should be pinched during administration. Following proper administration, a red indicator appears in the viewing window; the needle is not visible before, during, or after the injection. Patients who received naloxone in the out-of-hospital setting should seek immediate emergency medical assistance after the first dose due to the likelihood that respiratory and/or central nervous system depression will return. Repeat doses may be required until emergency medical assistance becomes available; a new device must be used as each device contains a single dose of naloxone.

Endotracheal (off-label route): There is only anecdotal support for this route of administration. May require a slightly higher dose than used in other routes. Dilute to 1 to 2 mL with normal saline; flush with 5 mL of saline and then administer 5 ventilations (AHA [Neumar 2010]).

Inhalation via nebulization (off-label route): Dilute 2 mg of naloxone with 3 mL of normal saline and administer via nebulizer face mask (Mycyk 2003; Weber 2012).

Intranasal:

Narcan Nasal Spray: Administer initial dose as soon as possible. Do not prime or test the device prior to administration. Administer in alternating nostrils with each dose. Place the patient in the supine position and provide support to the back of the neck to allow the head to tilt back. Following administration, turn the patient on their side. Each container contains a single intranasal spray, do not reuse; if repeat administration is necessary a new container must be used.

Alternate intranasal administration instructions using generic injectable solution: Administer total dose equally divided into each nostril using a mucosal atomization device (MAD) (AHA [Vanden Hoek 2010]; Kelly 2005; Robertson 2009). If a MAD is not available, the solution may be sprayed into the nares without a MAD; however, a significant amount of drug may be lost likely due to swallowing and subsequent first-pass metabolism (Dowling 2008; Robinson 2014).

Monitoring Parameters Respiratory rate, heart rate, blood pressure, temperature, level of consciousness, ABGs or pulse oximetry

Additional Information May contain methyl and propylparabens

Product Availability Naloxone (nasal spray): Narcan: FDA approved November 2015; availability anticipated early 2016. Consult prescribing information for additional information.

Dosage Forms Excipient information presented when available (limited, particularly for generics); consult specific product labeling. [DSC] = Discontinued product

Liquid, Nasal:

Narcan: 4 mg/0.1 mL (1 ea) [contains benzalkonium chloride, edetate disodium]

Solution, Injection, as hydrochloride:

Generic: 0.4 mg/mL (1 mL, 10 mL); 1 mg/mL (2 mL [DSC])

Solution, Injection, as hydrochloride [preservative free]:

Generic: 1 mg/mL (2 mL)

Solution Auto-injector, Injection, as hydrochloride:

Evzio: 0.4 mg/0.4 mL (0.4 mL)

◆ Naloxone and Buprenorphine *see* Buprenorphine and Naloxone *on page 267*

◆ Naloxone and Oxycodone *see* Oxycodone and Naloxone *on page 1362*

◆ Naloxone Hydrochloride *see* Naloxone *on page 1250*

◆ Naloxone Hydrochloride Dihydrate and Buprenorphine Hydrochloride *see* Buprenorphine and Naloxone *on page 267*

◆ Naloxone Hydrochloride Injection (Can) *see* Naloxone *on page 1250*

◆ Naloxone Hydrochloride Injection USP (Can) *see* Naloxone *on page 1250*

Naltrexone (nal TREKS one)

Brand Names: US ReVia; Vivitrol

Brand Names: Canada ReVia

Index Terms Naltrexone Hydrochloride

Pharmacologic Category Antidote; Opioid Antagonist

Use

Alcohol dependence: Treatment of alcohol dependence.

Opioid dependence: For the blockade of the effects of exogenously administered opioids.

Pregnancy Considerations Adverse events were observed in animal reproduction studies. Information related to the use of naltrexone during pregnancy is limited (Farid 2008).

Breast-Feeding Considerations Naltrexone is excreted into breast milk. Due to the potential for serious adverse reactions in the nursing infant, the manufacturer recommends a decision be made whether to discontinue nursing or to discontinue the drug, taking into account the importance of treatment to the mother.

Medication Guide Available Yes

Contraindications Hypersensitivity to naltrexone or any component of the formulation; opioid dependence or current use of opioid analgesics (including partial opioid agonists); acute opioid withdrawal; failure to pass naloxone challenge or positive urine screen for opioids

Warnings/Precautions Dose-related hepatocellular injury is possible; the margin of separation between the apparent safe and hepatotoxic doses appears to be ≤5-fold. Discontinue therapy if signs/symptoms of acute hepatitis develop. Clinicians should note that elevated transaminases may be a result of preexisting alcoholic liver disease, hepatitis B and/or C infection, or concomitant use of other hepatotoxic drugs; abrupt opioid withdrawal may also lead to acute liver injury. Therapy may precipitate withdrawal symptoms in patients addicted to opioids; patients should be opioid-free (including tramadol) for a minimum of 7-10 days; a naloxone challenge test may help to confirm patient is opioid-free prior to therapy if there is any suspicion since urinary opioid screen may not be sufficient proof. Patients transitioning from buprenorphine or methadone may be vulnerable to precipitation of withdrawal symptoms for as long as 2 weeks. Use of naltrexone does not eliminate or diminish withdrawal symptoms. Patients who had been treated with naltrexone may respond to lower opioid doses than previously used. This could result in potentially life-threatening opioid intoxication. Patients should be aware that they may be more sensitive to lower doses of opioids after naltrexone treatment is discontinued, after a missed dose, or near the end of the dosing interval. Warn patients that any attempt to overcome opioid blockade during naltrexone therapy, could potentially lead to fatal opioid overdose; the opioid competitive receptor blockade produced by naltrexone is potentially surmountable in the presence of large amounts of opioids. In naltrexone-treated patients requiring emergency pain management, consider alternatives to opioid therapy (eg, regional analgesia, nonopioid analgesics, general anesthesia). If opioid therapy is required for pain therapy, patients should be under the direct care of a trained anesthesia provider.

Suicidal thoughts, attempted suicide, and depression have been reported postmarketing; monitor closely. Hypersensitivity, including anaphylaxis, has been reported. Cases of eosinophilic pneumonia have been reported and should be considered in patients presenting with progressive hypoxia and dyspnea. Use with caution in patients with severe hepatic impairment (has not been studied; if coagulopathy presents, IM injection may cause hematoma formation). Use with caution in patients with moderate-to-severe renal impairment (has not been studied). Use IM injection with caution in patients with thrombocytopenia or any bleeding disorder (hemophilia and severe hepatic failure), and patients on anticoagulant therapy; bleeding/hematoma may occur from IM administration. Serious injection site reactions (eg, cellulitis, induration, hematoma, abscess, necrosis) have been reported with use, including severe cases requiring surgical debridement. Females appear to be at a higher risk. Patients should report any injection site pain, swelling, bruising, pruritus, or redness that does not improve (or worsens). For IM use only in the gluteal muscle; do **not** administer IV, SubQ, or into fatty tissue;

incorrect administration may increase the risk of injection site reactions. Vehicle used in the injectable naltrexone formulation (polylactide-co-glycolide microspheres) has rarely been associated with retinal artery occlusion in patients with abnormal arteriovenous anastomosis following injection of other drug products that also use the polylactide-co-glycolide microspheres vehicle.

Adverse Reactions Combined reporting of adverse events from oral and injectable formulations:

>10%:

Cardiovascular: Syncope (13%)

Central nervous system: Headache (3% to 25%), insomnia (3% to 14%), dizziness (4% to 13%), anxiety (2% to 12%), decreased energy (>10%), nervousness (4% to >10%)

Gastrointestinal: Nausea (10% to 33%), vomiting (3% to 14%), appetite decreased (14%), diarrhea (13%), abdominal pain (11%), abdominal cramping

Hepatic: ALT increased (13%)

Local: Injection site reaction (≤69%; includes bruising, induration, nodules, pain, pruritus, swelling, tenderness)

Neuromuscular & skeletal: CPK increased (11% to 39%), arthralgia (12%), myalgia (>10%)

Respiratory: Pharyngitis (7% to 11%)

1% to 10%:

Cardiovascular: Hypertension (5%)

Central nervous system: Suicidal ideation (≤10%), depression (8%), somnolence (2% to 4%), fatigue (4%), chills, energy increased, feeling down, irritability

Dermatologic: Skin rash (6% to 10%)

Endocrine & metabolic: Increased thirst, polydipsia

Gastrointestinal: Dry mouth (5%), toothache (4%), constipation

Genitourinary: Delayed ejaculation (<10%), impotency (<10%)

Hepatic: AST increased (2% to 10%), GGT increased (7%)

Neuromuscular & skeletal: Muscle cramps (8%), back pain (6%)

Miscellaneous: Influenza (5%)

<1% (Limited to important or life-threatening): Abnormality in thinking, acne vulgaris, alopecia, angina, anorexia, atrial fibrillation, blood pressure increased, cerebral aneurysm, chest tightness, cholecystitis, colitis, COPD, dehydration, delirium, depression, DVT, dysuria, ECG changes, edema, eosinophilia (transient), eosinophilic pneumonia, epistaxis, GI hemorrhage, hemorrhoids, hepatic insufficiency, hepatitis, HF, hypercholesterolemia, hyperkinesia, hypersensitivity reaction (includes anaphylaxis, angioedema, and urticaria), ischemic stroke, leukocytosis, lymphadenopathy, MI, opioid withdrawal, palpitation, pancreatitis, paralytic ileus, paranoia, PE, perirectal abscess, photophobia, pneumonia, rhinorrhea, rigors, seizure, shortness of breath, swelling of eye, tachycardia, thrombocytopenia, ulcer

Drug Interactions

Metabolism/Transport Effects None known.

Avoid Concomitant Use

Avoid concomitant use of Naltrexone with any of the following: Methylnaltrexone; Naloxegol

Increased Effect/Toxicity

Naltrexone may increase the levels/effects of: Naloxegol

The levels/effects of Naltrexone may be increased by: Methylnaltrexone

Decreased Effect

Naltrexone may decrease the levels/effects of: Analgesics (Opioid)

Preparation for Administration Injection: Prior to reconstitution, allow drug vial and provided diluent to reach room temperature (~45 minutes). Using the provided 1-inch *preparation* needle, reconstitute with 3.4 mL of the diluent and allow to dissolve by vigorously shaking the vial for ~1 minute. Mixed suspension will be milky white, free of clumps, and will move freely down the walls of the vial. Immediately after suspension, withdraw 4.2 mL of the suspension using the same preparation needle.

Prior to administration, replace the preparation needle with the appropriate size provided *administration* needle (use the 2-inch needle with the needle protection device for patients with a larger amount of subcutaneous tissue overlying the gluteal muscle; for very lean patients, the 1.5-inch needle may be appropriate; either needle may be used for patients with average body habitus). Prior to injection, remove any air bubbles and push on the plunger until 4 mL of the suspension remains in the syringe. Following reconstitution of the suspension, administer immediately.

Storage/Stability

Injection: Store unopened kit at 2°C to 8°C (36°F to 46°F). Kit may be kept at room temperature of ≤25°C (77°F) for ≤7 days prior to use; do not freeze. Following reconstitution of the suspension, administer immediately.

Tablet: Store at 20°C to 25°C (68°F to 77°F).

Mechanism of Action Naltrexone (a pure opioid antagonist) is a cyclopropyl derivative of oxymorphone similar in structure to naloxone and nalorphine (a morphine derivative); it acts as a competitive antagonist at opioid receptor sites, showing the highest affinity for mu receptors.

Pharmacodynamics/Kinetics

Duration: Oral: 50 mg: 24 hours; 100 mg: 48 hours; 150 mg: 72 hours; IM: 4 weeks

Absorption: Oral: Almost complete

Distribution: V_d: ~1350 L; widely throughout the body but considerable interindividual variation exists

Metabolism: Extensively metabolized via noncytochrome-mediated dehydrogenase conversion to 6-beta-naltrexol (primary metabolite) and related minor metabolites; glucuronide conjugates are also formed from naltrexone and its metabolites

Oral: Extensive first-pass effect

Protein binding: 21%

Bioavailability: Oral: Variable range (5% to 40%)

Half-life elimination: Oral: 4 hours; 6-beta-naltrexol: 13 hours; IM: naltrexone and 6-beta-naltrexol: 5-10 days (dependent upon erosion of polymer)

Time to peak, serum: Oral: ~60 minutes; IM: Biphasic: ~2 hours (first peak), ~2-3 days (second peak)

Excretion: Primarily urine (as metabolites and small amounts of unchanged drug)

Dosing

Adult & Geriatric Note: Do not initiate therapy until patient is opioid-free (including tramadol) for at least 7-10 days as determined by urinalysis; consider naloxone challenge test to confirm patient is opioid-free if there is any suspicion since urinary opioid screen may not be sufficient proof.

Alcohol dependence:

Oral: 50 mg daily; alternative maintenance regimens may be used and include: 50 mg on weekdays with a 100 mg dose on Saturday; 100 mg every other day; or 150 mg every 3 days (degree of blockade may be reduced with extended dosing interval regimens and doses >50 mg may increase risk of hepatocellular injury)

IM: 380 mg once every 4 weeks

Opioid dependence:

Oral: Initial: 25 mg; if no withdrawal signs occur, administer 50 mg/day thereafter; alternative maintenance regimens may be used and include: 50 mg on weekdays with a 100 mg dose on Saturday; 100 mg every other day; or 150 mg every 3 days (degree of blockade may be reduced with extended dosing interval regimens and doses >50 mg may increase risk of hepatocellular injury)

IM: 380 mg once every 4 weeks

Renal Impairment

Mild impairment: No dosage adjustment necessary.

Moderate-to-severe impairment: No dosage adjustment provided in manufacturer's labeling (has not been studied); use with caution since naltrexone and its primary metabolite are primarily excreted in urine.

Hepatic Impairment

Mild-to-moderate impairment: No dosage adjustment necessary.

Severe impairment: No dosage adjustment provided in manufacturer's labeling (has not been studied); naltrexone AUC increased ~5- and 10-fold in patients with compensated or decompensated hepatic cirrhosis respectively.

Administration

Oral: May be administered with or without food. Administration with food or after meals may minimize adverse gastrointestinal effects. Advise patient not to self-administer opioids while receiving naltrexone therapy.

IM: Vivitrol: Administer IM into the upper outer quadrant of the gluteal area; must inject dose using one of the provided needles for administration. Use either the 1.5-inch needle (for very lean patients) or the 2-inch needle (for patients with a larger amount of subcutaneous tissue overlying the gluteal muscle). Either needle may be used for patients with average body habitus. Avoid inadvertent injection into a blood vessel; do not administer IV, SubQ, or into fatty tissue (the risk of serious injection site reaction is increased if given incorrectly as a SubQ injection or into fatty tissue instead of the gluteal muscle). Injection should alternate between the 2 buttocks. Do not substitute any components of the dose-pack.

◀ **Monitoring Parameters** Liver function tests (baseline and periodic); monitor for opioid withdrawal, injection site reactions with IM administration, and depression and/or suicidal thinking

Test Interactions May cause cross-reactivity with some opioid immunoassay methods.

Dosage Forms Excipient information presented when available (limited, particularly for generics); consult specific product labeling.

Suspension Reconstituted, Intramuscular:
Vivitrol: 380 mg (1 ea)
Tablet, Oral, as hydrochloride:
ReVia: 50 mg [scored]
Generic: 50 mg

Naltrexone and Bupropion
(nal TREKS one & byoo PROE pee on)

Brand Names: US Contrave

Index Terms Bupropion and Naltrexone; Bupropion Hydrochloride and Naltrexone Hydrochloride

Pharmacologic Category Anorexiant; Antidepressant, Dopamine/Norepinephrine-Reuptake Inhibitor; Opioid Antagonist

Use Weight management: Adjunct to a reduced-calorie diet and increased physical activity for chronic weight management in adults with an initial body mass index (BMI) of ≥30 kg/m^2 or ≥27 kg/m^2 in the presence of at least one weight-related comorbid condition (eg, hypertension, type 2 diabetes mellitus, and/or dyslipidemia)

Limitations of use: The effect of naltrexone/bupropion on cardiovascular morbidity and mortality has not been established. The safety and effectiveness of naltrexone/bupropion in combination with other products intended for weight loss, including prescription drugs, over-the-counter drugs, and herbal preparations, have not been established.

Pregnancy Considerations Animal reproduction studies have not been conducted with this combination. Adverse fetal events following maternal use of bupropion during pregnancy have been reported in some studies. Weight-loss therapy is not recommended for pregnant women. Obese and overweight women should be encouraged to participate in weight reduction programs prior to attempting pregnancy; weight gain during pregnancy should be determined by their prepregnancy BMI and current guidelines (ADA, 2009; IOM, 2009). Use of this product is contraindicated in pregnant women.

Breast-Feeding Considerations Bupropion and naltrexone are excreted into breast milk. Breast-feeding is not recommended by the manufacturer.

Contraindications Hypersensitivity to bupropion, naltrexone, or any other component of the formulation; concomitant use of other bupropion-containing products; chronic opioid, opiate agonist (eg, methadone) or partial agonist (eg, buprenorphine) use; acute opioid withdrawal; uncontrolled hypertension; seizure disorder or a history of seizures; bulimia or anorexia nervosa; abrupt discontinuation of alcohol, benzodiazepines, barbiturates, and antiepileptic drugs; concomitant use of MAO inhibitors (concurrently or within 14 days of discontinuing the MAO inhibitor or naltrexone/bupropion); initiation of naltrexone/bupropion in a patient receiving linezolid or intravenous (IV) methylene blue; pregnancy

Warnings/Precautions [U.S. Boxed Warning]: Naltrexone/bupropion is not approved for use in the treatment of major depressive or psychiatric disorders; it contains bupropion the same active ingredient in some other antidepressant medications. Antidepressants increase the risk of suicidal thinking and behavior in children, adolescents, and young adults (18 to 24 years of age) with major depressive disorder (MDD) and other psychiatric disorders; consider risk prior to prescribing. Short-term studies of antidepressants did not show an increased risk in patients >24 years of age and showed a decreased risk in patients ≥65 years. Closely monitor patients for clinical worsening, suicidality, or unusual changes in behavior, particularly during the initial 1 to 2 months of therapy or during periods of dosage adjustments (increases or decreases); the patient's family or caregiver should be instructed to closely observe the patient and communicate condition with health care provider. A medication guide concerning the use of antidepressants should be dispensed with each prescription. The possibility of a suicide attempt is inherent in major depression and may persist until remission occurs. Worsening depression and severe abrupt suicidality that are not part of the presenting symptoms may require discontinuation or modification of drug therapy. Use caution in high-risk patients during initiation of therapy. Prescriptions should be written for the smallest quantity consistent with good patient care. The patient's family or caregiver should be alerted to monitor patients for the emergence of suicidality and associated behaviors such as anxiety, agitation, panic attacks, insomnia, irritability, hostility, impulsivity, akathisia, hypomania, and mania; patients should be instructed to notify their health care provider if any of these symptoms or worsening depression or psychosis occur.

Bupropion may precipitate a manic, mixed, or hypomanic episode; risk is increased in patients with bipolar disorder or who have risk factors for bipolar disorder. Screen patients for a history of bipolar disorder and the presence of risk factors including a family history of bipolar disorder, suicide, or depression. Naltrexone/bupropion is not FDA approved for bipolar depression. **[U.S. Boxed Warning]: Although naltrexone/bupropion is not approved for smoking cessation treatment, but serious neuropsychiatric events have occurred in patients taking bupropion for smoking cessation,** including changes in mood (eg, depression, mania), psychosis, hallucinations, paranoia, delusions, homicidal ideation, hostility, agitation, aggression, anxiety, panic, suicidal ideation, suicide attempt and completed suicide. **The majority of these reactions occurred during bupropion treatment; however some occurred during treatment discontinuation. A causal relationship is uncertain as depressed mood may be a symptom of nicotine withdrawal. Some cases also occurred in patients taking bupropion who continued to smoke. Observe all patients taking bupropion for neuropsychiatric reactions. Instruct patients to contact a health care provider if neuropsychiatric reactions occur.** Depression, suicide, attempted suicide, and suicidal ideation have also been reported with naltrexone use for the treatment of opioid dependence; however, no causal relationship has been demonstrated.

May precipitate symptoms of acute withdrawal in opioid-dependent patients. An opioid-free interval of a at least 7 to 10 days (including tramadol) is recommended for patients previously dependent on short-acting opioids (including tramadol); consider an opioid-free interval of up to 2 weeks in patients transitioning from buprenorphine or methadone. Patients who had been treated with naltrexone may respond to lower opioid doses than previously used. This could result in potentially life-threatening opioid intoxication. Warn patients that any attempt to overcome opioid blockade during naltrexone therapy, is dangerous and could potentially lead to fatal opioid overdose; the opioid competitive receptor blockade produced by naltrexone is potentially surmountable in the presence of large amounts of opioids. If chronic opiate therapy is required, treatment naltrexone/bupropion should be stopped; if intermittent opiate therapy is required, temporarily discontinue treatment naltrexone/bupropion and lower doses of opioids may be needed.

Bupropion may cause a dose-related risk of seizures. Use is contraindicated in patients with a seizure disorder or a history of seizures, current or past diagnosis of bulimia or anorexia nervosa or undergoing abrupt discontinuation of alcohol, benzodiazepines, barbiturates, and antiepileptic drugs. Use caution with concurrent use of antipsychotics, antidepressants, theophylline, systemic corticosteroids, stimulants (including cocaine), or hypoglycemic agents, or with excessive use of ethanol, benzodiazepines, sedative/hypnotics, or opioids. Use with caution in seizure-potentiating metabolic disorders (hypoglycemia, hyponatremia, severe hepatic impairment, and hypoxia), and in patients with an addiction to cocaine or stimulants, in patients withdrawing from sedatives, and in patients with a history of head trauma, severe stroke, arteriovenous malformation, or central nervous system tumor or infection. To minimize the risk of seizures, increase the dose gradually, administer the dose twice daily with no more than 2 tablets taken at a time, avoid administration with high-fat meals, skip missed doses, and limit the daily dose of to bupropion hydrochloride to ≤360 mg. Use of multiple bupropion formulations is contraindicated. Permanently discontinue if seizure occurs during therapy.

May elevate heart rate, blood pressure and cause hypertension; use is contraindicated in patients with uncontrolled hypertension. Events have been observed in patients with or without evidence of preexisting hypertension. Risks may be greater during the initial 3 months of therapy. Assess heart rate and blood pressure before initiating treatment and monitor periodically. Use with caution in patients with cardiovascular disease. Anaphylactoid/anaphylactic reactions have occurred, with symptoms of including pruritus, urticaria, angioedema, and dyspnea. Serious reactions have been (rarely) reported with bupropion, including erythema multiforme, Stevens-Johnson syndrome (SJS), and anaphylactic shock. Arthralgia, myalgia, and fever with rash and other symptoms suggestive of delayed hypersensitivity resembling serum sickness have been reported

with bupropion. Weight loss may increase the risk of hypoglycemia in patients with type 2 diabetes mellitus treated with insulin and/or insulin secretagogues. Monitor blood glucose levels at baseline and periodically during treatment. Consider decreases in doses for concurrent antidiabetic medications which are non-glucose-dependent; and make adjustments to antidiabetic drug regimens if hypoglycemia develops during treatment. Bupropion may cause mild pupillary dilation, which in susceptible individuals can lead to an episode of narrow-angle glaucoma. Consider evaluating patients who have not had an iridectomy for narrow-angle glaucoma risk factors. Cases of hepatitis, significant liver dysfunction, and transient, asymptomatic hepatic transaminase elevations have been observed with naltrexone use. Discontinue therapy if signs/ symptoms of acute hepatitis develop. Clinicians should note that elevated transaminases may be a result of preexisting alcoholic liver disease, hepatitis B and/or C infection, or concomitant use of other hepatotoxic drugs; abrupt opioid withdrawal may also lead to acute liver injury. Use with caution in patients with hepatic impairment; reduced doses are recommended. Use with caution in patients with mild renal impairment. Dosage reductions are necessary with moderate to severe impairment; avoid use in patients with end-stage renal disease. Use with caution in the elderly; may be at greater risk of drug accumulation during chronic dosing. Potentially significant drug-drug interactions may exist, requiring dose or frequency adjustment, additional monitoring, and/or selection of alternative therapy.

Adverse Reactions
>10%:
Central nervous system: Headache (18%), sleep disorder (14%)
Gastrointestinal: Nausea (33%), constipation (19%), vomiting (11%)

1% to 10%:
Cardiovascular: Hypertension (≤6%), increased blood pressure (≤6%), palpitations (2%), myocardial infarction (<2%), presyncope (<2%), tachycardia (<2%)
Central nervous system: Dizziness (10%), insomnia (9%; ≥65 years of age: 11%), depression (6%; ≥65 years of age: 7%), anxiety (4% to 6%), fatigue (4%), irritability (3%), disturbance in attention (<2% to 3%), abnormal dreams (<2%), agitation (<2%), altered mental status (<2%), amnesia (<2%), derealization (<2%), emotional lability (<2%), equilibrium disturbance (<2%), feeling abnormal (<2%), feeling hot (<2%), intention tremor (<2%), jitteriness (<2%), lethargy (<2%), memory impairment (<2%), nervousness (<2%), tension (<2%), vertigo (<2%)
Dermatologic: Hyperhidrosis (3%), alopecia (<2%)
Endocrine: Hot flash (4%), dehydration (<2%), increased thirst (<2%)
Gastrointestinal: Xerostomia (8%), diarrhea (7%), upper abdominal pain (4%), viral gastroenteritis (4%), abdominal pain (3%), dysgeusia (2%), cholecystitis (<2%), eructation (<2%), hematochezia (<2%), hernia (<2%), lower abdominal pain (<2%), motion sickness (<2%), swelling of lips (<2%)
Genitourinary: Urinary tract infection (3%), erectile dysfunction (<2%), irregular menses (<2%), urinary urgency (<2%), vaginal dryness (<2%), vaginal hemorrhage (<2%)
Hematologic & oncologic: Decreased hematocrit (<2%)
Hepatic: Increased liver enzymes (<2%)
Infection: Kidney infection (<2%), staphylococcal infection (<2%)
Neuromuscular & skeletal: Tremor (4%), strain (2%), herniated disk (<2%), jaw pain (<2%), weakness (<2%)
Otic: Tinnitus (3%)
Renal: Increased serum creatinine (<2%)
Respiratory: Pneumonia (<2%)
<1% (Limited to important or life-threatening): Hypoglycemia (concomitant use of antidiabetic medications), increased heart rate (resting), syncope

Drug Interactions
Metabolism/Transport Effects Refer to individual components.

Avoid Concomitant Use
Avoid concomitant use of Naltrexone and Bupropion with any of the following: MAO Inhibitors; Mequitazine; Methylnaltrexone; Naloxegol; Pimozide; Tamoxifen; Thioridazine

Increased Effect/Toxicity
Naltrexone and Bupropion may increase the levels/ effects of: Alcohol (Ethyl); ARIPiprazole; ARIPiprazole Lauroxil; AtoMOXetine; Brexpiprazole; Citalopram; CYP2D6 Substrates); Dapoxetine; DOXOrubicin (Conventional); DULoxetine; Eliglustat; Fesoterodine; FLUoxetine; FluvoxaMINE; Iloperidone; Lorcaserin; Mequitazine; Metoprolol; Naloxegol; Nebivolol; OCT2

Substrates; PARoxetine; Pimozide; Propafenone; Tamsulosin; Tetrabenazine; Thioridazine; Tricyclic Antidepressants; Vortioxetine

The levels/effects of Naltrexone and Bupropion may be increased by: Alcohol (Ethyl); Anti-Parkinson's Agents (Dopamine Agonist); CYP2B6 Inhibitors (Moderate); MAO Inhibitors; Methylnaltrexone; Mifepristone; Quazepam

Decreased Effect
Naltrexone and Bupropion may decrease the levels/ effects of: Analgesics (Opioid); Codeine; Iloperidone; Ioflupane I 123; Tamoxifen

The levels/effects of Naltrexone and Bupropion may be decreased by: Antihepaciviral Combination Products; CYP2B6 Inducers (Strong); Dabrafenib; Efavirenz; Isavuconazonium Sulfate; Lopinavir; Lumacaftor; Ritonavir

Storage/Stability Store at 25°C (77°F); excursions are permitted between 15°C and 30°C (59°F and 86°F).

Mechanism of Action Naltrexone is a pure opioid antagonist, and bupropion is a relatively weak inhibitor of the neuronal reuptake of dopamine and norepinephrine. The exact neurochemical effects of naltrexone/bupropion leading to weight loss are not fully understood. Effects may result from action on areas of the brain involved in the regulation of food intake: the hypothalamus (appetite regulatory center) and the mesolimbic dopamine circuit (reward system).

Pharmacodynamics/Kinetics See individual agents.

Dosing
Adult & Geriatric
Weight management: Oral:
Initial: One tablet (naltrexone 8 mg/bupropion 90 mg) once daily in the morning for 1 week; at week 2, increase to 1 tablet twice daily administered in the morning and evening and continue for 1 week; at week 3, increase to 2 tablets in the morning and 1 tablet in the evening and continue for 1 week; at week 4, increase to 2 tablets twice daily administered in the morning and evening and continue for the remainder of the treatment course.
Usual dosage: Two tablets (naltrexone 16 mg/bupropion 180 mg) twice daily (maximum dose: naltrexone 32 mg/bupropion 360 mg daily).

Concomitant Use with CYP2B6 inhibitors (eg, ticlopidine, clopidogrel): Maximum dose: 1 tablet (naltrexone 8 mg/bupropion 90 mg) twice daily

Discontinuation of therapy: If the patient has not lost at least 5% of baseline body weight after 12 weeks at the maintenance dosage, discontinue therapy; clinically meaningful weight loss is unlikely with continued treatment.

MAO inhibitor recommendations:
Switching to or from an MAO inhibitor antidepressant:
Allow 14 days to elapse between discontinuing an MAO inhibitor intended to treat depression and initiation of naltrexone/bupropion.
Allow 14 days to elapse between discontinuing naltrexone/bupropion and initiation of an MAO inhibitor intended to treat depression.
Use with reversible MAO inhibitors (such as linezolid or IV methylene blue):
Do not initiate naltrexone/bupropion in patients receiving linezolid or IV methylene blue; consider other interventions for psychiatric condition.
If urgent treatment with linezolid or IV methylene blue is required in a patient already receiving naltrexone/ bupropion and potential benefits outweigh potential risks, discontinue naltrexone/bupropion promptly and administer linezolid or IV methylene blue. Monitor for increased risk of hypertensive reactions for 2 weeks or until 24 hours after the last dose of linezolid or IV methylene blue, whichever comes first. May resume naltrexone/bupropion 24 hours after the last dose of linezolid or IV methylene blue (Wellbutrin prescribing information, 2013).

Renal Impairment
Mild impairment: There are no dosage adjustment provided in the manufacturer's labeling (has not been studied); use with caution.
Moderate or severe impairment: Maximum dose: One tablet (naltrexone 8 mg/bupropion 90 mg) twice daily
End-stage renal disease (ESRD): Use is not recommended.

Hepatic Impairment Maximum dose: One tablet (naltrexone 8 mg/bupropion 90 mg) daily

Dietary Considerations Do not administer with high-fat meals; may result in a significant increase in bupropion and naltrexone systemic exposure.

◄ **Administration** Administer twice daily doses in the morning and in the evening; do not administer with high-fat meals. Do not cut, chew, or crush tablets.

Monitoring Parameters Blood pressure and heart rate (baseline and periodic); blood glucose (baseline and periodic); weight; BMI; renal and liver function (base and periodic); mental status for depression, suicidal ideation (especially at the beginning of therapy or when doses are increased or decreased), anxiety, social functioning, mania, and panic attacks.

Dosage Forms Excipient information presented when available (limited, particularly for generics); consult specific product labeling.

Tablet Extended Release 12 Hour, Oral:

Contrave: Naltrexone hydrochloride 8 mg and bupropion hydrochloride 90 mg [contains edetate disodium, fd&c blue #2 aluminum lake]

♦ Naltrexone Hydrochloride *see* Naltrexone
on page 1252

♦ Namenda *see* Memantine *on page 1139*

♦ Namenda Titration Pak *see* Memantine *on page 1139*

♦ Namenda XR *see* Memantine *on page 1139*

♦ Namenda XR Titration Pack *see* Memantine
on page 1139

♦ Nanoparticle Albumin-Bound Paclitaxel *see* PACLitaxel (Protein Bound) *on page 1371*

♦ NAPA and NABZ *see* Sodium Phenylacetate and Sodium Benzoate *on page 1676*

Naphazoline (Nasal) (naf AZ oh leen)

Brand Names: US Privine® [OTC] [DSC]

Index Terms Naphazoline Hydrochloride

Pharmacologic Category Alpha$_1$ Agonist; Imidazoline Derivative

Use Temporary relief of nasal congestion associated with the common cold, upper respiratory allergies, or sinusitis

Dosing

Adult & Geriatric Nasal congestion (decongestant): Intranasal: 0.05%, instill 1-2 drops or sprays every 6 hours if needed; therapy should not exceed 3 days

Pediatric Nasal congestion (decongestant): Intranasal: Children >12 years: Refer to adult dosing.

Additional Information Complete prescribing information should be consulted for additional detail.

Dosage Forms Excipient information presented when available (limited, particularly for generics); consult specific product labeling. [DSC] = Discontinued product

Solution, intranasal, as hydrochloride [drops]:

Privine®: 0.05% (25 mL) [contains benzalkonium chloride] [DSC]

Solution, intranasal, as hydrochloride [spray]:

Privine®: 0.05% (20 mL) [contains benzalkonium chloride] [DSC]

Naphazoline (Ophthalmic) (naf AZ oh leen)

Brand Names: US Clear Eyes Redness Relief [OTC]

Brand Names: Canada Albalon; Clear Eyes; Diopticon; Naphcon Forte; Odan-Naphazoline; Redness Eye Drops; Refresh Redness Relief; Soothe Redness

Index Terms Naphazoline Hydrochloride

Pharmacologic Category Alpha$_1$ Agonist; Imidazoline Derivative; Ophthalmic Agent, Vasoconstrictor

Use Decrease in eye redness (vasoconstrictor):

Rx: Topical ocular vasoconstrictor.

OTC: Relief of redness of the eye due to minor irritation; temporary relief of burning and irritation due to dry eyes; as a protectant against further irritation or dryness of the eye.

Dosing

Adult & Geriatric Decrease in eye redness (vasoconstrictor): Ophthalmic:

Rx: 0.1% solution: 1 to 2 drops into conjunctival sac every 3 to 4 hours as needed

OTC: 0.012% or 0.03% solution: 1 to 2 drops into affected eye(s) up to 4 times daily

Renal Impairment There are no dosage adjustments provided in the manufacturer's labeling.

Hepatic Impairment There are no dosage adjustments provided in the manufacturer's labeling.

Additional Information Complete prescribing information should be consulted for additional detail.

Dosage Forms Excipient information presented when available (limited, particularly for generics); consult specific product labeling. [DSC] = Discontinued product

Solution, Ophthalmic, as hydrochloride:

Clear Eyes Redness Relief: 0.012% (6 mL) [contains benzalkonium chloride]

Generic: 0.1% (15 mL)

Naphazoline and Pheniramine
(naf AZ oh leen & fen NIR a meen)

Brand Names: US Naphcon-A [OTC]; Opcon-A [OTC]; Visine-A [OTC]

Brand Names: Canada Naphcon-A; Visine Advanced Allergy

Index Terms Pheniramine and Naphazoline

Pharmacologic Category Alkylamine Derivative; Alpha$_1$ Agonist; Histamine H$_1$ Antagonist; Histamine H$_1$ Antagonist, First Generation; Imidazoline Derivative; Ophthalmic Agent, Vasoconstrictor

Use Treatment of ocular congestion, irritation, and itching

Dosing

Adult & Geriatric Ophthalmic: 1-2 drops into the affected eye(s) up to 4 times/day

Pediatric Ophthalmic: Children ≥6 years: Refer to adult dosing.

Additional Information Complete prescribing information should be consulted for additional detail.

Dosage Forms Excipient information presented when available (limited, particularly for generics); consult specific product labeling.

Solution, ophthalmic:

Naphcon-A: Naphazoline hydrochloride 0.025% and pheniramine maleate 0.3% (5 mL) [contains benzalkonium chloride; 2 bottles/box], (15 mL) [contains benzalkonium chloride]

Opcon-A: Naphazoline hydrochloride 0.027% and pheniramine maleate 0.3% (15 mL) [contains benzalkonium chloride]

Visine-A: Naphazoline hydrochloride 0.025% and pheniramine maleate 0.3% (15 mL) [contains benzalkonium chloride]

Generic: Naphazoline hydrochloride 0.027% and pheniramine maleate 0.315% (15 mL)

♦ Naphazoline Hydrochloride *see* Naphazoline (Nasal)
on page 1256

♦ Naphazoline Hydrochloride *see* Naphazoline (Ophthalmic) *on page 1256*

♦ Naphcon-A [OTC] *see* Naphazoline and Pheniramine
on page 1256

♦ Naphcon-A (Can) *see* Naphazoline and Pheniramine
on page 1256

♦ Naphcon Forte (Can) *see* Naphazoline (Ophthalmic)
on page 1256

♦ Naprelan *see* Naproxen *on page 1256*

♦ Naproderm [DSC] *see* Naproxen *on page 1256*

♦ Naprosyn *see* Naproxen *on page 1256*

Naproxen (na PROKS en)

Brand Names: US Aleve [OTC]; All Day Pain Relief [OTC]; All Day Relief [OTC]; Anaprox; Anaprox DS; EC-Naprosyn; EnovaRX-Naproxen; Equipto-Naproxen; Flanax Pain Relief; Flanax Pain Relief [OTC]; Mediproxen [OTC]; Naprelan; Naproderm [DSC]; Naprosyn; Naproxen Comfort Pac; Naproxen DR; Naproxen Kit

Brand Names: Canada Aleve; Anaprox; Anaprox DS; Apo-Napro-Na; Apo-Napro-Na DS; Apo-Naproxen; Apo-Naproxen EC; Apo-Naproxen SR; Ava-Naproxen EC; Maxidol; Mylan-Naproxen EC; Naprelan; Naprosyn; Naproxen EC; Naproxen Sodium DS; Naproxen-NA; Naproxen-NA DF; Pediapharm Naproxen Suspension; PMS-Naproxen; PMS-Naproxen EC; PRO-Naproxen EC; Teva-Naproxen; Teva-Naproxen EC; Teva-Naproxen Sodium; Teva-Naproxen Sodium DS; Teva-Naproxen SR

Index Terms Naproxen Sodium

Pharmacologic Category Nonsteroidal Anti-inflammatory Drug (NSAID), Oral

Use

Acute gout/Ankylosing spondylitis/Bursitis/Juvenile arthritis/Juvenile rheumatoid arthritis/Osteoarthritis/Rheumatoid arthritis/Tendonitis (Rx products only): For the relief of the signs and symptoms of acute gout, ankylosing spondylitis, bursitis, juvenile arthritis (excluding ER tablets), juvenile rheumatoid arthritis (oral suspension only), osteoarthritis, rheumatoid arthritis, and tendonitis. Delayed-release naproxen is not recommended for initial treatment of acute pain.

Pain/Primary dysmenorrhea (Rx and OTC products): For the relief of mild to moderate pain and the treatment of primary dysmenorrhea. Delayed-release naproxen is not recommended for initial treatment of acute pain.

Pregnancy Considerations Adverse events were not observed in the initial animal reproduction studies; therefore, the manufacturer classifies naproxen as pregnancy category C. Naproxen crosses the placenta and can be detected in fetal tissue and the serum of newborn infants following *in utero* exposure. NSAID exposure during the first trimester is not strongly associated with congenital malformations; however, cardiovascular anomalies and cleft palate have been observed following NSAID exposure in some studies. The use of a NSAID close to conception may be associated with an increased risk of miscarriage. Nonteratogenic effects have been observed following NSAID administration during the third trimester including: Myocardial degenerative changes, prenatal constriction of the ductus arteriosus, fetal tricuspid regurgitation, failure of the ductus arteriosus to close postnatally; renal dysfunction or failure, oligohydramnios; gastrointestinal bleeding or perforation, increased risk of necrotizing enterocolitis; intracranial bleeding (including intraventricular hemorrhage), platelet dysfunction with resultant bleeding; pulmonary hypertension. Because they may cause premature closure of the ductus arteriosus, use of NSAIDs late in pregnancy should be avoided (use after 31 or 32 weeks gestation is not recommended by some clinicians). The Canadian labeling contraindicates use during the third trimester of pregnancy. The chronic use of NSAIDs in women of reproductive age may be associated with infertility that is reversible upon discontinuation of the medication. A registry is available for pregnant women exposed to autoimmune medications including naproxen. For additional information contact the Organization of Teratology Information Specialists, OTIS Autoimmune Diseases Study, at (877) 311-8972.

Breast-Feeding Considerations Small amounts of naproxen are excreted into breast milk. Naproxen has been detected in the urine of a breast-feeding infant. Breast-feeding is not recommended per the U.S. manufacturer labeling and is contraindicated per the Canadian manufacturer labeling. In a study which included 20 mother-infant pairs, there were two cases of drowsiness and one case of vomiting in the breast-fed infants. Maternal naproxen dose, duration, and relationship to breast-feeding were not provided.

Medication Guide Available Yes

Contraindications

Hypersensitivity to naproxen, aspirin, other NSAIDs, or any component of the formulation; treatment of perioperative pain in the setting of coronary artery bypass graft (CABG) surgery

Canadian labeling: Additional contraindications (not in U.S. labeling): Active peptic ulcers; active GI bleeding; cerebrovascular bleeding or other bleeding disorders; active GI inflammatory disease; severe liver impairment or active liver disease; severe renal impairment (Crcl <30 mL/minute) or deteriorating renal disease; severe uncontrolled heart failure; known hyperkalemia; third trimester of pregnancy; breast-feeding; inflammatory lesions or recent bleeding of the rectum or anus (suppository only); use in patients <16 years of age (suppository only); use in patients <18 years of age (naproxen enteric coated and sustained release tablets and naproxen sodium tablets); use in children <2 years (naproxen tablets and suspension).

Warnings/Precautions [U.S. Boxed Warning]: NSAIDs are associated with an increased risk of adverse cardiovascular thrombotic events, including MI and stroke. Risk may be increased with duration of use or preexisting cardiovascular risk factors or disease. Carefully evaluate individual cardiovascular risk profiles prior to prescribing. May cause new-onset hypertension or worsening of existing hypertension. Monitor blood pressure closely with initiation and during therapy. Use caution with fluid retention. Avoid use in heart failure (ACCF/AHA [Yancy, 2013]). Use the lowest effective dose for the shortest duration of time, consistent with individual patient goals, to reduce risk of cardiovascular or GI adverse events. Alternate therapies should be considered for patients at high risk. Concurrent administration of ibuprofen, and potentially other nonselective NSAIDs, may interfere with aspirin's cardioprotective effect. **[U.S. Boxed Warning]: Use is contraindicated for treatment of perioperative pain in the setting of coronary artery bypass graft (CABG) surgery.** Risk of MI and stroke may be increased with use following CABG surgery.

[U.S. Boxed Warning]: NSAIDs may increase risk of gastrointestinal irritation, inflammation, ulceration, bleeding, and perforation. These events may occur at any time during therapy and without warning. Risk for serious events is greater in elderly patients. Use caution with a history of GI disease (bleeding or ulcers). Canadian labeling contraindicates use with active peptic ulcers, GI bleeding, or inflammatory bowel disease. Use caution with concurrent therapy with aspirin, anticoagulants and/or corticosteroids, smoking, use of alcohol, the elderly or debilitated patients. When used concomitantly with aspirin, a substantial increase in the risk of gastrointestinal complications (eg, ulcer) occurs; concomitant gastroprotective therapy (eg, proton pump inhibitors) is recommended (Bhatt, 2008).

May increase the risk of aseptic meningitis, especially in patients with systemic lupus erythematosus (SLE) and mixed connective tissue disorders. Platelet adhesion and aggregation may be decreased; may prolong bleeding time; patients with coagulation disorders or who are receiving anticoagulants should be monitored closely. Anemia may occur; patients on long-term NSAID therapy should be monitored for anemia. Rarely, NSAID use may cause severe blood dyscrasias (eg, agranulocytosis, aplastic anemia, thrombocytopenia).

NSAID use may compromise existing renal function; dose-dependent decreases in prostaglandin synthesis may result from NSAID use, reducing renal blood flow which may cause renal decompensation. NSAID use may increase the risk for hyperkalemia (Canadian labeling contraindicates use in patients with known hyperkalemia). Patients with impaired renal function, dehydration, heart failure, liver dysfunction, those taking diuretics, and ACE inhibitors, and the elderly are at greater risk of renal toxicity and hyperkalemia. Rehydrate patient before starting therapy; monitor renal function closely. Not recommended for use in patients with advanced renal disease. Canadian labeling contraindicates use in severe renal impairment (CrCl <30 mL/minute) or deteriorating renal disease. Long-term NSAID use may result in renal papillary necrosis.

NSAIDs may cause serious skin adverse events including exfoliative dermatitis, Stevens-Johnson Syndrome (SJS) and toxic epidermal necrolysis (TEN); discontinue use at first sign of skin rash or hypersensitivity. Anaphylactoid reactions may occur, even without prior exposure; patients with "aspirin triad" (bronchial asthma, aspirin intolerance, rhinitis) may be at increased risk. Do not use in patients who experience bronchospasm, asthma, rhinitis, or urticaria with NSAID or aspirin therapy. Use caution in other forms of asthma.

Use with caution in patients with decreased hepatic function. Closely monitor patients with any abnormal LFT. Severe hepatic reactions (eg, fulminant hepatitis, liver failure) have occurred with NSAID use, rarely; discontinue if signs or symptoms of liver disease develop, or if systemic manifestations occur. Canadian labeling contraindicates use in severe impairment or with active liver disease.

NSAIDS may cause drowsiness, dizziness, blurred vision and other neurologic effects which may impair physical or mental abilities; patients must be cautioned about performing tasks which require mental alertness (eg, operating machinery or driving). Discontinue use with blurred or diminished vision and perform ophthalmologic exam. Monitor vision with long-term therapy. Withhold for at least 4-6 half-lives prior to surgical or dental procedures.

Use with caution in the elderly, particularly at higher doses; unbound plasma fraction increased. Dose adjustments may be necessary; avoid chronic use (unless alternative agents ineffective and patient can receive concomitant gastroprotective agent); nonselective oral NSAID use is associated with an increased risk of GI bleeding and peptic ulcer disease in older adults in high risk category (eg, >75 years or age or receiving concomitant oral/parenteral corticosteroids, anticoagulants, or antiplatelet agents) (Beers Criteria).

OTC labeling: Prior to self-medication, patients should contact healthcare provider if they have had recurring stomach pain or upset, ulcers, bleeding problems, asthma, high blood pressure, heart or kidney disease, other serious medical problems, are currently taking a diuretic, anticoagulant, other NSAIDs, or are ≥60 years of age. Recommended dosages and duration should not be exceeded, due to an increased risk of GI bleeding, MI, and stroke. Patients should stop use and consult a healthcare provider if symptoms get worse, newly appear, or continue; if an allergic reaction occurs; if feeling faint, vomit blood or have bloody/black stools; if having difficulty swallowing or heartburn, or if fever lasts for >3 days or pain >10 days. Consuming ≥3 alcoholic beverages/day or taking longer than recommended may increase the risk of GI bleeding. Not for self-medication (OTC use) in children <12 years of age. Canadian labeling contraindicates use of certain ▶

dosage forms based on age (refer to Contraindications for specific recommendations).

Adverse Reactions

1% to 10%:

Cardiovascular: Edema (3% to 9%), palpitations (<3%)

Central nervous system: Dizziness (≤9%), drowsiness (3% to 9%), headache (3% to 9%), vertigo (<3%)

Dermatologic: Pruritus (3% to 9%), skin rash (3% to 9%), ecchymoses (3% to 9%), diaphoresis (<3%)

Endocrine & metabolic: Fluid retention (3% to 9%), increased thirst (<3%)

Gastrointestinal: Abdominal pain (3% to 9%), constipation (3% to 9%), nausea (3% to 9%), heartburn (3% to 9%), diarrhea (<3%), dyspepsia (<3%), stomatitis (<3%), flatulence, gastrointestinal hemorrhage, gastrointestinal perforation, gastrointestinal ulcer, vomiting

Hematologic & oncologic: Hemolysis (3% to 9%), purpura (<3%), anemia, prolonged bleeding time

Hepatic: Increased liver enzymes

Ophthalmic: Visual disturbance (<3%)

Otic: Tinnitus (3% to 9%), auditory disturbance (<3%)

Renal: Renal function abnormality

Respiratory: Dyspnea (3% to 9%)

<1% (Limited to important or life-threatening): Abnormal dreams, agranulocytosis, alopecia, anaphylactoid reaction, anaphylaxis, angioedema, aphthous stomatitis, aseptic meningitis, asthma, blurred vision, cardiac arrhythmia, cardiac failure, cognitive dysfunction, colitis, coma, confusion, conjunctivitis, cystitis, depression, dysuria, eosinophilia, eosinophilic pneumonitis, erythema multiforme, exfoliative dermatitis, fever, glossitis, granulocytopenia, hallucination, hematemesis, hepatic failure, hepatitis, hepatotoxicity (idiosyncratic) (Chalasani, 2014), hyperglycemia, hypertension, hypoglycemia, hypotension, infection, interstitial nephritis, melena, jaundice, leukopenia, lymphadenopathy, menstrual disease, malaise, myalgia, myasthenia, myocardial infarction, oliguria, pancreatitis, pancytopenia, paresthesia, pneumonia, polyuria, proteinuria, rectal hemorrhage, renal failure, renal papillary necrosis, respiratory depression, sepsis, skin photosensitivity, Stevens-Johnson syndrome, tachycardia, seizure, syncope, thrombocytopenia, toxic epidermal necrolysis, vasculitis

Drug Interactions

Metabolism/Transport Effects Substrate of CYP1A2 (minor), CYP2C9 (minor); **Note:** Assignment of Major/Minor substrate status based on clinically relevant drug interaction potential

Avoid Concomitant Use

Avoid concomitant use of Naproxen with any of the following: Dexketoprofen; Floctafenine; Ketorolac (Nasal); Ketorolac (Systemic); Morniflumate; NSAID (COX-2 Inhibitor); Omacetaxine; Talniflumate; Urokinase

Increased Effect/Toxicity

Naproxen may increase the levels/effects of: 5-ASA Derivatives; Agents with Antiplatelet Properties; Aliskiren; Aminoglycosides; Anticoagulants; Apixaban; Bisphosphonate Derivatives; Collagenase (Systemic); CycloSPORINE (Systemic); Dabigatran Etexilate; Deferasirox; Deoxycholic Acid; Desmopressin; Digoxin; Drospirenone; Edoxaban; Eplerenone; Haloperidol; Ibritumomab; Lithium; Methotrexate; Nonsteroidal Anti-Inflammatory Agents; NSAID (COX-2 Inhibitor); Obinutuzumab; Omacetaxine; PEMEtrexed; Porfimer; Potassium-Sparing Diuretics; PRALAtrexate; Quinolone Antibiotics; Rivaroxaban; Salicylates; Tacrolimus (Systemic); Tenofovir Products; Thrombolytic Agents; Tositumomab and Iodine I 131 Tositumomab; Urokinase; Vancomycin; Verteporfin; Vitamin K Antagonists

The levels/effects of Naproxen may be increased by: ACE Inhibitors; Alcohol (Ethyl); Angiotensin II Receptor Blockers; Antidepressants (Tricyclic, Tertiary Amine); Corticosteroids (Systemic); CycloSPORINE (Systemic); Dasatinib; Dexketoprofen; Diclofenac (Systemic); Floctafenine; Glucosamine; Herbs (Anticoagulant/Antiplatelet Properties); Ibrutinib; Ketorolac (Nasal); Ketorolac (Systemic); Limaprost; Loop Diuretics; Morniflumate; Multivitamins/Fluoride (with ADE); Multivitamins/Minerals (with ADEK, Folate, Iron); Multivitamins/Minerals (with AE, No Iron); Omega-3 Fatty Acids; Pentosan Polysulfate Sodium; Pentoxifylline; Probenecid; Prostacyclin Analogues; Selective Serotonin Reuptake Inhibitors; Serotonin/Norepinephrine Reuptake Inhibitors; Sodium Phosphates; Talniflumate; Thiazide Diuretics; Tipranavir; Treprostinil; Vitamin E; Vitamin E (Oral)

Decreased Effect

Naproxen may decrease the levels/effects of: ACE Inhibitors; Aliskiren; Angiotensin II Receptor Blockers; Beta-Blockers; Eplerenone; HydrALAZINE; Loop Diuretics; Potassium-Sparing Diuretics; Prostaglandins (Ophthalmic); Salicylates; Selective Serotonin Reuptake Inhibitors; Thiazide Diuretics

The levels/effects of Naproxen may be decreased by: Bile Acid Sequestrants; Salicylates

Food Interactions Naproxen absorption rate/levels may be decreased if taken with food. Management: Administer with food, milk, or antacids to decrease GI adverse effects.

Storage/Stability Store at 15°C to 30°C (59°F to 86°F); suspension should not be exposed to excessive heat (>40°C [104°F]).

Mechanism of Action Reversibly inhibits cyclooxygenase-1 and 2 (COX-1 and 2) enzymes, which results in decreased formation of prostaglandin precursors; has antipyretic, analgesic, and anti-inflammatory properties

Other proposed mechanisms not fully elucidated (and possibly contributing to the anti-inflammatory effect to varying degrees), include inhibiting chemotaxis, altering lymphocyte activity, inhibiting neutrophil aggregation/activation, and decreasing proinflammatory cytokine levels.

Pharmacodynamics/Kinetics

Onset of action: Analgesic: 30 to 60 minutes

Duration: Analgesic: <12 hours

Absorption: Oral: Almost 100%

Distribution: 0.16 L/kg

Protein binding: >99% to albumin; increased free fraction in elderly

Metabolism: Hepatic to metabolites

Bioavailability: 95%

Half-life elimination: Normal renal function: 12 to 17 hours; Moderate-to-severe renal impairment: ~15 to 21 hours (Anttila, 1980)

Time to peak, serum:

Tablets, naproxen: 2 to 4 hours

Tablets, naproxen sodium: 1 to 2 hours

Tablets, delayed-release (empty stomach): 4 to 6 hours; range: 2 to 12 hours

Tablets, delayed-release (with food): 12 hours; range: 4 to 24 hours

Suspension: 1 to 4 hours

Suppository [Canadian product]: 2 to 3 hours

Excretion: Urine (95%; primarily as metabolites); feces (≤3%)

Dosing

Adult Note: Dosage expressed as naproxen base; 200 mg naproxen base is equivalent to 220 mg naproxen sodium. For relief of acute pain, naproxen sodium may be preferred due to more rapid absorption and onset; naproxen base may also be used however EC-Naprosyn is not recommended.

Ankylosing spondylitis, osteoarthritis, rheumatoid arthritis: Oral: 500 to 1,000 mg daily in 2 divided doses; in patients who require higher level of anti-inflammatory/analgesic activity and have tolerated lower doses, may increase to 1,500 mg/day for limited time period (<6 months)

Naproxen extended-release tablets: Initial: 750 to 1,000 mg once daily; in patients who require higher level of anti-inflammatory/analgesic activity and have tolerated lower doses, may temporarily increase to 1,500 mg once daily

Rectal suppository [Canadian product]: Insert one 500 mg suppository into the rectum once daily (**Note:** Suppository may be used to substitute for one oral dose in patients receiving 1,000 mg naproxen daily).

Gout, acute: Oral: Initial: 750 mg, followed by 250 mg every 8 hours until attack subsides

Naproxen extended-release tablets: Initial: 1,000 to 1,500 mg once daily followed by 1,000 mg once daily until attack subsides

Pain (mild to moderate), dysmenorrhea, acute tendonitis, bursitis: Oral: Initial: 500 mg, followed by 500 mg every 12 hours or 250 mg every 6 to 8 hours; maximum daily dose: Day 1: 1,250 mg; subsequent daily doses should not exceed 1,000 mg

Naproxen extended-release tablets: Oral: Initial: 1,000 mg once daily; may temporarily increase to 1,500 mg once daily if greater pain relief is needed. Dose should be subsequently reduced to a maximum of 1,000 mg daily.

Migraine, acute (off label use): Initial: 750 mg; an additional 250 to 500 mg may be given if needed (maximum: 1,250 mg in 24 hours) (Andersson, 1989; Nestvold, 1985).

OTC labeling: Pain, fever: 200 mg every 8 to 12 hours; if needed, may take 400 mg for the initial dose; maximum: 400 mg in any 8- to 12-hour period or 600 mg/24 hours

Geriatric Use with caution; dosage adjustment may be required. Refer to adult dosing.

Pediatric Note: Dosage expressed as naproxen base; 200 mg naproxen base is equivalent to 220 mg naproxen sodium.

Juvenile idiopathic arthritis: Children >2 years: Oral: **Note:** Oral suspension is recommended: 10 mg/kg/day in 2 divided doses (up to 15 mg/kg/day has been tolerated). Do not exceed 15 mg/kg/day.

OTC labeling: Pain, fever: Children ≥12 years: Oral: Refer to adult dosing.

Ankylosing spondylitis, osteoarthritis, rheumatoid arthritis: Adolescents ≥16 years: Rectal suppository [Canadian product]: Refer to adult dosing.

Renal Impairment CrCl <30 mL/minute
U.S. labeling: Use is not recommended.
Canadian labeling: Use is contraindicated.

Hepatic Impairment Manufacturer's labeling suggests that a reduced dose should be considered; use with caution in chronic disease (eg, alcoholic liver disease), particularly at higher doses; dose adjustment may be required. Canadian labeling contraindicates use in severe impairment or active liver disease.

Dietary Considerations Drug may cause GI upset, bleeding, ulceration, perforation; take with food or milk to minimize GI upset.

Administration
Oral: Administer with food, milk, or antacids to decrease GI adverse effects
Suspension: Shake suspension well before administration.
Tablet, delayed or extended release: Swallow tablet whole; do not break, crush, or chew.
Rectal suppository [Canadian product]: Insert suppository into rectum.

Monitoring Parameters Occult blood loss, periodic liver function test, CBC, BUN, serum creatinine; urine output; blood pressure (hypertensive patients); ophthalmic exam (for vision changes/disturbances)

Test Interactions Naproxen may interfere with 5-HIAA urinary assays; due to an interaction with m-dinitrobenzene, naproxen should be discontinued 72 hours before adrenal function testing if the Porter-Silber test is used. May interfere with urine detection of cannabinoids and barbiturates (false-positives).

Dosage Forms Considerations
EnovaRX-Naproxen and Equipto-Naproxen creams are compounded from a kit. Refer to manufacturer's package insert for compounding instructions.
Naproxen Comfort Pac kit contains naproxen tablets and Duraflex Comfort Gel
Flanax Pain Refief kit contains naproxen tablets and Flanax Liniment

Dosage Forms Excipient information presented when available (limited, particularly for generics); consult specific product labeling. [DSC] = Discontinued product
Capsule, Oral, as sodium:
  Aleve: 220 mg [contains brilliant blue fcf (fd&c blue #1)]
Cream, External:
  EnovaRX-Naproxen: 10% (60 g, 120 g) [contains cetyl alcohol]
  Equipto-Naproxen: 10% (120 g)
  Naproderm: 15% (60 g [DSC])
Kit, Combination:
  Flanax Pain Relief: 500 mg [contains cetearyl alcohol, cremophor el, propylparaben]
  Naproxen Comfort Pac: 500 mg [contains methylparaben, trolamine (triethanolamine)]
Suspension, Oral:
  Naprosyn: 125 mg/5 mL (480 mL)
  Generic: 125 mg/5 mL (500 mL)
Tablet, Oral:
  Naprosyn: 250 mg [DSC] [scored]
  Naprosyn: 375 mg [DSC]
  Naprosyn: 500 mg [scored]
  Naproxen Kit: 500 mg [scored]
  Generic: 250 mg, 375 mg, 500 mg
Tablet, Oral, as sodium:
  Aleve: 220 mg [contains fd&c blue #2 aluminum lake]
  All Day Pain Relief: 220 mg [contains fd&c blue #2 aluminum lake]
  All Day Pain Relief: 220 mg [gluten free; contains fd&c blue #2 aluminum lake]
  All Day Relief: 220 mg
  All Day Relief: 220 mg [contains fd&c blue #2 aluminum lake]
  All Day Relief: 220 mg [gluten free; contains fd&c blue #2 aluminum lake]
  Anaprox: 275 mg
  Anaprox DS: 550 mg [scored]
  Flanax Pain Relief: 220 mg [contains fd&c blue #2 (indigotine)]
  Mediproxen: 220 mg
  Generic: 220 mg, 275 mg, 550 mg
Tablet Delayed Release, Oral:
  EC-Naprosyn: 375 mg, 500 mg
  Naproxen DR: 375 mg, 500 mg

Tablet Extended Release 24 Hour, Oral, as sodium [strength expressed as base]:
  Naprelan: 375 mg, 500 mg, 750 mg
  Generic: 375 mg, 500 mg
Dosage Forms: Canada Note: Refer also to Dosage Forms. Combination kit is not available in Canada.
Excipient information presented when available (limited, particularly for generics); consult specific product labeling.
  Capsule, Oral, as sodium: Maxidol 220 mg
  Suppository, Rectal: 500 mg

♦ **Naproxen and Sumatriptan** see Sumatriptan and Naproxen on page 1720

♦ **Naproxen Comfort Pac** see Naproxen on page 1256

♦ **Naproxen DR** see Naproxen on page 1256

♦ **Naproxen EC (Can)** see Naproxen on page 1256

♦ **Naproxen Kit** see Naproxen on page 1256

♦ **Naproxen-NA (Can)** see Naproxen on page 1256

♦ **Naproxen-NA DF (Can)** see Naproxen on page 1256

♦ **Naproxen Sodium** see Naproxen on page 1256

♦ **Naproxen Sodium and Sumatriptan** see Sumatriptan and Naproxen on page 1720

♦ **Naproxen Sodium and Sumatriptan Succinate** see Sumatriptan and Naproxen on page 1720

♦ **Naproxen Sodium DS (Can)** see Naproxen on page 1256

♦ **Naramin [OTC]** see DiphenhydrAMINE (Systemic) on page 561

Naratriptan (NAR a trip tan)

Brand Names: US Amerge
Brand Names: Canada Amerge; Sandoz-Naratriptan; Teva-Naratriptan
Index Terms Naratriptan Hydrochloride
Pharmacologic Category Antimigraine Agent; Serotonin 5-HT$_{1B, 1D}$ Receptor Agonist
Use Migraines: Acute treatment of migraine attacks with or without aura in adults.
Pregnancy Considerations Adverse events were observed in animal reproduction studies. Pregnancy outcome information for naratriptan is available from a pregnancy registry sponsored by GlaxoSmithKline. As of October 2008, data was available for 55 infants/fetuses exposed to naratriptan, and seven exposed to both naratriptan and sumatriptan. Following naratriptan exposure, there was one infant born with a birth defect; this infant was also exposed to sumatriptan during the first trimester of pregnancy (Cunnington, 2009). The pregnancy registry was closed in January, 2012 and additional information may be obtained from the manufacturer (800-336-2176). Additional information related to the use of naratriptan in pregnancy is limited (Källén, 2011; Nezvalová-Henriksen, 2010; Nezvalová-Henriksen, 2012). Until additional information is available, other agents are preferred for the initial treatment of migraine in pregnancy (Da Silva, 2012; MacGregor, 2012; Williams, 2012).
Breast-Feeding Considerations It is not known if naratriptan is excreted in breast milk. Due to the potential for serious adverse reactions in the nursing infant, the manufacturer recommends a decision be made whether to discontinue nursing or to discontinue the drug, taking into account the importance of treatment to the mother.
Contraindications
Ischemic coronary artery disease (CAD) (angina pectoris, history of myocardial infarction [MI], or documented silent ischemia); coronary artery vasospasm, including Prinzmetal's angina; Wolff-Parkinson-White syndrome or arrhythmias associated with other cardiac accessory conduction pathway disorders; history of stroke, transient ischemic attack (TIA), or history of hemiplegic or basilar migraine; peripheral vascular disease; ischemic bowel disease; uncontrolled hypertension; recent use (within 24 hours) of another 5-HT$_1$ agonist, ergotamine-containing medication, or ergot-type medication (eg, dihydroergotamine or methysergide); severe renal impairment (CrCl <15 mL/minute) or severe hepatic impairment; hypersensitivity to naratriptan or any component of the formulation
Canadian labeling: Additional contraindications (not in U.S. labeling): Severe hypertension, cardiac arrhythmias (especially tachycardias); valvular heart disease, congenital heart disease, atherosclerotic disease; management of ophthalmoplegic migraine

Documentation of allergenic cross-reactivity for triptans is limited. However, because of similarities in chemical structure and/or pharmacologic actions, the possibility of cross-sensitivity cannot be ruled out with certainty.

Warnings/Precautions Use only if there is a clear diagnosis of migraine. Use is contraindicated in patients with severe hepatic or renal impairment. Do not give to patients with risk factors for CAD until a cardiovascular evaluation has been performed; if evaluation is satisfactory, the health care provider should administer the first dose (consider ECG monitoring) and cardiovascular status should be periodically re-evaluated. Use is contraindicated in patients with ischemic or vasospastic CAD and Wolff-Parkinson-White syndrome or arrhythmias associated with other cardiac accessory conduction pathway disorders. Additionally, the Canadian labeling contraindicates use in patients with valvular heart disease, cardiac arrhythmias (especially tachycardias) and congenital heart disease. Cardiac events (coronary artery vasospasm, transient ischemia, myocardial infarction, ventricular tachycardia/fibrillation, cardiac arrest, and death), cerebral/subarachnoid hemorrhage, stroke (some fatal), peripheral vascular ischemia, gastrointestinal vascular ischemia/infarction, splenic infarction, and Raynaud's syndrome have been reported with 5-HT$_1$ agonist administration. Partial vision loss and blindness (transient and permanent) have been reported with use of 5-HT$_1$ agonists; a causal relationship between these events and 5-HT$_1$ agonist administration has not been clearly determined. Patients who experience sensations of chest pain/pressure/tightness or symptoms suggestive of angina following dosing should be evaluated for coronary artery disease or Prinzmetal's angina before receiving additional doses; if dosing is resumed and similar symptoms recur, monitor with ECG. Significant elevation in blood pressure, including hypertensive crisis with acute impairment of organ systems, has been reported on rare occasions in patients with and without a history of hypertension; monitor blood pressure. Blood pressure increases may be more pronounced in the elderly. Use in patients with uncontrolled hypertension is contraindicated; the Canadian labeling also contraindicates use in patients with severe hypertension.

May cause CNS depression, such as dizziness, weakness, or drowsiness, which may impair physical or mental abilities; patients must be cautioned about performing tasks which require mental alertness (eg, operating machinery or driving). Only indicated for the acute treatment of migraine; not indicated for migraine prophylaxis, or for the treatment of cluster headache, hemiplegic, basilar, or ophthalmoplegic (Canadian labeling) migraine. Acute migraine agents (eg, triptans, opioids, ergotamine, or a combination of the agents) used for 10 or more days per month may lead to worsening of headaches (medication overuse headache); withdrawal treatment may be necessary in the setting of overuse. If a patient does not respond to the first dose, the diagnosis of migraine should be reconsidered; rule out underlying neurologic disease in patients with atypical headache and in patients with no prior history of migraine.

Potentially significant drug-drug interactions may exist, requiring dose or frequency adjustment, additional monitoring, and/or selection of alternative therapy. Symptoms of agitation, confusion, hallucinations, hyper-reflexia, myoclonus, shivering, and tachycardia may occur with concomitant proserotonergic drugs (ie, SSRIs/SNRIs or triptans) or agents which reduce naratriptan's metabolism. Concurrent use of serotonin precursors (eg, tryptophan) is not recommended. If concomitant administration with SSRIs is warranted, monitor closely, especially at initiation and with dose increases. Discontinue naratriptan if serotonin syndrome is suspected. Anaphylaxis, anaphylactoid, and hypersensitivity reactions (including angioedema) have occurred; may be life-threatening or fatal.

Adverse Reactions

1% to 10%:

Central nervous system: Pain (4%), fatigue (2%), dizziness (1% to 2%), drowsiness (1% to 2%), paresthesia (1% to 2%), hot and cold flashes (1%), sensation of pressure (1%; chest/neck/throat/jaw), vertigo (1%)

Gastrointestinal: Nausea (4% to 5%), vomiting (1%), xerostomia (1%)

Neuromuscular & skeletal: Neck pain (2%)

Ophthalmic: Photophobia (1%)

Respiratory: Constriction of the pharynx (2%), ENT infection (1%)

<1% (Limited to important or life-threatening): Abnormal bilirubin levels, abnormal hepatic function tests, anaphylactoid reaction, anaphylaxis, anemia, angina pectoris, angioedema, bradycardia, cerebral infarction, colonic ischemia, coronary artery vasospasm, depression, ECG changes (atrial fibrillation, atrial flutter, premature ventricular contractions, PR prolongation, or QTc prolongation), glycosuria, hallucination, heart murmur, hypersensitivity reaction (some cases severe, including circulatory collapse), hypertension, hypothyroidism, ischemic heart disease, ketonuria, myocardial infarction, palpitations, seizure, serotonin syndrome, skin rash, subarachnoid hemorrhage, subconjunctival hemorrhage, syncope, thrombocytopenia, transient ischemic attacks, ventricular fibrillation, ventricular tachycardia

Drug Interactions

Metabolism/Transport Effects None known.

Avoid Concomitant Use

Avoid concomitant use of Naratriptan with any of the following: Dapoxetine; Ergot Derivatives

Increased Effect/Toxicity

Naratriptan may increase the levels/effects of: Antipsychotic Agents; Droxidopa; Ergot Derivatives; Metoclopramide; Serotonin Modulators

The levels/effects of Naratriptan may be increased by: Antiemetics (5HT3 Antagonists); Antipsychotic Agents; Dapoxetine; Ergot Derivatives; Metaxalone; Tedizolid

Decreased Effect There are no known significant interactions involving a decrease in effect.

Storage/Stability Store at 20°C to 25°C (68°F to 77°F).

Mechanism of Action Selective agonist for serotonin (5-HT$_{1B}$ and 5-HT$_{1D}$ receptors) in cranial arteries; causes vasoconstriction and reduces sterile inflammation associated with antidromic neuronal transmission correlating with relief of migraine

Pharmacodynamics/Kinetics

Onset of action: ~1-2 hours (Bomhof, 1999; Tfelt-Hansen, 2000)

Absorption: Well absorbed

Distribution: V_{dss}: 170 L

Protein binding, plasma: 28% to 31%

Metabolism: Hepatic via CYP

Bioavailability: ~70%

Half-life, elimination: 6 hours; increased in renal impairment (moderate impairment; mean: 11 hours; range: 7-20 hours); increased in hepatic impairment (moderate impairment: 8-16 hours)

Time to peak: 2-3 hours

Excretion: Urine (50% of total dose as unchanged drug; 30% of total dose as metabolites)

Dosing

Adult Note: If the first dose is ineffective, diagnosis needs to be re-evaluated. The safety of treating >4 migraines/month has not been established.

Acute migraine: Oral: Initial: 1-2.5 mg; if headache recurs or does not fully resolve, a second dose may be administered after 4 hours (maximum: 5 mg daily).

Geriatric *U.S. labeling:* Refer to adult dosing. Dosing should generally start at the lower end of the dosing range due to possible increased incidence of hepatic, renal, and cardiac impairment.

Canadian labeling: Use is not recommended

Renal Impairment

Mild-to-moderate renal impairment:

U.S. labeling: Initial: 1 mg; do not exceed 2.5 mg in 24 hours.

Canadian labeling: Initial: 1 mg; do not exceed 2 mg in 24 hours

Severe renal impairment (CrCl <15 mL/minute): Use is contraindicated.

Hepatic Impairment

Mild-to-moderate hepatic impairment (Child-Pugh grade A or B):

U.S. labeling: Initial: 1 mg; do not exceed 2.5 mg in 24 hours

Canadian labeling: Initial: 1 mg; do not exceed 2 mg in 24 hours

Severe hepatic impairment (Child-Pugh grade C): Use is contraindicated.

Administration Administer orally as soon as symptoms appear; may take with or without food. Do **not** crush or chew tablet; swallow whole with water.

Monitoring Parameters Headache severity, blood pressure, signs/symptoms suggestive of angina; perform a cardiovascular evaluation in triptan-naïve patients who have multiple cardiovascular risk factors (eg, increased age, diabetes, hypertension, smoking, obesity, strong family history of CAD), monitor ECG with first dose in patients with multiple cardiovascular risk factors who have a negative cardiovascular evaluation and consider periodic cardiovascular evaluation in such patients if they are intermittent long-term users; signs/symptoms of serotonin syndrome and hypersensitivity reactions.

Dosage Forms Excipient information presented when available (limited, particularly for generics); consult specific product labeling.

Tablet, Oral:

Amerge: 1 mg, 2.5 mg

Generic: 1 mg, 2.5 mg

Extemporaneous Preparations A 0.5 mg/mL oral suspension may be made using tablets. Crush fifty 2.5 mg tablets and reduce to a fine powder. In small amounts, add 125 mL of Ora-Plus® and mix well after each addition. Transfer to a calibrated bottle, rinse mortar with vehicle, then add quantity of Ora-Sweet® or Ora-Sweet® SF sufficient to make 250 mL. Label "shake well" and "refrigerate". Stable 90 days refrigerated.

Nahata MC, Pai VB, and Hipple TF, *Pediatric Drug Formulations*, 5th ed, Cincinnati, OH: Harvey Whitney Books Co, 2004.

Natalizumab (na ta LIZ u mab)

Brand Names: US Tysabri
Brand Names: Canada Tysabri
Index Terms AN100226; Anti-4 Alpha Integrin; IgG4-Kappa Monoclonal Antibody
Pharmacologic Category Gastrointestinal Agent, Miscellaneous; Monoclonal Antibody, Selective Adhesion-Molecule Inhibitor
Use
Crohn disease: For inducing and maintaining clinical response and remission in adult patients with moderately to severely active Crohn disease with evidence of inflammation who have had an inadequate response to, or are unable to tolerate, conventional Crohn disease therapies and inhibitors of tumor necrosis factor-alpha (TNF-alpha).
Multiple sclerosis: As monotherapy for the treatment of patients with relapsing forms of multiple sclerosis (MS). Natalizumab increases the risk of PML. When initiating and continuing treatment with natalizumab, consider whether the expected benefit of natalizumab is sufficient to offset this risk.
Canada labeling: Treatment of relapsing forms of multiple sclerosis in patients who have had an inadequate response to, or are unable to tolerate, other therapies for multiple sclerosis.

Prescribing and Access Restrictions
US: Tysabri is deemed to have an approved REMS program. As a requirement of the REMS program, access to this medication is restricted. Patients must be enrolled in the Tysabri Outreach Unified Commitment to Health (TOUCH™) Prescribing Program (800-456-2255) to receive natalizumab (MS-TOUCH™ for multiple sclerosis or CD-TOUCH™ for Crohn disease). Healthcare providers must also register with the program in order to prescribe, dispense or administer natalizumab. Treatment must be reauthorized every 6 months. Natalizumab is available only through infusion centers registered with the TOUCH™ program; infusion center information is available at 1-800-456-2255.

Canada: Patients receiving natalizumab therapy for multiple sclerosis are to be enrolled in the Biogen Idec ONE Program™ (855-676-6300). This program is associated with the prescribing, administration, and monitoring of Canadian patients receiving natalizumab. Clinicians are educated on the appropriate use of natalizumab and are expected to discuss the benefits/risks of therapy. Clinicians should evaluate patients every 6 months during treatment.

Medication Guide Available Yes
Dosing
Adult & Geriatric
Multiple sclerosis: IV: 300 mg infused over 1 hour every 4 weeks
Crohn disease: IV: 300 mg infused over 1 hour every 4 weeks; discontinue if therapeutic benefit is not observed within initial 12 weeks of therapy
Concomitant use with corticosteroids: For patients who begin treatment while on chronic oral corticosteroids, begin tapering oral steroids when the onset of natalizumab therapeutic benefit is observed; discontinue use if patient cannot be tapered off of oral corticosteroids within 6 months of therapy initiation. If additional concomitant corticosteroids are required and exceed 3 months/year (in addition to initial corticosteroid taper), consider discontinuing therapy.
Concomitant use with immunosuppressants (eg, azathioprine, cyclosporine, 6-mercaptopurine, or methotrexate) or inhibitors of TNF-alpha: Avoid concomitant use.
Renal Impairment There are no dosage adjustments provided in manufacturer's labeling (has not been studied).
Hepatic Impairment There are no dosage adjustments provided in manufacturer's labeling (has not been studied). Discontinue use with jaundice or signs/symptoms of hepatic injury.
Additional Information Complete prescribing information should be consulted for additional detail.
Dosage Forms Excipient information presented when available (limited, particularly for generics); consult specific product labeling.
Concentrate, Intravenous [preservative free]:
Tysabri: 300 mg/15 mL (15 mL) [contains polysorbate 80]

Natamycin (na ta MYE sin)

Brand Names: US Natacyn
Brand Names: Canada Natacyn®
Index Terms Pimaricin
Pharmacologic Category Antifungal Agent, Ophthalmic
Use Treatment of blepharitis, conjunctivitis, and keratitis caused by susceptible fungi (*Aspergillus, Candida, Cephalosporium, Fusarium,* and *Penicillium*)
Dosing
Adult & Geriatric
Fungal keratitis: Ophthalmic: Instill 1 drop in conjunctival sac every 1-2 hours, after 3-4 days reduce to one drop 6-8 times/day; usual course of therapy is 2-3 weeks or until resolution of active fungal keratitis (may be useful to gradually reduce dosage at 4-7 day intervals to assure elimination of organism)
Fungal blepharitis or conjunctivitis: Ophthalmic: Instill 1 drop in conjunctival sac every 4-6 hours
Renal Impairment No dosage adjustment provided in manufacturer's labeling. However, dosage adjustment unlikely due to low systemic absorption.
Hepatic Impairment No dosage adjustment provided in manufacturer's labeling. However, dosage adjustment unlikely due to low systemic absorption.
Additional Information Complete prescribing information should be consulted for additional detail.
Dosage Forms Excipient information presented when available (limited, particularly for generics); consult specific product labeling.
Suspension, Ophthalmic:
Natacyn: 5% (15 mL)

Nateglinide (na te GLYE nide)

Brand Names: US Starlix
Brand Names: Canada Starlix
Pharmacologic Category Antidiabetic Agent, Meglitinide Analog

◄ **Use Type 2 diabetes mellitus:** For the treatment of adults with type 2 diabetes mellitus as an adjunct to diet and exercise to improve glycemic control.

Pregnancy Considerations Adverse events have been observed in animal reproduction studies. Information describing the effects of nateglinide on pregnancy outcomes is limited (Twaites 2007).

In women with diabetes, maternal hyperglycemia can be associated with congenital malformations as well as adverse effects in the fetus, neonate, and the mother (ACOG 2005; ADA 2015; Kitzmiller 2008; Metzger 2007). To prevent adverse outcomes, prior to conception and throughout pregnancy maternal blood glucose and HbA$_{1c}$ should be kept as close to target goals as possible but without causing significant hypoglycemia (ACOG 2013; ADA 2015; Blumer 2013; Kitzmiller 2008). Prior to pregnancy, effective contraception should be used until glycemic control is achieved (Kitzmiller 2008). Other agents are currently recommended to treat diabetes in pregnant women (ACOG 2013; Blumer 2013).

Breast-Feeding Considerations It is not known if nateglinide is excreted in breast milk. Breast-feeding is not recommended by the manufacturer.

Contraindications Hypersensitivity to nateglinide or any component of the formulation; type 1 diabetes; diabetic ketoacidosis (this condition should be treated with insulin)

Warnings/Precautions Use with caution in patients with moderate-to-severe hepatic impairment. Use caution in severe renal dysfunction, elderly, malnourished, or patients with adrenal/pituitary dysfunction; may be more susceptible to glucose-lowering effects. All oral hypoglycemic agents are capable of producing hypoglycemia. Proper patient selection, dosage, and instructions to the patients are important to avoid hypoglycemic episodes. Ethanol may increase the risk of hypoglycemia; instruct patients to avoid ethanol. It may be necessary to discontinue nateglinide and administer insulin if the patient is exposed to stress (eg, fever, trauma, infection, surgery). Indicated for adjunctive therapy with metformin; not to be used as a substitute for metformin monotherapy. Combination treatment with sulfonylureas is not recommended (no additional benefit). Patients not adequately controlled on oral agents which stimulate insulin release (eg, glyburide) should not be switched to nateglinide or have nateglinide added to therapy.

Adverse Reactions As reported with nateglinide monotherapy:

>10%: Respiratory: Upper respiratory infection (11%)

1% to 10%:

Central nervous system: Dizziness (4%)

Endocrine & metabolic: Hypoglycemia (2%), increased uric acid, weight gain

Neuromuscular & skeletal: Arthropathy (3%)

Respiratory: Flu-like symptoms (4%)

Miscellaneous:Accidental injury (3%)

Postmarketing and/or case reports (Limited to important or life-threatening): Cholestatic hepatitis, hypersensitivity reactions (including pruritus, rash, urticaria), increased liver enzymes, jaundice

Drug Interactions

Metabolism/Transport Effects Substrate of CYP2C9 (major), CYP3A4 (major), SLCO1B1; **Note:** Assignment of Major/Minor substrate status based on clinically relevant drug interaction potential; **Inhibits** CYP2C9 (weak)

Avoid Concomitant Use

Avoid concomitant use of Nateglinide with any of the following: Conivaptan; Fusidic Acid (Systemic); Idelalisib

Increased Effect/Toxicity

Nateglinide may increase the levels/effects of: Hypoglycemia-Associated Agents

The levels/effects of Nateglinide may be increased by: Alpha-Lipoic Acid; Androgens; Antidiabetic Agents; Conivaptan; CYP2C9 Inhibitors (Moderate); CYP2C9 Inhibitors (Strong); CYP3A4 Inhibitors (Moderate); CYP3A4 Inhibitors (Strong); Dasatinib; Eltrombopag; Fosaprepitant; Fusidic Acid (Systemic); Herbs (Hypoglycemic Properties); Idelalisib; Ivacaftor; Luliconazole; MAO Inhibitors; Mifepristone; Netupitant; Osimertinib; Palbociclib; Pegvisomant; Quinolone Antibiotics; Salicylates; Selective Serotonin Reuptake Inhibitors; Simeprevir; Stiripentol; Teriflunomide

Decreased Effect

The levels/effects of Nateglinide may be decreased by: Bosentan; CYP2C9 Inducers (Strong); CYP3A4 Inducers (Moderate); CYP3A4 Inducers (Strong); Dabrafenib; Deferasirox; Enzalutamide; Hyperglycemia-Associated Agents; Mitotane; Osimertinib; Quinolone Antibiotics; Siltuximab; St Johns Wort; Thiazide Diuretics; Tocilizumab

Food Interactions Rate of absorption is decreased and T$_{max}$ is delayed when taken with food. Food does not affect AUC. Multiple peak plasma concentrations may be observed if fasting. Not affected by composition of meal. Management: Administer 1-30 minutes prior to meals.

Storage/Stability Store at 25°C (77°F); excursions are permitted between 15°C and 30°C (59°F and 86°F).

Mechanism of Action Nonsulfonylurea hypoglycemic agent which blocks ATP-dependent potassium channels, depolarizing the membrane and facilitating calcium entry through calcium channels. Increased intracellular calcium stimulates insulin release from the pancreatic beta cells. Nateglinide-induced insulin release is glucose-dependent.

Pharmacodynamics/Kinetics

Onset of action: Insulin secretion: ~20 minutes

Peak effect: 1 hour

Duration: 4 hours

Absorption: Rapid

Distribution: 10 L

Protein binding: 98%, primarily to albumin

Metabolism: Hepatic via hydroxylation followed by glucuronide conjugation via CYP2C9 (70%) and CYP3A4 (30%) to metabolites

Bioavailability: 73%

Half-life elimination: 1.5 hours

Time to peak: ≤1 hour

Excretion: Urine (83%, 16% as unchanged drug); feces (10%)

Dosing

Adult & Geriatric Management of type 2 diabetes mellitus: Oral: Initial and maintenance dose: 120 mg 3 times daily, 1-30 minutes before meals; may be given alone or in combination with metformin or a thiazolidinedione. Patients close to HbA$_{1c}$ goal at initiation of therapy may be started at 60 mg 3 times daily

Renal Impairment

Mild to moderate impairment: No dosage adjustment necessary.

Severe impairment: No dosage adjustment necessary. Use with caution; may be more susceptible to glucose-lowering effects.

Hepatic Impairment

Mild impairment (Child-Pugh class A): No dosage adjustment necessary.

Moderate to severe impairment (Child-Pugh class B or C): No dosage adjustment provided in manufacturers labeling. Use with caution; has not been studied.

Dietary Considerations Nateglinide should be taken 1-30 minutes prior to meals. Scheduled dose should not be taken if meal is missed to avoid hypoglycemia. Dietary modification based on ADA recommendations is a part of therapy. Decreases blood glucose concentration. Hypoglycemia may occur. Must be able to recognize symptoms of hypoglycemia (sweating, dizziness, palpitations, increased appetite, trembling).

Administration Administer 1-30 minutes prior to meals. Scheduled dose should not be administered if a meal is missed to avoid hypoglycemia.

Monitoring Parameters Monitor weight and lipid profile. Monitor fasting blood glucose (periodically) and glycosylated hemoglobin (HbA$_{1c}$) levels (every 3 months) with a goal of decreasing these levels towards the normal range. During dose adjustment, fasting glucose can be used to determine response.

Reference Range

Recommendations for glycemic control in nonpregnant adults with diabetes (ADA, 2015):

HbA$_{1c}$: <7% (a more aggressive [<6.5%] or less aggressive [<8%] HbA$_{1c}$ goal may be targeted based on patient-specific characteristics)

Preprandial capillary plasma glucose: 80 to 130 mg/dL

Peak postprandial capillary blood glucose: <180 mg/dL

Recommendations for glycemic control in pediatric (all age groups) patients with type 1 diabetes (ADA, 2015):

HbA$_{1c}$: <7.5% (individualization may be appropriate based on patient-specific characteristics; <7% is reasonable if it can be achieved without excessive hypoglycemia)

Preprandial capillary plasma glucose: 90 to 130 mg/dL

Bedtime and overnight capillary blood glucose: 90 to 150 mg/dL

Additional Information An increase in weight was seen in nateglinide monotherapy, which was not seen when used in combination with metformin.

Dosage Forms Excipient information presented when available (limited, particularly for generics); consult specific product labeling.

Tablet, Oral:

Starlix: 60 mg, 120 mg

Generic: 60 mg, 120 mg

◆ **Natesto** *see* Testosterone *on page 1766*

Nebivolol (ne BIV oh lole)

Brand Names: US Bystolic
Brand Names: Canada Bystolic
Index Terms Nebivolol Hydrochloride
Pharmacologic Category Antihypertensive; Beta-Blocker, Beta-1 Selective
Use

Hypertension: Treatment of hypertension, alone or in combination with other agents
Guideline recommendations:

Hypertension: The 2014 guideline for the management of high blood pressure in adults (Eighth Joint National Committee [JNC 8]) recommends initiation of pharmacologic treatment to lower blood pressure for the following patients (JNC8 [James 2013]):
• Patients ≥60 years of age, with systolic blood pressure (SBP) ≥150 mm Hg or diastolic blood pressure (DBP) ≥90 mm Hg. Goal of therapy is SBP <150 mm Hg and DBP <90 mm Hg.
• Patients <60 years of age, with SBP ≥140 mm Hg or DBP ≥90 mm Hg. Goal of therapy is SBP <140 mm Hg and DBP <90 mm Hg.
• Patients ≥18 years of age with diabetes, with SBP ≥140 mm Hg or DBP ≥90 mm Hg. Goal of therapy is SBP <140 mm Hg and DBP <90 mm Hg.
• Patients ≥18 years of age with chronic kidney disease (CKD), with SBP ≥140 mm Hg or DBP ≥90 mm Hg. Goal of therapy is SBP <140 mm Hg and DBP <90 mm Hg.
Chronic kidney disease (CKD) and hypertension: Regardless of race or diabetes status, the use of an ACE inhibitor (ACEI) or angiotensin receptor blocker (ARB) as initial therapy is recommended to improve kidney outcomes. In the general nonblack population (without CKD) including those with diabetes, initial antihypertensive treatment should consist of a thiazide-type diuretic, calcium channel blocker, ACEI, or ARB. In the general black population (without CKD) including those with diabetes, initial antihypertensive treatment should consist of a thiazide-type diuretic or a calcium channel blocker **instead of** an ACEI or ARB.
Coronary artery disease (CAD) and hypertension: The American Heart Association, American College of Cardiology, and American Society of Hypertension (AHA/ACC/ASH) 2015 scientific statement for the treatment of hypertension in patients with CAD recommends the use of a beta blocker as part of a regimen in patients with hypertension and chronic stable angina with a history of prior MI. A BP target of <140/90 mm Hg is reasonable for the secondary prevention of cardiovascular events. A lower target BP (<130/80 mm Hg) may be appropriate in some individuals with CAD, previous MI, stroke or transient ischemic attack, or CAD risk equivalents (AHA/ACC/ASH [Rosendorff 2015]).

Dosing
Adult & Geriatric
Hypertension: Oral:
US labeling: Initial: 5 mg once daily; if initial response is inadequate, may be increased at 2-week intervals to a maximum dose of 40 mg once daily; usual dosage range (ASH/ISH [Weber, 2014]): 5 to 10 mg once daily
Canadian labeling: Initial: 5 mg once daily; if initial response is inadequate, may be increased at 2-week intervals to a maximum dose of 20 mg once daily; usual dosage range (ASH/ISH [Weber, 2014]): 5 to 10 mg once daily

Renal Impairment
CrCl 50 to 80 mL/minute: There are no dosage adjustments provided in the manufacturer's labeling; however, dose adjustment does not appear necessary. Following a single 5 mg dose in patients with CrCl 50 to 80 mL/minute, nebivolol clearance was unchanged.
CrCl 30 to 50 mL/minute: There are no dosage adjustments provided in the manufacturer's labeling; however, dose adjustment is likely not necessary. Following a single 5 mg dose in patients with moderate impairment, reduction in nebivolol clearance was negligible (~17%) (Shaw 2005).
CrCl <30 mL/minute: Initial: 2.5 mg once daily; if initial response is inadequate, may increase cautiously.
Hemodialysis: There are no dosage adjustments provided in the manufacturer's labeling (has not been studied). Due to lack of data, the Canadian labeling does not recommend use.

Hepatic Impairment
Mild impairment (Child-Pugh class A): There are no dosage adjustments provided in the manufacturer's labeling; use caution.
Moderate impairment (Child-Pugh class B): Initial: 2.5 mg once daily; if initial response is inadequate, may increase cautiously
Severe impairment (Child-Pugh class C): Use is contraindicated.

Additional Information Complete prescribing information should be consulted for additional detail.

Dosage Forms Excipient information presented when available (limited, particularly for generics); consult specific product labeling.
Tablet, Oral:
Bystolic: 2.5 mg, 5 mg, 10 mg, 20 mg [contains fd&c blue #2 aluminum lake, fd&c yellow #6 aluminum lake, polysorbate 80]

Necitumumab (ne si TOOM oo mab)

Brand Names: US Portrazza
Index Terms Anti-EGFR Monoclonal Antibody IMC-11F8; IMC-11F8; Portrazza
Pharmacologic Category Antineoplastic Agent, Epidermal Growth Factor Receptor (EGFR) Inhibitor; Antineoplastic Agent, Monoclonal Antibody
Use

Non-small cell lung cancer (squamous), metastatic: First-line treatment of metastatic squamous non-small cell lung cancer (NSCLC) in combination with gemcitabine and cisplatin
Limitations of use: Not indicated for treatment of non-squamous cell lung cancer.

Pregnancy Considerations Necitumumab is expected to cross the placenta. Based on animal data and the mechanism of action, necitumumab is expected to cause fetal harm if administered during pregnancy. Women of reproductive potential should use effective contraception during therapy and for 3 months after the last dose.

Breast-Feeding Considerations It is not known if necitumumab is excreted into breast milk; however, human IgG antibodies can be detected in breast milk. Due to the potential for serious adverse reactions in the nursing infant, breast-feeding is not recommended by the manufacturer during therapy or for 3 months after the last dose.

Contraindications There are no contraindications listed in the manufacturer's labeling.

Warnings/Precautions [US Boxed Warning]: Cardiopulmonary arrest and/or sudden death occurred in a small percentage of patients treated with necitumumab in combination with gemcitabine and cisplatin. Monitor serum electrolytes closely, including serum magnesium, potassium, and calcium, with aggressive replacement when warranted during and after necitumumab administration. Continue electrolyte monitoring for at least 8 weeks after the last dose. Some cardiopulmonary events were fatal; many of those patients had comorbid conditions (including a history of coronary artery disease). Patients with significant coronary artery disease, MI within 6 months, uncontrolled hypertension or uncontrolled heart failure were excluded from the squamous cell non-small cell lung cancer study. **[US Boxed Warning]: Hypomagnesemia occurred in a majority of patients receiving necitumumab in combination with gemcitabine and cisplatin; hypomagnesemia was severe in one-fifth of patients. Monitor for hypomagnesemia, hypocalcemia, and hypokalemia prior to each dose of necitumumab during treatment and for at least 8 weeks following completion of necitumumab. Withhold necitumumab for Grade 3 or 4 electrolyte abnormalities. Replete electrolytes as appropriate.** May resume treatment when hypomagnesemia and related electrolyte abnormalities are improved to grade 2 or lower. The median time to development of hypomagnesemia was 6 weeks after treatment initiation.

Dermatologic toxicity, including rash, dermatitis anceiform, acne, dry skin, pruritus, generalized rash, skin fissures, maculo-papular rash, and/or erythema occurs commonly; may be severe. Skin toxicity usually developed within the first 2 weeks of treatment and resolved within 17 weeks after onset. May require treatment interruption, dose reduction, or discontinuation. Patients should minimize exposure to the sun. Infusion-related reactions have been reported with necitumumab, usually after the first or second infusion. Premedication was not routinely administered prior to the first dose in the squamous cell NSCLC study. Monitor for signs/symptoms of infusion reaction. Discontinue for serious or life-threatening reactions. Venous and arterial thromboembolic events (VTE and ATE) were observed with necitumumab, including grades 3 and 4 events. The most common VTEs were deep vein thrombosis and pulmonary embolism and the most common ATEs were cerebral stroke and ischemia and MI. Discontinue necitumumab for serious or life-threatening VTE or ATE. The incidence of VTE may be higher in patients ≥70 years of age (compared to patients under age 70).

Necitumumab is not indicated for use in patients with nonsquamous NSCLC. In a study of necitumumab in combination with pemetrexed and cisplatin for the treatment of metastatic non-squamous NSCLC, patients experienced increased serious and fatal toxicities and cardiopulmonary arrest/sudden death within 30 days of the last dose of necitumumab (compared to pemetrexed and cisplatin without necitumumab).

Adverse Reactions Adverse reaction percentages reported as part of a combination regimen with gemcitabine and cisplatin.

>10%:

Central nervous system: Headache (11%)

Dermatologic: Skin toxicity (79%; grades 3/4: 8%), skin rash (44%; grades 3/4: 4%), acneiform eruption (15%; grades 3/4: 1%)

Endocrine & metabolic: Hypomagnesemia (43% to 83%; grades 3/4: 20%), hypocalcemia (45%; grades 3/4: 6%; with albumin corrected: 36%; grades 3/4: 4%), hypophosphatemia (31%; grades 3/4: 8%), hypokalemia (28%; grades 3/4: 5%), weight loss (13%)

Gastrointestinal: Vomiting (29%), diarrhea (16%), stomatitis (11%)

1% to 10%:

Cardiovascular: Venous thromboembolism (9%; grades 3/4: 5%), arterial thromboembolism (5%; grades 3/4: 4%), pulmonary embolism (5%), cardiorespiratory arrest (3%), deep vein thrombosis (2%), cerebrovascular accident (≤2%), ischemia (≤2%), myocardial infarction (1%)

Dermatologic: Acne vulgaris (9%), paronychia (7%), pruritus (7%), xeroderma (7%), skin fissure (5%)

Immunologic: Antibody development (4%; neutralizing: 1%)

Ophthalmic: Conjunctivitis (7%)

Respiratory: Hemoptysis (10%)

Miscellaneous: Infusion related reaction (2%; grade 3: <1%)

Drug Interactions

Metabolism/Transport Effects None known.

Avoid Concomitant Use There are no known interactions where it is recommended to avoid concomitant use.

Increased Effect/Toxicity There are no known significant interactions involving an increase in effect.

Decreased Effect There are no known significant interactions involving a decrease in effect.

Preparation for Administration Dilute for infusion in sodium chloride 0.9% to a total volume of 250 mL (do not use solutions containing dextrose). Gently invert to mix; do not shake.

Storage/Stability Store intact vials at 2°C to 8°C (36°F to 46°F). Do not freeze. Store in original carton to protect from light. Do not shake. Solutions diluted for infusion are stable for up to 4 hours at room temperature or 24 hours at 2°C to 8°C (36°F to 46°F); do not freeze or shake.

Mechanism of Action Necitumumab is a recombinant human IgG1 EGFR monoclonal antibody which binds (with a high affinity) to the ligand binding site of the EGFR receptor to prevent receptor activation and downstream signaling (Thatcher 2015).

Pharmacodynamics/Kinetics

Distribution: V_{dss}: 7 L

Half-life elimination: ~14 days

Dosing

Adult & Geriatric Note: For patients with a prior grade 1 or 2 infusion reaction, premedicate (prior to all subsequent necitumumab infusions) with diphenhydramine (or equivalent). For patients with a recurrent grade 1 or 2 infusion reaction, premedicate (prior to all subsequent necitumumab infusions) with diphenhydramine (or equivalent), acetaminophen, and dexamethasone (or equivalent).

Non-small cell lung cancer (squamous), metastatic: IV: 800 mg on days 1 and 8 of each 3-week treatment cycle (in combination with gemcitabine and cisplatin); continue until disease progression or unacceptable toxicity (Thatcher 2015).

In the study, gemcitabine and cisplatin were administered for a maximum of 6 cycles, while patients without disease progression continued necitumumab as single agent therapy (Thatcher 2015).

Renal Impairment There are no dosage adjustments provided in the manufacturer's labeling; however, based on pharmacokinetics, dosage adjustment is not likely necessary.

Hepatic Impairment

Mild to moderate impairment: There are no dosage adjustments provided in the manufacturer's labeling; however, based on pharmacokinetics, dosage adjustment is not likely necessary.

Severe impairment: There is no dosage adjustment provided in the manufacturer's labeling (has not been studied).

Adjustment for Toxicity

Dermatologic toxicity:

Grade 3 rash or acneiform rash: Withhold treatment until symptoms resolve to grade 2 or lower, then resume necitumumab with the dose reduced to 400 mg for at least 1 treatment cycle. If symptoms do not worsen, may increase the dose to 600 mg and then 800 mg in subsequent cycles.

Grade 3 rash or acneiform rash that does not resolve to grade 2 or lower within 6 weeks: Permanently discontinue.

Grade 3 rash or acneiform rash that worsens or is intolerable at the 400 mg dose: Permanently discontinue.

Grade 3 skin induration/fibrosis: Permanently discontinue.

Grade 4 dermatologic toxicity: Permanently discontinue.

Electrolyte abnormality: Grade 3 or 4 electrolyte abnormality: Withhold treatment; may resume when electrolyte abnormality has improved to grade 2 or lower (replete electrolytes as appropriate).

Infusion-related reactions:

Grade 1: Reduce infusion rate by 50%.

Grade 2: Interrupt infusion until signs/symptoms have resolved to grade 1 or 0, then resume with the rate reduced by 50% for all subsequent infusions.

Grade 3 or 4: Permanently discontinue.

Thromboembolic events: Serious or life-threatening VTE or ATE: Discontinue treatment.

Administration

IV: Infuse over 60 minutes using an infusion pump. Infuse through a separate line. Flush with sodium chloride 0.9% at the end of infusion. Monitor for infusion reactions; reduce infusion rate by 50% for grade 1 infusion reaction; interrupt infusion for grade 2 infusion reaction.

Necitumumab should be administered prior to gemcitabine and cisplatin (Thatcher 2015).

Monitoring Parameters Serum electrolytes, including magnesium, potassium, and calcium (prior to each dose during treatment and for at least 8 weeks following completion). Signs/symptoms of infusion-related reactions, dermatologic toxicity, and thromboembolism.

Dosage Forms Excipient information presented when available (limited, particularly for generics); consult specific product labeling.

Solution, Intravenous [preservative free]:

Portrazza: 800 mg/50 mL (50 mL) [contains mouse protein (murine) (hamster), polysorbate 80]

◆ Necon 0.5/35 *see* Ethinyl Estradiol and Norethindrone *on page 708*

◆ Necon 1/35 *see* Ethinyl Estradiol and Norethindrone *on page 708*

◆ Necon 1/50 *see* Norethindrone and Mestranol *on page 1300*

◆ Necon 7/7/7 *see* Ethinyl Estradiol and Norethindrone *on page 708*

◆ Necon 10/11 *see* Ethinyl Estradiol and Norethindrone *on page 708*

Nedocromil (ne doe KROE mil)

Brand Names: US Alocril
Brand Names: Canada Alocril®
Index Terms Nedocromil Sodium
Pharmacologic Category Mast Cell Stabilizer
Use Treatment of itching associated with allergic conjunctivitis
Dosing

Adult & Geriatric Allergic conjunctivitis: Ophthalmic: 1-2 drops in each eye twice daily throughout the period of exposure to allergen

Pediatric Allergic conjunctivitis: Ophthalmic: Children ≥3 years: Refer to adult dosing.

Renal Impairment No dosage adjustment provided in manufacturer's labeling. However, dosage adjustment unlikely due to low systemic absorption.

Hepatic Impairment No dosage adjustment provided in manufacturer's labeling. However, dosage adjustment unlikely due to low systemic absorption.

Additional Information Complete prescribing information should be consulted for additional detail.

Dosage Forms Excipient information presented when available (limited, particularly for generics); consult specific product labeling.

Solution, Ophthalmic, as sodium:

Alocril: 2% (5 mL) [contains benzalkonium chloride]

◆ Nedocromil Sodium *see* Nedocromil *on page 1265*

Nefazodone (nef AY zoe done)

Index Terms Nefazodone Hydrochloride; Serzone
Pharmacologic Category Antidepressant, Serotonin Reuptake Inhibitor/Antagonist
Use Depression: Treatment of depression
Medication Guide Available Yes
Dosing

Adult

Depression: Oral: Initial: 100 mg twice daily; alternatively depression treatment guidelines suggest starting doses of 50 to 100 mg daily (APA, 2010; Bauer 2013). Based on response and tolerability, gradually increase dose in increments of 100 to 200 mg daily (in 2 divided doses) and intervals of no less than 1 week to a usual dose of 150 to 600 mg daily in 2 divided doses

Discontinuation of therapy: Upon discontinuation of antidepressant therapy, gradually taper the dose to minimize the incidence of withdrawal symptoms and allow for the detection of re-emerging symptoms. Evidence supporting ideal taper rates is limited. APA and NICE guidelines suggest tapering therapy over at least several weeks with consideration to the half-life of the antidepressant; antidepressants with a shorter half-life may need to be tapered more conservatively. In addition for long-term treated patients, WFSBP guidelines recommend tapering over 4 to 6 months. If intolerable withdrawal symptoms occur following a dose reduction, consider resuming the previously prescribed dose and/ or decrease dose at a more gradual rate (APA, 2010; Bauer, 2002; Haddad, 2001; NCCMH, 2010; Schatzberg, 2006; Shelton, 2001; Warner, 2006).

MAO inhibitor recommendations:

Switching to or from an MAO inhibitor intended to treat psychiatric disorders:

Allow 14 days to elapse between discontinuing an MAO inhibitor intended to treat psychiatric disorders and initiation of nefazodone.

Allow 14 days to elapse between discontinuing nefazodone and initiation of an MAO inhibitor intended to treat psychiatric disorders.

Use with other MAO inhibitors (such as linezolid or IV methylene blue):

Do not initiate nefazodone in patients receiving linezolid or IV methylene blue; consider other interventions for psychiatric condition.

If urgent treatment with linezolid or IV methylene blue is required in a patient already receiving nefazodone and potential benefits outweigh potential risks, discontinue nefazodone promptly and administer linezolid or IV methylene blue. Monitor for serotonin syndrome for 2 weeks or until 24 hours after the last dose of linezolid or IV methylene blue, whichever comes first. May resume nefazodone 24 hours after the last dose of linezolid or IV methylene blue.

Geriatric Depression: Oral: Initial: 50 mg twice daily; gradually increase dose based on response and tolerability

Discontinuation of therapy: Refer to adult dosing.

MAO inhibitor recommendations: Refer to adult dosing.

Renal Impairment There are no dosage adjustments provided in the manufacturer's labeling; however, adjustment unlikely since renal impairment does not alter steady state nefazodone plasma concentrations.

Hepatic Impairment There are no dosage adjustments provided in the manufacturer's labeling; however, use with caution since the AUC of nefazodone and its metabolites are ~25% greater in patients with cirrhosis.

Additional Information Complete prescribing information should be consulted for additional detail.

Dosage Forms Excipient information presented when available (limited, particularly for generics); consult specific product labeling.

Tablet, Oral, as hydrochloride:

Generic: 50 mg, 100 mg, 150 mg, 200 mg, 250 mg

◆ Nefazodone Hydrochloride *see* Nefazodone *on page 1265*

Nelarabine (nel AY re been)

Brand Names: US Arranon
Brand Names: Canada Atriance
Index Terms 2-Amino-6-Methoxypurine Arabinoside; 506U78; GW506U78
Pharmacologic Category Antineoplastic Agent, Antimetabolite; Antineoplastic Agent, Antimetabolite (Purine Analog)
Use T-cell acute lymphoblastic leukemia/lymphoma: Treatment of relapsed or refractory T-cell acute lymphoblastic leukemia/lymphoma following at least 2 chemotherapy regimens.
Dosing

Adult & Geriatric T-cell acute lymphoblastic leukemia/lymphoma: IV: 1,500 mg/m²/dose on days 1, 3, and 5; repeat every 21 days until a transplant candidate, disease progression, or unacceptable toxicity.

Pediatric T-cell acute lymphoblastic leukemia/lymphoma: IV: 650 mg/m²/dose on days 1 through 5; repeat every 21 days until a transplant candidate, disease progression, or unacceptable toxicity.

Renal Impairment

CrCl ≥50 mL/minute: No dosage adjustment necessary.

CrCl <50 mL/minute: There are no dosage adjustments provided in the manufacturer's labeling, (although ARA-G clearance is decreased as renal function declines, data is insufficient for a dosing recommendation); monitor closely.

Hepatic Impairment There are no dosage adjustments provided in the manufacturer's labeling (has not been studied); closely monitor with severe impairment (total bilirubin >3 times ULN).

Adjustment for Toxicity

Neurologic toxicity ≥ grade 2: Discontinue treatment.

Hematologic or other (non-neurologic) toxicity: Consider treatment delay.

Additional Information Complete prescribing information should be consulted for additional detail.

Dosage Forms Excipient information presented when available (limited, particularly for generics); consult specific product labeling.

Solution, Intravenous:

Arranon: 5 mg/mL (50 mL)

◄ **Dosage Forms: Canada** Excipient information presented when available (limited, particularly for generics); consult specific product labeling.

Injection, solution:

Atriance: 5 mg/mL (50 mL)

Nelfinavir (nel FIN a veer)

Brand Names: US Viracept
Brand Names: Canada Viracept
Index Terms NFV
Pharmacologic Category Antiretroviral, Protease Inhibitor (Anti-HIV)
Use In combination with other antiretroviral therapy in the treatment of HIV infection

Dosing

Adult & Geriatric HIV infection: Oral: 750 mg 3 times daily or 1250 mg twice daily with meals in combination with other antiretroviral therapies. **Note:** The HHS Perinatal HIV Guidelines do not recommend the 3-times-daily dosing in pregnant women (HHS [perinatal] 2014).

Pediatric

HIV infection: Oral:

Children 2 to <13 years:

U.S. labeling:

Weight-directed dosing: 45 to 55 mg/kg twice daily or 25 to 35 mg/kg 3 times daily (maximum: 2500 mg daily)

Fixed dosing:

10 to 12 kg: 500 mg (2 tablets) twice daily **or** 250 mg (1 tablet) 3 times daily

13 to 18 kg: 750 mg (3 tablets) twice daily **or** 500 mg (2 tablets) 3 times daily

19 to 20 kg: 1000 mg (4 tablets) twice daily **or** 500 mg (2 tablets) 3 times daily

>20 kg: 1000 to 1250 mg (4 to 5 tablets) twice daily **or** 750 mg (3 tablets) 3 times daily

Canadian labeling: 25 to 30 mg/kg 3 times daily (maximum: 2500 mg daily).

Adolescents: Refer to adult dosing.

Renal Impairment There are no dosage adjustments provided in the manufacturer's labeling (has not been studied). However, since <2% excreted in urine a dosage reduction would not be expected. Guidelines suggest that no dosage adjustment is necessary (HHS [adult] 2015).

Hepatic Impairment

U.S. labeling:

Mild impairment (Child-Pugh class A): No dosage adjustment necessary.

Moderate to severe impairment (Child-Pugh class B or C): Use not recommended.

Canadian labeling: There is no dosage adjustment provided in the manufacturer's labeling; use with caution.

Additional Information Complete prescribing information should be consulted for additional detail.

Dosage Forms Excipient information presented when available (limited, particularly for generics); consult specific product labeling.

Tablet, Oral:

Viracept: 250 mg, 625 mg

◆ Nembutal *see* PENTobarbital *on page 1426*

◆ Nembutal Sodium (Can) *see* PENTobarbital *on page 1426*

◆ NeoCeuticals Post-Acne Fade [OTC] *see* Hydroquinone *on page 893*

◆ Neo DM [OTC] [DSC] *see* Chlorpheniramine, Phenylephrine, and Dextromethorphan *on page 378*

◆ Neo-Fradin [DSC] *see* Neomycin *on page 1266*

Neomycin (nee oh MYE sin)

Brand Names: US Neo-Fradin [DSC]
Index Terms Neomycin Sulfate
Pharmacologic Category Ammonium Detoxicant; Antibiotic, Aminoglycoside; Antibiotic, Topical

Use

Hepatic coma (portal-systemic encephalopathy): Adjunctive therapy in hepatic coma.

Surgical (perioperative) prophylaxis: Adjunctive therapy as part of a regimen for the suppression of the normal bacterial bowel flora (eg, preoperative bowel preparation), given concomitantly with enteric-coated erythromycin base.

Dosing

Adult & Geriatric

Surgical (perioperative) prophylaxis: Oral:

Manufacturer's labeling: 1 g at 1 PM, 2 PM, and 11 PM on the day preceding 8 AM surgery as an adjunct to mechanical cleansing of the bowel and oral erythromycin

Alternative recommendation: 1 g at 1 PM, 2 PM, and 11 PM on the day preceding 8 AM surgery combined with mechanical cleansing of the large intestine and oral erythromycin or metronidazole, and IV antibiotics on the day of surgery (Bratzler, 2013)

Hepatic encephalopathy: Oral: 4 to 12 g daily divided every 4 to 6 hours for 5 to 6 days

Chronic hepatic insufficiency: Oral: 4 g daily for an indefinite period

Pediatric

Surgical (perioperative) prophylaxis: Children and Adolescents: Oral: 15 mg/kg/dose for 3 doses administered over 10 hours (eg, at 1 PM, 2 PM, and 11 PM) on the the day preceding surgery; maximum dose: 1,000 mg; (Bratzler, 2013); used as an adjunct to mechanical cleansing of the intestine and in combination with erythromycin base or metronidazole and perioperative IV antibiotics

Renal Impairment There are no dosage adjustments provided in manufacturer's labeling; however, dosage reduction or discontinuation of therapy should be considered if a patient develops renal insufficiency. The risk of nephro- and/or ototoxicity is increased in patients with renal impairment.

Hepatic Impairment There are no dosage adjustments provided in manufacturer's labeling.

Additional Information Complete prescribing information should be consulted for additional detail.

Dosage Forms Excipient information presented when available (limited, particularly for generics); consult specific product labeling. [DSC] = Discontinued product

Solution, Oral, as sulfate:

Neo-Fradin: 25 mg/mL (480 mL [DSC])

Tablet, Oral, as sulfate:

Generic: 500 mg

Neomycin and Polymyxin B
(nee oh MYE sin & pol i MIKS in bee)

Brand Names: US Neosporin® G.U. Irrigant
Brand Names: Canada Neosporin® Irrigating Solution
Index Terms Polymyxin B and Neomycin
Pharmacologic Category Antibiotic, Topical; Genitourinary Irrigant
Use Short-term as a continuous irrigant or rinse in the urinary bladder to prevent bacteriuria and gram-negative rod septicemia associated with the use of indwelling catheters

Dosing

Adult & Geriatric Bladder irrigation: **Not for IV injection;** add 1 mL irrigant to 1 L isotonic saline solution and connect container to the inflow of lumen of 3-way catheter. Continuous irrigant or rinse in the urinary bladder for up to a maximum of 10 days with administration rate adjusted to patient's urine output; usually no more than 1 L of irrigant is used per day.

Pediatric Refer to adult dosing.

Additional Information Complete prescribing information should be consulted for additional detail.

Dosage Forms Excipient information presented when available (limited, particularly for generics); consult specific product labeling.

Solution, irrigation: Neomycin 40 mg and polymyxin B sulfate 200,000 units per 1 mL (1 mL, 20 mL)

Neosporin® G.U. Irrigant: Neomycin 40 mg and polymyxin sulfate B 200,000 units per 1 mL (1 mL, 20 mL)

◆ Neomycin, Bacitracin, and Polymyxin B *see* Bacitracin, Neomycin, and Polymyxin B (Ophthalmic) *on page 196*

◆ Neomycin, Bacitracin, and Polymyxin B *see* Bacitracin, Neomycin, and Polymyxin B (Topical) *on page 197*

◆ Neomycin, Bacitracin, Polymyxin B, and Hydrocortisone *see* Bacitracin, Neomycin, Polymyxin B, and Hydrocortisone (Ophthalmic) *on page 197*

◆ Neomycin, Bacitracin, Polymyxin B, and Hydrocortisone *see* Bacitracin, Neomycin, Polymyxin B, and Hydrocortisone (Topical) *on page 197*

Neomycin, Colistin, Hydrocortisone, and Thonzonium
(nee oh MYE sin, koe LIS tin, hye droe KOR ti sone, & thon ZOE nee um)

Brand Names: US Coly-Mycin® S; Cortisporin®-TC

Index Terms Colistin, Hydrocortisone, Neomycin, and Thonzonium; Hydrocortisone, Neomycin, Colistin, and Thonzonium; Thonzonium, Neomycin, Colistin, and Hydrocortisone

Pharmacologic Category Antibiotic, Otic; Antibiotic/Corticosteroid, Otic; Corticosteroid, Otic

Use Treatment of superficial and susceptible bacterial infections of the external auditory canal; for treatment of susceptible bacterial infections of mastoidectomy and fenestration cavities

Dosing

Adult & Geriatric Ear inflammation/infection: Otic:
Calibrated dropper: 5 drops in affected ear 3-4 times/day
Dropper bottle: 4 drops in affected ear 3-4 times/day
Note: Alternatively, a cotton wick may be inserted in the ear canal and saturated with suspension every 4 hours; wick should be replaced at least every 24 hours

Pediatric Ear inflammation/infection: Otic:
Calibrated dropper: 4 drops in affected ear 3-4 times/day
Dropper bottle: 3 drops in affected ear 3-4 times/day
Note: Alternatively, a cotton wick may be inserted in the ear canal and saturated with suspension every 4 hours; wick should be replaced at least every 24 hours

Renal Impairment No dosage adjustment provided in manufacturer's labeling. However, dosage adjustment unlikely due to low systemic absorption.

Hepatic Impairment No dosage adjustment provided in manufacturer's labeling. However, dosage adjustment unlikely due to low systemic absorption.

Additional Information Complete prescribing information should be consulted for additional detail.

Dosage Forms Excipient information presented when available (limited, particularly for generics); consult specific product labeling.
Suspension, otic [drops]:
Coly-Mycin® S: Neomycin 0.33%, colistin 0.3%, hydrocortisone acetate 1%, and thonzonium bromide 0.05% (5 mL) [contains thimerosal]
Cortisporin®-TC: Neomycin 0.33%, colistin 0.3%, hydrocortisone acetate 1%, and thonzonium bromide 0.05% (10 mL) [contains thimerosal]

Neomycin, Polymyxin B, and Dexamethasone
(nee oh MYE sin, pol i MIKS in bee, & deks a METH a sone)

Brand Names: US Maxitrol

Brand Names: Canada Dioptrol; Maxitrol

Index Terms Dexamethasone, Neomycin, and Polymyxin B; Polymyxin B, Neomycin, and Dexamethasone

Pharmacologic Category Antibiotic/Corticosteroid, Ophthalmic

Use Inflammatory ocular conditions: Management of corticosteroid-responsive inflammatory ocular conditions where bacterial infection or a risk of bacterial infection exists

Dosing

Adult & Geriatric

Inflammatory ocular conditions: Ophthalmic:
Suspension: Instill 1 to 2 drops into the conjunctival sac of the affected eye(s) 4 to 6 times daily. In severe disease, drops may be used hourly; frequency should decrease as signs and symptoms improve.
Ointment: Place ~1/2" ribbon in the conjunctival sac of the affected eye(s) 3 to 4 times daily
Note: If signs and symptoms do not improve after 2 days of treatment, the patient should be reevaluated.

Pediatric Inflammatory ocular conditions: Children ≥2 years and Adolescents: Ophthalmic: Suspension: Refer to adult dosing.

Renal Impairment There are no dosage adjustments provided in the manufacturer's labeling. However, dosage adjustment unlikely due to insignificant systemic absorption.

Hepatic Impairment There are no dosage adjustments provided in the manufacturer's labeling. However, dosage adjustment unlikely due to insignificant systemic absorption.

Additional Information Complete prescribing information should be consulted for additional detail.

Dosage Forms Excipient information presented when available (limited, particularly for generics); consult specific product labeling.
Ointment, ophthalmic: Neomycin 3.5 mg, polymyxin B sulfate 10,000 units, and dexamethasone 0.1% per g (3.5 g)
Maxitrol®: Neomycin 3.5 mg, polymyxin B sulfate 10,000 units, and dexamethasone 0.1% per g (3.5 g)

Suspension, ophthalmic [drops]: Neomycin 3.5 mg, polymyxin B sulfate 10,000 units, and dexamethasone 0.1% per 1 mL (5 mL)
Maxitrol®: Neomycin 3.5 mg, polymyxin B sulfate 10,000 units, and dexamethasone 0.1% per 1 mL (5 mL) [contains benzalkonium chloride]

Neomycin, Polymyxin B, and Gramicidin
(nee oh MYE sin, pol i MIKS in bee, & gram i SYE din)

Brand Names: US Neosporin® Ophthalmic Solution

Brand Names: Canada Neosporin®; Optimyxin Plus®

Index Terms Gramicidin, Neomycin, and Polymyxin B; Polymyxin B, Neomycin, and Gramicidin

Pharmacologic Category Antibiotic, Ophthalmic

Use Treatment of superficial ocular infection

Dosing

Adult & Geriatric Ophthalmic: Instill 1-2 drops 4-6 times/day or more frequently as required for severe infections
Pediatric Refer to adult dosing.

Additional Information Complete prescribing information should be consulted for additional detail.

Dosage Forms Excipient information presented when available (limited, particularly for generics); consult specific product labeling.
Solution, ophthalmic [drops]: Neomycin 1.75 mg, polymyxin B 10,000 units, and gramicidin 0.025 mg per 1 mL (10 mL)
Neosporin® Ophthalmic Solution: Neomycin 1.75 mg, polymyxin B 10,000 units, and gramicidin 0.025 mg per 1 mL (10 mL)

Neomycin, Polymyxin B, and Hydrocortisone (Ophthalmic)
(nee oh MYE sin, pol i MIKS in bee, & hye droe KOR ti sone)

Brand Names: Canada Cortimyxin

Index Terms Hydrocortisone, Neomycin, and Polymyxin B; Polymyxin B, Neomycin, and Hydrocortisone

Pharmacologic Category Antibiotic, Ophthalmic; Antibiotic/Corticosteroid, Ophthalmic; Corticosteroid, Ophthalmic

Use Ocular inflammatory conditions: Management of steroid-responsive inflammatory ocular conditions where bacterial infection or a risk of bacterial infection exists

Dosing

Adult & Geriatric Ocular inflammatory conditions: Ophthalmic: Instill 1 to 2 drops into affected eye(s) every 3 to 4 hours, or more frequently as required for severe infections Reevaluate patient if improvement not observed after 2 days of therapy. Monitor IOP if therapy exceeds 10 days

Pediatric Ocular inflammatory conditions: Children (off-label use): Ophthalmic: Instill 1 to 2 drops 3 to 4 hours into affected eye(s) has been used by some centers; dosing based on experience with other combination ophthalmic products with similar ingredients

Renal Impairment There are no dosage adjustments provided in the manufacturer's labeling. However, dosage adjustment unlikely due to low systemic absorption.

Hepatic Impairment There are no dosage adjustments provided in the manufacturer's labeling. However, dosage adjustment unlikely due to low systemic absorption.

Additional Information Complete prescribing information should be consulted for additional detail.

Dosage Forms Excipient information presented when available (limited, particularly for generics); consult specific product labeling.
Suspension, Ophthalmic:
Generic: 3.5-10000-1 (7.5 mL)

Neomycin, Polymyxin B, and Hydrocortisone (Otic)
(nee oh MYE sin, pol i MIKS in bee, & hye droe KOR ti sone)

Brand Names: US Cortisporin

Brand Names: Canada Cortimyxin; Cortisporin Otic

Index Terms Hydrocortisone, Neomycin, and Polymyxin B; Polymyxin B, Neomycin, and Hydrocortisone

Pharmacologic Category Antibiotic, Otic; Antibiotic/Corticosteroid, Otic; Corticosteroid, Otic

Use Otic infections: Treatment of superficial bacterial infections of the external auditory canal (otitis externa); treatment of infections of mastoidectomy and fenestration cavities (suspension only)

Dosing

Adult & Geriatric Note: Duration of use should be limited to 10 days unless otherwise directed by the health care provider.
Otic infections: Otic: Instill 4 drops 3 to 4 times daily; otic suspension is the preferred otic preparation.

Pediatric Note: Duration of use should be limited to 10 days unless otherwise directed by the health care provider.

Otic infections: Children ≥2 years and Adolescents: Otic: Instill 3 drops 3 to 4 times daily

Renal Impairment There are no dosage adjustments provided in the manufacturer's labeling. However, dosage adjustment unlikely due to low systemic absorption.

Hepatic Impairment There are no dosage adjustments provided in the manufacturer's labeling. However, dosage adjustment unlikely due to low systemic absorption.

Additional Information Complete prescribing information should be consulted for additional detail.

Dosage Forms Excipient information presented when available (limited, particularly for generics); consult specific product labeling.

Solution, Otic:
Cortisporin: 3.5-10000-1 (10 mL) [contains potassium metabisulfite]
Generic: Neomycin 3.5 mg, polymyxin B 10,000 units, and hydrocortisone 10 mg per 1 mL (10 mL)

Suspension, Otic:
Generic: 3.5-10000-1 (10 mL); Neomycin 3.5 mg, polymyxin B 10,000 units, and hydrocortisone 10 mg per 1 mL (10 mL)

Neomycin, Polymyxin B, and Hydrocortisone (Topical)
(nee oh MYE sin, pol i MIKS in bee, & hye droe KOR ti sone)

Brand Names: US Cortisporin
Brand Names: Canada Cortimyxin
Index Terms Hydrocortisone, Neomycin, and Polymyxin B; Polymyxin B, Neomycin, and Hydrocortisone
Pharmacologic Category Antibiotic, Topical; Antibiotic/Corticosteroid, Topical; Corticosteroid, Topical
Use Corticosteroid-responsive dermatoses with secondary infection: Treatment of corticosteroid-responsive dermatoses with secondary infection.
Dosing

Adult & Geriatric Corticosteroid-responsive dermatoses with secondary infection: Topical: Apply a thin layer 2 to 4 times daily. Therapy should be discontinued when control is achieved; if no improvement is seen, reassessment of diagnosis may be necessary

Pediatric Corticosteroid-responsive dermatoses with secondary infection: Topical: Children and Adolescents (off-label use): Some centers have used one application (a thin layer to affected areas) 2 to 4 times daily for up to 7 days. Therapy should be discontinued when control is achieved or after 7 days.

Renal Impairment There are no dosage adjustments provided in the manufacturer's labeling. However, dosage adjustment unlikely due to low systemic absorption.

Hepatic Impairment There are no dosage adjustments provided in the manufacturer's labeling. However, dosage adjustment unlikely due to low systemic absorption.

Additional Information Complete prescribing information should be consulted for additional detail.

Dosage Forms Excipient information presented when available (limited, particularly for generics); consult specific product labeling.

Cream, External:
Cortisporin: 0.5-0.5-10000 (7.5 g)

◆ Neomycin Sulfate see Neomycin on page 1266
◆ Neo-Polycin see Bacitracin, Neomycin, and Polymyxin B (Ophthalmic) on page 196
◆ Neo-Polycin HC see Bacitracin, Neomycin, Polymyxin B, and Hydrocortisone (Ophthalmic) on page 197
◆ NeoProfen see Ibuprofen on page 905
◆ Neoral see CycloSPORINE (Systemic) on page 459
◆ Neosar see Cyclophosphamide on page 455
◆ Neosporin® (Can) see Neomycin, Polymyxin B, and Gramicidin on page 1267
◆ Neosporin® G.U. Irrigant see Neomycin and Polymyxin B on page 1266
◆ Neosporin® Irrigating Solution (Can) see Neomycin and Polymyxin B on page 1266
◆ Neosporin® Ophthalmic Solution see Neomycin, Polymyxin B, and Gramicidin on page 1267
◆ Neosporin Original [OTC] see Bacitracin, Neomycin, and Polymyxin B (Topical) on page 197

Neostigmine (nee oh STIG meen)

Brand Names: US Bloxiverz; Prostigmin
Brand Names: Canada Prostigmin

Index Terms Neostigmine Bromide; Neostigmine Methylsulfate
Pharmacologic Category Acetylcholinesterase Inhibitor
Use

Myasthenia gravis (excluding Bloxiverz): Symptomatic control of myasthenia gravis

Postoperative bladder distention/Urinary retention (excluding Bloxiverz and Prostigmin tablets): Prevention and treatment of postoperative bladder distention and urinary retention after mechanical obstruction has been excluded.

Reversal of nondepolarizing muscle relaxants (excluding Prostigmin tablets): Reversal of effects of nondepolarizing neuromuscular blocking agents (eg, tubocurarine, or pancuronium) after surgery.

Dosing

Adult & Geriatric Note: Neostigmine (Prostigmin) tablets have been discontinued in the US for more than 1 year.

Myasthenia gravis: Diagnosis (off-label use): IM: 0.02 mg/kg as a single dose

Myasthenia gravis: Treatment:
Manufacturer's labeling:
Oral: Usual dose: 150 mg administered over a 24-hour period; interval between doses is of paramount importance and therapy is frequently required day and night. Dosage range: 15 to 375 mg daily in divided doses.
IM, SubQ: 0.5 mg; subsequent dosing based on individual patient response
Alternative recommendations (off-label dosing):
Oral: Initial: 15 mg every 8 hours; may increase every 1 to 2 days up to 375 mg daily maximum; interval between doses must be individualized to maximal response
IM, IV, SubQ: 0.5 to 2.5 mg every 1 to 3 hours as needed up to 10 mg/24 hours maximum

Reversal of nondepolarizing neuromuscular blockade after surgery:
Bloxiverz: IV: **Note:** An anticholinergic agent (atropine or glycopyrrolate) should be given prior to or in conjunction with neostigmine; in the presence of bradycardia, administer the anticholinergic prior to neostigmine. Peripheral nerve stimulation delivering train-of-four (TOF) stimulus must also be used to determine time of neostigmine initiation and need for additional doses.
Usual dose: 0.03 to 0.07 mg/kg generally achieves a TOF twitch ratio of 90% within 10 to 20 minutes of administration; maximum total dose: 0.07 mg/kg or 5 mg (whichever is less)
Dose selection guide:
The 0.03 mg/kg dose is recommended for reversal of NMBAs with shorter half-lives (eg, rocuronium); **or** when the first twitch response to the TOF stimulus is substantially >10% of baseline or when a second twitch is present.
The 0.07 mg/kg dose is recommended for NMBAs with longer half-lives (eg, vecuronium, pancuronium); **or** when the first twitch response is relatively weak (ie, not substantially >10% of baseline); or rapid recovery is needed.
Generic products: IV: 0.5 to 2 mg; repeat as required. Only in exceptional cases should the total dose exceed 5 mg. **Note:** Administer with atropine 0.6 to 1.2 mg in a separate syringe several minutes before neostigmine.

Postoperative urinary retention: IM, SubQ:
Prevention: 0.25 mg as soon as possible after operation; repeat every 4 to 6 hours for 2 to 3 days
Treatment: 0.5 mg; if urination does not occur within an hour, patient should be catheterized. After the bladder has emptied or patient has voided, continue 0.5 mg every 3 hours for at least 5 doses.

Postoperative bladder distention: IM, SubQ:
Prevention: 0.25 mg as soon as possible after operation; repeat every 4 to 6 hours for 2 to 3 days
Treatment: 0.5 mg as needed

Acute colonic pseudo-obstruction (Ogilvie syndrome) (off-label use): Adults: IV: 2 mg over 3 to 5 minutes (Ponec, 1999). **Note:** Administration over 60 minutes may reduce the incidence of bradycardia; however, efficacy may be reduced (Abeyta, 2001). Ensure atropine is available at the bedside to treat symptomatic neostigmine-induced bradycardia.

Pediatric Note: Neostigmine (Prostigmin) tablets have been discontinued in the US for more than 1 year.
Myasthenia gravis: Diagnosis (off-label use): Children: IM: 0.025 to 0.04 mg/kg as a single dose

Myasthenia gravis: Treatment (off-label use): Children:

Oral: 2 mg/kg/day, not to exceed 375 mg daily

IM, IV, SubQ: 0.01 to 0.04 mg/kg every 2 to 4 hours as needed

Reversal of nondepolarizing neuromuscular-blocking agents (NMBAs) after surgery (Bloxiverz): Infants, Children, and Adolescents: IV: Refer to adult dosing.

Note: An anticholinergic agent (atropine or glycopyrrolate) should be given prior to or in conjunction with neostigmine. Peripheral nerve stimulation delivering train-of-four (TOF) stimulus must also be used to determine time of neostigmine initiation and need for additional doses.

Renal Impairment

No dosage adjustment provided in manufacturer's labeling; however, the following adjustments have been recommended (Aronoff, 2007): Adults: Oral:

CrCl >50 mL/minute: No dosage adjustment necessary

CrCl 10 to 50 mL/minute: Administer 50% of normal dose.

CrCl <10 mL/minute: Administer 25% of normal dose.

Hemodialysis: No dosage adjustment necessary

Peritoneal dialysis: No dosage adjustment necessary

Continuous renal replacement therapy (CRRT): Administer 50% of normal dose

Hepatic Impairment No dosage adjustment provided in manufacturer's labeling.

Additional Information Complete prescribing information should be consulted for additional detail.

Product Availability Neostigmine (Prostigmin) tablets have been discontinued in the US for more than 1 year.

Dosage Forms Excipient information presented when available (limited, particularly for generics); consult specific product labeling. [DSC] = Discontinued product

Solution, Injection, as methylsulfate:

Prostigmin: 0.5 mg/mL (1 mL, 10 mL)

Generic: 0.5 mg/mL (10 mL); 1 mg/mL (10 mL)

Solution, Intravenous, as methylsulfate:

Bloxiverz: 5 mg/10 mL (10 mL); 10 mg/10 mL (10 mL) [contains phenol]

Generic: 5 mg/10 mL (10 mL); 10 mg/10 mL (10 mL)

Tablet, Oral, as bromide:

Prostigmin: 15 mg [DSC] [scored]

◆ Neostigmine Bromide see Neostigmine on page 1268

◆ Neostigmine Methylsulfate see Neostigmine on page 1268

◆ NeoStrata® HQ (Can) see Hydroquinone on page 893

◆ NeoStrata HQ Skin Lightening [OTC] see Hydroquinone on page 893

◆ Neo-Synephrine [DSC] see Phenylephrine (Systemic) on page 1442

◆ NEPA see Netupitant and Palonosetron on page 1269

Nepafenac (ne pa FEN ak)

Brand Names: US Ilevro; Nevanac

Brand Names: Canada Ilevro; Nevanac

Pharmacologic Category Nonsteroidal Anti-inflammatory Drug (NSAID), Ophthalmic

Use Treatment of pain and inflammation associated with cataract surgery

Dosing

Adult & Geriatric Pain, inflammation associated with cataract surgery: Ophthalmic:

Ilevro™: Instill 1 drop into affected eye(s) once daily, beginning 1 day prior to surgery, the day of surgery, and through the first 2 weeks of the postoperative period. Instill 1 additional drop 30-120 minutes prior to surgery.

Nevanac®: Instill 1 drop into affected eye(s) 3 times/day, beginning 1 day prior to surgery, the day of surgery, and through the first 2 weeks of the postoperative period

Pediatric Pain, inflammation associated with cataract surgery: Ophthalmic: Children ≥10 years and Adolescents: Refer to adult dosing.

Renal Impairment No dosage adjustment provided in manufacturer's labeling.

Hepatic Impairment No dosage adjustment provided in manufacturer's labeling.

Additional Information Complete prescribing information should be consulted for additional detail.

Dosage Forms Excipient information presented when available (limited, particularly for generics); consult specific product labeling.

Suspension, Ophthalmic:

Ilevro: 0.3% (1.7 mL, 3 mL) [contains benzalkonium chloride, edetate disodium, propylene glycol]

Nevanac: 0.1% (3 mL) [contains edentate disodium benzalkonium chloride]

◆ Neptazane see Methazolamide on page 1165

◆ Nerve Agent Antidote Kit see Atropine and Pralidoxime on page 179

◆ Nesacaine see Chloroprocaine on page 374

◆ Nesacaine-MPF see Chloroprocaine on page 374

Nesiritide (ni SIR i tide)

Brand Names: US Natrecor

Index Terms B-type Natriuretic Peptide (Human); hBNP; Natriuretic Peptide

Pharmacologic Category Natriuretic Peptide, B-Type, Human

Use Treatment of acutely decompensated heart failure (HF) with dyspnea at rest or with minimal activity

Dosing

Adult & Geriatric

Acute decompensated heart failure: IV: Initial: 2 mcg/kg (bolus optional); followed by continuous infusion at 0.01 mcg/kg/minute. **Note:** Should not be initiated at a dosage higher than initial recommended dose. There is limited experience with increasing the dose >0.01 mcg/kg/minute; in one trial, a limited number of patients received higher doses that were increased no faster than every 3 hours by 0.005 mcg/kg/minute (preceded by a bolus of 1 mcg/kg), up to a maximum of 0.03 mcg/kg/minute. Increases beyond the initial infusion rate should be limited to selected patients and accompanied by close hemodynamic and renal function monitoring.

Patients experiencing hypotension during the infusion: Infusion dose should be reduced or discontinued. Other measures to support blood pressure should be initiated (eg, IV fluids, Trendelenburg position). Hypotension may be prolonged (up to hours); once patient is stabilized, may attempt to restart at a lower dose (reduce previous infusion dose by 30% and omit bolus).

Maximum dosing weight: According to the manufacturer, the PRECEDENT Trial capped dosing weight at 160 kg and the VMAC Trial capped dosing weight at 175 kg. There are no specific guidelines on maximum dosing weight and clinical judgment should be used.

Renal Impairment No dosage adjustment necessary. Use cautiously in patients with renal impairment or those patients who rely on the renin-angiotensin-aldosterone system for renal perfusion. Monitor renal function closely.

Hepatic Impairment No dosage adjustment provided in manufacturer's labeling.

Additional Information Complete prescribing information should be consulted for additional detail.

Dosage Forms Excipient information presented when available (limited, particularly for generics); consult specific product labeling.

Solution Reconstituted, Intravenous:

Natrecor: 1.5 mg (1 ea)

◆ NESP see Darbepoetin Alfa on page 493

Netupitant and Palonosetron
(net UE pi tant & pal oh NOE se tron)

Brand Names: US Akynzeo

Index Terms NEPA; Palonosetron and Netupitant

Pharmacologic Category Antiemetic; Selective 5-HT$_3$ Receptor Antagonist; Substance P/Neurokinin 1 Receptor Antagonist

Use Chemotherapy-induced nausea and vomiting: Prevention of acute and delayed nausea and vomiting associated with initial and repeat courses of cancer chemotherapy, including, but not limited to, highly emetogenic chemotherapy.

Dosing

Adult

Highly-emetogenic chemotherapy (including cisplatin-based): Oral: One capsule ~1 hour prior to initiation of chemotherapy on day 1 (Gralla, 2014). **Note:** Antiemetic regimen also includes dexamethasone 12 mg orally ~30 minutes prior to initiation of chemotherapy on day 1, and 8 mg orally once daily on days 2 to 4.

Anthracycline and cyclophosphamide-based chemotherapy and chemotherapy not considered highly emetogenic: Oral: One capsule ~1 hour prior to initiation of chemotherapy on day 1 (Gralla, 2014). **Note:** Antiemetic regimen also includes dexamethasone 12 mg orally ~30 minutes prior to chemotherapy on day 1.

Geriatric No dosage adjustment necessary. Refer to adult dosing.

Renal Impairment

Mild or moderate impairment: No dosage adjustment is necessary.

Severe impairment or ESRD: Avoid use.

Hepatic Impairment

Mild or moderate impairment (Child-Pugh score 5 to 8): No dosage adjustment is necessary.

Severe impairment (Child-Pugh score >9): Avoid use.

Additional Information Complete prescribing information should be consulted for additional detail.

Dosage Forms Excipient information presented when available (limited, particularly for generics); consult specific product labeling.

Capsule, Oral:

Akynzeo: Netupitant 300 mg and palonosetron 0.5 mg

Nevirapine (ne VYE ra peen)

Brand Names: US Viramune; Viramune XR

Brand Names: Canada Auro-Nevirapine; Mylan-Nevirapine; Teva-Nevirapine; Viramune; Viramune XR

Index Terms NVP

Pharmacologic Category Antiretroviral, Reverse Transcriptase Inhibitor, Non-nucleoside (Anti-HIV)

Use In combination therapy with other antiretroviral agents for the treatment of HIV-1

Pregnancy Considerations Teratogenic effects were not observed in animal reproduction studies. Nevirapine has a high level of transfer across the human placenta. No increased risk of overall birth defects has been observed following first trimester exposure according to data collected by the antiretroviral pregnancy registry. Pharmacokinetics are not altered during pregnancy and dose adjustment is not needed. The HHS Perinatal HIV Guidelines consider nevirapine to be an alternative NNRTI for use in antiretroviral-naïve pregnant patients. Nevirapine may be initiated in pregnant women with a CD4$^+$ lymphocyte count <250/mm^3 or continued in women who are virologically suppressed and tolerating therapy once pregnancy is detected (regardless of CD4+ lymphocyte count); however, **do not** initiate therapy in pregnant women with a CD4$^+$ lymphocyte count >250/mm^3 unless the benefit of therapy clearly outweighs the risk. Elevated transaminase concentrations at baseline may increase the risk of toxicity; the monitoring recommendation for transaminase levels is generally the same as in nonpregnant women. Hypersensitivity reactions (including hepatic toxicity and rash) are more common in women on NNRTI.

Regardless of CD4 count or HIV RNA copy number, all HIV-infected pregnant women should receive a combination antiretroviral (ARV) drug regimen. A combination of antepartum, intrapartum, and infant ARV prophylaxis is recommended. ARV therapy should be started as soon as possible in women with symptomatic infection. Although earlier initiation may be more effective in reducing the perinatal transmission of HIV, initiation may be delayed until after 12 weeks gestation in women who do not require immediate treatment after careful consideration of maternal conditions (eg, nausea and vomiting) and the potential risks of first trimester fetal exposure for specific agents. A scheduled cesarean delivery at 38 weeks gestation is recommended for all women with HIV RNA >1000 copies/mL or unknown concentrations near delivery in order to decrease transmission. If ARV therapy must be interrupted for <24 hours during the peripartum period, stop then restart all medications simultaneously in order to decrease the chance of developing resistance. Long-term follow-up is recommended for all infants exposed to ARV medications. In couples who want to conceive, the HIV-infected partner should attain maximum viral suppression prior to conception.

Health care providers are encouraged to enroll pregnant women exposed to antiretroviral medications in the Antiretroviral Pregnancy Registry (1-800-258-4263 or www.-APRegistry.com). Health care providers caring for HIV-infected women and their infants may contact the National Perinatal HIV Hotline (888-448-8765) for clinical consultation (HHS [perinatal], 2014).

Breast-Feeding Considerations Nevirapine is excreted into breast milk and measurable in the serum of nursing infants. Maternal or infant antiretroviral therapy does not completely eliminate the risk of postnatal HIV transmission. In addition, multiclass resistant virus has been detected in breast-feeding infants despite maternal therapy. Therefore, in the United States, where formula is accessible, affordable, safe, and sustainable, and the risk of infant mortality due to diarrhea and respiratory infections is low, complete avoidance of breast-feeding by HIV-infected women is recommended to decrease potential transmission of HIV (HHS [perinatal], 2014).

Medication Guide Available Yes

Contraindications

Moderate-to-severe hepatic impairment (Child-Pugh class B or C); use in occupational or nonoccupational postexposure prophylaxis (PEP) regimens

Canadian labeling: Additional contraindications (not in US labeling): Clinically significant hypersensitivity to nevirapine or any component of the formulation; therapy rechallenge in patients with prior hypersensitivity reactions, severe rash, rash accompanied by constitutional symptoms, or clinical hepatitis due to nevirapine; severe hepatic dysfunction or AST or ALT >5 times ULN (pretreatment or during prior use of nevirapine); hereditary conditions of galactose intolerance (eg, galactosemia, Lapp lactase deficiency, glucose-galactose malabsorption); concomitant use of herbal products containing St John's wort

Warnings/Precautions Hazardous agent - use appropriate precautions for handling and disposal (NIOSH 2014 [group 2]).

[US Boxed Warning]: Severe hepatotoxic reactions may occur (fulminant and cholestatic hepatitis, hepatic necrosis) and, in some cases, have resulted in hepatic failure and death. The greatest risk of these reactions is within the initial 6 weeks of treatment. Patients with a history of chronic hepatitis (B or C) or increased baseline transaminase levels may be at increased risk of hepatotoxic reactions. Female gender and patients with increased CD4$^+$-cell counts may be at substantially greater risk of hepatic events (often associated with rash). Therapy in antiretroviral naive patients should not be started with elevated CD4$^+$-cell counts unless the benefit of therapy outweighs the risk of serious hepatotoxicity (adult/postpubertal females: CD4$^+$-cell counts >250 cells/mm^3; adult males: CD4$^+$-cell counts >400 cells/mm^3). Use with caution in patients with preexisting dysfunction; monitor closely for drug-induced hepatotoxicity. US labeling contraindicates use in patients with moderate-to-severe impairment (Child-Pugh class B or C). Canadian labeling contraindicates use in severe impairment.

[US Boxed Warning]: Severe life-threatening skin reactions (eg, Stevens-Johnson syndrome, toxic epidermal necrolysis, hypersensitivity reactions with rash and organ dysfunction), including fatal cases, have occurred. The greatest risk of these reactions is within the initial 6 weeks of treatment; intensive monitoring is required during the initial 18 weeks of therapy to detect potentially life-threatening dermatologic and hypersensitivity reactions. If a rash occurs within the first 18 weeks of therapy, immediately check serum transaminases. Risk is greatest in African-Americans, Asian, or Hispanic race/ethnicity or in females (DHHS, 2011). If a severe dermatologic or hypersensitivity reaction occurs,

nevirapine should be permanently discontinued; these events may include a severe rash, or a rash associated with fever, blisters, oral lesions, conjunctivitis, facial edema, muscle or joint aches, transaminase increases, general malaise, hepatitis, eosinophilia, granulocytopenia, lymphadenopathy, or renal dysfunction. Use of the 14-day lead-in dosing period is necessary to decrease the incidence of rash events. If nonsevere rash (in absence of transaminase elevations) occurs, do not increase dose until resolution of rash. If rash continues beyond 28 days, consider an alternative regimen. Coadministration of prednisone during the first 6 weeks of therapy increases incidence and severity of rash; concomitant prednisone is not recommended to prevent rash.

May cause redistribution of fat (eg, buffalo hump, peripheral wasting with increased abdominal girth, cushingoid appearance). Patients may develop immune reconstitution syndrome resulting in the occurrence of an inflammatory response to an indolent or residual opportunistic infection during initial HIV treatment or activation of autoimmune disorders (eg, Graves' disease, polymyositis, Guillain-Barré syndrome) later in therapy; further evaluation and treatment may be required. Rhabdomyolysis has been observed in conjunction with skin and/or hepatic adverse events during postmarketing surveillance. Termination of therapy is warranted with evidence of severe skin or liver toxicity.

Use with caution in patients taking strong CYP3A4 inhibitors, moderate or strong CYP3A4 inducers and major CYP3A4 substrates (see Drug Interactions); consider alternative agents that avoid or lessen the potential for CYP-mediated interactions. Concurrent use of St John's wort or efavirenz is not recommended; may decrease the therapeutic efficacy (St John's wort) or increase adverse effects (efavirenz). Canadian labeling contraindicates concurrent use with products containing St John's wort.

Nevirapine-based initial regimens should not be used in children <3 years of age if previously exposed to nevirapine during prevention of maternal-to-child transmission of HIV due to increased risk of resistance and treatment failure. Protease inhibitor-based initial regimens preferred in this population.

Due to rapid emergence of resistance, nevirapine should not be used as monotherapy or the only agent added to a failing regimen for the treatment of HIV. Consider alteration of antiretroviral therapies if disease progression occurs while patients are receiving nevirapine. Resistance may occur with a single mutation and cross-resistance may be conferred to other non-nucleoside reverse transcriptase inhibitors (HHS [adult], 2015).

Some dosage forms may contain polysorbate 80 (also known as Tweens). Hypersensitivity reactions, usually a delayed reaction, have been reported following exposure to pharmaceutical products containing polysorbate 80 in certain individuals (Isaksson, 2002; Lucente 2000; Shelley, 1995). Thrombocytopenia, ascites, pulmonary deterioration, and renal and hepatic failure have been reported in premature neonates after receiving parenteral products containing polysorbate 80 (Alade, 1986; CDC, 1984). See manufacturer's labeling.

Adverse Reactions Note: Potentially life-threatening nevirapine-associated adverse effects may present with the following symptoms: Abrupt onset of flu-like symptoms, abdominal pain, jaundice, or fever with or without rash; may progress to hepatic failure with encephalopathy. Skin rash is present in ~50% of cases.

>10%:

Dermatologic: Rash (1% to 7%; grade 1/2: 13%; grade 3/4: 2%)

Endocrine & metabolic: Cholesterol increased (240-300 mg/dL: 18% to 19%; >300 mg/dL: 3% to 4%), LDL increased (160-190 mg/dL: 15%; >190 mg/dL: 5%)

Hematologic: Neutropenia (4% to 13%; grades 3/4: 1% to 2%)

Hepatic: ALT increased (2.6-5 x ULN: 10% to 13%; ≥5.1 x ULN: 6% to 7%), symptomatic hepatic events (including hepatitis and hepatic failure: 2% to 11%; risk higher in ARV-naive women with CD4 counts >250 cells/mm^3 and ARV-naive men with CD4 counts >400 cells/mm^3)

1% to 10%:

Central nervous system: Fatigue (≤5%), headache (1% to 4%), fever (1% to 2%)

Gastrointestinal: Nausea (<1% to 9%), amylase increased (1.6-5 x ULN: 7% to 8%; ≥5.1 x ULN: <1%), abdominal pain (≤2%), diarrhea (≤2%)

Hepatic: AST increased (2.6-5 x ULN: 7% to 9%; ≥5.1 x ULN: 4% to 5%)

Neuromuscular & skeletal: Arthralgia (2%)

<1% (Limited to important or life-threatening): Allergic reactions, anaphylaxis, anemia, angioedema, bullous eruptions, cholestatic hepatitis, conjunctivitis, drug reaction with eosinophilia and systemic symptoms (DRESS), eosinophilia, fulminant hepatitis, granulocytopenia, hepatic necrosis, hypersensitivity syndrome, hypophosphatemia, immune reconstitution syndrome, jaundice, lymphadenopathy, oral lesions, redistribution/accumulation of body fat, renal dysfunction, rhabdomyolysis, Stevens-Johnson syndrome, toxic epidermal necrolysis, ulcerative stomatitis

Drug Interactions

Metabolism/Transport Effects Substrate of CYP2B6 (minor), CYP2D6 (minor), CYP3A4 (major); **Note:** Assignment of Major/Minor substrate status based on clinically relevant drug interaction potential; **Inhibits** CYP1A2 (weak), CYP2D6 (weak); **Induces** CYP2B6 (strong), CYP3A4 (weak)

Avoid Concomitant Use

Avoid concomitant use of Nevirapine with any of the following: Atazanavir; CarBAMazepine; Dolutegravir; Efavirenz; Elvitegravir; Etravirine; Itraconazole; Ketoconazole (Systemic); Rilpivirine; Simeprevir; St Johns Wort

Increased Effect/Toxicity

Nevirapine may increase the levels/effects of: Artesunate; Cyclophosphamide; Darunavir; Efavirenz; Etravirine; Rifabutin; Rilpivirine; TiZANidine

The levels/effects of Nevirapine may be increased by: Atazanavir; Darunavir; Efavirenz; Fluconazole; Osimertinib; Voriconazole

Decreased Effect

Nevirapine may decrease the levels/effects of: ARIPiprazole; Artemether; Artesunate; Atazanavir; CarBAMazepine; Caspofungin; Contraceptives (Estrogens); Contraceptives (Progestins); CYP2B6 Substrates; Dolutegravir; Efavirenz; Elvitegravir; Etravirine; Fosamprenavir; Hydrocodone; Indinavir; Itraconazole; Ketoconazole (Systemic); Lopinavir; Methadone; Nelfinavir; NiMODipine; Rifabutin; Rilpivirine; Rivaroxaban; Saquinavir; Saxagliptin; Simeprevir; Voriconazole

The levels/effects of Nevirapine may be decreased by: Bosentan; CarBAMazepine; CYP3A4 Inducers (Moderate); CYP3A4 Inducers (Strong); Dabrafenib; Deferasirox; Enzalutamide; Mitotane; Osimertinib; Rifabutin; Rifampin; Siltuximab; St Johns Wort; Tocilizumab

Storage/Stability Store at 25°C (77°F); excursion permitted to 15°C to 30°C (59°F to 86°F).

Mechanism of Action As a non-nucleoside reverse transcriptase inhibitor, nevirapine has activity against HIV-1 by binding to reverse transcriptase. It consequently blocks the RNA-dependent and DNA-dependent DNA polymerase activities including HIV-1 replication. It does not require intracellular phosphorylation for antiviral activity.

Pharmacodynamics/Kinetics

Absorption: >90%

Distribution: Widely; V$_d$: 1.2 L/kg; CSF penetration approximates 40% to 50% of plasma

Protein binding, plasma: ~60%

Metabolism: Extensively hepatic via CYP3A4 and CYP2B6 (hydroxylation to inactive compounds); may undergo enterohepatic recycling

Bioavailability: 93% (immediate release tablet); ~75% (extended release tablet [relative to immediate release]); 91% (oral solution)

Half-life elimination: Decreases over 2- to 4-week time with chronic dosing due to autoinduction (ie, half-life = 45 hours initially and decreases to 25-30 hours)

Time to peak, serum: Immediate release: 4 hours; Extended release:~24 hours

Excretion: Urine (~81%, primarily as metabolites, <3% as unchanged drug); feces (~10%)

Dosing

Adult & Geriatric HIV infection: Oral:

Note: Therapy in antiretroviral naive patients should not be initiated in patients with elevated CD4$^+$-cell counts unless the benefit of therapy outweighs the risk of serious hepatotoxicity (adult/postpubertal females: CD4$^+$-cell counts >250 cells/mm^3; adult males: CD4$^+$-cell counts >400 cells/mm^3).

Initial: *Immediate release:* 200 mg once daily for 14 days

Maintenance:

Immediate release: 200 mg twice daily (in combination with additional antiretroviral agents) if there is no rash or untoward effects during initial dosing period

Extended release: 400 mg once daily; maintenance therapy using the extended release must follow a 14-day initial dosing period (lead-in) using the immediate release formulation unless patient is already maintained on a nevirapine immediate release regimen

Note: If patient experiences a rash during the 14-day lead-in period, dose should not be increased until the rash has resolved. A lead-in period must always be done with immediate release formulation and regimen should not exceed 28 days; alternative treatment should be considered at that point. If a rash occurs within the first 18 weeks of therapy, immediately check serum transaminases. Discontinue if severe rash, rash with constitutional symptoms, or rash with elevated hepatic transaminases is noted. Coadministration of prednisone during the first 6 weeks of therapy increases incidence and severity of rash; concomitant prednisone is not recommended to prevent rash. Permanently discontinue if symptomatic hepatic events occur. If therapy with any formulation is interrupted for >7 days, restart with initial dose of immediate release formulation for 14 days.

Pediatric

HIV infection: Oral: **Note:** If patient experiences a rash during the 14-day lead-in period, dose should not be increased until the rash has resolved. A lead-in period must always be done with immediate release formulation and regimen should not exceed 28 days; alternative treatment should be considered at that point. If a rash occurs within the first 18 weeks of therapy, immediately check serum transaminases. Discontinue if severe rash, rash with constitutional symptoms, or rash with elevated hepatic transaminases is noted. Coadministration of prednisone during the first 6 weeks of therapy increases incidence and severity of rash; concomitant prednisone is not recommended to prevent rash. Permanently discontinue if symptomatic hepatic events occur. If therapy with any formulation is interrupted for >7 days, restart with initial dose of immediate release formulation for 14 days. Use of nevirapine in children <15 years of age is not approved in the Canadian labeling.

Manufacturer's labeling:

Infants and Children: *Immediate release:* 150 mg/m^2/dose once daily for first 14 days (maximum: 200 mg daily); increase dose to 150 mg/m^2/dose twice daily if no rash or untoward effects (maximum: 400 mg daily).

Children 6 to <18 years: *Extended release:* Dose based on body surface area (Mosteller formula); maintenance therapy using the extended release must follow a 14-day initial dosing period (lead-in) using the immediate release formulation unless patient is already maintained on a nevirapine immediate release regimen.

0.58 m^2 to 0.83 m^2: 200 mg once daily

0.84 m^2 to 1.16 m^2: 300 mg once daily

≥1.17 m^2: 400 mg once daily (do not exceed 400 mg daily)

Alternate recommendations (HHS [pediatric], 2014):

Note: Children <3 years of age: Nevirapine-based initial regimens should not be used in children previously exposed to nevirapine during prevention of maternal-to-child transmission of HIV

Children <8 years: *Immediate release:* 200 mg/m^2/dose once daily for first 14 days (maximum dose: 200 mg); increase dose to 200 mg/m^2/dose twice daily if no rash or untoward effects (maximum: 400 mg daily)

Children ≥8 years: *Immediate release:* 120-150 mg/m^2/dose once daily for 14 days (maximum dose: 200 mg); increase to 120-150 mg/m^2/dose twice daily if no rash or untoward effects (maximum: 400 mg daily)

Adolescents: *Immediate release:* Refer to adult dosing.

Prevention of perinatal HIV transmission (HHS [perinatal], 2014): **Note:** Nevirapine is used in combination with zidovudine in select situations (eg, infants born to mothers with only intrapartum therapy or no therapy). Use is not recommended in women receiving standard recommended antenatal antiretroviral prophylaxis.

Renal Impairment

Immediate release:

CrCl ≥20 mL/minute: No dosage adjustment necessary.

CrCl <20 mL/minute: There are no dosage adjustments provided in the manufacturer's labeling (has not been studied).

Extended release: There are no dosage adjustments provided in the manufacturer's labeling (has not been studied).

Hemodialysis: An additional 200 mg *immediate release* dose is recommended following dialysis.

Hepatic Impairment Permanently discontinue if symptomatic hepatic events occur.

US labeling:

Mild impairment (Child-Pugh class A):

Immediate release: There are no dosage adjustments provided in the manufacturer's labeling; use with caution.

Extended release: There are no dosage adjustments provided in the manufacturer's labeling (has not been studied).

Moderate-to-severe impairment (Child-Pugh class B or C): Use is contraindicated.

Canadian labeling:

Mild impairment (Child-Pugh class A): No dosage adjustment is necessary.

Moderate impairment (Child-Pugh class B): There are no dosage adjustments provided in the manufacturer's labeling. Use with caution.

Severe impairment (Child-Pugh class C): Use is contraindicated.

Administration Oral: May be administered with or without food; may be administered with an antacid or didanosine. Shake suspension gently prior to administration; the use of an oral dosing syringe is recommended, especially if the dose is ≤5 mL; if using a dosing cup, after administration, rinse cup with water and also administer rinse. Extended release tablets must be swallowed whole and not crushed, chewed, or divided.

Hazardous agent; use appropriate precautions for handling and disposal (NIOSH 2014 [group 2]).

Monitoring Parameters Monitor CBC and viral load. Baseline liver function tests should be obtained prior to nevirapine's initiation. HHS adult guidelines recommend serum transaminase monitoring every 2 weeks for the first 4 weeks of therapy, monthly for the first 18 weeks, then frequently thereafter. Patients receiving maintenance immediate release nevirapine who change to the extended release formulation should adhere to their regular monitoring schedule. HHS adult guidelines recommend serum transaminase monitoring every 2 weeks for the first 4 weeks of therapy, then monthly for 3 months, followed by every 3-4 months. HHS pediatric guidelines recommend serum transaminase monitoring every 2 weeks for the first 4 weeks of therapy, followed by every 4 months. Assess/evaluate AST/ALT immediately in any patients with a rash. Permanently discontinue if patient experiences severe rash, constitutional symptoms associated with rash, rash with elevated AST/ALT, or clinical hepatitis. Mild-to-moderate rash without AST/ALT elevation may continue treatment per discretion of prescriber. If mild-to-moderate urticarial rash, do not restart if treatment is interrupted.

Additional Information Patients should never be taking more than one form (ie, immediate release or extended release) of nevirapine concomitantly. Potential compliance problems, frequency of administration, and adverse effects should be discussed with patients before initiating therapy to help prevent the emergence of resistance. Early virologic failure was observed with tenofovir and didanosine delayed release capsules, plus either efavirenz or nevirapine; use caution in treatment-naive patients with high baseline viral loads. Due to rapid emergence of resistance, nevirapine should not be used as monotherapy or as the only agent added to a failing regimen for the treatment of HIV.

Dosage Forms Excipient information presented when available (limited, particularly for generics); consult specific product labeling.

Suspension, Oral:

Viramune: 50 mg/5 mL (240 mL) [contains methylparaben, propylparaben]

Generic: 50 mg/5 mL (240 mL)

Tablet, Oral:

Viramune: 200 mg [scored]

Generic: 200 mg

Tablet Extended Release 24 Hour, Oral:

Viramune XR: 100 mg, 400 mg

Generic: 100 mg, 400 mg

♦ Next Choice One Dose [DSC] *see* Levonorgestrel (Systemic) *on page 1064*

♦ Nexterone *see* Amiodarone *on page 94*

♦ NFV *see* Nelfinavir *on page 1266*

Niacin (NYE a sin)

Brand Names: US Niacin-50 [OTC]; Niacor; Niaspan; Slo-Niacin [OTC]
Brand Names: Canada Niaspan; Niaspan FCT; Niodan
Index Terms Nicotinic Acid; Vitamin B₃
Pharmacologic Category Antilipemic Agent, Miscellaneous; Vitamin, Water Soluble
Use Treatment of dyslipidemias (Fredrickson types IIa and IIb or primary hypercholesterolemia) as mono- or adjunctive therapy; to lower the risk of recurrent MI in patients with a history of MI and hyperlipidemia; to slow progression or promote regression of coronary artery disease; adjunctive therapy for severe hypertriglyceridemia in adult patients at risk of pancreatitis; dietary supplement
Pregnancy Considerations Animal reproduction studies have not been conducted. Water soluble vitamins cross the placenta. When used as a dietary supplement, niacin requirements may be increased in pregnant women compared to nonpregnant women (IOM, 1998). It is not known if niacin at lipid-lowering doses is harmful to the developing fetus. If a woman becomes pregnant while receiving niacin for primary hypercholesterolemia, niacin should be discontinued. If a woman becomes pregnant while receiving niacin for hypertriglyceridemia, the benefits and risks of continuing niacin should be assessed on an individual basis.
Breast-Feeding Considerations Niacin is excreted in breast milk. When used as a dietary supplement, niacin requirements may be increased in breast-feeding women compared to non-breast-feeding women (IOM, 1998). Due to the potential for serious adverse reactions in the breast-feeding infant, the manufacturer recommends a decision be made whether to discontinue breast-feeding or to discontinue the drug, taking into account the importance of treatment to the mother.
Contraindications Hypersensitivity to niacin, niacinamide, or any component of the formulation; active hepatic disease or significant or unexplained persistent elevations in hepatic transaminases; active peptic ulcer; arterial hemorrhage
Warnings/Precautions Prior to initiation, secondary causes for hypercholesterolemia (eg, poorly controlled diabetes mellitus, hypothyroidism) should be excluded; management with diet and other nonpharmacologic measures (eg, exercise or weight reduction) should be attempted prior to initiation. Use has not been evaluated in Fredrickson type I or III dyslipidemias. Use with caution in patients with unstable angina or in the acute phase of an MI or renal disease. In patients with preexisting coronary artery disease, the incidence of atrial fibrillation was observed more frequently in those receiving immediate release (crystalline) niacin as compared to placebo (Coronary Drug Project Research Group, 1975). Niacin should not be used if patient experiences new-onset atrial fibrillation during therapy (Stone, 2013). Niacin may increase fasting blood glucose, although clinical data suggest increases are generally modest (<5%) (Guyton, 2007). Use niacin with caution in patients with diabetes. Monitor glucose; adjustment of diet and/or hypoglycemic therapy may be necessary. Niacin should not be used if patient experiences persistent hyperglycemia during therapy (Stone, 2013). Use with caution in patients predisposed to gout; niacin should not be used if patient experiences acute gout during therapy (Stone, 2013).

Use with caution in patients with a past history of hepatic impairment and/or who consume substantial amounts of ethanol; contraindicated with active liver disease or unexplained persistent transaminase elevation. Niacin should not be used if hepatic transaminase elevations >2 to 3 times upper limit of normal occur during therapy (Stone, 2013). Rare cases of rhabdomyolysis have occurred during concomitant use with HMG-CoA reductase inhibitors. With concurrent use or if symptoms suggestive of myopathy occur, monitor creatine phosphokinase (CPK) and potassium; use with caution in patients with renal impairment, inadequately treated hypothyroidism, patients with diabetes or the elderly; risk for myopathy and rhabdomyolysis may be increased. May cause gastrointestinal distress, vomiting, diarrhea, or aggravate peptic ulcer. Gastrointestinal distress may be attenuated with a gradual increase in dose and administration with food. Use is contraindicated in patients with active peptic ulcer disease; use with caution in patients with a past history of peptic ulcer. Niacin should not be used if patient experiences unexplained abdominal pain or gastrointestinal symptoms

or unexplained weight loss during therapy (Stone, 2013). Dose-related reductions in platelet count and increases of prothrombin time may occur. Has been associated with small but statistically significant dose-related reductions in phosphorus levels. Monitor phosphorus levels periodically in patients at risk for hypophosphatemia.

Formulations of niacin (immediate release versus extended release) are not interchangeable (bioavailability varies); cases of severe hepatotoxicity, including fulminant hepatic necrosis, have occurred in patients who have substituted niacin products at equivalent doses. Patients should be initiated with low doses (eg, niacin extended release 500 mg at bedtime) with titration to achieve desired response. Flushing and pruritus, common adverse effects of niacin, may be attenuated with a gradual increase in dose, administering with food, avoidance of concurrent ingestion of ethanol or hot liquids, and/or by taking aspirin (adults: 325 mg) (Stone, 2013). May also use other NSAIDs according to the manufacturer. Flushing associated with extended release preparation is significantly reduced (Guyton, 2007). For immediate release preparations, may administer in 2 to 3 divided doses to reduce the frequency and severity. Niacin should not be used if patient experiences persistent severe cutaneous symptoms during therapy (Stone, 2013).

Potentially significant interactions may exist, requiring dose or frequency adjustment, additional monitoring, and/or selection of alternative therapy.
Adverse Reactions Frequency not defined.
Cardiovascular: Arrhythmias, atrial fibrillation, edema, flushing, hypotension, orthostasis, palpitation, syncope (rare), tachycardia
Central nervous system: Chills, dizziness, headache, insomnia, migraine, nervousness, pain
Dermatologic: Acanthosis nigricans, burning skin, dry skin, hyperpigmentation, maculopapular rash, pruritus, rash, skin discoloration, urticaria
Endocrine & metabolic: Glucose tolerance decreased, gout, phosphorous levels decreased, hyperuricemia
Gastrointestinal: Abdominal pain, amylase increased, diarrhea, dyspepsia, eructation, flatulence, nausea, peptic ulcers, vomiting
Hematologic: Platelet counts decreased
Hepatic: Hepatic necrosis (rare), hepatitis, jaundice, transaminases increased (dose-related), prothrombin time increased, total bilirubin increased
Neuromuscular & skeletal: CPK increased, leg cramps, myalgia, myasthenia, myopathy (with concurrent HMG-CoA reductase inhibitor), paresthesia, rhabdomyolysis (with concurrent HMG-CoA reductase inhibitor; rare), weakness
Ocular: Blurred vision, cystoid macular edema, toxic amblyopia
Respiratory: Cough, dyspnea
Miscellaneous: Diaphoresis, hypersensitivity reactions (rare; includes anaphylaxis, angioedema, laryngismus, vesiculobullous rash), LDH increased
Drug Interactions
Metabolism/Transport Effects None known.
Avoid Concomitant Use There are no known interactions where it is recommended to avoid concomitant use.
Increased Effect/Toxicity
Niacin may increase the levels/effects of: HMG-CoA Reductase Inhibitors

The levels/effects of Niacin may be increased by: Alcohol (Ethyl)
Decreased Effect
Niacin may decrease the levels/effects of: Antidiabetic Agents

The levels/effects of Niacin may be decreased by: Bile Acid Sequestrants
Storage/Stability
Niaspan: Store at 20°C to 25°C (68°F to 77°F).
Niacor: Store at 15°C to 30°C (59°F to 86°F).
Mechanism of Action Niacin (nicotinic acid) is bioconverted to nicotinamide which is further converted to nicotinamide adenine dinucleotide (NAD+) and the hydride equivalent (NADH) which are coenzymes necessary for tissue metabolism, lipid metabolism, and glycogenolysis (Belenky, 2006; Suave, 2008). The mechanism by which niacin (in lipid-lowering doses) affects plasma lipoproteins is not fully understood. It may involve several actions including partial inhibition of release of free fatty acids from adipose tissue, and increased lipoprotein lipase activity, which may increase the rate of chylomicron triglyceride removal from plasma. Ultimately, niacin reduces total cholesterol, apolipoprotein (apo) B, triglycerides, VLDL, LDL, lipoprotein (a), and increases HDL and other important components and subfractions (eg, LPA-I) (Kamanna, 2000)

Pharmacodynamics/Kinetics

Absorption: Immediate release formulation: Rapid and extensive. Extent of niacin ER absorption from niacin ER/lovastatin is increased (22% to 30%) with food.

Protein binding: <20% bound to serum proteins

Metabolism: Extensive first-pass metabolism; converted to nicotinamide adenine dinucleotide, nicotinuric acid (after conjugation with glycine), and other metabolites. At doses used to treat hyperlipidemia, metabolic pathways are saturable.

Half-life elimination: 20 to 48 minutes

Time to peak, serum: Immediate release formulation: 30 to 60 minutes; extended release formulation: 4 to 5 hours

Excretion: Urine 60% to 88% (unchanged drug [up to 12% recovered after multiple dosing] and metabolites)

Dosing

Adult & Geriatric Note: Formulations of niacin (regular release versus extended release) are not interchangeable.

Recommended daily allowances (National Academy of Sciences, 1998): Oral:

≥19 years: Females: 14 mg daily; Males: 16 mg daily

Pregnancy (all ages): 18 mg daily

Lactation (all ages): 17 mg daily

Dietary supplement (OTC labeling): Oral: 50 mg twice daily or 100 mg once daily. **Note:** Many over-the-counter formulations exist.

Hyperlipidemia: Oral:

Regular release formulation (Niacor): Initial: 250 mg once daily (with evening meal); increase frequency and/or dose every 4 to 7 days to desired response or first-level therapeutic dose (1.5 to 2 g daily in 2 to 3 divided doses); after 2 months, may increase at 2- to 4-week intervals to 3 g daily in 3 divided doses (maximum dose: 6 g daily in 3 divided doses). **Note:** Many over-the-counter formulations exist.

ACC/AHA Blood Cholesterol Guideline recommendations: Initial: 100 mg administered 3 times daily; increase dose gradually as tolerated to 3 g daily divided in 2 to 3 doses (Stone, 2013)

Sustained release (or controlled release) formulations: **Note:** Several over-the-counter formulations exist. Slo-Niacin: Usual dosage is 250 to 750 mg once daily, taken morning or evening, or as directed. Before using more than 500 mg daily, patient should consult health care provider.

Extended release formulation (Niaspan): Initial: 500 mg at bedtime for 4 weeks, then 1 g at bedtime for 4 weeks; adjust dose to response and tolerance; may increase daily dose every 4 weeks by not more than 500 mg daily to a maximum of 2 g daily. Recommended maintenance dose: 1,000 to 2,000 mg at bedtime.

ACC/AHA Blood Cholesterol Guideline recommendations: Initial: 500 mg once daily; increase dose gradually (ie, no sooner than at weekly intervals) over 4 to 8 weeks as tolerated to a maximum dose of 2 g once daily (Stone, 2013)

Pellagra (off-label use): Oral: 50 to 100 mg 3 to 4 times daily; maximum: 500 mg daily (Prousky 2003; Delgado-Sanchez 2008; DesGroseilliers 1976; Oldham 2012). Some experts prefer niacinamide for treatment due to more favorable side effect profile (Hegyi 2004; Jen 2010).

Pediatric Note: Formulations of niacin (regular release versus extended release) are not interchangeable.

Adequate intake (National Academy of Sciences, 1998): Oral:

0 to 5 months: 2 mg daily

6 to 11 months: 3 mg daily

Recommended daily allowances (National Academy of Sciences, 1998): Oral:

1 to 3 years: 6 mg daily

4 to 8 years: 8 mg daily

9 to 13 years: 12 mg daily

14 to 18 years: Females: 14 mg daily; Males: 16 mg daily

≥19 years: Refer to adult dosing.

Pellagra (off-label use) Oral: 50 to 100 mg 3 times daily. Some experts prefer niacinamide for treatment due to more favorable side effect profile (Hegyi 2004; Jen 2010).

Renal Impairment There are no dosage adjustments provided in the manufacturer's labeling (has not been studied); use with caution.

Hepatic Impairment There are no dosage adjustments provided in the manufacturer's labeling (has not been studied). Contraindicated in patients with significant or unexplained hepatic dysfunction, active liver disease or unexplained persistent transaminase elevations.

Adjustment for Toxicity Hepatic toxicity: Transaminases rise ≥3 times ULN, either persistent or if symptoms of nausea, fever, and/or malaise occur: Discontinue therapy.

Dietary Considerations Should be taken with meal; low-fat meal if treating hyperlipidemia. Avoid alcohol, hot drinks, and spicy foods around the time of niacin dose.

Administration Administer with food. To attenuate flushing symptoms, may premedicate with aspirin 325 mg administered 30 minutes before dose; avoid ingestion of hot liquids, alcohol, or spicy foods concurrently with niacin (Stone, 2013). May also use other NSAIDs to prevent flushing according to the manufacturer.

Niaspan: Administer at bedtime after a low-fat snack. Two of the 500 mg and one of the 1,000 mg tablet strengths are interchangeable, but three of the 500 mg and two of the 750 mg tablet strengths are not interchangeable. When switching from immediate-release tablet, initiate Niaspan with the recommended titration schedule. If therapy is interrupted for an extended period, dose should be retitrated.

Long-acting forms should not be crushed, broken, or chewed. Slo-Niacin may be broken along the score line. Do not substitute long-acting forms for immediate release ones.

Monitoring Parameters

2013 ACC/AHA Blood Cholesterol Guideline recommendations (Stone, 2013): Baseline hepatic transaminases, fasting blood glucose or hemoglobin A1c, and uric acid before initiation and repeat during uptitration to maintenance dose and every 6 months thereafter.

Manufacturer recommendations: Blood glucose (in diabetic patients); if on concurrent HMG-CoA reductase inhibitor, may periodically check CPK and serum potassium; liver function tests pretreatment, every 6-12 weeks for first year, then periodically (approximately every 6 months), monitor liver function more frequently if history of transaminase elevation with prior use; lipid profile; platelets (if on anticoagulants); PT (if on anticoagulants); uric acid (if predisposed to gout); phosphorus (if predisposed to hypophosphatemia)

Test Interactions False elevations in some fluorometric determinations of plasma or urinary catecholamines; false-positive urine glucose (Benedict's reagent)

Dosage Forms Excipient information presented when available (limited, particularly for generics); consult specific product labeling.

Capsule Extended Release, Oral:

Generic: 250 mg, 500 mg

Capsule Extended Release, Oral [preservative free]:

Generic: 250 mg, 500 mg

Tablet, Oral:

Niacin-50: 50 mg [starch free, sugar free, wheat free]

Niacor: 500 mg [scored]

Generic: 50 mg, 100 mg, 250 mg, 500 mg

Tablet, Oral [preservative free]:

Generic: 50 mg, 100 mg, 500 mg

Tablet Extended Release, Oral:

Niaspan: 500 mg, 750 mg, 1000 mg [contains fd&c yellow #6 aluminum lake]

Slo-Niacin: 250 mg [scored]

Slo-Niacin: 500 mg, 750 mg [scored; contains fd&c red #40]

Generic: 500 mg, 750 mg, 1000 mg

Tablet Extended Release, Oral [preservative free]:

Generic: 250 mg, 500 mg, 1000 mg

◆ Niacin-50 [OTC] see Niacin on page 1273

Niacinamide (nye a SIN a mide)

Index Terms Nicomide-T; Nicotinamide; Nicotinic Acid Amide; Vitamin B_3

Pharmacologic Category Vitamin, Water Soluble

Use Dietary supplement

Dosing

Adult & Geriatric Pellagra (off-label use): Oral: 100 mg every 6 hours for several days (or until resolution of major signs and symptoms), followed by 50 mg every 8-12 hours until skin lesions heal (Hegyi, 2004)

Pediatric Pellagra (off-label use): Oral: 10-50 mg every 6 hours until resolution of signs and symptoms (Hegyi, 2004)

Additional Information Complete prescribing information should be consulted for additional detail.

Dosage Forms Excipient information presented when available (limited, particularly for generics); consult specific product labeling.

Tablet, Oral:
Generic: 100 mg, 500 mg
Tablet, Oral [preservative free]:
Generic: 100 mg, 500 mg

Niacin and Lovastatin (NYE a sin & LOE va sta tin)

Brand Names: US Advicor
Index Terms Lovastatin and Niacin
Pharmacologic Category Antilipemic Agent, HMG-CoA Reductase Inhibitor; Antilipemic Agent, Miscellaneous
Use Primary hypercholesterolemia/mixed dyslipidemia: Treatment of primary hypercholesterolemia (heterozygous familial and nonfamilial) and mixed dyslipidemia (Fredrickson types IIa and IIb) in combination with a standard cholesterol-lowering diet.

Dosing

Adult & Geriatric Dosage forms are a fixed combination of niacin and lovastatin. Patients not currently on niacin extended release must start niacin extended release/lovastatin at the lowest dose.

Primary hypercholesterolemia/mixed dyslipidemia: Oral: Lowest dose: Niacin extended release 500 mg/lovastatin 20 mg once daily at bedtime with a low-fat snack; may increase by not more than 500 mg (niacin extended release) once daily at bedtime at 4-week intervals (maximum dose: niacin extended release 2000 mg/lovastatin 40 mg daily). **Note:** If therapy is interrupted for >7 days, reinstitution of therapy should begin with the lowest dose followed by retitration as needed.

Not for use as initial therapy of dyslipidemias. May be substituted for equivalent dose of Niaspan; however, manufacturer does not recommend direct substitution with other niacin products.

Dosage adjustment for lovastatin component with concomitant medications:
Amiodarone: Maximum recommended lovastatin dose: 40 mg daily
Danazol, diltiazem, dronedarone, or verapamil: Initial lovastatin dose: 10 mg daily (dosage unavailable with combination product; use separate components); Maximum recommended lovastatin dose: 20 mg daily

Renal Impairment
Mild to moderate impairment (CrCl ≥30 mL/minute): No dosage adjustment necessary
Severe impairment (CrCl <30 mL/minute): There are no dosage adjustments provided in the manufacturer's labeling; use doses of lovastatin >20 mg daily with caution

Hepatic Impairment There are no dosage adjustments provided in the manufacturer's labeling; contraindicated in active liver disease or unexplained persistent elevations of serum transaminases.

Additional Information Complete prescribing information should be consulted for additional detail.

Dosage Forms Excipient information presented when available (limited, particularly for generics); consult specific product labeling.

Tablet, variable release, oral:
Advicor 500/20: Niacin 500 mg [extended release] and lovastatin 20 mg [immediate release]
Advicor 750/20: Niacin 750 mg [extended release] and lovastatin 20 mg [immediate release]
Advicor 1000/20: Niacin 1000 mg [extended release] and lovastatin 20 mg [immediate release]
Advicor 1000/40: Niacin 1000 mg [extended release] and lovastatin 40 mg [immediate release]

◆ Niacor see Niacin on page 1273

◆ Niaspan see Niacin on page 1273

◆ Niaspan FCT (Can) see Niacin on page 1273

◆ Niastase (Can) see Factor VIIa (Recombinant) on page 733

◆ Niastase RT (Can) see Factor VIIa (Recombinant) on page 733

NiCARdipine (nye KAR de peen)

Brand Names: US Cardene IV; Cardene SR [DSC]
Index Terms Cardene; Nicardipine Hydrochloride
Pharmacologic Category Antianginal Agent; Antihypertensive; Calcium Channel Blocker; Calcium Channel Blocker, Dihydropyridine

Additional Appendix Information
Hypertension *on page 1996*
Use

Angina: Management of chronic stable angina (oral immediate-release product only)

Hypertension: Management of hypertension (oral immediate- and sustained-release products and IV); parenteral only for short-term use when oral treatment is not feasible or not desirable

The 2014 guideline for the management of high blood pressure in adults (JNC 8) recommends initiation of pharmacologic treatment to lower blood pressure for the following patients (JNC 8 [James 2013]):
• Patients ≥60 years of age with systolic blood pressure (SBP) ≥150 mm Hg or diastolic blood pressure (DBP) ≥90 mm Hg. Goal of therapy is SBP <150 mm Hg and DBP <90 mm Hg.
• Patients <60 years of age with SBP ≥140 mm Hg or DBP ≥90 mm Hg. Goal of therapy is SBP <140 mm Hg and DBP <90 mm Hg.
• Patients ≥18 years of age with diabetes with SBP ≥140 mm Hg or DBP ≥90 mm Hg. Goal of therapy is SBP <140 mm Hg and DBP <90 mm Hg.
• Patients ≥18 years of age with chronic kidney disease (CKD) with SBP ≥140 mm Hg or DBP ≥90 mm Hg. Goal of therapy is SBP <140 mm Hg and DBP <90 mm Hg.
In patients with chronic kidney disease (CKD), regardless of race or diabetes status, the use of an ACE inhibitor (ACEI) or angiotensin receptor blocker (ARB) as initial therapy is recommended to improve kidney outcomes. In the general nonblack population (without CKD) including those with diabetes, initial antihypertensive treatment should consist of a thiazide-type diuretic, calcium channel blocker, ACEI, or ARB. In the general black population (without CKD) including those with diabetes, initial antihypertensive treatment should consist of a thiazide-type diuretic or a calcium channel blocker instead of an ACEI or ARB.

Pregnancy Considerations Adverse events have been observed in some animal reproduction studies. Nicardipine has been used for the treatment of severe hypertension in pregnancy and preterm labor. Nicardipine crosses the placenta; changes in fetal heart rate, neonatal hypotension and neonatal acidosis have been observed following maternal use (rare; based on limited data). Adverse effects reported in pregnant women are generally similar to those reported in nonpregnant patients; however, pulmonary edema has been observed (Nij 2010). Untreated chronic maternal hypertension is also associated with adverse events in the fetus, infant, and mother. If treatment for hypertension during pregnancy is needed, other agents are preferred (ACOG 2013).

Breast-Feeding Considerations Nicardipine is minimally excreted in breast milk. In one study, peak milk concentrations ranged from 1.9 to 18.8 mcg/mL following oral maternal doses of 40 to 150 mg/day. The estimated exposure to the breast-feeding infant was calculated to be 0.073% of the weight-adjusted maternal oral dose or 0.14% of the weight-adjusted maternal IV dose. Breast-feeding is not recommended by some manufacturers.

Contraindications Hypersensitivity to nicardipine or any component of the formulation; advanced aortic stenosis

Warnings/Precautions Symptomatic hypotension with or without syncope can rarely occur; blood pressure must be lowered at a rate appropriate for the patient's clinical condition. Avoid systemic hypotension in acute cerebral infarction or hemorrhage. Tachycardia may occur; close monitoring of blood pressure and heart rate is required. Increased angina (frequency, duration, or severity) and/or MI has occurred with initiation or dosage titration of dihydropyridine calcium channel blockers. Reflex tachycardia may occur resulting in angina and/or MI in patients with obstructive coronary disease, especially in the absence of concurrent beta blockade. The most common side effect is peripheral edema (dose-dependent); occurs within 2 to 3 weeks of starting therapy. Use with caution in CAD (can cause increase in angina), mild to moderate aortic stenosis (may reduce coronary perfusion resulting in ischemia; use is contraindicated in patients with advanced aortic stenosis), and hypertrophic cardiomyopathy with outflow tract obstruction. The ACCF/AHA heart failure guidelines recommend to avoid use in patients with heart failure due to lack of benefit and/or worse outcomes with calcium channel blockers in general (Yancy 2013). To minimize infusion site reactions, peripheral infusion sites (for IV therapy) should be changed every 12 hours; use of small peripheral veins should be avoided. Use with caution in patients with hepatic impairment or reduced hepatic blood flow; consider lower starting dose and closely monitor response. Use with caution in patients with renal impairment; increase dose cautiously since clearance of nicardipine

is diminished in this population. Initiate at the low end of the dosage range in the elderly. Abrupt withdrawal may cause rebound angina in patients with CAD. Some dosage forms may contain propylene glycol; large amounts are potentially toxic and have been associated hyperosmolality, lactic acidosis, seizures and respiratory depression; use caution (AAP 1997; Zar 2007). Potentially significant drug-drug interactions may exist, requiring dose or frequency adjustment, additional monitoring, and/or selection of alternative therapy.

Adverse Reactions

1% to 10%:

Cardiovascular: Flushing (6% to 10%), pedal edema (dose related; 7% to 8%), exacerbation of angina pectoris (dose related; 6%), hypotension (IV 6%), palpitations (3% to 4%), tachycardia (1% to 4%), chest pain (IV 1%), extrasystoles (IV 1%), hemopericardium (IV 1%), hypertension (IV 1%), supraventricular tachycardia (IV 1%), edema (≤1%)

Central nervous system: Headache (6% to 15%), dizziness (4% to 7%), hypoesthesia (1%), intracranial hemorrhage (1%), pain (1%), somnolence (1%)

Dermatologic: Diaphoresis (1%), skin rash (≤1%)

Endocrine & metabolic: Hypokalemia (IV 1%)

Gastrointestinal: Nausea and vomiting (IV 5%), nausea (2%), dyspepsia (≤2%), abdominal pain (IV 1%), xerostomia (≤1%)

Genitourinary: Hematuria (1%)

Local: Injection site reaction (IV 1%), pain at injection site (IV 1%)

Neuromuscular & skeletal: Weakness (4% to 6%), myalgia (1%), paresthesia (1%)

<1% (Limited to important or life-threatening): Abnormal dreams, abnormal hepatic function tests, abnormal vision, angina pectoris, arthralgia, atrial fibrillation (not distinguishable from natural history of atherosclerotic vascular disease), cerebral ischemia (not distinguishable from natural history of atherosclerotic vascular disease), conjunctivitis, deep vein thrombophlebitis, depression, ECG abnormal, gingival hyperplasia, heart block (not distinguishable from natural history of atherosclerotic vascular disease), hot flash, hyperkinesia, hypersensitivity reaction, hypertonia, hypophosphatemia, hypotension (exertional; not distinguishable from natural history of atherosclerotic vascular disease), myocardial infarction (chronic therapy; may be due to disease progression), neck pain, nervousness, oxygen saturation decreased (possible pulmonary shunting), parotitis, pericarditis (not distinguishable from natural history of atherosclerotic vascular disease), peripheral vascular disease, respiratory tract disease, sinus node dysfunction (chronic therapy; may be due to disease progression), sustained tachycardia, thrombocytopenia, tinnitus, tremor, urinary frequency, ventricular extrasystoles, ventricular tachycardia, vertigo

Drug Interactions

Metabolism/Transport Effects Substrate of CYP1A2 (minor), CYP2C9 (minor), CYP2D6 (minor), CYP2E1 (minor), CYP3A4 (major), P-glycoprotein; **Note:** Assignment of Major/Minor substrate status based on clinically relevant drug interaction potential; **Inhibits** CYP2C19 (moderate), CYP2C9 (strong), CYP2D6 (moderate), CYP3A4 (weak), P-glycoprotein

Avoid Concomitant Use

Avoid concomitant use of NiCARdipine with any of the following: Bosutinib; Conivaptan; Fusidic Acid (Systemic); Idelalisib; PAZOPanib; Pimozide; Silodosin; Thioridazine; Topotecan; VinCRIStine (Liposomal)

Increased Effect/Toxicity

NiCARdipine may increase the levels/effects of: Afatinib; Amifostine; Antipsychotic Agents (Second Generation [Atypical]); ARIPiprazole; Atosiban; Bosentan; Bosutinib; Brentuximab Vedotin; Brexpiprazole; Calcium Channel Blockers (Nondihydropyridine); Carvedilol; Cilostazol; Citalopram; Colchicine; CYP2C19 Substrates; CYP2C9 Substrates; CYP2D6 Substrates; Dabigatran Etexilate; Diclofenac (Systemic); DOXOrubicin (Conventional); Dronabinol; DULoxetine; Edoxaban; Eliglustat; Everolimus; Fesoterodine; Flibanserin; Fosphenytoin; Highest Risk QTc-Prolonging Agents; Hydrocodone; Hypotension-Associated Agents; Lacosamide; Ledipasvir; Levodopa; Lomitapide; Magnesium Salts; Metoprolol; Moderate Risk QTc-Prolonging Agents; Naloxegol; Nebivolol; Neuromuscular-Blocking Agents (Nondepolarizing); NiMODipine; Nitroprusside; Ospemifene; Parecoxib; PAZOPanib; P-glycoprotein/ABCB1 Substrates; Phenytoin; Pimozide; Prucalopride; Ramelteon; Ranolazine; Rifaximin; Silodosin; Tacrolimus (Systemic); Tetrahydrocannabinol; Thioridazine; Topotecan; VinCRIStine (Liposomal)

The levels/effects of NiCARdipine may be increased by: Alfuzosin; Alpha1-Blockers; Antifungal Agents (Azole

Derivatives, Systemic); Aprepitant; Barbiturates; Brimonidine (Topical); Calcium Channel Blockers (Nondihydropyridine); Cannabis; Conivaptan; CycloSPORINE (Systemic); CYP3A4 Inhibitors (Moderate); CYP3A4 Inhibitors (Strong); Dapoxetine; Dasatinib; Diazoxide; Fluconazole; Fosaprepitant; Fusidic Acid (Systemic); Grapefruit Juice; Herbs (Hypotensive Properties); Idelalisib; Ivacaftor; Luliconazole; Macrolide Antibiotics; Magnesium Salts; Mifepristone; Molsidomine; Netupitant; Nicorandil; Obinutuzumab; Osimertinib; Palbociclib; Pentoxifylline; P-glycoprotein/ABCB1 Inhibitors; Phosphodiesterase 5 Inhibitors; Propafenone; Prostacyclin Analogues; Ranolazine; Simeprevir; Stiripentol

Decreased Effect

NiCARdipine may decrease the levels/effects of: Clopidogrel; Codeine; Tamoxifen; TraMADol

The levels/effects of NiCARdipine may be decreased by: Amphetamines; Barbiturates; Bosentan; Calcium Salts; CarBAMazepine; CYP3A4 Inducers (Moderate); CYP3A4 Inducers (Strong); Dabrafenib; Deferasirox; Efavirenz; Enzalutamide; Herbs (Hypertensive Properties); Melatonin; Methylphenidate; Mitotane; Nafcillin; Osimertinib; P-glycoprotein/ABCB1 Inducers; Phenytoin; Rifamycin Derivatives; Siltuximab; St Johns Wort; Tocilizumab; Yohimbine

Food Interactions Nicardipine average peak concentrations may be decreased if taken with food. Serum concentrations/toxicity of nicardipine may be increased by grapefruit juice. Management: Avoid grapefruit juice.

Preparation for Administration

IV: Vial: Dilute 25 mg vial with 240 mL of compatible solution to provide a 250 mL total volume solution and a final concentration of 0.1 mg/mL.

Premixed bags: No further dilution needed.

Storage/Stability

IV:

Premixed bags: Store at 20°C to 25°C (68°F to 77°F). Protect from light and excessive heat. Do not freeze.

Vials: Store at 20°C to 25°C (68°F to 77°F). Protect from light. Freezing does not adversely affect the product, but exposure to elevated temperatures should be avoided. Diluted solution (0.1 mg/mL) is stable at room temperature for 24 hours in glass or PVC containers. Stability has also been demonstrated at room temperature at concentrations up to 0.5 mg/mL in PVC containers for 24 hours or in glass containers for up to 7 days (Baaske 1996).

Oral: Store at room temperature. Protect from light.

Mechanism of Action Inhibits calcium ion from entering the "slow channels" or select voltage-sensitive areas of vascular smooth muscle and myocardium during depolarization, producing a relaxation of coronary vascular smooth muscle and coronary vasodilation; increases myocardial oxygen delivery in patients with vasospastic angina

Pharmacodynamics/Kinetics

Onset of action: IV: Within minutes (constant infusion)

Duration:

IV: ≤8 hours

Oral: Immediate release: ≤8 hours; Sustained release: 8 to 12 hours

Absorption: Oral: ~100%

Distribution: V_d: 8.3 L/kg

Protein binding: >95%

Metabolism: Hepatic; extensive first-pass effect (saturable)

Bioavailability: Oral: ~35%

Half-life elimination: Oral: Immediate release: 2 to 4 hours; Sustained release: 9 hours

Time to peak, serum: Oral: Immediate release: 30 to 120 minutes; Sustained release: 60 to 240 minutes

Excretion: Urine (49% to 60% as metabolites); feces (35% to 43% as metabolites)

Dosing

Adult Note: Cardene SR has been discontinued in the US for more than 1 year.

Angina: Immediate release: Oral: 20 mg 3 times daily; usual dosage: 20 to 40 mg 3 times daily (allow ≥3 days between dose increases)

Hypertension: Oral:

Immediate release: Initial: 20 mg 3 times daily; usual dosage: 20 to 40 mg 3 times daily (allow ≥3 days between dose increases)

Sustained release: Initial: 30 mg twice daily; usual dosage: 30 to 60 mg twice daily

Acute hypertension: IV: Initial: 5 mg/hour; may increase by 2.5 mg/hour every 5 minutes (for rapid titration) to every 15 minutes (for gradual titration) up to a maximum of 15 mg/hour; rapidly titrated patients, consider reduction to 3 mg/hour after response is achieved. Discontinue infusion if unacceptable hypotension or tachycardia occurs.

Arterial hypertension in acute ischemic stroke (off-label use [Jauch 2013]): IV:

Patient otherwise eligible for reperfusion treatment (eg, alteplase) except blood pressure (BP) >185/110 mm Hg: Initiate 5 mg/hour; titrate by 2.5 mg/hour at 5- to 15-minute intervals (maximum dose: 15 mg/hour). When goal BP obtained, adjust dose to maintain proper BP limits. If BP does not decline and remains >185/110 mm Hg, alteplase should not be administered.

Management of BP during and after reperfusion treatment (eg, alteplase) to maintain BP ≤180/105 mm Hg: If systolic BP >180 to 230 mm Hg or diastolic >105 to 120 mm Hg: Initiate 5 mg/hour; titrate by 2.5 mg/hour at 5- to 15-minute intervals (maximum dose: 15 mg/hour). If hypertension is refractory or diastolic BP >140 mm Hg, consider other IV antihypertensives (eg, nitroprusside).

Substitution for oral therapy (approximate equivalents):
20 mg every 8 hours oral, equivalent to 0.5 mg/hour IV infusion
30 mg every 8 hours oral, equivalent to 1.2 mg/hour IV infusion
40 mg every 8 hours oral, equivalent to 2.2 mg/hour IV infusion

Conversion to oral antihypertensive agent: Initiate oral antihypertensive at the same time that IV nicardipine is discontinued, if transitioning to oral nicardipine, start oral nicardipine 1 hour prior to IV discontinuation.

Geriatric Initiate at the low end of the dosage range. Specific guidelines for adjustment of nicardipine are not available, but careful monitoring is warranted and adjustment may be necessary.

Renal Impairment

Oral: Per the manufacturer: Initial: 20 mg 3 times daily (immediate release) or 30 mg twice daily (sustained release) with slow titration.

IV: There are no dosage adjustments provided in the manufacturer's labeling; titrate slowly with careful monitoring; dosage adjustment may be necessary.

Hepatic Impairment

Oral: Per the manufacturer: Initial: 20 mg twice daily (immediate release) with slow titration.

IV: There are no dosage adjustments provided in the manufacturer's labeling; titrate slowly with monitoring; dosage adjustment may be necessary.

Dietary Considerations Avoid grapefruit juice.

Usual Infusion Concentrations: Pediatric Note: Premixed solutions available

IV infusion: 100 mcg/mL

Usual Infusion Concentrations: Adult Note: Premixed solutions available

IV infusion: 25 mg in 250 mL (total volume) (concentration: 0.1 mg/mL) of D_5W, $D_5{}^1/_2NS$, D_5NS, D_5W with KCl 40 mEq, NS, or $^1/_2NS$

Administration

Oral: The total daily dose of immediate-release product may not automatically be equivalent to the daily sustained-release dose; use caution in converting. Administer without regards to meals; nicardipine sustained release administered with a meal may reduce the fluctuation in plasma levels. Do not chew or crush the sustained release formulation, swallow whole. Do not open or cut capsules.

IV:

Administer as a slow continuous infusion via central line or through a large peripheral vein. Peripheral venous irritation may be minimized by changing the site of infusion every 12 hours.

Premixed bags: Do not combine or run in the same line as other medications.

Monitoring Parameters Blood pressure, heart rate; consult individual institutional policies and procedures

Product Availability Cardene SR has been discontinued in the US for more than 1 year.

Dosage Forms Excipient information presented when available (limited, particularly for generics); consult specific product labeling. [DSC] = Discontinued product

Capsule, Oral, as hydrochloride:
Generic: 20 mg, 30 mg

Capsule Extended Release 12 Hour, Oral, as hydrochloride:
Cardene SR: 30 mg [DSC] [contains fd&c red #40]
Cardene SR: 45 mg [DSC], 60 mg [DSC] [contains fd&c blue #2 (indigotine)]

Solution, Intravenous, as hydrochloride:
Cardene IV: 20 mg (200 mL); 40 mg (200 mL); 2.5 mg/mL (10 mL [DSC])
Generic: 2.5 mg/mL (10 mL)

◆ **Nicardipine Hydrochloride** *see* NiCARdipine *on page 1275*

◆ NicAzelDoxy 30 [DSC] *see* Doxycycline *on page 601*
◆ NicAzelDoxy 60 [DSC] *see* Doxycycline *on page 601*
◆ Nicoderm (Can) *see* Nicotine *on page 1277*
◆ Nicoderm CQ [OTC] *see* Nicotine *on page 1277*
◆ Nicomide-T *see* Niacinamide *on page 1274*
◆ Nicorelief [OTC] *see* Nicotine *on page 1277*
◆ Nicorette [OTC] *see* Nicotine *on page 1277*
◆ Nicorette (Can) *see* Nicotine *on page 1277*
◆ Nicorette Mini [OTC] *see* Nicotine *on page 1277*
◆ Nicorette Plus (Can) *see* Nicotine *on page 1277*
◆ Nicorette Refill [OTC] [DSC] *see* Nicotine *on page 1277*
◆ Nicorette Starter Kit [OTC] *see* Nicotine *on page 1277*
◆ Nicotinamide *see* Niacinamide *on page 1274*

Nicotine (nik oh TEEN)

Brand Names: US Commit [OTC] [DSC]; Nicoderm CQ [OTC]; Nicorelief [OTC]; NICOrelief [OTC] [DSC]; Nicorette Mini [OTC]; Nicorette Refill [OTC] [DSC]; Nicorette Starter Kit [OTC]; Nicorette [OTC]; Nicotrol; Nicotrol NS; Thrive [OTC]

Brand Names: Canada Habitrol; Nicoderm; Nicorette; Nicorette Plus; Nicotrol

Index Terms Habitrol; Nicotine Patch

Pharmacologic Category Smoking Cessation Aid

Use Smoking cessation: Treatment to aid smoking cessation for the relief of nicotine withdrawal symptoms (including nicotine craving)

Pregnancy Considerations Adverse events have been observed in animal reproduction studies. Nicotine crosses the placenta (HHS 2014). Maternal smoking is associated with birth defects (HHS 2014; Hachshaw 2011); the incidence of birth defects following nicotine replacement therapy may be similar (limited data) (Dhalwani 2015). Nicotine exposure via cigarette smoke may cause increased ectopic pregnancy, low birth weight, increased risk of spontaneous abortion, increased perinatal mortality; increased aortic blood flow, increased heart rate, decreased uterine blood flow, and decreased breathing have been reported in the fetus. Smoking during pregnancy is associated with sudden infant death syndrome (SIDS), an increased risk of asthma, infantile colic, and childhood obesity (ACOG 2010; HHS 2014). Women who are pregnant should be encouraged not to smoke. The use of nicotine replacement products to aid in smoking cessation has not been adequately studied in pregnant women (amount of nicotine exposure is varied). Nonpharmacologic treatments are recommended. If the benefits of nicotine replacement therapy outweigh the unknown risks, it should be done under close supervision (ACOG, 2010).

Breast-Feeding Considerations Nicotine from cigarette smoke is found in breast milk and can be absorbed orally by the infant; hepatic clearance is likely lowest at birth. The amount of nicotine in breast milk from replacement products varies. Nicotine replacement therapy is considered to be compatible with breast feeding if the amount of nicotine is less than that received from smoking. Use of short acting products (gum, lozenges) is preferred (Sachs 2013). The manufacturer recommends caution be exercised when administering nicotine to breast-feeding women.

Contraindications

Hypersensitivity to nicotine or any component of the formulation.

OTC labeling: Nicorette lozenge: When used for self-medication, do not use if you are allergic to soya.

Warnings/Precautions Urge patients to stop smoking completely when initiating therapy. Nicotine can increase heart rate and blood pressure. The risk versus the benefits should be weighed in patients with cardiovascular or peripheral vascular diseases, specifically patients with a history of myocardial infarction and/or angina pectoris, serious cardiac arrhythmias, or vasospastic diseases (Buerger disease, Prinzmetal variant angina and Raynaud phenomena); use caution in patients with angina, hypertension, or recent MI. Discontinue use if irregular heartbeat or palpitations occur. Use caution in patients with accelerated hypertension due to the risk of malignant hypertension. Generally, avoid use during the immediate postmyocardial infarction period, in patients with serious arrhythmias, or with severe or worsening angina. Use with caution in patients with insulin-dependent diabetes, active peptic ulcer disease; severe hepatic impairment; hyperthyroidism; pheochromocytoma; severe renal impairment; use appropriate precautions for handling and disposal (EPA, P-listed).

OTC labeling: When used for self-medication, discontinue use and contact a health care provider if symptoms of nicotine overdose (eg, nausea, vomiting, dizziness, diarrhea, weakness, rapid heartbeat) or an allergic reaction (eg, difficulty breathing, rash) occurs.

Chewing gum and lozenge: When used for self-medication, consult a health care provider before use in patients on a sodium-restricted diet and in patients with a history of seizures. Discontinue chewing gum and consult a health care provider if mouth, teeth or jaw problems occur. Discontinue lozenge and consult a health care provider if mouth problems, persistent indigestion, or severe sore throat occurs.

Inhaler: Use with caution in patients with bronchospastic disease (eg, asthma, chronic pulmonary disease); may cause bronchospasm due to potential airway irritation; other forms of nicotine replacement may be preferred in patients with severe bronchospastic airway disease. Sustained use (beyond 6 months) by patients who quit smoking is not recommended.

Nasal spray: Use of nasal product is not recommended with chronic nasal disorders (eg, allergy, rhinitis, nasal polyps, and sinusitis). Exacerbations of bronchospasm has been reported in patients with preexisting asthma; use in patients with severe reactive airway disease is not recommended. Nasal mucosa irritation may occur. Sustained use (beyond 6 months) by patients who quit smoking is not recommended.

Transdermal patch: When used for self-medication, consult a health care provider before use in patients who have an allergy to adhesive tape or who have skin problems. Discontinue use and contact a health care provider if skin redness caused by the patch does not resolve after 4 days or if inflammation or rash occurs. If vivid dreams or other sleep disturbances occur, remove the patch at bedtime and apply another patch in the morning.

Adverse Reactions

Nasal spray/inhaler:
>10%:
Central nervous system: Headache (18% to 26%)
Gastrointestinal: Inhaler: Mouth/throat irritation (66%), dyspepsia (18%)
Respiratory: Inhaler: Cough (32%), rhinitis (23%)
1% to 10%:
Dermatologic: Acne (3%)
Endocrine & metabolic: Dysmenorrhea (3%)
Gastrointestinal: Flatulence (4%), gum problems (4%), diarrhea, hiccup, nausea, taste disturbance, tooth abrasions
Neuromuscular & skeletal: Back pain (6%), arthralgia (5%), jaw/neck pain
Respiratory: Nasal burning (nasal spray), sinusitis
Miscellaneous: Withdrawal symptoms
<1% (Limited to important or life-threatening): Allergy, amnesia, aphasia, bronchitis, bronchospasm, edema, migraine, numbness, pain, purpura, rash, sputum increased, vision abnormalities, xerostomia

Adverse events previously reported in prescription labeling for chewing gum, lozenge, and/or transdermal systems. Frequency not defined; may be product or dose specific:
Central nervous system: Concentration impaired, depression, dizziness, headache, insomnia, nervousness, pain
Gastrointestinal: Aphthous stomatitis, constipation, cough, diarrhea, dyspepsia, flatulence, gingival bleeding, glossitis, hiccups, jaw pain, nausea, salivation increased, stomatitis, taste perversion, tooth abrasions, ulcerative stomatitis, xerostomia
Dermatologic: Rash
Local: Application site reaction, local edema, local erythema
Neuromuscular & skeletal: Arthralgia, myalgia, paresthesia
Respiratory: Cough, sinusitis
Miscellaneous: Allergic reaction, diaphoresis

Drug Interactions

Metabolism/Transport Effects Substrate of CYP1A2 (minor), CYP2A6 (minor), CYP2B6 (minor), CYP2C19 (minor), CYP2C9 (minor), CYP2D6 (minor), CYP2E1 (minor), CYP3A4 (minor); **Note:** Assignment of Major/Minor substrate status based on clinically relevant drug interaction potential; **Inhibits** CYP2A6 (weak), CYP2E1 (weak)

Avoid Concomitant Use There are no known interactions where it is recommended to avoid concomitant use.

Increased Effect/Toxicity

Nicotine may increase the levels/effects of: Adenosine

The levels/effects of Nicotine may be increased by: Cimetidine; Varenicline

Decreased Effect There are no known significant interactions involving a decrease in effect.

Food Interactions Lozenge: Acidic foods/beverages decrease absorption of nicotine.

Storage/Stability Store at room temperature.
NicoDerm CQ: Dispose of used patches by folding sticky ends together; place in pouch and discard.
Nicorette gum, Nicorette lozenge and mini lozenge, Nicotrol: Protect from light. Wrap used pieces of gum in paper and discard.

Mechanism of Action Nicotine, a naturally occurring alkaloid, binds stereo-selectively to nicotinic-cholinergic receptors at the autonomic ganglia, in the adrenal medulla, at neuromuscular junctions, and in the brain. Two types of CNS effects are believed to be the basis of nicotine's positively reinforcing properties; a stimulating effect is exerted mainly in the cortex via the locus ceruleus and a reward effect is exerted in the limbic system. At low doses the stimulant effects predominate while at high doses the reward effects predominate.

Pharmacodynamics/Kinetics

Onset of action: Intranasal: More closely approximate the time course of plasma nicotine levels observed after cigarette smoking than other dosage forms (Svensson, 1987)
Absorption: Buccal mucosa, transdermal: Slow; Intranasal: ~53%; Inhaler: <5% reaches the lower respiratory tract
Distribution: 2 to 3 L/kg (Svensson, 1987)
Protein binding: 5% to 20% (Svensson, 1987)
Metabolism: Hepatic (major), kidney, and lung; >20 metabolites (primary metabolites are cotinine and trans-3-hydroxycotinine)
Half-life elimination: Transdermal: ~4 hours (Bannon, 1989); Intranasal: 1 to 2 hours; Oral inhalation: 1 to 2 hours
Time to peak, serum: Transdermal: ~2 to 8 hours (Bannon, 1989; DeVeaugh-Geiss, 2010); Intranasal: 4 to 15 minutes; Oral inhalation: ≤15 minutes; Gum: ~30 minutes (Svensson, 1987)
Excretion: Urine (~10% as unchanged)

Dosing

Adult & Geriatric

Tobacco cessation (patients should be advised to completely stop smoking upon initiation of therapy):

Gum: Chew 1 piece of gum when urge to smoke occurs. If strong or frequent cravings are present after 1 piece of gum, may use a second piece within the hour (do not continuously use one piece after the other). Patients who smoke their first cigarette within 30 minutes of waking should use the 4 mg strength; otherwise the 2 mg strength is recommended. Use according to the following 12-week dosing schedule:
Weeks 1 to 6: Chew 1 piece of gum every 1 to 2 hours (maximum: 24 pieces/day); to increase chances of quitting, chew at least 9 pieces/day during the first 6 weeks
Weeks 7 to 9: Chew 1 piece of gum every 2 to 4 hours (maximum: 24 pieces/day)
Weeks 10 to 12: Chew 1 piece of gum every 4 to 8 hours (maximum: 24 pieces/day)

Inhalation: Oral: Initial: Usually 6 to 16 cartridges per day; best effect was achieved by frequent continuous puffing (20 minutes); maximum: 16 cartridges/day; recommended duration of treatment is 3 months, after which patients may be weaned from the inhaler by gradual reduction of the daily dose over 6 to 12 weeks. Use beyond 6 months is not recommended (has not been studied).

Lozenge: Oral: 1 lozenge when urge to smoke occurs; do not use more than 1 lozenge at a time. Patients who smoke their first cigarette within 30 minutes of waking should use the 4 mg strength; otherwise the 2 mg strength is recommended. Use according to the following 12-week dosing schedule:
Weeks 1 to 6: 1 lozenge every 1 to 2 hours (maximum: 5 lozenges every 6 hours; 20 lozenges/day); to increase chances of quitting, use at least 9 lozenges/day during the first 6 weeks
Weeks 7 to 9: 1 lozenge every 2 to 4 hours (maximum: 5 lozenges every 6 hours; 20 lozenges/day)
Weeks 10 to 12: 1 lozenge every 4 to 8 hours (maximum: 5 lozenges every 6 hours; 20 lozenges/day)

Nasal: Spray: 1 to 2 doses/hour (each dose [2 sprays, one in each nostril] contains 1 mg of nicotine); do not exceed more than 5 doses (10 sprays) per hour [maximum: 40 mg/day (80 sprays)] or 3 months of treatment. **Note:** For best results, use at least the recommended minimum of 8 doses per day (less is unlikely to be effective).

Transdermal patch: Topical: **Note:** Adjustment may be required during initial treatment (move to higher dose if experiencing withdrawal symptoms; lower dose if side effects are experienced).

Patients smoking >10 cigarettes/day: Begin with step 1 (21 mg/day) for 6 weeks, **followed by** step 2 (14 mg/day) for 2 weeks; **finish with** step 3 (7 mg/day) for 2 weeks

Patients smoking ≤10 cigarettes/day: Begin with step 2 (14 mg/day) for 6 weeks, **followed by** step 3 (7 mg/day) for 2 weeks

Renal Impairment There are no dosage adjustments provided in the manufacturer's labeling (has not been studied). Only severe renal impairment should affect clearance of nicotine or its metabolites from circulation.

Hepatic Impairment There are no dosage adjustments provided in the manufacturer's labeling (has not been studied); because total system clearance of nicotine is dependent on hepatic blood flow, anticipate reduced clearance.

Dietary Considerations Some products may contain phenylalanine and/or sodium.

Administration

Gum: Chew slowly until it tingles, then place gum between cheek and gum until tingle is gone; repeat process until most of tingle is gone (~30 minutes). Do not eat or drink 15 minutes before using or while the gum is in mouth.

Lozenge: Do not chew or swallow; allow to dissolve slowly (~20 to 30 minutes); minimize swallowing and occasionally move lozenge from one side of the mouth to the other until completely dissolved. Do not eat or drink 15 minutes before using or while lozenge is in mouth.

Nasal spray: Prime pump prior to first use (pump 6 to 8 times until fine spray appears) or if it has not been used for 24 hours (pump 1 to 2 times). Blow nose prior to use. Tilt head back slightly and insert tip of bottle into nostril. Breathe through mouth and spray once in each nostril. Do not sniff, swallow, or inhale through the nose during administration. After administration, wait 2 to 3 minutes before blowing nose.

Oral Inhalation: Insert cartridge into inhaler and push hard until it pops into place. Replace mouthpiece and twist the top and bottom so that markings do not line up. Inhale deeply into the back of the throat or puff in short breaths. Nicotine in cartridge is used up after about 20 minutes of active puffing. Clean mouthpiece regularly with soap and water.

Transdermal patch: Apply new patch to nonhairy, clean, dry skin on the upper body or upper outer arm; each patch should be applied to a different site. Apply immediately after removing backing from patch; press onto skin for ~10 seconds. Patch may be worn for 16 or 24 hours. If cigarette cravings occur upon awakening, wear for 24 hours; if vivid dreams or other sleep disturbances occur, remove the patch at bedtime and apply a new patch in the morning. Do not cut patch; causes rapid evaporation, rendering the patch useless. Do not wear more than 1 patch at a time; do not leave patch on for more than 24 hours (may irritate skin). Wash hands after applying or removing patch. Discard patches by folding adhesive ends together, replace in pouch and dispose of properly in trash.

Hazardous agent; use appropriate precautions for handling and disposal (EPA, P-listed).

Monitoring Parameters Signs and symptoms of nicotine toxicity (eg, severe headache, dizziness, mental confusion, disturbed hearing and vision, abdominal pain; rapid, weak and irregular pulse; salivation, nausea, vomiting, diarrhea, cold sweat, weakness)

Additional Information A cigarette has 10-25 mg nicotine.

Dosage Forms Excipient information presented when available (limited, particularly for generics); consult specific product labeling. [DSC] = Discontinued product

Gum, Mouth/Throat, as polacrilex:
Nicorelief: 2 mg (50 ea, 110 ea)
Nicorelief: 2 mg (50 ea, 110 ea) [mint flavor]
Nicorelief: 4 mg (50 ea, 110 ea) [contains fd&c yellow #10 (quinoline yellow)]
Nicorelief: 4 mg (50 ea, 110 ea) [contains fd&c yellow #10 (quinoline yellow); mint flavor]
Nicorette: 2 mg (50 ea [DSC])
Nicorette: 2 mg (170 ea, 200 ea) [original flavor]
Nicorette: 2 mg (40 ea [DSC], 50 ea [DSC], 200 ea [DSC]) [contains menthol]
Nicorette: 2 mg (190 ea) [contains menthol; fresh mint flavor]
Nicorette: 2 mg (20 ea, 40 ea, 100 ea, 160 ea, 190 ea) [contains menthol; fruit flavor]
Nicorette: 2 mg (110 ea, 170 ea) [contains menthol; mint flavor]

Nicorette: 2 mg (40 ea [DSC]) [contains menthol, polysorbate 80]
Nicorette: 2 mg (20 ea, 100 ea, 160 ea, 190 ea) [contains menthol, polysorbate 80; cinnamon flavor]
Nicorette: 2 mg (20 ea, 100 ea, 160 ea, 190 ea) [contains menthol, polysorbate 80; mint flavor]
Nicorette: 4 mg (50 ea [DSC]) [contains fd&c yellow #10 (quinoline yellow)]
Nicorette: 4 mg (60 ea [DSC], 170 ea, 200 ea) [contains fd&c yellow #10 (quinoline yellow); original flavor]
Nicorette: 4 mg (100 ea, 160 ea, 190 ea) [contains fd&c yellow #10 (quinoline yellow), menthol, polysorbate 80; cinnamon flavor]
Nicorette: 4 mg (40 ea [DSC], 50 ea [DSC], 200 ea [DSC]) [contains fd&c yellow #10 aluminum lake, menthol]
Nicorette: 4 mg (100 ea, 190 ea) [contains fd&c yellow #10 aluminum lake, menthol; fresh mint flavor]
Nicorette: 4 mg (20 ea, 40 ea, 100 ea, 160 ea, 190 ea) [contains fd&c yellow #10 aluminum lake, menthol; fruit flavor]
Nicorette: 4 mg (110 ea, 170 ea) [contains fd&c yellow #10 aluminum lake, menthol; mint flavor]
Nicorette: 4 mg (40 ea [DSC]) [contains fd&c yellow #10 aluminum lake, menthol, polysorbate 80]
Nicorette: 4 mg (20 ea, 100 ea, 160 ea, 190 ea) [contains fd&c yellow #10 aluminum lake, menthol, polysorbate 80; mint flavor]
Nicorette Refill: 2 mg (192 ea [DSC], 216 ea [DSC])
Nicorette Refill: 2 mg (192 ea [DSC], 216 ea [DSC]) [contains menthol]
Nicorette Refill: 4 mg (192 ea [DSC], 216 ea [DSC]) [contains fd&c yellow #10 (quinoline yellow)]
Nicorette Refill: 4 mg (192 ea [DSC], 216 ea [DSC]) [contains fd&c yellow #10 aluminum lake, menthol]
Nicorette Starter Kit: 2 mg (110 ea) [original flavor]
Nicorette Starter Kit: 2 mg (100 ea) [contains menthol]
Nicorette Starter Kit: 4 mg (110 ea) [contains fd&c yellow #10 aluminum lake; original flavor]
Thrive: 2 mg (100 ea, 110 ea) [contains saccharin sodium]
Thrive: 4 mg (100 ea, 110 ea) [contains fd&c blue #2 (indigotine), saccharin sodium]
Generic: 2 mg (20 ea, 40 ea, 50 ea, 100 ea, 110 ea); 4 mg (20 ea, 40 ea, 50 ea, 100 ea, 110 ea)

Inhaler, Inhalation:
Nicotrol: 10 mg (168 ea) [contains menthol]

Kit, Transdermal:
Generic: 21-14-7 MG/24HR, 21-14-7 mg/24 hr

Lozenge, Mouth/Throat, as polacrilex:
Commit: 2 mg (48 ea [DSC], 72 ea [DSC], 108 ea [DSC])
Commit: 2 mg (48 ea [DSC]) [contains aspartame]
Commit: 4 mg (48 ea [DSC], 72 ea [DSC], 108 ea [DSC])
Commit: 4 mg (48 ea [DSC]) [contains aspartame]
NICOrelief: 2 mg (72 ea [DSC]); 4 mg (72 ea [DSC]) [contains aspartame; mint flavor]
Nicorette: 2 mg (72 ea, 81 ea) [cherry flavor]
Nicorette: 2 mg (108 ea) [contains aspartame]
Nicorette: 2 mg (27 ea, 72 ea, 81 ea, 168 ea) [contains aspartame, soy protein; mint flavor]
Nicorette: 4 mg (72 ea, 81 ea) [cherry flavor]
Nicorette: 4 mg (108 ea) [contains aspartame]
Nicorette: 4 mg (72 ea, 81 ea, 168 ea) [contains aspartame, soy protein; mint flavor]
Nicorette Mini: 2 mg (81 ea, 135 ea); 4 mg (81 ea, 135 ea)
Generic: 2 mg (24 ea, 27 ea, 72 ea [DSC]); 4 mg (24 ea, 27 ea, 72 ea [DSC])

Patch 24 Hour, Transdermal:
Nicoderm CQ: 7 mg/24 hr (14 ea); 14 mg/24 hr (7 ea [DSC], 14 ea, 21 ea); 21 mg/24 hr (7 ea, 14 ea, 21 ea)
Generic: 7 mg/24 hr (1 ea, 7 ea, 14 ea); 14 mg/24 hr (1 ea, 7 ea, 14 ea); 21 mg/24 hr (1 ea, 7 ea, 14 ea, 28 ea)

Solution, Nasal:
Nicotrol NS: 10 mg/mL (10 mL)

◆ Nicotine Patch *see* Nicotine *on page 1277*

◆ Nicotinic Acid *see* Niacin *on page 1273*

◆ Nicotinic Acid Amide *see* Niacinamide *on page 1274*

◆ Nicotrol *see* Nicotine *on page 1277*

◆ Nicotrol NS *see* Nicotine *on page 1277*

◆ Nidagel (Can) *see* MetroNIDAZOLE (Topical) *on page 1199*

◆ Nifediac CC *see* NIFEdipine *on page 1279*

◆ Nifedical XL *see* NIFEdipine *on page 1279*

NIFEdipine (nye FED i peen)

Brand Names: US Adalat CC; Afeditab CR; Nifediac CC; Nifedical XL; Procardia; Procardia XL

Brand Names: Canada Adalat XL; Apo-Nifed PA; Mylan-Nifedipine Extended Release; Nifedipine ER; PMS-Nifedipine; PMS-Nifedipine ER

Pharmacologic Category Antianginal Agent; Antihypertensive; Calcium Channel Blocker; Calcium Channel Blocker, Dihydropyridine

Additional Appendix Information

Hypertension *on page 1996*

Use

Management of chronic stable or vasospastic angina; treatment of hypertension (sustained release products only)

The 2014 guideline for the management of high blood pressure in adults (JNC 8) recommends initiation of pharmacologic treatment to lower blood pressure for the following patients (JNC 8 [James, 2013]):

• Patients ≥60 years of age with systolic blood pressure (SBP) ≥150 mm Hg or diastolic blood pressure (DBP) ≥90 mm Hg. Goal of therapy is SBP <150 mm Hg and DBP <90 mm Hg.

• Patients <60 years of age with SBP ≥140 mm Hg or DBP ≥90 mm Hg. Goal of therapy is SBP <140 mm Hg and DBP <90 mm Hg.

• Patients ≥18 years of age with diabetes with SBP ≥140 mm Hg or DBP ≥90 mm Hg. Goal of therapy is SBP <140 mm Hg and DBP <90 mm Hg.

• Patients ≥18 years of age with chronic kidney disease (CKD) with SBP ≥140 mm Hg or DBP ≥90 mm Hg. Goal of therapy is SBP <140 mm Hg and DBP <90 mm Hg.

In patients with chronic kidney disease (CKD), regardless of race or diabetes status, the use of an ACE inhibitor (ACEI) or angiotensin receptor blocker (ARB) as initial therapy is recommended to improve kidney outcomes. In the general nonblack population (without CKD) including those with diabetes, initial antihypertensive treatment should consist of a thiazide-type diuretic, calcium channel blocker, ACEI, or ARB. In the general black population (without CKD) including those with diabetes, initial antihypertensive treatment should consist of a thiazide-type diuretic or a calcium channel blocker instead of an ACEI or ARB.

Pregnancy Considerations Adverse events were observed in animal reproduction studies. Nifedipine crosses the placenta and small amounts can be detected in the urine of newborn infants (Manninen, 1991; Silberschmidt, 2008). An increase in perinatal asphyxia, cesarean delivery, prematurity, and intrauterine growth retardation have been reported following maternal use. Untreated chronic maternal hypertension is also associated with adverse events in the fetus, infant, and mother. If treatment for chronic hypertension during pregnancy is needed, nifedipine is one of the preferred agents (ACOG, 2013; SOGC [Magee, 2014]). Nifedipine is also recommended for the management of acute onset, severe hypertension (systolic BP ≥160 mm Hg or diastolic BP ≥110 mm Hg) with preeclampsia or eclampsia in pregnant and postpartum women (ACOG, 2015; Magee, 2014).

Nifedipine has also been evaluated for the treatment of preterm labor. Tocolytics may be used for the short-term (48 hour) prolongation of pregnancy to allow for the administration of antenatal steroids and should not be used prior to fetal viability or when the risks of use to the fetus or mother are greater than the risk of preterm birth (ACOG, 2012). Nifedipine is ineffective for maintenance tocolytic therapy (ACOG, 2012; Roos, 2013).

Breast-Feeding Considerations Nifedipine is excreted into breast milk. Reported concentrations are low and similar to those in the maternal serum (Ehrenkranz, 1989; Manninen, 1991; Penny, 1989). Breast-feeding is not recommended by the U.S. manufacturer (Canadian labeling contraindicates use). Nifedipine has been used for the treatment of Raynaud's phenomenon of the nipple in breast-feeding mothers (Barrett, 2013; Wu, 2012).

Contraindications

Hypersensitivity to nifedipine or any component of the formulation; concomitant use with strong CYP3A4 inducers (eg, rifampin); cardiogenic shock

Note: Considered contraindicated in patients with ST-elevation myocardial infarction (STEMI) (ACCF/AHA [O'Gara, 2013]).

Canadian labeling: Additional contraindications (not in U.S. labeling): Severe hypotension; patients with a Kock pouch (ileostomy after proctocolectomy; extended release tablets only); breast-feeding; pregnancy or women of childbearing potential. **Note:** SOGC and ACOG guidelines recommend nifedipine as a preferred agent for maternal hypertension (ACOG, 2013; SOGC [Magee, 2014]).

Warnings/Precautions Symptomatic hypotension with or without syncope can rarely occur; blood pressure must be lowered at a rate appropriate for the patient's clinical condition. **The use of immediate release nifedipine (sublingually or orally) in hypertensive emergencies and urgencies is neither safe nor effective.** Serious adverse events (eg, death, cerebrovascular ischemia, syncope, stroke, acute myocardial infarction, and fetal distress) have been reported. **Immediate release nifedipine should not be used for acute blood pressure reduction.**

Blood pressure lowering should be done at a rate appropriate for the patient's condition. Rapid drops in blood pressure can lead to arterial insufficiency. Increased angina and/or MI have occurred with initiation or dosage titration of dihydropyridine calcium channel blockers; use with caution in patients with obstructive coronary disease especially in the absence of concurrent beta-blockade. In patients with unstable angina/non-STEMI, the use of immediate-release nifedipine is not recommended except with concomitant beta-blockade (ACCF/AHA [Anderson, 2013]). Use with caution before major surgery. Cardiopulmonary bypass, intraoperative blood loss or vasodilating anesthesia may result in severe hypotension and/or increased fluid requirements. Consider withdrawing nifedipine (>36 hours) before surgery if possible.

The most common side effect is peripheral edema; occurs within 2-3 weeks of starting therapy. Reflex tachycardia may occur with use. Use with caution in severe aortic stenosis (especially with concomitant beta-adrenergic blocker), severe left ventricular dysfunction, renal impairment, hypertrophic cardiomyopathy (especially obstructive), concomitant therapy with beta-blockers or digoxin, and edema. The ACCF/AHA heart failure guidelines recommend to avoid use in patients with heart failure due to lack of benefit and/or worse outcomes with calcium channel blockers in general (Yancy, 2013). Use caution in patients with severe hepatic impairment. Clearance of nifedipine is reduced in cirrhotic patients leading to increased systemic exposure; monitor closely for adverse effects/toxicity and consider dose adjustments. Mild and transient elevations in liver function enzymes may be apparent within 8 weeks of therapy initiation. Abrupt withdrawal may cause rebound angina in patients with CAD. In the elderly, immediate release nifedipine should be avoided in due to potential to cause hypotension and risk of precipitating myocardial ischemia (Beers Criteria). Immediate release formulations should not be used to manage primary hypertension, adequate studies to evaluate outcomes have not been conducted. Avoid use of extended release tablets (Procardia XL) in patients with known stricture/narrowing of the GI tract. Adalat CC tablets contain lactose; do not use with galactose intolerance, Lapp lactase deficiency, or glucose-galactose malabsorption syndromes.

Potentially significant drug-drug interactions may exist, requiring dose or frequency adjustment, additional monitoring, and/or selection of alternative therapy.

Adverse Reactions

>10%:

Cardiovascular: Flushing (10% to 25%; extended release products 3% to 4%), peripheral edema (dose related 7% to 30%)

Central nervous system: Dizziness/lightheadedness/giddiness (10% to 27%), headache (10% to 23%)

Gastrointestinal: Nausea/heartburn (10% to 11%)

≥1% to 10%:

Cardiovascular: Palpitation (≤2% to 7%), transient hypotension (dose related 5%), CHF (2%)

Central nervous system: Nervousness/mood changes (≤2% to 7%), fatigue (6%), shakiness (≤2%), jitteriness (≤2%), sleep disturbances (≤2%), difficulties in balance (≤2%), fever (≤2%), chills (≤2%)

Dermatologic: Dermatitis (≤2%), pruritus (≤2%), urticaria (≤2%)

Endocrine & metabolic: Sexual difficulties (≤2%)

Gastrointestinal: Diarrhea (≤2%), constipation (≤2%), cramps (≤2%), flatulence (≤2%), gingival hyperplasia (≤10%)

Neuromuscular & skeletal: Muscle cramps/tremor (≤2% to 8%), weakness (<3%), inflammation (≤2%), joint stiffness (≤2%)

Ocular: Blurred vision (≤2%)

Respiratory: Cough/wheezing (6%), nasal congestion/sore throat (≤2% to 6%), chest congestion (≤2%), dyspnea (≤2%)

Miscellaneous: Diaphoresis (≤2%)

<1% (Limited to important or life-threatening): Agranulocytosis, allergic hepatitis, alopecia, anemia, angina, angioedema, aplastic anemia, arrhythmia, arthritis with positive ANA, bezoars (Procardia XL®), cerebral ischemia, depression, dysosmia, epistaxis, EPS, erectile dysfunction, erythema multiforme, erythromelalgia, exanthematous pustulosis, exfoliative dermatitis, facial edema,

gastroesophageal reflux, gastrointestinal obstruction (Procardia XL®), gastrointestinal ulceration (Procardia XL®), gynecomastia, hematuria, ischemia, leukopenia, lip cancer (Friedman, 2012), memory dysfunction, migraine, myalgia, myoclonus, nocturia, paranoid syndrome, parotitis, periorbital edema, photosensitivity, polyuria, purpura, Stevens-Johnson syndrome, syncope, tachycardia, taste perversion, thrombocytopenia, tinnitus, toxic epidermal necrolysis, transient blindness, ventricular arrhythmia

Reported with use of sublingual short-acting nifedipine: Acute MI, cerebrovascular ischemia, ECG changes, fetal distress, heart block, severe hypotension, sinus arrest, stroke, syncope

Drug Interactions

Metabolism/Transport Effects Substrate of CYP2D6 (minor), CYP3A4 (major); **Note:** Assignment of Major/Minor substrate status based on clinically relevant drug interaction potential; **Inhibits** CYP1A2 (weak), CYP2C9 (weak), CYP2D6 (weak)

Avoid Concomitant Use

Avoid concomitant use of NIFEdipine with any of the following: Conivaptan; CYP3A4 Inducers (Strong); Fusidic Acid (Systemic); Grapefruit Juice; Idelalisib; Phenytoin; St Johns Wort

Increased Effect/Toxicity

NIFEdipine may increase the levels/effects of: Amifostine; Antipsychotic Agents (Second Generation [Atypical]); ARIPiprazole; Atosiban; Beta-Blockers; Calcium Channel Blockers (Nondihydropyridine); Digoxin; DULoxetine; Hypotension-Associated Agents; Levodopa; Magnesium Salts; Neuromuscular-Blocking Agents (Nondepolarizing); Nitroprusside; Phenytoin; QuiNIDine; Tacrolimus (Systemic); TiZANidine; VinCRIStine; VinCRIStine (Liposomal)

The levels/effects of NIFEdipine may be increased by: Alcohol (Ethyl); Alfuzosin; Alpha1-Blockers; Antifungal Agents (Azole Derivatives, Systemic); Aprepitant; Barbiturates; Brimonidine (Topical); Calcium Channel Blockers (Nondihydropyridine); Cimetidine; Cisapride; Conivaptan; CycloSPORINE (Systemic); CYP3A4 Inhibitors (Moderate); CYP3A4 Inhibitors (Strong); Dapoxetine; Dasatinib; Diazoxide; Fluconazole; FLUoxetine; Fosaprepitant; Fusidic Acid (Systemic); Grapefruit Juice; Herbs (Hypotensive Properties); Idelalisib; Ivacaftor; Luliconazole; Macrolide Antibiotics; Magnesium Salts; Mifepristone; Molsidomine; Netupitant; Nicorandil; Obinutuzumab; Osimertinib; Palbociclib; Pentoxifylline; Phosphodiesterase 5 Inhibitors; Prostacyclin Analogues; QuiNIDine; Simeprevir; Stiripentol

Decreased Effect

NIFEdipine may decrease the levels/effects of: Clopidogrel; QuiNIDine

The levels/effects of NIFEdipine may be decreased by: Amphetamines; Barbiturates; Bosentan; Calcium Salts; CYP3A4 Inducers (Moderate); CYP3A4 Inducers (Strong); Dabrafenib; Deferasirox; Efavirenz; Herbs (Hypertensive Properties); Melatonin; Methylphenidate; Nafcillin; Osimertinib; Phenytoin; Siltuximab; St Johns Wort; Tocilizumab; Yohimbine

Food Interactions Nifedipine serum levels may be decreased if taken with food. Food may decrease the rate but not the extent of absorption of Procardia XL®. Increased nifedipine concentrations resulting in therapeutic and vasodilator side effects, including severe hypotension and myocardial ischemia, may occur if nifedipine is taken by patients ingesting grapefruit. Management: Avoid grapefruit/grapefruit juice.

Storage/Stability

Adalat CC, Afeditab CR, Procardia XL: Store below 30°C (86°F); protect from light and moisture.

Nifediac CC, Nifedical XL: Store at 25°C (77°F); excursions permitted to 15°C to 30°C (59°F to 86°F); protect from light and moisture.

Immediate release capsules (Procardia): Store at 15°C to 25°C (59°F to 77°F); prevent capsules from freezing; protect from light and moisture.

Mechanism of Action

Inhibits calcium ion from entering the "slow channels" or select voltage-sensitive areas of vascular smooth muscle and myocardium during depolarization, producing a relaxation of coronary vascular smooth muscle and coronary vasodilation; increases myocardial oxygen delivery in patients with vasospastic angina; also reduces peripheral vascular resistance, producing a reduction in arterial blood pressure.

Pharmacodynamics/Kinetics

Onset of action: Immediate release: ~20 minutes

Protein binding (concentration dependent): 92% to 98%

Metabolism: Hepatic via CYP3A4 to inactive metabolites

Bioavailability: Capsule: 40% to 77%; Sustained release: 65% to 89% relative to immediate release capsules; bioavailability increased with significant hepatic disease

Half-life elimination: Adults: Healthy: 2-5 hours; Cirrhosis: 7 hours; Elderly: 7 hours (extended release tablet)

Excretion: Urine (60% to 80% as inactive metabolites); feces

Dosing

Adult Dosage adjustments should occur at 7- to 14-day intervals to allow for adequate assessment of new dose; however, if clinically indicated, titration may be done more rapidly with appropriate monitoring; when switching from immediate-release to sustained-release formulations, use same total daily dose.

Chronic stable or vasospastic angina: Oral:

Immediate release: Initial: 10 mg 3 times daily; usual dose: 10 to 20 mg 3 times daily; coronary artery spasm may require up to 20 to 30 mg 3 to 4 times daily; single doses >30 mg and total daily doses >120 mg are rarely needed; maximum: 180 mg daily (U.S. labeling) or 120 mg daily (Canadian labeling); **Note:** Do not use for acute anginal episodes; may precipitate myocardial infarction

Extended release:

US labeling: Initial: 30 or 60 mg once daily; titrate as clinically indicated. Doses >90 mg daily should be used with caution and only if necessary (maximum: 120 mg daily)

Canadian labeling: Initial: 30 mg once daily; titrate as clinically indicated (maximum dose: 90 mg daily)

Hypertension: Oral: Extended release:

U.S. labeling: Initial: 30 or 60 mg once daily; usual dosage range (ASH/ISH [Weber, 2014]): 30 to 90 mg daily; maximum: 90 to 120 mg daily

Canadian labeling: Initial: 20 or 30 mg once daily; usual maintenance: 30 to 60 mg once daily (maximum: 90 mg daily)

Hypertension emergency in pregnancy (systolic BP ≥160 mm Hg or diastolic BP ≥110 mm Hg) (off-label dose): Oral: Immediate release: 10 mg; may repeat with a 20 mg dose in 20 minutes if needed. Also refer to administration protocols developed by the American College of Obstetricians and Gynecologists (ACOG, 2015).

High altitude pulmonary edema (off-label use; Luks, 2010): Oral:

Prevention: Extended release: 30 mg every 12 hours starting the day before ascent and may be discontinued after staying at the same elevation for 5 days or if descent initiated

Treatment: Extended release: 30 mg every 12 hours

Pulmonary hypertension (off-label use; Galie, 2004): Oral: Extended release: Initial: 30 mg twice daily; may increase cautiously to 120 to 240 mg daily

Raynaud's phenomenon (off-label use; Wigley, 2002): Oral: Extended release: Dosage range: 30 to 120 mg once daily

Geriatric Refer to adult dosing. In the management of hypertension, consider lower initial doses and titrate to response (Aronow, 2011).

Pediatric

High altitude pulmonary edema (off-label use; Pollard, 2001): Oral: **Note:** Treatment with NIFEdipine is only necessary if response to oxygen and/or descent is unsatisfactory; extended release preparation is preferred, but with proper dose and frequency adjustment: Immediate release: 0.5 mg/kg/dose (maximum: 20 mg/dose) every 8 hours

Hypertension (off-label use): Oral: Children 1 to 17 years: Extended release tablet: Initial: 0.2 to 0.5 mg/kg/day once daily or in 2 divided doses; maximum: 3 mg/kg/day up to 120 mg daily

Renal Impairment There are no dosage adjustments provided in manufacturer's labeling (has not been studied); the pharmacokinetics of nifedipine are not significantly influenced by the degree of renal impairment (only trace amounts of unchanged drug are found in urine).

Hemodialysis: Supplemental dose is not necessary.

Peritoneal dialysis effects: Supplemental dose is not necessary.

Hepatic Impairment There are no dosage adjustments provided in manufacturer's labeling (has not been studied); use with caution. Clearance of nifedipine is reduced in cirrhotic patients, which may lead to increased systemic exposure; monitor closely for adverse effects/toxicity and consider dose adjustments.

◄ **Dietary Considerations** Avoid grapefruit juice with all products.

Immediate release: Capsule is rapidly absorbed orally if it is administered without food, but may result in vasodilator side effects; if flushing is problematic, administration with low-fat meals may decrease. In general, can take with or without food.

Extended release: Adalat CC, Afeditab CR, Nifediac CC: Take on an empty stomach (manufacturer's labeling). Other extended release products may not have this recommendation; consult product labeling.

Administration

Immediate release: In general, may be administered with or without food.

Extended release: Tablets should be swallowed whole; do not crush, split, or chew.

Adalat CC, Afeditab CR, Nifediac CC: Administer on an empty stomach (per manufacturer). Other extended release products may not have this recommendation; consult product labeling.

Monitoring Parameters Heart rate, blood pressure, signs and symptoms of CHF, peripheral edema

Additional Information When measuring smaller doses from the liquid-filled capsules, consider the following concentrations (for Procardia) 10 mg capsule = 10 mg/0.34 mL; 20 mg capsule = 20 mg/0.45 mL; may be used preoperative to treat hypertensive urgency.

Considerable attention has been directed to potential increases in mortality and morbidity when short-acting nifedipine is used in treating hypertension. The rapid reduction in blood pressure may precipitate adverse cardiovascular events.

Short-acting nifedipine should not be used for acute anginal episodes since this may precipitate myocardial infarction. Extended-release formulations are preferred for the management of chronic or vasospastic angina (Poole-Wilson, 2004).

Equivalency of extended release formulation (Adalat CC): The manufacturer states that it is acceptable to interchange two 30 mg tablets with one 60 mg tablet to effectively deliver a 60 mg dose. However, it is not recommended to substitute one 90 mg tablet with three 30 mg tablets, since the resulting C_{max} is 29% higher compared to giving the single 90 mg tablet.

Dosage Forms Excipient information presented when available (limited, particularly for generics); consult specific product labeling. [DSC] = Discontinued product

Capsule, Oral:
Procardia: 10 mg
Generic: 10 mg, 20 mg
Tablet Extended Release 24 Hour, Oral:
Adalat CC: 30 mg, 60 mg, 90 mg
Afeditab CR: 30 mg, 60 mg
Nifediac CC: 30 mg, 60 mg
Nifediac CC: 90 mg [DSC] [contains tartrazine (fd&c yellow #5)]
Nifedical XL: 30 mg, 60 mg
Procardia XL: 30 mg, 60 mg, 90 mg
Generic: 30 mg, 60 mg, 90 mg

Extemporaneous Preparations A 4 mg/mL oral suspension may be made with liquid capsules (**Note:** Concentration inside capsule may vary depending on manufacturer. Procardia: 10 mg capsule contains a concentration of 10 mg/0.34 mL [29.4 mg/mL]). Puncture the top of twelve 10 mg liquid capsules with one needle to create a vent. Insert a second needle attached to a syringe and extract the liquid; transfer to a calibrated bottle and add sufficient quantity of a 1:1 mixture of Ora-Sweet and Ora-Plus to make 30 mL. Label "shake well". Stable 90 days under refrigeration or at room temperature.

Nahata MC, Morosco RS, and Willhite EA, "Stability of Nifedipine in Two Oral Suspensions Stored at Two Temperatures," *J Am Pharm Assoc*, 2002, 42(6):865-7.

◆ Nifedipine ER (Can) see NIFEdipine on page 1279
◆ Niferex see Polysaccharide-Iron Complex on page 1469
◆ Niftolid see Flutamide on page 791
◆ Nighttime Sleep Aid [OTC] see DiphenhydrAMINE (Systemic) on page 561
◆ Nikki see Ethinyl Estradiol and Drospirenone on page 702
◆ Nilandron see Nilutamide on page 1283

Nilotinib (nye LOE ti nib)

Brand Names: US Tasigna
Brand Names: Canada Tasigna
Index Terms AMN107; Nilotinib Hydrochloride Monohydrate

Pharmacologic Category Antineoplastic Agent, BCR-ABL Tyrosine Kinase Inhibitor; Antineoplastic Agent, Tyrosine Kinase Inhibitor

Use Chronic myelogenous leukemia:

Treatment of adults with newly diagnosed Philadelphia chromosome-positive chronic myelogenous leukemia (CML) in chronic phase.

Treatment of chronic- and accelerated-phase Philadelphia chromosome-positive CML in adults resistant or intolerant to prior therapy that included imatinib.

Medication Guide Available Yes

Dosing

Adult & Geriatric Note: If clinically indicated, may be administered in combination with hematopoietic growth factors (eg, erythropoietin, filgrastim) and with hydroxyurea or anagrelide.

Chronic myeloid leukemia (CML), Ph+, newly-diagnosed in chronic phase: Oral: 300 mg twice daily

CML, Ph+, resistant or intolerant in chronic or accelerated phase: Oral: 400 mg twice daily

Gastrointestinal stromal tumor (GIST), refractory (off-label use): Oral: 400 mg twice daily until disease progression or unacceptable toxicity (Reichardt, 2012)

Missed doses: If a dose is missed, do not make up, resume with next scheduled dose.

Dosage adjustment for concomitant CYP3A4 inhibitors/inducers:

CYP3A4 inhibitors: Avoid the concomitant use of a strong CYP3A4 inhibitor with nilotinib. If a strong CYP3A4 inhibitor is required, interruption of nilotinib treatment is recommended.

If therapy cannot be interrupted and concurrent use with a strong CYP3A4 inhibitor cannot be avoided:

US labeling: Consider reducing the nilotinib dose to 300 mg once daily in patients with resistant or intolerant Ph+ CML (chronic or accelerated phase) or to 200 mg once daily in newly-diagnosed chronic phase Ph+ CML, with careful monitoring, especially of the QT interval. When a strong CYP3A4 inhibitor is discontinued, allow a washout period prior to adjusting nilotinib dose upward.

Canadian labeling: There are no dosage adjustments provided in the manufacturer's labeling; use caution and monitor QT interval closely

CYP3A4 inducers: Avoid the concomitant use of a strong CYP3A4 inducer with nilotinib (based on pharmacokinetic parameters, an increased nilotinib dose is not likely to compensate for decreased exposure).

Renal Impairment There are no dosage adjustments provided in the manufacturer's labeling (has not been studied in patients with serum creatinine >1.5 times ULN); however, nilotinib and its metabolites have minimal renal excretion; dosage adjustments for renal dysfunction may not be necessary.

Hepatic Impairment

For hepatic impairment at treatment initiation: **Note:** Consider alternative therapies first if possible; recommendations vary by indication

US labeling:

Newly-diagnosed Ph+ CML in chronic phase: Mild-to-severe impairment (Child-Pugh class A, B, or C): Initial: 200 mg twice daily; may increase to 300 mg twice daily based on patient tolerability

Resistant or intolerant Ph+ CML in chronic or accelerated phase:

Mild-to-moderate impairment (Child-Pugh class A or B): Initial: 300 mg twice daily; may increase to 400 mg twice daily based on patient tolerability

Severe impairment (Child-Pugh class C): Initial: 200 mg twice daily; may increase to 300 mg twice daily and then further increase to 400 mg twice daily based on patient tolerability

Canadian labeling: No dosage adjustment necessary; use caution and monitor (including QT interval) closely.

For hepatotoxicity during treatment:

If bilirubin >3 times ULN (≥ grade 3): Withhold treatment, monitor bilirubin, resume treatment at 400 mg once daily when bilirubin returns to ≤1.5 times ULN (≤ grade 1)

If ALT or AST >5 times ULN (≥ grade 3): Withhold treatment, monitor transaminases, resume treatment at 400 mg once daily when ALT or AST returns to ≤2.5 times ULN (≤ grade 1)

Adjustment for Toxicity

Dosage adjustment for hematologic toxicity unrelated to underlying leukemia:

ANC <1000/mm^3 and/or platelets <50,000/mm^3: Withhold treatment, monitor blood counts

If ANC >1000/mm^3 and platelets >50,000/mm^3 within 2 weeks: Resume at prior dose

If ANC <1000/mm^3 and/or platelets <50,000/mm^3 for >2 weeks: Reduce dose to 400 mg once daily

Dosage adjustment for nonhematologic toxicity:

Amylase or lipase >2 times ULN (≥ grade 3): Withhold treatment, monitor serum amylase or lipase, resume treatment at 400 mg once daily when lipase or amylase returns to ≤1.5 times ULN (≤ grade 1)

Lipase increases in conjunction with abdominal symptoms: Withhold treatment and consider diagnostics to exclude pancreatitis.

Clinically-significant moderate or severe nonhematologic toxicity: Withhold treatment, upon resolution of toxicity, resume at 400 mg once daily; may escalate back to initial dose (300 mg twice daily or 400 mg twice daily depending on indication) if clinically appropriate.

Dosage adjustment for QT prolongation: Note: Repeat ECG ~7 days after any dosage adjustment.

QT$_c$ >480 msec: Withhold treatment, monitor and correct potassium and magnesium levels; review concurrent medications.

If QT$_c$F returns to <450 msec and to within 20 msec of baseline within 2 weeks: Resume at prior dose.

If QT$_c$F returns to 450 to 480 msec after 2 weeks: Reduce dose to 400 mg once daily.

If QT$_c$F >480 msec after dosage reduction to 400 mg once daily: Discontinue treatment.

Additional Information Complete prescribing information should be consulted for additional detail.

Dosage Forms Excipient information presented when available (limited, particularly for generics); consult specific product labeling.

Capsule, Oral:

Tasigna: 150 mg, 200 mg

♦ **Nilotinib Hydrochloride Monohydrate** see Nilotinib on page 1282

Nilutamide (ni LOO ta mide)

Brand Names: US Nilandron
Brand Names: Canada Anandron
Index Terms RU-23908
Pharmacologic Category Antineoplastic Agent, Antiandrogen
Use Prostate cancer, metastatic: Treatment of metastatic prostate cancer (in combination with surgical castration)
Dosing

Adult & Geriatric Prostate cancer, metastatic: Oral: 300 mg once daily (starting the same day or day after surgical castration) for 30 days, followed by 150 mg once daily. Consider therapy discontinuation in patients with evidence of disease progression.

Renal Impairment There are no dosage adjustments provided in the manufacturer's labeling.

Hepatic Impairment

Hepatic impairment at treatment initiation:

Mild or moderate impairment: There are no dosage adjustments provided in the manufacturer's labeling.

Severe impairment: Use is contraindicated.

Hepatotoxicity during treatment:

US labeling: ALT >2 times ULN or jaundice: Discontinue treatment.

Canadian labeling: Transaminases >3 times ULN: Interrupt treatment.

Additional Information Complete prescribing information should be consulted for additional detail.

Dosage Forms Excipient information presented when available (limited, particularly for generics); consult specific product labeling.

Tablet, Oral:

Nilandron: 150 mg

Dosage Forms: Canada Excipient information presented when available (limited, particularly for generics); consult specific product labeling.

Tablet, Oral:

Anandron: 50 mg

♦ **Nimbex** see Cisatracurium on page 394

NiMODipine (nye MOE di peen)

Brand Names: US Nymalize
Brand Names: Canada Nimotop
Index Terms Nimotop
Pharmacologic Category Calcium Channel Blocker; Calcium Channel Blocker, Dihydropyridine

Use Subarachnoid hemorrhage: For the improvement of neurological outcome by reducing the incidence and severity of ischemic deficits in adult patients with subarachnoid hemorrhage (SAH) from ruptured intracranial berry aneurysms regardless of their postictus neurological condition (ie, Hunt and Hess grades I to V)

Pregnancy Considerations Adverse events have been observed in animal reproduction studies. Nimodipine crosses the placenta (Belfort, 1994). Nimodipine has been evaluated for the management of pre-eclampsia (Belfort, 1994; Belfort, 2003), but it is not one of the agents currently recommended for severe intrapartum or postpartum hypertension associated with preeclampsia or eclampsia (ACOG, 2015).

Breast-Feeding Considerations Nimodipine is excreted into breast milk; two case reports note concentrations to be <1% of the weight-adjusted maternal dose (Carcas, 1996; Tonks, 1995). Breast-feeding is not recommended by the manufacturer.

Contraindications

US labeling:

Concomitant use with strong CYP3A4 inhibitors (eg, clarithromycin, telithromycin, delavirdine, indinavir, nelfinavir, ritonavir, saquinavir, ketoconazole, itraconazole, voriconazole, and nefazodone).

Nymalize: There are no contraindications listed in the manufacturer's labeling.

Canadian labeling: Hypersensitivity to nimodipine or any component of the formulation; concomitant use with phenobarbital, phenytoin, carbamazepine, or rifampin

Warnings/Precautions [U.S. Boxed Warning]: Nimodipine has inadvertently been administered IV when withdrawn from capsules into a syringe for subsequent nasogastric administration. Severe cardiovascular adverse events, including fatalities, have resulted; precautions (eg, adequate labeling, use of oral syringes) should be employed against such an event.

Increased angina and/or MI have occurred with initiation or dosage titration of calcium channel blockers. Reflex tachycardia may occur resulting in angina and/or MI in patients with obstructive coronary disease, especially in the absence of concurrent beta-blockade. Peripheral edema is a common adverse event; occurs within 2 to 3 weeks of starting therapy. Symptomatic hypotension with or without syncope can occur; blood pressure must be lowered at a rate appropriate for the patient's clinical condition. Monitor blood pressure closely during treatment. Use with caution in patients with cirrhosis due to the increased plasma concentrations of nimodipine and an increased risk of adverse reactions; a lower dose and close monitoring of blood pressure and heart rate is required. Intestinal pseudo-obstruction and ileus have been reported (rarely) during therapy.

Potentially significant drug-drug interactions may exist, requiring dose or frequency adjustment, additional monitoring, and/or selection of alternative therapy.

Adverse Reactions

1% to 10%:

Cardiovascular: Decreased blood pressure (4% to 5%), bradycardia (1%)

Central nervous system: Headache (1%)

Gastrointestinal: Nausea (1%)

<1% (Limited to important or life-threatening): Anemia, decreased platelet count, disseminated intravascular coagulation, edema, gastrointestinal hemorrhage, gastrointestinal pseudo-obstruction, hematoma, hepatitis, hypertension, increased lactate dehydrogenase, increased serum alkaline phosphatase, increased serum ALT, increased serum glucose, intestinal obstruction, jaundice, rebound vasospasm, thrombocytopenia

Drug Interactions

Metabolism/Transport Effects Substrate of CYP3A4 (major); **Note:** Assignment of Major/Minor substrate status based on clinically relevant drug interaction potential

Avoid Concomitant Use

Avoid concomitant use of NiMODipine with any of the following: Conivaptan; CYP3A4 Inducers (Strong); CYP3A4 Inhibitors (Strong); Fusidic Acid (Systemic); Grapefruit Juice; Idelalisib; St Johns Wort

Increased Effect/Toxicity

NiMODipine may increase the levels/effects of: Amifostine; Antipsychotic Agents (Second Generation [Atypical]); Atosiban; Calcium Channel Blockers (Nondihydropyridine); DULoxetine; Hypotension-Associated Agents; Levodopa; Magnesium Salts; Neuromuscular-Blocking Agents (Nondepolarizing); Nitroprusside; QuiNIDine; Tacrolimus (Systemic)

The levels/effects of NiMODipine may be increased by:
Alfuzosin; Alpha1-Blockers; Aprepitant; Barbiturates; Brimonidine (Topical); Calcium Channel Blockers (Nondihydropyridine); Cimetidine; Conivaptan; CycloSPORINE (Systemic); CYP3A4 Inhibitors (Moderate); CYP3A4 Inhibitors (Strong); CYP3A4 Inhibitors (Weak); Dapoxetine; Dasatinib; Diazoxide; Fluconazole; FLUoxetine; Fosaprepitant; Fusidic Acid (Systemic); Grapefruit Juice; Herbs (Hypotensive Properties); Idelalisib; Ivacaftor; Luliconazole; Macrolide Antibiotics; Magnesium Salts; Mifepristone; Molsidomine; Netupitant; Nicorandil; Obinutuzumab; Osimertinib; Palbociclib; Pentoxifylline; Phosphodiesterase 5 Inhibitors; Prostacyclin Analogues; QuiNIDine; Simeprevir; Stiripentol

Decreased Effect
NiMODipine may decrease the levels/effects of: Clopidogrel; QuiNIDine

The levels/effects of NiMODipine may be decreased by: Amphetamines; Barbiturates; Bosentan; Calcium Salts; CYP3A4 Inducers (Moderate); CYP3A4 Inducers (Strong); CYP3A4 Inducers (Weak); Dabrafenib; Deferasirox; Efavirenz; Herbs (Hypertensive Properties); Melatonin; Methylphenidate; Nafcillin; Osimertinib; Siltuximab; St Johns Wort; Tocilizumab; Yohimbine

Food Interactions Administration with a standard breakfast results in a 68% lower maximum plasma concentration and 38% lower bioavailability as compared to administration under fasted conditions. In addition, AUC and maximum plasma concentration were increased by an average of 51% and 24%, respectively, following administration of nimodipine with grapefruit juice (Fuhr, 1998). Management: Administer on an empty stomach, at least 1 hour before or 2 hours after meals. Avoid concurrent use of grapefruit juice and nimodipine.

Storage/Stability Store at 25°C (77°F); excursions are permitted to 15°C to 30°C (59°F to 86°F). Protect capsules from light and freezing. Protect solution from light and do not refrigerate.

Mechanism of Action Nimodipine shares the pharmacology of other calcium channel blockers; animal studies indicate that nimodipine has a greater effect on cerebral arterials than other arterials; this increased specificity may be due to the drug's increased lipophilicity and cerebral distribution as compared to nifedipine; inhibits calcium ion from entering the "slow channels" or select voltage sensitive areas of vascular smooth muscle and myocardium during depolarization

Pharmacodynamics/Kinetics
Protein binding: >95%
Metabolism: Extensively hepatic via CYP3A4; undergoes first-pass metabolism
Bioavailability: Capsule: 13%; Tablet [Canadian product]: 16% (range: 3% to 30%)
Half-life elimination: 1 to 2 hours; prolonged with renal impairment
Time to peak, serum: ~1 hour
Excretion: Urine (<1% as unchanged drug); feces

Dosing
Adult & Geriatric Note: For oral administration **ONLY.**
Subarachnoid hemorrhage: Oral: 60 mg every 4 hours for 21 consecutive days. **Note:** Start therapy within 96 hours of the onset of subarachnoid hemorrhage.
Renal Impairment No dosage adjustment provided in manufacturer's labeling. However, nimodipine undergoes minimal renal elimination and dose adjustment may not be necessary. Not removed by hemo- or peritoneal dialysis; supplemental dose is not necessary.
Hepatic Impairment Reduce dosage to 30 mg every 4 hours in patients with cirrhosis.

Administration For enteral administration ONLY. Life-threatening adverse events have occurred when administered parenterally. Administer on an empty stomach at least 1 hour before or 2 hours after meals.

Oral:
US labeling: Administer on an empty stomach at least 1 hour before or 2 hours after meals.
Canadian labeling: Administer without regards to meals; but administer consistently with or without meals. Tablet should be swallowed whole with an adequate amount of fluid (eg, glass of water). Do not crush tablet. Avoid alkaline mixtures for 2 hours before or after administration. Patient should not be lying down during administration.
Nasogastric (NG) or gastric tube administration:
Oral solution (Nymalize): Administer using the supplied oral syringe labeled **"ORAL USE ONLY"**. Following administration, refill the oral syringe with 20 mL of NS and flush any remaining contents from NG or gastric tube into the stomach.
Capsules: If the capsules cannot be swallowed, the liquid may be removed by making a hole in each end of the

capsule with an 18-gauge needle and extracting the contents into a syringe; transfer these contents into an oral syringe (amber-colored oral syringe preferred). It is strongly recommended that preparation be done in the pharmacy. Label oral syringe with **"WARNING: For ORAL use only"** or **"Not for IV use."** Follow with a flush of 30 mL NS.

Dosage Forms Excipient information presented when available (limited, particularly for generics); consult specific product labeling.
Capsule, Oral:
Generic: 30 mg
Solution, Oral:
Nymalize: 60 mg/20 mL (20 mL, 473 mL) [contains alcohol, usp, methylparaben, polyethylene glycol]
Dosage Forms: Canada Excipient information presented when available (limited, particularly for generics); consult specific product labeling.
Tablet, Oral:
Nimotop: 30 mg

♦ Nimotop *see* NiMODipine *on page 1283*

♦ Ninjacof-XG *see* Guaifenesin and Codeine *on page 861*

♦ Ninlaro *see* Ixazomib *on page 1008*

Nintedanib (nin TED a nib)

Brand Names: US Ofev
Brand Names: Canada Ofev
Index Terms BIBF1120; Nintedanib Esylate
Pharmacologic Category Tyrosine Kinase Inhibitor
Use Idiopathic pulmonary fibrosis: Treatment of idiopathic pulmonary fibrosis (IPF).
Pregnancy Considerations Adverse events were observed in animal reproduction studies. Women of reproductive potential should use adequate contraception; pregnancy should be avoided during therapy and for at least 3 months after the last dose.
Breast-Feeding Considerations It is not known if nintedanib is excreted in breast milk; however it is probable. Due to the potential for serious adverse reactions in the nursing infant, the manufacturer recommends a decision be made whether to discontinue nursing or to discontinue the drug, taking into account the importance of treatment to the mother.

Contraindications
There are no contraindications listed in the US manufacturer's labeling.
Canadian labeling: Hypersensitivity to nintedanib, peanut or soya or any component of the formulation; pregnancy
Warnings/Precautions Hazardous agent – use appropriate precautions for handling and disposal (meets NIOSH 2014 criteria). Arterial thromboembolic events, including MI, have been reported. Use caution in patients at high cardiovascular risk, including in patients with known coronary artery disease. Consider treatment interruption in patients who develop signs or symptoms of acute myocardial ischemia. Diarrhea, nausea, and vomiting may occur. Diarrhea occurred in over 50% of nintedanib-treated patients, and was generally mild to moderate. Treat with appropriate supportive care (eg, adequate hydration, antidiarrheals, antiemetics); dose reduction and/or treatment interruption may be required. If gastrointestinal events do not resolve, discontinue treatment. May increase the risk of GI perforation; only use in patients with risk of GI perforation if the benefit outweighs the risk. Use caution in patients with recent abdominal surgery. The Canadian labeling recommends waiting at least 4 weeks following abdominal surgery before initiating therapy. Discontinue in patients who develop GI perforation. Elevations of ALT, AST, GGT, alkaline phosphatase, and bilirubin have occurred; increases were reversible with dose modification/interruption. Obtain LFTs prior to treatment, monthly for 3 months, and every 3 months thereafter (or as clinically indicated).

May increase the risk of bleeding. Use in patients with known risk of bleeding only if the benefit outweighs the risk. Not recommended in patients with moderate or severe hepatic impairment (has not been studied). Patients should stop smoking prior to treatment and avoid smoking during therapy; smoking may decrease exposure to nintedanib. Potentially significant drug-drug interactions may exist, requiring dose or frequency adjustment, additional monitoring, and/or selection of alternative therapy.

Adverse Reactions
>10%:
Gastrointestinal: Diarrhea (62%), nausea (24%), abdominal pain (15%; includes abdominal tenderness, gastrointestinal pain, lower abdominal pain, upper abdominal pain), vomiting (12%), decreased appetite (11%)

Hepatic: Increased liver enzymes (14%; includes abnormal alanine aminotransferase, abnormal aspartate aminotransferase, abnormal gamma-glutamyl transferase, abnormal hepatic function tests, hepatic insufficiency, increased serum ALT, increased serum AST, increased gamma-glutamyl transferase, increased serum alkaline phosphatase, increased serum transaminases)

1% to 10%:

Cardiovascular: Hypertension (5%; includes hypertensive cardiomyopathy, hypertensive crisis), arterial thrombosis (3%), myocardial infarction (2%)

Central nervous system: Headache (8%)

Endocrine & metabolic: Weight loss (10%), hypothyroidism (1%)

Hematologic and oncologic: Hemorrhage (10%)

Respiratory: Bronchitis (1%)

<1% (Limited to important or life-threatening): Gastrointestinal perforation

Drug Interactions

Metabolism/Transport Effects Substrate of CYP3A4 (minor), P-glycoprotein; Note: Assignment of Major/Minor substrate status based on clinically relevant drug interaction potential

Avoid Concomitant Use

Avoid concomitant use of Nintedanib with any of the following: Combined Inducers of CYP3A4 and P-glycoprotein

Increased Effect/Toxicity

The levels/effects of Nintedanib may be increased by: Anticoagulants; Combined Inhibitors of CYP3A4 and P-glycoprotein; Lumacaftor; P-glycoprotein/ABCB1 Inhibitors; Ranolazine

Decreased Effect

The levels/effects of Nintedanib may be decreased by: Combined Inducers of CYP3A4 and P-glycoprotein; Lumacaftor; P-glycoprotein/ABCB1 Inducers; Pirfenidone

Storage/Stability Store at 25°C (77°F); excursions are permitted between 15°C and 30°C (59°F and 86°F). Protect from humidity and avoid excessive heat.

Mechanism of Action Inhibits multiple receptor tyrosine kinases (RTKs) and nonreceptor tyrosine kinases (nRTKs), including platelet-derived growth factor (PDGFR alpha and PDGFR beta); fibroblast growth factor receptor (FGFR1, FGFR2, FGFR3); vascular endothelial growth factor (VEGFR1, VEGFR2, and VEGFR3); and Fms-like tyrosine kinase-3 (FLT3). Nintedanib binds competitively to the adenosine triphosphate (ATP) binding pocket of these receptors and blocks the intracellular signaling which is crucial for the proliferation, migration, and transformation of fibroblasts.

Pharmacodynamics/Kinetics

Absorption: Food increases exposure ~20% and delays absorption

Distribution: V_{ss}: 1050 L

Protein binding: ~98%

Metabolism: Hydrolytic cleavage by esterases to free acid moiety BIBF 1202; which is then glucuronidated by UGT 1A1, UGT 1A7, UGT 1A8, and UGT 1A10 to BIBF 1202 glucuronide; CYP 3A4 (minor).

Bioavailability: ~5%

Half-life elimination: 9.5 hours

Time to peak, plasma: 2 hours (4 hours with food)

Excretion: Feces (~93%); urine (<1%)

Dosing

Adult & Geriatric

Idiopathic pulmonary fibrosis (IPF): Oral: 150 mg every 12 hours (maximum: 300 mg daily)

Missed dose: If a dose is missed, the next dose should be taken at the next scheduled time. Do not make up a missed dose.

Renal Impairment

*Mild to moderate impairment (CrCl ≥30 mL/minute):*No initial dosage adjustment necessary.

Severe impairment (CrCl <30 mL/minute): There are no dosage adjustments provided in the manufacturer's labeling (has not been studied)

Hepatic Impairment

Hepatic impairment at baseline:

Mild impairment: There are no dosage adjustments provided in the manufacturer's labeling (has not been studied); consider dose modification or discontinuation as needed.

Moderate to severe impairment: Use is not recommended (has not been studied).

Hepatotoxicity during treatment:

US labeling:

AST or ALT >3 times to <5 times ULN (without signs of severe liver damage): Interrupt treatment or reduce dosage to 100 mg every 12 hours. Once liver enzymes have returned to baseline values after treatment interruption, reintroduce therapy at 100 mg every 12 hours; may be subsequently

increased to 150 mg every 12 hours. If a patient does not tolerate 100 mg every 12 hours, discontinue treatment.

AST or ALT >5 times ULN or >3 times ULN with signs or symptoms of severe liver damage: Discontinue therapy.

Canadian labeling:

AST or ALT >3 times ULN (without signs of severe liver damage): Interrupt treatment or reduce dosage to 100 mg every 12 hours and monitor closely. Once liver enzymes have returned to baseline values after treatment interruption, reintroduce therapy at 100 mg every 12 hours; may be subsequently increased to 150 mg every 12 hours. If a patient does not tolerate 100 mg every 12 hours, discontinue treatment.

AST or ALT >3 times ULN with signs or symptoms of severe liver damage: Discontinue therapy.

Adjustment for Toxicity Gastrointestinal toxicity (eg, diarrhea, nausea, vomiting) or other adverse reactions/toxicity: Dose reduction or temporary interruption may be needed. Treatment may be resumed at 150 mg every 12 hours or 100 mg every 12 hours, which may subsequently be increased to 150 mg every 12 hours. If a patient does not tolerate 100 mg every 12 hours, discontinue treatment.

Dietary Considerations Take with food

Administration Oral: Administer with food. Swallow whole with liquid; do not chew or crush (bitter taste). Hazardous agent; use appropriate precautions for handling and disposal (meets NIOSH 2014 criteria).

Monitoring Parameters Obtain LFTs prior to treatment, monthly for 3 months, and every 3 months thereafter (or as clinically indicated). Monitor for gastrointestinal events (eg, diarrhea, nausea, vomiting), arterial thromboembolic events, bleeding, and gastrointestinal perforation.

Dosage Forms Excipient information presented when available (limited, particularly for generics); consult specific product labeling.

Capsule, Oral:

Ofev: 100 mg, 150 mg

◆ **Nintedanib Esylate** *see* Nintedanib *on page 1284*

◆ **Niodan (Can)** *see* Niacin *on page 1273*

◆ **Nipent** *see* Pentostatin *on page 1426*

◆ **Nipride (Can)** *see* Nitroprusside *on page 1291*

◆ **Niravam** *see* ALPRAZolam *on page 76*

Nisoldipine (nye SOL di peen)

Brand Names: US Sular

Pharmacologic Category Antihypertensive; Calcium Channel Blocker; Calcium Channel Blocker, Dihydropyridine

Use

Hypertension: Management of hypertension, alone or in combination with other antihypertensive agents

The 2014 guideline for the management of high blood pressure in adults (JNC 8) recommends initiation of pharmacologic treatment to lower blood pressure for the following patients (JNC 8 [James, 2013]):

• Patients ≥60 years of age with systolic blood pressure (SBP) ≥150 mm Hg or diastolic blood pressure (DBP) ≥90 mm Hg. Goal of therapy is SBP <150 mm Hg and DBP <90 mm Hg.

• Patients <60 years of age with SBP ≥140 mm Hg or DBP ≥90 mm Hg. Goal of therapy is SBP <140 mm Hg and DBP <90 mm Hg.

• Patients ≥18 years of age with diabetes with SBP ≥140 mm Hg or DBP ≥90 mm Hg. Goal of therapy is SBP <140 mm Hg and DBP <90 mm Hg.

• Patients ≥18 years of age with chronic kidney disease (CKD) with SBP ≥140 mm Hg or DBP ≥90 mm Hg. Goal of therapy is SBP <140 mm Hg and DBP <90 mm Hg.

In patients with chronic kidney disease (CKD), regardless of race or diabetes status, the use of an ACE inhibitor (ACEI) or angiotensin receptor blocker (ARB) as initial therapy is recommended to improve kidney outcomes. In the general nonblack population (without CKD) including those with diabetes, initial antihypertensive treatment should consist of a thiazide-type diuretic, calcium channel blocker, ACEI, or ARB. In the general black population (without CKD) including those with diabetes, initial antihypertensive treatment should consist of a thiazide-type diuretic or a calcium channel blocker instead of an ACEI or ARB.

Pregnancy Considerations Adverse events were not observed in animal reproduction studies when using doses that were not maternally toxic. Untreated chronic maternal hypertension is associated with adverse events in the fetus, infant, and mother. If treatment for hypertension ▶

during pregnancy is needed, other agents are preferred (ACOG, 2013).

Breast-Feeding Considerations It is not known if nisoldipine is excreted into breast milk. The manufacturer recommends a decision be made whether to discontinue nursing or to discontinue the drug, taking into account the importance of treatment to the mother.

Contraindications Hypersensitivity to nisoldipine, any component of the formulation, or other dihydropyridine calcium channel blockers

Warnings/Precautions With initiation or dosage titration of dihydropyridine calcium channel blockers, reflex tachycardia may occur resulting in angina and/or MI in patients with obstructive coronary disease especially in the absence of concurrent beta-blockade. Use with caution in patients with severe aortic stenosis, and hypertrophic cardiomyopathy with outflow tract obstruction. The ACCF/AHA heart failure guidelines recommend to avoid use in patients with heart failure due to lack of benefit and/or worse outcomes with calcium channel blockers in general (Yancy, 2013). Use with caution in hepatic impairment; lower starting dose required. The most common side effect is peripheral edema; occurs within 2-3 weeks of starting therapy. Symptomatic hypotension with or without syncope can rarely occur; blood pressure must be lowered at a rate appropriate for the patient's clinical condition. Some dosage forms contain tartrazine, which may cause allergic reactions in certain individuals (eg, aspirin hypersensitivity). Use with caution in patients >65 years of age; lower starting dose recommended.

Adverse Reactions

>10%:
Cardiovascular: Peripheral edema (dose related; 7% to 29%)
Central nervous system: Headache (22%)

1% to 10%:
Cardiovascular: Vasodilation (4%), palpitation (3%), angina exacerbation (2%), chest pain (2%)
Central nervous system: Dizziness (3% to 10%)
Dermatologic: Rash (2%)
Gastrointestinal: Nausea (2%)
Respiratory: Pharyngitis (5%), sinusitis (3%)

<1% (Limited to important or life-threatening): Alopecia, amblyopia, amnesia, anemia, anorexia, anxiety, appetite increased, arthralgia, arthritis, asthma, ataxia, atrial fibrillation, blepharitis, BUN increased, bruising, cellulitis, cerebral ischemia, colitis, conjunctivitis, creatinine increased, creatine kinase increased, CVA, depression, diabetes mellitus, diaphoresis, diarrhea, dreams abnormal, dyspepsia, dysphagia, dyspnea, dysuria, end inspiratory wheeze, epistaxis, exfoliative dermatitis, facial edema, fever, first-degree AV block, flu-like syndrome, gastritis, gastrointestinal hemorrhage, gingival hyperplasia, glaucoma, glossitis, gout, gynecomastia, heart failure (decompensated), hematuria, hepatomegaly, herpes simplex, herpes zoster; hypersensitivity reaction (eg, angioedema, shortness of breath, tachycardia, chest tightness, hypotension, and rash); hyper-/hypotension, hypertonia, hypoesthesia, hypokalemia, insomnia, jugular venous distention, keratoconjunctivitis, leukopenia, libido decreased, liver function tests abnormal, maculopapular rash, malaise, melena, migraine, mouth ulceration, myalgia, myasthenia, MI, myositis, nocturia, nonprotein nitrogen increased, orthostatic hypotension, paresthesia, petechiae, photosensitivity, pleural effusion, pruritus, pustular rash, rales, retinal detachment, skin discoloration, skin ulcer, somnolence, supraventricular tachycardia, syncope, systolic ejection murmur, taste disturbance, temporary unilateral loss of vision, tenosynovitis, thyroiditis, tremor; T-wave abnormalities on ECG (flattening, inversion, nonspecific changes); urinary frequency, urticaria, vaginal hemorrhage, venous insufficiency, ventricular extrasystoles, vertigo, vitreous floater, weight gain/loss, xerostomia

Drug Interactions

Metabolism/Transport Effects Substrate of CYP3A4 (major); **Note:** Assignment of Major/Minor substrate status based on clinically relevant drug interaction potential; **Inhibits** CYP1A2 (weak).

Avoid Concomitant Use

Avoid concomitant use of Nisoldipine with any of the following: Conivaptan; CYP3A4 Inducers (Moderate); CYP3A4 Inducers (Strong); CYP3A4 Inhibitors (Strong); Fusidic Acid (Systemic); Grapefruit Juice; Idelalisib

Increased Effect/Toxicity

Nisoldipine may increase the levels/effects of: Amifostine; Antipsychotic Agents (Second Generation [Atypical]); Atosiban; Calcium Channel Blockers (Nondihydropyridine); DULoxetine; Hypotension-Associated Agents; Levodopa; Magnesium Salts; Neuromuscular-Blocking Agents (Nondepolarizing); Nitroprusside; Tacrolimus (Systemic); TiZANidine

The levels/effects of Nisoldipine may be increased by: Alfuzosin; Alpha1-Blockers; Aprepitant; Barbiturates; Brimonidine (Topical); Calcium Channel Blockers (Nondihydropyridine); Cimetidine; Conivaptan; CycloSPORINE (Systemic); CYP3A4 Inhibitors (Moderate); CYP3A4 Inhibitors (Strong); Dapoxetine; Dasatinib; Diazoxide; Fluconazole; Fosaprepitant; Fusidic Acid (Systemic); Grapefruit Juice; Herbs (Hypotensive Properties); Idelalisib; Ivacaftor; Luliconazole; Macrolide Antibiotics; Magnesium Salts; Mifepristone; Molsidomine; Netupitant; Nicorandil; Obinutuzumab; Osimertinib; Palbociclib; Pentoxifylline; Phosphodiesterase 5 Inhibitors; Prostacyclin Analogues; Simeprevir; Stiripentol

Decreased Effect

Nisoldipine may decrease the levels/effects of: Clopidogrel

The levels/effects of Nisoldipine may be decreased by: Amphetamines; Barbiturates; Calcium Salts; CYP3A4 Inducers (Moderate); CYP3A4 Inducers (Strong); Deferasirox; Herbs (Hypertensive Properties); Melatonin; Methylphenidate; Osimertinib; Siltuximab; Tocilizumab; Yohimbine

Food Interactions Peak concentrations of nisoldipine may be significantly increased if taken with high-lipid foods; however, total exposure (AUC) may be reduced. Grapefruit juice has been shown to significantly increase the bioavailability of nisoldipine. Management: Take on an empty stomach 1 hour before or 2 hours after a meal. Avoid a high-fat diet. Avoid grapefruit products before and after dosing.

Storage/Stability Store at controlled room temperature of 20°C to 25°C (68°F to 77°F). Protect from light; protect from moisture.

Mechanism of Action As a dihydropyridine calcium channel blocker, structurally similar to nifedipine, nisoldipine impedes the movement of calcium ions into vascular smooth muscle and cardiac muscle. Dihydropyridines are potent vasodilators and are not as likely to suppress cardiac contractility and slow cardiac conduction as other calcium antagonists such as verapamil and diltiazem; nisoldipine is 5-10 times as potent a vasodilator as nifedipine.

Pharmacodynamics/Kinetics

Duration: >24 hours
Absorption: Well absorbed. Peak concentrations significantly increased with high-lipid meals; however, AUC is reduced.
Protein binding: >99%
Metabolism: Extensively hepatic; 1 active metabolite (10% of activity of parent); first-pass effect
Bioavailability: ~5%
Half-life elimination: 9-18 hours
Time to peak: 4-14 hours
Excretion: Urine (60% to 80% as inactive metabolites); feces

Dosing

Adult Hypertension: Oral:

Sular (Geomatrix delivery system): Oral: Initial: 17 mg once daily, then increase by 8.5 mg/week (or longer intervals) to attain adequate control of blood pressure
Usual dose range: 17-34 mg once daily; doses >34 mg once daily are not recommended

Nisoldipine extended-release tablet (original formulation): Initial: 20 mg once daily, then increase by 10 mg/week (or longer intervals) to attain adequate control of blood pressure
Usual dose range: 20-40 mg once daily; doses >60 mg once daily are not recommended

Conversion from nisoldipine extended-release (original formulation) to Sular Geomatrix delivery system:

Nisoldipine Extended Release Dosing Equivalency

Original Extended Release Formulation	Sular Extended Release (Geomatrix delivery system)
10 mg	8.5 mg
20 mg	17 mg
30 mg	25.5 mg
40 mg	34 mg

Geriatric Hypertension: Oral:

Sular (Geomatrix delivery system): Initial dose: 8.5 mg once daily; increase by 8.5 mg/week (or longer intervals) to attain adequate blood pressure control
Nisoldipine extended-release (original formulation): Initial dose: 10 mg once daily; increase by 10 mg/week (or longer intervals) to attain adequate blood pressure control.

Conversion from nisoldipine extended-release (original formulation) to Sular Geomatrix delivery system: Refer to adult dosing.

Renal Impairment

Mild to moderate impairment: No dosage adjustment necessary.

Severe impairment: No dosage adjustment provided in manufacturer's labeling.

Hepatic Impairment

Sular (Geomatrix delivery system): An initial dose exceeding 8.5 mg once daily is not recommended for patients with hepatic impairment.

Nisoldipine extended-release (original formulation): An initial dose exceeding 10 mg once daily is not recommended for patients with hepatic impairment.

Dietary Considerations Take on an empty stomach (1 hour before or 2 hours after a meal). Avoid grapefruit juice before and after dosing. Avoid grapefuit juice; avoid high-fat diet.

Administration Administer at the same time each day to ensure minimal fluctuation of serum levels. Avoid high-fat diet. Administer on an empty stomach (1 hour before or 2 hours after a meal). Swallow whole; do not crush, break, split, or chew.

Monitoring Parameters Blood pressure, heart rate

Dosage Forms Excipient information presented when available (limited, particularly for generics); consult specific product labeling.

Tablet Extended Release 24 Hour, Oral:
Sular: 8.5 mg
Sular: 17 mg [contains tartrazine (fd&c yellow #5)]
Sular: 34 mg
Generic: 8.5 mg, 17 mg, 20 mg, 25.5 mg, 30 mg, 34 mg, 40 mg

◆ Nitalapram see Citalopram on page 398

Nitazoxanide (nye ta ZOX a nide)

Brand Names: US Alinia
Index Terms NTZ
Pharmacologic Category Antiprotozoal
Use Treatment of diarrhea caused by *Cryptosporidium parvum* or *Giardia lamblia*
Dosing

Adult & Geriatric Diarrhea caused by *Cryptosporidium parvum* or *Giardia lamblia*: Oral suspension or tablets: 500 mg every 12 hours for 3 days

Clostridium difficile-associated diarrhea (off-label use): Oral suspension or tablets: 500 mg every 12 hours for 7 to 10 days (Musher 2006; Musher 2009)

Cryptosporidiosis-associated diarrhea in HIV-infected patients (off-label use): Oral: 500 to 1,000 mg twice daily for 14 days (must be used in conjunction with optimized ART, electrolyte replacement, and symptomatic treatment and rehydration) (HHS [OI adult 2015])

Pediatric

Diarrhea caused by *Cryptosporidium parvum* or *Giardia lamblia*: Oral: **Note:** May consider increasing duration up to 14 days in HIV-exposed/-infected patients with cryptosporidiosis (CDC 2009):

Children 1 to 3 years: Oral suspension: 100 mg every 12 hours for 3 days; may consider increasing duration up to 14 days in HIV-exposed/-infected pediatric patients with cryptosporidiosis (CDC 2009)

Children 4 to 11 years: Oral suspension: 200 mg every 12 hours for 3 days; may consider increasing duration up to 14 days in HIV-exposed/-infected pediatric patients with cryptosporidiosis (CDC 2009)

Children ≥12 years: Refer to adult dosing.

Cryptosporidiosis-associated diarrhea in HIV-infected patients (off-label use): Adolescents: Refer to adult dosing.

Renal Impairment There are no dosage adjustments provided in the manufacturer's labeling (has not been studied); use with caution.

Hepatic Impairment There are no dosage adjustments provided in the manufacturer's labeling (has not been studied); use with caution.

Additional Information Complete prescribing information should be consulted for additional detail.

Dosage Forms Excipient information presented when available (limited, particularly for generics); consult specific product labeling.

Suspension Reconstituted, Oral:
Alinia: 100 mg/5 mL (60 mL) [contains fd&c red #40, sodium benzoate; strawberry flavor]

Tablet, Oral:
Alinia: 500 mg [contains fd&c blue #2 aluminum lake, fd&c yellow #10 aluminum lake, fd&c yellow #6 aluminum lake, soybean lecithin]

◆ Nithiodote see Sodium Nitrite and Sodium Thiosulfate on page 1675

Nitisinone (ni TIS i known)

Brand Names: US Orfadin
Index Terms NTBC
Pharmacologic Category 4-Hydroxyphenylpyruvate Dioxygenase Inhibitor
Use Hereditary tyrosinemia type 1: Treatment of hereditary tyrosinemia type 1 (HT-1) as an adjunct to dietary restriction of tyrosine and phenylalanine
Prescribing and Access Restrictions Distributed by Orfadin4U comprehensive patient support program. Information regarding acquisition of product may be obtained by calling 877-473-3179. Additional information can be found at http://www.orfadin.com
Dosing

Adult & Geriatric Note: Must be used in conjunction with a diet restricted in tyrosine and phenylalanine.

Hereditary tyrosinemia type 1 (HT-1): Oral: Initial: 1 mg/kg/day in 2 divided doses

Dosing adjustment for inadequate response: Note: Inadequate response is defined as continued abnormal biological parameters (erythrocyte PBG-synthase activity, urine 5-ALA, and urine and plasma succinylacetone) despite treatment. Plasma succinylacetone may take up to 3 months to normalize after start of therapy. If the aforementioned parameters are not available, may use urine succinylacetone, liver function tests, alpha-fetoprotein, serum tyrosine, and serum phenylalanine to evaluate response (exceptions may include during initiation of therapy and exacerbations).

Abnormal biological parameters (erythrocyte PBG-synthase activity, urine 5-ALA, and urine succinylacetone) at 1 month: Increase dose to 1.5 mg/kg/day

Abnormal biological parameters (erythrocyte PBG-synthase activity, urine 5-ALA, and urine and plasma succinylacetone) at 3 months: Further increase to maximum dose of 2 mg/kg/day

Pediatric Note: Must be used in conjunction with a diet restricted in tyrosine and phenylalanine.

Hereditary tyrosinemia type 1 (HT-1): Oral: Children and Adolescents: Refer to adult dosing.

Renal Impairment There are no dosage adjustments provided in the manufacturer's labeling (has not been studied).

Hepatic Impairment There are no dosage adjustments provided in the manufacturer's labeling (has not been studied).

Additional Information Complete prescribing information should be consulted for additional detail.

Dosage Forms Excipient information presented when available (limited, particularly for generics); consult specific product labeling.

Capsule, Oral:
Orfadin: 2 mg, 5 mg, 10 mg

◆ Nitoman (Can) see Tetrabenazine on page 1772
◆ Nitro-Bid see Nitroglycerin on page 1289
◆ Nitro-Dur see Nitroglycerin on page 1289

Nitrofurantoin (nye troe fyoor AN toyn)

Brand Names: US Furadantin; Macrobid; Macrodantin
Brand Names: Canada Apo-Nitrofurantoin; Macrobid; Macrodantin; Novo-Furantoin; Teva-Nitrofurantoin
Pharmacologic Category Antibiotic, Miscellaneous
Use

Urinary tract infections: For the treatment of urinary tract infections (UTIs) when caused by susceptible strains of *Escherichia coli*, enterococci, *Staphylococcus aureus*, and certain susceptible strains of *Klebsiella* and *Enterobacter* species.

Acute cystitis: Nitrofurantoin monohydrate/macrocrystals: Indicated only for the treatment of acute uncomplicated UTIs (acute cystitis) caused by susceptible strains of *E. coli* or *Staphylococcus saprophyticus* in patients ≥12 years of age.

Pregnancy Considerations Adverse effects have not been observed in animal reproduction studies. Nitrofurantoin crosses the placenta (Perry, 1967) and maternal serum concentrations may be lower in pregnancy (Philipson, 1979). Current studies evaluating maternal use of nitrofurantoin during pregnancy and the development of birth defects have had mixed results (ACOG, 2011). An increased risk of neonatal jaundice was observed following maternal nitrofurantoin use during the last 30 days of pregnancy (Nordeng, 2013). Nitrofurantoin may be used to treat infections in pregnant women; use during the first

trimester should be limited to situations where no alternative therapies are available. Prescriptions should be written when clinically appropriate and for the shortest effective duration for confirmed infections (ACOG, 2011). Nitrofurantoin is contraindicated in pregnant patients at term (38-42 weeks gestation), during labor and delivery, or when the onset of labor is imminent due to the possibility of hemolytic anemia in the neonate. Alternative antibiotics should be considered in pregnant women with G-6-PD deficiency (Nordeng, 2013).

Breast-Feeding Considerations Trace amounts of nitrofurantoin can be detected in breast milk. Due to the potential for serious adverse reactions in the nursing infant, the manufacturer recommends a decision be made whether to discontinue nursing or to discontinue the drug, taking into account the importance of treatment to the mother. The therapeutic use of nitrofurantoin is contraindicated in neonates (<1 month of age) due to the possibility of hemolytic anemia caused by immature erythrocyte enzyme systems. In case reports, diarrhea was reported in two nursing infants and decreased milk volume was reported by one mother (dose, duration, relationship to breast-feeding not provided) (Ito, 1993).

Contraindications

Anuria, oliguria, or significant impairment of renal function (creatinine clearance [CrCl] <60 mL/minute or clinically significant elevated serum creatinine); previous history of cholestatic jaundice or hepatic dysfunction associated with prior nitrofurantoin use; hypersensitivity to drug or any component of the formulation.

Note: The manufacturer's contraindication in patients with CrCl <60 mL/minute has been challenged in the literature; limited data suggest that an alternative creatinine clearance threshold may be considered (Oplinger, 2013).

Because of the possibility of hemolytic anemia caused by immature erythrocyte enzyme systems (glutathione instability), the drug is contraindicated in pregnant patients at term (38 to 42 weeks gestation), during labor and delivery, or when the onset of labor is imminent; also contraindicated in neonates younger than 1 month of age.

Warnings/Precautions Use with caution in patients with G6PD deficiency (increased risk of hemolytic anemia). Urinary nitrofurantoin concentrations are variable in patients with impaired renal function. The manufacturer contraindicates use in CrCl <60 mL/minute; however, limited data suggest clinicians may consider using a lower threshold of CrCl ≥40 mL/minute when treatment is short term (≤1 week) for an uncomplicated UTI (Oplinger, 2013).

Use with caution if prolonged therapy is anticipated due to possible pulmonary toxicity. Acute, subacute, or chronic (usually after 6 months of therapy) pulmonary reactions (possibly fatal) have been observed in patients treated with nitrofurantoin; if these occur, discontinue therapy immediately; monitor closely for malaise, dyspnea, cough, fever, radiologic evidence of diffuse interstitial pneumonitis or fibrosis. Rare, but severe and sometimes fatal hepatic reactions (eg, cholestatic jaundice, hepatitis, hepatic necrosis) have been associated with nitrofurantoin (onset may be insidious); discontinue immediately if hepatitis occurs. Use is contraindicated in patients with a history of nitrofurantoin associated cholestatic jaundice or hepatic dysfunction. Monitor liver function test periodically. Has been associated with peripheral neuropathy (rare); risk may be increased in patients with anemia, renal impairment (CrCl <60 mL/minute), diabetes, vitamin B deficiency, debilitating disease, or electrolyte imbalance; use caution. Potentially significant drug-drug interactions may exist, requiring dose or frequency adjustment, additional monitoring, and/or selection of alternative therapy. Effects may be potentiated when used with other sedative drugs or ethanol. Use in the elderly, particularly females receiving long-term prophylaxis for recurrent UTIs, has been associated with an increased risk of hepatic and pulmonary toxicity, and peripheral neuropathy. In the elderly, avoid use for long-term suppression due to potential for pulmonary toxicity and availability of safer alternative agents (Beers Criteria). Use in the elderly, particularly females receiving long-term prophylaxis for recurrent UTIs, has also been associated with an increased risk of hepatic toxicity and peripheral neuropathy; monitor closely for toxicities during use. Prolonged use may result in fungal or bacterial superinfection, including *C. difficile*-associated diarrhea (CDAD) and pseudomembranous colitis; CDAD has been observed >2 months postantibiotic treatment. Use is contraindicated in children <1 month of age (at increased risk for hemolytic anemia). Not indicated for the treatment of pyelonephritis or perinephric abscesses. Postmarketing cases of optic neuritis have been reported.

Adverse Reactions Frequency not defined.

Cardiovascular: ECG changes (nonspecific ST/T wave changes, bundle branch block)

Central nervous system: Bulging fontanel (infants), chills, confusion, depression, dizziness, drowsiness, headache, malaise, numbness, paresthesia, peripheral neuropathy, pseudotumor cerebri, psychotic reaction, vertigo

Dermatologic: Alopecia, erythema multiforme, exfoliative dermatitis, pruritus, skin rash (eczematous, erythematous, maculopapular), Stevens-Johnson syndrome, urticaria

Endocrine & metabolic: Hyperphosphatemia

Gastrointestinal: Abdominal pain, anorexia, *Clostridium difficile* associated diarrhea, constipation, diarrhea, dyspepsia, flatulence, nausea, pancreatitis, pseudomembranous colitis, sialadenitis, vomiting

Genitourinary: Urine discoloration (brown)

Hematologic & oncologic: Agranulocytosis, aplastic anemia, eosinophilia, glucose-6-phosphate dehydrogenase deficiency anemia, granulocytopenia, hemoglobin decreased, hemolytic anemia, leukopenia, megaloblastic anemia, thrombocytopenia

Hepatic: Cholestatic jaundice, hepatitis, hepatic necrosis, increased serum transaminases

Hypersensitivity: Anaphylaxis, angioedema, hypersensitivity (including acute pulmonary hypersensitivity)

Infection: Superinfection (eg, *Pseudomonas* or *Candida*)

Neuromuscular & skeletal: Arthralgia, lupus-like syndrome, myalgia, weakness

Ophthalmic: Amblyopia, nystagmus, optic neuritis

Respiratory: Acute pulmonary reaction (symptoms include chills, chest pain, cough, dyspnea, fever, and eosinophilia), cough, cyanosis, dyspnea, pneumonitis, pulmonary fibrosis (with long-term use), pulmonary infiltration

Miscellaneous: Fever

Postmarketing and/or case reports (Limited to important or life-threatening): Hepatotoxicty (idiosyncratic) (Chalasani, 2014)

Drug Interactions

Metabolism/Transport Effects None known.

Avoid Concomitant Use

Avoid concomitant use of Nitrofurantoin with any of the following: BCG (Intravesical); Magnesium Trisilicate; Norfloxacin

Increased Effect/Toxicity

Nitrofurantoin may increase the levels/effects of: Eplerenone; Prilocaine; Sodium Nitrite; Spironolactone

The levels/effects of Nitrofurantoin may be increased by: Dapsone (Topical); Nitric Oxide; Probenecid

Decreased Effect

Nitrofurantoin may decrease the levels/effects of: BCG (Intravesical); BCG Vaccine (Immunization); Norfloxacin; Sodium Picosulfate; Typhoid Vaccine

The levels/effects of Nitrofurantoin may be decreased by: Magnesium Trisilicate

Food Interactions Nitrofurantoin serum concentrations may be increased if taken with food. Management: Administer with meals.

Storage/Stability

Capsules: Store at controlled room temperature, 15°C to 30°C (59°F to 86°F). Dispense in a tight container using a child-resistant closure.

Oral suspension: Avoid exposure to strong light, which may darken the drug. It is stable when stored between 20°C and 25°C (68°F and 77°F). Protect from freezing. Dispense in glass amber bottles.

Mechanism of Action Nitrofurantoin is reduced by bacterial flavoproteins to reactive intermediates that inactivate or alter bacterial ribosomal proteins leading to inhibition of protein synthesis, aerobic energy metabolism, DNA, RNA, and cell wall synthesis. Nitrofurantoin is bactericidal in urine at therapeutic doses. The broad-based nature of this mode of action may explain the lack of acquired bacterial resistance to nitrofurantoin, as the necessary multiple and simultaneous mutations of the target macromolecules would likely be lethal to the bacteria.

Pharmacodynamics/Kinetics

Absorption: Well absorbed; macrocrystalline form absorbed more slowly due to slower dissolution (causes less GI distress)

Distribution: V_d: 0.8 L/kg

Protein binding: 60% to 90%

Metabolism: Body tissues (except plasma) metabolize 60% of drug to inactive metabolites

Bioavailability: Increased with food by ~40%

Half-life elimination: 20-60 minutes; prolonged with renal impairment

Excretion:

Suspension: Urine (~40%) and feces (small amounts) as metabolites and unchanged drug

Macrocrystals: Urine (20% to 25% as unchanged drug)

Dosing

Adult

UTI treatment:

Furadantin, Macrodantin: Oral: 50-100 mg/dose every 6 hours; administer for 7 days or at least 3 days after obtaining sterile urine

Macrobid: Oral: 100 mg twice daily for 7 days

UTI prophylaxis (Furadantin, Macrodantin): Oral: 50-100 mg/dose at bedtime

Geriatric Avoid use; alternative agents preferred. Refer to adult dosing

Pediatric

UTI treatment:

Children >1 month (Furadantin, Macrodantin): Oral: 5-7 mg/kg/day in divided doses every 6 hours (maximum: 400 mg daily). Administer for 7 days or at least 3 days after obtaining sterile urine.

Children >12 years (Macrobid): Oral: Refer to adult dosing.

UTI prophylaxis: Children >1 month (Furadantin, Macrodantin): Oral: 1-2 mg/kg/day in divided doses every 12-24 hours (maximum: 100 mg daily) (*Red Book* [AAP] 2012)

Renal Impairment

CrCl ≥60 mL/minute: No dosage adjustment provided in manufacturer's labeling.

CrCl <60 mL/minute: Use is contraindicated. **Note:** Although more evidence is needed, limited data suggest clinicians consider use in patients with CrCl ≥40 mL/minute when treatment is short term (≤1 week) for an uncomplicated UTI (Oplinger, 2013)

Hepatic Impairment No dosage adjustment provided in manufacturer's labeling. Contraindicated in patients with a previous history of cholestatic jaundice or hepatic dysfunction associated with nitrofurantoin.

Dietary Considerations Take with meals to improve absorption and decrease adverse effects.

Administration Administer with meals to improve absorption and decrease adverse effects; suspension may be mixed with water, milk, fruit juice, or infant formula. Shake suspension well before use.

Monitoring Parameters Signs of pulmonary reaction; signs of numbness or tingling of the extremities; CBC, periodic liver function tests, periodic renal function tests with long-term use

Test Interactions False-positive urine glucose (Benedict's and Fehling's methods); no false positives with enzymatic tests

Dosage Forms Excipient information presented when available (limited, particularly for generics); consult specific product labeling. [DSC] = Discontinued product

Capsule, Oral:

Macrobid: 100 mg [contains brilliant blue fcf (fd&c blue #1), fd&c red #40, fd&c yellow #10 (quinoline yellow)]

Macrodantin: 50 mg, 100 mg [contains fd&c yellow #10 (quinoline yellow), fd&c yellow #6 (sunset yellow)]

Generic: 50 mg, 100 mg

Capsule, Oral, as macrocrystals:

Macrodantin: 25 mg

Macrodantin: 50 mg [DSC] [contains fd&c yellow #10 (quinoline yellow), fd&c yellow #6 (sunset yellow)]

Generic: 25 mg, 50 mg, 100 mg

Capsule, Oral, as monohydrate/macrocrystals:

Generic: 100 mg

Suspension, Oral:

Furadantin: 25 mg/5 mL (230 mL)

Generic: 25 mg/5 mL (230 mL, 240 mL)

◆ **Nitrogen Mustard** *see* Mechlorethamine (Systemic) *on page 1130*

Nitroglycerin (nye troe GLI ser in)

Brand Names: US Minitran; Nitro-Bid; Nitro-Dur; Nitro-Time; Nitrolingual; NitroMist; Nitronal; Nitrostat; Rectiv

Brand Names: Canada Minitran; Mylan-Nitro Sublingual Spray; Nitro-Dur; Nitroglycerin Injection, USP; Nitrol; Nitrostat; Rho-Nitro Pump Spray; Transderm-Nitro; Trinipatch

Index Terms Glyceryl Trinitrate; GTN; Nitroglycerol; Nitronal; NTG; TNG; Tridil

Pharmacologic Category Antianginal Agent; Antidote; Extravasation; Vasodilator

Additional Appendix Information

Hypertension *on page 1996*

Use Treatment or prevention of angina pectoris

Intravenous (IV) administration: Treatment or prevention of angina pectoris; acute decompensated heart failure (especially when associated with acute myocardial infarction); perioperative hypertension (especially during cardiovascular surgery); induction of intraoperative hypotension

Intra-anal administration (Rectiv ointment): Treatment of moderate-to-severe pain associated with chronic anal fissure

Pregnancy Considerations Animal reproduction studies have not been conducted with all products; adverse events were not observed in animal reproduction studies conducted using the ointment. Nitroglycerin crosses the placenta (David, 2000). Concentrations following application of a transdermal patch 0.4 mg/hour were low but detectable in the fetal serum (fetal/maternal ratio: 0.23) (Bustard, 2003). Nitroglycerin may be used in pregnancy when immediate relaxation of the uterus is needed (ACOG, 2006; Axemo, 1998; Chandraharan, 2005). Intravenous nitroglycerin may be used to treat pre-eclampsia with pulmonary edema (ESG, 2011).

Breast-Feeding Considerations It is not known if nitroglycerin is excreted in breast milk. The manufacturer recommends that caution be exercised when administering nitroglycerin to nursing women. Information related to the use of nitroglycerin and breast-feeding is limited (Böttiger, 2010; O'Sullivan, 2011).

Contraindications

Hypersensitivity to organic nitrates or any component of the formulation (includes adhesives for transdermal product); concurrent use with phosphodiesterase-5 (PDE-5) inhibitors (avanafil, sildenafil, tadalafil, or vardenafil); concurrent use with riociguat

Additional contraindications for IV product: Hypersensitivity to corn or corn products (solutions containing dextrose); constrictive pericarditis; pericardial tamponade; restrictive cardiomyopathy

Additional contraindications for sublingual product and rectal ointment: Early myocardial infarction (sublingual product only; see **Note**); increased intracranial pressure; severe anemia

Additional contraindications for translingual product: Increased intracranial pressure; severe anemia; acute circulatory failure or shock (Nitrolingual only)

Canadian labeling: Additional contraindications for transdermal patch (not in US labeling): Acute circulatory failure associated with marked hypotension (shock and states of collapse); orthostatic hypotension; myocardial insufficiency due to obstruction (eg, presence of aortic or mitral stenosis or of constrictive pericarditis); increased intracranial pressure; increased intraocular pressure; severe anemia

Note: According to the 2013 American College of Cardiology Foundation/American Heart Association (ACCF/AHA) guidelines of the management of ST-elevation myocardial infarction (STEMI) and the 2013 ACCF/AHA guidelines for the management of unstable angina/non-ST-elevation myocardial infarction, avoid nitrates in the following conditions: Hypotension (SBP <90 mm Hg or ≥30 mm Hg below baseline), marked bradycardia or tachycardia, and right ventricular infarction. Sublingual nitroglycerin may be used as initial treatment of ongoing chest pain in patients who may have STEMI or UA/NSTEMI (Anderson, 2013; O'Gara, 2013).

Warnings/Precautions Severe hypotension can occur. Use with caution in volume depletion, moderate hypotension, constrictive pericarditis, aortic or mitral stenosis, and extreme caution with inferior wall MI and suspected right ventricular involvement. The Canadian labeling contraindicates use in myocardial insufficiency due to obstruction such as constrictive pericarditis and aortic or mitral stenosis. According to the ACCF/AHA, avoid use in patients with severe hypotension (SBP <90 mm Hg or ≥30 mm Hg below baseline), marked bradycardia or tachycardia, and right ventricular MI (ACCF/AHA [Anderson, 2013]; ACCF/AHA [O'Gara, 2013]). Avoid use in patients with hypertrophic cardiomyopathy (HCM) with outflow tract obstruction; nitrates may reduce preload, exacerbating obstruction and cause hypotension or syncope and/or worsening of heart failure (ACCF/AHA [Gersh, 2011]).

Paradoxical bradycardia and increased angina pectoris can accompany hypotension. Orthostatic hypotension can also occur. Ethanol can accentuate this. Dose-related headaches may occur, especially during initial dosing. Tolerance does develop to nitrates and appropriate dosing is needed to minimize this (drug-free interval). Avoid use of long-acting agents in acute MI or acute HF; cannot easily reverse effects. Nitrates may aggravate angina caused by hypertrophic cardiomyopathy. Nitroglycerin may precipitate or aggravate increased intracranial pressure and subsequently may worsen clinical outcomes in patients with neurologic injury (eg, intracranial hemorrhage, traumatic brain injury). The Canadian labeling contraindicates use with increased intracranial pressure. Nitroglycerin transdermal patches may contain conducting metal (eg, aluminum); remove patch prior to MRI. Some dosage forms may contain propylene glycol; large amounts are potentially

toxic and have been associated hyperosmolality, lactic acidosis, seizures and respiratory depression; use caution (AAP, 1997; Zar, 2007). Potentially significant drug-drug interactions may exist, requiring dose or frequency adjustment, additional monitoring, and/or selection of alternative therapy.

Use caution when treating rectal anal fissures with nitroglycerin ointment formulation in patients with suspected or known significant cardiovascular disorders (eg, cardiomyopathies, heart failure, acute MI); intra-anal nitroglycerin administration may decrease systolic blood pressure and decrease arterial vascular resistance.

Adverse Reactions

Frequency not defined:

Cardiovascular: Bradycardia, flushing, hypotension, orthostatic hypotension, peripheral edema, syncope, tachycardia

Central nervous system: Headache (common), dizziness, lightheadedness

Gastrointestinal: Nausea, vomiting, xerostomia

Neuromuscular & skeletal: Paresthesia, weakness

Respiratory: Dyspnea, pharyngitis, rhinitis

Miscellaneous: Diaphoresis

<1% (Limited to important or life-threatening): Allergic reactions, anaphylactoid reaction, application site irritation (patch), blurred vision, cardiovascular collapse, contact dermatitis (ointment, patch), crescendo angina, exfoliative dermatitis, fixed drug eruption (ointment, patch), methemoglobinemia (rare; overdose), pallor, palpitation, rash, rebound hypertension, restlessness, shock, vertigo

Drug Interactions

Metabolism/Transport Effects None known.

Avoid Concomitant Use

Avoid concomitant use of Nitroglycerin with any of the following: Ergot Derivatives; Phosphodiesterase 5 Inhibitors; Riociguat

Increased Effect/Toxicity

Nitroglycerin may increase the levels/effects of: Amifostine; Antipsychotic Agents (Second Generation [Atypical]); DULoxetine; Ergot Derivatives; Hypotension-Associated Agents; Levodopa; Prilocaine; Riociguat; Rosiglitazone; Sodium Nitrite

The levels/effects of Nitroglycerin may be increased by: Alcohol (Ethyl); Alfuzosin; Barbiturates; Blood Pressure Lowering Agents; Brimonidine (Topical); Dapoxetine; Dapsone (Topical); Diazoxide; Herbs (Hypotensive Properties); Molsidomine; Nicorandil; Nitric Oxide; Obinutuzumab; Pentoxifylline; Phosphodiesterase 5 Inhibitors; Prostacyclin Analogues

Decreased Effect

Nitroglycerin may decrease the levels/effects of: Alteplase; Heparin

The levels/effects of Nitroglycerin may be decreased by: Ergot Derivatives

Preparation for Administration Nitronal (glyceryl trinitrate) 1 mg/mL (temporarily available in the U.S.):

To prepare a 100 **mcg**/mL solution: Withdraw 25 mL D$_5$W from a 250 mL bottle of D$_5$W and replace volume with 25 mg (25 mL) of Nitronal.

To prepare a 200 **mcg**/mL solution: Withdraw 50 mL D$_5$W from a 250 mL bottle of D$_5$W and replace volume with 50 mg (50 mL) of Nitronal.

Storage/Stability

IV solution: Doses should be made in glass bottles, EXCEL® or PAB® containers. Adsorption occurs to soft plastic (eg, PVC). Nitroglycerin diluted in D$_5$W or NS in glass containers is physically and chemically stable for 48 hours at room temperature and 7 days under refrigeration. In D$_5$W or NS in EXCEL®/PAB® containers it is physically and chemically stable for 24 hours at room temperature.

Sublingual tablets, slow-release capsules, topical ointment, and rectal ointment: Store at 20°C to 25°C (68°F to 77°F)

Transdermal patch: Store at 15°C to 30°C (59°F to 86°F)

Translingual spray: Store at 25°C (77°F); excursions permitted to 15°C to 30°C (59°F to 86°F). Do not forcefully open or burn container after use. Do not spray toward flames.

Mechanism of Action Nitroglycerin forms free radical nitric oxide. In smooth muscle, nitric oxide activates guanylate cyclase which increases guanosine 3'5' monophosphate (cGMP) leading to dephosphorylation of myosin light chains and smooth muscle relaxation. Produces a vasodilator effect on the peripheral veins and arteries with more prominent effects on the veins. Primarily reduces cardiac oxygen demand by decreasing preload (left ventricular end-diastolic pressure); may modestly reduce afterload; dilates coronary arteries and improves collateral flow to ischemic regions. For use in rectal fissures, intra-anal administration results in decreased sphincter tone and intra-anal pressure.

Pharmacodynamics/Kinetics

Onset of action: Sublingual tablet: 1 to 3 minutes; Translingual spray: Similar to sublingual tablet; Extended release: ~60 minutes; Topical: 15 to 30 minutes; Transdermal: ~30 minutes; IV: Immediate

Peak effect: Sublingual tablet: 5 minutes; Translingual spray: 4 to 10 minutes; Extended release: 2.5 to 4 hours; Topical: ~60 minutes; Transdermal: 120 minutes; IV: Immediate

Duration: Sublingual tablet: At least 25 minutes; Translingual spray: Similar to sublingual tablet; Extended release: 4 to 8 hours (Gibbons, 2002); Topical: 7 hours; Transdermal: 10 to 12 hours; IV: 3 to 5 minutes

Distribution: V$_d$: ~3 L/kg

Protein binding: 60%

Metabolism: Extensive first-pass effect; metabolized hepatically to glycerol di- and mononitrate metabolites via liver reductase enzyme; subsequent metabolism to glycerol and organic nitrate; nonhepatic metabolism via red blood cells and vascular walls also occurs

Half-life elimination: ~1 to 4 minutes

Excretion: Urine (as inactive metabolites)

Dosing

Adult & Geriatric Note: Hemodynamic and antianginal tolerance often develop within 24 to 48 hours of continuous nitrate administration. Nitrate-free interval (10 to 12 hours/day) is recommended to avoid tolerance development; gradually decrease dose in patients receiving NTG for prolonged period to avoid withdrawal reaction.

Angina/coronary artery disease:

Oral: 2.5 to 6.5 mg 3 to 4 times/day (maximum dose: 26 mg 4 times/day)

IV: 5 mcg/minute, increase by 5 mcg/minute every 3 to 5 minutes to 20 mcg/minute. If no response at 20 mcg/minute, may increase by 10 to 20 mcg/minute every 3 to 5 minutes (generally accepted maximum dose: 400 mcg/minute)

According to the 2013 ACCF/AHA guideline for the management of unstable angina/non-ST-elevation myocardial infarction (off-label dosing): Initial: 10 mcg/minute, increase by 10 mcg/minute every 3 to 5 minutes until relief of symptoms or blood pressure response noted; if no response at 20 mcg/minute, may increase by 10 mcg/minute and later by 20 mcg/minute may be used (Anderson, 2013). The 2013 ACCF/AHA guidelines for STEMI also recommend an initial dose of 10 mcg/minute with subsequent titration to desired blood pressure effect (O'Gara, 2013).

Sublingual: 0.3 to 0.6 mg every 5 minutes for maximum of 3 tablets in 15 minutes; may also use prophylactically 5 to 10 minutes prior to activities which may provoke an attack.

According to the 2013 ACCF/AHA guidelines for STEMI: If nitroglycerin is prescribed, advise the patient to take 1 dose promptly in response to chest pain. If pain is unrelieved or worsened 5 minutes after 1 dose, the patient should call 9-1-1 immediately (O'Gara, 2013).

Topical 2% ointment: 1/2" upon rising and 1/2" 6 hours later; if necessary, the dose may be doubled to 1" and subsequently doubled again to 2" if response is inadequate. Doses of 1/2" to 2" were used in clinical trials. Recommended maximum: 2 doses/day; include a nitrate free-interval ~10 to 12 hours/day.

Topical patch, transdermal: 0.2 to 0.4 mg/hour initially and titrate to doses of 0.4 to 0.8 mg/hour. Tolerance is minimized by using a patch-on period of 12 to 14 hours/day and patch-off period of 10 to 12 hours/day.

Translingual 0.4 mg/spray: 1 to 2 sprays onto or under tongue approximately every 5 minutes for maximum of 3 sprays in 15 minutes, may also be used prophylactically 5 to 10 minutes prior to activities which may provoke an angina attack

According to the 2013 ACCF/AHA guidelines for STEMI: If nitroglycerin is prescribed, advise the patient to take 1 dose promptly in response to chest pain. If pain is unrelieved or worsened 5 minutes after 1 dose, the patient should call 9-1-1 immediately (O'Gara, 2013).

Anal fissure, chronic (0.4% ointment): Intra-anal: 1 inch (equals 1.5 mg of nitroglycerin) every 12 hours for up to 3 weeks

Esophageal spastic disorders (off-label use): Sublingual: 0.3 to 0.6 mg (Swamy, 1977)

Extravasation (sympathomimetic vasopressors), treatment (alternative to phentolamine; off-label use): Based on limited data in neonates; optimal dosing has not been established: Topical 2% ointment: 4 mm/kg applied as a thin ribbon to the affected area has been reported in a case series; after 8 hours, if no improvement, the dose may be reapplied to the affected site (Wong, 1992). Application of a 1-inch strip on the affected site has also been described to be successful (Denkler, 1989); may also be considered for adults as an alternative to phentolamine (Hurst, 2004).

Gastroesophageal variceal hemorrhage (off-label use): IV infusion: Initial: 40 mcg/minute, increase by 40 mcg/minute every 15 minutes if systolic blood pressure is >90 to 100 mm Hg, up to a maximum of 400 mcg/minute (Garcia-Tsao, 2007; Gimson, 1986; Westaby, 1989). Coadminister with vasopressin and use at the highest effective dose for a maximum of 24 hours to minimize the development of adverse effects (Garcia-Tsao, 2007).

Uterine relaxation (off-label use): IV bolus: 100 to 200 mcg; may repeat dose every 2 minutes as necessary (Axemo, 1998; Chandraharan, 2005)

Pediatric Extravasation (sympathomimetic vasopressors), treatment (alternative to phentolamine; off-label use): Based on limited data in neonates; optimal dosing has not been established: Topical 2% ointment: 4 mm/kg applied as a thin ribbon to the affected area has been reported in a case series; after 8 hours, if no improvement, the dose may be reapplied to the affected site (Wong, 1992). Application of a 1-inch strip on the affected site has also been described to be successful (Denkler, 1989).

Renal Impairment There are no dosage adjustments provided in the manufacturer's labeling.

Hepatic Impairment There are no dosage adjustments provided in the manufacturer's labeling.

Usual Infusion Concentrations: Pediatric Note: Premixed solutions available

IV infusion: 100 **mcg**/mL, 200 **mcg**/mL, or 400 **mcg**/mL

Usual Infusion Concentrations: Adult Note: Premixed solutions available

IV infusion: 50 mg in 250 mL (concentration: 200 **mcg**/mL) **or** 100 mg in 250 mL (concentration: 400 **mcg**/mL) of D$_5$W

Administration

IV: Prepare in glass bottles, EXCEL or PAB containers. Adsorption occurs to soft plastic (eg, PVC); use administration sets intended for nitroglycerin. Administer via infusion pump.

Intra-anal ointment: Using a finger covering (eg, plastic wrap, surgical glove, finger cot), place finger beside 1 inch measuring guide on the box and squeeze ointment the length of the measuring line directly onto covered finger. Insert ointment into the anal canal using the covered finger up to first finger joint (do not insert further than the first finger joint) and apply ointment around the side of the anal canal. If intra-anal application is too painful, may apply the ointment to the outside of the anus. Wash hands following application.

Oral (extended release capsule): Swallow whole. Do not chew, break, or crush. Take with a full glass of water.

Sublingual: Do not chew, crush, or swallow sublingual tablet. Place under tongue and allow to dissolve. Alternately, may be placed in the buccal pouch.

Topical ointment: Wash hands prior to and after use. Application site should be clean, dry, and hair-free. Apply to chest or back with the applicator or dose-measuring paper. Spread in a thin layer over a 2.25 x 3.5 inch area. Do not rub into skin. Tape applicator into place.

Drug extravasation management, (treatment), sympathomimetic vasopressors (alternative to phentolamine) (off-label use): Stop vesicant infusion immediately and disconnect IV line (leave needle/cannula in place); gently aspirate extravasated solution from the IV line (do **NOT** flush the line); remove needle/cannula; elevate extremity. Apply nitroglycerin ointment as a thin ribbon to the affected area (Wong, 1992). May also apply dry warm compresses (Hurst, 2004).

Topical patch, transdermal: Application site should be clean, dry and hair-free. Remove patch after 12 to 14 hours. Rotate patch sites. Dispose of any used of unused patches by folding adhesive ends together, replace in pouch or sealed container and discard properly in trash, away from children and pets.

Translingual spray: Do not shake container. Prior to initial use, the pump must be primed by spraying 5 times (Nitrolingual) or 10 times (Nitromist) into the air. Priming sprays should be directed away from patient and others. Release spray onto or under tongue. Close mouth immediately after administration; do not inhale spray. Do not expectorate or rinse the mouth for 5 to 10 minutes following administration. Content of the container should be checked periodically; when the container is held upright, the end of the pump should be covered by the fluid in the bottle or the remaining sprays will not deliver the intended dose. If pump is unused for 6 weeks, a single priming spray (Nitrolingual) or 2 priming sprays (Nitromist) should be completed. If pump is unused for 3 months, re-prime with up to 5 sprays (Nitrolingual).

Monitoring Parameters Blood pressure, heart rate; consult individual institutional policies and procedures

Test Interactions IV formulation: Due to propylene glycol content, triglyceride assays dependent on glycerol oxidase may be falsely elevated.

Dosage Forms Excipient information presented when available (limited, particularly for generics); consult specific product labeling.

Aerosol Solution, Translingual:

NitroMist: 400 mcg/spray (4.1 g, 8.5 g) [contains menthol]

Generic: 400 mcg/spray (4.1 g, 8.5 g)

Capsule Extended Release, Oral:

Nitro-Time: 2.5 mg [contains brilliant blue fcf (fd&c blue #1), fd&c red #40, fd&c yellow #10 (quinoline yellow)]

Nitro-Time: 6.5 mg [contains brilliant blue fcf (fd&c blue #1), fd&c yellow #10 (quinoline yellow), fd&c yellow #6 (sunset yellow)]

Nitro-Time: 9 mg [contains fd&c yellow #10 (quinoline yellow), fd&c yellow #6 (sunset yellow)]

Generic: 2.5 mg, 6.5 mg, 9 mg

Ointment, Rectal:

Rectiv: 0.4% (30 g) [contains propylene glycol]

Ointment, Transdermal:

Nitro-Bid: 2% (1 g, 30 g, 60 g)

Patch 24 Hour, Transdermal:

Minitran: 0.1 mg/hr (30 ea); 0.2 mg/hr (30 ea); 0.4 mg/hr (30 ea); 0.6 mg/hr (30 ea)

Nitro-Dur: 0.1 mg/hr (30 ea, 100 ea); 0.2 mg/hr (30 ea, 100 ea); 0.3 mg/hr (1 ea, 30 ea, 100 ea); 0.4 mg/hr (30 ea, 100 ea); 0.6 mg/hr (30 ea, 100 ea); 0.8 mg/hr (30 ea, 100 ea)

Generic: 0.1 mg/hr (30 ea, 4350 ea); 0.2 mg/hr (30 ea, 4350 ea); 0.4 mg/hr (30 ea, 4350 ea); 0.6 mg/hr (30 ea, 4350 ea)

Solution, Intravenous:

Nitronal: 1 mg/mL (25 mL, 50 mL)

Generic: 25 mg (250 mL); 50 mg (250 mL, 500 mL); 100 mg (250 mL); 200 mg (500 mL); 5 mg/mL (10 mL)

Solution, Translingual:

Nitrolingual: 0.4 mg/spray (4.9 g, 12 g) [contains alcohol, usp]

Generic: 0.4 mg/spray (4.9 g, 12 g)

Tablet Sublingual, Sublingual:

Nitrostat: 0.3 mg, 0.4 mg, 0.6 mg

◆ Nitroglycerin Injection, USP (Can) *see* Nitroglycerin *on page 1289*

◆ Nitroglycerol *see* Nitroglycerin *on page 1289*

◆ Nitrol (Can) *see* Nitroglycerin *on page 1289*

◆ Nitrolingual *see* Nitroglycerin *on page 1289*

◆ NitroMist *see* Nitroglycerin *on page 1289*

◆ Nitronal *see* Nitroglycerin *on page 1289*

◆ Nitropress *see* Nitroprusside *on page 1291*

Nitroprusside (nye troe PRUS ide)

Brand Names: US Nitropress

Brand Names: Canada Nipride

Index Terms Nitroprusside Sodium; Sodium Nitroferricyanide; Sodium Nitroprusside

Pharmacologic Category Antihypertensive; Vasodilator

Additional Appendix Information

Hypertension *on page 1996*

Use Management of hypertensive crises; acute decompensated heart failure (HF); used for controlled hypotension to reduce bleeding during surgery

Pregnancy Considerations Animal studies have shown that nitroprusside may cross the placental barrier and result in fetal cyanide levels that are dose-related to maternal nitroprusside levels. However, information related to use in pregnancy is limited.

Breast-Feeding Considerations It is not known if nitroprusside is excreted in breast milk. Due to the potential for serious adverse reactions in the nursing infant, a decision should be made whether to discontinue nursing or to discontinue the drug, taking into account the importance of treatment to the mother.

◄ **Contraindications** Treatment of compensatory hypertension (aortic coarctation, arteriovenous shunting); to produce controlled hypotension during surgery in patients with known inadequate cerebral circulation or in moribund patients requiring emergency surgery; high output heart failure associated with reduced systemic vascular resistance (eg, septic shock); congenital optic atrophy or tobacco amblyopia

Warnings/Precautions [U.S. Boxed Warning] Excessive hypotension resulting in compromised perfusion of vital organs may occur; continuous blood pressure monitoring by experienced personnel is required. Except when used briefly or at low (<2 mcg/kg/minute) infusion rates, nitroprusside gives rise to large cyanide quantities. Do not use the maximum dose for more than 10 minutes; if blood pressure is not controlled by the maximum rate (ie, 10 mcg/kg/minute) after 10 minutes, discontinue infusion. Monitor for cyanide toxicity via acid-base balance and venous oxygen concentration; however, clinicians should note that these indicators may not always reliably indicate cyanide toxicity. Patients at risk of cyanide toxicity include those who are malnourished, have hepatic impairment, or those undergoing cardiopulmonary bypass, or therapeutic hypothermia (Rindone, 1992). Discontinue use of nitroprusside if signs and/or symptoms of cyanide toxicity (eg, metabolic acidosis, decreased oxygen saturation, bradycardia, confusion, convulsions) occur. Although not routinely done, sodium thiosulfate has been co-administered with nitroprusside using a 10:1 ratio of sodium thiosulfate to nitroprusside when higher doses of nitroprusside are used (eg, 4-10 mcg/kg/minute) for extended periods of time in order to prevent cyanide toxicity (Varon, 2008; Shulz, 2010); thiocyanate toxicity may still occur with this approach (Rindone, 1992). The use of other agents (eg, clevidipine, labetalol, nicardipine) should be considered if blood pressure is not controlled with nitroprusside. Use the lowest end of the dosage range with renal impairment. Cyanide toxicity may occur in patients with decreased liver function. Thiocyanate toxicity occurs in patients with renal impairment or those on prolonged infusions.

When nitroprusside is used for controlled hypotension during surgery, correct preexisting anemia and hypovolemia prior to use when possible. Use with extreme caution in patients with elevated intracranial pressure (head trauma, cerebral hemorrhage), myocardial infarction, severe renal impairment, hepatic failure, hypothyroidism. **[U.S. Boxed Warning]: Solution must be further diluted with 5% dextrose in water. Do not administer by direct injection.**

Adverse Reactions Frequency not defined.

Cardiovascular: Bradycardia, ECG changes, flushing, hypotension (excessive), palpitation, substernal distress, tachycardia

Central nervous system: Apprehension, dizziness, headache, intracranial pressure increased, restlessness

Dermatologic: Rash

Endocrine & metabolic: Metabolic acidosis (secondary to cyanide toxicity), hypothyroidism

Gastrointestinal: Abdominal pain, ileus, nausea, retching, vomiting

Hematologic: Methemoglobinemia, platelet aggregation decreased

Local: Injection site irritation

Neuromuscular & skeletal: Hyperreflexia (secondary to thiocyanate toxicity), muscle twitching

Ocular: Miosis (secondary to thiocyanate toxicity)

Otic: Tinnitus (secondary to thiocyanate toxicity)

Respiratory: Hyperoxemia (secondary to cyanide toxicity)

Miscellaneous: Cyanide toxicity, diaphoresis, thiocyanate toxicity

Drug Interactions

Metabolism/Transport Effects None known.

Avoid Concomitant Use There are no known interactions where it is recommended to avoid concomitant use.

Increased Effect/Toxicity

Nitroprusside may increase the levels/effects of: Amifostine; Antipsychotic Agents (Second Generation [Atypical]); DULoxetine; Hypotension-Associated Agents; Levodopa; Prilocaine; Sodium Nitrite

The levels/effects of Nitroprusside may be increased by: Alfuzosin; Barbiturates; Brimonidine (Topical); Calcium Channel Blockers; Dapsone (Topical); Diazoxide; Herbs (Hypotensive Properties); Molsidomine; Nicorandil; Nitric Oxide; Obinutuzumab; Pentoxifylline; Phosphodiesterase 5 Inhibitors; Prostacyclin Analogues

Decreased Effect

The levels/effects of Nitroprusside may be decreased by: Amphetamines; Herbs (Hypertensive Properties); Methylphenidate; Yohimbine

Preparation for Administration

Prior to administration, nitroprusside sodium should be further diluted by diluting 50 mg in 250-1000 mL of D₅W (preferred), LR, or NS.

Use only clear solutions; solutions of nitroprusside exhibit a color described as brownish, brown, brownish-pink, light orange, and straw. Solutions are highly sensitive to light. Exposure to light causes decomposition, resulting in a highly colored solution of orange, dark brown or blue. **A blue color indicates almost complete decomposition.** Do not use discolored solutions (eg, blue, green, red) or solutions in which particulate matter is visible.

Prepared solutions should be wrapped with aluminum foil or other opaque material to protect from light (do as soon as possible).

Storage/Stability Store the intact vial at 20°C to 25°C (68°F to 77°F). Protect from light.

Stability of parenteral admixture at room temperature (25°C) and at refrigeration temperature (4°C) is 24 hours.

Mechanism of Action Causes peripheral vasodilation by direct action on venous and arteriolar smooth muscle, thus reducing peripheral resistance; will increase cardiac output by decreasing afterload; reduces aortal and left ventricular impedance

Pharmacodynamics/Kinetics

Onset of action: Hypotensive effect: <2 minutes

Duration: Hypotensive effect: 1-10 minutes

Metabolism: Nitroprusside combines with hemoglobin to produce cyanide and cyanmethemoglobin. Cyanide detoxification occurs via rhodanase-mediated conversion of cyanide to thiocyanate; rhodanase couples cyanide molecules to sulfane sulfur groups from a sulfur donor (eg, thiosulfate, cystine, cysteine). This process has limited capacity and may become overwhelmed with large exposures once sulfur donor supplies are exhausted resulting in toxicity.

Half-life elimination: Nitroprusside, circulatory: ~2 minutes; Thiocyanate, elimination: ~3 days (may be doubled or tripled in renal failure)

Excretion: Urine (as thiocyanate)

Dosing

Adult & Geriatric

Acute hypertension: Initial: 0.3-0.5 mcg/kg/minute; may be titrated by 0.5 mcg/kg/minute every few minutes to achieve desired hemodynamic effect (Rhoney, 2009); maximum dose: 10 mcg/kg/minute. To avoid toxicity, some recommend a maximum dose of 2 mcg/kg/minute (Marik, 2007).

Acute decompensated heart failure: IV: Initial: 5-10 **mcg/minute**; may be titrated rapidly (eg, up to every 5 minutes) to achieve desired hemodynamic effect; usual dosage range: 5-300 **mcg/minute**. Doses >400 **mcg/minute** are not recommended due to minimal added benefit and increased risk for thiocyanate toxicity (HFSA, 2010).

Pediatric Acute hypertension: IV: Initial: 0.3-0.5 mcg/kg/minute; may be titrated every few minutes to achieve desired hemodynamic effect; maximum dose: 10 mcg/kg/minute (Hegenbarth, 2008; NHBPEP, 2005). Doses ≥1.8 mcg/kg/minute are associated with increased cyanide concentration in pediatric patients (Moffett, 2008); monitor cyanide levels with prolonged use (eg, >72 hours) (NHBPEP, 2005).

Renal Impairment No dosage adjustment provided in manufacturer's labeling. However, use in patients with renal impairment may lead to the accumulation of thiocyanate and subsequent toxicity; limit use.

Hepatic Impairment No dosage adjustment provided in manufacturer's labeling; due to the risk of cyanide toxicity, use with caution.

Usual Infusion Concentrations: Pediatric IV infusion: 100 **mcg/mL** or 200 **mcg/mL**

Usual Infusion Concentrations: Adult IV infusion: 50 mg in 250 mL (concentration: 200 **mcg/mL**) or 100 mg in 250 mL (concentration: 400 **mcg/mL**) of D₅W

Administration IV infusion only; infusion pump required; must be diluted prior to administration; not for direct injection. Due to potential for excessive hypotension, continuously monitor patient's blood pressure during therapy.

Monitoring Parameters Blood pressure, heart rate (cardiac monitor and blood pressure monitor required); monitor for cyanide and thiocyanate toxicity; monitor venous oxygen saturation; monitor acid-base status as acidosis can be the earliest sign of cyanide toxicity; monitor thiocyanate levels if requiring prolonged infusion (>3 days) or dose >3 mcg/kg/minute or patient has renal dysfunction; monitor cyanide blood levels (if available with appropriate turnaround time) in patients with decreased hepatic function

Consult individual institutional policies and procedures.

Reference Range Serum thiocyanate levels are not helpful in detecting toxicity. A level may be confirmatory if a patient is exhibiting signs and symptoms of thiocyanate toxicity. Initial signs of toxicity (eg, tinnitus) may be observed at levels >35 mcg/mL (manufacturer suggests 60 mcg/mL), but serious toxicity typically may not occur with levels <100 mcg/mL.

Dosage Forms Excipient information presented when available (limited, particularly for generics); consult specific product labeling.

Solution, Intravenous, as sodium:
Nitropress: 25 mg/mL (2 mL)

◆ **Nitroprusside Sodium** see Nitroprusside on page 1291

◆ **Nitrostat** see Nitroglycerin on page 1289

◆ **Nitro-Time** see Nitroglycerin on page 1289

Nivolumab (nye VOL ue mab)

Brand Names: US Opdivo
Brand Names: Canada Opdivo
Index Terms Anti-PD-1 Human Monoclonal Antibody MDX-1106; BMS-936558; MDX-1106; ONO-4538
Pharmacologic Category Antineoplastic Agent, Anti-PD-1 Monoclonal Antibody; Antineoplastic Agent, Monoclonal Antibody

Use

US labeling:

Melanoma, unresectable or metastatic: Treatment (as a single agent) of BRAF V600 wild-type unresectable or metastatic melanoma; unresectable or metastatic BRAF V600 mutation-positive melanoma with disease progression following ipilimumab and a BRAF inhibitor; treatment of BRAF V600 wild-type, unresectable, or metastatic melanoma (in combination with ipilimumab)

Non-small cell lung cancer, metastatic: Treatment of metastatic non-small cell lung cancer (NSCLC) that has progressed on or after platinum-based chemotherapy. Patients with EGFR or ALK genomic tumor aberrations should have disease progression (on approved EGFR- or ALK-directed therapy) prior to receiving nivolumab.

Renal cell cancer, clear cell (advanced): Treatment of advanced renal cell cancer in patients who have received prior anti-angiogenic therapy.

Canadian labeling:

Melanoma, unresectable or metastatic: Treatment of unresectable or metastatic BRAF V600 wild-type melanoma in previously untreated adults.

Pregnancy Considerations Adverse events were observed in animal reproduction studies. Nivolumab may be expected to cross the placenta; effects to the fetus may be greater in the second and third trimesters. Based on its mechanism of action, nivolumab is expected to cause fetal harm if used during pregnancy. Women of reproductive potential should use highly effective contraception during therapy and for at least 5 months after nivolumab treatment has been discontinued.

Breast-Feeding Considerations It is not known if nivolumab is excreted into breast milk. Due to the potential for serious adverse reactions in the nursing infant, the manufacturer recommends to discontinue nursing during treatment.

Medication Guide Available Yes

Contraindications There are no contraindications listed in the manufacturer's US labeling.

Canadian labeling: Hypersensitivity to nivolumab or any component of the formulation.

Warnings/Precautions Immune-mediated pneumonitis (severe pneumonitis or interstitial lung disease) has been observed, including cases which were fatal. Immune-mediated pneumonitis is defined as no other clear etiology and requiring corticosteroid use. The median time to development was 2.2 to 7.2 months (range: 2 days to 22.3 months) across several clinical trials. Some cases developed after nivolumab was discontinued for other reasons. With high-dose systemic corticosteroids (followed by a corticosteroid taper), all patients improved to grade 0 or 1; some patients with grade 2 or 3 pneumonitis had complete resolution (after completing corticosteroid therapy) and nivolumab was reinitiated without recurrence in some patients. Monitor for signs (with radiographic imaging) and symptoms of pneumonitis. May require treatment interruption, corticosteroid therapy, and/or permanent discontinuation. Grade 2 or higher pneumonitis should be managed with corticosteroids (prednisone 1 to 2 mg/kg daily or equivalent) followed by a corticosteroid taper. Withhold treatment until resolution for moderate (grade 2) immune-mediated pneumonitis; permanently discontinue for severe (grade 3) or life-threatening (grade 4) immune-mediated pneumonitis.

Diarrhea or colitis occurred commonly in patients receiving nivolumab (some cases were fatal). Immune-mediated colitis (defined as no other clear etiology and requiring corticosteroid use) including cases of grades 2 and 3 colitis occurred in some patients. The median time to onset of colitis was 1.4 to 5.1 months (range: 2 days to 19 months) from nivolumab initiation; some cases developed after nivolumab was discontinued for other reasons. In studies, the median duration of high-dose systemic corticosteroid therapy was 2.9 weeks to 1.4 months (range: 1 day to 7.4 months). Most patients with grade 2 or 3 immune-related colitis had complete resolution (improvement to grade 0); after resolution, nivolumab was reinitiated in some patients without recurrence, although was permanently discontinued in other patients. Monitor for signs and symptoms of colitis. May require treatment interruption, corticosteroid therapy, and/or permanent discontinuation. Severe colitis (grade 3) or life-threatening colitis (grade 4) should be managed with corticosteroids (prednisone 1 to 2 mg/kg daily or equivalent) followed by a corticosteroid taper. Moderate colitis (grade 2) of >5 days duration should be managed with corticosteroids (prednisone 0.5 to 1 mg/kg daily or equivalent) followed by a corticosteroid taper; may increase to prednisone 1 to 2 mg/kg daily (or equivalent) if colitis worsens or does not improve despite corticosteroid therapy. Permanently discontinue nivolumab for grade 4 colitis or diarrhea, or colitis that recurs upon reinitiation (single-agent therapy) or for severe or life-threatening colitis (grade 3 or 4) or for colitis that recurs upon reinitiation (in combination with ipilimumab).

ALT, AST, alkaline phosphatase, and total bilirubin elevations have occurred in nivolumab-treated patients. Immune-mediated hepatitis (defined as no other clear etiology and requiring corticosteroid use) occurred in patients receiving nivolumab; most cases included grade 2 and grade 3 hepatitis, although grade 4 toxicity also occurred. The time to onset ranged from ~2 weeks to ~8 months after nivolumab initiation (one case developed after nivolumab was discontinued for other reasons). Immune-mediated hepatitis was managed with high-dose systemic corticosteroids; liver function tests improved to grade 1 within 15 days of corticosteroid initiation in one trial. Immune-mediated hepatitis resolved and did not recur with continued corticosteroid use in some patients, although some patients experienced grade 3 recurrence and permanently discontinued treatment in a trial utilizing nivolumab as single-agent therapy. When used in combination with ipilimumab, several patients had complete resolution of hepatitis after completion of steroid therapy, and some patients had recurrence or worsening hepatitis when nivolumab and ipilimumab were restarted. Immune-mediated hepatitis recurred following nivolumab reinitiation in a NSCLC trial, leading to permanent nivolumab discontinuation. Monitor liver function at baseline and periodically for changes. Initiate corticosteroids (prednisone 1 to 2 mg/kg daily or equivalent) for grade 2 or higher transaminase elevations (with or without total bilirubin elevations). Withhold treatment for moderate (grade 2) immune-mediated hepatitis; permanently discontinue for severe (grade 3) or life-threatening (grade 4) immune-mediated hepatitis.

Creatinine elevations have occurred with nivolumab therapy. Immune-mediated nephritis (defined as ≥ grade 2 creatinine elevations with no other clear etiology and requiring corticosteroid use) may occur with nivolumab treatment. The time to onset for grade 2 or higher events ranged from ~1 week to ~12 months after nivolumab initiation; patients received high-dose systemic corticosteroids and treatment was withheld and discontinued. In clinical trials with single-agent nivolumab, immune-mediated nephritis resolved and did not recur with continued corticosteroid use in some patients, although other patients experienced ongoing renal dysfunction. In a clinical trial of nivolumab and ipilimumab combination therapy for the treatment of metastatic melanoma, immune-mediated renal dysfunction resolved with systemic corticosteroid use and interruption of nivolumab in one patient; another patient died with persistent renal dysfunction. Monitor serum creatinine at baseline and periodically during treatment. Initiate corticosteroids (prednisone 1 to 2 mg/kg daily or equivalent) followed by a corticosteroid taper for life-threatening (grade 4) serum creatinine elevation and permanently discontinue nivolumab. Withhold treatment for moderate (grade 2) and severe (grade 3) creatinine elevations and administer corticosteroids (prednisone 0.5 to 1 mg/kg daily or equivalent) followed by a corticosteroid taper; if toxicity worsens or does not improve, permanently discontinue and increase to prednisone 1 to 2 mg/kg daily (or equivalent).

In clinical trials, immune-mediated rash (including grade 2, 3, and 4 toxicity) was observed in patients receiving nivolumab (as a single agent or in combination with ipilimumab, although the incidence was higher with combination therapy). Fatal toxic epidermal necrolysis occurred rarely. In one study (combination therapy with ipilimumab), the time to onset of rash ranged from 1 day to 6.5 months; in a single-agent study the onset ranged from 2 days to 28.5 months. Among the patients with grade 3 rash who received nivolumab in combination with ipilimumab, several received systemic corticosteroid treatment and some patients had combination therapy withheld then reinitiated (with no recurrence of high-grade rash); all had resolution to ≤ grade 1 with no further corticosteroid requirements. Monitor closely; administer corticosteroids (prednisone 1 to 2 mg/kg/day or equivalent) for severe (grade 3) or life-threatening (grade 4) rash. Withhold treatment for grade 3 rash and permanently discontinue for life-threatening rash.

Type 1 diabetes mellitus may occur, including cases of new onset diabetes mellitus and diabetic ketoacidosis. The time to onset of diabetic ketoacidosis or diabetes mellitus ranged from 2.1 to 21.8 months. Monitor for hyperglycemia; administer insulin when clinically necessary. Withhold nivolumab for severe (grade 3) hyperglycemia until blood sugar has been appropriately controlled. Permanently discontinue for life-threatening (grade 4) hyperglycemia.

Immune-mediated encephalitis with both single-agent and combination nivolumab therapy may occur (rarely); may be fatal. Withhold nivolumab for new-onset moderate to severe neurologic signs/symptoms; evaluate to rule out infection or other neurologic causes. Brain MRI and/or lumbar puncture may be necessary. For confirmed immune-mediated encephalitis felt to be caused by nivolumab, administer corticosteroids (prednisone 1 to 2 mg/kg/day or equivalent), followed by a corticosteroid taper. Permanently discontinue if immune-mediated encephalitis occurs.

Hypophysitis may occur; over 10% of patients receiving nivolumab in combination with ipilimumab for metastatic melanoma developed grade 2 and 3 toxicity. Most patients received corticosteroids; combination therapy was restarted for the majority of the patients without worsening hypophysitis (several patients continued on corticosteroid therapy). The time to onset across several clinical trials ranged from 1.4 to 9.2 months. Monitor for signs/symptoms of hypophysitis. Administer corticosteroids (prednisone 1 mg/kg/day or equivalent) for grade 2 or higher toxicity. Withhold nivolumab for moderate (grade 2) or severe (grade 3) and permanently discontinue treatment for life-threatening (grade 4) hypophysitis. Adrenal insufficiency may occur; ~9% of patients receiving nivolumab in combination with ipilimumab developed adrenal insufficiency (including grade 3 toxicity). The median time to onset across two clinical trials was 3 to 5.8 months (range: 22 days to 20.9 months). Adrenal insufficiency occurred after treatment discontinuation in some patients. Toxicity resolved in several patients, some of whom remained on corticosteroid therapy; in two patients, combination therapy with nivolumab and ipilimumab was restarted and adrenal insufficiency did not recur. Monitor for signs/symptoms of adrenal insufficiency both during and after treatment. Administer corticosteroids (prednisone 1 to 2 mg/kg/day or equivalent) for severe (grade 3) or life-threatening (grade 4) adrenal insufficiency. Withhold nivolumab for moderate (grade 2) and permanently discontinue for severe (grade 3) or life-threatening (grade 4) toxicity.

Immune-mediated hyperthyroidism and hypothyroidism have occurred, mostly grades 1 and 2 hyper-/hypothyroidism (one patient receiving nivolumab in combination with ipilimumab experienced grade 3 autoimmune thyroiditis). The median onset for hyperthyroidism was ~1 to 3 months (range: Up to 14.2 months); most cases resolved (may require medical management, including corticosteroids and methimazole). Hypothyroidism occurred with a median onset of ~2 to 5 months (range: 1 day to 13.6 months). Most patients received subsequent nivolumab treatment (with or without ipilimumab) while continuing thyroid replacement therapy; in some patients, hypothyroidism completely resolved and levothyroxine was discontinued. Monitor thyroid function at baseline and for changes periodically during treatment (in one study patients were evaluated at baseline, treatment day 1, and every 6 weeks). Isolated hypothyroidism may be managed with hormone replacement therapy; initiate medical management to control hyperthyroidism. There are case reports of patients receiving nivolumab in combination with ipilimumab who developed hypothyroidism after resolution of grade 1 hyperthyroidism.

Other clinically relevant other immune-mediated disorders may occur; may develop after discontinuation of nivolumab. Immune-mediated adverse reactions observed included abducens nerve paresis, autoimmune neuropathy, demyelination, duodenitis, facial nerve paralysis, gastritis, Guillain-Barré syndrome, hypopituitarism, motor dysfunction, myasthenic syndrome, pancreatitis, polymyalgia rheumatic, sarcoidosis, systemic inflammatory response syndrome, uveitis, and vasculitis. If an immune-mediated adverse event is suspected, evaluate to exclude other causes. Based on symptom severity, withhold nivolumab, administer high-dose corticosteroids, and if appropriate, initiate hormone-replacement therapy. Upon improvement to grade 0 or 1, begin corticosteroid taper (over at least 1 month). After corticosteroid taper is completed and based on the severity of the reaction, may consider reinitiating nivolumab. Potentially significant drug-drug interactions may exist, requiring dose or frequency adjustment, additional monitoring, and/or selection of alternative therapy.

Adverse Reactions Frequency not always defined.

>10%:

Cardiovascular: Edema (17%; grade 3/4: 2%), chest pain (13%)

Central nervous system: Fatigue (50%; grade 3/4: 7%)

Dermatologic: Skin rash (16%; grade 3/4: <1%), pruritus (11%; grade 3/4: <1%)

Endocrine & metabolic: Hyponatremia (38%; grade 3/4: 10%), hypokalemia (20%; grade 3/4: 3%), hypomagnesemia (20%), hypercalcemia (20%; grade 3/4: 3%), hyperkalemia (18%; grade 3/4: 4%), hypocalcemia (18%; grade 3/4: 2%), weight loss (13%; grade 3/4: <1%)

Gastrointestinal: Decreased appetite (35%; grade 3/4: 3%), nausea (29%; grade 3/4: 2%), constipation (24%), colitis (≤21%, grades 3/4: 2%), diarrhea (18% to 21%; grade 3/4: 3%), vomiting (19%; grade 3/4: <1%), abdominal pain (16%; grade 3/4: 2%)

Hematologic & oncologic: Lymphocytopenia (47%; grade 3/4: 16%), anemia (28%; grade 3/4: 3%), thrombocytopenia (14%)

Hepatic: Increased serum AST (16%; grade 3/4: <1%), increased serum alkaline phosphatase (14%), increased serum ALT (12%)

Neuromuscular & skeletal: Musculoskeletal pain (36%; grade 3/4: 6%), weakness (19%; grade 3/4: 2%), arthralgia (13%)

Renal: Increased serum creatinine (22%)

Respiratory: Dyspnea (38%; grade 3/4: 9%), cough (32%; grade 3/4: 2%), pneumonia (10%; grade 3/4: 5%)

Miscellaneous: Fever (17%)

1% to 10%:

Cardiovascular: Vasculitis (<2%)

Central nervous system: Pain (10%; grade 3/4: 3%), peripheral sensory neuropathy (<10%), motor dysfunction (<2%), sixth nerve palsy (<2%), Guillain-Barre syndrome, myasthenia

Endocrine & metabolic: Hypothyroidism (4%), hyperthyroidism (2%), adrenocortical insufficiency (<2%), diabetic ketoacidosis, hypophysitis, pituitary insufficiency

Gastrointestinal: Pancreatitis (<2%)

Hepatic: Increased serum bilirubin (3%)

Neuromuscular & skeletal: Lambert-Eaton syndrome

Ophthalmic: Uveitis (<2%)

Respiratory: Bronchitis (<10%), upper respiratory tract infection (<10%), pneumonitis (6%)

<1% (Limited to important or life-threatening): Renal insufficiency

Drug Interactions

Metabolism/Transport Effects None known.

Avoid Concomitant Use

Avoid concomitant use of Nivolumab with any of the following: Belimumab

Increased Effect/Toxicity

Nivolumab may increase the levels/effects of: Belimumab

Decreased Effect There are no known significant interactions involving a decrease in effect.

Preparation for Administration Withdraw the required volume and transfer into an IV container. Dilute with either NS or D5W to a final concentration of 1 to 10 mg/mL. Mix by gentle inversion; do not shake.

Storage/Stability Store intact vials refrigerated at 2°C to 8°C (36°F to 46°F); do not freeze. Protect from light. Do not shake. After preparation, store the infusion solution at room temperature for no more than 4 hours (including infusion time) or refrigerated at 2°C to 8°C (36°F to 46°F) for up to 24 hours (including infusion time). Infusion must be completed within 24 hours of preparation. Do not freeze solutions prepared for infusion.

Mechanism of Action

Nivolumab is a fully human immunoglobulin G4 (IgG4) monoclonal antibody that selectively inhibits programmed cell death-1 (PD-1) activity by binding to the PD-1 receptor to block the ligands PD-L1 and PD-L2 from binding. The negative PD-1 receptor signaling that regulates T-cell activation and proliferation is therefore disrupted (Robert 2015). This releases PD-1 pathway-mediated inhibition of the immune response, including the antitumor immune response.

Combining nivolumab (anti-PD-1) with ipilimumab (anti-CTLA-4) results in enhanced T-cell function that is greater than that of either antibody alone, resulting in improved anti-tumor responses in metastatic melanoma.

Pharmacodynamics/Kinetics

Distribution: V_d: ~8 L (single-agent and combination therapy with ipilimumab)

Half-life elimination: ~27 days (single agent); ~25 days (combination therapy with ipilimumab)

Dosing

Adult & Geriatric

US labeling:

Melanoma, unresectable or metastatic: IV: 3 mg/kg once every 2 weeks (as a single agent) until disease progression or unacceptable toxicity (Robert 2015; Weber 2015).

Melanoma, unresectable or metastatic, first-line combination therapy: IV: 1 mg/kg once every 3 weeks (in combination with ipilimumab) for 4 doses, followed by 3 mg/kg once every 2 weeks (nivolumab monotherapy) until disease progression or unacceptable toxicity (Larkin 2015). **Note:** If nivolumab therapy is withheld, ipilimumab should also be withheld.

Non-small cell lung cancer, metastatic: IV: 3 mg/kg once every 2 weeks until disease progression or unacceptable toxicity (Borghaei 2015; Brahmer 2015).

Renal cell cancer, clear cell (advanced): IV: 3 mg/kg once every 2 weeks until disease progression or unacceptable toxicity (Motzer 2015)

Canadian labeling: Melanoma, unresectable or metastatic (BRAF V600 wild-type), first-line therapy: IV: 3 mg/kg once every 2 weeks (as a single agent), continue as long as benefiting clinically or until unacceptable toxicity occurs.

Renal Impairment

Renal impairment prior to treatment initiation:
US labeling: No dosage adjustment necessary.

Canadian labeling:
Mild to moderate impairment: No dosage adjustment necessary.

Severe impairment: There is no dosage adjustment provided in the manufacturer's labeling (insufficient data).

Renal toxicity during treatment:
US labeling:
Creatinine >1.5 to 6 times ULN or >1.5 times baseline: Withhold treatment; administer corticosteroids (prednisone 0.5 to 1 mg/kg daily or equivalent) followed by a corticosteroid taper; may resume therapy upon recovery to grade 0 or 1 toxicity. If toxicity worsens or does not improve, permanently discontinue and increase corticosteroid dose to prednisone 1 to 2 mg/kg daily (or equivalent).

Creatinine >6 times ULN or life-threatening: Permanently discontinue; initiate high-dose systemic corticosteroids (prednisone 1 to 2 mg/kg daily or equivalent) followed by a corticosteroid taper.

Canadian labeling:
Creatinine >1.5 to 3 times baseline or >1.5 to 3 times ULN: Withhold treatment and manage with corticosteroids (0.5 to 1 mg/kg methylprednisolone equivalent) followed by a taper; may resume therapy upon recovery to baseline and corticosteroid management is complete. If toxicity worsens or does not improve, permanently discontinue and increase corticosteroid dose (1 to 2 mg/kg methylprednisolone equivalent).

Creatinine >3 times baseline or >3 times ULN: Permanently discontinue; initiate high-dose systemic corticosteroids (1 to 2 mg/kg methylprednisolone equivalent).

Hepatic Impairment

Hepatic impairment prior to treatment initiation:
Mild impairment (total bilirubin ≤ ULN and AST > ULN or total bilirubin <1 to 1.5 times ULN and any AST): No dosage adjustment necessary.

Moderate (total bilirubin >1.5 to 3 times ULN and any AST) to severe (total bilirubin >3 times ULN and any AST) impairment: There are no dosage adjustments provided in the manufacturer's labeling (has not been studied).

Hepatotoxicity during treatment:
AST or ALT >3 to 5 times ULN or total bilirubin >1.5 to 3 times ULN: Withhold treatment; may resume therapy upon recovery to grade 0 or 1 toxicity.

AST or ALT >5 times ULN or total bilirubin >3 times ULN: Permanently discontinue.

Immune-mediated hepatitis:
Grade 2 or higher transaminase elevations (with or without total bilirubin elevations): Withhold treatment and initiate high-dose systemic corticosteroids (prednisone 1 to 2 mg/kg daily or equivalent)

Severe (grade 3) or life-threatening (grade 4): Permanently discontinue treatment and initiate high-dose systemic corticosteroids (prednisone 1 to 2 mg/kg daily or equivalent)

Adjustment for Toxicity

Withhold treatment for any of the following (may resume upon recovery to grade 0 or 1 toxicity):

Note: If receiving combination therapy with ipilimumab, when nivolumab is withheld, ipilimumab should also be withheld.

Adrenal insufficiency (grade 2)

Colitis:
Grade 2 colitis or diarrhea; for grade 2 colitis with a duration >5 days; also administer systemic corticosteroids (prednisone 0.5 to 1 mg/kg daily or equivalent) followed by a corticosteroid taper; may increase to prednisone 1 to 2 mg/kg daily (or equivalent) if colitis worsens or does not improve despite corticosteroid use

Grade 3 colitis or diarrhea (single-agent nivolumab); also administer systemic corticosteroids (prednisone 1 to 2 mg/kg daily or equivalent) followed by a corticosteroid taper

Diabetes mellitus, type 1 (grade 3 hyperglycemia); also administer insulin as clinically necessary

Hypophysitis (grade 2 or 3 [US labeling] or grade 2 [Canadian labeling]); also administer high-dose systemic corticosteroids (prednisone 1 mg/kg daily or equivalent)

Neurologic toxicity, new onset (moderate or severe)

Pneumonitis (grade 2); also administer high-dose systemic corticosteroids (prednisone 1 to 2 mg/kg daily or equivalent) followed by a corticosteroid taper

Rash (grade 3); also administer high-dose systemic corticosteroids (prednisone 1 to 2 mg/kg daily or equivalent)

Other immune-mediated toxicities; also administer high-dose systemic corticosteroids followed by a corticosteroid taper (over 1 month)

Other treatment-related toxicity (severe or grade 3, first occurrence)

Permanently discontinue for:

Adrenal insufficiency (grade 3 or 4); also administer high-dose systemic corticosteroids (prednisone 1 to 2 mg/kg daily or equivalent)

Colitis or diarrhea (grade 3, if in combination with ipilimumab) or colitis or diarrhea (grade 4); also administer high-dose systemic corticosteroids (prednisone 1 to 2 mg/kg daily or equivalent) followed by a corticosteroid taper

Colitis (recurrent)

Diabetes mellitus, type 1 (grade 4 hyperglycemia): also administer insulin as clinically necessary

Encephalitis (immune mediated); also administer high-dose systemic corticosteroids (prednisone 1 to 2 mg/kg daily or equivalent) followed by a corticosteroid taper

Hypophysitis (grade 4 [US labeling] or grade 3 or 4 [Canadian labeling]); also administer high-dose systemic corticosteroids (prednisone 1 mg/kg daily or equivalent)

Pneumonitis (grade 3 or 4); also administer high-dose systemic corticosteroids (prednisone 1 to 2 mg/kg daily or equivalent) followed by a corticosteroid taper

Rash (grade 4); also administer high-dose systemic corticosteroids (prednisone 1 to 2 mg/kg daily or equivalent)

Inability to reduce corticosteroid dose to prednisone ≤10 mg/day (or equivalent) within 12 weeks.

Other adverse reactions that are life-threatening or grade 4, severe or grade 3 adverse reactions that recur, or persistent grade 2 or 3 treatment-related toxicity lasts beyond 12 weeks.

Infusion-related reaction:

Mild or moderate reaction: Interrupt or slow the infusion rate

Severe or life-threatening reaction: Discontinue

Thyroid disorder (hyperthyroidism or hypothyroidism):
US labeling: There are no recommended dosage modifications.
Canadian labeling: Grade 4 hyperthyroidism: Permanently discontinue.

Administration
IV: Administer over 60 minutes through a line with a sterile, nonpyrogenic, low protein binding 0.2 to 1.2 micrometer in-line filter. Do not administer other medications through the same IV line. Flush IV line at the end of the infusion. Combination therapy with ipilimumab: When administered in combination with ipilimumab, infuse nivolumab first followed by ipilimumab on the same day. Use separate infusion bags and filters for each infusion. If nivolumab therapy is withheld, ipilimumab should also be withheld.

Monitoring Parameters Hepatic and renal function tests (baseline and periodic), thyroid function (baseline and periodically [eg, at treatment day 1 and every 6 weeks]); blood glucose. Monitor for signs/symptoms of adrenal insufficiency, hypophysitis, thyroid disorders, immune-mediated colitis, pneumonitis, rash, encephalitis; monitor for infusion reactions.

Dosage Forms Excipient information presented when available (limited, particularly for generics); consult specific product labeling.
Solution, Intravenous [preservative free]:
Opdivo: 40 mg/4 mL (4 mL); 100 mg/10 mL (10 mL) [contains polysorbate 80]

Nizatidine (ni ZA ti deen)

Brand Names: US Axid; Axid AR [OTC]
Brand Names: Canada Apo-Nizatidine; Axid; Gen-Nizatidine; Novo-Nizatidine; Nu-Nizatidine; PMS-Nizatidine
Pharmacologic Category Histamine H$_2$ Antagonist
Use Treatment and maintenance of duodenal ulcer; treatment of benign gastric ulcer; treatment of gastroesophageal reflux disease (GERD)

Dosing
Adult & Geriatric
Duodenal ulcer: Oral:
Treatment of active ulcer: 300 mg at bedtime or 150 mg twice daily
Maintenance of healed ulcer: 150 mg/day at bedtime
Gastric ulcer: Oral: 150 mg twice daily or 300 mg at bedtime
GERD: Oral: 150 mg twice daily
Helicobacter pylori eradication (off-label use): Oral: 150 mg twice daily (in combination with amoxicillin and clarithromycin [or bismuth, metronidazole, and tetracycline]) for 10 to 14 days (ACG [Chey 2007]; Graham 2003; Talley 1998).
Pediatric GERD (off-label use): Oral:
Children <12 years: 10 mg/kg/day in divided doses given twice daily; may not be as effective in children <12 years
Children ≥12 years: Refer to adult dosing.
Renal Impairment
Active treatment:
CrCl 20-50 mL/minute: 150 mg/day
CrCl <20 mL/minute: 150 mg every other day
Maintenance treatment:
CrCl 20-50 mL/minute: 150 mg every other day
CrCl <20 mL/minute: 150 mg every 3 days
Hepatic Impairment No dosage adjustment provided in manufacturer's labeling.
Additional Information Complete prescribing information should be consulted for additional detail.
Dosage Forms Excipient information presented when available (limited, particularly for generics); consult specific product labeling. [DSC] = Discontinued product
Capsule, Oral:
Axid: 150 mg [DSC], 300 mg
Generic: 150 mg, 300 mg
Solution, Oral:
Axid: 15 mg/mL (480 mL) [contains methylparaben, propylparaben, saccharin sodium; bubble-gum flavor]
Generic: 15 mg/mL (473 mL, 480 mL)
Tablet, Oral:
Axid AR: 75 mg

Nonoxynol 9 (non OKS i nole nine)

Brand Names: US Options Conceptrol [OTC]; Options Gynol II Contraceptive [OTC]; Shur-Seal Contraceptive [OTC]; Today Sponge [OTC]; VCF Vaginal Contraceptive [OTC]
Index Terms N-9
Pharmacologic Category Contraceptive; Spermicide
Use Contraception: Prevention of pregnancy
Dosing
Adult
Contraception: Females: Intravaginal: **Note:** If repeated intercourse takes place, additional application may be necessary. Prior to use, refer to specific product labeling for complete instructions.
Encare 100 mg: Unwrap and insert 1 suppository vaginally at least 10 minutes prior to intercourse; effective for 1 hour.
Options Conceptrol gel 4%: Insert 1 applicatorful (100 mg) vaginally immediately prior to intercourse; effective for 1 hour.
Options Gynol II gel 3%: Insert 1 applicatorful (150 mg) vaginally immediately prior to intercourse; effective for 1 hour. If used with a diaphragm, apply 1 applicatorful (approximately 1 teaspoonful) of gel onto dome of diaphragm and spread around the edge using fingertip prior to inserting. If intercourse occurs >6 hours after insertion, or if repeated intercourse occurs, additional application of gel is needed. Do not remove diaphragm to reapply; use applicator to apply gel, taking care not to dislodge the diaphragm.
Today: Insert 1 sponge (1,000 mg) vaginally prior to intercourse; allow to remain in place for 6 hours after intercourse before removing; effective for use up to 24 continuous hours. Do not leave in place for >30 hours.
VCF:
Film 28%: Insert 1 film vaginally at least 15 minutes, but no more than 3 hours, prior to intercourse. Insert new film for each act of intercourse or if more than 3 hours have elapsed.
Foam 12.5%: Insert 1 applicatorful no more than 1 hour prior to intercourse; effective for up to 1 hour.
Geriatric For use in women of reproductive potential; not for use in postmenopausal women.
Pediatric Contraception: Adolescents: Females: Intravaginal: Refer to adult dosing; not for use prior to menarche.
Renal Impairment There are no dosage adjustments provided in the manufacturer's labeling. Barrier contraceptives may not be appropriate for use in women in which the risk of pregnancy is unacceptable due to other health conditions, because of their relatively higher failure rate if not use correctly (CDC 2010).
Hepatic Impairment There are no dosage adjustments provided in the manufacturer's labeling. Barrier contraceptives may not be appropriate for use in women in which the risk of pregnancy is unacceptable due to other health conditions, because of their relatively higher failure rate if not use correctly (CDC 2010).
Additional Information Complete prescribing information should be consulted for additional detail.
Dosage Forms Excipient information presented when available (limited, particularly for generics); consult specific product labeling.
Film, Vaginal:
VCF Vaginal Contraceptive: 28% (3 ea, 6 ea, 9 ea) [contains glycerin, polyvinyl alcohol]
Foam, Vaginal:
VCF Vaginal Contraceptive: 12.5% (17 g) [hormone free; contains benzoic acid, cetyl alcohol, methylparaben, propylene glycol]

Gel, Vaginal:
 Options Conceptrol: 4% (2.55 g) [hormone free; contains methylparaben, propylene glycol]
 Options Gynol II Contraceptive: 3% (81 g) [hormone free; contains methylparaben, propylene glycol]
 Shur-Seal Contraceptive: 2% (24 ea)
 VCF Vaginal Contraceptive: 4% (2.55 g) [hormone free; contains edetate trisodium, methylparaben, propylene glycol, sodium benzoate]
Miscellaneous, Vaginal:
 Today Sponge: 1000 mg (3 ea) [contains benzoic acid, sodium metabisulfite]

◆ **Non-Pseudo Sinus Decongestant [OTC]** *see* Phenylephrine (Systemic) *on page 1442*

◆ **Nora-BE** *see* Norethindrone *on page 1298*

◆ **Noradrenaline** *see* Norepinephrine *on page 1297*

◆ **Noradrenaline Acid Tartrate** *see* Norepinephrine *on page 1297*

◆ **Norco** *see* Hydrocodone and Acetaminophen *on page 884*

◆ **Norcuron** *see* Vecuronium *on page 1881*

◆ **Norcuron® (Can)** *see* Vecuronium *on page 1881*

◆ **Nordeoxyguanosine** *see* Ganciclovir (Systemic) *on page 828*

◆ **Norditropin FlexPro** *see* Somatropin *on page 1686*

◆ **Norditropin Nordiflex (Can)** *see* Somatropin *on page 1686*

◆ **Norditropin NordiFlex Pen [DSC]** *see* Somatropin *on page 1686*

◆ **Norditropin Simplexx (Can)** *see* Somatropin *on page 1686*

◆ **Norel CS [OTC]** *see* Chlorpheniramine, Phenylephrine, and Dextromethorphan *on page 378*

◆ **Norelgestromin and Ethinyl Estradiol** *see* Ethinyl Estradiol and Norelgestromin *on page 707*

Norepinephrine (nor ep i NEF rin)

Brand Names: US Levophed
Brand Names: Canada Levophed®
Index Terms Levarterenol Bitartrate; Noradrenaline; Noradrenaline Acid Tartrate; Norepinephrine Bitartrate
Pharmacologic Category Alpha/Beta Agonist
Use Treatment of shock which persists after adequate fluid volume replacement; severe hypotension

Note: Recommended as the first-choice vasopressor for the treatment of sepsis and septic shock in adult patients (Dellinger, 2013)

Pregnancy Considerations Animal reproduction studies have not been conducted. Norepinephrine is an endogenous catecholamine and crosses the placenta (Minzter, 2010; Wang, 1999).

Breast-Feeding Considerations It is not known if norepinephrine is excreted in breast milk. The manufacturer recommends that caution be exercised when administering norepinephrine to nursing women.

Contraindications Hypersensitivity to norepinephrine, bisulfites (contains metabisulfite), or any component of the formulation; hypotension from hypovolemia except as an emergency measure to maintain coronary and cerebral perfusion until volume could be replaced; mesenteric or peripheral vascular thrombosis unless it is a lifesaving procedure; during anesthesia with cyclopropane (not available in U.S.) or halothane (not available in U.S.) anesthesia (risk of ventricular arrhythmias)

Warnings/Precautions Assure adequate circulatory volume to minimize need for vasoconstrictors. Avoid hypertension; monitor blood pressure closely and adjust infusion rate. Use with extreme caution in patients taking MAO-Inhibitors. Vesicant; ensure proper needle or catheter placement prior to and during infusion. Avoid extravasation; infuse into a large vein if possible. Avoid infusion into leg veins. Montior IV site closely. **[U.S. Boxed Warning]: If extravasation occurs, infiltrate the area with diluted phentolamine (5-10 mg in 10-15 mL of saline) with a fine hypodermic needle. Phentolamine should be administered as soon as possible after extravasation is noted to prevent sloughing/necrosis.** Product may contain sodium metabisulfite.

Adverse Reactions Frequency not defined.
Cardiovascular: Arrhythmias, bradycardia, peripheral (digital) ischemia
Central nervous system: Anxiety, headache (transient)
Local: Skin necrosis (with extravasation)
Respiratory: Dyspnea, respiratory difficulty

Drug Interactions
Metabolism/Transport Effects Substrate of COMT
Avoid Concomitant Use
Avoid concomitant use of Norepinephrine with any of the following: Ergot Derivatives; Inhalational Anesthetics; Iobenguane I 123
Increased Effect/Toxicity
Norepinephrine may increase the levels/effects of: Doxofylline; Droxidopa; Sympathomimetics

The levels/effects of Norepinephrine may be increased by: AtoMOXetine; Beta-Blockers; Cannabinoid-Containing Products; COMT Inhibitors; Ergot Derivatives; Hyaluronidase; Inhalational Anesthetics; Linezolid; MAO Inhibitors; Serotonin/Norepinephrine Reuptake Inhibitors; Tedizolid; Tricyclic Antidepressants
Decreased Effect
Norepinephrine may decrease the levels/effects of: Benzylpenicilloyl Polylysine; Iobenguane I 123; Ioflupane I 123

The levels/effects of Norepinephrine may be decreased by: Alpha1-Blockers; Spironolactone
Preparation for Administration Dilute with D_5W, D_5NS, or NS; dilution in NS is not recommended by the manufacturer; however, stability in NS has been demonstrated (Tremblay, 2008).
Storage/Stability Readily oxidized. Protect from light. Do not use if brown coloration. Stability of parenteral admixture at room temperature (25°C) is 24 hours.
Mechanism of Action Stimulates beta$_1$-adrenergic receptors and alpha-adrenergic receptors causing increased contractility and heart rate as well as vasoconstriction, thereby increasing systemic blood pressure and coronary blood flow; clinically, alpha effects (vasoconstriction) are greater than beta effects (inotropic and chronotropic effects)
Pharmacodynamics/Kinetics
Onset of action: IV: Very rapid-acting
Duration: vasopressor: 1-2 minutes
Metabolism: Via catechol-o-methyltransferase (COMT) and monoamine oxidase (MAO)
Excretion: Urine (84% to 96% as inactive metabolites)
Dosing
Adult & Geriatric Administration requires the use of an infusion pump.
 Note: Norepinephrine dosage is stated in terms of norepinephrine base.
 Hypotension/shock: Continuous IV infusion:
  Initial: 8-12 mcg/minute; titrate to desired response. Usual maintenance range: 2-4 mcg/minute; dosage range varies greatly depending on clinical situation. If patient remains hypotensive despite large doses, evaluate for occult hypovolemia and provide fluid resuscitation as appropriate.
  ACLS dosing range (weight-based dosing): Post cardiac arrest care: Initial: 0.1-0.5 mcg/**kg**/minute (7-35 mcg/minute in a 70 kg patient); titrate to desired response (AHA, 2010)
  Sepsis and septic shock (weight-based dosing): Range from clinical trials: 0.01-3 mcg/**kg**/minute (0.7-210 mcg/minute in a 70 kg patient) (Hollenberg, 2004)
Pediatric Administration requires the use of an infusion pump.
 Note: Norepinephrine dosage is stated in terms of norepinephrine base.
 Hypotension/shock: Continuous IV infusion: Initial: 0.05-0.1 mcg/kg/minute; titrate to desired effect; maximum dose: 2 mcg/kg/minute (AHA, 2010; Kleinman, 2007)
Renal Impairment No dosage adjustment provided in manufacturer's labeling.
Hepatic Impairment No dosage adjustment provided in manufacturer's labeling.
Usual Infusion Concentrations: Pediatric IV infusion: 8 **mcg/mL** or 16 **mcg/mL**
Usual Infusion Concentrations: Adult IV infusion: 4 mg in 250 mL (concentration: 16 **mcg/mL**) or 8 mg in 250 mL (concentration: 32 **mcg/mL**) of D_5W or NS
Administration Administer as a continuous infusion with the use of an infusion pump. Dilute prior to use. Administration via central line recommended (may cause severe ischemic necrosis if extravasated). Do not administer sodium bicarbonate (or any alkaline solution) through an IV line containing norepinephrine; inactivation of norepinephrine may occur.

Vesicant; ensure proper needle or catheter placement prior to and during infusion; avoid extravasation.

Extravasation management: If extravasation occurs, stop infusion immediately and disconnect (leave cannula/needle in place); gently aspirate extravasated solution (do **NOT** flush the line); remove needle/cannula; elevate extremity. Initiate phentolamine (or alternative) antidote. Apply dry warm compresses (Hurst, 2004).

Phentolamine (no longer available in the US): Dilute 5-10 mg in 10-15 mL NS and administer into extravasation site as soon as possible after extravasation (Peberdy, 2010) **or** dilute 5-10 mg in 10 mL NS and administer into extravasation area (within 12 hours of extravasation).

Alternatives to phentolamine:

Nitroglycerin topical 2% ointment (based on limited case reports in neonates/infants): Apply 4 mm/kg as a thin ribbon to the affected areas; may repeat after 8 hours if needed (Wong, 1992) **or** apply a 1-inch strip on the affected site (Denkler, 1989).

Terbutaline (based on limited case reports): Infiltrate extravasation area using a solution of terbutaline 1 mg diluted to 10 mL in NS (large extravasation site; administration volume varied from 3-10 mL) **or** 1 mg diluted in 1 mL NS (small/distal extravasation site; administration volume varied from 0.5-1 mL) (Stier, 1999).

Monitoring Parameters Blood pressure (or mean arterial pressure), heart rate; cardiac output (as appropriate), intravascular volume status, pulmonary capillary wedge pressure (as appropriate); monitor infusion site closely

Consult individual institutional policies and procedures.

Additional Information Norepinephrine dosage is stated in terms of norepinephrine base. Although the intravenous product vial designates the contents as norepinephrine bitartrate, the actual concentration shown is in terms of norepinephrine base 1 mg/mL.

Dosage Forms Excipient information presented when available (limited, particularly for generics); consult specific product labeling.

Solution, Intravenous [strength expressed as base]:
Levophed: 1 mg/mL (4 mL) [contains sodium metabisulfite]
Generic: 1 mg/mL (4 mL)

Solution, Intravenous [strength expressed as base, preservative free]:
Generic: 1 mg/mL (4 mL)

◆ Norepinephrine Bitartrate *see* Norepinephrine on page 1297

Norethindrone (nor ETH in drone)

Brand Names: US Aygestin; Camila; Deblitane; Errin; Heather; Jencycla; Jolivette; Lyza; Nor-QD; Nora-BE; Norlyroc; Ortho Micronor; Sharobel

Brand Names: Canada Micronor; Movisse; Norlutate

Index Terms Norethindrone Acetate; Norethisterone

Pharmacologic Category Contraceptive; Progestin

Use

Abnormal uterine bleeding *(norethindrone acetate):* Treatment of abnormal uterine bleeding due to hormonal imbalance in absence of organic pathology, such as submucous fibroids or uterine cancer

Amenorrhea, secondary *(norethindrone acetate):* Treatment of secondary amenorrhea

Contraception *(norethindrone):* Prevention of pregnancy

Endometriosis *(norethindrone acetate):* Treatment of endometriosis

Limitations of use:

Norethindrone is not indicated for emergency contraception.

Norethindrone acetate is not indicated for use with estrogen therapy in postmenopausal women for endometrial protection. Canadian labeling notes it is only appropriate for women with a uterus.

Pregnancy Considerations Use is contraindicated during pregnancy. First trimester exposure of progestins may cause genital abnormalities including hypospadias in male infants and mild virilization of external female genitalia. Changes in external genitalia have been reported in female infants exposed to norethindrone acetate (Fine 1963). Significant adverse events related to growth and development have not been observed following use of oral progestins in contraceptive doses (limited studies).

Norethindrone: Progestin-only contraceptives may be started immediately postpartum (CDC 2010; CDC 2013). A rapid return to fertility occurs when progestin-only contraceptives are discontinued.

Norethindrone acetate: The contraceptive dose of norethindrone acetate is not known. Barrier contraception is recommended to prevent unintended pregnancy (eg, when treating endometriosis) (Kaser 2012).

Breast-Feeding Considerations Following use as a contraceptive, small amounts of progestins are found in breast milk (1% to 6% of maternal serum concentration) and can be detected in infant plasma. Isolated reports of decreased milk production and very rare reports of jaundice in nursing infants have been noted. In general, adverse events related to infant growth and development have not been reported. The manufacturer of norethindrone acetate recommends that caution be used if administered to a nursing woman.

When used for contraception, may be started at any time postpartum in breast-feeding women (CDC 2010; CDC 2013).

Contraindications

Hypersensitivity to norethindrone or any component of the formulation; hepatic impairment or disease; breast cancer (known, suspected, or history of); undiagnosed abnormal genital bleeding; pregnancy

Norethindrone: Additional contraindications: Benign or malignant liver tumors

Norethindrone acetate:

Additional contraindications: DVT or PE (current or history of); active or recent history of arterial thromboembolic disease (eg, stroke, MI); as a diagnostic test for pregnancy

Additional contraindications in Canadian labeling: Estrogen or progestin dependant malignant tumor; partial or complete vision loss due to ophthalmic vascular disease; missed abortion

Warnings/Precautions Hazardous agent: Use appropriate precautions for handling and disposal (NIOSH 2014 [group 2]).

The use of combination hormonal contraceptives has been associated with a slight increase in the frequency of breast cancer; however, studies are not consistent. Data is insufficient to determine if progestin-only contraceptives also increase this risk. Norethindrone and norethindrone acetate are contraindicated in women with breast cancer. Not for use prior to menarche.

May have adverse effects on glucose tolerance; use caution in women with diabetes. May have adverse effects on lipid metabolism; use caution in women with hyperlipidemias. Use with caution in patients with a history of migraine. The use of estrogens and/or progestins may change the results of some laboratory tests (eg, coagulation factors, lipids, glucose tolerance, binding proteins). The dose, route, and the specific estrogen/progestin influence these changes. In addition, personal risk factors (eg, cardiovascular disease, smoking, diabetes, age) also contribute to adverse events; use of specific products may be contraindicated in women with certain risk factors.

Potentially significant drug-drug interactions may exist, requiring dose or frequency adjustment, additional monitoring, and/or selection of alternative therapy.

Norethindrone: Irregular menstrual bleeding patterns are common with progestin-only contraceptives; nonpharmacologic causes of abnormal bleeding should be ruled out. If follicular development occurs following use for contraception, follicles may grow and enlarge beyond the size attained in a normal cycle. May be asymptomatic or can be associated with mild abdominal pain; surgical intervention is rarely required. The possibility of ectopic pregnancy following use of a progestin-only contraceptive should be considered in patients with lower abdominal pain. Extremely rare hepatic adenomas and focal nodular hyperplasia resulting in fatal intra-abdominal hemorrhage have been reported in association with long-term combination oral contraceptive use. Data is insufficient to determine if progestin-only contraceptives also increase this risk. Use as a contraceptive is contraindicated in women with hepatic tumors. Progestin-only contraceptives may be used in women who smoke (CDC 2010). Because of an increased risk of cardiovascular disease, women using oral contraceptives should be strongly advised not to smoke. Progestin-only contraceptives contain less progestin than contained in estrogen/progestin–combined contraceptives. Risks associated with estrogen/progestin contraceptives should be considered for progestin-only products. Progestin-only contraceptives do not protect against HIV infection or other sexually transmitted diseases.

Norethindrone acetate: Risk factors for cardiovascular disorders include diabetes mellitus, hypercholesterolemia, hypertension, SLE, obesity, tobacco use, and/or history of venous thromboembolism (VTE). Risk factors should be managed appropriately. Discontinue if migraine, loss of vision, proptosis, diplopia or other visual disturbances occur; discontinue permanently if papilledema or retinal vascular lesions are observed on examination. Use with caution in patients with depression. Use with caution in

patients with diseases that may be exacerbated by fluid retention, including asthma, epilepsy, or cardiac or renal dysfunction.

Norethindrone acetate (Canadian labeling): Discontinue use with the onset of sudden enlargement, pain, or tenderness of preexisting uterine leiomyomata. Use caution with SLE; discontinue if signs of thromboembolism are present. Norlutate [Canadian product]): Avoid use in patients with rare hereditary problems of galactose intolerance, severe lactase deficiency, or glucose-galactose malabsorption.

Adverse Reactions Frequency not defined.

Cardiovascular: Cerebral embolism, cerebral thrombosis, deep vein thrombosis, edema, pulmonary embolism, retinal thrombosis

Central nervous system: Depression, dizziness, fatigue, headache, insomnia, migraine, emotional lability, nervousness

Dermatologic: Acne vulgaris, alopecia, chloasma, pruritus, skin rash, urticaria

Endocrine & metabolic: Amenorrhea, hirsutism, hypermenorrhea, menstrual disease, weight gain

Gastrointestinal: Abdominal pain, nausea, vomiting

Genitourinary: Breakthrough bleeding, breast hypertrophy, breast tenderness, cervical erosion, change in cervical secretions, decreased lactation, genital discharge, mastalgia, spotting, vaginal hemorrhage

Hypersensitivity: Anaphylaxis, hypersensitivity

Hepatic: Cholestatic jaundice, hepatitis, abnormal hepatic function tests

Neuromuscular & skeletal: Arm pain, leg pain

Ophthalmic: Optic neuritis (with or without vision loss)

Drug Interactions

Metabolism/Transport Effects Substrate of CYP3A4 (major); **Note:** Assignment of Major/Minor substrate status based on clinically relevant drug interaction potential; **Induces** CYP2C19 (weak/moderate)

Avoid Concomitant Use

Avoid concomitant use of Norethindrone with any of the following: Griseofulvin; Tranexamic Acid; Ulipristal

Increased Effect/Toxicity

Norethindrone may increase the levels/effects of: C1 inhibitors; Flibanserin; Selegiline; Thalidomide; Tranexamic Acid; Voriconazole

The levels/effects of Norethindrone may be increased by: Atazanavir; Boceprevir; Cobicistat; Herbs (Progestogenic Properties); Lopinavir; Metreleptin; Mifepristone; Osimertinib; Tipranavir; Voriconazole

Decreased Effect

Norethindrone may decrease the levels/effects of: Anticoagulants; Antidiabetic Agents; Fosamprenavir; Ulipristal; Vitamin K Antagonists

The levels/effects of Norethindrone may be decreased by: Acitretin; Aprepitant; Artemether; Barbiturates; Bexarotene (Systemic); Bile Acid Sequestrants; Bosentan; CarBAMazepine; CloBAZam; Colesevelam; CYP3A4 Inducers (Moderate); CYP3A4 Inducers (Strong); Dabrafenib; Darunavir; Deferasirox; Efavirenz; Enzalutamide; Eslicarbazepine; Exenatide; Felbamate; Fosamprenavir; Fosaprepitant; Fosphenytoin; Griseofulvin; LamoTRIgine; Lesinurad; Lopinavir; Lumacaftor; Metreleptin; Mifepristone; Mitotane; Mycophenolate; Nelfinavir; Nevirapine; Osimertinib; OXcarbazepine; Perampanel; Phenytoin; Primidone; Prucalopride; Retinoic Acid Derivatives; Rifamycin Derivatives; Rufinamide; Saquinavir; Siltuximab; St Johns Wort; Sugammadex; Telaprevir; Tocilizumab; Topiramate; Ulipristal

Storage/Stability Store at controlled room temperature.

Mechanism of Action Once absorbed, systemic disposition of norethindrone acetate (NETA) and norethindrone (NET) is the same.

NET is used in preparations for progestin-only contraception. NET suppresses ovulation, thickens cervical mucus (which inhibits sperm penetration), alters follicle-stimulating hormone (FSH) and luteinizing hormone (LH) concentrations, slows the movement of ovum through the fallopian tubes, and alters the endometrium.

Progestogens, such as NETA in the doses used for abnormal uterine bleeding, amenorrhea, and endometriosis, lead to atrophy of the endometrial tissue. They may also suppress new growth and implantation. Pain associated with endometriosis is decreased. When treating endometriosis, NETA may be used in combination with gonadotropin-releasing hormone agonists to decrease side effects from hypoestrogenism (ASRM 2014).

Pharmacodynamics/Kinetics

Absorption: Oral: Rapidly absorbed

Distribution: V_d: 4 L/kg

Protein binding: 61% to albumin; 36% to sex hormone-binding globulin (SHBG); SHBG capacity affected by plasma ethinyl estradiol levels (Orme 1983)

Metabolism: Oral: Norethindrone acetate is deacetylated to norethindrone; norethindrone undergoes hepatic reduction and conjugation; orally administered norethindrone is subject to first-pass effect (Orme 1983). In addition to forming glucuronide and sulfide conjugates, norethindrone is also metabolized to ethinyl estradiol (Kuhnz 1997; Orme 1983).

Bioavailability: 64% (Orme 1983)

Half-life elimination: ~8 to 9 hours

Time to peak: ~2 hours (varies by dose and use of concomitant estrogen (Orme 1983)

Excretion: Urine (>50% as metabolites); feces (20% to 40% as metabolites)

Dosing

Adult

Abnormal uterine bleeding and amenorrhea: Females: Oral: Norethindrone acetate: 2.5 to 10 mg/day for 5 to 10 days. Secretory transformation of the endometrium will occur when adequately primed with endogenous or exogenous estrogen. Withdrawal bleeding may be expected within 3 to 7 days after discontinuing norethindrone acetate. Canadian labeling recommends dosing to be initiated on the fifth day of the menstrual cycle and ending on the 25th day, assuming an interval of 28 days.

Contraception: Females: Oral: Norethindrone: 0.35 mg every day (no missed days)

Initial dose: Start on first day of menstrual period or the day after a miscarriage or abortion. If switching from a combined oral contraceptive, begin the day after finishing the last active combined tablet.

Missed dose: Take as soon as remembered. A back up method of contraception should be used for 48 hours if dose is taken ≥3 hours late.

Additional contraception dosing considerations (CDC 2013):

Initiation of therapy: May be started at any time in the menstrual cycle once it is determined that the woman is not pregnant. Back-up contraception is not needed if started within 5 days of onset of menstruation. If started >5 days after the onset of menstruation or at any time in a women experiencing amenorrhea (not postpartum), back up contraception should be used for 2 days.

Switching from a different contraceptive to a progestin-only contraceptive: May be started at any time if it is determined that the woman is not pregnant. Unless the woman abstains from sexual intercourse, a backup method of contraception is needed if it has been >5 days since menstrual bleeding has begun. When an additional method of contraception is needed, consider continuing the woman's previous method for 2 days after starting the progestin-only contraceptive.

Switching from an IUD to a progestin-only contraceptive: Continue the IUD for at least 2 days after the progestin-only contraceptive is started or advise the woman to abstain from sexual intercourse or use a barrier contraceptive for 2 days before removing the IUD. Alternately, an emergency contraceptive may be used at the time of IUD removal.

Endometriosis: Females: Oral: Norethindrone acetate: 5 mg/day for 14 days; increase at increments of 2.5 mg/day every 2 weeks to reach 15 mg/day; continue for 6 to 9 months or until breakthrough bleeding demands temporary termination

Pediatric Adolescents: Refer to adult dosing

Renal Impairment There are no dosage adjustments provided in the manufacturer's labeling.

Hepatic Impairment There are no dosage adjustments provided in the manufacturer's labeling. However, use is contraindicated in patients with hepatic tumors or impairment.

Dietary Considerations Should be taken at same time each day.

Administration

For oral administration. Administer at the same time each day.

When used for the prevention of pregnancy, a backup method of contraception should be used for 48 hours if dose is missed or taken ≥3 hours late. If vomiting or severe diarrhea occur within 3 hours of taking a dose, take another dose as soon as possible, then continue taking one dose daily and use a backup method of contraception (or avoid sexual intercourse) until 2 days after vomiting or diarrhea have resolved. Emergency contraception should be considered in the event of unprotected intercourse (CDC, 2013).

◄ Hazardous agent; use appropriate precautions for handling and disposal (NIOSH 2014 [group 2]).

Monitoring Parameters

Norethindrone: Contraception: Assessment of pregnancy status (prior to therapy); weight (optional; BMI at baseline may be helpful to monitor changes during therapy); assess potential health status changes at routine visits (CDC 2013).

Norethindrone acetate: Monitor patient for vision changes; signs or symptoms of depression; glycemic control in patients with diabetes; lipid profiles in patients being treated for hyperlipidemias. Canadian labeling recommends the first follow-up exam to be completed within 3 to 6 months after initiation of therapy and then at least yearly.

Regardless of indication, adequate diagnostic measures, including endometrial sampling, if indicated, should be performed to rule out malignancy in all cases of undiagnosed abnormal vaginal bleeding. Pathologist should be informed of therapy when submitting endometrial tissue for histologic evaluation.

Test Interactions Reduced response to metyrapone test. Progestin-only contraceptives may affect sex hormone binding globulin (decrease) or thyroxine concentrations (decrease; because of decreased thyroid binding globulin).

Dosage Forms Excipient information presented when available (limited, particularly for generics); consult specific product labeling.

Tablet, Oral:

Camila: 0.35 mg

Deblitane: 0.35 mg [contains fd&c blue #2 aluminum lake, fd&c red #40 aluminum lake, fd&c yellow #10 aluminum lake, soybean lecithin]

Errin: 0.35 mg

Heather: 0.35 mg [contains fd&c yellow #10 aluminum lake, fd&c yellow #6 aluminum lake]

Jencycla: 0.35 mg [contains brilliant blue fcf (fd&c blue #1), fd&c yellow #10 (quinoline yellow)]

Jolivette: 0.35 mg

Lyza: 0.35 mg [contains fd&c yellow #10 (quinoline yellow)]

Nor-QD: 0.35 mg

Nora-BE: 0.35 mg

Norlyroc: 0.35 mg

Ortho Micronor: 0.35 mg [contains fd&c yellow #10 (quinoline yellow)]

Sharobel: 0.35 mg [contains fd&c blue #1 aluminum lake, fd&c yellow #6 aluminum lake, soybean lecithin]

Generic: 0.35 mg

Tablet, Oral, as acetate:

Aygestin: 5 mg [scored]

Generic: 5 mg

Norethindrone and Mestranol
(nor eth IN drone & MES tra nole)

Brand Names: US Necon 1/50; Norinyl 1+50

Index Terms Mestranol and Norethindrone; Ortho Novum 1/50

Pharmacologic Category Contraceptive; Estrogen and Progestin Combination

Use Contraception: For the prevention of pregnancy

Limitations of use: Products containing the equivalent of estrogen 50 mcg should not be used unless medically indicated.

Dosing

Adult Females: Contraception: Oral: One tablet once daily

Schedule 1 (Sunday starter): Dose begins on first Sunday after onset of menstruation; if the menstrual period starts on Sunday, take first tablet that very same day. **With a Sunday start, an additional method of contraception should be used until after the first 7 days of consecutive administration.**

Schedule 2 (Day 1 starter): Dose starts on first day of menstrual cycle taking 1 tablet daily.

Missed or late doses (CDC, 2013):

If one dose is late (<24 hours since dose should have been taken) or if one dose is missed (24 to <48 hours since dose should have been taken): Take dose as soon as possible. Continue remaining doses at the usual time (even if that means 2 doses on the same day).

If ≥2 consecutive doses are missed (≥48 hours since dose should have been taken): Take the most recently missed dose as soon as possible, discard any other missed doses. Continue remaining doses at the usual time (even if that means taking 2 doses on the same day); use back-up contraception until hormonal pills have been taken for 7 consecutive days. If doses were missed during the last week of hormonal (active) tablets (eg, days 15 to 21 of a 28-day pack), omit the hormone-free interval by finishing the hormonal pills from the current pack and starting a new pack. If unable to start a new pack immediately, back up contraception is needed until hormonal pills from a new pack have been taken for 7 consecutive days. Consider use of emergency contraception in some situations (refer to guidelines for details).

Also refer to package insert for product specific information.

Pediatric Female: Contraception: Oral: See adult dosing; not to be used prior to menarche.

Renal Impairment There are no dosage adjustments provided in the manufacturer's labeling. Use with caution and monitor blood pressure closely.

Hepatic Impairment Use is contraindicated in patients with hepatic impairment.

Additional Information Complete prescribing information should be consulted for additional detail.

Dosage Forms Excipient information presented when available (limited, particularly for generics); consult specific product labeling.

Tablet, monophasic formulations:

Necon® 1/50: Norethindrone 1 mg and mestranol 0.05 mg [21 light blue tablets and 7 white inactive tablets] (28s)

Norinyl® 1+50: Norethindrone 1 mg and mestranol 0.05 mg [21 white tablets and 7 orange inactive tablets] (28s)

Nortriptyline (nor TRIP ti leen)

Brand Names: US Pamelor

Brand Names: Canada Apo-Nortriptyline; Ava-Nortriptyline; Aventyl; Dom-Nortriptyline; Norventyl; Nu-Nortriptyline; PMS-Nortriptyline; Teva-Nortriptyline

Index Terms Nortriptyline Hydrochloride

Pharmacologic Category Antidepressant, Tricyclic (Secondary Amine)

Use Depression: Treatment of symptoms of depression

Pregnancy Considerations Animal reproduction studies are inconclusive. Nortriptyline and its metabolites cross the human placenta and can be detected in cord blood (Loughhead, 2006). Tricyclic antidepressants may be associated with irritability, jitteriness, and convulsions (rare) in the neonate (Yonkers 2009).

The ACOG recommends that therapy for depression during pregnancy be individualized; treatment should incorporate the clinical expertise of the mental health clinician, obstetrician, primary healthcare provider, and pediatrician (ACOG 2008). According to the American Psychiatric Association (APA), the risks of medication treatment should be weighed against other treatment options and untreated depression. For women who discontinue antidepressant medications during pregnancy and who may be at high risk for postpartum depression, the medications can be restarted following delivery (APA 2010). Treatment algorithms have been developed by the ACOG and the APA for the management of depression in women prior to conception and during pregnancy (Yonkers 2009).

Breast-Feeding Considerations Nortriptyline is excreted into breast milk and the M/P ratio ranged from 0.87 to 3.71 in one case report (Matheson 1988). Based on available information, nortriptyline has not been detected in the serum of nursing infants; however, low levels of the active metabolite E-10-hydroxynortriptyline have been detected in the serum of newborns following breast-feeding (Wisner 1991). Based on information from one mother-infant pair, following maternal use of nortriptyline 125 mg/day, the estimated exposure to the breast-feeding infant would be 0.6% to 3% of the weight-adjusted maternal dose. Adverse events have not been reported in nursing infants. Infants should be monitored for signs of adverse events; routine monitoring of infant serum concentrations is not recommended (Fortinguerra 2009).

Medication Guide Available Yes

Contraindications Hypersensitivity to nortriptyline and similar chemical class, or any component of the formulation; use in a patient during the acute recovery phase of MI; use of MAO inhibitors intended to treat psychiatric disorders (concurrently or within 14 days of discontinuing either nortriptyline or the MAO inhibitor); initiation of nortriptyline in a patient receiving linezolid or intravenous methylene blue

Warnings/Precautions [US Boxed Warning]: Antidepressants increase the risk of suicidal thinking and behavior in children, adolescents, and young adults (18-24 years of age) with major depressive disorder (MDD) and other psychiatric disorders; consider risk prior to prescribing. Short-term studies did not show an increased risk in patients >24 years of age and showed a decreased risk in patients ≥65 years. Closely monitor for clinical worsening, suicidality, or unusual changes in behavior, particularly during the initial 1-2 months of therapy or during periods of dosage adjustments (increases or decreases); the patient's family or caregiver should be instructed to closely observe the patient and communicate condition with healthcare provider. A medication guide should be dispensed with each prescription. **Nortriptyline is not FDA approved for use in children.**

The possibility of a suicide attempt is inherent in major depression and may persist until remission occurs. Use caution in high-risk patients. Worsening depression and severe abrupt suicidality that are not part of the presenting symptoms may require discontinuation or modification of drug therapy. The patient's family or caregiver should be alerted to monitor patients for the emergence of suicidality and associated behaviors (such as agitation, irritability, hostility, impulsivity, and hypomania) and call healthcare provider.

May worsen psychosis in some patients or precipitate a shift to mania or hypomania in patients with bipolar disorder. Patients presenting with depressive symptoms should be screened for bipolar disorder. Monotherapy in patients with bipolar disorder should be avoided. **Nortriptyline is not FDA approved for the treatment of bipolar depression.**

Potentially life-threatening serotonin syndrome (SS) has occurred with serotonergic agents (eg, SSRIs, SNRIs), particularly when used in combination with other serotonergic agents (eg, triptans, TCAs, fentanyl, lithium, tramadol, buspirone, St John's wort, tryptophan) or agents that impair metabolism of serotonin (eg, MAO inhibitors intended to treat psychiatric disorders, other MAO inhibitors [ie, linezolid and intravenous methylene blue]). Discontinue treatment (and any concomitant serotonergic agent) immediately if signs/symptoms arise. TCAs may rarely cause bone marrow suppression; monitor for any signs of infection and obtain CBC if symptoms (eg, fever, sore throat) evident. The risk of sedation and orthostatic effects are low relative to other antidepressants. However, nortriptyline may result in impaired performance of tasks requiring alertness (eg, operating machinery or driving). The degree of anticholinergic blockade produced by this agent is moderate relative to other cyclic antidepressants, however, caution should still be used in patients with urinary retention, benign prostatic hyperplasia, narrow-angle glaucoma, xerostomia, visual problems, constipation, or history of bowel obstruction. May cause orthostatic hypotension (risk is low relative to other antidepressants) or conduction disturbances. Use with caution in patients with a history of cardiovascular disease (including previous MI, stroke, tachycardia, or conduction abnormalities). The risk conduction abnormalities with this agent is moderate relative to other antidepressants. CNS effects may be potentiated when used with other sedative drugs or ethanol.

Recommended by the manufacturer to discontinue prior to elective surgery; risks exist for drug interactions with anesthesia and for cardiac arrhythmias. However, definitive drug interactions have not been widely reported in the literature and continuation of tricyclic antidepressants is generally recommended as long as precautions are taken to reduce the significance of any adverse events that may occur (Pass 2004). May alter glucose regulation - use caution in patients with diabetes. Use caution in patients with a previous seizure disorder or condition predisposing to seizures such as brain damage, alcoholism, or concurrent therapy with other drugs which lower the seizure threshold. May increase the risks associated with electroconvulsive therapy. Bone fractures have been associated with antidepressant treatment. Consider the possibility of a fragility fracture if an antidepressant-treated patient presents with unexplained bone pain, point tenderness, swelling, or bruising (Rabenda 2013; Rizzoli 2012). Use with caution in patients with hepatic or renal dysfunction.

Use caution in elderly patients; may cause or exacerbate syndrome of inappropriate antidiuretic hormone secretion or hyponatremia; monitor sodium closely with initiation or dosage adjustments in older adults. May be inappropriate in older adults depending on comorbidities (eg, dementia, delirium) or in patients with a history of falls and fractures due to its potent anticholinergic effects (Beers Criteria).

Benzyl alcohol and derivatives: Some dosage forms may contain sodium benzoate/benzoic acid; benzoic acid (benzoate) is a metabolite of benzyl alcohol; large amounts of benzyl alcohol (≥99 mg/kg/day) have been associated with a potentially fatal toxicity ("gasping syndrome") in neonates; the "gasping syndrome" consists of metabolic acidosis, respiratory distress, gasping respirations, CNS dysfunction (including convulsions, intracranial hemorrhage), hypotension, and cardiovascular collapse (AAP ["Inactive" 1997]; CDC 1982); some data suggests that benzoate displaces bilirubin from protein binding sites (Ahlfors 2001); avoid or use dosage forms containing benzyl alcohol derivative with caution in neonates. See manufacturer's labeling.

Abrupt discontinuation or interruption of antidepressant therapy has been associated with a discontinuation syndrome. Symptoms arising may vary with antidepressant however commonly include nausea, vomiting, diarrhea, headaches, lightheadedness, dizziness, diminished appetite, sweating, chills, tremors, paresthesias, fatigue, somnolence, and sleep disturbances (eg, vivid dreams, insomnia). Greater risks for developing a discontinuation syndrome have been associated with antidepressants with shorter half-lives, longer durations of treatment, and abrupt discontinuation. For antidepressants of short or intermediate half-lives, symptoms may emerge within 2-5 days after treatment discontinuation and last 7-14 days (APA 2010; Fava 2006; Haddad 2001; Shelton 2001; Warner 2006).

Adverse Reactions Frequency not defined. Some reactions listed are based on reports for other agents in this same pharmacologic class and may not be specifically reported for nortriptyline.

Cardiovascular: Cardiac arrhythmia, cerebrovascular accident, edema, flushing, heart block, hypertension, hypotension, myocardial infarction, palpitations, tachycardia

Central nervous system: Agitation, anxiety, ataxia, confusion, delusions, disorientation, dizziness, drowsiness, drug fever, EEG pattern changes, extrapyramidal reaction, fatigue, hallucination, headache, hypomania, insomnia, nightmares, numbness, panic, peripheral neuropathy, psychosis (exacerbation), restlessness, seizure, tingling of extremities, tingling sensation, withdrawal symptoms

Dermatologic: Alopecia, diaphoresis (excessive), pruritus, skin photosensitivity, skin rash, urticaria

Endocrine & metabolic: Decreased libido, decreased serum glucose, galactorrhea, gynecomastia, increased libido, increased serum glucose, SIADH, weight gain, weight loss

Gastrointestinal: Abdominal cramps, anorexia, constipation, diarrhea, epigastric distress, melanoglossia, nausea, paralytic ileus, parotid gland enlargement, stomatitis, sublingual adenitis, unpleasant taste, vomiting, xerostomia

Genitourinary: Breast hypertrophy, impotence, nocturia, testicular swelling, urinary hesitance, urinary retention, urinary tract dilation

Hematologic & oncologic: Agranulocytosis, eosinophilia, petechia, purpura, thrombocytopenia

Hepatic: Abnormal hepatic function tests, cholestatic jaundice

Neuromuscular & skeletal: Tremor, weakness

Ophthalmic: Accommodation disturbance, blurred vision, eye pain, mydriasis

Otic: Tinnitus

Renal: Polyuria

Postmarketing and/or case reports (Limited to important or life-threatening): Angle-closure glaucoma, serotonin syndrome, suicidal ideation

Drug Interactions

Metabolism/Transport Effects Substrate of CYP1A2 (minor), CYP2C19 (minor), CYP2D6 (major), CYP3A4 (minor); **Note:** Assignment of Major/Minor substrate status based on clinically relevant drug interaction potential; **Inhibits** CYP2D6 (weak), CYP2E1 (weak)

Avoid Concomitant Use

Avoid concomitant use of Nortriptyline with any of the following: Aclidinium; Azelastine (Nasal); Cimetropium; Dapoxetine; Dronedarone; Eluxadoline; Glucagon; Glycopyrrolate; Glycopyrrolate (Oral Inhalation); Iobenguane I 123; Ipratropium (Oral Inhalation); Levosulpiride; Linezolid; MAO Inhibitors; Methylene Blue; Moxonidine; Orphenadrine; Paraldehyde; Potassium Chloride; Thalidomide; Tiotropium; Umeclidinium

Increased Effect/Toxicity

Nortriptyline may increase the levels/effects of: AbobotulinumtoxinA; Alcohol (Ethyl); Alpha-/Beta-Agonists (Direct-Acting); Alpha1-Agonists; Amphetamines; Analgesics (Opioid); Anticholinergic Agents; Antipsychotic Agents; ARIPiprazole; Azelastine (Nasal); Beta2-Agonists; Buprenorphine; Cimetropium; Citalopram; CNS Depressants; Desmopressin; Dronedarone; Eluxadoline; Escitalopram; Glucagon; Glycopyrrolate; Glycopyrrolate (Oral Inhalation); Highest Risk QTc-Prolonging Agents; Hydrocodone; Methotrimeprazine; Methylene Blue; Metyrosine; Mirabegron; Moderate Risk QTc-Prolonging Agents; Nicorandil; OnabotulinumtoxinA; Orphenadrine; Paraldehyde; Potassium Chloride; Pramipexole; QuiNIDine; Ramosetron; RimabotulinumtoxinB; ROPINIRole; Rotigotine; Serotonin Modulators; Sodium Phosphates; Sulfonylureas; Suvorexant; Thalidomide; Thiazide Diuretics; Tiotropium; Topiramate; TraMADol; Vitamin K Antagonists; Yohimbine; Zolpidem

The levels/effects of Nortriptyline may be increased by: Abiraterone Acetate; Aclidinium; Altretamine; Antiemetics (5HT3 Antagonists); Antipsychotic Agents; Brimonidine (Topical); BuPROPion; Cannabis; Cimetidine; Cinacalcet; Citalopram; Cobicistat; CYP2D6 Inhibitors (Moderate); CYP2D6 Inhibitors (Strong); Dapoxetine; Darunavir; Dexmethylphenidate; Doxylamine; Dronabinol; Droperidol; DULoxetine; Escitalopram; FLUoxetine; FluvoxaMINE; HydrOXYzine; Ipratropium (Oral Inhalation); Kava Kava; Linezolid; Lithium; Magnesium Sulfate; MAO Inhibitors; Metaxalone; Methotrimeprazine; Methylphenidate; Metoclopramide; Metyrosine; Mianserin; Mifepristone; Minocycline; Nabilone; Panobinostat; PARoxetine; Peginterferon Alfa-2b; Perampanel; Pramlintide; Protease Inhibitors; QuiNIDine; Rufinamide; Sertraline; Sodium Oxybate; Tapentadol; Tedizolid; Terbinafine (Systemic); Tetrahydrocannabinol; Thyroid Products; TraMADol; Umeclidinium; Valproate Products

Decreased Effect

Nortriptyline may decrease the levels/effects of: Acetylcholinesterase Inhibitors; Alpha1-Agonists; Alpha2-Agonists; Alpha2-Agonists (Ophthalmic); Gastrointestinal Agents (Prokinetic); Iobenguane I 123; Itopride; Levosulpiride; Moxonidine; Secretin

The levels/effects of Nortriptyline may be decreased by: Acetylcholinesterase Inhibitors; Barbiturates; CarBAMazepine; Peginterferon Alfa-2b; St Johns Wort

Storage/Stability Store at 20°C to 25°C (68°F to 77°F). Protect from light.

Mechanism of Action Traditionally believed to increase the synaptic concentration of serotonin and/or norepinephrine in the central nervous system by inhibition of their reuptake by the presynaptic neuronal membrane. However, additional receptor effects have been found including desensitization of adenyl cyclase, down regulation of beta-adrenergic receptors, and down regulation of serotonin receptors.

Pharmacodynamics/Kinetics

Onset of action: Therapeutic: 1-3 weeks

Distribution: V_d: 21 L/kg

Protein binding: 93% to 95%

Metabolism: Primarily hepatic; extensive first-pass effect

Half-life elimination: 28-31 hours

Time to peak, serum: 7-8.5 hours

Excretion: Urine (as metabolites and small amounts of unchanged drug); feces (small amounts)

Dosing

Adult

Depression: Oral: Initial: 25 mg 3 to 4 times/day; adjust dose based on response and tolerability up to 150 mg/day; total daily doses may be given once daily.

Chronic pain (off-label use): Oral: Initial: 10 to 25 mg once daily at bedtime; may increase as tolerated as soon as every 3 days up to 150 mg/day (APS,2008; Atkinson 1998; Orbai 2010). Patients with neuropathic pain and an inadequate response to nortriptyline alone may benefit from a combination with gabapentin (Gilron 2009).

Irritable bowel syndrome (off-label use): Oral: Initial: 10 mg once daily at bedtime; may gradually increase to a dose of 25 to 200 mg once daily (AGA [Drossman 2002]; Mertz 2003; Spiller 2007). May continue treatment for up to 6 to 12 months before tapering (AGA [Drossman 2002])

Myofascial pain (off-label use): Oral: Initial: 12.5 mg once daily at bedtime; may increase as tolerated up to 35 mg/day. If after 4 weeks at 25 to 35 mg/day there is no change in pain intensity, then consider alternative therapy (Haviv 2015).

Orofacial pain (off-label use): Oral: Initial: 10 to 30 mg once daily at bedtime; gradually titrated up to 100 mg/day as tolerated (Feinmann 1993; Romero-Reyes 2014).

Postherpetic neuralgia (off-label use): Oral: Initial: 10 to 20 mg once daily at bedtime; may increase as needed every 3 to 5 days in 10 mg once daily increments up to 160 mg/day (Raja 2002; Watson 1998).

Smoking cessation (off-label use): Oral: Initial: 25 mg once daily begun 10 to 28 days prior to selected "quit" date; titrate dose to 75 to 100 mg/day; continue therapy for ≥12 weeks after "quit" day (PHS 2008)

Discontinuation of therapy: Upon discontinuation of antidepressant therapy, gradually taper the dose to minimize the incidence of withdrawal symptoms and allow for the detection of re-emerging symptoms. Evidence supporting ideal taper rates is limited. APA and NICE guidelines suggest tapering therapy over at least several weeks with consideration to the half-life of the antidepressant; antidepressants with a shorter half-life may need to be tapered more conservatively. In addition for long-term treated patients, WFSBP guidelines recommend tapering over 4 to 6 months. If intolerable withdrawal symptoms occur following a dose reduction, consider resuming the previously prescribed dose and/or decrease dose at a more gradual rate (APA 2010; Bauer 2002; Haddad 2001; NCCMH 2010; Schatzberg 2006; Shelton 2001; Warner 2006).

MAO inhibitor recommendations:

Switching to or from an MAO inhibitor intended to treat psychiatric disorders:

Allow 14 days to elapse between discontinuing an MAO inhibitor intended to treat psychiatric disorders and initiation of nortriptyline.

Allow 14 days to elapse between discontinuing nortriptyline and initiation of an MAO inhibitor intended to treat psychiatric disorders.

Use with other MAO inhibitors (linezolid or IV methylene blue):

Do not initiate nortriptyline in patients receiving linezolid or IV methylene blue; consider other interventions for psychiatric condition.

If urgent treatment with linezolid or IV methylene blue is required in a patient already receiving nortriptyline and potential benefits outweigh potential risks, discontinue nortriptyline promptly and administer linezolid or IV methylene blue. Monitor for serotonin syndrome for 2 weeks or until 24 hours after the last dose of linezolid or IV methylene blue, whichever comes first. May resume nortriptyline 24 hours after the last dose of linezolid or IV methylene blue.

Geriatric

Depression: Oral: Initial: 30 to 50 mg/day, given as a single daily dose or in divided doses.

Discontinuation of therapy: Refer to adult dosing.

MAO inhibitor recommendations: Refer to adult dosing.

Renal Impairment There are no dosage adjustments provided in the manufacturer's labeling.

Hepatic Impairment Lower doses and slower titration are recommended dependent on individualization of dosage.

Monitoring Parameters Blood pressure and pulse rate (ECG, cardiac monitoring) prior to and during initial therapy in older adults; weight; blood levels are useful for therapeutic monitoring; suicide ideation (especially at the beginning of therapy or when doses are increased or decreased); signs/symptoms of serotonin syndrome

Reference Range

Plasma levels do not always correlate with clinical effectiveness

Therapeutic: 50-150 ng/mL (SI: 190-570 nmol/L)

Toxic: >500 ng/mL (SI: >1900 nmol/L)

Additional Information The maximum antidepressant effect of nortriptyline may not be seen for ≥2 weeks after initiation of therapy.

Dosage Forms Excipient information presented when available (limited, particularly for generics); consult specific product labeling.

Capsule, Oral:

Pamelor: 10 mg, 25 mg [contains fd&c yellow #10 (quinoline yellow), fd&c yellow #6 (sunset yellow)]

Pamelor: 50 mg

Pamelor: 75 mg [contains fd&c yellow #10 (quinoline yellow), fd&c yellow #6 (sunset yellow)]

Generic: 10 mg, 25 mg, 50 mg, 75 mg

Solution, Oral:

Generic: 10 mg/5 mL (473 mL)

Nystatin (Oral) (nye STAT in)

Brand Names: US Bio-Statin
Brand Names: Canada PMS-Nystatin
Pharmacologic Category Antifungal Agent, Oral Non-absorbed

Use Treatment of susceptible cutaneous, mucocutaneous, and oral cavity fungal infections normally caused by the *Candida* species

Dosing

Adult & Geriatric

Oral candidiasis: Suspension (swish and swallow): 400,000-600,000 units 4 times/day; swish in the mouth and retain for as long as possible (several minutes) before swallowing

Intestinal infections: Oral tablets: 500,000-1,000,000 units every 8 hours

Note: Powder for compounding: 1/8 teaspoon (500,000 units) to equal approximately 1/2 cup of water; give 4 times/day

Pediatric Oral candidiasis:

Suspension:

Premature infants: 100,000 units 4 times/day; paint suspension into recesses of the mouth

Infants: 200,000 units 4 times/day or 100,000 units to each side of mouth 4 times/day; paint suspension into recesses of the mouth

Children: 400,000-600,000 units 4 times/day; swish in the mouth and retain for as long as possible (several minutes) before swallowing

Powder for compounding: Children: Refer to adult dosing.

Renal Impairment No dosage adjustment provided in manufacturer's labeling.

Hepatic Impairment No dosage adjustment provided in manufacturer's labeling.

Additional Information Complete prescribing information should be consulted for additional detail.

Dosage Forms Excipient information presented when available (limited, particularly for generics); consult specific product labeling.

Capsule, Oral [preservative free]:

Bio-Statin: 500,000 units, 1,000,000 units [dye free]

Powder, Oral:

Bio-Statin: (1 ea)

Generic: (1 ea)

Suspension, Mouth/Throat:

Generic: 100,000 units/mL (5 mL, 60 mL, 473 mL, 480 mL)

Tablet, Oral:

Generic: 500,000 units

Nystatin (Topical) (nye STAT in)

Brand Names: US Nyamyc; Nyata; Nystop; Pedi-Dri [DSC]; Pediaderm AF Complete

Brand Names: Canada Nyaderm; Ratio-Nystatin

Pharmacologic Category Antifungal Agent, Topical

Use Fungal infections (cutaneous and mucocutaneous): Treatment of cutaneous and mucocutaneous fungal infections caused by *Candida albicans* and other susceptible *Candida* species.

Dosing

Adult & Geriatric Fungal infections (cutaneous and mucocutaneous): Topical: **Note:** Cream is usually preferred to ointment for intertriginous areas; very moist lesions are best treated with topical powder

Cream, ointment: Apply to the affected areas twice daily or as indicated until healing is complete

Powder: Apply to the affected areas 2 to 3 times daily until healing is complete

Pediatric Fungal infections (cutaneous and mucocutaneous): Infants, Children, and Adolescents: Topical: Refer to adult dosing.

Renal Impairment There are no dosage adjustments provided in the manufacturer's labeling. However, dosage adjustment unlikely due to low systemic absorption

Hepatic Impairment There are no dosage adjustments provided in the manufacturer's labeling. However, dosage adjustment unlikely due to low systemic absorption

Additional Information Complete prescribing information should be consulted for additional detail.

Dosage Forms Considerations

Nyata Kit contains nystatin powder and Curatin exfoliating serum.

Pediaderm AF Complete Kit contains nystatin cream and Pediaderm Diaper Defense cream.

Dosage Forms Excipient information presented when available (limited, particularly for generics); consult specific product labeling. [DSC] = Discontinued product

Cream, External:

Generic: 100,000 units/g (15 g, 30 g)

Kit, External:

Nyata: 100,000 units/g

Pediaderm AF Complete: 100,000 units/g [contains methylparaben, propylene glycol, propylparaben]

Ointment, External:

Generic: 100,000 units/g (15 g, 30 g)

Powder, External:

Nyamyc: 100,000 units/g (15 g, 30 g, 60 g)

Nystop: 100,000 units/g (15 g, 30 g, 60 g)

Pedi-Dri: 100,000 units/g (56.7 g [DSC])

Generic: 100,000 units/g (15 g, 30 g, 60 g)

Tablet, Vaginal:

Generic: 100,000 units [DSC]

Nystatin and Triamcinolone
(nye STAT in & trye am SIN oh lone)

Index Terms Mycolog-II; Triamcinolone and Nystatin

Pharmacologic Category Antifungal Agent, Topical; Corticosteroid, Topical

Use Treatment of cutaneous candidiasis

Dosing

Adult & Geriatric Cutaneous *Candida*: Topical: Apply sparingly to affected area(s) twice daily. Therapy should be discontinued when control is achieved or if symptoms persist for >25 days of therapy.

Pediatric Refer to adult dosing.

Additional Information Complete prescribing information should be consulted for additional detail.

Dosage Forms Excipient information presented when available (limited, particularly for generics); consult specific product labeling.

Cream: Nystatin 100,000 units and triamcinolone acetonide 0.1% (15 g, 30 g, 60 g)

Ointment: Nystatin 100,000 units and triamcinolone acetonide 0.1% (15 g, 30 g, 60 g)

◆ **Nystop** see Nystatin (Topical) *on page 1305*

◆ **Nytol [OTC]** see DiphenhydrAMINE (Systemic) *on page 561*

◆ **Nytol (Can)** see DiphenhydrAMINE (Systemic) *on page 561*

◆ **Nytol Extra Strength (Can)** see DiphenhydrAMINE (Systemic) *on page 561*

◆ **Nytol Maximum Strength [OTC]** see DiphenhydrAMINE (Systemic) *on page 561*

Obinutuzumab (oh bi nue TOOZ ue mab)

Brand Names: US Gazyva

Brand Names: Canada Gazyva

Index Terms GA101; R05072759; R7159

Pharmacologic Category Antineoplastic Agent, Anti-CD20; Antineoplastic Agent, Monoclonal Antibody

Use Chronic lymphocytic leukemia: Treatment of patients with previously untreated chronic lymphocytic leukemia (CLL) in combination with chlorambucil

Pregnancy Considerations Adverse effects were observed in animal reproduction studies. Monoclonal antibodies are known to cross the placenta. Based on the mechanism of action and on animal data, if exposure occurs during pregnancy, B-cell counts may be depleted and immunologic function may be affected in the neonate after birth. Administration of live vaccines to neonates and infants exposed *in utero* should be avoided until after B-cell recovery. The Canadian labeling recommends that women of child bearing potential use effective contraception during therapy and for 18 months after the last treatment.

Breast-Feeding Considerations It is not known if obinutuzumab is excreted into breast milk. However, endogenous human immunoglobulin can be detected in milk. Although antibodies in breast milk may not enter the nursing infant's circulations in substantial amounts, the US labeling recommends the decision to breast-feed during therapy should take into account the risk of exposure to the infant and the benefits of treatment to the mother. The Canadian labeling recommends discontinuing nursing during therapy and for 18 months after the last treatment.

Contraindications

US labeling: There are no contraindications listed in the manufacturer's labeling.

Canadian labeling: Known hypersensitivity (IgE mediated) to obinutuzumab or any component of the formulation.

Warnings/Precautions [US Boxed Warning]: Hepatitis B virus (HBV) reactivation may occur with use of CD20-directed cytolytic antibodies (including obinutuzumab) and may result in fulminant hepatitis, hepatic failure, and death. Screen all patients for HBV infection by measuring hepatitis B surface antigen (HBsAg) and hepatitis B core antibody (anti-HBc) prior to therapy initiation; monitor patients for clinical and laboratory signs of hepatitis or HBV during and for several months after treatment. Discontinue obinutuzumab (and concomitant chemotherapy) if viral hepatitis develops and initiate appropriate antiviral therapy.

Reactivation has occurred in patients who are HBsAg positive as well as in those who are HBsAg negative but are anti-HBc positive; HBV reactivation has also been observed in patients who had previously resolved HBV infection. HBV reactivation has been reported for other CD20-directed antibodies after therapy discontinuation. Reactivation of HBV replication is often followed by hepatitis. Use cautiously in patients who show evidence of prior HBV infection (eg, HBsAg positive [regardless of antibody status] or HBsAG negative but anti-HBc positive); consult with appropriate clinicians regarding monitoring and consideration of antiviral therapy before and/or during obinutuzumab treatment. The safety of resuming obinutuzumab treatment following HBV reactivation is not known; discuss reinitiation of therapy in patients with resolved HBV reactivation with physicians experienced in HBV management. American Society of Clinical Oncology (ASCO) provisional clinical opinion update on HBV screening recommendations (Hwang 2015): Patients receiving anti-CD20 antibodies are at high risk for HBV reactivation. Screen for HBV infection with HBsAG and anti-HBc tests prior to treatment initiation; either a total anti-HBc (with both immunoglobulin [IgG] and immunoglobulin [IgM]) or anti-HBc IgG test should be used to screen for chronic or unresolved HBV infection (do not use anti-HBc IgM as it may only confirm acute HBV infection). In addition, patients who have risk factors for HBV infection (eg, birthplace in a country with ≥2% HBV prevalence, household or sexual contact with HBV-infected patients, high-risk behaviors [eg, intravenous drug use], and HIV infection) should also be screened prior to beginning therapy. Initiate prophylactic antiviral therapy (utilizing antivirals with low rates of viral resistance) for HBsAg-positive/anti-HBc–positive patients (without delaying cancer therapy) and continue the antivirals during and for ~6 to 12 months after completing treatment. HBsAg-negative/anti-HBc–positive patients should be monitored for HBV reactivation with HBV DNA and ALT testing approximately every 3 months during treatment; antiviral therapy may be initiated prophylactically or begun promptly at the first sign of HBV reactivation.

[US Boxed Warning]: Progressive multifocal leukoencephalopathy (PML) resulting in death may occur with treatment. PML is due to JC virus infection. Consider PML in any patient with new onset or worsening neurological symptoms and if PML is suspected, discontinue obinutuzumab (consider discontinuation or dose reduction of any concomitant chemotherapy or immunosuppressive therapy) and evaluate promptly.

May cause severe and life-threatening infusion reactions; reactions may include bronchospasm, dyspnea, tachycardia, larynx and throat irritation, wheezing, laryngeal edema, flushing, hypertension, hypotension, fever, nausea, vomiting, diarrhea, headache and/or chills. Infusion reactions occur more frequently with the first 1,000 mg infused. Delayed reactions (up to 24 hours later) and reactions with subsequent infusions have occurred. Premedicate with acetaminophen, an antihistamine, and an IV glucocorticoid (dexamethasone or methylprednisolone) prior to infusion. Hydrocortisone has not been effective in reducing the rate of infusion reactions and is not recommended). Infusion reactions may require rate reduction, interruption of therapy, or treatment discontinuation. Monitor during the entire infusion; monitor patients with preexisting cardiac or pulmonary conditions closely. Due to the risk for hypotension, consider temporarily withholding antihypertensive therapies for 12 hours prior to, during, and for 1 hour after administration. Administer in a facility with immediate access to resuscitative measures (eg, glucocorticoids, epinephrine, bronchodilators, and/or oxygen). Serious cardiovascular events (some fatal) have been reported.

In clinical trials, grade 3 and 4 neutropenia and thrombocytopenia occurred when used in combination with chlorambucil. Neutropenia may have a late onset (>28 days after therapy completion) and/or be prolonged (duration >28 days). Monitor for signs/symptoms of infection; antimicrobial prophylaxis is recommended in neutropenic patients. Antiviral and/or antifungal prophylaxis should also be considered. In a small percentage of patients, thrombocytopenia occurred acutely (within 24 hours) after obinutuzumab administration; platelet transfusions may be necessary. Fatal hemorrhagic events during the first cycle have been reported; monitor frequently for thrombocytopenia and bleeding episodes, particularly during the initial cycle. Thrombocytopenia may require dose delays of obinutuzumab and chlorambucil and/or dose reductions of chlorambucil. Consider withholding platelet inhibitors, anticoagulants, or other medications which may increase bleeding risk (especially during the first cycle). Leukopenia and lymphopenia commonly occur. Monitor blood counts frequently throughout therapy. Bacterial, fungal, and new

or reactivated viral infections may occur during and/or following therapy; fatal infections have been reported. Do not administer to patients with an active infection. Patients with a history of recurrent or chronic infections may be at increased risk. Tumor lysis syndrome (TLS) has been reported with obinutuzumab (some cases fatal). Acute renal failure, hyperkalemia, hypocalcemia, hyperuricemia, and/or hyperphosphatemia may occur. Administer prophylaxis (antihyperuricemic therapy [eg, allopurinol or rasburicase] and hydration) in patients at high risk (high circulating lymphocyte counts [>25,000/mm³], high tumor burden, or renal impairment) prior to initiating obinutuzumab therapy (administer prior to each subsequent cycle if needed). Monitor lab parameters during initial treatment days in patients at risk for TLS. Correct electrolyte abnormalities; monitor renal function and hydration status, and administer supportive care, including dialysis as indicated. Administration of live virus vaccines during treatment (and until B-cell recovery) is not recommended; the safety and efficacy of immunization with live or attenuated viral vaccines during or after obinutuzumab therapy has not been determined. If obinutuzumab exposure occurs during pregnancy, the safety and timing of live virus vaccinations for the infant should be evaluated. Potentially significant drug-drug interactions may exist, requiring dose or frequency adjustment, additional monitoring, and/or selection of alternative therapy.

Adverse Reactions Adverse reactions reported in combination with chlorambucil. Frequency not always defined.

>10%:

Endocrine & metabolic: Hypocalcemia (37% to 38%; grades 3/4: 3%), hyperkalemia (14% to 33%; grades 3/4: 1 to 5%), hyponatremia (26% to 30%; grades 3/4: 7% to 8%), hypoalbuminemia (23%; grades 3/4: <1%), hypokalemia (15%; grade 3/4: 1%)

Hematologic & oncologic: Leukopenia (6% to 84%; grades 3/4: 4% to 37%), lymphocytopenia (80%; grades 3/4: 39% to 40%), neutropenia (38% to 78%; grades 3/4: 33% to 48%; onset ≥28 days after completion of treatment: 16%), thrombocytopenia (11% to 48%; grades 3/4: 10% to 13% onset within 24 hours of infusion: 4%), anemia (12% to 39%; grades 3/4: 5% to 10%)

Hepatic: Increased serum AST (27% to 29%; grades 3/4: 1% to 2%), increased serum ALT (27% to 28%; grades 3/4: 2%), increased serum alkaline phosphatase (18%)

Infection: Infection (38%; grades 3/4: 11%)

Neuromuscular & skeletal: Musculoskeletal signs and symptoms (18%; including pain)

Renal: Increased serum creatinine (30%; grades 3/4: <1%)

Miscellaneous: Infusion related reaction (initial infusion: 65% to 69%; grades 3/4: 20% to 21%; second infusion: 3%; subsequent infusions: <1%)

1% to 10%:

Cardiovascular: Thrombohemorrhagic event (4%), exacerbation of cardiac disease, flushing, hypertension, hypotension, tachycardia

Central nervous system: Chills, headache, progressive multifocal leukoencephalopathy

Endocrine & metabolic: Hyperphosphatemia, hyperuricemia

Gastrointestinal: Diarrhea (10%; grades 3/4: 2%), constipation (8%), vomiting

Genitourinary: Urinary tract infection (5% to 6%; grades 3/4: 1% to 2%)

Hematologic & oncologic: Tumor lysis syndrome (grades 3/4: 2%)

Hepatic: Increased liver enzymes (4%; may be secondary or exacerbated by premedications)

Infection: JCV (John Cunningham virus) infection, reactivation of HBV, renal infection (new or reactivation)

Neuromuscular & skeletal: Back pain (5%; grade 3/4: <1%)

Renal: Acute renal failure

Respiratory: Cough (10%), nasopharyngitis (6%; grades: <1%), bronchospasm, dyspnea, laryngeal edema, throat irritation, wheezing

Miscellaneous: Fever (9% to 10%; grades 3/4: <1%)

Drug Interactions

Metabolism/Transport Effects None known.

Avoid Concomitant Use

Avoid concomitant use of Obinutuzumab with any of the following: BCG (Intravesical); Belimumab; Deferiprone; Dipyrone; Natalizumab; Pimecrolimus; Tacrolimus (Topical); Tofacitinib; Vaccines (Live)

Increased Effect/Toxicity

Obinutuzumab may increase the levels/effects of: Amifostine; Antipsychotic Agents (Second Generation [Atypical]); Belimumab; Blood Pressure Lowering Agents; Deferiprone; DULoxetine; Fingolimod; Leflunomide; Natalizumab; Tofacitinib; Vaccines (Live)

The levels/effects of Obinutuzumab may be increased by: Agents with Antiplatelet Properties; Alfuzosin; Anticoagulants; Barbiturates; Brimonidine (Topical); Denosumab; Diazoxide; Dipyrone; Herbs (Hypotensive Properties); Molsidomine; Nicorandil; Pentoxifylline; Phosphodiesterase 5 Inhibitors; Pimecrolimus; Prostacyclin Analogues; Roflumilast; Tacrolimus (Topical); Trastuzumab

Decreased Effect

Obinutuzumab may decrease the levels/effects of: BCG (Intravesical); Coccidioides immitis Skin Test; Sipuleucel-T; Vaccines (Inactivated); Vaccines (Live)

The levels/effects of Obinutuzumab may be decreased by: Echinacea

Preparation for Administration

Cycle 1, day 1 and 2 doses (100 mg and 900 mg, respectively): Withdraw 40 mL of obinutuzumab solution from vial. Dilute 4 mL into a 100 mL infusion bag of NS (100 mg dose; use immediately). Dilute remaining 36 mL into a 250 mL NS infusion bag (900 mg dose, for use on day 2); store at 2°C to 8°C (36°F to 46°F) for up to 24 hours; use immediately after reaching room temperature. Gently invert to mix; do not shake or freeze.

Cycle 1 (day 8 and 15 doses) and cycles 2 through 6 (1000 mg): Withdraw 40 mL of obinutuzumab solution from vial. Dilute into a 250 mL NS infusion bag. Gently invert to mix; do not shake or freeze.

Do not use other diluents (eg, dextrose) to prepare the infusion. Final concentration for administration should be 0.4 to 4 mg/mL. May use PVC or non-PVC infusion bags.

Storage/Stability

Store intact vials at 2°C to 8°C (36°F to 46°F); do not freeze or shake. Protect from light. Diluted solutions for infusion should be used immediately. If not used immediately, the diluted solutions may be stored up to 24 hours at 2°C to 8°C (36°F to 46°F) followed by 48 hours (including infusion time) at room temperature of ≤30°C (≤86°F).

Mechanism of Action

Obinutuzumab is a glycoengineered type II anti-CD20 monoclonal antibody. The CD20 antigen is expressed on the surface of pre B- and mature B-lymphocytes; upon binding to CD20, obinutuzumab activates complement-dependent cytotoxicity, antibody-dependent cellular cytotoxicity and antibody-dependent cellular phagocytosis, resulting in cell death (Sehn 2012).

Pharmacodynamics/Kinetics

Distribution: V_d: ~3.9 L

Half-life elimination: ~29.7 days

Dosing

Adult & Geriatric Note: Premedication with acetaminophen, an antihistamine, and a glucocorticoid (dexamethasone or methylprednisolone) 30 to 60 minutes prior to treatment may be necessary (see Administration). Antihyperuricemic prophylaxis and adequate hydration are recommended for patients at risk for tumor lysis syndrome. Antimicrobial, antiviral, and antifungal prophylaxis may be considered in certain patients.

Chronic lymphocytic leukemia (CLL): IV:

Cycle 1: 100 mg on day 1, followed by 900 mg on day 2, followed by 1,000 mg weekly for 2 doses (days 8 and 15)

Cycles 2 through 6: 1,000 mg on day 1 every 28 days for 5 doses

Missed doses: Administer the missed dose as soon as possible; adjust dosing schedule accordingly. In some cases, patients who do not complete the day 1 cycle 1 dose may proceed to the day 2 cycle 1 treatment (if appropriate).

Renal Impairment

CrCl ≥30 mL/minute: There are no dosage adjustments provided in the US manufacturer's labeling; however, pharmacokinetics are not affected (based on pharmacokinetic analysis). The Canadian labeling recommends that no dosage adjustment is necessary.

CrCl <30 mL/minute: There are no dosage adjustments provided in the manufacturer's labeling (has not been studied)

Hepatic Impairment

There are no dosage adjustments provided in the manufacturer's labeling (has not been studied)

Adjustment for Toxicity

Hematologic: Grade 3 or 4 cytopenia: Consider treatment interruption

Infusion reactions:

Mild-to-moderate (Grades 1 and 2): Reduce infusion rate or interrupt infusion and manage symptoms as appropriate. Upon symptom resolution, continue or resume infusion. If no further infusion reaction symptoms occur, may resume infusion rate escalation as appropriate for the treatment cycle dose. Day 1 (cycle 1) infusion rate may be increased back up to a maximum of 25 mg/hour after 1 hour.

Severe (Grade 3): Interrupt therapy; manage symptoms as appropriate. Upon symptom resolution, may reinitiate infusion at no more than 50% of the rate at which the reaction occurred. If no further infusion reaction symptoms occur, may resume infusion rate escalation as appropriate for the treatment cycle dose. Day 1 (cycle 1) infusion rate may be increased back up to a maximum of 25 mg/hour after 1 hour. Permanently discontinue if ≥ grade 3 infusion-related symptoms occur upon rechallenge.

Life-threatening (Grade 4): Discontinue infusion immediately; permanently discontinue therapy.

Infection: Consider treatment interruption.

Other toxicity: Consider treatment interruption for ≥ grade 2 nonhematologic toxicity.

Administration

For IV infusion only. Do not administer IV push or as a bolus. Administer through a dedicated IV line; do not mix with or infuse with other medications. May use PVC or non-PVC administration sets. Premedication with acetaminophen, an antihistamine, and a glucocorticoid (dexamethasone or methylprednisolone) may be required to prevent infusion reactions (see below). In patients with neutropenia, antimicrobial prophylaxis is strongly recommended throughout the treatment period; antiviral and antifungal prophylaxis should be considered.

Premedication to prevent infusion reactions:

Cycle 1 (days 1 and 2): All patients should receive acetaminophen (650 to 1,000 mg) and an antihistamine (eg, diphenhydramine 50 mg) at least 30 minutes prior to infusion. In addition, an IV glucocorticoid (dexamethasone 20 mg or methylprednisolone 80 mg) should be administered at least 1 hour prior to infusion.

Cycle 1 (days 8 and 15), and cycles 2 through 6: All patients should receive acetaminophen 650 to 1,000 mg at least 30 minutes prior to infusion.

If patients experienced grade 1 or higher infusion-related reaction with previous infusion: Administer an antihistamine (eg, diphenhydramine 50 mg) in addition to acetaminophen at least 30 minutes prior to infusion.

If patients experienced a grade 3 infusion-related reaction with previous infusion **or** have a lymphocyte count >25,000 cells/mm³ prior to next treatment: Administer an IV glucocorticoid (dexamethasone 20 mg or methylprednisolone 80 mg) at least 1 hour prior to infusion, in addition to acetaminophen and an antihistamine at least 30 minutes prior to infusion.

Infusion rate:

Cycle 1 (day 1): Infuse at 25 mg/hour over 4 hours; do not increase the infusion rate

Cycle 1 (day 2): If no reaction to previous infusion, initiate infusion at 50 mg/hour for 30 minutes; if tolerated, may escalate rate in increments of 50 mg/hour every 30 minutes to a maximum rate of 400 mg/hour.

Cycle 1 (days 8 and 15), and cycles 2 through 6: If no reaction to previous infusion, initiate infusion at 100 mg/hour for 30 minutes; if tolerated, may escalate infusion rate in increments of 100 mg/hour every 30 minutes to a maximum rate of 400 mg/hour.

Monitoring Parameters

CBC with differential (at regular intervals), renal function, electrolytes, uric acid (if at risk for tumor lysis syndrome); hepatitis B screening in all patients (HBsAG and anti-HBc measurements) prior to therapy initiation. Hepatitis B virus (HBV) screening recommendations (American Society of Clinical Oncology provisional clinical opinion update [Hwang 2015]): Screen for HBV infection with hepatitis B surface antigen (HBsAG) and hepatitis B core antibody (anti-HBc) tests prior to treatment initiation; either a total anti-HBc (with both immunoglobulin G [IgG] and immunoglobulin M [IgM]) or anti-HBc IgG test should be used to screen for chronic or unresolved HBV infection (do not use anti-HBc IgM as it may only confirm acute HBV infection). HBsAg-negative/anti-HBc–positive patients should be monitored for HBV reactivation with HBV DNA and ALT testing approximately every 3 months during treatment.

Monitor for signs of active hepatitis B infection (during and for up to 12 months after therapy completion). Monitor for signs or symptoms of infusion reaction; signs of infection; fluid status; signs/symptoms of progressive multifocal leukoencephalopathy (PML; focal neurologic deficits, which may present as hemiparesis, visual field deficits, cognitive impairment, aphasia, ataxia, and/or cranial nerve deficits); evaluate for PML with brain MRI, lumbar puncture, and neurologist consultation.

Dosage Forms

Excipient information presented when available (limited, particularly for generics); consult specific product labeling.

Solution, Intravenous [preservative free]:

Gazyva: 1000 mg/40 mL (40 mL)

Ocriplasmin (ok ri PLAZ min)

Brand Names: US Jetrea
Brand Names: Canada Jetrea
Pharmacologic Category Ophthalmic Agent; Vitreolytic
Use Vitreomacular adhesion: Treatment of symptomatic vitreomacular adhesion (VMA)
Dosing
Adult & Geriatric Vitreomacular adhesion: Intravitreal: 0.125 mg once (as a single dose to the affected eye)
Renal Impairment There are no dosage adjustments provided in the manufacturer's labeling. However, dosage adjustment unlikely due to low systemic absorption.
Hepatic Impairment There are no dosage adjustments provided in the manufacturer's labeling. However, dosage adjustment unlikely due to low systemic absorption.
Additional Information Complete prescribing information should be consulted for additional detail.
Dosage Forms Excipient information presented when available (limited, particularly for generics); consult specific product labeling.
Solution, Intraocular [preservative free]:
Jetrea: 0.5 mg/0.2 mL (0.2 mL)

Octreotide (ok TREE oh tide)

Brand Names: US SandoSTATIN; SandoSTATIN LAR Depot
Brand Names: Canada Ocphyl; Octreotide Acetate Omega; Octreotide Injection; Sandostatin; Sandostatin LAR
Index Terms Longastatin; Octreotide Acetate
Pharmacologic Category Antidiarrheal; Antidote; Somatostatin Analog
Use
Acromegaly:
Injection solution: To reduce blood levels of growth hormone (GH) and insulin-like growth factor 1 (IGF-1) in patients with inadequate response to or who cannot be treated with surgical resection, pituitary irradiation, and bromocriptine mesylate at maximally tolerated doses; goal of therapy is to achieve normalization of GH and IGF-1 levels.
LAR depot suspension: Long-term maintenance treatment of acromegaly in patients with an inadequate response to surgery and/or radiotherapy (or for whom surgery/radiotherapy are not options) with a goal of therapy to reduce GH and IGF-1 levels to normal.
Carcinoid tumors:
Injection solution: Management of symptoms (diarrhea and flushing) in patients with metastatic carcinoid tumors.

LAR depot suspension: Long-term treatment of severe diarrhea and flushing episodes associated with metastatic carcinoid tumors.
Vasoactive intestinal peptide-secreting tumors:
Injection solution: Treatment of profuse watery diarrhea associated with vasoactive intestinal peptide-secreting tumors (VIPomas).
LAR depot suspension: Long-term treatment of profuse watery diarrhea associated with VIPomas.

Limitations of use: The effects of octreotide (injection solution and LAR depot suspension) on tumor size, rate of growth, and development of metastases in patients with carcinoid syndrome and VIPomas have not been determined.
Pregnancy Considerations Adverse events have not been observed in animal reproduction studies. Octreotide crosses the placenta and can be detected in the newborn at delivery (Caron 1995; Fassnacht 2001; Maffei 2010); data concerning use in pregnancy is limited. In case reports of acromegalic women who received normal doses of octreotide during pregnancy, no congenital malformations were reported. Because normalization of IGF-1 and GH may restore fertility in women with acromegaly, women of childbearing potential should use adequate contraception during treatment. Long-acting formulations should be discontinued ~2 months prior to a planned pregnancy; use short acting octreotide as needed until conception. Octreotide therapy may be considered in pregnant women with worsening symptoms if needed. Monitoring of IGF-1 and/or GH is not recommended during pregnancy (Katznelson 2014).
Breast-Feeding Considerations Octreotide is excreted in breast milk. In a case report, a woman was taking octreotide SubQ in doses up to 2400 mcg/day prior to and throughout pregnancy. Octreotide was measurable in the colostrum in concentrations similar to those in the maternal serum (Maffei 2010); however, oral absorption of octreotide is considered to be poor (Battershill, 1989). The manufacturer recommends that caution be exercised when administering octreotide to nursing women.
Contraindications Hypersensitivity to octreotide or any component of the formulation
Warnings/Precautions May impair gallbladder function; monitor patients for cholelithiasis. The incidence of gallbladder stone or biliary sludge increases with a duration of therapy of ≥12 months. Prophylactic cholecystectomy is recommended in patients with gastrointestinal or pancreatic neuroendocrine tumors undergoing abdominal surgery if octreotide treatment is planned (Oberg 2004). Use with caution in patients with renal and/or hepatic impairment; dosage adjustment may be required in patients receiving dialysis and in patients with established cirrhosis. Somatostatin analogs may affect glucose regulation. In type I diabetes, severe hypoglycemia may occur; in type II diabetes or patients without diabetes, hyperglycemia may occur. Insulin and other hypoglycemic medication requirements may change. Octreotide may worsen hypoglycemia in patients with insulinomas; use with caution. Do not use depot formulation for the treatment of sulfonylurea-induced hypoglycemia. Bradycardia, conduction abnormalities, and arrhythmia have been observed in acromegalic and carcinoid syndrome patients; use caution with CHF or concomitant medications that alter heart rate or rhythm. Cardiovascular medication requirements may change. Octreotide may enhance the adverse/toxic effects of other QTc-prolonging agents. May alter absorption of dietary fats; monitor for pancreatitis. May reduce excessive fluid loss in patients with conditions that cause such loss; monitor for elevations in zinc levels in such patients that are maintained on total parenteral nutrition (TPN). Chronic treatment has been associated with abnormal Schillings test; monitor vitamin B_{12} levels. Suppresses secretion of TSH; monitor for hypothyroidism.

Postmarketing cases of serious and fatal events, including hypoxia and necrotizing enterocolitis, have been reported with octreotide use in children (usually with serious underlying conditions), particularly in children <2 years of age. In studies with octreotide depot, the incidence of cholelithiasis in children is higher than the reported incidences for adults and efficacy was not demonstrated. Therapy may restore fertility; females of childbearing potential should use adequate contraception. Dosage adjustment may be necessary in the elderly; significant increases in elimination half-life have been observed in older adults. Vehicle used in depot injection (polylactide-co-glycolide microspheres) has rarely been associated with retinal artery occlusion in patients with abnormal arteriovenous anastomosis. Therapy with immediate release octreotide (solution) should be withheld 24 hours prior to administration of radiolabeled somatostatin analogs; the IM (depot) formulation should be withheld at least 2 months before

administration of radiolabeled somatostatin analogs (Oberg 2004). Potentially significant drug-drug interactions may exist, requiring dose or frequency adjustment, additional monitoring, and/or selection of alternative therapy.

Adverse Reactions Adverse reactions vary by route of administration and dosage form. Frequency of cardiac, endocrine, and gastrointestinal adverse reactions was generally higher in acromegalics.

>16%:

Cardiovascular: Sinus bradycardia (19% to 25%), chest pain (≤20%; non-depot formulations)

Central nervous system: Fatigue (1% to 32%), headache (6% to 30%), malaise (16% to 20%), fever (16% to 20%), dizziness (5% to 20%)

Dermatologic: Pruritus (≤18%)

Endocrine & metabolic: Hyperglycemia (2% to 27%)

Gastrointestinal: Abdominal pain (5% to 61%), loose stools (5% to 61%), nausea (5% to 61%), diarrhea (34% to 61%), flatulence (≤38%), cholelithiasis (13% to 38%; length of therapy dependent), biliary sludge (24%; length of therapy dependent), constipation (9% to 21%), vomiting (4% to 21%), biliary duct dilatation (12%)

Local: Injection site pain (2% to 50%; dose and formulation related)

Neuromuscular & skeletal: Back pain (1% to 27%), arthropathy (8% to 19%), myalgia (≤18%)

Respiratory: Upper respiratory infection (10% to 23%), dyspnea (≤20%; non-depot formulations)

Miscellaneous: Antibodies to octreotide (up to 25%; no efficacy change), flu symptoms (1% to 20%)

5% to 15%:

Cardiovascular: Hypertension (≤13%), conduction abnormalities (9% to 10%), arrhythmia (3% to 9%), palpitation, peripheral edema

Central nervous system: Pain (4% to 15%), anxiety, confusion, hypoesthesia, insomnia

Dermatologic: Rash (15%; depot formulation), alopecia (≤13%)

Endocrine & metabolic: Hypothyroidism (≤12%; non-depot formulations), goiter (≤8%; non-depot formulations)

Gastrointestinal: Dyspepsia (4% to 6%), feces discoloration (4% to 6%), steatorrhea (4% to 6%), tenesmus (4% to 6%), anorexia, cramping

Hematologic: Anemia (≤15%; non-depot formulations: <1%)

Neuromuscular & skeletal: Arthralgia, myalgia, paresthesia, rigors, weakness

Otic: Earache

Renal: Renal calculus

Respiratory: Cough, pharyngitis, rhinitis, sinusitis

Miscellaneous: Allergy, diaphoresis

1% to 4%:

Cardiovascular: Angina, cardiac failure, edema, flushing, hematoma, phlebitis

Central nervous system: Abnormal gait, amnesia, depression, dysphonia, hallucinations, nervousness, neuralgia, somnolence, vertigo

Dermatologic: Acne, bruising, cellulitis

Endocrine & metabolic: Hypoglycemia (2% to 4%), hypokalemia, hypoproteinemia, gout, cachexia, breast pain, impotence

Gastrointestinal: Colitis, diverticulitis, dysphagia, fat malabsorption, gastritis, gastroenteritis, gingivitis, glossitis, melena, stomatitis, taste perversion, xerostomia

Genitourinary: Incontinence, pollakiuria (non-depot formulations), urinary tract infection

Local: Injection site hematoma

Neuromuscular & skeletal: Hyperkinesia, hypertonia, joint pain, neuropathy, tremor

Ocular: Blurred vision, visual disturbance

Otic: Tinnitus

Renal: Albuminuria, renal abscess

Respiratory: Bronchitis, epistaxis

Miscellaneous: Bacterial infection, cold symptoms, moniliasis

<1% (Limited to important or life-threatening): Amenorrhea, anaphylactic shock, anaphylactoid reactions, aneurysm, aphasia, appendicitis, arthritis, ascending cholangitis, ascites, atrial fibrillation, basal cell carcinoma, Bell's palsy, biliary obstruction, breast carcinoma, cardiac arrest, cerebral vascular disorder, CHF, cholecystitis, cholestatic hepatitis, CK increased, deafness, diabetes insipidus, diabetes mellitus, fatty liver, galactorrhea, gallbladder polyp, GI bleeding, GI hemorrhage, GI ulcer, glaucoma, gynecomastia, hematuria, hepatitis, hypoadrenalism, hypoxia (children), intestinal obstruction, intracranial hemorrhage, intraocular pressure increased, ischemia, joint effusion, malignant hyperpyrexia, MI, migraine, necrotizing enterocolitis (neonates), nephrolithiasis, neuritis, oligomenorrhea, orthostatic hypotension, pancreatitis, pancytopenia, paresis, pituitary apoplexy, pleural effusion, pneumonia, pneumothorax, polymenorrhea, pulmonary embolism, pulmonary hypertension, pulmonary nodule, Raynaud's syndrome, renal failure, renal insufficiency, retinal vein thrombosis, seizures, status asthmaticus, suicide attempt, syncope, tachycardia, thrombocytopenia, thrombophlebitis, thrombosis, weight loss

Drug Interactions

Metabolism/Transport Effects None known.

Avoid Concomitant Use

Avoid concomitant use of Octreotide with any of the following: Ceritinib

Increased Effect/Toxicity

Octreotide may increase the levels/effects of: Bradycardia-Causing Agents; Bromocriptine; Ceritinib; Codeine; Highest Risk QTc-Prolonging Agents; Hypoglycemia-Associated Agents; Ivabradine; Lacosamide; Moderate Risk QTc-Prolonging Agents; Pegvisomant

The levels/effects of Octreotide may be increased by: Androgens; Antidiabetic Agents; Bretylium; Herbs (Hypoglycemic Properties); MAO Inhibitors; Mifepristone; Pegvisomant; Quinolone Antibiotics; Ruxolitinib; Salicylates; Selective Serotonin Reuptake Inhibitors; Tofacitinib

Decreased Effect

Octreotide may decrease the levels/effects of: Antidiabetic Agents; CycloSPORINE (Systemic)

The levels/effects of Octreotide may be decreased by: Quinolone Antibiotics

Food Interactions Octreotide may alter absorption of dietary fats. Management: Administer injections between meals to decrease GI effects.

Storage/Stability

Injection solution: Octreotide is a clear solution and should be stored at refrigerated temperatures between 2°C and 8°C (36°F and 46°F). Protect from light. May be stored at room temperature of 20°C to 30°C (68°F and 86°F) for up to 14 days when protected from light. Stable as a parenteral admixture in NS or D₅W for 24 hours. Discard multidose vials within 14 days after initial entry.

LAR depot suspension: Prior to dilution, store at refrigerated temperatures between 2°C and 8°C (36°F and 46°F). Protect from light. Additionally, the manufacturer reports that octreotide suspension may be stored at room temperature of 20°C to 25°C (68°F and 77°F) for up to 10 days when protected from light (data on file [Novartis 2011]). Depot drug product kit may be at room temperature for 30 to 60 minutes prior to use. Use suspension immediately after preparation.

Mechanism of Action Mimics natural somatostatin by inhibiting serotonin release, and the secretion of gastrin, VIP, insulin, glucagon, secretin, motilin, and pancreatic polypeptide. Decreases growth hormone and IGF-1 in acromegaly. Octreotide provides more potent inhibition of growth hormone, glucagon, and insulin as compared to endogenous somatostatin. Also suppresses LH response to GnRH, secretion of thyroid-stimulating hormone and decreases splanchnic blood flow.

Pharmacodynamics/Kinetics

Duration: SubQ: 6 to 12 hours

Absorption: SubQ: Rapid and complete; IM (depot formulation): Released slowly (via microsphere degradation in the muscle)

Distribution: V_d: 14 L (13 to 30 L in acromegaly)

Protein binding: 65%, primarily to lipoprotein (41% in acromegaly)

Metabolism: Extensively hepatic

Bioavailability: SubQ: 100%; IM: 60% to 63% of SubQ dose

Half-life elimination: 1.7 to 1.9 hours; Increased in elderly patients; Cirrhosis: Up to 3.7 hours; Fatty liver disease: Up to 3.4 hours; Renal impairment: Up to 3.1 hours

Time to peak, plasma: SubQ: 0.4 hours (0.7 hours acromegaly); IM: 1 hour

Excretion: Urine (32% as unchanged drug)

Dosing

Adult

Acromegaly:

SubQ, IV: Initial: 50 mcg 3 times/day; titrate to achieve growth hormone levels <5 ng/mL or IGF-I (somatomedin C) levels <1.9 units/mL in males and <2.2 units/mL in females. Usual effective dose: 100 mcg 3 times/day; range: 300 to 1,500 mcg/day. Doses above 300 mcg/day rarely result in additional benefit; if increased dose fails to provide additional benefit, the dose should be reduced. **Note:** Should be withdrawn yearly for a 4-week interval (8 weeks for depot injection) in patients who have received irradiation. Resume if levels increase and signs/symptoms recur.

▶

IM depot injection: Patients must be stabilized on subcutaneous octreotide for at least 2 weeks before switching to the long-acting depot. Upon switch: 20 mg IM intragluteally every 4 weeks for 3 months, then the dose may be modified based upon response.

Dosage adjustment for acromegaly: After 3 months of depot injections, the dosage may be continued or modified as follows:

GH ≤1 ng/mL, IGF-1 normal, and symptoms controlled: Reduce octreotide depot to 10 mg IM every 4 weeks

GH ≤2.5 ng/mL, IGF-1 normal, and symptoms controlled: Maintain octreotide depot at 20 mg IM every 4 weeks

GH >2.5 ng/mL, IGF-1 elevated, and/or symptoms uncontrolled: Increase octreotide depot to 30 mg IM every 4 weeks

Note: Patients not adequately controlled at a dose of 30 mg may increase dose to 40 mg every 4 weeks. Dosages >40 mg are not recommended.

Carcinoid tumors:

SubQ, IV: Initial 2 weeks: 100 to 600 mcg/day in 2 to 4 divided doses; usual range: 50 to 750 mcg/day (some patients may require up to 1,500 mcg/day); experience with doses above 750 mcg/day is limited.

IM depot injection: Patients must be stabilized on subcutaneous octreotide for at least 2 weeks before switching to the long-acting depot. Upon switch: 20 mg IM intragluteally every 4 weeks for 2 months, then the dose may be modified based upon response.

Note: Patients should continue to receive their SubQ injections for the first 2 weeks at the same dose in order to maintain therapeutic levels (some patients may require 3 to 4 weeks of continued SubQ injections). Patients who experience periodic exacerbations of symptoms may require temporary SubQ injections in addition to depot injections (at their previous SubQ dosing regimen) until symptoms have resolved.

Dosage adjustment for carcinoid tumors: After 2 months of depot injections, the dosage may be continued or modified as follows:

Increase to 30 mg IM every 4 weeks if symptoms are inadequately controlled

Decrease to 10 mg IM every 4 weeks, for a trial period, if initially responsive to 20 mg dose

Dosage >30 mg is not recommended

Vasoactive intestinal peptide tumors (VIPomas):

SubQ, IV: Initial 2 weeks: 200 to 300 mcg/day in 2 to 4 divided doses; titrate dose based on response/tolerance. Range: 150 to 750 mcg/day (doses >450 mcg/day are rarely required)

IM depot injection: Patients must be stabilized on subcutaneous octreotide for at least 2 weeks before switching to the long-acting depot. Upon switch: 20 mg IM intragluteally every 4 weeks for 2 months, then the dose may be modified based upon response.

Note: Patients receiving depot injection should continue to receive their SubQ injections for the first 2 weeks at the same dose in order to maintain therapeutic levels (some patients may require 3 to 4 weeks of continued SubQ injections). Patients who experience periodic exacerbations of symptoms may require temporary SubQ injections in addition to depot injections (at their previous SubQ dosing regimen) until symptoms have resolved.

Dosage adjustment for VIPomas: After 2 months of depot injections, the dosage may be continued or modified as follows:

Increase to 30 mg IM every 4 weeks if symptoms are inadequately controlled

Decrease to 10 mg IM every 4 weeks, for a trial period, if initially responsive to 20 mg dose

Dosage >30 mg is not recommended

Carcinoid crisis, prevention (off-label use): Immediate release octreotide solution (Oberg 2004):

Patients controlled with octreotide IM (depot) 20 to 30 mg: SubQ: 250 to 500 mcg within 1 to 2 hours prior to procedure.

Emergency surgery in somatostatin analog-naïve patients with functional neuroendocrine tumors:

IV bolus: 500 to 1000 mcg 1 to 2 hours prior to procedure **or**

SubQ: 500 mcg 1 to 2 hours prior to procedure

Intraoperative use for carcinoid crisis with hypotension: IV: 500 to 1,000 mcg bolus, repeat at 5 minute intervals until symptoms are controlled or IV: 500 to 1,000 mcg bolus followed by 50 to 200 mcg/hour continuous infusion during the procedure.

Postoperative dose (if supplemental doses required during procedure): IV: 50 to 200 mcg/hour continuous infusion for 24 hours, followed by resumption of the preoperative treatment schedule.

Diarrhea (off-label use): IV: Initial: 50 to 100 mcg every 8 hours; increase by 100 mcg/dose at 48-hour intervals; maximum dose: 500 mcg every 8 hours

Diarrhea (refractory) associated with chemotherapy (off-label use):

Low grade or uncomplicated: SubQ: 100 to 150 mcg every 8 hours (Benson 2004; Kornblau 2000)

Severe: Initial: SubQ: 100 to 150 mcg every 8 hours; may increase to 500 to 1500 mcg IV or SubQ every 8 hours (Kornblau 2000)

Complicated: IV, SubQ: Initial: 100 to 150 mcg 3 times/day or IV Infusion: 25 to 50 mcg/hour; may escalate to 500 mcg 3 times/day until controlled (Benson 2004)

Diarrhea associated with acute graft-versus-host disease (GVHD) (off-label use): IV: 500 mcg every 8 hours; discontinue within 24 hours of diarrhea resolution to avoid ileus; Maximum duration of therapy if diarrhea is not resolved: 7 days (Kornblau 2000)

Esophageal varices bleeding (off-label use): IV bolus: 25 to 100 mcg (usual bolus dose: 50 mcg) followed by continuous IV infusion of 25 to 50 mcg/hour for 2 to 5 days; may repeat bolus in first hour if hemorrhage not controlled (Corley 2001; Erstad 2001; Garcia-Tsao 2010)

Gastroenteropancreatic neuroendocrine tumors (off-label use):

IM (depot): 30 mg every 4 weeks until tumor progression or death (Rinke 2009) **or**

SubQ: Initial: 100 to 500 mcg 2 to 4 times daily (usually 150 mcg 3 times daily), may increase to response (symptom control) by doubling the dose every 3 to 4 days or a continuous subQ infusion of 1,000 to 2,000 mcg/day (Oberg 2004) **or**

IM (depot): Assure tolerability by initiating with the SubQ formulation for 3 to 7 days (and continue with SubQ for the first ~14 days after the initial IM depot dose). Then initiate IM (depot): 20 to 30 mg every 28 days (SubQ doses of 200 to 600 mcg/day should receive 20 mg IM and SubQ doses of 750 to 1,500 mcg/day should receive 30 mg IM); IM (depot) range: 20 to 60 mg every 28 days (Oberg 2004).

Malignant bowel obstruction (off-label use): SubQ: 200 to 900 mcg/day in 2 to 3 divided doses (Mercadante 2007; Mercadante 2012) or 300 mcg/day by continuous SubQ infusion (Mercadante 2000)

Sulfonylurea-induced hypoglycemia (off-label use):

Note: Although octreotide use has been advocated as a first line therapy, indications and dosing for octreotide are not firmly established (Glatstein 2012). Octreotide may reduce the incidence of recurrent hypoglycemia seen with dextrose-alone therapy (Fasano 2008). In addition, although subcutaneous administration is the preferred route, administration via intravenous bolus and intravenous infusion have also been described in the literature (Barkin 2013; Braatvedt 1997; Carr 2002; Crawford 2004; Dougherty 2010; Dougherty 2013; Fasano 2008; Graudins 1997; Green 2003; Hung 1997; McLaughlin 2000; Mordel 1998). Optimal care decisions should be made based upon patient-specific details. Repeat dosing, dose escalation, or initiation of a continuous infusion may be required in patients who experience recurrent hypoglycemia. Duration of treatment may exceed 24 hours.

SubQ: 50 to 75 mcg; repeat every 6 hours as needed based upon blood glucose concentrations (Fasano 2008; Howland 2011)

IV: Doses up to 125 mcg/hour have been used successfully (McLaughlin 2000)

Thymoma/thymic malignancies, advanced (off-label use): SubQ: 500 mcg 3 times daily; evaluate after 2 months, patients with remission (complete or partial) continued octreotide for up to a maximum of 12 months; patients with stable disease continued octreotide and also received prednisone for up to 12 months or until disease progression or unacceptable toxicity (Loehrer 2004).

Geriatric Refer to adult dosing. Elimination half-life is increased by 46% and clearance is decreased by 26%; dose adjustment may be required. Dosing should generally begin at the lower end of dosing range.

Pediatric Infants and Children:

Congenital hyperinsulinism (off-label use): SubQ: Initial: 2 to 10 mcg/kg/day; up to 40 mcg/kg/day have been used (Stanley 1997).

Secretory diarrhea (off-label use): IV, SubQ: Doses of 1 to 10 mcg/kg every 12 hours have been used in children beginning at the low end of the range and increasing by 0.3 mcg/kg/dose at 3-day intervals. Suppression of growth hormone (animal data) is of concern when used as long-term therapy.

Sulfonylurea-induced hypoglycemia (off-label use):
Note: Although octreotide use has been advocated as a first line therapy, indications and dosing for octreotide are not firmly established (Glatstein 2012). Octreotide may reduce the incidence of recurrent hypoglycemia seen with dextrose-alone therapy (Fasano 2008). In addition, although subcutaneous administration is the preferred route, administration via intravenous bolus and intravenous infusion have also been described in the literature (Barkin 2013; Braatvedt 1997; Carr 2002; Crawford 2004; Dougherty 2010; Dougherty 2013; Fasano 2008; Graudins 1997; Green 2003; Hung 1997; McLaughlin 2000; Mordel 1998). Optimal care decisions should be made based upon patient-specific details. Repeat dosing, dose escalation, or initiation of a continuous infusion may be required in patients who experience recurrent hypoglycemia. Duration of treatment may exceed 24 hours. SubQ: 1 to 1.25 mcg/kg; repeat in 6 hours as needed based upon blood glucose concentrations (Howland 2011). Children generally need only a single dose (Dougherty 2013).

Renal Impairment
Regular injection:
Mild to severe impairment: There are no dosage adjustments provided in the manufacturer's labeling.
Dialysis-dependent impairment: There are no specific dosage adjustments provided in the manufacturer's labeling; however, a dosage adjustment may be needed since clearance is reduced by ~50%.
Depot injection:
Mild to severe impairment: No dosage adjustment necessary.
Dialysis-dependent impairment: Initial dose: 10 mg IM every 4 weeks; titrate based upon response (clearance is reduced by ~50%)

Hepatic Impairment
Regular injection: There are no dosage adjustments provided in the manufacturer's labeling. Half-life is prolonged and total body clearance is decreased in patients with cirrhosis and fatty liver disease.
Depot injection: Patients with established cirrhosis of the liver: Initial dose: 10 mg IM every 4 weeks; titrate based upon response.

Dietary Considerations Schedule injections between meals to decrease GI effects. May alter absorption of dietary fats.

Usual Infusion Concentrations: Adult IV infusion: 500 mcg in 250 mL (concentration: 2 mcg/mL) of D_5W or NS

Administration
Regular injection formulation (do not use if solution contains particles or is discolored): Administer SubQ or IV; IV administration may be IV push (undiluted over 3 minutes), intermittent IV infusion (over 15 to 30 minutes), or continuous IV infusion (off-label route). In emergency situations (eg, carcinoid crisis), octreotide may be given as a rapid IV bolus.
SubQ: Use the concentration with smallest volume to deliver dose to reduce injection site pain. Rotate injection site; may bring to room temperature prior to injection.
Depot formulation: Administer IM intragluteal (avoid deltoid administration); alternate gluteal injection sites to avoid irritation. **Do not** administer Sandostatin LAR® intravenously or subcutaneously; must be administered immediately after mixing.

Monitoring Parameters
Acromegaly: Growth hormone, somatomedin C (IGF-1)
Carcinoid: 5-HIAA, plasma serotonin and plasma substance P
VIPomas: Vasoactive intestinal peptide
Chronic therapy: Thyroid function (baseline and periodic), vitamin B_{12} level, blood glucose, glycemic control and antidiabetic regimen (patients with diabetes mellitus); cardiac function (heart rate, ECG), zinc level (patients with excessive fluid loss maintained on TPN)

Reference Range Vasoactive intestinal peptide: <75 ng/L; levels vary considerably between laboratories

Dosage Forms Excipient information presented when available (limited, particularly for generics); consult specific product labeling.
Kit, Intramuscular:
SandoSTATIN LAR Depot: 10 mg, 20 mg, 30 mg
Solution, Injection:
SandoSTATIN: 50 mcg/mL (1 mL); 100 mcg/mL (1 mL)
SandoSTATIN: 200 mcg/mL (5 mL) [contains phenol]
SandoSTATIN: 500 mcg/mL (1 mL)
SandoSTATIN: 1000 mcg/mL (5 mL) [contains phenol]

Generic: 50 mcg/mL (1 mL); 100 mcg/mL (1 mL); 200 mcg/mL (5 mL); 1000 mcg/5 mL (5 mL); 500 mcg/mL (1 mL); 1000 mcg/mL (5 mL)
Solution, Injection [preservative free]:
Generic: 100 mcg/mL (1 mL); 500 mcg/mL (1 mL)

◆ Octreotide Acetate *see* Octreotide *on page 1308*
◆ Octreotide Acetate Omega (Can) *see* Octreotide *on page 1308*
◆ Octreotide Injection (Can) *see* Octreotide *on page 1308*
◆ Ocudox [DSC] *see* Doxycycline *on page 601*
◆ Ocufen *see* Flurbiprofen (Ophthalmic) *on page 791*
◆ Ocuflox *see* Ofloxacin (Ophthalmic) *on page 1314*
◆ Ocuflox® (Can) *see* Ofloxacin (Ophthalmic) *on page 1314*
◆ Odan-Naphazoline (Can) *see* Naphazoline (Ophthalmic) *on page 1256*
◆ Odan-Timol (Can) *see* Timolol (Ophthalmic) *on page 1790*
◆ O-desmethylvenlafaxine *see* Desvenlafaxine *on page 524*
◆ Odomzo *see* Sonidegib *on page 1690*
◆ ODV *see* Desvenlafaxine *on page 524*
◆ Oesclim (Can) *see* Estradiol (Systemic) *on page 681*

Ofatumumab (oh fa TOOM yoo mab)

Brand Names: US Arzerra
Brand Names: Canada Arzerra
Index Terms HuMax-CD20
Pharmacologic Category Antineoplastic Agent, Anti-CD20; Antineoplastic Agent, Monoclonal Antibody
Use
Chronic lymphocytic leukemia (CLL), previously untreated: Treatment of previously untreated CLL (in combination with chlorambucil) when fludarabine-based therapy is considered inappropriate
Chronic lymphocytic leukemia (CLL), refractory: Treatment of CLL refractory to fludarabine and alemtuzumab
Pregnancy Considerations Teratogenicity was not observed in animal reproduction studies, although prolonged depletion of circulating B cells was observed in animal offspring. The Canadian labeling recommends women of childbearing potential avoid pregnancy during and for 6 months after the last treatment.
Breast-Feeding Considerations It is not known if ofatumumab is excreted in human milk. However, human IgG is excreted in breast milk, and therefore, ofatumumab may also be excreted in milk. The effects of local GI and systemic exposure are unknown, therefore caution should be used in nursing women receiving ofatumumab.
Contraindications
U.S. labeling: There are no contraindications listed in the manufacturer's labeling.
Canadian labeling: Hypersensitivity to ofatumumab or any component of the formulation; presence or history of progressive multifocal leukoencephalopathy.
Warnings/Precautions [US Boxed Warning]: Hepatitis B virus (HBV) reactivation may occur in patients receiving CD20-directed antibody treatment, including ofatumumab; may result in fulminant hepatitis, hepatic failure, and death. Fatal cases of HBV have also occurred in patients not previously infected with HBV. Prior to initiating therapy, obtain hepatitis B surface antigen (HBsAg) and hepatitis B core antibody (anti-HBc) measurements in all patients; monitor for clinical and laboratory signs of hepatitis or HBV during and for several months after treatment. HBV reactivation has been reported up to 12 months after therapy discontinuation. Discontinue ofatumumab (and concomitant medications) if viral hepatitis develops and initiate appropriate antiviral therapy. Reactivation has occurred in patients who are HBsAg positive as well as in those who are HBsAg negative but are anti-HBc positive; HBV reactivation has also been observed in patients who had previously resolved HBV infection. Use cautiously in patients who show evidence of prior HBV infection (eg, HBsAg positive [regardless of antibody status] or HBsAG negative but anti-HBc positive); consult with appropriate clinicians regarding monitoring and consideration of antiviral therapy before and/or during ofatumumab treatment. The safety of resuming ofatumumab treatment following HBV reactivation is not known; discuss reinitiation of therapy in patients with resolved HBV reactivation with physicians experienced in HBV management. Bacterial, fungal, and other new or reactivated viral infections may occur during and/or following therapy; monitor closely for signs/symptoms of infection. Discontinue therapy for serious infections and treat appropriately.

American Society of Clinical Oncology (ASCO) provisional clinical opinion update on hepatitis B virus screening [Hwang, 2015]) recommendations: Patients receiving anti-CD20 antibodies are at high risk for hepatitis B virus (HBV) reactivation. Screen for HBV infection with hepatitis B surface antigen (HBsAG) and hepatitis B core antibody (anti-HBc) tests prior to treatment initiation; either a total anti-HBc (with both IgG and IgM) or anti-HBc IgG test should be used to screen for chronic or unresolved HBV infection (do not use anti-HBc IgM as it may only confirm acute HBV infection). In addition, patients who have risk factors for HBV infection (eg, birthplace in a country with ≥2% HBV prevalence, household or sexual contact with HBV infected patients, high-risk behaviors [eg, intravenous drug use], and HIV infection) should also be screened prior to beginning therapy. Initiate prophylactic antiviral therapy (utilizing antivirals with low rates of viral resistance) for HBsAg positive/anti-HBc positive patients (without delaying cancer therapy) and continue the antivirals during and for ~6 to 12 months after completing treatment. HBsAg negative/anti-HBc positive patients should be monitored for HBV reactivation with HBV DNA and ALT testing approximately every 3 months during treatment; antiviral therapy may be initiated prophylactically or begun promptly at the first sign of HBV reactivation.

May cause serious infusion reaction (some fatal); reactions may include bronchospasm, dyspnea, laryngeal edema, pulmonary edema, flushing, hypertension, hypotension, syncope, cardiac ischemia/infarction, acute coronary syndrome, arrhythmia, bradycardia, back pain, abdominal pain, fever, rash, urticaria, angioedema, cytokine release syndrome, and/or anaphylactoid/anaphylactic reactions. Infusion reactions occur more frequently with the first 2 infusions and may occur despite premedication. Premedicate prior to infusion with acetaminophen, an antihistamine, and a corticosteroid. Interrupt infusion for reaction of any severity and institute appropriate treatment; may require subsequent rate modification. Discontinue immediately and permanently if anaphylactic reaction occurs. Bowel obstruction and abdominal pain have been reported; patients presenting with abdominal pain should be assessed for presence of obstruction and treated appropriately.

[US Boxed Warning]: Progressive multifocal leukoencephalopathy (PML) resulting in death may occur with CD20-directed antibody treatment, including ofatumumab. Consider PML in any patient with new onset or worsening neurological symptoms, and if suspected, discontinue ofatumumab and evaluate promptly. Severe and prolonged (≥1 week) cytopenias (neutropenia, thrombocytopenia, and anemia) may occur. Grade 3 or 4 late-onset neutropenia (onset ≥42 days after last treatment dose) and/or prolonged neutropenia (not resolved 24 to 42 days after last dose) has been reported. Pancytopenia, agranulocytosis, and fatal neutropenic sepsis have occurred when used in combination with chlorambucil. Monitor blood counts regularly during and after treatment; more frequently if grade 3 or 4 cytopenias develop. Tumor lysis syndrome (TLS) has occurred in patients receiving ofatumumab; patients with a high tumor burden and/or high circulating lymphocyte counts (>25,000/mm³) are at increased risk for TLS. Administer prophylactic antihyperuricemic therapy and aggressive hydration beginning 12 to 24 hours prior to ofatumumab treatment. Correct electrolyte abnormalities; monitor renal function and hydration status.

Potentially significant drug-drug interactions may exist, requiring dose or frequency adjustment, additional monitoring, and/or selection of alternative therapy. Live vaccines should not be given to patients who have recently received ofatumumab; there is no data concerning secondary transmission; the ability to generate an immune response to any vaccine following treatment is unknown. Patients ≥65 years experienced a higher incidence of adverse reactions (compared with younger patients).

Adverse Reactions
>10%:
Central nervous system: Fatigue (15%)
Dermatologic: Skin rash (14%)
Gastrointestinal: Diarrhea (18%), nausea (11%)
Hematologic & oncologic: Neutropenia (≥ grade 3: 42%; grade 4: 18%; may be prolonged >2 weeks), anemia (16%; grades 3/4: 5%)
Infection: Infection (70%; includes bacterial, fungal, or viral; ≥ grade 3: 29%)
Respiratory: Pneumonia (23%), cough (19%), dyspnea (14%), bronchitis (11%), upper respiratory tract infection (11%)
Miscellaneous: Infusion related reaction (first infusion [300 mg]: 44%; second infusion [2000 mg]: 29%), fever (20%)

1% to 10%:
Cardiovascular: Peripheral edema (9%), hypertension (5%), hypotension (5%), tachycardia (5%)
Central nervous system: Chills (8%), insomnia (7%), headache (6%)
Dermatologic: Urticaria (8%), hyperhidrosis (5%)
Infection: Sepsis (8%), herpes zoster (6%)
Neuromuscular & skeletal: Back pain (8%), muscle spasm (5%)
Respiratory: Nasopharyngitis (8%), sinusitis (5%)
<1% (Limited to important or life-threatening): Angina pectoris, bacteremia, hemolytic anemia, hepatitis B (new onset or reactivation), hepatitis (cytolytic), hypoxia, interstitial pulmonary disease (infectious), intestinal obstruction, peritonitis, progressive multifocal leukoencephalopathy (PML), rigors, sepsis (neutropenic), septic shock, thrombocytopenia

Drug Interactions
Metabolism/Transport Effects None known.
Avoid Concomitant Use
Avoid concomitant use of Ofatumumab with any of the following: BCG (Intravesical); Belimumab; Natalizumab; Pimecrolimus; Tacrolimus (Topical); Tofacitinib; Vaccines (Live)

Increased Effect/Toxicity
Ofatumumab may increase the levels/effects of: Belimumab; Fingolimod; Leflunomide; Natalizumab; Tofacitinib; Vaccines (Live)

The levels/effects of Ofatumumab may be increased by: Denosumab; Pimecrolimus; Roflumilast; Tacrolimus (Topical); Trastuzumab

Decreased Effect
Ofatumumab may decrease the levels/effects of: BCG (Intravesical); Coccidioides immitis Skin Test; Sipuleucel-T; Vaccines (Inactivated); Vaccines (Live)

The levels/effects of Ofatumumab may be decreased by: Echinacea

Preparation for Administration Prepare all doses in 1000 mL NS. Begin infusion within 12 hours of preparation.
300 mg dose: Withdraw 15 mL from a 1000 mL NS bag. Add contents of 3 ofatumumab 100 mg vials to NS bag. Gently invert to mix; do not shake.
1000 mg dose: Withdraw 50 mL from a 1000 mL NS bag. Add contents of 1 ofatumumab 1000 mg vial. Gently invert to mix; do not shake.
2000 mg dose: Withdraw 100 mL from a 1000 mL NS bag. Add contents of 2 ofatumumab 1000 mg vials to NS bag. Gently invert to mix; do not shake.

Storage/Stability Store intact vials at 2°C to 8°C (36°F to 46°F); do not freeze. Protect from light. Diluted solutions for infusion must be started within 12 hours of preparation (may store at 2°C to 8°C [36°F to 46°F] if not used immediately); discard any remaining solution 24 hours after preparation.

Mechanism of Action Ofatumumab is a monoclonal antibody which binds specifically the extracellular (large and small) loops of the CD20 molecule (which is expressed on normal B lymphocytes and in B-cell CLL) resulting in potent complement-dependent cell lysis and antibody-dependent cell-mediated toxicity in cells that overexpress CD20.

Pharmacodynamics/Kinetics
Distribution: V_{dss}: 5.7 L (following repeated infusions)
Half-life elimination: 15.6 days (following repeated infusions)

Dosing
Adult & Geriatric Note: Premedicate with acetaminophen, an antihistamine, and a corticosteroid 30 to 120 minutes prior to treatment (see Administration).
Chronic lymphocytic leukemia (CLL), previously untreated: IV: Cycle 1 (cycle is 28 days): 300 mg on day 1, followed by 1000 mg on day 8; Subsequent cycles: 1000 mg on day 1 every 28 days; continue for at least 3 cycles until best response or a maximum of 12 cycles (in combination with chlorambucil)
CLL, refractory: IV: Initial dose: 300 mg week 1, followed 1 week later by 2000 mg once weekly for 7 doses (doses 2 to 8), followed 4 weeks later by 2000 mg once every 4 weeks for 4 doses (doses 9 to 12; for a total of 12 doses)

Renal Impairment
Mild or moderate impairment: There are no dosage adjustments provided in the U.S. manufacturer's labeling; however, there were no clinically relevant pharmacokinetic effects observed in patients with baseline CrCl ≥30 mL/minute. The Canadian labeling recommends that no dosage adjustment is necessary for CrCl >30 mL/minute.
Severe impairment: There are no dosage adjustments provided in the manufacturer's labeling.

Hepatic Impairment There are no dosage adjustments provided in the manufacturer's labeling (has not been studied).

Adjustment for Toxicity Infusion reaction: Interrupt infusion for infusion reaction (any severity). If the reaction resolves or remains at ≤ grade 2, resume with the following modifications (based on the grade of the initial reaction):

Grade 1 or 2 infusion reaction:

U.S. labeling: Resume at one-half of the previous rate; may increase (see Administration) based on patient tolerance.

Canadian labeling: Resume at one-half of the previous rate; may increase (see Administration) based on patient tolerance. If the infusion rate had not been increased above 12 mL/hour prior to interrupting therapy, resume infusion at 12 mL/hour; may then increase based on patient tolerance.

Grade 3 or 4 infusion reaction: Resume infusion at 12 mL/hour; may increase (see Administration) based on patient tolerance.

If reaction severity does not resolve to ≤ grade 2 despite management: Consider permanent discontinuation

Anaphylactic reaction: Discontinue permanently

Administration Do not administer IV push, IV bolus, or as a subcutaneous injection. Premedicate with acetaminophen, an antihistamine, and a corticosteroid 30 to 120 minutes prior to administration. Infuse in an environment equipped to monitor for and manage infusion reactions. Administer with infusion pump and administration set. Do not exceed infusion rates below. Do not mix with or infuse with other medications. Flush line before and after infusion with NS. Begin infusion within 12 hours of preparation. Interrupt infusion for any severity of infusion reaction; if the reaction resolves or remains at ≤ grade 2, may resume infusion (see Dosage Adjustment for Toxicity).

Previously untreated chronic lymphocytic leukemia:

Premedication: Premedicate with oral acetaminophen (1000 mg) or equivalent, an oral or IV antihistamine (eg, diphenhydramine 50 mg or cetirizine 10 mg orally or equivalent), and an IV corticosteroid (prednisolone 50 mg or equivalent). Full dose corticosteroid is recommended for the first 2 infusions; in the absence of infusion reaction ≥ grade 3, may gradually reduce or omit corticosteroid dose for subsequent infusions.

Cycle 1, day 1: Initiate infusion at 12 mL/hour for 30 minutes, if tolerated (no infusion reaction) increase to 25 mL/hour for 30 minutes, if tolerated, increase to 50 mL/hour for 30 minutes, if tolerated, increase to 100 mL/hour for 30 minutes, if tolerated, increase to 200 mL/hour for 30 minutes, if tolerated increase to 300 mL/hour for 30 minutes, if tolerated, increase to 400 mL/hour for remainder of infusion. Median duration of infusion: 5.2 hours.

Cycle 1, day 8 and cycles 2 to 12 (if no reaction to previous infusion): Initiate infusion at 25 mL/hour for 30 minutes, if tolerated (no infusion reaction) increase to 50 mL/hour for 30 minutes, if tolerated, increase to 100 mL/hour for 30 minutes, if tolerated, increase to 200 mL/hour for 30 minutes, if tolerated, increase to 400 mL/hour for remainder of infusion. Median duration of infusion: 4.2 to 4.4 hours.

Refractory chronic lymphocytic leukemia:

Premedication: Premedicate with oral acetaminophen (1000 mg) or equivalent, an oral or IV antihistamine (eg, diphenhydramine 50 mg or cetirizine 10 mg orally or equivalent), and an IV corticosteroid (prednisolone 100 mg or equivalent). Full dose corticosteroid is recommended for doses 1, 2, and 9; in the absence of infusion reaction ≥ grade 3, may gradually reduce or omit corticosteroid dose for doses 3 to 8; administer full or half corticosteroid dose with doses 10 to 12 if ≥ grade 3 reaction did not occur with dose 9.

Doses 1 and 2: Initiate infusion at 12 mL/hour for 30 minutes, if tolerated (no infusion reaction) increase to 25 mL/hour for 30 minutes, if tolerated, increase to 50 mL/hour for 30 minutes, if tolerated, increase to 100 mL/hour for 30 minutes, if tolerated, increase to 200 mL/hour for remainder of infusion. Median duration of infusion: 6.8 hours.

Doses 3 to 12: Initiate infusion at 25 mL/hour for 30 minutes, if tolerated (no infusion reaction) increase to 50 mL/hour for 30 minutes, if tolerated, increase to 100 mL/hour for 30 minutes, if tolerated, increase to 200 mL/hour for 30 minutes, if tolerated, increase to 400 mL/hour for remainder of infusion. Median duration of infusion: 4.2 to 4.4 hours.

Monitoring Parameters CBC with differential, renal function, electrolytes

Hepatitis B virus screening recommendations (ASCO provisional clinical opinion update [Hwang, 2015]): Screen for hepatitis B virus (HBV) infection with hepatitis B surface antigen (HBsAG) and hepatitis B core antibody (anti-HBc) tests prior to treatment initiation; either a total anti-HBc (with both IgG and IgM) or anti-HBc IgG test should be used to screen for chronic or unresolved HBV infection (do not use anti-HBc IgM as it may only confirm acute HBV infection). HBsAg negative/anti-HBc positive patients should be monitored for HBV reactivation with HBV DNA and ALT testing approximately every 3 months during treatment.

Signs of active hepatitis B infection (during and for up to 12 months after therapy completion); signs or symptoms of infusion reaction; signs of infection; fluid status; signs/symptoms of intestinal obstruction (eg, abdominal pain, repeated vomiting); signs/symptoms of progressive multifocal leukoencephalopathy (focal neurologic deficits, which may present as hemiparesis, visual field deficits, cognitive impairment, aphasia, ataxia, and/or cranial nerve deficits).

Dosage Forms Excipient information presented when available (limited, particularly for generics); consult specific product labeling.

Concentrate, Intravenous [preservative free]:

Arzerra: 100 mg/5 mL (5 mL); 1000 mg/50 mL (50 mL) [contains edetate disodium, mouse protein (murine) (hamster), polysorbate 80]

◆ Ofev see Nintedanib on page 1284

◆ Ofirmev see Acetaminophen on page 25

Ofloxacin (Systemic) (oh FLOKS a sin)

Brand Names: Canada Apo-Oflox; Novo-Ofloxacin

Pharmacologic Category Antibiotic, Fluoroquinolone

Use

Treatment of acute exacerbations of chronic bronchitis, community-acquired pneumonia, skin and skin structure infections (uncomplicated), urethral and cervical gonorrhea (acute, uncomplicated), urethritis and cervicitis (nongonococcal), mixed infections of the urethra and cervix, pelvic inflammatory disease (acute), cystitis (uncomplicated), urinary tract infections (complicated), prostatitis

Note: As of April 2007, the CDC no longer recommends the use of fluoroquinolones for the treatment of gonococcal disease.

Medication Guide Available Yes

Dosing

Adult & Geriatric

Cervicitis/urethritis (nongonococcal): Oral:

Nongonococcal: 300 mg every 12 hours for 7 days

Gonococcal (acute, uncomplicated): 400 mg as a single dose; **Note:** As of April 2007, the CDC no longer recommends the use of fluoroquinolones for the treatment of uncomplicated gonococcal disease.

Chronic bronchitis (acute exacerbation), community-acquired pneumonia, skin and skin structure infections (uncomplicated): Oral: 400 mg every 12 hours for 10 days

Pelvic inflammatory disease (acute): Oral: 400 mg every 12 hours for 10 to 14 days; **Note:** The CDC recommends use only if standard cephalosporin therapy is not feasible and community prevalence of quinolone-resistant gonococcal organisms is low. Culture sensitivity must be confirmed.

Prostatitis: Oral: 300 mg every 12 hours for 6 weeks

UTI: Oral:

Uncomplicated: 200 mg every 12 hours for 3 to 7 days

Complicated: 200 mg every 12 hours for 10 days

Epididymitis, nongonococcal (off-label use): Oral: 300 mg twice daily for 10 days (CDC, 2010); 200 mg twice daily for 14 days (Canadian STI Guidelines 2008)

Leprosy (multibacillary) (off-label use): Oral: 400 mg once daily (in combination with dapsone and rifampin) for 12 months (WHO 2012) **or** alternatively, 400 mg once monthly (in combination with monthly rifampin and minocycline) for 24 months (Villahermosa 2004; WHO 1998; WHO 2012).

Leprosy (paucibacillary) (off-label use):

Multiple-dose regimen: 400 mg once daily (in combination with rifampin) for 4 weeks (Balagon 2010).

Single-dose regimen: 400 mg as a single dose (in combination with single doses of rifampin and minocycline) (Manickam 2012). **Note:** Found to be less effective than standard WHO multiple drug therapy (WHO-MDT) for paucibacillary leprosy; should only be used if close follow-up of relapse is possible (Manickam 2012; Setia 2011).

Traveler's diarrhea (off-label use): Oral: 200 mg twice daily for 3 days (Hill 2006)

Renal Impairment Adults: Oral: After a normal initial dose, adjust as follows:

CrCl >50 mL/minute: No dosage adjustment necessary.

CrCl 20 to 50 mL/minute: Administer usual recommended dose every 24 hours.

CrCl <20 mL/minute: Administer half the usual recommended dose every 24 hours.

Intermittent hemodialysis (IHD): 100 to 200 mg after dialysis (Aronoff 2007)

Peritoneal dialysis: 200 mg every 24 hours (Aronoff 2007)

Continuous renal replacement therapy (CRRT): 300 mg every 24 hours (Aronoff 2007)

Hepatic Impairment

Mild to moderate impairment: There are no dosage adjustments provided in the manufacturer's labeling; use with caution.

Severe impairment (eg, cirrhosis with or without ascites): Maximum dose: 400 mg/day

Additional Information Complete prescribing information should be consulted for additional detail.

Dosage Forms Excipient information presented when available (limited, particularly for generics); consult specific product labeling. [DSC] = Discontinued product

Tablet, Oral:

Generic: 200 mg [DSC], 300 mg [DSC], 400 mg

Ofloxacin (Ophthalmic) (oh FLOKS a sin)

Brand Names: US Ocuflox

Brand Names: Canada Ocuflox®

Pharmacologic Category Antibiotic, Fluoroquinolone; Antibiotic, Ophthalmic

Use Treatment of superficial ocular infections involving the conjunctiva or cornea due to strains of susceptible organisms

Dosing

Adult

Conjunctivitis: Ophthalmic: Instill 1-2 drops in affected eye(s) every 2-4 hours for the first 2 days, then use 4 times/day for an additional 5 days.

Corneal ulcer: Ophthalmic: Instill 1-2 drops every 30 minutes while awake and every 4-6 hours after retiring for the first 2 days; beginning on day 3, instill 1-2 drops every hour while awake for 4-6 additional days; thereafter, 1-2 drops 4 times/day until clinical cure.

Pediatric

Conjunctivitis: Ophthalmic: Children ≥1 year: Refer to adult dosing.

Corneal ulcer: Ophthalmic: Children ≥1 year: Refer to adult dosing.

Renal Impairment No dosage adjustment provided in manufacturer's labeling. However, dosage adjustment unlikely due to low systemic absorption.

Hepatic Impairment No dosage adjustment provided in manufacturer's labeling. However, dosage adjustment unlikely due to low systemic absorption.

Additional Information Complete prescribing information should be consulted for additional detail.

Dosage Forms Excipient information presented when available (limited, particularly for generics); consult specific product labeling.

Solution, Ophthalmic:

Ocuflox: 0.3% (5 mL) [contains benzalkonium chloride]

Generic: 0.3% (5 mL, 10 mL)

Ofloxacin (Otic) (oh FLOKS a sin)

Index Terms Floxin Otic Singles

Pharmacologic Category Antibiotic, Fluoroquinolone; Antibiotic, Otic

Use Otitis externa, chronic suppurative otitis media, acute otitis media

Dosing

Adult

Otitis media, chronic suppurative with perforated tympanic membranes: Otic: Instill 10 drops (or the contents of 2 single-dose containers) into affected ear twice daily for 14 days

Otitis externa: Otic: Instill 10 drops (or the contents of 2 single-dose containers) into affected ear(s) once daily for 7 days

Pediatric Not for systemic use.

Acute otitis media with tympanotomy tubes: Otic: Children 1-12 years: Instill 5 drops (or the contents of 1 single-dose container) into affected ear twice daily for 10 days.

Otitis externa: Otic:

Children 6 months to 13 years: Instill 5 drops (or the contents of 1 single-dose container) into affected ear(s) once daily for 7 days

Children ≥13 years: Refer to adult dosing.

Otitis media, chronic suppurative with perforated tympanic membranes: Otic: Children >12 years: Refer to adult dosing.

Renal Impairment No dosage adjustment provided in manufacturer's labeling. However, dosage adjustment unlikely due to low systemic absorption.

Hepatic Impairment No dosage adjustment provided in manufacturer's labeling. However, dosage adjustment unlikely due to low systemic absorption.

Additional Information Complete prescribing information should be consulted for additional detail.

Dosage Forms Excipient information presented when available (limited, particularly for generics); consult specific product labeling.

Solution, Otic:

Generic: 0.3% (5 mL, 10 mL)

OLANZapine (oh LAN za peen)

Brand Names: US ZyPREXA; ZyPREXA Relprevv; ZyPREXA Zydis

Brand Names: Canada Abbott-Olanzapine ODT; Accel-Olanzapine; ACT Olanzapine; ACT Olanzapine ODT; Apo-Olanzapine; Apo-Olanzapine ODT; JAMP-Olanzapine ODT; Mar-Olanzapine; Mar-Olanzapine ODT; Mint-Olanzapine ODT; Mylan-Olanzapine; Mylan-Olanzapine ODT; Olanzapine for injection; Olanzapine ODT; PHL-Olanzapine; PHL-Olanzapine ODT; PMS-Olanzapine; PMS-Olanzapine ODT; RAN-Olanzapine; RAN-Olanzapine ODT; Riva-Olanzapine; Riva-Olanzapine ODT; Sandoz-Olanzapine; Sandoz-Olanzapine ODT; Teva-Olanzapine; Teva-Olanzapine OD; Zyprexa; Zyprexa Intramuscular; Zyprexa Zydis

Index Terms LY170053; Olanzapine Pamoate; Zyprexa Zydis

Pharmacologic Category Antimanic Agent; Second Generation (Atypical) Antipsychotic

Use

Oral: Treatment of the manifestations of schizophrenia; treatment of acute or mixed mania episodes associated with bipolar I disorder (as monotherapy or in combination with lithium or valproate); maintenance treatment of bipolar I disorder; in combination with fluoxetine for treatment-resistant or bipolar I depression

IM, extended-release (Zyprexa Relprevv): Treatment of schizophrenia

IM, short-acting (Zyprexa IntraMuscular): Treatment of acute agitation associated with schizophrenia and bipolar I mania

Pregnancy Considerations Adverse events were observed in animal reproduction studies. Olanzapine crosses the placenta and can be detected in cord blood at birth (Newport 2007). Information related to olanzapine use in pregnancy is limited (Goldstein 2000). Antipsychotic use during the third trimester of pregnancy has a risk for abnormal muscle movements (extrapyramidal symptoms [EPS] and/or withdrawal symptoms in newborns following delivery. Symptoms in the newborn may include agitation, feeding disorder, hypertonia, hypotonia, respiratory distress, somnolence, and tremor; these effects may be self-limiting or require hospitalization. Olanzapine may cause hyperprolactinemia, which may decrease reproductive function in both males and females.

The ACOG recommends that therapy during pregnancy be individualized; treatment with psychiatric medications during pregnancy should incorporate the clinical expertise of the mental health clinician, obstetrician, primary healthcare provider, and pediatrician. Safety data related to atypical antipsychotics during pregnancy is limited and routine use is not recommended. However, if a woman is inadvertently exposed to an atypical antipsychotic while pregnant, continuing therapy may be preferable to switching to a typical antipsychotic that the fetus has not yet been exposed to; consider risk:benefit (ACOG 2008). Evaluate risk factors for gestational diabetes and weight gain if considering use of olanzapine in a pregnant woman (NICE 2007).

Healthcare providers are encouraged to enroll women 18 to 45 years of age exposed to olanzapine during pregnancy in the Atypical Antipsychotics Pregnancy Registry (1-866-961-2388 or http://www.womensmentalhealth.org/pregnancyregistry).

Breast-Feeding Considerations Olanzapine is excreted into breast milk. At steady-state concentrations, it is estimated that a breast-fed infant may be exposed to ~2% of the maternal dose. In one study, the median time to peak milk concentration was ~5 hours after the maternal dose and serum concentrations in the nursing infants were low (<5 ng/mL; n=5) (Gardiner 2003). An increased risk of adverse events in nursing infants has not been reported (Gardiner 2003; Gilad 2011). Breast-feeding is not recommended by the manufacturer.

Prescribing and Access Restrictions As a requirement of the REMS program, only prescribers, healthcare facilities, and pharmacies registered with the Zyprexa Relprevv Patient Care Program are able to prescribe, distribute, or dispense Zyprexa Relprevv for patients who are enrolled in and meet all conditions of the program. Zyprexa Relprevv must be administered at a registered healthcare facility. Prescribers will need to be recertified every 3 years. Contact the Zyprexa Relprevv Patient Care Program at 1-877-772-9390.

Medication Guide Available Yes

Contraindications There are no contraindications listed in the manufacturer's labeling.

Canadian labeling: Hypersensitivity to olanzapine or any component of the formulation

Warnings/Precautions [US Boxed Warning]: Elderly patients with dementia-related psychosis treated with antipsychotics are at an increased risk of death compared with placebo. Most deaths appeared to be either cardiovascular (eg, heart failure, sudden death) or infectious (eg, pneumonia) in nature. In addition, an increased incidence of cerebrovascular effects (eg, transient ischemic attack, stroke) has been reported in studies of placebo-controlled trials of olanzapine in elderly patients with dementia-related psychosis. Use with caution in dementia with Lewy bodies; antipsychotics may worsen dementia symptoms and patients with dementia with Lewy bodies are more sensitive to the extrapyramidal side effects (APA, [Rabins 2007]). Olanzapine is not approved for the treatment of dementia-related psychosis.

May cause CNS depression, which impair physical and mental abilities; patients must be cautioned about performing tasks that require mental alertness (eg, operating machinery, driving). May be moderate to highly sedating in comparison with other antipsychotics (APA [Lehman 2004]); dose-related effects have been observed. Use caution in patients with cardiac disease. Use with caution in Parkinson disease, predisposition to seizures, or severe hepatic or renal disease. Life-threatening arrhythmias have occurred with therapeutic doses of some neuroleptics. May induce orthostatic hypotension; use caution with history of cardiovascular disease, hemodynamic instability, prior myocardial infarction, or ischemic heart disease. Dose-related increases in cholesterol and triglycerides have been noted. Use with caution in patients with preexisting abnormal lipid profile. Esophageal dysmotility and aspiration have been associated with antipsychotic use; use with caution in patients at risk of aspiration pneumonia. May cause dose-related increases in prolactin levels; clinical significance of hyperprolactinemia in patients with breast cancer or other prolactin-dependent tumors is unknown. Clinical manifestations of increased prolactin levels included menstrual-, sexual- and breast-related events. Significant dose-related weight gain (>7% of baseline weight) may occur; monitor waist circumference and BMI. Impaired core body temperature regulation may occur; caution with strenuous exercise, heat exposure, dehydration, and concomitant medication possessing anticholinergic effects.

Leukopenia, neutropenia, and agranulocytosis (sometimes fatal) have been reported in clinical trials and postmarketing reports with antipsychotic use; presence of risk factors (eg, preexisting low WBC or history of drug-induced leuko-/neutropenia) should prompt periodic blood count assessment. Discontinue therapy at first signs of blood dyscrasias or if absolute neutrophil count <1,000/mm^3.

May cause anticholinergic effects; use with caution in patients with decreased gastrointestinal motility, urinary retention, BPH, xerostomia, or narrow-angle glaucoma. Relative to other neuroleptics, olanzapine has a moderate potency of cholinergic blockade. May cause extrapyramidal symptoms (EPS), although risk of these reactions is lower relative to other neuroleptics. Risk of dystonia (and probably other EPS) may be greater with increased doses, use of conventional antipsychotics, males, and younger

patients. May be associated with neuroleptic malignant syndrome (NMS). May cause extreme and life-threatening hyperglycemia; use with caution in patients with diabetes or other disorders of glucose regulation; monitor. Olanzapine levels may be lower in patients who smoke. Smokers may require a daily dose 30% higher than nonsmokers in order to obtain an equivalent olanzapine concentration (Tsuda 2014); however, the manufacturer does not routinely recommend dosage adjustments.

Use in adolescent patients ≥13 years of age may result in increased weight gain and sedation, as well as greater increases in LDL cholesterol, total cholesterol, triglycerides, prolactin, and liver transaminase levels when compared with adults. Adolescent patients should be maintained on the lowest dose necessary. Use in elderly patients with dementia is associated with an increased risk of mortality and cerebrovascular accidents; avoid antipsychotic use for behavioral problems associated with dementia unless alternative nonpharmacologic therapies have failed and patient may harm self or others. In addition, use may cause or exacerbate syndrome of inappropriate antidiuretic hormone secretion or hyponatremia; monitor sodium closely with initiation or dosage adjustments in older adults. May also be inappropriate in older adults depending on comorbidities (eg, dementia, delirium) due to its potent anticholinergic effects (Beers Criteria).

The possibility of a suicide attempt is inherent in psychotic illness or bipolar disorder; use caution in high-risk patients during initiation of therapy. Prescriptions should be written for the smallest quantity consistent with good patient care.

Some dosage forms may contain polysorbate 80 (also known as Tweens). Hypersensitivity reactions, usually a delayed reaction, have been reported following exposure to pharmaceutical products containing polysorbate 80 in certain individuals (Isaksson 2002; Lucente 2000; Shelley 1995). Thrombocytopenia, ascites, pulmonary deterioration, and renal and hepatic failure have been reported in premature neonates after receiving parenteral products containing polysorbate 80 (Alade 1986; CDC 1984). See manufacturer's labeling.

There are two Zyprexa formulations for intramuscular injection: Zyprexa Relprevv is an extended-release formulation and Zyprexa Intramuscular is short-acting:

Extended-release IM injection (Zyprexa Relprevv): **[US Boxed Warning]: Sedation (including coma) and delirium (including agitation, anxiety, confusion, disorientation) have been observed following use of *Zyprexa Relprevv*.** Administer at a registered health care facility where patients should be continuously monitored (≥3 hours) for symptoms of olanzapine overdose; symptom development highest in first hour but may occur within or after 3 hours; risk of syndrome is cumulative with each injection; recovery expected by 72 hours. Upon determining alert status, patient should be escorted to their destination and not drive or operate heavy machinery for the remainder of the day.

Two unexplained deaths in patients who received *Zyprexa Relprevv* have been reported. The patients died 3 to 4 days after receiving an appropriate dose of the drug. Both patients were found to have high blood concentrations of olanzapine postmortem. It is unclear if these deaths were the result of postinjection delirium sedation syndrome (PDSS) (FDA Safety Communication 2013).

Zyprexa Relprevv is only available under a restricted distribution program. Only prescribers, health care facilities, and pharmacies registered with the program are able to prescribe, distribute, or dispense *Zyprexa Relprevv* for patients who are enrolled in and meet all conditions of the program.

Short-acting IM injection (Zyprexa IntraMuscular): Patients should remain recumbent if drowsy/dizzy until hypotension, bradycardia, and/or hypoventilation have been ruled out. Concurrent use of IM/IV benzodiazepines is not recommended (fatalities have been reported, though causality not determined).

Adverse Reactions

Oral: Unless otherwise noted, adverse events are reported for placebo-controlled trials in adult patients on monotherapy:

>10%:

Cardiovascular: Orthostatic hypotension (3% to ≥20%)

Central nervous system: Drowsiness (dose dependent; adolescents and adults 20% to 39%), extrapyramidal reaction (dose dependent; adults ≤32%; adolescents ≤10%), akathisia (adolescents and adults 3% to 27%), parkinsonian-like syndrome (14% to 20%; includes akinesia, cogwheel rigidity, extrapyramidal syndrome, hypertonia, hypokinesia, maked facies, and tremor), dizziness (adults 11% to 18%; adolescents 7% to 8%),

headache (adolescents 17%), fatigue (dose dependent; adolescents and adults 2% to 14%), insomnia (12%)

Endocrine & metabolic: Increased serum prolactin (adolescents 47%; adults 30%), weight gain (adults 5% to 6%; has been reported as high as 40%; adolescents 29% to 31%)

Gastrointestinal: Increased appetite (adolescents 17% to 29%; adults 3% to 6%), xerostomia (dose dependent; adults 3% to 22%; adolescents 4% to 7%), dyspepsia (adults 7% to 11%; adolescents 3%), constipation (adolescents and adults 4% to 11%)

Hepatic: Increased serum AST (adolescents 28%), decreased serum bilirubin (adolescents 22%), increased serum ALT (≥3 x ULN; adolescents and adults 5% to 12%)

Neuromuscular & skeletal: Weakness (dose dependent; 8% to 20%)

Miscellaneous: Accidental injury (12%)

1% to 10%:

Cardiovascular: Chest pain (3%), peripheral edema (3%), tachycardia (3%), hypertension (2%)

Central nervous system: Personality disorder (5% to 8%), abnormal gait (6%), hypertonia (3%), restlessness (adolescents 3%), falling (older adults ≥2%), articulation impairment (2%)

Endocrine & metabolic: Increased gamma-glutamyl transferase (adolescents 10%; adults 2%), increased uric acid (4%), menstrual disease (2%; including amenorrhea, hypomenorrhea, delayed menstruation, oligomenorrhea), breast changes (male and female adolescents ≤2%; including discharge, enlargement, galactorrhea, gynecomastia, lactation disorder)

Gastrointestinal: Abdominal pain (6%; adolescents), vomiting (≤4%; adolescents), diarrhea (3%; adolescents)

Genitourinary: Urinary incontinence (adults and older adults ≥2%), sexual disorder (2%; adolescents ≤1%; anorgasmia, delayed ejaculation, erectile dysfunction, changes in libido, abnormal orgasm, sexual dysfunction), urinary tract infection (2%)

Hematologic & oncologic: Bruise (5%)

Hepatic: Increased liver enzymes (adolescents ≤8%), increased serum alkaline phosphatase (≥1%)

Neuromuscular & skeletal: Tremor (4% to 7%; dose dependent), limb pain (adolescents and adults 5% to 6%), arthralgia (adults 5%; adolescents 2%), back pain (5%), muscle rigidity (2%; adolescents), dyskinesia (1%)

Ophthalmic: Amblyopia (3%)

Respiratory: Rhinitis (7%), cough (6%), nasopharyngitis (adolescents 4%), pharyngitis (4%), epistaxis (adolescents 3%), respiratory tract infection (adolescents 3%), sinusitis (adolescents 3%)

Miscellaneous: Fever (≤6%)

<1% (Limited to important or life-threatening): Accommodation disturbance, agranulocytosis, alopecia, anaphylactoid reaction, angioedema, ataxia, cerebrovascular accident, coma, confusion, diabetes mellitus, diabetic ketoacidosis, diabetic coma, hepatic injury (cholestatic or mixed), hepatitis, hyperbilirubinemia, hypercholesterolemia, hyperglycemia, hyperlipidemia, hypertriglyceridemia, hypoproteinemia, intestinal obstruction, jaundice, ketosis, leukocytosis (eosinophilia), leukopenia, liver steatosis, myopathy, neuroleptic malignant syndrome, neutropenia, osteoporosis, pancreatitis, priapism, pulmonary edema, pulmonary embolism, rhabdomyolysis, seizure, skin rash, suicidal tendencies, syncope, tardive dyskinesia, thrombocytopenia, tongue edema, transient ischemic attacks, urticaria, venous thrombosis, withdrawal syndrome

Injection: Frequency not always defined. Unless otherwise noted, adverse events are reported for placebo-controlled trials in adult patients on extended release IM injection (Zyprexa Relprevv). Also refer to adverse reactions noted with oral therapy.

Cardiovascular: Hypertension (2% to 3%), hypotension (short-acting solution for IM injection 2%), prolonged Q-T interval on ECG (2%), orthostatic hypotension (short-acting solution for IM injection 1%)

Central nervous system: Headache (13% to 18%), sedation (8% to 13%), drowsiness (both IM injection formulations 5% to 6%), akathisia (short-acting solution for IM injection 5%), dizziness (both IM injection formulations 4%), fatigue (3% to 4%), extrapyramidal reaction (solution for IM injection 2% to 4%), abnormality in thinking (3%), auditory hallucination (3%), parkinsonian-like syndrome (short-acting solution for IM injection 3%), restlessness (3%), pain (2% to 3%), abnormal dreams (2%), procedural pain (2%), sleep disorder (2%), dysarthria (1% to 2%)

Dermatologic: Acne vulgaris (2%)

Endocrine & metabolic: Weight gain (6% to 7%)

Gastrointestinal: Diarrhea (5% to 7%), vomiting (6%), xerostomia (2% to 6%), increased appetite (1% to 6%), nausea (long-acting IM formula 4% to 5%; short-acting solution for injection <1%), tooth infection (4%), toothache (3% to 4%), abdominal pain (3%), flatulence (1% to 2%)

Genitourinary: Vaginal discharge (4%)

Hepatic: Increased liver enzymes (3% to 4%)

Infection: Viral infection (2%)

Local: Pain at injection site (both IM injection formulations 1% to 4%), abscess at injection site

Neuromuscular & skeletal: Arthralgia (3%), back pain (5%), muscle spasm (1% to 3%), stiffness (4%), tremor (long-acting IM formula 3%; short-acting solution for injection 1%)

Otic: Otalgia (4%)

Respiratory: Cough (9%), nasal congestion (7%), nasopharyngitis (3% to 6%), upper respiratory tract infection (3% to 4%), pharyngolaryngeal pain (3%), sneezing (2%)

Miscellaneous: Fever (2%)

<1% (Limited to important or life-threatening): Delirium, increased creatine phosphokinase (short-acting solution for IM injection), postinjection delirium/sedation syndrome, syncope (short-acting solution for IM injection)

Drug Interactions

Metabolism/Transport Effects Substrate of CYP1A2 (major), CYP2D6 (minor); **Note:** Assignment of Major/Minor substrate status based on clinically relevant drug interaction potential; **Inhibits** CYP1A2 (weak), CYP2C19 (weak), CYP2C9 (weak), CYP2D6 (weak)

Avoid Concomitant Use

Avoid concomitant use of OLANZapine with any of the following: Aclidinium; Amisulpride; Azelastine (Nasal); Benzodiazepines; Cimetropium; Eluxadoline; Glucagon; Glycopyrrolate; Glycopyrrolate (Oral Inhalation); Ipratropium (Oral Inhalation); Levosulpiride; Metoclopramide; Orphenadrine; Paraldehyde; Potassium Chloride; Sulpiride; Thalidomide; Tiotropium; Umeclidinium

Increased Effect/Toxicity

OLANZapine may increase the levels/effects of: AbobotulinumtoxinA; Alcohol (Ethyl); Amisulpride; Analgesics (Opioid); Anticholinergic Agents; ARIPiprazole; Azelastine (Nasal); Benzodiazepines; Buprenorphine; Cimetropium; CNS Depressants; Eluxadoline; Glucagon; Glycopyrrolate; Glycopyrrolate (Oral Inhalation); Highest Risk QTc-Prolonging Agents; Hydrocodone; Mequitazine; Methotrimeprazine; Methylphenidate; Metyrosine; Mirabegron; Mirtazapine; Moderate Risk QTc-Prolonging Agents; OnabotulinumtoxinA; Orphenadrine; Paraldehyde; Potassium Chloride; Ramosetron; RimabotulinumtoxinB; Selective Serotonin Reuptake Inhibitors; Serotonin Modulators; Sulpiride; Suvorexant; Thalidomide; Thiazide Diuretics; Tiotropium; TiZANidine; Topiramate; Zolpidem

The levels/effects of OLANZapine may be increased by: Abiraterone Acetate; Acetylcholinesterase Inhibitors (Central); Aclidinium; Blood Pressure Lowering Agents; Brimonidine (Topical); Cannabis; CYP1A2 Inhibitors (Moderate); CYP1A2 Inhibitors (Strong); Deferasirox; Doxylamine; Dronabinol; Droperidol; FluvoxaMINE; HydrOXYzine; Ipratropium (Oral Inhalation); Kava Kava; LamoTRIgine; Lithium; Magnesium Sulfate; Methotrimeprazine; Methylphenidate; Metoclopramide; Metyrosine; Mianserin; Mifepristone; Minocycline; Nabilone; Peginterferon Alfa-2b; Perampanel; Pramlintide; Rufinamide; Serotonin Modulators; Sodium Oxybate; Tapentadol; Tetrahydrocannabinol; Umeclidinium; Vemurafenib

Decreased Effect

OLANZapine may decrease the levels/effects of: Acetylcholinesterase Inhibitors; Amphetamines; Antidiabetic Agents; Anti-Parkinson's Agents (Dopamine Agonist); Gastrointestinal Agents (Prokinetic); Itopride; Levosulpiride; Quinagolide; Secretin

The levels/effects of OLANZapine may be decreased by: Acetylcholinesterase Inhibitors; Antihepaciviral Combination Products; Cannabis; CYP1A2 Inducers (Strong); Cyproterone; Lithium; Osimertinib; Ritonavir; Teriflunomide; Valproate Products

Preparation for Administration

Injection, extended-release: Dilute as directed to final concentration of 150 mg/mL. Shake vigorously to mix; will form yellow, opaque suspension. Following reconstitution, suspension may be stored at room temperature and used within 24 hours. Shake vigorously to resuspend prior to administration. Use immediately once suspension is in syringe. Suspension may be irritating to skin; wear gloves during reconstitution. Do not mix diazepam, lorazepam, or haloperidol in the same syringe.

Injection, short-acting: Reconstitute 10 mg vial with 2.1 mL SWFI. Resulting solution is ~5 mg/mL. Use immediately (within 1 hour) following reconstitution. Discard any unused portion.

Storage/Stability

Injection, extended-release: Store at controlled room temperature, not to exceed 30°C (86°F).

Injection, short-acting: Store at 20°C to 25°C (68°F to 77°F); excursions permitted to 15°C to 30°C (59°F to 86°F); do not freeze. Protect from light.

Tablet and orally disintegrating tablet: Store at 20°C to 25°C (68°F to 77°F); excursions permitted to 15°C to 30°C (59°F to 86°F). Protect from light and moisture.

Mechanism of Action
Olanzapine is a second generation thienobenzodiazepine antipsychotic which displays potent antagonism of serotonin 5-HT$_{2A}$ and 5-HT$_{2C}$, dopamine D$_{1-4}$, histamine H$_1$, and alpha$_1$-adrenergic receptors. Olanzapine shows moderate antagonism of 5-HT$_3$ and muscarinic M$_{1-5}$ receptors, and weak binding to GABA-A, BZD, and beta-adrenergic receptors. Although the precise mechanism of action in schizophrenia and bipolar disorder is not known, the efficacy of olanzapine is thought to be mediated through combined antagonism of dopamine and serotonin type 2 receptor sites.

Pharmacodynamics/Kinetics

Absorption:

Oral: Well absorbed; not affected by food; tablets and orally disintegrating tablets are bioequivalent

Short-acting injection: Rapidly absorbed

Distribution: V$_d$: Extensive, 1000 L

Protein binding, plasma: 93% bound to albumin and alpha$_1$-glycoprotein

Metabolism: Highly metabolized via direct glucuronidation and cytochrome P450 mediated oxidation (CYP1A2, CYP2D6); 40% removed via first pass metabolism

Half-life elimination: 21 to 54 hours; ~1.5 times greater in elderly; Extended-release injection: ~30 days

Time to peak, plasma: Maximum plasma concentrations after IM administration are 5 times higher than maximum plasma concentrations produced by an oral dose.

Extended-release injection: ~7 days

Short-acting injection: 15 to 45 minutes

Oral: ~6 hours

Excretion: Urine (57%, 7% as unchanged drug); feces (30%)

Clearance: 40% increase in olanzapine clearance in smokers; 30% decrease in females

Dosing

Adult & Geriatric

Schizophrenia:

Oral: Initial: 5 to 10 mg once daily (increase to 10 mg once daily within 5 to 7 days); thereafter, adjust by 5 mg daily at 1-week intervals, up to a recommended maximum of 20 mg daily. Maintenance: 10 to 20 mg once daily. Doses up to 60 mg daily have been used in treatment-resistant schizophrenia; however, supporting evidence is limited (APA [Lehman, 2004]).

Special risk patients: Initial: 5 mg once daily is recommended in patients who are debilitated, who have a predisposition to hypotensive reactions, who exhibit a combination of factors that may result in slower metabolism of olanzapine (eg, nonsmoking female patients ≥65 years), or who may be more pharmacodynamically sensitive to olanzapine; increase dose with caution as clinically indicated.

Extended-release IM injection: **Note:** Establish tolerance to oral olanzapine prior to changing to extended-release IM injection. Maximum dose: 300 mg/2 weeks or 405 mg/4 weeks

Patients established on oral olanzapine 10 mg daily: Initial dose: 210 mg every 2 weeks for 4 doses or 405 mg every 4 weeks for 2 doses; Maintenance dose: 150 mg every 2 weeks or 300 mg every 4 weeks

Patients established on oral olanzapine 15 mg daily: Initial dose: 300 mg every 2 weeks for 4 doses; Maintenance dose: 210 mg every 2 weeks or 405 mg every 4 weeks

Patients established on oral olanzapine 20 mg daily: Initial and maintenance dose: 300 mg every 2 weeks

Special risk patients: Initial: 150 mg every 4 weeks is recommended in patients who are debilitated, who have a predisposition to hypotensive reactions, who exhibit a combination of factors that may result in slower metabolism of olanzapine (eg, nonsmoking female patients ≥65 years), or who may be more pharmacodynamically sensitive to olanzapine; increase dose with caution as clinically indicated.

Bipolar I (acute mixed or manic episodes: Oral:

Monotherapy: Initial: 10 to 15 mg once daily; increase by 5 mg daily at intervals of not less than 24 hours. Maintenance: 5 to 20 mg daily; recommended maximum dose: 20 mg daily.

Combination therapy (with lithium or valproate): Initial: 10 mg once daily; dosing range: 5 to 20 mg daily

Agitation (acute, associated with bipolar disorder or schizophrenia): Short-acting IM injection: Initial dose: 10 mg (a lower dose of 5 to 7.5 mg may be considered when clinical factors warrant); additional doses (up to 10 mg) may be considered; however, 2 hours after the initial dose and 4 hours after the second dose should be allowed between doses to evaluate response (maximum total daily dose: 30 mg)

Special risk patients: Consider a lower dose of 2.5 mg in patients who are debilitated, who have a predisposition to hypotensive reactions, or who may be more pharmacodynamically sensitive to olanzapine.

Depression:

Depression associated with bipolar disorder (in combination with fluoxetine): Oral: Initial: 5 mg in the evening; adjust as tolerated to usual range of 5 to 12.5 mg daily. See **"Note"**

Treatment-resistant depression (in combination with fluoxetine): Oral: Initial: 5 mg in the evening; adjust as tolerated to range of 5 to 20 mg daily. See **"Note"**

Note (olanzapine/fluoxetine combination [Symbyax]): When using individual components of fluoxetine with olanzapine rather than fixed dose combination product (Symbyax), approximate dosage correspondence is as follows:

Olanzapine 2.5 mg + fluoxetine 20 mg = Symbyax 3/25

Olanzapine 5 mg + fluoxetine 20 mg = Symbyax 6/25

Olanzapine 12.5 mg + fluoxetine 20 mg = Symbyax 12/25

Olanzapine 5 mg + fluoxetine 50 mg = Symbyax 6/50

Olanzapine 12.5 mg + fluoxetine 50 mg = Symbyax 12/50

Special risk patients: Initial: 2.5 to 5 mg once daily is recommended in patients who have a predisposition to hypotensive reactions, who have hepatic impairment, who exhibit a combination of factors that may result in slower metabolism of olanzapine (eg, female, elderly, nonsmoking status), or who may be more pharmacodynamically sensitive to olanzapine; increase dose with caution as clinically indicated.

Delirium (off-label use): Oral: 5 mg once daily for up to 5 days (NICE, 2010)

Post-traumatic stress disorder (off-label use): Oral: Initial: 5 to 10 mg daily; adjust dose based on response and tolerability every 1 to 2 weeks, up to 20 mg daily (Carey, 2012; Stein, 2002).

Prevention of chemotherapy-associated delayed nausea or vomiting (off-label use; in combination with a corticosteroid and serotonin [5-HT$_3$] antagonist): Oral: 10 mg once daily for 3 to 5 days, beginning on day 1 of chemotherapy **or** 5 mg once daily for 2 days before chemotherapy, followed by 10 mg once daily (beginning on the day of chemotherapy) for 3 to 8 days

Tourette syndrome (off-label use): Oral: Initial: 2.5 to 5 mg daily; increase gradually based on response and tolerability to a usual dosage range of 2.5 to 20 mg daily (Pringsheim, 2012; Roessner, 2011). After initial dosage, increments of 2.5 to 5 mg weekly or biweekly were commonly used for dosage adjustments in clinical trials up to a maximum dosage of 20 mg/day (Budman, 2001; Onofrj, 2000; Stamenkovic, 2000).

Pediatric

Bipolar I (acute mixed or manic episodes): Adolescents ≥13 years: Oral: Initial: 2.5 to 5 mg once daily; adjust by 2.5 to 5 mg daily to target dose of 10 mg daily; dosing range: 2.5 to 20 mg daily

Depression associated with bipolar I disorder (in combination with fluoxetine): Children and Adolescents 10 to 17 years: Oral: Initial: 2.5 mg once daily in the evening (in combination with fluoxetine); adjust dose, if needed, as tolerated; safety of doses >12 mg of olanzapine in combination with fluoxetine doses >50 mg has not been studied in pediatrics. Refer to adult dosing for **"Note"** for olanzapine/fluoxetine combination (Symbyax).

Schizophrenia: Adolescents ≥13 years: Oral: Initial: 2.5 to 5 mg once daily; adjust by 2.5 to 5 mg daily to target dose of 10 mg daily; dosing range: 2.5 to 20 mg daily

Tourette syndrome (off-label use): Children and Adolescents: Initial: 2.5 to 5 mg once daily; increase gradually based on response and tolerability to a usual dosage of 2.5 to 12.5 mg once daily (AACAP [Murphy 2013]; Pringsheim 2012). After initial dosage, increments of 2.5 to 5 mg weekly or biweekly were used for dosage adjustments in clinical trials up to a maximum dosage of 20 mg/day (McCracken 2008; Stephens 2004)

Renal Impairment No dosage adjustment necessary. Not removed by dialysis.

Hepatic Impairment There are no dosage adjustments provided in the manufacturer's labeling except when used in combination with fluoxetine (as separate components) the initial olanzapine dose should be limited to 2.5 to 5 mg daily. Use with caution (cases of hepatitis and liver injury have been reported with olanzapine use).

Dietary Considerations Tablets may be taken without regard to meals. Some products may contain phenylalanine.

Administration

Short-acting IM injection: **For IM administration only**; do not administer injection intravenously or subcutaneously; inject slowly, deep into muscle. If dizziness and/or drowsiness are noted, patient should remain recumbent until examination indicates postural hypotension and/or bradycardia are not a problem.

Extended-release IM injection: **For IM gluteal injection only**; do not administer IV or subcutaneously. After needle insertion into muscle, aspirate to verify that no blood appears. Do not massage injection site. Use diluent, syringes, and needles provided in convenience kit; obtain a new kit if aspiration of blood occurs.

Tablet: May be administered without regard to meals.

Orally-disintegrating: Remove from foil blister by peeling back (do not push tablet through the foil); place tablet in mouth immediately upon removal; tablet dissolves rapidly in saliva and may be swallowed with or without liquid. May be administered with or without food/meals.

Monitoring Parameters Mental status; vital signs (as clinically indicated); blood pressure (baseline; repeat 3 months after antipsychotic initiation, then yearly); weight, height, BMI, waist circumference (baseline; repeat at 4, 8, and 12 weeks after initiating or changing therapy, then quarterly; consider switching to a different antipsychotic for a weight gain ≥5% of initial weight); CBC (as clinically indicated; monitor frequently during the first few months of therapy in patients with preexisting low WBC or history of drug-induced leukopenia/neutropenia); electrolytes and liver function (annually and as clinically indicated); personal and family history of obesity, diabetes, dyslipidemia, hypertension, or cardiovascular disease (baseline; repeat annually); fasting plasma glucose level/HbA$_{1c}$ (baseline; repeat 3 months after starting antipsychotic, then yearly); fasting lipid panel (baseline; repeat 3 months after initiation of antipsychotic; if LDL level is normal repeat at 2-5 year intervals or more frequently if clinical indicated); changes in menstruation, libido, development of galactorrhea, erectile and ejaculatory function (at each visit for the first 12 weeks after the antipsychotic is initiated or until the dose is stable, then yearly); abnormal involuntary movements or parkinsonian signs (baseline; repeat weekly until dose stabilized for at least 2 weeks after introduction and for 2 weeks after any significant dose increase); tardive dyskinesia (every 12 months; high-risk patients every 6 months); ocular examination (yearly in patients >40 years; every 2 years in younger patients) (ADA 2004; Lehman 2004; Marder 2004)

Extended-release IM injection: Sedation/delirium for 3 hours after each dose

Dosage Forms Excipient information presented when available (limited, particularly for generics); consult specific product labeling.

Solution Reconstituted, Intramuscular:
ZyPREXA: 10 mg (1 ea) [contains tartaric acid]
Generic: 10 mg (1 ea)
Suspension Reconstituted, Intramuscular:
ZyPREXA Relprevv: 210 mg (1 ea); 300 mg (1 ea); 405 mg (1 ea) [contains polysorbate 80]
Tablet, Oral:
ZyPREXA: 2.5 mg, 5 mg, 7.5 mg, 10 mg
ZyPREXA: 15 mg [contains fd&c blue #2 aluminum lake]
ZyPREXA: 20 mg
Generic: 2.5 mg, 5 mg, 7.5 mg, 10 mg, 15 mg, 20 mg
Tablet Dispersible, Oral:
ZyPREXA Zydis: 5 mg, 10 mg, 15 mg, 20 mg [contains aspartame, methylparaben sodium, propylparaben sodium]
Generic: 5 mg, 10 mg, 15 mg, 20 mg

Dosage Forms: Canada Note: Refer to Dosage Forms. ZyPREXA Relprevv is not available in Canada.

◆ Olanzapine for injection (Can) see OLANZapine on page 1314

◆ Olanzapine ODT (Can) see OLANZapine on page 1314

◆ Olanzapine Pamoate see OLANZapine on page 1314

Olaparib (oh LAP a rib)

Brand Names: US Lynparza
Index Terms AZD2281; KU-0059436; PARP inhibitor AZD2281
Pharmacologic Category Antineoplastic Agent, PARP Inhibitor
Additional Appendix Information
Oral Dosages That Should Not Be Crushed on page 2003
Use Ovarian cancer, advanced: Treatment (monotherapy) of deleterious or suspected deleterious germline BRCA mutated (as detected by an approved test) advanced ovarian cancer in patients who have been treated with 3 or more prior lines of chemotherapy

Pregnancy Considerations Adverse events were observed in animal reproduction studies at doses less than human exposure. Based on its mechanism of action, olaparib may be expected to cause adverse events to the fetus. Women of reproductive potential should use highly effective contraception during therapy and for at least one month after treatment is discontinued.

Breast-Feeding Considerations It is not known if olaparib is excreted into breast milk. Due to the potential for serious adverse reactions in the nursing infant, the manufacturer recommends a decision be made to discontinue nursing or to discontinue the drug, taking into account the importance of treatment to the mother.

Prescribing and Access Restrictions Olaparib is available only through the designated specialty pharmacy Biologics, Inc. For further information on patient assistance, product availability, and prescribing instructions, please refer to the following website: http://myaccess360.com/hcp/reimbursement/Oncology.aspx?product=lynparza or call 1-844-275-2360.

Medication Guide Available Yes

Contraindications There are no contraindications listed in the manufacturer's labeling.

Warnings/Precautions Hazardous agent - use appropriate precautions for handling and disposal (meets NIOSH 2014 criteria). Anemia, neutropenia, thrombocytopenia and lymphopenia have been reported. Monitor complete blood counts at baseline and monthly thereafter; do not initiate olaparib until any hematologic toxicity caused by previous chemotherapy has resolved to ≤ grade 1. Myelodysplastic syndrome/acute myeloid leukemia (MDS/AML) has been reported (rarely) in a clinical trial of patients with deleterious or suspected deleterious germline BRCA-mutated advanced cancers receiving olaparib monotherapy. Most MDS/AML cases were fatal. The duration of therapy prior to development of the secondary cancers ranged from less than 6 months to greater than 2 years; all patients had received prior chemotherapy with platinum agents and/or other DNA-damaging medications. If prolonged hematologic toxicity occurs during therapy, interrupt treatment and monitor blood counts weekly until recovered; if counts do not recover to ≤ grade 1 after 4 weeks, further evaluation (including bone marrow and cytogenetic analyses) is necessary. If MDS/AML is confirmed, discontinue therapy.

Pneumonitis (including some fatalities) has occurred rarely. Interrupt treatment for new or worsening respiratory symptoms such as cough, dyspnea, fever, wheezing, or radiologic abnormalities; evaluate promptly. Discontinue treatment if pneumonitis is confirmed. Olaparib is associated with a moderate emetic potential; antiemetics are recommended to prevent nausea and vomiting. Potentially significant drug-drug interactions may exist, requiring dose or frequency adjustment, additional monitoring, and/or selection of alternative therapy.

Adverse Reactions Note: Frequency not always defined

≥10%:
Cardiovascular: Peripheral edema (10% to <20%)
Central nervous system: Fatigue (including weakness; 66% to 68%), headache (10% to 25%), dizziness (10% to <20%)
Dermatologic: Skin rash (10% to 25%)
Gastrointestinal: Nausea (64% to 75%), abdominal pain (43%), vomiting (32% to 43%), diarrhea (28% to 31%), dyspepsia (25%), decreased appetite (22% to 25%), dysgeusia (10% to 21%), constipation (10% to <20%)
Genitourinary: Urinary tract infection (10% to <20%)

Hematologic & oncologic: Decreased hemoglobin (85% to 90%; grades 3/4: 8% to 15%), increased MCV (57% to 85%), decreased absolute lymphocyte count (56%; grades 3/4: 17%), anemia (25% to 34%; grades 3/4: 4% to 18%), decreased neutrophils (25% to 32%; grades 3/4: 7% to 8%), decreased platelet count (26% to 30%; grades 3/4: 3% to 6%)

Neuromuscular & skeletal: Musculoskeletal pain (21% to 32%), myalgia (22% to 25%), back pain (10% to 25%)

Renal: Increased serum creatinine (26% to 30%)

Respiratory: Upper respiratory tract infection (26% to 43%), cough (10% to 21%), dyspnea (10% to <20%)

1% to ≤10%:

Cardiovascular: Hypertension, venous thrombosis (including pulmonary embolism)

Central nervous system: Anxiety, depression, insomnia, peripheral neuropathy

Dermatologic: Pruritus, xeroderma (including eczema)

Endocrine & metabolic: Hot flash, hyperglycemia, hypomagnesemia

Gastrointestinal: Stomatitis

Genitourinary: Dysuria, urinary incontinence, vulvovaginal disease

Hematologic & oncologic: Myelodysplastic syndrome (acute myeloid leukemia; 2%), leukopenia

Miscellaneous: Fever

<1% (Limited to important or life-threatening): Pneumonitis

Drug Interactions

Metabolism/Transport Effects Substrate of CYP3A4 (major), P-glycoprotein; **Note:** Assignment of Major/Minor substrate status based on clinically relevant drug interaction potential

Avoid Concomitant Use

Avoid concomitant use of Olaparib with any of the following: BCG (Intravesical); Bitter Orange; Conivaptan; CYP3A4 Inducers (Moderate); CYP3A4 Inducers (Strong); CYP3A4 Inhibitors (Moderate); CYP3A4 Inhibitors (Strong); Deferiprone; Dipyrone; Fusidic Acid (Systemic); Idelalisib

Increased Effect/Toxicity

Olaparib may increase the levels/effects of: CloZAPine; Deferiprone

The levels/effects of Olaparib may be increased by: Bitter Orange; Conivaptan; CYP3A4 Inhibitors (Moderate); CYP3A4 Inhibitors (Strong); Dasatinib; Dipyrone; Fosaprepitant; Fusidic Acid (Systemic); Idelalisib; Ivacaftor; Luliconazole; Osimertinib; Palbociclib; Simeprevir; Stiripentol

Decreased Effect

Olaparib may decrease the levels/effects of: BCG (Intravesical)

The levels/effects of Olaparib may be decreased by: CYP3A4 Inducers (Moderate); CYP3A4 Inducers (Strong); Deferasirox; Osimertinib; Siltuximab; Tocilizumab

Food Interactions Coadministration with grapefruit or Seville oranges may increase olaparib plasma concentrations. Management: Avoid concomitant administration with grapefruit or Seville oranges.

Storage/Stability Store at 25°C (77°F); excursions permitted from 15°C to 30°C (59°F to 86°F). Do not expose capsules to temperatures >40°C (104°F).

Mechanism of Action Olaparib is a poly (ADP-ribose) polymerase (PARP) enzyme inhibitor, including PARP1, PARP2, and PARP3. PARP enzymes are involved in DNA transcription, cell cycle regulation, and DNA repair. Olaparib is a potent oral PARP inhibitor which induces synthetic lethality in BRCA1/2 deficient tumor cells through the formation of double-stranded DNA breaks which cannot be accurately repaired, which leads to disruption of cellular homeostasis and cell death (Ledermann, 2012).

Pharmacodynamics/Kinetics

Absorption: Rapid; delayed with a high-fat meal (extent of absorption not significantly altered)

Distribution: 167 ± 196 L

Protein binding: ~82%

Metabolism: Primarily hepatic via CYP3A4; the majority of metabolism is through oxidation with some metabolites undergoing subsequent glucuronide or sulfate conjugation

Half-life elimination, terminal: 11.9 ± 4.8 hours

Time to peak: 1 to 3 hours

Excretion: Urine (44%, mostly metabolites); feces (42%, mostly metabolites)

Dosing

Adult & Geriatric Note: Administer only to patients with deleterious or suspected deleterious germline BRCA mutations, as detected by an approved test. Olaparib is associated with a moderate emetic potential; antiemetics are recommended to prevent nausea and vomiting.

Ovarian cancer, advanced: Oral: 400 mg twice daily until disease progression or unacceptable toxicity

Missed doses: If a dose is missed, administer the next dose at its scheduled time.

Dosage adjustment for concomitant therapy with CYP3A inhibitors: Avoid concomitant use with moderate or strong CYP3A inhibitors. Reduce dose to 200 mg twice daily if coadministration with a **moderate** CYP3A inhibitor cannot be avoided; reduce dose to 150 mg twice daily if coadministration with a **strong** CYP3A inhibitor cannot be avoided.

Renal Impairment

Mild impairment (CrCl 50 to 80 mL/minute): No dosage adjustment necessary; monitor closely for toxicity, as an increase in mean AUC has been observed in patients with mild impairment.

Moderate or severe impairment (CrCl <50 mL/minute): There are no dosage adjustments provided in the manufacturer's labeling (has not been studied).

Dialysis: There are no dosage adjustments provided in the manufacturer's labeling (has not been studied).

Hepatic Impairment There are no dosage adjustments provided in the manufacturer's labeling (has not been studied). Patients with bilirubin >1.5 times ULN and AST/ALT ≥2.5 times ULN (≥5 times ULN in the presence of liver metastases) were excluded from clinical trials.

Adjustment for Toxicity

Consider therapy interruption or dose reduction if adverse reactions occur. The recommended dose reduction is to 200 mg twice daily; if further reduction is required, reduce dose to 100 mg twice daily.

Pneumonitis: Discontinue

Secondary AML/MDS: Discontinue

Dietary Considerations Avoid grapefruit or Seville oranges.

Administration Olaparib is associated with a moderate emetic potential; antiemetics are recommended to prevent nausea and vomiting.

Oral: Swallow capsule whole; do not chew, dissolve, or open capsule. Do not administer if capsules appear deformed or show evidence of leakage.

Hazardous agent; use appropriate precautions for handling and disposal (meets NIOSH 2014 criteria).

Monitoring Parameters Complete blood count at baseline and monthly thereafter, or as clinically indicated (weekly until recovery for prolonged hematologic toxicity); monitor for signs/symptoms of AML/MDS and pneumonitis

Dosage Forms Excipient information presented when available (limited, particularly for generics); consult specific product labeling.

Capsule, Oral:

Lynparza: 50 mg

◆ Oleovitamin A *see* Vitamin A *on page 1905*

◆ Oleptro *see* TraZODone *on page 1834*

◆ Olestyr (Can) *see* Cholestyramine Resin *on page 381*

◆ Olex (Can) *see* Omeprazole *on page 1330*

Olmesartan (ole me SAR tan)

Brand Names: US Benicar

Brand Names: Canada Olmetec

Index Terms Olmesartan Medoxomil

Pharmacologic Category Angiotensin II Receptor Blocker; Antihypertensive

Use

Hypertension: Treatment of hypertension with or without concurrent use of other antihypertensive agents

Guideline recommendations:

Hypertension: The 2014 guideline for the management of high blood pressure in adults (Eighth Joint National Committee [JNC 8; James 2013]) recommends initiation of pharmacologic treatment to lower blood pressure for the following patients:

• Patients ≥60 years of age with systolic blood pressure (SBP) ≥150 mm Hg or diastolic blood pressure (DBP) ≥90 mm Hg. Goal of therapy is SBP <150 mm Hg and DBP <90 mm Hg.

• Patients <60 years of age with SBP ≥140 mm Hg or DBP ≥90 mm Hg. Goal of therapy is SBP <140 mm Hg and DBP <90 mm Hg.

• Patients ≥18 years of age with diabetes and SBP ≥140 mm Hg or DBP ≥90 mm Hg. Goal of therapy is SBP <140 mm Hg and DBP <90 mm Hg.

• Patients ≥18 years of age with chronic kidney disease (CKD) and SBP ≥140 mm Hg or DBP ≥90 mm Hg. Goal of therapy is SBP <140 mm Hg and DBP <90 mm Hg.

Chronic kidney disease (CKD) and hypertension: Regardless of race or diabetes status, the use of an ACE inhibitor (ACEI) or angiotensin receptor blocker (ARB) as initial therapy is recommended to improve kidney outcomes. In the general nonblack population (without CKD), including those with diabetes, initial antihypertensive treatment should consist of a thiazide-type diuretic, calcium channel blocker, ACEI, or ARB. In the general black population (without CKD), including those with diabetes, initial antihypertensive treatment should consist of a thiazide-type diuretic or a calcium channel blocker instead of an ACEI or ARB.

Coronary artery disease (CAD) and hypertension: The American Heart Association, American College of Cardiology, and American Society of Hypertension (AHA/ACC/ASH) 2015 scientific statement for the treatment of hypertension in patients with CAD recommends the use of an ARB (or ACE inhibitor) as part of a regimen in patients with hypertension and chronic stable angina if there is prior MI, LV systolic dysfunction, diabetes mellitus, or CKD. A BP target of <140/90 mm Hg is reasonable for the secondary prevention of cardiovascular events. A lower target BP (<130/80 mm Hg) may be appropriate in some individuals with CAD, previous MI, stroke or transient ischemic attack, or CAD risk equivalents (AHA/ACC/ASH [Rosendorff 2015]).

Pregnancy Considerations [U.S. Boxed Warning]: Drugs that act on the renin-angiotensin system can cause injury and death to the developing fetus. Discontinue as soon as possible once pregnancy is detected. The use of drugs which act on the renin-angiotensin system are associated with oligohydramnios. Oligohydramnios, due to decreased fetal renal function, may lead to fetal lung hypoplasia and skeletal malformations. Use is also associated with anuria, hypotension, renal failure, skull hypoplasia, and death in the fetus/neonate. The exposed fetus should be monitored for fetal growth, amniotic fluid volume, and organ formation. Infants exposed *in utero* should be monitored for hyperkalemia, hypotension, and oliguria (exchange transfusions or dialysis may be needed). These adverse events are generally associated with maternal use in the second and third trimesters.

Untreated chronic maternal hypertension is also associated with adverse events in the fetus, infant, and mother. The use of angiotensin II receptor blockers is not recommended to treat chronic uncomplicated hypertension in pregnant women and should generally be avoided in women of reproductive potential (ACOG, 2013).

Breast-Feeding Considerations It is not known if olmesartan is excreted into breast milk. Due to the potential for serious adverse reactions in the nursing infant, the manufacturer recommends a decision be made whether to discontinue nursing or to discontinue the drug, taking into account the importance of treatment to the mother.

Contraindications Concomitant use with aliskiren in patients with diabetes mellitus

Canadian labeling: Additional contraindications (not in U.S. labeling): Hypersensitivity to olmesartan or any component of the formulation; concomitant use with aliskiren in patients with moderate to severe renal impairment (GFR <60 mL/minute/1.73 m^2)

Documentation of allergenic cross-reactivity for angiotensin II receptor blockers is limited. However, because of similarities in chemical structure and/or pharmacologic actions, the possibility of cross-sensitivity cannot be ruled out with certainty.

Warnings/Precautions [U.S. Boxed Warning]: Drugs that act on the renin-angiotensin system can cause injury and death to the developing fetus. Discontinue as soon as possible once pregnancy is detected. May cause hyperkalemia; avoid potassium supplementation unless specifically required by healthcare provider. Avoid use or use a smaller dose in patients who are volume depleted; correct depletion first. May be associated with deterioration of renal function and/or increases in serum creatinine, particularly in patients with low renal blood flow (eg, renal artery stenosis, heart failure) whose glomerular filtration rate (GFR) is dependent on efferent arteriolar vasoconstriction by angiotensin II. Use with caution in unstented unilateral/bilateral renal artery stenosis. When unstented bilateral renal artery stenosis is present, use is generally avoided due to the elevated risk of deterioration in renal function unless possible benefits outweigh risks. Use with caution with preexisting renal insufficiency; significant aortic/mitral stenosis. Potentially significant drug-drug interactions may exist, requiring dose or frequency adjustment, additional monitoring, and/or selection of alternative therapy. In surgical patients on chronic angiotensin receptor blocker (ARB) therapy, intraoperative hypotension may occur with induction and maintenance of general anesthesia.

Symptoms of sprue-like enteropathy (ie, severe, chronic diarrhea with significant weight loss) has been reported; may develop months to years after treatment initiation with villous atrophy commonly found on intestinal biopsy. Once other etiologies have been excluded, discontinue treatment and consider other antihypertensive treatment. Clinical and histologic improvement was noted after treatment was discontinued in a case series of 22 patients (Ianiro, 2014; Rubio-Tapia, 2012).

Angioedema has been reported rarely with some angiotensin II receptor antagonists (ARBs) and may occur at any time during treatment (especially following first dose). It may involve the head and neck (potentially compromising airway) or the intestine (presenting with abdominal pain). Patients with idiopathic or hereditary angioedema or previous angioedema associated with ACE-inhibitor therapy may be at an increased risk. Prolonged frequent monitoring may be required, especially if tongue, glottis, or larynx are involved, as they are associated with airway obstruction. Patients with a history of airway surgery may have a higher risk of airway obstruction. Discontinue therapy immediately if angioedema occurs. Aggressive early management is critical. Intramuscular (IM) administration of epinephrine may be necessary. Do not readminister to patients who have had angioedema with ARBs.

Olmesartan has not been shown to be effective for hypertension in children younger than 6 years. Children younger than 1 year must not receive olmesartan for hypertension. The renin-angiotensin-aldosterone system plays a critical role in kidney development. Administering drugs that act directly on the renin-angiotensin-aldosterone system can have effects on the development of immature kidneys and alter normal renal development.

Adverse Reactions

1% to 10%:

Central nervous system: Dizziness (3%), headache

Endocrine & metabolic: Hyperglycemia, hypertriglyceridemia

Gastrointestinal: Diarrhea

Neuromuscular & skeletal: Back pain, CPK increased

Renal: Hematuria

Respiratory: Bronchitis, pharyngitis, rhinitis, sinusitis

Miscellaneous: Flu-like syndrome

<1% (Limited to important or life-threatening): Acute renal failure, alopecia, anaphylaxis, angioedema, arthritis, gastroenteritis, hypercholesterolemia, hyperkalemia, hyperlipidemia, hyperuricemia, liver enzymes increased, peripheral edema, rhabdomyolysis, serum creatinine increased, sprue-like symptoms, tachycardia

Drug Interactions

Metabolism/Transport Effects Substrate of SLCO1B1

Avoid Concomitant Use There are no known interactions where it is recommended to avoid concomitant use.

Increased Effect/Toxicity

Olmesartan may increase the levels/effects of: ACE Inhibitors; Amifostine; Antipsychotic Agents (Second Generation [Atypical]); Ciprofloxacin (Systemic); CycloSPORINE (Systemic); Drospirenone; DULoxetine; Hypotension-Associated Agents; Levodopa; Lithium; Nonsteroidal Anti-Inflammatory Agents; Potassium-Sparing Diuretics; Sodium Phosphates

The levels/effects of Olmesartan may be increased by: Alfuzosin; Aliskiren; Barbiturates; Brimonidine (Topical); Canagliflozin; Dapoxetine; Diazoxide; Eltrombopag; Eplerenone; Heparin; Heparin (Low Molecular Weight); Herbs (Hypotensive Properties); Molsidomine; Nicorandil; Obinutuzumab; Pentoxifylline; Phosphodiesterase 5 Inhibitors; Potassium Salts; Prostacyclin Analogues; Teriflunomide; Tolvaptan; Trimethoprim

Decreased Effect

The levels/effects of Olmesartan may be decreased by: Amphetamines; Colesevelam; Herbs (Hypertensive Properties); Methylphenidate; Nonsteroidal Anti-Inflammatory Agents; Yohimbine

Storage/Stability Store at 20°C to 25°C (68°F to 77°F).

Mechanism of Action As a selective and competitive, nonpeptide angiotensin II receptor antagonist, olmesartan blocks the vasoconstrictor and aldosterone-secreting effects of angiotensin II; olmesartan interacts reversibly at the AT1 and AT2 receptors of many tissues and has slow dissociation kinetics; its affinity for the AT1 receptor is 12,500 times greater than the AT2 receptor. Angiotensin II receptor antagonists may induce a more complete inhibition of the renin-angiotensin system than ACE inhibitors, they do not affect the response to bradykinin, and are less likely to be associated with nonrenin-angiotensin effects (eg, cough and angioedema). Olmesartan increases urinary flow rate and, in addition to being natriuretic and

kaliuretic, increases excretion of chloride, magnesium, uric acid, calcium, and phosphate.

Pharmacodynamics/Kinetics

Distribution: 17 L; does not cross the blood-brain barrier (animal studies)

Protein binding: 99%

Metabolism: Olmesartan medoxomil is hydrolyzed in the GI tract to active olmesartan. No further metabolism occurs.

Bioavailability: 26%

Half-life elimination: Terminal: 13 hours

Time to peak: 1 to 2 hours

Excretion: All as unchanged drug: Feces (50% to 65%); urine (35% to 50%)

Dosing

Adult Hypertension: Oral: Initial: 20 mg once daily; if initial response is inadequate, may be increased to 40 mg once daily after 2 weeks. Usual dosage range (ASH/ISH [Weber, 2014]): 20 to 40 mg daily. May administer with other antihypertensive agents if blood pressure inadequately controlled with olmesartan. Consider lower starting dose in patients with possible depletion of intravascular volume (eg, patients receiving diuretics).

Geriatric Hypertension: Oral: No initial dosage adjustment is necessary per labeling; however, may consider starting at 5 to 10 mg once daily (due to concomitant disease or age changes).

Pediatric Hypertension: Children 6 to 16 years: Oral:
20 kg to <35 kg: Initial: 10 mg once daily; if initial response inadequate after 2 weeks, dose may be increased (maximum: 20 mg once daily)

≥35 kg: Initial: 20 mg once daily; if initial response inadequate after 2 weeks, dose may be increased (maximum: 40 mg once daily)

Renal Impairment

U.S. labeling: Initial: No dosage adjustment is necessary for patients with moderate to severe renal impairment (creatinine clearance <40 mL/minute). However, AUC increased 3-fold in patients with CrCl <20 mL/minute; use with caution.

Canadian labeling:
Mild to moderate impairment: Maximum dose: 20 mg once daily

Severe impairment: There are no dosage adjustments provided in the manufacturer's labeling; use is not recommended.

Hepatic Impairment

U.S. labeling: Initial: No dosage adjustment is necessary for patients with moderate to severe hepatic dysfunction. Total drug exposure increased 60% in patients with moderate impairment.

Canadian labeling:
Mild impairment: No dosage adjustment is necessary.

Moderate impairment: Initial: Lower starting dose is recommended (maximum: 20 mg once daily)

Severe impairment: There are no dosage adjustment provided in the manufacturer's labeling; use is not recommended.

Dietary Considerations May be taken with or without food.

Administration May be administered with or without food.

Monitoring Parameters Blood pressure, electrolytes, serum creatinine, BUN, urinalysis

Dosage Forms Excipient information presented when available (limited, particularly for generics); consult specific product labeling.

Tablet, Oral, as medoxomil:
Benicar: 5 mg, 20 mg, 40 mg

Extemporaneous Preparations A 2 mg/mL oral suspension may be made with olmesartan tablets. Combine 50 mL purified water and twenty 20 mg tablets in an 8-ounce amber bottle and allow to stand for ≥5 minutes. Shake well for ≥1 minute, then allow to stand for ≥1 minute. Repeat shaking and standing process four additional times. Add 100 mL Ora-Sweet® and 50 mL Ora-Plus® to the suspension and shake well for ≥1 minute. Label "shake well" and "refrigerate". Stable for 28 days refrigerated.

Benicar® prescribing information, Daiichi Sankyo, Inc, Parsippany, NJ, 2010.

Olmesartan, Amlodipine, and Hydrochlorothiazide

(ole me SAR tan, am LOE di peen, & hye droe klor oh THYE a zide)

Brand Names: US Tribenzor™

Index Terms Amlodipine Besylate, Olmesartan Medoxomil, and Hydrochlorothiazide; Amlodipine, Hydrochlorothiazide, and Olmesartan; Hydrochlorothiazide, Olmesartan, and Amlodipine; Olmesartan, Hydrochlorothiazide, and Amlodipine

Pharmacologic Category Angiotensin II Receptor Blocker; Antianginal Agent; Antihypertensive; Calcium Channel Blocker; Calcium Channel Blocker, Dihydropyridine; Diuretic, Thiazide

Use Treatment of hypertension (not for initial therapy)

Dosing

Adult Note: Not for initial therapy. Dose is individualized; combination product may be substituted for individual components in patients currently maintained on all 3 agents separately or in patients not adequately controlled with any 2 of the following antihypertensive classes: Calcium channel blockers, angiotensin II receptor blockers, and diuretics.

Hypertension: Oral: Add-on/switch/replacement therapy: Amlodipine 5-10 mg, olmesartan 20-40 mg, and hydrochlorothiazide 12.5-25 mg once daily; dose may be titrated after 2 weeks of therapy. Maximum recommended daily dose: Amlodipine 10 mg/olmesartan 40 mg/hydrochlorothiazide 25 mg

Geriatric Patients ≥75 years of age should start amlodipine at 2.5 mg (combination product dosage form not available in this strength).

Renal Impairment
CrCl >30 mL/minute: No dosage adjustment necessary.
CrCl ≤30 mL/minute: Use of combination not recommended; contraindicated in patients with anuria

Hepatic Impairment
Mild-to-moderate hepatic impairment: No dosage adjustment provided in manufacturer's labeling. Use with caution.

Severe hepatic impairment: Use not recommended; initial daily dose of amlodipine is 2.5 mg (this dose of amlodipine is not available as a combination product).

Additional Information Complete prescribing information should be consulted for additional detail.

Dosage Forms Excipient information presented when available (limited, particularly for generics); consult specific product labeling.

Tablet, oral:
Tribenzor™: Olmesartan medoxomil 20 mg, amlodipine 5 mg, and hydrochlorothiazide 12.5 mg
Tribenzor™: Olmesartan medoxomil 40 mg, amlodipine 5 mg, and hydrochlorothiazide 12.5 mg
Tribenzor™: Olmesartan medoxomil 40 mg, amlodipine 5 mg, and hydrochlorothiazide 25 mg
Tribenzor™: Olmesartan medoxomil 40 mg, amlodipine 10 mg, and hydrochlorothiazide 12.5 mg
Tribenzor™: Olmesartan medoxomil 40 mg, amlodipine 10 mg, and hydrochlorothiazide 25 mg

◆ Olmesartan and Amlodipine see Amlodipine and Olmesartan on page 104

Olmesartan and Hydrochlorothiazide

(ole me SAR tan & hye droe klor oh THYE a zide)

Brand Names: US Benicar HCT

Brand Names: Canada Olmetec Plus

Index Terms Hydrochlorothiazide and Olmesartan Medoxomil; Olmesartan Medoxomil and Hydrochlorothiazide

Pharmacologic Category Angiotensin II Receptor Blocker; Diuretic, Thiazide

Use Treatment of hypertension (not recommended for initial treatment)

Dosing

Adult & Geriatric

Hypertension: Oral: Dosage must be individualized; may be titrated at 2- to 4-week intervals.

Replacement therapy: May be substituted for previously titrated dosages of the individual components.

Patients not controlled with single-agent therapy: Initiate by adding the lowest available dose of the alternative component (hydrochlorothiazide 12.5 mg or olmesartan 20 mg). Titrate to effect (maximum hydrochlorothiazide dose: 25 mg, maximum olmesartan dose: 40 mg).

Renal Impairment
CrCl >30 mL/minute: No dosage adjustment necessary.
CrCl ≤30 mL/minute: Use not recommended.

Hepatic Impairment No dosage adjustment necessary.

Additional Information Complete prescribing information should be consulted for additional detail.

Dosage Forms Excipient information presented when available (limited, particularly for generics); consult specific product labeling.

Tablet:
20/12.5: Olmesartan medoxomil 20 mg and hydrochlorothiazide 12.5 mg
40/12.5: Olmesartan medoxomil 40 mg and hydrochlorothiazide 12.5 mg
40/25: Olmesartan medoxomil 40 mg and hydrochlorothiazide 25 mg

Olodaterol (oh loe DA ter ol)

Brand Names: US Striverdi Respimat

Index Terms Olodaterol Hydrochloride

Pharmacologic Category Beta$_2$ Agonist; Beta$_2$-Adrenergic Agonist, Long-Acting

Use Chronic obstructive pulmonary disease: Long-term maintenance treatment of airflow obstruction in chronic obstructive pulmonary disease (COPD), including chronic bronchitis and/or emphysema

Pregnancy Considerations Adverse events were observed in some animal reproduction studies. Beta-agonists have the potential to affect uterine contractility if administered during labor.

Breast-Feeding Considerations Excretion of olodaterol into breast milk is unknown but likely. The manufacturer recommends that caution be used if administered to a nursing woman. The use of beta$_2$-receptor agonists are not considered a contraindication to breast-feeding (NAEPP, 2005).

Medication Guide Available Yes

Contraindications Monotherapy in the treatment of asthma (ie, use without a concomitant long-term asthma control medication). **Note:** Olodaterol is not FDA approved for treatment of asthma.

Documentation of allergenic cross-reactivity for sympathomimetics is limited. However, because of similarities in chemical structure and/or pharmacologic actions, the possibility of cross-sensitivity cannot be ruled out with certainty.

Warnings/Precautions [U.S. Boxed Warning]: Long-acting beta$_2$-agonists (LABAs) increase the risk of asthma-related deaths. The safety and efficacy of olodaterol in the treatment of asthma have not been established. In a large, randomized, placebo-controlled U.S. clinical trial (SMART, 2006), salmeterol was associated with an increase in asthma-related deaths (when added to usual asthma therapy); risk is considered a class effect among all LABAs. It is unknown if olodaterol increases asthma-related deaths. No data exist associating LABA use with an increased risk of death in patients with COPD. Rarely, paradoxical, life-threatening bronchospasm may occur with use of inhaled beta$_2$-agonists; distinguish from inadequate response, discontinue medication immediately, institute alternative therapy. Do **not** use for acute bronchospastic episodes of COPD; always prescribe olodaterol with an inhaled short-acting beta$_2$-agonist and educate patient on appropriate use. Do not initiate in patients with significantly worsening or acutely deteriorating COPD. Do not increase the olodaterol dose or frequency beyond what is recommended. Hypersensitivity reactions, including angioedema, may occur; discontinue therapy if patient develops an allergic reaction. Use with caution in patients with cardiovascular disease (arrhythmia, coronary insufficiency, hypertension, or HF); beta-agonists may cause elevation in blood pressure and heart rate. Beta$_2$-agonists may also produce electrocardiogram (ECG) changes (eg, T-wave flattening, QTc prolongation, ST segment depression). Use with caution in patients with diabetes mellitus; beta$_2$-agonists may increase serum glucose. Use with caution in patients with hyperthyroidism; may stimulate thyroid activity. Use with caution in patients with hypokalemia; beta$_2$-agonists may decrease serum potassium. Use with caution in patients with seizure disorders; beta$_2$-agonists may result in CNS stimulation/excitation. Potentially significant drug-drug interactions may exist, requiring dose or frequency adjustment, additional monitoring, and/or selection of alternative therapy. Do not use with other long-acting beta$_2$-agonists; deaths and significant cardiovascular effects have been reported with excessive sympathomimetic use.

Adverse Reactions

>10%:

Respiratory: Nasopharyngitis (11%)

1% to 10%:

Dermatologic: Skin rash (2%)

Genitourinary: Urinary tract infection (3%)

Neuromuscular & skeletal: Back pain (4%), arthralgia (2%)

Respiratory: Bronchitis (5%)

<1% (Limited to important or life-threatening): Asthma-related death, depression of ST segment on ECG, flattened T wave on ECG, hypersensitivity reaction (includes angioedema), hypokalemia (transient), increased serum glucose (high doses), increased diastolic blood pressure, increased pulse, increased systolic blood pressure, malignant neoplasm of lung, paradoxical bronchospasm, pneumonia, prolonged Q-T interval on ECG

Drug Interactions

Metabolism/Transport Effects Substrate of CYP2C8 (minor), CYP2C9 (minor), CYP3A4 (minor), UGT1A1, UGT1A7, UGT1A9, UGT2B7; **Note:** Assignment of Major/Minor substrate status based on clinically relevant drug interaction potential

Avoid Concomitant Use

Avoid concomitant use of Olodaterol with any of the following: Beta-Blockers (Nonselective); Iobenguane I 123; Long-Acting Beta2-Agonists; Loxapine

Increased Effect/Toxicity

Olodaterol may increase the levels/effects of: Atosiban; Doxofylline; Highest Risk QTc-Prolonging Agents; Long-Acting Beta2-Agonists; Loop Diuretics; Loxapine; Moderate Risk QTc-Prolonging Agents; Sympathomimetics; Thiazide Diuretics

The levels/effects of Olodaterol may be increased by: AtoMOXetine; Caffeine and Caffeine Containing Products; Cannabinoid-Containing Products; Linezolid; MAO Inhibitors; Mifepristone; Tedizolid; Theophylline Derivatives; Tricyclic Antidepressants

Decreased Effect

Olodaterol may decrease the levels/effects of: Iobenguane I 123

The levels/effects of Olodaterol may be decreased by: Beta-Blockers (Beta1 Selective); Beta-Blockers (Nonselective); Betahistine

Storage/Stability Store at 25°C (77°F); excursions are permitted between 15°C and 30°C (59°F and 86°F). Avoid freezing. Discard 3 months after cartridge is inserted into inhaler.

Mechanism of Action Long acting beta$_2$-receptor agonist; activates beta$_2$ airway receptors, resulting in the stimulation of intracellular adenyl cyclase and a subsequent increase in the synthesis of cyclic-3',5' adenosine monophosphate (cAMP). Elevated cAMP levels induce bronchodilation by relaxation of airway smooth muscle cells. Has much greater affinity for beta$_2$-receptors than for beta$_1$- or beta$_3$-receptors.

Pharmacodynamics/Kinetics

Onset of action: 5 minutes

Duration: 24 hours

Distribution: V_d: 1110 L

Protein binding: ~60%

Metabolism: Direct glucuronidation (UGT2B7, UGT1A1, 1A7, and 1A9) and O-demethylation (primarily CYP2C9 and 2C8)

Bioavailability: 30% (inhalation)

Half-life elimination: 7.5 hours

Time to peak: 10 to 20 minutes

Excretion: Urine (5% to 7% unchanged); feces

Dosing

Adult COPD: Inhalation: Two inhalations once daily (maximum: 2 inhalations per day.)

Geriatric Refer to adult dosing

Renal Impairment No dosage adjustment inecessary.

Hepatic Impairment

Mild to moderate impairment: No dosage adjustment necessary.

Severe impairment: There are no dosage adjustments provided in the manufacturer's labeling (has not been studied).

Administration For oral inhalation only. Prime inhaler prior to initial use or if not used for >21 days by pointing inhaler towards ground and actuating until aerosol cloud is seen, then repeat 3 additional times before use. If not used for >3 days (but ≤21 days), actuate once before use. To prepare inhaler for use after priming, refer to manufacturer labeling. When dose is ready to be administered, breathe in slowly through the mouth and press the dose release button; continue to breathe in slowly as long as possible, then hold breath for 10 seconds or for as long as comfortable. Repeat for second inhalation.

Monitoring Parameters FEV$_1$, FVC, and/or other pulmonary function tests; serum potassium, serum glucose; blood pressure, heart rate; CNS stimulation. Monitor for increased use of short-acting beta$_2$-agonist inhalers; may be marker of a deteriorating condition.

Dosage Forms Excipient information presented when available (limited, particularly for generics); consult specific product labeling.
Aerosol Solution, Inhalation:
Striverdi Respimat: 2.5 mcg/actuation (4 g) [contains benzalkonium chloride, edetate disodium]

◆ Olodaterol Hydrochloride see Olodaterol on page 1322

Olopatadine (Nasal) (oh la PAT a deen)

Brand Names: US Patanase
Index Terms Olopatadine Hydrochloride
Pharmacologic Category Histamine H$_1$ Antagonist; Histamine H$_1$ Antagonist, Second Generation; Piperidine Derivative
Use Treatment of the symptoms of seasonal allergic rhinitis
Dosing
Adult & Geriatric Seasonal allergic rhinitis: Intranasal: 2 sprays into each nostril twice daily
Pediatric Seasonal allergic rhinitis: Intranasal:
Children 6-11 years: 1 spray into each nostril twice daily
Children ≥12 years and Adolescents: Refer to adult dosing.
Renal Impairment No dosage adjustment necessary.
Hepatic Impairment No dosage adjustment necessary.
Additional Information Complete prescribing information should be consulted for additional detail.
Dosage Forms Considerations
Patanase 30.5 g bottles contain 240 sprays.
Dosage Forms Excipient information presented when available (limited, particularly for generics); consult specific product labeling.
Solution, Nasal:
Patanase: 0.6% (30.5 g) [contains benzalkonium chloride, edetate disodium]
Generic: 0.6% (30.5 g)

Olopatadine (Ophthalmic) (oh la PAT a deen)

Brand Names: US Pataday; Patanol; Pazeo
Brand Names: Canada ACT-Olopatadine; Apo-Olopatadine; CO Olopatadine; Pataday; Patanol; Sandoz-Olopatadine
Index Terms Olopatadine Hydrochloride
Pharmacologic Category Histamine H$_1$ Antagonist; Histamine H$_1$ Antagonist, Second Generation; Piperidine Derivative
Use Allergic conjunctivitis: Treatment of the signs and symptoms of allergic conjunctivitis
Dosing
Adult & Geriatric
Allergic conjunctivitis: Ophthalmic:
Pataday, Pazeo: Instill 1 drop into each affected eye once daily
Patanol: Instill 1 drop into each affected eye twice daily (allowing 6 to 8 hours between doses)
Pediatric
Allergic conjunctivitis: Ophthalmic:
Pataday, Pazeo: Children ≥2 years and Adolescents: Refer to adult dosing.
Patanol: Children ≥3 years and Adolescents: Refer to adult dosing.
Renal Impairment There are no dosage adjustments provided in the manufacturer's labeling. However, dosage adjustment unlikely due to low systemic absorption.
Hepatic Impairment There are no dosage adjustments provided in the manufacturer's labeling. However, dosage adjustment unlikely due to low systemic absorption.
Additional Information Complete prescribing information should be consulted for additional detail.
Dosage Forms Excipient information presented when available (limited, particularly for generics); consult specific product labeling.
Solution, Ophthalmic:
Pataday: 0.2% (2.5 mL) [contains benzalkonium chloride, edetate disodium]
Patanol: 0.1% (5 mL) [contains benzalkonium chloride]
Pazeo: 0.7% (2.5 mL) [contains benzalkonium chloride]
Generic: 0.1% (5 mL)

◆ Olopatadine Hydrochloride see Olopatadine (Nasal) on page 1323

◆ Olopatadine Hydrochloride see Olopatadine (Ophthalmic) on page 1323

Olsalazine (ole SAL a zeen)

Brand Names: US Dipentum
Brand Names: Canada Dipentum®

Index Terms Olsalazine Sodium
Pharmacologic Category 5-Aminosalicylic Acid Derivative
Use Maintenance of remission of ulcerative colitis in patients intolerant to sulfasalazine
Pregnancy Considerations Animal studies have demonstrated fetal developmental toxicities. There are no well-controlled studies in pregnant women. Use during pregnancy only if clearly necessary.
Breast-Feeding Considerations The active metabolite, 5-aminosalicylic acid may pass into breast milk. Diarrhea has been reported in breast-fed infants whose mothers took olsalazine.
Contraindications Hypersensitivity to olsalazine, salicylates, or any component of the formulation
Warnings/Precautions Diarrhea is a common adverse effect of olsalazine. May exacerbate symptoms of colitis. Use with caution in patients with renal or hepatic impairment. Use with caution in elderly patients. Use with caution in patients with severe allergies or asthma.
Adverse Reactions
>10%: Gastrointestinal: Diarrhea (11% to 17%; dose related)
1% to 10%:
Central nervous system: Depression (2%), dizziness/vertigo (1%)
Dermatologic: Rash (2%), pruritus (1%)
Gastrointestinal: Abdominal pain/cramps (10%), nausea (5%), bloating (2%), stomatitis (1%), vomiting (1%)
Neuromuscular & skeletal: Arthralgia (4%)
Respiratory: Upper respiratory infection (2%)
<1% (Limited to important or life-threatening): Alkaline phosphatase increased, Alopecia, ALT increased, anemia, angioedema, aplastic anemia, AST increased, bilirubin increased, blood in stool, blurred vision, bronchospasm, cholestatic hepatitis, cholestatic jaundice, chest pain, chills, cirrhosis, dehydration, dry eyes, dyspnea, dysuria, eosinophilia, epigastric discomfort, erythema, erythema nodosum, fever, flare of symptoms, flatulence, GGT increased, heart block (second degree), hematuria, hemolytic anemia, hepatitis, hepatic failure, hepatic necrosis, hot flashes, hypertension, impotence, insomnia, interstitial nephritis, interstitial pneumonia, irritability, jaundice, Kawasaki-like syndrome, LDH increased, leukopenia, lymphopenia, menorrhagia, mood swings, muscle cramps, myalgia, myocarditis, nephrotic syndrome, neutropenia, orthostatic hypotension, palpitation, pancreatitis, pancytopenia, paresthesia, pericarditis, peripheral edema, peripheral neuropathy, photosensitivity, proteinuria, rectal bleeding, rectal discomfort, reticulocytosis, rigors, tachycardia, thrombocytopenia, tinnitus, tremor, urinary frequency, watery eyes, xerostomia
Drug Interactions
Metabolism/Transport Effects None known.
Avoid Concomitant Use There are no known interactions where it is recommended to avoid concomitant use.
Increased Effect/Toxicity
Olsalazine may increase the levels/effects of: Heparin; Heparin (Low Molecular Weight); Thiopurine Analogs; Varicella Virus-Containing Vaccines

The levels/effects of Olsalazine may be increased by: Nonsteroidal Anti-Inflammatory Agents
Decreased Effect
Olsalazine may decrease the levels/effects of: Cardiac Glycosides
Storage/Stability Store at 20°C to 25°C (77°F); excursions permitted to 15°C to 30°C (59°F to 86°F).
Mechanism of Action Mesalamine (5-aminosalicylic acid) is the active component of olsalazine; the specific mechanism of action of mesalamine is unknown; however, it is thought that it modulates local chemical mediators of the inflammatory response, especially leukotrienes, and is also postulated to be a free radical scavenger or an inhibitor of tumor necrosis factor (TNF); action appears topical rather than systemic.
Pharmacodynamics/Kinetics
Absorption: <3%; very little intact olsalazine is systemically absorbed
Protein binding, plasma: >99%
Metabolism: Primarily via colonic bacteria to active drug, 5-aminosalicylic acid (5-ASA)
Half-life elimination: 54 minutes
Time to peak: ~1 hour
Excretion: Primarily feces; urine (<1%)
Dosing
Adult & Geriatric Ulcerative colitis: Oral: 1 g/day in 2 divided doses
Renal Impairment No dosage adjustment provided in manufacturer's labeling. Monitor patients with impaired renal function.

◀

Hepatic Impairment No dosage adjustment provided in manufacturer's labeling. Monitor patients with impaired hepatic function.

Dietary Considerations Take with food.

Administration Administer with food in evenly divided doses.

Monitoring Parameters CBC, hepatic function, renal function; stool frequency

Dosage Forms Excipient information presented when available (limited, particularly for generics); consult specific product labeling.

Capsule, Oral, as sodium:
Dipentum: 250 mg

♦ Olsalazine Sodium see Olsalazine on page 1323

♦ Olux see Clobetasol on page 412

♦ Olux-E see Clobetasol on page 412

♦ Olysio see Simeprevir on page 1657

Omacetaxine (oh ma se TAX een)

Brand Names: US Synribo

Index Terms CGX-625; HHT; Homoharringtonine; Omacetaxine Mepesuccinate

Pharmacologic Category Antineoplastic Agent, Cephalotaxine; Antineoplastic Agent, Protein Synthesis Inhibitor

Use Chronic myeloid leukemia: Treatment of chronic or accelerated phase chronic myeloid leukemia (CML) in adult patients resistant and/or intolerant to ≥2 tyrosine kinase inhibitors

Pregnancy Considerations Adverse events were observed in animal reproduction studies at doses less than the equivalent human dose (based on BSA). Based on the mechanism of action, omacetaxine may cause fetal harm if administered during pregnancy. Women of reproductive potential should avoid pregnancy during therapy. Omacetaxine may impair fertility in males.

Breast-Feeding Considerations It is not known if omacetaxine is excreted in breast milk. Due to the potential for serious adverse reactions in the nursing infant, the decision to discontinue omacetaxine or to discontinue breastfeeding should take into account the importance of treatment to the mother.

Medication Guide Available Yes

Contraindications There are no contraindications listed in the manufacturer's labeling.

Warnings/Precautions Hazardous agent: Use appropriate precautions for handling and disposal (NIOSH 2014 [group 1]). Grade 3/4 neutropenia, thrombocytopenia, and anemia commonly occur; generally reversible, although may require treatment delay and/or a reduction in the number of treatment days with future cycles. Myelosuppression may rarely be fatal. Monitor blood counts (in induction and maintenance cycles). Neutropenia may increase the risk for infection. Thrombocytopenia may increase the risk of bleeding; cerebrovascular hemorrhages have been reported (some fatal); gastrointestinal hemorrhages have occurred. Due to the increased risk of bleeding, avoid the use of anticoagulants, aspirin, and NSAIDs when the platelet count is <50,000/mm³. Patients ≥65 years of age are more likely to experience hematologic toxicity. Omacetaxine may induce glucose intolerance; hyperglycemia has been observed; hyperosmolar nonketotic hyperglycemia has been reported (case report). Monitor blood glucose frequently, especially in patients with diabetes or with risk factors for diabetes. Avoid use in patients with poorly controlled diabetes; may initiate after glycemic control has been established. Potentially significant interactions may exist, requiring dose or frequency adjustment, additional monitoring, and/or selection of alternative therapy.

Adverse Reactions

>10%:

Cardiovascular: Peripheral edema (16%)

Central nervous system: Fatigue (29% to 31%), headache (13% to 20%), chills (13%), insomnia (12%)

Dermatologic: Alopecia (15%), skin rash (11%)

Endocrine & metabolic: Uric acid increased (grades 3/4: 56% to 57%), hyperglycemia (grades 3/4: 10% to 15%; hyperosmolar nonketotic hyperglycemia <1%)

Gastrointestinal: Diarrhea (35% to 41%), nausea (29% to 35%), abdominal pain (16% to 23%), vomiting (12% to 15%), constipation (14%), anorexia (10% to 13%)

Hematologic: Thrombocytopenia (58% to 76%; grades 3/4: 49% to 88%), anemia 51% to 61%; grades 3/4: 36% to 80%), neutropenia (20% to 53%; grades 3/4: 18% to 81%), leukocytes decreased (grades 3/4: 61% to 72%), neutropenic fever (10% to 20%; grades 3/4: 10% to 16%), lymphopenia (17%; grades 3/4: 16%)

Local: Injection site reactions (22% to 35%; includes infusion related reaction, erythema, hematoma, hemorrhage, hypersensitivity, induration, inflammation, irritation, mass, edema, pruritus, and rash)

Neuromuscular & skeletal: Weakness (23% to 24%), arthralgia (19%), limb pain (11% to 13%), back pain (12%), myalgia (11%)

Renal: Creatinine increased (grades 3/4: 9% to 16%)

Respiratory: Epistaxis (11% to 17%), cough (≤16%), dyspnea (11%)

Miscellaneous: Infection (46% to 56%; grades 3/4: 11% to 20%), fever (25% to 29%)

1% to 10%:

Cardiovascular: Acute coronary syndrome, angina pectoris, arrhythmia, bradycardia, cerebral hemorrhage, chest pain, edema, hypertension, hypotension, palpitations, tachycardia, ventricular extrasystoles

Central nervous system: Anxiety, agitation, confusion, depression, dizziness, dysphonia, hyperthermia, hypoesthesia, lethargy, malaise, mental status change, pain, seizures

Dermatologic: Bruising, burning sensation, dry skin, erythema, hyperhidrosis, hyperpigmentation, petechiae, pruritus, purpura, skin exfoliation, skin lesions, skin ulceration

Endocrine & metabolic: Glucose decreased (grades 3/4: 6% to 8%), dehydration, diabetes mellitus, gout, hot flashes

Gastrointestinal: Abdominal distension, abnormal taste, anal fissure, aphthous stomatitis, appetite decreased, dyspepsia, dysphagia, gastritis, gastroesophageal reflux disease, GI bleeding, gingival bleeding, gingival pain, gingivitis, hemorrhoids, melena, mouth ulceration, mouth hemorrhage, mucosal inflammation, oral pain, stomatitis, xerostomia

Genitourinary: Dysuria

Hematologic: Bone marrow failure (10%; grades 3/4: 10%), hematoma

Hepatic: Bilirubin increased (grades 3/4: 6% to 9%), ALT increased (grades 3/4: 2% to 6%)

Neuromuscular & skeletal: Bone pain, muscle spasms, muscle weakness, musculoskeletal chest pain, musculoskeletal discomfort, musculoskeletal pain, paresthesia, sciatica, stiffness, tremor

Ocular: Blurred vision, cataract, conjunctival hemorrhage, conjunctivitis, diplopia, dry eyes, eye pain, eyelid edema, lacrimation increased

Otic: Ear hemorrhage, ear pain, tinnitus

Respiratory: Hemoptysis, nasal congestion, pharyngolaryngeal pain, rales, rhinorrhea, sinus congestion

Miscellaneous: Flu-like syndrome, hypersensitivity reactions, night sweats, transfusion reaction

Drug Interactions

Metabolism/Transport Effects Substrate of P-glycoprotein

Avoid Concomitant Use

Avoid concomitant use of Omacetaxine with any of the following: Anticoagulants; Aspirin; BCG (Intravesical); Natalizumab; Nonsteroidal Anti-Inflammatory Agents; Pimecrolimus; Tacrolimus (Topical); Tofacitinib; Vaccines (Live)

Increased Effect/Toxicity

Omacetaxine may increase the levels/effects of: Fingolimod; Leflunomide; Natalizumab; Tofacitinib; Vaccines (Live)

The levels/effects of Omacetaxine may be increased by: Anticoagulants; Aspirin; Denosumab; Nonsteroidal Anti-Inflammatory Agents; Pimecrolimus; Roflumilast; Tacrolimus (Topical); Trastuzumab

Decreased Effect

Omacetaxine may decrease the levels/effects of: Antidiabetic Agents; BCG (Intravesical); Coccidioides immitis Skin Test; Sipuleucel-T; Vaccines (Inactivated); Vaccines (Live)

The levels/effects of Omacetaxine may be decreased by: Echinacea

Preparation for Administration Hazardous agent: Use appropriate precautions for handling and disposal (NIOSH 2014 [group 1]). Avoid skin and eye contact; wear protective eyewear and gloves during handling and administration. Reconstitute each 3.5 mg vial with sodium chloride 0.9% (NS) 1 mL, resulting in a concentration of 3.5 mg/mL. Gently swirl until solution is clear (lyophilized powder dissolves completely in <1 minute).

Storage/Stability Store intact vials at 20°C to 25°C (68°F to 77°F); excursions are permitted between 15°C and 30°C (59°F and 86°F). Protect from light (intact vial and reconstituted solutions). Reconstituted solution should be used within 12 hours if stored at room temperature or within 6 days (144 hours) if refrigerated at 2°C to 8°C (36°F to 46°F).

Mechanism of Action Omacetaxine is a reversible protein synthesis inhibitor which binds to the A-site cleft of the ribosomal subunit to interfere with chain elongation and inhibit protein synthesis. It acts independently of BCR-ABL1 kinase-binding activity, and has demonstrated activity against tyrosine kinase inhibitor-resistant BCR-ABL mutations.

Pharmacodynamics/Kinetics

Onset:

Chronic phase CML: Mean time to major cytogenetic response: 3.5 months

Accelerated phase CML: Mean time to response: 2.3 months

Duration:

Chronic phase CML: Median duration of major cytogenetic response: 12.5 months

Accelerated phase CML: Median duration of major hematologic response: 4.7 months

Absorption: SubQ: Rapid (Nemunaitis, 2013)

Distribution: V_{dss}: 141 ± 93 L

Protein binding: ≤50%

Metabolism: Hydrolyzed by plasma esterases to 4'-DMHHT; minimal hepatic metabolism

Half-life elimination: ~6 hours

Time to peak: SubQ: ~30 minutes

Excretion: Urine (<15%)

Dosing

Adult & Geriatric Chronic myeloid leukemia (CML), chronic or accelerated phase: SubQ:

Induction: 1.25 mg/m² twice daily for 14 consecutive days of a 28-day treatment cycle; continue until hematologic response is achieved

Maintenance: 1.25 mg/m² twice daily for 7 consecutive days of a 28-day treatment cycle; continue until no longer achieving clinical treatment benefit

Missed doses: If a dose is missed, skip that dose and resume with the next regularly scheduled dose. Do not administer 2 doses at the same time to make up for a missed dose.

Renal Impairment There are no dosage adjustments provided in the manufacturer's labeling (has not been studied). Based on the minimal amount of unchanged drug excreted in the urine, dosage adjustment is not likely necessary (Nemunaitis, 2013).

Hepatic Impairment There are no dosage adjustments provided in the manufacturer's labeling (has not been studied).

Adjustment for Toxicity

Hematologic toxicity: May delay treatment cycles and/or reduce the number of treatment days during a cycle for hematologic toxicities.

Neutropenia grade 4 (ANC <500/mm³) or thrombocytopenia ≥ grade 3 (platelets <50,000/mm³) during a cycle: Delay the start of the next cycle until ANC ≥1000/mm³ and platelets ≥50,000/mm³ **AND** reduce the number of treatment days by 2 days (eg, reduce from 14 days to 12 days or reduce from 7 days to 5 days)

Nonhematologic toxicity: Manage symptomatically; interrupt and/or delay treatment until toxicity resolves.

Administration Administer subcutaneously at approximately 12 hour intervals. If home administration is to occur, advise patient on proper handling, storage conditions, administration, disposal, and clean-up of accidental spillage; ensure that the patient or patient's caregiver is an appropriate candidate for home administration.

Hazardous agent: Use appropriate precautions for handling and disposal (NIOSH 2014 [group 1]). Avoid skin and eye contact; wear protective eyewear and gloves during handling and administration.

Monitoring Parameters CBC with differential and platelets (weekly during induction and initial maintenance cycles, then every 2 weeks or as clinically indicated after initial maintenance cycles); blood glucose (frequently); signs/symptoms of infection; signs of bleeding

Dosage Forms Excipient information presented when available (limited, particularly for generics); consult specific product labeling.

Solution Reconstituted, Subcutaneous, as mepesuccinate [preservative free]:

Synribo: 3.5 mg (1 ea)

◆ Omacetaxine Mepesuccinate *see* Omacetaxine *on page 1324*

Omalizumab (oh mah lye ZOO mab)

Brand Names: US Xolair
Brand Names: Canada Xolair
Index Terms rhuMAb-E25

Pharmacologic Category Monoclonal Antibody, Anti-Asthmatic

Use

Asthma: Treatment of moderate to severe persistent asthma in adults and adolescents 12 years and older who have a positive skin test or *in vitro* reactivity to a perennial aeroallergen and whose symptoms are inadequately controlled with inhaled corticosteroids.

Guideline recommendations:

The 2007 National Asthma Education and Prevention Program asthma guidelines recommend use be considered as adjunctive therapy in patients with severe persistent asthma who have allergies and in patients with severe persistent asthma that is inadequately controlled with a combination of a high-dose inhaled corticosteroid and a long-acting beta₂-agonist (NAEPP 2007).

The Global Initiative for Asthma suggests use be considered as adjunctive therapy in patients with moderate or severe allergic asthma that is uncontrolled with a combination of a medium- to high-dose inhaled corticosteroid and a long-acting beta₂-agonist (GINA 2015).

Chronic idiopathic urticaria: Treatment of chronic idiopathic urticaria in adults and adolescents 12 years and older who remain symptomatic despite H_1 antihistamine treatment.

Pregnancy Considerations Adverse events have not been observed in animal reproduction studies. IgG molecules are known to cross the placenta. A registry has been established to monitor outcomes of women exposed to omalizumab during pregnancy or within 8 weeks prior to pregnancy (http://www.xolairpregnancyregistry.com or 866-496-5247).

Breast-Feeding Considerations It is not known if omalizumab is excreted in breast milk; however, IgG is excreted in human milk and excretion of omalizumab is expected. The manufacturer recommends that caution be exercised when administering omalizumab to breast-feeding women.

Medication Guide Available Yes

Contraindications Severe hypersensitivity reaction to omalizumab or any component of the formulation

Warnings/Precautions [U.S. Boxed Warning]: Anaphylaxis, including delayed-onset anaphylaxis, has been reported following administration; anaphylaxis may present as bronchospasm, hypotension, syncope, urticaria, and/or angioedema of the throat or tongue. Anaphylaxis has occurred after the first dose and in some cases >1 year after initiation of regular treatment. Due to the risk, patients should be observed closely for an appropriate time period after administration and should receive treatment only under direct medical supervision. Healthcare providers should be prepared to administer appropriate therapy for managing potentially life-threatening anaphylaxis. Patients should be instructed on identifying signs/symptoms of anaphylaxis and to seek immediate care if they arise. In postmarketing reports, anaphylaxis usually occurred with the first or second dose and with a time to onset of ≤60 minutes; however, reactions have been reported with subsequent doses (after 39 doses) and with a time to onset of up to 4 days after administration. Discontinue therapy following any severe reaction.

In rare cases, patients may present with systemic eosinophilia, sometimes presenting with clinical features of vasculitis consistent with Churg-Strauss syndrome, a condition which is often treated with systemic corticosteroid therapy. Healthcare providers should be alert to eosinophilia, vasculitic rash, worsening pulmonary symptoms, cardiac complications, and/or neuropathy presenting in their patients. A causal association between omalizumab and these underlying conditions has not been established. Reports of a constellation of symptoms including fever, arthritis or arthralgia, rash, and lymphadenopathy have been reported with postmarketing use (symptoms resemble those seen in patients experiencing serum sickness, although circulating immune complexes or a skin biopsy consistent with a Type III hypersensitivity reaction were not seen with these cases). Onset of symptoms generally occurred 1-5 days following the first or subsequent doses. Discontinue therapy in any patient reporting this constellation of signs/symptoms. Malignant neoplasms have been reported rarely with use in short-term studies; impact of long-term use is not known. Use caution with and monitor patients at high risk for parasitic (helminth) infections (risk of infection may be increased).

Therapy has not been shown to alleviate acute asthma exacerbations; do not use to treat acute bronchospasm or status asthmaticus. Do not use to treat forms of urticaria other than chronic idiopathic urticaria. Dosing for allergic ▶

asthma is based on body weight and pretreatment total IgE serum levels. IgE levels remain elevated up to 1 year following treatment; therefore, levels taken during treatment or for up to 1 year following treatment cannot and should not be used as a dosage guide. Dosing in chronic idiopathic urticaria is not dependent on serum IgE (free or total) level or body weight. Gradually taper systemic or inhaled corticosteroid therapy; do not discontinue corticosteroids abruptly following initiation of omalizumab therapy. The combined use of omalizumab and corticosteroids in patients with chronic idiopathic urticaria has not been evaluated. Potentially significant drug-drug interactions may exist, requiring dose or frequency adjustment, additional monitoring, and/or selection of alternative therapy.

Adverse Reactions

Asthma:

>10%: Local: Injection site reaction (45%; severe 12%; includes bruising, redness, warmth, burning, stinging, itching, hive formation, pain, indurations, mass, and inflammation). Most reactions occurred within 1 hour, lasted <8 days, and decreased in frequency with additional dosing.

1% to 10%:

Cardiovascular: Pulmonary embolism (≤3%), venous thrombosis (≤3%), myocardial infarction (2%), unstable angina pectoris (2%)

Central nervous system: Pain (7%), dizziness (3%), fatigue (3%)

Dermatologic: Dermatitis (2%), pruritus (2%)

Neuromuscular & skeletal: Arthralgia (8%), leg pain (4%), arm pain (2%), bone fracture (2%)

Otic: Otalgia (2%)

Chronic idiopathic urticaria:

>10%: Central nervous system: Headache (6% to 12%)

1% to 10%:

Cardiovascular: Peripheral edema (≥2%)

Central nervous system: Anxiety (≥2%), migraine (≥2%)

Dermatologic: Alopecia (≥2%)

Gastrointestinal: Toothache (≥2%)

Genitourinary: Urinary tract infection (≥2%)

Infection: Fungal infection (≥2%)

Local: Injection site reaction (3%)

Neuromuscular & skeletal: Arthralgia (3%), limb pain (≥2%), musculoskeletal pain (≥2%), myalgia (≥2%)

Respiratory: Nasopharyngitis (9%), sinusitis (5%), upper respiratory tract infection (3%), asthma (≥2%), oropharyngeal pain (≥2%), sinus headache (≥2%), cough (2%), viral upper respiratory tract infection (≤2%)

Miscellaneous: Fever (≥2%)

All indications: <1% (Limited to important or life-threatening): Alopecia, anaphylaxis, antibody development, arthritis, chest tightness, Churg-Strauss syndrome, lymphadenopathy, malignant neoplasm, pulmonary hypertension, syncope, thrombocytopenia, transient ischemic attacks

Drug Interactions

Metabolism/Transport Effects None known.

Avoid Concomitant Use

Avoid concomitant use of Omalizumab with any of the following: Belimumab; Loxapine

Increased Effect/Toxicity

Omalizumab may increase the levels/effects of: Belimumab; Loxapine

Decreased Effect There are no known significant interactions involving a decrease in effect.

Preparation for Administration Reconstitute using SWFI only; add SWFI 1.4 mL to upright vial using a 1-inch, 18-gauge needle on a 3 mL syringe and swirl gently for ~1 minute to evenly wet the powder; do not shake. Then gently swirl the upright vial for 5-10 seconds approximately every 5 minutes until dissolved; generally takes 15-20 minutes to dissolve completely. If it takes >20 minutes to dissolve completely, continue to swirl the upright vial for 5-10 seconds every 5 minutes until no gel-like particles are visible in the solution; do not use if contents are not completely dissolved after 40 minutes. Resulting solution is 150 mg/1.2 mL. Invert the vial for 15 seconds so the solution drains toward the stopper. Remove all of the solution by inserting a new 3 mL syringe with a 1-inch, 18-gauge needle into the inverted vial. Replace the 18-gauge needle with a 25-gauge needle for subcutaneous injection, and expel any air, bubbles, or excess solution to obtain the 1.2 mL dose.

Storage/Stability Prior to reconstitution, store under refrigeration at 2°C to 8°C (36°F to 46°F); product may be shipped at room temperature. Following reconstitution, protect from direct sunlight. May be stored for up to 8 hours if refrigerated or 4 hours if stored at room temperature.

Mechanism of Action

Asthma: Omalizumab is an IgG monoclonal antibody (recombinant DNA derived) which inhibits IgE binding to the high-affinity IgE receptor on mast cells and basophils. By decreasing bound IgE, the activation and release of mediators in the allergic response (early and late phase) is limited. Serum free IgE levels and the number of high-affinity IgE receptors are decreased. Long-term treatment in patients with allergic asthma showed a decrease in asthma exacerbations and corticosteroid usage.

Chronic idiopathic urticaria: Omalizumab binds to IgE and lowers free IgE levels. Subsequently, IgE receptors (FcεRI) on cells down-regulate. The mechanism by which these effects of omalizumab result in an improvement of chronic idiopathic urticaria symptoms is unknown.

Pharmacodynamics/Kinetics

Absorption: Slow following SubQ injection

Distribution: V_d: 78 ± 32 mL/kg

Metabolism: Degradation of IgG and omalizumab: IgE complexes by reticuloendothelial system and endothelial cells in the liver

Bioavailability: 62%

Half-life elimination: 26 days (asthma patients); 24 days (chronic idiopathic urticaria patients)

Time to peak: 7-8 days

Excretion: Primarily via hepatic degradation; intact IgG may be secreted in bile

Dosing

Adult & Geriatric Asthma: SubQ: Dose and frequency based on body weight and **pretreatment** total IgE serum levels. Dosing should be adjusted during therapy for significant changes in body weight. Dosing should **not** be adjusted based on total IgE levels taken during treatment or <1 year following interruption of therapy. If therapy has been interrupted for ≥1 year, total IgE levels may be re-evaluated for dosage determination.

Pretreatment serum IgE ≥30 to 100 units/mL:

U.S. labeling:

30 to 90 kg: 150 mg every 4 weeks

>90 to 150 kg: 300 mg every 4 weeks

Canadian labeling:

>20 to 90 kg: 150 mg every 4 weeks

>90 to 150 kg: 300 mg every 4 weeks

Pretreatment serum IgE >100 to 200 units/mL:

U.S. labeling:

30 to 90 kg: 300 mg every 4 weeks

>90 to 150 kg: 225 mg every 2 weeks

Canadian labeling:

>20 to 40 kg: 150 mg every 4 weeks

>40 to 90 kg: 300 mg every 4 weeks

>90 to 125 kg: 225 mg every 2 weeks

>125 to 150 kg: 300 mg every 2 weeks

Pretreatment serum IgE >200 to 300 units/mL:

U.S. labeling:

30 to 60 kg: 300 mg every 4 weeks

>60 to 90 kg: 225 mg every 2 weeks

>90 to 150 kg: 300 mg every 2 weeks

Canadian labeling:

>20 to 30 kg: 150 mg every 4 weeks

>30 to 60 kg: 300 mg every 4 weeks

>60 to 90 kg: 225 mg every 2 weeks

>90 to 125 kg: 300 mg every 2 weeks

>125 to 150 kg: 375 mg every 2 weeks

Pretreatment serum IgE >300 to 400 units/mL:

U.S. labeling:

30 to 70 kg: 225 mg every 2 weeks

>70 to 90 kg: 300 mg every 2 weeks

>90 kg: Do not administer dose

Canadian labeling:

>20 to 40 kg: 300 mg every 4 weeks

>40 to 70 kg: 225 mg every 2 weeks

>70 to 90 kg: 300 mg every 2 weeks

>90 kg: Do not administer dose

Pretreatment serum IgE >400 to 500 units/mL:

U.S. labeling:

30 to 70 kg: 300 mg every 2 weeks

>70 to 90 kg: 375 mg every 2 weeks

>90 kg: Do not administer dose

Canadian labeling:

>20 to 30 kg: 300 mg every 4 weeks

>30 to 50 kg: 225 mg every 2 weeks

>50 to 70 kg: 300 mg every 2 weeks

>70 to 90 kg: 375 mg every 2 weeks

>90 kg: Do not administer dose

Pretreatment serum IgE >500 to 600 units/mL:

U.S. labeling:

30 to 60 kg: 300 mg every 2 weeks

>60 to 70 kg: 375 mg every 2 weeks

>70 kg: Do not administer dose

Canadian labeling:
>20 to 30 kg: 300 mg every 4 weeks
>30 to 40 kg: 225 mg every 2 weeks
>40 to 60 kg: 300 mg every 2 weeks
>60 to 70 kg: 375 mg every 2 weeks
>70 kg: Do not administer dose
Pretreatment serum IgE >600 to 700 units/mL:
U.S. labeling:
30 to 60 kg: 375 mg every 2 weeks
>60 kg: Do not administer dose
Canadian labeling:
>20 to 40 kg: 225 mg every 2 weeks
>40 to 50 kg: 300 mg every 2 weeks
>50 to 60 kg: 375 mg every 2 weeks
>60 kg: Do not administer dose

Chronic idiopathic urticaria: SubQ: 150 or 300 mg every 4 weeks. Dosing is not dependent on serum IgE (free or total) level or body weight.

Pediatric Asthma/Chronic idiopathic urticaria: Adolescents ≥12 years: SubQ: Refer to adult dosing.

Renal Impairment There are no dosage adjustments provided in manufacturer's labeling.

Hepatic Impairment There are no dosage adjustments provided in manufacturer's labeling.

Adjustment for Toxicity
Severe hypersensitivity reaction or anaphylaxis: Discontinue treatment.
Fever, arthralgia, and rash: Discontinue treatment if this constellation of symptoms occurs.

Administration For SubQ injection only; doses >150 mg should be divided over more than one injection site (eg, 225 mg or 300 mg administered as two injections, 375 mg administered as three injections). Injections may take 5 to 10 seconds to administer (solution is slightly viscous). Administer only under direct medical supervision and observe patient for a minimum of 2 hours following administration of any dose given.

Monitoring Parameters Anaphylactic/hypersensitivity reactions, baseline serum total IgE; FEV$_1$, peak flow, and/or other pulmonary function tests; monitor for signs of infection

Test Interactions Total IgE levels are elevated for up to 1 year following treatment. Total serum IgE may be retested after interruption of therapy for 1 year or more.

Dosage Forms Excipient information presented when available (limited, particularly for generics); consult specific product labeling.
Solution Reconstituted, Subcutaneous [preservative free]:
Xolair: 150 mg (1 ea)

Ombitasvir, Paritaprevir, and Ritonavir
(om BIT as vir, par i TA pre vir, & ri TOE na vir)

Brand Names: US Technivie
Brand Names: Canada Technivie
Index Terms Paritaprevir, Ombitasvir, and Ritonavir; Ritonavir, Ombitasvir, and Paritaprevir
Pharmacologic Category Antihepaciviral, NS5A Inhibitor; Antihepaciviral, Protease Inhibitor (Anti-HCV); Cytochrome P-450 Inhibitor
Use Chronic hepatitis C: Treatment of chronic hepatitis C virus (HCV) genotype 4 infection without cirrhosis in combination with ribavirin.
Dosing
Adult & Geriatric
Chronic hepatitis C: Adults: Oral: **Note:** Ombitasvir, paritaprevir, and ritonavir are a fixed-dose combination tablet.
Genotype 4 without cirrhosis (used with concomitant ribavirin): 2 tablets once daily (every morning) with ribavirin for 12 weeks
Genotype 4 (treatment-naive) without cirrhosis (patients who cannot tolerate ribavirin): 2 tablets once daily (every morning) for 12 weeks
Renal Impairment
CrCl ≥15 mL/minute: No dosage adjustment necessary.
End-stage renal disease (ESRD) on dialysis: There are no dosage adjustments provided in the manufacturer's labeling (has not been studied).
Hepatic Impairment
Mild impairment (Child-Pugh class A): No dosage adjustment necessary.
Moderate to severe impairment (Child-Pugh class B or C): Use is contraindicated.
Adjustment for Toxicity
ALT >10 times ULN (persistent): Consider therapy discontinuation.
ALT increased along with signs or symptoms of hepatic inflammation, increasing direct bilirubin, alkaline phosphatase, or INR: Discontinue therapy.

Additional Information Complete prescribing information should be consulted for additional detail.
Dosage Forms Excipient information presented when available (limited, particularly for generics); consult specific product labeling.
Tablet, Oral:
Technivie: Ombitasvir 12.5 mg, paritaprevir 75 mg, and ritonavir 50 mg

Ombitasvir, Paritaprevir, Ritonavir, and Dasabuvir
(om BIT as vir, par i TA pre vir, ri TOE na vir, & da SA bue vir)

Brand Names: US Viekira Pak
Brand Names: Canada Holkira Pak
Index Terms Dasabuvir, Ombitasvir, Paritaprevir, and Ritonavir; Paritaprevir, Ombitasvir, Ritonavir, and Dasabuvir; Ritonavir, Ombitasvir, Paritaprevir, and Dasabuvir
Pharmacologic Category Antihepaciviral, NS5A Inhibitor; Antihepaciviral, Polymerase Inhibitor (Anti-HCV); Antihepaciviral, Protease Inhibitor (Anti-HCV); Cytochrome P-450 Inhibitor
Use Chronic hepatitis C: Treatment of genotype 1 chronic hepatitis C virus infection, with or without ribavirin, including patients with compensated cirrhosis.
Pregnancy Considerations Adverse events were not observed in animal reproduction studies. This combination product is contraindicated for use with ribavirin in pregnant women. Health care providers are encouraged to enroll pregnant women exposed to antiretroviral medications in the Antiretroviral Pregnancy Registry (1-800-258-4263 or http://www.APRegistry.com).
Breast-Feeding Considerations It is not known if the components of this combination are excreted into breast milk. According to the US labeling, the decision to breast-feed during therapy should take into account the risk of exposure to the infant and the benefits of treatment to the mother. The Canadian labeling recommends discontinuing nursing prior to initiating therapy. Mothers coinfected with HIV are discouraged from breast-feeding to decrease potential transmission of HIV (DHHS [perinatal] 2014).
Medication Guide Available Yes
Contraindications
Hypersensitivity (eg, toxic epidermal necrolysis, Stevens-Johnson syndrome) to any component of the formulation, including to ritonavir; moderate to severe hepatic impairment (Child-Pugh class B or C); concurrent use of drugs that are highly dependent on CYP3A for clearance and for which elevated plasma concentrations are associated with serious and/or life-threatening events; concurrent use of moderate or strong inducers of CYP3A, strong inducers of CYP2C8, or strong inhibitors of CYP2C8. Concurrent use of drugs that are contraindicated include, but are not necessarily limited to: alfuzosin, carbamazepine, colchicine, ergot derivatives (ergonovine, ergotamine, dihydroergotamine, methylergonovine), ethinyl estradiol-containing products, efavirenz, gemfibrozil, lovastatin, midazolam (oral), phenobarbital, phenytoin, pimozide, rifampin, sildenafil (when used for the treatment of pulmonary arterial hypertension [eg, Revatio]), simvastatin, St John's wort, triazolam. If used with ribavirin, contraindications of ribavirin also apply. See ribavirin prescribing information.
Canadian labeling: Additional contraindications (not in US labeling): Concomitant use with astemizole, avasimibe, bosentan, cisapride, etravirine, fusidic acid (oral formulation), modafinil, nafcillin, salmeterol, terfenadine
Warnings/Precautions Hepatic decompensation and hepatic failure, including liver transplantation and fatal cases, have been reported with ombitasvir, paritaprevir, ritonavir, and dasabuvir. Typically occurs between 1 and 4 weeks of treatment initiation; characterized by acute elevation of direct bilirubin, without ALT elevation, and signs and symptoms of hepatic decompensation. In patients with cirrhosis, monitor for clinical signs and symptoms of hepatic decompensation (eg, ascites, hepatic encephalopathy, variceal hemorrhage) and perform hepatic function testing (including direct bilirubin) at baseline, during the first 4 weeks of treatment initiation, and as indicated thereafter. Discontinue treatment in patients who develop signs/symptoms of hepatic decompensation. Elevations of hepatic enzymes (eg, ALT >5 times ULN) have been reported. Elevations are usually asymptomatic, occur within 4 weeks of treatment initiation, and decline within 2 to 8 weeks with continued dosing. Monitor hepatic enzymes during the first 4 weeks of treatment initiation and thereafter as clinically indicated. If ALT is elevated, repeat testing and continue to monitor closely; patients should contact their health care professional immediately if they experience onset of fatigue, weakness, lack of appetite, nausea and vomiting, jaundice, or discolored feces. Consider discontinuation if

ALT remains persistently >10 x ULN. Discontinue if ALT increase is accompanied by signs of hepatic inflammation, elevated direct bilirubin, alkaline phosphatase, or INR. Female patients taking ethinyl estradiol products are at increased risk. Avoid use in moderate to severe hepatic impairment (Child-Pugh class B or C). If used with concomitant ribavirin, contraindications of ribavirin, particularly pregnancy avoidance warnings, also apply (see ribavirin prescribing information).

Concomitant use of ethinyl estradiol-containing products is contraindicated; these products may be restarted approximately 2 weeks following completion of HCV therapy. Alternative methods of contraception (eg, nonhormonal methods, progestin only contraception) are recommended during therapy. Women using other estrogens (eg, estradiol, conjugated estrogens) should have hepatic enzymes tested during the first 4 weeks of treatment and as clinically indicated thereafter.

Potentially significant interactions may exist, requiring dose or frequency adjustment, additional monitoring, and/or selection of alternative therapy. Ritonavir, a component of the product, is also an HIV-1 protease inhibitor. In HCV/HIV coinfected patients, ritonavir can select for HIV-1 protease inhibitor resistance-associated substitutions. Any HCV/HIV-1 coinfected patients should also be taking a suppressive antiretroviral regimen to reduce resistance risk.

Adverse Reactions Incidences may include data from administration with and without ribavirin.

>10%:

Central nervous system: Fatigue (34%; patients with HCV/HIV-1 co-infection: 48%; liver transplant recipients: 50%); headache (liver transplant recipients: 44%; patients with HCV/HIV-1 co-infection: 16%), insomnia (5% to 26%)

Dermatologic: Dermatological reaction (7% to 24%; may include allergic dermatitis, contact dermatitis, dermal ulcer, dermatitis, desquamation, eczema, erythema, erythematous rash, exfoliative dermatitis, macular rash, maculopapular rash, papular rash, pruritic rash, psoriasis, skin photosensitivity, skin rash, urticaria), pruritus (7% to 18%)

Gastrointestinal: Diarrhea (liver transplant recipients: 26%), nausea (8% to 24%)

Hematologic & oncologic: Decreased hemoglobin (decrease to <8 g/dL: <1%; <10 g/dL: Liver transplant recipients: 29%, patients with HCV/HIV-1 co-infection: 11%)

Hepatic: Increased serum bilirubin (>2 x ULN; 2% to 15%; patients with HCV/HIV-1 co-infection: 54%); increased serum ALT (>5 x ULN; 1%; women taking concomitant ethinyl estradiol: 25%; women taking concomitant estrogens other than ethinyl estradiol: 3%)

Neuromuscular & skeletal: Weakness (4% to 14%; liver transplant recipients: 24%), muscle spasm (liver transplant recipients: 21%)

Respiratory: Cough (liver transplant recipients: 32%; patients with HCV/HIV-1 co-infection: 11%)

1% to 10%:

Central nervous system: Irritability (patients with HCV/HIV-1 co-infection: 10%)

Ophthalmic: Scleral icterus (patients with HCV/HIV-1 co-infection: 10%)

Respiratory: Dyspnea

<1% (Limited to important or life-threatening): Hepatic failure (in patients with underlying cirhosis; FDA Safety Alert, October 22, 2015), hypersensitivity reaction (including angioedema, tonue swelling, lip swelling), liver decompensation (in patients with underlying cirrhosis; FDA Safety Alert, October 22, 2015)

Drug Interactions

Metabolism/Transport Effects Substrate of BCRP, CYP2C8 (major), CYP2D6 (minor), CYP3A4 (major), P-glycoprotein, SLCO1B1, SLCO1B3; **Note:** Assignment of Major/Minor substrate status based on clinically relevant drug interaction potential; **Inhibits** BCRP, CYP3A4 (strong), P-glycoprotein, SLCO1B1, SLCO1B3, UGT1A1; **Induces** CYP1A2 (weak/moderate), CYP2C19 (weak/moderate)

Avoid Concomitant Use

Avoid concomitant use of Ombitasvir, Paritaprevir, Ritonavir, and Dasabuvir with any of the following: Ado-Trastuzumab Emtansine; Alfuzosin; Aprepitant; Astemizole; Avanafil; Axitinib; Barnidipine; Bosutinib; Bromocriptine; Cabozantinib; Ceritinib; Cisapride; Cobimetinib; Colchicine; Conivaptan; Crizotinib; CYP2C8 Inducers (Strong); CYP2C8 Inhibitors (Strong); CYP3A4 Inducers (Moderate); CYP3A4 Inducers (Strong); Dabrafenib; Dapoxetine; Darunavir; Domperidone; Dronedarone; Eletriptan; Eplerenone; Ergot Derivatives; Ethinyl Estradiol; Everolimus; Flibanserin; Fusidic Acid (Systemic); Halofantrine; Ibrutinib; Idelalisib; Irinotecan Products; Isavuconazonium Sulfate; Ivabradine; Lapatinib; Lercanidipine; Lomitapide; Lopinavir; Lovastatin; Lurasidone; Macitentan; Midazolam; Naloxegol; Nilotinib; NiMODipine; Nisoldipine; Olaparib; Osimertinib; Palbociclib; Pimozide; QuiNINE; Ranolazine; Red Yeast Rice; Regorafenib; Rilpivirine; Salmeterol; Silodosin; Simeprevir; Simvastatin; Sonidegib; Suvorexant; Tamsulosin; Terfenadine; Ticagrelor; Tolvaptan; Toremifene; Trabectedin; Triazolam; Ulipristal; Vemurafenib; VinCRIStine (Liposomal); Vorapaxar

Increased Effect/Toxicity

Ombitasvir, Paritaprevir, Ritonavir, and Dasabuvir may increase the levels/effects of: Ado-Trastuzumab Emtansine; Alfentanil; Alfuzosin; Alitretinoin (Systemic); Almotriptan; Alosetron; ALPRAZolam; Amiodarone; AmLODIPine; Apixaban; Aprepitant; ARIPiprazole; ARIPiprazole Lauroxil; Astemizole; AtorvaSTATin; Avanafil; Axitinib; Barnidipine; Bedaquiline; Bepridil; Bortezomib; Bosutinib; Brentuximab Vedotin; Brexpiprazole; Brinzolamide; Bromocriptine; Budesonide (Nasal); Budesonide (Oral Inhalation); Budesonide (Systemic); Budesonide (Topical); Buprenorphine; Cabazitaxel; Cabozantinib; Cannabis; Cariprazine; Ceritinib; Cilostazol; Cisapride; Clarithromycin; Cobimetinib; Colchicine; Conivaptan; Corticosteroids (Orally Inhaled); Corticosteroids (Systemic); Crizotinib; CycloSPORINE (Systemic); CYP3A4 Substrates; Dabrafenib; Daclatasvir; Dapoxetine; Dasatinib; Dienogest; Dofetilide; Domperidone; DOXOrubicin (Conventional); Dronabinol; Dronedarone; Drospirenone; Dutasteride; Eletriptan; Eliglustat; Eluxadoline; Eplerenone; Ergot Derivatives; Erlotinib; Estazolam; Etizolam; Everolimus; FentaNYL; Fesoterodine; Flecainide; Flibanserin; Fluticasone (Nasal); Fluticasone (Oral Inhalation); Fluvastatin; Gefitinib; GuanFACINE; Halofantrine; Hydrocodone; Ibrutinib; Iloperidone; Imatinib; Imidafenacin; Irinotecan Products; Isavuconazonium Sulfate; Ivabradine; Ivacaftor; Ixabepilone; Ketoconazole (Systemic); Lacosamide; Lapatinib; Lercanidipine; Levobupivacaine; Levomilnacipran; Linagliptin; Lomitapide; Lovastatin; Lumefantrine; Lurasidone; Macitentan; Maraviroc; MedroxyPROGESTERone; MethylPREDNISolone; Mexiletine; Midazolam; Mifepristone; Naloxegol; Nilotinib; NiMODipine; Nisoldipine; Olaparib; Osimertinib; Ospemifene; Oxybutynin; OxyCODONE; Palbociclib; Panobinostat; Parecoxib; Paricalcitol; PAZOPanib; Pimecrolimus; Pimozide; Pitavastatin; PONATinib; Pranlukast; Pravastatin; PrednisoLONE (Systemic); PredniSONE; Propafenone; QUEtiapine; QuiNIDine; QuiNINE; Ramelteon; Ranolazine; Red Yeast Rice; Regorafenib; Repaglinide; Retapamulin; Rilpivirine; Riociguat; RomiDEPsin; Rosuvastatin; Ruxolitinib; Salmeterol; Saxagliptin; Sildenafil; Silodosin; Simeprevir; Simvastatin; Sirolimus; Sonidegib; SORAfenib; Suvorexant; Tacrolimus (Systemic); Tacrolimus (Topical); Tadalafil; Tamsulosin; Tasimelteon; Terfenadine; Tetrahydrocannabinol; Ticagrelor; Tofacitinib; Tolterodine; Tolvaptan; Toremifene; Trabectedin; TraMADol; Triamcinolone (Systemic); Triazolam; Ulipristal; Vardenafil; Vemurafenib; Vilazodone; VinCRIStine (Liposomal); Vindesine; Vinorelbine; Vorapaxar; Zopiclone; Zuclopenthixol

The levels/effects of Ombitasvir, Paritaprevir, Ritonavir, and Dasabuvir may be increased by: Abiraterone Acetate; Atazanavir; Conivaptan; CYP2C8 Inhibitors (Moderate); CYP2C8 Inhibitors (Strong); CYP3A4 Inhibitors (Moderate); CYP3A4 Inhibitors (Strong); Deferasirox; Ethinyl Estradiol; Fusidic Acid (Systemic); Idelalisib; Ketoconazole (Systemic); Lopinavir; Luliconazole; Mifepristone; Netupitant

Decreased Effect

Ombitasvir, Paritaprevir, Ritonavir, and Dasabuvir may decrease the levels/effects of: BuPROPion; Darunavir; Ifosfamide; OLANZapine; Omeprazole; Prasugrel; Proguanil; Ticagrelor; Voriconazole

The levels/effects of Ombitasvir, Paritaprevir, Ritonavir, and Dasabuvir may be decreased by: CYP2C8 Inducers (Strong); CYP3A4 Inducers (Moderate); CYP3A4 Inducers (Strong); Deferasirox; Siltuximab; Tocilizumab

Food Interactions Moderate- to high-fat meals increased the AUC of ombitasvir ≤82%, paritaprevir ≤211%, ritonavir ≤49% and dasabuvir ≤30%, respectively. Management: Administer with a meal.

Storage/Stability Store at or below 30°C (86°F). Dispense in original carton.

Mechanism of Action

Combines 3 direct-acting hepatitis C virus antiviral agents with distinct mechanisms of action. Ombitasvir inhibits HCV NS5A, and interferes with viral RNA replication and virion assembly. Paritaprevir inhibits HCV NS3/4A protease and interferes with HCV coded polyprotein cleavage necessary for viral replication. Dasabuvir inhibits HCV

RNA-dependent RNA polymerase (encoded by the NS5B gene) which is also necessary for viral replication.

Ritonavir is not active against HCV. Ritonavir is a potent CYP3A inhibitor that increases peak and trough plasma drug concentrations of paritaprevir and overall drug exposure (ie, AUC).

Pharmacodynamics/Kinetics

Absorption: Dasabuvir: ~70%; Ombitasvir, paritaprevir, ritonavir: Not evaluated

Distribution:

Ombitasvir: V_d: 50.1 L

Paritaprevir: V_d: 16.7 L

Ritonavir: V_d: 21.5 L

Dasabuvir: V_d: 396 L

Protein binding: Ombitasvir: 99.9%; Paritaprevir: ~98%; Ritonavir: >99%; Dasabuvir: >99%

Metabolism:

Ombitasvir: Metabolized by amide hydrolysis and oxidative metabolism

Paritaprevir: Metabolized by CYP3A4 and to a lesser extent CYP3A5

Ritonavir: Metabolized by CYP3A and to a lesser extent CYP2D6

Dasabuvir: Metabolized by CYP2C8 and to a lesser extent CYP3A

Half-life elimination: Ombitasvir: 21 to 25 hours; Paritaprevir: 5.5 hours; Ritonavir: 4 hours; Dasabuvir 5.5 to 6 hours

Time to peak: Ombitasvir, paritaprevir, ritonavir, dasabuvir: 4 to 5 hours

Excretion:

Ombitasvir: Feces (~90%, mainly as unchanged drug) and urine (<2%, mainly as unchanged drug)

Paritaprevir: Feces (~88%, mainly as metabolites) and urine (~9%, mainly as metabolites)

Ritonavir: Feces (~86%) and urine (~11%)

Dasabuvir: Feces (~94%, mainly as metabolites) and urine (~2%, mainly as metabolites)

Dosing

Adult & Geriatric Chronic hepatitis C: Oral: **Note:** Regimen is a copackaged product; ombitasvir, paritaprevir, and ritonavir are a fixed-dose combination tablet; dasabuvir is an individual tablet.

Missed doses: May administer a missed dose if within 6 hours of regularly scheduled time (dasabuvir) or within 12 hours of regularly scheduled time (ombitasvir, paritaprevir, ritonavir). Otherwise, skip missed dose and resume at next scheduled time.

Genotype 1a, without cirrhosis (used with concomitant ribavirin):

Ombitasvir/paritaprevir/ritonavir tablet: Two tablets every morning for 12 weeks

Dasabuvir: 250 mg twice daily for 12 weeks

Genotype 1a, with cirrhosis (used with concomitant ribavirin):

US labeling: **Note:** Based on prior treatment history, some patients may be considered for a duration of therapy of 12 weeks.

Ombitasvir/paritaprevir/ritonavir tablet: Two tablets every morning for 24 weeks

Dasabuvir: 250 mg twice daily for 24 weeks

Canadian labeling:

Ombitasvir/paritaprevir/ritonavir tablet: Two tablets every morning for 12 weeks or for 24 weeks (if previous null response to pegylated interferon and ribavirin therapy)

Dasabuvir: 250 mg twice daily for 12 weeks or for 24 weeks (if previous null response to pegylated interferon and ribavirin therapy)

Genotype 1b, without cirrhosis:

Ombitasvir/paritaprevir/ritonavir tablet: Two tablets every morning for 12 weeks

Dasabuvir: 250 mg twice daily for 12 weeks

Genotype 1b, with cirrhosis (used with concomitant ribavirin):

Ombitasvir/paritaprevir/ritonavir tablet: Two tablets every morning for 12 weeks

Dasabuvir: 250 mg twice daily for 12 weeks

Genotype 1 (unknown subtype) or Genotype 1 (mixed infection) without cirrhosis (used with concomitant ribavirin):

Ombitasvir/paritaprevir/ritonavir tablet: Two tablets every morning for 12 weeks

Dasabuvir: 250 mg twice daily for 12 weeks

Genotype 1 (unknown subtype) or Genotype 1 (mixed infection) with cirrhosis (used with concomitant ribavirin):

Ombitasvir/paritaprevir/ritonavir tablet: Two tablets every morning for 24 weeks

Dasabuvir: 250 mg twice daily for 24 weeks

Genotype 1, liver transplant recipients, Metavir fibrosis score ≤2 (normal hepatic function, mild fibrosis) (regardless of genotype 1 subtype; used with concomitant ribavirin): **Note:** If calcineurin inhibitor used concomitantly, calcineurin inhibitor dosage adjustment is needed.

Ombitasvir/paritaprevir/ritonavir tablet: Two tablets every morning for 24 weeks

Dasabuvir: 250 mg twice daily for 24 weeks

Renal Impairment

Mild to severe impairment: No dosage adjustment necessary.

End stage renal disease (ESRD) on dialysis: There are no dosage adjustments provided in the manufacturer's labeling (has not been studied).

Hepatic Impairment

US labeling:

Mild impairment (Child-Pugh class A): No dosage adjustment necessary.

Moderate to severe impairment (Child-Pugh class B or C): Use is contraindicated.

Canadian labeling:

Mild impairment (Child-Pugh class A): No dosage adjustment necessary.

Moderate impairment (Child-Pugh class B): Use is not recommended.

Severe impairment (Child-Pugh class C): Use is contraindicated.

Dietary Considerations Take with a meal.

Administration Oral: Administer with a meal. The Canadian labeling recommends the tablets be swallowed whole and not crushed, chewed, or broken

Monitoring Parameters Baseline hepatic function tests and during the first 4 weeks of therapy, then periodically during therapy, especially in women taking concomitant estrogen products; serum HCV-RNA at baseline and at the end of treatment, during treatment follow-up, and when clinically indicated.

Dosage Forms Excipient information presented when available (limited, particularly for generics); consult specific product labeling.

Combination package:

Viekira Pak [28 day supply]:

Tablet, oral: Ombitasvir 12.5 mg, paritaprevir 75 mg, and ritonavir 50 mg (56s)

Tablet, oral: Dasabuvir 250 mg (56s)

♦ Omeclamox-Pak® *see* Omeprazole, Clarithromycin, and Amoxicillin *on page 1333*

♦ Omega 3 *see* Omega-3 Fatty Acids *on page 1329*

♦ Omega-3 2100 [OTC] *see* Omega-3 Fatty Acids *on page 1329*

♦ Omega-3-Acid Ethyl Esters *see* Omega-3 Fatty Acids *on page 1329*

♦ Omega-3 Fish Oil Ex St [OTC] *see* Omega-3 Fatty Acids *on page 1329*

♦ Omega-3 IQ [OTC] *see* Omega-3 Fatty Acids *on page 1329*

Omega-3 Fatty Acids (oh MEG a three FAT tee AS ids)

Brand Names: US Dialyvite Omega-3 Concentrate [OTC]; Expecta LIPIL [OTC] [DSC]; Fish Oil Ultra [OTC] [DSC]; High Potency Fish Oil [OTC] [DSC]; Lovaza; MarEPA [OTC] [DSC]; Marine Lipid Concentrate [OTC]; MaxEPA [OTC]; Maximum Red Krill [OTC]; Ocean Blue MiniCaps Omega-3 [OTC]; Omega Power [OTC]; Omega-3 2100 [OTC]; Omega-3 Fish Oil Ex St [OTC]; Omega-3 IQ [OTC]; Pro Nutrients Omega 3 [OTC]; Salmon Oil-1000 [OTC]; Sam-E.P.A. [OTC]; Sea-Omega 50 [OTC]; Systane Omega-3 Healthy Tears [OTC]; Vascepa

Index Terms AMR101; Docosahexaenoic Acid; Eicosapentaenoic Acid; Epanova; Ethyl Eicosapentaenoate; Ethyl Esters of Omega-3 Fatty Acids; Ethyl Icosapentate; Ethyl-Eicosapentaenoic Acid; Ethyl-EPA; Fish Oil; Icosapent Ethyl; Omega 3; Omega-3-Acid Ethyl Esters; Omtryg; P-OM3

Pharmacologic Category Antilipemic Agent, Omega-3 Fatty Acids

Use

Dietary supplement: As dietary supplements for patients at early risk of coronary artery disease primarily because of effects on platelets and lipids.

Note: The American Heart Association recommends that consumers without documented coronary heart disease eat a variety of fish, preferably oily fish (eg, salmon), at least twice a week. Fish oil supplements should only be considered for individuals with heart disease or high triglyceride levels in consultation with a physician (AHA, 2014).

Hypertriglyceridemia (Lovaza, Omtryg, Epanova, and Vascepa): As an adjunct to diet to reduce triglyceride levels in adults with severe (≥500 mg/dL) hypertriglyceridemia.

Note: The Endocrine Society recommends that omega-3 fatty acids may be considered for triglyceride levels >1000 mg/dL and may be used alone or in combination with HMG-CoA reductase inhibitors (Berglund, 2012). A number of OTC formulations containing omega-3 fatty acids are marketed as nutritional supplements; these do not have FDA-approved indications and may not contain the same amounts of the active ingredient.

Dosing

Adult & Geriatric

Hypertriglyceridemia: Oral:
Epanova: 2 g (2 capsules) or 4 g (4 capsules) once daily
Lovaza: 4 g (4 capsules) once daily or 2 g (2 capsules) twice daily
Omtryg: 4.8 g (4 capsules) once daily with meals or 2.4 g (2 capsules) twice daily with meals
Vascepa: 2 g (2 capsules) twice daily with or following meals

Treatment of IgA nephropathy (off-label use): Oral: Lovaza: 4 g (4 capsules) once daily (Donadio, 2001)

Renal Impairment There are no dosage adjustments provided in the manufacturer's labeling (has not been studied). EPA and DHA are not renally eliminated.

Hepatic Impairment There are no dosage adjustments provided in the manufacturer's labeling (has not been studied). Periodic monitoring of ALT and AST is recommended in patients with hepatic impairment.

Additional Information Complete prescribing information should be consulted for additional detail.

Product Availability

Epanova: FDA approved May 2014; anticipated availability is currently unknown.
Omtryg: FDA approved April 2014; anticipated availability is currently unknown.

Dosage Forms Considerations

Epanova: Each 1 g capsule contains at least 850 mg of polyunsaturated fatty acids, including multiple omega-3 fatty acids (EPA and DHA being the most abundant).

Lovaza, Omtryg: Each 1 g (Lovaza) or 1.2 g (Omtryg) capsule contains the combination of eicosapentaenoic acid (EPA; ~465 mg) and docosahexaenoic acid (DHA; ~375 mg) ethyl esters.

Vascepa: Icosapent ethyl contains ethyl esters of an omega-3 fatty acid, eicosapentaenoic acid (EPA), obtained from fish oil. It contains ≥96% EPA and does **not** contain docosahexaenoic acid (DHA). Historically, mixtures containing both EPA and DHA have increased LDL cholesterol in patients with severe hypertriglyceridemia. However, studies have suggested that icosapent ethyl has not caused significant increases in LDL cholesterol while significantly decreasing triglyceride levels (Bays, 2011; Miller, 2011).

Dosage Forms Excipient information presented when available (limited, particularly for generics); consult specific product labeling. [DSC] = Discontinued product

Capsule, Oral:
Dialyvite Omega-3 Concentrate: 600 mg
Expecta LIPIL: 200 mg [DSC]
Fish Oil Ultra: 1000 mg [DSC]
Lovaza: 1 g [contains soybean oil, tocopherol, dl-alpha]
MarEPA: 1000 mg [DSC]
Marine Lipid Concentrate: 240-360-5 MG-MG-UNIT
MaxEPA: 1000 mg
Ocean Blue MiniCaps Omega-3: 350 mg [gluten free, lactose free, sugar free; contains fd&c red #40, fd&c yellow #10 (quinoline yellow)]
Omega Power: 1050 mg [gluten free, lactose free, sugar free; contains fd&c red #40, fd&c yellow #10 (quinoline yellow); vanilla flavor]
Omega-3 2100: 1050 mg [odorless; orange flavor]
Vascepa: 1 g
Generic: 300 mg, 500 mg, 1000 mg, 1 g
Capsule, Oral [preservative free]:
High Potency Fish Oil: 500 mg [DSC] [dairy free, gluten free, lactose free, milk derivatives/products, no artificial color(s), no artificial flavor(s), soy free, sugar free, wheat free, yeast free]
Maximum Red Krill: 300 mg [gluten free; contains soybean oil]
Omega-3 Fish Oil Ex St: 880 mg [gluten free]
Salmon Oil-1000: 200 mg [corn free, rye free, starch free, sugar free, wheat free]
Sam-E.P.A.: 200-300 MG [dye free]
Sea-Omega 50: 1000 mg [cholesterol free, corn free, gluten free, milk derivatives/products, no artificial color(s), no artificial flavor(s), sodium free, starch free, sugar free, yeast free; contains soybeans (glycine max)]

Generic: 200 mg, 1000 mg, 1200 mg
Capsule Delayed Release, Oral:
Pro Nutrients Omega 3: 332.5 mg
Systane Omega-3 Healthy Tears: 500 mg [contains soybean oil]
Generic: 1000 mg
Tablet Chewable, Oral:
Omega-3 IQ: 240 mg [fruit flavor]

♦ Omega Power [OTC] *see* Omega-3 Fatty Acids on page 1329

Omeprazole (oh MEP ra zole)

Brand Names: US First-Omeprazole; Omeprazole+Syrspend SF Alka; PriLOSEC; PriLOSEC OTC [OTC]
Brand Names: Canada Apo-Omeprazole; Auro-Omeprazole; Ava-Omeprazole; Dom-Omeprazole DR; JAMP-Omeprazole DR; Losec; Mylan-Omeprazole; Olex; PMS-Omeprazole; PMS-Omeprazole DR; Q-Omeprazole; RAN-Omeprazole; ratio-Omeprazole; Riva-Omeprazole DR; Sandoz-Omeprazole; Teva-Omeprazole
Index Terms Omeprazole Magnesium
Pharmacologic Category Proton Pump Inhibitor; Substituted Benzimidazole
Use Short-term (4 to 8 weeks) treatment of active duodenal ulcer disease or active benign gastric ulcer; treatment of heartburn and other symptoms associated with gastroesophageal reflux disease (GERD) (up to 4 weeks); short-term (4 to 8 weeks) treatment of endoscopically-diagnosed erosive esophagitis; maintenance healing of erosive esophagitis; long-term treatment of pathological hypersecretory conditions (eg, Zollinger-Ellison syndrome); as part of a multidrug regimen for *H. pylori* eradication to reduce the risk of duodenal ulcer recurrence

OTC labeling: Short-term treatment of frequent, uncomplicated heartburn occurring ≥2 days/week

Pregnancy Considerations Adverse events have been observed in some animal reproduction studies. An increased risk of hypospadias was reported following maternal use of proton pump inhibitors (PPIs) during pregnancy (Anderka, 2012), but this was based on a small number of exposures and the same association was not found in another study (Erichsen, 2012). Most available studies have not shown an increased risk of major birth defects following maternal use of omeprazole during pregnancy (Diav-Citrin, 2005; Källén, 2001; Lalkin, 1998; Matok, 2012; Pasternak, 2010). When treating GERD in pregnancy, PPIs may be used when clinically indicated (Katz, 2013).

Breast-Feeding Considerations Omeprazole is excreted in breast milk. Milk concentrations of omeprazole were studied in a breast-feeding woman at 3 weeks postpartum. The mother had taken omeprazole 20 mg daily starting her 29th week of gestation and continued after delivery. Following administration of omeprazole 20 mg, peak concentrations in the maternal serum occurred 240 minutes after the dose and peak concentrations in the breast milk were 180 minutes after the dose. The concentrations of omeprazole detected in the breast milk were <7% of the highest maternal serum concentration (Marshall, 1998).The manufacturer recommends caution be used if administered to a nursing woman. The acidic content of the nursing infants' stomach may potentially inactivate any ingested omeprazole (Marshall, 1998).

Medication Guide Available Yes

Contraindications Hypersensitivity (eg, anaphylaxis, anaphylactic shock, angioedema, bronchospasm, acute interstitial nephritis, urticaria) to omeprazole, other substituted benzimidazole proton pump inhibitors, or any component of the formulation

Warnings/Precautions Use of proton pump inhibitors (PPIs) may increase the risk of gastrointestinal infections (eg, *Salmonella*, *Campylobacter*). Relief of symptoms does not preclude the presence of a gastric malignancy. Atrophic gastritis (by biopsy) has been noted with long-term omeprazole therapy. In long-term (2-year) studies in rats, omeprazole produced a dose-related increase in gastric carcinoid tumors. While available endoscopic evaluations and histologic examinations of biopsy specimens from human stomachs have not detected a risk from short-term exposure to omeprazole, further human data on the effect of sustained hypochlorhydria and hypergastrinemia are needed to rule out the possibility of an increased risk for the development of tumors in humans receiving long-term therapy. Use of PPIs may increase risk of *Clostridium difficile*-associated diarrhea (CDAD), especially in hospitalized patients; consider CDAD diagnosis in patients with persistent diarrhea that does not improve. Use the lowest dose and shortest duration of PPI therapy appropriate for the condition being treated.

PPIs may diminish the therapeutic effect of clopidogrel, thought to be due to reduced formation of the active metabolite of clopidogrel. The manufacturer of clopidogrel recommends either avoidance both omeprazole (even when scheduled 12 hours apart) and esomeprazole or use of a PPI with comparatively less effect on the active metabolite of clopidogrel (eg, pantoprazole). In contrast to these warnings, others have recommended the continued use of PPIs, regardless of the degree of inhibition, in patients with a history of GI bleeding or multiple risk factors for GI bleeding who are also receiving clopidogrel since no evidence has established clinically meaningful differences in outcome; however, a clinically significant interaction cannot be excluded in those who are poor metabolizers of clopidogrel (Abraham, 2010; Levine, 2011). Potentially significant interactions may exist, requiring dose or frequency adjustment, additional monitoring, and/or selection of alternative therapy.

Increased incidence of osteoporosis-related bone fractures of the hip, spine, or wrist may occur with PPI therapy. Patients on high-dose (multiple daily doses) or long-term (≥1 year) therapy should be monitored. Use the lowest effective dose for the shortest duration of time, use vitamin D and calcium supplementation, and follow appropriate guidelines to reduce risk of fractures in patients at risk. Acute interstitial nephritis has been observed in patients taking PPIs; may occur at any time during therapy and is generally due to an idiopathic hypersensitivity reaction. Discontinue if acute interstitial nephritis develops.

Hypomagnesemia, reported rarely, usually with prolonged PPI use of >3 months (most cases >1 year of therapy); may be symptomatic or asymptomatic; severe cases may cause tetany, seizures, and cardiac arrhythmias. Consider obtaining serum magnesium concentrations prior to beginning long-term therapy, especially if taking concomitant digoxin, diuretics, or other drugs known to cause hypomagnesemia; and periodically thereafter. Hypomagnesemia may be corrected by magnesium supplementation, although discontinuation of omeprazole may be necessary; magnesium levels typically return to normal within 1 week of stopping. Serum chromogranin A levels may be increased if assessed while patient on omeprazole; may lead to diagnostic errors related to neuroendocrine tumors.

Prolonged treatment (≥2 years) may lead to vitamin B_{12} malabsorption and subsequent vitamin B_{12} deficiency. The magnitude of the deficiency is dose-related and the association is stronger in females and those younger in age (<30 years); prevalence is decreased after discontinuation of therapy (Lam, 2013).

Decreased H. pylori eradication rates have been observed with short-term (≤7 days) combination therapy. The American College of Gastroenterology recommends 10 to 14 days of therapy (triple or quadruple) for eradication of H. pylori (Chey, 2007). Bioavailability may be increased in Asian populations and patients with hepatic dysfunction; consider dosage reductions, especially for maintenance healing of erosive esophagitis. Bioavailability may be increased in the elderly. When used for self-medication (OTC), do not use for >14 days.

Benzyl alcohol and derivatives: Some dosage forms may contain benzyl alcohol; large amounts of benzyl alcohol (≥99 mg/kg/day) have been associated with a potentially fatal toxicity ("gasping syndrome") in neonates; the "gasping syndrome" consists of metabolic acidosis, respiratory distress, gasping respirations, CNS dysfunction (including convulsions, intracranial hemorrhage), hypotension, and cardiovascular collapse (AAP ["Inactive" 1997]; CDC, 1982); some data suggests that benzoate displaces bilirubin from protein binding sites (Ahlfors, 2001); avoid or use dosage forms containing benzyl alcohol with caution in neonates. See manufacturer's labeling.

Adverse Reactions
1% to 10%:
Central nervous system: Headache (7%), dizziness (2%)
Dermatologic: Skin rash (2%)
Gastrointestinal: Abdominal pain (5%), diarrhea (4%), nausea (4%), flatulence (3%), vomiting (3%), acid regurgitation (2%), constipation (2%)
Neuromuscular & skeletal: Back pain (1%), weakness (1%)
Respiratory: Upper respiratory infection (2%), cough (1%)
<1% (Limited to important or life-threatening; adverse event occurrence may vary based on formulation): Abdominal swelling, abnormal dreams, aggression, agranulocytosis, allergic reactions, alopecia, anaphylaxis, anemia, angina pectoris, angioedema, anorexia, apathy, arthralgia, atrophic gastritis, benign gastric polyps, blurred vision, bone fracture, bradycardia, bronchospasm, chest pain, cholestatic hepatitis, Clostridium

difficile-associated diarrhea (CDAD), confusion, depression, dermatitis, diplopia, drowsiness, epistaxis, erythema multiforme, esophageal candidiasis, fecal discoloration, gastroduodenal carcinoids, glycosuria, gynecomastia, hallucinations, hematuria, hemolytic anemia, hepatic disease (hepatocellular, cholestatic, mixed), hepatic encephalopathy, hepatic failure, hepatic necrosis, hepatitis, hepatocellular hepatitis, hepatotoxicity (idiosyncratic) (Chalasani, 2014), hyperhidrosis, hypersensitivity, hypertension, hypocalcemia, hypoglycemia, hypokalemia, hypomagnesemia, hyponatremia, increased gamma glutamyl transferase, increased serum alkaline phosphatase, increased serum bilirubin, increased serum creatinine, increased serum transaminases, insomnia, interstitial nephritis, irritable bowel syndrome, jaundice, leg pain, leukocytosis, leukopenia, malaise, microscopic colitis, microscopic pyuria, mucosal atrophy (tongue), muscle cramps, myalgia, myasthenia, nervousness, neutropenia, ocular irritation, optic atrophy, optic neuritis, optic neuropathy (anterior ischemic), osteoporosis-related fracture, pain, palpitation, pancreatitis, pancytopenia, paresthesia, peripheral edema, petechiae, photophobia, pneumonia, proteinuria, pruritus, psychiatric disturbance, purpura, sleep disturbance, sore throat, Stevens-Johnson syndrome, stomatitis, tachycardia, testicular pain, thrombocytopenia, toxic epidermal necrolysis, tremor, urinary tract infection, urticaria, weight gain, xeroderma, xerophthalmia, xerostomia

Drug Interactions
Metabolism/Transport Effects Substrate of CYP2A6 (minor), CYP2C19 (major), CYP2C9 (minor), CYP2D6 (minor), CYP3A4 (minor); **Note:** Assignment of Major/Minor substrate status based on clinically relevant drug interaction potential; **Inhibits** CYP1A2 (weak), CYP2C19 (moderate), CYP2C9 (moderate), CYP2D6 (weak); **Induces** CYP1A2 (weak/moderate)

Avoid Concomitant Use
Avoid concomitant use of Omeprazole with any of the following: Clopidogrel; Dasatinib; Delavirdine; Erlotinib; Nelfinavir; PAZOPanib; Rifampin; Rilpivirine; Risedronate; St Johns Wort

Increased Effect/Toxicity
Omeprazole may increase the levels/effects of: Amphetamine; ARIPiprazole; Bosentan; Cannabis; Carvedilol; Cilostazol; Citalopram; CloZAPine; CycloSPORINE (Systemic); CYP2C19 Substrates; CYP2C9 Substrates; Dexmethylphenidate; Dextroamphetamine; Dronabinol; Escitalopram; Fosphenytoin; Methotrexate; Methylphenidate; Phenytoin; Raltegravir; Risedronate; Saquinavir; Tacrolimus (Systemic); Tetrahydrocannabinol; TiZANidine; Vitamin K Antagonists; Voriconazole

The levels/effects of Omeprazole may be increased by: Fluconazole; Ketoconazole (Systemic); Voriconazole

Decreased Effect
Omeprazole may decrease the levels/effects of: Atazanavir; Bisphosphonate Derivatives; Bosutinib; Cefditoren; Clopidogrel; CloZAPine; Cysteamine (Systemic); Dabigatran Etexilate; Dabrafenib; Dasatinib; Delavirdine; Erlotinib; Gefitinib; Indinavir; Iron Salts; Itraconazole; Ketoconazole (Systemic); Ledipasvir; Mesalamine; Multivitamins/Minerals (with ADEK, Folate, Iron); Mycophenolate; Nelfinavir; Nilotinib; PAZOPanib; Posaconazole; Rilpivirine; Riociguat; Risedronate

The levels/effects of Omeprazole may be decreased by: Antihepaciviral Combination Products; CYP2C19 Inducers (Strong); Dabrafenib; Enzalutamide; Fosphenytoin; Lumacaftor; Phenytoin; Rifampin; St Johns Wort; Tipranavir

Food Interactions Prolonged treatment (≥2 years) may lead to malabsorption of dietary vitamin B_{12} and subsequent vitamin B_{12} deficiency (Lam, 2013).

Preparation for Administration Granules for oral suspension: For oral administration, empty the contents of the 2.5 mg packet into 5 mL of water (10 mg packet into 15 mL of water); stir. For NG administration, add 5 mL of water into a catheter-tipped syringe, and then add the contents of a 2.5 mg packet (15 mL water for the 10 mg packet); shake. **Note:** Regardless of the route of administration, the suspension should be left to thicken for 2 to 3 minutes prior to administration.

Storage/Stability
Capsules, tablets: Store at 15°C to 30°C (59°F to 86°F). Protect from light and moisture.
Granules for oral suspension: Store at 25°C (77°F); excursions permitted to 15°C to 30°C (59°F to 86°F).

Powder for suspension (compounding kit): Prior to compounding, store at 15°C to 30°C (59°F to 86°F). Once compounded, the product is stable for 30 days under refrigeration [2°C to 8°C (36°F to 46°F)]; protect from light; protect from freezing.

OTC capsules: Store at 20°C to 25°C (68°F to 77°F); protect from moisture.

Mechanism of Action Proton pump inhibitor; suppresses gastric basal and stimulated acid secretion by inhibiting the parietal cell H+/K+ ATP pump

Pharmacodynamics/Kinetics

Onset of action: Antisecretory: ~1 hour

Peak effect: Within 2 hours

Duration: Up to 72 hours; 50% of maximum effect at 24 hours; after stopping treatment, secretory activity gradually returns over 3 to 5 days

Absorption: Rapid

Protein binding: ~95%

Metabolism: Hepatic via CYP2C19 primarily and (to a lesser extent) via 3A4 to hydroxy, desmethyl, and sulfone metabolites (all inactive); saturable first-pass effect

Bioavailability: Oral: ~30% to 40%; Hepatic dysfunction: ~100%; Asians: AUC increased up to fourfold compared to Caucasians

Half-life elimination: 0.5 to 1 hour; hepatic impairment: ~3 hours

Time to peak, plasma: 0.5 to 3.5 hours

Excretion: Urine (~77% as metabolites, very small amount as unchanged drug); feces

Dosing

Adult & Geriatric

Active duodenal ulcer: Oral: 20 mg once daily for 4 to 8 weeks

Gastric ulcers: Oral: 40 mg once daily for 4 to 8 weeks

Symptomatic GERD (without esophageal lesions): Oral: 20 mg once daily for up to 4 weeks

Erosive esophagitis: Oral: 20 mg once daily for 4 to 8 weeks; maintenance of healing: 20 mg once daily for up to 12 months total therapy (including treatment period of 4 to 8 weeks)

Helicobacter pylori **eradication:** Oral: Dose varies with regimen:

Manufacturer labeling: 40 mg once daily administered with clarithromycin 500 mg 3 times daily for 14 days **or** 20 mg twice daily administered with amoxicillin 1000 mg *and* clarithromycin 500 mg twice daily for 10 days. **Note:** Presence of ulcer at time of therapy initiation may necessitate an additional 14 to 18 days of omeprazole 20 mg daily (monotherapy) after completion of combination therapy.

American College of Gastroenterology guidelines (Chey, 2007):

Nonpenicillin allergy: 20 mg twice daily administered with amoxicillin 1000 mg *and* clarithromycin 500 mg twice daily for 10 to 14 days

Penicillin allergy: 20 mg twice daily administered with clarithromycin 500 mg *and* metronidazole 500 mg twice daily for 10 to 14 days **or** 20 mg once or twice daily administered with bismuth subsalicylate 525 mg *and* metronidazole 250 mg *plus* tetracycline 500 mg 4 times daily for 10 to 14 days

Pathological hypersecretory conditions: Oral: Initial: 60 mg once daily; doses up to 120 mg 3 times daily have been administered; administer daily doses >80 mg in divided doses

NSAID-induced ulcer treatment (off-label use): Oral: 20 mg once daily for 4 to 8 weeks; Maintenance: 20 mg once daily for up to 6 months (Hawkey, 1998)

NSAID-induced ulcer prophylaxis (off-label use): Oral: 20 mg once daily for up to 6 months (Cullen, 1998)

Stress ulcer prophylaxis, ICU patients (off-label use): Oral: 40 mg once daily (Levy, 1997) or may administer 40 mg loading dose followed by 20 to 40 mg once daily (ASHP, 1999). **Note:** Intended for patients with associated risk factors (eg, coagulopathy, mechanical ventilation for ≥48 hours, severe sepsis); discontinue use once risk factors have resolved (Dellinger, 2013). Omeprazole 20 mg via NG tube once daily may be less effective in some critically ill populations compared to 40 mg via NG tube once daily (Balaban, 1997).

Frequent heartburn (OTC labeling): Oral: 20 mg once daily for 14 days; treatment may be repeated after 4 months if needed

Pediatric

GERD or other acid-related disorders: Oral: Children 1 to 16 years:

5 kg to <10 kg: 5 mg once daily

10 kg to <20 kg: 10 mg once daily

≥20 kg: 20 mg once daily

Renal Impairment No dosage adjustment necessary.

Hepatic Impairment There are no dosage adjustments provided in the manufacturer's labeling. However, based on increased bioavailability, a dosage reduction should be considered, especially for maintenance of healing of erosive esophagitis.

Dietary Considerations Should be taken on an empty stomach; best if taken before breakfast.

Administration

Oral: Best if administered before breakfast.

Capsule: Should be swallowed whole; do not chew or crush. Delayed release capsule may be opened and contents added to 1 tablespoon of applesauce (use immediately after adding to applesauce); mixture should not be chewed or warmed.

Oral suspension: Following reconstitution, the suspension should be left to thicken for 2 to 3 minutes and administered within 30 minutes. If any material remains after administration, add more water, stir, and administer immediately.

Tablet: Should be swallowed whole; do not crush or chew.

Nasogastric/orogastric (NG/OG) tube administration:

Oral suspension (using packets): After removing a catheter-tip syringe plunger, add 5 mL of water to the syringe and the contents of a 2.5 mg packet (or 15 mL of water for the 10 mg packet). Immediately shake syringe and leave to thicken for 2 to 3 minutes; shake syringe again and within 30 minutes administer via NG or gastric tube (French size 6 or larger). Refill syringe with an equal amount of water, shake, and flush remaining contents through NG or gastric tube

Oral suspension (using capsules): The manufacturer of Prilosec® does not give recommendations for extemporaneous preparation of omeprazole capsules for NG/OG administration. Consider using the packets for oral suspension. If packets are unavailable, methods of preparation of capsules for NG/OG administration have been described (Balaban, 1997; Phillips, 1996). An extemporaneously prepared suspension with extended stability may also be used (DiGiacinto, 2000; Quercia, 1997; Sharma, 1999).

Monitoring Parameters Susceptibility testing is recommended in patients who fail *H. pylori*-eradication regimen.

Test Interactions Omeprazole may falsely elevate serum chromogranin A (CgA) levels. The increased CgA level may cause false-positive results in the diagnosis of a neuroendocrine tumor. Temporarily stop omeprazole ≥14 days prior to assessing CgA level; repeat level if initially elevated; use the same laboratory for all testing of CgA levels.

Dosage Forms Considerations First-Omeprazole and Omeprazole+Syrspend Alka oral suspensions are compounding kits. Refer to manufacturer's labeling for compounding instructions.

Dosage Forms Excipient information presented when available (limited, particularly for generics); consult specific product labeling.

Capsule Delayed Release, Oral:

PriLOSEC: 10 mg, 20 mg, 40 mg

Generic: 10 mg, 20 mg, 40 mg

Capsule Delayed Release, Oral, as magnesium [strength expressed as base]:

Generic: 20 mg

Packet, Oral, as magnesium [strength expressed as base]:

PriLOSEC: 2.5 mg (30 ea); 10 mg (30 ea)

Suspension, Oral:

First-Omeprazole: 2 mg/mL (90 mL, 150 mL, 300 mL) [contains benzyl alcohol, fd&c red #40, saccharin sodium; strawberry flavor]

Omeprazole+Syrspend SF Alka: 2 mg/mL (120 mL, 240 mL)

Omeprazole+Syrspend SF Alka: 2 mg/mL (100 mL) [cherry flavor]

Tablet Delayed Release, Oral:

Generic: 20 mg

Tablet Delayed Release, Oral, as magnesium [strength expressed as base]:

PriLOSEC OTC: 20 mg

PriLOSEC OTC: 20 mg [contains fd&c blue #2 aluminum lake, fd&c red #40 aluminum lake, saccharin sodium]

PriLOSEC OTC: 20 mg [contains fd&c blue #2 aluminum lake, fd&c red #40 aluminum lake, saccharin sodium; wild berry flavor]

Extemporaneous Preparations Note: More palatable omeprazole (2 mg/mL) suspensions are commercially available as compounding kits (First-Omeprazole, Omeprazole+Syrspend SF Alka Cherry Kit).

A 2 mg/mL oral omeprazole solution (Simplified Omeprazole Solution) may be made with five omeprazole 20 mg delayed release capsules and 50 mL sodium bicarbonate 8.4%. Empty capsules into beaker. Add sodium bicarbonate solution. Gently stir (about 15 minutes) until a white suspension forms. Transfer to amber-colored syringe or bottle. Stable for 14 days at room temperature or for 30 days refrigerated.

DiGiacinto JL, Olsen KM, Bergman KL, et al, "Stability of Suspension Formulations of Lansoprazole and Omeprazole Stored in Amber-Colored Plastic Oral Syringes," *Ann Pharmacother*, 2000, 34 (5):600-5.

Quercia R, Fan C, Liu X, et al, "Stability of Omeprazole in an Extemporaneously Prepared Oral Liquid," *Am J Health Syst Pharm*, 1997, 54(16):1833-6.

Sharma V, "Comparison of 24-hour Intragastric pH Using Four Liquid Formulations of Lansoprazole and Omeprazole," *Am J Health Syst Pharm*, 1999, 56(23 Suppl 4):18-21.

◆ Omeprazole, Amoxicillin, and Clarithromycin *see* Omeprazole, Clarithromycin, and Amoxicillin *on page 1333*

Omeprazole and Sodium Bicarbonate
(oh MEP ra zole & SOW dee um bye KAR bun ate)

Brand Names: US Zegerid; Zegerid OTC [OTC]
Index Terms Sodium Bicarbonate and Omeprazole
Pharmacologic Category Proton Pump Inhibitor; Substituted Benzimidazole
Use Short-term (4 to 8 weeks) treatment of active duodenal ulcer or active benign gastric ulcer; treatment of heartburn and other symptoms associated with gastroesophageal reflux disease (GERD) for up to 4 weeks; short-term (4 to 8 weeks) treatment of endoscopically diagnosed erosive esophagitis; maintenance healing of erosive esophagitis; reduction of risk of upper gastrointestinal bleeding in critically ill patients

OTC labeling: Short-term (2 weeks) treatment of frequent (2 days/week), uncomplicated heartburn
Medication Guide Available Yes
Dosing
Adult & Geriatric Note: Both strengths of Zegerid capsule and powder for oral suspension have identical sodium bicarbonate content, respectively. Do not substitute two 20 mg capsules/packets for one 40 mg dose.
Active duodenal ulcer: Oral: 20 mg once daily for 4 to 8 weeks
Gastric ulcers: Oral: 40 mg once daily for 4 to 8 weeks
Heartburn (OTC labeling): Oral: 20 mg once daily for 14 days. Do not take for >14 days or more often than every 4 months, unless instructed by healthcare provider.
Symptomatic GERD: Oral: 20 mg once daily for up to 4 weeks
Erosive esophagitis: Oral: 20 mg once daily for 4 to 8 weeks; maintenance of healing: 20 mg once daily for up to 12 months total therapy (including treatment period of 4 to 8 weeks)
Risk reduction of upper GI bleeding in critically ill patients (Zegerid powder for oral suspension): Oral:
Loading dose: Day 1: 40 mg every 6 to 8 hours for two doses
Maintenance dose: 40 mg daily for up to 14 days; therapy >14 days has not been evaluated
Renal Impairment No dosage adjustment necessary.
Hepatic Impairment There are no dosage adjustments provided in the manufacturer's labeling. However, based on increased bioavailability, a dosage reduction should be considered, especially for maintenance of healing of erosive esophagitis
Additional Information Complete prescribing information should be consulted for additional detail.
Dosage Forms Excipient information presented when available (limited, particularly for generics); consult specific product labeling.
Capsule, oral: Omeprazole 20 mg [immediate release] and sodium bicarbonate 1100 mg; omeprazole 40 mg [immediate release] and sodium bicarbonate 1100 mg
Zegerid: Omeprazole 20 mg [immediate release] and sodium bicarbonate 1100 mg [contains sodium 304 mg (13 mEq) per capsule]
Zegerid: Omeprazole 40 mg [immediate release] and sodium bicarbonate 1100 mg [contains sodium 304 mg (13 mEq) per capsule]
Zegerid OTC: Omeprazole 20 mg [immediate release] and sodium bicarbonate 1100 mg [contains sodium 303 mg (13 mEq) per capsule]

Powder for suspension, oral:
Zegerid: Omeprazole 20 mg and sodium bicarbonate 1680 mg per packet (30s) [contains sodium 460 mg (20 mEq) per packet]
Zegerid: Omeprazole 40 mg and sodium bicarbonate 1680 mg per packet (30s) [contains sodium 460 mg (20 mEq) per packet]

Omeprazole, Clarithromycin, and Amoxicillin
(oh MEP ra zole, kla RITH roe mye sin, & a moks i SIL in)

Brand Names: US Omeclamox-Pak®
Index Terms Amoxicillin, Clarithromycin, and Omeprazole; Clarithromycin, Amoxicillin, and Omeprazole; Omeprazole, Amoxicillin, and Clarithromycin
Pharmacologic Category Antibiotic, Macrolide Combination; Antibiotic, Penicillin; Gastrointestinal Agent, Miscellaneous; Proton Pump Inhibitor; Substituted Benzimidazole
Use *Helicobacter pylori* eradication: Eradication of *H. pylori* infection to reduce the risk of recurrent duodenal ulcer in adults with active or 1-year history of duodenal ulcer
Dosing
Adult & Geriatric *H. pylori* eradication: Oral: Omeprazole 20 mg (one capsule), clarithromycin 500 mg (one tablet), and amoxicillin 1,000 mg (two capsules) twice daily for 10 days. **Note:** If patient has an active duodenal ulcer at therapy initiation, an additional 18 days of omeprazole 20 mg once daily is recommended.
Renal Impairment Amoxicillin and clarithromycin pharmacokinetics are altered in renal impairment. The manufacturer's labeling suggests that prolonged dosing intervals for clarithromycin may be appropriate in severe renal impairment, but provides no recommendation in regards to amoxicillin.
Hepatic Impairment Avoid use in hepatic impairment.
Additional Information Complete prescribing information should be consulted for additional detail.
Dosage Forms Excipient information presented when available (limited, particularly for generics); consult specific product labeling.
Combination package, oral [each administration card contains]:
Omeclamox-Pak™:
Capsule, delayed release: Omeprazole: 20 mg (2s)
Tablet: Clarithromycin: 500 mg (2s)
Capsule: Amoxicillin: 500 mg (4s) [contains sodium ≤0.0052 mEq (0.119 mg)/capsule]

◆ Omeprazole Magnesium *see* Omeprazole *on page 1330*

◆ Omeprazole+Syrspend SF Alka *see* Omeprazole *on page 1330*

◆ Omnaris *see* Ciclesonide (Nasal) *on page 383*

◆ Omnaris HFA (Can) *see* Ciclesonide (Nasal) *on page 383*

◆ Omnicef *see* Cefdinir *on page 332*

◆ Omni Gel [OTC] *see* Fluoride *on page 782*

◆ Omnipred *see* PrednisoLONE (Ophthalmic) *on page 1496*

◆ Omnitarg *see* Pertuzumab *on page 1433*

◆ Omnitrope *see* Somatropin *on page 1686*

◆ Omtryg *see* Omega-3 Fatty Acids *on page 1329*

OnabotulinumtoxinA
(oh nuh BOT yoo lin num TOKS in aye)

Brand Names: US Botox; Botox Cosmetic
Brand Names: Canada Botox; Botox Cosmetic
Index Terms Botulinum Toxin Type A; BTX-A
Pharmacologic Category Neuromuscular Blocker Agent, Toxin; Ophthalmic Agent, Toxin
Use
Axillary hyperhidrosis (Botox): Treatment of severe primary axillary hyperhidrosis in adults not adequately managed with topical agents.
Cervical dystonia (Botox): Treatment of cervical dystonia in patients ≥16 years to reduce the severity of abnormal head position and neck pain.
Chronic migraine (Botox): Prophylaxis of chronic migraine headaches (≥15 days/month with headache lasting ≥4 hours/day) in adults.
Glabellar lines (Botox Cosmetic): Temporary improvement in the appearance of moderate to severe glabellar lines associated with corrugator and/or procerus muscle activity in adults.

◄ **Lateral canthal lines (Botox Cosmetic):** Temporary improvement in the appearance of moderate to severe lateral canthal lines associated with orbicularis oculi activity in adults.

Overactive bladder (Botox): Treatment of overactive bladder with symptoms of urge urinary incontinence, urgency, and frequency in adults who have an inadequate response to or who are intolerant to an anticholinergic medication.

Strabismus and blepharospasm associated with dystonia (Botox): Treatment of strabismus and blepharospasm associated with dystonia, including benign essential blepharospasm or VII nerve disorders, in patients ≥12 years.

Upper limb spasticity (Botox): Treatment of upper limb spasticity in adults to decrease the severity of increased muscle tone in elbow flexors (biceps), wrist flexors (flexor carpi radialis and flexor carpi ulnaris), finger flexors (flexor digitorum profundus and flexor digitorum sublimis), and thumb flexors (adductor pollicis and flexor pollicis longus).

Urinary incontinence due to detrusor overactivity (Botox): Treatment of urinary incontinence due to detrusor overactivity associated with a neurologic condition (eg, spinal cord injury [SCI], multiple sclerosis [MS]) in adults who have an inadequate response to or are intolerant of an anticholinergic medication.

Canadian labeling: Additional use (not in US labeling): Dynamic equinus foot deformity in pediatric cerebral palsy patients; treatment of forehead lines in adults

Medication Guide Available Yes

Dosing

Adult Note: The lowest recommended dose should be used when initiating treatment (regardless of indication). In adults treated for more than one indication, the maximum cumulative dose should be ≤400 units/3 months for Botox or ≤360 units/3 months for Botox Cosmetic. Canadian labeling recommends a maximum cumulative dose of 6 units/kg (up to 360 units) over 3 months in adult patients receiving additional treatment for noncosmetic indications.

Bladder dysfunction: Intradetrusor: **Note:** Prophylactic antimicrobial therapy (excluding aminoglycosides) should be administered 1 to 3 days prior to, on the day of, and for 1 to 3 days following onabotulinumtoxinA administration to decrease risk of urinary tract infection (UTI). Discontinue antiplatelet therapy at least 3 days prior to administration.

Detrusor overactivity associated with neurologic condition: 30 injections of 1 mL (recommended concentration: ~6.7 units/mL) for a total dose of 200 units/30 mL (maximum: 200 units); for the final injection, ~1 mL of sterile NS should be injected to ensure that the remaining medication in the needle is delivered to the bladder; may consider re-treatment with diminishing effect but no sooner than 12 weeks from previous administration (median time until second treatment in studies: 42 to 48 weeks).

Overactive bladder: 20 injections of 0.5 mL (recommended concentration: 10 units/mL) for a total dose of 100 units/10 mL (maximum: 100 units); for the final injection, ~1 mL of sterile NS should be injected to ensure that the remaining medication in the needle is delivered to the bladder; may consider re-treatment with diminishing effect but no sooner than 12 weeks from the previous administration (median time until second treatment in studies: ~24 weeks)

Blepharospasm: IM:

Botox: Initial dose: 1.25 to 2.5 units injected into the medial and lateral pretarsal orbicularis oculi of the upper lid and lateral pretarsal orbicularis oculi of lower lid

Dose may be increased up to twice the previous dose if the response from the initial dose lasted ≤2 months; maximum dose per site: 5 units. Tolerance may occur if treatments are given more often than every 3 months, but the effect is not usually permanent.

Cumulative dose:

US labeling: ≤200 units in 30-day period

Canadian labeling (not in US labeling): Botox: ≤200 units in 2-month period

Cervical dystonia: IM: For dosing guidance, the mean dose is 236 units (25th to 75th percentile range 198 to 300 units) divided among the affected muscles in patients previously treated with botulinum toxin (maximum: ≤50 units/site). Initial dose in previously untreated patients should be lower. Sequential dosing should be based on the patient's head and neck position, localization of pain, muscle hypertrophy, patient response, and previous adverse reactions. The total dose injected into the sternocleidomastoid muscles

should be ≤100 units to decrease the occurrence of dysphagia.

Canadian labeling (not in US labeling): IM: Botox: Effective range of 200 to 360 units has been used in clinical practice; administer no more frequently than every 2 months

Chronic migraine: IM: Administer 5 units/0.1 mL per site. Recommended total dose is 155 units once every 12 weeks. Each 155 unit dose should be equally divided and administered bilaterally, into 31 total sites as described below (refer to prescribing information for specific diagrams of recommended injection sites):

Corrugator: 5 units to each side (2 sites)

Procerus: 5 units (1 site only)

Frontalis: 10 units to each side (divided into 2 sites/side)

Temporalis: 20 units to each side (divided into 4 sites/side)

Occipitalis: 15 units to each side (divided into 3 sites/side)

Cervical paraspinal: 10 units to each side (divided into 2 sites/side)

Trapezius: 15 units to each side (divided into 3 sites/side)

Spasticity (focal): IM: Individualize dose based on patient size, extent, and location of muscle involvement, degree of spasticity, local muscle weakness, and response to prior treatment. In clinical trials used to support the FDA-approved labeling, total doses up to 400 units (Botox) were administered as separate injections typically divided among selected muscles; may repeat therapy at ≥3 months with appropriate dosage based upon the clinical condition of patient at time of re-treatment. Single session doses of ≤1,200 units (off-label dose) have been reported; however, safety and efficacy of routine use of doses >500 units has not been evaluated (Francisco, 2004). Single site doses of ≤400 units (off-label dose) in a lower limb (off-label use) have been reported (Nalysnyk, 2013).

Suggested guidelines for the treatment of upper limb spasticity. The lowest recommended starting dose should be used and ≤50 units/site should be administered. **Note:** Dose listed is total dose administered as individual or separate intramuscular injection(s):

Adductor pollicis: 20 units (1 site)

Biceps brachii: 100 to 200 units (divided into 4 sites)

Flexor digitorum profundus: 30 to 50 units (1 site)

Flexor digitorum sublimes: 30 to 50 units (1 site)

Flexor carpi radialis: 12.5 to 50 units (1 site)

Flexor carpi ulnaris: 12.5 to 50 units (1 site)

Flexor pollicis longus: 20 units (1 site)

Suggested guidelines for the treatment of stroke-related upper limb spasticity: *Canadian labeling:* **Note:** Dose listed is total dose administered as individual or separate intramuscular injection(s):

Adductor pollicis: 20 units (1 to 2 sites)

Biceps brachii: 100 to 200 units (up to 4 sites)

Flexor digitorum profundus: 15 to 50 units (1 to 2 sites)

Flexor digitorum sublimes: 15 to 50 units (1 to 2 sites)

Flexor carpi radialis: 15 to 60 units (1 to 2 sites)

Flexor carpi ulnaris: 10 to 50 units (1 to 2 sites)

Flexor pollicis longus: 20 units (1 to 2 sites)

Strabismus: IM: **Note:** Several minutes prior to injection, administration of local anesthetic and ocular decongestant drops are recommended.

Initial dose:

Vertical muscles and for horizontal strabismus <20 prism diopters: 1.25 to 2.5 units in any one muscle

Horizontal strabismus of 20 to 50 prism diopters: 2.5 to 5 units in any one muscle

Persistent VI nerve palsy ≥1 month: 1.25 to 2.5 units in the medial rectus muscle

Re-examine patients 7 to 14 days after each injection to assess the effect of that dose. Subsequent doses for patients experiencing incomplete paralysis of the target may be increased up to twice the previous administered dose. The maximum recommended dose as a single injection for any one muscle is 25 units. Do not administer subsequent injections until the effects of the previous dose are gone.

Primary axillary hyperhidrosis: Intradermal: 50 units/axilla. Injection area should be defined by standard staining techniques. Injections should be evenly distributed into multiple sites (10 to 15), administered in 0.1 to 0.2 mL aliquots, ~1 to 2 cm apart. May repeat when clinical effect diminishes.

Cosmetic uses:

Reduction of glabellar lines: Adults: IM: An effective dose is determined by gross observation of the patient's ability to activate the superficial muscles injected. The location, size, and use of muscles may vary markedly among individuals. Inject 0.1 mL (4 units) dose into each of five sites, two in each

corrugator muscle and one in the procerus muscle for a total dose 0.5 mL (20 units) administered no more frequently than every 3 to 4 months. **Note:** Treatment of adults >65 years is approved in the Canadian labeling.

Reduction of lateral canthus lines:

US labeling: Adults: IM: Inject 0.1 mL (4 units) into 3 injection sites per side (6 total injection points) in the lateral orbicularis oculi muscle for a total dose of 0.6 mL (24 units) administered no more frequently than every 3 months.

Canadian labeling: Adults: IM: Inject 2 to 6 units into each of 1 to 3 injection sites, lateral to the lateral orbital rim.

Reduction of forehead lines *(Canadian labeling; not in US labeling):* IM: Inject 2 to 6 units into each of four sites in the frontalis muscle every 1 to 2 cm along either side of forehead crease and 2 to 3 cm above eyebrows for total dose of 24 units.

Geriatric Initiate therapy at lowest recommended dose. Refer to adult dosing.

Pediatric Note: The lowest recommended dose should be used when initiating treatment (regardless of indication). Canadian labeling (not in US labeling) recommends a maximum cumulative dose of 6 units/kg (up to 200 units) over 3 months in pediatric patients receiving treatment for more than 1 indication.

Blepharospasm/strabismus: Children ≥12 years: Refer to adult dosing.

Cervical dystonia: Children ≥16 years: Refer to adult dosing.

Spasticity (cerebral palsy related [dynamic equinus foot deformity]): Botox: *Canadian labeling (not approved in US labeling):* Children ≥2 years: IM: 4 units/kg (total dose) divided into two injections into medial and lateral heads of the gastrocnemius of affected leg; if clinically indicated, may repeat every 2 months (maximum dose: 200 units); in diplegia, the recommended dose is 6 units/kg (total dose) divided between affected limbs

Renal Impairment There are no dosage adjustments provided in the manufacturer's labeling.

Hepatic Impairment There are no dosage adjustments provided in the manufacturer's labeling.

Additional Information Complete prescribing information should be consulted for additional detail.

Dosage Forms Excipient information presented when available (limited, particularly for generics); consult specific product labeling.

Solution Reconstituted, Injection:

Botox: 100 units (1 ea)

Solution Reconstituted, Injection [preservative free]:

Botox: 200 units (1 ea)

Solution Reconstituted, Intramuscular:

Botox Cosmetic: 100 units (1 ea) [contains albumin human]

Solution Reconstituted, Intramuscular [preservative free]:

Botox Cosmetic: 50 units (1 ea) [contains albumin human]

Dosage Forms: Canada Excipient information presented when available (limited, particularly for generics); consult specific product labeling.

Injection, powder for reconstitution [preservative free]:

Botox: Botulinum toxin A 50 units [contains albumin (human)], 100 units [contains albumin (human)], 200 units [contains albumin (human)]

Botox Cosmetic: Botulinum toxin A 50 units [contains albumin (human)], 100 units [contains albumin (human)], 200 units [contains albumin (human)]

Ondansetron (on DAN se tron)

Brand Names: US Zofran; Zofran ODT; Zuplenz

Brand Names: Canada ACT Ondansetron; Apo-Ondansetron; Ava-Ondansetron; Dom-Ondansetron; JAMP-Ondansetron; Mar-Ondansetron; Mint-Ondansetron; Mylan-Ondansetron; NAT-Ondansetron; Ondansetron Hydrochloride Dihydrate Injection; Ondansetron Injection; Ondansetron Injection USP; Ondansetron-Omega; Ondissolve ODF; PHL-Ondansetron; PMS-Ondansetron; RAN-Ondansetron; ratio-Ondansetron; Sandoz-Ondansetron; Sandoz-Ondansetron ODT; Septa-Ondansetron; Teva-Ondansetron; Zofran; Zofran ODT

Index Terms GR38032R; Ondansetron Hydrochloride

Pharmacologic Category Antiemetic; Selective 5-HT$_3$ Receptor Antagonist

Use

Cancer chemotherapy-induced nausea and vomiting:

IV: Prevention of nausea and vomiting associated with initial and repeat courses of emetogenic cancer chemotherapy (including high-dose cisplatin)

Oral:

Prevention of nausea and vomiting associated with highly emetogenic cancer chemotherapy (including cisplatin ≥50 mg/m^2).

Prevention of nausea and vomiting associated with initial and repeat courses of moderately emetogenic cancer chemotherapy.

Radiotherapy-associated nausea and vomiting: Oral: Prevention of nausea and vomiting associated with radiotherapy in patients receiving either total body irradiation, single high-dose fraction to the abdomen, or daily fractions to the abdomen.

Postoperative nausea and/or vomiting: IV and Oral: Prevention of postoperative nausea and/or vomiting (PONV). If nausea/vomiting occur in a patient who had not received prophylactic ondansetron, IV ondansetron may be administered to prevent further episodes.

Limitations of use: Routine prophylaxis for PONV in patients with minimal expectation of nausea and/or vomiting is not recommended, although use is recommended in patients when nausea and vomiting must be avoided in the postoperative period, even if the incidence of PONV is low.

Canadian labeling: Additional use (not in U.S. labeling): IV: Treatment of PONV

Pregnancy Considerations Teratogenic effects were not observed in animal reproduction studies. Ondansetron readily crosses the human placenta in the first trimester of pregnancy and can be detected in fetal tissue (Siu, 2006). The use of ondansetron for the treatment of nausea and vomiting of pregnancy (NVP) has been evaluated. Although a significant increase in birth defects has not been described in case reports and some studies (Ferreira, 2012; Pasternak, 2013), other studies have shown a possible association with ondansetron exposure and adverse fetal events (Anderka, 2012; Einarson, 2004). Additional studies are needed to determine safety to the fetus, particularly during the first trimester. Based on available data, use is generally reserved for severe NVP (hyperemesis gravidarum) or when conventional treatments are not effective (ACOG, 2004; Koren, 2012; Levicheck, 2002; Tan, 2011). Because a dose-dependent QT-interval prolongation occurs with use, the manufacturer recommends ECG monitoring in patients with electrolyte abnormalities (which can be associated with some cases of NVP; Koren, 2012). An international consensus panel recommends that 5-HT$_3$ antagonists (including ondansetron) should not be withheld in pregnant patients receiving chemotherapy for the treatment of gynecologic cancers, when chemotherapy is given according to general recommendations for chemotherapy use during pregnancy (Amant, 2010).

Breast-Feeding Considerations It is not known if ondansetron is excreted into breast milk. The U.S. manufacturer labeling recommends caution be used if administered to nursing women. The Canadian labeling recommends avoiding nursing during ondansetron treatment.

Contraindications Hypersensitivity to ondansetron or any component of the formulation; concomitant use of apomorphine

Warnings/Precautions Antiemetics are most effective when used prophylactically (Roila, 2010). If emesis occurs despite optimal antiemetic prophylaxis, reevaluate emetic risk, disease, concurrent morbidities and medications to assure antiemetic regimen is optimized (Basch, 2011). Does not stimulate gastric or intestinal peristalsis; may mask progressive ileus and/or gastric distension. Use with caution in patients allergic to other 5-HT$_3$ receptor antagonists; cross-reactivity has been reported.

Dose-dependent QT interval prolongation occurs with ondansetron use. Cases of torsade de pointes have also been reported to the manufacturer. Selective 5-HT$_3$ antagonists, including ondansetron, have been associated with a number of dose-dependent increases in ECG intervals (eg, PR, QRS duration, QT/QTc, JT), usually occurring 1 to 2 hours after IV administration. Single doses >16 mg ondansetron IV are no longer recommended due to the potential for an increased risk of QT prolongation. In most patients, these changes are not clinically relevant; however, when used in conjunction with other agents that prolong these intervals or in those at risk for QT prolongation, arrhythmia may occur. When used with agents that prolong the QT interval (eg, Class I and III antiarrhythmics) ▶

or in patients with cardiovascular disease, clinically relevant QT interval prolongation may occur resulting in torsade de pointes. Avoid ondansetron use in patients with congenital long QT syndrome. Use caution and monitor ECG in patients with other risk factors for QT prolongation (eg, medications known to prolong QT interval, electrolyte abnormalities [hypokalemia or hypomagnesemia], heart failure, bradyarrhythmias, and cumulative high-dose anthracycline therapy). IV formulations of 5-HT$_3$ antagonists have more association with ECG interval changes, compared to oral formulations. Dose limitations are recommended for patients with severe hepatic impairment (Child-Pugh class C); use with caution in mild-moderate hepatic impairment; clearance is decreased and half-life increased in hepatic impairment.

Serotonin syndrome has been reported with 5-HT$_3$ receptor antagonists, predominantly when used in combination with other serotonergic agents (eg, SSRIs, SNRIs, MAOIs, mirtazapine, fentanyl, lithium, tramadol, and/or methylene blue). Some of the cases have been fatal. The majority of serotonin syndrome reports due to 5-HT$_3$ receptor antagonist have occurred in a postanesthesia setting or in an infusion center. Serotonin syndrome has also been reported following overdose of ondansetron. Monitor patients for signs of serotonin syndrome, including mental status changes (eg, agitation, hallucinations, delirium, coma); autonomic instability (eg, tachycardia, labile blood pressure, diaphoresis, dizziness, flushing, hyperthermia); neuromuscular changes (eg, tremor, rigidity, myoclonus, hyperreflexia, incoordination); gastrointestinal symptoms (eg, nausea, vomiting, diarrhea); and/or seizures. If serotonin syndrome occurs, discontinue 5-HT$_3$ receptor antagonist treatment and begin supportive management. Potentially significant drug-drug interactions may exist, requiring dose or frequency adjustment, additional monitoring, and/or selection of alternative therapy. Orally disintegrating tablets contain phenylalanine.

Benzyl alcohol and derivatives: Some dosage forms may contain sodium benzoate/benzoic acid; benzoic acid (benzoate) is a metabolite of benzyl alcohol; large amounts of benzyl alcohol (≥99 mg/kg/day) have been associated with a potentially fatal toxicity ("gasping syndrome") in neonates; the "gasping syndrome" consists of metabolic acidosis, respiratory distress, gasping respirations, CNS dysfunction (including convulsions, intracranial hemorrhage), hypotension, and cardiovascular collapse (AAP ["Inactive" 1997]; CDC, 1982); some data suggests that benzoate displaces bilirubin from protein binding sites (Ahlfors, 2001); avoid or use dosage forms containing benzyl alcohol derivative with caution in neonates. See manufacturer's labeling.

Adverse Reactions Note: Percentages reported in adult patients unless otherwise specified.
>10%:
  Central nervous system: Headache (oral: 9% to 27%; IV: 17%), fatigue (oral: ≤9% to 13%), malaise (oral: ≤9% to 13%)
  Gastrointestinal: Constipation (6% to 11%)
1% to 10%:
  Central nervous system: Drowsiness (IV: ≤8%), sedation (IV: ≤8%), (dizziness (7%), agitation (oral: ≤6%), anxiety (oral: ≤6%), paresthesia (IV: 2%), sensation of cold (IV: 2%)
  Dermatologic: Pruritus (2% to 5%), skin rash (1%)
  Gastrointestinal: Diarrhea (oral: 6% to 7%; IV: Children 1 to 24 months of age: 2%)
  Genitourinary: Gynecologic disease (oral: 7%), urinary retention (oral: 5%)
  Hepatic: Increased serum ALT (>2 times ULN: 1% to 5%; transient), increased serum AST (>2 times ULN: 1% to 5%; transient)
  Local: Injection site reaction (IV: 4%; includes burning sensation at injection site, erythema at injection site, injection site pain)
  Respiratory: Hypoxia (oral: 9%)
  Miscellaneous: Fever (2% to 8%)
<1% (Limited to important or life-threatening): Abdominal pain, accommodation disturbance, atrial fibrillation, cardiorespiratory arrest (IV), depression of ST segment on ECG, dyspnea, extrapyramidal reaction (IV), flushing, hepatic failure (when used with other hepatotoxic medications), hiccups, hypersensitivity reaction, hypokalemia, hypotension, laryngospasm (IV), liver enzyme disorder, mucosal tissue reaction, myocardial infarction, neuroleptic malignant syndrome, positive lymphocyte transformation test, prolonged Q-T interval on ECG (dose dependent), second-degree atrioventricular block, serotonin syndrome, shock (IV), Stevens-Johnson syndrome, supraventricular tachycardia, syncope, tachycardia, tonic-clonic seizures, torsades de pointes, transient blindness (lasted ≤48 hours), transient blurred vision

(following infusion), vascular occlusive events, ventricular premature contractions, ventricular tachycardia, weakness

Drug Interactions
Metabolism/Transport Effects Substrate of CYP1A2 (minor), CYP2C9 (minor), CYP2D6 (minor), CYP2E1 (minor), CYP3A4 (major), P-glycoprotein; **Note:** Assignment of Major/Minor substrate status based on clinically relevant drug interaction potential; **Inhibits** CYP1A2 (weak), CYP2C9 (weak), CYP2D6 (weak)

Avoid Concomitant Use
Avoid concomitant use of Ondansetron with any of the following: Apomorphine; Highest Risk QTc-Prolonging Agents; Ivabradine; Mifepristone

Increased Effect/Toxicity
Ondansetron may increase the levels/effects of: Apomorphine; ARIPiprazole; Highest Risk QTc-Prolonging Agents; Moderate Risk QTc-Prolonging Agents; Panobinostat; Serotonin Modulators; TiZANidine

The levels/effects of Ondansetron may be increased by: Ivabradine; Mifepristone; P-glycoprotein/ABCB1 Inhibitors; QTc-Prolonging Agents (Indeterminate Risk and Risk Modifying); Ranolazine

Decreased Effect
Ondansetron may decrease the levels/effects of: Tapentadol; TraMADol

The levels/effects of Ondansetron may be decreased by: Bosentan; CYP3A4 Inducers (Moderate); CYP3A4 Inducers (Strong); Dabrafenib; Deferasirox; Enzalutamide; Mitotane; P-glycoprotein/ABCB1 Inducers; Siltuximab; St Johns Wort; Tocilizumab

Food Interactions Tablet: Food slightly increases the extent of absorption. Management: Administer without regard to meals.

Preparation for Administration Prior to IV infusion, dilute in 50 mL D$_5$W or NS.

Storage/Stability
Oral soluble film: Store between 20°C and 25°C (68°F and 77°F). Store pouches in cartons; keep film in individual pouch until ready to use.
Oral solution: Store between 15°C and 30°C (59°F and 86°F). Protect from light.
Tablet: Store between 2°C and 30°C (36°F and 86°F).
Vial: Store between 2°C and 30°C (36°F and 86°F). Protect from light. Stable when mixed in D$_5$W or NS for 48 hours at room temperature.
Premixed bag in D$_5$W: Store at 20°C to 25°C (68°F to 77°F), excursions permitted from 15°C to 30°C (59°F to 86°F); may refrigerate; avoid freezing and excessive heat; protect from light.

Mechanism of Action Selective 5-HT$_3$-receptor antagonist, blocking serotonin, both peripherally on vagal nerve terminals and centrally in the chemoreceptor trigger zone

Pharmacodynamics/Kinetics
Onset of action: ~30 minutes
Absorption: Oral: Well absorbed from GI tract
Distribution: V$_d$: Children: 1.9 to 3.7 L/kg
Protein binding, plasma: 70% to 76%
Metabolism: Extensively via hydroxylation, followed by glucuronide or sulfate conjugation; CYP1A2, CYP2D6, and CYP3A4 substrate; some demethylation occurs
Bioavailability: Oral: ~56% (some first pass metabolism)
Half-life elimination: Children <15 years: 2 to 7 hours; Adults: 3 to 6 hours
  Mild-to-moderate hepatic impairment (Child-Pugh classes A and B): Adults: 12 hours
  Severe hepatic impairment (Child-Pugh class C): Adults: 20 hours
Time to peak: Oral: ~2 hours; Oral soluble film: ~1 hour
Excretion: Urine (44% to 60% as metabolites, ~5% as unchanged drug); feces (~25%)

Dosing
Adult
  Prevention of chemotherapy-induced nausea and vomiting:
    U.S. labeling:
      Prevention of nausea and vomiting associated with emetogenic chemotherapy: IV: 0.15 mg/kg/dose (maximum: 16 mg/dose) administered over 15 minutes for 3 doses, beginning 30 minutes prior to chemotherapy, followed by subsequent doses 4 and 8 hours after the first dose
      Prevention of nausea and vomiting associated with highly emetogenic chemotherapy: Oral: 24 mg 30 minutes prior to the start of single-day chemotherapy

Prevention of nausea and vomiting associated with moderately emetogenic chemotherapy: Oral: 8 mg beginning 30 minutes before chemotherapy; repeat dose 8 hours after initial dose, then 8 mg every 12 hours for 1 to 2 days after chemotherapy completed

Canadian labeling:

Prevention of nausea and vomiting associated with highly emetogenic chemotherapy:

IV: 8 to 16 mg (maximum: 16 mg/dose) administered over 15 minutes at least 30 minutes prior to chemotherapy; may administer an additional 8 mg dose at 4 and 8 hours after the initial dose. May convert to oral therapy after the first 24 hours.

Oral: 8 mg every 8 hours for up to 5 days following chemotherapy; oral therapy is initiated after receiving 24 hours of IV ondansetron.

Prevention of nausea and vomiting associated with less emetogenic chemotherapy:

IV: 8 mg administered over 15 minutes at least 30 minutes prior to chemotherapy; may convert to oral therapy twice daily

Oral: 8 mg administered 1-2 hours prior to chemotherapy, followed by 8 mg orally twice daily for up to 5 days following chemotherapy

Guideline recommendations: **Prevention of chemotherapy-induced nausea and vomiting:**

American Society of Clinical Oncology (ASCO; Basch, 2011):

High emetic risk: Day(s) chemotherapy is administered (antiemetic regimen also includes dexamethasone and aprepitant or fosaprepitant):

IV: 8 mg or 0.15 mg/kg. **Note:** Single IV doses >16 mg are no longer recommended by the manufacturer due to the potential for QT prolongation.

Oral: 8 mg twice daily

Multinational Association of Supportive Care in Cancer (MASCC) and European Society of Medical Oncology (ESMO) (Roila, 2010):

Highly emetic chemotherapy (antiemetic regimen includes dexamethasone and aprepitant/fosaprepitant):

IV: 8 mg or 0.15 mg/kg as a single dose prior to chemotherapy. **Note:** Single IV doses >16 mg are no longer recommended by the manufacturer due to the potential for QT prolongation

Oral: 24 mg as a single dose prior to chemotherapy

Moderately emetic chemotherapy (antiemetic regimen includes dexamethasone [and aprepitant/fosaprepitant for AC chemotherapy regimen]):

IV: 8 mg or 0.15 mg/kg as a single dose prior to chemotherapy. **Note:** Single IV doses >16 mg are no longer recommended by the manufacturer due to the potential for QT prolongation.

Oral: 16 mg (as 8 mg twice daily)

Low emetic risk: Ondansetron (dose not specified) prior to chemotherapy on day 1

Prevention of radiation therapy-induced nausea and vomiting:

U.S. labeling:

Total body irradiation: Oral: 8 mg administered 1 to 2 hours before each daily fraction of radiotherapy

Single high-dose fraction radiotherapy to abdomen: Oral: 8 mg administered 1 to 2 hours before irradiation, then 8 mg every 8 hours after first dose for 1 to 2 days after completion of radiotherapy

Daily fractionated radiotherapy to abdomen: Oral: 8 mg administered 1 to 2 hours before irradiation, then 8 mg every 8 hours after first dose for each day of radiotherapy

Canadian labeling: Oral: 8 mg 1 to 2 hours prior to radiation followed by 8 mg every 8 hours for up to 5 days after a course of treatment

American Society of Clinical Oncology Antiemetic Guideline recommendations (Basch, 2011): Give before each fraction throughout radiation therapy for high emetic risk (continue for at least 24 hours after completion) and for moderate emetic risk. For low emetic risk, may give either as prevention or rescue; for minimal emetic risk, give as rescue (if rescue used for either low or minimal emetic risk, then prophylaxis should be given until the end of radiation therapy).

IV (off-label route/dosing): 8 mg or 0.15 mg/kg. **Note:** Single IV doses >16 mg are no longer recommended by the manufacturer due to the potential for QT prolongation.

Prevention of postoperative nausea and vomiting (PONV):

IM, IV (U.S. labeling) or IV (Canadian labeling): 4 mg as a single dose (over 2 to 5 minutes if giving IV) administered ~30 minutes before the end of

anesthesia (see **Note** below) or as treatment if vomiting occurs after surgery (Gan, 2007).

Note: The manufacturer recommends administration immediately before induction of anesthesia; however, this has been shown not to be as effective as administration at the end of surgery (Sun, 1997). Repeat doses given in response to inadequate control of nausea/vomiting from preoperative doses are generally ineffective.

Oral: 16 mg administered 1 hour prior to induction of anesthesia

Treatment of postoperative nausea and vomiting (Canadian labeling): IV: 4 mg as a single dose (preferably over 2 to 5 minutes, but not less than 30 seconds)

Treatment of severe or refractory hyperemesis gravidum (off-label use):

IV: 8 mg administered over 15 minutes every 12 hours (ACOG, 2004)

Oral: 8 mg every 12 hours (Levichek, 2002)

Geriatric

U.S. labeling: Oral, IV: No dosing adjustment required; refer to adult dosing.

Canadian labeling:

IV: Refer to adult dosing. **Note:** Not approved for post operative nausea/vomiting in elderly patients. In the prevention of nausea and vomiting associated with emetogenic chemotherapy, ECG monitoring should be considered in patients 65 to 74 years receiving higher initial dosing (eg, 16 mg); in patients ≥75 years, the initial dose should not exceed 8 mg; per usual adult dosing, may give 2 additional IV doses of 8 mg at least 4 hours apart (if third dose is needed, consider ECG monitoring).

Oral: No dosage adjustment required; refer to adult dosing.

Pediatric

Prevention of chemotherapy-induced nausea and vomiting:

U.S. labeling:

Prevention of nausea and vomiting associated with emetogenic chemotherapy: Infants ≥6 months, Children, and Adolescents: IV: 0.15 mg/kg/dose (maximum: 16 mg/dose) over 15 minutes for 3 doses, beginning 30 minutes prior to chemotherapy, followed by subsequent doses administered 4 and 8 hours after the first dose

Prevention of nausea and vomiting associated with moderately-emetogenic chemotherapy: Oral: Children 4 to 11 years: 4 mg 30 minutes before chemotherapy; repeat 4 and 8 hours after initial dose, then 4 mg every 8 hours for 1 to 2 days after chemotherapy completed

Children ≥12 years: Refer to adult dosing.

Canadian labeling:

Prevention of nausea and vomiting associated with emetogenic chemotherapy: Children 4 to 12 years:

IV: 3 to 5 mg/m^2 over 15 minutes at least 30 minutes prior to chemotherapy, then convert to oral therapy; continue for up to 5 days following chemotherapy

Oral: 4 mg every 8 hours for up to 5 days following chemotherapy; oral therapy is started after an IV dose is given prior to chemotherapy

Pediatric guideline recommendations:

Prevention of chemotherapy-induced nausea and vomiting (off-label dosing; Dupuis, 2013):

Highly emetogenic chemotherapy: Infants ≥1 month and Children <12 years: IV, Oral: 0.15 mg/kg/dose (5 mg/m^2/dose) prior to chemotherapy and then every 8 hours; maximum recommended IV dose: 16 mg. Antiemetic regimen also includes dexamethasone

Highly emetogenic chemotherapy: Children ≥12 years and Adolescents: IV, Oral: 0.15 mg/kg/dose (5 mg/m^2/dose) prior to chemotherapy and then every 8 hours; maximum recommended IV dose: 16 mg. Antiemetic regimen includes dexamethasone and if no known or suspected drug interactions, aprepitant

Moderately emetogenic chemotherapy: Infants ≥1 month, Children, and Adolescents: IV, Oral: 0.15 mg/kg/dose (5 mg/m^2/dose; maximum: 8 mg dose); prior to chemotherapy and then every 12 hours. Antiemetic regimen also includes dexamethasone.

Low emetogenicity chemotherapy: Infants ≥1 month, Children, and Adolescents: IV, Oral: 0.3 mg/kg/dose (10 mg/m^2/dose; maximum IV dose: 16 mg) prior to chemotherapy

Prevention of postoperative nausea and vomiting (PONV): *U.S. labeling:* Infants ≥1 month and Children ≤12 years: IV:

≤40 kg: 0.1 mg/kg as a single dose over 2 to 5 minutes

>40 kg: 4 mg as a single dose over 2 to 5 minutes

Renal Impairment No dosage adjustment necessary (there is no experience for oral ondansetron beyond day 1)

Hepatic Impairment

U.S. labeling:

Mild to moderate impairment: No dosage adjustment necessary.

Severe impairment (Child-Pugh class C):

IV: Day 1: Maximum daily dose: 8 mg (there is no experience beyond day 1)

Oral: Maximum daily dose: 8 mg

Canadian labeling:

Mild impairment: No dosage adjustment necessary.

Moderate to severe impairment: Maximum daily dose: 8 mg

Dietary Considerations Some products may contain phenylalanine.

Administration

Oral: Oral dosage forms should be administered 30 minutes prior to chemotherapy; 1 to 2 hours before radiotherapy; 1 hour prior to the induction of anesthesia

Orally-disintegrating tablets: Do not remove from blister until needed. Peel backing off the blister, do not push tablet through. Using dry hands, place tablet on tongue and allow to dissolve. Swallow with saliva.

Oral soluble film: Do not remove from pouch until immediately before use. Using dry hands, place film on top of tongue and allow to dissolve (4 to 20 seconds). Swallow with or without liquid. If using more than one film, each film should be allowed to dissolve completely before administering the next film.

IM: Should be administered undiluted.

IV:

IVPB: Infuse diluted solution over 15 to 30 minutes; 24-hour continuous infusions have been reported, but are rarely used.

Chemotherapy-induced nausea and vomiting: Give first dose 30 minutes prior to beginning chemotherapy.

IV push: Prevention of postoperative nausea and vomiting: Single doses may be administered IV injection as undiluted solution over at least 30 seconds but preferably over 2 to 5 minutes

Monitoring Parameters ECG (if applicable in high-risk or elderly patients); potassium, magnesium

Dosage Forms Excipient information presented when available (limited, particularly for generics); consult specific product labeling. [DSC] = Discontinued product

Film, Oral:

Zuplenz: 4 mg (1 ea, 10 ea); 8 mg (1 ea, 10 ea)

Solution, Injection:

Zofran: 40 mg/20 mL (20 mL) [contains methylparaben, propylparaben]

Generic: 4 mg/2 mL (2 mL); 40 mg/20 mL (20 mL)

Solution, Injection [preservative free]:

Generic: 4 mg/2 mL (2 mL)

Solution, Intravenous [preservative free]:

Generic: 32 mg (50 mL [DSC])

Solution, Oral:

Zofran: 4 mg/5 mL (50 mL) [strawberry flavor]

Generic: 4 mg/5 mL (50 mL)

Tablet, Oral:

Zofran: 4 mg, 8 mg

Generic: 4 mg, 8 mg, 24 mg

Tablet Dispersible, Oral:

Zofran ODT: 4 mg, 8 mg [contains aspartame, methylparaben sodium, propylparaben sodium; strawberry flavor]

Generic: 4 mg, 8 mg

Dosage Forms: Canada Refer to Dosage Forms. **Note:** Oral Film is not available in Canada.

Extemporaneous Preparations Note: Commercial oral solution is available (0.8 mg/mL)

If commercial oral solution is unavailable, a 0.8 mg/mL syrup may be made with ondansetron tablets, Ora-Plus® (Paddock), and any of the following syrups: Cherry syrup USP, Syrpalta® (HUMCO), Ora-Sweet® (Paddock), or Ora-Sweet® Sugar-Free (Paddock). Crush ten 8 mg tablets in a mortar and reduce to a fine powder (flaking of the tablet coating occurs). Add 50 mL Ora-Plus® in 5 mL increments, mixing thoroughly; mix while adding the chosen syrup in incremental proportions to **almost** 100 mL; transfer to a calibrated bottle, rinse mortar with syrup, and add sufficient quantity of syrup to make 100 mL. Label "shake well" and "refrigerate". Stable for 42 days refrigerated (Trissel, 1996).

Rectal suppositories: Calibrate a suppository mold for the base being used. Determine the displacement factor (DF) for ondansetron for the base being used (Fattibase® = 1.1; Polybase® = 0.6). Weigh the ondansetron tablet(s). Divide the tablet weight by the DF; this result is the weight of base displaced by the drug. Subtract the weight of base displaced from the calculated weight of base required for each suppository. Grind the ondansetron tablets in a mortar and reduce to a fine powder. Weigh out the appropriate weight of suppository base. Melt the base over a water bath (<55°C). Add the ondansetron powder to the suppository base and mix well. Pour the mixture into the suppository mold and cool. Stable for at least 30 days refrigerated (Tenjarla, 1998).

Tenjarla SN, Ward ES, and Fox JL, "Ondansetron Suppositories: Extemporaneous Preparation, Drug Release, Stability and Flux Through Rabbit Rectal Membrane," *Int J Pharm Compound*, 1998, 2(1):83-8.

Trissel LA, *Trissel's Stability of Compounded Formulations*, Washington, DC: American Pharmaceutical Association, 1996.

Opium Tincture (OH pee um TING chur)

Index Terms Deodorized Tincture of Opium (error-prone synonym); DTO (error-prone abbreviation); Opium Tincture, Deodorized; Tincture of Opium

Pharmacologic Category Analgesic, Opioid; Antidiarrheal

Use Diarrhea: Treatment of diarrhea in adults

Pregnancy Considerations Animal reproduction studies have not been conducted. Opium tincture contains morphine; refer to the Morphine (Systemic) monograph for additional information. In addition, this preparation contains large amounts of alcohol (19%).

Breast-Feeding Considerations Opium tincture contains morphine, which is excreted into breast milk; refer to the Morphine (Systemic) monograph for additional information. In addition, this preparation contains large amounts of alcohol (19%). The manufacturer recommends that caution be used if administered to a nursing woman.

Contraindications

Use in children; diarrhea caused by poisoning until the toxic material is eliminated from the GI tract

Documentation of allergenic cross-reactivity for opioids is limited. However, because of similarities in chemical structure and/or pharmacologic actions, the possibility of cross-sensitivity cannot be ruled out with certainty.

Warnings/Precautions May cause CNS depression, which may impair physical or mental abilities; patients must be cautioned about performing tasks which require mental alertness (eg, operating machinery or driving). Use with caution in patients with morbid obesity, adrenal insufficiency, hepatic impairment, biliary tract impairment, pancreatitis, head trauma, GI hemorrhage, thyroid dysfunction, prostatic hyperplasia/urinary stricture, respiratory disease, or a history of drug abuse. Avoid use in patients with CNS depression or coma as these patients are susceptible to intracranial effects of CO_2 retention. May cause hypotension; use with caution in patients with hypovolemia, cardiovascular disease (including acute MI), or with drugs which may exaggerate hypotensive effects (including phenothiazines or general anesthetics). May obscure diagnosis or clinical course of patients with acute abdominal conditions. Concurrent use of agonist/antagonist analgesics may precipitate withdrawal symptoms and/or reduced analgesic efficacy in patients following prolonged therapy with mu opioid agonists. Abrupt discontinuation following prolonged use may also lead to withdrawal symptoms. Use with caution in the elderly and debilitated patients; may be more sensitive to adverse effects. Potentially significant interactions may exist, requiring dose or frequency adjustment, additional monitoring, and/or selection of alternative therapy.

Do not confuse opium tincture with paregoric; opium tincture is 25 times more potent than paregoric; opium shares the toxic potential of opioid agonists, usual precautions of opioid agonist therapy should be observed; abrupt discontinuation after prolonged use may result in withdrawal symptoms. Infants <3 months of age are more susceptible to respiratory depression; if used (off-label), diluted doses are recommended and use with caution. Contraindicated for use in children according to the manufacturer. Opium tincture is not routinely used as a source of morphine to treat neonatal abstinence syndrome in infants exposed to chronic opioids *in utero*. If used, then dilution is necessary. In addition, use for this purpose may increase the risk of drug error and morphine overdose in the infant (AAP, 1998; Dow, 2012; Hudack, 2012).

Adverse Reactions Frequency not defined.

Cardiovascular: Bradycardia, hypotension, palpitations, peripheral vasodilation

Central nervous system: Central nervous system depression, depression, dizziness, drowsiness, drug dependence, headache, increased intracranial pressure, insomnia, malaise, restlessness

Gastrointestinal: Anorexia, biliary tract spasm, constipation, nausea, stomach cramps, vomiting

Genitourinary: Decreased urine output, genitourinary tract spasm

Hypersensitivity: Histamine release

Neuromuscular & skeletal: Weakness

Ophthalmic: Miosis

Respiratory: Respiratory depression

Limited to important or life-threatening: Hypogonadism (Brennan, 2013; Debono, 2011)

Drug Interactions

Metabolism/Transport Effects None known.

Avoid Concomitant Use

Avoid concomitant use of Opium Tincture with any of the following: Azelastine (Nasal); Eluxadoline; Mixed Agonist / Antagonist Opioids; Orphenadrine; Paraldehyde; Thalidomide

Increased Effect/Toxicity

Opium Tincture may increase the levels/effects of: Alcohol (Ethyl); Alvimopan; Azelastine (Nasal); CNS Depressants; Desmopressin; Diuretics; Eluxadoline; Hydrocodone; Methotrimeprazine; Metyrosine; Mirtazapine; Orphenadrine; Paraldehyde; Pramipexole; Ramosetron; ROPINIRole; Rotigotine; Selective Serotonin Reuptake Inhibitors; Suvorexant; Thalidomide; Zolpidem

The levels/effects of Opium Tincture may be increased by: Amphetamines; Anticholinergic Agents; Antipsychotic Agents (Phenothiazines); Brimonidine (Topical); Cannabis; Doxylamine; Dronabinol; Droperidol; HydrOXYzine; Kava Kava; Magnesium Sulfate; Methotrimeprazine; Minocycline; Nabilone; Perampanel; Rufinamide; Sodium Oxybate; Succinylcholine; Tapentadol; Tetrahydrocannabinol

Decreased Effect

Opium Tincture may decrease the levels/effects of: Pegvisomant

The levels/effects of Opium Tincture may be decreased by: Ammonium Chloride; Mixed Agonist / Antagonist Opioids; Naltrexone

Storage/Stability Store at 68°F to 77°F (20°C to 25°C). Protect from light.

Mechanism of Action Contains many opioid alkaloids including morphine; its mechanism for gastric motility inhibition is primarily due to this morphine content; it results in a decrease in digestive secretions, an increase in GI muscle tone, and therefore a reduction in GI propulsion

Pharmacodynamics/Kinetics

Absorption: Variable

Metabolism: Hepatic

Excretion: Urine

Dosing

Adult & Geriatric Note: Opium tincture contains morphine 10 mg/mL. Use caution in ordering, dispensing, and/or administering. The following doses are expressed in **mg** (milligram) dosing units of morphine.

Diarrhea: Oral: 6 **mg** of undiluted opium tincture (10 mg/mL) 4 times daily

Renal Impairment There are no dosage adjustments provided in the manufacturer's labeling.

Hepatic Impairment There are no dosage adjustments provided in the manufacturer's labeling; use with caution.

Monitoring Parameters Observe patient for excessive sedation, respiratory depression, implement safety measures, assist with ambulation; signs or symptoms of hypogonadism or hypoadrenalism (Brennan, 2013)

Test Interactions Increased aminotransferase [ALT/AST] (S)

Dosage Forms Excipient information presented when available (limited, particularly for generics); consult specific product labeling.

Tincture, Oral:

Generic: 10 mg/mL (1%) (118 mL, 473 mL)

Controlled Substance C-II

Oprelvekin (oh PREL ve kin)

Brand Names: US Neumega [DSC]

Index Terms IL-11; Interleukin-11; Recombinant Human Interleukin-11; Recombinant Interleukin-11; rhIL-11

Pharmacologic Category Biological Response Modulator; Human Growth Factor

Use Thrombocytopenia: Prevention of severe thrombocytopenia and to reduce the need for platelet transfusions following myelosuppressive chemotherapy for nonmyeloid malignancy in adults who are at high risk for thrombocytopenia

Dosing

Adult & Geriatric

Thrombocytopenia: SubQ: 50 mcg/kg once daily until postnadir platelet count ≥50,000/mm^3. Begin ~6 to 24 hours after the end of chemotherapy. In studies, doses were administered for 10 to 21 days (do not administer for more than 21 days). Discontinue at least 2 days prior to the next planned chemotherapy cycle.

Renal Impairment For dosage adjustment purposes, renal function may be estimated using the Cockcroft-Gault formula.

CrCl ≥30 mL/minute: No dosage adjustment necessary.

CrCl <30 mL/minute: Reduce dose to 25 mcg/kg once daily.

Hepatic Impairment There are no dosage adjustments provided in the manufacturer's labeling.

Additional Information Complete prescribing information should be consulted for additional detail.

Dosage Forms Excipient information presented when available (limited, particularly for generics); consult specific product labeling. [DSC] = Discontinued product

Solution Reconstituted, Subcutaneous [preservative free]:

Neumega: 5 mg (1 ea [DSC])

Oritavancin (or it a VAN sin)

Brand Names: US Orbactiv

Index Terms LY333328; Oritavancin Diphosphate

Pharmacologic Category Glycopeptide

Use Acute bacterial skin and skin structure infections: Treatment of adult patients with acute bacterial skin and skin structure infections (ABSSSI) caused by susceptible isolates of the following gram-positive microorganisms: *Staphylococcus aureus* (including methicillin-susceptible and methicillin-resistant isolates); *Streptococcus pyogenes; Streptococcus agalactiae; Streptococcus dysgalactiae, Streptococcus anginosus* group (including *S. anginosus, S. intermedius, S. constellatus*); and *Enterococcus faecalis* (vancomycin-susceptible isolates only)

Pregnancy Considerations Adverse events were not observed in animal reproduction studies.

Breast-Feeding Considerations It is not known if oritavancin is excreted into breast milk. The manufacturer recommends that caution be used if administered to a nursing woman.

Contraindications Hypersensitivity to oritavancin or any component of the formulation; use of intravenous unfractionated heparin for 48 hours after oritavancin administration (oritavancin falsely elevates aPTT for ~48 hours after administration)

Warnings/Precautions Serious hypersensitivity reactions have been reported (median onset in studies ~1.2 days). If an acute reaction occurs, discontinue infusion immediately and institute appropriate supportive care (median resolution ~2.4 days) Inquire about previous hypersensitivity reactions to glycopeptides; carefully monitor patients with a history of glycopeptide allergy. Infusion related reactions (pruritus, urticaria, flushing) have been reported. If reactions occur, consider slowing or interrupting infusion. In clinical trials, more cases of osteomyelitis were noted in patients treated with oritavancin. Monitor for signs and symptoms of osteomyelitis and institute appropriate alternate antibacterial therapy if warranted. Use may result in fungal or bacterial superinfection, including *C. difficile*-associated diarrhea (CDAD) and pseudomembranous colitis; CDAD has been observed >2 months postantibiotic treatment. Coadministration with warfarin may increase bleeding risk Use in patients on chronic warfarin therapy only when benefit is expected to outweigh risk; monitor frequently for signs of bleeding. Oritavancin has no independent coagulation system effects but artificially prolongs coagulation tests due to reagent reactions; use caution when interpreting results (see Test Interactions). Potentially significant drug-drug interactions may exist, requiring dose or frequency adjustment, additional monitoring, and/ or selection of alternative therapy.

Adverse Reactions

1% to 10%:

Cardiovascular: Tachycardia (3%), hypersensitivity angiitis (<2%), peripheral edema (<2%)

Central nervous system: Headache (7%), dizziness (3%)

Dermatologic: Erythema multiforme (<2%), pruritus (<2%), skin rash (<2%), urticaria (<2%)

Endocrine & metabolic: Hyperuricemia (<2%), hypoglycemia (<2%)

Gastrointestinal: Nausea (10%), vomiting (5%), diarrhea (4%)

Hematologic & oncologic: Anemia (<2%), eosinophilia (<2%)

Hepatic: Increased serum ALT (3%), increased serum AST (2%), increased total serum bilirubin (<2%)

Hypersensitivity: Angioedema (<2%)

Infection: Subcutaneous abscess (4%), limb abscess (≤4%)

Local: Injection site phlebitis (3%), injection site reaction (2%), erythema at injection site (<2%), extravasation (<2%), induration at injection site (<2%)

Neuromuscular & skeletal: Myalgia (<2%), osteomyelitis (<2%), tenosynovitis (<2%)

Respiratory: Bronchospasm (<2%), wheezing (<2%)

<1%, postmarketing, and/or case reports: *Clostridium difficile*-associated diarrhea, hypersensitivity reaction, INR abnormal, prolonged partial thromboplastin time, prolonged prothrombin time

Drug Interactions

Metabolism/Transport Effects Inhibits CYP2C19 (weak), CYP2C9 (weak)

Avoid Concomitant Use

Avoid concomitant use of Oritavancin with any of the following: BCG (Intravesical); Heparin

Increased Effect/Toxicity

Oritavancin may increase the levels/effects of: Vitamin K Antagonists

Decreased Effect

Oritavancin may decrease the levels/effects of: BCG (Intravesical); BCG Vaccine (Immunization); Heparin; Sodium Picosulfate; Typhoid Vaccine

Preparation for Administration Reconstitute each 400 mg vial with 40 mL of SWFI. Swirl gently to avoid foaming. The reconstituted vial contains 10 mg/mL oritavancin as a clear, colorless to pale yellow solution. Withdraw and discard 120 mL of fluid from a D_5W 1000 mL bag; withdraw 40 mL from each of 3 reconstituted vials and add to D_5W to bring the total bag volume to 1000 mL. (final solution concentration 1.2 mg/mL).

Storage/Stability Store intact vials at 20°C to 25°C (68°F to 77°F); excursions are permitted between 15°C and 30°C (59°F and 86°F). Reconstituted vials and diluted solution may be stored refrigerated at 2°C to 8°C (36°F to 46°F) for 12 hours or at room temperature 20°C to 25°C (68°F to 77°F) for 6 hours. The total time from reconstitution and dilution to completed administration should be ≤6 hours at room temperature or ≤12 hours if refrigerated.

Mechanism of Action Oritavancin is a lipoglycopeptide with concentration-dependent bactericidal activity. It inhibits cell wall biosynthesis by inhibiting the polymerization step by binding to stem peptides of peptidoglycan precursors, by inhibiting crosslinking by binding to bridging segments, and by disrupting bacterial membrane integrity, leading to cell death.

Pharmacodynamics/Kinetics

Distribution: V_d: 87.6 L

Protein binding: 85%

Metabolism: Not metabolized

Half-life elimination: 245 hours

Excretion: Feces and urine as unchanged drug (less than 1% and 5% in feces and urine, respectively, over two weeks postadministration)

Dosing

Adult & Geriatric Acute bacterial skin and skin structure infections (ABSSI): IV: 1200 mg as a single dose

Renal Impairment

CrCl ≥30 mL/minute: No dosage adjustment necessary.

CrCl <30 mL/minute: There are no dosage adjustments provided in the manufacturer's labeling (has not been studied); use with caution.

ESRD requiring hemodialysis: There are no dosage adjustments provided in the manufacturer's labeling (has not been studied); use with caution; not removed by hemodialysis.

Hepatic Impairment

Mild to moderate hepatic impairment (Child-Pugh class A or B): No dosage adjustment necessary.

Severe hepatic impairment (Child-Pugh class C): There are no dosage adjustments provided in the manufacturer's labeling (has not been studied); use with caution.

Administration IV: Infuse over 3 hours. If a common IV line is being used to administer other drugs in addition to oritavancin, the line should be flushed before and after each infusion with D_5W. If infusion-related reaction (pruritus, urticaria, flushing) occurs, consider slowing or interrupting infusion.

Monitoring Parameters Baseline serum urea nitrogen, serum creatinine, and liver function tests (AST, ALT, bilirubin). Monitor patients for any kind of infusion-related reactions (pruritus, urticaria, flushing), hypersensitivity reactions (especially in patients with reported glycopeptide allergy) and signs and symptoms of osteomyelitis.

Test Interactions Artificially prolongs coagulation tests (binds to and prevents action of phospholipid reagents), including activated clotting time (ACT), aPTT (48 hours), prothrombin time (24 hours) and international normalized ratio (24 hours). For patients requiring aPTT monitoring within 48 hours of a dose, consider a nonphospholipid dependent coagulation test (eg, Factor Xa [chromogenic] assay) or an alternative anticoagulant not requiring aPTT monitoring.

Dosage Forms Excipient information presented when available (limited, particularly for generics); consult specific product labeling.

Solution Reconstituted, Intravenous:
Orbactiv: 400 mg (1 ea, 3 ea)

♦ Oritavancin Diphosphate see Oritavancin on page 1340

♦ Orkambi see Lumacaftor and Ivacaftor on page 1114

Orlistat (OR li stat)

Brand Names: US Alli [OTC]; Xenical
Brand Names: Canada Xenical
Pharmacologic Category Lipase Inhibitor
Use Obesity management:
OTC: For weight loss in overweight adults when used along with a reduced-calorie and low-fat diet.
Rx: For obesity management, including weight loss and weight maintenance, when used in conjunction with a reduced-calorie diet; to reduce the risk for weight regain after prior weight loss.
Limitations of use: Orlistat is indicated for obese patients with an initial body mass index of ≥30 kg/m² or ≥27 kg/m² in the presence of other risk factors (eg, hypertension, diabetes, dyslipidemia).

Pregnancy Considerations Adverse events were not observed in animal reproduction studies. Although orlistat is minimally absorbed, weight-loss therapy is not recommended for pregnant women. Obese and overweight women should be encouraged to participate in weight reduction programs prior to attempting pregnancy; weight gain during pregnancy should be determined by their prepregnancy BMI and current guidelines (ADA, 2009; IOM, 2009). Use of orlistat is contraindicated in pregnant women.

Breast-Feeding Considerations Weight-loss therapy is generally not recommended for lactating women. Weight-loss programs which include physical activity and nutrition components should be discussed at the 6-week postpartum visit (ADA, 2009; IOM, 2009).

Contraindications Pregnancy; chronic malabsorption syndrome; cholestasis; hypersensitivity to orlistat or to any component of the formulation

Warnings/Precautions Cases of severe liver injury (some fatal) with hepatocellular necrosis or acute hepatic failure have been reported; liver transplantation has been required in some patients. Patients should be instructed to report any symptoms of hepatic dysfunction (eg, anorexia, pruritus, jaundice, dark urine, light colored stools, right upper quadrant pain); discontinue therapy and obtain liver function test immediately if symptoms occur. Advise patients to adhere to dietary guidelines; if taken with a diet high in fat (>30% total daily calories from fat) gastrointestinal adverse events may increase. Distribute daily fat intake over 3 main meals. If taken with any 1 meal very high in fat, the possibility of gastrointestinal effects increases. Counsel patients to take a multivitamin supplement that contains fat-soluble vitamins ≥2 hours before or after orlistat administration to ensure adequate nutrition; orlistat has been shown to reduce the absorption of some fat-soluble vitamins and beta-carotene. Increased levels of urinary oxalate following treatment may occur in some patients; cases of oxalate nephrolithiasis and oxalate nephropathy with renal failure have been reported. Monitor renal function in patients at risk for renal impairment; use with caution in patients with a history of hyperoxaluria or calcium oxalate nephrolithiasis. The potential exists for misuse in inappropriate patient populations (eg, patients with anorexia nervosa or bulimia) similar to any weight loss agent. In general, substantial weight loss may increase the

risk of cholelithiasis. Potentially significant interactions may exist, requiring dose or frequency adjustment, additional monitoring, and/or selection of alternative therapy.

Appropriate use: Prior to use, other causes for obesity (eg, hypothyroidism) should be ruled out. According to Endocrine Society practice guidelines, weight loss medication should be discontinued and alternative treatment considered if weight loss is <5% of body weight at 3 months or if safety/tolerability issues arise (Apovian, 2015).

Self-medication (OTC use): Prior to use, patients should contact their healthcare provider if they have ever had kidney stones, gall bladder disease, or pancreatitis. Patients taking medications for diabetes or thyroid disease, seizures, anticoagulants, or other weight-loss products should consult their healthcare provider or pharmacist before use. Patients who have had an organ transplant should not use orlistat. If severe and/or continuous abdominal pain, itching, yellowing of the eyes or skin, dark urine, or loss of appetite occurs, or seizure worsens, use should be discontinued and healthcare provider consulted.

Adverse Reactions The frequency of most adverse reactions (especially gastrointestinal effects) decreases over time. Frequency not always defined.
Cardiovascular: Pedal edema (≤3%)
Central nervous system: Headache (≤31%), fatigue (3% to 7%), anxiety (3% to 5%), sleep disorder (≤4%)
Dermatologic: Xeroderma (≤2%)
Endocrine & metabolic: Menstrual disease (≤10%), hypoglycemia (in patients with diabetes)
Gastrointestinal: Oily rectal leakage (4% to 27%), abdominal distress (≤26%), abdominal pain (≤26%), flatulence with discharge (2% to 24%), bowel urgency (3% to 22%), steatorrhea (6% to 20%), oily evacuation (2% to 12%), frequent bowel movements (3% to 11%), nausea (4% to 8%), fecal incontinence (2% to 8%), infectious diarrhea (≤5%), rectal pain (3% to 5%), gingival disease (4%), cholelithiasis (3%), abdominal distension (in patients with diabetes)
Genitourinary: Urinary tract infection (6% to 8%), vaginitis (3%)
Infection: Influenza (≤40%)
Neuromuscular & skeletal: Back pain (≤14%), leg pain (≤11%), myalgia (≤4%)
Otic: Otitis (4%)
Respiratory: Upper respiratory tract infection (38%), lower respiratory tract infection (≤8%)
<1% (Limited to important or life-threatening): Acute renal failure, bullous skin disease, calcium oxalate nephrolithiasis, hepatic failure, hepatitis, hypersensitivity, hypersensitivity angiitis, increased serum alkaline phosphatase, increased serum transaminases, kidney injury (acute), pancreatitis, renal disease (secondary to increased urinary oxalate excretion)

Drug Interactions
Metabolism/Transport Effects None known.
Avoid Concomitant Use There are no known interactions where it is recommended to avoid concomitant use.
Increased Effect/Toxicity
Orlistat may increase the levels/effects of: Warfarin
Decreased Effect
Orlistat may decrease the levels/effects of: Amiodarone; Anticonvulsants; CycloSPORINE (Systemic); Levothyroxine; Multivitamins/Fluoride (with ADE); Multivitamins/Minerals (with ADEK, Folate, Iron); Multivitamins/Minerals (with AE, No Iron); Paricalcitol; Propafenone; Vitamin D Analogs; Vitamins (Fat Soluble)

Storage/Stability Store at 25°C (77°F); excursions permitted to 15°C to 30°C (59°F to 86°F).

Mechanism of Action A reversible inhibitor of gastric and pancreatic lipases, thus inhibiting absorption of dietary fats by 30%.

Pharmacodynamics/Kinetics
Onset of action: 24-48 hours
Duration: 48-72 hours
Absorption: Minimal
Protein binding: >99% (lipoproteins and albumin)
Metabolism: Metabolized within the gastrointestinal wall; forms inactive metabolites
Half-life elimination: 1-2 hours
Time to peak, serum: ~8 hours
Excretion: Feces (~97%, 83% as unchanged drug); urine (<2%)

Dosing
Adult & Geriatric
Obesity management: Oral:
Xenical: 120 mg 3 times daily with each main meal containing fat (during or up to 1 hour after the meal); omit dose if meal is occasionally missed or contains no fat.
Alli: OTC labeling: 60 mg 3 times daily with each main meal containing fat (maximum dose: 180 mg daily).

◄ **Dosing adjustment with concomitant therapy:**
  Cyclosporine: Administer cyclosporine 3 hours after orlistat.
  Levothyroxine: Administer levothyroxine and orlistat at least 4 hours apart and monitor for changes in thyroid function.

Pediatric Obesity management (Xenical): Children ≥12 years and Adolescents: Refer to adult dosing.

Renal Impairment There are no dosage adjustments provided in the manufacturer's labeling (has not been studied). However, dosage adjustment unlikely due to low systemic absorption.

Hepatic Impairment There are no dosage adjustments provided in the manufacturer's labeling (has not been studied). However, dosage adjustment unlikely due to low systemic absorption.

Dietary Considerations Multivitamin supplements that contain fat-soluble vitamins should be taken once daily at least 2 hours before or after the administration of orlistat (ie, bedtime). Gastrointestinal effects of orlistat may increase if taken with any one meal very high in fat. Distribute daily intake of carbohydrates, fat (~30% of daily calories), and protein over three main meals.

Administration Administer during or up to 1 hour after each main meal containing fat; separate dose by at least 2 hours from multivitamin daily supplement. Omit dose if a meal is missed or contains no fat.

Monitoring Parameters BMI; diet (calorie and fat intake); serum glucose in patients with diabetes; thyroid function in patient with thyroid disease; liver function tests in patients exhibiting symptoms of hepatic dysfunction

Dosage Forms Excipient information presented when available (limited, particularly for generics); consult specific product labeling.
  Capsule, Oral:
    Alli: 60 mg [contains fd&c blue #2 (indigotine)]
    Xenical: 120 mg [contains fd&c blue #2 (indigotine)]

Orphenadrine (or FEN a dreen)

Brand Names: US Norflex
Brand Names: Canada Norflex™; Orphenace®; Rhoxal-orphendrine
Index Terms Orphenadrine Citrate
Pharmacologic Category Skeletal Muscle Relaxant
Use Treatment of muscle spasm associated with acute painful musculoskeletal conditions
Dosing
  Adult Muscle spasms:
    Oral: 100 mg twice daily
    IM, IV: 60 mg every 12 hours
  Geriatric Use caution; generally not recommended for use in the elderly.
  Renal Impairment No dosage adjustment provided in manufacturer's labeling.
  Hepatic Impairment No dosage adjustment provided in manufacturer's labeling.
  Additional Information Complete prescribing information should be consulted for additional detail.
  Dosage Forms Excipient information presented when available (limited, particularly for generics); consult specific product labeling.
    Solution, Injection, as citrate:
      Norflex: 30 mg/mL (2 mL) [contains sodium metabisulfite]
      Generic: 30 mg/mL (2 mL)
    Solution, Injection, as citrate [preservative free]:
      Generic: 30 mg/mL (2 mL)
    Tablet Extended Release 12 Hour, Oral, as citrate:
      Generic: 100 mg

Orphenadrine, Aspirin, and Caffeine (or FEN a dreen, AS pir in, & KAF een)

Index Terms Aspirin, Caffeine, and Orphenadrine; Aspirin, Orphenadrine, and Caffeine; Caffeine, Orphenadrine, and Aspirin; Norgesic
Pharmacologic Category Skeletal Muscle Relaxant
Use Relief of discomfort associated with skeletal muscular conditions
Dosing
  Adult Muscular pain/spasms: Oral: 1-2 tablets 3-4 times/day
  Geriatric Not recommended for use in the elderly; see individual agents

Renal Impairment No dosage adjustment provided in manufacturer's labeling.
Hepatic Impairment No dosage adjustment provided in manufacturer's labeling.
Additional Information Complete prescribing information should be consulted for additional detail.
Dosage Forms Excipient information presented when available (limited, particularly for generics); consult specific product labeling. [DSC] = Discontinued product
  Tablet: Orphenadrine citrate 25 mg, aspirin 385 mg, and caffeine 30 mg; orphenadrine citrate 50 mg, aspirin 770 mg, and caffeine 60 mg [DSC]

Oseltamivir (oh sel TAM i vir)

Brand Names: US Tamiflu
Brand Names: Canada Tamiflu

Pharmacologic Category Antiviral Agent; Neuraminidase Inhibitor

Use

Prophylaxis of influenza: Prophylaxis of influenza (A or B) infection in children ≥1 year of age and adults.

Treatment of influenza: Treatment of uncomplicated acute illness due to influenza (A or B) infection in children ≥2 weeks of age and adults who have been symptomatic for no more than 2 days.

The Advisory Committee on Immunization Practices (ACIP) recommends that **treatment** be considered for the following:

• Persons with severe, complicated or progressive illness
• Hospitalized persons
• Persons at higher risk for influenza complications:
 - Children <2 years of age (highest risk in children <6 months of age)
 - Adults ≥65 years of age
 - Persons with chronic disorders of the pulmonary (including asthma) or cardiovascular systems (except hypertension)
 - Persons with chronic metabolic diseases (including diabetes mellitus), hepatic disease, renal dysfunction, hematologic disorders (including sickle cell disease), or immunosuppression (including immunosuppression caused by medications or HIV)
 - Persons with neurologic/neuromuscular conditions (including conditions such as spinal cord injuries, seizure disorders, cerebral palsy, stroke, mental retardation, moderate to severe developmental delay, or muscular dystrophy) which may compromise respiratory function, the handling of respiratory secretions, or that can increase the risk of aspiration
 - Pregnant or postpartum women (≤2 weeks after delivery)
 - Persons <19 years of age on long-term aspirin therapy
 - American Indians and Alaskan Natives
 - Persons who are morbidly obese (BMI ≥40)
 - Residents of nursing homes or other chronic care facilities
• Use may also be considered for previously healthy, nonhigh-risk outpatients with confirmed or suspected influenza based on clinical judgment when treatment can be started within 48 hours of illness onset.

The ACIP recommends that **prophylaxis** be considered for the following:

• Postexposure prophylaxis may be considered for family or close contacts of suspected or confirmed cases, who are at higher risk of influenza complications, and who have not been vaccinated against the circulating strain at the time of the exposure.
• Postexposure prophylaxis may be considered for unvaccinated healthcare workers who had occupational exposure without protective equipment.
• Pre-exposure prophylaxis should only be used for persons at very high risk of influenza complications who cannot be otherwise protected at times of high risk for exposure.
• Prophylaxis should also be administered to all eligible residents of institutions that house patients at high risk when needed to control outbreaks.

The ACIP recommends that treatment and prophylaxis be given to children <1 year of age when indicated.

Pregnancy Considerations Adverse events were observed in some animal reproduction studies. Oseltamivir phosphate and its active metabolite oseltamivir carboxylate cross the placenta (Meijer, 2012). An increased risk of adverse neonatal or maternal outcomes has generally not been observed following maternal use of oseltamivir during pregnancy (CDC, 60[1], 2011; CDC, March 13, 2014).

Untreated influenza infection is associated with an increased risk of adverse events to the fetus and an increased risk of complications or death to the mother. Neuraminidase inhibitors are currently recommended for the treatment or prophylaxis of influenza in pregnant women and women up to 2 weeks postpartum (CDC 60 [1], 2011; CDC March 13, 2014; January 2015).

Breast-Feeding Considerations Low concentrations of oseltamivir and oseltamivir carboxylate (OC) have been detected in breast milk; levels are unlikely to lead to toxicity in a breast-fed infant. The manufacturer recommends that caution be used if administered to a nursing woman.

Influenza may cause serious illness in postpartum women and prompt evaluation for febrile respiratory illnesses is recommended (Louie, 2011).

Contraindications Hypersensitivity to oseltamivir or any component of the formulation

Warnings/Precautions Oseltamivir is not a substitute for the influenza virus vaccine. It has not been shown to prevent primary or concomitant bacterial infections that may occur with influenza virus. Use caution with renal impairment; dosage adjustment is required. Safety and efficacy for use in patients with chronic cardiac and/or kidney disease, severe hepatic impairment, or for treatment or prophylaxis in immunocompromised patients have not been established. Rare but severe hypersensitivity reactions, including anaphylaxis and severe dermatologic reactions (eg, Stevens-Johnson syndrome, erythema multiforme), have been associated with use. Discontinue use immediately if hypersensitivity occurs or is suspected and treat appropriately. Rare occurrences of neuropsychiatric events (including confusion, delirium, hallucinations, and/or self-injury) have been reported from postmarketing surveillance (primarily in pediatric patients); direct causation is difficult to establish (influenza infection may also be associated with behavioral and neurologic changes). Monitor closely for signs of any unusual behavior.

Antiviral treatment should begin within 48 hours of symptom onset. However, the CDC recommends that treatment may still be beneficial and should be started in hospitalized patients with severe, complicated or progressive illness if >48 hours. Treatment should not be delayed while awaiting results of laboratory tests for influenza. Nonhospitalized persons who are not at high risk for developing severe or complicated illness and who have a mild disease are not likely to benefit if treatment is started >48 hours after symptom onset. Nonhospitalized persons who are already beginning to recover do not need treatment. Oral suspension contains sorbitol (delivers ~2 g sorbitol per 75 mg dose) which is greater than the maximum daily limit for some patients; may cause diarrhea and dyspepsia; use with caution in patients with hereditary fructose intolerance. The Canadian labeling does not approve of use (treatment or prophylaxis) in infants <1 year of age.

Benzyl alcohol and derivatives: Some dosage forms may contain sodium benzoate/benzoic acid; benzoic acid (benzoate) is a metabolite of benzyl alcohol; large amounts of benzyl alcohol (≥99 mg/kg/day) have been associated with a potentially fatal toxicity ("gasping syndrome") in neonates; the "gasping syndrome" consists of metabolic acidosis, respiratory distress, gasping respirations, CNS dysfunction (including convulsions, intracranial hemorrhage), hypotension, and cardiovascular collapse (AAP ["Inactive" 1997]; CDC, 1982); some data suggests that benzoate displaces bilirubin from protein binding sites (Ahlfors, 2001); avoid or use dosage forms containing benzyl alcohol derivative with caution in neonates. See manufacturer's labeling.

Adverse Reactions

>10%: Gastrointestinal: Vomiting (2% to 15%)
1% to 10%:
 Gastrointestinal: Nausea (4% to 10%), abdominal pain (2% to 5%), diarrhea (1% to 3%)
 Ocular: Conjunctivitis (1%)
 Respiratory: Epistaxis (1%)
<1% (Limited to important or life-threatening): Allergy, anaphylactic/anaphylactoid reaction, angina, arrhythmia, confusion, erythema multiforme, fracture, gastrointestinal bleeding, hemorrhagic colitis, hepatitis, liver function tests abnormal, neuropsychiatric events, pseudomembranous colitis, pyrexia, seizure, Stevens-Johnson syndrome, swelling of face or tongue, toxic epidermal necrolysis

Drug Interactions

Metabolism/Transport Effects None known.

Avoid Concomitant Use There are no known interactions where it is recommended to avoid concomitant use.

Increased Effect/Toxicity
 The levels/effects of Oseltamivir may be increased by: Probenecid

Decreased Effect
 Oseltamivir may decrease the levels/effects of: Influenza Virus Vaccine (Live/Attenuated)

Preparation for Administration Oral suspension: Reconstitute with 55 mL of water to a final concentration of 6 mg/mL (to make 60 mL total suspension).

Storage/Stability

Capsules: Store at 25°C (77°F); excursions permitted to 15°C to 30°C (59°F to 86°F).

Oral suspension: Store powder for suspension at 25°C (77°F); excursions permitted to 15°C to 30°C (59°F to 86°F). Once reconstituted, store suspension under refrigeration at 2°C to 8°C (36°F to 46°F) or at room temperature; do not freeze. Use within 10 days of preparation if stored at room temperature or within 17 days of preparation if stored under refrigeration.

◄ **Mechanism of Action** Oseltamivir, a prodrug, is hydrolyzed to the active form, oseltamivir carboxylate (OC). OC inhibits influenza virus neuraminidase, an enzyme known to cleave the budding viral progeny from its cellular envelope attachment point (neuraminic acid) just prior to release.

Pharmacodynamics/Kinetics Note: Concurrent use of extracorporeal membrane oxygenation (ECMO): When used alone, ECMO has been shown not to impact oseltamivir carboxylate C_{max} and AUC in 2 small studies (Lemaitre, 2012; Mulla, 2013).

Absorption: Well absorbed

Distribution: V_d: 23 to 26 L (oseltamivir carboxylate); may be significantly increased in patients receiving ECMO (Lemaitre, 2012; Mulla, 2013)

Protein binding, plasma: Oseltamivir carboxylate: 3%; Oseltamivir: 42%

Metabolism: Hepatic (90%) to oseltamivir carboxylate; neither the parent drug nor active metabolite has any effect on the cytochrome P450 system

Bioavailability: 75% as oseltamivir carboxylate

Half-life elimination: Oseltamivir: 1 to 3 hours; Oseltamivir carboxylate: 6 to 10 hours

Excretion: Urine (>90% as oseltamivir carboxylate); feces

Dosing

Adult & Geriatric

Influenza prophylaxis: Oral: 75 mg once daily; initiate prophylaxis within 48 hours of contact with an infected individual; duration of prophylaxis: 10 days (manufacturer recommendation) or alternatively 7 days (CDC, 2012). During community outbreaks, duration of protection lasts for length of dosing period; safety and efficacy have been demonstrated for use up to 6 weeks in immunocompetent patients and safety has been demonstrated for use up to 12 weeks in patients who are immunocompromised.

Prophylaxis (institutional outbreak; CDC, 2012): Continue for ≥2 weeks and until ~7 days after identification of illness onset in the last patient

Influenza treatment: Oral: 75 mg twice daily initiated within 48 hours of onset of symptoms; usual duration of treatment: 5 days. However, optimal duration is uncertain for severe or complicated influenza. Consider longer duration (eg, >5 days) of therapy in severely ill patients who remain severely ill after 5 days of therapy. **Note:** Data suggest that increased doses (>150 mg daily) in critically ill patients is not necessary since blood concentrations of oseltamivir were comparable or higher compared to ambulatory patients given similar dosing regimens (Ariano, 2010; CDC [Influenza Antiviral Medications], 2014). Initiate as early as possible in any hospitalized patient with suspected/confirmed influenza regardless of the time of presentation from symptom onset (even if >48 hours) (CDC [Influenza Antiviral Medications], 2014); may be administered via naso- or orogastric tube in mechanically-ventilated patients (Taylor, 2008).

Critically ill: Concurrent use of extracorporeal membrane oxygenation (ECMO) alone: No dosage adjustment necessary (Lemaitre, 2012; Mulla, 2013).

Pediatric

Influenza prophylaxis: Oral: Initiate prophylaxis within 48 hours of contact with an infected individual

Manufacturer's labeling:

Children: 1 to 12 years:

≤15 kg: 30 mg once daily

>15 kg to ≤23 kg: 45 mg once daily

>23 kg to ≤40 kg: 60 mg once daily

>40 kg: 75 mg once daily

Adolescents ≥13 years: Refer to adult dosing.

Alternate recommendations:

American Academy of Pediatrics: Infants 0 to 11 months (off-label dosing; AAP, 2013): **Note:** Do not exceed maximum dose of weight-based dosing; see manufacturer's recommendation. Prophylaxis is not recommended for infants <3 months of age unless clinically critical.

0 to 8 months: 3 mg/kg/dose once daily

9 to 11 months: 3.5 mg/kg/dose once daily

Centers for Disease Control: Infants <12 months (off-label dosing; CDC, 2012): 3 mg/kg/dose once daily. **Note:** Do not exceed maximum dose of weight-based dosing; see manufacturer's recommendation. Prophylaxis is not recommended for infants <3 months of age unless clinically critical. The current CDC weight-based dosing recommendation is not intended for premature neonates.

Infectious Disease Society of America/Pediatric Infectious Disease Society: Infants and Children 3 to 23 months (off-label dosing; Bradley, 2011): **Note:** Do not exceed maximum dose of weight-based dosing; see manufacturer's recommendation.

3 to 8 months: 3 mg/kg/dose once daily

9 to 23 months: 3.5 mg/kg/dose once daily

Prophylaxis duration:

Individual/household exposure:

Manufacturer's labeling: 10 days

Alternate recommendations: 7 days (CDC, 2012); 10 days (AAP, 2013)

Community/institutional outbreak:

Manufacturer's labeling: May be used for up to 6 weeks

Alternate recommendations: Continue for ≥2 weeks and until ~7 days after identification of illness onset in the last patient (CDC, 2012) or until influenza activity in community subsides or immunity obtained from immunization (Bradley, 2011). During community outbreaks, duration of protection lasts for length of dosing period; safety and efficacy have been demonstrated for use up to 6 weeks in immunocompetent patients and safety has been demonstrated for use up to 12 weeks in patients who are immunocompromised.

Influenza treatment: Oral: Initiate treatment within 48 hours of onset of symptoms; usual duration of treatment is 5 days. However, optimal duration is uncertain for severe or complicated influenza. Consider longer duration (eg, >5 days) of therapy in severely ill patients who remain severely ill after 5 days of therapy. **Note:** Data suggest that increased doses in critically ill patients is not necessary since blood concentrations of oseltamivir were comparable or higher compared to ambulatory patients given similar dosing regimens (Ariano, 2010; CDC [Influenza Antiviral Medications], 2014). Initiate as early as possible in any hospitalized patient with suspected/confirmed influenza regardless of the time of presentation from symptom onset (even if >48 hours) (CDC [Influenza Antiviral Medications], 2014); may be administered via naso- or orogastric tube in mechanically-ventilated patients (Taylor, 2008).

U.S. manufacturer's labeling: **Note:** The following dosing is also supported by some clinicians (Bradley, 2011):

Infants ≥2 weeks: 3 mg/kg/dose twice daily

Children: 1 to 12 years:

≤15 kg: 30 mg twice daily

>15 kg to ≤23 kg: 45 mg twice daily

>23 kg to ≤40 kg: 60 mg twice daily

>40 kg: 75 mg twice daily

Adolescents ≥13 years: Refer to adult dosing.

Alternate recommendations:

American Academy of Pediatrics: Infants <12 months (off-label dosing; AAP, 2013): **Note:** Age defined as postmenstrual age (first day of mother's last period to birth plus the time elapsed after birth). Weight-based dosing recommendations for premature infants are lower than for term infants. Do not exceed maximum dose of weight-based dosing; see manufacturer's recommendation.

Infants, premature:

<38 weeks: 1 mg/kg/dose twice daily

38 to 40 weeks: 1.5 mg/kg/dose twice daily

>40 weeks: 3 mg/kg/dose twice daily

Infants, term:

0 to 8 months: 3 mg/kg/dose twice daily

9 to 11 months: 3.5 mg/kg/dose twice daily

Centers for Disease Control: Infants <2 weeks (off-label dosing; CDC, 2012): 3 mg/kg/dose twice daily. **Note:** Do not exceed maximum dose of weight-based dosing; see manufacturer's recommendation. The current CDC weight-based dosing recommendation is not intended for premature neonates.

Infectious Disease Society of America/Pediatric Infectious Disease Society: Infants and Children <24 months (off-label dosing; Bradley, 2011): **Note:** Do not exceed maximum dose of weight-based dosing; see manufacturer's recommendation.

Infants, premature: 1 mg/kg/dose twice daily

0 to 8 months: 3 mg/kg/dose twice daily

9 to 23 months: 3.5 mg/kg/dose twice daily

Renal Impairment

Treatment: Adults:

CrCl >60 mL/minute: No dosage adjustment necessary.

CrCl >30 to 60 mL/minute: 30 mg twice daily for 5 days

CrCl >10 to 30 mL/minute: 30 mg once daily for 5 days

End-stage renal disease (ESRD) not undergoing dialysis: Use is not recommended (has not been studied).

Prophylaxis: Adults:

U.S. labeling:

CrCl >60 mL/minute: No dosage adjustment necessary.

CrCl >30 to 60 mL/minute: 30 mg once daily

CrCl >10 to 30 mL/minute: 30 mg every other day

ESRD not undergoing dialysis: Use is not recommended (has not been studied).

Canadian labeling:

CrCl >60 mL/minute: No dosage adjustment necessary.

CrCl >30 to 60 mL/minute: 30 mg once daily for 10 to 14 days

CrCl 10 to 30 mL/minute: 30 mg every other day for 10 to 14 days

Intermittent hemodialysis (IHD) (CrCl ≤10 mL/minute): Adults:

Treatment: 30 mg after every hemodialysis session for 5 days. **Note:** Assumes three hemodialysis sessions in the 5-day period. Treatment may be initiated immediately if influenza symptoms develop during the 48 hours between hemodialysis sessions; however the post-hemodialysis dose should still be administered independently of the time of the initial dose administration.

Alternative recommendations: Treatment (AMMI Canada [Aoki, 2012]):

Low-flux hemodialysis: 30 mg after each dialysis session for 5 days

High-flux hemodialysis: 75 mg after each dialysis session for 5 days

Prophylaxis:

U.S. labeling: 30 mg after every other hemodialysis sessions for the recommended prophylaxis duration. **Note:** An initial dose may be administered prior to the start of dialysis.

Canadian labeling: An initial 30 mg dose may be given prior to dialysis if exposed during the 48 hours between dialysis sessions. To maintain therapeutic concentrations, administer 30 mg after every other dialysis session over a period of 10 to 14 days.

Children >1 year (off-label dose; Schreuder, 2010): Treatment:

≤15 kg: 7.5 mg after each hemodialysis session

>15 kg to ≤23 kg: 10 mg after each hemodialysis session

>23 kg to ≤40 kg: 15 mg after each hemodialysis session

>40 kg: 30 mg after each hemodialysis session

CAPD: Adults:

U.S. labeling: CrCl ≤10 mL/minute:

Treatment: 30 mg for one dose to provide a 5-day duration. Administer immediately after a dialysis exchange.

Prophylaxis: 30 mg once weekly for the recommended prophylaxis duration. Administer immediately after a dialysis exchange.

Canadian labeling:

Treatment: 30 mg once (prior to the start of dialysis) to provide a 5-day duration. Dose should be administered as soon as the determination has been made that treatment is necessary, regardless of when dialysis is scheduled.

Prophylaxis: 30 mg prior to start of dialysis, then 30 mg every 7 days for 10 to 14 days. Initial dose should be administered as soon as the determination has been made that prophylaxis is necessary, regardless of when dialysis is scheduled.

Continuous renal replacement therapy (CRRT) (high-flux):

Treatment (off-label dose; limited data): 30 mg once daily for 5 days or 75 mg every 48 hours to provide a 5-day duration (AMMI Canada [Aoki, 2012]; Ariano, 2010)

Prophylaxis (off-label): No data (AMMI Canada [Aoki, 2012])

Continuous veno-venous hemodialysis (CVVHD):

Adults: **Note:** Limited information available; optimal dosing has not been established: 150 mg twice daily administered via nasogastric or postpyloric feeding tube for suspected or confirmed H1N1 influenza demonstrated supratherapeutic oseltamivir carboxylate concentrations at effluent rates of 3,300 ± 919 mL/hour; the authors determined that the manufacturer recommended dosage of 75 mg once daily for patients with CrCl 10 to 30 mL/minute will likely achieve concentrations necessary to inhibit viral neuraminidase activity at these effluent rates; however, doses greater than 75 mg

once daily may be required when using higher effluent rates (Eyler, 2012).

CVVHD and concurrent use of ECMO: Adults: Lower oseltamivir carboxylate concentrations (~981 ng/mL) were observed as compared to those with the use of CVVHD alone (~2,760 ng/mL) when patients were administered 150 mg twice daily for suspected or confirmed H1N1 influenza (n=4; Eyler, 2012).

Hepatic Impairment

Mild-to-moderate impairment (Child-Pugh score ≤9): No dosage adjustment necessary.

Severe impairment: No dosage adjustment provided in manufacturer's labeling (has not been studied).

Obesity In adult morbidly obese patients (BMI >40 kg/m^2), systemic exposure of oseltamivir carboxylate was not reduced; therefore, no dosage adjustment is necessary (Thorne-Humphrey, 2011).

Dietary Considerations Take without regard to meals; take with food to improve tolerance.

Administration May be administered without regard to meals; take with food to improve tolerance.

Capsules may be opened and mixed with sweetened liquid (eg, chocolate syrup, corn syrup, caramel topping, light brown sugar dissolved in water). Administer oral suspension using the supplied oral syringe (exception: for children <1 year, a smaller volume [ie, <10 mL] oral syringe should be used in place of the supplied oral syringe to ensure accurate dosing); shake well before each use. If oral suspension is not available and/or appropriate strength of capsules are not available to mix with sweetened liquids, an extemporaneous preparation may be prepared (refer to Extemporaneous Preparations section of monograph for further details).

Mechanically ventilated critically ill patients: May administer via naso- or orogastric (NG/OG) tube. Dissolve powder from capsules in 20 mL of sterile water and inject down the NG/OG tube; follow with a 10 mL sterile water flush (Taylor, 2008).

Monitoring Parameters Signs or symptoms of unusual behavior, including attempts at self-injury, confusion, and/or delirium

Critically-ill patients: Repeat rRT-PCR or viral culture may help to determine on-going viral replication

Additional Information In clinical studies of the influenza virus, 1.3% of post-treatment isolates in adults and adolescents and 8.6% of isolates in children had decreased neuraminidase susceptibility *in vitro* to oseltamivir carboxylate.

The absence of symptoms does not rule out viral influenza infection and clinical judgment should guide the decision for therapy. Treatment should not be delayed while waiting for the results of diagnostic tests. Treatment should be considered for high-risk patients with symptoms despite a negative rapid influenza test when the illness cannot be contributed to another cause. Use of oseltamivir is not a substitute for vaccination (when available); susceptibility to influenza infection returns once therapy is discontinued.

Dosage Forms Excipient information presented when available (limited, particularly for generics); consult specific product labeling. [DSC] = Discontinued product

Capsule, Oral, as phosphate:

Tamiflu: 30 mg, 45 mg, 75 mg

Suspension Reconstituted, Oral, as base:

Tamiflu: 6 mg/mL (60 mL) [contains saccharin sodium, sodium benzoate; tutti-frutti flavor]

Suspension Reconstituted, Oral, as phosphate:

Tamiflu: 12 mg/mL (25 mL [DSC]) [contains saccharin sodium, sodium benzoate]

Extemporaneous Preparations

If the commercially prepared oral suspension is not available, the manufacturer provides the following compounding information to prepare a **6 mg/mL** suspension in emergency situations.

1. Place the specified amount of water into a polyethyleneterephthalate (PET) or glass bottle.

2. Carefully separate the capsule body and cap and pour the contents of the required number of 75 mg capsules into the PET or glass bottle.

3. Gently swirl the suspension to ensure adequate wetting of the powder for at least 2 minutes.

4. Slowly add the specified amount of vehicle to the bottle.

5. Close the bottle using a child-resistant cap and shake well for 30 seconds to completely dissolve the active drug.

6. Label "Shake Well Before Use."

Stable for 35 days at 2°C to 8°C (36°F to 46°F) or 5 days at 25°C (77°F). The Canadian labeling suggests that preparations made with water containing preservative (ie, 0.05% sodium benzoate) are stable for 49 days at 2°C to 8°C (36°F to 46°F) and 10 days at 25°C (77°F). Shake gently prior to use. Do **not** dispense with dosing device provided with commercially-available product.

Preparation of Oseltamivir 6 mg/mL Suspension

Body Weight	Total Volume per Patient[1]	# of 75 mg Capsules[2]	Required Volume of Water	Required Volume of Vehicle[2,3]	Treatment Dose (wt based)[4]	Prophylactic Dose (wt based)[4]
≤15 kg	75 mL	6	5 mL	69 mL	5 mL (30 mg) twice daily for 5 days	5 mL (30 mg) once daily for 10 days
16 to 23 kg	100 mL	8	7 mL	91 mL	7.5 mL (45 mg) twice daily for 5 days	7.5 mL (45 mg) once daily for 10 days
24 to 40 kg	125 mL	10	8 mL	115 mL	10 mL (60 mg) twice daily for 5 days	10 mL (60 mg) once daily for 10 days
≥41 kg	150 mL	12	10 mL	137 mL	12.5 mL (75 mg) twice daily for 5 days	12.5 mL (75 mg) once daily for 10 days

[1]Entire course of therapy.

[2]Based on total volume per patient.

[3]Acceptable vehicles are cherry syrup (Humco®), Ora-Sweet® SF, or simple syrup.

[4]Using 6 mg/mL suspension.

Canadian labeling:

Preparation of Oseltamivir 6 mg/mL Suspension

(using water with preservative (ie, 0.05% sodium benzoate)

Body Weight	Total Volume per Patient[1]	# of 75 mg Capsules[2]	Required Volume of Water (with preservative)	Treatment Dose (wt based)[2,3]	Prophylactic Dose (wt based)[2,3]
≤15 kg	75 mL	6	74 mL	5 mL (30 mg) twice daily for 5 days	5 mL (30 mg) once daily for 10 days
16 to 23 kg	100 mL	8	98 mL	7.5 mL (45 mg) twice daily for 5 days	7.5 mL (45 mg) once daily for 10 days
24 to 40 kg	125 mL	10	123 mL	10 mL (60 mg) twice daily for 5 days	10 mL (60 mg) once daily for 10 days
≥41 kg	150 mL	12	147 mL	12.5 mL (75 mg) twice daily for 5 days	12.5 mL (75 mg) once daily for 10 days

[1]Entire course of therapy.

[2]Using 6 mg/mL suspension.

[3]Measured dose should be mixed with an equal amount of sweetened liquid (eg, chocolate syrup, cherry syrup) to mask bitter taste.

◆ OSI-774 see Erlotinib on page 665

Osimertinib (oh si mer ti nib)

Brand Names: US Tagrisso

Index Terms AZD9291; Tagrisso

Pharmacologic Category Antineoplastic Agent, Epidermal Growth Factor Receptor (EGFR) Inhibitor; Antineoplastic Agent, Tyrosine Kinase Inhibitor

Use Non-small cell lung cancer, metastatic: Treatment of metastatic epidermal growth factor receptor (EGFR) T790M mutation-positive non-small cell lung cancer (NSCLC), as detected by an approved test, in patients who have progressed on or after EGFR tyrosine kinase inhibitor (TKI) therapy

Pregnancy Considerations Based on data from animal reproduction studies and the mechanism of action, use during pregnancy is expected to cause fetal harm. Women of reproductive potential should use effective contraception during therapy and for 6 weeks after the last dose. Males and female partners of reproductive potential should also use effective contraception during therapy and for 4 months after the last dose.

Breast-Feeding Considerations It is not known if osimertinib is excreted into breast milk. Because of the potential for serious adverse reactions in the nursing infant, breast-feeding is not recommended by the manufacturer during therapy or for 2 weeks after the last dose.

Prescribing and Access Restrictions Available through specialty pharmacies and distributors. Further information may be obtained from the manufacturer, Astra Zeneca, at 1-844-275-2360 or at https://www.tagrisso.com.

Contraindications There are no contraindications listed in the manufacturer's labeling.

Warnings/Precautions Hazardous agent – use appropriate precautions for handling and disposal (meets NIOSH 2014 criteria).

Interstitial lung disease (ILD) and pneumonitis was observed in clinical studies; some events were fatal. Withhold treatment with worsening respiratory symptoms (dyspnea, cough, fever) which may be indicative of ILD; permanently discontinue if ILD is confirmed.

Cardiomyopathy (cardiac failure, pulmonary edema, decreased ejection fraction, or stress cardiomyopathy) has been observed; some events were fatal. In patients who had baseline and at least one follow up assessment, a left ventricular ejection fraction (LVEF) decline of >10% and a drop to below 50% was noted. Assess LVEF (by echocardiogram or multigated acquisition [MUGA] scan) prior to treatment and then every 3 months while on treatment. Withhold treatment if ejection fraction decreases by 10% from baseline and is <50%. Permanently discontinue for symptomatic heart failure or persistent, asymptomatic left ventricular dysfunction that does not resolve within 4 weeks. Prolongation of the QTc interval may occur; QTc >500 msec and an increase from baseline of >60 msec have been reported. Patients with a baseline QTc of ≥470 were excluded from clinical trials. Monitor ECG and electrolytes periodically in patients with a history of long QTc syndrome, heart failure, electrolyte abnormalities, and/or those taking concurrent medications known to prolong the QTc interval. Permanently discontinue in patients who develop QTc interval prolongation with signs/symptoms of life-threatening arrhythmia.

Lymphopenia, thrombocytopenia, neutropenia, and anemia may occur (usually grades 1 and 2) with osimertinib. Diarrhea (usually grades 1 and 2) was observed in almost half the patients receiving osimertinib. Skin reactions, including rash, dry skin, and itching may occur. Nail toxicity may also occur. Potentially significant drug-drug interactions may exist, requiring dose or frequency adjustment, additional monitoring, and/or selection of alternative therapy. Confirm the presence of a T790M epidermal growth factor receptor (EGFR) mutation prior to treatment initiation. Information on diagnostic tests approved for detection of T790M EGFR mutations may be found at www.fda.gov/companiondiagnostics.

Adverse Reactions

>10%:

Central nervous system: Fatigue (14%), headache (10%)

Dermatologic: Skin rash (41%, including erythematous rash, macular rash, maculopapular rash, papular rash, pustular rash, erythema, folliculitis, acne vulgaris, dermatitis, dermatitis acneiform), xeroderma (31%), nail disease (25%), pruritus (14%)

Endocrine & metabolic: Hyponatremia (26%), hypermagnesemia (20%)

Gastrointestinal: Diarrhea (42%), nausea (17%), decreased appetite (16%), constipation (15%), stomatitis (12%)

Hematologic & oncologic: Lymphopenia (63%, grades 3/4: 3%), thrombocytopenia (54%, grades 3/4: 1%), anemia (44%, grades 3/4: <1%), neutropenia (33%, grades 3/4: 3%)

Neuromuscular & skeletal: Back pain (13%)

Ophthalmic: Eye disorder (19%, including dry eyes, blurred vision, keratitis, cataract, eye irritation, blepharitis, eye pain, increased lacrimation, vitreous floaters, <1% other ocular toxicity)

Respiratory: Cough (14%)

1% to 10%:

Cardiovascular: Venous thromboembolism (7%, including deep vein thrombosis, internal jugular thrombosis), cerebrovascular accident (3%), prolonged Q-T interval on EKG (≤3%; prolonged from baseline), pulmonary embolism (≤2%), reduced ejection fraction (<2%), cardiomyopathy (≤1%)

Respiratory: Pneumonia (≤4%; grade 3/4: 2%), interstitial pneumonitis (3%)

Drug Interactions

Metabolism/Transport Effects Substrate of BCRP, CYP3A4 (minor), P-glycoprotein; **Note:** Assignment of Major/Minor substrate status based on clinically relevant drug interaction potential; **Inhibits** BCRP

Avoid Concomitant Use
Avoid concomitant use of Osimertinib with any of the following: BCG (Intravesical); CYP3A4 Inducers (Strong); CYP3A4 Inhibitors (Strong); Deferiprone; Dipyrone; Highest Risk QTc-Prolonging Agents; Ivabradine; Mifepristone; Natalizumab; Pimecrolimus; St Johns Wort; Tacrolimus (Topical); Tofacitinib; Vaccines (Live)

Increased Effect/Toxicity
Osimertinib may increase the levels/effects of: CYP3A4 Substrates; Deferiprone; Fingolimod; Highest Risk QTc-Prolonging Agents; Leflunomide; Moderate Risk QTc-Prolonging Agents; Natalizumab; Tofacitinib; Vaccines (Live)

The levels/effects of Osimertinib may be increased by: CYP3A4 Inhibitors (Strong); Denosumab; Dipyrone; Ivabradine; Mifepristone; Pimecrolimus; QTc-Prolonging Agents (Indeterminate Risk and Risk Modifying); Roflumilast; Tacrolimus (Topical); Trastuzumab

Decreased Effect
Osimertinib may decrease the levels/effects of: BCG (Intravesical); Coccidioides immitis Skin Test; CYP1A2 Substrates; CYP3A4 Substrates; Sipuleucel-T; Vaccines (Inactivated); Vaccines (Live)

The levels/effects of Osimertinib may be decreased by: CYP3A4 Inducers (Strong); Echinacea; St Johns Wort

Preparation for Administration Hazardous agent; use appropriate precautions for handling and disposal (meets NIOSH 2014 criteria). For patients who have difficulty swallowing tablets, disperse tablet in ~50 mL of noncarbonated water (only), stir until tablet is completely dispersed and use immediately; rinse container with 120 to 240 mL water and drink or administer immediately. Do not crush, heat, or ultrisonicate during preparation. When it is necessary to manipulate the tablets (eg, to prepare an oral liquid), it is recommended to double glove, wear a protective gown, and prepare in a controlled device (NIOSH 2014).

Storage/Stability Store at 25°C (77°F); excursions are permitted between 15°C and 30°C (59°F and 86°F).

Mechanism of Action Osimertinib is an irreversible epidermal growth factor receptor (EGFR) tyrosine kinase inhibitor which binds to select mutant forms of EGFR, including T790M, L858R, and exon 19 deletion at lower concentrations than wild-type. Osimertinib is selective for sensitizing mutations and the T790M resistance mutation, which is the most common mechanism of resistance to EGFR tyrosine kinase inhibitors (Janne 2015).

Pharmacodynamics/Kinetics
Distribution: V_{ss}/F: 986 L
Protein binding: Binding is likely high
Metabolism: Hepatic; predominantly oxidation (via CYP3A4) and dealkylation to 2 active metabolites (AZ7550 and AZ5104)
Bioavailability: AUC is increased by 19% with a high-fat, high-calorie meal
Half-life, elimination: Mean (estimated): 48 hours
Time to peak: Median: 6 hours (range: 3 to 24 hours)
Excretion: Feces (68%; ~2% as unchanged drug); Urine (14%; ~2% as unchanged drug)

Dosing
Adult & Geriatric Note: T790M EGFR mutation status of tumor specimen should be confirmed prior to treatment initiation.

Non-small cell lung cancer, metastatic (T790M EGFR mutation-positive): Oral: 80 mg once daily until disease progression or unacceptable toxicity
Missed doses: If a dose is missed, do not make up the missed dose, take the next dose as scheduled.

Renal Impairment
CrCl 30 to 89 mL/minute: No dosage adjustment necessary.
CrCl <30 mL/minute and end stage renal disease: There are no dosage adjustments provided in the manufacturer's labeling (has not been studied).

Hepatic Impairment
Mild impairment (total bilirubin <ULN and AST 1 to 1.5 times ULN **or** total bilirubin 1 to 1.5 times ULN and any AST): No dosage adjustment necessary.
Moderate (total bilirubin 1.5 to 3 times ULN and any AST) or severe impairment (total bilirubin 3 to 10 times ULN and any AST): There are no dosage adjustments provided in the manufacturer's labeling (has not been studied).

Adjustment for Toxicity
Cardiotoxicity:
QTc interval >500 msec on at least 2 separate ECGs: Withhold treatment until QTc interval is <481 msec or recovers to baseline (if baseline QTc ≥481 msec) and then resume at a dose of 40 mg once daily.
QTc interval prolongation with signs/symptoms of life-threatening arrhythmia: Permanently discontinue.

Asymptomatic absolute decrease in left ventricular ejections fraction (LVEF) of 10% from baseline and below 50%: Withhold treatment for up to 4 weeks. If improved to baseline, resume treatment; if not improved to baseline, permanently discontinue.
Symptomatic heart failure: Permanently discontinue.
Pulmonary toxicity: Interstitial lung disease/pneumonitis: Permanently discontinue.
Other toxicities: Grade 3 or higher adverse reaction: Withhold treatment for up to 3 weeks. If improves to grade 2 or lower within 3 weeks, resume at either 80 mg once daily or 40 mg once daily. If not improved within 3 weeks, permanently discontinue.

Administration
Oral: May be administered with or without food.
For patients who have difficulty swallowing tablets, disperse tablet in ~50 mL of noncarbonated water (only), stir until tablet is completely dispersed and immediately swallow or administer through NG tube. Rinse container with 120 to 240 mL water and immediately drink or administer through NG tube. Do not crush, heat, or ultrasonicate during preparation.
Hazardous agent; use appropriate precautions for handling and disposal (meets NIOSH 2014 criteria). NIOSH recommends single gloving for administration of intact tablets (NIOSH 2014). Avoid exposure to crushed tablets. When it is necessary to manipulate the tablets (eg, to prepare an oral liquid), it is recommended to double glove, wear a protective gown, and prepare in a controlled device (NIOSH 2014).

Monitoring Parameters T790M epidermal growth factor receptor (EGFR) mutation status (prior to treatment). Monitor ECG and electrolytes periodically (in patients with a history of long QTc syndrome, heart failure, electrolyte abnormalities, and/or those taking concurrent medications known to prolong the QTc interval). Assess LVEF (by echocardiogram or multigated acquisition [MUGA] scan) prior to treatment and then every 3 months while on treatment. Monitor for signs/symptoms of interstitial lung disease or pneumonitis, dermatologic, and gastrointestinal toxicity.

Dosage Forms Excipient information presented when available (limited, particularly for generics); consult specific product labeling.
Tablet, Oral:
Tagrisso: 40 mg, 80 mg

◆ Osmitrol *see* Mannitol *on page 1124*
◆ Osmitrol® (Can) *see* Mannitol *on page 1124*
◆ OsmoPrep *see* Sodium Phosphates *on page 1677*

Ospemifene (os PEM i feen)

Brand Names: US Osphena
Index Terms FC1271a
Pharmacologic Category Selective Estrogen Receptor Modulator (SERM)
Use Treatment of moderate-to-severe dyspareunia due to vulvar and vaginal atrophy (VVA) of menopause
Pregnancy Considerations Adverse events were observed in animal reproduction studies. Use is contraindicated in women who are or may become pregnant. Ospemifene is currently approved only for the treatment of moderate-to-severe dyspareunia due to vulvar and vaginal atrophy (VVA) of menopause.
Breast-Feeding Considerations It is not known if ospemifene is excreted into breast milk.
Contraindications Hypersensitivity (eg, angioedema, urticaria, rash, pruritus) to ospemifene or any component of the formulation; undiagnosed abnormal vaginal bleeding; DVT or PE (current or history of); active or history of arterial thromboembolic disease (eg, stroke, MI); estrogen-dependent tumor (known or suspected); women who are or may become pregnant
Warnings/Precautions Hazardous agent: Use appropriate precautions for handling and disposal (meets NIOSH 2014 criteria). **[U.S. Boxed Warning]: The use of unopposed estrogen in women with an intact uterus is associated with an increased risk of endometrial cancer. The addition of a progestin to estrogen therapy may decrease the risk of endometrial hyperplasia, a precursor to endometrial cancer. Adequate diagnostic measures, including endometrial sampling if indicated, should be performed to rule out malignancy in postmenopausal women with undiagnosed abnormal vaginal bleeding. Ospemifene is an estrogen agonist/antagonist with agonistic effects on the endometrium.** For women with an intact uterus using an estrogen without a progestin, the risk of endometrial cancer is dependent upon dose and duration of therapy. Endometrial cancer was not reported in clinical studies of ospemifene (duration

≤52 weeks) and the use of progestins was not evaluated. Ospemifene was not studied in women with breast cancer. Use is not currently recommended in women with carcinoma of the breast (known, suspected or history of) and use is contraindicated with an estrogen-dependent tumor.

[U.S. Boxed Warning]: Using data from the Women's Health Initiative (WHI) studies, an increased risk of deep vein thrombosis (DVT) and stroke has been reported with oral conjugated estrogens. The following were reported with ospemifene in clinical trials lasting ≤15 months duration: thromboembolic stroke 0.72/1000 women (placebo 1.04/1000 women); hemorrhagic stroke 1.45/1000 women (placebo 0/1000 women); DVT 1.45/1000 women (placebo 1.04/1000 women). Risk factors for cardiovascular disorders, arterial vascular disorders and /or venous thromboembolism (VTE) should be managed appropriately. Risk factors include diabetes mellitus, hypercholesterolemia, hypertension, SLE, obesity, tobacco use, and/or history of VTE. Discontinue immediately if a VTE, thromboembolic or hemorrhagic stroke occur or are suspected.

[U.S. Boxed Warning]: Ospemifene should be used for the shortest duration possible consistent with treatment goals and risks for the individual woman.

Ospemifene has not been studied in patients with severe hepatic impairment; use is not recommended. Potentially significant interactions may exist, requiring dose or frequency adjustment, additional monitoring, and/or selection of alternative therapy. Consult drug interactions database for more detailed information. Whenever possible, discontinue at least 4-6 weeks prior to elective surgery associated with an increased risk of thromboembolism or during periods of prolonged immobilization.

Adverse Reactions

1% to 10%:
Dermatologic: Hyperhidrosis (2%)
Endocrine & metabolic: Hot flash (8%)
Genitourinary: Proliferative endometrium (9%), endometrial hyperplasia (without atypia, 6%), vaginal discharge (4%), genital discharge (1%)
Neuromuscular & skeletal: Muscle spasm (3%)
<1% (Limited to important or life-threatening): Deep vein thrombosis, endometrial polyps, hemorrhagic stroke, hypersensitivity, thrombotic stroke

Drug Interactions

Metabolism/Transport Effects Substrate of CYP2C19 (minor), CYP2C9 (major), CYP3A4 (major); **Note:** Assignment of Major/Minor substrate status based on clinically relevant drug interaction potential; **Inhibits** CYP2B6 (weak), CYP2C19 (weak), CYP2C8 (weak), CYP2C9 (weak), CYP2D6 (weak)

Avoid Concomitant Use

Avoid concomitant use of Ospemifene with any of the following: Amodiaquine; Estrogen Derivatives; Fluconazole; Selective Estrogen Receptor Modulators

Increased Effect/Toxicity

Ospemifene may increase the levels/effects of: Amodiaquine; ARIPiprazole

The levels/effects of Ospemifene may be increased by: CYP2C9 Inhibitors (Strong); CYP3A4 Inhibitors (Strong); Estrogen Derivatives; Fluconazole; Osimertinib; Selective Estrogen Receptor Modulators

Decreased Effect

The levels/effects of Ospemifene may be decreased by: Bosentan; CYP2C9 Inducers (Strong); CYP3A4 Inducers (Moderate); CYP3A4 Inducers (Strong); Dabrafenib; Deferasirox; Enzalutamide; Estrogen Derivatives; Mitotane; Osimertinib; Selective Estrogen Receptor Modulators; Siltuximab; St Johns Wort; Tocilizumab

Storage/Stability Store at controlled room temperature of 20°C to 25°C (68°F to 77°F); excursions permitted to 15°C to 30°C (59°F to 86°F).

Mechanism of Action Ospemifene is a selective estrogen receptor modulator (SERM); it activates estrogen pathways in some tissues and blocks estrogen pathways in others, and specifically has agonistic effects on the endometrium. In women with VVA, ospemifene was shown to improve vaginal changes associated with the decrease in natural estrogen production associated with menopause (improves vaginal maturation index, decreases vaginal pH) and significantly decreased the most bothersome moderate-to-severe subjective findings reported by women (vaginal dryness and dyspareunia) after 12 weeks of therapy (Bachmann, 2010).

Pharmacodynamics/Kinetics

Onset of action: A significant decrease in vaginal dryness and dyspareunia were observed after 12 weeks of therapy (Bachmann, 2010).
Distribution: V_d: 448 L
Protein binding: >99% bound to serum proteins

Metabolism: Hepatic via CYP3A4, 2C9, and 2C19; forms a metabolite (4-hydroxyospemifene)
Bioavailability: Increased approximately two- to threefold by food
Half-life elimination: ~26 hours
Time to peak: ~2 hours (range: 1-8 hours)
Excretion: Feces (75%); urine (7%; <0.2% as unchanged drug)

Dosing

Adult & Geriatric Dyspareunia, moderate-to-severe: Postmenopausal females: Oral: 60 mg once daily

Renal Impairment No dosage adjustment necessary.

Hepatic Impairment

Mild or moderate impairment (Child-Pugh class A or B): No dosage adjustment necessary.
Severe impairment (Child-Pugh class C): No dosage adjustment provided in manufacturer's labeling (has not been studied). Use is not recommended.

Administration Administer with food. Hazardous agent: Use appropriate precautions for handling and disposal (meets NIOSH 2014 criteria).

Monitoring Parameters Monitor for signs of endometrial cancer in female patients with uterus. Adequate diagnostic measures, including endometrial sampling, if indicated, should be performed to rule out malignancy in all cases of undiagnosed abnormal vaginal bleeding. Assess need for therapy at regular intervals. Monitor for signs/symptoms of stroke and VTE.

Dosage Forms Excipient information presented when available (limited, particularly for generics); consult specific product labeling.
Tablet, Oral:
Osphena: 60 mg

Oxacillin (oks a SIL in)

Brand Names: US Bactocill in Dextrose
Index Terms Methylphenyl Isoxazolyl Penicillin; Oxacillin Sodium
Pharmacologic Category Antibiotic, Penicillin
Use

Staphylococcal infections: Treatment of infections caused by penicillinase-producing staphylococci that have demonstrated susceptibility to the drug; empiric therapy in suspected cases of resistant staphylococcal infections.
Limitations of use: Oxacillin should not be used in infections caused by organisms susceptible to penicillin G.

Dosing

Adult Note: May contain a significant amount of sodium; consult product specific labeling for amount.
Endocarditis: IV: 2 g every 4 hours with gentamicin
Mild-to-moderate infections: IM, IV: 250 to 500 mg every 4 to 6 hours
Prosthetic joint infection: IV: 2 g every 4 hours with rifampin
Severe infections: IM, IV: 1 g every 4 to 6 hours
***Staphylococcus aureus,* methicillin-susceptible infections, including brain abscess, bursitis, erysipelas, mastitis, mastoiditis, osteomyelitis, perinephric abscess, pneumonia, pyomyositis, scalded skin syndrome, toxic shock syndrome:** IV: 2 g every 4 hours

Skin and soft tissue infections (IDSA [Stevens 2014]): IV:

Due to methicillin-susceptible Staphylococcus aureus (MSSA): 1 to 2 g every 4 hours for 7 to 14 days

Necrotizing infection due to MSSA (off-label use): 1 to 2 g every 4 hours; continue until further debridement is not necessary, patient has clinically improved, and patient is afebrile for 48 to 72 hours

Surgical site infections (trunk or extremity [away from axilla or perineum]) (off-label use): IV: 2 g every 6 hours (IDSA [Stevens 2014])

Geriatric Refer to adult dosing. **Note:** May contain a significant amount of sodium; consult product specific labeling for amount. The geriatric population may respond with a blunted natriuresis to salt loading. This may be clinically important in diseases such as congestive heart failure.

Pediatric Note: May contain a significant amount of sodium; consult product specific labeling for amount.

Community-acquired pneumonia (CAP) (IDSA/PIDS 2011), moderate-to-severe infection, *S. aureus* **(methicillin-susceptible) (preferred):** Infants >3 months and Children: IV: 150 to 200 mg/kg/day divided every 6-8 hours

Mild-to-moderate infections: IM, IV: 50 mg/kg/day in divided doses every 6 hours (maximum: 4 g daily)

Severe infections: Infants and Children: IM, IV: 100 mg/kg/day in divided doses every 4-6 hours (maximum: 12 g daily)

Skin and soft tissue infections (IDSA [Stevens 2014]): IV:

Due to methicillin-susceptible Staphylococcus aureus (MSSA): IV: 100 to 150 mg/kg/day in divided doses every 6 hours for 7 to 14 days

Necrotizing infection due to MSSA (off-label use): 200 mg/kg/day in divided doses every 6 hours; continue until further debridement is not necessary, patient has clinically improved, and patient is afebrile for 48 to 72 hours.

Renal Impairment There are no dosage adjustments provided in the manufacturer's labeling; however, manufacturer suggests considering a reduction in total dosage if renal impairment is known or suspected.

Hepatic Impairment There are no dosage adjustments provided in the manufacturer's labeling.

Additional Information Complete prescribing information should be consulted for additional detail.

Dosage Forms Excipient information presented when available (limited, particularly for generics); consult specific product labeling.

Solution, Intravenous:

Bactocill in Dextrose: 1 g/50 mL (50 mL); 2 g/50 mL (50 mL)

Solution Reconstituted, Injection:

Generic: 1 g (1 ea); 2 g (1 ea); 10 g (1 ea)

Solution Reconstituted, Injection [preservative free]:

Generic: 1 g (1 ea); 2 g (1 ea); 10 g (1 ea)

◆ Oxacillin Sodium *see* Oxacillin *on page 1348*

◆ Oxalatoplatin *see* Oxaliplatin *on page 1349*

◆ Oxalatoplatinum *see* Oxaliplatin *on page 1349*

Oxaliplatin (ox AL i pla tin)

Brand Names: US Eloxatin
Brand Names: Canada Eloxatin
Index Terms Diaminocyclohexane Oxalatoplatinum; L-OHP; Oxalatoplatin; Oxalatoplatinum
Pharmacologic Category Antineoplastic Agent, Alkylating Agent; Antineoplastic Agent, Platinum Analog
Use

Colon cancer, stage III (adjuvant therapy): Adjuvant treatment of stage III colon cancer (in combination with infusional fluorouracil and leucovorin) after complete resection of primary tumor.

Colorectal cancer, advanced: Treatment of advanced colorectal cancer (in combination with infusional fluorouracil and leucovorin).

Pregnancy Considerations Adverse events were observed in animal reproduction studies at one-tenth the equivalent human dose. Women of childbearing potential should be advised to avoid pregnancy and use effective contraception during treatment.

Canadian labeling: Use in pregnant women is contraindicated in the Canadian labeling. Males should be advised not to father children during and for up to 6 months following therapy. May cause permanent infertility in males. Prior to initiating therapy, advise males desiring to father children, to seek counseling on sperm storage.

Breast-Feeding Considerations It is not known if oxaliplatin is excreted in breast milk. Due to the potential for serious adverse reactions in the breast-feeding infant, the decision to discontinue breast-feeding or to discontinue oxaliplatin should take into account the benefits of treatment to the mother.

Contraindications

Hypersensitivity to oxaliplatin, other platinum-containing compounds, or any component of the formulation

Canadian labeling: Additional contraindications (not in US labeling): Pregnancy, breast-feeding; severe renal impairment (CrCl <30 mL/minute)

Warnings/Precautions Hazardous agent - use appropriate precautions for handling and disposal (NIOSH 2014 [group 1]). **[US Boxed Warning]: Anaphylactic/anaphylactoid reactions have been reported with oxaliplatin (may occur within minutes of administration); symptoms may be managed with epinephrine, corticosteroids, antihistamines,** and discontinuation; oxygen and bronchodilators have also been used (Kim 2009). Grade 3 or 4 hypersensitivity has been observed. Allergic reactions are similar to reactions reported with other platinum analogs, and may occur with any cycle. Reactions typically occur after multiple cycles; in retrospective reviews, reaction occurred at a median of 7 to 9 cycles, with an onset of 5 to 70 minutes (Kim 2009; Polyzos 2009). Symptoms may include bronchospasm (rare), erythema, hypotension (rare), pruritus, rash, and/or urticaria; previously-untreated patients have also experienced flushing, diaphoresis, diarrhea, shortness of breath, chest pain, hypotension, syncope, and disorientation. According to the manufacturer, rechallenge is contraindicated (deaths due to anaphylaxis have been associated with platinum derivatives). In patients rechallenged after mild hypersensitivity, reaction recurred at a higher level of severity; for patients with severe hypersensitivity, rechallenge (with 2 to 3 days of antihistamine and corticosteroid premedication, and prolongation of infusion time) allowed for 2 to 4 additional oxaliplatin cycles; however, rechallenge was not feasible in nearly two-thirds of patients due to the severity of the initial reaction (Polyzos 2009).

Two different types of peripheral sensory neuropathy may occur: First, an acute (within hours to 1 to 2 days), reversible (resolves within 14 days), with primarily peripheral symptoms that are often exacerbated by cold (may include pharyngolaryngeal dysesthesia); commonly recur with subsequent doses; avoid mucositis prophylaxis with ice chips, exposure to cold temperatures, or consumption of cold food/beverages during or within hours after oxaliplatin infusion. Cold-triggered neuropathy may last up to 7 days after oxaliplatin administration (Grothey 2011). Secondly, a more persistent (>14 days) presentation that often interferes with daily activities (eg, writing, buttoning, swallowing), these symptoms may improve in some patients upon discontinuing treatment. In a retrospective evaluation of patients treated with oxaliplatin for colorectal cancer, the incidence of peripheral sensory neuropathy was similar between diabetic and nondiabetic patients (Ramanathan 2010). Several retrospective studies (as well as a small, underpowered randomized trial) have suggested calcium and magnesium infusions before and after oxaliplatin administration may reduce incidence of cumulative sensory neuropathy; however, a recent abstract of an ongoing randomized, placebo-controlled, double-blind study in patients with colorectal cancer suggests there is no benefit of calcium and magnesium in preventing sensory neuropathy or in decreasing oxaliplatin discontinuation rates (Loprinzi 2013).

Grade 3 and 4 neutropenia occurs commonly with oxaliplatin in combination with fluorouracil and leucovorin; sepsis, neutropenic sepsis, and septic shock have been reported (some fatal). Delay treatment until neutrophils are ≥1500/mm³; withhold treatment for sepsis or septic shock. Reduce the dose after recovery from grade 4 neutropenia or neutropenic fever. QT prolongation and ventricular arrhythmias, including fatal torsades de pointes have been reported in postmarketing surveillance. ECG monitoring is recommend in patients with heart failure, bradyarrhythmias, concomitant medications known to cause QT prolongation (including class Ia and III antiarrhythmics), and electrolyte abnormalities. Avoid use in patients with congenital long QT syndrome. Monitor potassium and magnesium prior to and periodically during treatment; correct hypokalemia and hypomagnesemia prior to treatment initiation.

Oxaliplatin is associated with a moderate emetic potential; antiemetics are recommended to prevent nausea and vomiting (Basch 2011; Dupuis 2011; Roila 2010). Cases of reversible posterior leukoencephalopathy syndrome (RPLS) have been reported. Signs/symptoms include headache, mental status changes, seizure, blurred vision,

blindness and/or other vision changes; may be associated with hypertension; diagnosis is confirmed with brain imaging. May cause pulmonary fibrosis; withhold treatment for unexplained pulmonary symptoms (eg, crackles, dyspnea, nonproductive cough, pulmonary infiltrates) until interstitial lung disease or pulmonary fibrosis are excluded. Hepatotoxicity (including rare cases of hepatitis and hepatic failure) has been reported. Liver biopsy has revealed peliosis, nodular regenerative hyperplasia, sinusoidal alterations, perisinusoidal fibrosis, and veno-occlusive lesions; the presence of hepatic vascular disorders (including veno-occlusive disease) should be considered, especially in individuals developing portal hypertension or who present with increased liver function tests. Rhabdomyolysis (including fatal cases) has been reported with oxaliplatin; discontinue if signs/symptoms of rhabdomyolysis occur. Use caution with renal dysfunction; increased toxicity may occur; reduce initial dose in severe impairment. The Canadian labeling contraindicates use in severe renal impairment (CrCl <30 mL/minute). Potentially significant drug-drug interactions may exist, requiring dose or frequency adjustment, additional monitoring, and/or selection of alternative therapy. Elderly patients are more sensitive to some adverse events including diarrhea, dehydration, hypokalemia, leukopenia, fatigue and syncope. Oxaliplatin is an irritant with vesicant-like properties; ensure proper needle or catheter placement prior to and during infusion; avoid extravasation.

Adverse Reactions Percentages reported with monotherapy.

>10%:

Central nervous system: Peripheral neuropathy (may be dose limiting; 76% to 92%; acute 65%; grades 3/4: 5%; persistent 43%; grades 3/4: 3%), fatigue (61%), pain (14%), headache (13%), insomnia (11%)

Gastrointestinal: Nausea (64%), diarrhea (46%), vomiting (37%), abdominal pain (31%), constipation (31%), anorexia (20%), stomatitis (14%)

Hematologic & oncologic: Anemia (64%; grades 3/4: 1%), thrombocytopenia (30%; grades 3/4: 3%), leukopenia (13%)

Hepatic: Increased serum AST (54%; grades 3/4: 4%), increased serum ALT (36%; grades 3/4: 1%), increased serum bilirubin (13%; grades 3/4: 5%)

Neuromuscular & skeletal: Back pain (11%)

Respiratory: Dyspnea (13%), cough (11%)

Miscellaneous: Fever (25%)

1% to 10%:

Cardiovascular: Edema (10%), chest pain (5%), peripheral edema (5%), flushing (3%), thromboembolism (2%)

Central nervous system: Rigors (9%), dizziness (7%)

Dermatologic: Skin rash (5%), alopecia (3%), palmarplantar erythrodysesthesia (1%)

Endocrine & metabolic: Dehydration (5%), hypokalemia (3%)

Gastrointestinal: Dyspepsia (7%), dysgeusia (5%), flatulence (3%), hiccups (2%), mucositis (2%), gastroesophageal reflux disease (1%), dysphagia (acute 1% to 2%)

Genitourinary: Dysuria (1%)

Hematologic & oncologic: Neutropenia (7%)

Hypersensitivity: Hypersensitivity reaction (3%; includes urticaria, pruritus, facial flushing, shortness of breath, bronchospasm, diaphoresis, hypotension, syncope: grades 3/4: 2% to 3%)

Local: Injection site reaction (9%; redness/swelling/pain)

Neuromuscular & skeletal: Arthralgia (7%)

Ocular: Abnormal lacrimation (1%)

Renal: Increased serum creatinine (5% to 10%)

Respiratory: Upper respiratory tract infection (7%), rhinitis (6%), epistaxis (2%), pharyngitis (2%), pharyngolaryngeal dysesthesia (grades 3/4: 1% to 2%)

<1% (Limited to important or life-threatening; reported with mono- and combination therapy): Abnormal gait, acute renal failure, anaphylaxis, anaphylactic shock, anaphylactoid reaction, angioedema, aphonia, ataxia, blepharoptosis, cerebral hemorrhage, colitis, cranial nerve palsy, decreased deep tendon reflex, deafness, decreased visual acuity, diplopia, dysarthria, eosinophilic pneumonitis, fasciculations, febrile neutropenia, hematuria, hemolysis, hemolytic anemia (immuno-allergic), hemolytic-uremic syndrome, hemorrhage, hepatic failure, hepatic sinusoidal obstruction syndrome (SOS; veno-occlusive disease), hepatitis, hepatotoxicity, hypertension, hypomagnesemia, hypoxia, idiopathic noncirrhotic portal hypertension (nodular regenerative hyperplasia), increased INR, increased serum alkaline phosphatase, infusion related reaction (extravasation [including necrosis]), interstitial nephritis (acute), interstitial pulmonary disease, intestinal obstruction, laryngospasm, Lhermittes' sign, metabolic acidosis, muscle spasm, myoclonus, neutropenic enterocolitis, neutropenic

infection (sepsis), optic neuritis, pancreatitis, prolonged prothrombin time, purpura, rectal hemorrhage, renal tubular necrosis, reversible posterior leukoencephalopathy syndrome (RPLS), rhabdomyolysis, seizure, sepsis, temporary vision loss, thrombocytopenia (immuno-allergic), trigeminal neuralgia, visual field loss, voice disorder

Drug Interactions

Metabolism/Transport Effects Substrate of OCT2

Avoid Concomitant Use

Avoid concomitant use of Oxaliplatin with any of the following: BCG (Intravesical); Deferiprone; Dipyrone; Natalizumab; Pimecrolimus; Tacrolimus (Topical); Tofacitinib; Vaccines (Live)

Increased Effect/Toxicity

Oxaliplatin may increase the levels/effects of: CloZAPine; Deferiprone; Fingolimod; Highest Risk QTc-Prolonging Agents; Leflunomide; Moderate Risk QTc-Prolonging Agents; Natalizumab; Taxane Derivatives; Tofacitinib; Topotecan; Vaccines (Live)

The levels/effects of Oxaliplatin may be increased by: BuPROPion; Denosumab; Dipyrone; Mifepristone; Pimecrolimus; Roflumilast; Tacrolimus (Topical); Trastuzumab

Decreased Effect

Oxaliplatin may decrease the levels/effects of: BCG (Intravesical); Coccidioides immitis Skin Test; Fosphenytoin-Phenytoin; Sipuleucel-T; Vaccines (Inactivated); Vaccines (Live)

The levels/effects of Oxaliplatin may be decreased by: Echinacea

Preparation for Administration Hazardous agent; use appropriate precautions for handling and disposal (NIOSH 2014 [group 1]).

Do not prepare using a chloride-containing solution such as NaCl due to rapid conversion to monochloroplatinum, dichloroplatinum, and diaquoplatinum; all highly reactive in sodium chloride (Takimoto 2007). Do not use needles or administration sets containing aluminum during preparation.

Aqueous solution: Dilution with D_5W (250 or 500 mL) is required prior to administration.

Lyophilized powder: Use only SWFI or D_5W to reconstitute powder. To obtain final concentration of 5 mg/mL add 10 mL of diluent to 50 mg vial or 20 mL diluent to 100 mg vial. Gently swirl vial to dissolve powder. Dilution with D_5W (250 or 500 mL) is required prior to administration. Discard unused portion of vial.

Storage/Stability Store intact vials at room temperature of 25°C (77°F); excursions permitted to 15°C to 30°C (59°F to 86°F); do not freeze. Protect concentrated solution from light (store in original outer carton). According to the manufacturer, solutions diluted for infusion are stable up to 6 hours at room temperature of 20°C to 25°C (68°F to 77°F) or up to 24 hours under refrigeration at 2°C to 8°C (36°F to 46°F). Oxaliplatin solution diluted with D_5W to a final concentration of 0.7 mg/mL (polyolefin container) has been shown to retain >90% of the original concentration for up to 30 days when stored at room temperature or refrigerated; artificial light did not affect the concentration (Andre 2007). As this study did not examine sterility, refrigeration would be preferred to limit microbial growth. Solutions diluted for infusion do not require protection from light.

Mechanism of Action Oxaliplatin, a platinum derivative, is an alkylating agent. Following intracellular hydrolysis, the platinum compound binds to DNA forming cross-links which inhibit DNA replication and transcription, resulting in cell death. Cytotoxicity is cell-cycle nonspecific.

Pharmacodynamics/Kinetics

Distribution: V_d: 440 L

Protein binding: >90% primarily albumin and gamma globulin (irreversible binding to platinum)

Metabolism: Nonenzymatic (rapid and extensive), forms active and inactive derivatives

Half-life elimination: Terminal: 391 hours

Excretion: Urine (~54%); feces (~2%)

Dosing

Adult Note: Oxaliplatin is associated with a moderate emetic potential; antiemetics are recommended to prevent nausea and vomiting (Basch 2011; Dupuis 2011; Roila 2010).

Colorectal cancer (advanced): IV: 85 mg/m² every 2 weeks until disease progression or unacceptable toxicity (in combination with infusional fluorouracil/leucovorin)

Colon cancer, stage III (adjuvant therapy): IV: 85 mg/m² every 2 weeks for 6 months (12 cycles; in combination with infusional fluorouracil/leucovorin)

Colon/colorectal cancer (off-label doses or combinations): IV: 85 mg/m²/dose on days 1, 15, and 29 of an 8-week treatment cycle in combination with fluorouracil/leucovorin (Kuebler 2007) **or** 85 mg/m² every 2 weeks in combination with fluorouracil/leucovorin/irinotecan (Falcone 2007) **or** 130 mg/m² every 3 weeks in combination with capecitabine (Cassidy 2008; Haller 2011)

Biliary adenocarcinoma, advanced (off-label use): IV: GEMOX regimen: 100 mg/m² on day 2 every 2 weeks (in combination with gemcitabine) until disease progression or unacceptable toxicity (Andre 2004) **or** CAPOX regimen: 130 mg/m² on day 1 every 3 weeks (in combination with capecitabine) until disease progression or unacceptable toxicity (Nehls 2008)

Chronic lymphocytic leukemia, fludarabine-refractory (off-label use): IV: OFAR regimen: 25 mg/m²/day for 4 days every 4 weeks (in combination with fludarabine, cytarabine, and rituximab) for up to 6 cycles (Tsimberidou 2008)

Esophageal/gastric cancers (off-label use): IV: 130 mg/m² on day 1 every 3 weeks (in combination with epirubicin and either capecitabine or fluorouracil) for up to 8 cycles (Cunningham 2008) **or** 85 mg/m² on day 1 every 2 weeks (in combination with docetaxel, leucovorin, and fluorouracil) for up to 8 cycles (Al-Batran 2008) **or** 85 mg/m² on day 1 every 2 weeks (in combination with leucovorin and fluorouracil; FOLFOX4) for 6 cycles (Conroy 2010) **or**

Gastric cancer: IV: 130 mg/m² on day 1 every 3 weeks (in combination with capecitabine) for 8 cycles (Bang 2012)

Non-Hodgkin lymphoma, relapsed/refractory (off-label use): IV: 100 mg/m² on day 1 every 3 weeks (in combination with gemcitabine and rituximab) (Lopez 2008; Rodriguez 2007) **or** 130 mg/m² on day 1 every 3 weeks (in combination with cytarabine and dexamethasone) (Chau 2001)

Ovarian cancer, advanced (off-label use): IV: 130 mg/m² once every 3 weeks until disease progression or unacceptable toxicity (Dieras 2002; Piccart 2000)

Pancreatic cancer, advanced (off-label use): IV: 85 mg/m² every 2 weeks (in combination with fluorouracil, leucovorin, and irinotecan; FOLFIRINOX regimen) for up to 6 months (Conroy 2011) **or** 110 to 130 mg/m² on day 1 every 3 weeks (in combination with capecitabine) until disease progression or unacceptable toxicity (Xiong 2008)

Testicular cancer, refractory (off-label use): IV: 130 mg/m² every 3 weeks in combination with gemcitabine (De Georgi 2006; Kollmannsberger 2004; Pectasides 2004) **or** 130 mg/m² on day 1 every 3 weeks (in combination with gemcitabine and paclitaxel) for up to 8 cycles (Bokemeyer 2008)

Geriatric No dosage adjustment necessary. Refer to adult dosing.

Renal Impairment

Manufacturer's labeling:

US labeling:

CrCl ≥30 mL/minute: No dosage adjustment necessary.

CrCl <30 mL/minute: Reduce dose from 85 mg/m² to 65 mg/m².

Canadian labeling:

CrCl ≥50 mL/minute: No dosage adjustment necessary.

CrCl 30 to <50 mL/minute: No dosage adjustment necessary; monitor closely and reduce dose if toxicities occur.

CrCl <30 mL/minute: Use is contraindicated.

Alternate recommendations: CrCl ≥20 mL/minute: In a study with a limited number of patients with mild to moderate impairment, defined by the authors as CrCl 20 to 59 mL/minute (determined using 24-hour urine collection), oxaliplatin was well tolerated, suggesting a dose reduction may not be necessary in patients with CrCl ≥20 mL/minute receiving every-3-week dosing (dose range: 80 to 130 mg/m² every 3 weeks) (Takimoto 2003).

Hepatic Impairment Mild, moderate, or severe impairment: No dosage adjustment necessary (Doroshow 2003; Synold 2007).

Obesity *ASCO Guidelines for appropriate chemotherapy dosing in obese adults with cancer:* Utilize patient's actual body weight (full weight) for calculation of body surface area- or weight-based dosing, particularly when the intent of therapy is curative; manage regimen-related toxicities in the same manner as for nonobese patients; if a dose reduction is utilized due to toxicity, consider resumption of full weight-based dosing with subsequent

cycles, especially if cause of toxicity (eg, hepatic or renal impairment) is resolved (Griggs 2012).

Adjustment for Toxicity Acute toxicities: Longer infusion time (6 hours) may mitigate acute toxicities (eg, pharyngolaryngeal dysesthesia).

Neurosensory events:

Persistent (>7 days) grade 2 neurosensory events:

Adjuvant treatment of stage III colon cancer: Reduce dose to 75 mg/m²

Advanced colorectal cancer: Reduce dose to 65 mg/m²

Consider withholding oxaliplatin for grade 2 neuropathy lasting >7 days despite dose reduction.

Persistent (>7 days) grade 3 neurosensory events:

US labeling: Consider discontinuing oxaliplatin.

Canadian labeling:

Adjuvant treatment of stage III colon cancer: Discontinue oxaliplatin.

Advanced colorectal cancer: Reduce dose to 65 mg/m²; if not resolved prior to next cycle, then discontinue.

Persistent grade 4 neurosensory events (Canadian labeling): Advanced colorectal cancer: Discontinue oxaliplatin

Gastrointestinal toxicity (grade 3/4) occurring despite prophylactic treatment:

Adjuvant treatment of stage III colon cancer: Delay next dose until recovery from toxicity, then reduce dose to 75 mg/m².

Advanced colorectal cancer: Delay next dose until recovery from toxicity, then reduce dose to 65 mg/m².

Hematologic toxicity (grade 4 neutropenia [Canadian labeling: grade 3 or 4 neutropenia], febrile neutropenia, or grade 3/4 thrombocytopenia):

Adjuvant treatment of stage III colon cancer: Delay next dose until neutrophils recover to ≥1500/mm³ and platelets recover to ≥75,000/mm³, then reduce dose to 75 mg/m².

Advanced colorectal cancer: Delay next dose until neutrophils recover to ≥1500/mm³ and platelets recover to ≥75,000/mm³, then reduce dose to 65 mg/m².

Pulmonary toxicity (unexplained respiratory symptoms including nonproductive cough, dyspnea, crackles, pulmonary infiltrates): Discontinue until interstitial lung disease or pulmonary fibrosis have been excluded.

Rhabdomyolysis: Discontinue for signs/symptoms of rhabdomyolysis.

Sepsis or septic shock: Withhold treatment.

Administration Administer as IV infusion over 2 hours; extend infusion time to 6 hours for acute toxicities. Flush infusion line with D₅W prior to administration of any concomitant medication. Avoid mucositis prophylaxis with ice chips, exposure to cold temperatures, or consumption of cold food/beverages during or within hours after oxaliplatin infusion (may exacerbate acute neurological symptoms). Do not use needles or administration sets containing aluminum. When used in combination with a fluoropyrimidine (eg, 5-FU), infuse oxaliplatin first.

Oxaliplatin is associated with a moderate emetic potential; antiemetics are recommended to prevent nausea and vomiting (Basch 2011; Dupuis 2011; Roila 2010).

Irritant with vesicant-like properties; ensure proper needle or catheter placement prior to and during infusion. Avoid extravasation; monitor IV site for redness, swelling, or pain.

Extravasation management: If extravasation occurs, stop infusion immediately and disconnect (leave cannula/needle in place); gently aspirate extravasated solution (do **NOT** flush the line); remove needle/cannula; elevate extremity. Information conflicts regarding use of warm or cold compresses. Cold compresses could potentially precipitate or exacerbate peripheral neuropathy (de Lemos 2005).

Hazardous agent; use appropriate precautions for handling and disposal (NIOSH 2014 [group 1]).

Monitoring Parameters CBC with differential, blood chemistries, including serum creatinine, ALT, AST, and bilirubin (prior to each cycle), electrolytes, including potassium and magnesium (prior to and periodically during treatment); INR and prothrombin time (in patients on oral anticoagulant therapy); neurologic evaluation prior to each dose and periodically thereafter; hypersensitivity; respiratory effects; RPLS

◀ **Dosage Forms** Excipient information presented when available (limited, particularly for generics); consult specific product labeling. [DSC] = Discontinued product
Solution, Intravenous [preservative free]:
Eloxatin: 50 mg/10 mL (10 mL [DSC]); 100 mg/20 mL (20 mL [DSC]); 200 mg/40 mL (40 mL)
Generic: 50 mg/10 mL (10 mL); 100 mg/20 mL (20 mL)
Solution Reconstituted, Intravenous [preservative free]:
Generic: 50 mg (1 ea); 100 mg (1 ea)

◆ Oxandrin see Oxandrolone on page 1352

Oxandrolone (oks AN droe lone)

Brand Names: US Oxandrin
Pharmacologic Category Androgen
Use Adjunctive therapy to promote weight gain after weight loss following extensive surgery, chronic infections, or severe trauma, and in some patients who, without definite pathophysiologic reasons, fail to gain or to maintain normal weight; to offset protein catabolism with prolonged corticosteroid administration; relief of bone pain associated with osteoporosis
Dosing
Adult Weight gain (adjunct): Oral: 2.5-20 mg in divided doses 2-4 times daily based on individual response; a course of therapy of 2-4 weeks is usually adequate. This may be repeated intermittently as needed.
Geriatric Weight gain (adjunct): Oral: 5 mg twice daily
Pediatric Weight gain (adjunct): Oral: Children: Total daily dose: ≤0.1 mg/kg; may be repeated intermittently as needed
Renal Impairment No dosage adjustment provided in manufacturer's labeling; use with caution due to propensity to cause edema.
Hepatic Impairment No dosage adjustment provided in manufacturer's labeling; use with caution.
Additional Information Complete prescribing information should be consulted for additional detail.
Dosage Forms Excipient information presented when available (limited, particularly for generics); consult specific product labeling.
Tablet, Oral:
Oxandrin: 2.5 mg [scored]
Oxandrin: 10 mg
Generic: 2.5 mg, 10 mg
Controlled Substance C-III

Oxaprozin (oks a PROE zin)

Brand Names: US Daypro
Brand Names: Canada Apo-Oxaprozin
Pharmacologic Category Nonsteroidal Anti-inflammatory Drug (NSAID), Oral
Use Management of signs and symptoms of osteoarthritis, rheumatoid arthritis, and juvenile idiopathic arthritis (JIA)
Medication Guide Available Yes
Dosing
Adult & Geriatric Note: Individualize dosage to lowest effective dose for the shortest duration to minimize adverse effects.
Osteoarthritis, rheumatoid arthritis: Oral: 1200 mg once daily. **Note:** Patients with low body weight should start with 600 mg daily. A one-time loading dose of 1200-1800 mg (≤26 mg/kg) may be used when a quick onset of action is desired.
Maximum doses:
Patient <50 kg: Maximum: 1200 mg daily
Patient >50 kg with normal renal/hepatic function and low risk of peptic ulcer: Maximum: 1800 mg daily or 26 mg/kg/day (whichever is lower) in divided doses
Pediatric
Juvenile idiopathic arthritis (JIA): Oral:
Note: Individualize dosage to lowest effective dose for the shortest duration to minimize adverse effects.
Children 6-16 years:
22-31 kg: 600 mg once daily
32-54 kg: 900 mg once daily
≥55 kg: 1200 mg once daily
Renal Impairment In general, NSAIDs are not recommended for use in patients with advanced renal disease but the manufacturer of oxaprozin does provide some guidelines for adjustment in renal dysfunction.
Severe renal impairment or on dialysis: 600 mg once daily; may increase cautiously to 1200 mg daily with close monitoring.
Hepatic Impairment Use caution in patients with severe hepatic impairment.
Additional Information Complete prescribing information should be consulted for additional detail.

Dosage Forms Excipient information presented when available (limited, particularly for generics); consult specific product labeling.
Tablet, Oral:
Daypro: 600 mg [scored]
Generic: 600 mg

◆ Oxaydo see OxyCODONE on page 1357

Oxazepam (oks A ze pam)

Brand Names: Canada Apo-Oxazepam; Bio-Oxazepam; Novoxapram; Oxpam; Oxpram; PMS-Oxazepam; Riva-Oxazepam
Index Terms Serax
Pharmacologic Category Benzodiazepine
Use Management of anxiety disorders, including anxiety associated with depression; management of ethanol withdrawal
Dosing
Adult
Anxiety, mild-to-moderate: Oral: 10-15 mg 3-4 times daily
Anxiety, severe or associated with depression: Oral: 15-30 mg 3-4 times daily
Ethanol withdrawal: Oral: 15-30 mg 3-4 times daily
Geriatric Anxiety: Oral: Initial: 10 mg 3 times daily. If necessary, increase cautiously to 15 mg 3-4 times daily. Dose titration should be slow to evaluate sensitivity.
Pediatric Children >12 years and Adolescents: Refer to adult dosing.
Renal Impairment
No dosage adjustment provided in manufacturer's labeling
Hemodialysis: Not dialyzable (0% to 5%) (Greenblatt, 1981; Mokhlesi, 2003)
Hepatic Impairment No dosage adjustment provided in manufacturer's labeling; however, pharmacokinetic studies have shown that hepatic dysfunction is not expected to significantly decrease clearance (Furlan, 1999; Greenblatt, 1981).
Additional Information Complete prescribing information should be consulted for additional detail.
Dosage Forms Excipient information presented when available (limited, particularly for generics); consult specific product labeling.
Capsule, Oral:
Generic: 10 mg, 15 mg, 30 mg
Controlled Substance C-IV

OXcarbazepine (ox car BAZ e peen)

Brand Names: US Oxtellar XR; Trileptal
Brand Names: Canada Jamp-Oxcarbazepine; Trileptal
Index Terms GP 47680; OCBZ
Pharmacologic Category Anticonvulsant, Miscellaneous
Use
Partial seizures:
Immediate-release:
U.S labeling: Monotherapy or adjunctive therapy in the treatment of partial seizures in adults, as monotherapy in the treatment of partial seizures in children 4 years and older with epilepsy, and as adjunctive therapy in children 2 years and older with partial seizures.
Canadian labeling: Monotherapy or adjunctive therapy in the treatment of partial seizures in patients 6 years and older.
Extended-release: Adjunctive therapy in the treatment of partial seizures in adults and in children 6 to 17 years of age.
Pregnancy Considerations Adverse events have been observed in animal reproduction studies; therefore, the manufacturer classifies oxcarbazepine as pregnancy category C. Oxcarbazepine, the active metabolite MHD and the inactive metabolite DHD, crosses the placenta and can be detected in the newborn. An increased risk in the overall rate of major congenital malformations has not been observed following maternal use of oxcarbazepine. Available studies have not been large enough to determine if there is an increased risk of specific defects. In general, the risk of teratogenic effects is higher with AED polytherapy than monotherapy. Plasma concentrations of MHD gradually decrease due to physiologic changes which occur during pregnancy; patients should be monitored during pregnancy and postpartum. Oxcarbazepine may decrease plasma concentrations of hormonal contraceptives.

Patients exposed to oxcarbazepine during pregnancy are encouraged to enroll themselves into the NAAED Pregnancy Registry by calling 1-888-233-2334. Additional information is available at www.aedpregnancyregistry.org.

Breast-Feeding Considerations Oxcarbazepine and the active 10-hydroxy metabolite (MHD) are found in breast milk (small amounts). According to the manufacturer, the decision to continue or discontinue breast-feeding during therapy should take into account the risk of exposure to the infant and the benefits of treatment to the mother.

Medication Guide Available Yes

Contraindications Hypersensitivity to oxcarbazepine or any component of the formulation

Warnings/Precautions Hazardous agent - use appropriate precautions for handling and disposal (NIOSH 2014 [group 2]).

Antiepileptics are associated with an increased risk of suicidal behavior/thoughts with use (regardless of indication); patients should be monitored for signs/symptoms of depression, suicidal tendencies, and other unusual behavior changes during therapy and instructed to inform their healthcare provider immediately if symptoms occur.

Clinically-significant hyponatremia (serum sodium <125 mmol/L) may develop during oxcarbazepine use. Rare cases of anaphylaxis and angioedema have been reported, even after initial dosing; permanently discontinue should symptoms occur. Use caution in patients with previous hypersensitivity to carbamazepine (cross-sensitivity occurs in 25% to 30% of patients). Potentially serious, sometimes fatal, dermatologic reactions (eg, Stevens-Johnson, toxic epidermal necrolysis) and drug reaction with eosinophilia and systemic symptoms (DRESS) also known as multiorgan hypersensitivity reactions have been reported in adults and children; monitor for signs and symptoms of skin reactions and possible disparate manifestations associated with lymphatic, hepatic, renal, cardiovascular, and/or hematologic organ systems; discontinuation and conversion to alternate therapy may be required. Considering screening patients of Asian descent for the variant human leukocyte antigen (HLA) allele B*1502 prior to initiating therapy. This genetic variant has been associated with a significantly increased risk of developing Stevens-Johnson syndrome and/or toxic epidermal necrolysis in patients receiving carbamazepine. Structural similarity of oxcarbazepine to carbamazepine, available clinical evidence, and data from nonclinical studies showing a direct interaction of oxcarbazepine with the HLA-B*1502 protein suggest patients receiving oxcarbazepine may be at a similar risk. Consider avoiding use of oxcarbazepine in patients with a positive result. Screening is not recommending in low-risk populations or in current oxcarbazepine patients (risk usually during first few months of therapy). Clinical trials excluded patients with significant cardiovascular disease or ECG abnormalities; Canadian labeling recommends using caution with cardiac conduction abnormalities or concomitant drugs that depress atrioventricular (AV) conduction and to avoid use in patients with AV block. Monitor body weight/fluid retention in patients with HF; evaluate serum sodium in patients with worsening cardiac function or fluid retention.

Hepatitis and hepatic failure have been reported rarely (Hsu 2010; Trileptal Canadian product monograph 2013). Promptly evaluate any symptoms of hepatic dysfunction (eg, anorexia, nausea/vomiting, right upper quadrant pain, pruritus) and discontinue therapy immediately if significant abnormalities are confirmed. Agranulocytosis, leukopenia, and pancytopenia have been reported rarely. Discontinuation and conversion to alternate therapy may be required. Long term use has been associated with decreased bone mineral density, osteopenia, osteoporosis, and fractures.

As with all antiepileptic drugs, oxcarbazepine should be withdrawn gradually to minimize the potential of increased seizure frequency. Use of oxcarbazepine has been associated with CNS-related adverse events, most significant of these were cognitive symptoms including psychomotor slowing, difficulty with concentration, speech or language problems, somnolence or fatigue, and coordination abnormalities, including ataxia and gait disturbances. Single-dose studies show that half-life of the primary active metabolite is prolonged 3- to 4-fold and AUC is doubled in patients with CrCl <30 mL/minute; dose adjustment required in these patients. Potentially significant drug-drug interactions may exist, requiring dose or frequency adjustment, additional monitoring, and/or selection of alternative therapy. Oral suspension contains sorbitol; Canadian labeling recommends avoiding use in patients with fructose intolerance

Adverse Reactions Frequency not always defined. Incidence in children was similar.

>10%:
Central nervous system: Dizziness (20% to 49%), drowsiness (12% to 36%), headache (8% to 32%), ataxia (2% to 31%), abnormal gait (≤17%), fatigue (3% to 15%), vertigo (2% to 15%)
Gastrointestinal: Vomiting (7% to 36%), nausea (15% to 29%), abdominal pain (10% to 13%)
Neuromuscular & skeletal: Tremor (4% to 16%)
Ophthalmic: Diplopia (10% to 40%), nystagmus (3% to 26%), visual disturbance (1% to 14%)

1% to 10%:
Cardiovascular: Lower extremity edema (2%), hypotension (≤2%), bradycardia, cardiac failure, flushing, hypertension, orthostatic hypotension, palpitations, syncope, tachycardia
Central nervous system: Equilibrium disturbance (7%), nervousness (2% to 5%), amnesia (4%), emotional lability (4%), falling (4%), abnormality in thinking (≤4%), insomnia (2% to 4%), dysmetria (1% to 3%), speech disorder (1% to 3%), agitation (2%), confusion (2%), convulsions (2%), lack of concentration (2%), abnormal electroencephalogram (≤2%), feeling abnormal (≤2%), myasthenia (1% to 2%), aggressive behavior, anxiety, apathy, aphasia, aura, cerebral hemorrhage, delirium, delusion, depression, dystonia, euphoria extrapyramidal reaction, hemiplegia, hyperkinesia, hyperreflexia, hypertonia, hypokinesia, hyporeflexia, hypotonia, hysteria, impaired consciousness, intoxicated feeling, malaise, manic behavior, migraine, neuralgia, nightmares, oculogyric crisis, panic disorder, paralysis, personality disorder, precordial pain, psychosis, rigors, seizure (aggravated), stupor, voice disorder
Dermatologic: Skin rash (4%), diaphoresis (3%), acne vulgaris (1% to 2%), alopecia, contact dermatitis, eczema, erythematosus rash, facial rash, folliculitis, genital pruritus, maculopapular rash, miliaria, psoriasis, skin photosensitivity, urticaria, vitiligo
Endocrine & metabolic: Decreased serum sodium (<135 mEq/L: 7% to 9%), hyponatremia (1% to 3%), weight gain (2%), change in libido, hot flash, hyperglycemia, hypermenorrhea, hypocalcemia, hypoglycemia, hypokalemia, increased gamma-glutamyl transferase, intermenstrual bleeding, weight loss
Gastrointestinal: Diarrhea (7%), dyspepsia (≤6%), constipation (4% to 6%), dysgeusia (5%), xerostomia (3%), gastritis (≤3%), upper abdominal pain (≤3%), aphthous stomatitis, biliary colic, bloody stools, cholelithiasis, colitis, duodenal ulcer, dysphagia, enteritis, eructation, esophagitis, flatulence, gastric ulcer, gingival hemorrhage, gingival hyperplasia, hematemesis, hemorrhoids, hiccups, increased appetite, retching, sialadenitis, stomatitis
Genitourinary: Urinary frequency (2%), dysuria, hematuria, leukorrhea, priapism, urinary tract pain
Hematologic & oncologic: Bruise (2%), purpura, rectal hemorrhage, thrombocytopenia
Hepatic: Increased liver enzymes
Hypersensitivity: Hypersensitivity reaction (2%), angioedema
Neuromuscular & skeletal: Weakness (2% to 7%), back pain (4%), muscle spasm (2%), sprain (≤2%), right hypochondrium pain, systemic lupus erythematosus, tetany
Ophthalmic: Blurred vision (4%), accommodation disturbance (≤2%), blepharoptosis, cataract, conjunctival hemorrhage, hemianopia, mydriasis, ocular edema, photophobia, scotoma, xerophthalmia
Otic: Otitis externa, tinnitus
Renal: Nephrolithiasis, polyuria, renal pain
Respiratory: Rhinitis (5% to 10%), upper respiratory tract infection (7%), pulmonary infection (4%), epistaxis (4%), sinusitis (≤4%), nasopharyngitis (≤3%), pneumonia (2%), asthma, dyspnea, laryngismus, pleurisy
Miscellaneous: Fever (3%)
Postmarketing and/or case reports (Limited to important or life-threatening): Abnormal thyroid function test (decreased total T_4 and/or free T_4), acute generalized exanthematous pustulosis, agranulocytosis, anaphylaxis, aplastic anemia, bone fracture (long-term therapy), decreased bone mineral density (long-term therapy), DRESS syndrome, erythema multiforme, folate deficiency, hepatic failure, hepatitis (Hsu, 2010), hypersensitivity reaction, hypothyroidism, increased serum amylase, increased serum lipase, leukopenia, multiorgan hypersensitivity (eosinophilia, arthralgia, rash, fever, lymphadenopathy), osteopenia (long-term therapy), osteoporosis (long-term therapy), pancreatitis, pancytopenia, Stevens-Johnson syndrome, suicidal ideation, suicidal tendencies, toxic epidermal necrolysis

◄ **Drug Interactions**

Metabolism/Transport Effects Induces CYP3A4 (weak)

Avoid Concomitant Use

Avoid concomitant use of OXcarbazepine with any of the following: Dolutegravir; Elvitegravir; Eslicarbazepine; Ledipasvir; Rilpivirine; Selegiline; Sofosbuvir; Ulipristal

Increased Effect/Toxicity

OXcarbazepine may increase the levels/effects of: Fosphenytoin-Phenytoin; PHENobarbital; Selegiline

The levels/effects of OXcarbazepine may be increased by: Alcohol (Ethyl); Eslicarbazepine; Perampanel; Thiazide Diuretics

Decreased Effect

OXcarbazepine may decrease the levels/effects of: ARIPiprazole; Cobicistat; Contraceptives (Estrogens); Contraceptives (Progestins); Dolutegravir; Elvitegravir; Hydrocodone; Ledipasvir; NiMODipine; Perampanel; Rilpivirine; Saxagliptin; Sofosbuvir; Ulipristal

The levels/effects of OXcarbazepine may be decreased by: CarBAMazepine; Fosphenytoin-Phenytoin; Mefloquine; Mianserin; Orlistat; PHENobarbital; Valproate Products

Storage/Stability Store tablets and suspension at 25°C (77°F); excursions permitted to 15°C to 30°C (59°F to 86°F). Store suspension in the original container; use within 7 weeks of first opening container. Dispense extended release tablets in a tight, light-resistant container; protect from light and moisture.

Mechanism of Action Pharmacological activity results from both oxcarbazepine and its monohydroxy metabolite (MHD). Precise mechanism of anticonvulsant effect has not been defined. Oxcarbazepine and MHD block voltage-sensitive sodium channels, stabilizing hyperexcited neuronal membranes, inhibiting repetitive firing, and decreasing the propagation of synaptic impulses. These actions are believed to prevent the spread of seizures. Oxcarbazepine and MHD also increase potassium conductance and modulate the activity of high-voltage activated calcium channels.

Pharmacodynamics/Kinetics

Absorption: Complete

Distribution: MHD: V_d: 49 L

Protein binding, serum: MHD: ~40% (primarily to albumin)

Metabolism: Extensive to 10-monohydroxy metabolite (MHD; active); MHD is further glucuronidated or oxidized to a 10,11-dihydroxy metabolite (DHD; inactive)

Bioavailability: Immediate release: Decreased in children <8 years; increased in elderly >60 years

Half-life elimination: Immediate release: Parent drug: 2 hours; MHD: 9 hours; renal impairment (CrCl 30 mL/minute): MHD: 19 hours; Extended release: Parent drug: 7 to 11 hours; MHD: 9 to 11 hours

Clearance of MHD is increased in younger children (~80% in children 2-4 years of age) and approaches that of adults by ~13 years of age

Time to peak, serum (median): Immediate release: Tablets: 4.5 hours; Oral suspension: 6 hours

Excretion: Urine (95%, <1% as unchanged oxcarbazepine, 27% as unchanged MHD, 49% as MHD glucuronides); feces (<4%)

Dosing

Adult

Adjunctive therapy, partial seizures (epilepsy): Oral:

Immediate release (Trileptal): Initial: 600 mg daily in 2 divided doses; dose may be increased by as much as 600 mg/day increments at weekly intervals; recommended daily dose: 1200 mg daily in 2 divided doses. Although daily doses >1200 mg daily were somewhat more efficacious, most patients were unable to tolerate 2400 mg daily (due to CNS effects).

Extended release (Oxtellar XR): Initial: 600 mg once daily; dosage may be increased by 600 mg/day increments at weekly intervals. Recommended daily dose is 1200 to 2400 mg once daily. Although daily doses >1200 mg daily were somewhat more efficacious, most patients were unable to tolerate 2400 mg daily (due to CNS effects).

Conversion to monotherapy, partial seizures (epilepsy): Patients receiving concomitant antiepileptic drugs (AEDs): Oral: Immediate release (Trileptal): Initial: 600 mg daily in 2 divided doses while simultaneously reducing the dose of concomitant AEDs. Withdraw concomitant AEDs completely over 3 to 6 weeks, while increasing the oxcarbazepine dose in increments of 600 mg daily at weekly intervals, reaching the maximum oxcarbazepine dose (2400 mg daily) in about 2 to 4 weeks (lower doses have been effective in patients in whom monotherapy has been initiated).

Initiation of monotherapy, partial seizures (epilepsy): Patients not receiving prior AEDs: Oral: Immediate release (Trileptal): Initial: 600 mg daily in 2 divided doses. Increase dose by 300 mg daily every third day to a dose of 1200 mg daily. Higher dosages (2400 mg daily) have been shown to be effective in patients converted to monotherapy from other AEDs.

Conversion from immediate release (Trileptal) to extended release (Oxtellar XR): Higher doses of Oxtellar XR may be necessary.

Dosage adjustment with concomitant antiepileptic drugs (AEDs): Concomitant use with enzyme-inducing antiepileptic drugs (eg, carbamazepine, phenobarbital, phenytoin): Extended release (Oxtellar XR): Consider initiating dose at 900 mg once daily.

Neuropathic pain (off-label use): Oral: Initial: 300 mg/day; increase dose after 3 days to 300 mg twice daily, then adjust dose based on response and tolerability in increments of 300 mg every 5 days up to a maximum dose of 900 mg twice daily. Mean dose during clinical trial maintenance period was 1,445 mg/day (Dogra 2005).

Geriatric

Immediate release (Trileptal): Refer to adult dosing.

Extended release (Oxtellar XR): *Initial:* 300 mg or 450 mg once daily should be considered; dosage may be increased by 300 to 450 mg daily increments at weekly intervals to desired clinical response.

Pediatric

Adjunctive treatment, partial seizures (epilepsy): Oral:

Children 2 to 3 years (U.S. labeling): Immediate release (Trileptal):

Initial: 8 to 10 mg/kg/day, not to exceed 600 mg daily, given in 2 divided daily doses

Maintenance: The target maintenance dose should be achieved over 2 to 4 weeks, and is dependent upon patient weight (should not exceed 60 mg/kg/day given in 2 divided daily doses).

<20 kg: Consider initiating dose at 16 to 20 mg/kg/day; maximum maintenance dose should be achieved over 2 to 4 weeks and should not exceed 60 mg/kg/day

Children 4 to 16 years (U.S. labeling) or 6 to 16 years (Canadian labeling): Immediate release (Trileptal):

Initial: 8 to 10 mg/kg/day, not to exceed 600 mg daily, given in 2 divided daily doses

Maintenance: The target maintenance dose should be achieved over 2 weeks, and is dependent upon patient weight, according to the following:

20 to 29 kg: 900 mg daily in 2 divided doses

29.1 to 39 kg: 1200 mg daily in 2 divided doses

>39 kg: 1800 mg daily in 2 divided doses

Children 6 to 17 years: Extended release (Oxtellar XR):

Initial: 8 to 10 mg/kg once daily (not to exceed 600 mg daily in the first week)

Maintenance: The target maintenance dose should be achieved over 2 to 3 weeks with dose increases of 8 to 10 mg/kg/day increments at weekly intervals (maximum dosage incremental increase: 600 mg). Target maintenance dose depends on weight:

20 to 29 kg: 900 mg once daily

29.1 to 39 kg: 1200 mg once daily

>39 kg: 1800 mg once daily

Conversion to monotherapy, partial seizures (epilepsy): Patients receiving concomitant antiepileptic drugs (AEDs): Children 4 to 16 years (U.S. labeling) or 6 to 16 years (Canadian labeling): Oral: Immediate release (Trileptal): Initial: 8 to 10 mg/kg/day in twice daily divided doses, while simultaneously initiating the dose reduction of concomitant antiepileptic drugs; the concomitant drugs should be withdrawn over 3 to 6 weeks. Oxcarbazepine dose may be increased by a maximum of 10 mg/kg/day at weekly intervals. See below for recommended total daily dose by weight.

Initiation of monotherapy, partial seizures (epilepsy): Patients not receiving prior AEDs: Children 4 to 16 years (U.S. labeling) or 6 to 16 years (Canadian labeling): Oral: Immediate release (Trileptal): Initial: 8 to 10 mg/kg/day in twice daily divided doses; doses may be titrated by 5 mg/kg/day every third day. See below for recommended total daily dose by weight.

Range of maintenance doses by weight during monotherapy:

20 kg: 600 to 900 mg daily

25 to 30 kg: 900 to 1200 mg daily

35 to 40 kg: 900 to 1500 mg daily

45 kg: 1200 to 1500 mg daily

50 to 55 kg: 1200 to 1800 mg daily

60 to 65 kg: 1200 to 2100 mg daily

70 kg: 1500 to 2100 mg daily

Conversion from immediate release (Trileptal) to extended release (Oxtellar XR): Children ≥6 years and Adolescents: Refer to adult dosing.

Dosage adjustment with concomitant antiepileptic drugs (AEDs): Children ≥6 years and Adolescents: Refer to adult dosing.

Renal Impairment

Mild-to-moderate impairment: There are no dosage adjustments provided in the manufacturer's labeling.

Severe impairment (CrCl <30 mL/minute): Immediate release (Trileptal), Extended release (Oxtellar XR): Therapy should be initiated at one-half the usual starting dose (300 mg daily in adults) and increased slowly to achieve desired clinical response (eg, 300 to 450 mg daily at weekly intervals).

ESRD (on dialysis): Immediate release formulations should be used instead of extended release formulation.

Hepatic Impairment

Mild-to-moderate impairment: No dosage adjustments necessary.

Severe impairment:

Immediate release (Trileptal): There are no dosage adjustments provided in the manufacturer's labeling; use caution (has not been studied).

Extended release (Oxtellar XR): There are no dosage adjustments provided in the manufacturer's labeling; use is not recommended (has not been studied).

Administration

Immediate release: Administer twice daily without regard to meals.

Suspension: Prior to using for the first time, firmly insert the plastic adapter provided with the bottle. Cover adapter with child-resistant cap when not in use. Shake bottle for at least 10 seconds, remove child-resistant cap, and insert the oral dosing syringe provided to withdraw appropriate dose. Dose may be taken directly from oral syringe or may be mixed in a small glass of water immediately prior to swallowing. Rinse syringe with warm water after use and allow to dry thoroughly. Discard any unused portion after 7 weeks of first opening bottle.

Extended release: Administer once daily on an empty stomach at least 1 hour before or 2 hours after food. Swallow whole; do not cut, crush, or chew the tablets.

Hazardous agent; use appropriate precautions for handling and disposal (NIOSH 2014 [group 2]).

Monitoring Parameters Seizure frequency; serum sodium as deemed necessary (particularly during first 3 months of therapy); symptoms of CNS depression (dizziness, headache, somnolence); hypersensitivity reactions. Additional serum sodium monitoring recommended during maintenance treatment in patients receiving other medications known to decrease sodium levels, in patients with signs/symptoms of hyponatremia, and in patients with an increase in seizure frequency or severity. Periodic thyroid function tests (particularly pediatric patients) and CBC. Monitor for suicidality (eg, suicidal thoughts, depression, behavioral changes). Serum levels of concomitant antiepileptic drugs during titration as necessary.

Reference Range The metabolite of oxcarbazepine, 10-monohydroxy metabolite (MHD), is considered the active entity primarily responsible for the therapeutic effects. A number of studies have suggested optimal MHD concentrations for efficacy may range from 2 to 55 mcg/mL and some experts suggest a target range of 8 to 35 mcg/mL based on clinical experience; however, a clear correlation between plasma concentrations and therapeutic response has not been demonstrated. Therapeutic drug monitoring of MHD is not routinely warranted; however, it may be beneficial in optimizing seizure control in the following situations: Extremes of age, during pregnancy, to investigate the correlation between drug concentrations and toxicity especially with concurrent disease states such as renal impairment, to identify potential drug interactions, to assess reasons for therapeutic failure, or to rule out noncompliance (Bring 2008; May 2003).

Test Interactions Thyroid function tests; may depress serum T_4 without affecting T_3 levels or TSH

Additional Information At steady state, the extended release product administered once daily is not bioequivalent to the same daily dose of the immediate release formulation administered twice daily.

Dosage Forms Excipient information presented when available (limited, particularly for generics); consult specific product labeling.

Suspension, Oral:

Trileptal: 300 mg/5 mL (250 mL) [contains alcohol, usp, methyl hydroxybenzoate, propyl hydroxybenzoate, propylene glycol, saccharin sodium; lemon flavor]

Generic: 300 mg/5 mL (250 mL)

Tablet, Oral:

Trileptal: 150 mg, 300 mg, 600 mg [scored]

Generic: 150 mg, 300 mg, 600 mg

Tablet Extended Release 24 Hour, Oral:

Oxtellar XR: 150 mg, 300 mg, 600 mg

Oxiconazole (oks i KON a zole)

Brand Names: US Oxistat

Brand Names: Canada Oxistat®

Index Terms Oxiconazole Nitrate

Pharmacologic Category Antifungal Agent, Imidazole Derivative; Antifungal Agent, Topical

Use

Cream: Treatment of tinea pedis (athlete's foot), tinea cruris (jock itch), tinea corporis (ringworm), and tinea (pityriasis) versicolor

Lotion: Treatment of tinea pedis (athlete's foot), tinea cruris (jock itch), tinea corporis (ringworm)

Dosing

Adult & Geriatric

Tinea corporis/tinea cruris: Topical: Cream, lotion: Apply to affected areas 1-2 times daily for 2 weeks

Tinea pedis: Topical: Cream, lotion: Apply to affected areas 1-2 times daily for 1 month

Tinea versicolor: Topical: Cream: Apply to affected areas once daily for 2 weeks

Pediatric Tinea corporis, tinea cruris, tinea pedis, tinea versicolor: Children ≥12 years and Adolescents: Topical: Cream, lotion: Refer to adult dosing.

Additional Information Complete prescribing information should be consulted for additional detail.

Dosage Forms Excipient information presented when available (limited, particularly for generics); consult specific product labeling.

Cream, External:

Oxistat: 1% (30 g, 60 g, 90 g) [contains benzoic acid, cetyl alcohol, propylene glycol]

Lotion, External:

Oxistat: 1% (30 mL, 60 mL) [contains benzoic acid, cetyl alcohol, propylene glycol]

Oxybutynin (oks i BYOO ti nin)

Brand Names: US Ditropan XL; Gelnique; Oxytrol; Oxytrol For Women [OTC]

Brand Names: Canada Apo-Oxybutynin; Ditropan XL; Dom-Oxybutynin; Gelnique; Mylan-Oxybutynin; Oxybutyn; Oxybutynine; Oxytrol; PHL-Oxybutynin; PMS-Oxybutynin; Riva-Oxybutynin; Teva-Oxybutynin

Index Terms Ditropan; Oxybutynin Chloride

Pharmacologic Category Antispasmodic Agent, Urinary

Use Treatment of symptoms associated with overactive uninhibited neurogenic or reflex neurogenic bladder (eg, urgency, frequency, leakage, urge incontinence, dysuria); treatment of symptoms associated with detrusor overactivity due to a neurological condition (eg, spina bifida) (extended release tablet only)

Pregnancy Considerations Adverse events were not observed in animal reproduction studies.

◄ **Breast-Feeding Considerations** It is not known if oxybutynin is excreted into breast milk. The manufacturer recommends that caution be used if administered to a nursing woman. Suppression of lactation has been reported.

Contraindications Hypersensitivity to oxybutynin or any component of the formulation; patients with or at risk for uncontrolled narrow-angle glaucoma, urinary retention, gastric retention or conditions with severely decreased GI motility

OTC labeling: When used for self-medication, do not use if you have pain or burning when urinating, blood in urine, unexplained lower back or side pain, cloudy or foul-smelling urine; in males; age <18 years; only experience accidental urine loss when cough, sneeze, or laugh; diagnosis of urinary or gastric retention; glaucoma; hypersensitivity to oxybutynin.

Warnings/Precautions May cause hypersensitivity reactions, including anaphylaxis and angioedema. Cases of angioedema involving the face, lips, tongue, and/or larynx have been reported with oral oxybutynin; some cases have occurred after a single dose. Discontinue immediately if tongue, hypopharynx, or larynx is involved; promptly initiate appropriate management. Use with caution in patients with bladder outflow obstruction (may increase the risk of urinary retention), Parkinson disease (may aggravate symptoms of disease), treated angle-closure glaucoma (use is contraindicated in uncontrolled narrow-angle glaucoma), hyperthyroidism, coronary artery disease, heart failure, hypertension, cardiac arrhythmias, hepatic or renal impairment, prostatic hyperplasia (may cause urinary retention), hiatal hernia, myasthenia gravis, dementia, automonic neuropathy (may aggravate symptoms of decreased GI motility). Use with caution in patients with decreased GI motility or gastrointestinal obstructive disorders (eg, ulcerative colitis, intestinal atony, pyloric stenosis); may increase the risk of gastric retention. In patients with ulcerative colitis, use may decrease gastric motility to the point of increasing the risk of paralytic ileus or toxic megacolon. Use with caution in patients with gastroesophageal reflux or with medications that may exacerbate esophagitis (eg, bisphosphonates). May increase the risk of heat prostration. Anticholinergics may cause agitation, confusion, drowsiness, dizziness, hallucinations, headache, and/or blurred vision, which may impair physical or mental abilities; patients must be cautioned about performing tasks which require mental alertness (eg, operating machinery or driving). Dose reduction or discontinuation should be considered if CNS effects occur.

Potentially significant drug-drug interactions may exist, requiring dose or frequency adjustment, additional monitoring, and/or selection of alternative therapy. This medication is associated with potent anticholinergic properties which may be inappropriate in older adults depending on comorbidities (eg, dementia, delirium) (Beers Criteria).

The extended release formulation consists of drug within a nondeformable matrix; following drug release/absorption, the matrix/shell is expelled in the stool. The use of nondeformable products in patients with known stricture/narrowing of the GI tract has been associated with symptoms of obstruction. Transdermal patch may contain conducting metal (eg, aluminum); remove patch prior to MRI. When using the topical gel, cover treatment area with clothing after gel has dried to minimize transferring medication to others. Discontinue gel if skin irritation occurs. Gel contains ethanol; do not expose to open flame or smoking until gel has dried.

When used for self-medication (OTC), other causes of frequent urination (UTI, diabetes, early pregnancy, other serious conditions) may need to be considered prior to use. Patients should contact a health care provider if symptoms do not improve within 2 weeks of initial use or for new or worsening symptoms.

Adverse Reactions

Oral:

>10%:

Central nervous system: Dizziness (5% to 17%), drowsiness (6% to 14%)

Gastrointestinal: Xerostomia (35% to 71%; dose related), constipation (9% to 15%), nausea (5% to 12%)

1% to 10%:

Cardiovascular: Cardiac arrhythmia (sinus; 1% to <5%), decreased blood pressure (1% to <5%), edema (1% to <5%), flushing (1% to <5%), hypertension (1% to <5%), palpitations (1% to <5%), peripheral edema (1% to <5%)

Central nervous system: Headache (8%), nervousness (7%), insomnia (3% to 6%), confusion (1% to <5%), falling (1% to 5%), fatigue (1% to <5%), flank pain (1% to <5%), pain (1% to <5%)

Dermatologic: Pruritus (1% to <5%), xeroderma (1% to <5%)

Endocrine & metabolic: Fluid retention (1% to <5%), hyperglycemia (1% to <5%), increased thirst (1% to <5%)

Gastrointestinal: Diarrhea (1% to 8%), dyspepsia (5% to 6%), abdominal pain (1% to <5%), dysphagia (1% to <5%), eructation (1% to <5%), flatulence (1% to <5%), unpleasant taste (1% to <5%), vomiting (1% to <5%), gastroesophageal reflux disease (≤1%)

Genitourinary: Urinary hesitancy (2% to 9%), urinary tract infection (7%), urinary retention (1% to 6%), cystitis (1% to <5%), dysuria (1% to <5%), pollakiuria (1% to <5%)

Infection: Fungal infection (1% to <5%)

Neuromuscular & skeletal: Arthralgia (1% to <5%), back pain (1% to <5%), limb pain (1% to <5%), weakness (1% to <5%)

Ophthalmic: Blurred vision (4% to 10%), eye irritation (1% to <5%), keratoconjunctivitis sicca (1% to <5%), xerophthalmia (3%)

Respiratory: Asthma (1% to <5%), bronchitis (1% to <5%), cough (1% to <5%), dry throat (1% to <5%), hoarseness (1% to <5%), nasal congestion (1% to <5%), dry nose (1% to <5%), nasopharyngitis (1% to <5%), pharyngolaryngeal pain (1% to <5%), sinus congestion (1% to <5%), upper respiratory tract infection (1% to <5%)

Topical gel:

>10%:

Gastrointestinal: Xerostomia (8% to 12%)

Local: Application site reaction (6% to 14%; includes anesthesia, irritation, pain, papules)

1% to 10%:

Central nervous system: Dizziness (3%), fatigue (2%), headache (2%)

Dermatologic: Pruritus (1%)

Gastrointestinal: Constipation (1%)

Genitourinary: Urinary tract infection (7%)

Local: Application site erythema (4%), application site rash (3%), application site pruritus (2% to 3%), application site dermatitis (2%)

Ophthalmic: Blurred vision (<2%), xerophthalmia (<2%)

Respiratory: Nasopharyngitis (3%)

Transdermal:

>10%: Local: Application site pruritus (14% to 17%)

1% to 10%:

Dermatologic: Application site macules (3%)

Gastrointestinal: Xerostomia (4% to 10%), constipation (3%), diarrhea (3%)

Genitourinary: Dysuria (2%)

Local: Application site erythema (6% to 8%), application site vesicles (3%), application site rash (3%)

Ophthalmic: Visual disturbance (3%)

Postmarketing and/or case reports (Limited to important or life-threatening): Anaphylaxis, anorexia, cycloplegia, decreased gastrointestinal motility, glaucoma, hallucination, hypersensitivity reaction, impotence, suppressed lactation, memory impairment, mydriasis, psychotic reaction, prolonged Q-T interval on ECG, seizure, tachycardia

Drug Interactions

Metabolism/Transport Effects Substrate of CYP3A4 (minor); **Note:** Assignment of Major/Minor substrate status based on clinically relevant drug interaction potential; **Inhibits** CYP2C8 (weak), CYP2D6 (weak)

Avoid Concomitant Use

Avoid concomitant use of Oxybutynin with any of the following: Aclidinium; Amodiaquine; Cimetropium; Eluxadoline; Glucagon; Glycopyrrolate; Glycopyrrolate (Oral Inhalation); Ipratropium (Oral Inhalation); Levosulpiride; Potassium Chloride; Tiotropium; Umeclidinium

Increased Effect/Toxicity

Oxybutynin may increase the levels/effects of: AbobotulinumtoxinA; Amodiaquine; Analgesics (Opioid); Anticholinergic Agents; ARIPiprazole; Cannabinoid-Containing Products; Cimetropium; Eluxadoline; Glucagon; Glycopyrrolate; Glycopyrrolate (Oral Inhalation); Mirabegron; OnabotulinumtoxinA; Potassium Chloride; Ramosetron; RimabotulinumtoxinB; Thiazide Diuretics; Tiotropium; Topiramate

The levels/effects of Oxybutynin may be increased by: Aclidinium; Alcohol (Ethyl); CYP3A4 Inhibitors (Strong); Ipratropium (Oral Inhalation); Mianserin; Pramlintide; Umeclidinium

Decreased Effect

Oxybutynin may decrease the levels/effects of: Acetylcholinesterase Inhibitors; Gastrointestinal Agents (Prokinetic); Itopride; Levosulpiride; Secretin

The levels/effects of Oxybutynin may be decreased by: Acetylcholinesterase Inhibitors

Storage/Stability

Immediate release tablet and syrup: Store at 20°C to 25°C (68°F to 77°F). Protect from light.

Extended release tablet: Store at 25°C (77°F); excursions permitted to 15°C to 30°C (59°F to 86°F). Protect from moisture and humidity.

Topical gel (pump or sachets): Store at 25°C (77°F); excursions permitted to 15°C to 30°C (59°F to 86°F). Protect from moisture and humidity. Keep gel away from open flame. Do not store sachets outside the sealed pouch; apply immediately after removal from the protective pouch. Discard used sachets such that accidental application or ingestion by children, pets, or others is avoided.

Transdermal patch: Store at 20°C to 25°C (68°F to 77°F). Protect from moisture and humidity. Do not store outside the sealed pouch; apply immediately after removal from the protective pouch. Discard used patches such that accidental application or ingestion by children, pets, or others is avoided.

Mechanism of Action
Direct antispasmodic effect on smooth muscle, also inhibits the action of acetylcholine on smooth muscle (exhibits $1/5$ the anticholinergic activity of atropine, but has 4-10 times the antispasmodic activity); does not block effects at skeletal muscle or at autonomic ganglia; increases bladder capacity, decreases uninhibited contractions, and delays desire to void, therefore, decreases urgency and frequency

Pharmacodynamics/Kinetics

Onset of action: Oral: Immediate release: 30 to 60 minutes
Peak effect: 3 to 6 hours
Duration: Oral: Immediate release: 6 to 10 hours; Extended release: Up to 24 hours
Absorption: Oral: Rapid and well absorbed; Transdermal: High
Distribution: IV: V_d: 193 L
Protein binding: >99% primarily to alpha$_1$-acid glycoprotein
Metabolism: Hepatic via CYP3A4; Oral: High first-pass metabolism; forms active and inactive metabolites
Bioavailability: Oral: ~6%
Half-life elimination: IV: ~2 hours (parent drug), 7 to 8 hours (metabolites); Oral: Immediate release: ~2 to 3 hours; Extended release: ~13 hours; Transdermal: 30 to 64 hours
Time to peak, serum: Oral: Immediate release: ~60 minutes; Extended release: 4 to 6 hours; Transdermal: 24 to 48 hours
Excretion: Urine, as metabolites and unchanged drug (<0.1%)

Dosing

Adult Overactive bladder:

Oral:
Immediate release: 5 mg 2 to 3 times daily; maximum: 5 mg 4 times daily
Extended release: Initial: 5 to 10 mg once daily, adjust dose in 5 mg increments at weekly intervals; maximum: 30 mg once daily
Topical gel:
Gelnique 3%: Apply 3 pumps (84 mg) once daily
Gelnique 10%: Apply contents of 1 sachet (100 mg/g) once daily
Transdermal: Apply one 3.9 mg/day patch twice weekly (every 3 to 4 days)

Geriatric

Oral: Immediate release: Initial: 2.5 mg 2 to 3 times daily; increase cautiously
Topical gel, transdermal patch: Refer to adult dosing.

Pediatric Overactive bladder: Oral:

Children: >5 years: Immediate release: 5 mg twice daily; maximum: 5 mg 3 times daily
Children ≥6 years: Extended release: 5 mg once daily; adjust dose in 5 mg increments; maximum: 20 mg once daily

Renal Impairment No dosage adjustment provided in the manufacturer's labeling (not studied); use with caution.

Hepatic Impairment No dosage adjustment provided in the manufacturer's labeling (not studied); use with caution.

Dietary Considerations
Food causes a slight delay in the absorption of the oral solution and bioavailability is increased by ~25%. Absorption of the extended release tablet is not affected by food. May be taken without regard to meals.

Administration

Oral: Administer without regard to meals. Extended release tablets must be swallowed whole with liquid; do not crush, divide, or chew; take at approximately the same time each day.

Topical gel: For topical use only. Apply to clean, dry, intact skin on abdomen, thighs, or upper arms/shoulders. Wash hands after use. Cover treated area with clothing after gel has dried to prevent transfer of medication to others. Do not bathe, shower, or swim until 1 hour after gel applied. Do not apply to recently shaved skin.

Gelnique 3%: Prior to initial use, press pump 4 times to prime pump; discard any gel dispensed from pump during priming. Rotate application sites to avoid skin irritation.

Gelnique 10%: Rotate site; do not apply to same site on consecutive days.

Transdermal: Apply to clean, dry skin on abdomen, hip, or buttock. Select a new site for each new system (avoid reapplication to same site within 7 days). Wear patch under clothing; do not expose to sunlight.

Monitoring Parameters
Incontinence episodes, postvoid residual (PVR)

Test Interactions
May suppress the wheal and flare reactions to skin test antigens.

Dosage Forms
Excipient information presented when available (limited, particularly for generics); consult specific product labeling. [DSC] = Discontinued product

Gel, Transdermal:
Gelnique: 3% (92 g) [contains propylene glycol]
Gel, Transdermal, as chloride:
Gelnique: 10% (1 g) [contains alcohol, usp]
Patch Twice Weekly, Transdermal:
Oxytrol: 3.9 mg/24 hr (1 ea, 2 ea, 4 ea, 8 ea)
Oxytrol For Women: 3.9 mg/24 hr (8 ea); 3.9 mg/24hr (4 ea)
Syrup, Oral, as chloride:
Generic: 5 mg/5 mL (5 mL [DSC], 473 mL)
Tablet, Oral, as chloride:
Generic: 5 mg
Tablet Extended Release 24 Hour, Oral, as chloride:
Ditropan XL: 5 mg, 10 mg, 15 mg [contains polysorbate 80]
Generic: 5 mg, 10 mg, 15 mg

♦ **Oxybutynin Chloride** see Oxybutynin on page 1355
♦ **Oxybutynine (Can)** see Oxybutynin on page 1355
♦ **Oxycodan® (Can)** see Oxycodone and Aspirin on page 1362

OxyCODONE (oks i KOE done)

Brand Names: US Oxaydo; Oxecta [DSC]; OxyCONTIN; Roxicodone

Brand Names: Canada ACT Oxycodone CR; Apo-Oxycodone CR; Oxy.IR; OxyNEO; PMS-Oxycodone; PMS-Oxycodone CR; Supeudol

Index Terms Dihydrohydroxycodeinone; Oxaydo; Oxecta; Oxycodone Hydrochloride

Pharmacologic Category Analgesic, Opioid

Additional Appendix Information
Opioid Conversion Table and Morphine Equivalent Dose Table on page 1955

Use

Pain management:
Immediate release formulations: Management of moderate to severe pain where the use of an opioid analgesic is appropriate.

Extended release formulation: Management of pain severe enough to require daily, around-the-clock, long-term opioid treatment and for which alternative treatment options are inadequate.

Limitations of use: Because of the risks of addiction, abuse, and misuse with opioids, even at recommended doses, and because of the greater risks of overdose and death with extended-release opioid formulations, reserve oxycodone ER for use in patients for whom alternative treatment options (eg, nonopioid analgesics, immediate-release opioids) are ineffective, not tolerated, or would be otherwise inadequate to provide sufficient management of pain. Oxycodone ER is not indicated as an as-needed analgesic.

Pregnancy Considerations
Adverse events were observed in some animal reproduction studies. Opioids cross the placenta. Oxycodone should not be used immediately prior to or during labor. The Canadian labeling contraindicates use in pregnant women and during labor and delivery.

[US Boxed Warning]: Prolonged maternal use of opioids during pregnancy can cause neonatal withdrawal syndrome in the newborn which may be life-threatening if not recognized and treated according to protocols developed by neonatology experts. If prolonged opioid therapy is required in a pregnant woman, ensure treatment is available and warn patient

of risk to the neonate. If chronic opioid exposure occurs in pregnancy, adverse events in the newborn (including withdrawal) may occur; monitoring of the neonate is recommended. The minimum effective dose should be used if opioids are needed (Chou 2009). Neonatal abstinence syndrome following opioid exposure may present with autonomic (eg, fever, temperature instability), gastrointestinal (eg, diarrhea, vomiting, poor feeding/weight gain), or neurologic (eg, high-pitched crying, increased muscle tone, irritability, seizure, tremor) symptoms (Dow 2012; Hudak 2012).

Long-term opioid use may cause secondary hypogonadism, which may lead to sexual dysfunction or infertility (Brennan 2013).

Breast-Feeding Considerations Oxycodone is excreted into breast milk. Breast-feeding is not recommended in the US labeling and contraindicated in the Canadian labeling. Sedation and/or respiratory depression may occur in the infant; symptoms of opioid withdrawal may occur following the cessation of breast-feeding. Nursing infants exposed to large doses of opioids should be monitored for apnea and sedation. Use caution in a woman who may be an ultra-rapid metabolizer; oxycodone is a substrate for CYP2D6 and their nursing infants may be at higher risk for adverse events (Montgomery 2012).

Prescribing and Access Restrictions As a requirement of the REMS program, healthcare providers who prescribe OxyContin need to receive training on the proper use and potential risks of OxyContin. For training, please refer to http://www.oxycontinrems.com.

Medication Guide Available Yes

Contraindications

Hypersensitivity to oxycodone or any component of the formulation; significant respiratory depression; hypercarbia; acute or severe bronchial asthma; paralytic ileus (known or suspected); GI obstruction

Canadian labeling: Additional contraindications (not in US labeling): Hypersensitivity to other opioids; suspected surgical abdomen (eg, acute appendicitis or pancreatitis); any disease/condition that affects bowel transit; mild pain that can be managed with other pain medications (immediate release); mild, intermittent or short duration pain that can be managed with other pain medications or acute pain (extended release); chronic obstructive airway; status asthmaticus; cor pulmonale; acute alcoholism; delirium tremens; convulsive disorders; severe CNS depression; increased cerebrospinal or intracranial pressure; head injury; monoamine oxidase (MAO) inhibitors (concomitant use or within 14 days of therapy); pregnant women or during labor and delivery; breast-feeding

Warnings/Precautions May cause CNS depression, which may impair physical or mental abilities; patients must be cautioned about performing tasks which require mental alertness (eg, operating machinery or driving). Potentially significant drug-drug interactions may exist, requiring dose or frequency adjustment, additional monitoring, and/or selection of alternative therapy. Use with caution in patients with hypersensitivity reactions to other phenanthrene derivative opioid agonists (morphine, hydrocodone, hydromorphone, levorphanol, oxymorphone). Use with caution in pancreatitis (contraindicated in Canadian labeling) or biliary tract disease, acute alcoholism (contraindicated in Canadian labeling) (including delirium tremens), morbid obesity, adrenocortical insufficiency, history of seizure disorders (contraindicated in Canadian labeling), hypothyroidism (including myxedema), prostatic hyperplasia, urethral stricture, and toxic psychosis. Use with caution and monitor for respiratory depression in patients with significant chronic obstructive pulmonary disease or cor pulmonale (contraindicated in Canadian labeling), and patients having a substantially decreased respiratory reserve, hypoxia, or preexisting respiratory depression, particularly when initiating therapy and titrating with oxycodone; even therapeutic doses may decrease respiratory drive to the point of apnea. Consider the use of alternative nonopioid analgesics in these patients. May obscure diagnosis or clinical course of patients with acute abdominal conditions. Avoid use in patients with CNS depression/coma as these patients are susceptible to intracranial effects of CO_2 retention.

Use with caution in the elderly, debilitated, or cachectic patients, and hepatic or renal dysfunction. Hemodynamic effects (hypotension, orthostasis) may be exaggerated in patients with hypovolemia, concurrent vasodilating drugs, or in patients with head injury. Monitor for symptoms of hypotension following initiation or dose titration. Respiratory depressant effects and capacity to elevate CSF pressure may be exaggerated in presence of head injury, other intracranial lesion, or preexisting intracranial pressure. May cause constipation which may be problematic in patients with unstable angina and patients post-myocardial infarction. Concurrent use of mixed agonist/antagonist analgesics (eg, pentazocine, nalbuphine, butorphanol) or partial agonist (eg, buprenorphine) analgesics may precipitate withdrawal symptoms and/or reduced analgesic efficacy in patients following prolonged therapy with mu opioid agonists. Use with caution in the perioperative setting; individualize treatment when transitioning from parenteral to oral analgesics. Taper dose gradually when discontinuing.

Extended release tablets: Therapy should only be prescribed by healthcare professionals familiar with the use of potent opioids for chronic pain. **[US Boxed Warning]: May cause serious, life-threatening, or fatal respiratory depression. Monitor closely for respiratory depression, especially during initiation or dose escalation. Patients should swallow tablets whole; crushing, chewing, or dissolving can cause rapid release and a potentially fatal dose.** Carbon dioxide retention from opioid-induced respiratory depression can exacerbate the sedating effects of opioids. **[US Boxed Warning]: Use with all CYP3A4 inhibitors may result in increased effects and potentially fatal respiratory depression. In addition, discontinuation of a concomitant CYP 3A4 inducer may result in increased oxycodone concentrations. Monitor patients receiving any CYP 3A4 inhibitor or inducer.** Tablets may be difficult to swallow and could become lodged in throat; patients with swallowing difficulties may be at increased risk. Cases of intestinal obstruction or diverticulitis exacerbation have also been reported, including cases requiring medical intervention to remove the tablet; patients with an underlying GI disease (eg, esophageal cancer, colon cancer) may be at increased risk. **[US Boxed Warning]: Users are exposed to the risks of addiction, abuse, and misuse, potentially leading to overdose and death. Assess each patient's risk prior to prescribing; monitor all patients regularly for development of these behaviors or conditions.** Risk of opioid abuse is increased in patients with a history or family history of alcohol or drug abuse or mental illness. **[US Boxed Warning]: Accidental ingestion of even one dose, especially in children, can result in a fatal overdose of oxycodone. [US Boxed Warning]: Prolonged maternal use of opioids during pregnancy can cause neonatal withdrawal syndrome in the newborn which may be life-threatening if not recognized and treated according to protocols developed by neonatology experts. If prolonged opioid therapy is required in a pregnant woman, ensure treatment is available and warn patient of risk to the neonate.** Signs and symptoms include irritability, hyperactivity and abnormal sleep pattern, high pitched cry, tremor, vomiting, diarrhea and failure to gain weight. Onset, duration and severity depend on the drug used, duration of use, maternal dose, and rate of drug elimination by the newborn.

Oral solutions: **[US Boxed Warning]: Highly concentrated oral solution (20 mg/mL) should only be used in opioid tolerant patients (taking ≥30 mg/day of oxycodone or equivalent for ≥1 week). [US Boxed Warning]: Orders for oxycodone oral solutions (20 mg/mL or 5 mg/5 mL) should be clearly written to include the intended dose (in mg vs mL) and the intended product concentration to be dispensed to avoid potential dosing errors. Products should be stored out of reach of children; seek immediate medical care in the event of accidental ingestion.**

Benzyl alcohol and derivatives: Some dosage forms may contain sodium benzoate/benzoic acid; benzoic acid (benzoate) is a metabolite of benzyl alcohol; large amounts of benzyl alcohol (≥99 mg/kg/day) have been associated with a potentially fatal toxicity ("gasping syndrome") in neonates; the "gasping syndrome" consists of metabolic acidosis, respiratory distress, gasping respirations, CNS dysfunction (including convulsions, intracranial hemorrhage), hypotension, and cardiovascular collapse (AAP ["Inactive" 1997]; CDC 1982); some data suggests that benzoate displaces bilirubin from protein binding sites (Ahlfors 2001); avoid or use dosage forms containing benzyl alcohol derivative with caution in neonates. See manufacturer's labeling.

Adverse Reactions Unless otherwise noted, frequency of adverse reactions is shown as reported for adult patients receiving OxyContin.

>10%:

Central nervous system: Drowsiness (children and adolescents 11 to 16 years 1% to <5%; adults 23%), headache (children and adolescents 11 to 16 years 14%), dizziness (children ≥11 years, adolescents, and adults 9% to 13%)

Dermatologic: Pruritus (children ≥11 years, adolescents, and adults 6% to 13%)

Gastrointestinal: Constipation (children and adolescents 11 to 16 years 9%; adults 23%), nausea (children ≥11 years, adolescents, and adults 15% to 23%), vomiting (children ≥11 years, adolescents, and adults 12% to 21%)

Miscellaneous: Fever (children ≥11 years, adolescents, and adults 1% to 11%)

1% to 10%:

Cardiovascular: Orthostatic hypotension (1% to 5%), oxygen saturation decreased (children and adolescents 11 to 16 years 1% to <5%), tachycardia (children and adolescents 11 to 16 years 1% to <5%)

Central nervous system: Abnormal dreams (1% to 5%), abnormality in thinking (1% to 5%), anxiety (children ≥11 years, adolescents, and adults 1% to 5%), chills (children and adolescents 11 to 16 years 1% to 5%), confusion (1% to 5%), dysphoria (1% to 5%), euphoria (1% to 5%), insomnia (children ≥11 years, adolescents, and adults 1% to 5%), nervousness (1% to 5%), twitching (1% to 5%), agitation (children and adolescents 1% to <5%; adults <1%), depression (children and adolescents 1% to <5%; adults <1%), fatigue (children and adolescents 11 to 16 years 1% to <5%), hypoesthesia (children and adolescents 1% to <5%; adults <1%), lethargy (children and adolescents 11 to 16 years 1% to <5%), pain (children and adolescents 11 to 16 years 1% to <5%), paresthesia (children and adolescents 1% to <5%; adults <1%), procedural pain (children and adolescents 11 to 16 years 1% to <5%)

Dermatologic: Diaphoresis (5%), hyperhidrosis (children and adolescents 11 to 16 years 1% to <5%), skin rash (children ≥11 years, adolescents, and adults 1% to 5%)

Endocrine & metabolic: Hypochloremia (children and adolescents 11 to 16 years 1% to <5%), hyponatremia (children and adolescents 11 to 16 years 1% to <5%), weight loss (children and adolescents 11 to 16 years 1% to <5%)

Gastrointestinal: Xerostomia (6%), diarrhea (children ≥11 years, adolescents, and adults 1% to 6%), decreased appetite (children and adolescents 11 to 16 years 5%), abdominal pain (children ≥11 years, adolescents, and adults 1% to 5%), anorexia (1% to 5%), dyspepsia (1% to 5%), gastritis (1% to 5%), hiccups (1% to 5%), gastroesophageal reflux disease (children and adolescents 11 to 16 years 1% to <5%)

Genitourinary: Dysuria (children and adolescents 1% to <5%; adults <1%), urinary retention

Hematologic & oncologic: Decreased hemoglobin (children and adolescents 11 to 16 years 1% to <5%), decreased neutrophils (children and adolescents 11 to 16 years 1% to <5%), decreased platelet count (children and adolescents 11 to 16 years 1% to <5%), decreased red blood cells (children and adolescents 11 to 16 years 1% to <5%), febrile neutropenia (children and adolescents 11 to 16 years 1% to <5%), neutropenia (children and adolescents 11 to 16 years 1% to <5%)

Hepatic: Increased serum ALT (children and adolescents 11 to 16 years 1% to <5%)

Neuromuscular & skeletal: Weakness (children ≥11 years, adolescents, and adults 1% to 6%), limb pain (children and adolescents 11 to 16 years 1% to <5%), musculoskeletal pain (children and adolescents 11 to 16 years 1% to <5%)

Respiratory: Dyspnea (1% to 5%), oropharyngeal pain (children and adolescents 11 to 16 years 1% to <5%)

Miscellaneous: Seroma (children and adolescents 11 to 16 years 1% to <5%)

<1% (Limited to important or life-threatening): Abnormal stools (tablet in stool [some controlled release dosage forms]), amnesia, anaphylactoid reaction, chest pain, depression, depression of ST segment on ECG, diverticulitis (exacerbation), dysphagia (or other swallowing difficulties due to properties of controlled release tablets), edema (including facial and peripheral), emotional lability, hallucination, hematuria, histamine release, hyperalgesia, hyperkinesia, hypogonadism (Brennan 2013; Debono 2011), hyponatremia, hypotonia, increased intracranial pressure, intestinal obstruction, seizure, SIADH, speech disturbance, stomatitis, stupor, suicidal ideation, suicidal tendencies, syncope, urinary retention, withdrawal syndrome pressure, intestinal obstruction, malaise, paresthesia, seizure, SIADH, speech disturbance, stomatitis, stupor, syncope, urinary retention, withdrawal syndrome

Drug Interactions

Metabolism/Transport Effects Substrate of CYP2D6 (minor), CYP3A4 (major); **Note:** Assignment of Major/Minor substrate status based on clinically relevant drug interaction potential

Avoid Concomitant Use

Avoid concomitant use of OxyCODONE with any of the following: Azelastine (Nasal); Conivaptan; Eluxadoline; Fusidic Acid (Systemic); Idelalisib; Mixed Agonist / Antagonist Opioids; Orphenadrine; Paraldehyde; Thalidomide

Increased Effect/Toxicity

OxyCODONE may increase the levels/effects of: Alcohol (Ethyl); Alvimopan; Azelastine (Nasal); CNS Depressants; Desmopressin; Diuretics; Eluxadoline; Hydrocodone; Methotrimeprazine; Metyrosine; Mirtazapine; Orphenadrine; Paraldehyde; Pramipexole; Ramosetron; ROPINIRole; Rotigotine; Selective Serotonin Reuptake Inhibitors; Suvorexant; Thalidomide; Zolpidem

The levels/effects of OxyCODONE may be increased by: Amphetamines; Anticholinergic Agents; Antipsychotic Agents (Phenothiazines); Brimonidine (Topical); Cannabis; Conivaptan; CYP3A4 Inhibitors (Moderate); CYP3A4 Inhibitors (Strong); Dasatinib; Doxylamine; Dronabinol; Droperidol; Fosaprepitant; Fusidic Acid (Systemic); HydrOXYzine; Idelalisib; Ivacaftor; Kava Kava; Luliconazole; Magnesium Sulfate; MAO Inhibitors; Methotrimeprazine; Mifepristone; Minocycline; Nabilone; Osimertinib; Palbociclib; Perampanel; Rufinamide; Simeprevir; Sodium Oxybate; Stiripentol; Succinylcholine; Tapentadol; Tetrahydrocannabinol; Voriconazole

Decreased Effect

OxyCODONE may decrease the levels/effects of: Pegvisomant

The levels/effects of OxyCODONE may be decreased by: Ammonium Chloride; Bosentan; CYP3A4 Inducers (Moderate); CYP3A4 Inducers (Strong); Dabrafenib; Deferasirox; Enzalutamide; Mitotane; Mixed Agonist / Antagonist Opioids; Naltrexone; Osimertinib; Rifampin; Siltuximab; St Johns Wort; Tocilizumab

Storage/Stability Store at 25°C (77°F); excursions permitted between 15°C to 30°C (59°F to 86°F). Protect from light.

Mechanism of Action Binds to opiate receptors in the CNS, causing inhibition of ascending pain pathways, altering the perception of and response to pain; produces generalized CNS depression

Pharmacodynamics/Kinetics

Onset of action: Pain relief: Immediate release: 10 to 15 minutes

Peak effect: Immediate release: 0.5 to 1 hour

Duration: Immediate release: 3 to 6 hours; Extended release: ≤12 hours

Distribution: V_d: 2.6 L/kg; distributed to skeletal muscle, liver, intestinal tract, lungs, spleen, and brain

Protein binding: ~45%

Metabolism: Hepatically via CYP3A4 to noroxycodone (has weak analgesic), noroxymorphone, and alpha- and beta-noroxycodol. CYP2D6 mediated metabolism produces oxymorphone (has analgesic activity; low plasma concentrations), alpha- and beta-oxymorphol.

Bioavailability: Extended release, immediate release: 60% to 87%

Half-life elimination: Immediate release: 2 to 4 hours; Extended release: ~5 hours

Time to peak, plasma: Immediate release: 1.2 to 1.9 hours; Extended release: 4 to 5 hours

Excretion: Urine (~19% as parent; >64% as metabolites)

Dosing

Adult Pain management: Oral: **Note:** All doses should be titrated to appropriate effect. Reduced initial doses may be necessary in patients with adrenocortical insufficiency (eg, Addison disease), hypothyroidism, myxedema, severe respiratory impairment, toxic psychosis, prostatic hypertrophy or urethral stricture:

Immediate release: Initial: 5 to 15 mg every 4 to 6 hours as needed; dosing range: 5 to 20 mg per dose (APS 6th edition). For severe chronic pain, administer on a regularly scheduled basis, every 4 to 6 hours, at the lowest dose that will achieve adequate analgesia.

Extended release: **Note:** Oxycodone ER 60 mg and 80 mg strengths, a single dose >40 mg, or a total dose of >80 mg daily are for use only in opioid-tolerant patients. Opioid tolerance is defined as: Patients already taking at least 60 mg of oral morphine daily, 25 mcg of transdermal fentanyl per hour, 30 mg of oral oxycodone daily, 8 mg oral hydromorphone daily, or an equivalent dose of another opioid for at least 1 week.

Opioid naive (use as the first opioid analgesic or use in patients who are **not** opioid tolerant): Initial: 10 mg every 12 hours

Conversion from other oral oxycodone formulations to extended release oxycodone: Initiate extended release oxycodone with one-half the total daily oral oxycodone daily dose (mg/day) administered every 12 hours.

Conversion from other opioids to extended release oxycodone:

US labeling: Discontinue all other around-the-clock opioids when extended release oxycodone is initiated. Initiate with 10 mg every 12 hours. Substantial interpatient variability exists in relative potency. Therefore, it is safer to underestimate a patient's daily oral oxycodone requirement and provide breakthrough pain relief with rescue medication (eg, immediate release opioid) than to overestimate requirements.

Canadian labeling: Discontinue all other around-the-clock opioids when extended release oxycodone is initiated. Determine oral oxycodone equivalent daily dose (refer to manufacturer labeling for equivalent dosing conversion). Divide total daily oxycodone dose into 2 equal doses and administer every 12 hours.

Conversion from transdermal fentanyl to extended release oxycodone: For each 25 mcg/hour transdermal dose, substitute 10 mg extended release oxycodone every 12 hours; should be initiated 18 hours after the removal of the transdermal fentanyl patch

Conversion from methadone to extended release oxycodone: Close monitoring is required when converting methadone to another opioid. Ratio between methadone and other opioid agonists varies widely according to previous dose exposure. Methadone has a long half-life and can accumulate in the plasma.

Conversion from fixed-dose oxycodone/nonopioid combinations to extended release oxycodone: *Canadian labeling:*

If previous total daily dose of oxycodone in combination product was 5 to 25 mg, begin oxycodone extended release 10 to 20 mg every 12 hours.

If previous total daily dose of oxycodone in combination product was 30 to 45 mg, begin oxycodone extended release 20 to 30 mg every 12 hours.

If previous total daily dose of oxycodone in combination product was 50 to 60 mg, begin oxycodone extended release 30 to 40 mg every 12 hours.

If previous total daily dose of oxycodone in combination product was >60 mg, base dose on total daily dose of oxycodone.

Dose adjustment: Doses may be adjusted every 1 to 2 days; the total daily oxycodone dose may be increased by 25% to 50%. The total daily dose should be administered in divided doses every 12 hours. **Note:** Some clinicians have reported that in certain chronic pain patients, more frequent dosing (ie, every 8 hours) is required for effective pain relief (Gallagher 2007; Marcus 2004; Nicholson 2006), although dosing more frequently than every 12 hours is not recommended by the manufacturer, and safety and efficacy has not been established.

Dosage adjustment for concomitant therapy: Concomitant CNS depressants: Reduce usual initial oxycodone dose by 33% to 50%.

Discontinuation of therapy:

US labeling:

Immediate release: Decrease previous daily dose by 25% to 50% each day; monitor for signs/symptoms of withdrawal. If patient displays withdrawal symptoms, increase dose to previous dose and then reduce dose more slowly by increasing interval between dose reductions, decreasing amount of daily dose reduction, or both.

Extended release: Gradually titrate dose downward to prevent withdrawal signs/symptoms. Do not abruptly discontinue.

Canadian labeling: Decrease previous daily dose by 50% (administer in divided doses every 6 hours for 2 days [immediate release] or every 12 hours for 2 days [extended release]), then decrease dose by 25% every 2 days.

Dosage adjustment in debilitated patients (nonopioid tolerant):

Immediate release: Initial

US labeling: There are no dosage adjustments provided in the manufacturer's labeling; use caution.

Canadian labeling: There are no specific dosage adjustments provided in the manufacturer's labeling; however, a reduced dosage is recommended; use caution.

Extended release: Initial:

US labeling: Decrease dose by 33% to 50% of usual starting dose

Canadian labeling: There are no specific dosage adjustments provided in the manufacturer's labeling; however, a reduced dosage is recommended; use caution.

Geriatric Refer to adult dosing. Initiate therapy at low end of dosing range and use caution.

Pediatric Pain management: Children (off-label use): Oral: Immediate release, initial dose: 0.1 to 0.2 mg/kg/dose (moderate pain) or 0.2 mg/kg/dose (severe pain) (APS 6th edition). For severe chronic pain, administer on a regularly scheduled basis, every 4 to 6 hours, at the lowest dose that will achieve adequate analgesia.

Renal Impairment

US labeling: There are no dosage adjustments provided in the manufacturer's labeling. Serum concentrations are increased ~50% in patients with CrCl <60 mL/minute; adjust dose as clinically indicated.

Canadian labeling: Initial: Decrease dose to 33% to 50% of usual initial dose; titrate carefully.

Hepatic Impairment

Immediate release:

US labeling: Reduced initial doses may be necessary (use a conservative approach to initial dosing); adjust dose based on clinical situation.

Canadian labeling: Initial: Decrease dose to 33% to 50% of usual initial dose; titrate carefully.

Extended release: Initial: Decrease dose to 33% to 50% of usual starting dose; titrate carefully.

Dietary Considerations Instruct patient to avoid high-fat meals when taking some products (food has no effect on the reformulated OxyContin).

Administration Oral:

Extended release: **For oral use only.** Swallow tablet whole. Do not moisten, dissolve, cut, crush, break, or chew extended release tablets. Extended release tablets should be administered one at a time and each followed with water immediately after placing in the mouth. The Canadian labeling does not recommend administering via feeding tubes (eg, gastric, NG) due to potential for obstruction. The US labeling does not provide recommendations regarding administration via feeding tubes.

Immediate release: **For oral use only.** Must be swallowed whole with enough water to ensure complete swallowing immediately after placing in the mouth. The tablet should not be wet prior to placing in the mouth. Do not crush, chew, or dissolve the tablets. Oxecta product labeling does not recommend administering via feeding tubes (eg, gastric, NG) due to potential for obstruction. The formulation uses technology designed to discourage common methods of tampering to prevent misuse/abuse.

Appropriate laxatives should be administered to avoid the constipating side effects associated with use. Antiemetics may be needed for persistent nausea.

Monitoring Parameters Pain relief, respiratory and mental status, blood pressure; signs of misuse, abuse, and addiction; signs or symptoms of hypogonadism or hypoadrenalism (Brennan 2013)

Test Interactions Some quinolones may produce a false-positive urine screening result for opioids using commercially-available immunoassay kits. This has been demonstrated most consistently for levofloxacin and ofloxacin, but other quinolones have shown cross-reactivity in certain assay kits. Confirmation of positive opioid screens by more specific methods should be considered.

Additional Information Oxecta utilizes Acura Pharmaceutical's Aversion® technology which may help discourage misuse and abuse potential. Reduced abuse potential of Oxecta compared to other immediate-release oxycodone tablet formulations has not been proven; the FDA is requiring Pfizer to complete a post-approval epidemiological study to determine whether the formulation actually results in a decrease of misuse/abuse. In one clinical trial in nondependent recreational opioid users, the "drug-liking" responses and safety of crushed Oxecta tablets were compared to crushed immediate-release oxycodone tablets following the self-administered intranasal use. A small difference in "drug-liking" scores was observed, with lower scores reported in the crushed Oxecta group. In regards to safety, there was an increased incidence of nasopharyngeal and facial adverse events in the Oxecta group. In addition, there was decreased ability in the Oxecta group to completely administer the two crushed Oxecta tablets intranasally within a set time period. However, whether these differences translate into a significant clinical difference is unknown. Of note, pharmacokinetic studies showed that Oxecta is bioequivalent with oxycodone immediate-release tablets with no differences in T_{max} and half-life when administered in the fasted state.

Product Availability

Oxaydo: FDA approved immediate-release oxycodone product formulated to discourage abuse via snorting; availability anticipated in the third quarter of 2015.

Oxaydo is indicated for the management of acute and chronic moderate to severe pain where the use of an opioid analgesic is appropriate. Oxaydo is formerly known as Oxecta (Pfizer).

Dosage Forms Excipient information presented when available (limited, particularly for generics); consult specific product labeling. [DSC] = Discontinued product

Capsule, Oral, as hydrochloride:
Generic: 5 mg
Concentrate, Oral, as hydrochloride:
Generic: 20 mg/mL (30 mL); 100 mg/5 mL (15 mL, 30 mL)
Solution, Oral, as hydrochloride:
Generic: 5 mg/5 mL (5 mL, 15 mL, 473 mL, 500 mL)
Tablet, Oral, as hydrochloride:
Roxicodone: 5 mg [DSC]
Roxicodone: 5 mg [scored]
Roxicodone: 15 mg [scored; contains fd&c blue #2 (indigotine), fd&c yellow #10 (quinoline yellow)]
Roxicodone: 30 mg [DSC]
Roxicodone: 30 mg [scored]
Generic: 5 mg, 10 mg, 15 mg, 20 mg, 30 mg
Tablet Abuse-Deterrent, Oral, as hydrochloride:
Oxaydo: 5 mg, 7.5 mg
Oxecta: 5 mg [DSC], 7.5 mg [DSC]
Tablet ER 12 Hour Abuse-Deterrent, Oral, as hydrochloride:
OxyCONTIN: 10 mg, 15 mg, 20 mg, 30 mg, 40 mg, 60 mg
OxyCONTIN: 80 mg [contains fd&c blue #2 aluminum lake]
Generic: 10 mg, 20 mg, 40 mg, 80 mg

Dosage Forms: Canada Note: Refer also to Dosage Forms. Excipient information presented when available (limited, particularly for generics); consult specific product labeling.

Tablet, Oral, as hydrochloride:
Oxy IR: 5 mg, 10 mg, 20 mg
Supeudol: 5 mg, 10 mg, 20 mg
Tablet Controlled Release, Oral, as hydrochloride
OxyNeo: 10 mg, 15 mg, 20 mg, 30 mg, 40 mg, 60 mg, 80 mg

Controlled Substance C-II

Oxycodone and Acetaminophen
(oks i KOE done & a seet a MIN oh fen)

Brand Names: US Endocet; Percocet; Primlev; Roxicet; Xartemis XR; Xolox [DSC]
Brand Names: Canada Apo-Oxycodone/Acet; Endocet; Percocet; Percocet-Demi; PMS-Oxycodone-Acetaminophen; Ratio-Oxycocet; Rivacocet; Sandoz-Oxycodone/Acetaminophen
Index Terms Acetaminophen and Oxycodone; Tylox
Pharmacologic Category Analgesic Combination (Opioid); Analgesic, Opioid
Use
Acute pain (extended-release): Management of acute pain severe enough to require opioid treatment and for which alternative treatment options are inadequate.
Limitations of use: Because of the risks of addiction, abuse, misuse, overdose, and death with opioids, even at recommended doses, reserve extended-release (ER) for use in patients for whom alternative treatment options (eg, nonopioid analgesics) are ineffective, not tolerated, or would be otherwise inadequate.
Moderate to moderately severe pain (immediate release): Management of moderate to moderately-severe pain
Medication Guide Available Yes
Dosing
Adult Note: Initial dose is based on the **oxycodone** content; however, the maximum daily dose is based on the **acetaminophen** content.

Extended-release: Acute pain: Oral: Usual dose: 2 tablets every 12 hours; the second initial dose may be administered as early as 8 hours after the first initial dose if needed; subsequent doses are to be administered 2 tablets every 12 hours. Do not exceed acetaminophen 4 g daily. **NOTE:** Oxycodone/acetaminophen ER is not interchangeable with other oxycodone/acetaminophen products because of differing pharmacokinetic profiles that affect the frequency of administration.
Discontinuation: Do not stop abruptly in patients who may be physically dependent gradually decrease the dose by 50% every 2 to 4 days to prevent signs and symptoms of withdrawal.

Immediate release: Management of pain: Oral: Doses should be titrated to appropriate analgesic effects.
Manufacturer's labeling: Moderate to moderately severe pain: Initial dose, **based on oxycodone content**: 2.5-10 mg every 6 hours as needed. Titrate according to pain severity and individual response. Do not exceed acetaminophen 4 g daily.

Alternate recommendations (APS, 2008):
Moderate pain (off-label): Initial dose, **based on oxycodone content**: 5 mg. Doses typically given every 4-6 hours as needed; manufacturer's labeling recommends every 6 hours as needed. Do not exceed acetaminophen 4 g daily.
Severe pain (off-label): Initial dose, **based on oxycodone content**: 10-20 mg. Doses typically given every 4-6 hours as needed; manufacturer's labeling recommends every 6 hours as needed. Do not exceed acetaminophen 4 g daily.
Geriatric Management of pain: Oral:
No dosage adjustment provided in manufacturer's labeling; however, use with caution and consider decreasing the initial dose and/or increasing the frequency.
Severe pain (off-label dosing): **Immediate release:** Elderly >70 years: Consider decreasing the initial dose **(based on oxycodone content)** by 25% to 50%, then titrating the dose upward or downward as needed; monitor frequently during titration. Do not exceed acetaminophen 4 g daily (APS, 2008).
Pediatric Note: Initial dose is based on the **oxycodone** content; however, the maximum daily dose is based on the **acetaminophen** content.
Management of pain: Children and Adolescents (off-label; American Pain Society [APS], 2008): Oral: **Immediate-release:** Doses should be titrated to appropriate analgesic effects:
Moderate pain: Initial dose, based on oxycodone content: 0.1-0.2 mg/kg/dose. Doses typically given every 4-6 hours as needed; manufacturer's labeling recommends every 6 hours as needed; maximum initial oxycodone dose: 5 mg/dose. Do not exceed maximum daily acetaminophen dose: Children <45 kg: 90 mg/kg/day; Children ≥45 kg: 4000 mg daily
Severe pain: Initial dose, **based on oxycodone content**: 0.2 mg/kg/dose. Doses typically given every 4-6 hours as needed; manufacturer's labeling recommends every 6 hours as needed; maximum initial oxycodone dose: 10 mg. Do not exceed maximum daily acetaminophen dose: Children <45 kg: 90 mg/kg/day; Children ≥45 kg: 4000 mg daily
Renal Impairment
Extended-release: Initial dose: One tablet every 12 hours; adjust dose as needed.
Immediate-release: There are no dosage adjustments provided in manufacturer's labeling. Use with caution; reduced clearance in severe impairment may require dosage adjustment.
Hepatic Impairment
Extended-release: Initial dose: One tablet every 12 hours; adjust dose as needed.
Immediate-release: There are no dosage adjustments provided in manufacturer's labeling. Use with caution; reduced clearance in severe impairment may require dosage adjustment.
Additional Information Complete prescribing information should be consulted for additional detail.
Dosage Forms Excipient information presented when available (limited, particularly for generics); consult specific product labeling. [DSC] = Discontinued product
Capsule, Oral: 5/500: Oxycodone hydrochloride 5 mg and acetaminophen 500 mg [DSC]
Solution, Oral:
Roxicet: Oxycodone hydrochloride 5 mg and acetaminophen 325 mg per 5 mL (5 mL, 500 mL) [contains ethanol <0.5%; mint flavor]
Tablet, Oral: 2.5/325: Oxycodone hydrochloride 2.5 mg and acetaminophen 325 mg; 5/325: Oxycodone hydrochloride 5 mg and acetaminophen 325 mg; 7.5/325: Oxycodone hydrochloride 7.5 mg and acetaminophen 325 mg; 7.5/500: Oxycodone hydrochloride 7.5 mg and acetaminophen 500 mg [DSC]; 10/325: Oxycodone hydrochloride 10 mg and acetaminophen 325 mg; 10/650: Oxycodone hydrochloride 10 mg and acetaminophen 650 mg [DSC]
Endocet 2.5/325: Oxycodone hydrochloride 2.5 mg and acetaminophen 325 mg
Endocet 5/325 [scored]: Oxycodone hydrochloride 5 mg and acetaminophen 325 mg
Endocet 7.5/325: Oxycodone hydrochloride 7.5 mg and acetaminophen 325 mg
Endocet 7.5/500: Oxycodone hydrochloride 7.5 mg and acetaminophen 500 mg [DSC]
Endocet 10/325: Oxycodone hydrochloride 10 mg and acetaminophen 325 mg
Endocet 10/650: Oxycodone hydrochloride 10 mg and acetaminophen 650 mg [DSC]
Magnacet 5/400: Oxycodone hydrochloride 5 mg and acetaminophen 400 mg [DSC]
Magnacet 7.5/400: Oxycodone hydrochloride 7.5 mg and acetaminophen 400 mg [DSC]

Magnacet 10/400: Oxycodone hydrochloride 10 mg and acetaminophen 400 mg [DSC]

Percocet 2.5/325: Oxycodone hydrochloride 2.5 mg and acetaminophen 325 mg

Percocet 5/325 [scored]: Oxycodone hydrochloride 5 mg and acetaminophen 325 mg

Percocet 7.5/325: Oxycodone hydrochloride 7.5 mg and acetaminophen 325 mg

Percocet 7.5/500: Oxycodone hydrochloride 7.5 mg and acetaminophen 500 mg [DSC]

Percocet 10/325: Oxycodone hydrochloride 10 mg and acetaminophen 325 mg

Percocet 10/650: Oxycodone hydrochloride 10 mg and acetaminophen 650 mg [DSC]

Primlev 5/300: Oxycodone hydrochloride 5 mg and acetaminophen 300 mg

Primlev 7.5/300: Oxycodone hydrochloride 7.5 mg and acetaminophen 300 mg

Primlev 10/300: Oxycodone hydrochloride 10 mg and acetaminophen 300 mg

Roxicet 5/325 [scored]: Oxycodone hydrochloride 5 mg and acetaminophen 325 mg

Tablet, Extended Release, Oral:

Xartemis XR: Oxycodone hydrochloride 7.5 mg and acetaminophen 325 mg

Controlled Substance C-II

Oxycodone and Aspirin (oks i KOE done & AS pir in)

Brand Names: US Endodan; Percodan

Brand Names: Canada Endodan®; Oxycodan®; Percodan®

Index Terms Aspirin and Oxycodone

Pharmacologic Category Analgesic Combination (Opioid); Analgesic, Opioid

Use Management of moderate- to moderately-severe pain

Dosing

Adult & Geriatric Analgesic: Oral: One tablet every 6 hours as needed for pain; maximum aspirin dose should not exceed 4 g/day.

Pediatric Analgesic: Oral (dose based on total oxycodone content): Oxycodone 0.1-0.2 mg/kg/dose (maximum oxycodone: 5 mg/dose; maximum aspirin: 4 g/day). Doses should be given every 4-6 hours as needed (American Pain Society, 2008).

Renal Impairment Use with caution. Avoid use of aspirin in patients with CrCl <10 mL/minute.

Hepatic Impairment Use with caution. Avoid use of aspirin-containing products in severe impairment.

Additional Information Complete prescribing information should be consulted for additional detail.

Dosage Forms Excipient information presented when available (limited, particularly for generics); consult specific product labeling.

Tablet, Oral:

Endodan: Oxycodone hydrochloride 4.8355 mg and aspirin 325 mg [scored]

Percodan: Oxycodone hydrochloride 4.8355 mg and aspirin 325 mg [scored]

Generic: Oxycodone hydrochloride 4.8355 mg and aspirin 325 mg

Controlled Substance C-II

Oxycodone and Ibuprofen
(oks i KOE done & eye byoo PROE fen)

Index Terms Combunox; Ibuprofen and Oxycodone

Pharmacologic Category Analgesic Combination (Opioid); Analgesic, Opioid; Nonsteroidal Anti-inflammatory Drug (NSAID), Oral

Use Pain: Short-term (≤7 days) management of acute, moderate-to-severe pain

Medication Guide Available Yes

Dosing

Adult & Geriatric Pain: Oral: One oxycodone 5 mg/ibuprofen 400 mg tablet as needed (maximum: oxycodone 20 mg/ibuprofen 1600 mg per 24 hours); do not take for longer than 7 days

Pediatric Pain: Adolescents ≥14 years: Refer to adult dosing

Renal Impairment There are no dosage adjustments provided in the manufacturer's labeling (has not been studied). Not recommended in advanced renal disease.

Hepatic Impairment There are no dosage adjustments provided in the manufacturer's labeling (has not been studied).

Additional Information Complete prescribing information should be consulted for additional detail.

Dosage Forms Excipient information presented when available (limited, particularly for generics); consult specific product labeling.

Tablet: Oxycodone hydrochloride 5 mg and ibuprofen 400 mg

Controlled Substance C-II

Oxycodone and Naloxone
(oks i KOE done & nal OKS one)

Brand Names: Canada Targin

Index Terms Naloxone and Oxycodone; Oxycodone Hydrochloride and Naloxone Hydrochloride; Targiniq ER

Pharmacologic Category Analgesic, Opioid; Opioid Antagonist

Use

Pain: Management of moderate to severe pain requiring daily, around-the-clock, long-term opioid treatment and for which alternative treatment options are inadequate

Limitations of use: Reserve for use in patients whom alternative treatment options (eg, nonopioid analgesics or immediate-release opioids) are ineffective, not tolerated, or would be otherwise inadequate to provide sufficient management of pain. Not indicated as an as-needed analgesic; do not exceed recommended doses because higher doses may be associated with symptoms of opioid withdrawal or decreased analgesia.

Canadian labeling: Additional uses (not in U.S. labeling): Relief of opioid-induced constipation in patients who require an opioid

Pregnancy Considerations Animal reproduction studies have not been conducted with this combination. The Canadian labeling contraindicates use of this combination product during pregnancy and during labor and delivery. Also see individual agents.

Breast-Feeding Considerations Oxycodone is excreted in breast milk; it is not known if naloxone is excreted in breast milk. Breast feeding is not recommended by the manufacturer. The Canadian labeling contraindicates use of this combination product in nursing women. Also see individual agents.

Medication Guide Available Yes

Contraindications

Hypersensitivity to oxycodone, naloxone, or any component of the formulation; significant respiratory depression; acute or severe bronchial asthma in an unmonitored setting or in the absence of resuscitative equipment; known or suspected paralytic ileus and GI obstruction; moderate-to-severe hepatic impairment

Canadian labeling: Additional contraindications (not in U.S. labeling): Hypersensitivity to other opioids; rectal administration; suspected surgical abdomen (eg, acute appendicitis or pancreatitis); mild, intermittent, or short duration pain that can be managed with other pain medications; management of acute pain, including use in outpatient or day surgeries; management of perioperative pain; cor pulmonale; acute alcoholism, delirium tremens, and convulsive disorders; severe CNS depression, increased cerebrospinal or intracranial pressure, and head injury; concurrent use or use within 14 days of monoamine oxidase (MAO) inhibitors; opioid-dependent patients and for narcotic withdrawal treatment; use in women who are breast-feeding, pregnant, or during labor and delivery

Warnings/Precautions [U.S. Boxed Warning]: Serious, life-threatening, or fatal respiratory depression may occur with use of oxycodone/naloxone ER. Monitor for respiratory depression, especially during initiation of therapy or following a dose increase. To reduce the risk of respiratory depression, proper dosing and titration is essential. Overestimating the oxycodone/naloxone ER dose when converting patients from another opioid product can result in fatal overdose with the first dose.

[U.S. Boxed Warning]: Accidental ingestion of even one dose of oxycodone/naloxone ER, especially in children, can result in a fatal overdose of oxycodone.

[U.S. Boxed Warning]: Oxycodone/naloxone ER exposes patients and other users to the risks of opioid addiction, abuse, and misuse, which can lead to overdose and death. Assess each patient's risk prior to prescribing oxycodone/naloxone ER, and monitor all patients regularly for the development of these behaviors or conditions. Crushing, chewing, or dissolving the product can cause rapid release and absorption of a potentially fatal dose of oxycodone. Use with caution in patients with a history of drug abuse, acute alcoholism, or mental illness (eg, major depression); potential for drug dependency exists. Tolerance, psychological, and physical dependence may occur with prolonged use.

[U.S. Boxed Warning]: Concomitant use of oxycodone/ naloxone ER with CYP450 3A4 inhibitors may result in an increase in oxycodone plasma concentrations, which could increase or prolong adverse drug effects and may cause potentially fatal respiratory depression. In addition, discontinuation of a concomitantly used CYP450 3A4 inducer may result in an increase in oxycodone plasma concentration. Monitor patients receiving oxycodone/naloxone ER and any CYP3A4 inhibitor or inducer. Potentially significant interactions may exist requiring dose or frequency adjustment, additional monitoring, and/or selection of alternative therapy.

[U.S. Boxed Warning]: Prolonged use of oxycodone/ naloxone ER during pregnancy can result in neonatal opioid withdrawal syndrome, which may be life-threatening if not recognized and requires management according to protocols developed by neonatology experts. If opioid use is required for a prolonged period in a pregnant woman, advise the patient of the risk of neonatal opioid withdrawal syndrome and ensure appropriate treatment will be available.

Tablets must be swallowed whole; tablets that are broken, crushed, chewed, or dissolved may result in a rapid release and absorption of a potentially fatal dose of oxycodone. Do not exceed maximum recommended doses and limit use to patients in whom alternative treatment options (eg, nonopioid analgesics or immediate-release opioids) are ineffective, not tolerated, or otherwise inadequate to provide sufficient pain relief. Not indicated as an as-needed analgesic. Limit use of the 40 mg/20 mg tablet dosage form to patients with established tolerance to an opioid of comparable potency **(single doses >40 mg or daily doses >80 mg of oxycodone may cause fatal respiratory depression in patients who are not tolerant to the respiratory depressant effects of opioids)**. The Canadian labeling contraindicates rectal administration of this combination product and also does not indicate use in patients with cancer associated with peritoneal carcinomatosis or with sub-occlusive syndrome in advanced stages of pelvic and digestive cancer (not studied).

May cause CNS depression, which may impair physical or mental abilities; patients must be cautioned about performing tasks which require mental alertness (eg, operating machinery or driving). Use with extreme caution in patients with head injury, intracranial lesions, or elevated intracranial pressure; exaggerated elevation of ICP may occur. Avoid use in patients with impaired consciousness or coma.

May cause severe hypotension (including orthostatic hypotension and syncope); use with caution in patients with hypovolemia, cardiovascular disease (including acute MI), or drugs which may exaggerate hypotensive effects (including phenothiazines or general anesthetics). Monitor for symptoms of hypotension following initiation or dose titration; dose adjustment may be warranted. Avoid use in patients with circulatory shock.

Use with caution in patients with adrenocortical insufficiency, biliary tract impairment, pancreatitis, prostatic hyperplasia and/or urinary stricture, history of seizure disorders, thyroid dysfunction, toxic psychosis, and those who are morbidly obese. Use with caution in patients with preexisting respiratory compromise (hypoxia and/or hypercapnia), COPD or other obstructive pulmonary disease, and kyphoscoliosis or other skeletal disorder which may alter respiratory function; critical respiratory depression may occur, even at therapeutic dosages. Use with caution in debilitated patients and in the elderly; there is a greater potential for respiratory depression, even at therapeutic dosages.

Use with caution in patients with mild hepatic dysfunction; use is contraindicated with moderate-to-severe hepatic impairment. Use with caution in patients with renal dysfunction. May obscure diagnosis or clinical course of patients with acute abdominal conditions. Naloxone may cause diarrhea; patients should be instructed to report severe or persistent diarrhea lasting >3 days.

Opioids decrease bowel motility; monitor for decrease bowel motility in postoperative patients receiving opioids. The Canadian labeling contraindicates perioperative use (24 hours before or after surgery) of oxycodone/naloxone ER. Patients interrupting therapy to undergo pain-relieving procedures (eg, chordotomy) may require a dosage adjustment when resuming therapy after the postoperative recovery period.

Concurrent use of agonist/antagonist analgesics may precipitate withdrawal symptoms and/or reduced analgesic efficacy in patients following prolonged therapy with mu opioid agonists. Abrupt discontinuation following prolonged use may also lead to withdrawal symptoms. Do not abruptly stop oxycodone/naloxone ER; gradually decrease dose to prevent signs and symptoms of withdrawal.

Adverse Reactions
1% to 10%:
Cardiovascular: Peripheral edema (2% to 5%)
Central nervous system: Withdrawal syndrome (7%), fatigue (5%), headache (5%), depression (2%), dizziness (2%), drowsiness (1%), migraine (1%)
Dermatologic: Hyperhidrosis (7%), skin rash (1%)
Endocrine & metabolic: Increased serum glucose (2%), hyperglycemia (1%), hyperlipidemia (1%), hyperuricemia (1%), increased gamma-glutamyl transferase (1%)
Gastrointestinal: Nausea (3% to 8%), abdominal pain (<1% to 8%), anorexia (<1% to 8%), constipation (3% to 7%), vomiting (1% to 7%), xerostomia (3%), abdominal distention (2%), diarrhea (2%), gastroenteritis (2%)
Genitourinary: Urinary tract infection (4%)
Hematologic & oncologic: Anemia (5%), decreased hemoglobin (≤5%)
Infection: Viral infection (2%), influenza (1%)
Neuromuscular & skeletal: Weakness (7%), osteoarthritis (1%), tremor (1%)
Respiratory: Bronchitis (2%), sinusitis (1%)
<1% (Limited to important or life-threatening): Anal fissure, angina pectoris, anxiety, biliary obstruction, candidiasis, chest pain, cholelithiasis, deafness (unilateral), decreased platelet count, diverticulitis, eczema, ECG abnormality, erectile dysfunction, falling, first degree atrioventricular block, gastritis, gastroesophageal reflux disease, gastrointestinal hemorrhage, gout, hallucination, hemoptysis, hypersensitivity, hypertensive crisis, hypogonadism (Brennan, 2013; Debono, 2011), hyponatremia, hypophosphatemia, hypotension, increased blood pressure, increased heart rate, increased lactate dehydrogenase, increased liver enzymes, lipoma, loss of libido, memory impairment, neuromuscular blockade, nightmares, otitis externa, panic attack, paresthesia, periodontitis, photopsia, pneumonia, pollakiuria, polyneuropathy, respiratory depression, restless leg syndrome, right bundle branch block, stasis dermatitis, syncope, tenosynovitis, thrombophlebitis, thrombosis, tinnitus, tonic-clonic seizures, urinary incontinence, urinary retention, vaginal hemorrhage, weight loss

Drug Interactions
Metabolism/Transport Effects Refer to individual components.
Avoid Concomitant Use
Avoid concomitant use of Oxycodone and Naloxone with any of the following: Azelastine (Nasal); Conivaptan; Eluxadoline; Fusidic Acid (Systemic); Idelalisib; Methylnaltrexone; Mixed Agonist / Antagonist Opioids; Naloxegol; Orphenadrine; Paraldehyde; Thalidomide
Increased Effect/Toxicity
Oxycodone and Naloxone may increase the levels/ effects of: Alcohol (Ethyl); Alvimopan; Azelastine (Nasal); CNS Depressants; Desmopressin; Diuretics; Eluxadoline; Hydrocodone; Methotrimeprazine; Metyrosine; Mirtazapine; Naloxegol; Orphenadrine; Paraldehyde; Pramipexole; Ramosetron; ROPINIRole; Rotigotine; Selective Serotonin Reuptake Inhibitors; Suvorexant; Thalidomide; Zolpidem

The levels/effects of Oxycodone and Naloxone may be increased by: Amphetamines; Anticholinergic Agents; Antipsychotic Agents (Phenothiazines); Brimonidine (Topical); Cannabis; Conivaptan; CYP3A4 Inhibitors (Moderate); CYP3A4 Inhibitors (Strong); Dasatinib; Doxylamine; Dronabinol; Droperidol; Fosaprepitant; Fusidic Acid (Systemic); Idelalisib; Ivacaftor; Kava Kava; Luliconazole; Magnesium Sulfate; MAO Inhibitors; Methotrimeprazine; Methylnaltrexone; Mifepristone; Minocycline; Nabilone; Osimertinib; Palbociclib; Perampanel; Rufinamide; Simeprevir; Sodium Oxybate; Stiripentol; Succinylcholine; Tapentadol; Tetrahydrocannabinol; Voriconazole
Decreased Effect
Oxycodone and Naloxone may decrease the levels/ effects of: Pegvisomant

The levels/effects of Oxycodone and Naloxone may be decreased by: Ammonium Chloride; Bosentan; CYP3A4 Inducers (Moderate); CYP3A4 Inducers (Strong); Dabrafenib; Deferasirox; Enzalutamide; Mitotane; Mixed Agonist / Antagonist Opioids; Naltrexone; Osimertinib; Rifampin; Siltuximab; St Johns Wort; Tocilizumab
Storage/Stability Store at 15°C to 30°C (59°F to 86°F). Protect from light and moisture.

◄ **Mechanism of Action**

Oxycodone binds to opiate receptors in the CNS, causing inhibition of ascending pain pathways, altering the perception of and response to pain; produces generalized CNS depression; also binds to opiate receptors in peripheral organs including the gut to induce constipation.

Naloxone is a pure opioid antagonist that competes and displaces narcotics at opioid receptor sites, including gut opioid receptors, which counteracts opioid-induced constipation.

Pharmacodynamics/Kinetics Note: Pharmacokinetic parameters observed with oxycodone/naloxone controlled release formulation were similar to those observed with separate administration of controlled-release formulations of each agent (Smith, 2008).

Naloxone:

Bioavailability: Oral: <3%

Metabolism: Primarily hepatic via glucuronidation

Half-life elimination: ~4 to 17 hours

Excretion: Urine (as metabolites)

Oxycodone (controlled release):

Duration: ≤12 hours

Distribution: V_d: 2.6 L/kg; distributed to skeletal muscle, liver, intestinal tract, lungs, spleen, and brain

Protein binding: ~45% (Targin Canadian product monograph, 2013)

Metabolism: Hepatically via CYP3A4 to noroxycodone (has weak analgesic activity), noroxymorphone, and alpha- and beta-noroxycodol. CYP2D6 mediated metabolism produces oxymorphone (has analgesic activity; low plasma concentrations), alpha- and beta-oxymorphol. Analgesic activity of metabolites may be of little clinical significance

Bioavailability: 60% to 87% (**Note:** Proportional bioavailability of oxycodone 5 mg/naloxone 2.5 mg tablets to other tablet strengths has not been established)

Half-life elimination: ~4 to 5 hours

Time to peak, plasma: 3 to 4 hours

Excretion: Urine and feces (as parent drug and metabolites)

Dosing

Adult Moderate-to-severe pain: Oral:

U.S. labeling: **Note:** Oxycodone 40 mg/naloxone 20 mg tablets should only be used in opioid-tolerant patients. Do not exceed oxycodone 80 mg/naloxone 40 mg daily. Opioid tolerance is defined as: Patients already taking at least 60 mg of oral morphine daily, 25 mcg of transdermal fentanyl per hour, 30 mg of oral oxycodone daily, 8 mg oral hydromorphone daily, or an equivalent dose of another opioid for at least 1 week.

Opioid-naïve or not opioid tolerant: Initial: Oxycodone 10 mg/naloxone 5 mg every 12 hours

Converting from other opioids:

Currently on other oral oxycodone formulations: Administer 50% of the patient's total daily oral oxycodone dose as oxycodone/naloxone every 12 hours.

Currently on other oral opioids: Discontinue all other around-the-clock opioids; convert the patient's current total daily opioid dose(s) to an equivalent daily oral morphine dose (see manufacturer's labeling for conversion instructions). After equivalent daily oral morphine dose is determined, initiate oxycodone/naloxone as follows:

Oxycodone 10 mg/naloxone 5 mg every 12 hours (for patients with an equivalent daily oral morphine dose of 20 to <70 mg).

Oxycodone 20 mg/naloxone 10 mg every 12 hours (for patients with an equivalent daily oral morphine dose of 70 to <110 mg).

Oxycodone 30 mg/naloxone 15 mg every 12 hours (for patients with an equivalent daily oral morphine dose of 110 to <150 mg).

Oxycodone 40 mg/naloxone 20 mg every 12 hours (for patients with an equivalent daily oral morphine dose of 150 to 160 mg).

Currently on transdermal fentanyl: Initial: Oxycodone 10 mg/naloxone 5 mg every 12 hours substituted for each 25 mcg/hour fentanyl transdermal patch beginning 18 hours after removal of the transdermal fentanyl patch. Monitor closely during conversion.

Currently on transdermal buprenorphine: Initial: Oxycodone 10 mg/naloxone 5 mg every 12 hours for patients receiving transdermal buprenorphine (≤20 mcg/hour). Monitor closely during conversion.

Canadian labeling: **Note:** Oxycodone 5 mg/naloxone 2.5 mg tablets are intended for use in titration or dose adjustments. Multiple oxycodone 5 mg/naloxone 2.5 mg tablets should not be substituted for other tablet strengths. Oxycodone 40 mg/naloxone 20 mg tablets should only be used in opioid-tolerant patients. Do not exceed oxycodone 40 mg/naloxone 20 mg (single dose) or oxycodone 80 mg/naloxone 40 mg (daily dose).

Opioid-naive: Initial: Oxycodone 10 mg/naloxone 5 mg every 12 hours

Opioid-experienced:

Currently on other oral oxycodone formulations: Discontinue other oral oxycodone formulations and initiate oxycodone/naloxone at equivalent total daily dose of oxycodone administered in 2 equally divided doses every 12 hours

Currently on other opioids: Discontinue all other around-the-clock opioids. Initiate oxycodone/naloxone at the lowest available strength every 12 hours. Titrate dose as necessary to achieve adequate pain control with acceptable side effects. Adequate rescue medication should be available.

Dose adjustment:

U.S. labeling: Dose is individualized; titrate dose cautiously in increments of oxycodone 10 mg/naloxone 5 mg every 12 hours every 1 to 2 days until satisfactory response and acceptable adverse effects. Repeated pain at the end of the dosing interval may indicate the need for a dose adjustment rather than adjusting the dosing interval.

Canadian labeling: Dose is individualized; titrate dose cautiously every 1 to 2 days until satisfactory response and acceptable adverse effects. Repeated pain at the end of the dosing interval may indicate the need for a dose adjustment rather than adjusting the dosing interval.

Patients requiring rescue medication: Patients who experience breakthrough pain may require a rescue medication with an appropriate dose of an immediate-release analgesic. **Note:** Rescue medications used in clinical trials were immediate release oxycodone or combination products containing codeine.

U.S. labeling: No specific recommendations are made in the manufacturer's labeling.

Canadian labeling: Administer 1 dose of an immediate release opioid ~1/6 of the equivalent daily dose of oxycodone. Patients requiring >2 doses daily of rescue medication should have oxycodone/naloxone dose titrated upward every 1 to 2 days until satisfactory response is achieved (not to exceed recommended maximum dosing). Dosing interval (every 12 hours) should not be adjusted.

Discontinuation of therapy: Dose should be gradually tapered when no longer required in order to prevent withdrawal; do not abruptly discontinue.

U.S. labeling: See manufacturer's labeling for detailed instruction.

Canadian labeling: Decrease controlled release oxycodone dose by 50% of the previous daily dose (administered in 2 divided doses every 12 hours) for first 2 days, then reduce daily dose by 25% every 2 days.

Geriatric Refer to adult dosing. Initiate therapy at low end of dosing range; titrate dose cautiously to lowest dose that provides adequate pain relief with acceptable side effects.

Renal Impairment

U.S. labeling: Reduce dose to 50% the usual starting dose; titrate cautiously; consider use of alternative treatments without naloxone in patients with severe renal impairment.

Canadian labeling: There are no specific dosage adjustments provided in the manufacturer's labeling; however, a reduced dose is recommended; use with caution.

Hepatic Impairment

Mild impairment:

U.S. labeling: Initial: Reduce dose to 33% to 50% the usual starting dose; titrate cautiously.

Canadian labeling: There are no specific dosage adjustments provided in the manufacturer's labeling; however, a reduced dose is recommended; use with caution.

Moderate-to-severe impairment: Use is contraindicated.

Administration Oral: Administer with or without food. Swallow tablets whole one tablet at a time; do not break, crush, cut, chew, dissolve, or split. Breaking, chewing, crushing, cutting, dissolving, or splitting ER tablets will result in uncontrolled delivery of oxycodone and can lead to overdose or death. Tablets are not indicated for rectal administration; increased risk of adverse events due to enhanced rectal absorption.

Monitoring Parameters Pain relief; respiratory and mental status, blood pressure; constipation; signs of misuse, abuse, and addiction; signs or symptoms of hypogonadism or hypoadrenalism (Brennan, 2013)

Additional Information Compared to controlled release oxycodone, improved bowel function and similar efficacy in terms of pain relief have been observed with a controlled release formulation of oxycodone/naloxone (Ahmedzai, 2012; Löwenstein, 2010; Vondrackova, 2008).

Product Availability Targiniq ER: FDA approved July 2014; anticipated availability is currently unknown.

Dosage Forms: Canada Excipient information presented when available (limited, particularly for generics); consult specific product labeling.

Tablet, controlled release, oral:
Targin:
Oxycodone hydrochloride 5 mg and naloxone hydrochloride 2.5 mg
Oxycodone hydrochloride 10 mg and naloxone hydrochloride 5 mg
Oxycodone hydrochloride 20 mg and naloxone hydrochloride 10 mg
Oxycodone hydrochloride 40 mg and naloxone hydrochloride 20 mg

Controlled Substance C-II

◆ Oxycodone Hydrochloride *see* OxyCODONE *on page 1357*

◆ Oxycodone Hydrochloride and Naloxone Hydrochloride *see* Oxycodone and Naloxone *on page 1362*

◆ OxyCONTIN *see* OxyCODONE *on page 1357*

◆ Oxy.IR (Can) *see* OxyCODONE *on page 1357*

Oxymetholone (oks i METH oh lone)

Brand Names: US Anadrol-50
Pharmacologic Category Anabolic Steroid
Use Treatment of anemias caused by deficient red cell production
Dosing
Adult & Geriatric Note: The National Kidney Foundation does not recommend the use of androgens as an adjuvant to ESA treatment in anemic patients with chronic kidney disease (KDOQI, 2006).

Erythropoietic effects: Oral: 1-5 mg/kg/day once daily; usual effective dose: 1-2 mg/kg/day; give for a minimum trial of 3-6 months because response may be delayed
Pediatric Refer to adult dosing.
Renal Impairment No dosage adjustment provided in manufacturer's labeling. Use with caution due to risk of edema in patients with renal impairment.
Hepatic Impairment
Mild to moderate impairment: There are no dosage adjustments provided in the manufacturer's labeling.
Severe impairment: Use is contraindicated.
Additional Information Complete prescribing information should be consulted for additional detail.
Dosage Forms Excipient information presented when available (limited, particularly for generics); consult specific product labeling.
Tablet, Oral:
Anadrol-50: 50 mg [scored]
Controlled Substance C-III

Oxymorphone (oks i MOR fone)

Brand Names: US Opana; Opana ER
Index Terms Oxymorphone Hydrochloride
Pharmacologic Category Analgesic, Opioid
Additional Appendix Information
Opioid Conversion Table and Morphine Equivalent Dose Table *on page 1955*
Use Pain management:
Parenteral: Management of moderate-to-severe acute pain; analgesia during labor; preoperative medication; anesthesia support; relief of anxiety in patients with dyspnea associated with pulmonary edema secondary to acute left ventricular failure
Oral, regular release: Management of moderate-to-severe acute pain
Oral, extended release: Management of pain severe enough to require daily, around-the-clock, long-term opioid treatment and for which alternative treatment options are inadequate
Limitations of use: Because of the risks of addiction, abuse, and misuse with opioids, even at recommended doses, and because of the greater risks of overdose and death with ER opioid formulations, reserve oxymorphone ER for use in patients for whom alternative treatment options (eg, nonopioid analgesics, immediate-release opioids) are ineffective, not tolerated, or would be otherwise inadequate to provide sufficient pain management. Not indicated as an as-needed analgesic.

Pregnancy Considerations Adverse events were observed in some animal reproduction studies. Opioids cross the placenta. When used for pain relief during labor, opioids may temporarily affect the heart rate of the fetus (ACOG, 2002). Oxymorphone injection is indicated for analgesia during labor. Neonates should be monitored for respiratory depression.

[U.S. Boxed Warning]: Prolonged maternal use of opioids during pregnancy can cause neonatal withdrawal syndrome in the newborn which may be life-threatening if not recognized and treated according to protocols developed by neonatology experts. If prolonged opioid therapy is required in a pregnant woman, ensure treatment is available and warn patient of risk to the neonate. If chronic opioid exposure occurs in pregnancy, adverse events in the newborn (including withdrawal) may occur; monitoring of the neonate is recommended. The minimum effective dose should be used if opioids are needed (Chou, 2009). Neonatal abstinence syndrome following opioid exposure may present with autonomic (eg, fever, temperature instability), gastrointestinal (eg, diarrhea, vomiting, poor feeding/weight gain), or neurologic (eg, high-pitched crying, increased muscle tone, irritability, seizure, tremor) symptoms (Dow, 2012; Hudak, 2012).

Long-term opioid use may cause secondary hypogonadism, which may lead to sexual dysfunction or infertility (Brennan, 2013).

Breast-Feeding Considerations Some opioids can be found in breast milk. Withdrawal symptoms may be observed in breast-feeding infants when opioid analgesics are discontinued. The manufacturer recommends that caution be used if administered to a nursing woman. Nursing infants exposed to large doses of opioids should be monitored for apnea and sedation (Montgomery, 2012).
Medication Guide Available Yes
Contraindications Hypersensitivity to oxymorphone, other morphine analogs (phenanthrene derivatives), or any component of the formulation; paralytic ileus (known or suspected); moderate-to-severe hepatic impairment; severe respiratory depression (unless using immediate release or parenteral formulation in monitored setting with resuscitative equipment); acute/severe bronchial asthma; hypercarbia
Note: Parenteral formulation is also contraindicated in the treatment of upper airway obstruction and pulmonary edema due to a chemical respiratory irritant.
Warnings/Precautions An opioid-containing analgesic regimen should be tailored to each patient's needs and based upon the type of pain being treated (acute versus chronic), the route of administration, degree of tolerance for opioids (naive versus chronic user), age, weight, and patient comorbidities. The optimal analgesic dose varies widely among patients. Doses should be titrated to pain relief/prevention.

May cause CNS depression, which may impair physical or mental abilities; patients must be cautioned about performing tasks which require mental alertness (eg, operating machinery or driving). Potentially significant drug interactions may exist, requiring dose or frequency adjustment, additional monitoring, and/or selection of alternative therapy. Effects may be potentiated when used with other CNS depressants (eg, sedatives, anxiolytics, hypnotics, neuroleptics, other opioids). Use not recommended within 14 days of MAO inhibitors. Due to structural similarities, hypersensitivity to other phenanthrene-derivative opioid agonists (codeine, hydrocodone, hydromorphone, levorphanol, morphine) may result in similar hypersensitivity reaction if oxymorphone is used; therefore, the use of oxymorphone is contraindicated in patients with previous hypersensitivity to other phenanthrene derivatives. May cause respiratory depression. Use with caution and monitor for respiratory depression in patients with significant chronic obstructive pulmonary disease or cor pulmonale, and patients having a substantially decreased respiratory reserve, hypoxia, hypercarbia, or preexisting respiratory depression, particularly when initiating therapy and titrating with oxymorphone; even therapeutic doses may decrease respiratory drive to the point of apnea. Consider the use of alternative non-opioid analgesics in these patients. Use with caution in patients (particularly elderly, cachectic, or debilitated) with impaired respiratory function, adrenal disease, morbid obesity, seizure disorders, toxic psychosis, thyroid dysfunction, prostatic hyperplasia, or renal impairment. Use caution in mild hepatic dysfunction; use is contraindicated in moderate-to-severe hepatic impairment. Avoid use in patients with CNS depression or coma as these patients are susceptible to intracranial effects of CO_2 retention. Use only with extreme caution (if at all) in patients with head injury or increased intracranial pressure ▶

(ICP); potential to elevate ICP and/or blunt papillary response may be greatly exaggerated in these patients. Use with caution in patients with biliary tract dysfunction including acute pancreatitis; may cause constriction of sphincter of Oddi. May obscure diagnosis or clinical course of patients with acute abdominal conditions. May cause constipation which may be problematic in patients with unstable angina and patients post-myocardial infarction.

Oxymorphone shares the toxic potential of opioid agonists and usual precautions of opioid agonist therapy should be observed; may cause hypotension in patients with acute myocardial infarction, volume depletion, or concurrent drug therapy which may exaggerate vasodilation. The elderly may be particularly susceptible to adverse effects of opioids.

Concurrent use of mixed agonist/antagonist analgesics (eg, pentazocine, nalbuphine, butorphanol) or partial agonist (eg, buprenorphine) analgesics may precipitate withdrawal symptoms and/or reduced analgesic efficacy in patients following prolonged therapy with mu opioid agonists. Taper dose gradually when discontinuing.

Extended release tablets: **[U.S. Boxed Warning]: May cause serious, life-threatening, or fatal respiratory depression. Monitor closely for respiratory depression, especially during initiation or dose escalation. Patients should swallow tablets whole; crushing, chewing, or dissolving can cause rapid release and a potentially fatal dose.** Carbon dioxide retention from opioid-induced respiratory depression can exacerbate the sedating effects of opioids. Therapy should only be prescribed by healthcare professionals familiar with the use of potent opioids for chronic pain. **[U.S. Boxed Warning]: Users are exposed to the risks of addiction, abuse, and misuse, potentially leading to overdose and death. Assess each patient's risk prior to prescribing; monitor all patients regularly for development of these behaviors or conditions. Risk of opioid abuse is increased in patients with a history or family history of alcohol or drug abuse or mental illness.** Cases of thrombotic thrombocytopenic purpura (TTP) resulting in kidney failure (requiring dialysis) and death have been reported as a result of misuse by drug abusers injecting the extended-release tablets intravenously; tablets are intended for oral administration only. **[U.S. Boxed Warning]: Patients should not consume alcoholic beverages or medication containing ethanol while taking oxymorphone ER; ethanol may increase oxymorphone plasma levels resulting in a potentially fatal overdose. [U.S. Boxed Warning]: Accidental ingestion of even one dose, especially in children, can result in a fatal overdose of oxymorphone. [U.S. Boxed Warning]: Prolonged maternal use of opioids during pregnancy can cause neonatal withdrawal syndrome in the newborn which may be life-threatening if not recognized and treated according to protocols developed by neonatology experts. If prolonged opioid therapy is required in a pregnant woman,** ensure treatment is available and warn patient of risk to the neonate. Signs and symptoms include irritability, hyperactivity and abnormal sleep pattern, high pitched cry, tremor, vomiting, diarrhea and failure to gain weight. Onset, duration and severity depend on the drug used, duration of use, maternal dose, and rate of drug elimination by the newborn.

Adverse Reactions Incidence usually on higher end with extended release (ER) tablet.

>10%:
Central nervous system: Drowsiness (9% to 19%), dizziness (7% to 18%), headache (7% to 12%)
Dermatologic: Pruritus (8% to 15%)
Gastrointestinal: Nausea (19% to 33%), constipation (4% to 28%), vomiting (9% to 16%)
Miscellaneous: Fever (1% to 14%)

1% to 10%:
Cardiovascular: Edema (<10%), flushing (<10%), hypertension (<10%), hypotension (<10%), tachycardia (<10%)
Central nervous system: Depression (<10%), disorientation (<10%), lethargy (<10%), nervousness (<10%), restlessness (<10%), anxiety (1% to <10%), sedation (1% to <10%), fatigue (≤4%), insomnia (≤4%), confusion (3%)
Dermatologic: Diaphoresis (1% to <10%)
Endocrine & metabolic: Dehydration (<10%), weight loss (<10%)
Gastrointestinal: Abdominal distention (<10%), dyspepsia (<10%), flatulence (1% to <10%), xerostomia (1% to <10%), diarrhea (≤4%), abdominal pain (≤3%), decreased appetite (≤3%)
Neuromuscular & skeletal: Weakness (<10%)
Ophthalmic: Blurred vision (<10%)
Respiratory: Dyspnea (<10%), hypoxia (<10%)

<1% (Limited to important or life-threatening): Agitation, apnea (injection), atelectasis (injection), biliary colic, bradycardia, bronchospasm (injection), cold and clammy skin, dermatitis, difficulty in micturition, diplopia (injection), drug dependence, dysphoria, euphoria, hallucination, hot flash, hypersensitivity, hypersensitivity reaction, hypogonadism (Brennan, 2013; Debono, 2011), injection site reaction, intestinal obstruction, miosis, oliguria (injection), orthostatic hypotension, palpitations, respiratory depression, syncope, thrombotic thrombocytopenic purpura (inappropriate injection of ER tablet), ureteral spasm (injection), urinary retention, urticaria

Drug Interactions
Metabolism/Transport Effects None known.
Avoid Concomitant Use
Avoid concomitant use of Oxymorphone with any of the following: Azelastine (Nasal); Eluxadoline; MAO Inhibitors; Mixed Agonist / Antagonist Opioids; Orphenadrine; Paraldehyde; Thalidomide
Increased Effect/Toxicity
Oxymorphone may increase the levels/effects of: Alcohol (Ethyl); Alvimopan; Azelastine (Nasal); CNS Depressants; Desmopressin; Diuretics; Eluxadoline; Hydrocodone; MAO Inhibitors; Methotrimeprazine; Metyrosine; Mirtazapine; Orphenadrine; Paraldehyde; Pramipexole; Ramosetron; ROPINIRole; Rotigotine; Selective Serotonin Reuptake Inhibitors; Suvorexant; Thalidomide; Zolpidem

The levels/effects of Oxymorphone may be increased by: Amphetamines; Anticholinergic Agents; Antipsychotic Agents (Phenothiazines); Brimonidine (Topical); Cannabis; Doxylamine; Dronabinol; Droperidol; HydrOXYzine; Kava Kava; Magnesium Sulfate; Methotrimeprazine; Minocycline; Nabilone; Perampanel; Rufinamide; Sodium Oxybate; Succinylcholine; Tapentadol; Tetrahydrocannabinol
Decreased Effect
Oxymorphone may decrease the levels/effects of: Pegvisomant

The levels/effects of Oxymorphone may be decreased by: Ammonium Chloride; Mixed Agonist / Antagonist Opioids; Naltrexone
Food Interactions
Ethanol: Ethanol ingestion with extended-release tablets is specifically contraindicated due to possible accelerated release and potentially fatal overdose. Management: Avoid ethanol.
Food: When taken orally with a high-fat meal, peak concentration is 38% to 50% greater. Management: Both immediate-release and extended-release tablets should be taken 1 hour before or 2 hours after eating.
Storage/Stability Injection solution, tablet: Store at 25°C (77°F); excursions permitted to 15°C to 30°C (59°F to 86°F). Protect injection from light.
Mechanism of Action Oxymorphone hydrochloride is a potent opioid analgesic with uses similar to those of morphine. The drug is a semisynthetic derivative of morphine (phenanthrene derivative) and is closely related to hydromorphone chemically (Dilaudid®).
Pharmacodynamics/Kinetics
Onset of action: Parenteral: 5-10 minutes
Duration: Analgesic: Parenteral: 3-6 hours
Distribution: V_d: IV: 1.94-4.22 L/kg
Protein binding: 10% to 12%
Metabolism: Hepatic via glucuronidation to active and inactive metabolites
Bioavailability: Oral: ~10%
Half-life elimination: Oral: Immediate release: 7-9 hours; Extended release: 9-11 hours
Excretion: Urine (<1% as unchanged drug); feces
Dosing
Adult Analgesia: Note: Dosage must be individualized.
IM, SubQ: Initial: 1 to 1.5 mg; may repeat every 4 to 6 hours as needed
Labor analgesia: IM: 0.5 to 1 mg
IV: Initial: 0.5 mg
Oral:
Immediate release: Acute pain:
Opioid-naive: Initial: 5 to 10 mg every 4 to 6 hours as needed (American Pain Society [Miaskowski, 2008]). Dosage adjustment should be based on level of analgesia, side effects, pain intensity, and patient comorbidities.
Currently on stable dose of parenteral oxymorphone: Approximately 10 times the total daily parenteral requirement. The calculated total oral daily amount should be given in 4 to 6 equally divided doses.

Currently on other opioids: Use standard conversion chart to convert total daily dose of current opioid to oxymorphone equivalent. Generally start with one-half (1/2) the calculated total daily oxymorphone dosage and administer in divided doses every 4 to 6 hours.

Extended release: Chronic pain:

Opioid-naive (use as the first opioid analgesic or in patients who are not opioid tolerant): Initial: 5 mg every 12 hours.

Note: Opioid tolerance is defined as: Patients already taking at least 60 mg of oral morphine daily, 25 mcg of transdermal fentanyl per hour, 30 mg of oral oxycodone daily, 8 mg oral hydromorphone daily, 25 mg oral oxymorphone daily, or an equivalent dose of another opioid for at least 1 week.

Conversion from stable dose of parenteral oxymorphone to extended-release oxymorphone: Approximately 10 times the total daily parenteral requirement should be given in 2 divided doses as oxymorphone extended-release tablets (eg, [IV dose x 10] divided by 2). Due to patient variability, closely monitor patient for analgesia and adverse reactions upon conversion.

Conversion of stable dose of immediate-release oxymorphone to extended-release oxymorphone: Use same total daily dose. Administer one-half (1/2) of the daily dose of immediate-release oxymorphone as the extended-release formulation every 12 hours

Conversion from other oral opioids to extended-release oxymorphone: Discontinue all other around-the-clock opioids when extended release oxymorphone is initiated. Substantial interpatient variability exists in relative potency of opioids. Therefore, it is safer to underestimate a patient's daily oral oxymorphone requirement and provide breakthrough pain relief with rescue medication (eg, immediate release opioid) than to overestimate requirements. The conversion factors, per the manufacturer, in the chart (see table) provide an estimate to convert the daily dose of current opioid to an oxymorphone equivalent. Select the prior oral opioid, sum the current total daily dose, multiply by the conversion factor on the table to calculate the approximate oral oxymorphone daily dose, then divide daily dose by 2 to administer every 12 hours as oxymorphone extended release. Round down, if necessary, to the nearest strength available. For patients on a regimen of more than one opioid, calculate the approximate oral oxymorphone dose for each opioid and sum the totals to obtain the approximate total oxymorphone daily dose. For patients on a regimen of fixed-ratio opioid/nonopioid analgesic medications, only the opioid component of these medications should be used in the conversion. **Note:** The conversion factors in this conversion table are only to be used for the conversion from current opioid therapy to oxymorphone ER. Conversion factors in this table cannot be used to convert from oxymorphone ER to another opioid (doing so may lead to fatal overdose due to overestimation of the new opioid). This is not a table of equianalgesic doses. When converting from methadone to extended release oxymorphone, close monitoring is required. Ratio between methadone and other opioid agonists varies widely according to previous dose exposure. Methadone has a long half-life and can accumulate in the plasma.

Conversion Factors to Oxymorphone ER

Prior Oral Opioid	Approximate Oral Conversion Factor
Oxymorphone	1
Hydrocodone	0.5
Oxycodone	0.5
Methadone	0.5
Morphine	0.333

Titration and maintenance: Adjust therapy incrementally by 5 to 10 mg every 12 hours at intervals of every 3 to 7 days. Breakthrough pain may require a dose increase or rescue medication with an immediate-release analgesic.

Discontinuation of therapy: Gradually titrate dose downward every 2 to 4 days to prevent withdrawal signs/symptoms. Do not abruptly discontinue.

Geriatric Refer to adult dosing. **Note:** Initiate dosing at the lower end of the dosage range.

Renal Impairment CrCl <50 mL/minute: Reduce initial dosage of oral and parenteral formulations (bioavailability increased 57% to 65%). Begin therapy at lowest dose and titrate slowly with careful monitoring.

Hepatic Impairment

Mild impairment: Initiate with lowest possible dose and titrate slowly with careful monitoring.

Moderate to severe impairment: Use is contraindicated.

Dietary Considerations Immediate release and extended release tablets should be taken 1 hour before or 2 hours after eating.

Administration Oral: Administer immediate release and extended release tablets 1 hour before or 2 hours after eating. ER tablet should be swallowed whole; do not break, crush, dissolve, or chew.

Monitoring Parameters Respiratory rate, heart rate, blood pressure, CNS activity; signs or symptoms of hypogonadism or hypoadrenalism (Brennan, 2013)

Test Interactions Some quinolones may produce a false-positive urine screening result for opioids using commercially-available immunoassay kits. This has been demonstrated most consistently for levofloxacin and ofloxacin, but other quinolones have shown cross-reactivity in certain assay kits. Confirmation of positive opioid screens by more specific methods should be considered. May cause elevation in amylase (due to constriction of the sphincter of Oddi).

Dosage Forms Excipient information presented when available (limited, particularly for generics); consult specific product labeling. [DSC] = Discontinued product

Solution, Injection, as hydrochloride:

Opana: 1 mg/mL (1 mL)

Tablet, Oral, as hydrochloride:

Opana: 5 mg [contains fd&c blue #2 aluminum lake]

Opana: 10 mg [contains d&c red #30 aluminum lake]

Generic: 5 mg, 10 mg

Tablet ER 12 Hour Abuse-Deterrent, Oral, as hydrochloride:

Opana ER: 5 mg, 7.5 mg

Opana ER: 10 mg [contains fd&c yellow #6 (sunset yellow)]

Opana ER: 15 mg

Opana ER: 20 mg [contains brilliant blue fcf (fd&c blue #1), fd&c yellow #10 (quinoline yellow), fd&c yellow #6 (sunset yellow)]

Opana ER: 30 mg

Opana ER: 40 mg [contains fd&c yellow #10 (quinoline yellow), fd&c yellow #6 (sunset yellow)]

Tablet Extended Release 12 Hour, Oral, as hydrochloride:

Opana ER: 5 mg [DSC] [contains methylparaben, polysorbate 80]

Opana ER: 10 mg [DSC] [contains fd&c yellow #6 (sunset yellow), methylparaben, polysorbate 80]

Opana ER: 20 mg [DSC] [contains brilliant blue fcf (fd&c blue #1), fd&c yellow #10 (quinoline yellow), fd&c yellow #6 (sunset yellow), methylparaben, polysorbate 80]

Opana ER: 30 mg [DSC] [contains methylparaben, polysorbate 80]

Opana ER: 40 mg [DSC] [contains fd&c yellow #10 (quinoline yellow), fd&c yellow #6 (sunset yellow), methylparaben]

Generic: 5 mg, 7.5 mg, 10 mg, 15 mg, 20 mg, 30 mg, 40 mg

Controlled Substance C-II

◆ Oxymorphone Hydrochloride *see* Oxymorphone *on page 1365*

◆ OxyNEO (Can) *see* OxyCODONE *on page 1357*

Oxytocin (oks i TOE sin)

Brand Names: US Pitocin

Brand Names: Canada Oxytocin for injection

Index Terms Pit

Pharmacologic Category Oxytocic Agent

Use

Antepartum: Induction of labor in patients with a medical indication (eg, Rh problems, maternal diabetes, preeclampsia, at or near term); stimulation or reinforcement of labor (as in selected cases of uterine inertia); adjunctive therapy in management of incomplete or inevitable abortion

Postpartum: To produce uterine contractions during the third stage of labor and to control postpartum bleeding or hemorrhage.

Pregnancy Considerations [U.S. Boxed Warning]: To be used for medical rather than elective induction of labor. Animal reproduction studies have not been conducted. When used as indicated, teratogenic effects would not be expected. Nonteratogenic adverse reactions are reported in the neonate as well as the mother.

Breast-Feeding Considerations Endogenous levels of oxytocin naturally increase during breast-feeding.

Contraindications Hypersensitivity to oxytocin or any component of the formulation; significant cephalopelvic disproportion; unfavorable fetal positions or presentations (such as transverse lies); fetal distress when delivery is not imminent; hypertonic or hyperactive uterus; contraindicated vaginal delivery (invasive cervical cancer, active genital herpes, prolapse of the cord, cord presentation, total placenta previa, or vasa previa); obstetrical emergencies where surgical intervention is favored; where adequate uterine activity fails to achieve satisfactory progress

Warnings/Precautions Hazardous agent - use appropriate precautions for handling and disposal (NIOSH 2014 [group 3]). **[U.S. Boxed Warning]: To be used for medical rather than elective induction of labor.** Oxytocin is used to initiate or improve uterine contractions in order to achieve a vaginal delivery; it should only be used when medically needed for fetal or maternal reasons. Medical indications for labor induction may include Rh problems, maternal diabetes, preeclampsia at or near term, when delivery is in the best interest of mother or fetus, or premature rupture of membranes when delivery is indicated. Use is generally not recommended in the following conditions: Fetal distress, hydramnios, partial placenta previa, prematurity, borderline cephalopelvic disproportion, or conditions where there is a predisposition for uterine rupture (eg, previous major surgery on cervix or uterus, cesarean section, overdistention of the uterus, grand multiparity, past history of uterine sepsis or traumatic delivery). May produce intrinsic antidiuretic effect (ie, water intoxication). Severe water intoxication with convulsions, coma, and death may occur, particularly with large doses (40 to 50 milliunits/minute) or when given as a slow infusion over 24 hours and if the patient is receiving fluids by mouth. High doses or hypersensitivity to oxytocin may cause uterine hypertonicity, spasm, tetanic contraction, or rupture of the uterus. Intravenous preparations should be administered by adequately trained individuals familiar with its use and able to identify complications; continuous observation is necessary for all patients. Maternal deaths caused by hypertensive episodes, subarachnoid hemorrhage, or rupture of the uterus and fetal deaths have occurred with oxytocic medications when used for induction of labor or for augmentation in the first and second stages of labor.

Adverse Reactions Frequency not defined.

Fetus or neonate:

Cardiovascular: Arrhythmias (including premature ventricular contractions), bradycardia

Central nervous system: Brain or CNS damage (permanent), neonatal seizure

Hepatic: Neonatal jaundice

Ocular: Neonatal retinal hemorrhage

Miscellaneous: Fetal death, low Apgar score (5 minute)

Mother:

Cardiovascular: Arrhythmias (including premature ventricular contractions), hypertensive episodes

Gastrointestinal: Nausea, vomiting

Genitourinary: Pelvic hematoma, postpartum hemorrhage, uterine hypertonicity, tetanic contraction of the uterus, uterine rupture, uterine spasm

Hematologic: Afibrinogenemia (fatal)

Miscellaneous: Anaphylactic reaction, subarachnoid hemorrhage; severe water intoxication with convulsions, coma, and death is associated with a slow oxytocin infusion over 24 hours

Drug Interactions

Metabolism/Transport Effects None known.

Avoid Concomitant Use

Avoid concomitant use of Oxytocin with any of the following: Carboprost Tromethamine

Increased Effect/Toxicity

Oxytocin may increase the levels/effects of: Highest Risk QTc-Prolonging Agents; Moderate Risk QTc-Prolonging Agents

The levels/effects of Oxytocin may be increased by: Carboprost Tromethamine; Dinoprostone; Mifepristone; Misoprostol

Decreased Effect There are no known significant interactions involving a decrease in effect.

Preparation for Administration Hazardous agent; use appropriate precautions for handling and disposal (NIOSH 2014 [group 3]).

IV:

Induction or stimulation of labor: Add oxytocin 10 units to NS or LR 1,000 mL to yield a solution containing oxytocin 10 milliunits/mL. Rotate solution to mix.

Postpartum uterine bleeding: Add oxytocin 10 to 40 units to running IV infusion; maximum: 40 units to 1,000 mL.

Adjunctive management of abortion: Add oxytocin 10 units to 500 mL of a physiologic saline solution or D₅W.

Storage/Stability Store at 20°C to 25°C (68°F to 77°F).

Mechanism of Action Oxytocin stimulates uterine contraction by activating G-protein-coupled receptors that trigger increases in intracellular calcium levels in uterine myofibrils. Oxytocin also increases local prostaglandin production, further stimulating uterine contraction.

Pharmacodynamics/Kinetics

Onset of action: Uterine contractions: IM: 3 to 5 minutes; IV: ~1 minute

Duration: IM: 2 to 3 hours; IV: 1 hour

Half-life elimination: 1 to 6 minutes; decreased in late pregnancy and during lactation

Excretion: Urine (small amount unchanged)

Dosing

Adult Note: IV administration requires the use of an infusion pump.

Induction or stimulation of labor: IV: Initial: 0.5 to 1 milliunits/minute; gradually increase dose in increments of 1 to 2 milliunits/minute every 30 to 60 minutes until desired contraction pattern is established; dose may be decreased by similar increments after desired frequency of contractions is reached and labor has progressed to 5 to 6 cm dilation. Infusion rates up to 6 milliunits/minute provide oxytocin levels similar to those with spontaneous labor; rates >9 to 10 milliunits/minute are rarely required. Higher dose regimens (eg, initial dose 2 to 6 milliunits/minute) with larger incremental dose increases (eg, 1 to 6 milliunits/minute) have also been proposed; decrease or discontinue dose for abnormal or excessive uterine contractions (ACOG, 2009).

Note: Discontinue the oxytocin infusion immediately in the event of uterine hyperactivity and/or fetal distress. If uterine contractions become too powerful, the infusion can be stopped abruptly.

Postpartum uterine bleeding:

IM: 10 units after delivery of the placenta

IV: 10 to 40 units added to a running infusion solution depending on amount of infusion fluid remaining (maximum: 40 units in 1,000 mL of IV fluid); adjust infusion rate to sustain uterine contraction and control uterine atony

Adjunctive treatment of abortion: IV:

Incomplete, inevitable, or elective abortion: 10 units as an IV infusion after suction or a sharp curettage (used to help contract the uterus)

Midtrimester elective abortion: 10 to 20 milliunits/minute; maximum total dose: 30 units/12 hours (may decrease injection to abortion time)

Renal Impairment There are no dosage adjustments provided in the manufacturer's labeling.

Hepatic Impairment There are no dosage adjustments provided in the manufacturer's labeling.

Administration

Induction or stimulation of labor: Administer as an IV infusion (drip method) by use of an infusion pump; accurate control of the rate of infusion flow is essential.

Incomplete or inevitable abortion: Administer by IV infusion

Postpartum uterine bleeding: Administer by IV infusion or IM.

Hazardous agent; use appropriate precautions for handling and disposal (NIOSH 2014 [group 3]).

Monitoring Parameters Fluid intake and output during administration, uterine activity, blood pressure; electronic fetal monitoring

Dosage Forms Excipient information presented when available (limited, particularly for generics); consult specific product labeling.

Solution, Injection:

Pitocin: 10 units/mL (1 mL, 10 mL, 50 mL) [contains chlorobutanol (chlorobutol)]

Generic: 10 units/mL (1 mL, 10 mL, 30 mL)

◆ PA21 *see* Sucroferric Oxyhydroxide *on page 1704*
◆ Pacerone *see* Amiodarone *on page 94*

PACLitaxel (Conventional)
(pac li TAKS el con VEN sha nal)

Brand Names: Canada Apo-Paclitaxel; Paclitaxel for Injection; Paclitaxel Injection USP

Index Terms Conventional Paclitaxel; Onxyl; Taxol

Pharmacologic Category Antineoplastic Agent, Antimicrotubular; Antineoplastic Agent, Taxane Derivative

Use

Breast cancer: Adjuvant treatment of node-positive breast cancer; treatment of metastatic breast cancer after failure of combination chemotherapy or relapse within 6 months of adjuvant chemotherapy (prior therapy should have included an anthracycline)

Kaposi sarcoma (AIDS-related): Second-line treatment of AIDS-related Kaposi sarcoma

Non-small cell lung cancer: First-line treatment of non-small cell lung cancer (in combination with cisplatin) in patients who are not candidates for potentially curative surgery and/or radiation therapy

Ovarian cancer: Subsequent therapy for treatment of advanced ovarian cancer; first-line therapy of ovarian cancer (in combination with cisplatin)

Pregnancy Considerations Adverse events (embryotoxicity, fetal toxicity, and maternal toxicity) have been observed in animal reproduction studies at doses less than the recommended human dose. An *ex vivo* human placenta perfusion model illustrated that paclitaxel crossed the placenta at term. Placental transfer was low and affected by the presence of albumin; higher albumin concentrations resulted in lower paclitaxel placental transfer (Berveiller, 2012). Some pharmacokinetic properties of paclitaxel may be altered in pregnant women (van Hasselt, 2014). Women of childbearing potential should be advised to avoid becoming pregnant. A pregnancy registry is available for all cancers diagnosed during pregnancy at Cooper Health (877-635-4499).

Breast-Feeding Considerations Paclitaxel is excreted in breast milk (case report). The mother (3 months postpartum) was treated with paclitaxel 30 mg/m^2 (56.1 mg) and carboplatin once weekly for papillary thyroid cancer. Milk samples were obtained 4-316 hours after the infusion given at the sixth and final week of therapy. The average paclitaxel milk concentration over the testing interval was 0.78 mg/L. Although maternal serum concentrations were not noted in the report, the relative infant dose to a nursing infant was calculated to be ~17% of the maternal dose. Paclitaxel continued to be detected in breast milk when sampled at 172 hours after the dose and was below the limit of detection when sampled at 316 hours after the infusion (Griffin, 2012). Due to the potential for serious adverse reactions in a nursing infant, breast-feeding is not recommended.

Contraindications Hypersensitivity to paclitaxel, polyoxyl 35/polyoxyethylated castor oil (Cremophor EL), or any component of the formulation; treatment of solid tumors in patients with baseline neutrophil counts <1,500/mm^3; treatment of Kaposi sarcoma in patients with baseline neutrophil counts <1,000/mm^3.

Warnings/Precautions Hazardous agent - use appropriate precautions for handling and disposal (NIOSH 2014 [group 1]). **[US Boxed Warning]: Anaphylaxis and severe hypersensitivity reactions (dyspnea requiring bronchodilators, hypotension requiring treatment, angioedema, and/or generalized urticaria) have occurred in 2% to 4% of patients in clinical studies; premedicate with corticosteroids, diphenhydramine, and H$_2$ antagonists prior to infusion. Some reactions have been fatal despite premedication. If severe hypersensitivity occurs, stop infusion and do not rechallenge.** Minor hypersensitivity reactions (flushing, skin reactions, dyspnea, hypotension, or tachycardia) do not require interruption of treatment. Infusion-related hypotension, bradycardia, and/or hypertension may occur; frequent monitoring of vital signs is recommended, especially during the first hour of the infusion. Conventional paclitaxel formulations contain polyoxyl 35/polyoxyethylated castor oil (Cremophor EL) which is associated with hypersensitivity reactions. Formulations also contain dehydrated alcohol which may cause adverse CNS effects.

[US Boxed Warning]: Bone marrow suppression (primarily neutropenia; may be severe or result in infection) may occur. Monitor blood counts frequently. Do not administer if baseline neutrophil count is <1,500/mm^3 (for solid tumors) or <1,000/mm^3 (for patients with AIDS-related Kaposi sarcoma). Bone marrow suppression (usually neutropenia) is dose-dependent

and is the dose-limiting toxicity; neutrophil nadir is usually at a median of 11 days. Subsequent cycles should not be administered until neutrophils are >1,500/mm^3 (for solid tumors) and 1,000/mm^3 (for Kaposi sarcoma); platelets should recover to 100,000/mm^3. Reduce future doses by 20% for severe neutropenia (<500/mm^3 for 7 days or more) and consider the use of supportive therapy, including growth factor treatment.

Use extreme caution with hepatic dysfunction (myelotoxicity may be worsened in patients with total bilirubin >2 times ULN); dose reductions are recommended. Peripheral neuropathy may commonly occur; patients with pre-existing neuropathies from prior chemotherapy or coexisting conditions (eg, diabetes mellitus) may be at a higher risk; reduce dose by 20% for severe neuropathy. Rare but severe conduction abnormalities have been reported; conduct continuous cardiac monitoring during subsequent infusions for these patients. Elderly patients have an increased risk of toxicity (neutropenia, neuropathy, and cardiovascular events); use with caution. Intraperitoneal administration of paclitaxel is associated with a higher incidence of chemotherapy-related toxicity (Armstrong, 2006).

Paclitaxel is an irritant with vesicant-like properties; ensure proper needle or catheter placement prior to and during infusion; avoid extravasation. Injection site reactions are generally mild (skin discoloration, tenderness, erythema, or swelling) and occur more commonly with an extended infusion duration (eg, 24 hours); injection site reactions may be delayed (7 to 10 days). More severe reactions (phlebitis, cellulitis, skin exfoliation, necrosis, fibrosis, and induration) have also been reported. Recall skin reactions may occur despite administering through a different IV site. **[US Boxed Warning]: Should be administered under the supervision of an experienced cancer chemotherapy physician; administer in a facility sufficient to appropriately diagnose and manage complications.** Potentially significant drug-drug interactions may exist, requiring dose or frequency adjustment, additional monitoring, and/or selection of alternative therapy.

Adverse Reactions Percentages reported with single-agent therapy. **Note:** Myelosuppression is dose related, schedule related, and infusion-rate dependent (increased incidences with higher doses, more frequent doses, and longer infusion times) and, in general, rapidly reversible upon discontinuation.

>10%:

Cardiovascular: Flushing (28%), ECG abnormal (14% to 23%), edema (21%), hypotension (4% to 12%)

Dermatologic: Alopecia (87%), rash (12%)

Gastrointestinal: Nausea/vomiting (52%), diarrhea (38%), mucositis (17% to 35%; grades 3/4: up to 3%), stomatitis (15%; most common at doses >390 mg/m^2), abdominal pain (with intraperitoneal paclitaxel)

Hematologic: Neutropenia (78% to 98%; grade 4: 14% to 75%; onset 8-10 days, median nadir 11 days, recovery 15-21 days), leukopenia (90%; grade 4: 17%), anemia (47% to 90%; grades 3/4: 2% to 16%), thrombocytopenia (4% to 20%; grades 3/4: 1% to 7%), bleeding (14%)

Hepatic: Alkaline phosphatase increased (22%), AST increased (19%)

Local: Injection site reaction (erythema, tenderness, skin discoloration, swelling: 13%)

Neuromuscular & skeletal: Peripheral neuropathy (42% to 70%; grades 3/4: up to 7%), arthralgia/myalgia (60%), weakness (17%)

Renal: Creatinine increased (observed in KS patients only: 18% to 34%; severe: 5% to 7%)

Miscellaneous: Hypersensitivity reaction (31% to 45%; grades 3/4: up to 2%), infection (15% to 30%)

1% to 10%:

Cardiovascular: Bradycardia (3%), tachycardia (2%), hypertension (1%), rhythm abnormalities (1%), syncope (1%), venous thrombosis (1%)

Dermatologic: Nail changes (2%)

Hematologic: Febrile neutropenia (2%)

Hepatic: Bilirubin increased (7%)

Respiratory: Dyspnea (2%)

<1% (Limited to important or life-threatening): Anaphylaxis, arrhythmia, ataxia, atrial fibrillation, AV block, back pain, cardiac conduction abnormalities, cellulitis, CHF, chills, conjunctivitis, dehydration, enterocolitis, extravasation recall, hepatic encephalopathy, hepatic necrosis, induration, intestinal obstruction, intestinal perforation, interstitial pneumonia, ischemic colitis, lacrimation increased, maculopapular rash, malaise, MI, myocardial ischemia, necrotic changes and ulceration following extravasation, neuroencephalopathy, neutropenic enterocolitis, neutropenic typhlitis, ototoxicity (tinnitus and hearing loss), pancreatitis, paralytic ileus, phlebitis, pneumonitis, pruritus, pulmonary embolism, pulmonary fibrosis, radiation

recall, radiation pneumonitis, renal insufficiency, seizure, skin exfoliation, skin fibrosis, skin necrosis, Stevens-Johnson syndrome, supraventricular tachycardia, toxic epidermal necrolysis, ventricular tachycardia (asymptomatic), visual disturbances (scintillating scotomata)

Drug Interactions

Metabolism/Transport Effects Substrate of CYP2C8 (major), CYP3A4 (major), P-glycoprotein; **Note:** Assignment of Major/Minor substrate status based on clinically relevant drug interaction potential

Avoid Concomitant Use

Avoid concomitant use of PACLitaxel (Conventional) with any of the following: Atazanavir; BCG (Intravesical); Conivaptan; Deferiprone; Dipyrone; Fusidic Acid (Systemic); Idelalisib; Natalizumab; Pimecrolimus; SORAfenib; Tacrolimus (Topical); Tofacitinib; Vaccines (Live)

Increased Effect/Toxicity

PACLitaxel (Conventional) may increase the levels/effects of: Amifostine; Antineoplastic Agents (Anthracycline, Systemic); Antipsychotic Agents (Second Generation [Atypical]); Bexarotene (Systemic); CloZAPine; Deferiprone; DOXOrubicin (Conventional); DULoxetine; Fingolimod; Hypotension-Associated Agents; Leflunomide; Levodopa; Natalizumab; Tofacitinib; Trastuzumab; Vaccines (Live); Vinorelbine

The levels/effects of PACLitaxel (Conventional) may be increased by: Abiraterone Acetate; Alfuzosin; Aprepitant; Atazanavir; Barbiturates; Blood Pressure Lowering Agents; Brimonidine (Topical); Conivaptan; CYP2C8 Inhibitors (Moderate); CYP2C8 Inhibitors (Strong); CYP3A4 Inhibitors (Moderate); CYP3A4 Inhibitors (Strong); Dasatinib; Deferasirox; Denosumab; Diazoxide; Dipyrone; Fosaprepitant; Fusidic Acid (Systemic); Herbs (Hypotensive Properties); Idelalisib; Ivacaftor; Luliconazole; Mifepristone; Molsidomine; Netupitant; Nicorandil; Obinutuzumab; Osimertinib; Palbociclib; Pentoxifylline; P-glycoprotein/ABCB1 Inhibitors; Phosphodiesterase 5 Inhibitors; Pimecrolimus; Platinum Derivatives; Prostacyclin Analogues; Ranolazine; Roflumilast; Simeprevir; SORAfenib; Stiripentol; Tacrolimus (Topical)

Decreased Effect

PACLitaxel (Conventional) may decrease the levels/effects of: BCG (Intravesical); Coccidioides immitis Skin Test; Sipuleucel-T; Vaccines (Inactivated); Vaccines (Live)

The levels/effects of PACLitaxel (Conventional) may be decreased by: Bexarotene (Systemic); Bosentan; CYP2C8 Inducers (Strong); CYP3A4 Inducers (Moderate); CYP3A4 Inducers (Strong); Dabrafenib; Deferasirox; Echinacea; Enzalutamide; Mitotane; Osimertinib; P-glycoprotein/ABCB1 Inducers; Siltuximab; St Johns Wort; Tocilizumab; Trastuzumab

Preparation for Administration Hazardous agent; use appropriate precautions for handling and disposal (NIOSH 2014 [group 1]). Dilute for infusion in 250 to 1,000 mL D_5W, D_5LR, D_5NS, or NS to a concentration of 0.3 to 1.2 mg/mL, use a non-PVC container (glass or polyethylene). Chemotherapy dispensing devices (eg, Chemo Dispensing Pin) should not be used to withdraw paclitaxel from the vial; closed system transfer devices may not be compatible with undiluted paclitaxel.

Storage/Stability Store intact vials at room temperature of 20°C to 25°C (68°F to 77°F). Protect from light. Solutions diluted for infusion in D_5W and NS are stable for up to 27 hours at ambient temperature (~25°C).

Paclitaxel should be dispensed in either glass or non-PVC containers (eg, Excel/PAB). Use **nonpolyvinyl** (non-PVC) tubing (eg, polyethylene) to minimize leaching. Formulated in a vehicle known as polyoxyl 35/polyoxyethylated castor oil (Cremophor EL), which has been found to leach the plasticizer DEHP from polyvinyl chloride infusion bags or administration sets. Contact of the undiluted concentrate with plasticized polyvinyl chloride (PVC) equipment or devices is not recommended.

Mechanism of Action Paclitaxel promotes microtubule assembly by enhancing the action of tubulin dimers, stabilizing existing microtubules, and inhibiting their disassembly, interfering with the late G_2 mitotic phase, and inhibiting cell replication. In addition, the drug can distort mitotic spindles, resulting in the breakage of chromosomes. Paclitaxel may also suppress cell proliferation and modulate immune response.

Pharmacodynamics/Kinetics

V_{dss}: 24-hour infusion: 227 to 688 L/m^2; widely distributed into body fluids and tissues; affected by dose and duration of infusion

Protein binding: 89% to 98%

Metabolism: Hepatic via CYP2C8 and 3A4; forms metabolites (primarily 6α-hydroxypaclitaxel)

Half-life elimination:

3-hour infusion: Mean (terminal): ~13 to 20 hours

24-hour infusion: Mean (terminal): ~16 to 53 hours

Excretion: Feces (~71%; ~5% as unchanged drug); urine (~14%)

Dosing

Adult & Geriatric Note: Premedication with dexamethasone (20 mg orally at 12 and 6 hours prior to the dose [reduce dexamethasone dose to 10 mg orally with advanced HIV disease]), diphenhydramine (50 mg IV 30 to 60 minutes prior to the dose), and cimetidine, famotidine, or ranitidine (IV 30 to 60 minutes prior to the dose) is recommended.

Breast cancer, adjuvant treatment: IV: 175 mg/m² over 3 hours every 3 weeks for 4 cycles (administer sequentially following an anthracycline-containing regimen).

Breast cancer, metastatic or relapsed: IV: 175 mg/m² over 3 hours every 3 weeks

Non-small cell lung cancer: IV: 135 mg/m² over 24 hours every 3 weeks (in combination with cisplatin)

Ovarian cancer, advanced:

Previously treated: IV: 135 or 175 mg/m² over 3 hours every 3 weeks

Previously untreated: IV: 175 mg/m² over 3 hours every 3 weeks (in combination with cisplatin) or 135 mg/m² over 24 hours administered every 3 weeks (in combination with cisplatin)

Intraperitoneal (off-label route): 60 mg/m² on day 8 of a 21-day treatment cycle for 6 cycles, in combination with IV paclitaxel (135 mg/m² over 24 hours on day 1) and intraperitoneal cisplatin (Armstrong, 2006). **Note:** Administration of intraperitoneal paclitaxel should include the standard paclitaxel premedication regimen.

Previously untreated (off-label combination): IV: 175 mg/m² over 3 hours every 3 weeks (in combination with carboplatin) for 6 cycles, or 60 mg/m² over 1 hour weekly (in combination with carboplatin) for 18 weeks (Pignata, 2014)

Kaposi sarcoma, AIDS related: IV: 135 mg/m² over 3 hours every 3 weeks **or** 100 mg/m² over 3 hours every 2 weeks (due to dose-related toxicity, the 100 mg/m² dose should be used for patients with a lower performance status). **Note:** Reduce the dexamethasone premedication dose to 10 mg.

Bladder cancer, advanced or metastatic (off-label use): IV: 150 mg/m² every 2 weeks (in combination with gemcitabine) (Sternberg, 2001) **or** 200 mg/m² over 1 hour every 3 weeks (in combination with gemcitabine) for 6 cycles (Meluch, 2001)

Cervical cancer, advanced (off-label use): IV: 135 or 175 mg/m² every 3 weeks (in combination with bevacizumab and cisplatin) until disease progression or unacceptable toxicity (Tewari, 2014) **or** 175 mg/m² every 3 weeks (in combination with bevacizumab and topotecan) until disease progression or unacceptable toxicity (Tewari, 2014) **or** 135 mg/m² over 24 hours every 3 weeks (in combination with cisplatin) for 6 cycles (Monk, 2009; Moore, 2004).

Esophageal/gastric cancer, preoperative chemoradiation (off-label use): IV: 50 mg/m² on days 1, 8, 15, 22, and 29 (in combination with carboplatin and radiation therapy) followed by surgery within 4 to 6 weeks (van Hagen, 2012)

Head and neck cancers, advanced (off-label use): IV: 175 mg/m² over 3 hours every 3 weeks (in combination with cisplatin) for at least 6 cycles (Gibson, 2005)

Penile cancer, metastatic (off-label use): IV: 175 mg/m² over 3 hours every 3 to 4 weeks (in combination with ifosfamide and cisplatin) for 4 cycles (Pagliaro, 2010)

Small cell lung cancer, relapsed/refractory (off-label use): IV: 175 mg/m² over 3 hours every 3 weeks (as a single agent) for up to 5 cycles (Smit, 1998) **or** 80 mg/m² over 1 hour weekly for 6 weeks of an 8-week treatment cycle (as a single agent) until disease progression or unacceptable toxicity (Yamamoto, 2006)

Soft tissue sarcoma (angiosarcoma), advanced/unresectable (off-label use): IV: 80 mg/m² over 1 hour on days 1, 8, and 15 of a 4-week treatment cycle (as a single agent) for up to 6 cycles (Penel, 2008) **or** 135 to 175 mg/m² over 3 hours every 3 weeks (as a single agent) (Schlemmer, 2008) **or** 75 to 100 mg/m² once weekly (as a single agent) (Schlemmer, 2008)

Testicular germ cell tumors, relapsed/refractory (off-label use): IV: 80 mg/m² over 1 hour on days 1 and 8 of a 3-week treatment cycle (in combination with gemcitabine and oxaliplatin) for 2 cycles beyond best response and up to a maximum of 8 cycles (Bokemeyer, 2008) **or** 250 mg/m² over 24 hours on day 1 of a 3-week treatment cycle (in combination with ifosfamide, mesna, cisplatin, and filgrastim) for 4 cycles (Kondagunta,

2005) **or** 100 mg/m^2 over 1 hour on days 1, 8, and 15 of a 4-week treatment cycle (in combination with gemcitabine) for up to 6 cycles (Einhorn, 2007)

Thymoma/thymic carcinoma, advanced (off-label use): IV: 225 mg/m^2 over 3 hours every 3 weeks (in combination with carboplatin) for up to 6 cycles (Lemma, 2011)

Unknown primary adenocarcinoma (off-label use): IV: 200 mg/m^2 over 3 hours every 3 weeks (in combination with carboplatin) for 6 to 8 cycles (Briasoulis, 2000) **or** 200 mg/m^2 over 1 hour every 3 weeks (in combination with carboplatin and etoposide) for 4 to 8 cycles (Greco, 2000)

Renal Impairment There are no dosage adjustments provided in the manufacturer's labeling. Aronoff (2007) recommends no dosage adjustment necessary for adults with CrCl <50 mL/minute.

Hepatic Impairment Note: The manufacturer's labeling recommendations are based upon the patient's first course of therapy where the usual dose would be 135 mg/m^2 dose over 24 hours or the 175 mg/m^2 dose over 3 hours in patients with normal hepatic function. Dosage in subsequent courses should be based upon individual tolerance. Adjustments for other regimens are not available.

24-hour infusion:
Transaminases <2 times upper limit of normal (ULN) and bilirubin level ≤1.5 mg/dL: 135 mg/m^2

Transaminases 2 to <10 times ULN and bilirubin level ≤1.5 mg/dL: 100 mg/m^2

Transaminases <10 times ULN and bilirubin level 1.6 to 7.5 mg/dL: 50 mg/m^2

Transaminases ≥10 times ULN or bilirubin level >7.5 mg/dL: Avoid use

3-hour infusion:
Transaminases <10 times ULN and bilirubin level ≤1.25 times ULN: 175 mg/m^2

Transaminases <10 times ULN and bilirubin level 1.26 to 2 times ULN: 135 mg/m^2

Transaminases <10 times ULN and bilirubin level 2.01 to 5 times ULN: 90 mg/m^2

Transaminases ≥10 times ULN or bilirubin level >5 times ULN: Avoid use

Obesity *ASCO Guidelines for appropriate chemotherapy dosing in obese adults with cancer:* Utilize patient's actual body weight (full weight) for calculation of body surface area- or weight-based dosing, particularly when the intent of therapy is curative; manage regimen-related toxicities in the same manner as for nonobese patients; if a dose reduction is utilized due to toxicity, consider resumption of full weight-based dosing with subsequent cycles, especially if cause of toxicity (eg, hepatic or renal impairment) is resolved (Griggs, 2012).

Adjustment for Toxicity
Dosage modification for toxicity (solid tumors, including ovary, breast, and lung carcinoma): Courses of paclitaxel should not be repeated until the neutrophil count is ≥1,500/mm^3 and the platelet count is ≥100,000/mm^3; reduce dosage by 20% for patients experiencing severe peripheral neuropathy or severe neutropenia (neutrophil <500/mm^3 for a week or longer)

Dosage modification for immunosuppression in advanced HIV disease: Paclitaxel should not be given to patients with HIV if the baseline or subsequent neutrophil count is <1000 cells/mm^3. Additional modifications include: Reduce dosage of dexamethasone in premedication to 10 mg orally; reduce dosage by 20% in patients experiencing severe peripheral neuropathy or severe neutropenia (neutrophil <500/mm^3 for a week or longer); initiate concurrent hematopoietic growth factor (G-CSF) as clinically indicated

Administration
IV: Infuse over 3 or 24 hours (depending on indication/protocol); some off-label protocols use a 1-hour infusion. Infuse through a 0.22-micron in-line filter and polyethylene-lined (non-PVC) administration set. When administered as a part of a combination chemotherapy regimen, sequence of administration may vary by regimen; refer to specific protocol for sequence recommendation.

Premedication with dexamethasone (20 mg orally or IV at 12 and 6 hours before the dose; reduce to 10 mg with advanced HIV disease), diphenhydramine (50 mg IV 30 to 60 minutes prior to the dose), and cimetidine 300 mg, famotidine 20 mg, or ranitidine 50 mg (IV 30 to 60 minutes prior to the dose) is recommended.

Irritant with vesicant-like properties; avoid extravasation. Ensure proper needle or catheter position prior to administration.

Extravasation management: If extravasation occurs, stop infusion immediately and disconnect (leave cannula/needle in place); gently aspirate extravasated solution (do **NOT** flush the line); remove needle/cannula; initiate antidote (hyaluronidase); remove needle/cannula; elevate extremity. Information conflicts regarding the use of warm or cold compresses (Perez Fidalgo, 2012; Polovich, 2009).

Hyaluronidase: If needle/cannula still in place: Administer 1 to 6 mL (150 units/mL) into existing IV line; usual dose is 1 mL for each 1 mL of extravasated drug; if needle/cannula has been removed, inject subcutaneously in a clockwise manner around area of extravasation; may repeat several times over the next 3 to 4 hours (Ener, 2004).

Intraperitoneal (off-label route): Solution was prepared in warmed saline and infused as rapidly as possible through an implantable intraperitoneal catheter (Armstrong, 2006).

Hazardous agent; use appropriate precautions for handling and disposal (NIOSH 2014 [group 1]).

Monitoring Parameters CBC with differential and platelet count, liver and kidney function; monitor for hypersensitivity reactions, vital signs (frequently during the first hour of infusion), continuous cardiac monitoring (patients with conduction abnormalities); monitor infusion site during infusion.

Dosage Forms Considerations Paclitaxel injection contains polyoxyl 35/olyoxyethylated castor oil (Cremophor EL)

Dosage Forms Excipient information presented when available (limited, particularly for generics); consult specific product labeling.

Concentrate, Intravenous:
Generic: 100 mg/16.7 mL (16.7 mL); 30 mg/5 mL (5 mL); 150 mg/25 mL (25 mL); 300 mg/50 mL (50 mL)
Concentrate, Intravenous [preservative free]:
Generic: 100 mg/16.7 mL (16.7 mL); 30 mg/5 mL (5 mL); 300 mg/50 mL (50 mL)

PACLitaxel (Protein Bound)
(pac li TAKS el PROE teen bownd)

Brand Names: US Abraxane
Brand Names: Canada Abraxane for Injectable Suspension

Index Terms ABI-007; Albumin-Bound Paclitaxel; Albumin-Stabilized Nanoparticle Paclitaxel; nab-Paclitaxel; Nanoparticle Albumin-Bound Paclitaxel; Paclitaxel (Nanoparticle Albumin Bound); Paclitaxel, Albumin-Bound; Protein-Bound Paclitaxel

Pharmacologic Category Antineoplastic Agent, Antimicrotubular; Antineoplastic Agent, Taxane Derivative

Use
Breast cancer, metastatic: Treatment of refractory (metastatic) or relapsed (within 6 months of adjuvant therapy) breast cancer after failure of combination chemotherapy (including anthracycline-based therapy unless clinically contraindicated)

Non-small cell lung cancer (NSCLC): First-line treatment of locally advanced or metastatic NSCLC (in combination with carboplatin) in patients ineligible for curative surgery or radiation therapy

Pancreatic adenocarcinoma: First-line treatment of metastatic adenocarcinoma of the pancreas (in combination with gemcitabine)

Dosing
Adult & Geriatric Note: When administered as part of a combination chemotherapy regimen, sequence of administration may vary by regimen; refer to specific protocol for sequence of administration. Premedication is not generally necessary prior to paclitaxel (protein bound), but may be needed in patients with prior mild-to-moderate hypersensitivity reactions.

Breast cancer, metastatic: IV: 260 mg/m^2 every 3 weeks (Gradishar 2005)
Off-label dosing: IV: 100 to 150 mg/m^2 on days 1, 8, and 15 of a 28-day cycle (Gradishar 2009)

Non-small cell lung cancer (NSCLC), locally advanced or metastatic: IV: 100 mg/m^2 on days 1, 8, and 15 of each 21-day cycle (in combination with carboplatin) (Socinski 2012)

Pancreatic adenocarcinoma, metastatic: IV: 125 mg/m^2 on days 1, 8, and 15 of a 28-day cycle (in combination with gemcitabine) (Von Hoff 2013)

Melanoma, metastatic (off-label use): IV:
Previously treated patients: 100 mg/m^2 on days 1, 8, and 15 of a 28-day cycle; if tolerated, may increase dose by 25 mg/m^2 in cycle 2 and beyond (Hersh 2010)
Previously untreated patients: 150 mg/m^2 on days 1, 8, and 15 of a 28-day cycle (Hersh 2010)

Ovarian, fallopian tube, or primary peritoneal cancer, recurrent (off-label use): IV: 260 mg/m^2 on day 1 of a 21-day cycle for 6 to 8 cycles (Teneriello 2009) **or** 100 mg/m^2 on days 1, 8, and 15 of a 28-day cycle until disease progression or unacceptable toxicity (Coleman 2011)

Renal Impairment There are no dosage adjustments provided in the manufacturer's labeling (has not been studied).

Hepatic Impairment

Dosage adjustment for hepatic impairment at treatment initiation:

Breast cancer (every 3 week regimen):

Mild impairment (AST ≤10 times ULN and bilirubin >1 to ≤1.5 times ULN): No dosage adjustment is necessary.

Moderate impairment (AST ≤10 times ULN and bilirubin >1.5 to ≤3 times ULN): Reduce dose to 200 mg/m^2; may increase up to 260 mg/m^2 if the reduced dose is tolerated for 2 cycles

Severe impairment:

AST ≤10 times ULN and bilirubin >3 to ≤5 times ULN: Reduce dose to 200 mg/m^2; may increase up to 260 mg/m^2 in subsequent cycles if the reduced dose is tolerated for 2 cycles

AST >10 times ULN or bilirubin >5 times ULN: Use is not recommended (has not been studied).

Non-small cell lung cancer (NSCLC) regimen:

Mild impairment (AST ≤10 times ULN and bilirubin >1 to ≤1.5 times ULN): No dosage adjustment is necessary.

Moderate impairment (AST ≤10 times ULN and bilirubin >1.5 to ≤3 times ULN): Reduce dose to 80 mg/m^2; may increase up to 100 mg/m^2 in subsequent cycles if the reduced dose is tolerated for 2 cycles

Severe impairment:

AST ≤10 times ULN and bilirubin >3 to ≤5 times ULN: Reduce dose to 80 mg/m^2; may increase up to 100 mg/m^2 in subsequent cycles if the reduced dose is tolerated for 2 cycles

AST >10 times ULN or bilirubin >5 times ULN: Use is not recommended (has not been studied).

Pancreatic adenocarcinoma:

Mild impairment (AST ≤10 times ULN and bilirubin >1 to ≤1.5 times ULN): No dosage adjustment is necessary.

Moderate impairment (AST ≤10 times ULN and bilirubin >1.5 to ≤3 times ULN): Use is not recommended.

Severe impairment:

AST ≤10 times ULN and bilirubin >3 to ≤5 times ULN: Use is not recommended.

AST >10 times ULN or bilirubin >5 times ULN: Use is not recommended.

Dosage adjustment for hepatic impairment during treatment: AST >10 times ULN or bilirubin >5 times ULN: Withhold treatment

Obesity *ASCO Guidelines for appropriate chemotherapy dosing in obese adults with cancer:* Utilize patient's actual body weight (full weight) for calculation of body surface area- or weight-based dosing, particularly when the intent of therapy is curative; manage regimen-related toxicities in the same manner as for nonobese patients; if a dose reduction is utilized due to toxicity, consider resumption of full weight-based dosing with subsequent cycles, especially if cause of toxicity (eg, hepatic or renal impairment) is resolved (Griggs 2012).

Adjustment for Toxicity

Breast cancer (every 3 week regimen):

Severe neutropenia (<500 cells/mm^3) ≥1 week: Reduce dose to 220 mg/m^2 for subsequent courses

Recurrent severe neutropenia: Reduce dose to 180 mg/m^2 for subsequent courses

Sensory neuropathy

Grade 1 or 2: Dosage adjustment generally not required

Grade 3: Hold treatment until resolved to grade 1 or 2, then resume with reduced dose for all subsequent cycles

Severe sensory neuropathy: Reduce dose to 220 mg/m^2 for subsequent courses

Recurrent severe sensory neuropathy: Reduce dose to 180 mg/m^2 for subsequent courses

Non-small cell lung cancer (NSCLC):

Neutropenia: ANC <1500 cells/mm^3: Withhold therapy until ANC is ≥1500 cells/mm^3 on day 1 or ≥500 cells/mm^3 on days 8 or 15. Reduce dose upon therapy reinitiation if:

Neutropenic fever (ANC <500 cells/mm^3 with fever >38°C) **or** delay of next cycle by >7 days due to ANC <1500 cells/mm^3 **or** ANC <500 cells/mm^3 for >7 days:

First occurrence: Permanently reduce dose to 75 mg/m^2

Second occurrence: Permanently reduce dose to 50 mg/m^2

Third occurrence: Discontinue therapy.

Thrombocytopenia: Platelet count <100,000 cells/mm^3: Withhold therapy until platelet count is ≥100,000 cells/mm^3 on day 1 or ≥50,000 cells/mm^3 on days 8 or 15. Reduce dose upon therapy reinitiation if:

Platelet count <50,000 cells/mm^3:

First occurrence: Permanently reduce dose to 75 mg/m^2

Second occurrence: Discontinue therapy.

Sensory neuropathy: Withhold therapy for grade 3 or 4 peripheral neuropathy. Resume therapy at reduced doses when neuropathy resolves completely or improves to grade 1:

First occurrence: Permanently reduce dose to 75 mg/m^2

Second occurrence: Permanently reduce dose to 50 mg/m^2

Third occurrence: Discontinue therapy.

Pancreatic adenocarcinoma:

Note: Dose level reductions for toxicity:

Full dose: 125 mg/m^2

First dose reduction: 100 mg/m^2

Second dose reduction: 75 mg/m^2

If additional dose reduction is necessary: Discontinue.

Hematologic toxicity (neutropenia and/or thrombocytopenia):

Day 1: If ANC is <1500 cells/mm^3 or platelet count is <100,000 cells/mm^3: Withhold therapy until ANC is ≥1500 cells/mm^3 and platelet count is ≥100,000 cells/mm^3

Day 8:

If ANC is 500 to <1000 cells/mm^3 **or** platelet count is 50,000 to <75,000 cells/mm^3: Reduce 1 dose level

If ANC is <500 cells/mm^3 **or** platelet count is <50,000 cells/mm^3: Withhold day 8 dose

Day 15 (if day 8 doses were reduced or given without modification):

If ANC is 500 to <1000 cells/mm^3 **or** platelet count is 50,000 to <75,000 cells/mm^3: Reduce 1 dose level from day 8

If ANC is <500 cells/mm^3 **or** platelet count is <50,000 cells/mm^3: Withhold day 15 dose

Day 15 (if day 8 doses were withheld):

If ANC is ≥1000 cells/mm^3 **or** platelet count is ≥75,000 cells/mm^3: Reduce 1 dose level from day 1

If ANC is 500 to <1000 cells/mm^3 **or** platelet count is 50,000 to <75,000 cells/mm^3: Reduce 2 dose levels from day 1

If ANC is <500 cells/mm^3 **or** platelet count is <50,000 cells/mm^3: Withhold day 15 dose

Neutropenic fever: Withhold therapy for grade 3 or 4 fever. Resume therapy at next lower dose level when fever resolves and ANC is ≥1500 cells/mm^3.

Peripheral neuropathy: Withhold therapy for grade 3 or 4 peripheral neuropathy. Resume therapy at next lower dose level when neuropathy improves to ≤ grade 1.

Dermatologic toxicity: For grade 2 or 3 toxicity, reduce dose to next lower dose level; if toxicity persists, discontinue.

Gastrointestinal toxicity: Withhold therapy for grade 3 mucositis or diarrhea. Resume therapy at next lower dose level when improves to ≤ grade 1.

Additional Information Complete prescribing information should be consulted for additional detail.

Dosage Forms Excipient information presented when available (limited, particularly for generics); consult specific product labeling.

Suspension Reconstituted, Intravenous:

Abraxane: 100 mg (1 ea)

Palbociclib (pal boe SYE klib)

Brand Names: US Ibrance

Index Terms Palbociclib Isethionate; PD 0332991; PD-0332991; PD-332991

Pharmacologic Category Antineoplastic Agent, Cyclin-Dependent Kinase Inhibitor

Use Breast cancer, advanced (initial endocrine-based therapy): Treatment of estrogen receptor (ER)-positive, human epidermal growth factor receptor 2 (HER2)-negative advanced breast cancer (in combination with letrozole) in postmenopausal women as initial endocrine-based therapy for metastatic disease

Pregnancy Considerations Adverse events were observed in animal reproduction studies. Women of reproductive potential should use effective contraception during treatment and for at least 2 weeks after the last dose. Although not indicated for use in men, animal data suggests that palbociclib may affect male fertility.

Breast-Feeding Considerations It is not known if palbociclib is excreted into breast milk. Due to the potential for serious adverse reactions in the nursing infant, breast-feeding is not recommended by the manufacturer.

Prescribing and Access Restrictions Palbociclib is available through specialty pharmacies. For more information, refer to http://www.ibrance.com/getting-ibrance

Contraindications There are no contraindications listed in the manufacturer's labeling.

Warnings/Precautions Hazardous agent: Use appropriate precautions for handling and disposal (meets NIOSH 2014 criteria).

Neutropenia was commonly observed in clinical studies, including grades 3 and 4 neutropenia. The median time to the first neutropenia episode (any grade) was 15 days (range: 13 to 117 days); the median duration of grade 3 or higher neutropenia was 7 days. Leukopenia, anemia, lymphocytopenia, thrombocytopenia, and neutropenic fever have also been reported. Monitor blood counts; treatment interruption, delay, or dose reduction is recommended for grade 3 or 4 neutropenia.

Infections (including grades 3 and 4) were reported more frequently in patients receiving palbociclib and letrozole compared with those receiving only letrozole. Monitor for signs/symptoms of infection and manage appropriately. Pulmonary embolism was observed more frequently in patients receiving palbociclib and letrozole, compared to those receiving letrozole alone. Monitor for signs/symptoms of pulmonary embolism and manage appropriately. Nausea, vomiting, diarrhea, and stomatitis (generally grade 1 or 2) were reported from clinical studies. Potentially significant drug-drug interactions may exist, requiring dose or frequency adjustment, additional monitoring, and/or selection of alternative therapy.

Adverse Reactions Frequency not always defined.

>10%:
Central nervous system: Fatigue (41%; grade 3/4: 2%), peripheral neuropathy (13%)
Dermatologic: Alopecia (22%)
Gastrointestinal: Nausea (25%; grade 3: 2%), stomatitis (25%), diarrhea (21%; grade 3: 4%), decreased appetite (16%; grade 3: 1%), vomiting (15%)
Hematologic & oncologic: Abnormal absolute lymphocyte count (81%; grade 3: 17%; grade 4: 1%; decreased lymphocytes), neutropenia (75%; grade 3: 48%; grade 4: 6%), leukopenia (43%; grade 3: 19%), anemia (35%; grade 3: 5%; grade 4: 1%), thrombocytopenia (17%; grade 3: 2%)
Infection: Infection (55%; grade 3/4: 5%)
Neuromuscular & skeletal: Weakness (13%; grade 3: 2%)
Respiratory: Epistaxis (11%)
1% to 10%:
Cardiovascular: Pulmonary embolism (4% to 5%)
Respiratory: Upper respiratory tract infection (31%; grade 3: 1%)

Drug Interactions

Metabolism/Transport Effects Substrate of CYP3A4 (major); **Note:** Assignment of Major/Minor substrate status based on clinically relevant drug interaction potential; **Inhibits** CYP3A4 (weak)

Avoid Concomitant Use

Avoid concomitant use of Palbociclib with any of the following: BCG (Intravesical); Conivaptan; CYP3A4 Inducers (Moderate); CYP3A4 Inducers (Strong); CYP3A4 Inhibitors (Strong); Deferiprone; Dipyrone; Fusidic Acid (Systemic); Grapefruit Juice; Idelalisib; Natalizumab; Pimecrolimus; Pimozide; Tacrolimus (Topical); Tofacitinib; Vaccines (Live)

Increased Effect/Toxicity

Palbociclib may increase the levels/effects of: ARIPiprazole; CloZAPine; CYP3A4 Substrates; Deferiprone; Dofetilide; Fingolimod; Flibanserin; Hydrocodone; Leflunomide; Lomitapide; Natalizumab; NiMODipine; Pimozide; Tofacitinib; Vaccines (Live)

The levels/effects of Palbociclib may be increased by: Aprepitant; Conivaptan; CYP3A4 Inhibitors (Moderate); CYP3A4 Inhibitors (Strong); Dasatinib; Denosumab; Dipyrone; Fosaprepitant; Fusidic Acid (Systemic); Grapefruit Juice; Idelalisib; Ivacaftor; Luliconazole; Mifepristone; Netupitant; Osimertinib; Pimecrolimus; Roflumilast; Simeprevir; Stiripentol; Tacrolimus (Topical); Trastuzumab

Decreased Effect

Palbociclib may decrease the levels/effects of: BCG (Intravesical); Coccidioides immitis Skin Test; Sipuleucel-T; Vaccines (Inactivated); Vaccines (Live)

The levels/effects of Palbociclib may be decreased by: CYP3A4 Inducers (Moderate); CYP3A4 Inducers (Strong); Deferasirox; Echinacea; Osimertinib; Siltuximab; Tocilizumab

Food Interactions Coadministration with grapefruit may increase palbociclib plasma concentrations. Management: Avoid concomitant administration with grapefruit.

Storage/Stability Store at 20°C to 25°C (68°F to 77°F); excursions are permitted between 15°C and 30°C (59°F and 86°F).

Mechanism of Action Palbociclib is a reversible small molecule cyclin-dependent kinase (CDK) inhibitor which is selective for CDK 4 and 6. CDKs have a role in regulating progression through the cell cycle at the G1/S phase by blocking retinoblastoma (Rb) hyperphosphorylation (Finn, 2015). Palbociclib reduces proliferation of breast cancer cell lines by preventing progression from the G1 to the S cell cycle phase. The combination of palbociclib and letrozole provides for increased inhibition of Rb phosphorylation, downstream signaling, and tumor growth compared with each agent alone.

Pharmacodynamics/Kinetics

Absorption: Increased with high-fat, high-calorie food
Distribution: V_d (mean): 2,583 L
Protein binding: ~85%
Metabolism: Extensively hepatic; Major pathways: Oxidation and sulfonation, primarily by CYP3A and sulfotransferase (SULT) enzyme SULT2A1; Minor pathways: Acylation and glucuronidation
Bioavailability: Mean absolute bioavailability: 46%
Half-life elimination: 29 ± 5 hours
Time to peak: 6 to 12 hours
Excretion: Feces (~74%, primarily as metabolites); Urine (~18%; primarily as metabolites)

Dosing

Adult & Geriatric

Breast cancer, advanced, initial endocrine-based therapy: Females (HER-2 negative): Oral: 125 mg once daily for 21 days, followed by a 7-day rest period to complete a 28-day treatment cycle (in combination with continuous letrozole); continue until disease progression or unacceptable toxicity (Finn 2015).

Breast cancer, advanced, second-line endocrine-based therapy (off-label use): Females (HER-2 negative): Oral: 125 mg once daily for 21 days, followed by 7 days off, repeat every 28 days (in combination with fulvestrant [and goserelin if pre- or peri-menopausal]); continue until disease progression or unacceptable toxicity (Turner 2015).

Missed/vomited doses: If a dose is vomited or missed, an additional dose should not be taken that day. Resume dosing with the next scheduled daily dose.

Dosage adjustment for concomitant therapy:

Strong CYP3A4 inhibitors: Avoid concomitant use with strong CYP3A4 inhibitors (eg, azole antifungals, clarithromycin, nefazodone, protease inhibitors, telithromycin, verapamil, grapefruit or grapefruit juice) and consider alternatives with no or minimal CYP3A4 inhibition. If coadministration with a strong CYP3A4 inhibitor cannot be avoided, reduce palbociclib dose to 75 mg once daily. If the strong inhibitor is discontinued, increase palbociclib dose (after 3 to 5 inhibitor half-lives have elapsed) to the dose used prior to initiating the strong CYP3A4 inhibitor.

CYP3A4 inducers: Avoid concomitant use with moderate or strong CYP3A4 inducers.

Renal Impairment

Mild to moderate impairment (CrCl 30 to <90 mL/minute): There are no dosage adjustments provided in the manufacturer's labeling, although palbociclib exposure is not increased.

Severe impairment (CrCl <30 mL/minute): There are no dosage adjustments provided in the manufacturer's labeling (has not been studied).

◄ **Hepatic Impairment**
Mild impairment (total bilirubin ≤ULN and AST >ULN or total bilirubin >1 to 1.5 times ULN and any AST): There are no dosage adjustments provided in the manufacturer's labeling, although palbociclib exposure is not increased.

Moderate to severe impairment (total bilirubin >1.5 times ULN and any AST): There are no dosage adjustments provided in the manufacturer's labeling (has not been studied).

Adjustment for Toxicity May require treatment interruption/delay, dose reduction, or discontinuation for some adverse reactions. The recommended dose reduction (based on individual safety and tolerance) is to 100 mg daily; if further reduction is required, reduce dose to 75 mg daily. If dose reduction below 75 mg daily is required, discontinue treatment.

Hematologic toxicity (according to Common Toxicity Criteria for Adverse Events Version 4):
Grade 1 or 2: No dosage adjustment required.
Grade 3 (except lymphopenia unless associated with clinical events [eg, opportunistic infection]): No dosage adjustment required. Consider repeating CBC with differential one week later. Withhold initiation of the next cycle until ≤ grade 2.
Grade 3 (ANC 500/mm^3 to <1,000/mm^3) plus fever ≥38.5°C and/or infection: Withhold palbociclib treatment (and initiation of the next cycle) until resolved to ≤ grade 2. Resume at next lower dose upon restarting.
Grade 4 (except lymphopenia unless associated with clinical events [eg, opportunistic infection]): Withhold palbociclib treatment (and initiation of the next cycle) until resolved to ≤ grade 2. After resolution, resume at next lower dose.
Nonhematologic toxicity (according to Common Toxicity Criteria for Adverse Events Version 4):
Grade 1 or 2: No dosage adjustment required.
Grade 3 or higher (if persistent despite medical management): Withhold palbociclib until symptoms resolve to ≤ grade 1 or ≤ grade 2 (if toxicity is not a safety risk); after resolution, resume at the next lower dose.

Dietary Considerations Avoid grapefruit.

Administration Oral: Administer with food. Take at approximately the same time each day. Swallow whole, do not crush, chew, or open capsules prior to swallowing (do not ingest if capsules are broken, cracked, or not fully intact). Hazardous agent; use appropriate precautions for handling and disposal (meets NIOSH 2014 criteria).

Monitoring Parameters CBC with differential (prior to treatment initiation, every 2 weeks for first 2 cycles, then prior to each cycle, or as clinically indicated); monitor for signs/symptoms of infection and pulmonary embolism.

Dosage Forms Excipient information presented when available (limited, particularly for generics); consult specific product labeling.
Capsule, Oral:
Ibrance: 75 mg, 100 mg, 125 mg

◆ Palbociclib Isethionate *see* Palbociclib *on page 1372*
◆ Palgic [DSC] *see* Carbinoxamine *on page 311*

Palifermin (pal ee FER min)

Brand Names: US Kepivance
Brand Names: Canada Kepivance®
Index Terms AMJ 9701; Keratinocyte Growth Factor, Recombinant Human; rhKGF; rhu Keratinocyte Growth Factor; rHu-KGF
Pharmacologic Category Chemoprotective Agent; Keratinocyte Growth Factor
Use Decrease the incidence and duration of severe oral mucositis associated with hematologic malignancies in patients receiving myelotoxic therapy requiring hematopoietic stem cell support (when the preparative regimen is expected to result in mucositis ≥ grade 3 in most patients)

Note: Use (safety and efficacy) is not established for nonhematologic malignancies; use is not recommended with conditioning regimens containing melphalan 200 mg/m^2

Dosing
Adult & Geriatric Oral mucositis associated with hematopoietic stem cell transplant (HSCT) conditioning regimens: IV: 60 mcg/kg/day for 3 consecutive days before and 3 consecutive days after myelotoxic therapy; total of 6 doses (Spielberger, 2004)
Note: Administer first 3 doses prior to myelotoxic therapy, with the 3rd dose given 24-48 hours before beginning the myelotoxic conditioning regimen.

Administer the last 3 doses after completion of the conditioning regimen, with the first of these doses after but on the same day as HSCT infusion and at least 4 days after the most recent dose of palifermin.

Renal Impairment No dosage adjustment necessary.
Hepatic Impairment No dosage adjustment provided in the manufacturer's labeling (has not been studied).
Additional Information Complete prescribing information should be consulted for additional detail.
Dosage Forms Excipient information presented when available (limited, particularly for generics); consult specific product labeling.
Solution Reconstituted, Intravenous [preservative free]:
Kepivance: 6.25 mg (1 ea)

Paliperidone (pal ee PER i done)

Brand Names: US Invega; Invega Sustenna; Invega Trinza
Brand Names: Canada Invega; Invega Sustenna
Index Terms 9-hydroxy-risperidone; 9-OH-risperidone; Paliperidone Palmitate
Pharmacologic Category Second Generation (Atypical) Antipsychotic
Use
Schizophrenia: Treatment of schizophrenia
Schizoaffective disorder (oral and monthly IM paliperidone): Treatment of schizoaffective disorder as monotherapy and as an adjunct to mood stabilizers or antidepressants

Pregnancy Considerations Adverse events have not been observed in animal reproduction studies. Antipsychotic use during the third trimester of pregnancy has a risk for extrapyramidal symptoms (EPS) and/or withdrawal symptoms in newborns following delivery. Symptoms in the newborn may include agitation, feeding disorder, hypertonia, hypotonia, respiratory distress, somnolence, and tremor. These effects may be self-limiting and allow recovery within hours or days with no specific treatment, or they may be severe requiring prolonged hospitalization.

Paliperidone may cause hyperprolactinemia, which may decrease reproductive function in both males and females. Paliperidone is the active metabolite of risperidone; refer to Risperidone monograph for additional information.

The ACOG recommends that therapy during pregnancy be individualized; treatment with psychiatric medications during pregnancy should incorporate the clinical expertise of the mental health clinician, obstetrician, primary healthcare provider, and pediatrician. Safety data related to atypical antipsychotics during pregnancy is limited and routine use is not recommended. However, if a woman is inadvertently exposed to an atypical antipsychotic while pregnant, continuing therapy may be preferable to switching to a typical antipsychotic that the fetus has not yet been exposed to; consider risk:benefit (ACOG, 2008).

Healthcare providers are encouraged to enroll women 18 to 45 years of age exposed to paliperidone during pregnancy in the Atypical Antipsychotics Pregnancy Registry (1-866-961-2388 or http://www.womensmentalhealth.org/pregnancyregistry).

Breast-Feeding Considerations Paliperidone is excreted in breast milk. According to the manufacturer, the decision to continue or discontinue breast-feeding during therapy should take into account the risk of exposure to the infant and the benefits of treatment to the mother.

Contraindications Hypersensitivity to paliperidone, risperidone, or any component of the formulation

Warnings/Precautions [US Boxed Warning]: Elderly patients with dementia-related psychosis treated with antipsychotics are at an increased risk of death compared to placebo. Most deaths appeared to be either cardiovascular (eg, heart failure, sudden death) or infectious (eg, pneumonia) in nature. In addition, an increased incidence of cerebrovascular adverse effects (eg, transient ischemic attack, cerebrovascular accidents) has been reported in studies of placebo-controlled trials of risperidone (paliperidone is the primary active metabolite of risperidone) in elderly patients with dementia-related psychosis. Paliperidone is not approved for the treatment of dementia-related psychosis. In addition, patients with Lewy body dementia (LBD) may be more sensitive to CNS-related and extrapyramidal effects.

May cause CNS depression, which may impair physical or mental abilities; patients must be cautioned about performing tasks that require mental alertness (eg, operating machinery or driving). Use with caution in mild renal dysfunction; dose reduction recommended. Not recommended in patients with moderate to severe impairment.

Esophageal dysmotility and aspiration have been associated with antipsychotic use; use with caution in patients at risk of aspiration pneumonia (eg, Alzheimer disease).

Leukopenia, neutropenia, and agranulocytosis (sometimes fatal) have been reported in clinical trials and postmarketing reports with antipsychotic use; presence of risk factors (eg, preexisting low WBC or history of drug-induced leuko-/neutropenia) should prompt periodic blood count assessment. Discontinue therapy at first signs of blood dyscrasias or if absolute neutrophil count <1,000/mm^3.

Paliperidone is associated with increased prolactin levels; clinical significance of hyperprolactinemia in patients with breast cancer or other prolactin-dependent tumors is unknown. May alter temperature regulation. May mask toxicity of other drugs or conditions (eg, intestinal obstruction, Reye's syndrome, brain tumor) due to antiemetic effects. Priapism has been reported rarely with use. Hypersensitivity reactions, including anaphylactic reactions and angioedema, have been reported.

May cause orthostasis and syncope; use with caution in patients with known cardiovascular disease (heart failure, history of myocardial infarction or ischemia, conduction abnormalities), cerebrovascular disease, or conditions that predispose the patient to hypotension (dehydration, hypovolemia, and treatment with antihypertensive medications). May alter cardiac conduction; life-threatening arrhythmias have occurred with therapeutic doses of neuroleptics. Avoid use in combination with QTc-prolonging drugs. Avoid use in patients with congenital long QT syndrome and in patients with history of cardiac arrhythmia.

May cause extrapyramidal symptoms (EPS), including pseudoparkinsonism, acute dystonic reactions, akathisia, and tardive dyskinesia (risk of these reactions is low relative to other neuroleptics, and is dose dependent). Risk of dystonia (and probably other EPS) may be greater with increased doses, use of conventional antipsychotics, males, and younger patients. Risk of neuroleptic malignant syndrome (NMS) may be increased in patients with Parkinson disease or Lewy body dementia; monitor for symptoms of confusion, obtundation, postural instability and extrapyramidal symptoms. May cause hyperglycemia; in some cases may be extreme and associated with ketoacidosis, hyperosmolar coma, or death. All patients should be monitored for symptoms of hyperglycemia (eg, polydipsia, polyuria, polyphagia, weakness). Use with caution in patients with diabetes (or risk factors) or other disorders of glucose regulation; monitor for worsening of glucose control. Patients with risk factors for diabetes (eg, obesity or family history) should have a baseline fasting blood sugar (FBS) and periodically during treatment. Significant weight gain has been observed with antipsychotic therapy; incidence varies with product. Monitor waist circumference and BMI. May cause lipid abnormalities (LDL and triglycerides increased; HDL decreased). Few case reports describe intraoperative floppy iris syndrome (IFIS) in patients receiving risperidone and undergoing cataract surgery (Ford, 2011). IFIS has not been reported with paliperidone but caution is advised since it is the active metabolite of risperidone. Prior to cataract surgery, evaluate for prior or current paliperidone or risperidone use. The benefits or risks of interrupting paliperidone or risperidone prior to surgery have not been established; clinicians are advised to proceed with surgery cautiously.

The possibility of a suicide attempt is inherent in psychotic illness or bipolar disorder; use caution in high-risk patients during initiation of therapy. Prescriptions should be written for the smallest quantity consistent with good patient care.

Use in elderly patients with dementia is associated with an increased risk of mortality and cerebrovascular accidents; avoid antipsychotic use for behavioral problems associated with dementia unless alternative nonpharmacologic therapies have failed and patient may harm self or others. Paliperidone is not approved for the treatment of dementia-related psychosis. In addition, use may cause or exacerbate syndrome of inappropriate antidiuretic hormone secretion or hyponatremia; monitor sodium closely with initiation or dosage adjustments in older adults (Beers Criteria).

The tablet formulation consists of drug within a nonabsorbable shell that is expelled and may be visible in the stool. Use is not recommended in patients with preexisting severe gastrointestinal narrowing disorders. Patients with upper GI tract alterations in transit time may have increased or decreased bioavailability of paliperidone. Do not use in patients unable to swallow the tablet whole.

Adverse Reactions Unless otherwise noted, frequency of adverse effects is reported for the oral/IM formulation in adults. Frequency not always defined.

Cardiovascular: Tachycardia (3% to 14%), orthostatic hypotension (2% to 4%; dose dependent), bundle branch block (≤3%)

Central nervous system: Extrapyramidal reaction (adolescents 18% to 40%; adults ≤3% to 26%; dose dependent), drowsiness (adolescents 13% to 26%; adults 4% to 12%; dose dependent), parkinsonian-like syndrome (1% to 18%; dose dependent), akathisia (3% to 17%; dose dependent), headache (6% to 15%), dystonia (1% to 14%; dose dependent), agitation (≤10%), anxiety (≤9%), dizziness (2% to 6%), dysarthria (1% to 4%; dose dependent), fatigue (≤2% to 3%), lethargy (≤3%), sleep disorder (≤3%), tonic-clonic seizures

Dermatologic: Papular rash

Endocrine & metabolic: Increased serum prolactin (males: 42% to 46%; females: 27% to 32%), decreased HDL cholesterol (14%), abnormal triglycerides (5% to 13%), altered serum glucose (4% to 11%), blood cholesterol abnormal (4% to 11%), weight gain (6% to 19%; dose dependent), amenorrhea (≤6%), galactorrhea (≤4%), gynecomastia (≤3%)

Gastrointestinal: Vomiting (≤11%), nausea (4% to 8%), dyspepsia (5% to 6%), sialorrhea (≤6%; dose dependent), constipation (4% to 5%), abdominal pain (≤2% to 4%), increased appetite (2% to 3%), toothache (2% to 3%), xerostomia (2% to 3%), diarrhea (≤3%), swollen tongue (≤3%)

Genitourinary: Urinary tract infection (≤2% to 3%)

Hematologic & oncologic: Change in HDL (15% to 29%), change in LDL (4% to 14%)

Local: Injection site reaction (≤12%)

Neuromuscular & skeletal: Hyperkinesia (2% to 17%; dose dependent), tremor (3% to 12%), dyskinesia (adolescents and adults <1% to 9%), myalgia (≤4%; dose dependent), weakness (≤4%), back pain (1% to 3%), limb pain (≤3%), tongue paralysis (adolescents: ≤3%)

Ophthalmic: Blurred vision (≤3%)

Respiratory: Upper respiratory tract infection (2% to 10%), nasopharyngitis (adolescents and adults 2% to 5%; dose dependent), cough (2% to 3%; dose dependent), rhinitis (1% to 3%; dose dependent)

≤2% (Limited to important or life-threatening): Agranulocytosis, alopecia, anaphylaxis, antiemetic effect, aspiration pneumonia, atrial fibrillation, cerebrovascular accident, convulsions, deep vein thrombosis, diabetes mellitus, diabetic ketoacidosis, edema, epistaxis, erectile dysfunction, first degree atrioventricular block, hyperprolactinemia, hypertension, hypertonia, hypothermia, increased serum ALT, increased serum AST, insomnia, intestinal obstruction, intraoperative floppy iris syndrome, ischemia, jaundice, mania, neck stiffness, neuroleptic malignant syndrome, orthostatic dizziness, pancreatitis, postural orthostatic tachycardia, priapism, psychomotor agitation, pulmonary embolism, retrograde ejaculation, sedation, seizure, SIADH, sinus arrhythmia, sleep apnea, suicidal ideation, syncope, tardive dyskinesia, thrombocytopenia, thrombotic thrombocytopenic purpura, trismus, urinary incontinence, urinary retention, venous thromboembolism

Drug Interactions

Metabolism/Transport Effects Substrate of P-glycoprotein

Avoid Concomitant Use

Avoid concomitant use of Paliperidone with any of the following: Amisulpride; Azelastine (Nasal); Highest Risk QTc-Prolonging Agents; Ivabradine; Metoclopramide; Mifepristone; Moderate Risk QTc-Prolonging Agents; Orphenadrine; Paraldehyde; Sulpiride; Thalidomide

Increased Effect/Toxicity

Paliperidone may increase the levels/effects of: Alcohol (Ethyl); Amisulpride; Azelastine (Nasal); CNS Depressants; Highest Risk QTc-Prolonging Agents; Hydrocodone; Methotrimeprazine; Methylphenidate; Metyrosine; Orphenadrine; Paraldehyde; Selective Serotonin Reuptake Inhibitors; Serotonin Modulators; Sulpiride; Suvorexant; Thalidomide; Zolpidem

The levels/effects of Paliperidone may be increased by: Acetylcholinesterase Inhibitors (Central); Blood Pressure Lowering Agents; Brimonidine (Topical); Cannabis; Doxylamine; Dronabinol; Itraconazole; Ivabradine; Kava Kava; Lumacaftor; Magnesium Sulfate; Methotrimeprazine; Methylphenidate; Metoclopramide; Metyrosine; Mifepristone; Minocycline; Moderate Risk QTc-Prolonging Agents; Nabilone; Perampanel; P-glycoprotein/ABCB1 Inhibitors; QTc-Prolonging Agents (Indeterminate Risk and Risk Modifying); RisperiDONE; Rufinamide; Serotonin Modulators; Sodium Oxybate; Tapentadol; Tetrahydrocannabinol; Valproate Products

◄ **Decreased Effect**

Paliperidone may decrease the levels/effects of: Amphetamines; Antidiabetic Agents; Anti-Parkinson's Agents (Dopamine Agonist); Quinagolide

The levels/effects of Paliperidone may be decreased by: CarBAMazepine; Inducers of CYP3A4 (Strong) with P-glycoprotein; Lumacaftor; P-glycoprotein/ABCB1 Inducers; St Johns Wort

Storage/Stability

Oral, Monthly IM: Store at ≤25°C (77°F); excursions permitted to 15°C to 30°C (59°F to 86°F). Protect tablets from moisture.

3-month IM: Store at 20°C to 25°C (68°F to 77°F); excursions permitted to 15°C to 30°C (59°F to 86°F).

Mechanism of Action Paliperidone is considered a benzisoxazole atypical antipsychotic as it is the primary active metabolite of risperidone. As with other atypical antipsychotics, its therapeutic efficacy is believed to result from mixed central serotonergic and dopaminergic antagonism. The addition of serotonin antagonism to dopamine antagonism (classic neuroleptic mechanism) is thought to improve negative symptoms of psychoses and reduce the incidence of extrapyramidal side effects. Similar to risperidone, paliperidone demonstrates high affinity to α_1, D_2, H_1, and $5-HT_{2C}$ receptors, and low affinity for muscarinic and $5-HT_{1A}$ receptors. In contrast to risperidone, paliperidone displays nearly 10-fold lower affinity for α_2 and $5-HT_{2A}$ receptors, and nearly three- to fivefold less affinity for $5-HT_{1A}$ and $5-HT_{1D}$, respectively.

Pharmacodynamics/Kinetics

Absorption: IM: Slow release (Monthly: Begins on day 1 and continues up to 126 days; 3-month: Begins on day 1 and continues up to 18 months)

Distribution: V_d: Oral: 487 L; Monthly IM: 391 L; 3-month IM: 1960 L

Protein binding: 74%

Metabolism: Hepatic via CYP2D6 and 3A4 (limited role in elimination); minor metabolism (<10% each) via dealkylation, hydroxylation, dehydrogenation, and benzisoxazole scission

Bioavailability: Oral: 28%

Half-life elimination:

Oral: 23 hours; 24 to 51 hours with renal impairment (CrCl <80 mL/minute)

Monthly IM (following a single-dose administration): Range: 25 to 49 days

3-month IM: Deltoid injection range: 84 to 95 days; Gluteal injection range: 118 to 139 days

Time to peak, plasma: Oral: ~24 hours; Monthly IM: 13 days; 3-month IM: 30 to 33 days

Excretion: Urine (80%); feces (11%)

Dosing

Adult

US labeling:

Schizoaffective disorder:

Oral: Usual: 6 mg once daily in the morning; titration not required, though some may benefit from lower or higher doses (range: 3 to 12 mg daily). If exceeding 6 mg daily, increases of 3 mg daily are recommended at intervals of more than 4 days, up to a maximum of 12 mg daily.

Monthly IM: **Note:** Prior to initiation of monthly IM paliperidone, for patients naive to oral paliperidone or oral or injectable risperidone tolerability should be established with oral paliperidone or oral risperidone. Previous oral antipsychotics can be gradually discontinued at the time of initiation of monthly IM paliperidone. **Dosing based on paliperidone palmitate.**

Initiation of therapy:

Initial: 234 mg on treatment day 1 followed by 156 mg 1 week later with both doses administered in the deltoid muscle. The second dose may be administered 4 days before or after the weekly time point.

Maintenance: Following the 1-week initiation regimen, adjust the dose based on response and tolerability and begin a maintenance dose of 78 to 234 mg every month administered in either the deltoid or gluteal muscle (the 39 mg dose was not studied in schizoaffective disorder trials). The monthly maintenance dose may be administered 7 days before or after the monthly time point.

Conversion from oral paliperidone to monthly IM paliperidone: Initiate monthly IM paliperidone as described using the 1-week initiation regimen. Patients previously stabilized on oral doses can expect similar steady state exposure during maintenance treatment with monthly IM paliperidone using the following conversion:

Oral extended-release dose of 12 mg daily, then IM maintenance dose of 234 mg monthly

Oral extended-release dose of 6 mg daily, then IM maintenance dose of 117 mg monthly

Oral extended-release dose of 3 mg daily, then IM maintenance dose of 39 mg monthly

Conversion from other oral antipsychotics to monthly IM paliperidone: There is no systematically collected data to address switching patients from other oral antipsychotics to monthly IM paliperidone.

Switching from other long-acting injectable antipsychotics to monthly IM paliperidone: Initiate monthly IM paliperidone in the place of the next scheduled injection and continue at monthly intervals. The 1-week initiation regimen is not required in these patients.

Dosage adjustments: Adjustments may be made monthly (full effect from adjustments may not be seen for several months)

Missed second initiation dose:

If <4 weeks have elapsed since the first injection: Administer the missed dose (156 mg) in the deltoid as soon as possible, followed by a third dose of 117 mg in either the deltoid or gluteal muscle 5 weeks after the first injection (regardless of when the second injection was administered), then begin normal monthly maintenance dosing.

If ≥4 weeks and ≤7 weeks have elapsed since the first injection: Administer a dose of 156 mg in the deltoid as soon as possible, followed by another 156 mg dose in the deltoid 1 week later, then begin normal monthly maintenance dosing.

If >7 weeks has elapsed since the first injection: Therapy must be reinitiated following dosing recommendations for initiation of therapy.

Missed maintenance dose:

If ≥4 weeks and ≤6 weeks have elapsed since the last monthly injection: Administer the missed dose as soon as possible and continue therapy at monthly intervals.

If >6 weeks and ≤6 months have elapsed since the last monthly injection:

If the maintenance dose was <234 mg: Administer the same dose the patient was previously stabilized on in the deltoid as soon as possible, followed by a second equivalent dose in the deltoid 1 week later, then resume maintenance dose at monthly intervals.

If the maintenance dose was 234 mg: Administer a 156 mg dose in the deltoid as soon as possible, followed by a second dose of 156 mg in the deltoid 1 week later, then resume maintenance dose at monthly intervals.

If >6 months have elapsed since last monthly maintenance injection: Therapy must be reinitiated following dosing recommendations for initiation of therapy.

Schizophrenia:

Oral: Usual: 6 mg once daily in the morning; titration not required, though some may benefit from lower or higher doses (range: 3 to 12 mg daily). If exceeding 6 mg daily, increases of 3 mg daily are recommended no more frequently than every 5 days, up to a maximum of 12 mg daily.

IM:

Monthly paliperidone (Invega Sustenna): **Note:** Prior to initiation of monthly IM paliperidone, for patients naïve to oral paliperidone or oral or injectable risperidone tolerability should be established with oral paliperidone or oral risperidone. Previous oral antipsychotics can be gradually discontinued at the time of initiation of monthly IM paliperidone. **Dosing based on paliperidone palmitate.**

Initiation of therapy:

Initial: 234 mg on treatment day 1 followed by 156 mg 1 week later with both doses administered in the deltoid muscle. The second dose may be administered 4 days before or after the weekly time point.

Maintenance: Following the 1-week initiation regimen, begin a maintenance dose of 117 mg every month administered in either the deltoid or gluteal muscle. Some patients may benefit from higher or lower monthly maintenance doses (monthly maintenance dosage range: 39 to 234 mg). The monthly maintenance dose may be administered 7 days before or after the monthly time point.

Conversion from oral paliperidone to IM paliperidone:
Initiate IM therapy as described using the 1-week initiation regimen. Patients previously stabilized on oral doses can expect similar steady state exposure during maintenance treatment with IM therapy using the following conversion:
Oral extended-release dose of 12 mg daily, then IM maintenance dose of 234 mg monthly
Oral extended-release dose of 6 mg daily, then IM maintenance dose of 117 mg monthly
Oral extended-release dose of 3 mg daily, then IM maintenance dose of 39 to 78 mg monthly
Conversion from other oral antipsychotics to IM paliperidone: There is no systematically collected data to address switching patients from other oral antipsychotics to IM paliperidone.
Switching from other long-acting injectable antipsychotics to IM paliperidone: Initiate IM paliperidone in the place of the next scheduled injection and continue at monthly intervals. The 1-week initiation regimen is not required in these patients.
Dosage adjustments: Adjustments may be made monthly (full effect from adjustments may not be seen for several months)
Missed second initiation dose:
If <4 weeks have elapsed since the first injection: Administer the missed dose (156 mg) in the deltoid as soon as possible, followed by a third dose of 117 mg in either the deltoid or gluteal muscle 5 weeks after the first injection (regardless of when the second injection was administered), then begin normal monthly maintenance dosing.
If ≥4 weeks and ≤7 weeks have elapsed since the first injection: Administer a dose of 156 mg in the deltoid as soon as possible, followed by another 156 mg dose in the deltoid 1 week later, then begin normal monthly maintenance dosing.
If >7 weeks have elapsed since the first injection: Therapy must be reinitiated following dosing recommendations for initiation of therapy.
Missed maintenance dose:
If ≥4 weeks and ≤6 weeks have elapsed since the last monthly injection: Administer the missed dose as soon as possible and continue therapy at monthly intervals.
If >6 weeks and ≤6 months have elapsed since the last monthly injection:
If the maintenance dose was <234 mg: Administer the same dose the patient was previously stabilized on in the deltoid as soon as possible, followed by a second equivalent dose in the deltoid 1 week later, then resume maintenance dose at monthly intervals.
If the maintenance dose was 234 mg: Administer a 156 mg dose in the deltoid as soon as possible, followed by a second dose of 156 mg in the deltoid 1 week later, then resume maintenance dose at monthly intervals.
If >6 months have elapsed since last monthly maintenance injection: Therapy must be reinitiated following dosing recommendations for initiation of therapy.
Three-month paliperidone (Invega Trinza): **Note:** Three-month IM paliperidone is to be used only after monthly IM paliperidone (Invega Sustenna) has been established as adequate treatment for at least 4 months. The last 2 doses of monthly IM paliperidone should be the same dosage strength before starting 3-month IM paliperidone.
Conversion from monthly injection to 3-month injection: Initiate 3-month IM paliperidone when the next monthly IM paliperidone dose is scheduled. Base the 3-month dose on the previous monthly dose, using the equivalent 3.5 times higher dose. Three-month IM paliperidone may be administered up to 7 days before or after the next monthly dose date. Following the initial injection, administer every 3 months. Patients may be given the injection up to 2 weeks before or after the 3-month time point.
Monthly IM paliperidone (Invega Sustenna) 78 mg = 3-month IM paliperidone (Invega Trinza) 273 mg
Monthly IM paliperidone (Invega Sustenna) 117 mg = 3-month IM paliperidone (Invega Trinza) 410 mg
Monthly IM paliperidone (Invega Sustenna) 156 mg = 3-month IM paliperidone (Invega Trinza) 546 mg
Monthly IM paliperidone (Invega Sustenna) 234 mg = 3-month IM paliperidone (Invega Trinza) 819 mg

Conversion from 3-month IM paliperidone to monthly IM paliperidone: Initiate monthly IM paliperidone when the next 3-month IM paliperidone dose is scheduled. Base the monthly dose on the previous 3-month dose, using the equivalent 3.5 times lower dose. Following the initial injection, administer once monthly.
3-month IM paliperidone (Invega Trinza) 273 mg = Monthly IM paliperidone (Invega Sustenna) 78 mg
3-month IM paliperidone (Invega Trinza) 410 mg = Monthly IM paliperidone (Invega Sustenna) 117 mg
3-month IM paliperidone (Invega Trinza) 546 mg = Monthly IM paliperidone (Invega Sustenna) 156 mg
3-month IM paliperidone (Invega Trinza) 819 mg = Monthly IM paliperidone (Invega Sustenna) 234 mg
Conversion from 3-month IM paliperidone to paliperidone extended-release tablets: Initiate paliperidone extended release tablets 3 months after the last dose of 3-month IM paliperidone. Base the once daily extended-release tablet dose on the last 3-month injection dose and weeks since last administered. Use the following conversion.
If the last 3-month IM paliperidone dose was:
273 mg: 3 months to >24 weeks since the last dose = 3 mg paliperidone extended-release tablets
410 mg:
3 months to 24 weeks since the last dose = 3 mg paliperidone extended-release tablets
>24 weeks since the last dose = 6 mg paliperidone extended-release tablets
546 mg:
3 months to 18 weeks since the last dose = 3 mg paliperidone extended-release tablets
>18 weeks to 24 weeks since the last dose = 6 mg paliperidone extended-release tablets
>24 weeks since the last dose = 9 mg paliperidone extended-release tablets
819 mg:
3 months to 18 weeks since the last dose = 6 mg paliperidone extended-release tablets
>18 weeks to 24 weeks since the last dose = 9 mg paliperidone extended-release tablets
>24 weeks since the last dose = 12 mg paliperidone extended-release tablets
Dosage adjustments: Dosage adjustments can be made every 3 months in increments within the range of 273 to 819 mg based on response and tolerability. Due to the long-acting nature, the patient's response to an adjusted dose may not be apparent for several months.
Missed dose 3 ½ months to 4 months since last injection: Administer the previous 3-month dose as soon as possible and continue with normal dosing.
Missed dose 4 months to 9 months since last injection: Do not administer the next 3-month dose. If the last 3-month dose was:
273 mg: Administer 78 mg of monthly IM paliperidone (Invega Sustenna) into the deltoid muscle. Administer a second dose of 78 mg of monthly IM paliperidone (Invega Sustenna) one week later. One month following the second injection, administer 273 mg of 3-month IM paliperidone (Invega Trinza) into the deltoid or gluteal muscle and resume normal dosing at 3-month intervals.
410 mg: Administer 117 mg of monthly IM paliperidone (Invega Sustenna) into the deltoid muscle. Administer a second dose of 117 mg of monthly IM paliperidone (Invega Sustenna) one week later. One month following the second injection, administer 410 mg of 3-month IM paliperidone (Invega Trinza) into the deltoid or gluteal muscle and resume normal dosing at 3-month intervals.
546 mg: Administer 156 mg of monthly IM paliperidone (Invega Sustenna) into the deltoid muscle. Administer a second dose of 156mg of monthly IM paliperidone (Invega Sustenna) one week later. One month following the second injection, administer 546 mg of 3-month IM paliperidone (Invega Trinza) into the deltoid or gluteal muscle and resume normal dosing at 3-month intervals.
819 mg: Administer 156 mg of monthly IM paliperidone (Invega Sustenna) into the deltoid muscle. Administer a second dose of 156mg of monthly IM paliperidone (Invega Sustenna) one week later. One month following the second injection, administer 819 mg of 3-month IM paliperidone (Invega

Trinza) into the deltoid or gluteal muscle and resume normal dosing at 3-month intervals.

Missed dose longer than 9 months since last injection: Re-initiate treatment with monthly IM paliperidone (Invega Sustenna). Three-month IM paliperidone can be resumed after the patient has been adequately treated with monthly IM paliperidone for at least 4 months.

Canadian labeling:
Schizoaffective disorder:

Oral: Usual: 6 mg once daily in the morning; titration not required, though some may benefit from lower or higher doses (range: 3 to 12 mg daily). Dosage adjustments in increments or decrements of 3 mg daily are recommended at intervals of more than 5 days, maximum dose: 12 mg daily.

IM: Monthly paliperidone: **Note:** In patients naive to oral paliperidone or oral/injectable risperidone, tolerability should be established with oral paliperidone or oral risperidone prior to initiation of monthly IM paliperidone. Previous oral antipsychotics can be gradually discontinued at the time of initiation of monthly IM paliperidone. **Dosing based on paliperidone.**

Initiation of therapy:

Initial: 150 mg on treatment day 1 followed by 100 mg 1 week later (day 8) with both doses administered in the deltoid. The second dose may be administered up to 4 days before or after the weekly time point.

Maintenance: Following the 1-week initiation regimen, adjust the dose based on response and tolerability and begin a maintenance dose of 50 to 150 mg every month administered in either the deltoid or gluteal muscle. The monthly maintenance dose may be administered 7 days before or after the monthly time point.

Conversion from oral paliperidone to monthly IM paliperidone: Initiate monthly IM paliperidone as described using the 1-week initiation regimen. Patients previously stabilized on oral doses can expect similar steady state exposure during maintenance treatment with monthly IM paliperidone using the following conversion:

Oral extended-release dose of 12 mg daily, then IM maintenance dose of 150 mg monthly

Oral extended-release dose of 6 mg daily, then IM maintenance dose of 75 mg monthly

Oral extended-release dose of 3 mg daily, then IM maintenance dose of 25 to 50 mg monthly

Switching from other long-acting injectable antipsychotics (including Risperdal Consta) to monthly IM paliperidone: Initiate monthly IM paliperidone in the place of the next scheduled injection and continue at monthly intervals. The 1-week initiation regimen is not required in these patients.

Switching from injectable risperidone (Risperdal Consta) to monthly IM paliperidone:

Risperdal Consta dose of 25 mg every 2 weeks, then IM paliperidone maintenance dose of 50 mg monthly

Risperdal Consta dose of 37.5 mg every 2 weeks, then IM paliperidone maintenance dose of 75 mg monthly

Risperdal Consta dose of 50 mg every 2 weeks, then IM paliperidone maintenance dose of 100 mg monthly

Dosage adjustments: Adjustments may be made monthly (full effect from adjustments may not be seen for several months)

Missed second initiation dose:

If <4 weeks has elapsed since first injection: Administer the missed dose (100 mg) in the deltoid as soon as possible followed by a third dose of 75 mg in either the deltoid or gluteal muscle 5 weeks after the first injection (regardless of when the second injection was administered), then begin normal monthly maintenance dosing.

If 4 to 7 weeks have elapsed since first injection: Administer a dose of 100 mg in the deltoid as soon as possible, followed by another 100 mg dose in the deltoid 1 week later, then begin normal monthly maintenance dosing.

If >7 weeks has elapsed since the first injection: Therapy must be reinitiated following dosing recommendations for initiation of therapy.

Missed maintenance dose:

If <6 weeks have elapsed since the last monthly injection: Administer the missed dose as soon as possible and continue therapy at monthly intervals.

If >6 weeks and ≤6 months have elapsed since the last monthly injection:

If the maintenance dose was 25 to 100 mg: Administer the same dose the patient was previously stabilized on in the deltoid as soon as possible, followed by a second equivalent dose in the deltoid 1 week later, then resume maintenance dose at monthly intervals.

If the maintenance dose was 150 mg: Administer a 100 mg dose in the deltoid as soon as possible, followed by a second dose of 100 mg in the deltoid 1 week later, then resume maintenance dose at monthly intervals.

If >6 months have elapsed since last monthly maintenance injection: Therapy must be reinitiated following dosing recommendations for initiation of therapy.

Schizophrenia:

Oral: Usual: 6 mg once daily in the morning; titration not required, though some may benefit from lower or higher doses (range: 3 to 12 mg daily). Dosage adjustments in increments or decrements of 3 mg daily are recommended at intervals of more than 5 days, maximum dose: 12 mg daily.

IM: Monthly paliperidone: **Note:** In patients naive to oral paliperidone or oral/injectable risperidone, tolerability should be established with oral paliperidone or oral risperidone prior to initiation of monthly IM paliperidone. Previous oral antipsychotics can be gradually discontinued at the time of initiation of monthly IM paliperidone. **Dosing based on paliperidone.**

Initiation of therapy:

Initial: 150 mg on treatment day 1 followed by 100 mg 1 week later (day 8) with both doses administered in the deltoid. The second dose may be administered up to 4 days before or after the weekly time point.

Maintenance: Following the 1-week initiation regimen, begin a maintenance dose of 75 mg every month administered in either the deltoid or gluteal muscle. Some patients may benefit from higher or lower monthly maintenance doses (monthly maintenance dosage range: 25 to 150 mg). The monthly maintenance dose may be administered 7 days before or after the monthly time point.

Conversion from oral paliperidone to monthly IM paliperidone: Initiate monthly IM paliperidone as described using the 1-week initiation regimen. Patients previously stabilized on oral doses can expect similar steady state exposure during maintenance treatment with monthly IM paliperidone using the following conversion:

Oral extended-release dose of 12 mg daily, then IM maintenance dose of 150 mg monthly

Oral extended-release dose of 6 mg daily, then IM maintenance dose of 75 mg monthly

Oral extended-release dose of 3 mg daily, then IM maintenance dose of 25 to 50 mg monthly

Switching from other long-acting injectable antipsychotics (including Risperdal Consta) to monthly IM paliperidone: Initiate monthly IM paliperidone in the place of the next scheduled injection and continue at monthly intervals. The 1-week initiation regimen is not required in these patients.

Switching from injectable risperidone (Risperdal Consta) to monthly IM paliperidone:

Risperdal Consta dose of 25 mg every 2 weeks, then IM paliperidone maintenance dose of 50 mg monthly

Risperdal Consta dose of 37.5 mg every 2 weeks, then IM paliperidone maintenance dose of 75 mg monthly

Risperdal Consta dose of 50 mg every 2 weeks, then IM paliperidone maintenance dose of 100 mg monthly

Dosage adjustments: Adjustments may be made monthly (full effect from adjustments may not be seen for several months)

Missed second initiation dose:

If <4 weeks has elapsed since first injection: Administer the missed dose (100 mg) in the deltoid as soon as possible followed by a third dose of 75 mg in either the deltoid or gluteal muscle 5 weeks after the first injection (regardless of when the second injection was administered), then begin normal monthly maintenance dosing.

If 4 to 7 weeks have elapsed since first injection: Administer a dose of 100 mg in the deltoid as soon as possible, followed by another 100 mg dose in the deltoid 1 week later, then begin normal monthly maintenance dosing.

If >7 weeks has elapsed since the first injection: Therapy must be reinitiated following dosing recommendations for initiation of therapy.

Missed maintenance dose:

If <6 weeks have elapsed since the last monthly injection: Administer the missed dose as soon as possible and continue therapy at monthly intervals.

If >6 weeks and ≤6 months have elapsed since the last monthly injection:

If the maintenance dose was 25 to 100 mg: Administer the same dose the patient was previously stabilized on in the deltoid as soon as possible, followed by a second equivalent dose in the deltoid 1 week later, then resume maintenance dose at monthly intervals.

If the maintenance dose was 150 mg: Administer a 100 mg dose in the deltoid as soon as possible, followed by a second dose of 100 mg in the deltoid 1 week later, then resume maintenance dose at monthly intervals.

If >6 months have elapsed since last monthly maintenance injection: Therapy must be reinitiated following dosing recommendations for initiation of therapy.

Geriatric Refer to adult dosing. Additional monitoring of renal function and orthostatic blood pressure may be warranted.

Pediatric Schizophrenia: *US labeling:* Adolescents 12 to 17 years: Oral: Initial: 3 mg once daily; titration not required (no known benefit to efficacy from higher doses [ie, 6 mg daily for patients <51 kg and 12 mg daily for patients ≥51 kg]). If exceeding 3 mg daily, increases of 3 mg daily are recommended no more frequently than every 5 days.

Renal Impairment Clearance is decreased in renal impairment; adjust dose according to renal function:
Oral:

Mild impairment (CrCl 50 to 79 mL/minute): Initial dose: 3 mg once daily; maximum dose: 6 mg once daily

Moderate to severe impairment (CrCl 10 to 49 mL/minute): Initial dose: 1.5 mg once daily; maximum dose: 3 mg once daily

Severe impairment (CrCl <10 mL/minute): Use not recommended (has not been studied).

IM:

US labeling:

Mild impairment (CrCl 50 to 79 mL/minute):

Monthly IM paliperidone (Invega Sustenna): Initiation of therapy: 156 mg on treatment day 1, followed by 117 mg 1 week later with both doses administered in the deltoid, followed by a maintenance dose of 78 mg every month (administered in the deltoid or gluteal muscle)

Three-month IM paliperidone (Invega Trinza): Adjust dosage and stabilize the patient using the monthly IM injection, then transition to the 3-month IM injection.

Moderate to severe impairment (CrCl <50 mL/minute): Use not recommended

Canadian labeling:

Mild impairment (CrCl 50 to 79 mL/minute): Initiation of therapy: 100 mg on treatment day 1, followed by 75 mg 1 week later with both doses administered in the deltoid, followed by a maintenance dose of 50 mg every month (administered in the deltoid or gluteal muscle). Based on tolerability and/or response, maintenance dose may be adjusted within range of 25 to 100 mg.

Moderate to severe impairment (CrCl <50 mL/minute): Use not recommended

Hepatic Impairment Oral, IM (monthly, 3- month):

Mild to moderate impairment (Child-Pugh class A or B): No dosage adjustment necessary.

Severe impairment: There are no dosage adjustments provided in the manufacturer's labeling (has not been studied).

Administration

Oral: Administer in the morning without regard to meals. Extended release tablets should be swallowed whole with liquids; do not crush, chew, or divide.

IM Injection: Administer by IM route only as a single injection (do not divide); do not administer by any other route. Avoid inadvertent injection into vasculature.

Monthly paliperidone (Invega Sustenna): Prior to injection, shake syringe for **at least 10 seconds** to ensure a homogenous suspension. The 2 initial injections should be administered in the deltoid muscle using a 1 1/2 inch, 22-gauge needle for patients ≥90 kg, and a 1 inch, 23-gauge needle for patients <90 kg. The 2 initial deltoid intramuscular injections help attain therapeutic concentrations rapidly. Alternate deltoid injections (right and left deltoid muscle). The second dose may be administered

4 days before or after the weekly time point. Monthly maintenance doses can be administered in either the deltoid or gluteal muscle. Administer injections in the gluteal muscle using a 1 1/2 inch, 22-gauge needle (regardless of patient weight) in the upper-outer quadrant of the gluteal area. Alternate gluteal injections (right and left gluteal muscle). The monthly maintenance dose may be administered 7 days before or after the monthly time point.

Three-month paliperidone (Invega Trinza): Prior to injection, shake syringe for **at least 15 seconds** to ensure a homogenous suspension. **Inject within 5 minutes of shaking vigorously.** Inject slowly, deep into the deltoid or gluteal muscle. Must be administered using only the thin wall needles that are provided in the pack. Do **not** use needles from monthly IM paliperidone or other commercially-available needles to reduce the risk of blockage. Administer into the center of the deltoid muscle using a 1 1/2 inch, 22-gauge thin wall needle for patients ≥90 kg, and a 1 inch, 22-gauge thin wall needle for patients <90 kg. Alternate deltoid injections (right and left deltoid muscle). Administer injections in the gluteal muscle using a 1 1/2 inch, 22-gauge thin wall needle (regardless of patient weight) in the upper-outer quadrant of the gluteal area. Alternate gluteal injections (right and left gluteal muscle). In the event of an incompletely administered dose, do not re-inject the dose remaining in the syringe and do not administer another dose. Closely monitor and treat the patient with oral supplementation as clinically appropriate until the next scheduled 3-month injection.

Monitoring Parameters Mental status; vital signs (as clinically indicated); blood pressure (baseline; repeat 3 months after antipsychotic initiation, then yearly); weight, height, BMI, waist circumference (baseline; repeat at 4, 8, and 12 weeks after initiating or changing therapy, then quarterly; consider switching to a different antipsychotic for a weight gain ≥5% of initial weight); CBC (as clinically indicated; monitor frequently during the first few months of therapy in patients with preexisting low WBC or history of drug-induced leukopenia/neutropenia); electrolytes, renal and liver function (annually and as clinically indicated); personal and family history of obesity, diabetes, dyslipidemia, hypertension, or cardiovascular disease (baseline; repeat annually); fasting plasma glucose level/HbA$_{1c}$ (baseline; repeat 3 months after starting antipsychotic, then yearly); fasting lipid panel (baseline; repeat 3 months after initiation of antipsychotic; if LDL level is normal repeat at 2-5 year intervals or more frequently if clinical indicated); changes in menstruation, libido, development of galactorrhea, erectile and ejaculatory function (at each visit for the first 12 weeks after the antipsychotic is initiated or until the dose is stable, then yearly); abnormal involuntary movements or parkinsonian signs (baseline; repeat weekly until dose stabilized for at least 2 weeks after introduction and for 2 weeks after any significant dose increase); tardive dyskinesia (every 12 months; high-risk patients every 6 months); ocular examination (yearly in patients >40 years; every 2 years in younger patients) (ADA, 2004; Lehman, 2004; Marder, 2004).

Additional Information Invega is an extended release tablet based on the OROS osmotic delivery system. Water from the GI tract enters through a semipermeable membrane coating the tablet, solubilizing the drug into a gelatinous form which, through hydrophilic expansion, is then expelled through laser-drilled holes in the coating.

Dosage Forms Excipient information presented when available (limited, particularly for generics); consult specific product labeling.

Suspension, Intramuscular, as palmitate:

Invega Sustenna: 39 mg/0.25 mL (0.25 mL); 78 mg/0.5 mL (0.5 mL); 117 mg/0.75 mL (0.75 mL); 156 mg/mL (1 mL); 234 mg/1.5 mL (1.5 mL) [contains polyethylene glycol]

Invega Trinza: 410 mg/1.315 mL (1.315 mL); 273 mg/0.875 mL (0.875 mL); 546 mg/1.75 mL (1.75 mL); 819 mg/2.625 mL (2.625 mL) [contains polyethylene glycol]

Tablet Extended Release 24 Hour, Oral:

Invega: 1.5 mg, 3 mg, 6 mg, 9 mg

Generic: 1.5 mg, 3 mg, 6 mg, 9 mg

Dosage Forms: Canada Note: Refer also to Dosage Forms. Excipient information presented when available (limited, particularly for generics); consult specific product labeling.

Suspension, Intramuscular, as palmitate [strength expressed as base]:

Invega Sustenna: 50 mg/0.5 mL (0.5 mL), 75 mg/0.75 mL (0.75 mL), 100 mg/1 mL (1 mL), 150 mg/1.5 mL (1.5 mL) [contains polyethylene glycol]

◆ **Paliperidone Palmitate** see Paliperidone on page 1374

Palivizumab (pah li VIZ u mab)

Brand Names: US Synagis
Brand Names: Canada Synagis
Pharmacologic Category Monoclonal Antibody
Use Respiratory syncytial virus prophylaxis: Prevention of serious lower respiratory tract disease caused by respiratory syncytial virus (RSV) in pediatric patients at high risk of RSV disease. Safety and efficacy were established in infants with bronchopulmonary dysplasia (BPD), infants with a history of premature birth (≤35 weeks gestational age), and children with hemodynamically significant congenital heart disease (CHD).

The American Academy of Pediatrics (AAP, 2014) recommends RSV prophylaxis with palivizumab during RSV season for:
Infants born at ≤28 weeks 6 days gestational age and <12 months at the start of RSV season
Infants <12 months of age with chronic lung disease (CLD) of prematurity
Infants ≤12 months of age with hemodynamically significant congenital heart disease (CHD)
Infants and children <24 months of age with CLD of prematurity necessitating medical therapy (eg, supplemental oxygen, bronchodilator, diuretic, or chronic steroid therapy) within 6 months prior to the beginning of RSV season
AAP also suggests that palivizumab prophylaxis may be considered in the following circumstances:
Infants <12 months of age with congenital airway abnormality or neuromuscular disorder that decreases the ability to manage airway secretions
Infants <12 months of age with cystic fibrosis with clinical evidence of CLD and/or nutritional compromise
Children <24 months with cystic fibrosis with severe lung disease (previous hospitalization for pulmonary exacerbation in the first year of life or abnormalities on chest radiography or chest computed tomography that persist when stable) or weight for length less than the 10th percentile
Infants and children <24 months who are profoundly immunocompromised
Infants and children <24 months undergoing cardiac transplantation during RSV season

Limitations of use: Safety and efficacy have not been established for treatment of RSV disease.
Pregnancy Considerations Not for adult use; reproduction studies have not been conducted
Contraindications Significant prior hypersensitivity reaction to palivizumab or any component of the formulation
Warnings/Precautions Very rare cases of anaphylaxis, some fatal, have been observed following palivizumab. Rare cases of severe acute hypersensitivity reactions have also been reported. Use with caution after mild hypersensitivity reaction; permanently discontinue for severe hypersensitivity reaction. Safety and efficacy of palivizumab have not been demonstrated in the treatment of established RSV disease. Palivizumab is not recommended for the prevention of health care-associated RSV disease (AAP, 2014). Use with caution in patients with thrombocytopenia or any coagulation disorder; bleeding/hematoma may occur from IM administration.

Adverse Reactions
>10%:
Central nervous system: Fever (27%)
Dermatologic: Rash (12%)
1% to 10%: Miscellaneous: Antibody formation (1% to 2%)
<1% (Limited to important or life-threatening): Anaphylaxis (very rare - includes angioedema, dyspnea, hypotonia, pruritus, respiratory failure, unresponsiveness, urticaria); hypersensitivity reactions, injection site reactions, thrombocytopenia
Drug Interactions
Metabolism/Transport Effects None known.
Avoid Concomitant Use
Avoid concomitant use of Palivizumab with any of the following: Belimumab
Increased Effect/Toxicity
Palivizumab may increase the levels/effects of: Belimumab
Decreased Effect There are no known significant interactions involving a decrease in effect.
Preparation for Administration Do not shake, vigorously agitate, or dilute the solution. Administer immediately after withdrawal from the vial; discard unused portion.
Storage/Stability Store between 2°C and 8°C (36°F and 46°F) in original container; do not freeze. Extended storage information may be available; contact product manufacturer to obtain current recommendations.

Mechanism of Action Exhibits neutralizing and fusion-inhibitory activity against RSV; these activities inhibit RSV replication in laboratory and clinical studies
Pharmacodynamics/Kinetics
Bioavailability: 70%
Half-life elimination: 24.5 days
Dosing
Pediatric
Prevention of RSV: IM: Infants and Children <2 years: 15 mg/kg of body weight, monthly throughout RSV season (first dose administered prior to commencement of RSV season). **Note:** The American Academy of Pediatrics (AAP) recommends a maximum of 5 doses per season; if hospitalization occurs for breakthrough RSV infection, monthly prophylaxis should be discontinued for the remainder of that season (AAP, 2014).
Cardiopulmonary bypass patients: IM: Administer an additional dose as soon as possible after cardiopulmonary bypass procedure or at the conclusion of extracorporeal membrane oxygenation, even if <1 month from previous dose (AAP, 2014).
Renal Impairment There are no dosage adjustments provided in the manufacturer's labeling.
Hepatic Impairment There are no dosage adjustments provided in the manufacturer's labeling.
Administration IM injection should (preferably) be in the anterolateral aspect of the thigh; gluteal muscle should not be used routinely because of risk of damage to the sciatic nerve. Injection volumes over 1 mL should be administered as divided doses.
Monitoring Parameters Monitor for anaphylaxis or acute hypersensitivity reactions
Test Interactions May interfere (false negatives) with immunological-based RSV diagnostic tests (antigen detection) and viral culture assays; rely on reverse-transcriptase-polymerase chain reaction-based assays and clinical findings.
Dosage Forms Excipient information presented when available (limited, particularly for generics); consult specific product labeling.
Solution, Intramuscular [preservative free]:
Synagis: 50 mg/0.5 mL (0.5 mL); 100 mg/mL (1 mL) [contains glycine, histidine]

◆ Palladone *see* HYDROmorphone *on page 888*

Palonosetron (pal oh NOE se tron)

Brand Names: US Aloxi
Index Terms Palonosetron Hydrochloride; RS-25259; RS-25259-197
Pharmacologic Category Antiemetic; Selective 5-HT$_3$ Receptor Antagonist
Use
Chemotherapy-induced nausea and vomiting: Prevention of acute and delayed nausea and vomiting associated with initial and repeat courses in patients treated with moderately emetogenic cancer chemotherapy in adults; prevention of acute nausea and vomiting associated with initial and repeat courses in patients treated with highly emetogenic cancer chemotherapy in adults; prevention of acute nausea and vomiting associated with initial and repeat courses of emetogenic cancer chemotherapy (including highly emetogenic chemotherapy) in pediatric patients 1 month to <17 years.
Postoperative nausea and vomiting: Prevention of postoperative nausea and vomiting (PONV) for up to 24 hours following surgery in adults.
Limitations of use: Routine prophylaxis for PONV in patients with minimal expectation of nausea and/or vomiting is not recommended, although use is recommended in patients when nausea and vomiting must be avoided in the postoperative period, even if the incidence of PONV is low.
Pregnancy Considerations Adverse events have not been observed in animal reproduction studies. Use during pregnancy only if clearly needed.
Breast-Feeding Considerations It is not known if palonosetron is excreted in breast milk. Due to the potential for adverse reactions in the nursing infant, the manufacturer recommends a decision be made whether to discontinue nursing or to discontinue palonosetron, taking into account the importance of treatment to the mother.
Contraindications Hypersensitivity to palonosetron or any component of the formulation
Warnings/Precautions Hypersensitivity (including anaphylaxis) has been reported in patients with or without known hypersensitivity to other 5-HT$_3$ receptor antagonists. Serotonin syndrome has been reported with 5-HT$_3$ receptor antagonists, predominantly when used in combination with other serotonergic agents (eg, SSRIs, SNRIs, MAOIs, mirtazapine, fentanyl, lithium, tramadol, and/or

methylene blue). Some of the cases have been fatal. The majority of serotonin syndrome reports due to 5-HT$_3$ receptor antagonists have occurred in a post-anesthesia setting or in an infusion center. Serotonin syndrome has also been reported following overdose of another 5-HT$_3$ receptor antagonist. Monitor patients for signs of serotonin syndrome, including mental status changes (eg, agitation, hallucinations, delirium, coma); autonomic instability (eg, tachycardia, labile blood pressure, diaphoresis, dizziness, flushing, hyperthermia); neuromuscular changes (eg, tremor, rigidity, myoclonus, hyperreflexia, incoordination); gastrointestinal symptoms (eg, nausea, vomiting, diarrhea); and/or seizures. If serotonin syndrome occurs, discontinue 5-HT$_3$ receptor antagonist treatment and begin supportive management.

Although other selective 5-HT$_3$ receptor antagonists have been associated with dose-dependent increases in ECG intervals (eg, PR, QRS duration, QT/QTc, JT), palonosetron has not been shown to significantly affect the QT/QTc interval (Gonullu, 2012; Morganroth, 2008). Reduction in heart rate may occur with the 5-HT$_3$ antagonists, including palonosetron (Gonullu, 2012). Antiemetics are most effective when used prophylactically (Roila, 2010). Potentially significant drug-drug interactions may exist, requiring dose or frequency adjustment, additional monitoring, and/or selection of alternative therapy. If emesis occurs despite optimal antiemetic prophylaxis, re-evaluate emetic risk, disease, concurrent morbidities and medications to assure antiemetic regimen is optimized (Basch, 2011). For post-operative nausea and vomiting (PONV), may use for low expectation of PONV if it is essential to avoid nausea and vomiting in the postoperative period; use is not recommended if there is little expectation of nausea and vomiting.

Adverse Reactions Frequencies reported for both indications (chemotherapy-associated nausea and vomiting and postoperative nausea and vomiting) and in adults unless otherwise noted.

1% to 10%:
Cardiovascular: Prolonged Q-T interval on ECG (PONV 1% to 5%; chemotherapy-associated <1%), bradycardia (chemotherapy-associated 1%), sinus bradycardia (PONV: 1%), tachycardia (may be nonsustained; 1%), hypotension (≤1%)
Central nervous system: Headache (chemotherapy-associated: Adults 9%; infants, children, and adolescents <1%), anxiety (chemotherapy-associated: 1%), dizziness (infants, children, adolescents, and adults ≤1%)
Dermatologic: Pruritus (PONV: 1%)
Endocrine & metabolic: Hyperkalemia (chemotherapy-associated: 1%)
Gastrointestinal: Constipation (chemotherapy-associated: 5%), diarrhea (≤1%), flatulence (≤1%)
Genitourinary: Urinary retention (≤1%)
Hepatic: Increased serum ALT (≤1%; may be transient), increased serum AST (≤1%; may be transient)
Neuromuscular & skeletal: Weakness (chemotherapy-associated: 1%)
<1% (Limited to important or life-threatening): Amblyopia, anasarca, anemia, anorexia, arthralgia, chills, decreased appetite, decreased blood pressure, decreased gastrointestinal motility, decreased platelet count, dermatological disease (infants, children, and adolescents), distended vein, drowsiness, dyskinesia (infants, children, and adolescents), dyspepsia, epistaxis, erythema, euphoria, extrasystoles, eye irritation, flattened T wave on ECG, flu-like symptoms, hiccups, hot flash, hyperglycemia, hypersensitivity (very rare), hypertension, hypokalemia, hypoventilation, increased bilirubin (transient), increased liver enzymes, infusion site pain (infants, children, and adolescents), injection site reaction (very rare; includes burning sensation at injection site, discomfort at injection site, induration at injection site, pain at injection site), insomnia, ischemic heart disease, limb pain, metabolic acidosis, motion sickness, paresthesia, serotonin syndrome, sialorrhea, sinus arrhythmia, sinus tachycardia, supraventricular extrasystole, tinnitus, vein discoloration, ventricular premature contractions

Drug Interactions
Metabolism/Transport Effects Substrate of CYP1A2 (minor), CYP2D6 (minor), CYP3A4 (minor); **Note:** Assignment of Major/Minor substrate status based on clinically relevant drug interaction potential
Avoid Concomitant Use
Avoid concomitant use of Palonosetron with any of the following: Apomorphine
Increased Effect/Toxicity
Palonosetron may increase the levels/effects of: Apomorphine; Serotonin Modulators

Decreased Effect
Palonosetron may decrease the levels/effects of: Tapentadol; TraMADol
Storage/Stability Store intact vials at 20°C to 25°C (68°F to 77°F); excursions permitted to 15°C to 30°C (59°F to 86°F). Do not freeze. Protect from light. Solutions of 5 mcg/mL and 30 mcg/mL in NS, D$_5$W, D$_5^1/_2$NS, and D$_5$LR injection are stable for 48 hours at room temperature and 14 days under refrigeration (Trissel, 2004a).
Mechanism of Action Selective 5-HT$_3$ receptor antagonist, blocking serotonin, both on vagal nerve terminals in the periphery and centrally in the chemoreceptor trigger zone
Pharmacodynamics/Kinetics
Distribution: V$_d$: 8.3 ± 2.5 L/kg
Protein binding: ~62%
Metabolism: ~50% metabolized via CYP enzymes (and likely other pathways) to relatively inactive metabolites (N-oxide-palonosetron and 6-S-hydroxy-palonosetron); CYP1A2, 2D6, and 3A4 contribute to its metabolism
Half-life elimination: IV: Adults: ~40 hours; Children: ~20 to 30 hours
Excretion: Urine (80%; 40% as unchanged drug)
Dosing
Adult
Prevention of chemotherapy-induced nausea and vomiting: IV: 0.25 mg beginning ~30 minutes prior to the start of chemotherapy
Prevention of postoperative nausea and vomiting: IV: 0.075 mg immediately prior to anesthesia induction
Geriatric No dosage adjustment necessary. Refer to adult dosing.
Pediatric Prevention of chemotherapy-induced nausea and vomiting: Infants ≥1 month, Children, and Adolescents <17 years: IV: 20 **mcg**/kg (maximum dose: 1.5 **mg**) beginning ~30 minutes prior to the start of chemotherapy
Renal Impairment No dosage adjustment is necessary.
Hepatic Impairment No dosage adjustment is necessary.
Administration Flush IV line with NS prior to and following administration.
Prevention of chemotherapy-induced nausea and vomiting:
Children: Infuse over 15 minutes, beginning ~30 minutes prior to the start of chemotherapy
Adults: Infuse over 30 seconds, beginning ~30 minutes prior to the start of chemotherapy
Prevention of postoperative nausea and vomiting: Infuse over 10 seconds immediately prior to anesthesia induction
Dosage Forms Excipient information presented when available (limited, particularly for generics); consult specific product labeling.
Solution, Intravenous:
Aloxi: 0.25 mg/5 mL (5 mL) [contains edetate disodium]

◆ Palonosetron and Netupitant see Netupitant and Palonosetron on page 1269

◆ Palonosetron Hydrochloride see Palonosetron on page 1380

◆ Pal-Tizanidine (Can) see TiZANidine on page 1798

◆ 2-PAM see Pralidoxime on page 1486

Pamabrom (PAM a brom)

Pharmacologic Category Diuretic
Use Temporary relief of symptoms associated with premenstrual and menstrual periods (eg, bloating, water-weight gain, swelling, full feeling)
Dosing
Adult Premenstrual or menstrual symptoms: Oral: 50 mg after breakfast and then every 6 hours as needed (maximum: 200 mg/24 hours); should be taken 5-6 days prior to onset of menstrual period and continued until desired relief or end of period
Additional Information Complete prescribing information should be consulted for additional detail.

◆ Pamelor see Nortriptyline on page 1300

Pamidronate (pa mi DROE nate)

Brand Names: Canada Aredia; Pamidronate Disodium; Pamidronate Disodium Omega; PMS-Pamidronate
Index Terms Pamidronate Disodium
Pharmacologic Category Bisphosphonate Derivative
Use Hypercalcemia of malignancy: Treatment of moderate or severe hypercalcemia associated with malignancy, with or without bone metastases, in conjunction with adequate hydration.

Osteolytic bone metastases of breast cancer and osteolytic lesions of multiple myeloma: Treatment of osteolytic bone metastases of breast cancer and osteolytic lesions of multiple myeloma in conjunction with standard antineoplastic therapy.

Paget disease: Treatment of patients with moderate to severe Paget disease of bone.

Pregnancy Considerations Adverse events were observed in animal reproduction studies. It is not known if bisphosphonates cross the placenta, but fetal exposure is expected (Djokanovic, 2008; Stathopoulos, 2011). Bisphosphonates are incorporated into the bone matrix and gradually released over time. The amount available in the systemic circulation varies by dose and duration of therapy. Theoretically, there may be a risk of fetal harm when pregnancy follows the completion of therapy; however, available data have not shown that exposure to bisphosphonates during pregnancy significantly increases the risk of adverse fetal events (Djokanovic, 2008; Levy, 2009; Stathopoulos, 2011). Until additional data is available, most sources recommend discontinuing bisphosphonate therapy in women of reproductive potential as early as possible prior to a planned pregnancy; use in premenopausal women should be reserved for special circumstances when rapid bone loss is occurring (Bhalla, 2010; Pereira, 2012; Stathopoulos, 2011). Because hypocalcemia has been described following in utero bisphosphonate exposure, exposed infants should be monitored for hypocalcemia after birth (Djokanovic, 2008; Stathopoulos, 2011).

Breast-Feeding Considerations It is not known if pamidronate is excreted in breast milk. Pamidronate was not detected in the milk of a nursing woman receiving pamidronate 30 mg IV monthly (therapy started ~6 months postpartum). Following the first infusion, milk was pumped and collected for 0-24 hours and 25-48 hours, and each day pooled for analysis. Pamidronate readings were below the limit of quantification (<0.4 micromole/L). During therapy, breast milk was pumped and discarded for the first 48 hours following each infusion prior to resuming nursing. The infant was breast-fed >80% of the time; adverse events were not observed in the nursing infant (Simonoski, 2000). Monitoring the serum calcium concentrations of nursing infants is recommended (Stathopoulos, 2011). Due to the potential for serious adverse reactions in the nursing infant, the manufacturer recommends a decision be made whether to discontinue nursing or to discontinue the drug, taking into account the importance of treatment to the mother.

Contraindications Hypersensitivity to pamidronate, other bisphosphonates, or any component of the formulation

Warnings/Precautions Hazardous agent - use appropriate precautions for handling and disposal (meets NIOSH 2014 criteria). Osteonecrosis of the jaw (ONJ) has been reported in patients receiving bisphosphonates. Risk factors include invasive dental procedures (eg, tooth extraction, dental implants, boney surgery); a diagnosis of cancer, with concomitant chemotherapy, radiotherapy, or corticosteroids; poor oral hygiene, ill-fitting dentures; and comorbid disorders (anemia, coagulopathy, infection, preexisting dental disease). Most reported cases occurred after IV bisphosphonate therapy; however, cases have been reported following oral therapy. A dental exam and preventive dentistry should be performed prior to placing patients with risk factors on chronic bisphosphonate therapy. There is no evidence that discontinuing therapy reduces the risk of developing ONJ (Assael, 2009). The risk:benefit must be assessed by the treating physician and/or dentist/surgeon prior to any invasive dental procedure. Patients developing ONJ while on bisphosphonates should receive care by an oral surgeon.

Atypical femur fractures (after minimal or no trauma) have been reported. The fractures include subtrochanteric femur (bone just below the hip joint) and diaphyseal femur (long segment of the thigh bone). Some patients experience prodromal pain weeks or months before the fracture occurs. It is unclear if bisphosphonate therapy is the cause for these fractures. Patients receiving long-term (>3 to 5 years) bisphosphonate therapy may be at an increased risk. Consider discontinuing pamidronate in patients with a suspected femoral shaft fracture. Patients who present with thigh or groin pain in the absence of trauma should be evaluated. Infrequently, severe (and occasionally debilitating) musculoskeletal (bone, joint, and/or muscle) pain have been reported during bisphosphonate treatment. The onset of pain ranged from a single day to several months. Consider discontinuing therapy in patients who experience severe symptoms; symptoms usually resolve upon discontinuation. Some patients experienced recurrence when rechallenged with same drug or another bisphosphonate; avoid use in patients with a history of these symptoms in association with bisphosphonate therapy.

Initial or single doses have been associated with renal deterioration, progressing to renal failure and dialysis. Withhold pamidronate treatment (until renal function returns to baseline) in patients with evidence of renal deterioration. Glomerulosclerosis (focal segmental) with or without nephrotic syndrome has also been reported. Longer infusion times (>2 hours) may reduce the risk for renal toxicity, especially in patients with preexisting renal insufficiency. Single pamidronate doses should not exceed 90 mg. Patients with serum creatinine >3 mg/dL were not studied in clinical trials; limited data are available in patients with CrCl <30 mL/minute. Evaluate serum creatinine prior to each treatment. For the treatment of bone metastases, use is not recommended in patients with severe renal impairment; for renal impairment in indications other than bone metastases, use clinical judgment to determine if benefits outweigh potential risks.

Use has been associated with asymptomatic electrolyte abnormalities (including hypophosphatemia, hypokalemia, hypomagnesemia, and hypocalcemia). Rare cases of symptomatic hypocalcemia, including tetany have been reported. Patients with a history of thyroid surgery may have relative hypoparathyroidism; predisposing them to pamidronate-related hypocalcemia. Patients with preexisting anemia, leukopenia, or thrombocytopenia should be closely monitored during the first 2 weeks of treatment.

Hypercalcemia of malignancy (HCM): Adequate hydration is required during treatment (urine output ~2 L/day); avoid overhydration, especially in patients with heart failure.

Multiple myeloma: Patients with Bence-Jones proteinuria and dehydration should be adequately hydrated prior to therapy. The American Society of Clinical Oncology (ASCO) has also published guidelines on bisphosphonates use for prevention and treatment of bone disease in multiple myeloma (Kyle, 2007). Bisphosphonate (pamidronate or zoledronic acid) use is recommended in multiple myeloma patients with lytic bone destruction or compression spine fracture from osteopenia. Bisphosphonates may also be considered in patients with pain secondary to osteolytic disease, adjunct therapy to stabilize fractures or impending fractures, and for multiple myeloma patients with osteopenia but no radiographic evidence of lytic bone disease. Bisphosphonates are not recommended in patients with solitary plasmacytoma, smoldering (asymptomatic) or indolent myeloma, or monoclonal gammopathy of undetermined significance. The guidelines recommend monthly treatment for a period of 2 years. At that time, consider discontinuing in responsive and stable patients, and reinitiate if a new-onset skeletal-related event occurs. The ASCO guidelines are in alignment with the prescribing information for dosing, renal dose adjustments, infusion times, prevention and management of osteonecrosis of the jaw, and monitoring of laboratory parameter recommendations. According to the guidelines, in patients with extensive bone disease with existing severe renal disease (a serum creatinine >3 mg/dL or CrCl <30 mL/minute) pamidronate at a dose of 90 mg over 4 to 6 hours should be used (unless preexisting renal disease in which case a reduced initial dose should be considered). Monitor for albuminuria every 3 to 6 months; in patients with unexplained albuminuria >500 mg/24 hours, withhold the dose until level returns to baseline, then recheck every 3 to 4 weeks. Pamidronate may be reinitiated at a dose not to exceed 90 mg every 4 weeks with a longer infusion time of at least 4 hours.

Breast cancer (metastatic): The American Society of Clinical Oncology (ASCO) updated guidelines on the role of bone-modifying agents (BMAs) in the prevention and treatment of skeletal-related events for metastatic breast cancer patients (Van Poznak, 2011). The guidelines recommend initiating a BMA (denosumab, pamidronate, zoledronic acid) in patients with metastatic breast cancer to the bone. There is currently no literature indicating the superiority of one particular BMA. Optimal duration is not yet defined; however, the guidelines recommend continuing therapy until substantial decline in patient's performance status. The ASCO guidelines are in alignment with prescribing information for dosing, renal dose adjustments, infusion times, prevention and management of osteonecrosis of the jaw, and monitoring of laboratory parameter recommendations. BMAs are not the first-line therapy for pain. BMAs are to be used as adjunctive therapy for cancer-related bone pain associated with bone metastasis, demonstrating a modest pain control benefit. BMAs should be used in conjunction with agents such as NSAIDS, opioid and nonopioid analgesics, corticosteroids, radiation/surgery, and interventional procedures.

Adverse Reactions Note: Actual percentages may vary by indication and duration of infusion; treatment for multiple myeloma is associated with higher percentage.

>10%:

Central nervous system: Fatigue (≤37%), headache (≤26%), insomnia (≤22%)

Endocrine & metabolic: Hypophosphatemia (≤18%), hypokalemia (4% to 18%), hypocalcemia (≤3% to 17%), hypomagnesemia (10% to 12%)

Gastrointestinal: Nausea (≤54%), vomiting (≤36%), anorexia (≤26%), abdominal pain (≤23%), dyspepsia (≤23%)

Genitourinary: Urinary tract infection (≤19%)

Hematologic & oncologic: Anemia (≤43%), metastases (21% to 31%), granulocytopenia (≤20%)

Local: Infusion site reaction (≤18%; includes induration, pain, redness, and swelling)

Neuromuscular & skeletal: Myalgia (≤26%), weakness (≤22%), arthralgia (≤14%), osteonecrosis of the jaw (cancer patients: 1% to 11%)

Renal: Increased serum creatinine (≤19%)

Respiratory: Dyspnea (≤30%), cough (≤26%), upper respiratory tract infection (≤24%), sinusitis (≤16%), pleural effusion (≤11%)

Miscellaneous: Fever (18% to 39%; transient)

1% to 10%:

Cardiovascular: Atrial fibrillation (≤6%), hypertension (≤6%), syncope (≤6%), tachycardia (≤6%), atrial flutter (≤1%), cardiac failure (≤1%), edema (≤1%)

Central nervous system: Drowsiness (≤6%), psychosis (≤4%), seizure (≤2%)

Endocrine & metabolic: Hypothyroidism (≤6%)

Gastrointestinal: Constipation (≤6%), gastrointestinal hemorrhage (≤6%), diarrhea (≤1%), stomatitis (≤1%)

Genitourinary: Uremia (≤4%)

Hematologic & oncologic: Leukopenia (≤4%), neutropenia (≤1%), thrombocytopenia (≤1%)

Infection: Candidiasis (≤6%)

Neuromuscular & skeletal: Back pain, ostealgia

Respiratory: Rales (≤6%), rhinitis (≤6%)

<1% (Limited to important or life-threatening): Acute renal failure, anaphylactic shock, angioedema, cardiac failure, confusion, episcleritis, focal segmental glomerulosclerosis (including collapsing variant), hallucination (visual), hematuria, herpes virus infection (reactivation), hyperkalemia, hypernatremia, hypersensitivity reaction, hypervolemia, hypotension, inflammation at injection site, injection site phlebitis, iridocyclitis, iritis, left heart failure, lymphocytopenia, nephrotic syndrome, osteonecrosis (other than jaw), renal failure, renal insufficiency, scleritis, uveitis, xanthopsia

Drug Interactions

Metabolism/Transport Effects None known.

Avoid Concomitant Use There are no known interactions where it is recommended to avoid concomitant use.

Increased Effect/Toxicity

Pamidronate may increase the levels/effects of: Deferasirox

The levels/effects of Pamidronate may be increased by: Aminoglycosides; Nonsteroidal Anti-Inflammatory Agents; Systemic Angiogenesis Inhibitors; Thalidomide

Decreased Effect

The levels/effects of Pamidronate may be decreased by: Proton Pump Inhibitors

Preparation for Administration Hazardous agent; use appropriate precautions for handling and disposal (meets NIOSH 2014 criteria).

Powder for injection: Reconstitute by adding 10 mL of SWFI to each vial of lyophilized powder, the resulting solution will be 30 mg/10 mL or 90 mg/10 mL.

Pamidronate may be further diluted in 250 to 1000 mL of 0.45% or 0.9% sodium chloride or 5% dextrose. (The manufacturers recommend dilution in 1000 mL for hypercalcemia of malignancy, 500 mL for Paget's disease and bone metastases of myeloma, and 250 mL for bone metastases of breast cancer.)

Storage/Stability

Powder for reconstitution: Store at 20°C to 25°C (68°F to 77°F). The reconstituted solution is stable for 24 hours stored under refrigeration at 2°C to 8°C (36°F to 46°F). The diluted solution for infusion is stable at room temperature for up to 24 hours.

Solution for injection: Store at 20°C to 25°C (68°F to 77°F). The diluted solution for infusion is stable at room temperature for up to 24 hours.

Mechanism of Action Nitrogen-containing bisphosphonate; inhibits bone resorption and decreases mineralization by disrupting osteoclast activity (Gralow, 2009; Rogers, 2011)

Pharmacodynamics/Kinetics

Onset of action:

Hypercalcemia of malignancy (HCM): ≤24 hours for decrease in albumin-corrected serum calcium; maximum effect: ≤7 days

Paget disease: ~1 month for ≥50% decrease in serum alkaline phosphatase

Duration: HCM: 7 to 14 days; Paget disease: 1 to 372 days

Distribution: 38% to 70% over 120 hours

Metabolism: Not metabolized

Half-life elimination: 21 to 35 hours

Excretion: Biphasic; urine (30% to 62% as unchanged drug; lower in patients with renal dysfunction) within 120 hours

Dosing

Adult Note: Single doses should not exceed 90 mg.

Hypercalcemia of malignancy:

Moderate cancer-related hypercalcemia (corrected serum calcium: 12 to 13.5 mg/dL): 60 to 90 mg, as a single dose over 2 to 24 hours

Severe cancer-related hypercalcemia (corrected serum calcium: >13.5 mg/dL): 90 mg, as a single dose over 2 to 24 hours

Re-treatment in patients who show an initial complete or partial response (allow at least 7 days to elapse prior to re-treatment): May re-treat at the same dose if serum calcium does not return to normal or does not remain normal after initial treatment.

Multiple myeloma, osteolytic bone lesions: IV: 90 mg over 4 hours once monthly:

Lytic disease: American Society of Clinical Oncology (ASCO) guidelines: 90 mg over at least 2 hours once every 3 to 4 weeks for 2 years; discontinue after 2 years in patients with responsive and/or stable disease; resume therapy with new-onset skeletal-related events (Kyle, 2007)

Newly-diagnosed, symptomatic (off-label dose): 30 mg over 2.5 hours once monthly for at least 3 years (Gimsing, 2010)

Breast cancer, osteolytic bone metastases: IV: 90 mg over 2 hours once every 3 to 4 weeks

Paget's disease (moderate-to-severe): IV: 30 mg over 4 hours once daily for 3 consecutive days (total dose = 90 mg); may re-treat at initial dose if clinically indicated

Prevention of androgen deprivation-induced osteoporosis (off-label use): Males: IV: 60 mg over 2 hours once every 3 months (Smith, 2001)

Geriatric Refer to adult dosing. Begin at lower end of adult dosing range.

Renal Impairment Patients with serum creatinine >3 mg/dL were excluded from clinical trials; there are only limited pharmacokinetic data in patients with CrCl <30 mL/minute.

Manufacturer recommends the following guidelines:

Treatment of bone metastases: Use is not recommended in patients with severe renal impairment.

Renal impairment in indications other than bone metastases: Use clinical judgment to determine if benefits outweigh potential risks.

Multiple myeloma: American Society of Clinical Oncology (ASCO) guidelines (Kyle, 2007):

Severe renal impairment (serum creatinine >3 mg/dL or CrCl <30 mL/minute) and extensive bone disease: 90 mg over 4 to 6 hours. However, a reduced initial dose should be considered if renal impairment was preexisting.

Albuminuria >500 mg/24 hours (unexplained): Withhold dose until returns to baseline, then recheck every 3 to 4 weeks; consider reinitiating at a dose not to exceed 90 mg every 4 weeks and with a longer infusion time of at least 4 hours

Dosing adjustment in renal toxicity: In patients with bone metastases, treatment should be withheld for deterioration in renal function (increase of serum creatinine ≥0.5 mg/dL in patients with normal baseline [serum creatinine <1.4 mg/dL] or ≥1 mg/dL in patients with abnormal baseline [serum creatinine ≥1.4 mg/dL]). Resumption of therapy may be considered when serum creatinine returns to within 10% of baseline.

Hepatic Impairment

Mild to moderate impairment: No dosage adjustment necessary.

Severe impairment: There are no dosage adjustments provided in the manufacturer's labeling (has not been studied).

Dietary Considerations Multiple myeloma or metastatic bone lesions from solid tumors or Paget's disease: Take adequate daily calcium and vitamin D supplement (if patient is not hypercalcemic).

Administration IV: Infusion rate varies by indication. Longer infusion times (>2 hours) may reduce the risk for renal toxicity, especially in patients with preexisting renal insufficiency. The manufacturer recommends infusing over 2 to 24 hours for hypercalcemia of malignancy; over 2 hours for osteolytic bone lesions with metastatic breast cancer; and over 4 hours for Paget's disease and for osteolytic bone lesions with multiple myeloma. The ASCO guidelines for bisphosphonate use in multiple myeloma recommend infusing pamidronate over at least 2 hours; if therapy is withheld due to renal toxicity, infuse over at least 4 hours upon reintroduction of treatment after renal recovery (Kyle, 2007).

Hazardous agent; use appropriate precautions for handling and disposal (meets NIOSH 2014 criteria).

Monitoring Parameters Serum creatinine (prior to each treatment); serum electrolytes, including calcium, phosphate, magnesium, and potassium; CBC with differential; monitor for hypocalcemia for at least 2 weeks after therapy; dental exam and preventive dentistry prior to therapy for patients at risk of osteonecrosis, including all cancer patients; patients with preexisting anemia, leukopenia, or thrombocytopenia should be closely monitored during the first 2 weeks of treatment; in addition, monitor urine albumin every 3 to 6 months in multiple myeloma patients

Reference Range Calcium (total): Adults: 9 to 11 mg/dL (SI: 2.05 to 2.54 mmol/L), may slightly decrease with aging; Phosphorus: 2.5 to 4.5 mg/dL (SI: 0.81 to 1.45 mmol/L)

Test Interactions Bisphosphonates may interfere with diagnostic imaging agents such as technetium-99m-diphosphonate in bone scans.

Dosage Forms Excipient information presented when available (limited, particularly for generics); consult specific product labeling.
Solution, Intravenous, as disodium:
  Generic: 30 mg/10 mL (10 mL); 90 mg/10 mL (10 mL)
Solution, Intravenous, as disodium [preservative free]:
  Generic: 30 mg/10 mL (10 mL); 6 mg/mL (10 mL); 90 mg/10 mL (10 mL)
Solution Reconstituted, Intravenous, as disodium:
  Generic: 30 mg (1 ea); 90 mg (1 ea)

Pancrelipase (pan kre LYE pase)

Brand Names: US Creon; Pancreaze; Pancrelipase (Lip-Prot-Amyl); Pertzye; Ultresa; Viokace; Zenpep
Brand Names: Canada Cotazym; Creon; Pancrease MT; Ultrase; Ultrase MT; Viokace
Index Terms Amylase, Lipase, and Protease; Digestive Enzyme; Lipancreatin; Lipase, Protease, and Amylase; Pancrease MT; Pancreatic Enzymes; Pancrecarb MS-16; Pangestyme; Panocaps; Panokase; Protease, Lipase, and Amylase; Ultrase
Pharmacologic Category Enzyme
Use
Pancreatic insufficiency (exocrine): Treatment of exocrine pancreatic insufficiency caused by cystic fibrosis or other conditions. Creon is also approved for patients with chronic pancreatitis or pancreatectomy. Viokace, in combination with a proton-pump inhibitor, is approved for use in adults with exocrine pancreatic insufficiency caused by chronic pancreatitis or pancreatectomy.
Note: Viokace must be administered with a proton pump inhibitor (PPI) since it is not enteric coated.
Medication Guide Available Yes
Dosing
Adult & Geriatric Note: Dosing should not exceed recommended maximum dosage set forth by the Cystic Fibrosis Foundation Consensus Conferences Guidelines. Adjust dose based on body weight, clinical symptoms, and stool fat content. Allow several days between dose adjustments. Total daily dose reflects ~3 meals per day and 2 to 3 snacks per day, with half the mealtime dose given with a snack. Doses of lipase >2,500 units/kg/meal,

lipase >10,000 units/kg/**day**, or lipase >4,000 units/g fat daily should be used with caution and only with documentation of 3-day fecal fat measures. Doses of lipase >6,000 units/kg/meal are associated with colonic stricture and should be decreased.

Pancreatic insufficiency due to conditions such as cystic fibrosis: Oral (Creon, Pancreaze, Pertzye, Ultresa, Zenpep): Initial: Lipase 500 units/kg/meal. Dosage range: Lipase 500 to 2,500 units/kg/meal. Maximum: Lipase ≤2,500 units/kg/**meal or** lipase ≤10,000 units/kg/**day or** lipase <4,000 units/g of fat daily

Pancreatic insufficiency due to chronic pancreatitis or pancreatectomy: Oral:
Creon: Initial: Lipase 500 units/kg/meal with individualized dosage titrations. In one clinical trial, 72,000 units/meal while consuming ≥100 g of fat daily was used. Usually, half the prescribed dose for an individualized full meal should be given with each snack. Maximum: Lipase ≤2,500 units/kg/**meal or** lipase ≤10,000 units/kg/**day or** lipase <4,000 units/g of fat daily

Viokace (administer in combination with a proton pump inhibitor): Initial: Lipase 500 units/kg/meal with individualized dosage titration. In one clinical trial,125,280 units/meal while consuming ≥100 g of fat daily was used. Usually, half the prescribed dose for an individualized full meal should be given with each snack. Maximum: Lipase ≤2,500 units/kg/**meal or** lipase ≤10,000 units/kg/**day or** lipase <4,000 units/g of fat daily.

Pediatric Note: Dosing should not exceed recommended maximum dosage set forth by the Cystic Fibrosis Foundation Consensus Conferences Guidelines. Adjust dose based on body weight, clinical symptoms, and stool fat content. Allow several days between dose adjustments. Total daily dose reflects ~3 meals per day and 2 to 3 snacks per day, with half the mealtime dose given with a snack. Doses of lipase >2,500 units/kg/meal, lipase >10,000 units/kg/**day**, or lipase >4,000 units/g fat daily should be used with caution and only with documentation of 3-day fecal fat measures. Doses of lipase >6,000 units/kg/meal are associated with colonic stricture and should be decreased.

Pancreatic insufficiency due to conditions such as cystic fibrosis:
Infants ≤1 year (Creon, Pancreaze, Pancrelipase, Ultresa, Zenpep): Oral: Manufacturer's labeling: Lipase 2,000 to 4,000 units per 120 mL of formula or per breast-feeding based on available dosage form:
  Creon 3,000 units per 120 mL formula or per breast-feeding
  Pancreaze 2,600 units per 120 mL or per breast-feeding
  Pancrelipase 2,000 to 4,000 per 120 mL or per breast-feeding
  Ultresa 4,000 per 120 mL or per breast-feeding
  Zenpep: 3,000 units per 120 mL or per breast-feeding
Note: CF Guidelines recommend a dose of 2,000 to 5,000 units per feeding of formula, breast milk, or per breast-feeding (even if volume is <120 mL) for up to 2 years of age. Maximum daily dose: 10,000 lipase units/kg/day (Borowitz, 2009; Borowitz 2013).
Children >1 and <4 years (Pertzye [and weight ≥8 kg], Ultresa, Creon, Pancreaze, Zenpep): Oral: Initial: Lipase 1,000 units/kg/meal. Dosage range: Lipase 1,000 to 2,500 units/kg/meal. Maximum: Lipase ≤2,500 units/kg/**meal or** lipase ≤10,000 units/kg/**day or** lipase <4,000 units/g of fat daily
Children ≥4 years and Adolescents (Pertzye [and weight ≥16 kg], Ultresa, Creon, Pancreaze, Zenpep): Oral: Refer to adult dosing.

Renal Impairment There are no dosage adjustments provided in manufacturer's labeling. Use with caution.
Hepatic Impairment There are no dosage adjustments provided in manufacturer's labeling.
Additional Information Complete prescribing information should be consulted for additional detail.
Product Availability Ultresa (Lipase 4,000 USP units, protease 8,000 USP units, and amylase 8,000 USP units) capsules: FDA approved October 2014; availability anticipated in mid-2015. Consult prescribing information for additional information.
Dosage Forms Excipient information presented when available (limited, particularly for generics); consult specific product labeling.
Capsule, delayed release, bicarbonate buffered enteric coated microspheres, oral [porcine derived]:
  Pertzye: Lipase 8,000 USP units, protease 28,750 USP units, and amylase 30,250 USP units
  Pertzye: Lipase 16,000 USP units, protease 57,500 USP units, and amylase 60,500 USP units

Capsule, delayed release, enteric coated beads, oral [porcine derived]:
Pancrelipase (Lip-Prot-Amyl): Lipase 5000 USP units, protease 17,000 USP units, amylase 27,000 USP units
Zenpep: Lipase 3000 USP units, protease 10,000 USP units, and amylase 16,000 USP units
Zenpep: Lipase 5000 USP units, protease 17,000 USP units, and amylase 27,000 USP units
Zenpep: Lipase 10,000 USP units, protease 34,000 USP units, and amylase 55,000 USP units
Zenpep: Lipase 15,000 USP units, protease 51,000 USP units, and amylase 82,000 USP units
Zenpep: Lipase 20,000 USP units, protease 68,000 USP units, and amylase 109,000 USP units
Zenpep: Lipase 25,000 USP units, protease 85,000 USP units, and amylase 136,000 USP units
Zenpep: Lipase 40,000 USP units, protease 136,000 USP units, and amylase 218,000 USP units
Capsule, delayed release, enteric coated microspheres, oral [porcine derived]:
Creon: Lipase 3000 USP units, protease 9500 USP units, and amylase 15,000 USP units
Creon: Lipase 6000 USP units, protease 19,000 USP units, and amylase 30,000 USP units
Creon: Lipase 12,000 USP units, protease 38,000 USP units, and amylase 60,000 USP units
Creon: Lipase 24,000 USP units, protease 76,000 USP units, and amylase 120,000 USP units
Creon: Lipase 36,000 USP units, protease 114,000 USP units, and amylase 180,000 USP units
Capsule, delayed release, enteric coated microtablets, oral [porcine derived]:
Pancreaze: Lipase 4200 USP units, protease 10,000 USP units, and amylase 17,500 USP units
Pancreaze: Lipase 10,500 USP units, protease 25,000 USP units, and amylase 43,750 USP units
Pancreaze: Lipase 16,800 USP units, protease 40,000 USP units, and amylase 70,000 USP units
Pancreaze: Lipase 21,000 USP units, protease 37,000 USP units, and amylase 61,000 USP units
Capsule, delayed release, enteric coated minitablets, oral [porcine derived]:
Ultresa: Lipase 13,800 USP units, protease 27,600 USP units, and amylase 27,600 USP units
Ultresa: Lipase 20,700 USP units, protease 41,400 USP units, and amylase 41,400 USP units
Ultresa: Lipase 23,000 USP units, protease 46,000 USP units, and amylase 46,000 USP units
Tablet, oral [porcine derived]:
Viokace: Lipase 10,440 USP units, protease 39,150 USP units, and amylase 39,150 USP units
Viokace: Lipase 20,880 USP units, protease 78,300 USP units, and amylase 78,300 USP units

◆ Pancrelipase (Lip-Prot-Amyl) see Pancrelipase on page 1384

Pancuronium (pan kyoo ROE nee um)

Brand Names: Canada Pancuronium Bromide®
Index Terms Pancuronium Bromide; Pavulon [DSC]
Pharmacologic Category Neuromuscular Blocker Agent, Nondepolarizing
Use Facilitation of endotracheal intubation and relaxation of skeletal muscles during surgery; facilitation of mechanical ventilation in ICU patients; does not relieve pain or produce sedation
Pregnancy Considerations Animal reproduction studies have not been conducted. Small amounts of pancuronium cross the placenta (Daily, 1984). May be used short-term in cesarean section; reduced doses recommended in patients also receiving magnesium sulfate due to enhanced effects.
Contraindications Hypersensitivity to pancuronium, bromide, or any component of the formulation
Warnings/Precautions Ventilation must be supported during neuromuscular blockade. Elimination half-life is doubled due to reduced clearance of pancuronium and recovery is prolonged; use with caution in patients with renal and/or hepatic impairment (adjust dose appropriately); certain clinical conditions may result in potentiation or antagonism of neuromuscular blockade:
Antagonism: Respiratory alkalosis, hypercalcemia, demyelinating lesions, peripheral neuropathies, denervation, and muscle trauma
Potentiation: Electrolyte abnormalities (eg, severe hypocalcemia, severe hypokalemia, hypermagnesemia), neuromuscular diseases, metabolic acidosis, metabolic alkalosis, respiratory acidosis, Eaton-Lambert syndrome and myasthenia gravis

Resistance may occur in burn patients (≥20% of total body surface area), usually several days after the injury, and may persist for several months after wound healing. Resistance may occur in patients who are immobilized. Cross-sensitivity with other neuromuscular-blocking agents may occur; use extreme caution in patients with previous anaphylactic reactions. Use caution in the elderly.
[US Boxed Warning]: Should be administered by adequately trained individuals familiar with its use.

Benzyl alcohol and derivatives: Some dosage forms may contain benzyl alcohol; large amounts of benzyl alcohol (≥99 mg/kg/day) have been associated with a potentially fatal toxicity ("gasping syndrome") in neonates; the "gasping syndrome" consists of metabolic acidosis, respiratory distress, gasping respirations, CNS dysfunction (including convulsions, intracranial hemorrhage), hypotension, and cardiovascular collapse (AAP ["Inactive" 1997]; CDC, 1982); some data suggests that benzoate displaces bilirubin from protein binding sites (Ahlfors, 2001); avoid or use dosage forms containing benzyl alcohol with caution in neonates. See manufacturer's labeling.
Adverse Reactions Frequency not defined.
Cardiovascular: Elevation in pulse rate, elevated blood pressure and cardiac output, tachycardia, edema, skin flushing, circulatory collapse
Dermatologic: Rash, itching, erythema, burning sensation along the vein
Gastrointestinal: Excessive salivation
Neuromuscular & skeletal: Profound muscle weakness
Respiratory: Wheezing, bronchospasm
Miscellaneous: Hypersensitivity reaction
Postmarketing and/or case reports: Acute quadriplegic myopathy syndrome (prolonged use), anaphylactoid reactions, anaphylaxis, myositis ossificans (prolonged use)
Drug Interactions
Metabolism/Transport Effects None known.
Avoid Concomitant Use
Avoid concomitant use of Pancuronium with any of the following: QuiNINE
Increased Effect/Toxicity
Pancuronium may increase the levels/effects of: Cardiac Glycosides; Corticosteroids (Systemic); OnabotulinumtoxinA; RimabotulinumtoxinB

The levels/effects of Pancuronium may be increased by: AbobotulinumtoxinA; Aminoglycosides; Calcium Channel Blockers; Capreomycin; Clindamycin (Topical); Colistimethate; CycloSPORINE (Systemic); Fosphenytoin-Phenytoin; Inhalational Anesthetics; Ketorolac (Nasal); Ketorolac (Systemic); Lincosamide Antibiotics; Lithium; Loop Diuretics; Magnesium Salts; Minocycline; Polymyxin B; Procainamide; QuiNIDine; QuiNINE; Spironolactone; Tetracycline Derivatives; Theophylline Derivatives; Vancomycin
Decreased Effect
The levels/effects of Pancuronium may be decreased by: Acetylcholinesterase Inhibitors; Fosphenytoin-Phenytoin; Loop Diuretics; Theophylline Derivatives
Storage/Stability Refrigerate; however, stable for up to 6 months at room temperature.
Mechanism of Action Blocks neural transmission at the myoneural junction by binding with cholinergic receptor sites
Pharmacodynamics/Kinetics
Onset of effect: Peak effect: IV: 2-3 minutes
Duration (dose dependent): 60-100 minutes
Metabolism: Hepatic (30% to 45%); active metabolite 3-hydroxypancuronium ($\frac{1}{3}$ to $\frac{1}{2}$ the activity of parent drug)
Half-life elimination: 110 minutes
Excretion: Urine (55% to 70% as unchanged drug)
Dosing
Adult & Geriatric Administer IV; dose to effect; doses will vary due to interpatient variability
Surgery: Initial: 0.06-0.1 mg/kg or 0.05 mg/kg after initial dose of succinylcholine for intubation; maintenance dose: 0.01 mg/kg administered 60-100 minutes after initial dose and then 0.01 mg/kg every 25-60 minutes
Pretreatment/priming: 10% of intubating dose given 3-5 minutes before intubating dose
ICU paralysis (eg, facilitate mechanical ventilation) in select adequately sedated patients: 0.06-0.1 mg/kg bolus followed by either:
Continuous infusion: 1-2 **mcg/kg/minute** (0.06-0.12 **mg/kg/hour**) (Murray, 2002) **or** 0.8-1.7 **mcg/kg/minute** (0.048-0.102 **mg/kg/hour**) (Greenberg, 2013)
or
Intermittent bolus: 0.1-0.2 mg/kg every 1-3 hours
Pediatric Infants >1 month and Children: Refer to adult dosing.

Renal Impairment Elimination half-life is doubled, plasma clearance is reduced and rate of recovery is sometimes much slower. No dosage adjustment provided in manufacturer's labeling; however, the following adjustments have been recommended (Aronoff 2007):

CrCl >50 mL/minute: No dosage adjustment necessary.

CrCl 10-50 mL/minute: Administer 50% of normal dose.

CrCl <10 mL/minute: Avoid use.

Hemodialysis/peritoneal dialysis: Avoid use.

CRRT: Administer 50% of normal dose.

Hepatic Impairment Elimination half-life is doubled, plasma clearance is doubled, recovery time is prolonged, volume of distribution is increased (50%) and results in a slower onset, higher total dosage, and prolongation of neuromuscular blockade. Patients with liver disease may develop slow resistance to nondepolarizing muscle relaxant. Large doses may be required and problems may arise in antagonism.

Obesity Use ideal body weight for obese patients.

Administration May be administered undiluted by rapid IV injection

Monitoring Parameters Heart rate, blood pressure, assisted ventilation status; cardiac monitor, blood pressure monitor, and ventilator required

Additional Information Pancuronium is classified as a long-duration neuromuscular-blocking agent. Neuromuscular blockade will be prolonged in patients with decreased renal function. Pancuronium does not relieve pain or produce sedation. It may produce cumulative effect on duration of blockade. It produces tachycardia secondary to vagolytic activity and sympathetic stimulation.

Dosage Forms Excipient information presented when available (limited, particularly for generics); consult specific product labeling.

Solution, Intravenous, as bromide:

Generic: 1 mg/mL (10 mL); 2 mg/mL (2 mL, 5 mL)

◆ Pancuronium Bromide see Pancuronium on page 1385

◆ Pancuronium Bromide® (Can) see Pancuronium on page 1385

◆ Pandel see Hydrocortisone (Topical) on page 886

◆ Pangestyme see Pancrelipase on page 1384

◆ Panglobulin see Immune Globulin on page 927

Panitumumab (pan i TOOM yoo mab)

Brand Names: US Vectibix

Brand Names: Canada Vectibix

Index Terms ABX-EGF; MOAB ABX-EGF; Monoclonal Antibody ABX-EGF; rHuMAb-EGFr

Pharmacologic Category Antineoplastic Agent, Epidermal Growth Factor Receptor (EGFR) Inhibitor; Antineoplastic Agent, Monoclonal Antibody

Use

Colorectal cancer, metastatic: Treatment of patients with wild-type KRAS (exon 2 in codons 12 or 13) metastatic colorectal cancer (mCRC), either as first-line therapy in combination with FOLFOX (fluorouracil, leucovorin, and oxaliplatin) or as a single agent following disease progression after prior treatment with fluoropyrimidine-, oxaliplatin-, and irinotecan-containing chemotherapy regimens

Limitations of use: Panitumumab is not indicated for the treatment of patients with RAS-mutant mCRC or for whom RAS mutation status is unknown.

Pregnancy Considerations Animal reproduction studies have demonstrated adverse fetal effects. Based on animal studies, panitumumab may disrupt normal menstrual cycles. IgG is known to cross the placenta; therefore, it is possible the developing fetus may be exposed to panitumumab. Because panitumumab inhibits epidermal growth factor (EGF), a component of fetal development, adverse effects on pregnancy would be expected. Men and women of childbearing potential should use effective contraception during and for 6 months after treatment. In the US and Canada, women who become pregnant during panitumumab treatment are encouraged to enroll in Amgen's Pregnancy Surveillance Program (US: 1-800-772-6436; Canada: 1-866-512-6436).

Breast-Feeding Considerations It is not known if panitumumab is excreted in breast milk. The decision to discontinue panitumumab or discontinue breast-feeding should take into account the benefits of treatment to the mother. If breast-feeding is interrupted for panitumumab treatment, based on the half-life, breast-feeding should not be resumed for at least 2 months following the last dose. In the US and Canada, women who nurse during panitumumab treatment are encouraged to enroll in Amgen's Lactation Surveillance Program (US: 1-800-772-6436; Canada: 1-866-512-6436).

Contraindications

There are no contraindications listed in the manufacturer's US labeling.

Canadian labeling: History of severe or life-threatening hypersensitivity reactions to panitumumab or any component of the formulation.

Warnings/Precautions [US Boxed Warning]: Dermatologic toxicities have been reported in 90% of patients receiving single agent panitumumab and were severe (grade 3 or higher) in 15% of patients); may include dermatitis acneiform, pruritus, erythema, rash, skin exfoliation, paronychia, dry skin, and skin fissures. Severe skin toxicities may be complicated by infection, sepsis, necrotizing fasciitis, or abscesses. The median time to development of skin (or ocular) toxicity was 2 weeks, with resolution ~12 weeks after discontinuation. Monitor all dermatologic toxicities for development of inflammation or infection. Rare cases of Stevens-Johnson syndrome and toxic epidermal necrolysis have been reported; bullous mucocutaneous disease (life-threatening/fatal) have been observed. Withhold treatment for severe or life-threatening dermatologic or soft tissue toxicities associated with severe/life-threatening inflammatory or infectious complications; dermatologic toxicity may require dose reduction or permanent discontinuation. The severity of dermatologic toxicity is predictive for response; grades 2 to 4 skin toxicity correlates with improved progression free survival and overall survival, compared to grade 1 skin toxicity (Peeters, 2009; Van Cutsem, 2007). Patients should minimize sunlight exposure and wear sunscreen and protective clothing/hat; sunlight may exacerbate skin reactions. Keratitis and ulcerative keratitis (known risk factors for corneal perforation) have occurred. Monitor for evidence of ocular toxicity; interrupt or discontinue treatment for acute or worsening keratitis. Gastric mucosal and nail toxicities have also been reported.

Severe infusion reactions (bronchospasm, dyspnea, fever, chills, and hypotension) have been reported in ~1% of patients; fatal infusion reactions have been reported with postmarketing surveillance. Discontinue infusion for severe reactions; permanently discontinue in patients with persistent severe infusion reactions. Appropriate medical support for the management of infusion reactions should be readily available. Mild-to-moderate infusion reactions are managed by slowing the infusion rate.

Pulmonary fibrosis and interstitial lung disease have been observed (rarely) in clinical trials; fatalities have been reported. Interrupt treatment for acute onset or worsening of pulmonary symptoms; permanently discontinue treatment if interstitial lung disease is confirmed. Patients with a history of or evidence of interstitial pneumonitis or pulmonary fibrosis were excluded from most clinical trials; consider the benefits of therapy versus the risk of pulmonary complications in such patients. May cause diarrhea; the incidence and severity of chemotherapy-induced diarrhea and other toxicities (rash, electrolyte abnormalities, stomatitis) is increased with combination chemotherapy; severe diarrhea and dehydration (which may lead to acute renal failure) has been observed with panitumumab in combination with chemotherapy. In a study of bevacizumab with combination chemotherapy ± panitumumab, the use of panitumumab resulted in decreased progression-free and overall survival and significantly increased toxicity compared to regimens without panitumumab (Hecht, 2009). Toxicities included rash/acneiform dermatitis, diarrhea/dehydration, electrolyte disturbances, mucositis/stomatitis, and an increased incidence of pulmonary embolism. Magnesium and/or calcium depletion may occur during treatment (may be delayed; hypomagnesemia occurred ≥8 weeks after completion of panitumumab) and after treatment is discontinued; electrolyte repletion may be necessary; monitor for hypomagnesemia and hypocalcemia during treatment and for at least 8 weeks after completion. Hypokalemia has also been reported. Patients >65 years of age receiving panitumumab plus FOLFOX experienced a higher incidence of serious adverse events including severe diarrhea.

Patients with colorectal cancer with tumors with codons 12 and 13 (exon 2), codons 59 and 61 (exon 3), or codons 117 and 146 (exon 4) RAS (KRAS or NRAS) mutations are unlikely to benefit from EGFR inhibitor therapy. Panitumumab is not indicated patients with RAS mutation-positive metastatic colorectal cancer or patients in which RAS mutation status is unknown. Utilizing an anti-EGFR-directed antibody in patients whose tumors contain RAS mutations resulted in increased toxicity without clinical benefit. In a study of FOLFOX4 (fluorouracil, leucovorin and oxaliplatin) ± panitumumab, patients with a KRAS mutation who received panitumumab with FOLFOX4 experienced a significantly shortened progression-free survival (Douillard, 2010). In addition, a subset analysis of patients

with wild-type *KRAS* identified additional *RAS* (*KRAS* [exons 3 and 4] or *NRAS* [exons 2, 3, 4]) mutations; progression-free survival and overall survival were significantly shortened in patients with *RAS* mutations who received FOLFOX4 in combination with panitumumab (Douillard, 2013). The American Society of Clinical Oncology (ASCO) provisional clinical opinion (Allegra, 2009) recommends genotyping tumor tissue for KRAS mutation in all patients with metastatic colorectal cancer (genotyping may be done on archived specimens). An updated ASCO provisional clinical opinion recommends that all patients with metastatic colorectal cancer who are candidates for anti-EGFR therapy should be tested (in a certified lab) for mutations in both *KRAS* and *NRAS* exon 2 (codons 12 and 13), exon 3 (codons 59 and 61), and exon 4 (codons 117 and 146); anti-EGFR monoclonal antibody therapy should only be considered in patients whose tumors lack mutations after extended *RAS* testing (Allegra, 2015). Panitumumab is also reported to be ineffective in patients with BRAF V600E mutation (Di Nicolantonio, 2008).

Adverse Reactions
Monotherapy:
>10%:
Central nervous system: Fatigue (26%)
Dermatologic: Skin toxicity (90%; grades 3/4: 15%), erythema (66%; grades 3/4: 6%), pruritus (58%; grades 3/4: 3%), acneiform eruption (57%; grades 3/4: 7%), paronychia (25%; grades 3/4: 2%), rash (22%; grades 3/4: 1%), skin fissure (20%; grades 3/4: 1%), exfoliative dermatitis (18%; grades 3/4: 2%), acne vulgaris (14%; grades 3/4: 1%)
Endocrine & metabolic: Hypomagnesemia (grades 3/4: 7%)
Gastrointestinal: Nausea (23%), diarrhea (21%; grades 3/4: 2%), vomiting (19%)
Ophthalmic: Ocular toxicity (16%)
Respiratory: Dyspnea (18%), cough (15%)
Miscellaneous: Fever (17%)
1% to 10%:
Cardiovascular: Pulmonary embolism (1%)
Central nervous system: Chills (3%)
Dermatologic: Nail toxicity (10%), xeroderma (10%), desquamation (9%; grades 3/4: <1%), dermal ulcer (6%; grades 3/4: <1%), pustular rash (4%), papular rash (2%)
Endocrine & metabolic: Dehydration (3%)
Gastrointestinal: Mucositis (7%), stomatitis (7%), xerostomia (5%)
Immunologic: Antibody formation (≤5%)
Ophthalmic: Abnormal eyelash growth (6%), conjunctivitis (5%)
Respiratory: Epistaxis (4%), interstitial pulmonary disease (1%)
Miscellaneous: Infusion related reaction (3%; grades 3/4: <1%)
<1%: Hypersensitivity reaction, pulmonary fibrosis

Combination therapy with FOLFOX:
>10%:
Dermatologic: Skin rash (56%; grades 3/4: 17% to 26%), acneiform eruption (32%; grades 3/4: 10%), pruritus (23%; grades 3/4: <1%), paronychia (21%; grades 3/4: 3%), xeroderma (21%; grades 3/4: 2%), erythema (16%; grades 3/4: 2%), skin fissure (16%; grades 3/4: <1%), alopecia (15%), acne vulgaris (14%; grades 3/4: 3%)
Endocrine & metabolic: Hypomagnesemia (30%), hypokalemia (21%), weight loss (18%)
Gastrointestinal: Diarrhea (62%), anorexia (36%), abdominal pain (28%), stomatitis (27%), mucosal inflammation (25%)
Neuromuscular & skeletal: Weakness (25%)
Ophthalmic: Conjunctivitis (18%)
Respiratory: Epistaxis (14%)
1% to 10%:
Cardiovascular: Deep vein thrombosis (5%)
Central nervous system: Fatigue (≥1%), paresthesia (≥1%)
Dermatologic: Nail disorder (10%; grades 3/4: 1%), palmar-plantar erythrodysesthesia (9%; grades 3/4: 1%), cellulitis (3%)
Endocrine & metabolic: Dehydration (8%), hypocalcemia (6%)
Hypersensitivity: Hypersensitivity (≥1%)
Local: Localized infection (4%)
<1%: Antibody development

Postmarketing and/or case reports (Limited to important or life-threatening) (mono- and combination therapy): Abscess, angioedema, bullous skin disease (mucocutaneous), corneal ulcer, keratitis, necrotizing fasciitis, sepsis, skin necrosis, Stevens-Johnson syndrome, toxic epidermal necrolysis

Drug Interactions
Metabolism/Transport Effects None known.
Avoid Concomitant Use There are no known interactions where it is recommended to avoid concomitant use.
Increased Effect/Toxicity
Panitumumab may increase the levels/effects of: Porfimer; Verteporfin
Decreased Effect There are no known significant interactions involving a decrease in effect.
Preparation for Administration Inspect vial prior to use; solution is colorless but may contain a small amount of translucent-to-white amorphous panitumumab protein particles (will be removed with administration filter). Dilute in 100 mL (for doses ≤1000 mg) or 150 mL (doses >1000 mg) of normal saline to a final concentration of ≤10 mg/mL. Gently invert to mix; do not shake. Discard any unused portion remaining in the vial.
Storage/Stability Store intact vials in the original cartons under refrigeration at 2°C to 8°C (36°F to 46°F) until the time of use. Do not freeze; do not shake; protect from direct sunlight. Solution diluted for infusion should be used within 6 hours of preparation if stored at room temperature or within 24 hours of dilution if stored at 2°C to 8°C (36°F to 46°F); do not freeze.
Mechanism of Action Recombinant human IgG2 monoclonal antibody which binds specifically to the epidermal growth factor receptor (EGFR, HER1, c-ErbB-1) and competitively inhibits the binding of epidermal growth factor (EGF) and other ligands. Binding to the EGFR blocks phosphorylation and activation of intracellular tyrosine kinases, resulting in inhibition of cell survival, growth, proliferation and transformation. EGFR signal transduction may result in *KRAS* and *NRAS* wild-type activation; cells with *RAS* mutations appear to be unaffected by EGFR inhibition.
Pharmacodynamics/Kinetics Half-life elimination: ~7.5 days (range: 4 to 11 days)

Dosing
Adult & Geriatric
Colorectal cancer, metastatic, *KRAS* wild-type: IV: 6 mg/kg every 14 days as a single agent (Van Cutsem, 2007) or in combination with FOLFOX (fluorouracil, leucovorin, and oxaliplatin) (Douillard, 2010; Douillard, 2013); continue until disease progression or unacceptable toxicity (Douillard, 2010; Van Cutsem, 2007)
Colorectal cancer, metastatic, *KRAS* wild-type in combination with FOLFIRI (fluorouracil, leucovorin, and irinotecan; off-label combination): IV: 6 mg/kg every 14 days; continue until disease progression or unacceptable toxicity (Peeters, 2010)
Missed dose (Canadian labeling): Doses should be administered within 3 days before or after the scheduled dose (unless withheld for toxicity). If a dose is missed, administer as soon as possible; the next dose then should be administered on a new every 2 week schedule based on the day of the most recently administered dose.
Renal Impairment There are no dosage adjustments provided in the manufacturer's labeling (has not been studied).
Hepatic Impairment There are no dosage adjustments provided in the manufacturer's labeling (has not been studied).
Adjustment for Toxicity
Infusion reactions, mild-to-moderate (grade 1 or 2): Reduce the infusion rate by 50% for the duration of infusion.
Infusion reactions, severe (grade 3 or 4): Stop infusion; consider permanent discontinuation (depending on severity or persistence of reaction).
Dermatologic toxicity:
Grade 3 toxicity (first occurrence): Withhold 1 to 2 doses; if reaction improves to <grade 3, resume therapy at initial dose.
Grade 3 toxicity (second occurrence): Withhold 1 to 2 doses; if reaction improves to <grade 3, resume therapy at 80% of initial dose.
Grade 3 toxicity (third occurrence): Withhold 1 to 2 doses; if reaction improves to <grade 3, resume therapy at 60% of initial dose.
Grade 3 toxicity (fourth occurrence), grade 3 toxicity that does not recover to <grade 3 after withholding 1 or 2 doses, or grade 4 toxicity: Permanently discontinue.
Ocular toxicity (acute or worsening keratitis): Interrupt or discontinue treatment.
Pulmonary toxicity:
Acute onset or worsening pulmonary symptoms: Interrupt treatment.
Interstitial lung disease: Permanently discontinue treatment.

Administration IV: Administer via infusion pump; do not administer IV push or as a bolus. Doses ≤1000 mg, infuse over 1 hour; if first infusion is tolerated, subsequent doses may be administered over 30 to 60 minutes. Doses >1000 mg, infuse over 90 minutes. Administer through a low protein-binding 0.2 or 0.22 micrometer in-line filter. Flush line with NS before and after infusion; do not mix or administer with other medications. Reduce infusion rate by 50% for mild-to-moderate infusion reactions (grades 1 and 2); stop infusion for severe infusion reactions (grades 3 and 4) and consider permanent discontinuation. Appropriate medical support for the management of infusion reactions should be readily available.

Monitoring Parameters *KRAS* genotyping of tumor tissue. Monitor serum electrolytes, including magnesium and calcium (periodically during and for at least 8 weeks after therapy), and potassium. Monitor vital signs and temperature before, during, and after infusion. Monitor for skin toxicity, for evidence of ocular toxicity, and for acute onset or worsening pulmonary symptoms.

Dosage Forms Excipient information presented when available (limited, particularly for generics); consult specific product labeling.

Solution, Intravenous [preservative free]:
Vectibix: 100 mg/5 mL (5 mL); 400 mg/20 mL (20 mL)

Panobinostat (pan oh BIN oh stat)

Brand Names: US Farydak
Index Terms Faridak; LBH589; Panobinostat Lactate
Pharmacologic Category Antineoplastic Agent, Histone Deacetylase (HDAC) Inhibitor
Use Multiple myeloma: Treatment of multiple myeloma (in combination with bortezomib and dexamethasone) in patients who have received at least 2 prior regimens, including bortezomib and an immunomodulatory agent.

Pregnancy Considerations Adverse events were observed in animal reproduction studies. Pregnancy should be ruled out prior to treatment. Women of reproductive potential should avoid pregnancy and use an effective contraceptive during therapy and for 1 month after treatment. Males should use condoms during therapy and for 3 months after treatment.

Breast-Feeding Considerations It is not known if panobinostat is excreted into breast milk. Due to the potential for serious adverse reactions in the nursing infant, the manufacturer recommends a decision be made to discontinue nursing or to discontinue the drug, taking into account the importance of treatment to the mother.

Medication Guide Available Yes
Contraindications There are no contraindications listed in the manufacturer's labeling.
Warnings/Precautions Hazardous agent; use appropriate precautions for handling and disposal (meets NIOSH 2014 criteria).

[US Boxed Warning]: Severe diarrhea occurred in one-fourth of panobinostat treated patients. Monitor for symptoms, institute antidiarrheal treatment, interrupt panobinostat, and then reduce dose or discontinue panobinostat. Any grade diarrhea was reported in over two-thirds of patients, and may occur at any time. Monitor hydration status and serum electrolytes (including magnesium, potassium, and phosphate). Patients should have antidiarrheal medications available for use; begin antidiarrheal medications at the first sign of diarrhea, loose stools, or abdominal cramping. Interrupt panobinostat treatment for moderate diarrhea (4 to 6 stools per day). Panobinostat is associated with nausea and vomiting (moderate emetic potential); consider antiemetics to prevent nausea and vomiting. Some antiemetics known to prolong the QT interval (eg, dolasetron or ondansetron) may be used with frequent ECG monitoring.

[US Boxed Warning]: Severe and fatal cardiac ischemic events, severe arrhythmias, and ECG changes have occurred in patients receiving panobinostat. Arrhythmias may be exacerbated by electrolyte abnormalities. Obtain ECG and electrolytes at baseline and periodically during treatment as clinically indicated. ECG abnormalities including ST-segment depression and T-wave abnormalities have been observed. Monitor and correct electrolyte abnormalities as needed. Panobinostat may prolong the QT interval. Do not initiate treatment in patients with a QTcF >450 msec or with clinically significant baseline ST-segment or T-wave abnormalities. Interrupt treatment if QTcF increases to ≥480 msec; correct electrolyte abnormalities; if QT prolongation does not resolve, permanently discontinue panobinostat. Concomitant use with mediations known to prolong the QT interval is not recommended. Do not initiate panobinostat treatment in patients with a history of recent MI or unstable angina.

Severe thrombocytopenia, neutropenia and anemia have occurred; may require treatment interruption, dosage modification, discontinuation, transfusion or granulocyte colony-stimulating factor support. Monitor CBC with differential at baseline and during treatment; patients >65 years may require more frequent monitoring. Serious and fatal hemorrhage has occurred, including grade 3 and 4 hemorrhage. All patients with hemorrhage also experienced thrombocytopenia at the time of hemorrhage. Localized and systemic infections (including pneumonia, bacterial infections, invasive fungal infections, and viral infections) have been observed; infections may be severe (or fatal). Do not initiate treatment in patients with active infections. Monitor for sings/symptoms of infections during treatment. If infection occurs, begin appropriate management and consider interrupting or discontinuing panobinostat.

Hepatic dysfunction (transaminase and total bilirubin elevations) has been reported. Monitor liver function prior to and during treatment. If liver function tests are abnormal, consider dosage adjustments and monitor until liver function returns to normal or baseline. Initial dose should be reduced in patients with mild-to-moderate hepatic impairment; avoid use in patients with severe impairment. Potentially significant drug-drug/drug-food interactions may exist, requiring dose or frequency adjustment, additional monitoring, and/or selection of alternative therapy.

Adverse Reactions Frequency not always defined.
>10%:
Cardiovascular: Abnormal T waves on ECG (40%), peripheral edema (29%; grades 3/4: 2%), depression of ST segment on ECG (22%), cardiac arrhythmia (12%; grades 3/4: 3%)
Central nervous system: Fatigue (≤60%, grades 3/4: ≤25%), lethargy (≤60%; grades 3/4: ≤25%), malaise (≤60%; grades 3/4: ≤25%)
Endocrine & metabolic: Hypocalcemia (67%; grades 3/4: 5%), hypoalbuminemia (63%; grades 3/4: 2%), hypophosphatemia (63%; grades 3/4: 20%), hypokalemia (52%; grades 3/4: 18%), hyponatremia (49%; grades 3/4: 13%), hyperphosphatemia (29%; grades 3/4: 2%), hypermagnesemia (27%; grades 3/4: 5%), weight loss (12%; grades 3/4: 2%)
Gastrointestinal: Diarrhea (68%; grades 3/4: 25%), nausea (36%; grades 3/4: 6%), decreased appetite (28%; grades 3/4: 3%), vomiting (26%; grades 3/4: 7%)
Hematologic & oncologic: Thrombocytopenia (97%; grades 3/4: 67%), lymphocytopenia (82%; grades 3/4: 53%), leukopenia (81%; grades 3/4: 23%), neutropenia (75%; grades 3/4: 34%), anemia (62%; grades 3/4: 18%)
Hepatic: Hyperbilirubinemia (21%; grades 3/4: 1%)
Infection: Severe infection (31%; includes bacterial, fungal, and viral infections)
Neuromuscular & skeletal: Weakness (≤60%; grades ≥3: ≤25%)
Renal: Increased serum creatinine (41%; grades 3/4: 1%)
Miscellaneous: Fever (26%)
1% to 10%:
Cardiovascular: Hypertension (>2% to <10%), hypotension (>2% to <10%), orthostatic hypotension (>2% to <10%), palpitations (>2% to <10%), syncope (>2% to <10%), ischemic heart disease (4%), ECG changes, prolonged Q-T interval on ECG
Central nervous system: Chills (>2% to <10%), dizziness (>2% to <10%), headache (>2% to <10%), insomnia (>2% to <10%)
Dermatologic: Cheilitis (>2% to <10%), erythema (>2% to <10%), skin lesion (>2% to <10%), skin rash (>2% to <10%)
Endocrine & metabolic: Dehydration (>2% to <10%), fluid retention (>2% to <10%), hyperglycemia (>2% to <10%), hyperuricemia (>2% to <10%), hypomagnesemia (>2% to <10%), hypothyroidism (>2% to <10%)
Gastrointestinal: Abdominal distention (>2% to <10%), abdominal pain (>2% to <10%), colitis (>2% to <10%), dysgeusia (>2% to <10%), dyspepsia (>2% to <10%), flatulence (>2% to <10%), gastritis (>2% to <10%), gastrointestinal pain (>2% to <10%), xerostomia (>2% to <10%), gastrointestinal toxicity
Genitourinary: Urinary incontinence (>2% to <10%)
Hematologic & oncologic: Hemorrhage (grades 3/4: 4%)
Hepatic: Hepatitis B (>2% to <10%), increased serum alkaline phosphatase (>2% to <10%), increased aminotransferases, increased serum bilirubin
Infection: Sepsis (6%)
Neuromuscular & skeletal: Joint swelling (>2% to <10%), tremor (>2% to <10%)

Renal: Increased blood urea nitrogen (>2% to <10%), mean glomerular filtration rate decreased (>2% to <10%), renal failure (>2% to <10%)

Respiratory: Cough (>2% to <10%), dyspnea (>2% to <10%), rales (>2% to <10%), respiratory failure (>2% to <10%), wheezing (>2% to <10%)

Drug Interactions

Metabolism/Transport Effects Substrate of CYP2C19 (minor), CYP2D6 (minor), CYP3A4 (major), P-glycoprotein; **Note:** Assignment of Major/Minor substrate status based on clinically relevant drug interaction potential; **Inhibits** CYP2D6 (moderate)

Avoid Concomitant Use

Avoid concomitant use of Panobinostat with any of the following: BCG (Intravesical); Conivaptan; CYP3A4 Inducers (Strong); Fusidic Acid (Systemic); Grapefruit Juice; Highest Risk QTc-Prolonging Agents; Idelalisib; Ivabradine; Mifepristone; Natalizumab; Pimecrolimus; Pomegranate; Star Fruit; Tacrolimus (Topical); Thioridazine; Tofacitinib; Vaccines (Live)

Increased Effect/Toxicity

Panobinostat may increase the levels/effects of: CYP2D6 Substrates; DOXOrubicin (Conventional); Fesoterodine; Fingolimod; Highest Risk QTc-Prolonging Agents; Leflunomide; Metoprolol; Moderate Risk QTc-Prolonging Agents; Natalizumab; Nebivolol; Thioridazine; Tofacitinib; Vaccines (Live)

The levels/effects of Panobinostat may be increased by: Aprepitant; Conivaptan; CYP3A4 Inhibitors (Moderate); CYP3A4 Inhibitors (Strong); Dasatinib; Denosumab; Dolasetron; Fosaprepitant; Fusidic Acid (Systemic); Granisetron; Grapefruit Juice; Idelalisib; Ivabradine; Ivacaftor; Luliconazole; Mifepristone; Netupitant; Ondansetron; Palbociclib; Pimecrolimus; Pomegranate; QTc-Prolonging Agents (Indeterminate Risk and Risk Modifying); Roflumilast; Simeprevir; Star Fruit; Stiripentol; Tacrolimus (Topical); Trastuzumab

Decreased Effect

Panobinostat may decrease the levels/effects of: BCG (Intravesical); Coccidioides immitis Skin Test; Codeine; Sipuleucel-T; Tamoxifen; TraMADol; Vaccines (Inactivated); Vaccines (Live)

The levels/effects of Panobinostat may be decreased by: Bosentan; CYP3A4 Inducers (Moderate); CYP3A4 Inducers (Strong); Dabrafenib; Deferasirox; Echinacea; Siltuximab; St Johns Wort; Tocilizumab

Food Interactions Star fruit, pomegranate or pomegranate juice, and grapefruit or grapefruit juice may interfere with panobinostat metabolism. Management: Avoid star fruit, pomegranate or pomegranate juice, and grapefruit or grapefruit juice.

Storage/Stability Store at 20°C to 25°C (68°F to 77°F); excursions are permitted between 15°C and 30°C (59°F and 86°F). Store blister pack in original carton. Protect from light.

Mechanism of Action Panobinostat is a histone deacetylase (HDAC) inhibitor; inhibits enzymatic activity of HDACs resulting in increased acetylation of histone proteins. Accumulation of acetylated histones and other proteins induces cell cycle arrest and/or apoptosis of some transformed cells. Panobinostat has minimal activity in multiple myeloma as a single-agent; however, synergistic activity is demonstrated when combined with bortezomib and dexamethasone (San-Miguel 2014).

Pharmacodynamics/Kinetics

Protein binding: ~90% to plasma proteins

Metabolism: Extensive via reduction, hydrolysis, oxidation, and glucuronidation; CYP3A4 accounts for ~40% of elimination, CYP2D6 and CYP2C19 are minor pathways.

Bioavailability: ~21%; AUC is 16% lower (compared with fasting) when administered with a high-fat meal.

Half-life elimination: ~37 hours

Time to peak: Within 2 hours

Excretion: Feces (44% to 77%; <4% as unchanged drug); Urine (29% to 51%; <3% as unchanged drug)

Dosing

Adult & Geriatric Determine QTcF prior to the start of therapy and verify that QTcF <450 msec prior to panobinostat initiation. Baseline ANC should be at least 1,500/mm^3 and platelets at least 100,000/mm^3 prior to treatment. Panobinostat is associated with a moderate emetic potential; consider antiemetics to prevent nausea and vomiting.

Multiple myeloma: Adults: Oral: 20 mg once every other day for 3 doses each week during weeks 1 and 2 of a 21-day treatment cycle (eg, Monday, Wednesday, and Friday of weeks 1 and 2 only, rest during week 3) for up to 8 cycles (in combination with bortezomib and dexamethasone); treatment may continue (the same schedule for panobinostat; bortezomib and

dexamethasone schedules are modified) for an additional 8 cycles in patients experiencing clinical benefit and acceptable toxicity (San-Miguel 2014). The total duration of therapy may be up to 16 cycles (48 weeks).

Missed doses: Missed doses may be taken up to 12 hours after the scheduled time. Do not repeat the dose if vomiting occurs; patients should take the next usual scheduled dose.

Dosage adjustment for concomitant therapy:

CYP2D6 substrates: Avoid coadministration with sensitive CYP2D6 substrates (eg, atomoxetine, desipramine, dextromethorphan, metoprolol, nebivolol, perphenazine, tolterodine, venlafaxine) or CYP2D6 substrates that have a narrow therapeutic index (eg, thioridazine, pimozide).

Strong CYP3A inducers: Avoid concomitant use with strong CYP3A inducers.

Strong CYP3A inhibitors: Reduce the starting panobinostat dose to 10 mg with strong CYP3A inhibitors (eg, boceprevir, clarithromycin, conivaptin, indinavir, itraconazole, ketoconazole, lopinavir/ritonavir, nefazodone, nelfinavir, posaconazole, ritonavir, saquinavir, telaprevir, telithromycin, voriconazole).

Renal Impairment

Mild to severe impairment (CrCl <80 mL/minute): There are no dosage adjustments provided in the manufacturer's labeling. However, based on a pharmacokinetic study of a single 30 mg dose, renal impairment does not appear to impact panobinostat exposure in patients with mild, moderate, and severe renal impairment (excluding dialysis patients), and initial dosage adjustment is not necessary (Sharma 2015).

End-stage renal disease (ESRD) and ESRD on dialysis: There are no dosage adjustments provided in the manufacturer's labeling (has not been studied). The dialyzability of panobinostat is unknown.

Hepatic Impairment

Hepatic impairment *prior to* treatment:

Mild impairment (bilirubin ≤1 times ULN and AST >1 times ULN or bilirubin >1 to 1.5 times ULN and any AST): Reduce initial dose to 15 mg; monitor frequently for adverse events and adjust dose as needed for toxicity.

Moderate impairment (bilirubin >1.5 to 3 times ULN and any AST): Reduce initial dose to 10 mg; monitor frequently for adverse events and adjust dose as needed for toxicity.

Severe impairment: Avoid use.

Hepatic impairment *during* treatment: If liver function tests are abnormal, consider dosage adjustments and monitor until liver function returns to normal or baseline.

Adjustment for Toxicity If dose reductions are necessary, keep the same treatment schedule and reduce panobinostat dose in increments of 5 mg (from 20 mg to 15 mg, from 15 mg to 10 mg); if dose reduction below 10 mg 3 times a week is necessary, discontinue treatment.

Hematologic toxicity:

Thrombocytopenia:

Grade 3 (platelets <50,000/mm^3): No dosage adjustments are necessary; monitor platelets weekly.

Grade 3 (platelets <50,000/mm^3) with bleeding: Interrupt panobinostat treatment, monitor platelets weekly until platelets ≥50,000/mm^3 and then restart panobinostat at a reduced dose. (Interrupt bortezomib until platelets ≥75,000/mm^3; if only 1 dose omitted, restart bortezomib at the same dose; if ≥2 consecutive doses or doses within the same cycle are omitted, then restart bortezomib at a reduced dose.)

Grade 4 (platelets <25,000/mm^3): Interrupt panobinostat treatment, monitor platelets weekly until platelets ≥50,000/mm^3 and then restart panobinostat at a reduced dose. (Interrupt bortezomib until platelets ≥75,000/mm^3; if only 1 dose omitted, restart bortezomib at the same dose; if ≥2 consecutive doses or doses within the same cycle are omitted, then restart bortezomib at a reduced dose.)

Severe thrombocytopenia: Consider platelet transfusions. Discontinue panobinostat if thrombocytopenia does not improve despite treatment modifications or if repeated platelet transfusions are required.

Neutropenia:

Grade 3 (ANC 750 to 1,000/mm^3): No dosage adjustments are necessary.

Grade 3 (ANC 500 to 750/mm^3 [2 or more occurrences]): Interrupt panobinostat treatment until ANC ≥1,000/mm^3 and then restart at the same dose. (Bortezomib dosage adjustment is not necessary.)

◄

Grade 3 (ANC <1,000/mm^3) with neutropenic fever: Interrupt panobinostat treatment until neutropenic fever resolves and ANC ≥1,000/mm^3 and then restart at a reduced dose. (Interrupt bortezomib until neutropenic fever resolves and ANC ≥1,000/mm^3; if only 1 dose omitted, restart bortezomib at the same dose; if ≥2 consecutive doses or doses within the same cycle are omitted, then restart bortezomib at a reduced dose.)

Grade 4 (ANC <500/mm^3): Interrupt panobinostat treatment until ANC ≥1,000/mm^3 and then restart at a reduced dose. (Interrupt bortezomib until ANC ≥1,000/mm^3; if only 1 dose omitted, restart bortezomib at the same dose; if ≥2 consecutive doses or doses within the same cycle are omitted, then restart bortezomib at a reduced dose.)

Neutropenia, grade 3 or 4: Consider growth factor support or dose modification; if neutropenia does not improve or if severe infection occurs despite dose modification or growth factor support, discontinue panobinostat.

Anemia: Grade 3 (hemoglobin <8 g/dL): Interrupt panobinostat until hemoglobin ≥10 g/dL and then restart at a reduced dose.

Nonhematologic toxicity:

Cardiovascular: QTcF increase to ≥480 msec: Interrupt panobinostat treatment; correct electrolyte abnormalities. If QT prolongation does not resolve then permanently discontinue panobinostat.

Diarrhea:

First sign of abdominal cramping, loose stools, or onset of diarrhea: Begin antidiarrheal medication (eg, loperamide).

Grade 2 (moderate diarrhea; 4 to 6 stools per day): Interrupt panobinostat until resolved and then restart at the same dose. (Consider interruption of bortezomib until resolved and then restart at the same dose.)

Grade 3 (severe diarrhea; ≥7 stools per day, IV fluids or hospitalization required): Interrupt panobinostat treatment until resolved and then restart at a reduced dose. (Interrupt bortezomib until resolved and then restart at a reduced dose.)

Grade 4 (life-threatening): Permanently discontinue panobinostat. (Permanently discontinue bortezomib.)

Infection: Consider interrupting or discontinuing panobinostat.

Nausea or vomiting (panobinostat is associated with nausea and vomiting; consider prophylactic antiemetics):

Severe nausea (grades 3/4): Interrupt panobinostat treatment until resolved and then restart at a reduced dose.

Severe/life-threatening vomiting (grades 3/4): Interrupt panobinostat treatment until resolved and then restart at a reduced dose.

Other toxicities:

Grade 3 or 4 toxicity or recurrent grade 2 toxicity: Withhold panobinostat treatment until recovery to grade 1 or less and then restart at a reduced dose.

Recurrent grade 3 or 4 toxicity: Withhold panobinostat treatment until recovery to grade 1 or less and then restart at a reduced dose.

Dietary Considerations Avoid star fruit, pomegranate or pomegranate juice, and grapefruit or grapefruit juice.

Administration Panobinostat is associated with a moderate emetic potential; consider antiemetics to prevent nausea and vomiting. Administer orally at approximately the same time on scheduled days. May administer with or without food. Swallow capsule whole with a cup of water. Do not open, crush, or chew the capsules.

Hazardous agent; use appropriate precautions for handling and disposal (meets NIOSH 2014 criteria). Avoid exposure to crushed and/or broken capsules. Avoid direct skin or mucous membrane contact with powder inside the capsules; if contact occurs, wash thoroughly.

Monitoring Parameters CBC with differential and platelets (prior to treatment initiation then weekly or more often if clinically indicated during treatment); serum electrolytes, including potassium and magnesium prior to treatment and during treatment (in the clinical trial, electrolytes were monitored prior to the start of each cycle, after the fifth panobinostat dose in week 2 through cycle 8 and then at the beginning of cycles 9 to 16); liver function tests at baseline and regularly during treatment; pregnancy test (in women of reproductive potential, rule out pregnancy prior to and intermittently during treatment); ECG (prior to treatment initiation and periodically as clinically indicated during treatment); hydration status; monitor for gastrointestinal toxicity (eg, diarrhea, nausea, vomiting), signs/symptoms of hemorrhage and/or infection.

Dosage Forms Excipient information presented when available (limited, particularly for generics); consult specific product labeling.

Capsule, Oral:

Farydak: 10 mg [contains brilliant blue fcf (fd&c blue #1)]

Farydak: 15 mg, 20 mg

◆ Panobinostat Lactate *see* Panobinostat *on page 1388*

◆ Panocaps *see* Pancrelipase *on page 1384*

◆ Panokase *see* Pancrelipase *on page 1384*

◆ Panto I.V. (Can) *see* Pantoprazole *on page 1390*

◆ Pantoloc (Can) *see* Pantoprazole *on page 1390*

Pantoprazole (pan TOE pra zole)

Brand Names: US Protonix

Brand Names: Canada Abbott-Pantoprazole; ACT Pantoprazole; Apo-Pantoprazole; Dom-Pantoprazole; JAMP-Pantoprazole; Mar-Pantoprazole; Mint-Pantoprazole; Mylan-Pantoprazole; Panto I.V.; Pantoloc; Pantoprazole for Injection; Pantoprazole Magnesium; Pantoprazole Sodium for Injection; PMS-Pantoprazole; Priva-Pantoprazole; Ran-Pantoprazole; Riva-Pantoprazole; Sandoz-Pantoprazole; Tecta; Teva-Pantoprazole; Teva-Pantoprazole Magnesium

Index Terms Pantoprazole Magnesium; Pantoprazole Sodium

Pharmacologic Category Proton Pump Inhibitor; Substituted Benzimidazole

Use

Oral: Short-term (up to 8 weeks) treatment and maintenance of healing of erosive esophagitis associated with GERD; reduction in relapse rates of daytime and nighttime heartburn symptoms in GERD; hypersecretory disorders associated with Zollinger-Ellison syndrome or other GI hypersecretory disorders

IV: Short-term treatment (7-10 days) of patients with gastroesophageal reflux disease (GERD) and a history of erosive esophagitis; hypersecretory disorders associated with Zollinger-Ellison syndrome or other GI hypersecretory disorders

Canadian labeling: Additional use (not in US labeling): Oral: Peptic ulcer disease (eg, duodenal or gastric ulcer); adjunct treatment with antibiotics for *Helicobacter pylori* eradication; NSAID-induced ulcer prophylaxis (Pantoloc)

Pregnancy Considerations Adverse events have not been observed in animal reproduction studies. Most available studies have not shown an increased risk of major birth defects following maternal use of proton pump inhibitors during pregnancy (Diav-Citrin, 2005; Erichsen, 2012; Matok, 2012; Pasternak, 2010). When treating GERD in pregnancy, PPIs may be used when clinically indicated (Katz, 2013).

Breast-Feeding Considerations Pantoprazole is excreted in breast milk. The excretion of pantoprazole into breast milk was studied in a nursing woman, 10 months postpartum. Following a single dose of pantoprazole 40 mg, maternal milk and serum samples were obtained over 24 hours. Peak concentrations appeared in both the plasma and milk 2 hours after the dose. Pantoprazole concentrations in breast milk were below the limits of detection during most of the study period. Based on this single dose study, the authors calculated the expected exposure to a nursing infant to be 0.14% of the weight-adjusted maternal dose (Plante, 2004). Due to the potential for serious adverse reactions in the nursing infant, the manufacturer recommends a decision be made whether to discontinue nursing or to discontinue the drug, taking into account the importance of treatment to the mother; however, the acidic content of the nursing infants' stomach may potentially inactivate any ingested pantoprazole (Plante, 2004).

Medication Guide Available Yes

Contraindications Hypersensitivity (eg, anaphylaxis, anaphylactic shock, angioedema, bronchospasm, acute interstitial nephritis, urticaria) to pantoprazole, other substituted benzimidazole proton pump inhibitors, or any component of the formulation

Warnings/Precautions Use of proton pump inhibitors (PPIs) may increase the risk of gastrointestinal infections (eg, *Salmonella, Campylobacter*). Relief of symptoms does not preclude the presence of a gastric malignancy. Long-term pantoprazole therapy (especially in patients who were *H. pylori* positive) has caused biopsy-proven atrophic gastritis. Benign and malignant neoplasia has been observed in long-term rodent studies; while not reported in humans, the relevance of these findings in regards to tumorigenicity in humans is not known. Use of PPIs may increase risk of *Clostridium difficile*-associated diarrhea (CDAD), especially in hospitalized patients;

consider CDAD diagnosis in patients with persistent diarrhea that does not improve. Use the lowest dose and shortest duration of PPI therapy appropriate for the condition being treated. Prolonged treatment (≥2 years) may lead to vitamin B_{12} malabsorption and subsequent vitamin B_{12} deficiency. The magnitude of the deficiency is dose-related and the association is stronger in females and those younger in age (<30 years); prevalence is decreased after discontinuation of therapy (Lam, 2013).

Intravenous preparation contains edetate sodium (EDTA); use caution in patients who are at risk for zinc deficiency if other EDTA-containing solutions are coadministered. Some dosage forms may contain polysorbate 80 (also known as Tweens). Hypersensitivity reactions, usually a delayed reaction, have been reported following exposure to pharmaceutical products containing polysorbate 80 in certain individuals (Isaksson, 2002; Lucente 2000; Shelley, 1995). Thrombocytopenia, ascites, pulmonary deterioration, and renal and hepatic failure have been reported in premature neonates after receiving parenteral products containing polysorbate 80 (Alade, 1986; CDC, 1984). See manufacturer's labeling. Decreased H. pylori eradication rates have been observed with short-term (≤7 days) combination therapy. The American College of Gastroenterology recommends 10-14 days of therapy (triple or quadruple) for eradication of H. pylori (Chey, 2007).

PPIs may diminish the therapeutic effect of clopidogrel, thought to be due to reduced formation of the active metabolite of clopidogrel. The manufacturer of clopidogrel recommends either avoidance of both omeprazole (even when scheduled 12 hours apart) and esomeprazole or use of a PPI with comparatively less effect on the active metabolite of clopidogrel. Of the PPIs, pantoprazole has the lowest degree of CYP2C19 inhibition in vitro (Li, 2004) and has been shown to have less effect on conversion of clopidogrel to its active metabolite compared to omeprazole (Angiolillo, 2011). In contrast to these warnings, others have recommended the continued use of PPIs, regardless of the degree of inhibition, in patients with a history of GI bleeding or multiple risk factors for GI bleeding who are also receiving clopidogrel since no evidence has established clinically meaningful differences in outcome; however, a clinically-significant interaction cannot be excluded in those who are poor metabolizers of clopidogrel (Abraham, 2010; Levine, 2011). Potentially significant drug-drug interactions may exist, requiring dose or frequency adjustment, additional monitoring, and/or selection of alternative therapy.

Increased incidence of osteoporosis-related bone fractures of the hip, spine, or wrist may occur with PPI therapy. Patients on high-dose or long-term therapy (≥1 year) should be monitored. Use the lowest effective dose for the shortest duration of time, use vitamin D and calcium supplementation, and follow appropriate guidelines to reduce risk of fractures in patients at risk. Acute interstitial nephritis has been observed in patients taking PPIs; may occur at any time during therapy and is generally due to an idiopathic hypersensitivity reaction. Discontinue if acute interstitial nephritis develops. Thrombophlebitis and hypersensitivity reactions including anaphylaxis, Stevens-Johnson syndrome, and toxic epidermal necrolysis have been reported with IV administration.

Hypomagnesemia, reported rarely, usually with prolonged PPI use of >3 months (most cases >1 year of therapy); may be symptomatic or asymptomatic; severe cases may cause tetany, seizures, and cardiac arrhythmias. Consider obtaining serum magnesium concentrations prior to beginning long-term therapy, especially if taking concomitant digoxin, diuretics, or other drugs known to cause hypomagnesemia; and periodically thereafter. Hypomagnesemia may be corrected by magnesium supplementation, although discontinuation of pantoprazole may be necessary; magnesium levels typically return to normal within 2 weeks of stopping.

Some dosage forms may contain polysorbate 80 (also known as Tweens). Hypersensitivity reactions, usually a delayed reaction, have been reported following exposure to pharmaceutical products containing polysorbate 80 in certain individuals (Isaksson, 2002; Lucente 2000; Shelley, 1995). Thrombocytopenia, ascites, pulmonary deterioration, and renal and hepatic failure have been reported in premature neonates after receiving parenteral products containing polysorbate 80 (Alade, 1986; CDC, 1984). See manufacturer's labeling.

Adverse Reactions

>10%: Central nervous system: Headache (adults 12%; children >4%)

1% to 10%:

Cardiovascular: Facial edema (≤4%), edema (≤2%)

Central nervous system: Dizziness (≤4%), vertigo (≤4%), depression (≤2%)

Dermatologic: Skin rash (adults ≤2%; children >4%), urticaria (≤4%), pruritus (≤2%), skin photosensitivity (≤2%)

Endocrine & metabolic: Increased serum triglycerides (≤4%)

Gastrointestinal: Diarrhea (≤9%), abdominal pain (children >4%), vomiting (≥4%), constipation (≤4%), flatulence (children ≤4%), nausea (children ≤4%), xerostomia (≤2%)

Hematologic & oncologic: Leukopenia (≤2%), thrombocytopenia (≤2%)

Hepatic: Abnormal hepatic function tests (≤4%), hepatitis (≤2%)

Hypersensitivity: Hypersensitivity reaction (≤4%)

Local: Inflammation at injection site (≤2%)

Neuromuscular & skeletal: Arthralgia (≤4%), myalgia (≤4%), increased creatine phosphokinase (≤4%)

Ophthalmic: Blurred vision (≤2%)

Respiratory: Upper respiratory tract infection (children >4%)

Miscellaneous: Fever (adults ≤2%; children >4%)

<1% (Limited to important or life-threatening): Ageusia, agranulocytosis, albuminuria, anaphylaxis (including anaphylactic shock), anemia, angioedema, angina pectoris, aphthous stomatitis, atrial fibrillation, atrial flutter, atrophic gastritis, biliary colic, bone fracture, bursitis, candidiasis (gastrointestinal), cardiac arrhythmia, cardiac failure, cataract, cholecystitis, cholelithiasis, Clostridium difficile-associate diarrhea, colitis, contact dermatitis, cystitis, deafness, dehydration, diabetes mellitus, diplopia, duodenitis, dysmenorrhea, dysphagia, dysuria, ecchymoses, ECG abnormality, eosinophilia, epididymitis, epistaxis, erythema multiforme, exacerbation of asthma, extraocular palsy, fungal dermatitis, gastric ulcer, gastrointestinal carcinoma, gastrointestinal hemorrhage, gingivitis, glaucoma, glossitis, glycosuria, goiter, gout, hallucination, hematemesis, hematuria, hemorrhage, hepatic failure, hepatotoxicity (idiosyncratic) (Chalasani, 2014), hernia, hyperbilirubinemia, hyperesthesia, hypertension, hyperkinesia, hyperuricemia, hypokinesia, hypomagnesemia, hyponatremia, hypotension, impotence, increased gamma-glutamyl transferase, increased serum alkaline phosphatase, increased serum creatinine, interstitial nephritis, ischemic heart disease, jaundice, leukocytosis, lichenoid dermatitis, maculopapular rash, mastalgia, melena, myocardial infarction, neoplasm, nephrolithiasis, neuralgia, neuritis, optic neuropathy (including anterior ischemic), oral mucosa ulcer, ostealgia, palpitations, pancreatitis, pancytopenia, paresthesia, periodontitis, pneumonia, pyelonephritis, rectal hemorrhage, renal pain, retinal vascular disease, rhabdomyolysis, scrotal edema, seizure, Stevens-Johnson syndrome, stomatitis, syncope, tachycardia, tenosynovitis, thrombosis, tinnitus, tongue discoloration, toxic epidermal necrolysis, urethritis, visual disturbance

Drug Interactions

Metabolism/Transport Effects Substrate of CYP2C19 (major), CYP2D6 (minor), CYP3A4 (minor); **Note:** Assignment of Major/Minor substrate status based on clinically relevant drug interaction potential; **Inhibits** BCRP, CYP2C19 (weak); **Induces** CYP1A2 (weak/moderate)

Avoid Concomitant Use

Avoid concomitant use of Pantoprazole with any of the following: Dasatinib; Delavirdine; Erlotinib; Nelfinavir; PAZOPanib; Rilpivirine; Risedronate

Increased Effect/Toxicity

Pantoprazole may increase the levels/effects of: Amphetamine; Dexmethylphenidate; Dextroamphetamine; Methotrexate; Methylphenidate; PAZOPanib; Raltegravir; Risedronate; Saquinavir; Topotecan; Voriconazole

The levels/effects of Pantoprazole may be increased by: Fluconazole; Ketoconazole (Systemic); Voriconazole

Decreased Effect

Pantoprazole may decrease the levels/effects of: Atazanavir; Bisphosphonate Derivatives; Bosutinib; Cefditoren; Clopidogrel; Cysteamine (Systemic); Dabigatran Etexilate; Dabrafenib; Dasatinib; Delavirdine; Erlotinib; Gefitinib; Indinavir; Iron Salts; Itraconazole; Ketoconazole (Systemic); Ledipasvir; Mesalamine; Multivitamins/Minerals (with ADEK, Folate, Iron); Mycophenolate; Nelfinavir; Nilotinib; PAZOPanib; Posaconazole; Rilpivirine; Riociguat; Risedronate

The levels/effects of Pantoprazole may be decreased by: CYP2C19 Inducers (Strong); Dabrafenib; Enzalutamide; Lumacaftor; Tipranavir

Food Interactions Prolonged treatment (≥2 years) may lead to malabsorption of dietary vitamin B_{12} and subsequent vitamin B_{12} deficiency (Lam, 2013).

▶

◀ **Preparation for Administration** Reconstitute with 10 mL NS (final concentration 4 mg/mL). When administering by IV infusion, reconstituted solution may be added to 100 mL D₅W, NS, or LR.

Storage/Stability

Oral: Store tablet and oral suspension at 20°C to 25°C (68°F to 77°F); excursions permitted to 15°C to 30°C (59°F to 86°F).

IV: Prior to reconstitution, store at 20°C to 25°C (68°F to 77°F); excursions permitted to 15°C to 30°C (59°F to 86°F). Do not freeze. Protect from light prior to reconstitution; upon reconstitution, protection from light is not required. Per manufacturer's labeling, reconstituted solution is stable at room temperature for 6 hours; further diluted (admixed) solution should be stored at room temperature and used within 24 hours from the time of initial reconstitution. However, studies have shown that reconstituted solution (4 mg/mL) in polypropylene syringes is stable up to 96 hours at room temperature (Johnson, 2005). Upon further dilution, the admixed solution should be used within 96 hours from the time of initial reconstitution. The preparation should be stored at 3°C to 5°C (37°F to 41°F) if it is stored beyond 48 hours to minimize discoloration.

Mechanism of Action Suppresses gastric acid secretion by inhibiting the parietal cell H⁺/K⁺ ATP pump

Pharmacodynamics/Kinetics

Absorption: Rapid, well absorbed

Distribution: V_d: 11-24 L

Protein binding: 98%, primarily to albumin

Metabolism: Extensively hepatic; CYP2C19 (demethylation), CYP3A4; no evidence that metabolites have pharmacologic activity

Bioavailability: ~77%

Half-life elimination: 1 hour; increased to 3.5-10 hours with CYP2C19 deficiency

Time to peak: Oral: 2.5 hours

Excretion: Urine (71%); feces (18%)

Dosing

Adult & Geriatric

Erosive esophagitis associated with GERD:

Oral:

Treatment: 40 mg once daily for up to 8 weeks; an additional 8 weeks may be used in patients who have not healed after an 8-week course. **Note:** Canadian labeling recommends initial treatment for up to 4 weeks and an additional 4 weeks in patients who have not healed after the initial 4-week course. Lower doses (20 mg once daily) have been used successfully in mild GERD treatment (Dettmer, 1998).

Maintenance of healing: 40 mg once daily (US labeling) or 20 to 40 mg once daily (Canadian labeling); 20 mg once daily has been used successfully in maintenance of healing (Escourrou, 1999). **Note:** Has not been studied beyond 12 months.

IV: 40 mg once daily for 7 to 10 days

Hypersecretory disorders (including Zollinger-Ellison):

Oral: Initial: 40 mg twice daily; adjust dose based on patient needs; doses up to 240 mg daily have been administered

IV: 80 mg every 12 hours; adjust dose based on acid output measurements; 160 to 240 mg daily in divided doses has been used for a limited period (up to 7 days)

Prevention of rebleeding in peptic ulcer bleed (off-label use): *IV:*

Continuous infusion: Loading dose of 80 mg, followed by 8 mg/hour infusion for 72 hours (Barkun, 2010; Zargar, 2006).

Intermittent dosing: Loading dose of 80 mg followed by either 40 mg every 12 hours for 72 hours (Hung, 2007; Yamada, 2012) **or** 40 mg every 6 hours for 72 hours (Hsu, 2009). May also administer 40 mg every 12 hours for 72 hours without a loading dose (Yuksel, 2008).

Note: After completion, continue therapy with a single daily-dose oral PPI for a duration dictated by the underlying etiology (Barkun, 2010).

***Helicobacter pylori* eradication (off-label use in US):**

Oral:

American College of Gastroenterology guidelines (Chey, 2007):

Nonpenicillin allergy: 40 mg twice daily administered with amoxicillin 1000 mg *and* clarithromycin 500 mg twice daily for 10 to 14 days

Penicillin allergy: 40 mg twice daily administered with clarithromycin 500 mg *and* metronidazole 500 mg twice daily for 10 to 14 days **or** 40 mg once or twice daily administered with bismuth subsalicylate 525 mg *and* metronidazole 250 mg *plus* tetracycline 500 mg 4 times daily for 10 to 14 days

Canadian labeling: 40 mg twice daily administered with clarithromycin 500 mg twice daily *and* either metronidazole 500 mg **or** amoxicillin 1,000 mg twice daily for 7 days

Peptic ulcer disease (Canadian labeling): Oral: Treatment: 40 mg once daily for 2 weeks (duodenal ulcer) or 4 weeks (gastric ulcer); may extend therapy for an additional 2 or 4 weeks (based on indication) for inadequate healing

NSAID-induced ulcer prophylaxis (Canadian labeling): Oral: 20 mg once daily

Symptomatic GERD (Canadian labeling): Oral: Treatment: 40 mg once daily for up to 4 weeks; failure to achieve adequate symptom relief after the initial 4 weeks of therapy warrants further evaluation

Pediatric Erosive esophagitis associated with GERD: Oral:

Children <5 years: Dosage not established.

Children ≥5 years:

≥15 to <40 kg: 20 mg once daily for up to 8 weeks

≥40 kg: 40 mg once daily for up to 8 weeks

IV: Dosage not established

Renal Impairment No dosage adjustment necessary; pantoprazole is not removed by hemodialysis. Canadian labeling does not recommend use in combination therapy of *Helicobacter pylori* in patients with severe renal impairment (has not been studied).

Hepatic Impairment

US labeling: No dosage adjustment necessary; doses >40 mg daily have not been evaluated in patients with hepatic impairment.

Canadian labeling:

Mild-moderate impairment: No dosage adjustment necessary.

Severe impairment: IV, Oral: Manufacturer labeling suggests a maximum dose of 20 mg daily. Use in combination therapy of *Helicobacter pylori* is not recommended in patients with severe hepatic impairment (has not been studied).

Dietary Considerations

Oral: May be taken with or without food; best if taken before breakfast.

IV: Due to EDTA in preparation, zinc supplementation may be needed in patients prone to zinc deficiency.

Usual Infusion Concentrations: Adult IV infusion: 80 mg in 100 mL (concentration: 0.8 mg/mL) of D₅W or NS

Administration

IV: Flush IV line before and after administration. In-line filter not required.

2-minute infusion: The volume of reconstituted solution (4 mg/mL) to be injected may be administered intravenously over at least 2 minutes.

15-minute infusion: Infuse over 15 minutes at a rate not to exceed 7 mL/minute (3 mg/minute).

Continuous infusion: May also be administered as a continuous infusion for the prevention of rebleeding within peptic ulcer bleed (off-label use).

Oral:

Tablet: Should be swallowed whole, do not crush or chew. Best if taken before breakfast.

Delayed-release oral suspension: Should only be administered in apple juice or applesauce and taken ~30 minutes before a meal. Do not administer with any other liquid (eg, water) or foods.

Oral administration in **applesauce**: Sprinkle intact granules on 1 tablespoon of applesauce and swallow within 10 minutes of preparation.

Oral administration in **apple juice**: Empty intact granules into 5 mL of apple juice, stir for 5 seconds, and swallow immediately after preparation. Rinse container once or twice with apple juice and swallow immediately.

Nasogastric tube administration: Separate the plunger from the barrel of a 60 mL catheter tip syringe and connect to a ≥16 French nasogastric tube. Holding the syringe attached to the tubing as high as possible, empty the contents of the packet into barrel of the syringe, add 10 mL of apple juice and gently tap/shake the barrel of the syringe to help empty the syringe. Add an additional 10 mL of apple juice and gently tap/shake the barrel to help rinse. Repeat rinse with at least 2-10 mL aliquots of apple juice. No granules should remain in the syringe.

Monitoring Parameters Hypersecretory disorders: Acid output measurements, target level <10 mEq/hour (<5 mEq/hour if prior gastric acid-reducing surgery)

Test Interactions False-positive urine screening tests for tetrahydrocannabinol (THC) have been noted in patients receiving proton pump inhibitors, including pantoprazole.

Dosage Forms Excipient information presented when available (limited, particularly for generics); consult specific product labeling. [DSC] = Discontinued product

Packet, Oral:

Protonix: 40 mg (1 ea, 30 ea) [contains polysorbate 80]

Solution Reconstituted, Intravenous:

Protonix: 40 mg (1 ea) [contains edetate disodium]

Generic: 40 mg (1 ea [DSC])

Tablet Delayed Release, Oral:

Protonix: 20 mg, 40 mg

Generic: 20 mg, 40 mg

Dosage Forms: Canada Refer also to Dosage Forms.

Note: Oral packets are not available in Canada. Excipient information presented when available (limited, particularly for generics); consult specific product labeling.

Solution Reconstituted, Intravenous:

Panto IV: 40 mg [contains edetate disodium]

Tablet Enteric Coated, Oral, as sodium:

Pantoloc 20 mg, 40 mg

Tablet Enteric Coated, Oral, as magnesium:

Tecta: 40 mg

Extemporaneous Preparations A 2 mg/mL pantoprazole oral suspension may be made with pantoprazole tablets, sterile water, and sodium bicarbonate powder. Remove the Protonix® imprint from twenty 40 mg tablets with a paper towel dampened with ethanol (improves the look of product). Let tablets air dry. Crush the tablets in a mortar and reduce to a fine powder. Transfer to a 600 mL beaker, and add 340 mL sterile water. Place beaker on a magnetic stirrer. Add 16.8 g of sodium bicarbonate powder and stir for about 20 minutes until the tablet remnants have disintegrated. While stirring, add another 16.8 g of sodium bicarbonate powder and stir for about 5 minutes until powder has dissolved. Add enough sterile water for irrigation to bring the final volume to 400 mL. Mix well. Transfer to amber-colored bottle. Label "shake well" and "refrigerate". Stable for 62 days refrigerated.

Dentinger PJ, Swenson CF, and Anaizi NH, "Stability of Pantoprazole in an Extemporaneously Compounded Oral Liquid," *Am J Health Syst Pharm*, 2002, 59(10):953-6.

◆ Pantoprazole for Injection (Can) *see* Pantoprazole *on page 1390*

◆ Pantoprazole Magnesium *see* Pantoprazole *on page 1390*

◆ Pantoprazole Sodium *see* Pantoprazole *on page 1390*

◆ Pantoprazole Sodium for Injection (Can) *see* Pantoprazole *on page 1390*

◆ Pantothenyl Alcohol *see* Dexpanthenol *on page 531*

Papaverine (pa PAV er een)

Index Terms Papaverine Hydrochloride; Pavabid

Pharmacologic Category Vasodilator

Use Various vascular spasms associated with smooth muscle spasms as in myocardial infarction, angina, peripheral and pulmonary embolism, peripheral vascular disease; cerebral angiospastic states; visceral spasms (ureteral, biliary, and GI colic). **Note:** Labeled uses have fallen out of favor; safer and more effective alternatives are available.

Dosing

Adult & Geriatric Note: Labeled uses have fallen out of favor; safer and more effective alternatives are available. The manufacturer's labeling recommends the following dosing:

Arterial spasm: IM, IV: 30-120 mg; may repeat dose every 3 hours; if cardiac extrasystole occurs during use, may administer 2 doses 10 minutes apart

Renal Impairment No dosage adjustment provided in the manufacturer's labeling.

Hepatic Impairment No dosage adjustment provided in the manufacturer's labeling.

Additional Information Complete prescribing information should be consulted for additional detail.

Dosage Forms Excipient information presented when available (limited, particularly for generics); consult specific product labeling.

Solution, Injection, as hydrochloride:

Generic: 30 mg/mL (2 mL, 10 mL)

◆ Papaverine Hydrochloride *see* Papaverine *on page 1393*

Papillomavirus (9-Valent) Vaccine (Human, Recombinant)

(pap ih LO ma VYE rus nine VAY lent vak SEEN YU man ree KOM be nant)

Brand Names: US Gardasil 9

Index Terms HPV9

Pharmacologic Category Vaccine; Vaccine, Inactivated (Viral)

Additional Appendix Information

Immunization Administration Recommendations *on page 1974*

Immunization Schedules *on page 1979*

Use

Prevention of human papillomavirus infection:

Females 9 to 26 years of age:

For the prevention of the following diseases:

Cervical, vulvar, vaginal, and anal cancer caused by human papillomavirus (HPV) types 16, 18, 31, 33, 45, 52, and 58

Genital warts (condyloma acuminata) caused by HPV types 6 and 11

For the prevention of the following precancerous or dysplastic lesions caused by HPV types 6, 11, 16, 18, 31, 33, 45, 52, and 58:

Cervical intraepithelial neoplasia (CIN) grades 1, 2, and 3

Cervical adenocarcinoma in situ (AIS)

Vulvar intraepithelial neoplasia (VIN) grades 2 and 3

Vaginal intraepithelial neoplasia (VaIN) grades 2 and 3

Anal intraepithelial neoplasia (AIN) grades 1, 2, and 3

Males 9 through 15 years of age:

For the prevention of the following diseases:

Anal cancer caused by HPV types 16, 18, 31, 33, 45, 52, and 58

Genital warts (condyloma acuminata) caused by HPV types 6 and 11

For the prevention of the following precancerous or dysplastic lesions caused by HPV types 6, 11, 16, 18, 31, 33, 45, 52, and 58:

Anal intraepithelial neoplasia (AIN) grades 1, 2, and 3

The Advisory Committee on Immunization Practices (ACIP) recommends routine vaccination for females and males 11 to 12 years of age; can be administered as young as 9 years; catch-up vaccination is recommended for females 13 to 26 years of age and males 13 to 21 years of age. Vaccination for males 22 through 26 years of age is recommended if immunocompromised (including HIV) and for men who have sex with men and may be considered for any other male in this age group (CDC/ACIP [Petrosky 2015]).

Dosing

Adult

Immunization: IM: Females ≤26 years: 0.5 mL at 0, 2, and 6 months

CDC/ACIP recommended immunization schedule: 0.5 mL per dose for a total of 3 doses; administer the second and third doses at 2 and 6 months after initial dose. There should be a 1-month minimum interval between the first and second dose; a 3-month minimum interval between the second and third dose; a 6-month minimum interval between the first and third dose. Begin series in females ≤26 years or males ≤21 years if not previously vaccinated or completed the 3-dose series (typically administer first dose at age 11 to 12 years). Vaccination for males 22 through 26 years of age is recommended if immunocompromised (including HIV) and for men who have sex with men and may be considered for any other male in this age group. Second and third doses may be given after age 26 years to complete a previously initiated series (CDC/ACIP [Petrosky 2015]).

Pediatric

Immunization: IM:

Females: Children ≥9 years and Adolescents: 0.5 mL at 0, 2, and 6 months

Males: Children ≥9 years and, Adolescents ≤15 years: 0.5 mL at 0, 2, and 6 months

CDC/ACIP recommended immunization schedule: Children ≥9 years and Adolescents: IM: 0.5 mL per dose for a total of 3 doses administered as follows: Initial dose followed by a second dose at 1 to 2 months after initial and third doses at 6 months after the initial. Administer first dose at age 11 to 12 years although series may be initiated as early as 9 years of age. Minimum interval between first and second doses is 4 weeks; the minimum interval between the second and third dose is 12 weeks; the minimum interval between first and third doses is 24 weeks; begin series in females ages 13 to 26 years or males 13 to 21 years if not previously vaccinated or who have not completed the 3-dose

series. Males may also be vaccinated 22 through 26 years of age. Second and third doses may be given after age 26 years to complete a previously initiated series (CDC/ACIP [Petrosky 2015]).

Renal Impairment There are no dosage adjustments provided in the manufacturer's labeling.

Hepatic Impairment There are no dosage adjustments provided in the manufacturer's labeling.

Additional Information Complete prescribing information should be consulted for additional detail.

Dosage Forms Excipient information presented when available (limited, particularly for generics); consult specific product labeling.

Suspension, Intramuscular [preservative free]:

Gardasil 9: (0.5 mL) [contains polysorbate 80, yeast extract]

Suspension Prefilled Syringe, Intramuscular [preservative free]:

Gardasil 9: (0.5 mL) [contains polysorbate 80, yeast extract]

Papillomavirus (Types 6, 11, 16, 18) Vaccine (Human, Recombinant)

(pap ih LO ma VYE rus typs six e LEV en SIX teen AYE teen vak SEEN YU man ree KOM be nant)

Brand Names: US Gardasil

Brand Names: Canada Gardasil

Index Terms HPV Vaccine (Quadrivalent); HPV4; Human Papillomavirus Vaccine (Quadrivalent); Papillomavirus Vaccine, Recombinant; Quadrivalent Human Papillomavirus Vaccine

Pharmacologic Category Vaccine; Vaccine, Inactivated (Viral)

Additional Appendix Information

Immunization Administration Recommendations *on page 1974*

Immunization Schedules *on page 1979*

Use

Prevention of human papillomavirus infection:

US labeling:

Females 9 to 26 years of age:

For the prevention of the following diseases: Cervical, vulvar, vaginal, and anal cancer caused by HPV types 16 and 18; genital warts (condyloma acuminatum) caused by HPV types 6 and 11;

For the prevention of the following precancerous or dysplastic lesions caused by HPV types 6, 11, 16, and 18: Cervical intraepithelial neoplasia (CIN) grade 2/3 and cervical adenocarcinoma in situ; CIN grade 1; vulvar intraepithelial neoplasia grade 2 and 3; vaginal intraepithelial neoplasia grade 2 and 3; and anal intraepithelial neoplasia grades 1, 2, and 3.

Males 9 through 26 years of age:

For the prevention of the following diseases: Anal cancer caused by HPV types 16 and 18; genital warts (condyloma acuminata) caused by HPV types 6 and 11;

For the prevention of anal intraepithelial neoplasia grades 1, 2, and 3 caused by HPV types 6, 11, 16, and 18.

Limitations of use: Does not provide protection against vaccine HPV types to which a person has already been previously exposed, or HPV types not contained in the vaccine; does not prevent CIN grade 2/3 or worse in women >26 years of age. Not intended for the treatment of active external genital lesions or cervical, vulvar, vaginal, and anal cancers.

Canadian labeling:

Females ≥9 years and ≤26 years of age: Prevention of anal cancer caused by HPV types 16 and 18; anal intraepithelial neoplasia caused by HPV types 6, 11, 16, and 18

Females ≥9 years and ≤45 years of age: Prevention of cervical, vulvar, and vaginal cancer caused by HPV types 16 and 18; genital warts caused by HPV types 6 and 11; cervical adenocarcinoma *in situ*, vulvar, vaginal, or cervical intraepithelial neoplasia caused by HPV types 6, 11, 16, and 18

Males ≥9 years and ≤26 years of age: Prevention of anal cancer caused by HPV types 16 and 18; anal intraepithelial neoplasia caused by HPV types 6, 11, 16, and 18; genital warts caused by HPV types 6 and 11

The Advisory Committee on Immunization Practices (ACIP) recommends routine vaccination for females and males 11 to 12 years of age; can be administered as young as 9 years; catch-up vaccination is recommended for females 13 to 26 years of age and males 13 to 21 years of age. Vaccination for males 22 through 26 years of age is recommended if immunocompromised (including HIV) and

for men who have sex with men and may be considered for any other male in this age group (CDC/ACIP [Markowitz 2014]; CDC/ACIP [Strikas 2015]).

Medication Guide Available Yes

Dosing

Adult Immunization regimen:

US labeling: IM: Adults ≤26 years: 0.5 mL per dose for a total of 3 doses; administer the second and third doses at 2 and 6 months after initial dose

Canadian labeling: IM: Adults ≤45 years: 0.5 mL per dose for a total of 3 doses; administer the second and third doses at 2 and 6 months after initial dose

CDC/ACIP recommended immunization schedule: 0.5 mL per dose for a total of 3 doses; administer the second and third doses at 1 to 2 and 6 months after initial dose. There should be a 4-week minimum interval between the first and second dose; a 12-weeks minimum interval (16 weeks preferred) between the second and third dose; a 24-week minimum interval between the first and third dose. Begin series in females ≤26 years or males ≤21 years if not previously vaccinated or completed the 3-dose series (typically administer first dose at age 11 to 12 years). Vaccination for males 22 through 26 years of age is recommended if immunocompromised (including HIV) and for men who have sex with men and may be considered for any other male in this age group. Second and third doses may be given after age 26 years to complete a previously initiated series. The HPV vaccine series should be completed with the same product whenever possible (CDC/ACIP [Kim 2015]; CDC/ACIP [Markowitz 2014]).

Pediatric

Immunization: IM:

US labeling: Children ≥9 years and Adolescents: 0.5 mL per dose for a total of 3 doses; administer the second and third doses at 2 and 6 months after initial dose

Canadian labeling: Children ≥9 years and Adolescents: 0.5 mL per dose for a total of 3 doses; administer the second and third doses at 2 and 6 months after initial dose

CDC/ACIP recommended immunization schedule: 0.5 mL per dose for a total of 3 doses; administer the second and third doses at 1 to 2 and 6 months after initial dose. There should be a 4-week minimum interval between the first and second dose; a 12-weeks minimum interval (16 weeks preferred) between the second and third dose; a 24-week minimum interval between the first and third dose. Typically, administer first dose at age 11 to 12 years but may administer as young as 9 years; begin series in adolescents (≥13 years) if not previously vaccinated or who have not completed the 3-dose series (CDC/ACIP [Markowitz 2014]; CDC/ACIP [Strikas 2015]).

Renal Impairment There are no dosage adjustments provided in the manufacturer's labeling.

Hepatic Impairment There are no dosage adjustments provided in the manufacturer's labeling.

Additional Information Complete prescribing information should be consulted for additional detail.

Dosage Forms Excipient information presented when available (limited, particularly for generics); consult specific product labeling.

Injection, suspension [preservative free]:

Gardasil: HPV 6 L1 protein 20 mcg, HPV 11 L1 protein 40 mcg, HPV 16 L1 protein 40 mcg, and HPV 18 L1 protein 20 mcg per 0.5 mL (0.5 mL) [contains aluminum, polysorbate 80; manufactured using *S. cerevisiae* (baker's yeast)]

Papillomavirus (Types 16, 18) Vaccine (Human, Recombinant)

(pap ih LO ma VYE rus typs SIX teen AYE teen vak SEEN YU man ree KOM be nant)

Brand Names: US Cervarix

Brand Names: Canada Cervarix

Index Terms Bivalent Human Papillomavirus Vaccine; GSK-580299; HPV 16/18 L1 VLP/AS04 VAC; HPV Vaccine (Bivalent); HPV2; Human Papillomavirus Vaccine (Bivalent); Papillomavirus Vaccine, Recombinant

Pharmacologic Category Vaccine; Vaccine, Inactivated (Viral)

Additional Appendix Information

Immunization Administration Recommendations *on page 1974*

Immunization Schedules *on page 1979*

Use

Prevention of human papillomavirus infection:

US labeling: Prevention in females 9 to 25 years of age of the following diseases caused by oncogenic HPV types 16 and 18: Cervical cancer, cervical intraepithelial neoplasia (CIN) grade 2 or higher and adenocarcinoma in situ, and CIN grade 1.

The Advisory Committee on Immunization Practices (ACIP) recommends routine vaccination for females 11 to 12 years of age; can be administered as young as 9 years; catch-up vaccination is recommended for females 13 to 26 years of age (CDC/ACIP [Markowitz, 2014]; CDC/ACIP [Strikas, 2015]).

Canadian labeling: Females 9 through 45 years of age: Prevention of cervical cancer, cervical adenocarcinoma *in situ*, and cervical intraepithelial neoplasia caused by human papillomavirus (HPV) types 16, 18

The National Advisory Committee on Immunization (NACI) recommends routine vaccination for females between 9 and 26 years of age. It should not be administered in females <9 years but may be administered to females >26 years who are at ongoing risk of exposure (NACI [CCDR, 2012]).

Medication Guide Available Yes

Dosing

Adult Immunization: IM:

US labeling: Females ≤25 years: 0.5 mL at 0, 1, and 6 months

CDC/ACIP recommended immunization schedule: 0.5 mL per dose for a total of 3 doses; administer the second and third doses at 1 to 2 and 6 months after initial dose. There should be a 4-week minimum interval between the first and second dose; a 12-weeks minimum interval (16 weeks preferred) between the second and third dose; a 24-week minimum interval between the first and third dose. Begin series in females ≤26 years if not previously vaccinated or who have not completed the 3 dose series (typically administer first dose at age 11 to 12 years). If a female reaches 27 years of age before the vaccination series is complete, the remaining doses can be administered after age 26 years. Inadequate doses or doses received following a shorter than recommended dosing interval should be repeated. The HPV vaccine series should be completed with the same product whenever possible (CDC/ACIP [Kim, 2015]; CDC/ACIP [Markowitz, 2014]).

Canadian labeling: Females ≤45 years: 0.5 mL per dose for a total of 3 doses; administer the second and third doses at 1 and 6 months after initial dose; if necessary, may administer the second and third doses at 1 to 2.5 months and 5 to 12 months respectively after the initial dose.

Pediatric Immunization: IM:

US labeling: Children ≥9 years and Adolescents: Females: 0.5 mL per dose for a total of 3 doses; administer the second and third doses at 1 and 6 months after initial dose

CDC/ACIP recommended immunization schedule: 0.5 mL per dose for a total of 3 doses; administer the second and third doses at 1 to 2 and 6 months after initial dose. There should be a 4-week minimum interval between the first and second dose; a 12-weeks minimum interval (16 weeks preferred) between the second and third dose; a 24-week minimum interval between the first and third dose. Typically administer first dose to females at age 11 to 12 years but may administer as young as 9 years; begin series in female adolescents (≥13 years) if not previously vaccinated or who have not completed the 3-dose series. Inadequate doses or doses received following a shorter than recommended dosing interval should be repeated. The HPV vaccine series should be completed with the same product whenever possible (CDC/ACIP [Markowitz, 2014]; CDC/ACIP [Strikas, 2015]).

Canadian labeling: Children ≥9 years and Adolescents: Females: 0.5 mL per dose for a total of 3 doses; administer the second and third doses at 1 and 6 months after initial dose; if necessary, may administer the second and third doses at 1 to 2.5 months and 5 to 12 months respectively after the initial dose.

Renal Impairment There are no dosage adjustments provided in the manufacturer's labeling.

Hepatic Impairment There are no dosage adjustments provided in the manufacturer's labeling.

Additional Information Complete prescribing information should be consulted for additional detail.

Dosage Forms Excipient information presented when available (limited, particularly for generics); consult specific product labeling.

Injection, suspension [preservative free]:

Cervarix: HPV 16 L1 protein 20 mcg and HPV 18 L1 protein 20 mcg per 0.5 mL (0.5 mL) [contains aluminum, natural rubber/natural latex in prefilled syringe; manufactured using *Trichoplusia ni* (insect cells)]

◆ Papillomavirus Vaccine, Recombinant *see* Papillomavirus (Types 6, 11, 16, 18) Vaccine (Human, Recombinant) *on page 1394*

◆ Papillomavirus Vaccine, Recombinant *see* Papillomavirus (Types 16, 18) Vaccine (Human, Recombinant) *on page 1394*

◆ PAR-101 *see* Fidaxomicin *on page 765*

◆ Paracetamol *see* Acetaminophen *on page 25*

◆ Parafon Forte DSC *see* Chlorzoxazone *on page 381*

◆ Paraplatin *see* CARBOplatin *on page 312*

Parathyroid Hormone (par a THYE roid HOR mone)

Brand Names: US Natpara

Index Terms Natpara; PTH(1-84); Recombinant Human Parathyroid Hormone (1-84); rhPTH(1-84)

Pharmacologic Category Parathyroid Hormone Analog

Use

Hypoparathyroidism: Adjunct to calcium and vitamin D to control hypocalcemia in patients with hypoparathyroidism

Limitations of use: Because of the potential risk of osteosarcoma, recommended only for patients who cannot be well-controlled on calcium supplements and active forms of vitamin D alone; has not been studied in patients with hypoparathyroidism caused by calcium-sensing receptor mutations or in patients with acute postsurgical hypoparathyroidism

Pregnancy Considerations Adverse events were observed in animal reproduction studies.

Breast-Feeding Considerations It is not known if parathyroid hormone from this preparation is excreted into breast milk. According to the manufacturer, the decision breast-feed should take into account the risk of exposure to the infant and the benefits of treatment to the mother.

Prescribing and Access Restrictions As a requirement of the REMS program, access to this medication is restricted. Natpara is only available to certified health care prescribers and can only be dispensed by certified pharmacies under the Natpara REMS program. Further information is available at www.NATPARAREMS.com or by telephone at 1-855-NATPARA.

Medication Guide Available Yes

Contraindications There are no contraindications listed within the manufacturer's labeling.

Warnings/Precautions [US Boxed Warning]: In animal studies, parathyroid hormone has been associated with an increase in osteosarcoma; risk was dependent on both dose and duration. Avoid use in patients with an increased risk of osteosarcoma (including Paget disease, prior external beam or implant radiation therapy involving the skeleton, unexplained elevation of alkaline phosphatase, patients with open epiphyses, patients with hereditary disorders predisposing to osteosarcoma). Treatment should only be used in patients who cannot be well controlled on calcium supplements and active forms of vitamin D alone.

Severe hypercalcemia has been reported; the risk is highest during initiation of therapy and dose escalation. Monitor serum calcium concentrations and patients for signs and symptoms of hypercalcemia. Treat hypercalcemia as needed and consider temporary discontinuation or a reduction in dose if severe hypercalcemia occurs. Severe hypocalcemia has been reported and can occur at any time during therapy; the risk is highest when a dose is missed or when parathyroid hormone therapy is withheld or abruptly discontinued. Monitor serum calcium concentrations and patients for signs and symptoms of hypocalcemia. In patients who must have therapy interrupted or discontinued, resume treatment with or increase the dose of an active form of vitamin D and/or calcium supplements to prevent severe hypocalcemia.

In patients receiving calcium supplementation, maintain the same dose of calcium at initiation of parathyroid hormone therapy. In patients receiving active forms of vitamin D, reduce the dose of active vitamin D by 50% at initiation of parathyroid hormone therapy if serum calcium is >7.5 mg/dL. Active forms of vitamin D and calcium supplementation may require titration during parathyroid hormone therapy based on albumin-corrected serum

calcium concentrations; consult parathyroid hormone product labeling for more information.

Potentially significant drug-drug interactions may exist, requiring dose or frequency adjustment, additional monitoring, and/or selection of alternative therapy.

Adverse Reactions Frequency not always defined.

>10%:

Central nervous system: Paresthesia (31%), headache (25%), hypoesthesia (14%)

Endocrine & metabolic: Hypocalcemia (27%), hypercalcemia (19%)

Gastrointestinal: Diarrhea (12%), vomiting (12%)

Genitourinary: Hypercalciuria (11%)

Immunologic: Immunogenicity (6% to 16%; drug efficacy not affected)

Neuromuscular & skeletal: Arthralgia (11%)

1% to 10%:

Cardiovascular: Hypertension (6%)

Central nervous system: Peripheral pain (10%)

Endocrine & metabolic: Inhibited conversion of vitamin d3 to 25-hydroxy-d3 (6%)

Gastrointestinal: Upper abdominal pain (7%), facial numbness (6%)

Hematologic & oncologic: Osteosarcoma

Neuromuscular & skeletal: Neck pain (6%)

Respiratory: Upper respiratory tract infection (8%), sinusitis (7%)

Miscellaneous: Drug toxicity (risk when used concomitantly with digoxin and other drugs known to increase serum calcium)

Drug Interactions

Metabolism/Transport Effects None known.

Avoid Concomitant Use

Avoid concomitant use of Parathyroid Hormone with any of the following: Alendronate

Increased Effect/Toxicity

Parathyroid Hormone may increase the levels/effects of: Cardiac Glycosides

Decreased Effect

The levels/effects of Parathyroid Hormone may be decreased by: Alendronate

Preparation for Administration Reconstitute medication cartridge with provided mixing device. The mixing device can be used to reconstitute up to six medication cartridges.

Storage/Stability Prior to reconstitution, the dual-chamber medication cartridge should be stored in the package provided at 2°C to 8°C (36°F to 46°F). After reconstitution, the medication cartridge should be stored in the Q-Cliq pen at 2°C to 8°C (36°F to 46°F) for up to 14 days. Store away from heat and light. Discard reconstituted medication cartridges after 14 days. Do not freeze or shake or use if it has been frozen or shaken. The mixing device and empty Q-Cliq pen can be stored at room temperature.

Mechanism of Action Exogenous parathyroid hormone; parathyroid hormone raises serum calcium concentrations by increasing renal tubular calcium reabsorption, increasing intestinal calcium absorption, and by increasing bone turnover, which releases calcium into the circulation.

Pharmacodynamics/Kinetics

Onset of action: Peak effect: 10 to 12 hours

Duration: >24 hours

Distribution: V_{dss}: 5.35 L

Metabolism: Primarily hepatic; cleavage by cathepsins

Bioavailability: SubQ: 53%

Half-life elimination: ~3 hours

Time to peak: 5 to 30 minutes

Excretion: Renal (primarily by glomerular filtration)

Dosing

Adult

Hypoparathyroidism: SubQ: **Note:** Prior to initiation of therapy, confirm that the serum calcium concentration is >7.5 mg/dL and the 25-hydroxyvitamin D stores are sufficient (correct if insufficient)

Initial: 50 mcg once daily.

Dosage adjustment: **Note:** Active forms of vitamin D and calcium supplementation may require adjustment during parathyroid hormone therapy based on albumin-corrected serum calcium concentrations; consult parathyroid hormone product labeling for more information.

Serum calcium (albumin-corrected) cannot be maintained >8 mg/dL without an active form of vitamin D and/or calcium supplementation: Increase the parathyroid hormone dose in increments of 25 mcg/day every 4 weeks; maximum daily dose: 100 mcg/day

Serum calcium (albumin-corrected) repeatedly >9 mg/dL after discontinuation of active forms of vitamin D and calcium supplementation decreased to a dose sufficient to meet daily needs: May decrease the parathyroid hormone dose to a minimum of 25 mcg/day

Maintenance: Use the lowest dose required to prevent both hypocalcemia and hypercalciuria while maintaining albumin-corrected serum calcium concentrations at the lower half of the normal range (ie, between 8 and 9 mg/dL) without the need for active forms of vitamin D and with calcium supplementation sufficient to meet the patient's daily requirements.

Discontinuation or interruption of therapy: An abrupt interruption or discontinuation may result in severe hypocalcemia; resume treatment with or increase the dose of an active form of vitamin D and calcium supplementation (if indicated).

Missed dose: Administer parathyroid hormone as soon as reasonably feasible; additional calcium should be administered in the event of hypocalcemia.

Geriatric Dosing should start at the lower end of dosing range and titrate to response due to possible increased incidence of hepatic, renal, or cardiac impairment.

Renal Impairment

Mild to moderate impairment (CrCl ≥30 mL/minute): No dosage adjustment necessary.

Severe impairment (CrCl <30 mL/minute): There are no dosage adjustments provided in the manufacturer's labeling (has not been studied).

Dialysis: There are no dosage adjustments provided in the manufacturer's labeling (has not been studied).

Hepatic Impairment

Mild to moderate impairment (Child-Pugh class A or B): No dosage adjustment necessary.

Severe impairment (Child-Pugh class C): There are no dosage adjustments provided in the manufacturer's labeling (has not been studied).

Administration Administer subcutaneously into the thigh (alternate thighs each day) using the provided Q-Cliq pen. Follow instructions provided with the medication cartridges and the Q-Cliq pen to prepare the injection device for use. One Q-Cliq pen may be used for up to 2 years, with changing the reconstituted cartridge every 2 weeks. Patients and caregivers who will administer parathyroid hormone should receive appropriate training and instruction by a trained health care professional prior to first use.

Monitoring Parameters Total serum calcium (albumin-corrected) prior to therapy initiation, within 3 to 7 days following initiation or dosage adjustments until maintenance dose has been achieved, and periodically thereafter; urinary calcium excretion (after maintenance dose is achieved); signs and symptoms of hypo- and hypercalcemia

Dosage Forms Excipient information presented when available (limited, particularly for generics); consult specific product labeling.

Cartridge, Subcutaneous:

Natpara: 25 mcg (1 ea); 50 mcg (1 ea); 75 mcg (1 ea); 100 mcg (1 ea) [contains metacresol]

◆ Parathyroid Hormone (1-34) see Teriparatide on page 1765

◆ Parcaine [DSC] see Proparacaine on page 1515

◆ Parcopa [DSC] see Carbidopa and Levodopa on page 307

Paregoric (par e GOR ik)

Index Terms Camphorated Tincture of Opium (error-prone synonym)

Pharmacologic Category Analgesic, Opioid; Antidiarrheal

Use Diarrhea: Treatment of diarrhea

Dosing

Adult & Geriatric Note: Paregoric oral liquid contains morphine 2 mg/5 mL (0.4 mg/mL)

Diarrhea: Oral: 5 to 10 mL 1 to 4 times daily

Pediatric Note: Paregoric oral liquid contains morphine 2 mg/5 mL (0.4 mg/mL)

Diarrhea: Children and Adolescents: Oral: 0.25 to 0.5 mL/kg 1 to 4 times daily

Renal Impairment There are no dosage adjustments provided in the manufacturer's labeling. Use with caution in severe impairment.

Hepatic Impairment There are no dosage adjustments provided in the manufacturer's labeling. Use with caution in severe impairment.

Additional Information Complete prescribing information should be consulted for additional detail.

Dosage Forms Excipient information presented when available (limited, particularly for generics); consult specific product labeling.

Tincture, Oral:

Generic: 2 mg/5 mL (473 mL)

Controlled Substance C-III

◆ **Parenteral Nutrition** *see* Total Parenteral Nutrition on page 1818

Paricalcitol (pah ri KAL si tole)

Brand Names: US Zemplar
Brand Names: Canada Zemplar
Pharmacologic Category Vitamin D Analog
Use

IV: Prevention and treatment of secondary hyperparathyroidism associated with stage 5 chronic kidney disease (CKD)

Oral: Prevention and treatment of secondary hyperparathyroidism associated with stage 3 and 4 CKD and stage 5 CKD patients on hemodialysis or peritoneal dialysis

Pregnancy Considerations Adverse events were observed in some animal reproduction studies.

Breast-Feeding Considerations It is not known if paricalcitol is excreted in breast milk. Due to the potential for serious adverse reactions in the nursing infant, a decision should be made whether to discontinue nursing or to discontinue the drug, taking into account the importance of treatment to the mother.

Contraindications Hypersensitivity to paricalcitol or any component of the formulation; patients with evidence of vitamin D toxicity; hypercalcemia

Warnings/Precautions Excessive administration may lead to over suppression of PTH, hypercalcemia, hypercalciuria, hyperphosphatemia and adynamic bone disease. Acute hypercalcemia may increase risk of cardiac arrhythmias and seizures; use caution with cardiac glycosides as digitalis toxicity may be increased. Chronic hypercalcemia may lead to generalized vascular and other soft-tissue calcification. Phosphate and vitamin D (and its derivatives) should be withheld during therapy to avoid hypercalcemia. Risk of hypercalcemia may be increased by concomitant use of calcium-containing supplements and/or medications that increase serum calcium (eg, thiazide diuretics). Avoid regular administration of aluminum-containing preparations (eg, antacids, phosphate binders) to prevent aluminum overload and bone toxicity. Dialysate concentration of aluminum should be maintained at <10 mcg/L.

Adverse Reactions

>10%:

Gastrointestinal: Nausea (5% to 13%), diarrhea (7% to 12%)

Infection: Infection (bacterial, fungal, viral: 3% to 15%)

2% to 10%:

Cardiovascular: Hypertension (7%), edema (6% to 7%), hypotension (5%), palpitations (3%), chest pain (3%), peripheral edema (3%), syncope (3%)

Central nervous system: Pain (4% to 8%), dizziness (5% to 7%), chills (5%), insomnia (5%), vertigo (5%), headache (3% to 5%), anxiety (3%), depression (3%), fatigue (3%), malaise (3%)

Dermatologic: Skin rash (4% to 6%), dermal ulcer (3%), ecchymoses (3%)

Endocrine & metabolic: Hypervolemia (5%), dehydration (3%), hypoglycemia (3%)

Gastrointestinal: Vomiting (5% to 8%), gastrointestinal hemorrhage (5%), peritonitis (5%), constipation (4% to 5%), abdominal pain (4%), dyspepsia (3%), xerostomia (3%)

Genitourinary: Uremia (3%), urinary tract infection (3%)

Hypersensitivity: Hypersensitivity reaction (6%)

Infection: Influenza (5%), sepsis (3%)

Neuromuscular & skeletal: Arthralgia (5%), arthritis (5%), weakness (3% to 5%), back pain (3% to 4%), leg cramps (3%), muscle spasm (3%)

Respiratory: Nasopharyngitis (8%), pneumonia (5%), rhinitis (5%), oropharyngeal pain (4%), bronchitis (3%), cough (3%), sinusitis (3%)

Miscellaneous: Fever (3% to 5%)

<2% (Limited to important or life-threatening): Abnormal gait, abnormal hepatic function tests, anemia, angioedema (including laryngeal edema), atrial flutter, burning sensation of skin, cardiac arrest, cardiac arrhythmia, cerebrovascular accident, confusion, conjunctivitis, delirium, dysphagia, erectile dysfunction, extravasation reactions, gastritis, gastroesophageal reflux disease, glaucoma, hirsutism, hypercalciuria, hypercalcemia, hyperparathyroidism, hyperkalemia, hyperphosphatemia, hypocalcemia, hypoparathyroidism, increased serum creatinine, ischemic bowel disease, lymphadenopathy, malignant neoplasm of breast, myalgia, myoclonus, night sweats, ocular hyperemia, orthopnea, paresthesia, prolonged bleeding time, pruritus, pulmonary edema, rectal hemorrhage, upper respiratory tract infection, urticaria, vaginal infection, weight loss, wheezing

Drug Interactions

Metabolism/Transport Effects Substrate of CYP3A4 (minor); **Note:** Assignment of Major/Minor substrate status based on clinically relevant drug interaction potential

Avoid Concomitant Use

Avoid concomitant use of Paricalcitol with any of the following: Aluminum Hydroxide; Multivitamins/Fluoride (with ADE); Multivitamins/Minerals (with ADEK, Folate, Iron); Sucralfate; Vitamin D Analogs

Increased Effect/Toxicity

Paricalcitol may increase the levels/effects of: Aluminum Hydroxide; Cardiac Glycosides; Digoxin; Sucralfate; Vitamin D Analogs

The levels/effects of Paricalcitol may be increased by: Calcium Salts; CYP3A4 Inhibitors (Strong); Danazol; Multivitamins/Fluoride (with ADE); Multivitamins/Minerals (with ADEK, Folate, Iron); Thiazide Diuretics

Decreased Effect

The levels/effects of Paricalcitol may be decreased by: Bile Acid Sequestrants; Mineral Oil; Orlistat

Storage/Stability Store at 25°C (77°F); excursions permitted between 15°C to 30°C (59°F to 86°F).

Mechanism of Action Decreased renal conversion of vitamin D to its primary active metabolite (1,25-hydroxyvitamin D) in chronic renal failure leads to reduced activation of vitamin D receptor (VDR), which subsequently removes inhibitory suppression of parathyroid hormone (PTH) release; increased serum PTH (secondary hyperparathyroidism) reduces calcium excretion and enhances bone resorption. Paricalcitol is a synthetic vitamin D analog which binds to and activates the VDR in kidney, parathyroid gland, intestine and bone, thus reducing PTH levels and improving calcium and phosphate homeostasis.

Pharmacodynamics/Kinetics

Distribution: V_d:

Healthy subjects: Oral: 34 L; IV: 24 L

Stage 3 and 4 CKD: Oral: 44 to 46 L

Stage 5 CKD: Oral: 38 to 49 L; IV: 31 to 35 L

Protein binding: >99%

Metabolism: Hydroxylation and glucuronidation via hepatic and nonhepatic enzymes, including CYP24, CYP3A4, UGT1A4; forms metabolites (at least one active)

Bioavailability: Oral: 72% to 86% in healthy subjects

Half-life elimination:

Healthy subjects: Oral: 4 to 6 hours; IV: 5 to 7 hours

Stage 3 and 4 CKD: Oral: 17 to 20 hours

Stage 5 CKD (on HD or PD): Oral: 14 to 18 hours; IV: 14 to 15 hours

Time to peak, plasma: 3 hours: Delayed by food

Excretion: Healthy subjects: Feces (oral: 70%; IV: 63%); urine (oral: 18%, IV: 19%)

Dosing

Adult & Geriatric Note: In stage 3 to 5 CKD maintain Ca x P <55 mg^2/dL^2, reduce or interrupt dosing if recommended calcium phosphorus product (Ca x P) is exceeded or hypercalcemia is observed (K/DOQI Clinical Practice Guidelines, 2003).

Secondary hyperparathyroidism associated with chronic renal failure (stage 5 CKD):

IV: 0.04 to 0.1 mcg/kg (2.8 to 7 mcg) given as a bolus dose no more frequently than every other day at any time during dialysis; dose may be increased by 2 to 4 mcg every 2 to 4 weeks; doses as high as 0.24 mcg/kg (16.8 mcg) have been administered safely; the dose of paricalcitol should be adjusted based on serum intact PTH (iPTH) levels, as follows:

Same or increasing iPTH level: Increase paricalcitol dose

iPTH level decreased by <30%: Increase paricalcitol dose

iPTH level decreased by >30% and <60%: Maintain paricalcitol dose

iPTH level decrease by >60%: Decrease paricalcitol dose

iPTH level 1.5 to 3 times upper limit of normal: Maintain paricalcitol dose

Oral: Initial dose, in mcg, based on baseline iPTH level divided by 80. Administered 3 times weekly, no more frequently than every other day. **Note:** To reduce the risk of hypercalcemia initiate only after baseline serum calcium has been adjusted to ≤9.5 mg/dL.

Dose titration:

Titration dose (mcg) = Most recent iPTH level (pg/mL) divided by 80

Note: In situations where monitoring of iPTH, calcium, and phosphorus occurs less frequently than once per week, a more modest initial and dose titration rate may be warranted:

Modest titration dose (mcg) = Most recent iPTH level (pg/mL) divided by 100

Dosage adjustment for hypercalcemia or elevated Ca x P: Decrease calculated dose by 2 to 4 mcg. If further adjustment is required, dose should be reduced or interrupted until these parameters are normalized. If applicable, phosphate binder dosing may also be adjusted or withheld, or switched to a noncalcium-based phosphate binder

Secondary hyperparathyroidism associated with stage 3 and 4 CKD: Adults: Oral: Initial dose based on baseline serum iPTH:

iPTH ≤500 pg/mL: 1 mcg/day or 2 mcg 3 times/week
iPTH >500 pg/mL: 2 mcg/day or 4 mcg 3 times/week

Dosage adjustment based on iPTH level relative to baseline, adjust dose at 2- to 4-week intervals:

iPTH same or increased: Increase paricalcitol dose by 1 mcg/day or 2 mcg 3 times/week
iPTH decreased by <30%: Increase paricalcitol dose by 1 mcg/day or 2 mcg 3 times/week
iPTH decreased by ≥30% and ≤60%: Maintain paricalcitol dose
iPTH decreased by >60%: Decrease paricalcitol dose by 1 mcg/day* or 2 mcg 3 times/week
iPTH <60 pg/mL: Decrease paricalcitol dose by 1 mcg/day* or 2 mcg 3 times/week

*If patient is taking the lowest dose on a once-daily regimen, but further dose reduction is needed, decrease dose to 1 mcg 3 times/week. If further dose reduction is required, withhold drug as needed and restart at a lower dose and frequency. If applicable, calcium-phosphate binder dosing may also be adjusted or withheld, or switched to noncalcium-based binder.

Pediatric Secondary hyperparathyroidism associated with chronic renal failure (stage 5 CKD): IV: Children ≥5 years: Refer to adult dosing.

Renal Impairment No dosage adjustment necessary.

Hepatic Impairment
Mild to moderate impairment: No dosage adjustment necessary.
Severe impairment: No dosage adjustment provided in manufacturer's labeling (has not been studied).

Dietary Considerations May be taken with or without food. Some products may contain coconut or palm kernel oil.

Administration
Oral: May be administered with or without food. With the 3 times/week dosing schedule, doses should not be given more frequently than every other day.
IV: Administered as a bolus dose at anytime during dialysis. Doses should not be administered more often than every other day.

Monitoring Parameters
Signs and symptoms of vitamin D intoxication; signs and symptoms of hypercalcemia (eg, feeling tired, difficulty thinking clearly, loss of appetite, nausea, vomiting, constipation, increased thirst, increased urination, weight loss).
Serum calcium and phosphorus (closely monitor levels during dosage titration and after initiation of a strong CYP3A4 inhibitor):
IV: Twice weekly during initial phase, then at least monthly once dose established
Oral: At least every 2 weeks for initial 3 months or following dose adjustment, then monthly for 3 months, then every 3 months
Serum or plasma intact PTH (iPTH):
IV: Every 2 to 4 weeks, then every 3 months once dose established
Oral: At least every 2 weeks for 3 months or following dose adjustment, then monthly for 3 months, then every 3 months

Reference Range
Corrected total serum calcium (K/DOQI, 2003): CKD stages 3 and 4: 8.4 to 10.2 mg/dL (2.1 to 2.6 mmol/L); CKD stage 5: 8.4 to 9.5 mg/dL (2.1 to 2.37 mmol/L); KDIGO guidelines recommend maintaining normal ranges for all stages of CKD (3 to 5D) (KDIGO, 2009)
Phosphorus (K/DOQI, 2003):
CKD stages 3 and 4: 2.7 to 4.6 mg/dL (0.87 to 1.48 mmol/L) (adults); maintain within age-appropriate limits (children)
CKD stage 5 (including those treated with dialysis): 3.5 to 5.5 mg/dL (1.13 to 1.78 mmol/L) (children >12 years and adults); 4 to 6 mg/dL (1.29 to 1.94 mmol/L) (children 1 to 12 years)
KDIGO guidelines recommend maintaining normal ranges for CKD stages 3 to 5 and lowering elevated phosphorus levels toward the normal range for CKD stage 5D (KDIGO, 2009)

Serum calcium-phosphorus product (K/DOQI, 2003): CKD stage 3 to 5: <55 mg^2/dL^2 (children >12 years and adults); <65 mg^2/dL^2 (children ≤12 years)
PTH: Whole molecule, immunochemiluminometric assay (ICMA): 1.0 to 5.2 pmol/L; whole molecule, radioimmunoassay (RIA): 10.0 to 65.0 pg/mL; whole molecule, immunoradiometric, double antibody (IRMA): 1.0 to 6.0 pmol/L Target ranges by stage of chronic kidney disease (KDIGO, 2009): CKD stage 3 to 5: Optimal iPTH is unknown; maintain normal range (assay-dependent); CKD stage 5D: Maintain iPTH within 2 to 9 times the upper limit of normal for the assay used

Test Interactions In predialysis patients, paricalcitol may increase serum creatinine and therefore decrease the estimated GFR (eGFR).

Dosage Forms Excipient information presented when available (limited, particularly for generics); consult specific product labeling.
Capsule, Oral:
Zemplar: 1 mcg, 2 mcg, 4 mcg [contains alcohol, usp]
Generic: 1 mcg, 2 mcg, 4 mcg
Solution, Intravenous:
Zemplar: 2 mcg/mL (1 mL); 5 mcg/mL (1 mL, 2 mL) [contains alcohol, usp, propylene glycol]
Generic: 2 mcg/mL (1 mL); 5 mcg/mL (1 mL, 2 mL)

◆ Pariet (Can) see RABEprazole on page 1545
◆ Pariprazole see RABEprazole on page 1545
◆ Paritaprevir, Ombitasvir, and Ritonavir see Ombitasvir, Paritaprevir, and Ritonavir on page 1327
◆ Paritaprevir, Ombitasvir, Ritonavir, and Dasabuvir see Ombitasvir, Paritaprevir, Ritonavir, and Dasabuvir on page 1327
◆ Parlodel see Bromocriptine on page 255
◆ Parnate see Tranylcypromine on page 1829
◆ Parnate® (Can) see Tranylcypromine on page 1829
◆ Paroex see Chlorhexidine Gluconate on page 373

Paromomycin (par oh moe MYE sin)

Brand Names: Canada Humatin
Index Terms Paromomycin Sulfate
Pharmacologic Category Amebicide
Use
Intestinal amebiasis: Treatment of acute and chronic intestinal amebiasis (not effective for extraintestinal amebiasis).
Hepatic coma: Management (adjunctive) of hepatic coma.
Pregnancy Considerations Paromomycin is poorly absorbed when given orally. Information related to the use of paromomycin in pregnancy is limited (Kreutner 1981). Use may be considered for the treatment of giardiasis throughout pregnancy (Gardner 2001) or cryptosporidiosis after the first trimester (DHHS 2013) in pregnant women.
Breast-Feeding Considerations Paromomycin is poorly absorbed when given orally. Available information suggests that paromomycin may be used in nursing women when renal function is normal in both the mother and infant (Davidson 2009).
Contraindications Hypersensitivity to paromomycin or any component of the formulation; intestinal obstruction
Warnings/Precautions Use with caution in patients with impaired renal function or ulcerative bowel lesions (may lead to renal toxicity due to inadvertent absorption). Prolonged use may result in fungal or bacterial superinfection, including *C. difficile*-associated diarrhea (CDAD) and pseudomembranous colitis; CDAD has been observed >2 months postantibiotic treatment. Use in the absence of proven (or strongly suspected) susceptible infection is unlikely to provide benefit and may increase the risk for drug-resistance.
Adverse Reactions
1% to 10%: Gastrointestinal: Diarrhea, abdominal cramps, nausea, vomiting, heartburn
<1% (Limited to important or life-threatening): Enterocolitis (secondary), eosinophilia, ototoxicity, pruritus, rash, steatorrhea
Drug Interactions
Metabolism/Transport Effects None known.
Avoid Concomitant Use There are no known interactions where it is recommended to avoid concomitant use.
Increased Effect/Toxicity There are no known significant interactions involving an increase in effect.
Decreased Effect There are no known significant interactions involving a decrease in effect.
Storage/Stability Store at 20°C to 25°C (68°F to 77°F). Protect from moisture.

Mechanism of Action Acts directly on ameba; has anti-bacterial activity against normal and pathogenic organisms in the GI tract; interferes with bacterial protein synthesis by binding to 30S ribosomal subunits

Pharmacodynamics/Kinetics

Absorption: Poor oral absorption

Excretion: Feces (~100% as unchanged drug)

Dosing

Adult & Geriatric

Hepatic coma: Oral: 4 g daily in divided doses (at regular intervals) for 5 to 6 days

Intestinal amebiasis: Oral: 25 to 35 mg/kg/day in 3 divided doses for 5 to 10 days

Cryptosporidiosis-associated diarrhea in HIV-infected patients (off-label use): Oral: 500 mg 4 times daily for 14 to 21 days (must be used in conjunction with optimized ART, electrolyte replacement, and symptomatic treatment and rehydration) (HHS [OI adult 2015])

***Dientamoeba fragilis* (off-label use):** Oral: 25 to 35 mg/kg/day in 3 divided doses for 7 days (CDC 2012)

Pediatric

Intestinal amebiasis (acute and chronic): Children and Adolescents: Refer to adult dosing.

Cryptosporidiosis-associated diarrhea in HIV-infected patients (off-label use): Adolescents: Refer to adult dosing.

***Dientamoeba fragilis* (off-label use):** Children and Adolescents: Oral: 25-35 mg/kg/day in 3 divided doses for 7 days (CDC 2012; Vandenberg 2006)

Renal Impairment No dosage adjustment provided in the manufacturer's labeling (has not been studied).

Hepatic Impairment No dosage adjustment provided in the manufacturer's labeling (has not been studied).

Administration Administer orally with meals.

Dosage Forms Excipient information presented when available (limited, particularly for generics); consult specific product labeling.

Capsule, Oral:

Generic: 250 mg

◆ Paromomycin Sulfate *see* Paromomycin *on page 1398*

PARoxetine (pa ROKS e teen)

Brand Names: US Brisdelle; Paxil; Paxil CR; Pexeva

Brand Names: Canada Apo-Paroxetine; Auro-Paroxetine; CO Paroxetine; Dom-Paroxetine; JAMP-Paroxetine; Mylan-Paroxetine; Novo-Paroxetine; Paxil; Paxil CR; PHL-Paroxetine; PMS-Paroxetine; Q-Paroxetine; ratio-Paroxetine; Riva-Paroxetine; Sandoz-Paroxetine; Teva-Paroxetine

Index Terms Brisdelle; Paroxetine Hydrochloride; Paroxetine Mesylate

Pharmacologic Category Antidepressant, Selective Serotonin Reuptake Inhibitor

Use

Generalized anxiety disorder (immediate release): For the treatment of generalized anxiety disorder (GAD)

Major depressive disorder (immediate and controlled release): For the treatment of major depressive disorder (MDD)

Obsessive-compulsive disorder (immediate release): For the treatment of obsessions and compulsions in patients with obsessive-compulsive disorder (OCD)

Panic disorder (immediate and controlled release): For the treatment of panic disorder, with or without agoraphobia

Post-traumatic stress disorder (immediate release): For the treatment of post-traumatic stress disorder (PTSD)

Premenstrual dysphoric disorder (controlled release): For the treatment of premenstrual dysphoric disorder (PMDD)

Social anxiety disorder (immediate and controlled release): For the treatment of social anxiety disorder, also known as social phobia

Vasomotor symptoms of menopause (Brisdelle only): For the treatment of moderate to severe vasomotor symptoms associated with menopause

Pregnancy Considerations Studies in pregnant women have demonstrated a risk to the fetus. Paroxetine crosses the placenta. An increased risk of teratogenic effects, including cardiovascular defects, may be associated with maternal use of paroxetine or other SSRIs; however, available information is conflicting. Nonteratogenic effects in the newborn following SSRI/SNRI exposure late in the third trimester include respiratory distress, cyanosis, apnea, seizures, temperature instability, feeding difficulty, vomiting, hypoglycemia, hypo- or hypertonia, hyper-reflexia, jitteriness, irritability, constant crying, and tremor. Symptoms may be due to the toxicity of the SSRIs/SNRIs or a discontinuation syndrome and may be consistent with serotonin syndrome associated with SSRI treatment.

Persistent pulmonary hypertension of the newborn (PPHN) has also been reported with SSRI exposure. The long-term effects of *in utero* SSRI exposure on infant development and behavior are not known.

Due to pregnancy-induced physiologic changes, some pharmacokinetic parameters of paroxetine may be altered. The maternal CYP2D6 genotype also influences paroxetine plasma concentrations during pregnancy.

The manufacturer suggests discontinuing paroxetine or switching to another antidepressant unless the benefits of therapy justify continuing treatment during pregnancy; consider other treatment options for women who are planning to become pregnant. The ACOG recommends that therapy with SSRIs or SNRIs during pregnancy be individualized; treatment of depression during pregnancy should incorporate the clinical expertise of the mental health clinician, obstetrician, primary healthcare provider, and pediatrician. The ACOG also recommends that therapy with paroxetine be avoided during pregnancy if possible and that fetuses exposed in early pregnancy be assessed with a fetal echocardiography. According to the American Psychiatric Association (APA), the risks of medication treatment should be weighed against other treatment options and untreated depression. The use of paroxetine is not recommended as first line therapy during pregnancy. For women who discontinue antidepressant medications during pregnancy and who may be at high risk for postpartum depression, the medications can be restarted following delivery. Treatment algorithms have been developed by the ACOG and the APA for the management of depression in women prior to conception and during pregnancy. Menopausal vasomotor symptoms do not occur during pregnancy; therefore, the use of paroxetine for the treatment of menopausal vasomotor symptoms is contraindicated in pregnant women.

Breast-Feeding Considerations Paroxetine is excreted in breast milk and concentrations in the hindmilk are higher than in foremilk. Paroxetine has not been detected in the serum of nursing infants. Adverse reactions have been reported in nursing infants exposed to some SSRIs. The manufacturer recommends that caution be exercised when administering paroxetine to nursing women. Maternal use of an SSRI during pregnancy may cause delayed milk secretion. The American Academy of Breast-feeding Medicine suggests that paroxetine may be considered for the treatment of postpartum depression in appropriately selected women who are nursing. Mothers should be monitored for changes in symptoms and infants should be monitored for growth. The long-term effects on development and behavior have not been studied.

Medication Guide Available Yes

Contraindications Concurrent use with or within 14 days of MAOIs intended to treat psychiatric disorders; initiation in patients being treated with linezolid or methylene blue IV; concomitant use with pimozide or thioridazine; hypersensitivity to paroxetine or any of its inactive ingredients; pregnancy (Brisdelle only).

Warnings/Precautions Hazardous agent - use appropriate precautions for handling and disposal (NIOSH 2014 [group 3]). **[U.S. Boxed Warning]: Antidepressants increase the risk of suicidal thinking and behavior in children, adolescents, and young adults (18 to 24 years of age) with major depressive disorder (MDD) and other psychiatric disorders;** consider risk prior to prescribing. Short-term studies did not show an increased risk in patients >24 years of age and showed a decreased risk in patients ≥65 years. Closely monitor patients for clinical worsening, suicidality, or unusual changes in behavior, particularly during the initial 1 to 2 months of therapy or during periods of dosage adjustments (increases or decreases); the patient's family or caregiver should be instructed to closely observe the patient and communicate condition with healthcare provider. A medication guide concerning the use of antidepressants should be dispensed with each prescription. **Paroxetine is not FDA approved for use in children.**

The possibility of a suicide attempt is inherent in major depression and may persist until remission occurs. Use caution in high-risk patients. Worsening depression and severe abrupt suicidality that are not part of the presenting symptoms may require discontinuation or modification of drug therapy. The patient's family or caregiver should be alerted to monitor patients for the emergence of suicidality and associated behaviors (such as agitation, irritability, hostility, impulsivity, and hypomania) and call health care provider.

May worsen psychosis in some patients or precipitate a shift to mania or hypomania in patients with bipolar disorder. Patients presenting with depressive symptoms should be screened for bipolar disorder. Monotherapy in

patients with bipolar disorder should be avoided. **Paroxetine is not FDA approved for the treatment of bipolar depression.**

Potentially life-threatening serotonin syndrome (SS) has occurred with serotonergic agents (eg, SSRIs, SNRIs), particularly when used in combination with other serotonergic agents (eg, triptans, TCAs, fentanyl, lithium, tramadol, buspirone, St John's wort, tryptophan) or agents that impair metabolism of serotonin (eg, MAO inhibitors intended to treat psychiatric disorders, other MAO inhibitors [ie, linezolid and intravenous methylene blue]). Discontinue treatment (and any concomitant serotonergic agent) immediately if signs/symptoms arise.

Paroxetine may increase the risks associated with electroconvulsive therapy. Has a low potential to impair cognitive or motor performance - use caution when operating hazardous machinery or driving. Symptoms of agitation and/or restlessness may occur during initial few weeks of therapy. Low potential for sedation or anticholinergic effects relative to cyclic antidepressants. Bone fractures have been associated with SSRI treatment. Consider the possibility of a fragility fracture if an SSRI-treated patient presents with unexplained bone pain, point tenderness, swelling, or bruising.

Use caution in elderly patients; may be potentially inappropriate in patients with a history of falls or fractures, and may cause or exacerbate syndrome of inappropriate antidiuretic hormone secretion or hyponatremia; monitor sodium closely with initiation or dosage adjustments in older adults. Medication associated with potent anticholinergic properties which may be inappropriate in older adults depending on comorbidities (eg, dementia, delirium) (Beers Criteria).

Use caution in patients with a previous seizure disorder or condition predisposing to seizures such as brain damage or alcoholism. Use with caution in patients with hepatic dysfunction. May cause SIADH; volume depletion and/or diuretics may increase risk. Potentially significant drug-drug interactions may exist, requiring dose or frequency adjustment, additional monitoring, and/or selection of alternative therapy. Use with caution in patients with renal insufficiency or other concurrent illness (due to limited experience); dose reduction recommended with severe renal impairment. May cause or exacerbate sexual dysfunction. May cause mild pupillary dilation, which can lead to an episode of narrow-angle glaucoma in susceptible individuals. Consider evaluating patients who have not had an iridectomy for narrow-angle glaucoma risk factors. Avoid use in the first trimester of pregnancy. Menopausal vasomotor symptoms do not occur during pregnancy; therefore, the use of paroxetine for the treatment of menopausal vasomotor symptoms is contraindicated in pregnant women.

Brisdelle contains a lower dose than what is required for the treatment of psychiatric conditions. Patients who require paroxetine for the treatment of psychiatric conditions should discontinue Brisdelle and begin treatment with a paroxetine-containing medication which provides an adequate dosage.

Abrupt discontinuation or interruption of antidepressant therapy has been associated with a discontinuation syndrome. Symptoms arising may vary with antidepressant however commonly include nausea, vomiting, diarrhea, headaches, lightheadedness, dizziness, diminished appetite, sweating, chills, tremors, paresthesias, fatigue, somnolence, and sleep disturbances (eg, vivid dreams, insomnia). Greater risks for developing a discontinuation syndrome have been associated with antidepressants with shorter half-lives, longer durations of treatment, and abrupt discontinuation. For antidepressants of short or intermediate half-lives, symptoms may emerge within 2 to 5 days after treatment discontinuation and last 7 to 14 days (APA, 2010; Fava, 2006; Haddod, 2001; Shelton, 2001; Warner, 2006).

Some dosage forms may contain polysorbate 80 (also known as Tweens). Hypersensitivity reactions, usually a delayed reaction, have been reported following exposure to pharmaceutical products containing polysorbate 80 in certain individuals (Isaksson, 2002; Lucente 2000; Shelley, 1995). Thrombocytopenia, ascites, pulmonary deterioration, and renal and hepatic failure have been reported in premature neonates after receiving parenteral products containing polysorbate 80 (Alade, 1986; CDC, 1984). See manufacturer's labeling.

Adverse Reactions Frequency varies by dose and indication. Adverse reactions reported as a composite of all indications.

>10%:
Central nervous system: Drowsiness (15% to 24%), insomnia (11% to 24%), headache (6% to 18%), dizziness (6% to 14%)
Dermatologic: Diaphoresis (5% to 14%)
Endocrine & metabolic: Decreased libido (3% to 15%)
Gastrointestinal: Nausea (19% to 26%), xerostomia (9% to 18%), constipation (5% to 16%), diarrhea (9% to 12%)
Genitourinary: Ejaculatory disorder (13% to 28%)
Neuromuscular & skeletal: Weakness (12% to 22%), tremor (4% to 11%)

1% to 10%:
Cardiovascular: Vasodilatation (2% to 4%), chest pain (3%), palpitations (2% to 3%), hypertension (≥1%), tachycardia (≥1%)
Central nervous system: Nervousness (4% to 9%), anxiety (5%), fatigue (5%), agitation (3% to 5%), paresthesia (4%), abnormal dreams (3% to 4%), lack of concentration (3% to 4%), yawning (2% to 4%), depersonalization (≤3%), myoclonus (2% to 3%), amnesia (2%), chills (2%), emotional lability (≥1%), vertigo (≥1%), confusion (1%), myasthenia (1%)
Dermatologic: Skin rash (2% to 3%), pruritus (≥1%)
Endocrine & metabolic: Weight gain (≥1%)
Gastrointestinal: Decreased appetite (5% to 9%), dyspepsia (2% to 5%), flatulence (4%), abdominal pain (4%), nausea and vomiting (4%), increased appetite (2% to 4%), vomiting (2% to 3%), dysgeusia (2%)
Genitourinary: Male genital disease (10%), female genital tract disease (2% to 9%), impotence (2% to 9%), orgasm disturbance (2% to 9%), dysmenorrhea (5%), urinary frequency (2% to 3%), urinary tract infection (2%)
Infection: Infection (5% to 6%)
Neuromuscular & skeletal: Myalgia (2% to 4%), back pain (3%), myopathy (2%), arthralgia (≥1%)
Ophthalmic: Blurred vision (4%), visual disturbance (2% to 4%)
Otic: Tinnitus (≥1%)
Respiratory: Dyspnea (≤7%), pharyngitis (4%), sinusitis (≤4%), rhinitis (3%)

<1% (Limited to important or life-threatening): Abnormal erythrocytes, abnormal hepatic function tests, acute renal failure, adrenergic syndrome, agranulocytosis, akathisia, akinesia, anaphylactoid reaction, anaphylaxis, anemia (various), angina pectoris, angioedema, angle-closure glaucoma, aphasia, aphthous stomatitis, aplastic anemia, asthma, atrial fibrillation, bloody diarrhea, bone marrow aplasia, bradycardia, bronchitis, bulimia nervosa, bundle branch block, cardiac failure, cataract, cellulitis, cerebral ischemia, cerebrovascular accident, change in platelet count, cholelithiasis, colitis, deafness, dehydration, delirium, depression, diabetes mellitus, disorientation, drug dependence, dyskinesia, dysphagia, dystonia, eclampsia, emphysema, esophageal achalasia, exfoliative dermatitis, extrapyramidal reaction, fecal impaction, fungal dermatitis, gastroenteritis, goiter, Guillain-Barre syndrome, hallucination, hematemesis, hematologic disease, hematoma, hemoptysis, hemorrhage (eye, gingival, rectal, retinal, vaginal), hemorrhagic pancreatitis, hepatic failure, hepatic necrosis, hepatitis, hepatotoxicity, homicidal ideation, hyperbilirubinemia, hypercholesteremia, hypergammaglobulinemia, hyperglycemia, hyperhidrosis, hypersensitivity reaction, hyperthyroidism, hypoglycemia, hyponatremia, hypotension, hypothyroidism, immune thrombocytopenia, increased blood urea nitrogen, increased creatine phosphokinase, increased lactate dehydrogenase, increased serum alkaline phosphatase, intestinal obstruction, ischemic heart disease, jaundice, ketosis, low cardiac output, lymphadenopathy, meningitis, migraine, mydriasis, myelitis, myocardial infarction, neuroleptic malignant syndrome (Stevens, 2008), neuropathy, nodal arrhythmia, osteoarthritis, osteoporosis, pancreatitis, pancytopenia, peptic ulcer, peritonitis, phlebitis, pneumonia, prolonged bleeding time, pulmonary edema, pulmonary embolism, pulmonary fibrosis, pulmonary hypertension, restlessness, seizure, sepsis, serotonin syndrome, status epilepticus, Stevens-Johnson syndrome, suicidal ideation, suicidal tendencies, syncope, tetany, thrombophlebitis, thrombosis, torsades de pointes, toxic epidermal necrolysis, uncontrolled diabetes mellitus, vasculitis, ventricular arrhythmia, ventricular fibrillation, ventricular tachycardia, withdrawal syndrome (including increased dreaming/nightmares, muscle cramps/spasms/twitching, headache, nervousness/anxiety, fatigue/tiredness, restless feeling in legs, and trouble sleeping/insomnia)

Drug Interactions

Metabolism/Transport Effects Substrate of CYP2D6 (major); **Note:** Assignment of Major/Minor substrate status based on clinically relevant drug interaction potential; **Inhibits** CYP1A2 (weak), CYP2B6 (moderate), CYP2C19 (weak), CYP2C9 (weak), CYP2D6 (strong)

Avoid Concomitant Use

Avoid concomitant use of PARoxetine with any of the following: Dapoxetine; Dosulepin; Iobenguane I 123; Linezolid; MAO Inhibitors; Mequitazine; Methylene Blue; Pimozide; Tamoxifen; Thioridazine; Tryptophan; Urokinase

Increased Effect/Toxicity

PARoxetine may increase the levels/effects of: Agents with Antiplatelet Properties; Anticoagulants; Antidepressants (Serotonin Reuptake Inhibitor/Antagonist); Antipsychotic Agents; Apixaban; ARIPiprazole; ARIPiprazole Lauroxil; Asenapine; Aspirin; AtoMOXetine; Beta-Blockers; Blood Glucose Lowering Agents; Brexpiprazole; BusPIRone; CarBAMazepine; CloZAPine; Collagenase (Systemic); CYP2B6 Substrates; CYP2D6 Substrates; Dabigatran Etexilate; Deoxycholic Acid; Desmopressin; Dextromethorphan; Dosulepin; DOXOrubicin (Conventional); DULoxetine; Edoxaban; Eliglustat; Fesoterodine; Galantamine; Highest Risk QTc-Prolonging Agents; Ibritumomab; Iloperidone; Mequitazine; Methadone; Methylene Blue; Metoprolol; Mexiletine; Moderate Risk QTc-Prolonging Agents; Nebivolol; NSAID (COX-2 Inhibitor); NSAID (Nonselective); Obinutuzumab; Pimozide; Propafenone; Rivaroxaban; Salicylates; Serotonin Modulators; Tamsulosin; Tetrabenazine; Thiazide Diuretics; Thioridazine; Thrombolytic Agents; TiZANidine; Tositumomab and Iodine I 131 Tositumomab; TraMADol; Tricyclic Antidepressants; Urokinase; Vitamin K Antagonists; Vortioxetine

The levels/effects of PARoxetine may be increased by: Abiraterone Acetate; Alcohol (Ethyl); Analgesics (Opioid); Antiemetics (5HT3 Antagonists); Antipsychotic Agents; ARIPiprazole; Asenapine; BuPROPion; BusPIRone; Cimetidine; Clarithromycin; CNS Depressants; Cobicistat; CYP2D6 Inhibitors (Moderate); CYP2D6 Inhibitors (Strong); Dapoxetine; Dasatinib; DULoxetine; Glucosamine; Herbs (Anticoagulant/Antiplatelet Properties); Ibrutinib; Limaprost; Linezolid; Lithium; MAO Inhibitors; Metaxalone; Metoclopramide; Metyrosine; Mifepristone; Multivitamins/Fluoride (with ADE); Multivitamins/Minerals (with ADEK, Folate, Iron); Multivitamins/Minerals (with AE, No Iron); Omega-3 Fatty Acids; Panobinostat; Peginterferon Alfa-2b; Pentosan Polysulfate Sodium; Pentoxifylline; Pravastatin; Prostacyclin Analogues; Tedizolid; TraMADol; Tryptophan; Vitamin E; Vitamin E (Oral)

Decreased Effect

PARoxetine may decrease the levels/effects of: Aprepitant; Codeine; Cyclophosphamide; Fosaprepitant; Hydrocodone; Iloperidone; Iobenguane I 123; Ioflupane I 123; Tamoxifen; Thyroid Products

The levels/effects of PARoxetine may be decreased by: Aprepitant; CarBAMazepine; Cyproheptadine; Darunavir; Fosamprenavir; Fosaprepitant; NSAID (COX-2 Inhibitor); NSAID (Nonselective); Peginterferon Alfa-2b

Food Interactions Peak concentration is increased, but bioavailability is not significantly altered by food. Management: Administer without regard to meals.

Storage/Stability

Capsules: Store between 20°C and 25°C (68°F and 77°F); excursions permitted between 15°C and 30°C (59°F and 86°F). Protect from light and humidity.

Tablets: Store immediate-release tablets between 15°C and 30°C (59°F and 86°F) and controlled-release tablets at or below 25°C (77°F).

Suspension: Store at or below 25°C (77°F).

Mechanism of Action Paroxetine is a selective serotonin reuptake inhibitor, chemically unrelated to tricyclic, tetracyclic, or other antidepressants; presumably, the inhibition of serotonin reuptake from brain synapse stimulated serotonin activity in the brain

Pharmacodynamics/Kinetics

Onset of action: Depression: The onset of action is within a week; however, individual response varies greatly and full response may not be seen until 8-12 weeks after initiation of treatment.

Absorption: Completely absorbed following oral administration

Distribution: V_d: 8.7 L/kg (3-28 L/kg)

Protein binding: 93% to 95%

Metabolism: Extensively hepatic via CYP2D6 enzymes; primary metabolites are formed via oxidation and methylation of parent drug, with subsequent glucuronide/sulfate conjugation; nonlinear pharmacokinetics (via 2D6 saturation) may be seen with higher doses and longer duration of therapy. Metabolites exhibit ~2% potency of parent compound. C_{min} concentrations are 70% to 80% greater in the elderly compared to nonelderly patients; clearance is also decreased.

Half-life elimination: 21 hours (3-65 hours)

Time to peak:

Capsules: 3-8 hours

Tablets, oral suspension: Immediate release: 5.2-8.1 hours

Tablets: Controlled release: 6-10 hours

Excretion: Urine (64%, 2% as unchanged drug); feces (36% primarily via bile, <1% as unchanged drug)

Dosing

Adult

Major depressive disorder (MDD): Oral:

Paxil, Pexeva: Initial: 20 mg once daily, preferably in the morning; increase if needed by 10 mg/day increments at intervals of at least 1 week; maximum dose: 50 mg/day

Paxil CR: Initial: 25 mg once daily; increase if needed by 12.5 mg/day increments at intervals of at least 1 week; maximum dose: 62.5 mg/day

Generalized anxiety disorder (GAD) *(Paxil, Pexeva):* Oral: Initial: 20 mg once daily, preferably in the morning (if dose is increased, adjust in increments of 10 mg/day at 1-week intervals); doses of 20-50 mg/day were used in clinical trials, however, no greater benefit was seen with doses >20 mg.

Obsessive-compulsive disorder (OCD) *(Paxil, Pexeva):* Oral: Initial: 20 mg once daily, preferably in the morning; increase if needed by 10 mg/day increments at intervals of at least 1 week; recommended dose: 40 mg/day; range: 20-60 mg/day; maximum dose: 60 mg/day

Panic disorder: Oral:

Paxil, Pexeva: Initial: 10 mg once daily, preferably in the morning; increase if needed by 10 mg/day increments at intervals of at least 1 week; recommended dose: 40 mg/day; range: 10-60 mg/day; maximum dose: 60 mg/day

Paxil CR: Initial: 12.5 mg once daily; increase if needed by 12.5 mg/day at intervals of at least 1 week; maximum dose: 75 mg/day

Premenstrual dysphoric disorder (PMDD) *(Paxil CR):* Oral: Initial: 12.5 mg once daily in the morning; may be increased to 25 mg/day; dosing changes should occur at intervals of at least 1 week. May be given daily throughout the menstrual cycle or limited to the luteal phase.

Post-traumatic stress disorder (PTSD) *(Paxil):* Oral: Initial: 20 mg once daily, preferably in the morning; increase if needed by 10 mg/day increments at intervals of at least 1 week; range: 20-50 mg. Limited data suggest doses of 40 mg/day were not more efficacious than 20 mg/day.

Social anxiety disorder: Oral:

Paxil: Initial: 20 mg once daily, preferably in the morning; recommended dose: 20 mg/day; range: 20-60 mg/day; doses >20 mg may not have additional benefit

Paxil CR: Initial: 12.5 mg once daily, preferably in the morning; may be increased by 12.5 mg/day at intervals of at least 1 week; maximum dose: 37.5 mg/day

Vasomotor symptoms of menopause:

Brisdelle: 7.5 mg once daily at bedtime

Paxil CR (off-label use): 12.5-25 mg once daily (Stearns, 2003)

Discontinuation of therapy: Upon discontinuation of antidepressant therapy, gradually taper the dose to minimize the incidence of withdrawal symptoms and allow for the detection of re-emerging symptoms. Evidence supporting ideal taper rates is limited. APA and NICE guidelines suggest tapering therapy over at least several weeks with consideration to the half-life of the antidepressant; antidepressants with a shorter half-life may need to be tapered more conservatively. In addition for long-term treated patients, WFSBP guidelines recommend tapering over 4-6 months. If intolerable withdrawal symptoms occur following a dose reduction, consider resuming the previously prescribed dose and/or decrease dose at a more gradual rate (APA, 2010; Bauer, 2002; Haddad, 2001; NCCMH, 2010; Schatzberg, 2006; Shelton, 2001; Warner, 2006).

MAO inhibitor recommendations:

Switching to or from an MAO inhibitor intended to treat psychiatric disorders:

Allow 14 days to elapse between discontinuing an MAO inhibitor intended to treat psychiatric disorders and initiation of paroxetine.

Allow 14 days to elapse between discontinuing paroxetine and initiation of an MAO inhibitor intended to treat psychiatric disorders.

Use with other MAO inhibitors (linezolid or IV methylene blue):
Do not initiate paroxetine in patients receiving linezolid or IV methylene blue; consider other interventions for psychiatric condition.

If urgent treatment with linezolid or IV methylene blue is required in a patient already receiving paroxetine and potential benefits outweigh potential risks, discontinue paroxetine promptly and administer linezolid or IV methylene blue. Monitor for serotonin syndrome for 2 weeks or until 24 hours after the last dose of linezolid or IV methylene blue, whichever comes first. May resume paroxetine 24 hours after the last dose of linezolid or IV methylene blue.

Geriatric

Major depressive disorder (MDD), obsessive compulsive disorder (OCD), panic attack, social anxiety disorder:
Paxil, Pexeva: Oral: Initial: 10 mg/day; increase if needed by 10 mg/day increments at intervals of at least 1 week; maximum dose: 40 mg/day
Paxil CR: Initial: 12.5 mg/day; increase if needed by 12.5 mg/day increments at intervals of at least 1 week; maximum dose: 50 mg/day

Discontinuation of therapy: Refer to adult dosing.
MAO inhibitor recommendations: Refer to adult dosing.

Pediatric

Obsessive-compulsive disorder (OCD) (off-label use): Children and Adolescents 7-17 years: Oral: Initial: 10 mg daily; titrate every 7-14 days in increments of 10 mg daily as necessary to a maximum of 60 mg daily; trials have typically continued for a 10- to 12-week treatment course (Geller, 2004; Rosenberg, 1999)
Social anxiety disorder (off-label use): Children and Adolescents 8-17 years: Oral: Initial: 10 mg once daily; titrate at intervals of at least 7 days in increments of 10 mg daily; maximum daily dose: 50 mg daily; trials have typically continued for a 16-week treatment course (Wagner, 2004)

Discontinuation of therapy: Refer to adult dosing.
MAO inhibitor recommendations: Refer to adult dosing.

Renal Impairment Adults:

Brisdelle: No dosage adjustment necessary.
Paxil, Paxil CR, Pexeva:
CrCl 30-60 mL/minute: Plasma concentration is 2 times that seen in normal function. There are no dosage adjustments provided in manufacturer's labeling.
Severe impairment (CrCl <30 mL/minute): Mean plasma concentration is ~4 times that seen in normal function.
Paxil, Pexeva: Initial: 10 mg/day; increase if needed by 10 mg/day increments at intervals of at least 1 week; maximum dose: 40 mg/day
Paxil CR: Initial: 12.5 mg/day; increase if needed by 12.5 mg/day increments at intervals of at least 1 week; maximum dose: 50 mg/day

Hepatic Impairment Adults: In hepatic dysfunction, plasma concentration is 2 times that seen in normal function.
Brisdelle: No dosage adjustment necessary.
Paxil, Paxil CR, Pexeva:
Mild-to-moderate impairment: There are no dosage adjustments provided in manufacturer's labeling.
Severe impairment:
Paxil, Pexeva: Initial: 10 mg/day; increase if needed by 10 mg/day increments at intervals of at least 1 week; maximum dose: 40 mg/day
Paxil CR: Initial: 12.5 mg/day; increase if needed by 12.5 mg/day increments at intervals of at least 1 week; maximum dose: 50 mg/day

Dietary Considerations May be taken without regard to meals.

Administration May be administered without regard to meals. Paxil, Paxil CR, and Pexeva should preferentially be administered in the morning; whereas Brisdelle is recommended to be administered at bedtime. Do not crush, break, or chew controlled-release tablets or Pexeva tablets (film-coated).

Hazardous agent; use appropriate precautions for handling and disposal (NIOSH 2014 [group 3]).

Monitoring Parameters Mental status for depression, suicide ideation (especially at the beginning of therapy or when doses are increased or decreased), anxiety, social functioning, mania, panic attacks; signs/symptoms of serotonin syndrome; akathisia

Additional Information Paxil CR incorporates a degradable polymeric matrix (Geomatrix) to control dissolution rate over a period of 4-5 hours. An enteric coating delays the start of drug release until tablets have left the stomach.

Dosage Forms Excipient information presented when available (limited, particularly for generics); consult specific product labeling.
Capsule, Oral, as mesylate [strength expressed as base]:
Brisdelle: 7.5 mg [contains fd&c red #40, fd&c yellow #6 (sunset yellow)]
Suspension, Oral, as hydrochloride [strength expressed as base]:
Paxil: 10 mg/5 mL (250 mL) [contains fd&c yellow #6 aluminum lake, methylparaben, propylene glycol, propylparaben, saccharin sodium; orange flavor]
Tablet, Oral, as hydrochloride [strength expressed as base]:
Paxil: 10 mg, 20 mg [scored]
Paxil: 30 mg, 40 mg
Generic: 10 mg, 20 mg, 30 mg, 40 mg
Tablet, Oral, as mesylate [strength expressed as base]:
Pexeva: 10 mg
Pexeva: 20 mg [scored]
Pexeva: 30 mg, 40 mg
Tablet Extended Release 24 Hour, Oral, as hydrochloride [strength expressed as base]:
Paxil CR: 12.5 mg [contains fd&c yellow #10 aluminum lake, fd&c yellow #6 aluminum lake]
Paxil CR: 25 mg
Paxil CR: 37.5 mg [contains fd&c blue #2 aluminum lake]
Generic: 12.5 mg, 25 mg, 37.5 mg

Dosage Forms: Canada Note: Refer to Dosage Forms. Capsule, oral suspension, and tablet (as mesylate) are not available in Canada.

◆ Paroxetine Hydrochloride see PARoxetine on page 1399
◆ Paroxetine Mesylate see PARoxetine on page 1399
◆ PARP inhibitor AZD2281 see Olaparib on page 1318
◆ Parvolex (Can) see Acetylcysteine on page 31

Pasireotide (pas i REE oh tide)

Brand Names: US Signifor; Signifor LAR
Brand Names: Canada Signifor
Index Terms Pasireotide Diaspartate; SOM230
Pharmacologic Category Somatostatin Analog

Use

Acromegaly (Signifor LAR): Treatment of patients with acromegaly who have had an inadequate response to surgery and/or for whom surgery is not an option.
Cushing disease (Signifor): Treatment of Cushing disease in patients for whom pituitary surgery is not an option or has not been curative

Prescribing and Access Restrictions In Canada, patients must be enrolled in the Access Program for Signifor (Novartis Canada).

Medication Guide Available Yes

Dosing

Adult & Geriatric
Acromegaly (Signifor LAR): IM: Initial: 40 mg once every 28 days; for patients who have not normalized GH and/or IGF-1 levels after 3 months, increase to a maximum of 60 mg. If adverse reactions occur or IFG-1 level decreases to less than lower limit of normal, decrease dosage (temporarily or permanently) by 20 mg decrements.
Missed dose: If a dose is missed, dose may be given up to but no later than 14 days prior to the next dose.
Cushing disease (Signifor): SubQ:
Initial:
US labeling: 0.6 mg or 0.9 mg twice daily.
Canadian labeling: 0.6 mg twice daily.
Titrate based on response and tolerability. If adverse reactions occur, temporarily decrease dose by 0.3 mg increments. Recommended maintenance dosage range: 0.3 to 0.9 mg twice daily. **Note:** Maximum urinary free cortisol reductions are usually observed by 2 months of treatment. The Canadian labeling recommends to consider discontinuation if clinical improvement is not observed after 2 months of therapy.

Renal Impairment No dosage adjustment necessary.

Hepatic Impairment

Acromegaly (Signifor LAR):

Mild impairment (Child-Pugh class A): No dosage adjustment necessary.

Moderate hepatic impairment (Child-Pugh class B): Initial: 20 mg every 28 days (maximum: 40 mg every 28 days).

Severe hepatic impairment (Child-Pugh class C): Avoid use.

Cushing disease (Signifor):

Prior to initiation:

US labeling:

Mild impairment (Child-Pugh class A): No dosage adjustment necessary.

Moderate impairment (Child-Pugh class B): Initial: 0.3 mg twice daily (maximum: 0.6 mg twice daily)

Severe impairment (Child-Pugh class C): Use not recommended.

Canadian labeling:

Mild impairment (Child-Pugh class A): No dosage adjustment necessary.

Moderate or severe impairment (Child-Pugh class B or C): Use is contraindicated.

During therapy:

US labeling:

If ALT increases >3 times ULN or baseline value: Recheck ALT during recommended timeframe per recommendations in manufacturer's labeling for confirmation. If ALT level confirmed or increasing, interrupt therapy and investigate potential cause.

If any liver test ≥5 times ULN (with a normal baseline) OR >5 times the baseline value (with an abnormal baseline): Interrupt therapy and monitor liver tests more frequently per recommendations in manufacturer's labeling. If values return to normal or near normal, therapy may be reinitiated with extreme caution/monitoring only if another likely cause for hepatic effects is discovered.

Canadian labeling:

If ALT increases >3 times ULN to <5 times ULN: Recheck ALT in 48 hours and if value remains <5 times ULN, continue monitoring ALT every 48 hours. If levels increase >5 times ULN, discontinue therapy and do not reinitiate.

If ALT increases >5 times ULN or if ALT or AST increase >3 times ULN concurrently with an increased bilirubin >2 times ULN or if jaundice or other signs of clinically significant hepatic impairment: Discontinue therapy and investigate potential cause; monitor until resolution. Do not reinitiate therapy.

Additional Information Complete prescribing information should be consulted for additional detail.

Dosage Forms Excipient information presented when available (limited, particularly for generics); consult specific product labeling.

Solution, Subcutaneous:

Signifor: 0.3 mg/mL (1 mL); 0.6 mg/mL (1 mL); 0.9 mg/mL (1 mL)

Suspension Reconstituted, Intramuscular, as pamoate [strength expressed as base]:

Signifor LAR: 20 mg (1 ea); 40 mg (1 ea); 60 mg (1 ea)

Patiromer (pa TIR oh mer)

Brand Names: US Veltassa

Index Terms Patiromer Sorbitex Calcium

Pharmacologic Category Antidote

Use

Hyperkalemia: Treatment of hyperkalemia

Limitations of use: Patiromer should not be used as an emergency treatment for life-threatening hyperkalemia because of its delayed onset of action.

Pregnancy Considerations Patiromer is not absorbed systemically following oral administration. Use during pregnancy is not expected to result in significant exposure to the fetus.

Breast-Feeding Considerations Patiromer is not absorbed systemically following oral administration. Breast-feeding is not expected to result in significant exposure to a nursing child

Contraindications Hypersensitivity to patiromer or any component of the formulation

Warnings/Precautions [US Boxed Warning]: Patiromer binds many orally administered medications, which could decrease gastrointestinal absorption and lead to reduced efficacy. Administer other oral medications at least 6 hours before or 6 hours after patiromer. Choose patiromer or the other oral medication if adequate dosing separation is not possible. Avoid use in patients with severe constipation, bowel obstruction or impaction, including abnormal post-operative bowel motility disorders; patiromer may be ineffective and may worsen GI conditions. Patiromer binds to magnesium in the colon, which can lead to hypomagnesemia; monitor serum magnesium; consider magnesium supplementation if hypomagnesemia develops. Elderly patients may experience more gastrointestinal adverse reactions.

Adverse Reactions

1% to 10%:

Endocrine & metabolic: Hypomagnesemia (5% to 9%), hypokalemia (5%)

Gastrointestinal: Constipation (7%; transient), diarrhea (5%), abdominal distress (2%), flatulence (2%), nausea (2%)

<1% (Limited to important or life-threatening): Hypersensitivity reaction (including lip edema)

Drug Interactions

Metabolism/Transport Effects None known.

Avoid Concomitant Use There are no known interactions where it is recommended to avoid concomitant use.

Increased Effect/Toxicity There are no known significant interactions involving an increase in effect.

Decreased Effect There are no known significant interactions involving a decrease in effect.

Preparation for Administration Immediately prior to administration, add 30 mL of water to an empty glass or cup; empty entire contents of the packet(s) into the glass or cup and stir thoroughly. Add an additional 60 mL of water to the mixture; stir thoroughly (powder will not dissolve and the mixture will look cloudy). Do not heat (eg, microwave) or add to heated foods or liquids.

Storage/Stability Store at 2°C to 8°C (36°F to 46°F). If stored at room temperature (25°C ± 2°C [77°F ± 4°F]), use within 3 months of being taken out of the refrigerator. Avoid exposure to excessive heat above 40°C (104°F).

Mechanism of Action Patiromer, a non-absorbed, cation exchange polymer that contains a calcium-sorbitol counterion, increases fecal potassium excretion through binding of potassium in the lumen of the gastrointestinal tract, resulting in a reduction of serum potassium levels.

Pharmacodynamics/Kinetics

Absorption: Not systemically absorbed

Excretion: Feces

Dosing

Adult & Geriatric

Hyperkalemia: Oral: Initial: 8.4 g once daily; adjust dose at ≥1-week intervals in increments of 8.4 g (maximum dose: 25.2 g/day).

Renal Impairment No dosage adjustment necessary.

Hepatic Impairment There are no dosage adjustments provided in the manufacturer's labeling.

Dietary Considerations Take with food.

Administration Oral: Administer with food. Do not administer patiromer in its dry form. Following reconstitution, drink mixture immediately. If powder remains in the glass after drinking, add more water, stir, and drink immediately; repeat as needed to ensure the entire dose is administered. Do not heat patiromer (eg, microwave) or add to heated foods or liquids. When other oral medications are taken at the same time as patiromer, binding of the oral drug and patiromer in the gastrointestinal tract may occur. This may decrease absorption of the other oral drug and lead to loss of efficacy. Administer other oral medications at least 6 hours before or 6 hours after patiromer and monitor for clinical response and/or blood levels where possible.

Monitoring Parameters Serum potassium; serum magnesium.

Dosage Forms Excipient information presented when available (limited, particularly for generics); consult specific product labeling.

Packet, Oral:

Veltassa: 8.4 g (1 ea, 4 ea, 30 ea); 16.8 g (1 ea, 30 ea); 25.2 g (1 ea, 30 ea)

◆ Pazeo *see* Olopatadine (Ophthalmic) *on page 1323*

PAZOPanib (paz OH pa nib)

Brand Names: US Votrient
Brand Names: Canada Votrient
Index Terms GW786034; Pazopanib Hydrochloride
Pharmacologic Category Antineoplastic Agent, Tyrosine Kinase Inhibitor; Antineoplastic Agent, Vascular Endothelial Growth Factor (VEGF) Inhibitor
Use
Renal cell carcinoma, advanced: Treatment of advanced renal cell carcinoma
Soft tissue sarcoma, advanced: Treatment of advanced soft tissue sarcoma (in patients who have received prior chemotherapy)
Limitations of use: The efficacy of pazopanib for the treatment of adipocytic soft tissue sarcoma or gastrointestinal stromal tumors has not been demonstrated.
Pregnancy Considerations Adverse effects were observed in animal reproduction studies. Based on its mechanism of action, pazopanib would be expected to cause fetal harm if administered to a pregnant woman. Women of childbearing potential should avoid becoming pregnant during therapy.
Breast-Feeding Considerations It is not known if pazopanib is excreted in breast milk. According to the manufacturer, the decision to continue or discontinue breast-feeding during therapy should take into account the risk of exposure to the infant and the benefits of treatment to the mother.
Medication Guide Available Yes
Contraindications
There are no contraindications listed in the manufacturer's US labeling.
Canadian labeling: Hypersensitivity to pazopanib or any component of the formulation; use in pediatric patients <2 years of age (due to the antiangiogenic effects)
Warnings/Precautions Hazardous agent - use appropriate precautions for handling and disposal (NIOSH 2014 [group 1]). **[US Boxed Warning]: Severe and fatal hepatotoxicity (transaminase and bilirubin elevations) has been observed in studies. Monitor hepatic function and interrupt treatment, reduce dose, or discontinue as recommended.** Liver function testes should be monitored at baseline; at weeks 3, 5, 7, and 9; at months 3 and 4; and as clinically necessary, then periodically (after month 4). Transaminase elevations usually occur early in the treatment course. Use is not recommended in patients with preexisting severe hepatic impairment (bilirubin >3 times ULN with any ALT level); dosage reductions is recommended for preexisting moderate hepatic impairment (bilirubin >1.5 to 3 times ULN). Mild indirect (unconjugated) hyperbilirubinemia may occur in patients with Gilbert's syndrome; for patients with known Gilbert syndrome (only a mild indirect bilirubin elevation) and ALT >3 times ULN, follow isolated ALT elevation dosage modification recommendations.

Venous and arterial thromboembolism have been reported. DVT, pulmonary embolism, angina, transient ischemic attack, MI, and ischemic stroke were observed more frequently in the pazopanib group (versus placebo) in clinical trials. Fatalities were observed. Monitor for signs/symptoms of venous thrombotic events and pulmonary embolism. Use with caution in patients with a history of or an increased risk for these events. Use in patients with recent arteriothrombotic event (within 6 months) has not been studied and is not recommended. Thrombotic microangiopathy (TMA), including thrombotic thrombocytopenic purpura (TTP) and hemolytic uremic syndrome (HUS), has been observed in clinical studies. TMA has occurred with pazopanib monotherapy or when used in combination with bevacizumab or topotecan (off-label use); it typically occurs within 90 days of treatment initiation. Monitor for signs/symptoms and permanently discontinue in patients who develop TMA. Hemorrhagic events (including fatal events) have been reported. In clinical studies, the most common events in renal cell carcinoma patients were hematuria, epistaxis, hemoptysis, and rectal hemorrhage. Epistaxis, mouth hemorrhage, and anal hemorrhage were most common in soft tissue sarcoma patients. Use is not recommended in patients with a history of hemoptysis, cerebral hemorrhage or clinically significant gastrointestinal hemorrhage within 6 months (these populations were excluded from clinical trials).

May cause and/or worsen hypertension (hypertensive crisis has been observed); monitor frequently; blood pressure should be controlled prior to treatment initiation; antihypertensive therapy should be used if needed. Hypertension usually occurs early in the treatment course.

Dosage reduction may be necessary for hypertension that is persistent despite management with antihypertensive therapy; discontinue for hypertensive crisis, or for severe and persistent hypertension which is refractory to dose reduction and antihypertensive therapy. May cause new-onset or worsening of existing heart failure; baseline and periodic LVEF monitoring is recommended in patients at increased risk of heart failure (eg, prior anthracycline treatment). Concurrent hypertension may increase the risk for cardiac dysfunction. Monitor for signs/symptoms of heart failure. QTc prolongation, including torsade de pointes, has been observed; use caution in patients with a history of QTc prolongation, with medications known to prolong the QT interval, or with preexisting cardiac disease. Obtain baseline and periodic ECGs; correct electrolyte (potassium, calcium, and magnesium) abnormalities prior to and during treatment.

Gastrointestinal perforation and fistula (including fatal events) have been reported; monitor for symptoms of gastrointestinal perforation and fistula. Proteinuria has been reported with use. Obtain baseline and periodic urinalysis and 24-hour urine protein when clinically indicated. Dosage reduction may be necessary for significant proteinuria (≥3 g/24 hours); discontinue for recurrent proteinuria. Interstitial lung disease (ILD)/pneumonitis has been reported with pazopanib; may be fatal. Monitor for pulmonary symptoms which could indicate ILD/pneumonitis; discontinue if ILD or pneumonitis develop. Hypothyroidism has been reported with use; monitor thyroid function tests. Vascular endothelial growth factor (VEGF) receptor inhibitors are associated with impaired wound healing. Discontinue treatment at least 7 days prior to scheduled surgery; treatment reinitiation should be guided by clinical judgment. Discontinue if wound dehiscence occurs.

Patients with mild-to-moderate renal impairment (CrCl ≥30 mL/minute) were included in trials. There are no pharmacokinetic data in patients with severe renal impairment undergoing dialysis (peritoneal and hemodialysis); however, renal impairment is not expected to significantly influence pazopanib pharmacokinetics or exposure. Potentially significant drug-drug interactions may exist, requiring dose or frequency adjustment, additional monitoring, and/or selection of alternative therapy. Increased toxicity and mortality has been observed in trials evaluating concurrent use of pazopanib with other chemotherapeutic agents (pemetrexed, lapatinib). Pazopanib is not approved for use in combination with other chemotherapy.

Hand-foot skin reaction (HFSR) observed with tyrosine kinase inhibitors (TKIs) is distinct from hand-foot syndrome (palmar-plantar erythrodysesthesia) associated with traditional chemotherapy agents. HFSR due to TKIs is localized with defined hyperkeratotic lesions; symptoms include burning, dysesthesia, paresthesia, or tingling of the palms/soles, and generally occur within the first 2 to 4 weeks of treatment. Pressure and flexor areas may develop blisters (callus-like), dry/cracked skin, edema, erythema, desquamation, or hyperkeratosis. The incidence of hand-foot skin reaction (HFSR) is lower with pazopanib (compared to other tyrosine kinase inhibitors). Examine skin at baseline (remove calluses with pedicure prior to treatment) and with each visit; apply an emollient based moisturizer twice daily during treatment. If HSFR develops, consider changing moisturizer to a urea-based product; topical steroids may be utilized for the anti-inflammatory effect; avoid excessive friction or pressure to affected areas and avoid restrictive footwear. Temporary dose reduction or treatment interruption may be necessary (Appleby 2011).

Reversible posterior leukoencephalopathy syndrome (RPLS) has been reported (rarely); may be fatal. Monitor for neurological changes or symptoms (blindness, confusion, headache, lethargy, seizure, visual or neurologic disturbances); permanently discontinue pazopanib in patients who develop RPLS. Serious, including fatal, infections have been reported; monitor for signs and symptoms of infection. Temporarily or permanently discontinue therapy for serious infections as clinically indicated. Patients >60 years of age may be at greater risk for transaminase elevations (ALT >3 time ULN). Patients ≥65 years of age experienced increased incidences of grade 3 or 4 fatigue, hypertension, decreased appetite, and transaminase elevations and are at increased risk for hepatotoxicity. Pazopanib is not approved for use in pediatric patients. Based on its mechanism of action, organ growth and maturation during early postnatal development may be affected. May potentially cause serious adverse effects on organ development, particularly in children <2 years of age.

Adverse Reactions Frequency not always defined.

Cardiovascular: Hypertension (40% to 42%; grade 3: 4% to 7%, early in treatment), bradycardia (2% to 19%), peripheral edema (STS: 14%), cardiac insufficiency (11% to 13%), chest pain (5% to 10%; STS, grade 3: 2%), left ventricular systolic dysfunction (STS: 8%), venous thrombosis (1% to 5%), ischemia (2%), myocardial infarction (2%), prolonged Q-T interval on ECG (2%), facial edema (1%), transient ischemic attacks (1%), decreased left ventricular ejection fraction, hypertensive crisis

Central nervous system: Fatigue (19%, grade 3: 2%; STS: 65%, grades 3/4: 1% to 13%), tumor pain (STS: 29%, grade 3: 8%), headache (10%; STS: 23%, grade 3: 1%), dizziness (11%), insomnia (STS: 9%), voice disorder (4% to 8%), chills (STS: 5%), reversible posterior leukoencephalopathy syndrome

Dermatologic: Hair discoloration (38% to 39%, grade 3: <1%), exfoliative dermatitis (STS: 18%, grade 3: <1%), skin rash (8%), alopecia (8% to 12%), dermatological disease (STS: 11%, grade 3: 2%), hypopigmentation (STS, skin: 11%), palmar-plantar erythrodysesthesia (6%), skin depigmentation (3%), xeroderma (STS: 6%), nail disease (STS: 5%)

Endocrine & metabolic: Weight loss (9%, STS: 48%, grade 3: 4%), increased serum glucose (41% to 45%, grade 3: <1%), increased thyroid-stimulating hormone (TSH), decreased serum albumin (STS: 34%, grade 3: 1%), decreased serum phosphate (34%, grade 3: 4%), decreased serum sodium (31%, grade 3: 1% to 4%), decreased serum magnesium (26%, grades 3/4: ≤1%), decreased serum glucose (17%, grade 4: <1%), increased serum potassium (STS: 16%, grade 3: 1%), hypothyroidism (4% to 8%)

Gastrointestinal: Diarrhea (52% to 59%; grades 3/4: ≤5%), nausea (26%, grade 3: <1%; STS: 56%, grade 3: 3%), decreased appetite (STS: 40%, grade 3: 6%), anorexia (22%, grade 3: 2%), vomiting (21%, grades 3/4: ≤2%; STS: 33%, grade 3: 3%), dysgeusia (8%, STS: 28%), increased serum lipase (27%, grades 3/4: 4%), gastrointestinal pain (STS: 23%, grade 3: 3%), abdominal pain (11%, grade 3: 2%), mucositis (STS: 12%, grade 3: 2%), stomatitis (STS: 11%, grade 3: <1%), dyspepsia (5% to 7%), anal hemorrhage (2%), gastrointestinal perforation (1%)

Genitourinary: Proteinuria (1% to 9%), hematuria (4%)

Hematologic & oncologic: Leukopenia (37% to 44%; STS, grade 3: 1%), lymphocytopenia (31%; grades 3/4: ≤4%; STS: 43%, grade 3: 10%), thrombocytopenia (32% to 36%; grades 3/4: ≤3%; grade 4: ≤1%), neutropenia (33% to 34%; grades 3/4: ≤4%), hemorrhage (13% to 22%, including pulmonary, gastrointestinal, and genitourinary, grade 4: 1%, including intracranial, subarachnoid, and peritoneal), oral hemorrhage (3%), rectal hemorrhage (1%), hemolytic-uremic syndrome, thrombotic thrombocytopenic purpura

Hepatic: Increased serum AST (51% to 53%; grades 3/4: ≤7%), increased serum ALT (4% to 53%; grades 3/4: 2% to 10%), increased serum bilirubin (29% to 36%; grades 3/4: ≤3%), increased serum alkaline phosphatase (STS: 32%, grade 3: 3%), hepatotoxicity, severe hepatotoxicity

Infection: Serious infection

Neuromuscular & skeletal: Musculoskeletal pain (STS: 23%, grade 3: 2%), myalgia (STS: 23%, grade 3: 2%), weakness (14%, grade 3: 3%), arthralgia, muscle spasm

Ophthalmic: Blurred vision (STS: 5%)

Respiratory: Dyspnea (STS: 20%, grades 3/4: ≤5%), cough (STS: 17%), epistaxis (2% to 8%), pneumothorax (≤3%), hemoptysis (2%)

Miscellaneous: Tumor pain (29%), fistula (1%)

<1% (Limited to important or life-threatening): Cardiac disease, cerebral hemorrhage, cerebrovascular accident, congestive heart failure, interstitial pneumonitis, nephrotic syndrome, pancreatitis, retinal detachment, torsade de pointes

Drug Interactions

Metabolism/Transport Effects Substrate of BCRP, CYP1A2 (minor), CYP2C8 (minor), CYP3A4 (major), P-glycoprotein; **Note:** Assignment of Major/Minor substrate status based on clinically relevant drug interaction potential; **Inhibits** CYP2C8 (weak), CYP2D6 (weak), CYP3A4 (weak), SLCO1B1, UGT1A1

Avoid Concomitant Use

Avoid concomitant use of PAZOPanib with any of the following: Amodiaquine; BCG (Intravesical); BCRP/ABCG2 Inhibitors; Conivaptan; CYP3A4 Inducers (Strong); Fusidic Acid (Systemic); Grapefruit Juice; H2-Antagonists; Highest Risk QTc-Prolonging Agents; Idelalisib; Irinotecan Products; Ivabradine; Lapatinib; Mifepristone; Natalizumab; P-glycoprotein/ABCB1 Inhibitors; Pimecrolimus; Pimozide; Proton Pump Inhibitors; Tacrolimus (Topical); Tofacitinib; Vaccines (Live)

Increased Effect/Toxicity

PAZOPanib may increase the levels/effects of: Amodiaquine; ARIPiprazole; Bisphosphonate Derivatives; Fingolimod; Highest Risk QTc-Prolonging Agents; Hydrocodone; Irinotecan Products; Leflunomide; Moderate Risk QTc-Prolonging Agents; Natalizumab; NiMODipine; Pimozide; Tofacitinib; Vaccines (Live)

The levels/effects of PAZOPanib may be increased by: Aprepitant; BCRP/ABCG2 Inhibitors; Conivaptan; CYP3A4 Inhibitors (Moderate); CYP3A4 Inhibitors (Strong); Dasatinib; Denosumab; Fosaprepitant; Fusidic Acid (Systemic); Grapefruit Juice; HMG-CoA Reductase Inhibitors; Idelalisib; Ivabradine; Lapatinib; Luliconazole; Mifepristone; Netupitant; Palbociclib; P-glycoprotein/ABCB1 Inhibitors; Pimecrolimus; QTc-Prolonging Agents (Indeterminate Risk and Risk Modifying); Roflumilast; Stiripentol; Tacrolimus (Topical); Trastuzumab

Decreased Effect

PAZOPanib may decrease the levels/effects of: BCG (Intravesical); Coccidioides immitis Skin Test; Sipuleucel-T; Vaccines (Inactivated); Vaccines (Live)

The levels/effects of PAZOPanib may be decreased by: Antacids; Bosentan; CYP3A4 Inducers (Moderate); CYP3A4 Inducers (Strong); Deferasirox; Echinacea; H2-Antagonists; P-glycoprotein/ABCB1 Inducers; Proton Pump Inhibitors; Siltuximab; St Johns Wort; Tocilizumab

Food Interactions Systemic exposure of pazopanib is increased when administered with food (AUC twofold higher with a meal). Grapefruit juice may increase the levels/effects of pazopanib. Management: Take on an empty stomach 1 hour before or 2 hours after a meal. Maintain adequate nutrition and hydration, unless instructed to restrict fluid intake. Avoid grapefruit/grapefruit juice.

Storage/Stability Store at 20°C to 25°C (68°F to 77°F); excursions are permitted between 15°C and 30°C (59°F and 86°F).

Mechanism of Action Tyrosine kinase (multikinase) inhibitor; limits tumor growth via inhibition of angiogenesis by inhibiting cell surface vascular endothelial growth factor receptors (VEGFR-1, VEGFR-2, VEGFR-3), platelet-derived growth factor receptors (PDGFR-alpha and -beta), fibroblast growth factor receptor (FGFR-1 and -3), cytokine receptor (cKIT), interleukin-2 receptor inducible T-cell kinase, leukocyte-specific protein tyrosine kinase (Lck), and transmembrane glycoprotein receptor tyrosine kinase (c-Fms)

Pharmacodynamics/Kinetics

Protein binding: >99%

Metabolism: Hepatic; primarily via CYP3A4, minor metabolism via CYP1A2 and CYP2C8

Bioavailability: Rate and extent of bioavailability are increased with food and increased if tablets are crushed (do not crush tablets)

Half-life elimination: ~31 hours

Time to peak, plasma: 2 to 4 hours

Excretion: Feces (primarily); urine (<4%)

Dosing

Adult & Geriatric

Renal cell carcinoma (RCC), advanced: Oral: 800 mg once daily (Sternberg 2010)

Soft tissue sarcoma (STS), advanced: Oral: 800 mg once daily (Van Der Graaf 2012)

Thyroid cancer, advanced differentiated (off-label use): Oral: 800 mg once daily until disease progression or unacceptable toxicity (Bible 2010; Bible 2014)

Missed doses: If a dose is missed, do not take if <12 hours until the next dose.

Concomitant CYP3A4 inhibitors/inducers:

CYP3A4 inhibitors: Avoid concomitant strong CYP3A4 inhibitors (may increase pazopanib concentrations). If pazopanib must be administered concomitantly with a potent enzyme inhibitor, reduce pazopanib to 400 mg once daily with careful monitoring; further dosage reductions may be needed if adverse events occur.

CYP3A4 inducers: Avoid concomitant strong CYP3A4 inducers (may decrease pazopanib concentrations); use of pazopanib is not recommended in situations where the chronic use of a strong CYP3A4 inducer is required.

Renal Impairment No dosage adjustment necessary.

Hepatic Impairment

Preexisting impairment:

Mild (bilirubin ≤1.5 times ULN or ALT >ULN): No dosage adjustment required (Shibata 2013).

Moderate (bilirubin >1.5 to 3 times ULN): Consider alternative therapy or reduce to 200 mg once daily (maximum tolerated dose in patients with moderate hepatic impairment) (Shibata 2013).

Severe (bilirubin >3 times ULN with any ALT level): Use is not recommended.

During treatment:

Isolated ALT elevations 3 to 8 times ULN: Continue treatment, monitor liver function weekly until ALT returns to grade 1 or baseline.

Isolated ALT elevations >8 times ULN: Interrupt treatment until ALT returns to grade 1 or baseline. If therapy benefit is greater than the risk of hepatotoxicity, may reinitiate treatment at ≤400 mg once daily (with liver function monitored weekly for 8 weeks); permanently discontinue if ALT >3 times ULN occurs with reinitiation.

ALT >3 times ULN concurrently with bilirubin >2 times ULN: Permanently discontinue; monitor until resolution.

Gilbert syndrome with mild indirect bilirubin elevation and ALT >3 times ULN: Refer to isolated ALT elevations dosage recommendations above.

Adjustment for Toxicity

Initial dosage reduction: Note: Prior to dose reduction, temporarily discontinue therapy if 24-hour urine protein ≥3 g or for other toxicities when clinically indicated.

RCC: Reduce to 400 mg once daily

STS: Reduce to 600 mg once daily

Further modification: *RCC, STS:* Adjust dose in 200 mg increments or decrements based on individual tolerance; maximum dose: 800 mg

Hypertension: Manage as appropriate with antihypertensive therapy and interrupt treatment or reduce dose as clinically warranted.

Hypertension (severe, persistent, and refractory to antihypertensives and dose reduction) or evidence of hypertensive crisis: Discontinue treatment.

Infection, serious: Consider treatment interruption or discontinuation.

Proteinuria (24-hour urine protein ≥3 g): Interrupt treatment and reduce the dose.

Proteinuria (recurrent 24-hour urine protein ≥3 g refractory to dose reduction): Discontinue treatment.

Pulmonary toxicity: Interstitial lung disease (ILD) or pneumonitis: Discontinue treatment.

Reversible posterior leukoencephalopathy syndrome (RPLS): Permanently discontinue.

Thrombotic microangiopathy (TMA): Permanently discontinue.

Wound dehiscence: Discontinue treatment.

Dietary Considerations Avoid grapefruit juice.

Administration Administer on an empty stomach, 1 hour before or 2 hours after a meal. Do not crush tablet (rate of absorption may be increased; may affect systemic exposure).

Hazardous agent; use appropriate precautions for handling and disposal (NIOSH 2014 [group 1]).

Monitoring Parameters Monitor liver function tests at baseline; at weeks 3, 5, 7, and 9; at months 3 and 4; and as clinically necessary, then periodically after month 4 (US labeling) or at weeks 2, 4, 6, and 8 (Canadian labeling); months 3 and 4, and periodically thereafter (monitor more frequently if clinically indicated); serum electrolytes (eg, calcium, magnesium, potassium); urinalysis (for proteinuria; baseline and periodic), 24-hour urine protein (if clinically indicated); thyroid function (TSH and T$_4$ at baseline and TSH every 6 to 8 weeks during treatment [Appleby 2011]); blood pressure; ECG (baseline and periodic); LVEF (if at risk for cardiac dysfunction; baseline and periodic); signs/symptoms of gastrointestinal perforation or fistula, venous thrombotic events, pulmonary embolism, interstitial lung disease (ILD)/pneumonitis, infection, heart failure, or neurological changes.

Dosage Forms Excipient information presented when available (limited, particularly for generics); consult specific product labeling.

Tablet, Oral:

Votrient: 200 mg

Pegademase Bovine (peg A de mase BOE vine)

Brand Names: US Adagen

Brand Names: Canada Adagen

Pharmacologic Category Enzyme

Use Adenosine deaminase deficiency: For enzyme replacement therapy for adenosine deaminase (ADA) deficiency in infants to children of any age with severe combined immunodeficiency disease who are not suitable candidates for or who have failed bone marrow transplantation.

Dosing

Pediatric

Adenosine deaminase deficiency (enzyme replacement therapy): Infants, Children, and Adolescents: IM: Initial dosage: 10 units/kg for the first dose, 15 units/kg for the second dose, and 20 units/kg for the third dose; administer dose every 7 days; maintenance dose: 20 units/kg/week; increase by 5 units/kg/week if necessary; maximum single dose: 30 units/kg

Note: Dose should be individualized based on monitoring of plasma ADA activity levels and dATP content.

Renal Impairment There are no dosage adjustments provided in the manufacturer's labeling.

Hepatic Impairment There are no dosage adjustments provided in the manufacturer's labeling.

Additional Information Complete prescribing information should be consulted for additional detail.

Dosage Forms Excipient information presented when available (limited, particularly for generics); consult specific product labeling.
Solution, Intramuscular:
Adagen: 250 units/mL (1.5 mL)

♦ Pegalax (Can) *see* Polyethylene Glycol 3350 *on page 1465*

Pegaptanib (peg AP ta nib)

Brand Names: US Macugen
Brand Names: Canada Macugen
Index Terms EYE001; Pegaptanib Sodium
Pharmacologic Category Ophthalmic Agent; Vascular Endothelial Growth Factor (VEGF) Inhibitor
Use Macular degeneration: Treatment of neovascular (wet) age-related macular degeneration (AMD)
Dosing
Adult & Geriatric Age-related macular degeneration (AMD): Intravitreous injection: 0.3 mg into affected eye once every 6 weeks
Renal Impairment
U.S. labeling: No dosage adjustment provided in manufacturer's labeling.
Canadian labeling:
CrCl ≥30 mL/minute: No dosage adjustment necessary.
CrCl <20 mL/minute: No dosage adjustment provided in manufacturer's labeling (has not been studied).
ESRD requiring hemodialysis: No dosage adjustment provided in manufacturer's labeling (has not been studied).
Hepatic Impairment
U.S. labeling: No dosage adjustment provided in manufacturer's labeling.
Canadian labeling: Use has not been studied in patients with hepatic impairment.
Additional Information Complete prescribing information should be consulted for additional detail.
Dosage Forms Excipient information presented when available (limited, particularly for generics); consult specific product labeling.
Solution, Intraocular [preservative free]:
Macugen: 0.3 mg (0.09 mL)

♦ Pegaptanib Sodium *see* Pegaptanib *on page 1407*
♦ PEG-ASP *see* Pegaspargase *on page 1407*
♦ PEG-asparaginase *see* Pegaspargase *on page 1407*

Pegaspargase (peg AS par jase)

Brand Names: US Oncaspar
Index Terms L-asparaginase with Polyethylene Glycol; PEG-ASP; PEG-asparaginase; PEG-L-asparaginase; PEGLA; Polyethylene Glycol-L-asparaginase
Pharmacologic Category Antineoplastic Agent, Enzyme; Antineoplastic Agent, Miscellaneous
Use
Acute lymphoblastic leukemia and hypersensitivity to asparaginase: Treatment of acute lymphoblastic leukemia (ALL) in patients with hypersensitivity to native forms of L-asparaginase (as a component of a multiagent chemotherapy regimen)
Acute lymphoblastic leukemia, first-line: First-line treatment of ALL (as a component of a multiagent chemotherapy regimen)
Dosing
Adult & Geriatric Acute lymphoblastic leukemia (ALL): IM, IV: 2500 units/m^2 (as part of a combination chemotherapy regimen), do not administer more frequently than every 14 days
Pediatric Acute lymphoblastic leukemia (ALL): IM, IV: Refer to adult dosing.
Renal Impairment There are no dosage adjustments provided in the manufacturer's labeling.
Hepatic Impairment There are no initial dosage adjustments provided in the manufacturer's labeling. The following adjustments have been recommended (Stock 2011):
ALT/AST >3 to 5 times ULN: Continue therapy.
ALT/AST >5 to 20 times ULN: Delay next dose until transaminases <3 times ULN.
ALT/AST >20 times ULN: Discontinue therapy if it takes longer than 1 week for transaminases to return to <3 times ULN.
Direct bilirubin <3 mg/dL: Continue therapy.
Direct bilirubin 3.1 to 5 mg/dL: Hold pegaspargase and resume when direct bilirubin <2 mg/dL; consider switching to alternate asparaginase product.

Direct bilirubin >5 mg/dL: Discontinue pegaspargase; do not substitute other asparaginase products; do not make up for missed doses.
Adjustment for Toxicity The following adjustments have been recommended (Stock 2011):
Hyperammonemia-related fatigue: Continue therapy for grade 2 toxicity. If grade 3 toxicity occurs, reduce dose by 25%; resume full dose when toxicity ≤ grade 2 (make up for missed doses). If grade 4 toxicity occurs, reduce dose by 50%; resume full dose when toxicity ≤ grade 2 (make up for missed doses).
Hyperglycemia: Continue therapy for uncomplicated hyperglycemia. If hyperglycemia requires insulin therapy, hold pegaspargase (and any concomitant corticosteroids) until blood glucose controlled; resume dosing at prior dose level. For life-threatening hyperglycemia or toxicity requiring urgent intervention, hold pegaspargase (and corticosteroids) until blood glucose is controlled with insulin; resume pegaspargase and do not make up for missed doses.
Hypersensitivity reactions: May continue dosing for urticaria without bronchospasm, hypotension, edema, or need for parenteral intervention. If wheezing or other symptomatic bronchospasm with or without urticaria, angioedema, hypotension, and/or life-threatening hypersensitivity reactions occur, discontinue pegaspargase. Replace pegaspargase with asparaginase (Erwinia).
Hypertriglyceridemia: If serum triglyceride level <1,000 mg/dL, continue pegaspargase but monitor closely for pancreatitis. If triglyceride level >1,000 mg/dL, hold pegaspargase and monitor; resume therapy at prior dose level after triglyceride level returns to baseline.
Pancreatitis:
Asymptomatic amylase or lipase >3 times ULN (chemical pancreatitis) or radiologic abnormalities only: Continue pegaspargase and monitor levels closely.
Clinical pancreatitis (abdominal pain with amylase or lipase >3 times ULN for >3 days and/or development of pancreatic pseudocyst): Permanently discontinue pegaspargase.
Thrombosis and bleeding, CNS:
Thrombosis: Continue therapy for abnormal laboratory findings without a clinical correlate. If grade 3 toxicity occurs, discontinue therapy; if CNS signs/symptoms are fully resolved and further pegaspargase doses are required, may resume therapy at a lower dose and/or longer intervals between doses. Discontinue therapy for grade 4 toxicity.
Hemorrhage: Discontinue therapy; do not withhold therapy for abnormal laboratory findings without a clinical correlate. If grade 3 toxicity occurs, discontinue therapy; if CNS signs/symptoms are fully resolved and further pegaspargase doses are required, may resume therapy at a lower dose and/or longer intervals between doses. Discontinue therapy for grade 4 toxicity.
Thrombosis and bleeding, non-CNS:
Thrombosis: Continue therapy for abnormal laboratory findings without a clinical correlate. If grade 3 or 4 toxicity occurs, withhold therapy until acute toxicity and clinical signs resolve and anticoagulant therapy is stable or completed. Do not withhold therapy for abnormal laboratory findings without clinical correlate.
Hemorrhage: If grade 2 bleeding in conjunction with hypofibrinogenemia occurs, withhold therapy until bleeding ≤ grade 1. Do not withhold therapy for abnormal laboratory findings without clinical correlate. For grade 3 or 4 bleeding, withhold therapy until bleeding ≤ grade 1 and until acute toxicity and clinical signs resolve and coagulant replacement therapy is stable or completed.
Additional Information Complete prescribing information should be consulted for additional detail.
Dosage Forms Excipient information presented when available (limited, particularly for generics); consult specific product labeling.
Solution, Injection [preservative free]:
Oncaspar: 750 units/mL (5 mL)

♦ Pegasys *see* Peginterferon Alfa-2a *on page 1409*
♦ Pegasys ProClick *see* Peginterferon Alfa-2a *on page 1409*

Pegfilgrastim (peg fil GRA stim)

Brand Names: US Neulasta; Neulasta Onpro
Brand Names: Canada Neulasta
Index Terms G-CSF (PEG Conjugate); Granulocyte Colony Stimulating Factor (PEG Conjugate); Neulasta Onpro kit; Pegylated G-CSF; SD/01

◀ **Pharmacologic Category** Colony Stimulating Factor; Hematopoietic Agent

Use

Prevention of chemotherapy-induced neutropenia: To decrease the incidence of infection (as manifested by febrile neutropenia), in patients with nonmyeloid malignancies receiving myelosuppressive cancer chemotherapy associated with a clinically significant incidence of febrile neutropenia.

Limitation of use: Pegfilgrastim is not indicated for mobilization of peripheral blood progenitor cells for hematopoietic stem cell transplant.

Hematopoietic radiation injury syndrome (acute): To increase survival in patients acutely exposed to myelosuppressive doses of radiation.

Pregnancy Considerations Adverse events were observed in some animal reproduction studies.

Women who are exposed to Neulasta during pregnancy are encouraged to enroll in the Amgen Pregnancy Surveillance Program (800-772-6436).

Breast-Feeding Considerations It is not known if pegfilgrastim is excreted in breast milk. The manufacturer recommends that caution be exercised when administering pegfilgrastim to nursing women.

Contraindications Hypersensitivity (serious allergic reaction) to pegfilgrastim, filgrastim, or any component of the formulation

Warnings/Precautions Do not use pegfilgrastim in the period 14 days before to 24 hours after administration of cytotoxic chemotherapy because of the potential sensitivity of rapidly dividing myeloid cells to cytotoxic chemotherapy. Safety and efficacy have not been established with dose-dense chemotherapy regimens (Smith 2006). Not indicated for peripheral blood progenitor cell (PBPC) mobilization for hematopoietic stem cell transplantation.

Serious allergic reactions (including anaphylaxis) may occur, usually with the initial dose; may recur within days after discontinuation of initial antiallergic treatment. Permanently discontinue for severe reactions. Do not administer in patients with a history of serious allergic reaction to pegfilgrastim or filgrastim. Acute respiratory distress syndrome (ARDS) has been reported with use; evaluate patients with pulmonary symptoms such as fever, pulmonary infiltrates, or respiratory distress for ARDS. Discontinue pegfilgrastim if ARDS occurs. Rare cases of splenic rupture have been reported (some fatal); patients must be instructed to report left upper abdominal pain or shoulder pain. May precipitate sickle cell crises in patients with sickle cell disorders (severe and sometimes fatal sickle cell crises have occurred with filgrastim). The granulocyte-colony stimulating factor (G-CSF) receptor through which pegfilgrastim (and filgrastim) work has been located on tumor cell lines. May potentially act as a growth factor for any tumor type, including myeloid malignancies and myelodysplasia (pegfilgrastim is not approved for myeloid malignancies). Capillary leak syndrome (CLS), characterized by hypotension, hypoalbuminemia, edema, and hemoconcentration, may occur in patients receiving human granulocyte colony-stimulating factors (G-CSF), including pegfilgrastim. CLS episodes vary in frequency and severity. If CLS develops, monitor closely and manage symptomatically (may require intensive care). CLS may be life-threatening if treatment is delayed.

Leukocytosis (WBC ≥100,000/mm³) has been reported in patients receiving pegfilgrastim. Monitor complete blood counts during therapy. Glomerulonephritis has occurred, and generally resolved after pegfilgrastim dose reduction or discontinuation. Diagnosis was made by the presence of azotemia, microscopic and macroscopic hematuria, proteinuria, and renal biopsy. Evaluate if glomerulonephritis is suspected; if felt due to pegfilgrastim, consider dose reduction or therapy interruption.

The On-body injector contains an acrylic adhesive; may result in a significant reaction in patients who react to acrylic adhesives. A health care provider must fill the On-body injector prior to applying to the patient's skin. The On-body delivery system may be applied on the same day as chemotherapy administration as long as pegfilgrastim is delivered no less than 24 hours after chemotherapy is administered. The prefilled syringe provided in the On-body kit contains overfill to compensate for loss during delivery; do not use for manual subcutaneous injection (will result in higher than recommended dose). Do not use prefilled syringe intended for manual injection to fill the On-body injector; may result in lower than intended dose. The On-body injector is only for use with pegfilgrastim; do not use to deliver other medications. Do not expose the On-body injector to oxygen-rich environments (eg, hyperbaric chambers), MRI, x-ray (including airport x-ray), CT scan, or ultrasound (may damage injector system). Keep the On-body injector at least 4 inches away from electrical equipment, including cell phones, cordless phones, microwaves, and other common appliances (injector may not work properly).

Colony-stimulating factors may be considered in cancer patients with febrile neutropenia who are at high risk for infection-associated complications or who have prognostic factors indicative of a poor clinical outcome (eg, prolonged and severe neutropenia, age >65 years, hypotension, pneumonia, sepsis syndrome, presence of invasive fungal infection, uncontrolled primary disease, hospitalization at the time of fever development) (Freifeld 2011; Smith 2006). Colony-stimulating factors should not be routinely used for patients with neutropenia who are afebrile. Dose-dense regimens that require colony-stimulating factors should only be used within the context of a clinical trial or if supported by convincing evidence. The safety/efficacy of pegfilgrastim in the setting of dose-dense therapy has not been fully established (Smith 2015).

ASCO guidelines recommend that prophylactic colony-stimulating factors be used in patients ≥65 years with diffuse aggressive lymphoma treated with curative chemotherapy (eg, rituximab, cyclophosphamide, doxorubicin, vincristine, prednisone), especially if patients have comorbid conditions (Smith 2015). The 6 mg fixed dose should not be used in infants, children, and adolescents weighing <45 kg. CSF use in pediatric patients is typically directed by clinical pediatric protocols. ASCO Recommendations for the Use of WBC Growth Factors Clinical Practice Guideline Update states that CSFs may be reasonable as primary prophylaxis in pediatric patients when chemotherapy regimens with a high likelihood of febrile neutropenia are employed. Likewise, secondary CSF prophylaxis should be limited to high-risk patients. In pediatric cancers in which dose-intense chemotherapy (with a survival benefit) is used, CSFs should be given to facilitate chemotherapy administration. CSFs should not be used in the pediatric population for non-relapsed acute lymphoblastic or myeloid leukemia when no infection is present (Smith 2015). The On-body injector has not been studied for use in pediatrics. The packaging (needle cover) contains latex.

Adverse Reactions

Neuromuscular & skeletal: Ostealgia (31%), limb pain (9%)

<1% (Limited to important or life-threatening): Acute respiratory distress syndrome (ARDS), anaphylaxis, antibody development, capillary leak syndrome, glomerulonephritis, hypersensitivity angiitis, hypertonia, increased serum alkaline phosphatase, increased uric acid, leukocytosis, periorbital edema, peripheral edema, polyarthralgia, polymyalgia rheumatic, severe sickle cell crisis, splenic rupture, splenomegaly, Sweet syndrome

Drug Interactions

Metabolism/Transport Effects None known.

Avoid Concomitant Use There are no known interactions where it is recommended to avoid concomitant use.

Increased Effect/Toxicity There are no known significant interactions involving an increase in effect.

Decreased Effect

The levels/effects of Pegfilgrastim may be decreased by: Pegloticase

Preparation for Administration

Subcutaneous administration from the prefilled syringe: For doses of 6 mg, the prefilled syringe may be used. **Direct** administration of doses <6 mg using the prefilled syringe is not recommended by the manufacturer (it does not have graduation marks necessary for accurate measurement of doses other than 6 mg).

On-body injector: A health care provider must fill the On-body injector prior to applying to the patient's skin. The On-body delivery system may be applied on the same day as chemotherapy administration as long as pegfilgrastim is delivered no less than 24 hours after chemotherapy is administered.

The prefilled syringe provided in the On-body kit contains overfill to compensate for loss during delivery; do not use for manual subcutaneous injection (will result in higher than recommended dose). Do not use prefilled syringe intended for manual injection to fill the On-body injector; may result in lower than intended dose. The On-body injector has not been studied for use in pediatrics.

Storage/Stability Store under refrigeration at 2°C to 8°C (36°F to 46°F); do not freeze. If syringe for manual injection is inadvertently frozen, allow to thaw in refrigerator; discard if frozen more than one time. Protect from light. Do not shake. Allow to reach room temperature prior to injection. Prefilled syringe for manual injection may be kept at room temperature for up to 48 hours. The On-body injector kit should not be held at room temperature for longer than 12 hours prior to use (discard if stored at room temperature for >12 hours).

Mechanism of Action Stimulates the production, maturation, and activation of neutrophils, pegfilgrastim activates neutrophils to increase both their migration and cytotoxicity. Pegfilgrastim has a prolonged duration of effect relative to filgrastim and a reduced renal clearance.

Pharmacodynamics/Kinetics Half-life elimination: SubQ: Pediatrics (100 mcg/kg dose): 0 to 5 years: 30.1 ± 38.2 hours; 6 to 11 years: 20.2 ± 11.3 hours; 12 years and older: 21.2 ± 16 hours; Adults: 15 to 80 hours. Pharmacokinetics (in adults) were comparable between manual subcutaneous injection and the On-body injector system.

Dosing

Adult & Geriatric

Prevention of chemotherapy-induced neutropenia: SubQ: 6 mg once per chemotherapy cycle, beginning at least 24 hours after completion of chemotherapy; **Note:** Do not administer in the period between 14 days before and 24 hours after administration of cytotoxic chemotherapy.

Hematopoietic radiation injury syndrome (acute): SubQ: 6 mg once weekly for 2 doses. Obtain a baseline CBC prior to administration, but do not delay pegfilgrastim use if a CBC is not readily obtainable. Administer the first dose as soon as possible after suspected or confirmed radiation exposure greater than 2 gray (Gy). Administer the second dose 1 week after the first dose.

Pediatric

Prevention of chemotherapy-induced neutropenia:
Note: Do not administer in the period between 14 days before and 24 hours after administration of cytotoxic chemotherapy.

Children and Adolescents <45 kg: SubQ: Administer once per chemotherapy cycle, beginning at least 24 hours after completion of chemotherapy (dose and volume are based on patient weight). Maximum dose: 6 mg (Andre 2007; Borinstein 2009). **Note:** The prefilled syringe is not designed to allow for direct administration of doses less than 6 mg (0.6 mL). Due to the potential for dosing errors, the manufacturer does not recommend direct administration of doses less than 6 mg (0.6 mL); use caution to avoid dosing errors.
Patients <10 kg: 0.1 **mg/kg** (0.01 **mL/kg** volume)
Patients 10 to 20 kg: 1.5 **mg** (0.15 **mL** volume)
Patients 21 to 30 kg: 2.5 **mg** (0.25 **mL** volume)
Patients 31 to 44 kg: 4 **mg** (0.4 **mL** volume)
Children and Adolescents ≥45 kg: SubQ: 6 mg once per chemotherapy cycle, beginning at least 24 hours after completion of chemotherapy

Hematopoietic radiation injury syndrome (acute): Obtain a baseline CBC prior to administration, but do not delay pegfilgrastim use if a CBC is not readily obtainable. Administer the first dose as soon as possible after suspected or confirmed radiation exposure greater than 2 gray (Gy). Administer the second dose 1 week after the first dose.
Children and Adolescents <45 kg: SubQ: Administer 2 doses of pegfilgrastim one week apart (dose and volume are based on patient weight).
Patients <10 kg: 0.1 **mg/kg** (0.01 **mL/kg** volume)
Patients 10 to 20 kg: 1.5 **mg** (0.15 **mL** volume)
Patients 21 to 30 kg: 2.5 **mg** (0.25 **mL** volume)
Patients 31 to 44 kg: 4 **mg** (0.4 **mL** volume)
Children and Adolescents ≥45 kg: SubQ: 6 mg once weekly for 2 doses (the second dose should be administered 1 week after the first dose).

Renal Impairment No dosage adjustment necessary.

Hepatic Impairment There are no dosage adjustments provided in the manufacturer's labeling (has not been studied).

Administration Administer subcutaneously. Do not use 6 mg fixed dose in infants, children, or adolescents <45 kg (Smith 2006). Pegfilgrastim is available in prefilled syringes for manual subcutaneous administration or as a kit for use with the On-body injector. **Direct** administration of doses <6 mg using the prefilled syringe is not recommended by the manufacturer (it does not have graduation marks necessary for accurate measurement of doses other than 6 mg); use caution to avoid dosing errors.

Manual subcutaneous administration: Administer to outer upper arms, abdomen (except within 2 inches of navel), front middle thigh, or upper outer buttocks. Engage/activate needle guard following use to prevent accidental needlesticks

On-body injector: A health care provider must fill the On-body injector prior to applying to the patient's skin. Apply to intact, nonirritated skin on the back of the arm or abdomen (only use the back of the arm if caregiver is available to monitor On-body injection status). The On-body injector system will deliver pegfilgrastim over ~45 minutes approximately 27 hours after application. The On-body delivery system may be applied on the same day as chemotherapy administration as long as pegfilgrastim is delivered at least 24 hours after chemotherapy is administered. Keep the On-body injector dry for ~3 hours before dose delivery. A missed dose may occur if the On-body injector fails or leaks; if a dose is missed, administer a new dose by manual subcutaneous injection as soon as possible after discovery of missed dose. Do not expose the On-body injector to oxygen-rich environments (eg, hyperbaric chambers), MRI, x-ray (including airport x-ray), CT-scan, or ultrasound (may damage injector system). Keep the On-body injector at least 4 inches away from electrical equipment, including cell phones, cordless phones, microwaves, and other common appliances (injector may not work properly). The On-body injector has not been studied in pediatric patients. Refer to prescribing information for further details.

The prefilled syringe provided in the On-body kit contains overfill to compensate for loss during delivery; do not use for manual subcutaneous injection (will result in higher than recommended dose). Do not use prefilled syringe intended for manual injection to fill the On-body injector; may result in lower than intended dose. The On-body injector is only for use with pegfilgrastim; do not use to deliver other medications.

Monitoring Parameters

Chemotherapy-induced neutropenia: Complete blood count (with differential) and platelet count should be obtained prior to chemotherapy and as clinically necessary.

Hematopoietic radiation injury syndrome: CBC at baseline (do not delay administration if CBC not readily available); estimate absorbed radiation dose.

Evaluate fever, pulmonary infiltrates, and respiratory distress; evaluate for left upper abdominal pain, shoulder tip pain, or splenomegaly. Monitor for signs/symptoms of glomerulonephritis (azotemia, hematuria, proteinuria) and capillary leak syndrome (hypotension, hypoalbuminemia, edema and hemoconcentration). Monitor for sickle cell crisis (in patients with sickle cell anemia).

Test Interactions May interfere with bone imaging studies; increased hematopoietic activity of the bone marrow may appear as transient positive bone imaging changes

Dosage Forms Excipient information presented when available (limited, particularly for generics); consult specific product labeling.
Prefilled Syringe Kit, Subcutaneous [preservative free]:
Neulasta Onpro: 6 mg/0.6 mL (0.6 mL)
Solution, Subcutaneous [preservative free]:
Neulasta: 6 mg/0.6 mL (0.6 mL)

◆ PEG-IFN Alfa-2a *see* Peginterferon Alfa-2a *on page 1409*

◆ PEG-IFN Alfa-2b *see* Peginterferon Alfa-2b *on page 1411*

Peginterferon Alfa-2a
(peg in ter FEER on AL fa too aye)

Brand Names: US Pegasys; Pegasys ProClick
Brand Names: Canada Pegasys
Index Terms Interferon Alfa-2a (PEG Conjugate); PEG-IFN Alfa-2a; Pegylated Interferon Alfa-2a
Pharmacologic Category Interferon
Use

Chronic hepatitis B: Treatment of adults with hepatitis B e antigen (HBeAg)-positive and HBeAG-negative chronic hepatitis B virus (HBV) infection who have compensated liver disease and evidence of viral replication and liver inflammation

Chronic hepatitis C:
Combination therapy: Treatment of adults with chronic hepatitis C (CHC) with compensated liver disease as part of a combination regimen with other hepatitis C virus (HCV) antiviral drugs; treatment of pediatric patients 5 years and older with CHC and compensated liver disease in combination with ribavirin
Monotherapy (for patients with contraindications or who are intolerant to other HCV antiviral drugs): Treatment (as a single agent) of chronic hepatitis C in patients with compensated liver disease in patients with contraindications or significant intolerance to other HCV antiviral drugs
Limitations of use: Peginterferon alfa-2a alone or in combination with ribavirin without additional HCV antiviral drugs is not recommended for treatment of patients with chronic HCV who previously failed therapy with an interferon alfa. Peginterferon alfa-2a is not recommended for treatment of patients with CHC who have had solid organ transplantation.

Medication Guide Available Yes

Dosing
Adult & Geriatric
Chronic hepatitis C (monoinfection or coinfection with HIV): SubQ:
Manufacturer's labeling: 180 mcg once weekly for 48 weeks as monotherapy or in combination with ribavirin (Copegus). **Note:** Discontinue in patients with HCV (genotype 1) after 12 weeks if HCV RNA does not decrease by at least 2 log (compared to pretreatment) or if detectable HCV RNA is present at 24 weeks.

Duration of combination therapy: Monoinfection (based on genotype):
Genotypes 1, 2: Refer to the individual agents of HCV antiviral drugs
Genotypes 3: 24 weeks if peginterferon and ribavirin are used without other HCV antiviral drugs
Genotypes 4: 48 weeks if peginterferon and ribavirin are used without other HCV antiviral drugs
Genotypes 5, 6: No dosing recommendations provided; data insufficient

Duration of therapy: Coinfection with HIV: 48 weeks regardless of HCV genotype (if used without other HCV antiviral drugs). When used in combination with other antiviral drugs, refer to individual agents for duration of therapy

Alternative dosing:
Chronic hepatitis C (off-label uses; recommended regimens, AASLD/IDSA, 2014): Treatment naïve patients:
Genotype 1, 4, 5, or 6: Interferon eligible patients: 180 mcg once weekly in combination with sofosbuvir 400 mg once daily and ribavirin for 12 weeks:
<75 kg: Ribavirin 1000 mg daily
≥75 kg: Ribavirin 1200 mg daily
Chronic hepatitis C (off-label uses; recommended regimens, AASLD/IDSA, 2014): Treatment of **relapser** patients (non responders to a previous regimen of ribavirin and peginterferon **without** an HCV protease inhibitor):
Genotype 4, 5 or 6: Interferon eligible patients: 180 mcg once weekly in combination with sofosbuvir 400 mg once daily and ribavirin for 12 weeks:
<75 kg: Ribavirin 1000 mg daily
≥75 kg: Ribavirin 1200 mg daily
Chronic hepatitis C (off-label uses; recommended regimen, AASLD/IDSA, 2014): Treatment of **relapser** patients (non responders to a previous regimen of ribavirin and peginterferon **with or without** an HCV protease inhibitor):
Genotype 1: Interferon eligible patients: 180 mcg once weekly in combination with ribavirin for 12-24 weeks total and sofosbuvir 400 mg once daily for the first 12 weeks only
<75 kg: Ribavirin 1000 mg daily
≥75 kg: Ribavirin 1200 mg daily

Chronic hepatitis B: *SubQ:* 180 mcg once weekly for 48 weeks

Pediatric
Chronic hepatitis C: Children ≥5 years and Adolescents: SubQ: 180 mcg/1.73 m² x body surface area (BSA) once weekly (maximum dose: 180 mcg) with ribavirin (Copegus). **Note:** Children who reach their 18th birthday during treatment should remain on the pediatric regimen until completion of therapy.
Duration of therapy (based on genotype):
Genotypes 1, 4, 5, 6: 48 weeks
Genotypes 2, 3: 24 weeks

Renal Impairment
Adults:
CrCl ≥30 mL/minute: No dosage adjustment required.
CrCl <30 mL/minute: 135 mcg once weekly; monitor for toxicity
End-stage renal disease (ESRD) requiring hemodialysis: 135 mcg once weekly; monitor for toxicity. If severe adverse reactions or laboratory abnormalities occur, may reduce dose to 90 mcg once weekly until adverse reactions resolve; if intolerance persists after dosage adjustment, discontinue.
Children: There are no dosage adjustments provided in the manufacturer's labeling (has not been studied).

Hepatic Impairment
Hepatic impairment prior to initiation: Contraindicated in autoimmune hepatitis, hepatic decompensation (Child-Pugh >6 [class B and C]) in cirrhotic patients before treatment, and hepatic decompensation with Child-Pugh ≥6 in cirrhotic HCV patients coinfected with HIV before treatment.
Hepatic impairment during treatment:
Adults: **Note:** Immediately discontinue therapy if hepatic decompensation (Child-Pugh ≥6 [class B and C]) is observed.

HCV: ALT progressively rising above baseline: Decrease dose to 135 mcg once weekly **and** monitor LFTs more frequently. If ALT continues to rise despite dose reduction or ALT increase is accompanied by increased bilirubin or hepatic decompensation, discontinue therapy immediately. Therapy may resume after ALT flare subsides.
HBV:
ALT >5 x ULN: Consider decreasing dose to 135 mcg once weekly or temporarily discontinuing **and** monitor LFTs more frequently. If ALT continues to rise despite dose reduction or ALT increase is accompanied by increased bilirubin or hepatic decompensation, discontinue therapy immediately. Therapy may resume after ALT flare subsides.
ALT >10 x ULN: Consider discontinuing.
Children: HCV: **Note:** Immediately discontinue therapy if hepatic decompensation (Child-Pugh ≥6 [class B and C]) is observed.
ALT ≥5 but <10 x ULN: Decrease interferon dose to 135 mcg/1.73 m² x BSA once weekly. Monitor weekly; further modify dose if needed until ALT stabilizes or decreases.
ALT ≥10 x ULN (persistent): Discontinue treatment.

Adjustment for Toxicity Dosage modifications for adverse reactions and/or toxicity:
Children ≥5 years and Adolescents: HCV:
Moderate-to-severe adverse reactions: Decrease to 135 mcg/1.73 m² x BSA once weekly for initial dose reduction; further dose reductions to 90 mcg/1.73 m² x BSA once weekly or 45 mcg/1.73 m² x BSA once weekly may be necessary in some cases if reaction persists or recurs. Up to 3 dosing adjustments for toxicity may be made before discontinuation is considered.
Based on hematologic parameters:
ANC 750 to 999/mm³: Week 1 to 2: 135 mcg/1.73 m² x BSA once weekly; Weeks 3 to 48: No modification
ANC 500 to 749/mm³: Week 1 to 2: Delay or hold dose until ANC >750/mm³ then resume dose with 135 mcg/1.73 m² x BSA once weekly. Assess WBC weekly for 3 weeks to verify ANC >750/mm³; Weeks 3 to 48: 135 mcg/1.73 m² x BSA once weekly
ANC 250 to 499/mm³: Week 1 to 2: Delay or hold dose until ANC >750/mm³ then resume dose with 90 mcg/1.73 m² x BSA once weekly; Weeks 3 to 48: Delay or hold dose until ANC >750/mm³ then resume dose with 135 mcg/1.73 m² x BSA once weekly
ANC <250/mm³ (or febrile neutropenia): Discontinue treatment.
Platelet count <50,000/mm³: 90 mcg/1.73 m² x BSA once weekly
Depression (severity based on DSM-IV criteria [similar to adult dosing adjustment recommendations]):
Mild depression: No dosage adjustment required; evaluate once weekly by visit/phone call. If depression remains stable, continue weekly visits. If depression improves, resume normal visit schedule. For worsening depression, discontinue or reduce dosage to 90 mcg/1.73 m² x BSA once weekly or 135 mcg/1.73 m² x BSA once weekly. Consider psychiatric consultation.
Moderate depression: Decrease to 90 mcg/1.73 m² x BSA or 135 mcg/1.73 m² x BSA once weekly; evaluate once weekly with an office visit at least every other week. If depression remains stable, consider psychiatric evaluation and continue reduced dosing. If symptoms improve and remain stable for 4 weeks, resume normal visit schedule; continue reduced dosing or return to normal dose. For worsening depression, discontinue permanently and obtain immediate psychiatric consultation.
Severe depression: Discontinue permanently. Obtain immediate psychiatric consultation. Utilize follow-up psychiatric therapy as needed.

Adults: HCV, HBV:
Moderate-to-severe adverse reactions: Decrease to 135 mcg weekly for initial dose reduction; further dose reductions to 90 mcg weekly may be necessary in some cases if reaction persists or recurs.
Based on hematologic parameters:
ANC <750/mm³: 135 mcg once weekly
ANC <500/mm³: Suspend therapy until ANC >1,000/mm³, then restart at 90 mcg once weekly; monitor ANC
Platelet count <50,000/mm³: 90 mcg once weekly
Platelet count <25,000/mm³: Discontinue therapy
Depression (severity based on DSM-IV criteria):
Mild depression: No dosage adjustment required; evaluate once weekly by visit/phone call. If depression remains stable, continue weekly visits. If depression improves, resume normal visit schedule.

For worsening depression, discontinue or reduce dosage to 90 mcg or 135 mcg once weekly. Consider psychiatric consultation.

Moderate depression: Decrease to 90 mcg or 135 mcg once weekly; evaluate once weekly with an office visit at least every other week. If depression remains stable, consider psychiatric evaluation and continue with reduced dosing. If symptoms improve and remain stable for 4 weeks, resume normal visit schedule; continue reduced dosing or return to normal dose. For worsening depression, discontinue permanently and obtain immediate psychiatric consultation.

Severe depression: Discontinue permanently. Obtain immediate psychiatric consultation. Utilize follow-up psychiatric therapy as needed.

Additional Information Complete prescribing information should be consulted for additional detail.

Dosage Forms Excipient information presented when available (limited, particularly for generics); consult specific product labeling.

Kit, Subcutaneous [preservative free]:
Pegasys: 180 mcg/0.5 mL [contains benzyl alcohol]
Solution, Subcutaneous [preservative free]:
Pegasys: 180 mcg/mL (1 mL); 180 mcg/0.5 mL (0.5 mL) [contains benzyl alcohol, polysorbate 80]
Pegasys ProClick: 135 mcg/0.5 mL (0.5 mL) [contains benzyl alcohol, polysorbate 80]
Pegasys ProClick: 180 mcg/0.5 mL (0.5 mL) [contains benzyl alcohol]

Peginterferon Alfa-2b
(peg in ter FEER on AL fa too bee)

Brand Names: US Peg-Intron; Peg-Intron Redipen; Peg-Intron Redipen Pak 4; PegIntron; Sylatron
Brand Names: Canada PegIntron
Index Terms Interferon Alfa-2b (PEG Conjugate); PEG-IFN Alfa-2b; Pegylated Interferon Alfa-2b; Polyethylene Glycol Interferon Alfa-2b
Pharmacologic Category Antineoplastic Agent, Biological Response Modulator; Biological Response Modulator; Immunomodulator, Systemic; Interferon
Use
Chronic hepatitis C (CHC): Peg-Intron: Treatment of chronic hepatitis C (CHC) in compensated liver disease:
Combination therapy with ribavirin and an approved hepatitis C virus [HCV] NS3/4A protease inhibitor in adult patients with HCV genotype 1 infection.
Combination therapy with ribavirin in adult patients with HCV genotypes other than 1, in pediatric patients (3 to 17 years), or in patients with HCV genotype 1 with contraindications or intolerance to HCV NS3/4A protease inhibitor use.
Monotherapy in adult patients with contraindications or significant intolerance to ribavirin if previously untreated.
Limitations of use: Combination therapy with ribavirin provides substantially better response rates than monotherapy
Melanoma: Sylatron: Adjuvant treatment of melanoma (with microscopic or gross nodal involvement within 84 days of definitive surgical resection, including complete lymphadenectomy)
Medication Guide Available Yes
Dosing
Adult & Geriatric
Melanoma: SubQ: Initial: 6 mcg/kg/week for 8 doses; Maintenance: 3 mcg/kg/week for up to 5 years. **Note:** Premedicate with acetaminophen (500-1000 mg orally) 30 minutes prior to the first dose and as needed for subsequent doses thereafter.
Chronic hepatitis C (CHC): SubQ:
Manufacturer's labeling: **Note:** Discontinue after 12 weeks in patients with HCV (genotype 1) if HCV RNA does not decrease by at least 2 log (compared to pretreatment) or if detectable HCV RNA present at 24. Discontinuation is also recommended in patients who previously failed therapy (regardless of genotype) if detectable HCV RNA present at 12 or 24 weeks.
Combination therapy with ribavirin (treatment duration is 48 weeks for genotype 1, 24 weeks for genotypes 2 and 3, or 48 weeks for patients who previously failed therapy [regardless of genotype]): Initial dose (based on an average weekly dose of 1.5 mcg/kg):
<40 kg: 50 mcg once weekly (with ribavirin 800 mg/day)
40 to 50 kg: 64 mcg once weekly (with ribavirin 800 mg/day)
51 to 60 kg: 80 mcg once weekly (with ribavirin 800 mg/day)

61 to 65 kg: 96 mcg once weekly (with ribavirin 800 mg/day)
66 to 75 kg: 96 mcg once weekly (with ribavirin 1000 mg/day)
76 to 80 kg: 120 mcg once weekly (with ribavirin 1000 mg/day)
81 to 85 kg: 120 mcg once weekly (with ribavirin 1200 mg/day)
86 to 105 kg: 150 mcg once weekly (with ribavirin 1200 mg/day)
>105 kg: 1.5 mcg/kg once weekly (with ribavirin 1400 mg/day)
Monotherapy (duration of treatment is 1 year): Initial dose (based on average weekly dose of 1 mcg/kg):
≤45 kg: 40 mcg once weekly
46 to 56 kg: 50 mcg once weekly
57 to 72 kg: 64 mcg once weekly
73 to 88 kg: 80 mcg once weekly
89 to 106 kg: 96 mcg once weekly
107 to 136 kg: 120 mcg once weekly
137 to 160 kg: 150 mcg once weekly
Alternative dosing: **Note:** Current AASLD/IDSA recommendations do not specify a particular peginterferon (eg, 2a or 2b); however, guideline recommendations are based on clinical trials that used peginterferon alfa-2a. It is not known whether peginterferon alfa 2b could be used interchangeably. Please refer to http://www.hcvguidelines.org for additional information.
Pediatric Chronic hepatitis C (CHC):
Manufacturer labeling: Children 3 to 17 years: SubQ: Combination therapy with ribavirin: 60 mcg/m^2 once weekly; **Note:** Children who reach their 18th birthday during treatment should remain on the pediatric regimen. Treatment duration is 48 weeks for genotype 1, 24 weeks for genotypes 2 and 3. Discontinue combination therapy in patients with HCV (genotype 1) at 12 weeks if HCV-RNA does not decrease by at least 2 log (compared to pretreatment) or if detectable HCV-RNA present at 24 weeks.
American Association for the Study of Liver Diseases (AASLD) guideline recommendations (Ghany, 2009): Children 2-17 years: SubQ: Treatment of choice: Peginterferon alfa-2b 60 mcg/m^2 once weekly in combination with oral ribavirin 15 mg/kg/day for 48 weeks
Renal Impairment Chronic hepatitis C:
Peginterferon alfa-2b combination with ribavirin:
Adults: CrCl <50 mL/minute: Combination therapy with ribavirin is not recommended.
Children: Serum creatinine >2 mg/dL: Discontinue treatment.
Peginterferon alfa-2b monotherapy:
CrCl 30 to 50 mL/minute: Reduce dose by 25%
CrCl 10 to 29 mL/minute: Reduce dose by 50%
Hemodialysis: Reduce dose by 50%
Discontinue use if renal function declines during treatment.
Melanoma:
CrCl >50 mL/minute/1.73 m^2: No dosage adjustment is necessary.
CrCl 30 to 50 mL/minute/1.73 m^2: Reduce initial dose to 4.5 mcg/kg/week; reduce maintenance dose to 2.25 mcg/kg/week
CrCl <30 mL/minute/1.73 m^2 and ESRD on dialysis: Reduce initial dose to 3 mcg/kg/week; reduce maintenance dose to 1.5 mcg/kg/week
Hemodialysis: Following a single 1 mcg/kg/ dose, no clinically meaningful amount of peginterferon alfa-2b was removed during hemodialysis.
Hepatic Impairment
Decompensated liver disease or autoimmune hepatitis: Use is contraindicated.
Hepatic decompensation or severe hepatic injury during treatment (Child-Pugh score >6 [class B or C]): Discontinue immediately.
Adjustment for Toxicity
Melanoma:
Discontinue for any of the following: Persistent or worsening severe neuropsychiatric disorders (depression, psychosis, encephalopathy), grade 4 nonhematologic toxicity, new or worsening retinopathy, new-onset ventricular arrhythmia or cardiovascular decompensation, evidence of hepatic injury (severe) or hepatic decompensation (Child-Pugh score >6 [Class B or C]), development of hyper- or hypothyroidism or diabetes that cannot be effectively managed with medication, or inability to tolerate a dose of 1 mcg/kg/week
Temporarily withhold for any of the following: ANC <500/mm^3, platelets <50,000/mm^3, ECOG performance status (PS) ≥2, nonhematologic toxicity ≥ grade 3

May reinitiate at a reduced dose once ANC ≥500/mm³, platelets ≥50,000/mm³, ECOG PS at 0 to 1, and nonhematologic toxicity completely resolved or improved to grade 1.

Reduced dose schedule, Weeks 1 to 8:

First dose reduction (if prior dose 6 mcg/kg/week): 3 mcg/kg/week

Second dose reduction (if prior dose 3 mcg/kg/week): 2 mcg/kg/week

Third dose reduction (if prior dose 2 mcg/kg/week): 1 mcg/kg/week

Discontinue permanently if unable to tolerate 1 mcg/kg/week

Reduced dose schedule, Weeks 9 to 260:

First dose reduction (if prior dose 3 mcg/kg/week): 2 mcg/kg/week

Second dose reduction (if prior dose 2 mcg/kg/week): 1 mcg/kg/week

Discontinue permanently if unable to tolerate 1 mcg/kg/week

***Chronic hepatitis C:* Dosage adjustment for depression (severity based upon DSM-IV criteria):**

Mild depression: No dosage adjustment required; evaluate once weekly by visit/phone call. If depression remains stable, continue weekly visits. If depression improves, resume normal visit schedule. For worsening depression, see "Moderate depression" or "Severe depression" below.

Moderate depression: **Note:** Evaluate once weekly (visit or phone) with an office visit at least every other week. If depression remains stable, consider psychiatric evaluation and continue with reduced dosing. If symptoms improve and remain stable for 4 weeks, resume normal visit schedule; continue reduced dosing or return to normal dose. For worsening depression, see "Severe depression" below.

Children: Decrease peginterferon alfa-2b dose to 40 mcg/m²/week, may further decrease to 20 mcg/m²/week if needed

Adults:

Peginterferon alfa-2b combination therapy: Refer to adult weight-based dosage reduction with combination therapy for depression below

Peginterferon alfa-2b monotherapy: Refer to adult weight-based dosage reduction with monotherapy for depression below

Severe depression: Discontinue peginterferon alfa-2b and ribavirin permanently. Obtain immediate psychiatric consultation. Utilize followup psychiatric therapy as needed.

***Chronic hepatitis C:* Dosage adjustment in hematologic toxicity:**

Children:

Hemoglobin decrease ≥2 g/dL in any 4-week period and stable cardiac disease: Decrease peginterferon alfa-2b dose by 50%; decrease ribavirin dose by 200 mg daily (regardless of the patient's initial dose); monitor and evaluate weekly. If hemoglobin <8.5 g/dL any time after dose reduction or <12 g/dL after 4 weeks of dose reduction, permanently discontinue both peginterferon alfa-2b and ribavirin.

Hemoglobin 8.5 to <10 g/dL and no history of cardiac disease: Decrease ribavirin dose to 12 mg/kg/day; may further reduce to 8 mg/kg/day; no dosage adjustment necessary for peginterferon alfa-2b.

WBC 1000 to <1500/mm³, neutrophils 500 to <750/mm³, or platelets 50,000 to <70,000/mm³: Reduce peginterferon alfa-2b dose to 40 mcg/m²/week; may further reduce to 20 mcg/m²/week

Hemoglobin <8.5 g/dL, WBC <1000/mm³, neutrophils <500/mm³, or platelets <50,000/mm³: Permanently discontinue peginterferon alfa-2b and ribavirin

Adults:

Hemoglobin decrease ≥2 g/dL in any 4-week period and stable cardiac disease: Decrease peginterferon alfa-2b dose by 50%; decrease ribavirin dose by 200 mg daily. If hemoglobin <8.5 g/dL any time after dose reduction or <12 g/dL after 4 weeks of dose reduction, permanently discontinue both peginterferon alfa-2b and ribavirin.

Hemoglobin 8.5 to <10 g/dL and no history of cardiac disease: Decrease ribavirin dose by 200 mg daily (patients receiving 1400 mg daily should decrease dose by 400 mg daily [ie, first dose reduction to 1000 mg daily]); may further reduce ribavirin dose by additional 200 mg daily if needed. No dosage adjustment necessary for peginterferon alfa-2b.

WBC 1000 to <1500/mm³, neutrophils 500 to <750/mm³, or platelets 25,000 to <50,000/mm³:

Peginterferon alfa-2b combination therapy: Refer to adult weight-based dosage reduction with combination therapy for hematologic toxicity below.

Peginterferon alfa-2b monotherapy: Refer to adult weight-based dosage reduction monotherapy for hematologic toxicity below.

Hemoglobin <8.5 g/dL, WBC <1000/mm³, neutrophils <500/mm³, or platelets <25,000/mm³: Permanently discontinue peginterferon alfa-2b and ribavirin.

***Chronic hepatitis C:* Adult weight-based dosage reduction for depression or hematologic toxicity:**

Peginterferon alfa-2b combination therapy: Initially reduce to average weekly dose of 1 mcg/kg; may further reduce to average weekly dose of 0.5 mcg/kg if needed as follows:

<40 kg: 35 mcg once weekly; may further reduce to 20 mcg once weekly if needed

40 to 50 kg: 45 mcg once weekly; may further reduce to 25 mcg once weekly if needed

51 to 60 kg: 50 mcg once weekly; may further reduce to 30 mcg once weekly if needed

61 to 75 kg: 64 mcg once weekly; may further reduce to 35 mcg once weekly if needed

76 to 85 kg: 80 mcg once weekly; may further reduce to 45 mcg once weekly if needed

86 to 104 kg: 96 mcg once weekly; may further reduce to 50 mcg once weekly if needed

105 to 125 kg: 108 mcg once weekly; may further reduce to 64 mcg once weekly if needed

>125 kg: 135 mcg once weekly; may further reduce to 72 mcg once weekly if needed

Peginterferon alfa-2b monotherapy: Reduce to average weekly dose of 0.5 mcg/kg as follows:

≤45 kg: 20 mcg once weekly

46 to 56 kg: 25 mcg once weekly

57 to 72 kg: 30 mcg once weekly

73 to 88 kg: 40 mcg once weekly

89 to 106 kg: 50 mcg once weekly

107 to 136 kg: 64 mcg once weekly

≥137 kg: 80 mcg once weekly

Additional Information Complete prescribing information should be consulted for additional detail.

Dosage Forms Excipient information presented when available (limited, particularly for generics); consult specific product labeling. [DSC] = Discontinued product

Kit, Subcutaneous:

Sylatron: 4 x 200 mcg, 4 x 300 mcg, 4 x 600 mcg [DSC] [contains polysorbate 80]

Kit, Subcutaneous [preservative free]:

Peg-Intron: 50 mcg/0.5 mL, 80 mcg/0.5 mL, 120 mcg/0.5 mL, 150 mcg/0.5 mL

Peg-Intron Redipen: 50 mcg/0.5 mL, 80 mcg/0.5 mL, 120 mcg/0.5 mL, 150 mcg/0.5 mL

Peg-Intron Redipen Pak 4: 50 mcg/0.5 mL [DSC], 80 mcg/0.5 mL [DSC], 120 mcg/0.5 mL, 150 mcg/0.5 mL [DSC]

PegIntron: 50 mcg/0.5 mL, 80 mcg/0.5 mL, 120 mcg/0.5 mL, 150 mcg/0.5 mL [contains polysorbate 80]

Sylatron: 200 mcg, 300 mcg, 600 mcg [contains polysorbate 80]

Peginterferon Beta-1a
(peg inter FEER on BAY ta wun ay)

Brand Names: US Plegridy; Plegridy Starter Pack

Pharmacologic Category Biological Response Modulator; Immunomodulator, Systemic; Interferon

Use Multiple sclerosis: Treatment of patients with relapsing forms of multiple sclerosis

Medication Guide Available Yes

Dosing

Adult & Geriatric Multiple sclerosis: SubQ: Initial: 63 mcg on day 1; 94 mcg on day 15. Maintenance: 125 mcg every 14 days beginning on day 29. **Note:** Analgesics and/or antipyretics may help decrease flu-like symptoms during treatment.

Renal Impairment There are no dosage adjustments provided in the manufacturer's labeling; use with caution in severe renal impairment (CrCl <30 mL/minute).

Hepatic Impairment There are no dosage adjustments provided in the manufacturer's labeling.

Additional Information Complete prescribing information should be consulted for additional detail.

Dosage Forms Excipient information presented when available (limited, particularly for generics); consult specific product labeling.

Solution Pen-injector, Subcutaneous:
Plegridy: 125 mcg/0.5 mL (0.5 mL) [contains mouse protein (murine) (hamster)]
Plegridy Starter Pack: 63 mcg/0.5 mL & 94 mcg/0.5 mL (1 mL) [contains mouse protein (murine) (hamster)]

Solution Prefilled Syringe, Subcutaneous:
Plegridy: 125 mcg/0.5 mL (0.5 mL) [contains mouse protein (murine) (hamster)]
Plegridy Starter Pack: 63 mcg/0.5 mL & 94 mcg/0.5 mL (1 mL) [contains mouse protein (murine) (hamster)]

◆ Peg-Intron *see* Peginterferon Alfa-2b *on page 1411*

◆ PegIntron (Can) *see* Peginterferon Alfa-2b *on page 1411*

◆ Peg-Intron Redipen *see* Peginterferon Alfa-2b *on page 1411*

◆ Peg-Intron Redipen Pak 4 *see* Peginterferon Alfa-2b *on page 1411*

◆ PEGLA *see* Pegaspargase *on page 1407*

Pegloticase (peg LOE ti kase)

Brand Names: US Krystexxa
Index Terms PEG-Uricase; Pegylated Urate Oxidase; Polyethylene Glycol-Conjugated Uricase; Recombinant Urate Oxidase, Pegylated; Urate Oxidase, Pegylated
Pharmacologic Category Enzyme; Enzyme, Urate-Oxidase (Recombinant)
Use
Gout: Treatment of chronic gout in adult patients refractory to conventional therapy
Limitations of use: Not for the treatment of asymptomatic hyperuricemia
Pregnancy Considerations Adverse events have been observed in some animal reproduction studies.
Breast-Feeding Considerations It is not known if pegloticase is excreted in breast milk. The manufacturer does not recommend breast-feeding unless the potential benefit to the mother is greater than the possible risk to the infant.
Medication Guide Available Yes
Contraindications Glucose-6-phosphate dehydrogenase (G6PD) deficiency
Warnings/Precautions [US Boxed Warning]: Anaphylaxis and infusion reactions have been reported during and after administration; patients should be closely monitored during infusion and for an appropriate period of time after the infusion. Therapy should be administered in a health care facility by skilled medical personnel prepared for the immediate treatment of anaphylaxis. All patients should be premedicated with antihistamines and corticosteroids. Anaphylaxis may occur at any time during treatment (including the initial dose). Reactions generally occur within 2 hours of administration; however, delayed hypersensitivity reactions have also been reported. Infusion reactions are varied; symptoms range from chest pain, pruritus/urticaria, or dyspnea to a clinical presentation of anaphylaxis (eg, hemodynamic instability, perioral or lingual edema). If a less severe (nonanaphylactic) infusion reaction occurs, the infusion may be slowed, or stopped and restarted at a slower rate, at the physician's discretion. Risk of an infusion reaction is increased in patients whose uric acid is >6 mg/dL; therefore, **monitor serum uric acid concentrations prior to infusion and consider discontinuing treatment if concentrations exceed 6 mg/dL, particularly in the event of 2 consecutive concentrations >6 mg/dL.** Since oral antihyperuricemic agents may blunt the rise of serum uric acid levels, discontinue use prior to and do not initiate during the course of pegloticase therapy.

Therapy with antihyperuricemic agents commonly results in gout flare, particularly upon initiation due to rapid lowering of urate concentrations; gout flare-ups during treatment do not warrant discontinuation of therapy. Gout flare prophylaxis is recommended, using nonsteroidal anti-inflammatory agents (NSAID) or colchicines, unless contraindicated, beginning ≥1 week before initiation of pegloticase and continuing for at least 6 months. Exacerbation of heart failure has been observed in clinical trials; use caution in patients with preexisting heart failure. Due to the risk for hemolysis and methemoglobinemia, pegloticase is contraindicated in patients with G6PD deficiency. Patients at higher risk for G6PD deficiency (eg, African, Mediterranean) should be screened prior to therapy. Potential for immunogenicity exists with the use of therapeutic proteins. Antipegloticase antibodies and antiPEG antibodies commonly occurred during clinical trials in pegloticase-treated patients. High antipegloticase antibody

titers were associated with failure to maintain uric acid normalization and were also associated with a higher incidence of infusion reactions. Due to potential for immunogenicity, closely monitor patients who reinitiate therapy after discontinuing treatment for >4 weeks; patients may be at increased risk for anaphylaxis and infusion reactions.

Adverse Reactions
>10%:
Dermatologic: Bruising (11%), urticaria (11%)
Gastrointestinal: Nausea (12%)
Miscellaneous: Antibody formation (antipegloticase antibodies: 92%; antiPEG antibodies: 42%), gout flare (74% within the first 3 months), infusion reactions (26%)
1% to 10%:
Cardiovascular: Chest pain (6% to 10%)
Dermatologic: Erythema (10%), pruritus (10%)
Gastrointestinal: Constipation (6%), vomiting (5%)
Respiratory: Dyspnea (7%), nasopharyngitis (7%)
Miscellaneous: Anaphylaxis (≤7%)
Frequency not defined: Anemia, diarrhea, headache, muscle spasms, nephrolithiasis

Drug Interactions
Metabolism/Transport Effects None known.
Avoid Concomitant Use
Avoid concomitant use of Pegloticase with any of the following: Allopurinol; Febuxostat; Probenecid
Increased Effect/Toxicity
The levels/effects of Pegloticase may be increased by: Allopurinol; Febuxostat; Probenecid
Decreased Effect
Pegloticase may decrease the levels/effects of: Certolizumab Pegol; Pegademase Bovine; Pegaptanib; Pegaspargase; Pegfilgrastim; Peginterferon Alfa-2a; Peginterferon Alfa-2b; Pegvisomant
Preparation for Administration To prepare solution for administration, withdraw 1 mL (8 mg) and add to a 250 mL bag of NS or 1/2NS; invert bag several times to mix thoroughly (do **not** shake). Do not use vial if particulate matter is present or if solution is discolored (solution should be a clear and colorless). After withdrawal, discard any unused portion of the product remaining in the vial.
Storage/Stability Prior to use, vials must be stored in the carton to protect from light, and kept under refrigeration between 2°C to 8°C (36°F to 46°F) at all times. Do **not** shake or freeze.

Diluted solution may be stored up to 4 hours at 2°C to 8°C (36°F to 46°F). Diluted solution is also stable for 4 hours at room temperature of 20°C to 25°C (68°F to 77°F); however, refrigeration is preferred. The diluted solution should be protected from light, not frozen, and used within 4 hours of dilution. Prior to administration, allow the diluted solution to reach room temperature; do not warm to room temperature using any form of artificial heating such as a microwave or warm water bath.

Mechanism of Action Pegloticase is a pegylated recombinant form of urate-oxidase enzyme, also known as uricase (an enzyme normally absent in humans and high primates), which converts uric acid to allantoin (an inactive and water soluble metabolite of uric acid); it does not inhibit the formation of uric acid.

Pharmacodynamics/Kinetics
Onset of action: ~24 hours following the first dose, serum uric acid concentrations decreased
Duration: >300 hours (12.5 days)
Half-life elimination: Median: ~14 days
Excretion: Urine (as allantoin)

Dosing
Adult & Geriatric Note: Discontinue use of oral antihyperuricemic agents prior to initiating pegloticase and do not initiate during the course of therapy. Premedicate with antihistamines and corticosteroids. Gout flare prophylaxis with either NSAIDs or colchicine is also recommended, beginning at least 1 week prior to initiation and continuing for at least 6 months.

Gout: IV: 8 mg every 2 weeks
Renal Impairment No dosage adjustment necessary.
Hepatic Impairment There are no dosage adjustments provided in the manufacturer's labeling (has not been studied).

Administration Administer diluted solution by IV infusion over ≥120 minutes via gravity feed or an infusion pump or syringe-type pump. Do **not** administer by IV push or bolus. Administer in a healthcare setting by healthcare providers prepared to manage potential anaphylaxis. Monitor closely for infusion reactions during infusion and for an appropriate period of time after the infusion (anaphylaxis has been reported within 2 hours of the infusion). In the event or a less severe infusion reaction, infusion may be slowed, or stopped and restarted at a slower rate, based on the discretion of the physician.

◀ **Monitoring Parameters** Serum uric acid levels (prior to infusions; consider discontinuation if levels increase to >6 mg/dL, especially if two consecutive levels of >6 mg/dL are observed); infusion reactions and anaphylaxis (during infusion and post-infusion), G6PD deficiency screening (in patients at high risk for deficiency)

Reference Range

Uric acid, serum: An increase occurs during childhood
Adults:

Males: 3.4 to 7 mg/dL or slightly more
Females: 2.4 to 6 mg/dL or slightly more
Values >7 mg/dL are sometimes arbitrarily regarded as hyperuricemia, but there is no sharp line between normals on the one hand, and the serum uric acid of those with clinical gout. Normal ranges cannot be adjusted for purine ingestion, but high purine diet increases uric acid. Uric acid may be increased with body size, exercise, and stress.

Dosage Forms Excipient information presented when available (limited, particularly for generics); consult specific product labeling. [DSC] = Discontinued product
Solution, Intravenous:
Krystexxa: 8 mg/mL (1 mL [DSC])
Solution, Intravenous [preservative free]:
Krystexxa: 8 mg/mL (1 mL)

◆ PegLyte (Can) see Polyethylene Glycol-Electrolyte Solution on page 1466

◆ PEG-Uricase see Pegloticase on page 1413

Pegvisomant (peg VI soe mant)

Brand Names: US Somavert
Brand Names: Canada Somavert
Index Terms B2036-PEG
Pharmacologic Category Growth Hormone Receptor Antagonist
Use Acromegaly: Treatment of acromegaly in patients who have had an inadequate response to surgery or radiation therapy, or for whom these therapies are not appropriate.

Dosing

Adult & Geriatric Acromegaly: SubQ: Initial loading dose: 40 mg; maintenance dose: 10 mg once daily following initial loading dose; doses may be adjusted by 5 mg increments or decrements in 4- to 6-week intervals based on IGF-I concentrations (maximum maintenance dose: 30 mg daily)

Renal Impairment There are no dosage adjustments provided in the manufacturer's labeling (has not been studied).

Hepatic Impairment

At initiation of therapy:
Normal liver function test (LFT): Initiate therapy; monitor LFT monthly for first 6 months, quarterly for next 6 months, then biannually the following year.
Baseline LFT elevated but ≤3 x ULN: May initiate therapy with monthly evaluation of LFT for 1 year then biannually the following year.
Baseline LFT >3 times ULN: Do not initiate treatment without comprehensive work-up to determine cause; monitor closely if treatment is started.
With ongoing therapy:
LFT ≥3 x but <5 x ULN without signs/symptoms of hepatitis, hepatic injury, or increase in total bilirubin: Continue treatment, but monitor LFT weekly for further increases; perform comprehensive hepatic work-up to rule out alternative cause of hepatic dysfunction
LFT ≥5 x ULN or transaminase ≥3 x ULN associated with any increase in total bilirubin (with or without signs/symptoms of hepatitis or other liver injury): Discontinue immediately and perform comprehensive hepatic work-up. If LFTs return to normal, may cautiously consider restarting therapy with frequent LFT monitoring.
Signs or symptoms of hepatitis or hepatic injury: Perform comprehensive hepatic work-up; discontinue permanently if liver injury is confirmed.

Additional Information Complete prescribing information should be consulted for additional detail.

Dosage Forms Excipient information presented when available (limited, particularly for generics); consult specific product labeling.
Solution Reconstituted, Subcutaneous:
Somavert: 10 mg (1 ea); 15 mg (1 ea); 20 mg (1 ea); 25 mg (1 ea); 30 mg (1 ea)

◆ Pegylated DOXOrubicin Liposomal see DOXOrubicin (Liposomal) on page 597

◆ Pegylated G-CSF see Pegfilgrastim on page 1407

◆ Pegylated Interferon Alfa-2a see Peginterferon Alfa-2a on page 1409

◆ Pegylated Interferon Alfa-2b see Peginterferon Alfa-2b on page 1411

◆ Pegylated Liposomal DOXOrubicin see DOXOrubicin (Liposomal) on page 597

◆ Pegylated Liposomal DOXOrubicin Hydrochloride (Doxil, Caelyx) see DOXOrubicin (Liposomal) on page 597

◆ Pegylated Urate Oxidase see Pegloticase on page 1413

◆ PEGyLAX see Polyethylene Glycol 3350 on page 1465

◆ PeleVerus [OTC] see Sodium Chloride on page 1671

Pembrolizumab (pem broe LIZ ue mab)

Brand Names: US Keytruda
Brand Names: Canada Keytruda
Index Terms Anti-PD-1 Monoclonal Antibody MK-3475; Lambrolizumab; MK-3475; SCH 90045
Pharmacologic Category Antineoplastic Agent, Anti-PD-1 Monoclonal Antibody; Antineoplastic Agent, Monoclonal Antibody

Use

US labeling:

Melanoma, unresectable or metastatic: Treatment of unresectable or metastatic melanoma

Non-small cell lung cancer, metastatic: Treatment of metastatic non-small cell lung cancer in patients with PD-L1-expressing tumors (as determined by an approved test) who have disease progression on or after platinum-containing chemotherapy. Patients with EGFR or ALK genomic tumor aberrations should have disease progression (on approved EGFR- or ALK-directed therapy) prior to receiving pembrolizumab.

Canadian labeling: **Melanoma:** Treatment of unresectable or metastatic melanoma with disease progression following ipilimumab and if BRAF V600 mutation positive, a BRAF inhibitor or MEK inhibitor.

Pregnancy Considerations Animal reproduction studies have not been conducted. Immunoglobulins are known to cross the placenta; therefore fetal exposure to pembrolizumab is expected. Based on the mechanism of action, pembrolizumab may cause fetal harm if administered during pregnancy; an alteration in the immune response or immune mediated disorders may develop following in utero exposure. Women of reproductive potential should use highly effective contraception during therapy and for at least 4 months after treatment is complete.

Breast-Feeding Considerations It is not known if pembrolizumab is excreted into breast milk. The manufacturer recommends that breast-feeding be discontinued during therapy and for 4 months following the final dose. Immunoglobulins are excreted in breast milk; therefore pembrolizumab may be expected to appear in breast milk.

Medication Guide Available Yes

Contraindications

There are no contraindications listed in the manufacturer's US labeling.
Canadian labeling: Hypersensitivity to pembrolizumab or any component of the formulation.

Warnings/Precautions Immune-mediated pneumonitis has been observed, including fatal cases. For patients with melanoma, the median time to development was 4.3 months (range: ~2 days to ~19 months) and the median duration was 2.6 months (range: 2 days to ~15 months). Some patients required initial management with high-dose systemic corticosteroids, the median duration of initial corticosteroid therapy was 8 days (range: 1 to 34 days) followed by a corticosteroid taper. For patients with NSCLC, the median time to development was 1.7 months (range: 4 days to ~13 months) and the median duration was 1.2 months (range: 5 days to ~12 months). Some NSCLC patients had complete resolution of pneumonitis. May require treatment interruption, corticosteroid therapy (prednisone 1 to 2 mg/kg /day [or equivalent] followed by a taper, for grade 2 or higher pneumonitis), and/or permanent discontinuation. Monitor for signs and symptoms of pneumonitis; if pneumonitis is suspected, evaluate with radiographic imaging and administer systemic corticosteroids for grade 2 or higher pneumonitis. For NSCLC, pneumonitis occurred more frequently in patients with a history of asthma, COPD, or prior thoracic radiation.

Immune-mediated colitis has occurred, including cases of grade 2 to 4 colitis. The median time to onset of colitis was 3.4 months (range: 10 days to ~10 months) and the mediation duration was 1.4 months (range: 1 day to ~7 months) in patients with melanoma. In patients with NSCLC, the median time to onset was 1.6 months (range: ~1 to ~2 months) and the median duration was 16 days (range: 1 to ~6 weeks). In some melanoma patients, colitis was managed with high-dose systemic corticosteroids for a median duration of 6 days (range: 1 day to 5.3 months),

followed by a corticosteroid taper. Most patients with colitis experienced complete resolution. May require treatment interruption, systemic corticosteroid therapy, and/or permanent discontinuation. Monitor for signs and symptoms of colitis; administer systemic corticosteroids for grade 2 or higher colitis.

Immune-mediated hepatitis occurred (grades 2 to 4 hepatitis). The median onset for hepatitis was 26 days (range: 8 days to 21.4 months); the median duration was 1.2 months (range: 8 days to 4.7 months). Hepatitis resolved in most patients. Administer corticosteroids (prednisone 0.5 to 1 mg/kg/day [or equivalent] for grade 2 hepatitis, and prednisone 1 to 2 mg/kg/day [or equivalent] for grade 3 or higher, each followed by a taper), and withhold or discontinue therapy based on the severity of liver enzyme elevations. The median duration of high-dose corticosteroid therapy was 5 days (range: 1 to 14 days) followed by a taper. Monitor for liver function changes. May require treatment interruption, systemic corticosteroids (for grade 2 or higher toxicity), and/or permanent discontinuation.

Immune-mediated hypophysitis occurred (grades 2, 3, and 4). In patients with melanoma, the median time to onset was 3.3 months (range: 1 days to 7.2 months) and the median duration was 2.7 months (range 12 days to 12.7 months). The time to onset in NSCLC (1 patient) was 3.7 months. Monitor for signs/symptoms of hypophysitis (eg, hypopituitarism, adrenal insufficiency). May require treatment interruption, systemic corticosteroids, and hormone replacement (as clinically indicated), and/or permanent discontinuation.

Immune-mediated nephritis has occurred. The onset for autoimmune nephritis in melanoma patients was 5.1 months (range: 12 days to 12.8 months) and the median duration was 1.1 months (range: 3 days to 3.3 months). Grade 2 or higher nephritis should be managed with systemic corticosteroids (prednisone initial dose of 1 to 2 mg/kg/day [or equivalent], followed by a taper). The median duration of corticosteroid use was 15 days (range: 3 days to 1.6 months), followed by a taper. Nephritis resolved in some patients. Grade 2 or higher nephritis should be managed with systemic corticosteroids (prednisone initial dose of 1 to 2 mg/kg/day [or equivalent], followed by a taper). The median duration of corticosteroid use was 15 days (range: 3 days to 1.6 months), followed by a taper. Nephritis resolved in some patients. Monitor for renal function changes. May require treatment interruption, systemic corticosteroids (for grade 2 or higher toxicity), and/or permanent discontinuation.

Immune-mediated hyperthyroidism and hypothyroidism have occurred. The median onset for hyperthyroidism was 1.4 to 1.8 months (range: 1 day to ~22 months), and the median duration was 1.7 to 4.5 months (range: 1 day to ~13 months). Hyperthyroidism resolved in over two-thirds of melanoma patients. Hypothyroidism occurred with a median onset of 3.3 to 4.2 months (range: 5 days to 19 months) and median duration of 5.4 to 5.8 months (range: 6 days to 24.3 months). Hypothyroidism was generally managed with long-term thyroid hormone replacement therapy, although some patients only required short-term replacement therapy. Hypothyroidism did not require systemic corticosteroid therapy or discontinuation. Thyroid disorders may occur at any point in pembrolizumab therapy. Monitor for changes in thyroid function (at baseline, periodically during treatment and as clinically indicated) and for signs/symptoms of thyroid disorder. Administer thionamides and beta-blockers for hyperthyroidism as appropriate; may require treatment interruption and/or permanent discontinuation. Isolated hypothyroidism may be managed with replacement therapy (without corticosteroids and treatment interruption). Type 1 diabetes mellitus has occurred (including diabetic ketoacidosis). Insulin therapy may be required; if severe hyperglycemia is observed, administer antihyperglycemics and withhold pembrolizumab treatment until glucose control has been accomplished.

Other clinically relevant immune-mediated disorders have been observed, including rash, exfoliative dermatitis, bullous pemphigoid, uveitis, arthritis, vasculitis, myositis, Guillain-Barré syndrome, pancreatitis, hemolytic anemia, serum sickness, myasthenia gravis, and partial seizures (in a patient with inflammatory foci in brain parenchyma). If an immune-mediated adverse event is suspected, evaluate appropriately to confirm or exclude other causes; withhold treatment and administer systemic corticosteroids based on severity of reaction. Upon resolution to grade 0 or 1, initiate corticosteroid taper (continue tapering over at least 1 month). When reaction remains at grade 1 or less during taper may reinitiate pembrolizumab. Immune-mediated adverse reactions that do not resolve with systemic corticosteroids may be managed with other systemic

immunosuppressants (based on limited data). Discontinue permanently for severe or grade 3 immune-mediated adverse event that is recurrent or life-threatening. Infusion-related reactions (including severe and life-threatening cases) have occurred. Interrupt infusion for severe (grade 3) or life-threatening (grade 4) reactions; and permanently discontinue for severe (grade 3) or life-threatening (grade 4) infusion-related reactions.

Adverse Reactions

>10%:

Cardiovascular: Peripheral edema (17%; grade 3: 1%)

Central nervous system: Fatigue (47%; grade 3: 7%), headache (16%), chills (14%), insomnia (14%), dizziness (11%)

Dermatologic: Pruritus (30%), skin rash (29%), vitiligo (11%)

Endocrine & metabolic: Hyperglycemia (40%; grade 3: 1%; grade 4: 1%), hyponatremia (35%; grade 3: 9%), hypoalbuminemia (34%), hypertriglyceridemia (25%), hypocalcemia (24%; grade 3: 1%)

Gastrointestinal: Nausea (30%), decreased appetite (26%), constipation (21%), diarrhea (20%), vomiting (16%), abdominal pain (12%)

Hematologic & oncologic: Anemia (14% to 55%; grade 3: 5% to 7%; grade 4: 1%)

Hepatic: Increased serum AST (24%; grade 3: 1%; grade 4: 1%)

Neuromuscular & skeletal: Arthralgia (20%), limb pain (18%; grade 3: 1%), myalgia (14%; grade 3: 1%), back pain (12%; grade 3: 1%)

Respiratory: Cough (30%; grade 3: 1%), dyspnea (18%; grade 3: 2%), upper respiratory tract infection (11%; grade 3: 1%)

Miscellaneous: Fever (11%)

1% to 10%:

Dermatologic: Cellulitis (≥2%)

Endocrine & metabolic: Hypothyroidism (immune-mediated; 8%; grade 3: <1%), hyperthyroidism (immune-mediated; 1%; grade 2: <1%; grade 3: <1%)

Gastrointestinal: Colitis (including microscopic colitis: 1%; grade 2: <1%, grade 3: <1%)

Infection: Sepsis (≤10%)

Renal: Renal failure (≥2%)

Respiratory: Pneumonitis (3%; grade 2: 2%; grade 3: <1%), pneumonia (≥2%)

<1% (Limited to important or life-threatening): Adrenocortical insufficiency (immune-mediated), arthritis (immune-mediated), bullous pemphigoid, diabetic ketoacidosis, exfoliative dermatitis (immune-mediated), hemolytic anemia (immune-mediated), hepatitis (including autoimmune hepatitis; grade 4: <1%), hypophysitis (grade 2: <1%; grade 4: <1%), infusion related reaction, interstitial nephritis (with renal failure; grade 3: <1%; grade 4: <1%), Lambert-Eaton syndrome (immune-mediated), myositis (immune-mediated), nephritis (grade 2 autoimmune: <1%), optic neuritis (immune-mediated), pancreatitis (immune-mediated), partial epilepsy (immune-mediated; in a patient with inflammatory foci in brain parenchyma), rhabdomyolysis (immune-mediated), severe dermatitis, type 1 diabetes mellitus, uveitis (immune-mediated)

Drug Interactions

Metabolism/Transport Effects None known.

Avoid Concomitant Use There are no known interactions where it is recommended to avoid concomitant use.

Increased Effect/Toxicity There are no known significant interactions involving an increase in effect.

Decreased Effect There are no known significant interactions involving a decrease in effect.

Preparation for Administration

Injection solution (100 mg/4 mL vial): Withdraw appropriate volume from vial and transfer to IV bag containing 0.9% sodium chloride or D_5W; final concentration should be between 1 to 10 mg/mL. Mix by gently inverting bag. Discard unused portion of the vial.

Lyophilized powder (50 mg vial): Reconstitute by adding 2.3 mL SWFI along the vial wall (do not add directly to lyophilized powder); resulting vial concentration is 25 mg/mL. Slowly swirl vial; do not shake. Allow up to 5 minutes for bubbles to dissipate. Reconstituted solution is a clear to slightly opalescent and colorless to slightly yellow solution; discard if visible particles present. Withdraw appropriate volume from vial and transfer to IV bag containing 0.9% sodium chloride or D_5W final concentration should be between 1 to 10 mg/mL. Mix by gently inverting bag. Discard unused portion of the vial.

Storage/Stability Lyophilized powder (50 mg vial) and injection solution (100 mg/4 mL vial): Store intact vials refrigerated at 2°C to 8°C (36°F to 46°F); protect injection solution vials from light and do not shake or freeze. Reconstituted solutions and solutions diluted for infusion may be stored at room temperature for up to 6 hours (infusion must be completed within 6 hours of ▶

reconstitution) or refrigerated at 2°C to 8°C (36°F to 46°F) for no more than 24 hours from the time of reconstitution. Do not freeze. If refrigerated, allow to reach room temperature prior to administration.

Mechanism of Action Highly selective anti-PD-1 humanized monoclonal antibody which inhibits programmed cell death-1 (PD-1) activity by binding to the PD-1 receptor on T-cells to block PD-1 ligands (PD-L1 and PD-L2) from binding. Blocking the PD-1 pathway inhibits the negative immune regulation caused by PD-1 receptor signaling (Hamid, 2013). Anti-PD-1 antibodies (including pembrolizumab) reverse T-cell suppression and induce antitumor responses (Robert, 2014).

Pharmacodynamics/Kinetics
V_{dss}: 7.38 L
Half-life elimination: 27 days

Dosing

Adult & Geriatric

Melanoma, unresectable or metastatic: IV: 2 mg/kg once every 3 weeks until disease progression or unacceptable toxicity.

Non-small cell lung cancer, metastatic: IV: 2 mg/kg once every 3 weeks until disease progression or unacceptable toxicity.

Renal Impairment

US labeling: No dosage adjustment necessary. In a pharmacokinetic study, no difference in clearance was noted for patients with mild, moderate, or severe impairment (eGFR ≥15 mL/minute to 89 mL/minute) when compared to patients with normal renal function (eGFR ≥90 mL/minute); patients with eGFR <15 mL/minute were not studied.

Canadian labeling: •

Mild or moderate impairment: eGFR ≥30 mL/minute/1.73 m² to <90 mL/minute/1.73 m²: No dosage adjustment necessary.

Severe impairment: There are no dosage adjustments provided in the manufacturer's labeling.

Hepatic Impairment

*Hepatic impairment **prior** to treatment initiation:*

Mild impairment (total bilirubin ≤ULN and AST >ULN or total bilirubin >1 to 1.5 times ULN and any AST): No dosage adjustment necessary.

Moderate (total bilirubin >1.5 to 3 times ULN and any AST) to severe (total bilirubin >3 times ULN and any AST) impairment: There are no dosage adjustments provided in the manufacturer's labeling (has not been studied).

*Hepatotoxicity **during** treatment:* **Note:** For patients with baseline grade 2 ALT or AST abnormalities due to liver metastases, permanently discontinue if AST or ALT increases by ≥50% (relative to baseline) and persists at least 1 week.

AST or ALT >3 to 5 times ULN or total bilirubin >1.5 to 3 times ULN: Withhold treatment; may resume therapy upon recovery to grade 0 or 1 toxicity. Also administer corticosteroids (prednisone 0.5 to 1 mg/kg/day [or equivalent] followed by a taper).

AST or ALT >5 times ULN or total bilirubin >3 times ULN: Permanently discontinue. Also administer corticosteroids (prednisone 1 to 2 mg/kg/day [or equivalent] followed by a taper).

Adjustment for Toxicity

Withhold treatment for any of the following (may resume upon recovery to grade 0 or 1 toxicity):

Colitis, moderate (grade 2) or severe (grade 3); also administer corticosteroids (prednisone 1 to 2 mg/kg/day [or equivalent] followed by a taper).

Endocrinopathies:

Hyperglycemia, severe; also administer antihyperglycemics.

Hyperthyroidism, severe (grade 3) or life threatening (grade 4); manage with thionamides and beta-blockers as appropriate.

Hypophysitis, grade 2 (symptomatic); also administer corticosteroids (followed by a taper) and hormone replacement therapy if appropriate.

Nephritis, grade 2; also administer corticosteroids (prednisone 1 to 2 mg/kg/day [or equivalent] followed by a taper).

Pneumonitis, moderate (grade 2); also administer corticosteroids (prednisone 1 to 2 mg/kg/day [or equivalent] followed by a taper).

Other treatment-related toxicity, severe or grade 3; may require corticosteroids (based on severity). Upon improvement to grade 0 or 1, initiate corticosteroid taper and continue to taper over at least 1 month. Restart pembrolizumab if the adverse reaction remains at grade 0 or 1 following corticosteroid taper. May consider other systemic immunosuppressants if not controlled by corticosteroids (based on limited data).

Withhold (may resume upon recovery to grade 0 or 1 toxicity) or discontinue for:

Hyperthyroidism, severe (grade 3) or life-threatening (grade 4); manage with thionamides and beta-blockers as appropriate.

Hypophysitis, severe (grade 3) or life-threatening (grade 4); also administer corticosteroids and hormone replacement as appropriate.

Permanently discontinue for:

Adverse reactions that are life-threatening, persistent grade 2 or 3 adverse reaction (excluding endocrinopathies controlled with hormone replacement therapy) that does not recover to grade 0 or 1 within 12 weeks after the last pembrolizumab dose, or any recurrent severe or grade 3 treatment-related adverse reaction. Also administer corticosteroids (may consider other systemic immunosuppressants if not controlled by corticosteroids [based on limited data]).

Colitis, life-threatening (grade 4); also administer corticosteroids (prednisone 1 to 2 mg/kg/day [or equivalent] followed by a taper).

Immune mediated adverse reactions: Discontinue permanently if unable to reduce corticosteroid dose to prednisone ≤10 mg/day (or equivalent) within 12 weeks.

Infusion-related reaction, grade 3 or 4.

Nephritis, severe (grade 3) or life-threatening (grade 4); also administer corticosteroids (prednisone 1 to 2 mg/kg/day [or equivalent] followed by a taper).

Pneumonitis, severe (grade 3), life-threatening (grade 4), or moderate (grade 2) that recurs; also administer corticosteroids (prednisone 1 to 2 mg/kg/day [or equivalent] followed by a taper).

Administration IV: Infuse over 30 minutes through a 0.2 to 5 micron sterile, nonpyrogenic, low-protein binding inline or add-on filter. Do not infuse other medications through the same infusion line.

Monitoring Parameters PD-L1 expression status in patients with NSCLC; liver function tests (AST, ALT, and total bilirubin); renal function; thyroid function (at baseline, periodically during treatment and as clinically indicated); glucose; signs/symptoms of colitis, hypophysitis, thyroid disorders, pneumonitis, infusion reactions.

Dosage Forms Excipient information presented when available (limited, particularly for generics); consult specific product labeling.

Solution, Intravenous [preservative free]:
Keytruda: 100 mg/4 mL (4 mL) [contains polysorbate 80]
Solution Reconstituted, Intravenous [preservative free]:
Keytruda: 50 mg (1 ea) [contains polysorbate 80]

PEMEtrexed (pem e TREKS ed)

Brand Names: US Alimta
Brand Names: Canada Alimta
Index Terms LY231514; Pemetrexed Disodium
Pharmacologic Category Antineoplastic Agent, Antimetabolite; Antineoplastic Agent, Antimetabolite (Antifolate)

Use

Mesothelioma: Treatment of unresectable malignant pleural mesothelioma (in combination with cisplatin)

Non-small cell lung cancer (NSCLC), nonsquamous: Treatment of locally advanced or metastatic **non**squamous NSCLC (as initial treatment in combination with cisplatin, as single-agent maintenance treatment after 4 cycles of initial platinum-based double therapy, and single-agent treatment after prior chemotherapy)

Limitation of use: Not indicated for the treatment of **squamous** cell NSCLC

Pregnancy Considerations Adverse effects (embryotoxicity, fetotoxicity and teratogenicity) were observed in animal reproduction studies. Based on the mechanism of action, may cause fetal harm if administered to a pregnant woman. Women of childbearing potential should have a negative serum pregnancy test prior to treatment and should use effective contraceptive measures to avoid becoming pregnant during treatment. Irreversible infertility has been reported in males; prior to receiving treatment, males should be counseled on sperm storage. The Canadian labeling recommends that males receiving therapy use effective contraceptive measures and not father a child during, and for up to 6 months after therapy.

Breast-Feeding Considerations According to the manufacturer, the decision to continue or discontinue breast-feeding during therapy should take into account the risk of exposure to the infant and the benefits of treatment to the mother.

Contraindications Severe hypersensitivity to pemetrexed or any component of the formulation

Canadian labeling (additional contraindications; not in U.S. labeling): Concomitant yellow fever vaccine

Warnings/Precautions Hazardous agent - use appropriate precautions for handling and disposal (NIOSH 2014 [group 1]). Hypersensitivity (including anaphylaxis) has been reported with use. May cause bone marrow suppression (anemia, neutropenia, thrombocytopenia and/or pancytopenia); frequent laboratory monitoring is necessary (myelosuppression is often dose-limiting). Dose reductions in subsequent cycles may be required. Prophylactic folic acid and vitamin B$_{12}$ supplements are necessary to reduce hematologic and gastrointestinal toxicity and infection; initiate supplementation 1 week before the first dose of pemetrexed. Pretreatment with dexamethasone is necessary to reduce the incidence and severity of cutaneous reactions. Rarely, Stevens-Johnson syndrome and toxic epidermal necrolysis have been reported. Although the effect of third space fluid is not fully defined, studies have determined pemetrexed concentrations in patients with mild-to-moderate ascites/pleural effusions were similar to concentrations in trials of patients without third space fluid accumulation. Drainage of fluid from ascites/effusions may be considered, but is not likely necessary. Use caution with hepatic dysfunction not due to metastases; may require dose adjustment. Interstitial pneumonitis with respiratory insufficiency has been observed with use; interrupt therapy and evaluate promptly with progressive dyspnea and cough.

The manufacturer does not recommend use in patients with CrCl <45 mL/minute. Decreased renal function results in increased toxicity. Potentially significant drug-drug interactions may exist, requiring dose or frequency adjustment, additional monitoring, and/or selection of alternative therapy. Use caution in patients receiving concurrent nephrotoxins; may result in delayed pemetrexed clearance. NSAIDs may reduce the clearance of pemetrexed. In patients with CrCl 45-79 mL/minute, interruption of NSAID therapy may be necessary prior to, during, and immediately after pemetrexed therapy. Not indicated for use in patients with squamous cell NSCLC.

Adverse Reactions
>10%:
  Central nervous system: Fatigue (18% to 34%; dose-limiting)
  Dermatologic: Rash/desquamation (10% to 14%)
  Gastrointestinal: Nausea (12% to 31%), anorexia (19% to 22%), vomiting (6% to 16%), stomatitis (5% to 15%), diarrhea (5% to 13%)
  Hematologic: Anemia (15% to 19%; grades 3/4: 3% to 5%), leukopenia (6% to 12%; grades 3/4: 2% to 4%), neutropenia (6% to 11%; grades 3/4: 3% to 5%; dose-limiting; nadir: 8-10 days; recovery: 4-8 days after nadir)
  Respiratory: Pharyngitis (15%)
1% to 10%:
  Cardiovascular: Edema (1% to 5%)
  Central nervous system: Fever (1% to 8%)
  Dermatologic: Pruritus (1% to 7%), alopecia (1% to 6%), erythema multiforme (≤5%)
  Gastrointestinal: Constipation (1% to 6%), weight loss (1%), abdominal pain (≤5%)
  Hematologic: Thrombocytopenia (1% to 8%; grades 3/4: 2%; dose-limiting), febrile neutropenia (grades 3/4: 2%)
  Hepatic: ALT increased (8% to 10%; grades 3/4: ≤2%), AST increased (7% to 8%; grades 3/4: ≤1%)
  Neuromuscular & skeletal: Sensory neuropathy (≤9%), motor neuropathy (≤5%)
  Ocular: Conjunctivitis (≤5%), lacrimation increased (≤5%)
  Renal: Creatinine increased/creatinine clearance decreased (1% to 5%)
  Miscellaneous: Allergic reaction/hypersensitivity (≤5%), infection (≤5%), sepsis (1%)
<1% (Limited to important or life-threatening): Arrhythmia, colitis, dehydration, esophagitis, gastrointestinal obstruction, hemolytic anemia, hepatobiliary failure, hypertension, interstitial pneumonitis, pancreatitis, pancytopenia, peripheral ischemia, pulmonary embolism, radiation recall (median onset: 6 days; range: 1-35 days), renal failure, Stevens-Johnson syndrome, supraventricular arrhythmia, syncope, thrombosis/embolism, toxic epidermal necrolysis, ventricular tachycardia

Drug Interactions
Metabolism/Transport Effects None known.
Avoid Concomitant Use
  Avoid concomitant use of PEMEtrexed with any of the following: BCG (Intravesical); Deferiprone; Dipyrone; Natalizumab; Pimecrolimus; Tacrolimus (Topical); Tofacitinib; Vaccines (Live)
Increased Effect/Toxicity
  PEMEtrexed may increase the levels/effects of: CloZAPine; Deferiprone; Fingolimod; Leflunomide; Natalizumab; Tofacitinib; Vaccines (Live)

The levels/effects of PEMEtrexed may be increased by: Denosumab; Dipyrone; NSAID (Nonselective); Pimecrolimus; Roflumilast; Tacrolimus (Topical); Trastuzumab
Decreased Effect
  PEMEtrexed may decrease the levels/effects of: BCG (Intravesical); Coccidioides immitis Skin Test; Sipuleucel-T; Vaccines (Inactivated); Vaccines (Live)

The levels/effects of PEMEtrexed may be decreased by: Echinacea
Preparation for Administration Hazardous agent; use appropriate precautions for handling and disposal (NIOSH 2014 [group 1]). Reconstitute with NS (preservative free); add 4.2 mL to the 100 mg vial and 20 mL to the 500 mg vial, resulting in a 25 mg/mL concentration. Gently swirl. Solution may be colorless or green-yellow. Further dilute in 100 mL NS prior to infusion (the manufacturer recommends a total volume of 100 mL); may also dilute in D$_5$W (Zhang, 2006), although the manufacturer recommends NS.
Storage/Stability Store intact vials at room temperature of 25°C (77°F); excursions permitted to 15°C to 30°C (59°F to 86°F). Reconstituted solution in NS and infusion solutions (in D$_5$W or NS) are stable for 24 hours when refrigerated at 2°C to 8°C (36°F to 46°F). Concentrations at 25 mg/mL are stable in polypropylene syringes for 2 days at room temperature (23°C) (Zhang, 2005).
Mechanism of Action Antifolate; disrupts folate-dependent metabolic processes essential for cell replication. Inhibits thymidylate synthase (TS), dihydrofolate reductase (DHFR), glycinamide ribonucleotide formyltransferase (GARFT), and aminoimidazole carboxamide ribonucleotide formyltransferase (AICARFT), the enzymes involved in folate metabolism and DNA synthesis, resulting in inhibition of purine and thymidine nucleotide and protein synthesis.
Pharmacodynamics/Kinetics
Distribution: V$_{dss}$: 16.1 L
Protein binding: ~73% to 81%
Metabolism: Minimal
Half-life elimination: Normal renal function: 3.5 hours; CrCl 40 to 59 mL/minute: 5.3 to 5.8 hours
Excretion: Urine (70% to 90% as unchanged drug)
Dosing
Adult & Geriatric Note: Start vitamin supplements 1 week before initial pemetrexed dose: Folic acid 400 to 1000 mcg daily orally (begin 7 days prior to treatment initiation; continue daily during treatment and for 21 days after last pemetrexed dose) and vitamin B$_{12}$ 1000 mcg IM 7 days prior to treatment initiation and then every 3 cycles. Give dexamethasone 4 mg orally twice daily for 3 days, beginning the day before treatment to minimize cutaneous reactions. New treatment cycles should not begin unless ANC ≥1500/mm^3, platelets ≥100,000/mm^3, and CrCl ≥45 mL/minute.
Malignant pleural mesothelioma: IV: 500 mg/m^2 on day 1 of each 21-day cycle (in combination with cisplatin) **or** (off-label) in combination with carboplatin (Castagneto, 2008; Ceresoli, 2006) **or** (off-label) as single-agent therapy (Jassem, 2008; Taylor, 2008)

Non-small cell lung cancer, nonsquamous: IV:
  Initial treatment: 500 mg/m^2 on day 1 of each 21-day cycle (in combination with cisplatin)
  Maintenance or second-line treatment: 500 mg/m^2 on day 1 of each 21-day cycle (as a single-agent)
Bladder cancer, metastatic (off-label use): IV: 500 mg/m^2 on day 1 of each 21-day cycle until disease progression or unacceptable toxicity (Sweeney, 2006)
Cervical cancer, persistent or recurrent (off-label use): IV: 500 mg/m^2 on day 1 of each 21-day cycle until disease progression or unacceptable toxicity occurs (Lorusso, 2010) **or** 900 mg/m^2 on day 1 of each 21-day cycle (Miller, 2008)
Ovarian cancer, platinum-resistant (off-label use): IV: 500 mg/m^2 on day 1 of each 21-day cycle (Vergote, 2009)
Thymic malignancies, metastatic (off-label use): IV: 500 mg/m^2 on day 1 of each 21-day cycle for 6 cycles or until disease progression or unacceptable toxicity occurs (Loehrer, 2006)
Renal Impairment
Renal function may be estimated using the Cockcroft-Gault formula (using actual body weight) or glomerular filtration rate (GFR) measured by Tc99m-DPTA serum clearance.
CrCl ≥45 mL/minute: No dosage adjustment necessary.
CrCl <45 mL/minute: Use is not recommended (an insufficient number of patients have been studied for dosage recommendations).

◀

Concomitant NSAID use with renal dysfunction:
CrCl ≥80 mL/minute: No dosage adjustment necessary.
CrCl 45 to 79 mL/minute and NSAIDs with short half-lives (eg, ibuprofen, indomethacin, ketoprofen, ketorolac): Avoid NSAID for 2 days before, the day of, and for 2 days following a dose of pemetrexed.
Any creatinine clearance and NSAIDs with long half-lives (eg, nabumetone, naproxen, oxaprozin, piroxicam): Avoid NSAID for 5 days before, the day of, and 2 days following a dose of pemetrexed.

Hepatic Impairment Grade 3 (5.1 to 20 times ULN) **or** 4 (>20 times ULN) transaminase elevation during treatment: Reduce pemetrexed dose to 75% of previous dose (and cisplatin).

Obesity *ASCO Guidelines for appropriate chemotherapy dosing in obese adults with cancer:* Utilize patient's actual body weight (full weight) for calculation of body surface area- or weight-based dosing, particularly when the intent of therapy is curative; manage regimen-related toxicities in the same manner as for nonobese patients; if a dose reduction is utilized due to toxicity, consider resumption of full weight-based dosing with subsequent cycles, especially if cause of toxicity (eg, hepatic or renal impairment) is resolved (Griggs, 2012).

Adjustment for Toxicity
Toxicity: Discontinue if patient develops grade 3 or 4 toxicity after two dose reductions or immediately if grade 3 or 4 neurotoxicity develops
Hematologic toxicity: Upon recovery, reinitiate therapy
Nadir ANC <500/mm^3 and nadir platelets ≥50,000/mm^3: Reduce dose to 75% of previous dose of pemetrexed (and cisplatin)
Nadir platelets <50,000/mm^3 **without bleeding** (regardless of nadir ANC): Reduce dose to 75% of previous dose of pemetrexed (and cisplatin)
Nadir platelets <50,000/mm^3 **with bleeding** (regardless of nadir ANC): Reduce dose to 50% of previous dose of pemetrexed (and cisplatin)
Nonhematologic toxicity ≥ grade 3 (excluding neurotoxicity): Withhold treatment until recovery to baseline; upon recovery, reinitiate therapy as follows:
Grade 3 or 4 toxicity (excluding mucositis): Reduce dose to 75% of previous dose of pemetrexed (and cisplatin)
Grade 3 or 4 diarrhea or any diarrhea requiring hospitalization: Reduce dose to 75% of previous dose of pemetrexed (and cisplatin)
Grade 3 or 4 mucositis: Reduce pemetrexed dose to 50% of previous dose (continue cisplatin at 100% of previous dose)
Neurotoxicity:
Grade 0 to 1: Continue pemetrexed at 100% of previous dose (and cisplatin)
Grade 2: Continue pemetrexed at 100% of previous dose; reduce cisplatin dose to 50% of previous dose

Dietary Considerations Initiate folic acid supplementation 1 week before first dose of pemetrexed, continue for full course of therapy, and for 21 days after last dose. Institute vitamin B$_{12}$ 1 week before the first dose; administer every 9 weeks thereafter.

Administration IV: Infuse over 10 minutes. Hazardous agent; use appropriate precautions for handling and disposal (NIOSH 2014 [group 1]).

Monitoring Parameters CBC with differential and platelets (before each dose; monitor for nadir and recovery); serum creatinine, creatinine clearance, BUN, total bilirubin, ALT, AST (periodic); signs/symptoms of mucositis and diarrhea

Dosage Forms Excipient information presented when available (limited, particularly for generics); consult specific product labeling.
Solution Reconstituted, Intravenous:
Alimta: 100 mg (1 ea); 500 mg (1 ea)

◆ Pemetrexed Disodium *see* PEMEtrexed *on page 1416*

Penciclovir (pen SYE kloe veer)

Brand Names: US Denavir
Pharmacologic Category Antiviral Agent
Use Topical treatment of recurrent herpes simplex labialis (cold sores)
Dosing
Adult & Geriatric Herpes simplex labialis (cold sores): Topical: Apply cream at the first sign or symptom of cold sore (eg, tingling, swelling); apply every 2 hours during waking hours for 4 days.
Pediatric Herpes simplex labialis (cold sores): Children ≥12 years: Refer to adult dosing.
Additional Information Complete prescribing information should be consulted for additional detail.

Dosage Forms Excipient information presented when available (limited, particularly for generics); consult specific product labeling. [DSC] = Discontinued product
Cream, External:
Denavir: 1% (1.5 g [DSC], 5 g) [contains cetostearyl alcohol, propylene glycol]

PenicillAMINE (pen i SIL a meen)

Brand Names: US Cuprimine; Depen Titratabs
Brand Names: Canada Cuprimine®
Index Terms D-3-Mercaptovaline; D-Penicillamine; β,β-Dimethylcysteine
Pharmacologic Category Chelating Agent
Use Treatment of Wilson's disease, cystinuria; adjunctive treatment of severe, active rheumatoid arthritis
Canadian labeling: Additional use (not in U.S. labeling): Treatment of chronic lead poisoning
Dosing
Adult Note: Dose reduction to 250 mg/day may be considered prior to surgical procedures. May resume normal recommended dosing post-operatively once wound healing is complete.
Cystinuria: Oral: 1-4 g/day in 4 divided doses; usual dose: 2 g/day; initiation of therapy at 250 mg/day with gradual upward titration may reduce the risk of unwanted effects. **Note:** Adjust dose to limit cystine excretion to 100-200 mg/day (<100 mg/day with history of stone formation).
Lead poisoning: Oral: *Canadian labeling:* 900-1500 mg/day in 3 divided doses for 1-2 weeks, then 750 mg/day in divided doses until blood lead concentrations <60 mcg/dL or urinary lead excretion <500 mcg/L for 2 consecutive months.
Rheumatoid arthritis: Oral: Initial: 125-250 mg/day, may increase dose by 125-250 mg/day at 1- to 3-month intervals up to 1-1.5 g/day; discontinue in patients failing to improve after 3-4 months at these doses
Wilson's disease: Oral: **Note:** Dose that results in an initial 24-hour urinary copper excretion >2 mg/day should be continued for ~3 months; maintenance dose defined by amount resulting in <10 mcg serum free copper/dL.
Manufacturer's labeling: 750-1500 mg/day in divided doses; maximum dose: 2000 mg/day. **Note:** Limit daily dose to 750 mg/day (U.S. labeling) or 1000 mg/day (Canadian labeling) in pregnant women; if planned caesarian, limit dose to 250 mg/day during the last 6 weeks of pregnancy and postoperatively until wound healing is complete.
Alternate recommendations (off-label dosing): To increase tolerability, therapy may be initiated at 250-500 mg/day then titrated upward in 250 mg increments every 4-7 days; usual maintenance dose: 750-1000 mg/day in 2 divided doses; maximum: 1000-1500 mg/day in 2-4 divided doses. (American Association for the Study of Liver Diseases [AASLD] guidelines) (Roberts, 2008).
Geriatric Therapy should be initiated at low end of dosing range and titrated upward cautiously. Refer to adult dosing.
Pediatric Note: Dose reduction to 250 mg/day may be considered prior to surgical procedures. May resume normal recommended dosing postoperatively once wound healing is complete.
Cystinuria: Oral: 30 mg/kg/day in 4 divided doses; **Note:** Adjust dose to limit cystine excretion to 100-200 mg/day (<100 mg/day with history of stone formation).
Lead poisoning: Oral:
Canadian labeling: 30-40 mg/kg/day or 600-750 mg/m^2/day in 1-2 divided doses (maximum dose: 750 mg/day); treat until blood lead concentrations <40 mcg/dL for 2 consecutive months and at least 1 of the following: Decrease in erythrocyte protoporphyrin level to <3-5 times the average normal level or the excretion of coproporphyrin or delta-aminolevulinic acid decreases to the upper limit of normal.
Note: Manufacturer labeling recommends initiating therapy only in children who meet the following criteria: Asymptomatic, blood lead concentrations of 50-80 mcg/dL, erythrocyte protoporphyrin level >400-500 mcg/dL erythrocytes, excessive excretion of delta-aminolevulinic acid and/or coproporphyrin.
Alternate recommendations (off-label dosing): **Note:** The American Academy of Pediatrics (AAP) considers penicillamine a third-line agent for the management of lead poisoning (AAP, 2005; Chandran, 2010): 10-15 mg/kg/day for 4-12 weeks (Chandran, 2010). **Note:** The CDC recommends chelation treatment when blood lead concentrations are >45 mcg/dL (CDC, 2002). Children with blood lead concentrations

>70 mcg/dL or symptomatic lead poisoning should be treated with parenteral agents (AAP, 2005).

Wilson's disease (off-label dosing): Oral: 20 mg/kg/day in 2-3 divided doses, round off to the nearest 250 mg dose (American Association for the Study of Liver Diseases [AASLD] guidelines) (Roberts, 2008).

Note: Dose that results in an initial 24-hour urinary copper excretion >2 mg/day should be continued for ~3 months; maintenance dose defined by amount resulting in <10 mcg serum free copper/dL.

Rheumatoid arthritis (off-label use): Oral: Initial: 3 mg/kg/day (≤250 mg/day) for 3 months, then 6 mg/kg/day (≤500 mg/day) in divided doses twice daily for 3 months to a maximum of 10 mg/kg/day in 3-4 divided doses; maximum dose: 750 mg/day (Rosenberg, 1989)

Renal Impairment

Manufacturer's labeling: No dosage adjustment provided in manufacturer's labeling; however, the manufacturer labeling does suggest a cautious approach to dosing as this drug undergoes mainly renal elimination.

Alternate recommendations:

CrCl <50 mL/minute: Avoid use (Aronoff, 2007

Hemodialysis: Dialyzable; Administer 33% of usual dose (Aronoff, 2007); a dosing decrease from 250 mg/day to 250 mg 3 times/week after dialysis has been suggested in the treatment of rheumatoid arthritis (Swarup, 2004).

Hepatic Impairment No dosage adjustment provided in manufacturer's labeling; however, only a small fraction is metabolized hepatically.

Additional Information Complete prescribing information should be consulted for additional detail.

Dosage Forms Excipient information presented when available (limited, particularly for generics); consult specific product labeling.

Capsule, Oral:

Cuprimine: 250 mg [contains fd&c yellow #10 (quinoline yellow)]

Tablet, Oral:

Depen Titratabs: 250 mg [scored]

Penicillin G Benzathine
(pen i SIL in jee BENZ a theen)

Brand Names: US Bicillin L-A

Brand Names: Canada Bicillin L-A

Index Terms Benzathine Benzylpenicillin; Benzathine Penicillin G; Benzylpenicillin Benzathine

Pharmacologic Category Antibiotic, Penicillin

Use

Acute glomerulonephritis: Prophylaxis (secondary) in patients with a history of acute glomerulonephritis

Respiratory tract infections: Treatment of mild to moderate upper respiratory tract infections caused by streptococci susceptible to low, prolonged serum concentrations of penicillin G

Rheumatic fever and chorea: Prophylaxis (secondary) of rheumatic fever and/or chorea

Rheumatic heart disease: Prophylaxis (secondary) in patients with rheumatic heart disease

Syphilis and other venereal diseases: Treatment of syphilis, yaws, bejel, and pinta

Pregnancy Considerations Adverse events have not been observed in animal reproduction studies. Penicillin crosses the placenta and distributes into amniotic fluid. Maternal use of penicillins has generally not resulted in an increased risk of adverse fetal effects. Penicillin G is the drug of choice for treatment of syphilis during pregnancy.

Breast-Feeding Considerations Penicillins are excreted in breast milk. The manufacturer recommends that caution be exercised when administering penicillin to nursing women. Nondose-related effects could include modification of bowel flora and allergic sensitization.

Contraindications Hypersensitivity to penicillin(s) or any component of the formulation

Warnings/Precautions Use with caution in patients with impaired renal function, seizure disorder, or history of hypersensitivity to other beta-lactams. Serious anaphylactic reactions require immediate emergency treatment with epinephrine, oxygen, intravenous steroids and airway management (including intubation) as indicated. CDC and AAP do not currently recommend the use of penicillin G benzathine to treat congenital syphilis or neurosyphilis due to reported treatment failures and lack of published clinical data on its efficacy. Use only for infections susceptible to the low and very prolonged serum concentrations of benzathine penicillin G. Prolonged use may result in fungal or bacterial superinfection, including *C. difficile*-associated diarrhea (CDAD) and pseudomembranous colitis; CDAD has been observed >2 months postantibiotic treatment.

[U.S. Boxed Warning]: Not for intravenous use; cardiopulmonary arrest and death have occurred from inadvertent IV administration; administer by deep IM injection only; injection into or near an artery or nerve could result in severe neurovascular damage or permanent neurological damage. Quadriceps femoris fibrosis and atrophy have been reported after repeated IM injections of penicillin preparations into the anterolateral thigh. Extended duration of therapy or use associated with high serum concentrations may be associated with an increased risk for some adverse reactions.

Adverse Reactions Frequency not defined.

Cardiovascular: Cardiac arrest, cerebral vascular accident, cyanosis, gangrene, hypotension, pallor, palpitations, syncope, tachycardia, vasodilation, vasospasm, vasovagal reaction

Central nervous system: Anxiety, coma, confusion, dizziness, euphoria, fatigue, headache, nervousness, pain, seizure, somnolence

In addition, a syndrome of CNS symptoms has been reported which includes: Severe agitation with confusion, hallucinations (auditory and visual), and fear of death (Hoigne's syndrome); other symptoms include cyanosis, dizziness, palpitations, psychosis, seizures, tachycardia, taste disturbance, tinnitus

Gastrointestinal: Bloody stool, intestinal necrosis, nausea, vomiting

Genitourinary: Impotence, priapism

Hepatic: AST increased

Local: Injection site reactions: Abscess, atrophy, bruising, cellulitis, edema, hemorrhage, inflammation, lump, necrosis, pain, skin ulcer

Neuromuscular & skeletal: Arthritis exacerbation, joint disorder, neurovascular damage, numbness, periostitis, rhabdomyolysis, transverse myelitis, tremor, weakness

Ocular: Blindness, blurred vision

Renal: BUN increased, creatinine increased, hematuria, myoglobinuria, neurogenic bladder, proteinuria, renal failure

Miscellaneous: Diaphoresis, hypersensitivity reactions, Jarisch-Herxheimer reaction, lymphadenopathy, mottling, warmth

Drug Interactions

Metabolism/Transport Effects Substrate of OAT3

Avoid Concomitant Use

Avoid concomitant use of Penicillin G Benzathine with any of the following: BCG (Intravesical); Probenecid

Increased Effect/Toxicity

Penicillin G Benzathine may increase the levels/effects of: Methotrexate; Vitamin K Antagonists

The levels/effects of Penicillin G Benzathine may be increased by: Probenecid; Teriflunomide

Decreased Effect

Penicillin G Benzathine may decrease the levels/effects of: BCG (Intravesical); BCG Vaccine (Immunization); Mycophenolate; Sodium Picosulfate; Typhoid Vaccine

The levels/effects of Penicillin G Benzathine may be decreased by: Tetracycline Derivatives

Storage/Stability Store at 2°C to 8°C (36°F to 46°F); do not freeze. The following stability information has also been reported: May be stored at 25°C (77°F) for 7 days (Cohen, 2007).

Mechanism of Action Interferes with bacterial cell wall synthesis during active multiplication, causing cell wall death and resultant bactericidal activity against susceptible bacteria

Pharmacodynamics/Kinetics

Duration: 1 to 4 weeks (dose dependent); larger doses result in more sustained levels

Distribution: Highest levels in the kidney; lesser amounts in liver, skin, intestines

Protein Binding: ~60%

Absorption: IM: Slow

Excretion: Urine

Dosing

Adult & Geriatric

Usual dosage range: IM: 1.2 to 2.4 million units as a single dose

Upper respiratory infection, group A streptococci: IM: 1.2 million units as a single dose

Secondary prevention of glomerulonephritis: 1.2 million units every 4 weeks or 600,000 units twice monthly

Secondary prevention of rheumatic fever: 1.2 million units every 3 to 4 weeks or 600,000 units twice monthly (Gerber, 2009)

Pharyngitis, group A streptococci (IDSA guidelines): IM:

Acute treatment: 1.2 million units as a single dose (Shulman, 2012)

Chronic carrier treatment: 1.2 million units as a single dose in combination with oral rifampin (Shulman, 2012)

◀

Syphilis (CDC, 2010): IM:

Primary, Secondary, Early Latent (<1 year duration): 2.4 million units as a single dose

Late Latent, Latent with unknown duration: 2.4 million units once weekly for 3 doses

Neurosyphilis: Not indicated as single-drug therapy, but may be given once weekly for 3 weeks following IV treatment; refer to Penicillin G (Parenteral/Aqueous) monograph for dosing

Yaws, bejel, and pinta: IM: 1.2 million units as a single dose

Pediatric

Usual dosage range: IM: 50,000 units/kg as a single dose (maximum: 2.4 million units)

Upper respiratory infection, group A streptococci (eg, pharyngitis): Infants and Children: IM: Manufacturer's labeling:

<27.3 kg: 300,000 to 600,000 units as a single dose. Manufacturer labeling does not provide specific recommendation for children ≥27.3 kg.

For older children, a dose of 900,000 units as a single dose is recommended.

Primary prevention of rheumatic fever: Infants and Children: IM: ≤27 kg: 600,000 units as a single dose; >27 kg: 1.2 million units as a single dose (Gerber, 2009)

Secondary prevention of rheumatic fever: Infants and Children: IM: ≤27 kg: 600,000 units every 3-4 weeks; >27 kg: 1.2 million units every 3 to 4 weeks (Gerber, 2009)

Pharyngitis, group A streptococci (IDSA guidelines): Infants and Children: IM:

Acute treatment: <27 kg: 600,000 units as a single dose; ≥27 kg: 1.2 million units as a single dose (Shulman, 2012)

Chronic carrier treatment: <27 kg: 600,000 units as a single dose (in combination with oral rifampin); ≥27 kg: 1.2 million units as a single dose (in combination with oral rifampin) (Shulman, 2012)

Syphilis (CDC, 2010): IM:

Primary, Secondary, Early Latent (<1 year duration): Infants and Children: 50,000 units/kg as a single injection (maximum: 2.4 million units)

Late Latent, Latent with unknown duration: Children: 50,000 units/kg every week for 3 doses (maximum: 2.4 million units/dose)

Renal Impairment There are no dosage adjustments provided in the manufacturer's labeling; use with caution.

Hepatic Impairment There are no dosage adjustments provided in the manufacturer's labeling.

Administration IM: Warm to room temperature before administration to lessen the pain associated with injection. Administer by deep IM injection in the upper outer quadrant of the buttock; in children <2 years of age, IM injections should be made into the midlateral muscle of the thigh, not the gluteal region. Do not inject near an artery or a nerve; permanent neurological damage or gangrene may result. When doses are repeated, rotate the injection site. **Do not administer IV, intra-arterially, or SubQ.**

Monitoring Parameters Observe for signs and symptoms of anaphylaxis during first dose

Test Interactions Positive Coombs' [direct], false-positive urinary and/or serum proteins; false-positive or negative urinary glucose using Clinitest®

Dosage Forms Excipient information presented when available (limited, particularly for generics); consult specific product labeling.

Suspension, Intramuscular:

Bicillin L-A: 600,000 units/mL (1 mL); 1,200,000 units/2 mL (2 mL); 2,400,000 units/4 mL (4 mL) [contains methylparaben, propylparaben]

Penicillin G Benzathine and Penicillin G Procaine

(pen i SIL in jee BENZ a theen & pen i SIL in jee PROE kane)

Brand Names: US Bicillin® C-R; Bicillin® C-R 900/300

Index Terms Penicillin G Procaine and Benzathine Combined

Pharmacologic Category Antibiotic, Penicillin

Use May be used in specific situations in the treatment of streptococcal infections; primary prevention of rheumatic fever

Dosing

Adult & Geriatric Streptococcal infections: IM: 2.4 million units in a single dose

Pediatric

Streptococcal infections: IM:

Children:

<14 kg: 600,000 units in a single dose

14-27 kg: 900,000 units to 1.2 million units in a single dose

Children >27 kg: Refer to adult dosing.

Rheumatic fever, primary prevention (Bicillin® C-R 900/300): Children 6 months to 12 years: 1.2 million units as a single dose (Bass, 1976; Gerber, 2009). **Note:** The efficacy of this regimen for heavier patients is unknown.

Renal Impairment No dosage adjustment provided in manufacturer's labeling.

Hepatic Impairment No dosage adjustment provided in manufacturer's labeling.

Additional Information Complete prescribing information should be consulted for additional detail.

Dosage Forms Excipient information presented when available (limited, particularly for generics); consult specific product labeling. [DSC] = Discontinued product

Injection, suspension [prefilled syringe]:

Bicillin® C-R:

600,000 units: Penicillin G benzathine 300,000 units and penicillin G procaine 300,000 units per 1 mL (1 mL) [DSC]

1,200,000 units: Penicillin G benzathine 600,000 units and penicillin G procaine 600,000 units per 2 mL (2 mL)

2,400,000 units: Penicillin G benzathine 1,200,000 units and penicillin G procaine 1,200,000 units per 4 mL (4 mL) [DSC]

Bicillin® C-R 900/300: 1,200,000 units: Penicillin G benzathine 900,000 units and penicillin G procaine 300,000 units per 2 mL (2 mL)

Penicillin G (Parenteral/Aqueous)

(pen i SIL in jee, pa REN ter al, AYE kwee us)

Brand Names: US Pfizerpen-G

Brand Names: Canada Crystapen

Index Terms Benzylpenicillin Potassium; Benzylpenicillin Sodium; Crystalline Penicillin; Penicillin G Potassium; Penicillin G Sodium

Pharmacologic Category Antibiotic, Penicillin

Use Treatment of infections (including sepsis, pneumonia, pericarditis, endocarditis, meningitis, anthrax, botulism, gas gangrene, and tetanus) caused by susceptible organisms; active against some gram-positive organisms, generally not *Staphylococcus aureus*; some gram-negative organisms such as *Neisseria gonorrhoeae*, and some anaerobes and spirochetes

Pregnancy Considerations Adverse events have not been observed in animal reproduction studies. Penicillin crosses the placenta and distributes into amniotic fluid. Maternal use of penicillins has generally not resulted in an increased risk of adverse fetal effects. Penicillin G is the drug of choice for treatment of syphilis during pregnancy and penicillin G (parenteral/aqueous) is the drug of choice for the prevention of early-onset Group B Streptococcal (GBS) disease in newborns (consult current guidelines).

Breast-Feeding Considerations Very small amounts of penicillin G transfer into breast milk. Peak milk concentrations occur at approximately 1 hour after an IM dose and are higher if multiple doses are given. The manufacturer recommends that caution be exercised when administering penicillin to nursing women. Nondose-related effects could include modification of bowel flora and allergic sensitization.

Contraindications Hypersensitivity to penicillin or any component of the formulation

Warnings/Precautions Avoid intra-arterial administration or injection into or near major peripheral nerves or blood vessels since such injections may cause severe and/or permanent neurovascular damage; use with caution in patients with renal impairment (dosage reduction required), concomitant renal and hepatic impairment (further dosage adjustment may be required), preexisting seizure disorders, or with a history of hypersensitivity to cephalosporins. Prolonged use may result in fungal or bacterial superinfection, including *C. difficile*-associated diarrhea (CDAD) and pseudomembranous colitis; CDAD has been observed >2 months postantibiotic treatment. Serious and occasionally severe or fatal hypersensitivity (anaphylactoid) reactions have been reported in patients on penicillin therapy, especially with a history of beta-lactam hypersensitivity, history of sensitivity to multiple allergens, or previous IgE-mediated reactions (eg, anaphylaxis, angioedema, urticaria). Use with caution in asthmatic patients. Extended duration of therapy or use associated with high serum concentrations may be associated with an increased risk for some adverse reactions. Neonates may

have decreased renal clearance of penicillin and require frequent dosage adjustments depending on age. Product contains sodium and potassium; high doses of IV therapy may alter serum levels.

Adverse Reactions Frequency not defined.

Cardiovascular: Localized phlebitis, local thrombophlebitis

Central nervous system: Coma (high doses), hyperreflexia (high doses), myoclonus (high doses), seizure (high doses)

Dermatologic: Contact dermatitis, skin rash

Endocrine & metabolic: Electrolyte disturbance (high doses)

Gastrointestinal: Pseudomembranous colitis

Hematologic & oncologic: Neutropenia, positive direct Coombs test (rare, high doses)

Hypersensitivity: Anaphylaxis, hypersensitivity reaction (immediate and delayed), serum sickness

Immunologic: Jarisch-Herxheimer reaction

Local: Injection site reaction

Renal: Acute interstitial nephritis (high doses), renal tubular disease (high doses)

Drug Interactions

Metabolism/Transport Effects Substrate of OAT3

Avoid Concomitant Use

Avoid concomitant use of Penicillin G (Parenteral/Aqueous) with any of the following: BCG (Intravesical); Probenecid

Increased Effect/Toxicity

Penicillin G (Parenteral/Aqueous) may increase the levels/effects of: Methotrexate; Vitamin K Antagonists

The levels/effects of Penicillin G (Parenteral/Aqueous) may be increased by: Probenecid; Teriflunomide

Decreased Effect

Penicillin G (Parenteral/Aqueous) may decrease the levels/effects of: BCG (Intravesical); BCG Vaccine (Immunization); Mycophenolate; Sodium Picosulfate; Typhoid Vaccine

The levels/effects of Penicillin G (Parenteral/Aqueous) may be decreased by: Tetracycline Derivatives

Preparation for Administration

Intermittent IV: 5 million unit vial: Add 8.2 mL for a final concentration of 500,000 units/mL; add 3.2 mL for a final concentration of 1,000,000 units/mL. Dilute further to 50,000-145,000 units/mL prior to infusion.

Continuous IV infusion: 20 million unit vial: Add 11.5 mL for a final concentration of 1,000,000 units/mL. Dilute further in 1-2 L of infusion solution and administer over a 24-hour period.

Storage/Stability

Penicillin G potassium powder for injection should be stored below 86°F (30°C). Following reconstitution, solution may be stored for up to 7 days under refrigeration. Premixed bags for infusion should be stored in the freezer (-20°C or -4°F); frozen bags may be thawed at room temperature or in refrigerator. Once thawed, solution is stable for 14 days if stored in refrigerator or for 24 hours when stored at room temperature. Do not refreeze once thawed.

Penicillin G sodium powder for injection should be stored at controlled room temperature. Reconstituted solution may be stored under refrigeration for up to 3 days.

Mechanism of Action Interferes with bacterial cell wall synthesis during active multiplication, causing cell wall death and resultant bactericidal activity against susceptible bacteria

Pharmacodynamics/Kinetics

Distribution: Poor penetration across blood-brain barrier, despite inflamed meninges

Relative diffusion from blood into CSF: Poor unless meninges inflamed (exceeds usual MICs)

CSF:blood level ratio: Normal meninges: <1%; Inflamed meninges: 2% to 6%

Protein binding: 65%

Metabolism: Hepatic (30%) to penicilloic acid

Half-life elimination:

Neonates: <6 days old: 3.2-3.4 hours; 7-13 days old: 1.2-2.2 hours; >14 days old: 0.9-1.9 hours

Children and Adults: Normal renal function: 30-50 minutes

End-stage renal disease: 3.3-5.1 hours

Time to peak, serum: IM: ~30 minutes; IV: ~1 hour

Excretion: Urine (58% to 85% as unchanged drug)

Dosing

Adult & Geriatric

***Actinomyces* species:** IV: 10 to 20 million units/day divided every 4 to 6 hours for 4 to 6 weeks

***Clostridium* species:** IV:

Manufacturer's labeling: 20 million units/day in divided doses every 4 to 6 hours

Skin and soft tissue necrotizing infections (off-label use): 2 to 4 million units every 4 to 6 hours; use in

combination with clindamycin and continue until further debridement is not necessary, patient has clinically improved, and patient is afebrile for 48 to 72 hours (IDSA [Stevens 2014])

Corynebacterium diphtheriae: IV: 2 to 3 million units/day in divided doses every 4 to 6 hours for 10 to 12 days

Erysipelas: IV: 1 to 2 million units every 4 to 6 hours

Erysipelothrix: IV: 2 to 4 million units every 4 hours

Fascial space infections: IV: 2 to 4 million units every 4 to 6 hours with metronidazole

Leptospirosis: IV: 1.5 million units every 6 hours for 7 days

Listeria: IV: 15 to 20 million units/day in divided doses every 4 to 6 hours for 2 weeks (meningitis) or 4 weeks (endocarditis)

Lyme disease (meningitis): IV: 20 million units/day in divided doses

Neurosyphilis: IV: 18 to 24 million units/day in divided doses every 4 hours (or by continuous infusion) for 10 to 14 days (CDC 2006; CDC 2009; CDC 2010)

Prosthetic joint infection: IV:

Enterococcus spp *(penicillin-susceptible), streptococci (beta-hemolytic):* 20 to 24 million units daily continuous infusion every 24 hours or in divided doses every 4 hours for 4 to 6 weeks (Osmon 2013); **Note:** For penicillin-susceptible *Enterococcus* spp, consider addition of aminoglycoside.

Propionibacterium acnes: 20 million units daily continuous infusion every 24 hours or in divided doses every 4 hours for 4 to 6 weeks (Osmon 2013)

Streptococcus:

Brain abscess: IV: 18 to 24 million units/day in divided doses every 4 hours with metronidazole

Endocarditis or osteomyelitis: IV: 3 to 4 million units every 4 hours for at least 4 weeks

Group B streptococcus (neonatal prophylaxis): IV: 5 million units x 1 dose, then 2.5 to 3.0 million units every 4 hours until delivery (CDC 2010)

Skin infections, including skin and soft tissue necrotizing infections (off-label use): IV: 2 to 4 million units every 4 to 6 hours; use in combination with clindamycin for necrotizing infections and continue until further debridement is not necessary, patient has clinically improved, and patient is afebrile for 48 to 72 hours (IDSA [Stevens 2014])

Toxic shock: IV: 24 million units/day in divided doses with clindamycin

Streptococcal pneumonia: IV: 2 to 3 million units every 4 hours

Whipple's disease: IV: 2 million units every 4 hours for 2 weeks, followed by oral trimethoprim/sulfamethoxazole or doxycycline for 1 year

Relapse or CNS involvement: 4 million units every 4 hours for 4 weeks

Pediatric

Susceptible infections: IM, IV:

Infants ≥1 month and Children: 100,000 to 400,000 units/kg/day in divided doses every 4 to 6 hours (maximum dose: 24 million units/day)

Community-acquired pneumonia (CAP) (IDSA/PIDS 2011): IV: Infants and Children >3 months: **Note:** May consider addition of vancomycin or clindamycin to empiric therapy if community-acquired MRSA suspected. In children ≥5 years, a macrolide antibiotic should be added if atypical pneumonia cannot be ruled out.

Empiric treatment or *S. pneumoniae* (moderate-to-severe; MICs to penicillin ≤2.0 mcg/mL) (preferred): 200,000 to 250,000 units/kg/day divided every 4 to 6 hours

Group A *Streptococcus* (moderate-to-severe) (preferred): 100,000 to 250,000 units/kg/day divided every 4 to 6 hours

***Meningitis* (gonococcal):** IV: 250,000 units/kg/day in 4 divided doses

Moderate infections: IM, IV: 100,000 to 250,000 units/kg/day in 4 divided doses

Neurosyphilis: IV: 200,000 to 300,000 units/kg/day divided every 4 to 6 hours for 10 to 14 days (maximum dose: 24 million units/day)

Severe infections: IM, IV: 250,000 to 400,000 units/kg/day in divided doses every 4 to 6 hours (maximum dose: 24 million units/day)

Skin and soft tissue necrotizing infections due to *Clostridium* species (off-label use): IV: 60,000 to 100,000 units/kg every 6 hours; use in combination with clindamycin and continue until further debridement is not necessary, patient has clinically improved, and patient is afebrile for 48 to 72 hours (IDSA [Stevens 2014])

◀ **Streptococcal skin infections, including skin and soft tissue necrotizing infections (off-label use):** IV: 60,000 to 100,000 units/kg every 6 hours; use in combination with clindamycin for necrotizing infections and continue until further debridement is not necessary, patient has clinically improved, and patient is afebrile for 48 to 72 hours (IDSA [Stevens 2014])

Syphilis (congenital): IV:

Infants: 50,000 units/kg every 12 hours for first 7 days of life, then every 8 hours for a total of 10 days (CDC 2010)

Children: 50,000 units/kg every 4 to 6 hours for 10 days (CDC 2010)

Renal Impairment

Manufacturer's labeling:

Uremic patients with CrCl >10 mL/minute/1.73 m^2: Administer a normal dose followed by 50% of the normal dose every 4 to 5 hours

CrCl <10 mL/minute/1.73 m^2: Administer a normal dose followed by 50% of the normal dose every 8 to 10 hours

Alternate recommendation:

GFR >50 mL/minute: No dosage adjustments are necessary (Aronoff 2007).

GFR 10-50 mL/minute: Administer 75% of the normal dose (Aronoff 2007).

GFR <10 mL/minute: Administer 20% to 50% of the normal dose (Aronoff 2007).

Intermittent hemodialysis (IHD) (administer after hemodialysis on dialysis days) (Heintz 2009): Administer a normal dose followed by either 25% to 50% of normal dose every 4 to 6 hours **or** 50% to 100% of normal dose every 8 to 12 hours. For *mild-to-moderate* infections, administer 0.5 to 1 million units every 4 to 6 hours **or** 1 to 2 million units every 8 to 12 hours. For *neurosyphilis, endocarditis, or serious infections*, administer up to 2 million units every 4 to 6 hours; administer after dialysis on dialysis days **or** supplement with 500,000 units after dialysis. **Note:** Dosing dependent on the assumption of 3 times weekly, complete IHD sessions.

Continuous renal replacement therapy (CRRT) (Heintz 2009; Trotman 2005): Drug clearance is highly dependent on the method of renal replacement, filter type, and flow rate. Appropriate dosing requires close monitoring of pharmacologic response, signs of adverse reactions due to drug accumulation, as well as drug concentrations in relation to target trough (if appropriate). The following are general recommendations only (based on dialysate flow/ultrafiltration rates of 1 to 2 L/hour and minimal residual renal function) and should not supersede clinical judgment:

CVVH: Loading dose of 4 million units, followed by 2 million units every 4 to 6 hours

CVVHD: Loading dose of 4 million units, followed by 2 to 3 million units every 4 to 6 hours

CVVHDF: Loading dose of 4 million units, followed by 2 to 4 million units every 4 to 6 hours

Hepatic Impairment No dosage adjustment provided in manufacturer's labeling. However, the manufacturer's labeling recommends further adjustment of doses adjusted for renal impairment in patients with both renal and hepatic impairment.

Dietary Considerations Some products may contain potassium and/or sodium.

Administration

IM; Administer IM by deep injection in the upper outer quadrant of the buttock

IV: **Note:** The 20 million unit dosage form may be administered by continuous IV infusion only.

Intermittent IV: May be dissolved in small amounts of SWFI, NS, D$_5$W and administered peripherally as a 50,000-100,000 unit/mL solution. In fluid-restricted patients, 146,000 units/mL in SW results in a maximum recommended osmolality for peripheral infusion. Infuse over 15-30 minutes.

Continuous IV infusion: Determine the volume of fluid and rate of its administration required by the patient in a 24-hour period. Add the appropriate daily dosage of penicillin to this fluid. For example, if the daily dose is 10 million units and 2 L of fluid/day is required, add 5 million units to 1 L and adjust the rate of flow so the liter will be infused over 12 hours (83 mL/hour). Repeat steps (5 million units/L at 83 mL/hour) for the remaining 12 hours.

Monitoring Parameters Periodic electrolyte, hepatic, renal, cardiac and hematologic function tests during prolonged/high-dose therapy; observe for signs and symptoms of anaphylaxis during first dose

Test Interactions False-positive or negative urinary glucose determination using Clinitest®; positive Coombs' [direct]; false-positive urinary and/or serum proteins

Additional Information 1 million units is approximately equal to 625 mg.

Dosage Forms Excipient information presented when available (limited, particularly for generics); consult specific product labeling.

Solution, Intravenous, as potassium:

Generic: 20,000 units/mL (50 mL); 40,000 units/mL (50 mL); 60,000 units/mL (50 mL)

Solution Reconstituted, Injection, as potassium:

Pfizerpen-G: 5,000,000 units (1 ea); 20,000,000 units (1 ea)

Pfizerpen-G: 5,000,000 units (1 ea); 20,000,000 units (1 ea) [pyrogen free]

Generic: 5,000,000 units (1 ea); 20,000,000 units (1 ea)

Solution Reconstituted, Injection, as potassium [preservative free]:

Generic: 20,000,000 units (1 ea)

Solution Reconstituted, Injection, as sodium:

Generic: 5,000,000 units (1 ea)

◆ **Penicillin G Potassium** see Penicillin G (Parenteral/Aqueous) *on page 1420*

Penicillin G Procaine (pen i SIL in jee PROE kane)

Brand Names: Canada Pfizerpen-AS®; Wycillin®

Index Terms APPG; Aqueous Procaine Penicillin G; Procaine Benzylpenicillin; Procaine Penicillin G; Wycillin

Pharmacologic Category Antibiotic, Penicillin

Use

Anthrax, prophylaxis: To reduce the incidence of the disease following exposure to aerosolized *Bacillus anthracis.*

Anthrax, treatment: Treatment of anthrax, including postexposure inhalational disease due to aerosolized *B. anthracis.*

Diphtheria: As an adjunct to antitoxin for prevention of the carrier stage of diphtheria caused by susceptible *Corynebacterium diphtheriae.*

Endocarditis, subacute: Treatment of subacute bacterial endocarditis, only in extremely sensitive infections, caused by susceptible group A streptococci.

Erysipeloid: Treatment of erysipeloid caused by susceptible *Erysipelothrix rhusiopathiae.*

Fusospirochetosis: Treatment of fusospirochetosis (Vincent gingivitis and pharyngitis) in conjunction with dental care, and moderately severe infections of the oropharynx caused by susceptible fusiform bacilli and spirochetes.

Pneumococcal infection: Treatment of moderately severe infections of the respiratory tract caused by susceptible pneumococci.

Limitations of use: Severe pneumonia, empyema, bacteremia, pericarditis, meningitis, peritonitis, and arthritis of pneumococcal etiology are better treated with aqueous penicillin G during the acute stage.

Rat bite fever: Treatment of rat bite fever caused by susceptible *Streptobacillus moniliformis* and *Spirillum minus* organisms.

Skin and soft tissue infection: Treatment of moderately severe infections of the skin and soft tissues caused by susceptible staphylococci (penicillin G-susceptible).

Streptococcal infections: Treatment of moderately severe to severe infections of the upper respiratory tract, skin and soft tissue infections, scarlet fever, and erysipelas caused by susceptible streptococci (group A, without bacteremia).

Limitations of use: Some streptococcal groups, including group D (enterococcus), are resistant. Aqueous penicillin is recommended for streptococcal infections with bacteremia.

Syphilis: Treatment of syphilis (all stages) caused by susceptible *Treponema pallidum.*

Yaws, bejel, and pinta: Treatment of yaws, bejel, and pinta caused by susceptible organisms.

Limitations of use: When high, sustained serum levels are required, use aqueous penicillin G, either intramuscularly (IM) or intravenously (IV). Do not use in the treatment of beta-lactamase-producing organisms, which includes most strains of *Neisseria gonorrhea.*

Pregnancy Considerations Adverse events have not been observed in animal reproduction studies. Penicillin crosses the placenta and distributes into amniotic fluid. Maternal use of penicillins has generally not resulted in an increased risk of adverse fetal effects.

Breast-Feeding Considerations Penicillins are excreted in breast milk. The manufacturer recommends that caution be used when administering penicillin to nursing women. Nondose-related effects could include modification of bowel flora and allergic sensitization.

Contraindications Hypersensitivity to any penicillin or any component of the formulation.

Warnings/Precautions May need to modify dosage in patients with severe renal impairment or seizure disorders; avoid IV, intravascular, or intra-arterial administration of penicillin G procaine since severe and/or permanent neurovascular damage may occur. Serious and occasionally severe or fatal hypersensitivity (anaphylactic) reactions have been reported in patients on penicillin therapy, especially with a history of beta-lactam hypersensitivity, and/or sensitivity to multiple allergens. If an allergic reaction occurs, discontinue therapy and institute appropriate supportive measures. If there is a history of hypersensitivity to procaine, test with 0.1 mL of 1% or 2% procaine solution. If erythema, wheal, flare, or eruption occurs, patient may be sensitive to procaine; do not use penicillin G procaine in these patients. Treat sensitivity with supportive measures, including antihistamines. Immediate toxic reactions (eg, anxiety, confusion, agitation, depression, weakness, seizures, hallucinations, combativeness and expressed "fear of impending death") have been reported. Mental disturbance reactions are more common in patients receiving a large single dose (eg, 4.8 million units). Reactions are transient and last 15 to 30 minutes (eg, transverse myelitis with permanent paralysis, gangrene requiring digit or proximal extremity amputation, necrosis and sloughing at and surrounding the injection site) may occur. These reactions have occurred following injection into the deltoid, thigh or buttock areas. Other serious complications of suspected intravascular administration (eg, immediate distal and proximal pallor, mottling or cyanosis of the extremity around the injection site followed by bleb formation or severe edema requiring anterior and/or posterior compartment fasciotomy in the lower extremity) occur most often in infants and small children. If any evidence of blood supply compromise is noted, consult appropriate specialists promptly. Quadriceps femoris fibrosis and atrophy have been reported following repeated IM injections of penicillins into the anterolateral thigh. Extended duration of therapy or use associated with high serum concentrations may be associated with an increased risk for some adverse reactions. Prolonged use may result in fungal or bacterial superinfection, including *C. difficile*-associated diarrhea (CDAD) and pseudomembranous colitis; CDAD has been observed >2 months postantibiotic treatment. Do not use for the treatment of gonorrhea. Penicillin G procaine is not the same preparation as penicillin G benzathine-penicillin G procaine (eg, *Bicillin C-R*). Dispensing errors have occurred. Potentially significant drug-drug interactions may exist, requiring dose or frequency adjustment, additional monitoring, and/or selection of alternative therapy.

Adverse Reactions Frequency not defined.
Cardiovascular: Conduction disturbances, myocardial depression, vasodilation
Central nervous system: CNS stimulation, confusion, drowsiness, myoclonus, seizure
Hematologic: Hemolytic anemia, neutropenia, positive Coombs' reaction
Local: Pain at injection site, sterile abscess at injection site, thrombophlebitis
Renal: Interstitial nephritis
Miscellaneous: Hypersensitivity reactions, Jarisch-Herxheimer reaction, pseudoanaphylactic reactions, serum sickness

Drug Interactions
Metabolism/Transport Effects Substrate of OAT3
Avoid Concomitant Use
Avoid concomitant use of Penicillin G Procaine with any of the following: BCG (Intravesical); Probenecid
Increased Effect/Toxicity
Penicillin G Procaine may increase the levels/effects of: Methotrexate; Vitamin K Antagonists

The levels/effects of Penicillin G Procaine may be increased by: Probenecid; Teriflunomide
Decreased Effect
Penicillin G Procaine may decrease the levels/effects of: BCG (Intravesical); BCG Vaccine (Immunization); Mycophenolate; Sodium Picosulfate; Typhoid Vaccine

The levels/effects of Penicillin G Procaine may be decreased by: Tetracycline Derivatives
Storage/Stability Store at 2°C to 8°C (36°F to 46°F). Keep from freezing.
Mechanism of Action Inhibits bacterial cell wall synthesis by binding to one or more of the penicillin-binding proteins (PBPs); which in turn inhibits the final transpeptidation step of peptidoglycan synthesis in bacterial cell walls, thus inhibiting cell wall biosynthesis. Bacteria eventually lyse due to ongoing activity of cell wall autolytic enzymes (autolysins and murein hydrolases) while cell wall assembly is arrested.

Pharmacodynamics/Kinetics
Duration: Therapeutic: 15 to 24 hours
Absorption: IM: Slow
Distribution: High distribution in kidneys, lesser amounts in liver, skin and intestines. Very small levels found in CSF.
Protein binding: 60%
Time to peak, serum: ~4 hours
Excretion: Urine (60% to 90% as unchanged drug)
Dosing
Adult & Geriatric
Anthrax:
Inhalational (postexposure prophylaxis): IM: 1,200,000 units every 12 hours
Note: Not a preferred regimen (Hendricks 2014). Overall treatment duration should be 60 days. Available safety data suggest continued administration of penicillin G procaine for longer than 2 weeks may incur additional risk of adverse reactions. Clinicians may consider switching to effective alternative treatment for completion of therapy beyond 2 weeks (FDA 2001).
Cutaneous (treatment): IM: 600,000 to 1,000,000 units daily; Note: Not a preferred regimen (Hendricks 2014).
Diphtheria, adjunctive therapy with antitoxin: IM:
Manufacturer's labeling: 300,000 to 600,000 units daily. Alternate regimen (patients >10 kg): 600,000 units daily for 14 days (CDC 2014).
Diphtheria, carrier state: 300,000 units once daily for 10 days; Note: Penicillin G benzathine is preferred (CDC 2014).
Neurosyphilis (including ocular syphilis): IM:
Manufacturer's recommendations: 600,000 units daily for 10 to 15 days.
Alternate regimen: 2.4 million units daily with concomitant probenecid for 10 to 14 days; Note: Aqueous penicillin G IV is the preferred agent (CDC 2010).
Pneumococcal pneumonia (uncomplicated, moderately severe): IM: 600,000 to 1,000,000 units daily.
Staphylococcal infections (moderately severe to severe): IM: 600,000 to 1,000,000 units daily
Streptococcal infections (Group A; moderately severe to severe): IM: 600,000 to 1,000,000 units daily for a minimum of 10 days
Yaws: IM: 600,000 units daily. Note: Duration dependent upon the stage of disease; azithromycin is the preferred agent (Mitja 2015).
Pediatric
Anthrax, inhalational (postexposure prophylaxis): Infants, Children, and Adolescents: IM: 25,000 units/kg every 12 hours (maximum: 1,200,000 units/dose every 12 hours). Note: Not a preferred regimen (Bradley 2014). Overall treatment duration should be 60 days. Available safety data suggest continued administration of penicillin G procaine for longer than 2 weeks may incur additional risk for adverse reactions. Clinicians may consider switching to effective alternative treatment for completion of therapy beyond 2 weeks. (FDA 2001)
Diphtheria, adjunctive therapy with antitoxin: Infants, Children, and Adolescents: IM:
Manufacturer's labeling: 300,000 to 600,000 units daily.
Alternate regimen:
Patients ≤10 kg: 300,000 units daily for 14 days (CDC 2014).
Patients >10 kg: 600,000 units daily for 14 days (CDC 2014).
Diphtheria, carrier state: Infants, Children, and Adolescents: IM: 300,000 units once daily for 10 days; Note: Penicillin G benzathine is preferred (CDC 2014).
Syphilis (congenital) (<32 kg): Infants, Children, and Adolescents: IM: 50,000 units/kg once daily for 10 days; if more than 1 day of therapy is missed, the entire course should be restarted (CDC 2010)
Renal Impairment There are no dosage adjustments provided in the manufacturer's labeling, however, excretion is delayed with impaired renal function and dosage adjustments may be necessary. Use with caution.
Hepatic Impairment There are no dosage adjustments provided in the manufacturer's labeling.
Administration IM: Procaine suspension for deep IM injection only; do not inject in gluteal muscle in children <2 years of age; rotate the injection site; avoid IV, intravascular, or intra-arterial administration of penicillin G procaine since severe and/or permanent neurovascular damage may occur
Monitoring Parameters Hypersensitivity reactions with first dose, injection site reactions, mental status post injection, periodic renal and hematologic function tests with prolonged therapy.
Test Interactions Positive Coombs' [direct], false-positive urinary and/or serum proteins

Dosage Forms Excipient information presented when available (limited, particularly for generics); consult specific product labeling.

Suspension, Intramuscular:
Generic: 600,000 units/mL (1 mL, 2 mL)

◆ Penicillin G Procaine and Benzathine Combined see Penicillin G Benzathine and Penicillin G Procaine on page 1420

◆ Penicillin G Sodium see Penicillin G (Parenteral/Aqueous) on page 1420

Penicillin V Potassium
(pen i SIL in vee poe TASS ee um)

Brand Names: Canada Apo-Pen VK; Novo-Pen-VK; Nu-Pen-VK

Index Terms Pen VK; Phenoxymethyl Penicillin

Pharmacologic Category Antibiotic, Penicillin

Use Treatment of infections caused by susceptible organisms involving the respiratory tract, otitis media, sinusitis, skin, and soft tissues; prophylaxis in rheumatic fever

Pregnancy Considerations Penicillin crosses the placenta and distributes into amniotic fluid. Maternal use of penicillins has generally not resulted in an increased risk of adverse fetal effects. Due to pregnancy-induced physiologic changes, some pharmacokinetic parameters of penicillin V may be altered in the second and third trimester. Higher doses or increased dosing frequency may be required.

Breast-Feeding Considerations Penicillin V is excreted into breast milk (low concentrations) and may be detected in the urine of some breast-feeding infants. Loose stools and rash have been reported in nursing infants.

Contraindications Hypersensitivity to penicillin or any component of the formulation

Warnings/Precautions Use with caution in patients with severe renal impairment or history of seizures. Serious and occasionally severe or fatal hypersensitivity (anaphylactoid) reactions have been reported in patients on penicillin therapy, especially with a history of beta-lactam hypersensitivity, history of sensitivity to multiple allergens, or previous IgE-mediated reactions (eg, anaphylaxis, angioedema, urticaria). Use with caution in asthmatic patients. Extended duration of therapy or use associated with high serum concentrations may be associated with an increased risk for some adverse reactions. Prolonged use may result in fungal or bacterial superinfection, including *C. difficile*-associated diarrhea (CDAD) and pseudomembranous colitis; CDAD has been observed >2 months postantibiotic treatment.

Benzyl alcohol and derivatives: Some dosage forms may contain sodium benzoate/benzoic acid; benzoic acid (benzoate) is a metabolite of benzyl alcohol; large amounts of benzyl alcohol (≥99 mg/kg/day) have been associated with a potentially fatal toxicity ("gasping syndrome") in neonates; the "gasping syndrome" consists of metabolic acidosis, respiratory distress, gasping respirations, CNS dysfunction (including convulsions, intracranial hemorrhage), hypotension, and cardiovascular collapse (AAP ["Inactive" 1997]; CDC, 1982); some data suggests that benzoate displaces bilirubin from protein binding sites (Ahlfors 2001); avoid or use dosage forms containing benzyl alcohol derivative with caution in neonates. See manufacturer's labeling.

Adverse Reactions

>10%: Gastrointestinal: Melanoglossia, mild diarrhea, nausea, oral candidiasis, vomiting

<1% (Limited to important or life-threatening): Acute interstitial nephritis, convulsions, exfoliative dermatitis, hemolytic anemia, hypersensitivity reaction, positive Coombs' reaction, serum-sickness like reactions

Drug Interactions

Metabolism/Transport Effects None known.

Avoid Concomitant Use

Avoid concomitant use of Penicillin V Potassium with any of the following: BCG (Intravesical); Probenecid

Increased Effect/Toxicity

Penicillin V Potassium may increase the levels/effects of: Methotrexate; Vitamin K Antagonists

The levels/effects of Penicillin V Potassium may be increased by: Probenecid

Decreased Effect

Penicillin V Potassium may decrease the levels/effects of: BCG (Intravesical); BCG Vaccine (Immunization); Mycophenolate; Sodium Picosulfate; Typhoid Vaccine

The levels/effects of Penicillin V Potassium may be decreased by: Tetracycline Derivatives

Food Interactions Food decreases drug absorption rate; decreases drug serum concentration. Management: Take on an empty stomach 1 hour before or 2 hours after meals around-the-clock to promote less variation in peak and trough serum levels.

Storage/Stability Refrigerate suspension after reconstitution; discard after 14 days.

Mechanism of Action Inhibits bacterial cell wall synthesis by binding to one or more of the penicillin-binding proteins (PBPs); which in turn inhibits the final transpeptidation step of peptidoglycan synthesis in bacterial cell walls, thus inhibiting cell wall biosynthesis. Bacteria eventually lyse due to ongoing activity of cell wall autolytic enzymes (autolysins and murein hydrolases) while cell wall assembly is arrested.

Pharmacodynamics/Kinetics

Absorption: 60% to 73%

Distribution: Widely distributed to kidneys, liver, skin, tonsils, and into synovial, pleural, and pericardial fluids

Protein binding, plasma: 80%

Half-life elimination: 30 minutes; prolonged with renal impairment

Time to peak, serum: 0.5-1 hour

Excretion: Urine (as unchanged drug and metabolites)

Dosing

Adult & Geriatric

Actinomycosis: Oral:

Mild: 2000 to 4000 mg in 4 divided doses for 8 weeks

Surgical: 2000 to 4000 mg in 4 divided doses for 6 to 12 months (after IV penicillin G therapy of 4 to 6 weeks)

Bite wounds (animal) (off-label use): Oral: 500 mg 4 times daily in combination with dicloxacillin (IDSA [Stevens 2014])

Cutaneous anthrax, community-acquired (off-label use): 500 mg 4 times daily for 7 to 10 days (IDSA [Stevens 2014])

Cutaneous erysipeloid (off-label use): 500 mg 4 times daily for 7 to 10 days (IDSA [Stevens 2014])

Erysipelas: Oral: 500 mg 4 times daily

Fusospirochetosis (Vincent infection): 250 to 500 mg 3-4 times daily

Pharyngitis (streptococcal): Oral:

Manufacturer's labeling: 500 mg 3 to 4 times daily for 10 days

Acute treatment, group A streptococci (IDSA guidelines): 250 mg 4 times daily or 500 mg twice daily for 10 days (Shulman 2012)

Chronic carrier treatment, group A streptococcal (IDSA guidelines): 500 mg 4 times daily (maximum: 2000 mg daily) for 10 days in combination with oral rifampin (Shulman 2012)

Prophylaxis of recurrent rheumatic fever infections: Oral: 250 mg twice daily

Prosthetic joint infection (off-label use): *Chronic oral antimicrobial suppression (Enterococcus spp [penicillin-susceptible], streptococci [beta-hemolytic], Propionibacterium spp):* Oral: 500 mg 2 to 4 times daily (Osmon 2013)

Streptococcal skin infection: 250 to 500 mg every 6 hours (IDSA [Stevens 2014])

Pediatric

Community-acquired pneumonia (CAP) due to group A *Streptococcus*, mild infection or step-down therapy (preferred) (IDSA/PIDS 2011): Infants >3 months and Children: Oral: 50 to 75 mg/kg/day in 3 to 4 divided doses

Fusospirochetosis (Vincent infection): Children ≥12 years and Adolescents: Oral: Refer to adult dosing.

Pharyngitis (streptococcal) (IDSA guidelines): Children: Oral:

Acute treatment: 250 mg 2 to 3 times daily for 10 days

Chronic carrier treatment, group A streptococci: 50 mg/kg/day in 4 divided doses (maximum: 2000 mg daily) for 10 days in combination with oral rifampin (Shulman 2012)

Pharyngitis (streptococcal), acute treatment (IDSA guidelines): Adolescents: Refer to adult dosing.

Pneumococcal infection prophylaxis for anatomic or functional asplenia (eg, sickle cell disease [SCD]) (Kavanagh 2011; NHLBI 2014): Infants and Children: Oral:

Before 2 months of age (or as soon as SCD diagnosed or asplenia occurs) to <3 years of age: 125 mg twice daily

≥3 years: 250 mg twice daily; the decision to discontinue penicillin prophylaxis after 5 years of age in children who have not experienced invasive pneumococcal infection and have received recommended pneumococcal immunizations is patient and clinician dependent

Prophylaxis of recurrent rheumatic fever (secondary prevention): Oral: Refer to adult dosing.

Renal Impairment No dosage adjustment provided in manufacturer's labeling. Use with caution; excretion is prolonged in patients with renal impairment.

Hepatic Impairment No dosage adjustment provided in manufacturer's labeling.

Dietary Considerations Take on an empty stomach 1 hour before or 2 hours after meals.

Administration Administer on an empty stomach to increase oral absorption

Monitoring Parameters Periodic renal and hematologic function tests during prolonged therapy; monitor for signs of anaphylaxis during first dose

Test Interactions False-positive or negative urinary glucose determination using Clinitest®; positive Coombs' [direct]; false-positive urinary and/or serum proteins

Additional Information 0.7 mEq of potassium per 250 mg penicillin V; 250 mg equals 400,000 units of penicillin

Dosage Forms Excipient information presented when available (limited, particularly for generics); consult specific product labeling.

Solution Reconstituted, Oral:
Generic: 125 mg/5 mL (100 mL, 200 mL); 250 mg/5 mL (100 mL, 200 mL)
Tablet, Oral:
Generic: 250 mg, 500 mg

- ◆ Penlac *see* Ciclopirox *on page 384*
- ◆ Pentacel *see* Diphtheria and Tetanus Toxoids, Acellular Pertussis, Poliovirus and *Haemophilus* b Conjugate Vaccine *on page 567*
- ◆ Pentahydrate *see* Sodium Thiosulfate *on page 1682*
- ◆ Pentam ≥see Pentamidine (Systemic) *on page 1425*

Pentamidine (Systemic) (pen TAM i deen)

Brand Names: US Pentam
Index Terms Pentamidine Isethionate
Pharmacologic Category Antifungal Agent; Antiprotozoal

Use Treatment of pneumonia caused by *Pneumocystis jirovecii* pneumonia (PCP)

Dosing

Adult & Geriatric

Pneumocystis jirovecii **pneumonia (PCP), treatment:**
Manufacturer labeling: IM, IV: 4 mg/kg once daily for 14 to 21 days
HIV-infected patients (alternative to preferred therapy): IV: 4 mg/kg/dose once daily for 21 days; may reduce to 3 mg/kg/dose once daily if toxicity occurs (HHS [OI adult 2015])

Trypanosomiasis (off-label use): IM, IV: 4 mg/kg once daily for 7 to 10 days (CDC 2013)

Pediatric

Pneumocystis jirovecii **pneumonia (PCP), prophylaxis (primary and secondary) in oncology patients (including HSCT recipients) (off-label use): Note:** For patients intolerant to sulfamethoxazole and trimethoprim: Children ≥2 years and Adolescents: IV: 4 mg/kg/dose once a month (Kim 2008; Prasad 2007); in HSCT recipient, doses have been administered every 2 to 4 weeks (Tomblyn [CDC/IDSA 2009])

Pneumocystis jirovecii **pneumonia (PCP), treatment (moderate-severe disease): Note:** For patients who cannot tolerate or who fail to respond to 5 to 7 days of sulfamethoxazole and trimethoprim:
Manufacturer's labeling: Infants ≥5 months, Children, and Adolescents: IM, IV: 4 mg/kg/dose once daily for 14 to 21 days
HIV-exposed/-positive:
Infants and Children: IV: 4 mg/kg/dose once daily; if clinical improvement after 7 to 10 days of therapy, may change to an oral regimen to complete a 21-day course (HHS [OI pediatric 2013])
Adolescents: IV: Refer to adult dosing.
Non-HIV-exposed/-positive: Infants, Children, and Adolescents: IV: 3 to 4 mg/kg/dose once daily for 21 days (Bradley 2015)

Trypanosomiasis, treatment (non-CNS disease) (off-label use): Infants, Children, Adolescents, and Adults: IM, IV: 4 mg/kg/dose once daily for 7 to 10 days (Bradley 2015; CDC 2013; *Red Book* [AAP 2015])

Renal Impairment IV: The FDA-approved labeling recommends that caution should be used in patients with renal impairment; however, no specific dosage adjustment guidelines are available. The following guidelines have been used by some clinicians (Aronoff 2007):
Adults:
CrCl ≥10 mL/minute: No dosage adjustment necessary.
CrCl <10 mL/minute: Administer 4 mg/kg every 24 to 36 hours.

Children:
CrCl >30 mL/minute: No dosage adjustment necessary.
CrCl 10 to 30 mL/minute: Administer 4 mg/kg every 36 hours.
CrCl <10 mL/minute and peritoneal dialysis: Administer 4 mg/kg every 48 hours.
Hemodialysis: Administer 4 mg/kg every 48 hours, after dialysis on dialysis days.

Hepatic Impairment There are no dosage adjustments provided in the manufacturer's labeling (has not been studied). Use with caution.

Additional Information Complete prescribing information should be consulted for additional detail.

Dosage Forms Excipient information presented when available (limited, particularly for generics); consult specific product labeling.

Solution Reconstituted, Injection, as isethionate:
Pentam: 300 mg (1 ea)

Pentamidine (Oral Inhalation) (pen TAM i deen)

Brand Names: US Nebupent
Index Terms Pentamidine Isethionate
Pharmacologic Category Antifungal Agent; Antiprotozoal

Use Prevention of *Pneumocystis jirovecii* pneumonia (PCP) in high-risk, HIV-infected patients either with a history of PCP or with a CD4+ count ≤200/mm^3

Dosing

Adult & Geriatric

Pneumocystis jirovecii **pneumonia (PCP), prevention:** Primary or secondary prophylaxis (alternative to preferred therapy): Inhalation: 300 mg once every 4 weeks via Respirgard II nebulizer (HHS [OI adult 2015])

Pediatric

Pneumocystis jirovecii **pneumonia (PCP), prevention:**
Children ≥5 years (off-label population): Inhalation: 300 mg once every 4 weeks via Respirgard II nebulizer (HHS [OI pediatric 2013]; *Redbook* [AAP 2015]; Tomblyn 2009)
Adolescents (off-label population): Refer to adult dosing.

Renal Impairment There are no dosage adjustments provided in manufacturer's labeling (has not been studied). Use with caution.

Hepatic Impairment There are no dosage adjustments provided in manufacturer's labeling (has not been studied). Use with caution.

Additional Information Complete prescribing information should be consulted for additional detail.

Dosage Forms Excipient information presented when available (limited, particularly for generics); consult specific product labeling.

Solution Reconstituted, Inhalation, as isethionate:
Nebupent: 300 mg (1 ea)

- ◆ Pentamidine Isethionate *see* Pentamidine (Oral Inhalation) *on page 1425*
- ◆ Pentamidine Isethionate *see* Pentamidine (Systemic) *on page 1425*
- ◆ Pentamycetin® (Can) *see* Chloramphenicol *on page 371*
- ◆ Pentasa *see* Mesalamine *on page 1151*
- ◆ Pentasodium Colistin Methanesulfonate *see* Colistimethate *on page 443*
- ◆ Pentavalent Human-Bovine Reassortant Rotavirus Vaccine (PRV) *see* Rotavirus Vaccine *on page 1623*

Pentazocine (pen TAZ oh seen)

Brand Names: US Talwin
Brand Names: Canada Talwin
Index Terms Pentazocine Lactate
Pharmacologic Category Analgesic, Opioid; Analgesic, Opioid Partial Agonist

Additional Appendix Information
Opioid Conversion Table and Morphine Equivalent Dose Table *on page 1955*

Use Relief of moderate-to-severe pain; has also been used as a sedative prior to surgery and as a supplement to surgical anesthesia

Dosing

Adult

Analgesic:
IM, SubQ: 30-60 mg every 3-4 hours; do **not** exceed 60 mg/dose (maximum: 360 mg/day)
IV: 30 mg every 3-4 hours; do **not** exceed 30 mg/dose (maximum: 360 mg/day)

Labor pain:
IM: 30 mg once
IV: 20 mg every 2-3 hours as needed (maximum total dose: 60 mg)

Geriatric Use with caution; may be more sensitive to analgesic and sedative effects; decrease initial dose and monitor closely

Pediatric

Analgesia (off-label use): IM:
Children 5-8 years: 15 mg
Children: 9-14 years: 30 mg

Preoperative/preanesthetic: Children 1-16 years: IM: 0.5 mg/kg

Renal Impairment No dosage adjustment provided in manufacturer's labeling. Use with caution. The following guidelines have been used by some clinicians (Aronoff, 2007):
CrCl ≥50 mL/minute: No dosage adjustment necessary.
CrCl 10-50 mL/minute: Administer 75% of normal dose.
CrCl <10 mL/minute: Administer 50% of normal dose.

Hepatic Impairment No dosage adjustment provided in manufacturer's labeling. However, dosage adjustment may be necessary due to decreased metabolism and predisposition to adverse effects. Use with caution.

Additional Information Complete prescribing information should be consulted for additional detail.

Dosage Forms Excipient information presented when available (limited, particularly for generics); consult specific product labeling.
Solution, Injection:
Talwin: 30 mg/mL (1 mL)
Talwin: 30 mg/mL (10 mL) [contains methylparaben, sodium bisulfite]

Controlled Substance C-IV

♦ Pentazocine Lactate see Pentazocine on page 1425

PENTobarbital (pen toe BAR bi tal)

Brand Names: US Nembutal
Brand Names: Canada Nembutal Sodium
Index Terms Pentobarbital Sodium
Pharmacologic Category Anticonvulsant, Barbiturate; Barbiturate
Use Sedative/hypnotic; status epilepticus (refractory)
Dosing

Adult Note: Adjust dose based on patient's age, weight, and condition.

Hypnotic/sedative:
IM: 150 to 200 mg
IV: Initial: 100 mg; decrease dose for elderly or debilitated patients. If needed, may administer additional increments after at least 1 minute, up to a total dose of 200 to 500 mg

Barbiturate coma in severe brain injury patients/elevated intracranial pressure (off-label use; Bratton, 2007): IV: Loading dose: 10 mg/kg given over 30 minutes (or ≤25 mg/minute), followed by 5 mg/kg every hour for 3 doses; monitor blood pressure and respiratory rate. Maintenance infusion: Initial: 1 mg/kg/hour; may increase to 2 to 4 mg/kg/hour; maintain burst suppression on EEG.

Status epilepticus, refractory: IV: **Note:** Mechanical ventilation and cardiovascular monitoring required; titrate to cessation of electrographic seizures or burst suppression (NCS [Brophy, 2012]).

Neurocritical Care Society recommendations (NCS [Brophy, 2012]):
Loading dose: 5 to 15 mg/kg administered at a rate of ≤50 mg/minute, may give additional 5 to 10 mg/kg; follow with a continuous infusion.
Continuous infusion: 0.5 to 5 mg/kg/hour. If the patient experiences breakthrough status epilepticus while on continuous infusion, administer an additional 5 mg/kg bolus and increase infusion rate by 0.5 to 1 mg/kg/hour every 12 hours. **Note:** A period of at least 24 to 48 hours of electrographic control is recommended prior to withdrawing the continuous infusion; withdraw gradually to prevent recurrent status epilepticus

Geriatric Not recommended for use in the elderly; decrease dose if use becomes necessary.

Pediatric Note: Adjust dose based on patient's age, weight, and condition.

Hypnotic/sedative:
IM: 2 to 6 mg/kg; maximum: 100 mg/dose
IV: 1 to 6 mg/kg titrated in 1 to 2 mg/kg increments every 3 to 5 minutes to desired effect (Krauss, 2006)

Status epilepticus, refractory: IV: **Note:** Mechanical ventilation and cardiovascular monitoring required; titrate dose to cessation of electrographic seizures or burst suppression (NCS [Brophy, 2012]).

Neurocritical Care Society recommendations:
Loading dose: 5 to 15 mg/kg administered slowly (eg, over 60 to 120 minutes [maximum rate: 50 mg/minute]), may give additional 5 to 10 mg/kg; follow with a continuous infusion (NCS [Brophy, 2012]; Phelps, 2013).
Continuous infusion: 0.5 to 5 mg/kg/hour. If the patient experiences breakthrough status epilepticus while on continuous infusion, administer an additional 5 mg/kg bolus and increase infusion rate by 0.5 to 1 mg/kg/hour every 12 hours. **Note:** A period of at least 24 to 48 hours of electrographic control is recommended prior to withdrawing the continuous infusion; withdraw gradually to prevent recurrent status epilepticus (NCS [Brophy, 2012])

Renal Impairment No dosage adjustment provided in manufacturer's labeling. However, a reduced dosage in patients with renal dysfunction is recommended.

Hepatic Impairment No dosage adjustment provided in manufacturer's labeling. However, a reduced dosage in patients with liver dysfunction is recommended.

Additional Information Complete prescribing information should be consulted for additional detail.

Dosage Forms Excipient information presented when available (limited, particularly for generics); consult specific product labeling. [DSC] = Discontinued product
Solution, Injection, as sodium:
Nembutal: 50 mg/mL (20 mL [DSC], 50 mL [DSC])
Nembutal: 50 mg/mL (20 mL, 50 mL) [latex free; contains alcohol, usp, propylene glycol]

Controlled Substance C-II

♦ Pentobarbital Sodium see PENTobarbital on page 1426

Pentosan Polysulfate Sodium
(PEN toe san pol i SUL fate SOW dee um)

Brand Names: US Elmiron
Brand Names: Canada Elmiron®
Index Terms PPS
Pharmacologic Category Analgesic, Urinary
Use Relief of bladder pain or discomfort due to interstitial cystitis
Dosing

Adult & Geriatric Interstitial cystitis: Oral: 100 mg 3 times/day taken with water 1 hour before or 2 hours after meals

Note: Patients should be evaluated at 3 months and may be continued an additional 3 months if there has been no improvement and if there are no therapy-limiting side effects. **The risks and benefits of continued use beyond 6 months in patients who have not responded is not yet known.**

Pediatric Children ≥16 years: Refer to adult dosing.

Renal Impairment No dosage adjustment provided in manufacturer's labeling (has not been studied).

Hepatic Impairment No dosage adjustment provided in manufacturer's labeling (has not been studied). However, dosage adjustment may be necessary due to hepatic impairment impact on pharmacokinetics. Use with caution.

Additional Information Complete prescribing information should be consulted for additional detail.

Dosage Forms Excipient information presented when available (limited, particularly for generics); consult specific product labeling.
Capsule, Oral:
Elmiron: 100 mg [contains fd&c blue #1 aluminum lake, fd&c blue #2 aluminum lake, fd&c red #40 aluminum lake, fd&c yellow #10 aluminum lake]

Pentostatin (pen toe STAT in)

Brand Names: US Nipent
Brand Names: Canada Nipent
Index Terms 2'-Deoxycoformycin; Co-Vidarabine; dCF; Deoxycoformycin
Pharmacologic Category Antineoplastic Agent, Antimetabolite; Antineoplastic Agent, Antimetabolite (Purine Analog)
Use Hairy cell leukemia: Treatment (as a single-agent) of untreated and interferon-refractory hairy cell leukemia in patients with active disease (clinically significant anemia, neutropenia, thrombocytopenia, or disease-related symptoms)

Dosing

Adult & Geriatric

Hairy cell leukemia: IV: 4 mg/m² every 2 weeks. **Note:** The optimal duration has not been determined; in the absence of unacceptable toxicity, may continue until complete response is achieved or until 2 doses after complete response. Discontinue after 6 months if partial or complete response is not achieved.

Acute graft-versus-host disease (GVHD), steroid-refractory (off-label use): IV:

Initial therapy: 1.5 mg/m² days 1 to 3 and days 15 to 17 (in combination with corticosteroids) (Alousi, 2009)

Steroid-refractory disease: 1.5 mg/m² daily for 3 days; may repeat after 2 weeks if needed (Bolanos-Meade, 2005)

Chronic graft-versus-host disease (GVHD), steroid-refractory (off-label use): IV: 4 mg/m² once every 2 weeks; discontinue after 6 months for sustained objective response, or continue every 2 to 4 weeks for up to 12 months if still improving (Jacobsohn, 2007; Jacobsohn, 2009) **or** 4 mg/m² once every 2 weeks for 3 months (Wolff, 2011)

Chronic lymphocytic leukemia (CLL; off-label use): IV:

Previously treated: 4 mg/m² once every 3 weeks (in combination with cyclophosphamide and rituximab) for 6 cycles (Lamanna, 2006)

Previously untreated: 2 mg/m² once every 3 weeks (in combination with cyclophosphamide and rituximab) for 6 cycles (Kay, 2007)

Cutaneous T-cell lymphoma, mycosis fungoides/Sezary syndrome (off-label use): IV: 4 mg/m² once weekly for 3 weeks, then every 2 weeks for 6 weeks, then once monthly for a maximum of 6 months (Ho, 1999)

T-cell prolymphocytic leukemia, refractory (off-label use): IV: 4 mg/m² once weekly for 4 weeks then every 2 weeks until optimum response is achieved (Mercieca, 1994) **or** 4 mg/m² once weekly for 4 weeks then every 2 weeks (in combination with alemtuzumab) until complete or best response or up to a total of 14 doses (Ravandi, 2009)

Pediatric

Chronic graft-versus-host disease (GVHD), steroid-refractory: IV: 4 mg/m² once every 2 weeks; discontinue after 6 months for sustained objective response, or continue every 2 to 4 weeks for up to 12 months if still improving (Jacobsohn, 2007; Jacobsohn, 2009) **or** 4 mg/m² once every 2 weeks for 3 months (Wolff, 2011)

Renal Impairment There are no dosage adjustments provided in the manufacturer's labeling; although not adequately studied, two patients with CrCl 50 to 60 mL/minute achieved responses when treated with 2 mg/m²/dose. For renal toxicity *during* treatment, withhold for elevated serum creatinine and determine creatinine clearance. The following adjustments have also been recommended:

Kintzel, 1995:

CrCl 46 to 60 mL/minute: Administer 70% of dose

CrCl 31 to 45 mL/minute: Administer 60% of dose

CrCl <30 mL/minute: Consider use of alternative drug

Lathia, 2002:

CrCl ≥60 mL/minute: Administer 4 mg/m²/dose

CrCl 40 to 59 mL/minute: Administer 3 mg/m²/dose

CrCl 20 to 39 mL/minute: Administer 2 mg/m²/dose

Alousi, 2009; Jacobsohn, 2009; Poi, 2013 (for GVHD treatment):

CrCl 30 to 50 mL/minute/1.73 m²: Reduce dose by 50%

CrCl <30 mL/minute/1.73 m²: Withhold dose

Lamanna, 2006 (for previously treated CLL): Serum creatinine >2 mg/dL or 20% above patient's baseline: Withhold treatment until serum creatinine ≤2 mg/dL or returns to baseline, or until CrCl ≥50 mL/minute

Hepatic Impairment There are no dosage adjustments provided in the manufacturer's labeling.

Obesity

American Society of Clinical Oncology (ASCO) Guidelines for appropriate chemotherapy dosing in obese adults with cancer: Utilize patient's actual body weight (full weight) for calculation of body surface area- or weight-based dosing, particularly when the intent of therapy is curative; manage regimen-related toxicities in the same manner as for nonobese patients; if a dose reduction is utilized due to toxicity, consider resumption of full weight-based dosing with subsequent cycles, especially if cause of toxicity (eg, hepatic or renal impairment) is resolved (Griggs, 2012).

American Society for Blood and Marrow Transplantation (ASBMT) practice guideline committee position statement on chemotherapy dosing in obesity: Utilize actual body weight (full weight) for calculation of body surface area in pentostatin dosing for hematopoietic stem cell

---

transplant conditioning regimens in adults (Bubalo, 2014).

Adjustment for Toxicity

ANC <200/mm³ (with baseline ANC >500/mm³): Temporarily interrupt treatment until ANC returns to pre-dose levels.

CNS toxicity: Withhold treatment or discontinue.

Infection, active: Interrupt treatment until infection is controlled.

Rash: Severe rashes may require treatment interruption or discontinuation.

Other severe adverse reactions: Withhold treatment or discontinue.

Additional Information Complete prescribing information should be consulted for additional detail.

Dosage Forms Excipient information presented when available (limited, particularly for generics); consult specific product labeling. [DSC] = Discontinued product

Solution Reconstituted, Intravenous:

Nipent: 10 mg (1 ea)

Solution Reconstituted, Intravenous [preservative free]:

Generic: 10 mg (1 ea [DSC])

Pentoxifylline (pen toks IF i lin)

Brand Names: US TRENtal [DSC]

Brand Names: Canada Pentoxifylline SR

Index Terms Oxpentifylline; Trental

Pharmacologic Category Blood Viscosity Reducer Agent

Use

Intermittent claudication: Treatment of intermittent claudication on the basis of chronic occlusive arterial disease of the limbs.

Limitations of use: May improve function and symptoms, but not intended to replace more definitive therapy. **Note:** The American College of Chest Physicians (ACCP) discourages the use of pentoxifylline for the treatment of intermittent claudication refractory to exercise therapy (and smoking cessation) (Guyatt, 2012).

Dosing

Adult & Geriatric

Intermittent claudication: Oral: 400 mg 3 times daily; maximal therapeutic benefit may take 2 to 4 weeks to develop; recommended to maintain therapy for at least 8 weeks. May reduce to 400 mg twice daily if GI or CNS side effects occur; discontinue if side effects persist.

Note: Use for the treatment of intermittent claudication refractory to exercise therapy (and smoking cessation) has been discouraged by The American College of Chest Physicians (ACCP) (Guyatt, 2012).

Severe alcoholic hepatitis (Maddrey Discriminant Function [MDF] score ≥32, especially when corticosteroids contraindicated) (off-label use): Oral: 400 mg 3 times daily for 4 weeks (O'Shea, 2010)

Venous leg ulcer (off-label use): Oral: 400 mg 3 times daily (with compression therapy) (Jull, 2002; Robson, 2006)

Renal Impairment

Manufacturer's labeling: CrCl <30 mL/minute: 400 mg once daily

The following guidelines have been used by some clinicians:

Aronoff, 2007: Adults:

CrCl >50 mL/minute: 400 mg every 8 to 12 hours

CrCl 10-50 mL/minute: 400 mg every 12 to 24 hours

CrCl <10 mL minute: 400 mg every 24 hours

Hemodialysis: supplemental postdialysis dose is not necessary.

Peritoneal dialysis: 400 mg every 24 hours

Paap, 1996: Adults:

Moderate renal impairment (CrCl ~60 mL/minute): 400 mg twice daily.

Severe renal impairment (CrCl ~20 mL/minute): 400 mg once daily; further reduction may be required; Paap suggests 200 mg once daily, but with current products (extended or controlled release; unscored) may require adaptation to 400 mg once every other day.

Hepatic Impairment There are no dosage adjustments provided in manufacturer's labeling; use with caution.

Additional Information Complete prescribing information should be consulted for additional detail.

Dosage Forms Excipient information presented when available (limited, particularly for generics); consult specific product labeling. [DSC] = Discontinued product

Tablet Extended Release, Oral:

TRENtal: 400 mg [DSC] [contains benzyl alcohol]

Generic: 400 mg

◆ Pentoxifylline SR (Can) see Pentoxifylline on page 1427

◆ Pen VK *see* Penicillin V Potassium *on page 1424*

◆ PEP005 *see* Ingenol Mebutate *on page 952*

◆ Pepcid *see* Famotidine *on page 741*

◆ Pepcid AC (Can) *see* Famotidine *on page 741*

◆ Pepcid Complete (Can) *see* Famotidine *on page 741*

◆ Peptic guard (Can) *see* Famotidine *on page 741*

◆ Peptic Relief [OTC] *see* Bismuth Subsalicylate *on page 232*

◆ Pepto-Bismol [OTC] *see* Bismuth Subsalicylate *on page 232*

◆ Pepto-Bismol To-Go [OTC] *see* Bismuth Subsalicylate *on page 232*

Peramivir (pe RA mi veer)

Brand Names: US Rapivab
Index Terms BCX-1812; RWJ-270201
Pharmacologic Category Antiviral Agent; Neuraminidase Inhibitor

Use
Influenza: Treatment of acute, uncomplicated influenza in adults who have been symptomatic ≤2 days.
Limitations of use:
Efficacy has not been established for patients with serious influenza requiring hospitalization.
Efficacy is based on clinical trials in which influenza A was the predominant virus; a limited number of subjects with influenza B have been studied.

Pregnancy Considerations Adverse events were observed in some animal reproduction studies. Information related to the use of peramivir in pregnancy is limited (Hernandez 2011; Sorbello 2012). Based on information from one case, the pharmacokinetics of peramivir may be changed with pregnancy (Clay 2011).

Untreated influenza infection is associated with an increased risk of adverse events to the fetus and an increased risk of complications or death to the mother (CDC 62[07], 2013). Neuraminidase inhibitors are currently recommended for the treatment or prophylaxis of influenza in pregnant women and women up to 2 weeks postpartum (CDC 60[1], 2011; CDC March 13, 2014; CDC January 2015).

Breast-Feeding Considerations It is not known if peramivir is excreted into breast milk. According to the manufacturer, the decision to breast-feed during therapy should take into account the risk of exposure to the infant and the benefits of treatment to the mother. Influenza may cause serious illness in postpartum women and prompt evaluation for febrile respiratory illnesses is recommended (Louie 2011).

Contraindications There are no contraindications listed in the manufacturer's labeling.

Warnings/Precautions Rare serious skin reactions (eg, erythema multiforme, Stevens-Johnson syndrome)) have been reported. If skin reactions are suspected or occur, institute appropriate supportive treatment. Serious hypersensitivity reactions (eg, anaphylaxis, urticaria, angioedema) have been reported with other neuraminidase inhibitors. Although these reactions have not yet been observed with peramivir, discontinue infusion immediately and treat reaction if hypersensitivity is suspected. Rare occurrences of neuropsychiatric events (including abnormal behavior, delirium, and hallucinations), including fatalities, have been reported, primarily among pediatric patients. Onset is often abrupt and subsequent resolution is rapid. These events may occur in patients with encephalitis, encephalopathy, or in uncomplicated influenza. Closely monitor for signs of abnormal behavior. Emergence of resistance substitutions or other factors (eg, viral virulence) could decrease drug effectiveness. Consider available information on influenza drug susceptibility patterns/treatment effects when using; efficacy in patients with serious influenza requiring hospitalization has not been established. Has not been shown to prevent secondary serious bacterial infections occurring during influenza course; if bacterial infections occur, treat with antibiotics as appropriate. Elimination is primarily renal; dosage adjustment is required in renal impairment. Potentially significant drug-drug interactions may exist, requiring dose or frequency adjustment, additional monitoring, and/or selection of alternative therapy.

Adverse Reactions
1% to 10%:
Cardiovascular: Hypertension (2%)
Central nervous system: Insomnia (3%)
Endocrine: Increased serum glucose (>160 mg/dL: 5%)
Gastrointestinal: Diarrhea (8%), constipation (4%)
Hematologic and oncologic: Neutropenia (<1 x 10^9/L: 8%)

Hepatic: Increased serum ALT (>2.5 x ULN: 3%), increased serum AST (3%)
Neuromuscular & skeletal: Increased creatine phosphokinase (≥6 x ULN: 4%)
<1% (Limited to important or life-threatening): Abnormal behavior, delirium, erythema multiforme, exfoliative dermatitis, hallucination, skin rash, Stevens-Johnson syndrome

Drug Interactions
Metabolism/Transport Effects None known.
Avoid Concomitant Use There are no known interactions where it is recommended to avoid concomitant use.
Increased Effect/Toxicity There are no known significant interactions involving an increase in effect.
Decreased Effect
Peramivir may decrease the levels/effects of: Influenza Virus Vaccine (Live/Attenuated)

Preparation for Administration Dilute solution for injection in a compatible vehicle to a maximum volume of 100 mL. Administer immediately or store at 2°C to 8°C (36°F to 46°F) for up to 24 hours.

Storage/Stability Store intact vials at 20°C to 25°C (68°F to 77°F); excursions are permitted between 15°C and 30°C (59°F and 86°F).

Mechanism of Action Peramivir, a cyclopentane analogue, selectively inhibits the influenza virus neuraminidase enzyme, preventing the release of viral particles from infected cells.

Pharmacodynamics/Kinetics
Distribution: V_d: 12.56 L
Protein binding: <30%
Metabolism: Not significantly metabolized
Half-life elimination: ~20 hours
Excretion: Urine (~90% as unchanged drug)

Dosing
Adult & Geriatric Influenza (acute [≤2 days], uncomplicated): IV: 600 mg as a single dose
Renal Impairment Note: Renal function may be estimated using the Cockcroft-Gault formula.
CrCl ≥50 mL/minute: No dosage adjustment necessary.
CrCl 30 to 49 mL/minute: 200 mg as a single dose
CrCl 10 to 29 mL/minute: 100 mg as a single dose
End-stage renal disease requiring (ESRD) intermittent hemodialysis (IHD): 100 mg as a single dose, administered after dialysis

Hepatic Impairment There are no dosage adjustments provided in the manufacturer's labeling (has not been studied); however, not significantly metabolized hepatically.

Administration Administer as an intravenous infusion over 15 to 30 minutes.

Monitoring Parameters Baseline BUN and serum creatinine, neurologic abnormalities (eg, abnormal behavior), rash after administration.

Dosage Forms Excipient information presented when available (limited, particularly for generics); consult specific product labeling.
Solution, Intravenous [preservative free]:
Rapivab: 200 mg/20 mL (20 mL)

Perampanel (per AM pa nel)

Brand Names: US Fycompa
Brand Names: Canada Fycompa
Pharmacologic Category AMPA Glutamate Receptor Antagonist; Anticonvulsant, Miscellaneous

Use
Partial-onset seizures: Adjunctive therapy for the treatment of partial-onset seizures with or without secondarily generalized seizures in patients with epilepsy who are ≥12 years of age (US labeling) or adults (Canadian labeling).
Primary generalized tonic-clonic seizures: Adjunctive therapy for the treatment of primary generalized tonic-clonic seizures in patients with epilepsy who are ≥12 years of age (US labeling) or adults (Canadian labeling).

Pregnancy Considerations Adverse events have been observed in animal reproduction studies at doses equivalent to the human dose (based on BSA). Contraceptives containing levonorgestrel may be less effective; additional nonhormonal forms of contraception are recommended during perampanel therapy.

Patients exposed to perampanel during pregnancy are encouraged to enroll in the North American Antiepileptic Drug (NAAED) Pregnancy Registry by calling 1-888-233-2334. Additional information is available at www.aedpregnancyregistry.org.

Breast-Feeding Considerations It is not known if perampanel is excreted in breast milk. The manufacturer's US labeling recommends that caution be exercised when administering perampanel to nursing women. Due to the potential for serious adverse reactions in the nursing

infant, the Canadian labeling recommends a decision be made whether to discontinue nursing or to discontinue the drug, taking into account the importance of treatment to the mother.

Medication Guide Available Yes

Contraindications

There are no contraindications listed in manufacturer's US labeling.

Canadian labeling: Hypersensitivity to perampanel or any component of the formulation.

Warnings/Precautions [US Boxed Warning]: Dose-related serious and/or life-threatening neuropsychiatric events (including aggression, anger, homicidal ideation and threats, hostility, and irritability) have been reported most often occurring in first 6 weeks of therapy in patients with or without prior psychiatric history, prior aggressive behavior, or concomitant use of medications associated with hostility and aggression; monitor patients closely especially during dosage adjustments and when receiving higher doses. Adjust dose or immediately discontinue use if severe or worsening symptoms occur; permanently discontinue for persistent severe or worsening psychiatric symptoms or behaviors. Inform patients and caregivers to contact their healthcare provider immediately if they experience any atypical behavioral and/or mood changes while taking perampanel or after discontinuing perampanel. Concurrent use with alcohol has been associated with significantly worsened mood and increased anger; patients should avoid the use of alcohol during therapy. Pooled analysis of trials involving various antiepileptics (regardless of indication) showed an increased risk of suicidal thoughts/behavior (incidence rate: 0.43% treated patients compared to 0.24% of patients receiving placebo); risk observed as early as 1 week after initiation and continued through duration of trials (most trials ≤24 weeks). Monitor all patients for notable changes in behavior that might indicate suicidal thoughts or depression; notify healthcare provider immediately if symptoms occur. Dizziness, fatigue (including lethargy and weakness), gait disturbances (including abnormal coordination, ataxia, and balance disorder), and somnolence may occur during therapy; patients should be cautioned about performing tasks which require alertness (eg, operating machinery or driving). Concomitant use with CNS depressant (including alcohol) may increase the risk of CNS depression. Use caution if a CNS depressant must be used concurrently with perampanel. Not recommended for use in patients with severe hepatic impairment, severe renal impairment, or on hemodialysis; dosage adjustment recommended for mild-to-moderate hepatic impairment and consider slower titration in patients with moderate renal impairment. The Canadian labeling does not recommend use in patients with moderate or severe renal impairment or on hemodialysis. Use with extreme caution in patients who are at risk of falls (including head injuries and bone fracture); perampanel has been associated with falls and traumatic injury. Anticonvulsants should not be discontinued abruptly because of the possibility of increasing seizure frequency; therapy should be withdrawn gradually (≥1 week) to minimize the potential of increased seizure frequency, unless safety concerns require a more rapid withdrawal. Use caution in elderly due to increased risk of dizziness, gait or coordination disturbances, somnolence, fatigue-related events, and falls; proceed slowly with dosing titration in patients ≥65 years of age. Potentially significant drug-drug interactions may exist, requiring dose or frequency adjustment, additional monitoring, and/or selection of alternative therapy. Formulation may contain lactose.

Adverse Reactions Many adverse effects are dose-related. Frequency not always defined.

Cardiovascular: Peripheral edema (2%)

Central nervous system: Dizziness (16% to ≤47%), vertigo (3% to ≤47%), hostility (≤12% to ≤20%), aggressive behavior (2% to ≤20%), drowsiness (9% to 18%), abnormal gait (4% to 16%), fatigue (8% to 15%), headache (12% to 13%), irritability (2% to 12%), falling (5% to 10%), ataxia (≤8%), equilibrium disturbance (3% to 5%), anxiety (2% to 5%), dysarthria (1% to 4%), hypoesthesia (3%), hypersomnia (1% to 3%), anger (1% to 3%), memory impaired (2%), paresthesia (2%), confusion (1% to 2%), euphoria (≤2%), mood changes (1% to 2%), agitation, altered mental status, delusion, disorientation, emotional lability, homicidal ideation, paranoia, psychiatric disturbance (worsening)

Dermatologic: Skin rash (4%)

Endocrine & metabolic: Weight gain (4% to 9%), hyponatremia (2%)

Gastrointestinal: Vomiting (4% to 9%), nausea (6% to 8%), abdominal pain (5%), constipation (3%)

Genitourinary: Urinary tract infection (4%)

Hematologic & oncologic: Bruise (2% to 6%)

Neuromuscular & skeletal: Back pain (5%), sprain (4%), myalgia (3%), arthralgia (2% to 3%), limb pain (2% to 3%), musculoskeletal pain (2%), weakness (2%)

Ophthalmic: Blurred vision (3% to 4%), diplopia (3%)

Respiratory: Cough (4%), upper respiratory tract infection (4%), oropharyngeal pain (2%)

Miscellaneous: Head trauma (3%), laceration (2%), limb injury (1% to 2%)

<1% (limited to important or life-threatening): DRESS Syndrome, increased serum triglycerides, suicidal ideation

Drug Interactions

Metabolism/Transport Effects Substrate of CYP1A2 (minor), CYP2B6 (minor), CYP3A4 (major); **Note:** Assignment of Major/Minor substrate status based on clinically relevant drug interaction potential

Avoid Concomitant Use

Avoid concomitant use of Perampanel with any of the following: Alcohol (Ethyl); Azelastine (Nasal); CYP3A4 Inducers (Strong); Orphenadrine; Paraldehyde; St Johns Wort; Thalidomide

Increased Effect/Toxicity

Perampanel may increase the levels/effects of: Alcohol (Ethyl); Azelastine (Nasal); Buprenorphine; CNS Depressants; Hydrocodone; Methotrimeprazine; Metyrosine; Orphenadrine; OXcarbazepine; Paraldehyde; Pramipexole; ROPINIRole; Rotigotine; Selective Serotonin Reuptake Inhibitors; Suvorexant; Thalidomide; Zolpidem

The levels/effects of Perampanel may be increased by: Brimonidine (Topical); Cannabis; Dronabinol; Droperidol; Kava Kava; Magnesium Sulfate; Methotrimeprazine; Minocycline; Nabilone; Osimertinib; Rufinamide; Sodium Oxybate; Tapentadol; Tetrahydrocannabinol

Decreased Effect

Perampanel may decrease the levels/effects of: Contraceptives (Progestins)

The levels/effects of Perampanel may be decreased by: Bosentan; CarBAMazepine; CYP3A4 Inducers (Moderate); CYP3A4 Inducers (Strong); Dabrafenib; Deferasirox; Fosphenytoin; Mefloquine; Orlistat; Osimertinib; OXcarbazepine; Phenytoin; Siltuximab; St Johns Wort; Tocilizumab

Storage/Stability Store at 20°C to 25°C (68°F to 77°F); excursions permitted between 15°C to 30°C (59°F to 86°F).

Mechanism of Action The exact mechanism by which perampanel exerts antiseizure activity is not definitively known; it is a noncompetitive antagonist of the ionotropic alpha-amino-3-hydroxy-5-methyl-4-isoxazolepropionic acid (AMPA) glutamate receptor on postsynaptic neurons. Glutamate is a primary excitatory neurotransmitter in the central nervous center causing many neurological disorders from neuronal over excitation.

Pharmacodynamics/Kinetics

Absorption: Rapid and complete; food slows rate of absorption

Protein binding: ~95% to 96%; primarily albumin and alpha$_1$-acid glycoprotein

Metabolism: Extensive via primary oxidation mediated by CYP3A4/5, and to a lesser extent by CYP1A2 and CYP2B6, and sequential glucuronidation

Half-life elimination: ~105 hours

Time to peak: 0.5 to 2.5 hours; delayed 2 to 3 hours with food

Excretion: Feces (48%); urine (22%)

Dosing

Adult Note: Reduce the dosage in patients who experience serious psychiatric or behavioral reactions; discontinue immediately if symptoms are severe or worsening.

Partial-onset seizures (adjunct): Oral:

Patients **not** receiving enzyme-inducing AED regimens: Initial: 2 mg once daily at bedtime; may increase daily dose by 2 mg once daily no more frequently than at weekly intervals (US labeling) or 2-week intervals (Canadian labeling) based on response and tolerability. Recommended maintenance dose: 8 to 12 mg once daily at bedtime; some patients may respond to 4 mg once daily; 12 mg once daily has resulted in somewhat greater reductions in seizure rates in some patients but with substantial increase in side effects.

Patients receiving enzyme-inducing AED regimens (eg, phenytoin, carbamazepine, oxcarbazepine): Initial: 4 mg once daily at bedtime; may increase daily dose by 2 mg once daily no more frequently than at weekly intervals based on response and tolerability. Maintenance dose has not been established; highest dose used in clinical trials was 12 mg once daily.

Primary generalized tonic-clonic seizures (adjunct):
Oral:
Patients **not** receiving enzyme-inducing AED regimens: Initial: 2 mg once daily at bedtime; may increase dose by 2 mg once daily no more frequently than at weekly intervals (US labeling) or 2-week intervals (Canadian labeling) based on response and tolerability. Recommended maintenance dose: 8 mg once daily at bedtime; if tolerated and further seizure control is needed, may increase up to 12 mg once daily (maximum dose: 12 mg once daily).

Patients receiving enzyme-inducing AED regimens (eg, phenytoin, carbamazepine, oxcarbazepine): Initial 4 mg once daily at bedtime; may increase daily dose by 2 mg once daily no more frequently than at weekly intervals based on response and tolerability. Maintenance dose has not been established; highest dose used in clinical trials was 12 mg once daily.

Missed doses: Canadian labeling:
If a single dose is missed wait until next scheduled dose.

If >1 dose is missed for a continuous period of <3 weeks (patients not receiving enzyme-inducing AED regimens) or <1 week (patients receiving enzyme-inducing AED regimens), may consider resuming therapy at the previous dosage.

If therapy has been continuously omitted for periods longer than 3 weeks (patients not receiving enzyme-inducing AED regimens) or 1 week (patients receiving enzyme-inducing AED regimens), reinitiate therapy with initial dosing recommendations.

Geriatric Refer to adult dosing. Increase dose no more frequently than every 2 weeks.

Pediatric
US labeling:
Partial-onset seizures (adjunct): Children ≥12 years and Adolescents: Refer to adult dosing.
Primary generalized tonic-clonic seizures (adjunct): Children ≥12 years and Adolescents: Refer to adult dosing.
Canadian labeling: Not approved for use in patients <18 years of age.

Renal Impairment
US labeling:
CrCl ≥50 mL/minute: No dosage adjustment necessary.
CrCl 30 to 49 mL/minute: No dosage adjustment necessary; monitor closely and consider slower titration based on response and tolerability.
CrCl <30 mL/minute: Use not recommended (has not been studied).
Hemodialysis: Use not recommended (has not been studied).
Canadian labeling:
Mild impairment: No dosage adjustment necessary.
Moderate or severe impairment: Use not recommended (insufficient data in moderate impairment; has not been studied in severe impairment).
Hemodialysis: Use not recommended (has not been studied).

Hepatic Impairment
Mild impairment (Child-Pugh class A): Initial 2 mg once daily; may increase daily dose by 2 mg once daily no more frequently than every 2 weeks based on response and tolerability. Maximum: 6 mg once daily
Moderate impairment (Child-Pugh class B): Initial 2 mg once daily; may increase daily dose by 2 mg once daily no more frequently than every 2 weeks based on response and tolerability. Maximum: 4 mg once daily
Severe impairment (Child-Pugh class C): Use not recommended (has not been studied)

Administration Administer at bedtime without regard to food.

Monitoring Parameters Seizure frequency/duration; suicidality (eg, suicidal thoughts, depression, behavioral changes) during therapy and for at least 1 month after discontinuation; weight

Dosage Forms Excipient information presented when available (limited, particularly for generics); consult specific product labeling.
Tablet, Oral:
Fycompa: 2 mg, 4 mg, 6 mg, 8 mg
Fycompa: 10 mg, 12 mg [contains fd&c blue #2 aluminum lake]

Controlled Substance C-III

Perindopril (per IN doe pril)

Brand Names: US Aceon
Brand Names: Canada Coversyl
Index Terms Perindopril Erbumine
Pharmacologic Category Angiotensin-Converting Enzyme (ACE) Inhibitor; Antihypertensive
Use
Treatment of hypertension; reduction of cardiovascular mortality or nonfatal myocardial infarction in patients with stable coronary artery disease
Canadian labeling: Additional use (off-label use in US): Treatment of mild-moderate (NYHA I-III) heart failure (HF)

Guideline recommendations:
Hypertension: The 2014 guideline for the management of high blood pressure in adults (Eighth Joint National Committee [JNC 8]) recommends initiation of pharmacologic treatment to lower blood pressure for the following patients:
• Patients ≥60 years of age with systolic blood pressure (SBP) ≥150 mm Hg or diastolic blood pressure (DBP) ≥90 mm Hg. Goal of therapy is SBP <150 mm Hg and DBP <90 mm Hg.
• Patients <60 years of age with SBP ≥140 mm Hg or DBP is ≥90 mm Hg. Goal of therapy is SBP <140 mm Hg and DBP <90 mm Hg.
• Patients ≥18 years of age with diabetes and SBP ≥140 mm Hg or DBP ≥90 mm Hg. Goal of therapy is SBP <140 mm Hg and DBP <90 mm Hg.
• Patients ≥18 years of age with chronic kidney disease (CKD) and SBP ≥140 mm Hg or DBP ≥90 mm Hg. Goal of therapy is SBP <140 mm Hg and DBP <90 mm Hg.
Chronic kidney disease (CKD) and hypertension: Regardless of race or diabetes status, the use of an ACE inhibitor (ACEI) or angiotensin receptor blocker (ARB) as initial therapy is recommended to improve kidney outcomes. In the general nonblack population (without CKD) including those with diabetes, initial antihypertensive treatment should consist of a thiazide-type diuretic, calcium channel blocker, ACEI, or ARB. In the general black population (without CKD) including those with diabetes, initial antihypertensive treatment should consist of a thiazide-type diuretic or a calcium channel blocker **instead of** an ACEI or ARB.
Coronary artery disease (CAD) and hypertension: The American Heart Association, American College of Cardiology, and American Society of Hypertension (AHA/ACC/ASH) 2015 scientific statement for the treatment of hypertension in patients with CAD recommends the use of an ACE inhibitor (or an ARB) as part of a regimen in patients with hypertension and chronic stable angina if there is prior MI, LV systolic dysfunction, diabetes mellitus, or CKD. A BP target of <140/90 mm Hg is reasonable for the secondary prevention of cardiovascular events. A lower target BP (<130/80 mm Hg) may be appropriate in some individuals with CAD, previous MI, stroke or transient ischemic attack, or CAD risk equivalents (AHA/ACC/ASH [Rosendorff 2015]).
Heart failure: The ACCF/AHA 2013 heart failure guidelines recommend the use of ACE inhibitors, along with other guideline-directed medical therapies, to prevent HF in patients with a reduced ejection fraction who have a history of MI (stage B HF), to prevent HF in any patient with a reduced ejection fraction (stage B HF), or to treat those with HF and reduced ejection fraction (stage C HFrEF) (ACCF/AHA [Yancy 2013])

Pregnancy Considerations [U.S. Boxed Warning]: Drugs that act on the renin-angiotensin system can cause injury and death to the developing fetus. Discontinue as soon as possible once pregnancy is detected. Drugs that act on the renin-angiotensin system are associated with oligohydramnios. Oligohydramnios, due to decreased fetal renal function, may lead to fetal

lung hypoplasia and skeletal malformations. Their use in pregnancy is also associated with anuria, hypotension, renal failure, skull hypoplasia, and death in the fetus/neonate. Teratogenic effects may occur following maternal use of an ACE inhibitor during the first trimester, although this finding may be confounded by maternal disease. Because adverse fetal events are well documented with exposure later in pregnancy, ACE inhibitor use in pregnant women is not recommended (Seely 2014; Weber 2014). Infants exposed to an ACE inhibitor in utero should be monitored for hyperkalemia, hypotension, and oliguria. Oligohydramnios may not appear until after irreversible fetal injury has occurred. Exchange transfusions or dialysis may be required to reverse hypotension or improve renal function, although data related to the effectiveness in neonates is limited.

Chronic maternal hypertension itself is also associated with adverse events in the fetus/infant and mother. ACE inhibitors are not recommended for the treatment of uncomplicated hypertension in pregnancy (ACOG 2013) and they are specifically contraindicated for the treatment of hypertension and chronic heart failure during pregnancy by some guidelines (Regitz-Zagrosek 2011). In addition, ACE inhibitors should generally be avoided in women of reproductive age (ACOG, 2013). If treatment for hypertension or chronic heart failure in pregnancy is needed, other agents should be used (ACOG 2013; Regitz-Zagrosek 2011). In the Canadian product labeling, use is contraindicated in women who are pregnant or who are planning to become pregnant.

Breast-Feeding Considerations It is not known if perindopril is excreted in human breast milk. The US labeling recommends that caution be exercised when administering perindopril to nursing women. The Canadian labeling contraindicates use in nursing women.

Contraindications

Hypersensitivity to perindopril, any other ACE inhibitor, or any component of the formulation; angioedema related to previous treatment with an ACE inhibitor; history of hereditary/idiopathic angioedema; concomitant use with aliskiren in patients with diabetes mellitus

Canadian labeling: Additional contraindications (not in U.S. labeling): Concomitant use with aliskiren in patients with moderate-to-severe renal impairment (GFR <60 mL/minute/1.73 m^2); women who are pregnant, planning to become pregnant, or nursing; hereditary problems of galactose intolerance, glucose-galactose malabsorption, or the Lapp lactase deficiency (formulation contains lactose)

Warnings/Precautions Anaphylactic reactions may occur rarely with ACE inhibitors. At any time during treatment (especially following first dose), angioedema may occur rarely with ACE inhibitors; it may involve the head and neck (potentially compromising airway) or the intestine (presenting with abdominal pain). African-Americans and patients with idiopathic or hereditary angioedema may be at an increased risk. Risk may also be increased with concomitant use of mTOR inhibitor (eg, everolimus) therapy. Prolonged frequent monitoring may be required especially if tongue, glottis, or larynx are involved as they are associated with airway obstruction. Patients with a history of airway surgery may have a higher risk of airway obstruction. Aggressive early and appropriate management is critical. Use in patients with previous angioedema associated with ACE inhibitor therapy is contraindicated. Severe anaphylactoid reactions may be seen during hemodialysis (eg, CVVHD) with high-flux dialysis membranes (eg, AN69), and rarely, during low density lipoprotein apheresis with dextran sulfate cellulose. Rare cases of anaphylactoid reactions have been reported in patients undergoing sensitization treatment with hymenoptera (bee, wasp) venom while receiving ACE inhibitors.

Symptomatic hypotension with or without syncope can occur with ACE inhibitors (usually with the first several doses); effects are most often observed in volume-depleted patients; correct volume depletion prior to initiation; close monitoring of patient is required especially with initial dosing and dosing increases; blood pressure must be lowered at a rate appropriate for the patient's clinical condition. Initiation of therapy in patients with ischemic heart disease or cerebrovascular disease warrants close observation due to the potential consequences posed by falling blood pressure (eg, MI, stroke). Use with caution in hypertrophic cardiomyopathy with outflow tract obstruction and severe aortic stenosis. In patients on chronic ACE inhibitor therapy, intraoperative hypotension may occur with induction and maintenance of general anesthesia; use with caution before, during, or immediately after major surgery. Cardiopulmonary bypass, intraoperative blood loss, or vasodilating anesthesia increases endogenous renin release. Use of ACE inhibitors perioperatively will blunt angiotensin II formation and may result in hypotension. However, discontinuation of therapy prior to surgery is controversial. If continued preoperatively, avoidance of hypotensive agents during surgery is prudent (Hillis, 2011). **[U.S. Boxed Warning]: Drugs that act on the renin-angiotensin system can cause injury and death to the developing fetus. Discontinue as soon as possible once pregnancy is detected.**

Hyperkalemia may occur with ACE inhibitors; risk factors include renal dysfunction, diabetes mellitus, concomitant use of potassium-sparing diuretics, potassium supplements, and/or potassium-containing salts. Use cautiously, if at all, with these agents and monitor potassium closely. Cough may occur with ACE inhibitors. Other causes of cough should be considered (eg, pulmonary congestion in patients with heart failure) and excluded prior to discontinuation.

May be associated with deterioration of renal function and/or increases in serum creatinine, particularly in patients with low renal blood flow (eg, renal artery stenosis, heart failure) whose glomerular filtration rate (GFR) is dependent on efferent arteriolar vasoconstriction by angiotensin II; deterioration may result in oliguria, acute renal failure, and progressive azotemia. Small increases in serum creatinine may occur following initiation; consider discontinuation only in patients with progressive and/or significant deterioration in renal function. Use with caution in patients with unstented unilateral/bilateral renal artery stenosis. When unstented bilateral renal artery stenosis is present, use is generally avoided due to the elevated risk of deterioration in renal function unless possible benefits outweigh risks. Potentially significant drug-drug interactions may exist, requiring dose or frequency adjustment, additional monitoring, and/or selection of alternative therapy.

Rare toxicities associated with ACE inhibitors include cholestatic jaundice (which may progress to fulminant hepatic necrosis), agranulocytosis, neutropenia or leukopenia with myeloid hypoplasia. Patients with collagen vascular diseases (especially with concomitant renal impairment) or renal impairment alone may be at increased risk for hematologic toxicity; periodically monitor CBC with differential in these patients.

Adverse Reactions

>10%:

Central nervous system: Headache (24%)

Respiratory: Cough (incidence is higher in women, 3:1) (12%)

1% to 10%:

Cardiovascular: Edema (4%), chest pain (2%), ECG abnormal (2%), palpitation (1%)

Central nervous system: Dizziness (8%, less than placebo), sleep disorders (3%), depression (2%), fever (2%), nervousness (1%), somnolence (1%)

Dermatologic: Rash (2%)

Endocrine & metabolic: Hyperkalemia (1%, less than placebo), triglycerides increased (1%), menstrual disorder (1%)

Gastrointestinal: Diarrhea (4%), abdominal pain (3%), nausea (2%), vomiting (2%), dyspepsia (2%), flatulence (1%)

Genitourinary: Urinary tract infection (3%), sexual dysfunction (male 1%)

Hepatic: ALT increased (2%)

Neuromuscular & skeletal: Weakness (8%), back pain (6%), lower extremity pain (5%), upper extremity pain (3%), hypertonia (3%), paresthesia (2%), joint pain (1%), myalgia (1%), arthritis (1%), neck pain (1%)

Renal: Proteinuria (2%)

Respiratory: Upper respiratory tract infection (9%), sinusitis (5%), rhinitis (5%), pharyngitis (3%)

Otic: Tinnitus (2%), ear infection (1%)

Miscellaneous: Viral infection (3%), seasonal allergy (2%)

Note: Some reactions occurred at an incidence >1% but ≤ placebo.

<1% (Limited to important or life-threatening): Amnesia, anaphylaxis, angioedema, anxiety, AST increased, dyspnea, erythema, fluid retention, gout, leukopenia, migraine, MI, nephrolithiasis, neutropenia, orthostatic hypotension, pruritus, psychosocial disorder, pulmonary fibrosis, purpura, stroke, syncope, urinary retention, vertigo, visual hallucinations (Doane, 2013)

Additional adverse effects that have been reported with **ACE inhibitors** include agranulocytosis (especially in patients with renal impairment or collagen vascular disease), neutropenia, anemia, bullous pemphigoid, cardiac arrest, eosinophilic pneumonitis, exfoliative dermatitis, falls, hepatic failure, hyponatremia, jaundice, pancreatitis (acute), pancytopenia, pemphigus, psoriasis,

thrombocytopenia; decreases in creatinine clearance in some elderly hypertensive patients or those with chronic renal failure, and worsening of renal function in patients with bilateral renal artery stenosis or hypovolemic patients (diuretic therapy). In addition, a syndrome which may include fever, myalgia, arthralgia, interstitial nephritis, vasculitis, rash, eosinophilia and positive ANA, and elevated ESR has been reported with ACE inhibitors.

Drug Interactions

Metabolism/Transport Effects None known.

Avoid Concomitant Use

Avoid concomitant use of Perindopril with any of the following: Sacubitril

Increased Effect/Toxicity

Perindopril may increase the levels/effects of: Allopurinol; Amifostine; Antipsychotic Agents (Second Generation [Atypical]); AzaTHIOprine; Ciprofloxacin (Systemic); Drospirenone; DULoxetine; Ferric Gluconate; Gold Sodium Thiomalate; Grass Pollen Allergen Extract (5 Grass Extract); Hypotension-Associated Agents; Iron Dextran Complex; Levodopa; Lithium; Nonsteroidal Anti-Inflammatory Agents; Pregabalin; Sacubitril; Sodium Phosphates

The levels/effects of Perindopril may be increased by: Alfuzosin; Aliskiren; Angiotensin II Receptor Blockers; Barbiturates; Brimonidine (Topical); Canagliflozin; Dapoxetine; Diazoxide; DPP-IV Inhibitors; Eplerenone; Everolimus; Heparin; Heparin (Low Molecular Weight); Herbs (Hypotensive Properties); Loop Diuretics; Molsidomine; Nicorandil; Obinutuzumab; Pentoxifylline; Phosphodiesterase 5 Inhibitors; Potassium Salts; Potassium-Sparing Diuretics; Prostacyclin Analogues; Salicylates; Sirolimus; Temsirolimus; Thiazide Diuretics; TiZANidine; Tolvaptan; Trimethoprim

Decreased Effect

The levels/effects of Perindopril may be decreased by: Amphetamines; Aprotinin; Herbs (Hypertensive Properties); Icatibant; Lanthanum; Methylphenidate; Nonsteroidal Anti-Inflammatory Agents; Salicylates; Yohimbine

Food Interactions Perindopril active metabolite concentrations may be lowered if taken with food. Management: Administer prior to a meal.

Storage/Stability Store at room temperature of 20°C to 25°C (68°F to 77°F). Protect from moisture.

Mechanism of Action Perindopril is a prodrug for perindoprilat, which acts as a competitive inhibitor of angiotensin-converting enzyme (ACE); prevents conversion of angiotensin I to angiotensin II, a potent vasoconstrictor; results in lower levels of angiotensin II which, in turn, causes an increase in plasma renin activity and a reduction in aldosterone secretion

Pharmacodynamics/Kinetics

Onset of action: Peak effect: 1-2 hours

Protein binding: Perindopril: 60%; Perindoprilat: 10% to 20%

Metabolism: Hepatically hydrolyzed to active metabolite, perindoprilat (~17% to 20% of a dose) and other inactive metabolites

Bioavailability: Perindopril: 75%; Perindoprilat ~25% (~16% with food)

Half-life elimination: Parent drug: 1.5-3 hours; Metabolite: Effective: 3-10 hours, Terminal: 30-120 hours

Time to peak: Chronic therapy: Perindopril: 1 hour; Perindoprilat: 3-7 hours (maximum perindoprilat serum levels are 2-3 times higher and T_{max} is shorter following chronic therapy); CHF: Perindoprilat: 6 hours

Excretion: Urine (75%, 4% to 12% as unchanged drug)

Dosing

Adult

Heart failure (Canadian labeling; off-label use in U.S.): Oral: Initial: 2 mg once daily; if necessary, may titrate over 2-4 weeks to 4 mg once daily. The ACCF/AHA 2013 heart failure guidelines recommend an initial dose of 2 mg once daily with gradual dose titration to a target dose of 8-16 mg once daily (Yancy, 2013).

Hypertension: Oral: Initial: 4 mg/day but may be titrated to response; usual range: 4-8 mg/day (may be given in 2 divided doses); increase at 1- to 2-week intervals (maximum: 16 mg/day). **Note:** The Canadian labeling recommended maximum dose is 8 mg/day.

Concomitant therapy with diuretics: To reduce the risk of hypotension, discontinue diuretic, if possible, 2-3 days prior to initiating perindopril. If unable to stop diuretic, initiate perindopril at 2-4 mg/day (given in 1-2 divided doses) and monitor blood pressure closely for the first 2 weeks of therapy, and after any dose adjustment of perindopril or diuretic.

Stable coronary artery disease: Oral: Initial: 4 mg once daily for 2 weeks; then increase as tolerated to 8 mg once daily.

Geriatric

Hypertension: >65 years: Oral:

U.S. labeling: Initial: 4 mg/day; maintenance: 8 mg/day; experience with doses >8 mg/day is limited; may be given in 1-2 divided doses

Canadian labeling: Initial: 2 mg/day; if necessary may increase dose after 4 weeks to 4 mg/day; then to 8 mg/day (based on renal function); may be given in 1 or 2 divided doses.

ACCF/AHA Expert Consensus recommendations: Consider lower initial doses and titrating to response (Aronow, 2011)

Stable coronary artery disease: >70 years: Oral: Initial: 2 mg/day for 1 week; then increase as tolerated to 4 mg/day for 1 week; then increase as tolerated to 8 mg/day.

Renal Impairment

U.S. labeling:

CrCl >30 mL/minute: Initial: 2 mg/day; maintenance dosing not to exceed 8 mg/day

CrCl <30 mL/minute: Safety and efficacy not established.

Hemodialysis: Perindopril and its metabolites are dialyzable.

Canadian labeling:

CrCl ≥60 mL/minute: Initial: 4 mg/day; maintenance dosing not to exceed 8 mg/day

CrCl 30-60 mL/minute: 2 mg/day

CrCl 15-30 mL/minute: 2 mg every other day

Hemodialysis (CrCl <15 mL/minute): 2 mg on dialysis days (given after dialysis)

Hepatic Impairment No dosage adjustment provided in manufacturer's labeling. However, perindoprilat bioavailability is increased with hepatic impairment.

Administration Administer prior to a meal.

Monitoring Parameters Blood pressure; serum creatinine and potassium; if patient has collagen vascular disease and/or renal impairment, periodically monitor CBC with differential

2013 ACCF/AHA Heart Failure guideline recommendations: Within 1-2 weeks after initiation and periodically thereafter, reassess renal function and serum potassium especially in patients with preexisting hypotension, hyponatremia, diabetes mellitus, azotemia, or those taking potassium supplements (ACCF/AHA [Yancy, 2013]).

Additional Information *International considerations:* International products may be available as either the erbumine/tert-butylamine or arginine salt; dosages are expressed as salt strength: perindopril erbumine/tert-butylamine 4 mg is approximately equivalent to perindopril arginine 5 mg.

Dosage Forms Excipient information presented when available (limited, particularly for generics); consult specific product labeling. [DSC] = Discontinued product

Tablet, Oral, as erbumine:

Aceon: 2 mg [DSC], 4 mg [DSC]

Aceon: 4 mg [scored]

Aceon: 8 mg [DSC]

Aceon: 8 mg [scored]

Generic: 2 mg, 4 mg, 8 mg

Dosage Forms: Canada Excipient information presented when available (limited, particularly for generics); consult specific product labeling.

Tablet, Oral, as erbumine:

Coversyl: 2 mg, 4 mg, 8 mg

Permethrin (per METH rin)

Brand Names: US Acticin; Elimite

Brand Names: Canada Kwellada-P [OTC]; Nix [OTC]

Pharmacologic Category Antiparasitic Agent, Topical; Pediculocide; Scabicidal Agent

Use

Head lice (lotion/cream rinse): Treatment of head lice (*Pediculus humanus capitis*) and its nits (eggs).

Scabies (cream): Treatment of scabies (*Sarcoptes scabiei*) infestation.

Dosing
Adult
Head lice: Topical: Cream rinse/lotion: Prior to application, wash hair with conditioner-free shampoo; rinse with water and towel dry. Apply a sufficient amount of lotion or cream rinse to saturate the hair and scalp (especially behind the ears and nape of neck). Leave on hair for no longer than 10 minutes, then rinse off with warm water; remove remaining nits with nit comb. A single application is generally sufficient; however may repeat 7 days after first treatment if lice or nits are still present.

Scabies: Topical: Cream: Thoroughly massage cream (30 g for average adult) from head to soles of feet; leave on for 8-14 hours before removing (shower or bath); for infants and the elderly, also apply on the hairline, neck, scalp, temple, and forehead; may retreat if living mites are observed 14 days after first treatment; one application is generally curative.

Geriatric When treating scabies in elderly patients, also apply on the hairline, neck, scalp, temple, and forehead. Refer to adult dosing.

Pediatric
Head lice: Infants ≥2 months, Children, and Adolescents: Refer to adult dosing.

Scabies: Infants ≥2 month, Children, and Adolescents: Refer to adult dosing.

Renal Impairment There are no dosage adjustments provided in the manufacturer's labeling. Since topical permethrin is metabolized in the liver and excreted in the urine as inactive metabolites, there does not appear to be an increased risk of toxic reactions in patients with impaired renal function.

Hepatic Impairment There are no dosage adjustments provided in the manufacturer's labeling.

Additional Information Complete prescribing information should be consulted for additional detail.

Dosage Forms Excipient information presented when available (limited, particularly for generics); consult specific product labeling. [DSC] = Discontinued product
Cream, External:
  Acticin: 5% (60 g)
  Elimite: 5% (60 g) [contains formaldehyde solution]
  Generic: 5% (60 g)
Lotion, External:
  Generic: 1% (59 mL [DSC])

Perphenazine (per FEN a zeen)

Brand Names: Canada Apo-Perphenazine®
Index Terms Trilafon
Pharmacologic Category Antiemetic; First Generation (Typical) Antipsychotic
Use Treatment of schizophrenia; severe nausea and vomiting
Dosing
Adult
Schizophrenia: Oral:
Nonhospitalized: Initial: 4-8 mg 3 times/day; reduce dose as soon as possible to minimum effective dosage (maximum: 24 mg/day)
Hospitalized: 8-16 mg 2-4 times/day (maximum: 64 mg/day)
Nausea/vomiting: Oral: 8-16 mg/day in divided doses; reduce dose as soon as possible to minimum effective dosage (maximum: 24 mg/day)

Geriatric No dosage adjustment provided in manufacturer's labeling; however, initiate dosing at the lower end of the dosing range. Refer to adult dosing.

Renal Impairment 0% to 5% removed by hemodialysis (HD); no dosage adjustment provided in manufacturer's labeling.

Hepatic Impairment No dosage adjustment provided in manufacturer's labeling.

Additional Information Complete prescribing information should be consulted for additional detail.

Dosage Forms Excipient information presented when available (limited, particularly for generics); consult specific product labeling.
Tablet, Oral:
  Generic: 2 mg, 4 mg, 8 mg, 16 mg

◆ Perphenazine and Amitriptyline Hydrochloride see Amitriptyline and Perphenazine on page 101

◆ Persantine see Dipyridamole on page 570

◆ Persantine® (Can) see Dipyridamole on page 570

◆ Pertussis, Acellular (Adsorbed) see Diphtheria and Tetanus Toxoids, Acellular Pertussis, Poliovirus and Haemophilus b Conjugate Vaccine on page 567

Pertuzumab (per TU zoo mab)

Brand Names: US Perjeta
Brand Names: Canada Perjeta
Index Terms 2C4 Antibody; MOAB 2C4; Monoclonal Antibody 2C4; Omnitarg; rhuMAb-2C4
Pharmacologic Category Antineoplastic Agent, Anti-HER2; Antineoplastic Agent, Monoclonal Antibody
Use
US labeling:
Breast cancer, metastatic: Treatment of human epidermal growth factor receptor 2 (HER2)-positive metastatic breast cancer (in combination with trastuzumab and docetaxel) in patients who have not received prior anti-HER2 therapy or chemotherapy to treat metastatic disease.
Breast cancer, neoadjuvant treatment: Neoadjuvant treatment of locally advanced, inflammatory, or early stage HER2-positive, breast cancer (either greater than 2 cm in diameter or node positive) in combination with trastuzumab and docetaxel (as part of a complete treatment regimen for early breast cancer).
Limitations of use: The safety of pertuzumab as part of a doxorubicin-containing regimen has not been established; the safety of pertuzumab administered for more than 6 cycles for early breast cancer has not been established.
Canadian labeling: **Breast cancer, metastatic:** Treatment of human epidermal growth factor receptor 2 (HER2)-positive metastatic breast cancer (in combination with trastuzumab and docetaxel) in patients who have not received prior anti-HER2 therapy or chemotherapy to treat metastatic disease.

Pregnancy Considerations May cause fetal harm if administered during pregnancy. **[US Boxed Warning]: Pertuzumab exposure during pregnancy may result in embryo-fetal mortality and birth defects. Oligohydramnios, delayed fetal kidney development, and embryo-fetal death have been observed in animal reproduction studies. Advise patients of the risks and the need for effective contraception.** Verify pregnancy status prior to treatment initiation. Effective contraception should be used during therapy and for 7 months after the last dose (of pertuzumab in combination with trastuzumab) for women of childbearing potential. The Canadian labeling recommends that women of childbearing potential or male patients with female partners of childbearing potential use effective contraception during therapy and for 6 months after the last dose of pertuzumab. Advise patients to immediately report to healthcare provider if pregnancy is suspected during treatment. Effects during pregnancy are likely to occur in all 3 trimesters. If pertuzumab exposure occurs during pregnancy or exposure to pertuzumab in combination with trastuzumab occurs within 7 months prior to conception, healthcare providers should report the exposure to the Genentech Adverse Event Line (888-835-2555); monitor for oligohydramnios (if oligohydramnios occurs, fetal testing is indicated). Women exposed to pertuzumab during pregnancy or exposed to pertuzumab in combination with trastuzumab within 7 months prior to conception are encouraged to enroll in MotHER Pregnancy Registry (1-800-690-6720).

European Society for Medical Oncology (ESMO) guidelines for cancer during pregnancy recommend delaying treatment with HER2-targeted agents until after delivery in pregnant patients with HER2-positive disease (Peccatori, 2013).

Breast-Feeding Considerations It is not known if pertuzumab is excreted in human milk. Because many immunoglobulins are excreted in human milk, and the potential for serious adverse reactions in the nursing infant exists, the decision to discontinue breast-feeding or to discontinue pertuzumab should take into account the benefits of treatment to the mother. The extended half-life should be considered for decisions regarding breast-feeding after treatment is completed.

Contraindications Hypersensitivity to pertuzumab or any component of the formulation

Warnings/Precautions Hazardous agent - use appropriate precautions for handling and disposal (meets NIOSH 2014 criteria). **[US Boxed Warning]: May result in cardiac failure (clinical and subclinical). Assess left ventricular ejection fraction (LVEF) in all patients at baseline and during treatment. Discontinue for confirmed clinically significant decline in left ventricular function.** Decreases in LVEF are associated with HER-2 inhibitors, including pertuzumab. Patients who received prior anthracycline therapy or chest irradiation may be at an increased risk for cardiotoxicity. In studies of pertuzumab (versus placebo) in combination with trastuzumab and docetaxel for the treatment of metastatic breast

cancer, the rate of cardiotoxicity (LVEF decline or symptomatic LV systolic dysfunction) was not increased in the pertuzumab group when compared to placebo. In the neoadjuvant setting, the incidence of LV dysfunction was higher in patients treated with pertuzumab. In a study of pertuzumab, trastuzumab and docetaxel, compared with trastuzumab and docetaxel, the incidence of LVEF decline (of >10% decrease from baseline or to <50%) was 8.4% and 1.9%, respectively; LVEF recovered to ≥50% in all patients. In another neoadjuvant study, LVEF declines (of >10% decrease from baseline or to <50%) were noted in 6.9% to 16% of patients receiving various combinations and sequences of pertuzumab plus trastuzumab with FEC (fluorouracil, epirubicin, and cyclophosphamide), docetaxel, and/or carboplatin; LVEF recovered to ≥50% in most patients. Of note, patients with pretreatment LVEF ≤50%, CHF, LVEF decreases to <50% during prior trastuzumab treatment, or conditions which could impair LV function (eg, uncontrolled hypertension, recent MI, serious arrhythmia requiring treatment, or cumulative lifetime anthracycline exposure >360 mg/m^2 doxorubicin or its equivalent) were excluded from studies. Assess LVEF at baseline, every 3 months during treatment (metastatic patients) or every 6 weeks during treatment (neoadjuvant setting), and every 6 months after therapy discontinuation up to 24 months after the last dose of pertuzumab and/or trastuzumab. The US labeling recommends withholding pertuzumab and trastuzumab if LVEF <45% **or** 45% to 49% with a ≥10% absolute decline from baseline. The Canadian labeling recommends withholding pertuzumab and trastuzumab if LVEF <40% **or** 40% to 45% with ≥10% point decline from baseline. Repeat LVEF assessment in ~3 weeks; discontinue if LVEF has not improved or has declined further (unless potential benefits outweigh risks).

Infusion reactions (either during or on the day of infusion) have been associated with pertuzumab; commonly described as fever, chills, fatigue, headache, weakness, myalgia, hypersensitivity, abnormal taste or vomiting. The incidence of hypersensitivity/anaphylaxis was slightly higher in the group receiving pertuzumab (compared to placebo) in combination with trastuzumab and docetaxel. Monitor for 1 hour after the first infusion and for 30 minutes after subsequent infusions. For significant infusion reactions, interrupt or slow infusion rate; for severe infusion reactions, consider permanently discontinuing. Medications and equipment for the treatment of hypersensitivity should be available for immediate use during infusion. May cause fetal harm if administered during pregnancy. **[US Boxed Warning]: Pertuzumab exposure during pregnancy may result in embryo-fetal mortality and birth defects. Oligohydramnios, delayed fetal kidney development, and embryo-fetal death have been observed in animal reproduction studies. Advise patients of the risks and the need for effective contraception.** Verify pregnancy status prior to treatment initiation. Effective contraception should be used by all patients receiving pertuzumab during therapy and for 7 months after the last dose (of pertuzumab in combination with trastuzumab) in women of childbearing potential. The Canadian labeling recommends that women of childbearing potential or male patients with female partners of childbearing potential use effective contraception during therapy and for 6 months after the last dose of pertuzumab. Effects during pregnancy are likely to occur in any trimester.

Establish HER2 status prior to treatment; has only been studied in patients with evidence of HER2 overexpression, either as 3+ IHC (Dako Herceptest) or FISH amplification ratio ≥2 (Dako *HER2* FISH pharmDx test). Safety of combination or sequential therapy with doxorubicin-containing regimens has not been established. For early breast cancer, the safety of treatment beyond 6 cycles has not been determined.

Adverse Reactions Note: Reactions reported in combination therapy with trastuzumab and docetaxel unless otherwise noted.

>10%:

Central nervous system: Fatigue (26% to 38%), headache (11% to 21%), decreased left ventricular ejection fraction (8% to 16%), insomnia (8% to 13%), dizziness (3% to 13%)

Dermatologic: Alopecia (52% to 65%), skin rash (11% to 34%; grades 3/4: <1%), pruritus (4% to 14%), palmar-plantar erythrodysesthesia (11%), xeroderma (9% to 11%)

Gastrointestinal: Diarrhea (46% to 67%; grades 3/4: 5% to 8%), nausea (39% to 53%; monotherapy 24%), vomiting (13% to 36%; monotherapy 15%), decreased appetite (11% to 29%), constipation (23%), mucositis (20% to 28%), stomatitis (17% to 19%), dysgeusia (13% to 18%), abdominal pain (monotherapy 12%)

Hematologic & oncologic: Neutropenia (47% to 53%; grades 3/4: 43% to 49%), anemia (3% to 23%; grades 3/4: 3% to 4%), leukopenia (9% to 16%; grades 3/4: 5% to 12%), febrile neutropenia (8% to 14%; grades 3/4: 9% to 13%)

Hypersensitivity: Hypersensitivity (1% to 11%; grades 3/4: 2%)

Neuromuscular & skeletal: Weakness (15% to 26%), myalgia (11% to 23%), arthralgia (10% to 12%)

Respiratory: Upper respiratory tract infection (4% to 17%; grades 3/4: <1%), epistaxis (11%)

Miscellaneous: Fever (9% to 19%; grades 3/4: 1%), infusion reactions (13%; grades 3/4: <1%)

1% to 10%:

Cardiovascular: Left ventricular dysfunction (3% to 4%), peripheral edema (3% to 4%)

Central nervous system: Peripheral sensory neuropathy (8%; grades 3/4: 1%), peripheral neuropathy (1%)

Dermatologic: Nail disease (7%), paronychia (1% to 7%)

Gastrointestinal: Dyspepsia (8%), anorexia (monotherapy 5%)

Hematologic & oncologic: Thrombocytopenia (1%)

Hepatic: Increased serum ALT (3%)

Ophthalmic: Increased lacrimation (4% to 5%)

Respiratory: Dyspnea (5% to 8%), nasopharyngitis (7%), oropharyngeal pain (7%), cough (5%)

<1%, postmarketing, and/or case reports with combination therapy: Heart failure, pleural effusion, sepsis

Drug Interactions

Metabolism/Transport Effects None known.

Avoid Concomitant Use

Avoid concomitant use of Pertuzumab with any of the following: Belimumab

Increased Effect/Toxicity

Pertuzumab may increase the levels/effects of: Belimumab

Decreased Effect There are no known significant interactions involving a decrease in effect.

Preparation for Administration Hazardous agent; use appropriate precautions for handling and disposal (meets NIOSH 2014 criteria). Dilute in 250 mL NS only (do not use dextrose 5% solutions) in PVC or non-PVC (polyolefin) bags. Gently invert to mix; do not shake. Do not mix with other medications.

Storage/Stability Store intact vials at 2°C to 8°C (36°F to 46°F) until time of use. Protect from light. Do not freeze. Do not shake. Solutions diluted for infusion should be used immediately; if not used immediately, maybe stored at 2°C to 8°C (36°F to 46°F) for up to 24 hours.

Mechanism of Action Pertuzumab is a recombinant humanized monoclonal antibody which targets the extracellular human epidermal growth factor receptor 2 protein (HER2) dimerization domain. Inhibits HER2 dimerization and blocks HER downstream signaling halting cell growth and initiating apoptosis. Pertuzumab binds to a different HER2 epitope than trastuzumab so that when pertuzumab is combined with trastuzumab, a more complete inhibition of HER2 signaling occurs (Baselga, 2012).

Pharmacodynamics/Kinetics

Distribution: V$_d$: 5.12 L (Gianni, 2010)

Half-life elimination: Terminal: 18 days

Dosing

Adult & Geriatric Note: For pertuzumab, trastuzumab, and docetaxel combination regimens, pertuzumab and trastuzumab may be administered in any order; however, docetaxel should be given after pertuzumab and trastuzumab. Observe patients for 30 to 60 minutes after each pertuzumab infusion and before subsequent infusions of trastuzumab or docetaxel.

Breast cancer, metastatic HER2+: IV: 840 mg over 60 minutes followed by a maintenance dose of 420 mg over 30 to 60 minutes every 3 weeks until disease progression or unacceptable toxicity (in combination with trastuzumab and docetaxel) (Baselga, 2012; Swain, 2015).

Breast cancer, neoadjuvant treatment HER2+: Adults: IV: 840 mg over 60 minutes followed by a maintenance dose of 420 mg over 30 to 60 minutes every 3 weeks for 3 to 6 cycles; may be administered as one of the regimens below. Postoperatively, continue trastuzumab to complete 1 year of treatment.

Four preoperative cycles of pertuzumab, trastuzumab, and docetaxel, followed by 3 postoperative cycles of fluorouracil, epirubicin, and cyclophosphamide (FEC) (Gianni, 2012) **or**

Three preoperative cycles of FEC (alone) followed by 3 preoperative cycles of pertuzumab, trastuzumab, and docetaxel (Schneeweiss, 2013) **or**

Six preoperative cycles of pertuzumab, trastuzumab, docetaxel, and carboplatin (Schneeweiss, 2013)

Missed doses or delays: If <6 weeks has elapsed, administer the 420 mg maintenance dose; do not wait until the next planned dose. If ≥6 weeks has elapsed, readminister the 840 mg initial dose (over 60 minutes), and then follow with a maintenance dose of 420 mg (over 30 to 60 minutes) every 3 weeks.

Renal Impairment

CrCl ≥30 mL/minute: No dosage adjustment necessary.

CrCl <30 mL/minute: There are no dosage adjustments provided in the manufacturer's labeling (has not been studied).

Hepatic Impairment There are no dosage adjustments provided in the manufacturer's labeling (has not been studied).

Adjustment for Toxicity Note: Dose reductions are not recommended for pertuzumab; if trastuzumab is withheld, pertuzumab should also be withheld; if trastuzumab is discontinued, pertuzumab should be discontinued; pertuzumab and trastuzumab may be continued if docetaxel is discontinued.

Infusion-related reaction: Slow or interrupt the infusion

Serious hypersensitivity: Discontinue immediately

Cardiotoxicity:

US labeling: Left ventricular ejection fraction (LVEF) declines to <45% **or** LVEF 45% to 49% with ≥10% absolute decrease below pretreatment values: Withhold treatment (pertuzumab and trastuzumab) for at least 3 weeks; may resume if LVEF returns to >49% **or** to 45% to 49% with <10% absolute decrease below pretreatment values. If after a repeat assessment within ~3 weeks, LVEF has not improved (or has declined further), discontinue pertuzumab and trastuzumab (unless the benefit of treatment outweighs risks).

Canadian labeling: Left ventricular ejection fraction (LVEF) declines to <40% **or** LVEF 40% to 45% with ≥10% point decline from baseline: Withhold treatment (pertuzumab and trastuzumab) for at least 3 weeks; may resume if LVEF returns to >45% **or** to 40% to 45% with <10% decrease below pretreatment values. If after a repeat assessment within ~3 weeks, LVEF has not improved (or has declined further), discontinue pertuzumab and trastuzumab (unless the benefit of treatment outweighs risks).

Administration For IV infusion only, as a short infusion; infuse initial dose (840 mg) over 60 minutes; infuse maintenance dose (420 mg) over 30 to 60 minutes. Do not administer IV push or as a rapid bolus. Do not mix with other medications. For pertuzumab, trastuzumab, and docetaxel combination regimens, pertuzumab and trastuzumab may be administered in any order; however, docetaxel should be given after pertuzumab and trastuzumab. Observe patients for 30 to 60 minutes after each pertuzumab infusion and before subsequent infusions of trastuzumab or docetaxel.

Hazardous agent; use appropriate precautions for handling and disposal (meets NIOSH 2014 criteria).

Monitoring Parameters HER2 expression (either as 3+ IHC [Dako Herceptest™] or FISH amplification ratio ≥2 [Dako *HER*2 FISH pharmDx™ test]); pregnancy test; assess LVEF at baseline, every 3 months during treatment (more frequently for declines) in metastatic treatment and every 6 weeks for neoadjuvant treatment, and every 6 months following discontinuation for up to 24 months from the last dose of pertuzumab and/or trastuzumab); monitor for infusion reaction and hypersensitivity

Dosage Forms Excipient information presented when available (limited, particularly for generics); consult specific product labeling.

Solution, Intravenous [preservative free]:

Perjeta: 420 mg/14 mL (14 mL) [contains mouse protein (murine) (hamster)]

◆ Pertzye *see* Pancrelipase *on page 1384*

◆ Pethidine Hydrochloride *see* Meperidine *on page 1144*

◆ Pexeva *see* PARoxetine *on page 1399*

◆ PF-02341066 *see* Crizotinib *on page 450*

◆ PFA *see* Foscarnet *on page 813*

◆ Pfizerpen-AS® (Can) *see* Penicillin G Procaine *on page 1422*

◆ Pfizerpen-G *see* Penicillin G (Parenteral/Aqueous) *on page 1420*

◆ pFVIII *see* Antihemophilic Factor (Recombinant [Porcine Sequence]) *on page 133*

◆ PGE₁ *see* Alprostadil *on page 78*

◆ PGE₂ *see* Dinoprostone *on page 558*

◆ PGI₂ *see* Epoprostenol *on page 657*

◆ PGX *see* Epoprostenol *on page 657*

◆ Pharbedryl *see* DiphenhydrAMINE (Systemic) *on page 561*

◆ Pharbetol [OTC] *see* Acetaminophen *on page 25*

◆ Pharbetol Extra Strength [OTC] *see* Acetaminophen *on page 25*

◆ Pharmabase Barrier [OTC] *see* Zinc Oxide *on page 1929*

◆ Pharmorubicin (Can) *see* Epirubicin *on page 651*

◆ Pheburane (Can) *see* Sodium Phenylbutyrate *on page 1677*

◆ Phenadoz *see* Promethazine *on page 1510*

Phenazopyridine (fen az oh PEER i deen)

Brand Names: US Azo-Gesic [OTC]; Baridium [OTC]; Pyridium; Urinary Pain Relief [OTC]

Index Terms Phenazopyridine Hydrochloride; Phenylazo Diamino Pyridine Hydrochloride

Pharmacologic Category Analgesic, Urinary

Use Dysuria, symptomatic relief: Symptomatic relief of pain, burning, urgency, frequency, and other discomforts arising from irritation of the lower urinary tract mucosa caused by infection, trauma, surgery, endoscopic procedures, or the passage of sounds or catheters.

Dosing

Adult & Geriatric

Dysuria, symptomatic relief: Oral:

OTC labeling: Two tablets (190 mg) 3 times daily administered with or after meals for up to 2 days.

Rx labeling: 200 mg 3 times daily after meals for 2 days when used concomitantly with an antibacterial agent.

Pediatric Dysuria, symptomatic relief: Children ≥12 years and Adolescents: OTC labeling: Oral: Refer to adult dosing.

Renal Impairment Use is contraindicated.

Hepatic Impairment There are no dosage adjustments provided in the manufacturer's labeling.

Additional Information Complete prescribing information should be consulted for additional detail.

Dosage Forms Excipient information presented when available (limited, particularly for generics); consult specific product labeling.

Tablet, Oral, as hydrochloride:

Azo-Gesic: 95 mg

Baridium: 97.2 mg

Pyridium: 100 mg, 200 mg

Urinary Pain Relief: 95 mg

Generic: 95 mg, 100 mg, 200 mg

◆ Phenazopyridine Hydrochloride *see* Phenazopyridine *on page 1435*

Phenelzine (FEN el zeen)

Brand Names: US Nardil

Brand Names: Canada Nardil®

Index Terms Phenelzine Sulfate

Pharmacologic Category Antidepressant, Monoamine Oxidase Inhibitor

Use Symptomatic treatment of atypical, nonendogenous, or neurotic depression

Pregnancy Considerations Adverse events have been observed in animal reproduction studies. Information related to the use of phenelzine in pregnancy is limited (Frayne 2014; Gracious 1997; Pavy 1995).

Breast-Feeding Considerations It is not known if phenelzine is excreted in breast milk. According to the manufacturer, the decision to continue or discontinue breast-feeding during therapy should take into account the risk of exposure to the infant and the benefits of treatment to the mother.

Medication Guide Available Yes

Contraindications Hypersensitivity to phenelzine or any component of the formulation; congestive heart failure; pheochromocytoma; abnormal liver function tests or history of hepatic disease; renal disease or severe renal disease/impairment

Concurrent use of sympathomimetics (including amphetamines, cocaine, dopamine, epinephrine, methylphenidate, norepinephrine, or phenylephrine) and related compounds (methyldopa, levodopa, phenylalanine, tryptophan, or tyrosine), ophthalmic alpha₂-agonists (apraclonidine, brimonidine), CNS depressants, cyclobenzaprine, dextromethorphan, ethanol, meperidine, bupropion, or buspirone

At least 2 weeks should elapse between the discontinuation of serotoninergic agents (including SNRIs, SSRIs, and tricyclics) and other MAO inhibitors and the initiation of phenelzine. At least 5 weeks should elapse between ▶

the discontinuation of fluoxetine and the initiation of phenelzine. In all cases, a sufficient amount of time must be allowed for the clearance of the serotoninergic agent and any active metabolites prior to the initiation of phenelzine.

At least 2 weeks should elapse between the discontinuation of phenelzine and the initiation of the following agents: Serotoninergic agents (including SNRIs, SSRIs, fluoxetine, and tricyclics), bupropion, buspirone, and other antidepressants.

General anesthesia, spinal anesthesia (hypotension may be exaggerated). Use caution with local anesthetics containing sympathomimetic agents. Phenelzine should be discontinued ≥10 days prior to elective surgery.

Foods high in tyramine or dopamine content; foods and/or supplements containing tyrosine, phenylalanine, tryptophan, or caffeine

Warnings/Precautions [U.S. Boxed Warning]: Antidepressants increase the risk of suicidal thinking and behavior in children, adolescents, and young adults (18-24 years of age) with major depressive disorder (MDD) and other psychiatric disorders; consider risk prior to prescribing. Short-term studies did not show an increased risk in patients >24 years of age and showed a decreased risk in patients ≥65 years. Closely monitor for clinical worsening, suicidality, or unusual changes in behavior; the patient's family or caregiver should be instructed to closely observe the patient and communicate condition with healthcare provider. Such observation would generally include at least weekly face-to-face contact with patients or their family members or caregivers during the first 4 weeks of treatment, then every other week visits for the next 4 weeks, then at 12 weeks, and as clinically indicated beyond 12 weeks. Additional contact by telephone may be appropriate between face-to-face visits. Adults treated with antidepressants should be observed similarly for clinical worsening and suicidality, especially during the initial few months of a course of drug therapy, or at times of dose changes, either increases or decreases. A medication guide should be dispensed with each prescription. Phenelzine is not generally considered a first-line agent for the treatment of depression; phenelzine is typically used in patients who have failed to respond to other treatments. **Phenelzine is not FDA approved for the treatment of depression in children ≤16 years of age.**

The possibility of a suicide attempt is inherent in major depression and may persist until remission occurs. Monitor for worsening of depression or suicidality, especially during initiation of therapy (generally first 1-2 months) or with dose increases or decreases. Worsening depression and severe abrupt suicidality that are not part of the presenting symptoms may require discontinuation or modification of drug therapy. Use caution in high-risk patients during initiation of therapy. Prescriptions should be written for the smallest quantity consistent with good patient care. The patient's family or caregiver should be alerted to monitor patients for the emergence of suicidality and associated behaviors such as anxiety, agitation, panic attacks, insomnia, irritability, hostility, impulsivity, akathisia, hypomania, and mania; patients should be instructed to notify their healthcare provider if any of these symptoms or worsening depression occur.

May worsen psychosis in some patients or precipitate a shift to mania or hypomania in patients with bipolar disorder. Monotherapy in patients with bipolar disorder should be avoided. Patients presenting with depressive symptoms should be screened for bipolar disorder. Phenelzine is not FDA approved for the treatment of bipolar depression.

Sensitization to the effects of insulin may occur; monitor blood glucose closely in patients with diabetes. Use with caution in patients who have glaucoma, or hyperthyroidism. Cases of hypertensive crisis (sometimes fatal) have occurred; symptoms include: severe headache, nausea/vomiting, neck stiffness/soreness, photophobia, and sweating. Monitor blood pressure closely in all patients. Hypertensive crisis may occur with tyramine-, tryptophan-, or dopamine-containing foods. Phentolamine is recommended for the treatment of hypertensive crisis. Do not use with other MAO inhibitors or antidepressants. Do not use within 5 weeks of fluoxetine discontinuation or 2 weeks of other antidepressant discontinuation. Avoid products containing sympathomimetic stimulants or dextromethorphan. Concurrent use with antihypertensive agents may lead to exaggeration of hypotensive effects. May cause orthostatic hypotension; use with caution in patients with hypotension or patients who would not tolerate transient hypotensive episodes (cardiovascular or cerebrovascular disease); effects may be additive with other agents which cause orthostasis. Use with caution in patients at risk of seizures, or in patients receiving other drugs which may lower seizure threshold. Discontinue at least 48 hours prior

to myelography. May increase the risks associated with electroconvulsive therapy. Pyridoxine deficiency has occurred; symptoms include numbness and edema of hands; may respond to supplementation. Effects may be potentiated when used with other sedative drugs or ethanol.

Abrupt discontinuation or interruption of antidepressant therapy has been associated with a discontinuation syndrome. Symptoms arising may vary with antidepressant however commonly include nausea, vomiting, diarrhea, headaches, lightheadedness, dizziness, diminished appetite, sweating, chills, tremors, paresthesias, fatigue, somnolence, and sleep disturbances (eg, vivid dreams, insomnia). Greater risks for developing a discontinuation syndrome have been associated with antidepressants with shorter half-lives, longer durations of treatment, and abrupt discontinuation. More severe symptoms have also been associated with MAO inhibitors. For antidepressants of short or intermediate half-lives, symptoms may emerge within 2-5 days after treatment discontinuation and last 7-14 days (APA, 2010; Fava, 2006; Haddad, 2001; Shelton, 2001; Warner, 2006). According to the manufacturer, phenelzine use within 10 days prior to elective surgery is contraindicated. Currently, an MAO-safe anesthetic technique which excludes the use of meperidine and indirect-acting adrenergic agonists is recommended for patients requiring continued MAO inhibitor therapy (Huyse, 2006).

Adverse Reactions Frequency not defined.

Cardiovascular: Edema, orthostatic hypotension

Central nervous system: Anxiety (acute), ataxia, coma, delirium, dizziness, drowsiness, euphoria, fatigue, fever, headache, hyper-reflexia, hypersomnia, insomnia, mania, schizophrenia, seizure, twitching

Dermatologic: Pruritus, rash

Endocrine & metabolic: Decreased sexual ability (anorgasmia, ejaculatory disturbances, impotence), hypermetabolic syndrome, hypernatremia

Gastrointestinal: Constipation, weight gain, xerostomia

Genitourinary: Urinary retention

Hematologic: Leukopenia

Hepatic: Jaundice, necrotizing hepatocellular necrosis (rare), transaminases increased

Neuromuscular & skeletal: Myoclonia, paresthesia, tremor, weakness

Ocular: Blurred vision, glaucoma, nystagmus

Respiratory: Edema (glottis)

Miscellaneous: Diaphoresis, lupus-like syndrome, transient cardiac or respiratory depression (following ECT), withdrawal syndrome (nausea, vomiting, malaise)

Drug Interactions

Metabolism/Transport Effects Inhibits Monoamine Oxidase

Avoid Concomitant Use

Avoid concomitant use of Phenelzine with any of the following: Aclidinium; Alcohol (Ethyl); Alpha-/Beta-Agonists (Indirect-Acting); Alpha1-Agonists; Amphetamines; Anilidopiperidine Opioids; Antidepressants (Serotonin Reuptake Inhibitor/Antagonist); Apraclonidine; AtoMOXetine; Atropine (Ophthalmic); Bezafibrate; Buprenorphine; BuPROPion; BusPIRone; CarBAMazepine; Cimetropium; Cyclobenzaprine; Cyproheptadine; Dapoxetine; Dexmethylphenidate; Dextromethorphan; Diethylpropion; Eluxadoline; EPINEPHrine (Oral Inhalation); Glucagon; Glycopyrrolate; Glycopyrrolate (Oral Inhalation); HYDROmorphone; Ipratropium (Oral Inhalation); Isometheptene; Levonordefrin; Levosulpiride; Linezolid; Maprotiline; Meperidine; Mequitazine; Methyldopa; Methylene Blue; Methylphenidate; Mianserin; Mirtazapine; Moclobemide; Morphine (Liposomal); Morphine (Systemic); Oxymorphone; Pholcodine; Pizotifen; Potassium Chloride; Selective Serotonin Reuptake Inhibitors; Serotonin 5-HT1D Receptor Agonists; Serotonin/Norepinephrine Reuptake Inhibitors; Tapentadol; Tetrabenazine; Tetrahydrozoline (Nasal); Tianeptine; Tiotropium; Tricyclic Antidepressants; Tryptophan; Umeclidinium

Increased Effect/Toxicity

Phenelzine may increase the levels/effects of: AbobotulinumtoxinA; Alpha-/Beta-Agonists (Indirect-Acting); Alpha1-Agonists; Amifostine; Amphetamines; Analgesics (Opioid); Anticholinergic Agents; Antidepressants (Serotonin Reuptake Inhibitor/Antagonist); Antipsychotic Agents; Antipsychotic Agents (Second Generation [Atypical]); Apraclonidine; AtoMOXetine; Atropine (Ophthalmic); Beta2-Agonists; Betahistine; Bezafibrate; Blood Glucose Lowering Agents; Brimonidine (Ophthalmic); Brimonidine (Topical); BuPROPion; Cannabinoid-Containing Products; Cimetropium; Clemastine; Cyproheptadine; Dexmethylphenidate; Dextromethorphan; Diethylpropion; Domperidone; Doxapram; Doxylamine; Eluxadoline; EPINEPHrine (Nasal); EPINEPHrine (Oral Inhalation); Epinephrine (Racemic); EPINEPHrine

(Systemic); Glucagon; Glycopyrrolate; Glycopyrrolate (Oral Inhalation); Hydrocodone; HYDROmorphone; Hypotension-Associated Agents; Isometheptene; Levonordefrin; Linezolid; Lithium; Meperidine; Mequitazine; Methadone; Methyldopa; Methylene Blue; Methylphenidate; Metoclopramide; Mianserin; Mirabegron; Mirtazapine; Moclobemide; Morphine (Liposomal); Morphine (Systemic); Norepinephrine; OnabotulinumtoxinA; OxyCODONE; Pizotifen; Potassium Chloride; Ramosetron; Reserpine; RimabotulinumtoxinB; Selective Serotonin Reuptake Inhibitors; Serotonin 5-HT1D Receptor Agonists; Serotonin Modulators; Serotonin/Norepinephrine Reuptake Inhibitors; Succinylcholine; Tetrahydrozoline (Nasal); Thiazide Diuretics; Tiotropium; Topiramate; Tricyclic Antidepressants

The levels/effects of Phenelzine may be increased by: Aclidinium; Alcohol (Ethyl); Alfuzosin; Altretamine; Anilidopiperidine Opioids; Antiemetics (5HT3 Antagonists); Antipsychotic Agents; Barbiturates; Blood Pressure Lowering Agents; Brimonidine (Topical); Buprenorphine; BusPIRone; CarBAMazepine; COMT Inhibitors; Cyclobenzaprine; Dapoxetine; Diazoxide; Herbs (Hypotensive Properties); Ipratropium (Oral Inhalation); Levodopa; Maprotiline; Metaxalone; Molsidomine; Nicorandil; Obinutuzumab; Oxymorphone; Pentoxifylline; Pholcodine; Phosphodiesterase 5 Inhibitors; Pramlintide; Prostacyclin Analogues; Tapentadol; Tedizolid; Tetrabenazine; Tianeptine; TraMADol; Tryptophan; Umeclidinium

Decreased Effect

Phenelzine may decrease the levels/effects of: Acetylcholinesterase Inhibitors; Domperidone; Gastrointestinal Agents (Prokinetic); Itopride; Levosulpiride; Secretin

The levels/effects of Phenelzine may be decreased by: Acetylcholinesterase Inhibitors; Cyproheptadine; Domperidone

Food Interactions Concurrent ingestion of foods rich in tyramine, dopamine, tyrosine, phenylalanine, tryptophan, or caffeine may cause sudden and severe high blood pressure (hypertensive crisis or serotonin syndrome). Beverages containing tyramine (eg, hearty red wine and beer) may increase toxic effects. Management: Avoid tyramine-containing foods (aged or matured cheese, air-dried or cured meats including sausages and salamis; fava or broad bean pods, tap/draft beers, Marmite concentrate, sauerkraut, soy sauce, and other soybean condiments). Food's freshness is also an important concern; improperly stored or spoiled food can create an environment in which tyramine concentrations may increase. Avoid foods containing dopamine, tyrosine, phenylalanine, tryptophan, or caffeine. Avoid beverages containing tyramine.

Storage/Stability Store at 20°C to 25°C (68°F to 77°F). Protect from heat and light.

Mechanism of Action Thought to act by increasing endogenous concentrations of norepinephrine, dopamine, and serotonin through inhibition of the enzyme (monoamine oxidase) responsible for the breakdown of these neurotransmitters

Pharmacodynamics/Kinetics

Onset of action: Therapeutic: 2-4 weeks; geriatric patients receiving an average of 55 mg/day developed a mean platelet MAO activity inhibition of about 85%.

Duration: May continue to have a therapeutic effect and interactions 2 weeks after discontinuing therapy

Absorption: Well absorbed

Metabolism: Oxidized via monoamine oxidase (primary pathway) and acetylation (minor pathway)

Half-life elimination: 12 hours

Excretion: Urine (73% as metabolites)

Dosing

Adult Note: 45 mg phenelzine = 40 mg of isocarboxazid = 20 mg of tranylcypromine (Sheehan 1980)

Depression: Oral: Initial: 15 mg 3 times/day

Early phase: Increase rapidly, based on patient tolerance, to 60-90 mg/day (may take 4 weeks of 60 mg/day therapy before clinical response)

Maintenance: After maximum benefit is obtained, slowly reduce dose over several weeks; dose may be as low as 15 mg/day to 15 mg every other day

Discontinuation of therapy: Upon discontinuation of antidepressant therapy, gradually taper the dose to minimize the incidence of withdrawal symptoms and allow for the detection of re-emerging symptoms. Evidence supporting ideal taper rates is limited. APA and NICE guidelines suggest tapering therapy over at least several weeks with consideration to the half-life of the antidepressant; antidepressants with a shorter half-life and MAO inhibitors may need to be tapered more conservatively. In addition for long-term treated patients, WFSBP guidelines recommend tapering over

4-6 months. If intolerable withdrawal symptoms occur following a dose reduction, consider resuming the previously prescribed dose and/or decrease dose at a more gradual rate (APA, 2010; Bauer, 2002; Haddad, 2001; NCCMH, 2010; Schatzberg, 2006; Shelton, 2001; Warner, 2006).

MAO inhibitor recommendations:

Switching to or from an MAO inhibitor intended to treat psychiatric disorders:

Allow 14 days to elapse between discontinuing an alternative antidepressant without long half-life metabolites (eg, TCAs, paroxetine, fluvoxamine, venlafaxine) or MAO inhibitor intended to treat psychiatric disorders and initiation of phenelzine.

Allow 5 weeks to elapse between discontinuing fluoxetine (with long half-life metabolites) intended to treat psychiatric disorders and initiation of phenelzine.

Allow 14 days to elapse between discontinuing phenelzine and initiation of an alternative antidepressant or MAO inhibitor intended to treat psychiatric disorders.

Use with other MAO inhibitors (such as linezolid or IV methylene blue):

Do not initiate phenelzine in patients receiving linezolid or IV methylene blue; consider other interventions for psychiatric condition.

If urgent treatment with linezolid or IV methylene blue is required in a patient already receiving phenelzine and potential benefits outweigh potential risks, discontinue phenelzine promptly and administer linezolid or IV methylene blue. Monitor for serotonin syndrome for 2 weeks or until 24 hours after the last dose of linezolid or IV methylene blue, whichever comes first. May resume phenelzine 24 hours after the last dose of linezolid or IV methylene blue.

Geriatric Depression: Oral: Select dose with caution; generally initiating at the lower end of the dosing range; some clinicians recommend an initial dose of 7.5 mg, with dose increases of 7.5 mg/day every 4-8 days as tolerated to a usual therapeutic dose of 22.5-60 mg/day in older adults (Alexopoulos, 2004).

Discontinuation of therapy: Refer to adult dosing.

MAO inhibitor recommendations: Refer to adult dosing.

Renal Impairment

Mild to moderate impairment: No dosage adjustment provided in manufacturer's labeling.

Severe impairment: Use is contraindicated.

Hepatic Impairment Use is contraindicated.

Dietary Considerations Avoid tyramine-containing foods/beverages. Some examples include aged or matured cheese, air-dried or cured meats (including sausages and salamis), fava or broad bean pods, tap/draft beers, Marmite concentrate, sauerkraut, soy sauce and other soybean condiments. Food's freshness is also an important concern; improperly stored or spoiled food can create an environment where tyramine concentrations may increase.

Monitoring Parameters Blood pressure, heart rate; diet, weight; mood (if depressive symptoms), suicide ideation (especially during the initial months of therapy or when doses are increased or decreased)

Dosage Forms Excipient information presented when available (limited, particularly for generics); consult specific product labeling.

Tablet, Oral:

Nardil: 15 mg

Generic: 15 mg

◆ Phenelzine Sulfate *see* Phenelzine *on page 1435*

◆ Phenergan *see* Promethazine *on page 1510*

◆ Pheniramine and Naphazoline *see* Naphazoline and Pheniramine *on page 1256*

PHENobarbital (fee noe BAR bi tal)

Brand Names: US Luminal [DSC]

Brand Names: Canada PMS-Phenobarbital

Index Terms Luminal Sodium; Phenobarbital Sodium; Phenobarbitone; Phenylethylmalonylurea

Pharmacologic Category Anticonvulsant, Barbiturate; Barbiturate

Use Management of generalized tonic-clonic (grand mal), status epilepticus, and partial seizures; sedative/hypnotic

Note: Use to treat insomnia is not recommended (Schutte-Rodin 2008)

Pregnancy Considerations Barbiturates can be detected in the placenta, fetal liver, and fetal brain. Fetal and maternal blood concentrations may be similar following parenteral administration. An increased incidence of fetal abnormalities may occur following maternal use. The use of folic acid throughout pregnancy and vitamin K

during the last month of pregnancy is recommended; epilepsy itself, number of medications, genetic factors, or a combination of these probably influence the teratogenicity of anticonvulsant therapy. When used during the third trimester of pregnancy, withdrawal symptoms may occur in the neonate, including seizures and hyperirritability; symptoms of withdrawal may be delayed in the neonate up to 14 days after birth. Use during labor does not impair uterine activity; however, respiratory depression may occur in the newborn; resuscitation equipment should be available, especially for premature infants.

Breast-Feeding Considerations Phenobarbital is excreted into breast milk. Infantile spasms and other withdrawal symptoms have been reported following the abrupt discontinuation of breast-feeding.

Contraindications Hypersensitivity to barbiturates or any component of the formulation; marked hepatic impairment; dyspnea or airway obstruction; porphyria (manifest and latent); intra-arterial administration, subcutaneous administration (not recommended); use in patients with a history of sedative/hypnotic addiction; nephritic patients (large doses)

Warnings/Precautions Potential for drug dependency exists, abrupt cessation may precipitate withdrawal, including status epilepticus in epileptic patients. Do not administer in acute pain. Use caution in debilitated, renal or hepatic dysfunction, and pediatric patients. May cause paradoxical responses, including agitation and hyperactivity, particularly in acute pain and pediatric patients. Avoid use in the elderly due to risk of overdose with low dosages, tolerance to sleep effects, and increased risk of physical dependence (Beers Criteria). Use with caution in patients with depression or suicidal tendencies, or in patients with a history of drug abuse. Tolerance, psychological and physical dependence may occur with prolonged use. May cause CNS depression, which may impair physical or mental abilities. Effects with other sedative drugs or ethanol may be potentiated. May cause respiratory depression or hypotension, particularly when administered intravenously. Use with caution in hemodynamically unstable patients (hypovolemic shock, CHF) or patients with respiratory disease. Due to its long half-life and risk of dependence, phenobarbital is not recommended as a sedative in the elderly. Phenobarbital has been associated with cognitive deficits in children receiving chronic therapy for febrile seizures. Use with caution in patients with hypoadrenalism. Intra-arterial administration may cause reactions ranging from transient pain to gangrene and is contraindicated. Subcutaneous administration may cause tissue irritation (eg, redness, tenderness, necrosis) and is not recommended. Some dosage forms may contain propylene glycol; large amounts are potentially toxic and have been associated with hyperosmolality, lactic acidosis, seizures and respiratory depression; use caution (AAP 1997; Zar 2007).

Adverse Reactions Frequency not defined.

Cardiovascular: Bradycardia, hypotension, syncope

Central nervous system: Agitation, anxiety, ataxia, CNS excitation or depression, confusion, dizziness drowsiness, hallucinations, "hangover" effect, headache, hyperkinesia, impaired judgment, insomnia, lethargy, nervousness, nightmares, somnolence

Dermatologic: Exfoliative dermatitis, rash, Stevens-Johnson syndrome

Gastrointestinal: Nausea, vomiting, constipation

Hematologic: Agranulocytosis, thrombocytopenia, megaloblastic anemia

Local: Pain at injection site, thrombophlebitis with IV use

Renal: Oliguria

Respiratory: Laryngospasm, respiratory depression, apnea (especially with rapid IV use), hypoventilation

Miscellaneous: Gangrene with inadvertent intra-arterial injection

Drug Interactions

Metabolism/Transport Effects Substrate of CYP2C19 (major), CYP2C9 (minor), CYP2E1 (minor); **Note:** Assignment of Major/Minor substrate status based on clinically relevant drug interaction potential; **Induces** CYP1A2 (strong), CYP2A6 (strong), CYP2B6 (strong), CYP2C8 (strong), CYP2C9 (strong), CYP3A4 (strong), P-glycoprotein, UGT1A1

Avoid Concomitant Use

Avoid concomitant use of PHENobarbital with any of the following: Abiraterone Acetate; Antihepaciviral Combination Products; Apixaban; Apremilast; Aprepitant; Artemether; Axitinib; Azelastine (Nasal); Bedaquiline; Boceprevir; Bortezomib; Bosutinib; Cabozantinib; Cariprazine; Ceritinib; CloZAPine; Cobicistat; Cobimetinib; Crizotinib; Dabigatran Etexilate; Dabrafenib; Daclatasvir; Dienogest; Dolutegravir; Dronedarone; Eliglustat; Elvitegravir; Enzalutamide; Etravirine; Everolimus; Flibanserin; Hemin; Ibrutinib; Idelalisib; Irinotecan Products;

Isavuconazonium Sulfate; Itraconazole; Ivabradine; Ivacaftor; Ixazomib; Lapatinib; Ledipasvir; Lumefantrine; Lurasidone; Macitentan; Mianserin; Mifepristone; Naloxegol; Netupitant; NIFEdipine; Nilotinib; NiMODipine; Nintedanib; Nisoldipine; Olaparib; Ombitasvir, Paritaprevir, Ritonavir, and Dasabuvir; Orphenadrine; Osimertinib; Palbociclib; Panobinostat; Paraldehyde; PAZOPanib; Perampanel; Pirfenidone; PONATinib; Praziquantel; Ranolazine; Regorafenib; Rilpivirine; Rivaroxaban; Roflumilast; RomiDEPsin; Simeprevir; Sofosbuvir; Somatostatin Acetate; Sonidegib; SORAfenib; Stiripentol; Suvorexant; Tasimelteon; Telaprevir; Thalidomide; Ticagrelor; Tofacitinib; Tolvaptan; Toremifene; Trabectedin; Ulipristal; Vandetanib; Vemurafenib; VinCRIStine (Liposomal); Vorapaxar; Voriconazole

Increased Effect/Toxicity

PHENobarbital may increase the levels/effects of: Alcohol (Ethyl); Azelastine (Nasal); Blood Pressure Lowering Agents; Buprenorphine; Clarithromycin; CNS Depressants; Cyclophosphamide; Hydrocodone; Meperidine; Methotrimeprazine; Metyrosine; Orphenadrine; Paraldehyde; Pramipexole; Prilocaine; QuiNIDine; Rotigotine; Selective Serotonin Reuptake Inhibitors; Sodium Nitrite; Thalidomide; Thiazide Diuretics; Zolpidem

The levels/effects of PHENobarbital may be increased by: Brimonidine (Topical); Cannabis; Chloramphenicol; Clarithromycin; Cosyntropin; CYP2C19 Inhibitors (Moderate); CYP2C19 Inhibitors (Strong); Dapsone (Topical); Dexmethylphenidate; Doxylamine; Dronabinol; Droperidol; Felbamate; Fosphenytoin; HydrOXYzine; Kava Kava; Luliconazole; Magnesium Sulfate; Methotrimeprazine; Methylphenidate; Mianserin; Minocycline; Nabilone; Nitric Oxide; OXcarbazepine; Phenytoin; Primidone; QuiNINE; Rufinamide; Sodium Oxybate; Somatostatin Acetate; Tapentadol; Tetrahydrocannabinol; Valproate Products

Decreased Effect

PHENobarbital may decrease the levels/effects of: Abiraterone Acetate; Acetaminophen; Afatinib; Albendazole; Antihepaciviral Combination Products; Apixaban; Apremilast; Aprepitant; ARIPiprazole; ARIPiprazole Lauroxil; Artemether; Axitinib; Bazedoxifene; Bedaquiline; Bendamustine; Beta-Blockers; Boceprevir; Bortezomib; Bosutinib; Brentuximab Vedotin; Brexpiprazole; Cabozantinib; Calcium Channel Blockers; Canagliflozin; Cannabidiol; Cannabis; Cariprazine; Ceritinib; Chloramphenicol; Clarithromycin; CloZAPine; Cobicistat; Cobimetinib; Contraceptives (Estrogens); Contraceptives (Progestins); Corticosteroids (Systemic); Crizotinib; CycloSPORINE (Systemic); CYP1A2 Substrates; CYP2A6 Substrates; CYP2B6 Substrates; CYP2C8 Substrates; CYP2C9 Substrates; CYP3A4 Substrates; Dabigatran Etexilate; Dabrafenib; Daclatasvir; Dasatinib; Deferasirox; Dexamethasone (Systemic); Diclofenac (Systemic); Dienogest; Disopyramide; Dolutegravir; DOXOrubicin (Conventional); Doxycycline; Dronabinol; Dronedarone; Eliglustat; Elvitegravir; Enzalutamide; Erlotinib; Eslicarbazepine; Etizolam; Etoposide; Etoposide Phosphate; Etravirine; Everolimus; Exemestane; Felbamate; FentaNYL; Flibanserin; Fosphenytoin; Gefitinib; Griseofulvin; GuanFACINE; Hemin; Hydrocortisone (Systemic); Ibrutinib; Idelalisib; Imatinib; Irinotecan Products; Isavuconazonium Sulfate; Itraconazole; Ivabradine; Ivacaftor; Ixabepilone; Ixazomib; Lacosamide; LamoTRIgine; Lapatinib; Ledipasvir; Linagliptin; Lopinavir; Lumefantrine; Lurasidone; Macitentan; Maraviroc; Methadone; MethylPREDNISolone; MetroNIDAZOLE (Systemic); Mianserin; Mifepristone; Naloxegol; Netupitant; NIFEdipine; Nilotinib; NiMODipine; Nintedanib; Nisoldipine; Olaparib; Ombitasvir, Paritaprevir, Ritonavir, and Dasabuvir; Osimertinib; OXcarbazepine; Palbociclib; Paliperidone; Panobinostat; PAZOPanib; Perampanel; P-glycoprotein/ABCB1 Substrates; Phenytoin; Pirfenidone; PONATinib; Praziquantel; PrednisoLONE (Systemic); PredniSONE; Propacetamol; Propafenone; QUEtiapine; QuiNIDine; QuiNINE; Ranolazine; Regorafenib; Rilpivirine; Rivaroxaban; Roflumilast; Rolapitant; RomiDEPsin; Rufinamide; Saxagliptin; Simeprevir; Sofosbuvir; Sonidegib; SORAfenib; Stiripentol; SUNItinib; Suvorexant; Tadalafil; Tasimelteon; Telaprevir; Teniposide; Tetrahydrocannabinol; Ticagrelor; Tipranavir; Tofacitinib; Tolvaptan; Toremifene; Trabectedin; Treprostinil; Tricyclic Antidepressants; Ulipristal; Valproate Products; Vandetanib; Vemurafenib; Vilazodone; VinCRIStine (Liposomal); Vitamin K Antagonists; Vorapaxar; Voriconazole; Vortioxetine; Zaleplon; Zonisamide; Zuclopenthixol

The levels/effects of PHENobarbital may be decreased by: Amphetamines; Cholestyramine Resin; CYP2C19 Inducers (Strong); Darunavir; Folic Acid; Leucovorin Calcium-Levoleucovorin; Levomefolate; Lumacaftor; Mefloquine; Methylfolate; Mianserin; Multivitamins/Minerals

(with ADEK, Folate, Iron); Orlistat; Pyridoxine; Rifamycin Derivatives; Tipranavir

Food Interactions May cause decrease in vitamin D and calcium.

Storage/Stability

Elixir: Protect from light.

Injection: Protect from light. Not stable in aqueous solutions; use only clear solutions. Do not add to acidic solutions; precipitation may occur.

Mechanism of Action Long-acting barbiturate with sedative, hypnotic, and anticonvulsant properties. Barbiturates depress the sensory cortex, decrease motor activity, alter cerebellar function, and produce drowsiness, sedation, and hypnosis. In high doses, barbiturates exhibit anticonvulsant activity; barbiturates produce dose-dependent respiratory depression.

Pharmacodynamics/Kinetics

Onset of action: Oral: Hypnosis: 20 to 60 minutes; IV: ~5 minutes

Peak effect: IV: ~30 minutes

Duration: Oral: 6 to 10 hours; IV: 4 to 10 hours

Absorption: Oral: 70% to 90%

Protein binding: 20% to 45%; decreased in neonates

Metabolism: Hepatic via hydroxylation and glucuronide conjugation

Half-life elimination: Neonates: 45 to 500 hours; Infants: 20 to 133 hours; Children: 37 to 73 hours; Adults: 53 to 140 hours

Time to peak, serum: Oral: 1 to 6 hours

Excretion: Urine (20% to 50% as unchanged drug)

Dosing

Adult

Sedation:

IM, IV: 100 to 320 mg; larger doses may occasionally be necessary in persons with psychoses, and pronounced excitement, and in mental patients with insomnia. The effect of large doses must be closely watched. Maximum: 600 mg daily.

Oral: 30 to 120 mg daily in 2 to 3 divided doses; maximum: 400 mg daily

Status epilepticus: IV:

Neurocritical Care Society recommendation: 20 mg/kg (infused at 50 to 100 mg/minute); if necessary, may repeat once after 10 minutes with an additional 5 to 10 mg/kg (NCS [Brophy 2012]).

European Federation of Neurological Societies recommendation: 20 mg/kg (infused at 50 mg/minute); may administer additional boluses in the setting of an ICU. **Note:** EFNS recommends phenobarbital only for use in refractory complex partial status epilepticus (EFNS [Meierkord 2010]).

Note: Additional respiratory support may be required particularly when maximizing loading dose or if concurrent sedative therapy. Repeat doses administered sooner than 10 to 15 minutes may not allow adequate time for peak CNS concentrations to be achieved and may lead to CNS depression.

Seizures: Maintenance dose:

Manufacturer's labeling: Oral:

Elixir, oral solution: 60 to 200 mg daily

Tablets: 50 to 100 mg 2 or 3 times daily

Alternative dosing (limited data available) Usual dosing range: Oral, IV: **Note:** Dosage should be individualized based upon clinical response and serum concentration. Some centers have used: 1 to 3 mg/kg/day in divided doses or 50 to 100 mg 2 to 3 times daily

Alcohol withdrawal (off-label use):

IV: Initial dose of 260 mg, followed by subsequent doses of 130 mg as needed. Note: Clinical Institute Withdrawal Assessment (CIWA) scores were evaluated at 30 minute intervals in the clinical trial (Hendey 2011).

Oral: Fixed dose regimen of 60 mg 4 times daily on day 1, followed by 60 mg 3 times daily on day 2, 60 mg twice daily on day 3, and 30 mg twice daily on day 4. In addition, provide 60 mg as needed for breakthrough withdrawal symptoms (Mariani 2006; Rosenthal 1998). May also administer 130 mg IM as needed for more substantial withdrawal symptoms (eg, heart rate >120 bpm, SBP >150 mm Hg, marked agitation) (Rosenthal 1998).

Sedative/hypnotic withdrawal (off-label use): Several regimens have been evaluated:

Taper following dosage conversion: Initial daily requirement is determined by substituting phenobarbital in an equivalent dose to the baseline medication (clonazepam 1 mg = phenobarbital 60 mg was used in the study). Divided the calculated baseline total dose into 4 doses and administer every 6 hours for 2 days; then decrease the daily requirement by 10% per day over the next 10 days (Sullivan 1993).

Fixed dose taper: Initial 200 mg, followed by 100 mg every 4 hours for 5 doses, 60 mg every 4 hours for 4 doses, and then 60 mg every 8 hours for 3 doses (Kawasaki 2012).

Geriatric Geriatric patients should be started at the lowest recommended dose. Refer to adult dosing.

Pediatric

Sedation: Children: Oral: 2 mg/kg/**dose** 3 times daily; maximum dose: 40 mg

Alternative dosing (limited data available): IM, Oral: 2 to 3 mg/kg/day in divided doses every 8 to 12 hours (Nelson 1996)

Status epilepticus: Initial: Infants, Children, and Adolescents: IV:

American Academy of Pediatrics recommendation: 20 mg/kg (maximum dose: 1000 mg) over 10 minutes; if necessary, may repeat dose after 15 minutes (maximum total dose: 40 mg/kg) (AAP [Hegenbarth 2008]).

Neurocritical Care Society recommendation: 20 mg/kg (infused at 50 to 100 mg/minute); if necessary, may repeat once after 10 minutes with an additional 5 to 10 mg/kg (NCS [Brophy 2012]).

Manufacturer's labeling: 15 to 20 mg/kg over 10 to 15 minutes.

Note: Additional respiratory support may be required particularly when maximizing loading dose or if concurrent sedative therapy. Repeat doses administered sooner than 10 to 15 minutes may not allow adequate time for peak CNS concentrations to be achieved and may lead to CNS depression.

Seizures: Maintenance dose: Oral, IV:

Manufacturer's labeling: Infants, Children, and Adolescents: Oral: 3 to 6 mg/kg/day

Alternative dosing (limited data available) (Geurinni 2006; Kliegman 2011):

Initial: Oral, IV:

Infants and Children ≤5 years: 3 to 5 mg/kg/day in 1 to 2 divided doses

Children >5 years: 2 to 3 mg/kg/day in 1 to 2 divided doses

Adolescents: 1 to 3 mg/kg/day in 1 to 2 divided doses (Nelson 1996)

Usual dosing range: Oral, IV: **Note:** Dosage should be individualized based upon clinical response and serum concentration; once daily doses usually administered at bedtime in children and adolescents. Some centers have used:

Infants: 5 to 6 mg/kg/day in 1 to 2 divided doses

Children:

1 to 5 years: 6 to 8 mg/kg/day in 1 to 2 divided doses

5 to 12 years: 4 to 6 mg/kg/day in 1 to 2 divided doses

Adolescents: 1 to 3 mg/kg/day in 1 to 2 divided doses or 50 to 100 mg 2 to 3 times daily

Renal Impairment No specific dosage adjustment provided in manufacturer's labeling; reduced doses are recommended. The following guidelines have been used by some clinicians (Aronoff 2007):

Adults:

CrCl ≥10 mL/minute: No dosage adjustment necessary.

CrCl <10 mL/minute: Administer every 12 to 16 hours.

Hemodialysis (moderately dialyzable [20% to 50%]): Administer dose before dialysis and 50% of dose after dialysis.

Peritoneal dialysis: Administer 50% of normal dose.

CRRT: Administer normal dose and monitor levels.

Infants, Children, and Adolescents: **Note:** Renally adjusted dose recommendations are based on doses of 3 to 7 mg/kg/day every 12 to 24 hours

GFR ≥10 mL/minute/1.73 m^2: No dosage adjustment necessary.

GFR <10 mL/minute/1.73 m^2: Decrease normal dose by 50% and administer every 24 hours

Intermittent hemodialysis: Moderately dialyzable (20% to 50%): Supplemental dose may be needed during and after dialysis depending on individual seizure threshold

Peritoneal dialysis (PD): 40% to 50% removed; amount varies depending on number of cycles

Continuous renal replacement therapy (CRRT): Monitor serum concentrations; a case report suggests that clearance and volume of distribution increased with CVVH; more frequent and higher dosing may be necessary in some cases (Pasko 2004)

Hepatic Impairment There are no dosage adjustments provided in the manufacturer's labeling; reduced doses are recommended. Phenobarbital exposure is increased with hepatic impairment; use with caution

◄ **Dietary Considerations** Vitamin D: Loss in vitamin D due to malabsorption; increase intake of foods rich in vitamin D. Supplementation of vitamin D and/or calcium may be necessary. Injection may contain sodium.

Administration
May be administered IV, IM or orally.

According to the manufacturer, rapid IV administration >60 mg/minute in adults and >30 mg/minute in children should be avoided. In the setting of status epilepticus, the Neurocritical Care Society and the European Federation of Neurological Societies recommends administration at a rate of 50 to 100 mg/minute (EFNS [Meierkord 2010]; NCS [Brophy 2012]). Avoid extravasation. Intra-arterial injection is contraindicated. Avoid subcutaneous administration.

For IM administration, inject deep into muscle. Do not exceed 5 mL per injection site due to potential for tissue irritation

Monitoring Parameters Phenobarbital serum concentrations, mental status, CBC, LFTs, seizure activity

Reference Range
Therapeutic:
Infants and Children: 15 to 40 mcg/mL (SI: 65 to 172 micromole/L)
Adults: 20 to 40 mcg/mL (SI: 86 to 172 micromole/L)
Toxic: >40 mcg/mL (SI: >172 micromole/L)
Toxic concentration: Slowness, ataxia, nystagmus: 35 to 80 mcg/mL (SI: 150 to 344 micromole/L)
Coma with reflexes: 65 to 117 mcg/mL (SI: 279 to 502 micromole/L)
Coma without reflexes: >100 mcg/mL (SI: >430 micromole/L)

Test Interactions Assay interference of LDH

Additional Information Injectable solutions contain propylene glycol.

Phenobarbital tablets are also available from some generic manufacturers in strengths that are exactly equivalent to fractional grain strengths: 16.2 mg ($^1/_4$ grain), 32.4 mg ($^1/_2$ grain), 64.8 mg (1 grain). To avoid medication errors, do not prescribe phenobarbital in grains.

Dosage Forms Excipient information presented when available (limited, particularly for generics); consult specific product labeling. [DSC] = Discontinued product
Elixir, Oral:
Generic: 20 mg/5 mL (5 mL [DSC], 7.5 mL [DSC], 15 mL [DSC], 473 mL)
Solution, Oral:
Generic: 20 mg/5 mL (473 mL)
Solution, Injection, as sodium:
Luminal: 130 mg/mL (1 mL [DSC]) [contains alcohol, usp]
Generic: 65 mg/mL (1 mL); 130 mg/mL (1 mL)
Tablet, Oral:
Generic: 15 mg, 16.2 mg, 30 mg, 32.4 mg, 60 mg, 64.8 mg, 97.2 mg, 100 mg

Controlled Substance C-IV

Extemporaneous Preparations An alcohol-free 10 mg/mL phenobarbital oral suspension may be made from tablets and one of two different vehicles (a 1:1 mixture of Ora-Plus® and Ora-Sweet® or a 1:1 mixture of Ora-Plus® and Ora-Sweet® SF). Crush ten phenobarbital 60 mg tablets in a glass mortar and reduce to a fine powder. Mix 30 mL of Ora-Plus® and 30 mL of either Ora-Sweet® or Ora-Sweet® SF; stir vigorously. Add 15 mL of the vehicle to the powder and mix to a uniform paste. Transfer the mixture to a 2 ounce amber plastic prescription bottle. Rinse mortar and pestle with 15 mL of the vehicle; transfer to bottle. Repeat, then add quantity of vehicle sufficient to make 60 mL. Label "shake well." May mix dose with chocolate syrup (1:1 volume) immediately before administration to mask the bitter aftertaste. Stable for 115 days when stored in amber plastic prescription bottles at room temperature.
Cober M and Johnson CE, "Stability of an Extemporaneously Prepared Alcohol-Free Phenobarbital Suspension," *Am J Health Syst Pharm*, 2007, 64(6):644-6.

◆ Phenobarbital, Hyoscyamine, Atropine, and Scopolamine see Hyoscyamine, Atropine, Scopolamine, and Phenobarbital *on page 900*

◆ Phenobarbital Sodium see PHENobarbital *on page 1437*

◆ Phenobarbitone see PHENobarbital *on page 1437*

◆ Phenoptin see Sapropterin *on page 1636*

Phenoxybenzamine (fen oks ee BEN za meen)

Brand Names: US Dibenzyline
Index Terms Phenoxybenzamine Hydrochloride
Pharmacologic Category Alpha$_1$ Blocker; Antidote
Use Symptomatic management of pheochromocytoma

Dosing
Adult & Geriatric
Pheochromocytoma, hypertension: Oral: Initial: 10 mg twice daily, increase by 10 mg every other day until optimal blood pressure response is achieved; usual range: 20-40 mg 2-3 times/day. Doses up to 240 mg/day have been reported (Kinney, 2000).
Micturition disorders (off-label use): Oral: 10-20 mg 1-2 times/day
Pediatric Pheochromocytoma, hypertension (off-label uses): Oral: Initial: 0.25-1 mg/kg/day (maximum: 10 mg); increase slowly to blood pressure control
Renal Impairment No dosage adjustment provided in manufacturer's labeling. Use with caution.
Hepatic Impairment No dosage adjustment provided in manufacturer's labeling.
Additional Information Complete prescribing information should be consulted for additional detail.
Dosage Forms Excipient information presented when available (limited, particularly for generics); consult specific product labeling.
Capsule, Oral, as hydrochloride:
Dibenzyline: 10 mg [contains fd&c yellow #6 (sunset yellow)]
Generic: 10 mg

◆ Phenoxybenzamine Hydrochloride see Phenoxybenzamine *on page 1440*

◆ Phenoxymethyl Penicillin see Penicillin V Potassium *on page 1424*

Phentermine (FEN ter meen)

Brand Names: US Adipex-P; Suprenza
Index Terms Phentermine Hydrochloride
Pharmacologic Category Anorexiant; Central Nervous System Stimulant; Sympathomimetic
Use Short-term (few weeks) adjunct therapy in obese patients with an initial body mass index (BMI) ≥30 kg/m^2 or ≥27 kg/m^2 in the presence of other risk factors (eg, diabetes, hyperlipidemia, controlled hypertension); therapy should be used in conjunction with a comprehensive weight management program.

Dosing
Adult & Geriatric Note: Dosing is presented in terms of the salt, phentermine hydrochloride (not as phentermine base).
Obesity (short-term adjunct): Oral:
Capsule, tablet: 15-37.5 mg daily given in 1-2 divided doses. Individualize to achieve adequate response with lowest effective dose.
Orally disintegrating tablet (ODT): One tablet (15-37.5 mg daily) every morning. Individualize to achieve adequate response with lowest effective dose.
Pediatric Children >16 years: Refer to adult dosing.
Renal Impairment No dosage adjustment provided in manufacturer's labeling (has not been studied). Phentermine is excreted in the urine and systemic exposure may be increased in renal impairment; use with caution.
Hepatic Impairment No dosage adjustment provided in manufacturer's labeling (has not been studied).
Additional Information Complete prescribing information should be consulted for additional detail.
Dosage Forms Excipient information presented when available (limited, particularly for generics); consult specific product labeling.
Capsule, Oral, as hydrochloride:
Adipex-P: 37.5 mg
Generic: 15 mg, 30 mg, 37.5 mg
Tablet, Oral, as hydrochloride:
Adipex-P: 37.5 mg [scored; contains brilliant blue fcf (fd&c blue #1)]
Generic: 37.5 mg
Tablet Dispersible, Oral, as hydrochloride:
Suprenza: 15 mg [contains fd&c blue #1 aluminum lake, fd&c yellow #5 aluminum lake]
Suprenza: 30 mg [contains fd&c yellow #5 aluminum lake]
Suprenza: 37.5 mg [contains fd&c blue #1 aluminum lake]

Controlled Substance C-IV

◆ Phentermine Hydrochloride see Phentermine *on page 1440*

Phentolamine (fen TOLE a meen)

Brand Names: US OraVerse
Brand Names: Canada OraVerse; Rogitine
Index Terms Phentolamine Mesylate; Regitine [DSC]

Pharmacologic Category Alpha$_1$ Blocker; Antidote, Extravasation; Antihypertensive

Additional Appendix Information

Hypertension *on page 1996*

Use Diagnosis of pheochromocytoma via the phentolamine-blocking test (see **"Note"**); prevention and management of hypertensive episodes associated with pheochromocytoma resulting from stress or manipulation during the perioperative period; prevention and treatment of dermal necrosis/sloughing after extravasation of norepinephrine

OraVerse: Reversal of soft tissue anesthesia and the associated functional deficits resulting from a local dental anesthetic containing a vasoconstrictor

Note: The phentolamine-blocking test for the diagnosis of pheochromocytoma has largely been supplanted by the measurement of catecholamine concentrations and catecholamine metabolites (eg, metanephrine) in the plasma and urine; reserve phentolamine for cases when additional confirmation is necessary to determine diagnosis.

Pregnancy Considerations Adverse events were observed in some oral animal reproduction studies. Diagnosing and treating pheochromocytoma is critical for favorable maternal and fetal outcomes (Schenker, 1971; Schenker, 1982).

Breast-Feeding Considerations It is not known if phentolamine is excreted in breast milk. Due to the potential for serious adverse reaction in the nursing infant, the decision to discontinue phentolamine or discontinue breast-feeding during treatment should take in account the benefits of treatment to the mother.

Contraindications

Hypersensitivity to phentolamine, any component of the formulation, or related compounds; MI (or history of MI), coronary insufficiency, angina, or other evidence suggestive of coronary artery disease

Canadian labeling: Additional contraindications (not in US labeling): Hypotension

OraVerse:

US labeling: There are no contraindications listed in the manufacturer's labeling.

Canadian labeling: Hypersensitivity to phentolamine or any component of the formulation.

Warnings/Precautions MI, cerebrovascular spasm, and cerebrovascular occlusion have been reported following administration, usually associated with hypotensive episodes. Tachycardia and cardiac arrhythmias may occur. Discontinue if symptoms of angina occur or worsen. The use of phentolamine as a blocking agent in the screening of patients with hypertension has predominantly been replaced with urinary/biochemical assays; phentolamine use should be reserved for situations where additional confirmation is necessary and after risks associated with use have been considered. Potentially significant drug-drug interactions may exist, requiring dose or frequency adjustment, additional monitoring, and/or selection of alternative therapy.

Adverse Reactions Frequency not always defined.

Cardiovascular: Tachycardia (OraVerse ≤6%), bradycardia (OraVerse ≤4%), hypertension (OraVerse <3%), cerebrovascular occlusion, hypotension, myocardial infarction

Central nervous system: Headache (OraVerse ≤6%), mouth pain (OraVerse <3%) paresthesia (OraVerse <3%; mild, transient), cerebrovascular spasm

Dermatologic: Facial swelling (OraVerse <3%), pruritus (OraVerse <3%)

Gastrointestinal: Diarrhea (OraVerse <3%), upper abdominal pain (OraVerse <3%), vomiting (OraVerse <3%), nausea

Local: Pain at injection site (OraVerse 4% to 6%)

Neuromuscular & skeletal: Jaw pain (OraVerse <3%)

Postmarketing and/or case reports (Limited to important or life-threatening): Cardiac arrhythmia, orthostatic hypotension

Drug Interactions

Metabolism/Transport Effects None known.

Avoid Concomitant Use

Avoid concomitant use of Phentolamine with any of the following: Alpha1-Blockers

Increased Effect/Toxicity

Phentolamine may increase the levels/effects of: Alpha1-Blockers; Amifostine; Antipsychotic Agents (Second Generation [Atypical]); Calcium Channel Blockers; DULoxetine; Hypotension-Associated Agents; Levodopa

The levels/effects of Phentolamine may be increased by: Barbiturates; Beta-Blockers; Brimonidine (Topical); Dapoxetine; Diazoxide; Herbs (Hypotensive Properties); Molsidomine; Nicorandil; Obinutuzumab; Pentoxifylline; Phosphodiesterase 5 Inhibitors; Prostacyclin Analogues

Decreased Effect

Phentolamine may decrease the levels/effects of: Alpha-/Beta-Agonists; Alpha1-Agonists

The levels/effects of Phentolamine may be decreased by: Amphetamines; Herbs (Hypertensive Properties); Methylphenidate; Yohimbine

Preparation for Administration Powder for injection: Reconstitute 5 mg vial with 1 mL sterile water for injection. For treatment of extravasation, further dilute 5 to 10 mg in 10 mL of normal saline (manufacturer's recommendation) or in 10 to 15 mL of saline (Peberdy, 2010).

Storage/Stability

Powder for injection: Store intact vials 20°C to 25°C (68°F to 77°F). Reconstituted solution should be used immediately after preparation (per manufacturer).

Solution for injection (OraVerse): Store at 20°C to 25°C (68°F to 77°F); brief excursions permitted between 15°C to 30°C (59°F to 86°F). Protect from heat and light. Do not freeze.

Mechanism of Action Competitively blocks alpha-adrenergic receptors (nonselective) to produce brief antagonism of circulating epinephrine and norepinephrine to reduce hypertension caused by alpha effects of these catecholamines and minimizes tissue injury due to extravasation of these and other sympathomimetic vasoconstrictors (eg, dopamine, phenylephrine); also has a positive inotropic and chronotropic effect on the heart thought to be due to presynaptic alpha-2 receptor blockade which results in release of presynaptic norepinephrine (Hoffman, 1980)

OraVerse: Causes vasodilation and increased blood flow in injection area via alpha-adrenergic blockade to accelerate reversal of soft tissue anesthesia

Pharmacodynamics/Kinetics

Onset of action: IM: 15 to 20 minutes; IV: 1 to 2 minutes (Chobanian, 2003)

Peak effect: OraVerse: 10 to 20 minutes

Duration: IM: 30 to 45 minutes; IV: 10 to 30 minutes (Chobanian, 2003)

Metabolism: Hepatic

Half-life elimination: IV: 19 minutes

Excretion: Urine (~13% as unchanged drug)

Dosing

Adult & Geriatric

Extravasation of norepinephrine, management (manufacturer's labeling): Local infiltration: Inject 5 or 10 mg (diluted in 10 mL 0.9% sodium chloride) into extravasation area (as soon as extravasation is noted but within 12 hours of extravasation).

Extravasation of sympathomimetic vasopressors, management (off-label use): Infiltrate extravasation site with 5 or 10 mg diluted in 10 to 15 mL 0.9% sodium chloride as soon as possible after extravasation (Peberdy, 2010).

Diagnosis of pheochromocytoma (phentolamine-blocking test): Note: The phentolamine-blocking test for the diagnosis of pheochromocytoma has largely been supplanted by the measurement of catecholamine concentrations and catecholamine metabolites (eg, metanephrine) in the plasma and urine; reserve phentolamine for cases when additional confirmation is necessary to determine diagnosis: IM, IV: 5 mg

Hypertensive episodes associated with pheochromocytoma, prevention and management: Note: In the perioperative period, the use of other agents may be preferred due to slow onset of action and prolonged duration of phentolamine in comparison to the other agents (eg, nitroprusside) (Miller, 2010).

Preoperative: IM, IV: 5 mg given 1 to 2 hours before surgery and repeat if needed.

Intraoperative: IV: Administer 5 mg as indicated to prevent or control paroxysms of hypertension, tachycardia, respiratory depression, seizure, or other effects associated with epinephrine intoxication resulting from tumor manipulation or other stressor (eg, intubation) (Miller, 2010).

Hypertensive crisis (off-label use): Note: Generally used in the setting of catecholamine excess (eg, pheochromocytoma) (Marik, 2007): IV: 1 to 5 mg bolus; maximum single dose: 15 mg. A continuous infusion may be administered after initial bolus dosing (eg, 1 mg/hour titrated to blood pressure response) to a maximum infusion rate of 40 mg/hour (McMillian, 2011).

Reversal of oral soft tissue (lip, tongue) anesthesia (OraVerse): Infiltration or block technique: Submucosal oral injection: **Note:** Dose is based upon the number of cartridges of local anesthetic administered. Infiltration or block injection:

0.2 mg if one-half cartridge of anesthesia was administered

0.4 mg if 1 cartridge of anesthesia was administered

0.8 mg if 2 cartridges of anesthesia were administered

◀ **Pediatric**

Extravasation of norepinephrine, management (manufacturer's labeling): Local infiltration: Inject 5 to 10 mg (diluted in 10 mL 0.9% sodium chloride) into extravasation area (as soon as extravasation is noted but within 12 hours of extravasation).

Extravasation of sympathomimetic vasopressors, management (off-label use): Infiltrate extravasation site with 5 to 10 mg diluted in 10 to 15 mL 0.9% sodium chloride as soon as possible after extravasation (Peberdy, 2010).

Diagnosis of pheochromocytoma (phentolamine-blocking test): Note: The phentolamine-blocking test for the diagnosis of pheochromocytoma has largely been supplanted by the measurement of catecholamine concentrations and catecholamine metabolites (eg, metanephrine) in the plasma and urine; reserve phentolamine for cases when additional confirmation is necessary to determine diagnosis.
IM: 3 mg
IV: 1 mg

Hypertensive episodes associated with pheochromocytoma, prevention and management: Note: In the perioperative period, the use of other agents may be preferred due to slow onset of action and prolonged duration of phentolamine in comparison to the other agents (eg, nitroprusside) (Miller, 2010).

Preoperative: IM, IV: 1 mg given 1 to 2 hours before surgery and repeat if needed.

Intraoperative: IV: Administer 1 mg as indicated to prevent or control paroxysms of hypertension, tachycardia, respiratory depression, seizure, or other effects associated with epinephrine intoxication resulting from tumor manipulation or other stressor (eg, intubation) (Miller, 2010).

Reversal of oral soft tissue (lip, tongue) anesthesia (OraVerse): Infiltration or block technique: Submucosal oral injection:
Children: 15 to 30 kg: 0.2 mg maximum dose
Children >30 kg and <12 years: 0.4 mg maximum dose
Children >30 kg and ≥12 years: Refer to adult dosing.

Renal Impairment There are no dosage adjustments provided in manufacturer's labeling.

Hepatic Impairment There are no dosage adjustments provided in manufacturer's labeling.

Administration

Extravasation management (treatment), sympathomimetic vasopressors: Stop vesicant infusion immediately and disconnect IV line (leave needle/cannula in place); gently aspirate extravasated solution from the IV line (do **NOT** flush the line); remove needle/cannula; elevate extremity. Inject phentolamine 5 to 10 mg/10 mL saline into extravasation site (as soon as possible but within 12 hours of extravasation). AHA recommends diluting 5 to 10 mg in 10 to 15 mL saline and administering into the site (Peberdy, 2010).

Pheochromocytoma diagnosis: Patient should be supine throughout test, preferable in a quiet, dark room. Blood pressure should be monitored every 10 minutes for at least 30 minutes, delay phentolamine administration until after blood pressure is stable (at an untreated, hypertensive level). A drop in blood pressure >35 mm Hg (systolic) and >25 mm Hg (diastolic) is considered a positive response. If blood pressure is elevated, unchanged, or decrease is <35 mm Hg (systolic) and <25 mm Hg (diastolic), then response is negative. Confirm positive response with other diagnostic measure. Negative responses do not exclude a pheochromocytoma diagnosis, particularly in patients with paroxysmal hypertension where an incidence of false negatives is high.

IM: After IM injection, monitor blood pressure every 5 minutes for 35 to 40 minutes. Blood pressure drops to above parameters within 20 minutes are considered positive.

IV: Inject rapidly (after venous response to venipuncture has subsided); then monitor blood pressure immediately after injection, every 30 seconds for 3 minutes, then every minute for 7 minutes. Maximum response is generally achieved within 2 minutes; duration may last 15 to 30 minutes (although return to prior blood pressure may be sooner).

Pheochromocytoma-associated hypertensive episode: Administer IM or IV 1 to 2 hours prior to surgery and repeat during surgery (IV) if necessary.

Reversal of oral soft tissue (lip, tongue) anesthesia (OraVerse): Submucosal oral injection: Use the same location and dental technique employed for administration of the local anesthetic.

Hypertensive crisis (off-label use): Administer as an IV bolus (Marik, 2007); may follow with a continuous IV infusion (McMillian, 2011).

Monitoring Parameters Blood pressure, heart rate; monitor and document extravasation site; monitor patient for orthostasis; assist patient with ambulation

Dosage Forms Excipient information presented when available (limited, particularly for generics); consult specific product labeling. [DSC] = Discontinued product
Solution, Injection, as mesylate:
Generic: 5 mg/mL (1 mL [DSC])
Solution, Injection, as mesylate [preservative free]:
OraVerse: 0.4 mg/1.7 mL (1.7 mL) [contains edetate disodium; dental cartridge]
Solution Reconstituted, Injection, as mesylate:
Generic: 5 mg (1 ea [DSC])

◆ Phentolamine Mesylate *see* Phentolamine *on page 1440*

◆ Phenylalanine Mustard *see* Melphalan *on page 1137*

◆ Phenylazo Diamino Pyridine Hydrochloride *see* Phenazopyridine *on page 1435*

Phenylephrine (Systemic) (fen il EF rin)

Brand Names: US Contac-D [OTC] [DSC]; Little Colds Decongestant [OTC]; Medi-Phenyl [OTC]; Nasal Decongestant PE Max St [OTC]; Nasal Decongestant [OTC]; Neo-Synephrine [DSC]; Non-Pseudo Sinus Decongestant [OTC]; PediaCare Childrens Decongest [OTC] [DSC]; Sudafed PE Childrens [OTC]; Sudafed PE Maximum Strength [OTC]; Sudogest PE [OTC]; Vazculep

Index Terms Phenylephrine Hydrochloride

Pharmacologic Category Alpha-Adrenergic Agonist

Use Treatment of hypotension, vascular failure in shock (see **"Note"**); as a vasoconstrictor in regional analgesia; as a decongestant [OTC]

Note: Not recommended for routine use in the treatment of septic shock (SCCM [Dellinger, 2013]).

Pregnancy Considerations Animal reproduction studies have not been conducted. Phenylephrine crosses the placenta at term. Maternal use of phenylephrine during the first trimester of pregnancy is not strongly associated with an increased risk of fetal malformations; maternal dose and duration of therapy were not reported in available publications. Phenylephrine is available over-the-counter (OTC) for the symptomatic relief of nasal congestion. Decongestants are not the preferred agents for the treatment of rhinitis during pregnancy. Oral phenylephrine should be avoided during the first trimester of pregnancy; short-term use (<3 days) of intranasal phenylephrine may be beneficial to some patients although its safety during pregnancy has not been studied. Phenylephrine injection is used at delivery for the prevention and/or treatment of maternal hypotension associated with spinal anesthesia in women undergoing cesarean section. Phenylephrine may be associated with a more favorable fetal acid base status than ephedrine; however, overall fetal outcomes appear to be similar. Nausea or vomiting may be less with phenylephrine than ephedrine but is also dependent upon blood pressure control. Phenylephrine may be preferred in the absence of maternal bradycardia.

Breast-Feeding Considerations It is not known if phenylephrine is excreted into breast milk. The manufacturer recommends that caution be exercised when administering phenylephrine to nursing women.

Contraindications Hypersensitivity to phenylephrine or any component of the formulation
Injection: Severe hypertension; ventricular tachycardia
Vazculep: There are no contraindications listed in the manufacturer's labeling.
OTC labeling (Oral): When used for self-medication: Use with or within 14 days of MAO inhibitor therapy

Warnings/Precautions Some products contain sulfites which may cause allergic reactions in susceptible individuals. Use with extreme caution in patients taking MAO inhibitors. Use with caution in patients with hyperthyroidism.

Intravenous: Phenylephrine may cause severe bradycardia (likely baroreflex mediated) and reduced cardiac output due to an increase in cardiac afterload especially in patients with preexisting cardiac dysfunction (Goertz 1993; Yamazaki 1982). May also precipitate angina in patients with severe coronary artery disease and increase pulmonary arterial pressure. Use with caution in patients with preexisting bradycardia, partial heart block, myocardial disease, or severe coronary artery disease. Avoid or use with extreme caution in patients with heart failure or cardiogenic shock; increased systemic vascular resistance may significantly reduce cardiac output. Avoid use in patients with hypertension (contraindicated in severe hypertension); monitor blood pressure closely and adjust infusion rate. Assure adequate circulatory volume to

minimize need for vasoconstrictors. Vesicant; ensure proper needle or catheter placement prior to and during infusion; avoid extravasation. **[US Boxed Warning]: Should be administered by adequately trained individuals familiar with its use.** Acidosis may reduce the efficacy of phenylephrine; correct acidosis prior to or during use of phenylephrine. Patients with autonomic dysfunction (eg, spinal cord injury) may exhibit an exaggerated increase in blood pressure response to phenylephrine.

Oral: When used for self-medication (OTC), use caution with asthma, bowel obstruction/narrowing, hyperthyroidism, diabetes mellitus, cardiovascular disease, ischemic heart disease, hypertension, increased intraocular pressure, prostatic hyperplasia or in the elderly. Notify healthcare provider if symptoms do not improve within 7 days or are accompanied by fever. Discontinue and contact healthcare provider if nervousness, dizziness, or sleeplessness occur.

Benzyl alcohol and derivatives: Some dosage forms may contain sodium benzoate/benzoic acid; benzoic acid (benzoate) is a metabolite of benzyl alcohol; large amounts of benzyl alcohol (≥99 mg/kg/day) have been associated with a potentially fatal toxicity ("gasping syndrome") in neonates; the "gasping syndrome" consists of metabolic acidosis, respiratory distress, gasping respirations, CNS dysfunction (including convulsions, intracranial hemorrhage), hypotension, and cardiovascular collapse (AAP ["Inactive" 1997]; CDC 1982); some data suggests that benzoate displaces bilirubin from protein binding sites (Ahlfors 2001); avoid or use dosage forms containing benzyl alcohol derivative with caution in neonates. See manufacturer's labeling.

Adverse Reactions Frequency not defined.

Injection:

Cardiovascular: Cardiac arrhythmia (rare), exacerbation of angina, hypertension, hypertensive crisis, ischemia, localized blanching, low cardiac output, peripheral vasoconstriction (severe), reflex bradycardia, visceral vasoconstriction (severe), worsening of heart failure

Central nervous system: Anxiety, dizziness, excitability, headache, insomnia, nervousness, paresthesia, precordial pain (or discomfort), restlessness

Dermatologic: Pallor, piloerection, pruritus

Endocrine & metabolic: Metabolic acidosis

Gastrointestinal: Epigastric pain, gastric irritation, nausea, vomiting

Genitourinary: Decreased renal blood flow, decreased urine output

Hypersensitivity: Hypersensitivity reaction (including skin rash, urticaria, leukopenia, agranulocytosis, thrombocytopenia)

Local: Extravasation which may lead to necrosis and sloughing of surrounding tissue

Neuromuscular & skeletal: Neck pain, tremor, weakness

Ophthalmic: Blurred vision

Respiratory: Dyspnea, exacerbation of pulmonary arterial hypertension, respiratory distress

Oral: Central nervous system: Anxiety, dizziness, excitability, headache, insomnia, nervousness, restlessness

Drug Interactions

Metabolism/Transport Effects None known.

Avoid Concomitant Use

Avoid concomitant use of Phenylephrine (Systemic) with any of the following: Ergot Derivatives; Hyaluronidase; Iobenguane I 123; MAO Inhibitors

Increased Effect/Toxicity

Phenylephrine (Systemic) may increase the levels/effects of: Doxofylline; Sympathomimetics

The levels/effects of Phenylephrine (Systemic) may be increased by: Acetaminophen; AtoMOXetine; Cannabinoid-Containing Products; Ergot Derivatives; Hyaluronidase; Linezolid; MAO Inhibitors; Propacetamol; Tedizolid; Tricyclic Antidepressants

Decreased Effect

Phenylephrine (Systemic) may decrease the levels/effects of: Benzylpenicilloyl Polylysine; FentaNYL; Iobenguane I 123; Ioflupane I 123

The levels/effects of Phenylephrine (Systemic) may be decreased by: Alpha1-Blockers; Tricyclic Antidepressants

Preparation for Administration Solution for injection:

IV infusion: May dilute 10 mg in 500 mL NS or D5W (Vazculep preferred dilution). May also dilute 50 mg in 500 mL NS, 100 mg in 500 mL NS, or 1250 mg in 500 mL NS (Gupta 2004; Weber 1970).

IV injection: May dilute with SWFI, NS, or D5W to a concentration of 1 mg/mL. May also prepare a 0.1 mg/mL solution for bolus administration. **Note:** Vazculep prescribing information recommends preparation of 0.1 mg/mL solution for bolus administration.

Storage/Stability

Solution for injection: Store vials at controlled room temperature of 15°C to 25°C (59°F to 77°F). Protect from light. Do not use solution if brown or contains a precipitate.

IV infusion: Concentrations of 0.1 and 0.2 mg/mL in NS are stable for at least 14 days at room temperature of 25°C (77°F) (Gupta 2004). Dilution of 2.5 mg/mL in NS retained potency for at least 24 hours at 22°C (Weber 1970). Vazculep: Do not hold diluted solutions for longer than 4 hours at room temperature or 24 hours refrigerated.

Stability in syringes: Concentration of 0.1 mg/mL in NS (polypropylene syringes) is stable for at least 30 days at -20°C (-4°F), 3°C to 5°C (37°F to 41°F), or 23°C to 25°C (73.4°F to 77°F) (Kiser 2007). Vazculep: Do not hold diluted solutions for longer than 4 hours at room temperature or 24 hours refrigerated.

Oral: Store at controlled room temperature of 15°C to 25°C (59°F to 77°F). Protect from light.

Mechanism of Action Potent, direct-acting alpha-adrenergic agonist with virtually no beta-adrenergic activity; produces systemic arterial vasoconstriction. Such increases in systemic vascular resistance result in dose dependent increases in systolic and diastolic blood pressure and reductions in heart rate and cardiac output especially in patients with heart failure.

Pharmacodynamics/Kinetics

Onset of action:

Blood pressure increase/vasoconstriction: IM, SubQ: 10 to 15 minutes; IV: Immediate

Nasal decongestant: Oral: 15 to 30 minutes (Kollar 2007)

Duration:

Blood pressure increase/vasoconstriction: IM: 1 to 2 hours; IV: ~15 to 20 minutes; SubQ: 50 minutes

Nasal decongestant: Oral: ≤4 hours (Kollar 2007)

Absorption: Oral: Rapid and complete (Kanfer 1993)

Distribution: V_d: Initial: 26 to 61 L; V_{dss}: 184 to 543 L (mean: 340 L) (Hengstmann 1982)

Metabolism: Hepatic via oxidative deamination (Oral: 24%; IV: 50%); Undergoes sulfation (Oral [mostly within gut wall]: 46%; IV: 8%) and some glucuronidation; forms inactive metabolites (Kanfer 1993)

Bioavailability: Oral: ≤38% (Hengstmann 1982; Kanfer 1993)

Half-life elimination: Alpha phase: ~5 minutes; Terminal phase: 2 to 3 hours (Hengstmann 1982; Kanfer 1993)

Time to peak: Oral: 0.75 to 2 hours (Kanfer 1993)

Excretion: Urine (mostly as inactive metabolites)

Dosing

Adult & Geriatric

Hypotension/shock: Note: The Society of Critical Care Medicine (SCCM) does not recommend phenylephrine for septic shock except in the following circumstances: Norepinephrine (preferred first-line agent) is associated with serious arrhythmias, cardiac output is known to be high and blood pressure persistently low, or when the combination of inotrope/vasopressor and low-dose vasopressin failed to achieve target mean arterial pressure and phenylephrine is used as salvage therapy (SCCM [Dellinger 2013]).

IV bolus: 100 to 500 mcg/dose every 10 to 15 minutes as needed (initial dose should not exceed 500 mcg)

IV infusion: Initial dose: 100 to 180 mcg/minute, **or alternatively,** 0.5 mcg/kg/minute; titrate to desired response. Dosing ranges between 0.4 to 9.1 mcg/kg/minute have been reported when treating septic shock (Gregory 1991).

ACLS guideline recommendations (to treat severe hypotension [eg, systolic blood pressure <70 mm Hg] and low total peripheral resistance): Initial dose: 0.5 to 2 mcg/kg/minute; titrate to effect (AHA [Peberdy 2010]).

Hypotension during anesthesia:

IV bolus: 40 to 100 mcg/dose every 1 to 2 minutes as needed (total dose should not exceed 200 mcg)

IV infusion: Initial dose: 10 to 35 mcg/minute adjusted according to blood pressure goal (not to exceed 200 mcg/minute)

Nasal congestion: *Oral:* OTC labeling: 10 mg every 4 hours as needed for ≤7 days (maximum: 60 mg/24 hours)

Pediatric

Hypotension/shock: Note: The Society of Critical Care Medicine (SCCM) does not recommend phenylephrine for septic shock except in the following circumstances: Norepinephrine (preferred first-line agent) is associated with serious arrhythmias, cardiac output is known to be high and blood pressure persistently low, or when the combination of inotrope/vasopressor and low-dose vasopressin failed to achieve target mean arterial pressure and phenylephrine is used as salvage therapy (SCCM [Dellinger 2013]).

IV bolus: 5 to 20 mcg/kg/dose every 10 to 15 minutes as needed

IV infusion: 0.1 to 0.5 mcg/kg/minute

Nasal congestion: *Oral:* OTC labeling:

4 to <6 years: 2.5 mg every 4 hours as needed for ≤7 days (maximum: 15 mg/24 hours)

6 to <12 years: 5 mg every 4 hours as needed for ≤7 days (maximum: 30 mg/24 hours)

≥12 years: Refer to adult dosing.

Dietary Considerations Some products may contain phenylalanine and/or sodium.

Usual Infusion Concentrations: Pediatric IV infusion: 20 **mcg**/mL, 40 **mcg**/mL, or 60 **mcg**/mL

Usual Infusion Concentrations: Adult IV infusion: 10 mg in 500 mL (concentration: 20 **mcg**/mL) of D_5W or NS, 50 mg in 500 mL (concentration: 100 **mcg**/mL) of NS, **or** 100 mg in 500 mL (concentration: 200 **mcg**/mL) of NS

Other institutions may use concentrations of 40 **mcg**/mL **or** 160 **mcg**/mL; however, stability information is not available for these concentrations.

Administration

IV:

Hypotension/shock: May be administered as an intermittent IV bolus over 20 to 30 seconds or via continuous infusion (after diluting). When administering as a continuous infusion, central line administration is preferred. IV infusions require an infusion pump.

Hypotension during anesthesia: Administer as an IV bolus over 20 to 30 seconds.

Vesicant; ensure proper needle or catheter placement prior to and during infusion; avoid extravasation.

Extravasation management: If extravasation occurs, stop infusion immediately and disconnect (leave cannula/needle in place); gently aspirate extravasated solution (do **NOT** flush the line); remove needle/cannula; elevate extremity. Initiate phentolamine (or alternative antidote). Apply dry warm compresses (Hurst 2004).

Phentolamine (no longer available in the US): Dilute 5 to 10 mg in 10 to 15 mL NS and administer into extravasation site as soon as possible after extravasation (AHA [Peberdy 2010]).

Alternatives to phentolamine:

Nitroglycerin topical 2% ointment (based on limited case reports in neonates/infants): Apply 4 mm/kg as a thin ribbon to the affected areas; may repeat after 8 hours if needed (Wong 1992) **or** apply a 1-inch strip on the affected site (Denkler 1989).

Terbutaline (based on limited case reports): Infiltrate extravasation area using a solution of terbutaline 1 mg diluted to 10 mL in NS (large extravasation site; administration volume varied from 3 to 10 mL) **or** 1 mg diluted in 1 mL NS (small/distal extravasation site; administration volume varied from 0.5 to 1 mL) (Stier 1999).

Monitoring Parameters Blood pressure (or mean arterial pressure), heart rate; cardiac output (as appropriate), intravascular volume status, pulmonary capillary wedge pressure (as appropriate); monitor infusion site closely

Consult individual institutional policies and procedures.

Product Availability

Vazculep (10 mg/mL injection): FDA approved July 2014; anticipated availability is currently unknown.

Vazculep is indicated for the treatment of clinically important hypotension resulting primarily from vasodilation in the setting of anesthesia.

Dosage Forms Excipient information presented when available (limited, particularly for generics); consult specific product labeling. [DSC] = Discontinued product

Liquid, Oral, as hydrochloride:

Little Colds Decongestant: 2.5 mg/mL (30 mL) [alcohol free, dye free, saccharin free; contains sodium benzoate; grape flavor]

Solution, Injection, as hydrochloride:

Neo-Synephrine: 10 mg/mL (1 mL [DSC]) [contains sodium metabisulfite]

Generic: 10 mg/mL (1 mL, 5 mL, 10 mL)

Solution, Intravenous, as hydrochloride:

Vazculep: 10 mg/mL (1 mL, 5 mL, 10 mL) [contains sodium metabisulfite]

Solution, Oral, as hydrochloride:

PediaCare Childrens Decongest: 2.5 mg/5 mL (118 mL [DSC]) [contains edetate disodium, fd&c red #40, sodium benzoate]

Sudafed PE Childrens: 2.5 mg/5 mL (118 mL) [alcohol free, sugar free; contains edetate disodium, fd&c red #40, sodium benzoate; berry flavor]

Tablet, Oral, as hydrochloride:

Contac-D: 10 mg [DSC] [contains fd&c red #40 aluminum lake]

Medi-Phenyl: 5 mg

Nasal Decongestant: 10 mg [contains fd&c blue #2 (indigotine), fd&c red #40, fd&c yellow #6 aluminum lake]

Nasal Decongestant PE Max St: 10 mg [pseudoephedrine free; contains fd&c red #40 aluminum lake]

Non-Pseudo Sinus Decongestant: 10 mg [contains fd&c red #40 aluminum lake, fd&c yellow #6 aluminum lake]

Sudafed PE Maximum Strength: 10 mg [contains fd&c red #40 aluminum lake, fd&c yellow #10 aluminum lake, fd&c yellow #6 aluminum lake]

Sudafed PE Maximum Strength: 10 mg [contains fd&c red #40 aluminum lake, fd&c yellow #6 aluminum lake]

Sudafed PE Maximum Strength: 10 mg [pseudoephedrine free; contains fd&c red #40 aluminum lake, fd&c yellow #10 aluminum lake, fd&c yellow #6 aluminum lake]

Sudogest PE: 10 mg [contains fd&c red #40]

♦ Phenylephrine and Chlorpheniramine *see* Chlorpheniramine and Phenylephrine *on page 376*

♦ Phenylephrine and Cyclopentolate *see* Cyclopentolate and Phenylephrine *on page 455*

♦ Phenylephrine and Dextromethorphan *see* Dextromethorphan and Phenylephrine *on page 535*

♦ Phenylephrine and Diphenhydramine *see* Diphenhydramine and Phenylephrine *on page 564*

♦ Phenylephrine, Chlorpheniramine, and Dextromethorphan *see* Chlorpheniramine, Phenylephrine, and Dextromethorphan *on page 378*

♦ Phenylephrine Hydrochloride *see* Phenylephrine (Systemic) *on page 1442*

♦ Phenylephrine Hydrochloride and Diphenhydramine Hydrochloride *see* Diphenhydramine and Phenylephrine *on page 564*

♦ Phenylephrine Hydrochloride and Guaifenesin *see* Guaifenesin and Phenylephrine *on page 862*

♦ Phenylephrine Tannate and Diphenhydramine Tannate *see* Diphenhydramine and Phenylephrine *on page 564*

♦ Phenylethylmalonylurea *see* PHENobarbital *on page 1437*

♦ Phenyl Salicylate, Methenamine, Methylene Blue, Benzoic Acid, and Hyoscyamine *see* Methenamine, Phenyl Salicylate, Methylene Blue, Benzoic Acid, and Hyoscyamine *on page 1166*

♦ Phenyl Salicylate, Methenamine, Methylene Blue, Sodium Biphosphate, and Hyoscyamine *see* Methenamine, Sodium Phosphate Monobasic, Phenyl Salicylate, Methylene Blue, and Hyoscyamine *on page 1166*

♦ Phenytek *see* Phenytoin *on page 1444*

Phenytoin (FEN i toyn)

Brand Names: US Dilantin; Dilantin Infatabs; Phenytek; Phenytoin Infatabs

Brand Names: Canada Dilantin; Novo-Phenytoin; Taro-Phenytoin; Tremytoine Inj

Index Terms Dilantin; Diphenylhydantoin; DPH; Phenytoin Sodium; Phenytoin Sodium, Extended; Phenytoin Sodium, Prompt

Pharmacologic Category Anticonvulsant, Hydantoin

Use Seizures: Control of generalized tonic-clonic and complex partial (psychomotor, temporal lobe) seizures; prevention and treatment of seizures occurring during or following neurosurgery

Pregnancy Considerations Phenytoin crosses the placenta (Harden and Pennell 2009). An increased risk of congenital malformations and adverse outcomes may occur following *in utero* phenytoin exposure. Reported malformations include orofacial clefts, cardiac defects, dysmorphic facial features, nail/digit hypoplasia, growth abnormalities including microcephaly, and mental deficiency. Isolated cases of malignancies (including neuroblastoma) and coagulation defects in the neonate (may be life threatening) following delivery have also been reported. Maternal use of phenytoin should be avoided when possible to decrease the risk of cleft palate and poor cognitive outcomes. Polytherapy may also increase the risk of congenital malformations; monotherapy is

recommended (Harden and Meader 2009). The maternal use of folic acid throughout pregnancy is recommended to reduce the risk of major congenital malformations (Harden and Pennell 2009).

Total plasma concentrations of phenytoin are decreased in the mother during pregnancy; unbound plasma (free) concentrations are also decreased and plasma clearance is increased. Due to pregnancy-induced physiologic changes, women who are pregnant may require dose adjustments of phenytoin in order to maintain clinical response; monitoring during pregnancy should be considered (Harden and Pennell 2009). For women with epilepsy who are planning a pregnancy in advance, baseline serum concentrations should be measured once or twice prior to pregnancy during a period when seizure control is optimal. Monitoring can then be continued once each trimester during pregnancy and postpartum; more frequent monitoring may be needed in some patients. Monitoring of unbound plasma concentrations is recommended (Patsalos 2008). In women taking phenytoin who are trying to avoid pregnancy, potentially significant interactions may exist with hormone-containing contraceptives; consult drug interactions database for more detailed information.

Patients exposed to phenytoin during pregnancy are encouraged to enroll themselves into the North American Antiepileptic Drug (NAAED) Pregnancy Registry by calling 1-888-233-2334. Additional information is available at https:\\aedpregnancyregistry.org.

Breast-Feeding Considerations Phenytoin is excreted in breast milk; however, the amount to which the infant is exposed is considered small. The manufacturers of phenytoin do not recommend breast-feeding during therapy.

Medication Guide Available Yes

Contraindications
Hypersensitivity to phenytoin, other hydantoins, or any component of the formulation; concurrent use of delavirdine

IV: Sinus bradycardia, sinoatrial block, second- and third-degree heart block, Adams-Stokes syndrome

Warnings/Precautions Hazardous agent - use appropriate precautions for handling and disposal (NIOSH 2014 [group 2]).

Antiepileptics are associated with an increased risk of suicidal behavior/thoughts with use (regardless of indication); patients should be monitored for signs/symptoms of depression, suicidal tendencies, and other unusual behavior changes during therapy and instructed to inform their healthcare provider immediately if symptoms occur.

[US Boxed Warning]: Phenytoin must be administered slowly. Intravenous administration should not exceed 50 mg/minute in adult patients. In pediatric patients, intravenous administration rate should not exceed 1-3 mg/kg/minute or 50 mg/minute whichever is slower. Hypotension and severe cardiac arrhythmias (eg, heart block, ventricular tachycardia, ventricular fibrillation) may occur with rapid administration; adverse cardiac events have been reported at or below the recommended infusion rate. Cardiac monitoring is necessary during and after administration of intravenous phenytoin; reduction in rate of administration or discontinuation of infusion may be necessary. For nonemergency use, intravenous phenytoin should be administered more slowly; the use of oral phenytoin should be used whenever possible. Vesicant (intravenous administration); ensure proper catheter or needle position prior to and during infusion; avoid extravasation; IV form may cause soft tissue irritation and inflammation, and skin necrosis at IV site; avoid IV administration in small veins. The "purple glove syndrome" (ie, discoloration with edema and pain of distal limb) may occur following peripheral IV administration of phenytoin; may or may not be associated with drug extravasation; symptoms may resolve spontaneously; however, skin necrosis and limb ischemia may occur; interventions such as fasciotomies, skin grafts, and amputation (rare) may be required. Use with caution in patients with porphyria; discontinue if rash or lymphadenopathy occurs; a spectrum of hematologic effects have been reported with use (eg, agranulocytosis, leukopenia, granulocytopenia, thrombocytopenia, and pancytopenia) with or without bone marrow suppression) and may be fatal; use with caution in patients with hepatic dysfunction, hypothyroidism, or underlying cardiac disease; IV use is contraindicated in patients with sinus bradycardia, sinoatrial block, or second- and third-degree heart block; use with caution in elderly or debilitated patients, or in any condition associated with low serum albumin levels, which will increase the free fraction of phenytoin in the serum and, therefore, the pharmacologic response. Plasma concentrations of phenytoin sustained above the optimal range may produce confusional states referred to as delirium, psychosis, or encephalopathy, or

rarely, irreversible cerebellar dysfunction. Measure plasma phenytoin concentrations at the first sign of acute toxicity; dosage reduction is indicated if phenytoin concentrations are excessive; if symptoms persist, discontinue administration. Anticonvulsants should not be discontinued abruptly because of the possibility of increasing seizure frequency; therapy should be withdrawn gradually to minimize the potential of increased seizure frequency, unless safety concerns require a more rapid withdrawal.

Severe reactions, including toxic epidermal necrolysis (TEN) and Stevens-Johnson syndrome (some fatal) have been reported; the onset of symptoms is usually within 28 days of treatment, but can occur later. Discontinue phenytoin if there are any signs of rash and evaluate for signs and symptoms of drug reaction with eosinophilia and systemic symptoms (DRESS). Data suggests a genetic susceptibility for serious skin reactions in patients of Asian descent. Asian patients with the variant HLA-B*1502 may be at an increased risk of developing Stevens-Johnson syndrome and/or TEN. **Note:** Carbamazepine, another antiepileptic with a chemical structure similar to phenytoin, includes in the manufacturer labeling a recommendation to screen patients of Asian descent for the HLA-B*1502 allele prior to initiating therapy; this is not a current recommendation in the phenytoin manufacturer labeling. Patients with a positive result should avoid phenytoin. Potentially serious, sometimes fatal multiorgan hypersensitivity reactions (also known as drug reaction with eosinophilia and systemic symptoms [DRESS]) have been reported with some antiepileptic drugs; including phenytoin; monitor for signs and symptoms of possible manifestations associated with lymphatic, hepatic, renal, and/or hematologic organ systems; gradual discontinuation and conversion to alternate therapy may be required. Chronic use of phenytoin has been associated with decreased bone mineral density (osteopenia, osteoporosis, and osteomalacia) and bone fractures. Chronic use may result in decreased vitamin D concentrations due to hepatic enzyme induction and may lead to vitamin D deficiency, hypocalcemia and hypophosphatemia; monitor as appropriate and consider implementing vitamin D and calcium supplementation. Cases of acute hepatotoxicity, including infrequent cases of acute hepatic failure, have been reported. Other manifestations include jaundice, hepatomegaly, elevated serum transaminase levels, leukocytosis, and eosinophilia. The clinical course of acute phenytoin hepatotoxicity ranges from prompt recovery to fatal outcomes. Immediately discontinue phenytoin in patients who develop acute hepatotoxicity and do not readminister. Consider alternative therapy in patients who have experienced hypersensitivity to structurally similar drugs such as carboxamides (eg, carbamazepine), barbiturates, succinimides, and oxazolidinediones (eg, trimethadione). Lymphadenopathy may occur (local or generalized), including benign lymph node hyperplasia, pseudolymphoma, lymphoma, and Hodgkin disease; cause and effect relationship has not been established. Use with caution in patients with diabetes mellitus; phenytoin may inhibit insulin release and increase serum glucose in patients with diabetes. Phenytoin is not indicated for the treatment of absence seizures or seizures due to hypoglycemia or other metabolic causes. Potentially significant interactions may exist, requiring dose or frequency adjustment, additional monitoring, and/or selection of alternative therapy.

Benzyl alcohol and derivatives: Some dosage forms may contain sodium benzoate/benzoic acid; benzoic acid (benzoate) is a metabolite of benzyl alcohol; large amounts of benzyl alcohol (≥99 mg/kg/day) have been associated with a potentially fatal toxicity ("gasping syndrome") in neonates; the "gasping syndrome" consists of metabolic acidosis, respiratory distress, gasping respirations, CNS dysfunction (including convulsions, intracranial hemorrhage), hypotension, and cardiovascular collapse (AAP ["Inactive" 1997]; CDC 1982); some data suggests that benzoate displaces bilirubin from protein binding sites (Ahlfors 2001); avoid or use dosage forms containing benzyl alcohol derivative with caution in neonates. See manufacturer's labeling.

Propylene glycol: Some dosage forms may contain propylene glycol; large amounts are potentially toxic and have been associated hyperosmolality, lactic acidosis, seizures and respiratory depression; use caution (AAP 1997; Zar 2007).

Adverse Reactions Frequency not defined.
Cardiovascular: Atrial conduction depression (IV administration), bradycardia (IV administration), cardiac arrhythmia (IV administration), circulatory shock (IV administration), hypotension (IV administration), periarteritis nodosa, ventricular conduction depression (IV adminsitration), ventricular fibrillation (IV administration)

Central nervous system: Ataxia, confusion, dizziness, drowsiness, headache, insomnia, mood changes, nervousness, paresthesia, peripheral neuropathy (associated with chronic treatment), slurred speech, twitching, vertigo

Dermatologic: Bullous dermatitis, exfoliative dermatitis, hypertrichosis, morbilliform rash (most common), scarlatiniform rash, skin or other tissue necrosis (IV administration), skin rash, toxic epidermal necrolysis

Endocrine & metabolic: Hyperglycemia, vitamin D deficiency (associated with chronic treatment)

Gastrointestinal: Constipation, dysgeusia (metallic taste), gingival hyperplasia, nausea, enlargement of facial features (lips), vomiting

Genitourinary: Peyronie's disease

Hematologic & oncologic: Agranulocytosis, granulocytopenia, Hodgkin lymphoma, immunoglobulin abnormality, leukopenia, lymphadenopathy, macrocytosis, malignant lymphoma, megaloblastic anemia, pancytopenia, pseudolymphoma, purpuric dermatitis, thrombocytopenia

Hepatic: Acute hepatic failure, hepatic injury, hepatitis, toxic hepatitis

Hypersensitivity: Anaphylaxis

Immunologic: DRESS syndrome

Local: Injection site reaction ("purple glove syndrome"; edema, discoloration, and pain distal to injection site), local inflammation (IV administration), local irritation (IV administration), localized tenderness (IV administration), local tissue necrosis (IV administration)

Neuromuscular & skeletal: Coarsening of facial features, osteomalacia, systemic lupus erythematosus, tremor

Ophthalmic: Nystagmus

Miscellaneous: Fever, tissue sloughing (IV administration)

<1% (Limited to important or life-threatening): Dyskinesia, hepatotoxicity (idiosyncratic) (Chalasani 2014)

Drug Interactions

Metabolism/Transport Effects Substrate of CYP2C19 (major), CYP2C9 (major), CYP3A4 (minor); **Note:** Assignment of Major/Minor substrate status based on clinically relevant drug interaction potential; **Induces** CYP2B6 (strong), CYP2C19 (strong), CYP2C8 (strong), CYP2C9 (strong), CYP3A4 (strong), P-glycoprotein, UGT1A1

Avoid Concomitant Use

Avoid concomitant use of Phenytoin with any of the following: Abiraterone Acetate; Antihepaciviral Combination Products; Apixaban; Apremilast; Aprepitant; Artemether; Axitinib; Azelastine (Nasal); Bedaquiline; Boceprevir; Bortezomib; Bosutinib; Cabozantinib; Cariprazine; Ceritinib; CloZAPine; Cobicistat; Cobimetinib; Crizotinib; Dabigatran Etexilate; Dabrafenib; Daclatasvir; Delavirdine; Dienogest; Dolutegravir; Dronedarone; Eliglustat; Elvitegravir; Enzalutamide; Etravirine; Everolimus; Flibanserin; Ibrutinib; Idelalisib; Irinotecan Products; Isavuconazonium Sulfate; Itraconazole; Ivabradine; Ivacaftor; Ixazomib; Lapatinib; Ledipasvir; Lumefantrine; Lurasidone; Macitentan; Mifepristone; Naloxegol; Netupitant; NIFEdipine; Nilotinib; NiMODipine; Nintedanib; Nisoldipine; Olaparib; Ombitasvir, Paritaprevir, Ritonavir, and Dasabuvir; Orphenadrine; Osimertinib; Palbociclib; Panobinostat; Paraldehyde; PAZOPanib; PONATinib; Praziquantel; Ranolazine; Regorafenib; Rilpivirine; Rivaroxaban; Roflumilast; RomiDEPsin; Simeprevir; Sofosbuvir; Sonidegib; SORAfenib; Stiripentol; Suvorexant; Tasimelteon; Telaprevir; Thalidomide; Ticagrelor; Tofacitinib; Tolvaptan; Toremifene; Trabectedin; Uliprista; Vandetanib; Vemurafenib; VinCRIStine (Liposomal); Vorapaxar

Increased Effect/Toxicity

Phenytoin may increase the levels/effects of: Azelastine (Nasal); Buprenorphine; Chloramphenicol; Clarithromycin; CNS Depressants; Cyclophosphamide; Fosamprenavir; Hydrocodone; Lithium; Methotrexate; Methotrimeprazine; Metyrosine; Neuromuscular-Blocking Agents (Nondepolarizing); Orphenadrine; Paraldehyde; PHENobarbital; Pramipexole; Prilocaine; ROPINIRole; Rotigotine; Selective Serotonin Reuptake Inhibitors; Sodium Nitrite; Thalidomide; Vitamin K Antagonists; Zolpidem

The levels/effects of Phenytoin may be increased by: Alcohol (Ethyl); Amiodarone; Antifungal Agents (Azole Derivatives, Systemic); Benzodiazepines; Brimonidine (Topical); Calcium Channel Blockers; Cannabis; Capecitabine; CarBAMazepine; Carbonic Anhydrase Inhibitors; CeFAZolin; Chloramphenicol; Chlorpheniramine; Cimetidine; Clarithromycin; Cosyntropin; CYP2C19 Inhibitors (Moderate); CYP2C19 Inhibitors (Strong); CYP2C9 Inhibitors (Moderate); CYP2C9 Inhibitors (Strong); Dapsone (Topical); Delavirdine; Dexamethasone (Systemic); Dexketoprofen; Dexmethylphenidate; Disulfiram; Doxylamine; Dronabinol; Droperidol; Efavirenz; Eslicarbazepine; Ethosuximide; Felbamate; Floxuridine; Fluconazole; Fluorouracil (Systemic); Fluorouracil

(Topical); FLUoxetine; FluvoxaMINE; Halothane; HydrOXYzine; Isoniazid; Kava Kava; Luliconazole; Lumacaftor; Magnesium Sulfate; Methotrimeprazine; Methylphenidate; MetroNIDAZOLE (Systemic); Miconazole (Oral); Minocycline; Nabilone; NIFEdipine; Nitric Oxide; Omeprazole; OXcarbazepine; Rufinamide; Sertraline; Sodium Oxybate; Sulfamethoxazole; Tacrolimus (Systemic); Tapentadol; Tegafur; Telaprevir; Tetrahydrocannabinol; Ticlopidine; Topiramate; TraZODone; Trimethoprim; Vitamin K Antagonists

Decreased Effect

Phenytoin may decrease the levels/effects of: Abiraterone Acetate; Acetaminophen; Afatinib; Albendazole; Amiodarone; Antifungal Agents (Azole Derivatives, Systemic); Antihepaciviral Combination Products; Apixaban; Apremilast; Aprepitant; ARIPiprazole; ARIPiprazole Lauroxil; Artemether; Axitinib; Bazedoxifene; Bedaquiline; Boceprevir; Bortezomib; Bosutinib; Brentuximab Vedotin; Brexpiprazole; Busulfan; Cabozantinib; Calcium Channel Blockers; Canagliflozin; Cannabidiol; Cannabis; CarBAMazepine; Cariprazine; Caspofungin; Ceritinib; Chloramphenicol; Clarithromycin; CloZAPine; Cobicistat; Cobimetinib; Contraceptives (Estrogens); Contraceptives (Progestins); Corticosteroids (Systemic); Crizotinib; CycloSPORINE (Systemic); CYP2B6 Substrates; CYP2C19 Substrates; CYP2C8 Substrates; CYP2C9 Substrates; CYP3A4 Substrates; Dabigatran Etexilate; Dabrafenib; Daclatasvir; Dasatinib; Deferasirox; Delavirdine; Dexamethasone (Systemic); Diclofenac (Systemic); Dienogest; Disopyramide; Dolutegravir; Doxofylline; DOXOrubicin (Conventional); Doxycycline; Dronabinol; Dronedarone; Efavirenz; Eliglustat; Elvitegravir; Enzalutamide; Erlotinib; Eslicarbazepine; Ethosuximide; Etoposide; Etoposide Phosphate; Etravirine; Everolimus; Exemestane; Ezogabine; Felbamate; FentaNYL; Flibanserin; Flunarizine; Gefitinib; GuanFACINE; HMG-CoA Reductase Inhibitors; Hydrocortisone (Systemic); Ibrutinib; Idelalisib; Imatinib; Irinotecan Products; Isavuconazonium Sulfate; Itraconazole; Ivabradine; Ivacaftor; Ixabepilone; Ixazomib; Lacosamide; LamoTRIgine; Lapatinib; Ledipasvir; Levodopa; Linagliptin; Loop Diuretics; Lopinavir; Lumefantrine; Lurasidone; Macitentan; Maraviroc; Mebendazole; Meperidine; Methadone; Methyl PREDNISolone; MetroNIDAZOLE (Systemic); Metyrapone; Mexiletine; Mianserin; Mifepristone; Naloxegol; Nelfinavir; Netupitant; Neuromuscular-Blocking Agents (Nondepolarizing); NIFEdipine; Nilotinib; NiMODipine; Nintedanib; Nisoldipine; Olaparib; Ombitasvir, Paritaprevir, Ritonavir, and Dasabuvir; Omeprazole; Osimertinib; OXcarbazepine; Palbociclib; Paliperidone; Panobinostat; PAZOPanib; Perampanel; P-glycoprotein/ABCB1 Substrates; PONATinib; Praziquantel; PrednisoLONE (Systemic); PredniSONE; Primidone; Propacetamol; Propafenone; QUEtiapine; QuiNIDine; QuiNINE; Ranolazine; Regorafenib; Rilpivirine; Ritonavir; Rivaroxaban; Roflumilast; Rolapitant; RomiDEPsin; Rufinamide; Saxagliptin; Sertraline; Simeprevir; Sirolimus; Sofosbuvir; Sonidegib; SORAfenib; SUNItinib; Suvorexant; Tacrolimus (Systemic); Tadalafil; Tasimelteon; Telaprevir; Temsirolimus; Teniposide; Tetrahydrocannabinol; Theophylline Derivatives; Thyroid Products; Ticagrelor; Tipranavir; Tofacitinib; Tolvaptan; Topiramate; Topotecan; Toremifene; Trabectedin; TraZODone; Treprostinil; Trimethoprim; Uliprista; Valproate Products; Vandetanib; Vemurafenib; Vilazodone; VinCRIStine; VinCRIStine (Liposomal); Vorapaxar; Vortioxetine; Zaleplon; Zonisamide; Zuclopenthixol

The levels/effects of Phenytoin may be decreased by: Alcohol (Ethyl); Amphetamines; Bleomycin; CarBAMazepine; Ciprofloxacin (Systemic); Colesevelam; CYP2C9 Inducers (Strong); Darunavir; Dexamethasone (Systemic); Diazoxide; Enzalutamide; Folic Acid; Fosamprenavir; Leucovorin Calcium-Levoleucovorin; Levomefolate; Lopinavir; Lumacaftor; Mefloquine; Methotrexate; Methylfolate; Mianserin; Multivitamins/Minerals (with ADEK, Folate, Iron); Nelfinavir; Orlistat; PHENobarbital; Platinum Derivatives; Pyridoxine; Rifampin; Ritonavir; Stiripentol; Theophylline Derivatives; Tipranavir; Valproate Products; Vigabatrin; VinCRIStine; Vindesine

Food Interactions

Ethanol:

Acute use: Ethanol inhibits metabolism of phenytoin and may also increase CNS depression. Management: Monitor patients. Caution patients about effects.

Chronic use: Ethanol stimulates metabolism of phenytoin. Management: Monitor patients.

Food: If phenytoin is administered with enteral feeding preparations and/or related nutritional supplements, serum concentrations of phenytoin may be decreased. Management: Do not administer phenytoin concomitantly with an enteral feeding preparation.

Preparation for Administration Hazardous agent; use appropriate precautions for handling and disposal (NIOSH 2014 [group 2]).

IV: May be further diluted in NS to a final concentration ≥5 mg/mL; infusion must be completed within 4 hours after preparation. Do not refrigerate.

Storage/Stability

Capsule, tablet: Store at 20°C to 25°C (68°F to 77°F). Protect capsules from light. Protect capsules and tablets from moisture.

Oral suspension: Store at 20°C to 25°C (68°F to 77°F); do not freeze. Protect from light.

Solution for injection: Store at 15°C to 30°C (59°F to 86°F). Use only clear solutions free of precipitate and haziness; slightly yellow solutions may be used. Precipitation may occur if solution is refrigerated and may dissolve at room temperature.

Mechanism of Action Stabilizes neuronal membranes and decreases seizure activity by increasing efflux or decreasing influx of sodium ions across cell membranes in the motor cortex during generation of nerve impulses; prolongs effective refractory period and suppresses ventricular pacemaker automaticity, shortens action potential in the heart

Pharmacodynamics/Kinetics

Onset of action: IV: ~0.5 to 1 hour

Absorption: Oral: Slow

Distribution: V_d:

Neonates: Premature: 1 to 1.2 L/kg; Full-term: 0.8 to 0.9 L/kg

Infants: 0.7 to 0.8 L/kg

Children: 0.7 L/kg

Adults: 0.6 to 0.7 L/kg

Protein binding:

Neonates: ≥80% (≤20% free)

Infants: ≥85% (≤15% free)

Adults: 90% to 95%

Others: Decreased protein binding

Disease states resulting in a decrease in serum albumin concentration: Burns, hepatic cirrhosis, nephrotic syndrome, pregnancy, cystic fibrosis

Disease states resulting in an apparent decrease in affinity of phenytoin for serum albumin: Renal failure, jaundice (severe), other drugs (displacers), hyperbilirubinemia (total bilirubin >15 mg/dL), CrCl <25 mL/minute (unbound fraction is increased two- to threefold in uremia)

Metabolism: Follows dose-dependent capacity-limited (Michaelis-Menten) pharmacokinetics with increased V_{max} (ie, metabolic capacity) in infants >6 months of age and children versus adults; major metabolite (via oxidation), HPPA, undergoes enterohepatic recirculation

Bioavailability: Formulation dependent

Half-life elimination: Range: 7 to 42 hours; **Note:** Elimination is not first-order (ie, follows Michaelis-Menten pharmacokinetics); half-life increases with increasing phenytoin concentrations; best described using parameters such as V_{max} (metabolic capacity) and Km (constant equal to the concentration at which the rate of metabolism is $1/2$ of V_{max}).

Time to peak, serum (formulation dependent): Oral: Extended-release capsule: 4 to 12 hours; Immediate release preparation: 1.5 to 3 hours

Excretion: Urine (<5% as unchanged drug); as glucuronides

Clearance: Highly variable, dependent upon intrinsic hepatic function and dose administered; increased clearance and decreased serum concentrations with febrile illness

Dosing

Adult Note: Phenytoin base (eg, oral suspension, chewable tablets) contains ~8% more drug than phenytoin sodium (~92 mg base is equivalent to 100 mg phenytoin sodium). Dosage adjustments and closer serum monitoring may be necessary when switching dosage forms.

Status epilepticus: IV:

Neurocritical Care Society recommendation: Loading dose: 20 mg/kg at a maximum rate of 50 mg/minute; if necessary, may give an additional dose of 5 to 10 mg/kg 10 minutes after the loading dose (NCS [Brophy 2012])

Manufacturer recommendation: Loading dose: 10 to 15 mg/kg at a maximum rate of 50 mg/minute; initial maintenance dose: IV or Oral: 100 mg every 6 to 8 hours

Anticonvulsant: Oral:

Immediate release:

Tablet: Initial: 100 mg 3 times daily, individualize dosage with dosage adjustments at no less than 7- to 10-day intervals; maintenance dose: 300 to 400 mg/day; an increase to 600 mg/day may be necessary

Suspension: Initial: 125 mg 3 times daily, individualize dosage with dosage adjustments at no less than 7- to 10-day intervals; an increase to 625 mg/day may be necessary

Extended release:

Loading dose: 1 g divided into 3 doses (400, 300, 300 mg) administered at 2-hour intervals; begin maintenance dosage 24 hours after loading dose. **Note:** Do not use loading dose regimen in patients with a history of renal or hepatic disease. Reserve for patients who require rapid steady state serum levels, when IV administration is not desirable, and for patients in a clinic or hospital setting where phenytoin levels can be closely monitored.

Initial dosage (treatment naïve): 100 mg 3 times daily; adjust dosage at no less than 7- to 10-day intervals

Maintenance dose: 100 mg 3 to 4 times daily, doses up to 200 mg 3 times a day may be necessary. May consider converting patients established on 100 mg 3 times daily to 300 mg once daily

Geriatric Clearance is decreased in geriatric patients; lower doses or less frequent dosing may be required.

Pediatric Note: Phenytoin base (eg, oral suspension, chewable tablets) contains ~8% more drug than phenytoin sodium (~92 mg base is equivalent to 100 mg phenytoin sodium). Dosage adjustments and closer serum monitoring may be necessary when switching dosage forms.

Status epilepticus: Infants, Children, Adolescents: IV:

Neurocritical Care Society recommendation: Loading dose: 20 mg/kg at a maximum rate of 1 mg/kg/minute; if necessary, may give an additional dose of 5 to 10 mg/kg 10 minutes after the loading dose (NCS [Brophy 2012])

Manufacturer recommendation: Loading dose: 15 to 20 mg/kg, followed by maintenance therapy

Anticonvulsant (nonemergent use): Oral:

Immediate release: Children and Adolescents: Tablet and suspension: Initial: 5 mg/kg/day in 2 to 3 equally divided doses, individualize dosage with dosage adjustments at no less than 7- to 10-day intervals; maintenance dose: 4 to 8 mg/kg/day (maximum: 300 mg/day). Some experts suggest higher maintenance doses may be necessary in infant and young children (range: 8 to 10 mg/kg/day in divided doses) (Guerrini 2006).

Extended release: Children and Adolescents: Initial: 5 mg/kg/day in 2 or 3 equally divided doses, individualize dosage with dosage adjustments at no less than 7- to 10-day intervals; maintenance dose: 4 to 8 mg/kg/day (maximum: 300 mg/day)

Renal Impairment There are no dosage adjustments provided in the manufacturer's labeling; <5% excreted as unchanged drug. Serum concentration may be difficult to interpret in renal failure. Monitoring of free (unbound) concentrations or adjustment to allow interpretation is recommended.

Hepatic Impairment There are no dosage adjustments provided in the manufacturer's labeling; undergoes hepatic metabolism and clearance may be decreased. Monitor free phenytoin levels closely. Dosage adjustments may be necessary.

Obesity

Adults: Evidence from one small study in adult patients (N=24) with obesity (range: 71 to 197 kg) demonstrated that the volume of distribution (V_d) was 0.68 ± 0.03 L/kg (range: 0.53 to 0.85 L/kg) and distribution into weight in excess of IBW is disproportionately greater (by a factor of 1.33) (Abernethy 1985). Based on this evidence, the following dosing strategies have been suggested:

Loading dose:

14 mg/kg (IBW) + 19 mg/kg (weight in excess of IBW); maximum dose: 2 g (Abernethy 1985; Erstad 2004)

For example: For a patient with a total body weight (TBW) of 300 lb (136 kg) and an IBW of 73 kg Loading dose = 14 mg/kg (73 kg) + 19 mg/kg (136 kg minus 73 kg) = 2219 mg; administer the maximum dose of 2,000 mg

OR

May also target a specific concentration (eg, 15 to 20 mg/L) by using the V_d obtained from patients with obesity (Abernethy 1985; Burton 2006). Therefore, the concentration desired (in mg/L) may be multiplied by this V_d (obesity) (in L) which is

determined using the patient's total and ideal body weights.

V_d (obesity) = 0.65 L/kg (IBW) + 1.33 (TBW – IBW)

Loading dose = Calculated V_d (obesity) (target concentration)

For example: For a patient with a total body weight (TBW) of 300 lb (136 kg) and an IBW of 73 kg

V_d (obesity) = 0.65 L/kg (73 kg) + 1.33 (136 kg – 73 kg) = 131 L; then,

Loading dose = 131 L x 15 mg/L = 1,965 mg

Maintenance dose: Base on ideal body weight if using weight-based regimens or use conventional daily doses with adjustments based upon therapeutic drug monitoring and clinical effectiveness. (Abernethy 1985; Erstad 2002; Erstad 2004)

Note: Additional data are necessary to further define dosing strategies in the obese patient.

Dietary Considerations

Folic acid: Phenytoin may decrease mucosal uptake of folic acid; to avoid folic acid deficiency and megaloblastic anemia, some clinicians recommend giving patients on anticonvulsants prophylactic doses of folic acid and cyanocobalamin. Folic acid 0.5 mg/day has been shown to reduce the incidence of phenytoin-induced gingival overgrowth in children (Arya 2011). However, folate supplementation may increase seizures in some patients (dose dependent). Discuss with healthcare provider prior to using any supplements.

Calcium: Hypocalcemia has been reported in patients taking prolonged high-dose therapy with an anticonvulsant. Some clinicians have given an additional 4000 units/week of vitamin D (especially in those receiving poor nutrition and getting no sun exposure) to prevent hypocalcemia.

Vitamin D: Phenytoin interferes with vitamin D metabolism and osteomalacia may result; may need to supplement with vitamin D

Tube feedings: Tube feedings decrease phenytoin absorption. To avoid decreased serum levels with continuous NG feeds, hold feedings for 1-2 hours prior to and 1-2 hours after phenytoin administration, if possible. The manufacturer recommends not to administer concomitantly with an enteral feeding preparation. There is a variety of opinions on how to administer phenytoin with enteral feedings. Be **consistent** throughout therapy.

Injection may contain sodium.

Administration

Oral:

Immediate release: Divide daily dose into 2 to 3 doses per day; if the daily dosage cannot be divided equally, take the larger dose before retiring.

Chewable tablets: May chew thoroughly before being swallowing or swallow whole.

Suspension: Shake well prior to use; measure and administer dose using a calibrated oral dosing syringe (or other accurate dose-measuring device). Absorption is impaired when phenytoin suspension is given concurrently to patients who are receiving continuous nasogastric feedings. A method to resolve this interaction is to divide the daily dose of phenytoin and withhold the administration of nutritional supplements for 1 to 2 hours before and after each phenytoin dose. The manufacturer recommends not to administer concomitantly with an enteral feeding preparation.

Extended release: Usually dosed every 12 hours; however, in patients with sufficiently long half-life, may be dosed every 24 hours.

IM: **Avoid** IM administration due to severe risk of local tissue destruction and necrosis; use **fos**phenytoin if IM administration necessary (Boucher 1996; Meek 1999). The manufacturer's labeling includes IM administration; however, in general the IM route should be avoided and should **NOT** be used for status epilepticus.

IV: Fosphenytoin may be considered for loading in patients who are in status epilepticus, hemodynamically unstable, or develop hypotension/bradycardia with IV administration of phenytoin. Although, phenytoin may be administered by direct IV injection, it is preferable that phenytoin be administered via infusion pump either undiluted or diluted in normal saline as an IV piggyback (IVPB) to prevent exceeding the maximum infusion rate (monitor closely for extravasation during infusion). The maximum rate of IV administration is 50 mg/minute in adults. Highly sensitive patients (eg, elderly, patients with preexisting cardiovascular conditions) should receive phenytoin more slowly (eg, 20 mg/minute) (Meek 1999). In neonates, the manufacturer recommends a maximum rate of 1 to 3 mg/kg/minute; however, a lower maximum rate of 0.5 to 1 mg/kg/minute is used clinically (Sankar 2010; Shields 1989). An in-line 0.22 to 0.55 micron filter is recommended for IVPB solutions due to the potential for precipitation of the solution. Following IV administration, NS should be injected through the same needle or IV catheter to prevent irritation.

SubQ: SubQ administration is **not** recommended because of the possibility of local tissue damage (due to high pH).

Vesicant; ensure proper needle or catheter placement prior to and during IV infusion. Avoid extravasation.

Extravasation management: If extravasation occurs, stop infusion immediately and disconnect (leave needle/cannula in place); gently aspirate extravasated solution (do **NOT** flush the line); remove needle/cannula; elevate extremity. There is conflicting information regarding an antidote; some sources recommend not to use an antidote (Montgomery 1999 [pediatric reference]), while other sources recommend hyaluronidase.

Hyaluronidase (if appropriate): SubQ: Administer four separate 0.2 mL injections of a 15 units/mL solution (using a 25-gauge needle) into area of extravasation (Sokol 1998)

Hazardous agent; use appropriate precautions for handling and disposal (NIOSH 2014 [group 2]).

Monitoring Parameters CBC, liver function; suicidality (eg, suicidal thoughts, depression, behavioral changes); plasma phenytoin concentrations (if available, free phenytoin concentrations should be obtained in patients with renal impairment and/or hypoalbuminemia; if free phenytoin concentrations are unavailable, the adjusted total concentration may be determined based upon equations in adult patients). Trough concentrations are generally recommended for routine monitoring.

Additional monitoring with IV use: Continuous cardiac monitoring (rate, rhythm, blood pressure) and observation during administration recommended; blood pressure and pulse should be monitored every 15 minutes for 1 hour after administration (Meek, 1999); infusion site reactions

Consult individual institutional policies and procedures.

Reference Range Timing of serum samples: Because it is slowly absorbed, peak blood levels may occur 4 to 8 hours after ingestion of an oral dose. The serum half-life varies with the dosage and the drug follows Michaelis-Menten kinetics. The average adult half-life is about 24 hours. Steady-state concentrations are reached in 5 to 10 days.

Children and Adults: Toxicity is measured clinically, and some patients require levels outside the suggested therapeutic range

Therapeutic range:

Total phenytoin: 10 to 20 mg/L (SI: 40 to 79 micromole/L) (children and adults), 8 to 15 mg/L (SI: 32 to 59 micromole/L) (neonates)

Concentrations of 5 to 10 mg/L (SI: 20 to 40 micromole/L) may be therapeutic for some patients but concentrations <5 mg/L (SI: <20 micromole/L) are not likely to be effective

50% of patients show decreased frequency of seizures at concentrations >10 mg/L (SI: >40 micromole/L)

86% of patients show decreased frequency of seizures at concentrations >15 mg/L (SI: >59 micromole/L)

Add another anticonvulsant if satisfactory therapeutic response is not achieved with a phenytoin concentration of 20 mg/L (SI: 79 micromole/L)

Free phenytoin: 1 to 2.5 mg/L (SI: 4 to 10 micromole/L)

Total phenytoin:

Toxic: >30 mg/L (SI: >119 micromole/L)

Lethal: >100 mg/L (SI: >396 micromole/L)

When to draw levels (Winter 2010):

Key points: Time of sampling is dependent on the disease state being treated and the clinical condition of the patient. Trough concentrations are generally recommended for routine monitoring. However, timing of sampling is not as critical in patients receiving the extended-release dosage form because the slow absorption minimizes the fluctuations between peak and trough concentrations.

After a loading dose:

First concentration: It is prudent to draw within 2 to 3 days of therapy initiation to ensure that the patient's metabolism is not remarkably altered. Alternatively, if rapid therapeutic levels are needed, a level may be drawn 2 hours after completion of an IV loading dose (Meek 1999) or 24 hours after administration of an oral loading dose (Osborn 1987) to aid in determining maintenance dose or need to reload.

Second concentration: Draw within 5 to 8 days of therapy initiation with subsequent doses of phenytoin adjusted accordingly

If plasma concentrations have not changed over a 3- to 5-day period, monitoring interval may be increased to once weekly in the acute clinical setting. In stable patients requiring long-term therapy, generally monitor levels at 3- to 12-month intervals

Adjustment of serum concentration: See tables.

Note: Although it is ideal to obtain free phenytoin concentrations to assess serum concentrations in patients with hypoalbuminemia or renal failure (CrCl ≤10 mL/minute), it may not always be possible. If free phenytoin concentrations are unavailable, the following equations may be utilized in adult patients.

Adjustment of Serum Concentration in Adults With Low Serum Albumin

Measured Total Phenytoin Concentration mg/L (micromole/L)	Patient's Serum Albumin (g/dL)			
	3.5	3	2.5	2
	Adjusted Total Phenytoin Concentration mg/L[1] (micromole/L)			
5 (20)	6 (24)	7 (28)	8 (32)	10 (40)
10 (40)	13 (51.5)	14 (55)	17 (67)	20 (79)
15 (59)	19 (75)	21 (83)	25 (99)	30 (119)

[1]Adjusted concentration = measured total concentration divided by [(0.2 x albumin) + 0.1].

Adjustment of Serum Concentration in Adults With Renal Failure (CrCl ≤10 mL/min)

Measured Total Phenytoin Concentration mg/L (micromole/L)	Patient's Serum Albumin (g/dL)				
	4	3.5	3	2.5	2
	Adjusted Total Phenytoin Concentration mg/L[1] (micromole/L)				
5 (20)	10 (40)	11 (44)	13 (51.5)	14 (55)	17 (67)
10 (40)	20 (79)	22 (87)	25 (99)	29 (115)	33 (131)
15 (59)	30 (119)	33 (131)	38 (150)	43 (170)	50 (198)

[1]Adjusted concentration = measured total concentration divided by [(0.1 x albumin) + 0.1].

Test Interactions Falsely high plasma phenytoin concentrations may occur when measured by immunoanalytical techniques (eg, TD_X, TD_XFL_X, Emit 2000). Phenytoin may produce falsely low results for serum concentrations of T_4, and dexamethasone or metyrapone tests. Phenytoin may cause increased serum levels of glucose, alkaline phosphatase, and gamma glutamyl transpeptidase (GGT).

Dosage Forms Considerations

The capsule dosage form represents *Extended Phenytoin Sodium Capsules,* USP, a designation differentiating the drug from *Prompt Phenytoin Sodium Capsules,* USP (no longer available) as the extended form was characterized by a slow and extended rate of absorption when the two were compared.

Dosage Forms Excipient information presented when available (limited, particularly for generics); consult specific product labeling.

Capsule, Oral, as sodium:
Dilantin: 30 mg [contains fd&c yellow #10 (quinoline yellow)]
Dilantin: 100 mg
Phenytek: 200 mg, 300 mg [contains brilliant blue fcf (fd&c blue #1), fd&c blue #1 aluminum lake, fd&c blue #2 aluminum lake, fd&c red #40 aluminum lake, fd&c yellow #10 aluminum lake]
Generic: 100 mg, 200 mg, 300 mg
Solution, Injection, as sodium:
Generic: 50 mg/mL (2 mL, 5 mL)
Suspension, Oral:
Dilantin: 125 mg/5 mL (237 mL) [orange-vanilla flavor]
Generic: 125 mg/5 mL (4 mL, 237 mL)
Tablet Chewable, Oral:
Dilantin Infatabs: 50 mg [scored]
Phenytoin Infatabs: 50 mg [scored; contains fd&c yellow #10 aluminum lake, fd&c yellow #6 aluminum lake, saccharin sodium]
Generic: 50 mg

Physostigmine (fye zoe STIG meen)

Index Terms Eserine Salicylate; Physostigmine Salicylate; Physostigmine Sulfate

Pharmacologic Category Acetylcholinesterase Inhibitor; Antidote

Use Reversal of central nervous system anticholinergic syndrome

Note: Physostigmine should only be used to reverse toxic, life-threatening delirium caused by pure anticholinergic agents (ie, atropine, diphenhydramine, dimenhydrinate, *Atropa belladonna* [deadly nightshade], or jimson weed [*Datura* spp]). Consultation with a clinical toxicologist or poison control center is recommended in patients who require physostigmine administration.

Dosing

Adult & Geriatric Reversal of toxic anticholinergic effects: Note: When administering by IV injection, administer no faster than 1 mg/minute to prevent bradycardia, respiratory distress, and seizures from too rapid administration.

IM, IV: Initial: 0.5-2 mg; may repeat every 10-30 minutes until response occurs. Subsequent doses may be required to manage life-threatening anticholinergic effects (Krenzelok, 2010).

Pediatric Reversal of toxic anticholinergic effects: Note: Reserve for life-threatening situations only. When administering by IV injection, administer no faster than 0.5 mg/minute to prevent bradycardia, respiratory distress, and seizures from too rapid administration.

IM, IV: Initial: 0.02 mg/kg; may repeat every 5-10 minutes until response occurs (maximum total dose: 2 mg)

Renal Impairment No dosage adjustment provided in manufacturer's labeling.

Hepatic Impairment No dosage adjustment provided in manufacturer's labeling.

Additional Information Complete prescribing information should be consulted for additional detail.

Dosage Forms Excipient information presented when available (limited, particularly for generics); consult specific product labeling.
Solution, Injection, as salicylate:
Generic: 1 mg/mL (2 mL)

Phytonadione (fye toe na DYE one)

Brand Names: US Mephyton

Brand Names: Canada AquaMEPHYTON; Konakion; Mephyton

Index Terms Methylphytyl Napthoquinone; Phylloquinone; Phytomenadione; Vitamin K; Vitamin K_1

Pharmacologic Category Vitamin, Fat Soluble

Additional Appendix Information
Reversal of Oral Anticoagulants on page 1959

Use Prevention and treatment of hypoprothrombinemia caused by vitamin K antagonist (VKA)-induced (eg, warfarin-induced) or other drug-induced vitamin K deficiency, altered activity, or altered metabolism; hypoprothrombinemia caused by malabsorption or inability to synthesize vitamin K; prophylaxis and treatment of hemorrhagic disease of the newborn

Pregnancy Considerations Animal reproduction studies have not been conducted. Phytonadione crosses the placenta in limited concentrations (Kazzi, 1990). The dietary requirements of vitamin K are the same in pregnant and nonpregnant women (IOM, 2000). In general, medications used as antidotes should take into consideration the health and prognosis of the mother; antidotes should be administered to pregnant women if there is a clear indication for use and should not be withheld because of fears of teratogenicity (Bailey, 2003).

Breast-Feeding Considerations Small amounts of dietary vitamin K can be detected in breast milk and the dietary requirements of vitamin K are the same in nursing and non-nursing women (IOM, 2000). Information following the use of phytonadione has not been located. The manufacturer recommends caution be used if phytonadione is administered to a nursing woman.

Contraindications Hypersensitivity to phytonadione or any component of the formulation

Warnings/Precautions [US Boxed Warning]: Severe reactions resembling hypersensitivity reactions (eg, anaphylaxis) have occurred rarely during or immediately after IV administration (even with proper dilution and rate of administration); some patients had no previous exposure to phytonadione. Some injectable dosage forms contain polyoxyethylated castor oil (Cremophor EL) which is associated with hypersensitivity reactions. Anaphylactoid reactions typically occurred when patients received large IV doses administered rapidly with formulations containing polyethoxylated castor oil (also called polyoxyethylated castor oil); proper dosing, dilution, and administration will minimize risk (Ageno, 2012; Riegert-Johnson, 2002). Limit IV administration to situations where an alternative route of administration is not feasible and the benefit of therapy outweighs the risk of hypersensitivity reactions. Allergic reactions have also occurred with IM and SubQ injections, albeit less frequently. In obstructive jaundice or with biliary fistulas concurrent administration of bile salts is necessary. Manufacturers recommend the SubQ route over other parenteral routes. SubQ is less predictable when compared to the oral route. The American College of Chest Physicians recommends the IV route in patients with major bleeding secondary to warfarin. The IV route should be restricted to emergency situations where oral phytonadione cannot be used. Efficacy is delayed regardless of route of administration; patient management may require other treatments in the interim. In patients receiving a therapeutic vitamin K antagonist (VKA) (eg, warfarin), administer a dose of phytonadione that will quickly lower the INR into a safe range without causing resistance to warfarin. High phytonadione doses may lead to warfarin resistance for at least one week. Patients with LAAR-induced coagulopathy require much larger doses and longer treatment durations (up to months) after exposure compared to that needed to reverse VKA-induced coagulopathy. Use with caution in neonates, especially premature infants; severe hemolytic anemia, jaundice, and hyperbilirubinemia have been reported with larger than recommended doses (10 to 20 mg). In liver disease, if initial doses do not reverse coagulopathy then higher doses are unlikely to have any effect. Ineffective in hereditary hypoprothrombinemia.

Benzyl alcohol and derivatives: Some dosage forms may contain benzyl alcohol; large amounts of benzyl alcohol (≥99 mg/kg/day) have been associated with a potentially fatal toxicity ("gasping syndrome") in neonates; the "gasping syndrome" consists of metabolic acidosis, respiratory distress, gasping respirations, CNS dysfunction (including convulsions, intracranial hemorrhage), hypotension, and cardiovascular collapse (AAP ["Inactive" 1997]; CDC, 1982); some data suggests that benzoate displaces bilirubin from protein binding sites (Ahlfors, 2001); avoid or use dosage forms containing benzyl alcohol with caution in neonates. See manufacturer's labeling.

The parenteral product may contain aluminum; toxic aluminum concentrations may be seen with high doses, prolonged use, or renal dysfunction. Premature neonates are at higher risk due to immature renal function and aluminum intake from other parenteral sources. Parenteral aluminum exposure of >4 to 5 mcg/kg/day is associated with CNS and bone toxicity; tissue loading may occur at

lower doses (Federal Register, 2002). See manufacturer's labeling.

Some dosage forms may contain polysorbate 80 (also known as Tweens). Hypersensitivity reactions, usually a delayed reaction, have been reported following exposure to pharmaceutical products containing polysorbate 80 in certain individuals (Isaksson, 2002; Lucente 2000; Shelley, 1995). Thrombocytopenia, ascites, pulmonary deterioration, and renal and hepatic failure have been reported in premature neonates after receiving parenteral products containing polysorbate 80 (Alade, 1986; CDC, 1984). See manufacturer's labeling.

Adverse Reactions Frequency not defined.

Cardiovascular: Cyanosis, flushing, hyper-/hypotension

Central nervous system: Dizziness

Dermatologic: Erythematous skin eruptions, pruritus, scleroderma-like lesions

Endocrine & metabolic: Hyperbilirubinemia (newborn; greater than recommended doses)

Gastrointestinal: Abnormal taste

Local: Injection site reactions

Respiratory: Dyspnea

Miscellaneous: Diaphoresis, hypersensitivity reactions, nonimmunologic anaphylaxis (formerly known as anaphylactoid reaction), sweating

Drug Interactions

Metabolism/Transport Effects None known.

Avoid Concomitant Use There are no known interactions where it is recommended to avoid concomitant use.

Increased Effect/Toxicity There are no known significant interactions involving an increase in effect.

Decreased Effect

Phytonadione may decrease the levels/effects of: Vitamin K Antagonists

The levels/effects of Phytonadione may be decreased by: Mineral Oil; Orlistat

Preparation for Administration Dilute injection solution in preservative-free NS, D_5W, or D_5NS. To reduce the incidence of anaphylactoid reaction upon IV administration, dilute dose in a minimum of 50 mL of compatible solution and administer using an infusion pump over at least 20 minutes (Ageno, 2012).

Storage/Stability

Injection: Store at 15°C to 30°C (59°F to 86°F). Protect from light. **Note:** Store Hospira product at 20°C to 25°C (68°F to 77°F).

Oral: Store tablets at 15°C to 30°C (59°F to 86°F). Protect from light.

Mechanism of Action Promotes liver synthesis of clotting factors (II, VII, IX, X); however, the exact mechanism as to this stimulation is unknown. Menadiol is a water soluble form of vitamin K; phytonadione has a more rapid and prolonged effect than menadione; menadiol sodium diphosphate (K_4) is half as potent as menadione (K_3).

Pharmacodynamics/Kinetics

Onset of action: Increased coagulation factors: Oral: 6-10 hours; IV: 1-2 hours

Peak effect: INR values return to normal: Oral: 24-48 hours; IV: 12-14 hours

Absorption: Oral: From intestines in presence of bile; SubQ: Variable

Metabolism: Rapidly hepatic

Excretion: Urine and feces

Dosing

Adult & Geriatric Note: According to the manufacturer, SubQ is the preferred parenteral route; IM route should be avoided due to the risk of hematoma formation; IV route should be restricted for emergency use only. The American College of Chest Physicians (ACCP) recommends the IV route in patients with major bleeding secondary to use of vitamin K antagonists (VKAs).

Adequate intake (AI): Oral: Males: 120 mcg/day; Females: 90 mcg/day

Hypoprothrombinemia due to drugs (other than coumarin derivatives) or factors limiting absorption or synthesis: Oral, SubQ, IM, IV: Initial: 2.5-25 mg (rarely up to 50 mg)

Vitamin K deficiency (supratherapeutic INR) secondary to VKAs (eg, warfarin) (off-label dose):

If INR above therapeutic range to <4.5 (no evidence of bleeding): Lower or hold next VKA dose and monitor frequently; when INR approaches desired range, resume VKA dosing with a lower dose (Patriquin, 2011).

If INR 4.5-10 (no evidence of bleeding): The 2012 ACCP guidelines recommend against routine phytonadione (aka, vitamin K) administration in this setting (Guyatt, 2012). Previously, the 2008 ACCP guidelines recommended if no risk factors for bleeding exist, to omit next 1 or 2 VKA doses, monitor INR more frequently, and resume with an appropriately adjusted

VKA dose when INR in desired range; may consider administering vitamin K orally 1-2.5 mg if other risk factors for bleeding exist (Hirsh, 2008). Others have recommended consideration of vitamin K 1 mg orally or 0.5 mg IV (Patriquin, 2011).

If INR >10 (no evidence of bleeding): The 2012 ACCP guidelines recommend administration of oral vitamin K (dose not specified) in this setting (Guyatt, 2012). Previously, the 2008 ACCP guidelines recommended to hold warfarin, administer vitamin K orally 2.5-5 mg, expect INR to be reduced within 24-48 hours, monitor INR more frequently and give additional vitamin K at an appropriate dose if necessary; resume warfarin at an appropriately adjusted dose when INR is in desired range (Hirsh, 2008). Others have recommended consideration of vitamin K 2-2.5 mg orally or 0.5-1 mg IV (Patriquin, 2011).

If minor bleeding at any INR elevation: Hold warfarin, may administer vitamin K orally 2.5-5 mg, monitor INR more frequently, may repeat dose after 24 hours if INR correction incomplete; resume warfarin at an appropriately adjusted dose when INR is in desired range (Patriquin, 2011).

If major bleeding at any INR elevation: The 2012 ACCP guidelines recommend administration of four-factor prothrombin complex concentrate (PCC) and IV vitamin K 5-10 mg in this setting (Guyatt, 2012). The only available four-factor PCC in the U.S. is Kcentra. Other four-factor PCCs **not** available in the U.S. include Beriplex P/N, Cofact, and Octaplex. Bebulin VH and Profilnine SD **do not** contain adequate levels of factor VII and are considered **three**-factor PCCs. Previously, the 2008 ACCP guidelines recommended to hold warfarin, administer vitamin K 10 mg by slow IV infusion and supplement with PCC depending on the urgency of the situation; IV vitamin K may be repeated every 12 hours (Hirsh, 2008).

Note: Use of high doses of vitamin K (eg, 10-15 mg) may cause warfarin resistance for ≥1 week. During this period of resistance, heparin or low-molecular-weight heparin (LMWH) may be given until INR responds (Ansell, 2008).

Preprocedural/surgical INR normalization in patients receiving warfarin (routine use): Oral: 1-2.5 mg once administered on the day before surgery; recheck INR on day of procedure/surgery (Douketis, 2012). Others have recommended the use of vitamin K 1 mg orally for mild INR elevations (ie, INR 3.0-4.5) (Patriquin, 2011).

Pediatric Note: According to the manufacturer, SubQ is the preferred parenteral route; IM route should be avoided due to the risk of hematoma formation; IV route should be restricted for emergency use only. The American College of Chest Physicians (ACCP) recommends the IV route in patients with major bleeding secondary to use of vitamin K antagonists (VKAs).

Adequate intake (AI): Oral:

Infants:

0-6 months: 2 **mcg**/day

7-12 months: 2.5 **mcg**/day

Children:

1-3 years: 30 **mcg**/day

4-8 years: 55 **mcg**/day

9-13 years: 60 **mcg**/day

14-18 years: 75 **mcg**/day

Hemorrhagic disease of the newborn:

Prophylaxis: IM: 0.5-1 mg within 1 hour of birth

Treatment: IM, SubQ: 1 mg/dose/day; higher doses may be necessary if mother has been receiving oral anticoagulants

Vitamin K deficiency (supratherapeutic INR) secondary to vitamin K antagonists (VKAs) (eg, warfarin) (off-label use): Infants and Children: *Excessively prolonged INR (usually INR >8; no significant bleeding):* **Note:** Limited data available: IV: 0.03 mg/kg/dose; maximum dose: 1 mg (Bolton-Maggs, 2002); if significant bleeding, consider use of fresh frozen plasma, prothrombin complex concentrates, or recombinant factor VIIa (Monagle, 2012).

Renal Impairment No dosage adjustment provided in manufacturer's labeling.

Hepatic Impairment No dosage adjustment provided in manufacturer's labeling.

Administration

IV administration: Infuse slowly; rate of infusion should not exceed 1 mg/minute. Alternatively, dilute dose in a minimum of 50 mL of compatible solution and administer using an infusion pump over at least 20 minutes (Ageno, 2012). The injectable route should be used only if the oral route is not feasible or there is a greater urgency to reverse anticoagulation.

Oral: The parenteral formulation may also be used for small oral doses (eg, 1 mg) or situations in which tablets cannot be swallowed (Crowther, 2000; O'Connor, 1986).

Monitoring Parameters PT, INR; monitor for hypersensitivity reactions if administering IV.

Dosage Forms Considerations Injectable products may contain alcohol, benzyl alcohol, polysorbate 80, propylene glycol, or polyoxyethylated/polyethoxylated castor oil (Cremophor EL).

Dosage Forms Excipient information presented when available (limited, particularly for generics); consult specific product labeling.

Injection, aqueous colloidal: 1 mg/0.5 mL (0.5 mL); 10 mg/mL (1 mL)

Injection, aqueous colloidal [preservative free]: 1 mg/0.5 mL (0.5 mL)

Tablet, oral: 100 mcg

Mephyton®: 5 mg [scored]

Extemporaneous Preparations A 1 mg/mL oral suspension may be made with tablets. Crush six 5 mg tablets in a mortar and reduce to a fine powder. Add 5 mL each of water and methylcellulose 1% and mix to a uniform paste. Mix while adding sorbitol in incremental proportions to almost 30 mL; transfer to a calibrated bottle, rinse mortar with sorbitol, and add quantity of sorbitol sufficient to make 30 mL. Label "shake well" and "refrigerate". Stable for 3 days.

Nahata MC and Hipple TF, *Pediatric Drug Formulations*, 3rd ed, Cincinnati, OH: Harvey Whitney Books Co, 1997.

Note: The parenteral formulation may also be used for small oral doses (eg, 1 mg) or situations in which tablets cannot be swallowed (Crowther, 2000; O'Connor, 1986).

◆ PI₃K Delta Inhibitor CAL-101 *see* Idelalisib *on page 911*

◆ PIC 200 [OTC] *see* Polysaccharide-Iron Complex *on page 1469*

◆ Picato *see* Ingenol Mebutate *on page 952*

◆ Picodan (Can) *see* Sodium Picosulfate, Magnesium Oxide, and Citric Acid *on page 1680*

◆ Picoflo (Can) *see* Sodium Picosulfate, Magnesium Oxide, and Citric Acid *on page 1680*

◆ Pico-Salax® (Can) *see* Sodium Picosulfate, Magnesium Oxide, and Citric Acid *on page 1680*

◆ Pidorubicin *see* Epirubicin *on page 651*

◆ Pidorubicin Hydrochloride *see* Epirubicin *on page 651*

Pilocarpine (Systemic) (pye loe KAR peen)

Brand Names: US Salagen

Brand Names: Canada Salagen®

Index Terms Pilocarpine Hydrochloride

Pharmacologic Category Cholinergic Agonist

Use Symptomatic treatment of xerostomia caused by salivary gland hypofunction resulting from radiotherapy for cancer of the head and neck or Sjögren's syndrome

Dosing

Adult & Geriatric Xerostomia: Oral:

Following head and neck cancer: 5 mg 3 times/day, titration up to 10 mg 3 times/day may be considered for patients who have not responded adequately; do not exceed 2 tablets/dose

Sjögren's syndrome: 5 mg 4 times/day

Renal Impairment No dosage adjustment necessary.

Hepatic Impairment

Mild impairment (Child-Pugh score 5-6): No dosage adjustment necessary.

Moderate impairment (Child-Pugh score 7-9): 5 mg twice daily regardless of indication; adjust dose based on response and tolerability

Severe impairment (Child-Pugh score >10): Not recommended.

Additional Information Complete prescribing information should be consulted for additional detail.

Dosage Forms Excipient information presented when available (limited, particularly for generics); consult specific product labeling.

Tablet, Oral, as hydrochloride:

Salagen: 5 mg

Salagen: 7.5 mg [contains fd&c blue #2 aluminum lake]

Generic: 5 mg, 7.5 mg

Pilocarpine (Ophthalmic) (pye loe KAR peen)

Brand Names: US Isopto Carpine; Pilopine HS

Brand Names: Canada Diocarpine; Isopto® Carpine; Pilopine HS®

Index Terms Pilocarpine Hydrochloride

Pharmacologic Category Ophthalmic Agent, Antiglaucoma; Ophthalmic Agent, Miotic

Use Management of chronic simple glaucoma, chronic and acute angle-closure glaucoma

Dosing

Adult & Geriatric

Glaucoma: Ophthalmic:

Solution: Instill 1-2 drops up to 6 times/day; adjust the concentration and frequency as required to control elevated intraocular pressure.

Gel: Instill 0.5" ribbon into lower conjunctival sac once daily at bedtime.

To counteract the mydriatic effects of sympathomimetic agents (off-label use): Ophthalmic: *Solution:* Instill 1 drop of a 1% solution in the affected eye.

Renal Impairment No dosage adjustment provided in manufacturer's labeling.

Hepatic Impairment No dosage adjustment provided in manufacturer's labeling.

Additional Information Complete prescribing information should be consulted for additional detail.

Dosage Forms Excipient information presented when available (limited, particularly for generics); consult specific product labeling.

Gel, Ophthalmic, as hydrochloride:

Pilopine HS: 4% (4 g) [contains benzalkonium chloride, edetate disodium]

Solution, Ophthalmic, as hydrochloride:

Isopto Carpine: 1% (15 mL); 2% (15 mL); 4% (15 mL)

Generic: 1% (15 mL); 2% (15 mL); 4% (15 mL)

◆ Pilocarpine Hydrochloride *see* Pilocarpine (Ophthalmic) *on page 1452*

◆ Pilocarpine Hydrochloride *see* Pilocarpine (Systemic) *on page 1452*

◆ Pilopine HS *see* Pilocarpine (Ophthalmic) *on page 1452*

◆ Pilopine HS® (Can) *see* Pilocarpine (Ophthalmic) *on page 1452*

◆ Pimaricin *see* Natamycin *on page 1261*

Pimecrolimus (pim e KROE li mus)

Brand Names: US Elidel

Brand Names: Canada Elidel

Pharmacologic Category Calcineurin Inhibitor; Immunosuppressant Agent; Topical Skin Product

Use Atopic dermatitis: Second-line therapy for short-term and noncontinuous long-term treatment of mild to moderate atopic dermatitis in nonimmunocompromised patients 2 years and older who have failed to respond adequately to other topical prescription treatments, or when those treatments are not advisable.

Pregnancy Considerations Adverse events were not observed in animal reproduction studies following topical application.

Breast-Feeding Considerations It is not known if pimecrolimus is excreted in breast milk. Due to the potential for serious adverse reactions in the nursing infant, the manufacturer recommends a decision be made whether to discontinue nursing or to discontinue the drug, taking into account the importance of treatment to the mother.

Medication Guide Available Yes

Contraindications Hypersensitivity to pimecrolimus or any component of the formulation

Warnings/Precautions Hazardous agent; use appropriate precautions for handling and disposal (meets NIOSH 2014 criteria). **[US Boxed Warning]: Topical calcineurin inhibitors (including pimecrolimus) have been associated with rare cases of lymphoma and skin malignancy.** Avoid use on malignant or premalignant skin conditions (eg, cutaneous T-cell lymphoma). **[US Boxed Warning]: Continuous long-term use of calcineurin inhibitors (including pimecrolimus) should be avoided and application of cream should be limited to areas of involvement with atopic dermatitis. Safety of intermittent use for >1 year has not been established.** Diagnosis should be reconfirmed if sign/symptoms do not improve within 6 weeks of treatment.

May cause local symptoms (eg, burning, pruritus, soreness, stinging) during first few days of treatment; usually self-resolving as atopic dermatitis lesions heal. Should not be used in immunocompromised patients, including patients on concomitant systemic immunosuppressive therapy. Patients with atopic dermatitis are predisposed to skin infections; therapy has been associated with an increased risk of developing eczema herpeticum, varicella zoster, and herpes simplex. Do not apply to areas of active bacterial or viral infection; local infections at the treatment site should be resolved prior to therapy. Skin papilloma (warts) have been observed with use; discontinue use if there is worsening of skin papillomas or they do not respond to conventional treatment. Pimecrolimus may be

associated with development of lymphadenopathy; possible infectious causes should be investigated. Discontinue use in patients with unknown cause of lymphadenopathy or acute infectious mononucleosis. Not recommended for use in patients with skin disease which may increase the potential for systemic absorption (eg, Netherton's syndrome). Avoid artificial or natural sunlight exposure, even when pimecrolimus is not on the skin. Safety not established in patients with generalized erythroderma. **[US Boxed Warning]: The use of pimecrolimus in children <2 years of age is not recommended,** particularly since the effect on immune system development is unknown.

Benzyl alcohol and derivatives: Some dosage forms may contain benzyl alcohol; large amounts of benzyl alcohol (≥99 mg/kg/day) have been associated with a potentially fatal toxicity ("gasping syndrome") in neonates; the "gasping syndrome" consists of metabolic acidosis, respiratory distress, gasping respirations, CNS dysfunction (including convulsions, intracranial hemorrhage), hypotension, and cardiovascular collapse (AAP ["Inactive" 1997]; CDC, 1982); some data suggests that benzoate displaces bilirubin from protein binding sites (Ahlfors, 2001); avoid or use dosage forms containing benzyl alcohol with caution in neonates. See manufacturer's labeling.

Adverse Reactions

>10%:

Central nervous system: Headache (children and adolescents 11% to 25%; adults 7%), fever (children and adolescents 13%; adults 1%)

Infection: Influenza (3% to 13%)

Local: Local burning (adults 26%; children and adolescents 2% to 8%; tends to resolve/improve as lesions resolve), application site reaction (adults 15%; children and adolescents 2%)

Respiratory: Nasopharyngitis (infants, children, and adolescents 10% to 27%; adults 8%), upper respiratory tract infection (children and adolescents 14% to 19%; adults 4%), cough (children and adolescents 9% to 16%; adults 2%), bronchitis (children and adolescents ≤11%; adults ≤2%)

1% to 10%:

Dermatologic: Folliculitis (adults 6%; children and adolescents 1%), skin infection (5% to 6%), impetigo (4%), warts (children and adolescents ≤3%), acne vulgaris (≤2%), herpes simplex dermatitis (≤2%), molluscum contagiosum (children and adolescents ≤2%), urticaria (≤1%)

Gastrointestinal: Diarrhea (children and adolescents 1% to 8%; adults ≤2%), gastroenteritis (children and adolescents ≤7%; adults 2%), vomiting (1% to 4%), constipation (children and adolescents ≤4%), abdominal pain (≤3%), toothache (≤3%), nausea (1% to 2%)

Genitourinary: Dysmenorrhea (1% to 2%)

Hypersensitivity: Hypersensitivity (3% to 5%)

Infection: Viral infection (children and adolescents ≤7%), herpes simplex infection (≤4%), bacterial infection (1% to 2%), staphylococcal infection (1% to 2%), varicella (≤1%)

Local: Local irritation (adults ≤6%; children and adolescents ≤1%), local pruritus (1% to 6%), localized erythema (≤2%)

Neuromuscular & skeletal: Arthralgia (≤2%), back pain (≤2%)

Ocular: Conjunctivitis (≤2% to 3%), eye infection (≤1%)

Otic: Otic infection (1% to 6%), otitis media (1% to 3%)

Respiratory: Sore throat (4% to 8%), pharyngitis (children and adolescents 1% to 8%; adults 1%), tonsillitis (children and adolescents ≤6%; adults <1%), asthma (3% to 4%), asthma aggravated (children and adolescents ≤4%), streptococcal pharyngitis (children and adolescents 3%), nasal congestion (1% to 3%), sinusitis (1% to 3%), epistaxis (≤3%), dyspnea (≤2%), flu-like symptoms (≤2%), pneumonia (≤2%), rhinitis (≤2%), rhinorrhea (children and adolescents ≤2%), viral upper respiratory tract infection (≤2%), wheezing (children and adolescents ≤1%)

Miscellaneous: Laceration (children and adolescents ≤2%)

<1% (Limited to important or life-threatening): Anaphylaxis, angioedema, eczema (herpeticum), lymphadenopathy, malignant neoplasm (basal cell carcinoma, squamous cell carcinoma, malignant melanoma, malignant lymphoma), skin discoloration

Drug Interactions

Metabolism/Transport Effects Substrate of CYP3A4 (minor); **Note:** Assignment of Major/Minor substrate status based on clinically relevant drug interaction potential

Avoid Concomitant Use

Avoid concomitant use of Pimecrolimus with any of the following: Immunosuppressants

Increased Effect/Toxicity

Pimecrolimus may increase the levels/effects of: Immunosuppressants

The levels/effects of Pimecrolimus may be increased by: CYP3A4 Inhibitors (Moderate); CYP3A4 Inhibitors (Strong)

Decreased Effect There are no known significant interactions involving a decrease in effect.

Storage/Stability Store at 25°C (77°F); excursions permitted to 15°C to 30°C (59°F to 86°F); do not freeze.

Mechanism of Action Penetrates inflamed epidermis to inhibit T cell activation by blocking transcription of proinflammatory cytokine genes such as interleukin-2, interferon gamma (Th1-type), interleukin-4, and interleukin-10 (Th2-type). Pimecrolimus binds to the intracellular protein FKBP-12, inhibiting calcineurin, which blocks cytokine transcription and inhibits T-cell activation. Prevents release of inflammatory cytokines and mediators from mast cells *in vitro* after stimulation by antigen/IgE.

Pharmacodynamics/Kinetics Absorption: Poor when applied to 13% to 62% body surface area in adults treated for atopic dermatitis for up to a year; detectable blood levels were observed in a higher proportion of children, as compared to adults. Does not penetrate psoriatic plaque (Menter, 2009)

Dosing

Adult & Geriatric

Atopic dermatitis (mild-to-moderate): Topical: Apply thin layer to affected area twice daily. **Note:** Limit application to involved areas. Discontinue use when symptoms have resolved; re-evaluate if symptoms persist >6 weeks.

Oral lichen planus (off-label use): Topical: Apply twice daily for 1 month (Passeron, 2007; Volz, 2008)

Psoriasis (off-label use): Topical: Apply twice daily (Gribetz, 2004; Menter, 2009)

Pediatric Atopic dermatitis (mild-to-moderate): Children ≥2 years and Adolescents: Topical: Refer to adult dosing.

Administration Apply a thin layer to affected skin. Limit application to areas of involvement. Do not use with occlusive dressings. Burning at the application site is most common in first few days; improves as atopic dermatitis improves. Discontinue use when symptoms have resolved; re-evaluate if symptoms persist >6 weeks. Moisturizers may be applied after use of pimecrolimus cream. Wash hands after use.

Oral lichen planus (off-label use): Apply to affected oral mucosa, cover with a thin layer of gauze to delay dilution with saliva (Volz, 2008). Eating, drinking or chewing gum was not allowed for 30 minutes after application (Passeron, 2007).

Hazardous agent; use appropriate precautions for handling and disposal (meets NIOSH 2014 criteria).

Dosage Forms Excipient information presented when available (limited, particularly for generics); consult specific product labeling.

Cream, External:

Elidel: 1% (30 g, 60 g, 100 g) [contains benzyl alcohol, cetyl alcohol, propylene glycol]

Pimozide (PI moe zide)

Brand Names: US Orap

Brand Names: Canada Apo-Pimozide; Orap; PMS-Pimozide

Pharmacologic Category First Generation (Typical) Antipsychotic

Use Suppression of severe motor and phonic tics in patients with Tourette's disorder who have failed to respond satisfactorily to standard treatment

Dosing

Adult Note: An ECG should be performed baseline and periodically thereafter, especially during dosage adjustment.

Tourette disorder: Oral: Initial: 1 to 2 mg/day in divided doses, then increase dosage as needed every other day; maximum dose: 10 mg/day or 0.2 mg/kg/day (whichever is less); **Note:** If therapy requires exceeding dose of 4 mg/day, CYP2D6 geno-/phenotyping should be performed; CYP2D6 poor metabolizers should be dose titrated in ≥14-day increments and should not receive doses in excess of 4 mg/day.

Delusional parasitosis (off-label): Oral: Initial: 0.5 to 2 mg once daily. Increase dose based on response and tolerability in 1 mg increments every 3 to 7 days up to a usual dosage of 2 to 4 mg daily (doses up to 12 mg daily have been studied, however manufacturer labeling recommends a maximum dose of 10 mg/day or 0.2 mg/kg/day). Consider taper of therapy in ▶

decrements of ≥1 mg weekly after adequate relief of symptoms for 1 month; assess for return of symptoms and need for continued long-term treatment (Lorenzo 2004). Additional data may be necessary to further define the role of pimozide in this condition.

Geriatric Note: An ECG should be performed baseline and periodically thereafter, especially during dosage adjustment.

Tourette disorder: Oral: Recommend initial dose of 1 mg/day; periodically attempt gradual reduction of dose to determine if tic persists; follow up for 1 to 2 weeks before concluding the tic is a persistent disease phenomenon and not a manifestation of drug withdrawal. **Note:** An ECG should be performed baseline and periodically thereafter, especially during dosage adjustment.

Pediatric Note: An ECG should be performed baseline and periodically thereafter, especially during dosage adjustment.

Tourette disorder: Oral:

Children 2 to 12 years: Initial: 0.05 mg/kg preferably once at bedtime; may be increased every third day to a maximum of 0.2 mg/kg/day (do not exceed 10 mg/day); usual range: 2 to 4 mg/day. **Note:** If therapy requires exceeding dose of 0.05 mg/kg/day, CYP2D6 geno-/phenotyping should be performed; CYP2D6 poor metabolizers should be dose titrated in ≥14-day increments and should not receive doses in excess of 0.05 mg/kg/day.

Children >12 years and Adolescents: Refer to adult dosing.

Renal Impairment No dosage adjustment provided in manufacturer's labeling. Use with caution.

Hepatic Impairment No dosage adjustment provided in manufacturer's labeling. Use with caution.

Adjustment for Toxicity

ECG changes:

Children: QTc prolongation >0.47 seconds or >25% above baseline: Decrease dose.

Adults: QTc prolongation >0.52 seconds or >25% above baseline: Decrease dose.

NMS syndrome: Discontinue (monitor carefully if therapy is reinitiated).

Tardive dyskinesia signs/symptoms: Consider discontinuing.

Additional Information Complete prescribing information should be consulted for additional detail.

Dosage Forms Excipient information presented when available (limited, particularly for generics); consult specific product labeling.

Tablet, Oral:

Orap: 1 mg, 2 mg [scored]

Generic: 1 mg, 2 mg

Dosage Forms: Canada Excipient information presented when available (limited, particularly for generics); consult specific product labeling.

Tablet, Oral: 2 mg, 4 mg [scored]

◆ Pimtrea see Ethinyl Estradiol and Desogestrel on page 701

◆ Pin-X [OTC] see Pyrantel Pamoate on page 1530

Pindolol (PIN doe lole)

Brand Names: Canada Apo-Pindol; Dom-Pindolol; PMS-Pindolol; Sandoz-Pindolol; Teva-Pindolol; Visken

Pharmacologic Category Antihypertensive; Beta-Blocker With Intrinsic Sympathomimetic Activity

Use

US labeling: **Hypertension:** Treatment of hypertension, alone or in combination with other agents

The 2014 guideline for the management of high blood pressure in adults (Eighth Joint National Committee [JNC 8]) recommends initiation of pharmacologic treatment to lower blood pressure for the following patients:

• Patients ≥60 years of age with systolic blood pressure (SBP) ≥150 mm Hg or diastolic blood pressure (DBP) ≥90 mm Hg. Goal of therapy is SBP <150 mm Hg and DBP <90 mm Hg.

• Patients <60 years of age with SBP ≥140 mm Hg or DBP ≥90 mm Hg. Goal of therapy is SBP <140 mm Hg and DBP <90 mm Hg.

• Patients ≥18 years of age with diabetes and SBP ≥140 mm Hg or DBP ≥90 mm Hg. Goal of therapy is SBP <140 mm Hg and DBP <90 mm Hg.

• Patients ≥18 years of age with chronic kidney disease (CKD) and SBP ≥140 mm Hg or DBP ≥90 mm Hg. Goal of therapy is SBP <140 mm Hg and DBP <90 mm Hg.

In patients with CKD, regardless of race or diabetes status, the use of an ACE inhibitor (ACEI) or angiotensin receptor blocker (ARB) as initial therapy is recommended to improve kidney outcomes. In the general nonblack population (without CKD) including those with diabetes, initial antihypertensive treatment should consist of a thiazide-type diuretic, calcium channel blocker, ACEI, or ARB. In the general black population (without CKD) including those with diabetes, initial antihypertensive treatment should consist of a thiazide-type diuretic or a calcium channel blocker **instead of** an ACEI or ARB.

Canadian labeling:

Angina pectoris: Prophylaxis of angina pectoris

Hypertension: Treatment of hypertension, alone or in combination with other agents

Dosing

Adult

Angina pectoris: *Canadian labeling:* Oral: Initial: 5 mg 3 times daily; increase as necessary every 1 to 2 weeks. Usual maintenance dose: 15 to 40 mg daily in 3 or 4 divided doses (maximum daily dose: 40 mg).

Hypertension:

US labeling: Oral: Initial: 5 mg twice daily; increase as necessary by 10 mg daily every 3 to 4 weeks (maximum daily dose: 60 mg).

Canadian labeling: Oral: Initial: 5 mg twice daily; increase as necessary by 10 mg daily every 1 to 2 weeks. Usual maintenance dose: 15 to 45 mg daily (maximum daily dose: 45 mg). If daily maintenance dose is ≤20 mg daily, may give as single dose in the morning; if >30 mg daily, administer in 3 divided doses.

Antidepressant augmentation (off-label use): Oral: 2.5 to 5 mg 3 times daily (Ballesteros 2004; Geretsegger 2008; Portella 2011)

Atrial fibrillation (rate control) (off-label use): Initial: 5 mg twice daily; may increase at weekly intervals to 15 mg twice daily. May use in combination with digoxin (James 1989).

Geriatric Refer to adult dosing. Use with caution.

Renal Impairment

US labeling: There are no dosage adjustments provided in the manufacturer's labeling. In uremic patients, use with caution due to significantly decreased clearance.

Canadian labeling: No dosage adjustment necessary in mild or moderate impairment; manufacturer suggests that a reduced dose may be necessary in severe impairment but does not provide specific dosing recommendations.

Hepatic Impairment

US labeling: There are no dosage adjustments provided in the manufacturer's labeling. In cirrhotic patients, use with caution due to significantly prolonged elimination half-life (may be 10 times as long compared to normal patients).

Canadian labeling: No dosage adjustment necessary in mild or moderate impairment; manufacturer suggests that a reduced dose may be necessary in severe impairment but does not provide specific dosing recommendations.

Additional Information Complete prescribing information should be consulted for additional detail.

Dosage Forms Excipient information presented when available (limited, particularly for generics); consult specific product labeling.

Tablet, Oral:

Generic: 5 mg, 10 mg

Dosage Forms: Canada Excipient information presented when available (limited, particularly for generics); consult specific product labeling.

Tablet, Oral:

Generic: 5 mg, 10 mg, 15 mg

◆ Pink Bismuth see Bismuth Subsalicylate on page 232

◆ Pink Bismuth [OTC] see Bismuth Subsalicylate on page 232

◆ Pinnacaine Otic [DSC] see Benzocaine on page 217

Pioglitazone (pye oh GLI ta zone)

Brand Names: US Actos

Brand Names: Canada Accel-Pioglitazone; ACH-Pioglitazone; ACT Pioglitazone; Actos; Apo-Pioglitazone; Auro-Pioglitazone; Dom-Pioglitazone; JAMP-Pioglitazone; Mint-Pioglitazone; Mylan-Pioglitazone; PHL-Pioglitazone; PMS-Pioglitazone; PRO-Pioglitazone; RAN-Pioglitazone; ratio-Pioglitazone; Sandoz-Pioglitazone; Teva-Pioglitazone; Van-Pioglitazone

Pharmacologic Category Antidiabetic Agent, Thiazolidinedione

Use Type 2 diabetes mellitus (noninsulin dependent, NIDDM), monotherapy or combination therapy: Adjunct to diet and exercise, to improve glycemic control

Medication Guide Available Yes

Dosing
Adult & Geriatric Type 2 diabetes: Oral:
Initial:
U.S. labeling: Monotherapy or combination therapy: 15-30 mg once daily
Patients with heart failure (NYHA Class I or II): Monotherapy or combination therapy: 15 mg once daily
Note: Not recommended in patients with symptomatic heart failure
Canadian labeling: Monotherapy or combination therapy (with a sulfonylurea or metformin): 15-30 mg once daily
Dosage titration: If response is inadequate based on HbA$_{1c}$, the dosage may be increased in 15 mg increments with careful monitoring of adverse effects (eg, weight gain, edema, signs/symptoms of heart failure); maximum recommended dose: 45 mg once daily
Dosage adjustment for hypoglycemia with combination therapy:
With an insulin secretagogue (eg, sulfonylurea): Decrease the insulin secretagogue dose.
With insulin: Decrease insulin dose by 10% to 25%
Dosage adjustment with strong CYP2C8 inhibitors (eg, gemfibrozil): Maximum recommended dose: 15 mg once daily
Renal Impairment No dosage adjustment necessary.
Hepatic Impairment No dosage adjustment necessary (mean AUC values are unaffected in Child-Pugh grade B/C compared to healthy subjects); however, liver injury has been associated with use.
U.S. labeling:
Prior to initiation: Evaluate liver tests (ALT, AST, alkaline phosphatase, total bilirubin) and if abnormal, initiate with caution.
During therapy: If liver injury is suspected (eg, fatigue, jaundice, dark urine): Interrupt therapy, measure serum liver tests, and investigate possible etiologies:
If ALT >3 x ULN **and** without alternative etiologies: Do not reinitiate therapy.
If ALT >3 x ULN **and** total bilirubin >2 x ULN **and** without alternative etiologies: Do not reinitiate therapy (these patients are at increased risk for severe drug-induced hepatotoxicity).
If ALT elevated (but <3 x ULN) **or** total bilirubin elevated (but <2 x ULN) **and** with an alternative etiology: May reinitiate with caution.
Canadian labeling:
Severe hepatic impairment: Use is contraindicated.
Prior to initiation:
If ALT >2.5 x ULN or clinical evidence of active liver disease: Do not initiate therapy.
If ALT 1-2.5 x ULN: Initiate therapy with caution and investigate etiology of liver enzyme elevation.
During therapy:
If ALT levels >3 x ULN: Recheck levels immediately and if ALT elevation >3 x ULN persists, discontinue therapy.
If ALT 1-2.5 x ULN: Continue therapy with caution and investigate etiology of liver enzyme elevation.
Additional Information Complete prescribing information should be consulted for additional detail.
Dosage Forms Excipient information presented when available (limited, particularly for generics); consult specific product labeling.
Tablet, Oral:
Actos: 15 mg, 30 mg, 45 mg
Generic: 15 mg, 30 mg, 45 mg

Pioglitazone and Glimepiride
(pye oh GLI ta zone & GLYE me pye ride)

Brand Names: US Duetact
Index Terms Glimepiride and Pioglitazone; Glimepiride and Pioglitazone Hydrochloride
Pharmacologic Category Antidiabetic Agent, Sulfonylurea; Antidiabetic Agent, Thiazolidinedione
Use Diabetes mellitus, type 2: Management of type 2 diabetes mellitus (noninsulin dependent, NIDDM) as an adjunct to diet and exercise in adult patients already treated with a thiazolidinedione and a sulfonylurea or who have inadequate control on either agent alone
Medication Guide Available Yes
Dosing
Adult
Diabetes mellitus, type 2: Oral: Initial dose should be based on current dose of pioglitazone and/or sulfonylurea.
Patients inadequately controlled on **glimepiride** alone: Initial dose: Pioglitazone 30 mg/glimepiride 2 mg or pioglitazone 30 mg/glimepiride 4 mg once daily

Patients inadequately controlled on **pioglitazone** alone: Initial dose: Pioglitazone 30 mg/glimepiride 2 mg once daily
Patients currently on sulfonylurea monotherapy (other than glimepiride) or switching from combination therapy of pioglitazone plus a sulfonylurea (other than glimepiride): Initial: Pioglitazone 30 mg/glimepiride 2 mg once daily. When converting patients from other sulfonylureas with longer half-lives (eg, chlorpropamide) to glimepiride, observe patient carefully for 1 to 2 weeks due to overlapping hypoglycemic effects.
Patients with systolic dysfunction (eg, NYHA Class I and II): Initiate only after patient has been safely titrated to 30 mg of pioglitazone. Initial dose: Pioglitazone 30 mg/glimepiride 2 mg once daily.
Dosage adjustment: Dosage may be increased up to a maximum dose of pioglitazone 45 mg/glimepiride 8 mg once daily based on effectiveness and tolerability. Dosage adjustments in patients with systolic dysfunction should be done carefully and patient monitored for symptoms of worsening heart failure.
Geriatric Initiate and adjust dose conservatively; observe carefully for hypoglycemia. Refer to adult dosing.
Renal Impairment Initiate and adjust dose conservatively; observe carefully for hypoglycemia.
Hepatic Impairment Initiate cautiously in patients with abnormal LFTs. During treatment, if ALT levels elevate >3 times ULN, interrupt treatment; do not restart unless another etiology for the hepatic abnormality is found. If ALT >3 times the reference range with serum total bilirubin >2 times the reference range without alternative etiologies, do not restart therapy.
Additional Information Complete prescribing information should be consulted for additional detail.
Dosage Forms Excipient information presented when available (limited, particularly for generics); consult specific product labeling.
Tablet: 30/2: Pioglitazone 30 mg and glimepiride 2 mg; 30/4: Pioglitazone 30 mg and glimepiride 4 mg
Duetact:
30 mg/2 mg: Pioglitazone 30 mg and glimepiride 2 mg
30 mg/4 mg: Pioglitazone 30 mg and glimepiride 4 mg

Pioglitazone and Metformin
(pye oh GLI ta zone & met FOR min)

Brand Names: US Actoplus Met; Actoplus Met XR
Index Terms Metformin Hydrochloride and Pioglitazone Hydrochloride
Pharmacologic Category Antidiabetic Agent, Biguanide; Antidiabetic Agent, Thiazolidinedione
Use Type 2 diabetes mellitus: As an adjunct to diet and exercise to improve glycemic control in adults with type 2 diabetes mellitus when treatment with both pioglitazone and metformin is appropriate.
Medication Guide Available Yes
Dosing
Adult
Diabetes mellitus, type 2: Oral:
Immediate release tablet:
Initial: Pioglitazone 15 mg/metformin 500 mg twice daily **or** pioglitazone 15 mg/metformin 850 mg tablets once daily
Patients with heart failure (NYHA Class I or II): Initial: Pioglitazone 15 mg/metformin 500 mg once daily **or** pioglitazone 15 mg/metformin 850 mg once daily. **Note:** Not recommended in patients with symptomatic heart failure.
Inadequately controlled on metformin monotherapy: Pioglitazone 15 mg/metformin 500 mg twice daily or pioglitazone 15 mg/metformin 850 mg once or twice daily (depending on the dose of metformin already being taken).
Inadequately controlled on pioglitazone monotherapy: Pioglitazone 15 mg/metformin 500 twice daily or pioglitazone 15 mg/metformin 850 mg once daily.
Dose titration: If necessary, may titrate gradually with careful monitoring of adverse effects (eg, weight gain, edema, signs/symptoms of heart failure). Maximum daily dose: Pioglitazone 45 mg/metformin 2,550 mg. **Note:** Metformin daily doses >2,000 mg may be better tolerated if given 3 times daily.
Extended-release tablet: Initial (includes patients with NYHA Class I or II heart failure): Pioglitazone 15 to 30 mg/metformin 1,000 mg once daily. If necessary, titrate gradually with careful monitoring of adverse effects (eg, weight gain, edema, signs/symptoms of heart failure). Maximum daily dose: Pioglitazone 45 mg/metformin 2,000 mg.

Inadequately controlled on metformin or pioglitazone monotherapy: Pioglitazone 15 mg/metformin 1,000 mg twice daily or pioglitazone 30 mg/metformin 1,000 mg once daily.

Dosage adjustment for hypoglycemia with combination therapy:
With an insulin secretagogue (eg, sulfonylurea): Decrease the insulin secretagogue dose.
With insulin: Decrease insulin dose by 10% to 25%.
Dosage adjustment with strong CYP2C8 inhibitors (eg, gemfibrozil): Maximum recommended dose: Pioglitazone 15 mg and metformin 850 mg daily (immediate release) or pioglitazone 15 mg/metformin 1,000 mg daily (extended release).
Geriatric *Immediate-release or extended-release tablet:* Refer to adult dosing. The initial and maintenance dosing should be conservative, due to the potential for decreased renal function (monitor). Generally, elderly patients should not be titrated to the maximum; do not use in patients ≥80 years of age unless normal renal function has been established.
Renal Impairment Immediate-release or variable-release tablet:
*Manufacturer's labeling:*Serum creatinine (SCr) ≥1.5 mg/dL (males) or ≥1.4 mg/dL (females) or abnormal CrCl (not defined): Use is contraindicated.
Alternate recommendations: **Note:** The United Kingdom National Institute for Health and Clinical Excellence (NICE) Guidelines recommend prescribing metformin with caution in those patients who are at risk of sudden deterioration in renal function and at risk of an estimated glomerular filtration rate (eGFR) <45 mL/minute/1.73 m^2 (NICE, 2008]). Some evidence suggests that use of metformin is unsafe when eGFR <30 mL/minute/1.73 m^2 (calculated using MDRD) (Shaw, 2007). A review of the available data by members of the American Diabetes Association proposed the following recommendations based on eGFR (Lipska, 2011):
eGFR ≥60 mL/minute/1.73 m^2: No contraindications, monitor renal function annually
eGFR ≥45 to <60 mL/minute/1.73 m^2: Continue use; monitor renal function every 3 to 6 months
eGFR ≥30 to <45 mL/minute/1.73 m^2: In patients currently receiving metformin, use with caution, consider dosage reduction (eg, 50% reduction or 50% of maximal dose), monitor renal function every 3 months. Do not initiate therapy in patients with eGFR <45 mL/minute/1.73 m^2
eGFR <30 mL/minute/1.73 m^2: Discontinue use
Hepatic Impairment Immediate-release or variable-release tablet: The manufacturer recommends to avoid metformin since liver disease is considered a risk factor for the development of lactic acidosis during metformin therapy. However, continued use of metformin in diabetics with liver dysfunction, including cirrhosis, has been used successfully and may be associated with a survival benefit in carefully selected patients; use cautiously in patients at risk for lactic acidosis (eg, renal impairment, alcohol use) (Brackett, 2010; Zhang, 2014). Use of pioglitazone should be done with caution or avoided.
Additional Information Complete prescribing information should be consulted for additional detail.
Dosage Forms Excipient information presented when available (limited, particularly for generics); consult specific product labeling.
Tablet, oral: 15/500: Pioglitazone 15 mg and metformin hydrochloride 500 mg; 15/850: Pioglitazone 15 mg and metformin hydrochloride 850 mg
Actoplus Met:
15/500: Pioglitazone 15 mg and metformin hydrochloride 500 mg
15/850: Pioglitazone 15 mg and metformin hydrochloride 850 mg
Tablet, variable release, oral:
Actoplus Met XR:
15/1000: Pioglitazone 15 mg [immediate release] and metformin hydrochloride 1000 mg [extended release]
30/1000: Pioglitazone 30 mg [immediate release] and metformin hydrochloride 1000 mg [extended release]

Piperacillin and Tazobactam
(pi PER a sil in & ta zoe BAK tam)

Brand Names: US Zosyn
Brand Names: Canada AJ-PIP/TAZ; Piperacillin and Tazobactam for Injection; Tazocin
Index Terms Piperacillin and Tazobactam Sodium; Piperacillin Sodium and Tazobactam Sodium; Tazobactam and Piperacillin
Pharmacologic Category Antibiotic, Penicillin

Use
Moderate to severe bacterial infections: For the treatment of patients with moderate to severe infections caused by susceptible isolates of the designated bacteria in the following conditions.
Community-acquired pneumonia: Treatment of moderate severity community-acquired pneumonia (CAP) caused by beta-lactamase-producing strains of *Haemophilus influenzae*. IDSA/ATS guidelines only recommend piperacillin/tazobactam for CAP caused by *P. aeruginosa* or due to aspiration (Mandell 2007).
Intra-abdominal infections: Treatment of appendicitis complicated by rupture or abscess and peritonitis caused by beta-lactamase-producing strains of *Escherichia coli*, *Bacteroides fragilis*, *Bacteroides ovatus*, *Bacteroides thetaiotaomicron*, or *Bacteroides vulgatus*.
Nosocomial pneumonia: Treatment of moderate to severe nosocomial pneumonia caused by beta-lactamase-producing strains of *Staphylococcus aureus* and by piperacillin/tazobactam-susceptible *Acinetobacter baumanii*, *H. influenzae*, *Klebsiella pneumoniae*, and *Pseudomonas aeruginosa* (nosocomial pneumonia caused by *P. aeruginosa* should be treated in combination with an aminoglycoside).
Pelvic infections: Treatment of postpartum endometriosis or pelvic inflammatory disease caused by beta-lactamase-producing strains of *E. coli*.
Skin and skin structure infections: Treatment of skin and skin structure infections, including cellulitis, cutaneous abscesses, and ischemic/diabetic foot infections caused by beta-lactamase-producing strains of *S. aureus*.
Pregnancy Considerations Adverse events have not been observed in animal reproduction studies. Piperacillin and tazobactam both cross the placenta and are found in the fetal serum, placenta, amniotic fluid, and fetal urine. When used during pregnancy, the clearance and volume of distribution of piperacillin/tazobactam are increased; half-life and AUC are decreased (Bourget, 1998). Piperacillin/tazobactam is approved for the treatment of postpartum gynecologic infections, including endometritis or pelvic inflammatory disease, caused by susceptible organisms.
Breast-Feeding Considerations Low concentrations of piperacillin are excreted in breast milk; information for tazobactam is not available. The manufacturer recommends that caution be used when administering piperacillin/tazobactam to nursing women. Nondose-related effects could include modification of bowel flora.
Contraindications Hypersensitivity to penicillins, cephalosporins, beta-lactamase inhibitors, or any component of the formulation
Warnings/Precautions Serious and occasionally severe or fatal hypersensitivity (anaphylactic/anaphylactoid) reactions have been reported in patients on penicillin therapy, especially with a history of beta-lactam hypersensitivity, history of sensitivity to multiple allergens, or previous IgE-mediated reactions (eg, anaphylaxis, angioedema, urticaria). Serious skin reactions, including toxic epidermal necrolysis (TEN) and Stevens-Johnson syndrome (SJS), acute exanthematous pustulosis, and drug reaction with eosinophilia and systemic symptoms (DRESS) have been reported. If a skin rash develops, monitor closely. Discontinue if lesions progress.

Bleeding disorders have been observed, particularly in patients with renal impairment; discontinue if thrombocytopenia or bleeding occurs. Leukopenia/neutropenia may occur; appears to be reversible and most frequently associated with prolonged administration. Assess hematologic parameters periodically, especially with prolonged (≥21 days) use.

Assess electrolytes periodically in patients with low potassium reserves, especially those receiving cytotoxic therapy or diuretics. Due to sodium load and to the adverse effects of high serum concentrations of penicillins, dosage modification is required in patients with impaired or underdeveloped renal function; use with caution in patients with seizures or in patients with history of beta-lactam allergy; associated with an increased incidence of rash and fever in cystic fibrosis patients. Use may result in fungal or bacterial superinfection, including *C. difficile*-associated diarrhea (CDAD) and pseudomembranous colitis; CDAD has been observed >2 months postantibiotic treatment.

Potentially significant drug-drug interactions may exist, requiring dose or frequency adjustment, additional monitoring, and/or selection of alternative therapy.
Adverse Reactions Frequency not always defined.
Cardiovascular: Phlebitis (1%), flushing (≤1%), hypotension (≤1%), thrombophlebitis (≤1%)

Central nervous system: Headache (8%), insomnia (7%), rigors (≤1%)

Dermatologic: Skin rash (4%), pruritus (3%), purpura (≤1%)

Endocrine & metabolic: Hypoglycemia (≤1%), decreased serum albumin, decreased serum glucose, decreased serum total protein, electrolyte disturbance (increases and decreases in sodium, potassium, and calcium), hyperglycemia, hypokalemia, increased gamma-glutamyl transferase

Gastrointestinal: Diarrhea (11%), constipation (8%), nausea (7%), dyspepsia (3%), vomiting (3%), abdominal pain (1%), pseudomembranous colitis (≤1%)

Hematologic & oncologic: Decreased hematocrit, decreased hemoglobin, eosinophilia, leukopenia, neutropenia, positive direct Coombs test, prolonged bleeding time, prolonged partial thromboplastin time, prolonged prothrombin time, thrombocythemia, thrombocytopenia

Hepatic: Increased serum alkaline phosphatase, increased serum ALT, increased serum AST, increased serum bilirubin

Hypersensitivity: Anaphylaxis (≤1%)

Infection: Candidiasis (2%)

Local: Local irritation (3%), injection site reaction (≤1%)

Neuromuscular & skeletal: Arthralgia (≤1%), myalgia (≤1%)

Renal: Increased blood urea nitrogen, increased serum creatinine

Respiratory: Epistaxis (≤1%)

<1%, postmarketing, and/or case reports (Limited to important and life-threatening): Acute generalized exanthemous pustulosis, agranulocytosis, *Clostridium difficile* associated diarrhea, convulsions, DRESS syndrome, erythema multiforme, hemolytic anemia, hypersensitivity reaction, jaundice, pancytopenia, shock, Stevens-Johnson syndrome, toxic epidermal necrolysis

Drug Interactions

Metabolism/Transport Effects None known.

Avoid Concomitant Use

Avoid concomitant use of Piperacillin and Tazobactam with any of the following: BCG (Intravesical); Probenecid

Increased Effect/Toxicity

Piperacillin and Tazobactam may increase the levels/effects of: Flucloxacillin [Floxacillin]; Methotrexate; Vancomycin; Vecuronium; Vitamin K Antagonists

The levels/effects of Piperacillin and Tazobactam may be increased by: Probenecid

Decreased Effect

Piperacillin and Tazobactam may decrease the levels/effects of: Aminoglycosides; BCG (Intravesical); BCG Vaccine (Immunization); Mycophenolate; Sodium Picosulfate; Typhoid Vaccine

The levels/effects of Piperacillin and Tazobactam may be decreased by: Tetracycline Derivatives

Preparation for Administration Reconstitute single-dose vials with 5 mL of diluent per 1 g of piperacillin and then further dilute to a volume of 50 to 150 mL. Reconstitute pharmacy bulk vials with 152 mL of diluent to yield a concentration of piperacillin 200 mg/mL and tazobactam 25 mg/mL; transfer reconstituted solution and further dilute to a volume of 50 to 150 mL for administration. Thaw galaxy containers at 20°C to 25°C (68°F to 77°F) or 2°C to 8°C (36°F to 46°F).

Storage/Stability

Vials: Store intact vials at 20°C to 25°C (68°F to 77°F). Use single-dose or bulk vials immediately after reconstitution. Discard any unused portion after 24 hours if stored at 20°C to 25°C (68°F to 77°F) or after 48 hours if stored at 2°C to 8°C (36°F to 46°F). Do not freeze vials after reconstitution. Stability in IV bags has been demonstrated for up to 24 hours at room temperature and up to 1 week at refrigerated temperature. Stability in an ambulatory IV infusion pump has been demonstrated for a period of 12 hours at room temperature.

Galaxy containers: Store at or below -20°C (-4°F). The thawed solution is stable for 14 days at 2°C to 8°C (36°F to 46°F) or 24 hours at 20°C to 25°C (68°F to 77°F). Do not refreeze.

Mechanism of Action Piperacillin inhibits bacterial cell wall synthesis by binding to one or more of the penicillin-binding proteins (PBPs); which in turn inhibits the final transpeptidation step of peptidoglycan synthesis in bacterial cell walls, thus inhibiting cell wall biosynthesis. Bacteria eventually lyse due to ongoing activity of cell wall autolytic enzymes (autolysins and murein hydrolases) while cell wall assembly is arrested. Piperacillin exhibits time-dependent killing. Tazobactam inhibits many beta-lactamases, including staphylococcal penicillinase and Richmond-Sykes types 2, 3, 4, and 5, including extended spectrum enzymes; it has only limited activity against class 1 beta-lactamases other than class 1C types.

Pharmacodynamics/Kinetics

Distribution: Well into lungs, intestinal mucosa, uterus, ovary, fallopian tube, interstitial fluid, gallbladder, and bile; penetration into CSF is low in subjects with noninflamed meninges

Protein binding: Piperacillin and tazobactam: ~30%

Metabolism:

Piperacillin: Desethyl metabolite (weak activity)

Tazobactam: Inactive metabolite

Half-life elimination: Piperacillin and tazobactam: 0.7-1.2 hours (unaffected by dose or duration of infusion)

Time to peak, plasma: Immediately following completion of 30-minute infusion

Excretion: Clearance of both piperacillin and tazobactam are directly proportional to renal function

Piperacillin: Urine (68% as unchanged drug); feces (10% to 20%)

Tazobactam: Urine (80% as unchanged drug; remainder as inactive metabolite)

Dialysis: Hemodialysis removes 30% to 40% of a piperacillin/tazobactam dose; peritoneal dialysis removes 6% of piperacillin and 21% of tazobactam

Dosing

Adult & Geriatric Note: Dosing presented is based on traditional infusion method (IV infusion over 30 minutes) unless otherwise specified as the extended infusion method (IV infusion over 4 hours [off-label method]).

Usual dosage range: IV: 3.375 g every 6 hours or 4.5 g every 6 to 8 hours; maximum: 18 g daily

Extended infusion method (off-label dosing): 3.375 to 4.5 g IV over 4 hours every 8 hours (Kim 2007; Shea 2009); an alternative regimen of 4.5 g IV over 3 hours every 6 hours has also been described (Kim 2007)

Indication-specific dosing:

Appendicitis, diverticulitis, intra-abdominal abscess, peritonitis: IV: 3.375 g every 6 hours for 7 to 10 days

Pneumonia:

Community-acquired pneumonia (CAP): IV: 3.375 g every 6 hours for 7 to 10 days. **Note:** IDSA/ATS guidelines only recommend piperacillin/tazobactam for CAP caused by *P. aeruginosa* or due to aspiration (Mandell 2007).

Nosocomial pneumonia: IV: 4.5 g every 6 hours for 7 to 14 days (when used empirically, combination with an aminoglycoside or antipseudomonal fluoroquinolone is recommended; consider discontinuation of additional agent if *P. aeruginosa* is not isolated) (ATS 2005).

Skin and soft tissue infection: IV: 3.375 g every 6 hours for 7 to 10 days. **Note:** For severe diabetic foot infections, recommended treatment duration is up to 4 weeks depending on severity of infection and response to therapy (Lipsky 2012).

Necrotizing infections (off-label use): IV:3.375 g every 6 to 8 hours (in combination with vancomycin for empiric therapy); continue until further debridement is not necessary, patient has clinically improved, and patient is afebrile for 48 to 72 hours (IDSA [Stevens 2014]).

Bite wounds (animal) (off-label use): IV: 3.375 g every 6 to 8 hours (IDSA [Stevens 2014])

Intra-abdominal infection, complicated (off-label use): IV: 3.375 g every 6 hours for 4 to 7 days (provided source controlled). **Note:** Increase to 3.375 g every 4 hours or 4.5 g every 6 hours if *P. aeruginosa* is suspected. Not recommended for mild-to-moderate, community-acquired intra-abdominal infections due to risk of toxicity and the development of resistant organisms (Solomkin 2010).

Surgical (perioperative) prophylaxis (off-label use): IV: 3.375 g within 60 minutes prior to surgery. Doses may be repeated in 2 hours if procedure is lengthy or if there is excessive blood loss (Bratzler 2013).

Surgical site infections (intestinal or genitourinary tract) (off-label use): IV: 3.375 g every 6 hours or 4.5 g every 8 hours (IDSA [Stevens 2014])

Pediatric Note: Piperacillin and tazobactam is a combination product; each 3.375 g vial contains 3 g piperacillin sodium and 0.375 g tazobactam sodium in an 8:1 ratio. Dosage recommendations in **pediatric** patients are based on the **piperacillin** component. Dosing presented is based on traditional infusion method (IV infusion over 30 minutes) unless otherwise specified as the extended infusion method (IV infusion over 4 hours [off-label method]).

Usual dosage range: IV:

Infants 2 to 9 months: 80 mg piperacillin/kg/dose every 8 hours (Red Book [AAP] 2012):

Infants >9 months, Children, and Adolescents: 100 mg piperacillin/kg/dose every 8 hours (maximum dose: 16 g piperacillin/day) (Red Book [AAP] 2012):

Children and Adolescents: Extended-infusion method: Limited data available: 100 mg piperacillin/kg/dose infused over 4 hours 3 times daily. Dosing based on a prospective, observational study (n=332) in a single children's hospital comparing the extended interval method to traditional dosing (Nichols 2012).

Indication-specific dosing: Infants, Children, and Adolescents: **Note:** In pediatric patients, dosage recommendations are based on the **piperacillin** component. Dosing is presented in mg/kg/**dose** and mg/kg/**day**; use caution.

Appendicitis, peritonitis:

Infants 2 to 9 months: IV: 80 mg piperacillin/kg/dose every 8 hours

Infants >9 months, Children, and Adolescents ≤40 kg: IV: 100 mg piperacillin/kg/dose every 8 hours (maximum: 3,000 mg piperacillin/dose)

Children and Adolescents >40 kg: Refer to adult dosing.

Cystic fibrosis, pseudomonal lung infections (off-label use):

Standard dosing: IV: 240 to 400 mg piperacillin/kg/**day** divided every 8 hours (Kliegman, 2011); others have used 350 to 400 mg/kg/**day** divided every 4 hours in early piperacillin trials (Zobell, 2013).

High-dose: Limited data available: IV: 450 mg piperacillin/kg/**day** every 4 to 6 hours or 600 mg piperacillin/kg/**day** divided every 4 hours has been described from early studies of piperacillin alone; usual maximum daily dose: 18 to 24 g piperacillin/**day**. **Note:** Piperacillin doses >600 mg/kg/day or an extended duration of therapy (>14 days) have been associated with dose-related adverse effects including serum sickness, immune-mediated hemolytic anemia and bone marrow suppression (Zobell 2013).

Intra-abdominal infection, complicated (off-label use): IV: 200 to 300 mg piperacillin/kg/day divided every 6 to 8 hours (maximum dose: 12 g piperacillin/day) (Solomkin, 2010).

Skin and soft tissue necrotizing infections (off-label use): IV: 60 to 75 mg piperacillin/kg every 6 hours (in combination with vancomycin for empiric therapy); continue until further debridement is not necessary, patient has clinically improved, and patient is afebrile for 48 to 72 hours. (IDSA [Stevens 2014])

Surgical (perioperative) prophylaxis (off-label use): **Note:** Doses may be repeated in 2 hours if procedure is lengthy or if there is excessive blood loss (Bratzler 2013): IV:

Infants 2 to 9 months: 80 mg piperacillin/kg within 60 minutes prior to surgical incision (maximum: 3,000 mg piperacillin/dose)

Infants >9 months, Children, and Adolescents ≤40 kg: 100 mg piperacillin/kg within 60 minutes prior to surgical incision (maximum: 3,000 mg piperacillin/dose).

Children and Adolescents >40 kg: Refer to adult dosing.

Renal Impairment

Adults:

Traditional infusion method (ie, IV infusion over 30 minutes): Manufacturer's labeling:

CrCl >40 mL/minute: No dosage adjustment necessary.

CrCl 20 to 40 mL/minute: Administer 2.25 g every 6 hours (3.375 g every 6 hours for nosocomial pneumonia)

CrCl <20 mL/minute: Administer 2.25 g every 8 hours (2.25 g every 6 hours for nosocomial pneumonia)

Note: Some clinicians suggest adjusting the dose at CrCl ≤20 mL/minute (rather than CrCl <40 mL/minute) in patients receiving either traditional or extended-infusion methods, particularly if treating serious gram-negative infections (empirically or definitively) (Patel 2010).

Extended infusion method (off-label dosing): CrCl ≤20 mL/minute: 3.375 g IV over 4 hours every 12 hours (Patel 2010)

End-stage renal disease (ESRD):

Intermittent hemodialysis (IHD): IV: 2.25 g every 12 hours (2.25 g every 8 hours for nosocomial pneumonia). **Note:** Dosing dependent on the assumption of 3 times/week, complete IHD sessions. Administer scheduled doses after hemodialysis on dialysis days; if next regularly scheduled dose is not due

right after dialysis session, administer an additional dose of 0.75 g after the dialysis session.

Peritoneal dialysis (PD): 2.25 g every 12 hours (2.25 g every 8 hours for nosocomial pneumonia).

Continuous renal replacement therapy (CRRT) (Heintz 2009; Trotman 2005): Drug clearance is highly dependent on the method of renal replacement, filter type, and flow rate. Appropriate dosing requires close monitoring of pharmacologic response, signs of adverse reactions due to drug accumulation, as well as drug concentrations in relation to target trough (if appropriate). The following are general recommendations only (based on dialysate flow/ultrafiltration rates of 1 to 2 L/hour and minimal residual renal function) and should not supersede clinical judgment (Trotman 2005):

CVVH: 2.25 to 3.375 g every 6 to 8 hours

CVVHD: 2.25 to 3.375 g every 6 hours

CVVHDF: 3.375 g every 6 hours

Note: Higher dose of 3.375 g should be considered when treating resistant pathogens (especially *Pseudomonas* spp); alternative recommendations suggest dosing of 4.5 g every 8 hours (Valtonen 2001); regardless of regimen, there is some concern of tazobactam (TAZ) accumulation, given its lower clearance relative to piperacillin (PIP). Some clinicians advocate dosing with PIP to alternate with PIP/TAZ, particularly in CVVH-dependent patients, to lessen this concern.

Infants, Children, and Adolescents: There are no dosage adjustments provided in the manufacturer's labeling; however, the following adjustments have been recommended (Aronoff, 2007): Dosing based on a usual dose of 200 to 300 mg piperacillin/kg/day in divided doses every 6 hours.

GFR >50 mL/minute/1.73 m^2: No dosage adjustment necessary.

GFR 30 to 50 mL/minute/1.73 m^2: 35 to 50 mg piperacillin/kg/dose every 6 hours

GFR <30 mL/minute/1.73 m^2: 35 to 50 mg piperacillin/kg/dose every 8 hours

End-stage renal disease (ESRD) on intermittent hemodialysis (IHD): Hemodialysis removes 30% to 40% of a piperacillin/tazobactam dose: 50 to 75 mg piperacillin/kg/dose every 12 hours

Peritoneal dialysis (PD): Peritoneal dialysis removes 21% of tazobactam and 6% of piperacillin: 50 to 75 mg piperacillin/kg/dose every 12 hours

Continuous renal replacement therapy (CRRT): 35 to 50 mg piperacillin/kg/dose every 8 hours

Hepatic Impairment No dosage adjustment necessary.

Dietary Considerations Some products may contain sodium.

Administration Administer by IV infusion over 30 minutes. For extended infusion administration (off-label dosing), administer over 3-4 hours (Kim 2007; Shea 2009).

Some penicillins (eg, carbenicillin, ticarcillin, and piperacillin) have been shown to inactivate aminoglycosides *in vitro*. This has been observed to a greater extent with tobramycin and gentamicin, while amikacin has shown greater stability against inactivation. Concurrent use of these agents may pose a risk of reduced antibacterial efficacy *in vivo*, particularly in the setting of profound renal impairment. However, definitive clinical evidence is lacking. If combination penicillin/aminoglycoside therapy is desired in a patient with renal dysfunction, separation of doses (if feasible), and routine monitoring of aminoglycoside levels, CBC, and clinical response should be considered. **Note:** Reformulated Zosyn containing EDTA has been shown to be compatible *in vitro* for Y-site infusion with amikacin and gentamicin diluted in NS or D$_5$W (applies **only** to specific concentrations and varies by product; consult manufacturer's labeling). Reformulated Zosyn containing EDTA is **not** compatible with tobramycin.

Monitoring Parameters Creatinine, BUN, CBC with differential, PT, PTT, serum electrolytes, LFTs, urinalysis; signs of bleeding; monitor for signs of anaphylaxis during first dose

Test Interactions Positive Coombs' [direct] test; false positive reaction for urine glucose using copper-reduction method (Clinitest); may result in false positive results with the Platelia *Aspergillus* enzyme immunoassay (EIA)

Some penicillin derivatives may accelerate the degradation of aminoglycosides *in vitro*, leading to a potential underestimation of aminoglycoside serum concentration.

Dosage Forms Excipient information presented when available (limited, particularly for generics); consult specific product labeling.

Note: 8:1 ratio of piperacillin sodium/tazobactam sodium

Infusion [premixed iso-osmotic solution]:

Zosyn: 2.25 g: Piperacillin 2 g and tazobactam 0.25 g (50 mL) [contains edetate disodium, sodium 130 mg (5.68 mEq)]

Zosyn: 3.375 g: Piperacillin 3 g and tazobactam 0.375 g (50 mL) [contains edetate disodium, sodium 195 mg (8.52 mEq)]

Zosyn: 4.5 g: Piperacillin 4 g and tazobactam 0.5 g (100 mL) [contains edetate disodium, sodium 260 mg (11.36 mEq)]

Injection, powder for reconstitution: 2.25 g: Piperacillin 2 g and tazobactam 0.25 g; 3.375 g: Piperacillin 3 g and tazobactam 0.375 g; 4.5 g: Piperacillin 4 g and tazobactam 0.5 g; 40.5 g: Piperacillin 36 g and tazobactam 4.5 g

Zosyn: 2.25 g: Piperacillin 2 g and tazobactam 0.25 g [contains edetate disodium, sodium 130 mg (5.68 mEq)]

Zosyn: 3.375 g: Piperacillin 3 g and tazobactam 0.375 g [contains edetate disodium, sodium 195 mg (8.52 mEq)]

Zosyn: 4.5 g: Piperacillin 4 g and tazobactam 0.5 g [contains edetate disodium, sodium 260 mg (11.36 mEq)]

Zosyn: 40.5 g: Piperacillin 36 g and tazobactam 4.5 g [contains edetate disodium, sodium 2340 mg (102.24 mEq); bulk pharmacy vial]

◆ Piperacillin and Tazobactam for Injection (Can) *see* Piperacillin and Tazobactam *on page 1456*

◆ Piperacillin and Tazobactam Sodium *see* Piperacillin and Tazobactam *on page 1456*

◆ Piperacillin Sodium and Tazobactam Sodium *see* Piperacillin and Tazobactam *on page 1456*

◆ Piperazine Estrone Sulfate *see* Estropipate *on page 695*

◆ Piperonyl Butoxide and Pyrethrins *see* Pyrethrins and Piperonyl Butoxide *on page 1531*

◆ Pirmella 1/35 *see* Ethinyl Estradiol and Norethindrone *on page 708*

◆ Pirmella 7/7/7 *see* Ethinyl Estradiol and Norethindrone *on page 708*

Piroxicam (peer OKS i kam)

Brand Names: US Feldene

Brand Names: Canada Apo-Piroxicam; Dom-Piroxicam; PMS-Piroxicam; PMS-Piroxicam Suppositories; Teva-Piroxicam

Pharmacologic Category Nonsteroidal Anti-inflammatory Drug (NSAID), Oral

Use

Arthritis: Relief of signs and symptoms of osteoarthritis and rheumatoid arthritis.

Canadian labeling: Additional use (not in U.S. labeling): Symptomatic treatment of ankylosing spondylitis

Medication Guide Available Yes

Dosing

Adult Note: Individualize dosage to lowest effective dose for the shortest duration to minimize adverse effects.

Osteoarthritis, rheumatoid arthritis: *US labeling:* Oral: 20 mg once daily.

Ankylosing spondylitis, osteoarthritis, rheumatoid arthritis: *Canadian labeling:* Oral, Rectal suppository: 10 to 20 mg daily in 1 to 2 divided doses (maximum dose: 20 mg daily)

Geriatric Refer to adult dosing. Initiate therapy cautiously at low end of dosing range.

Renal Impairment

Mild to moderate impairment:

US labeling: There are no dosage adjustments provided in the manufacturer's labeling.

Canadian labeling: There are no specific dosage adjustments provided in the manufacturer's labeling; however, a dosage reduction is recommended. Caution and close monitoring is advised for patients with CrCl <60 mL/minute. Use is contraindicated in patients with deteriorating renal disease.

Severe impairment:

US labeling: Use is not recommended (has not been studied); if therapy must be initiated, close monitoring is recommended.

Canadian labeling: Use is contraindicated in severe impairment (CrCl <30 mL/minute) or in patients with deteriorating renal disease.

Hepatic Impairment There are no specific dosage adjustments provided in the manufacturer's labeling; however, a dosage reduction is recommended. **Note:** Canadian labeling contraindicates use in severe impairment or in patients with active liver disease.

Additional Information Complete prescribing information should be consulted for additional detail.

Dosage Forms Excipient information presented when available (limited, particularly for generics); consult specific product labeling.

Capsule, Oral:

Feldene: 10 mg, 20 mg

Generic: 10 mg, 20 mg

Dosage Forms: Canada Note: Refer also to Dosage Forms. Excipient information presented when available (limited, particularly for generics); consult specific product labeling.

Suppository, Rectal: 10 mg, 20 mg

◆ *p*-Isobutylhydratropic Acid *see* Ibuprofen *on page 905*

◆ Pit *see* Oxytocin *on page 1367*

Pitavastatin (pi TA va sta tin)

Brand Names: US Livalo

Index Terms Pitavastatin Calcium

Pharmacologic Category Antilipemic Agent, HMG-CoA Reductase Inhibitor

Use Primary hyperlipidemia and mixed dyslipidemia: Adjunct to dietary therapy to reduce elevations in total cholesterol (TC), LDL-C, apolipoprotein B (Apo B), and triglycerides (TG), and to increase low HDL-C in patients with primary hyperlipidemia and mixed dyslipidemia

Dosing

Adult & Geriatric

Primary hyperlipidemia and mixed dyslipidemia: Oral: Initial: 2 mg once daily; may be increased to maximum 4 mg once daily

Note: Doses should be individualized according to the baseline LDL-cholesterol levels, the recommended goal of therapy, and patient response; adjustments should be made at intervals of 4 weeks.

Prevention of cardiovascular disease (off-label use): ACC/AHA Blood Cholesterol Guideline recommendations to reduce the risk of atherosclerotic cardiovascular disease (ASCVD) (Stone, 2013): Adults ≥21 years: Oral:

Primary prevention:

LDL-C ≥190 mg/dL: High intensity therapy necessary; use alternate statin therapy (eg, atorvastatin or rosuvastatin)

Type 1 or 2 diabetes and age 40-75 years: Moderate intensity therapy: 2-4 mg once daily

Type 1 or 2 diabetes, age 40-75 years, and an estimated 10-year ASCVD risk ≥7.5%: High intensity therapy necessary; use alternate statin therapy (eg, atorvastatin or rosuvastatin)

Age 40-75 years and an estimated 10-year ASCVD risk ≥7.5%: Moderate to high intensity therapy: 2-4 mg once daily or consider using high intensity statin therapy (eg, atorvastatin or rosuvastatin)

Secondary prevention:

Patient has clinical ASCVD (eg, coronary heart disease, stroke/TIA, or peripheral arterial disease presumed to be of atherosclerotic origin) or is post-CABG (AHA [Kulik, 2015]) **and:**

Age ≤75 years: High intensity therapy necessary; use alternate statin therapy (eg, atorvastatin or rosuvastatin)

Age >75 years or not a candidate for high intensity therapy: Moderate intensity therapy: 2-4 mg once daily

Dosage adjustment with concomitant medications:

Erythromycin: Pitavastatin dose should not exceed 1 mg once daily

Rifampin: Pitavastatin dose should not exceed 2 mg once daily

Renal Impairment

CrCl 15-60 mL/minute/1.73 m² (not receiving hemodialysis): Initial: 1 mg once daily; maximum: 2 mg once daily

ESRD: Initial: 1 mg once daily; maximum: 2 mg once daily

Hepatic Impairment Contraindicated in active liver disease or in patients with unexplained persistent elevations of serum transaminases.

Adjustment for Toxicity

Severe muscle symptoms or fatigue: Promptly discontinue use; evaluate CPK, creatinine, and urinalysis for myoglobinuria (Stone, 2013).

Mild to moderate muscle symptoms: Discontinue use until symptoms can be evaluated; evaluate patient for conditions that may increase the risk for muscle symptoms (eg, hypothyroidism, reduced renal or hepatic function, rheumatologic disorders such as polymyalgia rheumatica, steroid myopathy, vitamin D deficiency, or primary muscle diseases). Upon resolution, resume the original or lower dose of pitavastatin. If muscle symptoms recur, discontinue pitavastatin use. After muscle symptom resolution, may then use a low dose of a different statin; gradually increase if tolerated. In the absence of continued statin use, if muscle symptoms or elevated CPK continues after 2 months, consider other causes of muscle symptoms. If determined to be due to another condition aside from statin use, may resume statin therapy at the original dose (Stone, 2013).

Additional Information Complete prescribing information should be consulted for additional detail.

Dosage Forms Excipient information presented when available (limited, particularly for generics); consult specific product labeling.
Tablet, Oral:
Livalo: 1 mg, 2 mg, 4 mg

Plerixafor (pler IX a fore)

Brand Names: US Mozobil
Brand Names: Canada Mozobil
Index Terms AMD3100; LM3100
Pharmacologic Category Hematopoietic Agent; Hematopoietic Stem Cell Mobilizer
Use Peripheral stem cell mobilization: Mobilization of hematopoietic stem cells (HSC) for collection and subsequent autologous transplantation (in combination with filgrastim) in patients with non-Hodgkin lymphoma (NHL) and multiple myeloma (MM)

Dosing

Adult & Geriatric Note: Dosing is based on actual body weight. Begin plerixafor after patient has received filgrastim (10 mcg/kg once daily) for 4 days; plerixafor, filgrastim, and apheresis should be continued daily until sufficient cell collection up to a maximum of 4 days.

Hematopoietic stem cell mobilization (in non-Hodgkin lymphoma and multiple myeloma): SubQ: Administer ~11 hours prior to apheresis
US labeling:
Patients ≤83 kg: 20 mg fixed dose **or** 0.24 mg/kg once daily for up to 4 consecutive days
Patients >83 kg: 0.24 mg/kg once daily for up to 4 consecutive days; maximum dose: 40 mg daily
Canadian labeling: 0.24 mg/kg once daily for up to 4 consecutive days; maximum dose: 40 mg daily
Renal Impairment Note: Creatinine clearance estimate based on Cockcroft-Gault formula:
US labeling:
CrCl >50 mL/minute: No dosage adjustment necessary.
CrCl ≤50 mL/minute:
Patients ≤83 kg: 13 mg fixed dose **or** 0.16 mg/kg once daily
Patients >83 kg and <160 kg: 0.16 mg/kg once daily; maximum dose: 27 mg daily
Hemodialysis: There are no dosage adjustments provided in the manufacturer's labeling (has not been studied).

Canadian labeling:
CrCl >50 mL/minute: No dosage adjustment necessary
CrCl 20 to 50 mL/minute: 0.16 mg/kg once daily; maximum dose: 27 mg daily
CrCl <20 mL/minute and hemodialysis: There are no dosage adjustments provided in the manufacturer's labeling (has not been studied).
Hepatic Impairment There are no dosage adjustments provided in the manufacturer's labeling.
Obesity The manufacturer recommends calculating the dose based on actual weight for patients weighing up to 175% of ideal body weight (maximum dose: 40 mg daily). Dosing in patients >175% of ideal body weight has not been studied.
Additional Information Complete prescribing information should be consulted for additional detail.
Dosage Forms Excipient information presented when available (limited, particularly for generics); consult specific product labeling.
Solution, Subcutaneous [preservative free]:
Mozobil: 24 mg/1.2 mL (1.2 mL)

Pneumococcal Conjugate Vaccine (13-Valent)

(noo moe KOK al KON ju gate vak SEEN, thur TEEN vay lent)

Brand Names: US Prevnar 13
Brand Names: Canada Prevnar 13
Index Terms PCV13; Pneumococcal 13-Valent Conjugate Vaccine
Pharmacologic Category Vaccine; Vaccine, Inactivated (Bacterial)
Additional Appendix Information
Immunization Administration Recommendations *on page 1974*

Immunization Schedules *on page 1979*

Use
U.S. labeling:
Immunization of infants ≥6 weeks, children, and adolescents through 17 years against *Streptococcus pneumoniae* infection caused by serotypes included in the vaccine

Immunization of infants ≥6 weeks and children through 5 years against otitis media caused by *Streptococcus pneumoniae* serotypes 4, 6B, 9V, 14, 18C, 19F, and 23F

Immunization of adults ≥50 years against pneumococcal pneumonia and invasive disease caused by *Streptococcus pneumoniae* serotypes included in the vaccine

Canadian labeling:

Immunization of infants ≥6 weeks, children, and adolescents through 17 years against invasive disease caused by *Streptococcus pneumoniae* serotypes included in the vaccine

Immunization of adults ≥18 years against pneumococcal pneumonia and invasive disease caused by *Streptococcus pneumoniae* serotypes included in the vaccine

The Advisory Committee on Immunization Practices (ACIP) recommends routine vaccination for the following (ACIP [Kobayashi 2015]; CDC/ACIP [Nuorti 2010]):

All infants and children age 2 to 59 months

Children 60 to 71 months with underlying medical conditions including:

Immunocompetent children with chronic heart disease (particularly cyanotic congenital heart disease and heart failure), chronic lung disease (including asthma if treated with high dose corticosteroids), diabetes, cerebrospinal fluid leaks, or cochlear implants

Children with functional or anatomic asplenia, including sickle cell disease or other hemoglobinopathies, congenital or acquired asplenia, or splenic dysfunction.

Children with immunocompromising conditions including congenital immunodeficiency (includes B or T cell deficiency, compliment deficiencies and phagocytic disorders; excludes chronic granulomatous disease), HIV infection, chronic renal failure, nephrotic syndrome, leukemia, lymphoma, Hodgkin disease, generalized malignancies, solid organ transplant, or other diseases requiring immunosuppressive drugs (including long term systemic corticosteroids and radiation therapy)

Children who received ≥1 dose of PCV7

Note: Routine use is not recommended for healthy children ≥5 years.

Children ≥6 years and Adolescents ≤18 years (CDC/ACIP, 62[25] 2013), and Adults ≥19 years (CDC/ACIP, 61[40] 2012): The ACIP also recommends routine vaccination for persons with the following underlying medical conditions:

Immunocompetent persons with cerebrospinal fluid leaks or cochlear implants

Persons with functional or anatomic asplenia, including sickle cell disease or other hemoglobinopathies, congenital or acquired asplenia

Persons with immunocompromising conditions including congenital or acquired immunodeficiency (includes B or T cell deficiency, compliment deficiencies and phagocytic disorders; excludes chronic granulomatous disease), HIV infection, chronic renal failure, nephrotic syndrome, leukemia, lymphoma, Hodgkin disease, generalized malignancies, solid organ transplant, multiple myeloma, or other diseases requiring immunosuppressive drugs (including long term systemic corticosteroids and radiation therapy)

All adults ≥65 years (CDC/ACIP [Tomczyk 2014])

Medication Guide Available Yes

Dosing

Adult

Immunization:

US labeling: Adults ≥50 years: IM: 0.5 mL as a single dose.

Canadian labeling: Adults ≥18 years (including those at high risk of infection [eg, sickle cell disease, HIV infection] or previously vaccinated with a pneumococcal polysaccharide vaccine): IM: 0.5 mL as a single dose (PCV13 should be administered prior to pneumococcal polysaccharide vaccine if sequential administration is considered).

Alternative recommendations:

Adults 19 to <65 years with specified underlying medical conditions: IM: 0.5 mL as a single dose

Note: Which vaccines are indicated (pneumococcal conjugate vaccine [PCV 13] and/or pneumococcal polysaccharide vaccine [PPSV23]) is dependent on previous pneumococcal vaccination history; some medical conditions do not require PCV13 [see guidelines for details] (ACIP [Kobayashi 2015]; CDC/ACIP [Kim 2015]):

Pneumococcal vaccine-naive or vaccination status unknown: Administer PCV13 followed by PPSV23 at least 8 weeks later

Previously received PPSV23 but not PCV13: Administer PCV13 ≥1 year after the PPSV23 dose

Previously received PCV13 but not PPSV23: No additional PCV 13 doses are needed

Revaccination: Administration of additional doses is not recommended for adults (CDC/ACIP [Kim 2015]).

Adults ≥65 years: IM: 0.5 mL as a single dose

Note: All patients should receive both pneumococcal conjugate vaccine (PCV13) and pneumococcal polysaccharide vaccine (PPSV23) (ACIP [Kobayashi 2015]; CDC/ACIP [Tomczyk 2014]):

Pneumococcal vaccine-naive or vaccination status unknown: Administer PCV13 followed by PPSV23 ≥1 year later (minimum interval of 8 weeks for certain high-risk groups)

Previously received PPSV23 (at age ≥65 years) but not PCV13: Administer PCV13 ≥1 year after the last dose of PPSV23

Previously received PPSV23 (at age <65 years) but not PCV13: Administer PCV13 ≥1 year after the last dose of PPSV23; administer PPSV23 ≥1 year later (minimum interval of 8 weeks for certain high-risk groups) and at least 5 years after the last PPSV23 dose

Previously received PCV13: No additional PCV13 doses are needed

HSCT, autologous or allogeneic (Canadian labeling): IM: 0.5 mL for a total of 4 doses with first dose administered 3 to 6 months after HSCT followed by second and third doses administered at least 1 month apart and then a booster dose 6 months after the third dose.

Geriatric Immunization:

Adults ≥65 years: All patients should receive both pneumococcal conjugate vaccine (PCV 13) and pneumococcal polysaccharide vaccine (PPSV23) (ACIP [Kobayashi 2015]; CDC/ACIP [Tomczyk 2014]):

Pneumococcal vaccine-naïve: IM: Administer PCV13 0.5 ml as a single dose, followed by PPSV23 ≥1 year later (minimum interval of 8 weeks for certain high-risk groups)

Previously received pneumococcal polysaccharide vaccine (PPSV23):

Received at age <65 years: IM: Administer PCV13 0.5 mL as a single dose ≥1 year after the last dose of PPSV23, followed by PPSV23 at least ≥1 year later (minimum interval of 8 weeks for certain high-risk groups) and at least 5 years after the last dose of PPSV23

Received at age ≥65 years: IM: Administer PCV13 0.5 mL as a single dose ≥1 year after the last dose of PPSV23; no additional doses of PPSV23 are needed for routine vaccination

Previously received PCV13: No additional PCV13 doses are needed

Pediatric

Primary immunization: IM: *Infants and Children 6 weeks to 15 months:* 0.5 mL/dose for a total of 4 doses. The first dose may be given as young as 6 weeks of age, but is typically given at 8 weeks (2 months). The 3 remaining doses are usually given at 4, 6, and 12 to 15 months. The recommended dosing interval is 4 to 8 weeks. The minimum interval between doses in children <1 year is 1 month. The minimum interval between the third and fourth dose is 8 weeks.

Alternative recommendations [Canadian National Advisory Committee on Immunizations (NACI) 2012-2014]: Healthy infants: May consider a total of three 0.5 mL doses with the first dose administered at 2 months, the second dose at 4 months of age and a third dose at 12 months.

Catch-up Immunization (previously unvaccinated with PCV13): *Infants ≥7 months, Children, and Adolescents:*

Infants 7 to 11 months: 0.5 mL for a total of 3 doses; first 2 doses at least 4 weeks apart, followed by a third dose after the 1-year birthday (12 to 15 months), separated from the second dose by at least 8 weeks

Children 12 to 23 months: 0.5 mL for a total of 2 doses, separated by at least 8 weeks

Healthy Children 24 to 59 months: 0.5 mL as a single dose

Children 24 to 71 months with an underlying medical condition: 0.5 mL for a total of 2 doses, separated by 8 weeks (CDC/ACIP [Nuorti 2010])

Children 6 through 17 years: 0.5 mL as a single dose. If PCV7 was previously administered, give PCV13 ≥8 weeks after that dose

Canadian labeling: Children >1 year (previous completed vaccination with PCV7): IM: 0.5 mL as a single dose in the second year of life

HSCT, autologous or allogeneic (Canadian labeling): Children ≥2 years and Adolescents: Refer to adult dosing.

Renal Impairment There are no dosage adjustments provided in the manufacturer's labeling.

Hepatic Impairment There are no dosage adjustments provided in the manufacturer's labeling.

Additional Information Complete prescribing information should be consulted for additional detail.

Dosage Forms Excipient information presented when available (limited, particularly for generics); consult specific product labeling.

Injection, suspension:

Prevnar 13: 2 mcg of each capsular saccharide for serotypes 1, 3, 4, 5, 6A, 7F, 9V, 14, 18C, 19A, 19F, and 23F, and 4 mcg of serotype 6B [bound to diphtheria CRM_{197} protein ~34 mcg] per 0.5 mL (0.5 mL) [contains aluminum, polysorbate 80, and yeast]

Pneumococcal Polysaccharide Vaccine (23-Valent)

(noo moe KOK al pol i SAK a ride vak SEEN, TWEN tee three VAY lent)

Brand Names: US Pneumovax 23

Brand Names: Canada Pneumo 23; Pneumovax 23

Index Terms 23-Valent Pneumococcal Polysaccharide Vaccine; 23PS; Pneumococcal Polysaccharide Vaccine (Polyvalent); PPSV; PPSV23; PPV23

Pharmacologic Category Vaccine; Vaccine, Inactivated (Bacterial)

Additional Appendix Information

Immunization Administration Recommendations *on page 1974*

Immunization Schedules *on page 1979*

Use

Pneumococcal disease prevention: Active immunization of children ≥2 years and persons ≥50 years who are at increased risk for pneumococcal disease caused by the 23 serotypes included in the vaccine.

The Advisory Committee on Immunization Practices (ACIP) recommends routine vaccination for patients with the following underlying medical conditions (ACIP [Kobayashi 2015]; CDC/ACIP 59[34] 2010; CDC/ACIP 61[40] 2012; CDC/ACIP [Nuorti 2010]; CDC/ACIP [Tomczyk 2014]):

Children ≥2 years of age, adolescents, and adults 19 to 64 years with functional or anatomic asplenia, including sickle cell disease or other hemoglobinopathies, congenital or acquired asplenia, splenic dysfunction, or splenectomy

Immunocompetent children ≥2 years of age and adolescents with chronic heart disease (particularly cyanotic congenital heart disease and heart failure), chronic lung disease (including asthma if treated with high dose corticosteroids), diabetes, cerebrospinal fluid leaks, or cochlear implants

Immunocompetent adults 19 to 64 years with chronic heart disease (including heart failure and cardiomyopathies; excluding hypertension), chronic lung disease (including COPD, emphysema, and asthma), diabetes, cerebrospinal fluid leaks, cochlear implants, alcoholism, chronic liver disease, cirrhosis, and cigarette smokers

Immunocompromised children ≥2 years of age, adolescents, and adults 19 to 64 years with congenital or acquired immunodeficiency (includes B or T cell deficiency, compliment deficiencies and phagocytic disorders; excludes chronic granulomatous disease), HIV infection, chronic renal failure, nephrotic syndrome, leukemia, lymphoma, Hodgkin disease, generalized malignancies, solid organ transplant, multiple myeloma, or other diseases requiring immunosuppressive drugs (including long-term systemic corticosteroids and radiation therapy)

All adults ≥65 years of age

Medication Guide Available Yes

Dosing

Adult

Immunization: Adults 19 to <65 years with specified underlying medical conditions: IM, SubQ: 0.5 mL as a single dose. **Note:** Some medical conditions do not require pneumococcal conjugate vaccine (PCV13) [see guidelines for details] (ACIP [Kobayashi 2015]; CDC/ACIP [Kim 2015]):

Primary vaccination:

Pneumococcal vaccine-naive or vaccination status unknown: Administer PCV13 followed by pneumococcal polysaccharide vaccine (PPSV23) at least 8 weeks later

Previously received PPSV23 but not PCV13: No additional PPSV23 doses needed for primary vaccination; administer PCV13 ≥1 year after the last PPSV23 dose was received

Previously received PCV13 but not PPSV23: Administer PPSV23 at least 8 weeks after PCV13

Revaccination: Adults 19 to 64 years with functional or anatomic asplenia, chronic renal failure or nephrotic syndrome, or who are immunocompromised: One PPSV23 revaccination dose ≥5 years after first dose of PPSV23 and ≥8 weeks after PCV13. **Note:** If PPSV23 is given before PCV13, the minimum interval is 1 year (ACIP [Kobayashi 2015]; CDC 61[40] 2012; CDC/ACIP 59[34] 2010).

Geriatric

Immunization: Adults ≥65 years: IM, SubQ: 0.5 mL as a single dose. **Note:** All patients should receive both pneumococcal conjugate vaccine (PCV 13) and pneumococcal polysaccharide vaccine (PPSV23) (ACIP [Kobayashi 2015]; CDC/ACIP [Tomczyk 2014]):

Pneumococcal vaccine-naive or vaccination status unknown: Administer PCV13 followed by PPSV23 ≥1 year later (minimum interval of 8 weeks for certain high-risk groups)

Previously received PPSV23 (at age <65 years) but not PCV13: Administer PCV13 ≥1 year after the last dose of PPSV23; administer PPSV23 ≥1 year later (minimum interval of 8 weeks for certain high-risk groups) and at least 5 years after the last PPSV23 dose

Previously received PPSV23 (at age ≥65 years) but not PCV13: No additional PPSV23 doses are needed; administer PCV13 ≥1 year after the last dose of PPSV23

Previously received PCV13 but not PPSV23: Administer PPSV23 ≥1 year after the PCV13 dose (minimum interval of 8 weeks for certain high-risk groups) or as soon as possible if this time window has passed

Pediatric

Immunization: Children ≥2 years and Adolescents: IM, SubQ: 0.5 mL as a single dose

Primary vaccination: Children ≥2 years and Adolescents with specified underlying medical conditions: One dose of pneumococcal polysaccharide vaccine (PPSV23) should be given at ≥2 years of age. Immunization with pneumococcal conjugate vaccine (PCV13) should be completed prior to PPSV23 as recommended. The minimum interval between PCV13 and PPSV23 is 8 weeks (CDC/ACIP [Nuorti 2010]).

Revaccination: Children ≥2 years and Adolescents with functional or anatomic asplenia, those who are immunocompromised, and others with high-risk medical conditions [see guidelines for details]: One revaccination dose ≥5 years after the first dose of PPSV23. Revaccination of immunocompetent individuals is generally not recommended (CDC/ACIP [Strikas 2015]).

Renal Impairment There are no dosage adjustments provided in the manufacturer's labeling.

Hepatic Impairment There are no dosage adjustments provided in the manufacturer's labeling.

Additional Information Complete prescribing information should be consulted for additional detail.

Dosage Forms Excipient information presented when available (limited, particularly for generics); consult specific product labeling.

Injection, solution:

Pneumovax 23: 25 mcg each of 23 capsular polysaccharide isolates/0.5 mL (0.5 mL, 2.5 mL)

Podophyllum Resin (po DOF il um REZ in)

Brand Names: US Podocon

Brand Names: Canada Podofilm®

Index Terms Mandrake; May Apple; Podophyllin

Pharmacologic Category Keratolytic Agent

Use Topical treatment of soft external genital (venereal) warts (condylomata acuminata); compound benzoin tincture generally is used as the medium for topical application

Dosing

Adult & Geriatric Condylomata acuminatum: Topical: Applied by physician only.

Pediatric Refer to adult dosing.

Additional Information Complete prescribing information should be consulted for additional detail.

Dosage Forms Excipient information presented when available (limited, particularly for generics); consult specific product labeling.

Solution, External:
Podocon: 25% (15 mL)

Polidocanol (pol i DOE kuh nol)

Brand Names: US Asclera; Varithena
Pharmacologic Category Sclerosing Agent
Use Varicose veins:

Asclera: To treat uncomplicated spider veins (varicose veins 1 mm or less in diameter) and uncomplicated reticular veins (varicose veins 1 to 3 mm in diameter) in the lower extremity.

Varithena: To treat incompetent great saphenous veins, accessory saphenous veins, and visible varicosities of the great saphenous vein system above and below the knee.

Dosing

Adult Varicose veins: IV:

Asclera:

Reticular veins (1 to 3 mm diameter): 0.1 to 0.3 mL of 1% solution per injection (maximum: 10 mL per session); may repeat in 7 to 14 days

Spider veins (≤1 mm diameter): 0.1 to 0.3 mL of 0.5% solution per injection (maximum: 10 mL per session); may repeat in 7 to 14 days

Varithena: *Great saphenous veins and accessory saphenous veins:* 5 mL of 1% solution per injection (maximum: 15 mL per session); may repeat in ≥5 days

Renal Impairment There are no dosage adjustments provided in manufacturer's labeling.

Hepatic Impairment There are no dosage adjustments provided in manufacturer's labeling.

Additional Information Complete prescribing information should be consulted for additional detail.

Dosage Forms Excipient information presented when available (limited, particularly for generics); consult specific product labeling.

Foam, Intravenous:
Varithena: 180 mg/18 mL (45 mL) [contains alcohol, usp]
Solution, Intravenous [preservative free]:
Asclera: 0.5% (2 mL); 1% (2 mL) [contains alcohol, usp]

◆ Polio Vaccine *see* Poliovirus Vaccine (Inactivated) *on page 1465*

◆ Poliovirus, Inactivated (IPV) *see* Diphtheria and Tetanus Toxoids, Acellular Pertussis, and Poliovirus Vaccine *on page 566*

◆ Poliovirus, Inactivated (IPV) *see* Diphtheria and Tetanus Toxoids, Acellular Pertussis, Poliovirus and *Haemophilus* b Conjugate Vaccine *on page 567*

Poliovirus Vaccine (Inactivated)
(POE lee oh VYE rus vak SEEN, in ak ti VAY ted)

Brand Names: US IPOL
Brand Names: Canada Imovax Polio
Index Terms Enhanced-Potency Inactivated Poliovirus Vaccine; IPV; Polio Vaccine; Salk Vaccine
Pharmacologic Category Vaccine; Vaccine, Inactivated (Viral)
Additional Appendix Information

Immunization Administration Recommendations *on page 1974*

Immunization Schedules *on page 1979*

Use Poliovirus prevention:

Active immunization of infants (≥6 weeks [US labeling]; ≥2 months [Canadian labeling]), children, adolescents, and adults for prevention of poliomyelitis caused by poliovirus types 1, 2, and 3.

US labeling: Infants (as young as 6 weeks), children, adolescents, and adults

Canadian labeling: Infants (as young as 2 months), children, adolescents, and adults

The Advisory Committee on Immunization Practices (ACIP) recommends routine vaccination for the following:
• All infants and children (first dose given at 2 months of age) (CDC/ACIP, 58[30] 2009)

Routine immunization of adults in the United States is generally not recommended. Adults with previous wild poliovirus disease, who have never been immunized, or those who are incompletely immunized may receive inactivated poliovirus vaccine if they fall into one of the following categories (CDC/ACIP [Prevots 2000]):
• Travelers to regions or countries where poliomyelitis is endemic or epidemic
• Healthcare workers in close contact with patients who may be excreting poliovirus
• Laboratory workers handling specimens that may contain poliovirus
• Members of communities or specific population groups with diseases caused by wild poliovirus
• Incompletely vaccinated or unvaccinated adults in a household or with other close contact with children receiving oral poliovirus (may be at increased risk of vaccine associated paralytic poliomyelitis)

Medication Guide Available Yes

Dosing

Adult & Geriatric Immunization: IM, SubQ:

Previously unvaccinated: Administer 0.5 mL per dose for a total of 3 doses given as follows: Two 0.5 mL doses administered at 1- to 2-month intervals, followed by a third dose 6-12 months later. If <3 months, but at least 2 months are available before protection is needed, 3 doses may be administered at least 1 month apart. If administration must be completed within 1 to 2 months, give 2 doses at least 1 month apart. If <1 month is available, give 1 dose.

Incompletely vaccinated: Adults with at least 1 previous dose of OPV, <3 doses of IPV, or a combination of OPV and IPV equaling <3 doses, administer at least one 0.5 mL dose of IPV. Additional doses to complete the series may be given if time permits.

Completely vaccinated and at increased risk of exposure: One 0.5 mL dose

Pediatric Immunization: IM, SubQ:

Primary immunization: Infants and Children 6 weeks to 47 months: Administer three 0.5 mL doses, at 2, 4, and 6 to 18 months

Booster dose: Children 4 to 6 years: 0.5 mL as a single dose; Minimum interval between booster and previous dose is 6 months. The final (booster) dose should be given at ≥4 years, regardless of the number of previous doses. If the final dose is not given at 4 to 6 years, it should be given as soon as feasible (CDC/ACIP 2009).

Note: Use of the minimum age and minimum intervals (4 weeks) during the first 6 months of life should only be done when the vaccine recipient is at risk for imminent exposure to circulating poliovirus (shorter intervals and earlier start dates may lead to lower seroconversion) (CDC/ACIP 2009).

Renal Impairment There are no dosage adjustments provided in the manufacturer's labeling.

Hepatic Impairment There are no dosage adjustments provided in the manufacturer's labeling.

Additional Information Complete prescribing information should be consulted for additional detail.

Dosage Forms Excipient information presented when available (limited, particularly for generics); consult specific product labeling.

Injection, suspension:
IPOL: Type 1 poliovirus 40 D-antigen units, type 2 poliovirus 8 D-antigen units, and type 3 poliovirus 32 D-antigen units per 0.5 mL (0.5 mL, 5 mL) [contains 2-phenoxyethanol, formaldehyde, calf serum protein, neomycin (may have trace amounts), streptomycin (may have trace amounts), and polymyxin B (may have trace amounts)]

◆ Polocaine *see* Mepivacaine *on page 1145*

◆ Polocaine® (Can) *see* Mepivacaine *on page 1145*

◆ Polocaine-MPF *see* Mepivacaine *on page 1145*

◆ Polycin *see* Bacitracin and Polymyxin B (Ophthalmic) *on page 196*

◆ Polycin B [DSC] *see* Bacitracin and Polymyxin B (Ophthalmic) *on page 196*

◆ Polycitra *see* Citric Acid, Sodium Citrate, and Potassium Citrate *on page 400*

◆ Polycitra K *see* Potassium Citrate and Citric Acid *on page 1481*

◆ Polyethylene Glycol-L-asparaginase *see* Pegaspargase *on page 1407*

Polyethylene Glycol 3350
(pol i ETH i leen GLY kol 3350)

Brand Names: US GaviLAX [OTC]; GlycoLax [OTC]; HealthyLax [OTC]; MiraLax [OTC]; PEGyLAX

Brand Names: Canada Lax-A-Day; Peg 3350; Pegalax; Relaxa

Index Terms Macrogol; PEG

Pharmacologic Category Laxative, Osmotic

Use Occasional constipation: Treatment of occasional constipation

Dosing

Adult & Geriatric

Occasional constipation: Oral: 17 g (~1 heaping tablespoon) dissolved in 120 to 240 mL (4 to 8 ounces) of beverage, once daily; do not use for >1 to 2 weeks (product specific) unless directed by health care provider

Canadian labeling (not in US labeling): Oral: 17 g (~1 heaping tablespoon) dissolved in 240 mL (8 ounces) of beverage once daily; do not use for >1 week unless directed by health care provider

Bowel preparation before colonoscopy (off-label use): Oral: 17 g (~1 heaping tablespoon) in 240 mL (8 ounces) of clear liquid every 10 minutes until 2,000 mL of volume are consumed (start within 6 hours after administering bisacodyl delayed-release tablets or magnesium citrate) (ASCRS/ASGE/SAGES [Wexner 2006])

Pediatric

Occasional constipation (off-label use):

Infants, Children, and Adolescents <17 years: Oral: 0.2 to 0.8 g/kg/day (NASPGHAN [Tabbers 2014]); higher initial dose of 1 g/kg has been suggested (Loening-Baucke 2004; Pashankar 2001); maximum daily dose: 17 g/day. **Note:** Dosage should be individualized to achieved desired effect, infants and young children may require higher doses than school-aged children (Loening-Buck 2004; Pashankar 2001)

Adolescents ≥17 years: Refer to adult dosing.

Bowel preparation before colonoscopy (off-label use): Adolescents ≥17 years: Refer to adult dosing.

Renal Impairment There are no dosage adjustments provided in the manufacturer's labeling.

Hepatic Impairment There are no dosage adjustments provided in the manufacturer's labeling.

Additional Information Complete prescribing information should be consulted for additional detail.

Dosage Forms Excipient information presented when available (limited, particularly for generics); consult specific product labeling.

Packet, Oral:

HealthyLax: (1 ea, 14 ea)

MiraLax: (1 ea, 10 ea, 12 ea, 24 ea)

Generic: (1 ea, 14 ea, 30 ea, 100 ea)

Powder, Oral:

GaviLAX: (238 g, 510 g)

GlycoLax: (119 g, 255 g, 527 g)

MiraLax: (1 ea, 119 g, 238 g, 510 g)

PEGyLAX: (527 g)

Generic: 17 g/dose (119 g, 238 g, 510 g); (119 g, 238 g, 250 g, 255 g, 500 g, 510 g, 527 g, 850 g)

Dosage Forms: Canada Excipient information presented when available (limited, particularly for generics); consult specific product labeling.

Powder, Oral: 17 g/dose (238 g, 510 g)

Sachet, Oral: 17 g/sachet (4 ea, 14 ea)

◆ Polyethylene Glycol-Conjugated Uricase *see* Pegloticase *on page 1413*

Polyethylene Glycol-Electrolyte Solution
(pol i ETH i leen GLY kol ee LEK troe lite soe LOO shun)

Brand Names: US Colyte; GaviLyte-C; GaviLyte-G; GaviLyte-N; GoLYTELY; MoviPrep; NuLYTELY; TriLyte

Brand Names: Canada Colyte; Klean-Prep; PegLyte

Index Terms Electrolyte Lavage Solution

Pharmacologic Category Laxative, Osmotic

Use Bowel cleansing prior to colonoscopy or barium enema X-ray examination

Pregnancy Considerations Animal reproduction studies have not been conducted. Information related to the use of polyethylene glycol-electrolyte solution in pregnancy is limited (Neri, 2004). Colonoscopy in pregnant women is generally reserved for strong indications or life-threatening emergencies; until additional safety data for polyethylene glycol-electrolyte solution is available, other agents may be preferred for this purpose (Siddiqui, 2006; Wexner, 2006).

Breast-Feeding Considerations It is not known if polyethylene glycol-electrolyte solution is excreted into breast milk. Significant changes in the mother's fluid or electrolyte balance would not be expected with most products.

Medication Guide Available Yes

Contraindications Hypersensitivity to polyethylene glycol or any component of the formulation; ileus, gastrointestinal obstruction, gastric retention, bowel perforation, toxic colitis, toxic megacolon

Warnings/Precautions Evaluate patients with symptoms of bowel obstruction or perforation (nausea, vomiting, abdominal pain or distension) prior to use; if a patient develops severe bloating, distention or abdominal pain during administration, slow the rate of administration or temporarily discontinue use until the symptoms subside. Correct electrolyte abnormalities in patients prior to use. No additional ingredients or flavors (other than the flavor packets provided) should be added to the polyethylene glycol-electrolyte solution.

Fluid and electrolyte disturbances can lead to arrhythmias, seizures, and renal impairment. Advise patients to maintain adequate hydration before, during, and after treatment. If patient becomes dehydrated or experiences significant vomiting after treatment, consider post-colonoscopy lab tests (electrolytes, creatinine, and BUN). Serious arrhythmias have been reported (rarely) with the use of ionic osmotic laxative products. Use with caution in patients who may be at risk of cardiac arrhythmias (eg, patients with a history of prolonged QT, uncontrolled arrhythmias, recent MI, unstable angina, CHF, or cardiomyopathy). Consider pre-dose and post-colonoscopy ECGs in these patients. Generalized tonic-clonic seizures and/or loss of consciousness have occurred rarely in patients with no prior history of seizures. Seizures resolved with the correction of fluid and electrolyte abnormalities. Use with caution in patients with a history of seizures or who are at an increased risk of seizures (eg, concomitant administration of medications that lower the seizures threshold, patients withdrawing from alcohol or benzodiazepines) and in patients with known or suspected hyponatremia or low serum osmolality.

Cases of ischemic colitis have been reported; concomitant use of stimulant laxatives may increase the risk and is not recommended. The potential for mucosal aphthous ulcerations as a result of the bowel preparation should be considered, especially when evaluating colonoscopy results in patients with known or suspected inflammatory bowel disease. Use with caution in patients with severe ulcerative colitis. Use with caution in patients with renal impairment and/or in patients taking medications that may adversely affect renal function (eg, diuretics, NSAIDs, ACE inhibitors, ARBs). Patients with impaired renal function should be instructed to remain adequately hydrated; consider pre-dose and post-colonoscopy lab tests (electrolytes, creatinine, BUN) in these patients. Observe unconscious or semiconscious patients with impaired gag reflex or those who are otherwise prone to regurgitation or aspiration during administration; use with caution.

MoviPrep: Use with caution in patients with G6PD deficiency (especially patients with an active infection, history of hemolysis, or taking concomitant medications known to precipitate hemolytic reactions) due to the presence of sodium ascorbate and ascorbic acid in the formulation. Contains phenylalanine.

Use in patients <2 years of age may result in hypoglycemia, dehydration, and hypokalemia; use with caution and monitor closely. Use with caution in patients >60 years of age; serious adverse events have been reported (eg, asystole, esophageal perforation, chest infiltration following vomiting and aspiration, Mallory-Weiss tear with GI bleeding, pulmonary edema with sudden dyspnea).

Adverse Reactions

>10%:

Central nervous system: Sleep disorder (35%; evening prep vs oral sodium phosphate solution [90 mL]), rigors (34%; evening prep vs oral sodium phosphate solution [90 mL]), malaise (18% to 27%; MoviPrep split dose vs 4 L PEG with electrolytes [18%]; evening dose vs oral sodium phosphate solution [90 mL] [53%])

Endocrine & metabolic: Increased thirst (<47%)

Gastrointestinal: Abdominal distention (<60%; evening prep vs oral sodium phosphate solution [90 mL]), anorectal pain (<52%; evening prep vs oral sodium phosphate solution [90 mL]), bloating (≤50%), nausea (14% to ≤50%; split dose vs 4 L PEG with electrolytes [20%]; evening prep vs oral sodium phosphate solution [90 mL] [47%]), abdominal pain (6% to 39%; evening prep vs oral sodium phosphate solution [90 mL] [32%]; split dose vs PEG with electrolytes [6%]), hunger (30%; evening prep vs oral sodium phosphate solution [90 mL]), vomiting (7% to 12%; evening MoviPrep vs oral sodium phosphate solution (90 mL) [8%]; split dose vs PEG with electrolytes [13%])

1% to 10%:
Central nervous system: Dizziness (3% to 7%; evening prep vs oral sodium phosphate solution [90 mL]), headache (2%; evening prep vs oral sodium phosphate solution [90 mL])
Endocrine & metabolic: Hypokalemia (children 0%; evening prep vs oral sodium phosphate solution [90 mL] [6%])
Gastrointestinal: Dyspepsia (1% to 3%)
Frequency not defined, postmarketing, and/or case reports: Anaphylaxis, angioedema, aspiration, asystole (older adults >60 years), chest tightness, esophageal perforation (older adults >60 years), hypersensitivity reaction, ischemic colitis, Mallory-Weiss syndrome (older adults >60 years), pulmonary edema (older adults >60 years), rhinorrhea, seizure, shock, tightness in chest and throat, upper gastrointestinal hemorrhage (older adults >60 years), urticaria

Drug Interactions
Metabolism/Transport Effects None known.
Avoid Concomitant Use There are no known interactions where it is recommended to avoid concomitant use.
Increased Effect/Toxicity There are no known significant interactions involving an increase in effect.
Decreased Effect There are no known significant interactions involving a decrease in effect.

Preparation for Administration
CoLyte, GaviLyte-C, GaviLyte-G, GaviLyte-N, GoLYTELY, NuLYTELY, TriLyte: Using the container provided, add lukewarm water (may use tap water) up to the 4 L water mark; shake vigorously several times to ensure dissolution of the powder. No additional ingredients or flavors should be added to the solution (other than the flavor packets provided).
MoviPrep: Mix the contents of pouch A and pouch B (one each) in container provided. Add lukewarm water to fill line (~1 L); mix the solution until dissolved. No additional ingredients or flavors should be added to the solution.

Concentrations for reconstituted solutions:
CoLyte, GaviLyte-C: When dissolved in sufficient water to make 4 L, the final solution contains PEG-3350 18 mmol/L, sodium 125 mmol/L, sulfate 80 mmol/L, chloride 35 mmol/L, bicarbonate 20 mmol/L, and potassium 10 mmol/L
GaviLyte-G, GoLYTELY: When dissolved in sufficient water to make 4 L, the final solution contains PEG-3350 17.6 mmol/L, sodium 125 mmol/L, sulfate 40 mmol/L, chloride 35 mmol/L, bicarbonate 20 mmol/L, and potassium 10 mmol/L
GaviLyte-N, NuLYTELY, TriLyte: When dissolved in sufficient water to make 4 L, the final solution contains PEG-3350 31.3 mmol/L, sodium 65 mmol/L, chloride 53 mmol/L, bicarbonate 17 mmol/L, and potassium 5 mmol/L.

Storage/Stability
CoLyte, GaviLyte-C, GaviLyte-G, GaviLyte-N, GoLYTELY, NuLYTELY, TriLyte: Prior to reconstitution, store at 25°C (77°F); excursions permitted to 15°C to 30°C (59°F to 86°F). Refrigerate reconstituted solution. Use within 48 hours of preparation; discard any unused portion.
MoviPrep: Prior to reconstitution, store at 20°C to 25°C (68°F to 77°F); excursions permitted to 15°C to 30°C (59°F to 86°F). Refrigerate reconstituted solution in an upright position. Use within 24 hours of preparation; discard any unused portion.

Mechanism of Action Induces catharsis by strong electrolyte and osmotic effects
Pharmacodynamics/Kinetics Onset of effect: Oral: ~1 hour

Dosing
Adult & Geriatric
Bowel cleansing:
CoLyte, GaviLyte-C, GaviLyte-G, GaviLyte-N, GoLYTELY, NuLYTELY, TriLyte:
Oral: 240 mL (8 oz) every 10 minutes until 4 L are consumed or the rectal effluent is clear; rapid drinking of each portion is preferred to drinking small amounts continuously
Nasogastric: 20-30 mL/minute until 4 L are administered or the rectal effluent is clear
MoviPrep: Oral: Administer 2 L total with an additional 1 L of clear fluid prior to colonoscopy as follows:
Split dose (2 day regimen) (preferred method):
Dose 1: Evening before colonoscopy (10-12 hours before dose 2): 240 mL (8 oz) every 15 minutes until 1 L (entire contents of container) is consumed. Then fill container with 480 mL (16 oz) of clear liquid and consume prior to going to bed.
Dose 2: On the morning of the colonoscopy (beginning at least 3.5 hours prior to procedure): 240 mL (8 oz) every 15 minutes until 1 L (entire contents of

container) is consumed. Then fill container with 480 mL (16 oz) of clear liquid and consume at least 2 hours before the procedure.
Evening only dose (1 day regimen) (alternate method):
Dose 1: Evening before colonoscopy (at least 3.5 hours before bedtime): 240 mL (8 oz) every 15 minutes until 1 L (entire contents of container) is consumed
Dose 2: ~90 minutes after starting dose 1: 240 mL (8 oz) every 15 minutes until 1 L (entire contents of container) is consumed. Then fill container with 1 L (32 oz) of clear liquid and consume all of the liquid prior to going to bed.
Whole bowel irrigation (off-label use; AACT, 2004): Nasogastric: 1500-2000 mL/hour until the rectal effluent is clear. **Note:** Continue treatment at least until the rectal effluent is clear; treatment duration may be extended based on corroborative evidence of continued presence of poisons in the GI tract as determined by radiographic means or the presence of the poison in the effluent.

Pediatric
Bowel cleansing: Infants ≥6 months, Children, and Adolescents: GaviLyte-N, NuLYTELY, TriLyte: Oral, Nasogastric: 25 mL/kg/hour until the rectal effluent is clear (maximum total dose: 4 L)
Whole bowel irrigation (off-label use; AACT, 2004): Nasogastric:
Infants ≥9 months and Children <6 years: 500 mL/hour until the rectal effluent is clear
Children ≥6 years: 1000 mL/hour until the rectal effluent is clear
Adolescents: 1500-2000 mL/hour until the rectal effluent is clear
Note: Continue treatment at least until the rectal effluent is clear; treatment duration may be extended based on corroborative evidence of continued presence of poisons in the GI tract as determined by radiographic means or the presence of the poison in the effluent.

Renal Impairment No dosage adjustment provided in manufacturer's labeling. Use with caution due to risks of fluid and electrolyte abnormalities.
Hepatic Impairment No dosage adjustment provided in manufacturer's labeling (has not been studied).

Dietary Considerations
CoLyte, GaviLyte-C, GaviLyte-G, GaviLyte-N, GoLYTELY, NuLYTELY, TriLyte: Ideally, the patient should fast for ~3-4 hours prior to administration, but in no case should solid food be given for at least 2 hours before the solution is given. Some products contain aspartame which is metabolized to phenylalanine.
MoviPrep: Patient should not eat solid food from start of solution administration until after colonoscopy. Patient may have clear liquid soup/plain yogurt for dinner; finish at least 1 hour before start of colon prep. MoviPrep contains phenylalanine.

Administration
Oral: Rapid drinking of each portion is preferred to drinking small amounts continuously. No additional ingredients or flavors (other than the flavor packets provided) should be added to the polyethylene glycol-electrolyte solution. Chilling the solution may improve palatability; administration of a chilled solution is **not** recommended in infants. Oral medications should not be administered within 1 hour of start of therapy.

Nasogastric administration: CoLyte, GaviLyte-C, GaviLyte-G, GaviLyte-N, GoLYTELY, NuLYTELY, TriLyte: The solution may be administered via nasogastric tube for bowel cleansing and whole bowel irrigation (preferred route; off-label use) in patients who are unwilling or unable to drink the solution.
Monitoring Parameters Electrolytes, serum glucose, BUN, urine osmolality; children <2 years of age should be monitored for hypoglycemia, dehydration, hypokalemia

Whole bowel irrigation (off-label use; AACT, 2004): Rectal effluent (continue until clear or the poison is completely removed)
Dosage Forms Excipient information presented when available (limited, particularly for generics); consult specific product labeling.
Powder, for solution, oral: PEG 3350 240 g, sodium sulfate 22.72 g, sodium bicarbonate 6.72 g, sodium chloride 5.84 g, and potassium chloride 2.98 g (4000 mL); PEG 3350 236 g, sodium sulfate 22.74 g, sodium bicarbonate 6.74 g, sodium chloride 5.86 g, and potassium chloride 2.97 g (4000 mL); PEG 3350 240 g, sodium bicarbonate 5.72 g, sodium chloride 11.2 g, and potassium chloride 1.48 g (4000 mL); PEG 3350 420 g, sodium bicarbonate 5.72 g, sodium chloride 11.2 g, and potassium chloride 1.48 g (4000 mL)

Colyte: PEG 3350 227.1 g, sodium sulfate 21.5 g, sodium bicarbonate 6.36 g, sodium chloride 5.53 g, and potassium chloride 2.82 g (3785 mL) [supplied with cherry, lemon lime, and orange flavor packs]

Colyte: PEG 3350 240 g, sodium sulfate 22.72 g, sodium bicarbonate 6.72 g, sodium chloride 5.84 g, and potassium chloride 2.98 g (4000 mL) [supplied with cherry, citrus berry, lemon lime, orange, and pineapple flavor packs]

GaviLyte-C: PEG 3350 240 g, sodium sulfate 22.72 g, sodium bicarbonate 6.72 g, sodium chloride 5.84 g, and potassium chloride 2.98 g (4000 mL) [supplied with lemon flavor packet]

GaviLyte-G: PEG 3350 236 g, sodium sulfate 22.74 g, sodium bicarbonate 6.74 g, sodium chloride 5.86 g, and potassium chloride 2.97 g (4000 mL) [supplied with lemon flavor packet]

GaviLyte-N: PEG 3350 420 g, sodium bicarbonate 5.72 g, sodium chloride 11.2 g, and potassium chloride 1.48 g (4000 mL) [supplied with lemon flavor packet]

GoLYTELY: PEG 3350 227.1 g, sodium sulfate 21.5 g, sodium bicarbonate 6.36 g, sodium chloride 5.53 g, and potassium chloride 2.82 g per packet (1s) [regular flavor; makes 1 gallon of solution after mixing]

GoLYTELY: PEG 3350 236 g, sodium sulfate 22.74 g, sodium bicarbonate 6.74 g, sodium chloride 5.86 g, and potassium chloride 2.97 g (4000 mL) [regular and pineapple flavor]

MoviPrep: Pouch A: PEG 3350 100g, sodium sulfate 7.5 g, sodium chloride 2.69 g, potassium chloride 1.02 g; Pouch B: Ascorbic acid 4.7 g, sodium ascorbate 5.9 g (1000 mL) [contains phenylalanine 131 mg/treatment; lemon flavor; packaged with 2 of Pouch A and 2 of Pouch B in carton and a disposable reconstitution container]

NuLYTELY: PEG 3350 420 g, sodium bicarbonate 5.72 g, sodium chloride 11.2 g, and potassium chloride 1.48 g (4000 mL) [supplied with cherry, lemon-lime, orange, and pineapple flavor packs]

TriLyte: PEG 3350 420 g, sodium bicarbonate 5.72 g, sodium chloride 11.2 g, and potassium chloride 1.48 g (4000 mL) [supplied with cherry, citrus berry, lemon lime, orange, and pineapple flavor packs]

◆ Polyethylene Glycol Interferon Alfa-2b see Peginterferon Alfa-2b on page 1411

◆ Poly-Iron 150 [OTC] see Polysaccharide-Iron Complex on page 1469

Poly-L-Lactic Acid (POL i el LAK tik AS id)

Brand Names: US Sculptra®; Sculptra® Aesthetic
Index Terms New-Fill®; PLA
Pharmacologic Category Cosmetic Agent, Implant
Use Restoration and/or correction of facial lipoatrophy in patients with HIV; correction of shallow to deep nasolabial fold contour deficiencies and other facial wrinkles in immunocompetent patients
Dosing
Adult & Geriatric
Facial wrinkles (Sculptra® Aesthetic): Intradermal: 0.1-0.2 mL per individual injection to a maximum of 2.5 mL per nasolabial fold as a single treatment; may repeat treatment at ≥3 week intervals up to 4 times
Lipoatrophy (Sculptra®): Intradermal or SubQ: ~0.05-0.2 mL per individual injection depending on technique used; ~20 injections may be needed per cheek. Treatment should be individualized. Separate treatments by ≥2 weeks. Typical course involves 3-6 treatments. Supplemental injections may be needed. Do not overfill contour deficiency. For patients with severe facial fat loss, the average treatment requires ~1 vial per cheek area per treatment.
Additional Information Complete prescribing information should be consulted for additional detail.
Dosage Forms Excipient information presented when available (limited, particularly for generics); consult specific product labeling.
Injection, powder for suspension:
Sculptra®, Sculptra® Aesthetic: Poly-L-lactic acid USP

Polymyxin B (pol i MIKS in bee)

Index Terms Polymyxin B Sulfate
Pharmacologic Category Antibiotic, Irrigation; Antibiotic, Miscellaneous
Use Treatment of acute infections caused by susceptible strains of *Pseudomonas aeruginosa*; parenteral use of polymyxin B has mainly been replaced by less toxic antibiotics, reserved for life-threatening infections caused by

organisms resistant to the preferred drugs (eg, pseudomonal meningitis - intrathecal administration)
Dosing
Adult & Geriatric
Ear canal infections (external): Otic (in combination with other drugs): Instill 1-2 drops, 3-4 times daily; should be used sparingly to avoid accumulation of excess debris.
Bladder irrigation (in combination with 57 mg neomycin sulfate): Continuous irrigant or rinse in the urinary bladder for up to 10 days using 20 mg (equal to 200,000 units) added to 1 L of normal saline; usually no more than 1 L of irrigant is used per day unless urine flow rate is high; administration rate is adjusted to patient's urine output.
Ocular infections: Ophthalmic: A concentration of 0.1% to 0.25% is administered as 1-3 drops every hour, then increasing the interval as response indicates to 1-3 drops 4-6 times daily.
Systemic infections:
IM: 25,000-30,000 units/kg/day divided every 4-6 hours
IV: 15,000-25,000 units/kg/day divided every 12 hours
Intrathecal: 50,000 units daily for 3-4 days, then every other day for at least 2 weeks
Note: Total daily dose should not exceed 2,000,000 units.
Topical irrigation or topical solution: 500,000 units/L of normal saline; maximum daily dose should not exceed 2,000,000 units.
Selective gastrointestinal tract decontamination (off-label use): Oral: 1,000,000 units orally 4 times daily for 2 days prior to surgery through post-operative day 3 in combination with tobramycin and amphotericin B (Roos, 2011).
Pediatric
Ear canal infections (external): Children ≥2 years and Adolescents: Otic: Refer to adult dosing.
Systemic infections:
Infants and Children <2 years:
IM: Up to 40,000 units/kg/day divided every 6 hours (not routinely recommended due to pain at injection sites)
IV: Up to 40,000 units/kg/day divided every 12 hours
Intrathecal: 20,000 units daily for 3-4 days, then 25,000 units every other day for at least 2 weeks after CSF cultures are negative and CSF (glucose) has returned to within normal limits
Children ≥2 years and Adolescents: Refer to adult dosing.
Renal Impairment
For individuals with renal impairment, the manufacturer's labeling recommends a dosage reduction so that the dose does not exceed 15,000 units/kg/day.
The following adjustments have been used by some clinicians (modified from Hoeprich, 1970): IV, IM:
Loading dose (first day of therapy): CrCl <80 mL/minute: 25,000 units/kg in 2 equally divided doses every 12 hours
Subsequent dosage:
CrCl 30-80 mL/minute: 10,000-15,000 units/kg in 2 equally divided doses every 12 hours
CrCl <30 mL/minute: 10,000-15,000 units/kg every 2-3 days
Anuric patients: 10,000 units/kg every 5-7 days
Hemodialysis, peritoneal dialysis (Cunha, 1988): Adults: IM: 250,000 units every 24 hours; no supplemental dose necessary.
Note: Some data suggest that renal adjustment may not be necessary since total body clearance of polymyxin B is not altered in the setting of renal impairment and nonrenal pathways are primarily responsible for elimination (Zavascki, 2008). These authors suggest that renal dosage adjustment recommendations should await further data from larger clinical trials.
Hepatic Impairment No dosage adjustment provided in manufacturer's labeling.
Additional Information Complete prescribing information should be consulted for additional detail.
Dosage Forms Excipient information presented when available (limited, particularly for generics); consult specific product labeling.
Solution Reconstituted, Injection:
Generic: 500,000 units (1 ea)
Solution Reconstituted, Injection [preservative free]:
Generic: 500,000 units (1 ea)

◆ Polymyxin B and Bacitracin see Bacitracin and Polymyxin B (Ophthalmic) on page 196

◆ Polymyxin B and Bacitracin see Bacitracin and Polymyxin B (Topical) on page 196

◆ Polymyxin B and Neomycin see Neomycin and Polymyxin B on page 1266

- Polymyxin B and Trimethoprim see Trimethoprim and Polymyxin B on page 1847
- Polymyxin B, Bacitracin, and Neomycin see Bacitracin, Neomycin, and Polymyxin B (Ophthalmic) on page 196
- Polymyxin B, Bacitracin, and Neomycin see Bacitracin, Neomycin, and Polymyxin B (Topical) on page 197
- Polymyxin B, Bacitracin, Neomycin, and Hydrocortisone see Bacitracin, Neomycin, Polymyxin B, and Hydrocortisone (Ophthalmic) on page 197
- Polymyxin B, Bacitracin, Neomycin, and Hydrocortisone see Bacitracin, Neomycin, Polymyxin B, and Hydrocortisone (Topical) on page 197
- Polymyxin B, Neomycin, and Dexamethasone see Neomycin, Polymyxin B, and Dexamethasone on page 1267
- Polymyxin B, Neomycin, and Gramicidin see Neomycin, Polymyxin B, and Gramicidin on page 1267
- Polymyxin B, Neomycin, and Hydrocortisone see Neomycin, Polymyxin B, and Hydrocortisone (Ophthalmic) on page 1267
- Polymyxin B, Neomycin, and Hydrocortisone see Neomycin, Polymyxin B, and Hydrocortisone (Otic) on page 1267
- Polymyxin B, Neomycin, and Hydrocortisone see Neomycin, Polymyxin B, and Hydrocortisone (Topical) on page 1268
- Polymyxin B Sulfate see Polymyxin B on page 1468
- Polymyxin E see Colistimethate on page 443
- Polynuclear Iron (III)-Oxyhydroxide (pn-FeOOH) see Sucroferric Oxyhydroxide on page 1704

Polysaccharide-Iron Complex
(pol i SAK a ride-EYE ern KOM pleks)

Brand Names: US EZFE 200 [OTC]; Ferrex 150 [OTC]; Ferric x-150 [OTC]; FerUS [OTC] [DSC]; iFerex 150 [OTC]; Myferon 150 [OTC]; NovaFerrum 50 [OTC]; NovaFerrum Pediatric Drops [OTC]; Nu-Iron [OTC]; PIC 200 [OTC]; Poly-Iron 150 [OTC]
Index Terms Iron-Polysaccharide Complex; Niferex
Pharmacologic Category Iron Salt
Use Iron deficiency anemia: Management (prevention and treatment) of iron deficiency anemia
Dosing
Adult & Geriatric
Dietary Reference Intake: Dose is RDA presented as elemental iron unless otherwise noted (IOM, 2001):
19-50 years: Males: 8 mg daily; Females: 18 mg daily; Pregnant females: 27 mg daily; Lactating females: 9 mg daily
≥50 years: 8 mg daily

Iron deficiency anemia: Oral: 150-300 mg daily
Pediatric
Dietary Reference Intake: Dose is RDA presented as elemental iron unless otherwise noted (IOM, 2001):
0-6 months: 0.27 mg daily (adequate intake)
7-12 months: 11 mg daily
1-3 years: 7 mg daily
4-8 years: 10 mg daily
9-13 years: 8 mg daily
14-18 years: Males: 11 mg daily; Females: 15 mg daily; Pregnant females: 27 mg daily; Lactating females: 10 mg daily

Iron deficiency anemia: Oral:
Infants and Children <4 years: 15 mg daily
Children ≥12 years: 50 mg daily
Additional Information Complete prescribing information should be consulted for additional detail.
Dosage Forms Excipient information presented when available (limited, particularly for generics); consult specific product labeling. [DSC] = Discontinued product
Capsule, Oral:
EZFE 200: 200 mg [non-toxic; contains brilliant blue fcf (fd&c blue #1), fd&c red #40, fd&c yellow #10 (quinoline yellow)]
Ferrex 150: 150 mg [contains fd&c blue #1 aluminum lake, fd&c red #40 aluminum lake, fd&c yellow #5 aluminum lake]
Ferric x-150: 150 mg [contains brilliant blue fcf (fd&c blue #1), fd&c red #40, tartrazine (fd&c yellow #5)]
FerUS: 150 mg [DSC]
iFerex 150: 150 mg [contains brilliant blue fcf (fd&c blue #1), fd&c red #40, fd&c yellow #10 (quinoline yellow)]
Myferon 150: 150 mg
NovaFerrum 50: 50 mg
Nu-Iron: 150 mg [contains brilliant blue fcf (fd&c blue #1), fd&c red #40]

PIC 200: 200 mg
Poly-Iron 150: 150 mg
Liquid, Oral:
NovaFerrum Pediatric Drops: 15 mg/mL (120 mL) [alcohol free, dye free, gluten free, lactose free, sodium free, sugar free; contains sodium benzoate; raspberry-grape flavor]

- Polysporin [OTC] see Bacitracin and Polymyxin B (Topical) on page 196
- Polytrim® see Trimethoprim and Polymyxin B on page 1847
- Polytrim™ (Can) see Trimethoprim and Polymyxin B on page 1847
- P-OM3 see Omega-3 Fatty Acids on page 1329

Pomalidomide (poe ma LID oh mide)

Brand Names: US Pomalyst
Brand Names: Canada Pomalyst
Index Terms CC-4047
Pharmacologic Category Angiogenesis Inhibitor; Antineoplastic Agent; Immunomodulator, Systemic
Use Multiple myeloma, relapsed/refractory: Treatment of multiple myeloma (in combination with dexamethasone) in patients who have received at least 2 prior therapies, including lenalidomide and a proteasome inhibitor, and have demonstrated disease progression on or within 60 days of completion of the last therapy.
Pregnancy Considerations [US Boxed Warning]: Pomalidomide is an analogue of thalidomide (a known human teratogen) and may cause severe birth defects or embryo-fetal death if taken during pregnancy. Pomalidomide cannot be used in women who are pregnant or may become pregnant during therapy. Obtain 2 negative pregnancy tests prior to initiation of treatment; 2 forms of contraception (or abstain from heterosexual intercourse) must be used at least 4 weeks prior to, during, and for ≥4 weeks after pomalidomide treatment (and during treatment interruptions) in females of reproductive potential. In order to decrease the risk of embryo-fetal exposure, pomalidomide is available only through a restricted distribution program (Pomalyst REMS). In Canada, distribution is restricted to physicians, pharmacists, and patients registered with the RevAid program.

Studies in animals have shown evidence of fetal abnormalities and use is contraindicated in women who are or may become pregnant. Women of childbearing potential should be treated only if they are able to comply with the conditions of the Pomalyst REMS Program (US) or RevAid program (Canada). Reliable contraception is required even with a history of infertility (unless due to hysterectomy or if ≥24 consecutive months postmenopausal (natural). Reliable methods of birth control include one highly effective method (eg, tubal ligation, IUD, hormonal [birth control pills, injections, hormonal patches, vaginal rings, or implants], or partner's vasectomy) and one additional effective method (eg, male latex or synthetic condom, diaphragm, or cervical cap). Pregnancy tests should be performed 10 to 14 days (US labeling) or 7 to 14 days (Canadian labeling) and 24 hours prior to beginning therapy; weekly for the first 4 weeks and then every 4 weeks (every 2 weeks if menstrual cycle irregular) thereafter and during therapy interruptions for at least 4 weeks after discontinuation. Pomalidomide must be immediately discontinued for a missed period, abnormal pregnancy test or abnormal menstrual bleeding; refer patient to a reproductive toxicity specialist if pregnancy occurs during treatment. Pomalidomide is present in the semen of males taking this medication. Males (including those vasectomized) should use a latex or synthetic condom during any sexual contact with women of childbearing age during treatment, during treatment interruptions, and for 28 days after discontinuation. Male patients should not donate sperm. Any suspected fetal exposure should be reported in the US to the FDA via the MedWatch program (1-800-332-1088) and to Celgene Corporation (1-888-423-5436) and in Canada to Celgene (1-888-738-2341).
Breast-Feeding Considerations It is not known if pomalidomide is excreted into breast milk. Due to the potential for serious adverse reactions in the nursing infant, a decision should be made to discontinue nursing or to discontinue treatment with pomalidomide, taking into account the importance of treatment to the mother.
Prescribing and Access Restrictions As a requirement of the REMS program, access to this medication is restricted. Pomalidomide is approved for marketing in the US only under a Food and Drug Administration (FDA) approved, restricted distribution program called Pomalyst REMS (celgeneriskmanagement.com or 1-888-423-5436).

Prescribers and pharmacies must be certified with the program to prescribe or dispense pomalidomide; patients must comply with the program requirements. No more than a 4-week supply should be dispensed. Prescriptions must be filled within 7 days (for females of reproductive potential) or within 30 days (for all other patients) after the authorization number is obtained. Subsequent prescriptions may be filled only if fewer than 7 days of therapy remain on the previous prescription. A new prescription is required for further dispensing (a telephone prescription may not be accepted). Pregnancy testing with a sensitivity of at least 50 milliunits/mL is required for females of childbearing potential.

In Canada, pomalidomide is only available through a restricted distribution program called RevAid. Only physicians and pharmacists registered with the program are authorized to prescribe or dispense pomalidomide. Patients must also be registered and meet all conditions of the program. Two negative pregnancy tests with a sensitivity of at least 25 milliunits/mL are required prior to initiating therapy in women of childbearing potential. Further information is available at 1-888-738-2431 or www.RevAid.ca.

Medication Guide Available Yes

Contraindications Pregnancy

Canadian labeling: Additional contraindications (not in US labeling): Hypersensitivity to pomalidomide, thalidomide, lenalidomide, or any component of the formulation; breast-feeding; women of childbearing potential not using 2 effective means of contraception; male patients unable to comply with required contraceptive measures

Warnings/Precautions Hazardous agent - use appropriate precautions for handling and disposal (meets NIOSH 2014 criteria). Due to the embryo-fetal risk, pomalidomide is only available through a restricted program under the Pomalyst REMS program. Pomalidomide should only be prescribed to patients who can understand and comply with the conditions of the Pomalyst REMS program. Prescribers and pharmacies must be certified with the REMS program. In Canada, pomalidomide is only available through the restricted RevAid program. Prescribers and pharmacists must be registered with the program to prescribe and dispense pomalidomide; patients must also be registered and meet all conditions of the program.

[US Boxed Warning]: Pomalidomide is a thalidomide (human teratogen) analog and may cause severe life-threatening birth defects or embryo-fetal deaths; use is contraindicated in pregnancy. Pregnancy must be excluded prior to therapy initiation with 2 negative pregnancy tests; prevent pregnancy during therapy with 2 reliable forms of contraception (or abstain from heterosexual intercourse) beginning 4 weeks prior to, during and for 4 weeks after pomalidomide therapy (and during treatment interruptions) in females of reproductive potential. In order to decrease the risk of embryo-fetal exposure, pomalidomide is available only through a restricted distribution program (Pomalyst REMS). Reliable methods of birth control include one highly effective method (eg, tubal ligation, IUD, hormonal [birth control pills, injections, hormonal patches, vaginal rings, or implants], or partner's vasectomy) and one additional effective method (eg, male latex or synthetic condom, diaphragm, or cervical cap). Males taking pomalidomide must use a latex or synthetic condom during any sexual contact with a woman of childbearing potential during therapy and for up to 28 days after treatment discontinuation, even if successfully vasectomized. Patients should not donate blood during pomalidomide treatment and for 1 month after therapy discontinuation; male patients receiving pomalidomide must not donate sperm.

Neutropenia, anemia, and thrombocytopenia were frequently reported in clinical trials; neutropenia was the most frequently reported grade 3/4 adverse event, followed by anemia and thrombocytopenia. Neutropenic fever has also been reported. Monitor complete blood counts weekly for the first 8 weeks of therapy and monthly or as clinically indicated thereafter; may require therapy interruption, reduction and/or discontinuation. Acute myelogenous leukemia (AML) as a secondary malignancy has been reported in patients receiving pomalidomide in the investigational treatment of condition(s) other than multiple myeloma. **[US Boxed Warning]: Venous and arterial thromboembolic events such as deep vein thrombosis (DVT), pulmonary embolism (PE), MI, and stroke have occurred during pomalidomide therapy. Clinical trials utilized antithrombotic prophylaxis. Thromboprophylaxis is recommended; and should be based on assessment of the patient's underlying risk factors.** Arterial thrombotic events also included cerebrovascular

ischemia and ischemic heart disease. Monitor for signs/symptoms of thromboembolism (shortness of breath, chest pain, or arm or leg swelling) and advise patients to promptly seek medical attention should symptoms occur. May cause dizziness and/or confusion; caution patients to avoid tasks that require mental alertness (eg, operating machinery or driving). Avoid concomitant medications which may exacerbate dizziness and confusion. Angioedema and severe dermatologic reactions have been reported. Discontinue (permanently) for angioedema, skin exfoliation, bullae, or any other severe dermatologic toxicity. Use with caution in patients with a prior history of serious hypersensitivity reactions to thalidomide or lenalidomide; such patients were excluded from pomalidomide clinical trials and may therefore be at risk for hypersensitivity reactions when administered pomalidomide. Peripheral and sensory neuropathy occurred in clinical trials, including some cases of grade 3 neuropathy, although no cases of grade 4 neuropathy were observed. Monitor closely for signs/symptoms of neuropathy; may require therapy interruption, dose modification and/or discontinuation.

Interstitial lung disease (ILD) and related events (eg,pneumonitis) have been reported. Acute onset or unexplained worsening of pulmonary symptoms may require further evaluation to exclude ILD. The Canadian labeling recommends interruption of therapy for suspected ILD; if ILD is confirmed, treat appropriately and consider benefits/risks of pomalidomide prior to resuming therapy. Safety and efficacy have not been evaluated in patients with renal or hepatic impairment. Pomalidomide is hepatically metabolized; avoid use in patients with serum bilirubin >2 mg/dL and AST/ALT >3 times ULN (has not been studied). Hepatic failure (with fatalities) has been reported; elevated bilirubin and ALT have also been observed; monitor liver function tests; interrupt treatment and reduce dose if liver enzymes are elevated. Pomalidomide and its metabolites are excreted by the kidneys; avoid use in patients with serum creatinine >3 mg/dL (has not been studied). The Canadian labeling recommends avoiding use if CrCl <45 mL/minute. Patients with a high tumor burden may be at risk for tumor lysis syndrome; monitor closely; institute appropriate management for hyperuricemia. Potentially significant drug-drug interactions may exist, requiring dose or frequency adjustment, additional monitoring, and/or selection of alternative therapy. Cigarette smoking may induce CYP1A2 mediated metabolism of pomalidomide, potentially reducing its systemic exposure and efficacy.

Adverse Reactions Frequency not always defined.

Cardiovascular: Peripheral edema (25%), angina pectoris, congestive cardiac failure, hypotension, myocardial infarction, septic shock, syncope

Central nervous system: Fatigue (≤58%), peripheral neuropathy (22%), dizziness (22%; grades 3/4: <5%), neuropathy (18%; grades 3/4: 2%), headache (15%), anxiety (13%), confusion (12%; grades 3/4: 6%), chills (10%), insomnia (7%), pain (6%), altered mental status, depression, falling, non-cardiac chest pain

Dermatologic: Skin rash (21%), pruritus (15%), xeroderma (9%), hyperhidrosis (8%), cellulitis

Endocrine & metabolic: Hypercalcemia (22%; grades 3/4: 10%), hypokalemia (12%; grades 3/4: <5%), hyperglycemia (11%; grades 3/4: <5%), hyponatremia (11%; grades 3/4: <5%), dehydration (<10%; grade 3/4: 5%), hypocalcemia (6%), weight gain (≤5%)

Gastrointestinal: Constipation (36%), nausea (36%), diarrhea (35%), decreased appetite (23%), weight loss (15%), vomiting (14%), weight loss (15%), abdominal pain, *clostridium difficile*, increased serum alanine aminotransferase

Genitourinary: Urinary tract infection (10%, grades 3/4: 2%), urosepsis

Hematologic & oncologic: Neutropenia (53%; grades 3/4: 48%), anemia (38%; grades 3/4: 23%), thrombocytopenia (26%; grades 3/4: 22%), leukopenia (13%; grades 3/4: 7%), febrile neutropenia (<10%), lymphocytopenia (4%; grades 3/4: 2%), decreased hemoglobin

Infection: Sepsis (<10%), bacteremia, pneumonia due to *Streptococcal* species, viral infection

Neuromuscular & skeletal: Weakness (≤58%), back pain (35%), musculoskeletal chest pain (23%), muscle spasm (22%), arthralgia (17%), myasthenia (14%), musculoskeletal pain (12%), ostealgia (12%), tremor (10%), limb pain (8%), fracture, vertebral compression fracture

Renal: Increased serum creatinine (19%), renal failure (15%)

Respiratory: Upper respiratory tract infection (37%), dyspnea (36%), pneumonia (28%), epistaxis (17%), cough (17%), productive cough (9%), oropharyngeal pain (6%), bronchospasm, lobar pneumonia, pulmonary infection

Miscellaneous: Fever (23%), night sweats (5%), failure to thrive, multi-organ failure, physical health deterioration

<1% (Limited to important or life-threatening: Acute myelocytic leukemia, hyperbilirubinemia, hyperkalemia, hypersensitivity reaction, increased liver enzymes, increased serum ALT, interstitial pulmonary disease, neutropenic sepsis, pancytopenia, pelvic pain, *Pneumocystis jiroveci* pneumonia, respiratory syncytial virus infection, tumor lysis syndrome, urinary retention, vertigo

Drug Interactions

Metabolism/Transport Effects Substrate of CYP1A2 (major), CYP2C19 (minor), CYP2D6 (minor), CYP3A4 (minor), P-glycoprotein; **Note:** Assignment of Major/Minor substrate status based on clinically relevant drug interaction potential

Avoid Concomitant Use

Avoid concomitant use of Pomalidomide with any of the following: Abatacept; Anakinra; Azelastine (Nasal); BCG (Intravesical); Canakinumab; Certolizumab Pegol; CYP1A2 Inhibitors (Strong); Deferiprone; Dipyrone; Natalizumab; Orphenadrine; Paraldehyde; Pimecrolimus; Rilonacept; Tacrolimus (Topical); Thalidomide; Tocilizumab; Tofacitinib; Vaccines (Live); Vedolizumab

Increased Effect/Toxicity

Pomalidomide may increase the levels/effects of: Abatacept; Alcohol (Ethyl); Anakinra; Azelastine (Nasal); Bisphosphonate Derivatives; Buprenorphine; Canakinumab; Certolizumab Pegol; CloZAPine; CNS Depressants; Deferiprone; Fingolimod; Hydrocodone; Leflunomide; Methotrimeprazine; Metyrosine; Mirtazapine; Natalizumab; Orphenadrine; Paraldehyde; Pramipexole; Rilonacept; ROPINIRole; Rotigotine; Selective Serotonin Reuptake Inhibitors; Suvorexant; Thalidomide; Tofacitinib; Vaccines (Live); Vedolizumab; Zolpidem

The levels/effects of Pomalidomide may be increased by: Abiraterone Acetate; Brimonidine (Topical); Cannabis; CYP1A2 Inhibitors (Moderate); CYP1A2 Inhibitors (Strong); Deferasirox; Denosumab; Dipyrone; Doxylamine; Dronabinol; Droperidol; HydrOXYzine; Kava Kava; Magnesium Sulfate; Methotrimeprazine; Minocycline; Nabilone; Peginterferon Alfa-2b; Perampanel; Pimecrolimus; Roflumilast; Rufinamide; Sodium Oxybate; Tacrolimus (Topical); Tapentadol; Tetrahydrocannabinol; Tocilizumab; Trastuzumab; Vemurafenib

Decreased Effect

Pomalidomide may decrease the levels/effects of: BCG (Intravesical); Coccidioides immitis Skin Test; Sipuleucel-T; Vaccines (Inactivated); Vaccines (Live)

The levels/effects of Pomalidomide may be decreased by: Cannabis; CYP1A2 Inducers (Strong); Cyproterone; Echinacea; Osimertinib; Teriflunomide

Storage/Stability Store at 20°C to 25°C (68°F to 77°F); excursions permitted to 15°C to 30°C (59°F to 86°F).

Mechanism of Action Induces cell cycle arrest and apoptosis directly in multiple myeloma cells; enhances T cell- and natural killer (NK) cell-mediated cytotoxicity; inhibits production of proinflammatory cytokines tumor necrosis factor-α (TNF-α), IL-1, IL-6, and IL-12; inhibits angiogenesis (Zhu 2013)

Pharmacodynamics/Kinetics

Absorption: Rapid; slowed by food. Canadian labeling suggests that the overall effect of food on extent of absorption is minimal (AUC decreased 8%).

Distribution: V_{dss}: 62 to 138 L; semen distribution is ~67% of plasma levels

Protein binding: 12% to 44%

Metabolism: Hepatic via CYP1A2 and CYP3A4; CYP2C19 and CYP2D6 (minor)

Half-life elimination: ~9.5 hours (healthy subjects); ~7.5 hours (multiple myeloma patients)

Time to peak: 2 to 3 hours

Excretion: Urine (73%; 2% as unchanged drug); feces (15%; 8% as unchanged drug)

Dosing

Adult Note: ANC should be ≥500 cells/mm³ (US labeling) or ≥1,000 cells/mm³ (Canadian labeling) and platelets ≥50,000 cells/mm³ prior to initiating new cycles of therapy.

Multiple myeloma, relapsed/refractory: Oral:

4 mg once daily on days 1 to 21 of 28-day cycles (in combination with dexamethasone); continue until disease progression or unacceptable toxicity (Richardson 2014; San Miguel 2013).

Dosage adjustment for concomitant therapy with strong CYP1A2 inhibitors in the presence of strong CYP3A4 and P-gp inhibitors:

US labeling: Avoid concomitant use of strong CYP1A2 inhibitors. If concomitant use of strong CYP1A2 inhibitors in the presence of strong CYP3A4 and P-gp inhibitors cannot be avoided, reduce the pomalidomide dose by 50%.

Canadian labeling: Avoid concomitant use of strong CYP1A2 and CYP3A4 inhibitors together. There are no dosage adjustments provided in the manufacturer's labeling when concomitant use cannot be avoided; monitor closely if used in combination with a strong CYP1A2 inhibitor.

Geriatric Refer to adult dosing. The Canadian labeling recommends reducing the dosage of concurrent dexamethasone by 50% in patients >75 years of age.

Renal Impairment Serum creatinine >3 mg/dL (US labeling) or CrCl <45 mL/minute (Canadian labeling): Avoid use (has not been studied).

Hepatic Impairment

Hepatic impairment prior to treatment: Bilirubin >2 mg/dL and AST/ALT >3 times ULN: Avoid use (has not been studied).

Hepatic impairment during treatment: If liver enzymes are elevated, stop pomalidomide and evaluate; after liver enzymes return to baseline, may consider restarting at a lower dose.

Adjustment for Toxicity

Hematologic:

If ANC <500 cells/mm³ (or ANC <1,000 cells/mm³ with fever ≥38.5°C) and/or platelets <25,000 cells/mm³: Interrupt therapy and follow weekly CBCs. When ANC ≥500 cells/mm³ (US labeling) or ≥1,000 cells/mm³ (Canadian labeling) and/or platelets ≥50,000 cells/mm³: Resume dosing at 3 mg once daily.

For each subsequent drop of ANC <500 cells/mm³ and/or platelets <25,000 cells/mm³: Interrupt therapy. When ANC ≥500 cells/mm³ (US labeling) or ≥1,000 cells/mm³ (Canadian labeling) and/or platelets ≥50,000 cells/mm³: Resume dosing at 1 mg less than the previous dose. If toxicities occur at 1 mg daily dose, discontinue treatment.

Nonhematologic: If grade 3 or 4 toxicity occurs, interrupt therapy until resolved to ≤ grade 2; if appropriate, may restart therapy at 1 mg less than the previous dose. If toxicities occur at 1 mg daily dose, discontinue treatment.

Dermatologic toxicity:

Angioedema, skin exfoliation, bullae, or any other severe dermatologic toxicity: Permanently discontinue.

Canadian labeling: Grade 2 to 3 skin rash: Consider treatment interruption or discontinuation; may consider reinitiation only if potential benefits outweigh potential risks.

Pulmonary toxicity (Canadian labeling): Interrupt therapy for signs/symptoms of interstitial lung disease (ILD); if ILD is confirmed, may resume therapy only after evaluating benefit/risks.

Administration Swallow whole; do not break, chew, or open the capsules.

US labeling: Administer on an empty stomach with water (at least 2 hours before or 2 hours after a meal).

Canadian labeling: Administer without regard to meals.

Missed doses: May administer a missed dose if within 12 hours of usual dosing time. If >12 hours, skip the dose for that day and resume usual dosing the following day. Do not take 2 doses to make up for a skipped dose.

Hazardous agent; use appropriate precautions for handling and disposal (meets NIOSH 2014 criteria). NIOSH recommends single gloving for administration of intact capsules (NIOSH 2014).

Monitoring Parameters CBC with differential and platelets weekly for the first 8 weeks and monthly or as clinically necessary thereafter; renal function (ie, serum creatinine, creatinine clearance); liver function tests (monthly); monitor for signs/symptoms of thromboembolism, neuropathy, and tumor lysis syndrome (in patients at risk), and for acute or worsening pulmonary symptoms suggestive of interstitial lung disease. Consider thyroid function tests (TSH recommended at baseline and every 2 to 3 months during treatment for structurally similar medications [Hamnvik 2011]).

Women of childbearing potential: Pregnancy test 10 to 14 days (US labeling) or 7 to 14 days (Canadian labeling) **and** 24 hours prior to initiating therapy, weekly during the first month, then monthly thereafter in women with regular menstrual cycles or every 2 weeks in women with irregular menstrual cycles. Pregnancy tests should be continued for at least 4 weeks after discontinuation.

Dosage Forms Excipient information presented when available (limited, particularly for generics); consult specific product labeling.

Capsule, Oral:

Pomalyst: 1 mg, 2 mg, 3 mg [contains fd&c blue #2 (indigotine)]

Pomalyst: 4 mg [contains brilliant blue fcf (fd&c blue #1), fd&c blue #2 (indigotine)]

◆ Pomalyst see Pomalidomide on page 1469

PONATinib (poe NA ti nib)

Brand Names: US Iclusig

Index Terms AP24534; Ponatinib Hydrochloride

Pharmacologic Category Antineoplastic Agent, BCR-ABL Tyrosine Kinase Inhibitor; Antineoplastic Agent, Tyrosine Kinase Inhibitor

Use

Acute lymphoblastic leukemia: Treatment of Philadelphia chromosome-positive acute lymphoblastic leukemia (Ph+ ALL) in patients who are T315I-positive or for whom no other tyrosine kinase inhibitor therapy is indicated.

Chronic myeloid leukemia: Treatment of chronic myeloid leukemia (CML) in chronic, accelerated, or blast phase in patients who are T315I-positive or for whom no other tyrosine kinase inhibitor therapy is indicated.

Pregnancy Considerations Adverse events were observed in animal reproduction studies when administered in doses lower than or equivalent to the normal human dose. Based on its mechanism of action, adverse effects on pregnancy would be expected. Women of childbearing potential should be advised to avoid pregnancy during therapy.

Breast-Feeding Considerations It is not known if ponatinib is excreted in breast milk. Due to the potential for serious adverse reactions in the nursing infant, a decision should be made to discontinue nursing or to discontinue the drug, taking into account the importance of treatment to the mother.

Prescribing and Access Restrictions Patient access and support is available through the ARIAD PASS program. Information regarding program enrollment may be found at http://www.ariadpass.com or by calling 1-855-447-PASS (7277).

Medication Guide Available Yes

Contraindications There are no contraindications listed in the manufacturer's labeling.

Warnings/Precautions Hazardous agent - use appropriate precautions for handling and disposal (meets NIOSH 2014 criteria). **[US Boxed Warning]: Arterial and venous thrombosis and occlusions have occurred in ponatinib-treated patients. Events included fatal myocardial infarction (MI), stroke, stenosis of large arterial vessels of the brain, severe peripheral vascular disease, and the need for urgent revascularization procedures; incidents were observed in patients with and without cardiovascular risk factors (including patients ≤50 years of age). Monitor closely for thromboembolism/ vascular occlusion; interrupt or discontinue therapy immediately for vascular occlusion. Consider risk: benefit ratio when deciding to restart therapy.** Fatal and life-threatening vascular occlusion may occur within 2 weeks of therapy initiation and is not dose dependent (events have occurred at doses as low as 15 mg daily), and may cause recurrent or multisite occlusion. Increasing age and a prior history of ischemia, hypertension, diabetes, or hyperlipidemia are risk factors for development of ponatinib-associated vascular occlusion. Many patients required a revascularization procedure (cerebrovascular, coronary, and peripheral arterial) due to serious arterial thrombosis/occlusion. MI and coronary artery occlusion may result in heart failure due to myocardial ischemia. Peripheral arterial occlusive events, including fatal mesenteric artery occlusion and life-threatening peripheral arterial disease, have occurred. Some patients have required amputation due to digital or distal extremity necrosis. Venous thromboembolism, including deep vein thrombosis, pulmonary embolism, superficial thrombophlebitis, and retinal vein thrombosis, have been reported. May require dosage adjustment or discontinuation. Monitor for signs/ symptoms of arterial or venous thromboembolism.

[US Boxed Warning]: Serious heart failure (HF) or left ventricular dysfunction, including fatalities, were reported in clinical trials. Monitor for signs/symptoms of HF; interrupt or discontinue ponatinib therapy for new or worsening HF. Treat as clinically warranted if HF develops. Consider ponatinib discontinuation in the event of serious HF. Cardiac arrhythmias (bradyarrhythmias and tachyarrhythmias) have also been reported. Symptomatic bradyarrhythmia which required pacemaker implantation occurred in a few patients; other rhythms identified were complete heart block, sick sinus syndrome, and atrial fibrillation with bradycardia and pauses. Tachyarrhythmias reported include atrial fibrillation (most common), atrial flutter, supraventricular tachycardia, and atrial tachycardia; some events required hospitalization. Monitor for sign/ symptoms of bradycardia (fainting, dizziness, chest pain) and tachycardia (palpitations, dizziness). May require therapy interruption. Treatment-emergent hypertension developed in over half of ponatinib-treated patients; symptomatic hypertension or hypertensive crisis were reported in several patients, requiring urgent intervention. Blood pressure may worsen in patients with preexisting hypertension. Monitor blood pressure closely, and manage elevated pressures as clinically indicated. May require therapy interruption, dosage reduction, or discontinuation if hypertension is resistant to medical management. Renal artery stenosis (associated with worsening, labile, or treatment-resistant hypertension) has occurred in some patients receiving ponatinib. Evaluate for renal artery stenosis for hypertension that significantly worsens, is labile, or treatment-resistant.

[US Boxed Warning]: Liver failure and death resulting from ponatinib-induced hepatotoxicity were observed; monitor liver function prior to and at least monthly (or as clinically indicated) during treatment. Hepatotoxicity may require treatment interruption (followed by dose reduction) or discontinuation. One case of fulminant hepatic failure leading to death occurred within 1 week of therapy initiation; acute liver failure has also occurred. Treatment may result in ALT and/or AST elevations, and may be irreversible. A single-dose (30 mg) pharmacokinetic study found that ponatinib exposure was not increased in patients with hepatic impairment (Child-Pugh class A, B, or C) as compared to patients with normal hepatic function. While generally well tolerated, patients with hepatic impairment did have an increased overall incidence of adverse reactions (eg, gastrointestinal disorders, pancreatitis). Monitor closely when administering to patients with impaired hepatic function. The starting dose should be reduced in patients with hepatic impairment.

Severe myelosuppression (grade 3 or 4) was commonly observed in clinical trials, and the incidence was greater in patients with accelerated or blast phase CML and Ph+ ALL. Monitor blood counts closely; may require therapy interruption and/or dosage reduction. Hemorrhagic events occurred commonly in ponatinib-treated patients, including serious events such as cerebral and gastrointestinal hemorrhages; fatalities were reported. Serious bleeding episodes occurred more frequently in patients with accelerated or blast phase CML, and Ph+ ALL; most patients had grade 4 thrombocytopenia. Monitor platelet levels closely and for signs/symptoms of bleeding, and interrupt therapy if necessary.

Treatment-related lipase elevations and clinical pancreatitis occurred in clinical studies; the majority of cases resolved within 2 weeks of therapy interruption or dose reduction. Monitor serum lipase every 2 weeks for the first 2 months and monthly thereafter or as clinically indicated; more frequent monitoring may be considered in patients with a history of pancreatitis or alcohol abuse. Monitor for clinical signs of pancreatitis, such as abdominal symptoms; interrupt therapy if necessary. Do not reinitiate treatment until complete resolution of symptoms and lipase level is <1.5 times ULN. Serious gastrointestinal perforation (fistula) occurred very rarely; monitor for signs/symptoms of perforation and/or fistula. Serious fluid retention events, including fatality due to brain edema (very rare), were observed in ponatinib-treated patients. Peripheral edema, pleural effusions, and pericardial effusions were commonly seen; effusions and ascites were less common. Monitor patients for fluid retention; may require therapy interruption, dosage reduction, or discontinuation.

Peripheral and cranial neuropathy have been reported. Peripheral neuropathy, paresthesia, hypoesthesia, and hyperesthesia occurred most frequently; cranial neuropathy occurred rarely. In one-third of patients who experienced symptoms, neuropathy developed during the first month of therapy. Monitor for signs/symptoms of neuropathy; consider interrupting treatment if neuropathy develops. Serious ocular events such as blindness and blurred

vision have occurred with ponatinib use. Macular edema, retinal vein occlusion, and retinal hemorrhage have been reported in a small percentage of patients; conjunctival or corneal irritation, dry eye, or eye pain occurred more frequently. Other toxicities include cataracts, glaucoma, iritis, iridocyclitis, and ulcerative keratitis. Perform comprehensive ophthalmic exams prior to therapy initiation and periodically during treatment.

Hyperuricemia and serious tumor lysis syndrome (rare) were reported. Patients should receive adequate hydration and be monitored for elevated uric acid levels and/or the development of tumor lysis syndrome. Correct elevated uric acid levels prior to initiating therapy. As ponatinib inhibits VEGF activity, therapy may impair wound healing. Hold therapy for at least 1 week prior to major surgery; resume therapy post procedure based on clinical judgment of appropriate wound healing. Potentially significant drug-drug interactions may exist, requiring dose or frequency adjustment, additional monitoring, and/or selection of alternative therapy. Patients ≥65 years of age may be more likely to experience weakness, decreased appetite, dyspnea, increased lipase, muscle spasms, peripheral edema, and thrombocytopenia; monitor closely. Cautious dose selection is recommended based on greater frequency of decreased hepatic, renal, or cardiac function, and of concomitant disease or other drug therapy.

Adverse Reactions

>10%:
Cardiovascular: Hypertension (53% to 71%), peripheral edema (13% to 22%; grades 3/4: ≤1%), arterial ischemia (3% to 20%; grades 3/4: ≤11%; including cardiac, cerebrovascular, and peripheral-vascular ischemia), cardiac failure (6% to 15%; including congestive heart failure, reduced ejection fraction, pulmonary edema, cardiogenic shock, cardiorespiratory arrest, right ventricular failure), myocardial infarction (12%)
Central nervous system: Fatigue or weakness (31% to 39%), headache (25% to 39%), pain (6% to 16%), chills (7% to 13%), insomnia (7% to 12%), dizziness (3% to 11%)
Dermatologic: Skin rash (34% to 54%), xeroderma (24% to 39%), cellulitis (≤11%)
Endocrine & metabolic: Increased serum glucose (58%), decreased serum phosphate (57%), decreased serum calcium (52%), decreased serum sodium (29%), decreased serum glucose (24%), decreased serum potassium (16%), increased serum potassium (15%), decreased serum bicarbonate (11%)
Gastrointestinal: Abdominal pain (34% to 49%), constipation (24% to 47%), increased serum lipase (41%; grades 3/4: 15%), nausea (22% to 32%), decreased appetite (8% to 31%), diarrhea (13% to 26%), vomiting (13% to 24%), stomatitis (9% to 23%), weight loss (5% to 13%), gastrointestinal hemorrhage (2% to 11%; grades 3/4: ≤6%)
Genitourinary: Urinary tract infection (≤12%)
Hematologic & oncologic: Neutropenia (grades 3/4: 24% to 63%), leukopenia (grades 3/4: 14% to 63%), thrombocytopenia (grades 3/4: 36% to 57%), anemia (grades 3/4: 9% to 55%), bone marrow depression (severe grade 3 or 4: 48%), lymphocytopenia (grades 3/4: 10% to 37%), febrile neutropenia (1% to 25%), hemorrhage (24%; including cerebral hemorrhage and gastrointestinal hemorrhage)
Hepatic: Increased serum ALT (53%; grades 3/4: 8%), increased serum AST (41%; grades 3/4: 4%), increased serum alkaline phosphatase (37%), decreased serum albumin (28%), increased serum bilirubin (19%)
Infection: Sepsis (1% to 22%)
Miscellaneous: Fever (23% to 32%)
Neuromuscular & skeletal: Arthralgia (13% to 31%), myalgia (6% to 22%), limb pain (9% to 17%), back pain (11% to 16%), peripheral neuropathy (6% to 16%; including burning sensation), muscle spasm (5% to 13%), ostealgia (9% to 12%)
Respiratory: Dyspnea (6% to 21%), pleural effusion (3% to 19%; grades 3/4: ≤3%), cough (6% to 18%), pneumonia (3% to 13%), nasopharyngitis (3% to 12%), upper respiratory tract infection (≤11%)
1% to 10%:
Cardiovascular: Peripheral ischemia (8%), supraventricular tachycardia (5%), venous thromboembolism (5%), atrial fibrillation (4%), pericardial effusion (1% to 3%), cerebral hemorrhage (2%), bradycardia (1%; symptomatic)
Endocrine & metabolic: Increased serum sodium (10%), hyperuricemia (7%), increased serum calcium (5%), increased serum triglycerides (3%)
Gastrointestinal: Pancreatitis (6%; grade 3: 5%), increased serum amylase (3%)

Ophthalmic: Blurred vision (6%), retinal toxicity (3%, including macular edema, retinal vein occlusion, retinal hemorrhage)
Renal: Increased serum creatinine (7%)
Frequency not defined:
Cardiovascular: Cerebrovascular accident
Gastrointestinal: Mouth pain, oral mucosa ulcer, oropharyngeal pain, throat ulcer, tongue ulcer
Ophthalmic: Cataract, conjunctival irritation, corneal ulcer, dry eye syndrome, eye pain, glaucoma, iridocyclitis, iritis, keratitis
<1% (Limited to important or life-threatening): Acute hepatic failure, ascites, atrial flutter, atrial tachycardia, cerebral edema, complete atrioventricular block, gastrointestinal fistula, gastrointestinal perforation, mesenteric artery occlusion, pulmonary embolism, retinal vein thrombosis, sick sinus syndrome, tumor lysis syndrome (serious)

Drug Interactions

Metabolism/Transport Effects Substrate of BCRP, CYP2C8 (minor), CYP2D6 (minor), CYP3A4 (minor), P-glycoprotein; **Note:** Assignment of Major/Minor substrate status based on clinically relevant drug interaction potential; **Inhibits** BCRP, BSEP, P-glycoprotein

Avoid Concomitant Use
Avoid concomitant use of PONATinib with any of the following: BCG (Intravesical); CYP3A4 Inducers (Strong); Deferiprone; Dipyrone; St Johns Wort

Increased Effect/Toxicity
PONATinib may increase the levels/effects of: CloZAPine; Deferiprone

The levels/effects of PONATinib may be increased by: CYP3A4 Inhibitors (Strong); Dipyrone; Grapefruit Juice

Decreased Effect
PONATinib may decrease the levels/effects of: BCG (Intravesical)

The levels/effects of PONATinib may be decreased by: CYP3A4 Inducers (Strong); St Johns Wort

Storage/Stability Store at 20°C to 25°C (68°F to 77°F); excursions permitted between 15°C to 30°C (59°F to 86°F).

Mechanism of Action Ponatinib is a pan-BCR-ABL tyrosine kinase inhibitor with *in vitro* activity against cells expressing native or mutant BCR-ABL (including T315I); it also inhibits VEGFR, FGFR, PDGFR, EPH, and SRC kinases, as well as KIT, RET, TIE2, and FLT3.

Pharmacodynamics/Kinetics

Absorption: Plasma concentrations not affected by food
Distribution: V_d: 1223 L
Protein binding: >99% to plasma proteins
Metabolism: Primarily hepatic through CYP3A4; CYP2C8, CYP2D6, and CYP3A5 are also involved in metabolism. Phase II metabolism occurs via esterases and/or amidases.
Half-life elimination: ~24 hours (range: 12 to 66 hours)
Time to peak: ≤6 hours
Excretion: Feces (~87%); urine (~5%)

Dosing

Adult & Geriatric Note: The optimal ponatinib dose has not been identified. Consider discontinuing therapy if no response has occurred by 3 months (90 days) of therapy.
Acute lymphoblastic leukemia (ALL), Philadelphia chromosome-positive (Ph+), T315I-positive or in patients for whom no other tyrosine kinase inhibitor therapy is indicated: Oral: Initial: 45 mg once daily
Chronic myeloid leukemia (CML); chronic, accelerated, or blast phase), T315I-positive or in patients for whom no other tyrosine kinase inhibitor therapy is indicated: Oral: Initial: 45 mg once daily; consider reducing the dose for patients in chronic or accelerated phase who have achieved a major cytogenetic response

Dosage adjustment for strong CYP3A inhibitors: Reduce ponatinib dose to 30 mg once daily when administered with concomitant strong CYP3A inhibitors (eg, boceprevir, clarithromycin, conivaptan, grapefruit juice, indinavir, itraconazole, ketoconazole, lopinavir/ritonavir, nefazodone, nelfinavir, posaconazole, ritonavir, saquinavir, telaprevir, telithromycin, voriconazole).

Renal Impairment There are no dosage adjustments provided in the manufacturer's labeling (has not been studied); although renal excretion is not a major excretion route for ponatinib.

Hepatic Impairment
Hepatic impairment prior to treatment initiation: Mild-to-severe impairment (Child-Pugh class A, B, or C): Initial: 30 mg once daily; monitor closely for toxicity.

Hepatotoxicity during treatment:

AST or ALT >3 times ULN (≥ grade 2): If toxicity occurs at a dose of 45 mg daily, interrupt therapy; upon recovery to ≤ grade 1 (<3 times ULN), resume therapy at 30 mg daily. If toxicity occurs at a dose of 30 mg daily, interrupt therapy; upon recovery to ≤ grade 1, resume therapy at 15 mg daily. If toxicity occurs at a dose of 15 mg daily, discontinue therapy.

ALT or AST ≥3 times ULN with bilirubin >2 times ULN and alkaline phosphatase <2 times ULN: Discontinue therapy.

Adjustment for Toxicity

Hematologic: ANC <1000/mm^3 or platelets <50,000/mm^3:

First occurrence: Interrupt therapy; upon recovery of ANC to ≥1500/mm^3 and platelets to ≥75,000/mm^3, resume therapy at 45 mg daily.

Second occurrence: Interrupt therapy; upon recovery of ANC to ≥1500/mm^3 and platelets to ≥75,000/mm^3, resume therapy at a reduced dose of 30 mg daily.

Third occurrence: Interrupt therapy; upon recovery of ANC to ≥1500/mm^3 and platelets to ≥75,000/mm^3, resume therapy at a reduced dose of 15 mg daily.

Nonhematologic toxicity:

Arterial or venous occlusive reactions: Interrupt therapy; do not resume ponatinib in the event of serious occlusive events unless the potential benefit of therapy outweighs the risk of recurrent occlusions and other treatment options are not available.

Pancreatitis and lipase elevations:

Asymptomatic grade 1 or 2 serum lipase elevation: Consider interrupting therapy or dose reduction.

Asymptomatic grade 3 or 4 serum lipase elevation (>2 times ULN) or asymptomatic radiologic pancreatitis (grade 2): If toxicity occurs at a dose of 45 mg daily, interrupt therapy; upon recovery to ≤ grade 1 (<1.5 times ULN), resume therapy at a reduced dose of 30 mg daily. If toxicity occurs at a dose of 30 mg daily, interrupt therapy; upon recovery to ≤ grade 1, resume therapy at a reduced dose of 15 mg daily. If toxicity occurs at a dose of 15 mg daily, discontinue therapy.

Symptomatic grade 3 pancreatitis: If toxicity occurs at a dose of 45 mg daily, interrupt therapy; upon recovery of serum lipase elevation to ≤ grade 1 and complete symptom resolution, resume therapy at a reduced dose of 30 mg daily. If toxicity occurs at a dose of 30 mg daily, interrupt therapy; upon recovery of serum lipase elevation to ≤ grade 1 and complete symptom resolution, resume therapy at a reduced dose of 15 mg daily. If toxicity occurs at a dose of 15 mg daily, discontinue therapy.

Grade 4 pancreatitis: Discontinue therapy.

Other nonhematologic toxicities: For serious reactions (other than arterial or venous occlusion), modify the dose or interrupt treatment; do not restart therapy until symptom resolution or unless the benefit of therapy outweighs the risk of recurrent toxicity.

Dietary Considerations Avoid grapefruit juice.

Administration Administer with or without food. Swallow tablets whole (do not crush or dissolve). Hazardous agent; use appropriate precautions for handling and disposal (meets NIOSH 2014 criteria). NIOSH recommends single gloving for administration of intact tablets (NIOSH 2014).

Monitoring Parameters CBC with differential and platelets every 2 weeks for the first 3 months, then monthly or as clinically needed; liver function tests at baseline and at least monthly thereafter or more frequently if clinically warranted; serum lipase every 2 weeks for the first 2 months and monthly thereafter (more frequently in patients with a history of pancreatitis or alcohol abuse); serum electrolytes and uric acid; monitor cardiac function, blood pressure, signs/symptoms of arterial/venous occlusion or thromboembolism, hemorrhage, fluid retention, pancreatitis (clinical signs), gastrointestinal perforation/fistula, hepatotoxicity (jaundice, anorexia, bleeding, bruising); comprehensive ocular exam at baseline and periodically; signs/symptoms of neuropathy

Dosage Forms Excipient information presented when available (limited, particularly for generics); consult specific product labeling.

Tablet, Oral:

Iclusig: 15 mg, 45 mg

◆ Ponatinib Hydrochloride *see* PONATinib *on page 1472*

◆ Ponstan (Can) *see* Mefenamic Acid *on page 1134*

◆ Ponstel *see* Mefenamic Acid *on page 1134*

◆ Pontocaine [DSC] *see* Tetracaine (Systemic) *on page 1772*

◆ Pontocaine [DSC] *see* Tetracaine (Topical) *on page 1773*

◆ Pontocaine (Can) *see* Tetracaine (Systemic) *on page 1772*

◆ Pontocaine (Can) *see* Tetracaine (Topical) *on page 1773*

Porfimer (POR fi mer)

Brand Names: US Photofrin

Brand Names: Canada Photofrin

Index Terms CL-184116; Dihematoporphyrin Ether; Porfimer Sodium

Pharmacologic Category Antineoplastic Agent, Miscellaneous

Use

Barrett esophagus: Ablation of high-grade dysplasia in Barrett esophagus (in patients who do not undergo esophagectomy)

Endobronchial cancer: Treatment of microinvasive endobronchial non-small cell lung cancer (NSCLC) in patients for whom surgery and radiation therapy are not indicated; reduction of obstruction and symptom palliation in patients with obstructing (partial or complete) endobronchial NSCLC

Esophageal cancer: Palliation of obstructing (partial or complete) esophageal cancer (in patients who cannot be treated satisfactorily with laser therapy)

Canadian labeling: Additional use (not in US labeling: Second-line treatment of recurrent, superficial papillary bladder cancer

Dosing

Adult & Geriatric

Photodynamic therapy in esophageal cancer or endobronchial non-small cell lung cancer: IV: 2 mg/kg, followed by endoscopic exposure to the appropriate laser light and debridement; repeat courses must be separated by at least 30 days (delay subsequent treatment for insufficient healing) for a maximum of 3 courses

Photodynamic therapy in Barrett esophagus dysplasia: IV: 2 mg/kg, followed by endoscopic exposure to the appropriate laser light; repeat courses must be separated by at least 90 days (delay subsequent treatment for insufficient healing) for a maximum of 3 courses

Photodynamic therapy in papillary bladder cancer (Canadian labeling; not in U.S. labeling): IV: 2 mg/kg, followed by cystoscopic exposure to the appropriate laser light. **Note:** Repeat dosing is not recommended due to increased risk of bladder contracture.

Renal Impairment There are no dosage adjustments provided in the manufacturer's labeling (has not been studied).

Hepatic Impairment There are no dosage adjustments provided in the manufacturer's labeling (has not been studied).

Additional Information Complete prescribing information should be consulted for additional detail.

Dosage Forms Excipient information presented when available (limited, particularly for generics); consult specific product labeling.

Solution Reconstituted, Intravenous, as sodium [preservative free]:

Photofrin: 75 mg (1 ea)

Dosage Forms: Canada Excipient information presented when available (limited, particularly for generics); consult specific product labeling.

Injection, powder for reconstitution, as sodium:

Photofrin®: 15 mg

◆ Porfimer Sodium *see* Porfimer *on page 1474*

◆ Portia *see* Ethinyl Estradiol and Levonorgestrel *on page 703*

◆ Portrazza *see* Necitumumab *on page 1263*

Posaconazole (poe sa KON a zole)

Brand Names: US Noxafil

Brand Names: Canada Posanol

Index Terms SCH 56592

Pharmacologic Category Antifungal Agent, Oral

Additional Appendix Information

Oral Dosages That Should Not Be Crushed *on page 2003*

Use

Prophylaxis of invasive *Aspergillus* and *Candida* infections: Suspension and delayed-release tablets (13 years and older) and injection (18 years and older): Prophylaxis of invasive *Aspergillus* and *Candida* infections in patients who are at high risk of developing these infections due to being severely immunocompromised (eg, hematopoietic stem cell transplant [HSCT] recipients with graft-versus-host disease [GVHD] or those with prolonged

neutropenia secondary to chemotherapy for hematologic malignancies).

Oropharyngeal candidiasis: Suspension (13 years and older): Treatment of oropharyngeal candidiasis (including patients refractory to itraconazole and/or fluconazole)

Canadian labeling: Additional use (not in US labeling): **Invasive Aspergillus and Candida infections:** Suspension and delayed-release tablets (13 years and older) and injection (18 years and older): Treatment of invasive aspergillosis in patients refractory to or intolerant of itraconazole or amphotericin B

Pregnancy Considerations Adverse events have been observed in animal reproduction studies.

Breast-Feeding Considerations It is not known if posaconazole is excreted in breast milk. Due to the potential for serious adverse reactions in the nursing infant, the manufacturer recommends a decision be made to discontinue nursing or the drug, taking into account the importance of treatment to the mother.

Contraindications

Coadministration with sirolimus, ergot alkaloids (eg, ergotamine, dihydroergotamine), HMG-CoA reductase inhibitors that are primarily metabolized through CYP3A4 (eg, atorvastatin, lovastatin, simvastatin), or CYP3A4 substrates that prolong the QT interval (eg, pimozide, quinidine); hypersensitivity to posaconazole, other azole antifungal agents, or any component of the formulation.

Canadian labeling: Additional contraindications (not in US labeling): Coadministration with terfenadine, astemizole, or cisapride (each drug is no longer marketed in Canada).

Warnings/Precautions The delayed-release tablet and oral suspension are not to be used interchangeably due to dosing differences for each formulation. Hepatic dysfunction has occurred, ranging from mild/moderate increases of ALT, AST, alkaline phosphatase, total bilirubin, and/or clinical hepatitis to severe reactions (cholestasis, hepatic failure including death). Consider discontinuation of therapy in patients who develop clinical evidence of liver disease that may be secondary to posaconazole. Elevations in liver function tests have been generally reversible after posaconazole has been discontinued; some cases resolved without drug interruption. More severe reactions have been observed in patients with underlying serious medical conditions (eg, hematologic malignancy) and primarily with suspension total daily doses of 800 mg. Monitor liver function tests at baseline and periodically during therapy. If increases occur, monitor for severe hepatic injury development. Use caution in patients with an increased risk of arrhythmia (long QT syndrome, concurrent QTc-prolonging drugs, drugs metabolized through CYP3A4, hypokalemia). Correct electrolyte abnormalities (eg, potassium, magnesium, and calcium) before initiating therapy. Potentially significant drug-drug interactions may exist, requiring dose or frequency adjustment, additional monitoring, and/or selection of alternative therapy.

US labeling contraindicates use in patients with hypersensitivity to other azole antifungal agents; Canadian labeling does not contraindicate use, but recommends using caution in hypersensitivity with other azole antifungal agents; cross-reaction may occur, but has not been established. Consider alternative therapy or closely monitor for breakthrough fungal infections in patients receiving drugs that decrease absorption or increase the metabolism of posaconazole or in any patient unable to eat or tolerate an oral liquid nutritional supplement or acidic carbonated beverage (eg, ginger ale). Do not give IV formulation as an intravenous bolus injection. Avoid/limit use of IV formulation in patients with eGFR <50 mL/minute/1.73 m^2; injection contains excipient cyclodextrin (sulfobutyl ether beta-cyclodextrin [SBECD]), which may accumulate; consider using oral posaconazole in these patients unless benefit of injection outweighs the risk. Evaluate renal function (particularly serum creatinine) at baseline and periodically during therapy. If increases occur, consider oral therapy. Monitor for breakthrough fungal infections. Patients weighing >120 kg may have lower plasma drug exposure; monitor closely for breakthrough fungal infections. Oral suspension contains glucose; patients with rare glucose-galactose malabsorption may require alternative agents.

Benzyl alcohol and derivatives: Some dosage forms may contain sodium benzoate/benzoic acid; benzoic acid (benzoate) is a metabolite of benzyl alcohol; large amounts of benzyl alcohol (≥99 mg/kg/day) have been associated with a potentially fatal toxicity ("gasping syndrome") in neonates; the "gasping syndrome" consists of metabolic acidosis, respiratory distress, gasping respirations, CNS dysfunction (including convulsions, intracranial hemorrhage), hypotension, and cardiovascular collapse (AAP

["Inactive" 1997]; CDC 1982); some data suggests that benzoate displaces bilirubin from protein binding sites (Ahlfors 2001); avoid or use dosage forms containing benzyl alcohol derivative with caution in neonates. See manufacturer's labeling.

Polysorbate 80: Some dosage forms may contain polysorbate 80 (also known as Tweens). Hypersensitivity reactions, usually a delayed reaction, have been reported following exposure to pharmaceutical products containing polysorbate 80 in certain individuals (Isaksson 2002; Lucente 2000; Shelley 1995). Thrombocytopenia, ascites, pulmonary deterioration, and renal and hepatic failure have been reported in premature neonates after receiving parenteral products containing polysorbate 80 (Alade 1986; CDC 1984). See manufacturer's labeling.

Adverse Reactions Note: Unless otherwise specified, incidences represent adverse reactions identified with oral formulations; systemic includes oral and intravenous routes. Percentages reflect data from use in comparator trials with multiple concomitant conditions and medications; some adverse reactions may be due to underlying condition(s).

>10%:

Cardiovascular: Thrombophlebitis (intravenous via peripheral venous catheter: 60%), hypertension (systemic: 8% to 18%), peripheral edema (systemic: 12% to 16%), edema (9% to 15%), hypotension (14%), tachycardia (12%)

Central nervous system: Headache (systemic: 8% to 28%), rigors (≤20%), fatigue (systemic: 3% to 17%), insomnia (1% to 17%), chills (systemic: 10% to 16%), lower extremity edema (15%), dizziness (11%), pain (1% to 11%)

Dermatologic: Skin rash (systemic: 15% to 24%), pruritus (11%)

Endocrine & metabolic: Hypokalemia (systemic: ≤30%), hypomagnesemia (systemic: 10% to 18%), weight loss (1% to 14%), hyperglycemia (11%), dehydration (1% to 11%)

Gastrointestinal: Diarrhea (systemic: 10% to 42%), nausea (systemic: 2% to 38%), vomiting (systemic: 7% to 29%), abdominal pain (systemic: 5% to 27%), constipation (systemic: 8% to 21%), anorexia (2% to 19%), mucositis (14% to 17%), stomatitis (14%), decreased appetite (systemic: 10% to 12%), oral candidiasis (1% to 12%), upper abdominal pain (systemic: 6% to 11%)

Hematologic & oncologic: Thrombocytopenia (systemic: <5% to 29%), anemia (systemic: 2% to 25%), neutropenia (4% to 23%), febrile neutropenia (20%), petechia (systemic: 8% to 11%)

Hepatic: Increased serum ALT (<5% to 17%)

Infection: Bacteremia (18%), herpes simplex infection (3% to 15%), cytomegalovirus disease (14%)

Neuromuscular & skeletal: Musculoskeletal pain (16%), weakness (2% to 13%), arthralgia (11%)

Respiratory: Cough (systemic: 3% to 25%), dyspnea (systemic: 1% to 20%), epistaxis (systemic: 14% to 17%), pharyngitis (12%)

Miscellaneous: Fever (systemic: 6% to 45%)

1% to 10%:

Cardiovascular: Pulmonary embolism (<5%), torsades de pointes (<5%)

Central nervous system: Anxiety (9%), paresthesia (<5%)

Dermatologic: Diaphoresis (2% to 10%)

Endocrine & metabolic: Hypocalcemia (9%), adrenocortical insufficiency (<5%)

Gastrointestinal: Dyspepsia (10%)

Genitourinary: Vaginal hemorrhage (10%)

Hematologic & oncologic: Hemolytic-uremic syndrome (<5%), thrombotic thrombocytopenic purpura (<5%)

Hepatic: Hyperbilirubinemia (<5% to 10%), increased serum AST (3% to <5%), hepatic failure (<5%), hepatitis (<5%), hepatomegaly (<5%), jaundice (<5%), increased liver enzymes (<5%), increased serum alkaline phosphatase (1% to 3%)

Hypersensitivity: Hypersensitivity reaction (<5%)

Neuromuscular & skeletal: Back pain (10%)

Renal: Acute renal failure (<5%)

Respiratory: Pneumonia (3% to 10%), upper respiratory tract infection (7%)

<1% (Limited to important or life-threatening): Atrial fibrillation, cholestasis, hypersensitivity, prolonged Q-T interval on ECG, reduced ejection fraction, syncope

Drug Interactions

Metabolism/Transport Effects Inhibits CYP3A4 (strong)

Avoid Concomitant Use

Avoid concomitant use of Posaconazole with any of the following: Ado-Trastuzumab Emtansine; Alfuzosin; Aprepitant; Astemizole; AtorvaSTATin; Avanafil; Axitinib; Barnidipine; Bosutinib; Bromocriptine; Cabozantinib;

Ceritinib; Cisapride; Cobimetinib; Conivaptan; Crizotinib; Dabrafenib; Dapoxetine; Dihydroergotamine; Dofetilide; Domperidone; Dronedarone; Efavirenz; Eletriptan; Eplerenone; Ergoloid Mesylates; Ergonovine; Ergotamine; Everolimus; Flibanserin; Halofantrine; Ibrutinib; Irinotecan Products; Isavuconazonium Sulfate; Ivabradine; Lapatinib; Lercanidipine; Lomitapide; Lovastatin; Lumacaftor; Lurasidone; Macitentan; Methadone; Methylergonovine; Naloxegol; Nilotinib; NiMODipine; Nisoldipine; Olaparib; Osimertinib; Palbociclib; Pimozide; QuiNIDine; Ranolazine; Red Yeast Rice; Regorafenib; Saccharomyces boulardii; Salmeterol; Silodosin; Simeprevir; Simvastatin; Sirolimus; Sonidegib; Suvorexant; Tamsulosin; Terfenadine; Ticagrelor; Tolvaptan; Toremifene; Trabectedin; Ulipristal; Vemurafenib; VinCRIStine (Liposomal); Vorapaxar

Increased Effect/Toxicity

Posaconazole may increase the levels/effects of: Ado-Trastuzumab Emtansine; Alfuzosin; Alitretinoin (Systemic); Almotriptan; Alosetron; Antineoplastic Agents (Vinca Alkaloids); Apixaban; Aprepitant; ARIPiprazole; ARIPiprazole Lauroxil; Astemizole; Atazanavir; AtorvaSTATin; Avanafil; Axitinib; Barnidipine; Bedaquiline; Boceprevir; Bortezomib; Bosentan; Bosutinib; Brentuximab Vedotin; Brexpiprazole; Brinzolamide; Bromocriptine; Budesonide (Nasal); Budesonide (Oral Inhalation); Budesonide (Systemic); Budesonide (Topical); BusPIRone; Busulfan; Cabazitaxel; Cabozantinib; Calcium Channel Blockers; Cannabis; Cariprazine; Ceritinib; Cilostazol; Cisapride; Cobimetinib; Colchicine; Conivaptan; Corticosteroids (Orally Inhaled); Corticosteroids (Systemic); Crizotinib; CycloSPORINE (Systemic); CYP3A4 Substrates; Dabrafenib; Daclatasvir; Dapoxetine; Dasatinib; Dienogest; Digoxin; Dihydroergotamine; DOCEtaxel; Dofetilide; Domperidone; DOXOrubicin (Conventional); Dronabinol; Dronedarone; Drospirenone; Dutasteride; Eletriptan; Eliglustat; Enzalutamide; Eplerenone; Ergoloid Mesylates; Ergonovine; Ergotamine; Erlotinib; Estazolam; Etizolam; Etravirine; Everolimus; FentaNYL; Fesoterodine; Flibanserin; Fluticasone (Nasal); Fluticasone (Oral Inhalation); Fosamprenavir; Fosphenytoin; Gefitinib; GlipiZIDE; GuanFACINE; Halofantrine; Highest Risk QTc-Prolonging Agents; Hydrocodone; Ibrutinib; Idelalisib; Iloperidone; Imatinib; Imidafenacin; Irinotecan Products; Isavuconazonium Sulfate; Ivabradine; Ivacaftor; Ixabepilone; Lacosamide; Lapatinib; Lercanidipine; Levobupivacaine; Levomilnacipran; Lomitapide; Losartan; Lovastatin; Lurasidone; Macitentan; Maraviroc; MedroxyPROGESTERone; Methadone; Methylergonovine; MethylPREDNISolone; Mifepristone; Moderate Risk QTc-Prolonging Agents; Naloxegol; Nilotinib; NiMODipine; Nisoldipine; Olaparib; Osimertinib; Ospemifene; Oxybutynin; OxyCODONE; Palbociclib; Panobinostat; Parecoxib; Paricalcitol; PAZOPanib; Phenytoin; Pimecrolimus; Pimozide; PONATinib; Pranlukast; PredniSOLONE (Systemic); PredniSONE; Propafenone; QUEtiapine; QuiNIDine; Ramelteon; Ranolazine; Red Yeast Rice; Regorafenib; Repaglinide; Retapamulin; Rifamycin Derivatives; Rilpivirine; Ritonavir; RomiDEPsin; Ruxolitinib; Salmeterol; Saxagliptin; Sildenafil; Silodosin; Simeprevir; Simvastatin; Sirolimus; Solifenacin; Sonidegib; SORAfenib; SUNItinib; Suvorexant; Tacrolimus (Systemic); Tacrolimus (Topical); Tadalafil; Tamsulosin; Tasimelteon; Telaprevir; Temsirolimus; Terfenadine; Tetrahydrocannabinol; Ticagrelor; Tofacitinib; Tolterodine; Tolvaptan; Toremifene; Trabectedin; TraMADol; Ulipristal; Vardenafil; Vemurafenib; Vilazodone; VinCRIStine (Liposomal); Vitamin K Antagonists; Vorapaxar; Zopiclone; Zuclopenthixol

The levels/effects of Posaconazole may be increased by: Boceprevir; Etravirine; Mifepristone; Telaprevir

Decreased Effect

Posaconazole may decrease the levels/effects of: Amphotericin B; Ifosfamide; Prasugrel; Saccharomyces boulardii; Ticagrelor

The levels/effects of Posaconazole may be decreased by: Didanosine; Efavirenz; Etravirine; Fosamprenavir; Fosphenytoin; H2-Antagonists; Lumacaftor; Metoclopramide; Phenytoin; Proton Pump Inhibitors; Rifamycin Derivatives; Sucralfate

Food Interactions
Bioavailability increased ~3 times when posaconazole suspension was administered with a nonfat meal or an oral liquid nutritional supplement; increased ~4 times when administered with a high-fat meal. Following administration of posaconazole delayed-release tablets, the AUC increased 51% when given with a high-fat meal compared with a fasted state. Management: Suspension must be administered with or within 20 minutes of a full meal, an oral liquid nutritional supplement, or an acidic carbonated beverage (eg, ginger ale). Take tablet with food. Consider alternative antifungal therapy in patients with inadequate oral intake or severe diarrhea/vomiting.

Preparation for Administration
IV: Equilibrate the refrigerated vial to room temperature. Contents of vial should be withdrawn and admixed with D_5W, D_5W with KCl 20 mEq, D_5NS, $D_51/2NS$, 1/2NS, or NS to achieve a concentration of 1 to 2 mg/mL. The admixed solution may be colorless to yellow. Color variations in this range do not affect potency. Admixture should be used immediately; may be stored for up to 24 hours between 2°C and 8°C (36°F and 46°F).

Storage/Stability
Suspension: Store at 25°C (77°F); excursions are permitted between 15°C and 30°C (59°F and 86°F). Do not freeze. The Canadian labeling recommends to discard 4 weeks after opening.

Tablets: Store between 20°C and 25°C (68°F and 77°F); excursions are permitted between 15°C and 30°C (59°F and 86°F).

Injection: Store at 2°C to 8°C (36°F to 46°F).

Mechanism of Action
Interferes with fungal cytochrome P450 (lanosterol-14α-demethylase) activity, decreasing ergosterol synthesis (principal sterol in fungal cell membrane) and inhibiting fungal cell membrane formation.

Pharmacodynamics/Kinetics
Absorption: Coadministration of the tablets or oral suspension with food or coadministration of the oral suspension with liquid nutritional supplements and/or acidic carbonated beverages (eg, ginger ale) increases absorption; fasting states do not provide sufficient absorption to ensure adequate plasma concentrations.

Distribution: V_d: Oral: 287 L; Injection: ~261 L

Protein binding: >98%; predominantly bound to albumin

Metabolism: Not significantly metabolized; 17% undergoes non-CYP-mediated metabolism, primarily via hepatic glucuronidation into metabolites

Half-life elimination: Suspension: 35 hours (range: 20 to 66 hours); Tablets: 26 to 31 hours; Injection: ~27 hours

Time to peak, plasma: Suspension: ~3 to 5 hours; Tablets: ~4 to 5 hours

Excretion: Feces 71% (~66% of the total dose as unchanged drug); urine 13% (<0.2% of the total dose as unchanged drug)

Dosing
Adult & Geriatric Note: The delayed-release tablet and oral suspension are not to be used interchangeably due to dosing differences for each formulation.

Aspergillosis, invasive:
Prophylaxis:
Oral:
Suspension: 200 mg 3 times daily; duration of therapy is based on recovery from neutropenia or immunosuppression. In patients with acute myelogenous leukemia (AML) or myelodysplastic syndromes (MDS), posaconazole was initiated at the time of chemotherapy initiation (or if receiving anthracyclines, 24 hours after the last anthracycline dose) and was continued until recovery from neutropenia, until complete remission, or for up to 12 weeks, whichever occurred first (Cornely 2007). The Canadian labeling recommends initiating posaconazole in patients with AML or MDS several days before the anticipated onset of neutropenia and continuing for 7 days after the neutrophil count rises above 500/mm³. In patients with graft-versus-host disease (GVHD) receiving immunosuppressive therapy, posaconazole was continued for 112 days (Ullmann 2007), although the optimal duration in GVHD has not been fully defined (Tomblyn 2009).

Tablets (delayed release): Initial: 300 mg twice daily on day 1; Maintenance dose: 300 mg once daily on day 2 and thereafter. Duration is based on recovery from neutropenia or immunosuppression. The Canadian labeling recommends initiating posaconazole in patients with AML or MDS several days before the anticipated onset of neutropenia and continuing for 7 days after the neutrophil count rises above 500/mm³.

Missed doses: Take as soon as remembered. If it is <12 hours until the next dose, skip the missed does and return to the regular schedule. Do not double doses.

IV: Loading dose: 300 mg twice a day on day 1; maintenance dose: 300 mg once daily on day 2 and thereafter. Duration is based on recovery from neutropenia or immunosuppression. The Canadian labeling recommends initiating posaconazole in patients with AML or MDS several days before the anticipated onset of neutropenia and continuing for 7 days after the neutrophil count rises above 500/mm³.

Treatment (refractory to or intolerant of conventional therapy):

US off-label use: Oral: Suspension: 200 mg 4 times daily initially; after disease stabilization, may decrease frequency to 400 mg twice daily (Walsh 2007). **Note:** Duration of therapy should be a minimum of 6 to 12 weeks or throughout period of immunosuppression and until lesions have resolved (Walsh 2008). Duration of therapy in HIV-infected patients should be until infection resolution and CD4 count >200 cells/mm³ (HHS [OI adult 2015])

Canadian labeling:

Oral:

Suspension: 400 mg twice daily; in patients unable to tolerate food or nutritional supplement, administer 200 mg 4 times daily; duration of therapy is based on severity of underlying disease, recovery from immunosuppression, and clinical response.

Tablets (delayed release): Initial: 300 mg twice daily on day 1; Maintenance dose: 300 mg once daily; duration of therapy is based on disease severity, recovery from immunosuppression, and clinical response.

IV: Loading dose: 300 mg twice daily on day 1; Maintenance dose: 300 mg once daily on day 2 and thereafter. Duration of therapy is based on disease severity, recovery from immunosuppression, and clinical response.

Candidal infections:

US labeling:

Prophylaxis:

Oral:

Suspension: 200 mg 3 times daily; duration of therapy is based on recovery from neutropenia or immunosuppression

Tablets (delayed release): Oral: Initial: 300 mg twice daily on day 1; Maintenance dose: 300 mg once daily on day 2 and thereafter; duration of therapy is based on recovery from neutropenia or immunosuppression

Missed doses: Take as soon as remembered. If it is <12 hours until the next dose, skip the missed does and return to the regular schedule. Do not double doses.

IV: Initial: 300 mg twice daily on day 1; Maintenance dose: 300 mg once daily on day 2 and thereafter; duration of therapy is based on recovery from neutropenia or immunosuppression.

Treatment: Oral: Suspension:

Oropharyngeal infection: Initial: 100 mg twice daily on day 1; Maintenance: 100 mg once daily on day 2 and thereafter for 13 days

Refractory oropharyngeal infection:

Manufacturer's labeling: 400 mg twice daily; duration of therapy is based on underlying disease and clinical response

Alternate dosing: HIV-infected patients (alternative to fluconazole or azole refractory): 400 mg twice daily on day 1, then 400 mg once daily for 7 to 14 days for initial episodes (continue for 28 days in azole refractory patients) (HHS [OI adult 2015])

Esophageal infection in HIV-infected patients (azole refractory) (off-label use): 400 mg twice daily for 28 days. **Note:** If patient has frequent or severe recurrences, may continue for suppressive therapy; consider discontinuing when CD4 >200/mm³ (HHS [OI adult 2015])

Canadian labeling:

Prophylaxis: Note: Initiate posaconazole in patients with AML or MDS several days before the anticipated onset of neutropenia and continue therapy for 7 days after the neutrophil count rises above 500/mm³.

Oral:

Suspension: 200 mg 3 times daily; duration of therapy is based on recovery from neutropenia or immunosuppression.

Tablets (delayed release): Initial: 300 mg twice daily on day 1; Maintenance dose: 300 mg once daily on day 2 and thereafter; duration of therapy is based on recovery from neutropenia or immunosuppression.

Injection: IV: Initial: 300 mg twice daily on day 1; Maintenance dose: 300 mg once daily on day 2 and thereafter; duration of therapy is based on recovery from neutropenia or immunosuppression.

Treatment: Oral: Suspension: Oropharyngeal infection: Initial: 100 mg twice daily for 1 day; Maintenance: 100 mg once daily for 13 days

Coccidioidomycosis in HIV-infected patients (alternative to preferred therapy) (off-label use; HHS [OI adult 2015]): Oral:

Mild infections (eg, focal pneumonia): 200 to 400 mg twice daily; patients who complete initial therapy should be considered for lifelong suppressive therapy.

Chronic suppressive therapy: 200 mg twice daily

Mucormycosis (off-label use): Suspension: Oral: 800 mg daily in 2 or 4 divided doses; duration of therapy is based on response and risk of relapse due to immunosuppression (Greenberg 2006)

Cryptococcal infections:

Pulmonary, nonimmunosuppressed (off-label use): 400 mg twice daily. **Note:** Fluconazole is considered first-line treatment (Perfect 2010).

Salvage treatment of relapsed infection (off-label use): 400 mg twice daily (or 200 mg 4 times daily) for 10 to 12 weeks. **Note:** Salvage treatment should only be started after an appropriate course of an induction regimen (Perfect 2010).

Pediatric Note: The delayed-release tablet and oral suspension are not to be used interchangeably due to dosing differences for each formulation.

Aspergillosis, invasive (prophylaxis): Oral: Adolescents ≥13 years: Refer to adult dosing.

Candidal infections: Oral: Adolescents ≥13 years: Refer to adult dosing.

Coccidioidomycosis in HIV-infected patients (alternative to preferred therapy) (off-label use): Adolescents: Oral: Refer to adult dosing.

Primary antifungal prophylaxis in allogeneic HSCT with grades 2 to 4 acute graft-versus-host-disease (GVHD) or chronic extensive GVHD (guideline recommendation): Adolescents ≥13 years: Oral: Suspension: 200 mg 3 times daily beginning with GVHD diagnosis, continue until GVHD resolves (Science 2014)

Primary antifungal prophylaxis in AML or MDS in centers with a high local incidence of mold infections (alternative to fluconazole; guideline recommendation): Adolescents ≥13 years: Oral: Suspension: 200 mg 3 times daily during chemotherapy-associated neutropenia (Science 2014)

Renal Impairment

Delayed-release tablets and oral suspension:

eGFR 20 to 80 mL/minute/1.73 m²: No dosage adjustment necessary.

eGFR <20 mL/minute/1.73 m²: No dosage adjustment necessary; however, monitor for breakthrough fungal infections due to variability in posaconazole exposure.

Intravenous infusion:

eGFR ≥50 mL/minute/1.73 m²: No dosage adjustment recommended

eGFR <50 mL/minute/1.73 m²: Avoid use unless risk/benefit has been assessed; the intravenous vehicle (cyclodextrin) may accumulate. Monitor serum creatinine levels; if increases occur, consider oral therapy.

Hepatic Impairment

US labeling:

Preexisting mild-to-severe impairment (Child-Pugh class A, B, or C): No dosage adjustment necessary.

Hepatotoxicity during treatment: There are no dosage adjustments provided in the manufacturer's labeling; consider discontinuing therapy.

Canadian labeling: There are no dosage adjustments provided in the manufacturer's labeling; use with caution in severe impairment.

Dietary Considerations

Tablets (delayed release): US labeling recommends taking with food. Canadian labeling indicates that the tablet may be taken with or without food.

Suspension: Give during or within 20 minutes following a full meal, liquid nutritional supplement, or an acidic carbonated beverage (eg, ginger ale).

Consider alternative antifungal therapy in patients with inadequate oral intake or severe diarrhea/vomiting; if alternative therapy is not an option, closely monitoring for breakthrough fungal infections.

Adequate posaconazole absorption from GI tract and subsequent plasma concentrations are dependent on food for efficacy. Lower average plasma concentrations have been associated with an increased risk of treatment failure.

Administration

Suspension: Oral: Shake well before use. Administer with provided measured dosing spoon during or within 20 minutes following a full meal; patients who are unable to eat a full meal may take each dose with an oral liquid nutritional supplement; or acidic carbonated beverage (eg, ginger ale). Consider an alternative antifungal in patients unable to eat a full meal or tolerate a liquid nutritional supplement or acidic carbonated beverage

and who do not have the option of taking the delayed-release tablet or injection. Dosing spoon should be rinsed clean with water after each use and before storage. The oral suspension and delayed-release tablet are not to be used interchangeably due to dosing differences for each formulation.

Tablets (delayed release): Oral: Swallow tablets whole; do not divide, crush, dissolve, or chew. The US labeling recommends to administer with food. The Canadian labeling indicates that the tablet may be administered with or without food. Use only for prophylaxis indication (preferred oral formulation for this indication because it generally provides higher plasma drug exposures than oral suspension under both fed and fasted conditions). The delayed-release tablet and oral suspension are not to be used interchangeably due to dosing differences for each formulation.

Closely monitor patients with severe diarrhea or vomiting for breakthrough fungal infections.

Injection: Infuse over 90 minutes via a central venous line. Do not administer IV push or bolus. Must be infused through an in-line filter (0.22-micron polyethersulfone [PES] or polyvinylidene difluoride [PVDF]). Infusion through a peripheral line should only be used as a one-time infusion over 30 minutes in a patient who will be receiving a central venous line for subsequent doses, or to bridge a period during which a central venous line is to be replaced or is in use for another infusion. Note: In clinical trials, multiple peripheral infusions given through the same vein resulted in infusion-site reactions.

Monitoring Parameters Hepatic function (eg, AST/ALT, alkaline phosphatase and bilirubin) prior to initiation and during treatment; renal function, especially in patients on IV therapy if eGFR <50 mL/minute/1.73 m^2; electrolyte disturbances (eg, calcium, magnesium, potassium); CBC; breakthrough fungal infections; adequate oral intake

Dosage Forms Excipient information presented when available (limited, particularly for generics); consult specific product labeling.

Solution, Intravenous:
Noxafil: 300 mg/16.7 mL (16.7 mL) [contains edetate disodium]

Suspension, Oral:
Noxafil: 40 mg/mL (105 mL) [contains polysorbate 80, sodium benzoate; cherry flavor]

Tablet Delayed Release, Oral:
Noxafil: 100 mg

◆ Posanol (Can) see Posaconazole on page 1474

Potassium Acetate (poe TASS ee um AS e tate)

Pharmacologic Category Electrolyte Supplement, Parenteral

Use Potassium deficiency; to avoid chloride when high concentration of potassium is needed, source of bicarbonate

Dosing

Adult & Geriatric IV doses should be incorporated into the patient's maintenance IV fluids, intermittent IV potassium administration should be reserved for severe depletion situations and requires ECG monitoring; doses listed as mEq of potassium

Treatment of hypokalemia: IV: 40-100 mEq/day
IV intermittent infusion (must be diluted prior to administration):
5-10 mEq/dose (maximum: 40 mEq/dose) to infuse over 2-3 hours (maximum: 40 mEq over 1 hour)
Note: Continuous cardiac monitor recommended for rates >0.5 mEq/kg/hour

Potassium dosage/rate of infusion guidelines:
Serum potassium >2.5 mEq/L: Maximum infusion rate: 10 mEq/hour; maximum concentration: 40 mEq/L; maximum 24-hour dose: 200 mEq
Serum potassium <2.5 mEq/L: Maximum infusion rate: 40 mEq/hour; maximum concentration: 80 mEq/L; maximum 24-hour dose: 400 mEq

Pediatric IV doses should be incorporated into the patient's maintenance IV fluids, intermittent IV potassium administration should be reserved for severe depletion situations and requires ECG monitoring; doses listed as mEq of potassium.
Note: Use caution in premature neonates; potassium acetate for injection contains aluminum.

Treatment of hypokalemia: IV: 2-5 mEq/kg/day
IV intermittent infusion (must be diluted prior to administration): 0.5-1 mEq/kg/dose (maximum: 30 mEq/dose) to infuse at 0.3-0.5 mEq/kg/hour (maximum: 1 mEq/kg/hour)
Note: Continuous cardiac monitor recommended for rates >0.5 mEq/kg/hour

Potassium dosage/rate of infusion guidelines:
Serum potassium >2.5 mEq/L: Maximum infusion rate: 10 mEq/hour; maximum concentration: 40 mEq/L; maximum 24-hour dose: 200 mEq
Serum potassium <2.5 mEq/L: Maximum infusion rate: 40 mEq/hour; maximum concentration: 80 mEq/L; maximum 24-hour dose: 400 mEq

Renal Impairment No dosage adjustment provided in manufacturer's labeling. Use caution; potassium acetate injection may increase serum aluminum and/or potassium.

Hepatic Impairment No dosage adjustment provided in manufacturer's labeling. Use with caution.

Additional Information Complete prescribing information should be consulted for additional detail.

Dosage Forms Excipient information presented when available (limited, particularly for generics); consult specific product labeling.
Solution, Intravenous:
Generic: 2 mEq/mL (20 mL, 50 mL, 100 mL); 4 mEq/mL (50 mL)

Potassium Acid Phosphate
(poe TASS ee um AS id FOS fate)

Brand Names: US K-Phos

Index Terms Potassium Phosphate Monobasic

Pharmacologic Category Urinary Acidifying Agent

Use To acidify the urine to lower urinary calcium concentrations; reduce odor and rash caused by ammonia in urine; to increase the antibacterial activity of methenamine

Dosing

Adult & Geriatric Urine acidification: Oral: 1000 mg 4 times daily

Renal Impairment No dosage adjustment provided in manufacturer's labeling. Use with caution. Contraindicated in patients with severe impairment (<30% of normal function) or with hyperphosphatemia or hyperkalemia.

Hepatic Impairment No dosage adjustment provided in manufacturer's labeling. Use with caution.

Additional Information Complete prescribing information should be consulted for additional detail.

Dosage Forms Considerations

500 mg of potassium acid phosphate = elemental potassium 144 mg = potassium 3.7 mEq = potassium 3.7 mmol

500 mg of potassium acid phosphate = elemental phosphorus 114 mg = phosphorus 3.7 mmol

Dosage Forms Excipient information presented when available (limited, particularly for generics); consult specific product labeling.
Tablet, Oral:
K-Phos: 500 mg [scored]

Potassium Bicarbonate and Potassium Chloride
(poe TASS ee um bye KAR bun ate & poe TASS ee um KLOR ide)

Index Terms K-Lyte/Cl; Potassium Bicarbonate and Potassium Chloride (Effervescent)

Pharmacologic Category Electrolyte Supplement, Oral

Use Treatment or prevention of hypokalemia

Dosing

Adult & Geriatric Hypokalemia: Oral:
Prevention: 16-24 mEq/day in 2-4 divided doses
Treatment: 40-100 mEq/day in 2-4 divided doses

Pediatric Oral: 1-4 mEq/kg/24 hours in divided doses as required to maintain normal serum potassium

Renal Impairment No dosage adjustment provided in manufacturer's labeling. However, patients with chronic renal failure require serum potassium monitoring and appropriate dosage adjustment.

Hepatic Impairment No dosage adjustment provided in manufacturer's labeling.

Additional Information Complete prescribing information should be consulted for additional detail.

Dosage Forms Excipient information presented when available (limited, particularly for generics); consult specific product labeling.
Tablet for solution, oral [effervescent]: Potassium chloride 25 mEq [potassium bicarbonate 0.5 g and potassium chloride 1.5 g]

◆ Potassium Bicarbonate and Potassium Chloride (Effervescent) see Potassium Bicarbonate and Potassium Chloride on page 1478

Potassium Bicarbonate and Potassium Citrate
(poe TASS ee um bye KAR bun ate & poe TASS ee um SIT rate)

Brand Names: US Effer-K; K-Effervescent; K-Prime; K-Vescent; Klor-Con/EF

Index Terms Potassium Bicarbonate and Potassium Citrate (Effervescent)

Pharmacologic Category Electrolyte Supplement, Oral

Use Treatment or prevention of hypokalemia, particularly when it is necessary to avoid chloride or the acid/base status requires bicarbonate

Dosing

Adult & Geriatric Note: Doses expressed as mEq of potassium.

Normal daily requirement: 40-100 mEq/day or 1-2 mEq/kg/day (off-label dose; Mirtallo, 2004)

Hypokalemia: Oral:
Prevention: 10-80 mEq/day in 1-4 divided doses
Treatment: 40-100 mEq/day in 2-4 divided doses. **Note:** For asymptomatic mild hypokalemia, generally recommended to limit doses to 20-25 mEq/dose to avoid GI discomfort.

Renal Impairment No dosage adjustment provided in manufacturer's labeling. However, patients with chronic renal failure require serum potassium monitoring and appropriate dosage adjustment.

Hepatic Impairment No dosage adjustment provided in manufacturer's labeling.

Additional Information Complete prescribing information should be consulted for additional detail.

Dosage Forms Considerations Strength expressed in terms of mEqs of potassium

Dosage Forms Excipient information presented when available (limited, particularly for generics); consult specific product labeling. [DSC] = Discontinued product
Tablet Effervescent, Oral:
Effer-K: 10 mEq
Effer-K: 10 mEq [contains fd&c red #40; cherry-vanilla flavor]
Effer-K: 20 mEq
Effer-K: 20 mEq [scored; contains fd&c red #40, fd&c yellow #6 (sunset yellow); orange cream flavor]
Effer-K: 25 mEq [lime flavor]
Effer-K: 25 mEq [contains fd&c red #40, fd&c red #40 aluminum lake, saccharin; cherry berry flavor]
Effer-K: 25 mEq [contains fd&c yellow #10 (quinoline yellow), fd&c yellow #10 aluminum lake, saccharin; lemon citrus flavor]
Effer-K: 25 mEq [contains fd&c yellow #6 (sunset yellow), fd&c yellow #6 aluminum lake, saccharin; orange flavor]
Effer-K: 25 mEq [contains saccharin; unflavored flavor]
K-Effervescent: 25 mEq [orange flavor]
K-Prime: 25 mEq [contains fd&c yellow #6 (sunset yellow), fd&c yellow #6 aluminum lake, saccharin; orange flavor]
K-Vescent: 25 mEq [orange flavor]
Klor-Con/EF: 25 mEq [DSC] [contains fd&c yellow #6 (sunset yellow), fd&c yellow #6 aluminum lake, saccharin]
Klor-Con/EF: 25 mEq [DSC] [contains fd&c yellow #6 (sunset yellow), fd&c yellow #6 aluminum lake, saccharin; orange flavor]
Klor-Con/EF: 25 mEq [sugar free; contains fd&c yellow #6 (sunset yellow), fd&c yellow #6 aluminum lake, saccharin]
Klor-Con/EF: 25 mEq [sugar free; contains fd&c yellow #6 (sunset yellow), fd&c yellow #6 aluminum lake, saccharin; orange flavor]
Generic: 25 mEq

◆ Potassium Bicarbonate and Potassium Citrate (Effervescent) *see* Potassium Bicarbonate and Potassium Citrate *on page 1479*

Potassium Chloride (poe TASS ee um KLOR ide)

Brand Names: US K-Lor [DSC]; K-Sol; K-Tab; K-Vescent [DSC]; Klor-Con; Klor-Con 10; Klor-Con M10; Klor-Con M15; Klor-Con M20; Klor-Con Sprinkle; Micro-K

Brand Names: Canada Apo-K; K-10; K-Dur; Micro-K Extencaps; Roychlor; Slo-Pot; Slow-K

Index Terms KCl; Kdur

Pharmacologic Category Electrolyte Supplement, Oral; Electrolyte Supplement, Parenteral

Use Treatment or prevention of hypokalemia

Pregnancy Considerations Reproduction studies have not been conducted. Potassium requirements are the same in pregnant and nonpregnant women. Adverse events have not been observed following use of potassium supplements in healthy women with normal pregnancies.

Use caution in pregnant women with other medical conditions (eg, pre-eclampsia; may be more likely to develop hyperkalemia) (IOM, 2004). Potassium supplementation (that does not cause maternal hyperkalemia) would not be expected to cause adverse fetal events.

Breast-Feeding Considerations Potassium is excreted into breast milk (IOM, 2004). The normal content of potassium in human milk is ~13 mEq/L. Supplementation (that does not cause maternal hyperkalemia) would not be expected to affect normal concentrations.

Contraindications Hypersensitivity to any component of the formulation; hyperkalemia. In addition, solid oral dosage forms are contraindicated in patients in whom there is a structural, pathological, and/or pharmacologic cause for delay or arrest in passage through the GI tract.

Warnings/Precautions Close monitoring of serum potassium concentrations is needed to avoid hyperkalemia. Use with caution in patients with renal impairment, cardiac disease, acid/base disorders, or potassium-altering conditions/disorders. Use with caution in digitalized patients or patients receiving concomitant medications or therapies that increase potassium (eg, ACEI, potassium-sparing diuretics, potassium containing salt substitutes). Do **NOT** administer undiluted or IV push; inappropriate parenteral administration may be fatal. Always administer potassium further diluted; refer to appropriate dilution and administration rate recommendations. Vesicant/irritant (at concentrations >0.1 mEq/mL); ensure proper catheter or needle position prior to and during infusion; avoid extravasation. Pain and phlebitis may occur during parenteral infusion requiring a decrease in infusion rate or potassium concentration. Avoid administering potassium diluted in dextrose solutions during initial therapy; potential for transient decreases in serum potassium due to intracellular shift of potassium from dextrose-stimulated insulin release. May cause GI upset (eg, nausea, vomiting, diarrhea, abdominal pain, discomfort) and lead to GI ulceration, bleeding, perforation, and/or obstruction. Oral liquid preparations (not solid) should be used in patients with esophageal compression or delayed gastric emptying.

Adverse Reactions Frequency not defined.
Dermatologic: Rash
Endocrine & metabolic: Hyperkalemia
Gastrointestinal: Abdominal pain/discomfort, diarrhea, flatulence, GI bleeding (oral), GI obstruction (oral), GI perforation (oral), nausea, vomiting

Drug Interactions

Metabolism/Transport Effects None known.

Avoid Concomitant Use
Avoid concomitant use of Potassium Chloride with any of the following: Anticholinergic Agents; Glycopyrrolate

Increased Effect/Toxicity
Potassium Chloride may increase the levels/effects of: ACE Inhibitors; Aliskiren; Angiotensin II Receptor Blockers; Potassium-Sparing Diuretics

The levels/effects of Potassium Chloride may be increased by: Anticholinergic Agents; Eplerenone; Glycopyrrolate; Heparin; Heparin (Low Molecular Weight); Nicorandil

Decreased Effect There are no known significant interactions involving a decrease in effect.

Preparation for Administration Parenteral: Potassium must be diluted prior to parenteral administration. The concentration of infusion may be dependent on patient condition and specific institution policy. Some clinicians recommend that the maximum concentration for peripheral infusion is 10 mEq/100 mL and 20-40 mEq/100 mL for central infusions.

Storage/Stability
Capsule: MicroK: Store between 20°C to 25°C (68°F to 77°F).
Powder for oral solution: Klor-Con: Store at room temperature of 15°C to 30°C (59°F to 86°F).
Solution for injection: Store at 25°C (77°F); do not freeze; avoid excessive heat. Use only clear solutions. When admixed in most common infusion solutions, potassium chloride is stable indefinitely (ie, until the labeled expiration date of the infusion solution).
Tablet: K-Tab: Store below 30°C (86°F).

Mechanism of Action Potassium is the major cation of intracellular fluid and is essential for the conduction of nerve impulses in heart, brain, and skeletal muscle; contraction of cardiac, skeletal and smooth muscles; maintenance of normal renal function, acid-base balance, carbohydrate metabolism, and gastric secretion

Pharmacodynamics/Kinetics
Absorption: Well absorbed from upper GI tract
Distribution: Enters cells via active transport from extracellular fluid
Excretion: Primarily urine; skin and feces (small amounts); most intestinal potassium reabsorbed

Dosing

Adult & Geriatric IV doses should be incorporated into the patient's maintenance IV fluids; intermittent IV potassium administration should be reserved for severe depletion situations in patients undergoing ECG monitoring. Doses expressed as mEq of potassium.

Normal daily requirements: *Oral, IV:* 40-80 mEq/day
Prevention of hypokalemia: *Oral:* 20-40 mEq/day in 1-2 divided doses
Treatment of hypokalemia:
Oral:
Mild to moderate hypokalemia: **Note:** If deficits are severe or ongoing losses are great, IV route should be considered.
Manufacturer's labeling: Usual dose: 40 to 100 mEq daily in divided doses; limit single doses to 20 to 25 mEq/dose to avoid GI discomfort.
Alternate dosing: Some clinicians initiate treatment with 10 to 20 mEq given 2 to 4 times per day (20 to 80 mEq/day), depending upon the severity of the hypokalemia. Total daily doses up to 120 mEq may be necessary as determined by laboratory assessment, patient symptoms and/or ongoing losses (Brophy, 2014).
Severe hypokalemia: Some clinicians initiate treatment with 40 mEq given 3 to 4 times per day; may also administer 20 mEq every 2 to 3 hours in conjunction with IV potassium administration with careful monitoring.
IV intermittent infusion: Peripheral or central line: ≤10 mEq/hour; repeat as needed based on frequently obtained lab values; central line infusion and continuous ECG monitoring highly recommended for infusions >10 mEq/hour.
Potassium dosage/rate of infusion general guidelines (per product labeling): **Note:** High variability exists in dosing/infusion rate recommendations; therapy guided by patient condition and specific institutional guidelines.
Serum potassium >2.5 to 3.5 mEq/L: Maximum infusion rate: 10 mEq/hour; maximum concentration: 40 mEq/L; maximum 24-hour dose: 200 mEq
Serum potassium <2.5 mEq/L or symptomatic hypokalemia (excluding emergency treatment of cardiac arrest): Maximum infusion rate (central line only): 40 mEq/hour in presence of continuous ECG monitoring and frequent lab monitoring; In selected situations, patients may require up to 400 mEq/24 hours.

Pediatric IV doses should be incorporated into the patient's maintenance IV fluids; intermittent IV potassium administration should be reserved for severe depletion situations in patients undergoing ECG monitoring. Doses expressed as mEq of potassium.

Normal daily requirements: *Oral, IV:* 1-2 mEq/kg/day
Prevention of hypokalemia: *Oral:* 1-2 mEq/kg/day in 1-2 divided doses
Treatment of hypokalemia:
Oral: 1-2 mEq/kg initially, then as needed based on frequently obtained lab values. If deficits are severe or ongoing losses are great, IV route should be considered.
IV intermittent infusion: 0.5-1 mEq/kg/dose (maximum dose: 40 mEq). If infusion exceeds 0.5 mEq/kg/hour, physician should be at bedside and patient should have continuous ECG monitoring; repeat as needed based on frequently obtained lab values.

Renal Impairment No dosage adjustment provided in manufacturer's labeling. Use caution; potassium acetate injection may increase serum aluminum and/or potassium.

Hepatic Impairment No dosage adjustment provided in manufacturer's labeling.

Dietary Considerations Administer with plenty of fluid to decrease stomach irritation and discomfort. Some dietary sources of potassium include leafy green vegetables (eg, spinach, cabbage), tomatoes, cucumbers, zucchini, fruits (eg, apples, oranges, and bananas), root vegetables (eg, carrots, radishes), beans, and peas.

Administration

Parenteral: Potassium must be diluted prior to parenteral administration. Do not administer IV push. In general, the dose, concentration of infusion and rate of administration may be dependent on patient condition and specific institution policy. Some clinicians recommend that the maximum concentration for peripheral infusion is 10 mEq/100 mL and maximum rate of administration for peripheral infusion is 10 mEq/hour (Kraft, 2005). ECG monitoring is recommended for peripheral or central infusions >10 mEq/hour in adults (Kraft, 2005). Concentrations and rates of infusion may be greater with central

line administration. Concentrations of 20 to 40 mEq/100 mL at a maximum rate of 40 mEq/hour via central line have been safely administered (Hamill, 1991; Kruse, 1990)

Vesicant/irritant (at concentrations >0.1 mEq/mL); ensure proper needle or catheter placement prior to and during IV infusion. Avoid extravasation.

Extravasation management: If extravasation occurs, stop infusion immediately and disconnect (leave needle/cannula in place); gently aspirate extravasated solution (do **NOT** flush the line); initiate hyaluronidase antidote; remove needle/cannula; apply dry cold compresses (Hurst, 2004); elevate extremity.
Hyaluronidase: Intradermal or SubQ: Inject a total of 1 mL (15 units/mL) as five separate 0.2 mL injections (using a 25-gauge needle) into area of extravasation at the leading edge in a clockwise manner (MacCara, 1983; Zenk, 1981).

Oral: Oral dosage forms should be taken with meals and a full glass of water or other liquid to minimize the risk of GI irritation. Prescribing information for the various oral preparations recommend that no more than 20 mEq or 25 mEq should be given as single dose.
Capsule: MicroK: Swallow whole, do not chew. Capsules may also be opened and contents sprinkled on a spoonful of applesauce or pudding and should be swallowed immediately without chewing.
Powder: Klor-Con: Dissolve one packet in 4-5 ounces of water or other beverage prior to administration.
Tablet:
K-Tab, Kaon-Cl, Klor-Con: Swallow tablets whole; do not crush, chew, or suck on tablet.
Klor-Con M: Swallow tablets whole; do not crush, chew, or suck on tablet. Tablet may also be broken in half and each half swallowed separately; the whole tablet may be dissolved in ~4 ounces of water (allow ~2 minutes to dissolve, stir well and drink immediately)

Monitoring Parameters Serum potassium, chloride, magnesium (to facilitate potassium repletion), cardiac monitor (if intermittent infusion or potassium infusion rates 0.5 mEq/kg/hour in children or >10 mEq/hour in adults); to assess adequate replacement, repeat serum potassium level 2-4 hours after dose

Reference Range Note: Reference ranges may vary depending on the laboratory
Serum potassium: 3.5-5.2 mEq/L

Dosage Forms Considerations 750 mg potassium chloride = elemental potassium 390 mg = potassium 10 mEq = potassium 10 mmol

Dosage Forms Excipient information presented when available (limited, particularly for generics); consult specific product labeling. [DSC] = Discontinued product
Capsule Extended Release, Oral:
Klor-Con Sprinkle: 8 mEq [contains brilliant blue fcf (fd&c blue #1)]
Klor-Con Sprinkle: 10 mEq [contains fd&c red #40, fd&c yellow #10 (quinoline yellow)]
Micro-K: 8 mEq, 10 mEq
Generic: 8 mEq, 10 mEq
Liquid, Oral:
Generic: 20 mEq/15 mL (10%) (473 mL); 40 mEq/15 mL (20%) (473 mL)
Packet, Oral:
K-Lor: 20 mEq (30 ea [DSC], 100 ea [DSC])
K-Vescent: 20 mEq (100 ea [DSC])
Klor-Con: 20 mEq (1 ea, 30 ea, 100 ea); 25 mEq (30 ea, 100 ea) [sugar free; contains fd&c yellow #6 (sunset yellow); fruit flavor]
Generic: 20 mEq (1 ea, 30 ea, 100 ea)
Solution, Intravenous:
Generic: 5 mEq (250 mL); 10 mEq (500 mL, 1000 mL); 20 mEq (1000 mL); 30 mEq (1000 mL); 40 mEq (1000 mL); 0.4 mEq/mL (50 mL); 10 mEq/100 mL (100 mL); 10 mEq/50 mL (50 mL); 20 mEq/100 mL (100 mL); 20 mEq/50 mL (50 mL); 30 mEq/100 mL (100 mL [DSC]); 40 mEq/100 mL (100 mL); 2 mEq/mL (5 mL, 10 mL, 15 mL, 20 mL, 30 mL, 250 mL); 20 mEq/L (1000 mL); 40 mEq/L (1000 mL)
Solution, Oral:
K-Sol: 20 mEq/15 mL (10%) (473 mL) [alcohol free, dye free, sugar free; contains methylparaben, propylene glycol, propylparaben, saccharin sodium]
K-Sol: 40 mEq/15 mL (20%) (473 mL) [alcohol free, sugar free; contains fd&c red #40, saccharin sodium, sodium benzoate]
Generic: 20 MEQ/15ML (10%) (30 mL); 20 mEq/15 mL (10%) (15 mL, 30 mL, 473 mL, 3800 mL); 40 mEq/15 mL (20%) (15 mL [DSC], 473 mL)

Tablet Extended Release, Oral:

K-Tab: 8 mEq, 10 mEq [contains fd&c yellow #10 (quinoline yellow)]

K-Tab: 20 mEq

Klor-Con: 8 mEq [contains fd&c blue #1 aluminum lake, fd&c blue #2 aluminum lake]

Klor-Con 10: 10 mEq [contains fd&c yellow #10 aluminum lake, fd&c yellow #6 aluminum lake]

Klor-Con M10: 10 mEq

Klor-Con M15: 15 mEq [scored]

Klor-Con M20: 20 mEq [scored]

Generic: 8 mEq, 10 mEq, 20 mEq

Potassium Citrate and Citric Acid
(poe TASS ee um SIT rate & SI trik AS id)

Brand Names: US Cytra-K; Virtrate-K

Index Terms Citric Acid and Potassium Citrate; Polycitra K

Pharmacologic Category Alkalinizing Agent, Oral

Use

Acidosis: Treatment of acidosis in certain renal tubular disorders.

Gout (adjuvant): As an adjuvant to uricosurics in gout therapy.

Systemic alkalinizer: Alkalinizing agent in conditions where long-term maintenance of alkaline urine is desirable.

Dosing

Adult & Geriatric Systemic alkalinizer, Acidosis, Gout (adjuvant): Oral:

Powder: One packet dissolved in water 4 times daily; adjust dose to urinary pH

Solution: 10 to 30 mL 4 times daily; adjust dose based on urinary pH

Pediatric Systemic alkalinizer, Acidosis: Children and Adolescents: Oral: Solution: 5 to 15 mL 4 times daily; adjust dose based on urinary pH

Renal Impairment There are no dosage adjustments provided in manufacturer's labeling. Use is contraindicated in patients with anuria or severe renal impairment with oliguria or azotemia.

Hepatic Impairment There are no dosage adjustments provided in manufacturer's labeling.

Additional Information Complete prescribing information should be consulted for additional detail.

Dosage Forms Excipient information presented when available (limited, particularly for generics); consult specific product labeling. [DSC] = Discontinued product

Powder for solution, oral:

Cytra-K: Potassium citrate monohydrate 3300 mg and citric acid monohydrate 1002 mg per packet (100s) [sugar free; fruit-punch flavor; each packet contains potassium 30 mEq equivalent to bicarbonate 30 mEq]

Solution, oral:

Cytra-K: Potassium citrate monohydrate 1100 mg and citric acid monohydrate 334 mg per 5 mL (480 mL) [ethanol free, sugar free; contains propylene glycol; cherry flavor; contains potassium 2 mEq/mL equivalent to bicarbonate 2 mEq /mL]

Virtrate-K: Potassium citrate monohydrate 1100 mg and citric acid monohydrate 334 mg per 5 mL (480 mL) [sugar free; contains propylene glycol; cherry flavor; contains potassium 2 mEq/mL equivalent to bicarbonate 2 mEq /mL]

Generic: Potassium citrate monohydrate 1100 mg and citric acid monohydrate 334 mg per 5 mL (473 mL)

◆ Potassium Citrate, Citric Acid, and Sodium Citrate *see* Citric Acid, Sodium Citrate, and Potassium Citrate *on page 400*

Potassium Gluconate
(poe TASS ee um GLOO coe nate)

Brand Names: US K-99 [OTC]

Pharmacologic Category Electrolyte Supplement, Oral

Use Dietary supplement

Dosing

Adult & Geriatric Dietary supplement: Oral: One tablet daily

Renal Impairment No dosage adjustment provided in manufacturer's labeling.

Hepatic Impairment No dosage adjustment provided in manufacturer's labeling.

Additional Information Complete prescribing information should be consulted for additional detail.

Dosage Forms Considerations 1 g potassium gluconate = elemental potassium 167 mg = potassium 4.3 mEq = potassium 4.3 mmol

Dosage Forms Excipient information presented when available (limited, particularly for generics); consult specific product labeling.

Capsule, Oral [preservative free]:

K-99: 595 mg [dye free, sugar free, yeast free]

Tablet, Oral:

Generic: 2 mEq, 2.5 mEq

Tablet, Oral [strength expressed as base]:

Generic: 80 mg

Potassium Iodide (poe TASS ee um EYE oh dide)

Brand Names: US SSKI; ThyroShield [OTC]

Index Terms KI; Saturated Potassium Iodide Solution; Saturated Solution of Potassium Iodide

Pharmacologic Category Antidote; Antithyroid Agent; Expectorant

Use Expectorant for the symptomatic treatment of chronic pulmonary diseases complicated by mucous; block thyroidal uptake of radioactive isotopes of iodine in a nuclear radiation emergency

Dosing

Adult & Geriatric

RDA: 150 mcg (iodine)

Expectorant (SSKI®): Oral: 300-600 mg (0.3-0.6 mL) 3-4 times daily

Thyroid block following nuclear radiation emergency (iOSAT™, ThyroSafe®, ThyroShield®): Includes pregnant/lactating women: Oral: 130 mg once daily, continue for 10-14 days or as directed by public officials (until risk of exposure has passed or other measures are implemented)

Thyroidectomy preparation (off-label use): Oral: 50-100 mg (1-2 drops **or** 0.05-0.1 mL SSKI®) 3 times daily; administer for 10 days before surgery; if not euthyroid prior to surgery, consider concurrent beta-blockade (eg, propranolol) in the immediate preoperative period to reduce the risk of thyroid storm (Bahn, 2011)

Sporotrichosis (cutaneous, lymphocutaneous; off-label use) (SSKI®): Oral: Initial: 5 drops 3 times daily; increase to 40-50 drops 3 times daily as tolerated until 2-4 weeks after lesions have resolved (usual duration 3-6 months) (Kauffman, 2007)

Thyroid gland protection during radiopharmaceutical use (off-label use): Oral: Tablet: 130 mg once daily **or** Solution (SSKI®): 4 drops 3 times daily (Bexxar® prescribing information, 2012). **Note:** Begin at 1-48 hours prior to exposure. Continue potassium iodide after radiopharmaceutical administration until risk of exposure has diminished (treatment duration and time of initiation is dependent on the radiopharmaceutical, consult specific protocol).

Thyrotoxic crisis/thyroid storm (off-label use): Oral: **Note:** Administer at least 1-2 hours after antithyroid drug administration: 250 mg (5 drops **or** 0.25 mL SSKI®) every 6 hours (Bahn, 2011)

Pediatric

Thyroid block following nuclear radiation emergency (iOSAT™, ThyroSafe®, ThyroShield®): Dosing should continue for 10-14 days or as directed by public officials (until risk of exposure has passed or other measures are implemented): Oral:

Infants ≤1 month: 16.25 mg once daily

Infants >1 month to Children ≤3 years: 32.5 mg once daily

Children >3 to ≤12 years: 65 mg once daily

Children >12-18 years weighing <68 kg: 65 mg once daily

Children >12-18 years weighing ≥68 kg: 130 mg once daily

Thyroidectomy preparation (off-label use): Oral: 150-350 mg (3-7 drops **or** 0.15-0.35 mL SSKI®) 3 times daily; administer for 10 days before surgery; if not euthyroid prior to surgery, consider concurrent beta-blockade (eg, propranolol) in the immediate preoperative period to reduce the risk of thyroid storm (Bahn, 2011)

Thyroid gland protection during radiopharmaceutical use (off-label use): Oral (Giammarile, 2008; Olivier, 2003):

Infants <5 kg: 16 mg once daily

Children 1 month to 3 years or 5-15 kg: 32 mg once daily

Children 3-13 years or 15-50 kg: 65 mg once daily

Children >13 years or >50 kg: 130 mg once daily

Note: Begin at 1-48 hours prior to exposure. Continue potassium iodide after radiopharmaceutical administration until risk of exposure has diminished (treatment duration and time of initiation is dependent on the radiopharmaceutical, consult specific protocol).

Thyrotoxic crisis/thyroid storm (off-label use): Oral:
Note: Administer at least 1-2 hours after antithyroid drug administration:
Infants: 100 mg (2 drops **or** 0.1 mL SSKI®) 4 times daily (Eyal, 2008)
Children: 250 mg (5 drops **or** 0.25 mL SSKI®) 2-4 times daily (Eyal, 2008)

Renal Impairment No dosage adjustment provided in the manufacturer's labeling.

Hepatic Impairment No dosage adjustment provided in the manufacturer's labeling.

Additional Information Complete prescribing information should be consulted for additional detail.

Dosage Forms Excipient information presented when available (limited, particularly for generics); consult specific product labeling.
Solution, Oral:
SSKI: 1 g/mL (30 mL, 237 mL)
ThyroShield: 65 mg/mL (30 mL) [contains brilliant blue fcf (fd&c blue #1), fd&c red #40, methylparaben, propylene glycol, propylparaben, saccharin sodium; black raspberry flavor]

Potassium Iodide and Iodine
(poe TASS ee um EYE oh dide & EYE oh dine)

Index Terms Iodine and Potassium Iodide; Lugol's Solution; Strong Iodine Solution

Pharmacologic Category Antiseptic, Topical; Antithyroid Agent

Use Topical antiseptic

Dosing

Adult & Geriatric

Antiseptic: Topical: Apply directly to area(s) requiring antiseptic.

RDA: 150 mcg (iodine)

Preparation for thyroidectomy (off-label use): Oral: 5-7 drops (0.25-0.35 mL) 3 times daily; administer for 10 days before surgery; if not euthyroid prior to surgery, consider concurrent beta-blockade (eg, propranolol) in the immediate preoperative period to reduce the risk of thyroid storm (Bahn, 2011)

Thyrotoxic crisis (off-label use): Oral: 4-8 drops every 6-8 hours; begin administration ≥1 hour following the initial dose of either propylthiouracil or methimazole (Nayak, 2006)

Thyroid gland protection during radiopharmaceutical use (off-label use): Oral: 20 drops 3 times daily has been recommended (Bexxar® prescribing information, 2012)
Note: Initiate 1-48 hours prior to radiopharmaceutical exposure and continue after radiopharmaceutical administration until risk of exposure has diminished (treatment initiation time and duration is dependent on the radiopharmaceutical agent used, consult specific protocol or labeling.

Pediatric Thyrotoxic crisis (off-label use): Oral: 4-8 drops 3 times daily; begin therapy preferably 2 hours following the initial dose of propylthiouracil or alternatively, methimazole (Eyal, 2008)

Renal Impairment No dosage adjustment provided in manufacturer's labeling.

Hepatic Impairment No dosage adjustment provided in manufacturer's labeling.

Additional Information Complete prescribing information should be consulted for additional detail.

Dosage Forms Excipient information presented when available (limited, particularly for generics); consult specific product labeling.
Solution, oral: Potassium iodide 100 mg/mL and iodine 50 mg/mL (473 mL)
Solution, topical: Potassium iodide 100 mg/mL and iodine 50 mg/mL (8 mL)

Potassium Phosphate (poe TASS ee um FOS fate)

Brand Names: US Neutra-Phos®-K [OTC] [DSC]

Index Terms Phosphate, Potassium

Pharmacologic Category Electrolyte Supplement, Parenteral

Use Treatment and prevention of hypophosphatemia; **Note:** The concomitant amount of potassium must be calculated into the total electrolyte content. For each 1 mmol of phosphate, ~1.5 mEq of potassium will be administered. Therefore, if ordering 30 mmol of potassium phosphate, the patient will receive ~45 mEq of potassium.

Pregnancy Considerations Reproduction studies have not been conducted. Phosphorus requirements are the same in pregnant and nonpregnant women (IOM, 1997). Although this product is not used for potassium supplementation, adverse events have not been observed

following use of potassium supplements in healthy women with normal pregnancies. Use caution in pregnant women with other medical conditions (eg, pre-eclampsia; may be more likely to develop hyperkalemia) (IOM, 2004).

Breast-Feeding Considerations Phosphorus, sodium, and potassium are normal constituents of human milk.

Contraindications Hyperphosphatemia, hyperkalemia, hypocalcemia

Warnings/Precautions Close monitoring of serum potassium concentrations is needed to avoid hyperkalemia. Use with caution in patients with renal insufficiency, cardiac disease, metabolic alkalosis. Use with caution in digitalized patients and patients receiving concomitant potassium-altering therapies. Parenteral potassium may cause pain and phlebitis, requiring a decrease in infusion rate or potassium concentration. Vesicant/irritant (may depend on concentration); ensure proper catheter or needle position prior to and during infusion; avoid extravasation. The parenteral product may contain aluminum; toxic aluminum concentrations may be seen with high doses, prolonged use, or renal dysfunction. Premature neonates are at higher risk due to immature renal function and aluminum intake from other parenteral sources. Parenteral aluminum exposure of >4 to 5 mcg/kg/day is associated with CNS and bone toxicity; tissue loading may occur at lower doses (Federal Register, 2002). See manufacturer's labeling.

Adverse Reactions Frequency not defined.
Cardiovascular: Arrhythmia, bradycardia, chest pain, ECG changes, edema, heart block, hypotension
Central nervous system: Listlessness, mental confusion, tetany (with large doses of phosphate)
Endocrine & metabolic: Hyperkalemia
Gastrointestinal: Diarrhea, nausea, stomach pain, vomiting
Genitourinary: Urine output decreased
Local: Phlebitis
Neuromuscular & skeletal: Paralysis, paresthesia, weakness
Renal: Acute renal failure
Respiratory: Dyspnea

Drug Interactions

Metabolism/Transport Effects None known.

Avoid Concomitant Use There are no known interactions where it is recommended to avoid concomitant use.

Increased Effect/Toxicity
Potassium Phosphate may increase the levels/effects of: ACE Inhibitors; Aliskiren; Angiotensin II Receptor Blockers; Potassium-Sparing Diuretics

The levels/effects of Potassium Phosphate may be increased by: Eplerenone; Heparin; Heparin (Low Molecular Weight); Nicorandil

Decreased Effect
The levels/effects of Potassium Phosphate may be decreased by: Antacids; Calcium Salts; Iron Salts; Magnesium Salts; Multivitamins/Minerals (with ADEK, Folate, Iron); Sucralfate

Food Interactions Avoid administering with oxalate (berries, nuts, chocolate, beans, celery, tomato) or phytate-containing foods (bran, whole wheat).

Preparation for Administration In general, the dose, concentration of infusion, and rate of administration may be dependent on patient condition and specific institution policy. Intermittent infusion doses of potassium phosphate are typically prepared in 100-250 mL of NS or D_5W (usual phosphate concentration range: 0.15-0.6 mmol/mL) (Charron, 2003; Rosen, 1995). Suggested maximum concentrations:
Central line administration: 26.8 mmoL potassium phosphate/100 mL (40 mEq potassium/100 mL)
Peripheral line administration: 6.7 mmoL potassium phosphate/100 mL (10 mEq potassium/100 mL)

Observe the vial for the presence of translucent visible particles. Do not use vial if particles are present. Dilute in a compatible IV fluid. **Note:** Due to the potential presence of particulates, American Regent, Inc recommends the use of a 5 micron filter when preparing IV potassium phosphate-containing solutions (Important Drug Administration Information, American Regent, 2011); a similar recommendation has not been noted by other manufacturers.

Storage/Stability Store intact vials at 20°C to 25°C (68°F to 77°F); excursions permitted between 15°C and 30°C (59°F and 86°F).

Mechanism of Action
Phosphorus in the form of organic and inorganic phosphate has a variety of important biochemical functions in the body and is involved in many significant metabolic and enzymatic reactions in almost all organs and tissues. It exerts a modifying influence on the steady state of calcium levels, a buffering effect on acid-base equilibrium and a primary role in the renal excretion of hydrogen ion.

Potassium is the major cation of intracellular fluid and is essential for the conduction of nerve impulses in heart, brain, and skeletal muscle; contraction of cardiac, skeletal and smooth muscles; maintenance of normal renal function, acid-base balance, carbohydrate metabolism, and gastric secretion.

Dosing

Adult & Geriatric Note: If phosphate repletion is required and a phosphate product is not available at your institution, consider the use of sodium glycerophosphate pentahydrate (Glycophos) as a suitable substitute. Concentration and dosing are different from FDA-approved products; use caution when switching between products. Refer to Sodium Glycerophosphate Pentahydrate monograph.

Caution: The concomitant amount of potassium must be calculated into the total electrolyte content. For each 1 mmol of phosphate, ~1.5 mEq of potassium will be administered. Therefore, if ordering 30 mmol of potassium phosphate, the patient will receive ~45 mEq of potassium. With orders for IV phosphate, there is considerable confusion associated with the use of millimoles (mmol) versus milliequivalents (mEq) to express the phosphate requirement. The most reliable method of ordering IV phosphate is by millimoles, then specifying the potassium or sodium salt. Doses listed as mmol of phosphate.

Acute treatment of hypophosphatemia: Repletion of severe hypophosphatemia should be done IV because large doses of oral phosphate may cause diarrhea and intestinal absorption may be unreliable. Reserve intermittent IV infusion for severe depletion situations; may require continuous cardiac monitoring depending on potassium administration rate. Guidelines differ based on degree of illness, need/use of parenteral nutrition, and severity of hypophosphatemia. If potassium >4.0 mEq/L consider phosphate replacement strategy without potassium (eg, sodium phosphates). Patients with severe renal impairment were excluded from phosphate supplement trials. **Note:** 1 mmol phosphate = 31 mg phosphorus; 1 mg phosphorus = 0.032 mmol phosphate.

General replacement guidelines (Lentz, 1978):
Low dose, if serum phosphate losses are recent and uncomplicated: Initial: 0.08 mmol/kg over 6 hours
Intermediate dose, if serum phosphorus level <1 mg/dL (<0.32 mmol/L): Initial: 0.16 mmol/kg per dose over 6 hours
Note: The initial dose may be increased by 25% to 50% if the patient is symptomatic secondary to hypophosphatemia and lowered by 25% to 50% if the patient is hypercalcemic. Do not exceed the maximum dose of 0.24 mmol/kg/dose (or 16.9 mmol for a 70-kg patient).

Critically-ill adult patients receiving concurrent enteral/parenteral nutrition (Brown, 2006; Clark, 1995): Note: Round doses to the nearest 7.5 mmol for ease of preparation. If administering with phosphate-containing parenteral nutrition, do not exceed 15 mmol/L within parenteral nutrition.
Low dose, serum phosphorus level 2.3-3 mg/dL (0.74-0.96 mmol/L): 0.16-0.32 mmol/kg over 4-6 hours
Intermediate dose, serum phosphorus level 1.6-2.2 mg/dL (0.51-0.71 mmol/L): 0.32-0.64 mmol/kg over 4-6 hours
High dose, serum phosphorus <1.5 mg/dL (<0.5 mmol/L): 0.64-1 mmol/kg over 8-12 hours
Obesity: May use adjusted body weight for patients weighing >130% of ideal body weight (and BMI <40 kg/m^2) by using [IBW + 0.25 (actual body weight - IBW)].

Parenteral nutrition: IV: 10-15 mmol/1000 kcal (Hicks, 2001) **or** 20-40 mmol/24 hours (Mirtallo, 2004 [ASPEN guidelines])

Pediatric Note: If phosphate repletion is required and a phosphate product is not available at your institution, consider the use of sodium glycerophosphate pentahydrate (Glycophos) as a suitable substitute. Concentration and dosing are different from FDA-approved products; use caution when switching between products. Refer to Sodium Glycerophosphate Pentahydrate monograph.

Caution: The concomitant amount of potassium must be calculated into the total electrolyte content. For each 1 mmol of phosphate, ~1.5 mEq of potassium will be administered. Therefore, if ordering 30 mmol of potassium phosphate, the patient will receive ~45 mEq of potassium. With orders for IV phosphate, there is considerable confusion associated with the use of millimoles (mmol) versus milliequivalents

(mEq) to express the phosphate requirement. The most reliable method of ordering IV phosphate is by millimoles, then specifying the potassium or sodium salt. Doses listed as mmol of phosphate.

Intermittent IV infusion should be reserved for severe depletion situations; may require continuous cardiac monitoring depending on potassium administration rate. It is difficult to determine total body phosphorus deficit. There are no prospective studies of parenteral phosphate replacement in children. The following weight-based guidelines for **adult** dosing may be cautiously employed in pediatric patients. Guidelines differ based on degree of illness, use of TPN, and severity of hypophosphatemia. **Note:** 1 mmol phosphate = 31 mg phosphorus; 1 mg phosphorus = 0.032 mmol phosphate.

General replacement guidelines (Lentz, 1978):
Low dose, if serum phosphate losses are recent and uncomplicated: Initial: 0.08 mmol/kg over 6 hours
Intermediate dose, if serum phosphorus level <1 mg/dL (<0.32 mmol/L): Initial: 0.16 mmol/kg per dose over 6 hours
Note: The initial dose may be increased by 25% to 50% if the patient is symptomatic secondary to hypophosphatemia and lowered by 25% to 50% if the patient is hypercalcemic. Do not exceed the maximum dose of 0.24 mmol/kg/dose (or 16.9 mmol for a 70-kg patient).
Critically-ill adult patients receiving concurrent enteral/parenteral nutrition (Brown, 2006; Clark, 1995): Note: Round doses to the nearest 7.5 mmol for ease of preparation. If administering with phosphate-containing parenteral nutrition, do not exceed 15 mmol/L within parenteral nutrition.
Low dose, serum phosphorus level 2.3-3 mg/dL (0.74-0.96 mmol/L): 0.16-0.32 mmol/kg over 4-6 hours
Intermediate dose, serum phosphorus level 1.6-2.2 mg/dL (0.51-0.71 mmol/L): 0.32-0.64 mmol/kg over 4-6 hours
High dose, serum phosphorus <1.5 mg/dL (<0.5 mmol/L): 0.64-1 mmol/kg over 8-12 hours
Obesity: May use adjusted body weight for patients weighing >130% of ideal body weight (and BMI <40 kg/m^2) by using [IBW + 0.25 (actual body weight - IBW)].

Parenteral nutrition:
Infants and Children: 0.5-2 mmol/kg/24 hours (Mirtallo, 2004 [ASPEN guidelines])
Children >50 kg and Adolescents: 10-40 mmol/24 hours (Mirtallo, 2004 [ASPEN guidelines])
Obesity Refer to indication-specific dosing for obesity-related information (may not be available for all indications).

Administration Injection must be diluted in appropriate IV solution and volume prior to administration. In general, the dose, concentration of infusion, and rate of administration may be dependent on patient condition and specific institution policy. Must consider administration precautions for phosphate and potassium when prescribing. **Note:** Due to the potential presence of translucent visible particles, American Regent, Inc recommends the use of a 0.22 micron in-line filter for IV administration (1.2 micron filter if admixture contains lipids) (Important Drug Administration Information, American Regent, 2011); a similar recommendation has not been noted by other manufacturers.

For adult patients with severe symptomatic hypophosphatemia (ie, <1.5 mg/dL), may administer at rates up to 15 mmol phosphate/hour (this rate will deliver potassium at 22.5 mEq/hour) (Charron 2003; Rosen 1995). Potassium infusion rates >10 mEq/hour should be administered via central line (minimizes burning and phlebitis). ECG monitoring is recommended for potassium infusions >10 mEq/hour in adults or >0.5 mEq/kg/hour in children. In patients with renal dysfunction and/or less severe hypophosphatemia, slower administration rates (eg, over 4 to 6 hours) or oral repletion is recommended.

Vesicant/irritant (may depend on concentration); ensure proper needle or catheter placement prior to and during IV infusion. Avoid extravasation.

Extravasation management: If extravasation occurs, stop infusion immediately and disconnect (leave needle/cannula in place); gently aspirate extravasated solution (do **NOT** flush the line); initiate hyaluronidase antidote; remove needle/cannula; apply dry cold compresses (Hurst 2004); elevate extremity.

Hyaluronidase: Intradermal or SubQ: Inject a total of 1 mL (15 units/mL) as five separate 0.2 mL injections (using a 25-gauge needle) into area of extravasation at the leading edge in a clockwise manner (MacCara 1983; Zenk 1981).

Monitoring Parameters Serum potassium, calcium, phosphorus, magnesium (to facilitate potassium repletion); cardiac monitor (if intermittent infusion or potassium infusion rates >0.5 mEq/kg/hour in children or >10 mEq/hour in adults); to assess adequate replacement, repeat serum potassium and phosphorus levels 2-4 hours after dose

Reference Range Note: Reference ranges may vary depending on the laboratory

Serum calcium: 8.4-10.2 mg/dL

Serum phosphorus: Both low and high ends of the normal range are higher in children than in adults.

Infants: 4.5-7.5 mg/dL (1.45-2.42 mmol/L)
Children: ~4-6 mg/dL (1.29-1.94 mmol/L)
Adults: 2.5-4.5 mg/dL (0.81-1.45 mmol/L)
Serum potassium: 3.5-5.2 mEq/L

Dosage Forms Considerations

Potassium 4.4 mEq is equivalent to potassium 170 mg

Phosphorous 3 mmol is equivalent to phosphorus 93 mg

Dosage Forms Excipient information presented when available (limited, particularly for generics); consult specific product labeling.

Injection, solution: Potassium 4.4 mEq and phosphorus 3 mmol per mL (5 mL, 15 mL, 50 mL) [equivalent to potassium 170 mg and elemental phosphorus 93 mg per mL]

Potassium Phosphate and Sodium Phosphate

(poe TASS ee um FOS fate & SOW dee um FOS fate)

Brand Names: US Av-Phos 250 Neutral; K-Phos Neutral; K-Phos No. 2; Phos-NaK; Phospha 250 Neutral; Virt-Phos 250 Neutral

Index Terms Neutra-Phos; Sodium Phosphate and Potassium Phosphate

Pharmacologic Category Electrolyte Supplement, Oral

Use

Phosphate supplement: As a phosphorus supplement

Urinary acidification: To increase urinary phosphate and pyrophosphate

K-Phos No. 2: Urinary acidifier for patients with elevated urinary pH to help keep calcium soluble and reduce odor and rash caused by ammoniacal urine; increases the antibacterial activity of methenamine.

Dosing

Adult & Geriatric Note: Dosage expressed in terms of elemental phosphorus.

Phosphate supplement: Oral: 250 to 500 mg 4 times daily

Urinary acidification (K-Phos No. 2): Oral: 250 mg 4 times daily; may be increased to 250 mg every 2 hours when the urine is difficult to acidify (maximum: 2,000 mg/day)

Pediatric Phosphate supplement: Note: Dosage expressed in terms of elemental phosphorus: Children ≥4 years and Adolescents: Oral: 250 mg 4 times daily

Renal Impairment There are no dosage adjustment provided in the manufacturer's labeling. Use with caution. Contraindicated in patients with severe impairment (<30% of normal function).

Hepatic Impairment There are no dosage adjustments provided in the manufacturer's labeling. Use with caution.

Additional Information Complete prescribing information should be consulted for additional detail.

Dosage Forms Excipient information presented when available (limited, particularly for generics); consult specific product labeling.

Powder for solution, oral:

Phos-NaK: Dibasic potassium phosphate, monobasic potassium phosphate, dibasic sodium phosphate, and monobasic sodium phosphate per packet (100s) [sugar free; equivalent to elemental phosphorus 250 mg (8 mmol), sodium 160 mg (6.9 mEq), and potassium 280 mg (7.1 mEq) per packet; fruit flavor]

Tablet, oral:

Av-Phos 250 Neutral: Monobasic potassium phosphate 155 mg, dibasic sodium phosphate 852 mg, and monobasic sodium phosphate 130 mg [equivalent to elemental phosphorus 250 mg (8 mmol), sodium 298 mg (13 mEq), and potassium 45 mg (1.1 mEq)]

K-Phos Neutral: Monobasic potassium phosphate 155 mg, dibasic sodium phosphate 852 mg, and monobasic sodium phosphate 130 mg [equivalent to elemental phosphorus 250 mg (8 mmol), sodium 298 mg (13 mEq), and potassium 45 mg (1.1 mEq)]

K-Phos No. 2: Potassium acid phosphate 305 mg and sodium acid phosphate 700 mg [equivalent to elemental phosphorus 250 mg (8 mmol), sodium 134 mg (5.8 mEq), and potassium 88 mg (2.3 mEq)]

Phospha 250 Neutral: Monobasic potassium phosphate 155 mg, dibasic sodium phosphate 852 mg, and monobasic sodium phosphate 130 mg [equivalent to elemental phosphorus 250 mg (8 mmol), sodium 298 mg (13 mEq), and potassium 45 mg (1.1 mEq)]

Virt-Phos 250 Neutral: Monobasic potassium phosphate 155 mg, dibasic sodium phosphate 852 mg, and monobasic sodium phosphate 130 mg [equivalent to elemental phosphorus 250 mg (8 mmol), sodium 298 mg (13 mEq), and potassium 45 mg (1.1 mEq)]

◆ Potassium Phosphate Monobasic *see* Potassium Acid Phosphate *on page 1478*

◆ Potassium Sulfate, Magnesium Sulfate, and Sodium Sulfate *see* Sodium Phosphate, Potassium Sulfate, and Magnesium Sulfate *on page 1681*

◆ Potassium Sulfate, Sodium Sulfate, and Magnesium Sulfate *see* Sodium Phosphate, Potassium Sulfate, and Magnesium Sulfate *on page 1681*

◆ Potiga *see* Ezogabine *on page 731*

◆ PPD *see* Tuberculin Tests *on page 1850*

◆ PPI-0903 *see* Ceftaroline Fosamil *on page 344*

◆ PPI-0903M *see* Ceftaroline Fosamil *on page 344*

◆ PPS *see* Pentosan Polysulfate Sodium *on page 1426*

◆ PPSV *see* Pneumococcal Polysaccharide Vaccine (23-Valent) *on page 1464*

◆ PPSV23 *see* Pneumococcal Polysaccharide Vaccine (23-Valent) *on page 1464*

◆ PPV23 *see* Pneumococcal Polysaccharide Vaccine (23-Valent) *on page 1464*

◆ PR-171 *see* Carfilzomib *on page 315*

◆ Pradaxa *see* Dabigatran Etexilate *on page 473*

PRALAtrexate (pral a TREX ate)

Brand Names: US Folotyn

Index Terms PDX

Pharmacologic Category Antineoplastic Agent, Antimetabolite; Antineoplastic Agent, Antimetabolite (Antifolate)

Use Peripheral T-cell lymphoma: Treatment of relapsed or refractory peripheral T-cell lymphoma (PTCL)

Pregnancy Considerations Adverse effects were observed in animal reproduction studies. May cause fetal harm if administered to a pregnant woman.

Breast-Feeding Considerations It is not known if pralatrexate is excreted in breast milk. Due to the potential for serious adverse reactions in the nursing infant, a decision should be made to discontinue breast-feeding or to discontinue pralatrexate, taking into account the benefits of treatment to the mother.

Contraindications There are no contraindications listed in the manufacturer's labeling.

Warnings/Precautions Hazardous agent - use appropriate precautions for handling and disposal (NIOSH 2014 [group 1]). May cause bone marrow suppression (thrombocytopenia, neutropenia and anemia); may require dosage modification; monitor blood counts. Mucositis, including stomatitis or mucosal inflammation of gastrointestinal and genitourinary tracts, may occur; monitor weekly; may require dosage modification. Prophylactic folic acid and vitamin B_{12} supplements are necessary to reduce hematologic toxicity and treatment-related mucositis. Severe and potentially fatal dermatologic reactions, including skin exfoliation, ulceration, and toxic epidermal necrolysis (TEN) have been reported. Skin reaction may be progressive; severity may increase with continued treatment; may also involve skin and subcutaneous tissues which are affected by lymphoma; monitor all dermatologic reactions closely; withhold or discontinue treatment for severe dermatologic reaction.

Pralatrexate may cause tumor lysis syndrome (TLS); monitor closely, if TLS develops, treat for associated complications. Use with caution in patients with moderate-to-severe renal impairment (has not been studied in patients with renal impairment); monitor renal function and for systemic toxicity due to increased exposure. Concurrent use with drugs with substantial renal clearance (eg, NSAIDs, sulfamethoxazole/trimethoprim) may result in delayed pralatrexate clearance. Liver function test abnormalities have been observed with use; monitor liver function; persistent abnormalities may indicate hepatotoxicity and may require dosage modification or discontinuation.

Patients with moderate-to-severe renal impairment are at risk for increased exposure and toxicity. Avoid use in patients with end-stage renal disease (ESRD), including patients undergoing dialysis (unless the potential benefit outweighs potential risks); serious adverse reactions, including toxic epidermal necrolysis and mucositis were reported in patients with ESRD undergoing dialysis. Monitor renal function and for systemic toxicity due to increased exposure. Potentially significant drug-drug interactions may exist, requiring dose or frequency adjustment, additional monitoring, and/or selection of alternative therapy.

Adverse Reactions

>10%:

Cardiovascular: Edema (30%)

Central nervous system: Fatigue (36%), fever (32%)

Dermatologic: Rash (15%; grades 3/4: 0%), pruritus (14%; grade 3: 2%; grade 4: 0%)

Endocrine & metabolic: Hypokalemia (15%)

Gastrointestinal: Mucositis (70%; grade 3: 17%; grade 4: 4%), nausea (40%), constipation (33%), vomiting (25%), diarrhea (21%), anorexia (15%), abdominal pain (12%)

Hematologic: Thrombocytopenia (41%; grade 3: 14%; grade 4: 19%), anemia (34%; grade 3: 15%; grade 4: 2%), neutropenia (24%; grade 3: 13%; grade 4: 7%), leukopenia (11%; grade 3: 3%; grade 4: 4%)

Hepatic: Transaminases increased (13%; grade 3: 5%; grade 4: 0%)

Neuromuscular & skeletal: Limb pain (12%), back pain (11%)

Respiratory: Cough (28%), epistaxis (26%), dyspnea (19%), pharyngolaryngeal pain (14%)

Miscellaneous: Night sweats (11%), infection

1% to 10%:

Cardiovascular: Tachycardia (10%)

Endocrine & metabolic: Dehydration (serious >3%)

Hematologic: Neutropenic fever (serious >3%)

Neuromuscular & skeletal: Weakness (10%)

Respiratory: Upper respiratory infection (10%)

Miscellaneous: Sepsis (serious >3%)

<1% (Limited to important or life-threatening): Bowel obstruction, cardiopulmonary arrest, lymphopenia, odynophagia, pancytopenia, skin exfoliation, skin ulceration, toxic epidermal necrolysis (TEN), tumor lysis syndrome (TLS)

Drug Interactions

Metabolism/Transport Effects Substrate of BCRP

Avoid Concomitant Use

Avoid concomitant use of PRALAtrexate with any of the following: BCG (Intravesical); Natalizumab; Pimecrolimus; Tacrolimus (Topical); Tofacitinib; Vaccines (Live)

Increased Effect/Toxicity

PRALAtrexate may increase the levels/effects of: Fingolimod; Leflunomide; Natalizumab; Tofacitinib; Vaccines (Live)

The levels/effects of PRALAtrexate may be increased by: Denosumab; Nonsteroidal Anti-Inflammatory Agents; Pimecrolimus; Probenecid; Roflumilast; Salicylates; Sulfamethoxazole; Tacrolimus (Topical); Trastuzumab; Trimethoprim

Decreased Effect

PRALAtrexate may decrease the levels/effects of: BCG (Intravesical); Coccidioides immitis Skin Test; Sapropterin; Sipuleucel-T; Vaccines (Inactivated); Vaccines (Live)

The levels/effects of PRALAtrexate may be decreased by: Echinacea

Preparation for Administration Hazardous agent; use appropriate precautions for handling and disposal (NIOSH 2014 [group 1]). Withdraw into syringe for administration; do not dilute (manufacturer recommends immediate use after placing in syringe). Discard unused portion in the vial.

Storage/Stability Store intact vials refrigerated at 2°C to 8°C (36°F to 46°F). Store in original carton to protect from light until use. Unopened vials (stored in the original carton) are stable for up to 72 hours at room temperature (discard after 72 hours).

Mechanism of Action Antifolate analog; inhibits DNA, RNA, and protein synthesis by selectively entering cells expressing reduced folate carrier (RFC-1), is polyglutamylated by folylpolyglutamate synthetase (FPGS) and then competes for the DHFR-folate binding site to inhibit dihydrofolate reductase (DHFR)

Pharmacodynamics/Kinetics

Distribution: *S*-diastereomer: 105 L; *R*-diastereomer: 37 L

Protein binding: ~67%

Half-life elimination: 12 to 18 hours

Excretion: Urine (~34% as unchanged drug)

Dosing

Adult & Geriatric Note: Initiate vitamin supplements before initial pralatrexate dose: Folic acid 1 to 1.25 mg/day orally beginning 10 days prior to initial pralatrexate dose; continue during treatment and for 30 days after last pralatrexate dose; vitamin B_{12} 1,000 mcg IM within 10 weeks prior to initial pralatrexate dose and every 8 to 10 weeks thereafter (after initial dose, B_{12} may be administered on the same day as pralatrexate).

Prior to administering any dose, mucositis should be ≤ grade 1 and absolute neutrophil count (ANC) should be ≥1,000/mm³; platelets should be ≥100,000/mm³ for the first dose and ≥50,000/mm³ for subsequent doses

Peripheral T-cell lymphoma (PTCL), relapsed or refractory: IV: 30 mg/m² once weekly for 6 weeks of a 7-week treatment cycle; continue until disease progression or unacceptable toxicity (O'Connor, 2011)

Cutaneous T-cell lymphoma, relapsed or refractory (off-label use): IV: 15 mg/m² once weekly for 3 weeks of a 4-week treatment cycle (Horwitz, 2012)

Renal Impairment

Moderate-to-severe renal impairment: Exposure and toxicities may be increased; monitor for toxicities and adjust dose accordingly.

End-stage renal disease (ESRD), including dialysis-dependent: Avoid use (unless the potential benefit outweighs risks).

Hepatic Impairment Patients with total bilirubin >1.5 mg/dL, AST or ALT >2.5 times the upper limit of normal (ULN), or ALT or AST >5 times ULN if documented hepatic lymphoma involvement were excluded from clinical trials. Persistent abnormalities may indicate hepatotoxicity requiring dosage modification:

Grade 3 (AST or ALT >5 to 20 times ULN or bilirubin >3 to 10 times ULN): Omit dose; decrease to 20 mg/m² when recovers to ≤ grade 2

Grade 4 (AST or ALT >20 times ULN or bilirubin >10 times ULN): Discontinue treatment.

Obesity *ASCO Guidelines for appropriate chemotherapy dosing in obese adults with cancer:* Utilize patient's actual body weight (full weight) for calculation of body surface area- or weight-based dosing, particularly when the intent of therapy is curative; manage regimen-related toxicities in the same manner as for nonobese patients; if a dose reduction is utilized due to toxicity, consider resumption of full weight-based dosing with subsequent cycles, especially if cause of toxicity (eg, hepatic or renal impairment) is resolved (Griggs, 2012).

Adjustment for Toxicity Severe or intolerable adverse events may require dose omission, reduction or interruption. Do not make up omitted doses at the end of a cycle; do not re-escalate dose after a reduction due to toxicity.

Hematologic toxicity:

Platelets:

<50,000/mm³ (for 1-week duration): Omit dose; continue at previous dose if platelets recover within 1 week

<50,000/mm³ (for 2-week duration): Omit dose; decrease to 20 mg/m² if platelets recover within 2 weeks

<50,000/mm³ (for 3-week duration): Discontinue treatment.

ANC:

500 to 1,000/mm³ without fever (for 1-week duration): Omit dose; continue at previous dose if ANC recovers within 1 week

500 to 1,000/mm³ with fever **or** ANC <500/mm³ (for 1-week duration): Omit dose, give filgrastim or sargramostim support; continue at previous dose (with growth factor support) if ANC recovers within 1 week

500 to 1,000/mm³ with fever **or** ANC <500/mm³ (recurrent or for 2-week duration): Omit dose and give filgrastim or sargramostim support; decrease to 20 mg/m² (with growth factor support) if ANC recovers within 2 weeks

500 to 1,000/mm³ with fever **or** ANC <500/mm³ (second recurrence or for 3 week duration): Discontinue treatment.

Nonhematologic toxicity: Mucositis (on day of treatment):

Grade 2: Omit dose; continue at previous dose when recovers to ≤ grade 1

Grade 3 or recurrent grade 2: Omit dose and decrease to 20 mg/m² when recovers to ≤ grade 1

Grade 4: Discontinue treatment.

Nonhematologic toxicity (other than mucositis):

Grade 3: Omit dose; decrease to 20 mg/m² when recovers to ≤ grade 2

Grade 4: Discontinue treatment.

◀ **Administration** Administer IV push (undiluted) over 3 to 5 minutes into the line of a free-flowing normal saline IV

Hazardous agent; use appropriate precautions for handling and disposal (NIOSH 2014 [group 1]).

Monitoring Parameters CBC with differential (baseline and weekly), serum chemistries, including renal and liver function tests (prior to the first and fourth doses in each cycle); mucositis severity (baseline and weekly); monitor for signs of tumor lysis syndrome and for dermatologic reactions

Dosage Forms Excipient information presented when available (limited, particularly for generics); consult specific product labeling.

Solution, Intravenous [preservative free]:
Folotyn: 20 mg/mL (1 mL); 40 mg/2 mL (2 mL)

Pralidoxime (pra li DOKS eem)

Brand Names: US Protopam Chloride

Index Terms 2-PAM; 2-Pyridine Aldoxime Methochloride; 2PAM; Pralidoxime Chloride

Pharmacologic Category Antidote

Use Treatment of muscle weakness and/or respiratory depression secondary to poisoning due to organophosphate anticholinesterase pesticides and chemicals (eg, nerve agents); control of overdose of anticholinesterase medications used to treat myasthenia gravis (ambenonium, neostigmine, pyridostigmine)

Dosing

Adult & Geriatric

Anticholinesterase overdose (eg, neostigmine, pyridostigmine): IV: 1000-2000 mg; followed by increments of 250 mg every 5 minutes as needed

Organophosphate poisoning: Note: Use in conjunction with atropine; a response to atropine should be established before pralidoxime is administered. IM or SubQ administration should be considered when IV administration is not feasible:

IV: Loading dose: 1000-2000 mg; Maintenance: Repeat bolus of 1000-2000 mg after 1 hour and repeated every 10-12 hours thereafter, as needed. Alternatively, administer a loading dose of 30 mg/kg followed by a maintenance infusion of 8 mg/kg/hour (off-label dose; Roberts, 2007).

IM:

Mild symptoms: 600 mg; repeat as needed for persistent mild symptoms every 15 minutes to a maximum total dose of 1800 mg; may administer doses in rapid succession if severe symptoms develop

Severe symptoms: 600 mg; repeat twice in rapid succession to deliver a total dose of 1800 mg

Persistent symptoms: May repeat the entire series (1800 mg) beginning ~1 hour after administration of the last injection

Pediatric Organophosphate poisoning: Note: Use in conjunction with atropine; a response to atropine should be established before pralidoxime is administered. IM or SubQ administration should be considered when IV administration is not feasible:

IV:

Children and Adolescents ≤16 years: Loading dose: 20-50 mg/kg (maximum: 2000 mg/dose); Maintenance infusion: 10-20 mg/kg/hour; alternatively, a repeat bolus of 20-50 mg/kg (maximum: 2000 mg/dose) may be administered after 1 hour and repeated every 10-12 hours thereafter, as needed

Adolescents >16 years: Refer to adult dosing.

IM:

Children <40 kg:

Mild symptoms: 15 mg/kg; repeat as needed for persistent mild symptoms every 15 minutes to a maximum total dose of 45 mg/kg; may administer doses in rapid succession if severe symptoms develop

Severe symptoms: 15 mg/kg; repeat twice in rapid succession to deliver a total dose of 45 mg/kg

Persistent symptoms: May repeat the entire series (45 mg/kg) beginning ~1 hour after administration of the last injection

Children ≥40 kg and Adolescents: Refer to adult dosing.

Renal Impairment No specific dosage adjustment provided in manufacturer's labeling; however, because pralidoxime is excreted in the urine, dosage reduction is recommended in patients with renal impairment.

Hepatic Impairment No dosage adjustment provided in the manufacturer's labeling; undergoes hepatic metabolism.

Additional Information Complete prescribing information should be consulted for additional detail.

Dosage Forms Excipient information presented when available (limited, particularly for generics); consult specific product labeling.

Solution Auto-injector, Intramuscular, as chloride:
Generic: 600 mg/2 mL (2 mL)

Solution Reconstituted, Intravenous, as chloride:
Protopam Chloride: 1 g (1 ea)

◆ Pralidoxime and Atropine see Atropine and Pralidoxime on page 179

◆ Pralidoxime Chloride see Pralidoxime on page 1486

◆ Praluent see Alirocumab on page 70

◆ PramCort see Pramoxine and Hydrocortisone on page 1489

Pramipexole (pra mi PEKS ole)

Brand Names: US Mirapex; Mirapex ER

Brand Names: Canada ACT-Pramipexole; Apo-Pramipexole; Auro-Pramipexole; Ava-Pramipexole; Dom-Pramipexole; Mirapex; Mylan-Pramipexole; PMS-Pramipexole; Sandoz-Pramipexole; Teva-Pramipexole

Index Terms Pramipexole Dihydrochloride Monohydrate

Pharmacologic Category Anti-Parkinson's Agent, Dopamine Agonist

Use

Parkinson disease: Treatment of Parkinson disease.

Restless legs syndrome (immediate release only): Treatment of moderate to severe primary restless legs syndrome (RLS).

Pregnancy Considerations Adverse events were observed in animal reproduction studies. Information related to the use of pramipexole for the treatment of Parkinson's disease (Benbir, 2013; Mucchiut 2004) or restless legs syndrome (RLS) (Dostal, 2013) in pregnant women is limited. Current guidelines note that the available information is insufficient to make a recommendation for the treatment of RLS in pregnant women (Aurora, 2012).

Breast-Feeding Considerations It is not known if pramipexole is excreted into breast milk; however, pramipexole inhibits prolactin secretion in humans and may potentially inhibit lactation. Due to the potential for serious adverse reactions in the nursing infant, the manufacturer recommends a decision be made whether to discontinue nursing or to discontinue the drug, taking into account the importance of treatment to the mother.

Contraindications There are no contraindications listed in the manufacturer's labeling.

Warnings/Precautions Caution should be taken in patients with renal impairment; dose adjustment may be necessary. Extended-release tablets are not recommended for use in patients with CrCl <30 mL/minute or ESRD requiring hemodialysis. May cause or exacerbate dyskinesias; use caution in patients with preexisting dyskinesias. May cause orthostatic hypotension; Parkinson disease patients appear to have an impaired capacity to respond to a postural challenge. Use with caution in patients at risk of hypotension or where transient hypotensive episodes would be poorly tolerated. Parkinson patients being treated with dopaminergic agonists ordinarily require careful monitoring for signs and symptoms of postural hypotension, especially during dose escalation. May cause hallucinations (visual, auditory, or mixed), particularly in older patients. May cause or exacerbate mental status and behavioral changes, which may be severe, including psychotic-like behavior during treatment or after starting or increasing the dose; manifestations may include paranoid ideation, delusions, hallucinations, confusion, psychotic-like behavior, disorientation, aggressive behavior, agitation, and delirium. Avoid use in patients with a major psychotic disorder. Dopaminergic therapy has been reported to cause symptoms resembling neuroleptic malignant syndrome (altered consciousness, autonomic instability, elevated temperature, and muscular rigidity) associated with rapid dose reduction, discontinuation, or changes in therapy; taper dose to decrease risk of hyperpyrexia and confusion.

Dopamine agonists have been associated with compulsive behaviors and/or loss of impulse control, which has manifested as pathological gambling, compulsive buying, libido increases (hypersexuality), binge eating, and/or other intense urges. Causality has not been established, and controversy exists as to whether this phenomenon is related to the underlying disease, prior behaviors/addictions and/or drug therapy. Dose reduction or discontinuation of therapy has been reported to reverse these behaviors in some, but not all cases. Risk for melanoma development is increased in Parkinson disease patients; drug causation or factors contributing to risk have not been

established. Patients should be monitored closely and periodic skin examinations should be performed.

Taper gradually when discontinuing therapy in Parkinson disease; dopaminergic agents have been associated with a syndrome resembling neuroleptic malignant syndrome on abrupt withdrawal or significant dosage reduction after long-term use. Ergot-derived dopamine agonists have been associated with fibrotic complications (eg, retroperitoneal fibrosis, pleural effusion, pleural thickening, pulmonary infiltrates, cardiac valvulopathy). Although pramipexole is not an ergot, there have been postmarketing reports of possible fibrotic complications (peritoneal, pleural, pulmonary) with pramipexole; monitor closely for signs and symptoms of fibrosis. Discontinuation of therapy may resolve complications, but not in all cases.

Pramipexole has been associated with somnolence, particularly at higher dosages (>1.5 mg/day). In addition, patients have reported falling asleep while engaging in activities of daily living; this has been reported to occur without significant warning signs; some of these events had been reported one year after the initiation of therapy. Before initiating treatment, advise patients of the potential to develop drowsiness, and inquire about factors that may increase the risk (eg, concomitant sedating medications and/or alcohol, presence of sleep disorders, concomitant medications that increase pramipexole plasma levels). Patients must be cautioned about performing tasks which require mental alertness (eg, operating machinery, driving). Monitor for daytime somnolence or preexisting sleep disorder; discontinue if significant daytime sleepiness or episodes of falling asleep occur; if a decision is made to continue therapy, advise patients not to drive and to avoid other potentially dangerous activities. Pramipexole has been associated with somnolence. Use caution in elderly patients because they may be more sensitive to these adverse drug reactions.

Pathologic degenerative changes were observed in the retinas of albino rats during studies with this agent, but were not observed in the retinas of albino mice or in other species. The significance of these data for humans remains uncertain. Augmentation (earlier onset of symptoms in the evening/afternoon, increase and/or spread of symptoms to other extremities) or rebound (worsening of symptoms following treatment cessation with greater intensity than before treatment initiation) may occur in some RLS patients. Potentially significant interactions may exist, requiring dose or frequency adjustment, additional monitoring, and/or selection of alternative therapy.

Adverse Reactions Actual frequency may be dependent on dose and/or formulation. All adverse reactions are as reported for Parkinson disease unless otherwise noted.
>10%:
Cardiovascular: Orthostatic hypotension (3% to 53%; dose related)
Central nervous system: Drowsiness (Parkinson disease: 9% to 36%; dose related; restless leg syndrome: 6%), extrapyramidal reaction (28%), insomnia (Parkinson disease: 4% to 27%; restless leg syndrome: 13%), dizziness (2% to 26%), hallucination (5% to 17%), headache (restless leg syndrome: 16%; Parkinson disease: 4% to 7%), worsening of restless leg syndrome (augmentation; 12%), abnormal dreams (Parkinson disease: 11%; restless leg syndrome: 8%)
Gastrointestinal: Nausea (Parkinson disease: 11% to 28%; dose related; restless leg syndrome: 11% to 27%), constipation (Parkinson disease: 6% to 14%; dose related; restless leg syndrome: 4%)
Neuromuscular & skeletal: Dyskinesia (17% to 47%), weakness (3% to 14%)
Miscellaneous: Accidental injury (17%)
1% to 10%:
Cardiovascular: Peripheral edema (2% to 8%), edema (4% to 5%), chest pain (3%)
Central nervous system: Worsening of restless leg syndrome (rebound; 10%), confusion (4% to 10%), fatigue (restless leg syndrome: 7% to 9%; Parkinson disease: 6%), dystonia (2% to 8%), abnormal gait (7%), hypertonia (7%), amnesia (4% to 6%; dose related), narcolepsy (2% to 6%), falling (4%), impulse control disorder (3% to 4%; eg, binge eating, hypersexuality, pathological gambling, shopping), vertigo (2% to 4%), hypoesthesia (3%), abnormality in thinking (2% to 3%), akathisia (2% to 3%), malaise (2% to 3%), sleep disorder (1% to 3%), equilibrium disturbance (2%), paranoia (2%), depression (2%), delusions (2%), myasthenia (1%), myoclonus (1%)
Dermatologic: Dermatological disease (2%)
Endocrine & metabolic: Weight loss (2%), decreased libido (1%)

Gastrointestinal: Xerostomia (Parkinson disease: 4% to 7%; restless leg syndrome: 3%), diarrhea (restless leg syndrome: 1% to 7%; Parkinson disease: 2%), anorexia (4% to 5%), vomiting (4%), upper abdominal pain (3% to 4%), dyspepsia (3%), increased appetite (2% to 3%), dysphagia (2%), sialorrhea (2%), abdominal distress (1% to 2%)
Genitourinary: Urinary frequency (6%), urinary tract infection (4%), impotence (2%), urinary incontinence (2%)
Infection: Influenza (restless leg syndrome: 3% to 7%)
Neuromuscular & skeletal: Limb pain (restless leg syndrome: 3% to 7%), muscle spasm (5%), arthritis (3%), tremor (3%), back pain (2% to 3%), bursitis (2%), muscle twitching (2%), elevated creatinine phosphokinase (1%)
Ophthalmic: Accommodation disturbance (4%), visual disturbance (3%), diplopia (1%)
Respiratory: Nasal congestion (restless leg syndrome: 3% to 6%), dyspnea (4%), cough (3%), rhinitis (3%), pneumonia (2%)
Miscellaneous: Fever (1%)
<1% (Limited to important or life-threatening): Aggressive behavior, agitation, altered mental status, behavioral changes, cardiac failure, delirium, delusions, disorientation, fibrothorax, increased libido, paranoia, peritoneal fibrosis, psychotic symptoms, pulmonary fibrosis, rhabdomyolysis, SIADH, syncope

Drug Interactions
Metabolism/Transport Effects None known.
Avoid Concomitant Use
Avoid concomitant use of Pramipexole with any of the following: Amisulpride; Sulpiride
Increased Effect/Toxicity
Pramipexole may increase the levels/effects of: Amifostine; BuPROPion; DULoxetine; Hypotension-Associated Agents; Levodopa

The levels/effects of Pramipexole may be increased by: Alcohol (Ethyl); Alfuzosin; Blood Pressure Lowering Agents; Brimonidine (Topical); Cimetidine; CNS Depressants; Diazoxide; Herbs (Hypotensive Properties); Methylphenidate; Molsidomine; Nicorandil; Obinutuzumab; Pentoxifylline; Phosphodiesterase 5 Inhibitors; Prostacyclin Analogues
Decreased Effect
Pramipexole may decrease the levels/effects of: Amisulpride; Antipsychotic Agents (First Generation [Typical]); Sulpiride

The levels/effects of Pramipexole may be decreased by: Amisulpride; Antipsychotic Agents (First Generation [Typical]); Antipsychotic Agents (Second Generation [Atypical]); Metoclopramide; Sulpiride
Food Interactions Food intake does not affect the extent of drug absorption although the time to maximal plasma concentration is delayed when taken with a meal. Management: Administer without regard to meals.
Storage/Stability Store at 25°C (77°F); excursions permitted to 15°C to 30°C (59°F to 86°F). Protect from light and high humidity.
Mechanism of Action Pramipexole is a nonergot dopamine agonist with specificity for the D_2 subfamily dopamine receptor, and has also been shown to bind to D_3 and D_4 receptors. By binding to these receptors, it is thought that pramipexole can stimulate dopamine activity on the nerves of the striatum and substantia nigra.
Pharmacodynamics/Kinetics
Absorption: Rapid
Distribution: V_d: 500 L
Protein binding: ~15%
Metabolism: Negligible (<10%)
Bioavailability: Immediate release: >90%; Extended release (as compared to immediate release): 100%
Half-life elimination: 8.5 hours; Elderly: 12 hours
Time to peak, serum: Immediate release: ~2 hours; Extended release: 6 hours
Excretion: Urine (90% as unchanged drug)
Dosing
Adult & Geriatric Note: Retitration of dose should be considered for any significant interruption in therapy.
Parkinson disease: Oral:
Immediate release: Initial: 0.125 mg 3 times daily, increase gradually every 5 to 7 days; maintenance (usual): 0.5 to 1.5 mg 3 times daily
Discontinuation of therapy: Reduce dose by 0.75 mg per day until daily dose is equivalent to 0.75 mg once daily, then reduce by 0.375 mg per day thereafter
Extended release: Initial: 0.375 mg once daily; increase gradually not more frequently than every 5 to 7 days to 0.75 mg once daily and then (if necessary) by 0.75 mg per dose; maximum: 4.5 mg once daily.

Discontinuation of therapy: Reduce dose by 0.75 mg per day until daily dose is equivalent to 0.75 mg once daily, then reduce by 0.375 mg per day thereafter.

Converting from immediate release to extended release: May initiate extended-release tablet the morning after the last immediate-release evening tablet is taken. The total daily dose should remain the same.

Restless legs syndrome: Oral: *Immediate release:* Initial: 0.125 mg once daily 2 to 3 hours before bedtime. Dose may be doubled every 4 to 7 days up to 0.5 mg once daily. **Note:** If augmentation occurs, dose earlier in the day.

Discontinuation of therapy: No gradual dose reduction recommended in manufacturer's labeling; however, worsening of symptoms may occur with abrupt discontinuation.

Bipolar depression (off-label use): Oral: *Immediate release:* Initial: 0.125 mg given 2 to 3 times daily; increase gradually by 0.125 to 0.25 mg daily every 3 to 7 days to a target range of 1 to 3 mg/day given in 2 to 3 divided doses. In clinical trials, the average dose was 1.7 mg/day and maximum dose allowed was 4.5 or 5 mg/day. Used in combination with mood stabilizers (Goldberg 2004; Zarate 2004).

Fibromyalgia (off-label use): Oral: *Immediate release:* Initial: 0.25 mg once daily at bedtime; may be increased weekly by 0.25 mg/day increments up to 4.5 mg daily as a single bedtime dose. **Note:** Study evaluated use in patients receiving concomitant medications (Holman 2005).

Renal Impairment

Parkinson disease: *Immediate release:*

CrCl >50 mL/minute: No dosage adjustment necessary.

CrCl 30 to 50 mL/minute: Initial: 0.125 mg twice daily (maximum: 0.75 mg 3 times daily)

CrCl 15 to 29 mL/minute: Initial: 0.125 mg once daily (maximum: 1.5 mg once daily)

CrCl <15 mL/minute: There are no dosage adjustments provided in the manufacturer's labeling (has not been studied).

ESRD requiring hemodialysis: There are no dosage adjustments provided in the manufacturer's labeling (has not been studied).

Parkinson disease: *Extended release:*

CrCl >50 mL/minute: No dosage adjustment necessary.

CrCl 30 to 50 mL/minute: Initial: 0.375 mg every other day; may increase to 0.375 mg once daily no sooner than 1 week after initiation. If necessary, may increase by 0.375 mg per dose not more frequently than every 7 days; maximum recommended dose: 2.25 mg once daily

CrCl <30 mL/minute: Use not recommended.

ESRD requiring hemodialysis: Use not recommended.

Restless legs syndrome: *Immediate release:*

CrCl >60 mL/minute: No dosage adjustment necessary.

CrCl 20 to 60 mL/minute: No dosage adjustment necessary; however, duration between titration should be increased to 14 days.

CrCl <20 mL/minute: There are no dosage adjustments provided in the manufacturer's labeling (has not been studied).

Hepatic Impairment Immediate release and extended release: There are no dosage adjustments provided in the manufacturer's labeling (has not been studied); however, no adjustment expected since undergoes minimal hepatic metabolism.

Dietary Considerations May be taken with or without food. May be taken with food to decrease nausea.

Administration Doses should be titrated gradually to avoid the onset of intolerable side effects. The dosage should be increased to achieve a maximum therapeutic effect, balanced against the side effects of dyskinesia, hallucinations, somnolence, and dry mouth. Administer with or without food; administer with food to decrease nausea. Extended-release tablets should be swallowed whole and not chewed, crushed, or divided. For RLS, administer 2 to 3 hours before bedtime; if augmentation occurs, dose earlier in the day.

Monitoring Parameters Blood pressure, heart rate (especially during dose escalation); body weight changes; CNS depression, fall risk, behavior changes (eg, compulsive behaviors); periodic skin examinations.

Dosage Forms Excipient information presented when available (limited, particularly for generics); consult specific product labeling.

Tablet, Oral, as dihydrochloride monohydrate:
Mirapex: 0.125 mg
Mirapex: 0.25 mg, 0.5 mg [scored]
Mirapex: 0.75 mg
Mirapex: 1 mg, 1.5 mg [scored]

Generic: 0.125 mg, 0.25 mg, 0.5 mg, 0.75 mg, 1 mg, 1.5 mg

Tablet Extended Release 24 Hour, Oral, as dihydrochloride monohydrate:
Mirapex ER: 0.375 mg, 0.75 mg, 1.5 mg, 2.25 mg, 3 mg, 3.75 mg, 4.5 mg
Generic: 0.375 mg, 0.75 mg, 1.5 mg, 2.25 mg, 3 mg, 4.5 mg

♦ Pramipexole Dihydrochloride Monohydrate *see* Pramipexole *on page 1486*

Pramlintide (PRAM lin tide)

Brand Names: US SymlinPen 120; SymlinPen 60

Index Terms Pramlintide Acetate

Pharmacologic Category Amylinomimetic; Antidiabetic Agent

Use Type 1 and type 2 diabetes: Adjunct treatment in patients with type 1 or type 2 diabetes who use mealtime insulin therapy and who have failed to achieve desired glucose control despite optimal insulin therapy.

Pregnancy Considerations Adverse events have been observed in animal reproduction studies. Based on *in vitro* data, pramlintide has a low potential to cross the placenta.

In women with diabetes, maternal hyperglycemia can be associated with congenital malformations as well as adverse effects in the fetus, neonate, and the mother (ACOG 2005; ADA 2015; Kitzmiller 2008; Metzger 2007). To prevent adverse outcomes, prior to conception and throughout pregnancy maternal blood glucose and HbA$_{1c}$ should be kept as close to target goals as possible but without causing significant hypoglycemia (ACOG 2013; ADA 2015; Blumer 2013; Kitzmiller 2008). Prior to pregnancy, effective contraception should be used until glycemic control is achieved (Kitzmiller 2008). Other agents are currently recommended to treat diabetes in pregnant women (ACOG 2013; Blumer 2013).

Breast-Feeding Considerations It is not known if pramlintide is excreted in breast milk. The manufacturer recommends that pramlintide be used in nursing women only when the potential benefit to the mother outweighs the possible risk to the infant.

Medication Guide Available Yes

Contraindications Serious hypersensitivity to pramlintide or any component of the formulation; confirmed diagnosis of gastroparesis; hypoglycemia unawareness

Warnings/Precautions [U.S. Boxed Warning]: Coadministration with insulin may induce severe hypoglycemia (usually within 3 hours following administration); coadministration with insulin therapy is an approved indication but does require an initial dosage reduction of insulin and frequent pre and post blood glucose monitoring to reduce risk of severe hypoglycemia. Concurrent use of other glucose-lowering agents may increase risk of hypoglycemia. Avoid use in patients with poor compliance with their insulin regimen and/or blood glucose monitoring. Do not use in patients with HbA$_{1c}$ levels more than 9%, recurrent episodes of severe hypoglycemia requiring assistance during the past 6 months, or hypoglycemia unawareness; obtain detailed history of glucose control (eg, HbA$_{1c}$, incidence of hypoglycemia, glucose monitoring, and medication compliance) and body weight before initiating therapy. Use caution in patients with visual or dexterity impairment. Use caution when driving or operating heavy machinery until effects on blood sugar are known. Potentially significant drug-drug interactions may exist, requiring dose or frequency adjustment, additional monitoring, and/or selection of alternative therapy. Avoid use in patients with conditions or concurrent medications likely to impair gastric motility (eg, anticholinergics); do not use in patients requiring medication(s) to stimulate gastric emptying. Injection site reactions, including erythema, edema, or pruritus, may occur; usually resolve in a few days to weeks. According to the manufacturer and the Centers for Disease Control and Prevention (CDC), pen-shaped injection devices should never be used for more than one person (even when the needle is changed) because of the risk of transmission of blood-borne pathogens. The injection device should be clearly labeled with individual patient information to ensure that the correct pen is used (CDC, 2012).

Adverse Reactions

>10%:

Central nervous system: Headache (5% to 13%)

Endocrine & metabolic: Severe hypoglycemia (type 1 diabetes ≤17%)

Gastrointestinal: Nausea (28% to 48%), anorexia (≤17%), vomiting (7% to 11%)

Miscellaneous: Accidental injury (8% to 14%)

1% to 10%:

Central nervous system: Fatigue (3% to 7%), dizziness (2% to 6%)

Endocrine & metabolic: Severe hypoglycemia (type 2 diabetes ≤8%)

Gastrointestinal: Abdominal pain (2% to 8%)

Hypersensitivity: Hypersensitivity reaction (≤6%)

Neuromuscular & skeletal: Arthralgia (2% to 7%)

Respiratory: Cough (2% to 6%), pharyngitis (3% to 5%)

Postmarketing and/or case reports (Limited to important or life-threatening): Injection site reaction, pancreatitis

Drug Interactions

Metabolism/Transport Effects None known.

Avoid Concomitant Use There are no known interactions where it is recommended to avoid concomitant use.

Increased Effect/Toxicity

Pramlintide may increase the levels/effects of: Anticholinergic Agents; Hypoglycemia-Associated Agents; Insulin

The levels/effects of Pramlintide may be increased by: Alpha-Lipoic Acid; Androgens; MAO Inhibitors; Pegvisomant; Quinolone Antibiotics; Salicylates; Selective Serotonin Reuptake Inhibitors

Decreased Effect

The levels/effects of Pramlintide may be decreased by: Hyperglycemia-Associated Agents; Quinolone Antibiotics; Thiazide Diuretics

Storage/Stability Store at 2°C to 8°C (36°F to 46°F); do not freeze. After initial use, may be kept refrigerated or at room temperature ≤30°C (≤86°F); discard after 30 days. Protect from light.

Mechanism of Action Synthetic analog of human amylin cosecreted with insulin by pancreatic beta cells; reduces postprandial glucose increases via the following mechanisms: 1) prolongation of gastric emptying time, 2) reduction of postprandial glucagon secretion, and 3) reduction of caloric intake through centrally-mediated appetite suppression

Pharmacodynamics/Kinetics

Duration: ~3 hours

Protein binding: ~60%

Metabolism: Primarily renal to des-lys^1 pramlintide (active metabolite)

Bioavailability: ~30% to 40%

Half-life elimination: ~48 minutes

Time to peak, plasma: 20 minutes

Excretion: Primarily urine

Dosing

Adult & Geriatric Note: When initiating pramlintide, reduce current mealtime insulin dose (including premixed preparations) by 50% to avoid hypoglycemia. If pramlintide is discontinued for any reason, restart therapy with same initial titration protocol. If a dose is missed, wait until the next scheduled dose and administer the usual amount.

Type 1 diabetes mellitus: SubQ: Initial: 15 mcg immediately prior to major meals; titrate in 15 mcg increments every 3 days (if no significant nausea occurs) to target dose of 30 to 60 mcg prior to major meals (consider discontinuation if intolerant of 30 mcg dose)

Type 2 diabetes mellitus: SubQ: Initial: 60 mcg immediately prior to major meals; after 3 days, increase to 120 mcg prior to each major meal if no significant nausea occurs (if nausea occurs at 120 mcg dose, reduce to 60 mcg)

Renal Impairment

CrCl ≥15 mL/minute: No dosage adjustment necessary.

End-stage renal disease [ESRD]: There are no dosage adjustments provided in the manufacturer's labeling (has not been studied).

Hepatic Impairment There are no dosage adjustments provided in the manufacturer's labeling (has not been studied); however, need for adjustment not likely since undergoes minimal hepatic metabolism.

Dietary Considerations Dietary modification based on ADA recommendations is a part of therapy; pramlintide to be administered prior to major meals consisting of ≥250 Kcal or ≥30 g carbohydrates

Administration Subcutaneous: Do not mix with insulins; administer subcutaneously into abdominal or thigh areas at sites distinct from concomitant insulin injections (do not administer into arm due to variable absorption); rotate injection sites frequently. Allow solution to reach room temperature before administering; may reduce injection site reactions. For oral medications in which a rapid onset of action is desired, administer 1 hour before, or 2 hours after pramlintide, if possible.

Monitoring Parameters Prior to initiating therapy: HbA$_{1c}$, hypoglycemic history, body weight. During therapy: Pre- and postprandial and bedtime serum glucose, HbA$_{1c}$, signs and symptoms of hypoglycemia

Reference Range

Recommendations for glycemic control in nonpregnant adults with diabetes (ADA, 2015):

HbA$_{1c}$: <7% (a more aggressive [<6.5%] or less aggressive [<8%] HbA$_{1c}$ goal may be targeted based on patient-specific characteristics)

Preprandial capillary plasma glucose: 80 to 130 mg/dL

Peak postprandial capillary blood glucose: <180 mg/dL

Recommendations for glycemic control in pediatric (all age groups) patients with type 1 diabetes (ADA, 2015):

HbA$_{1c}$: <7.5% (individualization may be appropriate based on patient-specific characteristics; <7% is reasonable if it can be achieved without excessive hypoglycemia)

Preprandial capillary plasma glucose: 90 to 130 mg/dL

Bedtime and overnight capillary blood glucose: 90 to 150 mg/dL

Dosage Forms Excipient information presented when available (limited, particularly for generics); consult specific product labeling.

Solution Pen-injector, Subcutaneous, as acetate:

SymlinPen 60: 1500 mcg/1.5 mL (1.5 mL) [contains metacresol]

SymlinPen 120: 2700 mcg/2.7 mL (2.7 mL) [contains metacresol]

◆ Pramlintide Acetate *see* Pramlintide *on page 1488*

◆ Pramosone *see* Pramoxine and Hydrocortisone *on page 1489*

◆ Pramosone E *see* Pramoxine and Hydrocortisone *on page 1489*

◆ Pramox HC (Can) *see* Pramoxine and Hydrocortisone *on page 1489*

Pramoxine and Hydrocortisone
(pra MOKS een & hye droe KOR ti sone)

Brand Names: US Analpram E; Analpram HC; Epifoam; Novacort; PramCort; Pramosone; Pramosone E; ProCort; ProctoFoam HC; Zypram [DSC]

Brand Names: Canada Pramox HC; Proctofoam-HC

Index Terms Hydrocortisone and Pramoxine; Pramoxine Hydrochloride and Hydrocortisone Acetate

Pharmacologic Category Anesthetic/Corticosteroid

Use Dermatoses: Relief of inflammatory and pruritic manifestations of corticosteroid-responsive dermatoses

Dosing

Adult & Geriatric Dermatoses: Topical, rectal: Apply to affected areas 3 to 4 times daily.

Pediatric Dermatoses: Infants, Children, and Adolescents: Topical, rectal: Refer to adult dosing.

Renal Impairment There are no dosage adjustments provided in the manufacturer's labeling.

Hepatic Impairment There are no dosage adjustments provided in the manufacturer's labeling.

Additional Information Complete prescribing information should be consulted for additional detail.

Dosage Forms Excipient information presented when available (limited, particularly for generics); consult specific product labeling.

Aerosol, foam, rectal:

ProctoFoam HC: Pramoxine hydrochloride 1% and hydrocortisone acetate 1% (10 g)

Aerosol, foam, topical:

Epifoam: Pramoxine hydrochloride 1% and hydrocortisone acetate 1% (10 g)

Cream, topical: Pramoxine hydrochloride 1% and hydrocortisone acetate 1% (30 g); pramoxine hydrochloride 1% and hydrocortisone acetate 2.5% (30 g)

Analpram Advanced Kit: Pramoxine hydrochloride 1% and hydrocortisone acetate 2.5% [kit includes Analpram HC cream, diosmiplex (Vasculera) tablets, AloeClean wipes, and applicators]

Analpram E Kit: Pramoxine hydrochloride 1% and hydrocortisone acetate 2.5% (4 g, 30 g) [kit includes Prax wipes]

Analpram HC: Pramoxine hydrochloride 1% and hydrocortisone acetate 1% (4 g, 30 g); pramoxine hydrochloride 1% and hydrocortisone acetate 2.5% (4 g, 30 g)

PramCort: Pramoxine hydrochloride 1% and hydrocortisone acetate 1% (30 g) [contains propylene glycol]

Pramosone: Pramoxine hydrochloride 1% and hydrocortisone acetate 1% (30 g, 60 g); pramoxine hydrochloride 1% and hydrocortisone acetate 2.5% (30 g, 60 g)

Pramosone E: Pramoxine hydrochloride 1% and hydrocortisone acetate 2.5% (30 g, 60 g)

ProCort: Pramoxine hydrochloride 1.15% and hydrocortisone acetate 1.85% (60 g)

Zypram: Pramoxine hydrochloride 1% and hydrocortisone acetate 2.35% (30 g [DSC]) [contains benzyl alcohol, propylene glycol]

Gel, topical:

Novacort: Pramoxine hydrochloride 1% and hydrocortisone acetate 2% (29 g) [contains aloe, benzyl alcohol, propylene glycol]

Lotion, topical:

Analpram-HC: Pramoxine hydrochloride 1% and hydrocortisone acetate 2.5% (60 mL)

Pramosone: Pramoxine hydrochloride 1% and hydrocortisone acetate 1% (60 mL, 120 mL, 240 mL); pramoxine hydrochloride 1% and hydrocortisone acetate 2.5% (60 mL, 120 mL)

Ointment, topical:

Pramosone: Pramoxine hydrochloride 1% and hydrocortisone acetate 1% (30 g); pramoxine hydrochloride 1% and hydrocortisone acetate 2.5% (30 g)

◆ Pramoxine Hydrochloride and Hydrocortisone Acetate *see* Pramoxine and Hydrocortisone *on page 1489*

◆ PrandiMet *see* Repaglinide and Metformin *on page 1570*

◆ Prandin *see* Repaglinide *on page 1569*

◆ Prascion *see* Sulfur and Sulfacetamide *on page 1716*

◆ Prascion FC *see* Sulfur and Sulfacetamide *on page 1716*

◆ Prascion RA *see* Sulfur and Sulfacetamide *on page 1716*

Prasugrel (PRA soo grel)

Brand Names: US Effient
Brand Names: Canada Effient
Index Terms CS-747; LY-640315; Prasugrel Hydrochloride
Pharmacologic Category Antiplatelet Agent; Antiplatelet Agent, Thienopyridine
Additional Appendix Information
Oral Antiplatelet Comparison Chart *on page 1963*
Use Acute coronary syndrome to be managed with percutaneous coronary intervention (PCI): To reduce the rate of thrombotic cardiovascular events (including stent thrombosis) in patients who are to be managed with PCI for unstable angina (UA), non-ST-segment elevation MI (NSTEMI), or ST-elevation MI (STEMI).
Medication Guide Available Yes
Dosing
Adult Acute coronary syndrome (ACS): Oral:

Percutaneous coronary intervention (PCI) for ACS: Loading dose: 60 mg administered promptly (as soon as coronary anatomy is known) and no later than 1 hour after PCI; Maintenance dose: 10 mg once daily (in combination with aspirin 75 to 325 mg/day; 81 mg/day recommended [Levine, 2011]). For patients with STEMI, a loading dose may also be administered if PCI is performed >24 hours after treatment with a fibrin-specific thrombolytic (ie, alteplase, reteplase, tenecteplase) (ACCF/AHA [O'Gara, 2013]).

Duration of prasugrel (in combination with aspirin) after stent placement: **Premature interruption of therapy may result in stent thrombosis, MI, and death.** According to the ACCF/AHA/SCAI PCI guidelines, those with ACS receiving either stent type (bare metal [BMS] or drug-eluting stent [DES]) or those receiving a DES for a non-ACS indication, prasugrel for at least 12 months is recommended (ACCF/AHA/SCAI [Levine, 2011]). The ACCF/AHA guidelines for the management of UA/NSTEMI recommend up to 12 months of prasugrel in patients with ACS who receive a BMS (ACCF/AHA [Anderson, 2013]). A duration >12 months may be considered in patients with DES placement. Recent data has demonstrated that continued dual antiplatelet therapy for a total of 30 months (compared to 12 months) significantly reduced the risk of stent thrombosis and major adverse cardiovascular/cerebrovascular events but was associated with a higher risk of bleeding (Mauri, 2014). Those receiving a BMS for a non-ACS indication should be given at least 1 month and ideally up to 12 months; if patient is at increased risk of bleeding, give for a minimum of 2 weeks (ACCF/AHA/SCAI [Levine, 2011]).

Maintenance dosing in low body weight (ie, <60 kg) individuals: Due to a higher incidence of bleeding in patients weighing <60 kg, a maintenance dose of 5 mg once daily may be considered. In aspirin-treated patients weighing <60 kg (mean: 56.4 ± 3.7 kg) with stable coronary artery disease, the use of prasugrel 5 mg once daily was shown to reduce platelet reactivity to a similar extent as prasugrel 10 mg administered once daily to patients >60 kg (mean: 84.7 ± 14.9 kg); clinical events were not evaluated (Erlinge, 2012). In patients with ACS (medically managed) treated with

aspirin, a 5 mg daily maintenance dose (after a 30 mg loading dose) in patients <60 kg did not demonstrate a significant difference in the composite primary end point of death from cardiovascular causes, MI, or stroke compared to patients >60 kg treated with a 10 mg maintenance dose; bleeding risk was not increased (Roe, 2012).

Conversion from clopidogrel to prasugrel: Beginning 24 hours after the last clopidogrel dose (loading or maintenance), may initiate prasugrel 10 mg once daily or a 60 mg loading dose followed in 24 hours with 10 mg once daily (Angiolillo, 2010; Payne, 2008; Wiviott, 2007).

Geriatric Refer to adult dosing. Patients ≥75 years: Use not recommended; may be considered in high-risk situations (eg, patients with diabetes or history of MI).

Renal Impairment No dosage adjustment necessary.

Hepatic Impairment

Mild to moderate hepatic impairment (Child-Pugh class A and B): No dosage adjustment necessary for mild-to-moderate hepatic impairment.

Severe hepatic impairment (Child-Pugh class C): No dosage adjustment provided in manufacturer's labeling (has not been studied).

Additional Information Complete prescribing information should be consulted for additional detail.

Dosage Forms Excipient information presented when available (limited, particularly for generics); consult specific product labeling.

Tablet, Oral:
Effient: 5 mg, 10 mg

◆ Prasugrel Hydrochloride *see* Prasugrel *on page 1490*

◆ Pravachol *see* Pravastatin *on page 1490*

Pravastatin (prav a STAT in)

Brand Names: US Pravachol
Brand Names: Canada ACT Pravastatin; Apo-Pravastatin; Dom-Pravastatin; JAMP-Pravastatin; Mint-Pravastatin; Mylan-Pravastatin; PHL-Pravastatin; PMS-Pravastatin; Pravachol; RAN-Pravastatin; Riva-Pravastatin; Sandoz-Pravastatin; Teva-Pravastatin
Index Terms Pravastatin Sodium
Pharmacologic Category Antilipemic Agent, HMG-CoA Reductase Inhibitor
Use Use with dietary therapy for the following:

Primary prevention of coronary events: In hypercholesterolemic patients without established coronary heart disease to reduce cardiovascular morbidity (myocardial infarction, coronary revascularization procedures) and mortality.

Secondary prevention of cardiovascular events in patients with established coronary heart disease: To slow the progression of coronary atherosclerosis; to reduce cardiovascular morbidity (myocardial infarction, coronary vascular procedures) and to reduce mortality; to reduce the risk of stroke and transient ischemic attacks

Primary and secondary prevention of atherosclerotic cardiovascular disease (ASCVD) according to the American College of Cardiology/American Heart Association: To reduce the risk of ASCVD in patients with clinical ASCVD (eg, coronary heart disease, stroke/TIA, or peripheral arterial disease presumed to be of atherosclerotic origin) who are greater than 75 years of age or not a candidate for high-intensity statin therapy; in patients without clinical ASCVD if LDL-C is 190 mg/dL or greater and not a candidate for high-intensity statin therapy; in patients without clinical ASCVD who have type 1 or type 2 diabetes and are between 40 and 75 years of age; in patients with an estimated 10-year ASCVD risk 7.5% or greater and who are between 40 and 75 years of age (Stone, 2013). The American Heart Association (AHA) recommends statin therapy (unless contraindicated) for all coronary artery bypass graft (CABG) surgery patients to help maintain long-term graft patency and help obtain the highest level of physical health and quality of life (AHA [Kulik, 2015]). Specific recommendations from the Kidney Disease: Improving Global Outcomes (KDIGO) organization have also been released for patients with chronic kidney disease (KDIGO [Tonelli, 2013]).

Hyperlipidemias: Reduce elevations in total cholesterol, LDL-C, apolipoprotein B, and triglycerides (elevations of 1 or more components are present in Fredrickson type IIa, IIb, III, and IV hyperlipidemias)

Heterozygous familial hypercholesterolemia (HeFH): In pediatric patients, 8-18 years of age, with HeFH having LDL-C ≥190 mg/dL **or** LDL ≥160 mg/dL with positive family history of premature cardiovascular disease (CVD) or 2 or more CVD risk factors in the pediatric patient

Pregnancy Considerations Adverse events were observed in some animal reproduction studies. Pravastatin was found to cross the placenta in an *ex vivo* study using term human placentas (Nanovskaya, 2013). There are reports of congenital anomalies following maternal use of HMG-CoA reductase Inhibitors in pregnancy; however, maternal disease, differences in specific agents used, and the low rates of exposure limit the interpretation of the available data (Godfrey, 2012; Lecarpentier, 2012). Cholesterol biosynthesis may be important in fetal development; serum cholesterol and triglycerides increase normally during pregnancy. The discontinuation of lipid lowering medications temporarily during pregnancy is not expected to have significant impact on the long term outcomes of primary hypercholesterolemia treatment.

Use of pravastatin is contraindicated in pregnancy. HMG-CoA reductase Inhibitors should be discontinued prior to pregnancy (ADA, 2013). If treatment of dyslipidemias is needed in pregnant women or in women of reproductive age, other agents are preferred (Berglund, 2012; Stone, 2013). The manufacturer recommends administration to women of childbearing potential only when conception is highly unlikely and patients have been informed of potential hazards.

Breast-Feeding Considerations A small amount of pravastatin is excreted into breast milk. Data is available from eight lactating females administered pravastatin 20 mg twice daily for 2.5 days. After the fifth dose, maximum maternal serum concentrations were ~40 ng/mL (pravastatin) and ~26 ng/mL (metabolite) and maximum milk concentrations were ~3.9 ng/mL (pravastatin) and ~2.1 ng/mL (metabolite). Maximum milk concentrations were detected ~3 hours after the dose (Pan, 1988). Due to the potential for serious adverse reactions in a nursing infant, use while breast-feeding is contraindicated by the manufacturer.

Contraindications Hypersensitivity to pravastatin or any component of the formulation; active liver disease; unexplained persistent elevations of serum transaminases; pregnancy; breast-feeding

Warnings/Precautions Secondary causes of hyperlipidemia should be ruled out prior to therapy. Liver function must be monitored by periodic laboratory assessment. Rhabdomyolysis with acute renal failure has occurred. Risk may be increased with concurrent use of other drugs which may cause rhabdomyolysis (including colchicine, gemfibrozil, fibric acid derivatives, or niacin at doses ≥1 g/day). Discontinue in any patient in which CPK levels are markedly elevated (>10 times ULN) or if myopathy is suspected/diagnosed. Immune-mediated necrotizing myopathy (IMNM), an autoimmune-mediated myopathy, has been reported (rarely) with HMG-CoA reductase inhibitor therapy. IMNM presents as proximal muscle weakness with elevated CPK levels, which persists despite discontinuation of HMG-CoA reductase inhibitor therapy; additionally, muscle biopsy may show necrotizing myopathy with limited inflammation; immunosuppressive therapy (eg, corticosteroids, azathioprine) may be used for treatment. The manufacturer recommends temporary discontinuation for elective major surgery, acute medical or surgical conditions, or in any patient experiencing an acute or serious condition predisposing to renal failure (eg, sepsis, hypotension, trauma, uncontrolled seizures). Based on current research and clinical guidelines (Fleisher, 2009), HMG-CoA reductase inhibitors should be continued in the perioperative period. Postoperative discontinuation of statin therapy is associated with an increased risk of cardiac morbidity and mortality. Use with caution in patients with advanced age, these patients are predisposed to myopathy. Use caution in patients with previous liver disease or heavy ethanol use. If serious hepatotoxicity with clinical symptoms and/or hyperbilirubinemia or jaundice occurs during treatment, interrupt therapy. If an alternate etiology is not identified, do not restart pravastatin. Liver enzyme tests should be obtained at baseline and as clinically indicated; routine periodic monitoring of liver enzymes is not necessary. Increases in HbA$_{1c}$ and fasting blood glucose have been reported with HMG-CoA reductase inhibitors; however, the benefits of statin therapy far outweigh the risk of dysglycemia. Treatment in patients <8 years of age is not recommended.

Adverse Reactions As reported in short-term trials; safety and tolerability with long-term use were similar to placebo 1% to 10%:

Cardiovascular: Chest pain (4%)

Central nervous system: Headache (2% to 6%), fatigue (4%), dizziness (1% to 3%)

Dermatologic: Rash (4%)

Gastrointestinal: Nausea/vomiting (7%), diarrhea (6%), heartburn (3%)

Genitourinary: Cystitis (interstitial; Huang 2015)

Hepatic: Increased transaminases (>3x normal on two occasions: 1%)

Neuromuscular & skeletal: Myalgia (2%)

Respiratory: Cough (3%)

Miscellaneous: Influenza (2%)

<1% (Limited to important or life-threatening): Allergy, amnesia (reversible), anaphylaxis, angioedema, cholestatic jaundice, cirrhosis, cognitive impairment (reversible), confusion (reversible), cranial nerve dysfunction, dermatomyositis, erythema multiforme, ESR increase, fulminant hepatic necrosis, gynecomastia, hemolytic anemia, hepatitis, hepatoma, lens opacity, libido change, lupus erythematosus-like syndrome, memory disturbance (reversible), memory impairment (reversible), muscle weakness, myopathy, neuropathy, pancreatitis, paresthesia, peripheral nerve palsy, polymyalgia rheumatica, positive ANA, purpura, rhabdomyolysis, Stevens-Johnson syndrome, taste disturbance, tremor, vasculitis, vertigo

Additional class-related events or case reports (not necessarily reported with pravastatin therapy): Angioedema, cataracts, depression, diabetes mellitus (new onset), dyspnea, eosinophilia, erectile dysfunction, facial paresis, hypersensitivity reaction, immune-mediated necrotizing myopathy (IMNM), impaired extraocular muscle movement, impotence, increased blood glucose, increased glycosylated hemoglobin (HbA$_{1c}$), increased transaminases, interstitial lung disease, leukopenia, malaise, memory loss, ophthalmoplegia, paresthesia, peripheral neuropathy, photosensitivity, psychic disturbance, skin discoloration, thrombocytopenia, thyroid dysfunction, toxic epidermal necrolysis, vomiting

Drug Interactions

Metabolism/Transport Effects Substrate of CYP3A4 (minor), P-glycoprotein, SLCO1B1; **Note:** Assignment of Major/Minor substrate status based on clinically relevant drug interaction potential; **Inhibits** CYP2C9 (weak), CYP2D6 (weak)

Avoid Concomitant Use

Avoid concomitant use of Pravastatin with any of the following: Fusidic Acid (Systemic); Gemfibrozil; Red Yeast Rice

Increased Effect/Toxicity

Pravastatin may increase the levels/effects of: ARIPiprazole; CycloSPORINE (Systemic); DAPTOmycin; PARoxetine; PAZOPanib; Trabectedin; Vitamin K Antagonists

The levels/effects of Pravastatin may be increased by: Acipimox; Antihepaciviral Combination Products; Bezafibrate; Boceprevir; Ciprofibrate; Clarithromycin; Colchicine; CycloSPORINE (Systemic); Daclatasvir; Darunavir; Eltrombopag; Erythromycin (Systemic); Fenofibrate and Derivatives; Fusidic Acid (Systemic); Gemfibrozil; Itraconazole; Niacin; Niacinamide; Raltegravir; Red Yeast Rice; Sacubitril; Simeprevir; Telaprevir; Telithromycin; Teriflunomide

Decreased Effect

Pravastatin may decrease the levels/effects of: Lanthanum

The levels/effects of Pravastatin may be decreased by: Antacids; Bile Acid Sequestrants; Efavirenz; Fosphenytoin; Nelfinavir; Phenytoin; Rifamycin Derivatives; Saquinavir

Storage/Stability Store at 25°C (77°F); excursions permitted to 15°C to 30°C (59°F to 86°F). Protect from moisture and light.

Mechanism of Action Pravastatin is a competitive inhibitor of 3-hydroxy-3-methylglutaryl coenzyme A (HMG-CoA) reductase, which is the rate-limiting enzyme involved in *de novo* cholesterol synthesis. In addition to the ability of HMG-CoA reductase inhibitors to decrease levels of high-sensitivity C-reactive protein (hsCRP), they also possess pleiotropic properties including improved endothelial function, reduced inflammation at the site of the coronary plaque, inhibition of platelet aggregation, and anticoagulant effects (de Denus, 2002; Ray, 2005).

Pharmacodynamics/Kinetics

Onset of action: Several days

Peak effect: 4 weeks

Absorption: Rapidly absorbed; average absorption 34%

Protein binding: 50%

Metabolism: Hepatic multiple metabolites; primary metabolite is 3α-hydroxy-iso-pravastatin (2.5% to 10% activity of parent drug)

Bioavailability: 17%

Half-life elimination: 77 hours (including all metabolites); pravastatin: ~2-3 hours (Pan, 1990); 3α-hydroxy-iso-pravastatin: ~1.5 hours (Gustavson, 2005)

Time to peak, serum: 1-1.5 hours

Excretion: Feces (70%); urine (≤20%, 8% as unchanged drug)

Dosing

Adult & Geriatric Note: Doses should be individualized according to the baseline LDL-cholesterol levels, the recommended goal of therapy, and patient response; adjustments should be made at intervals of 4 weeks or more; doses may need adjusted based on concomitant medications

Hyperlipidemias, primary prevention of coronary events, secondary prevention of cardiovascular events (also see ACC/AHA Blood Cholesterol Guideline recommendations): Oral: Initial: 40 mg once daily; titrate dosage to response (usual range: 10-80 mg) (maximum dose: 80 mg once daily)

Prevention of cardiovascular disease: ACC/AHA Blood Cholesterol Guideline recommendations to reduce the risk of atherosclerotic cardiovascular disease (ASCVD) (Stone, 2013): Adults ≥21 years: Oral:

Primary prevention:

LDL-C ≥190 mg/dL: High intensity therapy necessary; use alternate statin therapy (eg, atorvastatin or rosuvastatin)

Type 1 or 2 diabetes and age 40-75 years: Moderate intensity therapy: 40-80 mg once daily

Type 1 or 2 diabetes, age 40-75 years, and an estimated 10-year ASCVD risk ≥7.5%: High intensity therapy necessary; use alternate statin therapy (eg, atorvastatin or rosuvastatin)

Age 40-75 years and an estimated 10-year ASCVD risk ≥7.5%: Moderate to high intensity therapy: 40-80 mg once daily or consider using high intensity statin therapy (eg, atorvastatin or rosuvastatin)

Secondary prevention:

Patient has clinical ASCVD (eg, coronary heart disease, stroke/TIA, or peripheral arterial disease presumed to be of atherosclerotic origin) or is post-CABG (AHA [Kulik 2015]) **and:**

Age ≤75 years: High intensity therapy necessary; use alternate statin therapy (eg, atorvastatin or rosuvastatin)

Age >75 years or not a candidate for high intensity therapy: Moderate intensity therapy: 40-80 mg once daily

Dosage adjustment for pravastatin with concomitant medications:

Clarithromycin: Limit daily pravastatin dose to 40 mg/day

Cyclosporine: Initial: 10 mg pravastatin daily, titrate with caution (maximum dose: 20 mg/day)

Pediatric

Heterozygous familial hypercholesterolemia (HeFH): Oral: Children:

8-13 years: 20 mg/day

14-18 years: 40 mg/day

Dosage adjustment for pravastatin with concomitant medications (clarithromycin, cyclosporine): Refer to adult dosing.

Note: Doses should be individualized according to the baseline LDL-cholesterol levels, the recommended goal of therapy, and patient response; adjustments should be made at intervals of 4 weeks or more; doses may need adjusted based on concomitant medications

Renal Impairment Significant impairment: Initial dose: 10 mg/day

Hepatic Impairment Contraindicated in active liver disease or in patients with unexplained persistent elevations of serum transaminases.

Adjustment for Toxicity

Severe muscle symptoms or fatigue: Promptly discontinue use; evaluate CPK, creatinine, and urinalysis for myoglobinuria (Stone, 2013).

Mild to moderate muscle symptoms: Discontinue use until symptoms can be evaluated; evaluate patient for conditions that may increase the risk for muscle symptoms (eg, hypothyroidism, reduced renal or hepatic function, rheumatologic disorders such as polymyalgia rheumatica, steroid myopathy, vitamin D deficiency, primary muscle diseases). Upon resolution, resume the original or lower dose of pravastatin. If muscle symptoms recur, discontinue pravastatin use. After muscle symptom resolution, may then use a low dose of a different statin; gradually increase if tolerated. In the absence of continued statin use, if muscle symptoms or elevated CPK continues after 2 months, consider other causes of muscle symptoms. If determined to be due to another condition aside from statin use, may resume statin therapy at the original dose (Stone, 2013).

Dietary Considerations May be taken without regard to meals. Before initiation of therapy, patients should be placed on a standard cholesterol-lowering diet for 6 weeks and the diet should be continued during drug therapy.

Red yeast rice contains variable amounts of several compounds that are structurally similar to HMG-CoA reductase inhibitors, primarily monacolin K (or mevinolin) which is structurally identical to lovastatin; concurrent use of red yeast rice with HMG-CoA reductase inhibitors may increase the incidence of adverse and toxic effects (Lapi, 2008; Smith, 2003).

Administration May be administered without regard to meals.

Monitoring Parameters

2013 ACC/AHA Blood Cholesterol Guideline recommendations (Stone, 2013):

Lipid panel (total cholesterol, HDL, LDL, triglycerides): Baseline lipid panel; fasting lipid profile within 4-12 weeks after initiation or dose adjustment and every 3-12 months (as clinically indicated) thereafter. If 2 consecutive LDL levels are <40 mg/dL, consider decreasing the dose.

Hepatic transaminase levels: Baseline measurement of hepatic transaminase levels (ie, ALT); measure hepatic function if symptoms suggest hepatotoxicity (eg, unusual fatigue or weakness, loss of appetite, abdominal pain, dark-colored urine or yellowing of skin or sclera) during therapy.

CPK: CPK should not be routinely measured. Baseline CPK measurement is reasonable for some individuals (eg, family history of statin intolerance or muscle disease, clinical presentation, concomitant drug therapy that may increase risk of myopathy). May measure CPK in any patient with symptoms suggestive of myopathy (pain, tenderness, stiffness, cramping, weakness, or generalized fatigue).

Evaluate for new-onset diabetes mellitus during therapy; if diabetes develops, continue statin therapy and encourage adherence to a heart-healthy diet, physical activity, a healthy body weight, and tobacco cessation.

If patient develops a confusional state or memory impairment, may evaluate patient for nonstatin causes (eg, exposure to other drugs), systemic and neuropsychiatric causes, and the possibility of adverse effects associated with statin therapy.

Manufacturer's labeling: Liver enzyme tests at baseline and repeated when clinically indicated. **Upon initiation or titration, lipid panel should be analyzed at intervals of 4 weeks or more.**

Dosage Forms Excipient information presented when available (limited, particularly for generics); consult specific product labeling.

Tablet, Oral, as sodium:

Pravachol: 20 mg, 40 mg, 80 mg

Generic: 10 mg, 20 mg, 40 mg, 80 mg

◆ Pravastatin Sodium *see* Pravastatin *on page 1490*

◆ Praxbind *see* IdaruCIZUMAB *on page 910*

◆ Praxis ASA EC 81 Mg Daily Dose (Can) *see* Aspirin *on page 157*

Praziquantel (pray zi KWON tel)

Brand Names: US Biltricide

Brand Names: Canada Biltricide

Pharmacologic Category Anthelmintic

Use Helminths: Treatment of infections caused by the following: All species of *Schistosoma* (eg, *Schistosoma mekongi, S. japonicum, S. mansoni, S. hematobium*) and the liver flukes *Clonorchis sinensis/Opisthorchis viverrini*

Dosing

Adult & Geriatric

Schistosomiasis: Oral: 20 mg/kg/dose 3 times daily at 4- to 6-hour intervals for 1 day

Clonorchiasis/opisthorchiasis: Oral:

Manufacturer's labeling: 25 mg/kg/dose 3 times daily at 4- to 6-hour intervals for 1 day

Alternate recommendations (off-label dose): 25 mg/kg/dose 3 times daily for 2 days (*Drugs for Parasitic Infections* 2013)

Cysticercosis (off-label use): Oral: 50 mg/kg/day divided every 8 hours for 14 days (Takayanagui, 2004)

Tapeworms (off-label use): Oral: 5-10 mg/kg as a single dose (25 mg/kg for *Hymenolepis nana*) (Liu, 1996)

Pediatric Children ≥4 years and Adolescents: Refer to adult dosing.

Renal Impairment No dosage adjustment necessary.

Hepatic Impairment There are no dosage adjustments provided in manufacturer's labeling. However, total drug exposure in moderate-to-severe impairment is increased.

Additional Information Complete prescribing information should be consulted for additional detail.

Dosage Forms Excipient information presented when available (limited, particularly for generics); consult specific product labeling.

Tablet, Oral:

Biltricide: 600 mg [scored]

Prazosin (PRAZ oh sin)

Brand Names: US Minipress

Brand Names: Canada Apo-Prazo; Minipress; Teva-Prazosin

Index Terms Furazosin; Prazosin Hydrochloride

Pharmacologic Category Alpha$_1$ Blocker; Antihypertensive

Additional Appendix Information

Hypertension *on page 1996*

Use

Hypertension: Treatment of hypertension

The 2014 guideline for the management of high blood pressure in adults (Eighth Joint National Committee [JNC 8]) does **not** recommend the use of prazosin in the treatment of hypertension (James 2013).

Dosing

Adult

Hypertension:

US labeling: Oral: Initial: 1 mg/dose 2 or 3 times daily, increased slowly to usual dosage range of 6 to 15 mg/day in divided doses or alternatively, 1 to 5 mg twice daily (ASH/ISH [Weber 2014]). Dose may be increased up to 20 mg/day in divided doses; however, some patients may benefit from up to 40 mg/day in divided doses.

Concomitant diuretics or other antihypertensives: When adding a diuretic or other antihypertensive, decrease prazosin dose to 1 or 2 mg 3 times daily and retitrate.

Canadian labeling: Oral:

Immediate release: Initial: 0.5 mg 2 or 3 times daily for ≥3 days; may increase to 1 mg 2 or 3 times daily for ≥3 days and then further increase gradually per response/tolerability to a maximum of 20 mg/day in 2 or 3 divided doses.

Concomitant diuretics or other antihypertensives: Initial: 0.5 mg at bedtime; may increase to 0.5 mg 2 or 3 times daily; increase gradually for patients already on other diuretics or other antihypertensive agents. When adding a diuretic or other antihypertensive agent to prazosin therapy, reduce prazosin dose to 1 or 2 mg 2 or 3 times daily and retitrate.

Extended release: Initial: 2.5 mg once daily; increase slowly over 7 to 14 days per response/tolerability up to a maximum of 20 mg once daily. Monitor response to ensure adequate blood pressure control throughout 24-hour period. Patients receiving immediate-release prazosin as monotherapy or concurrently with other antihypertensives may be switched to extended-release prazosin at an equivalent dose or nearest higher total daily dose.

PTSD-related nightmares and sleep disruption (off-label use): Oral: Initial: 1 mg at bedtime; after 2 to 3 days increase dose to 2 mg at bedtime, then adjust dosage based on response and tolerability in 1 to 2 mg increments every 7 days up to a maximum of 15 mg/day (Raskind, 2003; Raskind, 2007; Taylor, 2008). (Titration as rapid as every 2 to 3 days has been evaluated [Taylor, 2008]). Usual dose range: 3 to 15 mg at bedtime (APA [Benedek, 2009])

Raynaud phenomenon (off-label use): Oral: Initial: 0.5 to 1 mg once daily (at bedtime) **or** 0.5 mg twice daily; gradually adjust dose based on response and tolerability up 12 mg/day in 2 to 3 divided doses (Nielson, 1983; Russell, 1985; Wollersheim, 1988)

Geriatric Refer to adult dosing. In the management of hypertension, consider lower initial doses and titrate to response (Aronow 2011).

Pediatric

Hypertension (off-label use): Oral: Children: Initial: 0.05 to 0.1 mg/kg/day in 3 divided doses; maximum: 0.5 mg/kg/day (not to exceed 20 mg) (NHBPEP, Fourth Report)

Canadian labeling: Children ≥12 years and Adolescents: Oral: Refer to adult dosing.

Renal Impairment

US labeling: There are no dosage adjustments provided in the manufacturer's labeling.

Canadian labeling: Moderate to severe impairment: Immediate release: Initial: 0.5 mg daily; increase dose gradually.

Hepatic Impairment There are no dosage adjustments provided in the manufacturer's labeling.

Additional Information Complete prescribing information should be consulted for additional detail.

Dosage Forms Excipient information presented when available (limited, particularly for generics); consult specific product labeling.

Capsule, Oral:

Minipress: 1 mg, 2 mg, 5 mg

Generic: 1 mg, 2 mg, 5 mg

Dosage Forms: Canada Excipient information presented when available (limited, particularly for generics); consult specific product labeling.

Tablet, Oral:

Minipress: 1 mg, 2 mg, 5 mg

Tablet Extended Release 24 Hour, Oral, as hydrochloride:

Minipress XL: 2.5 mg, 5 mg

◆ Prazosin Hydrochloride *see* Prazosin *on page 1493*

◆ Precedex *see* Dexmedetomidine *on page 529*

◆ Precise [OTC] *see* Methyl Salicylate and Menthol *on page 1187*

◆ Precose *see* Acarbose *on page 24*

◆ Predator [OTC] *see* Lidocaine (Topical) *on page 1074*

◆ Pred Forte *see* PrednisoLONE (Ophthalmic) *on page 1496*

◆ Pred-G *see* Prednisolone and Gentamicin *on page 1496*

◆ Pred Mild *see* PrednisoLONE (Ophthalmic) *on page 1496*

Prednicarbate (pred ni KAR bate)

Brand Names: US Dermatop

Brand Names: Canada Dermatop

Pharmacologic Category Corticosteroid, Topical

Additional Appendix Information

Topical Corticosteroids *on page 1952*

Use Dermatoses: Relief of the inflammatory and pruritic manifestations of corticosteroid-responsive dermatoses (medium potency topical corticosteroid)

Dosing

Adult & Geriatric Steroid-responsive dermatoses: Topical: Cream, ointment: Apply a thin film to affected area twice daily. Therapy should be discontinued when control is achieved; if no improvement is seen within 2 weeks, reassessment of diagnosis may be necessary.

Pediatric

Steroid-responsive dermatoses: Topical:

Cream: Children ≥1 year and Adolescents: Refer to adult dosing.

Ointment: Children ≥10 year and Adolescents: Refer to adult dosing.

Additional Information Complete prescribing information should be consulted for additional detail.

Dosage Forms Excipient information presented when available (limited, particularly for generics); consult specific product labeling.

Cream, External:

Dermatop: 0.1% (60 g) [contains cetostearyl alcohol, edetate disodium]

Generic: 0.1% (15 g, 60 g)

Ointment, External:

Dermatop: 0.1% (60 g) [contains propylene glycol]

Generic: 0.1% (15 g, 60 g)

PrednisoLONE (Systemic) (pred NISS oh lone)

Brand Names: US AsmalPred Plus [DSC]; AsmalPred [DSC]; Flo-Pred; Millipred; Millipred DP; Millipred DP 12-Day; Orapred ODT; Orapred [DSC]; Pediapred; Prelone; Veripred 20

Brand Names: Canada Hydeltra T.B.A.; Novo-Prednisolone; Pediapred

Index Terms Prednisolone Sodium Phosphate; Prelone

Pharmacologic Category Corticosteroid, Systemic

Additional Appendix Information

Corticosteroids Systemic Equivalencies *on page 1950*

Use Treatment of endocrine disorders, rheumatic disorders, collagen diseases, allergic diseases, respiratory diseases, hematologic disorders, neoplastic diseases, edematous states, and gastrointestinal diseases; resolution of acute exacerbations of multiple sclerosis; management of fulminating or disseminated tuberculosis and trichinosis; acute or chronic solid organ rejection

Pregnancy Considerations Adverse events have been observed with corticosteroids in animal reproduction studies. Prednisolone crosses the placenta; prior to reaching the fetus, prednisolone is converted by placental enzymes to prednisone. As a result, the amount of prednisolone

reaching the fetus is ~8-10 times lower than the maternal serum concentration (healthy women at term; similar results observed with preterm pregnancies complicated by HELLP syndrome) (Beitins 1972; van Runnard Heimel 2005). Some studies have shown an association between first trimester systemic corticosteroid use and oral clefts (Park-Wyllie 2000; Pradat 2003). Systemic corticosteroids may also influence fetal growth (decreased birth weight); however, information is conflicting (Lunghi 2010). Hypoadrenalism may occur in newborns following maternal use of corticosteroids in pregnancy; monitor.

When systemic corticosteroids are needed in pregnancy, it is generally recommended to use the lowest effective dose for the shortest duration of time, avoiding high doses during the first trimester (Leachman 2006; Lunghi 2010; Makol 2011; Østensen 2009). Inhaled corticosteroids are preferred for the treatment of asthma during pregnancy. Oral corticosteroids, such as prednisolone, may be used for the treatment of severe persistent asthma if needed; the lowest dose administered on alternate days (if possible) should be used (NAEPP 2005). Prednisolone may be used to treat women during pregnancy who require therapy for congenital adrenal hyperplasia (Speiser 2010). Topical agents are preferred for managing atopic dermatitis in pregnancy; for severe symptomatic or recalcitrant atopic dermatitis, a short course of prednisolone may be used during the third trimester (Koutroulis 2011).

Women exposed to prednisolone during pregnancy for the treatment of an autoimmune disease may contact the OTIS Autoimmune Diseases Study at 877-311-8972.

Breast-Feeding Considerations Prednisolone is excreted into breast milk. In one study (n=6), milk concentrations were 5% to 25% of the maternal serum concentration with peak concentrations occurring ~1 hour after the maternal dose. The milk/plasma ratio was found to be 0.2 with doses ≥30 mg/day and 0.1 with doses <30 mg/day. Following a maternal dose of prednisolone 80 mg/day, it was calculated that a breast-feeding infant would ingest <0.1% of the maternal dose (Ost 1985). One manufacturer notes that when used systemically, maternal use of corticosteroids have the potential to cause adverse events in a nursing infant (eg, growth suppression, interfere with endogenous corticosteroid production) and therefore caution should be used when administered to nursing women. In order to decrease potential exposure to a nursing infant, one manufacturer recommends administering the dose after nursing, at the time of day with the longest interval between feeds. Other sources recommend waiting 4 hours after the maternal dose before breast-feeding (Bae 2012; Leachman 2006; Makol 2011; Ost 1985). Other guidelines note that maternal use of systemic corticosteroids is not a contraindication to breast-feeding (NAEPP 2005).

Contraindications Hypersensitivity to prednisolone or any component of the formulation; acute superficial herpes simplex keratitis; live or attenuated virus vaccines (with immunosuppressive doses of corticosteroids); systemic fungal infections; varicella

Warnings/Precautions May cause hypercorticism or suppression of hypothalamic-pituitary-adrenal (HPA) axis, particularly in younger children or in patients receiving high doses for prolonged periods. HPA axis suppression may lead to adrenal crisis. Withdrawal and discontinuation of a corticosteroid should be done slowly and carefully. Particular care is required when patients are transferred from systemic corticosteroids to inhaled products due to possible adrenal insufficiency or withdrawal from steroids, including an increase in allergic symptoms. Patients receiving >20 mg per day of prednisone (or equivalent) may be most susceptible. Fatalities have occurred due to adrenal insufficiency in asthmatic patients during and after transfer from systemic corticosteroids to aerosol steroids; aerosol steroids do **not** provide the systemic steroid needed to treat patients having trauma, surgery, or infections.

Acute myopathy has been reported with high dose corticosteroids, usually in patients with neuromuscular transmission disorders; may involve ocular and/or respiratory muscles; monitor creatine kinase; recovery may be delayed. Corticosteroid use may cause psychiatric disturbances, including depression, euphoria, insomnia, mood swings, and personality changes. Preexisting psychiatric conditions may be exacerbated by corticosteroid use. Prolonged use of corticosteroids may also increase the incidence of secondary infection, mask acute infection (including fungal infections), prolong or exacerbate viral infections, or limit response to vaccines. Exposure to chickenpox should be avoided; corticosteroids should not be used to treat ocular herpes simplex. Corticosteroids should not be used for cerebral malaria or viral hepatitis. Close observation is required in patients with latent tuberculosis and/or TB reactivity; restrict use in active TB (only

in conjunction with antituberculosis treatment). Prolonged use of corticosteroids may result in glaucoma; cataract formation may occur. Prolonged treatment with corticosteroids has been associated with the development of Kaposi's sarcoma (case reports); if noted, discontinuation of therapy should be considered.

Use with caution in patients with thyroid disease, hepatic impairment, renal impairment, cardiovascular disease, diabetes, glaucoma, cataracts, myasthenia gravis, patients at risk for osteoporosis, patients at risk for seizures, or GI diseases (diverticulitis, peptic ulcer, ulcerative colitis) due to perforation risk. Avoid ethanol may enhance gastric mucosal irritation. Use caution following acute MI (corticosteroids have been associated with myocardial rupture). Because of the risk of adverse effects, systemic corticosteroids should be used cautiously in the elderly in the smallest possible effective dose for the shortest duration. Withdraw therapy with gradual tapering of dose. May affect growth velocity; growth should be routinely monitored in pediatric patients. Potentially significant drug-drug interactions may exist, requiring dose or frequency adjustment, additional monitoring, and/or selection of alternative therapy.

Benzyl alcohol and derivatives: Some dosage forms may contain sodium benzoate/benzoic acid; benzoic acid (benzoate) is a metabolite of benzyl alcohol; large amounts of benzyl alcohol (≥99 mg/kg/day) have been associated with a potentially fatal toxicity ("gasping syndrome") in neonates; the "gasping syndrome" consists of metabolic acidosis, respiratory distress, gasping respirations, CNS dysfunction (including convulsions, intracranial hemorrhage), hypotension, and cardiovascular collapse (AAP ["Inactive" 1997]; CDC 1982); some data suggests that benzoate displaces bilirubin from protein binding sites (Ahlfors 2001); avoid or use dosage forms containing benzyl alcohol derivative with caution in neonates. See manufacturer's labeling.

Propylene glycol: Some dosage forms may contain propylene glycol; large amounts are potentially toxic and have been associated hyperosmolality, lactic acidosis, seizures, and respiratory depression; use caution (AAP 1997; Zar 2007).

Adverse Reactions Frequency not defined.

Cardiovascular: Cardiomyopathy, CHF, edema, facial edema, hypertension

Central nervous system: Headache, insomnia, malaise, nervousness, pseudotumor cerebri, psychic disorders, seizure, vertigo

Dermatologic: Bruising, facial erythema, hirsutism, petechiae, skin test reaction suppression, thin fragile skin, urticaria

Endocrine & metabolic: Carbohydrate tolerance decreased, Cushing's syndrome, diabetes mellitus, growth suppression, hyperglycemia, hypernatremia, hypokalemia, hypokalemic alkalosis, menstrual irregularities, negative nitrogen balance, pituitary adrenal axis suppression

Gastrointestinal: Abdominal distention, increased appetite, indigestion, nausea, pancreatitis, peptic ulcer, ulcerative esophagitis, weight gain

Hepatic: LFTs increased (usually reversible)

Neuromuscular & skeletal: Arthralgia, aseptic necrosis (humeral/femoral heads), fractures, muscle mass decreased, muscle weakness, osteoporosis, steroid myopathy, tendon rupture, weakness

Ocular: Cataracts, exophthalmus, eyelid edema, glaucoma, intraocular pressure increased, irritation

Respiratory: Epistaxis

Miscellaneous: Diaphoresis increased, impaired wound healing

<1% (Limited to important or life-threatening): Venous thrombosis (Johannesdottir, 2013)

Drug Interactions

Metabolism/Transport Effects Substrate of CYP3A4 (minor); **Note:** Assignment of Major/Minor substrate status based on clinically relevant drug interaction potential

Avoid Concomitant Use

Avoid concomitant use of PrednisoLONE (Systemic) with any of the following: Aldesleukin; BCG (Intravesical); Indium 111 Capromab Pendetide; Mifepristone; Natalizumab; Pimecrolimus; Tacrolimus (Topical); Tofacitinib

Increased Effect/Toxicity

PrednisoLONE (Systemic) may increase the levels/ effects of: Acetylcholinesterase Inhibitors; Amphotericin B; Androgens; Ceritinib; CycloSPORINE (Systemic); Deferasirox; Fingolimod; Leflunomide; Loop Diuretics; Natalizumab; Nicorandil; NSAID (COX-2 Inhibitor); NSAID (Nonselective); Quinolone Antibiotics; Thiazide Diuretics; Tofacitinib; Vaccines (Live); Warfarin

The levels/effects of PrednisoLONE (Systemic) may be increased by: Aprepitant; Boceprevir; CycloSPORINE (Systemic); CYP3A4 Inhibitors (Strong); Denosumab; Estrogen Derivatives; Fosaprepitant; Indacaterol; Mifepristone; Neuromuscular-Blocking Agents (Nondepolarizing); Pimecrolimus; Ritonavir; Roflumilast; Salicylates; Tacrolimus (Topical); Telaprevir; Trastuzumab

Decreased Effect

PrednisoLONE (Systemic) may decrease the levels/effects of: Aldesleukin; Antidiabetic Agents; BCG (Intravesical); Calcitriol (Systemic); Coccidioides immitis Skin Test; Corticorelin; CycloSPORINE (Systemic); Hyaluronidase; Indium 111 Capromab Pendetide; Isoniazid; Salicylates; Sipuleucel-T; Telaprevir; Urea Cycle Disorder Agents; Vaccines (Inactivated); Vaccines (Live)

The levels/effects of PrednisoLONE (Systemic) may be decreased by: Antacids; Bile Acid Sequestrants; Carbimazole; CYP3A4 Inducers (Strong); Echinacea; Methimazole; Mifepristone; Mitotane

Storage/Stability

Flo-Pred: Store at 20°C to 25°C (68°F to 77°F). Flo-Pred™ should be dispensed in the original container (to avoid loss of formulation during transfer).

Millipred: Store at 20°C to 25°C (68°F to 77°F).

Orapred ODT: Store at 20°C to 25°C (68°F to 77°F) in blister pack. Protect from moisture.

Orapred, Veripred 20: 2°C to 8°C (36°F to 46°F).

Pediapred: 4°C to 25°C (39°F to 77°F); may be refrigerated.

Mechanism of Action

Decreases inflammation by suppression of migration of polymorphonuclear leukocytes and reversal of increased capillary permeability; suppresses the immune system by reducing activity and volume of the lymphatic system

Pharmacodynamics/Kinetics

Duration: 18-36 hours

Protein binding (concentration dependent): 65% to 91%; decreased in elderly

Metabolism: Primarily hepatic, but also metabolized in most tissues, to inactive compounds

Half-life elimination: 3.6 hours; End-stage renal disease: 3-5 hours

Excretion: Primarily urine (as glucuronides, sulfates, and unconjugated metabolites)

Dosing

Adult Dose depends upon condition being treated and response of patient. Oral dosage expressed in terms of prednisolone base. Consider alternate day therapy for long-term therapy. Discontinuation of long-term therapy requires gradual withdrawal by tapering the dose. Patients undergoing unusual stress while receiving corticosteroids, should receive increased doses prior to, during, and after the stressful situation.

Usual dose (range): Oral: 5 to 60 mg daily
Asthma exacerbations:
Global Initiative for Asthma guidelines (GINA 2015): Management in primary care or acute care facility: 1 mg/kg/day (maximum: 50 mg daily) as a single daily dose usually given for 5 to 7 days
National Asthma Education and Prevention Program guidelines (NAEPP 2007):
Asthma exacerbations (emergency care or hospital doses): 40 to 80 mg/day in a single dose or in 2 divided doses until peak expiratory flow is 70% of predicted or personal best
Short-course outpatient "burst" (acute asthma): 40 to 60 mg/day in a single dose or in 2 divided doses for 5 to 10 days. **Note:** Burst should be continued until symptoms resolve and peak expiratory flow is at least 80% of personal best; usually requires 3 to 10 days of treatment; longer treatment may be required
Long-term treatment: 7.5 to 60 mg daily given as a single dose in the morning or every other day as needed for asthma control
Rheumatoid arthritis: Oral: Initial: 5 to 7.5 mg daily, adjust dose as necessary
Multiple sclerosis: Oral: 200 mg daily for 1 week followed by 80 mg every other day for 1 month
Acute exacerbations of chronic obstructive pulmonary disease (COPD) (off-label use): Oral: 30 to 40 mg daily for 10 to 14 days (GOLD guidelines 2013)
Bell's palsy (off-label use): Oral: 60 mg once daily for 5 days, then taper dose downward by 10 mg daily for 5 days (total treatment duration: 10 days) (Engstrom 2008; Berg 2012) **or** 50 mg daily (in 1 or 2 divided doses) for 10 days (begin within 72 hours of onset of symptoms) (Baugh 2013; Sullivan 2007)
Severe alcoholic hepatitis (Maddrey Discriminant Function [MDF] score ≥32) (off-label use): Oral: 40 mg daily for 28 days, followed by a 2-week taper (O'Shea 2010)

Dosing adjustment in hyperthyroidism: Prednisolone dose may need to be increased to achieve adequate therapeutic effects.

Geriatric Use lowest effective adult dose. Dose depends upon condition being treated and response of patient; alternate day dosing may be attempted in some disease states.

Pediatric Dose depends upon condition being treated and response of patient; dosage for infants and children should be based on severity of the disease and response of the patient rather than on strict adherence to dosage indicated by age, weight, or body surface area. Oral dosage expressed in terms of prednisolone base. Consider alternate day therapy for long-term therapy. Discontinuation of long-term therapy requires gradual withdrawal by tapering the dose. Patients undergoing unusual stress while receiving corticosteroids, should receive increased doses prior to, during, and after the stressful situation.

Asthma exacerbations:
Global Initiative for Asthma guidelines (GINA 2015): Management in primary care or acute care facility:
Children ≤2 years: 1 to 2 mg/kg/day (maximum: 20 mg daily) for up to 5 days
Children 3 to 5 years: 1 to 2 mg/kg/day (maximum: 30 mg daily) for up to 5 days
Children 6 to 11 years: 1 to 2 mg/kg/day (maximum: 40 mg daily) usually given for 3 to 5 days
Children ≥12 years and Adolescents: Refer to adult dosing.
National Asthma Education and Prevention Program guidelines (NAEPP 2007):
Children <12 years:
Asthma exacerbations (emergency care or hospital doses): 1 to 2 mg/kg/day in 2 divided doses (maximum: 60 mg/day) until peak expiratory flow is 70% of predicted or personal best
Short-course "burst" (acute asthma): 1 to 2 mg/kg/day in single dose or 2 divided doses for 3 to 10 days; maximum dose: 60 mg/day. **Note:** Burst should be continued until symptoms resolve or patient achieves peak expiratory flow 80% of personal best; usually requires 3 to 10 days of treatment; longer treatment may be required
Long-term treatment: 0.25 to 2 mg/kg/day given as a single dose in the morning or every other day as needed for asthma control; maximum dose: 60 mg/day
Children ≥12 years and Adolescents: Refer to adult dosing.
Anti-inflammatory or immunosuppressive dose: Oral: 0.1 to 2 mg/kg/day in divided doses 1 to 4 times daily
Nephrotic syndrome: Oral:
Initial (first 3 episodes): 2 mg/kg/day **or** 60 mg/m^2/day (maximum: 80 mg daily) in divided doses 3 to 4 times daily until urine is protein free for 3 consecutive days (maximum: 28 days); followed by 1 to 1.5 mg/kg/dose **or** 40 mg/m^2/dose given every other day for 4 weeks
Maintenance (for frequent relapses): 0.5 to 1 mg/kg/dose given every other day for 3-6 months
Bell's palsy (off-label use): Adolescents ≥16 years: Oral: 50 mg daily (in 1 or 2 divided doses) for 10 days; treatment should begin within 72 hours of onset of symptoms (Baugh 2013; Sullivan 2007)

Dosing adjustment in hyperthyroidism: Refer to adult dosing.

Renal Impairment No dosage adjustment provided in manufacturer's labeling. Use with caution.
Hemodialysis: Slightly dialyzable (5% to 20%); administer dose posthemodialysis
Peritoneal dialysis: Supplemental dose is not necessary
Hepatic Impairment No dosage adjustment provided in manufacturer's labeling.

Dietary Considerations Should be taken after meals or with food or milk to decrease GI effects; increase dietary intake of pyridoxine, vitamin C, vitamin D, folate, calcium, and phosphorus.

Administration Administer oral formulation with food or milk to decrease GI effects.
Flo-Pred: Administer using the provided calibrated syringe (supplied by manufacturer) to accurately measure the dose. Syringe should be washed prior to next use.
Orapred ODT: Do not break or use partial tablet. Remove tablet from blister pack just prior to use. May swallow whole or allow to dissolve on tongue.

Monitoring Parameters Blood pressure; blood glucose, electrolytes; intraocular pressure (use >6 weeks); bone mineral density; growth in children

Test Interactions Response to skin tests

Dosage Forms Considerations

Orapred oral solution contains fructose.

Orapred ODT dispersible tablets contain sucrose.

Prelone oral syrup contains sucrose.

Dosage Forms Excipient information presented when available (limited, particularly for generics); consult specific product labeling. [DSC] = Discontinued product

Solution, Oral, as base:

Generic: 15 mg/5 mL (240 mL, 480 mL)

Solution, Oral, as sodium phosphate [strength expressed as base]:

AsmalPred: 15 mg/5 mL (89 mL [DSC]) [contains alcohol, usp, sodium benzoate]

AsmalPred Plus: 15 mg/5 mL (237 mL [DSC]) [contains alcohol, usp, sodium benzoate]

Millipred: 10 mg/5 mL (237 mL) [alcohol free, dye free; contains edetate disodium, methylparaben, saccharin sodium; grape flavor]

Orapred: 15 mg/5 mL (20 mL [DSC], 237 mL [DSC]) [dye free; contains alcohol, usp, sodium benzoate; grape flavor]

Pediapred: 5 mg/5 mL (120 mL) [alcohol free, dye free, sugar free; contains edetate disodium, methylparaben; raspberry flavor]

Veripred 20: 20 mg/5 mL (237 mL) [alcohol free, dye free; contains edetate disodium, methylparaben, saccharin sodium; grape flavor]

Generic: 15 mg/5 mL (237 mL, 473 mL [DSC]); 25 mg/5 mL (237 mL); 5 mg/5 mL (120 mL)

Suspension, Oral, as acetate [strength expressed as base]:

Flo-Pred: 15 mg/5 mL (30 mL) [contains butylparaben, disodium edta, propylene glycol; cherry flavor]

Syrup, Oral, as base:

Prelone: 15 mg/5 mL (240 mL) [contains alcohol, usp, benzoic acid, brilliant blue fcf (fd&c blue #1), fd&c red #40, propylene glycol, saccharin sodium; cherry flavor]

Generic: 15 mg/5 mL (240 mL, 480 mL)

Tablet, Oral, as base:

Millipred: 5 mg [scored; contains fd&c yellow #10 (quinoline yellow), fd&c yellow #6 (sunset yellow), sodium benzoate]

Millipred DP: 5 mg [scored; contains fd&c yellow #10 (quinoline yellow), fd&c yellow #6 (sunset yellow), sodium benzoate]

Millipred DP 12-Day: 5 mg [scored; contains fd&c yellow #10 (quinoline yellow), fd&c yellow #6 (sunset yellow), sodium benzoate]

Tablet Dispersible, Oral, as sodium phosphate [strength expressed as base]:

Orapred ODT: 10 mg, 15 mg, 30 mg [grape flavor]

Generic: 10 mg, 15 mg, 30 mg

PrednisoLONE (Ophthalmic) (pred NISS oh lone)

Brand Names: US Omnipred; Pred Forte; Pred Mild

Brand Names: Canada Minims Prednisolone Sodium Phosphate; PMS-Prednisolone Sodium Phosphate Forte; Pred Forte; Pred Mild; Ratio-Prednisolone; Sandoz Prednisolone

Index Terms Econopred; Prednisolone Acetate, Ophthalmic; Prednisolone Sodium Phosphate, Ophthalmic

Pharmacologic Category Corticosteroid, Ophthalmic

Use

Corneal injury: Treatment of corneal injury from chemical or thermal burns (excluding Pred Forte) or to radiation burns or penetration of foreign bodies (excluding Pred Forte, Pred Mild).

Ophthalmic inflammatory conditions: Treatment of steroid-responsive inflammatory conditions of the palpebral and bulbar conjunctiva, cornea, and anterior segment of the globe such as acne rosacea, allergic conjunctivitis, cyclitis, herpes zoster keratitis, iritis, superficial punctate keratitis, and selected infective conjunctivitis.

Dosing

Adult & Geriatric

Ophthalmic inflammatory conditions/corneal injury: Ophthalmic:

Prednisolone acetate: Instill 1 to 2 drops in the affected eye(s) 2 to 4 times daily. During the initial 24 to 48 hours, the dosing frequency may be increased if necessary. If signs and symptoms fail to improve after 2 days, re-evaluate. Do not discontinue therapy prematurely; withdraw therapy with gradual tapering of dose in chronic conditions.

Prednisolone sodium phosphate: Instill 1 to 2 drops into conjunctival sac hour during the day and every 2 hours at night until satisfactory response is obtained, then use 1 drop every 4 hours; subsequent reduction to 1 drop 3 to 4 times daily may be adequate. Do not discontinue therapy prematurely; withdraw therapy with gradual tapering of dose in chronic conditions.

Pediatric Ophthalmic inflammation, treatment: Children and Adolescents (off-label use): Ophthalmic: Prednisolone acetate 1%: Limited data available: Instill 1 to 2 drops into conjunctival sac 3 to 6 times daily. If signs and symptoms fail to improve after 2 days, re-evaluate. Initiate with more frequent dosing, and decrease as clinically indicated. If signs and symptoms fail to improve after 2 days, re-evaluate (Wilson, 2009).

Renal Impairment There are no dosage adjustments provided in the manufacturer's labeling.

Hepatic Impairment There are no dosage adjustments provided in the manufacturer's labeling.

Additional Information Complete prescribing information should be consulted for additional detail.

Dosage Forms Excipient information presented when available (limited, particularly for generics); consult specific product labeling.

Solution, Ophthalmic, as sodium phosphate:

Generic: 1% (10 mL)

Suspension, Ophthalmic, as acetate:

Omnipred: 1% (5 mL, 10 mL) [contains benzalkonium chloride, edetate disodium, polysorbate 80]

Pred Forte: 1% (1 mL, 5 mL, 10 mL, 15 mL) [contains benzalkonium chloride, edetate disodium, polysorbate 80, sodium bisulfite]

Pred Mild: 0.12% (5 mL, 10 mL)

Generic: 1% (5 mL, 10 mL, 15 mL)

◆ Prednisolone Acetate, Ophthalmic see PrednisoLONE (Ophthalmic) on page 1496

Prednisolone and Gentamicin
(pred NIS oh lone & jen ta MYE sin)

Brand Names: US Pred-G

Index Terms Gentamicin and Prednisolone

Pharmacologic Category Antibiotic/Corticosteroid, Ophthalmic

Use Inflammatory ocular conditions and superficial ocular infections: Treatment of steroid responsive inflammatory ocular conditions where either a superficial bacterial ocular infection or the risk of bacterial ocular infection exists

Dosing

Adult & Geriatric Inflammatory conditions and superficial ocular infections: Ophthalmic:

Ointment: Apply 1/2 inch ribbon into the conjunctival sac of the affected eye(s) 1 to 3 times per day

Suspension: Instill 1 drop into the conjunctival sac of the affected eye(s) 2 to 4 times per day; during the initial 24 to 48 hours, the dosing frequency may be increased if necessary up to 1 drop every hour

Note: If signs and symptoms do not improve after 2 days of treatment, the patient should be re-evaluated.

Renal Impairment There are no dosage adjustments provided in the manufacturer's labeling

Hepatic Impairment There are no dosage adjustments provided in the manufacturer's labeling

Additional Information Complete prescribing information should be consulted for additional detail.

Dosage Forms Excipient information presented when available (limited, particularly for generics); consult specific product labeling. [DSC] = Discontinued product

Ointment, ophthalmic:

Pred-G: Prednisolone acetate 0.6% and gentamicin sulfate 0.3% (3.5 g)

Suspension, ophthalmic:

Pred-G: Prednisolone acetate 1% and gentamicin sulfate 0.3% (5 mL) [contains benzalkonium chloride]

◆ Prednisolone and Sulfacetamide see Sulfacetamide and Prednisolone on page 1708

◆ Prednisolone Sodium Phosphate see PrednisoLONE (Systemic) on page 1493

◆ Prednisolone Sodium Phosphate, Ophthalmic see PrednisoLONE (Ophthalmic) on page 1496

PredniSONE (PRED ni sone)

Brand Names: US Deltasone; PredniSONE Intensol; Rayos

Brand Names: Canada Apo-Prednisone; JAA-Prednisone; Teva-Prednisone; Winpred

Index Terms Deltacortisone; Deltadehydrocortisone; Deltasone

Pharmacologic Category Corticosteroid, Systemic

Additional Appendix Information

Corticosteroids Systemic Equivalencies on page 1950

Use

Allergic states: Control of severe or incapacitating allergic conditions intractable to adequate trials of conventional treatment in drug hypersensitivity reactions, seasonal or perennial allergic rhinitis; serum sickness.

Dermatologic diseases: Atopic dermatitis; bullous dermatitis herpetiformis; contact dermatitis; exfoliative dermatitis/erythroderma; mycosis fungoides; pemphigus; severe erythema multiforme (Stevens-Johnson syndrome).

Immediate-release only: Severe psoriasis, severe seborrheic dermatitis.

Endocrine disorders: Congenital adrenal hyperplasia; hypercalcemia of malignancy; nonsuppurative thyroiditis; primary or secondary adrenocortical insufficiency (hydrocortisone or cortisone is the first choice; synthetic analogues may be used in conjunction with mineralocorticoids where applicable; in infancy, mineralocorticoid supplementation is of particular importance).

GI diseases: During acute episodes in regional enteritis (Crohn disease) and ulcerative colitis.

Hematologic disorders: Acquired (autoimmune) hemolytic anemia; congenital (erythroid) hypoplastic anemia/Diamond-Blackfan anemia; idiopathic thrombocytopenic purpura in adults; secondary thrombocytopenia in adults.

Delayed-release only: Pure red cell aplasia.

Immediate-release only: Erythroblastopenia (red blood cell anemia).

Neoplastic diseases:

Delayed-release only: Treatment of acute leukemia and aggressive lymphomas.

Immediate-release only: Palliative management of leukemias and lymphomas in adults; acute leukemia of childhood.

Nervous system (delayed-release only): Acute exacerbations of multiple sclerosis; cerebral edema associated with primary or metastatic brain tumor, craniotomy, or head injury.

Ophthalmic diseases:

Delayed-release only: Severe acute and chronic allergic and inflammatory processes involving the eye and its adnexa, such as sympathetic ophthalmia; uveitis and ocular inflammatory conditions unresponsive to topical steroids.

Immediate-release only: Severe acute and chronic allergic and inflammatory processes involving the eye and its adnexa, such as allergic conjunctivitis, allergic corneal marginal ulcers, anterior segment inflammation, chorioretinitis, diffuse posterior uveitis and choroiditis, herpes zoster ophthalmicus, iridocyclitis, iritis, keratitis, optic neuritis, sympathetic ophthalmia.

Renal diseases: To induce a diuresis or remission of proteinuria in the nephrotic syndrome, without uremia, of the idiopathic type or that is caused by lupus erythematosus.

Respiratory diseases: Aspiration pneumonitis; asthma; fulminating or disseminated pulmonary tuberculosis when used concurrently with appropriate chemotherapy; symptomatic sarcoidosis.

Delayed-release only: Acute exacerbations of chronic obstructive pulmonary disease (COPD); allergic bronchopulmonary aspergillosis; hypersensitivity pneumonitis; idiopathic bronchiolitis obliterans with organizing pneumonia; idiopathic eosinophilic pneumonias; idiopathic pulmonary fibrosis; *Pneumocystis carinii* pneumonia (PCP) associated with hypoxemia occurring in an HIV-positive individual who is also under treatment with appropriate anti-PCP antibiotics.

Immediate-release only: Berylliosis; Loeffler syndrome not manageable by other means.

Rheumatic disorders:

Maintenance therapy:

Delayed-release only: During an exacerbation or as maintenance therapy in selected cases of ankylosing spondylitis, dermatomyositis/polymyositis, polymyalgia rheumatica, psoriatic arthritis, relapsing polychondritis, rheumatoid arthritis including juvenile rheumatoid arthritis, Sjögren syndrome, systemic lupus erythematosus, vasculitis.

Immediate-release only: During an exacerbation or as maintenance therapy in selected cases of acute rheumatic carditis, systemic dermatomyositis (polymyositis), systemic lupus erythematosus.

Short-term therapy:

Delayed release only: As adjunctive therapy for short-term administration in acute gouty arthritis.

Immediate-release only: As adjunctive therapy for short-term administration in acute and subacute bursitis; acute gouty arthritis; acute nonspecific tenosynovitis; ankylosing spondylitis; epicondylitis; posttraumatic osteoarthritis; psoriatic arthritis; rheumatoid arthritis including juvenile rheumatoid arthritis; synovitis of osteoarthritis.

Miscellaneous: Trichinosis with neurologic or myocardial involvement; tuberculous meningitis with subarachnoid block or impending block when used concurrently with appropriate antituberculous chemotherapy.

Delayed-release only: Acute or chronic solid organ rejection.

Pregnancy Considerations Adverse events have been observed with corticosteroids in animal reproduction studies. Prednisone and its metabolite, prednisolone, cross the human placenta. In the mother, prednisone is converted to the active metabolite prednisolone by the liver. Prior to reaching the fetus, prednisolone is converted by placental enzymes back to prednisone. As a result, the level of prednisone remaining in the maternal serum and reaching the fetus are similar; however, the amount of prednisolone reaching the fetus is ~8-10 times lower than the maternal serum concentration (healthy women at term) (Beitins, 1972). Some studies have shown an association between first trimester systemic corticosteroid use and oral clefts (Park-Wyllie 2000; Pradat 2003). Systemic corticosteroids may also influence fetal growth (decreased birth weight); however, information is conflicting (Lunghi 2010). Hypoadrenalism may occur in newborns following maternal use of corticosteroids in pregnancy; monitor.

When systemic corticosteroids are needed in pregnancy, it is generally recommended to use the lowest effective dose for the shortest duration of time, avoiding high doses during the first trimester (Leachman 2006; Lunghi 2010; Makol 2011; Østensen 2009). Inhaled corticosteroids are preferred for the treatment of asthma during pregnancy. Oral corticosteroids, such as prednisone, may be used for the treatment of severe persistent asthma if needed; the lowest dose administered on alternate days (if possible) should be used (NAEPP 2005). Prednisone may be used to treat lupus nephritis in pregnant women who have active nephritis or substantial extrarenal disease activity (Hahn 2012).

Pregnant women exposed to prednisone for antirejection therapy following a transplant may contact the National Transplantation Pregnancy Registry (NTPR) at 215-955-4820. Women exposed to prednisone during pregnancy for the treatment of an autoimmune disease (eg, rheumatoid arthritis) may contact the OTIS Autoimmune Diseases Study at 877-311-8972.

Breast-Feeding Considerations Prednisone and its metabolite, prednisolone, are found in low concentrations in breast milk. Following a maternal dose of 10 mg (n=1), milk concentrations were measured ~2 hours after the maternal dose (prednisone 0.0016 mcg/mL; prednisolone 0.0267 mcg/mL) (Katz, 1975). In a study which included six mother/infant pairs, adverse events were not observed in nursing infants (maternal prednisone dose not provided) (Ito, 1993).

The manufacturer notes that when used systemically, maternal use of corticosteroids has the potential to cause adverse events in a nursing infant (eg, growth suppression, interfere with endogenous corticosteroid production) and therefore, a decision should be made whether to discontinue nursing or to discontinue the drug, taking into account the importance of treatment to the mother. If there is concern about exposure to the infant, some guidelines recommend waiting 4 hours after the maternal dose of an oral systemic corticosteroid before breast-feeding in order to decrease potential exposure to the nursing infant (based on a study using prednisolone) (Bae 2011; Leachman 2006; Makol 2011; Ost, 1985). Other guidelines note that maternal use of prednisone is not a contraindication to breast-feeding (NAEPP 2005).

Contraindications Hypersensitivity to prednisone or any component of the formulation; administration of live or live attenuated vaccines with immunosuppressive doses of prednisone; systemic fungal infections

Documentation of allergenic cross-reactivity for corticosteroids is limited. However, because of similarities in chemical structure and/or pharmacologic actions, the possibility of cross-sensitivity cannot be ruled out with certainty.

Warnings/Precautions May cause hypercorticism or suppression of hypothalamic-pituitary-adrenal (HPA) axis, particularly in younger children or in patients receiving high doses for prolonged periods. HPA axis suppression may lead to adrenal crisis. Withdrawal and discontinuation of a corticosteroid should be done slowly and carefully. Particular care is required when patients are transferred from

systemic corticosteroids to inhaled products due to possible adrenal insufficiency or withdrawal from steroids, including an increase in allergic symptoms. Patients receiving >20 mg per day of prednisone (or equivalent) may be most susceptible. Fatalities have occurred due to adrenal insufficiency in asthmatic patients during and after transfer from systemic corticosteroids to aerosol steroids; aerosol steroids do **not** provide the systemic steroid needed to treat patients having trauma, surgery, or infections.

Acute myopathy has been reported with high dose corticosteroids, usually in patients with neuromuscular transmission disorders; may involve ocular and/or respiratory muscles; monitor creatine kinase; recovery may be delayed. Prolonged use of corticosteroids may increase the incidence of secondary infection, mask acute infection (including fungal infections), prolong or exacerbate viral infections, or limit response to inactivated vaccines. Exposure to chickenpox or measles should be avoided. Corticosteroids should not be used to treat viral hepatitis or cerebral malaria. Close observation is required in patients with latent tuberculosis and/or TB reactivity; restrict use in active TB (only fulminating or disseminated TB in conjunction with antituberculosis treatment). Amebiasis should be ruled out in any patient with recent travel to tropic climates or unexplained diarrhea prior to initiation of corticosteroids. Prolonged treatment with corticosteroids has been associated with the development of Kaposi sarcoma (case reports); if noted, discontinuation of therapy should be considered (Goedert 2002). Use with caution in patients with cataracts and/or glaucoma; increased intraocular pressure, open-angle glaucoma, and cataracts have occurred with prolonged use. Use with caution in patients with a history of ocular herpes simplex; corneal perforation has occurred; do not use in active ocular herpes simplex. Consider routine eye exams in chronic users. Corticosteroid use may cause psychiatric disturbances, including severe depression, euphoria, insomnia, mood swings, and personality changes, to frank psychotic manifestations. Preexisting psychiatric conditions may be exacerbated by corticosteroid use. Rare cases of anaphylactoid reactions have been observed in patients receiving corticosteroids.

Use with caution in patients with HF, hypertension, diabetes, GI diseases (diverticulitis, fresh intestinal anastomoses, active or latent peptic ulcer, ulcerative colitis [nonspecific]), hepatic impairment, myasthenia gravis, MI, patients with or who are at risk for osteoporosis, renal impairment, seizure disorders or thyroid disease. May affect growth velocity; growth and development should be routinely monitored in pediatric patients. Because of the risk of adverse effects, systemic corticosteroids should be used cautiously in the elderly in the smallest possible effective dose for the shortest duration.

Withdraw therapy with gradual tapering of dose. Increased mortality was observed in patients receiving high-dose IV methylprednisolone; high-dose corticosteroids should not be used for the management of head injury. Potentially significant drug-drug interactions may exist, requiring dose or frequency adjustment, additional monitoring, and/or selection of alternative therapy.

Benzyl alcohol and derivatives: Some dosage forms may contain sodium benzoate/benzoic acid; benzoic acid (benzoate) is a metabolite of benzyl alcohol; large amounts of benzyl alcohol (≥99 mg/kg/day) have been associated with a potentially fatal toxicity ("gasping syndrome") in neonates; the "gasping syndrome" consists of metabolic acidosis, respiratory distress, gasping respirations, CNS dysfunction (including convulsions, intracranial hemorrhage), hypotension, and cardiovascular collapse (AAP ["Inactive" 1997]; CDC, 1982); some data suggests that benzoate displaces bilirubin from protein binding sites (Ahlfors 2001); avoid or use dosage forms containing benzyl alcohol derivative with caution in neonates. See manufacturer's labeling.

Propylene glycol: Some dosage forms may contain propylene glycol; large amounts are potentially toxic and have been associated hyperosmolality, lactic acidosis, seizures, and respiratory depression; use caution (AAP ["Inactive" 1997]; Zar 2007).

Adverse Reactions Frequency not defined.

Cardiovascular: Congestive heart failure (in susceptible patients), hypertension

Central nervous system: Emotional instability, headache, intracranial pressure increased (with papilledema), psychic derangements (including euphoria, insomnia, mood swings, personality changes, severe depression), seizure, vertigo

Dermatologic: Bruising, facial erythema, petechiae, thin fragile skin, urticaria, wound healing impaired

Endocrine & metabolic: Adrenocortical and pituitary unresponsiveness (in times of stress), carbohydrate intolerance, Cushing's syndrome, diabetes mellitus, fluid retention, growth suppression (in children), hypokalemic alkalosis, hypothyroidism enhanced, menstrual irregularities, negative nitrogen balance due to protein catabolism, potassium loss, sodium retention

Gastrointestinal: Abdominal distension, pancreatitis, peptic ulcer (with possible perforation and hemorrhage), ulcerative esophagitis

Hepatic: ALT increased, AST increased, alkaline phosphatase increased

Neuromuscular & skeletal: Aseptic necrosis of femoral and humeral heads, muscle mass loss, muscle weakness, osteoporosis, pathologic fracture of long bones, steroid myopathy, tendon rupture (particularly Achilles tendon), vertebral compression fractures

Ocular: Exophthalmos, glaucoma, intraocular pressure increased, posterior subcapsular cataracts

Miscellaneous: Allergic reactions, anaphylactic reactions, diaphoresis, hypersensitivity reactions, infections, Kaposi's sarcoma

<1% (Limited to important or life-threatening): Venous thrombosis (Johannesdottir, 2013)

Drug Interactions

Metabolism/Transport Effects Substrate of CYP3A4 (minor); **Note:** Assignment of Major/Minor substrate status based on clinically relevant drug interaction potential; **Induces** CYP2C19 (weak/moderate)

Avoid Concomitant Use

Avoid concomitant use of PredniSONE with any of the following: Aldesleukin; BCG (Intravesical); Indium 111 Capromab Pendetide; Mifepristone; Natalizumab; Pimecrolimus; Tacrolimus (Topical); Tofacitinib

Increased Effect/Toxicity

PredniSONE may increase the levels/effects of: Acetylcholinesterase Inhibitors; Amphotericin B; Androgens; Ceritinib; CycloSPORINE (Systemic); Deferasirox; Fingolimod; Leflunomide; Loop Diuretics; Natalizumab; Nicorandil; NSAID (COX-2 Inhibitor); NSAID (Nonselective); Quinolone Antibiotics; Thiazide Diuretics; Tofacitinib; Vaccines (Live); Warfarin

The levels/effects of PredniSONE may be increased by: Aprepitant; Boceprevir; CycloSPORINE (Systemic); CYP3A4 Inhibitors (Strong); Denosumab; Estrogen Derivatives; Fluconazole; Fosaprepitant; Indacaterol; Mifepristone; Neuromuscular-Blocking Agents (Nondepolarizing); Pimecrolimus; Ritonavir; Roflumilast; Salicylates; Tacrolimus (Topical); Telaprevir; Trastuzumab

Decreased Effect

PredniSONE may decrease the levels/effects of: Aldesleukin; Antidiabetic Agents; BCG (Intravesical); Calcitriol (Systemic); Coccidioides immitis Skin Test; Corticorelin; CycloSPORINE (Systemic); Hyaluronidase; Indium 111 Capromab Pendetide; Isoniazid; Salicylates; Sipuleucel-T; Telaprevir; Urea Cycle Disorder Agents; Vaccines (Inactivated); Vaccines (Live)

The levels/effects of PredniSONE may be decreased by: Antacids; Bile Acid Sequestrants; CYP3A4 Inducers (Strong); Echinacea; Mifepristone; Mitotane; Somatropin; Tesamorelin

Storage/Stability

Store at 25°C (77°F); excursions permitted to 15°C to 30°C (59°F to 86°F). Protect from light and moisture.

Oral solution, concentrate: Discard opened bottle after 90 days.

Mechanism of Action Decreases inflammation by suppression of migration of polymorphonuclear leukocytes and reversal of increased capillary permeability; suppresses the immune system by reducing activity and volume of the lymphatic system; suppresses adrenal function at high doses. Antitumor effects may be related to inhibition of glucose transport, phosphorylation, or induction of cell death in immature lymphocytes. Antiemetic effects are thought to occur due to blockade of cerebral innervation of the emetic center via inhibition of prostaglandin synthesis.

Pharmacodynamics/Kinetics

Absorption: 50% to 90% (may be altered in hepatic failure, chronic renal failure, inflammatory bowel disease, hyperthyroidism, and in the elderly) (Frey 1990)

Protein binding (concentration dependent): <50% (Frey 1990)

Metabolism: Hepatic to metabolite prednisolone (active)

Half-life elimination: 2 to 3 hours

Time to peak: Oral:

Immediate-release tablet: 2 hours; Delayed-release tablet: 6 to 6.5 hours

Excretion: Urine (as conjugates)

Dosing

Adult **General dosing range:** Oral: Initial: 5 to 60 mg daily; **Note:** Dose depends upon condition being treated and response of patient. Consider alternate day therapy for long-term therapy. Discontinuation of long-term therapy requires gradual withdrawal by tapering the dose.

Prednisone taper (other regimens also available):

Day 1: 30 mg divided as 10 mg before breakfast, 5 mg at lunch, 5 mg at dinner, 10 mg at bedtime

Day 2: 5 mg at breakfast, 5 mg at lunch, 5 mg at dinner, 10 mg at bedtime

Day 3: 5 mg 4 times daily (with meals and at bedtime)

Day 4: 5 mg 3 times daily (breakfast, lunch, bedtime)

Day 5: 5 mg 2 times daily (breakfast, bedtime)

Day 6: 5 mg before breakfast

Indication-specific dosing:

Acute asthma (NAEPP 2007): Oral: 40 to 60 mg per day for 3 to 10 days; administer as single or 2 divided doses

Acute exacerbations of chronic obstructive pulmonary disease (COPD) (off-label use for immediate release products; off-label dose): Oral: 40 mg once daily for 5 days (GOLD 2014).

Acute gout (ACR guidelines [Khanna 2012]): Oral: Initial: ≥0.5 mg/kg for 5 to 10 days

Anaphylaxis, adjunctive treatment (Lieberman 2005): Oral: 0.5 mg/kg

Antineoplastic: Oral: Usual range: 10 mg daily to 100 mg/m^2/day (depending on indication). **Note:** Details concerning dosing in combination regimens should also be consulted.

Autoimmune hepatitis (off-label use; Czaja 2002): Oral: Initial treatment: 60 mg daily for 1 week, *followed by* 40 mg daily for 1 week, *then* 30 mg daily for 2 weeks, *then* 20 mg daily. Half this dose should be given when used in combination with azathioprine.

Bell palsy (off-label use): Oral: 60 mg daily for 5 days, followed by a 5-day taper. Treatment should begin within 72 hours of onset of symptoms (Baugh 2013).

Crohn disease, moderate/severe (off-label use): Oral: 40 to 60 mg daily until resolution of symptoms and resumption of weight gain (usual duration: 7 to 28 days) (Lichtenstein 2009)

Dermatomyositis/polymyositis: Oral: 1 mg/kg daily (range: 0.5 to 1.5 mg/kg/day), often in conjunction with steroid-sparing therapies; depending on response/tolerance, consider slow tapering after 2 to 8 weeks depending on response; taper regimens vary widely, but often involve 5 to 10 mg decrements per week and may require 6 to 12 months to reach a low once-daily or every-other-day dose to prevent disease flare (Briemberg 2003; Hengstman 2009; Iorizzo 2008; Wiendl 2008)

Giant cell arteritis (off-label use): Oral: Initial: 40 to 60 mg daily; typically requires 1 to 2 years of treatment, but may begin to taper after 2 to 3 months; alternative dosing of 30 to 40 mg daily has demonstrated similar efficacy (Hiratzka 2010)

Graves ophthalmopathy prophylaxis (off-label use): Oral: 0.4 to 0.5 mg/kg/day, starting 1 to 3 days after radioactive iodine treatment, and continued for 1 month, then gradually taper over 2 months (Bahn 2011)

Herpes zoster (off-label use; Dworkin 2007): Oral: 60 mg daily for 7 days, *followed by* 30 mg daily for 7 days, *then* 15 mg daily for 7 days

Immune thrombocytopenia (ITP) (American Society of Hematology, 1997): Oral: 1 to 2 mg/kg/day

Lupus nephritis, induction (Hahn 2012): Oral:

Class III-IV lupus nephritis: 0.5 to 1 mg/kg/day (after glucocorticoid pulse) tapered after a few weeks to lowest effective dose, in combination with an immunosuppressive agent

Class V lupus nephritis: 0.5 mg/kg/day for 6 months in combination mycophenolate mofetil; if not improved after 6 months, use 0.5 to 1 mg/kg/day (after a glucocorticoid pulse) for an additional 6 months in combination with cyclophosphamide

Multiple sclerosis, acute exacerbations: Oral: 200 mg daily for 1 week, followed by 80 mg every other day for 1 month.

***Pneumocystis* pneumonia (adjunctive therapy) in HIV-infected patients (off-label dose):** Oral: 40 mg twice daily for 5 days beginning as early as possible and within 72 hours of PCP therapy, followed by 40 mg once daily on days 6 through 10, then 20 mg once daily on days 11 through 21 (HHS [OI adult 2015])

Polymyalgia rheumatica (off-label dose): Oral: Evidence to support an optimal dose and duration are lacking; recommendations provided are general guidelines only. Individualize therapy using the minimum effective dose and duration (Dejaco [EULAR/ACR 2015]):

Initial: Dosage range: 12.5 to 25 mg daily; consider higher doses within this range for patients at high risk of relapse and low risk of adverse events; consider lower doses within this range for patients with high risk factors for side effects (eg, diabetes, osteoporosis, glaucoma). Single daily doses are preferred over divided daily doses. Avoid initial doses ≤7.5 mg/day or >30 mg/day.

Tapering: For initial dosing, taper to a dose of 10 mg/day within 4 to 8 weeks. If relapse occurs, increase dosing to the prerelapse dose and gradually taper back to the dose which relapse occurred within 4 to 8 weeks. Once remission is achieved (initial or relapse therapy), taper daily dose by 1 mg every 4 weeks (or by 1.25 mg decrements if using schedules such as 10 mg and 7.5 mg on alternate days) until discontinuation.

Prostate cancer, metastatic (off-label use): Oral: 5 mg twice daily (in combination with abiraterone) until disease progression or unacceptable toxicity (de Bono 2011; Ryan 2015) **or** 10 mg once daily (in combination with cabazitaxel) for up to 10 cycles (de Bono 2010) **or** 5 mg twice daily (in combination with docetaxel) for up to 10 cycles (Berthold 2008; Tannock 2004).

Rheumatoid arthritis (American College of Rheumatology 2002): Oral: ≤10 mg daily

Subacute thyroiditis (off-label use): Oral: 40 mg daily for 1 to 2 weeks; gradually taper over 2 to 4 weeks or longer depending on clinical response. **Note:** NSAIDs should be considered first-line therapy in such patients (Bahn 2011).

Takayasu arteritis (off-label use): Oral: Initial: 40 to 60 mg daily; taper to lowest effective dose when ESR and CRP levels are normal; usual duration: 1 to 2 years (Hiratzka 2010)

Thyrotoxicosis (type II amiodarone-induced; off-label use): Oral: 40 mg daily for 14 to 28 days; gradually taper over 2 to 3 months depending on clinical response (Bahn 2011)

Tuberculosis, severe, paradoxical reactions (off-label dose, AIDS*info* guidelines 2008): Oral: 1 mg/kg/day, gradually reduce after 1 to 2 weeks

Geriatric Refer to adult dosing; use the lowest effective dose.

Pediatric

General dosing range: Oral: Refer to adult dosing. **Note:** Dose depends upon condition being treated and response of patient; dosage for infants and children should be based on severity of the disease and response of the patient rather than on strict adherence to dosage indicated by age, weight, or body surface area. Consider alternate day therapy for long-term therapy. Discontinuation of long-term therapy requires gradual withdrawal by tapering the dose.

Indication-specific dosing:

Acute asthma (NAEPP 2007): Oral:

0 to 11 years 1 to 2 mg/kg/day for 3 to 10 days (maximum: 60 mg daily)

≥12 years: Refer to Adults dosing

Autoimmune hepatitis (off-label use; Czaja 2002): Oral: Initial treatment: 2 mg/kg/day for 2 weeks (maximum: 60 mg daily), followed by a taper over 6 to 8 weeks to a dose of 0.1 to 0.2 mg/kg/day or 5 mg daily

Bell palsy (off-label use): Adolescents ≥16 years: Oral: 60 mg daily for 5 days, followed by a 5-day taper. Treatment should begin within 72 hours of onset of symptoms (Baugh 2013).

Nephrotic syndrome (Pediatric Nephrology Panel recommendations [Hogg 2000]): Oral: Initial: 2 mg/kg daily or 60 mg/m^2/day given every day in 1 to 3 divided doses (maximum: 80 mg daily) until urine is protein free or for 4 to 6 weeks; followed by maintenance dose: 2 mg/kg/dose or 40 mg/m^2/dose given every other day in the morning; gradually taper and discontinue after 4 to 6 weeks. **Note:** No definitive treatment guidelines exist. Dosing is dependent on institution protocols and individual response.

***Pneumocystis* pneumonia (adjunctive therapy) in HIV-infected patients (off-label dose; AIDS*info* guidelines 2008):** Oral:

Children: 1 mg/kg twice daily for 5 days, *followed by* 0.5 to 1 mg/kg twice daily for 5 days, *followed by* 0.5 mg/kg once daily for 11 to 21 days

Adolescents: Refer to adult dosing.

◀ **Renal Impairment Dosing adjustment in renal impairment:** There are no dosage adjustments provided in the manufacturer's labeling.

Hemodialysis effects: Supplemental dose is not necessary.

Hepatic Impairment There are no dosage adjustments provided in the manufacturer's labeling.

Dietary Considerations May require increased dietary intake of pyridoxine, vitamin C, vitamin D, folate, calcium, and phosphorus; may require decreased dietary intake of sodium and potassium supplementation

Administration

Administer after meals or with food or milk to decrease GI upset. May administer antacids between meals to help prevent peptic ulcers.

Delayed-release tablets: Swallow whole; do not break, divide, crush, or chew.

Oral solution, concentrate: Administer only with provided calibrated dropper.

Monitoring Parameters Blood pressure; weight; serum glucose; electrolytes; growth in pediatric patients; presence of infection, bone mineral density; assess HPA axis suppression (eg, ACTH stimulation test, morning plasma cortisol test, urinary free cortisol test); Hgb; occult blood loss; chest x-ray (at regular intervals during prolonged therapy); IOP with therapy >6 weeks.

Test Interactions Decreased response to skin tests

Additional Information Tapering of corticosteroids after a short course of therapy (<7-10 days) is generally not required unless the disease/inflammatory process is slow to respond. Tapering after prolonged exposure is dependent upon the individual patient, duration of corticosteroid treatments, and size of steroid dose. Recovery of the HPA axis may require several months. Subtle but important HPA axis suppression may be present for as long as several months after a course of as few as 10-14 days duration. Testing of HPA axis (cosyntropin) may be required, and signs/symptoms of adrenal insufficiency should be monitored in patients with a history of use.

Dosage Forms Excipient information presented when available (limited, particularly for generics); consult specific product labeling.

Concentrate, Oral:

PredniSONE Intensol: 5 mg/mL (30 mL) [contains alcohol, usp; unflavored flavor]

Solution, Oral:

Generic: 5 mg/5 mL (5 mL, 120 mL, 500 mL)

Tablet, Oral:

Deltasone: 20 mg [scored; contains fd&c yellow #10 aluminum lake, fd&c yellow #6 aluminum lake]

Generic: 1 mg, 2.5 mg, 5 mg, 10 mg, 20 mg, 50 mg

Tablet Delayed Release, Oral:

Rayos: 1 mg, 2 mg, 5 mg

◆ PredniSONE Intensol *see* PredniSONE *on page 1496*

Pregabalin (pre GAB a lin)

Brand Names: US Lyrica

Brand Names: Canada ACT Pregabalin; Apo-Pregabalin; Auro-Pregabalin; Dom-Pregabalin; GD-Pregabalin; JAMP-Pregabalin; Lyrica; Mar-Pregabalin; Mint-Pregabalin; MYL Pregabalin; PMS-Pregabalin; RAN-Pregabalin; Riva-Pregabalin; Sandoz-Pregabalin; Teva-Pregabalin

Index Terms CI-1008; S-(+)-3-isobutylgaba

Pharmacologic Category Analgesic, Miscellaneous; Anticonvulsant, Miscellaneous

Use Management of neuropathic pain associated with diabetic peripheral neuropathy or with spinal cord injury; management of postherpetic neuralgia; adjunctive therapy for partial-onset seizure disorder; management of fibromyalgia

Pregnancy Considerations Adverse events have been observed in animal reproduction studies. In addition, male-mediated teratogenicity has been observed in animal reproduction studies; implications in humans are not defined. Impaired male and female fertility has been noted in animal studies. Pregabalin crosses the human placenta (Ohman, 2011). Outcome data following maternal use of pregabalin during pregnancy is limited (Veiby, 2014).

Patients exposed to pregabalin during pregnancy are encouraged to enroll themselves into the North American Antiepileptic Drug (NAAED) Pregnancy Registry by calling 1-888-233-2334. Additional information is available at www.aedpregnancyregistry.org.

Breast-Feeding Considerations Pregabalin is excreted in breast milk (Ohman, 2011). Due to the potential for serious adverse reactions in the nursing infant, the manufacturer recommends that a decision be made whether to discontinue nursing or to discontinue the drug, taking into account the importance of treatment to the mother.

Medication Guide Available Yes

Contraindications Hypersensitivity to pregabalin or any component of the formulation

Warnings/Precautions Antiepileptics are associated with an increased risk of suicidal behavior/thoughts with use (regardless of indication); patients should be monitored for signs/symptoms of depression, suicidal tendencies, and other unusual behavior changes during therapy and instructed to inform their healthcare provider immediately if symptoms occur.

Angioedema has been reported; may be life threatening; use with caution in patients with a history of angioedema episodes. Concurrent use with other drugs known to cause angioedema (eg, ACE inhibitors) may increase risk. Hypersensitivity reactions, including skin redness, blistering, hives, rash, dyspnea, and wheezing have been reported; discontinue treatment of hypersensitivity occurs. Dizziness and somnolence are commonly reported; effects generally occur shortly after initiation and occur more frequently at higher doses. Patients must be cautioned about performing tasks which require mental alertness (eg, operating machinery or driving). Visual disturbances (blurred vision, decreased acuity and visual field changes) have been associated with pregabalin therapy; patients should be instructed to notify their physician if these effects are noted.

Pregabalin has been associated with increases in CPK and rare cases of rhabdomyolysis. Patients should be instructed to notify their prescriber if unexplained muscle pain, tenderness, or weakness, particularly if fever and/or malaise are associated with these symptoms. Use may cause peripheral edema or weight gain; use with caution in patients with heart failure (NYHA Class III or IV) due to limited data in this patient population. In addition, effect on weight gain/edema may be additive with the thiazolidinedione class of antidiabetic agents; use caution when coadministering these agents, particularly in patients with prior cardiovascular disease. May decrease platelet count or prolong PR interval.

Has been noted to be tumorigenic (increased incidence of hemangiosarcoma) in animal studies; significance of these findings in humans is unknown. Pregabalin has been associated with discontinuation symptoms following abrupt cessation, and increases in seizure frequency (when used as an antiepileptic) may occur. Should not be discontinued abruptly; dosage tapering over at least 1 week is recommended. Use caution in renal impairment; dosage adjustment required.

Adverse Reactions Note: Frequency of adverse effects may be influenced by dose or concurrent therapy. In add-on trials in epilepsy, frequency of CNS and adverse effects were higher than those reported in pain management trials. Range noted below is inclusive of all trials.

>10%:

Cardiovascular: Peripheral edema (≤16%)

Central nervous system: Dizziness (8% to 45%), somnolence (4% to 36%), ataxia (1% to 20%), headache (5% to 14%), fatigue (5% to 11%)

Gastrointestinal: Weight gain (≤16%), xerostomia (1% to 15%)

Neuromuscular & skeletal: Tremor (≤11%)

Ocular: Blurred vision (1% to 12%), diplopia (≤12%)

Miscellaneous: Infection (3% to 14%), accidental injury (2% to 11%)

1% to 10%:

Cardiovascular: Edema (≤8%), chest pain (1% to 4%), hypertension (2%), hypotension (2%)

Central nervous system: Neuropathy (2% to 9%), thinking abnormal (≤9%), confusion (≤7%), euphoria (≤7%), speech disorder (≤7%), attention disturbance (4% to 6%), amnesia (≤6%), incoordination (≤6%), pain (2% to 5%), insomnia (4%), memory impaired (1% to 4%), vertigo (1% to 4%), hypoesthesia (2% to 3%), feeling abnormal (1% to 3%), anxiety (2%), lethargy (1% to 2%), drunk feeling (1% to 2%), disorientation (≤2%), depersonalization (≥1%), fever (≥1%), hypertonia (≥1%), sedation (≥1%), stupor (≥1%), nervousness (≤1%)

Dermatologic: Decubitus ulcer (3%), facial edema (≤3%), bruising (≥1%), pruritus (≥1%)

Endocrine & metabolic: Fluid retention (2% to 3%), hypoglycemia (1% to 3%), libido decreased (≥1%)

Gastrointestinal: Constipation (≤10%), appetite increased (2% to 7%), nausea (5%), flatulence (≤3%), vomiting (1% to 3%), abdominal distension (2%), abdominal pain (≥1%), gastroenteritis (≥1%)

Genitourinary: Incontinence (≤3%), anorgasmia (≥1%), impotence (≥1%), urinary frequency (≥1%)

Hematologic: Thrombocytopenia (≥1%)

Neuromuscular & skeletal: Balance disorder (2% to 9%), abnormal gait (≤8%), weakness (2% to 7%), arthralgia (3% to 6%), twitching (≤5%), muscle spasm (2% to 4%), back pain (≤4%), myoclonus (≤4%), CPK increased (3%), neck pain (3%), pain in extremity (3%), joint swelling (2%), paresthesia (2%), leg cramps (≥1%), myalgia (≥1%), myasthenia (1%)

Ocular: Visual abnormalities (≤5%), eye disorder (≤2%), conjunctivitis (≥1%), nystagmus (≥1%)

Otic: Otitis media (≥1%), tinnitus (≥1%)

Respiratory: Nasopharyngitis (8%), sinusitis (4% to 7%), pharyngolaryngeal pain (1% to 3%), bronchitis (≤3%), dyspnea (≤3%)

Miscellaneous: Flu-like syndrome (1% to 2%), allergic reaction (≥1%)

<1% (Limited to important or life-threatening): Abnormal ejaculation, abscess, acute renal failure, addiction, agitation, albuminuria, alopecia, amenorrhea, anaphylactoid reaction, anemia, angioedema, anisocoria, apathy, aphasia, aphthous stomatitis, apnea, arthrosis, ascites, atelectasis, bladder cancer, blepharitis, blindness, bronchiolitis, cellulitis, cerebellar syndrome, cervicitis, chills, cholecystitis, cholelithiasis, chondrodystrophy, circumoral paresthesia, cogwheel rigidity, colitis, coma, corneal ulcer, crystalluria (urate), delirium, delusions, diarrhea, dry eyes, dysarthria, dysautonomia, dyskinesia, dysmenorrhea, dysphagia, dyspareunia, dystonia, dysuria, eczema, encephalopathy, eosinophilia, epididymitis, esophageal ulcer, esophagitis, exfoliative dermatitis, exophthalmos, extraocular palsy, extrapyramidal syndrome, eye hemorrhage, female lactation, gastritis, GI hemorrhage, glomerulitis, glucose tolerance decreased, granuloma, Guillain-Barré syndrome, gynecomastia, hallucinations, heart failure, hematuria, hirsutism, hostility, hyperacusis, hyperalgesia, hyperesthesia, hyper-/hypokinesia; hypersensitivity (including skin redness, blistering, hives, rash, dyspnea, and wheezing); hypotonia, intracranial hypertension, iritis, keratitis, keratoconjunctivitis, libido increased, laryngismus, leukopenia, leukorrhea, leukocytosis, lichenoid dermatitis, lung edema, lung fibrosis, lymphadenopathy, malaise, manic reaction, melanosis, melena, miosis, mouth ulcer, mydriasis, myelofibrosis, neck rigidity, nephritis, neuralgia, night blindness, ocular hemorrhage, oliguria, ophthalmoplegia, optic atrophy, pancreatitis, papilledema, paranoid reaction, parosmia, pelvic pain, periodontal abscess, peripheral neuritis, personality disorder, photophobia, photosensitivity, polycythemia, postural hypotension, prothrombin decreased, psychotic depression, ptosis, pulmonary edema, pulmonary fibrosis, purpura, pyelonephritis, rash (vesiculobullous, petechial, purpuric, pustular); rectal hemorrhage, renal calculus, retinal edema, retinal vascular disorder, retroperitoneal fibrosis, rhabdomyolysis, schizophrenic reaction, shock, skin atrophy, skin necrosis, skin nodule, skin ulcer, ST depression, Stevens-Johnson syndrome, subcutaneous nodule, suicide, suicide attempt, syncope, taste loss, taste perversion, thrombocythemia, thrombophlebitis, tongue edema, torticollis, trismus, urinary retention, urticaria, uveitis, ventricular fibrillation

Drug Interactions

Metabolism/Transport Effects None known.

Avoid Concomitant Use

Avoid concomitant use of Pregabalin with any of the following: Azelastine (Nasal); Orphenadrine; Paraldehyde; Thalidomide

Increased Effect/Toxicity

Pregabalin may increase the levels/effects of: Alcohol (Ethyl); Antidiabetic Agents (Thiazolidinedione); Azelastine (Nasal); Buprenorphine; CNS Depressants; Hydrocodone; Methotrimeprazine; Metyrosine; Mirtazapine; Orphenadrine; Paraldehyde; Pramipexole; ROPINIRole; Rotigotine; Selective Serotonin Reuptake Inhibitors; Suvorexant; Thalidomide; Zolpidem

The levels/effects of Pregabalin may be increased by: ACE Inhibitors; Brimonidine (Topical); Cannabis; Doxylamine; Dronabinol; Droperidol; HydrOXYzine; Kava Kava; Magnesium Sulfate; Methotrimeprazine; Minocycline; Nabilone; Perampanel; Rufinamide; Sodium Oxybate; Tapentadol; Tetrahydrocannabinol

Decreased Effect

The levels/effects of Pregabalin may be decreased by: Mefloquine; Mianserin; Orlistat

Storage/Stability Store at 25°C (77°F); excursions permitted to 15°C to 30°C (59°F to 86°F).

Mechanism of Action Binds to alpha$_2$-delta subunit of voltage-gated calcium channels within the CNS and modulates calcium influx at the nerve terminals, thereby inhibiting excitatory neurotransmitter release including glutamate, norepinephrine (noradrenaline), serotonin, dopamine, substance P, and calcitonin gene-related peptide (Gajraj, 2007; McKeage, 2009). Although structurally related to GABA, it does not bind to GABA or benzodiazepine receptors. Exerts antinociceptive and anticonvulsant activity. Pregabalin may also affect descending noradrenergic and serotonergic pain transmission pathways from the brainstem to the spinal cord.

Pharmacodynamics/Kinetics

Onset of action: Pain management: Effects may be noted as early as the first week of therapy.

Distribution: V_d: 0.5 L/kg

Protein binding: 0%

Metabolism: Negligible

Bioavailability: >90%

Half-life elimination: 6.3 hours

Time to peak, plasma: 1.5 hours (3 hours with food)

Excretion: Urine (90% as unchanged drug; minor metabolites)

Dosing

Adult & Geriatric Note: When discontinuing, taper off gradually over at least 1 week.

Fibromyalgia: Oral:

U.S. labeling: Initial: 150 mg daily in divided doses (75 mg twice daily); may be increased to 300 mg daily (150 mg twice daily) within 1 week based on tolerability and effect; may be further increased to 450 mg daily (225 mg twice daily). Maximum dose: 450 mg daily (dosages up to 600 mg daily were evaluated with no significant additional benefit and an increase in adverse effects)

Canadian labeling: Initial: 150 mg daily in divided doses (75 mg twice daily); may be increased to 300 mg daily (150 mg twice daily) after 1 week based on tolerability and effect; may be further increased to 450 mg daily (225 mg twice daily). The manufacturer labeling suggests that patients with severe ongoing symptoms may receive up to a maximum of 600 mg daily (300 mg twice daily). However, dosages up to 600 mg daily have been evaluated with no significant additional benefit and an increase in adverse effects.

Neuropathic pain, diabetes-associated: Oral:

U.S. labeling: Initial: 150 mg daily in divided doses (50 mg 3 times daily); may be increased within 1 week based on tolerability and effect; maximum dose: 300 mg daily in 3 divided doses (dosages up to 600 mg daily were evaluated with no significant additional benefit and an increase in adverse effects)

Canadian labeling: Initial: 150 mg daily in divided doses (50 mg 3 times daily or 75 mg twice daily); may be increased after 1 week based on tolerability and effect to 300 mg daily (150 mg twice daily). The manufacturer labeling suggests that patients with severe ongoing symptoms may receive up to a maximum of 600 mg daily (300 mg twice daily). However, dosages up to 600 mg daily have been evaluated with no significant additional benefit and an increase in adverse effects.

Neuropathic pain, spinal cord injury associated: Oral: Initial: 150 mg daily in divided doses (75 mg twice daily); may be increased to 300 mg daily (150 mg twice daily) within 1 week based on tolerability and effect; further titration to 600 mg daily (300 mg twice daily) after 2-3 weeks may be considered in patients who do not experience sufficient relief of pain provided they are able to tolerate pregabalin. Maximum dose: 600 mg daily

Partial-onset seizures (adjunctive therapy): Oral: Initial: 150 mg daily in divided doses (75 mg twice daily or 50 mg 3 times daily); may be increased based on tolerability and effect (optimal titration schedule has not been defined). Maximum dose: 600 mg daily

Postherpetic neuralgia: Oral: Initial: 150 mg daily in divided doses (75 mg twice daily or 50 mg 3 times daily); may be increased to 300 mg daily within 1 week based on tolerability and effect; further titration (to 600 mg daily) after 2-4 weeks may be considered in patients who do not experience sufficient relief of pain provided they are able to tolerate pregabalin. Maximum dose: 600 mg daily

Renal Impairment Renal function may be estimated using the Cockcroft-Gault formula. Then determine recommended dosage regimen based on the indication-specific total daily dose for normal renal function (CrCl ≥60 mL/minute). For example, if the indication-specific daily dose is 450 mg daily for normal renal function, the daily dose should be reduced to 225 mg daily (in 2-3 divided doses) for a creatinine clearance of 30-60 mL/minute (see table).

Pregabalin Renal Impairment Dosing

CrCl (mL/minute)	Total Pregabalin Daily Dose (mg/day)				Dosing Frequency
≥60 (normal renal function)	150	300	450	600	2-3 divided doses
30-60	75	150	225	300	2-3 divided doses
15-30	25-50	75	100-150	150	1-2 divided doses
<15	25	25-50	50-75	75	Single daily dose

Posthemodialysis supplementary dosage (as a single additional dose):
25 mg/day schedule: Single supplementary dose of 25 mg or 50 mg
25-50 mg/day schedule: Single supplementary dose of 50 mg or 75 mg
50-75 mg/day schedule: Single supplementary dose of 75 mg or 100 mg
75 mg/day schedule: Single supplementary dose of 100 mg or 150 mg

Hepatic Impairment No dosage adjustment provided in manufacturer's labeling. However, no adjustment expected since undergoes minimal hepatic metabolism.

Dietary Considerations May be taken with or without food.

Administration May be administered with or without food.

Monitoring Parameters Measures of efficacy (pain intensity/seizure frequency); degree of sedation; symptoms of myopathy or ocular disturbance; weight gain/edema; skin integrity (in patients with diabetes); suicidality (eg, suicidal thoughts, depression, behavioral changes)

Dosage Forms Excipient information presented when available (limited, particularly for generics); consult specific product labeling.

Capsule, Oral:

Lyrica: 25 mg, 50 mg, 75 mg, 100 mg, 150 mg, 200 mg, 225 mg, 300 mg

Solution, Oral:

Lyrica: 20 mg/mL (473 mL) [contains methylparaben, propylparaben]

Controlled Substance C-V

Primaquine (PRIM a kween)

Index Terms Primaquine Phosphate; Prymaccone

Pharmacologic Category Aminoquinoline (Antimalarial); Antimalarial Agent

Use

Malaria: For the radical cure (prevention of relapse) of vivax malaria

Canadian labeling: Additional use (not in US labeling): For the radical cure (prevention of relapse) of ovale malaria

Pregnancy Considerations Animal reproduction studies have not been conducted. Primaquine use is not recommended in pregnant women (CDC 2013). Consult current CDC guidelines for the treatment of malaria during pregnancy.

Breast-Feeding Considerations It is not known if primaquine is excreted in breast milk. If therapy is needed, the mother and infant should be tested for G6PD deficiency; primaquine may be used in breast-feeding mothers and infants with normal G6PD levels and concentrations (CDC 2012).

Contraindications

Use in acutely ill patients who have a tendency to develop granulocytopenia (eg, rheumatoid arthritis, SLE); concurrent use with other medications causing hemolytic anemia or myeloid bone marrow suppression; concurrent use with or recent use of quinacrine

Canadian labeling: Additional contraindications (not in US labeling): Hypersensitivity to primaquine or any component of the formulation

Documentation of allergenic cross-reactivity for aminoquinolines is limited. However, because of similarities in chemical structure and/or pharmacologic actions, the possibility of cross-sensitivity cannot be ruled out with certainty.

Warnings/Precautions Use with caution in patients with G6PD deficiency (hemolytic anemia may occur), NADH methemoglobin reductase deficiency (methemoglobinemia may occur); do not exceed recommended dosage and duration. Moderate to severe hemolytic reactions may occur in individuals with G6PD deficiency and personal or familial history of favism. Geographic regions with a high prevalence of G6PD deficiency (eg, Africa, southern Europe, Mediterranean region, Middle East, southeast Asia, Oceania) are associated with a higher incidence of hemolytic anemia. Promptly discontinue with signs of hemolytic anemia (darkening of urine, marked fall in hemoglobin or erythrocyte count). The CDC recommends screening for G6PD deficiency prior to therapy initiation (CDC 2013). Anemia, methemoglobinemia, and leukopenia have been associated with primaquine use; monitor during treatment. Immediately discontinue if marked darkening of the urine or sudden decrease in hemoglobin concentration or leukocyte count occurs.

May cause QT prolongation; monitor ECG in patients with cardiac disease, long QT syndrome, a history of ventricular arrhythmias, uncorrected hypokalemia and/or hypomagnesemia, or bradycardia (<50 beats per minute), and during concomitant administration with QT interval prolonging agents. Some dosage forms may contain polysorbate 80 (also known as Tweens). Hypersensitivity reactions, usually a delayed reaction, have been reported following exposure to pharmaceutical products containing polysorbate 80 in certain individuals (Isaksson 2002; Lucente 2000; Shelley 1995). Thrombocytopenia, ascites, pulmonary deterioration, and renal and hepatic failure have been reported in premature neonates after receiving parenteral products containing polysorbate 80 (Alade 1986; CDC 1984). See manufacturer's labeling. Potentially significant

drug-drug interactions may exist, requiring dose or frequency adjustment, additional monitoring, and/or selection of alternative therapy.

Adverse Reactions Frequency not defined.

Cardiovascular: Cardiac arrhythmias, prolonged Q-T interval on ECG

Gastrointestinal: Abdominal cramps, epigastric distress, nausea, vomiting

Hematologic & oncologic: Anemia, hemolytic anemia (in patients with G6PD deficiency), leukopenia, methemoglobinemia (in NADH-methemoglobin reductase-deficient individuals)

Ophthalmic: Accommodation disturbance

Drug Interactions

Metabolism/Transport Effects Substrate of CYP2D6 (major), CYP3A4 (major); **Note:** Assignment of Major/Minor substrate status based on clinically relevant drug interaction potential; **Inhibits** CYP1A2 (strong), CYP2D6 (weak); **Induces** CYP1A2 (weak/moderate)

Avoid Concomitant Use

Avoid concomitant use of Primaquine with any of the following: Agomelatine; Artemether; DULoxetine; Highest Risk QTc-Prolonging Agents; Ivabradine; Lumefantrine; Mefloquine; Mifepristone; Pomalidomide; Tasimelteon; TiZANidine

Increased Effect/Toxicity

Primaquine may increase the levels/effects of: Agomelatine; Antipsychotic Agents (Phenothiazines); ARIPiprazole; Bendamustine; Beta-Blockers; Cardiac Glycosides; CloZAPine; CYP1A2 Substrates; Dapsone (Systemic); Dapsone (Topical); DULoxetine; Highest Risk QTc-Prolonging Agents; Lumefantrine; Mefloquine; Moderate Risk QTc-Prolonging Agents; Pentoxifylline; Pirfenidone; Pomalidomide; Prilocaine; Rasagiline; Sodium Nitrite; Tasimelteon; TiZANidine

The levels/effects of Primaquine may be increased by: Abiraterone Acetate; Artemether; Cobicistat; CYP2D6 Inhibitors (Moderate); CYP2D6 Inhibitors (Strong); Dapsone (Systemic); Darunavir; Ivabradine; Mefloquine; Mifepristone; Nitric Oxide; Panobinostat; Peginterferon Alfa-2b; QTc-Prolonging Agents (Indeterminate Risk and Risk Modifying)

Decreased Effect

Primaquine may decrease the levels/effects of: Anthelmintics

The levels/effects of Primaquine may be decreased by: Bosentan; CYP3A4 Inducers (Moderate); CYP3A4 Inducers (Strong); Dabrafenib; Deferasirox; Enzalutamide; Mitotane; Peginterferon Alfa-2b; Siltuximab; St Johns Wort; Tocilizumab

Storage/Stability Store at 25°C (77°F); excursions permitted to 15°C to 30°C (59°F to 86°F). Protect from light.

Mechanism of Action Primaquine is an antiprotozoal agent active against exoerythrocytic stages of *Plasmodium ovale* and *P. vivax*, also active against the primary exoerythrocytic stages of *P. falciparum* and gametocytes of *Plasmodia*; disrupts mitochondria and binds to DNA

Pharmacodynamics/Kinetics

Absorption: Well absorbed

Metabolism: Hepatic to carboxyprimaquine (active)

Half-life elimination: 3 to 6 hours

Time to peak, serum: 1 to 3 hours

Excretion: Urine (small amounts as unchanged drug)

Dosing

Adult & Geriatric Note: The CDC requires screening for G6PD deficiency prior to initiating treatment with primaquine. Dosage expressed as mg of base (15 mg base = 26.3 mg primaquine phosphate).

Malaria: Oral:

Treatment or prevention of relapse of P. vivax malaria (US labeling): 15 mg once daily in combination with chloroquine for 14 days (maximum dose: 15 mg/day)

Treatment or prevention of relapse of P. vivax or P. ovale malaria (Canadian labeling): 15 mg once daily for 14 days (maximum dose: 15 mg/day); for the prevention of delayed primary attacks and relapse of in individuals who have returned home from areas where these plasmodial species are endemic, initiate therapy during the last 2 weeks of, or immediately following therapy with chloroquine or another suitable antimalarial agent. The manufacturer suggests that higher dosing or extended therapy may be required for resistant *P. vivax* but does not provide specific recommendations.

Treatment of uncomplicated P. vivax and P. ovale malaria (off-label use): 30 mg once daily for 14 days with chloroquine or hydroxychloroquine; alternative regimen (for mild G6PD deficiency or as an alternative to daily regimen): 45 mg once weekly for 8 weeks (use only after consultation with an infectious disease/ tropical medicine expert) (CDC 2013)

Chemoprophylaxis (off-label use): 30 mg once daily; start 1 to 2 days prior to travel and continue for 7 days after departure from malaria-endemic area (CDC Yellow Book 2014)

Presumptive antirelapse therapy for P. vivax and P. ovale malaria (off-label use): 30 mg once daily for 14 days after departure from malaria-endemic area (CDC Yellow Book 2014)

***Pneumocystis* pneumonia (PCP) treatment in HIV-infected patients (alternative to preferred therapy) (off-label use):** Oral: 30 mg once daily for 21 days (in combination with clindamycin) (HHS [OI adult 2015])

Pediatric Note: The CDC requires screening for G6PD deficiency prior to initiating treatment with primaquine. Dosage expressed as mg of base (15 mg base = 26.3 mg primaquine phosphate).

Malaria: Oral:

Treatment or prevention of relapse of P. vivax or P. ovale malaria (Canadian labeling): Children and Adolescents: 0.39 mg/kg once daily for 14 days (maximum: 15 mg/day)

Treatment of uncomplicated P. vivax and P. ovale malaria (off-label use): 0.5 mg/kg (maximum: 30 mg/day) daily for 14 days with chloroquine or hydroxychloroquine (CDC 2013)

Chemoprophylaxis (off-label use): 0.5 mg/kg once daily (maximum dose: 30 mg/day); start 1 to 2 days prior to travel and continue for 7 days after departure from malaria-endemic area (CDC Yellow Book 2014)

Presumptive antirelapse therapy for P. vivax and P. ovale malaria (off-label use): 0.5 mg/kg (maximum dose: 30 mg/day) once daily for 14 days after departure from malaria-endemic area (CDC Yellow Book 2014)

***Pneumocystis* pneumonia (PCP) treatment in HIV-infected patients (alternative to preferred therapy) (off-label use) (alternative to preferred therapy):**

Children: 0.3 mg/kg once daily for 21 days (in combination with clindamycin) (HHS [OI pediatric 2013])

Adolescents: Refer to adult dosing.

Renal Impairment There are no dosage adjustments provided in the manufacturer's labeling.

Hepatic Impairment There are no dosage adjustments provided in the manufacturer's labeling.

Administration Administer with meals to decrease adverse GI effects. If patient vomits within 30 minutes of taking a dose, then they should repeat the dose (CDC 2013).

Monitoring Parameters Periodic CBC, visual color check of urine, glucose, electrolytes; if hemolysis suspected, monitor CBC, haptoglobin, peripheral smear, urinalysis dipstick for occult blood, G6PD deficiency screening (prior to initiating treatment; CDC recommendation); ECG (in patients at risk for QT prolongation)

Dosage Forms Excipient information presented when available (limited, particularly for generics); consult specific product labeling.

Tablet, Oral, as phosphate:

Generic: 26.3 mg

Extemporaneous Preparations A 6 mg base/5 mL oral suspension may be made using tablets. Crush ten 15 mg base tablets and reduce to a fine powder. In small amounts, add a total of 10 mL Carboxymethylcellulose 1.5% and mix to a uniform paste; mix while adding Simple Syrup, NF to **almost** 125 mL; transfer to a calibrated bottle, rinse mortar with vehicle, and add quantity of vehicle sufficient to make 125 mL. Label "shake well" and "refrigerate". Stable 7 days.

Nahata MC, Pai VB, and Hipple TF, *Pediatric Drug Formulations*, 5th ed, Cincinnati, OH: Harvey Whitney Books Co, 2004.

◆ Primaquine Phosphate see Primaquine on page 1502

◆ Primatene Mist see EPINEPHrine (Systemic) on page 647

◆ Primaxin (Can) see Imipenem and Cilastatin on page 923

◆ Primaxin I.M. [DSC] see Imipenem and Cilastatin on page 923

◆ Primaxin I.V. see Imipenem and Cilastatin on page 923

Primidone (PRI mi done)

Brand Names: US Mysoline

Brand Names: Canada Apo-Primidone

Index Terms Desoxyphenobarbital; Primaclone

Pharmacologic Category Anticonvulsant, Miscellaneous; Barbiturate

Use Management of grand mal, psychomotor, and focal seizures

Pregnancy Considerations Primidone and its metabolites (PEMA, phenobarbital, and p-hydroxyphenobarbital) cross the placenta; neonatal serum concentrations at birth are similar to those in the mother. Withdrawal symptoms may occur in the neonate and may be delayed due to the long half-life of primidone and its metabolites. Use may be associated with birth defects and adverse events; the use of folic acid throughout pregnancy and vitamin K during the last month of pregnancy is recommended. Epilepsy itself, number of medications, genetic factors, or a combination of these probably influence the teratogenicity of anticonvulsant therapy.

Patients exposed to primidone during pregnancy are encouraged to enroll themselves into the NAAED Pregnancy Registry by calling 1-888-233-2334. Additional information is available at www.aedpregnancyregistry.org.

Breast-Feeding Considerations Primidone and its metabolites (PEMA, phenobarbital, and p-hydroxyphenobarbital) are found in breast milk (variable concentrations). The manufacturer recommends discontinuing breast-feeding if undue drowsiness and somnolence occur in the newborn.

Medication Guide Available Yes

Contraindications Hypersensitivity to phenobarbital; porphyria

Warnings/Precautions Antiepileptics are associated with an increased risk of suicidal behavior/thoughts with use (regardless of indication); patients should be monitored for signs/symptoms of depression, suicidal tendencies, and other unusual behavior changes during therapy and instructed to inform their healthcare provider immediately if symptoms occur.

Use with caution in patients with renal or hepatic impairment, pulmonary insufficiency; abrupt withdrawal may precipitate status epilepticus. Potential for drug dependency exists. Do not administer to patients in acute pain. Use caution in elderly, debilitated, or pediatric patients - may cause paradoxical responses. May cause CNS depression, which may impair physical or mental abilities. Patients must cautioned about performing tasks which require mental alertness (eg, operating machinery or driving). Effects with other sedative drugs or ethanol may be potentiated. Use with caution in patients with depression or suicidal tendencies, or in patients with a history of drug abuse. Tolerance or psychological and physical dependence may occur with prolonged use. Primidone's active metabolite, phenobarbital, has been associated with cognitive deficits in children receiving chronic therapy for febrile seizures. Use with caution in patients with hypoadrenalism.

Benzyl alcohol and derivatives: Some dosage forms may contain sodium benzoate/benzoic acid; benzoic acid (benzoate) is a metabolite of benzyl alcohol; large amounts of benzyl alcohol (≥99 mg/kg/day) have been associated with a potentially fatal toxicity ("gasping syndrome") in neonates; the "gasping syndrome" consists of metabolic acidosis, respiratory distress, gasping respirations, CNS dysfunction (including convulsions, intracranial hemorrhage), hypotension, and cardiovascular collapse (AAP ["Inactive" 1997]; CDC, 1982); some data suggests that benzoate displaces bilirubin from protein binding sites (Ahlfors, 2001); avoid or use dosage forms containing benzyl alcohol derivative with caution in neonates. See manufacturer's labeling.

Adverse Reactions Frequency not defined.

Central nervous system: Ataxia, drowsiness, emotional disturbances, fatigue, hyperirritability, suicidal ideation, vertigo

Dermatologic: Morbilliform skin eruptions

Gastrointestinal: Anorexia, nausea, vomiting

Genitourinary: Impotence

Hematologic: Agranulocytosis, granulocytopenia, megaloblastic anemia (idiosyncratic), red cell aplasia/hypoplasia

Ocular: Diplopia, nystagmus

Drug Interactions

Metabolism/Transport Effects Induces CYP1A2 (strong), CYP2B6 (strong), CYP2C8 (strong), CYP2C9 (strong), CYP3A4 (strong), P-glycoprotein

Avoid Concomitant Use

Avoid concomitant use of Primidone with any of the following: Abiraterone Acetate; Antihepaciviral Combination Products; Apixaban; Apremilast; Aprepitant; Artemether; Axitinib; Azelastine (Nasal); Bedaquiline; Boceprevir; Bortezomib; Bosutinib; Cabozantinib; Cariprazine; Ceritinib; CloZAPine; Cobicistat; Cobimetinib; Crizotinib; Dabigatran Etexilate; Dabrafenib; Daclatasvir; Dienogest; Dolutegravir; Dronedarone; Eliglustat; Enzalutamide; Etravirine; Everolimus; Flibanserin; Ibrutinib; Idelalisib; Irinotecan Products; Isavuconazonium Sulfate; Itraconazole; Ivabradine; Ivacaftor; Ixazomib; Lapatinib; Ledipasvir; Lumefantrine; Lurasidone; Macitentan; Mifepristone; Naloxegol; Netupitant; NIFEdipine; Nilotinib; NiMODipine; Nintedanib; Nisoldipine; Olaparib; Ombitasvir, Paritaprevir, Ritonavir, and Dasabuvir; Orphenadrine; Osimertinib; Palbociclib; Panobinostat; Paraldehyde; PAZOPanib; Perampanel; Pirfenidone; PONATinib; Praziquantel; Ranolazine; Regorafenib; Rilpivirine; Rivaroxaban; Roflumilast; RomiDEPsin; Simeprevir; Sofosbuvir; Sonidegib; SORAfenib; Suvorexant; Tasimelteon; Telaprevir; Thalidomide; Ticagrelor; Tofacitinib; Tolvaptan; Toremifene; Trabectedin; Ulipristal; Vandetanib; Vemurafenib; VinCRIStine (Liposomal); Vorapaxar

Increased Effect/Toxicity

Primidone may increase the levels/effects of: Alcohol (Ethyl); Azelastine (Nasal); Barbiturates; Buprenorphine; Clarithromycin; CNS Depressants; Cyclophosphamide; Hydrocodone; Methotrimeprazine; Metyrosine; Orphenadrine; Paraldehyde; Pramipexole; Rotigotine; Selective Serotonin Reuptake Inhibitors; Thalidomide; Valproate Products; Zolpidem

The levels/effects of Primidone may be increased by: Brimonidine (Topical); Cannabis; Carbonic Anhydrase Inhibitors; Clarithromycin; Cosyntropin; Dexmethylphenidate; Doxylamine; Dronabinol; Droperidol; Felbamate; HydrOXYzine; Kava Kava; Magnesium Sulfate; Methotrimeprazine; Methylphenidate; Minocycline; Nabilone; Sodium Oxybate; Tapentadol; Tetrahydrocannabinol; Valproate Products

Decreased Effect

Primidone may decrease the levels/effects of: Abiraterone Acetate; Afatinib; Antihepaciviral Combination Products; Apixaban; Apremilast; Aprepitant; ARIPiprazole; ARIPiprazole Lauroxil; Artemether; Axitinib; Bazedoxifene; Bedaquiline; Bendamustine; Boceprevir; Bortezomib; Bosutinib; Brentuximab Vedotin; Brexpiprazole; Cabozantinib; Canagliflozin; Cannabidiol; Cannabis; Cariprazine; Ceritinib; Clarithromycin; CloZAPine; Cobicistat; Cobimetinib; Contraceptives (Progestins); Corticosteroids (Systemic); Crizotinib; CYP1A2 Substrates; CYP2B6 Substrates; CYP2C8 Substrates; CYP2C9 Substrates; CYP3A4 Substrates; Dabigatran Etexilate; Dabrafenib; Daclatasvir; Dasatinib; Dexamethasone (Systemic); Diclofenac (Systemic); Dienogest; Dolutegravir; DOXOrubicin (Conventional); Dronabinol; Dronedarone; Eliglustat; Enzalutamide; Erlotinib; Eslicarbazepine; Etizolam; Etoposide; Etoposide Phosphate; Etravirine; Everolimus; Exemestane; Felbamate; FentaNYL; Flibanserin; Gefitinib; GuanFACINE; Hydrocortisone (Systemic); Ibrutinib; Idelalisib; Imatinib; Irinotecan Products; Isavuconazonium Sulfate; Itraconazole; Ivabradine; Ivacaftor; Ixabepilone; Ixazomib; LamoTRIgine; Lapatinib; Ledipasvir; Linagliptin; Lumefantrine; Lurasidone; Macitentan; Maraviroc; Methadone; MethylPREDNISolone; MetroNIDAZOLE (Systemic); Mifepristone; Naloxegol; Netupitant; NIFEdipine; Nilotinib; NiMODipine; Nintedanib; Nisoldipine; Olaparib; Ombitasvir, Paritaprevir, Ritonavir, and Dasabuvir; Osimertinib; Palbociclib; Paliperidone; Panobinostat; PAZOPanib; Perampanel; P-glycoprotein/ABCB1 Substrates; Pirfenidone; PONATinib; Praziquantel; PrednisoLONE (Systemic); PredniSONE; Propafenone; QUEtiapine; QuiNIDine; Ranolazine; Regorafenib; Rilpivirine; Rivaroxaban; Roflumilast; Rolapitant; RomiDEPsin; Rufinamide; Saxagliptin; Simeprevir; Sofosbuvir; Sonidegib; SORAfenib; SUNItinib; Suvorexant; Tadalafil; Tasimelteon; Telaprevir; Tetrahydrocannabinol; Ticagrelor; Tofacitinib; Tolvaptan; Toremifene; Trabectedin; Treprostinil; Ulipristal; Vandetanib; Vemurafenib; Vilazodone; VinCRIStine (Liposomal); Vorapaxar; Vortioxetine; Zaleplon; Zuclopenthixol

The levels/effects of Primidone may be decreased by: Carbonic Anhydrase Inhibitors; Folic Acid; Fosphenytoin; Leucovorin Calcium-Levoleucovorin; Levomefolate; Mefloquine; Methylfolate; Orlistat; Phenytoin

Food Interactions Protein-deficient diets increase duration of action of primidone.

Storage/Stability Store at 20°C to 25°C (68°F to 77°F).

Mechanism of Action Decreases neuron excitability, raises seizure threshold similar to phenobarbital; primidone has two active metabolites, phenobarbital and phenylethylmalonamide (PEMA); PEMA may enhance the activity of phenobarbital

Pharmacodynamics/Kinetics

Absorption: 60% to 80%

Distribution: Adults: V_d: 0.6 L/kg

Protein binding: 30%

Metabolism: Hepatic to phenobarbital (active) by oxidation and to phenylethylmalonamide (PEMA; active) by scission of the heterocyclic ring

Half-life elimination (age dependent): Primidone: Mean: 5-15 hours (variable); PEMA: 16 hours (variable)

Time to peak, serum: ~3 hours (variable)

Excretion: Urine (40% as unchanged drug; the remainder is unconjugated PEMA, phenobarbital and its metabolites)

Dosing

Adult & Geriatric

Seizure disorders (grand mal, psychomotor, and focal):

Oral: Days 1 to 3: 100 to 125 mg/day at bedtime; days 4 to 6: 100 to 125 twice daily; days 7 to 9: 100 to 125 mg 3 times daily; usual dose: 750 to 1,500 mg/day in divided doses 3 to 4 times/day with maximum dosage of 2 g/day

Patients already receiving other anticonvulsants: Initial: 100 to 125 mg at bedtime; gradually increase to maintenance dose as other drug is gradually decreased, continue until desired level obtained or other drug completely withdrawn. If goal is monotherapy, conversion should be completed over ≥2 weeks.

Essential tremor (off-label use): Initial: 50 to 62.5 mg once daily; increase dose gradually based on response and tolerability in increments of 62.5 to 125 mg every 1 to 3 days or by 250 mg every week and administer in 2 to 3 divided doses (Findley 1985; Gorman 1986; Koller 1986; Sasso 1988). Usual dosage: 250 to 750 mg/day (Zappia 2013); maximum: 750 mg/day (AAN [Zesiewicz 2005]).

Note: Lower maintenance doses (250 mg daily) have been found to be equally or more effective than higher doses (750 mg daily) with fewer adverse effects (Koller 1986; Serrano-Duenas 2003). However, lower initial doses (as low as 7.5 mg/day) and more gradual titration schedules have not been found to improve tolerability (O'Suilleabhain 2002).

Pediatric Seizure disorders (grand mal, psychomotor, and focal): Oral:

Children <8 years: Initial: Days 1-3: 50 mg/day given at bedtime; days 4-6: 50 mg twice daily; days 7-9: 100 mg twice daily; usual dose: 375-750 mg/day in 3-4 divided doses (10-25 mg/kg/day)

Children ≥8 years: Refer to adult dosing.

Renal Impairment Adults: No dosage adjustment provided in manufacturer's labeling. However, the following guidelines have been used by some clinicians (Aronoff, 2007): **Note:** Avoid in renal failure if possible; due to active metabolites with long half-lives and complex kinetics:

CrCl ≥50 mL/minute: Administer every 12 hours

CrCl 10 to 50 mL/minute: Administer every 12 to 24 hours

CrCl <10 mL/minute: Administer every 24 hours

Hemodialysis: Administer dose postdialysis

Hepatic Impairment No dosage adjustment provided in manufacturer's labeling. However, increased side effects may occur in severe liver disease; monitor plasma levels and adjust dose accordingly.

Dietary Considerations Folic acid: Low erythrocyte and CSF folate concentrations. Megaloblastic anemia has been reported. To avoid folic acid deficiency and megaloblastic anemia, some clinicians recommend giving patients on anticonvulsants prophylactic doses of folic acid and cyanocobalamin.

Monitoring Parameters Serum primidone and phenobarbital concentration, neurological status. Due to CNS effects, monitor closely when initiating drug in elderly. Monitor CBC and sequential multiple analysis-12 (SMA-12) at 6-month intervals to compare with baseline obtained at start of therapy. Monitor for suicidality (eg, suicidal thoughts, depression, behavioral changes). Since elderly metabolize phenobarbital at a slower rate than younger adults, it is suggested to measure both primidone and phenobarbital levels together.

Reference Range Therapeutic: Children <5 years: 7-10 mcg/mL (SI: 32-46 micromole/L); Adults: 5-12 mcg/mL (SI: 23-55 micromole/L); toxic effects rarely present with levels <10 mcg/mL (SI: 46 micromole/L) if phenobarbital concentrations are low. Dosage of primidone is adjusted with reference mostly to the phenobarbital level; Toxic: >15 mcg/mL (SI: >69 micromole/L)

Dosage Forms Excipient information presented when available (limited, particularly for generics); consult specific product labeling.

Tablet, Oral:

Mysoline: 50 mg, 250 mg [scored]

Generic: 50 mg, 250 mg

Dosage Forms: Canada Excipient information presented when available (limited, particularly for generics); consult specific product labeling.

Tablet, oral:

Apo-Primidone®: 125 mg, 250 mg

Probenecid (proe BEN e sid)

Brand Names: Canada Benuryl

Index Terms Benemid [DSC]

Pharmacologic Category Uricosuric Agent

Use Treatment of hyperuricemia associated with gout or gouty arthritis; prolongation and elevation of beta-lactam plasma levels (eg, uncomplicated gonococcal infection)

Dosing

Adult & Geriatric

Hyperuricemia with gout: Oral: 250 mg twice daily for 1 week; may increase to 500 mg twice daily; if needed, may increase to a maximum of 2 g/day (increase dosage in 500 mg increments every 4 weeks). If serum uric acid levels are within normal limits and gout attacks have been absent for 6 months, daily dosage may be reduced by 500 mg every 6 months.

Prolong penicillin serum levels: Oral: 500 mg 4 times/day. **Note:** Dosing per manufacturer, see indication-specific dosing.

Gonorrhea, uncomplicated infections of cervix, urethra, and rectum: Oral: 1 g once with cefoxitin 2 g IM (CDC, 2010)

Pelvic inflammatory disease (off-label use): Oral: 1 g once with cefoxitin 2 g IM plus doxycycline (CDC, 2010)

Neurosyphilis (off-label use): Oral: 500 mg 4 times/day with procaine penicillin 2.4 million units/day IM for 10-14 days (CDC, 2010). **Note:** Penicillin G aqueous IV is the preferred agent.

Pediatric

Note: Contraindicated in children <2 years of age.

Prolong penicillin serum levels: Oral: Children 2-14 years: Initial: 25 mg/kg, then 40 mg/kg/day in 4 divided doses (maximum: 500 mg/dose)

Treatment of gonorrhea: >50 kg: Refer to adult dosing.

Renal Impairment CrCl <30 mL/minute: Avoid use.

Hepatic Impairment No dosage adjustment provided in manufacturer's labeling.

Additional Information Complete prescribing information should be consulted for additional detail.

Dosage Forms Excipient information presented when available (limited, particularly for generics); consult specific product labeling.

Tablet, Oral:

Generic: 500 mg

Procainamide (pro KANE a mide)

Brand Names: Canada Apo-Procainamide; Procainamide Hydrochloride Injection, USP; Procan SR
Index Terms PCA (error-prone abbreviation); Procainamide Hydrochloride; Procaine Amide Hydrochloride; Procanbid; Pronestyl
Pharmacologic Category Antiarrhythmic Agent, Class Ia
Additional Appendix Information
Adult ACLS Algorithms *on page 1993*
Pediatric ALS (PALS) Algorithms *on page 1990*
Use
Intravenous: Treatment of life-threatening ventricular arrhythmias
Oral [Canadian product]: Treatment of supraventricular arrhythmias. **Note:** In the treatment of atrial fibrillation, use only when preferred treatment is ineffective or cannot be used. Use in paroxysmal atrial tachycardia when reflex stimulation or other measures are ineffective.
Dosing
Adult Dose must be titrated to patient's response.
Antiarrhythmic:
IM: 50 mg/kg/day divided every 3 to 6 hours **or** 0.5 to 1 g every 4 to 8 hours (Koch-Weser, 1971)
IV:
Loading dose: 15 to 18 mg/kg administered as slow infusion over 25 to 30 minutes **or** 100 mg/dose at a rate not to exceed 50 mg/minute repeated every 5 minutes as needed to a total dose of 1 g.
Hemodynamically stable monomorphic VT or pre-excited atrial fibrillation (ACLS, 2010): Loading dose: Infuse 20 to 50 mg/minute **or** 100 mg every 5 minutes until arrhythmia controlled, hypotension occurs, QRS complex widens by 50% of its original width, or total of 17 mg/kg is given. Follow with a continuous infusion of 1 to 4 mg/minute. **Note:** Not recommended for use in ongoing ventricular fibrillation (VF) or pulseless ventricular tachycardia (VT) due to prolonged administration time and uncertain efficacy.
Maintenance dose: 1 to 4 mg/minute by continuous infusion. Maintenance infusions should be reduced by one-third in patients with moderate renal or cardiac impairment and by two-thirds in patients with severe renal or cardiac impairment.
Oral [Canadian product]: Sustained release formulation (Procan SR®): Maintenance: 50 mg/kg/24 hours given in divided doses every 6 hours
Suggested Procan SR® maintenance dose:
<55 kg: 500 mg every 6 hours
55 to 91 kg: 750 mg every 6 hours
>91 kg: 1000 mg every 6 hours
Geriatric Refer to adult dosing. Initiate doses at lower end of dosage range.
Pediatric Must be titrated to patient's response:
Arrhythmias:
IM: 20 to 30 mg/kg/day divided every 4 to 6 hours; maximum: 4 g/day
IV:
Load: 3 to 6 mg/kg/dose over 5 minutes not to exceed 100 mg/dose; may repeat every 5 to 10 minutes to maximum of 15 mg/kg/load
Maintenance as continuous IV infusion: 20 to 80 mcg/kg/minute; maximum: 2 g/24 hours
Possible VT (PALS, 2010): IV; I.O.: 15 mg/kg over 30 to 60 minutes
Renal Impairment
Oral [Canadian product]:
Manufacturer's labeling: Manufacturer recommends increasing dosing interval; specific interval increase not described
Alternate dosing:
CrCl >50 mL/minute: No dosage adjustment necessary (Bauer, 2008)
CrCl 10 to 50 mL/minute: Reduce initial daily dose by 25% to 50% (Bauer, 2008)
CrCl <10 mL/minute: Reduce initial daily dose by 50% to 75% (Bauer, 2008). Monitor procainamide/NAPA concentrations closely.
IV:
Manufacturer's labeling: Manufacturer recommends dosage reduction; specific dosage reduction not described, however, close monitoring of procainamide and NAPA concentrations and clinical effectiveness recommended
Alternate dosing:
CrCl >50 mL/minute: No dosage adjustment necessary (Bauer, 2008)
CrCl 10–50 mL/minute: Reduce continuous infusion dose by 25% to 50% (Bauer, 2008)

CrCl <10 mL/minute: Reduce continuous infusion dose by 50% to 75% (Bauer, 2008). Monitor procainamide/NAPA concentrations closely.
Dialysis:
Procainamide: Moderately hemodialyzable (20% to 50%); NAPA: Not dialyzable (0% to 5%): Monitor procainamide/N-acetylprocainamide (NAPA) concentrations; supplementation may be necessary (Aronoff, 2007)
Procainamide/NAPA: Not peritoneal dialyzable (0% to 5%) (Aronoff, 2007)
Continuous renal replacement therapy (CRRT): In patients with chronic kidney disease receiving CRRT, reduce maintenance dose by 50%. In patients with anuria receiving CRRT, further dosage reduction may be required; use of an initial 1 mg/minute continuous infusion dose has been suggested. Monitor procainamide/NAPA concentrations closely (Mohamed, 2013).
Hepatic Impairment
Manufacturer's labeling: Manufacturer recommends reduction in frequency of administration; specific frequency reduction not described; however, close monitoring of procainamide and NAPA concentrations and clinical effectiveness recommended.
Alternate dosing (Bauer, 2008):
Oral [Canadian product]:
Child-Pugh score 8–10: Reduce initial daily dose by 25%. Monitor procainamide/NAPA concentrations closely.
Child-Pugh score >10: Reduce initial daily dose by 50%. Monitor procainamide/NAPA concentrations closely.
IV:
Child-Pugh score 8–10: Reduce continuous infusion dose by 25%. Monitor procainamide/NAPA concentrations closely.
Child-Pugh score >10: Reduce continuous infusion dose by 50%. Monitor procainamide/NAPA concentrations closely.
Additional Information Complete prescribing information should be consulted for additional detail.
Dosage Forms Excipient information presented when available (limited, particularly for generics); consult specific product labeling.
Solution, Injection, as hydrochloride:
Generic: 100 mg/mL (10 mL); 500 mg/mL (2 mL)
Dosage Forms: Canada Excipient information presented when available (limited, particularly for generics); consult specific product labeling.
Tablet, sustained release, oral, as hydrochloride:
Procan SR®: 250 mg, 500 mg, 750 mg

◆ Procainamide Hydrochloride *see* Procainamide *on page 1506*

◆ Procainamide Hydrochloride Injection, USP (Can) *see* Procainamide *on page 1506*

◆ Procaine Amide Hydrochloride *see* Procainamide *on page 1506*

◆ Procaine Benzylpenicillin *see* Penicillin G Procaine *on page 1422*

◆ Procaine Penicillin G *see* Penicillin G Procaine *on page 1422*

◆ Procanbid *see* Procainamide *on page 1506*

◆ Procan SR (Can) *see* Procainamide *on page 1506*

Procarbazine (proe KAR ba zeen)

Brand Names: US Matulane
Brand Names: Canada Matulane; Natulan
Index Terms Benzmethyzin; Ibenzmethyzin; N-Methylhydrazine; PCB; PCZ; Procarbazine Hydrochloride
Pharmacologic Category Antineoplastic Agent, Alkylating Agent
Use Treatment of Hodgkin lymphoma
Dosing
Adult Note: Procarbazine is associated with a high emetic potential; antiemetics are recommended to prevent nausea and vomiting (Roila, 2010). The manufacturer suggests that an estimated lean body mass be used in obese patients and patients with rapid weight gain due to edema, ascites, or abnormal fluid retention.

Hodgkin lymphoma:
MOPP regimen: While procarbazine is approved as part of the MOPP regimen, the MOPP regimen is generally no longer used due to improved toxicity profiles with other combination regimens used in the treatment of Hodgkin lymphoma.

BEACOPP, standard or escalated regimen (off-label dosing): Oral: 100 mg/m^2 days 1 to 7 every 21 days (in combination with bleomycin, etoposide, doxorubicin, cyclophosphamide, vincristine, and prednisone) for 8 cycles (Diehl, 2003)

Non-Hodgkin lymphomas (NHL; off-label use):

CEPP regimen: Oral: 60 mg/m^2 days 1 to 10 every 28 days (in combination with cyclophosphamide, etoposide and prednisone) (Chao, 1990)

PEP-C regimen: Oral: 50 mg daily at bedtime (length of induction cycle depends on phase of treatment and blood counts; frequency may vary based on tolerance in maintenance cycle; in combination with prednisone, etoposide, and cyclophosphamide) (Coleman, 2008)

CNS tumors, anaplastic oligodendroglioma/oligoastrocytoma (off-label use): *PCV regimen:* Oral: 60 mg/m^2 days 8 to 21 every 6 weeks (in combination with lomustine and vincristine) for 6 cycles (van den Bent, 2006) **or** 75 mg/m^2 days 8-21 every 6 weeks (in combination with lomustine and vincristine) for up to 4 cycles (Cairncross, 2006).

Primary CNS lymphoma (off-label use): Oral: 100 mg/m^2 for 7 days in cycles 1, 3, and 5 (in combination with methotrexate [high-dose], vincristine, methotrexate [intrathecal], leucovorin, dexamethasone, cytarabine [high-dose], and whole brain radiation) (DeAngelis, 2002).

Geriatric Refer to adult dosing; use with caution.

Pediatric Note: Procarbazine is associated with a high emetic potential; antiemetics are recommended to prevent nausea and vomiting (Dupuis, 2011). The manufacturer suggests that an estimated lean body mass be used in obese patients and patients with rapid weight gain due to edema, ascites, or abnormal fluid retention.

Hodgkin lymphoma:

MOPP regimen: While procarbazine is approved as part of the MOPP regimen, the MOPP regimen is generally no longer used due to improved toxicity profiles with other combination regimens used in the treatment of Hodgkin lymphoma.

BEACOPP regimen (off-label dosing): Oral: 100 mg/m^2 days 0 to 6 of a 21-day treatment cycle (in combination with bleomycin, etoposide, doxorubicin, cyclophosphamide, vincristine, and prednisone) for 4 cycles (Kelley, 2011).

Renal Impairment No dosage adjustment provided in manufacturer's labeling; use with caution; may result in increased toxicity. However, because predominantly inactive metabolites are excreted via the kidneys, dosage adjustment is not necessary (Kintzel, 1995).

Hepatic Impairment No dosage adjustment provided in manufacturer's labeling; use with caution; may result in increased toxicity. The following adjustments have been reported in literature:

Floyd, 2006:

Transaminases 1.6-6 times ULN: Administer 75% of dose

Transaminases >6 times ULN: Use clinical judgment

Serum bilirubin >5 mg/dL or transaminases >3 times ULN: Avoid use

King, 2001: Serum bilirubin >5 mg/dL or transaminases >180 units/L: Avoid use

Obesity *ASCO Guidelines for appropriate chemotherapy dosing in obese adults with cancer:* Utilize patient's actual body weight (full weight) for calculation of body surface area- or weight-based dosing, particularly when the intent of therapy is curative; manage regimen-related toxicities in the same manner as for nonobese patients; if a dose reduction is utilized due to toxicity, consider resumption of full weight-based dosing with subsequent cycles, especially if cause of toxicity (eg, hepatic or renal impairment) is resolved (Griggs, 2012). **Note:** The manufacturer suggests that an estimated lean body mass be used in obese patients and patients with rapid weight gain due to edema, ascites, or abnormal fluid retention.

Adjustment for Toxicity Withhold treatment (promptly) for any of the following: CNS toxicity (eg, paresthesia, confusion, neuropathy), hematologic toxicity (WBC <4000/mm^3 or platelets <100,000/mm^3), hypersensitivity, gastrointestinal toxicities (stomatitis, diarrhea), and hemorrhage or bleeding.

Additional Information Complete prescribing information should be consulted for additional detail.

Dosage Forms Excipient information presented when available (limited, particularly for generics); consult specific product labeling.

Capsule, Oral, as hydrochloride:

Matulane: 50 mg

◆ Procarbazine Hydrochloride *see* Procarbazine on page 1506

◆ Procardia *see* NIFEdipine on page 1279
◆ Procardia XL *see* NIFEdipine on page 1279
◆ PRO-Cefadroxil (Can) *see* Cefadroxil on page 328
◆ PRO-Cefuroxime (Can) *see* Cefuroxime on page 353
◆ ProCentra *see* Dextroamphetamine on page 532
◆ Procet-30 (Can) *see* Acetaminophen and Codeine on page 28
◆ Procetofene *see* Fenofibrate and Derivatives on page 746
◆ Prochieve *see* Progesterone on page 1510

Prochlorperazine (proe klor PER a zeen)

Brand Names: US Compazine; Compro

Brand Names: Canada Apo-Prochlorperazine; Nu-Prochlor; PMS-Prochlorperazine; Sandoz-Prochlorperazine

Index Terms Chlormeprazine; Compazine; Prochlorperazine Edisylate; Prochlorperazine Maleate; Prochlorperazine Mesylate

Pharmacologic Category Antiemetic; First Generation (Typical) Antipsychotic

Use Management of severe nausea and vomiting; psychotic disorders, including schizophrenia and anxiety **(Note:** Not a recommended therapy by schizophrenia treatment guidelines [Hasan 2012; Lehman 2004]); nonpsychotic anxiety

Pregnancy Considerations Jaundice or hyper- or hyporeflexia have been reported in newborn infants following maternal use of phenothiazines. Antipsychotic use during the third trimester of pregnancy has a risk for abnormal muscle movements (extrapyramidal symptoms [EPS]) and withdrawal symptoms in newborns following delivery. Symptoms in the newborn may include agitation, feeding disorder, hypertonia, hypotonia, respiratory distress, somnolence, and tremor; these effects may be self-limiting or require hospitalization. Use may interfere with pregnancy tests, causing false positive results. Prochlorperazine has been used for the treatment of nausea and vomiting associated with pregnancy (Levicheck 2002; Mahadevan 2006); however, other agents may be preferred (ACOG 2004).

Breast-Feeding Considerations Other phenothiazines are excreted in human milk; excretion of prochlorperazine is not known.

Contraindications

Hypersensitivity to prochlorperazine or any component of the formulation (cross-reactivity between phenothiazines may occur); coma or presence of large amounts of CNS depressants (eg, alcohol, opioids, barbiturates); postoperative management of nausea/vomiting following pediatric surgery; use in infants and children <2 years or <9 kg; pediatric conditions for which dosage has not been established

Documentation of allergic cross-reactivity for phenothiazines is limited. However, because of similarities in chemical structure and/or pharmacologic actions, the possibility of cross-sensitivity cannot be ruled out with certainty.

Canadian labeling: Additional contraindications (not in US labeling): Presence of circulatory collapse; severe cardiovascular disorders; altered state of consciousness; concomitant use of high dose hypnotics; severe depression; presence of blood dyscrasias, hepatic or renal impairment, or pheochromocytoma; suspected or established subcortical brain damage with or without hypothalamic damage

Warnings/Precautions [US Boxed Warning]: Elderly patients with dementia-related psychosis treated with antipsychotics are at an increased risk of death (compared to placebo). This was based on analyses of 17 placebo-controlled trials (duration ~10 weeks), predominantly in patients taking atypical antipsychotics which revealed a risk of death in drug-treated patients between 1.6 and 1.7 times the risk of death in placebo-treated patients. Over the course of a typical 10-week controlled trial, the rate of death in drug-treated patients was ~4.5% compared with ~2.6% in the placebo group. Although the causes of death varied, most deaths appeared to be either cardiovascular (eg, heart failure, sudden death) or infectious (eg, pneumonia) in nature. Observational studies suggest that, similar to atypical antipsychotic drugs, treatment with conventional antipsychotic drugs may increase mortality, although the extent to which increased mortality may be attributed to the antipsychotic drug as opposed to some characteristic(s) of the patients is not clear. Prochlorperazine is not approved for the treatment of dementia-related psychosis.

Prochlorperazine may cause extrapyramidal symptoms (EPS), including pseudoparkinsonism, acute dystonic reactions, akathisia, and tardive dyskinesia. Risk of dystonia (and possibly other EPS) may be greater with increased doses, use of conventional antipsychotics, males, and younger patients. Risk of tardive dyskinesia and potential for irreversibility often associated with total cumulative dose and therapy duration and may also be increased in elderly patients (particularly elderly women); antipsychotics may also mask signs/symptoms of tardive dyskinesia. Consider therapy discontinuation with signs/symptoms of tardive dyskinesia. Antipsychotic use has been associated with esophageal dysmotility and aspiration; use with caution in patients at risk of pneumonia (ie, Alzheimer's disease).

May be sedating and impair physical or mental abilities; use with caution in disorders where CNS depression is a feature. Use with caution in Parkinson's disease; hemodynamic instability; predisposition to seizures; subcortical brain damage; and in severe cardiac, hepatic, or renal disease. Canadian labeling contraindicates use in patients with severe cardiac disease, hepatic or renal impairment, subcortical brain damage, and circulatory collapse. May alter temperature regulation, obscure intestinal obstruction or brain tumor or mask toxicity of other drugs. May alter cardiac conduction. Hypotension may occur following administration, particularly when parenteral form is used or in high dosages. May cause orthostatic hypotension; use with caution in patients at risk of this effect or in those who would not tolerate transient hypotensive episodes (cerebrovascular disease, cardiovascular disease, hypovolemia, or concurrent medication use which may predispose to hypotension/bradycardia).

Leukopenia, neutropenia, and agranulocytosis (sometimes fatal) have been reported in clinical trials and postmarketing reports with antipsychotic use; presence of risk factors (eg, preexisting low WBC or history of drug-induced leuko-/neutropenia) should prompt periodic blood count assessment. Discontinue therapy at first signs of blood dyscrasias or if absolute neutrophil count <1000/mm^3.

Due to its potent anticholinergic effects, may be inappropriate in older adults depending on comorbidities (eg, dementia, delirium) (Beers Criteria). Use with caution in patients with decreased gastrointestinal motility, urinary retention, BPH, xerostomia, visual problems, or narrow-angle glaucoma (screening is recommended). Use caution with exposure to heat. May cause pigmentary retinopathy, and lenticular and corneal deposits, particularly with prolonged therapy. Use associated with increased prolactin levels; clinical significance of hyperprolactinemia in patients with breast cancer or other prolactin-dependent tumors is unknown. Avoid use in patients with signs/symptoms suggestive of Reye's syndrome. Children with acute illness or dehydration are more susceptible to neuromuscular reactions; use cautiously. May be associated with neuroleptic malignant syndrome (NMS). Some dosage forms may contain sodium sulfite.

Benzyl alcohol and derivatives: Some dosage forms may contain benzyl alcohol; large amounts of benzyl alcohol (≥99 mg/kg/day) have been associated with a potentially fatal toxicity ("gasping syndrome") in neonates; the "gasping syndrome" consists of metabolic acidosis, respiratory distress, gasping respirations, CNS dysfunction (including convulsions, intracranial hemorrhage), hypotension, and cardiovascular collapse (AAP ["Inactive" 1997]; CDC 1982); some data suggests that benzoate displaces bilirubin from protein binding sites (Ahlfors 2001); avoid or use dosage forms containing benzyl alcohol with caution in neonates. See manufacturer's labeling. Potentially significant drug-drug interactions may exist, requiring dose or frequency adjustment, additional monitoring, and/or selection of alternative therapy.

Adverse Reactions Reported with prochlorperazine or other phenothiazines. Frequency not defined.

Cardiovascular: Cardiac arrest, cerebral edema, hypotension, peripheral edema, Q-wave distortions, sudden death, T-wave distortions

Central nervous system: Agitation, altered cerebrospinal fluid proteins, catatonia, coma, cough reflex suppressed, dizziness, drowsiness, fever (mild [IM]), headache, hyperpyrexia, impairment of temperature regulation, insomnia, neuroleptic malignant syndrome (NMS), oculogyric crisis, opisthotonos, restlessness, seizure, somnolence, tremulousness

Dermatologic: Angioedema, contact dermatitis, epithelial keratopathy, erythema, eczema, exfoliative dermatitis, itching, photosensitivity, skin pigmentation, urticaria

Endocrine & metabolic: Amenorrhea, galactorrhea, gynecomastia, glucosuria, hyper-/hypoglycemia, lactation, libido (changes in), menstrual irregularity

Gastrointestinal: Appetite increased, atonic colon, constipation, ileus, nausea, obstipation, vomiting, weight gain, xerostomia

Genitourinary: Ejaculating dysfunction, ejaculatory disturbances, impotence, priapism, urinary retention

Hematologic: Agranulocytosis, aplastic anemia, eosinophilia, hemolytic anemia, leukopenia, pancytopenia, thrombocytopenic purpura

Hepatic: Biliary stasis, cholestatic jaundice, hepatotoxicity

Neuromuscular & skeletal: Dystonias (torticollis, carpopedal spasm, trismus, protrusion of tongue); extrapyramidal symptoms (pseudoparkinsonism, akathisia, dystonias, tardive dyskinesia, hyperreflexia); SLE-like syndrome, tremor

Ocular: Blurred vision, lenticular/corneal deposits, miosis, mydriasis, pigmentary retinopathy

Respiratory: Asthma, laryngeal edema, nasal congestion

Miscellaneous: Allergic reactions, asphyxia, diaphoresis

Drug Interactions

Metabolism/Transport Effects None known.

Avoid Concomitant Use

Avoid concomitant use of Prochlorperazine with any of the following: Aclidinium; Amisulpride; Azelastine (Nasal); Cimetropium; Dofetilide; Dronedarone; Eluxadoline; Glucagon; Glycopyrrolate; Glycopyrrolate (Oral Inhalation); Ipratropium (Oral Inhalation); Levosulpiride; Metoclopramide; Orphenadrine; Paraldehyde; Potassium Chloride; Sulpiride; Thalidomide; Tiotropium; Umeclidinium

Increased Effect/Toxicity

Prochlorperazine may increase the levels/effects of: AbobotulinumtoxinA; Alcohol (Ethyl); Amisulpride; Analgesics (Opioid); Anticholinergic Agents; Antidepressants (Serotonin Reuptake Inhibitor/Antagonist); Azelastine (Nasal); Beta-Blockers; Buprenorphine; Cimetropium; CNS Depressants; Dofetilide; Dronedarone; Eluxadoline; Glucagon; Glycopyrrolate; Glycopyrrolate (Oral Inhalation); Hydrocodone; Mequitazine; Methotrimeprazine; Methylphenidate; Metyrosine; Mirabegron; Mirtazapine; OnabotulinumtoxinA; Orphenadrine; Paraldehyde; Porfimer; Potassium Chloride; Ramosetron; RimabotulinumtoxinB; Selective Serotonin Reuptake Inhibitors; Serotonin Modulators; Sulpiride; Suvorexant; Thalidomide; Thiazide Diuretics; Thiopental; Tiotropium; Topiramate; Verteporfin; Zolpidem

The levels/effects of Prochlorperazine may be increased by: Acetylcholinesterase Inhibitors (Central); Aclidinium; Antidepressants (Serotonin Reuptake Inhibitor/Antagonist); Antimalarial Agents; Beta-Blockers; Brimonidine (Topical); Cannabis; Deferoxamine; Doxylamine; Dronabinol; Droperidol; HydrOXYzine; Ipratropium (Oral Inhalation); Kava Kava; Lithium; Magnesium Sulfate; Methotrimeprazine; Methylphenidate; Metoclopramide; Metyrosine; Mianserin; Minocycline; Nabilone; Perampanel; Pramlintide; Rufinamide; Serotonin Modulators; Sodium Oxybate; Tapentadol; Tetrabenazine; Tetrahydrocannabinol; Umeclidinium

Decreased Effect

Prochlorperazine may decrease the levels/effects of: Acetylcholinesterase Inhibitors; Amphetamines; Anti-Parkinson's Agents (Dopamine Agonist); Gastrointestinal Agents (Prokinetic); Itopride; Levosulpiride; Quinagolide; Secretin

The levels/effects of Prochlorperazine may be decreased by: Acetylcholinesterase Inhibitors; Antacids; Anti-Parkinson's Agents (Dopamine Agonist); Lithium

Storage/Stability

Injection:

Edisylate: Store at 20°C to 25°C (68°F to 77°F); do not freeze. Protect from light. Clear or slightly yellow solutions may be used.

Mesylate (Canadian availability; not available in US): Store at 15°C to 30°C (59°F to 86°F). Protect from light. Do not use if solution is discolored or hazy.

IV infusion: Injection may be diluted in 50 to 100 mL NS or D_5W.

Suppository: Store at 20°C to 25°C (68°F to 77°F). Do not remove from wrapper until ready to use.

Tablet: Store at 20°C to 25°C (68°F to 77°F). Protect from light.

Mechanism of Action Prochlorperazine is a piperazine phenothiazine antipsychotic which blocks postsynaptic mesolimbic dopaminergic D_1 and D_2 receptors in the brain, including the chemoreceptor trigger zone; exhibits a strong alpha-adrenergic and anticholinergic blocking effect and depresses the release of hypothalamic and hypophyseal hormones; believed to depress the reticular activating system, thus affecting basal metabolism, body temperature, wakefulness, vasomotor tone and emesis

Pharmacodynamics/Kinetics

Onset of action: Oral: 30 to 40 minutes; IM: 10 to 20 minutes; Rectal: ~60 minutes

Peak antiemetic effect: IV: 30 to 60 minutes

Duration: Rectal: 3 to 12 hours; IM, Oral: 3 to 4 hours

Distribution: V_d: 1400 to 1548 L (Taylor 1987)

Metabolism: Primarily hepatic; N-desmethyl prochlorperazine (major active metabolite)

Bioavailability: Oral: 12.5% (Isah 1991)

Half-life elimination: Oral: 6 to 10 hours (single dose), 14 to 22 hours (repeated dosing) (Isah 1991); IV: 6 to 10 hours (Isah 1991; Taylor 1987)

Excretion: Mainly in feces

Dosing

Adult Note: Injection solution mesylate formulation has Canadian availability (not available in US).

Antiemetic:

Oral (tablet): 5 to 10 mg 3 to 4 times/day; usual maximum: 40 mg/day; larger doses may rarely be required

IM (as edisylate): 5 to 10 mg every 3 to 4 hours; usual maximum: 40 mg/day

IM (as mesylate): 5 to 10 mg 2 to 3 times/day; usual maximum: 40 mg/day

IV (as edisylate): 2.5 to 10 mg; maximum: 10 mg/dose or 40 mg/day; may repeat dose every 3 to 4 hours as needed

Rectal:

US labeling: 25 mg twice daily

Canadian labeling: 5 to 10 mg 3 to 4 times/day

Surgical nausea/vomiting: Note: Should not exceed 40 mg/day

IM (as edisylate): 5 to 10 mg 1 to 2 hours before anesthesia induction or to control symptoms during or after surgery; may repeat once if necessary

IM (as mesylate): 5 to 10 mg 1 to 2 hours before anesthesia induction; may repeat once if needed during surgery; postoperatively: 5 to 10 mg every 3 to 4 hours as needed up to maximum of 40 mg daily

IV (as edisylate): 5 to 10 mg 15 to 30 minutes before anesthesia induction or to control symptoms during or after surgery; may repeat once if necessary

IV (as mesylate): 20 mg/L of IV solution during surgery or postoperatively; usual maximum: 30 mg daily

Rectal (off-label use; Golembiewski 2005): 25 mg

Antipsychotic:

Oral: 5 to 10 mg 3 to 4 times/day; titrate dose slowly every 2 to 3 days; doses up to 150 mg/day may be required in some patients for treatment of severe disturbances

IM (as edisylate): Initial: 10 to 20 mg; if necessary repeat initial dose every 2 to 4 hours to gain control; more than 3 to 4 doses are rarely needed. If parenteral administration is still required; give 10 to 20 mg every 4 to 6 hours; convert to oral therapy as soon as possible.

IM (as mesylate): Initial: 10 to 20 mg; if necessary repeat initial dose every 2 to 4 hours to gain control; more than 3 to 4 doses are rarely needed; convert to oral therapy as soon as possible.

Nonpsychotic anxiety: *Oral (tablet):* Usual dose: 5 mg 3 to 4 times/day; do not exceed 20 mg/day or administer >12 weeks

Geriatric Initiate at lower end of dosage range; titrate slowly and cautiously. Refer to adult dosing.

Pediatric Note: Injection solution mesylate formulation has Canadian availability (not available in US).

Use is contraindicated in children <9 kg or <2 years.

Antiemetic:

Oral (therapy >1 day usually not required):

9 to 13 kg: 2.5 mg 1 to 2 times/day as needed (maximum: 7.5 mg/day)

>13 to 18 kg: 2.5 mg 2 to 3 times/day as needed (maximum: 10 mg/day)

>18 to 39 kg: 2.5 mg 3 times/day or 5 mg 2 times/day as needed (maximum: 15 mg/day)

IM (as edisylate): 0.13 mg/kg/dose; convert to oral therapy as soon as possible

IM (as mesylate): 0.14 mg/kg/dose; convert to oral therapy at equivalent or greater dose (if necessary) as soon as possible

Antipsychotic: Children 2 to 12 years:

Oral: 2.5 mg 2 to 3 times/day; do not give more than 10 mg the first day; increase dosage as needed to maximum daily dose of 20 mg for 2 to 5 years and 25 mg for 6 to 12 years

IM (as edisylate): 0.13 mg/kg/dose; convert to oral therapy as soon as possible

IM (as mesylate): 0.14 mg/kg/dose; convert to oral therapy at equivalent or greater dose (if necessary) as soon as possible

Renal Impairment

US labeling: There are no dosage adjustments provided in the manufacturer's labeling.

Canadian labeling: Use is contraindicated.

Hepatic Impairment

US labeling: There are no dosage adjustments provided in the manufacturer's labeling; systemic exposure may be increased as drug undergoes hepatic metabolism.

Canadian labeling: Use is contraindicated.

Dietary Considerations Increase dietary intake of riboflavin; should be administered with food or water. Rectal suppositories may contain coconut and palm oil.

Administration

IM: Inject by deep IM into outer quadrant of buttocks.

IV: May be administered by slow IV push at a rate not exceeding 5 mg/minute or by IV infusion. Do not administer as a bolus injection. To reduce the risk of hypotension, patients receiving IV prochlorperazine must remain lying down and be observed for at least 30 minutes following administration. Avoid skin contact with injection solution, contact dermatitis has occurred. Do not dilute with any diluent containing parabens as a preservative.

Oral: Administer tablet without regard to meals.

Rectal: Do not remove from wrapper until ready to use.

Monitoring Parameters Mental status; vital signs (as clinically indicated); weight, height, BMI, waist circumference (baseline; at every visit for the first 6 months; quarterly with stable antipsychotic dose); CBC (as clinically indicated; monitor frequently during the first few months of therapy in patients with preexisting low WBC or history of drug-induced leukopenia/neutropenia); electrolytes and liver function (annually and as clinically indicated); fasting plasma glucose level/HbA$_{1c}$ (baseline, then yearly; in patients with diabetes risk factors or if gaining weight repeat 4 months after starting antipsychotic, then yearly); lipid panel (baseline; repeat every 2 years if LDL level is normal; repeat every 6 months if LDL level is >130 mg/dL); changes in menstruation, libido, development of galactorrhea, erectile and ejaculatory function (at each visit for the first 12 weeks after the antipsychotic is initiated or until the dose is stable, then yearly); abnormal involuntary movements or parkinsonian signs (baseline; repeat weekly until dose stabilized for at least 2 weeks after introduction and for 2 weeks after any significant dose increase); tardive dyskinesia (every 6 months; high-risk patients every 3 months); visual changes (inquire yearly); ocular examination (yearly in patients >40 years; every 2 years in younger patients) (ADA 2004; Lehman 2004; Marder 2004).

Test Interactions False-positives for phenylketonuria, pregnancy

Additional Information Not recommended as an antipsychotic due to inferior efficacy compared to other phenothiazines.

Dosage Forms Excipient information presented when available (limited, particularly for generics); consult specific product labeling.

Solution, Injection, as edisylate [strength expressed as base]:

Generic: 5 mg/mL (2 mL, 10 mL)

Suppository, Rectal:

Compazine: 25 mg (12 ea)

Compro: 25 mg (12 ea)

Generic: 25 mg (12 ea, 1000 ea)

Tablet, Oral, as maleate [strength expressed as base]:

Compazine: 5 mg, 10 mg

Generic: 5 mg, 10 mg

Dosage Forms: Canada Excipient information presented when available (limited, particularly for generics); consult specific product labeling.

Injection, solution, as mesylate [strength expressed as base]: 5 mg/mL (2 mL)

Suppository, rectal: 10 mg (10s)

Progesterone (proe JES ter one)

Brand Names: US Crinone; Endometrin; First-Progesterone VGS 100; First-Progesterone VGS 200; First-Progesterone VGS 25; First-Progesterone VGS 400; First-Progesterone VGS 50; Prometrium
Brand Names: Canada Crinone; Endometrin; Prometrium
Index Terms Pregnenedione; Prochieve; Progestin
Pharmacologic Category Progestin
Use

Oral: Prevention of endometrial hyperplasia in nonhysterectomized, postmenopausal women who are receiving conjugated estrogen tablets; secondary amenorrhea

IM: Amenorrhea; abnormal uterine bleeding due to hormonal imbalance

Intravaginal gel: Part of assisted reproductive technology (ART) for infertile women with progesterone deficiency; secondary amenorrhea

Vaginal insert: Part of ART for infertile women with progesterone deficiency

Dosing
Adult & Geriatric Females:
Amenorrhea: IM: 5 to 10 mg/day for 6 to 8 consecutive days
Amenorrhea, secondary:
Intravaginal gel: 45 mg (4% gel) every other day for 6 doses; if response is inadequate, may increase to 90 mg (8% gel) at same schedule
Oral: 400 mg every evening for 10 days
ART in patients who require progesterone supplementation:
Intravaginal gel: 90 mg (8% gel) once daily. If pregnancy occurs, may continue treatment for 10 to 12 weeks.
Intravaginal insert: 100 mg 2 to 3 times daily starting at oocyte retrieval and continuing for up to 10 weeks.
ART in patients with partial or complete ovarian failure:
Intravaginal gel: 90 mg (8% gel) twice daily. If pregnancy occurs, continue treatment for 10 to 12 weeks.
Endometrial hyperplasia prevention (in postmenopausal women with a uterus who are receiving daily conjugated estrogen tablets): Oral: 200 mg as a single daily dose every evening for 12 days sequentially per 28-day cycle
Functional uterine bleeding: IM: 5 to 10 mg/day for 6 doses
Prevention of spontaneous preterm delivery (singleton pregnancy and prior preterm birth or short cervix) (off-label use): Intravaginal gel: 90 mg (8% gel) once daily (Hassan, 2011; O'Brien, 2009). Treatment initiation is recommended before or at gestational week 24 (ACOG, 2012).

Renal Impairment
Injection, oral: There are no dosage adjustments provided in the manufacturer's labeling (has not been studied). Use with caution.
Intravaginal gel, insert: There are no dosage adjustments provided in the manufacturer's labeling.

Hepatic Impairment Use is contraindicated in liver dysfunction or disease.
Additional Information Complete prescribing information should be consulted for additional detail.
Dosage Forms Considerations Progesterone cream 10% and vaginal suppositories are compounding kits. Refer to manufacturer's labeling for compounding instructions.
Dosage Forms Excipient information presented when available (limited, particularly for generics); consult specific product labeling.
Capsule, Oral:
 Prometrium: 100 mg, 200 mg [contains peanut oil]
 Generic: 100 mg, 200 mg
Cream, Transdermal:
 Generic: 10% (60 g)
Gel, Vaginal:
 Crinone: 4% (1.125 g); 8% (1.125 g)
Insert, Vaginal:
 Endometrin: 100 mg (21 ea)
Oil, Intramuscular:
 Generic: 50 mg/mL (10 mL)
Suppository, Vaginal:
 First-Progesterone VGS 25: 25 mg (30 ea)
 First-Progesterone VGS 50: 50 mg (30 ea)
 First-Progesterone VGS 100: 100 mg (30 ea)
 First-Progesterone VGS 200: 200 mg (30 ea)
 First-Progesterone VGS 400: 400 mg (30 ea)

Promethazine (proe METH a zeen)

Brand Names: US Phenadoz; Phenergan; Promethegan
Brand Names: Canada Bioniche Promethazine; Histantil; Phenergan; PMS-Promethazine
Index Terms Promethazine Hydrochloride
Pharmacologic Category Antiemetic; Histamine H_1 Antagonist; Histamine H_1 Antagonist, First Generation; Phenothiazine Derivative
Use

Allergic conditions: Perennial and seasonal allergic rhinitis; vasomotor rhinitis; allergic conjunctivitis due to inhalant allergens and foods; mild, uncomplicated allergic skin manifestations of urticaria and angioedema; amelioration of allergic reactions to blood or plasma; dermographism; anaphylactic reactions, as adjunctive therapy to epinephrine and other standard measures, after the acute manifestations have been controlled

Antiemetic: Prevention and control of nausea and vomiting associated with certain types of anesthesia and surgery; antiemetic therapy in postoperative patients

Motion sickness: Active and prophylactic treatment of motion sickness

Postoperative adjunct: Adjunctive therapy with analgesics and/or anesthesia

Sedation: Preoperative, postoperative, and obstetric sedation; for sedation, relief of apprehension, and production of light sleep from which the patient can be easily aroused

Pregnancy Considerations Adverse effects have not been observed in animal reproduction studies. Promethazine crosses the placenta. Maternal promethazine use has generally not resulted in an increased risk of birth defects. Platelet aggregation may be inhibited in newborns following maternal use of promethazine within 2 weeks of delivery. Promethazine is used for the treatment of nausea and vomiting of pregnancy (refer to current guidelines). Promethazine is also indicated for use during labor for obstetric sedation and may be used alone or as an adjunct to opioid analgesics.

Breast-Feeding Considerations It is not known if promethazine is excreted in breast milk. According to the manufacturer, the decision to continue or discontinue breast-feeding during therapy should take into account the risk of exposure to the infant and the benefits of treatment to the mother. Antihistamines may decrease maternal serum prolactin concentrations when administered prior to the establishment of nursing.

Contraindications Hypersensitivity or idiosyncratic reaction to promethazine, other phenothiazines, or any component of the formulation; coma; treatment of lower respiratory tract symptoms, including asthma; children <2 years of age; intra-arterial or subcutaneous administration

Warnings/Precautions [US Boxed Warning]: Respiratory depression, including fatalities, have been reported in children <2 years of age. Contraindicated in children <2 years of age. In children ≥2 years, use the lowest possible dose; other drugs with respiratory depressant effects should be avoided. Antiemetics are not recommended for the treatment of uncomplicated vomiting in pediatric patients; limit use to prolonged vomiting of known etiology. Avoid use in children who may have Reye syndrome or hepatic disease as adverse reactions caused by promethazine may be confused with signs of primary disease.

[US Boxed Warning]: Promethazine injection can cause severe tissue injury (including gangrene) regardless of the route of administration. Tissue irritation and damage may result from perivascular extravasation, unintentional intra-arterial administration, and intraneuronal or perineuronal infiltration. In addition to gangrene, adverse events reported include tissue necrosis, abscesses, burning, pain, erythema, edema, paralysis, severe spasm of distal vessels, phlebitis, thrombophlebitis, venous thrombosis, sensory loss, and palsies. Surgical intervention including fasciotomy, skin graft, and/or amputation have been necessary in some cases. The preferred route of administration is by deep intramuscular (IM) injection. Subcutaneous administration is contraindicated. Discontinue intravenous injection immediately with onset of pain and evaluate for arterial injection or perivascular extravasation. Although there is no proven successful management of unintentional intra-arterial injection or perivascular extravasation, sympathetic block and heparinization have been used in the acute management of unintentional intra-arterial injection based on results from animal studies. Vesicant; for IV administration (**not** the preferred route of administration), ensure proper needle or catheter placement prior to and during administration; avoid extravasation.

Avoid use in patients with compromised respiratory function or in patients at risk for respiratory failure (eg, COPD, sleep apnea); may lead to potentially fatal respiratory depression. Impaired core body temperature regulation may occur; caution with strenuous exercise, heat exposure, dehydration, and concomitant medication possessing anticholinergic effects. May cause CNS depression, which may impair physical or mental abilities; patients must be cautioned about performing tasks that require mental alertness (eg, operating machinery or driving). Use with caution in bone marrow suppression. Use with caution in patients with hepatic impairment; cholestatic jaundice has been reported with use. Use with caution in patients at risk of seizures, including those with a history of seizures, head trauma, brain damage, alcoholism, or concurrent therapy with medications which may lower seizure threshold. May alter cardiac conduction (life-threatening arrhythmias have occurred with therapeutic doses of phenothiazines). May cause orthostatic hypotension; use with caution in patients at risk of this effect or in those who would not tolerate transient hypotensive episodes (cerebrovascular disease, cardiovascular disease, hypovolemia, or concurrent medication use which may predispose to hypotension/bradycardia). May cause photosensitivity; avoid prolonged sun exposure. Potentially significant interactions may exist, requiring dose or frequency adjustment, additional monitoring, and/or selection of alternative therapy.

May cause anticholinergic effects (constipation, xerostomia, blurred vision, urinary retention); use with caution in patients with decreased gastrointestinal motility, pyloroduodenal obstruction, urinary retention, bladder neck obstruction, BPH, xerostomia, or visual problems. Use with caution in cardiovascular disease, narrow angle glaucoma, Parkinson disease, myasthenia gravis. May cause extrapyramidal symptoms, including pseudoparkinsonism, acute dystonic reactions, akathisia, and tardive dyskinesia. May be associated with neuroleptic malignant syndrome (NMS). In the elderly, avoid use of this potent anticholinergic agent due to increased risk of confusion, dry mouth, constipation, and other anticholinergic effects; clearance decreases in patients of advanced age (Beers Criteria). Injection may contain sodium metabisulfite.

Some dosage forms may contain sodium benzoate/benzoic acid; benzoic acid (benzoate) is a metabolite of benzyl alcohol; large amounts of benzyl alcohol (≥99 mg/kg/day) have been associated with a potentially fatal toxicity ("gasping syndrome") in neonates; the "gasping syndrome" consists of metabolic acidosis, respiratory distress, gasping respirations, CNS dysfunction (including convulsions, intracranial hemorrhage), hypotension and cardiovascular collapse (AAP 1997; CDC 1982); some data suggests that benzoate displaces bilirubin from protein binding sites (Ahlfors 2001); avoid or use dosage forms containing benzyl alcohol derivative with caution in neonates. See manufacturer's labeling.

Adverse Reactions Frequency not defined.

Cardiovascular: Bradycardia, hyper-/hypotension, nonspecific QT changes, orthostatic hypotension, tachycardia,

Central nervous system: Agitation akathisia, catatonic states, confusion, delirium, disorientation, dizziness, drowsiness, dystonias, euphoria, excitation, extrapyramidal symptoms, faintness, fatigue, hallucinations, hysteria, insomnia, lassitude, pseudoparkinsonism, tardive dyskinesia, nervousness, neuroleptic malignant syndrome, nightmares, sedation, seizure, somnolence

Dermatologic: Angioneurotic edema, dermatitis, photosensitivity, skin pigmentation (slate gray), urticaria

Endocrine & metabolic: Amenorrhea, breast engorgement, gynecomastia, hyperglycemia, lactation

Gastrointestinal: Constipation, nausea, vomiting, xerostomia

Genitourinary: Ejaculatory disorder, impotence, urinary retention

Hematologic: Agranulocytosis, leukopenia, thrombocytopenia, thrombocytopenic purpura

Hepatic: Jaundice

Local: Abscess, distal vessel spasm, gangrene, injection site reactions (burning, edema, erythema, pain), palsies, paralysis, phlebitis, sensory loss, thrombophlebitis, tissue necrosis, venous thrombosis

Neuromuscular & skeletal: Incoordination, tremor

Ocular: Blurred vision, corneal and lenticular changes, diplopia, epithelial keratopathy, pigmentary retinopathy

Otic: Tinnitus

Respiratory: Apnea, asthma, nasal congestion, respiratory depression

Drug Interactions

Metabolism/Transport Effects Substrate of CYP2B6 (major), CYP2D6 (major); **Note:** Assignment of Major/Minor substrate status based on clinically relevant drug interaction potential; **Inhibits** CYP2D6 (weak)

Avoid Concomitant Use

Avoid concomitant use of Promethazine with any of the following: Aclidinium; Azelastine (Nasal); Cimetropium; Dapoxetine; Eluxadoline; Glucagon; Glycopyrrolate; Glycopyrrolate (Oral Inhalation); Ipratropium (Oral Inhalation); Levosulpiride; Metoclopramide; Orphenadrine; Paraldehyde; Potassium Chloride; Thalidomide; Tiotropium; Umeclidinium

Increased Effect/Toxicity

Promethazine may increase the levels/effects of: AbobotulinumtoxinA; Alcohol (Ethyl); Analgesics (Opioid); Anticholinergic Agents; Antipsychotic Agents; ARIPiprazole; Azelastine (Nasal); Buprenorphine; Cimetropium; CNS Depressants; Eluxadoline; Glucagon; Glycopyrrolate; Glycopyrrolate (Oral Inhalation); Highest Risk QTc-Prolonging Agents; Hydrocodone; Methotrimeprazine; Mirabegron; Moderate Risk QTc-Prolonging Agents; OnabotulinumtoxinA; Orphenadrine; Paraldehyde; Potassium Chloride; Pramipexole; Ramosetron; RimabotulinumtoxinB; ROPINIRole; Rotigotine; Serotonin Modulators; Suvorexant; Thalidomide; Thiazide Diuretics; Tiotropium; Topiramate; Zolpidem

The levels/effects of Promethazine may be increased by: Abiraterone Acetate; Aclidinium; Antiemetics (5HT3 Antagonists); Antipsychotic Agents; Brimonidine (Topical); Cannabis; Cobicistat; CYP2B6 Inhibitors (Moderate); CYP2D6 Inhibitors (Moderate); CYP2D6 Inhibitors (Strong); Dapoxetine; Darunavir; Doxylamine; Dronabinol; Droperidol; HydrOXYzine; Ipratropium (Oral Inhalation); Kava Kava; Magnesium Sulfate; Metaxalone; Methotrimeprazine; Metoclopramide; Metyrosine; Mianserin; Mifepristone; Minocycline; Nabilone; Panobinostat; Peginterferon Alfa-2b; Perampanel; Pramlintide; Quazepam; Rufinamide; Sodium Oxybate; Tapentadol; Tedizolid; Tetrahydrocannabinol; Umeclidinium

Decreased Effect

Promethazine may decrease the levels/effects of: Acetylcholinesterase Inhibitors; EPINEPHrine (Nasal); EPINEPHrine (Oral Inhalation); Epinephrine (Racemic); EPINEPHrine (Systemic); Gastrointestinal Agents (Prokinetic); Itopride; Levosulpiride; Secretin

The levels/effects of Promethazine may be decreased by: Acetylcholinesterase Inhibitors; CYP2B6 Inducers (Strong); Dabrafenib; Lumacaftor; Peginterferon Alfa-2b

Preparation for Administration Parenteral: IV: Although IV administration should be avoided, promethazine has been administered IV in select patients. Solution for injection may be administered at a maximum concentration of 25 mg/mL; however, to minimize phlebitis further dilution is recommended. Some have suggested further diluting the 25 mg/mL with 10 to 20 mL NS (ISMP 2006).

Storage/Stability

Injection, oral solution, tablets: Store between 20°C and 25°C (68°F and 77°F). Protect from light.

Suppositories: Store refrigerated between 2°C and 8°C (36°F and 46°F).

Mechanism of Action Phenothiazine derivative; blocks postsynaptic mesolimbic dopaminergic receptors in the brain; exhibits a strong alpha-adrenergic blocking effect and depresses the release of hypothalamic and hypophyseal hormones; competes with histamine for the H_1-receptor; muscarinic-blocking effect may be responsible for antiemetic activity; reduces stimuli to the brainstem reticular system

Pharmacodynamics/Kinetics

Onset of action: Oral, IM: ~20 minutes; IV: ~5 minutes

Duration: Usually 4 to 6 hours (up to 12 hours)

Absorption: Oral: Rapid and complete; large first pass effect limits systemic bioavailability (Sharma, 2003)

Distribution: V_d: Syrup: 98 L/kg (range: 17 to 277 L/kg) (Strenkoski-Nox, 2000)

Metabolism: Hepatic; hydroxylation via CYP2D6 and N-demethylation via CYP2B6; significant first-pass effect (Sharma, 2003)

Bioavailability: Oral: ~25% (Sharma, 2003)

Half-life elimination: IM: ~10 hours; IV: 9 to 16 hours; Suppositories: 16 to 19 hours (range: 4 to 34 hours) (Strenkoski-Nox, 2000)

Time to maximum serum concentration: Suppositories: 6.7 to 8.6 hours; Syrup: 4.4 hours (Strenkoski-Nox, 2000)

Excretion: Urine

Dosing

Adult & Geriatric

Allergic conditions:

Oral, rectal: 25 mg at bedtime **or** 12.5 mg before meals and at bedtime (usual range: 6.25 to 12.5 mg 3 times daily)

IM, IV: 25 mg, may repeat in 2 hours when necessary; switch to oral route as soon as feasible

Antiemetic: Oral, IM, IV, rectal: 12.5 to 25 mg every 4 to 6 hours as needed

Motion sickness: Oral, rectal: Initial: 25 mg 30 to 60 minutes before departure; repeat 8 to 12 hours later as needed; maintenance: 25 mg twice daily.

Obstetrics (labor) analgesia adjunct: IM, IV: Early labor: 50 mg; Established labor: 25 to 75 mg in combination with analgesic at reduced dosage; may repeat every 4 hours for up to 2 additional doses (maximum: 100 mg/day while in labor)

Pre-/postoperative analgesia/hypnotic adjunct: IM, IV: 25 to 50 mg in combination with analgesic or hypnotic (at reduced dosage)

Sedation: Oral, IM, IV, rectal: 25 to 50 mg/dose

Pediatric

Allergic conditions: Children ≥2 years: Oral, rectal: 0.1 mg/kg/dose (maximum: 12.5 mg) every 6 hours during the day and 0.5 mg/kg/dose (maximum: 25 mg) at bedtime as needed

Antiemetic: Children ≥2 years: Oral, IM, IV, rectal: 0.25 to 1 mg/kg 4 to 6 times/day as needed (maximum: 25 mg/dose)

Motion sickness: Children ≥2 years: Oral, rectal: 0.5 mg/kg/dose 30 minutes to 1 hour before departure, then every 12 hours as needed (maximum dose: 25 mg twice daily)

Preoperative analgesia/hypnotic adjunct: Children ≥2 years: IM, IV: 1.1 mg/kg in combination with an analgesic or hypnotic (at reduced dosage) and with an atropine-like agent (at appropriate dosage). **Note:** Promethazine dosage should not exceed half of suggested adult dosage.

Sedation: Children ≥2 years: Oral, IM, IV, rectal: 12.5 to 25 mg at bedtime or preoperatively (maximum: 25 mg/dose)

Renal Impairment There are no dosage adjustments provided in the manufacturer's labeling.

Hepatic Impairment

Adults: There are no dosage adjustments provided in the manufacturer's labeling; use with caution (cholestatic jaundice has been reported with use).

Children ≥2 years and Adolescents: The manufacturer recommends avoiding use in pediatric patients with signs and symptoms of hepatic disease (extrapyramidal symptoms caused by promethazine may be confused with CNS signs of hepatic disease).

Dietary Considerations Increase dietary intake of riboflavin.

Administration

Oral: Administer with food, water, or milk to decrease GI distress. Measure and administer prescribed dose of oral solution using dosing syringe, dosing spoon, or dosing cup.

Parenteral: Not for SubQ administration; promethazine is a chemical irritant which may produce necrosis.

IM: Preferred route of administration; administer as a deep IM injection

IV: IV use should be avoided when possible since severe tissue damage has occurred with IV administration; in selected patients, promethazine has been diluted and infused at a maximum rate of 25 mg/minute. To minimize phlebitis, consider administering over 10 to 15 minutes, limiting initial dose to 1/4 or 1/2 the usual dose (eg, in adults 6.25 to 12.5 mg), further diluting the 25 mg/mL strength in 10 to 20 mL NS, and administering through a large bore vein (not hand or wrist) or via a running IV line at port farthest from patient's vein (ISMP 2006).

Vesicant; ensure proper needle or catheter placement prior to and during infusion; avoid extravasation. Discontinue immediately if burning or pain occurs with administration; evaluate for inadvertent arterial injection or extravasation.

Extravasation management: If extravasation occurs, stop infusion immediately and disconnect (leave cannula/needle in place); gently aspirate extravasated solution (do **NOT** flush the line); remove needle/cannula; elevate extremity. Apply dry cold compresses (Hurst 2004).

Monitoring Parameters Relief of symptoms, mental status; signs and symptoms of tissue injury (burning or pain at injection site, phlebitis, edema) with IV administration

Test Interactions Pregnancy tests (hCG-based) may result in false-negatives or false-positives; increased serum glucose may be seen with glucose tolerance tests; may result in false-positives with urine detection of amphetamine/methamphetamine (Melanson 2006); may alter the flare response in intradermal allergen tests (Melanson 2006)

Dosage Forms Excipient information presented when available (limited, particularly for generics); consult specific product labeling. [DSC] = Discontinued product

Solution, Injection, as hydrochloride:

Phenergan: 50 mg/mL (1 mL [DSC])

Phenergan: 50 mg/mL (1 mL) [contains edetate disodium, phenol, sodium metabisulfite]

Phenergan: 25 mg/mL (1 mL) [pyrogen free; contains edetate disodium, phenol, sodium metabisulfite]

Generic: 25 mg/mL (1 mL); 50 mg/mL (1 mL)

Solution, Oral, as hydrochloride:

Generic: 6.25 mg/5 mL (118 mL, 473 mL)

Suppository, Rectal, as hydrochloride:

Phenadoz: 12.5 mg (12 ea); 25 mg (12 ea)

Phenergan: 12.5 mg (12 ea); 25 mg (12 ea); 50 mg (12 ea)

Promethegan: 12.5 mg (12 ea); 25 mg (12 ea, 1000 ea); 50 mg (12 ea)

Generic: 12.5 mg (1 ea, 12 ea); 25 mg (1 ea, 12 ea); 50 mg (12 ea)

Syrup, Oral, as hydrochloride:
Generic: 6.25 mg/5 mL (118 mL, 473 mL)
Tablet, Oral, as hydrochloride:
Generic: 12.5 mg, 25 mg, 50 mg

Promethazine and Codeine
(proe METH a zeen & KOE deen)

Index Terms Codeine and Promethazine
Pharmacologic Category Analgesic, Opioid; Antitussive; Histamine H₁ Antagonist; Histamine H₁ Antagonist, First Generation; Phenothiazine Derivative
Use Cough and upper respiratory symptoms: Temporary relief of coughs and upper respiratory symptoms associated with allergy or the common cold
Dosing
Adult Upper respiratory symptoms: Oral: 5 mL (promethazine 6.25 mg/codeine 10 mg) every 4 to 6 hours (maximum: 30 mL [promethazine 37.5 mg/codeine 60 mg] per 24 hours)
Geriatric Refer to adult dosing. Use with caution; consider using decreased dose.
Pediatric Cough and upper respiratory symptoms: Oral:
Children 6 to <12 years: 2.5 to 5 mL (promethazine 3.125 to 6.25 mg/codeine 5 to 10 mg) every 4 to 6 hours (maximum: 30 mL [promethazine 37.5 mg/codeine 60 mg] per 24 hours)
Children ≥12 years and Adolescents: Refer to adult dosing.
Renal Impairment There are no specific dosage adjustments provided in the manufacturer's labeling. Use with caution; reduce initial dose in significant renal impairment.
Hepatic Impairment
Adults: There are no dosage adjustments provided in the manufacturer's labeling. Cholestatic jaundice has been reported with promethazine use and codeine clearance may be reduced. Use with caution; reduce initial dose in significant hepatic impairment.
Children ≥6 years and Adolescents: Avoid use in pediatric patients with signs and symptoms of hepatic disease (extrapyramidal symptoms caused by promethazine may be confused with CNS signs of hepatic disease).
Additional Information Complete prescribing information should be consulted for additional detail.
Dosage Forms Excipient information presented when available (limited, particularly for generics); consult specific product labeling.
Syrup, oral: Promethazine hydrochloride 6.25 mg and codeine phosphate 10 mg per 5 mL (5 mL, 118 mL, 473 mL)
Controlled Substance C-V

Promethazine and Dextromethorphan
(proe METH a zeen & deks troe meth OR fan)

Index Terms Dextromethorphan and Promethazine
Pharmacologic Category Antitussive; Histamine H₁ Antagonist; Histamine H₁ Antagonist, First Generation; Phenothiazine Derivative
Use Temporary relief of coughs and upper respiratory symptoms associated with allergy or the common cold
Dosing
Adult & Geriatric Cough and upper respiratory symptoms: Oral: 5 mL every 4 to 6 hours; maximum: 30 mL in 24 hours
Pediatric Cough and upper respiratory symptoms: Oral: Children:
2 to <6 years: 1.25 to 2.5 mL every 4 to 6 hours; maximum: 10 mL in 24 hours
6 to <12 years: 2.5 to 5 mL every 4 to 6 hours; maximum: 20 mL in 24 hours
≥12 years and Adolescents: Refer to adult dosing
Renal Impairment There are no dosage adjustments provided in the manufacturer's labeling.
Hepatic Impairment
Adults: There are no dosage adjustments provided in the manufacturer's labeling; use with caution (cholestatic jaundice has been reported with use).
Children ≥2 years and Adolescents: The manufacturer recommends to avoid use in pediatric patients with signs and symptoms of hepatic disease (extrapyramidal symptoms caused by promethazine may be confused with CNS signs of hepatic disease).
Additional Information Complete prescribing information should be consulted for additional detail.

Dosage Forms Excipient information presented when available (limited, particularly for generics); consult specific product labeling.
Syrup: Promethazine hydrochloride 6.25 mg and dextromethorphan hydrobromide 15 mg per 5 mL (120 mL, 480 mL)

Propafenone (pro PAF en one)

Brand Names: US Rythmol; Rythmol SR
Brand Names: Canada Apo-Propafenone; Mylan-Propafenone; PMS-Propafenone; Rythmol
Index Terms Propafenone Hydrochloride
Pharmacologic Category Antiarrhythmic Agent, Class Ic
Use Treatment of life-threatening ventricular arrhythmias; to prolong the time to recurrence of paroxysmal atrial fibrillation/flutter (PAF) or paroxysmal supraventricular tachycardia (PSVT) in patients with disabling symptoms without structural heart disease
Extended release capsule: Prolong the time to recurrence of symptomatic atrial fibrillation in patients without structural heart disease
Pregnancy Considerations Adverse events were observed in some animal reproduction studies. Propafenone and its metabolite cross the placenta and can be detected in the newborn (Libardoni 1991). Guidelines are available for use during pregnancy. Until more information is available, generally reserved for use when other agents are not effective (Regitz-Zagrosek 2011).
Breast-Feeding Considerations Propafenone is excreted in breast milk. Due to the potential for serious adverse reactions in the nursing infant, the manufacturer recommends a decision be made whether to discontinue nursing or to discontinue the drug, taking into account the importance of treatment to the mother.
Contraindications
Hypersensitivity to propafenone or any component of the formulation; sinoatrial, AV, and intraventricular disorders of impulse generation and/or conduction (except in patients with a functioning artificial pacemaker); Brugada syndrome, sinus bradycardia; cardiogenic shock; uncompensated cardiac failure; marked hypotension; bronchospastic disorders or severe obstructive pulmonary disease; uncorrected electrolyte abnormalities
Canadian labeling: Additional contraindications (not in US labeling): MI within past 3 months; severe hepatic impairment; myasthenia gravis; concurrent use with ritonavir
Warnings/Precautions [US Boxed Warning]: In the Cardiac Arrhythmia Suppression Trial (CAST), recent (>6 days but <2 years ago) myocardial infarction patients with asymptomatic, non-life-threatening ventricular arrhythmias did not benefit and may have been harmed by attempts to suppress the arrhythmia with flecainide or encainide. An increased mortality or nonfatal cardiac arrest rate (7.7%) was seen in the active treatment group compared with patients in the placebo group (3%). The applicability of the CAST results to other populations is unknown. Antiarrhythmic agents should be reserved for patients with life-threatening ventricular arrhythmias.

Can cause life-threatening drug-induced arrhythmias, including ventricular fibrillation, ventricular tachycardia, asystole, and torsade de pointes (Hii, 1991). The manufacturer notes that propafenone may increase the QT interval; however, due to QRS prolongation; changes in the QT interval are difficult to interpret. In an evaluation of propafenone (450 mg/day) in healthy individuals compared to other selected antiarrhythmic agents, propafenone did not affect repolarization time (eg, QT, QTc, JT, JTc) only depolarization time (ie, QRS interval) (Sarubbi, 1998). Monitor for proarrhythmic effects, and when necessary, adjust dose to prevent QTc prolongation. Initiation of propafenone may unmask Brugada syndrome; obtain ECG after treatment initiation and discontinue if ECG indicative of Brugada syndrome.

In the treatment of atrial fibrillation in the elderly, avoid antiarrhythmics as first-line treatment. In older adults, data suggests rate control may provide more benefits than risks compared to rhythm control for most patients (Beers Criteria).

Slows atrioventricular conduction, potentially leading to first degree AV block; degree of PR interval prolongation and increased QRS duration are dose and concentration related. Avoid in patients with conduction disturbances (unless functioning pacemaker present).

May alter pacing and sensing thresholds of artificial pacemakers. Propafenone use may be considered in patients with obstructive lung disease who do not have bronchospasm (AHA/ACC/HRS [January, 2014]). Use in patients with bronchospastic disease or severe obstructive lung disease is contraindicated.

Avoid use in patients with heart failure; similar agents have been shown to increase mortality in this population; may precipitate or exacerbate condition. Use is contraindicated in patients with uncorrected electrolyte abnormalities. Correct electrolyte disturbances, especially hypokalemia or hypomagnesemia, prior to use and throughout therapy. Hepatic abnormalities (including fulminant hepatitis and fatalities) have been reported. Administer cautiously in significant hepatic or renal dysfunction. The Canadian labeling contraindicates use in severe hepatic impairment. Use with caution in patients with myasthenia gravis; may exacerbate condition; the Canadian labeling contraindicates use in patients with myasthenia gravis. May cause dizziness, fatigue, blurred vision; caution patients about performing dangerous tasks (eg, driving, operating machinery). Agranulocytosis has been reported; generally occurring within the first 2 months of therapy. Upon therapy discontinuation, WBC usually normalized by 14 days. Positive ANA titers have been reported. Titers have decreased with and without propafenone discontinuation. Positive titers have not usually been associated with clinical symptoms, although at least one case of drug induced lupus erythematosus has been reported. Consider therapy discontinuation in symptomatic patients with positive ANA titers. Potentially significant drug-drug interactions may exist, requiring dose or frequency adjustment, additional monitoring, and/or selection of alternative therapy.

Adverse Reactions

1% to 10%:

Cardiovascular: New or worsened arrhythmia (proarrhythmic effect) (2% to 10%), angina (2% to 5%), CHF (1% to 4%), ventricular tachycardia (1% to 3%), palpitation (1% to 3%), AV block (first-degree) (1% to 3%), syncope (1% to 2%), increased QRS interval (1% to 2%), chest pain (1% to 2%), PVCs (1% to 2%), bradycardia (1% to 2%), edema (0% to 1%), bundle branch block (0% to 1%), atrial fibrillation (1%), hypotension (0% to 1%), intraventricular conduction delay (0% to 1%)

Central nervous system: Dizziness (4% to 15%), fatigue (2% to 6%), headache (2% to 5%), ataxia (0% to 2%), insomnia (0% to 2%), anxiety (1% to 2%), drowsiness (1%)

Dermatologic: Rash (1% to 3%)

Gastrointestinal: Nausea/vomiting (2% to 11%), unusual taste (3% to 23%), constipation (2% to 7%), dyspepsia (1% to 3%), diarrhea (1% to 3%), xerostomia (1% to 2%), anorexia (1% to 2%), abdominal pain (1% to 2%), flatulence (0% to 1%)

Neuromuscular & skeletal: Tremor (0% to 1%), arthralgia (0% to 1%), weakness (1% to 2%)

Ocular: Blurred vision (1% to 6%)

Respiratory: Dyspnea (1% to 5%)

Miscellaneous: Diaphoresis (1%)

<1% (Limited to important or life-threatening): Agranulocytosis, alopecia, amnesia, anemia, apnea, AV block (second or third degree), asystole, AV dissociation, cardiac arrest, cholestasis (0.1%), coma, confusion, CHF, depression, granulocytopenia, hepatitis (0.03%), hyperglycemia, impotence, increased bleeding time, leukopenia, lupus erythematosus, mania, memory loss, nephrotic syndrome, paresthesia, peripheral neuropathy, pruritus, psychosis, purpura, renal failure, seizure (0.3%), SIADH, sinus node dysfunction, thrombocytopenia, tinnitus, torsade de pointes, ventricular fibrillation, vertigo

Drug Interactions

Metabolism/Transport Effects Substrate of CYP1A2 (minor), CYP2D6 (minor), CYP3A4 (minor); **Note:** Assignment of Major/Minor substrate status based on clinically relevant drug interaction potential; **Inhibits** CYP1A2 (weak), CYP2D6 (weak)

Avoid Concomitant Use

Avoid concomitant use of Propafenone with any of the following: Amiodarone; Antiarrhythmic Agents (Class Ia); Antiarrhythmic Agents (Class III); Ceritinib; FLUoxetine; Fosamprenavir; Highest Risk QTc-Prolonging Agents; Ivabradine; Mifepristone; QuiNIDine; Ritonavir; Saquinavir; Tipranavir

Increased Effect/Toxicity

Propafenone may increase the levels/effects of: Antiarrhythmic Agents (Class Ia); Antiarrhythmic Agents (Class III); ARIPiprazole; Beta-Blockers; Bradycardia-Causing Agents; Cardiac Glycosides; Ceritinib; CYP2D6 Inhibitors (Moderate); FLUoxetine; Highest Risk QTc-Prolonging Agents; Lacosamide; Moderate Risk QTc-Prolonging Agents; Propranolol; Theophylline Derivatives; TiZANidine; Venlafaxine; Vitamin K Antagonists

The levels/effects of Propafenone may be increased by: Amiodarone; Antihepaciviral Combination Products; Boceprevir; Bretylium; Cimetidine; CYP2D6 Inhibitors (Strong); CYP3A4 Inhibitors (Moderate); CYP3A4 Inhibitors (Strong); FLUoxetine; FluvoxaMINE; Fosamprenavir; Ivabradine; Mifepristone; Mirabegron; PARoxetine; QTc-Prolonging Agents (Indeterminate Risk and Risk Modifying); QuiNIDine; Ritonavir; Ruxolitinib; Saquinavir; Sertraline; Telaprevir; Tipranavir; Tofacitinib

Decreased Effect

The levels/effects of Propafenone may be decreased by: CYP3A4 Inducers (Strong); Etravirine; Orlistat; St Johns Wort

Food Interactions

Administration of food with single-dose propafenone increased propafenone serum concentrations and bioavailability; however, with multidose administration, propafenone bioavailability was not significantly different between fed and fasted states. Management: Administer without regard to meals.

Propafenone serum concentrations may be increased with concomitant use of grapefruit juice. Management: Avoid concomitant use of grapefruit juice.

Storage/Stability Store at 25°C (77°F); excursions permitted to 15°C to 30°C (59°F to 86°F).

Mechanism of Action Propafenone is a class 1c antiarrhythmic agent which possesses local anesthetic properties, blocks the fast inward sodium current, and slows the rate of increase of the action potential. Prolongs conduction and refractoriness in all areas of the myocardium, with a slightly more pronounced effect on intraventricular conduction; it prolongs effective refractory period, reduces spontaneous automaticity and exhibits some beta-blockade activity.

Pharmacodynamics/Kinetics

Absorption: Well absorbed

Distribution: V_d: Adults: 252 L

Protein binding: 95% to alpha$_1$-acid glycoprotein

Metabolism: Hepatic via CYP2D6, CYP3A4 and CYP1A2 to two active metabolites (5-hydroxypropafenone and N-depropylpropafenone) then ultimately to glucuronide or sulfate conjugates. Two genetically determined metabolism groups exist (extensive and poor metabolizers); 10% of Caucasians are poor metabolizers. Exhibits nonlinear pharmacokinetics; when dose is increased from 300-900 mg/day, serum concentrations increase tenfold; this nonlinearity is thought to be due to saturable first-pass effect.

Bioavailability: Immediate release (IR): 150 mg: 3.4%; 300 mg: 10.6%; relative bioavailability of extended release (ER) capsule is less than IR tablet; the bioavailability of an ER capsule regimen of 325 mg twice-daily regimen approximates an IR tablet regimen of 150 mg 3 times/day.

Half-life elimination: Extensive metabolizers: 2-10 hours; Poor metabolizers: 10-32 hours

Time to peak, serum: IR: 3.5 hours; ER: 3-8 hours

Excretion: Urine (<1% unchanged; remainder as glucuronide or sulfate conjugates); feces

Dosing

Adult & Geriatric Note: Patients who exhibit significant widening of QRS complex or second- or third-degree AV block may need dose reduction.

Atrial fibrillation (to prevent recurrence): Oral:

Extended release capsule: Initial: 225 mg every 12 hours; dosage increase may be made at a minimum of 5-day intervals; may increase to 325 mg every 12 hours; if further increase is necessary, may increase to 425 mg every 12 hours

Immediate release tablet: Initial: 150 mg every 8 hours; dosage increase may be made at minimum of 3- to 4-day intervals, may increase to 225 mg every 8 hours; if further increase is necessary, may increase to 300 mg every 8 hours

Paroxysmal supraventricular tachycardia (to prevent recurrence), ventricular arrhythmias: Oral: *Immediate release tablet:* Initial: 150 mg every 8 hours (US labeling) or 300 mg every 12 hours (Canadian labeling); dosage increase may be made at minimum of 3- to 4-day intervals, may increase to 225 mg every 8 hours; if further increase is necessary, may increase to 300 mg every 8 hours

Paroxysmal atrial fibrillation, pharmacologic cardioversion (off-label use): Oral: *Immediate release tablet:* Outpatient: "Pill-in-the-pocket" dose: 450 mg (weight <70 kg), 600 mg (weight ≥70 kg). May not repeat in ≤24 hours (Alboni, 2004; AHA/ACC/HRS [January, 2014]). **Note:** An initial inpatient cardioversion trial should have been successful before sending patient home on this approach. Patient must be taking an AV nodal-blocking agent (eg, beta-blocker, nondihydropyridine calcium channel blocker) prior to initiation of antiarrhythmic.

Renal Impairment

There are no dosage adjustments provided in the manufacturer's labeling; however, 50% of propafenone metabolites (some active) are excreted in the urine; some data suggest that no dosage adjustment is necessary (Burgess, 1989; Fromm, 1994); however, use with caution.

Hemodialysis/CVVH: Minimally dialyzable (Burgess, 1989; Seto, 1999); supplemental dose not necessary

Hepatic Impairment

US labeling: There are no dosage adjustment provided in the manufacturer's labeling; however, dosage reduction should be considered as drug undergoes hepatic metabolism. Use with caution.

Canadian labeling:

Mild to moderate impairment: Initial: 150 mg once daily; dosage increase may be made at minimum of 4-day intervals to 150 mg twice daily, then to 150 mg every 8 hours; if further increase is necessary, may increase to 300 mg every 12 hours

Severe impairment: Use is contraindicated.

Administration

Oral: Capsules should be swallowed whole; do not crush or chew; may be taken without regard to meals.

The Canadian labeling recommends the tablet be swallowed whole with liquid and to be administered with food.

Monitoring Parameters ECG, blood pressure, pulse (particularly at initiation of therapy)

Dosage Forms Excipient information presented when available (limited, particularly for generics); consult specific product labeling.

Capsule Extended Release 12 Hour, Oral, as hydrochloride:

Rythmol SR: 225 mg, 325 mg, 425 mg [contains soybean lecithin]

Generic: 225 mg, 325 mg, 425 mg

Tablet, Oral, as hydrochloride:

Rythmol: 150 mg, 225 mg [scored]

Generic: 150 mg, 225 mg, 300 mg

Dosage Forms: Canada Excipient information presented when available (limited, particularly for generics); consult specific product labeling.

Tablet, Oral, as hydrochloride:

Rythmol: 150 mg, 300 mg [scored]

◆ Propafenone Hydrochloride *see* Propafenone *on page 1513*

Propantheline (proe PAN the leen)

Index Terms Propantheline Bromide
Pharmacologic Category Anticholinergic Agent
Use Adjunctive treatment of peptic ulcer
Dosing

Adult Antisecretory (off-label use), antispasmodic: Oral: 15 mg 3 times/day before meals or food and 30 mg at bedtime

Geriatric Antisecretory (off-label use): 7.5 mg 3 times/day before meals and at bedtime; increase as necessary to a maximum of 30 mg 3 times/day

Pediatric

Antisecretory (off-label use): Oral: 1-2 mg/kg/day in 3-4 divided doses

Antispasmodic: Oral: 2-3 mg/kg/day in divided doses every 4-6 hours and at bedtime

Renal Impairment No dosage adjustment provided in manufacturer's labeling.

Hepatic Impairment No dosage adjustment provided in manufacturer's labeling.

Additional Information Complete prescribing information should be consulted for additional detail.

Dosage Forms Excipient information presented when available (limited, particularly for generics); consult specific product labeling.

Tablet, Oral, as bromide:

Generic: 15 mg

◆ Propantheline Bromide *see* Propantheline *on page 1515*

Proparacaine (proe PAR a kane)

Brand Names: US Alcaine; Parcaine [DSC]
Brand Names: Canada Alcaine®; Diocaine®
Index Terms Proparacaine Hydrochloride; Proxymetacaine
Pharmacologic Category Local Anesthetic, Ophthalmic
Use Topical anesthesia for tonometry, gonioscopy; suture removal from cornea; removal of corneal foreign body; short operative procedure involving the cornea and conjunctiva
Dosing

Adult & Geriatric

Short corneal and conjunctival procedures: Ophthalmic: Instill 1 drop in eye(s) every 5-10 minutes for 5-7 doses

Tonometry, gonioscopy, suture removal: Ophthalmic: Instill 1-2 drops in eye(s) just prior to procedure

Pediatric Children and Adolescents: Refer to adult dosing

Renal Impairment No dosage adjustment provided in manufacturer's labeling.

Hepatic Impairment No dosage adjustment provided in manufacturer's labeling.

Additional Information Complete prescribing information should be consulted for additional detail.

Dosage Forms Excipient information presented when available (limited, particularly for generics); consult specific product labeling. [DSC] = Discontinued product

Solution, Ophthalmic, as hydrochloride:

Alcaine: 0.5% (15 mL) [contains benzalkonium chloride]

Parcaine: 0.5% (15 mL [DSC])

Generic: 0.5% (15 mL)

Proparacaine and Fluorescein
(proe PAR a kane & FLURE e seen)

Brand Names: US Flucaine
Index Terms Fluorescein and Proparacaine
Pharmacologic Category Diagnostic Agent; Local Anesthetic
Use For use in ophthalmic procedures when a topical disclosing agent is needed along with an anesthetic
Dosing

Adult & Geriatric

Short corneal and conjunctival surgical procedures requiring deep ophthalmic anesthesia: Ophthalmic: Instill 1 drop in each eye every 5-10 minutes for 5-7 doses

Tonometry, gonioscopy, foreign body or suture removal: Ophthalmic: Instill 1-2 drops in each eye just prior to procedure

Renal Impairment No dosage adjustment provided in manufacturer's labeling.

Hepatic Impairment No dosage adjustment provided in manufacturer's labeling.

Additional Information Complete prescribing information should be consulted for additional detail.

Dosage Forms Excipient information presented when available (limited, particularly for generics); consult specific product labeling. [DSC] = Discontinued product

Solution, ophthalmic: Proparacaine hydrochloride 0.5% and fluorescein sodium 0.25% (5 mL)

Flucaine: Proparacaine hydrochloride 0.5% and fluorescein sodium 0.25% (5 mL)

◆ Proparacaine Hydrochloride *see* Proparacaine *on page 1515*
◆ Propecia *see* Finasteride *on page 769*

◆ Propine® (Can) *see* Dipivefrin *on page 570*
◆ PRO-Pioglitazone (Can) *see* Pioglitazone *on page 1454*

Propofol (PROE po fole)

Brand Names: US Diprivan; Fresenius Propoven
Brand Names: Canada Diprivan; PMS-Propofol; Propofol Injection; Propofol-II Injection
Pharmacologic Category General Anesthetic
Use Induction of anesthesia in patients ≥3 years of age; maintenance of anesthesia in patients >2 months of age; in adults, for monitored anesthesia care sedation during procedures; in adults, for sedation in intubated, mechanically-ventilated ICU patients

Note: Consult local regulations and individual institutional policies and procedures.
Pregnancy Considerations Propofol crosses the placenta and may be associated with neonatal CNS and respiratory depression. Propofol is not recommended by the manufacturer for obstetrics, including cesarean section deliveries.
Breast-Feeding Considerations Propofol is excreted in breast milk. Breast-feeding is not recommended by the manufacturer. A green discoloration to the breast milk was noted in a woman following administration of propofol during surgery for removal of an ectopic pregnancy. Although other medications were also administered, propofol was detected in the milk and assumed to be the cause; resolution of this effect occurred within 48 hours after surgery (Birkholz, 2009).
Contraindications Hypersensitivity to propofol or any component of the formulation; hypersensitivity to eggs, egg products, soybeans, or soy products; when general anesthesia or sedation is contraindicated

Note: Fresenius Propoven is also contraindicated in patients who are hypersensitive to peanuts. In July 2012, the FDA initiated temporary importation of Fresenius Propoven 1% (propofol) injection into the U.S. market to address a propofol shortage.
Warnings/Precautions May rarely cause hypersensitivity, anaphylaxis, anaphylactoid reactions, angioedema, bronchospasm, and erythema; medications for the treatment of hypersensitivity reactions should be available for immediate use. Use with caution in patients with history of hypersensitivity/anaphylactic reaction to peanuts; a low risk of crossreactivity between soy and peanuts may exist. Use is contraindicated in patients who are hypersensitive to eggs, egg products, soybeans, or soy products. The major cardiovascular effect of propofol is hypotension especially if patient is hypovolemic or if bolus dosing is used; use with caution in patients who are hemodynamically unstable, hypovolemic, or have abnormally low vascular tone (eg, sepsis). Use requires careful patient monitoring, should only be used by experienced personnel who are not actively engaged in the procedure or surgery. If used in a nonintubated and/or non–mechanically ventilated patient, qualified personnel and appropriate equipment for rapid institution of respiratory and/or cardiovascular support must be immediately available. Use to induce moderate (conscious) sedation in patients warrants monitoring equivalent to that seen with deep anesthesia. Consult local regulations and individual institutional policies and procedures.

Use a lower induction dose, a slower maintenance rate of administration, and avoid rapidly administered boluses in the elderly, debilitated, or ASA-PS (American Society of Anesthesiologists - Physical Status) 3/4 patients to reduce the incidence of unwanted cardiorespiratory depressive events. Use caution in patients with severe cardiac disease (ejection fraction <50%) or respiratory disease; may have more profound adverse cardiovascular responses to propofol. Use caution in patients with a history of epilepsy or seizures; seizure may occur during recovery phase. Use caution in patients with increased intracranial pressure or impaired cerebral circulation; substantial decreases in mean arterial pressure and subsequent decreases in cerebral perfusion pressure may occur; consider continuous infusion or administer as a slow bolus. In most cases, propofol does not significantly affect the QT interval (Staikou, 2014). However, prolongation of the QT interval, usually within normal limits, has occurred in case reports and small prospective studies and may be dose dependent (Hume-Smith, 2008; Kim, 2008; McConachie, 1989; Saarnivaara, 1990; Saarinvaara, 1993; Sakabe, 2002). Shortening of the QT interval has also occurred (Erdil, 2009; Tanskanen, 2002).

Propofol-related infusion syndrome (PRIS) is a serious side effect with a high mortality rate (up to 33%) characterized by dysrhythmia (eg, bradycardia or tachycardia), heart failure, hyperkalemia, lipemia, metabolic acidosis, and/or rhabdomyolysis or myoglobinuria with subsequent renal failure. Risk factors include poor oxygen delivery, sepsis, serious cerebral injury, and the administration of high doses of propofol (usually doses >83 mcg/kg/minute or >5 mg/kg/hour for >48 hours), but has also been reported following large dose, short term infusions during surgical anesthesia. PRIS has also been reported with lower-dose infusions (Chukwuemeka, 2006; Merz, 2006). The onset of the syndrome is rapid, occurring within 4 days of initiation. Alternate sedative therapy should be considered for patients with escalating doses of vasopressors or inotropes, when cardiac failure occurs during high-dose propofol infusion, when metabolic acidosis is observed, or in whom lengthy and/or high-dose sedation is needed (Barr, 2013; Corbett, 2008).

Because propofol is formulated within a 10% fat emulsion, hypertriglyceridemia is an expected side effect. Patients who develop hypertriglyceridemia (eg, >500 mg/dL) are at risk of developing pancreatitis. An alternative sedative agent should be employed if significant hypertriglyceridemia occurs. Use with caution in patients with preexisting pancreatitis; use of propofol may exacerbate this condition. Use caution in patients with preexisting hyperlipidemia as evidenced by increased serum triglyceride levels or serum turbidity. Transient local pain may occur during IV injection; perioperative myoclonia has occurred. Propofol should only be used in pregnancy if clearly needed. Not recommended for use in obstetrics, including cesarean section deliveries. Safety and efficacy in pediatric intensive care unit patients have not been established. Concurrent use of fentanyl and propofol in pediatric patients may result in bradycardia.

Concomitant use with opioids may lead to increased sedative or anesthetic effects of propofol, more pronounced decreases in systolic, diastolic, and mean arterial pressures and cardiac output; lower doses of propofol may be needed. In addition, fentanyl may cause serious bradycardia when used with propofol in pediatric patients. Alfentanil use with propofol has precipitated seizure activity in patients without any history of epilepsy. Discontinue opioids and paralytic agents prior to weaning. Avoid abrupt discontinuation prior to weaning or daily wake up assessments. Abrupt discontinuation can result in rapid awakening, anxiety, agitation, and resistance to mechanical ventilation; wean the infusion rate so the patient awakens slowly. Propofol lacks analgesic properties; pain management requires specific use of analgesic agents, at effective dosages, propofol must be titrated separately from the analgesic agent.

Propofol vials and prefilled syringes have the potential to support the growth of various microorganisms despite product additives intended to suppress microbial growth. To limit the potential for contamination, recommendations in product labeling for handling and administering propofol should be strictly adhered to. Some formulations may contain edetate disodium which may lead to decreased zinc levels in patients with prolonged therapy (>5 days) or a predisposition to zinc deficiency (eg, burns, diarrhea, or sepsis). A holiday from propofol infusion should take place after 5 days of therapy to allow for evaluation and necessary replacement of zinc. Some formulations may contain sulfites.

Benzyl alcohol and derivatives: Some dosage forms may contain benzyl alcohol; large amounts of benzyl alcohol (≥99 mg/kg/day) have been associated with a potentially fatal toxicity ("gasping syndrome") in neonates; the "gasping syndrome" consists of metabolic acidosis, respiratory distress, gasping respirations, CNS dysfunction (including convulsions, intracranial hemorrhage), hypotension, and cardiovascular collapse (AAP ["Inactive" 1997]; CDC, 1982); some data suggests that benzoate displaces bilirubin from protein binding sites (Ahlfors, 2001); avoid or use dosage forms containing benzyl alcohol with caution in neonates. See manufacturer's labeling.
Adverse Reactions
>10%:
  Cardiovascular: Hypotension (children 17%; adults 3% to 26%)
  Central nervous system: Movement (children 17%; adults 3% to 10%)
  Local: Injection site burning, stinging, or pain (children 10%; adults 18%)
  Respiratory: Apnea lasting 30-60 seconds (children 10%; adults 24%), apnea lasting >60 seconds (children 5%; adults 12%)

1% to 10%:
  Cardiovascular: Hypertension (children 8%), arrhythmia (1% to 3%), bradycardia (1% to 3%), cardiac output decreased (1% to 3%; concurrent opioid use increases incidence), tachycardia (1% to 3%)
  Dermatologic: Pruritus (1% to 3%), rash (children 5%; adults 1% to 3%)
  Endocrine & metabolic: Hypertriglyceridemia (3% to 10%)
  Respiratory: Respiratory acidosis during weaning (3% to 10%)
<1% (Limited to important or life-threatening): Agitation, amblyopia, anaphylaxis, anaphylactoid reaction, anticholinergic syndrome, asystole, atrial arrhythmia, bigeminy, cardiac arrest, chills, cough, dizziness, delirium, discoloration (green [urine, hair, or nailbeds]), extremity pain, fever, flushing, hemorrhage, hypersalivation, hypertonia, hypomagnesemia, hypoxia, infusion site reactions (including pain, swelling, blisters and/or tissue necrosis following accidental extravasation); laryngospasm, leukocytosis, lung function decreased, myalgia, myoclonia (rarely including convulsions and opisthotonos), nausea, pancreatitis, paresthesia, phlebitis, postoperative unconsciousness with or without increase in muscle tone, premature atrial contractions, premature ventricular contractions, pulmonary edema, propofol-related infusion syndrome, rhabdomyolysis, somnolence, syncope, thrombosis, urine cloudy, vision abnormality, wheezing

Drug Interactions

Metabolism/Transport Effects Substrate of CYP1A2 (minor), CYP2A6 (minor), CYP2B6 (major), CYP2C19 (minor), CYP2C9 (minor), CYP2D6 (minor), CYP2E1 (minor), CYP3A4 (minor); **Note:** Assignment of Major/Minor substrate status based on clinically relevant drug interaction potential; **Inhibits** CYP1A2 (weak), CYP2C9 (weak), CYP2D6 (weak), CYP2E1 (weak), CYP3A4 (weak)

Avoid Concomitant Use
Avoid concomitant use of Propofol with any of the following: Azelastine (Nasal); Orphenadrine; Paraldehyde; Pimozide; Thalidomide

Increased Effect/Toxicity
Propofol may increase the levels/effects of: Alcohol (Ethyl); Amifostine; Antipsychotic Agents (Second Generation [Atypical]); ARIPiprazole; Azelastine (Nasal); Buprenorphine; CNS Depressants; DULoxetine; Flibanserin; Highest Risk QTc-Prolonging Agents; Hydrocodone; Hypotension-Associated Agents; Levodopa; Lomitapide; Methotrimeprazine; Metyrosine; Midazolam; Mirtazapine; Moderate Risk QTc-Prolonging Agents; NiMODipine; Orphenadrine; Paraldehyde; Pimozide; Pramipexole; ROPINIRole; Ropivacaine; Rotigotine; Selective Serotonin Reuptake Inhibitors; Suvorexant; Thalidomide; TiZANidine; Zolpidem

The levels/effects of Propofol may be increased by: Alfentanil; Alfuzosin; Barbiturates; Blood Pressure Lowering Agents; Brimonidine (Topical); Cannabis; CYP2B6 Inhibitors (Moderate); Diazoxide; Doxylamine; Dronabinol; Droperidol; Herbs (Hypotensive Properties); HydrOXYzine; Kava Kava; Magnesium Sulfate; Methotrimeprazine; Midazolam; Mifepristone; Minocycline; Molsidomine; Nabilone; Nicorandil; Obinutuzumab; Pentoxifylline; Perampanel; Phosphodiesterase 5 Inhibitors; Prostacyclin Analogues; Quazepam; Rifampin; Rufinamide; Sodium Oxybate; Tapentadol; Tetrahydrocannabinol

Decreased Effect There are no known significant interactions involving a decrease in effect.

Food Interactions
Edetate disodium, an ingredient of propofol emulsion, may lead to decreased zinc levels in patients on prolonged therapy (>5 days) or those predisposed to deficiency (burns, diarrhea, and/or major sepsis). Management: Zinc replacement therapy may be needed.

Preparation for Administration
Does not need to be diluted; however, propofol may be further diluted in 5% dextrose in water to a concentration of ≥2 mg/mL.

Storage/Stability
Store between 4°C to 22°C (40°F to 72°F); refrigeration is not required. Do not freeze. If transferred to a syringe or other container prior to administration, use within 6 hours. If used directly from vial/prefilled syringe, use within 12 hours. If diluted in 5% dextrose stable for 8 hours at room temperature. Shake well before use. Do not use if there is evidence of separation of phases of emulsion.

Mechanism of Action
Propofol is a short-acting, lipophilic intravenous general anesthetic. The drug is unrelated to any of the currently used barbiturate, opioid, benzodiazepine, arylcyclohexylamine, or imidazole intravenous anesthetic agents. Propofol causes global CNS depression, presumably through agonism of GABA$_A$ receptors and perhaps reduced glutamatergic activity through NMDA receptor blockade.

Pharmacodynamics/Kinetics
Onset of action: Anesthetic: Bolus infusion (dose dependent): 9 to 51 seconds (average 30 seconds)
Duration (dose and rate dependent): 3 to 10 minutes
Distribution: V_d: 2 to 10 L/kg; after a 10-day infusion, V_d approaches 60 L/kg; decreased in the elderly
Protein binding: 97% to 99%
Metabolism: Hepatic to water-soluble sulfate and glucuronide conjugates (~50%)
Half-life elimination: Biphasic: Initial: 40 minutes; Terminal: 4 to 7 hours (after 10-day infusion, may be up to 1 to 3 days)
Excretion: Urine (~88% as metabolites, 40% as glucuronide metabolite); feces (<2%)

Dosing

Adult Consult local regulations and individual institutional policies and procedures. Dosage must be individualized based on total body weight and titrated to the desired clinical effect. Wait at least 3 to 5 minutes between dosage adjustments to clinically assess drug effects. Smaller doses are required when used with opioids; the following are general dosing guidelines:

General anesthesia: Note: Increase dose in patients with chronic alcoholism (Fassoulaki, 1993); decrease dose with acutely intoxicated (alcoholic) patients.
Induction of general anesthesia:
  Healthy adults, ASA-PS 1 or 2, <55 years: IV: 2 to 2.5 mg/kg (~40 mg every 10 seconds until onset of induction)
  Debilitated, ASA-PS 3 or 4: Refer to geriatric dosing.
Maintenance of general anesthesia:
  Healthy adults, ASA-PS 1 or 2, <55 years:
    IV infusion: Initial: 100 to 200 mcg/kg/minute (or 6 to 12 mg/kg/hour) for 10 to 15 minutes; usual maintenance infusion rate: 50 to 100 mcg/kg/minute (or 3 to 6 mg/kg/hour) to optimize recovery time.
    IV intermittent bolus: 25 to 50 mg increments as needed
  Debilitated, ASA-PS 3 or 4: IV Infusion: Refer to geriatric dosing.

Monitored anesthesia care sedation:
  Healthy adults, ASA-PS 1 or 2, <55 years: Slow IV infusion: 100 to 150 mcg/kg/minute (or 6 to 9 mg/kg/hour) for 3 to 5 minutes or slow injection: 0.5 mg/kg over 3 to 5 minutes followed by IV infusion of 25 to 75 mcg/kg/minute (or 1.5 to 4.5 mg/kg/hour) or incremental bolus doses: 10 mg or 20 mg
  Debilitated or ASA-PS 3 or 4 patients: Use 80% of healthy adult dose

ICU sedation in intubated mechanically-ventilated patients: Avoid rapid bolus injection; individualize dose and titrate to response.
  Continuous infusion: Initial: 5 mcg/kg/minute (or 0.3 mg/kg/hour); increase by 5 to 10 mcg/kg/minute (or 0.3 to 0.6 mg/kg/hour) every 5 to 10 minutes until desired sedation level is achieved; usual maintenance: 5 to 50 mcg/kg/minute (or 0.3 to 3 mg/kg/hour); reduce dose after adequate sedation established and adjust to response (eg, evaluate frequently to use minimum dose for sedation). Daily interruption with retitration or a light target level of sedation is recommended to minimize prolonged sedative effects (Barr, 2013).
  Elderly, debilitated, or ASA-PS 3 or 4 patients: Refer to geriatric dosing.

Postoperative nausea and vomiting (PONV), rescue therapy (off-label use): IV: 15 to 20 mg, may be repeated (Gan 2004; SAA [Gan 2007]; Unlugenc 2004).

Status epilepticus, refractory (off-label use): IV: **Note:** Mechanical ventilation and cardiovascular monitoring required; titrate dose to cessation of electrographic seizures or burst suppression (NCS [Brophy, 2012]).
  Neurocritical Care Society recommendations (NCS [Brophy, 2012]):
    Loading dose: 1 to 2 mg/kg with initiation of a continuous infusion.

Continuous infusion: Initial: 20 mcg/kg/minute (1.2 mg/kg/**hour**). If the patient experiences break-through status epilepticus while on continuous infusion, increase infusion rate by 5 to 10 mcg/kg/minute (0.3 to 0.6 mg/kg/**hour**) every 5 minutes (may also administer a 1 mg/kg bolus dose with continuous infusion titration); dosage range: 30 to 200 mcg/kg/minute (1.8 to 12 mg/kg/**hour**). **Note:** Use caution with doses >80 mcg/kg/minute (>4.8 mg/kg/**hour**) for >48 hours. Prior to withdrawal, a period of at least 24 to 48 hours of electrographic control is recommended; withdraw gradually to prevent recurrent status epilepticus.

Geriatric Consult local regulations and individual institutional policies and procedures. Dosage must be individualized based on total body weight and titrated to the desired clinical effect. Wait at least 3 to 5 minutes between dosage adjustments to clinically assess drug effects. Smaller doses are required when used with opioids; the following are general dosing guidelines:

General anesthesia: Note: Increase dose in patients with chronic alcoholism (Fassoulaki, 1993); decrease dose with acutely intoxicated (alcoholic) patients.
Induction of general anesthesia: Elderly, debilitated, ASA-PS 3 or 4: IV: 1 to 1.5 mg/kg (~20 mg every 10 seconds until onset of induction)
Maintenance of general anesthesia: Elderly, debilitated, ASA-PS 3 or 4: IV infusion: 50 to 100 mcg/kg/minute (or 3 to 6 mg/kg/**hour**)
Monitored anesthesia care sedation: Elderly, debilitated, ASA-PS 3 or 4: IV: Use 80% of healthy adult dose
ICU sedation in intubated mechanically-ventilated patients: Avoid rapid bolus injection; individualize dose and titrate to response:
Continuous infusion: Elderly, debilitated, ASA-PS 3 or 4: Use 80% of healthy adult dose; reduce dose after adequate sedation established and adjust to response (eg, evaluate frequently to use minimum dose for sedation). Daily interruption with retitration or a light target level of sedation is recommended to minimize prolonged sedative effects (Barr, 2013).

Pediatric Consult local regulations and individual institutional policies and procedures. Dosage must be individualized based on total body weight and titrated to the desired clinical effect. Wait at least 3 to 5 minutes between dosage adjustments to clinically assess drug effects. Smaller doses are required when used with opioids; the following are general dosing guidelines:

General anesthesia: Note: Increase dose in patients with chronic alcoholism (Fassoulaki, 1993); decrease dose with acutely intoxicated (alcoholic) patients.
Induction of general anesthesia: IV: Healthy children 3 to 16 years, ASA-PS 1 or 2: 2.5 to 3.5 mg/kg over 20 to 30 seconds; use a lower dose for children ASA-PS 3 or 4
Maintenance of general anesthesia: IV infusion: Healthy children 2 months to 16 years, ASA-PS 1 or 2: 125 to 300 mcg/kg/minute (or 7.5 to 18 mg/kg/**hour**); after 30 minutes, if clinical signs of light anesthesia are absent, decrease the infusion rate. Children ≤5 years may require larger infusion rates compared to older children.
Status epilepticus, refractory (off-label use): IV: **Note:** Mechanical ventilation and cardiovascular monitoring required; titrate dose to cessation of electrographic seizures or burst suppression (NCS [Brophy, 2012]).
Neurocritical Care Society recommendations (NCS [Brophy, 2012]):
Loading dose: 1 to 2 mg/kg with initiation of a continuous infusion.
Continuous infusion: Initial: 20 mcg/kg/minute (1.2 mg/kg/**hour**). If the patient experiences break-through status epilepticus while on continuous infusion, increase infusion rate by 5 to 10 mcg/kg/minute (0.3 to 0.6 mg/kg/**hour**) every 5 minutes (may also administer a 1 mg/kg bolus dose with continuous infusion titration); dosage range: 30 to 200 mcg/kg/minute (1.8 to 12 mg/kg/**hour**). **Note:** Use caution with doses >80 mcg/kg/minute (>4.8 mg/kg/**hour**) for >48 hours. Prior to withdrawal, a period of at least 24 to 48 hours of electrographic control is recommended; withdraw gradually to prevent recurrent status epilepticus.

Renal Impairment No dosage adjustment necessary.
Hepatic Impairment No dosage adjustment necessary.
Dietary Considerations Propofol is formulated in an oil-in-water emulsion. If on parenteral nutrition, may need to adjust the amount of lipid infused. Propofol emulsion contains 1.1 kcal/mL. Soybean fat emulsion is used as a vehicle for propofol. Formulations also contain egg phosphatide and glycerol.

Administration Consult local regulations and individual institutional policies and procedures. Strict aseptic technique must be maintained in handling although a preservative has been added. Do not use if contamination is suspected. Do not administer through the same IV catheter with blood or plasma. Tubing and any unused portions of propofol vials should be discarded after 12 hours.

To reduce pain associated with injection, use larger veins of forearm or antecubital fossa; lidocaine IV (1 mL of a 1% solution) may also be used prior to administration or it may be added to propofol immediately before administration in a quantity not to exceed 20 mg lidocaine per 200 mg propofol. Do not use filter <5 micron for administration.

Monitoring Parameters Cardiac monitor, blood pressure, oxygen saturation (during monitored anesthesia care sedation), arterial blood gas (with prolonged infusions). With prolonged infusions (eg, ICU sedation), monitor for metabolic acidosis, hyperkalemia, rhabdomyolysis or elevated CPK, hepatomegaly, and progression of cardiac and renal failure.

ICU sedation: Assess and adjust sedation according to scoring system (Richmond Agitation-Sedation Scale [RASS] or Sedation-Agitation Scale [SAS]) (Barr, 2013); assess CNS function daily. Serum triglyceride levels should be obtained prior to initiation of therapy and every 3-7 days thereafter, especially if receiving for >48 hours with doses exceeding 50 mcg/kg/minute (Devlin, 2005); use intravenous port opposite propofol infusion or temporarily suspend infusion and flush port prior to blood draw.

Diprivan®: Monitor zinc levels in patients predisposed to deficiency (burns, diarrhea, major sepsis) or after 5 days of treatment.

Dosage Forms Excipient information presented when available (limited, particularly for generics); consult specific product labeling.
Emulsion, Intravenous:
Diprivan: 10 mg/mL (10 mL, 20 mL, 50 mL, 100 mL) [contains edetate disodium, egg phospholipids (egg lecithin), glycerin, soybean oil]
Generic: 10 mg/mL (20 mL, 50 mL, 100 mL)
Emulsion, Intravenous [preservative free]:
Fresenius Propoven: 10 mg/mL (20 mL, 50 mL, 100 mL) [contains egg phosphatides, soybean oil]
Generic: 10 mg/mL (20 mL, 50 mL, 100 mL)

◆ Propofol-II Injection (Can) *see* Propofol *on page 1516*
◆ Propofol Injection (Can) *see* Propofol *on page 1516*

Propranolol (proe PRAN oh lole)

Brand Names: US Hemangeol; Inderal LA; Inderal XL; InnoPran XL
Brand Names: Canada Apo-Propranolol; Dom-Propranolol; Inderal; Inderal LA; Novo-Pranol; Nu-Propranolol; PMS-Propranolol; Propranolol Hydrochloride Injection, USP; Teva-Propranolol
Index Terms Hemangeol; Inderal; Propranolol Hydrochloride
Pharmacologic Category Antianginal Agent; Antiarrhythmic Agent, Class II; Antihypertensive; Beta-Adrenergic Blocker, Nonselective
Use Management of hypertension; angina pectoris; pheochromocytoma; essential tremor; supraventricular arrhythmias (such as atrial fibrillation and flutter, AV nodal re-entrant tachycardias), ventricular tachycardias (catecholamine-induced arrhythmias, digoxin toxicity); prevention of myocardial infarction; migraine headache prophylaxis; symptomatic treatment of obstructive hypertrophic cardiomyopathy (formerly known as hypertrophic subaortic stenosis); treatment of proliferating infantile hemangioma requiring systemic therapy (Hemangeol only)

Guideline recommendations:
Hypertension: The 2014 guideline for the management of high blood pressure in adults (JNC 8) recommends initiation of pharmacologic treatment to lower blood pressure for the following patients (JNC8 [James 2013]):
• Patients ≥60 years of age, with systolic blood pressure (SBP) ≥150 mm Hg or diastolic blood pressure (DBP) ≥90 mm Hg. Goal of therapy is SBP <150 mm Hg and DBP <90 mm Hg.
• Patients <60 years of age, with SBP ≥140 mm Hg or DBP ≥90 mm Hg. Goal of therapy is SBP <140 mm Hg and DBP <90 mm Hg.
• Patients ≥18 years of age with diabetes, with SBP ≥140 mm Hg or DBP ≥90 mm Hg. Goal of therapy is SBP <140 mm Hg and DBP <90 mm Hg.

• Patients ≥18 years of age with chronic kidney disease (CKD), with SBP ≥140 mm Hg or DBP ≥90 mm Hg. Goal of therapy is SBP <140 mm Hg and DBP <90 mm Hg.

Chronic kidney disease (CKD) and hypertension: Regardless of race or diabetes status, the use of an ACE inhibitor (ACEI) or angiotensin receptor blocker (ARB) as initial therapy is recommended to improve kidney outcomes. In the general nonblack population (without CKD) including those with diabetes, initial antihypertensive treatment should consist of a thiazide-type diuretic, calcium channel blocker, ACEI, or ARB. In the general black population (without CKD) including those with diabetes, initial antihypertensive treatment should consist of a thiazide-type diuretic or a calcium channel blocker **instead of** an ACEI or ARB. Beta-blockers are no longer recommended as first-line therapy in the general patient population.

Coronary artery disease (CAD) and hypertension: The American Heart Association, American College of Cardiology, and American Society of Hypertension (AHA/ACC/ASH) 2015 scientific statement for the treatment of hypertension in patients with CAD recommends the use of a beta blocker as part of a regimen in patients with hypertension and chronic stable angina with a history of prior MI. A BP target of <140/90 mm Hg is reasonable for the secondary prevention of cardiovascular events. A lower target BP (<130/80 mm Hg) may be appropriate in some individuals with CAD, previous MI, stroke or transient ischemic attack, or CAD risk equivalents (AHA/ACC/ASH [Rosendorff 2015]).

Pregnancy Considerations Adverse events have been observed in some animal reproduction studies; therefore, the manufacturer classifies propranolol as pregnancy category C. Propranolol crosses the placenta and is measurable in the newborn serum following maternal use during pregnancy. In a cohort study, an increased risk of cardiovascular defects was observed following maternal use of beta-blockers during pregnancy. Intrauterine growth restriction (IUGR), small placentas, as well as fetal/neonatal bradycardia, hypoglycemia, and/or respiratory depression have been observed following *in utero* exposure to beta-blockers as a class. Adequate facilities for monitoring infants at birth should be available. Untreated chronic maternal hypertension and pre-eclampsia are also associated with adverse events in the fetus, infant, and mother. The peak maternal serum concentrations of propranolol and the active metabolite 4-hydroxypropranolol do not change during pregnancy; peak serum concentrations of naphthoxylactic acid are lower in the third trimester when compared to postpartum. Propranolol is recommended for use in the management of thyrotoxicosis in pregnancy. Propranolol has been evaluated for the treatment of hypertension in pregnancy, but other agents may be more appropriate for use. Propranolol has also been used in the management of hypertrophic obstructive cardiomyopathy in pregnancy and has been studied for use as an adjunctive agent in the management of dysfunctional labor (dystocia).

Breast-Feeding Considerations Propranolol is excreted into breast milk with peak concentrations occurring ~2-3 hours after an oral dose. The inactive metabolites of propranolol have also been detected in breast milk. The manufacturer recommends that caution be exercised when administering propranolol to nursing women. Due to immature hepatic metabolism in newborns, breast-feeding infants should be monitored for adverse events.

Prescribing and Access Restrictions Prescriptions for Hemangeol may be obtained via the Hemangeol Patient Access program. Visit http://www.hemangeol.com/hcp/hemangeol-direct/ or call 855-618-4950 for ordering information.

Contraindications

Hypersensitivity to propranolol, beta-blockers, or any component of the formulation; uncompensated congestive heart failure (unless the failure is due to tachyarrhythmias being treated with propranolol), cardiogenic shock; severe sinus bradycardia, sick sinus syndrome, or heart block greater than first-degree (except in patients with a functioning artificial pacemaker); bronchial asthma

Hemangeol (additional contraindications): Premature infants with corrected age <5 weeks; infants weighing <2 kg; heart rate <80 bpm; blood pressure <50/30 mm Hg; pheochromocytoma; history of bronchospasm

Warnings/Precautions Consider preexisting conditions such as sick sinus syndrome before initiating. Administer cautiously in compensated heart failure and monitor for a worsening of the condition (efficacy of propranolol in HF has not been demonstrated). **[US Boxed Warning]: Beta-blocker therapy should not be withdrawn abruptly (particularly in patients with CAD), but gradually tapered to avoid acute tachycardia, hypertension, and/or ischemia.** Beta-blockers without alpha1-adrenergic receptor blocking activity should be avoided in patients with Prinzmetal variant angina (Mayer 1998). Chronic beta-blocker therapy should not be routinely withdrawn prior to major surgery. May precipitate or aggravate symptoms of arterial insufficiency in patients with PVD and Raynaud's disease; use with caution and monitor for progression of arterial obstruction. Bradycardia may be observed more frequently in elderly patients (>65 years of age); dosage reductions may be necessary. Potentially significant drug-drug interactions may exist, requiring dose or frequency adjustment, additional monitoring, and/or selection of alternative therapy. Cigarette smoking may decrease plasma levels of propranolol by increasing metabolism. Patients should be advised to avoid smoking.

Use cautiously in patients with diabetes because it can mask prominent hypoglycemic symptoms. May mask signs of hyperthyroidism (eg, tachycardia); if hyperthyroidism is suspected, carefully manage and monitor; abrupt withdrawal may exacerbate symptoms of hyperthyroidism or precipitate thyroid storm. May alter thyroid-function tests. Use with caution in myasthenia gravis or psychiatric disease (may cause CNS depression). Use cautiously in renal and hepatic dysfunction; dosage adjustment may be required in hepatic impairment. In general, patients with bronchospastic disease should not receive beta-blockers; if used at all, should be used cautiously with close monitoring. Adequate alpha-blockade is required prior to use of any beta-blocker for patients with untreated pheochromocytoma. May induce or exacerbate psoriasis. Use caution with history of severe anaphylaxis to allergens; patients taking beta-blockers may become more sensitive to repeated challenges. Treatment of anaphylaxis (eg, epinephrine) in patients taking beta-blockers may be ineffective or promote undesirable effects.

Considerations when treating infantile hemangioma: Bradycardia and/or hypotension may occur or be worsened; monitor heart rate and blood pressure after propranolol initiation or increase in dose; discontinue treatment if severe (<80 bpm) or symptomatic bradycardia or hypotension (systolic blood pressure <50 mm Hg) occurs. Infants with large facial infantile hemangioma should be investigated for potential arteriopathy associated with PHACE syndrome prior to propranolol therapy; decreases in blood pressure caused by propranolol may increase risk of stroke in PHACE syndrome patients with cerebrovascular anomalies. May potentiate hypoglycemia and/or mask signs and symptoms. Withhold the dose in infants or children who are not feeding regularly or who are vomiting; discontinue therapy and seek immediate treatment if hypoglycemia occurs. May cause bronchospasm. Interrupt therapy in infants or children with lower respiratory tract infection associated with dyspnea or wheezing.

Adverse Reactions Frequency not always defined.

Cardiovascular: Cold extremities (infants: 7% to 8%), angina pectoris, atrioventricular conduction disturbance, bradycardia, cardiogenic shock, congestive heart failure, hypotension, ineffective myocardial contractions, syncope

Central nervous system: Sleep disorder (infants: 16% to 18%), agitation (infants: 5% to 9%), fatigue (5% to 7%), dizziness (4% to 7%), nightmares (infants: 2% to 6%), irritability (infants: 1% to 6%), drowsiness (infants: 1% to 5%), amnesia, carpal tunnel syndrome (rare), catatonia, cognitive dysfunction, confusion, hypersomnia, lethargy, paresthesia, psychosis, vertigo

Dermatologic: Changes in nails, contact dermatitis, dermal ulcer, eczematous rash, erosive lichen planus, hyperkeratosis, pruritus, skin rash

Endocrine & metabolic: Hyperglycemia, hyperkalemia, hyperlipidemia, hypoglycemia

Gastrointestinal: Diarrhea (infants: 5% to 6%), abdominal pain (infants: ≤4%), decreased appetite (infants: 3% to 4%), constipation (1% to 3%), anorexia, stomach discomfort

Genitourinary: Oliguria (rare), proteinuria (rare)

Hematologic & oncologic: Immune thrombocytopenia, thrombocytopenia

Hepatic: Increased serum alkaline phosphatase, increased serum transaminases

Neuromuscular & skeletal: Arthropathy, oculomucocutaneous syndrome, polyarthritis

Ophthalmic: Conjunctival hyperemia, decreased visual acuity, mydriasis

Renal: Increased blood urea nitrogen, interstitial nephritis (rare)

◀

Respiratory: Bronchitis (infants: 8% to 13%; associated with cough, fever, diarrhea, and vomiting), bronchiolitis (infants; associated with cough, fever, diarrhea, and vomiting), bronchospasm, dyspnea, pulmonary edema, wheezing

Miscellaneous: Ulcer

<1% (Limited to important or life-threatening): Agranulocytosis, alopecia, arterial insufficiency, arterial mesenteric thrombosis, decreased heart rate (infants), decreased serum glucose (infants), depression, emotional lability, epigastric distress, erythema multiforme, fever combined with generalized ache, sore throat, laryngospasm, and respiratory distress), hallucination, hypersensitivity reaction (including anaphylaxis, anaphylactoid reaction), impotence, insomnia, ischemic colitis, lupus-like syndrome, myotonia, myopathy, nonthrombocytopenic purpura, peripheral arterial disease (exacerbation), Peyronie's disease, pharyngitis, psoriasiform eruption, purpura, Raynaud's phenomenon, second degree atrioventricular block (infants; in a patient with an underlying conduction disorder), slightly clouded sensorium, Stevens-Johnson syndrome, systemic lupus erythematosus, temporary amnesia, tingling of extremities (hands), toxic epidermal necrolysis, urticaria, visual disturbance, weakness, xerophthalmia

Drug Interactions

Metabolism/Transport Effects Substrate of CYP1A2 (major), CYP2C19 (minor), CYP2D6 (major), CYP3A4 (minor); **Note:** Assignment of Major/Minor substrate status based on clinically relevant drug interaction potential; **Inhibits** CYP1A2 (weak), CYP2D6 (weak), P-glycoprotein

Avoid Concomitant Use

Avoid concomitant use of Propranolol with any of the following: Beta2-Agonists; Bosutinib; Ceritinib; Floctafenine; Methacholine; PAZOPanib; Rivastigmine; Silodosin; Topotecan; VinCRIStine (Liposomal)

Increased Effect/Toxicity

Propranolol may increase the levels/effects of: Afatinib; Alpha-/Beta-Agonists (Direct-Acting); Alpha1-Blockers; Alpha2-Agonists; Amifostine; Antipsychotic Agents (Phenothiazines); Antipsychotic Agents (Second Generation [Atypical]); ARIPiprazole; Bosutinib; Bradycardia-Causing Agents; Brentuximab Vedotin; Bupivacaine; Cardiac Glycosides; Ceritinib; Cholinergic Agonists; Colchicine; Dabigatran Etexilate; Disopyramide; Doxofylline; DOXOrubicin (Conventional); DULoxetine; Edoxaban; Ergot Derivatives; Everolimus; Fingolimod; Grass Pollen Allergen Extract (5 Grass Extract); Hypotension-Associated Agents; Insulin; Ivabradine; Lacosamide; Ledipasvir; Levodopa; Lidocaine (Systemic); Lidocaine (Topical); Mepivacaine; Methacholine; Midodrine; Naloxegol; PAZOPanib; P-glycoprotein/ABCB1 Substrates; Prucalopride; Ranolazine; Rifaximin; Rizatriptan; Silodosin; Sulfonylureas; TiZANidine; Topotecan; VinCRIStine (Liposomal); ZOLMitriptan

The levels/effects of Propranolol may be increased by: Abiraterone Acetate; Acetylcholinesterase Inhibitors; Alcohol (Ethyl); Alpha2-Agonists; Aminoquinolines (Antimalarial); Amiodarone; Anilidopiperidine Opioids; Antipsychotic Agents (Phenothiazines); Barbiturates; Bretylium; Brimonidine (Topical); Calcium Channel Blockers (Nondihydropyridine); Cobicistat; CYP1A2 Inhibitors (Moderate); CYP1A2 Inhibitors (Strong); CYP2D6 Inhibitors (Moderate); CYP2D6 Inhibitors (Strong); Darunavir; Deferasirox; Diazoxide; Dipyridamole; Disopyramide; Dronedarone; Floctafenine; FluvoxaMINE; Herbs (Hypotensive Properties); Lacidipine; Molsidomine; Nicorandil; NIFEdipine; Obinutuzumab; Panobinostat; Peginterferon Alfa-2b; Pentoxifylline; Phosphodiesterase 5 Inhibitors; Propafenone; Prostacyclin Analogues; QuiNIDine; Regorafenib; Reserpine; Rivastigmine; Ruxolitinib; Selective Serotonin Reuptake Inhibitors; Tofacitinib; Vemurafenib; Zileuton

Decreased Effect

Propranolol may decrease the levels/effects of: Beta2-Agonists; Lacidipine; Theophylline Derivatives

The levels/effects of Propranolol may be decreased by: Alcohol (Ethyl); Amphetamines; Barbiturates; Bile Acid Sequestrants; Cannabis; CYP1A2 Inducers (Strong); Cyproterone; Herbs (Hypertensive Properties); Methylphenidate; Nonsteroidal Anti-Inflammatory Agents; Osimertinib; Peginterferon Alfa-2b; Rifamycin Derivatives; Teriflunomide; Yohimbine

Food Interactions

Ethanol: Ethanol may increase or decrease plasma levels of propranolol. Reports are variable and have shown both enhanced as well as inhibited hepatic metabolism (of propranolol). Management: Caution advised with consumption of ethanol and monitor for heart rate and/or blood pressure changes.

Food: Propranolol serum levels may be increased if taken with food. Protein-rich foods may increase bioavailability; a change in diet from high carbohydrate/low protein to low carbohydrate/high protein may result in increased oral clearance. Management: Tablets (immediate release) should be taken on an empty stomach. Capsules (extended release) may be taken with or without food, but be consistent with regard to food.

Storage/Stability

Injection: Store at 20°C to 25°C (68°F to 77°F); protect from freezing or excessive heat. Once diluted, propranolol is stable for 24 hours at room temperature in D_5W or NS. Protect from light. Solution has a maximum stability at pH of 3 and decomposes rapidly in alkaline pH.

Capsule, tablet, oral solution: Store at controlled room temperature; protect from freezing or excessive heat. Protect from light and moisture. Dispense Hemangeol in original container; discard 2 months after first opening.

Mechanism of Action

Nonselective beta-adrenergic blocker (class II antiarrhythmic); competitively blocks response to beta$_1$- and beta$_2$-adrenergic stimulation which results in decreases in heart rate, myocardial contractility, blood pressure, and myocardial oxygen demand. Nonselective beta-adrenergic blockers (propranolol, nadolol) reduce portal pressure by producing splanchnic vasoconstriction (beta$_2$ effect) thereby reducing portal blood flow.

Pharmacodynamics/Kinetics

Onset of action: Beta-blockade: Oral: 1 to 2 hours

Duration: Immediate release: 6 to 12 hours; Extended-release formulations: ~24 to 27 hours

Absorption: Oral: Rapid and complete

Distribution: V_d: 4 L/kg (adults)

Protein binding: Newborns: 68%; Adults: ~90% (S-isomer primarily to alpha$_1$-acid glycoprotein; R-isomer primarily to albumin)

Metabolism: Hepatic via CYP2D6, and CYP1A2 to 4-hydroxypropranolol (active) and inactive compounds; extensive first-pass effect

Bioavailability: ~25% reaches systemic circulation due to high first-pass metabolism; protein-rich foods increase bioavailability by ~50%

Half-life elimination: Infants: ~3.5 hours (Hemangeol); Children: 3.9 to 6.4 hours; Adults: Immediate release formulation: 3 to 6 hours; Extended-release formulations: 8 to 10 hours

Time to peak: Immediate release: Adults: 1 to 4 hours; Infants: ≤2 hours (Hemangeol); Extended-release formulations: ~6 to 14 hours

Excretion: Metabolites are excreted primarily in urine (96% to 99%); <1% excreted in urine as unchanged drug

Dosing

Adult

Essential tremor: Oral: Immediate-release formulations: 40 mg twice daily initially; maintenance doses: Usually 120 to 320 mg/day

Hypertension: Oral:

Immediate-release formulations: 40 mg twice daily; increase dosage every 3 to 7 days; usual dose: 120 to 240 mg divided in 2 to 3 doses/day; maximum daily dose: 640 mg; usual dosage range (ASH/ISH [Weber 2014]): 40 to 160 mg twice daily

Extended-release formulations:

Inderal LA: Initial: 80 mg once daily; usual maintenance: 120 to 160 mg once daily; maximum daily dose: 640 mg

Inderal XL, InnoPran XL: Initial: 80 mg once daily at bedtime; if initial response is inadequate, may be increased at 2 to 3 week intervals to a maximum daily dose of 120 mg

Migraine headache prophylaxis: Oral:

Immediate-release formulations: Initial: 80 mg/day divided every 6 to 8 hours; increase by 20 to 40 mg/dose every 3 to 4 weeks to a maximum of 160 to 240 mg/day given in divided doses every 6 to 8 hours; if satisfactory response not achieved within 6 weeks of starting therapy, drug should be withdrawn gradually over several weeks

Inderal LA: Initial: 80 mg once daily; effective dose range: 160 to 240 mg once daily

Obstructive hypertrophic cardiomyopathy: Oral:

Immediate-release formulations: 20 to 40 mg 3 to 4 times/day

Inderal LA: 80 to 160 mg once daily

Pheochromocytoma: Oral: Immediate-release formulations: 30 to 60 mg/day in divided doses

Post-MI mortality reduction: Oral: Immediate-release formulations: Initial: 40 mg 3 times/day; usual dosage range: 180 to 240 mg/day in 3 to 4 divided doses

Stable angina: Oral:

Immediate-release formulations: 80 to 320 mg/day in doses divided 2 to 4 times/day

Inderal LA: Initial: 80 mg once daily; maximum dose: 320 mg once daily

Tachyarrhythmias:

Oral: Immediate-release formulations: 10 to 30 mg/dose every 6 to 8 hours or a usual maintenance dose of 10 to 40 mg three or four times daily for rate control in patients with atrial fibrillation (AHA/ACC/HRS [January 2014]).

IV: 1 to 3 mg/dose slow IVP; repeat every 2-5 minutes up to a total of 5 mg; titrate initial dose to desired response. **Note:** Once response achieved or maximum dose administered, additional doses should not be given for at least 4 hours.

or

0.5 to 1 mg over 1 minute; may repeat, if necessary, up to a total maximum dose of 0.1 mg/kg (ACLS guidelines 2010)

or

1 mg over 1 minute; may be repeated every 2 minutes up to 3 doses for rate control in patients with atrial fibrillation (AHA/ACC/HRS [January 2014]).

Akathisia, antipsychotic-induced (off-label use): Oral: Immediate-release formulations: Initial: 10 mg twice daily **or** 10 mg 3 times daily; adjust dose based on response and tolerability up to 120 mg/day (Adler 1986; Adler 1993; Kane 2009; Kramer 1989). Treatment guidelines recommend doses of 30 to 90 mg/day (APA [Lehman 2004]; WFSBP [Hasan 2013].

Performance anxiety (off-label use): Oral: Immediate-release formulations: 40 mg 60 to 90 minutes prior to anxiety-provoking event (Hartley 1983). Additional data may be necessary to further define the role of propranolol in this condition.

Thyroid storm (off-label use):

Oral: Immediate-release formulations: 60 to 80 mg every 4 hours; may consider the use of an intravenous shorter-acting beta-blocker (ie, esmolol) (Bahn 2011)

IV: 0.5 to 1 mg administered over 10 minutes every 3 hours (Gardner 2011)

Thyrotoxicosis (off-label use): Oral: Immediate-release formulations: 10 to 40 mg/dose every 6 to 8 hours; may also consider administering extended or sustained release formulations (Bahn 2011)

Tremor, lithium-induced (off-label use): Oral: Immediate-release formulations: 30 to 80 mg/day in divided doses; adjust dose based on response and tolerability (Gelenberg 1995; Kirk 1973; Lapierre 1976). Additional data may be necessary to further define the role of propranolol in this condition.

Variceal hemorrhage prophylaxis (off-label use) (AASLD [Garcia-Tsao 2007]): Oral:

Primary prophylaxis: Immediate-release formulations: Initial: 20 mg twice daily; adjust to maximal tolerated dose. **Note:** Risk factors for hemorrhage include Child-Pugh class B/C or variceal red wale markings on endoscopy.

Secondary prophylaxis: Immediate-release formulations: Initial: 20 mg twice daily; adjust to maximal tolerated dose

Geriatric

IV: Use caution; initiate at lower end of the dosing range.

Oral:

Hypertension: Consider lower initial doses and titrate to response (Aronow 2011)

Tachyarrhythmias: Immediate-release formulations: Initial: 10 mg twice daily; increase dosage every 3 to 7 days; usual dose range: 10 to 320 mg/day given in 1 to 2 divided doses.

Refer to adult dosing for additional uses.

Pediatric

Proliferating infantile hemangioma (Hemangeol): Infants ≥2 kg: Oral: **Note:** Initiate treatment at age 5 weeks to 5 months; doses should be administered at least 9 hours apart. Refer to product labeling for detailed weight-based dosing tabulation.

Week 1: 0.15 mL/kg (~0.6 mg/kg) twice daily

Week 2: 0.3 mL/kg (~1.1 mg/kg) twice daily

Week 3 (maintenance): 0.4 mL/kg (~1.7 mg/kg) twice daily; maintain this dose for 6 months. Readjust dose periodically as the child's weight increases. Treatment may be reinitiated if hemangiomas recur.

Hypertension (off-label use): Children and Adolescents: Oral: Immediate-release formulations: Initial: 1 to 2 mg/kg/day divided in 2 to 3 doses/day; titrate dose to effect; maximum dose: 4 mg/kg/day up to 640 mg/day; sustained-release formulation may be dosed once daily (NHBPEP 2004; NHLBI 2011).

Thyrotoxicosis (off-label use): Adolescents: Oral: Refer to adult dosing.

Renal Impairment There are no dosage adjustments provided in the manufacturer's labeling. However, renal impairment increases systemic exposure to propranolol. Use with caution.

Not dialyzable (0% to 5%); supplemental dose is not necessary.

Peritoneal dialysis effects: Supplemental dose is not necessary.

Hepatic Impairment There are no dosage adjustments provided in the manufacturer's labeling. However, hepatic impairment increases systemic exposure to propranolol. Use with caution.

Dietary Considerations Tablets (immediate release) should be taken on an empty stomach; capsules (extended release) may be taken with or without food, but should always be taken consistently (with food or on an empty stomach). Hemangeol should be administered during or right after a feeding to reduce the risk of hypoglycemia; skip dose if child is not eating or is vomiting.

Administration

IV: IV dose is much smaller than oral dose. When administered acutely for cardiac treatment, monitor ECG and blood pressure. May administer by rapid infusion (IV push) at a rate of 1 mg/minute or by slow infusion over ~30 minutes. Necessary monitoring for surgical patients who are unable to take oral beta-blockers (prolonged ileus) has not been defined. Some institutions require monitoring of baseline and postinfusion heart rate and blood pressure when a patient's response to beta-blockade has not been characterized (ie, the patient's initial dose or following a change in dose). Consult individual institutional policies and procedures. Do not crush long-acting oral forms.

Oral: Tablets (immediate release) should be taken on an empty stomach; capsules (extended release) may be taken with or without food, but should always be taken consistently (with food or on an empty stomach). Do not crush long-acting oral forms.

Hemangeol should be administered during or right after a feeding to reduce the risk of hypoglycemia; skip dose if child is not eating or is vomiting. Administer doses at least 9 hours apart. Do not shake Hemangeol before use. Administer Hemangeol directly into the child's mouth using the supplied oral dosing syringe; if needed, may be diluted with a small quantity of milk or fruit juice and given in a baby's bottle.

Monitoring Parameters Acute cardiac treatment: Monitor ECG, heart rate, and blood pressure with IV administration; heart rate and blood pressure with oral administration

Consult individual institutional policies and procedures.

Hemangeol: Monitor heart rate and blood pressure for 2 hours after initiation or dose increases.

Dosage Forms Excipient information presented when available (limited, particularly for generics); consult specific product labeling.

Capsule Extended Release 24 Hour, Oral, as hydrochloride:

Inderal LA: 60 mg, 80 mg, 120 mg, 160 mg [contains brilliant blue fcf (fd&c blue #1)]

Inderal XL: 80 mg, 120 mg

InnoPran XL: 80 mg, 120 mg

Generic: 60 mg, 80 mg, 120 mg, 160 mg

Solution, Intravenous, as hydrochloride:

Generic: 1 mg/mL (1 mL)

Solution, Oral, as hydrochloride:

Hemangeol: 4.28 mg/mL (120 mL) [alcohol free, paraben free, sugar free; contains saccharin sodium]

Generic: 20 mg/5 mL (500 mL); 40 mg/5 mL (500 mL)

Tablet, Oral, as hydrochloride:

Generic: 10 mg, 20 mg, 40 mg, 60 mg, 80 mg

◆ Propranolol Hydrochloride *see* Propranolol *on page 1518*

◆ Propranolol Hydrochloride Injection, USP (Can) *see* Propranolol *on page 1518*

◆ Propylene Glycol Diacetate, Acetic Acid, and Hydrocortisone *see* Acetic Acid, Propylene Glycol Diacetate, and Hydrocortisone *on page 31*

◆ 2-Propylpentanoic Acid *see* Valproic Acid and Derivatives *on page 1861*

Propylthiouracil (proe pil thye oh YOOR a sil)

Brand Names: Canada Propyl-Thyracil

Index Terms PTU (error-prone abbreviation)

Pharmacologic Category Antithyroid Agent; Thioamide

Use Hyperthyroidism: Treatment of hyperthyroidism in patients with Graves' disease or toxic multinodular goiter who are intolerant of methimazole and for whom surgery or radioactive iodine therapy is not an appropriate treatment

regimen; amelioration of hyperthyroid symptoms in preparation for thyroidectomy or radioactive iodine therapy (in patients who are intolerant of methimazole).

Pregnancy Considerations Propylthiouracil has been found to readily cross the placenta. Teratogenic effects have not been observed; however, nonteratogenic adverse effects, including fetal and neonatal hypothyroidism, goiter, and hyperthyroidism, have been reported following maternal propylthiouracil use. The transfer of thyroid-stimulating immunoglobulins can stimulate the fetal thyroid in utero and transiently after delivery and may increase the risk of fetal or neonatal hyperthyroidism (De Groot 2012; Peleg 2002).

Antithyroid treatment is recommended for the control of hyperthyroidism during pregnancy (Casey 2006; De Groot 2012). Uncontrolled maternal hyperthyroidism may result in adverse neonatal outcomes (eg, prematurity, low birth weight) and adverse maternal outcomes (eg, preeclampsia, congestive heart failure, stillbirth, and abortion). To prevent adverse fetal and maternal events, normal maternal thyroid function should be maintained prior to conception and throughout pregnancy (De Groot 2012).

[US Boxed Warning]: Because of the risk of fetal abnormalities associated with methimazole, propylthiouracil may be the treatment of choice when an antithyroid drug is indicated during or just prior to the first trimester of pregnancy. Due to an increased risk of liver toxicity, use of methimazole may be preferred during the second and third trimesters. If drug therapy is changed, maternal thyroid function should be monitored after 2 weeks and then every 2 to 4 weeks (De Groot 2012). Propylthiouracil, along with other medications, is used for the treatment of thyroid storm in pregnant women (ACOG 2015).

The pharmacokinetics of propylthiouracil are not significantly changed during pregnancy; however, the severity of hyperthyroidism may fluctuate throughout pregnancy (DeGroot 2012; Sitar 1979; Sitar 1982). Doses of propylthiouracil may be decreased as pregnancy progresses and discontinued weeks to months prior to delivery.

Breast-Feeding Considerations Propylthiouracil is excreted in human breast milk; however, the infant dose is considered low and unlikely to affect infant thyroid hormones. The American Thyroid Association considers doses <300 mg/day to be safe during breast-feeding (Stagnaro-Green 2011).

Medication Guide Available Yes

Contraindications

Hypersensitivity to propylthiouracil or any component of the formulation

Canadian labeling: Additional contraindications (not in US labeling): Breast-feeding

Warnings/Precautions Hazardous agent - use appropriate precautions for handling and disposal (NIOSH 2014 [group 2]).

[US Boxed Warning]: Severe liver injury and acute liver failure (sometimes fatal) have been reported and have included cases requiring liver transplantation in adult and pediatric patients, including pregnant women. Reserve propylthiouracil for patients who cannot tolerate methimazole and in whom radioactive iodine therapy or surgery are not appropriate treatments for the management of hyperthyroidism. Routine liver function test monitoring may not reduce risk due to unpredictable and rapid onset. Patients should be counseled to recognize and report symptoms suggestive of hepatic dysfunction (eg, anorexia, pruritus, right upper quadrant pain), especially in first 6 months of treatment, which should prompt immediate discontinuation.

[US Boxed Warning]: Due to the risk of fetal abnormalities associated with methimazole, propylthiouracil may be the treatment of choice when an antithyroid drug is indicated during or just prior to the first trimester of pregnancy.

May cause significant bone marrow depression; the most severe manifestation is agranulocytosis (usually occurs within first 3 months of therapy). Aplastic anemia, thrombocytopenia, and leukopenia may also occur. Use with caution in patients receiving other drugs known to cause myelosuppression (particularly agranulocytosis); discontinue if significant bone marrow suppression occurs, particularly agranulocytosis or aplastic anemia.

A lupus-like syndrome (including splenomegaly and vasculitis) may occur. Interstitial pneumonitis has been reported; discontinue if this reaction occurs. Has been associated with nephritis and glomerulonephritis, sometimes leading to acute renal failure. ANCA-positive vasculitis or leukocytoclastic vasculitis may occur; discontinue in

patients who develop vasculitis during therapy. May cause hypoprothrombinemia and bleeding. Monitoring is recommended, especially before surgical procedures. May cause hypothyroidism; routinely monitor TSH and free T_4 levels, adjust dose to maintain euthyroid state. Dermatologic toxicity may occur; discontinue in the presence of exfoliative dermatitis.

Potentially significant interactions may exist, requiring dose or frequency adjustment, additional monitoring, and/or selection of alternative therapy.

Adverse Reactions Frequency not defined.

Cardiovascular: Edema, periarteritis, vasculitis (ANCA-positive, cutaneous, leukocytoclastic)

Central nervous system: Drowsiness, drug fever, headache, neuritis, paresthesia, vertigo

Dermatologic: Alopecia, dermal ulcer, erythema nodosum, exfoliative dermatitis, pruritus, skin pigmentation, skin rash, Stevens-Johnson syndrome, toxic epidermal necrolysis, urticaria

Gastrointestinal: Ageusia, dysgeusia, nausea, salivary gland disease, stomach pain, vomiting

Hematologic & oncologic: Agranulocytosis, aplastic anemia, granulocytopenia, hemorrhage, hypoprothrombinemia, leukopenia, lymphadenopathy, splenomegaly, thrombocytopenia

Hepatic: Acute hepatic failure, hepatitis, hepatotoxicity (idiosyncratic) (Chalasani 2014), jaundice

Neuromuscular & skeletal: Arthralgia, lupus-like syndrome, myalgia

Renal: Acute renal failure, glomerulonephritis, nephritis

Respiratory: Interstitial pneumonitis, pulmonary alveolar hemorrhage

Miscellaneous: Fever

Drug Interactions

Metabolism/Transport Effects None known.

Avoid Concomitant Use

Avoid concomitant use of Propylthiouracil with any of the following: BCG (Intravesical); Deferiprone; Dipyrone; Sodium Iodide I131

Increased Effect/Toxicity

Propylthiouracil may increase the levels/effects of: Cardiac Glycosides; CloZAPine; Deferiprone; Theophylline Derivatives

The levels/effects of Propylthiouracil may be increased by: Dipyrone

Decreased Effect

Propylthiouracil may decrease the levels/effects of: BCG (Intravesical); Sodium Iodide I131; Vitamin K Antagonists

Storage/Stability Store at 15°C to 30°C (59°F to 86°F).

Mechanism of Action Inhibits the synthesis of thyroid hormones by blocking the conversion of thyroxine to triiodothyronine in peripheral tissues (does not inactivate existing thyroxine and triiodothyronine stores in circulating blood and the thyroid and does not interfere with replacement thyroid hormones.

Pharmacodynamics/Kinetics

Duration: 12 to 24 hours (Clark 2006)

Distribution: Concentrated in the thyroid gland (Clark 2006)

Protein binding: 80% to 85% (Clark 2006)

Metabolism: Hepatic

Bioavailability: 53% to 88% (Clark 2006)

Half-life elimination: ~1 hour (Clark 2006)

Time to peak, serum: 1 to 2 hours (Clark 2006)

Excretion: Urine (35%; primarily as metabolites)

Dosing

Adult

Hyperthyroidism: Oral:

US labeling: Initial: 300 mg daily in 3 equally divided doses (~8-hour intervals); 400 mg daily in patients with severe hyperthyroidism and/or very large goiters; an occasional patient will require 600 to 900 mg daily; usual maintenance: 100 to 150 mg daily in 3 equally divided doses

Canadian labeling: Initial: 50 to 100 mg every 8 hours; may increase up to a maximum of 500 mg daily; some patients may require initial doses up to 900 mg daily. May reduce dose (euthyroid usually occurs after 6 to 8 weeks) by 1/3 every 4 to 6 weeks to a maintenance dose of 50 mg 2 or 3 times daily. **Note:** Administer doses >300 mg daily every 4 to 6 hours.

Graves' disease (off-label dosing): Oral: Initial: 50 to 150 mg (depending on severity) 3 times daily to restore euthyroidism; maintenance: 50 mg 2 to 3 times daily for a total of 12 to 18 months, then tapered or discontinued if TSH is normal at that time (Bahn 2011)

Thyrotoxic crisis/thyroid storm (off-label dosing): Oral: **Note:** Recommendations vary widely and have not been evaluated in comparative trials. Typical dosing is 800 to 1,200 mg/day given as 200 to 300 mg every 4 to 6 hours; some clinicians advocate an initial loading dose of 600 to 1,000 mg. After initial response, dose

may be reduced gradually to a maintenance dosage (100 to 600 mg/day in divided doses) (Goldberg 2003; Nayak 2006). The American Thyroid Association and the American Association of Clinical Endocrinologists recommend 500 to 1,000 mg loading dose followed by 250 mg every 4 hours (Bahn 2011).

Duration of therapy: Clinical improvement generally occurs in 1 to 3 months, after which dosage reduction may be employed (to prevent hypothyroidism), with discontinuation considered after 12 to 18 months of therapy. Thyroid function should be monitored every 2 months thereafter for 6 months until remission is confirmed, followed by annual evaluations (Cooper 2005).

Pediatric Hyperthyroidism: *Canadian labeling:* Oral: (generally not recommended for use in children unless alternative therapies are not appropriate):
Initial dose guideline: 150 mg/m^2/day
Children 6 to 10 years: 50 to 150 mg daily in 3 equally divided doses (~8-hour intervals)
Children >10 years and Adolescents: 150 to 300 mg daily in 3 equally divided doses (~8-hour intervals)
Maintenance dose (general): 50 mg twice daily (when euthyroid)

Renal Impairment There are no dosage adjustments provided in the manufacturer's labeling.

Hepatic Impairment There are no dosage adjustments provided in the manufacturer's labeling.

Administration Administer orally in 3 equally divided doses at approximately 8 hour intervals. Administer doses >300 mg/day divided every 4 to 6 hours (Canadian labeling).

Hazardous agent; use appropriate precautions for handling and disposal (NIOSH 2014 [group 2]). Avoid exposure to crushed or broken tablets; if it is necessary to manipulate the tablets (eg, to prepare an oral solution), it is recommended to double glove, wear a protective gown, and prepare in a controlled device. Disposable gloves should be worn when handling tablets or suspension for administration; health care providers should also wear a protective gown (NIOSH 2014).

Monitoring Parameters CBC with differential, prothrombin time (especially before surgical procedures), liver function tests (bilirubin, alkaline phosphatase, ALT, AST), and thyroid function tests (TSH, T$_3$, T$_4$) every 4 to 6 weeks until euthyroid; periodic blood counts are recommended for chronic therapy

Reference Range Normal laboratory values:
Total T$_4$: 5 to 12 mcg/dL
Serum T$_3$: 90 to 185 ng/dL
Free thyroxine index (FT$_4$ I): 6 to 10.5
TSH: 0.5 to 4.0 microunits/mL

Additional Information Preferred over methimazole in thyroid storm due to inhibition of peripheral conversion as well as synthesis of thyroid hormone.

Graves' hyperthyroidism: Elevated T$_3$ may be the sole indicator of inadequate treatment. Elevated TSH indicates excessive antithyroid treatment. Monitoring of TSH is a poor indicator of treatment effectiveness, as levels may remain suppressed for months, despite euthyroid state (Cooper 2005).

A potency ratio of methimazole to propylthiouracil of at least 20-30:1 is recommended when changing from one drug to another (eg, 300 mg of propylthiouracil would be roughly equivalent to 10-15 mg of methimazole) (Bahn 2011).

Dosage Forms Excipient information presented when available (limited, particularly for generics); consult specific product labeling.
Tablet, Oral:
Generic: 50 mg

Extemporaneous Preparations Hazardous agent; use appropriate precautions for handling and disposal (NIOSH 2014 [group 2]). When manipulating tablets, NIOSH recommends double gloving, a protective gown, and preparation in a controlled device; if not prepared in a controlled device, respiratory and eye protection as well as ventilated engineering controls are recommended (NIOSH 2014).

A 5 mg/mL oral suspension may be made with tablets and a 1:1 mixture of Ora-Plus and Ora-Sweet. Crush twenty 50 mg propylthiouracil tablets in a mortar and reduce to a fine powder. Add small portions of vehicle and mix to a uniform paste; mix while adding vehicle in incremental proportions to **almost** 200 mL; transfer to a calibrated bottle, rinse mortar with vehicle, and add quantity of vehicle sufficient to make 200 mL. Label "shake well" and "refrigerate". Stable for 91 days refrigerated (preferred) and 70 days at room temperature.
Nahata MC, Pai VB, and Hipple TF, *Pediatric Drug Formulations*, 5th ed, Cincinnati, OH: Harvey Whitney Books Co, 2004.

Protamine (PROE ta meen)

Index Terms Protamine Sulfate
Pharmacologic Category Antidote
Additional Appendix Information
Reversal of Oral Anticoagulants *on page 1959*
Use Treatment of heparin overdosage; neutralize heparin during surgery or dialysis procedures
Pregnancy Considerations Animal reproduction studies have not been conducted. In general, medications used as antidotes should take into consideration the health and prognosis of the mother; antidotes should be administered to pregnant women if there is a clear indication for use and should not be withheld because of fears of teratogenicity (Bailey, 2003). Protamine sulfate may be used during delivery to reduce the risk of bleeding following maternal use of heparin or low molecular weight heparin (LMWH) (Bates, 2012).
Breast-Feeding Considerations It is not known if protamine is excreted in breast milk. The manufacturer recommends that caution be exercised when administering protamine to nursing women.
Contraindications Hypersensitivity to protamine or any component of the formulation
Warnings/Precautions May not be totally effective in some patients following cardiac surgery despite adequate doses. May cause hypersensitivity reaction in patients (have epinephrine 1:1000 and resuscitation equipment available). **[U.S. Boxed Warning]: Hypotension, cardiovascular collapse, noncardiogenic pulmonary edema, pulmonary vasoconstriction, and pulmonary hypertension may occur. Risk factors for such events include: use of high doses or overdose, repeated doses, previous protamine administration (including protamine-containing drugs), fish allergy, vasectomy, severe left ventricular dysfunction, abnormal preoperative pulmonary hemodynamics.** Too rapid administration can cause severe hypotensive and anaphylactoid-like reactions. Heparin rebound associated with anticoagulation and bleeding has been reported to occur occasionally; symptoms typically occur 8-9 hours after protamine administration, but may occur as long as 18 hours later.
Adverse Reactions Frequency not defined.
Cardiovascular: Sudden fall in blood pressure, bradycardia, flushing, hypotension
Central nervous system: Lassitude
Gastrointestinal: Nausea, vomiting
Hematologic: Hemorrhage
Respiratory: Dyspnea, pulmonary hypertension
Miscellaneous: Hypersensitivity reactions

◄

Drug Interactions

Metabolism/Transport Effects None known.

Avoid Concomitant Use There are no known interactions where it is recommended to avoid concomitant use.

Increased Effect/Toxicity There are no known significant interactions involving an increase in effect.

Decreased Effect There are no known significant interactions involving a decrease in effect.

Storage/Stability Refrigerate; do not freeze. Stable for at least 2 weeks at room temperature. Preservative-free formulation does not require refrigeration.

Mechanism of Action Combines with strongly acidic heparin to form a stable complex (salt) neutralizing the anticoagulant activity of both drugs

Pharmacodynamics/Kinetics

Onset of action: IV: Heparin neutralization: ~5 minutes

Half-life elimination: ~7 minutes

Dosing

Adult & Geriatric

Heparin neutralization: IV: Protamine dosage is determined by the dosage of heparin; 1 mg of protamine neutralizes ~100 units of heparin; maximum dose: 50 mg

Note: When heparin is given as a continuous IV infusion, only heparin given in the preceding several hours should be considered when administering protamine. For example, a patient receiving heparin at 1250 units/hour will require ~30 mg of protamine for reversal of heparin given in the last 2-2.5 hours (Garcia, 2012).

Heparin overdosage, following intravenous administration: IV: Since blood heparin concentrations decrease rapidly **after** administration, adjust the protamine dosage depending upon the duration of time since heparin administration as follows: See table.

Time Elapsed	Dose of Protamine (mg) to Neutralize 100 units of Heparin
Immediate	1-1.5
30-60 min	0.5-0.75
>2 h	0.25-0.375

Heparin overdosage, following SubQ injection: IV: 1-1.5 mg protamine per 100 units heparin; this may be done by a portion of the dose (eg, 25-50 mg) given slowly IV followed by the remaining portion as a continuous infusion over 8-16 hours (the expected absorption time of the SubQ heparin dose) (Caravati 2004).

LMWH overdose (off-label use): IV: **Note:** Anti-Xa activity is never completely neutralized (maximum: ~60% to 75%). Excessive protamine doses may worsen bleeding potential.

Enoxaparin (Lovenox® prescribing information, 2011):

Enoxaparin administered in ≤8 hours: Dose of protamine should equal the dose of enoxaparin administered. Therefore, 1 mg of protamine sulfate neutralizes 1 mg of enoxaparin.

Enoxaparin administered in >8 hours or if it has been determined that a second dose of protamine is required (eg, if aPTT measured 2-4 hours after the first dose remains prolonged or if bleeding continues): 0.5 mg of protamine sulfate for every 1 mg of enoxaparin administered

Dalteparin or tinzaparin (Fragmin® prescribing information, 2010; Innohep® prescribing information, 2010): 1 mg protamine for each 100 anti-Xa units of dalteparin or tinzaparin; if PTT prolonged 2-4 hours after first dose (or if bleeding continues), consider additional dose of 0.5 mg for each 100 anti-Xa units of dalteparin or tinzaparin.

Pediatric Refer to adult dosing.

Renal Impairment No dosage adjustment provided in manufacturer's labeling.

Hepatic Impairment No dosage adjustment provided in manufacturer's labeling.

Administration For IV use only; **incompatible** with cephalosporins and penicillins; administer slow IVP (50 mg over 10 minutes); rapid IV infusion causes hypotension; inject without further dilution over 1-3 minutes; maximum of 50 mg in any 10-minute period

Monitoring Parameters Coagulation test, aPTT or ACT, cardiac monitor and blood pressure monitor required during administration

Dosage Forms Excipient information presented when available (limited, particularly for generics); consult specific product labeling.

Solution, Intravenous, as sulfate:

Generic: 10 mg/mL (5 mL, 25 mL)

Solution, Intravenous, as sulfate [preservative free]:

Generic: 10 mg/mL (5 mL, 25 mL)

◆ Protamine Sulfate *see* Protamine *on page 1523*

◆ Protease, Lipase, and Amylase *see* Pancrelipase *on page 1384*

◆ Proteasome Inhibitor MLN9708 *see* Ixazomib *on page 1008*

◆ Protein C *see* Protein C Concentrate (Human) *on page 1524*

◆ Protein-Bound Paclitaxel *see* PACLitaxel (Protein Bound) *on page 1371*

Protein C Concentrate (Human)
(PROE teen cee KON suhn trate HYU man)

Brand Names: US Ceprotin

Index Terms Protein C

Pharmacologic Category Blood Product Derivative; Enzyme; Protein C

Use Severe congenital protein C deficiency: Prevention and treatment of venous thrombosis and purpura fulminans in adults and pediatric patients with severe congenital protein C deficiency.

Dosing

Adult Patient variables (including age, clinical condition, severity of protein C deficiency, and plasma levels of protein C) will influence dosing and duration of therapy. Individualize frequency, duration, and dose based on protein C activity and patient pharmacokinetic profile.

Severe congenital protein C deficiency: IV:

Acute episode/short-term prophylaxis: Initial dose: 100 to 120 units/kg (for determination of recovery and half-life)

Subsequent 3 doses: 60 to 80 units/kg every 6 hours (adjust to maintain peak protein C activity of 100%)

Maintenance dose: 45 to 60 units/kg every 6 or 12 hours (adjust to maintain recommended maintenance trough protein C activity levels >25%)

Long-term prophylaxis: Maintenance dose: 45 to 60 units/kg every 12 hours (recommended maintenance trough protein C activity levels >25%)

Note: Maintain target peak protein C activity of 100% during acute episodes and short-term prophylaxis. After resolution of the acute episode or for long-term prophylaxis, maintain trough levels of protein C activity >25%. Higher peak levels of protein C may be necessary in prophylactic therapy of patients at increased risk for thrombosis (eg, infection, trauma, surgical intervention). If a patient is switched to an oral anticoagulant, continue protein C replacement until stable anticoagulation is obtained. Initiate the oral anticoagulant at a low dose and adjust incrementally, rather than using a standard loading dose.

Pediatric Patient variables (including age, clinical condition, severity of protein C deficiency, and plasma levels of protein C) will influence dosing and duration of therapy. Individualize frequency, duration, and dose based on protein C activity and patient pharmacokinetic profile.

Severe congenital protein C deficiency: Infants, Children, and Adolescents: IV: Refer to adult dosing.

Note: Maintain target peak protein C activity of 100% during acute episodes and short-term prophylaxis. After resolution of the acute episode or for long-term prophylaxis, maintain trough levels of protein C activity >25%. Higher peak levels of protein C may be necessary in prophylactic therapy of patients at increased risk for thrombosis (eg, infection, trauma, surgical intervention). If a patient is switched to an oral anticoagulant, continue protein C replacement until stable anticoagulation is obtained. Initiate the oral anticoagulant at a low dose and adjust incrementally, rather than using a standard loading dose.

Renal Impairment There are no dosage adjustments provided in the manufacturer's labeling (has not been studied); monitor closely for sodium overload.

Hepatic Impairment There are no dosage adjustments provided in the manufacturer's labeling (has not been studied).

Additional Information Complete prescribing information should be consulted for additional detail.

Dosage Forms Excipient information presented when available (limited, particularly for generics); consult specific product labeling.

Solution Reconstituted, Intravenous [preservative free]:

Ceprotin: 500 units (1 ea); 1000 units (1 ea) [contains albumin human, heparin, mouse protein (murine) (hamster)]

◆ Prothrombin Complex Concentrate (Caution: Confusion-prone synonym) *see* Factor IX Complex (Human) [(Factors II, IX, X)] *on page 734*

◆ Prothrombin Complex Concentrate (Caution: Confusion-prone synonym) *see* Prothrombin Complex Concentrate (Human) [(Factors II, VII, IX, X), Protein C, and Protein S] *on page 1525*

Prothrombin Complex Concentrate (Human) [(Factors II, VII, IX, X), Protein C, and Protein S]

(PRO throm bin KOM pleks KON cen trate HYU man FAK ters too SEV en nyne ten PROE teen cee & PROE teen ess)

Brand Names: US Kcentra

Brand Names: Canada Beriplex P/N; Octaplex

Index Terms 4 Factor PCC; 4-Factor PCC; Beriplex P/N; Confidex; Four-Factor PCC; PCC (Caution: Confusion-prone synonym); Prothrombin Complex Concentrate (Caution: Confusion-prone synonym)

Pharmacologic Category Blood Product Derivative; Hemostatic Agent; Prothrombin Complex Concentrate (PCC)

Additional Appendix Information

Reversal of Oral Anticoagulants *on page 1959*

Use Bleeding, treatment and prophylaxis: Urgent reversal of acquired coagulation factor deficiency induced by vitamin K antagonist (VKA) (eg, warfarin) therapy in patients with acute major bleeding or a need for an urgent surgery/invasive procedure

Pregnancy Considerations Animal reproduction studies have not been conducted. Parvovirus B19 or hepatitis A, which may be present in plasma-derived products, may affect a pregnant woman more seriously than a nonpregnant woman.

Breast-Feeding Considerations It is not known if prothrombin complex concentrate is excreted in breast milk. The manufacturer recommends that PCC be administered only if clearly needed when treating a nursing woman.

Contraindications

Kcentra, Beriplex P/N [Canadian product]: Hypersensitivity (ie, anaphylaxis or severe systemic reaction) to prothrombin complex concentrate (PCC) or any component of the formulation including factors II, VII, IX, X, protein C and S, antithrombin III and human albumin; disseminated intravascular coagulation (DIC); known heparin-induced thrombocytopenia (product contains heparin).

Octaplex [Canadian product]: Hypersensitivity to prothrombin complex concentrate (PCC) or any component of the formulation; heparin-induced thrombocytopenia type II or known allergy to heparin (product contains heparin); non-life-threatening bleeding episodes in individuals with recent myocardial infarction, high risk of thrombosis, or angina pectoris; non-life-threatening bleeding episodes in individuals with untreated disseminated intravascular coagulation (DIC) who can be given fresh frozen plasma (FFP); coagulation disorders due to chronic liver disease or liver transplantation; bleeding associated with hepatic parenchyme disorders, esophageal varices, or major hepatic surgery; immunoglobulin A (IgA) deficiency, with known antibodies against IgA

Warnings/Precautions [US Boxed Warning]: Because patients being treated with vitamin K antagonist (VKA) therapy have an underlying risk of or a diagnosed thromboembolic disease state, administration of prothrombin complex concentrate (PCC) may predispose the patient to a thromboembolic complication. Benefits of reversing VKA therapy should be weighed against the potential risk of a thromboembolic event. Resumption of anticoagulation should occur once the risk of thromboembolism outweighs the risk of acute bleeding. Fatal and nonfatal arterial and venous thromboembolic complications and DIC have been reported; closely monitor for thromboembolic events during and after administration. Use has not been evaluated in patients who have experienced a thromboembolic event, MI, DIC, CVA, TIA, unstable angina, or severe peripheral vascular disease within the prior 3 months. Administration of PCC may exacerbate underlying hypercoagulable states in recipients of vitamin K antagonists.

Prothrombin complex concentrate (Human) [(Factors II, VII, IX, X), Protein C, Protein S] (Kcentra, Beriplex P/N [Canadian product], and Octaplex [Canadian product]) contains therapeutic levels of factor VII component and should not be confused with Factor IX complex (Human) [Factors II, IX, X] (Bebulin, Profilnine) which contains low or nontherapeutic levels of factor VII. Hypersensitivity reaction (eg, angioedema, bronchospasm, dyspnea, flushing, hypotension, nausea/vomiting, pulmonary edema, urticaria, tachycardia, tachypnea) may occur; if serious reaction occurs, discontinue administration and begin appropriate treatment. Since severe hypersensitivity and anaphylactic reactions may rarely occur with use;

immediate medical treatment (including epinephrine 1:1,000) should be readily available in the event of a severe reaction. May consider prophylactic treatment (eg, antihistamines, glucocorticoids) in patients predisposed to allergies. Formulations contain heparin.

Product of human plasma; may potentially contain infectious agents which could transmit disease. Screening of donors, as well as testing and/or inactivation or removal of certain viruses, reduces the risk. Infections thought to be transmitted by this product should be reported to the manufacturer. Beriplex P/N and Octaplex [Canadian products] labeling recommends consideration of hepatitis A and hepatitis B vaccination for all patients receiving regular/repeated administration of human plasma-derived prothrombin complex products.

Hepatic synthesis of the prothrombin complex (Factors II, VII, IX and X) coagulation factors is vitamin K dependent. Severe hepatic dysfunction, inadequate absorption of vitamin K (eg, pancreatic disorders, diarrhea) or vitamin K antagonist therapy or overdose may lead to coagulation factor deficiencies. In patients with an acquired deficiency of the vitamin K-dependent coagulation factors, administer PCC only if a rapid correction (eg, emergency surgery, major bleeding) is necessary. If not indicated and caused by Vitamin K antagonist therapy, coagulation factor deficiencies may be managed by reducing or discontinuing therapy of the vitamin K antagonist and/or administration of vitamin K.

Octaplex [Canadian product]: Development of antibodies to one or more of the human prothrombin factors may occur rarely, resulting in an inadequate clinical response; monitor for signs of antibody formation. Product labeling recommends monitoring antithrombin (AT) levels in patients being treated for bleeding as a result of chronic liver disease or liver transplantation. If AT levels are deficient, AT should be administered concomitantly with PCC. No clinical data are available for use of PCC to treat bleeding due to liver parenchyme disorders, major liver surgery, or esophageal varices; use of PCC for these indications is contraindicated and the preferred method of treatment is fresh frozen plasma (FFP).

Adverse Reactions

1% to 10%:

Cardiovascular: Hypotension (5% to 7%), tachycardia (3% to 5%), atrial fibrillation (4%), hypertension (1% to 3%), pulmonary embolism (≤2%), pulmonary edema (2%), cerebrovascular accident (1% to 2%), arteriovenous fistula site complication (clot, ≤1%), chest pain (1%), deep vein thrombosis (1%), venous thrombosis (calf, 1%; radial vein: ≤1%), thrombosis (microthrombosis of toes, ≤1%)

Central nervous system: Headache (1% to 8%), insomnia (1% to 5%), intracranial hemorrhage (3%), mental status changes (3%)

Endocrine & metabolic: Hypervolemia (1% to 6%), hypokalemia (2% to 5%)

Gastrointestinal: Nausea and vomiting (4% to 6%), constipation (2%), diarrhea (2%)

Hematologic and oncologic: Anemia (3% to 6%), prolonged bleeding time (skin laceration, contusion, subcutaneous hematoma, 4%)

Hepatic: Increased serum transaminases (1%)

Immunologic: Antibody development (parvovirus B19 seropositive, 3%)

Local: Burning sensation at injection site (1%)

Neuromuscular & skeletal: Arthralgia (4%)

Respiratory: Pleural effusion (4%), respiratory distress (2% to 4%), rales (1%)

Postmarketing and/or case reports (Limited to important or life-threatening): Angioedema, arterial thrombosis, bronchospasm, disseminated intravascular coagulation, hypersensitivity reaction, myocardial infarction, peripheral ischemia, thromboembolic complications, thrombosis, transient ischemic attacks, venous insufficiency

Preparation for Administration Kcentra, Beriplex P/N [Canadian product], or Octaplex [Canadian product]: Prior to reconstitution, allow diluent (SWFI) and prothrombin complex concentrate (PCC) vials to warm to room temperature. Aseptically push the plastic spike at the blue end of the Mix2Vial transfer set through the center of the stopper of the diluent vial. After carefully removing only the clear package from the Mix2Vial transfer set, invert the diluent vial with the transfer set still attached and push the plastic spike through the center of the stopper of PCC vial; diluent will automatically transfer. While still attached, gently swirl PCC vial to ensure product is dissolved; do not shake. Disconnect the 2 vials; contents of PCC vial are now available for removal by screwing a syringe onto the transfer set. Inject appropriate amount of air into vial, invert vial, and withdraw amount needed. Remove syringe from transfer set and attach an administration set to the syringe.

Note: Kcentra vials may contain differing amounts of factor IX units per vial. The exact amount of factor IX units in each vial should be used when calculating and preparing the total dose to be administered. Overdosage errors have occurred when the dose has been improperly calculated. (ISMP 2014)

Storage/Stability

Kcentra, Beriplex P/N [Canadian product]: Store at 2°C to 25°C (36°F to 77°F); do not freeze. Protect from light. Reconstituted product may be stored at 2°C to 25°C (36°F to 77°F) and used within 4 hours (Kcentra) or 3 hours (Beriplex P/N) following reconstitution. If cooled, warm to 20°C to 25°C (68°F to 77°F) prior to administration.

Octaplex [Canadian product]: Store at 2°C to 25°C (36°F to 77°F); do not freeze. Protect from light. Reconstituted solution should be administered immediately, but may be stored for up to 8 hours at 2°C to 25°C (36°F to 77°F) if sterility is maintained.

Mechanism of Action

Prothrombin complex concentrate provides an increase in the levels of the vitamin K-dependent coagulation factors (II, VII, IX, and X) with the addition of protein C and protein S. Coagulation factors II, IX, and X are part of the intrinsic coagulation pathway, while factor VII is part of the extrinsic coagulation pathway. In the *extrinsic* pathway, damaged blood vessels release endothelial tissue factor (TF) which complexes with factor VII to form TF-factor VIIa. Within the *intrinsic* pathway, factor IX is converted to IXa. Factor IXa (as well as TF-factor VIIa) converts factor X to factor Xa in the final common pathway of coagulation. Factor Xa activates prothrombin (factor II) into thrombin (IIa) which converts fibrinogen into fibrin resulting in clot formation. Proteins C and S are vitamin K-dependent inhibiting enzymes involved in regulating the coagulation process. Protein S serves as a cofactor for protein C which is converted to activated protein C (APC). APC is a serine protease which inactivates factors Va and VIIIa, limiting thrombotic formation.

Pharmacodynamics/Kinetics

Onset of action: Rapid; significant INR decline within 10 minutes

Duration: ~6 to 8 hours

Distribution: V_{dss}: Factor II: 71.4 mL/kg; Factor VII: 45 mL/kg; Factor IX: 114.3 mL/kg; Factor X: 55.5 mL/kg; Protein C: 62.2 mL/kg; Protein S: 78.8 mL/kg

Half-life elimination: Factor II: 48 to 60 hours; Factor VII: 1.5 to 6 hours; Factor IX: 20 to 24 hours; Factor X: 24 to 48 hours; Protein C: 1.5 to 6 hours; Protein S: 24 to 48 hours

Note: Half-lives may be significantly reduced in severe hepatocellular damage, DIC, or extended catabolic metabolism.

Dosing

Adult & Geriatric Note: Prothrombin complex concentrate (Human) [(Factors II, VII, IX, X), Protein C, Protein S] (Kcentra, Beriplex P/N [Canadian product], and Octaplex [Canadian product]) contains therapeutic levels of factor VII component and should not be confused with Factor IX complex (Human) [Factors II, IX, X] (Bebulin, Profilnine) which contains low or nontherapeutic levels of factor VII.

Kcentra, Beriplex P/N [Canadian product]: **Vitamin K antagonist (VKA) reversal in patients with acute major bleeding or need for an urgent surgery/invasive procedure:** IV: Individualize dosing based on current pre-dose INR. Dosage is expressed in units of factor IX activity. Administer with vitamin K concurrently. Repeat dosing is not recommended (has not been studied).

Pretreatment INR: 2 to <4: Administer 25 units/kg; maximum dose: 2,500 units

Pretreatment INR: 4 to 6: Administer 35 units/kg; maximum dose: 3,500 units

Pretreatment INR: >6: Administer 50 units/kg; maximum dose: 5,000 units

Octaplex [Canadian product]: **Bleeding/perioperative prophylaxis of bleeding during vitamin K antagonist therapy:** Individualized dosing based on severity of disorder, extent and location of bleeding, and clinical status of patient. IV: Approximate doses required for normalization of INR (≤1.2 within 1 hour); dosage is expressed in units of factor IX activity:

Pretreatment INR: 2 to 2.5: Administer 22.5 to 32.5 units/kg; maximum dose: 3,000 units (or 120 mL)

Pretreatment INR: 2.5 to 3: Administer 32.5 to 40 units/kg; maximum dose: 3,000 units (or 120 mL)

Pretreatment INR: 3 to 3.5: Administer 40 to 47.5 units/kg; maximum dose: 3,000 units (or 120 mL)

Pretreatment INR: >3.5: Administer >47.5 units/kg; maximum dose: 3,000 units (or 120 mL)

With the correction of vitamin K antagonist-induced impairment of hemostasis in patients who have been treated concomitantly with an appropriate vitamin K dose, repeat dosing with PCC is usually not necessary.

Pediatric Octaplex [Canadian product]: Adolescents ≥17 years: Refer to adult dosing.

Renal Impairment There are no dosage adjustments provided in the manufacturer's labeling.

Hepatic Impairment There are no dosage adjustments provided in the manufacturer's labeling.

Obesity Kcentra, Beriplex [Canadian product]: In patients weighing >100 kg; do not exceed maximum dose recommended according to pretreatment INR.

Administration

Kcentra, Beriplex P/N [Canadian product]: IV: Administer at room temperature at a rate of 0.12 mL/kg/minute (~3 **units**/kg/minute); do **not** exceed 8.4 mL/minute (~210 **units**/minute). Do not allow blood to enter into syringe; since fibrin clot formation may occur.

Octaplex [Canadian product]: IV: Administer at a rate of 1 mL/minute initially, followed by 2 to 3 mL/minute. Reduce infusion rate or interrupt infusion if patient's pulse rate increases significantly.

Monitoring Parameters

Kcentra: INR (baseline and at 30 minutes post dose); clinical response during and after treatment; signs of thromboembolism

Octaplex [Canadian product]: Coagulation factor assays, protein C, protein S, aPTT, PT, INR, CBC, AT, D-dimer, fibrinogen; development of circulating coagulation factor antibodies (inhibitors); heart rate (before and during administration)

Test Interactions aPTT (formulation contains heparin)

Dosage Forms Considerations

Kcentra, Beriplex P/N [Canadian product]: **Note:** Potency on the vial label is expressed in terms of the Factor IX nominal strength (500 units or 1,000 units). Consult individual vial labels for exact potency within each vial.

Total active ingredient composition of 500 unit vial is:
Factor II: 380 to 800 units
Factor VII: 200 to 500 units
Factor IX: 400 to 620 units (Kcentra) or 500 units (Beriplex P/N)
Factor X: 500 to 1,020 units
Protein C: 420 to 820 units
Protein S: 240 to 680 units

Total active ingredient composition of 1,000 unit vial is:
Factor II: 760 to 1,600 units
Factor VII: 400 to 1,000 units
Factor IX: 800 to 1,240 units (Kcentra) or 1,000 units (Beriplex P/N)
Factor X: 1,000 to 2,040 units
Protein C: 840 to 1,640 units
Protein S: 480 to 1,360 units

Octaplex [Canadian product]: **Note:** Potency on the vial label is expressed in terms of the Factor IX nominal strength (500 units or 1,000 units). Consult individual vial labels for exact potency within each vial.

Total active ingredient composition of 500 unit vial is:
Factor II: 280 to 760 units
Factor VII: 180 to 480 units
Factor IX: 500 units
Factor X: 360 to 600 units
Protein C: 260 to 620 units
Proteins S: 240 to 640 units

Total active ingredient composition of 1,000 unit vial is:
Factor II: 560 to 1,520 units
Factor VII: 360 to 960 units
Factor IX: 1,000 units
Factor X: 720 to 1,200 units
Protein C: 520 to 1,240 units
Protein S: 480 to 1,280 units

Dosage Forms Excipient information presented when available (limited, particularly for generics); consult specific product labeling.

Kit, Intravenous [preservative free]:
Kcentra: ~500 units, ~1000 units [pyrogen free; contains albumin human, heparin]

Dosage Forms: Canada Excipient information presented when available (limited, particularly for generics); consult specific product labeling.

Kit, Intravenous [preservative free]:
Beriplex P/N: 500 units, 1000 units [pyrogen free, contains albumin human, heparin; packaged with diluent]
Octaplex: 500 units, 1000 units [contains heparin, polysorbate 80; packaged with diluent]

◆ Protonix *see* Pantoprazole *on page 1390*

◆ Protopam Chloride *see* Pralidoxime *on page 1486*

◆ Protopic *see* Tacrolimus (Topical) *on page 1729*

◆ Protopic® (Can) *see* Tacrolimus (Topical) *on page 1729*

♦ PRO-Topiramate (Can) *see* Topiramate *on page 1810*

♦ Pro-Triazide (Can) *see* Hydrochlorothiazide and Triamterene *on page 884*

♦ Protrin DF (Can) *see* Sulfamethoxazole and Trimethoprim *on page 1710*

Protriptyline (proe TRIP ti leen)

Brand Names: US Vivactil [DSC]
Index Terms Protriptyline Hydrochloride; Vivactil
Pharmacologic Category Antidepressant, Tricyclic (Secondary Amine)
Use Depression: Treatment of depression
Medication Guide Available Yes
Dosing

Adult Depression: Oral: Initial: 10 to 20 mg daily divided in 3 to 4 doses; gradually increase based on response and tolerability to a usual dose of 20 to 60 mg/day in 3 to 4 divided doses; maximum 60 mg/day (APA, 2010; Bauer, 2013)

Discontinuation of therapy: Upon discontinuation of antidepressant therapy, gradually taper the dose to minimize the incidence of withdrawal symptoms and allow for the detection of re-emerging symptoms. Evidence supporting ideal taper rates is limited. APA and NICE guidelines suggest tapering therapy over at least several weeks with consideration to the half-life of the antidepressant; antidepressants with a shorter half-life may need to be tapered more conservatively. In addition for long-term treated patients, WFSBP guidelines recommend tapering over 4-6 months. If intolerable withdrawal symptoms occur following a dose reduction, consider resuming the previously prescribed dose and/or decrease dose at a more gradual rate (APA, 2010; Bauer, 2002; Haddad, 2001; NCCMH, 2010; Schatzberg, 2006; Shelton, 2001; Warner, 2006).

MAO inhibitor recommendations:
Switching to or from an MAO inhibitor intended to treat psychiatric disorders:
Allow 14 days to elapse between discontinuing an MAO inhibitor intended to treat psychiatric disorders and initiation of protriptyline.
Allow 14 days to elapse between discontinuing protriptyline and initiation of an MAO inhibitor intended to treat psychiatric disorders.
Use with other MAO inhibitors (such as linezolid or IV methylene blue):
Do not initiate protriptyline in patients receiving linezolid or IV methylene blue; consider other interventions for psychiatric condition.
If urgent treatment with linezolid or IV methylene blue is required in a patient already receiving protriptyline and potential benefits outweigh potential risks, discontinue protriptyline promptly and administer linezolid or IV methylene blue. Monitor for serotonin syndrome for 2 weeks or until 24 hours after the last dose of linezolid or IV methylene blue, whichever comes first. May resume protriptyline 24 hours after the last dose of linezolid or IV methylene blue.

Geriatric Depression: Oral: Initial: 15 mg daily in 3 divided doses; gradually increase based on response and tolerability; maximum 60 mg/day. **Note:** Monitor cardiovascular system closely if daily dose exceeds 20 mg.
Discontinuation of therapy: Refer to adult dosing.
MAO inhibitor recommendations: Refer to adult dosing.

Pediatric Depression: Adolescents: Oral: Initial: 15 mg daily in 3 divided doses; gradually increase based on response and tolerability; maximum 60 mg/day. **Note:** Controlled clinical trials have not shown tricyclic antidepressants to be superior to placebo for the treatment of children and adolescents; not recommended as a first-line medication (Dopheide, 2006; Wagner, 2005).
Discontinuation of therapy: Refer to adult dosing.
MAO inhibitor recommendations: Refer to adult dosing.

Renal Impairment There are no dosage adjustments provided in the manufacturer's labeling.
Hepatic Impairment There are no dosage adjustments provided in the manufacturer's labeling.

Additional Information Complete prescribing information should be consulted for additional detail.

Dosage Forms Excipient information presented when available (limited, particularly for generics); consult specific product labeling. [DSC] = Discontinued product
Tablet, Oral, as hydrochloride:
Vivactil: 5 mg [DSC] [contains fd&c red #40, fd&c yellow #6 (sunset yellow)]
Vivactil: 10 mg [DSC] [contains fd&c yellow #10 (quinoline yellow)]
Generic: 5 mg, 10 mg

♦ Protriptyline Hydrochloride *see* Protriptyline *on page 1527*

♦ Protylol (Can) *see* Dicyclomine *on page 545*

♦ PRO-Valacyclovir (Can) *see* ValACYclovir *on page 1858*

♦ Provenge *see* Sipuleucel-T *on page 1662*

♦ Proventil HFA *see* Albuterol *on page 57*

♦ Provera *see* MedroxyPROGESTERone *on page 1131*

♦ Provera-Pak (Can) *see* MedroxyPROGESTERone *on page 1131*

♦ PRO-Verapamil SR (Can) *see* Verapamil *on page 1889*

♦ Provigil *see* Modafinil *on page 1222*

♦ Provil [OTC] *see* Ibuprofen *on page 905*

♦ Provir *see* Crofelemer *on page 452*

♦ Provisc *see* Hyaluronate and Derivatives *on page 879*

♦ Provocholine *see* Methacholine *on page 1159*

♦ Proxymetacaine *see* Proparacaine *on page 1515*

♦ PROzac *see* FLUoxetine *on page 786*

♦ Prozac (Can) *see* FLUoxetine *on page 786*

♦ PROzac Weekly *see* FLUoxetine *on page 786*

♦ Prozena [DSC] *see* Lidocaine (Topical) *on page 1074*

♦ PRP-OMP (PedvaxHIB) *see* Haemophilus b Conjugate Vaccine *on page 866*

♦ PRP-T (ActHIB) *see* Haemophilus b Conjugate Vaccine *on page 866*

♦ PRP-T (Hiberix) *see* Haemophilus b Conjugate Vaccine *on page 866*

♦ Prudoxin *see* Doxepin (Topical) *on page 592*

♦ Prussian Blue *see* Ferric Hexacyanoferrate *on page 761*

♦ Prymaccone *see* Primaquine *on page 1502*

♦ 23PS *see* Pneumococcal Polysaccharide Vaccine (23-Valent) *on page 1464*

♦ PS-341 *see* Bortezomib *on page 243*

Pseudoephedrine (soo doe e FED rin)

Brand Names: US Childrens Silfedrine [OTC]; Decongestant 12Hour Max St [OTC]; Decongestant [OTC] [DSC]; ElixSure Congestion [OTC]; Genaphed [OTC]; Nasal Decongestant [OTC]; Nexafed [OTC]; Psudatabs [OTC]; Shopko Nasal Decongestant Max [OTC]; Shopko Nasal Decongestant [OTC]; Simply Stuffy [OTC]; Sudafed 12 Hour [OTC]; Sudafed 24 Hour [OTC]; Sudafed Childrens [OTC]; Sudafed [OTC]; Sudanyl [OTC]; SudoGest 12 Hour [OTC]; SudoGest [OTC]; Suphedrine [OTC]; Unifed [OTC] [DSC]; Zephrex-D [OTC]
Brand Names: Canada Balminil Decongestant; Benylin® D for Infants; Contac® Cold 12 Hour Relief Non Drowsy; Drixoral® ND; Eltor®; PMS-Pseudoephedrine; Pseudofrin; Robidrine®; Sudafed® Decongestant
Index Terms d-Isoephedrine Hydrochloride; Pseudoephedrine Hydrochloride; Pseudoephedrine Sulfate; Sudafed
Pharmacologic Category Alpha/Beta Agonist; Decongestant
Use Temporary symptomatic relief of nasal congestion due to common cold, upper respiratory allergies, and sinusitis; also promotes nasal or sinus drainage
Dosing

Adult Nasal congestion: General dosing guidelines: Oral: Immediate release: 60 mg every 4-6 hours; Extended release: 120 mg every 12 hours **or** 240 mg every 24 hours; maximum: 240 mg/24 hours

Geriatric Nasal congestion: Use caution in this population; initiate using immediate release formulation: 30-60 mg every 6 hours as needed

Pediatric Nasal congestion: General dosing guidelines: Oral:
Children:
4-5 years: 15 mg every 4-6 hours; maximum: 60 mg/24 hours
6-12 years: 30 mg every 4-6 hours; maximum: 120 mg/24 hours
>12 years: Refer to adult dosing.
Renal Impairment No dosage adjustment provided in manufacturer's labeling.

Hepatic Impairment No dosage adjustment provided in manufacturer's labeling.

Additional Information Complete prescribing information should be consulted for additional detail.

Dosage Forms Excipient information presented when available (limited, particularly for generics); consult specific product labeling. [DSC] = Discontinued product

Gel, Oral, as hydrochloride:

ElixSure Congestion: 15 mg/5 mL (120 mL) [alcohol free; contains brilliant blue fcf (fd&c blue #1), carbomer 934p, propylene glycol, propylparaben; grape bubblegum flavor]

Liquid, Oral, as hydrochloride:

Childrens Silfedrine: 15 mg/5 mL (118 mL, 237 mL) [grape flavor]

Nasal Decongestant: 30 mg/5 mL (118 mL) [contains fd&c red #40, methylparaben, saccharin sodium, sodium benzoate; raspberry flavor]

Sudafed Childrens: 15 mg/5 mL (118 mL) [alcohol free, sugar free; contains brilliant blue fcf (fd&c blue #1), edetate disodium, fd&c red #40, menthol, polyethylene glycol, saccharin sodium, sodium benzoate; grape flavor]

Unifed: 30 mg/5 mL (120 mL [DSC], 480 mL [DSC], 3840 mL [DSC])

Syrup, Oral, as hydrochloride:

Nasal Decongestant: 30 mg/5 mL (473 mL) [contains fd&c red #40, methylparaben, saccharin sodium, sodium benzoate; raspberry flavor]

Generic: 30 mg/5 mL (118 mL [DSC])

Tablet, Oral, as hydrochloride:

Decongestant: 30 mg [DSC]

Genaphed: 30 mg

Nasal Decongestant: 30 mg [contains fd&c red #40 aluminum lake, fd&c yellow #6 aluminum lake]

Nasal Decongestant: 30 mg [contains fd&c red #40 aluminum lake, polysorbate 80]

Psudatabs: 30 mg [contains fd&c red #40, fd&c yellow #10 (quinoline yellow), fd&c yellow #6 (sunset yellow)]

Shopko Nasal Decongestant Max: 30 mg [contains fd&c red #40 aluminum lake]

Simply Stuffy: 30 mg

Sudafed: 30 mg

Sudafed: 30 mg [contains fd&c red #40 aluminum lake, fd&c yellow #10 aluminum lake, fd&c yellow #6 aluminum lake]

Sudanyl: 30 mg

SudoGest: 30 mg [contains fd&c red #40 aluminum lake, fd&c yellow #10 aluminum lake, fd&c yellow #6 aluminum lake]

SudoGest: 30 mg [contains fd&c red #40 aluminum lake, fd&c yellow #6 aluminum lake]

SudoGest: 60 mg [scored]

Suphedrine: 30 mg

Generic: 30 mg, 60 mg

Tablet Abuse-Deterrent, Oral, as hydrochloride:

Nexafed: 30 mg

Zephrex-D: 30 mg

Tablet Extended Release 12 Hour, Oral, as hydrochloride:

Decongestant 12Hour Max St: 120 mg [contains polysorbate 80]

Shopko Nasal Decongestant: 120 mg

Sudafed 12 Hour: 120 mg

Sudafed 12 Hour: 120 mg [contains fd&c blue #1 aluminum lake]

SudoGest 12 Hour: 120 mg

Generic: 120 mg

Tablet Extended Release 24 Hour, Oral, as hydrochloride:

Sudafed 24 Hour: 240 mg

♦ Pseudoephedrine and Chlorpheniramine *see* Chlorpheniramine and Pseudoephedrine *on page 377*

♦ Pseudoephedrine and Desloratadine *see* Desloratadine and Pseudoephedrine *on page 520*

Pseudoephedrine and Dextromethorphan
(soo doe e FED rin & deks troe meth OR fan)

Brand Names: US Pedia Relief Cough and Cold [OTC]; Sudafed® Children's Cold & Cough [OTC]

Brand Names: Canada Balminil DM D; Benylin® DM-D; Koffex DM-D; Novahistex® DM Decongestant; Novahistine® DM Decongestant; Robitussin® Childrens Cough & Cold

Index Terms Dextromethorphan and Pseudoephedrine

Pharmacologic Category Antitussive/Decongestant

Use Temporary symptomatic relief of nasal congestion and cough due to common cold, hay fever, upper respiratory allergies

Dosing

Adult & Geriatric Relief of nasal congestion and cough:

General dosing guidelines base on pseudoephedrine component: Oral: 60 mg every 4-6 hours (maximum: 240 mg/24 hours)

Product-specific dosing: Oral: Sudafed® Children's Cold & Cough: 20 mL every 4 hours (maximum: 80 mL/24 hours)

Pediatric Relief of nasal congestion and cough:

General dosing guidelines base on pseudoephedrine component: Oral:

Children 2-6 years: 15 mg every 4-6 hours (maximum: 60 mg/24 hours)

Children 6-12 years: 30 mg every 4-6 hours (maximum: 120 mg/24 hours)

Children ≥12 years and Adults: 60 mg every 4-6 hours (maximum: 240 mg/24 hours)

Product-specific dosing: Oral:

Children 2-6 years (Sudafed® Children's Cold & Cough): 5 mL every 4 hours (maximum: 20 mL/24 hours)

Children 6-12 years (Sudafed® Children's Cold & Cough): 10 mL every 4 hours (maximum: 40 mL/24 hours)

Children ≥12 years: Refer to adult dosing.

Additional Information Complete prescribing information should be consulted for additional detail.

Dosage Forms Excipient information presented when available (limited, particularly for generics); consult specific product labeling.

Liquid:

Sudafed® Children's Cold & Cough: Pseudoephedrine hydrochloride 15 mg and dextromethorphan hydrobromide 5 mg per 5 mL (120 mL) [alcohol free, sugar free; contains sodium benzoate; cherry berry flavor]

Syrup:

Pedia Relief Cough and Cold: Pseudoephedrine hydrochloride 15 mg and dextromethorphan hydrobromide 7.5 mg per 5 mL (120 mL) [cherry flavor]

♦ Pseudoephedrine and Fexofenadine *see* Fexofenadine and Pseudoephedrine *on page 765*

♦ Pseudoephedrine and Guaifenesin *see* Guaifenesin and Pseudoephedrine *on page 863*

Pseudoephedrine and Ibuprofen
(soo doe e FED rin & eye byoo PROE fen)

Brand Names: US Advil Cold & Sinus [OTC]

Brand Names: Canada Advil Cold & Sinus; Advil Cold & Sinus Daytime; Children's Advil Cold; Sudafed Sinus Advance

Index Terms Ibuprofen and Pseudoephedrine

Pharmacologic Category Decongestant/Analgesic

Use Cold, sinus, and flu symptoms: Temporary relief of common cold, sinus, and flu symptoms (including nasal congestion, sinus pressure, headache, minor body aches and pains, and fever)

Dosing

Adult Cold, sinus, and flu symptoms: Oral: One capsule/tablet (pseudoephedrine 30 mg/ibuprofen 200 mg) every 4 to 6 hours while symptoms persist; may increase to 2 tablets/capsules (pseudoephedrine 60 mg/ibuprofen 400 mg) every 4 to 6 hours if symptoms (maximum: 6 tablets/capsules per 24 hours [pseudoephedrine 180 mg/ibuprofen 1,200 mg per 24 hours]).

Geriatric Refer to adult dosing; use with caution.

Pediatric Cold, sinus, and flu symptoms: Children ≥12 years and Adolescents Refer to adult dosing.

Renal Impairment There are no dosage adjustments provided in the manufacturer's labeling; use with caution

Hepatic Impairment There are no dosage adjustments provided in the manufacturer's labeling; use with caution

Additional Information Complete prescribing information should be consulted for additional detail.

Dosage Forms Excipient information presented when available (limited, particularly for generics); consult specific product labeling.

Capsule, liquid filled, Oral:

Advil Cold & Sinus: Pseudoephedrine hydrochloride 30 mg and ibuprofen 200 mg [solubilized ibuprofen as free acid and potassium salt; contains potassium 20 mg/capsule and coconut oil]

Tablet, Oral:

Advil Cold & Sinus: Pseudoephedrine hydrochloride 30 mg and ibuprofen 200 mg

Generic: Pseudoephedrine hydrochloride 30 mg and ibuprofen 200 mg

Psyllium (SIL i yum)

Brand Names: US Dietary Fiber Laxative [OTC]; Evac [OTC]; Fiber Therapy [OTC]; Geri-Mucil [OTC]; Konsyl [OTC]; Konsyl-D [OTC]; Laxmar Natural Vegetable Laxat [OTC] [DSC]; MetaFiber [OTC] [DSC]; Metamucil Multi-Health Fiber [OTC]; Natural Fiber Therapy [OTC]; Natural Fiber [OTC]; Natural Psyllium Fiber [OTC] [DSC]; Natural Psyllium Seed [OTC]; Natural Vegetable Fiber [OTC]; Reguloid [OTC]; Sorbulax [OTC]

Brand Names: Canada Metamucil®

Index Terms Plantago Seed; Plantain Seed; Psyllium Husk; Psyllium Hydrophilic Mucilloid

Pharmacologic Category Antidiarrheal; Fiber Supplement; Laxative, Bulk-Producing

Use OTC labeling: Dietary fiber supplement; treatment of occasional constipation; reduce risk of coronary heart disease (CHD)

Dosing

Adult & Geriatric General dosing guidelines; consult specific product labeling.

Adequate intake for total fiber: Oral: **Note:** The definition of "fiber" varies; however, the soluble fiber in psyllium is only one type of fiber which makes up the daily recommended intake of total fiber.

Adults 19-50 years: Males: 38 g/day; Females: 25 g/day

Adults ≥51 years: Males: 30 g/day; Females: 21 g/day

Pregnancy: 28 g/day

Lactation: 29 g/day

Constipation: Oral: Psyllium: 2.5-30 g per day in divided doses

Reduce risk of CHD: Oral: Soluble fiber ≥7 g (psyllium seed husk ≥10.2 g) per day (DHHS, 1998)

Pediatric General dosing guidelines; consult specific product labeling.

Adequate intake for total fiber: Oral: **Note:** The definition of "fiber" varies; however, the soluble fiber in psyllium is only one type of fiber which makes up the daily recommended intake of total fiber.

Children 1-3 years: 19 g/day

Children 4-8 years: 25 g/day

Children 9-13 years: Males: 31 g/day; Females: 26 g/day

Children 14-18 years: Males: 38 g/day; Females: 26 g/day

Constipation: Oral:

Children 6-11 years: Psyllium: 1.25-15 g per day in divided doses

Children ≥12 years: Refer to adult dosing.

Reduce risk of CHD: Oral: Children ≥12 years: Refer to adult dosing.

Additional Information Complete prescribing information should be consulted for additional detail.

Dosage Forms Considerations Psyllium hydrophilic mucilloid 3.4 g is equivalent to 2 g Soluble fiber

Dosage Forms Excipient information presented when available (limited, particularly for generics); consult specific product labeling. [DSC] = Discontinued product

Capsule, Oral:

Konsyl: 520 mg [gluten free, sugar free]

Natural Fiber: 0.52 g

Reguloid: 0.52 g [contains fd&c yellow #6 aluminum lake]

Packet, Oral:

Konsyl: 28.3% (1 ea) [gluten free, kosher certified; contains fd&c yellow #10 (quinoline yellow), fd&c yellow #6 (sunset yellow)]

Konsyl: 28.3% (30 ea) [gluten free, kosher certified; contains fd&c yellow #10 (quinoline yellow), fd&c yellow #6 (sunset yellow); orange flavor]

Konsyl: 60.3% (1 ea, 30 ea) [gluten free, kosher certified, sugar free; contains aspartame, fd&c yellow #6 (sunset yellow); orange flavor]

Konsyl: 100% (1 ea, 30 ea, 100 ea) [gluten free, kosher certified, sugar free; bland flavor]

Metamucil MultiHealth Fiber: 58.12% (1 ea, 30 ea, 44 ea) [gluten free, sugar free; contains aspartame, fd&c yellow #6 (sunset yellow); orange flavor]

Powder, Oral:

Dietary Fiber Laxative: 28.3% (283 g, 300 g, 425 g, 660 g) [contains fd&c yellow #6 (sunset yellow)]

Fiber Therapy: 58.6% (283 g) [sugar free; contains aspartame, fd&c yellow #6 (sunset yellow)]

Geri-Mucil: 68% (368 g)

Geri-Mucil: 68% (368 g) [contains fd&c yellow #6 aluminum lake]

Geri-Mucil: 68% (284 g) [sugar free]

Geri-Mucil: 68% (283 g) [sugar free; contains aspartame, fd&c yellow #6 aluminum lake]

Konsyl: 28.3% (538 g) [gluten free, kosher certified; contains fd&c yellow #10 (quinoline yellow), fd&c yellow #6 (sunset yellow); orange flavor]

Konsyl: 30.9% (397 g) [gluten free, kosher certified; contains fd&c yellow #6 (sunset yellow); orange flavor]

Konsyl: 60.3% (450 g) [gluten free, kosher certified, sugar free; contains aspartame, fd&c yellow #6 (sunset yellow); orange flavor]

Konsyl: 71.67% (300 g) [gluten free, kosher certified, sugar free; bland flavor]

Konsyl: 100% (300 g, 450 g) [gluten free, kosher certified, sugar free]

Konsyl: 100% (300 g, 450 g) [gluten free, kosher certified, sugar free; bland flavor]

Konsyl: 60.3% (283 g) [sugar free; contains aspartame, fd&c yellow #6 (sunset yellow); orange flavor]

Konsyl-D: 52.3% (325 g [DSC]) [flavor free]

Konsyl-D: 52.3% (397 g, 500 g [DSC]) [flavor free; sweet flavor]

Laxmar Natural Vegetable Laxat: 58.6% (397 g [DSC]) [sugar free]

MetaFiber: 30.9% (368 g [DSC]); 48% (368 g [DSC]) [contains sucrose]

MetaFiber: 30.9% (398 g [DSC]); 48.57% (398 g [DSC]) [stimulant free]

MetaFiber: 58.6% (284 g [DSC]) [stimulant free, sugar free]

Metamucil MultiHealth Fiber: 58.6% (425 g [DSC]) [gluten free, sugar free; contains aspartame, brilliant blue fcf (fd&c blue #1), fd&c red #40]

Metamucil MultiHealth Fiber: 63% (660 g) [gluten free, sugar free]

Natural Fiber Therapy: 30.9% (368 g, 539 g); 48.57% (368 g, 538 g)

Natural Psyllium Fiber: 58.6% (368 g [DSC])

Natural Psyllium Fiber: 58.6% (368 g [DSC]) [contains fd&c yellow #6 aluminum lake]

Natural Psyllium Seed: 100% (480 g) [animal products free, gelatin free, gluten free, kosher certified, lactose free, no artificial color(s), no artificial flavor(s), starch free, sugar free, yeast free]

Natural Vegetable Fiber: 30.9% (368 g [DSC]) [contains fd&c yellow #6 (sunset yellow)]

Natural Vegetable Fiber: 48.57% (368 g)

Natural Vegetable Fiber: 58.6% (283 g [DSC]) [sugar free; contains aspartame, fd&c yellow #6 (sunset yellow)]

Natural Vegetable Fiber: 63% (283 g [DSC]) [sugar free]

Reguloid: 48.57% (369 g, 540 g)

Reguloid: 28.3% (369 g, 540 g) [contains fd&c yellow #6 (sunset yellow), fd&c yellow #6 aluminum lake; orange flavor]

Reguloid: 58.6% (284 g, 426 g) [sugar free; natural flavor]

Reguloid: 58.6% (284 g, 426 g) [sugar free; contains aspartame, fd&c yellow #6 (sunset yellow), fd&c yellow #6 aluminum lake]

Sorbulax: 100% (420 g)

Powder, Oral [preservative free]:

Evac: (480 g) [dye free]

Pyrantel Pamoate (pi RAN tel PAM oh ate)

Brand Names: US Pamix [OTC]; Pin-X [OTC]; Reeses Pinworm Medicine [OTC]

Brand Names: Canada Combantrin

Pharmacologic Category Anthelmintic

Use Pinworms: Treatment of pinworms caused by *Enterobius vermicularis* (alternative agent; not preferred therapy)

Dosing

Adult & Geriatric Note: Dose is expressed as pyrantel base; not preferred therapy since newer treatments are available.

Enterobius vermicularis **(pinworm):** Oral: 11 mg/kg administered as a single dose; maximum: 1 g per dose

Ancylostoma duodenale **and** *Necator americanus* **(hookworms) (off-label use):** Oral: 11 mg/kg (maximum: 1 g/dose) administered once daily for 3 days (Bethony 2006; Drugs for Parasitic Infections 2013; Kappagoda 2011)

Moniliformis **(off-label use):** Oral: 11 mg/kg administered as a single dose; repeat twice 2 weeks apart (Drugs for Parasitic Infections 2013)

Trichostrongylus **(off-label use):** Oral: 11 mg/kg administered as a single dose; maximum: 1 g per dose (Drugs for Parasitic Infections 2013)

Pediatric Children ≥2 years and Adolescents: Refer to adult dosing.

Renal Impairment There are no dosage adjustments provided in the manufacturer's labeling.

Hepatic Impairment There are no dosage adjustments provided in the manufacturer's labeling; use with caution.

Additional Information Complete prescribing information should be consulted for additional detail.

Dosage Forms Excipient information presented when available (limited, particularly for generics); consult specific product labeling.

Suspension, Oral [strength expressed as base]:

Pamix: 50 mg/mL (30 mL, 60 mL, 240 mL)

Pin-X: 50 mg/mL (30 mL, 60 mL) [sugar free; contains methylparaben, propylene glycol, propylparaben, saccharin sodium, sodium benzoate; caramel flavor]

Reeses Pinworm Medicine: 50 mg/mL (30 mL) [contains saccharin sodium, sodium benzoate]

Tablet, Oral [strength expressed as base]:

Reeses Pinworm Medicine: 62.5 mg [scored]

Tablet Chewable, Oral [strength expressed as base]:

Pin-X: 250 mg [scored; contains aspartame, fd&c yellow #6 aluminum lake; orange flavor]

Pyrazinamide (peer a ZIN a mide)

Brand Names: Canada Tebrazid™

Index Terms Pyrazinoic Acid Amide

Pharmacologic Category Antitubercular Agent

Use Adjunctive treatment of tuberculosis in combination with other antituberculosis agents

Pregnancy Considerations Teratogenic effects have not been observed in animal reproduction studies. Due to the risk of tuberculosis to the fetus, treatment is recommended when the probability of maternal disease is moderate to high. Although not recommended as the initial treatment regimen, the use of pyrazinamide during pregnancy is recommended by The World Health Organization (Blumberg, 2003).

Breast-Feeding Considerations Low concentrations of pyrazinamide have been detected in breast milk; concentrations are less than maternal plasma concentration (Holdiness, 1984). The amount of drug in breast milk is considered insufficient for the treatment of tuberculosis in breast-fed infants.

Contraindications Hypersensitivity to pyrazinamide or any component of the formulation; acute gout; severe hepatic damage

Warnings/Precautions Use with caution in patients with a history of alcoholism, renal failure, chronic gout, diabetes mellitus, or porphyria. Dose-related hepatotoxicity ranging from transient ALT/AST elevations to jaundice, hepatitis and/or liver atrophy (rare) has occurred. Use with caution in patients receiving concurrent medications associated with hepatotoxicity (particularly with rifampin). The 2-month rifampin-pyrazinamide regimen for the treatment of latent tuberculosis infection (LTBI) has been associated with severe and fatal liver injuries; incidence increased with pyrazinamide doses >30 mg/kg/day. The Infectious Diseases Society of America and Centers for Disease Control and Prevention recommend that the 2-month rifampin-pyrazinamide regimen should not generally be used in patients with LTBI.

Adverse Reactions

1% to 10%:

Central nervous system: Malaise

Gastrointestinal: Anorexia, nausea, vomiting

Neuromuscular & skeletal: Arthralgia, myalgia

<1% (Limited to important or life-threatening): Acne, angioedema (rare), anticoagulant effect, dysuria, fever, gout, hepatotoxicity, interstitial nephritis, itching, photosensitivity, porphyria, rash, sideroblastic anemia, thrombocytopenia, urticaria

Drug Interactions

Metabolism/Transport Effects None known.

Avoid Concomitant Use There are no known interactions where it is recommended to avoid concomitant use.

Increased Effect/Toxicity

Pyrazinamide may increase the levels/effects of: CycloSPORINE (Systemic); Rifampin

Decreased Effect

Pyrazinamide may decrease the levels/effects of: Benzbromarone

Storage/Stability Store at controlled room temperature of 15°C to 30°C (59°F to 86°F).

Mechanism of Action Converted to pyrazinoic acid in susceptible strains of *Mycobacterium* which lowers the pH of the environment; exact mechanism of action has not been elucidated

Pharmacodynamics/Kinetics Bacteriostatic or bactericidal depending on drug's concentration at infection site

Absorption: Well absorbed

Distribution: Widely into body tissues and fluids including liver, lung, and CSF

Relative diffusion from blood into CSF: Adequate with or without inflammation (exceeds usual MICs)

CSF:blood level ratio: Inflamed meninges: 100%

Protein binding: 50%

Metabolism: Hepatic

Half-life elimination: 9-10 hours

Time to peak, serum: Within 2 hours

Excretion: Urine (4% as unchanged drug)

Dosing

Adult Tuberculosis treatment: Oral: **Note:** Used as part of a multidrug regimen. Treatment regimens consist of an initial 2-month phase, followed by a continuation phase of 4 or 7 additional months; pyrazinamide is administered in the initial phase of treatment.

Suggested dosing based on lean body weight (Blumberg, 2003; CDC, 2003):

Daily therapy:

40-55 kg: 1000 mg

56-75 kg: 1500 mg

76-90 kg: 2000 mg (maximum dose regardless of weight)

Twice weekly directly observed therapy (DOT):

40-55 kg: 2000 mg

56-75 kg: 3000 mg

76-90 kg: 4000 mg (maximum dose regardless of weight)

Three times/week DOT:

40-55 kg: 1500 mg

56-75 kg: 2500 mg

76-90 kg: 3000 mg (maximum dose regardless of weight)

Pediatric Tuberculosis treatment: Oral: **Note:** Used as part of a multidrug regimen. Treatment regimens consist of an initial 2-month phase, followed by a continuation phase of 4 or 7 additional months; pyrazinamide is administered in the initial phase of treatment.
HIV negative (CDC, 2003):
Daily therapy: 15-30 mg/kg/day (maximum: 2 g/day)
Twice weekly directly observed therapy (DOT): 50 mg/kg/dose (maximum: 2 g/dose)
HIV-exposed/-infected: Daily therapy: 20-40 mg/kg/dose once daily (maximum: 2 g/day) (CDC, 2009)

Renal Impairment Adults: CrCl <30 mL/minute or receiving hemodialysis: Treatment of TB: 25-35 mg/kg/dose 3 times per week administered after dialysis (Blumberg, 2003; CDC, 2003)

Hepatic Impairment No dosage adjustment provided in manufacturer's labeling. Use is contraindicated in cases of severe hepatic impairment.

Monitoring Parameters Periodic liver function tests, serum uric acid, sputum culture, chest x-ray 2-3 months into treatment and at completion

Test Interactions Reacts with Acetest® and Ketostix® to produce pinkish-brown color

Dosage Forms Excipient information presented when available (limited, particularly for generics); consult specific product labeling.
Tablet, Oral:
Generic: 500 mg

Extemporaneous Preparations A 100 mg/mL oral suspension may be made with tablets. Crush two-hundred pyrazinamide 500 mg tablets and mix with a suspension containing 500 mL methylcellulose 1% and 500 mL simple syrup. Add to this a suspension containing one-hundred forty crushed pyrazinamide tablets in 350 mL methylcellulose 1% and 350 mL simple syrup to make 1.7 L suspension. Label "shake well" and "refrigerate". Stable for 60 days refrigerated (preferred) and 45 days at room temperature.
Nahata MC, Morosco RS, and Peritre SP, "Stability of Pyrazinamide in Two Suspensions," *Am J Health Syst Pharm,* 1995, 52(14):1558-60.

◆ **Pyrazinoic Acid Amide** *see* Pyrazinamide *on page 1530*

Pyrethrins and Piperonyl Butoxide
(pye RE thrins & pi PER oh nil byo TOKS ide)

Brand Names: US A-200 Lice Treatment Kit [OTC]; A-200 Maximum Strength [OTC]; LiceMD [OTC]; Licide [OTC]; Pronto Complete Lice Removal System [OTC]; Pronto Plus Lice Killing Mousse Plus Vitamin E [OTC]; Pronto Plus Lice Killing Mousse Shampoo Plus Natural Extracts and Oils [OTC]; Pronto Plus Warm Oil Treatment and Conditioner [OTC]; RID Maximum Strength [OTC]

Brand Names: Canada Pronto Lice Control; R & C II; R & C Shampoo/Conditioner; RID Mousse

Index Terms Piperonyl Butoxide and Pyrethrins

Pharmacologic Category Antiparasitic Agent, Topical; Pediculocide; Shampoo, Pediculocide

Use *Pediculus humanus* infestations: Treatment of *Pediculus humanus* infestations (head lice, body lice, pubic lice, and their eggs)

Dosing
Adult & Geriatric Treatment of *Pediculus humanus* infestations: Topical: Apply to dry hair and/or other infested area; allow to remain on area for 10 minutes and then wash and rinse; repeat treatment in 7 to 10 days.

Pediatric Treatment of *Pediculus humanus* infestations: Children ≥2 years and Adolescents: Topical: Refer to adult dosing.

Renal Impairment There are no dosage adjustments provided in the manufacturer's labeling

Hepatic Impairment There are no dosage adjustments provided in the manufacturer's labeling

Additional Information Complete prescribing information should be consulted for additional detail.

Dosage Forms Excipient information presented when available (limited, particularly for generics); consult specific product labeling.
Kit:
A-200 Lice Treatment Kit:
Shampoo: Pyrethrins 0.33% and piperonyl butoxide 4% (120 mL)
Solution [spray; for bedding; not for human or animal use]: Permethrin 0.5% (180 mL)
[packaged with nit removal comb]
LiceMD:
Gel: Pyrethrins 0.33% and piperonyl butoxide 4% (118 mL)
[packaged with non medicated shampoo, nit removal comb, and gloves]

Pronto Complete Lice Removal System:
Shampoo: Pyrethrins 0.33% and piperonyl butoxide 4% (60 mL)
Solution, topical: Benzalkonium chloride 0.1% (60 mL) [lice egg remover antiseptic] [packaged with household furniture spray and nit removal comb]
Oil, topical:
Pronto Plus Warm Oil Treatment and Conditioner: Pyrethrins 0.33% and piperonyl butoxide 4% (36 mL) [fruity herbal scent; packaged with nit removal comb]
Shampoo:
A-200 Maximum Strength: Pyrethrins 0.33% and piperonyl butoxide 4% (60 mL, 120 mL) [contains benzyl alcohol; packaged with nit removal comb]
Licide: Pyrethrins 0.33% and piperonyl butoxide 4% (120 mL) [packaged with nit removal comb; also available in a kit containing shampoo, household spray, and nit removal comb]
Pronto Plus Lice Killing Mousse Shampoo Plus Natural Extracts and Oils: Pyrethrins 0.33% and piperonyl butoxide 4% (60 mL) [packaged with nit removal comb]
Pronto Plus Lice Killing Mousse Shampoo Plus Vitamin E: Pyrethrins 0.33% and piperonyl butoxide 4% (120 mL) [blue mousse shampoo; contains vitamin E; packaged with nit removal comb]
RID Maximum Strength: Pyrethrins 0.33% and piperonyl butoxide 4% (60 mL, 120 mL, 180 mL, 240 mL) [packaged with nit removal comb; also available in a kit containing shampoo, gel, and furniture spray]

◆ **Pyri 500 [OTC]** *see* Pyridoxine *on page 1533*
◆ **2-Pyridine Aldoxime Methochloride** *see* Pralidoxime *on page 1486*
◆ **Pyridium** *see* Phenazopyridine *on page 1435*

Pyridostigmine (peer id oh STIG meen)

Brand Names: US Mestinon; Regonol
Brand Names: Canada Mestinon; Mestinon-SR
Index Terms Pyridostigmine Bromide
Pharmacologic Category Acetylcholinesterase Inhibitor
Use
Myasthenia gravis (oral only): Treatment of myasthenia gravis.
Reversal of nondepolarizing muscle relaxants (injection only): Reversal agent or antagonist to the neuromuscular blocking effects of nondepolarizing muscle relaxants.
Military use: Pretreatment for Soman nerve gas exposure
Pregnancy Considerations Adverse events were not observed in animal reproduction studies. Pyridostigmine may cross the placenta (Buckley 1968). Use of pyridostigmine may be continued during pregnancy for the treatment of myasthenia gravis (Skie 2010; Norwood 2013) and its use should be continued during labor (Norwood 2013). Transient neonatal myasthenia gravis may occur in 10% to 20% of neonates due to placental transfer of maternal antibodies (Skie 2010; Varner 2013).

In general, medications used as antidotes should take into consideration the health and prognosis of the mother; antidotes should be administered to pregnant women if there is a clear indication for use and should not be withheld because of fears of teratogenicity (Bailey 2003).

Breast-Feeding Considerations Pyridostigmine is excreted in breast milk (Hardell 1992). The manufacturer recommends that caution be exercised when administering pyridostigmine to nursing women.

Information is available from two mothers using pyridostigmine for myasthenia gravis throughout pregnancy and postpartum. Maternal doses ranged from 180 mg to 300 mg/day. Milk concentrations averaged ≤0.1% of the weight adjusted maternal dose (n=2); infant plasma concentrations were less than the limit of quantification (<2 ng/mL; n=1) (Hardell 1992). Disease exacerbations may occur in nursing women with poorly controlled myasthenia gravis due to fatigue associated with breast-feeding. Babies born to women with myasthenia gravis may have feeding difficulties due to transient myasthenia gravis of the newborn (Norwood 2013). Nursing infants should be monitored for fatigue associated with transient neonatal myasthenia gravis (Varner 2013), however current guidelines note that nursing is not contraindicated in women taking pyridostigmine for myasthenia gravis (Norwood 2013).

Contraindications Hypersensitivity to pyridostigmine, anticholinesterase agents, or any component of the formulation; mechanical intestinal or urinary obstruction

Documentation of allergenic cross-reactivity for anticholinergic muscle stimulants is limited. However, because of similarities in chemical structure and/or pharmacologic actions, the possibility of cross-sensitivity cannot be ruled out with certainty.

Warnings/Precautions Symptoms of excess cholinergic activity may occur (eg, salivation, sweating, urinary incontinence). Overdosage may result in cholinergic crisis (eg, muscle weakness), which must be distinguished from myasthenic crisis; discontinue immediately in the presence of cholinergic crisis. Hypersensitivity reactions may occur; have atropine and epinephrine ready to treat hypersensitivity reactions. Inadequate reversal induced by nondepolarizing muscle relaxants is possible; manage with manual or mechanical ventilation until recovery is adequate (additional doses not recommended). Failure to produce prompt (within 30 minutes) reversal of neuromuscular blockade may occur in the presence of extreme debilitation, carcinomatosis, or with concomitant use of certain broad-spectrum antibiotics, or anesthetic agents and other drugs which enhance neuromuscular blockade or cause respiratory depression.

Use with caution in patients with bradycardia or other cardiac arrhythmias, glaucoma, renal impairment, asthma, bronchospastic disease, COPD, or bromide sensitivity. Potentially significant interactions may exist, requiring dose or frequency adjustment, additional monitoring, and/or selection of alternative therapy.

Injection not indicated for use in neonates; may contain benzyl alcohol which has been associated with "gasping syndrome" in neonates. Injection must be administered by trained personnel; use of peripheral nerve stimulation to monitor neuromuscular function recovery and continuous patient observation until recovery of normal respiration is recommended. To counteract anticholinergic effects, use of glycopyrrolate or atropine sulfate simultaneously with or prior to administration is recommended. Adequate facilities should be available for cardiopulmonary resuscitation when testing and adjusting dose for myasthenia gravis.

Military use: Only for pretreatment for exposure to Soman; discontinue pyridostigmine at the first sign of Soman exposure (do not administer pyridostigmine after Soman exposure); atropine and pralidoxime must be administered after Soman exposure (pyridostigmine pretreatment offers no benefit against Soman unless atropine and pralidoxime are administered once symptoms of poisoning appear). Use in conjunction with protective garments, including gas mask, hood and overgarments.

Adverse Reactions Frequency not defined.

Cardiovascular: Arrhythmias (especially bradycardia), AV block, cardiac arrest, decreased carbon monoxide, flushing, hypotension, nodal rhythm, nonspecific ECG changes, syncope, tachycardia

Central nervous system: Convulsions, dizziness, drowsiness, dysphonia, headache, loss of consciousness

Dermatologic: Skin rash, thrombophlebitis (IV), urticaria

Gastrointestinal: Abdominal pain, diarrhea, dysphagia, flatulence, hyperperistalsis, nausea, salivation, stomach cramps, vomiting

Genitourinary: Urinary urgency

Neuromuscular & skeletal: Arthralgia, dysarthria, fasciculations, muscle cramps, myalgia, spasms, weakness

Ocular: Amblyopia, lacrimation, small pupils

Respiratory: Bronchial secretions increased, bronchiolar constriction, bronchospasm, dyspnea, laryngospasm, respiratory arrest, respiratory depression, respiratory muscle paralysis

Miscellaneous: Allergic reactions, anaphylaxis, diaphoresis increased

Drug Interactions

Metabolism/Transport Effects None known.

Avoid Concomitant Use There are no known interactions where it is recommended to avoid concomitant use.

Increased Effect/Toxicity

Pyridostigmine may increase the levels/effects of: Beta-Blockers; Cholinergic Agonists; Succinylcholine

The levels/effects of Pyridostigmine may be increased by: Corticosteroids (Systemic)

Decreased Effect

Pyridostigmine may decrease the levels/effects of: Anticholinergic Agents; Neuromuscular-Blocking Agents (Nondepolarizing)

The levels/effects of Pyridostigmine may be decreased by: Anticholinergic Agents; Dipyridamole; Methocarbamol

Preparation for Administration Myasthenic crisis (off-label use): *Continuous infusion:* May dilute 25 mg in 100 mL of D_5W (Saltis 1993).

Storage/Stability

Store at 25°C (77°F); excursions permitted to 15°C to 30°C (59°F to 86°F); protect from light.

Military use: Store between 2°C and 8°C (36°F to 46°F); protect from light. Discard 3 months after issue. Do not dispense after removal from the refrigerator for more than a total of 3 months.

Mechanism of Action Inhibits destruction of acetylcholine by acetylcholinesterase which facilitates transmission of impulses across myoneural junction

Pharmacodynamics/Kinetics

Onset of action: Within 30 minutes (Maggi 2011)

Duration: 3 to 4 hours in the daytime (Maggi 2011)

Absorption: Oral: Very poor

Distribution: 19 ± 12 L

Metabolism: Hepatic

Bioavailability: 10% to 20%

Half-life elimination:

Oral: 3 hours; renal failure: ≤6 hours

IV: ~1.5 hours (Aquilonius 1980)

Time to peak, plasma: Oral: ~1 to 3 hours

Excretion: Urine (75%)

Dosing

Adult & Geriatric

Myasthenia gravis:

Oral: Highly individualized dosing ranges:

Immediate-release: 60 to 1,500 mg/day, usually 600 mg/day divided into 5 to 6 doses, spaced to provide maximum relief

Sustained release: 180 to 540 mg once or twice daily (doses separated by at least 6 hours); **Note:** It may be necessary to use immediate-release therapy in conjunction with sustained-release therapy.

IM, IV (off-label use): To supplement during labor and postpartum, during myasthenic crisis, or when oral therapy is impractical: ~1/30th of oral dose; observe patient closely for cholinergic reactions. IM route preferred due to significant complications (eg, cardiac arrest) observed with the IV route (Maggi 2011; Varner 2013). May also administer as a continuous infusion for myasthenic crisis.

Continuous infusion: IV: 1 to 2 mg/hour with gradual titration in increments of 0.5 to 1 mg/hour, up to a maximum rate of 4 mg/hour (Berrouschot 1997; Saltis 1993)

Reversal of nondepolarizing muscle relaxants: IV: 0.1 to 0.25 mg/kg/dose (onset to peak effect is dose-dependent; return of twitch height to 90% of control occurs within ~6 minutes; full recovery usually occurs within 15 to 30 minutes)

Note: The monitoring of muscle twitch response to peripheral nerve stimulation is advised; administer pyridostigmine after spontaneous recovery of neuromuscular function has begun. Atropine sulfate or glycopyrrolate IV should be administered immediately prior to or simultaneously with pyridostigmine to minimize side effects. Inadequate reversal is possible; manage by manual or mechanical ventilation until recovery is judged adequate (additional doses are not recommended).

Soman nerve gas exposure, pretreatment (military use): Note: Do not administer pyridostigmine after Soman exposure; if taken immediately before exposure (eg, when gas attack alarm is given) or at the same time, it is not expected to be effective and may exacerbate the effects of a sub-lethal exposure to Soman.

Oral: 30 mg every 8 hours beginning several hours prior to exposure; discontinue at first sign of Soman exposure, then immediately begin atropine and pralidoxime.

Pediatric

Myasthenia gravis (off-label use):

Note: Limited data available; dosage should be adjusted such that larger doses administered prior to time of greatest fatigue.

Oral: Immediate release: 1 mg/kg/dose every 4 to 6 hours; maximum daily dose: 7 mg/kg/day divided in 5 to 6 doses; (Usual daily dose: 600 mg/day; doses as high as 1,500 mg/day have been used) (Andrews 1998; Maggi 2011)

IM, IV: 0.05 to 0.15 mg/kg/dose (maximum dose: 10 mg) (Kleigman 2007). IM route preferred due to significant complications (eg, cardiac arrest) observed with the IV route (Maggi 2011).

Renal Impairment There are no dosage adjustments provided in the manufacturer's labeling. However, lower initial doses dosages may be required due to prolonged elimination in renal impairment.

Hepatic Impairment There are no dosage adjustments provided in the manufacturer's labeling.

Administration Do **not** crush sustained release tablet. For myasthenic crisis (off-label use), may administer IM, slow IV push, or as a continuous infusion (Maggi 2011; Saltis 1993).

Monitoring Parameters ECG, blood pressure, and heart rate especially with IV use; observe for cholinergic reactions (eg, nausea, vomiting, diarrhea, increased salivation), particularly when administered IV; consult individual institutional policies and procedures

Dosage Forms Excipient information presented when available (limited, particularly for generics); consult specific product labeling.

Solution, Intravenous, as bromide:
Regonol: 10 mg/2 mL (2 mL) [contains benzyl alcohol]
Syrup, Oral, as bromide:
Mestinon: 60 mg/5 mL (473 mL) [contains alcohol, usp, brilliant blue fcf (fd&c blue #1), fd&c red #40, sodium benzoate; raspberry flavor]
Tablet, Oral, as bromide:
Mestinon: 60 mg [scored]
Generic: 60 mg
Tablet Extended Release, Oral, as bromide:
Mestinon: 180 mg [scored]
Generic: 180 mg

◆ Pyridostigmine Bromide *see* Pyridostigmine *on page 1531*

Pyridoxine (peer i DOKS een)

Brand Names: US Neuro-K-250 T.D. [OTC]; Neuro-K-250 Vitamin B6 [OTC]; Neuro-K-50 [OTC]; Neuro-K-500 [OTC]; Pyri 500 [OTC]

Index Terms B6; B_6; Pyridoxine Hydrochloride; Vitamin B_6

Pharmacologic Category Vitamin, Water Soluble

Use Prevention and treatment of vitamin B_6 deficiency

Pregnancy Considerations Water soluble vitamins cross the placenta. Maternal pyridoxine plasma concentrations may decrease as pregnancy progresses and requirements may be increased in pregnant women (IOM 1998). Pyridoxine is used to treat nausea and vomiting of pregnancy (Neibyl 2010). In general, medications used as antidotes should take into consideration the health and prognosis of the mother; antidotes should be administered to pregnant women if there is a clear indication for use and should not be withheld because of fears of teratogenicity (Bailey 2003).

Breast-Feeding Considerations Pyridoxine is found in breast milk and concentrations vary by maternal intake. Pyridoxine requirements are increased in nursing women compared to non-nursing women (IOM 1998). Possible inhibition of lactation at doses >600 mg/day when taken immediately postpartum (Foukas 1973).

Contraindications Hypersensitivity to pyridoxine or any component of the formulation

Warnings/Precautions Severe, permanent peripheral neuropathies have been reported; neurotoxicity is more common with long-term administration of large doses (>2 g/day). Dependence and withdrawal may occur with doses >200 mg/day. Single vitamin deficiency is rare; evaluate for other deficiencies. The parenteral product may contain aluminum; toxic aluminum concentrations may be seen with high doses, prolonged use, or renal dysfunction. Premature neonates are at higher risk due to immature renal function and aluminum intake from other parenteral sources. Parenteral aluminum exposure of >4 to 5 mcg/kg/day is associated with CNS and bone toxicity; tissue loading may occur at lower doses (Federal Register 2002). See manufacturer's labeling.

Pharmacy supply of emergency antidotes: Guidelines suggest that at least 8-24 g be stocked. This is enough to treat 1 patient weighing 100 kg for an initial 8- to 24-hour period. In areas where tuberculosis is common, hospitals should consider stocking 24 g. This is enough to treat 1 patient for 24 hours (Dart 2009).

Adverse Reactions Frequency not defined.

Central nervous system: Headache, seizure (following very large IV doses), somnolence
Endocrine & metabolic: Acidosis, folic acid decreased
Gastrointestinal: Nausea
Hepatic: AST increased
Neuromuscular & skeletal: Neuropathy, paresthesia
Miscellaneous: Allergic reactions

Drug Interactions

Metabolism/Transport Effects None known.

Avoid Concomitant Use There are no known interactions where it is recommended to avoid concomitant use.

Increased Effect/Toxicity There are no known significant interactions involving an increase in effect.

Decreased Effect

Pyridoxine may decrease the levels/effects of: Altretamine; Barbiturates; Fosphenytoin; Levodopa; Phenytoin

Storage/Stability Injection: Store at 20°C to 25°C (68°F to 77°F). Protect from light.

Mechanism of Action Precursor to pyridoxal, which functions in the metabolism of proteins, carbohydrates, and fats; pyridoxal also aids in the release of liver and muscle-stored glycogen and in the synthesis of GABA (within the central nervous system) and heme

Pharmacodynamics/Kinetics

Absorption: Enteral, parenteral: Well absorbed
Metabolism: Hepatic to pyridoxal phosphate and pyridoxamine phosphate (active forms)
Half-life elimination: Biologic: 15-20 days
Excretion: Urine

Dosing

Adult & Geriatric

Recommended daily allowance (RDA): Oral (IOM 1998):
19-50 years: 1.3 mg
≥51 years:
Females: 1.5 mg
Males: 1.7 mg
Pregnancy: 1.9 mg
Lactation: 2 mg

Dietary deficiency: IM, IV: 10-20 mg/day for 3 weeks, followed by oral therapy. Doses up to 600 mg/day may be needed with pyridoxine dependency syndrome.

Gyromitrin-containing mushroom (false morel) overdose/toxicity (treatment/prophylaxis) (off-label use): IV: 25 mg/kg over 15-30 minutes; repeat dose as needed to control seizures (Diaz 2005; Lheureux 2005)

Nausea and vomiting of pregnancy (off-label use): Oral: 10 to 25 mg every 8 hours (Neibyl 2010)

Neurological toxicities (ie, seizures, coma) associated with isoniazid overdose (prevention) (off-label use): IV: Asymptomatic patients who present within 2 hours of ingesting a potentially toxic amount of isoniazid should receive a prophylactic dose of pyridoxine (Hernon 2015). Dosing recommendations are the same as for the treatment of symptomatic patients.

Neurological toxicities (ie, seizures, coma) associated with isoniazid overdose (treatment) (off-label use): IV:

Acute ingestion of known amount: Initial: A total dose of pyridoxine equal to the amount of isoniazid ingested (maximum dose: 5 g); administer at a rate of 0.5 to 1 g/minute until seizures stop or the maximum initial dose has been administered; may repeat every 5 to 10 minutes as needed to control persistent seizure activity and/or CNS toxicity. If seizures stop prior to the administration of the calculated initial dose, infuse the remaining pyridoxine over 4 to 6 hours (Howland 2015; Morrow 2006).

Acute ingestion of unknown amount: Initial: 5 g; administer at a rate of 0.5 to 1 g/minute; may repeat every 5 to 10 minutes as needed to control persistent seizure activity and/or CNS toxicity (Howland 2015; Morrow 2006)

Peripheral neuropathy associated with isoniazid therapy for *Mycobacterium tuberculosis* (prevention): Oral: 25 to 50 mg/day (CDC [Kaplan 2009])

Pediatric

Adequate Intake (AI): Oral (IOM 1998): Infants:
1-6 months: 0.1 mg/day
7-12 months: 0.3 mg/day

Recommended daily allowance (RDA): Oral (IOM 1998): Children:
1-3 years: 0.5 mg
4-8 years: 0.6 mg
9-13 years: 1 mg
14-18 years:
Females: 1.5 mg
Males: 1.3 mg

Gyromitrin-containing mushroom (false morel) overdose/toxicity (treatment/prophylaxis) (off-label use): Children and Adolescents: Refer to adult dosing.

Neurological toxicities (ie, seizures, coma) associated with isoniazid overdose (prevention) (off-label use): Refer to adult dosing.

Neurological toxicities (ie, seizures, coma) associated with isoniazid overdose (treatment) (off-label use): IV: Children and Adolescents:

Acute ingestion of known amount: Initial: A total dose of pyridoxine equal to the amount of isoniazid ingested (maximum dose: 70 mg/kg, up to 5 g); administer at a rate of 0.5 to 1 g/minute until seizures stop or the maximum initial dose has been administered; may repeat every 5 to 10 minutes as needed to control persistent seizure activity and/or CNS toxicity. If seizures stop prior to the administration of the calculated ▶

initial dose, infuse the remaining pyridoxine over 4 to 6 hours (Howland 2015; Morrow 2006).

Acute ingestion of unknown amount: Initial: 70 mg/kg (maximum dose: 5 g); administer at a rate of 0.5 to 1 g/minute; may repeat every 5 to 10 minutes as needed to control persistent seizure activity and/or CNS toxicity (Howland 2015; Morrow 2006; Santucci 1999)

Administration Burning may occur at the injection site after IM administration.

Gyromitrin-containing mushroom (false morel) overdose/toxicity (treatment/prophylaxis) (off-label use): Administer dose over 15 to 30 minutes (Lheureux 2005).

Isoniazid toxicity (off-label use): Initial doses should be administered at a rate of 0.5 to 1 g/minute. If the parenteral formulation is not available, anecdotal reports suggest that pyridoxine tablets may be crushed and made into a slurry and given at the same dose orally or via nasogastric (NG) tube (Hernon 2015). Oral administration is not recommended for acutely poisoned patients with seizure activity.

Monitoring Parameters For treatment of isoniazid or Gyromitrin-containing mushroom toxicity: Anion gap, arterial blood gases, electrolytes, neurological exam, seizure activity

Reference Range Over 50 ng/mL (SI: 243 nmol/L) (varies considerably with method). A broad range is ~25-80 ng/mL (SI: 122-389 nmol/L). HPLC method for pyridoxal phosphate has normal range of 3.5-18 ng/mL (SI: 17-88 nmol/L).

Test Interactions False positive urobilinogen spot test using Ehrlich's reagent

Dosage Forms Excipient information presented when available (limited, particularly for generics); consult specific product labeling.

Capsule, Oral, as hydrochloride:
Neuro-K-250 T.D.: 250 mg [corn free, rye free, starch free, sugar free, wheat free]
Solution, Injection, as hydrochloride:
Generic: 100 mg/mL (1 mL)
Tablet, Oral, as hydrochloride:
Neuro-K-50: 50 mg
Neuro-K-500: 500 mg
Neuro-K-250 Vitamin B6: 250 mg
Pyri 500: 500 mg
Generic: 25 mg, 50 mg, 100 mg, 250 mg
Tablet, Oral, as hydrochloride [preservative free]:
Generic: 25 mg, 50 mg, 100 mg
Tablet Extended Release, Oral, as hydrochloride:
Generic: 200 mg

Extemporaneous Preparations A 1 mg/mL oral solution may be made using pyridoxine injection. Withdraw 100 mg (1 mL of a 100 mg/mL injection) from a vial with a needle and syringe; add to 99 mL simple syrup in an amber bottle. Label "refrigerate". Stable for 30 days refrigerated.

Nahata MC, Pai VB, and Hipple TF, *Pediatric Drug Formulations*, 5th ed, Cincinnati, OH: Harvey Whitney Books Co, 2004.

◆ Pyridoxine and Doxylamine *see* Doxylamine and Pyridoxine *on page 606*

◆ Pyridoxine, Folic Acid, and Cyanocobalamin *see* Folic Acid, Cyanocobalamin, and Pyridoxine *on page 805*

◆ Pyridoxine Hydrochloride *see* Pyridoxine *on page 1533*

Pyrimethamine (peer i METH a meen)

Brand Names: US Daraprim
Brand Names: Canada Daraprim [DSC]
Pharmacologic Category Antimalarial Agent
Use

Malaria chemoprophylaxis: Chemoprophylaxis of malaria due to susceptible strains of plasmodia.
Limitations of use: Resistance to pyrimethamine is prevalent worldwide; it is not suitable as a prophylactic agent for travelers to most areas.

Malaria treatment: Treatment (in combination with a sulfonamide) of acute malaria due to susceptible strains of plasmodia.

Toxoplasmosis: Treatment of toxoplasmosis (in combination with a sulfonamide).

Pregnancy Considerations Adverse events have been observed in animal reproduction studies. If administered during pregnancy (ie, for toxoplasmosis), supplementation of folate is strongly recommended. Pregnancy should be avoided during therapy.

Breast-Feeding Considerations Pyrimethamine enters breast milk and may result in significant systemic concentrations in breast-fed infants. The effect of concurrent therapy with sulfonamide or dapsone (frequently used with pyrimethamine as combination treatment) must be considered.

Prescribing and Access Restrictions As of June 2015, pyrimethamine is no longer available in retail pharmacies in the United States. It is only available through a special pharmacy program (http://www.daraprimdirect.com/healthcare-providers).

Contraindications Hypersensitivity to pyrimethamine or any component of the formulation; megaloblastic anemia secondary to folate deficiency

Warnings/Precautions Administer leucovorin calcium to prevent hematologic complications due to pyrimethamine-induced folic acid deficiency-state; continue leucovorin during therapy and for 1 week after therapy is discontinued (to account for the long half-life of pyrimethamine) (HHS [OI pediatric, 2013]. Megaloblastic anemia, leukopenia, thrombocytopenia, and pancytopenia have been reported; most commonly with high doses. Monitor CBC and platelets twice weekly in patients receiving high-dose therapy (eg, when used for toxoplasmosis treatment). Use with caution in patients with impaired renal or hepatic function or with possible G6PD deficiency. Use caution in patients with seizure disorders or possible folate deficiency (eg, malabsorption syndrome, pregnancy, alcoholism). Potentially significant interactions may exist, requiring dose or frequency adjustment, additional monitoring, and/or selection of alternative therapy.

Adverse Reactions Frequency not defined.
Cardiovascular: Arrhythmias (large doses)
Dermatologic: Erythema multiforme, rash, Stevens-Johnson syndrome, toxic epidermal necrolysis
Gastrointestinal: Anorexia, atrophic glossitis, vomiting
Hematologic: Leukopenia, megaloblastic anemia, pancytopenia, pulmonary eosinophilia, thrombocytopenia
Genitourinary: Hematuria
Miscellaneous: Anaphylaxis

Drug Interactions
Metabolism/Transport Effects Inhibits CYP2C9 (moderate)
Avoid Concomitant Use
Avoid concomitant use of Pyrimethamine with any of the following: Artemether; Lumefantrine
Increased Effect/Toxicity
Pyrimethamine may increase the levels/effects of: Antipsychotic Agents (Phenothiazines); Bosentan; Cannabis; Carvedilol; CYP2C9 Substrates; Dapsone (Systemic); Dapsone (Topical); Dronabinol; Lumefantrine; Tetrahydrocannabinol

The levels/effects of Pyrimethamine may be increased by: Artemether; Dapsone (Systemic)
Decreased Effect
The levels/effects of Pyrimethamine may be decreased by: Methylfolate
Storage/Stability Store at 15°C to 25°C (59°F to 77°F). Protect from light.
Mechanism of Action Inhibits parasitic dihydrofolate reductase, resulting in inhibition of vital tetrahydrofolic acid synthesis
Pharmacodynamics/Kinetics
Absorption: Well absorbed
Protein binding: 87%
Half-life elimination: 80 to 95 hours (White, 1985)
Time to peak, serum: 2 to 6 hours
Excretion: Urine (16% to 32%)
Dosing
Adult & Geriatric

Isosporiasis (*Isospora belli* infection) in HIV-infected patients (off-label use; HHS [OI adult 2015]): Oral:
Treatment (alternative to trimethoprim-sulfamethoxazole): 50 to 75 mg once daily in combination with leucovorin calcium
Chronic maintenance (secondary prophylaxis): 25 mg once daily in combination with leucovorin calcium

Malaria chemoprophylaxis: Oral: 25 mg once weekly. **Note:** Current CDC recommendations for malaria prophylaxis do not include the use of pyrimethamine (CDC 2014); resistance to pyrimethamine is prevalent worldwide.

Malaria treatment (non-*falciparum* malaria; use in conjunction with a sulfonamide [eg, sulfadoxine]): Oral: 25 mg daily for 2 days; following clinical cure, administer a once-weekly chemoprophylaxis regimen for ≥10 weeks. **Note:** Pyrimethamine use alone is **not** recommended; if circumstances arise where it must be used alone in semi-immune patients, give adults 50 mg daily for 2 days; then (following clinical cure) administer a once-weekly chemoprophylaxis regimen for ≥10 weeks

Note: Pyrimethamine use alone is **not** recommended; if circumstances arise where it must be used alone in semi-immune patients, give adults 50 mg daily for 2 days; then (following clinical cure) administer a once-weekly chemoprophylaxis regimen for ≥10 weeks.

Pneumocystis pneumonia (PCP) in HIV-infected patients (off-label use; HHS [OI adult 2015]): Oral:
Primary prophylaxis (alternative to trimethoprim-sulfamethoxazole): 50 or 75 mg once weekly in combination with dapsone and leucovorin calcium; **or** 25 mg once daily in combination with atovaquone and leucovorin calcium
Chronic maintenance (secondary prophylaxis; alternative to trimethoprim-sulfamethoxazole): 50 to 75 mg once weekly in combination with dapsone and leucovorin calcium; **or** 25 mg once daily in combination with atovaquone and leucovorin calcium

Toxoplasmosis treatment: Oral: 50 to 75 mg/day for 1 to 3 weeks depending on patient's tolerance and response, then may reduce dose by 50% and continue for 4 to 5 weeks; use with a sulfonamide in combination with leucovorin calcium

Toxoplasmosis in HIV-infected patients (off-label; HHS [OI adult 2015]): Oral:
Primary prophylaxis (alternative to trimethoprim sulfamethoxazole): 50 or 75 mg once weekly in combination with dapsone and leucovorin calcium; **or** 25 mg once daily in combination with atovaquone and leucovorin calcium (HHS [OI adult 2015])
Chronic maintenance therapy (secondary prophylaxis): 25 to 50 mg once daily in combination with sulfadiazine and leucovorin calcium (preferred); **or** 25 to 50 mg once daily in combination with clindamycin and leucovorin calcium; **or** 25 mg once daily in combination with atovaquone and leucovorin calcium (HHS [OI adult 2015])
Treatment of Toxoplasma gondii encephalitis: 200 mg as a single dose, followed by 50 mg (<60 kg) or 75 mg (≥60 kg) daily, in combination with sulfadiazine and leucovorin calcium for at least 6 weeks (preferred); **or** 200 mg as a single dose, followed by 50 mg (<60 kg) or 75 mg (≥60 kg) daily in combination with leucovorin calcium plus clindamycin or atovaquone or azithromycin. **Note:** Pyrimethamine is no longer available in retail pharmacies in the US and is only available through a special pharmacy program. According to the HHS Guidelines for the prevention and treatment of opportunistic infections in the HIV-infected adults and adolescents, if there is a delay in procuring pyrimethamine for patients with suspected or documented toxoplasmosis who do not have a history of sulfa allergy, trimethoprim-sulfamethoxazole should be used in place of pyrimethamine-containing regimens until pyrimethamine is available (HHS [OI adult, 2015]).

Pediatric

Isosporiasis (*Isospora belli* infection) in HIV-infected patients (off-label use): Adolescents: Refer to adult dosing.

Malaria chemoprophylaxis: Oral: Begin prophylaxis before entering endemic area: **Note:** Current CDC recommendations for malaria prophylaxis do not include the use of pyrimethamine (CDC 2014); resistance to pyrimethamine is prevalent worldwide.
Infants and Children <4 years: 6.25 mg once weekly
Children 4 to 10 years: 12.5 mg once weekly
Children >10 years and Adolescents: Refer to adult dosing.

Malaria treatment (non-*falciparum* malaria; use in conjunction with a sulfonamide [eg, sulfadoxine]): Oral: **Note:** Current CDC recommendations for malaria treatment do not include the use of pyrimethamine (CDC 2013); resistance to pyrimethamine is prevalent worldwide.
Children ≥4 years and Adolescents: 25 mg daily for 2 days; following clinical cure, administer a once weekly chemoprophylaxis regimen for ≥10 weeks
Note: Pyrimethamine use alone is **not** recommended; if circumstances arise where it must be used alone in semi-immune patients, give children >10 years and adolescents 50 mg daily for 2 days (children 4 to 10 years of age receive 25 mg daily for 2 days), then (following clinical cure) administer a once-weekly chemoprophylaxis regimen for ≥10 weeks

Pneumocystis pneumonia (PCP) in HIV-infected patients (off-label use): Adolescents: Refer to adult dosing.

Toxoplasmosis treatment: Oral: Loading dose: 1 mg/kg/day divided into 2 equal daily doses for 2 to 4 days, then may decrease dose to 0.5 mg/kg/day divided into 2 doses for 4 weeks; use with a sulfonamide and leucovorin calcium

Toxoplasmosis in HIV-infected patients (off-label): Oral:
Primary prophylaxis:
Infants and Children: 1 mg/kg/day (or 15 mg/m²) once daily (maximum: 25 mg), with dapsone or atovaquone, in combination with oral leucovorin calcium (HHS [OI pediatric 2013])
Adolescents: Refer to adult dosing.
Chronic maintenance therapy (secondary prophylaxis):
Infants and Children: 1 mg/kg/day (or 15 mg/m²) once daily (maximum: 25 mg) given with sulfadiazine (or atovaquone or clindamycin), in combination with oral leucovorin calcium (HHS [OI pediatric 2013])
Adolescents: Refer to adult dosing.
Treatment of congenital toxoplasmosis: Infants and Children: Loading dose: 2 mg/kg/day once daily for 2 days, then 1 mg/kg once daily for 2 to 6 months, followed by 1 mg/kg administered 3 times weekly, in combination with leucovorin calcium and sulfadiazine (treatment duration: 12 months) (HHS [OI pediatric 2013])
Treatment of acquired toxoplasmosis: Infants and Children: Acute induction: Loading dose: 2 mg/kg once daily (maximum: 50 mg/day) for 3 days, then 1 mg/kg/day once daily (maximum: 25 mg/day), with sulfadiazine or clindamycin in combination with leucovorin calcium (treatment duration: ≥6 weeks) (HHS [OI pediatric 2013])
Treatment of Toxoplasma gondii encephalitis: Adolescents: Refer to adult dosing.

Renal Impairment There are no dosage adjustments provided in the manufacturer's labeling. Use with caution.

Hepatic Impairment There are no dosage adjustments provided in the manufacturer's labeling. Use with caution.

Dietary Considerations Take with meals.

Administration Oral: Administer with meals to minimize GI distress.

Monitoring Parameters CBC, including platelet counts twice weekly with high-dose therapy (eg, when used for toxoplasmosis treatment; frequency not defined for lower doses); liver and renal function

Dosage Forms Excipient information presented when available (limited, particularly for generics); consult specific product labeling.
Tablet, Oral:
  Daraprim: 25 mg [scored]

Dosage Forms: Canada Excipient information presented when available (limited, particularly for generics); consult specific product labeling. [DSC] = Discontinued product
Tablet, Oral:
  Daraprim: 25 mg [DSC]

Extemporaneous Preparations A 2 mg/mL oral suspension may be made with tablets and a 1:1 mixture of Simple Syrup, NF and methylcellulose 1%. Crush forty 25 mg tablets in a mortar and reduce to a fine powder. Add small portions of vehicle and mix to a uniform paste; mix while adding vehicle in incremental proportions to **almost** 500 mL; transfer to a calibrated bottle, rinse mortar with vehicle, and add quantity of vehicle sufficient to make 500 mL. Label "shake well" and "refrigerate". Stable for 91 days.
Nahata MC, Pai VB, and Hipple TF, *Pediatric Drug Formulations*, 5th ed, Cincinnati, OH: Harvey Whitney Books Co, 2004.

Quazepam (KWAZ e pam)

Brand Names: US Doral
Brand Names: Canada Doral
Pharmacologic Category Benzodiazepine
Use Insomnia: For the treatment of insomnia characterized by difficulty in falling asleep, frequent nocturnal awakenings, and/or early morning
Medication Guide Available Yes
Dosing
Adult Hypnotic: Oral: Initial: 7.5 mg at bedtime; in some patients, the dose may be increased to 15 mg if necessary for efficacy.
Geriatric Dosing should be cautious; begin at lower end of dosing range (ie, 7.5 mg)
Renal Impairment No dosage adjustment provided in manufacturer's labeling.
Hepatic Impairment No dosage adjustment provided in manufacturer's labeling.
Additional Information Complete prescribing information should be consulted for additional detail.
Dosage Forms Excipient information presented when available (limited, particularly for generics); consult specific product labeling.
Tablet, Oral:
Doral: 15 mg [contains fd&c yellow #6 aluminum lake]
Generic: 15 mg
Controlled Substance C-IV

QUEtiapine (kwe TYE a peen)

Brand Names: US SEROquel; SEROquel XR
Brand Names: Canada Abbott-Quetiapine; ACT-Quetiapine; Apo-Quetiapine; Auro-Quetiapine; Dom-Quetiapine; JAMP-Quetiapine; Mar-Quetiapine; Mylan-Quetiapine; PHL-Quetiapine; PMS-Quetiapine; PRO-Quetiapine; Quetiapine XR; RAN-Quetiapine; Riva-Quetiapine; Sandoz-Quetiapine; Sandoz-Quetiapine XRT; Seroquel; Seroquel XR; Teva-Quetiapine; Teva-Quetiapine XR
Index Terms Quetiapine Fumarate
Pharmacologic Category Second Generation (Atypical) Antipsychotic
Use
Bipolar disorder: Acute treatment of manic (both immediate release and extended release [ER]) or mixed (ER only) episodes associated with bipolar I disorder, both as monotherapy and as an adjunct to lithium or divalproex; maintenance treatment of bipolar I disorder, as an adjunct to lithium or divalproex; acute treatment of depressive episodes associated with bipolar disorder

Major depressive disorder (ER only): Adjunctive therapy to antidepressants for the treatment of major depressive disorder.

Schizophrenia: Treatment of schizophrenia.

Pregnancy Considerations Adverse events were observed in animal reproduction studies. Quetiapine crosses the placenta and can be detected in cord blood (Newport 2007). Congenital malformations have not been observed in humans (based on limited data). Antipsychotic use during the third trimester of pregnancy has a risk for abnormal muscle movements (extrapyramidal symptoms [EPS]) and/or withdrawal symptoms in newborns following delivery. Symptoms in the newborn may include agitation, feeding disorder, hypertonia, hypotonia, respiratory distress, somnolence, and tremor; these effects may be self-limiting or require hospitalization. Quetiapine may cause hyperprolactinemia, which may decrease reproductive function in both males and females.

Treatment algorithms have been developed by the ACOG and the APA for the management of depression in women prior to conception and during pregnancy (Yonkers 2009). The ACOG recommends that therapy during pregnancy be individualized; treatment with psychiatric medications during pregnancy should incorporate the clinical expertise of the mental health clinician, obstetrician, primary healthcare provider, and pediatrician. Safety data related to atypical antipsychotics during pregnancy is limited and routine use is not recommended. However, if a woman is inadvertently exposed to an atypical antipsychotic while pregnant, continuing therapy may be preferable to switching to a typical antipsychotic that the fetus has not yet been exposed to; consider risk:benefit (ACOG 2008).

Healthcare providers are encouraged to enroll women 18-45 years of age exposed to quetiapine during pregnancy in the Atypical Antipsychotics Pregnancy Registry (1-866-961-2388 or http://www.womensmentalhealth.org/pregnancyregistry).

Breast-Feeding Considerations Quetiapine is excreted into breast milk. Based on information from 8 mother-infant pairs, concentrations of quetiapine in breast milk have been reported from undetectable to 170 mcg/L. The estimated exposure to the breast-feeding infant would be up to 0.1 mg/kg/day (relative infant dose up to 0.43% based on a weight adjusted maternal dose of 400 mg/day). Due to the potential for serious adverse reactions in the nursing infant, the manufacturer recommends a decision be made whether to discontinue nursing or to discontinue the drug, taking into account the importance of treatment to the mother.

Medication Guide Available Yes
Contraindications Hypersensitivity to quetiapine or any component of the formulation

Warnings/Precautions [US Boxed Warning]: Antidepressants increase the risk of suicidal thinking and behavior in children, adolescents, and young adults (18-24 years of age) with major depressive disorder (MDD) and other psychiatric disorders; consider risk prior to prescribing. Short-term studies did not show an increased risk in patients >24 years of age and showed a decreased risk in patients ≥65 years. Closely monitor all patients for clinical worsening, suicidality, or unusual changes in behavior; particularly during the initial 1-2 months of therapy or during periods of dosage adjustments (increased or decreases); the patient's family or caregiver should be instructed to closely observe the patient and communicate condition with healthcare provider. A medication guide concerning the use of antidepressants should be dispensed with each prescription. **Quetiapine is not approved in the U.S. for use in children <10 years of age.**

May precipitate a shift to mania or hypomania in patients with bipolar disorder. Patients presenting with depressive symptoms should be screened for bipolar disorder; the screening should include a detailed psychiatric history covering a family history of suicide, bipolar disorder, and depression. Quetiapine is approved in the US for the treatment of bipolar depression. Pharmacologic treatment for pediatric bipolar I disorder or schizophrenia should be initiated only after thorough diagnostic evaluation and a careful consideration of potential risks vs benefits. If a pharmacologic agent is initiated, it should be a component of a total treatment program including psychological, educational and social interventions. Increased blood pressure (including hypertensive crisis) has been reported in children and adolescents; monitor blood pressure at baseline and periodically during use.

Leukopenia, neutropenia, and agranulocytosis (sometimes fatal) have been reported with antipsychotic use; presence of risk factors (eg, preexisting low WBC or history of drug-induced leuko-/neutropenia) should prompt periodic blood count assessment. Discontinue therapy at first signs of blood dyscrasias or if absolute neutrophil count <1000/mm^3.

May cause orthostatic hypotension; use with caution in patients at risk of this effect or in those who would not tolerate transient hypotensive episodes (cerebrovascular disease, cardiovascular disease, dehydration, hypovolemia, or concurrent medication use which may predispose to hypotension/bradycardia) especially during the initial dose titration period. Use has been associated with QT prolongation; postmarketing reports have occurred in patients with concomitant illness, quetiapine overdose, or who were receiving concomitant therapy known to increase QT interval or cause electrolyte imbalance. Avoid use in patients at increased risk of torsade de pointes/sudden death (eg, hypokalemia, hypomagnesemia, history of cardiac arrhythmias, congenital prolongation of QT interval, concomitant medications with QTc interval-prolonging properties). Use with caution in patients at increased risk of QT prolongation (eg, cardiovascular disease, heart failure, cardiac hypertrophy, elderly, family history of QT prolongation). May cause hyperglycemia; in some cases may be extreme and associated with ketoacidosis, hyperosmolar coma, or death. All patients should be monitored for symptoms of hyperglycemia (eg, polydipsia, polyuria, polyphagia, weakness) and undergo a fasting blood glucose test if symptoms develop during treatment. Patients with risk factors for diabetes (eg, obesity or family history) should have a baseline fasting blood sugar (FBS) and periodically during treatment. Use with caution in patients with preexisting abnormal lipid profile. Significant weight gain has been observed with antipsychotic therapy; incidence varies with product. Monitor waist circumference and BMI.

[US Boxed Warning]: Elderly patients with dementia-related psychosis treated with antipsychotics are at an increased risk of death compared to placebo. Most deaths appeared to be either cardiovascular (eg, heart failure, sudden death) or infectious (eg, pneumonia) in nature. Use with caution in dementia with Lewy bodies; antipsychotics may worsen dementia symptoms and patients with dementia with Lewy bodies are more sensitive to the extrapyramidal side effects. Relative to other antipsychotics quetiapine has a lower propensity to cause extrapyramidal side effects (APA, [Rabins 2007]). Quetiapine is not approved for the treatment of dementia-related psychosis. Avoid antipsychotic use for behavioral problems associated with dementia unless alternative non-pharmacologic therapies have failed and patient may harm self or others. In addition, use may cause or exacerbate syndrome of inappropriate antidiuretic hormone secretion or hyponatremia; monitor sodium closely with initiation or dosage adjustments in older adults (Beers Criteria).

May cause dose-related decreases in thyroid levels, including cases requiring thyroid replacement therapy. Measure both TSH and free T$_4$, along with clinical assessment, at baseline and follow-up to determine thyroid status; measurement of TSH alone may not be accurate (exact mechanism of quetiapine's effect on the thyroid axis is unknown). Due to anticholinergic effects, use with caution in patients with decreased gastrointestinal motility, urinary retention, BPH, xerostomia, visual problems, and narrow-angle glaucoma. Relative to other antipsychotics, quetiapine has a moderate potency of cholinergic blockade. May cause extrapyramidal symptoms (EPS) and/or tardive dyskinesia. Risk of dystonia (and probably other EPS) may be greater with increased doses, use of conventional antipsychotics, males, and younger patients. Impaired core body temperature regulation may occur; caution with strenuous exercise, heat exposure, dehydration, and concomitant medication possessing anticholinergic effects. Use may be associated with neuroleptic malignant syndrome (NMS); monitor for mental status changes, fever, muscle rigidity and/or autonomic instability. Rare cases have been reported with quetiapine. Esophageal dysmotility and aspiration have been associated with antipsychotic use; use with caution in patients at risk of aspiration pneumonia (eg, Alzheimer disease). Development of cataracts has been observed in animal studies; lens changes have been observed in humans during long-term treatment. Lens examination, such as a slit-lamp exam, on initiation of therapy and every 6 months thereafter is recommended by manufacturer. Use caution with Parkinson disease, history of seizures, and renal impairment. Use caution with hepatic impairment; may cause elevations of liver enzymes. May cause CNS depression,

which may impair physical or mental abilities; patients must be cautioned about performing tasks that require mental alertness (eg, operating machinery or driving). Anaphylactic reactions have been reported with use. May increase prolactin levels; clinical significance of hyperprolactinemia in patients with breast cancer or other prolactin-dependent tumors is unknown. Potentially significant drug-drug interactions may exist, requiring dose or frequency adjustment, additional monitoring, and/or selection of alternative therapy. May cause withdrawal symptoms (rare) with abrupt cessation; gradually taper dose during discontinuation.

Adverse Reactions Actual frequency may be dependent upon dose and/or indication. Unless otherwise noted, frequency of adverse effects is reported for adult patients; spectrum and incidence of adverse effects similar in children (with significant exceptions noted).

>10%:
  Cardiovascular: Hypertension (diastolic; children and adolescents 41%; adults 2%), systolic hypertension (children and adolescents 15%), tachycardia (1% to 11%)
  Central nervous system: Drowsiness (16% to 57%), headache (17% to 21%), agitation (6% to 20%), dizziness (7% to 19%), fatigue (3% to 14%), extrapyramidal reaction (1% to 13%)
  Endocrine & metabolic: Weight gain (dose related; 3% to 28%), increased serum triglycerides (≥200 mg/dL, 8% to 22%), decreased HDL cholesterol (≤40 mg/dL, 6% to 20%), total cholesterol increased (≥240 mg/dL, 7% to 18%), increased LDL cholesterol (≥160 mg/dL, 4% to 12%), hyperglycemia (≥200 mg/dL post glucose challenge or fasting glucose ≥126 mg/dL, 2% to 3%)
  Gastrointestinal: Xerostomia (7% to 44%; children and adolescents 4% to 10%), increased appetite (2% to 12%), constipation (2% to 11%)

1% to 10%:
  Cardiovascular: Orthostatic hypotension (2% to 7%; children and adolescents <1%), palpitations (4%), peripheral edema (4%), increased heart rate (2% to 4%), hypotension (3%), hypertension (1% to 2%), syncope (1% to 2%)
  Central nervous system: Pain (7%), drug-induced Parkinson's disease (2% to ≤6%), lethargy (5%), dysarthria (2% to 5%), irritability (2% to 5%), akathisia (1% to 5%), hypertonia (4%), twitching (4%), anxiety (2% to 4%), abnormal dreams (2% to 3%), hypersomnia (2% to 3%), paresthesia (2% to 3%), aggressive behavior (children and adolescents 1% to 3%), depression (1% to 3%), dystonic reaction (1% to 3%), abnormality in thinking (2%), ataxia (2%), confusion (2%), decreased mental acuity (2%), disorientation (2%), disturbance in attention (2%), falling (2%), hypoesthesia (2%), lack of concentration (2%), migraine (2%), restless leg syndrome (2%), restlessness (2%), vertigo (2%)
  Dermatologic: Skin rash (4%), acne vulgaris (children and adolescents 2% to 3%), diaphoresis (2%), pallor (children and adolescents 1% to 2%)
  Endocrine & metabolic: Hyperprolactinemia (4%), increased thirst (children and adolescents 2%), decreased libido (≤2%), hypothyroidism (≤2%)
  Gastrointestinal: Nausea (5% to 10%), vomiting (1% to 8%), dyspepsia (dose related; 2% to 7%), abdominal pain (1% to 7%), gastroenteritis (2% to 4%), toothache (2% to 3%), anorexia (1% to 3%), periodontal abscess (adolescents 1% to 3%), decreased appetite (2%), dysphagia (2%), flatulence (2%), gastroesophageal reflux disease (2%)
  Genitourinary: Pollakiuria (2%), urinary tract infection (2%)
  Hematologic & oncologic: Neutropenia (≤2%), leukopenia (≥1%)
  Hepatic: Increased serum transaminases (1% to 6%)
  Hypersensitivity: Seasonal allergy (2%)
  Neuromuscular & skeletal: Weakness (1% to 10%), tremor (2% to 8%), back pain (1% to 5%), dyskinesia (3% to 4%), arthralgia (1% to 4%), muscle rigidity (3%), muscle spasm (1% to 3%), stiffness (children and adolescents 1% to 3%), limb pain (2%), myalgia (2%), neck pain (2%)
  Ophthalmic: Blurred vision (1% to 4%), amblyopia (2% to 3%)
  Otic: Otalgia (2%)
  Respiratory: Pharyngitis (4% to 6%), nasal congestion (3% to 6%), rhinitis (3% to 4%), epistaxis (adolescents 3%), sinus congestion (2% to 3%), upper respiratory tract infection (2% to 3%), cough (≥1% to 3%), dyspnea (≥1% to 3%), sinus headache (2%), sinusitis (2%), influenza (1% to 2%)
  Miscellaneous: Fever (2%)

◀ <1% (Limited to important or life-threatening): Abnormality of blepharitis, abnormal T waves on ECG, accommodation, acute hepatic failure, acute renal failure, agranulocytosis, alcohol intolerance, amenorrhea, amnesia, anemia, angina pectoris, apathy, aphasia, arthritis, atrial fibrillation, atrioventricular block, bone pain, bruxism, buccoglossal syndrome, bundle branch block, cardiac failure, cardiomyopathy, cataract, catatonic reaction, cerebrovascular accident, choreoathetosis, cyanosis, cystitis, deafness, deep vein thrombophlebitis, dehydration, delirium, delusions, depersonalization, diabetes mellitus, dysmenorrhea, dysuria, ecchymosis, eosinophilia, facial edema, first degree atrioventricular block, flattened T wave on ECG, galactorrhea, glossitis, hemiplegia, hemolysis, hepatic injury (cholestatic or mixed), hepatitis (with or without jaundice), hyperkinesia, hyperlipemia, hypersensitivity, hyperthyroidism, hyperventilation, hypochromic anemia, hypoglycemia, increased creatinine phosphokinase, increased gamma-glutamyl transferase, increased libido, increased QRS duration, increased salivation, increased serum alkaline phosphatase, increased ST segment on ECG, intestinal obstruction, irregular pulse, leukocytosis, leukorrhea, liver steatosis, lymphadenopathy, malaise, manic reaction, melena, myasthenia, myocarditis, myoclonus, neuralgia, neuroleptic malignant syndrome, orchitis, pancreatitis, paranoid reaction, pathological fracture, pelvic pain, pneumonia, priapism, prolonged Q-T interval on ECG, pruritus, psoriasis, psychosis, rectal hemorrhage, rhabdomyolysis, seborrhea, seizure, SIADH, stomatitis, ST segment changes on ECG, stupor, subdural hematoma, suicidal ideation, tardive dyskinesia, thrombocytopenia, thrombophlebitis, tongue edema, uterine hemorrhage, vaginal hemorrhage, vaginitis, vasodilatation, vulvovaginal moniliasis, vulvovaginitis, widened QRS complex on ECG

Drug Interactions

Metabolism/Transport Effects Substrate of CYP2D6 (minor), CYP3A4 (major); **Note:** Assignment of Major/Minor substrate status based on clinically relevant drug interaction potential

Avoid Concomitant Use

Avoid concomitant use of QUEtiapine with any of the following: Aclidinium; Amisulpride; Azelastine (Nasal); Cimetropium; Clarithromycin; Conivaptan; Eluxadoline; Fusidic Acid (Systemic); Glucagon; Glycopyrrolate; Glycopyrrolate (Oral Inhalation); Highest Risk QTc-Prolonging Agents; Idelalisib; Ipratropium (Oral Inhalation); Ivabradine; Levosulpiride; Methadone; Metoclopramide; Mifepristone; Moderate Risk QTc-Prolonging Agents; Orphenadrine; Paraldehyde; Potassium Chloride; Sulpiride; Thalidomide; Tiotropium; Umeclidinium

Increased Effect/Toxicity

QUEtiapine may increase the levels/effects of: AbobotulinumtoxinA; Alcohol (Ethyl); Amisulpride; Analgesics (Opioid); Anticholinergic Agents; Azelastine (Nasal); CarBAMazepine; Cimetropium; CNS Depressants; Eluxadoline; Glucagon; Glycopyrrolate; Glycopyrrolate (Oral Inhalation); Highest Risk QTc-Prolonging Agents; Hydrocodone; Methadone; Methotrimeprazine; Methylphenidate; Metyrosine; OnabotulinumtoxinA; Orphenadrine; Paraldehyde; Potassium Chloride; Ramosetron; RimabotulinumtoxinB; Selective Serotonin Reuptake Inhibitors; Serotonin Modulators; St Johns Wort; Sulpiride; Suvorexant; Thalidomide; Thiazide Diuretics; Tiotropium; Topiramate; Zolpidem

The levels/effects of QUEtiapine may be increased by: Acetylcholinesterase Inhibitors (Central); Aclidinium; Aprepitant; Blood Pressure Lowering Agents; Brimonidine (Topical); Cannabis; Clarithromycin; Conivaptan; CYP3A4 Inhibitors (Moderate); CYP3A4 Inhibitors (Strong); Doxylamine; Dronabinol; Fosaprepitant; Fusidic Acid (Systemic); Idelalisib; Ipratropium (Oral Inhalation); Ivabradine; Ivacaftor; Kava Kava; Luliconazole; Magnesium Sulfate; Methadone; Methotrimeprazine; Methylphenidate; Metoclopramide; Metyrosine; Mifepristone; Minocycline; Moderate Risk QTc-Prolonging Agents; Nabilone; Netupitant; Palbociclib; Perampanel; Pramlintide; QTc-Prolonging Agents (Indeterminate Risk and Risk Modifying); Ritonavir; Rufinamide; Serotonin Modulators; Simeprevir; Sodium Oxybate; Stiripentol; Tapentadol; Tetrahydrocannabinol; Umeclidinium

Decreased Effect

QUEtiapine may decrease the levels/effects of: Acetylcholinesterase Inhibitors; Amphetamines; Antidiabetic Agents; Anti-Parkinson's Agents (Dopamine Agonist); Gastrointestinal Agents (Prokinetic); Itopride; Levosulpiride; Quinagolide; Secretin

The levels/effects of QUEtiapine may be decreased by: Acetylcholinesterase Inhibitors; Bosentan; CarBAMazepine; CYP3A4 Inducers (Moderate); CYP3A4 Inducers (Strong); Dabrafenib; Deferasirox; Enzalutamide; Mitotane; Siltuximab; St Johns Wort; Tocilizumab

Food Interactions In healthy volunteers, administration of quetiapine (immediate release) with food resulted in an increase in the peak serum concentration and AUC by 25% and 15%, respectively, compared to the fasting state. Administration of the extended release formulation with a high-fat meal (~800-1000 calories) resulted in an increase in peak serum concentration by 44% to 52% and AUC by 20% to 22% for the 50 mg and 300 mg tablets; administration with a light meal (≤300 calories) had no significant effect on the C_{max} or AUC. Management: Administer without food or with a light meal (≤300 calories).

Storage/Stability Store at 25°C (77°F); excursions permitted between 15°C and 30°C (59°F and 86°F).

Mechanism of Action Quetiapine is a dibenzothiazepine atypical antipsychotic. It has been proposed that this drug's antipsychotic activity is mediated through a combination of dopamine type 2 (D_2) and serotonin type 2 (5-HT$_2$) antagonism. It is an antagonist at multiple neurotransmitter receptors in the brain: Serotonin 5-HT$_{1A}$ and 5-HT$_2$, dopamine D_1 and D_2, histamine H_1, and adrenergic alpha$_1$- and alpha$_2$-receptors; but appears to have no appreciable affinity at cholinergic muscarinic and benzodiazepine receptors. Norquetiapine, an active metabolite, differs from its parent molecule by exhibiting high affinity for muscarinic M1 receptors.

Antagonism at receptors other than dopamine and 5-HT$_2$ with similar receptor affinities may explain some of the other effects of quetiapine. The drug's antagonism of histamine H_1-receptors may explain the somnolence observed. The drug's antagonism of adrenergic alpha$_1$-receptors may explain the orthostatic hypotension observed.

Pharmacodynamics/Kinetics

Absorption: Rapidly absorbed following oral administration; high-fat meals (800 to 1000 calories) increase C_{max} 8% and AUC 2% of quetiapine XR; light meals (300 calories) had no effect.

Distribution: V_d: 6 to 14 L/kg

Protein binding, plasma: 83%

Metabolism: Primarily hepatic; via CYP3A4; forms the metabolite N-desalkyl quetiapine (active) and two inactive metabolites

Bioavailability: 100% (relative to oral solution)

Half-life elimination:

Mean: Terminal: Quetiapine: ~6 hours; Extended release: ~7 hours

Metabolite: N-desalkyl quetiapine: 12 hours

Time to peak, plasma: Immediate release: 1.5 hours; Extended release: 6 hours

Excretion: Urine (73% as metabolites, <1% of total dose as unchanged drug); feces (20%)

Dosing

Adult

Bipolar disorder: Oral:

Depressive episodes: **Note:** In clinical trials, doses up to 600 mg/day were not associated with any further benefit compared to 300 mg/day.

Immediate release: Initial: 50 mg once daily at bedtime on day 1; increase to 100 mg once daily on day 2, further increase by 100 mg daily each day until 300 mg once daily is reached by day 4. Usual dose: 300 mg once daily; maximum dose: 300 mg once daily.

Extended release: Initial: 50 mg once daily on day 1; increase to 100 mg once daily on day 2, further increase by 100 mg once daily until 300 mg once daily is reached by day 4. Usual dose: 300 mg once daily; maximum dose: 300 mg once daily (US labeling) or 600 mg once daily (Canadian labeling).

Mania (monotherapy or as an adjunct to lithium or divalproex): Immediate release: Initial: 50 mg twice daily on day 1, further increase by 100 mg daily (administered twice daily) until 200 mg twice daily is reached by day 4; may further increase to 800 mg daily by day 6 in increments of ≤200 mg daily. Usual dosage range: 400 to 800 mg daily; maximum dose: 800 mg daily.

Manic or mixed (monotherapy or as an adjunct to lithium or divalproex): Extended release: Initial: 300 mg once daily on day 1; increase to 600 mg once daily on day 2 then adjust dose to between 400 to 800 mg once daily on day 3; usual dosage range: 400 to 800 mg once daily; maximum dose: 800 mg once daily.

Maintenance therapy (adjunct to lithium or divalproex): Immediate release or extended release: Usual dosage range: 400 to 800 mg daily; maximum dose: 800 mg daily. **Note:** In the maintenance phase, patients generally continue on the same dose on which they were stabilized. Average time of stabilization was 15 weeks in clinical trials. During maintenance treatment, periodically reassess need for continued therapy and the appropriate dose.

Major depressive disorder (adjunct to antidepressants): Oral: Extended release: Initial: 50 mg once daily on days 1 and 2; increase to 150 mg once daily on day 3. Usual dosage range: 150 to 300 mg daily; maximum dose: 300 mg once daily.

Schizophrenia: Oral:

Immediate release: Initial: 25 mg twice daily; increase in increments of 25 to 50 mg divided 2 to 3 times daily on days 2 and 3 to a range of 300 to 400 mg daily in 2 to 3 divided doses by day 4. Further adjustments as needed at intervals of at least 2 days in increments of 25 to 50 mg twice daily. Usual dosage range: 150 to 750 mg daily; maximum dose: 750 mg daily.

Extended release: Initial: 300 mg once daily; increase in increments of up to 300 mg once daily (in intervals of ≥1 day). Usual dosage range: 400 to 800 mg once daily; maximum dose: 800 mg once daily.

Maintenance therapy (monotherapy): Extended release: Usual dosage range: 400 to 800 mg once daily; maximum dose: 800 mg once daily. **Note:** During maintenance treatment, periodically reassess need for continued therapy and the appropriate dose.

Generalized anxiety disorder, monotherapy (off-label): Oral: Extended release: Initial: 50 mg once daily at bedtime; based on response and tolerability, after 3 days increase dose to 150 mg once daily at bedtime; further dosage adjustments up to 300 mg once daily at bedtime may be considered after at least 2 days of 150 mg daily (Bandelow 2010; Katzman 2011; Merideth 2012).

ICU delirium (off-label use): Oral: Immediate release: Initial: 50 mg twice daily; may increase as necessary on a daily basis in increments of 50 mg twice daily to a maximum dose of 400 mg daily (Devlin 2010)

Obsessive-compulsive disorder, treatment-resistant (augmentation; off-label use): Oral: Immediate release: Initial: 25 to 50 mg once daily; increased gradually based on response and tolerability up to 400 mg/day (Atmaca 2002; Denys 2004; Fineberg 2005).

Post-traumatic stress disorder (off-label use): Oral: Immediate release: Initial: 25 mg at bedtime; increase dose at 25 mg increments every 1 to 2 days up to 100 mg at bedtime by the end of week 1; further adjust dose based on response and tolerability at increments of 25 mg/day or up to 100 mg/week, to a maximum dose of 400 mg/day administered in 1 or 2 divided doses. Average dose in clinical trials: 100 to 200 mg/day (range 25 to 400 mg/day) (Ahearn 2006; Hamner 2003; Kozaric-Kovacic 2007).

Switching from immediate release to extended release: May convert patients from immediate release to extended release tablets at the equivalent total daily dose and administer once daily; individual dosage adjustments may be necessary.

Reinitiation of treatment: Patients who have discontinued therapy for >1 week should generally be retitrated following reinitiation of therapy; patients who have discontinued <1 week, can generally be reinitiated on their previous maintenance dose

Dosage adjustment for concomitant therapy:

Concomitant use with a strong CYP3A4 inhibitor (eg, ketoconazole, itraconazole, indinavir, ritonavir, nefazodone): Immediate release or extended release: Decrease quetiapine to one-sixth of the original dose; when strong CYP3A4 inhibitor is discontinued, increase quetiapine by sixfold.

Concomitant use with a strong CYP3A4 inducer (eg, phenytoin, carbamazepine, rifampin, St John's wort): Immediate release or extended release: Increase quetiapine up to fivefold of the original dose when combined with chronic treatment (>7 or 14 days) of a strong CYP3A4 inducer; titrate based on clinical response and tolerance; when the strong CYP3A4 inducer is discontinued, decrease quetiapine to the original dose within 7 to 14 days.

Geriatric

Bipolar disorder or schizophrenia: Oral: Immediate release and extended release: Initial: 50 mg daily; may increase in increments of 50 mg daily to an effective dose, based on individual clinical response and tolerability

Major depressive disorder (adjunct to antidepressants): Oral:

US labeling: Extended release: 50 mg once daily; may increase by 50 mg once daily to an effective dose, based on individual clinical response and tolerability

Canadian labeling: Extended release: 50 mg once daily on days 1 to 3, based on response and tolerability, may increase to 100 mg/day on day 4 and 150 mg/day on day 8

Psychosis/agitation related to Alzheimer disease and other dementias (off-label use): Oral: Immediate release: Initial: 12.5 to 50 mg daily; if necessary, gradually increase based on response and tolerability not to exceed 200 to 300 mg daily. Consider periodic dosage adjustments to reduce or discontinue therapy as clinically indicated (APA [Rabins 2007]; Fujikawa 2004; McManus 1999; Scharre 2002).

Psychosis in Parkinson disease (off-label use): Oral: Immediate release: Initial: 25 mg daily in 1 to 2 divided doses; adjust dose gradually based on response and tolerability up to 200 mg daily; mean dose in clinical trials was ~91 mg daily (Merims 2006; Morgante 2004). Additional data may be necessary to further define the role of quetiapine in this condition.

Switching from immediate release to extended release: Refer to adult dosing.

Reinitiation of treatment: Refer to adult dosing.

Dosage adjustment for concomitant therapy: Refer to adult dosing.

Pediatric Note: Not approved for use in pediatric patients <18 years in Canadian labeling.

Bipolar disorder: Children ≥10 years and Adolescents ≤17 years: Oral: *Mania (monotherapy):*

Immediate release: Initial: 25 mg twice daily on day 1; increase to 50 mg twice daily on day 2, then increase by 100 mg daily (administered twice daily) each day until 200 mg twice day is reached on day 5. May further increase up to 600 mg daily in increments of ≤100 mg daily. Usual dosage range: 400 to 600 mg daily; maximum: 600 mg daily. **Note:** Total daily doses may also be divided into 3 doses per day, based on response and tolerability.

Extended release: Initial: 50 mg once daily on day 1; increase to 100 mg once daily on day 2, further increase by 100 mg once daily until 400 mg once daily is reached on day 5. Usual dosage range: 400 to 600 mg once daily; maximum dose: 600 mg once daily.

Schizophrenia: Adolescents 13 to ≤17 years: Oral:

Immediate release: Initial: 25 mg twice daily on day 1; increase to 50 mg twice daily on day 2, further increase by 100 mg daily each day (divided twice daily) until 400 mg twice daily is reached on day 5. May further increase up to 800 mg daily in increments of ≤100 mg daily. Usual dosage range: 400 to 800 mg daily; maximum dose: 800 mg daily. **Note:** Total daily doses may also be divided into 3 doses per day, based on response and tolerability.

Extended release: Initial: 50 mg once daily on day 1; increase to 100 mg once daily on day 2, further increase by 100 mg once daily until 400 mg once daily is reached on day 5. Usual dosage range: 400 to 800 mg once daily; maximum dose: 800 mg once daily.

Switching from immediate release to extended release: Refer to adult dosing.

Reinitiation of treatment: Refer to adult dosing.

Dosage adjustment for concomitant therapy: Refer to adult dosing.

Renal Impairment No dosage adjustment necessary.

Hepatic Impairment

Immediate release tablet: Initial: 25 mg daily, increase dose by 25 to 50 mg daily to effective dose, based on individual clinical response and tolerability

Extended release tablet: Initial: 50 mg once daily; increase dose by 50 mg once daily to effective dose, based on individual clinical response and tolerability

Dietary Considerations Administer extended release tablet without food or with a light meal (≤300 calories).

Administration

Oral:

Immediate release tablet: Administer with or without food.

Extended release tablet: Administer without food or with a light meal (≤300 calories), preferably in the evening. Swallow tablet whole; do not break, crush, or chew.

Nasogastric/enteral tube (off-label route): Hold tube feeds for 30 minutes before administration; flush with 25 mL of sterile water. Crush dose using immediate-release formulation, mix in 10 mL water and administer via NG/ enteral tube; follow with a 50 mL flush of sterile water (Devlin 2010).

Monitoring Parameters Mental status; vital signs (as clinically indicated); blood pressure (baseline; repeat 3 months after antipsychotic initiation, then yearly, particularly in children and adolescents); weight, height, BMI, waist circumference (baseline; repeat at 4, 8, and 12 weeks after initiating or changing therapy, then quarterly; consider switching to a different antipsychotic for a weight gain ≥5% of initial weight); CBC (as clinically indicated; monitor frequently during the first few months of therapy in patients with preexisting low WBC or history of drug-induced leukopenia/neutropenia); electrolytes and liver function (annually and as clinically indicated); TSH, free T_4, and thyroid clinical assessment (baseline and follow-up); fasting plasma glucose level/HbA$_{1c}$ (baseline; repeat 3 months after starting antipsychotic, then yearly); fasting lipid panel (baseline; repeat 3 months after initiation of antipsychotic; if LDL level is normal, repeat at 2-5 year intervals or more frequently if clinically indicated); changes in menstruation, libido, development of galactorrhea, erectile and ejaculatory function (at each visit for the first 12 weeks after the antipsychotic is initiated or until the dose is stable, then yearly); abnormal involuntary movements or parkinsonian signs (baseline; repeat weekly until dose stabilized for at least 2 weeks after introduction and for 2 weeks after any significant dose increase); tardive dyskinesia (every 12 months; high-risk patients every 6 months); lens examination, such as a slit-lamp exam, on initiation of therapy and every 6 months is recommended by manufacturer; alternatively, experts suggest it may be reasonable to inquire yearly about visual changes and perform ocular examinations yearly in patients >40 years or every 2 years in younger patients (ADA 2004; Lehman 2004; Marder 2004).

Test Interactions May interfere with urine detection of methadone (false-positives); may cause false-positive serum TCA screen

Dosage Forms Excipient information presented when available (limited, particularly for generics); consult specific product labeling.

Tablet, Oral:
SEROquel: 25 mg, 50 mg, 100 mg, 200 mg, 300 mg, 400 mg
Generic: 25 mg, 50 mg, 100 mg, 200 mg, 300 mg, 400 mg

Tablet Extended Release 24 Hour, Oral:
SEROquel XR: 50 mg, 150 mg, 200 mg, 300 mg, 400 mg

Quinapril (KWIN a pril)

Brand Names: US Accupril
Brand Names: Canada Accupril; Apo-Quinapril; GD-Quinapril; PMS-Quinapril
Index Terms Quinapril Hydrochloride
Pharmacologic Category Angiotensin-Converting Enzyme (ACE) Inhibitor; Antihypertensive

Use
Heart failure: Adjunctive treatment of heart failure (HF)
Hypertension: Treatment of hypertension

Guideline recommendations:
Heart failure: The ACCF/AHA 2013 heart failure guidelines recommend the use of ACE inhibitors, along with other guideline directed medical therapies, to prevent HF in patients with a reduced ejection fraction who have a history of MI (stage B HF), to prevent HF in any patient with a reduced ejection fraction (stage B HF), or to treat those with HF and reduced ejection fraction (stage C HFrEF) (ACCF/AHA [Yancy, 2013]).

Hypertension: The 2014 guideline for the management of high blood pressure in adults (Eighth Joint National Committee [JNC 8]) recommends initiation of pharmacologic treatment to lower blood pressure for the following patients:

• Patients ≥60 years of age with systolic blood pressure (SBP) ≥150 mm Hg or diastolic blood pressure (DBP) ≥90 mm Hg. Goal of therapy is SBP <150 mm Hg and DBP <90 mm Hg.

• Patients <60 years of age with SBP ≥140 mm Hg or DBP is ≥90 mm Hg. Goal of therapy is SBP <140 mm Hg and DBP <90 mm Hg.

• Patients ≥18 years of age with diabetes and SBP ≥140 mm Hg or DBP ≥90 mm Hg. Goal of therapy is SBP <140 mm Hg and DBP <90 mm Hg.

• Patients ≥18 years of age with chronic kidney disease (CKD) and SBP ≥140 mm Hg or DBP ≥90 mm Hg. Goal of therapy is SBP <140 mm Hg and DBP <90 mm Hg.

Chronic kidney disease (CKD) and hypertension: Regardless of race or diabetes status, the use of an ACE inhibitor (ACEI) or angiotensin receptor blocker (ARB) as initial therapy is recommended to improve kidney outcomes. In the general nonblack population (without CKD) including those with diabetes, initial antihypertensive treatment should consist of a thiazide-type diuretic, calcium channel blocker, ACEI, or ARB. In the general black population (without CKD) including those with diabetes, initial antihypertensive treatment should consist of a thiazide-type diuretic or a calcium channel blocker **instead of** an ACEI or ARB.

Coronary artery disease (CAD) and hypertension: The American Heart Association, American College of Cardiology and American Society of Hypertension (AHA/ACC/ASH) 2015 scientific statement for the treatment of hypertension in patients with CAD recommends the use of an ACE inhibitor (or an ARB) as part of a regimen in patients with hypertension and chronic stable angina if there is prior MI, LV systolic dysfunction, diabetes mellitus, or CKD. A BP target of <140/90 mm Hg is reasonable for the secondary prevention of cardiovascular events. A lower target BP (<130/80 mm Hg) may be appropriate in some individuals with CAD, previous MI, stroke or transient ischemic attack, or CAD risk equivalents (AHA/ACC/ASH [Rosendorff 2015]).

Pregnancy Considerations [U.S. Boxed Warning]: Drugs that act on the renin-angiotensin system can cause injury and death to the developing fetus. Discontinue as soon as possible once pregnancy is detected. Quinapril crosses the placenta. Drugs that act on the renin-angiotensin system are associated with oligohydramnios. Oligohydramnios, due to decreased fetal renal function, may lead to fetal lung hypoplasia and skeletal malformations. The use of these drugs in pregnancy is also associated with anuria, hypotension, renal failure, skull hypoplasia, and death in the fetus/neonate. Teratogenic effects may occur following maternal use of an ACE inhibitor during the first trimester, although this finding may be confounded by maternal disease. Because adverse fetal events are well documented with exposure later in pregnancy, ACE inhibitor use in pregnant women is not recommended (Seely 2014; Weber 2014). Infants exposed to an ACE inhibitor in utero should be monitored for hyperkalemia, hypotension, and oliguria. Oligohydramnios may not appear until after irreversible fetal injury has occurred. Exchange transfusions or dialysis may be required to reverse hypotension or improve renal function, although data related to the effectiveness in neonates is limited.

Chronic maternal hypertension itself is also associated with adverse events in the fetus/infant and mother. ACE inhibitors are not recommended for the treatment of uncomplicated hypertension in pregnancy (ACOG 2013) and they are specifically contraindicated for the treatment of hypertension and chronic heart failure during pregnancy by some guidelines (Regitz-Zagrosek 2011). In addition, ACE inhibitors should generally be avoided in women of reproductive age (ACOG 2013). If treatment for hypertension or chronic heart failure in pregnancy is needed, other agents should be used (ACOG 2013; Regitz-Zagrosek 2011). In the Canadian product labeling, use is contraindicated in women who are pregnant, who are planning to become pregnant, or who are of child bearing potential and not using effective contraception.

Breast-Feeding Considerations Quinapril is excreted in breast milk. The manufacturer recommends that caution be exercised when administering quinapril to nursing women. The Canadian labeling contraindicates use in nursing women.

Contraindications
Hypersensitivity to quinapril or any component of the formulation; angioedema related to previous treatment with an ACE inhibitor; concomitant use with aliskiren in patients with diabetes mellitus.

Documentation of allergenic cross-reactivity for ACE inhibitors is limited. However, because of similarities in chemical structure and/or pharmacologic actions, the possibility of cross-sensitivity cannot be ruled out with certainty.

Canadian labeling: Additional contraindications (not in U.S. labeling): Women who are pregnant, intend to become pregnant, or of childbearing potential and not using adequate contraception; breast-feeding; concomitant use with aliskiren, angiotensin receptor blockers (ARBs),

or other ACE inhibitors in patients with moderate-to-severe renal impairment (GFR <60 mL/minute/1.73 m²), hyperkalemia (>5 mmol/L), or congestive heart failure who are hypotensive; concomitant use with angiotensin receptor blockers (ARBs) or other ACE inhibitors in diabetic patients with end organ damage; hereditary problems of galactose intolerance, glucose-galactose malabsorption or Lapp lactase deficiency

Warnings/Precautions Anaphylactic reactions may occur rarely with ACE inhibitors. At any time during treatment (especially following first dose) angioedema may occur rarely with ACE inhibitors; it may involve the head and neck (potentially compromising airway) or the intestine (presenting with abdominal pain). African-Americans and patients with idiopathic or hereditary angioedema may be at an increased risk. Risk may also be increased with concomitant use of mTOR inhibitor (eg, everolimus) therapy. Prolonged frequent monitoring may be required especially if tongue, glottis, or larynx are involved as they are associated with airway obstruction. Patients with a history of airway surgery may have a higher risk of airway obstruction. Aggressive early and appropriate management is critical. Use in patients with previous angioedema associated with ACE inhibitor therapy is contraindicated. Severe anaphylactoid reactions may be seen during hemodialysis (eg, CVVHD) with high-flux dialysis membranes (eg, AN69), and rarely, during low density lipoprotein apheresis with dextran sulfate cellulose. Rare cases of anaphylactoid reactions have been reported in patients undergoing sensitization treatment with hymenoptera (bee, wasp) venom while receiving ACE inhibitors. Formulation may contain lactose.

Symptomatic hypotension with or without syncope can occur with ACE inhibitors (usually with the first several doses); effects are most often observed in volume-depleted patients; close monitoring of patient is required especially with initial dosing and dosing increases; blood pressure must be lowered at a rate appropriate for the patient's clinical condition. Initiation of therapy in patients with ischemic heart disease or cerebrovascular disease warrants close observation due to the potential consequences posed by falling blood pressure (eg, MI, stroke). Use with caution in hypertrophic cardiomyopathy with outflow tract obstruction and severe aortic stenosis. In patients on chronic ACE inhibitor therapy, intraoperative hypotension may occur with induction and maintenance of general anesthesia; use with caution before, during, or immediately after major surgery. Cardiopulmonary bypass, intraoperative blood loss, or vasodilating anesthesia increases endogenous renin release. Use of ACE inhibitors perioperatively will blunt angiotensin II formation and may result in hypotension. However, discontinuation of therapy prior to surgery is controversial. If continued preoperatively, avoidance of hypotensive agents during surgery is prudent (Hillis, 2011). **[U.S. Boxed Warning]: Drugs that act on the renin-angiotensin system can cause injury and death to the developing fetus. Discontinue as soon as possible once pregnancy is detected.**

Hyperkalemia may occur with ACE inhibitors; risk factors include renal dysfunction, diabetes mellitus, concomitant use of potassium-sparing diuretics, potassium supplements, and/or potassium-containing salts. Use cautiously, if at all, with these agents and monitor potassium closely. Cough may occur with ACE inhibitors. Other causes of cough should be considered (eg, pulmonary congestion in patients with heart failure) and excluded prior to discontinuation.

May be associated with deterioration of renal function and/or increases in serum creatinine, particularly in patients with low renal blood flow (eg, renal artery stenosis, heart failure) whose glomerular filtration rate (GFR) is dependent on efferent arteriolar vasoconstriction by angiotensin II; deterioration may result in oliguria, acute renal failure, and progressive azotemia. Small increases in serum creatinine may occur following initiation; consider discontinuation only in patients with progressive and/or significant deterioration in renal function. Use with caution in patients with unstented unilateral/bilateral renal artery stenosis. When unstented bilateral renal artery stenosis is present, use is generally avoided due to the elevated risk of deterioration in renal function unless possible benefits outweigh risks. Potentially significant drug-drug interactions may exist, requiring dose or frequency adjustment, additional monitoring, and/or selection of alternative therapy.

Rare toxicities associated with ACE inhibitors include cholestatic jaundice (which may progress to fulminant hepatic necrosis), agranulocytosis, neutropenia, or leukopenia with myeloid hypoplasia. Patients with collagen vascular diseases (especially with concomitant renal impairment) or renal impairment alone may be at increased risk for hematologic toxicity; periodically monitor CBC with differential in these patients.

Adverse Reactions Note: Frequency ranges include data from hypertension and heart failure trials. Higher rates of adverse reactions have generally been noted in patients with CHF. However, the frequency of adverse effects associated with placebo is also increased in this population.

1% to 10%:
Cardiovascular: Hypotension (3%), chest pain (2%), first-dose hypotension (up to 3%)
Central nervous system: Dizziness (4% to 8%), headache (2% to 6%), fatigue (3%)
Dermatologic: Rash (1%)
Endocrine & metabolic: Hyperkalemia (2%)
Gastrointestinal: Vomiting/nausea (1% to 2%), diarrhea (1.7%)
Neuromuscular & skeletal: Myalgias (2% to 5%), back pain (1%)
Renal: BUN/serum creatinine increased (2%, transient elevations may occur with a higher frequency), worsening of renal function (in patients with bilateral renal artery stenosis or hypovolemia)
Respiratory: Upper respiratory symptoms, cough (2% to 4%; up to 13% in some studies), dyspnea (2%)
<1% (Limited to important or life-threatening): Acute renal failure, agranulocytosis, alopecia, amblyopia, anaphylactoid reaction, angina, angioedema, arrhythmia, cerebrovascular accident, depression, dermatopolymyositis, eosinophilic pneumonitis, exfoliative dermatitis, gastrointestinal hemorrhage, heart failure, hemolytic anemia, hepatitis, hyperkalemia, hypertensive crisis, impotence, insomnia, MI, orthostatic hypotension, pancreatitis, pemphigus, photosensitivity, shock, stroke, syncope, thrombocytopenia, viral infection, visual hallucinations (Doane, 2013)
A syndrome which may include fever, myalgia, arthralgia, interstitial nephritis, vasculitis, rash, eosinophilia and positive ANA, and elevated ESR has been reported with ACE inhibitors. In addition, pancreatitis, hepatic necrosis, neutropenia, and/or agranulocytosis (particularly in patients with collagen-vascular disease or renal impairment) have been associated with many ACE inhibitors.

Drug Interactions
Metabolism/Transport Effects None known.
Avoid Concomitant Use
Avoid concomitant use of Quinapril with any of the following: Sacubitril
Increased Effect/Toxicity
Quinapril may increase the levels/effects of: Allopurinol; Amifostine; Antipsychotic Agents (Second Generation [Atypical]); AzaTHIOprine; Drospirenone; DULoxetine; Ferric Gluconate; Gold Sodium Thiomalate; Grass Pollen Allergen Extract (5 Grass Extract); Hypotension-Associated Agents; Iron Dextran Complex; Levodopa; Lithium; Nonsteroidal Anti-Inflammatory Agents; Pregabalin; Sacubitril; Sodium Phosphates

The levels/effects of Quinapril may be increased by: Alfuzosin; Aliskiren; Angiotensin II Receptor Blockers; Barbiturates; Brimonidine (Topical); Canagliflozin; Dapoxetine; Diazoxide; DPP-IV Inhibitors; Eplerenone; Everolimus; Heparin; Heparin (Low Molecular Weight); Herbs (Hypotensive Properties); Loop Diuretics; Molsidomine; Nicorandil; Obinutuzumab; Pentoxifylline; Phosphodiesterase 5 Inhibitors; Potassium Salts; Potassium-Sparing Diuretics; Prostacyclin Analogues; Salicylates; Sirolimus; Temsirolimus; Thiazide Diuretics; TiZANidine; Tolvaptan; Trimethoprim
Decreased Effect
Quinapril may decrease the levels/effects of: Quinolone Antibiotics; Tetracycline Derivatives

The levels/effects of Quinapril may be decreased by: Amphetamines; Aprotinin; Herbs (Hypertensive Properties); Icatibant; Lanthanum; Methylphenidate; Nonsteroidal Anti-Inflammatory Agents; Salicylates; Yohimbine
Storage/Stability Store at 15°C to 30°C (59°F to 86°F). Protect from light.
Mechanism of Action Competitive inhibitor of angiotensin-converting enzyme (ACE); prevents conversion of angiotensin I to angiotensin II, a potent vasoconstrictor; results in lower levels of angiotensin II which causes an increase in plasma renin activity and a reduction in aldosterone secretion; a CNS mechanism may also be involved in hypotensive effect as angiotensin II increases adrenergic outflow from CNS; vasoactive kallikreins may be decreased in conversion to active hormones by ACE inhibitors, thus reducing blood pressure

Pharmacodynamics/Kinetics
Onset of action: 1 hour

Duration: 24 hours

Absorption: Quinapril: ≥60%

Protein binding: Quinapril: 97%; Quinaprilat: 97%

Metabolism: Rapidly hydrolyzed to quinaprilat, the active metabolite

Half-life elimination: Quinapril: 0.8 hours; Quinaprilat: 3 hours; increases as CrCl decreases

Time to peak, serum: Quinapril: 1 hour; Quinaprilat: ~2 hours

Excretion: Urine (50% to 60% primarily as quinaprilat)

Dosing
Adult

Heart failure: Oral: Initial: 5 mg twice daily, titrated at weekly intervals to 20 to 40 mg daily in 2 divided doses; target dose: 20 mg twice daily (ACCF/AHA [Yancy, 2013])

Canadian labeling: Initial: 5 mg once daily; as tolerated, may double daily dose (eg, 10 mg once daily) at weekly intervals to a maximum of 40 mg daily given in 2 divided doses.

Hypertension: Oral: Initial: 10 to 20 mg once daily in patients not on diuretics, adjust according to blood pressure response at peak (2 to 6 hours post dose) and trough blood levels; initial dose may be reduced to 5 mg in patients receiving diuretics if the diuretic is continued. Usual dose range (ASH/ISH [Weber, 2014]): 10 to 40 mg once daily. **Note:** The Canadian labeling recommends a maximum dose of 40 mg daily.

Geriatric

Heart failure: Refer to adult dosing.

Hypertension: Oral: Initial: 10 mg once daily; titrate to optimal response.

Pediatric Hypertension (off-label use): Children and Adolescents: Oral: Initial 5 to 10 mg once daily; maximum: 80 mg daily (National High Blood Pressure Education Program Working Group on High Blood Pressure in Children and Adolescents, 2004)

Renal Impairment Lower initial doses should be used; after initial dose (if tolerated), administer initial dose twice daily; may be increased at weekly intervals to optimal response:

Heart failure: Oral: Initial:

CrCl >30 mL/minute: Administer 5 mg daily

CrCl 10 to 30 mL/minute: Administer 2.5 mg daily

CrCl <10 mL/minute: There are no dosage adjustments provided in manufacturer's labeling.

Hypertension: Oral: Initial:

CrCl >60 mL/minute: Administer 10 mg daily

CrCl 30 to 60 mL/minute: Administer 5 mg daily

CrCl 10 to 30 mL/minute: Administer 2.5 mg daily

CrCl <10 mL/minute: There are no dosage adjustments provided in manufacturer's labeling.

Hepatic Impairment There are no dosage adjustments provided in manufacturer's labeling (has not been studied).

Administration Administer without regard to meals.

Monitoring Parameters Blood pressure; serum creatinine and potassium; if patient has collagen vascular disease and/or renal impairment, periodically monitor CBC with differential

2013 ACCF/AHA Heart Failure guideline recommendations: Within 1-2 weeks after initiation and periodically thereafter, reassess renal function and serum potassium especially in patients with preexisting hypotension, hyponatremia, diabetes mellitus, azotemia, or those taking potassium supplements (ACCF/AHA [Yancy, 2013]).

Dosage Forms Excipient information presented when available (limited, particularly for generics); consult specific product labeling.

Tablet, Oral:

Accupril: 5 mg [scored; contains magnesium carbonate]

Accupril: 10 mg, 20 mg, 40 mg [contains magnesium carbonate]

Generic: 5 mg, 10 mg, 20 mg, 40 mg

Extemporaneous Preparations A 1 mg/mL quinapril oral suspension may be made with tablets, K-Phos® Neutral (equivalent to 250 mg elemental phosphorus, 13 mEq sodium, and 1.1 mEq potassium per tablet), Bicitra®, and Ora-Sweet SF™. Place ten quinapril 20 mg tablets in an amber plastic prescription bottle (eg, 240 mL). In a separate container, prepare a buffer solution by crushing one K-Phos® Neutral tablet and dissolving it in 100 mL sterile water for irrigation. Add 30 mL of the prepared K-Phos® buffer solution to the quinapril tablets. Shake for at least 2 minutes, then remove cap and allow the concentrate to stand for 15 minutes, then shake the concentrate again for an additional minute. Add 30 mL of Bicitra® and shake for 2 minutes. Add quantity sufficient of Ora-Sweet SF® (~140 mL) to make 200 mL and shake the suspension. Store in amber plastic prescription bottles; label "shake well" and "refrigerate." Stable for 28 days refrigerated (Freed, 2005).

Freed A, Silbering SB, Kolodsick KJ, et al, "The Development and Stability Assessment of Extemporaneous Pediatric Formulations of Accupril," *Int J Pharm*, 2005, 304(1-2):135-44.

◆ Quinapril Hydrochloride *see* Quinapril *on page 1540*

◆ Quinate (Can) *see* QuiNIDine *on page 1542*

◆ Quinidex *see* QuiNIDine *on page 1542*

QuiNIDine (KWIN i deen)

Brand Names: Canada Apo-Quinidine; BioQuin Durules; Novo-Quinidin; Quinate

Index Terms Quinidex; Quinidine Gluconate; Quinidine Polygalacturonate; Quinidine Sulfate

Pharmacologic Category Antiarrhythmic Agent, Class Ia; Antimalarial Agent

Use

Quinidine gluconate and sulfate salts: Conversion and prevention of relapse into atrial fibrillation and/or flutter; suppression of ventricular arrhythmias. **Note:** Due to proarrhythmic effects, use should be reserved for life-threatening arrhythmias. Moreover, the use of quinidine has largely been replaced by more effective/safer antiarrhythmic agents and/or nonpharmacologic therapies (eg, radiofrequency ablation).

Quinidine gluconate (IV formulation): Conversion of atrial fibrillation/flutter and ventricular tachycardia. **Note:** The use of IV quinidine gluconate for these indications has been replaced by more effective/safer antiarrhythmic agents (eg, amiodarone and procainamide).

Quinidine gluconate (IV formulation) and quinidine sulfate: Treatment of malaria (*Plasmodium falciparum*)

Pregnancy Considerations Animal reproduction studies have not been conducted. Quinidine crosses the placenta and can be detected in the amniotic fluid, cord blood, and neonatal serum. Quinidine is indicated for use in the treatment of severe malaria infection in pregnant women (CDC, 2011; Smereck, 2011) and has also been used to treat arrhythmias in pregnancy when other agents are ineffective (European Society of Cardiology, 2003).

Breast-Feeding Considerations Quinidine can be detected in breast milk at concentrations slightly lower than those in the maternal serum. The manufacturer recommends avoiding use in nursing women.

Contraindications Hypersensitivity to quinidine or any component of the formulation; thrombocytopenia; thrombocytopenic purpura; myasthenia gravis; heart block greater than first degree; idioventricular conduction delays (except in patients with a functioning artificial pacemaker); those adversely affected by anticholinergic activity; concurrent use of quinolone antibiotics which prolong QT interval, cisapride, amprenavir, or ritonavir

Warnings/Precautions Monitor for proarrhythmic effects; may cause QT prolongation and subsequent torsade de pointes. Monitor and adjust dose to prevent QTc prolongation. Avoid use in patients with diagnosed or suspected congenital long QT syndrome. Correct hypokalemia before initiating therapy. Hypokalemia may worsen toxicity. **[U.S. Boxed Warning]: Antiarrhythmic drugs have not been shown to enhance survival in non-life-threatening ventricular arrhythmias and may increase mortality; the risk is greatest with structural heart disease. Quinidine may increase mortality in treatment of atrial fibrillation/flutter.** May precipitate or exacerbate HF. Reduce dosage in hepatic impairment. Use may cause digoxin-induced toxicity (adjust digoxin's dose). Use caution with concurrent use of other antiarrhythmics. Hypersensitivity reactions can occur. Can unmask sick sinus syndrome (causes bradycardia); use with caution in patients with heart block. In older adults, the manufacturer of the injectable product suggests initaiting therapy of low end of the dosage range.

Has been associated with severe hepatotoxic reactions, including granulomatous hepatitis. Hemolysis may occur in patients with G6PD (glucose-6-phosphate dehydrogenase) deficiency. Different salt products are not interchangeable.

Adverse Reactions Frequency not always defined.

Cardiovascular: Palpitations (7%), angina pectoris (6%), cardiac arrhythmia (3%; new or worsened; proarrhythmic effect), ECG abnormality (3%), cerebral ischemia (2%), prolonged Q-T interval on ECG (modest prolongation is common; however, excessive prolongation is rare and indicates toxicity), syncope

Central nervous system: Dizziness (3% to 15%), fatigue (7%), headache (3% to 7%), disturbed sleep (3%), nervousness (2%), ataxia (1%)

Dermatologic: Skin rash (5% to 6%)

Gastrointestinal: Diarrhea (24% to 35%), gastrointestinal distress (upper; 22%), nausea and vomiting (3%), esophagitis

Neuromuscular & skeletal: Weakness (2% to 5%), tremor (2%)

Ophthalmic: Visual disturbance (3%)

Miscellaneous: Fever (6%)

<1% (Limited to important or life-threatening): Acute psychosis, agranulocytosis, angioedema, arthralgia, bradycardia (exacerbated, in sick sinus syndrome), bronchospasm, cerebrovascular insufficiency (possibly resulting in ataxia, apprehension, and seizure), cinchonism (may include tinnitus, high-frequency hearing loss, deafness, vertigo, blurred vision, diplopia, photophobia, headache, confusion, and delirium; usually associated with chronic toxicity but may occur after brief exposure to a moderate dose), depression, dyschromia, exfoliative dermatitis, granulomatous hepatitis, hemolytic anemia, hepatotoxicity, immune thrombocytopenia, increased creatine phosphokinase, lupus-like syndrome, lymphadenopathy, optic neuritis, pneumonitis, psoriaform eruption, Sjogren's syndrome, skin photosensitivity, thrombocytopenia, torsades de pointes, uveitis, vasculitis, ventricular fibrillation, ventricular tachycardia (including paradoxical, during atrial fibrillation/flutter), visual field loss

Drug Interactions

Metabolism/Transport Effects Substrate of CYP2C9 (minor), CYP2E1 (minor), CYP3A4 (major), P-glycoprotein; **Note:** Assignment of Major/Minor substrate status based on clinically relevant drug interaction potential; **Inhibits** CYP2C9 (weak), CYP2D6 (strong), CYP3A4 (weak), P-glycoprotein

Avoid Concomitant Use

Avoid concomitant use of QuiNIDine with any of the following: Amiodarone; Antifungal Agents (Azole Derivatives, Systemic); Bosutinib; Conivaptan; Crizotinib; Enzalutamide; Erythromycin (Systemic); Fingolimod; Fusidic Acid (Systemic); Haloperidol; Highest Risk QTc-Prolonging Agents; Idelalisib; Ivabradine; Lopinavir; Mefloquine; Mequitazine; Mifepristone; Moderate Risk QTc-Prolonging Agents; Nelfinavir; PAZOPanib; Pimozide; Propafenone; Ritonavir; Saquinavir; Silodosin; Tamoxifen; Thioridazine; Tipranavir; Topotecan; VinCRIStine (Liposomal)

Increased Effect/Toxicity

QuiNIDine may increase the levels/effects of: Afatinib; ARIPiprazole; ARIPiprazole Lauroxil; AtoMOXetine; Bosutinib; Brentuximab Vedotin; Brexpiprazole; Calcium Channel Blockers (Dihydropyridine); Cardiac Glycosides; Colchicine; CYP2D6 Substrates; Dabigatran Etexilate; Dalfampridine; Dapoxetine; Dextromethorphan; DOXOrubicin (Conventional); DULoxetine; Edoxaban; Everolimus; Fesoterodine; Flibanserin; FluvoxaMINE; Haloperidol; Highest Risk QTc-Prolonging Agents; Ledipasvir; Lomitapide; Mefloquine; Mequitazine; Metoprolol; Naloxegol; Nebivolol; Neuromuscular-Blocking Agents; NiMODipine; PAZOPanib; P-glycoprotein/ABCB1 Substrates; Pimozide; Propafenone; Propranolol; Prucalopride; Rifaximin; Silodosin; Tamsulosin; Thioridazine; Topotecan; TraMADol; Tricyclic Antidepressants; Verapamil; VinCRIStine (Liposomal); Vitamin K Antagonists; Vortioxetine

The levels/effects of QuiNIDine may be increased by: Amiodarone; Antacids; Antifungal Agents (Azole Derivatives, Systemic); Aprepitant; Atazanavir; Boceprevir; Calcium Channel Blockers (Dihydropyridine); Carbonic Anhydrase Inhibitors; Cimetidine; Cobicistat; Conivaptan; Crizotinib; CYP3A4 Inhibitors (Moderate); CYP3A4 Inhibitors (Strong); Darunavir; Diltiazem; Erythromycin (Systemic); Fingolimod; FluvoxaMINE; Fosamprenavir; Fosaprepitant; Fosphenytoin; Fusidic Acid (Systemic); Haloperidol; Idelalisib; Indinavir; Ivabradine; Ivacaftor; Lopinavir; Luliconazole; Lurasidone; Mifepristone; Moderate Risk QTc-Prolonging Agents; Nelfinavir; Netupitant; Ombitasvir, Paritaprevir, and Ritonavir; Ombitasvir, Paritaprevir, Ritonavir, and Dasabuvir; Palbociclib; P-glycoprotein/ABCB1 Inhibitors; PHENobarbital; QTc-Prolonging Agents (Indeterminate Risk and Risk Modifying); Reserpine; Ritonavir; Saquinavir; Simeprevir; Stiripentol; Telaprevir; Tipranavir; Tricyclic Antidepressants; Verapamil

Decreased Effect

QuiNIDine may decrease the levels/effects of: Codeine; Dihydrocodeine; Hydrocodone; Tamoxifen; TraMADol

The levels/effects of QuiNIDine may be decreased by: Bosentan; Calcium Channel Blockers (Dihydropyridine); CYP3A4 Inducers (Moderate); CYP3A4 Inducers (Strong); Dabrafenib; Deferasirox; Enzalutamide; Etravirine; Fosphenytoin; Kaolin; Mitotane; P-glycoprotein/ABCB1 Inducers; PHENobarbital; Phenytoin; Potassium-Sparing Diuretics; Primidone; Rifamycin Derivatives; Siltuximab; St Johns Wort; Sucralfate; Tocilizumab

Food Interactions Changes in dietary salt intake may alter the rate and extent of quinidine absorption. Quinidine serum levels may be increased if taken with food. Food has a variable effect on absorption of sustained release formulation. The rate of absorption of quinidine may be decreased following the ingestion of grapefruit juice. Excessive intake of fruit juice or vitamin C may decrease urine pH and result in increased clearance of quinidine with decreased serum concentration. Alkaline foods may result in increased quinidine serum concentrations. Management: Avoid changes in dietary salt intake. Grapefruit juice should be avoided. Take around-the-clock to avoid variation in serum levels and with food or milk to avoid GI irritation.

Storage/Stability

Solution for injection: Store at room temperature of 25°C (77°F).

Tablets: Store at controlled room temperature of 20°C to 25°C (68°F to 77°F). Protect from light.

Mechanism of Action Class Ia antiarrhythmic agent; depresses phase O of the action potential; decreases myocardial excitability and conduction velocity, and myocardial contractility by decreasing sodium influx during depolarization and potassium efflux in repolarization; also reduces calcium transport across cell membrane

Pharmacodynamics/Kinetics

Distribution: V_d: Adults: 2 to 3 L/kg, decreased with congestive heart failure (0.5 L/kg), malaria; increased with cirrhosis

Protein binding: Newborns: 50% to 70%; Adults: 80% to 88%

Binds mainly to alpha$_1$-acid glycoprotein and to a lesser extent albumin; protein-binding changes may occur in periods of stress due to increased alpha$_1$-acid glycoprotein concentrations (eg, acute myocardial infarction) or in certain disease states due to decreased alpha$_1$-acid glycoprotein concentrations (eg, cirrhosis, hyperthyroidism, malnutrition)

Metabolism: Extensively hepatic (50% to 90%) to inactive compounds

Bioavailability: Sulfate: ~70% with wide variability between patients (45% to 100%); Gluconate: 70% to 80%

Half-life elimination, plasma: Children: 3 to 4 hours; Adults: 6 to 8 hours; prolonged with elderly, cirrhosis, and congestive heart failure

Time to peak, serum: Sulfate: 2 hours; Gluconate: 3 to 6 hours

Excretion: Urine (15% to 25% as unchanged drug)

Dosing

Adult Note: Dosage expressed in terms of the salt: 267 mg of quinidine gluconate = 200 mg of quinidine sulfate.

Atrial fibrillation/flutter (pharmacological conversion): Oral: **Note:** Discontinue use if at any time during therapy, the QRS complex widens to 130% of its pretreatment duration, the QTc interval widens to 130% of its pretreatment duration and is >500 msecs, P waves disappear, or the patient develops significant tachycardia, symptomatic bradycardia, or hypotension; consider other means of cardioversion (eg, direct current cardioversion). Discontinue if sinus rhythm is not restored in a reasonable amount of time. For patients with structural heart disease or other risk factors for toxicity, initiate or dose-adjust in a setting where continuous monitoring and resuscitation are available. Monitor patients for 2 to 3 days once the appropriate dose has been achieved.

Immediate release formulations: Quinidine sulfate: Initial: 400 mg/dose every 6 hours; if after 4 or 5 doses there is no conversion, may increase cautiously to desired effect

Extended release formulations:

Quinidine sulfate: Initial: 300 mg every 8 to 12 hours; the dose may be increased cautiously to desired effect

Quinidine gluconate: Initial: 648 mg every 8 hours; if after 3 or 4 doses there is no conversion, may increase cautiously to desired effect.

or

Initial: 324 mg every 8 hours for 2 days; then 648 mg every 12 hours for 2 days; then 648 mg every 8 hours for up to 4 days. The 4 day stretch may come at one of the lower doses if a lower dose is the highest tolerated dosing regimen.

Maintenance of sinus rhythm in patients with paroxysmal atrial fibrillation/flutter or life-threatening ventricular arrhythmias: Oral: **Note:** Dosing regimens for suppression of life-threatening ventricular arrhythmias have not been adequately studied. Reduce total daily dose if at any time during therapy, the QRS complex widens to 130% of its pretreatment duration, the QTc interval widens to 130% of its pretreatment duration and is >500 msecs, P waves disappear, or the patient develops significant tachycardia, symptomatic bradycardia, or hypotension. For patients with structural heart disease or other risk factors for toxicity, initiate or dose-adjust in a setting where continuous monitoring and resuscitation are available. Monitor patients for 2 to 3 days once the appropriate dose has been achieved.

Immediate release formulations: Quinidine sulfate: Initial: 200 mg every 6 hours; the dose may be increased cautiously to desired effect.

Extended release formulations:

Quinidine sulfate: Initial: 300 mg every 8 to 12 hours; the dose may be increased cautiously to desired effect

Quinidine gluconate: Initial: 324 mg every 8 to 12 hours; the dose may be increased cautiously to desired effect. Usual dose range according to the AHA/ACC/HRS guidelines for management of atrial fibrillation: 324 to 648 mg every 8 hours (AHA/ACC/HRS [January, 2014]).

Severe malaria, treatment: IV (quinidine gluconate): 10 mg/kg infused over 60 to 120 minutes followed by 0.02 mg/kg/minute continuous infusion for ≥24 hours; alternatively, may administer 24 mg/kg loading dose over 4 hours, followed by 12 mg/kg over 4 hours every 8 hours (beginning 8 hours after initiation of the loading dose); complete treatment with oral quinine once parasite density <1% and patient can receive oral medication; total duration of treatment (quinidine/quinine): 3 days (Africa or South America) or 7 days (Southeast Asia); use in combination with doxycycline, tetracycline or clindamycin (CDC malaria guidelines, 2009). **Note:** Close monitoring, including telemetry, required.

Geriatric

Oral: Refer to adult dosing.

IV: Refer to adult dosing. Initiate therapy at the low end of the dosage range.

Pediatric Note: Dosage expressed in terms of the salt: 267 mg of quinidine gluconate = 200 mg of quinidine sulfate.

Severe malaria, treatment: Children: IV (quinidine gluconate): 10 mg/kg infused over 60 to 120 minutes followed by 0.02 mg/kg/minute continuous infusion for ≥24 hours; alternatively, may administer 24 mg/kg loading dose over 4 hours, followed by 12 mg/kg over 4 hours every 8 hours (beginning 8 hours after initiation of the loading dose); complete treatment with oral quinine once parasite density <1% and patient can receive oral medication; total duration of treatment (quinidine/quinine): 3 days (Africa or South America) or 7 days (Southeast Asia); use in combination with doxycycline, tetracycline or clindamycin (CDC malaria guidelines, 2009). **Note:** Close monitoring, including telemetry, required.

Renal Impairment No dosage adjustment provided in manufacturer's labeling. Use with caution. The following guidelines have been used by some clinicians (Aronoff, 2007): Oral:

CrCl ≥10 mL/minute: No dosage adjustment necessary.

CrCl <10 mL/minute: Administer 75% of normal dose.

Hemodialysis: Dose following hemodialysis.

Peritoneal dialysis: Supplemental dose is not necessary.

CRRT: No dosage adjustment required; monitor serum concentrations.

Hepatic Impairment No dosage adjustment provided in manufacturer's labeling. Use with caution due to reduced clearance.

Dietary Considerations Administer with food or milk to decrease gastrointestinal irritation. Avoid changes in dietary salt intake.

Usual Infusion Concentrations: Adult IV infusion: Quinidine gluconate: 800 mg in 50 mL (concentration: 16 mg/mL) of D_5W

Administration Administer around-the-clock to promote less variation in peak and trough serum levels

Oral: Do not crush, chew, or break sustained release dosage forms. Some preparations of quinidine gluconate extended release tablets may be split in half to facilitate dosage titration; tablets are not scored.

Parenteral: Minimize use of PVC tubing to enhance bioavailability; shorter tubing lengths are recommended by the manufacturer

Monitoring Parameters Cardiac monitor required during IV administration; CBC, liver and renal function tests, should be routinely performed during long-term administration

Consult individual institutional policies and procedures.

Reference Range Therapeutic: 2 to 5 mcg/mL (SI: 6.2 to 15.4 micromole/L). Patient-dependent therapeutic response occurs at levels of 3 to 6 mcg/mL (SI: 9.2 to 18.5 micromole/L). Optimal therapeutic level is method dependent; >6 mcg/mL (SI: >18 micromole/L).

Dosage Forms Excipient information presented when available (limited, particularly for generics); consult specific product labeling.

Solution, Injection, as gluconate:
Generic: 80 mg/mL (10 mL)
Tablet, Oral, as sulfate:
Generic: 200 mg, 300 mg
Tablet Extended Release, Oral, as gluconate:
Generic: 324 mg
Tablet Extended Release, Oral, as sulfate:
Generic: 300 mg

Extemporaneous Preparations A 10 mg/mL oral liquid preparation may be made with tablets and one of three different vehicles (cherry syrup, a 1:1 mixture of Ora-Sweet® and Ora-Plus®, or a 1:1 mixture of Ora-Sweet® SF and Ora-Plus®). Crush six 200 mg tablets in a mortar and reduce to a fine powder. Add 15 mL of the chosen vehicle and mix to a uniform paste; mix while adding vehicle in incremental proportions to **almost** 120 mL; transfer to a calibrated bottle, rinse mortar with vehicle, and add quantity of vehicle sufficient to make 120 mL. Label "shake well" and "protect from light". Stable for 60 days when stored in amber plastic prescription bottles in the dark at room temperature or refrigerated.

Allen LV and Erickson MA, "Stability of Bethanechol Chloride, Pyrazinamide, Quinidine Sulfate, Rifampin, and Tetracycline in Extemporaneously Compounded Oral Liquids," *Am J Health Syst Pharm*, 1998, 55(17):1804-9.

◆ Quinidine and Dextromethorphan *see* Dextromethorphan and Quinidine *on page 535*

◆ Quinidine Gluconate *see* QuiNIDine *on page 1542*

◆ Quinidine Polygalacturonate *see* QuiNIDine *on page 1542*

◆ Quinidine Sulfate *see* QuiNIDine *on page 1542*

QuiNINE (KWYE nine)

Brand Names: US Qualaquin

Brand Names: Canada Apo-Quinine; Novo-Quinine; Quinine-Odan

Index Terms Quinine Sulfate

Pharmacologic Category Antimalarial Agent

Use In conjunction with other antimalarial agents, treatment of uncomplicated chloroquine-resistant *P. falciparum* malaria

Medication Guide Available Yes

Dosing

Adult & Geriatric Note: Actual duration of quinine treatment for malaria may be dependent upon the geographic region or pathogen. Dosage expressed in terms of the salt; 1 capsule Qualaquin = 324 mg of quinine sulfate = 269 mg of base; Canadian products contain 200 mg of quinine sulfate = 167 mg of base or 300 mg of quinine sulfate = 250 mg of base.

Treatment of uncomplicated chloroquine-resistant *P. falciparum* malaria: Oral:

CDC guidelines: 648 mg every 8 hours for 3 to 7 days. Tetracycline, doxycycline, or clindamycin should also be given.

Canadian labeling: 600 mg every 8 hours for 3 to 7 days. **Note:** Use in combination with tetracycline, doxycycline, or clindamycin.

Treatment of uncomplicated chloroquine-resistant *P. vivax* malaria (off-label use; CDC guidelines): Oral: 648 mg every 8 hours for 3 to 7 days. Tetracycline or doxycycline plus primaquine should also be given.

Babesiosis (off-label use): Oral: 650 mg every 6 to 8 hours for 7 to 10 days with clindamycin (Vannier 2012; Wormser 2006). **Note:** Relapsing infection may require at least 6 weeks of therapy (Vannier 2012).

Pediatric Note: Actual duration of quinine treatment for malaria may be dependent upon the geographic region or pathogen. Dosage expressed in terms of the salt; 1 capsule Qualaquin = 324 mg of quinine sulfate = 269 mg of base; Canadian products contain 200 mg of quinine sulfate = 167 mg of base or 300 mg of quinine sulfate = 250 mg of base.

Treatment of uncomplicated chloroquine-resistant *P. falciparum* malaria:

CDC guidelines: Oral: 30 mg/kg/day in divided doses every 8 hours for 3 to 7 days. Tetracycline, doxycycline, or clindamycin (consider risk versus benefit of using tetracycline or doxycycline in children <8 years) should also be given.

Canadian labeling: **Note:** Use in combination with tetracycline, doxycycline, or clindamycin.

Children and Adolescents <16 years: 9 mg/kg (maximum: 600 mg) every 8 hours for 3 to 7 days (consider risk versus benefit of using tetracycline or doxycycline in children <8 years)

Adolescents ≥16 years: Refer to adult dosing.

Treatment of uncomplicated chloroquine-resistant *P. vivax* malaria (off-label use; CDC guidelines): Oral: 30 mg/kg/day in divided doses every 8 hours for 3 to 7 days. Tetracycline or doxycycline (consider risk versus benefit of using tetracycline or doxycycline in children <8 years) plus primaquine should also be given.

Renal Impairment

US labeling:

Mild or moderate impairment: There are no dosage adjustments provided in the manufacturer's labeling (has not been studied); use caution.

Severe chronic impairment (not on dialysis): Initial dose: 648 mg followed by 324 mg every 12 hours

Canadian labeling:

Mild or moderate impairment: There are no dosage adjustments provided in the manufacturer's labeling; use caution

Severe chronic impairment: Initial dose: 600 mg followed by 300 mg every 12 hours for 7 days

Alternative recommendations (Aronoff 2007): **Note:** Dosage adjustments are not recommended in cases of severe malaria

GFR >50 mL/minute: No dosage adjustment necessary.

GFR 10 to 50 mL/minute: Administer every 8 to 12 hours

GFR <10 mL/minute: Administer every 24 hours

Intermittent hemodialysis: Administer dose after dialysis. **Note:** Clearance of ~6.5% achieved within 1 hour of hemodialysis.

Peritoneal dialysis: Dose as for GFR <10 mL/minute

CRRT: Dose as for GFR 10 to 50 mL/minute

Hepatic Impairment

US labeling:

Mild to moderate impairment (Child-Pugh classes A and B): No dosing adjustment required; monitor closely.

Severe impairment (Child-Pugh class C): Avoid use.

Canadian labeling: There are no dosage adjustments provided in the manufacturer's labeling; use with caution and monitor closely.

Additional Information Complete prescribing information should be consulted for additional detail.

Dosage Forms Excipient information presented when available (limited, particularly for generics); consult specific product labeling.

Capsule, Oral, as sulfate:

Qualaquin: 324 mg

Generic: 324 mg

Dosage Forms: Canada Excipient information presented when available (limited, particularly for generics); consult specific product labeling.

Capsule, Oral, as sulfate: 200 mg [equivalent to quinine base 167 mg], 300 mg [equivalent to quinine base 250 mg]

♦ Quinine-Odan (Can) see QuiNINE on page 1544

♦ Quinine Sulfate see QuiNINE on page 1544

♦ Quinol see Hydroquinone on page 893

Quinupristin and Dalfopristin
(kwi NYOO pris tin & dal FOE pris tin)

Brand Names: US Synercid®
Brand Names: Canada Synercid®
Index Terms Dalfopristin and Quinupristin; RP-59500
Pharmacologic Category Antibiotic, Streptogramin
Use Treatment of complicated skin and skin structure infections caused by methicillin-susceptible *Staphylococcus aureus* or *Streptococcus pyogenes*
Dosing
Adult & Geriatric
Complicated skin and skin structure infection: IV: 7.5 mg/kg every 12 hours for at least 7 days
Bacteremia, MRSA (persistent, vancomycin failure) (off-label use): IV: 7.5 mg/kg every 8 hours (Liu, 2011)
Pediatric Children ≥12 years: Refer to adult dosing.
Renal Impairment No dosage adjustment necessary.

Hepatic Impairment No dosage adjustment provided in manufacturer's labeling. However, pharmacokinetic data suggest dosage adjustment may be necessary.

Additional Information Complete prescribing information should be consulted for additional detail.

Dosage Forms Excipient information presented when available (limited, particularly for generics); consult specific product labeling.

Injection, powder for reconstitution:

Synercid®: 500 mg: Quinupristin 150 mg and dalfopristin 350 mg

♦ Quixin see Levofloxacin (Ophthalmic) on page 1063

♦ Quixin [DSC] see Levofloxacin (Ophthalmic) on page 1063

♦ QVA149 see Indacaterol and Glycopyrrolate on page 934

♦ Qvar see Beclomethasone (Systemic) on page 204

♦ QVAR (Can) see Beclomethasone (Systemic) on page 204

♦ R & C II (Can) see Pyrethrins and Piperonyl Butoxide on page 1531

♦ R & C Shampoo/Conditioner (Can) see Pyrethrins and Piperonyl Butoxide on page 1531

♦ R-1569 see Tocilizumab on page 1802

♦ R7159 see Obinutuzumab on page 1305

♦ R207910 see Bedaquiline on page 207

♦ R05072759 see Obinutuzumab on page 1305

♦ RabAvert see Rabies Vaccine on page 1547

RABEprazole (ra BEP ra zole)

Brand Names: US Aciphex; AcipHex Sprinkle
Brand Names: Canada Apo-Rabeprazole; Pariet; Pat-Rabeprazole; PMS-Rabeprazole EC; PRO-Rabeprazole; Rabeprazole EC; RAN-Rabeprazole; Riva-Rabeprazole EC; Sandoz-Rabeprazole; Teva-Rabeprazole EC
Index Terms Pariprazole
Pharmacologic Category Proton Pump Inhibitor; Substituted Benzimidazole
Use
Duodenal ulcers: Short-term (4 weeks or fewer) treatment in the healing and symptomatic relief of duodenal ulcers in adults.
Gastroesophageal reflux disease:
Erosive or ulcerative: Short-term (4 to 8 weeks) treatment in the healing and symptomatic relief of erosive or ulcerative gastroesophageal reflux disease (GERD) in adults; for maintaining healing and reduction in relapse rates of heartburn symptoms in adults with erosive or ulcerative GERD.
Symptomatic: Treatment of symptomatic GERD for up to 4 weeks in adults, up to 8 weeks in children ≥12 years and adolescents, and up to 12 weeks in children 1 to 11 years of age.
***Helicobacter pylori* eradication:** In combination with amoxicillin and clarithromycin as a 3-drug regimen for the treatment of adults with *H. pylori* infection and duodenal ulcer disease (active or history of within the past 5 years) to eradicate *H. pylori*.
Pathological hypersecretory conditions: Long-term treatment of pathological hypersecretory conditions, including Zollinger-Ellison syndrome in adults.

Canadian labeling: Additional uses (not in U.S. labeling): Treatment of nonerosive reflux disease (NERD); treatment of gastric ulcers

Pregnancy Considerations Adverse events have not been observed in animal reproduction studies. Available studies have not shown an increased risk of major birth defects following maternal use of proton pump inhibitors during pregnancy; however, information specific to rabeprazole is limited (Pasternak, 2010); most information available for omeprazole. When treating GERD in pregnancy, PPIs may be used when clinically indicated (Katz, 2013).

Breast-Feeding Considerations It is not known if rabeprazole is excreted in breast milk. The manufacturer recommends that caution be exercised when administering rabeprazole to nursing women.

Medication Guide Available Yes

Contraindications Hypersensitivity (eg, anaphylaxis, anaphylactic shock, angioedema, bronchospasm, acute interstitial nephritis, urticaria) to rabeprazole, other substituted benzimidazole proton pump inhibitors, or any component of the formulation

◀ **Warnings/Precautions** Use of proton pump inhibitors (PPIs) may increase the risk of gastrointestinal infections (eg, *Salmonella, Campylobacter*). Use caution in severe hepatic impairment. Relief of symptoms with rabeprazole does not preclude the presence of a gastric malignancy. Use of PPIs may increase risk of *Clostridium difficile*-associated diarrhea (CDAD), especially in hospitalized patients; consider CDAD diagnosis in patients with persistent diarrhea that does not improve. Use the lowest dose and shortest duration of PPI therapy appropriate for the condition being treated. Decreased *H. pylori* eradication rates have been observed with short-term (≤7 days) combination therapy. The American College of Gastroenterology recommends 10 to 14 days of therapy (triple or quadruple) for eradication of *H. pylori* (Chey, 2007).

PPIs may diminish the therapeutic effect of clopidogrel, thought to be due to reduced formation of the active metabolite of clopidogrel. The manufacturer of clopidogrel recommends either avoidance of both omeprazole (even when scheduled 12 hours apart) and esomeprazole or use of a PPI with comparatively less effect on the active metabolite of clopidogrel. Avoidance of rabeprazole appears prudent due to potent *in vitro* CYP2C19 inhibition (Li, 2004) and lack of sufficient comparative *in vivo* studies with other PPIs. In contrast to these warnings, others have recommended the continued use of PPIs, regardless of the degree of inhibition, in patients with a history of GI bleeding or multiple risk factors for GI bleeding who are also receiving clopidogrel since no evidence has established clinically meaningful differences in outcome; however, a clinically-significant interaction cannot be excluded in those who are poor metabolizers of clopidogrel (Abraham, 2010; Levine, 2011). Potentially significant drug-drug interactions may exist, requiring dose or frequency adjustment, additional monitoring, and/or selection of alternative therapy.

Increased incidence of osteoporosis-related bone fractures of the hip, spine, or wrist may occur with PPI therapy. Patients on high-dose (multiple daily doses) or long-term therapy (≥1 year) should be monitored. Acute interstitial nephritis has been observed in patients taking PPIs; may occur at any time during therapy and is generally due to an idiopathic hypersensitivity reaction. Discontinue if acute interstitial nephritis develops. Use the lowest effective dose for the shortest duration of time, use vitamin D and calcium supplementation, and follow appropriate guidelines to reduce risk of fractures in patients at risk.

Hypomagnesemia, reported rarely, usually with prolonged PPI use of >3 months (most cases >1 year of therapy); may be symptomatic or asymptomatic; severe cases may cause tetany, seizures, and cardiac arrhythmias. Consider obtaining serum magnesium concentrations prior to beginning long-term therapy, especially if taking concomitant digoxin, diuretics, or other drugs known to cause hypomagnesemia; and periodically thereafter. Hypomagnesemia may be corrected by magnesium supplementation, although discontinuation of rabeprazole may be necessary; magnesium levels typically return to normal within 1 week of stopping.

Prolonged treatment (≥2 years) may lead to vitamin B_{12} malabsorption and subsequent vitamin B_{12} deficiency. The magnitude of the deficiency is dose-related and the association is stronger in females and those younger in age (<30 years); prevalence is decreased after discontinuation of therapy (Lam, 2013).

Adverse Reactions Frequency not always defined.

1% to 10%:
Cardiovascular: Peripheral edema
Central nervous system: Headache (2% to 10%), pain (3%), dizziness
Gastrointestinal: Diarrhea (2% to 5%), nausea (2% to 5%), abdominal pain (4%), vomiting (4%), flatulence (3%), constipation (2%), xerostomia
Hepatic: Hepatic encephalopathy, hepatitis, increased liver enzymes
Infection: Increased susceptibility to infection (2%)
Neuromuscular & skeletal: Arthralgia, myalgia
Respiratory: Pharyngitis (3%)
<1% (Limited to important or life-threatening): Agranulocytosis, albuminuria, alopecia, amblyopia, anaphylaxis, anemia, angioedema, bone fracture, bullous rash, cholecystitis, cholelithiasis, *Clostridium difficile* associated diarrhea (CDAD), colitis, coma, delirium, disorientation, erythema multiforme, gynecomastia, hematuria, hemolytic anemia, hepatotoxicity (idiosyncratic) (Chalasani, 2014), hyperammonemia, hypersensitivity reaction, hypertension, hypokalemia, hypomagnesemia, hyponatremia, increased thyroid stimulating hormone level, interstitial nephritis, jaundice, leukocytosis, leukopenia, melena, migraine, neutropenia, osteoporosis, palpitation,

pancreatitis, pancytopenia, pathological fracture due to osteoporosis, pneumonia, rhabdomyolysis, sinus bradycardia, Stevens-Johnson syndrome, thrombocytopenia, toxic epidermal necrolysis

Drug Interactions

Metabolism/Transport Effects Substrate of CYP2C19 (major); CYP3A4 (major); **Note:** Assignment of Major/Minor substrate status based on clinically relevant drug interaction potential; **Inhibits** CYP2C19 (weak), CYP2C8 (moderate), CYP2D6 (weak)

Avoid Concomitant Use

Avoid concomitant use of RABEprazole with any of the following: Amodiaquine; Dasatinib; Delavirdine; Erlotinib; Nelfinavir; PAZOPanib; Rilpivirine; Risedronate

Increased Effect/Toxicity

RABEprazole may increase the levels/effects of: Amodiaquine; Amphetamine; ARIPiprazole; CYP2C8 Substrates; Dexmethylphenidate; Dextroamphetamine; Methotrexate; Methylphenidate; Raltegravir; Risedronate; Saquinavir; Tacrolimus (Systemic); Voriconazole

The levels/effects of RABEprazole may be increased by: Fluconazole; Ketoconazole (Systemic); Osimertinib; Voriconazole

Decreased Effect

RABEprazole may decrease the levels/effects of: Atazanavir; Bisphosphonate Derivatives; Bosutinib; Cefditoren; Clopidogrel; Cysteamine (Systemic); Dabigatran Etexilate; Dabrafenib; Dasatinib; Delavirdine; Erlotinib; Gefitinib; Indinavir; Iron Salts; Itraconazole; Ketoconazole (Systemic); Ledipasvir; Mesalamine; Multivitamins/Minerals (with ADEK, Folate, Iron); Mycophenolate; Nelfinavir; Nilotinib; PAZOPanib; Posaconazole; Rilpivirine; Riociguat; Risedronate

The levels/effects of RABEprazole may be decreased by: Bosentan; CYP2C19 Inducers (Strong); CYP3A4 Inducers (Moderate); CYP3A4 Inducers (Strong); Dabrafenib; Deferasirox; Enzalutamide; Mitotane; Osimertinib; Siltuximab; St Johns Wort; Tipranavir; Tocilizumab

Food Interactions Prolonged treatment (≥2 years) may lead to malabsorption of dietary vitamin B_{12} and subsequent vitamin B_{12} deficiency (Lam, 2013).

Storage/Stability Store at 25°C (77°F); excursions are permitted between 15°C and 30°C (59°F and 86°F). Protect from moisture.

Mechanism of Action Potent proton pump inhibitor; suppresses gastric acid secretion by inhibiting the parietal cell H+/K+ ATP pump

Pharmacodynamics/Kinetics

Onset of action: Within 1 hour
Duration: 24 hours
Absorption: Oral: Well absorbed within 1 hour
Protein binding, serum: ~96%
Metabolism: Hepatic via CYP3A and 2C19 to inactive metabolites
Bioavailability: Tablet: ~52%
Half-life elimination (dose dependent): 1 to 2 hours
Time to peak, plasma: Tablet: 2 to 5 hours; Capsule: 1 to 6.5 hours
Excretion: Urine (90% primarily as thioether carboxylic acid metabolites); remainder in feces

Dosing

Adult & Geriatric

Duodenal ulcer: Oral: 20 mg once daily for ≤4 weeks; additional therapy may be required for some patients.

Gastric ulcers: *Canadian labeling:* Oral: 20 mg once daily up to 6 weeks; additional therapy may be required for some patients.

Gastroesophageal reflux disease (GERD):

Erosive or ulcerative GERD: Treatment: 20 mg once daily for 4 to 8 weeks; if inadequate response, may repeat up to an additional 8 weeks; maintenance: 20 mg once daily.

Canadian labeling: 20 mg once daily for 4 weeks; if inadequate response, may repeat for an additional 4 weeks (lack of symptom control after 4 weeks warrants further evaluation); maintenance: 10 mg once daily (maximum: 20 mg once daily).

Symptomatic GERD: Treatment: 20 mg once daily for 4 weeks; if inadequate response, may repeat for an additional 4 weeks.

Canadian labeling: 10 mg once daily (maximum: 20 mg once daily) for 4 weeks; lack of symptom control after 4 weeks warrants further evaluation.

Helicobacter pylori **eradication:** Oral:

Manufacturer labeling: 20 mg twice daily administered with amoxicillin 1000 mg *and* clarithromycin 500 mg twice daily for 7 days

American College of Gastroenterology guidelines (Chey, 2007):

Nonpenicillin allergy: 20 mg twice daily administered with amoxicillin 1000 mg *and* clarithromycin 500 mg twice daily for 10 to 14 days

Penicillin allergy: 20 mg twice daily administered with clarithromycin 500 mg *and* metronidazole 500 mg twice daily for 10 to 14 days **or** 20 mg once or twice daily administered with bismuth subsalicylate 525 mg *and* metronidazole 250 mg *plus* tetracycline 500 mg 4 times daily for 10 to 14 days

Hypersecretory conditions: Oral: 60 mg once daily; dose may need to be adjusted as necessary. Doses as high as 100 mg once daily and 60 mg twice daily have been used, and continued as long as necessary (up to 1 year in some patients).

Nonerosive reflux disease (NERD): *Canadian labeling:* Oral: Treatment: 10 mg (maximum: 20 mg once daily) for 4 weeks; lack of symptom control after 4 weeks warrants further evaluation

Pediatric

Gastroesophageal reflux disease (GERD):

Children 1 to 11 years: Oral:

<15 kg: 5 mg once daily for ≤12 weeks; if inadequate response may increase to 10 mg once daily.

≥15 kg: 10 mg once daily for ≤12 weeks.

Children ≥12 years and Adolescents: Oral: 20 mg once daily for ≤8 weeks.

Renal Impairment No dosage adjustment necessary.

Hepatic Impairment

Mild-to-moderate: No dosage adjustment necessary.

Severe: There are no dosage adjustments provided in the manufacturer's labeling (has not been studied). Use with caution.

Dietary Considerations

Capsules: Take 30 minutes before a meal.

Tablets: May be taken with or without food. However, when used for the healing of duodenal ulcers, it is best if taken after breakfast. When used for the eradication of *Helicobacter pylori*, take with the morning and evening meals.

Administration May be administered with an antacid.

Capsules: Administer 30 minutes before a meal. Open capsule and sprinkle contents on a small amount of soft food (eg, applesauce, fruit or vegetable based baby food, yogurt) or empty contents into a small amount of liquid (eg, infant formula, apple juice, pediatric electrolyte solution); food or liquid should be at or below room temperature. Do not chew or crush granules; administer whole dose within 15 minutes of preparation (do not store for future use).

Tablets: May be administered with or without food. However, when used for the healing of duodenal ulcers, administration after breakfast is recommended. When used for the eradication of *H. pylori*, administration with the morning and evening meals is recommended. Swallow tablets whole; do not crush, split, or chew.

Monitoring Parameters Magnesium levels in patients on long-term treatment or those taking digoxin, diuretics, or other drugs that cause hypomagnesemia; susceptibility testing recommended in patients who fail *H. pylori* eradication regimen.

Dosage Forms Excipient information presented when available (limited, particularly for generics); consult specific product labeling.

Capsule Sprinkle, Oral, as sodium:

AcipHex Sprinkle: 5 mg [contains fd&c blue #2 aluminum lake]

AcipHex Sprinkle: 10 mg [contains fd&c yellow #6 (sunset yellow)]

Tablet Delayed Release, Oral, as sodium:

Aciphex: 20 mg

Generic: 20 mg

Dosage Forms: Canada Excipient information presented when available (limited, particularly for generics); consult specific product labeling.

Note: Sprinkle capsules are not available in Canada

Tablet, delayed release, enteric coated, as sodium:

Pariet: 10 mg, 20 mg

◆ Rabeprazole EC (Can) *see* RABEprazole *on page 1545*

Rabies Immune Globulin (Human)
(RAY beez i MYUN GLOB yoo lin, HYU man)

Brand Names: US HyperRAB S/D; Imogam Rabies-HT

Brand Names: Canada HyperRAB S/D; Imogam Rabies Pasteurized

Index Terms HRIG; RIG

Pharmacologic Category Blood Product Derivative; Immune Globulin

Additional Appendix Information

Immunization Administration Recommendations *on page 1974*

Immunization Schedules *on page 1979*

Use

Rabies exposure: Part of postexposure prophylaxis of persons with suspected rabies exposure. Provides passive immunity until active immunity with rabies vaccine is established. Not for use in persons with a history of vaccination (preexposure or postexposure prophylaxis) and documentation of antibody response. Each exposure to possible rabies infection should be individually evaluated.

Factors to consider include: species of biting animal, circumstances of biting incident (provoked vs unprovoked bite), type of exposure to rabies infection (bite vs nonbite), vaccination status of biting animal, presence of rabies in the region. See product information for additional details.

Dosing

Adult & Geriatric Postexposure prophylaxis: Local wound infiltration/IM: 20 units/kg in a single dose, RIG should always be administered as part of rabies vaccine regimen. If anatomically feasible, the full rabies immune globulin dose should be infiltrated around and into the wound(s); remaining volume should be administered IM at a site distant from the vaccine administration site. If rabies vaccine was initiated without rabies immune globulin, rabies immune globulin may be administered through the seventh day after the administration of the first dose of the vaccine (day 0). Administration of RIG is not recommended after the seventh day post vaccine since an antibody response to the vaccine is expected during this time period.

Note: Not recommended for use in persons with a history of rabies vaccination (preexposure or postexposure prophylaxis) and documentation of antibody response.

Pediatric Refer to adult dosing.

Renal Impairment There are no dosage adjustments provided in manufacturer's labeling.

Hepatic Impairment There are no dosage adjustments provided in manufacturer's labeling.

Additional Information Complete prescribing information should be consulted for additional detail.

Dosage Forms Excipient information presented when available (limited, particularly for generics); consult specific product labeling.

Injectable, Intramuscular:

Imogam Rabies-HT: 150 units/mL (2 mL, 10 mL)

Injectable, Intramuscular [preservative free]:

HyperRAB S/D: 150 units/mL (2 mL, 10 mL)

Rabies Vaccine (RAY beez vak SEEN)

Brand Names: US Imovax Rabies; RabAvert

Brand Names: Canada Imovax Rabies; RabAvert

Index Terms HDCV; Human Diploid Cell Cultures Rabies Vaccine; PCEC; Purified Chick Embryo Cell

Pharmacologic Category Vaccine, Inactivated (Viral)

Additional Appendix Information

Immunization Administration Recommendations *on page 1974*

Immunization Schedules *on page 1979*

Use Pre-exposure and postexposure vaccination against rabies

The Advisory Committee on Immunization Practices (ACIP) recommends a primary course of prophylactic immunization (pre-exposure vaccination) for the following:

• Persons with continuous risk of infection, including rabies research laboratory and biologics production workers

• Persons with frequent risk of infection in areas where rabies is enzootic, including rabies diagnostic laboratory workers, cavers, veterinarians and their staff, and animal control and wildlife workers; persons who frequently handle bats

• Persons with infrequent risk of infection, including veterinarians and animal control staff with terrestrial animals in areas where rabies infection is rare, veterinary students, and travelers visiting areas where rabies is enzootic and immediate access to medical care and biologicals is limited

The ACIP recommends the use of postexposure vaccination for a particular person be assessed by the severity and likelihood versus the actual risk of acquiring rabies. Consideration should include the type of exposure, epidemiology of rabies in the area, species of the animal, circumstances of the incident, and the availability of the

exposing animal for observation or rabies testing. Post-exposure vaccination is used in both previously vaccinated and previously unvaccinated individuals.

Medication Guide Available Yes

Dosing

Adult & Geriatric

Pre-exposure vaccination: IM: A total of 3 doses, 1 mL each, on days 0, 7, and 21-28.

Note: Prolonging the interval between doses does not interfere with immunity achieved after the concluding dose of the basic series.

Postexposure vaccination: All postexposure treatment should begin with immediate cleansing of the wound with soap and water

Persons not previously immunized as above: IM: 5 doses (1 mL each) on days 0, 3, 7, 14, 28. In addition, patients should receive rabies immune globulin with the first dose (day 0). **Note:** A regimen of 4 doses (1 mL each) on days 0, 3, 7, 14 may be used in persons who are not immunosuppressed (ACIP recommendations, 2010).

Persons who have previously received postexposure prophylaxis with rabies vaccine, received a recommended IM pre-exposure series of rabies vaccine or have a previously documented rabies antibody titer considered adequate: IM: Two doses (1 mL each) on days 0 and 3; do not administer rabies immune globulin

Booster (for persons with continuous or frequent risk of infection): IM: 1 mL based on antibody titers

Pediatric Refer to adult dosing.

Renal Impairment No dosage adjustment provided in manufacturer's labeling.

Hepatic Impairment No dosage adjustment provided in manufacturer's labeling.

Additional Information Complete prescribing information should be consulted for additional detail.

Dosage Forms Excipient information presented when available (limited, particularly for generics); consult specific product labeling.

Injectable, Intramuscular [preservative free]:

Imovax Rabies: 2.5 units/mL (1 ea) [contains albumin human, neomycin sulfate]

Suspension Reconstituted, Intramuscular:

RabAvert: 2.5 units (1 ea) [contains albumin human, chicken protein, edetate disodium, gelatin (bovine), neomycin]

Raloxifene (ral OKS i feen)

Brand Names: US Evista

Brand Names: Canada ACT Raloxifene; Apo-Raloxifene; Evista; PMS-Raloxifene; Teva-Raloxifene

Index Terms Keoxifene Hydrochloride; Raloxifene Hydrochloride

Pharmacologic Category Selective Estrogen Receptor Modulator (SERM)

Use Prevention and treatment of osteoporosis in postmenopausal women; risk reduction for invasive breast cancer in postmenopausal women with osteoporosis and in postmenopausal women with high risk for invasive breast cancer

Pregnancy Considerations Adverse events were observed in in animal reproduction studies. Raloxifene is contraindicated for use in women who are or may become pregnant.

Breast-Feeding Considerations It is not known if raloxifene is excreted into breast milk. Breast-feeding is contraindicated by the manufacturer.

Medication Guide Available Yes

Contraindications History of or current venous thromboembolic disorders (including DVT, PE, and retinal vein thrombosis); pregnancy or women who could become pregnant; breast-feeding

Warnings/Precautions Hazardous agent - use appropriate precautions for handling and disposal (NIOSH 2014 [group 2]).

[U.S. Boxed Warning]: May increase the risk for DVT or PE; use contraindicated in patients with history of or current venous thromboembolic disorders. Use with caution in patients at high risk for venous thromboembolism; the risk for DVT and PE are higher in the first 4 months of treatment. Discontinue at least 72 hours prior to and during prolonged immobilization (postoperative recovery or prolonged bedrest). **[U.S. Boxed Warning]: The risk of death due to stroke may be increased in women with coronary heart disease or in women at risk for coronary events;** use with caution in patients with cardiovascular disease. Not be used for the prevention of cardiovascular disease. Use caution with moderate-to-severe renal dysfunction, hepatic impairment, unexplained uterine bleeding, and in women with a history of elevated triglycerides in response to treatment with oral estrogens (or estrogen/progestin). Safety with concomitant estrogen therapy has not been established. Safety and efficacy in premenopausal women or men have not been established. Not indicated for treatment of invasive breast cancer, to reduce the risk of recurrence of invasive breast cancer or to reduce the risk of noninvasive breast cancer. The efficacy (for breast cancer risk reduction) in women with inherited BRCA1 and BRCA1 mutations has not been established.

Adverse Reactions Note: Raloxifene has been associated with increased risk of thromboembolism (DVT, PE) and superficial thrombophlebitis; risk is similar to reported risk of HRT

>10%:

Cardiovascular: Peripheral edema (3% to 14%)

Endocrine & metabolic: Hot flashes (8% to 29%)

Neuromuscular & skeletal: Arthralgia (11% to 16%), leg cramps/muscle spasm (6% to 12%)

Miscellaneous: Flu syndrome (14% to 15%), infection (11%)

1% to 10%:

Cardiovascular: Chest pain (3%), venous thromboembolism (1% to 2%)

Central nervous system: Insomnia (6%)

Dermatologic: Rash (6%)

Endocrine & metabolic: Breast pain (4%)

Gastrointestinal: Weight gain (9%), abdominal pain (7%), vomiting (5%), flatulence (2% to 3%), cholelithiasis (≤3%), gastroenteritis (≤3%)

Genitourinary: Vaginal bleeding (6%), leukorrhea (3%), urinary tract disorder (3%), uterine disorder (3%), vaginal hemorrhage (3%), endometrial disorder (≤3%)

Neuromuscular & skeletal: Myalgia (8%), tendon disorder (4%)

Respiratory: Bronchitis (10%), sinusitis (10%), pharyngitis (8%), pneumonia (3%), laryngitis (≤2%)

Miscellaneous: Diaphoresis (8%)

<1% (Limited to important or life-threatening): Apolipoprotein A-1 increased, apolipoprotein B decreased, death related to VTE, fibrinogen decreased, hypertriglyceridemia (in women with a history of increased triglycerides in response to oral estrogens), intermittent claudication, LDL cholesterol decreased, lipoprotein decreased, retinal vein occlusion, stroke related to VTE, superficial thrombophlebitis, total serum cholesterol decreased

Drug Interactions

Metabolism/Transport Effects None known.

Avoid Concomitant Use

Avoid concomitant use of Raloxifene with any of the following: Ospemifene

Increased Effect/Toxicity

Raloxifene may increase the levels/effects of: Ospemifene

Decreased Effect

Raloxifene may decrease the levels/effects of: Levothyroxine; Ospemifene

The levels/effects of Raloxifene may be decreased by: Bile Acid Sequestrants

Storage/Stability Store at controlled room temperature of 20°C to 25°C (68°F to 77°F); excursions permitted to 15°C to 30°C (59°F to 86°F).

Mechanism of Action A selective estrogen receptor modulator (SERM), meaning that it affects some of the same receptors that estrogen does, but not all, and in some instances, it antagonizes or blocks estrogen; it acts like estrogen to prevent bone loss and has the potential to block some estrogen effects in the breast and uterine

tissues. Raloxifene decreases bone resorption, increasing bone mineral density and decreasing fracture incidence.

Pharmacodynamics/Kinetics
Onset of action: 8 weeks

Absorption: Rapid; ~60%

Distribution: 2348 L/kg

Protein binding: >95% to albumin and α-glycoprotein; does not bind to sex-hormone-binding globulin

Metabolism: Hepatic, extensive first-pass effect; metabolized to glucuronide conjugates

Bioavailability: ~2%

Half-life elimination: 28-33 hours

Excretion: Primarily feces; urine (<0.2% as unchanged drug; <6% as glucuronide conjugates)

Dosing
Adult & Geriatric
Osteoporosis: Females: Oral: 60 mg once daily

Invasive breast cancer risk reduction: Female: Oral: 60 mg once daily for 5 years per ASCO guidelines (Visvanathan, 2009)

Renal Impairment No dosage adjustment provided in manufacturer's labeling. Use caution in moderate-to-severe impairment.

Hepatic Impairment No dosage adjustment provided in manufacturer's labeling (has not been studied). Use with caution.

Dietary Considerations May be taken without regard to meals. Osteoporosis prevention or treatment: Ensure adequate calcium and vitamin D intake; if dietary intake is inadequate, dietary supplementation is recommended. Women and men should consume:

Calcium: 1000 mg/day (men: 50 to 70 years) **or** 1200 mg/day (women ≥51 years and men ≥71 years) (IOM, 2011; NOF [Cosman 2014])

Vitamin D: 800 to 1000 int. units daily (men and women ≥50 years) (NOF [Cosman 2014]). Recommended Dietary Allowance (RDA): 600 int. units daily (men and women ≤70 years) **or** 800 int. units daily (men and women ≥71 years) (IOM, 2011).

Administration May be administered without regard to meals.

Hazardous agent; use appropriate precautions for handling and disposal (NIOSH 2014 [group 2]).

Monitoring Parameters Lipid profile; adequate diagnostic measures, including endometrial sampling, if indicated, should be performed to rule out malignancy in all cases of undiagnosed abnormal vaginal bleeding

Osteoporosis: Bone mineral density (BMD) should be evaluated 1 to 2 years after initiating therapy and every 2 years thereafter (NOF [Cosman 2014]); annual measurements of height and weight; serum calcium and 25 (OH)D; may consider monitoring biochemical markers of bone turnover

Reference Range
Calcium (total): Adults: 9 to 11 mg/dL (2.05 to 2.54 mmol/L), may slightly decrease with aging

Phosphorus: 2.5 to 4.5 mg/dL (0.81 to 1.45 mmol/L)

Vitamin D: There is no clear consensus on a reference range for total serum 25(OH)D concentrations or the validity of this level as it relates clinically to bone health. In addition, there is significant variability in the reporting of serum 25(OH)D levels as a result of different assay types in use; however, the following ranges have been suggested:

Adults (IOM, 2011): Sufficient levels in practically all persons: ≥20 ng/mL (50 nmol/L); concern for risk of toxicity: >50 ng/mL (125 nmol/L)

Osteoporosis patients (NOF [Cosman 2014]): Recommended level to reach and maintain: ~30 ng/mL (75 nmol/L)

Additional Information The decrease in estrogen-related adverse effects with the selective estrogen-receptor modulators in general and raloxifene in particular should improve compliance and decrease the incidence of cardiovascular events and fractures while not increasing breast cancer.

Oncology Comment: The American Society of Clinical Oncology (ASCO) guidelines for breast cancer risk reduction (Visvanathan, 2009) recommend raloxifene (for 5 years) as an option to reduce the risk of ER-positive invasive breast cancer in postmenopausal women with a 5-year projected risk (based on NCI trial model) of ≥1.66%, or with lobular carcinoma *in situ*. Raloxifene should not be used in premenopausal women. Women with osteoporosis may use raloxifene beyond 5 years of treatment. According to the NCCN breast cancer risk reduction guidelines (v.2.2009), raloxifene is only recommended for postmenopausal women (≥35 years of age), and is equivalent to tamoxifen although, raloxifene has a better adverse event

profile; however, tamoxifen is superior in reducing the risk on noninvasive breast cancer.

Dosage Forms Excipient information presented when available (limited, particularly for generics); consult specific product labeling.

Tablet, Oral, as hydrochloride:

Evista: 60 mg

Generic: 60 mg

◆ Raloxifene Hydrochloride *see* Raloxifene *on page 1548*

Raltegravir (ral TEG ra vir)

Brand Names: US Isentress

Brand Names: Canada Isentress

Index Terms MK-0518; RAL

Pharmacologic Category Antiretroviral, Integrase Inhibitor (Anti-HIV)

Use HIV infection:

U.S. labeling: Treatment of HIV-1 infection in combination with other antiretroviral agents in patients 4 weeks and older and weighing at least 3 kg

Canadian labeling: Treatment of HIV-1 infection in combination with other antiretroviral agents in patients ≥2 years of age

Pregnancy Considerations Adverse events were observed in some animal reproduction studies. Raltegravir has high transfer across the human placenta and can be detected in neonatal serum after delivery. Standard doses appear to be appropriate in pregnant women. The DHHS Perinatal HIV Guidelines consider raltegravir to be an alternative for use in antiretroviral-naïve pregnant patients when drug interactions with protease inhibitors are a concern. Because of its ability to rapidly suppress viral load, some experts have suggested using raltegravir in late pregnancy in women who have high viral loads; however, this use is not routinely recommended at this time. Reversible elevation of liver enzymes occurred in a patient who initiated raltegravir late in pregnancy; monitor liver enzymes if used during pregnancy.

Regardless of CD4 count or HIV RNA copy number, all HIV-infected pregnant women should receive a combination antiretroviral (ARV) drug regimen. A combination of antepartum, intrapartum, and infant ARV prophylaxis is recommended. ARV therapy should be started as soon as possible in women with symptomatic infection. Although earlier initiation may be more effective in reducing the perinatal transmission of HIV, initiation may be delayed until after 12 weeks gestation in women who do not require immediate treatment after careful consideration of maternal conditions (eg, nausea and vomiting) and the potential risks of first trimester fetal exposure for specific agents. A scheduled cesarean delivery at 38 weeks gestation is recommended for all women with HIV RNA >1000 copies/mL or unknown concentrations near delivery in order to decrease transmission. If ARV therapy must be interrupted for <24 hours during the peripartum period, stop then restart all medications simultaneously in order to decrease the chance of developing resistance. Long-term follow-up is recommended for all infants exposed to ARV medications. In couples who want to conceive, the HIV-infected partner should attain maximum viral suppression prior to conception.

Health care providers are encouraged to enroll pregnant women exposed to antiretroviral medications in the Antiretroviral Pregnancy Registry (1-800-258-4263 or www.APRegistry.com). Health care providers caring for HIV-infected women and their infants may contact the National Perinatal HIV Hotline (888-448-8765) for clinical consultation (HHS [perinatal], 2014).

Breast-Feeding Considerations It is not known if raltegravir is excreted into breast milk. Maternal or infant antiretroviral therapy does not completely eliminate the risk of postnatal HIV transmission. In addition, multiclass-resistant virus has been detected in breast-feeding infants despite maternal therapy. Therefore, in the United States, where formula is accessible, affordable, safe, and sustainable, and the risk of infant mortality due to diarrhea and respiratory infections is low, complete avoidance of breast-feeding by HIV-infected women is recommended to decrease potential transmission of HIV (HHS [perinatal], 2014).

Contraindications

There are no contraindications listed in the manufacturer's labeling.

Canadian labeling: Hypersensitivity to raltegravir or any other component of the formulation

Warnings/Precautions Patients may develop immune reconstitution syndrome resulting in the occurrence of an inflammatory response to an indolent or residual opportunistic infection during initial HIV treatment or activation of autoimmune disorders (eg, Graves' disease, polymyositis, Guillain-Barré syndrome) later in therapy; further evaluation and treatment may be required. Severe, life-threatening or fatal cases of Stevens-Johnson syndrome and toxic epidermal necrolysis have been reported. Hypersensitivity reactions (rash [may occur with fever, fatigue, malaise, conjunctivitis, or other constitutional symptoms], organ dysfunction and/or hepatic failure) have also been reported. Discontinue immediately if a severe skin reaction or hypersensitivity symptoms develop. Monitor liver transaminases and start supportive therapy. Myopathy and rhabdomyolysis have been reported; use caution in patients with risk factors for CK elevations and/or skeletal muscle abnormalities. Potentially significant drug-drug interactions may exist, requiring dose or frequency adjustment, additional monitoring, and/or selection of alternative therapy. Avoid use as a boosted PI replacement in antiretroviral experienced patients with documented resistance to nucleoside reverse transcriptase inhibitors. Raltegravir plus darunavir/ritonavir should not be used in adolescent and adult HIV-1 patients with a pre-ART CD4 count <200 cells/mm^3 and/or HIV RNA>100,000 copies/mL (HHS [adult] 2015).

Chewable tablet contains phenylalanine. Raltegravir film-coated tablets and chewable tablets or oral suspension are not bioequivalent and are not substitutable on a mg/mg basis.

Adverse Reactions
>10%:
Hepatic: Increased serum ALT (1% to 11%; incidence higher with hepatitis B and/or C coinfection)
2% to 10%:
Central nervous system: Insomnia (4%), headache (2% to 4%), dizziness (2%), fatigue (2%)
Endocrine & metabolic: Increased serum glucose (126 to 250 mg/dL: 7% to 10%; 251 to 500 mg/dL: 2% to 3%)
Gastrointestinal: Increased serum lipase (2% to 5%), increased serum amylase (2% to 4%), nausea (3%)
Hematologic: Abnormal absolute neutrophil count (2% to 3%), thrombocytopenia (1% to 3%)
Hepatic: Increased serum AST (1% to 9%; incidence higher with hepatitis B and/or C coinfection), hyperbilirubinemia (<1% to 6%), increased serum alkaline phosphatase (<1% to 2%)
Neuromuscular & skeletal: Increased creatine phosphokinase (10 to 19.9 x ULN: 4%; ≥20 x ULN: 3%)
<2% (Limited to important or life-threatening): Anemia, cerebellar ataxia, depression (particularly in subjects with a preexisting history of psychiatric illness), drug rash with eosinophilia and systemic symptoms (DRESS; Perry, 2013), gastritis, hepatic failure, hepatitis, hypersensitivity, myopathy, nephrolithiasis, psychomotor agitation (children; grade 3), renal failure, rhabdomyolysis, Stevens-Johnson syndrome, suicidal ideation, toxic epidermal necrolysis

Drug Interactions
Metabolism/Transport Effects Substrate of UGT1A1
Avoid Concomitant Use
Avoid concomitant use of Raltegravir with any of the following: Aluminum Hydroxide; Magnesium Salts
Increased Effect/Toxicity
Raltegravir may increase the levels/effects of: Fibric Acid Derivatives; HMG-CoA Reductase Inhibitors; Zidovudine

The levels/effects of Raltegravir may be increased by: Proton Pump Inhibitors; Rifapentine
Decreased Effect
Raltegravir may decrease the levels/effects of: Fosamprenavir

The levels/effects of Raltegravir may be decreased by: Aluminum Hydroxide; Fosamprenavir; Magnesium Salts; Rifabutin; Rifampin; Rifapentine; Tipranavir
Food Interactions Variable absorption depending upon meal type (low- vs high-fat meal) and dosage form. Management: Raltegravir was administered without regard to meals in clinical trials.
Storage/Stability
Store at 20°C to 25°C (68°F to 77°F); excursions are permitted between 15°C and 30°C (59°F and 86°F).
Chewable tablets: Store in the original package; keep desiccant in the bottle to protect from moisture.
Oral suspension: Store in the original container; do not open foil packet until ready for reconstitution and use.
Mechanism of Action Incorporation of viral DNA into the host cell's genome is required to produce a self-replicating provirus and propagation of infectious virion particles. The viral cDNA strand produced by reverse transcriptase is subsequently processed and inserted into the human genome by the enzyme HIV-1 integrase (encoded by the pol gene of HIV). Raltegravir inhibits the catalytic activity of integrase, thus preventing integration of the proviral gene into human DNA.

Pharmacodynamics/Kinetics
Absorption: Film-coated tablet: AUC increased twofold with high-fat meal; Chewable tablet: AUC decreased by ~6% with high-fat meal (not clinically significant); Oral suspension: The effect of food was not studied
Protein binding: ~83%
Metabolism: Primarily hepatic glucuronidation mediated by UGT1A1
Bioavailability: Film-coated tablet: Not established; however, chewable tablet and oral suspension have higher bioavailability compared to film-coated tablet
Half-life elimination: ~9 hours
Time to peak, plasma: Film-coated tablet: ~3 hours
Excretion: Feces (~51%, as unchanged drug); urine (~32%; 9% as unchanged drug)

Dosing
Adult & Geriatric
HIV treatment: Oral: Film-coated tablet: 400 mg twice daily. Raltegravir is a component of a recommended initial regimen with tenofovir plus emtricitabine (or lamivudine) in ART-naive patients (HHS [adult] 2015).
Occupational HIV postexposure, prophylaxis (off-label use): Oral: Film-coated tablet: 400 mg twice daily for 4 weeks with concomitant emtricitabine/tenofovir. Recommended as preferred therapy (Kuhar, 2013).

Dosage adjustment for rifampin coadministration: 800 mg twice daily
Pediatric HIV treatment: Oral: **Note:** Raltegravir film-coated tablets and chewable tablets or oral suspension are not bioequivalent and are not substitutable on a mg/mg basis
U.S. labeling:
Infants ≥4 weeks and Children (≥3 to <25 kg): Weight-based dosing based on ~6 mg/kg/dose twice daily (maximum dose: 600 mg/day [chewable tablet]; 200 mg/day [oral suspension]).
3 to <4 kg: 20 mg twice daily (oral suspension)
4 to <6 kg: 30 mg twice daily (oral suspension)
6 to <8 kg: 40 mg twice daily (oral suspension)
8 to <11 kg: 60 mg twice daily (oral suspension)
11 to <14 kg: 80 mg twice daily (oral suspension) or 75 mg twice daily (chewable tablet) (see **"Note"**)
14 to <20 kg: 100 mg twice daily (oral suspension or chewable tablet) (see **"Note"**)
20 to <25 kg: 150 mg twice daily (chewable tablet)
Note: Infants and Children ≥4 weeks who are between 11 and <20 kg may use either the chewable tablet or the oral suspension. Patients can remain on the oral suspension as long as their weight is <20 kg.
Children and Adolescents ≥25 kg: **Note:** If unable to swallow a tablet, chewable tablets may be used. Raltegravir is a component of a recommended initial regimen with tenofovir plus emtricitabine (or lamivudine) in adolescent ART-naive patients (HHS [adult] 2015).
Film-coated tablet: Refer to adult dosing.
Chewable tablet: Weight-based dosing based on ~6 mg/kg/dose twice daily (maximum dose: 600 mg/day).
25 to <28 kg: 150 mg twice daily (see **"Note"**)
28 to <40 kg: 200 mg twice daily (see **"Note"**)
≥40 kg: 300 mg twice daily (see **"Note"**)
Note: May use either weight-based dosing (chewable tablet) or adult dosing (film-coated tablet).
Canadian labeling: Chewable tablet: Children 2 to <12 years (maximum dose: 600 mg/day):
7 to <10 kg: 50 mg twice daily
10 to <14 kg: 75 mg twice daily
14 to <20 kg: 100 mg twice daily
20 to <28 kg: 150 mg twice daily
28 to <40 kg: 200 mg twice daily
≥40 kg: 300 mg twice daily

Dosage adjustment for rifampin coadministration: There are no data to guide dose adjustment in patients <18 years of age.
Renal Impairment
Mild, moderate, and severe impairment: No dosage adjustment necessary.
End-stage renal disease (ESRD) on intermittent hemodialysis (IHD): Dose after dialysis on dialysis days.

Hepatic Impairment

Mild-to-moderate impairment: No dosage adjustment necessary.

Severe impairment: There are no dosage adjustments provided in manufacturer's labeling (has not been studied).

Dietary Considerations Some products may contain phenylalanine.

Administration May be administered without regard to meals.

Chewable tablets: May be chewed or swallowed whole; the 100 mg chewable tablet may be divided into equal halves.

Film-coated tablets: Must be swallowed whole.

Oral suspension: Open foil packet of drug (100 mg). Measure 5 mL water in provided mixing cup. Pour packet contents into 5 mL water, close lid and swirl for 30-60 seconds. Do not turn the mixing cup upside down. Once mixed, measure recommended suspension dose with an oral syringe. Administer within 30 minutes of mixing with water. Discard any remaining suspension in the trash.

Monitoring Parameters Viral load, CD4 count, lipid profile

HIV occupational postexposure prophylaxis (PEP) (Kuhar, 2013): Documented HIV test (at baseline and 6 weeks, 12 weeks and 6 months after exposure); if confirmation that a fourth generation HIV p2 antigen-HIV antibody test is being used, monitor at baseline, 6 weeks and 4 months after exposure. CBC, renal and hepatic function assessments at baseline and 2 weeks after exposure (minimum recommendations, others dictated by clinical assessment)

Dosage Forms Excipient information presented when available (limited, particularly for generics); consult specific product labeling.

Packet, Oral:

Isentress: 100 mg (60 ea) [contains polyethylene glycol; banana flavor]

Tablet, Oral:

Isentress: 400 mg [contains polyethylene glycol]

Tablet Chewable, Oral:

Isentress: 25 mg [contains aspartame, saccharin sodium; orange banana flavor]

Isentress: 100 mg [scored; contains aspartame, saccharin sodium; orange banana flavor]

Ramelteon (ra MEL tee on)

Brand Names: US Rozerem

Index Terms TAK-375

Pharmacologic Category Hypnotic, Miscellaneous; Melatonin Receptor Agonist

Use Treatment of insomnia characterized by difficulty with sleep onset

Pregnancy Considerations Animal studies have demonstrated teratogenic effects. May cause disturbances of reproductive hormonal regulation (eg, disruption of menses or decreased libido). There are no adequate and well-controlled studies in pregnant women.

Breast-Feeding Considerations It is not known if ramelteon is excreted in breast milk. The manufacturer recommends that caution be exercised when administering ramelteon to nursing women.

Medication Guide Available Yes

Contraindications History of angioedema with previous ramelteon therapy (do not rechallenge); concurrent use with fluvoxamine

Warnings/Precautions Symptomatic treatment of insomnia should be initiated only after careful evaluation of potential causes of sleep disturbance. Failure of sleep disturbance to resolve after a reasonable period of treatment may indicate psychiatric and/or medical illness. Because of the rapid onset of action, administer immediately prior to bedtime or after the patient has gone to bed and is having difficulty falling asleep. Hypnotics/sedatives have been associated with abnormal thinking and behavior changes including decreased inhibition, aggression, bizarre behavior, agitation, hallucinations, and depersonalization. These changes may occur unpredictably and may indicate previously unrecognized psychiatric disorders; evaluate appropriately. Postmarketing studies have indicated that the use of hypnotic/sedative agents (including ramelteon) for sleep has been associated with hypersensitivity reactions including anaphylaxis as well as angioedema. Do not rechallenge patients who have developed angioedema with ramelteon therapy. An increased risk for hazardous sleep-related activities such as sleep-driving; cooking and eating food, and making phone calls while asleep have also been noted. Use caution with preexisting depression or other psychiatric conditions. Caution when using with other CNS depressants; avoid engaging in hazardous activities or activities requiring mental alertness. Not recommended for use in patients with severe sleep apnea or COPD. Use caution with moderate hepatic impairment; not recommended in patients with severe impairment. May cause disturbances of hormonal regulation. Use caution when administered concomitantly with strong CYP1A2 inhibitors.

Adverse Reactions

1% to 10%:

Central nervous system: Dizziness (4% to 5%), somnolence (3% to 5%), fatigue (3% to 4%), insomnia worsened (3%), depression (2%)

Endocrine & metabolic: Serum cortisol decreased (1%)

Gastrointestinal: Nausea (3%), taste perversion (2%)

Neuromuscular & skeletal: Myalgia (2%), arthralgia (2%)

Respiratory: Upper respiratory infection (3%)

Miscellaneous: Influenza (1%)

Postmarketing and/or case reports: Anaphylaxis, angioedema, complex sleep-related behavior (sleep-driving, cooking or eating food, making phone calls), prolactin levels increased, testosterone levels decreased

Drug Interactions

Metabolism/Transport Effects Substrate of CYP1A2 (major), CYP2C19 (minor), CYP3A4 (minor); Note: Assignment of Major/Minor substrate status based on clinically relevant drug interaction potential

Avoid Concomitant Use

Avoid concomitant use of Ramelteon with any of the following: Azelastine (Nasal); FluvoxaMINE; Orphenadrine; Paraldehyde; Sodium Oxybate; Thalidomide

Increased Effect/Toxicity

Ramelteon may increase the levels/effects of: Alcohol (Ethyl); Azelastine (Nasal); Buprenorphine; CNS Depressants; Hydrocodone; Methotrimeprazine; Metyrosine; Mirtazapine; Orphenadrine; Paraldehyde; Pramipexole; ROPINIRole; Rotigotine; Selective Serotonin Reuptake Inhibitors; Sodium Oxybate; Suvorexant; Thalidomide; Zolpidem

The levels/effects of Ramelteon may be increased by: Abiraterone Acetate; Brimonidine (Topical); Cannabis; CYP1A2 Inhibitors (Moderate); CYP1A2 Inhibitors (Strong); CYP2C9 Inhibitors (Strong); CYP3A4 Inhibitors (Strong); Deferasirox; Doxylamine; Dronabinol; Droperidol; Fluconazole; FluvoxaMINE; HydrOXYzine; Kava Kava; Magnesium Sulfate; Methotrimeprazine; Minocycline; Nabilone; Peginterferon Alfa-2b; Perampanel; Rufinamide; Tapentadol; Tetrahydrocannabinol; Vemurafenib

Decreased Effect

The levels/effects of Ramelteon may be decreased by: Rifamycin Derivatives

Food Interactions Taking with high-fat meal delays T_{max} and increases AUC (~31%). Management: Do not take with a high-fat meal.

Storage/Stability Store at 25°C (77°F); excursions permitted to 15°C to 30°C (59°F to 86°F). Protect from moisture.

Mechanism of Action Potent, selective agonist of melatonin receptors MT_1 and MT_2 (with little affinity for MT_3) within the suprachiasmic nucleus of the hypothalamus, an area responsible for determination of circadian rhythms and synchronization of the sleep-wake cycle. Agonism of MT_1 is thought to preferentially induce sleepiness, while MT_2 receptor activation preferentially influences regulation of circadian rhythms. Ramelteon is eightfold more selective for MT_1 than MT_2 and exhibits nearly sixfold higher affinity for MT_1 than melatonin, presumably allowing for enhanced effects on sleep induction.

Pharmacodynamics/Kinetics

Onset of action: 30 minutes

Absorption: Rapid; high-fat meal delays T_{max} and increases AUC (~31%)

Distribution: 74 L

Protein binding: ~82%

Metabolism: Extensive first-pass effect; oxidative metabolism primarily through CYP1A2 and to a lesser extent through CYP2C and CYP3A4; forms active metabolite (M-II)

Bioavailability: Absolute: 1.8%

Half-life elimination: Ramelteon: 1-2.6 hours; M-II: 2-5 hours

Time to peak, plasma: Median: 0.5-1.5 hours

Excretion: Primarily as metabolites: Urine (84%); feces (4%)

Dosing

Adult & Geriatric Insomnia: Oral: One 8 mg tablet within 30 minutes of bedtime

Renal Impairment No dosage adjustment necessary.

Hepatic Impairment

Mild-to-moderate impairment: No dosage adjustment necessary. Use with caution.

Severe impairment: Use is not recommended.

Dietary Considerations Do not take with high-fat meal.

◄ **Administration** Do not administer with a high-fat meal. Swallow tablet whole; do not break.

Dosage Forms Excipient information presented when available (limited, particularly for generics); consult specific product labeling.

Tablet, Oral:

Rozerem: 8 mg

Ramipril (RA mi pril)

Brand Names: US Altace

Brand Names: Canada ACT Ramipril; Altace; Apo-Ramipril; Auro-Ramipri; Dom-Ramipril; JAMP-Ramipril; Mar-Ramipril; Mint-Ramipril; Mylan-Ramipril; PMS-Ramipril; Pro-Ramipril; RAN-Ramipril; ratio-Ramipril; Sandoz-Ramipril; Teva-Ramipril

Pharmacologic Category Angiotensin-Converting Enzyme (ACE) Inhibitor; Antihypertensive

Use

Heart failure post-myocardial infarction: Treatment of heart failure (HF) after myocardial infarction (MI)

Hypertension: Treatment of hypertension, alone or in combination with thiazide diuretics

Reduction in risk of MI, stroke, and death from cardiovascular causes: To reduce the risk of MI, stroke, and death in patients ≥55 years of age at high risk of developing major cardiovascular events

Guideline recommendations:

Heart failure: The 2013 American College of Cardiology Foundation/American Heart Association (ACCF/AHA) heart failure guidelines recommend the use of ACE inhibitors, along with other guideline-directed medical therapies, to prevent HF in patients with a reduced ejection fraction who have a history of MI (stage B HF), to prevent HF in any patient with a reduced ejection fraction (stage B HF), or to treat those with HF and reduced ejection fraction (stage C HFrEF) (Yancy, 2013)

Hypertension: The 2014 guideline for the management of high blood pressure in adults (Eighth Joint National Committee [JNC 8]) recommends initiation of pharmacologic treatment to lower blood pressure for the following patients:

• Patients ≥60 years of age with systolic blood pressure (SBP) ≥150 mm Hg or diastolic blood pressure (DBP) ≥90 mm Hg. Goal of therapy is SBP <150 mm Hg and DBP <90 mm Hg.

• Patients <60 years of age with SBP ≥140 mm Hg or DBP is ≥90 mm Hg. Goal of therapy is SBP <140 mm Hg and DBP <90 mm Hg.

• Patients ≥18 years of age with diabetes and SBP ≥140 mm Hg or DBP ≥90 mm Hg. Goal of therapy is SBP <140 mm Hg and DBP <90 mm Hg.

• Patients ≥18 years of age with chronic kidney disease (CKD) and SBP ≥140 mm Hg or DBP ≥90 mm Hg. Goal of therapy is SBP <140 mm Hg and DBP <90 mm Hg.

Chronic kidney disease (CKD) and hypertension: Regardless of race or diabetes status, the use of an ACE inhibitor (ACEI) or angiotensin receptor blocker (ARB) as initial therapy is recommended to improve kidney outcomes. In the general nonblack population (without CKD) including those with diabetes, initial antihypertensive treatment should consist of a thiazide-type diuretic, calcium channel blocker, ACEI, or ARB. In the general black population (without CKD) including those with diabetes, initial antihypertensive treatment should consist of a thiazide-type diuretic or a calcium channel blocker **instead of** an ACEI or ARB.

Coronary artery disease (CAD) and hypertension: The American Heart Association, American College of Cardiology and American Society of Hypertension (AHA/ACC/ASH) 2015 scientific statement for the treatment of hypertension in patients with CAD recommends the use of an ACE inhibitor (or an ARB) as part of a regimen in patients with hypertension and chronic stable angina if there is prior MI, LV systolic dysfunction, diabetes mellitus, or CKD. A BP target of <140/90 mm Hg is reasonable for the secondary prevention of cardiovascular events. A lower target BP (<130/80 mm Hg) may be appropriate in some individuals with CAD, previous MI, stroke or transient ischemic attack, or CAD risk equivalents (AHA/ACC/ASH [Rosendorff 2015]).

STEMI: The 2013 ACCF/AHA guidelines for the management of patients with ST-elevation myocardial infarction (STEMI) state that an ACE inhibitor should be initiated within the first 24 hours after STEMI in patients with anterior MI, heart failure, or left ventricular ejection fraction (LVEF) ≤0.4. It is also reasonable to initiate an ACE inhibitor in all patients with STEMI (O'Gara, 2013).

Pregnancy Considerations [US Boxed Warning]: Drugs that act on the renin-angiotensin system can cause injury and death to the developing fetus. Discontinue as soon as possible once pregnancy is detected. Ramipril crosses the placenta. Drugs that act on the renin-angiotensin system are associated with oligo-hydramnios. Oligohydramnios, due to decreased fetal renal function, may lead to fetal lung hypoplasia and skeletal malformations. The use of these drugs in pregnancy is also associated with anuria, hypotension, renal failure, skull hypoplasia, and death in the fetus/neonate. Teratogenic effects may occur following maternal use of an ACE inhibitor during the first trimester, although this finding may be confounded by maternal disease. Because adverse fetal events are well documented with exposure later in pregnancy, ACE inhibitor use in pregnant women is not recommended (Seely 2014; Weber 2014). Infants exposed to an ACE inhibitor in utero should be monitored for hyperkalemia, hypotension, and oliguria. Oligohydramnios may not appear until after irreversible fetal injury has occurred. Exchange transfusions or dialysis may be required to reverse hypotension or improve renal function, although data related to the effectiveness in neonates is limited.

Chronic maternal hypertension itself is also associated with adverse events in the fetus/infant and mother. ACE inhibitors are not recommended for the treatment of uncomplicated hypertension in pregnancy (ACOG 2013) and they are specifically contraindicated for the treatment of hypertension and chronic heart failure during pregnancy by some guidelines (Regitz-Zagrosek 2011). In addition, ACE inhibitors should generally be avoided in women of reproductive age (ACOG 2013). If treatment for hypertension or chronic heart failure in pregnancy is needed, other agents should be used (ACOG 2013; Regitz-Zagrosek 2011).

Breast-Feeding Considerations Ramipril and its metabolites were not detected in breast milk following a single oral dose of 10 mg. It is not known if multiple doses will produce detectable levels. Breast-feeding is not recommended by the manufacturer.

Contraindications Hypersensitivity to ramipril or any component of the formulation; prior hypersensitivity (including angioedema) to ACE inhibitors; concomitant use with aliskiren in patients with diabetes mellitus

Warnings/Precautions Anaphylactic reactions may occur rarely with ACE inhibitors. At any time during treatment (especially following first dose) angioedema may occur rarely with ACE inhibitors; it may involve the head and neck (potentially compromising airway) or the intestine (presenting with abdominal pain). African-Americans and patients with idiopathic or hereditary angioedema may be at an increased risk. Risk may also be increased with concomitant use of mTOR inhibitor (eg, everolimus) therapy. Prolonged frequent monitoring may be required especially if tongue, glottis, or larynx are involved as they are associated with airway obstruction. Patients with a history of airway surgery may have a higher risk of airway obstruction. Aggressive early and appropriate management is critical. Use in patients with previous angioedema associated with ACE inhibitor therapy is contraindicated. Severe anaphylactoid reactions may be seen during hemodialysis (eg, CVVHD) with high-flux dialysis membranes (eg, AN69), and rarely, during low density lipoprotein apheresis with dextran sulfate cellulose. Rare cases of anaphylactoid reactions have been reported in patients undergoing sensitization treatment with hymenoptera (bee, wasp) venom while receiving ACE inhibitors.

Symptomatic hypotension with or without syncope can occur with ACE inhibitors (usually with the first several doses); effects are most often observed in volume-depleted patients; close monitoring of patient is required especially with initial dosing and dosing increases; blood pressure must be lowered at a rate appropriate for the patient's clinical condition. Initiation of therapy in patients with ischemic heart disease or cerebrovascular disease warrants close observation due to the potential consequences posed by falling blood pressure (eg, MI, stroke). Use with caution in hypertrophic cardiomyopathy with outflow tract obstruction and severe aortic stenosis. In patients on chronic ACE inhibitor therapy, intraoperative hypotension may occur with induction and maintenance of general anesthesia; use with caution before, during, or immediately after major surgery. Cardiopulmonary bypass, intraoperative blood loss, or vasodilating anesthesia increases endogenous renin release. Use of ACE inhibitors perioperatively will blunt angiotensin II formation and may result in hypotension. However, discontinuation of therapy prior to surgery is controversial. If continued

preoperatively, avoidance of hypotensive agents during surgery is prudent (Hillis, 2011). **[U.S. Boxed Warning]: Drugs that act on the renin-angiotensin system can cause injury and death to the developing fetus. Discontinue as soon as possible once pregnancy is detected.**

Hyperkalemia may occur with ACE inhibitors; risk factors include renal dysfunction, diabetes mellitus, concomitant use of potassium-sparing diuretics, potassium supplements, and/or potassium containing salts. Use cautiously, if at all, with these agents and monitor potassium closely. Cough may occur with ACE inhibitors. Other causes of cough should be considered (eg, pulmonary congestion in patients with heart failure) and excluded prior to discontinuation.

May be associated with deterioration of renal function and/ or increases in serum creatinine, particularly in patients with low renal blood flow (eg, renal artery stenosis, heart failure) whose glomerular filtration rate (GFR) is dependent on efferent arteriolar vasoconstriction by angiotensin II; deterioration may result in oliguria, acute renal failure, and progressive azotemia. Small increases in serum creatinine may occur following initiation; consider discontinuation only in patients with progressive and/or significant deterioration in renal function. Use with caution in patients with unstented unilateral/bilateral renal artery stenosis. When unstented bilateral renal artery stenosis is present, use is generally avoided due to the elevated risk of deterioration in renal function unless possible benefits outweigh risks. Potentially significant drug-drug interactions may exist, requiring dose or frequency adjustment, additional monitoring, and/or selection of alternative therapy.

Rare toxicities associated with ACE inhibitors include cholestatic jaundice (which may progress to fulminant hepatic necrosis), agranulocytosis, neutropenia, or leukopenia with myeloid hypoplasia. Patients with collagen vascular diseases (especially with concomitant renal impairment) or renal impairment alone may be at increased risk for hematologic toxicity; periodically monitor CBC with differential in these patients.

Adverse Reactions Note: Frequency ranges include data from hypertension and heart failure trials. Higher rates of adverse reactions have generally been noted in patients with CHF. However, the frequency of adverse effects associated with placebo is also increased in this population.

>10%: Respiratory: Cough increased (7% to 12%)
1% to 10%:
Cardiovascular: Hypotension (11%), angina (up to 3%), orthostatic hypotension (2%), syncope (up to 2%)
Central nervous system: Headache (1% to 5%), dizziness (2% to 4%), fatigue (2%), vertigo (up to 2%)
Endocrine & metabolic: Hyperkalemia (1% to 10%)
Gastrointestinal: Nausea/vomiting (1% to 2%)
Neuromuscular & skeletal: Chest pain (noncardiac) (1%)
Renal: Renal dysfunction (1%), serum creatinine increased (1% to 2%), BUN increased (<1% to 3%); transient increases of creatinine and/or BUN may occur more frequently
Respiratory: Cough (estimated 1% to 10%)
<1% (Limited to important or life-threatening): Agranulocytosis, amnesia, anaphylactoid reaction, angioedema, arrhythmia, bone marrow depression, convulsions, depression, dysphagia, eosinophilia, erythema multiforme, hearing loss, hemolytic anemia, hepatitis, hypersensitivity reactions (urticaria, rash, fever), impotence, insomnia, MI, neuropathy, onycholysis, pancreatitis, pancytopenia, pemphigoid, pemphigus, photosensitivity, proteinuria, Stevens-Johnson syndrome, symptomatic hypotension, thrombocytopenia, toxic epidermal necrolysis, visual hallucinations (Doane, 2013)
Worsening of renal function may occur in patients with bilateral renal artery stenosis or in hypovolemia. In addition, a syndrome which may include fever, myalgia, arthralgia, interstitial nephritis, vasculitis, rash, eosinophilia and positive ANA, and elevated ESR has been reported with ACE inhibitors. Risk of pancreatitis and/or agranulocytosis may be increased in patients with collagen vascular disease or renal impairment.

Drug Interactions
Metabolism/Transport Effects None known.
Avoid Concomitant Use
Avoid concomitant use of Ramipril with any of the following: Sacubitril; Telmisartan
Increased Effect/Toxicity
Ramipril may increase the levels/effects of: Allopurinol; Amifostine; Antipsychotic Agents (Second Generation [Atypical]); AzaTHIOprine; Ciprofloxacin (Systemic); Drospirenone; DULoxetine; Ferric Gluconate; Gold Sodium Thiomalate; Grass Pollen Allergen Extract (5 Grass Extract); Hypotension-Associated Agents; Iron Dextran Complex; Levodopa; Lithium; Nonsteroidal Anti-Inflammatory Agents; Pregabalin; Sacubitril; Sodium Phosphates

The levels/effects of Ramipril may be increased by: Alfuzosin; Aliskiren; Angiotensin II Receptor Blockers; Barbiturates; Brimonidine (Topical); Canagliflozin; Dapoxetine; Diazoxide; DPP-IV Inhibitors; Eplerenone; Everolimus; Heparin; Heparin (Low Molecular Weight); Herbs (Hypotensive Properties); Loop Diuretics; Molsidomine; Nicorandil; Obinutuzumab; Pentoxifylline; Phosphodiesterase 5 Inhibitors; Potassium Salts; Potassium-Sparing Diuretics; Prostacyclin Analogues; Salicylates; Sirolimus; Telmisartan; Temsirolimus; Thiazide Diuretics; TiZANidine; Tolvaptan; Trimethoprim

Decreased Effect
The levels/effects of Ramipril may be decreased by: Amphetamines; Aprotinin; Herbs (Hypertensive Properties); Icatibant; Lanthanum; Methylphenidate; Nonsteroidal Anti-Inflammatory Agents; Salicylates; Yohimbine

Storage/Stability Store at 15°C to 30°C (59°F to 86°F). Ramipril mixed with applesauce, apple juice, or water may be stored at room temperature for up to 24 hours or for up to 48 hours under refrigeration.

Mechanism of Action Ramipril is an ACE inhibitor which prevents the formation of angiotensin II from angiotensin I and exhibits pharmacologic effects that are similar to captopril. Ramipril must undergo enzymatic saponification by esterases in the liver to its biologically active metabolite, ramiprilat. The pharmacodynamic effects of ramipril result from the high-affinity, competitive, reversible binding of ramiprilat to angiotensin-converting enzyme, thus preventing the formation of the potent vasoconstrictor angiotensin II. This isomerized enzyme-inhibitor complex has a slow rate of dissociation, which results in high potency and a long duration of action; a CNS mechanism may also be involved in the hypotensive effect as angiotensin II increases adrenergic outflow from CNS; vasoactive kallikreins may be decreased in conversion to active hormones by ACE inhibitors, thus reducing blood pressure

Pharmacodynamics/Kinetics
Onset of action: 1-2 hours
Duration: 24 hours
Absorption: Well absorbed (50% to 60%)
Distribution: Plasma levels decline in a triphasic fashion; rapid decline is a distribution phase to peripheral compartment, plasma protein and tissue ACE (half-life: 2-4 hours); second phase is an apparent elimination phase representing the clearance of free ramiprilat (half-life: 9-18 hours); and final phase is the terminal elimination phase representing the equilibrium phase between tissue binding and dissociation
Protein binding: Ramipril: 73%; Ramiprilat: 56%
Metabolism: Hepatic to the active form, ramiprilat
Bioavailability: Ramipril: 28%; Ramiprilat: 44%
Half-life elimination: Ramiprilat: Effective: 13-17 hours; Terminal: >50 hours
Time to peak, serum: Ramipril: ~1 hour; Ramiprilat: 2-4 hours
Excretion: Urine (60%) and feces (40%) as parent drug and metabolites

Dosing
Adult Note: Consider discontinuation or dose reduction of concomitant diuretic when initiating ramipril. If diuretic cannot be discontinued or dose reduced, consider reduced initial ramipril dose. Monitor blood pressure closely until stabilized.
Heart failure post-myocardial infarction: Oral: Initial: 2.5 mg twice daily (patient should be monitored for at least 2 hours after initial dose and for at least an additional hour after blood pressure has stabilized); may reduce dose to 1.25 mg twice daily for hypotension. Reduce the dose of any concomitant diuretics, if possible. Continue initial dose for one week then titrate upward every 3 weeks as tolerated to target dose of 5 mg twice daily.
Heart failure (off-label use): Oral: Initial: 1.25 to 2.5 mg once daily; target dose: 10 mg once daily (ACCF/AHA [Yancy, 2013])
Hypertension: Oral: Initial dose in patients not receiving a diuretic is 2.5 mg once daily; titrate to effect. Usual maintenance (per the manufacturer): 2.5 to 20 mg daily in 1 or 2 divided doses (consider twice daily administration for patients unable to maintain adequate blood pressure control with once daily administration). Usual dosage range (ASH/ISH [Weber, 2014]): 5 to 10 mg daily

Reduction in risk of MI, stroke, and death from cardiovascular causes: Oral: Initial: 2.5 mg once daily for 1 week, then 5 mg once daily for the next 3 weeks, then increase as tolerated to 10 mg once daily (may be given as divided dose in hypertensive or recently post-MI patients)

Dosage adjustment for patients with volume depletion: Initial: 1.25 mg once daily; titrate as tolerated to effect

Geriatric Refer to adult dosing. Adjust for renal function for elderly since glomerular filtration rates are decreased; may see exaggerated hypotensive effects if renal clearance is not considered.

In the management of hypertension, consider lower initial doses and titrate to response (Aronow, 2011).

Renal Impairment

CrCl >40 mL/minute: No dosage adjustment necessary.
CrCl <40 mL/minute: Administer 25% of normal dose.
Renal artery stenosis: Initial: 1.25 mg once daily; titrate as tolerated to effect
Renal failure and heart failure post-MI: Initial: 1.25 mg once daily, may increase to 1.25 mg twice daily and then up to 2.5 mg twice daily as tolerated
Renal failure and hypertension: Initial: 1.25 mg once daily, titrated as tolerated to effect; maximum: 5 mg daily

Hepatic Impairment No dosage adjustment provided in manufacturer's labeling; discontinue use for jaundice or marked elevation of hepatic enzymes.

Administration Swallow capsule whole; may open the capsule and the mix contents with 120 mL of water, apple juice, or applesauce.

Monitoring Parameters Blood pressure; serum creatinine and potassium; if patient has collagen vascular disease and/or renal impairment, periodically monitor CBC with differential

2013 ACCF/AHA Heart Failure guideline recommendations: Within 1-2 weeks after initiation and periodically thereafter, reassess renal function and serum potassium especially in patients with preexisting hypotension, hyponatremia, diabetes mellitus, azotemia, or those taking potassium supplements (ACCF/AHA [Yancy, 2013]).

Test Interactions Positive Coombs' [direct]; may cause false-positive results in urine acetone determinations using sodium nitroprusside reagent

Dosage Forms Excipient information presented when available (limited, particularly for generics); consult specific product labeling.

Capsule, Oral:
Altace: 1.25 mg
Altace: 2.5 mg [contains fd&c red #40, fd&c yellow #10 (quinoline yellow)]
Altace: 5 mg [contains brilliant blue fcf (fd&c blue #1), fd&c red #40]
Altace: 10 mg [contains brilliant blue fcf (fd&c blue #1)]
Generic: 1.25 mg, 2.5 mg, 5 mg, 10 mg

Dosage Forms: Canada Note: Also refer to Dosage Forms. Excipient information presented when available (limited, particularly for generics); consult specific product labeling.

Capsule, Oral:
Altace: 15 mg
Tablet, Oral: 1.25 mg, 2.5 mg, 5 mg, 10 mg

Ramucirumab (ra mue SIR ue mab)

Brand Names: US Cyramza
Brand Names: Canada Cyramza
Index Terms IMC-1121B
Pharmacologic Category Antineoplastic Agent, Monoclonal Antibody; Antineoplastic Agent, Vascular Endothelial Growth Factor (VEGF) Inhibitor; Antineoplastic Agent, Vascular Endothelial Growth Factor Receptor 2 (VEGFR2) Inhibitor

Use

US labeling:

Colorectal cancer, metastatic: Treatment (in combination with FOLFIRI [irinotecan, leucovorin, and fluorouracil]) of metastatic colorectal cancer (mCRC) in patients with disease progression on or after prior therapy with bevacizumab, oxaliplatin, and a fluoropyrimidine.

Gastric cancer, advanced or metastatic: Treatment (single-agent or in combination with paclitaxel) of advanced or metastatic gastric or gastroesophageal junction adenocarcinoma in patients with disease progression on or following fluoropyrimidine- or platinum-containing chemotherapy

Non-small cell lung cancer, metastatic: Treatment (in combination with docetaxel) of metastatic non-small cell lung cancer (NSCLC) in patients with disease progression on or after platinum-based chemotherapy. Patients with EGFR or ALK genomic tumor aberrations should have disease progression on FDA-approved therapy for these aberrations prior to receiving ramucirumab.

Canadian labeling: **Gastric cancer, advanced or metastatic:** Treatment (single-agent or in combination with paclitaxel) of advanced or metastatic gastric or gastroesophageal junction adenocarcinoma in patients with disease progression on or following fluoropyrimidine- or platinum-containing chemotherapy.

Pregnancy Considerations Ramucirumab inhibits angiogenesis, which is of critical importance to human fetal development. Based on the mechanism of action, ramucirumab may cause fetal harm if administered during pregnancy. Women of reproductive potential should use effective contraception during and for at least 3 months after the last ramucirumab dose. Ramucirumab may impair fertility in women.

Breast-Feeding Considerations It is not known if ramucirumab is excreted in breast milk. Immunoglobulins are excreted in breast milk, and it is assumed that ramucirumab may appear in breast milk. Due to the potential for serious adverse reactions in the nursing infant, breastfeeding is not recommended by the manufacturer.

Contraindications

There are no contraindications listed in the manufacturer's US labeling.

Canadian labeling: Hypersensitivity to ramucirumab or any component of the formulation.

Warnings/Precautions [US Boxed Warning]: Ramucirumab is associated with an increased risk of hemorrhage and gastrointestinal hemorrhage, which may be severe or sometimes fatal. Discontinue ramucirumab permanently in patients who experience serious bleeding. Patients receiving NSAIDs were excluded from some clinical trials; the risk of gastric hemorrhage in patients with gastric tumors receiving NSAIDs is not known. In addition, NSCLC patients receiving therapeutic anticoagulation or chronic NSAID or other antiplatelet therapy (other than aspirin), or with radiograph evidence of major airway or blood vessel involvement or intratumor cavitation were also excluded from the clinical study; the risk of pulmonary hemorrhage in such patients is not known. Serious and fatal arterial thrombotic events, including MI, cardiac arrest, cerebrovascular accident, and cerebral ischemia, have occurred with ramucirumab. Discontinue permanently in patients who experience serious arterial thrombotic events.

Ramucirumab is associated with infusion-related reactions (may be severe), generally occurring with the first or second dose. Symptoms of infusion reactions have included chills, flushing, hypotension, bronchospasm, dyspnea, hypoxia, wheezing, chest pain/tightness, supraventricular tachycardia, back pain/spasms, rigors/tremors, and/or paresthesia. Monitor for infusion reaction symptoms during infusion; discontinue immediately and permanently for grade 3 or 4 reactions. Administer in a facility equipped to manage infusion reactions. May cause and/or worsen hypertension; the incidence of severe hypertension is increased with ramucirumab. Blood pressure (BP) should be controlled prior to treatment initiation. Monitor BP every 2 weeks (more frequently if indicated) during treatment. If severe hypertension occurs, temporarily withhold until medically controlled. Discontinue permanently if medically significant hypertension cannot be controlled with antihypertensive therapy or in patients with hypertensive crisis or hypertensive encephalopathy. Ramucirumab is associated with proteinuria (may be severe). Monitor proteinuria during treatment by urine dipstick and/or urinary protein creatinine ratio for the development of and/or worsening of proteinuria. Withhold treatment for urine protein levels ≥2 g/24 hours. Discontinue permanently for urine protein >3 g/24 hours or for nephrotic syndrome.

[US Boxed Warning]: Ramucirumab may increase the risk of gastrointestinal perforation, a potentially fatal event. Discontinue permanently in patients who experience a gastrointestinal perforation. Cases of reversible posterior leukoencephalopathy syndrome (RPLS) have been reported (may be fatal). Symptoms of RPLS include headache, seizure, confusion, lethargy, blindness and/or other vision, or neurologic disturbances. Confirm diagnosis of RPLS with MRI; discontinue ramucirumab with confirmed RPLS diagnosis. Resolution of symptoms may occur within days after discontinuation, although neurologic sequelae may remain in some patients. **[US Boxed Warning]: Impaired wound healing can occur with antibodies inhibiting the VEGF pathway. Discontinue ramucirumab in patients with impaired wound healing. Withhold ramucirumab prior to surgery and discontinue in patients who develop wound healing**

complications. Following surgery, use clinical judgment to resume based on adequate wound healing. If wound healing complications develop during treatment, withhold ramucirumab until wound is fully healed. Ramucirumab was not studied in patients with serious or nonhealing wounds. Clinical deterioration, including new onset or worsening encephalopathy, ascites, or hepatorenal syndrome has been reported in patients with Child-Pugh class B or C cirrhosis receiving ramucirumab. Use in patients with Child-Pugh class B or C cirrhosis only if the potential benefits outweigh the potential risks. Hypothyroidism has been observed; monitor thyroid function during treatment.

A higher incidence of neutropenia and thrombocytopenia were observed when ramucirumab was used in combination with paclitaxel (compared to paclitaxel with placebo); monitor CBC with differential when used in combination with paclitaxel. Antiangiogenic medications may increase the risk for heart failure (HF); events consistent with HF have been reported with ramucirumab. Use with caution in patients with known (or at risk of) coronary artery disease. Ramucirumab may enhance the cardiotoxicity of other chemotherapy with cardiotoxic potential (Cyramza Canadian labeling 2015).

Adverse Reactions As reported with monotherapy. Frequency not always defined.

Cardiovascular: Hypertension (16%; grades 3/4: 8%), arterial thrombosis (including myocardial infarction, cardiac arrest, cerebrovascular accident, and cerebral ischemia; 2%)

Central nervous system: Headache (9%)

Dermatologic: Skin rash (4%)

Endocrine & metabolic: Hyponatremia (6%)

Gastrointestinal: Diarrhea (14%), intestinal obstruction (2%)

Genitourinary: Proteinuria (8% to 17%; grade ≥3: 1%)

Hematologic & oncologic: Decreased red blood cells (requiring transfusion; 11%), neutropenia (5%), anemia (4%), hemorrhage (2% to 4%)

Immunologic: Antibody development (3%; neutralizing: 1%)

Respiratory: Epistaxis (5%)

Miscellaneous: Infusion related reaction (≤16%; reactions minimized with premedications)

<1% and frequency not defined (Limited to important or life-threatening): Gastrointestinal perforation, reversible posterior leukoencephalopathy syndrome

Drug Interactions

Metabolism/Transport Effects None known.

Avoid Concomitant Use

Avoid concomitant use of Ramucirumab with any of the following: Belimumab

Increased Effect/Toxicity

Ramucirumab may increase the levels/effects of: Belimumab; Bisphosphonate Derivatives

Decreased Effect There are no known significant interactions involving a decrease in effect.

Preparation for Administration Dilute total dose in NS 250 mL prior to administration (the manufacturer recommends a final volume of 250 mL). Do not use dextrose containing solutions. Invert gently to mix thoroughly; do not shake. Discard unused portion of the vial.

Storage/Stability Store intact vials at 2°C to 8°C (36°F to 46°F); do not freeze. Retain in original carton to protect from light. Do not shake. Solutions diluted for infusion may be stored at 2°C to 8°C (36°F to 46°F) for no longer than 24 hours (do not freeze) or may be stored for 4 hours at room temperature (below 25°C [77°F]); do not shake diluted product.

Mechanism of Action Ramucirumab is a recombinant monoclonal antibody which inhibits vascular endothelial growth factor receptor 2 (VEGFR2). Ramucirumab has a high affinity for VEGFR2 (Spratlin, 2010), binding to it and blocking binding of VEGFR ligands, VEGF-A, VEGF-C, and VEGF-D to inhibit activation of VEGFR2, thereby inhibiting ligand-induced proliferation and migration of endothelial cells. VEGFR2 inhibition results in reduced tumor vascularity and growth (Fuchs, 2014).

Pharmacodynamics/Kinetics Half-life elimination: 14 days

Dosing

Adult & Geriatric Note: Premedicate prior to infusion with an IV H₁ antagonist (for patients who experienced a grade 1 or 2 infusion reaction with a prior infusion, also premedicate with dexamethasone or equivalent and acetaminophen).

US labeling:

Colorectal cancer, metastatic: IV: 8 mg/kg every 2 weeks in combination with FOLFIRI (irinotecan, leucovorin, and fluorouracil); continue until disease progression or unacceptable toxicity.

Gastric cancer, advanced or metastatic: IV: 8 mg/kg every 2 weeks as a single agent or in combination with paclitaxel; continue until disease progression or unacceptable toxicity.

Non-small cell lung cancer, metastatic: IV: 10 mg/kg on day 1 every 21 days in combination with docetaxel; continue until disease progression or unacceptable toxicity

Canadian labeling: **Gastric cancer, advanced or metastatic:** Adults: IV: 8 mg/kg every 2 weeks as a single agent or in combination with paclitaxel; continue until disease progression or unacceptable toxicity.

Renal Impairment No dosage adjustment necessary.

Hepatic Impairment

Mild impairment (normal bilirubin with AST > ULN or total bilirubin >1 to 1.5 times ULN and any AST): No dosage adjustment necessary.

Moderate impairment (total bilirubin >1.5 to 3 times ULN and any AST): No dosage adjustment necessary.

Severe impairment (total bilirubin >3 times ULN and any AST): There are no dosage adjustments provided in the manufacturer's labeling (has not been studied). Use in patients with Child-Pugh class B or C cirrhosis only if the potential benefits outweigh the potential risks.

Adjustment for Toxicity

Infusion-related reaction:

Grade 1 or 2: Reduce infusion rate by 50%

Grade 3 or 4: Permanently discontinue

Hypertension:

Severe hypertension: Interrupt infusion until controlled with medical management

Severe hypertension, uncontrolled: Permanently discontinue

Proteinuria:

Urine protein ≥2 g/24 hours (first dose reduction): Withhold treatment; when urine protein returns to <2 g/24 hours, reinitiate at a reduced dose of 6 mg/kg (if initial dose was 8 mg/kg) or 8 mg/kg (if initial dose was 10 mg/kg)

Recurrent urine protein ≥2 g/24 hours (second dose reduction): Withhold treatment; when urine protein returns to <2 g/24 hours, reinitiate at a reduced dose of 5 mg/kg (if first dose reduction was to 6 mg/kg) or 6 mg/kg (if first dose reduction was to 8 mg/kg)

Urine protein >3 g/24 hours: Discontinue permanently

Nephrotic syndrome: Discontinue permanently

Arterial thrombotic events: Discontinue permanently

Bleeding, grade 3 or 4: Discontinue permanently

Gastrointestinal perforation: Discontinue permanently

Reversible posterior leukoencephalopathy syndrome (RPLS): Discontinue permanently for confirmed diagnosis

Wound healing complications: Withhold treatment prior to surgery; do not reinitiate until the surgical wound is fully healed. If wound healing complications develop during treatment, withhold ramucirumab until the wound is fully healed.

Administration Premedicate prior to infusion with an IV H₁ antagonist; for patients who experienced a grade 1 or 2 infusion reaction with a prior infusion, also premedicate with dexamethasone (or equivalent) and acetaminophen.

Infuse over 60 minutes through a separate infusion line using an infusion pump; the use of a 0.22 micron protein sparing filter is recommended. Do not administer as an IV push or bolus. Flush the line with NS after infusion is complete. Do not infuse in the same IV line with electrolytes or other medications. Administer ramucirumab prior to docetaxel, paclitaxel, or FOLFIRI if administering in combination. Monitor for infusion reaction; reduce infusion rate (by 50%) for grade 1 or 2 infusion reaction; discontinue permanently for grade 3 or 4 infusion reaction.

Monitoring Parameters Liver function tests; urine protein (by urine dipstick and/or urinary protein creatinine ratio); thyroid function; CBC with differential (when used as a part of combination chemotherapy); blood pressure (every 2 weeks; more frequently if indicated); signs/symptoms of infusion-related reactions (during infusion); signs/symptoms of arterial thromboembolic events, bleeding/hemorrhage, gastrointestinal perforation, wound healing impairment, and reversible posterior leukoencephalopathy syndrome

Dosage Forms Excipient information presented when available (limited, particularly for generics); consult specific product labeling.

Solution, Intravenous [preservative free]:

Cyramza: 100 mg/10 mL (10 mL); 500 mg/50 mL (50 mL) [contains polysorbate 80]

Ranibizumab (ra ni BIZ oo mab)

Brand Names: US Lucentis
Brand Names: Canada Lucentis
Index Terms rhuFabV2
Pharmacologic Category Angiogenesis Inhibitor; Monoclonal Antibody; Ophthalmic Agent; Vascular Endothelial Growth Factor (VEGF) Inhibitor

Use

Diabetic retinopathy: Treatment of diabetic retinopathy (nonproliferative diabetic retinopathy [NPDR]), proliferative diabetic retinopathy [PDR]) in patients with diabetic macular edema (DME)

Macular degeneration: Treatment of neovascular (wet) age-related macular degeneration (AMD)

Macular edema: Treatment of macular edema following retinal vein occlusion (RVO); diabetic macular edema (DME)

Choroidal neovascularization secondary to pathologic myopia: *Canadian labeling:* Additional use (not in US labeling): Treatment of visual impairment due to choroidal neovascularization (CNV) secondary to pathologic myopia

Dosing

Adult & Geriatric

Age-related macular degeneration (AMD): Intravitreal:

U.S. labeling: 0.5 mg once a month (approximately every 28 days). Frequency may be reduced (eg, 4 to 5 injections over 9 months) after the first 3 injections or may be reduced after the first 4 injections to once every 3 months if monthly injections are not feasible.

Canadian labeling: 0.5 mg once a month. Frequency may be reduced after the first 3 injections to once every 3 months if monthly injections are not feasible.

Note: A regimen averaging 4 to 5 doses over 9 months is expected to maintain visual acuity and an every-3-month dosing regimen has reportedly resulted in a ~5 letter (1 line) loss of visual acuity over 9 months, as compared to monthly dosing which may result in an additional ~1 to 2 letter gain.

Choroidal neovascularization secondary to pathologic myopia: Intravitreal: *Canadian labeling:* Initial: 0.5 mg; may repeat 0.5 mg dose at monthly intervals if clinically indicated.

Diabetic macular edema (DME): Intravitreal:

U.S. labeling: 0.3 mg once a month (approximately every 28 days)

Canadian labeling: 0.5 mg once a month until achievement of stable visual acuity for 3 consecutive months. Upon discontinuation, may resume monthly therapy if monitoring identifies a loss of visual acuity.

Diabetic retinopathy (DR): Adults: Intravitreal: 0.3 mg once a month (approximately every 28 days)

Macular edema following retinal vein occlusion (RVO): Intravitreal: 0.5 mg once a month (approximately every 28 days). **Note:** Canadian labeling recommends continuing therapy until achievement of stable visual acuity for 3 consecutive months; upon discontinuation, may resume monthly therapy if monitoring identifies a loss of visual acuity.

Renal Impairment No dosage adjustment necessary.

Hepatic Impairment There are no dosage adjustments provided in the manufacturer's labeling. However, significant systemic exposure is not expected.

Additional Information Complete prescribing information should be consulted for additional detail.

Dosage Forms Excipient information presented when available (limited, particularly for generics); consult specific product labeling.

Solution, Intraocular [preservative free]:

Lucentis: 0.3 mg/0.05 mL (0.05 mL); 0.5 mg/0.05 mL (0.05 mL)

Dosage Forms: Canada Excipient information presented when available (limited, particularly for generics); consult specific product labeling.

Solution, Intraocular [preservative free]:

Lucentis: 10 mg/mL (0.23 mL)

Ranitidine (ra NI ti deen)

Brand Names: US Acid Reducer Maximum Strength [OTC] [DSC]; Acid Reducer [OTC]; Deprizine FusePaq; GoodSense Acid Reducer [OTC]; Ranitidine Acid Reducer [OTC]; Zantac; Zantac 150 Maximum Strength [OTC]; Zantac 75 [OTC]; Zantac EFFERdose [DSC]; Zantac in NaCl [DSC]

Brand Names: Canada Acid Reducer; ACT Ranitidine; Apo-Ranitidine; Dom-Ranitidine; Myl-Ranitidine; Mylan-Ranitidine; PHL-Ranitidine; PMS-Ranitidine; RAN-Ranitidine; Ranitidine Injection, USP; Riva-Ranitidine; Sandoz-Ranitidine; Teva-Ranitidine; Zantac; Zantac 75; Zantac Maximum Strength Non-Prescription

Index Terms Ranitidine Hydrochloride

Pharmacologic Category Histamine H_2 Antagonist

Use

Oral:

Duodenal ulcer: Short-term treatment of active duodenal ulcer and maintenance therapy after the healing of acute ulcers.

Erosive esophagitis: Treatment of endoscopically diagnosed erosive esophagitis; for the maintenance of healing of erosive esophagitis.

Gastric ulcer: Short-term treatment of active, benign gastric ulcer and maintenance therapy after the healing of acute ulcer.

Gastroesophageal reflux disease: Treatment of gastroesophageal reflux disease (GERD).

Pathological hypersecretory conditions: Treatment of pathological hypersecretory conditions (eg, Zollinger-Ellison syndrome, systemic mastocytosis).

Heartburn (OTC only): Relief and prevention of heartburn associated with acid indigestion and sour stomach.

Injection:

Duodenal ulcers: Indicated in some hospitalized patients with intractable duodenal ulcers.

Pathological hypersecretory conditions: Indicated in some hospitalized patients with pathological hypersecretory conditions (eg, Zollinger-Ellison).

Patients not able to take oral medication: As an alternative to the oral dosage form for short-term use in patients who are unable to take oral medication.

Pregnancy Considerations Adverse events were not observed in animal reproduction studies. Ranitidine crosses the placenta (Armentano, 1989). Histamine H_2 antagonists have been evaluated for the treatment of gastroesophageal reflux disease (GERD) as well as gastric and duodenal ulcers during pregnancy. If needed, ranitidine is the agent of choice (Cappell 2003; Richter 2003). Histamine H_2 antagonists may be used for aspiration prophylaxis prior to cesarean delivery (ASA 2007).

Breast-Feeding Considerations Ranitidine is excreted into breast milk. The manufacturer recommends that caution be exercised when administering ranitidine to nursing women. Peak milk concentrations of ranitidine occur ~5.5 hours after the dose (case report) (Kearns, 1985).

Contraindications

Hypersensitivity to ranitidine or any component of the formulation

OTC labeling: When used for self-medication (OTC), do not use if trouble or pain when swallowing food, vomiting with blood, or bloody or black stools, allergic to ranitidine or other acid reducers. Do not use with other acid reducers. Do not use 150 mg tablet with kidney disease without medical advice.

Documentation of allergenic cross-reactivity for histamine H$_2$ antagonists is limited. However, because of similarities in chemical structure and/or pharmacologic actions, the possibility of cross-sensitivity cannot be ruled out with certainty.

Warnings/Precautions Rare cases of reversible confusion have been associated with ranitidine; usually elderly or severely ill patients, or in patients with renal or hepatic impairment. Elevation in ALT levels has occurred with higher doses (≥100 mg) or prolonged IV therapy (≥5 days); monitor ALT levels daily for the remainder of treatment. Use with caution in patients with hepatic impairment (ranitidine undergoes hepatic metabolism). Ranitidine is primarily excreted renally; dosage adjustment is recommended in patients with renal impairment. Avoid use in patients with history of acute porphyria (may precipitate attacks). Prolonged treatment (≥2 years) may lead to vitamin B$_{12}$ malabsorption and subsequent vitamin B$_{12}$ deficiency. The magnitude of the deficiency is dose-related and the association is stronger in females and those younger in age (<30 years); prevalence is decreased after discontinuation of therapy (Lam 2013). Symptoms of GI distress may be associated with a variety of conditions; symptomatic response to H$_2$ antagonists does not rule out the potential for significant pathology (eg, malignancy).

Use of gastric acid inhibitors, including proton pump inhibitors and H$_2$ blockers, has been associated with an increased risk for development of acute gastroenteritis and community-acquired pneumonia in pediatric patients (Canani 2006). Rapid IV administration has been associated with bradycardia (rare), usually in patients with predisposing risk factors for cardiac rhythm disorders. Do not exceed the recommended IV administration rate(s). Ranitidine syrup may contain up to 7.5% alcohol.

When used for self-medication (OTC), notify health care provider before use if any of the following are present: Frequent chest pain; frequent wheezing particularly with heartburn; nausea/vomiting; unexplained weight loss; stomach pain; heartburn longer than 3 months; heartburn with light-headedness, sweating, or dizziness; chest pain or shoulder pain with shortness of breath; sweating or pain that spreads to arms, neck, or shoulders; light-headedness. Stop use and notify health care provider if heartburn continues, worsens, or lasts longer than 14 days.

Potentially significant interactions may exist, requiring dose or frequency adjustment, additional monitoring, and/or selection of alternative therapy.

Adverse Reactions Frequency not defined.

Cardiovascular: Asystole, atrioventricular block, bradycardia (with rapid IV administration), premature ventricular beats, tachycardia, vasculitis

Central nervous system: Agitation, dizziness, depression, hallucinations, headache, insomnia, malaise, mental confusion, somnolence, vertigo

Dermatologic: Alopecia, erythema multiforme, rash

Endocrine & metabolic: Prolactin levels increased

Gastrointestinal: Abdominal discomfort/pain, constipation, diarrhea, nausea, necrotizing enterocolitis (VLBW neonates; Guillet, 2006), pancreatitis, vomiting

Hematologic: Acquired immune hemolytic anemia, acute porphyritic attack, agranulocytosis, aplastic anemia, granulocytopenia, leukopenia, pancytopenia, thrombocytopenia

Hepatic: Cholestatic hepatitis, hepatic failure, hepatitis, jaundice

Local: Transient pain, burning or itching at the injection site

Neuromuscular & skeletal: Arthralgia, involuntary motor disturbance, myalgia

Ocular: Blurred vision

Renal: Acute interstitial nephritis, serum creatinine increased

Respiratory: Pneumonia (causal relationship not established)

Miscellaneous: Anaphylaxis, angioneurotic edema, hypersensitivity reactions (eg, bronchospasm, fever, eosinophilia)

Drug Interactions

Metabolism/Transport Effects Substrate of CYP1A2 (minor), CYP2C19 (minor), CYP2D6 (minor), OCT2, P-glycoprotein; **Note:** Assignment of Major/Minor substrate status based on clinically relevant drug interaction potential; **Inhibits** CYP1A2 (weak), CYP2D6 (weak)

Avoid Concomitant Use

Avoid concomitant use of Ranitidine with any of the following: Dasatinib; Delavirdine; PAZOPanib; Risedronate

Increased Effect/Toxicity

Ranitidine may increase the levels/effects of: ARIPiprazole; Dexmethylphenidate; Doxofylline; Methylphenidate; Procainamide; Risedronate; Saquinavir; Sulfonylureas; TiZANidine; Varenicline; Warfarin

The levels/effects of Ranitidine may be increased by: BuPROPion; Lumacaftor; P-glycoprotein/ABCB1 Inhibitors; Ranolazine

Decreased Effect

Ranitidine may decrease the levels/effects of: Atazanavir; Bosutinib; Cefditoren; Cefpodoxime; Cefuroxime; Cysteamine (Systemic); Dabrafenib; Dasatinib; Delavirdine; Erlotinib; Fosamprenavir; Gefitinib; Indinavir; Iron Salts; Itraconazole; Ketoconazole (Systemic); Ledipasvir; Mesalamine; Multivitamins/Minerals (with ADEK, Folate, Iron); Nelfinavir; Nilotinib; PAZOPanib; Posaconazole; Prasugrel; Rilpivirine

The levels/effects of Ranitidine may be decreased by: Lumacaftor; P-glycoprotein/ABCB1 Inducers

Food Interactions Prolonged treatment (≥2 years) may lead to malabsorption of dietary vitamin B$_{12}$ and subsequent vitamin B$_{12}$ deficiency (Lam 2013).

Preparation for Administration

Continuous infusion: Dilute in D$_5$W or other compatible IV solution; for Zollinger-Ellison patients, dilute in D$_5$W or other compatible IV solution to a maximum concentration of 2.5 mg/mL.

Intermittent bolus injection: Dilute in NS or other compatible IV solution to a maximum concentration of 2.5 mg/mL (20 mL).

Intermittent infusion: Dilute in D$_5$W or other compatible IV solution to a maximum concentration of 0.5 mg/mL (100 mL).

IM: No dilution necessary.

Storage/Stability

Capsules, tablets: Store between 20°C and 25°C (68°F and 77°F). Protect from light. Protect from moisture.

Injection: Store intact vials between 4°C and 25°C (39°F to 77°F); excursion permitted to 30°C (86°F). Protect from light; do not freeze. Avoid excessive heat (brief exposure up to 40°C does not affect the product). Undiluted solution is a clear, colorless to yellow color; slight darkening does not affect potency. Stable for 48 hours at room temperature when diluted for infusion in commonly used IV solutions (eg, NS, D$_5$W, D$_{10}$W, Ringer's lactate injection, sodium bicarbonate 5% injection).

Suspension (Deprizine FusePaq): Store unused kit between 15°C and 30°C (59°F and 86°F); store reconstituted suspension between 2°C and 8°C (36°F and 46°F). The final suspension is stable for 8 weeks.

Syrup: Store between 4°C and 25°C (39°F and 77°F). Protect from light.

Mechanism of Action Competitive inhibition of histamine at H$_2$-receptors of the gastric parietal cells, which inhibits gastric acid secretion, gastric volume, and hydrogen ion concentration are reduced. Does not affect pepsin secretion, pentagastrin-stimulated intrinsic factor secretion, or serum gastrin.

Pharmacodynamics/Kinetics

Absorption: Oral: 50%; IM: Rapid

Distribution: V$_d$: Normal renal function: ~1.4 L/kg; CrCl 25 to 35 mL/minute: 1.76 L/kg

Protein binding: ~15%

Metabolism: Hepatic (minor) to N-oxide, S-oxide, and N-desmethyl metabolites

Bioavailability: Oral tablets: ~50%; IM: 90% to 100%

Half-life elimination:

Oral: Normal renal function: 2.5 to 3 hours

IV: Normal renal function: 2 to 2.5 hours; CrCl 25 to 35 mL/minute: 4.8 hours

Time to peak, serum: Oral: 2 to 3 hours; IM: ≤15 minutes

Excretion: Urine (as unchanged drug): Oral: 30%, IV: 70%; feces (as metabolites)

Dosing

Adult

Duodenal ulcer:

Oral: Treatment: 150 mg twice daily, or 300 mg once daily after the evening meal or at bedtime; maintenance of healing: 150 mg once daily at bedtime

IM: 50 mg every 6 to 8 hours

IV:

Intermittent bolus or infusion: 50 mg every 6 to 8 hours (if increased doses are necessary utilize more frequent administration up to a maximum of 400 mg/day).

Continuous IV infusion: 6.25 mg/hour

Erosive esophagitis: Oral: Treatment: 150 mg 4 times daily; maintenance of healing: 150 mg twice daily

Gastric ulcer, benign: Oral: 150 mg twice daily; maintenance of healing: 150 mg once daily at bedtime

Gastroesophageal reflux disease (GERD): Oral: 150 mg twice daily

Heartburn prevention or relief (OTC labeling): Oral:

Prevention: 75 to 150 mg 30 to 60 minutes before eating food or drinking beverages that cause heartburn (maximum: 2 doses/day); do not use for more than 14 days

Relief of symptoms: 75 mg to 150 mg up to twice daily (maximum: 2 doses/day); do not use for more than 14 days

Pathological hypersecretory conditions:

Oral: 150 mg twice daily; adjust dose or frequency as clinically indicated; doses of up to 6 g/day have been used in patients with severe disease

IM: 50 mg every 6 to 8 hours

IV:

Continuous IV infusion: 6.25 mg/hour

Continuous infusion for Zollinger-Ellison: Initial: 1 mg/kg/hour; measure gastric acid output at 4 hours, if >10 mEq or if patient is symptomatic, increase dose in increments of 0.5 mg/kg/hour; doses of up to 2.5 mg/kg/hour (or 220 mg/hour) have been used

Intermittent bolus or infusion: 50 mg every 6 to 8 hours (if increased doses are necessary utilize more frequent administration up to a maximum of 400 mg/day)

Patients not able to take oral medication:

IM: 50 mg every 6 to 8 hours

IV:

Intermittent bolus or infusion: 50 mg every 6 to 8 hours (if increased doses are necessary utilize more frequent administration up to a maximum of 400 mg/day)

Continuous IV infusion: 6.25 mg/hour

Anaphylaxis, adjunct therapy (off-label use): IV: 50 mg/dose; should not be used as monotherapy or as first line therapy (AAAAI/ACAAI [Lieberman 2010])

Premedication to prevent taxane hypersensitivity (off-label use): IV: 50 mg administered 30 minutes prior to paclitaxel administration (along with dexamethasone and diphenhydramine) (Lee 2009)

Stress ulcer prophylaxis, ICU patients (off-label use) (ASHP 1999): Note: Intended for patients with associated risk factors (eg, coagulopathy, mechanical ventilation for >48 hours, severe sepsis); discontinue use once risk factors have resolved. The Surviving Sepsis Campaign guidelines suggest the use of proton pump inhibitors rather than H_2 antagonist therapy (Dellinger 2013). Oral, nasogastric (NG) tube: 150 mg twice daily; may administer a 300 mg loading dose prior to maintenance dosing (Pemberton 1993)

IV: Intermittent bolus: 50 mg every 6 to 8 hours (Cook 1998; Geus 1993)

Geriatric Refer to adult dosing (use caution with dose selection).

Pediatric

Duodenal ulcer:

Oral:

Treatment:

Infants, Children, and Adolescents ≤16 years: 4 to 8 mg/kg/day divided twice daily; maximum: 300 mg/day

Adolescents >16 years: Refer to adult dosing

Maintenance of healing:

Infants, Children, and Adolescents ≤16 years: 2 to 4 mg/kg once daily; maximum: 150 mg/day

Adolescents >16 years: Refer to adult dosing.

IM: Adolescents >16 years: Refer to adult dosing.

IV:

Infants, Children, and Adolescents ≤16 years: 2 to 4 mg/kg/day divided every 6 to 8 hours; maximum dose: 50 mg/dose

Adolescents >16 years: Refer to adult dosing.

Gastric ulcer: Oral:

Treatment:

Infants, Children, and Adolescents ≤16 years: 4 to 8 mg/kg/day divided twice daily; maximum: 300 mg/day

Adolescents >16 years: Refer to adult dosing

Maintenance of healing:

Infants, Children, and Adolescents ≤16 years: 2 to 4 mg/kg once daily; maximum: 150 mg/day

Adolescents >16 years: Refer to adult dosing.

Gastroesophageal reflux disease (GERD) or erosive esophagitis: Oral:

Infants, Children, and Adolescents ≤16 years: 5 to 10 mg/kg/day divided twice daily; maximum: 300 mg/day

Adolescents >16 years: Refer to adult dosing.

Heartburn prevention or relief (OTC labeling):

Prevention: Children ≥12 years and Adolescents: Oral: 75 to 150 mg 30 to 60 minutes before eating food or drinking beverages that cause heartburn (maximum: 2 doses/day); do not use for more than 14 days

Relief of symptoms: Children ≥12 years and Adolescents: Oral: 75 to 150 mg up to twice daily (maximum: 2 doses/day); do not use for more than 14 days

Patients not able to take oral medication:

Infants, Children, and Adolescents <16 years: IV: 2 to 4 mg/kg/day divided every 6 to 8 hours; maximum dose: 50 mg/dose

Adolescents ≥16 years: IV: Refer to adult dosing.

Pathological hypersecretory conditions: Adolescents >16 years: Refer to adult dosing.

Anaphylaxis, adjunct therapy (off-label use): Infants, Children, and Adolescents: IV: 1 mg/kg/dose; maximum dose: 50 mg/dose; **Note:** Should not be used as monotherapy or as first line therapy (AAAAI/ACAAI [Lieberman 2010])

Renal Impairment

Adults:

CrCl ≥50 mL/minute: No dosage adjustment necessary.

CrCl <50 mL/minute:

Oral: 150 mg every 24 hours; adjust dose cautiously if needed

IV: 50 mg every 18 to 24 hours; adjust dose cautiously if needed

Hemodialysis: Adjust dosing schedule so that dose is scheduled to coincide with the end of hemodialysis.

Stress ulcer prophylaxis (ASHP 1999): CrCl <50 mL/minute:

Oral, nasogastric (NG) tube: 150 mg 1 to 2 times daily

IV: Intermittent bolus: 50 mg every 12 to 24 hours

Pediatrics (Aronoff 2007):

Oral: Based on a usual dose of 2 to 6 mg/kg/day divided every 8 to 12 hours

GFR >50 mL/minute/1.73 m^2: No dosage adjustment necessary.

GFR 30 to 50 mL/minute/1.73 m^2: 2 mg/kg/dose every 12 hours

GFR 10 to 29 mL/minute/1.73 m^2: 1 mg/kg/dose every 12 hours

GFR <10 mL/minute/1.73 m^2: 1 mg/kg/dose every 24 hours

Hemodialysis: 1 mg/kg/dose every 24 hours

Peritoneal dialysis: 1 mg/kg/dose every 24 hours

Continuous renal replacement therapy: 2 mg/kg/dose every 12 hours

Parenteral (IV): Based on a usual dose of 2 to 4 mg/kg/day divided every 6 to 24 hours

GFR >50 mL/minute/1.73 m^2: No dosage adjustment necessary.

GFR 30 to 50 mL/minute/1.73 m^2: 1 mg/kg/dose every 12 hours

GFR 10 to 29 mL/minute/1.73 m^2: 0.5 mg/kg/dose every 12 hours

GFR <10 mL/minute/1.73 m^2: 0.5 mg/kg/dose every 24 hours

Hemodialysis: 0.5 mg/kg/dose every 24 hours

Peritoneal dialysis: 0.5 mg/kg/dose every 24 hours

Continuous renal replacement therapy: 1 mg/kg/dose every 12 hours

Hepatic Impairment There are no dosage adjustments provided in the manufacturer's labeling; use with caution.

Dietary Considerations Some products may contain phenylalanine and/or sodium. Oral dosage forms may be taken with or without food.

Usual Infusion Concentrations: Pediatric IV infusion: 0.5 mg/mL

Usual Infusion Concentrations: Adult IV infusion: 50 mg in 50 mL (concentration: 1 mg/mL) **or** 500 mg in 250 mL (concentration: 2 mg/mL) of D_5W or NS

Administration

Injection may be administered IM or IV:

IM: Injection is administered undiluted

IV: Must be diluted; may be administered intermittent bolus, intermittent IV infusion, or continuous IV infusion

Intermittent bolus: Manufacturer recommends a maximum rate of administration of 10 mg/minute (infuse over at least 5 minutes); however, in adults may also be administered at a maximum rate of 25 mg/minute (or over 2 minutes) if necessary (Coursin 1988; Goelzer 1988; Smith 1987).

Intermittent IV infusion: Administer over a maximum rate of 2.5 to 3.5 mg/minute (infuse over at least 15 to 20 minutes)

Continuous IV infusion: Administer at a rate of 6.25 mg/hour; for Zollinger-Ellison patients, administer at a rate of 1 mg/**kg**/hour (infusion rates as high as 220 mg/hour have been used).

Monitoring Parameters AST, ALT, serum creatinine; occult blood with GI bleeding, signs/symptoms of peptic ulcer disease; when used to prevent stress-related GI bleeding, measure the intragastric pH and try to maintain pH >4; when used for Zollinger-Ellison syndrome, monitor gastric acid secretion (goal: <10 mEq/hour); signs of confusion

Test Interactions False-positive urine protein using Multistix.

Dosage Forms Considerations Deprizine FusePaq is a compounding kit for the preparation of an oral suspension. Refer to manufacturer's labeling for compounding instructions.

Dosage Forms Excipient information presented when available (limited, particularly for generics); consult specific product labeling. [DSC] = Discontinued product
Capsule, Oral:
  Generic: 150 mg, 300 mg
Solution, Injection:
  Zantac: 50 mg/2 mL (2 mL); 150 mg/6 mL (6 mL); 1000 mg/40 mL (40 mL) [contains phenol]
  Generic: 50 mg/2 mL (2 mL); 150 mg/6 mL (6 mL); 1000 mg/40 mL (40 mL)
Solution, Intravenous [preservative free]:
  Zantac in NaCl: 50 mg (50 mL [DSC])
Suspension Reconstituted, Oral:
  Deprizine FusePaq: 22.4 mg/mL (250 mL) [contains sodium benzoate]
Syrup, Oral:
  Zantac: 15 mg/mL (480 mL [DSC]) [contains alcohol, usp, butylparaben, propylparaben, saccharin sodium; peppermint flavor]
  Generic: 15 mg/mL (10 mL, 473 mL, 474 mL, 480 mL); 75 mg/5 mL (473 mL, 480 mL [DSC]); 150 mg/10 mL (10 mL)
Tablet, Oral:
  Acid Reducer: 75 mg, 150 mg
  Acid Reducer: 150 mg [sodium free, sugar free]
  Acid Reducer: 75 mg [DSC] [sugar free]
  Acid Reducer Maximum Strength: 150 mg [DSC] [sugar free; contains fd&c yellow #6 (sunset yellow)]
  GoodSense Acid Reducer: 75 mg [gluten free]
  Ranitidine Acid Reducer: 75 mg
  Zantac 75: 75 mg
  Zantac: 150 mg, 300 mg
  Zantac 150 Maximum Strength: 150 mg
  Zantac 150 Maximum Strength: 150 mg [sodium free, sugar free; contains brilliant blue fcf (fd&c blue #1); mint flavor]
  Generic: 75 mg, 150 mg, 300 mg
Tablet Effervescent, Oral:
  Zantac EFFERdose: 25 mg [DSC] [contains aspartame, sodium benzoate]

◆ Ranitidine Acid Reducer [OTC] *see* Ranitidine *on page 1556*
◆ Ranitidine Hydrochloride *see* Ranitidine *on page 1556*
◆ Ranitidine Injection, USP (Can) *see* Ranitidine *on page 1556*
◆ RAN-Lansoprazole (Can) *see* Lansoprazole *on page 1032*
◆ RAN-Letrozole (Can) *see* Letrozole *on page 1048*
◆ RAN-Levetiracetam (Can) *see* LevETIRAcetam *on page 1056*
◆ RAN-Lisinopril (Can) *see* Lisinopril *on page 1088*
◆ RAN-Losartan (Can) *see* Losartan *on page 1107*
◆ RAN-Memantine (Can) *see* Memantine *on page 1139*
◆ RAN-Metformin (Can) *see* MetFORMIN *on page 1156*
◆ RAN-Montelukast (Can) *see* Montelukast *on page 1229*
◆ RAN-Olanzapine (Can) *see* OLANZapine *on page 1314*
◆ RAN-Olanzapine ODT (Can) *see* OLANZapine *on page 1314*

Ranolazine (ra NOE la zeen)

Brand Names: US Ranexa
Pharmacologic Category Antianginal Agent; Cardiovascular Agent, Miscellaneous
Use Chronic angina: Treatment of chronic angina
  Note: According to the 2012 ACCF/AHA/ACP/AATS/PCNA/SCAI/STS guidelines for patients with stable ischemic heart disease, ranolazine may be useful when prescribed as a substitute for beta blockers for relief of symptoms if initial treatment with beta blockers leads to unacceptable side effects, is less effective, or if initial treatment with beta blockers is contraindicated. May also be used in combination with beta blockers, for relief of symptoms when initial treatment with beta blockers is not successful (Fihn 2012).

Pregnancy Considerations Adverse events have been observed in animal reproduction studies.
Breast-Feeding Considerations It is not known if ranolazine is excreted into breast milk. According to the manufacturer, the decision to breastfeed during therapy should take into account the risk of exposure to the infant and the benefits of treatment to the mother.
Contraindications Hepatic cirrhosis; concurrent strong CYP3A inhibitors; concurrent CYP3A inducers
Warnings/Precautions Ranolazine has been shown to prolong QT interval in a dose/plasma concentration-related manner. Cirrhotic patients with mild to moderate hepatic impairment demonstrated a 3-fold increase in QT prolongation. The incidence of symptomatic arrhythmias was similar to placebo in one trial (Morrow 2007). Risk versus benefit should be assessed in patients maintained on a higher dose (>2,000 mg/day) or exposure, concurrent use of other QT-prolonging drugs, potassium-channel variants known to cause QT prolongation, family history of or congenital long QT syndrome, or known acquired QT interval prolongation. Ranolazine plasma levels increase in patients with mild and moderate hepatic impairment; use is contraindicated in patients with hepatic cirrhosis. Acute renal failure has been observed in some patients with severe renal impairment (CrCl <30 mL/minute); if acute renal failure develops (marked increase in serum creatinine associated with increased BUN), discontinue ranolazine and manage appropriately. Monitor renal function periodically in patients with moderate to severe renal impairment; particularly for increases in serum creatinine accompanied by increased BUN. In a renal impairment study, patients with severe impairment exhibited an initial elevation in diastolic blood pressure (~12 to 17 mm Hg at day 3), however this diminished to ~4 mm Hg increase by day 5 (Jerling 2005); consider monitoring blood pressure in patients with renal dysfunction. Ranolazine has not been evaluated in patients requiring dialysis.

Ranolazine will not relieve acute angina episode and has not demonstrated benefit in acute coronary syndrome. Potentially significant drug-drug interactions may exist, requiring dose or frequency adjustment, additional monitoring, and/or selection of alternative therapy. Use is contraindicated with inducers and strong inhibitors of CYP3A. Use with caution in patients ≥75 years of age; they may experience more adverse events (including serious adverse events) and drug discontinuations due to adverse events.

Adverse Reactions
>0.5% to 10%:
  Cardiovascular: Bradycardia (≤4%), hypotension (≤4%), orthostatic hypotension (≤4%), palpitation (≤4%), peripheral edema (≤4%), prolonged QT interval on ECG (>500 msec: ≤1%)
  Central nervous system: Headache (≤6%), dizziness (6%; may be dose-related), confusion (≤4%), vertigo (≤4%), syncope (≤4%)
  Dermatologic: Hyperhidrosis (≤4%)
  Gastrointestinal: Constipation (5%), abdominal pain (≤4%), anorexia (≤4%), dyspepsia (≤4%), nausea (≤4%; dose related), vomiting (≤4%), xerostomia (≤4%)
  Genitourinary: Hematuria (≤4%)
  Neuromuscular: Weakness (≤4%)
  Ophthalmic: Blurred vision (≤4%)
  Otic: Tinnitus (≤4%)
  Respiratory: Dyspnea (≤4%)
≤0.5% (Limited to important or life-threatening): Angioedema, decreased glycosylated hemoglobin, decreased T-wave amplitude, dysuria, eosinophilia, hallucination, hypoesthesia, increased blood urea nitrogen, increased serum creatinine, leukopenia, pancytopenia, paresthesia, pruritus, pulmonary fibrosis, renal failure, thrombocytopenia, torsade de pointes (case report [Morrow, 2007]), tremor, T-wave changes (notched), urinary retention, urine discoloration
Drug Interactions
  Metabolism/Transport Effects Substrate of CYP2D6 (minor), CYP3A4 (major), P-glycoprotein; **Note:** Assignment of Major/Minor substrate status based on clinically relevant drug interaction potential; **Inhibits** CYP2D6 (weak), CYP3A4 (weak), P-glycoprotein
  Avoid Concomitant Use
    Avoid concomitant use of Ranolazine with any of the following: Antifungal Agents (Azole Derivatives, Systemic); Bosutinib; Conivaptan; CYP3A4 Inducers (Moderate); CYP3A4 Inducers (Strong); CYP3A4 Inhibitors (Strong); Fusidic Acid (Systemic); Idelalisib; PAZOPanib; Pimozide; Rifampin; Silodosin; St Johns Wort; Topotecan; VinCRIStine (Liposomal)

Increased Effect/Toxicity

Ranolazine may increase the levels/effects of: Afatinib; ARIPiprazole; AtorvaSTATin; Bosutinib; Brentuximab Vedotin; Colchicine; Dabigatran Etexilate; Digoxin; DOX-Orubicin (Conventional); Edoxaban; Everolimus; Flibanserin; Highest Risk QTc-Prolonging Agents; Hydrocodone; Ledipasvir; Lomitapide; Lovastatin; MetFORMIN; Moderate Risk QTc-Prolonging Agents; Naloxegol; NiMODipine; PAZOPanib; P-glycoprotein/ABCB1 Substrates; Pimozide; Prucalopride; Rifaximin; Silodosin; Simvastatin; Tacrolimus (Systemic); Topotecan; VinCRIStine (Liposomal)

The levels/effects of Ranolazine may be increased by: Antifungal Agents (Azole Derivatives, Systemic); Calcium Channel Blockers (Nondihydropyridine); Conivaptan; CYP3A4 Inhibitors (Moderate); CYP3A4 Inhibitors (Strong); Dasatinib; Fosaprepitant; Fusidic Acid (Systemic); Idelalisib; Ivacaftor; Luliconazole; Mifepristone; Osimertinib; Palbociclib; P-glycoprotein/ABCB1 Inhibitors; Simeprevir; Stiripentol

Decreased Effect

The levels/effects of Ranolazine may be decreased by: CYP3A4 Inducers (Moderate); CYP3A4 Inducers (Strong); Deferasirox; Osimertinib; P-glycoprotein/ABCB1 Inducers; Rifampin; Siltuximab; St Johns Wort; Tocilizumab

Food Interactions Grapefruit, grapefruit juice, or grapefruit-containing products may increase the serum concentration of ranolazine. Management: Avoid grapefruit-containing products or dose adjustment of ranolazine may is required.

Storage/Stability Store at 25°C (77°F); excursions permitted to 15°C to 30°C (59°F to 86°F).

Mechanism of Action Ranolazine exerts antianginal and anti-ischemic effects without changing hemodynamic parameters (heart rate or blood pressure). At therapeutic levels, ranolazine inhibits the late phase of the inward sodium channel (late I_{Na}) in ischemic cardiac myocytes during cardiac repolarization reducing intracellular sodium concentrations and thereby reducing calcium influx via Na^+-Ca^{2+} exchange. Decreased intracellular calcium reduces ventricular tension and myocardial oxygen consumption. It is thought that ranolazine produces myocardial relaxation and reduces anginal symptoms through this mechanism although this is uncertain. At higher concentrations, ranolazine inhibits the rapid delayed rectifier potassium current (I_{Kr}) thus prolonging the ventricular action potential duration and subsequent prolongation of the QT interval.

Pharmacodynamics/Kinetics

Absorption: Highly variable

Protein binding: ~62%

Metabolism: Extensive; Hepatic via CYP3A (major) and 2D6 (minor); intestines

Bioavailability: Tablet: 76% (compared to solution)

Half-life elimination: Ranolazine: Terminal: 7 hours; Metabolites (activity undefined): 6 to 22 hours

Time to peak, plasma: 2 to 5 hours

Excretion: Primarily urine (75% mostly as metabolites; <5% as unchanged drug); feces (25% mostly as metabolites; <5% as unchanged drug)

Dosing

Adult Note: May be used with beta-blockers, nitrates, calcium channel blockers, antiplatelet therapy, lipid-lowering therapy, angiotensin-converting enzyme (ACE) inhibitors, and angiotensin-receptor blockers.

Chronic angina: Oral: Initial: 500 mg twice daily; may increase to 1,000 mg twice daily as needed (based on symptoms); maximum recommended dose: 1,000 mg twice daily

Missed doses: If a dose is missed, it should be taken at the next scheduled time; the next dose should not be doubled.

Dosage adjustment for ranolazine with concomitant medications:

Diltiazem, erythromycin, fluconazole, verapamil, and other moderate CYP3A inhibitors: Ranolazine dose should not exceed 500 mg twice daily

CYP3A inducers or strong CYP3A inhibitors: Concomitant use is contraindicated

P-glycoprotein inhibitors (eg, cyclosporine): Titrate ranolazine based on clinical response

Geriatric Refer to adult dosing. Select dose cautiously, starting at the lower end of the dosing range.

Renal Impairment There are no dosage adjustments provided in the manufacturer's labeling. However, plasma ranolazine levels increased ~40% to 50% in patients with varying degrees of renal dysfunction. Discontinue if acute renal failure develops during treatment. Ranolazine has not been evaluated in patients requiring dialysis, although it is unlikely to be removed by hemodialysis due to plasma protein binding.

Hepatic Impairment There are no dosage adjustments provided in the manufacturer's labeling. Use is contraindicated with hepatic cirrhosis.

Dietary Considerations Limit the use of grapefruit juice; the ranolazine dose should not exceed 500 mg twice daily when taken with grapefruit juice or grapefruit-containing products.

Administration Oral: Administer with or without meals. Swallow tablet whole; do not crush, break, or chew.

Monitoring Parameters Baseline and follow up ECG to evaluate QT interval; monitor renal function periodically in patients with moderate to severe renal impairment, particularly for increases in serum creatinine accompanied by increased BUN; consider monitoring blood pressure in patients with renal dysfunction; correct and maintain serum potassium in normal limits

Dosage Forms Excipient information presented when available (limited, particularly for generics); consult specific product labeling.

Tablet Extended Release 12 Hour, Oral:

Ranexa: 500 mg, 1000 mg

Rasagiline (ra SA ji leen)

Brand Names: US Azilect

Brand Names: Canada Azilect

Index Terms AGN 1135; Rasagiline Mesylate; TVP-1012

Pharmacologic Category Anti-Parkinson's Agent, MAO Type B Inhibitor

Use Parkinson disease: Treatment of Parkinson disease

Pregnancy Considerations Adverse effects have been observed in animal reproduction studies.

Breast-Feeding Considerations It is not known if rasagiline is excreted in breast milk. The manufacturer recommends caution be exercised when administering rasagiline to nursing women.

Contraindications Concomitant use of an MAO inhibitor (including selective MAO-B inhibitors), meperidine, methadone, propoxyphene, or tramadol within 14 days of rasagiline; concomitant use with cyclobenzaprine, dextromethorphan, or St John's wort

Warnings/Precautions Hazardous agent - use appropriate precautions for handling and disposal (NIOSH 2014 [group 2]).

May cause exacerbation of hypertension; monitor for new onset hypertension or hypertension not adequately controlled after starting rasagiline. Medication adjustment may be necessary if blood pressure elevation is sustained. In patients taking recommended doses of rasagiline, dietary restriction of most tyramine-containing products is not necessary; however, certain foods (eg, aged cheeses) may contain high amounts (>150 mg) of tyramine and could lead to hypertensive crisis. Avoid concomitant use with foods high in tyramine. Rasagiline is a selective inhibitor of MAO-B at the recommended doses; however, MAO-B selectivity diminishes in a dose-related manner above the recommended daily doses. May cause orthostatic hypotension, particularly in combination with levodopa. Orthostatic hypotension occurs most frequently during the first 2 months of therapy and decreases over time.

Serotonin syndrome (SS) has been reported with concomitant antidepressant (eg, SSRI, SNRI, TCA, tetracyclic and triazolopyridine antidepressants) use; concomitant use is not recommended within 14 days of rasagiline administration (within 5 weeks for antidepressants with long half-lives such as fluoxetine). SS has also been reported with concomitant use of MAO inhibitors (including selective MAO-B inhibitors), meperidine, methadone, propoxyphene, and tramadol; concomitant use within 14 days of rasagiline administration is contraindicated. A symptom complex resembling neuroleptic malignant syndrome (NMS) has been reported in association with rapid dose reduction, withdrawal of, or changes in drugs that increase central dopaminergic tone. Discontinue treatment (and any concomitant antidepressants) immediately if signs/symptoms arise. According to many of the MAO inhibitors manufacturers, use within 10 days prior to elective surgery is contraindicated. Currently, an MAO-safe anesthetic technique which excludes the use of meperidine and indirect-acting adrenergic agonists is recommended for patients requiring continued MAO inhibitor therapy (Huyse, 2006).

Somnolence and falling asleep while engaged in activities of daily living (including operation of motor vehicles) have been reported; some cases reported that there were no warning signs for the onset of symptoms. Symptom onset may occur well after initiation of treatment; some events have occurred >1 year after initiation of rasagiline. Prior to treatment initiation evaluate for factors that may increase these risks such as concomitant sedating medications, the presence of sleep disorders, and concomitant medications that increase rasagiline plasma levels (eg, ciprofloxacin). Monitor for drowsiness or sleepiness. If significant daytime sleepiness or episodes of falling asleep during activities that require active participation occurs (eg, driving, conversations, eating), discontinue rasagiline. There is insufficient information to suggest that dose reductions will eliminate these symptoms. If therapy is continued, advise patient to avoid driving and other potentially dangerous activities.

Dyskinesia, exacerbation of preexisting dyskinesia, or increased dopaminergic side effects may occur when used as an adjunct to levodopa. Decreasing the dose of levodopa may mitigate these side effects. May cause new or worsening mental status and behavioral changes, which may be severe, including paranoid ideation, delusions, hallucinations, confusion, psychotic-like behavior, disorientation, aggressive behavior, agitation, and delirium after starting or increasing the dose of rasagiline. Intense urges to gamble or spend money, increased sexual urges, binge eating, and/or other intense urges, as well as the inability to control these urges have also been reported. Monitor for these symptoms. If symptoms develop, consider dose reduction or discontinue of therapy. Avoidance of use is recommended in patients with major psychotic disorder due to the risk of exacerbating psychosis with an increase in central dopaminergic tone. Many treatments for psychosis that decrease central dopaminergic tone may also decrease the effectiveness of rasagiline.

Risk of melanoma may be increased with rasagiline, although increased risk has been associated with Parkinson's disease itself; patients should have regular and frequent skin examinations. Use with caution in patients with mild hepatic impairment; dose reduction recommended. Avoid use in patients with moderate-to-severe hepatic impairment. Potentially significant drug-drug interactions may exist, requiring dose or frequency adjustment, additional monitoring, and/or selection of alternative therapy. Hazardous agent - use appropriate precautions for handling and disposal (NIOSH, 2012).

Adverse Reactions Unless otherwise noted, the following adverse reactions are as reported for monotherapy. Spectrum of adverse events was generally similar with adjunctive therapy, though the incidence tended to be higher. Frequency not always defined.
>10%:
  Cardiovascular: Orthostatic hypotension (adjunctive therapy 3% to 13%, adjunctive therapy dose-related 6% to 9%; adjunctive therapy, 1 mg dose 3%; mild to moderate systolic blood pressure decrease [≥20 mmHg], 1 mg dose 44%; mild to moderate diastolic blood pressure decrease [≥10 mmHg], 1 mg dose 40%; severe diastolic blood pressure decrease [≥20 mmHg], 1 mg dose 9%; severe systolic blood pressure decrease [≥40 mmHg], 1 mg dose 7%), hypotension (3% post-treatment [systolic <90 mmHg or diastolic <50 mmHg combined with significant decrease from baseline, systolic >30 mmHg or diastolic >20 mmHg])
  Central nervous system: Headache (14%; adjunctive therapy 6% to 11%)
  Gastrointestinal: Nausea (adjunctive therapy 6% to 12%)
  Neuromuscular & skeletal: Dyskinesia (adjunctive therapy 18%)
  Miscellaneous: Trauma (adjunctive therapy 8% to 12%)
1% to 10%:
  Cardiovascular: Peripheral edema (7%), increased blood pressure (adjunctive therapy, significant increase, >180 mmHg systolic or >100 mmHg diastolic 4%; adjunctive therapy, post-treatment [>180 mmHg systolic or >100 mmHg diastolic combined with significant increase from baseline >30 mmHg systolic or >20 mmHg diastolic] 2%), angina, bundle branch block, chest pain
  Central nervous system: Dizziness (7%), drowsiness (adjunctive therapy 4% to 6%), ataxia (adjunctive therapy 3% to 6%), depression (5%), falling (5%; adjunctive therapy 6% to 12%), abnormal dreams (adjunctive therapy 1% to 4%), dystonia (adjunctive therapy 2% to 3%), malaise (2%), paresthesia (2%; adjunctive therapy 2% to 5%), insomnia (adjunctive therapy 4%), hallucinations (1%; adjunctive therapy 4% to 5%), myasthenia (adjunctive therapy 2%), vertigo (2%), anxiety
  Dermatologic: Skin rash (adjunctive therapy 3% to 6%), ecchymosis (2%; adjunctive therapy 2% to 5%), diaphoresis (adjunctive therapy 2% to 3%), alopecia, skin carcinoma, vesiculobullous rash
  Endocrine & metabolic: Weight loss (adjunctive therapy, dose-related 2% to 9%), impotence, libido decreased
  Gastrointestinal: Constipation (adjunctive therapy 4% to 9%), dyspepsia (7%; adjunctive therapy 4% to 5%), diarrhea (adjunctive therapy 5% to 7%), vomiting (adjunctive therapy 4% to 7%), xerostomia (adjunctive therapy, dose-related 2% to 6%), abdominal pain (adjunctive therapy 2% to 5%), anorexia (adjunctive therapy 2% to 5%), gastroenteritis (3%), gingivitis (adjunctive therapy 1% to 2%), hernia (adjunctive therapy 1% to 2%), gastrointestinal hemorrhage
  Genitourinary: Hematuria, urinary incontinence
  Hematologic and oncologic: Hemorrhage (adjunctive therapy 1% to 2%), leukopenia
  Hepatic: Liver function tests increased
  Infection: Infection (adjunctive therapy 2% to 3%)
  Neuromuscular & skeletal: Arthralgia (7%; adjunctive therapy 5% to 8%), back pain (adjunctive therapy 4%), neck pain (2%; adjunctive therapy 1% to 3%), tenosynovitis (adjunctive therapy 1% to 3%), arthritis (2%), abnormal gait, hyperkinesias, hypertonia, neuropathy, weakness
  Ophthalmic: Conjunctivitis (3%)
  Renal: Albuminuria
  Respiratory: Flu-like symptoms (5%), dyspnea (adjunctive therapy 3% to 5%), cough (adjunctive therapy 4%), upper respiratory tract infection (adjunctive therapy 4%), rhinitis (3%), asthma
  Miscellaneous: Fever (3%), allergic reaction
<1% (Limited to important or life-threatening): Acute kidney failure, aggressive behavior, agitation, amyotrophy, aphasia, apnea, arterial thrombosis, atrial arrhythmia, atrioventricular block, bigeminy, blepharitis, blepharoptosis, blindness, cardiac failure, cerebral hemorrhage, cerebral ischemia, deafness, deep vein thrombophlebitis, delirium, delusions, diplopia, disorientation, dysautonomia, dysesthesia, emphysema, esophageal ulcer, exacerbation of hypertension, excessive daytime sleepiness (including during operation of motor vehicles), exfoliative dermatitis, facial paralysis, gastric ulcer, genitourinary disorders, glaucoma, gynecomastia, hematemesis, hemiplegia, hostility, hypocalcemia, hypotension (while supine), impulse control disorder (pathological gambling, hypersexuality, intense urges to spend money, binge eating, and/or other intense urges and the inability to control the urges), interstitial pneumonitis, intestinal

obstruction, intestinal perforation, intestinal stenosis, jaundice, keratitis, large intestine perforation, laryngeal edema, laryngismus, leukoderma, leukorrhea, macrocytic anemia, manic depressive reaction, mania, megacolon, menstrual abnormalities, myelitis, myocardial infarction, nephrolithiasis, neuralgia, neuritis, (a complex resembling) neuroleptic malignant syndrome (associated with rapid dose reduction, withdrawal of or changes in medication; includes autonomic insufficiency, hyperthermia, impaired consciousness, muscle rigidity), nocturia, oral paresthesia, osteonecrosis, paranoia, personality disorder, pleural effusion, pneumothorax, polyuria, psychiatric disturbance (new or worsening mental status and behavioral changes that may be severe, including psychotic-like behavior during or after starting or increasing doses), psychoneurosis, psychotic symptoms, psychotic depression, pulmonary fibrosis, purpura, retinal degeneration, retinal detachment, seizure, strabismus, stupor, thrombocythemia, tongue edema, ventricular fibrillation, ventricular tachycardia, vestibular disturbance, visual field defect, vulvovaginal candidiasis

Drug Interactions

Metabolism/Transport Effects Substrate of CYP1A2 (major); **Note:** Assignment of Major/Minor substrate status based on clinically relevant drug interaction potential; **Inhibits** Monoamine Oxidase

Avoid Concomitant Use

Avoid concomitant use of Rasagiline with any of the following: Alcohol (Ethyl); Alpha-/Beta-Agonists (Indirect-Acting); Alpha1-Agonists; Amphetamines; Anilidopiperidine Opioids; Antidepressants (Serotonin Reuptake Inhibitor/Antagonist); Apraclonidine; AtoMOXetine; Atropine (Ophthalmic); Bezafibrate; Buprenorphine; BuPROPion; BusPIRone; CarBAMazepine; Cyclobenzaprine; Cyproheptadine; Dapoxetine; Dexmethylphenidate; Dextromethorphan; Diethylpropion; EPINEPHrine (Oral Inhalation); HYDROmorphone; Isometheptene; Levonordefrin; Linezolid; Maprotiline; Meperidine; Mequitazine; Methyldopa; Methylene Blue; Methylphenidate; Mianserin; Mirtazapine; Moclobemide; Morphine (Liposomal); Morphine (Systemic); Oxymorphone; Pholcodine; Pizotifen; Selective Serotonin Reuptake Inhibitors; Serotonin 5-HT1D Receptor Agonists; Serotonin/Norepinephrine Reuptake Inhibitors; Tapentadol; Tetrabenazine; Tetrahydrozoline (Nasal); Tricyclic Antidepressants; Tryptophan

Increased Effect/Toxicity

Rasagiline may increase the levels/effects of: Alpha-/Beta-Agonists (Indirect-Acting); Alpha1-Agonists; Amifostine; Amphetamines; Antidepressants (Serotonin Reuptake Inhibitor/Antagonist); Antipsychotic Agents; Antipsychotic Agents (Second Generation [Atypical]); Apraclonidine; AtoMOXetine; Atropine (Ophthalmic); Beta2-Agonists; Betahistine; Bezafibrate; Blood Glucose Lowering Agents; Brimonidine (Ophthalmic); Brimonidine (Topical); BuPROPion; Cyproheptadine; Dexmethylphenidate; Dextromethorphan; Diethylpropion; Domperidone; Doxapram; EPINEPHrine (Nasal); EPINEPHrine (Oral Inhalation); Epinephrine (Racemic); EPINEPHrine (Systemic); Hydrocodone; HYDROmorphone; Hypotension-Associated Agents; Isometheptene; Levonordefrin; Linezolid; Lithium; Meperidine; Mequitazine; Methadone; Methyldopa; Methylene Blue; Methylphenidate; Metoclopramide; Mianserin; Mirtazapine; Moclobemide; Morphine (Liposomal); Morphine (Systemic); Norepinephrine; OxyCODONE; Pizotifen; Reserpine; Selective Serotonin Reuptake Inhibitors; Serotonin 5-HT1D Receptor Agonists; Serotonin Modulators; Serotonin/Norepinephrine Reuptake Inhibitors; Tetrahydrozoline (Nasal); Tricyclic Antidepressants

The levels/effects of Rasagiline may be increased by: Abiraterone Acetate; Alcohol (Ethyl); Alfuzosin; Altretamine; Anilidopiperidine Opioids; Antiemetics (5HT3 Antagonists); Antipsychotic Agents; Barbiturates; Blood Pressure Lowering Agents; Brimonidine (Topical); Buprenorphine; BusPIRone; CarBAMazepine; COMT Inhibitors; Cyclobenzaprine; CYP1A2 Inhibitors (Moderate); CYP1A2 Inhibitors (Strong); Dapoxetine; Deferasirox; Diazoxide; Herbs (Hypotensive Properties); Levodopa; Maprotiline; Metaxalone; Molsidomine; Nicorandil; Obinutuzumab; Oxymorphone; Peginterferon Alfa-2b; Pentoxifylline; Pholcodine; Phosphodiesterase 5 Inhibitors; Prostacyclin Analogues; Tapentadol; Tedizolid; Tetrabenazine; TraMADol; Tryptophan; Vemurafenib

Decreased Effect

Rasagiline may decrease the levels/effects of: Domperidone; Pipamperone [INT]

The levels/effects of Rasagiline may be decreased by: Cannabis; CYP1A2 Inducers (Strong); Cyproheptadine; Cyproterone; Domperidone; Osimertinib; Pipamperone [INT]; Teriflunomide

Food Interactions Concurrent ingestion of foods rich in tyramine, dopamine, tyrosine, phenylalanine, tryptophan, or caffeine may cause sudden and severe high blood pressure (hypertensive crisis or serotonin syndrome). Management: Avoid foods containing high amounts (>150 mg) of tyramine (aged or matured cheese, air-dried or cured meats including sausages and salamis; fava or broad bean pods, tap/draft beers, Marmite concentrate, sauerkraut, soy sauce, and other soybean condiments). Food's freshness is also an important concern; improperly stored or spoiled food can create an environment in which tyramine concentrations may increase. Avoid these foods during and for 2 weeks after discontinuation of medication. Avoid foods containing dopamine, tyrosine, phenylalanine, tryptophan, or caffeine.

Storage/Stability Store at 25°C (77°F); excursions permitted to 15°C to 30°C (59°F to 86°F).

Mechanism of Action Potent, irreversible and selective inhibitor of brain monoamine oxidase (MAO) type B, which plays a major role in the catabolism of dopamine. Inhibition of dopamine depletion in the striatal region of the brain reduces the symptomatic motor deficits of Parkinson's disease. There is also experimental evidence of rasagiline conferring neuroprotective effects (antioxidant, antiapoptotic), which may delay onset of symptoms and progression of neuronal deterioration.

Pharmacodynamics/Kinetics

Duration: ~1 week (irreversible inhibition)

Absorption: Rapid

Protein binding: 88% to 94%, primarily to albumin

Metabolism: Hepatic N-dealkylation and/or hydroxylation via CYP1A2 to multiple inactive metabolites

Distribution: V_{dss}: 87 L

Bioavailability: ~36%

Half-life elimination: ~3 hours (no correlation with biologic effect due to irreversible inhibition)

Time to peak, plasma: ~1 hour

Excretion: Urine (62%, <1% of total dose as unchanged drug); feces (7%)

Dosing

Adult & Geriatric Parkinson disease: Oral:

Monotherapy or adjunctive therapy (not including levodopa): 1 mg once daily (maximum: 1 mg once daily)

Adjunctive therapy with levodopa: Initial: 0.5 mg once daily; may increase to 1 mg once daily based on response and tolerability (maximum: 1 mg once daily)

Note: When added to existing levodopa therapy, a dose reduction of levodopa may be required to avoid exacerbation of dyskinesias; typical dose reductions of ~9% to 13% were employed in clinical trials.

Dose reduction with concomitant ciprofloxacin or other CYP1A2 inhibitors: Maximum dose: 0.5 mg once daily

Renal Impairment

US labeling:

Mild to moderate impairment: No dosage adjustment necessary.

Severe impairment: There are no dosage adjustments provided in the manufacturer's labeling (has not been studied).

Canadian labeling:

Mild impairment: No dosage adjustment necessary.

Moderate to severe impairment: Use is not recommended (manufacturer cites lacks of safety data)

Hepatic Impairment

Mild impairment (Child-Pugh score 5 to 6): Maximum dose: 0.5 mg once daily

Moderate to severe impairment (Child-Pugh score 7 to 15): Use is not recommended.

Dietary Considerations May be taken without regard to meals. Avoid products containing high amounts of tyramine (>150 mg), such as aged cheeses (eg, Stilton cheese). Restriction of tyramine-containing products with lower amounts (<150 mg) of tyramine is not necessary in patients taking recommended doses. Some examples of tyramine-containing products include aged or matured cheese, air-dried or cured meats (including sausages and salamis), fava or broad bean pods, tap/draft beers, Marmite concentrate, sauerkraut, soy sauce and other soybean condiments. Food's freshness is also an important concern; improperly stored or spoiled food can create an environment where tyramine concentrations may increase.

Administration Administer without regard to meals.

Hazardous agent; use appropriate precautions for handling and disposal (NIOSH 2014 [group 2]).

Monitoring Parameters Blood pressure; symptoms of parkinsonism; new or worsening mental status and behavioral changes; somnolence and falling asleep during activities of daily living; skin examination for presence of melanoma (higher incidence in Parkinson's patients- drug causation not established)

Additional Information When adding rasagiline to levodopa/carbidopa, the dose of the latter can usually be decreased. Studies are investigating the use of rasagiline in early Parkinson's disease to slow the progression of the disease.

Dosage Forms Excipient information presented when available (limited, particularly for generics); consult specific product labeling.

Tablet, Oral:
Azilect: 0.5 mg, 1 mg

◆ Rasagiline Mesylate *see* Rasagiline *on page 1560*

Rasburicase (ras BYOOR i kayse)

Brand Names: US Elitek
Brand Names: Canada Fasturtec
Index Terms Recombinant Urate Oxidase; Urate Oxidase
Pharmacologic Category Enzyme; Enzyme, Urate-Oxidase (Recombinant)
Use

Hyperuricemia associated with malignancy: Initial management of uric acid levels in pediatric and adult patients with leukemia, lymphoma, and solid tumor malignancies receiving chemotherapy expected to result in tumor lysis and elevation of plasma uric acid
Limitations of use: Indicated only for a single course of treatment

Pregnancy Considerations Adverse effects were observed in animal reproduction studies. Use during pregnancy only if the benefit to the mother outweighs the potential risk to the fetus.

Breast-Feeding Considerations It is not known if rasburicase is excreted in breast milk. Due to the potential for serious adverse reactions in the nursing infant, a decision should be made to discontinue breast-feeding or the drug, taking into account the benefits of treatment to the mother. The Canadian labeling does not recommend use in breastfeeding women.

Contraindications History of anaphylaxis or severe hypersensitivity to rasburicase or any component of the formulation; history of hemolytic reaction or methemoglobinemia associated with rasburicase; glucose-6-phosphatase dehydrogenase (G6PD) deficiency

Warnings/Precautions [US Boxed Warning]: Severe hypersensitivity reactions (including anaphylaxis) have been reported; immediately and permanently discontinue in patients developing serious hypersensitivity reaction; reactions may occur at any time during treatment, including the initial dose. Signs and symptoms of hypersensitivity may include bronchospasm, chest pain/tightness, dyspnea, hypotension, hypoxia, shock, or urticaria. The safety and efficacy of more than one course of administration has not been established. **[US Boxed Warning]: Due to the risk for hemolysis (<1%), rasburicase is contraindicated in patients with G6PD deficiency; discontinue immediately and permanently in any patient developing hemolysis. Patients at higher risk for G6PD deficiency (eg, African or Mediterranean descent) should be screened prior to therapy;** severe hemolytic reactions occurred within 2 to 4 days of rasburicase initiation. **[US Boxed Warning]: Methemoglobinemia has been reported (<1%). Discontinue immediately and permanently in any patient developing methemoglobinemia;** initiate appropriate treatment (eg, transfusion, methylene blue) if methemoglobinemia occurs.

[US Boxed Warning]: Enzymatic degradation of uric acid in blood samples will occur if left at room temperature, which may interfere with serum uric acid measurements; specific guidelines for the collection of plasma uric acid samples must be followed, including collection in prechilled tubes with heparin anticoagulant, immediate ice water bath immersion and assay within 4 hours. Patients at risk for tumor lysis syndrome should receive appropriate IV hydration as part of uric acid management; however, alkalinization (with sodium bicarbonate) concurrently with rasburicase is not recommended (Coiffier 2008). Rasburicase is immunogenic and can elicit an antibody response; efficacy may be reduced with subsequent courses of therapy.

Adverse Reactions

>10%:
Cardiovascular: Peripheral edema (50%)
Central nervous system: Headache (26%), anxiety (24%)
Dermatologic: Rash (13%; serious: <1%)

Endocrine & metabolic: Hypophosphatemia (17%), hypervolemia (12%)
Gastrointestinal: Nausea (27% to 58%), vomiting (38% to 50%), abdominal pain (20% to 22%), constipation (20%), diarrhea (20%), mucositis (15%)
Hepatic: Hyperbilirubinemia (16%), increased serum ALT (11%)
Immunologic: Antibody development (children: 11%; IgE: 6%), development of IgG antibodies (18%; neutralizing 8%)
Infection: Sepsis (12%; serious: 5%)
Respiratory: Pharyngolaryngeal pain (14%)
Miscellaneous: Fever (46%)
1% to 10%:
Cardiovascular: Ischemic heart disease (≥2%), supraventricular arrhythmia (≥2%)
Endocrine & metabolic: Hyperphosphatemia (10%)
Gastrointestinal: Gastrointestinal infection (≥2%)
Hematologic & oncologic: Pulmonary hemorrhage (≥2%)
Hypersensitivity: Hypersensitivity (4%)
Infection: Infection (abdominal, ≥2%)
Respiratory: Respiratory failure (≥2%)
<1% (Limited to important or life-threatening): Anaphylaxis, hemolysis, methemoglobinemia, seizure

Drug Interactions

Metabolism/Transport Effects None known.
Avoid Concomitant Use There are no known interactions where it is recommended to avoid concomitant use.
Increased Effect/Toxicity There are no known significant interactions involving an increase in effect.
Decreased Effect There are no known significant interactions involving a decrease in effect.

Preparation for Administration Reconstitute with provided diluent (use 1 mL diluent for the 1.5 mg vial and 5 mL diluent for the 7.5 mg vial). Mix by gently swirling; do **not** shake or vortex. Discard if discolored or containing particulate matter. Total dose should be further diluted in NS to a final volume of 50 mL. Do not use filters during reconstitution or administration.

Storage/Stability The lyophilized drug product and the diluent for reconstitution should be stored at 2°C to 8°C (36°F to 46°F); do not freeze. Protect from light. Reconstituted solution and solution diluted for infusion may be stored for up to 24 hours at 2°C to 8°C (36°F to 46°F). Discard unused product.

Mechanism of Action Rasburicase is a recombinant urate-oxidase enzyme, which converts uric acid to allantoin (an inactive and soluble metabolite of uric acid); it does not inhibit the formation of uric acid.

Pharmacodynamics/Kinetics

Onset: Uric acid levels decrease within 4 hours of initial administration
Distribution: Children: 110 to 127 mL/kg; Adults: 76 to 138 mL/kg
Half-life elimination: ~16 to 23 hours

Dosing

Adult & Geriatric Hyperuricemia associated with malignancy: IV: 0.2 mg/kg once daily for up to 5 days (US labeling [use beyond 5 days or administration of more than 1 course is not recommended]) or up to 7 days (Canadian labeling) **or**
Alternate dosing (off-label; Coiffier 2008): 0.05 to 0.2 mg/kg once daily for 1 to 7 days (average of 2 to 3 days) with the duration of treatment dependent on plasma uric acid levels and clinical judgment (patients with significant tumor burden may require an increase to twice daily); the following dose levels are recommended based on risk of tumor lysis syndrome (TLS):
High risk: 0.2 mg/kg once daily (duration is based on plasma uric acid levels)
Intermediate risk: 0.15 mg/kg once daily (duration is based on plasma uric acid levels)
Low risk: 0.1 mg/kg once daily (duration is based on clinical judgment); a dose of 0.05 mg/kg was used effectively in one trial
Single-dose rasburicase (off-label dosing; based on limited data): 0.15 mg/kg (Campara 2009; Liu 2005) **or** 3 to 7.5 mg as a single dose (Hutcherson 2006; McBride 2013; McDonnell 2006; Reeves 2008; Trifilio 2006); repeat doses (1.5 to 6 mg) may be needed based on serum uric acid levels
Prevention in high-risk patients with hematologic malignancies (off-label dosing): 3 mg as a single dose (Jones, 2015)

Pediatric Hyperuricemia associated with malignancy: IV: 0.2 mg/kg once daily for up to 5 days (US labeling [use beyond 5 days or administration of more than 1 course is not recommended]) or up to 7 days (Canadian labeling) **or**

Alternate dosing (off-label; Coiffier 2008): 0.05 to 0.2 mg/kg once daily for 1 to 7 days (average of 2 to 3 days) with the duration of treatment dependent on plasma uric acid levels and clinical judgment (patients with significant tumor burden may require an increase to twice daily); the following dose levels are recommended based on risk of tumor lysis syndrome (TLS):

High risk: 0.2 mg/kg once daily (duration is based on plasma uric acid levels)

Intermediate risk: 0.15 mg/kg once daily (duration is based on plasma uric acid levels); may consider managing initially with a single dose

Low risk: 0.1 mg/kg once daily (duration is based on clinical judgment); a dose of 0.05 mg/kg was used effectively in one trial

Single-dose rasburicase (off-label dosing; based on limited data): 0.15 mg/kg; additional doses may be needed based on serum uric acid levels (Liu 2005)

Prevention in high-risk patients with hematologic malignancies (off-label dosing): 0.2 mg/kg as a single dose (Jones, 2015)

Renal Impairment There are no dosage adjustments provided in the manufacturer's labeling.

Hepatic Impairment There are no dosage adjustments provided in the manufacturer's labeling.

Administration

IV infusion over 30 minutes; do **not** administer as a bolus infusion. Do **not** filter during infusion. If not possible to administer through a separate line, IV line should be flushed with at least 15 mL saline prior to and following rasburicase infusion.

The optimal timing of rasburicase administration (with respect to chemotherapy administration) is not specified in the US labeling. In some studies, chemotherapy was administered 4 to 24 hours after the first rasburicase dose (Cortes 2010; Kikuchi 2009; Vadhan-Raj 2012); however, rasburicase generally may be administered irrespective of chemotherapy timing. The Canadian labeling recommends initiating chemotherapy as soon as 4 hours after rasburicase administration.

Monitoring Parameters Plasma uric acid levels (4 hours after rasburicase administration, then every 6 to 8 hours until TLS resolution); CBC, G6PD deficiency screening (in patients at high risk for deficiency); monitor for hypersensitivity

Test Interactions Specific handling procedures must be followed to prevent the degradation of uric acid in plasma samples. Blood must be collected in prechilled tubes containing heparin anticoagulant. Samples must then be **immediately** immersed and maintained in an ice water bath. Prepare samples by centrifugation in a precooled centrifuge (4°C). Samples must be analyzed within 4 hours of collection.

Dosage Forms Excipient information presented when available (limited, particularly for generics); consult specific product labeling.

Solution Reconstituted, Intravenous:

Elitek: 1.5 mg (1 ea); 7.5 mg (1 ea)

◆ ratio-Trazodone (Can) *see* TraZODone *on page 1834*

◆ ratio-Valproic (Can) *see* Valproic Acid and Derivatives *on page 1861*

Raxibacumab (rax i BAK ue mab)

Index Terms ABthrax

Pharmacologic Category Antidote; Monoclonal Antibody

Use Treatment of inhalational anthrax following exposure to *Bacillus anthracis* in combination with appropriate antimicrobial therapy; prophylaxis of inhalational anthrax when alternative therapies are unavailable or not appropriate

Prescribing and Access Restrictions Raxibacumab is not available for general public use. All supplies are currently owned by the federal government for inclusion in the Strategic National Stockpile and for use by the U.S. military.

Dosing

Adult & Geriatric Anthrax, prophylaxis or treatment: IV: 40 mg/kg as a single dose

Note: Administer diphenhydramine 25-50 mg (may administer oral or IV depending on the proximity to start of raxibacumab infusion) ≤1 hour prior to administration of raxibacumab to reduce the risk of infusion reactions. Must be administered in combination with antimicrobial therapy.

Pediatric Anthrax, prophylaxis or treatment: Children and Adolescents: IV: **Note:** Administer diphenhydramine (may administer oral or IV depending on the proximity to start of raxibacumab infusion) ≤1 hour prior to administration of raxibacumab to reduce the risk of infusion reactions. Must be administered in combination with antimicrobial therapy.

≤15 kg: 80 mg/kg as a single dose
>15 kg to 50 kg: 60 mg/kg as a single dose
>50 kg: 40 mg/kg as a single dose

Renal Impairment No dosage adjustment provided in manufacturer's labeling. However, dosage adjustment unlikely as clearance is nonrenal.

Hepatic Impairment No dosage adjustment provided in manufacturer's labeling (has not been studied).

Additional Information Complete prescribing information should be consulted for additional detail.

Dosage Forms Excipient information presented when available (limited, particularly for generics); consult specific product labeling.

Injection, solution: 50 mg/mL (34 mL) [contains polysorbate 80, sucrose 10 mg/mL]

◆ Rayos *see* PredniSONE *on page 1496*

◆ Razadyne *see* Galantamine *on page 826*

◆ Razadyne ER *see* Galantamine *on page 826*

◆ 6R-BH4 *see* Sapropterin *on page 1636*

◆ Reactine (Can) *see* Cetirizine *on page 364*

◆ Rea-Lo [OTC] *see* Urea *on page 1853*

◆ Rea Lo 39 *see* Urea *on page 1853*

◆ Rea Lo 40 *see* Urea *on page 1853*

◆ Rebetol *see* Ribavirin (Systemic) *on page 1574*

◆ Rebif *see* Interferon Beta-1a *on page 969*

◆ Rebif Rebidose *see* Interferon Beta-1a *on page 969*

◆ Rebif Rebidose Titration Pack *see* Interferon Beta-1a *on page 969*

◆ Rebif Titration Pack *see* Interferon Beta-1a *on page 969*

◆ Reclast *see* Zoledronic Acid *on page 1934*

◆ Reclipsen *see* Ethinyl Estradiol and Desogestrel *on page 701*

◆ Recombinant α-L-Iduronidase (Glycosaminoglycan α-L-Iduronohydrolase) *see* Laronidase *on page 1037*

◆ Recombinant C1 Inhibitor *see* C1 Inhibitor (Recombinant) *on page 277*

◆ Recombinant Desulfatohirudin *see* Desirudin *on page 519*

◆ Recombinant Granulocyte-Macrophage Colony Stimulating Factor *see* Sargramostim *on page 1637*

◆ Recombinant Hirudin *see* Desirudin *on page 519*

◆ Recombinant Human Deoxyribonuclease *see* Dornase Alfa *on page 587*

◆ Recombinant Human Interleukin-2 *see* Aldesleukin *on page 60*

◆ Recombinant Human Interleukin-11 *see* Oprelvekin *on page 1339*

◆ Recombinant Human Parathyroid Hormone (1-34) *see* Teriparatide *on page 1765*

◆ Recombinant Human Parathyroid Hormone (1-84) *see* Parathyroid Hormone *on page 1395*

◆ Recombinant Human Platelet-Derived Growth Factor B *see* Becaplermin *on page 204*

◆ Recombinant Human Thyrotropin *see* Thyrotropin Alfa *on page 1784*

◆ Recombinant Interleukin-11 *see* Oprelvekin *on page 1339*

◆ Recombinant Methionyl-Human Leptin *see* Metreleptin *on page 1195*

◆ Recombinant Urate Oxidase *see* Rasburicase *on page 1563*

◆ Recombinant Urate Oxidase, Pegylated *see* Pegloticase *on page 1413*

◆ Recombinate *see* Antihemophilic Factor (Recombinant) *on page 132*

◆ Recombivax HB *see* Hepatitis B Vaccine (Recombinant) *on page 876*

◆ Recort Plus [OTC] *see* Hydrocortisone (Topical) *on page 886*

◆ Rectacort-HC [DSC] *see* Hydrocortisone (Topical) *on page 886*

◆ RectiCare [OTC] *see* Lidocaine (Topical) *on page 1074*

◆ Rectiv *see* Nitroglycerin *on page 1289*

◆ Rederm [OTC] *see* Hydrocortisone (Topical) *on page 886*

◆ Redness Eye Drops (Can) *see* Naphazoline (Ophthalmic) *on page 1256*

◆ Reedy-Atorvastatin (Can) *see* AtorvaSTATin *on page 169*

◆ Reeses Pinworm Medicine [OTC] *see* Pyrantel Pamoate *on page 1530*

◆ Refenesen [OTC] *see* GuaiFENesin *on page 860*

◆ Refenesen 400 [OTC] *see* GuaiFENesin *on page 860*

◆ Refenesen DM [OTC] *see* Guaifenesin and Dextromethorphan *on page 861*

◆ Refenesen™ PE [OTC] *see* Guaifenesin and Phenylephrine *on page 862*

◆ Refenesen Plus [OTC] *see* Guaifenesin and Pseudoephedrine *on page 863*

◆ Refissa *see* Tretinoin (Topical) *on page 1841*

◆ Refresh Eye Itch Relief [OTC] [DSC] *see* Ketotifen (Ophthalmic) *on page 1018*

◆ Refresh Redness Relief (Can) *see* Naphazoline (Ophthalmic) *on page 1256*

◆ Regitine [DSC] *see* Phentolamine *on page 1440*

◆ Reglan *see* Metoclopramide *on page 1188*

◆ REGN727 *see* Alirocumab *on page 70*

◆ Regonol *see* Pyridostigmine *on page 1531*

Regorafenib (re goe RAF e nib)

Brand Names: US Stivarga
Brand Names: Canada Stivarga
Index Terms BAY 73-4506
Pharmacologic Category Antineoplastic Agent, Tyrosine Kinase Inhibitor; Antineoplastic Agent, Vascular Endothelial Growth Factor (VEGF) Inhibitor

Use

Colorectal cancer, metastatic: Treatment of metastatic colorectal cancer in patients previously treated with fluoropyrimidine-, oxaliplatin-, and irinotecan-based chemotherapy, anti-VEGF therapy, and anti-EGFR therapy (if *KRAS* wild type)

Gastrointestinal stromal tumors: Treatment of locally-advanced, unresectable, or metastatic gastrointestinal stromal tumor (GIST) in patients previously treated with imatinib and sunitinib

Pregnancy Considerations In animal reproduction studies, teratogenic effects were observed with doses less than the equivalent human dose. Based on the mechanism of action, regorafenib may cause fetal harm if administered during pregnancy. Patients (male and female) should use effective contraception during therapy and for at least 2 months following treatment.

Breast-Feeding Considerations It is not known if regorafenib is excreted into breast milk. Due to the potential for serious adverse reactions in the nursing infant, a decision should be made to discontinue regorafenib or to discontinue breast-feeding during therapy, taking into account the benefits of treatment to the mother.

Prescribing and Access Restrictions Regorafenib is available only through the REACH support program. Information regarding program enrollment may be found at http://www.stivarga-us.com/hcp/mcrc/support.html or by calling 1-866-639-2827.

Contraindications There are no contraindications listed in the manufacturer's US labeling.

Canadian labeling: Hypersensitivity to regorafenib, any component of the formulation, or sorafenib.

Warnings/Precautions Hazardous agent - use appropriate precautions for handling and disposal (meets NIOSH 2014 criteria). Myocardial ischemia and infarction were observed at a higher incidence than placebo in a clinical trial. Interrupt therapy in patients who develop new or acute onset ischemia or infarction; resume only if the benefit of therapy outweighs the cardiovascular risk. Hand-foot skin reaction (HFSR), also known as palmar-plantar erythrodysesthesia (PPE), and rash were commonly seen in clinical trials; erythema multiforme and Stevens Johnson syndrome were also observed more frequently in regorafenib-treated patients. Toxic epidermal necrolysis occurred rarely. Onset of dermatologic toxicity typically occurs in the first cycle of treatment. Therapy interruptions, dosage reductions, and/or discontinuation may be necessary depending on the severity and persistence. Supportive treatment may be of benefit for symptomatic relief. Gastrointestinal perforation or fistula has occurred in a small number of patients treated with regorafenib; some cases were fatal. Monitor for signs/symptoms of perforation (fever, abdominal pain with constipation, and/or nausea/vomiting); permanently discontinue therapy if perforation or fistula develop. The incidence of hemorrhage was increased with regorafenib. Hemorrhage of the respiratory, gastrointestinal, or genitourinary tracts was observed in trials; some cases were fatal. Permanently discontinue in patients who experience severe or life-threatening bleeding. In patients receiving concomitant warfarin, monitor INR frequently.

[U.S. Boxed Warning]: Severe and sometimes fatal hepatotoxicity has been observed in clinical trials. Monitor hepatic function at baseline and during treatment. Interrupt therapy for hepatotoxicity; dose reductions or discontinuation are necessary depending on the severity and persistence. Hepatocyte necrosis with lymphocyte infiltration has been demonstrated with liver biopsy. Regorafenib is primarily eliminated hepatically. Closely monitor for adverse effects in patients with mild or moderate impairment; use is not recommended in severe hepatic impairment.

Elevated blood pressure was observed in clinical trials (onset typically in the first cycle of therapy); ensure blood pressure is adequately controlled prior to initiation. Monitor blood pressure weekly for the first 6 weeks and monthly thereafter or as clinically indicated; if hypertension develops, interrupt therapy or permanently discontinue for severe or uncontrolled hypertension. Hypertensive crisis has occurred in some patients. Reversible posterior leukoencephalopathy syndrome (RPLS) occurred very rarely in regorafenib-treated patients; evaluate promptly if symptoms (eg, seizures, headache, visual disturbances, confusion, or altered mental function) occur. Discontinue if diagnosis is confirmed. Regorafenib inhibits vascular endothelial growth factor, which may lead to impaired wound healing. Stop therapy at least 2 weeks prior to scheduled surgery; resume regorafenib postsurgery based on clinical judgment of wound healing; discontinue therapy if wound dehiscence occurs.

Potentially significant drug-drug or drug-food interactions may exist, requiring dose or frequency adjustment, additional monitoring, and/or selection of alternative therapy.

Adverse Reactions

>10%:

Cardiovascular: Hypertension (30% to 59%; grade ≥3: 8% to 28%)

Central nervous system: Fatigue (52% to 64%), voice disorder (30% to 39%), pain (29%), headache (10% to 16%)

Dermatologic: Palmar-plantar erythrodysesthesia (45% to 67%; grade ≥3: 17% to 22%), skin rash (26% to 30%; grade ≥3: 6% to 7%), alopecia (8% to 24%)

Endocrine & metabolic: Hypocalcemia (17% to 59%), hypophosphatemia (55% to 57%), weight loss (14% to 32%), hyponatremia (30%), increased amylase (26%), hypokalemia (21% to 26%), hypothyroidism (4% to 18%)

Gastrointestinal: Diarrhea (43% to 47%), decreased appetite (31% to 47%), increased serum lipase (14% to 46%), mucositis (33% to 40%), nausea (20%), vomiting (17%)

Hematologic & oncologic: Anemia (79%; grade 3: 5%; grade 4: 1%), lymphocytopenia (30% to 54%; grade 3: 8% to 9%), thrombocytopenia (13% to 41%; grade 3: 1% to 2%; grade 4: <1%), increased INR (24%), hemorrhage (11% to 21%; grade ≥3: 2% to 4%), neutropenia (3% to 16%; grade 3: 1%)

Hepatic: Increased serum AST (58% to 65%; grade 3: 5%; grade 4: 1%), increased serum ALT (45%; grade 3: 4% to 5%; grade 4: 1%), hyperbilirubinemia (33% to 45%)

Infection: Infection (31% to 32%; grade ≥3: 5% to 9%)

Neuromuscular & skeletal: Stiffness (14%)

Renal: Proteinuria (33% to 60%)

Miscellaneous: Fever (21% to 28%)

1% to 10%:

Cardiovascular: Ischemic heart disease (≤1%), myocardial infarction (≤1%)

Gastrointestinal: Dysgeusia (8%), xerostomia (5%), gastrointestinal fistula (≤2%), gastrointestinal perforation (≤2%), gastroesophageal reflux disease (1%)

Hepatic: Hepatic failure (≤2%)

Neuromuscular & skeletal: Tremor (2%)

Respiratory: Dyspnea (2%)

<1% (Limited to important or life-threatening): Bradycardia, erythema multiforme, hepatic injury (severe), hypersensitivity reaction, hypertensive crisis, reversible posterior leukoencephalopathy syndrome, Stevens-Johnson syndrome, toxic epidermal necrolysis

Drug Interactions

Metabolism/Transport Effects Substrate of CYP3A4 (major), UGT1A9; **Note:** Assignment of Major/Minor substrate status based on clinically relevant drug interaction potential; **Inhibits** BCRP, P-glycoprotein, UGT1A1, UGT1A9

Avoid Concomitant Use

Avoid concomitant use of Regorafenib with any of the following: Conivaptan; CYP3A4 Inducers (Strong); CYP3A4 Inhibitors (Strong); Fusidic Acid (Systemic); Grapefruit Juice; Idelalisib; Irinotecan Products; St Johns Wort

Increased Effect/Toxicity

Regorafenib may increase the levels/effects of: Beta-Blockers; Bisphosphonate Derivatives; Calcium Channel Blockers (Nondihydropyridine); Digoxin; Irinotecan Products; Ivabradine

The levels/effects of Regorafenib may be increased by: Aprepitant; Conivaptan; CYP3A4 Inhibitors (Moderate); CYP3A4 Inhibitors (Strong); Dasatinib; Fosaprepitant; Fusidic Acid (Systemic); Grapefruit Juice; Idelalisib; Ivacaftor; Luliconazole; Mifepristone; Netupitant; Osimertinib; Palbociclib; Simeprevir; Stiripentol; Warfarin

Decreased Effect

The levels/effects of Regorafenib may be decreased by: Bosentan; CYP3A4 Inducers (Moderate); CYP3A4 Inducers (Strong); Dabrafenib; Deferasirox; Osimertinib; Siltuximab; St Johns Wort; Tocilizumab

Food Interactions Regorafenib serum concentrations may be altered when taken with grapefruit or grapefruit juice. Management: Avoid concurrent use.

Storage/Stability Store at 25°C (77°F); excursions permitted to 15°C to 30°C (59°F to 86°F). Store tablets in the original bottle and protect from moisture (do not remove the desiccant); keep container tightly closed. Discard any unused tablets 7 weeks after opening the bottle.

Mechanism of Action Regorafenib is a multikinase inhibitor; it targets kinases involved with tumor angiogenesis, oncogenesis, and maintenance of the tumor microenvironment which results in inhibition of tumor growth. Specifically, it inhibits VEGF receptors 1-3, KIT, PDGFR-alpha, PDGFR-beta, RET, FGFR1 and 2, TIE2, DDR2, TrkA, Eph2A, RAF-1, BRAF, BRAF^{V600E}, SAPK2, PTK5, and Abl.

Pharmacodynamics/Kinetics

Absorption: A high-fat meal increased the mean AUC of the parent drug by 48% compared to the fasted state and decreased the mean AUC of the M-2 (N-oxide) and M-5 (N-oxide and N-desmethyl) active metabolites by 20% and 51%, respectively. A low-fat meal increased the mean AUC of regorafenib, M-2, and M-5 by 36%, 40% and 23%, respectively (as compared to the fasted state).

Protein binding: 99.5% (active metabolites M-2 and M-5 are also highly protein bound)

Metabolism: Hepatic via CYP3A4 and UGT1A9, primarily to active metabolites M-2 (N-oxide) and M-5 (N-oxide and N-desmethyl)

Bioavailability: Tablets: 69%; Oral solution: 83%

Half-life elimination: Regorafenib: 28 hours (range: 14 to 58 hours); M-2 metabolite: 25 hours (range: 14 to 32 hours); M-5 metabolite: 51 hours (range: 32 to 70 hours)

Time to peak: 4 hours

Excretion: Feces (71%; 47% as parent compound; 24% as metabolites); Urine (19%)

Dosing

Adult & Geriatric

Colorectal cancer, metastatic: Oral: 160 mg once daily for the first 21 days of each 28-day cycle; continue until disease progression or unacceptable toxicity (Grothey, 2013)

Gastrointestinal stromal tumor (GIST), locally-advanced, unresectable, or metastatic: Oral: 160 mg once daily for the first 21 days of each 28-day cycle; continue until disease progression or unacceptable toxicity (Demetri, 2013)

Missed doses: Do not administer 2 doses on the same day to make up for a missed dose from the previous day.

Renal Impairment

Preexisting mild impairment (CrCl 60 to 89 mL/minute): No dosage adjustment necessary.

Preexisting moderate impairment (CrCl 30 to 59 mL/minute): There are no dosage adjustments provided in the manufacturer's labeling (limited pharmacokinetic data available).

Preexisting severe impairment (CrCl <30 mL/minute): There are no dosage adjustments provided in the manufacturer's labeling (has not been studied).

Hepatic Impairment

Preexisting mild or moderate impairment (Child-Pugh Class A or B): No dosage adjustment necessary; closely monitor for adverse effects.

Preexisting severe impairment (Child-Pugh Class C): Use is not recommended (has not been studied).

Hepatotoxicity during treatment:

Grade 3 AST and/or ALT elevation: Withhold dose until recovery. If benefit of treatment outweighs toxicity risk, resume therapy at a reduced dose of 120 mg once daily.

AST or ALT >20 times ULN: Discontinue permanently.

AST or ALT >3 times ULN **and** bilirubin >2 times ULN: Discontinue permanently.

Recurrence of AST or ALT >5 times ULN despite dose reduction to 120 mg: Discontinue permanently.

Adjustment for Toxicity

Dermatologic:

Grade 2 hand-foot skin reaction (HFSR; palmar-plantar erythrodysesthesia [PPE]) of any duration: Reduce dose to 120 mg once daily for first occurrence. If grade 2 HFSR recurs at this dose, further reduce the dose to 80 mg once daily. Interrupt therapy for grade 2 HFSR that is recurrent or fails to improve within 7 days in spite of dosage reduction.

Grade 3 HFSR: Interrupt therapy for a minimum of 7 days. Upon recovery, reduce dose to 120 mg once daily. If grade 2 to 3 toxicity recurs at this dose, further reduce dose to 80 mg once daily upon recovery. Interrupt therapy for grade 2 to 3 HFSR that is recurrent or fails to improve within 7 days in spite of dosage reduction.

Recurrent or persistent HFSR at 80 mg once daily: Discontinue treatment.

Hypertension: Grade 2 (symptomatic): Interrupt therapy.

Other toxicity: Any grade 3 or 4 adverse reaction (other than hepatotoxicity): Interrupt therapy; upon recovery, reduce dose to 120 mg once daily. If any grade 3 or 4 adverse reaction occurs while on this reduced dose, may further reduce dose to 80 mg once daily upon recovery. For any grade 4 adverse reaction, only resume therapy if the benefit outweighs the risk. Permanently discontinue therapy if unable to tolerate 80 mg once daily.

Gastrointestinal perforation/fistula: Discontinue permanently.

Hemorrhage (severe or life-threatening): Discontinue permanently.

Reversible posterior leukoencephalopathy syndrome (RPLS): Discontinue.

Wound dehiscence: Discontinue.

Dietary Considerations Take after a low-fat meal (containing <600 calories and <30% fat). Avoid grapefruit juice.

Administration Take at the same time each day. Swallow tablet whole with water after a low-fat meal (containing <600 calories and <30% fat). Hazardous agent; use appropriate precautions for handling and disposal (meets NIOSH 2014 criteria).

Monitoring Parameters Monitor for hand-foot skin reaction (HFSR)/palmar-plantar erythrodysesthesia (PPE); signs/symptoms of cardiac ischemia or infarction; bleeding; signs/symptoms of GI perforation or fistula; signs/symptoms of reversible posterior leukoencephalopathy syndrome (severe headaches, seizure, confusion, or change in vision). Monitor for impaired wound healing. Obtain liver function tests at baseline, every 2 weeks during the first 2 months of treatment, then monthly or more frequently if clinically necessary (weekly until improvement if liver function tests are elevated). Monitor blood pressure weekly for the first 6 weeks of therapy and with every subsequent cycle, or more frequently if indicated. CBC with differential and platelets and serum electrolytes (baseline and periodic). Monitor INR more frequently if receiving warfarin.

Dosage Forms Excipient information presented when available (limited, particularly for generics); consult specific product labeling.

Tablet, Oral:

Stivarga: 40 mg [contains soybean lecithin]

Remifentanil (rem i FEN ta nil)

Brand Names: US Ultiva

Brand Names: Canada Remifentanil Hydrochloride for Injection

Index Terms GI87084B

Pharmacologic Category Analgesic, Opioid; Anilidopiperidine Opioid

Use Analgesic for use during the induction and maintenance of general anesthesia; for continued analgesia into the immediate postoperative period; analgesic component of monitored anesthesia

Pregnancy Considerations Adverse events were not observed in animal reproduction studies. Remifentanil has been shown to cross the placenta; fetal and maternal concentrations may be similar.

Breast-Feeding Considerations It is not known if remifentanil is excreted into breast milk. The manufacturer recommends that caution be used if administered to a nursing woman. Remifentanil has a limited duration of action; use may be appropriate for breast-feeding women undergoing short procedures (Montgomery, 2012).

Contraindications Not for intrathecal or epidural administration, due to the presence of glycine in the formulation; hypersensitivity to remifentanil, fentanyl, or fentanyl analogs, or any component of the formulation

Warnings/Precautions Remifentanil is not recommended as the sole agent for induction of anesthesia, because the loss of consciousness cannot be assured. Due to the high incidence of apnea, hypotension, respiratory depression, tachycardia and muscle rigidity remifentanil should only be administered by individuals specifically trained in the use of anesthetic agents and should not be used in diagnostic or therapeutic procedures outside the monitored anesthesia setting; resuscitative and intubation equipment should be readily available. May cause hypotension; use with caution in patients with hypovolemia, cardiovascular disease (including acute MI), or drugs which may exaggerate hypotensive effects (including phenothiazines or general anesthetics). Shares the toxic potentials of opioid agonists, and precautions of opioid agonist therapy should be observed. In patients <55 years of age, intraoperative awareness has been reported when used with propofol rates of ≤75 mcg/kg/minute.

Rapid IV infusion (single dose >1 mcg/kg over 30-60 seconds and infusion rates >0.1 mcg/kg/minute) should only be used during maintenance of general anesthesia; may result in skeletal muscle and chest wall rigidity, impaired ventilation, or respiratory distress/arrest; nondepolarizing skeletal muscle relaxant may be required. Chest wall rigidity may resolve by decreasing the infusion rate or temporarily stopping the infusion. Inadequate clearing of IV tubing following remifentanil administration could result in chest wall rigidity, respiratory depression, and apnea when another fluid is administered through the same line. Interruption of an infusion will result in offset of effects within 5-10 minutes; the discontinuation of remifentanil infusion should be preceded by the establishment of adequate postoperative analgesia orders, especially for patients in whom postoperative pain is anticipated. Use caution in the morbidly obese. Use with caution in patients with a history of drug abuse or acute alcoholism; potential for drug dependency exists. Tolerance, psychological and physical dependence may occur with prolonged use.

Adverse Reactions Frequency of adverse events may vary based on surgical procedures and rate of infusion.

>10%:

Cardiovascular: Hypotension (2% to 19%), bradycardia (1% to 7%; dose dependent)

Central nervous system: Headache (<2% to 18%)

Dermatologic: Pruritus (<2% to 18%)

Gastrointestinal: Nausea (<36% to 44%), vomiting (<16% to 22%)

Neuromuscular & skeletal: Muscle rigidity (<1% to 11%; includes chest wall rigidity)

1% to 10%:

Cardiovascular: Hypertension (1% to 2%; dose dependent), tachycardia (≤1%; dose dependent), flushing (1%)

Central nervous system: Fever (<5%), dizziness (<5%), postoperative pain (<2%), chills (1%), agitation (≤1%)

Local: Pain at injection site (1%)

Respiratory: Respiratory depression (<7%), apnea (<3%), hypoxia (≤1%)

Miscellaneous: Diaphoresis (6%), shivering (<5%), warm sensation (1%)

<1% (Limited to important or life-threatening): Abdominal discomfort, amnesia, anaphylaxis, anxiety, arrhythmias, awareness under anesthesia without pain, bronchitis, bronchospasm, chest pain, confusion, constipation, cough, CPK increased, diarrhea, disorientation, dysphagia, dysphoria, dyspnea, dysuria, ECG changes, electrolyte disorders, erythema, gastroesophageal reflux, hallucinations, heart block, heartburn, hiccups, hyperglycemia, ileus, incontinence, involuntary movement, laryngospasm, leukocytosis, liver dysfunction, lymphopenia, nasal congestion, nightmares, nystagmus, oliguria, paresthesia, pharyngitis, pleural effusion, prolonged emergence from anesthesia, pulmonary edema, rales, rapid awakening from anesthesia, rash, rhinorrhea, rhonchi, seizure, sleep disturbance, stridor, syncope, temperature regulation impaired, thrombocytopenia, tremors, twitching, urine retention, urticaria, xerostomia

Drug Interactions

Metabolism/Transport Effects None known.

Avoid Concomitant Use

Avoid concomitant use of Remifentanil with any of the following: Azelastine (Nasal); Eluxadoline; MAO Inhibitors; Mixed Agonist / Antagonist Opioids; Orphenadrine; Paraldehyde; Thalidomide

Increased Effect/Toxicity

Remifentanil may increase the levels/effects of: Alcohol (Ethyl); Alvimopan; Amifostine; Antipsychotic Agents (Second Generation [Atypical]); Azelastine (Nasal); Beta-Blockers; Calcium Channel Blockers (Nondihydropyridine); CNS Depressants; Desmopressin; Diuretics; DULoxetine; Eluxadoline; Hydrocodone; Hypotension-Associated Agents; Levodopa; MAO Inhibitors; Methotrimeprazine; Metyrosine; Mirtazapine; Orphenadrine; Paraldehyde; Pramipexole; Ramosetron; ROPINIRole; Rotigotine; Selective Serotonin Reuptake Inhibitors; Suvorexant; Thalidomide; Zolpidem

The levels/effects of Remifentanil may be increased by: Alfuzosin; Amphetamines; Anticholinergic Agents; Antipsychotic Agents (Phenothiazines); Barbiturates; Blood Pressure Lowering Agents; Brimonidine (Topical); Cannabis; Diazoxide; Doxylamine; Dronabinol; Droperidol; Herbs (Hypotensive Properties); HydrOXYzine; Kava Kava; Magnesium Sulfate; Methotrimeprazine; Minocycline; Molsidomine; Nabilone; Nicorandil; Obinutuzumab; Pentoxifylline; Perampanel; Phosphodiesterase 5 Inhibitors; Prostacyclin Analogues; Rufinamide; Sodium Oxybate; Succinylcholine; Tapentadol; Tetrahydrocannabinol

Decreased Effect

Remifentanil may decrease the levels/effects of: Pegvisomant

The levels/effects of Remifentanil may be decreased by: Ammonium Chloride; Mixed Agonist / Antagonist Opioids; Naltrexone

Preparation for Administration Prepare solution by adding 1 mL of diluent per 1 mg of remifentanil. Shake well. Further dilute to a final concentration of 20, 25, 50, or 250 mcg/mL.

Storage/Stability Prior to reconstitution, store at 2°C to 25°C (36°F to 77°F). Stable for 24 hours at room temperature after reconstitution and further dilution to concentrations of 20-250 mcg/mL (4 hours if diluted with LR).

Mechanism of Action Binds with stereospecific mu-opioid receptors at many sites within the CNS, increases pain threshold, alters pain reception, inhibits ascending pain pathways

Pharmacodynamics/Kinetics

Onset of action: IV: 1-3 minutes

Distribution: V_d: 100 mL/kg; increased in children

Protein binding: ~70% (primarily alpha$_1$ acid glycoprotein)

Metabolism: Rapid via blood and tissue esterases

Half-life elimination (dose dependent): Terminal: 10-20 minutes; effective: 3-10 minutes

Excretion: Urine

Dosing

Adult Anesthesia: IV continuous infusion:

Induction of anesthesia: 0.5-1 mcg/kg/minute; if endotracheal intubation is to occur in <8 minutes, an initial dose of 1 mcg/kg may be given over 30-60 seconds

Coronary bypass surgery: 1 mcg/kg/minute

Maintenance of anesthesia: Supplemental bolus dose of 1 mcg/kg may be administered every 2-5 minutes. Consider increasing concomitant anesthetics with infusion rate >1 mcg/kg/minute. Infusion rate can be titrated upward in increments of 25% to 100% or downward in decrements of 25% to 50%. May titrate every 2-5 minutes.

With nitrous oxide (66%): 0.4 mcg/kg/minute (range: 0.1-2 mcg/kg/minute)

With isoflurane: 0.25 mcg/kg/minute (range: 0.05-2 mcg/kg/minute)

With propofol: 0.25 mcg/kg/minute (range: 0.05-2 mcg/kg/minute)

Coronary bypass surgery: 1 mcg/kg/minute (range: 0.125-4 mcg/kg/minute); supplemental dose: 0.5-1 mcg/kg

Continuation as an analgesic in immediate postoperative period: 0.1 mcg/kg/minute (range: 0.025-0.2 mcg/kg/minute). Infusion rate may be adjusted every 5 minutes in increments of 0.025 mcg/kg/minute. Bolus doses are not recommended. Infusion rates >0.2 mcg/kg/minute are associated with respiratory depression.

Coronary bypass surgery, continuation as an analgesic into the ICU: 1 mcg/kg/minute (range: 0.05-1 mcg/kg/minute)

Analgesic component of monitored anesthesia care:

Note: Supplemental oxygen is recommended:

Single IV dose given 90 seconds prior to local anesthetic:

Remifentanil alone: 1 mcg/kg over 30-60 seconds

With midazolam: 0.5 mcg/kg over 30-60 seconds

Continuous infusion beginning 5 minutes prior to local anesthetic:

Remifentanil alone: 0.1 mcg/kg minute

With midazolam: 0.05 mcg/kg/minute

Continuous infusion given after local anesthetic:

Remifentanil alone: 0.05 mcg/kg/minute (range: 0.025-0.2 mcg/kg/minute)

With midazolam: 0.025 mcg/kg/minute (range: 0.025-0.2 mcg/kg/minute)

Note: Following local or anesthetic block, infusion rate should be decreased to 0.05 mcg/kg/minute; rate adjustments of 0.025 mcg/kg/minute may be done at 5-minute intervals

Critically-ill patients (off-label dose): Loading dose: 1.5 mcg/kg; followed by 0.008-0.25 mcg/kg/minute (**or** 0.5-15 mcg/kg/**hour**) (SCCM [Barr, 2013])

Geriatric Elderly patients have an increased sensitivity to effect of remifentanil; doses should be decreased by 50% and titrated. Refer to adult dosing.

Pediatric

Maintenance of anesthesia with nitrous oxide (70%): Children Birth to 2 months: Continuous IV infusion: 0.4 mcg/kg/minute (range: 0.4-1 mcg/kg/minute); supplemental bolus dose of 1 mcg/kg may be administered, smaller bolus dose may be required with potent inhalation agents, potent neuraxial anesthesia, significant comorbidities, significant fluid shifts, or without atropine

pretreatment. Clearance in neonates is highly variable; dose should be carefully titrated.

Maintenance of anesthesia with halothane, sevoflurane, or isoflurane: Continuous IV infusion: Children 1-12 years: 0.25 mcg/kg/minute (range: 0.05-1.3 mcg/kg/minute); supplemental bolus dose of 1 mcg/kg may be administered every 2-5 minutes. Consider increasing concomitant anesthetics with infusion rate >1 mcg/kg/minute. Infusion rate can be titrated upward in increments up to 50% or titrated downward in decrements of 25% to 50%. May titrate every 2-5 minutes.

Renal Impairment No dosage adjustment necessary.

Hepatic Impairment No dosage adjustment necessary.

Obesity Dose should be based on ideal body weight (IBW) in obese patients (>30% over IBW).

Administration An infusion device should be used to administer continuous infusions. During the maintenance of general anesthesia, IV boluses may be administered over 30-60 seconds. Injections should be given into IV tubing close to the venous cannula; tubing should be cleared after treatment to prevent residual effects when other fluids are administered through the same IV line.

Monitoring Parameters Respiratory and cardiovascular status, blood pressure, heart rate

Additional Information Ultra short-acting opioid that is unique compared to other short-acting opioids. This agent is not considered suitable as the sole agent for induction; remifentanil should be used in combination with other induction agents. Bolus doses are not recommended for sedation cases and in treatment of postoperative pain due to risk of respiratory depression and muscle rigidity. Due to remifentanil's short duration of action, when postoperative pain is anticipated, discontinuation of an infusion of remifentanil should be preceded by an adequate postoperative analgesic (ie, fentanyl, morphine).

Dosage Forms Excipient information presented when available (limited, particularly for generics); consult specific product labeling.

Solution Reconstituted, Intravenous [preservative free]:
Ultiva: 1 mg (1 ea); 2 mg (1 ea); 5 mg (1 ea)

Controlled Substance C-II

Repaglinide (re PAG li nide)

Brand Names: US Prandin

Brand Names: Canada ACT-Repaglinide; Apo-Repaglinide; Auro-Repaglinide; GlucoNorm; PMS-Repaglinide; Sandoz-Repaglinide

Pharmacologic Category Antidiabetic Agent, Meglitinide Analog

Use Diabetes mellitus, type 2: Management of type 2 diabetes mellitus (noninsulin dependent, NIDDM) as an adjunct to diet and exercise; may be used in combination with metformin or thiazolidinediones (US labeling) or metformin or rosiglitazone (Canadian labeling)

Pregnancy Considerations Adverse events have been observed in some animal reproduction studies. Repaglinide was shown to have a low potential to cross the placenta using an *ex vivo* perfusion model (Tertti 2011). Information describing the effects of repaglinide on pregnancy outcomes is limited.

In women with diabetes, maternal hyperglycemia can be associated with congenital malformations as well as adverse effects in the fetus, neonate, and the mother (ACOG 2005; ADA 2015; Kitzmiller 2008; Metzger 2007). To prevent adverse outcomes, prior to conception and throughout pregnancy maternal blood glucose and HbA$_{1c}$ should be kept as close to target goals as possible but without causing significant hypoglycemia (ACOG 2013; ADA 2015; Blumer 2013; Kitzmiller 2008). Prior to pregnancy, effective contraception should be used until glycemic control is achieved (Kitzmiller 2008). Other agents are currently recommended to treat diabetes in pregnant women (ACOG 2013; Blumer 2013).

Breast-Feeding Considerations It is not known if repaglinide is excreted in breast milk. Due to the potential for serious adverse reactions in the nursing infant, the manufacturer recommends a decision be made whether to discontinue nursing or to discontinue the drug, taking into account the importance of treatment to the mother.

Contraindications

Hypersensitivity to repaglinide or any component of the formulation; diabetic ketoacidosis, with or without coma; type 1 diabetes (insulin dependent, IDDM); concurrent gemfibrozil therapy

Canadian labeling: Additional contraindications (not in US labeling): Severe hepatic impairment; concurrent use with clopidogrel

Warnings/Precautions Use with caution in patients with hepatic impairment; the Canadian labeling contraindicates use in severe impairment. Use caution in severe renal dysfunction, elderly, debilitated, malnourished, or patients with adrenal/pituitary dysfunction; may be more susceptible to glucose-lowering effects. May cause hypoglycemia; appropriate patient selection, dosage, and patient education are important to avoid hypoglycemic episodes. Ethanol may increase risk of hypoglycemia; instruct patients to avoid ethanol. It may be necessary to discontinue repaglinide and administer insulin if the patient is exposed to stress (fever, trauma, infection, surgery). Theoretically, repaglinide may increase cardiovascular events as observed in some studies using oral hypoglycemic drugs, but there are no long-term studies assessing this concern. Not indicated for use in combination with NPH insulin as there have been case reports of myocardial ischemia; further evaluation required to assess the safety of this combination. Potentially significant drug-drug interactions may exist, requiring dose or frequency adjustment, additional monitoring, and/or selection of alternative therapy.

Adverse Reactions

>10%:
Central nervous system: Headache (9% to 11%)
Endocrine & metabolic: Hypoglycemia (16% to 31%)
Respiratory: Upper respiratory tract infection (10% to 16%)

1% to 10%:
Cardiovascular: Ischemia (4%), chest pain (2% to 3%)
Gastrointestinal: Diarrhea (4% to 5%), constipation (2% to 3%)
Genitourinary: Urinary tract infection (2% to 3%)
Neuromuscular & skeletal: Back pain (5% to 6%), arthralgia (3% to 6%)
Respiratory: Sinusitis (3% to 6%), bronchitis (2% to 6%)
Miscellaneous: Allergy (1% to 2%)

<1% (Limited to important or life-threatening): Anaphylactoid reaction, arrhythmia, hemolytic anemia, hepatic dysfunction (severe), hepatitis, hypertension, leukopenia, MI, pancreatitis, Stevens-Johnson syndrome, thrombocytopenia, visual disturbances (transient)

Drug Interactions

Metabolism/Transport Effects Substrate of CYP2C8 (major), CYP3A4 (major), SLCO1B1; **Note:** Assignment of Major/Minor substrate status based on clinically relevant drug interaction potential

Avoid Concomitant Use

Avoid concomitant use of Repaglinide with any of the following: Atazanavir; Gemfibrozil

Increased Effect/Toxicity

Repaglinide may increase the levels/effects of: Hypoglycemia-Associated Agents

The levels/effects of Repaglinide may be increased by: Abiraterone Acetate; Alpha-Lipoic Acid; Androgens; Antidiabetic Agents; Atazanavir; Clopidogrel; CycloSPORINE (Systemic); CYP2C8 Inhibitors (Moderate); CYP2C8 Inhibitors (Strong); CYP3A4 Inhibitors (Strong); Deferasirox; Eltrombopag; Gemfibrozil; Herbs (Hypoglycemic Properties); Macrolide Antibiotics; MAO Inhibitors; Mifepristone; Osimertinib; Pegvisomant; Quinolone Antibiotics; Salicylates; Selective Serotonin Reuptake Inhibitors; Telaprevir; Teriflunomide; Trimethoprim

Decreased Effect

The levels/effects of Repaglinide may be decreased by: Bosentan; CYP2C8 Inducers (Strong); CYP3A4 Inducers (Moderate); CYP3A4 Inducers (Strong); Dabrafenib; Enzalutamide; Hyperglycemia-Associated Agents; Mitotane; Osimertinib; Quinolone Antibiotics; Rifampin; Siltuximab; St Johns Wort; Thiazide Diuretics; Tocilizumab

Food Interactions When given with food, the AUC of repaglinide is decreased. Taking medication without eating may cause hypoglycemia. Management: Administer 15-30 minutes prior to a meal. If a meal is skipped, skip dose for that meal.

Storage/Stability Do not store above 25°C (77°F). Protect from moisture.

◀ **Mechanism of Action** Nonsulfonylurea hypoglycemic agent which blocks ATP-dependent potassium channels, depolarizing the membrane and facilitating calcium entry through calcium channels. Increased intracellular calcium stimulates insulin release from the pancreatic beta cells. Repaglinide-induced insulin release is glucose-dependent.

Pharmacodynamics/Kinetics

Onset of action: Single dose: Increased insulin levels: ~15-60 minutes

Duration: 4-6 hours

Absorption: Rapid and complete

Distribution: V_d: 31 L

Protein binding, plasma: >98% to albumin

Metabolism: Hepatic via CYP3A4 and CYP2C8 isoenzymes and glucuronidation to inactive metabolites

Bioavailability: ~56%

Half-life elimination: ~1 hour

Time to peak, plasma: ~1 hour

Excretion: Feces (~90%, <2% as unchanged drug); Urine (~8%, 0.1% as unchanged drug)

Dosing

Adult & Geriatric

Diabetes mellitus, type 2: Oral:

Patients not previously treated or whose HbA$_{1c}$ is <8%: Initial: 0.5 mg before each meal

Patients previously treated with blood glucose-lowering agents whose HbA$_{1c}$ is ≥8%: Initial: 1 or 2 mg before each meal.

Dose adjustment: Determine dosing adjustments by blood glucose response, usually fasting blood glucose. Double the preprandial dose up to 4 mg until satisfactory blood glucose response is achieved. At least 1 week should elapse to assess response after each dose adjustment.

Dose range: 0.5-4 mg taken with meals. Repaglinide may be dosed preprandially 2, 3, or 4 times/day in response to changes in the patient's meal pattern. Maximum recommended daily dose: 16 mg.

Patients receiving other oral hypoglycemic agents: When repaglinide is used to replace therapy with other oral hypoglycemic agents, it may be started the day after the final dose is given. Observe patients carefully for hypoglycemia because of potential overlapping of drug effects. When transferred from longer half-life sulfonylureas (eg, chlorpropamide), close monitoring may be indicated for up to ≥1 week.

Combination therapy: If repaglinide monotherapy does not result in adequate glycemic control, metformin or a thiazolidinedione may be added. Or, if metformin or thiazolidinedione therapy does not provide adequate control, repaglinide may be added. The starting dose and dose adjustments for combination therapy are the same as repaglinide monotherapy. Carefully adjust the dose of each drug to determine the minimal dose required to achieve the desired pharmacologic effect. Failure to do so could result in an increase in the incidence of hypoglycemic episodes. Use appropriate monitoring of FPG and HbA$_{1c}$ measurements to ensure that the patient is not subjected to excessive drug exposure or increased probability of secondary drug failure. If glucose is not achieved after a suitable trial of combination therapy, consider discontinuing these drugs and using insulin.

Renal Impairment

US labeling:

CrCl ≥40 mL/minute: No dosage adjustment necessary.

CrCl 20 to 40 mL/minute: Initial: 0.5 mg with meals; titrate carefully.

CrCl <20 mL/minute: There are no dosage adjustments provided in the manufacturer's labeling (has not been studied).

Hemodialysis: There are no dosage adjustments provided in the manufacturer's labeling (has not been studied).

Canadian labeling: Initial: No dosage adjustment necessary; titrate carefully.

Hepatic Impairment There are no dosage adjustments provided in the manufacturer's labeling. Use with caution; use conservative initial and maintenance doses and longer intervals between dosage adjustments. The Canadian labeling contraindicates use in severe impairment.

Dietary Considerations Take repaglinide 15-30 minutes before meals. Individualized medical nutrition therapy (MNT) based on ADA recommendations is an integral part of therapy. May cause hypoglycemia. Must be able to recognize symptoms of hypoglycemia (palpitations, tachycardia, sweaty palms, diaphoresis, lightheadedness).

Administration Oral: Administer 15 minutes before meals; however, time may vary from immediately preceding a meal to as long as 30 minutes before a meal. If the patient misses a meal or is unable to take anything by mouth, repaglinide should not be administered to avoid hypoglycemia. Patients consuming extra meals should be instructed to add a dose for the extra meal.

Monitoring Parameters Monitor fasting blood glucose (periodically) and glycosylated hemoglobin (HbA$_{1c}$) levels (every 3 months) with a goal of decreasing these levels towards the normal range. During dose adjustment, fasting glucose can be used to determine response.

Reference Range

Recommendations for glycemic control in nonpregnant adults with diabetes (ADA, 2015):

HbA$_{1c}$: <7% (a more aggressive [<6.5%] or less aggressive [<8%] HbA$_{1c}$ goal may be targeted based on patient-specific characteristics)

Preprandial capillary plasma glucose: 80 to 130 mg/dL

Peak postprandial capillary blood glucose: <180 mg/dL

Recommendations for glycemic control in pediatric (all age groups) patients with type 1 diabetes (ADA, 2015):

HbA$_{1c}$: <7.5% (individualization may be appropriate based on patient-specific characteristics; <7% is reasonable if it can be achieved without excessive hypoglycemia)

Preprandial capillary plasma glucose: 90 to 130 mg/dL

Bedtime and overnight capillary blood glucose: 90 to 150 mg/dL

Dosage Forms Excipient information presented when available (limited, particularly for generics); consult specific product labeling.

Tablet, Oral:

Prandin: 0.5 mg, 1 mg, 2 mg

Generic: 0.5 mg, 1 mg, 2 mg

Dosage Forms: Canada Excipient information presented when available (limited, particularly for generics); consult specific product labeling.

Tablet, Oral:

Gluconorm: 0.5 mg, 1 mg, 2 mg

Repaglinide and Metformin

(re PAG li nide & met FOR min)

Brand Names: US PrandiMet

Index Terms Metformin and Repaglinide; Repaglinide and Metformin Hydrochloride

Pharmacologic Category Antidiabetic Agent, Biguanide; Antidiabetic Agent, Meglitinide Analog

Use Management of type 2 diabetes mellitus (noninsulin dependent, NIDDM), as an adjunct to diet and exercise, in patients currently receiving or not adequately controlled on metformin and/or a meglitinide

Dosing

Adult & Geriatric Type 2 diabetes mellitus: Oral: **Note:** Daily doses should be divided and given 2-3 times daily with meals (maximum single dose: 4 mg/dose [repaglinide], 1000 mg/dose [metformin]; maximum daily dose: 10 mg/day [repaglinide], 2500 mg/day [metformin])

Patients currently taking repaglinide and metformin: Initial doses should be based on (but not exceeding) the patient's current doses of repaglinide and metformin; titrate as needed to the maximum daily dose to achieve targeted glycemic control

Patients inadequately controlled on metformin alone: Initial dose: Repaglinide 1 mg/metformin 500 mg twice daily with meals. Titrate slowly to reduce the risk of repaglinide-induced hypoglycemia.

Patients inadequately controlled on a meglitinide alone: Initial dose: Metformin 500 mg twice daily plus repaglinide at a dose similar to (but not exceeding) the patient's current dose. Titrate slowly to reduce the risk of metformin-induced gastrointestinal adverse effects.

Renal Impairment

Manufacturer's labeling: Serum creatinine (SCr) ≥1.5 mg/dL (males) or ≥1.4 mg/dL (females) or abnormal CrCl (not defined): Use is contraindicated.

Alternate recommendations: **Note:** The United Kingdom National Institute for Health and Clinical Excellence (NICE) Guidelines recommends prescribing metformin with caution in those patients who are at risk of sudden deterioration in renal function and at risk of an estimated glomerular filtration rate (eGFR) <45 mL/minute/1.73 m^2 (NICE, 2008). Some evidence suggests that use of metformin is unsafe when eGFR <30 mL/minute/1.73 m^2 (calculated using MDRD) (Shaw, 2007). A review of the available data by members of the American Diabetes Association proposed the following recommendations based on eGFR (Lipska, 2011):

eGFR ≥60 mL/minute/1.73 m^2: No contraindications, monitor renal function annually

eGFR ≥45 to <60 mL/minute/1.73 m²: Continue use; monitor renal function every 3 to 6 months

eGFR ≥30 to <45 mL/minute/1.73 m²: In patients currently receiving metformin, use with caution, consider dosage reduction (eg, 50% reduction or 50% of maximal dose), monitor renal function every 3 months. Do not initiate therapy in patients with eGFR <45 mL/minute/1.73 m²

eGFR <30 mL/minute/1.73 m²: Discontinue use

Hepatic Impairment The manufacturer recommends to avoid metformin since liver disease is considered a risk factor for the development of lactic acidosis during metformin therapy. However, continued use of metformin in diabetics with liver dysfunction, including cirrhosis, has been used successfully and may be associated with a survival benefit in carefully selected patients; use cautiously in patients at risk for lactic acidosis (eg, renal impairment, alcohol use) (Brackett, 2010; Zhang, 2014). Repaglinide should be used with caution in patients with hepatic impairment.

Additional Information Complete prescribing information should be consulted for additional detail.

Dosage Forms Excipient information presented when available (limited, particularly for generics); consult specific product labeling.

Tablet, Oral:

PrandiMet®:

1/500: Repaglinide 1 mg and metformin hydrochloride 500 mg

2/500: Repaglinide 2 mg and metformin hydrochloride 500 mg

Generic:

1/500: Repaglinide 1 mg and metformin hydrochloride 500 mg

2/500: Repaglinide 2 mg and metformin hydrochloride 500 mg

Reserpine (re SER peen)

Pharmacologic Category Central Monoamine-Depleting Agent; Rauwolfia Alkaloid

Use

Agitated psychotic states: Treatment of agitated psychotic states (schizophrenia)

Hypertension: Management of mild to moderate hypertension

Note: According to the Eighth Joint National Committee (JNC 8) guidelines, reserpine is **not** recommended for the initial treatment of hypertension (James, 2013).

Dosing

Adult

Hypertension:

Manufacturer's labeling: Initial: 0.5 mg/day for 1-2 weeks; maintenance: 0.1-0.25 mg/day

Note: Clinically, the need for a "loading" period (as recommended by the manufacturer) is not well supported, and alternative dosing is preferred.

Alternative dosing (off-label): Initial: 0.1 mg once daily; adjust as necessary based on response.

Usual dose range (ASH/ISH [Weber, 2014]): 0.1-0.25 mg once daily

Schizophrenia: Dosing recommendations vary; initial dose recommendations generally range from 0.05-0.25 mg (although manufacturer recommends 0.5 mg once daily initially). May be increased in increments of 0.1-0.25 mg

Geriatric Oral: Initial: 0.05 mg once daily increasing by 0.05 mg every week as necessary; full antihypertensive effects may take as long as 3 weeks (Beers Criteria: Avoid doses >0.25 mg daily)

Pediatric Children: Hypertension: 0.01-0.02 mg/kg/24 hours divided every 12 hours; maximum dose: 0.25 mg/day (not recommended in children)

Renal Impairment No dosage adjustment provided in manufacturer's labeling. The following dosing adjustments have been used by some clinicians (Aronoff, 2007):

CrCl <10 mL/minute: Avoid use.

Hemodialysis, peritoneal dialysis: Not removed by hemo- or peritoneal dialysis; supplemental dose is not necessary.

Hepatic Impairment No dosage adjustment provided in manufacturer's labeling.

Additional Information Complete prescribing information should be consulted for additional detail.

Dosage Forms Excipient information presented when available (limited, particularly for generics); consult specific product labeling.

Tablet, Oral:

Generic: 0.1 mg, 0.25 mg

Retapamulin (re te PAM ue lin)

Brand Names: US Altabax

Pharmacologic Category Antibiotic, Pleuromutilin; Antibiotic, Topical

Use Impetigo: Treatment of impetigo due to *Staphylococcus aureus* (methicillin-susceptible isolates only) or *Streptococcus pyogenes* in adults and pediatric patients 9 months and older.

Dosing

Adult & Geriatric

Impetigo: Topical: Apply a thin layer to affected area twice daily for 5 days (maximum; total treatment area should not exceed 100 cm² total body surface area).

Pediatric

Impetigo: Infants ≥9 months, Children, and Adolescents: Topical: Apply a thin layer to affected area twice daily for 5 days (maximum: total treatment area should not exceed 2% of total body surface area).

Renal Impairment There are no dosage adjustments provided in the manufacturer's labeling. However, dosage adjustment unlikely due to low systemic absorption.

Hepatic Impairment There are no dosage adjustments provided in the manufacturer's labeling. However, dosage adjustment unlikely due to low systemic absorption.

Additional Information Complete prescribing information should be consulted for additional detail.

Dosage Forms Excipient information presented when available (limited, particularly for generics); consult specific product labeling.

Ointment, External:

Altabax: 1% (15 g, 30 g)

Rh₀(D) Immune Globulin
(ar aych oh (dee) i MYUN GLOB yoo lin)

Brand Names: US HyperRHO S/D; MICRhoGAM Ultra-Filtered Plus; RhoGAM Ultra-Filtered Plus; Rhophylac; WinRho SDF

Brand Names: Canada WinRho SDF

Index Terms Anti-D Immunoglobulin; RhIG; Rho(D) Immune Globulin (Human); RhoIGIV; RhoIVIM

Pharmacologic Category Blood Product Derivative; Immune Globulin

Use

Immune thrombocytopenia (ITP):

Rhophylac: To increase platelet counts in Rh₀ (D) positive nonsplenectomized adults with chronic ITP.

WinRho SDF: To increase platelet counts in Rho (D) positive nonsplenectomized patients with the following conditions: acute ITP (children), chronic ITP (adults and children), or ITP secondary to HIV infection (adults and children).

Pregnancy and other obstetric conditions:

Prevention of rhesus (Rh) isoimmunization in an Rh-incompatible pregnancy. All products are for use in Rh₀(D) negative mothers who are not already sensitized to the Rh₀(D) factor. An Rh-incompatible pregnancy is assumed if the fetus/baby is either Rh₀(D) positive or Rh₀(D) unknown or if the father is either Rh₀(D) positive or Rh₀(D) unknown. Use is not needed if the father or baby is conclusively Rh₀(D) negative. Product specific indications are as follows based on the above criteria:

HyperRHO S/D Full Dose: For antepartum prophylaxis at ~28 weeks gestation; for administration within 72 hours of birth for the prevention of hemolytic disease of the newborn; for administration within 72 hours of spontaneous or induced abortion, ruptured tubal pregnancy, amniocentesis or abdominal trauma.

HyperRHO S/D Mini Dose: For administration within 3 hours (or as soon as possible) of spontaneous or induced abortion up to 12 weeks' gestation.

MICRhoGAM Ultra-Filtered Plus: For administration within 72 hours of actual or threatened termination of pregnancy (spontaneous or induced) up to and including 12 weeks' gestation.

RhoGAM Ultra-Filtered Plus: For antepartum prophylaxis at 26 to 28 weeks' gestation; for administration within 72 hours of birth for prevention of hemolytic disease of the newborn; for administration within 72 hours of amniocentesis, chorionic villus sampling (CVS), percutaneous umbilical blood sampling (PUBS), abdominal trauma or obstetrical manipulation, ectopic pregnancy, threatened pregnancy loss after 12 weeks' gestation (with continuation of pregnancy), pregnancy termination (spontaneous or induced) after 12 weeks' gestation.

Rhophylac: For antepartum prophylaxis at 28 to 30 weeks' gestation; for administration within 72 hours of birth for the prevention of hemolytic disease of the newborn; for administration within 72 hours of obstetric complications including miscarriage, abortion, threatened abortion, ectopic pregnancy or hydatiform mole, transplacental hemorrhage resulting from antepartum hemorrhage; for administration within 72 hours of invasive procedures during pregnancy including amniocentesis, chorionic biopsy, or obstetric manipulative procedures such as external version or abdominal trauma.

WinRho SDF: For antepartum prophylaxis at 28 weeks' gestation; for administration within 72 hours of birth for the prevention of hemolytic disease of the newborn; for administration following obstetric complications including miscarriage, abortion, threatened abortion, ectopic pregnancy or hydatiform mole, transplacental hemorrhage resulting from antepartum hemorrhage; for administration following invasive procedures during pregnancy including amniocentesis, chorionic biopsy, or obstetric manipulative procedures such as external version or abdominal trauma.

Transfusion:

HyperRHO S/D Full Dose, MICRhoGAM Ultra-Filtered Plus, RhoGAM Ultra-Filtered Plus, Rhophylac, and WinRho SDF: To prevent isoimmunization in Rh₀(D) negative individuals who have been transfused with Rh₀(D) positive red blood cells or blood components containing red blood cells.

Dosing

Adult

Note: Rh₀(D) immune globulin 300 mcg has traditionally been referred to as a "full dose". Potency and dosing recommendations may also be expressed in international units by comparison to the WHO anti-Rh₀(D) standard where 1 mcg = 5 international units

Immune thrombocytopenia (ITP):

Rhophylac: IV: 50 mcg/kg

WinRho SDF: IV:

Initial: 50 mcg/kg as a single injection, or can be given as a divided dose on separate days. If hemoglobin is <10 g/dL: Dose should be reduced to 25 to 40 mcg/kg.

Subsequent dosing: 25 to 60 mcg/kg can be used if required to increase platelet count; frequency of dosing is dependent upon clinical response

Maintenance dosing if patient **did respond** to initial dosing: 25 to 60 mcg/kg based on platelet count and hemoglobin concentration

Maintenance dosing if patient **did not respond** to initial dosing:

Hemoglobin <8 g/dL: Alternative treatment should be used

Hemoglobin 8 to 10 g/dL: Redose between 25 to 40 mcg/kg

Hemoglobin >10 g/dL: Redose between 50 to 60 mcg/kg

Rh₀(D) suppression: Note: In general, a 300 mcg dose will suppress the immune response to a fetal-maternal hemorrhage with ≤15 mL of Rh-positive RBC. If exposure to >15 mL of Rh-positive RBC is suspected, an appropriate dose should be calculated. If the first dose is administered early in pregnancy, additional doses may be needed to ensure adequate levels of passively acquired anti-D at delivery (ACOG 1999). If delivery occurs within 3 weeks after the last antepartum dose, a postpartum dose may be withheld, but testing for fetal-maternal hemorrhage of >15 mL should be performed (ACOG 1999).

Pregnancy prophylaxis: Note: if antepartum prophylaxis is indicated, the mother may also need a postpartum dose if the infant is Rh-positive.

Antepartum prophylaxis:

HyperRHO S/D Full Dose: IM: 300 mcg at ~28 weeks' gestation.

RhoGAM: IM: 300 mcg at 26 to 28 weeks' gestation; if delivery does not occur within 12 weeks after the dose, a second 300 mcg dose is recommended. If the first dose is prior to 26 weeks' gestation, administer every 12 weeks to ensure adequate levels of passively acquired anti-D. If delivery occurs within 3 weeks after the last antepartum dose, a postpartum dose may be withheld, but testing for fetal-maternal hemorrhage of >15 mL should be performed.

Rhophylac: IM, IV: 300 mcg at 28 to 30 weeks' gestation.

WinRho SDF: IM, IV: 300 mcg at 28 weeks' gestation. If the first dose is administered early in pregnancy, administer every 12 weeks to ensure adequate levels of passively acquired anti-D.

Postpartum prophylaxis:

HyperRHO S/D Full Dose: IM: 300 mcg provides sufficient antibody if volume of Rh-positive RBC exposure is ≤15 mL. If exposure to >15 mL of Rh-positive RBC is suspected, an appropriate dose should be calculated (see dosing for excessive fetomaternal hemorrhage). The dose should be administered within 72 hours of delivery, but may provide some benefit if given later.

RhoGAM: IM: 300 mcg provides sufficient antibody if volume of Rh-positive RBC exposure is ≤15 mL. If exposure to >15 mL of Rh-positive RBC is suspected, an appropriate dose should be calculated. The dose should be administered within 72 hours of delivery.

Rhophylac: IM, IV: 300 mcg provides sufficient antibody if volume of Rh-positive RBC exposure is ≤15 mL. If exposure to >15 mL of Rh-positive RBC is suspected, an appropriate dose should be calculated (see dosing for excessive fetomaternal hemorrhage). The dose should be administered within 72 hours of delivery.

WinRho SDF: IM, IV: 120 mcg. The dose should be administered within 72 hours of delivery but may be given up to 28 days after delivery.

Other pregnancy/obstetric conditions:

Abdominal trauma:

HyperRHO S/D Full Dose: IM: 300 mcg following abdominal trauma in the second or third trimester. If exposure to >15 mL of Rh-positive RBC is suspected, an appropriate dose should be calculated (see dosing for excessive fetomaternal hemorrhage).

RhoGam: IM: 300 mcg within 72 hours following abdominal trauma or obstetrical manipulation occurring at ≥13 weeks' gestation. If exposure to >15 mL of Rh-positive RBC is suspected, an appropriate dose should be calculated.

Rhophylac: IV, IM: 300 mcg within 72 hours of complication. If exposure to >15 mL of Rh-positive RBC is suspected, an appropriate dose should be calculated (see dosing for excessive fetomaternal hemorrhage).

Amniocentesis:

HyperRHO S/D Full Dose: IM: 300 mcg at 15 to 18 weeks' gestation or during the third trimester. If exposure to >15 mL of Rh-positive RBC is suspected, an appropriate dose should be calculated (see dosing for excessive fetomaternal hemorrhage).

RhoGam: IM: 300 mcg within 72 hours of a procedure occurring at ≥13 weeks' gestation. If exposure to >15 mL of Rh-positive RBC is suspected, an appropriate dose should be calculated.

Rhophylac: IV, IM: 300 mcg within 72 hours of procedure. If exposure to >15 mL of Rh-positive RBC is suspected, an appropriate dose should be calculated (see dosing for excessive fetomaternal hemorrhage).

WinRho SDF: IV, IM: 300 mcg immediately after amniocentesis occurring before 34 weeks' gestation; repeat dose every 12 weeks during pregnancy. Administer 120 mcg within 72 hours of amniocentesis occurring after 34 weeks' gestation.

Ectopic pregnancy:

HyperRHO S/D Full Dose: IM: 300 mcg for complications occurring at ≥13 weeks' gestation. If exposure to >15 mL of Rh-positive RBC is suspected, an appropriate dose should be calculated (see dosing for excessive fetomaternal hemorrhage).

RhoGam: IM: 300 mcg within 72 hours of complications occurring at ≥13 weeks' gestation. If exposure to >15 mL of Rh-positive RBC is suspected, an appropriate dose should be calculated.

Rhophylac: IV, IM: 300 mcg within 72 hours of complication. If exposure to >15 mL of Rh-positive RBC is suspected, an appropriate dose should be calculated (see dosing for excessive fetomaternal hemorrhage).

Termination of pregnancy (spontaneous or induced):

HyperRHO S/D Mini Dose: IM: 50 mcg within 3 hours or as soon as possible following spontaneous or induced abortion occurring <13 weeks' gestation; administer within 72 hours of termination if prompt administration is not possible.

HyperRHO S/D Full Dose: IM: 300 mcg following miscarriage or abortion occurring ≥13 weeks' gestation. If exposure to >15 mL of Rh-positive RBC is suspected, an appropriate dose should be calculated (see dosing for excessive fetomaternal hemorrhage).

MICRhoGAM: IM: 50 mcg within 72 hours of actual or threatened termination occurring <13 weeks' gestation.

RhoGAM: IM: 300 mcg within 72 hours following spontaneous or induced termination occurring ≥13 weeks' gestation. If exposure to >15 mL of Rh-positive RBC is suspected, an appropriate dose should be calculated.

Rhophylac: IV, IM: 300 mcg within 72 hours of miscarriage or abortion. If exposure to >15 mL of Rh-positive RBC is suspected, an appropriate dose should be calculated (see dosing for excessive fetomaternal hemorrhage).

WinRho SDF: IV, IM: 120 mcg within 72 hours of abortion occurring after 34 weeks' gestation.

Threatened pregnancy loss with continuation of pregnancy:

HyperRHO S/D Full Dose: IM: 300 mcg following threatened loss at any time during pregnancy; administer as soon as possible. If exposure to >15 mL of Rh-positive RBC is suspected, an appropriate dose should be calculated (see dosing for excessive fetomaternal hemorrhage).

RhoGAM: IM: 300 mcg within 72 hours following threatened loss ≥13 weeks' gestation. If exposure to >15 mL of Rh-positive RBC is suspected, an appropriate dose should be calculated.

Rhophylac: IV, IM: 300 mcg within 72 hours of threatened abortion. If exposure to >15 mL of Rh-positive RBC is suspected, an appropriate dose should be calculated (see dosing for excessive fetomaternal hemorrhage).

WinRho SDF: IV, IM: 300 mcg immediately following a threatened abortion occurring any time during pregnancy

Additional invasive/manipulative procedures or obstetric complications:

RhoGam: IM: 300 mcg within 72 hours of chorionic villus sampling or percutaneous umbilical blood sampling ≥13 weeks' gestation. If exposure to >15 mL of Rh-positive RBC is suspected, an appropriate dose should be calculated.

Rhophylac: IV, IM: 300 mcg within 72 hours of procedures such as chorionic biopsy or external version, or within 72 hours of complications such as hydatidiform mole, or transplacental hemorrhage resulting from antepartum hemorrhage. If exposure to >15 mL of Rh-positive RBC is suspected, an appropriate dose should be calculated (see dosing for excessive fetomaternal hemorrhage).

WinRho SDF: IV, IM: 300 mcg immediately after chorionic villus sampling before 34 weeks' gestation; repeat dose every 12 weeks during pregnancy. Administer 120 mcg within 72 hours of manipulation occurring after 34 weeks' gestation.

Dosing for excessive fetomaternal hemorrhage:

HyperRHO S/D Full Dose: IM: When exposure to >15 mL Rh-positive RBC or >30 mL whole blood is suspected, a fetal red cell count should be calculated. The fetal RBC volume is then divided by 15 mL, providing the number of 300 mcg doses (vials/syringes) to administer. If the dose calculated results in a fraction, round up to the next higher whole 300 mcg dose (vial/syringe).

Rhophylac: IV, IM: When exposure to >15 mL Rh-positive RBC, administer 300 mcg; in addition, administer 20 mcg per mL fetal RBC in excess of 15 mL if bleeding can be quantified or an additional 300 mcg if excess bleeding cannot be quantified. Total dose should be administered within 72 hours of complication.

Transfusion: Note: Actual dose is based upon volume of blood/blood product exposure.

WinRho SDF: Administer within 72 hours after exposure of incompatible blood transfusion.

IV: Calculate dose as follows; administer 600 mcg every 8 hours until the total dose is administered:

Exposure to Rh$_o$(D) positive whole blood: 9 mcg/mL blood

Exposure to Rh$_o$(D) positive red blood cells: 18 mcg/mL cells

IM: Calculate dose as follows; administer 1,200 mcg every 12 hours until the total dose is administered:

Exposure to Rh$_o$(D) positive whole blood: 12 mcg/mL blood

Exposure to Rh$_o$(D) positive red blood cells: 24 mcg/mL cells

HyperRHO S/D Full Dose: IM: Multiply the volume of Rh-positive whole blood administered by the hematocrit of the donor unit to equal the volume of RBCs transfused. The volume of RBCs is then divided by 15 mL, providing the number of 300 mcg doses (vials/syringes) to administer. If the dose calculated results in a fraction, round up to the next higher whole 300 mcg dose (vial/syringe). Administer as soon as possible and within 72 hours after an incompatible transfusion.

MICRhoGAM: IM: <2.5 mL of Rh-positive red blood cell exposure: 50 mcg. Administer within 72 hours after an incompatible transfusion.

RhoGAM: IM:

2.5 to 15 mL Rh-positive red blood cell exposure: 300 mcg. Administer within 72 hours after an incompatible transfusion.

>15 mL Rh-positive red blood cell exposure: 20 mcg per mL of Rh-positive red blood cell exposure. Multiple doses may be given at the same time or spaced at intervals; total dose must be given within 72 hours of exposure.

Rhophylac: IM, IV: 20 mcg per 2 mL transfused blood or 20 mcg per mL erythrocyte concentrate. Administer within 72 hours after an incompatible transfusion.

Geriatric Refer to adult dosing. Patients >65 years of age with a concurrent comorbid condition may be at increased risk of developing acute hemolytic reactions. Fatal outcomes associated with IVH have occurred most frequently in those >65 years. Use with caution; consider starting at lower doses.

Pediatric Immune thrombocytopenia (ITP): Children and Adolescents: WinRho SDF: Refer to adult dosing.

Renal Impairment There are no dosage adjustments provided in the manufacturer's labeling.

Hepatic Impairment There are no dosage adjustments provided in the manufacturer's labeling.

Additional Information Complete prescribing information should be consulted for additional detail.

Dosage Forms Excipient information presented when available (limited, particularly for generics); consult specific product labeling. [DSC] = Discontinued product

Solution, Injection:

WinRho SDF: 2500 units/2.2 mL (2.2 mL); 5000 units/4.4 mL (4.4 mL); 1500 units/1.3 mL (1.3 mL); 15,000 units/13 mL (13 mL)

Solution, Injection [preservative free]:

WinRho SDF: 2500 units/2.2 mL (2.2 mL); 5000 units/4.4 mL (4.4 mL); 1500 units/1.3 mL (1.3 mL); 15,000 units/13 mL (13 mL) [contains polysorbate 80]

Solution Prefilled Syringe, Injection [preservative free]:

Rhophylac: 1500 units/2 mL (2 mL)

Solution Prefilled Syringe, Intramuscular:

HyperRHO S/D: 250 units (1 ea [DSC])

Solution Prefilled Syringe, Intramuscular [preservative free]:

HyperRHO S/D: 250 units (1 ea); 1500 units (1 ea) [latex free]

MICRhoGAM Ultra-Filtered Plus: 250 units (1 ea) [latex free, thimerosal free; contains polysorbate 80]

RhoGAM Ultra-Filtered Plus: 1500 units (1 ea) [latex free, thimerosal free; contains polysorbate 80]

Ribavirin (Systemic) (rye ba VYE rin)

Brand Names: US Copegus; Rebetol; Ribasphere; Ribasphere RibaPak

Brand Names: Canada Ibavyr

Index Terms RTCA; Tribavirin

Pharmacologic Category Antihepaciviral, Nucleoside (Anti-HCV)

Use

Oral capsule: In combination with interferon alfa 2b (pegylated or nonpegylated) injection for the treatment of chronic hepatitis C in interferon alfa-naive or experienced-patients with compensated liver disease. Patients likely to fail re-treatment after a prior failed course include previous nonresponders, those who received previous pegylated interferon treatment, patients who have significant bridging fibrosis or cirrhosis, or those with genotype 1 infection.

Oral solution: In combination with interferon alfa-2b (pegylated or nonpegylated) injection for the treatment of chronic hepatitis C in interferon alfa-naive or experienced patients ≥3 years of age with compensated liver disease. Patients likely to fail re-treatment after a prior failed course include previous nonresponders, those who received previous pegylated interferon treatment, patients who have significant bridging fibrosis or cirrhosis, or those with genotype 1 infection.

Oral tablet: In combination with peginterferon alfa-2a for the treatment of adults (Copegus, Moderiba, Ribasphere) and patients ≥5 years of age (Copegus and Moderiba) with chronic HCV infection who have compensated liver disease and have not previously been treated with interferon alpha, and in adult chronic hepatitis C patients coinfected with HIV

Pregnancy Considerations [US Boxed Warning]: Use is contraindicated in pregnant women or male partners of pregnant women. Significant teratogenic and/or embryocidal effects have been observed in all animal species with adequate studies. Avoid pregnancy in female patients and female partners of male patients during therapy by using two effective forms of contraception; continue contraceptive measures for at least 6 months after completion of therapy. A negative pregnancy test is required immediately before initiation, monthly during therapy, and for 6 months after treatment is discontinued. If patient or female partner becomes pregnant during treatment, she should be counseled about potential risks of exposure.

Health care providers and patients are encouraged to enroll women exposed to ribavirin during pregnancy or within 6 months after treatment in the Ribavirin Pregnancy Registry (800-593-2214).

Breast-Feeding Considerations It is not known if ribavirin is excreted in breast milk. Due to the potential for serious adverse reactions in the nursing infant, the manufacturer recommends that a decision be made whether to discontinue nursing or to discontinue the drug, taking into account the importance of treatment to the mother.

Medication Guide Available Yes

Contraindications

Oral formulations: Hypersensitivity to ribavirin or any component of the formulation; women who are pregnant or may become pregnant; males whose female partners are pregnant; patients with hemoglobinopathies (eg, thalassemia major, sickle cell anemia); concomitant use with didanosine

Ribasphere capsules and Rebetol capsules/solution: Additional contraindications: Patients with a CrCl <50 mL/minute

Oral combination therapy with alfa interferons: Autoimmune hepatitis, hepatic decompensation (Child-Pugh score >6; class B and C) in cirrhotic chronic hepatitis C monoinfected patients prior to treatment, hepatic decompensation (Child-Pugh score ≥6) in cirrhotic chronic hepatitis C patients coinfected with HIV prior to treatment. Also refer to individual monographs for Interferon Alfa-2b

(Intron A), Peginterferon Alfa-2b, and Peginterferon Alfa-2a (Pegasys) for additional contraindication information.

Warnings/Precautions Hazardous agent - use appropriate precautions for handling and disposal (NIOSH 2014 [group 3]).

Oral: Safety and efficacy have not been established in patients who have received organ transplants, or been coinfected with hepatitis B or HIV (ribavirin tablets may be used in adult HIV-coinfected patients unless CD4+ cell count is ≤100 cells/microliter and HIV-1 RNA <5,000 cells/mm³). Hemoglobin at initiation must be ≥12 g/dL (women) or ≥13 g/dL (men) in CHC monoinfected patients and ≥11 g/dL (women) or ≥12 g/dL (men) in CHC and HIV coinfected patients. Oral ribavirin should not be used for adenovirus, RSV, influenza or parainfluenza infections. Severe psychiatric events have occurred including depression and suicidal/homicidal ideation during combination therapy. Avoid use in patients with a psychiatric history; discontinue if severe psychiatric symptoms occur. Acute hypersensitivity reactions (eg, anaphylaxis, angioedema, bronchoconstriction, and urticaria) have been observed with ribavirin and alfa interferon combination therapy. Severe cutaneous reactions, including Stevens-Johnson syndrome and exfoliative dermatitis have been reported (rarely) with ribavirin and alfa interferon combination therapy; discontinue with signs or symptoms of severe skin reactions. Use with caution in patients with renal impairment; dosage adjustment or discontinuation may be required. Elderly patients are more susceptible to adverse effects; use caution.

[US Boxed Warning]: Monotherapy not effective for chronic hepatitis C infection.

[US Boxed Warning]: Hemolytic anemia is the primary clinical toxicity of oral therapy; anemia associated with ribavirin may worsen underlying cardiac disease and lead to fatal and nonfatal myocardial infarctions. Avoid use in patients with significant/unstable cardiac disease. Anemia usually occurs within 1 to 2 weeks of therapy initiation; observed in ~10% to 13% of patients when alfa interferons were combined with ribavirin. Assess cardiac function before initiation of therapy. If patient has underlying cardiac disease, assess electrocardiogram prior to and periodically during treatment. If any deterioration in cardiovascular status occurs, discontinue therapy. Use caution in patients with baseline risk of severe anemia. Assess hemoglobin and hematocrit at baseline and, at minimum, weeks 2 and 4 of therapy since initial drop may be significant. Patients with renal dysfunction and/or those >50 years of age should be carefully assessed for development of anemia. Pancytopenia and bone marrow suppression have been reported with the combination of ribavirin, interferon, and azathioprine. Use caution in pulmonary disease; pulmonary symptoms have been associated with administration. Discontinue therapy if evidence of hepatic decompensation is observed. Use caution in patients with sarcoidosis (exacerbation reported). Dental and periodontal disorders have been reported with ribavirin and interferon therapy; patients should be instructed to brush teeth twice daily and have regular dental exams. Serious ophthalmologic disorders have occurred with combination therapy. All patients require an eye exam at baseline; those with preexisting ophthalmologic disorders (eg, diabetic or hypertensive retinopathy) require periodic follow up. Delay in weight and height increases have been noted in children treated with combination therapy for CHC. In clinical studies, decreases were noted in weight and height for age z-scores and normative growth curve percentiles. Following treatment, rebound growth and weight gain occurred in most patients; however, a small percentage did not. Long-term data indicate that combination therapy may inhibit growth resulting in reduced adult height. Growth should be closely monitored in pediatric patients during therapy and post-treatment for growth catch-up.

[US Boxed Warning]: Significant teratogenic and/or embryocidal effects have been observed in all animal studies. Use is contraindicated in pregnant women or male partners of pregnant women. Avoid pregnancy in female patients and female partners of male patients during therapy by using two effective forms of contraception; continue contraceptive measures for at least 6 months after completion of therapy. The manufacturer recommends that pregnant health care workers take precautions to limit exposure to ribavirin aerosol.

Benzyl alcohol and derivatives: Some dosage forms may contain sodium benzoate/benzoic acid; benzoic acid (benzoate) is a metabolite of benzyl alcohol; large amounts of benzyl alcohol (≥99 mg/kg/day) have been associated with a potentially fatal toxicity ("gasping syndrome") in neonates; the "gasping syndrome" consists of metabolic acidosis, respiratory distress, gasping respirations, CNS dysfunction (including convulsions, intracranial hemorrhage), hypotension, and cardiovascular collapse (AAP ["Inactive" 1997]; CDC 1982); some data suggests that benzoate displaces bilirubin from protein binding sites (Ahlfors 2001); avoid or use dosage forms containing benzyl alcohol derivative with caution in neonates. See manufacturer's labeling.

Adverse Reactions

All adverse reactions are documented while receiving combination therapy with alfa interferons; percentages as reported in adults unless noted, most common pediatric adverse reactions were similar to adults; asterisked (*) percentages are those similar to interferon therapy alone:

>10%:

Central nervous system: Fatigue (60% to 70% [30% in pediatric patients])*, headache (43% to 66%)*, fever (32% to 55%)*, insomnia (26% to 41% [9% in pediatric patients]), depression (20% to 36%)*, irritability (23% to 33%), dizziness (14% to 26%), impaired concentration (10% to 21%)*, pain (≤13%), emotional lability (7% to 12%)*, anxiety (11%)

Dermatologic: Alopecia (27% to 36% [17% in pediatric patients]), pruritus (13% to 29% [11% in pediatric patients]), rash (5% to 28%), dry skin (10% to 24%), dermatitis (≤16%)

Endocrine and metabolic: Growth suppression (pediatric) percentile decrease (≥15 percentiles: weight 43%; height 25%), hyperuricemia (33% to 38%)

Gastrointestinal: Nausea (25% to 47% [18% in pediatric patients]), anorexia (21% to 32%), weight decrease (10% to 29%), vomiting (9% to 25%)*, diarrhea (10% to 22%), dyspepsia (6% to 16%), abdominal pain (8% to 13% [21% in pediatric patients]), xerostomia (≤12%), RUQ pain (≤12%)

Hematologic: Leukopenia (6% to 45%), neutropenia (8% to 42%; grade 4: 2% to 11%; 40% with HIV coinfection), hemoglobin decreased (11% to 35%), anemia (11% to 17%), thrombocytopenia (<1% to 15%), lymphopenia (12% to 14%), hemolytic anemia (10% to 13%)

Hepatic: Bilirubin increase (10% to 32%)

Local: Injection site reaction (36% to 58%), inflammation at injection site (18% to 25%)

Neuromuscular & skeletal: Decreased linear skeletal growth (including lagging weight gain; 70% in pediatric patients), myalgia (40% to 64% [17% in pediatric patients])*, rigors (25% to 48%), arthralgia (21% to 34%)*, musculoskeletal pain (19% to 28% [35% in pediatric patients])

Respiratory: Upper respiratory tract infection (60% in pediatric patients), dyspnea (13% to 26%), cough (7% to 23%), pharyngitis (≤13%), sinusitis (≤12%)*

Miscellaneous: Flu-like syndrome (13% to 18% [up to 91% in pediatric patients])*, viral infection (≤12%), diaphoresis (≤11%)

1% to 10%:

Cardiovascular: Chest pain (5% to 9%)*, flushing (≤4%)

Central nervous system: Mood alteration (≤6%; 9% with HIV coinfection), agitation (5% to 8%), nervousness (6%)*, memory impairment (≤6%), malaise (≤6%), suicidal ideation (adolescents: 2%; adults: 1%)

Dermatologic: Eczema (4% to 5%)

Endocrine & metabolic: Menstrual disorder (≤7%), hypothyroidism (≤5%)

Gastrointestinal: Taste perversion (4% to 9%), constipation (5%)

Hepatic: Hepatomegaly (4%), transaminases increased (1% to 3%), hepatic decompensation (2% with HIV coinfection)

Neuromuscular & skeletal: Weakness (9% to 10%), back pain (5%)

Ocular: Blurred vision (≤6%), conjunctivitis (≤5%)

Respiratory: Rhinitis (≤8%), exertional dyspnea (≤7%)

Miscellaneous: Fungal infection (≤6%), bacterial infection (3% to 5%)

<1% (Limited to important or life-threatening): Aggression, angina, aplastic anemia, arrhythmia; autoimmune disorders (systemic lupus erythematosus, rheumatoid arthritis, sarcoidosis); bone marrow suppression, cerebral hemorrhage, cholangitis, colitis, coma, corneal ulcer, dehydration, diabetes mellitus, drug abuse relapse/overdose, exfoliative dermatitis, fatty liver, hearing impairment/loss, gastrointestinal bleeding, gout, hallucination, hepatic dysfunction, hyper-/hypothyroidism, hypersensitivity (including anaphylaxis, angioedema, bronchoconstriction, and urticaria), macular edema, myositis, optic neuritis, papilledema, pancreatitis, peptic ulcer, peripheral neuropathy, pneumonitis, psychosis, psychotic disorder, pulmonary dysfunction, pulmonary embolism, pulmonary infiltrates, pure red cell aplasia, retinal artery/vein thrombosis, retinal detachment, retinal hemorrhage, retinopathy,

sarcoidosis exacerbation; skin reactions (erythema multiforme, exfoliative dermatitis, urticaria, vesiculobullous eruptions); Stevens-Johnson syndrome, suicide, thrombotic thrombocytopenic purpura, thyroid function test abnormalities; transplant rejection (kidney, liver); vision loss

Note: Incidence of headache, fever, suicidal ideation, and vomiting are higher in children.

Drug Interactions

Metabolism/Transport Effects None known.

Avoid Concomitant Use

Avoid concomitant use of Ribavirin (Systemic) with any of the following: Didanosine

Increased Effect/Toxicity

Ribavirin (Systemic) may increase the levels/effects of: AzaTHIOprine; Didanosine; Reverse Transcriptase Inhibitors (Nucleoside)

The levels/effects of Ribavirin (Systemic) may be increased by: Interferons (Alfa); Zidovudine

Decreased Effect

Ribavirin (Systemic) may decrease the levels/effects of: Influenza Virus Vaccine (Live/Attenuated)

Food Interactions High-fat meal increases the AUC and C_{max}. Management: Capsule (in combination with peginterferon alfa-2b) and tablet should be administered with food. Other dosage forms and combinations should be taken consistently in regards to food.

Storage/Stability Oral: Store at 25°C (77°F); excursions permitted between 15°C and 30°C (59°F and 86°F). Solution may also be refrigerated at 2°C to 8°C (36°F to 46°F).

Mechanism of Action Inhibits replication of RNA and DNA viruses; inhibits influenza virus RNA polymerase activity and inhibits the initiation and elongation of RNA fragments resulting in inhibition of viral protein synthesis

Pharmacodynamics/Kinetics

Distribution: Oral capsule: Single dose: V_d: 2,825 L; distribution significantly prolonged in the erythrocyte (16 to 40 days), which can be used as a marker for intracellular metabolism

Protein binding: Oral: None

Metabolism: Hepatically and intracellularly (forms active metabolites); may be necessary for drug action

Bioavailability: Oral: 64%

Half-life elimination, plasma: Adults: Oral:

Capsule, single dose: 24 hours in healthy adults, 44 hours with chronic hepatitis C infection (increases to ~298 hours at steady state)

Tablet, single dose: ~120 to 170 hours

Time to peak, serum: Oral capsule: Multiple doses: 3 hours; Tablet: 2 hours

Excretion: Oral capsule: Urine (61%), feces (12%)

Dosing

Adult & Geriatric *Manufacturer's labeling:*

Chronic hepatitis C monoinfection (in combination with peginterferon alfa-2b): *Oral capsule, oral solution (Rebetol, Ribasphere):* **Note:** Recommended therapy duration [manufacturer labeling]: Genotype 1: 48 weeks; genotypes 2,3: 24 weeks); recommended therapy duration for patients who previously failed therapy: 48 weeks [regardless of genotype])

<66 kg: 800 mg daily (400 mg in the morning and evening)

66 to 80 kg: 1,000 mg daily (400 mg in the morning, 600 mg in the evening)

81 to 105 kg: 1,200 mg daily (600 mg in the morning, 600 mg in the evening)

>105 kg: 1,400 mg daily (600 mg in the morning, 800 mg in the evening)

Chronic hepatitis C monoinfection (in combination with interferon alfa-2b): *Oral capsule (Rebetol, Ribasphere):* **Note:** Individualized therapy duration [manufacturer labeling] 24 to 48 weeks:

≤75 kg: 1,000 mg daily (400 mg in the morning, 600 mg in the evening)

>75 kg: 1,200 mg daily (600 mg in the morning, 600 mg in the evening)

Chronic hepatitis C monoinfection (in combination with peginterferon alfa-2a): *Oral tablet (Copegus, Moderiba, Ribasphere):*

Genotype 1, 4:

<75 kg: 1,000 mg daily in 2 divided doses for 48 weeks

≥75 kg: 1,200 mg daily in 2 divided doses for 48 weeks

Genotype 2, 3: 800 mg daily in 2 divided doses for 24 weeks

Chronic hepatitis C coinfection with HIV (in combination with peginterferon alfa-2a): *Oral tablet (Copegus, Moderiba, Ribasphere):* 800 mg daily in 2 divided doses for 48 weeks (regardless of genotype)

Alternative recommendations: **Note:** *AALSD/IDSA guidelines do not specify which peginterferon is preferred but in clinical trials cited peginterferon alfa 2a was used.*

Chronic hepatitis C (off-label regimens; recommended by AASLD/IDSA 2014): Treatment-naive patients:

Genotype 1:

Interferon eligible patients: in combination with sofosbuvir and peginterferon alfa

<75 kg: 1,000 mg daily in 2 divided doses for 12 weeks

≥75 kg: 1,200 mg daily in 2 divided doses for 12 weeks

Interferon-ineligible patients: in combination with sofosbuvir and simeprevir: **Note: Ribavirin therapy is optional** in these patients:

<75 kg: 1,000 mg daily in 2 divided doses for 12 weeks

≥75 kg: 1,200 mg daily in 2 divided doses for 12 weeks

Genotype 2: Regardless of interferon eligibility: in combination with sofosbuvir

<75 kg: 1,000 mg daily in 2 divided doses for 12 weeks

≥75 kg: 1,200 mg daily in 2 divided doses for 12 weeks

Genotype 3: Regardless of interferon eligibility: in combination with sofosbuvir

<75 kg: 1,000 mg daily in 2 divided doses for 24 weeks

≥75 kg: 1,200 mg daily in 2 divided doses for 24 weeks

Genotype 4:

Interferon eligible patients: in combination with sofosbuvir and peginterferon alfa

<75 kg: 1,000 mg daily in 2 divided doses for 12 weeks

≥75 kg: 1,200 mg daily in 2 divided doses for 12 weeks

Interferon-ineligible patients: in combination with sofosbuvir:

<75 kg: 1,000 mg daily in 2 divided doses for 24 weeks

≥75 kg: 1,200 mg daily in 2 divided doses for 24 weeks

Genotype 5 or 6: Interferon eligible patients: in combination with sofosbuvir and peginterferon alfa

<75 kg: 1,000 mg daily in 2 divided doses for 12 weeks

≥75 kg: 1,200 mg daily in 2 divided doses for 12 weeks

Chronic hepatitis C (off-label regimens; recommended by AASLD/IDSA 2014): Treatment of relapser patients (nonresponders to a previous regimen of ribavirin and peginterferon alfa *without* an HCV protease inhibitor):

Genotype 1: Regardless of interferon eligibility: in combination with sofosbuvir and simeprevir:

Ribavirin therapy is optional in these patients:

<75 kg: 1,000 mg daily in 2 divided doses for 12 weeks

≥75 kg: 1,200 mg daily in 2 divided doses for 12 weeks

Genotype 2: Regardless of interferon eligibility: in combination with sofosbuvir

<75 kg: 1,000 mg daily in 2 divided doses for 12 weeks

≥75 kg: 1,200 mg daily in 2 divided doses for 12 weeks

Note: Patients with cirrhosis may benefit from extension of treatment to 16 weeks.

Genotype 3: Regardless of interferon eligibility: in combination with sofosbuvir

<75 kg: 1,000 mg daily in 2 divided doses for 24 weeks

≥75 kg: 1,200 mg daily in 2 divided doses for 24 weeks

Genotype 4: Interferon eligible patients: in combination with sofosbuvir and weekly peginterferon alfa

<75 kg: 1,000 mg daily in 2 divided doses for 12 weeks

≥75 kg: 1,200 mg daily in 2 divided doses for 12 weeks

Genotype 5 or 6: Interferon eligible patients: in combination with sofosbuvir and weekly peginterferon alfa

<75 kg: 1,000 mg daily in 2 divided doses for 12 weeks

≥75 kg: 1,200 mg daily in 2 divided doses for 12 weeks

Chronic hepatitis C (off-label regimens; recommended by AASLD/IDSA 2014): Treatment of relapser patients (nonresponders to a previous regimen of ribavirin and peginterferon alfa *with or without* an HCV protease inhibitor):
Genotype 1: **Note:** Alternative regimen (AALSD/IDSA 2014)
Interferon eligible patients: in combination with sofosbuvir for the first 12 weeks and peginterferon alfa for the entire regimen:
<75 kg: 1,000 mg daily in 2 divided doses for 12 to 24 weeks total
≥75 kg: 1,200 mg daily in 2 divided doses for 12 to 24 weeks total

Pediatric
Chronic hepatitis C monoinfection (in combination with pegylated or nonpegylated interferon alfa-2b):
Children ≥3 years: *Oral capsule or solution (Rebetol, Ribasphere):* **Note:** Oral solution should be used in children <47 kg, or those unable to swallow capsules. Children who start treatment prior to age 18 years should continue on pediatric dosing regimen through therapy completion. Recommended therapy duration (manufacturer labeling): Genotypes 2,3: 24 weeks; all other genotypes: 48 weeks
Oral capsule, oral solution dosing recommendations:
<47 kg: 15 mg/kg/day in 2 divided doses (morning and evening) as oral solution
47 to 59 kg: 800 mg daily (400 mg in morning and evening)
60 to 73 kg: 1,000 mg daily (400 mg in morning and 600 mg in the evening)
>73 kg: 1,200 mg daily (600 mg in morning and evening)
Alternative recommendations: American Association for the Study of Liver Diseases (AASLD) guidelines: Children 2 to 17 years with chronic hepatitis C infection (Ghany 2009): Treatment of choice: Ribavirin 15 mg/kg daily (in combination with weekly SubQ peginterferon alfa-2b) for 48 weeks

Chronic hepatitis C monoinfection (in combination with peginterferon alfa-2a):
Children ≥5 years and Adolescents: *Oral tablet (Copegus, Moderiba):* **Note:** Assess child's ability to swallow tablet; children who start treatment prior to age 18 years should continue on pediatric dosing regimen through therapy completion. Recommended therapy duration (manufacturer labeling): Genotypes 2,3: 24 weeks; all other genotypes: 48 weeks
23 to 33 kg: 400 mg daily (200 mg in the morning and evening)
34 to 46 kg: 600 mg daily (200 mg in the morning and 400 mg in the evening)
47 to 59 kg: 800 mg daily (400 mg in the morning and evening)
60 to 74 kg: 1,000 mg daily (400 mg in the morning and 600 mg in the evening)
≥75 kg: 1,200 mg daily (600 mg in the morning and evening)

Renal Impairment CHC infection: Oral:
Rebetol capsules/solution, Ribasphere capsules:
Adults:
CrCl ≥50 mL/minute: No dosage adjustments necessary.
CrCl <50 mL/minute: Use is contraindicated.
Children: Serum creatinine >2 mg/dL: Permanently discontinue treatment.
Ribasphere tablets: Adults:
CrCl ≥50 mL/minute: No dosage adjustments necessary.
CrCl <50 mL/minute: Use is not recommended.
Copegus and Moderiba tablets: Adults:
CrCl >50 mL/minute: No dosage adjustments necessary.
CrCl 30 to 50 mL/minute: Alternate 200 mg and 400 mg every other day.
CrCl <30 mL/minute: 200 mg once daily.
ESRD requiring hemodialysis: 200 mg once daily.
Note: The dose of Copegus and Moderiba should not be further modified in patients with renal impairment. If severe adverse reactions or laboratory abnormalities develop it should be discontinued, if appropriate, until the adverse reactions resolve or decrease in severity. If abnormalities persist after restarting, therapy should be discontinued.

Hepatic Impairment CHC infection: Hepatic decompensation (Child-Pugh class B and C): Manufacturer's labeling: Oral tablets: Use contraindicated.

Adjustment for Toxicity
Notes:
Children and Adolescents: Once a laboratory abnormality or clinical adverse event has resolved, the ribavirin dose may be increased, based on clinical judgment, to its original assigned dose. Initiate restart at 50% of the full dose.
Adults: Once ribavirin has been withheld due to clinical adverse event or laboratory abnormality, an attempt can be made to restart ribavirin, in divided doses, at 600 mg daily, with a further ribavirin increase to 800 mg daily. Increasing the ribavirin dose to its original assigned dose (1,000 to 1,200 mg daily) is not recommended.

Patient **without** cardiac history:
Hemoglobin 8.5 to <10 g/dL:
Children ≥3 years: Oral capsules, oral solution:
First reduction: Decrease to 12 mg/kg/day
Second reduction: Decrease to 8 mg/kg/day
Children ≥5 years and Adolescents: Oral tablets (Copegus, Moderiba):
23 to 33 kg: Decrease dose to 200 mg daily (in the morning)
34 to 59 kg: Decrease dose to 400 mg daily (200 mg in the morning and evening)
≥60 kg: Decrease dose to 600 mg daily (200 mg in the morning and 400 mg in the evening)
Adults:
Oral capsules, oral solution:
First reduction: ≤105 kg: Decrease by 200 mg daily; >105 kg: Decrease by 400 mg daily
Second reduction: Decrease by an additional 200 mg daily (not weight-based)
Oral tablets: Decrease dose to 600 mg daily (200 mg in the morning, 400 mg in the evening)
Hemoglobin <8.5 g/dL: Children, Adolescents, and Adults: Oral capsules, solution, tablets: Permanently discontinue treatment.
WBC <1,000 mm^3, neutrophils <500 mm^3: Children and Adults: Oral capsules, solution: Permanently discontinue treatment.
Platelets <50 x 10^9/L: Children: Oral capsules, solution: Permanently discontinue treatment.
Platelets <25 x 10^9/L: Adults: Oral capsules, solution: Permanently discontinue treatment.
Laboratory abnormalities or adverse reactions other than decreased hemoglobin: Children ≥5 years, Adolescents, and Adults: Oral tablets (Moderiba): Refer to dose modification guidelines in the manufacturer's labeling.

Patient **with** stable cardiac history:
Hemoglobin has decreased ≥2 g/dL during any 4-week period of treatment:
Children and Adolescents: Oral capsules, solution: Decrease ribavirin by 200 mg daily (regardless of the patient's initial dose); decrease peginterferon alfa-2b dose by 50%; monitor and evaluate weekly. If hemoglobin <8.5 g/dL any time after dose reduction or <12 g/dL after 4 weeks of dose reduction, permanently discontinue treatment.
Children ≥5 years and Adolescents: Oral tablets (Copegus, Moderiba):
23 to 33 kg: Decrease dose to 200 mg daily (in the morning)
34 to 59 kg: Decrease dose to 400 mg daily (200 mg in the morning and evening)
≥60 kg: 600 mg daily (200 mg in the morning, 400 mg in the evening)
Note: If hemoglobin <8.5 g/dL any time after dose reduction or <12 g/dL after 4 weeks of dose reduction, permanently discontinue treatment.
Hemoglobin has decreased ≥2 g/dL during any 4-week period of treatment: Adults:
Oral capsules, solution: Decrease dose by 200 mg daily; decrease peginterferon alfa-2b by 50%. If hemoglobin <8.5 g/dL any time after dose reduction or <12 g/dL after 4 weeks of dose reduction, permanently discontinue treatment.
Oral tablets: Decrease dose to 600 mg daily (200 mg in the morning, 400 mg in the evening). If hemoglobin <8.5 g/dL any time after dose reduction or <12 g/dL after 4 weeks of dose reduction, permanently discontinue treatment.
Hemoglobin <8.5 g/dL: Children, Adolescents, and Adults: Oral capsules, solution, tablets: Permanently discontinue treatment.
WBC <1,000 mm^3, neutrophils <500 mm^3: Children and Adults: Oral capsules, solution: Permanently discontinue treatment.
Platelets <50 x 10^9/L: Children: Oral capsules, solution: Permanently discontinue treatment.

Platelets <25 x 10^9/L: Adults: Oral capsules, solution: Permanently discontinue treatment.

Laboratory abnormalities or adverse reactions other than decreased hemoglobin: Children ≥5 years, Adolescents, and Adults: Oral tablets (Moderiba): Refer to dose modification guidelines in the manufacturer's labeling.

Dietary Considerations Capsules, solution, and tablets should be taken with food.

Administration Oral:

Capsule: Administer with food. Capsule should not be opened, crushed, chewed, or broken.

Solution: Administer with food. Use oral solution for children <47 kg, or those who cannot swallow capsules.

Tablet: Administer with food.

Hazardous agent; use appropriate precautions for handling and disposal (NIOSH 2014 [group 3]).

Monitoring Parameters

Pretreatment hematological and biochemical tests are recommended for all patients; dental exam, ECG (if preexisting cardiac abnormalities or disease) and ophthalmic exam (also periodically during treatment for those with preexisting ophthalmologic disorders) are also recommended. In adults, hematologic tests should be at treatment weeks 2 and 4, biochemical tests at week 4, and TSH at week 12. In pediatric patients, monitor growth closely during and after treatment.

Pregnancy screening (in woman of childbearing age) and pregnancy tests monthly during and for 6 months after treatment discontinuation.

In pediatric clinical studies, hematologic and biochemical assessments were made at weeks 1, 3, 5 and 8, then every 4 weeks thereafter. Growth velocity and weight should also be monitored during and periodically after treatment discontinuation.

Baseline values used in adult clinical trials in combination with alfa interferons:

Platelet count ≥90,000/mm^3 (75,000/mm^3 for cirrhosis or 70,000/mm^3 for coinfection with HIV)

ANC ≥1500/mm^3

Hemoglobin ≥12 g/dL for women and ≥13 g/dL for men (11 g/dL for HIV coinfected women and 12 g/dL for HIV coinfected men)

TSH and T$_4$ within normal limits or adequately controlled

CD4$^+$ cell count ≥200 cells/microL or CD4$^+$ cell count 100-200 cells/microL and HIV-1 RNA <5000 copies/mL for coinfection with HIV

Serum HCV RNA (pretreatment, week 12 and week 24, and 24 weeks after completion of therapy). **Note:** Discontinuation of therapy may be considered after 12 weeks in patients with HCV (genotypes 1,4) who fail to achieve an early virologic response (EVR) (defined as ≥2-log decrease in HCV RNA compared to pretreatment) or after 24 weeks with detectable HCV RNA. Treat patients with HCV (genotypes 2,3) for 24 weeks (if tolerated) and then evaluate HCV RNA levels (Ghany 2009).

Reference Range

Rapid virological response (RVR): Absence of detectable HCV RNA after 4 weeks of treatment

Early viral response (EVR): ≥2-log decrease in HCV RNA after 12 weeks of treatment

End of treatment response (ETR): Absence of detectable HCV RNA at end of the recommended treatment period

Sustained treatment response (STR) or sustained virologic response (SVR): Absence of HCV RNA in the serum 6 months following completion of full treatment course

Dosage Forms Excipient information presented when available (limited, particularly for generics); consult specific product labeling.

Capsule, Oral:

Rebetol: 200 mg

Ribasphere: 200 mg

Generic: 200 mg

Solution, Oral:

Rebetol: 40 mg/mL (100 mL) [contains propylene glycol, sodium benzoate; bubble-gum flavor]

Tablet, Oral:

Copegus: 200 mg

Ribasphere: 200 mg [contains fd&c blue #2 aluminum lake]

Ribasphere: 400 mg, 600 mg [contains fd&c blue #1 aluminum lake]

Ribasphere RibaPak: Ribasphere RibaPak 800: 400 mg AM dose, 400 mg PM dose, Ribasphere RibaPak 1200: 600 mg AM dose, 600 mg PM dose, Ribasphere RibaPak 1000: 600 mg AM dose, 400 mg PM dose [contains fd&c blue #1 aluminum lake]

Ribasphere RibaPak: Ribasphere RibaPak 600: 200 mg AM dose, 400 mg PM dose [contains fd&c blue #1 aluminum lake, fd&c blue #2 aluminum lake]

Generic: 200 mg

Ribavirin (Oral Inhalation) (rye ba VYE rin)

Brand Names: US Virazole

Brand Names: Canada Virazole

Index Terms RTCA; Tribavirin

Pharmacologic Category Antiviral Agent

Use Respiratory syncytial virus: Treatment of hospitalized infants and young children with respiratory syncytial virus (RSV) infections; specially indicated for treatment of severe lower respiratory tract RSV infections in patients with an underlying compromising condition (prematurity, cardiopulmonary disease, or immunosuppression)

Pregnancy Considerations Use is contraindicated in females who are or may become pregnant. **[US Boxed Warning]: Significant teratogenic and/or embryocidal effects have been observed in all animal species with adequate studies.** The manufacturer recommends that pregnant health care workers take precautions to limit exposure to ribavirin aerosol; potential occupational exposure may be greatest if administration is via oxygen tent or hood, and lower if administered via mechanical ventilation. The minimum interval following exposure to ribavirin inhalation prior to pregnancy is not known.

Breast-Feeding Considerations It is not known if ribavirin is excreted in breast milk.

Contraindications Hypersensitivity to ribavirin or any component of the formulation; women who are pregnant or may become pregnant

Warnings/Precautions Hazardous agent - use appropriate precautions for handling and disposal (NIOSH 2014 [group 3]).

[US Boxed Warning]: Use with caution in patients requiring assisted ventilation because precipitation of the drug in the respiratory equipment may interfere with safe and effective patient ventilation; sudden deterioration of respiratory function has been observed; monitor carefully in patients with COPD and asthma for deterioration of respiratory function.

[US Boxed Warning]: Sudden respiratory deterioration has been observed during the initiation of aerosolized ribavirin in infants; carefully monitor during treatment. If deterioration of respiratory function occurs, stop treatment; reinstitute with extreme caution, continuous monitoring, and consider concomitant administration of bronchodilators.

[US Boxed Warning]: Significant teratogenic and/or embryocidal effects have been observed in all animal species with adequate studies. Use is contraindicated in pregnant women. The manufacturer recommends that pregnant health care workers take precautions to limit exposure to ribavirin aerosol.

Adverse Reactions

1% to 10%:

Central nervous system: Fatigue, headache, insomnia

Gastrointestinal: Nausea, anorexia

Hematologic: Anemia

<1%: Hypotension, cardiac arrest, digitalis toxicity, conjunctivitis, mild bronchospasm, worsening of respiratory function, apnea

Note: Incidence of adverse effects (approximate) in healthcare workers: Headache (51%); conjunctivitis (32%); rhinitis, nausea, rash, dizziness, pharyngitis, and lacrimation (10% to 20%); bronchospasm and/or chest pain (case reports in individuals with underlying airway disease)

Drug Interactions

Metabolism/Transport Effects None known.

Avoid Concomitant Use

Avoid concomitant use of Ribavirin (Oral Inhalation) with any of the following: Didanosine

Increased Effect/Toxicity

Ribavirin (Oral Inhalation) may increase the levels/effects of: AzaTHIOprine; Didanosine; Reverse Transcriptase Inhibitors (Nucleoside)

The levels/effects of Ribavirin (Oral Inhalation) may be increased by: Interferons (Alfa); Zidovudine

Decreased Effect

Ribavirin (Oral Inhalation) may decrease the levels/effects of: Influenza Virus Vaccine (Live/Attenuated)

Preparation for Administration Hazardous agent; use appropriate precautions for handling and disposal (NIOSH 2014 [group 3]).

Continuous aerosolization: Per the manufacturer, reconstitute 6 g vial with at least 75 mL of preservative free sterile water for injection or inhalation; shake vial well to mix. Transfer vial contents to the clean, sterile 500 mL SPAG-2 reservoir and further dilute to a final volume of 300 mL with preservative free sterile water for injection or inhalation; final concentration: 20 mg/mL. Alternatively,

sterile NS has been used for dilution rather than sterile water to achieve a near isotonic solution (Meert 1994). Intermittent aerosolization: Reconstitute 6 g vial with 100 mL of preservative free sterile water; final concentration: 60 mg/mL (Englund 1994).

Storage/Stability Store vials in a dry place at 15°C to 30°C (59°F to 86°F). Reconstituted solution is stable for 24 hours at room temperature.

Mechanism of Action Inhibits replication of RNA and DNA viruses; inhibits influenza virus RNA polymerase activity and inhibits the initiation and elongation of RNA fragments resulting in inhibition of viral protein synthesis

Pharmacodynamics/Kinetics

Absorption: Inhalation: Systemic; dependent upon respiratory factors and method of drug delivery; maximal absorption occurs with the use of aerosol generator via endotracheal tube; highest concentrations in respiratory tract and erythrocytes

Bioavailability: Oral: 64%

Half-life elimination, plasma: Children: Inhalation: 6.5 to 11 hours

Time to peak, serum: Inhalation: At end of inhalation period

Excretion: Inhalation: Urine (40% as unchanged drug and metabolites)

Dosing

Adult & Geriatric

RSV infection in hematopoietic cell or heart/lung transplant recipients (off-label use): Aerosol inhalation: RSV infection in hematopoietic cell or heart/lung transplant recipients (off-label use): 2 g (over 2 hours) every 8 hours (Boeckh 2007; Liu 2010)

Note: Heart/lung transplant recipients also received IVIG, methylprednisolone and palivizumab. Dosage and protocol may be institution specific. (Boeckh 2007; Chemaly 2006; Liu 2010).

Pediatric

RSV infection: Note: Due to potential toxic effects of exposed healthcare workers and variable efficacy results in trials, the AAP recommends against routine use of ribavirin to treat RSV; use should be reserved for patients with documented, potentially life-threatening disease (Red Book [AAP 2015]).

Infants and Children: Aerosol inhalation: Use with Viratek small particle aerosol generator (SPAG-2). **Note:** Dose actually delivered to the patient will depend on patient's minute ventilation.

Continuous aerosolization: 6 g administered over 12 to 18 hours/day for 3 to 7 days

Intermittent aerosolization: 2 g over 2 hours 3 times daily in nonmechanically ventilated patients for 3 to 7 days has been used to permit easier accessibility for patient care and limit environmental exposure of healthcare worker. Due to apparent increased potential for crystallization of the high-dose 60 mg/mL solution around areas of turbulent flow such as bends in tubing or connector pieces, use of high-dose therapy in individuals with an endotracheal tube in place is not recommended (Englund 1994).

Renal Impairment There are no dosage adjustments provided in the manufacturer's labeling (has not been studied).

Hepatic Impairment There are no dosage adjustments provided in the manufacturer's labeling (has not been studied).

Administration Inhalation: Ribavirin should be administered in well-ventilated rooms (at least 6 air changes/hour). In mechanically-ventilated patients, ribavirin can potentially be deposited in the ventilator delivery system depending on temperature, humidity, and electrostatic forces; this deposition can lead to malfunction or obstruction of the expiratory valve, resulting in inadvertently high positive end-expiratory pressures. The use of one-way valves in the inspiratory lines, a breathing circuit filter in the expiratory line, and frequent monitoring and filter replacement have been effective in preventing these problems. Solutions in SPAG-2 unit should be discarded at least every 24 hours and when the liquid level is low before adding newly reconstituted solution. Should not be mixed with other aerosolized medication.

Hazardous agent; use appropriate precautions for handling and disposal (NIOSH 2014 [group 3]).

Monitoring Parameters Respiratory function, hemoglobin, reticulocyte count, CBC with differential, I & O

Dosage Forms Excipient information presented when available (limited, particularly for generics); consult specific product labeling.

Solution Reconstituted, Inhalation [preservative free]:

Virazole: 6 g (1 ea)

Riboflavin (RYE boe flay vin)

Brand Names: US B-2-400 [OTC]

Index Terms Lactoflavin; Vitamin B_2; Vitamin G

Pharmacologic Category Vitamin, Water Soluble

Use Dietary supplement

Dosing

Adult & Geriatric

Dietary supplement: Oral: 100 mg once or twice daily

Recommended daily intake:

≥19 years: Females: 1.1 mg; Males: 1.3 mg

Pregnancy: 1.4 mg

Lactation 1.6 mg

Pediatric Oral:

Adequate intake:

1-6 months: 0.3 mg/day

7-12 months: 0.4 mg/day

Recommended daily intake:

1-3 years: 0.5 mg

4-8 years: 0.6 mg

9-13 years: 0.9 mg

14-18 years: Females: 1 mg; Males: 1.3 mg

Additional Information Complete prescribing information should be consulted for additional detail.

Dosage Forms Excipient information presented when available (limited, particularly for generics); consult specific product labeling.

Capsule, Oral:

B-2-400: 400 mg

Generic: 50 mg

Tablet, Oral:

Generic: 25 mg, 50 mg, 100 mg

Tablet, Oral [preservative free]:

Generic: 100 mg

◆ Ridaura see Auranofin on page 180

◆ Ridaura® (Can) see Auranofin on page 180

◆ RID Maximum Strength [OTC] see Pyrethrins and Piperonyl Butoxide on page 1531

◆ RID Mousse (Can) see Pyrethrins and Piperonyl Butoxide on page 1531

Rifabutin (rif a BYOO tin)

Brand Names: US Mycobutin

Brand Names: Canada Mycobutin

Index Terms Ansamycin

Pharmacologic Category Antibiotic, Miscellaneous; Antitubercular Agent

Use *Mycobacterium avium* **complex (MAC), prophylaxis:** Prevention of disseminated MAC disease in patients with advanced human immunodeficiency virus (HIV) infection

Pregnancy Considerations Adverse events were seen in some animal reproduction studies.

Breast-Feeding Considerations In the United States, where formula is accessible, affordable, safe, and sustainable, and the risk of infant mortality due to diarrhea and respiratory infections is low, complete avoidance of breast-feeding by HIV-infected women is recommended to decrease potential transmission of HIV (DHHS [perinatal] 2011).

Contraindications Clinically significant hypersensitivity to rifabutin, other rifamycins, or any component of the formulation

Warnings/Precautions Rifabutin must not be administered for MAC prophylaxis to patients with active tuberculosis since its use may lead to the development of tuberculosis that is resistant to both rifabutin and rifampin. Caution if active TB in the HIV-positive patient may present atypically (ie, negative PPD or extrapulmonary manifestations). Uveitis may occur; carefully monitor patients when used in combination with macrolides or azole antifungals. If uveitis is suspected, refer patient to an ophthalmologist and consider temporarily discontinuing treatment. May be associated with neutropenia and/or thrombocytopenia (rarely); consider periodic monitoring of hematologic parameters and discontinue permanently if signs of thrombocytopenia (eg, petechial rash) (HHS [OI adult 2015]). Use with caution in patients with renal impairment; dosage reduction recommended in severe renal impairment (CrCl <30 mL/minute). Use with caution in patients with hepatic impairment; discontinue in patients with AST >3 x ULN (symptomatic) or ≥5 x ULN (regardless of symptoms) or if significant bilirubin and/or alkaline phosphatase elevations occur (HHS [OI adult 2015]). Hypersensitivity reactions, including anaphylaxis, hypotension, urticaria, angioedema, acute bronchospasm, conjunctivitis, thrombocytopenia, neutropenia, and flu-like syndrome may occur with rifamycins. Discontinue use

and administer supportive care if hypersensitivity occurs. Prolonged use may result in fungal or bacterial super-infection, including *C. difficile*-associated diarrhea (CDAD) and pseudomembranous colitis; CDAD has been observed >2 months postantibiotic treatment. May cause brown/orange discoloration of urine, feces, saliva, sweat, tears, sputum, and skin. Remove soft contact lenses during therapy since permanent staining may occur. Potentially significant drug-drug interactions may exist, requiring dose or frequency adjustment, additional monitoring, and/or selection of alternative therapy.

Adverse Reactions

>10%:

Dermatologic: Skin rash (11%)

Genitourinary: Discoloration of urine (30%)

Hematologic & oncologic: Neutropenia (25%), leukopenia (10% to 17%)

1% to 10%:

Gastrointestinal: Nausea (≤6%), abdominal pain (4%), dysgeusia (3%), dyspepsia (3%), eructation (3%), vomiting (≤3%), flatulence (2%)

Hematologic & oncologic: Thrombocytopenia (5%)

Neuromuscular & skeletal: Myalgia (2%)

Miscellaneous: Fever (2%)

<1% (Limited to important or life-threatening): Abnormal T waves on ECG, agranulocytosis, aphasia, bronchospasm, *clostridium difficile* associated diarrhea, confusion, corneal deposits, flu-like symptoms, granulocytopenia, hemolysis, hepatitis, hypersensitivity, jaundice, lymphocytopenia, myositis, pancytopenia, paresthesia, pseudomembranous colitis, seizure, thrombotic thrombocytopenic purpura, uveitis

Drug Interactions

Metabolism/Transport Effects Substrate of CYP1A2 (minor), CYP3A4 (major); **Note:** Assignment of Major/Minor substrate status based on clinically relevant drug interaction potential; **Induces** CYP3A4 (strong)

Avoid Concomitant Use

Avoid concomitant use of Rifabutin with any of the following: Abiraterone Acetate; Antihepaciviral Combination Products; Apixaban; Apremilast; Aprepitant; Artemether; Atovaquone; Axitinib; BCG (Intravesical); Bedaquiline; Boceprevir; Bortezomib; Bosutinib; Cabozantinib; Cariprazine; Ceritinib; CloZAPine; Cobimetinib; Crizotinib; Dabrafenib; Daclatasvir; Delavirdine; Dienogest; Dronedarone; Eliglustat; Elvitegravir; Enzalutamide; Everolimus; Flibanserin; Ibrutinib; Idelalisib; Irinotecan Products; Isavuconazonium Sulfate; Itraconazole; Ivabradine; Ivacaftor; Ixazomib; Lapatinib; Ledipasvir; Lumefantrine; Lurasidone; Macitentan; Mifepristone; Mycophenolate; Naloxegol; Netupitant; NIFEdipine; Nilotinib; NiMODipine; Nisoldipine; Olaparib; Osimertinib; Palbociclib; Panobinostat; PAZOPanib; Perampanel; PONATinib; Praziquantel; Ranolazine; Regorafenib; Rivaroxaban; Roflumilast; RomiDEPsin; Simeprevir; Sofosbuvir; Sonidegib; SORAfenib; Suvorexant; Tasimelteon; Telaprevir; Ticagrelor; Tofacitinib; Tolvaptan; Toremifene; Trabectedin; Ulipristal; Vandetanib; Vemurafenib; VinCRIStine (Liposomal); Vorapaxar; Voriconazole

Increased Effect/Toxicity

Rifabutin may increase the levels/effects of: Clarithromycin; Clopidogrel; Darunavir; Fosamprenavir; Ifosfamide; Isoniazid; Lopinavir; Pitavastatin

The levels/effects of Rifabutin may be increased by: Antifungal Agents (Azole Derivatives, Systemic); Atazanavir; Boceprevir; Clarithromycin; Darunavir; Delavirdine; Elvitegravir; Fosamprenavir; Indinavir; Lopinavir; Macrolide Antibiotics; Nelfinavir; Nevirapine; Ritonavir; Saquinavir; Telaprevir; Tipranavir; Voriconazole

Decreased Effect

Rifabutin may decrease the levels/effects of: Abiraterone Acetate; Alfentanil; Antifungal Agents (Azole Derivatives, Systemic); Antihepaciviral Combination Products; Apixaban; Apremilast; Aprepitant; ARIPiprazole; ARIPiprazole Lauroxil; Artemether; Atovaquone; Axitinib; Barbiturates; BCG (Intravesical); BCG Vaccine (Immunization); Bedaquiline; Boceprevir; Bortezomib; Bosutinib; Brentuximab Vedotin; Brexpiprazole; Buprenorphine; BusPIRone; Cabozantinib; Calcium Channel Blockers; Cannabidiol; Cannabis; Cariprazine; Ceritinib; Clarithromycin; CloZAPine; Cobimetinib; Contraceptives (Estrogens); Contraceptives (Progestins); Corticosteroids (Systemic); Crizotinib; CycloSPORINE (Systemic); CYP3A4 Substrates; Dabrafenib; Daclatasvir; Dapsone (Systemic); Dasatinib; Delavirdine; Dexamethasone (Systemic); Dienogest; DOXOrubicin (Conventional); Dronabinol; Dronedarone; Efavirenz; Eliglustat; Elvitegravir; Enzalutamide; Erlotinib; Etizolam; Etoposide; Etoposide Phosphate; Etravirine; Everolimus; Exemestane; FentaNYL; Flibanserin; Gefitinib; GuanFACINE; HMG-CoA Reductase Inhibitors; Hydrocodone; Hydrocortisone (Systemic); Ibrutinib; Idelalisib; Ifosfamide; Imatinib;

Indinavir; Irinotecan Products; Isavuconazonium Sulfate; Itraconazole; Ivabradine; Ivacaftor; Ixabepilone; Ixazomib; Lapatinib; Ledipasvir; Linagliptin; Lumefantrine; Lurasidone; Macitentan; Maraviroc; MethylPREDNISolone; Mifepristone; Morphine (Systemic); Mycophenolate; Naloxegol; Nelfinavir; Netupitant; Nevirapine; NIFEdipine; Nilotinib; NiMODipine; Nisoldipine; Olaparib; Osimertinib; Palbociclib; Panobinostat; PAZOPanib; Perampanel; PONATinib; Praziquantel; PrednisoLONE (Systemic); PredniSONE; Propafenone; QUEtiapine; QuiNIDine; Raltegravir; Ramelteon; Ranolazine; Regorafenib; Rilpivirine; Rivaroxaban; Roflumilast; Rolapitant; RomiDEPsin; Saquinavir; Saxagliptin; Simeprevir; Sodium Picosulfate; Sofosbuvir; Sonidegib; SORAfenib; SUNItinib; Suvorexant; Tacrolimus (Systemic); Tadalafil; Tamoxifen; Tasimelteon; Telaprevir; Temsirolimus; Tetrahydrocannabinol; Ticagrelor; Tofacitinib; Tolvaptan; Toremifene; Trabectedin; Typhoid Vaccine; Ulipristal; Vandetanib; Vemurafenib; Vilazodone; VinCRIStine (Liposomal); Vitamin K Antagonists; Vorapaxar; Voriconazole; Vortioxetine; Zaleplon; Zolpidem; Zuclopenthixol

The levels/effects of Rifabutin may be decreased by: Bosentan; CYP3A4 Inducers (Moderate); CYP3A4 Inducers (Strong); Deferasirox; Efavirenz; Mitotane; Nevirapine; Siltuximab; St Johns Wort; Tocilizumab

Food Interactions High-fat meal may decrease the rate but not the extent of absorption. Management: May administer with meals.

Storage/Stability Store at 25°C (77°F); excursions permitted to 15°C to 30°C (59°F to 86°F).

Mechanism of Action Inhibits DNA-dependent RNA polymerase at the beta subunit which prevents chain initiation

Pharmacodynamics/Kinetics

Absorption: Readily, 53%

Distribution: V_d: 9.3 L/kg

Protein binding: 85%

Metabolism: To 5 metabolites; predominantly 25-O-desacetyl-rifabutin (antimicrobial activity equivalent to parent drug; contributes ≤10% of antimicrobial activity) and 31-hydroxy-rifabutin

Bioavailability: Absolute: HIV: 20%

Half-life elimination: Terminal: 45 hours (range: 16 to 69 hours)

Time to peak, serum: 2 to 4 hours

Excretion: Urine (53% as metabolites); feces (30%)

Dosing

Adult & Geriatric

Mycobacterium avium **complex (MAC) disease (disseminated) in HIV-infected patients:** Oral:

Prophylaxis: Manufacturer's labeling: 300 mg once daily or 150 mg twice daily with food to reduce gastrointestinal upset

Treatment (off-label use): 300 mg once daily as optional adjunct therapy with clarithromycin or azithromycin (plus ethambutol) (HHS [OI adult 2015])

Tuberculosis (off-label use): Oral:

Latent tuberculosis (LTBI) treatment (to prevent TB) in HIV-infected patients: Daily dose based on concomitant ART for 4 months (HHS [OI adult 2015]) **Note:** LTBI treatment is recommended in HIV-infected patients testing positive for LTBI (but have no evidence of TB disease or no prior history of treatment for active or LTBI) **or** in HIV-infected close contacts of anyone who has infectious TB (regardless of screening tests for LTBI). LTBI treatment is not associated with clinical benefit or recommended in HIV infected patients who are anergic and who have not had recent contact with anyone with infectious TB (HHS [OI adult 2015])

Treatment of active TB (may be used as a substitute for rifampin):

Non-HIV-infected patients: 300 mg once daily or intermittently 2 to 3 times weekly as part of multidrug regimen (ATS /CDC/IDSA 2003).

HIV-infected patients (and not receiving protease inhibitors, efavirenz, rilpivirine or elvitegravir/cobicistat/emtricitabine/tenofovir): 5 mg/kg/day (usual dose: 300 mg) once daily or intermittently 3 times weekly as part of a multidrug regimen (HHS [OI adult 2015]).

Pediatric

Mycobacterium avium complex disease in HIV-exposed/-infected patients (off-label use): Oral:

Prophylaxis for recurrence of Mycobacterium avium complex (MAC): Infants and Children: 5 mg/kg (maximum dose: 300 mg) once daily as an optional add-on to primary therapy of clarithromycin and ethambutol (CDC 2009).

Prophylaxis for first episode of MAC: Children ≥6 years: 300 mg once daily (CDC 2009).

Treatment of severe MAC:
Infants and Children: 10 to 20 mg/kg (maximum dose: 300 mg) once daily, in addition to primary therapy of clarithromycin and ethambutol (CDC 2009).
Adolescents (disseminated disease): Refer to adult dosing.

Tuberculosis, treatment of active disease (as an alternative/substitute for rifampin) (off-label use): Oral:
Infants and Children: HIV-exposed/-infected patients: 10 to 20 mg/kg (maximum dose: 300 mg) once daily or intermittently 2 to 3 times weekly (CDC 2009).
Adolescents:
Non-HIV-infected patients: Adolescents ≥15 years or >40 kg: Refer to adult dosing.
HIV-infected patients (and not receiving protease inhibitors, efavirenz, rilpivirine or elvitegravir/cobicistat/emtricitabine/tenofovir): Refer to adult dosing.
Tuberculosis, LTBI treatment (to prevent TB) in HIV-infected patients (alternative to preferred therapy) (off-label use): Adolescents: Refer to adult dosing.

Renal Impairment
CrCl ≥30 mL/minute: No dosage adjustment necessary.
CrCl <30 mL/minute: Reduce dose by 50%

Hepatic Impairment
Mild impairment: No dosage adjustment necessary.
Moderate to severe impairment: There are no dosage adjustments provided in manufacturer's labeling (has not been studied).

Dietary Considerations May be taken with meals.

Administration May be administered with meals to minimize nausea or vomiting.

Monitoring Parameters Periodic liver function tests, CBC with differential, platelet count, signs/symptoms of hypersensitivity or uveitis

Dosage Forms Excipient information presented when available (limited, particularly for generics); consult specific product labeling.
Capsule, Oral:
Mycobutin: 150 mg
Generic: 150 mg

Extemporaneous Preparations A 20 mg/mL rifabutin oral suspension may be made with capsules and a 1:1 mixture of Ora-Sweet® and Ora-Plus®. Empty the the powder from eight 150 mg rifabutin capsules into a glass mortar; add 20 mL of vehicle and mix to a uniform paste. Mix while adding vehicle in incremental proportions to **almost** 60 mL; transfer to a calibrated bottle, rinse mortar with vehicle, and add quantity of vehicle sufficient to make 60 mL. Label "shake well". Stable for 12 weeks at 4°C, 25°C, 30°C, and 40°C.
Haslam JL, Egodage KL, Chen Y, et al, "Stability of Rifabutin in Two Extemporaneously Compounded Oral Liquids," *Am J Health Syst Pharm*, 1999, 56(4):333-6.

◆ Rifadin *see* Rifampin *on page 1581*
◆ Rifampicin *see* Rifampin *on page 1581*

Rifampin (rif AM pin)

Brand Names: US Rifadin
Brand Names: Canada Rifadin; Rofact
Index Terms Rifampicin
Pharmacologic Category Antibiotic, Miscellaneous; Antitubercular Agent
Use Management of active tuberculosis in combination with other agents; elimination of meningococci from the nasopharynx in asymptomatic carriers
Pregnancy Considerations Adverse events have been observed in animal reproduction studies. Rifampin crosses the human placenta. Due to the risk of tuberculosis to the fetus, treatment is recommended when the probability of maternal disease is moderate to high (ATC/CDC 2003). Postnatal hemorrhages have been reported in the infant and mother with administration during the last few weeks of pregnancy.
Breast-Feeding Considerations Rifampin is excreted in breast milk (Vorherr 1974). Due to the potential for serious adverse reactions in the nursing infant, the manufacturer recommends a decision be made whether to discontinue nursing or to discontinue the drug, taking into account the importance of treatment to the mother. The CDC does not consider rifampin a contraindication to breast-feeding (ATC/CDC 2003).
Contraindications Hypersensitivity to rifampin, any rifamycins, or any component of the formulation; concurrent use of atazanavir, darunavir, fosamprenavir, ritonavir/saquinavir, ritonavir, or tipranavir
Warnings/Precautions Use with caution and modify dosage in patients with liver impairment; observe for hyperbilirubinemia; discontinue therapy if this in conjunction with clinical symptoms or any signs of significant hepatocellular damage develop. Use with caution in patients receiving

concurrent medications associated with hepatotoxicity. Use with caution in patients with a history of alcoholism (even if ethanol consumption is discontinued during therapy). Since rifampin since rifampin has enzyme-inducing properties, porphyria exacerbation is possible; use with caution in patients with porphyria; do not use for meningococcal disease, only for short-term treatment of asymptomatic carrier states

Regimens of >600 mg once or twice weekly in adults have been associated with a high incidence of adverse reactions including a flu-like syndrome, hypersensitivity, thrombocytopenia, leukopenia, and anemia. Urine, feces, saliva, sweat, tears, and CSF may be discolored to red/orange; remove soft contact lenses during therapy since permanent staining may occur. Do not administer IV form via IM or SubQ routes; restart infusion at another site if extravasation occurs. Prolonged use may result in fungal or bacterial superinfection, including *C. difficile*-associated diarrhea (CDAD) and pseudomembranous colitis; CDAD has been observed >2 months postantibiotic treatment. Monitor for compliance in patients on intermittent therapy.

Adverse Reactions
1% to 10%:
Dermatologic: Rash (1% to 5%)
Gastrointestinal (1% to 2%): Anorexia, cramps, diarrhea, epigastric distress, flatulence, heartburn, nausea, pseudomembranous colitis, pancreatitis, vomiting
Hepatic: LFTs increased (up to 14%)
Frequency not defined:
Cardiovascular: Edema, flushing
Central nervous system: Ataxia, behavioral changes, concentration impaired, confusion, dizziness, drowsiness, fatigue, fever, headache, numbness, psychosis
Dermatologic: Pemphigoid reaction, pruritus, urticaria
Endocrine & metabolic: Adrenal insufficiency, menstrual disorders
Hematologic: Agranulocytosis (rare), DIC, eosinophilia, hemoglobin decreased, hemolysis, hemolytic anemia, leukopenia, thrombocytopenia (especially with high-dose therapy)
Hepatic: Hepatitis (rare), jaundice
Neuromuscular & skeletal: Myalgia, osteomalacia, weakness
Ocular: Exudative conjunctivitis, visual changes
Renal: Acute renal failure, BUN increased, hemoglobinuria, hematuria, interstitial nephritis, uric acid increased
Miscellaneous: Flu-like syndrome

Drug Interactions
Metabolism/Transport Effects Substrate of P-glycoprotein, SLCO1B1; **Inhibits** SLCO1B1; **Induces** CYP1A2 (strong), CYP2A6 (strong), CYP2B6 (strong), CYP2C19 (strong), CYP2C8 (strong), CYP2C9 (strong), CYP3A4 (strong), P-glycoprotein, UGT1A1

Avoid Concomitant Use
Avoid concomitant use of Rifampin with any of the following: Abiraterone Acetate; Antihepaciviral Combination Products; Apixaban; Apremilast; Aprepitant; Artemether; Atazanavir; Atovaquone; Axitinib; BCG (Intravesical); Bedaquiline; Boceprevir; Bortezomib; Bosutinib; Cabozantinib; Cariprazine; Ceritinib; CloZAPine; Cobicistat; Cobimetinib; Crizotinib; Dabigatran Etexilate; Dabrafenib; Daclatasvir; Darunavir; Delavirdine; Dienogest; Diltiazem; Dronedarone; Edoxaban; Eliglustat; Elvitegravir; Enzalutamide; Esomeprazole; Etravirine; Everolimus; Fimasartan; Flibanserin; Fosamprenavir; Ibrutinib; Idelalisib; Indinavir; Irinotecan Products; Isavuconazonium Sulfate; Itraconazole; Ivabradine; Ivacaftor; Ixazomib; Lapatinib; Ledipasvir; Lopinavir; Lumefantrine; Lurasidone; Macitentan; Mifepristone; Mycophenolate; Naloxegol; Nelfinavir; Netupitant; NIFEdipine; Nilotinib; NiMODipine; Nintedanib; Nisoldipine; Olaparib; Ombitasvir; Paritaprevir; Ritonavir, and Dasabuvir; Omeprazole; Osimertinib; Palbociclib; Panobinostat; PAZOPanib; Perampanel; Pirfenidone; PONATinib; Praziquantel; QuiNINE; Ranolazine; Regorafenib; Rilpivirine; Ritonavir; Rivaroxaban; Roflumilast; RomiDEPsin; Saquinavir; Simeprevir; Sofosbuvir; Sonidegib; SORAfenib; Suvorexant; Tasimelteon; Telaprevir; Ticagrelor; Tipranavir; Tofacitinib; Tolvaptan; Toremifene; Trabectedin; Uliprstal; Vandetanib; Vemurafenib; VinCRIStine (Liposomal); Vorapaxar; Voriconazole

Increased Effect/Toxicity
Rifampin may increase the levels/effects of: Bosentan; Clarithromycin; Clopidogrel; Cyclophosphamide; Eluxadoline; Fexofenadine; Fimasartan; Isoniazid; Leflunomide; Lopinavir; Pitavastatin; Propofol; RomiDEPsin; Saquinavir

◀

The levels/effects of Rifampin may be increased by: Antifungal Agents (Azole Derivatives, Systemic); Clarithromycin; Delavirdine; Eltrombopag; Lumacaftor; Macrolide Antibiotics; P-glycoprotein/ABCB1 Inhibitors; Pyrazinamide; Teriflunomide; Voriconazole

Decreased Effect

Rifampin may decrease the levels/effects of: Abiraterone Acetate; Afatinib; Alfentanil; Amiodarone; Antidiabetic Agents (Thiazolidinedione); Antifungal Agents (Azole Derivatives, Systemic); Antihepaciviral Combination Products; Apixaban; Apremilast; Aprepitant; ARIPiprazole; ARIPiprazole Lauroxil; Artemether; Atazanavir; Atovaquone; Axitinib; Barbiturates; Bazedoxifene; BCG (Intravesical); BCG Vaccine (Immunization); Bedaquiline; Bendamustine; Beta-Blockers; Boceprevir; Bortezomib; Bosentan; Bosutinib; Brentuximab Vedotin; Brexpiprazole; Buprenorphine; BusPIRone; Cabozantinib; Calcium Channel Blockers; Canagliflozin; Cannabidiol; Cannabis; Cariprazine; Caspofungin; Ceritinib; Chloramphenicol; Citalopram; Clarithromycin; CloZAPine; Cobicistat; Cobimetinib; Contraceptives (Estrogens); Contraceptives (Progestins); Corticosteroids (Systemic); Crizotinib; CycloSPORINE (Systemic); CYP1A2 Substrates; CYP2A6 Substrates; CYP2B6 Substrates; CYP2C19 Substrates; CYP2C8 Substrates; CYP2C9 Substrates; CYP3A4 Substrates; Dabigatran Etexilate; Dabrafenib; Daclatasvir; Dapsone (Systemic); Darunavir; Dasatinib; Deferasirox; Delavirdine; Dexamethasone (Systemic); Diclofenac (Systemic); Dienogest; Diltiazem; Disopyramide; Dolutegravir; DOXOrubicin (Conventional); Doxycycline; Dronabinol; Dronedarone; Edoxaban; Efavirenz; Eliglustat; Elvitegravir; Enzalutamide; Erlotinib; Esomeprazole; Etoposide; Etoposide Phosphate; Etravirine; Everolimus; Exemestane; FentaNYL; Fexofenadine; Flibanserin; Fosamprenavir; Fosaprepitant; Fosphenytoin; Gefitinib; GuanFACINE; HMG-CoA Reductase Inhibitors; Hydrocodone; Hydrocortisone (Systemic); Ibrutinib; Idelalisib; Imatinib; Indinavir; Irinotecan Products; Isavuconazonium Sulfate; Itraconazole; Ivabradine; Ivacaftor; Ixabepilone; Ixazomib; LamoTRIgine; Lapatinib; Ledipasvir; Linagliptin; Lopinavir; Losartan; Lumefantrine; Lurasidone; Macitentan; Maraviroc; Methadone; MethylPREDNISolone; Mifepristone; Mirabegron; Morphine (Systemic); Mycophenolate; Naloxegol; Nelfinavir; Netupitant; Nevirapine; NIFEdipine; Nilotinib; NiMODipine; Nintedanib; Nisoldipine; Nitrazepam; Olaparib; Ombitasvir, Paritaprevir, Ritonavir, and Dasabuvir; Omeprazole; Osimertinib; OxyCODONE; Palbociclib; Paliperidone; Panobinostat; PAZOPanib; Perampanel; P-glycoprotein/ABCB1 Substrates; Phenytoin; Pirfenidone; PONATinib; Prasugrel; Praziquantel; PrednisoLONE (Systemic); PredniSONE; Propafenone; QUEtiapine; QuiNIDine; QuiNINE; Raltegravir; Ramelteon; Ranolazine; Regorafenib; Repaglinide; Rilpivirine; Ritonavir; Rivaroxaban; Roflumilast; Rolapitant; Saquinavir; Saxagliptin; Simeprevir; Sirolimus; Sodium Picosulfate; Sofosbuvir; Sonidegib; SORAfenib; Sulfonylureas; SUNItinib; Suvorexant; Tacrolimus (Systemic); Tadalafil; Tamoxifen; Tasimelteon; Telaprevir; Temsirolimus; Terbinafine (Systemic); Tetrahydrocannabinol; Thyroid Products; Ticagrelor; Tipranavir; Tofacitinib; Tolvaptan; Toremifene; Trabectedin; Treprostinil; Typhoid Vaccine; Ulipristal; Valproate Products; Vandetanib; Vemurafenib; Vilazodone; VinCRIStine (Liposomal); Vorapaxar; Voriconazole; Vortioxetine; Zaleplon; Zidovudine; Zolpidem; Zuclopenthixol

The levels/effects of Rifampin may be decreased by: Lumacaftor; P-glycoprotein/ABCB1 Inducers

Food Interactions Food decreases the extent of absorption; rifampin concentrations may be decreased if taken with food. Management: Administer on an empty stomach with a glass of water (ie, 1 hour prior to, or 2 hours after meals or antacids).

Preparation for Administration Reconstitute vial with 10 mL SWFI. Prior to injection, dilute in appropriate volume of a compatible solution (eg, 100 mL D$_5$W).

Storage/Stability Store capsules and intact vials at 25°C (77°F); excursions permitted to 15°C to 30°C (59°F to 86°F); avoid excessive heat (>40°C [104°F]). Protect the intact vials from light. Reconstituted vials are stable for 24 hours at room temperature.

Stability of parenteral admixture at room temperature (25°C [77°F]) is 4 hours for D$_5$W and 24 hours for NS.

Mechanism of Action Inhibits bacterial RNA synthesis by binding to the beta subunit of DNA-dependent RNA polymerase, blocking RNA transcription

Pharmacodynamics/Kinetics

Duration: ≤24 hours

Absorption: Oral: Well absorbed; food may delay or slightly reduce peak

Distribution: Highly lipophilic; crosses blood-brain barrier well

Relative diffusion from blood into CSF: Adequate with or without inflammation (exceeds usual MICs)

CSF:blood level ratio: Inflamed meninges: 25%

Protein binding: 80%

Metabolism: Hepatic; undergoes enterohepatic recirculation

Half-life elimination: 3-4 hours; prolonged with hepatic impairment; End-stage renal disease: 1.8-11 hours

Time to peak, serum: Oral: 2-4 hours

Excretion: Feces (60% to 65%) and urine (~30%) as unchanged drug

Dosing

Adult & Geriatric

Tuberculosis, active: Oral, IV: **Note:** A four-drug regimen (isoniazid, rifampin, pyrazinamide, and ethambutol) is preferred for the initial, empiric treatment of TB. When the drug susceptibility results are available, the regimen should be altered as appropriate.

Daily therapy: 10 mg/kg/day (maximum: 600 mg/day)

Directly observed therapy (DOT): 10 mg/kg (maximum: 600 mg) administered 2 or 3 times/week (*MMWR*, 2003)

Tuberculosis, latent infection (LTBI): As an alternative to isoniazid: Oral, IV: 10 mg/kg/day (maximum: 600 mg/day) for 4 months. **Note:** Combination with pyrazinamide should not generally be offered (*MMWR*, Aug 8, 2003).

Endocarditis, prosthetic valve due to MRSA (off-label use): Oral, IV: 300 mg every 8 hours for at least 6 weeks (combine with vancomycin for the entire duration of therapy and gentamicin for the first 2 weeks) (Liu, 2011)

***H. influenzae* prophylaxis (off-label use):** Oral, IV: 600 mg every 24 hours for 4 days

Leprosy (off-label use): Oral, IV:

Multibacillary: 600 mg once monthly for 24 months in combination with ofloxacin and minocycline

Paucibacillary: 600 mg once monthly for 6 months in combination with dapsone

Single lesion: 600 mg as a single dose in combination with ofloxacin 400 mg and minocycline 100 mg

Meningococcal meningitis prophylaxis (off-label use): Oral, IV: 600 mg every 12 hours for 2 days

Meningitis *(Pneumococcus* or *Staphylococcus)* (off-label use): Oral, IV: 600 mg once daily

Nasal carriers of *Staphylococcus aureus* (off-label use): Oral, IV: 600 mg/day for 5-10 days; **Note: Must use in combination with at least one other systemic antistaphylococcal antibiotic.** Not recommended as first-line drug for decolonization; evidence is weak for use in patients with recurrent infections (Liu, 2011).

Nontuberculous mycobacterium *(M. kansasii)* (off-label use): Oral, IV: 10 mg/kg/day (maximum: 600 mg/day) for duration to include 12 months of culture-negative sputum; typically used in combination with ethambutol and isoniazid

Pharyngeal chronic carriers of group A streptococci, treatment (off-label use; IDSA guidelines): Oral: 20 mg/kg/day once daily (maximum: 600 mg daily) for the last 4 days of treatment when combined with oral penicillin V **or** 20 mg/kg/day in 2 divided doses (maximum: 600 mg daily) for 4 days when combined with intramuscular benzathine penicillin G (Shulman, 2012)

Prosthetic joint infection (off-label use): *Staphylococci (oxacillin-susceptible or -resistant):* Oral:

Debridement and prosthesis retention or following 1-stage exchange, acute treatment: 300-450 mg every 12 hours in combination with an IV antistaphylococcal antibiotic for 2-6 weeks (Osmon, 2013)

Debridement and prosthesis retention or following 1-stage exchange, chronic treatment:

Total ankle, elbow, hip, or shoulder arthroplasty: 300-450 mg every 12 hours in combination with an oral antistaphylococcal antibiotic for 3 months (Osmon, 2013)

Total knee arthroplasty: 300-450 mg every 12 hours in combination with an oral antistaphylococcal antibiotic for 6 months (Osmon, 2013)

Following resection arthroplasty with or without planned staged reimplantation: 300-450 mg every 12 hours in combination with an IV antistaphylococcal antibiotics for 4-6 weeks (Osmon, 2013)

***Staphylococcus aureus* infections, adjunctive therapy (off-label use):** Oral, IV: 600 mg once daily or 300-450 mg every 12 hours with other antibiotics. **Note:** Must be used in combination with another antistaphylococcal antibiotic to avoid rapid development of resistance (Liu, 2011).

Pediatric

Tuberculosis, active: Oral, IV:

Infants and Children <12 years:

Daily therapy: 10-20 mg/kg/day usually as a single dose (maximum: 600 mg/day)

Twice weekly directly observed therapy (DOT): 10-20 mg/kg (maximum: 600 mg)

See "Note" in adult dosing.

Tuberculosis, latent infection (LTBI): As an alternative to isoniazid: Children: 10-20 mg/kg/day (maximum: 600 mg/day) for 6 months

***H. influenzae* prophylaxis (off-label use):** Oral, IV: Infants and Children: 20 mg/kg/day every 24 hours for 4 days, not to exceed 600 mg/dose

Meningococcal prophylaxis (off-label use): Oral:

<1 month: 10 mg/kg/day in divided doses every 12 hours for 2 days

Infants and Children: 20 mg/kg/day in divided doses every 12 hours for 2 days (maximum: 600 mg/dose)

Nasal carriers of *Staphylococcus aureus* (off-label use): Oral, IV: 15 mg/kg/day divided every 12 hours for 5-10 days; **Note: Must use in combination with at least one other systemic antistaphylococcal antibiotic.** Not recommended as first-line drug for decolonization; evidence is weak for use in patients with recurrent infections (Liu, 2011).

Pharyngeal chronic carriers of group A streptococci, treatment (off-label use; IDSA guidelines): Children and Adolescents: Refer to adult dosing.

Renal Impairment No dosage adjustment necessary.

Poorly dialyzed; no supplemental dose or dosage adjustment necessary, including patients on intermittent hemodialysis, peritoneal dialysis, or continuous renal replacement therapy (eg, CVVHD).

Hepatic Impairment No dosage adjustment provided in manufacturer's labeling.

Dietary Considerations Rifampin should be taken on an empty stomach.

Administration

IV: Administer IV preparation by slow IV infusion over 30 minutes to 3 hours at a final concentration not to exceed 6 mg/mL. Do **not** administer IM or SubQ. Avoid extravasation.

Oral: Administer on an empty stomach (ie, 1 hour prior to, or 2 hours after meals or antacids) to increase total absorption. The compounded oral suspension must be shaken well before using. May mix contents of capsule with applesauce or jelly.

Monitoring Parameters Periodic (baseline and every 2-4 weeks during therapy) monitoring of liver function (AST, ALT, bilirubin), CBC, mental status, sputum culture, chest x-ray 2-3 months into treatment

Test Interactions May interfere with urine detection of opioids (false-positive); positive Coombs' reaction [direct], rifampin inhibits standard assay's ability to measure serum folate and B_{12}; transient increase in LFTs and decreased biliary excretion of contrast media

Dosage Forms Excipient information presented when available (limited, particularly for generics); consult specific product labeling.

Capsule, Oral:

Rifadin: 150 mg, 300 mg

Generic: 150 mg, 300 mg

Solution Reconstituted, Intravenous:

Rifadin: 600 mg (1 ea)

Generic: 600 mg (1 ea)

Extemporaneous Preparations A rifampin 1% w/v suspension (10 mg/mL) may be made with capsules and one of four syrups (Syrup NF, simple syrup, Syrpalta® syrup, or raspberry syrup). Empty the contents of four 300 mg capsules or eight 150 mg capsules onto a piece of weighing paper. If necessary, crush contents to produce a fine powder. Transfer powder to a 4-ounce amber glass or plastic prescription bottle. Rinse paper and spatula with 20 mL of chosen syrup and add the rinse to bottle; shake vigorously. Add 100 mL syrup to the bottle and shake vigorously. Label "shake well". Stable for 4 weeks at room temperature or refrigerated.

A 25 mg/mL oral suspension may be made with capsules and cherry syrup concentrate diluted 1:4 with simple syrup, NF. Empty the contents of ten 300 mg capsules into a mortar and reduce to a fine powder. Add 20 mL of the vehicle and mix to a uniform paste; mix while adding the vehicle in incremental proportions to **almost** 120 mL; transfer to a calibrated bottle, rinse mortar with vehicle, and add quantity of vehicle sufficient to make 120 mL. Label "shake well" and "refrigerate". Stable for 28 days refrigerated (preferred) or at room temperature.

Nahata MC, Pai VB, and Hipple TF, *Pediatric Drug Formulations*, 5th ed, Cincinnati, OH: Harvey Whitney Books Co, 2004.

Rifapentine (rif a PEN teen)

Brand Names: US Priftin

Pharmacologic Category Antitubercular Agent

Use

Active pulmonary tuberculosis: Treatment of active pulmonary tuberculosis caused by *Mycobacterium tuberculosis* in adults and children 12 years and older; must be used in combination with one or more antituberculosis drugs to which the isolate is susceptible.

Limitations of use: Rifapentine should not be used once weekly in the continuation phase regimen in combination with isoniazid in HIV-infected patients with active pulmonary tuberculosis because of a higher rate of failure and/or relapse with rifampin-resistant organisms. Rifapentine has not been studied as part of the initial phase treatment regimen in HIV-infected patients with active pulmonary tuberculosis.

Latent tuberculosis infection: Treatment of latent tuberculosis infection caused by *Mycobacterium tuberculosis*, in combination with isoniazid, in adults and children 2 years and older at high risk of progression to tuberculosis disease. To identify candidates for latent tuberculosis infection treatment, refer to Centers for Disease Control and Prevention (CDC) guidelines for current recommendations.

Limitations of use: Rifapentine in combination with isoniazid is not recommended for individuals presumed to be exposed to rifamycin- or isoniazid-resistant *M. tuberculosis*.

Pregnancy Considerations Adverse events have been observed in animal reproduction studies. Information related to the use of rifapentine in pregnant women is limited. Postnatal hemorrhages have been reported in the infant and mother with rifampin (another rifamycin) administration during the last few weeks of pregnancy. Due to the risk of tuberculosis to the fetus, treatment is recommended when the probability of maternal disease is moderate to high. The CDC does not recommend rifapentine as part of the treatment regimen due to insufficient data in pregnant women (CDC, 2003).

Breast-Feeding Considerations It is not known if rifapentine is excreted in breast milk. Because of the potential for serious adverse reactions in the nursing infant, the manufacturer recommends a decision be made whether to discontinue nursing or the drug, taking into account the importance of treatment to the mother. Rifapentine may discolor breast milk red-orange.

Medication Guide Available Yes

Contraindications Hypersensitivity to rifapentine, other rifamycins, or any component of the formulation

Warnings/Precautions Patients with abnormal liver tests and/or liver disease should only be given rifapentine when absolutely necessary and under strict medical supervision. Monitoring of liver function tests (eg, serum transaminases) should be carried out prior to therapy and then every 2 to 4 weeks during therapy. Combination therapy should be discontinued if ALT is ≥5 times the upper limit of normal (ULN) even in the absence of liver dysfunction symptoms or ≥3 times ULN in the presence of symptoms (CDC, 2012). Use is not recommended in patients with porphyria; exacerbation is possible due to enzyme-inducing properties. Hypersensitivity reactions, including anaphylaxis, may occur. Discontinue therapy and administer supportive measures if hypersensitivity occurs.

Use of rifapentine during the **initial phase** of treatment in HIV-seropositive patients has not been evaluated. Rifapentine should not be used during the **continuation phase** of treatment in HIV-seropositive patients; a higher rate of failure and/ or relapse with rifampin-resistant organisms has been reported. Use with caution in patients with cavitary pulmonary lesions and/or positive sputum cultures after initial treatment phase and patients with bilateral pulmonary disease; higher relapse rates may occur in these patients. Rifapentine may produce a red-orange discoloration of body tissues/fluids including skin, teeth, tongue, urine, feces, saliva, sputum, tears, sweat, and cerebral spinal fluid. Contact lenses may become permanently stained; remove soft contact lenses during therapy. Advise patients with dentures that permanent staining of dentures may occur.

Prolonged use may result in fungal or bacterial superinfection, including *C. difficile*-associated diarrhea (CDAD) and pseudomembranous colitis; CDAD has been observed >2 months postantibiotic treatment. Compliance with dosing regimen is absolutely necessary for successful drug therapy. Potentially significant interactions may exist, requiring dose or frequency adjustment, additional monitoring, and/or selection of alternative therapy.

Adverse Reactions Frequency may vary based on treatment phase; adverse reaction data is based on rifapentine combination therapy.

>10%:
Endocrine & metabolic: Hyperuricemia (≤32%; most likely due to pyrazinamide from initiation phase)
Genitourinary: Pyuria (11% to 22%), hematuria (10% to 18%), urinary tract infection (7% to 13%)
Hematologic & oncologic: Neutropenia (6% to 13%), lymphocytopenia (3% to 13%), anemia (2% to 11%)

1% to 10%:
Cardiovascular: Chest pain (3% to 6%), edema (1%)
Central nervous system: Pain (3% to 6%), headache (≤3%), dizziness (1%), fatigue (≤1%)
Dermatologic: Diaphoresis (2% to 5%), skin rash (3% to 4%), acne vulgaris (≤3%), pruritus (≤3%), maculopapular rash (≤2%)
Endocrine & metabolic: Hypoglycemia (5% to 10%), hyperglycemia (1% to 4%), increased nonprotein nitrogen (1% to 3%), gout (1%), hyperphosphatemia (1%)
Gastrointestinal: Anorexia (3% to 4%), nausea (≤3%), constipation (1% to 2%), dyspepsia (1% to 2%), abdominal pain (≤2%), diarrhea (≤2%), vomiting (≤2%), hemorrhoids (1%)
Genitourinary: Casts in urine (4% to 8%), cystitis (1%)
Hematologic & oncologic: Leukopenia (4% to 7%), thrombocytosis (≤6%), leukocytosis (2% to 3%), neutrophilia (1% to 3%), thrombocythemia (1% to 3%), polycythemia (≤2%), lymphadenopathy (≤1%)
Hepatic: Increased serum ALT (2% to 7%), increased serum AST (2% to 6%), hepatotoxicity (≤2%)
Hypersensitivity: Hypersensitivity reaction (≤4%; children & adolescents 1%)
Infection: Influenza (3% to 8%), herpes zoster (1%), infection (1%)
Neuromuscular & skeletal: Back pain (4% to 7%), arthralgia (≤4%), osteoarthrosis (1%), tremor (1%)
Ophthalmic: Conjunctivitis (≤3%)
Respiratory: Hemoptysis (2% to 8%), cough (3% to 6%), bronchitis (3%), pharyngitis (1% to 2%), epistaxis (1%), pleurisy (1%)
Miscellaneous: Accidental injury (1% to 5%), fever (≤1%)
<1% (Limited to important or life-threatening): Ageusia, allergic skin reaction, alopecia, anaphylaxis, asthma, azotemia, confusion, convulsions, depression, diabetes mellitus, disorientation, dysuria, enlargement of salivary glands, erythematous rash, esophagitis, fungal infection, gastritis, hematoma, hepatitis, hepatomegaly, hyperbilirubinemia, hypercalcemia, hyperhidrosis, hyperkalemia, hyperlipidemia, increased blood urea nitrogen, increased serum alkaline phosphatase, jitteriness, laryngeal edema, laryngitis, leukorrhea, lymphocytosis, myalgia, myasthenia, myositis, oropharyngeal pain, orthostatic hypotension, palpitations, pancreatitis, paresthesia, pericarditis, peripheral neuropathy, pneumonitis, pulmonary fibrosis, pulmonary tuberculosis (exacerbation), purpura, pyelonephritis, rhabdomyolysis, seizure, skin discoloration, suicidal ideation, syncope, tachycardia, thrombosis, urinary incontinence, vaginal hemorrhage, vaginitis, viral infection, voice disorder, vulvovaginal candidiasis, weight gain, weight loss

Drug Interactions
Metabolism/Transport Effects Induces CYP2C8 (strong), CYP2C9 (strong), CYP3A4 (strong)
Avoid Concomitant Use
Avoid concomitant use of Rifapentine with any of the following: Abiraterone Acetate; Antihepaciviral Combination Products; Apixaban; Apremilast; Aprepitant; Artemether; Atovaquone; Axitinib; Bedaquiline; Boceprevir; Bortezomib; Bosutinib; Cabozantinib; Cariprazine; Ceritinib; CloZAPine; Cobicistat; Cobimetinib; Crizotinib; Dabrafenib; Daclatasvir; Darunavir; Delavirdine; Dienogest; Dronedarone; Eliglustat; Elvitegravir; Enzalutamide; Etravirine; Everolimus; Flibanserin; Ibrutinib; Idelalisib; Irinotecan Products; Isavuconazonium Sulfate; Itraconazole; Ivabradine; Ivacaftor; Ixazomib; Lapatinib; Ledipasvir; Lumefantrine; Lurasidone; Macitentan; Mifepristone; Mycophenolate; Naloxegol; Netupitant; NIFEdipine; Nilotinib; NiMODipine; Nisoldipine; Olaparib; Ombitasvir, Paritaprevir, Ritonavir, and Dasabuvir; Osimertinib; Palbociclib; Panobinostat; PAZOPanib; Perampanel; PONATinib; Praziquantel; Ranolazine; Regorafenib; Rilpivirine; Rivaroxaban; Roflumilast; RomiDEPsin; Simeprevir; Sofosbuvir; Sonidegib; SORAfenib; Suvorexant; Tasimelteon; Telaprevir; Ticagrelor; Tofacitinib; Tolvaptan; Toremifene; Trabectedin; Uliprystal; Vandetanib; Vemurafenib; VinCRIStine (Liposomal); Vorapaxar; Voriconazole

Increased Effect/Toxicity
Rifapentine may increase the levels/effects of: Clarithromycin; Clopidogrel; Ifosfamide; Isoniazid; Pitavastatin; Raltegravir

The levels/effects of Rifapentine may be increased by: Antifungal Agents (Azole Derivatives, Systemic); Clarithromycin; Delavirdine; Voriconazole

Decreased Effect
Rifapentine may decrease the levels/effects of: Abiraterone Acetate; Alfentanil; Antifungal Agents (Azole Derivatives, Systemic); Antihepaciviral Combination Products; Apixaban; Apremilast; Aprepitant; ARIPiprazole; ARIPiprazole Lauroxil; Artemether; Atovaquone; Axitinib; Barbiturates; Bedaquiline; Beta-Blockers; Boceprevir; Bortezomib; Bosutinib; Brentuximab Vedotin; Brexpiprazole; Buprenorphine; BusPIRone; Cabozantinib; Calcium Channel Blockers; Cannabidiol; Cannabis; Cariprazine; Ceritinib; Clarithromycin; CloZAPine; Cobicistat; Cobimetinib; Contraceptives (Estrogens); Contraceptives (Progestins); Corticosteroids (Systemic); Crizotinib; CycloSPORINE (Systemic); CYP2C8 Substrates; CYP2C9 Substrates; CYP3A4 Substrates; Dabrafenib; Daclatasvir; Dapsone (Systemic); Darunavir; Dasatinib; Delavirdine; Dexamethasone (Systemic); Diclofenac (Systemic); Dienogest; DOXOrubicin (Conventional); Dronabinol; Dronedarone; Eliglustat; Elvitegravir; Enzalutamide; Erlotinib; Etizolam; Etoposide; Etoposide Phosphate; Etravirine; Everolimus; Exemestane; FentaNYL; Flibanserin; Gefitinib; GuanFACINE; HMG-CoA Reductase Inhibitors; Hydrocodone; Hydrocortisone (Systemic); Ibrutinib; Idelalisib; Ifosfamide; Imatinib; Irinotecan Products; Isavuconazonium Sulfate; Itraconazole; Ivabradine; Ivacaftor; Ixabepilone; Ixazomib; Lapatinib; Ledipasvir; Linagliptin; Lumefantrine; Lurasidone; Macitentan; Maraviroc; Methadone; MethylPREDNISolone; Mifepristone; Morphine (Systemic); Mycophenolate; Naloxegol; Netupitant; NIFEdipine; Nilotinib; NiMODipine; Nisoldipine; Olaparib; Ombitasvir, Paritaprevir, Ritonavir, and Dasabuvir; Osimertinib; Palbociclib; Panobinostat; PAZOPanib; Perampanel; PONATinib; Praziquantel; PrednisoLONE (Systemic); PredniSONE; Propafenone; QUEtiapine; QuiNIDine; Raltegravir; Ramelteon; Ranolazine; Regorafenib; Rilpivirine; Rivaroxaban; Roflumilast; Rolapitant; RomiDEPsin; Saxagliptin; Simeprevir; Sofosbuvir; Sonidegib; SORAfenib; SUNItinib; Suvorexant; Tacrolimus (Systemic); Tadalafil; Tamoxifen; Tasimelteon; Telaprevir; Temsirolimus; Tetrahydrocannabinol; Ticagrelor; Tofacitinib; Tolvaptan; Toremifene; Trabectedin; Treprostinil; Uliprystal; Vandetanib; Vemurafenib; Vilazodone; VinCRIStine (Liposomal); Vorapaxar; Voriconazole; Vortioxetine; Zaleplon; Zidovudine; Zolpidem; Zuclopenthixol

Food Interactions High-fat meals increase AUC and maximum serum concentration by 40% to 50%. Management: Administer with meals.

Storage/Stability Store at 25°C (77°F); excursions permitted to 15°C to 30°C (59°F to 86°F). Protect from excessive heat and humidity.

Mechanism of Action Inhibits DNA-dependent RNA polymerase in susceptible strains of *Mycobacterium tuberculosis* (MTB) (but not in mammalian cells). Rifapentine is bactericidal against both intracellular and extracellular MTB organisms.

Pharmacodynamics/Kinetics
Absorption: High-fat meals increase AUC and C_{max} by 40% to 50%.
Distribution: V_d: ~70 L
Protein binding: Rifapentine: ~98%, primarily to albumin; 25-desacetyl rifapentine: ~93%
Metabolism: Hepatic; hydrolyzed by an esterase enzyme to form the active metabolite 25-desacetyl rifapentine
Bioavailability: 70%
Half-life elimination: Rifapentine: ~17 hours; 25-desacetyl rifapentine: ~24 hours
Time to peak, serum: 3 to 10 hours
Excretion: Feces (70%); urine (17%, primarily as metabolites)

Dosing
Adult & Geriatric
Active pulmonary tuberculosis: Oral: **Rifapentine should not be used alone**; initial phase should include a 3- to 4-drug regimen
Initial phase: 600 mg twice weekly (with an interval ≥72 hours between doses) by directly observed therapy (DOT) for 2 months
Continuation phase: 600 mg once weekly by DOT for 4 months
Latent tuberculosis infection: Oral: Use once weekly for 3 months; **Note:** Must be administered under DOT and given in combination with isoniazid (maximum dose: 900 mg).
25.1 to 32 kg: 600 mg
32.1 to 50 kg: 750 mg
>50 kg: 900 mg

Pediatric

Active pulmonary tuberculosis: Children ≥12 years and Adolescents: Oral: Refer to adult dosing.

Latent tuberculosis infection: Children ≥2 years and Adolescents: Oral: Use once weekly for 3 months; **Note:** Must be administered under direct observation therapy (DOT) and given in combination with isoniazid (maximum dose: 900 mg):

10 to 14 kg: 300 mg

14.1 to 25 kg: 450 mg

25.1 to 32 kg: 600 mg

32.1 to 50 kg: 750 mg

>50 kg: 900 mg

Renal Impairment There are no dosage adjustments provided in the manufacturer's labeling (has not been studied).

Hepatic Impairment There are no dosage adjustments provided in the manufacturer's labeling; use with caution. Pharmacokinetics in varying degrees of hepatic impairment were similar to those in healthy volunteers.

Dietary Considerations Take with food.

Administration Administer with meals. For patients who cannot swallow tablets, the tablets may be crushed and added to a small amount of semi-solid food and consumed immediately.

Monitoring Parameters Patients with preexisting hepatic problems should have liver function tests monitored (eg, serum transaminases) prior to therapy and then every 2 to 4 weeks during therapy. In treatment of latent infection with rifapentine and isoniazid combination therapy, patients with HIV infection, liver disorders, immediate postpartum (≤3 months after delivery), or regular ethanol use should have liver function (at least alanine aminotransferase [ALT]) monitored prior to therapy and then at subsequent clinical visits whose baseline testing is abnormal or for others at risk for liver disease (CDC, 2012).

Test Interactions Rifampin has been shown to inhibit standard microbiological assays for serum folate and vitamin B$_{12}$; this should be considered for rifapentine; therefore, alternative assay methods should be considered.

Additional Information Rifapentine has been studied in patients with tuberculosis receiving a 6-month short-course intensive regimen approval. Outcomes were based on 6-month follow-up treatment observed in clinical trial 008 as a surrogate for the 2-year follow-up generally accepted as evidence for efficacy in the treatment of pulmonary tuberculosis. In a study of rifapentine and isoniazid given weekly by direct observation therapy for 12 weeks in latent tuberculosis, the regimen was as effective as 36 weeks of daily isoniazid alone and had higher treatment completion rates (Sterling, 2011). CDC recommends the combination of rifapentine and isoniazid once weekly for 12 weeks as an equal alternative to daily isoniazid for 9 months (CDC, 2011).

Dosage Forms Excipient information presented when available (limited, particularly for generics); consult specific product labeling.

Tablet, Oral:

Priftin: 150 mg [contains disodium edta, fd&c blue #2 aluminum lake]

Rifaximin (rif AX i min)

Brand Names: US Xifaxan

Pharmacologic Category Antibiotic, Miscellaneous

Use

Hepatic encephalopathy: Reduction in the risk of overt hepatic encephalopathy recurrence in adults

Irritable bowel syndrome with diarrhea: Treatment of irritable bowel syndrome with diarrhea (IBS-D) in adults

Traveler's diarrhea: Treatment of traveler's diarrhea caused by noninvasive strains of E. coli in adults and pediatric patients ≥12 years of age

Limitations of use: Rifaximin should not be used in patients with diarrhea complicated by fever or blood in the stool or diarrhea caused by pathogens other than E. coli.

Pregnancy Considerations Adverse events have been observed in some animal reproduction studies. Due to the limited oral absorption of rifaximin in patients with normal hepatic function, exposure to the fetus is expected to be low.

Breast-Feeding Considerations It is not known if rifaximin is excreted in human milk. Due to the potential for serious adverse reactions in the nursing infant, the manufacturer recommends a decision be made whether to discontinue nursing or to discontinue the drug, taking into account the importance of treatment to the mother. Because of the limited oral absorption of rifaximin in

patients with normal hepatic function, exposure to the nursing infant is expected to be low.

Contraindications Hypersensitivity to rifaximin, other rifamycin antibiotics, or any component of the formulation

Warnings/Precautions Hypersensitivity reactions (eg, exfoliative dermatitis, rash, urticaria, flushing, angioneurotic edema, pruritus, anaphylaxis) have occurred; these events have occurred as early as within 15 minutes of drug administration. Efficacy has not been established for the treatment of diarrhea due to pathogens other than E. coli, including C. jejuni, Shigella and Salmonella. Consider alternative therapy if symptoms persist or worsen after 24 to 48 hours of treatment. Not for treatment of systemic infections; <1% is absorbed orally. Prolonged use may result in fungal or bacterial superinfection, including C. difficile-associated diarrhea (CDAD) and pseudomembranous colitis; CDAD has been observed >2 months post-antibiotic treatment. Use caution in severe hepatic impairment (Child-Pugh class C); efficacy for prevention of encephalopathy has not been established in patients with a Model for End-Stage Liver Disease (MELD) score >25. Potentially significant drug-drug interactions may exist, requiring dose or frequency adjustment, additional monitoring, and/or selection of alternative therapy. Some dosage forms may contain propylene glycol; large amounts are potentially toxic and have been associated hyperosmolality, lactic acidosis, seizures, and respiratory depression; use caution (AAP 1997; Zar 2007).

Adverse Reactions Frequency of adverse events generally higher following treatment for hepatic encephalopathy (HE). Percentages are presented for HE unless otherwise stated.

>10%:

Cardiovascular: Peripheral edema (15%)

Central nervous system: Dizziness (13%), fatigue (12%)

Hepatic: Ascites (11%)

Gastrointestinal: Nausea (14%; irritable bowel syndrome with diarrhea 2% to 3%)

2% to 10%:

Central nervous system: Headache (travelers' diarrhea 10%), depression (7%)

Dermatological: Pruritus (9%), skin rash (5%)

Gastrointestinal: Abdominal pain (>2% to 9%), pseudomembranous colitis (<5%; travelers' diarrhea or irritable bowel syndrome with diarrhea <2%)

Hematologic & oncologic: Anemia (8%)

Hepatic: Increased serum ALT (irritable bowel syndrome with diarrhea 2%)

Neuromuscular & skeletal: Muscle spasm (9%), arthralgia (6%), increased creatine phosphokinase (<5%; travelers' diarrhea or irritable bowel syndrome with diarrhea <2%)

Respiratory: Nasopharyngitis (7%), dyspnea (6%), epistaxis (>2% to 5%)

Miscellaneous: Fever (6%)

All indications: <2% (Limited to important or life-threatening): Anaphylaxis, Clostridium difficile associated diarrhea, exfoliative dermatitis, hypersensitivity reaction

Drug Interactions

Metabolism/Transport Effects Substrate of CYP3A4 (minor), P-glycoprotein, SLCO1A2, SLCO1B1, SLCO1B3; **Note:** Assignment of Major/Minor substrate status based on clinically relevant drug interaction potential; **Inhibits** P-glycoprotein, SLCO1A2, SLCO1B1, SLCO1B3

Avoid Concomitant Use

Avoid concomitant use of Rifaximin with any of the following: BCG (Intravesical)

Increased Effect/Toxicity

The levels/effects of Rifaximin may be increased by: CycloSPORINE (Systemic); P-glycoprotein/ABCB1 Inhibitors

Decreased Effect

Rifaximin may decrease the levels/effects of: BCG (Intravesical); BCG Vaccine (Immunization); Sodium Picosulfate

Storage/Stability Store at 20°C to 25°C (68°F to 77°F); excursions permitted to 15°C to 30°C (59°F to 86°F).

Mechanism of Action Rifaximin inhibits bacterial RNA synthesis by binding to bacterial DNA-dependent RNA polymerase.

Pharmacodynamics/Kinetics

Absorption: Oral:

Traveler's diarrhea: Low

Hepatic encephalopathy: Increased absorption in patients with Child-Pugh class C compared with patients with Child-Pugh class A

Protein binding: Healthy subjects: ~68%; Hepatic impairment: 62%

Metabolism: Extensive, mainly by CYP3A

Half-life elimination: Healthy subjects: ~6 hours; IBS-D patients: 6 hours

Time to peak: Healthy subjects and ISB-D patients: ~1 hour

Excretion: Feces (~97% as unchanged drug); urine (<1%)

Dosing

Adult & Geriatric

Hepatic encephalopathy: Oral:

Reduction of overt hepatic encephalopathy recurrence: 550 mg 2 times daily. **Note:** Supporting clinical trial evaluated efficacy over 6-month treatment period.

Treatment of hepatic encephalopathy (off-label use): 400 mg every 8 hours for 5 to 10 days (Mas 2003)

Irritable bowel syndrome with diarrhea (IBS-D): Oral: 550 mg 3 times daily for 14 days; may be retreated up to 2 times with the same dosing regimen if symptoms recur.

Traveler's diarrhea: Oral: 200 mg 3 times daily for 3 days

Clostridium difficile-associated diarrhea (off-label use): Oral: 200 to 400 mg 2 to 3 times daily for 14 days (Johnson 2007)

Pediatric Traveler's diarrhea: Oral: Children ≥12 years and Adolescents: Refer to adult dosing.

Renal Impairment There are no dosage adjustments provided in the manufacturer's labeling (has not been studied).

Hepatic Impairment No dosage adjustment necessary. Use with caution in severe impairment (Child-Pugh class C); however, systemic absorption is limited and pharmacokinetic parameters are highly variable.

Dietary Considerations May be taken with or without food.

Administration Oral: Administer with or without food.

Monitoring Parameters Hypersensitivity reactions, temperature, blood in stool, change in symptoms; monitor changes in mental status in hepatic encephalopathy

Dosage Forms Excipient information presented when available (limited, particularly for generics); consult specific product labeling.

Tablet, Oral:

Xifaxan: 200 mg, 550 mg [contains edetate disodium]

Extemporaneous Preparations A 20 mg/mL oral suspension may be made using tablets. Crush six 200 mg tablets and reduce to a fine powder. Add 30 mL of a 1:1 mixture of Ora-Sweet® and Ora-Plus® or a 1:1 mixture of Ora-Sweet® SF and Ora-Plus®; mix well while adding the vehicle in geometric proportions to **almost** 60 mL; transfer to a calibrated bottle, rinse mortar with vehicle, and add quantity of vehicle sufficient to make 60 mL. Label "shake well". Stable 60 days at room temperature.

Cober MP, Johnson CE, Lee J, et al, "Stability of Extemporaneously Prepared Rifaximin Oral Suspensions," *Am J Health Syst Pharm*, 2010, 67(4):287-89.

♦ rIFN beta-1a *see* Interferon Beta-1a *on page 969*

♦ rIFN beta-1b *see* Interferon Beta-1b *on page 972*

♦ RIG *see* Rabies Immune Globulin (Human) *on page 1547*

Rilonacept (ri LON a sept)

Brand Names: US Arcalyst

Pharmacologic Category Interleukin-1 Inhibitor

Use Cryopyrin-associated periodic syndromes: For the treatment of cryopyrin-associated periodic syndromes, including familial cold autoinflammatory syndrome and Muckle-Wells syndrome in adults and children 12 years and older.

Dosing

Adult & Geriatric Cryopyrin-associated periodic syndromes: SubQ:

Initial: 320 mg given as 2 separate injections (160 mg [2 **mL**] per injection) on the same day at 2 different sites

Maintenance: 160 mg once weekly. **Note:** Begin maintenance dose 1 week following loading dose; do not administer more frequently than once weekly.

Pediatric Cryopyrin-associated periodic syndromes: SubQ:

Children ≥12 years and Adolescents <18 years:

Initial: 4.4 mg/kg (maximum loading dose: 320 mg) given as 1 to 2 separate injections (maximum single injection: 160 mg [2 **mL**]); if multiple injections are necessary, administer on the same day at 2 different sites

Maintenance: 2.2 mg/kg (maximum dose: 160 mg) once weekly. **Note:** Begin maintenance dose 1 week following loading dose; do not administer more frequently than once weekly.

Adolescents ≥18 years: Refer to adult dosing.

Renal Impairment There are no dosage adjustments provided in the manufacturer's labeling (has not been studied).

Hepatic Impairment There are no dosage adjustments provided in manufacturer's labeling (has not been studied).

Additional Information Complete prescribing information should be consulted for additional detail.

Dosage Forms Excipient information presented when available (limited, particularly for generics); consult specific product labeling.

Solution Reconstituted, Subcutaneous [preservative free]: Arcalyst: 220 mg (1 ea) [contains polyethylene glycol]

Rilpivirine (ril pi VIR een)

Brand Names: US Edurant

Brand Names: Canada Edurant

Index Terms TMC278

Pharmacologic Category Antiretroviral, Reverse Transcriptase Inhibitor, Non-nucleoside (Anti-HIV)

Use HIV-1 infection: Treatment of HIV-1 infections in antiretroviral treatment-naive patients with HIV-1 RNA ≤100,000 copies/mL at the start of therapy in combination with at least 2 other antiretroviral agents

Pregnancy Considerations Adverse events have not been observed in animal reproduction studies. Available data in pregnant women are insufficient and the DHHS Perinatal HIV Guidelines do not recommend use unless other alternatives are not available. Hypersensitivity reactions (including hepatic toxicity and rash) are more common in women on NNRTI therapy; it is not known if pregnancy increases this risk.

Regardless of CD4 count or HIV RNA copy number, all HIV-infected pregnant women should receive a combination antiretroviral (ARV) drug regimen. A combination of antepartum, intrapartum, and infant ARV prophylaxis is recommended. ARV therapy should be started as soon as possible in women with symptomatic infection. Although earlier initiation may be more effective in reducing the perinatal transmission of HIV, initiation may be delayed until after 12 weeks gestation in women who do not require immediate treatment after careful consideration of maternal conditions (eg, nausea and vomiting) and the potential risks of first trimester fetal exposure for specific agents. A scheduled cesarean delivery at 38 weeks gestation is recommended for all women with HIV RNA >1000 copies/mL or unknown concentrations near delivery in order to decrease transmission. If ARV therapy must be interrupted for <24 hours during the peripartum period, stop then restart all medications simultaneously in order to decrease the chance of developing resistance. Long-term follow-up is recommended for all infants exposed to ARV medications. In couples who want to conceive, the HIV-infected partner should attain maximum viral suppression prior to conception.

Health care providers are encouraged to enroll pregnant women exposed to antiretroviral medications in the Antiretroviral Pregnancy Registry (1-800-258-4263 or www.APRegistry.com). Health care providers caring for HIV-infected women and their infants may contact the National Perinatal HIV Hotline (888-448-8765) for clinical consultation (HHS [perinatal], 2014).

Breast-Feeding Considerations It is not known if rilpivirine is excreted into breast milk. Maternal or infant antiretroviral therapy does not completely eliminate the risk of postnatal HIV transmission. In addition, multiclass-resistant virus has been detected in breast-feeding infants despite maternal therapy. Therefore, in the United States, where formula is accessible, affordable, safe, and sustainable, and the risk of infant mortality due to diarrhea and respiratory infections is low, complete avoidance of breast-feeding by HIV-infected women is recommended to decrease potential transmission of HIV (HHS [perinatal], 2014). Similarly, the Canadian labeling does not recommend use in nursing women.

Contraindications

Coadministration with anticonvulsants (carbamazepine, oxcarbazepine, phenobarbital, phenytoin), antimycobacterials (rifampin, rifapentine), proton pump inhibitors (esomeprazole, lansoprazole, omeprazole, pantoprazole, rabeprazole), systemic dexamethasone (more than a single dose), or St John's wort.

Canadian labeling: Additional contraindications (not in US labeling): Hypersensitivity to rilpivirine or any component of the formulation

Warnings/Precautions Hypersensitivity and severe skin reactions have been reported, including severe rash or rash accompanied by fever, blisters, mucosal involvement, conjunctivitis, facial edema, angioedema, hepatitis or eosinophilia, or drug reaction with eosinophilia and systemic symptoms (DRESS) with rilpivirine-containing regimens. Some skin reactions were accompanied by constitutional

symptoms (eg, fever); other skin reactions were associated with organ dysfunction (eg, hepatic serum biochemistry elevations). In clinical trials, treatment-related rashes ≥ grade 2 were reported in 3% of patients. Most rashes were Grade 1 or 2 and occurred within the first 4 to 6 weeks of therapy. No Grade 4 rashes were reported. Monitor laboratory parameters and clinical status; discontinue if any hypersensitivity or skin rash develop. May cause depressive disorders (depression, depressed mood, dysphoria, mood changes, negative thoughts, suicide attempts, or suicidal ideation); monitor for changes and need for intervention. Causes hepatotoxicity; patients with significant transaminase elevations or hepatitis B or C prior to treatment may be at greater risk; has occurred in a few adult patients with no prior hepatic disease or risk factors. Baseline and periodic laboratory LFT evaluation during therapy is recommended. May cause redistribution of fat (eg, buffalo hump, peripheral wasting with increased abdominal girth, cushingoid appearance). Patients may develop immune reconstitution syndrome resulting in the occurrence of an inflammatory response to an indolent or residual opportunistic infection during initial HIV treatment or activation of autoimmune disorders (eg, Graves' disease, polymyositis, Guillain-Barré syndrome) later in therapy; further evaluation and treatment may be required.

Potentially significant interactions may exist, requiring dose or frequency adjustment, additional monitoring, and/or selection of alternative therapy. Doses >25 mg daily (ie, 75 mg daily, 300 mg daily) have been associated with QTc prolongation; use caution when coadministering with a drug with a known risk of torsades de pointes (HHS [adult] 2015). Do not use in adolescent and adult HIV-1 patients with a pre-ART of CD4 count <200 cells/mm^3 and/or HIV RNA >100,000 copies/mL (HHS [adult] 2015).

Adverse Reactions

>10%:

Central nervous system: Depression (5% to 9%; children and adolescents: 19%), headache (3%; children and adolescents: 19%), drowsiness (children and adolescents: 14%)

Endocrine & metabolic: Decreased plasma cortisol (7%; children and adolescents: 20%; decrease from baseline via ACTH stimulation test; clinical significance is unknown), increased serum cholesterol (7% to 17%), increased LDL cholesterol (5% to 14%)

Gastrointestinal: Nausea (1%; children and adolescents: 11%)

Hepatic: Increased serum ALT (5% to 18%), increased serum AST (4% to 16%)

1% to 10%:

Central nervous system: Dizziness (1%; children and adolescents: 8%), insomnia (3%), abnormal dreams (2%), fatigue (2%)

Dermatologic: Skin rash (3% to 6%)

Endocrine & metabolic: Increased serum triglycerides (2%)

Gastrointestinal: Abdominal pain (2%; children and adolescents: 8%), vomiting (1%; children and adolescents: 6%)

Hepatic: Increased serum bilirubin (3% to 5%)

Renal: Increased serum creatinine (1% to 6%)

<1% (Limited to important or life-threatening): Conjunctivitis, DRESS syndrome, hepatitis, hypersensitivity reaction, localized vesiculation, nephrotic syndrome, suicidal ideation

Drug Interactions

Metabolism/Transport Effects Substrate of CYP3A4 (major); **Note:** Assignment of Major/Minor substrate status based on clinically relevant drug interaction potential

Avoid Concomitant Use

Avoid concomitant use of Rilpivirine with any of the following: Antihepaciviral Combination Products; CarBAMazepine; Dexamethasone (Systemic); Efavirenz; Etravirine; Fosphenytoin; OXcarbazepine; PHENobarbital; Phenytoin; Primidone; Proton Pump Inhibitors; Reverse Transcriptase Inhibitors (Non-Nucleoside); Rifamycin Derivatives; St Johns Wort

Increased Effect/Toxicity

Rilpivirine may increase the levels/effects of: Efavirenz; Etravirine; Highest Risk QTc-Prolonging Agents; Moderate Risk QTc-Prolonging Agents

The levels/effects of Rilpivirine may be increased by: Antihepaciviral Combination Products; Boceprevir; CYP3A4 Inhibitors (Strong); Darunavir; Ketoconazole (Systemic); Lopinavir; Macrolide Antibiotics; Mifepristone; Osimertinib; Reverse Transcriptase Inhibitors (Non-Nucleoside); Simeprevir

Decreased Effect

Rilpivirine may decrease the levels/effects of: CarBAMazepine; Didanosine; Efavirenz; Etravirine; Ketoconazole (Systemic); Methadone

The levels/effects of Rilpivirine may be decreased by: Antacids; Bosentan; CarBAMazepine; CYP3A4 Inducers (Moderate); CYP3A4 Inducers (Strong); Dabrafenib; Deferasirox; Dexamethasone (Systemic); Didanosine; Enzalutamide; Fosphenytoin; H2-Antagonists; Mitotane; Osimertinib; OXcarbazepine; PHENobarbital; Phenytoin; Primidone; Proton Pump Inhibitors; Reverse Transcriptase Inhibitors (Non-Nucleoside); Rifabutin; Rifamycin Derivatives; Siltuximab; St Johns Wort; Tocilizumab

Food Interactions

Absorption increased by ~40% when taken with a normal-to high-calorie meal. Management: Administer with a normal- to high-calorie meal. Administration with a protein supplement drink alone does not increase absorption.

Grapefruit products: Grapefruit products may inhibit CYP3A4-mediated metabolism of rilpivirine and increase its exposure. Management: Avoid grapefruit products during therapy; if these products are consumed monitor for increased effects/toxicity.

Storage/Stability Store at 25°C (77°F); excursions permitted to 15°C to 30°C (59°F to 86°F). Keep in original container; protect from light.

Mechanism of Action As a non-nucleoside reverse transcriptase inhibitor, rilpivirine has activity against HIV-1 by binding to reverse transcriptase. It consequently blocks the RNA-dependent and DNA-dependent DNA polymerase activities, including HIV-1 replication. It does not require intracellular phosphorylation for antiviral activity.

Pharmacodynamics/Kinetics

Absorption: Increased 40% with a meal (normal-to-high calorie)

Protein binding: 99.7% (primarily albumin)

Metabolism: Hepatic, primarily by CYP3A4

Half-life elimination: ~50 hours

Time to peak, plasma: 4 to 5 hours

Excretion: Feces (85%, ~25% as unchanged drug); urine (~6%; <1% as unchanged drug)

Dosing

Adult

HIV-1 infection: Patients ≥35 kg: Oral: 25 mg once daily.

Dosage adjustment for concomitant therapy with rifabutin: Increase to 50 mg once daily in patients on concomitant rifabutin. Decrease to 25 mg once daily when rifabutin is stopped.

Pediatric

HIV-1 infection: Children ≥12 years and Adolescents ≥35 kg: Refer to adult dosing.

Dosage adjustment for concomitant therapy with rifabutin: Refer to adult dosing.

Renal Impairment

Mild or moderate renal impairment: No dosage adjustment necessary.

Severe or end-stage renal impairment (ESRD): Use with caution; no dosage adjustment necessary (HHS [adult] 2015).

Hemodialysis/peritoneal dialysis: Due to extensive protein binding, significant removal by hemodialysis or peritoneal dialysis is unlikely.

Hepatic Impairment

Mild to moderate impairment (Child-Pugh class A or B): No dosage adjustment necessary.

Severe impairment (Child-Pugh class C): There are no dosage adjustments provided in the manufacturer's labeling (has not been studied). Department of Health and Human Services (HHS) HIV treatment guidelines also have no dosage recommendation (HHS [adult] 2015). The Canadian labeling recommends avoiding use due to lack of data.

Dietary Considerations Take with a normal- to high-calorie meal. Taking with a protein supplement drink alone does not increase absorption.

Administration Swallow tablet whole with water. Administer with a normal- to high-calorie meal. Taking with a protein supplement drink alone does not increase absorption.

Monitoring Parameters Cholesterol, triglycerides, hepatic transaminases; signs of skin rash, fever, and/or hypersensitivity reactions, signs and symptoms of infection

Additional Information Rilpivirine has been shown in several studies to be noninferior to efavirenz in treatment-naive HIV-1 patients. Efficacy data in clinical studies exist for up to 96 weeks. Patients with CD4+ counts <200 cells/mm^3 (regardless of HIV-1 RNA at the start of therapy) are more likely to experience virologic failure (defined as HIV-1 RNA ≥50 copies/mL) than patients with CD4+ counts ≥200 cells/mm^3. Additionally, patients with

increased HIV-1 viral loads at treatment initiation (HIV-1 RNA >100,000 copies/mL) are more likely to develop virologic failure. Increased viral load patients also are more likely to develop rilpivirine-resistance, tenofovir and emtricitabine/lamivudine resistance and NNRTI class cross-resistance. Rilpivirine resistance patterns are very similar to those of etravirine (including cross resistance with single substitutions at K101P, Y181I, and Y181V) (Azijn, 2010). In rilpivirine-treated patients who experience virologic failure, rilpivirine-resistant mutations are very common (HHS [adult] 2015).

Dosage Forms Excipient information presented when available (limited, particularly for generics); consult specific product labeling.
Tablet, Oral:
Edurant: 25 mg

◆ Rilpivirine, Emtricitabine, and Tenofovir Disoproxil Fumarate see Emtricitabine, Rilpivirine, and Tenofovir Disoproxil Fumarate on page 636

◆ Rilutek see Riluzole on page 1588

◆ Rilutek® (Can) see Riluzole on page 1588

Riluzole (RIL yoo zole)

Brand Names: US Rilutek
Brand Names: Canada Apo-Riluzole®; Mylan-Riluzole; Rilutek®
Index Terms 2-Amino-6-Trifluoromethoxy-benzothiazole; RP-54274
Pharmacologic Category Glutamate Inhibitor
Use Treatment of amyotrophic lateral sclerosis (ALS); riluzole can extend survival or time to tracheostomy
Pregnancy Considerations Impaired fertility, decreased implantation, increased intrauterine death, and adverse effects on offspring growth and viability were observed in animal studies. There are no adequate or well-controlled studies in pregnant women.
Breast-Feeding Considerations It is not known if riluzole is excreted in breast milk. Breast-feeding is not recommended by the manufacturer.
Contraindications Severe hypersensitivity reactions to riluzole or any component of the formulation
Warnings/Precautions Among 4000 patients given riluzole for ALS, there were 3 cases of marked neutropenia (ANC <500/mm^3), all seen within the first 2 months of treatment. Interstitial lung disease (primarily hypersensitivity pneumonitis) has occurred, requires prompt evaluation and possible discontinuation. Use with caution in patients with concomitant renal insufficiency. Use with caution in patients with current evidence or history of abnormal liver function; do not administer if baseline liver function tests are elevated. May cause elevations in transaminases (usually transient). May cause elevations in transaminases (usually transient) within first 3 months of therapy; discontinue if ALT levels are ≥5 times upper limit of normal or if jaundice develops. The elderly or female patients may have decreased clearance of riluzole; use with caution. May cause dizziness or somnolence; caution should be used performing tasks which require alertness (operating machinery or driving). Effects may be potentiated when used with other sedative drugs or ethanol.

Adverse Reactions
>10%:
Gastrointestinal: Nausea (16%)
Neuromuscular & skeletal: Weakness (19%)
1% to 10%:
Cardiovascular: Hypertension (5%), peripheral edema (3%), tachycardia (3%)
Central nervous system: Dizziness (4%), somnolence (2%), vertigo (2%), malaise (1%)
Dermatologic: Pruritus (4%), eczema (2%), exfoliative dermatitis (1%)
Gastrointestinal: Abdominal pain (5%), vomiting (4%), flatulence (3%), oral moniliasis (1%), stomatitis (1%), tooth caries (1%)
Genitourinary: Urinary tract infection (3%), dysuria (1%)
Hepatic: Liver function tests increased (8% >3 x ULN; 2% >5 x ULN)
Neuromuscular & skeletal: Arthralgia (4%), paresthesia (circumoral; 2%), tremor (1%)
Respiratory: Lung function decreased (10%), cough increased (3%)
<1% (Limited to important or life-threatening): Alkaline phosphatase increased, amblyopia, anaphylactoid reaction, anaphylaxis, angioedema, aplastic anemia, arthrosis, asthma, ataxia, bone necrosis, bradycardia, bundle branch block, cataract, cerebral hemorrhage, deafness, dementia, diabetes mellitus, diabetes insipidus, edema, erythema multiforme, extrapyramidal syndrome, facial paralysis, gastrointestinal hemorrhage, gastrointestinal ulcer, GGT increased, glaucoma, hallucination, heart failure, hematemesis, hematuria, hemoptysis, hepatitis, hypercalcemia, hypokalemia, hypokinesia, hyponatremia, hypotension, hypersensitivity pneumonitis, interstitial lung disease, jaundice, LDH increased, leukocytosis, leukopenia, lymphadenopathy, mania, myoclonus, neutropenia, osteoporosis, pancreatitis, peripheral neuritis, pleural effusion, pseudomembranous colitis, purpura, respiratory acidosis, seizure, subarachnoid hemorrhage, thrombosis, urinary retention, urticaria, uterine hemorrhage, ventricular fibrillation, ventricular tachycardia

Drug Interactions
Metabolism/Transport Effects Substrate of CYP1A2 (major); **Note:** Assignment of Major/Minor substrate status based on clinically relevant drug interaction potential
Avoid Concomitant Use There are no known interactions where it is recommended to avoid concomitant use.
Increased Effect/Toxicity There are no known significant interactions involving an increase in effect.
Decreased Effect
The levels/effects of Riluzole may be decreased by: Cannabis; CYP1A2 Inducers (Strong); Cyproterone; Osimertinib; Teriflunomide
Food Interactions A high-fat meal decreases absorption of riluzole (decreasing AUC by 20% and peak blood levels by 45%). Charbroiled food may increase riluzole elimination. Management: Administer at the same time each day, at least 1 hour before or 2 hours after a meal.
Storage/Stability Store at 20°C to 25°C (68°F to 77°F). Protect from bright light.
Mechanism of Action Mechanism of action is not known. Pharmacologic properties include inhibitory effect on glutamate release, inactivation of voltage-dependent sodium channels; and ability to interfere with intracellular events that follow transmitter binding at excitatory amino acid receptors
Pharmacodynamics/Kinetics
Absorption: ~90%; high-fat meal decreases AUC by 20% and peak blood levels by 45%
Protein binding, plasma: 96%, primarily to albumin and lipoproteins
Metabolism: Extensively hepatic to six major and a number of minor metabolites via CYP1A2 dependent hydroxylation and glucuronidation
Bioavailability: Oral: Absolute: ~60%
Half-life elimination: 12 hours
Excretion: Urine (90%; 85% as metabolites, 2% as unchanged drug) and feces (5%) within 7 days
Dosing
Adult & Geriatric
ALS treatment: Oral: 50 mg every 12 hours; no increased benefit can be expected from higher daily doses, but adverse events are increased.
Dosage adjustment in smoking: Cigarette smoking is known to induce CYP1A2; patients who smoke cigarettes would be expected to eliminate riluzole faster. There is no information, however, on the effect of, or need for, dosage adjustment in these patients.
Renal Impairment No dosage adjustment provided in manufacturer's labeling. Use with caution.
Hepatic Impairment No dosage adjustment provided in manufacturer's labeling. Use with caution.
Dietary Considerations Take at least 1 hour before or 2 hours after a meal.
Administration Administer at the same time each day, at least 1 hour before or 2 hours after a meal.
Monitoring Parameters Monitor serum aminotransferases including ALT levels before and during therapy. Evaluate serum ALT levels every month during the first 3 months of therapy, every 3 months during the remainder of the first year and periodically thereafter. Evaluate ALT levels more frequently in patients who develop elevations. Maximum increases in serum ALT usually occurred within 3 months after the start of therapy and were usually transient when <5 times ULN (upper limits of normal). Discontinue therapy if ALT levels are ≥5 times upper limit of normal or if jaundice develops.

In trials, if ALT levels were <5 times ULN, treatment continued and ALT levels usually returned to below 2 times ULN within 2-6 months. There is no experience with continued treatment of ALS patients once ALT values exceed 5 times ULN.
Dosage Forms Excipient information presented when available (limited, particularly for generics); consult specific product labeling.
Tablet, Oral:
Rilutek: 50 mg
Generic: 50 mg

RimabotulinumtoxinB
(rime uh BOT yoo lin num TOKS in bee)

Brand Names: US Myobloc
Index Terms Botulinum Toxin Type B
Pharmacologic Category Neuromuscular Blocker Agent, Toxin
Use Treatment of cervical dystonia (spasmodic torticollis)
Medication Guide Available Yes
Dosing
Adult & Geriatric Cervical dystonia: IM: Initial: 2500-5000 units divided among the affected muscles in patients **previously treated** with botulinum toxin; initial dose in **previously untreated** patients should be lower. Subsequent dosing should be optimized according to patient's response.
Pediatric Not established in pediatric patients
Renal Impairment No dosage adjustment provided in manufacturer's labeling.
Hepatic Impairment No dosage adjustment provided in manufacturer's labeling.
Additional Information Complete prescribing information should be consulted for additional detail.
Dosage Forms Excipient information presented when available (limited, particularly for generics); consult specific product labeling.
Solution, Intramuscular [preservative free]:
Myobloc: 2500 units/0.5 mL (0.5 mL); 5000 units/mL (1 mL); 10,000 units/2 mL (2 mL) [contains albumin human]

Rimantadine (ri MAN ta deen)

Brand Names: US Flumadine
Brand Names: Canada Flumadine®
Index Terms Rimantadine Hydrochloride
Pharmacologic Category Antiviral Agent; Antiviral Agent, Adamantane
Use Prophylaxis (adults and children >1 year of age) and treatment (adults) of influenza A viral infection (per manufacturer labeling; also refer to current ACIP guidelines for recommendations during current flu season)

Note: In certain circumstances, the ACIP recommends use of rimantadine in combination with oseltamivir for the treatment or prophylaxis of influenza A infection when resistance to oseltamivir is suspected.

Dosing
Adult
Prophylaxis of influenza A: Oral: 100 mg twice daily
Note: Prophylaxis (institutional outbreak): In order to control outbreaks in institutions, if influenza A virus subtyping is unavailable and oseltamivir resistant viruses are circulating, rimantadine may be used in combination with oseltamivir if zanamivir cannot be used. Treatment should continue for ≥2 weeks and until ~10 days after illness onset in the last patient (CDC, 2011; Harper, 2009).
Treatment of influenza A: Oral: 100 mg twice daily
Geriatric Prophylaxis or treatment of influenza A: Oral: 100 mg daily in the elderly (≥65 years), including elderly nursing home patients.
Pediatric
Prophylaxis of influenza A: Oral:
Children:
1-9 years: 5 mg/kg/day in 1-2 divided doses; maximum: 150 mg/day
≥10 years and <40 kg: 5 mg/kg/day in 2 divided doses (CDC, 2011)
≥10 years and ≥40 kg: Refer to adult dosing.
Prophylaxis (institutional outbreak): Refer to adult dosing.
Treatment of influenza A: Oral: Children ≥17 years: Refer to adult dosing.
Renal Impairment
CrCl ≥30 mL/minute: No dosage adjustment necessary.
CrCl <30 mL/minute: Maximum: 100 mg daily
Hepatic Impairment Severe dysfunction: Maximum: 100 mg daily
Additional Information Complete prescribing information should be consulted for additional detail.
Dosage Forms Excipient information presented when available (limited, particularly for generics); consult specific product labeling. [DSC] = Discontinued product
Tablet, Oral, as hydrochloride:
Flumadine: 100 mg [DSC]
Flumadine: 100 mg [contains fd&c yellow #6 (sunset yellow), fd&c yellow #6 aluminum lake]
Generic: 100 mg

◆ **Rimantadine Hydrochloride** *see* Rimantadine *on page 1589*

Rimexolone (ri MEKS oh lone)

Brand Names: US Vexol
Brand Names: Canada Vexol
Pharmacologic Category Corticosteroid, Ophthalmic
Use Ophthalmic inflammatory conditions: Treatment of postoperative inflammation following ocular surgery; treatment of anterior uveitis
Dosing
Adult & Geriatric
Anterior uveitis: Ophthalmic: Instill 1 to 2 drops in conjunctival sac of affected eye every hour during waking hours for the first week, then 1 drop every 2 hours during waking hours of the second week, and then taper until uveitis is resolved
Postoperative ocular inflammation: Ophthalmic: Instill 1 to 2 drops in conjunctival sac of affected eye 4 times daily beginning 24 hours after surgery and continuing through the first 2 weeks of the postoperative period
Renal Impairment There are no dosage adjustments provided in the manufacturer's labeling.
Hepatic Impairment There are no dosage adjustments provided in the manufacturer's labeling.
Additional Information Complete prescribing information should be consulted for additional detail.
Dosage Forms Excipient information presented when available (limited, particularly for generics); consult specific product labeling.
Suspension, Ophthalmic:
Vexol: 1% (5 mL, 10 mL)

◆ **Rinnovi Nail System [DSC]** *see* Urea *on page 1853*

Riociguat (rye oh SIG ue at)

Brand Names: US Adempas
Brand Names: Canada Adempas
Index Terms Adempas; BAY 63-2521
Pharmacologic Category Soluble Guanylate Cyclase (sGC) Stimulator
Use
Chronic thromboembolic pulmonary hypertension: Treatment of adults with persistent/recurrent chronic thromboembolic pulmonary hypertension (CTEPH) (WHO group 4) after surgical treatment or inoperable CTEPH to improve exercise capacity and WHO functional class
Pulmonary arterial hypertension: Treatment of adults with pulmonary artery hypertension (PAH) (WHO group 1) to improve exercise capacity, improve WHO functional class and to delay clinical worsening
Pregnancy Considerations Reproduction studies in animals have shown evidence of fetal abnormalities and use is contraindicated in women who are or may become pregnant. **[U.S. Boxed Warnings]: Riociguat may cause fetal harm if given to pregnant women. Riociguat is available to females only through the restricted Adempas Risk Evaluation and Mitigation Strategy (REMS) Program. All females of reproductive potential should have a negative pregnancy test prior to beginning therapy and testing should continue monthly during treatment and one month after discontinuing therapy. Females of childbearing potential should not become pregnant during therapy or for 1 month following discontinuation riociguat.** All females regardless of their reproductive potential must be enrolled in the REMS program; prescribers and pharmacies must also be enrolled in the program. Females of reproductive potential must be able to comply with pregnancy testing and contraception requirements of the program. Women may use one highly effective form of contraception (intrauterine device, contraceptive implant, or tubal sterilization) or a combination of methods (hormonal contraceptive with a barrier method or two barrier methods). A hormonal contraceptive or barrier method must be used in addition to a partner's vasectomy, if that method is chosen. Females should be counseled on pregnancy prevention and planning and instructed to notify their prescriber immediately if a pregnancy should occur. Women with pulmonary arterial hypertension (PAH) are encouraged to avoid pregnancy (Badesch, 2007; McLaughlin, 2009).
Breast-Feeding Considerations It is not known if riociguat is excreted into breast milk. Due to the potential for adverse reactions in the nursing infant, the manufacturer recommends a decision be made whether to discontinue nursing or to discontinue the drug, taking into account the importance of treatment to the mother. The Canadian labeling contraindicates use in breast-feeding women.

Prescribing and Access Restrictions As a requirement of the REMS program, access to this medication is restricted. Female patients, prescribers, and pharmacies must register and be active in the Adempas REMS Program. Additional information, including certified pharmacies, is provided at www.adempasREMS.com or by calling 1-855-423-3672.

Contraindications Pregnancy; coadministration with nitrates or nitric oxide donors (eg, amyl nitrite) in any form; concomitant administration with phosphodiesterase (PDE) inhibitors, including specific PDE-5 inhibitors (eg, sildenafil, tadalafil, vardenafil) or nonspecific PDE inhibitors (eg, dipyridamole, theophylline)

Canadian labeling: Additional contraindications (not in U.S. labeling): Hypersensitivity to riociguat or any component of the formulation; breast-feeding

Warnings/Precautions Hazardous agent – use appropriate precautions for handling and disposal (meets NIOSH 2014 criteria). Reduces blood pressure. Use with caution in patients at increased risk for symptomatic hypotension or ischemia (eg, patients with hypovolemia, severe left ventricular outflow obstruction, resting hypotension, autonomic dysfunction) or concurrent use of antihypertensives or strong CYP and P-gp/BCRP inhibitors. Consider initiating at a lower dose for patients at risk of hypotension and/or dose reduction if hypotension develops. The Canadian labeling recommends avoiding use in patients with systolic blood pressure <95 mm Hg at initiation of therapy (has not been studied). Patients must be cautioned about performing tasks which require mental alertness (eg, operating machinery or driving). Serious bleeding has been observed; consider periodic monitoring for bleeding.

Use is not recommended in patients with pulmonary veno-occlusive disease (PVOD). Discontinue in any patient with pulmonary edema suggestive of PVOD. Use with caution in patients with renal and hepatic impairment. The Canadian labeling does not recommend use in patients with severe hepatic impairment (Child-Pugh class C) and patients with CrCl <15 mL/minute or receiving dialysis (has not been studied).

[U.S. Boxed Warning] May cause fetal harm if given to pregnant women. All females of reproductive potential should have a negative pregnancy test prior to beginning therapy and testing should continue monthly during treatment and one month after discontinuing therapy. Females of childbearing potential should not become pregnant during therapy or for 1 month following discontinuation of riociguat. Women may use one highly effective form of contraception (intrauterine device, contraceptive implant, or tubal sterilization) or a combination of methods (hormonal contraceptive with a barrier method or two barrier methods). A hormonal contraceptive or barrier method must be used in addition to a partner's vasectomy, if that method is chosen. Females should be counseled on pregnancy prevention and planning and instructed to notify their prescriber immediately if a pregnancy should occur. **[U.S. Boxed Warning]: Riociguat is available to females only through the restricted Adempas Risk Evaluation and Mitigation Strategy (REMS) Program.** All females, regardless of their reproductive potential, must be enrolled in the REMS program; prescribers and pharmacies must also be enrolled in the program. Females of reproductive potential must be able to comply with pregnancy testing and contraception requirements of the program. Call 855-4-ADEMPAS or visit www.AdempasREMS.com for more information.

Riociguat concentrations are 50% to 60% lower in patients who smoke compared to nonsmokers; consider titrating dose to >2.5 mg 3 times daily, if tolerated. A decreased dose may be necessary in patients who stop smoking during therapy. Potentially significant drug-drug interactions may exist, requiring dose or frequency adjustment, additional monitoring, and/or selection of alternative therapy.

Adverse Reactions Frequency not always defined.

Cardiovascular: Hypotension (3% to 10%; Ghofrani, 2013), palpitations, peripheral edema

Central nervous system: Headache (27%), dizziness (20%)

Gastrointestinal: Dyspepsia (13% to 19%; Ghofrani, 2013), nausea (14%), diarrhea (12%), vomiting (10%), gastritis (2% to 6%; Ghofrani, 2013), constipation (5%), gastroesophageal reflux disease (5%), abdominal distention, dysphagia

Hematologic & oncologic: Anemia (7%), major hemorrhage (2%; including vaginal hemorrhage, catheter site hemorrhage, subdural hematoma, hematemesis, and intra-abdominal hemorrhage)

Respiratory: Hemoptysis (1%), epistaxis, nasal congestion

Drug Interactions

Metabolism/Transport Effects Substrate of BCRP, CYP2C8 (major), CYP3A4 (major), P-glycoprotein; **Note:** Assignment of Major/Minor substrate status based on clinically relevant drug interaction potential

Avoid Concomitant Use

Avoid concomitant use of Riociguat with any of the following: Amyl Nitrite; Dipyridamole; Doxofylline; Ibudilast; Phosphodiesterase 5 Inhibitors; Theophylline Derivatives; Vasodilators (Organic Nitrates)

Increased Effect/Toxicity

Riociguat may increase the levels/effects of: Amifostine; Antipsychotic Agents (Second Generation [Atypical]); DULoxetine; Hypotension-Associated Agents; Levodopa

The levels/effects of Riociguat may be increased by: Alfuzosin; Amyl Nitrite; Anagrelide; Antihepaciviral Combination Products; Apremilast; Barbiturates; Blood Pressure Lowering Agents; Brimonidine (Topical); Cilostazol; Cobicistat; Diazoxide; Dipyridamole; Doxofylline; Eltrombopag; Herbs (Hypotensive Properties); Ibudilast; Itraconazole; Ketoconazole (Systemic); Milrinone; Molsidomine; Obinutuzumab; Osimertinib; Pentoxifylline; P-glycoprotein/ABCB1 Inhibitors; Phosphodiesterase 5 Inhibitors; Prostacyclin Analogues; Protease Inhibitors; Ranolazine; Roflumilast; Rolapitant; Teriflunomide; Theophylline Derivatives; Vasodilators (Organic Nitrates)

Decreased Effect

The levels/effects of Riociguat may be decreased by: Antacids; Bosentan; CYP2C8 Inducers (Strong); CYP3A4 Inducers (Moderate); CYP3A4 Inducers (Strong); Dabrafenib; Deferasirox; Enzalutamide; Mitotane; Osimertinib; P-glycoprotein/ABCB1 Inducers; Proton Pump Inhibitors; Siltuximab; St Johns Wort; Tocilizumab

Storage/Stability Store at 25°C (77°F); excursions are permitted from 15°C to 30°C (59°F to 86°F).

Mechanism of Action Riociguat has a dual mode of action. It sensitizes soluble guanylate cyclase (sGC) to endogenous nitric oxide (NO) by stabilizing the NO-sGC binding. Riociguat also directly stimulates sGC independent of NO. Riociguat stimulates the NO-sGC-cGMP pathway and leads to increased generation of cGMP with subsequent vasodilation.

Pharmacodynamics/Kinetics

Distribution: ~30 L

Protein binding: Plasma: ~95%

Metabolism: Mainly cleared by metabolism by CYP1A1, CYP3A, CYP2C8 and CYP2J2. Formation of the major active metabolite, M1, is catalyzed by CYP1A1, which is inducible by polycyclic aromatic hydrocarbons such as those present in cigarette smoke. M1 is only 1/3 to 1/10 as potent as the parent drug and is further metabolized to the inactive N-glucuronide. Plasma concentrations of M1 in patients with pulmonary arterial hypertension are about half those for riociguat.

Bioavailability: ~94%

Half-life elimination: Patients: 12 hours; Healthy subjects: 7 hours

Time to peak, plasma: 1.5 hours

Excretion: Feces (~53%); urine (~40%)

Dosing

Adult Chronic thromboembolic pulmonary hypertension, pulmonary arterial hypertension: Oral: Initial: 1 mg 3 times daily; may initiate dose at 0.5 mg 3 times daily in patients who may not tolerate the hypotensive effects. If tolerated, may increase the dose by 0.5 mg 3 times daily if systolic blood pressure remains >95 mm Hg and the patient has no signs or symptoms of hypotension; increase dose at intervals of ≥2 weeks. Maximum dose: 2.5 mg 3 times daily.

Missed doses: If a dose is missed, continue with the next regularly scheduled dose. If therapy is interrupted for ≥3 days, retitration is required.

Dosage adjustment for concurrent use in patients receiving strong multi-pathway CYP and P-gp/BCRP inhibitors (eg, azole antifungals or protease inhibitors):
  U.S. labeling: Consider a starting dose of 0.5 mg 3 times daily.
  Canadian labeling: Concomitant use is not recommended.

Dosage adjustment for patients who smoke: Dose may be titrated to >2.5 mg 3 times daily, if tolerated. A decreased dose may be necessary in patients who stop smoking during therapy.

Geriatric Refer to adult dosing. Use with caution; riociguat exposure is increased.

Renal Impairment

CrCl ≥15 mL/minute: No dosage adjustment provided in manufacturer's labeling.

CrCl <15 mL/minute: No dosage adjustment provided in manufacturer's labeling (has not been studied). Canadian labeling recommends avoiding use.

Dialysis: No dosage adjustment provided in manufacturer's labeling (has not been studied). Canadian labeling recommends avoiding use.

Hepatic Impairment

Mild to moderate hepatic impairment (Child-Pugh class A and B): No dosage adjustment provided in manufacturer's labeling.

Severe hepatic impairment (Child-Pugh class C): No dosage adjustment provided in manufacturer's labeling (has not been studied). Canadian labeling recommends avoiding use.

Adjustment for Toxicity

Hypotension:

U.S. labeling: Decrease dose by 0.5 mg 3 times daily if hypotensive effects are not tolerated.

Canadian labeling: If SBP <95 mm Hg and no signs/symptoms of hypotension may maintain current dose. If SBP is <95 mm Hg and signs/symptoms of hypotension are present, hold the next 3 doses and if clinically appropriate, resume 24 hours later by decreasing dose by 0.5 mg 3 times daily.

Pulmonary edema: Consider the possibility of pulmonary veno-occlusive disease (PVOD); if confirmed discontinue treatment with riociguat.

Administration

Oral: Administer with or without food.

Hazardous agent; use appropriate precautions for handling and disposal (meets NIOSH 2014 criteria).

Monitoring Parameters Monitor blood pressure and signs and symptoms of hypotension. Monitor for significant peripheral edema and improvements in pulmonary function and exercise tolerance. Women of childbearing potential must have a negative pregnancy test prior to the initiation of therapy, monthly during treatment, and 1 month after discontinuation of therapy.

Dosage Forms Excipient information presented when available (limited, particularly for generics); consult specific product labeling.

Tablet, Oral:

Adempas: 0.5 mg, 1 mg, 1.5 mg, 2 mg, 2.5 mg

◆ Riomet see MetFORMIN on page 1156

◆ Riopan Plus see Magaldrate and Simethicone on page 1118

Risedronate (ris ED roe nate)

Brand Names: US Actonel; Atelvia

Brand Names: Canada Actonel; Actonel DR; Apo-Risedronate; Auro-Risedronate; Dom-Risedronate; JAMP-Risedronate; Mylan-Risedronate; PMS-Risedronate; ratio-Risedronate; Riva-Risedronate; Sandoz-Risedronate; Teva-Risedronate

Index Terms Risedronate Sodium

Pharmacologic Category Bisphosphonate Derivative

Use

Actonel: Treatment of Paget disease of the bone; treatment and prevention of glucocorticoid-induced osteoporosis; treatment and prevention of osteoporosis in postmenopausal women; treatment of osteoporosis in men

Atelvia: Treatment of osteoporosis in postmenopausal women

Pregnancy Considerations Adverse events were observed in some animal reproduction studies. It is not known if bisphosphonates cross the placenta, but fetal exposure is expected (Djokanovic, 2008; Stathopoulos, 2011). Bisphosphonates are incorporated into the bone matrix and gradually released over time. The amount available in the systemic circulation varies by dose and duration of therapy. Theoretically, there may be a risk of fetal harm when pregnancy follows the completion of therapy; however, available data have not shown that exposure to bisphosphonates during pregnancy significantly increases the risk of adverse fetal events (Djokanovic, 2008; Levy, 2009; Stathopoulos, 2011). Until additional data is available, most sources recommend discontinuing bisphosphonate therapy in women of reproductive potential as early as possible prior to a planned pregnancy; use in premenopausal women should be reserved for special circumstances when rapid bone loss is occurring (Bhalla, 2010; Pereira, 2012; Stathopoulos, 2011). Because hypocalcemia has been described following *in utero* bisphosphonate exposure, exposed infants

should be monitored for hypocalcemia after birth (Djokanovic, 2008; Stathopoulos, 2011).

Breast-Feeding Considerations It is not known if risedronate is excreted into breast milk. Due to the potential for serious adverse reactions in the nursing infant, the manufacturer recommends a decision be made whether to discontinue nursing or to discontinue the drug, taking into account the importance of treatment to the mother.

Medication Guide Available Yes

Contraindications Hypersensitivity to risedronate, bisphosphonates, or any component of the formulation; hypocalcemia; inability to stand or sit upright for at least 30 minutes; abnormalities of the esophagus (eg, stricture, achalasia) which delay esophageal emptying

Warnings/Precautions Bisphosphonates may cause upper gastrointestinal disorders such as dysphagia, esophagitis, esophageal ulcer, and gastric ulcer; risk increases in patients unable to comply with dosing instructions. Use with caution in patients with dysphagia, esophageal disease, gastritis, duodenitis, or ulcers (may worsen underlying condition). Discontinue if new or worsening symptoms occur. Use caution in patients with renal impairment (not recommended in patients with a CrCl <30 mL/minute). Hypocalcemia must be corrected before therapy initiation with risedronate. Ensure adequate calcium and vitamin D intake, especially for patients with Paget's disease in whom the pretreatment rate of bone turnover may be greatly elevated.

Bisphosphonate therapy has been associated with osteonecrosis, primarily of the jaw. Risk factors for osteonecrosis of the jaw (ONJ) include invasive dental procedures (eg, tooth extraction, dental implants, boney surgery); a diagnosis of cancer, with concomitant chemotherapy or corticosteroids; poor oral hygiene, ill-fitting dentures; and comorbid disorders (anemia, coagulopathy, infection, pre-existing dental disease); risk may increase with duration of bisphosphonate use. Most reported cases occurred after IV bisphosphonate therapy; however, cases have been reported following oral therapy. A dental exam and preventive dentistry should be performed prior to placing patients with risk factors on chronic bisphosphonate therapy. The manufacturer's labeling states that discontinuing bisphosphonates in patients requiring invasive dental procedures may reduce the risk of ONJ. However, other experts suggest that there is no evidence that discontinuing therapy reduces the risk of developing ONJ (Assael, 2009). The risk:benefit must be assessed by the treating physician and/or dentist/surgeon prior to any invasive dental procedure. Patients developing ONJ while on bisphosphonates should receive care by an oral surgeon.

Atypical femur fractures have been reported in patients receiving bisphosphonates for treatment/prevention of osteoporosis. The fractures include subtrochanteric femur (bone just below the hip joint) and diaphyseal femur (long segment of the thigh bone). Some patients experience prodromal pain weeks or months before the fracture occurs. It is unclear if bisphosphonate therapy is the cause for these fractures, although the majority of cases have been reported in patients taking bisphosphonates. Patients receiving long-term (>3 to 5 years) therapy may be at an increased risk. Discontinue bisphosphonate therapy in patients who develop a femoral shaft fracture.

Infrequently, severe (and occasionally debilitating) bone, joint, and/or muscle pain have been reported during bisphosphonate treatment. The onset of pain ranged from a single day to several months. Consider discontinuing therapy in patients who experience severe symptoms; symptoms usually resolve upon discontinuation. Some patients experienced recurrence when rechallenged with same drug or another bisphosphonate; avoid use in patients with a history of these symptoms in association with bisphosphonate therapy.

In the management of osteoporosis, re-evaluate the need for continued therapy periodically; the optimal duration of treatment has not yet been determined. Consider discontinuing after 3 to 5 years of use in patients at low-risk for fracture; following discontinuation, re-evaluate fracture risk periodically. When using for glucocorticoid-induced osteoporosis, evaluate sex steroid hormonal status prior to treatment initiation; consider appropriate hormone replacement if necessary. Not approved for use in pediatric patients with osteogenesis imperfecta due to lack of efficacy in reducing the risk of fracture. Potentially significant drug-drug interactions may exist, requiring dose or frequency adjustment, additional monitoring, and/or selection of alternative therapy.

◀ **Adverse Reactions** Frequency may vary with product, dose, and indication.

>10%:

Cardiovascular: Hypertension (11%)

Central nervous system: Headache (3% to 18%)

Dermatologic: Skin rash (8% to 12%)

Gastrointestinal: Gastrointestinal disease (perforations, ulcers, or bleeding; 51%), diarrhea (5% to 20%), nausea (4% to 13%), abdominal pain (2% to 12%)

Genitourinary: Urinary tract infection (11%)

Infection: Infection (31%)

Neuromuscular & skeletal: Arthralgia (7% to 33%), back pain (6% to 28%)

1% to 10%:

Cardiovascular: Peripheral edema (8%), chest pain (7%), cardiac arrhythmia (2%)

Central nervous system: Depression (7%), dizziness (3% to 7%)

Endocrine & metabolic: Increased parathyroid hormone (8% to 9%; >1.5 x ULN: ≤2%), hypocalcemia (≤5%), hypophosphatemia (<3% decrease from baseline)

Gastrointestinal: Dyspepsia (4% to 8%), constipation (3% to 7%), vomiting (2% to 5%), gastritis (1% to 3%), gastroesophageal reflux disease (1% to 2%), duodenitis (≤1%), glossitis (≤1%)

Genitourinary: Benign prostatic hyperplasia (5%), nephrolithiasis (3%)

Hypersensitivity: Acute phase reaction-like symptoms (≤8%; includes fever, influenza-like illness)

Infection: Influenza (6% to 7%)

Neuromuscular & skeletal: Arthropathy (7%), myalgia (1% to 7%), limb pain (2% to 4%), musculoskeletal pain (2%), muscle spasm (1% to 2%)

Ophthalmic: Cataract (7%)

Respiratory: Flu-like symptoms (10%), pharyngitis (6%), rhinitis (6%), bronchitis (4%), upper respiratory tract infection (3% to 4%)

<1% (Limited to important or life-threatening): Esophageal ulcer, esophagitis, exacerbation of asthma, gastric ulcer, hypersensitivity reaction, osteonecrosis (primarily of the jaw), Stevens-Johnson syndrome, toxic epidermal necrolysis

Drug Interactions

Metabolism/Transport Effects None known.

Avoid Concomitant Use

Avoid concomitant use of Risedronate with any of the following: H2-Antagonists; Proton Pump Inhibitors

Increased Effect/Toxicity

Risedronate may increase the levels/effects of: Deferasirox

The levels/effects of Risedronate may be increased by: Aminoglycosides; H2-Antagonists; Nonsteroidal Anti-Inflammatory Agents; Proton Pump Inhibitors; Systemic Angiogenesis Inhibitors

Decreased Effect

The levels/effects of Risedronate may be decreased by: Antacids; Calcium Salts; Iron Salts; Magnesium Salts; Multivitamins/Minerals; Multivitamins/Minerals (with ADEK, Folate, Iron); Multivitamins/Minerals (with AE, No Iron); Proton Pump Inhibitors

Food Interactions Food reduces absorption (similar to other bisphosphonates); mean oral bioavailability is decreased when given with food. Management: Administer immediate release tablet with at least 6 oz of plain water (not mineral water) ≥30 minutes before the first food or drink of the day other than water. Administer delayed release tablet with at least 4 ounces of plain water immediately after breakfast.

Storage/Stability Store at room temperature of 20°C to 25°C (68°F to 77°F).

Mechanism of Action A bisphosphonate which inhibits bone resorption via actions on osteoclasts or on osteoclast precursors; decreases the rate of bone resorption, leading to an indirect increase in bone mineral density. In Paget's disease, characterized by disordered resorption and formation of bone, inhibition of resorption leads to an indirect decrease in bone formation; but the newly-formed bone has a more normal architecture.

Pharmacodynamics/Kinetics

Onset of action: May require weeks

Absorption: Rapid

Distribution: V_d: 13.8 L/kg

Protein binding: ~24%

Metabolism: None

Bioavailability: Poor, ~0.54% to 0.75%

Half-life elimination: Initial: 1.5 hours; Terminal: 480 to 561 hours

Time to peak, serum: 1 to 3 hours

Excretion: Urine (up to 85%); feces (as unabsorbed drug)

Dosing

Adult & Geriatric Note: Patients should receive supplemental calcium and vitamin D if dietary intake is inadequate. Consider discontinuing after 3 to 5 years of use for osteoporosis in patients at low-risk for fracture.

Paget disease of bone: Oral: *Immediate release tablet:* 30 mg once daily for 2 months

Note: Re-treatment may be considered (following post-treatment observation of at least 2 months) if relapse occurs, or if treatment fails to normalize serum alkaline phosphatase. For re-treatment, the dose and duration of therapy are the same as for initial treatment. No data are available on more than one course of retreatment. The Endocrine Society guidelines suggest retreatment may be required between 1 and 5 years (Singer, 2014).

Osteoporosis (postmenopausal): Oral:

Immediate release tablet: Prevention and treatment: 5 mg once daily **or** 35 mg once weekly **or** 150 mg once a month

Delayed release tablet: Treatment: 35 mg once weekly

Osteoporosis (males) treatment: Oral: *Immediate release tablet:* 35 mg once weekly

Osteoporosis (glucocorticoid-induced) prevention and treatment: Oral: *Immediate release tablet:* 5 mg once daily

Missed doses: Immediate release tablet:

Once-weekly: If a once-weekly dose is missed, it should be given the next morning after remembered; may then return to the original once-weekly schedule (original scheduled day of the week), however, do not give 2 doses on the same day.

Monthly (150 mg once monthly): If 150 mg once-monthly dose is missed, it should be given the next morning after remembered if the next month's scheduled dose is >7 days away. If the next month's scheduled dose is within 7 days, wait until the next month's scheduled dose. For either scenario, may then return to the original monthly schedule (original scheduled day of the month). Do not give >150 mg within 7 days.

Renal Impairment

CrCl ≥30 mL/minute: No dosage adjustment necessary.

CrCl <30 mL/minute: Use is not recommended

Hepatic Impairment No dosage adjustment provided in manufacturer's labeling (has not been studied). However, dosage adjustment unlikely because risendronate is not metabolized by the liver.

Dietary Considerations Ensure adequate calcium and vitamin D intake; if dietary intake is inadequate, dietary supplementation is recommended. Women and men should consume:

Calcium: 1000 mg/day (men: 50 to 70 years) **or** 1200 mg/day (women ≥51 years and men ≥71 years) (IOM, 2011; NOF [Cosman 2014])

Vitamin D: 800 to 1000 int. units daily (men and women ≥50 years) (NOF [Cosman 2014]). Recommended Dietary Allowance (RDA): 600 int. units daily (men and women ≤70 years) **or** 800 int. units daily (men and women ≥71 years) (IOM, 2011).

Take immediate release tablet with at least 6 oz of **plain water** (not mineral water) ≥30 minutes before the first food or drink of the day other than water. Take delayed release tablet with at least 4 ounces of **plain water** immediately **after** breakfast.

Administration Note: Avoid administration of oral calcium supplements, antacids, magnesium supplements/laxatives, and iron preparations within 30 minutes of risedronate administration.

Immediate release tablet: Risedronate immediate release tablets must be taken on an empty stomach with a full glass (6 to 8 oz) of **plain water** (not mineral water) at least 30 minutes before any food, drink, or other medications orally to avoid interference with absorption. Patient must remain sitting upright or standing for at least 30 minutes after taking (to reduce esophageal irritation). Tablet should be swallowed whole; do not crush or chew.

Delayed release tablet: Risedronate delayed release tablets must be taken with at least 4 oz of **plain water** (not mineral water) immediately after breakfast. Patient must remain sitting upright or standing for at least 30 minutes after taking (to reduce esophageal irritation). Tablet should be swallowed whole; do not cut, split, crush, or chew.

Monitoring Parameters

Osteoporosis: Bone mineral density (BMD) should be evaluated 1 to 2 years after initiating therapy and every 2 years thereafter (NOF [Cosman 2014] in patients with combined risedronate and glucocorticoid treatment, BMD should be made at initiation and repeated after 6 to 12 months; annual measurements of height and weight,

assessment of chronic back pain; serum calcium and 25 (OH)D; consider measuring biochemical markers of bone turnover

Paget disease: Alkaline phosphatase at 6 to 12 weeks for initial response to treatment (when bone turnover will have shown a substantial decline) and potentially at 6 months (maximal suppression of high bone turnover); following treatment completion, monitor at ~6- to 12-month intervals (Singer, 2014); monitoring more specific biochemical markers of bone turnover (eg, serum P1NP, NTX, serum beta-CTx) is generally only warranted in patients with Paget disease who have abnormal liver or biliary tract function or when early assessment of response to treatment is needed (eg, spinal compression, very active disease) (Singer, 2014); serum calcium and 25(OH)D; pain

Reference Range
Calcium (total): Adults: 9 to 11 mg/dL (2.05 to 2.54 mmol/L), may slightly decrease with aging

Phosphorus: 2.5 to 4.5 mg/dL (0.81 to 1.45 mmol/L)

Vitamin D: There is no clear consensus on a reference range for total serum 25(OH)D concentrations or the validity of this level as it relates clinically to bone health. In addition, there is significant variability in the reporting of serum 25(OH)D levels as a result of different assay types in use; however, the following ranges have been suggested:

Adults (IOM, 2011): Sufficient levels in practically all persons: ≥20 ng/mL (50 nmol/L); concern for risk of toxicity: >50 ng/mL (125 nmol/L)

Osteoporosis patients (NOF [Cosman 2014]): Recommended level to reach and maintain: ~30 ng/mL (75 nmol/L)

Test Interactions Bisphosphonates may interfere with diagnostic imaging agents such as technetium-99m-diphosphonate in bone scans.

Dosage Forms Excipient information presented when available (limited, particularly for generics); consult specific product labeling.

Tablet, Oral, as sodium:
Actonel: 5 mg, 30 mg, 35 mg
Actonel: 150 mg [contains fd&c blue #2 aluminum lake]
Generic: 5 mg, 30 mg, 35 mg, 150 mg

Tablet Delayed Release, Oral, as sodium:
Atelvia: 35 mg [contains edetate disodium]
Generic: 35 mg

RisperiDONE (ris PER i done)

Brand Names: US RisperDAL; RisperDAL Consta; RisperDAL M-TAB; RisperiDONE M-TAB

Brand Names: Canada ACT Risperidone; Apo-Risperidone; Ava-Risperidone; Dom-Risperidone; JAMP-Risperidone; Mar-Risperidone; Mint-Risperidone; Mylan-Risperidone; Mylan-Risperidone ODT; PHL-Risperidone; PMS-Risperidone; PMS-Risperidone ODT; PRO-Risperidone; RAN-Risperidone; ratio-Risperidone; Risperdal; Risperdal Consta; Risperdal M-Tab; Riva-Risperidone; Sandoz-Risperidone; Teva-Risperidone

Index Terms Risperdal M-Tab

Pharmacologic Category Antimanic Agent; Second Generation (Atypical) Antipsychotic

Use
Oral: Treatment of schizophrenia; treatment of acute mania or mixed episodes associated with bipolar I disorder (as monotherapy in children or adults, or in combination with lithium or valproate in adults); treatment of irritability/aggression associated with autistic disorder

Canadian labeling: Additional use (not in US labeling): Short-term treatment of aggression or psychotic symptoms in patients with severe dementia of the Alzheimer type unresponsive to nonpharmacologic therapy and when there is risk of harm to self or others.

Injection: Treatment of schizophrenia; maintenance treatment of bipolar I disorder in adults as monotherapy or in combination with lithium or valproate

Pregnancy Considerations Adverse events were observed in animal reproduction studies. In human studies, risperidone and its metabolite cross the placenta (Newport, 2007). An increased risk of teratogenic effects has not been observed following maternal use of risperidone (limited data) (Coppola, 2007). Agenesis of the corpus callosum has been noted in one case report of an infant exposed in utero; relationship to risperidone exposure is not known. Antipsychotic use during the third trimester of pregnancy has a risk for extrapyramidal symptoms (EPS) and/or withdrawal symptoms in newborns following delivery. Symptoms in the newborn may include agitation, feeding disorder, hypertonia, hypotonia, respiratory distress, somnolence, and tremor. These effects may be self-limiting and allow recovery within hours or days with no specific treatment, or they may be severe requiring prolonged hospitalization. When using Risperdal® Consta®, patients should notify healthcare provider if they become or intend to become pregnant during therapy or within 12 weeks of last injection. Risperidone may cause hyperprolactinemia, which may decrease reproductive function in both males and females.

The ACOG recommends that therapy during pregnancy be individualized; treatment with psychiatric medications during pregnancy should incorporate the clinical expertise of the mental health clinician, obstetrician, primary healthcare provider, and pediatrician. Safety data related to atypical antipsychotics during pregnancy is limited and routine use is not recommended. However, if a woman is inadvertently exposed to an atypical antipsychotic while pregnant, continuing therapy may be preferable to switching to a typical antipsychotic that the fetus has not yet been exposed to; consider risk:benefit (ACOG, 2008).

Healthcare providers are encouraged to enroll women 18 to 45 years of age exposed to risperidone during pregnancy in the Atypical Antipsychotics Pregnancy Registry (1-866-961-2388 or http://www.womensmentalhealth.org/pregnancyregistry).

Breast-Feeding Considerations Risperidone and its metabolite are excreted in breast milk. Due to the potential for serious adverse reactions in the nursing infant, the manufacturer recommends a decision be made whether to discontinue nursing or to discontinue the drug, taking into account the importance of treatment to the mother. It is also recommended that women using Risperdal Consta not breast-feed during therapy or for 12 weeks after the last injection.

Contraindications Hypersensitivity to risperidone or any component of the formulation

Warnings/Precautions Hazardous agent - use appropriate precautions for handling and disposal (NIOSH 2014 [group 2]).

[US Boxed Warning]: Elderly patients with dementia-related psychosis treated with antipsychotics are at an increased risk of death compared to placebo. Most deaths appeared to be either cardiovascular (eg, heart failure, sudden death) or infectious (eg, pneumonia) in nature. In addition, an increased incidence of cerebrovascular effects (eg, transient ischemic attack, cerebrovascular accidents) has been reported in studies of placebo-controlled trials of risperidone in elderly patients with dementia-related psychosis. Use with caution in dementia with Lewy bodies; antipsychotics may worsen dementia symptoms and patients with dementia with Lewy bodies are more sensitive to the extrapyramidal side effects (APA [Rabins, 2007]). Risperidone is not approved for the treatment of dementia-related psychosis. The Canadian labeling indicates risperidone (oral) for short-term use in severe Alzheimer dementia to manage aggression and psychotic symptoms. Careful assessment of risk factors for stroke or existing cardiovascular morbidities is required prior to initiation.

Leukopenia, neutropenia, and agranulocytosis (sometimes fatal) have been reported in clinical trials and postmarketing reports with antipsychotic use; presence of risk factors (eg, preexisting low WBC or history of drug-induced leuko-/neutropenia) should prompt periodic blood count assessment. Discontinue therapy at first signs of blood dyscrasias or if absolute neutrophil count <1,000/mm^3.

Low to moderately sedating, use with caution in disorders where CNS depression is a feature. Use with caution in Parkinson disease; antipsychotics may aggravate the motor disturbances of Parkinson disease (APA [Rabins, 2007]). Caution in patients with predisposition to seizures. Use with caution in renal or hepatic dysfunction; dose reduction recommended. Esophageal dysmotility and aspiration have been associated with antipsychotic use; use with caution in patients at risk of aspiration pneumonia (ie, Alzheimer's disease). Risperidone is associated with greater increases in prolactin levels as compared to other antipsychotic agents; clinical significance of hyperprolactinemia in patients with breast cancer or other prolactin-dependent tumors is unknown. May alter temperature regulation. May mask toxicity of other drugs or conditions

◄ (eg, intestinal obstruction, Reyes syndrome, brain tumor) due to antiemetic effects. Neutropenia has been reported with antipsychotic use, including fatal cases of agranulocytosis. Preexisting myelosuppression (disease or drug-induced) increases risk and these patients should have frequent CBC monitoring; decreased blood counts in absence of other causative factors should prompt discontinuation of therapy.

Use with caution in patients with cardiovascular diseases (eg, heart failure, history of myocardial infarction or ischemia, cerebrovascular disease, conduction abnormalities). May cause orthostatic hypotension; use with caution in patients at risk of this effect (eg, concurrent medication use which may predispose to hypotension/bradycardia or presence of hypovolemia) or in those who would not tolerate transient hypotensive episodes. May alter cardiac conduction (low risk relative to other neuroleptics); life-threatening arrhythmias have occurred with therapeutic doses of neuroleptics.

May cause anticholinergic effects (confusion, agitation, constipation, xerostomia, blurred vision, urinary retention); therefore, they should be used with caution in patients with decreased gastrointestinal motility, urinary retention, BPH, xerostomia, or visual problems (including narrow-angle glaucoma). Relative to other neuroleptics, risperidone has a low potency of cholinergic blockade. Few case reports describe intraoperative floppy iris syndrome (IFIS) in patients receiving risperidone and undergoing cataract surgery (Ford, 2011). Prior to cataract surgery, evaluate for prior or current risperidone use. The benefits or risks of interrupting risperidone prior to surgery have not been established; clinicians are advised to proceed with surgery cautiously.

May cause extrapyramidal symptoms, including pseudoparkinsonism, acute dystonic reactions, akathisia, and tardive dyskinesia. Risk of dystonia (and possibly other EPS) may be greater with increased doses, use of conventional antipsychotics, males, and younger patients. Risk of tardive dyskinesia and potential for irreversibility may be increased in elderly patients (particularly women), prolonged therapy, and higher total cumulative dose. Risk of neuroleptic malignant syndrome (NMS) may be increased in patients with Parkinson's disease or Lewy body dementia; monitor for symptoms of confusion, obtundation, postural instability and extrapyramidal symptoms. May cause hyperglycemia; in some cases may be extreme and associated with ketoacidosis, hyperosmolar coma, or death. Use with caution in patients with diabetes or other disorders of glucose regulation; monitor for worsening of glucose control. Dyslipidemia has been reported with atypical antipsychotics; risk profile may differ between agents. Discrepant results have been reported in clinical trials, regarding lipid changes associated with risperidone (American Diabetes Association, 2004). Significant weight gain has been observed with antipsychotic therapy; incidence varies with product. Monitor waist circumference and BMI. Rare cases of priapism have been reported.

Use in elderly patients with dementia is associated with an increased risk of mortality and cerebrovascular accidents; avoid antipsychotic use for behavioral problems associated with dementia unless alternative nonpharmacologic therapies have failed and patient may harm self or others. In addition, use may cause or exacerbate syndrome of inappropriate antidiuretic hormone secretion or hyponatremia; monitor sodium closely with initiation or dosage adjustments in older adults (Beers Criteria).

The possibility of a suicide attempt is inherent in psychotic illness or bipolar disorder; use caution in high-risk patients during initiation of therapy. Prescriptions should be written for the smallest quantity consistent with good patient care. Long-term effects on growth or sexual maturation have not been evaluated. Vehicle used in injectable suspension (polylactide-co-glycolide microspheres) has rarely been associated with retinal artery occlusion in patients with abnormal arteriovenous anastomosis; not for intravenous use; administer only as an intramuscular injection.

Potentially significant drug-drug interactions may exist, requiring dose or frequency adjustment, additional monitoring, and/or selection of alternative therapy. Benzyl alcohol and derivatives: Some dosage forms may contain sodium benzoate/benzoic acid; benzoic acid (benzoate) is a metabolite of benzyl alcohol; large amounts of benzyl alcohol (≥99 mg/kg/day) have been associated with a potentially fatal toxicity ("gasping syndrome") in neonates; the "gasping syndrome" consists of metabolic acidosis, respiratory distress, gasping respirations, CNS dysfunction (including convulsions, intracranial hemorrhage), hypotension, and cardiovascular collapse (AAP ["Inactive" 1997]; CDC, 1982); some data suggests that benzoate displaces bilirubin from protein binding sites (Ahlfors, 2001); avoid or use dosage forms containing benzyl alcohol derivative with caution in neonates. See manufacturer's labeling.

Adverse Reactions

>10%:

Central nervous system: Sedation (children 12% to 63%; adults 5% to 11%), parkinsonian-like syndrome (children 6% to 62%; adults 8% to 25%), drowsiness (adults 5% to 41%; children 4% to 11%), insomnia (≤32%), fatigue (children 18% to 31%; adults 1% to 9%), headache (12% to 21%), anxiety (≤8% to 16%), dizziness (3% to 16%), drooling (children 12%; adults <4%), akathisia (5% to 11%)

Endocrine & metabolic: Weight gain (≥7% kg increase from baseline: children 8% to 33%; adults 4% to 21%)

Gastrointestinal: Increased appetite (children 4% to 44%; adults 4%), vomiting (children 10% to 20%; adults <4%), constipation (5% to 17%), abdominal pain (children 6% to 16%; adults <4%), nausea (5% to 16%)

Genitourinary: Urinary incontinence (children 16%; adults <4%)

Neuromuscular & skeletal: Tremor (adults ≤24%; children ≤11%)

Respiratory: Nasopharyngitis (children 19%; adults ≤4%), cough (children ≤17%; adults ≤4%), rhinorrhea (children 12%; adults <4%)

Miscellaneous: Fever (children 16%; adults 1% to 2%)

1% to 10%:

Cardiovascular: Bradycardia (<4%), bundle branch block (<4%), buttock pain (<4%), chest pain (<4%), ECG changes (<4%), facial edema (<4%), first degree atrioventricular block (<4%), hypotension (<4%), orthostatic hypotension (<4%), palpitations (<4%), paresthesia (<4%), prolonged Q-T interval on ECG (<4%), tachycardia (adults <4%; children <1%), hypertension (≤3%), peripheral edema (≤3%), syncope (1% to 2%)

Central nervous system: Dystonia (2% to 6%), abnormal gait (4%), pain (1% to 4%), decreased attention span (≤4%), agitation (<4%), ataxia (<4%), depression (<4%), disturbed sleep (<4%), falling (<4%), lethargy (<4%), malaise (<4%), nervousness (<4%), orthostatic dizziness (<4%), seizure (<4%), tardive dyskinesia (<4%), vertigo (<4%), hypoesthesia (≤2%)

Dermatologic: Skin rash (<4% to 8%), eczema (<4%), pruritus (<4%), skin sclerosis (<4%), xeroderma (≤3%), acne vulgaris (<1% to 2%)

Endocrine & metabolic: Increased thirst (children ≤7%; adults <1%), weight loss (≤4%), amenorrhea (4%), decreased libido (<4%), galactorrhea (<4%), gynecomastia (<4%), hyperglycemia (<4%), hyperprolactinemia (<4%), increased gamma-glutamyl transferase (<4%), oligomenorrhea (<4%)

Gastrointestinal: Xerostomia (≤7% to 10%), dyspepsia (3% to 10%), sialorrhea (1% to 10%), diarrhea (<4% to 8%), decreased appetite (≤6%), anorexia (<4%), gastritis (<4%), gastroenteritis (<4%), toothache (≤3%)

Genitourinary: Menstruation (≤4%), cystitis (<4%), ejaculatory disorder (<4%), erectile dysfunction (<4%), glycosuria (<4%), irregular menses (<4%), mastalgia (<4%), sexual disorder (<4%), urinary tract infection (<4%)

Hematologic & oncologic: Anemia (<4%), neutropenia (<4%)

Hepatic: Increased serum ALT (<4%), increased serum AST (<4%)

Hypersensitivity: Hypersensitivity (<4%)

Infection: Infection (<4%), influenza (<4%), localized infection (<4%), subcutaneous abscess (<4%), viral infection (<4%)

Local: Induration at injection site (<4%), injection site reaction (<4%), pain at injection site (<4%), swelling at injection site (<4%)

Neuromuscular & skeletal: Limb pain (2% to 6%), dyskinesia (adults ≤6%; children <1%), back pain (≤4%), arthralgia (2% to 4%), abnormal posture (<4%), akinesia (<4%), hypokinesia (<4%), musculoskeletal chest pain (<4%), myalgia (<4%), neck pain (<4%), weakness (<4%), increased creatine phosphokinase (≤2%)

Ophthalmic: Blurred vision (2% to 7%), conjunctivitis (<4%), reduced visual acuity (<4%)

Otic: Otalgia (≤4%), otic infection (<4%)

Respiratory: Nasal congestion (≤6% to 10%), pharyngolaryngeal pain (3% to 10%), rhinitis (<4% to 9%), respiratory tract infection (≤6% to 8%), bronchitis (<4%), dyspnea (<4%), flu-like symptoms (<4%), pharyngitis (<4%), pneumonia (<4%), sinusitis (<4%), epistaxis (≤2%), sinus congestion (≤2%)

<1% (Limited to important or life-threatening): Abnormal erythrocytes, abscess at injection site, acariasis, agranulocytosis, alopecia, anaphylaxis, angioedema, apnea, aspiration, atrial fibrillation, atrial premature contractions, cardiorespiratory arrest, cerebral ischemia,

cerebrovascular accident, cholestatic hepatitis, cholinergic syndrome, coma, cyst, delirium, depression of ST segment on ECG, dermal ulcer, diabetes mellitus, diabetic coma, diabetic ketoacidosis, disruption of body temperature regulation, diverticulitis, esophageal motility disorder, eye infection, fecal incontinence, fecaloma, glaucoma, granulocytopenia, hematoma, hemorrhage, hepatic failure, hepatic injury, hyperkeratosis, hyperthermia, hypertonia, hypertriglyceridemia, hyperuricemia, hypoglycemia, hypokalemia, hyponatremia, hypothermia, impaired consciousness, increased serum cholesterol, intestinal obstruction, intraoperative floppy iris syndrome, leukocytosis, leukopenia, leukorrhea, lower respiratory tract infection, lymphadenopathy, mania, migraine, myocardial infarction, myocarditis, neuroleptic malignant syndrome, nystagmus, ocular hyperemia, pancreatitis, Pelger-Huët anomaly, phlebitis, pituitary neoplasm, precocious puberty, priapism, pulmonary embolism, renal insufficiency, retinal artery occlusion, retrograde ejaculation, rhabdomyolysis, SIADH, sleep apnea, swelling of eye, synostosis, thrombocytopenia, thrombophlebitis, thrombotic thrombocytopenic purpura, tissue necrosis, tongue paralysis, torticollis, transient ischemic attacks, unresponsive to stimuli, urinary retention, ventricular premature contractions, ventricular tachycardia, water intoxication, withdrawal syndrome

Drug Interactions

Metabolism/Transport Effects Substrate of CYP2D6 (major), CYP3A4 (minor), P-glycoprotein; **Note:** Assignment of Major/Minor substrate status based on clinically relevant drug interaction potential; **Inhibits** CYP2D6 (weak)

Avoid Concomitant Use

Avoid concomitant use of RisperiDONE with any of the following: Aclidinium; Amisulpride; Azelastine (Nasal); Cimetropium; Eluxadoline; Glucagon; Glycopyrrolate; Glycopyrrolate (Oral Inhalation); Ipratropium (Oral Inhalation); Levosulpiride; Metoclopramide; Orphenadrine; Paraldehyde; Potassium Chloride; Sulpiride; Thalidomide; Tiotropium; Umeclidinium

Increased Effect/Toxicity

RisperiDONE may increase the levels/effects of: AbobotulinumtoxinA; Alcohol (Ethyl); Amisulpride; Analgesics (Opioid); Anticholinergic Agents; ARIPiprazole; Azelastine (Nasal); Buprenorphine; Cimetropium; CNS Depressants; Eluxadoline; Glucagon; Glycopyrrolate; Glycopyrrolate (Oral Inhalation); Highest Risk QTc-Prolonging Agents; Hydrocodone; Mequitazine; Methotrimeprazine; Methylphenidate; Metyrosine; Mirabegron; Mirtazapine; Moderate Risk QTc-Prolonging Agents; OnabotulinumtoxinA; Orphenadrine; Paliperidone; Paraldehyde; Potassium Chloride; Ramosetron; RimabotulinumtoxinB; Selective Serotonin Reuptake Inhibitors; Serotonin Modulators; Sulpiride; Suvorexant; Thalidomide; Thiazide Diuretics; Tiotropium; Topiramate; Zolpidem

The levels/effects of RisperiDONE may be increased by: Abiraterone Acetate; Acetylcholinesterase Inhibitors (Central); Aclidinium; Blood Pressure Lowering Agents; Brimonidine (Topical); Cannabis; Cobicistat; CYP2D6 Inhibitors (Moderate); CYP2D6 Inhibitors (Strong); Darunavir; Doxylamine; Dronabinol; Droperidol; HydrOXYzine; Ipratropium (Oral Inhalation); Kava Kava; Lithium; Loop Diuretics; Lumacaftor; Magnesium Sulfate; Methotrimeprazine; Methylphenidate; Metoclopramide; Metyrosine; Mianserin; Mifepristone; Minocycline; Nabilone; Panobinostat; Peginterferon Alfa-2b; Perampanel; P-glycoprotein/ABCB1 Inhibitors; Pramlintide; Ranolazine; Rufinamide; Selective Serotonin Reuptake Inhibitors; Serotonin Modulators; Sodium Oxybate; Tapentadol; Tetrahydrocannabinol; Umeclidinium; Valproate Products; Verapamil

Decreased Effect

RisperiDONE may decrease the levels/effects of: Acetylcholinesterase Inhibitors; Amphetamines; Antidiabetic Agents; Anti-Parkinson's Agents (Dopamine Agonist); Gastrointestinal Agents (Prokinetic); Itopride; Levosulpiride; Quinagolide; Secretin

The levels/effects of RisperiDONE may be decreased by: Acetylcholinesterase Inhibitors; CarBAMazepine; Lithium; Lumacaftor; Peginterferon Alfa-2b; P-glycoprotein/ABCB1 Inducers

Food Interactions Oral solution is not compatible with beverages containing tannin or pectinate (cola or tea). Management: Administer oral solution with water, coffee, orange juice, or low-fat milk.

Preparation for Administration Hazardous agent; use appropriate precautions for handling and disposal (NIOSH 2014 [group 2]).

Risperdal Consta: Do not substitute any components of the dose pack. Bring to room temperature for ≥30 minutes prior to reconstitution (do not warm any other way). Reconstitute with provided diluent only. Refer to the manufacturer's labeling for device assembly and reconstitution instructions. Do not store suspension after reconstitution; administer immediately after reconstitution.

Storage/Stability

Injection: Risperdal Consta: Store at 2°C to 8°C (36°F to 46°F) and protect from light. May be stored at 25°C (77°F) for up to 7 days prior to administration; do not expose unrefrigerated product to temperatures above 77°F (25°C). Following reconstitution, administer immediately (do not store for future use).

Oral solution, tablet: Store at 15°C to 25°C (59°F to 77°F). Protect from light and moisture. Keep orally-disintegrating tablets sealed in foil pouch until ready to use. Do not freeze solution.

Mechanism of Action Risperidone is a benzisoxazole atypical antipsychotic with mixed serotonin-dopamine antagonist activity that binds to 5-HT$_2$-receptors in the CNS and in the periphery with a very high affinity; binds to dopamine-D$_2$ receptors with less affinity. The binding affinity to the dopamine-D$_2$ receptor is 20 times lower than the 5-HT$_2$ affinity. The addition of serotonin antagonism to dopamine antagonism (classic neuroleptic mechanism) is thought to improve negative symptoms of psychoses and reduce the incidence of extrapyramidal side effects. Alpha$_1$, alpha$_2$ adrenergic, and histaminergic receptors are also antagonized with high affinity. Risperidone has low to moderate affinity for 5-HT$_{1C}$, 5-HT$_{1D}$, and 5-HT$_{1A}$ receptors, weak affinity for D$_1$ and no affinity for muscarinics or beta$_1$ and beta$_2$ receptors

Pharmacodynamics/Kinetics

Absorption:

Oral: Rapid and well absorbed; food does not affect rate or extent

Injection: <1% absorbed initially; main release occurs at ~3 weeks and is maintained from 4 to 6 weeks

Distribution: V$_d$: 1 to 2 L/kg

Protein binding, plasma: Risperidone 90%; 9-hydroxyrisperidone: 77%

Metabolism: Extensively hepatic via CYP2D6 to 9-hydroxyrisperidone (similar pharmacological activity as risperidone); *N*-dealkylation is a second minor pathway

Bioavailability: Oral: 70%; Tablet (relative to solution): 94%; orally-disintegrating tablets and oral solution are bioequivalent to tablets

Half-life elimination: Active moiety (risperidone and its active metabolite 9-hydroxyrisperidone)

Oral: 20 hours (mean)

Extensive metabolizers: Risperidone: 3 hours; 9-hydroxyrisperidone: 21 hours

Poor metabolizers: Risperidone: 20 hours; 9-hydroxyrisperidone: 30 hours

Injection: 3 to 6 days; related to microsphere erosion and subsequent absorption of risperidone

Time to peak, plasma: Oral: Risperidone: Within 1 hour; 9-hydroxyrisperidone: Extensive metabolizers: 3 hours; Poor metabolizers: 17 hours

Excretion: Urine (70%); feces (14%)

Dosing

Adult Note: When reinitiating treatment after discontinuation, the initial titration schedule should be followed. Limiting initial dose to 2 mg daily (in 1 or 2 divided doses) may reduce the risk of orthostatic hypotension/syncope.

Bipolar mania: *Oral:* Recommended starting dose: 2 to 3 mg once daily; if needed, adjust dose by 1 mg daily in intervals ≥24 hours; dosing range: 1 to 6 mg daily.

Maintenance: No dosing recommendation available for treatment >3 weeks duration

Bipolar I maintenance: *IM (Risperdal Consta):* 25 mg every 2 weeks; if unresponsive, some may benefit from larger doses (37.5 to 50 mg); maximum dose: 50 mg every 2 weeks. Dosage adjustments should not be made more frequently than every 4 weeks. A lower initial dose of 12.5 mg may be appropriate in some patients (eg, demonstrated poor tolerability to other psychotropic medications).

Note: Oral risperidone (or other antipsychotic) should be administered with the initial injection of Risperdal Consta and continued for 3 weeks (then discontinued) to maintain adequate therapeutic plasma concentrations prior to main release phase of risperidone from injection site. When switching from depot administration to a short-acting formulation, administer short-acting agent in place of the next regularly-scheduled depot injection.

Schizophrenia:

Oral: Initial: 2 mg daily in 1 to 2 divided doses; may be increased by 1 to 2 mg daily at intervals ≥24 hours to a recommended dosage range of 4 to 8 mg daily; may be given as a single daily dose once maintenance dose is achieved; daily dosages >6 mg do not appear to confer any additional benefit, and the incidence of extrapyramidal symptoms is higher than with lower doses. Further dose adjustments should be made in increments/decrements of 1 to 2 mg daily on a weekly basis. Dose range studied in clinical trials: 4 to 16 mg daily. Maintenance: Recommended dosage range: 2 to 8 mg daily

IM (Risperdal Consta): Initial: 25 mg every 2 weeks; if unresponsive, some may benefit from larger doses (37.5 to 50 mg); maximum dose: 50 mg every 2 weeks. Dosage adjustments should not be made more frequently than every 4 weeks. A lower initial dose of 12.5 mg may be appropriate in some patients (eg, demonstrated poor tolerability to other psychotropic medications).

Note: Oral risperidone (or other antipsychotic) should be administered with the initial injection of Risperdal Consta and continued for 3 weeks (then discontinued) to maintain adequate therapeutic plasma concentrations prior to main release phase of risperidone from injection site. When switching from depot administration to a short-acting formulation, administer short-acting agent in place of the next regularly-scheduled depot injection.

Major depressive disorder (adjunct to antidepressants; off-label use): Oral: Initial: 0.25 mg to 0.5 mg daily; slowly adjust dose based on response and tolerability up to 3 mg/day (Keitner 2009; Mahmoud 2007; Rapaport 2006; Reeves 2008). Average doses in clinical trials were 1.2 to 1.6 mg/day (Komossa 2010)

Post-traumatic stress disorder (PTSD) (off-label use): *Oral:* Initial: 0.5 to 1 mg at bedtime or 0.5 mg twice daily; may adjust dose based on response and tolerability to a maximum of 8 mg daily; total daily dose may be given in 2 or 3 divided doses. Average dose in clinical trials: 1.25 to 3.75 mg daily (Bandelow 2008; Bartzokis 2005; Hamner 2003; Padala 2006; Reich 2004; Rothbaum 2008).

Tourette's syndrome (off-label use): *Oral:* Initial: 0.25 mg once daily; increase gradually based on response and tolerability up to a usual dosage of 0.25 to 6 mg daily (Pringsheim 2012; Roessner 2011). Dosage adjustments in clinical trials were commonly in increments of <0.5 mg twice daily and at intervals ≥3 days (Bruggeman 2001; Dion 2002; Scahill 2003).

Geriatric

Oral: **Note:** Limiting initial dose to 1 mg daily (in 2 divided doses) may reduce the risk of orthostatic hypotension/syncope. Additional monitoring of renal function and orthostatic blood pressure may be warranted. If once-daily dosing in the elderly or debilitated patient is considered, a twice-daily regimen should be used to titrate to the target dose, and this dose should be maintained for 2 to 3 days prior to attempts to switch to a once-daily regimen.

US labeling: Initial: 0.5 mg twice daily; titration should progress slowly in increments of no more than 0.5 mg twice daily; increases to dosages >1.5 mg twice daily should occur at intervals of ≥1 week.

Canadian labeling: Schizophrenia: Initial: 0.25 mg twice daily; titrate slowly to a maximum dose of 3 mg daily Psychosis/agitation related to Alzheimer disease and other dementias (labeled indication in Canada; off-label use in US):

Canadian labeling: Severe Alzheimer dementia (short-term management): Initial: 0.25 mg twice daily; titrate in increments of 0.25 mg every 2 to 4 days as needed. Most patients respond optimally to 0.5 mg twice daily; maximum dose: 2 mg daily in 2 divided doses. Consider periodic dosage adjustments or therapy discontinuation as clinically indicated.

Alternative recommendations: Initial: 0.25 to 1 mg daily; if necessary, gradually increase based on response and tolerability not to exceed 2 mg once daily. Doses >1 mg daily are associated with higher rates of extrapyramidal symptoms. Consider periodic dosage adjustments to reduce or discontinue therapy as clinically indicated (APA [Rabins 2007]; Brodaty 2003; De Deyn 1999; Katz 1999; Schneider 2006; Sultzer 2008).

IM (Risperdal Consta): 25 mg every 2 weeks; a lower initial dose of 12.5 mg may be appropriate in some patients.

Note: Oral risperidone (or other antipsychotic) should be administered with the initial injection of Risperdal Consta and continued for 3 weeks (then discontinued)

to maintain adequate therapeutic plasma concentrations prior to main release phase of risperidone from injection site. When switching from depot administration to a short-acting formulation, administer short-acting agent in place of the next regularly-scheduled depot injection.

Pediatric Note: When reinitiating treatment after discontinuation, the initial titration schedule should be followed. Use in patients <18 years of age is not recommended in the Canadian labeling.

Autism: Children ≥5 years and Adolescents: *Oral:*

<15 kg: Use with caution; specific dosing recommendations not available

15 to <20 kg: Initial: 0.25 mg daily; may increase dose to 0.5 mg daily after ≥4 days, maintain dose for ≥14 days. In patients not achieving sufficient clinical response, may increase dose by 0.25 mg daily in ≥2-week intervals. Doses ranging from 0.5 to 3 mg daily have been evaluated; however, therapeutic effect reached plateau at 1 mg daily in clinical trials. Following clinical response, consider gradually lowering dose. May be administered once daily or in divided doses twice daily.

≥20 kg: Initial: 0.5 mg daily; may increase dose to 1 mg daily after ≥4 days, maintain dose for ≥14 days. In patients not achieving sufficient clinical response, may increase dose by 0.5 mg daily in ≥2-week intervals. Doses ranging from 0.5 to 3 mg daily have been evaluated; however, therapeutic effect reached plateau at 2.5 mg daily (3 mg daily in children >45 kg) in clinical trials. Following clinical response, consider gradually lowering dose. May be administered once daily or in divided doses twice daily.

Bipolar mania: Children and Adolescents 10 to 17 years: *Oral:* Initial: 0.5 mg once daily; dose may be adjusted in increments of 0.5 to 1 mg daily at intervals ≥24 hours to a dose of 1 to 2.5 mg daily. Doses ranging from 0.5 to 6 mg daily have been evaluated; however doses >2.5 mg daily do not confer additional benefit and are associated with increased adverse events.

Maintenance: No dosing recommendation available for treatment >3 weeks duration

Schizophrenia: Adolescents 13 to 17 years: *Oral:* Initial: 0.5 mg once daily; dose may be adjusted in increments of 0.5 to 1 mg daily at intervals ≥24 hours to a dose of 3 mg daily. Doses ranging from 1 to 6 mg daily have been evaluated, however, doses >3 mg daily do not confer additional benefit and are associated with increased adverse events.

Tourette's syndrome (off-label use):

Children and Adolescents: Initial: 0.125 to 0.5 mg once daily; increase gradually based on response and tolerability up to a usual dosage of 0.75 to 3 mg daily (AACAP [Murphy 2013]; Pringsheim 2012). Dosage adjustments in clinical trials were commonly in increments of <0.5 mg twice daily and at intervals ≥3 days; doses up to 4 mg daily have been evaluated in children and up to 6 mg daily in adolescents (Bruggeman 2001; Dion 2002; Ghanizadeh 2014; Gilbert 2004; Scahill 2003).

Renal Impairment Adults: **Note:** Limiting initial dose to 1 mg daily (in 2 divided doses) may reduce the risk of orthostatic hypotension/syncope.

Oral:

US labeling:

Mild or moderate impairment (CrCl ≥30 mL/minute): There are no dosage adjustments provided in the manufacturer's labeling. However, clearance may be decreased and doses should be reduced in patients with renal disease.

Severe impairment (CrCl <30 mL/minute): Initial: 0.5 mg twice daily; titrate slowly in increments of no more than 0.5 mg twice daily; increases to dosages >1.5 mg twice daily should occur at intervals of ≥1 week. Clearance of the active moiety is decreased by 60% in patients with moderate-to-severe renal disease (CrCl <60 mL/minute) compared to healthy subjects.

Canadian labeling: Mild to severe impairment: Initial: 0.5 mg twice daily; titrate slowly in increments of no more than 0.5 mg twice daily. Increases to dosages >1.5 mg twice daily should occur at intervals of ≥1 week. Slower titrations may be appropriate in some patients.

IM: Initiate with **oral** dosing (0.5 mg twice daily for 1 week then 2 mg daily for 1 week); if tolerated, begin 25 mg **IM** every 2 weeks; continue oral dosing for 3 weeks after the first IM injection. An initial IM dose of 12.5 mg may also be considered.

Hepatic Impairment Adults: **Note:** Limiting initial doses to 1 mg daily (in 2 divided doses) may reduce the risk of orthostatic hypotension/syncope.

Oral:

US labeling:

Mild or moderate impairment (Child-Pugh class A or B): There are no dosage adjustments provided in the manufacturer's labeling. However, based on pharmacokinetics, doses should be reduced in patients with liver disease.

Severe impairment (Child-Pugh class C): Initial: 0.5 mg twice daily; titration should progress slowly in increments of no more than 0.5 mg twice daily; increases to dosages >1.5 mg twice daily should occur at intervals of ≥1 week. The mean free fraction of risperidone in plasma was increased by 35% in patients with hepatic impairment compared to healthy subjects.

Canadian labeling: Schizophrenia and related psychotic disorders: Mild to severe impairment (Child–Pugh Class A, B, or C): Initial: 0.25 mg to 0.5 mg twice daily; titrate slowly in increments of 0.5 mg twice daily up to maximum dose of 1mg to 2 mg twice daily. Increases to dosages >1.5 mg twice daily should occur at intervals of ≥1 week.

IM: Initiate with **oral** dosing (0.5 mg twice daily for 1 week then 2 mg daily for 1 week); if tolerated, begin 25 mg **IM** every 2 weeks; continue oral dosing for 3 weeks after the first IM injection. An initial IM dose of 12.5 mg may also be considered.

Dietary Considerations May be taken without regard to meals. Some products may contain phenylalanine.

Administration

Oral: May be administered without regard to meals.

Oral solution can be administered directly from the provided pipette or may be mixed with water, coffee, orange juice, or low-fat milk, but is **not compatible** with cola or tea.

In children or adolescents experiencing somnolence, half the daily dose may be administered twice daily **or** the once-daily dose may be administered at bedtime.

Risperdal M-Tab should not be removed from blister pack until administered. Do not push tablet through foil (tablet may become damaged); peel back foil to expose tablet. Using dry hands, place immediately on tongue. Tablet will dissolve within seconds, and may be swallowed with or without liquid. Do not split or chew.

IM: Shake syringe vigorously just before injection. Administer IM into either the deltoid muscle or the upper outer quadrant of the gluteal area. Not for intravenous use; administer only IM; avoid inadvertent injection into vasculature. Injection should alternate between the two arms or buttocks. Do not combine two different dosage strengths into one single administration. Do not substitute any components of the dose-pack; administer with needle provided (1-inch needle for deltoid administration or 2-inch needle for gluteal administration).

Hazardous agent; use appropriate precautions for handling and disposal (NIOSH 2014 [group 2]).

Monitoring Parameters Mental status; vital signs (as clinically indicated); blood pressure (baseline; repeat 3 months after antipsychotic initiation, then yearly); weight, height, BMI, waist circumference (baseline; repeat at 4, 8, and 12 weeks after initiating or changing therapy, then quarterly; consider switching to a different antipsychotic for a weight gain ≥5% of initial weight); CBC (as clinically indicated; monitor frequently during the first few months of therapy in patients with preexisting low WBC or history of drug-induced leukopenia/neutropenia); electrolytes, renal and liver function (annually and as clinically indicated); personal and family history of obesity, diabetes, dyslipidemia, hypertension, or cardiovascular disease (baseline; repeat annually); fasting plasma glucose level/HbA$_{1c}$ (baseline; repeat 3 months after starting antipsychotic, then yearly); fasting lipid panel (baseline; repeat 3 months after initiation of antipsychotic; if LDL level is normal repeat at 2 to 5 year intervals or more frequently if clinical indicated); changes in menstruation, libido, development of galactorrhea, erectile and ejaculatory function (at each visit for the first 12 weeks after the antipsychotic is initiated or until the dose is stable, then yearly); abnormal involuntary movements or parkinsonian signs (baseline; repeat weekly until dose stabilized for at least 2 weeks after introduction and for 2 weeks after any significant dose increase); tardive dyskinesia (every 12 months; high-risk patients every 6 months); ocular examination (yearly in patients >40 years; every 2 years in younger patients) (ADA, 2004; Lehman, 2004; Marder, 2004).

Additional Information Risperdal Consta is an injectable formulation of risperidone using the extended release Medisorb® drug-delivery system; small polymeric microspheres degrade slowly, releasing the medication at a controlled rate.

Dosage Forms Excipient information presented when available (limited, particularly for generics); consult specific product labeling.

Solution, Oral:

RisperDAL: 1 mg/mL (30 mL) [contains benzoic acid]

Generic: 1 mg/mL (30 mL)

Suspension Reconstituted, Intramuscular:

RisperDAL Consta: 12.5 mg (1 ea); 25 mg (1 ea); 37.5 mg (1 ea); 50 mg (1 ea)

Tablet, Oral:

RisperDAL: 0.25 mg, 0.5 mg, 1 mg

RisperDAL: 2 mg [contains fd&c yellow #6 aluminum lake]

RisperDAL: 3 mg [contains fd&c yellow #10 (quinoline yellow)]

RisperDAL: 4 mg [contains fd&c blue #2 aluminum lake, fd&c yellow #10 (quinoline yellow)]

Generic: 0.25 mg, 0.5 mg, 1 mg, 2 mg, 3 mg, 4 mg

Tablet Dispersible, Oral:

RisperDAL M-TAB: 0.5 mg, 1 mg, 2 mg, 3 mg, 4 mg [contains aspartame, peppermint oil (mentha piperita oil)]

RisperiDONE M-TAB: 0.5 mg, 1 mg, 2 mg, 3 mg, 4 mg [contains aspartame]

Generic: 0.25 mg, 0.5 mg, 1 mg, 2 mg, 3 mg, 4 mg

◆ **RisperiDONE M-TAB** *see* RisperiDONE *on page 1593*

◆ **Ritalin** *see* Methylphenidate *on page 1180*

◆ **Ritalin LA** *see* Methylphenidate *on page 1180*

◆ **Ritalin SR [DSC]** *see* Methylphenidate *on page 1180*

◆ **Ritalin SR (Can)** *see* Methylphenidate *on page 1180*

Ritonavir (ri TOE na veer)

Brand Names: US Norvir

Brand Names: Canada Norvir

Pharmacologic Category Antiretroviral, Protease Inhibitor (Anti-HIV)

Use Treatment of HIV infection; should always be used as part of a multidrug regimen

Pregnancy Considerations Adverse events were observed in animal reproduction studies only with doses which were also maternally toxic. Ritonavir has a low level of transfer across the human placenta; no increased risk of overall birth defects has been observed following first trimester exposure according to data collected by the antiretroviral pregnancy registry. Early studies have shown lower plasma levels during pregnancy compared to postpartum, however dosage adjustment is not needed when used as a low-dose booster in pregnant women. The DHHS Perinatal HIV Guidelines consider ritonavir to be a preferred protease inhibitor (PI) for use during pregnancy when used as a booster for other Pis (not recommended as a single protease inhibitor in ART naïve pregnant women). The oral solution contains alcohol and therefore may not be the best formulation for use in pregnancy. A small increased risk of preterm birth has been associated with maternal use of protease inhibitor-based combination antiretroviral (ARV) therapy during pregnancy; however, the benefits of use generally outweigh this risk and Pls should not be withheld if otherwise recommended. Hyperglycemia, new onset of diabetes mellitus, or diabetic ketoacidosis have been reported with protease inhibitors; it is not clear if pregnancy increases this risk.

Regardless of CD4 count or HIV RNA copy number, all HIV-infected pregnant women should receive a combination antiretroviral ARV drug regimen. A combination of antepartum, intrapartum, and infant ARV prophylaxis is recommended. ARV therapy should be started as soon as possible in women with symptomatic infection. Although earlier initiation may be more effective in reducing the perinatal transmission of HIV, initiation may be delayed until after 12 weeks gestation in women who do not require immediate treatment after careful consideration of maternal conditions (eg, nausea and vomiting) and the potential risks of first trimester fetal exposure for specific agents. A scheduled cesarean delivery at 38 weeks gestation is recommended for all women with HIV RNA >1000 copies/mL or unknown concentrations near delivery in order to decrease transmission. If ARV therapy must be interrupted for <24 hours during the peripartum period, stop then restart all medications simultaneously in order to decrease the chance of developing resistance. Long-term follow-up is recommended for all infants exposed to ARV medications. In couples who want to conceive, the HIV-infected partner should attain maximum viral suppression prior to conception.

Health care providers are encouraged to enroll pregnant women exposed to antiretroviral medications in the Antiretroviral Pregnancy Registry (1-800-258-4263 or ▶

www.APRegistry.com). Health care providers caring for HIV-infected women and their infants may contact the National Perinatal HIV Hotline (888-448-8765) for clinical consultation (HHS [perinatal], 2014).

Breast-Feeding Considerations It is not known if ritonavir is excreted into breast milk; serum concentrations in nursing infants were undetectable at 12 weeks of age. Maternal or infant antiretroviral therapy does not completely eliminate the risk of postnatal HIV transmission. In addition, multiclass-resistant virus has been detected in breast-feeding infants despite maternal therapy. Therefore, in the United States, where formula is accessible, affordable, safe, and sustainable, and the risk of infant mortality due to diarrhea and respiratory infections is low, complete avoidance of breast-feeding by HIV-infected women is recommended to decrease potential transmission of HIV (HHS [perinatal], 2014).

Contraindications

Hypersensitivity to ritonavir or any component of the formulation; concurrent alfuzosin, amiodarone, cisapride, dihydroergotamine, ergonovine, ergotamine, flecainide, lovastatin, methylergonovine, midazolam (oral), pimozide, propafenone, quinidine, sildenafil (when used for the treatment of pulmonary arterial hypertension [eg, Revatio]), simvastatin, St John's wort, triazolam, and voriconazole (when ritonavir ≥800 mg/day)

Canadian labeling: Additional contraindications (not in US labeling): Concurrent use with astemizole, bepridil, fusidic acid, methylergonovine, midazolam, rivaroxaban, voriconazole (regardless of ritonavir dose), salmeterol, terfenadine, or vardenafil

Warnings/Precautions [US Boxed Warning]: Ritonavir may interact with many medications, including antiarrhythmics, ergot alkaloids, and sedatives/hypnotics, resulting in potentially serious and/or life-threatening adverse events. Some interactions may require dose or frequency adjustment, additional monitoring, and/or selection of alternative therapy. Pancreatitis has been observed (including fatalities); use with caution in patients with increased triglycerides; monitor serum lipase and amylase and for gastrointestinal symptoms. Increases in total cholesterol and triglycerides have been reported; screening should be done prior to therapy and periodically throughout treatment. Temporary or permanent discontinuation may be clinically indicated.

Protease inhibitors have been associated with a variety of hypersensitivity events (some severe), including rash, anaphylaxis (rare), angioedema, bronchospasm, erythema multiforme, toxic epidermal necrolysis, and/or Stevens-Johnson syndrome (rare). It is generally recommended to discontinue treatment if severe rash or moderate symptoms accompanied by other systemic symptoms occur. Use with caution in patients with cardiomyopathy, ischemic heart disease, preexisting conduction abnormalities, or structural heart disease; may be at increased risk of conduction abnormalities (eg, second- or third-degree AV block). Ritonavir has been associated with AV block due to prolongation of PR interval; use caution with drugs that prolong the PR interval. Use with caution in patients with hemophilia A or B; increased bleeding during protease inhibitor therapy has been reported and additional Factor VIII may be needed. Changes in glucose tolerance, hyperglycemia, exacerbation of diabetes, DKA, and new-onset diabetes mellitus have been reported in patients receiving protease inhibitors. May be associated with fat redistribution (buffalo hump, increased abdominal girth, breast engorgement, facial atrophy, and dyslipidemia). Immune reconstitution syndrome may develop resulting in the occurrence of an inflammatory response to an indolent or residual opportunistic infection during initial HIV treatment or activation of autoimmune disorders (eg, Graves' disease, polymyositis, Guillain-Barré syndrome) later in therapy; further evaluation and treatment may be required. May cause hepatitis or exacerbate preexisting hepatic dysfunction (including fatalities); use with caution in patients with hepatitis B or C, cirrhosis, or those with high baseline transaminases; consider increased monitoring of transaminases in these patients. Norvir® tablets are **not** bioequivalent to Norvir® capsules. Gastrointestinal side effects (eg, nausea, vomiting, abdominal pain, diarrhea) or paresthesias may be more common when patients are switching from the capsule to the tablet formulation due to a higher C_{max} (26% increase) observed with the tablet formulation compared to the capsule. These side effects should decrease as therapy is continued.

Oral solution contains ethanol and propylene glycol; healthcare providers should pay special attention to accurate calculation, measurement, and administration of dose; ethanol competitively inhibits propylene glycol metabolism; preterm infants may be at increased risk of toxicity due to decreased ability to metabolize propylene glycol.

Postmarketing adverse reactions (cardiac toxicity, lactic acidosis, renal failure, CNS depression, respiratory complications, acute renal failure including fatalities) have been reported in preterm neonates receiving ritonavir-containing solutions. Do not use in neonates with a postmenstrual age (first day of mother's last menstrual period to birth plus elapsed time after birth) <44 weeks, unless benefit outweighs risk and neonate is closely monitored (serum creatinine and osmolality, CNS depression, renal toxicity, lactic acidosis, cardiac conduction abnormalities, hemolysis).

Adverse Reactions Percentages as reported for combined experiences in both treatment-naive and experienced adults unless otherwise noted:

>10%:
  Cardiovascular: Flushing (13%)
  Central nervous system: Paresthesia (3% to 51%), fatigue (46%), dizziness (3% to 16%)
  Dermatologic: Skin rash (≤28%), pruritus (12%)
  Endocrine & metabolic: Hypercholesterolemia (3%; >240 mg/dL: 37% to 45%), increased serum triglycerides (9%; >800 mg/dL: 17% to 34%; >1500 mg/dL: 1% to 13%)
  Gastrointestinal: Diarrhea (15% to 68%), nausea (26% to 57%), vomiting (14% to 32%), abdominal pain (6% to 26%), dysgeusia (7% to 16%) dyspepsia (≤12%)
  Hepatic: Increased gamma-glutamyl transferase (5% to 20%)
  Neuromuscular & skeletal: Musculoskeletal pain (arthralgia and back pain, ≤19%), weakness (10% to 15%), increased creatine phosphokinase (4% to 12%)
  Respiratory: Cough (22%), oropharyngeal pain (16%)
2% to 10%:
  Cardiovascular: Edema (including peripheral edema, ≤6%), hypertension (≤3%), syncope (1% to 3%), vasodilatation (2%)
  Central nervous system: Peripheral neuropathy (10%), headache (6% to 7%), confusion (3%), disturbance in attention (3%), drowsiness (2% to 3%), insomnia (2% to 3%), depression (2%), anxiety (≤2%), malaise (1% to 2%)
  Dermatologic: Acne vulgaris (4%), diaphoresis (2% to 3%)
  Endocrine & metabolic: Increased uric acid (≤4%), lipodystrophy (acquired, 3%)
  Gastrointestinal: Anorexia (2% to 8%), flatulence (1% to 8%), increased serum amylase (grades 3/4; pediatric: 7%), throat irritation (local, 2% to 3%), gastrointestinal hemorrhage (≤2%)
  Hematologic & oncologic: Neutropenia (grades 3/4; pediatric: 9%), thrombocytopenia (<2%; grades 3/4; pediatric: 5%), anemia (<2%; grades 3/4; pediatric: 4%)
  Hepatic: Increased serum AST (6% to 10%), increased serum ALT (8% to 9%), hepatitis (≤9%)
  Hypersensitivity: Hypersensitivity reaction (≤8%)
  Neuromuscular & skeletal: Myalgia (2% to 9%)
  Ophthalmic: Blurred vision (6%)
  Renal: Polyuria (4%)
  Respiratory: Pharyngitis (≤1% to 3%)
  Miscellaneous: Fever (1% to 5%)
<2% (Limited to important or life-threatening): Adrenal suppression, adrenocortical cortex insufficiency, anaphylaxis, amnesia, angioedema, aphasia, asthma, atrioventricular block (first, second, or third degree), cachexia, cerebral ischemia, chest pain, cholestatic jaundice, coma, Cushing's syndrome, dementia, depersonalization, diabetes mellitus, diabetic ketoacidosis, esophageal ulcer, gastroenteritis, gastroesophageal reflux disease, gout, hallucination, hematologic disease (myeloproliferative), hemorrhage (in patients with hemophilia A or B), hepatic coma, hepatitis, hepatomegaly, hepatosplenomegaly, hyperglycemia, hypotension, hypothermia, hypoventilation, immune reconstitution syndrome, intestinal obstruction, leukemia (acute myeloblastic), leukopenia, lymphadenopathy, lymphocytosis, malignant melanoma, manic behavior, myocardial infarction, neuropathy, orthostatic hypotension, palpitations, pancreatitis, paralysis, pneumonia, prolongation P-R interval on ECG, prolonged Q-T interval on ECG, pseudomembranous colitis, rectal hemorrhage, redistribution of body fat, renal failure, renal insufficiency, right bundle branch block, seizure, Stevens-Johnson syndrome, subdural hematoma, syncope, tachycardia, torsades de pointes, toxic epidermal necrolysis, ulcerative colitis, vasospasm, venous thrombosis (cerebral)

Drug Interactions

Metabolism/Transport Effects Substrate of CYP1A2 (minor), CYP2B6 (minor), CYP2D6 (minor), CYP3A4 (major), P-glycoprotein; **Note:** Assignment of Major/Minor substrate status based on clinically relevant drug interaction potential; **Inhibits** CYP2C19 (weak), CYP2C8 (strong), CYP2C9 (weak), CYP2D6 (strong), CYP2E1

(weak), CYP3A4 (strong), P-glycoprotein, SLCO1B1; **Induces** CYP1A2 (weak/moderate), CYP2C9 (weak/moderate)

Avoid Concomitant Use

Avoid concomitant use of Ritonavir with any of the following: Ado-Trastuzumab Emtansine; Alfuzosin; Amiodarone; Amodiaquine; Aprepitant; Astemizole; Atovaquone; Avanafil; Axitinib; Barnidipine; Bosutinib; Bromocriptine; Cabozantinib; Ceritinib; Cisapride; Cobimetinib; Conivaptan; Crizotinib; Dabrafenib; Dapoxetine; Disulfiram; Domperidone; Dronedarone; Eletriptan; Enzalutamide; Eplerenone; Ergot Derivatives; Everolimus; Flecainide; Flibanserin; Fluticasone (Nasal); Fusidic Acid (Systemic); Halofantrine; Ibrutinib; Irinotecan Products; Isavuconazonium Sulfate; Ivabradine; Lapatinib; Lercanidipine; Lomitapide; Lovastatin; Lurasidone; Macitentan; Mequitazine; MetroNIDAZOLE (Systemic); Midazolam; Naloxegol; Nilotinib; NiMODipine; Nisoldipine; Olaparib; Ombitasvir, Paritaprevir, Ritonavir, and Dasabuvir; Osimertinib; Palbociclib; PAZOPanib; Pimozide; Propafenone; QuiNIDine; QuiNINE; Ranolazine; Red Yeast Rice; Regorafenib; Rifampin; Rivaroxaban; Salmeterol; Silodosin; Simeprevir; Simvastatin; Sonidegib; St Johns Wort; Suvorexant; Tamoxifen; Tamsulosin; Terfenadine; Thioridazine; Ticagrelor; Tolvaptan; Topotecan; Toremifene; Trabectedin; Triazolam; Ulipristal; Vemurafenib; VinCRIStine (Liposomal); Vorapaxar; Voriconazole

Increased Effect/Toxicity

Ritonavir may increase the levels/effects of: Ado-Trastuzumab Emtansine; Afatinib; Alfuzosin; Alitretinoin (Systemic); Almotriptan; Alosetron; ALPRAZolam; Amiodarone; Amodiaquine; Apixaban; Aprepitant; ARIPiprazole; ARIPiprazole Lauroxil; Astemizole; AtoMOXetine; AtorvaSTATin; Avanafil; Axitinib; Barnidipine; Bedaquiline; Bortezomib; Bosentan; Bosutinib; Brentuximab Vedotin; Brexpiprazole; Brinzolamide; Bromocriptine; Budesonide (Nasal); Budesonide (Oral Inhalation); Budesonide (Systemic); Budesonide (Topical); Cabazitaxel; Cabozantinib; Calcium Channel Blockers (Nondihydropyridine); Cannabis; CarBAMazepine; Cariprazine; Ceritinib; Cilostazol; Cisapride; Clarithromycin; Clorazepate; Cobimetinib; Colchicine; Conivaptan; Corticosteroids (Orally Inhaled); Corticosteroids (Systemic); Crizotinib; Cyclophosphamide; CycloSPORINE (Systemic); CYP2C8 Substrates; CYP2D6 Substrates; CYP3A4 Substrates; Dabigatran Etexilate; Dabrafenib; Daclatasvir; Dapoxetine; Dasatinib; Diazepam; Dienogest; Digoxin; Disulfiram; Domperidone; DOXOrubicin (Conventional); Dronabinol; Dronedarone; Drospirenone; DULoxetine; Dutasteride; Edoxaban; Efavirenz; Eletriptan; Eliglustat; Eluxadoline; Enfuvirtide; Enzalutamide; Eplerenone; Ergot Derivatives; Erlotinib; Estazolam; Etizolam; Everolimus; FentaNYL; Fesoterodine; Flecainide; Flibanserin; Flurazepam; Fluticasone (Nasal); Fluticasone (Oral Inhalation); Fusidic Acid (Systemic); GuanFACINE; Halofantrine; Highest Risk QTc-Prolonging Agents; Hydrocodone; Ibrutinib; Idelalisib; Iloperidone; Imatinib; Imidafenacin; Irinotecan Products; Isavuconazonium Sulfate; Itraconazole; Ivabradine; Ivacaftor; Ixabepilone; Ketoconazole (Systemic); Lacosamide; Lapatinib; Ledipasvir; Lercanidipine; Levobupivacaine; Levomilnacipran; Linagliptin; Lomitapide; Lovastatin; Lurasidone; Macitentan; Maraviroc; MedroxyPROGESTERone; Meperidine; Mequitazine; MethylPREDNISolone; Metoprolol; MetroNIDAZOLE (Systemic); Midazolam; Mifepristone; Moderate Risk QTc-Prolonging Agents; Naloxegol; Nebivolol; Nefazodone; Nilotinib; NiMODipine; Nintedanib; Nisoldipine; Olaparib; Ombitasvir, Paritaprevir, Ritonavir, and Dasabuvir; Osimertinib; Ospemifene; Oxybutynin; OxyCODONE; Palbociclib; Panobinostat; Parecoxib; Paricalcitol; PAZOPanib; P-glycoprotein/ABCB1 Substrates; Pimecrolimus; Pimozide; Pioglitazone; PONATinib; Pranlukast; PredniSOLONE (Systemic); PredniSONE; Propafenone; Protease Inhibitors; Prucalopride; QUEtiapine; QuiNIDine; QuiNINE; Ramelteon; Ranolazine; Red Yeast Rice; Regorafenib; Retapamulin; Rifabutin; Rifaximin; Rilpivirine; Riociguat; Rivaroxaban; RomiDEPsin; Rosuvastatin; Ruxolitinib; Salmeterol; Saxagliptin; Sildenafil; Silodosin; Simeprevir; Simvastatin; Sonidegib; SORAfenib; Suvorexant; Tacrolimus (Systemic); Tacrolimus (Topical); Tadalafil; Tamsulosin; Tasimelteon; Telaprevir; Temsirolimus; Terfenadine; Tetrabenazine; Tetrahydrocannabinol; Thioridazine; Ticagrelor; Tofacitinib; Tolterodine; Tolvaptan; Topotecan; Toremifene; Trabectedin; TraMADol; TraZODone; Treprostinil; Triamcinolone (Systemic); Triazolam; Ulipristal; Vardenafil; Vemurafenib; Vilazodone; VinBLAStine; VinCRIStine; VinCRIStine (Liposomal); Vindesine; Vinorelbine; Vorapaxar; Vortioxetine; Zolpidem; Zopiclone; Zuclopenthixol

The levels/effects of Ritonavir may be increased by: ARIPiprazole; Clarithromycin; Delavirdine; Efavirenz; Enfuvirtide; Fusidic Acid (Systemic); Mifepristone; P-glycoprotein/ABCB1 Inhibitors; Posaconazole; QuiNINE; Simeprevir

Decreased Effect

Ritonavir may decrease the levels/effects of: Abacavir; Antidiabetic Agents; Atovaquone; Boceprevir; BuPROPion; Canagliflozin; Clarithromycin; Codeine; Contraceptives (Estrogens); Deferasirox; Delavirdine; Etravirine; Fosphenytoin; Hydrocodone; Ifosfamide; Iloperidone; LamoTRIgine; Meperidine; Methadone; OLANZapine; Phenytoin; Prasugrel; Proguanil; QuiNINE; Tamoxifen; Telaprevir; Ticagrelor; TraMADol; Valproate Products; Voriconazole; Warfarin; Zidovudine

The levels/effects of Ritonavir may be decreased by: Boceprevir; CarBAMazepine; CYP3A4 Inducers (Moderate); CYP3A4 Inducers (Strong); Fosphenytoin; Garlic; Mitotane; Phenytoin; Rifampin; Siltuximab; St Johns Wort; Tocilizumab

Food Interactions Food enhances absorption. Management: Manufacturer recommends taking with food. Maintain adequate hydration, unless instructed to restrict fluid intake.

Storage/Stability

Capsule: Store under refrigeration at 2°C to 8°C (36°F to 46°F); may be left out at room temperature of <25°C (<77°F) if used within 30 days. Protect from light. Avoid exposure to excessive heat.

Solution: Store at room temperature at 20°C to 25°C (68°F to 77°F); do not refrigerate. Avoid exposure to excessive heat. Keep cap tightly closed.

Tablet: Store at ≤30°C (86°F); exposure to temperatures ≤50°C (122°F) permitted for ≤7 days. Exposure to high humidity outside of the original container (or a USP equivalent container) for >2 weeks is not recommended.

Mechanism of Action Binds to the site of HIV-1 protease activity and inhibits cleavage of viral Gag-Pol polyprotein precursors into individual functional proteins required for infectious HIV. This results in the formation of immature, noninfectious viral particles.

Pharmacodynamics/Kinetics

Absorption: Variable; increased with food; In the fed state, mean C_{max} of the tablet formulation increased by 26% compared to the capsule.

Distribution: High concentrations in serum and lymph nodes; V_d: 0.16 to 0.66 L/kg

Protein binding: 98% to 99%

Metabolism: Hepatic via CYP3A4 and 2D6; five metabolites, low concentration of an active metabolite (M-2) achieved in plasma (oxidative)

Half-life elimination: 3 to 5 hours

Time to peak, plasma: Oral solution: 2 hours (fasted); 4 hours (nonfasted)

Excretion: Urine (~11%, ~4% as unchanged drug); feces (~86%, ~34% as unchanged drug)

Dosing

Adult & Geriatric Note: Must be given in combination with other antiretroviral agents. Norvir tablets are **not** bioequivalent to Norvir capsules. Patients who take ritonavir capsules may experience more GI adverse reactions such as nausea, vomiting, abdominal pain, or diarrhea when switching from the capsule to the tablet because of the greater maximum plasma concentration (C_{max}) achieved with the tablet compared with the capsule.

Treatment of HIV infection: Manufacturer's labeling: Oral (**Note:** Not recommended as the primary protease inhibitor in any regimen (HHS [adult] 2015): 600 mg twice daily. May consider dose titration schedule to reduce the risk of treatment related adverse events; initiate at a dose of 300 mg twice daily, then increase by 100 mg twice daily every 2 to 3 days to recommended dosage of 600 mg twice daily (maximum: 600 mg twice daily). The Canadian labeling recommends completing titration within 14 days.

Pharmacokinetic "booster" in combination with other protease inhibitors (off-label use): Oral: 100 to 400 mg daily in 1 to 2 divided doses (HHS [adult] 2015) **Note:** Used to boost the darunavir component of a recommended initial regimen (coadministered with tenofovir and emtricitabine [or lamivudine]) in ART-naïve patients (HHS [adult] 2015). In patients without evidence of PI resistance, once-daily booster-dosing of 100 mg ritonavir may be preferred to 200 mg daily due to less gastrointestinal and metabolic adverse events. Refer to individual protease inhibitor monographs; specific dosage recommendations often require adjustment of both agents.

Pediatric Note: Must be given in combination with other antiretroviral agents. Norvir tablets are **not** bioequivalent to Norvir capsules. Patients who take ritonavir capsules may experience more GI adverse reactions such as nausea, vomiting, abdominal pain, or diarrhea when switching from the capsule to the tablet because of the greater maximum plasma concentration (C_{max}) achieved with the tablet compared with the capsule.

Treatment of HIV infection:

US labeling:

Infants >1 month and Children: Oral: Initiate dose at 250 mg/m^2/dose twice daily; titrate dose upward every 2 to 3 days by 50 mg/m^2 twice daily to recommended dosage of 350 to 400 mg/m^2/dose twice daily (maximum dose: 600 mg twice daily). If 400 mg/m^2/dose twice daily is not tolerated, the highest tolerated dose may be used for maintenance therapy. **Note:** Oral solution should not be administered to neonates before a postmenstrual age (first day of mother's last period to birth plus the time elapsed after birth) <44 weeks.

Adolescents: Refer to adult dosing.

Canadian labeling:

Children ≥2 years and Adolescents ≤16 years: Initiate dose at 250 mg/m^2/dose twice daily; titrate dose upward every 2 to 3 days by 50 mg/m^2 twice daily to recommended dosage of 400 mg/m^2/dose twice daily (maximum dose: 600 mg twice daily). If 400 mg/m^2/dose twice daily is not tolerated, the highest tolerated dose may be used for maintenance therapy.

Adolescents ≥17 years: Refer to adult dosing.

Renal Impairment No dosage adjustment necessary.

Hepatic Impairment

US labeling:

Mild to moderate impairment (Child-Pugh class A or B): No dosage adjustment necessary; however, ritonavir levels may be decreased in moderate impairment and patient response should be monitored.

Severe impairment (Child-Pugh class C): Not recommended (has not been studied).

Canadian labeling:

Mild impairment (Child-Pugh class A): No dosage adjustment necessary.

Moderate or severe impairment (Child-Pugh class B or C): There are no dosage adjustments provided in the manufacturer's labeling.

Dietary Considerations Oral solution contains 43% ethanol by volume. Consider ethanol content of all medications being administered; monitor for toxicity particularly in pediatric patients.

Administration Oral: Administer all formulations with food, per the manufacturer. DHHS guidelines recommend administering the tablets with food and administering capsules or oral solution with food, if possible, to improve tolerability (HHS [adult] 2015). Liquid formulations usually have an unpleasant taste. Consider mixing it with chocolate milk or a liquid nutritional supplement and taking within 60 minutes. Whenever possible, administer oral solution with calibrated dosing syringe. Dosage cups should be washed immediately with soap and hot water after use to remove drug residue and then be allowed to dry prior to next use. Shake solution well before use. Tablets should be swallowed whole; do not chew, break, or crush.

Monitoring Parameters Triglycerides, cholesterol, CBC, LFTs, CPK, uric acid, basic HIV monitoring, viral load, CD4 count, glucose, serum amylase and lipase

Additional Information Potential compliance problems, frequency of administration and adverse effects should be discussed with patients before initiating therapy to help prevent the emergence of resistance.

Dosage Forms Excipient information presented when available (limited, particularly for generics); consult specific product labeling.

Capsule, Oral:

Norvir: 100 mg [contains alcohol, usp]

Solution, Oral:

Norvir: 80 mg/mL (240 mL) [contains alcohol, usp, fd&c yellow #6 (sunset yellow), propylene glycol, saccharin sodium; peppermint-caramel flavor]

Tablet, Oral:

Norvir: 100 mg

◆ Ritonavir and Lopinavir *see* Lopinavir and Ritonavir *on page 1098*

◆ Ritonavir, Ombitasvir, and Paritaprevir *see* Ombitasvir, Paritaprevir, and Ritonavir *on page 1327*

◆ Ritonavir, Ombitasvir, Paritaprevir, and Dasabuvir *see* Ombitasvir, Paritaprevir, Ritonavir, and Dasabuvir *on page 1327*

◆ Rituxan *see* RiTUXimab *on page 1600*

RiTUXimab (ri TUK si mab)

Brand Names: US Rituxan

Brand Names: Canada Rituxan

Index Terms Anti-CD20 Monoclonal Antibody; C2B8 Monoclonal Antibody; IDEC-C2B8

Pharmacologic Category Antineoplastic Agent, Anti-CD20; Antineoplastic Agent, Monoclonal Antibody; Anti-rheumatic Miscellaneous; Immunosuppressant Agent; Monoclonal Antibody

Use

Treatment of CD20-positive non-Hodgkin lymphomas (NHL):

Relapsed or refractory, low-grade or follicular B-cell NHL (as a single agent)

Follicular B-cell NHL, previously untreated (in combination with first-line chemotherapy, and as single-agent maintenance therapy if response to first-line rituximab with chemotherapy)

Nonprogressing, low-grade B-cell NHL (as a single agent after first-line CVP treatment)

Diffuse large B-cell NHL, previously untreated (in combination with CHOP chemotherapy [or other anthracycline-based regimen])

Treatment of CD20-positive chronic lymphocytic leukemia (CLL) (in combination with fludarabine and cyclophosphamide)

Treatment of moderately- to severely-active rheumatoid arthritis (in combination with methotrexate) in adult patients with inadequate response to one or more TNF antagonists

Treatment of granulomatosis with polyangiitis (GPA; Wegener's granulomatosis) (in combination with glucocorticoids)

Treatment of microscopic polyangiitis (MPA) (in combination with glucocorticoids)

Pregnancy Considerations Animal reproduction studies have demonstrated adverse effects including decreased (reversible) B-cells and immunosuppression. Rituximab crosses the placenta and can be detected in the newborn. In one infant born at 41 weeks gestation, *in utero* exposure occurred from week 16-37; rituximab concentrations were higher in the neonate at birth (32,095 ng/mL) than the mother (9750 ng/mL) and still measurable at 18 weeks of age (700 ng/mL infant; 500 ng/mL mother) (Friedrichs, 2006).

B-cell lymphocytopenia lasting <6 months may occur in exposed infants. Limited information is available following maternal use of rituximab for the treatment of lymphomas and hematologic disorders (Ton, 2011). Retrospective case reports of inadvertent pregnancy during rituximab treatment collected by the manufacturer (often combined with concomitant teratogenic therapies) describe premature births and infant hematologic abnormalities and infections; no specific pattern of birth defects has been observed (limited data) (Chakravarty, 2010). Use is not recommended to treat non-life-threatening maternal conditions (eg, rheumatoid arthritis) during pregnancy (Makol, 2011; Østensen, 2008) and other agents are preferred for treating lupus nephritis in pregnant women (Hahn, 2012).

Effective contraception should be used during and for 12 months following treatment. Healthcare providers are encouraged to enroll women with rheumatoid arthritis exposed to rituximab during pregnancy in the Mother-ToBabyAutoImmune Diseases Study by contacting the Organization of Teratology Information Specialists (OTIS) (877-311-8972).

Breast-Feeding Considerations It is not known if rituximab is excreted in human milk. However, human IgG is excreted in breast milk, and therefore, rituximab may also be excreted in milk. Although rituximab would not be expected to enter the circulation of a nursing infant in significant amounts, the decision to discontinue rituximab or discontinue breast-feeding should take into account the benefits of treatment to the mother.

Medication Guide Available Yes

Contraindications There are no contraindications listed in the FDA-approved manufacturer's labeling.

Canadian labeling (not in U.S. labeling): Type 1 hypersensitivity or anaphylactic reaction to murine proteins, Chinese Hamster Ovary (CHO) cell proteins, or any component of the formulation; patients who have or have had progressive multifocal leukoencephalopathy (PML)

Warnings/Precautions [U.S. Boxed Warning]: Severe (occasionally fatal) infusion-related reactions have been reported, usually with the first infusion; fatalities have been reported within 24 hours of infusion; monitor closely during infusion; discontinue for severe

reactions and provide medical intervention for grades 3 or 4 infusion reactions. Reactions usually occur within 30-120 minutes and may include hypotension, angioedema, bronchospasm, hypoxia, urticaria, and in more severe cases pulmonary infiltrates, acute respiratory distress syndrome, myocardial infarction, ventricular fibrillation, cardiogenic shock and/or anaphylaxis. Risk factors associated with fatal outcomes include chronic lymphocytic leukemia, female gender, mantle cell lymphoma, or pulmonary infiltrates. Closely monitor patients with a history of prior cardiopulmonary reactions or with preexisting cardiac or pulmonary conditions and patients with high numbers of circulating malignant cells (>25,000/mm^3). Prior to infusion, premedicate patients with acetaminophen and an antihistamine (and methylprednisolone for patients with RA). Discontinue infusion for severe reactions; treatment is symptomatic. Medications for the treatment of hypersensitivity reactions (eg, bronchodilators, epinephrine, antihistamines, corticosteroids) should be available for immediate use. Discontinue infusion for serious or life-threatening cardiac arrhythmias. Perform cardiac monitoring during and after the infusion in patients who develop clinically significant arrhythmias or who have a history of arrhythmia or angina. Mild-to-moderate infusion-related reactions (eg, chills, fever, rigors) occur frequently and are typically managed through slowing or interrupting the infusion. Infusion may be resumed at a 50% infusion rate reduction upon resolution of symptoms. Due to the potential for hypotension, consider withholding antihypertensives 12 hours prior to treatment.

[U.S. Boxed Warning]: Hepatitis B virus (HBV) reactivation may occur with use and may result in fulminant hepatitis, hepatic failure, and death. Screen all patients for HBV infection by measuring hepatitis B surface antigen (HBsAG) and hepatitis B core antibody (anti-HBc) prior to therapy initiation; monitor patients for clinical and laboratory signs of hepatitis or HBV during and for several months after treatment. Discontinue rituximab (and concomitant medications) if viral hepatitis develops and initiate appropriate antiviral therapy. Reactivation has occurred in patients who are HBsAg positive as well as in those who are HBsAg negative but are anti-HBc positive; HBV reactivation has also been observed in patients who had previously resolved HBV infection. HBV reactivation has been reported up to 24 months after therapy discontinuation. Use cautiously in patients who show evidence of prior HBV infection (eg, HBsAg positive [regardless of antibody status] or HBsAg negative but anti-HBc positive); consult with appropriate clinicians regarding monitoring and consideration of antiviral therapy before and/or during rituximab treatment. The safety of resuming rituximab treatment following HBV reactivation is not known; discuss reinitiation of therapy in patients with resolved HBV reactivation with physicians experienced in HBV management.

[U.S. Boxed Warning]: Progressive multifocal leukoencephalopathy (PML) due to JC virus infection has been reported with rituximab use; may be fatal. Cases were reported in patients with hematologic malignancies receiving rituximab either with combination chemotherapy, or with hematopoietic stem cell transplant. Cases were also reported in patients receiving rituximab for autoimmune diseases who had received prior or concurrent immunosuppressant therapy. Onset may be delayed, although most cases were diagnosed within 12 months of the last rituximab dose. A retrospective analysis of patients (n=57) diagnosed with PML following rituximab therapy, found a median of 16 months (following rituximab initiation), 5.5 months (following last rituximab dose), and 6 rituximab doses preceded PML diagnosis. Clinical findings included confusion/disorientation, motor weakness/hemiparesis, altered vision/speech, and poor motor coordination with symptoms progressing over weeks to months (Carson, 2009). Promptly evaluate any patient presenting with neurological changes; consider neurology consultation, brain MRI and lumbar puncture for suspected PML. Discontinue rituximab in patients who develop PML; consider reduction/discontinuation of concurrent chemotherapy or immunosuppressants. Avoid use if severe active infection is present. Serious and potentially fatal bacterial, fungal, and either new or reactivated viral infections may occur during treatment and after completing rituximab. Infections have been observed in patients with prolonged hypogammaglobulinemia, defined as hypogammaglobulinemia >11 months after rituximab exposure; monitor immunoglobulin levels as necessary. Associated new or reactivated viral infections have included cytomegalovirus, herpes simplex virus, parvovirus B19, varicella zoster virus, West Nile virus, and hepatitis B and C. Discontinue rituximab in patients who develop other serious infections and initiate appropriate anti-infective treatment.

Tumor lysis syndrome leading to acute renal failure requiring dialysis (some fatal) may occur 12-24 hours following the first dose when used as a single agent in the treatment of NHL. Hyperkalemia, hypocalcemia, hyperuricemia, and/or hyperphosphatemia may occur. Administer prophylaxis (antihyperuricemic therapy, hydration) in patients at high risk (high numbers of circulating malignant cells ≥25,000/mm^3 or high tumor burden). May cause fatal renal toxicity in patients with hematologic malignancies. Patients who received combination therapy with cisplatin and rituximab for NHL experienced renal toxicity during clinical trials; this combination is not an approved treatment regimen. Monitor for signs of renal failure; discontinue rituximab with increasing serum creatinine or oliguria. Correct electrolyte abnormalities; monitor hydration status.

[U.S. Boxed Warning]: Severe and sometimes fatal mucocutaneous reactions (lichenoid dermatitis, paraneoplastic pemphigus, Stevens-Johnson syndrome, toxic epidermal necrolysis and vesiculobullous dermatitis) have been reported; onset has been variable but has occurred as early as the first day of exposure. Discontinue in patients experiencing severe mucocutaneous skin reactions; the safety of re-exposure following mucocutaneous reactions has not been evaluated. Use caution with preexisting cardiac or pulmonary disease, or prior cardiopulmonary events. Rheumatoid arthritis patients are at increased risk for cardiovascular events; monitor closely during and after each infusion. Elderly patients are at higher risk for cardiac (supraventricular arrhythmia) and pulmonary adverse events (pneumonia, pneumonitis). Abdominal pain, bowel obstruction, and perforation (rarely fatal) have been reported with an average onset of symptoms of ~6 days (range: 1-77 days); complaints of abdominal pain or repeated vomiting should be evaluated, especially if early in the treatment course. Live vaccines should not be given concurrently with rituximab; there is no data available concerning secondary transmission of live vaccines with or following rituximab treatment. RA patients should be brought up to date with nonlive immunizations (following current guidelines) at least 4 weeks before initiating therapy; evaluate risks of therapy delay versus benefit (of nonlive vaccines) for NHL patients. Safety and efficacy of rituximab in combination with biologic agents or disease-modifying antirheumatic drugs (DMARDs) other than methotrexate have not been established. Rituximab is not recommended for use in RA patients who have not had prior inadequate response to TNF antagonists. Safety and efficacy of re-treatment for RA have not been established. The safety of concomitant immunosuppressants other than corticosteroids has not been evaluated in patients with granulomatosis with polyangiitis (GPA; Wegener's granulomatosis) or microscopic polyangiitis (MPA) after rituximab-induced B-cell depletion. There are only limited data on subsequent courses of rituximab for GPA or MPA; safety and efficacy of re-treatment have not been established.

Some dosage forms may contain polysorbate 80 (also known as Tweens). Hypersensitivity reactions, usually a delayed reaction, have been reported following exposure to pharmaceutical products containing polysorbate 80 in certain individuals (Isaksson, 2002; Lucente 2000; Shelley, 1995). Thrombocytopenia, ascites, pulmonary deterioration, and renal and hepatic failure have been reported in premature neonates after receiving parenteral products containing polysorbate 80 (Alade, 1986; CDC, 1984). See manufacturer's labeling.

Adverse Reactions Note: Patients treated with rituximab for rheumatoid arthritis (RA) may experience fewer adverse reactions.
>10%:
  Cardiovascular: Peripheral edema (8% to 16%), hypertension (6% to 12%)
  Central nervous system: Fever (5% to 53%), fatigue (13% to 39%), chills (3% to 33%), headache (17% to 19%), insomnia (≤14%), pain (12%)
  Dermatologic: Rash (10% to 17%; grades 3/4: 1%), pruritus (5% to 17%), angioedema (11%; grades 3/4: 1%)
  Gastrointestinal: Nausea (8% to 23%), diarrhea (10% to 17%), abdominal pain (2% to 14%), weight gain (11%)
  Hematologic: Cytopenias (grades 3/4: ≤48%; may be prolonged), lymphopenia (48%; grades 3/4: 40%; median duration: 14 days), anemia (8% to 35%; grades 3/4: 3%), leukopenia (NHL: 14%; grades 3/4: 4%; CLL: grades 3/4: 23%; GPA/MPA: 10%), neutropenia (NHL: 14%; grades 3/4: 4% to 6%; median duration: 13 days; CLL: grades 3/4: 30% to 49%), neutropenic fever (CLL: grades 3/4: 9% to 15%), thrombocytopenia (12%; grades 3/4: 2% to 11%)
  Hepatic: ALT increased (≤13%)

Neuromuscular & skeletal: Neuropathy (≤30%), weakness (2% to 26%), muscle spasm (≤17%), arthralgia (6% to 13%)

Respiratory: Cough (13%), rhinitis (3% to 12%), epistaxis (≤11%)

Miscellaneous: Infusion-related reactions (lymphoma: First dose 77%; decreases with subsequent infusions; may include angioedema, bronchospasm, chills, dizziness, fever, headache, hyper-/hypotension, myalgia, nausea, pruritus, rash, rigors, urticaria, and vomiting; reactions reported are lower [first infusion: 32%] in RA; CLL: 59%; grades 3/4: 7% to 9%; GPA/MPA: 12%); infection (19% to 62%; grades 3/4: 4%; bacterial: 19%; viral 10%; fungal: 1%), human antichimeric antibody (HACA) positive (1% to 23%), night sweats (15%)

1% to 10%:

Cardiovascular: Hypotension (10%; grades 3/4: 2%), flushing (5%)

Central nervous system: Dizziness (10%), anxiety (2% to 5%), migraine (RA: 2%)

Dermatologic: Urticaria (2% to 8%)

Endocrine & metabolic: Hyperglycemia (9%)

Gastrointestinal: Vomiting (10%), dyspepsia (RA: 3%)

Neuromuscular & skeletal: Back pain (10%), myalgia (10%), paresthesia (2%)

Respiratory: Dyspnea (≤10%), throat irritation (2% to 9%), bronchospasm (8%), dyspnea (7%), upper respiratory tract infection (RA: 7%), sinusitis (6%)

Miscellaneous: LDH increased (7%)

Postmarketing and/or case reports: Acute renal failure, anaphylactoid reaction/anaphylaxis, angina, aplastic anemia, ARDS, arrhythmia, bowel obstruction/perforation, bronchiolitis obliterans, cardiac failure, cardiogenic shock, encephalomyelitis, fatal infusion-related reactions, fulminant hepatitis, gastrointestinal perforation, hemolytic anemia, hepatic failure, hepatitis, hepatitis B reactivation, hyperviscosity syndrome (in Waldenström's macroglobulinemia), hypogammaglobulinemia (prolonged), hypoxia, interstitial pneumonitis, laryngeal edema, lichenoid dermatitis, lupus-like syndrome, marrow hypoplasia, MI, mucositis, mucocutaneous reaction, neutropenia (late-onset occurring >40 days after last dose), optic neuritis, pancytopenia (prolonged), paraneoplastic pemphigus (uncommon), pleuritis, pneumonia, pneumonitis, polyarticular arthritis, polymyositis, posterior reversible encephalopathy syndrome (PRES), progressive multifocal leukoencephalopathy (PML), pure red cell aplasia, renal toxicity, reversible posterior leukoencephalopathy syndrome (RPLS), serum sickness, Stevens-Johnson syndrome, supraventricular arrhythmia, systemic vasculitis, toxic epidermal necrolysis, tuberculosis reactivation, tumor lysis syndrome, uveitis, vasculitis with rash, ventricular fibrillation, ventricular tachycardia, vesiculobullous dermatitis, viral reactivation (includes JC virus, cytomegalovirus, herpes simplex virus, parvovirus B19, varicella zoster virus, West Nile virus, and hepatitis C), wheezing

Drug Interactions

Metabolism/Transport Effects None known.

Avoid Concomitant Use

Avoid concomitant use of RiTUXimab with any of the following: Abatacept; BCG (Intravesical); Belimumab; Certolizumab Pegol; Deferiprone; Dipyrone; Natalizumab; Pimecrolimus; Tacrolimus (Topical); Tofacitinib; Vaccines (Live)

Increased Effect/Toxicity

RiTUXimab may increase the levels/effects of: Abatacept; Belimumab; Certolizumab Pegol; CloZAPine; Deferiprone; Fingolimod; Leflunomide; Natalizumab; Tofacitinib; Vaccines (Live)

The levels/effects of RiTUXimab may be increased by: Denosumab; Dipyrone; Pimecrolimus; Roflumilast; Tacrolimus (Topical); Trastuzumab

Decreased Effect

RiTUXimab may decrease the levels/effects of: BCG (Intravesical); Coccidioides immitis Skin Test; Sipuleucel-T; Vaccines (Inactivated); Vaccines (Live)

The levels/effects of RiTUXimab may be decreased by: Echinacea

Preparation for Administration Withdraw necessary amount of rituximab and dilute to a final concentration of 1-4 mg/mL with 0.9% sodium chloride or 5% dextrose in water. Gently invert the bag to mix the solution. Do not shake.

Storage/Stability Store intact vials refrigerated at 2°C to 8°C (36°F to 46°F); do not freeze. Do not shake. Protect vials from direct sunlight. Solutions for infusion are stable at 2°C to 8°C (36°F to 46°F) for 24 hours and at room temperature for an additional 24 hours.

Mechanism of Action Rituximab is a monoclonal antibody directed against the CD20 antigen on B-lymphocytes. CD20 regulates cell cycle initiation; and, possibly, functions as a calcium channel. Rituximab binds to the antigen on the cell surface, activating complement-dependent B-cell cytotoxicity; and to human Fc receptors, mediating cell killing through an antibody-dependent cellular toxicity. B-cells are believed to play a role in the development and progression of rheumatoid arthritis. Signs and symptoms of RA are reduced by targeting B-cells and the progression of structural damage is delayed.

Pharmacodynamics/Kinetics

Duration: Detectable in serum 3-6 months after completion of treatment; B-cell recovery begins ~6 months following completion of treatment; median B-cell levels return to normal by 12 months following completion of treatment

Absorption: IV: Immediate and results in a rapid and sustained depletion of circulating and tissue-based B cells

Distribution: RA: 3.1 L; GPA/MPA: 4.5 L

Half-life elimination:

CLL: Median terminal half-life: 32 days (range: 14-62 days)

NHL: Median terminal half-life: 22 days (range: 6-52 days)

RA: Mean terminal half-life: 18 days (range: 5-78 days)

GPA/MPA: 23 days (range: 9-49 days)

Excretion: Uncertain; may undergo phagocytosis and catabolism in the reticuloendothelial system (RES)

Dosing

Adult & Geriatric Note: Details concerning dosing in combination regimens should also be consulted. Pretreatment with acetaminophen and an antihistamine is recommended for all indications. For oncology uses, antihyperuricemic therapy and aggressive hydration are recommended for patients at risk for tumor lysis syndrome (high tumor burden or lymphocytes >25,000/mm^3). In patients with CLL, *Pneumocystis jirovecii* pneumonia (PCP) and antiherpetic viral prophylaxis is recommended during treatment (and for up to 12 months following treatment). In patients with granulomatosis with polyangiitis (GPA) and microscopic polyangiitis (MPA), PCP prophylaxis is recommended during and for 6 months after rituximab treatment. For patients with RA, premedication with methylprednisolone 100 mg IV (or equivalent) is recommended 30 minutes prior to each dose.

Chronic lymphocytic leukemia (CLL): IV infusion: 375 mg/m^2 on the day prior to fludarabine/cyclophosphamide in cycle 1, then 500 mg/m^2 on day 1 (every 28 days) of cycles 2-6

Granulomatosis with polyangiitis (GPA; Wegener's granulomatosis): IV infusion: 375 mg/m^2 once weekly for 4 doses (in combination with methylprednisolone IV for 1-3 days followed by daily prednisone)

Non-Hodgkin lymphoma (NHL; relapsed/refractory, low-grade or follicular CD20-positive, B-cell): IV infusion: 375 mg/m^2 once weekly for 4 or 8 doses

Re-treatment following disease progression: 375 mg/m^2 once weekly for 4 doses

NHL (diffuse large B-cell): IV infusion: 375 mg/m^2 given on day 1 of each chemotherapy cycle for up to 8 doses

NHL (follicular, CD20-positive, B-cell, previously untreated): IV infusion: 375 mg/m^2 given on day 1 of each chemotherapy cycle for up to 8 doses

Maintenance therapy (as a single agent, in patients with partial or complete response to rituximab plus chemotherapy; begin 8 weeks after completion of combination chemotherapy): IV infusion: 375 mg/m^2 every 8 weeks for 12 doses

NHL (nonprogressing, low-grade, CD20-positive, B-cell, after 6-8 cycles of first line CVP are completed): IV infusion: 375 mg/m^2 once weekly for 4 doses every 6 months for a maximum of 16 doses

NHL: Combination therapy with ibritumomab: IV infusion: 250 mg/m^2 IV day 1; repeat in 7-9 days with ibritumomab

Canadian labeling: **NHL, low grade or follicular:** IV infusion:

Initial: 375 mg/m^2 once weekly for 4 doses (as a single agent) **or** 375 mg/m^2 on day 1 of each 21-day cycle for 8 cycles (in combination with CVP chemotherapy)

Maintenance (responding to induction therapy): 375 mg/m^2 every 3 months until disease progression or up to a maximum of 2 years

Rheumatoid arthritis: IV infusion: 1000 mg on days 1 and 15 in combination with methotrexate; subsequent courses may be administered every 24 weeks (based on clinical evaluation), if necessary may be repeated no sooner than every 16 weeks

Microscopic polyangiitis (MPA): IV infusion: 375 mg/m^2 once weekly for 4 doses (in combination with methylprednisolone IV for 1-3 days followed by daily prednisone)

Chronic graft-versus-host disease (GVHD), refractory (off-label use): IV infusion: 375 mg/m^2 once weekly for 4 doses (Cutler, 2006)

Idiopathic thrombocytopenic purpura (ITP; off-label use): IV infusion: 375 mg/m^2 once weekly for 4 doses (Arnold, 2007; Godeau, 2008)

Hodgkin lymphoma (off-label use): IV infusion: 375 mg/m^2 once weekly for 4 weeks (Ekstrand, 2003; Schulz, 2008)

Idiopathic membranous nephropathy (IMN), resistant (off-label use): IV infusion: 375 mg/m^2 once weekly for 4 doses with re-treatment at 6 months (Fervenza, 2010) **or** 1000 mg on days 1 and 15 (Fervenza, 2008) **or** 375 mg/m^2 single doses titrated to B cell response (Cravedi, 2007)

Lupus nephritis, refractory (off-label use): IV infusion: 375 mg/m^2 once weekly for 4 doses (Melander, 2009) **or** 500-1000 mg on days 1 and 15 (Vigna-Perez, 2006)

Pemphigus vulgaris, refractory (off-label use): IV infusion: 375 mg/m^2 once weekly of weeks 1, 2, and 3 of a 4-week cycle, repeat for 1 additional cycle, then 1 dose per month for 4 months (total of 10 doses in 6 months) (Ahmed, 2006)

Post-transplant lymphoproliferative disorder (off-label use): IV infusion: 375 mg/m^2 once weekly for 4 doses (Choquet, 2006)

Thrombotic thrombocytopenic purpura (TTP), relapsed/refractory (off-label use): IV infusion: 375 mg/m^2 once weekly for 4 doses (Scully, 2007; Scully, 2011)

Waldenström's macroglobulinemia (off-label use): IV infusion: 375 mg/m^2 once weekly for 4 weeks (Dimopoulos, 2002)

Pediatric Note: Pretreatment with acetaminophen and an antihistamine is recommended.

Autoimmune hemolytic anemia (AIHA; off-label use): IV infusion: 375 mg/m^2 once weekly for 2-4 doses (Zecca, 2003)

Chronic immune thrombocytopenia (ITP; off-label use): IV infusion: 375 mg/m^2 once weekly for 4 doses (Parodi, 2009; Wang, 2005)

Nephrotic syndrome, severe, refractory (off-label use): IV infusion: 375 mg/m^2 once weekly for 1-4 doses has been used in small case series, case reports, and retrospective analyses, including reports of successful remission induction of severe or refractory nephrotic syndromes that are poorly responsive to standard therapies (Dello Strologo, 2009; Fujinaga, 2010; Guigonis, 2008; Prytula, 2010)

Renal Impairment No dosage adjustment provided in manufacturer's labeling (has not been studied).

Hepatic Impairment No dosage adjustment provided in manufacturer's labeling (has not been studied).

Administration Note: Some pediatric protocols utilize an alternate rituximab administration rate. Refer to specific protocol for administration rate guidelines.

Do **not** administer IV push or bolus. If a reaction occurs, slow or stop the infusion. If the reaction abates, restart infusion at 50% of the previous rate. Discontinue infusion in the event of serious or life-threatening cardiac arrhythmias.

IV: Initial infusion: Start rate of 50 mg/hour; if there is no reaction, increase the rate by 50 mg/hour increments every 30 minutes, to a maximum rate of 400 mg/hour.

Subsequent infusions:

Standard infusion rate: If patient tolerated initial infusion, start at 100 mg/hour; if there is no reaction, increase the rate by 100 mg/hour increments every 30 minutes, to a maximum rate of 400 mg/hour.

Accelerated infusion rate (90 minutes): For patients with previously untreated follicular NHL and diffuse large B-cell NHL who are receiving a corticosteroid as part of their combination chemotherapy regimen, have a circulating lymphocyte count <5000/mm^3, or have no significant cardiovascular disease. After tolerance has been established (no grade 3 or 4 infusion-related event) at the recommended infusion rate in cycle 1, a rapid infusion rate may be used beginning with cycle 2. The daily corticosteroid, acetaminophen, and diphenhydramine are administered prior to treatment, then the rituximab dose is administered over 90 minutes, with 20% of the dose administered over the first 30 minutes and the remaining 80% is given over 60 minutes (Sehn, 2007). If the 90-minute infusion in cycle 2 is tolerated, the same rate may be used for the remainder of the treatment regimen (through cycles 6 or 8).

Monitoring Parameters CBC with differential and platelets (obtain at weekly to monthly intervals and more frequently in patients with cytopenias, or at 2-4 month intervals in rheumatoid arthritis patients, GPA and MPA), peripheral CD20$^+$ cells; HAMA/HACA titers (high levels may increase the risk of allergic reactions); renal function, fluid balance; vital signs; monitor for infusion reactions, cardiac monitoring during and after infusion in rheumatoid arthritis patients and in patients with preexisting cardiac disease or if arrhythmias develop during or after subsequent infusions.

Screen all patients for HBV infection prior to therapy initiation (eg, HBsAG and anti-HBc measurements). In addition, carriers and patients with evidence of current infection or recovery from prior hepatitis B infection should be monitored closely for clinical and laboratory signs of HBV reactivation and/or infection during therapy and for up to 2 years following completion of treatment. High-risk patients should be screened for hepatitis C (per NCCN NHL guidelines v.2.2013).

Complaints of abdominal pain, especially early in the course of treatment, should prompt a thorough diagnostic evaluation and appropriate treatment. Signs or symptoms of progressive multifocal leukoencephalopathy (focal neurologic deficits, which may present as hemiparesis, visual field deficits, cognitive deficits, aphasia, ataxia, and/or cranial nerve deficits. If PML is suspected, obtain brain MRI scan and lumbar puncture.

Dosage Forms Excipient information presented when available (limited, particularly for generics); consult specific product labeling.

Solution, Intravenous [preservative free]:
Rituxan: 10 mg/mL (10 mL, 50 mL) [contains polysorbate 80]

Rivaroxaban (riv a ROX a ban)

Brand Names: US Xarelto; Xarelto Starter Pack
Brand Names: Canada Xarelto
Index Terms BAY 59-7939
Pharmacologic Category Anticoagulant; Anticoagulant, Factor Xa Inhibitor
Additional Appendix Information
Oral Anticoagulant Comparison Chart *on page 1957*
Reversal of Oral Anticoagulants *on page 1959*
Use
Deep vein thrombosis prophylaxis: Postoperative thromboprophylaxis of deep vein thrombosis (DVT) which may lead to pulmonary embolism in patients undergoing knee or hip replacement surgery.
Deep vein thrombosis treatment: Treatment of DVT.
Nonvalvular atrial fibrillation: Prevention of stroke and systemic embolism in patients with nonvalvular atrial fibrillation (AF).
Note: The 2014 American Heart Association/American College of Cardiology/Heart Rhythm Society guidelines for the management of AF recommend oral anticoagulation for patients with nonvalvular AF or atrial flutter with prior stroke, TIA, or a CHA_2DS_2-VASc score ≥2. As an alternative to warfarin, rivaroxaban may also be used for 3 weeks prior and 4 weeks after cardioversion in patients with AF or atrial flutter of ≥48 hours duration or when the duration is unknown. (January 2014).
Pulmonary embolism treatment: Treatment of pulmonary embolism.
Reduction in the risk (secondary prevention) of recurrent deep vein thrombosis and/or pulmonary embolism: Reduction in the risk of recurrence of DVT and pulmonary embolism following initial 6 months of treatment for DVT and/or pulmonary embolism.
Pregnancy Considerations Use during pregnancy is contraindicated in the Canadian labeling.

Adverse events were observed in animal reproduction studies. Based on ex-vivo data, rivaroxaban crosses the placenta (Bapat 2015). Information related to the use of rivaroxaban during pregnancy (Hoeltzenbein 2015) and postpartum (Rudd 2015) is limited. Data are insufficient to evaluate the safety of oral factor Xa inhibitors during pregnancy; use during pregnancy should be avoided (Guyatt 2012). Use may increase the risk of pregnancy related hemorrhage. Clinicians should note that the anticoagulant effect cannot be easily monitored or readily reversed. Prompt clinical evaluation is warranted with any unexplained decrease in hemoglobin, hematocrit or blood pressure, or fetal distress. Pregnancy planning should be discussed if use is needed in women of reproductive potential.

Breast-Feeding Considerations Use in breast-feeding mothers is contraindicated in the Canadian labeling.

It is not known if rivaroxaban is excreted into breast milk. Due to the potential for serious adverse reactions in the nursing infant, the decision to discontinue rivaroxaban or to discontinue breast-feeding during therapy should take into account the benefits of treatment to the mother; use of alternative anticoagulants is preferred (Guyatt 2012).
Medication Guide Available Yes
Contraindications Severe hypersensitivity to rivaroxaban or any component of the formulation; active pathological bleeding

Canadian labeling: Additional contraindications (not in U.S. labeling): Hepatic disease (including Child-Pugh classes B and C) associated with coagulopathy and clinically relevant bleeding risk; lesions or conditions at increased risk of clinically significant bleeding (eg, hemorrhagic or ischemic cerebral infarction, spontaneous or acquired impairment of hemostasis, active peptic ulcer disease with recent bleeding); concomitant systemic treatment with strong CYP3A4 and P-glycoprotein (P-gp) inhibitors (eg, ketoconazole, itraconazole, posaconazole, ritonavir); concomitant use with any other anticoagulant including unfractionated heparin (except at doses used to maintain central venous or arterial catheter patency), low molecular weight heparins (eg, enoxaparin, dalteparin) or heparin derivatives (eg, fondaparinux); concomitant use with warfarin, dabigatran, or apixaban except when switching therapy to or from rivaroxaban; pregnancy; lactation
Warnings/Precautions Most common complication is bleeding; major hemorrhages (eg, intracranial, GI, retinal, epidural hematoma, adrenal bleeding) have been reported. Certain patients are at increased risk of bleeding; risk factors include bacterial endocarditis, congenital or acquired bleeding disorders, thrombocytopenia, recent puncture of large vessels or organ biopsy, stroke, intracerebral surgery, or other neuraxial procedure, severe uncontrolled hypertension, renal impairment, recent major surgery, recent major bleeding (intracranial, GI, intraocular, or pulmonary), concomitant use of drugs that affect hemostasis, and advanced age. Monitor for signs and symptoms of bleeding. Prompt clinical evaluation is warranted with any unexplained decrease in hemoglobin or blood pressure. **Note:** No specific antidote exists for rivaroxaban reversal; not dialyzable due to high plasma protein binding. Protamine sulfate and vitamin K are not expected to affect the anticoagulant activity of rivaroxaban. The use of activated prothrombin complex concentrate (aPCC) or recombinant factor VIIa has not been evaluated. The use of a four-factor PCC (Cofact, not available in the U.S.) in healthy subjects has been shown to reverse the anticoagulant effect (ie, normalize the prothrombin time) of rivaroxaban (Eerenberg 2011).

[US Boxed Warning]: Spinal or epidural hematomas may occur with neuraxial anesthesia (epidural or spinal anesthesia) or spinal puncture in patients who are anticoagulated; may result in long-term or permanent paralysis. The risk of spinal/epidural hematoma is increased with the use of indwelling epidural catheters, concomitant administration of other drugs that affect hemostasis (eg, NSAIDS, platelet inhibitors, other anticoagulants), in patients with a history of traumatic or repeated epidural or spinal punctures, or a history of spinal deformity or spinal surgery. Monitor for signs of neurologic impairment (eg, midline back pain, numbness/weakness of legs, bowel/bladder dysfunction); prompt diagnosis and treatment are necessary. In patients who are anticoagulated or pharmacologic thromboprophylaxis is anticipated, assess risks versus benefits prior to neuraxial interventions. The optimal timing between the administration of rivaroxaban and neuraxial procedures is not known. Placement or removal of an epidural catheter or lumbar puncture is best performed when the anticoagulant effect of rivaroxaban is low. European guidelines recommend waiting at least 22 to 26 hours following the last rivaroxaban dose when using prophylactic dosing (eg, 10 mg once daily) before catheter placement or lumbar puncture (Gogarten 2010). When higher doses are used (eg, 20 mg once daily), some suggest avoidance of neuraxial procedures for at least 48 hours (Rosencher 2013). In patients who have received neuraxial anesthesia concurrently with rivaroxaban (usually in patients undergoing knee or hip replacement surgery), avoid removal of epidural catheter for at least 18 hours following the last rivaroxaban dose; avoid rivaroxaban administration for at least 6 hours following epidural catheter removal; if traumatic puncture occurs, avoid rivaroxaban administration for at least 24 hours. In addition to these and other clinical variables, consider renal function and the age of the patient (elderly patients exhibit a prolonged rivaroxaban

half-life [11 to 13 hours]) (Kubitza 2010; Rosencher 2013). The Canadian labeling recommends avoiding doses >10 mg in patients with a postoperative indwelling epidural catheter.

[US Boxed Warning]: As with any oral anticoagulant in the absence of adequate alternative anticoagulation, an increased risk of thrombotic events (including stroke) may occur with premature discontinuation of rivaroxaban. Consider the addition of alternative anticoagulant therapy when discontinuing rivaroxaban for reasons other than pathological bleeding or completion of a course of therapy. An increased rate of stroke was observed during the transition from rivaroxaban to warfarin in clinical trials in atrial fibrillation patients. In a post-hoc analysis of the ROCKET AF trial, patients who temporarily (>3 days) or permanently discontinued anticoagulation, the risk of stroke or non-CNS embolism was similar with rivaroxaban as compared to warfarin (Patel 2013).

Avoid use in patients with moderate to severe hepatic impairment (Child-Pugh classes B and C) or in coagulopathy with any hepatic disease associated with coagulopathy. Use with caution in patients with moderate renal impairment (CrCl 30 to 49 mL/minute) when used for postoperative thromboprophylaxis including patients receiving concomitant drug therapy that may increase rivaroxaban systemic exposure and those with deteriorating renal function. Monitor for any signs or symptoms of blood loss. Avoid use in severe renal impairment (DVT/PE, postoperative thromboprophylaxis: CrCl <30 mL/minute; nonvalvular atrial fibrillation: CrCl <15 mL/minute) since rivaroxaban exposure is expected to increase; discontinue use in patients who develop acute renal failure. According to the AHA/ACC/HRS, may consider dose reduction in patients with nonvalvular AF and moderate to severe chronic kidney disease (CKD), although safety and efficacy of this approach has not been established (AHA/ACC/HRS [January 2014]). Use with caution in the elderly. Elderly patients exhibit higher rivaroxaban concentrations compared to younger patients due primarily to reduced clearance. Overall, efficacy of rivaroxaban in the elderly (age ≥65 years) was similar to that of patients <65 years of age. Both thrombotic and bleeding events were higher in the elderly; however, the risk to benefit profile was favorable among all age groups.

Potentially significant drug-drug interactions may exist, requiring dose or frequency adjustment, additional monitoring, and/or selection of alternative therapy. In patients with renal impairment, concomitant use of rivaroxaban with combined P-gp and weak or moderate CYP3A4 inhibitors should only occur if the potential benefit outweighs the risk of bleeding. Formulation contains lactose; use is not recommended in patients with lactose or galactose intolerance (eg, Lapp lactase deficiency, glucose-galactose malabsorption).

Discontinue rivaroxaban at least 24 hours prior to surgery/invasive procedures. Some have recommended to discontinue rivaroxaban 3 days prior to a procedure in patients with a CrCl ≥50 mL/minute or 5 days prior in patients with a CrCl <50 mL/minute (Wysokinski 2012). The risk of bleeding should be weighed against the urgency of the procedure; reinitiate when adequate hemostasis has been achieved unless oral therapy cannot be administered then consider administration of a parenteral anticoagulant. Safety and efficacy have not been established in patients with prosthetic heart valves or significant rheumatic heart disease (eg, mitral stenosis); use is not recommended. Non-valvular atrial fibrillation is defined as atrial fibrillation that occurs in the absence of rheumatic mitral valve disease, mitral valve repair, or prosthetic heart valve (AHA/ACC/HRS [January 2014]). Rivaroxaban is **not** recommended as an alternative to unfractionated heparin in the treatment of acute pulmonary embolism in hemodynamically unstable patients or patients requiring thrombolysis or pulmonary embolectomy.

Adverse Reactions Frequency not always defined.
Central nervous system: Fatigue (1%), syncope (1%)
Dermatologic: Wound secretion (3%), pruritus (2%), skin blister (1%)
Gastrointestinal: Nausea (1% to 3%), abdominal pain (2%), dyspepsia (1%), toothache (1%)
Genitourinary: Urinary tract infection (1%)
Hematologic & oncologic: Hemorrhage (DVT prophylaxis: 5% to 6% [major: <1%]; DVT/PE treatment: 28% [major: ≤1%]), pulmonary hemorrhage (with and without bronchiectasis)
Hepatic: Increased serum transaminases (>3 x ULN: 2% [Watkins 2011])
Neuromuscular & skeletal: Back pain (4%), limb pain (2%), osteoarthritis (2%), muscle spasm (1%)

Respiratory: Oropharyngeal pain (1%), sinusitis (1%)
<1% (Limited to important or life-threatening): Agranulocytosis, cholestasis, decreased hemoglobin (≥2 g/dL), dysuria, ecchymoses, epidural hematoma, gastrointestinal hemorrhage, hemiparesis, hemophthalmos, hepatitis, hepatic injury (Liakoni 2014), hypermenorrhea, hypersensitivity, hypotension, increased amylase, increased blood urea nitrogen, increased lactate dehydrogenase, increased serum alkaline phosphatase, increased serum creatinine, increased serum lipase, intracranial hemorrhage, jaundice, retroperitoneal hemorrhage, Stevens-Johnson syndrome, subdural hematoma, tachycardia, thrombocytopenia (<100,000/mm^3 or <50% baseline)

Drug Interactions
Metabolism/Transport Effects Substrate of CYP2J2 (minor), CYP3A4 (major), P-glycoprotein; **Note:** Assignment of Major/Minor substrate status based on clinically relevant drug interaction potential

Avoid Concomitant Use
Avoid concomitant use of Rivaroxaban with any of the following: Anticoagulants; Apixaban; CYP3A4 Inducers (Strong); Dabigatran Etexilate; Edoxaban; Hemin; Inhibitors of CYP3A4 (Strong) and P-glycoprotein; Omacetaxine; St Johns Wort; Urokinase; Vorapaxar

Increased Effect/Toxicity
Rivaroxaban may increase the levels/effects of: Collagenase (Systemic); Deferasirox; Deoxycholic Acid; Ibritumomab; Nintedanib; Obinutuzumab; Omacetaxine; Tositumomab and Iodine I 131 Tositumomab

The levels/effects of Rivaroxaban may be increased by: Agents with Antiplatelet Properties; Anticoagulants; Antiplatelet Agents (P2Y12 Inhibitors); Apixaban; Aspirin; Clarithromycin; Dabigatran Etexilate; Dasatinib; Edoxaban; Erythromycin (Systemic); Fusidic Acid (Systemic); Hemin; Herbs (Anticoagulant/Antiplatelet Properties); Ibrutinib; Inhibitors of CYP3A4 (Moderate) and P-glycoprotein; Inhibitors of CYP3A4 (Strong) and P-glycoprotein; Limaprost; Nonsteroidal Anti-Inflammatory Agents; NSAID (Nonselective); Omega-3 Fatty Acids; Osimertinib; Pentosan Polysulfate Sodium; Prostacyclin Analogues; Salicylates; Sugammadex; Thrombolytic Agents; Tibolone; Tipranavir; Urokinase; Vitamin E; Vitamin E (Oral); Vorapaxar

Decreased Effect
Rivaroxaban may decrease the levels/effects of: Factor X (Human)

The levels/effects of Rivaroxaban may be decreased by: Bosentan; CYP3A4 Inducers (Moderate); CYP3A4 Inducers (Strong); Dabrafenib; Deferasirox; Estrogen Derivatives; Nevirapine; Osimertinib; Progestins; Siltuximab; St Johns Wort; Tocilizumab

Food Interactions Grapefruit juice may increase levels/effects of rivaroxaban. Management: Use caution.

Storage/Stability Store at 25°C (77°F); excursions permitted to 15°C to 30°C (59°F to 86°F).

Mechanism of Action Inhibits platelet activation and fibrin clot formation via direct, selective and reversible inhibition of factor Xa (FXa) in both the intrinsic and extrinsic coagulation pathways. FXa, as part of the prothrombinase complex consisting also of factor Va, calcium ions, factor II and phospholipid, catalyzes the conversion of prothrombin to thrombin. Thrombin both activates platelets and catalyzes the conversion of fibrinogen to fibrin.

Pharmacodynamics/Kinetics
Absorption: Rapid
Distribution: V_{dss}: ~50 L
Protein binding: ~92% to 95% (primarily to albumin)
Metabolism: Hepatic via CYP3A4/5 and CYP2J2
Bioavailability: Absolute bioavailability: 10 mg dose: ~80% to 100%; 20 mg dose: ~66% (fasting; increased with food)
Half-life elimination: Terminal: 5 to 9 hours; Elderly: 11 to 13 hours
Time to peak, plasma: 2 to 4 hours
Excretion: Urine (66% primarily via active tubular secretion [36% as unchanged drug; 30% as inactive metabolites]); feces (28% [7% as unchanged drug; 21% as inactive metabolites])

Dosing
Adult & Geriatric Note: Extremes of body weight (<50 kg or >120 kg) do not significantly influence rivaroxaban exposure (Kubitza 2007).
Deep vein thrombosis (DVT), pulmonary embolism (PE) treatment: Oral: Initial: 15 mg twice daily with food for 21 days followed by 20 mg once daily with food. **Note:** The American College of Chest Physicians (ACCP) recommends anticoagulant treatment for 3 months in patients with provoked DVT or ≥3 months with unprovoked DVT (duration depends on bleeding risk) (Guyatt 2012). Canadian labeling recommends continuation of treatment for at least 3 months if first

episode of DVT is secondary to transient risk factors (eg, recent trauma, surgery, immobilization) and an extended duration of treatment if patient has permanent risk factors or idiopathic DVT/PE.

Reduction in the risk (secondary prevention) of recurrent DVT/PE after an initial 6 months of treatment: Oral: 20 mg once daily with food; duration of treatment in the EINSTEIN-Extension Study was 6 to 12 months in addition to the initial treatment duration of 6 to 12 months (EINSTEIN Investigators 2010).

Postoperative DVT thromboprophylaxis: Oral: **Note:** Initiate therapy after hemostasis has been established, 6 to 10 hours postoperatively.

Knee replacement: 10 mg once daily; recommended total duration of therapy: 12 to 14 days; ACCP recommendation: Minimum of 10 to 14 days; extended duration of up to 35 days suggested (Guyatt 2012).

Hip replacement: 10 mg once daily; total duration of therapy: 35 days; ACCP recommendation: Minimum of 10 to 14 days; extended duration of up to 35 days suggested (Guyatt 2012).

Nonvalvular atrial fibrillation (to prevent stroke and systemic embolism): Oral: 20 mg once daily with the evening meal.

Conversion:

Conversion *from* warfarin: Discontinue warfarin and initiate rivaroxaban as soon as INR falls to <3.0 (U.S. labeling) or ≤2.5 (Canadian labeling)

Conversion *to* warfarin: **Note:** Rivaroxaban affects INR; therefore, initial INR measurements after initiating warfarin may be unreliable.

U.S. labeling: Discontinue rivaroxaban and initiate both warfarin and a parenteral anticoagulant at the time the next dose of rivaroxaban would have been taken (other approaches to this conversion may be acceptable).

Canadian labeling: Continue rivaroxaban concomitantly with warfarin until INR ≥2.0 and then discontinue rivaroxaban. **Note:** Caution must be employed with this strategy given the lack of an antidote for rivaroxaban reversal. During the first 2 days of concomitant therapy, usual doses of warfarin may be given without INR testing. Thereafter, while on concomitant therapy, measure INR daily just prior to the next scheduled rivaroxaban dose, as appropriate. After rivaroxaban has been discontinued, INR testing may be done at least 24 hours after the last rivaroxaban dose.

Conversion *from* continuous infusion unfractionated heparin: Initiate rivaroxaban at the time of heparin discontinuation

Conversion *to* continuous infusion unfractionated heparin: Discontinue rivaroxaban and initiate continuous infusion unfractionated heparin at the time the next dose of rivaroxaban would have been taken.

Conversion *from* anticoagulants (other than warfarin and continuous infusion unfractionated heparin):

U.S. labeling: Discontinue current anticoagulant and initiate rivaroxaban ≤2 hours prior to the next regularly scheduled evening dose of the discontinued anticoagulant.

Canadian labeling: Discontinue current anticoagulant and initiate rivaroxaban ≤2 hours prior to the next regularly scheduled evening dose of the discontinued anticoagulant; patients previously receiving prophylactic doses of anticoagulant may initiate rivaroxaban ≥6 hours after last prophylactic dose.

Conversion *to* other anticoagulants (other than warfarin): Discontinue rivaroxaban and initiate the anticoagulant at the time the next dose of rivaroxaban would have been taken

Renal Impairment Note: Clinical trials evaluating safety and efficacy utilized the Cockcroft-Gault formula with the use of actual body weight (weight range of patients enrolled in clinical trials: 33 to 209 kg) (data on file; Janssen Pharmaceuticals Inc 2012).

DVT, PE, reduction of the risk of recurrent DVT/PE:
US labeling:
CrCl ≥30 mL/minute: There are no dosage adjustments provided in manufacturer's labeling.
CrCl <30 mL/minute: Avoid use.

Canadian labeling:
CrCl ≥30 mL/minute: No dosage adjustment necessary.
CrCl <30 mL/minute: Avoid use.

Nonvalvular atrial fibrillation:
US labeling:
CrCl >50 mL/minute: No dosage adjustment necessary.

CrCl 15 to 50 mL/minute: 15 mg once daily with the evening meal. According to the AHA/ACC/HRS, may consider dose reduction in patients with moderate to severe chronic kidney disease (CKD), although safety and efficacy of this approach has not been established (AHA/ACC/HRS [January 2014]).

CrCl <15 mL/minute: Avoid use. **Note:** In patients with severe or end-stage chronic kidney disease, warfarin remains the anticoagulant of choice (AHA/ACC/HRS [January 2014]).

ESRD requiring hemodialysis: Avoid use. **Note:** In patients with severe or end-stage chronic kidney disease, warfarin remains the anticoagulant of choice (AHA/ACC/HRS [January 2014]).

Canadian labeling:
CrCl ≥50 mL/minute: No dosage adjustment necessary.
CrCl 30 to 49 mL/minute: 15 mg once daily
CrCl <30 mL/minute: Avoid use.

Postoperative thromboprophylaxis:
CrCl >50 mL/minute: No dosage adjustment necessary.
CrCl 30 to 50 mL/minute: No dosage adjustment necessary; use with caution.
CrCl <30 mL/minute: Avoid use.
ESRD requiring hemodialysis: Avoid use.

Hepatic Impairment
US labeling:
Mild hepatic impairment (Child-Pugh class A): There are no dosage adjustments provided in manufacturer's labeling. Limited data indicates pharmacokinetics and pharmacodynamic response were similar to healthy subjects.

Moderate to severe hepatic impairment (Child-Pugh class B or C) and patients with any hepatic disease associated with coagulopathy: Avoid use.

Canadian labeling:
Mild hepatic impairment (Child-Pugh class A): There are no dosage adjustments provided in the manufacturer's labeling. Limited data indicate pharmacokinetics and pharmacodynamic response were similar to healthy subjects.

Moderate impairment (Child-Pugh class B): There are no dosage adjustments provided in the manufacturer's labeling; use with caution. Limited data indicate a significant increase in pharmacodynamic response and pharmacokinetics (eg, increased AUC [~2.3-fold for total and ~2.6-fold for unbound] and C_{max} [27% for total and 38% for unbound]).

Severe hepatic impairment (Child-Pugh class C): There are no dosage adjustments provided in the manufacturer's labeling (has not been studied).

Hepatic impairment (including Child-Pugh class B and C) associated with coagulopathy, and having clinically relevant bleeding risk: Use is contraindicated.

Obesity Body weight >120 kg did not significantly influence rivaroxaban exposure (Kubitza 2007). Clinical outcomes in postoperative thromboprophylaxis trials were also not affected by weight (up to 190 kg) (Turpie 2011). Therefore, dosage adjustment is not required.

Administration Administer doses ≥15 mg/day with food; dose of 10 mg/day may be administered without regard to meals. For nonvalvular atrial fibrillation, administer with the evening meal. For patients who cannot swallow whole tablets, the tablets (all strengths) may be crushed and mixed with applesauce immediately prior to use; immediately follow administration of the 15 mg and 20 mg tablets with food (10 mg tablets may be administered without regards to food).

For nasogastric/gastric feeding tube administration, the tablets (all strengths) may be crushed and mixed in 50 mL of water; administer the suspension within 4 hours of preparation and follow administration of the 15 mg and 20 mg tablets immediately with enteral feeding (10 mg tablets may be administered without regards to food). Avoid administration distal to the stomach; a decrease in the AUC and C_{max} (29% and 56%, respectively) was observed when rivaroxaban was delivered to the proximal small intestine; further decreases may be seen with delivery to the distal small intestine or ascending colon.

Missed doses: Patients receiving 15 mg twice daily dosing who miss a dose should take a dose immediately to ensure 30 mg of rivaroxaban is administered per day (two 15 mg tablets may be taken together); resume therapy the following day as previously taken. Patients receiving once-daily dosing who miss a dose should take a dose as soon as possible on the same day; resume therapy the following day as previously taken.

Monitoring Parameters Routine monitoring of coagulation tests not required; in major clinical trials, monitoring of coagulation tests (eg, aPTT, PT/INR, or antifactor Xa activity) did not occur. Prothrombin time (PT) or antifactor Xa activity may be used to detect presence of rivaroxaban (neither is intended to be used for dosage adjustment). However, variability exists among PT assays and even more so when converted to INR. Therefore, antifactor Xa activity measurement is the preferred test (Asmis 2012; Barrett 2010; Kubitza 2005). A therapeutic range has not been defined, and dosage adjustment based on results has not been established.

CBC with differential; renal function prior to initiation, when clinically indicated, and at least annually (AHA/ACC/HRS [January 2014]); hepatic function

Test Interactions Prolongs activated partial thromboplastin time (aPTT), HepTest®, and Russell viper venom time

Dosage Forms Excipient information presented when available (limited, particularly for generics); consult specific product labeling.
Tablet, Oral:
Xarelto: 10 mg, 15 mg, 20 mg
Tablet Therapy Pack, Oral:
Xarelto Starter Pack: 15 mg (42s) and 20 mg (9s) (51 ea)

♦ Riva-Sertraline (Can) see Sertraline on page 1649

♦ Riva-Simvastatin (Can) see Simvastatin on page 1659

♦ Rivasol (Can) see Zinc Sulfate on page 1929

♦ Rivasone (Can) see Betamethasone (Topical) on page 224

♦ Riva-Sotalol (Can) see Sotalol on page 1694

Rivastigmine (ri va STIG meen)

Brand Names: US Exelon
Brand Names: Canada Apo-Rivastigmine; Exelon; Med-Rivastigmine; Mint-Rivastigmine; Mylan-Rivastigmine; Novo-Rivastigmine; PMS-Rivastigmine; ratio-Rivastigmine; Sandoz-Rivastigmine
Index Terms ENA 713; Rivastigmine Tartrate; SDZ ENA 713
Pharmacologic Category Acetylcholinesterase Inhibitor (Central)
Use
Alzheimer dementia:
Oral: Treatment of mild to moderate dementia of the Alzheimer type.
Transdermal: Treatment of mild, moderate, and severe dementia of the Alzheimer type.
Parkinson disease dementia: Treatment of mild to moderate dementia associated with Parkinson disease. **Note:** Use of the transdermal patch in treatment of Parkinson-related dementia is not approved in the Canadian labeling.
Pregnancy Considerations Adverse events have not been observed in animal reproduction studies.
Breast-Feeding Considerations It is not known if rivastigmine is excreted in breast milk. Due to the potential for serious adverse reactions in the nursing infant, the manufacturer recommends a decision be made whether to discontinue nursing or to discontinue the drug, taking into account the importance of treatment to the mother.
Contraindications
Hypersensitivity to rivastigmine, other carbamate derivatives, or any component of the formulation; history of application-site reactions with rivastigmine patch
Canadian labeling: Additional contraindications (not in US labeling): Severe hepatic impairment; history of severe skin reactions (eg, allergic dermatitis [disseminated], Stevens-Johnson syndrome) with oral or transdermal rivastigmine
Warnings/Precautions Significant nausea/vomiting/diarrhea or anorexia/weight loss/decreased appetite are associated with use; occurs more frequently in women and during the titration phase. The incidence and severity of these reactions are dose-related; dehydration may result from prolonged vomiting or diarrhea. Monitor weight during therapy. Therapy should be initiated at lowest dose and titrated; if treatment is interrupted for >3 days, reinstate at the lowest daily dose. May have vagotonic effects which may cause bradycardia and/or heart block with or without a history of cardiac disease. Alzheimer treatment guidelines consider bradycardia to be a relative contraindication for use of centrally-active cholinesterase inhibitors. Postmarketing cases of overdose (including fatalities) have been reported in association with medication errors/improper use of rivastigmine transdermal patches. No more than 1 patch should be applied daily and existing patch must be removed prior to applying new patch.

Disseminated allergic dermatitis has been reported following both oral and transdermal administration. Discontinue use of all routes of rivastigmine therapy in patients who develop disseminated allergic dermatitis. Use of the transdermal patch may result in allergic contact dermatitis; discontinue therapy if an intense local reaction occurs (eg, increasing erythema, edema, papules, vesicles) and if symptoms do not improve after 48 hours of patch removal. If therapy is still required, oral rivastigmine may be used following negative allergy testing; some patients may not be able to take rivastigmine in any form. Postmarketing reports of disseminated hypersensitivity skin reactions have occurred with use of oral or transdermal products; discontinue use of all rivastigmine therapy in these cases.

Use caution in patients with a history of peptic ulcer disease or concurrent NSAID use; may increase gastric acid secretion. Monitor for active or occult bleeding. Use caution in patients with sick-sinus syndrome, bradycardia or other supraventricular conduction conditions, urinary obstruction, seizure disorders, or pulmonary conditions such as asthma or COPD. May exacerbate or induce extrapyramidal symptoms; worsening of symptoms (eg, tremor) in patients with Parkinson disease has been observed. May cause CNS depression, which may impair physical or mental abilities; patients must be cautioned about performing tasks that require mental alertness (eg, operating machinery or driving). Systemic exposure may be increased in patients <50 kg and decreased in patients >100 kg. Consider dose reduction if toxicities develop in patients <50 kg (oral and transdermal). Potentially significant drug-drug interactions may exist, requiring dose or frequency adjustment, additional monitoring, and/or selection of alternative therapy. Nicotine increases the clearance of rivastigmine by 23%.

Adverse Reactions Many concentration-related effects are reported at a lower frequency by transdermal route.
>10%:
Central nervous system: Dizziness (oral: 6% to 21%; transdermal: ≤6%), headache (oral: 4% to 17%; transdermal ≤4%), agitation (transdermal: 1% to 14%), falling (6% to 12%)
Endocrine & metabolic: Weight loss (3% to 26%)
Gastrointestinal: Nausea (oral: 17% to 47%; transdermal: 2% to 10%), vomiting (oral: 13% to 31%; transdermal: 3% to 9%), diarrhea (oral: 5% to 19%; transdermal: ≤7%), anorexia (oral: ≤17%; transdermal: ≤3%), abdominal pain (oral: 13%; transdermal: 2%)
Local: Application site erythema (transdermal: 1% to 13%)
Neuromuscular & skeletal: Tremor (oral: 4% to 23%; transdermal: 7%)
1% to 10%:
Cardiovascular: Hypertension (1% to 3%), syncope (oral: 3%)
Central nervous system: Fatigue (oral: 4% to 9%; transdermal: 2% to 4%), insomnia (1% to 9%), confusion (oral: 8%), depression (2% to 6%), drowsiness (4% to 6%), malaise (oral: 5%), anxiety (1% to 5%), hallucination (2% to 5%), abnormal gait (transdermal: 4%), psychomotor agitation (transdermal: 1% to 3%), aggressive behavior (1% to 3%), exacerbation of Parkinson's disease (oral: 1% to 3%), cogwheel rigidity (oral: 1% to 3%), restlessness (oral: 1% to 3%), drug-induced Parkinson's disease (oral: 2%)
Dermatologic: Diaphoresis (oral: 2% to 4%)
Endocrine & metabolic: Dehydration (1% to 2%)
Gastrointestinal: Dyspepsia (oral: 9%), decreased appetite (≤9%), upper abdominal pain (≤4%), sialorrhea (oral: 1% to 2%)
Genitourinary: Urinary tract infection (1% to 10%), urinary incontinence (≤3%)
Local: Application site pruritus (transdermal: ≤5%), application site irritation (transdermal: ≤3%), application site rash (transdermal: 2%)
Neuromuscular & skeletal: Weakness (2% to 6%;), bradykinesia (3% to 4%), hypokinesia (1% to 4%), dyskinesia (3%)
<1% (Limited to important or life-threatening): Atrial fibrillation, atrioventricular block, bradycardia, dystonia, edema, extrapyramidal reaction, gastrointestinal hemorrhage, hepatic failure, hepatitis, hyperacidity, hypersensitivity reaction, seizure, severe vomiting (with esophageal rupture; following inappropriate reinitiation of dose), sick-sinus syndrome, skin blister, Stevens-Johnson syndrome, tachycardia

Drug Interactions
Metabolism/Transport Effects None known.
Avoid Concomitant Use
Avoid concomitant use of Rivastigmine with any of the following: Beta-Blockers; Ceritinib; Metoclopramide

Increased Effect/Toxicity

Rivastigmine may increase the levels/effects of: Antipsychotic Agents; Beta-Blockers; Bradycardia-Causing Agents; Ceritinib; Cholinergic Agonists; Ivabradine; Lacosamide; Metoclopramide; Succinylcholine

The levels/effects of Rivastigmine may be increased by: Bretylium; Corticosteroids (Systemic); Ruxolitinib; Tofacitinib

Decreased Effect

Rivastigmine may decrease the levels/effects of: Anticholinergic Agents; Neuromuscular-Blocking Agents (Nondepolarizing)

The levels/effects of Rivastigmine may be decreased by: Anticholinergic Agents; Dipyridamole

Food Interactions Food delays absorption by 90 minutes, lowers C_{max} by 30% and increases AUC by 30%. Management: Administer with meals.

Storage/Stability

Oral: Store at 25°C (77°F); excursions are permitted between 15°C and 30°C (59°F and 86°F); do not freeze oral solution. Store solution in an upright position. Stable at room temperature for up to 4 hours when solution is mixed with cold fruit juice or soda.

Transdermal patch: Store at 25°C (77°F); excursions are permitted between 15°C and 30°C (59°F and 86°F). Patches should be kept in sealed pouch until use.

Mechanism of Action A deficiency of cortical acetylcholine is thought to account for some of the symptoms of Alzheimer disease and the dementia of Parkinson disease; rivastigmine increases acetylcholine in the central nervous system through reversible inhibition of its hydrolysis by cholinesterase

Pharmacodynamics/Kinetics

Duration: Anticholinesterase activity (CSF): ~10 hours (6 mg oral dose)

Absorption: Oral: Fasting: Rapid and complete within 1 hour; Transdermal patch: Within 30 to 60 minutes

Distribution: V_d: 1.8 to 2.7 L/kg; penetrates blood-brain barrier (CSF levels are ~40% of plasma levels following oral administration)

Protein binding: 40%

Metabolism: Extensively via cholinesterase-mediated hydrolysis in the brain; metabolite undergoes N-demethylation and/or sulfate conjugation hepatically; CYP minimally involved; linear kinetics at 3 mg twice daily, but nonlinear at higher doses

Bioavailability: Oral: 36%

Half-life elimination: Oral: 1.5 hours; Transdermal patch: ~3 hours (after removal)

Time to peak: Oral: 1 hour; Transdermal patch: 8 to 16 hours following first dose

Excretion: Urine (97% as metabolites); feces (0.4%)

Dosing

Adult

Note: Exelon oral solution and capsules are bioequivalent.

Note: Exelon oral solution has been discontinued in the US for more than 1 year.

Alzheimer dementia, mild to moderate:

Oral: Initial: 1.5 mg twice daily; may increase by 3 mg daily (1.5 mg/dose) every 2 weeks based on tolerability (maximum recommended dose: 6 mg twice daily)

Low body weight: Careful titration and monitoring should be performed in patients with low body weight. In patients <50 kg, monitor closely for toxicities (eg, excessive nausea, vomiting), and consider reducing the dose if such toxicities develop.

Note: If GI adverse events occur, discontinue treatment for several doses then restart at the same or next lower dosage level; antiemetics have been used to control GI symptoms. If dosing is interrupted for ≤3 days, restart the treatment at the same or lower dose and titrate as previously described.

Transdermal patch:

US labeling: Initial: Apply 4.6 mg/24 hours patch once daily; if well tolerated, may titrate (no sooner than every 4 weeks) to 9.5 mg/24 hours (continue as long as therapeutically beneficial), and then to 13.3 mg/24 hours (maximum dose); doses >13.3 mg/24 hours have not been shown to be more effective and are associated with significant increases in adverse events. Recommended effective dose: Apply 9.5 mg/24 hours or 13.3 mg/24 hours patch once daily; remove old patch and replace with a new patch every 24 hours

Canadian labeling: Initial: Apply 4.6 mg/24 hours patch once daily; if well tolerated, may titrate (no sooner than after 4 weeks) to 9.5 mg/24 hours (continue as long as therapeutically beneficial). Further titration to 13.3 mg/24 hours (maximum dose)

may be considered in patients with moderately severe disease.

Low body weight: Careful titration and monitoring should be performed in patients with low body weight. In patients <50 kg, monitor closely for toxicities (eg, excessive nausea, vomiting) and consider reducing the maintenance dose to 4.6 mg/24 hour if such toxicities develop.

Note: If dosing is interrupted for ≤3 days, restart treatment with the same or a lower strength patch. If interrupted for >3 days, reinitiate at 4.6 mg/24 hours and titrate (no sooner than every 4 weeks) to lowest effective maintenance dose.

Conversion from oral therapy: If oral daily dose <6 mg, switch to 4.6 mg/24 hours patch; if oral daily dose 6-12 mg, switch to 9.5 mg/24 hours patch. Apply patch on the day following last oral dose.

Alzheimer dementia, severe: *Transdermal patch:* Initial: Apply 4.6 mg/24 hours patch once daily. Titrate dose as recommended for transdermal dosing for mild-to-moderate Alzheimer's dementia. Recommended effective dose: Apply 13.3 mg/24 hours patch once daily; remove old patch and replace with a new patch every 24 hours

Low body weight: Careful titration and monitoring should be performed in patients with low body weight. In patients <50 kg, monitor closely for toxicities (eg, excessive nausea, vomiting) and consider reducing the maintenance dose to 4.6 mg/24 hours if such toxicities develop.

Note: If dosing is interrupted for ≤3 days, restart treatment with the same or a lower strength patch. If interrupted for >3 days, reinitiate at 4.6 mg/24 hour and titrate (no sooner than every 4 weeks) to lowest effective maintenance dose.

Parkinson-related dementia, mild to moderate:

Oral: Initial: 1.5 mg twice daily; may increase by 3 mg daily (1.5 mg per dose) every 4 weeks based on tolerability (maximum recommended dose: 6 mg twice daily)

Low body weight: Careful titration and monitoring should be performed in patients with low body weight. In patients <50 kg, monitor closely for toxicities (eg, excessive nausea, vomiting) and consider reducing the dose if such toxicities develop.

Note: If GI adverse events occur, discontinue treatment for several doses then restart at the same or next lower dosage level; antiemetics have been used to control GI symptoms. If dosing is interrupted for ≤3 days, restart the treatment at the same or lower dose and titrate as previously described.

Transdermal patch: Initial: If well tolerated, may titrate (no sooner than every 4 weeks) to 9.5 mg/24 hours (continue as long as therapeutically beneficial), and then to 13.3 mg/24 hours (maximum dose); doses >13.3 mg/24 hours have not been shown to be more effective and are associated with significant increases in adverse events. Recommended effective dose: Apply 9.5 mg/24 hours or 13.3 mg/24 hours patch once daily; remove old patch and replace with a new patch every 24 hours. **Note:** Use of the transdermal patch in treatment of Parkinson-related dementia is not approved in the Canadian labeling.

Low body weight: Careful titration and monitoring should be performed in patients with low body weight. In patients <50 kg, monitor closely for toxicities (eg, excessive nausea, vomiting) and consider reducing the maintenance dose to 4.6 mg/24 hour if such toxicities develop.

Note: If dosing is interrupted for ≤3 days, restart treatment with the same or a lower strength patch. If interrupted for >3 days, reinitiate at 4.6 mg/24 hours and titrate (no sooner than every 4 weeks) to lowest effective maintenance dose.

Lewy body dementia (off-label use): *Oral:* Initial: 1.5 mg twice daily; may increase by 3 mg daily (1.5 mg per dose) every 2 weeks based on tolerability up to a maximum of 6 mg twice daily (titration lasted up to 8 weeks); study duration was 23 weeks (McKeith, 2000). An extension study was conducted in a limited number of patients (at the same dose) for up to 96 weeks (Grace, 2001).

Geriatric Following oral administration, clearance is significantly lower in patients >60 years of age, but dosage adjustments are not recommended. Age was not associated with exposure in patients treated transdermally. Titrate dose to individual's tolerance. Refer to adult dosing. **Note:** Canadian labeling recommends an initial oral dose of 1.5 mg once daily in patients >85 years of age with low body weight (<50 kg) or serious comorbidities, with a slower titration rate than used for adults.

Renal Impairment
US labeling:
Oral: Moderate to severe impairment (CrCl ≤50 mL/minute): There are no dosage adjustments provided in the manufacturer's labeling; patients may only be able to tolerate lower doses.
Transdermal: No dosage adjustment necessary.
Canadian labeling:
Oral: Initial dose: 1.5 mg once daily; titrate dose at a rate slower than recommended for adults with normal renal function.
Transdermal: No dosage adjustment necessary.

Hepatic Impairment
US labeling:
Oral:
Mild to moderate impairment (Child-Pugh class A and B): There are no dosage adjustments provided in the manufacturer's labeling; clearance is reduced and patients may require lower doses.
Severe impairment (Child-Pugh class C): There are no dosage adjustments provided in the manufacturer's labeling (has not been studied).
Transdermal:
Mild to moderate impairment (Child-Pugh class A and B): Initial and maximum dose: 4.6 mg/24 hours
Severe impairment (Child-Pugh class C): There are no dosage adjustments provided in the manufacturer's labeling (has not been studied).
Canadian labeling:
Oral:
Mild to moderate impairment (Child-Pugh class A and B): Initial dose: 1.5 mg once daily; titrate dose at a rate slower than recommended for adults with normal hepatic function.
Severe impairment (Child-Pugh class C): Use is contraindicated.
Transdermal:
Mild to moderate impairment (Child-Pugh class A and B): There are no dosage adjustments provided in the manufacturer's labeling; titrate dose cautiously
Severe impairment (Child-Pugh class C): Use is contraindicated.

Administration
Oral: Administer with meals (breakfast and dinner). Capsule should be swallowed whole. Liquid form, which is available for patients who cannot swallow capsules, can be swallowed directly from syringe or mixed with water, soda, or cold fruit juice. Stir well and drink within 4 hours of mixing.
Topical: Apply transdermal patch to upper or lower back (alternatively, may apply to upper arm or chest). Do not use patch if the pouch seal is broken or if the patch is cut, altered, or damaged. Avoid reapplication to same spot of skin for 14 days (eg, may rotate sections of back). Apply to clean, dry, and hairless skin. Patch should be pressed down firmly by applying pressure with the hand over the entire patch for at least 30 seconds, making sure edges stick well. Do not apply to red, irritated, or broken skin. Avoid areas of recent application of lotion or powder. After removal, fold patch to press adhesive surfaces together, place in previously saved pouch, and discard. Avoid eye contact; wash hands after handling patch. Remove old patch and replace with a new patch every 24 hours (at the same time each day). If a dose is missed or if the patch falls off, apply a new patch immediately and replace the following day at the usual application time. Avoid exposing the patch to external sources of heat (eg, sauna, excessive light) for prolonged periods of time. No more than 1 patch should be applied daily and existing patch must be removed prior to applying new patch. Discard any used or unused patches by folding adhesive sides together and dispose of in trash away from children and pets.

Monitoring Parameters Cognitive function at periodic intervals, symptoms of GI intolerance, weight

Product Availability Note: Exelon oral solution has been discontinued in the US for more than 1 year.

Dosage Forms Excipient information presented when available (limited, particularly for generics); consult specific product labeling. [DSC] = Discontinued product
Capsule, Oral:
Exelon: 1.5 mg, 3 mg, 4.5 mg, 6 mg
Generic: 1.5 mg, 3 mg, 4.5 mg, 6 mg
Patch 24 Hour, Transdermal:
Exelon: 4.6 mg/24 hr (1 ea, 30 ea); 9.5 mg/24 hr (1 ea, 30 ea); 13.3 mg/24 hr (1 ea, 30 ea)
Generic: 4.6 mg/24 hr (30 ea); 9.5 mg/24 hr (30 ea); 13.3 mg/24 hr (30 ea)
Solution, Oral:
Exelon: 2 mg/mL (120 mL [DSC])

◆ Rivastigmine Tartrate *see* Rivastigmine *on page 1607*

◆ Riva-Terbinafine (Can) *see* Terbinafine (Systemic) *on page 1759*
◆ Riva-Valacyclovir (Can) *see* ValACYclovir *on page 1858*
◆ Riva-Venlafaxine XR (Can) *see* Venlafaxine *on page 1886*
◆ Riva-Verapamil SR (Can) *see* Verapamil *on page 1889*
◆ Riva-Zolmitriptan (Can) *see* ZOLMitriptan *on page 1938*
◆ Rivotril (Can) *see* ClonazePAM *on page 419*
◆ Rixubis *see* Factor IX (Recombinant) *on page 738*

Rizatriptan (rye za TRIP tan)

Brand Names: US Maxalt; Maxalt-MLT
Brand Names: Canada ACT Rizatriptan; ACT Rizatriptan ODT; Apo-Rizatriptan; Apo-Rizatriptan RPD; Dom-Rizatriptan RDT; JAMP-Rizatriptan; JAMP-Rizatriptan IR; Mar-Rizatriptan; Maxalt; Maxalt RPD; Mint-Rizatriptan ODT; Mylan-Rizatriptan ODT; NAT-Rizatriptan ODT; PMS-Rizatriptan RDT; Riva-Rizatriptan ODT; Rizatriptan ODT; Rizatriptan RDT; Sandoz-Rizatriptan ODT; Teva-Rizatriptan ODT; Van-Rizatriptan

Index Terms MK462

Pharmacologic Category Antimigraine Agent; Serotonin 5-HT$_{1B, 1D}$ Receptor Agonist

Use Acute treatment of migraine with or without aura

Pregnancy Considerations Adverse events were observed in animal reproduction studies. Information related to rizatriptan use in pregnancy is limited (Källén, 2011; Nezvalová-Henriksen, 2010; Nezvalová-Henriksen, 2012).

A pregnancy registry has been established to monitor outcomes of women exposed to rizatriptan during pregnancy (800-986-8999). Preliminary data from the pregnancy registry (prospectively collected from 65 live births 1998-2004) does not show an increased risk of congenital malformations (Fiore, 2005). Until additional information is available, other agents are preferred for the initial treatment of migraine in pregnancy (Da Silva, 2012; MacGregor, 2012; Williams, 2012).

Breast-Feeding Considerations It is not known if rizatriptan is excreted in breast milk. The manufacturer recommends that caution be exercised when administering rizatriptan to nursing women.

Contraindications Hypersensitivity to rizatriptan or any component of the formulation; documented ischemic heart disease or other significant cardiovascular disease; coronary artery vasospasm (including Prinzmetal's angina); history of stroke or transient ischemic attack; peripheral vascular disease; ischemic bowel disease; uncontrolled hypertension; basilar or hemiplegic migraine; during or within 2 weeks of MAO inhibitors; during or within 24 hours of treatment with another 5-HT$_1$ agonist, or an ergot-containing or ergot-type medication (eg, methysergide, dihydroergotamine)

Warnings/Precautions Only indicated for treatment of acute migraine; not for the prevention of migraines or the treatment of cluster headache. If a patient does not respond to the first dose, the diagnosis of migraine should be reconsidered. Coronary artery vasospasm, transient ischemia, myocardial infarction, ventricular tachycardia/fibrillation, cardiac arrest, and death have been reported with 5-HT$_1$ agonist administration. Patients who experience sensations of chest pain/pressure/tightness or symptoms suggestive of angina following dosing should be evaluated for coronary artery disease or Prinzmetal's angina before receiving additional doses; if dosing is resumed and similar symptoms recur, monitor with ECG. Should not be given to patients who have risk factors for CAD (eg, hypertension, hypercholesterolemia, smoker, obesity, diabetes, strong family history of CAD, menopause, male >40 years of age) without adequate cardiac evaluation. Patients with suspected CAD should have cardiovascular evaluation to rule out CAD before considering use; if cardiovascular evaluation is "satisfactory," first dose should be given in the healthcare provider's office (consider ECG monitoring). Periodic evaluation of cardiovascular status should be done in all patients. Significant elevation in blood pressure, including hypertensive crisis, has also been reported on rare occasions in patients with and without a history of hypertension. Cerebral/subarachnoid hemorrhage, stroke, peripheral vascular ischemia, gastrointestinal ischemia/infarction, splenic infarction and Raynaud's syndrome have been reported with 5-HT$_1$ agonist administration. Use is contraindicated in patients with a history of stroke or transient ischemic attack. Rarely, partial vision loss and blindness (transient and permanent) have been reported with 5-HT$_1$ agonists.

Use with caution in elderly or patients with hepatic or renal impairment (including dialysis patients). Symptoms of agitation, confusion, hallucinations, hyper-reflexia, myoclonus, shivering, and tachycardia may occur with concomitant proserotonergic drugs (eg, SSRIs/SNRIs or triptans) or agents which reduce rizatriptan's metabolism. Concurrent use of serotonin precursors (eg, tryptophan) is not recommended. If concomitant administration with SSRIs is warranted, monitor closely, especially at initiation and with dose increases. Acute migraine agents (eg, triptans, opioids, ergotamine, or a combination of the agents) used for 10 or more days per month may lead to worsening of headaches (medication overuse headache); withdrawal treatment may be necessary in the setting of overuse. Maxalt-MLT tablets contain phenylalanine.

Adverse Reactions
1% to 10%:
Cardiovascular: Chest pain (<2% to 3%), flushing (>1%), palpitation (>1%)
Central nervous system: Dizziness (4% to 9%), somnolence (4% to 8%), fatigue (adults 4% to 7%; children >1%), pain (3%), headache (≤2%), euphoria (>1%), hypoesthesia (>1%)
Dermatologic: Skin flushing
Gastrointestinal: Nausea (4% to 6%), xerostomia (3%), abdominal discomfort (children >1%), diarrhea (>1%), vomiting (>1%)
Neuromuscular & skeletal: Weakness (4% to 7%), paresthesia (3% to 4%); neck, throat, and jaw pain/tightness/pressure (≤2%), tremor (>1%)
Respiratory: Dyspnea (>1%)
Miscellaneous: Feeling of heaviness (<1% to 2%)
<1% (Limited to important or life-threatening): Anaphylaxis/anaphylactoid reactions, angina, angioedema, blurred vision, bradycardia, confusion, edema, hallucination (children), hearing impairment, hypertensive crisis, memory impairment, MI, myocardial ischemia, pruritus, seizure, syncope, tachycardia, tinnitus, tongue edema, toxic epidermal necrolysis, vasospasm, vertigo, wheezing

Drug Interactions
Metabolism/Transport Effects None known.
Avoid Concomitant Use
Avoid concomitant use of Rizatriptan with any of the following: Dapoxetine; Ergot Derivatives; MAO Inhibitors
Increased Effect/Toxicity
Rizatriptan may increase the levels/effects of: Antipsychotic Agents; Droxidopa; Ergot Derivatives; Metoclopramide; Serotonin Modulators

The levels/effects of Rizatriptan may be increased by: Antiemetics (5HT3 Antagonists); Antipsychotic Agents; Dapoxetine; Ergot Derivatives; MAO Inhibitors; Metaxalone; Propranolol
Decreased Effect There are no known significant interactions involving a decrease in effect.
Food Interactions Food delays absorption. Management: Administer without regard to meals.
Storage/Stability Store at room temperature of 15°C to 30°C (59°F to 86°F); orally disintegrating tablets should be stored in blister pack until administration.
Mechanism of Action Selective agonist for serotonin (5-HT$_{1B}$ and 5-HT$_{1D}$ receptors) in cranial arteries; causes vasoconstriction and reduces sterile inflammation associated with antidromic neuronal transmission correlating with relief of migraine
Pharmacodynamics/Kinetics
Onset of action: Most patients have response to treatment within 2 hours
Distribution: V$_d$: Females: 110 L; Males 140 L
Protein binding: 14%
Metabolism: Via monoamine oxidase-A; forms metabolites; significant first-pass metabolism
Bioavailability: ~45%
Half-life elimination: 2-3 hours
Time to peak: Maxalt®: 1-1.5 hours (delayed up to 0.7 hour with Maxalt-MLT®)
Excretion: Urine (82%, 14% as unchanged drug); feces (12%)
Dosing
Adult & Geriatric Note: In patients with risk factors for coronary artery disease, following adequate evaluation to establish the absence of coronary artery disease, the initial dose should be administered in a setting where response may be evaluated (physician's office or similarly staffed setting). ECG monitoring may be considered.

Migraine: Oral: 5-10 mg, repeat after 2 hours if significant relief is not attained; maximum: 30 mg/24 hours
Dose adjustment with concomitant propranolol therapy: 5 mg/dose (maximum: 15 mg/24 hours)

Pediatric Note: In patients with risk factors for coronary artery disease, following adequate evaluation to establish the absence of coronary artery disease, the initial dose should be administered in a setting where response may be evaluated (physician's office or similarly staffed setting). ECG monitoring may be considered.

Migraine: Oral: Children 6-17 years: **Note:** Safety and efficacy of multiple rizatriptan doses in a 24-hour period have not been established for pediatric patients.
<40 kg: 5 mg as a single dose
≥40 kg: 10 mg as a single dose
Dose adjustment with concomitant propranolol therapy:
<40 kg: Use not recommended
≥40 kg: 5 mg as a single dose (maximum: 5 mg/24 hours)
Renal Impairment No dosage adjustment provided in manufacturer's labeling; however, the AUC was 44% greater in patients on hemodialysis.
Hepatic Impairment No dosage adjustment provided in manufacturer's labeling; however, plasma concentrations are increased by 30% in patients with moderate hepatic dysfunction.
Dietary Considerations Some products may contain phenylalanine.
Administration May be administered with or without food. For orally-disintegrating tablets (Maxalt-MLT®), patient should be instructed to place tablet on tongue and allow to dissolve. Dissolved tablet will be swallowed with saliva.
Monitoring Parameters Headache severity, signs/symptoms suggestive of angina; consider monitoring blood pressure, heart rate, and/or ECG with first dose in patients with likelihood of unrecognized coronary disease, such as patients with significant hypertension, hypercholesterolemia, obese patients, patients with diabetes, smokers with other risk factors or strong family history of coronary artery disease
Dosage Forms Excipient information presented when available (limited, particularly for generics); consult specific product labeling.
Tablet, Oral:
Maxalt: 5 mg, 10 mg
Generic: 5 mg, 10 mg
Tablet Dispersible, Oral:
Maxalt-MLT: 5 mg, 10 mg [contains aspartame; peppermint flavor]
Generic: 5 mg, 10 mg

◆ Robitussin Peak Cold Cough + Chest Congestion DM [OTC] *see* Guaifenesin and Dextromethorphan *on page 861*

◆ Robitussin Peak Cold Maximum Strength Cough + Chest Congestion DM [OTC] *see* Guaifenesin and Dextromethorphan *on page 861*

◆ Robitussin Peak Cold Sugar-Free Cough + Chest Congestion DM [OTC] *see* Guaifenesin and Dextromethorphan *on page 861*

◆ Rocaltrol *see* Calcitriol *on page 284*

◆ Rocephin *see* CefTRIAXone *on page 349*

Rocuronium (roe kyoor OH nee um)

Brand Names: US Zemuron
Brand Names: Canada Rocuronium Bromide Injection; Zemuron
Index Terms ORG 9426; Rocuronium Bromide
Pharmacologic Category Neuromuscular Blocker Agent, Nondepolarizing
Use Neuromuscular blockade: As an adjunct to general anesthesia to facilitate rapid sequence and routine tracheal intubation and to provide skeletal muscle relaxation during surgery or mechanical ventilation.
Pregnancy Considerations Teratogenic effects were not observed in animal reproduction studies. Rocuronium crosses the placenta; umbilical venous plasma levels are ~18% of the maternal concentration following a maternal dose of 0.6 mg/kg (Abouleish, 1994). The manufacturer does not recommend use for rapid sequence induction during cesarean section.
Breast-Feeding Considerations Information related to rocuronium use and breast-feeding has not been located. If present in breast milk, oral absorption by a nursing infant would be expected to be minimal (Lee, 1993).
Contraindications Hypersensitivity (eg, anaphylaxis) to rocuronium, other neuromuscular-blocking agents, or any component of the formulation
Warnings/Precautions Use with caution in patients with cardiovascular disease and pulmonary disease; ventilation must be supported during neuromuscular blockade; certain clinical conditions may result in potentiation or antagonism of neuromuscular blockade:

Potentiation: Electrolyte abnormalities (eg, severe hypocalcemia, severe hypokalemia, hypermagnesemia), cachexia, neuromuscular diseases, metabolic acidosis, metabolic alkalosis, respiratory acidosis, Eaton-Lambert syndrome, and myasthenia gravis

Antagonism: Respiratory alkalosis, hypercalcemia, demyelinating lesions, peripheral neuropathies, denervation, and muscle trauma

Use with caution in patients with hepatic impairment; clinical duration may be prolonged. Resistance may occur in burn patients (≥20% of total body surface area), usually several days after the injury, and may persist for several months after wound healing. Cross-sensitivity with other neuromuscular-blocking agents may occur; use is contraindicated in patients with previous anaphylactic reactions to other neuromuscular blockers. Use with caution in patients with pulmonary hypertension or valvular heart disease. Use caution in the elderly. Should be administered by adequately trained individuals familiar with its use. Use appropriate anesthesia, pain control, and sedation. In patients requiring long-term administration in the ICU, tolerance to rocuronium may develop; use of a peripheral nerve stimulator to monitor drug effects is strongly recommended. Additional doses of rocuronium or any other neuromuscular-blocking agent should be avoided unless definite excessive response to nerve stimulation is present.

Some patients may experience prolonged recovery of neuromuscular function after administration (especially after prolonged use). Patients should be adequately recovered prior to extubation. Other factors associated with prolonged recovery should be considered (eg, corticosteroid use, patient condition). In addition to prolonging recovery from neuromuscular blockade, concomitant use with corticosteroids has been associated with development of acute quadriplegic myopathy syndrome (AQMS). Current guidelines recommend neuromuscular blockers be discontinued as soon as possible in patients receiving corticosteroids or interrupted daily until necessary to restart them based on clinical condition (Murray, 2002). Numerous drugs either *antagonize* (eg, acetylcholinesterase inhibitors) or *potentiate* (eg, calcium channel blockers, certain antimicrobials, inhalation anesthetics, lithium, magnesium salts, procainamide, and quinidine) the effects of neuromuscular blockade; use with caution in patients receiving these agents. Immediate treatment (including

epinephrine 1:1000) for anaphylactoid and/or hypersensitivity reactions should be available during use. Not recommended by the manufacturer for rapid sequence intubation in pediatric patients; however, it has been used successfully in clinical trials for this indication. If extravasation occurs, local irritation may ensue; discontinue administration immediately and restart in another vein.

Adverse Reactions Frequency not always defined.

Cardiovascular: Increased peripheral vascular resistance (abdominal aortic surgery: 24%, frequency not defined during other procedures), tachycardia (≤5%; incidence greater in children), hypertension, transient hypotension

Hypersensitivity: Anaphylaxis

<1% (Limited to important or life-threatening): Anaphylactoid reaction, asthma, cardiac arrhythmia, ECG abnormality, hiccups, injection site edema, nausea, vomiting

Drug Interactions

Metabolism/Transport Effects None known.

Avoid Concomitant Use

Avoid concomitant use of Rocuronium with any of the following: QuiNINE

Increased Effect/Toxicity

Rocuronium may increase the levels/effects of: Cardiac Glycosides; Corticosteroids (Systemic); OnabotulinumtoxinA; RimabotulinumtoxinB

The levels/effects of Rocuronium may be increased by: AbobotulinumtoxinA; Aminoglycosides; Calcium Channel Blockers; Capreomycin; Clindamycin (Topical); Colistimethate; CycloSPORINE (Systemic); Fosphenytoin-Phenytoin; Inhalational Anesthetics; Ketorolac (Nasal); Ketorolac (Systemic); Lincosamide Antibiotics; Lithium; Loop Diuretics; Magnesium Salts; Minocycline; Polymyxin B; Procainamide; QuiNIDine; QuiNINE; Spironolactone; Tetracycline Derivatives; Vancomycin

Decreased Effect

The levels/effects of Rocuronium may be decreased by: Acetylcholinesterase Inhibitors; Fosphenytoin-Phenytoin; Loop Diuretics

Preparation for Administration May be diluted in D5NS, D5W, LR or NS at concentrations up to 5 mg/mL; use within 24 hours of preparation.

Storage/Stability Store unopened/undiluted vials under refrigeration at 2°C to 8°C (36°F to 46°F); do not freeze. When stored at room temperature (25°C [77°F]), it is stable for 60 days; once opened, use within 30 days. Dilutions up to 5 mg/mL in 0.9% sodium chloride, dextrose 5% in water, 5% dextrose in sodium chloride 0.9%, or lactated Ringer's are stable for up to 24 hours at room temperature.

Mechanism of Action Blocks acetylcholine from binding to receptors on motor endplate inhibiting depolarization

Pharmacodynamics/Kinetics

Onset of action: Good intubation conditions within 1-2 minutes (depending on dose administered); maximum neuromuscular blockade within 4 minutes

Duration: ~30 minutes (with standard doses, increases with higher doses and inhalational anesthetic agents; patient age dependent)

Distribution: V_d: ~0.25 L/kg

Protein binding: ~30%

Metabolism: Minimally hepatic; 17-desacetylrocuronium (5% to 10% activity of parent drug)

Half-life elimination: 66 to 144 minutes

Excretion: Feces (31%); urine (26%) (Proost, 2000)

Dosing

Adult & Geriatric Dose to effect; doses will vary due to interpatient variability. Dosing also dependent on anesthetic technique and age of patient.

Rapid sequence intubation: IV: 0.6 to 1.2 mg/kg

Obesity: In adult patients with morbid obesity (BMI >40 kg/m^2), the use of 1.2 mg/kg using ideal body weight (IBW) provided a short onset of action and excellent or good intubating conditions at 60 seconds in one study (Gaszynski, 2011).

Tracheal intubation: IV:

Initial: 0.45 to 0.6 mg/kg; administration of 0.3 mg/kg may also provide optimal conditions for tracheal intubation (Barclay, 1997)

Obesity: May use ideal body weight (IBW) for morbidly obese (BMI >40 kg/m^2) adult patients (Leykin, 2004); onset time may be slightly delayed using IBW. The manufacturer recommends dosing based on actual body weight in all obese patients.

Maintenance for continued surgical relaxation: 0.1 to 0.2 mg/kg; repeat as needed **or** a continuous infusion of 10 to 12 **mcg**/kg/**minute** (0.6 to 0.72 **mg**/kg/**hour**) only after recovery of neuromuscular function is evident; infusion rates have ranged from 4 to 16 mcg/kg/**minute** (0.24 to 0.96 **mg**/kg/**hour**)

Note: Inhaled anesthetic agents prolong the duration of action of rocuronium. Use lower end of the dosing range; redosing interval guided by monitoring with a peripheral nerve stimulator.

Preinduction defasciculation (off-label use): IV: 0.03 to 0.06 mg/kg given 1.5 to 3 minutes before administration of succinylcholine (Harvey, 1998; Martin, 1998)

ICU paralysis (eg, facilitate mechanical ventilation) in adequately sedated patients (off-label use): Initial bolus dose: 0.6 to 1 mg/kg, then a continuous IV infusion of 8 to 12 **mcg**/kg/**minute** (0.48 to 0.72 **mg/kg/hour**); monitor depth of blockade every 2 to 3 hours initially until stable dose, then every 8 to 12 hours; adjust rate of administration by 10% increments according to peripheral nerve stimulation response or desired clinical response (Greenberg, 2013; Murray, 2002; Rudis, 1996; Sparr, 1997; Warr, 2011).

Note: When possible, minimize depth and duration of paralysis. Stopping the infusion for some time until forced to restart based on patient condition is recommended to reduce post-paralytic complications (eg, acute quadriplegic myopathy syndrome [AQMS]) (Murray, 2002).

Intermittent dosing has also been described with an initial loading dose of 50 mg followed by 25 mg given when peripheral nerve stimulation returns (Sparr, 1997).

Pediatric Dose to effect; doses will vary due to interpatient variability. Dosing also dependent on anesthetic technique and age of patient.

Neonates, Infants, Children, and Adolescents: **Note:** In general, onset is shortened and duration is prolonged as dose increases. Duration is shortest in children >2 to ≤11 years and longest in neonates and infants.

Tracheal intubation: IV: 0.45 mg/kg or 0.6 mg/kg
Maintenance for continued surgical relaxation: IV: 0.075 to 0.15 mg/kg; redosing interval is guided by monitoring with a peripheral nerve stimulator **or** 7 to 12 **mcg**/kg/**minute** (0.42 to 0.72 **mg**/kg/**hour**) as a continuous infusion; use lower end of the continuous infusion dosing range for neonates and the upper end for children >2 to ≤11 years

Rapid sequence intubation (off-label use): IV: 0.9 mg/kg or 1.2 mg/kg. Not recommended, per the manufacturer, for rapid sequence intubation in pediatric patients; however, it has been used successfully in clinical trials for this indication in children >1 year (Cheng, 2002; Fuchs-Buder, 1996; Mazurek, 1998; Naguib, 1997).

Renal Impairment No dosage adjustment necessary. Duration of neuromuscular blockade may vary in patients with renal impairment.

Hepatic Impairment No dosage adjustment provided in manufacturer's labeling. However, dosage reductions may be necessary in patients with liver disease; duration of neuromuscular blockade may be prolonged due to increased volume of distribution. When rapid sequence intubation is required in adult patients with ascites, a dose on the higher end of the dosage range may be necessary to achieve adequate neuromuscular blockade.

Obesity Refer to indication-specific dosing for obesity-related information (may not be available for all indications).

Administration Administer IV only; may be administered as a bolus injection (undiluted) or via a continuous infusion.

Monitoring Parameters Peripheral nerve stimulator measuring twitch response, heart rate, blood pressure, assisted ventilation status

Additional Information Rocuronium is classified as an intermediate-duration neuromuscular-blocking agent. Do not mix in the same syringe with barbiturates. Rocuronium does not relieve pain or produce sedation.

Dosage Forms Excipient information presented when available (limited, particularly for generics); consult specific product labeling.
Solution, Intravenous, as bromide:
Zemuron: 50 mg/5 mL (5 mL); 100 mg/10 mL (10 mL)
Generic: 50 mg/5 mL (5 mL); 100 mg/10 mL (10 mL)
Solution, Intravenous, as bromide [preservative free]:
Generic: 50 mg/5 mL (5 mL); 100 mg/10 mL (10 mL)

◆ *Rocuronium Bromide see Rocuronium on page 1611*
◆ *Rocuronium Bromide Injection (Can) see Rocuronium on page 1611*
◆ *Rofact (Can) see Rifampin on page 1581*

Roflumilast (roe FLUE mi last)

Brand Names: US Daliresp
Brand Names: Canada Daxas

Pharmacologic Category Phosphodiesterase-4 Enzyme Inhibitor

Use Chronic obstructive pulmonary disease: To reduce the risk of chronic obstructive pulmonary disease (COPD) exacerbations in patients with severe COPD associated with chronic bronchitis and a history of exacerbations

Pregnancy Considerations Adverse events were observed in some animal reproduction studies. The Canadian labeling recommends avoiding use during pregnancy and in women of childbearing potential not using adequate contraception.

Breast-Feeding Considerations It is not known if roflumilast can be detected in breast milk; however, excretion into human breast milk is likely. Breast-feeding is not recommended by the manufacturer.

Medication Guide Available Yes

Contraindications Moderate or severe hepatic impairment (Child-Pugh class B or C)

Canadian labeling: Additional contraindication (not in U.S. labeling): Hypersensitivity to roflumilast or any component of the formulation

Warnings/Precautions Not indicated for relieving acute bronchospasms or for use as monotherapy of COPD; use only as adjunctive therapy to bronchodilator therapy. Neuropsychiatric effects (eg, anxiety, depression) have been reported with use; rarely, suicidal behavior/ideation and completed suicide were reported. Avoid use in patients with a history of depression with suicidal behavior/ideations; instruct patients/caregivers to report psychiatric symptoms and consider discontinuation of therapy in such patients. Systemic exposure may be increased in patients with mild hepatic impairment; use in moderate to severe impairment is contraindicated.

May cause weight loss and/or diarrhea (sometimes severe); weight loss usually observed within 6 months of initiating therapy and diarrhea within 4 weeks. Instruct patients to monitor weight regularly. Avoid initiation of therapy or discontinue therapy with unexplained/pronounced weight loss. Potentially significant drug-drug interactions may exist, requiring dose or frequency adjustment, additional monitoring, and/or selection of alternative therapy. May contain lactose; the Canadian labeling recommends avoiding use in patients with galactose intolerance, Lapp lactase deficiency, or glucose-galactose malabsorption. The Canadian labeling recommends avoiding use in patients with cancer (excluding basal cell carcinoma), heart failure (NYHA III/IV), severe acute infection, immunosuppression, or immunosuppressive therapy (excludes short-term systemic corticosteroid use for COPD exacerbation).

Adverse Reactions
2% to 10%:
Central nervous system: Headache (4%), dizziness (2%), insomnia (2%)
Endocrine & metabolic: Weight loss (5% to 10% of body weight: 8% to 20%; >10% loss: 7%)
Gastrointestinal: Diarrhea (10%), nausea (5%), decreased appetite (2%)
Infection: Influenza (3%)
Neuromuscular & skeletal: Back pain (3%)
<2% (Limited to important or life-threatening): Abdominal pain, anemia, arthritis, atrial fibrillation, depression, dysgeusia, epistaxis, gastritis, gastroesophageal reflux disease, gynecomastia, hematochezia, hypersensitivity, increased gamma-glutamyl transferase, increased lactate dehydrogenase, increased serum AST, lung carcinoma, muscle spasm, myalgia, myasthenia, pancreatitis, paresthesia, prostate carcinoma, renal failure, respiratory tract infection, rhinitis, sinusitis, suicidal ideation, suicidal tendencies, suicide completed, supraventricular cardiac arrhythmia, urinary tract infection

Drug Interactions
Metabolism/Transport Effects Substrate of CYP1A2 (minor), CYP3A4 (major); **Note:** Assignment of Major/Minor substrate status based on clinically relevant drug interaction potential

Avoid Concomitant Use
Avoid concomitant use of Roflumilast with any of the following: CYP3A4 Inducers (Strong); Loxapine; Rifampin

Increased Effect/Toxicity
Roflumilast may increase the levels/effects of: Immunosuppressants; Loxapine; Riociguat

The levels/effects of Roflumilast may be increased by: Cimetidine; Ciprofloxacin (Systemic); FluvoxaMINE

Decreased Effect
The levels/effects of Roflumilast may be decreased by: Bosentan; CYP3A4 Inducers (Moderate); CYP3A4 Inducers (Strong); Dabrafenib; Deferasirox; Rifampin; St Johns Wort

Storage/Stability Store at 20°C to 25°C (68°F to 77°F), excursions permitted from 15°C to 30°C (59°F to 86°F).

Mechanism of Action Roflumilast and its active N-oxide metabolite selectively inhibit phosphodiesterase-4 (PDE4) leading to an accumulation of cyclic AMP (cAMP) within inflammatory and structural cells important in the pathogenesis of COPD. Anti-inflammatory effects include suppression of cytokine release and inhibition of lung infiltration by neutrophils and other leukocytes. Pulmonary remodeling and mucociliary malfunction are also attenuated.

Pharmacodynamics/Kinetics

Distribution: V_d: 2.9 L/kg

Protein binding: 99%; N-oxide metabolite: 97%

Metabolism: Hepatic via CYP3A4 and CYP1A2 to active N-oxide metabolite; also undergoes conjugation

Bioavailability: ~80%

Half-life elimination: 17 hours; N-oxide metabolite: 30 hours

Time to peak: ~1 hour (delayed by food); N-oxide metabolite: ~8 hours

Excretion: Urine (~70% as metabolites)

Dosing

Adult & Geriatric COPD: Oral: 500 mcg once daily

Renal Impairment No dosage adjustment necessary.

Hepatic Impairment

Mild impairment (Child-Pugh class A): No dosage adjustment necessary. Use with caution; 500 mcg once daily dose has not been evaluated in mild impairment.

Moderate-to-severe impairment (Child-Pugh class B or C): Use is contraindicated.

Administration Administer without regard to meals.

Monitoring Parameters Liver function tests. Measure weight regularly during therapy

Dosage Forms Excipient information presented when available (limited, particularly for generics); consult specific product labeling.

Tablet, Oral:

Daliresp: 500 mcg

Dosage Forms: Canada Excipient information presented when available (limited, particularly for generics); consult specific product labeling.

Tablet, oral:

Daxas: 500 mcg

Rolapitant (roe LA pi tant)

Brand Names: US Varubi

Index Terms Rolapitant Hydrochloride; Rolapitant Monohydrate Hydrochloride; SCH-619734

Pharmacologic Category Antiemetic; Substance P/Neurokinin 1 Receptor Antagonist

Use Chemotherapy-induced nausea and vomiting (CINV), prevention: Prevention of delayed nausea and vomiting associated with initial and repeat courses of emetogenic cancer chemotherapy, including, but not limited to, highly-emetogenic chemotherapy in adults (in combination with other antiemetic agents).

Pregnancy Considerations Adverse events were observed in some animal reproduction studies.

Breast-Feeding Considerations It is not known if rolapitant is excreted into breast milk. According to the manufacturer, the decision to breast-feed during therapy should take into account the risk of exposure to the infant and the benefits of treatment to the mother.

Contraindications Concurrent use of thioridazine (a CYP2D6 substrate)

Warnings/Precautions Avoid use in patients with severe hepatic impairment; if use cannot be avoided, monitor for adverse reactions related to rolapitant. Potentially significant drug-drug interactions may exist, requiring dose or frequency adjustment, additional monitoring, and/or selection of alternative therapy. Rolapitant's inhibitory effect on CYP2D6 may persist for at least 7 days (or longer); increased plasma concentrations of certain CYP2D6 substrates may result in QT prolongation and torsades de pointes. Monitor for adverse reactions if concomitant use with CYP2D6 substrates with a narrow therapeutic index cannot be avoided. Avoid concurrent use with pimozide; concurrent use with thioridazine is contraindicated.

Adverse Reactions Clinical trials were conducted in patients receiving combination therapy with a 5-HT3 receptor antagonist and dexamethasone. It is not possible to correlate frequency of adverse events with rolaprepitant alone.

1% to 10%:

Central nervous system: Dizziness (6%)

Gastrointestinal: Decreased appetite (9%), hiccups (5%), dyspepsia (4%), stomatitis (4%), abdominal pain (3%)

Genitourinary: Urinary tract infection (4%)

Hematologic & oncologic: Neutropenia (7% to 9%), anemia (3%)

Drug Interactions

Metabolism/Transport Effects Substrate of CYP3A4 (major); **Note:** Assignment of Major/Minor substrate status based on clinically relevant drug interaction potential; **Inhibits** BCRP, CYP2B6 (weak), CYP2C8 (weak), CYP2D6 (moderate), P-glycoprotein

Avoid Concomitant Use

Avoid concomitant use of Rolapitant with any of the following: Amodiaquine; Bosutinib; PAZOPanib; Pimozide; Silodosin; Thioridazine; Topotecan; VinCRIStine (Liposomal)

Increased Effect/Toxicity

Rolapitant may increase the levels/effects of: Afatinib; Amodiaquine; ARIPiprazole; BCRP/ABCG2 Substrates; Bosutinib; Brentuximab Vedotin; Brexpiprazole; Colchicine; CYP2D6 Substrates; Dabigatran Etexilate; DOXOrubicin (Conventional); Edoxaban; Eliglustat; Everolimus; Fesoterodine; Ledipasvir; Metoprolol; Naloxegol; Nebivolol; PAZOPanib; P-glycoprotein/ABCB1 Substrates; Pimozide; Prucalopride; Ranolazine; Rifaximin; Silodosin; Thioridazine; Topotecan; VinCRIStine (Liposomal)

The levels/effects of Rolapitant may be increased by: Osimertinib; Propafenone

Decreased Effect

Rolapitant may decrease the levels/effects of: Codeine; Tamoxifen; TraMADol

The levels/effects of Rolapitant may be decreased by: Bosentan; CYP3A4 Inducers (Moderate); CYP3A4 Inducers (Strong); Dabrafenib; Deferasirox; Enzalutamide; Mitotane; Osimertinib; Siltuximab; St Johns Wort; Tocilizumab

Storage/Stability Store at 20°C to 25°C (68°F to 77°F); excursions are permitted between 15°C and 30°C (59°F and 86°F)

Mechanism of Action Rolapitant prevents delayed nausea and vomiting associated with emetogenic chemotherapy by selectively and competitively inhibiting the substance P/neurokinin 1 (NK_1) receptor.

Pharmacodynamics/Kinetics

Distribution: V_d/F: 387 L

Protein binding: 99.8%

Metabolism: Hepatic; primarily by CYP3A4 to form active metabolite M19 (major)

Half-life elimination: ~7 days (range: 169 to 183 hours)

Time to peak: ~4 hours

Excretion: Feces (73%); urine (~14%; primarily as metabolites)

Dosing

Adult & Geriatric

Chemotherapy-induced nausea and vomiting (prevention): Oral: **Note:** Do not administer rolapitant at less than 2-week intervals. No dosage adjustment for concomitant dexamethasone is required.

Highly emetogenic chemotherapy (cisplatin-based): 180 mg administered ~1 to 2 hours prior to chemotherapy on day 1 only (in combination with dexamethasone given on days 1, 2, 3, and 4 and a 5-HT₃ receptor antagonist given on day 1)

Moderately emetogenic chemotherapy and anthracycline/cyclophosphamide combinations: 180 mg administered ~1 to 2 hours prior to chemotherapy on day 1 only (in combination with dexamethasone given on day 1 and a 5-HT₃ receptor antagonist given as appropriate based the agent selected)

Renal Impairment

CrCl 30 to 90 mL/minute: There are no dosage adjustments provided in the manufacturer's labeling; however, based on pharmacokinetics, dosage adjustment is not likely necessary.

CrCl <30 ml/minute and end-stage renal disease (ESRD): There are no dosage adjustments provided in the manufacturer's labeling (has not been studied).

Hepatic Impairment

Child-Pugh classes A and B: No dosage adjustment is necessary.

Child-Pugh class C: Avoid use if possible (has not been studied); if use cannot be avoided, monitor closely for adverse reactions related to rolapitant.

Administration Administer orally ~1 to 2 hours prior to each chemotherapy cycle (on day 1 only). May be administered without regard to meals.

Monitoring Parameters If concomitant use with CYP2D6 substrates with a narrow therapeutic index cannot be avoided, monitor for adverse reactions.

Dosage Forms Excipient information presented when available (limited, particularly for generics); consult specific product labeling.

Tablet, Oral:

Varubi: 90 mg [contains fd&c blue #2 aluminum lake]

◆ Rolapitant Hydrochloride see Rolapitant on page 1613

◆ Rolapitant Monohydrate Hydrochloride see Rolapitant on page 1613

◆ Rolene (Can) see Betamethasone (Topical) on page 224

◆ Romazicon [DSC] see Flumazenil on page 780

◆ Romazicon (Can) see Flumazenil on page 780

RomiDEPsin (roe mi DEP sin)

Brand Names: US Istodax
Index Terms Depsipeptide; FK228; FR901228
Pharmacologic Category Antineoplastic Agent, Histone Deacetylase (HDAC) Inhibitor
Use
Cutaneous T-cell lymphoma: Treatment of cutaneous T-cell lymphoma (CTCL) in patients who have received at least one systemic prior therapy
Peripheral T-cell lymphoma: Treatment of peripheral T-cell lymphoma (PTCL) in patients who have received at least one prior therapy
Pregnancy Considerations Adverse events were observed in animal reproduction studies. Based on the mechanism of action, romidepsin may cause fetal harm if administered during pregnancy.

Breast-Feeding Considerations It is not known if romidepsin is excreted in breast milk. Due to the potential for serious adverse reactions in the nursing infant, the manufacturer recommends a decision be made whether to discontinue nursing or to discontinue the drug, taking into account the importance of treatment to the mother.

Contraindications There are no contraindications listed in the manufacturer's labeling.

Warnings/Precautions Hazardous agent - use appropriate precautions for handling and disposal (NIOSH 2014 [group 1]). Anemia, leukopenia, neutropenia, lymphopenia and thrombocytopenia may occur; may require dosage modification; monitor blood counts during treatment. Serious infections (occasionally fatal), including pneumonia, sepsis, and viral reactivation (eg, Epstein Barr and hepatitis B) have occurred during or within 30 days of treatment. Monitor patients with a history of hepatitis B infections closely for viral reactivation; consider antiviral prophylaxis. Epstein Barr reactivation leading to liver failure has also been reported, with ganciclovir antiviral prophylaxis failure in one case. The risk of life-threatening infection may be increased in patients who have received prior with antilymphocytic monoclonal antibodies or who have disease involvement in the bone marrow. QTc prolongation has been observed; use caution in patients with a history of QTc prolongation, congenital long QT syndrome, with medications known to prolong the QT interval, or with preexisting cardiac disease. Obtain baseline and periodic ECG (12-lead); monitor and correct electrolyte (potassium, magnesium, and calcium) abnormalities prior to and during treatment. T-wave and ST-segment changes have also been reported. Use with caution in patients with moderate-to-severe hepatic impairment or end-stage renal disease. Tumor lysis syndrome (TLS) has been observed; closely monitor patients with advanced disease and/or with a high tumor burden (risk of TLS may be higher); if TLS occurs, initiate appropriate treatment. Potentially significant drug-drug interactions may exist, requiring dose or frequency adjustment, additional monitoring, and/or selection of alternative therapy.

Adverse Reactions
>10%:
Cardiovascular: ST-T wave changes (2% to 63%), hypotension (7% to 23%)
Central nervous system: Fatigue (53% to 77%), fever (20% to 47%), headache (15% to 34%), chills (11% to 17%)
Dermatologic: Pruritus (7% to 31%), dermatitis/exfoliative dermatitis (4% to 27%)
Endocrine & metabolic: Hypocalcemia (4% to 52%), hyperglycemia (2% to 51%), hypoalbuminemia (3% to 48%), hyperuricemia (≤33%), hypomagnesemia (22% to 28%), hypermagnesemia (≤27%), hypophosphatemia (≤27%), hypokalemia (6% to 20%), hyponatremia (≤20%)

Gastrointestinal: Nausea (56% to 86%; grades 3/4: 2% to 6%), anorexia (23% to 54%), vomiting (34% to 52%; grades 3/4: ≤10%), taste alteration (15% to 40%), constipation (12% to 40%), diarrhea (20% to 36%), weight loss (10% to 15%), abdominal pain (13% to 14%)
Hematologic: Anemia (19% to 72%; grades 3/4: 3% to 28%), thrombocytopenia (17% to 72%; grades 3/4: ≤36%), neutropenia (11% to 66%; grades 3/4: 4% to 47%), lymphopenia (4% to 57%; grades 3/4: ≤37%), leukopenia (4% to 55%; grades 3/4: ≤45%)
Hepatic: AST increased (3% to 28%), ALT increased (3% to 22%)
Neuromuscular & skeletal: Weakness (53% to 77%)
Respiratory: Cough (18% to 21%), dyspnea (13% to 21%)
Miscellaneous: Infection (46% to 54%; grades 3/4: 11% to 33%)
1% to 10%:
Cardiovascular: Peripheral edema (6% to 10%), tachycardia (≤10%), chest pain, DVT, edema, QT prolongation, supraventricular arrhythmia, syncope, ventricular arrhythmia
Dermatologic: Cellulitis
Endocrine & metabolic: Dehydration
Gastrointestinal: Stomatitis (6% to 10%)
Hematologic: Neutropenic fever
Hepatic: Hyperbilirubinemia
Respiratory: Hypoxia, pneumonia, pneumonitis, pulmonary embolism
Miscellaneous: Central line infection, hypersensitivity, sepsis, tumor lysis syndrome (1% to 2%)
<1% (Limited to important or life-threatening): Acute renal failure, acute respiratory distress syndrome, atrial fibrillation, bacteremia, candida infection, cardiopulmonary failure, cardiogenic shock, Epstein-Barr virus reactivation, multiorgan failure, septic shock

Drug Interactions
Metabolism/Transport Effects Substrate of CYP3A4 (major), P-glycoprotein; **Note:** Assignment of Major/Minor substrate status based on clinically relevant drug interaction potential; **Inhibits** BSEP

Avoid Concomitant Use
Avoid concomitant use of RomiDEPsin with any of the following: BCG (Intravesical); CYP3A4 Inducers (Strong); Deferiprone; Dexamethasone (Systemic); Dipyrone; Natalizumab; Pimecrolimus; Rifampin; St Johns Wort; Tacrolimus (Topical); Tofacitinib; Vaccines (Live)

Increased Effect/Toxicity
RomiDEPsin may increase the levels/effects of: CloZAPine; Deferiprone; Fingolimod; Highest Risk QTc-Prolonging Agents; Leflunomide; Moderate Risk QTc-Prolonging Agents; Natalizumab; Tofacitinib; Vaccines (Live); Warfarin

The levels/effects of RomiDEPsin may be increased by: CYP3A4 Inhibitors (Strong); Denosumab; Dipyrone; Mifepristone; Osimertinib; P-glycoprotein/ABCB1 Inhibitors; Pimecrolimus; Ranolazine; Rifampin; Roflumilast; Tacrolimus (Topical); Trastuzumab

Decreased Effect
RomiDEPsin may decrease the levels/effects of: BCG (Intravesical); Coccidioides immitis Skin Test; Sipuleucel-T; Vaccines (Inactivated); Vaccines (Live)

The levels/effects of RomiDEPsin may be decreased by: Bosentan; CYP3A4 Inducers (Moderate); CYP3A4 Inducers (Strong); Dabrafenib; Deferasirox; Dexamethasone (Systemic); Echinacea; Osimertinib; P-glycoprotein/ABCB1 Inducers; Siltuximab; St Johns Wort; Tocilizumab

Food Interactions Grapefruit juice may increase the levels/effects of romidepsin. Management: Avoid grapefruit juice.

Preparation for Administration Hazardous agent; use appropriate precautions for handling and disposal (NIOSH 2014 [group 1]). Reconstitute each 10 mg vial with 2 mL of supplied diluent to a reconstituted concentration of 5 mg/mL; swirl until dissolved. (**Note:** Although the reconstituted vial contains a final volume of 2 mL, due to the viscosity of the reconstituted solution, a total volume <2 mL [usually ~1.6-1.8 mL] can be withdrawn from each vial.) Further dilute in 500 mL normal saline; compatible with polyvinyl chloride (PVC), ethylene vinyl acetate (EVA), polyethylene (PE) and glass infusion containers.

Storage/Stability Store intact vials at room temperature of 20°C to 25°C (68°F to 77°F); excursions are permitted between 15°C and 30°C (59°F and 86°F). The reconstituted solution is stable for 8 hours at room temperature. Solutions diluted for infusion are stable for 24 hours at room temperature; however, the manufacturer recommends use as soon as possible after dilution.

Mechanism of Action Histone deacetylase inhibitor; catalyzes acetyl group removal from protein lysine residues (including histone and transcription factors). Inhibition of histone deacetylase results in accumulation of acetyl groups, leading to alterations in chromatin structure and transcription factor activation causing termination of cell growth (induces arrest in cell cycle at G_1 and G_2/M phases) leading to cell death.

Pharmacodynamics/Kinetics

Protein binding: 92% to 94%; primarily to α_1-acid glycoprotein

Metabolism: Hepatic, primarily via CYP3A4, minor metabolism from CYP3A5, 1A1, 2B6, and 2C19

Half-life elimination: ~3 hours

Dosing

Adult & Geriatric

Cutaneous T-cell lymphoma: IV: 14 mg/m² days 1, 8, and 15 of a 28-day treatment cycle; repeat cycle as long as benefit continues and treatment is tolerated.

Peripheral T-cell lymphoma: IV: 14 mg/m² days 1, 8, and 15 of a 28-day treatment cycle; repeat cycle as long as benefit continues and treatment is tolerated.

Renal Impairment There are no dosage adjustments provided in the manufacturer's labeling (has not been studied). However, dosage adjustment is not likely necessary since pharmacokinetics are unaffected by renal impairment. Use with caution in patients with end-stage renal disease (has not been studied).

Hepatic Impairment

Mild impairment: There are no dosage adjustments provided in the manufacturer's labeling. However, mild hepatic impairment does not significantly influence the pharmacokinetics of romidepsin.

Moderate or severe impairment: There are no dosage adjustments provided in the manufacturer's labeling. Use with caution.

Obesity *American Society of Clinical Oncology (ASCO) Guidelines for appropriate chemotherapy dosing in obese adults with cancer:* Utilize patient's actual body weight (full weight) for calculation of body surface area- or weight-based dosing, particularly when the intent of therapy is curative; manage regimen-related toxicities in the same manner as for nonobese patients; if a dose reduction is utilized due to toxicity, consider resumption of full weight-based dosing with subsequent cycles, especially if cause of toxicity (eg, hepatic or renal impairment) is resolved (Griggs, 2012).

Adjustment for Toxicity

Nonhematologic toxicity (excluding alopecia):

Grade 2 or 3: Delay treatment until toxicity returns to ≤ grade 1 or baseline, may restart at 14 mg/m²

Grade 4 or recurrent grade 3 toxicity: Delay treatment until toxicity returns to ≤ grade 1 or baseline, permanently reduce dose to 10 mg/m²

Recurrent grade 3 or 4 toxicity despite dosage reduction: Discontinue treatment

Hematologic toxicity:

Grade 3 or 4 neutropenia or thrombocytopenia: Delay treatment until ANC ≥1500/mm³ and/or platelets ≥75,000/mm³ or baseline, may restart at 14 mg/m²

Grade 4 febrile neutropenia or thrombocytopenia requiring platelet transfusion: Delay treatment until toxicity returns to ≤ grade 1 or baseline, permanently reduce dose to 10 mg/m²

Dietary Considerations Avoid grapefruit juice.

Administration Infuse over 4 hours. Although romidepsin has a low emetic potential, antiemetics to prevent nausea and vomiting were used in clinical trials (Piekarz, 2009; Piekarz, 2011).

Hazardous agent; use appropriate precautions for handling and disposal (NIOSH 2014 [group 1]).

Monitoring Parameters Serum electrolytes (baseline and periodic; especially potassium and magnesium); CBC with differential and platelets, ECG (baseline and periodic; in patients with significant cardiovascular disease, congenital long QT syndrome, and in patients taking QT-prolonging medications); signs/symptoms of infection or tumor lysis syndrome

Dosage Forms Excipient information presented when available (limited, particularly for generics); consult specific product labeling.

Solution Reconstituted, Intravenous:

Istodax: 10 mg (1 ea) [contains alcohol, usp, propylene glycol]

RomiPLOStim (roe mi PLOE stim)

Brand Names: US Nplate

Brand Names: Canada Nplate

Index Terms AMG 531

Pharmacologic Category Colony Stimulating Factor; Hematopoietic Agent; Thrombopoietic Agent

Use

Chronic immune thrombocytopenia: Treatment of thrombocytopenia in patients with chronic immune thrombocytopenia (ITP) who have had insufficient response to corticosteroids, immune globulin, or splenectomy

Limitations of use: Should be used only when the degree of thrombocytopenia and clinical condition increase the risk for bleeding; should not be used in attempt to normalize platelet counts; **not** indicated for the treatment of thrombocytopenia due to myelodysplastic syndrome or any cause of thrombocytopenia other than chronic ITP.

Pregnancy Considerations Adverse events have been observed in animal reproduction studies. Use during pregnancy only if the potential benefit to the mother outweighs the potential risk to the fetus.

Women exposed to romiplostim during pregnancy are encouraged to enroll in the Nplate pregnancy (1-800-772-6436). In Canada, women who become pregnant during treatment are encouraged to enroll in Amgen's Pregnancy Surveillance Program (1-866-512-6436).

Breast-Feeding Considerations It is not known if romiplostim is excreted in breast milk. Due to the potential for serious adverse reactions in the nursing infant, the manufacturer recommends a decision be made to discontinue breast-feeding or to discontinue romiplostim, taking into account the importance of treatment to the mother. In Canada, women who nurse during treatment are encouraged to enroll in Amgen's Lactation Surveillance Program (1-866-512-6436).

Medication Guide Available Yes

Contraindications There are no contraindications listed in the US labeling.

Canadian labeling: Hypersensitivity to romiplostim or any component of the formulation; known history of sensitivity or allergy to any *E. coli*-derived product.

Warnings/Precautions May increase the risk for bone marrow reticulin formation or progression; this formation may improve upon discontinuation of therapy. Thromboembolism or thrombotic complications may occur with increased platelets; follow dosage adjustment recommendations to minimize the risk for thrombotic or thromboembolic complications; use with caution in patients with a history of cerebrovascular disease. Progression from existing myelodysplastic syndrome (MDS) to acute myeloid leukemia (AML) has been observed in clinical trials studying romiplostim for severe thrombocytopenia associated with MDS (not an approved indication); a higher percentage of patients receiving romiplostim experienced transformation to AML (compared to placebo). An increase in the percentage of circulating myeloblasts in peripheral blood counts was also noted (both in patients who progressed to AML and in those who did not); blast cells decreased to baseline after discontinuation in some patients.

Indicated only when the degree of thrombocytopenia and clinical conditions increase the risk for bleeding; use the lowest dose necessary to achieve and maintain platelet count ≥50,000/mm³. Do not use to normalize platelet counts. Discontinue if platelet count does not respond to a level to avoid clinically important bleeding after 4 weeks at the maximum recommended dose. May be used in combination with other therapies for ITP, including corticosteroids, danazol, azathioprine, immune globulin, or Rho (D) immune globulin; not indicated for the treatment of thrombocytopenia due to any cause other than chronic ITP. Reduce dose or discontinue ITP medications when platelet count ≥50,000/mm³. Lack of response or failure to maintain platelet response should trigger investigation in to causative factors, including neutralizing antibodies to romiplostim.

Overdose may result in thrombotic/thromboembolic complications due to excessive platelet levels; underdose may result in lack of platelet response and potential for bleeding. Use caution when calculating dose and appropriate volume for administration (volume may be very small; administer with syringe that allows for 0.01 mL graduations).

Upon discontinuation of therapy, rebound thrombocytopenia and risk of bleeding may develop. Severity may be greater than pretreatment level; monitor CBCs and platelet counts weekly for at least 2 weeks after discontinuation.

Use with caution in patients with chronic liver disease; portal vein thrombosis has been reported in these patients.

Adverse Reactions

>10%:

Central nervous system: Headache (35%), dizziness (17%), insomnia (16%)

Gastrointestinal: Abdominal pain (11%)

Hematologic: Circulating myeloblasts increased (MDS patients: 17%)

Neuromuscular & skeletal: Arthralgia (26%), myalgia (14%), limb pain (13%)

1% to 10%:

Gastrointestinal: Dyspepsia (7%)

Hematologic: Rebound thrombocytopenia (7%), AML (MDS patients: 4% to 6%), bone marrow reticulin formation/deposition (4%)

Neuromuscular & skeletal: Shoulder pain (8%), paresthesia (6%)

Miscellaneous: Antibody formation (romiplostim 6%; TPO 4%)

<1% (Limited to important or life-threatening): Angioedema, erythromelalgia, hypersensitivity, marrow fibrosis with collagen, thromboembolism, thrombotic complications

Drug Interactions

Metabolism/Transport Effects None known.

Avoid Concomitant Use There are no known interactions where it is recommended to avoid concomitant use.

Increased Effect/Toxicity There are no known significant interactions involving an increase in effect.

Decreased Effect There are no known significant interactions involving a decrease in effect.

Preparation for Administration Reconstitute with only preservative free SWFI (add 0.72 mL to 250 mcg vial or 1.2 mL to 500 mcg vial). Do not use bacteriostatic water for injection. Gently invert vial and swirl; do not shake. Usually dissolves within 2 minutes.

Storage/Stability Store intact vials refrigerated at 2°C to 8°C (36°F to 46°F); do not freeze. Protect from light. Store in original carton until use. Reconstituted solution may be stored at room temperature of 25°C (77°F) or refrigerated at 2°C to 8°C (36°F to 46°F) for up to 24 hours prior to administration. Protect reconstituted solution from light; discard any unused portion.

Mechanism of Action Thrombopoietin (TPO) peptide mimetic which increases platelet counts in ITP by binding to and activating the human TPO receptor.

Pharmacodynamics/Kinetics

Onset of action: Platelet count increase: SubQ: 4 to 9 days (Wang, 2004); Peak platelet count increase: Days 12 to 16 (Wang, 2004)

Duration: Platelet counts return to baseline by day 28 (Wang, 2004)

Absorption: SubQ: Slow (Wang, 2004)

Half-life elimination: Median: 3.5 days (range: 1 to 34 days)

Time to peak, plasma: SubQ: Median: 14 hours (range: 7 to 50 hours)

Dosing

Adult & Geriatric Note: Initial dose is based on actual body weight. Use the lowest dose sufficient to maintain platelet count ≥50,000/mm³ as necessary to reduce the risk of bleeding. Adjust dose based on platelet count response; discontinue if platelet count does not respond to a level that avoids clinically important bleeding after 4 weeks at the maximum recommended dose. Do not use to normalize platelet counts.

Chronic immune thrombocytopenia (ITP): SubQ: Initial: 1 mcg/kg once weekly; adjust dose by 1 mcg/kg/week increments to achieve platelet count ≥50,000/mm³ and to reduce the risk of bleeding; Maximum dose: 10 mcg/kg/week (median dose needed to achieve response in clinical trials: 2 mcg/kg)

Dosage adjustment recommendations:

Platelet count <50,000/mm³:

US labeling: Increase weekly dose by 1 mcg/kg

Canadian labeling: Increase weekly dose by 1 mcg/kg every 1 to 2 weeks

Platelet count >200,000/mm³ for 2 consecutive weeks: Reduce weekly dose by 1 mcg/kg

Platelet count >400,000/mm³: Withhold dose; assess platelet count weekly; when platelet count <200,000/mm³, resume with the weekly dose reduced by 1 mcg/kg

Renal Impairment There are no dosage adjustments provided in the manufacturer's labeling (has not been studied).

Hepatic Impairment There are no dosage adjustments provided in the manufacturer's labeling (has not been studied).

Dietary Considerations Some products may contain sucrose.

Administration Administer SubQ. Administration volume may be small; use appropriate syringe (with graduations to 0.01 mL) for administration. Verify calculations, final concentration, and volume drawn up for administration.

Monitoring Parameters CBC with differential and platelets (baseline, during treatment [weekly until platelet response stable for at least 4 weeks then monthly] and weekly for at least 2 weeks following discontinuation or completion of treatment)

Evaluate for neutralizing antibodies in patients with inadequate response (blood samples may be submitted to the manufacturer for assay [1-800-772-6436]).

Reference Range Target platelet count of 50,000-200,000/mm³; platelet life span: 8-11 days

Additional Information Restricted access to Nplate was previously a REMS requirement via the Nplate NEXUS (Network of Experts Understanding and Supporting Nplate and Patients) program. Patients, prescribers, and pharmacies were required to be enrolled in this program. However, the FDA eliminated this REMS requirement in December 2011. There is currently no restricted access to obtaining Nplate.

Dosage Forms Excipient information presented when available (limited, particularly for generics); consult specific product labeling.

Solution Reconstituted, Subcutaneous [preservative free]: Nplate: 250 mcg (1 ea); 500 mcg (1 ea)

♦ Romycin [DSC] see Erythromycin (Ophthalmic) on page 672

ROPINIRole (roe PIN i role)

Brand Names: US Requip; Requip XL

Brand Names: Canada ACT-Ropinirole; JAMP-Ropinirole; PMS-Ropinirole; RAN-Ropinirole; Requip

Index Terms Ropinirole Hydrochloride

Pharmacologic Category Anti-Parkinson's Agent, Dopamine Agonist

Use

Parkinson disease: Treatment of Parkinson disease

Restless legs syndrome (immediate release only): Treatment of moderate to severe primary restless legs syndrome (RLS)

Pregnancy Considerations Adverse events have been observed in animal reproduction studies. Information related to the use of ropinirole for the treatment of restless legs syndrome (RLS) in pregnant women is limited. Current guidelines note that the available information is insufficient to make a recommendation for use in pregnant women (Aurora, 2012; Dostal, 2013).

Breast-Feeding Considerations It is not known if ropinirole is excreted into breast milk. Ropinirole inhibits prolactin secretion in humans and may potentially inhibit lactation. The manufacturer recommends that caution be exercised when administering ropinirole to nursing women.

Contraindications Hypersensitivity to ropinirole or any component of the formulation

Warnings/Precautions May cause orthostatic hypotension; Parkinson disease patients appear to have an impaired capacity to respond to a postural challenge. Use with caution in patients at risk of hypotension (such as those receiving antihypertensive or antiarrhythmic drugs) or where transient hypotensive episodes would be poorly tolerated (cardiovascular disease or cerebrovascular disease). Parkinson patients being treated with dopaminergic agonists ordinarily require careful monitoring for signs and symptoms of postural hypotension, especially during dose escalation, and should be informed of this risk. Syncope, sometimes associated with bradycardia, was observed in association with ropinirole in both Parkinson disease patients and patients with RLS.

Use with caution in patients with preexisting dyskinesia, hepatic impairment or ESRD on dialysis (use in patients with severe renal impairment and who are not undergoing regular hemodialysis is not recommended in the Canadian labeling). May cause hallucinations, particularly in older patients. May also cause or exacerbate mental status and behavioral changes, which may be severe, including psychotic-like behavior during treatment or after starting or increasing the dose; manifestations may include paranoid ideation, delusions, hallucinations, confusion, psychotic-like behavior, disorientation, aggressive behavior, agitation, and delirium. Avoid use in patients with a major psychotic disorder; may exacerbate psychosis.

Patients have reported falling asleep while engaging in activities of daily living; this has been reported to occur without significant warning signs; some of these events had been reported one year after the initiation of therapy. Ropinirole has also been associated with somnolence. Before initiating treatment, advise patients of the potential to develop drowsiness, and inquire about factors that may increase the risk (eg, concomitant sedating medications and/or alcohol, presence of sleep disorders, concomitant

medications that increase pramipexole plasma levels). Patients must be cautioned about performing tasks which require mental alertness (eg, operating machinery or driving). Monitor for daytime somnolence or preexisting sleep disorder; discontinue if significant daytime sleepiness or episodes of falling asleep occur; if a decision is made to continue therapy, advise patients not to drive and to avoid other potentially dangerous activities.

Has been associated with compulsive behaviors and/or loss of impulse control, which has manifested as pathological gambling, libido increases (hypersexuality), compulsive buying, binge or compulsive eating and/or other intense urges. Dose reduction or discontinuation of therapy has been reported to reverse these behaviors in some, but not all cases. Risk for melanoma development is increased in Parkinson disease patients; drug causation or factors contributing to risk have not been established. Patients should be monitored closely and periodic skin examinations should be performed.

Augmentation (earlier onset of symptoms in the evening/afternoon, increase and/or spread of symptoms to other extremities) or rebound (shifting of symptoms to early morning hours) may occur in some RLS patients. Consider dosage adjustment or discontinuation of treatment if augmentation or rebound symptoms occur. Pathologic degenerative changes were observed in the retinas of albino rats during studies with this agent, but were not observed in the retinas of albino mice or in other species. The significance of these data for humans remains uncertain.

Taper gradually when discontinuing therapy in Parkinson disease; dopaminergic agents have been associated with a syndrome resembling neuroleptic malignant syndrome on abrupt withdrawal or significant dosage reduction after long-term use. Ergot-derived dopamine agonists have been associated with fibrotic complications (eg, pericarditis, retroperitoneal fibrosis, pleural effusion, pleural thickening, pulmonary infiltrates, cardiac valvulopathy). Although ropinirole is not an ergot, there have been postmarketing reports of possible fibrotic complications (pleural effusion, pleural fibrosis, interstitial lung disease, and cardiac valvulopathy) with ropinirole; monitor closely for signs and symptoms of fibrosis. Discontinuation of therapy may resolve complications, but not in all cases. The elderly may be prone to an increased risk of adverse drug reactions. Extended release ropinirole is designed to release medication over a 24-hour period; if rapid gastrointestinal transit occurs, there may be risk of incomplete release of medication and medication residue being passed in the stool. Potentially significant drug-drug interactions may exist, requiring dose or frequency adjustment, additional monitoring, and/or selection of alternative therapy.

Adverse Reactions

Frequency not always defined. Data inclusive of trials in early Parkinson disease (without levodopa) and Restless Legs Syndrome.

>10%:

Cardiovascular: Hypotension (including orthostatic; 2% to 25%), syncope (1% to 12%)

Central nervous system: Drowsiness (11% to 40%), dizziness (6% to 40%), fatigue (including weakness, malaise; 9% to 16%)

Gastrointestinal: Nausea (immediate release: 40% to 60%; extended release: 19%), vomiting (11% to 12%)

Infection: Viral infection (11%)

1% to 10%:

Cardiovascular: Lower extremity edema (7%), dependent edema (6%), hypertension (5%), chest pain (4%), flushing (3%), palpitations (3%), peripheral ischemia (3%), atrial fibrillation (2%), extrasystoles (2%), peripheral edema (2%), tachycardia (2%)

Central nervous system: Pain (8%), headache (extended release: 6%), confusion (5%), hallucination (5%; dose related), hypoesthesia (4%), amnesia (3%), paresthesia (3%), yawning (3%), lack of concentration (2%), vertigo (2%), falling, insomnia

Dermatologic: Diaphoresis (6%), hyperhidrosis (3%)

Gastrointestinal: Dyspepsia (4% to 10%), abdominal pain (3% to 7%), constipation (5%), xerostomia (3% to 5%), diarrhea (5%), anorexia (4%), flatulence (3%)

Genitourinary: Urinary tract infection (5%), impotence (3%)

Hepatic: Increased serum alkaline (3%)

Infection: Influenza (3%)

Neuromuscular & skeletal: Arthralgia (4%), limb pain (3%), muscle cramps (3%), hyperkinesia (2%), muscle spasm, myalgia

Ophthalmic: Visual disturbance (6%), eye disease (3%), xerophthalmia (2%)

Respiratory: Nasopharyngitis (9%), pharyngitis (6%), rhinitis (4%), sinusitis (4%), bronchitis (3%), cough (3%), dyspnea (3%), nasal congestion (2%)

Miscellaneous: Fever

Advanced Parkinson disease (with levodopa):

>10%:

Cardiovascular: Decreased diastolic blood pressure (orthostatic; ≥10 mm Hg: 63%; ≥20 mm Hg: 10%; semi-supine; ≥20 mm Hg: 25%), systolic hypotension (orthostatic; ≥20 mm Hg: 38%; semi-supine; ≥40 mm Hg: 10%); decreased blood pressure (combined systolic and diastolic; orthostatic; mild to moderate: 23%), decreased heart rate (≥15 beats/minute: 19% to 24%), increased heart rate (≥15 beats/minute: 23%; ≥30 beats/minute: 2%)

Central nervous system: Dizziness (immediate release: 26%; extended release: 8%), drowsiness (immediate release: 20%, extended release: 7%), headache (17%)

Gastrointestinal: Nausea (immediate release: 30%; extended-release: 11%)

Neuromuscular & skeletal: Dyskinesia (immediate release: 34%; extended-release: 13%; dose related)

1% to 10%:

Cardiovascular: Systolic hypertension (≥40 mm Hg: 8% to 9%), hypotension (≤7%; including orthostatic), peripheral edema (4%), syncope (1% to 3%), hypertension (3%; dose related), bradycardia

Central nervous system: Hallucination (6% to 10%; dose related), falling (2% to 10%; dose related), confusion (9%), anxiety (2% to 6%), amnesia (5%), nervousness (5%), pain (5%), paresthesia (5%), vertigo (4%), abnormal dreams (3%), paresis (3%)

Dermatologic: Diaphoresis (5% to 7%)

Endocrine & metabolic: Weight loss (2%)

Gastrointestinal: Abdominal pain (6% to 9%), vomiting (7%), constipation (4% to 6%), diarrhea (3% to 5%), xerostomia (2% to 5%), dysphagia (2%), flatulence (2%), sialorrhea (2%)

Genitourinary: Urinary tract infection (6%), pyuria (2%), urinary incontinence (2%)

Hematologic: Anemia (2%)

Infection: Viral infection

Neuromuscular & skeletal: Arthralgia (7%), tremor (6%), hypokinesia (5%), arthritis (3%), back pain (3%)

Ophthalmic: Diplopia (2%)

Respiratory: Upper respiratory tract infection (9%), dyspnea (3%), nasopharyngitis (≥2%)

Miscellaneous: Increased drug level (7%)

Postmarketing and/or case reports (Limited to important or life-threatening): Heart valve disease, hypersensitivity reaction (angioedema, pruritus), impulse control disorder (eg, pathological gambling, hypersexuality, binge eating), interstitial pulmonary disease, mental status changes, pleural effusion

Drug Interactions

Metabolism/Transport Effects Substrate of CYP1A2 (major), CYP3A4 (minor); **Note:** Assignment of Major/Minor substrate status based on clinically relevant drug interaction potential; **Inhibits** CYP1A2 (weak), CYP2D6 (weak)

Avoid Concomitant Use

Avoid concomitant use of ROPINIRole with any of the following: Amisulpride; Sulpiride

Increased Effect/Toxicity

ROPINIRole may increase the levels/effects of: Amifostine; BuPROPion; DULoxetine; Hypotension-Associated Agents; Levodopa; TiZANidine

The levels/effects of ROPINIRole may be increased by: Abiraterone Acetate; Alcohol (Ethyl); Alfuzosin; Blood Pressure Lowering Agents; Brimonidine (Topical); Ciprofloxacin (Systemic); CNS Depressants; CYP1A2 Inhibitors (Moderate); CYP1A2 Inhibitors (Strong); Deferasirox; Diazoxide; Estrogen Derivatives; Herbs (Hypotensive Properties); Methylphenidate; Molsidomine; Nicorandil; Obinutuzumab; Peginterferon Alfa-2b; Pentoxifylline; Phosphodiesterase 5 Inhibitors; Prostacyclin Analogues; Vemurafenib

Decreased Effect

ROPINIRole may decrease the levels/effects of: Amisulpride; Antipsychotic Agents (First Generation [Typical]); Sulpiride

The levels/effects of ROPINIRole may be decreased by: Amisulpride; Antipsychotic Agents (First Generation [Typical]); Antipsychotic Agents (Second Generation [Atypical]); Cannabis; CYP1A2 Inducers (Strong); Cyproterone; Metoclopramide; Osimertinib; Sulpiride; Teriflunomide

Storage/Stability Store at room temperature. Protect from light and moisture.

Mechanism of Action Ropinirole has a high relative *in vitro* specificity and full intrinsic activity at the D_2 and D_3 dopamine receptor subtypes, binding with higher affinity to D_3 than to D_2 or D_4 receptor subtypes; relevance of D_3 receptor binding in Parkinson disease is unknown. Ropinirole has moderate *in vitro* affinity for opioid receptors. Ropinirole and its metabolites have negligible *in vitro* affinity for dopamine D_1, 5-HT$_1$, 5-HT$_2$, benzodiazepine, GABA, muscarinic, alpha$_1$-, alpha$_2$-, and beta-adrenoreceptors. Although precise mechanism of action of ropinirole is unknown, it is believed to be due to stimulation of postsynaptic dopamine D_2-type receptors within the caudate putamen in the brain. Ropinirole caused decreases in systolic and diastolic blood pressure at doses >0.25 mg. The mechanism of ropinirole-induced postural hypotension is believed to be due to D_2-mediated blunting of the noradrenergic response to standing and subsequent decrease in peripheral vascular resistance.

Pharmacodynamics/Kinetics

Absorption: Immediate release: Rapid

Distribution: V_d: 7.5 L/kg

Protein binding: 40%

Metabolism: Extensively hepatic via CYP1A2 to inactive metabolites; first-pass effect

Bioavailability: Absolute: 45% to 55%

Half-life elimination: ~6 hours

Time to peak: Immediate release: ~1-2 hours; Extended release: 6-10 hours; T_{max} increased by 2.5-3 hours when taken with a high-fat meal

Excretion: Urine (<10% as unchanged drug, 60% as metabolites)

Dosing

Adult

Parkinson disease: Oral:

Immediate-release tablet: The dosage should be increased to achieve a maximum therapeutic effect, balanced against the principal side effects of nausea, dizziness, somnolence and dyskinesia. Recommended starting dose is 0.25 mg 3 times/day; based on individual patient response, the dosage should be titrated with weekly increments as described below:
  • Week 1: 0.25 mg 3 times/day; total daily dose: 0.75 mg
  • Week 2: 0.5 mg 3 times/day; total daily dose: 1.5 mg
  • Week 3: 0.75 mg 3 times/day; total daily dose: 2.25 mg
  • Week 4: 1 mg 3 times/day; total daily dose: 3 mg
  Note: After week 4, if necessary, daily dosage may be increased by 1.5 mg/day on a weekly basis up to a dose of 9 mg/day, and then by up to 3 mg/day weekly to a total of 24 mg/day. If a significant interruption in therapy with ropinirole occurs, retitration may be warranted.

Parkinson disease discontinuation taper: Gradually taper over 7 days as follows: reduce frequency of administration from 3 times daily to twice daily for 4 days, then reduce to once daily for remaining 3 days.

Extended release tablet: Initial: 2 mg once daily for 1-2 weeks, followed by increases of 2 mg/day at weekly or longer intervals based on therapeutic response and tolerability (maximum: 24 mg/day; **Note:** If a significant interruption in therapy with ropinirole occurs, retitration may be warranted. When discontinuing gradually taper over 7 days.

Restless legs syndrome (RLS): Oral: Immediate release tablets: Initial: 0.25 mg once daily 1-3 hours before bedtime. Dose may be increased after 2 days to 0.5 mg daily, and after 7 days to 1 mg daily. Dose may be further titrated upward in 0.5 mg increments every week until reaching a daily dose of 3 mg during week 6. Daily dose may be increased to a maximum of 4 mg beginning week 7.
  Note: If a significant interruption in therapy with ropinirole occurs, retitration may be warranted. Doses up to 4 mg per day may be discontinued without tapering.

Converting from ropinirole immediate release tablets to ropinirole extended-release tablets: Choose a once daily extended-release dose that most closely matches current immediate-release daily dose.

Geriatric Titrate dose to clinical response. Refer to adult dosing.

Renal Impairment

Moderate renal impairment (CrCl 30 to 50 mL/minute): No dosage adjustment necessary.

Severe renal impairment (CrCl <30 mL/minute): There are no dosage adjustments provided in the manufacturer's labeling (has not been studied). Use with caution. **Note:** The Canadian labeling recommends to avoid use in patients with severe renal impairment and who are not undergoing regular hemodialysis.

ESRD requiring hemodialysis:

Immediate release:

Parkinson disease: Initial: 0.25 mg 3 times daily; may titrate dose upward based on tolerability and efficacy (maximum dose: 18 mg daily); postdialysis supplemental doses are not required

Restless legs syndrome: Initial: 0.25 mg once daily; may titrate dose upward based on tolerability and efficacy (maximum dose: 3 mg daily); postdialysis supplemental doses are not required

Extended release: Initial: 2 mg once daily; may titrate dose upward based on tolerability and efficacy (maximum dose: 18 mg daily); postdialysis supplemental doses are not required

Hepatic Impairment There are no dosage adjustments provided in the manufacturer's labeling (has not been studied). Titrate with caution.

Administration Administer without regard to meals. Swallow extended-release tablet whole; do not crush, split, or chew.

Monitoring Parameters Blood pressure (orthostatic); daytime alertness; CNS depression, fall risk, behavior changes (eg, compulsive behaviors); periodic skin examinations

Additional Information If therapy with a drug known to be a potent inhibitor of CYP1A2 is stopped or started during treatment with ropinirole, adjustment of ropinirole dose may be required. Ropinirole binds to melanin-containing tissues (ie, eyes, skin) in pigmented rats. After a single dose, long-term retention of drug was demonstrated, with a half-life in the eye of 20 days; not known if ropinirole accumulates in these tissues over time.

Dosage Forms Excipient information presented when available (limited, particularly for generics); consult specific product labeling.

Tablet, Oral:

Requip: 0.25 mg, 0.5 mg, 1 mg, 2 mg, 3 mg, 4 mg, 5 mg [contains fd&c blue #2 aluminum lake, fd&c yellow #6 aluminum lake, polysorbate 80]

Generic: 0.25 mg, 0.5 mg, 1 mg, 2 mg, 3 mg, 4 mg, 5 mg

Tablet Extended Release 24 Hour, Oral:

Requip XL: 2 mg, 4 mg, 6 mg, 8 mg, 12 mg [contains fd&c blue #2 aluminum lake, fd&c yellow #6 aluminum lake]

Generic: 2 mg, 4 mg, 6 mg, 8 mg, 12 mg

◆ Ropinirole Hydrochloride *see* ROPINIRole *on page 1616*

Ropivacaine (roe PIV a kane)

Brand Names: US Naropin

Brand Names: Canada Naropin; Ropivacaine Hydrochloride Injection, USP

Index Terms Ropivacaine Hydrochloride

Pharmacologic Category Local Anesthetic

Use

Acute pain management: For acute pain management administered as an epidural continuous infusion, intermittent bolus (eg, postoperative or labor), or local infiltration.

Surgical anesthesia: For the production of local or regional anesthesia for surgery administered as an epidural block, including cesarean section, major nerve block, or local infiltration.

Dosing

Adult Dose varies with procedure, onset and depth of anesthesia desired, vascularity of tissues, duration of anesthesia, and condition of patient: A test dose of short-acting local anesthetic containing epinephrine (eg, 3 to 5 mL) should be administered prior to induction of complete block with ropivacaine. Incremental ropivacaine dosing is recommended. Adults:

Surgical anesthesia:

Lumbar epidural block for surgery:
  15 to 30 **mL** of 0.5% solution
  15 to 25 **mL** of 0.75% solution
  15 to 20 **mL** of 1% solution

Lumbar epidural block for cesarean section:
  20 to 30 **mL** of 0.5% solution
  15 to 20 **mL** dose of 0.75% solution

Thoracic epidural block:
  5 to 15 **mL** dose of 0.5% solution
  5 to 15 **mL** dose of 0.75% solution

Major nerve block:
  35 to 50 **mL** dose of 0.5% solution
  10 to 40 **mL** dose of 0.75% solution

Field block: 1 to 40 **mL** dose of 0.5% solution

Labor pain management: Lumbar epidural: Initial: 10 to 20 mL 0.2% solution; continuous infusion dose: 6 to 14 mL/hour of 0.2% solution with incremental injections of 10 to 15 mL/hour of 0.2% solution

Postoperative pain management:
Peripheral nerve block: Continuous infusion dose: 5 to 10 mL/hour of 0.2% solution (Bagry, 2008; Klein, 2000)

Lumbar or thoracic epidural: Continuous infusion dose: 6 to 14 mL/hour of 0.2% solution

Infiltration/minor nerve block:
1 to 100 mL dose of 0.2% solution
1 to 40 mL dose of 0.5% solution

Geriatric Refer to adult dosing. Use with caution; initial dose reductions may be necessary.

Renal Impairment There are no dosage adjustments provided in the manufacturer's labeling. However, ropivacaine and its metabolites are renally excreted, and the risk of toxic reactions may be greater.

Hepatic Impairment There are no dosage adjustments provided in the manufacturer's labeling. Use with caution; ropivacaine undergoes hepatic metabolism and patients may be at a greater risk for developing toxic drug levels.

Additional Information Complete prescribing information should be consulted for additional detail.

Dosage Forms Excipient information presented when available (limited, particularly for generics); consult specific product labeling.

Solution, Injection, as hydrochloride [preservative free]:
Naropin: 2 mg/mL (10 mL, 20 mL, 100 mL, 200 mL); 5 mg/mL (20 mL, 30 mL, 100 mL, 200 mL); 7.5 mg/mL (20 mL); 10 mg/mL (10 mL, 20 mL)
Generic: 2 mg/mL (10 mL, 20 mL); 5 mg/mL (30 mL); 7.5 mg/mL (20 mL); 10 mg/mL (10 mL, 20 mL)

◆ Ropivacaine Hydrochloride see Ropivacaine on page 1618

◆ Ropivacaine Hydrochloride Injection, USP (Can) see Ropivacaine on page 1618

◆ Rosadan see MetroNIDAZOLE (Topical) on page 1199

◆ Rosanil see Sulfur and Sulfacetamide on page 1716

◆ Rosasol (Can) see MetroNIDAZOLE (Topical) on page 1199

Rosiglitazone (roh si GLI ta zone)

Brand Names: US Avandia
Brand Names: Canada Avandia
Pharmacologic Category Antidiabetic Agent, Thiazolidinedione
Use Type 2 diabetes: Adjunct to diet and exercise to improve glycemic control in adults with type 2 diabetes mellitus (noninsulin dependent, NIDDM); may be used as monotherapy or in combination with metformin or a sulfonylurea.
Limitations of use: Should not be used in patients with type 1 diabetes mellitus or diabetic ketoacidosis; use with insulin is not recommended.
Prescribing and Access Restrictions Health Canada requires written informed consent for new and current patients receiving rosiglitazone.
Medication Guide Available Yes
Dosing
Adult & Geriatric Type 2 diabetes: Oral: **Note:** All patients should be initiated at the lowest recommended dose.
Initial: 4 mg daily as a single daily dose or in divided doses twice daily. If response is inadequate after 8-12 weeks of treatment, the dosage may be increased to 8 mg daily (maximum dose) as a single daily dose or in divided doses twice daily. In clinical trials, the 4 mg twice-daily regimen resulted in the greatest reduction in fasting plasma glucose and HbA$_{1c}$.
Note: When used in combination therapy with other hypoglycemic agents, a dose reduction of the concurrent agent may be necessary if hypoglycemia occurs. The Canadian labeling recommends a maximum rosiglitazone dose of 4 mg daily when used in combination with a sulfonylurea.
Renal Impairment No dosage adjustment necessary.
Hepatic Impairment There are no dosage adjustments provided in the manufacturer's labeling. Clearance is significantly lower in hepatic impairment; therapy should not be initiated if the patient exhibits active liver disease or increased transaminases (ALT >2.5 times the upper limit of normal) at baseline.
Additional Information Complete prescribing information should be consulted for additional detail.

Dosage Forms Excipient information presented when available (limited, particularly for generics); consult specific product labeling.
Tablet, Oral:
Avandia: 2 mg, 4 mg, 8 mg

Rosiglitazone and Glimepiride
(roh si GLI ta zone & GLYE me pye ride)

Brand Names: US Avandaryl [DSC]
Index Terms Glimepiride and Rosiglitazone Maleate
Pharmacologic Category Antidiabetic Agent, Sulfonylurea; Antidiabetic Agent, Thiazolidinedione
Use Diabetes mellitus, type 2: Adjunct to diet and exercise to improve glycemic control in adults with type 2 diabetes mellitus (noninsulin dependent, NIDDM)
Medication Guide Available Yes
Dosing
Adult
Diabetes mellitus, type 2: Oral: **Note:** Rosiglitazone dose should be initiated at the lowest recommended dose.
Initial: Rosiglitazone 4 mg and glimepiride 1 mg once daily **or** rosiglitazone 4 mg and glimepiride 2 mg once daily (for patients previously treated with a sulfonylurea or rosiglitazone)
Patients switching from combination therapy of rosiglitazone and glimepiride as separate tablets: Use current dose.
Titration: Carefully titrate dose in debilitated or malnourished patients and in patients with adrenal insufficiency.
Dose adjustment in patients previously on sulfonylurea monotherapy: May take 2 weeks to observe decreased blood glucose and 2 to 3 months to see full effects of rosiglitazone component. If not adequately controlled after 8 to 12 weeks, increase daily dose of rosiglitazone component.
Dose adjustment in patients previously on rosiglitazone monotherapy: If not adequately controlled after 1 to 2 weeks, increase daily dose of glimepiride component in ≤2 mg increments in 1 to 2 week intervals.
Maximum dose: Rosiglitazone 8 mg and glimepiride 4 mg once daily
Geriatric Rosiglitazone 4 mg and glimepiride 1 mg once daily; carefully titrate dose.
Renal Impairment Rosiglitazone 4 mg and glimepiride 1 mg once daily; carefully titrate dose.
Hepatic Impairment Rosiglitazone 4 mg and glimepiride 1 mg once daily; carefully titrate dose. Therapy should not be initiated if the patient exhibits symptoms of active liver disease or increased transaminases (ALT >2.5 times the upper limit of normal) at baseline since clearance is significantly lower in hepatic impairment. During therapy, if ALT >3 times ULN, reevaluate levels promptly and discontinue if elevation persists or if jaundice occurs at any time during use.
Additional Information Complete prescribing information should be consulted for additional detail.
Dosage Forms Excipient information presented when available (limited, particularly for generics); consult specific product labeling.
Tablet, Oral:
Avandaryl: 4 mg/1 mg: Rosiglitazone 4 mg and glimepiride 1 mg [DSC]
Avandaryl: 4 mg/2 mg: Rosiglitazone 4 mg and glimepiride 2 mg [DSC]
Avandaryl: 4 mg/4 mg: Rosiglitazone 4 mg and glimepiride 4 mg [DSC]
Avandaryl: 8 mg/2 mg: Rosiglitazone 8 mg and glimepiride 2 mg [DSC]
Avandaryl: 8 mg/4 mg: Rosiglitazone 8 mg and glimepiride 4 mg [DSC]

Rosiglitazone and Metformin
(roh si GLI ta zone & met FOR min)

Brand Names: US Avandamet
Brand Names: Canada Avandamet
Index Terms Metformin and Rosiglitazone; Metformin Hydrochloride and Rosiglitazone Maleate; Rosiglitazone Maleate and Metformin Hydrochloride
Pharmacologic Category Antidiabetic Agent, Biguanide; Antidiabetic Agent, Thiazolidinedione
Use
Type 2 diabetes: Adjunct to diet and exercise to improve glycemic control in adults with type 2 diabetes mellitus (noninsulin dependent, NIDDM).

Limitations of use: Should not be used in patients with type 1 diabetes mellitus or diabetic ketoacidosis; use with insulin is not recommended.

Prescribing and Access Restrictions Health Canada requires written informed consent for new and current patients receiving rosiglitazone.

Medication Guide Available Yes

Dosing

Adult Type 2 diabetes mellitus: Oral: **Note:** Daily dose should be divided. Rosiglitazone dose should be initiated at the lowest recommended dose.

Patients inadequately controlled on diet and exercise alone: Initial dose: Rosiglitazone 2 mg and metformin 500 mg once or twice daily. Patients with HbA$_{1c}$ >11% or fasting plasma glucose (FPG) >270 mg/dL: Initial: Rosiglitazone 2 mg and metformin 500 mg twice daily may be considered. If not adequately controlled after 4 weeks, the dose may be increased in increments of rosiglitazone 2 mg and metformin 500 mg per day given in divided doses.

Patients inadequately controlled on metformin alone: Initial dose: Rosiglitazone 4 mg daily plus current dose of metformin

Patients inadequately controlled on rosiglitazone alone: Initial dose: Metformin 1000 mg daily plus current dose of rosiglitazone

Patients switching from combination therapy of rosiglitazone and metformin as separate tablets: Use current dose

Titration:

Dose adjustment after rosiglitazone dosage increase: If not adequately controlled after 8 to 12 weeks, increase daily dose of rosiglitazone component in 4 mg increments.

Dose adjustment after metformin dosage increase: If not adequately controlled after 1 to 2 weeks, increase daily dose of metformin component in 500 mg increments.

Maximum daily dose: Rosiglitazone 8 mg/metformin 2000 mg.

Geriatric The initial and maintenance dosing should be conservative, due to the potential for decreased renal function (monitor). Generally, elderly patients should not be titrated to the maximum. Do not use in patients ≥80 years unless normal renal function has been established.

Renal Impairment

Manufacturer's labeling:

Serum creatinine (SCr) ≥1.5 mg/dL (males) or ≥1.4 mg/dL (females): Use is contraindicated

Abnormal CrCl (US labeling: Not defined; Canadian labeling: <60 mL/minute): Use is contraindicated

Alternate recommendations: Note: The United Kingdom National Institute for Health and Clinical Excellence (NICE) Guidelines recommend prescribing metformin with caution in those patients who are at risk of sudden deterioration in renal function and at risk of an estimated glomerular filtration rate (eGFR) <45 mL/minute/1.73 m^2 (NICE 2008). Some evidence suggests that use of metformin is unsafe when eGFR <30 mL/minute/1.73 m^2 (calculated using MDRD) (Shaw 2007). A review of the available data by members of the American Diabetes Association proposed the following recommendations based on eGFR (Lipska 2011):

eGFR ≥60 mL/minute/1.73 m^2: No contraindications, monitor renal function annually

eGFR ≥45 to <60 mL/minute/1.73 m^2: Continue use; monitor renal function every 3 to 6 months

eGFR ≥30 to <45 mL/minute/1.73 m^2: In patients currently receiving metformin, use with caution, consider dosage reduction (eg, 50% reduction or 50% of maximal dose), monitor renal function every 3 months. Do not initiate therapy in patients with eGFR <45 mL/minute/1.73 m^2.

eGFR <30 mL/minute/1.73 m^2: Discontinue use

Hepatic Impairment The manufacturer recommends to avoid metformin since liver disease is considered a risk factor for the development of lactic acidosis during metformin therapy. However, continued use of metformin in diabetics with liver dysfunction, including cirrhosis, has been used successfully and may be associated with a survival benefit in carefully selected patients; use cautiously in patients at risk for lactic acidosis (eg, renal impairment, alcohol use) (Brackett 2010; Zhang 2014). Do not initiate rosiglitazone therapy with active liver disease or ALT >2.5 times the upper limit of normal.

Additional Information Complete prescribing information should be consulted for additional detail.

Dosage Forms Excipient information presented when available (limited, particularly for generics); consult specific product labeling.

Tablet, Oral:

Avandamet: 2/500: Rosiglitazone 2 mg and metformin hydrochloride 500 mg [DSC]

Avandamet: 4/500: Rosiglitazone 4 mg and metformin hydrochloride 500 mg [DSC]

Avandamet: 2/1000: Rosiglitazone 2 mg and metformin hydrochloride 1000 mg

Avandamet: 4/1000: Rosiglitazone 4 mg and metformin hydrochloride 1000 mg [DSC]

Dosage Forms: Canada Note: Refer also to dosage forms.

Excipient information presented when available (limited, particularly for generics); consult specific product labeling.

Tablet, Oral:

Avandamet: 1/500: Rosiglitazone 1 mg and metformin hydrochloride 500 mg

◆ Rosiglitazone Maleate and Metformin Hydrochloride see Rosiglitazone and Metformin on page 1619

◆ Rosone (Can) see Betamethasone (Topical) on page 224

◆ Rosula Wash see Sulfur and Sulfacetamide on page 1716

Rosuvastatin (roe soo va STAT in)

Brand Names: US Crestor

Brand Names: Canada ACT-Rosuvastatin; Apo-Rosuvastatin; Crestor; Dom-Rosuvastatin; Jamp-Rosuvastatin; Mar-Rosuvastatin; Med-Rosuvastatin; Mint-Rosuvastatin; Mylan-Rosuvastatin; PMS-Rosuvastatin; RAN-Rosuvastatin; Riva-Rosuvastatin; Sandoz-Rosuvastatin; Teva-Rosuvastatin

Index Terms Rosuvastatin Calcium

Pharmacologic Category Antilipemic Agent, HMG-CoA Reductase Inhibitor

Use

Heterozygous familial hypercholesterolemia in pediatric patients: Adjunct to diet to reduce total cholesterol, low-density lipoprotein cholesterol (LDL-C), and apolipoprotein B (apo B) levels in children and adolescent males and females who are at least 1 year postmenarche and are 8 to 17 years of age with heterozygous familial hypercholesteremia if after an adequate trial of diet therapy the following findings are present: LDL-C more than 190 mg/dL or more than 160 mg/dL and there is a positive family history of premature cardiovascular (CV) disease or 2 or more other CV disease risk factors.

Homozygous familial hypercholesterolemia: To reduce LDL-C, total cholesterol, and apo B in adults with homozygous familial hypercholesterolemia as an adjunct to other lipid-lowering treatments (eg, LDL apheresis) or alone if such treatments are unavailable.

Hyperlipidemia and mixed dyslipidemia: Adjunctive therapy to diet to reduce elevated total cholesterol, LDL-C, apo B, non–high-density lipoprotein cholesterol (non-HDL-C), and triglyceride levels, and to increase HDL-C in adult patients with primary hyperlipidemia or mixed dyslipidemia.

Hypertriglyceridemia: Adjunct to diet for the treatment of adults with hypertriglyceridemia.

Primary dysbetalipoproteinemia (type III hyperlipoproteinemia): Adjunct to diet for the treatment of patients with primary dysbetalipoproteinemia (type III hyperlipoproteinemia).

Prevention of cardiovascular disease:

Primary prevention: To reduce the risk of stroke, myocardial infarction, or arterial revascularization procedures in patients without clinically evident coronary heart disease or lipid abnormalities but with all of the following: 1) an increased risk of cardiovascular disease based on age ≥50 years old in men and ≥60 years old in women, 2) hsCRP ≥2 mg/L, and 3) the presence of at least one additional cardiovascular disease risk factor such as hypertension, low HDL-C, smoking, or a family history of premature coronary heart disease.

Secondary prevention: Adjunctive therapy to diet to slow the progression of atherosclerosis in adults as part of a treatment strategy to lower total cholesterol and LDL-C to target levels.

Primary and secondary prevention of atherosclerotic cardiovascular disease (ASCVD) according to the American College of Cardiology/American Heart Association: To reduce the risk of ASCVD in patients with clinical ASCVD (eg, coronary heart disease, stroke/TIA, or peripheral arterial disease presumed to be of atherosclerotic origin); in patients without clinical ASCVD if

LDL-C is 190 mg/dL or greater; in patients without clinical ASCVD who have type 1 or type 2 diabetes and are between 40 and 75 years of age; in patients with an estimated 10-year ASCVD risk 7.5% or greater and who are between 40 and 75 years of age (Stone 2013). The American Heart Association (AHA) recommends statin therapy (unless contraindicated) for all coronary artery bypass graft (CABG) surgery patients to help maintain long-term graft patency and help obtain the highest level of physical health and quality of life (AHA [Kulik 2015]). Specific recommendations from the Kidney Disease: Improving Global Outcomes (KDIGO) organization have also been released for patients with chronic kidney disease (KDIGO [Tonelli 2013]).

Pregnancy Considerations Adverse events have been observed in some animal reproduction studies. There are reports of congenital anomalies following maternal use of HMG-CoA reductase inhibitors in pregnancy; however, maternal disease, differences in specific agents used, and the low rates of exposure limit the interpretation of the available data (Godfrey 2012; Lecarpentier 2012). Cholesterol biosynthesis may be important in fetal development; serum cholesterol and triglycerides increase normally during pregnancy. The discontinuation of lipid lowering medications temporarily during pregnancy is not expected to have significant impact on the long term outcomes of primary hypercholesterolemia treatment.

Use of rosuvastatin is contraindicated in pregnancy. HMG-CoA reductase inhibitors should be discontinued prior to pregnancy (ADA 2013). If treatment of dyslipidemias is needed in pregnant women or in women of reproductive age, other agents are preferred (Berglund 2012; Stone 2013). The manufacturer recommends administration to women of childbearing potential only when conception is highly unlikely and patients have been informed of potential hazards.

Breast-Feeding Considerations It is not known if rosuvastatin is excreted in breast milk. Due to the potential for serious adverse reactions in a nursing infant, use while breast-feeding is contraindicated by the manufacturer.

Contraindications

Known hypersensitivity to any component of the formulation; active liver disease or unexplained persistent elevations of serum transaminases; pregnancy; breast-feeding.

Canadian labeling: Additional contraindications (not in US labeling): Concomitant administration of cyclosporine; use of 40 mg dose in Asian patients, patients with predisposing risk factors for myopathy/rhabdomyolysis (eg, hereditary muscle disorders, history of myotoxicity with other HMG-CoA reductase inhibitors, concomitant use with fibrates or niacin, severe hepatic impairment, severe renal impairment [CrCl <30 mL/minute/1.73 m²], hypothyroidism, alcohol abuse)

Warnings/Precautions Secondary causes of hyperlipidemia should be ruled out prior to therapy. Rosuvastatin has not been studied when the primary lipid abnormality is chylomicron elevation (Fredrickson types I and V). Post-marketing reports of fatal and nonfatal hepatic failure are rare. If serious hepatotoxicity with clinical symptoms and/or hyperbilirubinemia or jaundice occurs during treatment, interrupt therapy. If an alternate etiology is not identified, do not restart rosuvastatin. Liver enzyme tests should be obtained at baseline and as clinically indicated; routine periodic monitoring of liver enzymes is not necessary. Use with caution in patients who consume large amounts of ethanol or have a history of liver disease; use is contraindicated with active liver disease or unexplained transaminase elevations. Hematuria (microscopic) and proteinuria have been observed; more commonly reported in adults receiving rosuvastatin 40 mg daily, but typically transient and not associated with a decrease in renal function. Consider dosage reduction if unexplained hematuria and proteinuria persists. HMG-CoA reductase inhibitors may cause rhabdomyolysis with acute renal failure and/or myopathy. Discontinue in any patient in which CPK levels are markedly elevated (>10 times ULN) or if myopathy is suspected/diagnosed. This risk is dose-related and is increased with concurrent use of other lipid-lowering medications (fibric acid derivatives or niacin doses ≥1 g/day), other interacting drugs, drugs associated with myopathy (eg, colchicine), age ≥65 years, female gender, certain subgroups of Asian ancestry, uncontrolled hypothyroidism, and renal dysfunction. Dose reductions may be necessary. Immune-mediated necrotizing myopathy (IMNM), an autoimmune-mediated myopathy, has been reported (rarely) with HMG-CoA reductase inhibitor therapy. IMNM presents as proximal muscle weakness with elevated CPK levels, which persists despite discontinuation of HMG-CoA reductase inhibitor therapy; additionally, muscle biopsy may show necrotizing myopathy with limited inflammation; immunosuppressive therapy (eg, corticosteroids, azathioprine) may be useful for treatment.

The manufacturer recommends temporary discontinuation for elective major surgery, acute medical or surgical conditions, or in any patient experiencing an acute or serious condition predisposing to renal failure (eg, sepsis, dehydration, electrolyte disorders, hypotension, trauma, uncontrolled seizures). Based on current research and clinical guidelines (Fleisher 2009), HMG-CoA reductase inhibitors should be continued in the perioperative period. Patients should be instructed to report unexplained muscle pain, tenderness, weakness, or dark urine; in Canada, concomitant use with cyclosporine or niacin is contraindicated, and rosuvastatin at a dose of 40 mg/day in Asian patients is contraindicated. Small increases in HbA₁c (mean: ~0.1%) and fasting blood glucose have been reported with rosuvastatin; however, the benefits of statin therapy far outweigh the risk of dysglycemia.

Potentially significant interactions may exist, requiring dose or frequency adjustment, additional monitoring, and/or selection of alternative therapy. Consult drug interactions database for more detailed information. Dosage adjustment required in patients with a CrCl <30 mL/minute/1.73 m² and not receiving hemodialysis (contraindicated in the Canadian labeling). Use with caution in elderly patients as they are more predisposed to myopathy.

Adverse Reactions

>10%: Neuromuscular & skeletal: Myalgia (2% to 13%)

1% to 10%:

Central nervous system: Headache (6% to 9%), dizziness (4%)

Endocrine & metabolic: Diabetes mellitus (new onset: 3%)

Gastrointestinal: Nausea (4% to 6%), constipation (3% to 5%)

Genitourinary: Cystitis (interstitial; Huang 2015)

Hepatic: Increased serum ALT (2%; >3 times ULN)

Neuromuscular & skeletal: Arthralgia (4% to 10%), increased creatine phosphokinase (3%; >10 x ULN: Children 3%), weakness (5%)

<1% (Limited to important or life-threatening): Abnormal thyroid function test, cognitive dysfunction (reversible; includes amnesia, confusion, memory impairment), depression, elevated glycosylated hemoglobin (HbA₁c), gynecomastia, hematuria (microscopic), hepatic failure, hepatitis, hypersensitivity reaction (including angioedema, pruritus, skin rash, urticaria), immune-mediated necrotizing myopathy, increased gamma-glutamyl transferase, increased serum alkaline phosphatase, increased serum bilirubin, increased serum glucose, increased serum transaminases, jaundice, myoglobinuria, myopathy, myositis, pancreatitis, peripheral neuropathy, proteinuria (dose related), renal failure, rhabdomyolysis, sleep disorder (including insomnia and nightmares), thrombocytopenia

Drug Interactions

Metabolism/Transport Effects Substrate of BCRP, CYP2C9 (minor), CYP3A4 (minor), SLCO1B1; **Note:** Assignment of Major/Minor substrate status based on clinically relevant drug interaction potential

Avoid Concomitant Use

Avoid concomitant use of Rosuvastatin with any of the following: Fusidic Acid (Systemic); Gemfibrozil; Ledipasvir; Red Yeast Rice

Increased Effect/Toxicity

Rosuvastatin may increase the levels/effects of: DAPTOmycin; PAZOPanib; Trabectedin; Vitamin K Antagonists

The levels/effects of Rosuvastatin may be increased by: Acipimox; Amiodarone; Bezafibrate; Boceprevir; Ciprofibrate; Clopidogrel; Colchicine; CycloSPORINE (Systemic); Daclatasvir; Dronedarone; Eltrombopag; Eluxadoline; Fenofibrate and Derivatives; Fusidic Acid (Systemic); Gemfibrozil; Itraconazole; Ledipasvir; Niacin; Niacinamide; Ombitasvir, Paritaprevir, Ritonavir, and Dasabuvir; Protease Inhibitors; Raltegravir; Red Yeast Rice; Rolapitant; Sacubitril; Simeprevir; Telaprevir; Teriflunomide

Decreased Effect

Rosuvastatin may decrease the levels/effects of: Lanthanum

The levels/effects of Rosuvastatin may be decreased by: Antacids; Eslicarbazepine

Storage/Stability Store between 20°C and 25°C (68°F to 77°F). Protect from moisture.

Mechanism of Action Inhibitor of 3-hydroxy-3-methylglutaryl coenzyme A (HMG-CoA) reductase, the rate-limiting enzyme in cholesterol synthesis (reduces the production of mevalonic acid from HMG-CoA); this then results in a compensatory increase in the expression of LDL receptors

on hepatocyte membranes and a stimulation of LDL catabolism. In addition to the ability of HMG-CoA reductase inhibitors to decrease levels of high-sensitivity C-reactive protein (hsCRP), they also possess pleiotropic properties including improved endothelial function, reduced inflammation at the site of the coronary plaque, inhibition of platelet aggregation, and anticoagulant effects (de Denus 2002; Ray 2005).

Pharmacodynamics/Kinetics
Onset of action: Within 1 week; maximal at 4 weeks

Distribution: V_d: 134 L

Protein binding: 88%

Metabolism: Hepatic (10%), via CYP2C9 (1 active metabolite identified: N-desmethyl rosuvastatin, one-sixth to one-half the HMG-CoA reductase activity of the parent compound)

Bioavailability: 20% (high first-pass extraction by liver)
Asian patients have been noted to have increased bioavailability.

Half-life elimination: 19 hours

Time to peak, plasma: 3-5 hours

Excretion: Feces (90%), primarily as unchanged drug

Dosing
Adult & Geriatric Note: Doses should be individualized according to the baseline LDL-cholesterol levels, the recommended goal of therapy, and patient response; adjustments should be made at intervals of 4 weeks or more.

Hyperlipidemia, mixed dyslipidemia, hypertriglyceridemia, primary dysbetalipoproteinemia, slowing progression of atherosclerosis, primary prevention of cardiovascular disease: Oral:

Initial dose:

General dosing: 10 to 20 mg once daily; 20 mg once daily may be used in patients with severe hyperlipidemia (LDL >190 mg/dL) and aggressive lipid targets (McKenney 2009)

Conservative dosing: Patients requiring less aggressive treatment or predisposed to myopathy (including patients of Asian descent): 5 mg once daily

Titration: After initiation or upon titration, analyze lipid levels within 2 to 4 weeks (peak, steady-state lowering effects usually seen between 4 to 6 weeks [McKenney 2009]) and adjust dose accordingly; dosing range: 5 to 40 mg daily (maximum dose: 40 mg once daily)

Note: The 40 mg dose should be reserved for patients who have not achieved goal cholesterol levels on a dose of 20 mg daily, including patients switched from another HMG-CoA reductase inhibitor.

Homozygous familial hypercholesterolemia (FH):
Oral: Initial: 20 mg once daily (maximum dose: 40 mg daily)

Prevention of cardiovascular disease: ACC/AHA Blood Cholesterol Guideline recommendations to reduce the risk of atherosclerotic cardiovascular disease (ASCVD) (Stone 2013): Adults ≥21 years: Oral:

Primary prevention:

LDL-C ≥190 mg/dL: High-intensity therapy: 20 to 40 mg once daily.

Type 1 or 2 diabetes and age 40 to 75 years: Moderate-intensity therapy: 5 to 10 mg once daily.

Type 1 or 2 diabetes, age 40 to 75 years, and an estimated 10-year ASCVD risk ≥7.5%: High intensity therapy: 20 to 40 mg once daily

Age 40 to 75 years and an estimated 10-year ASCVD risk ≥7.5%: Moderate- to high-intensity therapy: 5 to 40 mg once daily

Secondary prevention:

Patient has clinical ASCVD (eg, coronary heart disease, stroke/TIA, or peripheral arterial disease presumed to be of atherosclerotic origin) or is post-CABG (AHA [Kulik 2015]) **and:**

Age ≤75 years: High-intensity therapy: 20 to 40 mg once daily.

Age >75 years or not a candidate for high-intensity therapy: Moderate-intensity therapy: 5 to 10 mg once daily.

Dosage adjustment for rosuvastatin with concomitant medications: Oral:

US labeling:

Cyclosporine: Rosuvastatin dose should not exceed 5 mg once daily

Gemfibrozil: Avoid concurrent use; if unable to avoid concurrent use, initiate rosuvastatin at 5 mg once daily; dose should not exceed 10 mg once daily

Atazanavir/ritonavir, lopinavir/ritonavir, or simeprevir: Initiate rosuvastatin at 5 mg once daily; dose should not exceed 10 mg once daily

Canadian labeling:

Cyclosporine: Concomitant use is contraindicated

Gemfibrozil: Rosuvastatin dose should not exceed 20 mg daily

Dosage adjustment for hematuria and/or persistent, unexplained proteinuria while on 40 mg daily: Reduce dose and evaluate causes.

Pediatric Note: Doses should be individualized according to the baseline LDL-cholesterol levels, the recommended goal of therapy, and patient response; adjustments should be made at intervals of 4 weeks or more.

Heterozygous familial hypercholesterolemia (HeFH):

US labeling: Children and Adolescents 8 to 17 years (females >1 year postmenarche): Oral:

Children 8 to <10 years: 5 to 10 mg once daily; safety and efficacy of dosages above 10 mg daily not established

Children and Adolescents 10 to 17 years: 5 to 20 mg once daily; safety and efficacy of dosages above 20 mg daily not established

Dosage adjustment for rosuvastatin with concomitant cyclosporine, gemfibrozil, atazanavir/ritonavir, lopinavir/ritonavir, or simeprevir: Refer to adult dosing.

Canadian labeling: Children and Adolescents 10 to 17 years (females >1 year postmenarche): Oral: 5 to 10 mg once daily; maximum: 10 mg daily

Renal Impairment
CrCl ≥30 mL/minute/1.73 m^2: No dosage adjustment necessary.

CrCl <30 mL/minute/1.73 m^2: Initial: 5 mg once daily; maximum: 10 mg once daily

Hepatic Impairment
US labeling: Manufacturer labeling does not provide specific dosing recommendations; however, systemic exposure may be increased in patients with liver disease (increased AUC and C_{max}); use is contraindicated in active liver disease or unexplained transaminase elevations.

Canadian labeling:

Active hepatic disease or unexplained persistent transaminase >3 x ULN: Use is contraindicated.

Mild-to-moderate impairment: No dosage adjustment necessary.

Severe impairment: Initial: 5 mg daily. Maximum: 20 mg once daily.

Adjustment for Toxicity
Severe muscle symptoms or fatigue: Promptly discontinue use; evaluate CPK, creatinine, and urinalysis for myoglobinuria (Stone 2013).

Mild to moderate muscle symptoms: Discontinue use until symptoms can be evaluated; evaluate patient for conditions that may increase the risk for muscle symptoms (eg, hypothyroidism, reduced renal or hepatic function, rheumatologic disorders such as polymyalgia rheumatica, steroid myopathy, vitamin D deficiency, or primary muscle diseases). Upon resolution, resume the original or lower dose of rosuvastatin. If muscle symptoms recur, discontinue rosuvastatin use. After muscle symptom resolution, may then use a low dose of a different statin; gradually increase if tolerated. In the absence of continued statin use, if muscle symptoms or elevated CPK continues after 2 months, consider other causes of muscle symptoms. If determined to be due to another condition aside from statin use, may resume statin therapy at the original dose (Stone 2013).

Dietary Considerations Red yeast rice contains variable amounts of several compounds that are structurally similar to HMG-CoA reductase inhibitors, primarily monacolin K (or mevinolin) which is structurally identical to lovastatin; concurrent use of red yeast rice with HMG-CoA reductase inhibitors may increase the incidence of adverse and toxic effects (Lapi 2008; Smith 2003).

Administration Administer with or without food. May be taken at any time of the day; swallow tablet whole.

Monitoring Parameters
2013 ACC/AHA Blood Cholesterol Guideline recommendations (Stone 2013):

Lipid panel (total cholesterol, HDL, LDL, triglycerides): Baseline lipid panel; fasting lipid profile within 4-12 weeks after initiation or dose adjustment and every 3-12 months (as clinically indicated) thereafter. If 2 consecutive LDL levels are <40 mg/dL, consider decreasing the dose.

Hepatic transaminase levels: Baseline measurement of hepatic transaminase levels (ie, ALT); measure hepatic function if symptoms suggest hepatotoxicity (eg, unusual fatigue or weakness, loss of appetite, abdominal pain, dark-colored urine or yellowing of skin or sclera) during therapy.

CPK: CPK should not be routinely measured. Baseline CPK measurement is reasonable for some individuals (eg, family history of statin intolerance or muscle disease, clinical presentation, concomitant drug therapy that may increase risk of myopathy). May measure CPK in any patient with symptoms suggestive of myopathy (pain, tenderness, stiffness, cramping, weakness, or generalized fatigue).

Evaluate for new-onset diabetes mellitus during therapy; if diabetes develops, continue statin therapy and encourage adherence to a heart-healthy diet, physical activity, a healthy body weight, and tobacco cessation.

If patient develops a confusional state or memory impairment, may evaluate patient for nonstatin causes (eg, exposure to other drugs), systemic and neuropsychiatric causes, and the possibility of adverse effects associated with statin therapy.

Manufacturer's labeling: Liver enzyme tests at baseline and repeated when clinically indicated. Upon initiation or titration, lipid panel should be analyzed within 2 to 4 weeks.

Dosage Forms Excipient information presented when available (limited, particularly for generics); consult specific product labeling.

Tablet, Oral:

Crestor: 5 mg, 10 mg, 20 mg, 40 mg

◆ Rosuvastatin Calcium *see* Rosuvastatin *on page 1620*
◆ Rotarix *see* Rotavirus Vaccine *on page 1623*
◆ RotaTeq *see* Rotavirus Vaccine *on page 1623*

Rotavirus Vaccine (ROE ta vye rus vak SEEN)

Brand Names: US Rotarix; RotaTeq
Brand Names: Canada Rotarix; RotaTeq
Index Terms Human Rotavirus Vaccine, Attenuated (HRV); Pentavalent Human-Bovine Reassortant Rotavirus Vaccine (PRV); Rotavirus Vaccine, Pentavalent; RV1 (Rotarix); RV5 (RotaTeq)
Pharmacologic Category Vaccine; Vaccine, Live (Viral)
Additional Appendix Information

Immunization Administration Recommendations *on page 1974*

Immunization Schedules *on page 1979*

Use

Rotavirus gastroenteritis prevention:

Rotarix: Prevention of rotavirus gastroenteritis in infants 6 to 24 weeks of age caused by the serotypes G1,G3, G4, and G9 when administered as a 2-dose series.

RotaTeq: Prevention of rotavirus gastroenteritis in infants 6 to 32 weeks of age caused by the serotypes G1, G2, G3, and G4 when administered as a 3-dose series.

The Advisory Committee on Immunization Practices (ACIP) recommends routine vaccination of all infants (CDC/ACIP [Cortese, 2009]).

Medication Guide Available Yes

Dosing

Pediatric Prevention of rotavirus gastroenteritis: Oral:

Manufacturer's labeling:

Infants 6 to 24 weeks of age: Rotarix: A total of two 1 mL doses (U.S. labeling) or two 1.5 mL doses (Canadian labeling), the first dose given at 6 weeks of age, followed by the second dose given ≥4 weeks later. The 2-dose series should be completed by 24 weeks of age.

Infants 6 to 32 weeks of age: RotaTeq: A total of three 2 mL doses, the first dose given at 6 to 12 weeks of age, followed by subsequent doses at 4- to 10-week intervals. Administer all doses by 32 weeks of age.

ACIP recommendations (CDC/ACIP [Cortese, 2009]):

The first dose can be given at 6 to 14 weeks of age. The series should not be started in infants ≥15 weeks. The final dose in the series should be administered by 8 months 0 days of age. The minimum interval between doses is 4 weeks. RotaTeq should be given in 3 doses administered at 2-, 4-, and 6 months of age. Rotarix should be given in 2 doses administered at 2- and 4 months of age. For infants inadvertently administered rotavirus vaccine at ≥15 weeks of age, the vaccine series may be completed according to schedule. The ACIP recommends to complete the vaccine series with the same product whenever possible. If continuing with same product will cause vaccination to be deferred, or if product used previously is unknown, vaccination should be completed with the product available. If RotaTeq was used in any previous doses, or if the specific product used was unknown, a total of 3 doses should be given. Infants who have had rotavirus gastroenteritis before getting the full course of vaccine should still initiate or complete the recommended schedule; initial infection provides only partial immunity.

Renal Impairment There are no dosage adjustments provided in the manufacturer's labeling.

Hepatic Impairment There are no dosage adjustments provided in the manufacturer's labeling.

Additional Information Complete prescribing information should be consulted for additional detail.

Dosage Forms Excipient information presented when available (limited, particularly for generics); consult specific product labeling.

Powder, for suspension, oral [preservative free; human derived]:

Rotarix: G1P[8] ≥10^6 CCID$_{50}$ per 1 mL [contains sorbitol, sucrose; supplied with diluent which may contain natural rubber/natural latex in packaging]

Solution, oral [preservative free; bovine and human derived]:

RotaTeq: G1 ≥2.2 x 10^6 infectious units, G2 ≥2.8 x 10^6 infectious units, G3 ≥2.2 x 10^6 infectious units, G4 ≥2 x 10^6 infectious units, and P1A [8] ≥2.3 x 10^6 infectious units per 2 mL (2 mL) [contains sucrose]

Dosage Forms: Canada Excipient information presented when available (limited, particularly for generics); consult specific product labeling.

Suspension, oral [human derived]:

Rotarix: ≥10^6 CCID$_{50}$ per 1.5 mL (1.5 mL)

◆ Rotavirus Vaccine, Pentavalent *see* Rotavirus Vaccine *on page 1623*

Rotigotine (roe TIG oh teen)

Brand Names: US Neupro
Brand Names: Canada Neupro
Index Terms N-0923
Pharmacologic Category Anti-Parkinson's Agent, Dopamine Agonist
Use

Parkinson disease: For the treatment of Parkinson disease.

Restless legs syndrome: For the treatment of moderate to severe primary restless legs syndrome.

Pregnancy Considerations Adverse events have been observed in animal reproduction studies. The Canadian labeling does not recommend use in pregnant women.

Breast-Feeding Considerations It is not known if rotigotine is excreted in breast milk. Rotigotine decreases prolactin secretion and lactation may be inhibited. The manufacturer recommends that caution be exercised when administering rotigotine to nursing women. The Canadian labeling recommends discontinuing breast-feeding in women who require therapy.

Contraindications Hypersensitivity to rotigotine or any component of the formulation

Warnings/Precautions Use is commonly associated with somnolence. In addition, falling asleep during activities of daily living, including while driving, has also been reported and may occur without significant warning signs. Monitor for daytime somnolence or preexisting sleep disorder. Patients must be cautioned about performing tasks which require mental alertness (eg, operating machinery or driving). Use with caution in patients receiving other CNS depressants or psychoactive agents; discontinue if significant daytime sleepiness or episodes of falling asleep occur. Effects with other sedative drugs or ethanol may be potentiated.

Dopamine agonists may cause orthostatic hypotension and syncope; Parkinson disease patients appear to have an impaired capacity to respond to a postural challenge. Use with caution in patients at risk of hypotension (such as those receiving antihypertensive drugs) or where transient hypotensive episodes would be poorly tolerated (cardiovascular disease or cerebrovascular disease). Parkinson disease and restless legs syndrome (RLS) patients being treated with dopaminergic agonists ordinarily require careful monitoring for signs and symptoms of postural hypotension, especially during dose escalation, and should be informed of this risk. Weight gain and fluid retention have been reported, primarily associated with development of peripheral edema in Parkinson disease patients; use caution and monitor for weight gain in patients with concomitant illnesses (eg, heart failure or renal insufficiency). Therapy has also been associated with increases in blood pressure (may be significant), and increased heart rate; use caution in preexisting cardiovascular disease.

Dopamine agonists have been associated with compulsive behaviors and/or loss of impulse control, which has manifested as pathological gambling, libido increases (hypersexuality), and/or binge eating. Causality has not been established, and controversy exists as to whether this

phenomenon is related to the underlying disease, prior behaviors/addictions and/or drug therapy. Dose reduction or discontinuation of therapy has been reported to reverse these behaviors in some, but not all cases.

In RLS patents, augmentation (earlier onset of symptoms each day and/or an overall increase in symptom severity) or rebound (considered to be an end of dose effect) may occur.

Use with caution in patients with preexisting dyskinesia; therapy may cause or exacerbate dyskinesia. Therapy may also cause hallucinations (dose-related) and other psychotic like behaviors (eg, agitation, delirium, delusions, aggression); in general, avoid use in patients with preexisting major psychotic disorders. Risk for melanoma development is increased in Parkinson's disease patients; drug causation or factors contributing to risk have not been established. Patients receiving therapy for any indication should be monitored closely and periodic skin examinations should be performed. Other dopaminergic agents have been associated with a syndrome resembling neuroleptic malignant syndrome on withdrawal and/or significant dosage reduction. Taper treatment when discontinuing therapy; do not stop abruptly. Rare cases of pleural effusion, pleural thickening, pulmonary infiltrates, retroperitoneal fibrosis, pericarditis and/or cardiac valvulopathy have been reported in patients treated with ergot-derived dopamine agonists. The potential of rotigotine, a nonergot-derived dopamine agonist, to cause similar fibrotic complications is unknown. Discontinuation of therapy may resolve complications, but not in all cases.

Patch contains aluminum; remove patch prior to magnetic resonance imaging or cardioversion to avoid skin burns. Patch also contains sodium metabisulfite which may cause allergic reaction in susceptible individuals. Dose-dependent application site reactions, potentially severe, have been observed; daily rotation of application sites has been shown to decrease incidence of reactions. If a generalized (nonapplication site) skin reaction occurs; discontinue therapy. Avoid exposure of application site to any direct external heat sources (eg, hair dryers, heating pads, electric blankets, saunas, hot tubs, direct sunlight); heat exposure has not been studied with the rotigotine patch, but an increase in the rate and extent of absorption has been observed with other transdermal products.

Adverse Reactions
>10%:

Cardiovascular: Systolic hypotension (13% to 32%), peripheral edema (dose related; 3% to 14%)

Central nervous system: Drowsiness (dose related; 5% to 32%), orthostatic hypotension (8% to 29%), dizziness (5% to 23%), headache (10% to 21%), fatigue (6% to 18%), sleep disorder (disturbance in initiating/maintaining sleep; dose related; 2% to 14%), malaise (≤14%), hallucination (dose related; 3% to 13%), insomnia (7% to 11%)

Dermatologic: Hyperhidrosis (dose related; 1% to 11%)

Endocrine & metabolic: Decreased serum glucose (1% to 15%)

Gastrointestinal: Nausea (dose related; 15% to 48%), vomiting (dose related; 2% to 20%)

Hematologic & oncologic: Decreased hematocrit (8% to 17%), decreased hemoglobin (8% to 15%)

Local: Application site reaction (dose related; 21% to 46%)

Neuromuscular & skeletal: Dyskinesia (dose related; 14% to 17%), weakness (≤14%), arthralgia (8% to 11%)

1% to 10%:

Cardiovascular: Increased diastolic blood pressure (4% to 8%), systolic hypertension (5%), hypertension (dose related; 1% to 5%), atrioventricular block (3%), abnormal T waves on ECG (≤3%), syncope

Central nervous system: Abnormal dreams (dose related; 1% to 7%), nightmares (dose related; 3% to 5%), depression (2% to 5%), paresthesia (dose related; 4%), vertigo (3% to 4%), equilibrium disturbance (2% to 3%), irritability (1% to 3%), sleep attacks (dose related; 1% to 2%)

Dermatologic: Pruritus (4% to 9%), erythema (dose related; 2% to 6%)

Endocrine & metabolic: Weight gain (2% to 9%), change in libido (4% to 6%), hot flash (3% to 4%), low serum ferritin (dose related; 2%), menstrual disorder (1% to 2%)

Gastrointestinal: Constipation (5% to 9%), anorexia (2% to 9%), xerostomia (dose related; 7%), diarrhea (5% to 7%), dyspepsia (dose related; 2% to 3%), viral gastroenteritis (1% to 2%)

Genitourinary: Change in WBC count (urine, ≤3%)

Hematologic & oncologic: Basal cell carcinoma (3%), leukocyturia (3%)

Infection: Herpes simplex infection (3%)

Neuromuscular & skeletal: Tremor (4%), muscle spasm (dose related; 3% to 4%)

Ophthalmic: Visual disturbance (3% to 5%)

Otic: Tinnitus (2% to 3%)

Renal: Increased blood urea nitrogen (3% to 11%)

Respiratory: Nasopharyngitis (8% to 10%), cough (3%), nasal congestion (3%), sinus congestion (2% to 3%), sinusitis (dose related; 2% to 3%)

Miscellaneous: Hiccups (dose related; 2% to 3%)

<1% (Limited to important or life-threatening): Confusion, delirium, delusions, impulse control disorder, increased creatine phosphokinase, neuroleptic malignant syndrome, paranoia, psychotic symptoms

Drug Interactions
Metabolism/Transport Effects None known.

Avoid Concomitant Use
Avoid concomitant use of Rotigotine with any of the following: Amisulpride

Increased Effect/Toxicity
Rotigotine may increase the levels/effects of: Amifostine; BuPROPion; DULoxetine; Hypotension-Associated Agents; Levodopa

The levels/effects of Rotigotine may be increased by: Alcohol (Ethyl); Alfuzosin; Blood Pressure Lowering Agents; Brimonidine (Topical); CNS Depressants; Diazoxide; Herbs (Hypotensive Properties); Methylphenidate; Molsidomine; Nicorandil; Obinutuzumab; Pentoxifylline; Phosphodiesterase 5 Inhibitors; Prostacyclin Analogues

Decreased Effect
Rotigotine may decrease the levels/effects of: Amisulpride; Antipsychotic Agents (First Generation [Typical])

The levels/effects of Rotigotine may be decreased by: Amisulpride; Antipsychotic Agents (First Generation [Typical]); Antipsychotic Agents (Second Generation [Atypical]); Metoclopramide

Storage/Stability Store at 20°C to 25°C (68°F to 77°F); excursions are permitted between 15°C and 30°C (59°F and 86°F). Store in original pouch until application.

Mechanism of Action Rotigotine is a nonergot dopamine agonist with specificity for D_3-, D_2-, and D_1-dopamine receptors. Although the precise mechanism of action of rotigotine is unknown, it is believed to be due to stimulation of postsynaptic dopamine D_2-type auto receptors within the substantia nigra in the brain, leading to improved dopaminergic transmission in the motor areas of the basal ganglia, notably the caudate nucleus/putamen regions.

Pharmacodynamics/Kinetics
Distribution: V_d: ~84 L/kg

Protein binding: ~90%

Metabolism: Extensive via conjugation and N-dealkylation; multiple CYP isoenzymes, sulfotransferases, and two UDP-glucuronosyltransferases involved in catalyzing the metabolism

Half-life elimination: After removal of patch: ~5 to 7 hours

Time to peak, plasma: 15 to 18 hours; can occur 4 to 27 hours post application

Excretion: Urine (~71% as inactive conjugates and metabolites, <1% as unchanged drug); feces (~23%)

Dosing
Adult & Geriatric
Parkinson disease: Topical: Transdermal:
Early-stage: Initial: Apply 2 mg/24 hours patch once daily; may increase by 2 mg/24 hours weekly, based on clinical response and tolerability; lowest effective dose: 4 mg/24 hours (maximum dose: 6 mg/24 hours [U.S. labeling] or 8 mg/24 hours [Canadian labeling])

Advanced-stage: Initial: Apply 4 mg/24 hours patch once daily; may increase by 2 mg/24 hours weekly, based on clinical response and tolerability. Recommended dose: 8 mg/24 hours; in clinical trials maximum doses up to 16 mg/24 hours were used.

Discontinuation of treatment in Parkinson's disease: Decrease by ≤2 mg/24 hours preferably every other day until withdrawal complete

Restless legs syndrome (RLS): Topical: Transdermal: Initial: Apply 1 mg/24 hours patch once daily; may increase by 1 mg/24 hours weekly, based on clinical response and tolerability; lowest effective dose: 1 mg/24 hours (maximum dose: 3 mg/24 hours)

Discontinuation of treatment for RLS: Decrease by 1 mg/24 hours preferably every other day until withdrawal complete

Renal Impairment
Mild-to-severe impairment (CrCl ≥15 mL/minute): No dosage adjustment necessary.

End-stage renal disease (ESRD) requiring hemodialysis: No dosage adjustment necessary.

Hepatic Impairment

Mild-to-moderate hepatic impairment (Child-Pugh class A or B): No dosage adjustment necessary.

Severe hepatic impairment: There are no dosage adjustments provided in manufacturer's labeling (has not been studied).

Administration Transdermal patch: Apply patch to clean, dry, hairless area of intact healthy skin on the front of the abdomen, thigh, hip, flank, shoulder, or upper arm at approximately the same time daily. Remove from pouch immediately before use and press patch firmly in place on skin for 30 seconds. Application sites should be rotated on a daily basis. Do not apply to same application site more than once every 14 days or apply patch to oily, irritated or damaged skin. Avoid exposing patch to external heat sources (eg, heating pad, electric blanket, heat lamp, hot tub, direct sunlight). If applied to hairy area, shave ≥3 days prior to applying patch. If patch falls off, immediately apply a new one to a new site.

Monitoring Parameters Blood pressure (including orthostatic); daytime alertness; periodic skin evaluations (melanoma development)

Additional Information In April 2008, Neupro was removed from the market following a recall due to the formation of rotigotine crystals (resembling snowflakes) on the patch. The crystallization resulted in decreased drug available for absorption and altered efficacy. Reintroduction of a reformulated Neupro into the U.S. market was announced in 2012.

Dosage Forms Excipient information presented when available (limited, particularly for generics); consult specific product labeling.

Patch 24 Hour, Transdermal:

Neupro: 1 mg/24 hr (30 ea); 2 mg/24 hr (30 ea); 3 mg/24 hr (30 ea); 4 mg/24 hr (30 ea); 6 mg/24 hr (30 ea); 8 mg/24 hr (30 ea) [contains sodium metabisulfite]

Rufinamide (roo FIN a mide)

Brand Names: US Banzel
Brand Names: Canada Banzel
Index Terms CGP 33101; E 2080; RUF 331; Xilep
Pharmacologic Category Anticonvulsant, Triazole Derivative

Use Lennox-Gastaut syndrome: Adjunctive treatment of seizures associated with Lennox-Gastaut syndrome in adults and children 1 year and older

Pregnancy Considerations Adverse effects were seen in animal reproduction studies. Hormonal contraceptives may be less effective with concurrent rufinamide use; additional forms of nonhormonal contraceptives should be used.

Patients exposed to rufinamide during pregnancy are encouraged to enroll themselves into the AED Pregnancy Registry by calling 1-888-233-2334. Additional information is available at www.aedpregnancyregistry.org.

Breast-Feeding Considerations Excretion into breast milk is unknown, but may be expected. Due to the potential for serious adverse reactions in the nursing infant, the manufacturer recommends a decision be made whether to discontinue nursing or to discontinue the drug, taking into account the importance of treatment to the mother.

Medication Guide Available Yes

Contraindications Patients with familial short QT syndrome

Canadian labeling: Additional contraindications (not in U.S. labeling): Family history of short QT syndrome; presence or history of short QT interval; hypersensitivity to rufinamide, triazole derivatives, or any component of the formulation

Warnings/Precautions Has been associated with shortening of the QT interval. Use caution in patients receiving concurrent medications that shorten the QT interval. Contraindicated in patients with familial short-QT syndrome (Canadian labeling also contraindicates use in patients with a family history of short QT syndrome or presence or history of short QT interval). Use has been associated with CNS-related adverse events, most significant of these were cognitive symptoms (including somnolence or fatigue) and coordination abnormalities (including ataxia, dizziness, and gait disturbances). Caution patients about performing tasks which require mental alertness (eg, operating machinery or driving).

Potentially serious, sometimes fatal, multiorgan hypersensitivity reactions (also known as drug reaction with eosinophilia and systemic symptoms [DRESS]) have been reported. Monitor for signs and symptoms (eg, fever, rash, lymphadenopathy, eosinophilia) in association with other organ system involvement (eg, hepatitis, nephritis, hematological abnormalities, myocarditis, myositis). Evaluate immediately if signs or symptoms are present. Discontinuation and conversion to alternate therapy may be required. Potentially serious, sometimes fatal, dermatologic reactions including Stevens-Johnson syndrome (SJS) have been reported; monitor for signs and symptoms of skin reactions; discontinuation and conversion to alternate therapy may be required. Potentially significant drug-drug interactions may exist, requiring dose or frequency adjustment, additional monitoring, and/or selection of alternative therapy.

Antiepileptics are associated with an increased risk of suicidal behavior/thoughts with use (regardless of indication); patients should be monitored for signs/symptoms of depression, suicidal tendencies, and other unusual behavior changes during therapy and instructed to inform their healthcare provider immediately if symptoms occur. Use with caution in patients with mild-to-moderate hepatic impairment; use in not recommended in patients with severe hepatic impairment. Anticonvulsants should not be discontinued abruptly because of the possibility of increasing seizure frequency; therapy should be withdrawn gradually to minimize the potential of increased seizure frequency, unless safety concerns require a more rapid withdrawal. Reducing dose by ~25% every two days was effective in trials. Decreased white blood cell count has been reported during treatment. Some dosage forms may contain propylene glycol; large amounts are potentially toxic and have been associated hyperosmolality, lactic acidosis, seizures, and respiratory depression; use caution (AAP, 1997; Zar, 2007).

Adverse Reactions

>10%:

Cardiovascular: Shortened QT interval (46% to 65%; dose related)

Central nervous system: Headache (adults 27%, children 16%), drowsiness (11% to 24%), dizziness (3% to 19%), fatigue (9% to 16%)

Gastrointestinal: Vomiting (children 17%, adults 5%), nausea (7% to 12%)

1% to 10%:

Central nervous system: Ataxia (4% to 5%), status epilepticus (≤4%), aggressive behavior (children 3%), anxiety (adults 3%), disturbance in attention (children 3%), hyperactivity (children 3%), vertigo (adults 3%), abnormal gait (1% to 3%), convulsions (children 2%)

Dermatologic: Skin rash (children 4%), pruritus (children 3%)

Gastrointestinal: Decreased appetite (children 5%), constipation (adults 3%), dyspepsia (adults 3%), upper abdominal pain (3%), increased appetite (≥1%)

Hematologic & oncologic: Leukopenia (4%), anemia (1%)

Infection: Influenza (children 5%)

Neuromuscular & skeletal: Tremor (adults 6%), back pain (adults 3%)

Ophthalmic: Diplopia (4% to 9%), blurred vision (adults 6%), nystagmus (adults 6%)

Otic: Otic infection (children 3%), pollakiuria (1%)

Respiratory: Nasopharyngitis (children 5%), bronchitis (children 3%), sinusitis (children 3%)

<1% (Limited to important or life-threatening): Atrioventricular block (first degree), bundle branch block (right), dysuria, hematuria, hypersensitivity (multiorgan), iron-deficiency anemia, lymphadenopathy, nephrolithiasis, neutropenia, nocturia, polyuria, Stevens-Johnson syndrome, suicidal ideation, thrombocytopenia, urinary incontinence

Drug Interactions

Metabolism/Transport Effects Inhibits CYP2E1 (weak); **Induces** CYP3A4 (weak)

Avoid Concomitant Use There are no known interactions where it is recommended to avoid concomitant use.

Increased Effect/Toxicity

Rufinamide may increase the levels/effects of: CNS Depressants; Fosphenytoin; PHENobarbital; Phenytoin

The levels/effects of Rufinamide may be increased by: Alcohol (Ethyl); Valproate Products

Decreased Effect

Rufinamide may decrease the levels/effects of: ARIPiprazole; CarBAMazepine; Ethinyl Estradiol; Hydrocodone; NiMODipine; Norethindrone; Saxagliptin

The levels/effects of Rufinamide may be decreased by: CarBAMazepine; Fosphenytoin; PHENobarbital; Phenytoin; Primidone

Food Interactions Food increases the absorption of rufinamide. Management: Take with food.

Storage/Stability Store at 25°C (77°F); excursions permitted to 15°C to 30°C (59°F to 86°F). Protect tablets from moisture. Discard oral suspension within 90 days after opening; cap of bottle fits over the adapter.

Mechanism of Action A triazole-derivative antiepileptic whose exact mechanism is unknown. *In vitro*, it prolongs the inactive state of the sodium channels, thereby limiting repetitive firing of sodium-dependent action potentials mediating anticonvulsant effects.

Pharmacodynamics/Kinetics

Absorption: Slow; extensive ≥85%; increased with food

Distribution: V_d: ~50 L

Protein binding: 34%, primarily to albumin (27%)

Metabolism: Extensively via carboxylesterase-mediated hydrolysis of the carboxylamide group to CGP 47292 (inactive metabolite); weak inhibitor of CYP2E1 and weak inducer of CYP3A4

Bioavailability: Extent decreased with increased dose; oral tablets and oral suspension are bioequivalent

Half-life elimination: ~6 to 10 hours

Time to peak, plasma: 4 to 6 hours

Excretion: Urine (85%, ~66% as CGP 47292, 2% as unchanged drug)

Dosing

Adult Lennox-Gastaut syndrome (adjunctive): Oral:

US labeling: Initial: 400 to 800 mg daily in 2 equally divided doses; increase dose by 400 to 800 mg daily every other day to a maximum dose of 3,200 mg daily in 2 equally divided doses

Canadian labeling:

<30 kg: Initial: 200 mg daily in 2 equally divided doses; increase dose by 5 mg/kg/day every 2 weeks until satisfactory control (maximum dose: 1,300 mg daily)

≥30 kg: Initial: 400 mg daily in 2 equally divided doses; increase dose by 5 mg/kg/day every 2 weeks until satisfactory control (maximum dose: 30 to 50 kg: 1,800 mg daily; 50.1 to 70 kg: 2,400 mg daily; ≥70.1 kg: 3,200 mg daily). **Note:** Dose was increased as frequently as every other day in clinical trials.

Note: Discontinue therapy gradually to minimize the potential of increased seizure frequency, unless safety concerns require a more rapid withdrawal. Reducing dose by approximately 25% every 2 days was effective in trials.

Dosage adjustment for concomitant medications: Valproate:

US labeling: Initial rufinamide dose should be <400 mg daily

Canadian labeling: Initial rufinamide dose should be less than the initial daily recommended dosage; however, a specific dosage recommendation is not included in the manufacturer's labeling.

Geriatric Refer to adult dosing. Initiate at the low end of the dosing range; use with caution.

Pediatric Lennox-Gastaut syndrome (adjunctive): Oral:

US labeling:

Children and Adolescents <17 years: Initial: 10 mg/kg/day in 2 equally divided doses; increase dose by ~10 mg/kg every other day to a maximum dose of 45 mg/kg/day, not to exceed 3,200 mg daily in 2 equally divided doses

Adolescents ≥17 years: Refer to adult dosing.

Canadian labeling: Children ≥4 years and Adolescents:

<30 kg: Initial: 200 mg daily in 2 equally divided doses; increase dose by 5 mg/kg/day every 2 weeks until satisfactory control (maximum dose: 1,300 mg daily)

≥30 kg: Initial: 400 mg daily in 2 equally divided doses; increase dose by 5 mg/kg/day every 2 weeks until satisfactory control (maximum dose: 30 to 50 kg: 1,800 mg daily; 50.1 to 70 kg: 2,400 mg daily; ≥70.1 kg: 3,200 mg daily). **Note:** Dose was increased as frequently as every other day in clinical trials.

Note: Discontinue therapy gradually to minimize the potential of increased seizure frequency, unless safety concerns require a more rapid withdrawal. Reducing dose by approximately 25% every 2 days was effective in trials.

Dosage adjustment for concomitant medications: Valproate:

US labeling: Initial rufinamide dose should be <10 mg/kg/day

Canadian labeling: Initial rufinamide dose should be less than the initial daily recommended dosage; however, a specific dosage recommendation is not included in the manufacturer's labeling.

Renal Impairment

CrCl <30 mL/minute: No dosage adjustment necessary.

Hemodialysis: There are no dosage adjustments provided in the manufacturer's labeling. However, consider dosage adjustment for loss of drug.

Hepatic Impairment

Mild to moderate impairment (Child-Pugh score 5 to 9): Use with caution.

Severe impairment (Child-Pugh score 10 to 15): There are no dosage adjustments provided in the manufacturer's labeling (has not been studied); use is not recommended.

Dietary Considerations Take with food.

Administration Administer with food. Tablets may be swallowed whole, split in half, or crushed. Oral suspension should be administered using the provided adapter and calibrated oral syringe; shake well before each dose.

Monitoring Parameters Seizure (frequency and duration); serum levels of concurrent anticonvulsants; suicidality (eg, suicidal thoughts, depression, behavioral changes); rash (may indicate multi-organ hypersensitivity reactions)

Dosage Forms Excipient information presented when available (limited, particularly for generics); consult specific product labeling. [DSC] = Discontinued product

Suspension, Oral:

Banzel: 40 mg/mL (460 mL) [contains methylparaben, propylene glycol, propylparaben; orange flavor]

Tablet, Oral:

Banzel: 200 mg, 400 mg [scored]

Dosage Forms: Canada Excipient information presented when available (limited, particularly for generics); consult specific product labeling.

Tablet, oral:

Banzel: 100 mg [scored]

Extemporaneous Preparations A 40 mg/mL oral suspension may be made using tablets. Crush twelve 400 mg tablets (or twenty-four 200 mg tablets) and reduce to a fine powder. Add 60 mL of Ora-Plus® in incremental proportions until a smooth suspension is obtained; then mix well while adding 60 mL of Ora-Sweet® or Ora-Sweet® SF; transfer to a calibrated bottle. Label "shake well". Stable 90 days at room temperature.

Hutchinson DJ, Liou Y, Best R, et al, "Stability of Extemporaneously Prepared Rufinamide Oral Suspensions," *Ann Pharmacother*, 2010, 44(3):462-5.

◆ Rulox [OTC] *see* Aluminum Hydroxide, Magnesium Hydroxide, and Simethicone *on page 85*

Ruxolitinib (rux oh LI ti nib)

Brand Names: US Jakafi

Brand Names: Canada Jakavi

Index Terms INCB 18424; INCB018424; INCB424; Ruxolitinib Phosphate

Pharmacologic Category Antineoplastic Agent, Janus Associated Kinase Inhibitor; Antineoplastic Agent, Tyrosine Kinase Inhibitor; Janus Associated Kinase Inhibitor

Use

US labeling:

Myelofibrosis: Treatment of intermediate or high-risk myelofibrosis, including primary myelofibrosis, post-polycythemia vera (post-PV) myelofibrosis and post-essential thrombocythemia (post-ET) myelofibrosis

Polycythemia vera: Treatment of polycythemia vera with an inadequate response to or intolerance to hydroxyurea

Canadian labeling:

Myelofibrosis: Treatment of splenomegaly and/or its associated symptoms in adult patients with primary myelofibrosis, post-PV myelofibrosis or post-ET myelofibrosis

Pregnancy Considerations Increased resorptions (late) and reduced fetal weights were observed in animal reproduction studies. The Canadian labeling recommends avoiding use during pregnancy and that women of childbearing potential and male patients use effective contraception during therapy.

Breast-Feeding Considerations It is not known if ruxolitinib is excreted in breast milk. According to the manufacturer, due to the potential for serious adverse reactions in the nursing infant, a decision should be made to discontinue ruxolitinib or to discontinue breast-feeding during therapy, taking into account the benefits of treatment to the mother.

Prescribing and Access Restrictions Available through specialty/network pharmacies. Further information may be obtained from the manufacturer, Incyte, at 1-855-452-5234 or at www.Jakafi.com.

Contraindications

There are no contraindications listed in the manufacturer's U.S. labeling.

Canadian labeling: Hypersensitivity to ruxolitinib or any component of the formulation or container; history of or current progressive multifocal leukoencephalopathy

Warnings/Precautions Hazardous agent - use appropriate precautions for handling and disposal (meets NIOSH 2014 criteria). Hematologic toxicity, including thrombocytopenia, anemia and neutropenia may occur; may require dosage modification; monitor complete blood counts at baseline, every 2 to 4 weeks during dose stabilization, and then as clinically necessary. Thrombocytopenia is generally reversible with treatment interruption or dose reduction; platelet transfusions may be administered during treatment if clinically indicated. Anemia may require blood transfusion; may consider dose modification. Neutropenia (ANC <500/mm³) is generally reversible and managed by treatment interruption.

Serious bacterial, mycobacterial (including tuberculosis), fungal, or viral infections have occurred. Active serious infections should be resolved prior to treatment initiation. Monitor for infections (including signs/symptoms of active tuberculosis and herpes zoster) during treatment. Prompt treatment is recommended if symptoms of active tuberculosis and/or herpes zoster infection develop. Evaluate for tuberculosis risk factors prior to treatment initiation; patients at higher risk for tuberculosis (prior residence/travel to countries with a high tuberculosis prevalence, close contacts with active tuberculosis, or history of latent or active tuberculosis where adequate treatment course cannot be confirmed) should be tested for latent infection. For patients with evidence of tuberculosis (active or latent), decide risk-benefit of continuing treatment. Progressive multifocal leukoencephalopathy (PML) has been reported; discontinue and evaluate if suspected. May require initial dosage reduction for hepatic impairment; in patients with myelofibrosis, avoid use if platelets <50,000/mm³ and with hepatic impairment (any degree). May require initial dosage reduction for renal impairment. Avoid use in patients with ESRD not requiring dialysis; in patients with myelofibrosis, avoid use if platelets <50,000/mm³ and with moderate-to-severe renal impairment. Ruxolitinib is not removed by dialysis, however, some active metabolites may be removed. On dialysis days, patients are advised to take their dose following dialysis sessions. Potentially significant drug-drug interactions may exist, requiring dose or frequency adjustment, additional monitoring, and/or selection of alternative therapy. Discontinue treatment in myelofibrosis patients after 6 months if no reduction in spleen size or no improvement in symptoms. Consider gradually tapering off if discontinuing for reasons other than thrombocytopenia. Within ~1 week after discontinuation, symptoms of myelofibrosis generally return to pretreatment levels. Acute relapse of myelofibrosis symptoms (eg, fever, respiratory distress, hypotension, DIC, multiorgan failure), splenomegaly, worsening cytopenias, hemodynamic compensation, and septic shock-like syndrome have been reported with treatment tapering or discontinuation (Tefferi, 2011). Symptoms generally return over approximately 1 week. Evaluate and treat any intercurrent illness and consider restarting or increasing dose. Consider gradually tapering off if discontinuing for reasons other than thrombocytopenia or neutropenia. Patients should not interrupt/discontinue treatment without consulting healthcare provider.

Non-melanoma skin cancers (basal cell, squamous cell, and Merkel cell carcinoma) have been reported in patients who have received ruxolitinib; periodic skin examinations should be performed.

Adverse Reactions

>10%:

Central nervous system: Dizziness (15% to 18%), headache (15% to 16%), fatigue (15%), insomnia (12%) (Verstovsek 2012)

Dermatologic: Bruise (23%), pruritus (14%)

Endocrine & metabolic: Increased serum cholesterol (17% to 35%), hypertriglyceridemia (15%)

Gastrointestinal: Diarrhea (15%), abdominal pain (15%)

Hematologic & oncologic: Anemia (72% to 96%; grade 3: ≤34%; grade 4: ≤11%), thrombocytopenia (27% to 70%; grade 3: 5% to 9%; grade 4: ≤4%), neutropenia (3% to 19%; grade 3: 5%; grade 4: ≤2%)

Hepatic: Increased serum ALT (25%; grade 3: <1%), increased serum AST (17% to 23%)

Neuromuscular & skeletal: Muscle spasm (12%)

Respiratory: Dyspnea (13%)

1% to 10%:

Cardiovascular: Edema (8%), hypertension (<6%)

Endocrine & metabolic: Weight gain (≤7%)

Gastrointestinal: Constipation (8%), nausea (6%), flatulence (5%), vomiting

Genitourinary: Urinary tract infection (≤9%)

Infection: Herpes zoster (2% yo 6%)

Neuromuscular & skeletal: Weakness (7%)

Respiratory: Nasopharyngitis (9%), cough (8%), epistaxis (6%)

<1% (Limited to important or life-threatening): Bradycardia, disseminated intravascular coagulation, fever, hemorrhagic diathesis, hypotension, multi-organ failure, myelofibrosis (symptom exacerbation), progressive multifocal leukoencephalopathy, prolonged Q-T interval on ECG, respiratory distress, systolic hypertension, tuberculosis, withdrawal syndrome

Drug Interactions

Metabolism/Transport Effects Substrate of CYP3A4 (major); **Note:** Assignment of Major/Minor substrate status based on clinically relevant drug interaction potential

Avoid Concomitant Use

Avoid concomitant use of Ruxolitinib with any of the following: BCG (Intravesical); Conivaptan; Deferiprone; Dipyrone; Fusidic Acid (Systemic); Idelalisib; Natalizumab; Pimecrolimus; Tacrolimus (Topical); Tofacitinib; Vaccines (Live)

Increased Effect/Toxicity

Ruxolitinib may increase the levels/effects of: Bradycardia-Causing Agents; CloZAPine; Deferiprone; Fingolimod; Leflunomide; Natalizumab; Tofacitinib; Vaccines (Live)

The levels/effects of Ruxolitinib may be increased by: Aprepitant; Conivaptan; CYP3A4 Inhibitors (Moderate); CYP3A4 Inhibitors (Strong); Dasatinib; Denosumab; Dipyrone; Fluconazole; Fosaprepitant; Fusidic Acid (Systemic); Grapefruit Juice; Idelalisib; Ivacaftor; Luliconazole; Mifepristone; Netupitant; Osimertinib; Palbociclib; Pimecrolimus; Roflumilast; Simeprevir; Stiripentol; Tacrolimus (Topical); Trastuzumab

Decreased Effect

Ruxolitinib may decrease the levels/effects of: BCG (Intravesical); Coccidioides immitis Skin Test; Sipuleucel-T; Vaccines (Inactivated); Vaccines (Live)

The levels/effects of Ruxolitinib may be decreased by: Bosentan; CYP3A4 Inducers (Moderate); CYP3A4 Inducers (Strong); Dabrafenib; Deferasirox; Echinacea; Enzalutamide; Mitotane; Osimertinib; Siltuximab; St Johns Wort; Tocilizumab

Food Interactions Grapefruit juice may increase the effects of ruxolitinib. Management: Avoid grapefruit juice.

Storage/Stability Store at 20°C to 25°C (68°F to 77°F); excursions are permitted between 15°C and 30°C (59°F and 86°F).

Mechanism of Action Kinase inhibitor which selectively inhibits Janus Associated Kinases (JAKs), JAK1 and JAK2. JAK1 and JAK2 mediate signaling of cytokine and growth factors responsible for hematopoiesis and immune function; JAK mediated signaling involves recruitment of STATs (signal transducers and activators of transcription) to cytokine receptors which leads to modulation of gene expression. In myelofibrosis and polycythemia vera, JAK1/2 activity is dysregulated; ruxolitinib modulates the affected JAK1/2 activity.

Pharmacodynamics/Kinetics

Absorption: Rapid

Distribution: V_d: Myelofibrosis: 72 L; Polycythemia vera: 75 L

Protein binding: ~97%; primarily to albumin

Metabolism: Hepatic, primarily via CYP3A4 (and minimally CYP2C9); forms active metabolites responsible for 20% to 50% of activity

Half-life elimination: Ruxolitinib: 2.8 to 3 hours (hepatic impairment: 4 to 5 hours); Ruxolitinib + metabolites: ~6 hours

Time to peak: Within 1 to 2 hours

Excretion: Urine (74%, <1% as unchanged drug); feces (22%, <1% as unchanged drug)

Dosing

Adult Note: Consider gradually tapering off (by 5 mg twice daily each week) if discontinuing for reasons other than thrombocytopenia.

Myelofibrosis: Oral: Initial dose (based on platelet count, titrate dose thereafter based on efficacy and safety):

Platelets >200,000/mm³: 20 mg twice daily

Platelets 100,000 to 200,000/mm³: 15 mg twice daily

Platelets 50,000 to <100,000/mm³: 5 mg twice daily

Dosage modification based on response in patients with baseline platelet count ≥100,000/mm³ prior to initial treatment with ruxolitinib: For insufficient response (with adequate platelet and neutrophil counts), may increase the dose in 5 mg twice daily increments to a maximum dose of 25 mg twice daily. Do not increase during initial 4 weeks and no more frequently than every 2 weeks. Discontinue treatment after 6 months if no reduction in spleen size or no improvement in symptoms. When discontinuing for reasons other than thrombocytopenia, consider gradually tapering by ~5 mg twice daily per week.

Dose increases may be considered if meet all of the following situations:

- Failure to achieve either a 50% reduction (from baseline) in palpable spleen length or a 35% reduction (from baseline) in spleen volume (measured by CT or MRI)
- Platelet count >125,000/mm³ at 4 weeks (and never <100,000/mm³)
- Absolute neutrophil count (ANC) >750/mm³

Dosage modification for bleeding requiring intervention (regardless of platelet count): Interrupt treatment until bleeding resolved; may consider resuming at the prior dose if the underlying cause of bleeding has resolved or at a reduced dose if the underlying cause of bleeding persists.

Dosage modification based on response in patients with baseline platelet 50,000 to <100,000/mm³ prior to initial treatment with ruxolitinib: For insufficient response (with adequate platelet and neutrophil counts), may increase the dose in 5 mg daily increments to a maximum dose of 10 mg twice daily. Do not increase during initial 4 weeks and no more frequently than every 2 weeks. Discontinue treatment after 6 months if no reduction in spleen size or no improvement in symptoms.

Dose increases may be considered if meet all of the following situations:

- Platelet count remains ≥40,000/mm³ and did not decrease more than 20% in prior 4 weeks
- Absolute neutrophil count (ANC) >1,000/mm³
- No adverse event or hematological toxicity resulting in dose reduction or interruption occurred in prior 4 weeks

Polycythemia vera: Oral: Initial dose: 10 mg twice daily (titrate dose based on efficacy and safety)

Dose modification due to insufficient response: If response is insufficient and platelet, hemoglobin, and neutrophil counts are adequate, the dose may be increased in 5 mg twice daily increments to a maximum of 25 mg twice daily, Do not increase dose in the first 4 weeks of treatment and not more frequently than every 2 weeks. Consider dose increases in patients who meet all of the following conditions:

- Inadequate efficacy demonstrated by one or more of the following: Continued need for phlebotomy, WBC >ULN of normal range, platelet count >ULN of normal range, or palpable spleen that is reduced by <25% from baseline.
- Platelet count ≥140,000/mm³
- Hemoglobin ≥12 g/dL
- ANC ≥1,500/mm³

Dosage adjustment with concomitant strong CYP3A4 inhibitors (eg, azole antifungals, clarithromycin, conivaptin, grapefruit juice, mibefradil, nefazodone, protease inhibitors, telithromycin) and fluconazole (≤200 mg):

US labeling: **Note:** Avoid concomitant use with fluconazole doses >200 mg daily.

Myelofibrosis: Initial dose:

Platelets ≥100,000/mm³: 10 mg twice daily.

Platelets 50,000/mm³ to <100,000/mm³: 5 mg once daily.

Polycythemia vera: Initial dose: 5 mg twice daily

Patients stabilized on ruxolitinib ≥10 mg twice daily: Reduce dose by 50% (rounded up to the closest available tablet strength).

Patients stabilized on ruxolitinib 5 mg twice daily: Reduce dose to 5 mg once daily.

Patients stabilized on ruxolitinib 5 mg once daily: Avoid strong CYP3A4 inhibitors or fluconazole or interrupt treatment for the duration of strong CYP3A4 inhibitor or fluconazole use.

Monitor closely and further adjust dose based on safety and efficacy.

Dosage adjustment with concomitant strong CYP3A4 inhibitors or concomitant moderate CYP2C9 and CYP3A4 inhibitors (Canadian labeling): Initial dose: 10 mg twice daily (~50% of the dose, rounded to the closest available strength); monitor hematologic parameters more frequently (eg, twice weekly) and titrate dose based on safety and efficacy. Avoid concomitant use if platelets <100,000/mm³. If used concomitantly with fluconazole, do not exceed fluconazole 200 mg/day.

Renal Impairment

U.S. labeling:

Myelofibrosis:

CrCl 15 to 59 mL/minute and platelets >150,000/mm³: No dosage adjustment is necessary.

CrCl 15 to 59 mL/minute and platelets 100,000 to 150,000/mm³: Initial dose: 10 mg twice daily; additional dose adjustments should be made with careful monitoring.

CrCl 15 to 59 mL/minute and platelets 50,000 to <100,000/mm³: Initial dose: 5 mg once daily; additional dose adjustments should be made with careful monitoring.

CrCl 15 to 59 mL/minute and platelets <50,000/mm³: Avoid use.

End-stage renal disease (ESRD) on dialysis and platelets 100,000 to 200,000/mm³: Initial dose: 15 mg once after dialysis; administer subsequent doses after dialysis on dialysis days. Additional dose adjustments should be made with frequent monitoring.

ESRD on dialysis and platelets >200,000/mm³: Initial dose: 20 mg once after dialysis; administer subsequent doses after dialysis on dialysis days. Additional dose adjustments should be made with frequent monitoring.

ESRD not requiring dialysis: Avoid use.

Polycythemia vera:

CrCl 15 to 59 mL/minute and any platelet count: Initial: 5 mg twice daily. Additional dose adjustments should be made with frequent monitoring.

End-stage renal disease (ESRD) on dialysis: Initial dose: 10 mg once after dialysis; additional dose adjustments should be made with careful monitoring

ESRD not requiring dialysis: Avoid use.

Canadian labeling:

CrCl <50 mL/minute and platelets ≥100,000/mm³: Initial dose: 10 mg twice daily; additional dose adjustments should be made with careful monitoring.

CrCl <50 mL/minute and platelets <100,000/mm³: Avoid use

ESRD on dialysis and platelets 100,000 to 200,000/mm³: Initial dose: 15 mg; administer subsequent doses after dialysis on dialysis days. Additional dose adjustments should be made with careful monitoring.

ESRD on dialysis and platelets >200,000/mm³: Initial dose: 20 mg; administer subsequent doses after dialysis on dialysis days. Additional dose adjustments should be made with careful monitoring.

Hepatic Impairment

U.S. labeling:

Myelofibrosis:

Mild-to-severe impairment (Child-Pugh class A, B, or C) and platelets >150,000/mm³: No dosage adjustment is necessary.

Mild-to-severe impairment (Child-Pugh class A, B, or C) and platelets 100,000 to 150,000/mm³: Initial dose: 10 mg twice daily; additional dose adjustments should be made with careful monitoring.

Mild-to-severe impairment (Child-Pugh class A, B, or C) and platelets 50,000 to <100,000/mm³: Initial dose: 5 mg once daily; additional dose adjustments should be made with careful monitoring.

Mild-to-severe impairment (Child-Pugh class A, B, or C) and platelets <50,000/mm³: Avoid use.

Polycythemia vera: Mild-to-severe impairment (Child-Pugh class A, B, or C) and any platelet count: Initial dose: 5 mg twice daily; additional dose adjustments should be made with careful monitoring.

Canadian labeling:

Hepatic impairment and platelets ≥100,000/mm³: Initial dose: 10 mg twice daily; additional dose adjustments should be made with careful monitoring.

Hepatic impairment and platelets <100,000/mm³: Avoid use.

Adjustment for Toxicity

Myelofibrosis:

Dosage modification for treatment interruption:

U.S. labeling:

If baseline platelet count ≥100,000/mm³ prior to initial treatment with ruxolitinib and:

Platelets <50,000/mm³ and ANC <500/mm³: Interrupt treatment; upon platelet recovery (to ≥50,000/mm³) or ANC recovery (to ≥750/mm³), dosing may be restarted or increased based on the following platelet or ANC levels

Platelets ≥125,000/mm³: Dose should be at least 5 mg twice daily below the dose at treatment interruption, up to a maximum of 20 mg twice daily

Platelets 100,000 to <125,000/mm³: Dose should be at least 5 mg twice daily below the dose at treatment interruption, up to a maximum of 15 mg twice daily

Platelets 75,000 to <100,000/mm³: Dose should be at least 5 mg twice daily below the dose at treatment interruption, up to a maximum of 10 mg twice daily for at least 2 weeks; may increase to 15 mg twice daily if stable

Platelets 50,000 to <75,000/mm³: 5 mg twice daily for at least 2 weeks; may increase to 10 mg twice daily if stable

Platelets <50,000/mm³: Continue to withhold treatment

ANC ≥750/mm³: Resume at 5 mg once daily or 5 mg twice daily below the largest dose in the week prior to treatment interruption, whichever is greater

Note: Long-term maintenance at 5 mg twice daily has not demonstrated responses; limit use of the dose level to patients where the benefits outweigh risks

If baseline platelet count 50,000 to <100,000/mm³ prior to initial treatment with ruxolitinib and:

Platelets <25,000/mm³ and ANC <500/mm³: Interrupt treatment; upon platelet recovery (to ≥35,000/mm³) or ANC recovery (to ≥750/mm³), resume at 5 mg once daily or 5 mg twice daily below the largest dose in the week prior to treatment interruption, whichever is greater

Note: Long-term maintenance at 5 mg twice daily has not demonstrated responses; limit use of the dose level to patients where the benefits outweigh risks

Canadian labeling: Platelets <50,000/mm³ or ANC <500 mm³: Interrupt treatment; upon recovery of platelets to ≥50,000/mm³ or ANC to ≥500/mm³, dosing may be restarted at 5 mg twice daily and then gradually titrated based on blood cell counts.

Dosage reduction for thrombocytopenia in patients with baseline platelet count ≥100,000/mm³ prior to initial treatment with ruxolitinib:

Platelet Count	Dose at Time of Thrombocytopenia				
	25 mg twice/day	20 mg twice/day	15 mg twice/day	10 mg twice/day	5 mg twice/day
	New Dose	New Dose	New Dose	New Dose	New Dose
100,000 to <125,000/mm³	20 mg twice/day	15 mg twice/day	No change	No change	No change
75,000 to <100,000/mm³	10 mg twice/day	10 mg twice/day	10 mg twice/day	No change	No change
50,000 to <75,000/mm³	5 mg twice/day	5 mg twice/day	5 mg twice/day	5 mg twice/day	No change
<50,000/mm³	Hold dose	Hold dose	Hold dose	Hold dose	Hold dose

Note: Long-term maintenance at 5 mg twice daily has not demonstrated responses; limit use of the dose level to patients where the benefits outweigh risks

Dosage reduction for thrombocytopenia in patients with baseline platelet 50,000 to <100,000/mm³ prior to initial treatment with ruxolitinib:

Platelets 25,000 to <35,000/mm³ **and** platelet count decreased <20% during prior 4 weeks:

If current daily dose >5 mg: Reduce dose by 5 mg once daily

If current dose 5 mg once daily: Continue 5 mg once daily

Platelets 25,000 to <35,000/mm³ **and** platelet count decreased ≥20% during prior four weeks:

If current daily dose >10 mg: Reduce dose by 5 mg twice daily

If current dose 5 mg twice daily: Reduce dose to 5 mg once daily

If current dose 5 mg once daily: Continue 5 mg once daily

Platelets <25,000 mm³: Continue to withhold treatment

Note: Long-term maintenance at 5 mg twice daily has not demonstrated responses; limit use of the dose level to patients where the benefits outweigh risks

Polycythemia vera:

Hematologic toxicity:

Hemoglobin ≥12 g/dL AND platelets ≥100,000/mm³: No dosage adjustment necessary.

Hemoglobin 10 to <12 g/dL AND platelets 75,000 to <100,000/mm³: Consider dosage adjustment to avoid dose interruptions due to anemia and thrombocytopenia.

Hemoglobin 8 to <10 g/dL OR platelets 50,000 to <75,000/mm³: Reduce dose by 5 mg twice daily; for patients currently receiving 5 mg twice daily, reduce dose to 5 mg once daily.

Hemoglobin <8 g/dL OR platelets <50,000/mm³ OR ANC <1,000/mm³: Interrupt dosing.

Dosage reduction following treatment interruption (use the most severe category of hemoglobin, platelets or ANC to determine reinitiation dose):

Hemoglobin <8 g/dL OR platelets <50,000/mm³ OR ANC <1,000/mm³: Continue to hold.

Hemoglobin 8 to <10 g/dL OR platelets 50,000 to <75,000/mm³ OR ANC 1,000 to <1,500/mm³: Restart at a maximum of 5 mg twice daily (continue treatment for at least 2 weeks, if stable, then may increase dose by 5 mg twice daily) or no more than 5 mg twice daily less than the dose that resulted in dose interruption

Hemoglobin 10 to <12 g/dL OR platelets 75,000 to <100,000/mm³ OR ANC 1,500 to <2,000/mm³: Restart at a maximum of 10 mg twice daily (continue treatment for at least 2 weeks, if stable, then may increase dose by 5 mg twice daily) or no more than 5 mg twice daily less than the dose that resulted in dose interruption

Hemoglobin ≥12 g/dL OR platelets ≥100,000/mm³ OR ANC ≥2,000/mm³: Restart at a maximum of 15 mg twice daily (continue treatment for at least 2 weeks, if stable, then may increase dose by 5 mg twice daily) or no more than 5 mg twice daily less than the dose that resulted in dose interruption

Note: If dose interruption was required while receiving 5 mg twice daily, may restart at 5 mg twice daily or 5 mg once daily (but not higher) once hemoglobin is ≥10 g/dL, platelets are ≥75,000/mm³, and ANC is ≥1,500/mm³

Dose management after restarting treatment: After restarting following a dose interruption, the dose may be titrated, although the maximum total daily dose should not exceed 5 mg less than the dose resulting in the interruption (unless dose interruption following phlebotomy-associated anemia, in which case the maximum total daily dose is not limited).

Dietary Considerations Avoid grapefruit juice (may increase the effects of ruxolitinib).

Administration Oral:

U.S. labeling: May be administered orally with or without food. If a dose is missed, return to the usual dosing schedule and do **not** administer an additional dose.

If unable to ingest tablets, may administer through a nasogastric (NG) tube (≥8 Fr): Suspend 1 tablet in ~40 mL water and stir for ~10 minutes and administer (within 6 hours after dispersion) with appropriate syringe; rinse NG tube with ~75 mL water (effect of enteral tube feeding on ruxolitinib exposure has not been evaluated)

Canadian labeling: May be administered orally with or without food. Tablet should be swallowed whole and not be cut, broken, dissolved, crushed, or chewed. If a dose is missed, return to the usual dosing schedule and do not administer an additional dose.

Hazardous agent; use appropriate precautions for handling and disposal (meets NIOSH 2014 criteria). NIOSH recommends single gloving for administration of intact tablets (NIOSH 2014).

Monitoring Parameters CBC (baseline, every 2 to 4 weeks until dose stabilized, then as clinically indicated), renal function, hepatic function. Perform periodic skin examinations monitor for signs/symptoms of infection. Additional Canadian labeling recommendations include tuberculin skin test and/or interferon-gamma release assay prior to initiation, ECG at baseline and then periodically during therapy, and heart rate and blood pressure during therapy.

Dosage Forms Excipient information presented when available (limited, particularly for generics); consult specific product labeling.

Tablet, Oral:

Jakafi: 5 mg, 10 mg, 15 mg, 20 mg, 25 mg

Extemporaneous Preparations Hazardous agent; use appropriate precautions for handling and disposal (meets NIOSH 2014 criteria). When compounding an oral liquid or suspension, NIOSH recommends double gloving, a protective gown, and preparation in a controlled device; if not prepared in a controlled device, respiratory and eye protection as well as ventilated engineering controls are recommended (NIOSH 2014).

A suspension for nasogastric administration may be prepared with tablets. Place one tablet into ~40 mL water; stir for approximately 10 minutes. Administer within 6 hour after preparation.

Jakafi (ruxolitinib) [prescribing information]. Wilmington, DE: Incyte Corporation; December 2014.

Sacrosidase (sak ROE si dase)

Brand Names: US Sucraid

Brand Names: Canada Sucraid®

Pharmacologic Category Enzyme, Gastrointestinal

Use Oral replacement therapy in sucrase deficiency, as seen in congenital sucrase-isomaltase deficiency (CSID)

Prescribing and Access Restrictions Sucraid® is not available in retail pharmacies or via mail-order pharmacies. To obtain the product, please refer to http://www.sucraid.net/how-to-order-sucraid or call 1-866-740-2743.

Dosing

Adult & Geriatric Congenital sucrase-isomaltase deficiency (CSID): Oral: 17,000 units (2 mL) per meal or snack. Doses should be diluted with 2-4 oz of cold or room temperature water, milk, or formula. Approximately one-half of the dose should be taken before and the remainder of a dose taken during each meal or snack.

Pediatric Congenital sucrase-isomaltase deficiency (CSID):

Infants ≥5 months and Children ≤15 kg: Oral: 8500 units (1 mL) per meal or snack. Doses should be diluted with 2-4 oz of cold or room temperature water, milk, or formula. Approximately one-half of the dose should be taken before and the remainder of a dose taken during each meal or snack.

Children >15 kg and Adolescents: Refer to adult dosing.

Renal Impairment No dosage adjustment provided in manufacturer's labeling.

Hepatic Impairment No dosage adjustment provided in manufacturer's labeling.

Additional Information Complete prescribing information should be consulted for additional detail.

Dosage Forms Excipient information presented when available (limited, particularly for generics); consult specific product labeling.

Solution, Oral:

Sucraid: 8500 units/mL (118 mL) [contains papain]

Sacubitril and Valsartan (sak UE bi tril & val SAR tan)

Brand Names: US Entresto

Brand Names: Canada Entresto

Index Terms LCZ696; Valsartan and Sacubitril

Pharmacologic Category Angiotensin II Receptor Blocker; Neprilysin Inhibitor

Use

US labeling:

Heart failure: Reduce the risk of cardiovascular death and hospitalization for heart failure in patients with chronic heart failure (NYHA Class II-IV) and reduced ejection fraction; usually administered in conjunction with other heart failure therapies, in place of an angiotensin-converting enzyme (ACE) inhibitor or other angiotensin II receptor blocker (ARB)

Note: Prior to enrollment in the PARADIGM-HF clinical trial, patients were already receiving a stable dose of an ACE inhibitor or ARB at daily doses equivalent to at least 10 mg of enalapril (McMurray 2014).

Canadian labeling:

Heart failure: Reduce the risk of cardiovascular death and hospitalization for heart failure in patients with chronic heart failure (NYHA Class II or III) and reduced ejection fraction; should be administered in conjunction with other heart failure therapies, in place of an angiotensin-converting enzyme (ACE) inhibitor or other angiotensin II receptor blocker (ARB).

Pregnancy Considerations [US Boxed Warning]: Drugs that act on the renin-angiotensin system can cause injury and death to the developing fetus. Discontinue as soon as possible once pregnancy is detected. Refer to the Valsartan monograph for additional information.

Breast-Feeding Considerations It is not known if sacubitril or valsartan are found in breast milk. Due to the potential for serious adverse reactions in the nursing infant, breast feeding is not recommended by the manufacturer.

Contraindications

Hypersensitivity to sacubitril, valsartan, or any component of the formulation; history of angioedema related to previous ACE inhibitor or ARB therapy; concomitant use or use within 36 hours of ACE inhibitors; concomitant use of aliskiren in patients with diabetes

Canadian labeling: Additional contraindications (not in US labeling): Recent symptomatic hypotension prior to initiation of treatment with sacubitril/valsartan; history of hereditary or idiopathic angioedema; concomitant use of aliskiren in patients with moderate to severe renal impairment (eGFR <60 mL/minute/1.73 m^2); pregnancy.

Warnings/Precautions [US Boxed Warning]: Drugs that act on the renin-angiotensin system can cause injury and death to the developing fetus. Discontinue as soon as possible once pregnancy is detected. Angioedema has been reported rarely with some

angiotensin II receptor antagonists (ARBs) and may occur at any time during treatment (especially following first dose). It may involve the head and neck (potentially compromising airway) or the intestine (presenting with abdominal pain). Patients with idiopathic or hereditary angioedema or previous angioedema associated with ACE-inhibitor therapy may be at an increased risk. Prolonged frequent monitoring may be required, especially if tongue, glottis, or larynx are involved, as they are associated with airway obstruction. Patients with a history of airway surgery may have a higher risk of airway obstruction. Discontinue therapy immediately if angioedema occurs. Aggressive early management is critical. Intramuscular (IM) administration of epinephrine may be necessary. Do not readminister to patients who have had angioedema with ARBs. Hyperkalemia may occur; risk factors include renal dysfunction, diabetes mellitus, hypoaldosteronism, high potassium diet, concomitant use of aliskiren (contraindicated), potassium-sparing diuretics, potassium supplements, and/or potassium containing salts. Use cautiously, if at all, with these agents and monitor potassium closely. During the initiation of therapy, hypotension may occur, particularly in patients with heart failure or post-MI patients. Symptomatic hypotension may occur upon initiation in patients who are salt- or volume-depleted (eg, those treated with high-dose diuretics); correct volume depletion prior to administration or initiate at a lower dose. This transient hypotensive response is not a contraindication to further treatment with sacubitril and valsartan. May be associated with deterioration of renal function and/or increases in serum creatinine, particularly in patients with low renal blood flow (eg, renal artery stenosis, heart failure) whose glomerular filtration rate (GFR) is dependent on efferent arteriolar vasoconstriction by angiotensin II; deterioration may result in oliguria, acute renal failure, and progressive azotemia. Small increases in serum creatinine may occur following initiation; consider discontinuation only in patients with progressive and/or significant deterioration in renal function. Use with caution in patients with significant aortic/mitral stenosis, and patients with unstented unilateral/bilateral renal artery stenosis. When unstented bilateral renal artery stenosis is present, use is generally avoided due to the elevated risk of deterioration in renal function unless possible benefits outweigh risks. Use with caution in preexisting renal insufficiency; reduce initial dosage for severe impairment (eGFR <30 mL/minute/1.73 m^2). The Canadian labeling recommends avoiding use in patients with eGFR <30 mL/minute/1.73 m^2. Use with caution and reduce dosage in patients with moderate hepatic impairment; use is not recommended in patients with severe hepatic impairment. Use caution when initiating in heart failure; may need to adjust dose, and/or concurrent diuretic therapy, because of valsartan-induced hypotension. Careful monitoring of BUN, serum creatinine, and potassium is necessary especially if preexisting renal disease exists. In patients on chronic angiotensin receptor blocker (ARB) therapy, intraoperative hypotension may occur with induction and maintenance of general anesthesia; however, discontinuation of therapy prior to surgery is controversial. If continued preoperatively, avoidance of hypotensive agents during surgery is prudent (Hillis 2011). Potentially significant drug-drug interactions may exist, requiring dose or frequency adjustment, additional monitoring, and/or selection of alternative therapy.

Adverse Reactions

>10%

Cardiovascular: Hypotension (18%)

Endocrine & metabolic: Hyperkalemia (4% to 16%)

Renal: Increased (>50% rise) serum creatinine (1% to 16%)

1% to 10%:

Cardiovascular: Orthostatic hypotension (2%)

Central nervous system: Dizziness (6%), falling (2%)

Hematologic & oncologic: Decreased hematocrit (≤5%), decreased hemoglobin (≤5%)

Hypersensitivity: Angioedema (black patients: 2%; others: <1%)

Renal: Renal failure (5%)

Respiratory: Cough (9%)

Drug Interactions

Metabolism/Transport Effects Refer to individual components.

Avoid Concomitant Use

Avoid concomitant use of Sacubitril and Valsartan with any of the following: ACE Inhibitors

Increased Effect/Toxicity

Sacubitril and Valsartan may increase the levels/effects of: Amifostine; Antipsychotic Agents (Second Generation [Atypical]); Ciprofloxacin (Systemic); CycloSPORINE (Systemic); Drospirenone; DULoxetine; HMG-CoA Reductase Inhibitors; Hydrochlorothiazide; Hypotension-Associated Agents; Levodopa; Lithium; Nonsteroidal Anti-Inflammatory Agents; Potassium-Sparing Diuretics; Sodium Phosphates

The levels/effects of Sacubitril and Valsartan may be increased by: ACE Inhibitors; Alfuzosin; Aliskiren; Barbiturates; Blood Pressure Lowering Agents; Brimonidine (Topical); Canagliflozin; Dapoxetine; Diazoxide; Eltrombopag; Eplerenone; Heparin; Heparin (Low Molecular Weight); Herbs (Hypotensive Properties); Hydrochlorothiazide; Molsidomine; Nicorandil; Obinutuzumab; Pentoxifylline; Phosphodiesterase 5 Inhibitors; Potassium Salts; Prostacyclin Analogues; Teriflunomide; Tolvaptan; Trimethoprim

Decreased Effect

The levels/effects of Sacubitril and Valsartan may be decreased by: Amphetamines; Herbs (Hypertensive Properties); Methylphenidate; Nonsteroidal Anti-Inflammatory Agents; Yohimbine

Storage/Stability Store at 25°C (77°F); excursions permitted between 15°C and 30°C (59°F and 86°F). Protect from moisture.

Mechanism of Action

Sacubitril: Prodrug that inhibits neprilysin (neutral endopeptidase [NEP]) through the active metabolite LBQ657, leading to increased levels of peptides, including natriuretic peptides.

Valsartan: Produces direct antagonism of the angiotensin II (AT2) receptors. Displaces angiotensin II from the AT1 receptor; antagonizes AT1-induced vasoconstriction, aldosterone release, catecholamine release, arginine vasopressin release, water intake, and hypertrophic responses.

Pharmacodynamics/Kinetics

Distribution: V_d: Sacubitril: 103 L; Valsartan: 75 L

Protein binding: 94% to 97%

Metabolism:

Sacubitril: Converted to active metabolite LBQ657 by esterases; LBQ657 is not further metabolized to a significant extent

Valsartan: Minimally metabolized (~20%; <10% as a hydroxyl metabolite)

Bioavailability: Sacubitril: >60%

Half-life elimination: Sacubitril: 1.4 hours; LBQ657: 11.5 hours; Valsartan: 9.9 hours

Time to peak: Sacubitril: 0.5 hours; LBQ657: 2 hours; Valsartan: 1.5 hours

Excretion:

Sacubitril: Urine (52% to 68%, primarily as LBQ657); feces (37% to 48%, primarily as LBQ657)

Valsartan: Urine (~13%, parent drug and metabolites); feces (86%, parent drug and metabolites)

Dosing

Adult

US labeling: Note: Entresto contains sacubitril (24 mg, 49 mg, or 97 mg) and valsartan (26 mg, 51 mg, or 103 mg). Use caution when prescribing since dosing in clinical trials was based on the total amount of both components (ie, 24/26 mg, 49/51 mg and 97/103 mg were referred to as 50 mg, 100 mg, and 200 mg, respectively). To reduce the risk of errors, include the doses of both ingredients (eg, Entresto 24/26 mg) when prescribing Entresto. The valsartan in Entresto is more bioavailable than the valsartan in other marketed tablet formulations; valsartan 26 mg, 51 mg, and 103 mg in Entresto is equivalent to valsartan 40 mg, 80 mg, and 160 mg in other marketed tablet formulations, respectively.

Heart failure: Oral: *Patients previously taking >10 mg/day of enalapril or >160 mg/day of valsartan or equivalent dose of another ACE inhibitor or ARB:* Initial: Sacubitril 49 mg and valsartan 51 mg twice daily. Double the dose as tolerated after 2 to 4 weeks to the target maintenance dose of sacubitril 97 mg and valsartan 103 mg twice daily. **Note:** Concomitant use of an ACE inhibitor is contraindicated; allow a 36 hour washout period when switching from or to an ACE inhibitor.

Patients previously taking low doses of an ACE inhibitor (≤10 mg/day of enalapril or an equivalent dose of another ACE inhibitor)or ARB (≤160 mg/day of valsartan or an equivalent dose of another ARB): Initial: Sacubitril 24 mg and valsartan 26 mg twice daily. Double the dose as tolerated every 2 to 4 weeks to the target maintenance dose of sacubitril 97 mg and valsartan 103 mg twice daily.

*Patients **not** currently taking an ACE inhibitor or an ARB:* Initial: Sacubitril 24 mg and valsartan 26 mg twice daily. Double the dose as tolerated every 2 to 4 weeks to the target maintenance dose of sacubitril 97 mg and valsartan 103 mg twice daily.

Canadian labeling: **Note:** Use caution when prescribing since dosing in clinical trials was based on the total amount of both components (ie, 48.6/51.4 mg and 97.2/102.8 mg were referred to as 100 mg, and 200 mg respectively). To reduce the risk of errors, include the doses of both ingredients when prescribing Entresto. The valsartan in Entresto is more bioavailable than the valsartan in other marketed tablet formulations; valsartan 26 mg, 51 mg, and 103 mg in Entresto is equivalent to valsartan 40 mg, 80 mg, and 160 mg in other marketed tablet formulations, respectively.

Heart failure: Adults: Oral: Initial: Sacubitril 48.6 mg and valsartan 51.4 mg twice daily. Increase the dose as tolerated after 2 to 4 weeks to the target maintenance dose of sacubitril 97.2 mg and valsartan 102.8 mg twice daily. If tolerability becomes an issue, consider temporary down-titration or interruption of therapy. **Note:** Concomitant use of an ACE inhibitor is contraindicated; allow a 36 hour washout period when switching from or to an ACE inhibitor.

Patients with risk factors for hypotension or with low systolic blood pressure: Initial: Consider sacubitril 24.3 mg and valsartan 25.7 mg twice daily. Increase the dose as tolerated every 2 to 4 weeks to the target maintenance dose of sacubitril 97.2 mg and valsartan 102.8 mg twice daily.

Geriatric *US labeling:* Refer to adult dosing.

Canadian labeling:

<75 years: Refer to adult dosing.

≥75 years: Initial: Consider sacubitril 24.3 mg and valsartan 25.7 mg twice daily. Increase the dose as tolerated every 2 to 4 weeks to the target maintenance dose of sacubitril 97.3 mg and valsartan 102.8 mg twice daily.

Renal Impairment

US labeling:

Estimated glomerular filtration rate (eGFR) ≥30 mL/minute/1.73 m^2: No dosage adjustment necessary.

eGFR <30 mL/minute/1.73 m^2: Initial: Sacubitril 24 mg and valsartan 26 mg twice daily

Canadian labeling:

Estimated glomerular filtration rate (eGFR) ≥30 mL/minute/1.73 m^2: No dosage adjustment necessary.

eGFR <30 mL/minute/1.73 m^2: Use is not recommended.

Hepatic Impairment

US labeling:

Mild impairment (Child-Pugh class A): No dosage adjustment necessary.

Moderate impairment (Child-Pugh class B): Initial: Sacubitril 24 mg and valsartan 26 mg twice daily

Severe impairment (Child-Pugh class C): Use not recommended (has not been studied).

Canadian labeling:

Mild impairment (Child-Pugh class A): No dosage adjustment necessary.

Moderate impairment (Child-Pugh class B): Initial: Sacubitril 24.3 mg and valsartan 25.7 mg twice daily.

Severe impairment (Child-Pugh class C): Use is not recommended (has not been studied).

Administration Oral: Administer with or without food.

Monitoring Parameters Baseline and periodic serum potassium, renal function, BP.

2013 ACCF/AHA Heart Failure guideline recommendations: Within 1 to 2 weeks after initiation of an ARB, reassess blood pressure (including postural blood pressure changes), renal function, and serum potassium; follow closely after dose changes. Patients with systolic blood pressure <80 mm Hg, low serum sodium, diabetes mellitus, and impaired renal function should be closely monitored (Yancy, 2013). **Note:** Sacubitril/valsartan was not available for use at the time of the publication of these guidelines.

Dosage Forms Excipient information presented when available (limited, particularly for generics); consult specific product labeling.

Tablet, Oral:

Entresto: Sacubitril 24 mg and valsartan 26 mg, Sacubitril 49 mg and valsartan 51 mg, Sacubitril 97 mg and valsartan 103 mg

Dosage Forms: Canada Excipient information presented when available (limited, particularly for generics); consult specific product labeling.

Tablet, Oral:

Entresto: Sacubitril 24.3 mg and valsartan 25.7 mg, Sacubitril 48.6 mg and valsartan 51.4 mg, Sacubitril 97.2 mg and valsartan 102.8 mg

◆ Safetussin® CD [OTC] *see* Dextromethorphan and Phenylephrine *on page 535*

◆ Safe Tussin DM [OTC] *see* Guaifenesin and Dextromethorphan *on page 861*

◆ Safe Wash [OTC] *see* Sodium Chloride *on page 1671*

◆ Safyral *see* Ethinyl Estradiol, Drospirenone, and Levomefolate *on page 712*

◆ SAHA *see* Vorinostat *on page 1913*

◆ Saizen *see* Somatropin *on page 1686*

◆ Saizen Click.Easy *see* Somatropin *on page 1686*

◆ Salagen *see* Pilocarpine (Systemic) *on page 1452*

◆ Salagen® (Can) *see* Pilocarpine (Systemic) *on page 1452*

◆ Salazopyrin (Can) *see* SulfaSALAzine *on page 1714*

◆ Salazopyrin En-Tabs (Can) *see* SulfaSALAzine *on page 1714*

◆ Salbutamol *see* Albuterol *on page 57*

◆ Salbutamol and Ipratropium *see* Ipratropium and Albuterol *on page 978*

◆ Salbutamol HFA (Can) *see* Albuterol *on page 57*

◆ Salbutamol Sulphate *see* Albuterol *on page 57*

◆ Salcatonin *see* Calcitonin *on page 282*

◆ Salicylazosulfapyridine *see* SulfaSALAzine *on page 1714*

◆ Salicylsalicylic Acid *see* Salsalate *on page 1634*

◆ Saline *see* Sodium Chloride *on page 1671*

◆ Saline Flush ZR *see* Sodium Chloride *on page 1671*

◆ Saline Mist Spray [OTC] *see* Sodium Chloride *on page 1671*

◆ Saljet [OTC] *see* Sodium Chloride *on page 1671*

◆ Saljet Rinse [OTC] *see* Sodium Chloride *on page 1671*

◆ Salk Vaccine *see* Poliovirus Vaccine (Inactivated) *on page 1465*

Salmeterol (sal ME te role)

Brand Names: US Serevent Diskus

Brand Names: Canada Serevent Diskhaler Disk; Serevent Diskus

Index Terms Salmeterol Xinafoate

Pharmacologic Category Beta$_2$ Agonist; Beta$_2$-Adrenergic Agonist, Long-Acting

Use

Asthma/Bronchospasm: Treatment of asthma and the prevention of bronchospasm (only as concomitant therapy with a long-term asthma control medication, such as an inhaled corticosteroid), in patients 4 years and older with reversible obstructive airway disease, including patients with symptoms of nocturnal asthma.

Chronic obstructive pulmonary disease: Maintenance treatment of bronchospasm associated with chronic obstructive pulmonary disease (COPD) (including emphysema and chronic bronchitis).

Exercise-induced bronchospasm: Prevention of exercise-induced bronchospasm (EIB) in patients 4 years and older (monotherapy may be indicated in patients without persistent asthma).

Limitations of use: Salmeterol is not indicated for the relief of acute bronchospasm.

Pregnancy Considerations Adverse events were observed in some animal reproduction studies. Beta-agonists have the potential to affect uterine contractility if administered during labor.

Uncontrolled asthma is associated with adverse events on pregnancy (increased risk of perinatal mortality, preeclampsia, preterm birth, low birth weight infants). Although data related to its use in pregnancy is limited, salmeterol may be used when a long-acting beta agonist is needed to treat moderate persistent or severe persistent asthma in pregnant women (NAEPP, 2005).

Breast-Feeding Considerations It is not known if salmeterol is excreted into breast milk. The manufacturer recommends that caution be exercised when administering salmeterol to nursing women. The use of beta$_2$-receptor agonists are not considered a contraindication to breast-feeding (NAEPP, 2005).

Medication Guide Available Yes

Contraindications

Hypersensitivity to salmeterol or any component of the formulation (milk proteins); monotherapy in the treatment of asthma (ie, use without a concomitant long-term asthma control medication, such as an inhaled corticosteroid); treatment of status asthmaticus or other acute episodes of asthma or COPD

Canadian labeling: Additional contraindications (not in U.S. labeling): Presence of tachyarrhythmias

Documentation of allergenic cross-reactivity for sympatho-mimetics is limited. However, because of similarities in chemical structure and/or pharmacologic actions, the possibility of cross-sensitivity cannot be ruled out with certainty.

Warnings/Precautions Asthma treatment: **[U.S. Boxed Warning]: Long-acting beta₂-agonists (LABAs) increase the risk of asthma-related deaths. Salmeterol should only be used in asthma patients as adjuvant therapy in patients who are currently receiving but are not adequately controlled on a long-term asthma control medication (ie, an inhaled corticosteroid).** Mono-therapy with an LABA is contraindicated in the treatment of asthma. In a large, randomized, placebo-controlled U.S. clinical trial (SMART, 2006), salmeterol was associated with an increase in asthma-related deaths (when added to usual asthma therapy); risk is considered a class effect among all LABAs. Data are not available to determine if the addition of an inhaled corticosteroid lessens this increased risk of death associated with LABA use. Assess patients at regular intervals once asthma control is main-tained on combination therapy to determine if step-down therapy is appropriate and the LABA can be discontinued (without loss of asthma control), and the patient can be maintained on an inhaled corticosteroid. LABAs are not appropriate in patients whose asthma is adequately con-trolled on low- or medium-dose inhaled corticosteroids. Do **not** use for acute bronchospasm. Short-acting beta₂-ago-nist (eg, albuterol) should be used for acute symptoms and symptoms occurring between treatments. Do **not** initiate in patients with significantly worsening or acutely deteriorat-ing asthma; reports of severe (sometimes fatal) respiratory events have been reported when salmeterol has been initiated in this situation. Corticosteroids should not be stopped or reduced when salmeterol is initiated. During initiation, watch for signs of worsening asthma. Patients must be instructed to use short-acting beta₂-agonists (eg, albuterol) for acute asthmatic or COPD symptoms and to seek medical attention in cases where acute symptoms are not relieved or a previous level of response is dimin-ished. The need to increase frequency of use of short-acting beta₂-agonist may indicate deterioration of asthma, and treatment must not be delayed. Because LABAs may disguise poorly controlled persistent asthma, frequent or chronic use of LABAs for exercise-induced bronchospasm is discouraged by the NIH Asthma Guidelines (NIH, 2007). Salmeterol should not be used more than twice daily; do not use with other long-acting beta₂-agonists. **[U.S. Boxed Warning]: LABAs may increase the risk of asthma-related hospitalization in pediatric and adolescent patients.** In general, a combination product containing a LABA and an inhaled corticosteroid is preferred in patients <18 years of age to ensure compliance.

COPD treatment: Appropriate use: Do **not** use for acute episodes of COPD. Do **not** initiate in patients with signifi-cantly worsening or acutely deteriorating COPD. Data are not available to determine if LABA use increases the risk of death in patients with COPD. Canadian labeling suggest concurrent use of oral or inhaled corticosteroids may not be necessary in COPD because the role of inhaled cortico-steroids is less well established; concurrent use should be determined by the treating physician.

Use caution in patients with cardiovascular disease (eg, arrhythmia, coronary insufficiency, or hypertension), seiz-ure disorders, diabetes, hyperthyroidism, hepatic impair-ment, or hypokalemia. Beta-agonists may cause elevation in blood pressure, heart rate, CNS stimulation/excitation, increase serum glucose, decrease serum potassium, increase risk of arrhythmia, and electrocardiogram (ECG) changes, such as flattening of the T wave, prolongation of the QTc interval, and ST segment depression.

Immediate hypersensitivity reactions (urticaria, angioe-dema, rash, bronchospasm) bronchospasm, hypotension) including anaphylaxis have been reported. There have been reports of laryngeal spasm, irritation, swelling (stridor, choking) with use. Salmeterol should not be used more than twice daily; do not exceed recommended dose; do not use with other long-acting beta₂-agonists; serious adverse events have been associated with excessive use of inhaled sympathomimetics. Rarely, paradoxical broncho-spasm, which may be life threatening, may occur with use of inhaled bronchodilating agents; this should be distin-guished from inadequate response. Potentially significant drug-drug interactions may exist, requiring dose or fre-quency adjustment, additional monitoring, and/or selection of alternative therapy (consult drug interactions database for more detailed information). Powder for oral inhalation contains lactose; very rare anaphylactic reactions have been reported in patients with severe milk protein allergy.

Adverse Reactions

>10%:
Central nervous system: Headache (13% to 17%)
Neuromuscular & skeletal: Pain (1% to 12%)
1% to 10%:
Cardiovascular: Hypertension (4%), edema (1% to 3%), pallor
Central nervous system: Dizziness (4%), sleep disturb-ance (1% to 3%), fever (1% to 3%), anxiety (1% to 3%), migraine (1% to 3%)
Dermatologic: Rash (1% to 4%), contact dermatitis (1% to 3%), eczema (1% to 3%), urticaria (3%), photo-dermatitis (1% to 2%)
Endocrine & metabolic: Hyperglycemia (1% to 3%)
Gastrointestinal: Throat irritation (7%), nausea (1% to 3%), dyspepsia (1% to 3%), dental pain (1% to 3%), gastrointestinal infection (1% to 3%), oropharyngeal candidiasis (1% to 3%), xerostomia (1% to 3%)
Hepatic: Liver enzymes increased
Neuromuscular & skeletal: Muscular cramps/spasm (3%), articular rheumatism (1% to 3%), arthralgia (1% to 3%), joint pain (1% to 3%), muscular stiffness (1% to 3%), paresthesia (1% to 3%), rigidity (1% to 3%)
Ocular: Keratitis/conjunctivitis (1% to 3%)
Respiratory: Nasal congestion (4% to 9%), tracheitis/bronchitis (7%), pharyngitis (≤6%), cough (5%), influ-enza (5%), viral respiratory tract infection (5%), sinusitis (4% to 5%), rhinitis (4% to 5%), asthma (3% to 4%)
<1% (Limited to important or life-threatening): Abdominal pain, agitation, aggression, anaphylactic reaction (some in patients with severe milk allergy [Diskus®]), angioe-dema, aphonia, arrhythmia, atrial fibrillation, cataracts, chest congestion, chest tightness, choking, contusions, Cushing syndrome, Cushingoid features, depression, dysmenorrhea, dyspnea, earache, ecchymoses, edema (facial, oropharyngeal), eosinophilic conditions, glau-coma, growth velocity reduction in children/adolescents, hypercorticism, hypersensitivity reaction (immediate and delayed), hypokalemia, hypothyroidism, intraocular pres-sure increased, laryngeal spasm/irritation, irregular men-struation, myositis, oropharyngeal irritation, osteoporosis, pallor, paradoxical bronchospasm, paradoxical tracheitis, paranasal sinus pain, PID, QTc prolongation, restless-ness, stridor, supraventricular tachycardia, syncope, tremor, vaginal candidiasis, vaginitis, vulvovaginitis, rare cases of vasculitis (Churg-Strauss syndrome), ventricular tachycardia, weight gain

Drug Interactions

Metabolism/Transport Effects Substrate of CYP3A4 (major); **Note:** Assignment of Major/Minor substrate sta-tus based on clinically relevant drug interaction potential

Avoid Concomitant Use
Avoid concomitant use of Salmeterol with any of the following: Beta-Blockers (Nonselective); Conivaptan; CYP3A4 Inhibitors (Strong); Fusidic Acid (Systemic); Idelalisib; Iobenguane I 123; Long-Acting Beta2-Ago-nists; Loxapine; Telaprevir; Tipranavir

Increased Effect/Toxicity
Salmeterol may increase the levels/effects of: Atosiban; Doxofylline; Highest Risk QTc-Prolonging Agents; Long-Acting Beta2-Agonists; Loop Diuretics; Loxapine; Moder-ate Risk QTc-Prolonging Agents; Sympathomimetics; Thiazide Diuretics

The levels/effects of Salmeterol may be increased by: Aprepitant; AtoMOXetine; Cannabinoid-Containing Prod-ucts; Conivaptan; CYP3A4 Inhibitors (Moderate); CYP3A4 Inhibitors (Strong); Dasatinib; Fosaprepitant; Fusidic Acid (Systemic); Idelalisib; Ivacaftor; Linezolid; Luliconazole; MAO Inhibitors; Mifepristone; Netupitant; Osimertinib; Palbociclib; Simeprevir; Stiripentol; Tedi-zolid; Telaprevir; Tipranavir; Tricyclic Antidepressants

Decreased Effect
Salmeterol may decrease the levels/effects of: Ioben-guane I 123

The levels/effects of Salmeterol may be decreased by: Beta-Blockers (Beta1 Selective); Beta-Blockers (Nonse-lective); Betahistine; Osimertinib

Storage/Stability Store at 68°F and 77°F (20°C and 25°C); excursions are permitted between 59°F and 86°F (15°C and 30°C). Protect from direct heat or sunlight. Store Diskus in the unopened foil pouch and only open when ready for use; stable for 6 weeks after removal from foil pouch.

Mechanism of Action Relaxes bronchial smooth muscle by selective action on beta₂-receptors with little effect on heart rate; salmeterol acts locally in the lung.

Pharmacodynamics/Kinetics

Onset of action: Asthma: 30-48 minutes, COPD: 2 hours
Peak effect: Asthma: 3 hours, COPD: 2-5 hours
Duration: 12 hours
Absorption: Systemic: Inhalation: Undetectable to poor

Protein binding: 96%
Metabolism: Hepatic; hydroxylated via CYP3A4
Half-life elimination: 5.5 hours
Time to peak, serum: ~20 minutes
Excretion: Feces (60%); urine (25%)

Dosing

Adult & Geriatric Note: Do not use for the relief of acute bronchospasm.

Asthma/Bronchospasm (maintenance and prevention): Inhalation: One inhalation twice daily (~12 hours apart); maximum: 1 inhalation twice daily. **Note:** For asthma control, long acting beta$_2$-agonists (LABAs) should be used in combination with inhaled corticosteroids and not as monotherapy.

COPD (maintenance): Inhalation: One inhalation twice daily (~12 hours apart); maximum: 1 inhalation twice daily

Exercise-induced bronchospasm (prevention): Inhalation: One inhalation at least 30 minutes prior to exercise; additional doses should not be used for 12 hours; should not be used in individuals already receiving salmeterol twice daily. **Note:** Because LABAs may disguise poorly controlled persistent asthma, frequent or chronic use of LABAs for exercise-induced bronchospasm is discouraged by the Asthma Guidelines (NAEPP, 2007).

Pediatric Note: Do not use for the relief of acute bronchospasm.

Asthma/Bronchospasm (maintenance/prevention) and exercise-induced bronchospasm (prevention): Inhalation: Children ≥4 years and Adolescents: Refer to adult dosing.

Renal Impairment There are no dosage adjustments provided in the manufacturer's labeling.

Hepatic Impairment There are no dosage adjustments provided in the manufacturer's labeling (has not been studied). Use with caution.

Dietary Considerations Some products may contain lactose; very rare anaphylactic reactions have been reported in patients with severe milk protein allergy.

Administration For oral inhalation route only. Before inhaling the dose, breath out fully; do not exhale into the Diskus device; activate and use only in a level, horizontal position. Inhale quickly and deeply through the Diskus; hold breath for about 10 seconds or for as long as comfortable and exhale slowly. Do not use with a spacer device or wash mouthpiece; Diskus should be kept dry. Discard device 6 weeks after removal from foil pouch or when the dose counter reads "0" (whichever comes first).

Monitoring Parameters FEV$_1$, peak flow, and/or other pulmonary function tests; blood pressure, heart rate; CNS stimulation; serum glucose, serum potassium. Monitor for increased use of short-acting beta$_2$-agonist inhalers; may be marker of a deteriorating asthma condition.

Dosage Forms Excipient information presented when available (limited, particularly for generics); consult specific product labeling.
Aerosol Powder Breath Activated, Inhalation:
Serevent Diskus: 50 mcg/dose (28 ea, 60 ea) [contains lactose]

Dosage Forms: Canada Excipient information presented when available (limited, particularly for generics); consult specific product labeling.
Powder for oral inhalation:
Serevent Diskhaler Disk: Salmeterol xinafoate 50 mcg (60s) [delivers 50 mcg/inhalation; contains lactose]

Salsalate (SAL sa late)

Brand Names: US Disalcid
Index Terms Disalicylic Acid; Salicylsalicylic Acid
Pharmacologic Category Salicylate

Use Rheumatic disorders: Treatment of signs and symptoms of osteoarthritis, rheumatoid arthritis, and related rheumatic disorders

Dosing

Adult Rheumatic disorders: Oral: **Note:** Use the lowest effective dose for the shortest duration; after observing the response to initial therapy, adjust dose as needed. Usual dose: 3 g per day in 2 to 3 divided doses

Geriatric Refer to adult dosing. May require lower dosage.

Renal Impairment There are no dosage adjustments provided in the manufacturer's labeling. Use is not recommended in patients with advanced renal disease.

Hepatic Impairment There are no dosage adjustments provided in the manufacturer's labeling.

Additional Information Complete prescribing information should be consulted for additional detail.

Dosage Forms Excipient information presented when available (limited, particularly for generics); consult specific product labeling.
Tablet, Oral:
Disalcid: 500 mg, 750 mg
Generic: 500 mg, 750 mg

Sapropterin (sap roe TER in)

Brand Names: US Kuvan
Brand Names: Canada Kuvan
Index Terms 6R-BH4; Phenoptin; Sapropterin Dihydro-
chloride; Tetrahydrobiopterin
Pharmacologic Category Enzyme Cofactor
Use Hyperphenylalaninemia: To reduce blood phenylala-
nine (PHE) levels in patients with hyperphenylalaninemia
caused by tetrahydrobiopterin (BH4)-responsive phenyl-
ketonuria in conjunction with a PHE-restricted diet.
Dosing
Adult & Geriatric
Hyperphenylalaninemia: Oral:
Initial:
US labeling: 10 to 20 mg/kg once daily
Canadian labeling: 10 mg/kg once daily
Maintenance: Adjust dose after 1 month based on blood
phenylalanine levels (if phenylalanine levels do not
decrease from baseline after initiating 10 mg/kg,
increase dose to 20 mg/kg once daily); discontinue if
phenylalanine levels do not decrease after 1 month of
treatment at 20 mg/kg/day (nonresponder). Mainte-
nance range: 5 to 20 mg/kg once daily

Missed dose: A missed dose should be taken as soon as
possible, but 2 doses should not be taken on the
same day.
Pediatric
Hyperphenylalaninemia:
US labeling:
Infants and Children ≥1 month to 6 years: Initial:
10 mg/kg once daily; adjust after 1 month based on
blood phenylalanine levels (if phenylalanine levels
do not decrease from baseline after initiating
10 mg/kg, increase dose to 20 mg/kg once daily);
discontinue if phenylalanine levels do not decrease
after 1 month of treatment at 20 mg/kg/day (nonresponder). Maintenance range: 5 to 20 mg/kg once
daily
Children ≥7 years and Adolescents: Refer to adult
dosing.
Canadian labeling: Children ≥4 years and Adolescents:
Refer to adult dosing.
Renal Impairment There are no dosage adjustments
provided in manufacturer's labeling (has not been
studied). Use with caution.

Hepatic Impairment There are no dosage adjustments
provided in manufacturer's labeling (has not been
studied). Use with caution.
Additional Information Complete prescribing information
should be consulted for additional detail.
Dosage Forms Excipient information presented when
available (limited, particularly for generics); consult specific
product labeling.
Packet, Oral, as dihydrochloride:
Kuvan: 100 mg (1 ea, 30 ea); 500 mg (1 ea, 30 ea)
Tablet Soluble, Oral, as dihydrochloride:
Kuvan: 100 mg
Dosage Forms: Canada Refer to Dosage Forms. **Note:**
Powder (packet) for oral solution is not available in Can-
ada.

♦ Sapropterin Dihydrochloride *see* Sapropterin
on page 1636

Saquinavir (sa KWIN a veer)

Brand Names: US Invirase
Brand Names: Canada Invirase
Index Terms Fortovase; Saquinavir Mesylate; SQV
Pharmacologic Category Antiretroviral, Protease Inhib-
itor (Anti-HIV)
Use HIV-1 infection: Treatment of HIV-1 infection in adults
(>16 years); used in combination with ritonavir and other
antiretroviral agents
Medication Guide Available Yes
Dosing
Adult Note: ECG should be done prior to starting therapy;
do not initiate therapy if pretreatment QT interval >450
msec. Saquinavir should always be used with concomitant ritonavir.
HIV-1 infection: Oral: 1,000 mg twice daily given in
combination with ritonavir 100 mg twice daily. This
combination should be given together and within 2
hours after a full meal in combination with a nucleoside
analog. For patients already taking ritonavir 100 mg
twice daily as part of their antiretroviral regimen, no
additional ritonavir is needed.
Treatment-naive patients: Canadian labeling (not in US
labeling): Initial: Saquinavir 500 mg twice daily given
in combination with ritonavir 100 mg twice daily for 7
days. Maintenance: Saquinavir 1,000 mg twice daily
given in combination with ritonavir 100 mg twice daily.
Patients with recent exposure (without washout) to a
ritonavir or non-nucleoside reverse transcriptase
inhibitor based regimen may receive usual initial dosing (ie, saquinavir 1,000 mg twice daily in combination
with ritonavir 100 mg twice daily).
Geriatric Clinical studies did not include sufficient numbers of patients ≥65 years of age. Use caution due to
increased frequency of organ dysfunction.
Pediatric
HIV-1 infection: Oral:
Children ≥2 years and Adolescents <16 years (off-label
dosing) (HHS [pediatric] 2015):
5 kg to <15 kg: Saquinavir 50 mg/kg/dose (maximum
single dose: 1,000 mg) **plus** ritonavir 3 mg/kg/dose
twice daily
15 kg to <40 kg: Saquinavir 50 mg/kg/dose (maximum
single dose: 1,000 mg) **plus** ritonavir 2.5 mg/kg/dose
twice daily
≥40 kg: Saquinavir 1,000 mg **plus** ritonavir 100 mg
twice daily
Adolescents >16 years: Refer to adult dosing.
Renal Impairment No dosage adjustment necessary;
use with caution in severe renal impairment or ESRD.
Hepatic Impairment
Mild to moderate impairment (Child-Pugh classes A and
B): No dosage adjustment necessary.
Severe impairment (Child-Pugh class C): Use is contra-
indicated.
Additional Information Complete prescribing information
should be consulted for additional detail.
Dosage Forms Excipient information presented when
available (limited, particularly for generics); consult specific
product labeling.
Capsule, Oral:
Invirase: 200 mg
Tablet, Oral:
Invirase: 500 mg

Sargramostim (sar GRAM oh stim)

Brand Names: US Leukine
Brand Names: Canada Leukine
Index Terms GM-CSF; GMCSF; Granulocyte-Macrophage Colony Stimulating Factor; Prokine; Recombinant Granulocyte-Macrophage Colony Stimulating Factor; rhuGM-CSF
Pharmacologic Category Colony Stimulating Factor; Hematopoietic Agent
Use

Acute myeloid leukemia (AML; following induction chemotherapy): To shorten time to neutrophil recovery and to reduce the incidence of severe and life-threatening infections and infections resulting in death following induction chemotherapy in older adults (≥55 years of age)

Bone marrow transplant (allogeneic or autologous) failure or engraftment delay: For graft failure or engraftment delay in patients who have undergone allogeneic or autologous bone marrow transplantation, to prolong survival (survival benefit may be greater in patients with autologous bone marrow transplant failure or engraftment delay, no previous total body irradiation, malignancy other than leukemia, or multiple organ failure score ≤2)

Myeloid reconstitution after allogeneic bone marrow transplantation: To accelerate myeloid recovery in patients undergoing allogeneic bone marrow transplant from HLA-matched related donors (safe and effective in accelerating myeloid engraftment, reducing the incidence of bacteremia and other culture-positive infections, and shortening the median hospitalization duration)

Myeloid reconstitution after autologous bone marrow transplantation: To accelerate myeloid recovery following transplantation in non-Hodgkin lymphoma (NHL), acute lymphoblastic leukemia (ALL), Hodgkin lymphoma patients undergoing autologous bone marrow transplant (safe and effective in accelerating myeloid engraftment, reducing the median duration of antibiotic administration, reducing the median duration of infectious episodes, and shortening the median hospitalization duration)

Peripheral stem cell transplantation (autologous), mobilization and post-transplant: Mobilization of hematopoietic progenitor cells for collection by leukapheresis (increases the number of progenitor cells capable of engraftment and may lead to more rapid engraftment); to accelerate myeloid reconstitution following peripheral blood progenitor cell transplantation

Pregnancy Considerations Animal reproduction studies have not been conducted.

Breast-Feeding Considerations It is not known if sargramostim is excreted in breast milk. Breast-feeding is not recommended by the manufacturer.

Contraindications Hypersensitivity to sargramostim, yeast-derived products, or any component of the formulation; concurrent (24 hours preceding/following) use with myelosuppressive chemotherapy or radiation therapy; patients with excessive (≥10%) leukemic myeloid blasts in bone marrow or peripheral blood

Warnings/Precautions Simultaneous administration or administration 24 hours preceding/following cytotoxic chemotherapy or radiotherapy is contraindicated due to the sensitivity of rapidly dividing hematopoietic progenitor cells. If there is a rapid increase in blood counts (ANC >20,000/mm³, WBC >50,000/mm³, or platelets >500,000/mm³), decrease the dose by 50% or discontinue therapy. Excessive blood counts should fall to normal within 3 to 7 days after the discontinuation of therapy. Monitor CBC with differential twice weekly during treatment. Limited response to sargramostim may be seen in patients who have received bone marrow purged by chemical agents which do not preserve an adequate number of responsive hematopoietic progenitors (eg, <1.2 x 10⁴/kg progenitors). In patients receiving autologous bone marrow transplant, response to sargramostim may be limited if extensive radiotherapy to the abdomen or chest or multiple myelotoxic agents were administered prior to transplantation. May potentially act as a growth factor for any tumor type, particularly myeloid malignancies; caution should be exercised when using in any malignancy with myeloid characteristics. Discontinue use if disease progression occurs during treatment.

Anaphylaxis or other serious allergic reactions have been reported; discontinue immediately and initiate appropriate therapy if a serious allergic or anaphylactic reaction occurs. A "first-dose effect", characterized by respiratory distress, hypoxia, flushing, hypotension, syncope, and/or tachycardia, may occur (rarely) with the first dose of a cycle and resolve with appropriate symptomatic treatment; symptoms do not usually occur with subsequent doses within that cycle. Sequestration of granulocytes in pulmonary circulation and dyspnea have been reported; monitor respiratory symptoms during and following IV infusion. Decrease infusion rate by 50% if dyspnea occurs; discontinue the infusion if dyspnea persists despite reduction in the rate of administration. Subsequent doses may be administered at the standard rate with careful monitoring. Use with caution in patients with hypoxia or preexisting pulmonary disease. Edema, capillary leak syndrome, pleural and/or pericardial effusion have been reported; fluid retention has been shown to be reversible with dosage reduction or discontinuation of sargramostim with or without concomitant use of diuretics. Use with caution in patients with preexisting fluid retention, pulmonary infiltrates, or congestive heart failure; may exacerbate fluid retention.

Use with caution in patients with preexisting cardiac disease. Reversible transient supraventricular arrhythmias have been reported, especially in patients with a history of arrhythmias. Use with caution in patients with hepatic impairment (hyperbilirubinemia and elevated transaminases have been observed) or renal impairment (serum creatinine elevations have been observed). Monitor hepatic and renal function at least every other week in patients with history of impairment.

Benzyl alcohol and derivatives: Some dosage forms may contain benzyl alcohol; large amounts of benzyl alcohol (≥99 mg/kg/day) have been associated with a potentially fatal toxicity ("gasping syndrome") in neonates; the "gasping syndrome" consists of metabolic acidosis, respiratory distress, gasping respirations, CNS dysfunction (including convulsions, intracranial hemorrhage), hypotension, and cardiovascular collapse (AAP ["Inactive" 1997]; CDC, 1982); some data suggests that benzoate displaces bilirubin from protein binding sites (Ahlfors, 2001); avoid or use dosage forms containing benzyl alcohol with caution in neonates. See manufacturer's labeling.

Adverse Reactions
>10%:
Cardiovascular: Hypertension (34%), edema (13% to 25%), pericardial effusion (4% to 25%), thrombosis (19%), chest pain (15%), peripheral edema (11%), tachycardia (11%)
Central nervous system: Malaise (57%), headache (26%), chills (25%), anxiety (11%), insomnia (11%)
Dermatologic: Skin rash (44% to 77%), pruritus (23%)
Endocrine & metabolic: Weight loss (37%), hyperglycemia (25%), hypercholesterolemia (17%), hypomagnesemia (15%)
Gastrointestinal: Diarrhea (81% to 89%), nausea (58% to 70%), vomiting (46% to 70%), gastric ulcer (50%), abdominal pain (38%), anorexia (13%), hematemesis (13%), dysphagia (11%), gastrointestinal hemorrhage (11%)
Hepatic: Hyperbilirubinemia (30%)
Neuromuscular & skeletal: Weakness (66%), ostealgia (21%), arthralgia (11% to 21%), myalgia (18%)
Ophthalmic: Retinal hemorrhage (11%)
Renal: Increased blood urea nitrogen (23%), increased serum creatinine (15%)
Respiratory: Pharyngitis (23%), epistaxis (17%), dyspnea (15%)
Miscellaneous: Fever (81%)
1% to 10%:
Immunologic: Antibody development (2%)
Respiratory: Pleural effusion (1%)
<1% (Limited to important or life-threatening): Anaphylaxis, capillary leak syndrome, cardiac arrhythmia, eosinophilia, hypoxia, leukocytosis, liver function impairment (transient), pericarditis, prolonged prothrombin time, respiratory distress, rigors, sore throat, supraventricular cardiac arrhythmia, syncope, thrombocythemia, thrombophlebitis

Drug Interactions
Metabolism/Transport Effects None known.
Avoid Concomitant Use There are no known interactions where it is recommended to avoid concomitant use.
Increased Effect/Toxicity
Sargramostim may increase the levels/effects of: Bleomycin

The levels/effects of Sargramostim may be increased by: Cyclophosphamide
Decreased Effect There are no known significant interactions involving a decrease in effect.

Preparation for Administration
Powder for injection: May be reconstituted with 1 mL of preservative free SWFI or bacteriostatic water for injection. Direct the diluent toward the side of the vial and gently swirl to reconstitute; do not shake. Do not mix the contents of vials which have been reconstituted with different diluents.
SubQ: May be administered without further dilution.

IV: Further dilution with NS is required. If the final sargramostim concentration is <10 mcg/mL, 1 mg of human albumin per 1 mL of NS should be added (eg, add 1 mL of 5% human albumin per 50 mL of NS).

Storage/Stability Store intact vials at 2°C to 8°C (36°F to 46°F); do not freeze. Do not shake.

Solution for injection: May be stored for up to 20 days at 2°C to 8°C (36°F to 46°F) once the vial has been entered. Discard remaining solution after 20 days.

Powder for injection: Preparations made with SWFI should be administered as soon as possible, and discarded within 6 hours of reconstitution. Solutions reconstituted with bacteriostatic water may be stored for up to 20 days at 2°C to 8°C (36°F to 46°F); do not freeze. When combining previously reconstituted solutions with freshly reconstituted solutions, administer within 6 hours following preparation; the contents of vials reconstituted with different diluents should not be mixed together.

Mechanism of Action Stimulates proliferation, differentiation and functional activity of neutrophils, eosinophils, monocytes, and macrophages.

Pharmacodynamics/Kinetics

Duration: WBCs return to baseline within 1 to 2 weeks of discontinuing drug

Half-life elimination: IV: ~60 minutes; SubQ: ~2.7 hours

Time to peak, serum: SubQ: 1 to 3 hours

Dosing

Adult & Geriatric Note: May round the dose to the nearest vial size (Ozer, 2000).

Acute myeloid leukemia (following induction chemotherapy): Adults ≥55 years: IV: 250 mcg/m^2/day (infused over 4 hours) starting approximately on day 11 or 4 days following the completion of induction chemotherapy (if day 10 bone marrow is hypoplastic with <5% blasts), continue until ANC >1500/mm^3 for 3 consecutive days or a maximum of 42 days. If WBC >50,000/mm^3 and/or ANC >20,000/mm^3, interrupt treatment or reduce the dose by 50%.

If a second cycle of chemotherapy is necessary, administer ~4 days after the completion of chemotherapy if the bone marrow is hypoplastic with <5% blasts

Discontinue sargramostim immediately if leukemic regrowth occurs. If a severe adverse reaction occurs, reduce the dose by 50% or temporarily discontinue the dose until the reaction abates.

Bone marrow transplantation (allogeneic or autologous) failure or engraftment delay: IV: 250 mcg/m^2/day (infused over 2 hours) for 14 days; If engraftment has not occurred after 7 days off sargramostim, may repeat. If engraftment still has not occurred after 7 days off sargramostim, a third course of 500 mcg/m^2/day for 14 days may be attempted. If there is still no improvement, it is unlikely that further dose escalation will be of benefit.

If a severe adverse reaction occurs, reduce the dose by 50% or temporarily discontinue the dose until the reaction abates

If blast cells appear or disease progression occurs, discontinue treatment

If WBC >50,000/mm^3 and/or ANC >20,000 cells/mm^3, interrupt treatment or reduce the dose by 50%.

Myeloid reconstitution after allogeneic or autologous bone marrow transplantation: IV: 250 mcg/m^2/day (infused over 2 hours), begin 2 to 4 hours after the marrow infusion and ≥24 hours after chemotherapy or radiotherapy, when the post marrow infusion ANC is <500 /mm^3, and continue until ANC >1500 /mm^3 for 3 consecutive days. If WBC >50,000/mm^3 and/or ANC >20,000/mm^3, interrupt treatment or reduce the dose by 50%.

If a severe adverse reaction occurs, reduce dose by 50% or temporarily discontinue the dose until the reaction abates

If blast cells appear or progression of the underlying disease occurs, discontinue treatment

Peripheral stem cell transplantation (autologous), mobilization: IV, SubQ: 250 mcg/m^2/day IV (infused over 24 hours) or SubQ once daily; continue the same dose throughout peripheral blood progenitor cell collection. If WBC >50,000/mm^3, reduce the dose by 50%.

Note: The optimal schedule for peripheral blood progenitor cell collection has not been established (usually begun by day 5 and performed daily until protocol specified targets are achieved). If adequate numbers of progenitor cells are not collected, consider other mobilization therapy.

Peripheral stem cell transplantation (autologous), post-transplant: IV, SubQ: 250 mcg/m^2/day IV (infused over 24 hours) or SubQ once daily beginning immediately following infusion of progenitor cells; continue until ANC is >1500/mm^3 for 3 consecutive days.

Primary prophylaxis of neutropenia in patients receiving chemotherapy (outside transplant and AML) or who are at high risk for neutropenic fever (off-label use): SubQ: 250 mcg/m^2/day (may round to the nearest vial size [Ozer, 2000]) beginning at least 24 hours after chemotherapy administration; continue until ANC >2000 to 3000/mm^3 (Smith, 2006).

Treatment of radiation-induced myelosuppression of the bone marrow (off-label use): SubQ: 250 mcg/m^2/day; continue until ANC >1000/mm^3 (Smith, 2006; Waselenko, 2004).

Renal Impairment There are no dosage adjustments provided in the manufacturer's labeling.

Hepatic Impairment There are no dosage adjustments provided in the manufacturer's labeling.

Administration Sargramostim is administered as a subcutaneous injection or intravenous infusion.

IV: Infuse over 2 hours, 4 hours or 24 hours (indication specific). An in-line membrane filter should **NOT** be used for intravenous administration.

SubQ: Administer undiluted; rotate injection sites, avoiding navel/waistline.

Monitoring Parameters CBC with differential (twice weekly during treatment), renal/liver function tests (at least every 2 weeks in patients displaying renal or hepatic dysfunction prior to treatment initiation); pulmonary function; vital signs; hydration status; weight

Test Interactions May interfere with bone imaging studies; increased hematopoietic activity of the bone marrow may appear as transient positive bone imaging changes

Dosage Forms Excipient information presented when available (limited, particularly for generics); consult specific product labeling. [DSC] = Discontinued product

Solution, Injection:

Leukine: 500 mcg/mL (1 mL [DSC]) [contains benzyl alcohol]

Solution Reconstituted, Intravenous [preservative free]:

Leukine: 250 mcg (1 ea)

Saxagliptin (sax a GLIP tin)

Brand Names: US Onglyza

Brand Names: Canada Onglyza

Index Terms BMS-477118

Pharmacologic Category Antidiabetic Agent, Dipeptidyl Peptidase IV (DPP-IV) Inhibitor

Use Diabetes mellitus, type 2: As an adjunct to diet and exercise to improve glycemic control in adults with type 2 diabetes mellitus (noninsulin dependent, NIDDM) as monotherapy or in combination therapy.

Pregnancy Considerations Adverse events were not observed in animal reproduction studies, except with doses that were also maternally toxic. In women with diabetes, maternal hyperglycemia can be associated with congenital malformations as well as adverse effects in the fetus, neonate, and the mother (ACOG 2005; ADA 2015; Kitzmiller 2008; Metzger 2007). To prevent adverse outcomes, prior to conception and throughout pregnancy maternal blood glucose and HbA$_{1c}$ should be kept as close to target goals as possible but without causing significant hypoglycemia (ACOG 2013; ADA 2015; Blumer 2013; Kitzmiller 2008). Prior to pregnancy, effective contraception should be used until glycemic control is achieved (Kitzmiller 2008). Other agents are currently recommended to treat diabetes in pregnant women (ACOG 2013; Blumer 2013).

Breast-Feeding Considerations It is not known if saxagliptin is excreted in breast milk. The US labeling recommends that caution be exercised when administering saxagliptin to nursing women. The Canadian labeling does not recommend use in nursing women.

Medication Guide Available Yes

Contraindications

Hypersensitivity (eg, anaphylaxis, angioedema, exfoliative skin conditions) to saxagliptin or any component of the formulation

Canadian labeling: Additional contraindications (not in U.S. labeling): Diabetic ketoacidosis, diabetic coma/precoma, type 1 diabetes mellitus

Warnings/Precautions Use with caution in patients with moderate-to-severe renal dysfunction, end-stage renal disease (ESRD) requiring hemodialysis, and in patients taking strong CYP3A4/5 inhibitors (eg, atazanavir, clarithromycin, indinavir, itraconazole, nefazodone, nelfinavir, ritonavir, saquinavir, telithromycin [also see Drug Interactions]); dosing adjustment required. No specific recommendations regarding patients with heart failure are provided in the U.S. manufacturer labeling. Initial clinical trials included only a limited number of patients with heart failure (HF). However, recent data from a large multi-center, randomized, double-blind, placebo-controlled trial in patients with type 2 diabetes with a history of, or at risk for, cardiovascular events demonstrated an increased risk of hospitalization for HF especially during the first 12 months of therapy for patients with elevated levels of natriuretic peptides, previous HF, or chronic kidney disease (Scirica 2013; Scirica 2014).

Severe and disabling arthralgia has been reported with DPP-IV inhibitor use; onset may occur within one day to years after treatment initiation and may resolve with discontinuation of therapy. Some patients may experience a recurrence of symptoms if DPP-IV inhibitor therapy resumed. Hypersensitivity reactions, including anaphylaxis, angioedema, and/or exfoliative dermatologic reactions have been reported; discontinue if signs/symptoms of severe hypersensitivity reactions occur. Cases of acute pancreatitis have been reported; discontinue immediately if suspected. Contains lactose; Canadian labeling recommends avoiding use in patients with galactose intolerance, Lapp lactase deficiency, or glucose-galactose malabsorption syndromes. Saxagliptin is not indicated for use in patients with type 1 diabetes mellitus (insulin dependent, IDDM) or for the treatment of diabetic ketoacidosis (DKA). Potentially significant interactions may exist, requiring dose or frequency adjustment, additional monitoring, and/ or selection of alternative therapy.

Adverse Reactions Frequencies and adverse reactions reported with monotherapy unless otherwise noted.

1% to 10%:
Cardiovascular: Peripheral edema (≤4%; incidence increased in conjunction with thiazolidinediones: ≤8%)
Central nervous system: Headache (7%)
Endocrine & metabolic: Hypoglycemia (≤6%; incidence increased in conjunction with insulin secretagogues: ≤15%)
Gastrointestinal: Abdominal pain (2%), gastroenteritis (2%), vomiting (2%)
Genitourinary: Urinary tract infection (7%)
Hematologic: Lymphocytopenia (≤2%; dose related)
Hypersensitivity: Hypersensitivity reaction (2%; including facial edema and urticaria)
Respiratory: Sinusitis (3%)
<1% (important or life-threatening): Acute pancreatitis, anaphylaxis, angioedema, exfoliative dermatitis, immune thrombocytopenia, increased creatine phosphokinase, increased serum creatinine, severe arthralgia (FDA Safety Alert, Aug 28, 2015), skin rash

Drug Interactions
Metabolism/Transport Effects Substrate of CYP3A4 (major), P-glycoprotein; **Note:** Assignment of Major/Minor substrate status based on clinically relevant drug interaction potential

Avoid Concomitant Use
Avoid concomitant use of Saxagliptin with any of the following: Conivaptan; Fusidic Acid (Systemic); Idelalisib

Increased Effect/Toxicity
Saxagliptin may increase the levels/effects of: ACE Inhibitors; Hypoglycemia-Associated Agents; Insulin; Sulfonylureas

The levels/effects of Saxagliptin may be increased by: Alpha-Lipoic Acid; Androgens; Aprepitant; Conivaptan; CYP3A4 Inhibitors (Moderate); CYP3A4 Inhibitors (Strong); Dasatinib; Fosaprepitant; Fusidic Acid (Systemic); Idelalisib; Ivacaftor; Luliconazole; Lumacaftor; MAO Inhibitors; Mifepristone; Netupitant; Osimertinib; Palbociclib; Pegvisomant; P-glycoprotein/ABCB1 Inhibitors; Quinolone Antibiotics; Ranolazine; Salicylates; Selective Serotonin Reuptake Inhibitors; Simeprevir; Stiripentol

Decreased Effect
The levels/effects of Saxagliptin may be decreased by: CYP3A4 Inducers; Hyperglycemia-Associated Agents; Lumacaftor; Osimertinib; P-glycoprotein/ABCB1 Inducers; Quinolone Antibiotics; Thiazide Diuretics

Storage/Stability Store at 20°C to 25°C (68°F to 77°F); excursions permitted between 15°C to 30°C (59°F to 86°F).

Mechanism of Action Saxagliptin inhibits dipeptidyl peptidase IV (DPP-IV) enzyme resulting in prolonged active incretin levels. Incretin hormones (eg, glucagon-like peptide-1 [GLP-1] and glucose-dependent insulinotropic polypeptide [GIP]) regulate glucose homeostasis by increasing insulin synthesis and release from pancreatic beta cells and decreasing glucagon secretion from pancreatic alpha cells. Decreased glucagon secretion results in decreased hepatic glucose production. Under normal physiologic circumstances, incretin hormones are released by the intestine throughout the day and levels are increased in response to a meal; incretin hormones are rapidly inactivated by the DPP-IV enzyme.

Pharmacodynamics/Kinetics
Duration: 24 hours
Protein binding: Negligible
Metabolism: Hepatic via CYP3A4/5 to 5-hydroxy saxagliptin (active; ~50% potency of the parent compound)
Half-life elimination: Saxagliptin: 2.5 hours; 5-hydroxy saxagliptin: 3.1 hours
Time to peak, plasma: Saxagliptin: 2 hours; 5-hydroxy saxagliptin: 4 hours
Excretion: Urine (75%, 24% of the total dose as saxagliptin, 36% of the total dose as 5-hydroxy saxagliptin); feces (22%)

Dosing
Adult & Geriatric
Diabetes mellitus, type 2: Oral: 2.5 to 5 mg once daily (*US labeling*) or 5 mg once daily (*Canadian labeling*)
Concomitant use with strong CYP3A4/5 inhibitors (eg, atazanavir, clarithromycin, indinavir, itraconazole, ketoconazole, nefazodone, nelfinavir, ritonavir, saquinavir, telithromycin):
US labeling: 2.5 mg once daily
Canadian labeling: There are no dosage adjustments provided in the manufacturer's labeling; concurrent administration of single dose saxagliptin (100 mg) and ketoconazole increased saxagliptin systemic exposure 145% and decreased exposure to saxagliptin's major metabolite by 88%.
Concomitant use with insulin or insulin secretagogues: Reduced dose of insulin or insulin secretagogues (eg, sulfonylureas) may be needed

Renal Impairment Note: Renal function may be estimated using the Cockcroft-Gault formula or the MDRD formula for dosage adjustment purposes.
Mild impairment (CrCl >50 mL/minute): No dosage adjustment necessary.
Moderate to severe impairment (CrCl ≤50 mL/minute): 2.5 mg once daily.
ESRD requiring hemodialysis:
U.S. labeling: 2.5 mg once daily; administer postdialysis
Canadian labeling: Use is not recommended.
Peritoneal dialysis: There are no dosage adjustments provided in the manufacturer's labeling (has not been studied).

Hepatic Impairment
U.S. labeling: Mild-to-severe impairment: No dosage adjustment necessary.
Canadian labeling:
Mild impairment: There are no dosage adjustments provided in manufacturer's labeling.
Moderate to severe impairment: Use is not recommended (lack of clinical experience).

Dietary Considerations Individualized medical nutrition therapy (MNT) is an integral part of therapy (ADA 2013).

Administration May be administered without regard to meals. Swallow whole; do not split or cut tablets.

Monitoring Parameters Plasma glucose, HbA_{1c}, renal function (prior to initiation of therapy and periodically thereafter); signs/symptoms of pancreatitis

Reference Range
Recommendations for glycemic control in nonpregnant adults with diabetes (ADA 2015):
HbA_{1c}: <7% (a more aggressive [<6.5%] or less aggressive [<8%] HbA_{1c} goal may be targeted based on patient-specific characteristics)
Preprandial capillary plasma glucose: 80 to 130 mg/dL
Peak postprandial capillary blood glucose: <180 mg/dL

Recommendations for glycemic control in pediatric (all age groups) patients with type 1 diabetes (ADA 2015):
HbA_{1c}: <7.5% (individualization may be appropriate based on patient-specific characteristics; <7% is reasonable if it can be achieved without excessive hypoglycemia)
Preprandial capillary plasma glucose: 90 to 130 mg/dL
Bedtime and overnight capillary blood glucose: 90 to 150 mg/dL

Dosage Forms Excipient information presented when available (limited, particularly for generics); consult specific product labeling.

Tablet, Oral:

Onglyza: 2.5 mg, 5 mg

Saxagliptin and Metformin
(sax a GLIP tin & met FOR min)

Brand Names: US Kombiglyze XR
Brand Names: Canada Komboglyze
Index Terms Metformin and Saxagliptin; Metformin Hydrochloride and Saxagliptin; Saxagliptin and Metformin Hydrochloride
Pharmacologic Category Antidiabetic Agent, Biguanide; Antidiabetic Agent, Dipeptidyl Peptidase IV (DPP-IV) Inhibitor
Use Management of type 2 diabetes mellitus (noninsulin dependent, NIDDM) as an adjunct to diet and exercise when treatment with both saxagliptin and metformin is appropriate
Medication Guide Available Yes
Dosing
Adult

Diabetes mellitus, type 2: Oral:

US labeling: Initial doses should be based on current dose of saxagliptin and metformin; daily doses should be given once daily with the evening meal. Maximum: Saxagliptin 5 mg/metformin 2000 mg daily

Patients inadequately controlled on metformin alone: Initial dose: Saxagliptin 2.5-5 mg daily plus current dose of metformin. **Note:** Patients who require saxagliptin 2.5 mg (eg, dose adjusted for concomitant use of strong CYP3A4/5 inhibitors) and metformin >1000 mg should not be switched to the combination product.

Patients inadequately controlled on saxagliptin alone: Initial dose: Metformin 500 mg daily plus saxagliptin 5 mg daily. **Note:** Metformin-naive patients currently receiving saxagliptin 2.5 mg daily (eg, dose adjusted for concomitant use of strong CYP3A4/5 inhibitors) should not be switched to the combination product.

Concomitant use with strong CYP3A4/5 inhibitors: Maximum: Saxagliptin 2.5 mg/metformin 1000 mg daily

Concomitant use with insulin or insulin secretagogues: Reduced dose of insulin or insulin secretagogues (eg, sulfonylureas) may be needed.

Canadian labeling: Initial doses should be based on current dose of saxagliptin and metformin; daily dose should be divided into 2 equal doses given with meals. Maximum: Saxagliptin 5 mg/metformin 2000 mg daily

Patients inadequately controlled on metformin alone: Initial dose: Saxagliptin 2.5 mg twice daily plus current dose of metformin.

Concomitant use with insulin: Reduced dose of insulin may be needed.

Geriatric Refer to adult dosing. The initial and maintenance dosing should be conservative, due to the potential for decreased renal function (monitor). Do not use in patients ≥80 years of age unless normal renal function has been established.

Renal Impairment

Manufacturer's labeling:

Serum creatinine (SCr) ≥1.5 mg/dL (males) or ≥1.4 mg/dL (females): Use is contraindicated

Abnormal CrCl (US labeling: Not defined; Canadian labeling: <60 mL/minute): Use is contraindicated

Alternate recommendations: Note: The United Kingdom National Institute for Health and Clinical Excellence (NICE) Guidelines recommend prescribing metformin with caution in those patients who are at risk of sudden deterioration in renal function and at risk of an estimated glomerular filtration rate (eGFR) <45 mL/minute/1.73 m^2 (NICE 2008). Some evidence suggests that use of metformin is unsafe when eGFR <30 mL/minute/1.73 m^2 (calculated using MDRD) (Shaw 2007). A review of the available data by members of the American Diabetes Association proposed the following recommendations based on eGFR (Lipska 2011):

eGFR ≥60 mL/minute/1.73 m^2: No contraindications, monitor renal function annually

eGFR ≥45 to <60 mL/minute/1.73 m^2: Continue use; monitor renal function every 3 to 6 months

eGFR ≥30 to <45 mL/minute/1.73 m^2: In patients currently receiving metformin, use with caution, consider dosage reduction (eg, 50% reduction or 50% of maximal dose), monitor renal function every 3 months. Do not initiate therapy in patients with eGFR <45 mL/minute/1.73 m^2.

eGFR <30 mL/minute/1.73 m^2: Discontinue use

Hepatic Impairment

US labeling: The manufacturer recommends to avoid metformin since liver disease is considered a risk factor for the development of lactic acidosis during metformin therapy. However, continued use of metformin in diabetics with liver dysfunction, including cirrhosis, has been used successfully and may be associated with a survival benefit in carefully selected patients; use cautiously in patients at risk for lactic acidosis (eg, renal impairment, alcohol use) (Brackett 2010; Zhang 2014).

Canadian labeling: Use is not recommended with clinical or laboratory evidence of disease and contraindicated in the presence of moderate-to-severe impairment.

Additional Information Complete prescribing information should be consulted for additional detail.

Dosage Forms Excipient information presented when available (limited, particularly for generics); consult specific product labeling.

Tablet, variable release, oral:

Kombiglyze XR 2.5/1000: Saxagliptin 2.5 mg [immediate release] and metformin hydrochloride 1000 mg [extended release]

Kombiglyze XR 5/500: Saxagliptin 5 mg [immediate release] and metformin hydrochloride 500 mg [extended release]

Kombiglyze XR 5/1000: Saxagliptin 5 mg [immediate release] and metformin hydrochloride 1000 mg [extended release]

Dosage Forms: Canada Excipient information presented when available (limited, particularly for generics); consult specific product labeling.

Tablet, oral:

Komboglyze 2.5/500: Saxagliptin 2.5 mg [immediate release] and metformin hydrochloride 500 mg [immediate release]

Komboglyze 2.5/850: Saxagliptin 2.5 mg [immediate release] and metformin hydrochloride 850 mg [immediate release]

Komboglyze 2.5/1000: Saxagliptin 2.5 mg [immediate release] and metformin hydrochloride 1000 mg [immediate release]

Scopolamine (Systemic) (skoe POL a meen)

Brand Names: US Transderm-Scop
Brand Names: Canada Buscopan; Scopolamine Hydrobromide Injection; Transderm-V
Index Terms Hyoscine Butylbromide; Scopolamine Base; Scopolamine Butylbromide; Scopolamine Hydrobromide
Pharmacologic Category Anticholinergic Agent
Use

Scopolamine base: Transdermal: Prevention of nausea/vomiting associated with motion sickness and recovery from anesthesia and surgery

Scopolamine hydrobromide: Injection: Preoperative medication to produce amnesia, sedation, tranquilization, antiemetic effects, and decrease salivary and respiratory secretions

Scopolamine butylbromide [Canadian product]: Oral/injection: Treatment of smooth muscle spasm of the genitourinary or gastrointestinal tract; injection may also be used prior to radiological/diagnostic procedures to prevent spasm

Pregnancy Considerations Adverse events were observed in some animal reproduction studies. Scopolamine crosses the placenta; may cause respiratory depression and/or neonatal hemorrhage when used during pregnancy. Transdermal scopolamine has been used as an adjunct to epidural anesthesia for cesarean delivery without adverse CNS effects on the newborn. Parenteral administration does not increase the duration of labor or affect uterine contractions. Except when used prior to cesarean section, use during pregnancy only if the benefit to the mother outweighs the potential risk to the fetus.

Breast-Feeding Considerations Scopolamine is excreted into breast milk. The manufacturer recommends caution be used if scopolamine is administered to a nursing woman.

Contraindications

Transdermal, oral: Hypersensitivity to scopolamine, other belladonna alkaloids, or any component of the formulation; narrow-angle glaucoma

Injection: Hypersensitivity to scopolamine, other belladonna alkaloids, or any component of the formulation; narrow-angle glaucoma; chronic lung disease (repeated administration)

Canadian labeling: Additional contraindications (not in U.S. labeling):

Oral: Glaucoma, megacolon, myasthenia gravis, obstructive prostatic hypertrophy

Injection:

Hyoscine butylbromide: Untreated narrow-angle glaucoma; megacolon, prostatic hypertrophy with urinary retention; stenotic lesions of the GI tract; myasthenia gravis; tachycardia, angina, or heart failure; IM administration in patients receiving anticoagulant therapy

Scopolamine hydrobromide: Glaucoma or predisposition to narrow-angle glaucoma; paralytic ileus; prostatic hypertrophy; pyloric obstruction; tachycardia secondary to cardiac insufficiency or thyrotoxicosis

Warnings/Precautions Use with caution in patients with coronary artery disease, tachyarrhythmias, heart failure, hypertension, or hyperthyroidism; evaluate tachycardia prior to administration. Use caution in hepatic or renal impairment; adverse CNS effects occur more often in these patients. Use injectable and transdermal products with caution in patients with prostatic hyperplasia or urinary retention. Discontinue if patient reports unusual visual disturbances or pain within the eye. Use caution in GI obstruction, hiatal hernia, reflux esophagitis, and ulcerative colitis. Use with caution in patients with a history of seizure or psychosis; may exacerbate these conditions. Lower doses (0.1mg) may have vagal mimetic effects (eg, increase vagal tone causing paradoxical bradycardia).

Anaphylaxis including episodes of shock has been reported following parenteral administration; observe for signs/symptoms of hypersensitivity following parenteral administration. Patients with a history of allergies or asthma may be at increased risk of hypersensitivity reactions. Adverse events (including dizziness, headache, nausea, vomiting) may occur following abrupt discontinuation of large doses or in patients with Parkinson's disease; adverse events may also occur following removal of the transdermal patch although symptoms may not appear until ≥24 hours after removal.

Idiosyncratic reactions may rarely occur; patients may experience acute toxic psychosis, agitation, confusion, delusions, hallucinations, paranoid behavior, and rambling speech. May cause CNS depression, which may impair physical or mental abilities; patients must be cautioned about performing tasks which require mental alertness (eg, operating machinery or driving). Effects with other sedative drugs or ethanol may be potentiated.

Transdermal patch may contain conducting metal (eg, aluminum); remove patch prior to MRI. Use of the transdermal product in patients with open-angle glaucoma may necessitate adjustments in glaucoma therapy.

Scopolamine (hyoscine) hydrobromide should not be interchanged with scopolamine butylbromide formulations; dosages are not equivalent.

Avoid use in the elderly due to potent anticholinergic adverse effects and uncertain effectiveness (Beers Criteria). Use with caution in infants and children since they may be more susceptible to adverse effects of scopolamine. Tablets may contain sucrose; avoid use of tablets in patients who are fructose intolerant.

Adverse Reactions Frequency not defined.

Cardiovascular: Bradycardia, flushing, orthostatic hypotension, tachycardia

Central nervous system: Acute toxic psychosis (rare), agitation (rare), ataxia, confusion, delusion (rare), disorientation, dizziness, drowsiness, fatigue, hallucination (rare), headache, irritability, loss of memory, paranoid behavior (rare), restlessness, sedation

Dermatologic: Drug eruptions, dry skin, dyshidrosis, erythema, pruritus, rash, urticaria

Endocrine & metabolic: Thirst

Gastrointestinal: Constipation, diarrhea, dry throat, dysphagia, nausea, vomiting, xerostomia

Genitourinary: Dysuria, urinary retention

Neuromuscular & skeletal: Tremor, weakness

Ocular: Accommodation impaired, blurred vision, conjunctival infection, cycloplegia, dryness, glaucoma (narrow-angle), increased intraocular pain, itching, photophobia, pupil dilation, retinal pigmentation

Respiratory: Dry nose, dyspnea

Miscellaneous: Anaphylaxis (rare), anaphylactic shock (rare), angioedema, diaphoresis decreased, heat intolerance, hypersensitivity reactions

Drug Interactions

Metabolism/Transport Effects None known.

Avoid Concomitant Use

Avoid concomitant use of Scopolamine (Systemic) with any of the following: Aclidinium; Azelastine (Nasal); Cimetropium; Eluxadoline; Glucagon; Glycopyrrolate; Glycopyrrolate (Oral Inhalation); Ipratropium (Oral Inhalation); Levosulpiride; Orphenadrine; Paraldehyde; Potassium Chloride; Thalidomide; Tiotropium; Umeclidinium

Increased Effect/Toxicity

Scopolamine (Systemic) may increase the levels/effects of: AbobotulinumtoxinA; Alcohol (Ethyl); Analgesics (Opioid); Anticholinergic Agents; Azelastine (Nasal); Buprenorphine; Cimetropium; CNS Depressants; Eluxadoline; Glucagon; Glycopyrrolate; Glycopyrrolate (Oral Inhalation); Hydrocodone; Methotrimeprazine; Metyrosine; Mirabegron; Mirtazapine; OnabotulinumtoxinA; Orphenadrine; Paraldehyde; Potassium Chloride; Pramipexole; Ramosetron; RimabotulinumtoxinB; ROPINIRole; Rotigotine; Selective Serotonin Reuptake Inhibitors; Suvorexant; Thalidomide; Thiazide Diuretics; Tiotropium; Topiramate; Zolpidem

The levels/effects of Scopolamine (Systemic) may be increased by: Aclidinium; Brimonidine (Topical); Cannabis; Doxylamine; Dronabinol; Droperidol; HydrOXYzine; Ipratropium (Oral Inhalation); Kava Kava; Magnesium Sulfate; Methotrimeprazine; Mianserin; Minocycline; Nabilone; Perampanel; Pramlintide; Rufinamide; Sodium Oxybate; Tapentadol; Tetrahydrocannabinol; Umeclidinium

Decreased Effect

Scopolamine (Systemic) may decrease the levels/effects of: Acetylcholinesterase Inhibitors; Gastrointestinal Agents (Prokinetic); Itopride; Levosulpiride; Secretin

The levels/effects of Scopolamine (Systemic) may be decreased by: Acetylcholinesterase Inhibitors

Preparation for Administration Solution for injection:

IM: Butylbromide: No dilution required.

IV:

Butylbromide: No dilution is necessary prior to injection.

Hydrobromide: Dilute with an equal volume of sterile water.

Storage/Stability

Solution for injection:

Butylbromide [Canadian product]: Store at room temperature. Do not freeze. Protect from light and heat. Stable in D_5W, $D_{10}W$, NS, Ringer's solution, and LR for up to 8 hours.

Hydrobromide: Store at room temperature of 20°C to 25°C (68°F to 77°F). Protect from light. Avoid acid solutions; hydrolysis occurs at pH <3.

Tablet [Canadian product]: Store at room temperature. Protect from light and heat.

Transdermal system: Store at 20°C to 25°C (68°F to 77°F).

Mechanism of Action Blocks the action of acetylcholine at parasympathetic sites in smooth muscle, secretory glands and the CNS; increases cardiac output, dries secretions, antagonizes histamine and serotonin; at usual recommended doses, causes blockade of muscarinic receptors at the cardiac SA-node and is parasympatholytic (ie, blocks vagal activity increasing heart rate)

Pharmacodynamics/Kinetics

Onset of action: Oral, IM: 0.5 to 1 hour; IV: 10 minutes; Transdermal: 6 to 8 hours

Duration: IM, IV, SubQ: 4 hours

Absorption: IM, SubQ: Rapid; Oral: Quaternary salts (butyl-bromide) are poorly absorbed (local concentrations in the GI tract following oral dosing may be high)

Distribution: V_d: Butylbromide: 128 L

Protein binding: Butylbromide: ~4% (albumin)

Metabolism: Hepatic

Bioavailability: Oral: 8%

Half-life elimination: Butylbromide: ~5 to 11 hours; Hydro-bromide: ~1 to 4 hours; Scopolamine base: 9.5 hours

Time to peak: Hydrobromide: IM: ~20 minutes, SubQ: ~15 minutes; Butylbromide: Oral: ~2 hours; Scopolamine base: Transdermal: 24 hours

Excretion: Urine (<10%, as parent drug and metabolites); IV: Butylbromide: Urine (42% to 61% [half as parent drug]), feces (28% to 37%)

Dosing

Adult Note: Scopolamine injection is no longer available in the US.

Note: Scopolamine (hyoscine) hydrobromide should not be interchanged with scopolamine butylbromide formulations. Dosages are not equivalent.

Scopolamine base:

Preoperative: Transdermal patch: Apply 1 patch to hairless area behind ear the night before surgery or 1 hour prior to cesarean section (apply no sooner than 1 hour before surgery to minimize newborn exposure); remove 24 hours after surgery

Motion sickness: Transdermal patch: Apply 1 patch to hairless area behind the ear at least 4 hours prior to exposure and every 3 days as needed; effective if applied as soon as 2 to 3 hours before anticipated need, best if 12 hours before

Chemotherapy-induced nausea and vomiting, breakthrough (off-label use): Apply 1 patch every 72 hours (NCCN Antiemesis guidelines v.1.2012)

Scopolamine hydrobromide:

Antiemetic: SubQ: 0.6 to 1 mg

Preoperative: IM, IV, SubQ: 0.3 to 0.65 mg

Sedation, tranquilization: IM, IV, SubQ:

U.S. labeling: 0.6 mg 3 to 4 times/day

Canadian labeling: 0.3 to 0.6 mg 3 to 4 times/day

Scopolamine butylbromide [Canadian product]: *Gastrointestinal/genitourinary spasm:*

Oral: Acute therapy: 10 to 20 mg daily (1 to 2 tablets); prolonged therapy: 10 mg (1 tablet) 3 to 5 times/day; maximum: 60 mg/day

IM, IV, SubQ: 10 to 20 mg; maximum: 100 mg/day

Geriatric Lower dosages may be required. Refer to adult dosing.

Pediatric Note: Scopolamine injection is no longer available in the US.

Scopolamine hydrobromide:

Antiemetic: SubQ: 0.006 mg/kg

Preoperative: IM, IV, SubQ:

Children 6 months to 3 years: 0.1 to 0.15 mg

Children 3 to 6 years: 0.2-0.3 mg

Renal Impairment No dosage adjustment provided in manufacturer's labeling. However, caution is recommended due to increased risks of adverse effects.

Hepatic Impairment No dosage adjustment provided in manufacturer's labeling. However, caution is recommended due to increased risks of adverse effects.

Administration Note: Butylbromide or hydrobromide may be administered by IM, IV, or SubQ injection.

IM: **Butylbromide:** Intramuscular injections should be administered 10-15 minutes prior to radiological/diagnostic procedures.

IV:

Butylbromide: No dilution is necessary prior to injection; inject at a rate of 1 mL/minute

Hydrobromide: Dilute with an equal volume of sterile water and administer by direct IV; inject over 2-3 minutes

Oral: Tablet should be swallowed whole and taken with a full glass of water.

Transdermal: Apply to hairless area of skin behind the ear. Wash hands before and after applying the disc to avoid drug contact with eyes. Do not use any patch that has been damaged, cut, or manipulated in any way. Topical patch is programmed to deliver 1 mg over 3 days. Once applied, do not remove the patch for 3 full days (motion sickness). When used postoperatively for nausea/vomiting, the patch should be removed 24 hours after surgery. If patch becomes displaced, discard and apply a new patch. Dispose of used or unused patches in the trash out of reach from children and pets.

Monitoring Parameters Body temperature, heart rate, urinary output, intraocular pressure

Test Interactions Interferes with gastric secretion test

Product Availability Scopolamine injection is no longer available in the US.

Dosage Forms Excipient information presented when available (limited, particularly for generics); consult specific product labeling.

Patch 72 Hour, Transdermal:

Transderm-Scop: 1.5 mg (1 ea, 4 ea, 10 ea, 24 ea)

Solution, Injection, as hydrobromide:

Generic: 0.4 mg/mL (1 mL)

Dosage Forms: Canada Note: Refer also to Dosage Forms

Excipient information presented when available (limited, particularly for generics); consult specific product labeling.

Tablet, oral, as butylbromide:

Buscopan: 10 mg

Solution, Injection, as butylbromide:

Buscopan: 20 mg/mL (1 mL)

Secobarbital (see koe BAR bi tal)

Brand Names: US Seconal

Index Terms Quinalbarbitone Sodium; Secobarbital Sodium

Pharmacologic Category Barbiturate

Use Preanesthetic agent; short-term treatment of insomnia

Dosing

Adult

Insomnia (hypnotic): Oral: Usual: 100 mg at bedtime.

Note: Limit to short-term use only; efficacy for sleep induction and maintenance is lost after 14 days.

Preoperative sedation: Oral: 200-300 mg 1-2 hours before procedure

Geriatric Refer to adult dosing. Manufacturer's labeling recommends a dose reduction, but does not provide specific dosing recommendations.

Renal Impairment No specific dosage adjustment provided in manufacturer's labeling. However, a dosage reduction is recommended. Slightly dialyzable (5% to 20%).

Hepatic Impairment No dosage adjustment provided in manufacturer's labeling. However, dosage reduction is recommended.

Additional Information Complete prescribing information should be consulted for additional detail.

Dosage Forms Excipient information presented when available (limited, particularly for generics); consult specific product labeling.

Capsule, Oral, as sodium:

Seconal: 100 mg [contains fd&c yellow #10 (quinoline yellow)]

Controlled Substance C-II

◆ Secobarbital Sodium see Secobarbital on page 1642

◆ Seconal see Secobarbital on page 1642

◆ Sectral see Acebutolol on page 24

◆ Sectral® (Can) see Acebutolol on page 24

Secukinumab (sek ue KIN ue mab)

Brand Names: US Cosentyx; Cosentyx Sensoready Pen
Brand Names: Canada Cosentyx
Index Terms AIN457; Cosentyx
Pharmacologic Category Antipsoriatic Agent; Interleukin-17A Receptor Antagonist; Monoclonal Antibody
Use Plaque psoriasis: Treatment of moderate to severe plaque psoriasis in adult patients who are candidates for systemic therapy or phototherapy.
Pregnancy Considerations Adverse events were not observed in animal reproduction studies. In general, maternal use of monoclonal antibodies during pregnancy may increase the risk of infection to the exposed infant or interfere with vaccine administration in the newborn (Mervic, 2014). Other agents are currently preferred for the treatment of plaque psoriasis in pregnant women (Hsu, 2012).
Breast-Feeding Considerations It is not known if secukinumab is excreted in breast milk. The manufacturer recommends that caution be used if administered to a nursing woman.
Medication Guide Available Yes
Contraindications Serious hypersensitivity reaction to secukinumab or any component of the formulation
Warnings/Precautions Secukinumab may increase the risk of infections. A higher rate of infections was observed with secukinumab treatment in clinical trials, including nasopharyngitis, upper respiratory tract infection, and mucocutaneous candida infection; the incidence appeared to be dose-dependent. Use with caution in patients with a chronic infection or a history of recurrent infection. In patients who develop a serious infection, monitor closely and discontinue use until the infection resolves. Patients should be evaluated for tuberculosis infection prior to initiating therapy; do not initiate therapy in patients with an active tuberculosis infection. Consider antituberculosis therapy if an adequate course of treatment cannot be confirmed in patients with a history of latent or active tuberculosis. Monitor all patients for signs and symptoms of active tuberculosis during and after treatment. Patients should be brought up to date with all immunizations before initiating therapy. Live vaccines should not be given concurrently; non-live vaccines administered during secukinumab therapy may not elicit an immune response sufficient to prevent disease.

Treatment with secukinumab may cause exacerbations of Crohn disease; monitor patients with active Crohn disease closely. Urticaria and anaphylaxis have been reported; discontinue immediately if signs develop and initiate appropriate treatment. Some dosage forms may contain dry natural rubber (latex).

Adverse Reactions Note: Frequency not always defined.
>10%:
Infection: Infection (29% to 48%)
Respiratory: Nasopharyngitis (11% to 12%)
1% to 10%:
Dermatologic: Urticaria (≤1%), candidiasis
Gastrointestinal: Diarrhea (3% to 4%), mucocutaneous candidiasis (1%), oral herpes (≤1%)
Hypersensitivity: Anaphylaxis, hypersensitivity
Infection: Serious infection (≤1%), herpes virus infection, staphylococcal infection
Respiratory: Upper respiratory tract infection (3%), pharyngitis (1%), rhinitis (1%), rhinorrhea (≤1%)
<1% (Limited to important or life-threatening): Conjunctivitis, exacerbation of Crohn disease, immunogenicity, impetigo, increased serum transaminases, inflammatory bowel disease, neutropenia, oral candidiasis, otitis externa, otitis media, sinusitis, tinea pedis, tonsillitis
Drug Interactions
Metabolism/Transport Effects None known.

Avoid Concomitant Use
Avoid concomitant use of Secukinumab with any of the following: BCG (Intravesical); Belimumab; Natalizumab; Pimecrolimus; Tacrolimus (Topical); Tofacitinib; Vaccines (Live)
Increased Effect/Toxicity
Secukinumab may increase the levels/effects of: Belimumab; Fingolimod; Leflunomide; Natalizumab; Tofacitinib; Vaccines (Live)

The levels/effects of Secukinumab may be increased by: Denosumab; Pimecrolimus; Roflumilast; Tacrolimus (Topical); Trastuzumab
Decreased Effect
Secukinumab may decrease the levels/effects of: BCG (Intravesical); Coccidioides immitis Skin Test; Sipuleucel-T; Vaccines (Inactivated); Vaccines (Live)

The levels/effects of Secukinumab may be decreased by: Echinacea
Preparation for Administration
Remove vial from the refrigerator and allow to stand for 15 to 30 minutes to reach room temperature. Reconstitute by slowly injecting 1 mL of sterile water onto the powder. Tilt the vial approximately 45 degrees and gently rotate between the fingertips for approximately 1 minute; do not shake or invert. Let the vial sit at room temperature for 10 minutes to allow for dissolution (foaming may occur). Tilt the vial approximately 45 degrees and gently rotate between the fingertips for approximately 1 minute again; do not shake or invert. Allow the vial to stand undisturbed at room temperature for approximately 5 minutes. The reconstituted solution should be essentially free of visible particles, clear to opalescent, and colorless to slightly yellow. Do not use if the lyophilized powder has not fully dissolved or if the liquid contains visible particles, is cloudy, or discolored.
The Sensoready pen or prefilled syringe should be removed from the refrigerator and allowed to stand for 15 to 30 minutes to reach room temperature prior to administration.
Storage/Stability Store intact vials, Sensoready pens, and prefilled syringes refrigerated at 2°C to 8°C (36°F to 46°F). Protect from light; keep in original carton. Do not freeze or shake. After reconstitution of the vial, use the solution immediately or store in the refrigerator at 2°C to 8°C (36°F to 46°F) for up to 24 hours. Do not freeze. The Sensoready pen or prefilled syringe may be stored at room temperature for up to an hour immediately prior to administration. Discard any unused portion.
Mechanism of Action Secukinumab is a human IgG1 monoclonal antibody that selectively binds to the interleukin-17A (IL-17A) cytokine and inhibits its interaction with the IL-17 receptor. IL-17A is a naturally occurring cytokine involved in normal inflammatory and immune responses. Secukinumab inhibits the release of proinflammatory cytokines and chemokines.
Pharmacodynamics/Kinetics Note: Weight: Secukinumab clearance and volume of distribution increase as body weight increases.
Distribution: V_d: 7.1 to 8.6 L
Metabolism: Expected to be degraded into small peptides and amino acids via catabolic pathways similar to that which is seen with endogenous IgG
Bioavailability: 55% to 77%
Half-life elimination: 22 to 31 days
Time to peak: ~6 days
Dosing
Adult & Geriatric
Plaque psoriasis: SubQ: 300 mg once weekly at weeks 0, 1, 2, 3, and 4 followed by 300 mg every 4 weeks. Some patients may only require 150 mg per dose.
Renal Impairment There are no dosage adjustments provided in the manufacturer's labeling (has not been studied).
Hepatic Impairment There are no dosage adjustments provided in the manufacturer's labeling (has not been studied).

Administration SubQ: Allow to reach room temperature prior to injection. Inject into the front of thighs, lower abdomen (≥2 inches away from the navel) or outer upper arms; administer each injection at a different anatomic location than a previous injection and avoid areas where the skin is tender, bruised, erythematous, indurated, or affected by psoriasis, or where there are scars or stretch marks. The Sensoready pen or prefilled syringe may be self-injected by the patient following proper training in SubQ injection technique; the lyophilized powder is to be administered by health care providers only.
Monitoring Parameters Signs and symptoms of infection, active tuberculosis (during and after treatment), and exacerbations of Crohn's disease

◀ **Dosage Forms** Excipient information presented when available (limited, particularly for generics); consult specific product labeling.

Solution Auto-injector, Subcutaneous [preservative free]:
Cosentyx Sensoready Pen: 150 mg/mL (1 mL) [contains mouse protein (murine) (hamster), polysorbate 80]
Solution Prefilled Syringe, Subcutaneous [preservative free]:
Cosentyx: 150 mg/mL (1 mL) [contains mouse protein (murine) (hamster), polysorbate 80]

◆ Secura Antifungal [OTC] *see* Miconazole (Topical) *on page 1201*

◆ Secura Antifungal Extra Thick [OTC] *see* Miconazole (Topical) *on page 1201*

◆ Seebri Breezhaler (Can) *see* Glycopyrrolate *on page 850*

◆ Seebri Neohaler *see* Glycopyrrolate *on page 850*

◆ Selax [OTC] (Can) *see* Docusate *on page 578*

◆ Select 1/35 (Can) *see* Ethinyl Estradiol and Norethindrone *on page 708*

Selegiline (se LE ji leen)

Brand Names: US Eldepryl; Emsam; Zelapar
Brand Names: Canada Apo-Selegiline; Dom-Selegiline; Mylan-Selegiline; PMS-Selegiline; Teva-Selegiline
Index Terms Deprenyl; L-Deprenyl; Selegiline Hydrochloride
Pharmacologic Category Anti-Parkinson's Agent, MAO Type B Inhibitor; Antidepressant, Monoamine Oxidase Inhibitor
Use
Parkinson disease: Adjunct in the management of patients with Parkinson disease being treated with levodopa/carbidopa who exhibit deterioration in the quality of their response to therapy (oral products)
Major depressive disorder: Treatment of major depressive disorder (transdermal product)
Pregnancy Considerations Adverse events were observed in some animal reproduction studies.
Breast-Feeding Considerations It is not known if selegiline is excreted in breast milk. Due to the potential for serious adverse reactions in the nursing infant, breastfeeding is not recommended by the manufacturer.
Medication Guide Available Yes
Contraindications Hypersensitivity to selegiline or any component of the formulation; concomitant use of meperidine

Orally disintegrating tablet: Additional contraindications: Use with meperidine, methadone, propoxyphene, tramadol, MAO inhibitors (concurrently or within 14 days of discontinuing selegiline or one of these medications); use with St. John's wort, cyclobenzaprine, or dextromethorphan

Transdermal: Additional contraindications: Pheochromocytoma; use of carbamazepine, serotonin reuptake inhibitors (including SSRIs and SNRIs), clomipramine, imipramine, meperidine, tramadol, propoxyphene, methadone, pentazocine, and dextromethorphan (concurrently, within 2 weeks of selegiline discontinuation, or selegiline use within 4 to 5 half-lives (approximately 1 week; 5 weeks for fluoxetine) of discontinuation of the contraindicated drug); patients <12 years of age

Warnings/Precautions Antidepressants increase the risk of suicidal thinking and behavior in children, adolescents, and young adults in short-term studies. Short-term studies did not show an increased risk in patients >24 years of age and showed a decreased risk in patients ≥65 years. Closely monitor patients for clinical worsening, and emergence of suicidal thoughts and behaviors, particularly during the initial 1 to 2 months of therapy or during periods of dosage adjustments (increases or decreases); the patient's family or caregiver should be instructed to closely observe the patient and communicate condition with health care provider. A medication guide concerning the use of antidepressants should be dispensed with each prescription. Transdermal selegiline is not FDA approved for use in children <12 years of age.

The possibility of a suicide attempt is inherent in major depression and may persist until remission occurs. Worsening depression and severe abrupt suicidality that are not part of the presenting symptoms may require discontinuation or modification of drug therapy. Use caution in high-risk patients during initiation of therapy. Prescriptions should be written for the smallest quantity consistent with good patient care. The patient's family or caregiver should be alerted to monitor patients for the emergence of suicidality and associated behaviors such as anxiety, agitation, panic attacks, insomnia, irritability, hostility, impulsivity, akathisia, hypomania, and mania; patients should be instructed to notify their healthcare provider if any of these symptoms or worsening depression or psychosis occur.

Dopaminergic agents used for Parkinson disease or restless legs syndrome have been associated with compulsive behaviors and/or loss of impulse control, which has manifested as pathological gambling, libido increases (hypersexuality), uncontrolled spending of money, binge eating, and/or other intense urges. Causality has not been established, and controversy exists as to whether this phenomenon is related to the underlying disease, prior behaviors/addictions and/or drug therapy. Dose reduction or discontinuation of therapy has been reported to reverse these behaviors in some, but not all cases. The orally disintegrating tablets may cause new or worsening mental status and behavioral changes including hallucinations and psychotic-like behavior with initiation of therapy, after dose increases, or during the course of therapy. Symptoms may consist of paranoid ideation, delusions, hallucinations, confusion, psychotic-like behavior, disorientation, aggressive behavior, agitation, and delirium. Avoid use in patients with a major psychotic disorder. The transdermal product may precipitate a shift to mania or hypomania in patients with bipolar disorder. Monotherapy in patients with bipolar disorder should be avoided. Patients presenting with depressive symptoms should be screened for bipolar disorder, including a family history of suicide, bipolar disorder, and depression. **Selegiline is not FDA approved for the treatment of bipolar depression.** The orally disintegrating tablet may cause somnolence and episodes of sudden sleep onset, which may impair physical or mental abilities. Elderly patients, patients with current sleep disorders, and patients with concomitant sedating medications are at greatest risk. Patients must be cautioned about performing tasks that require mental alertness (eg, operating machinery or driving). Discontinue if significant daytime sleepiness or episodes of falling asleep occur; if a decision is made to continue therapy, advise patients not to drive and to avoid other potentially dangerous activities. The orally disintegrating tablet may potentiate the dopaminergic side effects of levodopa and cause dyskinesia or exacerbate preexisting dyskinesia requiring a reduction of the dose of levodopa.

Orally disintegrating tablet may cause orthostatic hypotension; use with caution in patients at risk of this effect or in those who would not tolerate transient hypotensive episodes (cerebrovascular disease, cardiovascular disease, hypovolemia, or concurrent medication use which may predispose to hypotension/bradycardia). Incidence may also be increased in older adults and when titrating to the 2.5 mg dosage in patients taking the orally disintegrating tablet. Monitor patients for new onset or exacerbation of hypertension. Risk for melanoma development is increased in Parkinson disease patients; drug causation or factors contributing to risk have not been established. Patients should be monitored closely and periodic skin examinations should be performed. Orally disintegrating tablets may cause irritation of buccal mucosa including swallowing pain, mouth pain, discrete areas of focal reddening, multiple foci of reddening, edema, and/or ulceration. Elderly patients have a greater incidence of adverse effects with orally disintegrating products. Use oral products with caution in patients with renal impairment; orally disintegrating tablets are not recommended in patients with severe renal impairment (CrCl <30 mL/minute) and ESRD. Use oral products with caution in patients with hepatic impairment; dosage adjustments may be necessary with orally disintegrating tablets in patients with mild to moderate hepatic impairment (Child-Pugh class A and B); orally disintegrating tablets are not recommended in patients with severe hepatic impairment (Child-Pugh class C).

Potentially life-threatening serotonin syndrome (SS) has occurred with serotonergic agents (eg, SSRIs, SNRIs) when used in combination with other serotonergic agents (eg, triptans, TCAs, fentanyl, lithium, tramadol, buspirone, St John's wort, tryptophan) or agents that impair metabolism of serotonin (eg, MAO inhibitors intended to treat psychiatric disorders, other MAO inhibitors [ie, linezolid and intravenous methylene blue]). Monitor patients closely for signs of SS such as mental status changes (eg, agitation, hallucinations, delirium, coma); autonomic instability (eg, tachycardia, labile blood pressure, diaphoresis); neuromuscular changes (eg, tremor, rigidity, myoclonus); GI symptoms (eg, nausea, vomiting, diarrhea); and/or seizures. Discontinue treatment (and any concomitant serotonergic agent) immediately if signs/symptoms arise. Potentially significant interactions may exist, requiring dose or frequency adjustment, additional monitoring, and/or selection of alternative therapy. Do not use the orally

disintegrating product concurrently with other selegiline products; wait at least 14 days from discontinuation before initiating treatment with another selegiline dosage form. Transdermal patches may contain conducting metal (eg, aluminum); remove patch prior to MRI. Avoid exposure of application site and surrounding area to direct external heat sources (eg, heating pads, electric blankets, heat lamps, saunas, hot tubs); may increase drug absorption. Some products may contain phenylalanine.

Nonselective MAO inhibition occurs with transdermal delivery and is necessary for antidepressant efficacy. Hypertensive crisis as a result of ingesting tyramine-rich foods is always a concern with nonselective MAO inhibition. Although transdermal delivery minimizes inhibition of MAO-A in the gut, there is limited data with higher transdermal doses; dietary modifications are recommended with doses >6 mg/24 hours. Discontinue therapy immediately if hypertensive crisis occurs. With the oral product, MAO-B selective inhibition should not pose a problem with tyramine-containing products as long as the typical oral doses are employed, however, rare hypertensive reactions have been reported. Increased risk of nonselective MAO inhibition occurs with oral capsule/tablet doses >10 mg/day or orally disintegrating tablet doses >2.5 mg/day.

Abrupt discontinuation or interruption of antidepressant therapy has been associated with a discontinuation syndrome. Symptoms arising may vary with antidepressant however commonly include nausea, vomiting, diarrhea, headaches, lightheadedness, dizziness, diminished appetite, sweating, chills, tremors, paresthesias, fatigue, somnolence, and sleep disturbances (eg, vivid dreams, insomnia). Less common symptoms include electric shock-like sensations, cardiac arrhythmias (more common with tricyclic antidepressants), myalgias, parkinsonism, arthralgias, and balance difficulties. Psychological symptoms may also emerge such as agitation, anxiety, akathisia, panic attacks, irritability, aggressiveness, worsening of mood, dysphoria, mood lability, hyperactivity, mania/hypomania, depersonalization, decreased concentration, slowed thinking, confusion, and memory or concentration difficulties. Greater risks for developing a discontinuation syndrome have been associated with antidepressants with shorter half-lives, longer durations of treatment, and abrupt discontinuation. More severe symptoms have also been associated with MAO inhibitors. For antidepressants of short or intermediate half-lives, symptoms may emerge within 2 to 5 days after treatment discontinuation and last 7 to 14 days (APA, 2010; Fava, 2006; Haddad, 2001; Shelton, 2001; Warner, 2006). According to many MAO inhibitor manufacturers, use within 10 days prior to elective surgery is contraindicated. Currently, an MAO-safe anesthetic technique which excludes the use of meperidine and indirect-acting adrenergic agonists is recommended for patients requiring continued MAO inhibitor therapy (Huyse, 2006).

Adverse Reactions Unless otherwise noted, the percentage of adverse events is reported for the transdermal patch (Note: ODT = orally disintegrating tablet, Oral = capsule/tablet):

>10%:
Central nervous system: Headache (18%; ODT 7%; oral 4%), insomnia (12%; ODT 7%), dizziness (oral 14%; ODT 11%)

Gastrointestinal: Nausea (oral 20%; ODT 11%)

Local: Application site reaction (24%)

1% to 10%:
Cardiovascular: Hypotension (including postural 3% to 10%), palpitation (oral 2%), chest pain (≥1%; ODT 2%), hypertension (≥1%; ODT 3%), peripheral edema (≥1%)

Central nervous system: Pain (ODT 8%; oral 2%), hallucinations (oral 6%; ODT 4%), confusion (oral 6%; ODT 4%), vivid dreams (oral 4%), ataxia (ODT 3%), somnolence (ODT 3%), lethargy (oral 2%), agitation (≥1%), amnesia (≥1%), paresthesia (≥1%), thinking abnormal (≥1%), depression (<1%; ODT 2%)

Dermatologic: Rash (4%), bruising (≥1%; ODT 2%), pruritus (≥1%), acne (≥1%)

Endocrine & metabolic: Weight loss (5%; oral 2%), hypokalemia (ODT 2%), sexual side effects (≤1%)

Gastrointestinal: Diarrhea (9%; ODT 2%; oral 2%), xerostomia (8%; oral 6%; ODT 4%), stomatitis (ODT 5%), abdominal pain (oral 8%), dyspepsia (4%; ODT 5%), dysphagia (ODT 2%), dental caries (ODT 2%), constipation (≥1%; ODT 4%), flatulence (≥1%; ODT 2%), anorexia (≥1%), gastroenteritis (≥1%), taste perversion (≥1%; ODT 2%), vomiting (≥1%; ODT 3%)

Genitourinary: Urinary retention (oral 2%), dysmenorrhea (≥1%), metrorrhagia (≥1%), UTI (≥1%), urinary frequency (≥1%)

Neuromuscular & skeletal: Dyskinesia (ODT 6%), back pain (ODT 5%; oral 2%), ataxia (<1%; ODT 3%), leg cramps (ODT 3%; oral 2%), myalgia (≥1%; ODT 3%), neck pain (≥1%), tremor (<1%; ODT 3%)

Otic: Tinnitus (≥1%)

Respiratory: Rhinitis (ODT 7%), pharyngitis (3%; ODT 4%), sinusitis (3%), cough (≥1%), bronchitis (≥1%), dyspnea (<1%; ODT 3%)

Miscellaneous: Diaphoresis (≥1%)

Oral and/or transdermal patch: <1% or frequency not defined (limited to important or life-threatening): Abnormal liver function tests, alkaline phosphatase increased, appetite increased, arrhythmia, asthma, ataxia, atrial fibrillation, bacterial infection, behavior/mood changes, bilirubinemia, bradycardia, bradykinesia, breast neoplasm (female), breast pain, chorea, circumoral paresthesia, colitis, dehydration, delusions, depersonalization, depression, emotional lability, epistaxis, eructation, euphoria, face edema, fever, fungal infection, gastritis, generalized spasm, glossitis, heat stroke, hematuria (female), hernia, hostility, hypercholesterolemia, hyperesthesia, hyperglycemia, hyperkinesias, hypertonia, hypoglycemic reaction, hyponatremia, impulsive/compulsive behaviors (eg, pathological gambling, hypersexuality, binge eating), kidney calculus (female), lactate dehydrogenase increased, laryngismus, leukocytosis, leukopenia, libido increased, loss of balance, lymphadenopathy, maculopapular rash, manic reaction, melena, MI, migraine, moniliasis, myasthenia, myoclonus, neoplasia, neurosis, osteoporosis, otitis external, palpitation, paranoid reaction, parasitic infection, parosmia, pelvic pain, periodontal abscess, peripheral vascular disorder, pneumonia, polyuria (female), prostatic hyperplasia, rectal hemorrhage, salivation increased, skin hypertrophy, skin benign neoplasm, suicide attempt, syncope, tachycardia, tenosynovitis, tongue edema, twitching, urinary retention, urinary urgency (male and female), urination impaired (male), urticaria, vaginal hemorrhage, vaginal moniliasis, vaginitis, vasodilatation, vertigo, vesiculobullous rash, viral infection, visual field defect

Drug Interactions

Metabolism/Transport Effects Substrate of CYP1A2 (minor), CYP2A6 (minor), CYP2B6 (major), CYP2C8 (minor), CYP2D6 (minor), CYP3A4 (minor); Note: Assignment of Major/Minor substrate status based on clinically relevant drug interaction potential; **Inhibits** CYP1A2 (weak), CYP2A6 (weak), CYP2C19 (weak), CYP2D6 (weak), CYP2E1 (weak), Monoamine Oxidase

Avoid Concomitant Use

Avoid concomitant use of Selegiline with any of the following: Alcohol (Ethyl); Alpha-/Beta-Agonists (Indirect-Acting); Alpha1-Agonists; Amphetamines; Anilidopiperidine Opioids; Antidepressants (Serotonin Reuptake Inhibitor/Antagonist); Apraclonidine; AtoMOXetine; Atropine (Ophthalmic); Bezafibrate; Buprenorphine; BuPROPion; BusPIRone; CarBAMazepine; Cyclobenzaprine; Cyproheptadine; Dapoxetine; Dexmethylphenidate; Dextromethorphan; Diethylpropion; EPINEPHrine (Oral Inhalation); HYDROmorphone; Isometheptene; Levonordefrin; Linezolid; Maprotiline; Meperidine; Mequitazine; Methyldopa; Methylene Blue; Methylphenidate; Mianserin; Mirtazapine; Moclobemide; Morphine (Liposomal); Morphine (Systemic); OXcarbazepine; Oxymorphone; Pholcodine; Pizotifen; Selective Serotonin Reuptake Inhibitors; Serotonin 5-HT1D Receptor Agonists; Serotonin/Norepinephrine Reuptake Inhibitors; Tapentadol; Tetrabenazine; Tetrahydrozoline (Nasal); Tricyclic Antidepressants; Tryptophan

Increased Effect/Toxicity

Selegiline may increase the levels/effects of: Alpha-/Beta-Agonists (Indirect-Acting); Alpha1-Agonists; Amifostine; Amphetamines; Antidepressants (Serotonin Reuptake Inhibitor/Antagonist); Antipsychotic Agents; Antipsychotic Agents (Second Generation [Atypical]); Apraclonidine; ARIPiprazole; AtoMOXetine; Atropine (Ophthalmic); Beta2-Agonists; Betahistine; Bezafibrate; Blood Glucose Lowering Agents; Brimonidine (Ophthalmic); Brimonidine (Topical); BuPROPion; Cyproheptadine; Dexmethylphenidate; Dextromethorphan; Diethylpropion; Domperidone; Doxapram; EPINEPHrine (Nasal); EPINEPHrine (Oral Inhalation); Epinephrine (Racemic); EPINEPHrine (Systemic); Hydrocodone; HYDROmorphone; Hypotension-Associated Agents; Isometheptene; Levonordefrin; Linezolid; Lithium; Meperidine; Mequitazine; Methadone; Methyldopa; Methylene Blue; Methylphenidate; Metoclopramide; Mianserin; Mirtazapine; Moclobemide; Morphine (Liposomal); Morphine (Systemic); Norepinephrine; OxyCODONE; Pizotifen; Reserpine; Selective Serotonin Reuptake Inhibitors; Serotonin 5-HT1D Receptor Agonists; Serotonin Modulators; Serotonin/Norepinephrine Reuptake Inhibitors; ▶

Tetrahydrozoline (Nasal); TiZANidine; Tricyclic Antidepressants

The levels/effects of Selegiline may be increased by: Alcohol (Ethyl); Alfuzosin; Altretamine; Anilidopiperidine Opioids; Antiemetics (5HT3 Antagonists); Antipsychotic Agents; Barbiturates; Blood Pressure Lowering Agents; Brimonidine (Topical); Buprenorphine; BusPIRone; CarBAMazepine; COMT Inhibitors; Contraceptives (Estrogens); Contraceptives (Progestins); Cyclobenzaprine; CYP2B6 Inhibitors (Moderate); Dapoxetine; Diazoxide; Herbs (Hypotensive Properties); Levodopa; Maprotiline; Metaxalone; Molsidomine; Nicorandil; Obinutuzumab; OXcarbazepine; Oxymorphone; Pentoxifylline; Pholcodine; Phosphodiesterase 5 Inhibitors; Prostacyclin Analogues; Quazepam; Tapentadol; Tedizolid; Tetrabenazine; TraMADol; Tryptophan

Decreased Effect

Selegiline may decrease the levels/effects of: Domperidone; Ioflupane I 123; Pipamperone [INT]

The levels/effects of Selegiline may be decreased by: CYP2B6 Inducers (Strong); Cyproheptadine; Dabrafenib; Domperidone; Lumacaftor; Pipamperone [INT]

Food Interactions Concurrent ingestion of foods rich in tyramine, dopamine, tyrosine, phenylalanine, tryptophan, or caffeine may cause sudden and severe high blood pressure (hypertensive crisis or serotonin syndrome). Beverages containing tyramine (eg, hearty red wine and beer) may increase toxic effects. Management: Avoid tyramine-containing foods (aged or matured cheese, air-dried or cured meats including sausages and salamis; fava or broad bean pods, tap/draft beers, Marmite concentrate, sauerkraut, soy sauce, and other soybean condiments). Food's freshness is also an important concern; improperly stored or spoiled food can create an environment in which tyramine concentrations may increase. Avoid foods containing dopamine, tyrosine, phenylalanine, tryptophan, or caffeine. Avoid beverages containing tyramine.

Storage/Stability

Capsule, tablet, transdermal: Store at 20°C to 25°C (68°F to 77°F). Store patch in sealed pouch and apply immediately after removal.

Orally disintegrating tablet: Store at 25°C (77°F); excursions permitted to 15°C to 30°C (59°F to 86°F). Use within 3 months of opening pouch and immediately after opening individual blister.

Mechanism of Action Potent, irreversible inhibitor of monoamine oxidase (MAO). Plasma concentrations achieved via administration of oral dosage forms in recommended doses confer selective inhibition of MAO type B, which plays a major role in the metabolism of dopamine; selegiline may also increase dopaminergic activity by interfering with dopamine reuptake at the synapse. When administered transdermally in recommended doses, selegiline achieves higher blood levels and effectively inhibits both MAO-A and MAO-B, which blocks catabolism of other centrally active biogenic amine neurotransmitters.

Pharmacodynamics/Kinetics

Onset of action: Therapeutic: Oral: Within 1 hour

Duration: Oral: 24 to 72 hours

Absorption:

Orally disintegrating tablet: Rapid; greater bioavailability than capsule/tablet. Food decreases C_{max} and AUC ~60%.

Transdermal: 25% to 30% (of total selegiline content) over 24 hours

Protein binding: ~90%; up to 85% (orally disintegrating tablet)

Metabolism: Hepatic, primarily via CYP2B6, CYP3A4, and CYP2A6 (minor) to active (N-desmethylselegiline, amphetamine, methamphetamine) and inactive metabolites

Half-life elimination: Oral: 10 hours; Transdermal: 18 to 25 hours

Excretion: Urine (primarily metabolites); feces

Dosing

Adult

Parkinson disease:

Capsule/tablet: 5 mg twice daily with breakfast and lunch

Orally disintegrating tablet: Initial: 1.25 mg once daily for at least 6 weeks; may increase to 2.5 mg once daily based on clinical response and tolerability (maximum: 2.5 mg once daily)

Depression: Transdermal: Initial: 6 mg/24 hours once daily; may titrate based on clinical response in increments of 3 mg/day every 2 weeks up to a maximum of 12 mg/24 hours

Discontinuation of therapy: Upon discontinuation of antidepressant therapy, gradually taper the dose to minimize the incidence of withdrawal symptoms and allow for the detection of re-emerging symptoms. Evidence supporting ideal taper rates is limited. APA and NICE guidelines suggest tapering therapy over at least several weeks with consideration to the half-life of the antidepressant; antidepressants with a shorter half-life and MAO inhibitors may need to be tapered more conservatively. In addition for long-term treated patients, WFSBP guidelines recommend tapering over 4-6 months. If intolerable withdrawal symptoms occur following a dose reduction, consider resuming the previously prescribed dose and/or decrease dose at a more gradual rate (APA, 2010; Bauer, 2002; Haddad, 2001; NCCMH, 2010; Schatzberg, 2006; Shelton, 2001; Warner, 2006).

MAO inhibitor recommendations:

Switching to or from an MAO inhibitor intended to treat psychiatric disorders:

Allow 14 days (or a time equal to 4 to 5 half-lives of the drug) to elapse between discontinuing an alternative antidepressant without long half-life metabolites (eg, TCAs, paroxetine, fluvoxamine, venlafaxine) or MAO inhibitor intended to treat psychiatric disorders and initiation of selegiline.

Allow 5 weeks to elapse between discontinuing fluoxetine (with long half-life metabolites) intended to treat psychiatric disorders and initiation of selegiline.

Allow 14 days to elapse between discontinuing selegiline and initiation of an alternative antidepressant or MAO inhibitor intended to treat psychiatric disorders.

Use with other MAO inhibitors (such as linezolid or IV methylene blue):

Do not initiate selegiline in patients receiving linezolid or IV methylene blue; consider other interventions for psychiatric condition.

If urgent treatment with linezolid or IV methylene blue is required in a patient already receiving selegiline and potential benefits outweigh potential risks, discontinue selegiline promptly and administer linezolid or IV methylene blue. Monitor for serotonin syndrome for 2 weeks or until 24 hours after the last dose of linezolid or IV methylene blue, whichever comes first. May resume selegiline 24 hours after the last dose of linezolid or IV methylene blue.

Geriatric

Parkinson disease:

Capsule/tablet: ≤5 mg/day (when combined with levodopa) is recommended by some clinicians to decrease the enhanced dopaminergic side effects (Olanow, 2001)

Orally disintegrating tablet: Refer to adult dosing

Depression: Transdermal: 6 mg/24 hours

Discontinuation of therapy: Refer to adult dosing.

MAO inhibitor recommendations: Refer to adult dosing.

Pediatric ADHD (off-label use): Children and Adolescents: Oral: 5-15 mg/day (Jankovic, 1993)

Discontinuation of therapy: Refer to adult dosing.

MAO inhibitor recommendations: Refer to adult dosing.

Renal Impairment

Oral:

Capsules/tablets: There are no dosage adjustments provided in the manufacturer's labeling (has not been studied). Use with caution.

Orally disintegrating tablet:

Mild to moderate impairment (CrCl 30 to 89 mL/minute): No dosage adjustment necessary.

Severe impairment (CrCl <30 mL/minute): Use is not recommended.

End-stage renal disease: Use is not recommended.

Transdermal:

eGFR ≥15 mL/minute/1.73 m^2: No dosage adjustment necessary.

eGFR <15 mL/minute/1.73 m^2: There are no dosage adjustments provided in the manufacturer's labeling (has not been studied).

ESRD requiring dialysis: There are no dosage adjustments provided in the manufacturer's labeling (has not been studied).

Hepatic Impairment

Oral:

Capsules/tablets: There are no dosage adjustments provided in the manufacturer's labeling (has not been studied). Use with caution.

Orally disintegrating tablet:

Mild to moderate impairment (Child-Pugh class A and B): No dosage adjustment necessary.

Severe impairment (Child-Pugh class C): Use is not recommended.

Transdermal:
Mild to moderate impairment (Child-Pugh class A and B): No dosage adjustment necessary.
Severe impairment (Child-Pugh class C): There are no dosage adjustments provided in the manufacturer's labeling (has not been studied).

Dietary Considerations Avoid or limit tyramine-containing foods/beverages (product and/or dose-dependent). Some examples include aged or matured cheese, air-dried or cured meats (including sausages and salamis), fava or broad bean pods, tap/draft beers, Marmite concentrate, sauerkraut, soy sauce and other soybean condiments. Food's freshness is also an important concern; improperly stored or spoiled food can create an environment where tyramine concentrations may increase.

Transdermal: 9 mg/24 hours or 12 mg/24 hours: Avoid tyramine-rich foods or beverages beginning the first day of treatment or for 2 weeks after discontinuation or dose reduction to 6 mg/24 hours.
Orally disintegrating tablet: Do not take with food or liquid. Some products may contain phenylalanine.

Administration

Oral: Orally disintegrating tablet: Administer in morning before breakfast; place on top of tongue and allow to dissolve. Avoid food or liquid 5 minutes before and after administration.

Topical: Transdermal: Apply to clean, dry, intact skin to the upper torso (below the neck and above the waist), upper thigh, or outer surface of the upper arm. Avoid exposure of application site to external heat source, which may increase the amount of drug absorbed. Do not apply to skin that is hairy, oily, irritated, broken, scarred, or calloused. Apply at the same time each day and rotate application sites. Wash hands with soap and water after handling. Avoid touching the sticky side of the patch. Avoid tyramine-rich foods and beverages beginning on the first day of 9 mg/24 hours or 12 mg/24 hours doses; avoid tyramine-rich foods and beverages for 2 weeks following a dose reduction to 6 mg/24 hours or discontinuation of 9 mg/24 hours or 12 mg/hours. Discard any used or unused patches by folding adhesive ends together, replace in pouch or sealable container and discard properly in trash away from children and pets.

Monitoring Parameters Blood pressure; symptoms of parkinsonism; general mood and behavior (increased anxiety, presence of mania or agitation); suicidal ideation (especially at the beginning of therapy or when doses are increased or decreased); periodic skin examinations

Test Interactions May interfere with urine detection of amphetamine/methamphetamine (false-positive).

Additional Information When adding selegiline to levodopa/carbidopa, the dose of the latter can usually be decreased.

Dosage Forms Excipient information presented when available (limited, particularly for generics); consult specific product labeling.
Capsule, Oral, as hydrochloride:
Eldepryl: 5 mg
Generic: 5 mg
Patch 24 Hour, Transdermal:
Emsam: 6 mg/24 hr (30 ea); 9 mg/24 hr (30 ea); 12 mg/24 hr (30 ea)
Tablet, Oral, as hydrochloride:
Generic: 5 mg
Tablet Dispersible, Oral, as hydrochloride:
Zelapar: 1.25 mg [contains aspartame; grapefruit flavor]
Dosage Forms: Canada Note: Refer to Dosage Forms. Capsule, dispersible tablet, and transdermal patch are not available in Canada.

Selenium (se LEE nee um)

Brand Names: US Aqueous Selenium [OTC]; Oceanic Selenium [OTC]; Se Aspartate [OTC]; Se-100 [OTC]; Se-Plus Protein [OTC]; Selenicaps-200 [OTC]; Selenimin [OTC]; Selenimin-200 [OTC]
Pharmacologic Category Trace Element, Parenteral
Use Trace metal supplement
Dosing
Adult & Geriatric Nutritional supplement:
Oral:
Recommended daily allowance (RDA):
Adults: 55 mcg/day
Pregnancy: 60 mcg/day
Lactation: 70 mcg/day

IV in TPN solutions:
Metabolically stable: 20-40 mcg/day
Deficiency from prolonged TPN support: 100 mcg/day
Pediatric Nutritional supplement:
Oral:
Adequate intake (AI):
1-6 months: 15 mcg/day
7-12 months: 20 mcg/day
Recommended daily allowance (RDA):
1-3 years: 20 mcg/day
4-8 years: 30 mcg/day
9-13 years 40 mcg/day
≥14 years: 55 mcg/day
IV in TPN solutions: 3 mcg/kg/day
Additional Information Complete prescribing information should be consulted for additional detail.
Dosage Forms Excipient information presented when available (limited, particularly for generics); consult specific product labeling.
Capsule, Oral:
Selenicaps-200: 200 mcg [corn free, no artificial color(s), rye free, sugar free, wheat free, yeast free]
Capsule, Oral [preservative free]:
Se-100: 100 mcg [dye free, yeast free]
Liquid, Oral:
Aqueous Selenium: 95 mcg/drop (15 mL) [contains sodium benzoate]
Solution, Intravenous:
Generic: 40 mcg/mL (10 mL)
Tablet, Oral:
Oceanic Selenium: 50 mcg, 200 mcg [animal products free, gelatin free, gluten free, kosher certified, lactose free, no artificial color(s), no artificial flavor(s), starch free, sugar free, yeast free]
Se Aspartate: 50 mcg
Se-Plus Protein: 200 mcg
Selenimin: 125 mcg [corn free, rye free, starch free, sugar free, wheat free]
Selenimin-200: 200 mcg [corn free, rye free, starch free, sugar free, wheat free, yeast free]
Generic: 50 mcg, 200 mcg
Tablet, Oral [preservative free]:
Generic: 50 mcg, 200 mcg
Tablet Extended Release, Oral [preservative free]:
Generic: 200 mcg

Selenium Sulfide (se LEE nee um SUL fide)

Brand Names: US Anti-Dandruff [OTC]; Dandrex [OTC]; Selsun [DSC]; Tersi
Brand Names: Canada Versel®
Pharmacologic Category Topical Skin Product
Use Treatment of itching and flaking of the scalp associated with dandruff, to control scalp seborrheic dermatitis; treatment of tinea versicolor
Dosing
Adult & Geriatric
Dandruff, seborrhea: Topical: Massage 5-10 mL of shampoo into wet scalp, leave on scalp 2-3 minutes, rinse thoroughly. Usually 2 applications each week for 2 weeks will provide control. After this, may repeat at less frequent intervals (eg, once weekly, every 2-4 weeks). Rub foam into affected skin twice daily.
Tinea versicolor: Topical: Apply the 2.5% lotion to affected area and lather with small amounts of water; leave on skin for 10 minutes, then rinse thoroughly; apply every day for 7 days; rub foam into affected skin twice daily
Additional Information Complete prescribing information should be consulted for additional detail.
Dosage Forms Excipient information presented when available (limited, particularly for generics); consult specific product labeling. [DSC] = Discontinued product
Foam, External:
Tersi: 2.25% (70 g) [contains trolamine (triethanolamine)]
Lotion, External:
Selsun: 2.5% (120 mL [DSC])
Generic: 2.5% (118 mL, 120 mL)
Shampoo, External:
Anti-Dandruff: 1% (207 mL) [contains brilliant blue fcf (fd&c blue #1), menthol]
Dandrex: 1% (240 mL)

Selexipag (se LEX i pag)

Brand Names: US Uptravi
Index Terms ACT-293987; NS-304
Pharmacologic Category Prostacyclin; Prostacyclin IP Receptor Agonist; Vasodilator

Use Pulmonary arterial hypertension: Treatment of pulmonary arterial hypertension (PAH) (WHO Group I) to delay disease progression and reduce the risk of hospitalization for PAH

Pregnancy Considerations Adverse events have not been observed in animal reproduction studies. Women with pulmonary arterial hypertension (PAH) are encouraged to avoid pregnancy (McLaughlin 2009).

Breast-Feeding Considerations It is not known if selexipag is excreted in breast milk. Due to the potential for serious adverse reactions in the nursing infant, the manufacturer recommends a decision be made to discontinue nursing or to discontinue the drug, taking into account the importance of treatment to the mother.

Contraindications There are no contraindications listed in the manufacturer's labeling.

Warnings/Precautions If signs of pulmonary edema occur, consider the possibility of associated pulmonary veno-occlusive disease (PVOD). If PVOD is confirmed, discontinue treatment. Use with caution in patients with moderate hepatic impairment (dosage modification is recommended); avoid use in patients with severe hepatic impairment. Potentially significant drug-drug interactions may exist, requiring dose or frequency adjustment, additional monitoring, and/or selection of alternative therapy.

Adverse Reactions

>10%:
Cardiovascular: Flushing (12%)
Central nervous system: Headache (65%)
Dermatologic: Skin rash (11%)
Gastrointestinal: Diarrhea (42%), nausea (33%), vomiting (18%)
Neuromuscular & skeletal: Jaw pain (26%), limb pain (17%), myalgia (16%), arthralgia (11%)

1% to 10%:
Endocrine & metabolic: Hyperthyroidism (1%)
Gastrointestinal: Decreased appetite (6%)
Hematologic & oncologic: Decreased hemoglobin (below 10 g/dL: 9%), anemia (8%)

Drug Interactions

Metabolism/Transport Effects Substrate of BCRP, CYP2C8 (major), CYP3A4 (minor), SLCO1B1, SLCO1B3; **Note:** Assignment of Major/Minor substrate status based on clinically relevant drug interaction potential

Avoid Concomitant Use
Avoid concomitant use of Selexipag with any of the following: CYP2C8 Inhibitors (Strong)

Increased Effect/Toxicity
The levels/effects of Selexipag may be increased by: Abiraterone Acetate; CYP2C8 Inhibitors (Moderate); CYP2C8 Inhibitors (Strong); Deferasirox; Lumacaftor; Mifepristone

Decreased Effect
The levels/effects of Selexipag may be decreased by: Lumacaftor

Storage/Stability Store at 20°C to 25°C (68°F to 77°F); excursions permitted to 15°C and 30°C (59°F and 86°F).

Mechanism of Action Selexipag is a selective prostacyclin IP receptor agonist. Prostacyclin is produced in the endothelial cells and induces vasodilation; also inhibits platelet aggregation. Patients with pulmonary arterial hypertension appear to have a dysregulation in the prostacyclin metabolic pathways (Galie 2013).

Pharmacodynamics/Kinetics

Absorption: Rapid (Kaufmann 2015)
Protein binding: ~99%; to albumin and alpha-1 acid glycoprotein
Metabolism: Hepatic via CYP3A4, CYP2C8, UGT1A3 and UGT2B7; hydrolyzed by carboxylesterase 1 to the active metabolite, ACT-333679, which is a major contributor to the activity (Kaufmann, 2015); the active metabolite is then glucuronidated
Half-life elimination: Terminal: Selexipag: 0.8 to 2.5 hours; Active metabolite: 6.2 to 13.5 hours
Time to peak: Selexipag: 1 to 3 hours; Active metabolite: 3 to 4 hours; Delayed with food
Excretion: Feces (~93%); urine (12%; as inactive metabolites)

Dosing

Adult & Geriatric Pulmonary arterial hypertension: Oral: Initial: 200 mcg twice daily; increase by 200 mcg twice daily, usually at weekly intervals, to the highest tolerated dose (maximum dose: 1,600 mcg twice daily). If a dose is not tolerated, reduce dose to previously tolerated dose.
Missed dose: If dose is missed, take dose as soon as possible unless the next dose is within the next 6 hours. If ≥3 days of treatment are missed, restart at a lower dose and then retitrate.

Renal Impairment
Glomerular filtration rate (estimated) ≥15 mL/minute/1.73 m²: No dosage adjustment necessary.
Dialysis patients or glomerular filtration rate (estimated) <15 mL/minute/1.73 m²: There are no dosage adjustments provided in the manufacturer's labeling (has not been studied).

Hepatic Impairment
Mild hepatic impairment (Child-Pugh class A): No dosage adjustment necessary.
Moderate hepatic impairment (Child-Pugh class B): Initial: 200 mcg once daily; may increase by 200 mcg once daily at weekly intervals, as tolerated.
Severe hepatic impairment (Child-Pugh class C): Avoid use.

Administration Oral: Administer with or without food; tolerability may be improved when taken with food. Swallow tablets whole; do not split, crush, or chew.

Monitoring Parameters Liver function tests. Monitor for signs of pulmonary edema and for improvements in pulmonary function, exercise tolerance, and quality of life.

Product Availability Uptravi: FDA approved December 2015; anticipated availability is early January 2016

Dosage Forms Excipient information presented when available (limited, particularly for generics); consult specific product labeling.
Tablet, Oral:
Uptravi: 200 mcg, 400 mcg, 600 mcg, 800 mcg, 1000 mcg, 1200 mcg, 1400 mcg, 1600 mcg
Tablet Therapy Pack, Oral:
Uptravi: 200 mcg (140s) and 800 mcg (60s) (200 ea)

◆ Seroquel XR (Can) see QUEtiapine on page 1536
◆ Serostim see Somatropin on page 1686

Sertaconazole (ser ta KOE na zole)

Brand Names: US Ertaczo
Index Terms Sertaconazole Nitrate
Pharmacologic Category Antifungal Agent, Imidazole Derivative; Antifungal Agent, Topical
Use Tinea pedis: For the topical treatment of interdigital tinea pedis in immunocompetent patients 12 years of age and older, caused by *Trichophyton rubrum, Trichophyton mentagrophytes,* and *Epidermophyton floccosum.*
Dosing
Adult & Geriatric Tinea pedis: Topical: Apply between toes and to surrounding healthy skin twice daily for 4 weeks
Pediatric Tinea pedis: Topical: Children ≥12 years and Adolescents: Refer to adult dosing.
Additional Information Complete prescribing information should be consulted for additional detail.
Dosage Forms Excipient information presented when available (limited, particularly for generics); consult specific product labeling. [DSC] = Discontinued product
Cream, External, as nitrate:
Ertaczo: 2% (30 g [DSC], 60 g) [contains methylparaben]

◆ Sertaconazole Nitrate see Sertaconazole on page 1649

Sertraline (SER tra leen)

Brand Names: US Zoloft
Brand Names: Canada ACT Sertraline; Apo-Sertraline; Auro-Sertraline; Dom-Sertraline; GD-Sertraline; JAMP-Sertraline; Mar-Sertraline; MINT-Sertraline; Mylan-Sertraline; PHL-Sertraline; PMS-Sertraline; Q-Sertraline; Ran-Sertraline; ratio-Sertraline; Riva-Sertraline; Sandoz-Sertraline; Teva-Sertraline; Zoloft
Index Terms Sertraline Hydrochloride
Pharmacologic Category Antidepressant, Selective Serotonin Reuptake Inhibitor
Use
Major depressive disorder: Treatment of major depressive disorder (MDD) in adults.
Obsessive-compulsive disorder: Treatment of obsessions and compulsions in patients with obsessive-compulsive disorder (OCD).
Panic disorder: Treatment of panic disorder in adults with or without agoraphobia.
Post-traumatic stress disorder: Treatment of post-traumatic stress disorder (PTSD) in adults.
Premenstrual dysphoric disorder: Treatment of premenstrual dysphoric disorder (PMDD) in adults.
Social anxiety disorder: Treatment of social anxiety disorder (social phobia) in adults.
Pregnancy Considerations Adverse events have been observed in animal reproduction studies. Sertraline crosses the human placenta. An increased risk of teratogenic effects, including cardiovascular defects, may be associated with maternal use of sertraline or other SSRIs; however, available information is conflicting. Nonteratogenic effects in the newborn following SSRI/SNRI exposure late in the third trimester include respiratory distress, cyanosis, apnea, seizures, temperature instability, feeding difficulty, vomiting, hypoglycemia, hypo- or hypertonia, hyper-reflexia, jitteriness, irritability, constant crying, and tremor. Symptoms may be due to the toxicity of the SSRIs/SNRIs or a discontinuation syndrome and may be consistent with serotonin syndrome associated with SSRI treatment. Persistent pulmonary hypertension of the newborn (PPHN) has also been reported with SSRI exposure. The long-term effects of *in utero* SSRI exposure on infant development and behavior are not known.

Due to pregnancy-induced physiologic changes, women who are pregnant may require adjusted doses of sertraline to achieve euthymia. The ACOG recommends that therapy with SSRIs or SNRIs during pregnancy be individualized; treatment of depression during pregnancy should incorporate the clinical expertise of the mental health clinician, obstetrician, primary healthcare provider, and pediatrician. According to the American Psychiatric Association (APA), the risks of medication treatment should be weighed against other treatment options and untreated depression. For women who discontinue antidepressant medications during pregnancy and who may be at high risk for postpartum depression, the medications can be restarted following delivery. Treatment algorithms have been developed by the ACOG and the APA for the management of depression in women prior to conception and during pregnancy.

Breast-Feeding Considerations Sertraline and desmethylsertraline are excreted in breast milk. Adverse events have been reported in nursing infants exposed to some SSRIs. The American Academy of Breast-feeding Medicine suggests that sertraline may be considered for the treatment of postpartum depression in appropriately selected women who are nursing. Infants exposed to sertraline while breast-feeding generally receive a low relative dose and serum concentrations are not detectable in most infants. Sertraline concentrations in the hindmilk are higher than in foremilk. If the benefits of the mother receiving the sertraline and breast-feeding outweigh the risks, the mother may consider pumping and discarding breast milk with the feeding 7-9 hours after the daily dose to decrease sertraline exposure to the infant. The long-term effects on development and behavior have not been studied. The manufacturer recommends that caution be exercised when administering sertraline to nursing women. Maternal use of an SSRI during pregnancy may cause delayed milk secretion.
Medication Guide Available Yes
Contraindications
Use of MAOIs intended to treat psychiatric disorders (concurrently or within 14 days of stopping an MAOI or sertraline); concurrent use with pimozide; initiation in patients treated with linezolid or methylene blue IV; hypersensitivity to sertraline or any component of the formulation; concurrent use with disulfiram (oral concentrate only).
Documentation of allergenic cross-reactivity for SSRIs is limited. However, because of similarities in chemical structure and/or pharmacologic actions, the possibility of cross-sensitivity cannot be ruled out with certainty.
Warnings/Precautions [U.S. Boxed Warning]: Antidepressants increase the risk of suicidal thinking and behavior in children, adolescents, and young adults (18 to 24 years of age) with major depressive disorder (MDD) and other psychiatric disorders; consider risk prior to prescribing. Short-term studies did not show an increased risk in patients >24 years of age and showed a decreased risk in patients ≥65 years. Closely monitor patients for clinical worsening, suicidality, or unusual changes in behavior, particularly during the initial 1 to 2 months of therapy or during periods of dosage adjustments (increases or decreases); the patient's family or caregiver should be instructed to closely observe the patient and communicate condition with healthcare provider. A medication guide concerning the use of antidepressants should be dispensed with each prescription. **Sertraline is not FDA approved for use in children with major depressive disorder (MDD). However, it is approved for the treatment of obsessive-compulsive disorder (OCD) in children ≥6 years of age.**

The possibility of a suicide attempt is inherent in major depression and may persist until remission occurs. Use caution in high-risk patients. Worsening depression and severe abrupt suicidality that are not part of the presenting symptoms may require discontinuation or modification of drug therapy. The patient's family or caregiver should be alerted to monitor patients for the emergence of suicidality and associated behaviors (such as agitation, irritability, hostility, impulsivity, and hypomania) and call healthcare provider.

May precipitate a mixed/manic episode in patients at risk for bipolar disorder. Use with caution in patients with a family history of bipolar disorder, mania, or hypomania. Patients presenting with depressive symptoms should be screened for bipolar disorder. **Sertraline is not FDA approved for the treatment of bipolar depression.**

Potentially life-threatening serotonin syndrome (SS) has occurred with serotonergic agents (eg, SSRIs, SNRIs), particularly when used in combination with other serotonergic agents (eg, triptans, TCAs, fentanyl, lithium, tramadol, buspirone, St John's wort, tryptophan) or agents that impair metabolism of serotonin (eg, MAO inhibitors intended to treat psychiatric disorders, other MAO inhibitors [ie, linezolid and intravenous methylene blue]). Discontinue treatment (and any concomitant serotonergic agent) immediately if signs/symptoms arise. Has a very low potential to impair cognitive or motor performance. However, caution patients regarding activities requiring alertness until response to sertraline is known. Does not appear to potentiate the effects of alcohol, however, ethanol use is not advised.

Use caution in patients with a previous seizure disorder or condition predisposing to seizures such as brain damage, alcoholism, or concurrent therapy with other drugs which lower the seizure threshold. May increase the risks associated with electroconvulsive therapy. May cause mild pupillary dilation which in susceptible individuals can lead

to an episode of narrow-angle glaucoma. Consider evaluating patients who have not had an iridectomy for narrow-angle glaucoma risk factors. Use with caution in patients with hepatic dysfunction and in elderly patients. May cause hyponatremia/SIADH (elderly at increased risk); volume depletion (diuretics may increase risk). Use caution in elderly patients; may be potentially inappropriate in patients with a history of falls or fractures, and may cause or exacerbate syndrome of inappropriate antidiuretic hormone secretion or hyponatremia; monitor sodium closely with initiation or dosage adjustments in older adults (Beers Criteria). Sertraline acts as a mild uricosuric; use with caution in patients at risk of uric acid nephropathy. Use with caution in patients where weight loss is undesirable. May cause or exacerbate sexual dysfunction. Potentially significant drug-drug interactions may exist, requiring dose or frequency adjustment, additional monitoring, and/or selection of alternative therapy.

Use oral concentrate formulation with caution in patients with latex sensitivity; dropper dispenser contains dry natural rubber. Some dosage forms may contain polysorbate 80 (also known as Tweens). Hypersensitivity reactions, usually a delayed reaction, have been reported following exposure to pharmaceutical products containing polysorbate 80 in certain individuals (Isaksson, 2002; Lucente 2000; Shelley, 1995). Thrombocytopenia, ascites, pulmonary deterioration, and renal and hepatic failure have been reported in premature neonates after receiving parenteral products containing polysorbate 80 (Alade, 1986; CDC, 1984). See manufacturer's labeling.

Monitor growth in pediatric patients. Given their lower body weight, lower doses are advisable in pediatric patients in order to avoid excessive plasma levels, despite slightly greater metabolism efficiency than adults.

Abrupt discontinuation or interruption of antidepressant therapy has been associated with a discontinuation syndrome. Symptoms arising may vary with antidepressant however commonly include nausea, vomiting, diarrhea, headaches, lightheadedness, dizziness, diminished appetite, sweating, chills, tremors, paresthesias, fatigue, somnolence, and sleep disturbances (eg, vivid dreams, insomnia). Greater risks for developing a discontinuation syndrome have been associated with antidepressants with shorter half-lives, longer durations of treatment, and abrupt discontinuation. For antidepressants of short or intermediate half-lives, symptoms may emerge within 2 to 5 days after treatment discontinuation and last 7 to 14 days (APA, 2010; Fava, 2006; Haddad, 2001; Shelton, 2001; Warner, 2006).

Adverse Reactions

>10%:

Central nervous system: Insomnia (12% to 28%), headache (25%), dizziness (6% to 17%), fatigue (10% to 16%), drowsiness (2% to 15%)

Dermatologic: Diaphoresis (4% to 11%)

Endocrine & metabolic: Decreased libido (1% to 11%)

Gastrointestinal: Nausea (13% to 30%), diarrhea (13% to 24%), xerostomia (6% to 16%), dyspepsia (6% to 13%), anorexia (3% to 11%)

Genitourinary: Ejaculatory disorder (7% to 19%)

Neuromuscular & skeletal: Tremor (<1% to 11%)

1% to 10%:

Cardiovascular: Chest pain (≥1%), palpitations (≥1%)

Central nervous system: Malaise (7% to 9%), pain (3% to 6%), agitation (1% to 6%), nervousness (5%), paresthesia (2%), aggressive behavior (children ≥2%), hypertonia (≥1%), hypoesthesia (≥1%), yawning (≥1%), anxiety

Dermatologic: Skin rash (3%)

Endocrine & metabolic: Weight gain (≥1%)

Gastrointestinal: Constipation (5% to 8%), abdominal pain (6% to 7%), vomiting (4%), increased appetite (≥1%)

Genitourinary: Urinary incontinence (children ≥2%), impotence (≥1%)

Hematologic & oncologic: Purpura (children ≥2%)

Neuromuscular & skeletal: Hyperkinesia (children ≥2%), back pain (≥1%), myalgia (≥1%), weakness (≥1%)

Ophthalmic: Visual disturbance (3%)

Otic: Tinnitus (3%)

Respiratory: Epistaxis (children ≥2%), sinusitis (children ≥2%), rhinitis (≥1%)

Miscellaneous: Fever (children ≥2%)

<1% (Limited to important or life-threatening): Acute renal failure, agranulocytosis, altered platelet function, anaphylactoid reaction, angle-closure glaucoma, aplastic anemia, apnea, ataxia, atrial arrhythmia, atrioventricular block, bradycardia, cerebrovascular spasm, choreoathetosis, colitis, coma, cystitis, depression, diverticulitis, dystonia, edema, esophagitis, extrapyramidal reaction, hematuria, hemoptysis, hepatic failure, hepatitis,

hepatomegaly, hypertension, hypoglycemia, hyponatremia, increased INR, increased serum bilirubin, increased serum transaminases, leukopenia, myocardial infarction, neuroleptic malignant syndrome (Stevens, 2008), oculogyric crisis, orthostatic hypotension, pancreatitis, peptic ulcer bleed, peripheral ischemia, proctitis, prolonged Q-T interval on ECG, pulmonary hypertension, pyelonephritis, rectal hemorrhage, serotonin syndrome, SIADH, Stevens-Johnson syndrome, suicidal ideation, thrombocytopenia, torsades de pointes, urinary frequency, ventricular tachycardia, withdrawal syndrome

Drug Interactions

Metabolism/Transport Effects Substrate of CYP2B6 (minor), CYP2C19 (minor), CYP2C9 (minor), CYP2D6 (minor), CYP3A4 (minor); **Note:** Assignment of Major/Minor substrate status based on clinically relevant drug interaction potential; **Inhibits** CYP1A2 (weak), CYP2B6 (moderate), CYP2C19 (moderate), CYP2C8 (weak), CYP2C9 (weak), CYP2D6 (moderate)

Avoid Concomitant Use

Avoid concomitant use of Sertraline with any of the following: Amodiaquine; Dapoxetine; Disulfiram; Dosulepin; Iobenguane I 123; Linezolid; MAO Inhibitors; Methylene Blue; Pimozide; Thioridazine; Tryptophan; Urokinase

Increased Effect/Toxicity

Sertraline may increase the levels/effects of: Agents with Antiplatelet Properties; Amodiaquine; Anticoagulants; Antidepressants (Serotonin Reuptake Inhibitor/Antagonist); Antipsychotic Agents; Apixaban; ARIPiprazole; Aspirin; Beta-Blockers; Blood Glucose Lowering Agents; Brexpiprazole; BusPIRone; CarBAMazepine; Cilostazol; Citalopram; CloZAPine; Collagenase (Systemic); CYP2B6 Substrates; CYP2C19 Substrates; CYP2D6 Substrates; Dabigatran Etexilate; Deoxycholic Acid; Desmopressin; Dextromethorphan; Dosulepin; DOXOrubicin (Conventional); Edoxaban; Eliglustat; Fesoterodine; Fosphenytoin; Galantamine; Highest Risk QTc-Prolonging Agents; Ibritumomab; Methadone; Methylene Blue; Metoprolol; Moderate Risk QTc-Prolonging Agents; Nebivolol; NSAID (COX-2 Inhibitor); NSAID (Nonselective); Obinutuzumab; Phenytoin; Pimozide; Propafenone; RisperiDONE; Rivaroxaban; Salicylates; Serotonin Modulators; Thiazide Diuretics; Thioridazine; Thrombolytic Agents; TiZANidine; Tositumomab and Iodine I 131 Tositumomab; TraMADol; Tricyclic Antidepressants; Urokinase; Vitamin K Antagonists

The levels/effects of Sertraline may be increased by: Alcohol (Ethyl); Analgesics (Opioid); Antiemetics (5HT3 Antagonists); Antipsychotic Agents; BusPIRone; Cimetidine; CNS Depressants; Dapoxetine; Dasatinib; Disulfiram; Erythromycin (Systemic); Glucosamine; Grapefruit Juice; Herbs (Anticoagulant/Antiplatelet Properties); Ibrutinib; Limaprost; Linezolid; Lithium; MAO Inhibitors; Metaxalone; Metoclopramide; Metyrosine; Mifepristone; Multivitamins/Fluoride (with ADE); Multivitamins/Minerals (with ADEK, Folate, Iron); Multivitamins/Minerals (with AE, No Iron); Omega-3 Fatty Acids; Pentosan Polysulfate Sodium; Pentoxifylline; Prostacyclin Analogues; Tedizolid; Tipranavir; TraMADol; Tryptophan; Vitamin E; Vitamin E (Oral)

Decreased Effect

Sertraline may decrease the levels/effects of: Clopidogrel; Codeine; Cyclophosphamide; Iobenguane I 123; Ioflupane I 123; Tamoxifen; Thyroid Products

The levels/effects of Sertraline may be decreased by: CarBAMazepine; Cyproheptadine; Darunavir; Efavirenz; Fosphenytoin; NSAID (COX-2 Inhibitor); NSAID (Nonselective); Phenytoin

Food Interactions Sertraline average peak serum levels may be increased if taken with food. Management: Administer consistently with or without food.

Preparation for Administration Oral concentrate: Must be diluted before use. **Immediately before administration**, use the dropper provided to measure the required amount of concentrate; mix with 4 ounces (1/2 cup) of water, ginger ale, lemon/lime soda, lemonade, or orange juice only. Do not mix with any other liquids than these. The dose should be taken immediately after mixing; do not mix in advance. A slight haze may appear after mixing; this is normal.

Storage/Stability Store at 25°C (77°F); excursions are permitted between 15°C and 30°C (59°F and 86°F).

Mechanism of Action Antidepressant with selective inhibitory effects on presynaptic serotonin (5-HT) reuptake and only very weak effects on norepinephrine and dopamine neuronal uptake. *In vitro* studies demonstrate no significant affinity for adrenergic, cholinergic, GABA, dopaminergic, histaminergic, serotonergic, or benzodiazepine receptors.

Pharmacodynamics/Kinetics

Onset of action: Depression: The onset of action is within a week, however, individual response varies greatly and full response may not be seen until 8-12 weeks after initiation of treatment.

Absorption: Area under the plasma concentration time curve (AUC) slightly increased and mean peak plasma concentrations (C_{max}) 25% greater when administered with food.

Protein binding: 98%

Metabolism: Hepatic; may involve CYP2C19 and CYP2D6; extensive first pass metabolism; forms metabolite N-desmethylsertraline (APA, 2010)

Bioavailability: Bioavailability of tablets and solution are equivalent

Half-life elimination: Sertraline: 26 hours; N-desmethylsertraline: 66 hours (range: 62-104 hours)

Time to peak, plasma: Sertraline: 4.5-8.4 hours

Excretion: Urine and feces

Dosing

Adult

Depression/obsessive-compulsive disorder: Oral: Initial: 50 mg daily. **Note:** May increase daily dose, at intervals of not less than 1 week, to a maximum of 200 mg daily.

Panic disorder, post-traumatic stress disorder (PTSD), social anxiety disorder: Oral: Initial: 25 mg once daily; increased after 1 week to 50 mg once daily; maximum dose: 200 mg daily

Premenstrual dysphoric disorder (PMDD): Oral: 50 mg daily either daily throughout menstrual cycle **or** limited to the luteal phase of menstrual cycle. Patients not responding to 50 mg daily may benefit from dose increases (50 mg increments per menstrual cycle) up to 150 mg daily when dosing throughout menstrual cycle **or** up to 100 mg day when dosing during luteal phase only. If a 100 mg daily dose has been established with luteal phase dosing, a 50 mg daily titration step for 3 days should be utilized at the beginning of each luteal phase dosing period.

Binge-eating disorder (off-label use): Oral: Initial: 25 mg daily after lunch for 3 days; increase at 25 mg increments every 3 days based on response and tolerability. Usual dose range: 100-200 mg daily. Maximum dose: 200 mg daily (Leombruni P, 2008).

Bulimia nervosa (off-label use): Oral: Initial: 50 mg daily; increase at 50 mg increments each week based on response and tolerability. Maximum dose: 200 mg daily (Milano 2004; Sloan 2003).

Generalized anxiety disorder (GAD) off-label use: Oral: Initial dose: 25 mg once daily for 1 week; increase based on response and tolerability. Maximum dose: 200 mg daily (Ball 2005; Brawman, 2006; Dahl, 2005).

Discontinuation of therapy: Upon discontinuation of antidepressant therapy, gradually taper the dose to minimize the incidence of withdrawal symptoms and allow for the detection of re-emerging symptoms. Evidence supporting ideal taper rates is limited. APA and NICE guidelines suggest tapering therapy over at least several weeks with consideration to the half-life of the antidepressant; antidepressants with a shorter half-life may need to be tapered more conservatively. In addition for long-term treated patients, WFSBP guidelines recommend tapering over 4-6 months. If intolerable withdrawal symptoms occur following a dose reduction, consider resuming the previously prescribed dose and/or decrease dose at a more gradual rate (APA, 2010; Bauer, 2002; Haddad, 2001; NCCMH, 2010; Schatzberg, 2006; Shelton, 2001; Warner, 2006).

MAO inhibitor recommendations:

Switching to or from an MAO inhibitor intended to treat psychiatric disorders:

Allow 14 days to elapse between discontinuing an MAO inhibitor intended to treat psychiatric disorders and initiation of sertraline.

Allow 14 days to elapse between discontinuing sertraline and initiation of an MAO inhibitor intended to treat psychiatric disorders.

Use with other MAO inhibitors (linezolid or IV methylene blue):

Do not initiate sertraline in patients receiving linezolid or IV methylene blue; consider other interventions for psychiatric condition.

If urgent treatment with linezolid or IV methylene blue is required in a patient already receiving sertraline and potential benefits outweigh potential risks, discontinue sertraline promptly and administer linezolid or IV methylene blue. Monitor for serotonin syndrome for 2 weeks or until 24 hours after the last dose of linezolid or IV methylene blue, whichever comes first. May resume sertraline 24 hours after the last dose of linezolid or IV methylene blue.

Pediatric

Obsessive-compulsive disorder (OCD):

Children 6-12 years: Oral: Initial: 25 mg once daily. **Note:** May increase daily dose, at intervals of not less than 1 week, to a maximum of 200 mg daily.

Adolescents 13-17 years: Oral: Initial: 50 mg once daily. **Note:** May increase daily dose, at intervals of not less than 1 week, to a maximum of 200 mg daily.

Depression (off-label use):

Children 6-12 years: Oral: Initial: 12.5-25 mg once daily; titrate dose upwards if clinically needed; may increase by 25-50 mg daily increments at intervals of at least 1 week; mean final dose in 21 children (8-18 years of age) was 100 ± 53 mg or 1.6 mg/kg/day (n=11); range: 25-200 mg daily; maximum dose: 200 mg daily (Dopheide, 2006; Tierney, 1995); avoid excessive dosing

Adolescents 13-17 years: Oral: Initial 25-50 mg once daily; titrate dose upwards if clinically needed; may increase by 50 mg daily increments at intervals of at least 1 week; mean final dose in 13 adolescents was 110 ± 50 mg or about 2 mg/kg/day (McConville, 1996); in another study using a slower titration, the mean dose at week 6 was 93 mg (n=41) and at week 10 was 127 mg (n=34) (Ambrosini, 1999); range: 25-200 mg daily; maximum dose: 200 mg daily (Dopheide, 2006).

Discontinuation of therapy: Refer to adult dosing.

MAO inhibitor recommendations: Refer to adult dosing.

Renal Impairment No dosage adjustment is provided in manufacturer's labeling; however, sertraline pharmacokinetics does not appear to be affected by renal impairment.

Hepatic Impairment No specific dosage adjustment provided in manufacturer's labeling (has not been studied). Use with caution due to extensive hepatic metabolism and risk of increased exposure. A lower dose or less frequent dosing is recommended.

Administration Administer once daily either in the morning or evening; if somnolence is noted, administer at bedtime.

Oral concentrate: Must be diluted immediately before use. **Note:** Use with caution in patients with latex sensitivity; dropper dispenser contains dry natural rubber.

Monitoring Parameters Weight, height, BMI (longitudinal monitoring); mental status for depression, suicide ideation (especially at the beginning of therapy or when doses are increased or decreased), anxiety, social functioning, mania, panic attacks, or other unusual changes in behavior; signs/symptoms of serotonin syndrome.

Test Interactions May interfere with urine detection of benzodiazepines (false-positive)

Dosage Forms Excipient information presented when available (limited, particularly for generics); consult specific product labeling.

Concentrate, Oral:

Zoloft: 20 mg/mL (60 mL) [contains alcohol, usp, menthol]

Generic: 20 mg/mL (60 mL)

Tablet, Oral:

Zoloft: 25 mg [scored; contains fd&c blue #1 aluminum lake, fd&c red #40 aluminum lake, fd&c yellow #10 aluminum lake, polysorbate 80]

Zoloft: 50 mg [scored; contains fd&c blue #2 aluminum lake]

Zoloft: 100 mg [scored; contains polysorbate 80]

Generic: 25 mg, 50 mg, 100 mg

Dosage Forms: Canada Excipient information presented when available (limited, particularly for generics); consult specific product labeling.

Capsule, Oral: 25 mg, 50 mg, 100 mg

◆ Sertraline Hydrochloride see Sertraline on page 1649

◆ Serzone see Nefazodone on page 1265

◆ Setlakin see Ethinyl Estradiol and Levonorgestrel on page 703

Sevelamer (se VEL a mer)

Brand Names: US Renagel; Renvela

Brand Names: Canada Renagel; Renvela

Index Terms Sevelamer Carbonate; Sevelamer Hydrochloride

Pharmacologic Category Phosphate Binder

Use Reduction or control of serum phosphorous in patients with chronic kidney disease on hemodialysis

Pregnancy Considerations Adverse events were observed in animal reproduction studies. Sevelamer is not absorbed systemically; however, it may cause a reduction in the absorption of some vitamins.

Breast-Feeding Considerations Sevelamer is not absorbed systemically; however, it may cause a reduction in the absorption of some vitamins.

Contraindications Bowel obstruction

Warnings/Precautions Use with caution in patients with gastrointestinal disorders including dysphagia, swallowing disorders, severe gastrointestinal motility disorders (including constipation), or major gastrointestinal surgery. May cause reductions in vitamin D, E, K, or folic acid absorption. May bind to some drugs in the gastrointestinal tract and decrease their absorption; when changes in absorption of oral medications may have significant clinical consequences (such as antiarrhythmic and antiseizure medications), these medications should be taken at least 1 hour before or 3 hours after a dose of sevelamer. Tablets should not be taken apart or chewed; broken or crushed tablets will rapidly expand in water/saliva and may be a choking hazard.

Adverse Reactions

>10%:

Endocrine & metabolic: Metabolic acidosis (children: 34% [Pieper, 2006]); adults: Frequency not defined)

Gastrointestinal: Vomiting (22%), nausea (20%), diarrhea (19%), dyspepsia (16%)

1% to 10%:

Endocrine & metabolic: Hypercalcemia (5% to 7%)

Gastrointestinal: Abdominal pain (9%), constipation (8%), flatulence (8%), peritonitis (peritoneal dialysis: 8%)

Postmarketing and/or case reports: Fecal impaction, intestinal obstruction (rare), intestinal perforation (rare)

Drug Interactions

Metabolism/Transport Effects None known.

Avoid Concomitant Use There are no known interactions where it is recommended to avoid concomitant use.

Increased Effect/Toxicity There are no known significant interactions involving an increase in effect.

Decreased Effect

Sevelamer may decrease the levels/effects of: Calcitriol (Systemic); Cholic Acid; CycloSPORINE (Systemic); Levothyroxine; Mycophenolate; Quinolone Antibiotics; Tacrolimus (Systemic)

Food Interactions May cause reductions in vitamin D, E, K, or folic acid absorption. Management: Must be administered with meals. Consider vitamin supplementation.

Preparation for Administration Powder for oral suspension: Mix powder with water prior to administration. The 0.8 g packet should be mixed with 30 mL of water and the 2.4 g packet should be mixed with 60 mL of water (multiple packets may be mixed together using the appropriate amount of water).

Storage/Stability Store at controlled room temperature of 25°C (77°F); excursions permitted to 15°C to 30°C (59°F to 86°F). Protect from moisture.

Mechanism of Action Sevelamer (a polymeric compound) binds phosphate within the intestinal lumen, limiting absorption and decreasing serum phosphate concentrations without altering calcium, aluminum, or bicarbonate concentrations.

Pharmacodynamics/Kinetics

Onset of action: Reduction in serum phosphorus has been demonstrated after 1-2 weeks (Burke, 1997; Chertow, 1997).

Absorption: Not systemically absorbed

Excretion: Feces

Dosing

Adult & Geriatric Note: The dosing of sevelamer carbonate and sevelamer hydrochloride are similar; when switching from one product to another, the same dose (on a mg per mg basis) should be utilized.

Control of serum phosphorous: Oral:

Patients not taking a phosphate binder: 800-1600 mg 3 times/day with meals; the initial dose may be based on serum phosphorous levels:

>5.5 mg/dL to <7.5 mg/dL: 800 mg 3 times/day

≥7.5 mg/dL to <9.0 mg/dL: 1200-1600 mg 3 times/day

≥9.0 mg/dL: 1600 mg 3 times/day

Maintenance dose adjustment based on serum phosphorous concentration (goal range of 3.5-5.5 mg/dL; maximum dose studied was equivalent to 13 g/day [sevelamer hydrochloride] or 14 g/day [sevelamer carbonate]):

>5.5 mg/dL: Increase by 400-800 mg per meal at 2-week intervals

3.5-5.5 mg/dL: Maintain current dose

<3.5 mg/dL: Decrease by 400-800 mg per meal

Dosage adjustment when switching between phosphate-binder products: 667 mg of calcium acetate is equivalent to ~800 mg sevelamer (carbonate or hydrochloride)

Conversion based on dose per meal:

Calcium acetate 667 mg: Convert to 800 mg Renagel/Renvela

Calcium acetate 1334 mg: Convert to 1600 mg as Renagel/Renvela (800 mg tablets x 2) or 1200 mg as Renagel (400 mg tablets x 3)

Calcium acetate 2001 mg: Convert to 2400 mg as Renagel/Renvela (800 mg tablets x 3) or 2000 mg as Renagel (400 mg tablets x 5)

Pediatric Control of serum phosphorous (off-label use): Oral: In a pilot study of 17 pediatric patients aged 11.8 ± 3.7 years on hemodialysis (n=3) or peritoneal dialysis (n=14), initial doses of 121 ± 50 mg/kg/day (4.5 ± 5 g/day) were used. Doses were adjusted based on the serum phosphorus with final doses of 163 ± 46 mg/kg (6.7 ± 2.4 g/day) without any adverse effects (Mahdavi, 2003). In a study of 18 patients aged 0.9-18 years with chronic kidney disease, a mean dose of 140 ± 86 mg/kg/day (5.38 ± 3.24 g/day) resulted in good phosphorus control with minimal adverse effects. Initial doses were based on prior phosphate-binder dose and were adjusted based on the serum phosphorus (Pieper, 2006).

Renal Impairment No dosage adjustment provided in manufacturer's labeling (has not been studied).

Hepatic Impairment No dosage adjustment provided in manufacturer's labeling.

Dietary Considerations Take with meals. Reduced levels of folic acid, and vitamins D, E, and K may occur; most hemodialysis patients in clinical trials received vitamin supplementation.

Administration Must be administered with meals.

Powder for oral suspension: Stir vigorously to suspend mixture just prior to drinking; powder does not dissolve. Drink within 30 minutes of preparing and resuspend just prior to drinking.

Tablets: Swallow whole; do not crush, chew, or break.

Monitoring Parameters

Serum chemistries, including bicarbonate and chloride

Serum calcium and phosphorus: Frequency of measurement may be dependent upon the presence and magnitude of abnormalities, the rate of progression of CKD, and the use of treatments for CKD-mineral and bone disorders (KDIGO, 2009):

CKD stage 3: Every 6-12 months

CKD stage 4: Every 3-6 months

CKD stage 5 and 5D: Every 1-3 months

Periodic 24-hour urinary calcium and phosphorus; magnesium; alkaline phosphatase every 12 months or more frequently in the presence of elevated PTH; creatinine, BUN, albumin; intact parathyroid hormone (iPTH) every 3-12 months depending on CKD severity

Reference Range

Corrected total serum calcium (K/DOQI, 2003): CKD stages 3 and 4: 8.4-10.2 mg/dL (2.1-2.6 mmol/L); CKD stage 5: 8.4-9.5 mg/dL (2.1-2.37 mmol/L); KDIGO guidelines recommend maintaining normal ranges for all stages of CKD (3-5D) (KDIGO, 2009)

Phosphorus (K/DOQI, 2003):

CKD stages 3 and 4: 2.7-4.6 mg/dL (0.87-1.48 mmol/L) (adults); maintain within age-appropriate limits (children)

CKD stage 5 (including those treated with dialysis): 3.5-5.5 mg/dL (1.13-1.78 mmol/L) (children >12 years and adults); 4-6 mg/dL (1.29-1.94 mmol/L) (children 1-12 years)

KDIGO guidelines recommend maintaining normal ranges for CKD stages 3-5 and lowering elevated phosphorus levels toward the normal range for CKD stage 5D (KDIGO, 2009)

Serum calcium-phosphorus product (K/DOQI, 2003): CKD stage 3-5: <55 mg^2/dL^2 (children >12 years and adults); <65 mg2/dL2 (children ≤12 years)

PTH: Whole molecule, immunochemiluminometric assay (ICMA): 1.0-5.2 pmol/L; whole molecule, radioimmunoassay (RIA): 10.0-65.0 pg/mL; whole molecule, immunoradiometric, double antibody (IRMA): 1.0-6.0 pmol/L

Target ranges by stage of chronic kidney disease (KDIGO, 2009): CKD stage 3-5: Optimal iPTH is unknown; maintain normal range (assay-dependent); CKD stage 5D: Maintain iPTH within 2-9 times the upper limit of normal for the assay used

Dosage Forms Excipient information presented when available (limited, particularly for generics); consult specific product labeling. [DSC] = Discontinued product
Packet, Oral, as carbonate:
Renvela: 0.8 g (1 ea, 90 ea); 2.4 g (1 ea, 90 ea) [citrus flavor]
Tablet, Oral, as carbonate:
Renvela: 800 mg
Generic: 800 mg [DSC]
Tablet, Oral, as hydrochloride:
Renagel: 400 mg, 800 mg

- ◆ Sevelamer Carbonate *see* Sevelamer *on page 1651*
- ◆ Sevelamer Hydrochloride *see* Sevelamer *on page 1651*
- ◆ SfRowasa *see* Mesalamine *on page 1151*
- ◆ SGN-35 *see* Brentuximab Vedotin *on page 250*
- ◆ Sharobel *see* Norethindrone *on page 1298*
- ◆ Shingles Vaccine *see* Zoster Vaccine *on page 1944*
- ◆ Shohl's Solution (Modified) *see* Sodium Citrate and Citric Acid *on page 1673*
- ◆ Shopko Athletes Foot [OTC] *see* Clotrimazole (Topical) *on page 428*
- ◆ Shopko Nasal Decongestant [OTC] *see* Pseudoephedrine *on page 1527*
- ◆ Shopko Nasal Decongestant Max [OTC] *see* Pseudoephedrine *on page 1527*
- ◆ Shur-Seal Contraceptive [OTC] *see* Nonoxynol 9 *on page 1296*
- ◆ Sig-Enalapril (Can) *see* Enalapril *on page 636*
- ◆ Signifor *see* Pasireotide *on page 1402*
- ◆ Signifor LAR *see* Pasireotide *on page 1402*
- ◆ Silace [OTC] *see* Docusate *on page 578*
- ◆ Siladryl Allergy [OTC] *see* DiphenhydrAMINE (Systemic) *on page 561*
- ◆ Silapap Children's [OTC] *see* Acetaminophen *on page 25*
- ◆ Silapap Infant's [OTC] *see* Acetaminophen *on page 25*

Sildenafil (sil DEN a fil)

Brand Names: US Revatio; Viagra
Brand Names: Canada ACT-Sildenafil; Apo-Sildenafil; GD-Sildenafil; Jamp-Sildenafil; M-Sildenafil; Mint-Sildenafil; MYL-Sildenafil; PMS-Sildenafil; RAN-Sildenafil; ratio-Sildenafil R; Revatio; Sandoz-Sildenafil; Teva-Sildenafil; Viagra
Index Terms Sildenafil Citrate; UK92480
Pharmacologic Category Phosphodiesterase-5 Enzyme Inhibitor
Use
Pulmonary arterial hypertension: Revatio: Treatment of pulmonary arterial hypertension (PAH) (WHO Group I; efficacy established predominately in patients with WHO/NYHA functional class II and III) in adults to improve exercise ability and delay clinical worsening.
Note: Based on the 2007 American College of Chest Physicians (ACCP) Evidence-Based Clinical Practice Guidelines on Medical Therapy for Pulmonary Hypertension, in patients with pulmonary arterial hypertension (NYHA functional class II and III) who are not candidates for, or who have failed, calcium channel blocker therapy, sildenafil is an effective and recommended treatment option in the management of this condition. The level of evidence for NYHA functional class IV is low and therefore cannot be recommended for routine use in this population. The 2009 American College of Cardiology Foundation/American Heart Association (ACCF/AHA) Expert Consensus Document on Pulmonary Hypertension and the 5th World Symposium on Pulmonary Hypertension (WSPH) suggests the use of oral phosphodiesterase type 5 inhibitors (when appropriate) in patients with WHO Group I pulmonary arterial hypertension (ie, idiopathic PAH and PAH related to connective tissue disease or anorexigens) as an alternative to an endothelin receptor antagonist in lower risk (WHO functional class II and III) patients who did not have a positive acute vasodilator testing. First-line therapy in patients with higher risk (WHO functional class IV) continues to be intravenous prostacyclin therapy; however, if the patient is not a candidate for intravenous prostacyclin therapy, the use of other therapies including phosphodiesterase-5 inhibitors should be considered (ACCF/AHA [McLaughlin, 2009]; ACCP [Badesch, 2007]; WSPH [Gaile, 2013]).

Erectile dysfunction: Viagra: Treatment of erectile dysfunction (ED)

Pregnancy Considerations Adverse events were not observed in animal reproduction studies. Information related to the use of sildenafil for the treatment of pulmonary arterial hypertension (PAH) in pregnant women is limited (Hsu, 2011). Current guidelines recommend that women with PAH use effective contraception and avoid pregnancy (Badesch, 2007; McLaughlin, 2009). Less than 0.001% appears in the semen.
Breast-Feeding Considerations It is not known if sildenafil is excreted in breast milk. The manufacturer recommends that caution be exercised when administering sildenafil to nursing women.
Contraindications
Hypersensitivity to sildenafil or any component of the formulation; concurrent use (regularly/intermittently) of organic nitrates in any form (eg, nitroglycerin, isosorbide dinitrate); concomitant use of riociguat (a guanylate cyclase stimulator).
According to the manufacturers of protease inhibitors (atazanavir, darunavir, fosamprenavir, indinavir, lopinavir/ritonavir, nelfinavir, ritonavir, saquinavir, tipranavir): Concurrent use with a protease inhibitor regimen when sildenafil is used for pulmonary artery hypertension (eg, Revatio).
Canadian labeling: Additional contraindications (not in US labeling): Prior episode of non-arteritic anterior ischemic optic neuropathy (NAION).
Warnings/Precautions Decreases in blood pressure may occur due to vasodilator effects; use with caution in patients with left ventricular outflow obstruction (aortic stenosis, hypertrophic obstructive cardiomyopathy), those on antihypertensive therapy, with resting hypotension (BP <90/50 mm Hg), fluid depletion, or autonomic dysfunction; may be more sensitive to hypotensive actions. Patients should be hemodynamically stable prior to initiating therapy at the lowest possible dose. Use with caution in patients with uncontrolled hypertension (>170/110 mm Hg); life-threatening arrhythmias, stroke or MI within the last 6 months; cardiac failure or coronary artery disease causing unstable angina; safety and efficacy have not been studied in these patients. There is a degree of cardiac risk associated with sexual activity; therefore, physicians should consider the cardiovascular status of their patients prior to initiating any treatment for erectile dysfunction. If pulmonary edema occurs when treating pulmonary arterial hypertension (PAH), consider the possibility of pulmonary veno-occlusive disease (PVOD); continued use is not recommended in patient with PVOD. Substantial consumption of ethanol may increase the risk of hypotension and orthostasis. Lower ethanol consumption has not been associated with significant changes in blood pressure or increase in orthostatic symptoms. Have patients avoid or limit ethanol consumption.

Sildenafil should be used with caution in patients with anatomical deformation of the penis (angulation, cavernosal fibrosis, or Peyronie's disease) and in patients who have conditions which may predispose them to priapism (sickle cell anemia, multiple myeloma, leukemia). All patients should be instructed to seek medical attention if erection persists >4 hours. Painful erection >6 hours in duration has been reported rarely.

Vision loss, including permanent loss of vision, may occur and be a sign of nonarteritic anterior ischemic optic neuropathy (NAION). Risk may be increased with history of vision loss. Other risk factors for NAION include low cup-to-disc ratio ("crowded disc"), coronary artery disease, diabetes, hypertension, hyperlipidemia, smoking, and age >50 years. The Canadian labeling contraindicates use in patients with a prior episode of NAION. May cause dose-related impairment of color discrimination. Use caution in patients with retinitis pigmentosa; a minority have genetic disorders of retinal phosphodiesterases (no safety information available). Sudden decrease or loss of hearing has been reported; hearing changes may be accompanied by tinnitus and dizziness. A direct relationship between therapy and vision or hearing loss has not been determined.

The potential underlying causes of erectile dysfunction should be evaluated prior to treatment. Potentially significant drug-drug interactions may exist, requiring dose or frequency adjustment, additional monitoring, and/or selection of alternative therapy. Use of sildenafil is contraindicated in patients currently taking nitrate preparations. However, when nitrate administration becomes medically necessary, the ACCF/AHA 2013 guidelines on treatment of ST-segment elevation MI and the ACCF/AHA 2012 guidelines on treatment of unstable angina/non ST-segment elevation MI support administration of nitrates only if 24 hours have elapsed after use of sildenafil (ACCF/AHA [Anderson, 2013]; ACCF/AHA [O'Gara,

◀ 2013]). Hypersensitivity reactions, including anaphylactic reaction and anaphylactic shock, have been reported.

Avoid abrupt discontinuation, especially if used as monotherapy in PAH as exacerbation may occur. Use caution in patients with bleeding disorders or with active peptic ulcer disease; safety has not been established. Efficacy has not be established for treatment of pulmonary hypertension associated with sickle cell disease. Use with caution in the elderly, or patients with renal or hepatic dysfunction; dose adjustment may be needed. Use of Revatio, especially chronic use, is not recommended in children. After 2 years of treatment, increased mortality was seen in a long-term (median treatment exposure: 4.6 years) study at higher doses (20-80 mg [depending upon weight] 3 times/day) (Barst, 2012a; Barst, 2012b).

Benzyl alcohol and derivatives: Some dosage forms may contain sodium benzoate/benzoic acid; benzoic acid (benzoate) is a metabolite of benzyl alcohol; large amounts of benzyl alcohol (≥99 mg/kg/day) have been associated with a potentially fatal toxicity ("gasping syndrome") in neonates; the "gasping syndrome" consists of metabolic acidosis, respiratory distress, gasping respirations, CNS dysfunction (including convulsions, intracranial hemorrhage), hypotension, and cardiovascular collapse (AAP ["Inactive" 1997]; CDC, 1982); some data suggests that benzoate displaces bilirubin from protein binding sites (Ahlfors, 2001); avoid or use dosage forms containing benzyl alcohol derivative with caution in neonates. See manufacturer's labeling. Oral suspensions may be available in multiple concentrations (commercially available: 10 mg/mL; extemporaneous preparation: 2.5 mg/mL); dosing should be presented in mg of sildenafil; use extra precaution when verifying product formulation and calculation of dose volumes. The 2 mL oral syringe provided by the manufacturer only provides measurements for fixed doses of 5 mg and 20 mg; for patients not receiving either of these fixed doses, an appropriate-size calibrated oral syringe will need to be dispensed.

Adverse Reactions Based upon normal doses for either indication or route. (Adverse effects such as flushing, diarrhea, myalgia, and visual disturbances may be increased with adult doses >100 mg/24 hours.)

>10%:
Cardiovascular: Flushing (10% to 19%)
Central nervous system: Headache (16% to 46%)
Gastrointestinal: Dyspepsia (3% to 17%; dose related)
Ophthalmic: Visual disturbance (2% to 11%; including vision color changes, blurred vision, and photophobia; dose related)
Respiratory: Epistaxis (9% to 13%)

2% to 10%:
Central nervous system: Insomnia (≤7%), dizziness (2% to 4%), paresthesia (≤3%)
Dermatologic: Erythema (6%), skin rash (1% to 3%)
Gastrointestinal: Diarrhea (3% to 9%), gastritis (≤3%), nausea (2% to 3%)
Genitourinary: Urinary tract infection (3%)
Hepatic: Increased liver enzymes (2% to 10%)
Neuromuscular & skeletal: Myalgia (2% to 7%), back pain (3% to 4%)
Respiratory: Nasal congestion (4% to 9%), exacerbation of dyspnea (≤7%), nasal congestion (4%), rhinitis (4%), sinusitis (3%)
Miscellaneous: Fever (6%)

<2% (Limited to important or life-threatening): Abnormal hepatic function tests, absent reflexes, amnesia (transient global), anemia, anorgasmia, anterior chamber eye hemorrhage, anterior ischemic optic neuropathy, arthritis, auditory impairment, basal cell carcinoma (Loeb 2015), breast hypertrophy, burning sensation of eyes, cardiac failure, cataract, cerebrovascular hemorrhage, colitis, cystitis, depression, diaphoresis, diplopia, dry eye syndrome, dysphagia, ECG abnormality, ejaculatory disorder, exfoliative dermatitis, falling, gastroenteritis, genital edema, gingivitis, glossitis, gout, herpes simplex infection, hyperglycemia, hypernatremia, hypersensitivity reaction, hypertension, hypertonia, hypoglycemia, increased bronchial secretions, increased intraocular pressure, ischemic heart disease, laryngitis, leukopenia, malignant melanoma (Li 2014; Loeb 2015), migraine, myasthenia, mydriasis, myocardial infarction, neuralgia, neuropathy, orthostatic hypotension, otalgia, peripheral edema, pharyngitis, photophobia, priapism, prolonged erection, pulmonary hemorrhage, rectal hemorrhage, retinal edema, retinal hemorrhage, retinal vascular disease, rupture of tendon, seizure, severe sickle cell crisis (vaso-occlusive crisis in patients with pulmonary hypertension

associated with sickle cell disease), skin photosensitivity, stomatitis, syncope, synovitis, tachycardia, transient ischemic attacks, unstable diabetes, urinary incontinence, ventricular arrhythmia, vitreous detachment, vitreous traction

Drug Interactions

Metabolism/Transport Effects Substrate of CYP1A2 (minor), CYP2C19 (minor), CYP2C9 (minor), CYP2D6 (minor), CYP2E1 (minor), CYP3A4 (major); **Note:** Assignment of Major/Minor substrate status based on clinically relevant drug interaction potential; **Inhibits** CYP2C9 (weak)

Avoid Concomitant Use
Avoid concomitant use of Sildenafil with any of the following: Alprostadil; Amyl Nitrite; Boceprevir; Conivaptan; Dapoxetine; Fusidic Acid (Systemic); Idelalisib; Molsidomine; Phosphodiesterase 5 Inhibitors; Riociguat; Telaprevir; Vasodilators (Organic Nitrates)

Increased Effect/Toxicity
Sildenafil may increase the levels/effects of: Alpha1-Blockers; Alprostadil; Amyl Nitrite; Blood Pressure Lowering Agents; Bosentan; Phosphodiesterase 5 Inhibitors; Riociguat; Vasodilators (Organic Nitrates)

The levels/effects of Sildenafil may be increased by: Alcohol (Ethyl); Aprepitant; Boceprevir; Conivaptan; CYP3A4 Inhibitors (Moderate); CYP3A4 Inhibitors (Strong); Dapoxetine; Dasatinib; Erythromycin (Systemic); Fluconazole; Fosaprepitant; Fusidic Acid (Systemic); Idelalisib; Itraconazole; Ivacaftor; Ketoconazole (Systemic); Lorcaserin; Luliconazole; Mifepristone; Molsidomine; Netupitant; Osimertinib; Palbociclib; Posaconazole; Protease Inhibitors; Sapropterin; Simeprevir; Stiripentol; Telaprevir; Voriconazole

Decreased Effect
The levels/effects of Sildenafil may be decreased by: Bosentan; CYP3A4 Inducers (Moderate); CYP3A4 Inducers (Strong); Dabrafenib; Deferasirox; Enzalutamide; Etravirine; Mitotane; Osimertinib; Siltuximab; St Johns Wort; Tocilizumab

Food Interactions Grapefruit juice may increase serum levels/toxicity of sildenafil. Management: Avoid grapefruit juice.

Storage/Stability
Tablets/injection: Store at 20°C to 25°C (68°F to 77°F); excursions are permitted to 15°C to 30°C (59°F to 86°F).
Oral suspension: Store unreconstituted powder below 30°C (86°F); protect from moisture. Store reconstituted oral suspension below 30°C (86°F) or at 2°C to 8°C (36°F to 46°F). Do not freeze. Discard unused Revatio oral suspension after 60 days.

Mechanism of Action
Erectile dysfunction: Does not directly cause penile erections, but affects the response to sexual stimulation. The physiologic mechanism of erection of the penis involves release of nitric oxide (NO) in the corpus cavernosum during sexual stimulation. NO then activates the enzyme guanylate cyclase, which results in increased levels of cyclic guanosine monophosphate (cGMP), producing smooth muscle relaxation and inflow of blood to the corpus cavernosum. Sildenafil enhances the effect of NO by inhibiting phosphodiesterase type 5 (PDE-5), which is responsible for degradation of cGMP in the corpus cavernosum; when sexual stimulation causes local release of NO, inhibition of PDE-5 by sildenafil causes increased levels of cGMP in the corpus cavernosum, resulting in smooth muscle relaxation and inflow of blood to the corpus cavernosum; at recommended doses, it has no effect in the absence of sexual stimulation.
Pulmonary arterial hypertension (PAH): Inhibits phosphodiesterase type 5 (PDE-5) in smooth muscle of pulmonary vasculature where PDE-5 is responsible for the degradation of cyclic guanosine monophosphate (cGMP). Increased cGMP concentration results in pulmonary vasculature relaxation; vasodilation in the pulmonary bed and the systemic circulation (to a lesser degree) may occur.

Pharmacodynamics/Kinetics
Onset of action: ~60 minutes
Duration: 2-4 hours
Absorption: Rapid; slower with a high-fat meal
Distribution: V_{dss}: 105 L
Protein binding, plasma: ~96%
Metabolism: Hepatic via CYP3A4 (major) and CYP2C9 (minor route); forms N-desmethyl metabolite (active)
Bioavailability: 41% (25% to 63%)

Half-life elimination: ~4 hours; the elderly and those with severe renal impairment have reduced clearance of sildenafil and its active N-desmethyl metabolite

Time to peak: 30-120 minutes; delayed by 60 minutes with a high-fat meal

Excretion: Feces (~80%); urine (~13%)

Dosing

Adult

Erectile dysfunction (Viagra): Oral: Usual dose: 50 mg once daily 1 hour (range: 30 minutes to 4 hours) before sexual activity as needed; dosing range: 25 to 100 mg once daily; maximum recommended dose: 100 mg once daily.

Pulmonary arterial hypertension (PAH) (Revatio):
IV: 2.5 mg or 10 mg 3 times daily
Oral: 5 mg or 20 mg 3 times daily, taken 4 to 6 hours apart; maximum recommended dose: 20 mg 3 times daily

Dosage considerations for patients stable on alpha-blockers: Viagra: Initial: 25 mg

Dosage adjustment for concomitant use of potent CYP34A inhibitors:
Revatio:
Strong CYP3A inhibitors (eg, itraconazole, ketoconazole): Not recommended
Protease inhibitors: Concurrent use is contraindicated
Viagra:
Strong CYP3A inhibitors (eg, itraconazole, ketoconazole) or erythromycin: Starting dose of 25 mg should be considered
Protease inhibitors: Maximum sildenafil dose: 25 mg every 48 hours

Geriatric Elderly >65 years: Use with caution.
Erectile dysfunction (Viagra): Starting dose of 25 mg should be considered.
PAH (Revatio): Refer to adult dosing.

Renal Impairment
CrCl ≥30 mL/minute:
Revatio: No dosage adjustment necessary.
Viagra: No dosage adjustment recommended.
CrCl <30 mL/minute:
Revatio: No dosage adjustment necessary.
Viagra: Starting dose of 25 mg should be considered.

Hepatic Impairment
Mild to moderate impairment (Child-Pugh classes A and B):
Revatio: No dosage adjustment necessary.
Viagra: Starting dose of 25 mg should be considered.
Severe impairment (Child-Pugh class C):
Revatio: There are no dosage adjustments provided in manufacturer's labeling (has not been studied).
Viagra: Starting dose of 25 mg should be considered.

Dietary Considerations Avoid grapefruit juice.

Administration

Revatio: Administer doses at least 4 to 6 hours apart. Shake oral suspension well for ≥10 seconds before administering dose; do not mix with any other medication or additional flavoring agent. Administer injection as an IV bolus.

Viagra: Administer with or without food 30 minutes to 4 hours before sexual activity

Monitoring Parameters PAH: Monitor blood pressure and pulse when used concurrently with medications that lower blood pressure; monitor for pulmonary edema

Additional Information Sildenafil is ~10 times more selective for PDE-5 as compared to PDE6. This enzyme is found in the retina and is involved in phototransduction. At higher plasma levels, interference with PDE6 is believed to be the basis for changes in color vision noted in some patients.

Dosage Forms Excipient information presented when available (limited, particularly for generics); consult specific product labeling.
Solution, Intravenous:
Revatio: 10 mg/12.5 mL (12.5 mL)
Generic: 10 mg/12.5 mL (12.5 mL)
Suspension Reconstituted, Oral:
Revatio: 10 mg/mL (112 mL) [contains sodium benzoate]
Tablet, Oral:
Revatio: 20 mg
Viagra: 25 mg, 50 mg, 100 mg [contains fd&c blue #2 aluminum lake]
Generic: 20 mg

Extemporaneous Preparations Note: Commercial oral suspension is available (10 mg/mL)

A 2.5 mg/mL sildenafil citrate oral suspension may be made with tablets and either a 1:1 mixture of methylcellulose 1% and simple syrup NF or a 1:1 mixture of Ora-Sweet and Ora-Plus. Crush thirty sildenafil 25 mg tablets (Viagra) in a mortar and reduce to a fine powder. Add small portions of chosen vehicle and mix to a uniform paste; mix while adding vehicle in incremental proportions to **almost** 300 mL; transfer to a graduated cylinder, rinse mortar with vehicle, and add quantity of vehicle sufficient to make 300 mL. Store in amber plastic bottles and label "shake well". Stable for 90 days at room temperature or refrigerated.

Nahata MC, Morosco RS, and Brady MT, "Extemporaneous Sildenafil Citrate Oral Suspensions for the Treatment of Pulmonary Hypertension in Children," *Am J Health-Syst Pharm*, 2006, 63(3):254-7.

◆ Sildenafil Citrate *see* Sildenafil *on page 1653*

◆ Silenor *see* Doxepin (Systemic) *on page 590*

◆ Silexin [OTC] *see* Guaifenesin and Dextromethorphan *on page 861*

◆ Silkis (Can) *see* Calcitriol *on page 284*

Silodosin (SI lo doe sin)

Brand Names: US Rapaflo
Brand Names: Canada Rapaflo®
Index Terms KMD 3213
Pharmacologic Category Alpha₁ Blocker
Use Treatment of signs and symptoms of benign prostatic hyperplasia (BPH)

Dosing

Adult & Geriatric BPH: Oral: 8 mg once daily with a meal

Renal Impairment
CrCl >50 mL/minute: No dosage adjustment necessary.
CrCl 30-50 mL/minute: 4 mg once daily.
CrCl <30 mL/minute: Use is contraindicated.

Hepatic Impairment
Mild-to-moderate impairment (Child-Pugh class A or B): No dosage adjustment necessary.
Severe impairment (Child-Pugh class C): Use is contraindicated (has not been studied).

Additional Information Complete prescribing information should be consulted for additional detail.

Dosage Forms Excipient information presented when available (limited, particularly for generics); consult specific product labeling.
Capsule, Oral:
Rapaflo: 4 mg, 8 mg

◆ Silphen Cough [OTC] *see* DiphenhydrAMINE (Systemic) *on page 561*

◆ Siltussin DAS [OTC] *see* GuaiFENesin *on page 860*

◆ Siltussin DM [OTC] *see* Guaifenesin and Dextromethorphan *on page 861*

◆ Siltussin DM DAS [OTC] *see* Guaifenesin and Dextromethorphan *on page 861*

◆ Siltussin SA [OTC] *see* GuaiFENesin *on page 860*

Siltuximab (sil TUX i mab)

Brand Names: US Sylvant
Brand Names: Canada Sylvant
Index Terms CNTO 328
Pharmacologic Category Antineoplastic Agent, Monoclonal Antibody; Interleukin-6 Receptor Antagonist
Use Castleman disease: Treatment of multicentric Castleman disease (MCD) in patients who are human immunodeficiency virus (HIV) negative and human herpesvirus-8 (HHV-8) negative

Limitations of use: Has not been studied in patients with MCD who are HIV positive or HHV-8 positive because in a nonclinical study, siltuximab did not bind to virally produced IL-6

Pregnancy Considerations Adverse events were not observed in animal reproduction studies. However, decreased globulin levels were detected in the pregnant animals and their offspring. Infants born to pregnant women treated with siltuximab may be at increased risk for infection. Use during pregnancy only if the potential benefit outweighs the possible risk to the fetus. Women of childbearing potential should use effective contraception during and for 3 months following treatment discontinuation.

Breast-Feeding Considerations It is not known if siltuximab is excreted in breast milk. Because many immunoglobulins are excreted in breast milk and the potential for adverse reactions in the nursing infant exists, the manufacturer recommends a decision be made to discontinue nursing or to discontinue the drug, taking into account the importance of treatment to the mother.

Contraindications Severe hypersensitivity to siltuximab or any component of the formulation

Warnings/Precautions Discontinue infusion immediately (and permanently) if signs of anaphylaxis occur; do not reinitiate therapy. Discontinue in patients with severe infusion reaction, severe allergic reactions, or cytokine release syndromes. If a mild to moderate infusion reaction develops, temporarily discontinue the infusion; if the reaction resolves, may reinitiate at a lower infusion rate. Consider premedication with acetaminophen, antihistamines, and corticosteroids. If infusion-related reactions recur despite appropriate premedication and infusion rate reduction, discontinue therapy. Administer in a setting equipped to provide resuscitation equipment; medications for the treatment of hypersensitivity reactions (eg, bronchodilators, epinephrine, antihistamines, and corticosteroids) should be readily available. Siltuximab may mask signs and symptoms of infection, including signs of acute inflammation (eg, fever, C-reactive protein elevation). Do not administer to patients with severe infections (until infection resolves); monitor closely for infections and initiate appropriate anti-infective therapy if needed. If infection develops, withhold therapy until resolved. Siltuximab administration may result in elevated hemoglobin levels in patients with multicentric Castleman disease; monitor blood counts prior to each dose for the first 12 months and every 3 dosing cycles thereafter, or as clinically necessary. May require therapy interruption. Gastrointestinal perforation has been observed in clinical trials. Use with caution in patients at risk for perforation; promptly evaluate concerning symptoms. Do not administer live vaccines to patients receiving siltuximab; IL-6 inhibition may interfere with immune response to vaccination. Approved for use only in patients who are HIV negative and HHV-8 negative. Siltuximab was not studied in patients positive for these disease states due to the lack of drug binding to virally produced IL-6 in a nonclinical study. Potentially significant drug-drug interactions may exist, requiring dose or frequency adjustment, additional monitoring, and/or selection of alternative therapy.

Adverse Reactions

\>10%:

Cardiovascular: Peripheral edema (16%)

Central nervous system: Fatigue (21%; long-term exposure)

Dermatologic: Pruritus (28%), skin rash (28%)

Endocrine & metabolic: Weight gain (19%), hyperuricemia (11%)

Gastrointestinal: Diarrhea (32%; long-term exposure), abdominal pain (12%)

Neuromuscular & skeletal: Arthralgia (21%; long-term exposure), limb pain (21%; long-term exposure)

Respiratory: Upper respiratory tract infection (26%; long-term exposure: 63%)

1% to 10%:

Cardiovascular: Hypotension (4% to 6%; grades 3/4: 2% [anaphylactic reaction])

Central nervous system: Headache (8%)

Dermatologic: Eczema (4%), psoriasis (4%), skin hyperpigmentation (4%), xeroderma (4%)

Endocrine & metabolic: Hypertriglyceridemia (8%), dehydration (4%), hypercholesterolemia (4%)

Gastrointestinal: Constipation (8%), decreased appetite (4%)

Hematologic & oncologic: Thrombocytopenia (9%)

Renal: Renal insufficiency (8%)

Respiratory: Lower respiratory tract infection (8%), oropharyngeal pain (8%)

Miscellaneous: Infusion related reaction (5%)

<1% (Limited to important or life-threatening): Anaphylaxis

Drug Interactions

Metabolism/Transport Effects None known.

Avoid Concomitant Use

Avoid concomitant use of Siltuximab with any of the following: BCG (Intravesical); Belimumab; Natalizumab; Pimecrolimus; Tacrolimus (Topical); Tofacitinib; Vaccines (Live)

Increased Effect/Toxicity

Siltuximab may increase the levels/effects of: Belimumab; Fingolimod; Leflunomide; Natalizumab; Tofacitinib; Vaccines (Live)

The levels/effects of Siltuximab may be increased by: Denosumab; Pimecrolimus; Roflumilast; Tacrolimus (Topical); Trastuzumab

Decreased Effect

Siltuximab may decrease the levels/effects of: BCG (Intravesical); Coccidioides immitis Skin Test; CYP3A4 Substrates; Sipuleucel-T; Vaccines (Inactivated); Vaccines (Live)

The levels/effects of Siltuximab may be decreased by: Echinacea

Preparation for Administration Allow intact vials to come to room temperature (~30 minutes) and remain at room temperature for the duration of preparation. Reconstitute with 5.2 mL (100 mg vial) or 20 mL (400 mg vial) SWFI to a final concentration of 20 mg/mL; gently swirl to fully dissolve powder (usually takes <60 minutes). Do not shake or swirl vigorously. Must further dilute within 2 hours to 250 mL with D5W (infusion bag must be made of polyvinyl chloride [PVC], polyolefin [PO], polypropylene [PP], or polyethylene [PE], or PE bottles may be used. After all solids are completely dissolved, remove a volume equal to the total calculated dose volume of reconstituted siltuximab from the bag of D5W; slowly add the appropriate volume of reconstituted siltuximab solution to the infusion bag and gently invert to mix. Complete infusion within 4 hours of dilution of the reconstituted solution to the infusion bag.

Storage/Stability Store intact vials at 2°C to 8°C (36°F to 46°F); protect from light. Reconstituted solution should be further diluted for infusion within 2 hours; complete infusion within 4 hours of dilution of the reconstituted solution to the infusion container. Discard any unused portion of the reconstituted solution or solution diluted for infusion.

Mechanism of Action Chimeric monoclonal antibody which binds with high affinity and specificity to IL-6; prevents IL-6 from binding to both soluble and membrane-bound IL-6 receptors. Overproduction of IL-6 may lead to systemic manifestations in multicentric Castleman disease (MCD) patients by inducing C-reactive protein (CRP) synthesis (Kurzrock, 2010). Lowering serum IL-6 levels may improve systemic symptoms of Castleman disease.

Pharmacodynamics/Kinetics

Distribution: 4.5 L

Half-life elimination: ~21 days (range: 14.2 to 29.7 days)

Dosing

Adult & Geriatric Note: Consider delaying first dose if ANC <1000/mm^3, platelets <75,000/mm^3, and hemoglobin ≥17 g/dL; subsequent doses may be delayed if ANC <1000/mm^3, platelets <50,000/mm^3, and hemoglobin ≥17 g/dL. Do not reduce dose.

Castleman disease, multicentric (in patients who are HIV negative and HHV-8 negative): IV: 11 mg/kg over 1 hour every 3 weeks until treatment failure

Renal Impairment

CrCl ≥15 mL/minute: No initial dosage adjustment is necessary.

CrCl <15 mL/minute: There are no dosage adjustments provided in the manufacturer's labeling (has not been studied).

End-stage renal disease (ESRD): There are no dosage adjustments provided in the manufacturer's labeling (has not been studied).

Hepatic Impairment

Mild to moderate impairment (Child Pugh class A or B): No initial dosage adjustment is necessary.

Severe impairment (Child Pugh class C): There are no dosage adjustments provided in the manufacturer's labeling (has not been studied).

Adjustment for Toxicity

Hematologic toxicity: ANC <1000/mm^3, platelets <50,000/mm^3, and hemoglobin ≥17 g/dL: Consider delaying treatment until ANC ≥1000/mm^3, platelets ≥50,000/mm^3, and hemoglobin <17 g/dL

Anaphylaxis, cytokine release syndromes, and/or severe infusion-related or allergic reactions: Discontinue permanently.

Infection, severe: Withhold treatment until infection resolves.

Administration Administer IV over 1 hour using administration sets lined with polyvinyl chloride (PVC), polyurethane (PU), or polyethylene (PE), which contain a 0.2 micron inline polyethersulfone (PES) filter. Do not infuse in the same line with other medications. Complete infusion within 4 hours of dilution of the reconstituted solution to the infusion container.

Monitoring Parameters Monitor complete blood count with differential prior to each dose for the first 12 months and every 3 dosing cycles thereafter, or as clinically necessary; monitor for anaphylaxis and signs/symptoms of infusion-related, allergic, or cytokine release reactions; monitor for infection and signs/symptoms of gastrointestinal perforation.

Dosage Forms Excipient information presented when available (limited, particularly for generics); consult specific product labeling.

Solution Reconstituted, Intravenous [preservative free]:

Sylvant: 100 mg (1 ea); 400 mg (1 ea) [contains mouse protein (murine) (hamster), polysorbate 80]

◆ Silvadene see Silver Sulfadiazine on page 1657

◆ Silver Bullet Suppository [OTC] (Can) *see* Bisacodyl
on page 231

Silver Nitrate (SIL ver NYE trate)

Index Terms AgNO₃

Pharmacologic Category Antibiotic, Topical; Cauterizing Agent, Topical; Topical Skin Product, Antibacterial

Use Astringent, cauterization of wounds, germicidal, removal of granulation tissue, corns, and warts

Dosing

Adult & Geriatric Antiseptic, wound cauterization: Topical:

Sticks: Apply to mucous membranes and other moist skin surfaces only on area to be treated

Topical solution: Usual: Apply a cotton applicator dipped in solution on the affected area 2-3 times/week for 2-3 weeks.

Pediatric Antiseptic, wound cauterization: Topical: Refer to adult dosing.

Additional Information Complete prescribing information should be consulted for additional detail.

Dosage Forms Excipient information presented when available (limited, particularly for generics); consult specific product labeling.

Applicator sticks, topical: Silver nitrate 75% and potassium nitrate 25%

Solution, topical: 0.5% (960 mL); 10% (30 mL); 25% (30 mL); 50% (30 mL)

Silver Sulfadiazine (SIL ver sul fa DYE a zeen)

Brand Names: US Silvadene; SSD; Thermazene [DSC]
Brand Names: Canada Flamazine®
Pharmacologic Category Antibiotic, Topical
Use Prevention and treatment of infection in second and third degree burns

Dosing

Adult & Geriatric Antiseptic, burns: Topical: Apply once or twice daily

Pediatric Refer to adult dosing.

Additional Information Complete prescribing information should be consulted for additional detail.

Dosage Forms Excipient information presented when available (limited, particularly for generics); consult specific product labeling. [DSC] = Discontinued product

Cream, External:

Silvadene: 1% (20 g, 25 g, 50 g, 85 g, 400 g, 1000 g) [contains methylparaben, propylene glycol]

SSD: 1% (25 g, 50 g, 85 g, 400 g) [contains cetyl alcohol, methylparaben, propylene glycol]

Thermazene: 1% (20 g [DSC], 50 g [DSC], 85 g [DSC], 400 g [DSC], 1000 g [DSC]) [contains methylparaben, propylene glycol]

Generic: 1% (20 g, 25 g, 50 g, 85 g, 400 g)

Simeprevir (sim E pre vir)

Brand Names: US Olysio
Brand Names: Canada Galexos
Index Terms TMC435
Pharmacologic Category Antihepaciviral, Protease Inhibitor (Anti-HCV)

Use

Chronic hepatitis C: Treatment of genotype 1 or 4 chronic hepatitis C (in combination with other antihepacivirals)

Limitations of use: Not for use as monotherapy; when used in combination with peginterferon alfa and ribavirin, screening patients with HCV genotype 1a infection for the presence of virus with the NS3 Q80k polymorphism is strongly recommended (if detected, consider alternative therapy); not recommended for use in patients who have previously failed a simeprevir-containing regimen or another regimen containing HCV protease inhibitors.

Pregnancy Considerations Adverse events were observed in animal reproduction studies. Women of reproductive potential should use effective contraception during therapy. Treatment of HCV is not recommended for women who are already pregnant (AASLD, 2014).

If simeprevir is used in combination with ribavirin all warnings related to the use of ribavirin and pregnancy and/or contraception should be followed. Current guidelines note that ribavirin should not be used in pregnant women and males with female partners who are pregnant. A negative pregnancy test is required before initiation. Female patients (and their male partners) as well as male patients (and their female partners) should use two forms of effective contraception during therapy and for 6 months after therapy is discontinued. Pregnancy testing should be done at appropriate intervals (AASLD, 2014).

Breast-Feeding Considerations It is not known if simeprevir is excreted into breast milk. Due to the potential for serious adverse reactions in the nursing infant, the manufacturer recommends a decision be made whether to discontinue nursing or to discontinue the drug, taking into account the importance of treatment to the mother.

Contraindications

There are no contraindications listed in the manufacturer's labeling, however, all contraindications to other antihepaciviral drugs used in combination with simeprevir for the treatment of chronic hepatitis C infection also apply to their use in a simeprevir-containing regimen; refer to each monograph for individual product contraindications

Canadian labeling: Additional contraindications (not in U.S. labeling): Hypersensitivity to simeprevir or any component of the formulation

Warnings/Precautions Reduced sustained virologic response (SVR) rates of simeprevir in combination with peginterferon alfa and ribavirin were observed in patients infected with hepatitis C genotype 1a with an NS3 Q80K polymorphism at baseline compared to patients without the polymorphism; consider alternative therapy in these patients. Test hepatitis C genotype 1a patients treated with simeprevir in combination with peginterferon alfa and ribavirin prior to treatment initiation for the Q80K polymorphism; consider testing in hepatitis C genotype 1a patients treated with simeprevir in combination with sofosbuvir (AASLD/IDSA, 2014).

Hepatic decompensation and failure (including fatal cases) have been reported, most cases in patients with current advanced and/or decompensated cirrhosis; liver transaminases should be monitored at baseline and as clinically indicated. Modest bilirubin level increases, not impacting hepatic function, have been reported; monitoring at baseline and as clinically indicated is recommended, especially if marked increases occur (eg, total bilirubin >2.5 times the ULN); discontinue if elevation is accompanied by liver transaminase increases or clinical signs or symptoms of hepatic decompensation (eg, fatigue, weakness, lack of appetite, nausea and vomiting, jaundice, discolored feces).

Higher simeprevir exposures have been associated with an increased risk of adverse effects (including increased bilirubin, rash, and photosensitivity) in people of East Asian ancestry. An appropriate dose in these patients has not been determined. Use with caution. Rash has been typically observed within first 4 weeks of therapy initiation but may occur at any time. Severe rashes and rash requiring discontinuation have occurred in combination with peginterferon alfa and ribavirin. If a patient experiences a mild to moderate rash, follow for progression and/or development of mucosal signs (eg, oral lesions, conjunctivitis) or systemic symptoms. If rash becomes severe, discontinue simeprevir and monitor for rash resolution. Avoid excessive sunlight, tanning devices, and take precautions to limit exposure (eg, loose fitting clothing, sunscreen); may cause moderate to severe phototoxicity reactions (exaggerated sunburn appearance, burning, erythema, exudation, blistering, and edema). Most reactions have occurred within the first 4 weeks of therapy. Discontinue use if photosensitivity occurs and monitor until the reaction resolves. If therapy is to be continued in a patient who has experienced photosensitivity, expert consultation is advised. Contains a sulfonamide moiety. In patients with a history of sulfa allergy, no increased incidence of rash or photosensitivity has been reported, although the risk of reaction (or potential severity) cannot be excluded. Discontinue if signs of hypersensitivity are noted.

US manufacturer's labeling does not recommend use in moderate or severe hepatic impairment (Child-Pugh class B or C). Do not administer in combination with peginterferon and ribavirin patients with decompensated cirrhosis (moderate to severe hepatic impairment [Child-Pugh class B or C]). Combination therapy with ribavirin may cause birth defects; avoid pregnancy in females and female partners of male patients. Combination therapy with ribavirin is contraindicated in pregnancy. Use 2 effective forms of contraception during treatment and for 6 months after completion of treatment. Do not use as monotherapy. See other agents for additional warnings and precautions associated with their use. Safety and efficacy have not been established in patients who have received liver transplants, who have HCV genotypes other than genotype 1, or who have failed to respond to other HCV direct-acting inhibitors or on repeated courses of simeprevir. Potentially significant drug-drug interactions may exist, requiring dose or frequency adjustments, additional monitoring, and/or selection of alternative therapy. Symptomatic bradycardia (some requiring pacemaker intervention) has occurred in patients receiving amiodarone and sofosbuvir in combination with another direct acting antiviral, including simeprevir. Fatal cardiac arrest occurred in a patient receiving a

sofosbuvir (eg, ledipasvir/sofosbuvir) combination product. Bradycardia generally occurred within hours to days following coadministration; however, some cases have occurred 2 weeks following the initiation of HCV treatment. The risk of bradycardia may be increased in patients taking beta blockers or patients with underlying cardiac comorbidities and/or advanced liver disease. Bradycardia generally resolves following discontinuation of HCV treatment. Coadministration of amiodarone with simeprevir and sofosbuvir in combination is not recommended. However, if patients have no treatment alternatives, patients should be counseled about the interaction and have in-patient cardiac monitoring for the first 48 hours of coadministration followed by daily outpatient or self-monitoring of heart rate for at least the first 2 weeks of treatment. Due to the long half-life of amiodarone, cardiac monitoring (as described) is also recommended if amiodarone was discontinued just prior to beginning treatment with sofosbuvir and simeprevir. Patients should seek medical attention immediately if they experience fainting or near-fainting, dizziness, lightheadedness, malaise, weakness, excessive tiredness, shortness of breath, chest pains, confusion, or memory problems. Formulation contains lactose; the Canadian labeling recommends avoiding use in patients with rare hereditary disturbances of galactose intolerance (severe lactase deficiency or glucose-galactose malabsorption).

Adverse Reactions Percentages reported for combination therapy with peginterferon alfa and ribavirin (Peg-IFN-alfa and RBV) unless otherwise noted.

>10%:

Central nervous system: Fatigue (with sofosbuvir 25%), headache (with sofosbuvir 21%), dizziness (with sofosbuvir 16%), insomnia (with sofosbuvir 14%)

Dermatologic: Skin rash (with Peg-IFN-alfa and RBV 28%; including erythema, eczema, rash maculopapular, urticaria, toxic skin eruption, dermatitis exfoliative, cutaneous vasculitis, photosensitivity reaction), pruritus (with Peg-IFN-alfa and RBV 22%; with sofosbuvir 11%)

Gastrointestinal: Nausea (with Peg-IFN-alfa and RBV 22%; with sofosbuvir 21%), diarrhea (with sofosbuvir 16%)

Hepatic: Increased serum bilirubin (<50%)

Neuromuscular & skeletal: Myalgia (16%)

Respiratory: Dyspnea (12%)

1% to 10%:

Dermatologic: Skin photosensitivity (with sofosbuvir 7%; with Peg-IFN-alfa and RBV 5%; grade 3: 1%)

Hepatic: Increased serum alkaline phosphatase (<4%)

Drug Interactions

Metabolism/Transport Effects Substrate of CYP3A4 (major), P-glycoprotein, SLCO1B1; **Note:** Assignment of Major/Minor substrate status based on clinically relevant drug interaction potential; **Inhibits** CYP1A2 (weak), P-glycoprotein, SLCO1B1

Avoid Concomitant Use

Avoid concomitant use of Simeprevir with any of the following: Bosutinib; Cisapride; Conivaptan; CycloSPORINE (Systemic); CYP3A4 Inducers (Moderate); CYP3A4 Inducers (Strong); CYP3A4 Inhibitors (Moderate); CYP3A4 Inhibitors (Strong); Erythromycin (Systemic); Fusidic Acid (Systemic); Idelalisib; Ledipasvir; Milk Thistle; Nevirapine; PAZOPanib; Protease Inhibitors; Silodosin; St Johns Wort; Topotecan; VinCRIStine (Liposomal).

Increased Effect/Toxicity

Simeprevir may increase the levels/effects of: Afatinib; AtorvaSTATin; Bosutinib; Brentuximab Vedotin; Cisapride; Colchicine; CycloSPORINE (Systemic); CYP3A4 Substrates; Dabigatran Etexilate; Digoxin; DOXOrubicin (Conventional); Edoxaban; Everolimus; Ledipasvir; Lovastatin; Midazolam; Naloxegol; PAZOPanib; P-glycoprotein/ABCB1 Substrates; Phosphodiesterase 5 Inhibitors; Pitavastatin; Porfimer; Pravastatin; Protease Inhibitors; Prucalopride; Ranolazine; Rifaximin; Rilpivirine; Rosuvastatin; Silodosin; Simvastatin; Tenofovir Disoproxil Fumarate; TiZANidine; Topotecan; Triazolam; Verteporfin; VinCRIStine (Liposomal).

The levels/effects of Simeprevir may be increased by: Conivaptan; CycloSPORINE (Systemic); CYP3A4 Inhibitors (Moderate); CYP3A4 Inhibitors (Strong); Dasatinib; Eltrombopag; Erythromycin (Systemic); Fosaprepitant; Fusidic Acid (Systemic); Idelalisib; Ivacaftor; Ledipasvir; Luliconazole; Milk Thistle; Osimertinib; Palbociclib; Protease Inhibitors; Stiripentol; Teriflunomide

Decreased Effect

The levels/effects of Simeprevir may be decreased by: CYP3A4 Inducers (Moderate); CYP3A4 Inducers (Strong); Deferasirox; Escitalopram; Nevirapine; Osimertinib; Siltuximab; St Johns Wort; Tenofovir Disoproxil Fumarate; Tocilizumab

Storage/Stability Store below 30°C (86°F). Store in the original bottle. Protect from light.

Mechanism of Action Simeprevir is an inhibitor of HCV NS3/4A protease, a protease that is essential for viral replication. It is considered a direct-acting antiviral treatment for HCV, also called a specifically targeted antiviral therapy for HCV (STAT-C).

Pharmacodynamics/Kinetics

Absorption: Food enhances absorption.

Protein binding: >99% (albumin and alpha 1-acid glycoprotein)

Metabolism: Primarily oxidative metabolism by CYP3A4 (and possibly CYP2C8 and CYP2C19) to unchanged drug and metabolites (minor).

Bioavailability: 62% (single dose under fed conditions)

Half-life elimination: Plasma: 10 to 13 hours (healthy volunteers); 41 hours (HCV-infected patients)

Time to peak, serum: 4 to 6 hours

Excretion: Feces (~91%); urine (<1%)

Dosing

Adult & Geriatric Note: If other antihepaciviral treatment (sofosbuvir or peginterferon and ribavirin) is discontinued for any reason, simeprevir must also be discontinued. Do not reduce simeprevir dosage or interrupt therapy; if therapy must be interrupted due to adverse reactions or inadequate response, do not reinitiate.

Treatment of chronic hepatitis C (CHC): Oral:

Manufacturer's labeling: 150 mg once daily (in combination with sofosbuvir or peginterferon alfa and ribavirin). Treatment duration is indication and response-specific.

Missed dose: If a dose is missed within 12 hours of the time it is usually taken, take as soon as possible. If more than 12 hours have passed since the dose is usually taken, do not take the missed dose and the patient should resume the usual schedule.

Treatment-naive or treatment-experienced (includes prior relapse patients, prior partial responders, and prior null responders who failed previous interferon-based therapy) (HCV genotype 1, mono-infected) when used with sofosbuvir: **Note:** No treatment stopping rules apply to the combination of simeprevir with sofosbuvir:

US labeling:

Patients without cirrhosis: Weeks 1 to 12: Dual therapy: Simeprevir 150 mg once daily

Patients with cirrhosis: Weeks 1 to 24: Dual therapy: Simeprevir 150 mg once daily

Canadian labeling:

Patients without cirrhosis: Weeks 1 to 12: Dual therapy: Simeprevir 150 mg once daily

Patients with cirrhosis: Weeks 1 to 12: Dual therapy: Simeprevir 150 mg once daily. Note: May consider up to 24 weeks treatment duration

Treatment-naive or prior relapse patients (HCV genotype 1 or 4) when used with peginterferon alfa and ribavirin (including those with or without cirrhosis who are mono-infected and those patients without cirrhosis who are co-infected with HIV): **Note:** Prior relapsers include patients with an undetectable HCV-RNA upon completion of treatment (prior interferon-based regimen) but with detectable HCV-RNA during the follow up period.

Weeks 1 to 12: Triple therapy: Simeprevir 150 mg once daily

HCV-RNA **detectable** (level ≥25 units/mL) at week 4: Discontinue simeprevir, peginterferon alfa, and ribavirin (treatment determined to be inadequate).

Weeks 13 to 23 (based on HCV-RNA results at week 12):

HCV-RNA **undetectable** (level <25 units/mL) at week 12: Discontinue simeprevir (treatment completed). Dual therapy: Peginterferon alfa and ribavirin only (through week 24)

HCV-RNA **detectable** (level ≥25 units/mL) at week 12: Discontinue simeprevir (treatment completed), peginterferon alfa, and ribavirin (treatment determined to be inadequate).

Week 24 (based on HCV-RNA results at week 24):

HCV-RNA **undetectable** (level <25 units/mL) at week 24: Dual therapy: Peginterferon alfa and ribavirin only (through week 24)

HCV-RNA **detectable** (level ≥25 units/mL) at week 24: Discontinue peginterferon alfa and ribavirin (treatment determined to be inadequate).

Treatment-naive or prior relapse patients (HCV genotype 1 or 4) with cirrhosis who are co-infected with HIV when used with peginterferon alfa and ribavirin: **Note:** Prior relapsers include patients with an undetectable HCV-RNA upon completion of treatment (prior interferon-based regimen) but with detectable HCV-RNA during the follow up period.

Weeks 1 to 12: Triple therapy: Simeprevir 150 mg daily

HCV-RNA **detectable** (level ≥25 units/mL) at week 4: Discontinue simeprevir, peginterferon alfa, and ribavirin (treatment determined to be inadequate).

HCV-RNA **undetectable** (level <25 units/mL) at week 12: Discontinue simeprevir (treatment completed). Dual therapy: Peginterferon alfa and ribavirin only (through week 48)

Weeks 13 to 48 (based on HCV-RNA results at weeks 12 and 24):

HCV-RNA **detectable** (level ≥25 units/mL) at week 12: Discontinue simeprevir (treatment completed) and peginterferon alfa and ribavirin (treatment determined to be inadequate).

HCV-RNA **undetectable** (level <25 units/mL) at week 24: Discontinue simeprevir (treatment was completed after week 12). Dual therapy: Peginterferon alfa and ribavirin only (through week 48)

HCV-RNA **detectable** (level ≥25 units/mL) at week 24: Discontinue peginterferon alfa, and ribavirin (treatment determined to be inadequate).

Previously treated patients (HCV genotype 1 or 4; partial response or null responders including those with or without cirrhosis and those who are mono-infected or with HIV co-infection when used with peginterferon alfa and ribavirin: **Note:** Partial response includes patients with a ≥2-log$_{10}$ HCV-RNA decrease at week 12 but detectable HCV-RNA at the end of prior interferon-based therapy. Prior null responders include patients with a <2-log$_{10}$ HCV-RNA decrease at week 12 during interferon-based therapy.

Weeks 1 to 12: Triple therapy: Simeprevir 150 mg daily

HCV-RNA **detectable** (level ≥25 units/mL) at week 4: Discontinue simeprevir, peginterferon alfa, and ribavirin (treatment determined to be inadequate).

HCV-RNA **undetectable** (level <25 units/mL) at week 12: Discontinue simeprevir (treatment completed). Dual therapy: Peginterferon alfa and ribavirin only (through week 48)

Weeks 13 to 48 (based on HCV-RNA results at weeks 12 and 24):

HCV-RNA **detectable** (level ≥25 units/mL) at week 12: Discontinue simeprevir (treatment completed) and peginterferon alfa and ribavirin (treatment determined to be inadequate).

HCV-RNA **undetectable** (level <25 units/mL) at week 24: Discontinued simeprevir (treatment was completed after week 12). Dual therapy: Peginterferon alfa and ribavirin only (through week 48)

HCV-RNA **detectable** (level ≥25 units/mL) at week 24: Discontinue peginterferon alfa, and ribavirin (treatment determined to be inadequate).

Alternative dosing:

Treatment-naive patients: Patients who cannot receive peginterferon: Genotype 1a (off-label regimen): 150 mg once daily with sofosbuvir and ribavirin for 12 weeks (without cirrhosis) or 24 weeks (with cirrhosis). **Note:** A recommended regimen (AASLD/IDSA, 2014)

Relapsed chronic hepatitis C patients (nonresponders to a previous regimen of ribavirin and peginterferon alfa without an HCV protease inhibitor): Genotype 1 patients (off-label regimen): 150 mg once daily with sofosbuvir and with ribavirin for 12 weeks (without cirrhosis) or 24 weeks (with cirrhosis). **Note:** A recommended regimen (AASLD/IDSA, 2014).

Renal Impairment No dosage adjustment necessary. Not studied in patients with CrCl ≤30 mL/minute or with end-stage renal disease (ESRD), including those requiring hemodialysis.

Hepatic Impairment

Mild impairment (Child-Pugh class A): No dosage adjustment necessary.

Moderate or severe impairment (Child-Pugh class B or C): Use is not recommended. Do not administer in combination with peginterferon and ribavirin in patients with decompensated cirrhosis.

Administration Oral: Administer with food. Administer concurrently with peginterferon alfa and ribavirin or sofosbuvir. Maintain adequate fluid intake/hydration. Swallow capsules whole; do not chew, crush, break, cut, or dissolve the capsule.

Monitoring Parameters

Bilirubin, liver enzymes (at baseline and during therapy as clinically indicated), and uric acid at baseline and periodically when clinically indicated

Serum HCV-RNA at baseline, weeks 4, 12, and 24, at end of treatment, during treatment follow-up, and when clinically indicated

Pretreatment and monthly pregnancy tests up to 6 months following discontinuation of therapy for women of child-bearing age

Dosage Forms Excipient information presented when available (limited, particularly for generics); consult specific product labeling.

Capsule, Oral:

Olysio: 150 mg

◆ Simethicone, Aluminum Hydroxide, and Magnesium Hydroxide *see* Aluminum Hydroxide, Magnesium Hydroxide, and Simethicone *on page 85*

◆ Simethicone and Loperamide Hydrochloride *see* Loperamide and Simethicone *on page 1098*

◆ Simethicone and Magaldrate *see* Magaldrate and Simethicone *on page 1118*

◆ Simply Allergy [OTC] *see* DiphenhydrAMINE (Systemic) *on page 561*

◆ Simply Sleep [OTC] *see* DiphenhydrAMINE (Systemic) *on page 561*

◆ Simply Sleep (Can) *see* DiphenhydrAMINE (Systemic) *on page 561*

◆ Simply Stuffy [OTC] *see* Pseudoephedrine *on page 1527*

◆ Simponi *see* Golimumab *on page 852*

◆ Simponi Aria *see* Golimumab *on page 852*

◆ Simponi I.V. (Can) *see* Golimumab *on page 852*

◆ Simulect *see* Basiliximab *on page 201*

Simvastatin (sim va STAT in)

Brand Names: US Zocor

Brand Names: Canada ACT-Simvastatin; Apo-Simvastatin; Auro-Simvastatin; Dom-Simvastatin; JAMP-Simvastatin; Mar-Simvastatin; Mint-Simvastatin; Mylan-Simvastatin; PHL-Simvastatin; PMS-Simvastatin; Q-Simvastatin; RAN-Simvastatin; Riva-Simvastatin; Sandoz-Simvastatin; Simvastatin-Odan; Teva-Simvastatin; Zocor

Pharmacologic Category Antilipemic Agent, HMG-CoA Reductase Inhibitor

Use Used with dietary therapy for the following:

Secondary prevention of cardiovascular events in hypercholesterolemic patients with established coronary heart disease (CHD) or at high risk for CHD: To reduce cardiovascular morbidity (myocardial infarction, coronary/noncoronary revascularization procedures) and mortality; to reduce the risk of stroke

Hyperlipidemias: To reduce elevations in total cholesterol (total-C), LDL-C, apolipoprotein B, triglycerides, and VLDL-C, and to increase HDL-C in patients with primary hypercholesterolemia (elevations of 1 or more components are present in Fredrickson type IIa, IIb, III, and IV hyperlipidemias); treatment of homozygous familial hypercholesterolemia

Heterozygous familial hypercholesterolemia (HeFH): In adolescent patients (10-17 years of age, females >1 year postmenarche) with HeFH having LDL-C ≥190 mg/dL or LDL-C ≥160 mg/dL with positive family history of premature cardiovascular disease (CVD), or 2 or more CVD risk factors in the adolescent patient

Primary and secondary prevention of atherosclerotic cardiovascular disease (ASCVD) according to the American College of Cardiology/American Heart Association: To reduce the risk of ASCVD in patients with clinical ASCVD (eg, coronary heart disease, stroke/TIA, or peripheral arterial disease presumed to be of atherosclerotic origin) who are greater than 75 years of age or not a candidate for high-intensity statin therapy; in patients without clinical ASCVD if LDL-C is 190 mg/dL or greater and not a candidate for high-intensity statin therapy; in patients without clinical ASCVD who have type 1 or type 2 diabetes and are between 40 and 75 years of age; in patients with an estimated 10-year ASCVD risk 7.5% or greater and who are between 40 and 75 years of age (Stone, 2013). The American Heart Association (AHA) recommends statin therapy (unless contraindicated) for all coronary artery bypass graft (CABG) surgery patients to help maintain long-term graft patency and help obtain the highest level of physical health and quality of life (AHA [Kulik, 2015]). Specific recommendations from the Kidney Disease: Improving Global Outcomes (KDIGO) organization have also been released for patients with chronic kidney disease (KDIGO [Tonelli, 2013]).

Pregnancy Considerations Adverse events were not observed in animal reproduction studies. There are reports of congenital anomalies following maternal use of HMG-CoA reductase inhibitors in pregnancy; however, maternal disease, differences in specific agents used, and the low rates of exposure limit the interpretation of the available

data (Godfrey, 2012; Lecarpentier, 2012). Cholesterol biosynthesis may be important in fetal development; serum cholesterol and triglycerides increase normally during pregnancy. The discontinuation of lipid lowering medications temporarily during pregnancy is not expected to have significant impact on the long term outcomes of primary hypercholesterolemia treatment.

Use of simvastatin is contraindicated in pregnancy. HMG-CoA reductase inhibitors should be discontinued prior to pregnancy (ADA, 2013). If treatment of dyslipidemias is needed in pregnant women or in women of reproductive age, other agents are preferred (Berglund, 2012; Stone, 2013). The manufacturer recommends administration to women of childbearing potential only when conception is highly unlikely and patients have been informed of potential hazards.

Breast-Feeding Considerations It is not known if simvastatin is excreted into breast milk. Due to the potential for serious adverse reactions in a nursing infant, breast-feeding is contraindicated by the manufacturer.

Contraindications Hypersensitivity to simvastatin or any component of the formulation; active liver disease; unexplained persistent elevations of serum transaminases; concomitant use of strong CYP3A4 inhibitors (eg, clarithromycin, erythromycin, itraconazole, ketoconazole, nefazodone, posaconazole, voriconazole, protease inhibitors [including boceprevir and telaprevir], telithromycin, cobicistat-containing products), cyclosporine, danazol, and gemfibrozil; pregnancy; breast-feeding

Warnings/Precautions Secondary causes of hyperlipidemia should be ruled out prior to therapy. Liver enzyme tests should be obtained at baseline and as clinically indicated; routine periodic monitoring of liver enzymes is not necessary. Use with caution in patients who consume large amounts of ethanol or have a history of liver disease; use is contraindicated with active liver disease and with unexplained transaminase elevations. Rhabdomyolysis with acute renal failure has occurred. Risk of rhabdomyolysis is dose-related and increased with high doses (80 mg), concurrent use of lipid-lowering agents which may also cause rhabdomyolysis (other fibrates or niacin doses ≥1 g/day), or moderate-to-strong CYP3A4 inhibitors (eg, amiodarone, grapefruit juice in large quantities, or verapamil), age ≥65 years, female gender, uncontrolled hypothyroidism, and renal dysfunction. In Chinese patients, do not use high-dose simvastatin (80 mg) if concurrently taking niacin ≥1 g/day; may increase risk of myopathy. Immune-mediated necrotizing myopathy (IMNM), an autoimmune-mediated myopathy, has been reported (rarely) with HMG-CoA reductase inhibitor therapy. IMNM presents as proximal muscle weakness with elevated CPK levels, which persists despite discontinuation of HMG-CoA reductase inhibitor therapy; additionally, muscle biopsy may show necrotizing myopathy with limited inflammation; immunosuppressive therapy (eg, corticosteroids, azathioprine) may be used for treatment. Concomitant use of simvastatin with some drugs may require cautious use, may not be recommended, may require dosage adjustments, or may be contraindicated. If concurrent use of a contraindicated interacting medication is unavoidable, treatment with simvastatin should be suspended during use or consider the use of an alternative HMG-CoA reductase inhibitor void of CYP3A4 metabolism. Monitor closely if used with other drugs associated with myopathy (eg, colchicine). Increases in HbA1c and fasting blood glucose have been reported with HMG-CoA reductase inhibitors; however, the benefits of statin therapy far outweigh the risk of dysglycemia. The manufacturer recommends temporary discontinuation for elective major surgery, acute medical or surgical conditions, or in any patient experiencing an acute or serious condition predisposing to renal failure (eg, sepsis, hypotension, trauma, uncontrolled seizures). Based on current research and clinical guidelines (Fleisher, 2009), HMG-CoA reductase inhibitors should be continued in the perioperative period. Use with caution in patients with severe renal impairment; initial dosage adjustment is necessary; monitor closely.

Adverse Reactions Frequency not always defined.

Cardiovascular: Atrial fibrillation (6%), edema (3%)

Central nervous system: Headache (3% to 7%), vertigo (5%)

Dermatologic: Eczema (5%)

Gastrointestinal: Abdominal pain (7%), constipation (2% to 7%), gastritis (5%), nausea (5%)

Genitourinary: Cystitis (interstitial; Huang 2015)

Hepatic: Increased transaminases (>3 x ULN; 1%)

Neuromuscular & skeletal: Increased CPK (>3 x normal; 5%), myalgia (4%)

Respiratory: Upper respiratory infections (9%), bronchitis (7%)

<1% (Limited to important or life-threatening): Alopecia, amnesia (reversible), anaphylaxis, anemia, angioedema, arthralgia, arthritis, chills, cognitive impairment (reversible), confusion (reversible), depression, dermatomyositis, diabetes mellitus (new onset), diarrhea, dizziness, dryness of skin/mucous membranes, dyspepsia, dyspnea, eosinophilia, erythema multiforme, fever, flatulence, flushing, hemolytic anemia, hepatic failure, hepatitis, hypersensitivity reaction, increased alkaline phosphatase, increased blood glucose, increased ESR, increased GGT, increased glycosylated hemoglobin (HbA1c), jaundice, leukopenia, malaise, memory disturbance (reversible), memory impairment (reversible), muscle cramps, nail changes, nodules, pancreatitis, paresthesia, peripheral neuropathy, photosensitivity, polymyalgia rheumatica, positive ANA, pruritus, purpura, rash, rhabdomyolysis, skin discoloration, Stevens-Johnson syndrome, systemic lupus erythematosus-like syndrome, thrombocytopenia, toxic epidermal necrolysis, urticaria, vasculitis, vomiting, weakness

Additional class-related events or case reports (not necessarily reported with simvastatin therapy): Alteration in taste, anorexia, anxiety, cataracts, cholestatic jaundice, cirrhosis, decreased libido, depression, erectile dysfunction/impotence, facial paresis, fatty liver, fulminant hepatic necrosis, gynecomastia, hepatoma, hyperbilirubinemia, immune-mediated necrotizing myopathy (IMNM), impaired extraocular muscle movement, increased bilirubin, increased CPK (>10 x normal), interstitial lung disease, ophthalmoplegia, peripheral nerve palsy, psychic disturbance, renal failure (secondary to rhabdomyolysis), thyroid dysfunction, tremor, vertigo

Drug Interactions

Metabolism/Transport Effects Substrate of CYP3A4 (major), SLCO1B1; **Note:** Assignment of Major/Minor substrate status based on clinically relevant drug interaction potential; **Inhibits** CYP2C8 (weak), CYP2C9 (weak), CYP2D6 (weak)

Avoid Concomitant Use

Avoid concomitant use of Simvastatin with any of the following: Amodiaquine; Boceprevir; Clarithromycin; Conivaptan; CycloSPORINE (Systemic); CYP3A4 Inhibitors (Strong); Danazol; Erythromycin (Systemic); Fusidic Acid (Systemic); Gemfibrozil; Grapefruit Juice; Idelalisib; Mifepristone; Protease Inhibitors; Red Yeast Rice; Telaprevir; Telithromycin

Increased Effect/Toxicity

Simvastatin may increase the levels/effects of: Amodiaquine; ARIPiprazole; DAPTOmycin; Diltiazem; PAZOPanib; Trabectedin; Vitamin K Antagonists

The levels/effects of Simvastatin may be increased by: Acipimox; Amiodarone; AmLODIPine; Aprepitant; Azithromycin (Systemic); Bezafibrate; Boceprevir; Ciprofibrate; Clarithromycin; Colchicine; Conivaptan; CycloSPORINE (Systemic); CYP3A4 Inhibitors (Moderate); CYP3A4 Inhibitors (Strong); Cyproterone; Daclatasvir; Danazol; Dasatinib; Diltiazem; Dronedarone; Eltrombopag; Erythromycin (Systemic); Fenofibrate and Derivatives; Fluconazole; Fosaprepitant; Fusidic Acid (Systemic); Gemfibrozil; Grapefruit Juice; Green Tea; Idelalisib; Imatinib; Ivacaftor; Lercanidipine; Lomitapide; Luliconazole; Mifepristone; Netupitant; Niacin; Niacinamide; Osimertinib; Palbociclib; Protease Inhibitors; QuiNINE; Raltegravir; Ranolazine; Red Yeast Rice; Sacubitril; Simeprevir; Stiripentol; Telaprevir; Telithromycin; Teriflunomide; Ticagrelor; Verapamil

Decreased Effect

Simvastatin may decrease the levels/effects of: Lanthanum

The levels/effects of Simvastatin may be decreased by: Antacids; Bosentan; CYP3A4 Inducers (Moderate); CYP3A4 Inducers (Strong); Dabrafenib; Deferasirox; Efavirenz; Enzalutamide; Eslicarbazepine; Etravirine; Fosphenytoin; Mitotane; Osimertinib; Phenytoin; Rifampin Derivatives; Siltuximab; St Johns Wort; Tocilizumab

Food Interactions Simvastatin serum concentration may be increased when taken with grapefruit juice. Management: Avoid concurrent intake of large quantities of grapefruit juice (>1 quart/day).

Storage/Stability Tablets should be stored in tightly-closed containers at temperatures between 5°C to 30°C (41°F to 86°F).

Mechanism of Action Simvastatin is a methylated derivative of lovastatin that acts by competitively inhibiting 3-hydroxy-3-methylglutaryl-coenzyme A (HMG-CoA) reductase, the enzyme that catalyzes the rate-limiting step in cholesterol biosynthesis. In addition to the ability of HMG-CoA reductase inhibitors to decrease levels of high-sensitivity C-reactive protein (hsCRP), they also possess pleiotropic properties including improved endothelial function,

reduced inflammation at the site of the coronary plaque, inhibition of platelet aggregation, and anticoagulant effects (de Denus, 2002; Ray, 2005).

Pharmacodynamics/Kinetics
Onset of action: >3 days
Peak effect: 2 weeks
Absorption: 85%
Protein binding: ~95%
Metabolism: Hepatic via CYP3A4; extensive first-pass effect
Bioavailability: <5%
Half-life elimination: Unknown
Time to peak: 1.3 to 2.4 hours
Excretion: Feces (60%); urine (13%)

Dosing
Adult Note: Doses should be individualized according to the baseline LDL-cholesterol levels, the recommended goal of therapy, and the patient's response; adjustments should be made at intervals of 4 weeks or more; doses may need adjusted based on concomitant medications

Note: Dosing limitation: Simvastatin 80 mg is limited to patients that have been taking this dose for >12 consecutive months without evidence of myopathy and are not currently taking or beginning to take a simvastatin dose-limiting or contraindicated interacting medication. If patient is unable to achieve low-density lipoprotein-cholesterol (LDL-C) goal using the 40 mg dose of simvastatin, increasing to 80 mg dose is not recommended. Instead, switch patient to an alternative LDL-C-lowering treatment providing greater LDL-C reduction.

Homozygous familial hypercholesterolemia: Oral: 40 mg once daily in the evening

Prevention of cardiovascular events (also see ACC/AHA Blood Cholesterol Guideline recommendations), hyperlipidemias: Oral: 10 to 20 mg once daily in the evening; range: 5 to 40 mg/day
Patients requiring only moderate reduction of LDL-C: May be started at 5 to 10 mg once daily in the evening; adjust to achieve recommended LDL-C goal.
Patients requiring reduction of >40% of LDL-C: May be started at 40 mg once daily in the evening; adjust to achieve recommended LDL-C goal.
Patients with CHD or at high risk for cardiovascular events (patients with diabetes, PVD, history of stroke or other cerebrovascular disease): Dosing should be started at 40 mg once daily in the evening; start simultaneously with diet therapy.

Prevention of cardiovascular disease: ACC/AHA Blood Cholesterol Guideline recommendations to reduce the risk of atherosclerotic cardiovascular disease (ASCVD) (Stone, 2013): Adults ≥21 years: Oral:
Primary prevention:
LDL-C ≥190 mg/dL: High intensity therapy necessary; use alternate statin therapy (eg, atorvastatin or rosuvastatin)
Type 1 or 2 diabetes and age 40 to 75 years: Moderate intensity therapy: 20 to 40 mg once daily
Type 1 or 2 diabetes, age 40 to 75 years, and an estimated 10-year ASCVD risk ≥7.5%: High intensity therapy necessary; use alternate statin therapy (eg, atorvastatin or rosuvastatin)
Age 40 to 75 years and an estimated 10-year ASCVD risk ≥7.5%: Moderate to high intensity therapy: 20 to 40 mg once daily or consider using high intensity statin therapy (eg, atorvastatin or rosuvastatin)
Secondary prevention:
Patient has clinical ASCVD (eg, coronary heart disease, stroke/TIA, or peripheral arterial disease presumed to be of atherosclerotic origin) or is post-CABG (AHA [Kulik, 2015]) **and**:
Age ≤75 years: High intensity therapy necessary; use alternate statin therapy (eg, atorvastatin or rosuvastatin)
Age >75 years or not a candidate for high intensity therapy: Moderate intensity therapy: 20 to 40 mg once daily

Dosage adjustment for simvastatin with concomitant medications: Note: Patients currently tolerating and requiring a dose of simvastatin 80 mg who require initiation of an interacting drug with a dose cap for simvastatin should be switched to an alternative statin with less potential for drug-drug interaction.
Amiodarone, amlodipine, or ranolazine: Simvastatin dose should **not** exceed 20 mg/day
Diltiazem, dronedarone, or verapamil: Simvastatin dose should **not** exceed 10 mg/day
Lomitapide: Reduce simvastatin dose by 50% when initiating lomitapide. Simvastatin dose should not

exceed 20 mg/day (or 40 mg daily for those who previously tolerated simvastatin 80 mg daily for ≥1 year without evidence of muscle toxicity)

Dosage adjustment in Chinese patients on niacin doses ≥1 g/day:
US labeling: Use caution with simvastatin doses exceeding 20 mg/day; because of an increased risk of myopathy, do not administer simvastatin 80 mg concurrently.
Canadian labeling: Concomitant use is not recommended in Chinese and other Asian patients.
Geriatric Oral: Initial: Maximum reductions in LDL-cholesterol may be achieved with daily dose ≤20 mg.
Pediatric HeFH: Oral: Children 10 to 17 years (females >1 year postmenarche): 10 mg once daily in the evening; range: 10 to 40 mg/day (maximum: 40 mg/day)

Dosage adjustment with concomitant medications: With concomitant amiodarone, amlodipine, diltiazem, dronedarone, lomitapide, ranolazine, or verapamil: Refer to adult dosing.
Note: Doses should be individualized according to the baseline LDL-cholesterol levels, the recommended goal of therapy, and the patient's response; adjustments should be made at intervals of 4 weeks or more; doses may need adjusted based on concomitant medications

Renal Impairment Manufacturer's recommendations:
Mild to moderate renal impairment: No dosage adjustment necessary; simvastatin does not undergo significant renal excretion.
Severe renal impairment: CrCl <30 mL/minute: Initial: 5 mg/day with close monitoring.

Hepatic Impairment Use is contraindicated in the setting of active liver disease.

Adjustment for Toxicity
Severe muscle symptoms or fatigue: Promptly discontinue use; evaluate CPK, creatinine, and urinalysis for myoglobinuria (Stone, 2013).
Mild to moderate muscle symptoms: Discontinue use until symptoms can be evaluated; evaluate patient for conditions that may increase the risk for muscle symptoms (eg, hypothyroidism, reduced renal or hepatic function, rheumatologic disorders such as polymyalgia rheumatica, steroid myopathy, vitamin D deficiency, or primary muscle diseases). Upon resolution, resume the original or lower dose of simvastatin. If muscle symptoms recur, discontinue simvastatin use. After muscle symptom resolution, may then use a low dose of a different statin; gradually increase if tolerated. In the absence of continued statin use, if muscle symptoms or elevated CPK continues after 2 months, consider other causes of muscle symptoms. If determined to be due to another condition aside from statin use, may resume statin therapy at the original dose (Stone, 2013).

Dietary Considerations May be taken without regard to meals. Red yeast rice contains variable amounts of several compounds that are structurally similar to HMG-CoA reductase inhibitors, primarily monacolin K (or mevinolin) which is structurally identical to lovastatin; concurrent use of red yeast rice with HMG-CoA reductase inhibitors may increase the incidence of adverse and toxic effects (Lapi, 2008; Smith, 2003).

Administration May be administered without regard to meals. Administer in the evening for maximal efficacy.

Monitoring Parameters *2013 ACC/AHA Blood Cholesterol Guideline recommendations (Stone, 2013):*
Lipid panel (total cholesterol, HDL, LDL, triglycerides): Baseline lipid panel; fasting lipid profile within 4 to 12 weeks after initiation or dose adjustment and every 3 to 12 months (as clinically indicated) thereafter. If 2 consecutive LDL levels are <40 mg/dL, consider decreasing the dose.
Hepatic transaminase levels: Baseline measurement of hepatic transaminase levels (ie, ALT); measure hepatic function if symptoms suggest hepatotoxicity (eg, unusual fatigue or weakness, loss of appetite, abdominal pain, dark-colored urine or yellowing of skin or sclera) during therapy.
CPK: CPK should not be routinely measured. Baseline CPK measurement is reasonable for some individuals (eg, family history of statin intolerance or muscle disease, clinical presentation, concomitant drug therapy that may increase risk of myopathy). May measure CPK in any patient with symptoms suggestive of myopathy (pain, tenderness, stiffness, cramping, weakness, or generalized fatigue).
Evaluate for new-onset diabetes mellitus during therapy; if diabetes develops, continue statin therapy and encourage adherence to a heart-healthy diet, physical activity, a healthy body weight, and tobacco cessation.

If patient develops a confusional state or memory impairment, may evaluate patient for nonstatin causes (eg, exposure to other drugs), systemic and neuropsychiatric causes, and the possibility of adverse effects associated with statin therapy.

Manufacturer's labeling: Liver enzyme tests at baseline and repeated when clinically indicated. Measure CPK when myopathy is being considered or may measure CPK periodically in high risk patients (eg, drug-drug interaction). Lipid panel should be analyzed after 4 weeks of therapy and periodically thereafter.

Dosage Forms Excipient information presented when available (limited, particularly for generics); consult specific product labeling.

Tablet, Oral:
Zocor: 5 mg, 10 mg, 20 mg, 40 mg, 80 mg
Generic: 5 mg, 10 mg, 20 mg, 40 mg, 80 mg

◆ Simvastatin and Ezetimibe *see* Ezetimibe and Simvastatin *on page 731*

◆ Simvastatin and Sitagliptin *see* Sitagliptin and Simvastatin *on page 1667*

◆ Simvastatin-Odan (Can) *see* Simvastatin *on page 1659*

◆ Sinemet *see* Carbidopa and Levodopa *on page 307*

◆ Sinemet CR *see* Carbidopa and Levodopa *on page 307*

◆ Sinequan *see* Doxepin (Systemic) *on page 590*

◆ Singulair *see* Montelukast *on page 1229*

Sipuleucel-T (si pu LOO sel tee)

Brand Names: US Provenge
Index Terms APC8015; Prostate Cancer Vaccine, Cell-Based
Pharmacologic Category Cellular Immunotherapy, Autologous
Additional Appendix Information
Immunization Administration Recommendations *on page 1974*
Immunization Schedules *on page 1979*
Use Prostate cancer, metastatic: Treatment of asymptomatic or minimally symptomatic metastatic castrate-resistant (hormone-refractory) prostate cancer.
Prescribing and Access Restrictions Patients may receive Sipuleucel-T at a participating site. Physicians must go through an inservice and register to prescribe the treatment; patients must also complete an enrollment form. Information on registration and enrollment is available at 1-877-336-3736.
Dosing
Adult & Geriatric Note: Premedicate with oral acetaminophen 650 mg and an antihistamine (eg, diphenhydramine 50 mg) ~30 minutes prior to infusion. For autologous use only. Do not infuse until confirmation of product release has been received from the company.

Prostate cancer, metastatic: IV: Each dose contains ≥50 million autologous CD54+ cells (obtained through leukapheresis) activated with PAP-GM-CSF; administer doses at ~2-week intervals for a total of 3 doses (Kantoff, 2010). If unable to receive a scheduled infusion, an additional leukapheresis procedure will be necessary prior to continuing a course of treatment.
Renal Impairment There are no dosage adjustments provided in the manufacturer's labeling.
Hepatic Impairment There are no dosage adjustments provided in the manufacturer's labeling.
Adjustment for Toxicity Acute infusion reaction: Interrupt or slow infusion rate (depending on the severity of infusion reaction); may require acetaminophen, IV H$_1$ and/or H$_2$ antagonists, or low-dose meperidine to manage acute symptoms.
Additional Information Complete prescribing information should be consulted for additional detail.
Dosage Forms Excipient information presented when available (limited, particularly for generics); consult specific product labeling.
Suspension, Intravenous [preservative free]:
Provenge: (250 mL)

◆ Sirdalud *see* TiZANidine *on page 1798*

Sirolimus (sir OH li mus)

Brand Names: US Rapamune
Brand Names: Canada Rapamune
Index Terms Rapamycin
Pharmacologic Category Immunosuppressant Agent; mTOR Kinase Inhibitor

Use
Lymphangioleiomyomatosis: Treatment of lymphangioleiomyomatosis. Therapeutic drug monitoring is recommended for all patients receiving sirolimus.
Renal transplantation: Prophylaxis of organ rejection in patients receiving renal transplants (in low-to-moderate immunologic risk patients in combination with cyclosporine and corticosteroids with cyclosporine withdrawn 2 to 4 months after transplant, and in high immunologic risk patients in combination with cyclosporine and corticosteroids for the first year after transplant). Therapeutic drug monitoring is recommended for all patients receiving sirolimus. High immunologic risk renal transplant patients are defined (per the manufacturer's labeling) as Black transplant recipients and/or repeat renal transplant recipients who lost a previous allograft based on an immunologic process and/or patients with high PRA (panel-reactive antibodies; peak PRA level >80%).
Limitations of use (renal transplantation): Cyclosporine withdrawal has not been studied in patients with Banff grade 3 acute rejection or vascular rejection prior to cyclosporine withdrawal, patients who are dialysis-dependent, patients with serum creatinine >4.5 mg/dL, Black patients, patients with multiorgan transplants or secondary transplants, or those with high levels of PRA. In patients at high immunologic risk, the safety and efficacy of sirolimus used in combination with cyclosporine and corticosteroids have not been studied beyond 1 year; therefore, after the first 12 months following transplantation, consider any adjustments to the immunosuppressive regimen on the basis of the clinical status of the patient. The safety and efficacy of sirolimus have not been established in patients younger than 13 years or in pediatric renal transplant patients younger than 18 years who are considered at high immunologic risk. The safety and efficacy of de novo use of sirolimus without cyclosporine have not been established in renal transplant patients. The safety and efficacy of conversion from calcineurin inhibitors to sirolimus in maintenance renal transplant patients have not been established.
Pregnancy Considerations Adverse events have been observed in animal reproduction studies. Effective contraception must be initiated before therapy with sirolimus and continued for 12 weeks after discontinuation.

The National Transplantation Pregnancy Registry (NTPR, Temple University) is a registry for pregnant women taking immunosuppressants following any solid organ transplant. The NTPR encourages reporting of all immunosuppressant exposures during pregnancy in transplant recipients at 1-877-955-6877.
Breast-Feeding Considerations It is not known if sirolimus is excreted in breast milk. Due to the potential for serious adverse reactions in the nursing infant, the manufacturer recommends a decision be made whether to discontinue nursing or to discontinue the drug, taking into account the importance of treatment to the mother.
Medication Guide Available Yes
Contraindications Hypersensitivity to sirolimus or any component of the formulation
Warnings/Precautions Hazardous agent - use appropriate precautions for handling and disposal (NIOSH 2014 [group 2]).

[US Boxed Warning]: Immunosuppressive agents, including sirolimus, increase the risk of infection and may be associated with the development of lymphoma. Immune suppression may also increase the risk of opportunistic infections including activation of latent viral infections (including BK virus-associated nephropathy), fatal infections, and sepsis. Prophylactic treatment for *Pneumocystis jirovecii* pneumonia (PCP) should be administered for 1 year post-transplant; prophylaxis for cytomegalovirus (CMV) should be taken for 3 months post-transplant in patients at risk for CMV. Progressive multifocal leukoencephalopathy (PML), an opportunistic CNS infection caused by reactivation of the JC virus, has been reported in patients receiving immunosuppressive therapy, including sirolimus. Clinical findings of PML include apathy, ataxia, cognitive deficiency, confusion, and hemiparesis; promptly evaluate any patient presenting with neurological changes; consider decreasing the degree of immunosuppression with consideration to the risk of organ rejection in transplant patients.

[US Boxed Warning]: Sirolimus is not recommended for use in liver or lung transplantation. Bronchial anastomotic dehiscence cases have been reported in lung transplant patients when sirolimus was used as part of an immunosuppressive regimen; most of these reactions were fatal. Studies indicate an association with an increased risk of hepatic artery thrombosis

(HAT), graft failure, and increased mortality (with evidence of infection) in liver transplant patients when sirolimus is used in combination with cyclosporine and/or tacrolimus. Most cases of HAT occurred within 30 days of transplant.

In renal transplant patients, de novo use without cyclosporine has been associated with higher rates of acute rejection. Sirolimus should be used in combination with cyclosporine (and corticosteroids) initially when used in renal transplant patients. Cyclosporine may be withdrawn in low-to-moderate immunologic risk patients after 2 to 4 months, in conjunction with an increase in sirolimus dosage. In high immunologic risk patients, use in combination with cyclosporine and corticosteroids is recommended for the first year. Safety and efficacy of combination therapy with cyclosporine in high immunologic risk patients has not been studied beyond 12 months of treatment; adjustment of immunosuppressive therapy beyond 12 months should be considered based on clinical judgment. Monitor renal function closely when combined with cyclosporine; consider dosage adjustment or discontinue in patients with increasing serum creatinine.

May increase serum creatinine and decrease GFR. Use caution when used concurrently with medications which may alter renal function. May delay recovery of renal function in patients with delayed allograft function. Increased urinary protein excretion has been observed when converting renal transplant patients from calcineurin inhibitors to sirolimus during maintenance therapy. A higher level of proteinuria prior to sirolimus conversion correlates with a higher degree of proteinuria after conversion. In some patients, proteinuria may reach nephrotic levels; nephrotic syndrome (new onset) has been reported. Increased risk of BK viral-associated nephropathy which may impair renal function and cause graft loss; consider decreasing immunosuppressive burden if evidence of deteriorating renal function.

Use caution with hepatic impairment; a reduction in the maintenance dose is recommended. Has been associated with an increased risk of fluid accumulation and lymphocele; peripheral edema, lymphedema, ascites, and pleural and pericardial effusions (including significant effusions and tamponade) were reported; use with caution in patients in whom fluid accumulation may be poorly tolerated, such as in cardiovascular disease (heart failure or hypertension) and pulmonary disease. Cases of interstitial lung disease (ILD) (eg, pneumonitis, bronchiolitis obliterans organizing pneumonia [BOOP], pulmonary fibrosis) have been observed (some fatal); may be associated with pulmonary hypertension (including pulmonary arterial hypertension) and risk may be increased with higher trough levels. ILD may resolve with dose reduction or discontinuation of therapy. Potentially significant drug-drug interactions may exist, requiring dose or frequency adjustment, additional monitoring, and/or selection of alternative therapy. Concurrent use with a calcineurin inhibitor (cyclosporine, tacrolimus) may increase the risk of calcineurin inhibitor-induced hemolytic uremic syndrome/thrombotic thrombocytopenic purpura/thrombotic microangiopathy (HUS/TTP/TMA). Immunosuppressants may affect response to vaccination. Therefore, during treatment with sirolimus, vaccination may be less effective. The use of live vaccines should be avoided.

Hypersensitivity reactions, including anaphylactic/anaphylactoid reactions, angioedema, exfoliative dermatitis, and hypersensitivity vasculitis have been reported. Concurrent use with other drugs known to cause angioedema (eg, ACE inhibitors) may increase risk. Immunosuppressant therapy is associated with an increased risk of skin cancer; limit sun and ultraviolet light exposure; use appropriate sun protection. May increase serum lipids (cholesterol and triglycerides); use with caution in patients with hyperlipidemia; monitor cholesterol/lipids; if hyperlipidemia occurs, follow current guidelines for management (diet, exercise, lipid lowering agents); antihyperlipidemic therapy may not be effective in normalizing levels. May be associated with wound dehiscence and impaired healing; use caution in the perioperative period. Patients with a body mass index (BMI) >30 kg/m^2 are at increased risk for abnormal wound healing.

Sirolimus tablets and oral solution are not bioequivalent, due to differences in absorption. Clinical equivalence was seen using 2 mg tablet and 2 mg solution. It is not known if higher doses are also clinically equivalent. Monitor sirolimus levels if changes in dosage forms are made. Some dosage forms may contain propylene glycol; large amounts are potentially toxic and have been associated hyperosmolality, lactic acidosis, seizures, and respiratory depression; use caution (AAP, 1997; Zar 2007). [US Boxed Warning]: Should only be used by physicians

experienced in immunosuppressive therapy and management of transplant patients. Adequate laboratory and supportive medical resources must be readily available. Sirolimus concentrations are dependent on the assay method (eg, chromatographic and immunoassay) used; assay methods are not interchangeable. Variations in methods to determine sirolimus whole blood concentrations, as well as interlaboratory variations, may result in improper dosage adjustments, which may lead to subtherapeutic or toxic levels. Determine the assay method used to assure consistency (or accommodations if changes occur), and for monitoring purposes, be aware of alterations to assay method or reference range and that values from different assays may not be interchangeable.

Adverse Reactions Incidence of many adverse effects is dose related. Reported events exclusive to renal transplant patients unless otherwise noted. Frequency not always defined.

Cardiovascular: Peripheral edema (≥20% to 58%, LAM and renal transplants), hypertension (49%), edema (18% to 20%), chest pain (LAM), deep vein thrombosis, pulmonary embolism, tachycardia

Central nervous system: Headache (≥20% to 34%, LAM and renal transplants), pain (29% to 33%), dizziness (LAM)

Dermatologic: Acne vulgaris (≥20% to 22%, LAM and renal transplants), skin rash (10% to 20%)

Endocrine & metabolic: Hypertriglyceridemia (45% to 57%), hypercholesterolemia (≥20% to 46%, LAM and renal transplants), amenorrhea, diabetes mellitus, hypermenorrhea, hypervolemia, hypokalemia, increased lactate dehydrogenase, menstrual disease, ovarian cyst

Gastrointestinal: Constipation (36% to 38%), abdominal pain (≥20% to 36%, LAM and renal transplants), diarrhea (≥20% to 35%, LAM and renal transplants), nausea (≥20% to 31%, LAM and renal transplants), stomatitis (3% to >20%)

Genitourinary: Urinary tract infection (33%)

Hematologic & oncologic: Anemia (23% to 33%), thrombocytopenia (14% to 30%), lymphoproliferative disorder (≤3%; including lymphoma), skin carcinoma (≤3%; includes basal cell carcinoma, squamous cell carcinoma, melanoma), hemolytic-uremic syndrome, leukopenia, lymphocele, thrombotic thrombocytopenic purpura

Infection: Herpes simplex infection, herpes zoster, sepsis

Neuromuscular & skeletal: Arthralgia (25% to 31%), myalgia (LAM), osteonecrosis

Renal: Increased serum creatinine (39% to 40%), pyelonephritis

Respiratory: Nasopharyngitis (LAM), epistaxis, pneumonia, upper respiratory tract infection (LAM)

Miscellaneous: Wound healing impairment

<3% (Limited to important or life-threatening): Ascites, azoospermia, cardiac tamponade, cytomegalovirus, dehiscence (fascial), Epstein-Barr infection, exfoliative dermatitis, focal segmental glomerulosclerosis, hepatic necrosis, hepatotoxicity, hyperglycemia, hypersensitivity angiitis, hypersensitivity reaction, hypophosphatemia, incisional hernia, interstitial pulmonary disease (dose related; includes pneumonitis, pulmonary fibrosis, and bronchiolitis obliterans organizing pneumonia with no identified infectious etiology), lymphedema, mycobacterium infection, nephrotic syndrome, neutropenia, pancreatitis, pancytopenia, pericardial effusion, pleural effusion, pneumonia due to Pneumocystis carinii, progressive multifocal leukoencephalopathy, proteinuria, pseudomembranous colitis, pulmonary alveolitis, pulmonary hemorrhage, renal disease (BK virus-associated), reversible posterior leukoencephalopathy syndrome, tuberculosis, weight loss, wound dehiscence

Drug Interactions

Metabolism/Transport Effects Substrate of CYP3A4 (major), P-glycoprotein; **Note:** Assignment of Major/Minor substrate status based on clinically relevant drug interaction potential

Avoid Concomitant Use

Avoid concomitant use of Sirolimus with any of the following: BCG (Intravesical); Conivaptan; Crizotinib; Deferiprone; Dipyrone; Enzalutamide; Fusidic Acid (Systemic); Idelalisib; Mifepristone; Natalizumab; Pimecrolimus; Posaconazole; Tacrolimus (Systemic); Tacrolimus (Topical); Tofacitinib; Vaccines (Live); Voriconazole

Increased Effect/Toxicity

Sirolimus may increase the levels/effects of: ACE Inhibitors; CloZAPine; CycloSPORINE (Systemic); Deferiprone; Fingolimod; Leflunomide; Natalizumab; Tacrolimus (Systemic); Tacrolimus (Topical); Tofacitinib; Vaccines (Live)

The levels/effects of Sirolimus may be increased by: Aprepitant; Boceprevir; Clotrimazole (Topical); Conivaptan; Crizotinib; CycloSPORINE (Systemic); CYP3A4 Inhibitors (Moderate); CYP3A4 Inhibitors (Strong);

Dasatinib; Denosumab; Dipyrone; Fluconazole; Fosaprepitant; Fusidic Acid (Systemic); Idelalisib; Itraconazole; Ivacaftor; Ketoconazole (Systemic); Luliconazole; Macrolide Antibiotics; Mifepristone; Nelfinavir; Netupitant; Ombitasvir, Paritaprevir, Ritonavir, and Dasabuvir; Osimertinib; Palbociclib; P-glycoprotein/ABCB1 Inhibitors; Pimecrolimus; Posaconazole; Ranolazine; Roflumilast; Stiripentol; Tacrolimus (Systemic); Tacrolimus (Topical); Telaprevir; Trastuzumab; Voriconazole

Decreased Effect

Sirolimus may decrease the levels/effects of: Antidiabetic Agents; BCG (Intravesical); Coccidioides immitis Skin Test; Sipuleucel-T; Tacrolimus (Systemic); Vaccines (Inactivated); Vaccines (Live)

The levels/effects of Sirolimus may be decreased by: Bosentan; CYP3A4 Inducers (Moderate); CYP3A4 Inducers (Strong); Dabrafenib; Deferasirox; Echinacea; Efavirenz; Enzalutamide; Fosphenytoin; Mitotane; Osimertinib; P-glycoprotein/ABCB1 Inducers; Phenytoin; Rifampin; Siltuximab; St Johns Wort; Tocilizumab

Food Interactions Grapefruit juice may decrease clearance of sirolimus. Ingestion with high-fat meals decreases peak concentrations but increases AUC by 23% to 35%. Management: Avoid grapefruit juice. Take consistently (either with or without food) to minimize variability.

Storage/Stability

Oral solution: Store at 2°C to 8°C (36°F to 46°F). Protect from light. A slight haze may develop in refrigerated solutions, but the quality of the product is not affected. After opening, solution should be used within 1 month. If necessary, may be stored at temperatures up to 25°C (77°F) for ≤15 days after opening. Product may be stored in amber syringe for a maximum of 24 hours (at room temperature or refrigerated). Discard syringe after single use. Solution should be used immediately following dilution.

Tablet: Store at 20°C to 25°C (68°F to 77°F). Protect from light.

Mechanism of Action Sirolimus inhibits T-lymphocyte activation and proliferation in response to antigenic and cytokine stimulation and inhibits antibody production. Its mechanism differs from other immunosuppressants. Sirolimus binds to FKBP-12, an intracellular protein, to form an immunosuppressive complex which inhibits the regulatory kinase, mTOR (mechanistic target of rapamycin). This inhibition suppresses cytokine mediated T-cell proliferation, halting progression from the G1 to the S phase of the cell cycle. It inhibits acute rejection of allografts and prolongs graft survival.

In lymphangioleiomyomatosis, the mTOR signaling pathway is activated through the loss of the tuberous sclerosis complex (TSC) gene function (resulting in cellular proliferation and release of lymphangiogenic growth factors). By inhibiting the mTOR pathway, sirolimus prevents the proliferation of lymphangioleiomyomatosis cells.

Pharmacodynamics/Kinetics

Absorption: Rapid

Distribution: 12 L/kg (range: 4 to 20 L/kg)

Protein binding: ~92%, primarily to albumin

Metabolism: Extensive; in intestinal wall via P-glycoprotein and hepatic via CYP3A4 to 7 major metabolites

Bioavailability: Oral solution: 14%; Oral tablet: 18%

Half-life elimination: Mean: 62 hours (range: 46 to 78 hours); extended in hepatic impairment (Child-Pugh class A or B) to 113 hours

Time to peak: Oral solution: 1 to 3 hours; Tablet: 1 to 6 hours

Excretion: Feces (91% due to P-glycoprotein-mediated efflux into gut lumen); urine (2%)

Dosing

Adult & Geriatric

Low-to-moderate immunologic risk renal transplant patients: Oral:

<40 kg: Loading dose: 3 mg/m^2 on day 1, followed by maintenance dosing of 1 mg/m^2 once daily

≥40 kg: Loading dose: 6 mg on day 1; maintenance: 2 mg once daily

High immunologic risk renal transplant patients: Oral: Loading dose: Up to 15 mg on day 1; maintenance: 5 mg/day; obtain trough concentration between days 5 to 7 and adjust accordingly. Continue concurrent cyclosporine/sirolimus/corticosteroid therapy for 1 year following transplantation. Further adjustment of the regimen must be based on clinical status.

Dosage adjustment for renal transplantation: Sirolimus dosages should be adjusted to maintain trough concentrations within desired range based on risk and concomitant therapy. Maximum daily dose: 40 mg. Dosage should be adjusted at intervals of 7 to 14 days to account for the long half-life of sirolimus. In general, dose proportionality may be assumed. New sirolimus dose **equals** current dose **multiplied by** (target concentration **divided by** current concentration). **Note:** If large dose increase is required, consider loading dose calculated as:

Loading dose **equals** (new maintenance dose **minus** current maintenance dose) **multiplied by** 3

Maximum dose in 1 day: 40 mg; if required dose is >40 mg (due to loading dose), divide loading dose over 2 days. Whole blood concentrations should not be used as the sole basis for dosage adjustment (monitor clinical signs/symptoms, tissue biopsy, and laboratory parameters).

Maintenance therapy after withdrawal of cyclosporine: Cyclosporine withdrawal is not recommended in high immunological risk patients. Following 2 to 4 months of combined therapy, withdrawal of cyclosporine may be considered in low-to-moderate immunologic risk patients. Cyclosporine should be discontinued over 4 to 8 weeks, and a necessary increase in the dosage of sirolimus (up to fourfold) should be anticipated due to removal of metabolic inhibition by cyclosporine and to maintain adequate immunosuppressive effects. Dose-adjusted trough target concentrations are typically 16 to 24 ng/mL for the first year post-transplant and 12 to 20 ng/mL thereafter (measured by chromatographic methodology).

Lymphangioleiomyomatosis: Adults: Oral: Initial: 2 mg once daily. Obtain trough concentration in 10 to 20 days; adjust dose to maintain a target concentration of 5 to 15 ng/mL.

Dosage adjustment for lymphangioleiomyomatosis: Once the maintenance dose is adjusted, further adjustments should be made at 7 to 14 day intervals to account for the long half-life of sirolimus. In general, dose proportionality may be assumed. New sirolimus dose **equals** current dose **multiplied by** (target concentration **divided by** current concentration). Once a stable dose is achieved, trough concentrations should be assessed at least every 3 months.

Graft-versus-host disease (GVHD): Oral:

GVHD prophylaxis (off-label use): 12 mg loading dose on day -3, followed by 4 mg daily (target trough level: 3 to 12 ng/mL); taper off after 6 to 9 months (Armand 2008; Cutler 2007)

Treatment of refractory acute GVHD (off-label use): 4 to 5 mg/m^2 for 14 days (no loading dose) (Benito 2001)

Treatment of chronic GVHD (off-label use): 6 mg loading dose, followed by 2 mg daily (target trough level: 7 to 12 ng/mL) for 6 to 9 months (Couriel 2005)

Heart transplantation (off-label use): Oral: **Note:** The use of sirolimus in the immediate post-cardiac transplant period (ie, de novo heart transplant) as a primary immunosuppressant has fallen out of favor due to adverse effects (eg, impaired wound healing and infection); however, patients may be converted to sirolimus from a calcineurin inhibitor (after at least 6 months from time of transplant [Costanzo 2010]) or may have sirolimus added to a calcineurin inhibitor to prevent or minimize further transplant related vasculopathy or renal toxicity due to calcineurin inhibitor use.

Conversion from a calcineurin inhibitor (CNI) (ie, cyclosporine, tacrolimus): Reduce cyclosporine by 25 mg twice daily or tacrolimus by 1 mg twice daily followed by initiation of sirolimus 1 mg once daily; adjust sirolimus dose to target trough level of 8 to 14 ng/mL, withdraw CNI, repeat biopsy 2 weeks after CNI withdrawal (Topilsky 2012). Alternatively, maintain CNI concentrations and initiate sirolimus 1 mg once daily for 1 week; adjust sirolimus to target trough levels of 10 to 15 ng/mL over 2 weeks, then reduce CNI to target 50% of therapeutic concentrations and after 2 weeks evaluate for rejection. If no rejection, continue same regimen for an additional month, then reduce CNI to 25% of therapeutic concentrations with repeat biopsy 2 weeks later; if no rejection, may discontinue CNI after 2 weeks and continue to maintain sirolimus trough levels of 10 to 15 ng/mL (usual doses required to maintain target levels: 1 to 8 mg daily) (Kushwaha 2005).

Conversion from antiproliferative drug (ie, azathioprine or mycophenolate) while maintaining calcineurin inhibitor: Upon discontinuation of antiproliferative, administer sirolimus 6 mg loading dose followed by 2 mg once daily titrated to a target trough level of 4 to 15 ng/mL (Mancini 2003) or 4 to 12 ng/mL per ISHLT recommendations (Costanzo 2010).

Renal angiomyolipoma (off-label use): Oral: Initial: 0.5 mg/m^2 once daily titrated to a target trough level of 3 to 6 ng/mL (may increase to target trough level of 6 to 10 ng/mL if <10% reduction in lesion diameters at 2 months) for 2 years (Davies 2011)

Pediatric Low-to-moderate immunologic risk renal transplant patients: Adolescents ≥13 years: Oral: Refer to adult dosing.

Renal Impairment No dosage adjustment is necessary. However, adjustment of regimen (including discontinuation of therapy) should be considered when used concurrently with cyclosporine and elevated or increasing serum creatinine is noted.

Hepatic Impairment
Loading dose: No dosage adjustment is necessary.
Maintenance dose:
Mild to moderate impairment (Child-Pugh classes A and B): Reduce maintenance dose by ~33%.
Severe impairment (Child-Pugh class C): Reduce maintenance dose by ~50%.

Administration Initial dose should be administered as soon as possible after transplant. Sirolimus should be taken 4 hours after oral cyclosporine (Neoral or Gengraf). Should be administered consistently (either with or without food).

Solution: Mix (by stirring vigorously) with at least 2 ounces of water or orange juice. No other liquids should be used for dilution. Patient should drink diluted solution immediately. The cup should then be refilled with an additional 4 ounces of water or orange juice, stirred vigorously, and the patient should drink the contents at once.
Tablet: Do not crush, split, or chew.

Hazardous agent; use appropriate precautions for handling and disposal (NIOSH 2014 [group 2]).

Monitoring Parameters Monitor LFTs and CBC during treatment. Monitor sirolimus levels in all patients (especially in pediatric patients, patients ≥13 years of age weighing <40 kg, patients with hepatic impairment, or on concurrent potent inhibitors or inducers of CYP3A4 or P-gp, and/or if cyclosporine dosing is markedly reduced or discontinued), and when changing dosage forms of sirolimus. Also monitor serum cholesterol and triglycerides, blood pressure, serum creatinine, and urinary protein. Serum drug concentrations should be determined 3 to 4 days after loading doses and 7 to 14 days after dosage adjustments for renal transplant patients; however, these concentrations should not be used as the sole basis for dosage adjustment, especially during withdrawal of cyclosporine (monitor clinical signs/symptoms, tissue biopsy, and laboratory parameters). Monitor serum trough concentration 10 to 20 days after initiating therapy for lymphangioleiomyomatosis and 7 to 14 days after dosage adjustments. Once a stable dose is achieved, trough concentrations should be assessed at least every 3 months. **Note:** Concentrations and ranges are dependent on and will vary with assay methodology (chromatographic or immunoassay); assay methods are not interchangeable.

Reference Range Note: Sirolimus concentrations are dependent on the assay method (eg, chromatographic and immunoassay) used; assay methods are not interchangeable. Determine the assay method used to assure consistency (or accommodations if changes occur) and for monitoring purposes, be aware of alterations to assay method or reference range.

Serum trough concentration goals for renal transplantation (based on HPLC methods):
Concomitant cyclosporine: 4 to 12 ng/mL
Low-to-moderate immunologic risk (after cyclosporine withdrawal): 16 to 24 ng/mL for the first year after transplant; after 1 year: 12 to 20 ng/mL
High immunologic risk (with cyclosporine): 10 to 15 ng/mL

Note: Trough concentrations vary based on clinical context and use of additional immunosuppressants. The following represents typical ranges.
When combined with tacrolimus and mycophenolate mofetil (MMF) without steroids: 6 to 8 ng/mL
As a substitute for tacrolimus (starting 4 to 8 weeks post-transplant), in combination with MMF and steroids: 8 to 12 ng/mL
Following conversion from tacrolimus to sirolimus >6 months post-transplant due to chronic allograft nephropathy: 4 to 6 ng/mL

Serum trough concentrations for heart transplantation (off-label use):
With calcineurin inhibitor (eg, cyclosporine): 4 to 12 ng/mL (Costanzo 2010)
Without calcineurin inhibitor: 10 to 15 ng/mL (Raichlin 2007a; Raichlin 2007b)
Following conversion from cyclosporine or tacrolimus to sirolimus: Initial (maintained until completion of conversion [~2 weeks]): 8 to 14 ng/mL (Topilsky 2012) **or** 9 to 15 ng/mL (Zuckermann 2012); Maintenance: 10 to 15 ng/mL (Kushwaha 2005) **or** 7 to 15 ng/mL (Zuckermann 2012)
Serum trough concentrations for lymphangioleiomyomatosis: 5 to 15 ng/mL
Serum trough concentrations for GVHD prophylaxis in allogeneic stem cell transplant (off-label use): 3 to 12 ng/mL (Armand 2008; Cutler 2007)
Serum trough concentrations for advanced chordoma (off-label use): 15 to 20 ng/mL (Stacchiotti 2009)
Serum trough concentrations for renal angiomyolipoma (off-label use): 3 to 6 ng/mL; may increase to 6 to 10 ng/mL if <10% reduction in lesion diameters at 2 months (Davies 2011)

Dosage Forms Excipient information presented when available (limited, particularly for generics); consult specific product labeling.
Solution, Oral:
Rapamune: 1 mg/mL (60 mL) [contains alcohol, usp]
Tablet, Oral:
Rapamune: 0.5 mg, 1 mg, 2 mg
Generic: 0.5 mg, 1 mg, 2 mg

◆ **Sirop Docusate De Sodium [OTC] (Can)** see Docusate on page 578

◆ **Sirturo** see Bedaquiline on page 207

SitaGLIPtin (sit a GLIP tin)

Brand Names: US Januvia
Brand Names: Canada Januvia
Index Terms MK-0431; Sitagliptin Phosphate
Pharmacologic Category Antidiabetic Agent, Dipeptidyl Peptidase IV (DPP-IV) Inhibitor
Additional Appendix Information
Oral Dosages That Should Not Be Crushed on page 2003
Use Diabetes mellitus, type 2: As an adjunct to diet and exercise to improve glycemic control in adults with type 2 diabetes mellitus (noninsulin dependent) as monotherapy or combination therapy.
Pregnancy Considerations Adverse events have not been observed in animal reproduction studies.

In women with diabetes, maternal hyperglycemia can be associated with congenital malformations as well as adverse effects in the fetus, neonate, and the mother (ACOG 2005; ADA 2015; Kitzmiller 2008; Metzger 2007). To prevent adverse outcomes, prior to conception and throughout pregnancy maternal blood glucose and HbA$_{1c}$ should be kept as close to target goals as possible but without causing significant hypoglycemia (ACOG 2013; ADA 2015; Blumer 2013; Kitzmiller 2008). Prior to pregnancy, effective contraception should be used until glycemic control is achieved (Kitzmiller 2008). Other agents are currently recommended to treat diabetes in pregnant women (ACOG 2013; Blumer 2013).

Health care providers are encouraged to enroll women exposed to sitagliptin during pregnancy in the registry (1-800-986-8999).
Breast-Feeding Considerations It is not known if sitagliptin is excreted in breast milk. The US labeling recommends that caution be exercised when administering sitagliptin to breast-feeding women. The Canadian labeling does not recommend use in breast-feeding women.
Medication Guide Available Yes
Contraindications Serious hypersensitivity (eg, anaphylaxis, angioedema) to sitagliptin or any component of the formulation
Warnings/Precautions Avoid use in type 1 diabetes mellitus (insulin dependent) and diabetic ketoacidosis due to lack of efficacy in these populations. Monitor blood glucose closely; dosage adjustments of insulin or insulin secretagogues may be necessary. Worsening renal function, including acute renal failure, sometimes requiring dialysis has been reported. Use with caution in patients with moderate to severe renal dysfunction and end-stage renal disease (ESRD) requiring hemodialysis or peritoneal dialysis; dosing adjustment required. Canadian labeling recommends against use in patients with severe hepatic impairment.

Severe and disabling arthralgia has been reported with DPP-IV inhibitor use; onset may occur within one day to years after treatment initiation and may resolve with discontinuation of therapy. Some patients may experience a recurrence of symptoms if DPP-IV inhibitor therapy resumed. Serious hypersensitivity reactions, including anaphylaxis, angioedema, and exfoliative skin reactions, such as Stevens-Johnson syndrome, have been reported; discontinue if signs/symptoms of hypersensitivity reactions occur. Use with caution if patient has experienced angioedema with other dipeptidyl peptidase IV (DPP-IV) inhibitor use. Cases of acute pancreatitis (including hemorrhagic and necrotizing with some fatalities) have been reported with use; monitor for signs/symptoms of pancreatitis. Discontinue use immediately if pancreatitis is suspected and initiate appropriate management. Use with caution in patients with a history of pancreatitis (not known if this population is at greater risk).

No specific recommendations regarding patients with cardiovascular disease (including heart failure) are provided in the US labeling (Canadian labeling recommends against use in the heart failure population). Clinical trials included only a limited number of patients with heart failure. In one large randomized, double-blinded trial in patients with type 2 diabetes and established cardiovascular disease (history of major CAD, ischemic cerebrovascular disease, or atherosclerotic peripheral arterial disease), the occurrence of the primary composite cardiovascular outcome (cardiovascular death, nonfatal MI, nonfatal stroke, or hospitalization for unstable angina) was found to be noninferior to placebo. In addition, the rate of hospitalization for heart failure did not differ between the two groups (Green 2015). Diabetes self-management education is essential to maximize the effectiveness of therapy. Potentially significant interactions may exist, requiring dose or frequency adjustment, additional monitoring, and/or selection of alternative therapy.

Adverse Reactions Reported with monotherapy.

1% to 10%:

Cardiovascular: Peripheral edema (2%)

Endocrine & metabolic: Hypoglycemia (1%)

Gastrointestinal: Diarrhea (4%), constipation (3%), nausea (2%)

Neuromuscular & skeletal: Osteoarthritis (1%)

Respiratory: Nasopharyngitis (5%), pharyngitis (1%), upper respiratory tract infection (viral; 1%)

<1% (important or life-threatening): Acne rosacea, acute pancreatitis (including hemorrhagic or necrotizing forms with some fatalities), acute renal failure (possibly requiring dialysis), anaphylaxis, anemia, angioedema, bundle branch block, depression, erectile dysfunction, exfoliative dermatitis, gastritis (*Helicobacter*), gastroesophageal reflux disease, hypertension, hypersensitivity, hypersensitivity vasculitis, hypotension, increased liver enzymes, liver steatosis, migraine, orthostatic hypotension, peripheral neuropathy, renal insufficiency, severe arthralgia (FDA Safety Alert, Aug 28, 2015), Stevens-Johnson syndrome

Drug Interactions

Metabolism/Transport Effects Substrate of P-glycoprotein

Avoid Concomitant Use There are no known interactions where it is recommended to avoid concomitant use.

Increased Effect/Toxicity

SitaGLIPtin may increase the levels/effects of: ACE Inhibitors; Digoxin; Hypoglycemia-Associated Agents; Insulin; Sulfonylureas

The levels/effects of SitaGLIPtin may be increased by: Alpha-Lipoic Acid; Androgens; Lumacaftor; MAO Inhibitors; Pegvisomant; P-glycoprotein/ABCB1 Inhibitors; Quinolone Antibiotics; Ranolazine; Salicylates; Selective Serotonin Reuptake Inhibitors

Decreased Effect

The levels/effects of SitaGLIPtin may be decreased by: Hyperglycemia-Associated Agents; Lumacaftor; P-glycoprotein/ABCB1 Inducers; Quinolone Antibiotics; Thiazide Diuretics

Storage/Stability Store at 20°C to 25°C (68°F to 77°F); excursions permitted to 15°C to 30°C (59°F to 86°F).

Mechanism of Action Sitagliptin inhibits dipeptidyl peptidase IV (DPP-IV) enzyme resulting in prolonged active incretin levels. Incretin hormones (eg, glucagon-like peptide-1 [GLP-1] and glucose-dependent insulinotropic polypeptide [GIP]) regulate glucose homeostasis by increasing insulin synthesis and release from pancreatic beta cells and decreasing glucagon secretion from pancreatic alpha cells. Decreased glucagon secretion results in decreased hepatic glucose production. Under normal physiologic circumstances, incretin hormones are released by the intestine throughout the day and levels are increased in

response to a meal; incretin hormones are rapidly inactivated by the DPP-IV enzyme.

Pharmacodynamics/Kinetics

Absorption: Rapid

Distribution: ~198 L

Protein binding: 38%

Metabolism: Not extensively metabolized; minor metabolism via CYP3A4 and 2C8 to metabolites (inactive) suggested by *in vitro* studies

Bioavailability: ~87%

Half-life elimination: 12.4 hours

Time to peak, plasma: 1 to 4 hours

Excretion: Urine 87% (~79% as unchanged drug, 16% as metabolites); feces 13%

Dosing

Adult

Diabetes mellitus, type 2: Oral: 100 mg once daily

Concomitant use with insulin and/or insulin secretagogues (eg, sulfonylureas): Reduced dose of insulin and/or insulin secretagogues may be needed.

Renal Impairment

CrCl ≥50 mL/minute: No dosage adjustment necessary.

CrCl ≥30 to <50 mL/minute (approximate SCr of >1.7 to ≤3 mg/dL [males] or >1.5 to ≤2.5 mg/dL [females]): 50 mg once daily

CrCl <30 mL/minute (approximate SCr of >3 mg/dL [males] or >2.5 mg/dL [females]): 25 mg once daily

ESRD requiring hemodialysis or peritoneal dialysis: 25 mg once daily; administer without regard to timing of hemodialysis

Hepatic Impairment

Mild to moderate impairment (Child-Pugh classes A and B): No dosage adjustment necessary.

Severe impairment (Child-Pugh class C):

US labeling: There are no dosage adjustments provided in the manufacturer's labeling (has not been studied).

Canadian labeling: Use is not recommended.

Dietary Considerations Individualized medical nutrition therapy (MNT) based on American Diabetes Association (ADA) recommendations is an integral part of therapy.

Administration Administer without regard to meals.

Monitoring Parameters HbA$_{1c}$, serum glucose; renal function prior to initiation and periodically during treatment

Reference Range

Recommendations for glycemic control in nonpregnant adults with diabetes (ADA 2015):

HbA$_{1c}$: <7% (a more aggressive [<6.5%] or less aggressive [<8%] HbA$_{1c}$ goal may be targeted based on patient-specific characteristics)

Preprandial capillary plasma glucose: 80 to 130 mg/dL

Peak postprandial capillary blood glucose: <180 mg/dL

Recommendations for glycemic control in pediatric (all age groups) patients with type 1 diabetes (ADA 2015):

HbA$_{1c}$: <7.5% (individualization may be appropriate based on patient-specific characteristics; <7% is reasonable if it can be achieved without excessive hypoglycemia)

Preprandial capillary plasma glucose: 90 to 130 mg/dL

Bedtime and overnight capillary blood glucose: 90 to 150 mg/dL

Dosage Forms Excipient information presented when available (limited, particularly for generics); consult specific product labeling.

Tablet, Oral:

Januvia: 25 mg, 50 mg, 100 mg

Sitagliptin and Metformin

(sit a GLIP tin & met FOR min)

Brand Names: US Janumet; Janumet XR

Brand Names: Canada Janumet; Janumet XR

Index Terms Metformin and Sitagliptin; Sitagliptin Phosphate and Metformin Hydrochloride

Pharmacologic Category Antidiabetic Agent, Biguanide; Antidiabetic Agent, Dipeptidyl Peptidase IV (DPP-IV) Inhibitor

Use Diabetes mellitus, type 2: As an adjunct to diet and exercise to improve glycemic control in adults with type 2 diabetes mellitus when treatment with both sitagliptin and metformin is appropriate

Medication Guide Available Yes

Dosing

Adult Note: Patients receiving concomitant insulin and/or insulin secretagogues (eg, sulfonylureas) may require dosage adjustments of these agents.

Diabetes mellitus, type 2: Oral: Initial doses should be based on current dose of sitagliptin and metformin.

Patients inadequately controlled on metformin alone: Initial dose:

Immediate release: Sitagliptin 100 mg daily plus current daily dose of metformin given in 2 equally divided doses; maximum: sitagliptin 100 mg/metformin 2000 mg daily. **Note:** The US labeling recommends patients currently receiving metformin 850 mg twice daily receive an initial dose of sitagliptin 50 mg and metformin 1000 mg twice daily.

Extended release: Sitagliptin 100 mg daily plus current daily dose of metformin given once daily; maximum: sitagliptin 100 mg/metformin 2000 mg daily. **Note:** The US labeling recommends patients currently receiving immediate release metformin 850-1000 mg twice daily receive an initial dose of sitagliptin 100 mg and metformin 2000 mg once daily.

Patients inadequately controlled on sitagliptin alone: Initial dose: **Note:** Patients currently receiving a renally-adjusted dose of sitagliptin should not be switched to a combination product.

Immediate release: Metformin 1000 mg daily plus sitagliptin 100 mg daily given in 2 equally divided doses

Extended release: Metformin 1000 mg and sitagliptin 100 mg once daily

Conversion from immediate release to extended release: Convert using same total daily dose (up to the maximum recommended dose), but adjust frequency as indicated for immediate (twice daily) or extended (once daily) release products.

Patients inadequately controlled on combination metformin and either pioglitazone, a sulfonylurea, or insulin: Canadian labeling (not in US labeling): Sitagliptin 100 mg daily plus current daily dose of metformin given in 2 equally divided doses. If taking insulin or a sulfonylurea concomitantly with sitagliptin/metformin, the dosage of insulin or sulfonylurea may need adjusted.

Patients inadequately controlled on combination therapy with sitagliptin and insulin: Canadian labeling (not in US labeling): Sitagliptin 100 mg daily plus metformin (dose based on glycemic control) given in 2 equally divided doses. Insulin dose may need adjusted.

Dosing adjustment: Metformin component may be gradually increased up to the maximum dose. Maximum dose: Sitagliptin 100 mg/metformin 2000 mg daily

Geriatric Refer to adult dosing. The initial and maintenance dosing should be conservative, due to the potential for decreased renal function (monitor). Do not use in patients ≥80 years of age unless normal renal function has been established.

Renal Impairment

US labeling:

Serum creatinine (SCr) ≥1.5 mg/dL (males) or ≥1.4 mg/dL (females): Use is contraindicated.

Abnormal CrCl (US labeling: Not defined; Canadian labeling: <60 mL/minute): Use is contraindicated.

Canadian labeling: Use is contraindicated in renal impairment (serum creatinine ≥136 micromol/L [males] or ≥124 micromol/L [females], or CrCl <60 mL/minute)

Alternate recommendations: **Note:** The United Kingdom National Institute for Health and Clinical Excellence (NICE) Guidelines recommend prescribing metformin with caution in those patients who are at risk of sudden deterioration in renal function and at risk of an estimated glomerular filtration rate (eGFR) <45 mL/minute/1.73 m^2 (NICE, 2008). Some evidence suggests that use of metformin is unsafe when eGFR <30 mL/minute/1.73 m^2 (calculated using MDRD) (Shaw, 2007). A review of the available data by members of the American Diabetes Association proposed the following recommendations based on eGFR (Lipska, 2011):

eGFR ≥60 mL/minute/1.73 m^2: No contraindications, monitor renal function annually

eGFR ≥45 to <60 mL/minute/1.73 m^2: Continue use; monitor renal function every 3 to 6 months. **Note:** The manufacturer's labeling for sitagliptin recommends a maximum dose of 50 mg once daily in patients with CrCl 30 to <50 mL/minute.

eGFR ≥30 to <45 mL/minute/1.73 m^2: In patients currently receiving metformin, use with caution, consider dosage reduction (eg, 50% reduction or 50% of maximal dose), monitor renal function every 3 months. Do not initiate therapy in patients with eGFR <45 mL/minute/1.73 m^2. **Note:** The manufacturer's labeling for sitagliptin recommends a maximum dose of 50 mg once daily in patients with CrCl 30 to <50 mL/minute.

eGFR <30 mL/minute/1.73 m^2: Discontinue use

Hepatic Impairment

US labeling: The manufacturer recommends to avoid metformin since liver disease is considered a risk factor for the development of lactic acidosis during metformin therapy. However, continued use of metformin in diabetics with liver dysfunction, including cirrhosis, has been used successfully and may be associated with a survival benefit in carefully selected patients; use cautiously in patients at risk for lactic acidosis (eg, renal impairment, alcohol use) (Brackett, 2010; Zhang, 2014). Use of sitagliptin in patients with severe hepatic impairment has not been studied.

Canadian labeling: Use is not recommended with clinical or laboratory evidence of disease and contraindicated in the presence of severe impairment.

Additional Information Complete prescribing information should be consulted for additional detail.

Dosage Forms Excipient information presented when available (limited, particularly for generics); consult specific product labeling.

Tablet, oral:

Janumet 50/500: Sitagliptin 50 mg and metformin hydrochloride 500 mg

Janumet 50/1000: Sitagliptin 50 mg and metformin hydrochloride 1000 mg

Tablet, extended release, oral:

Janumet XR: 50/500: Sitagliptin 50 mg and metformin hydrochloride 500 mg

Janumet XR: 50/1000: Sitagliptin 50 mg and metformin hydrochloride 1000 mg

Janumet XR: 100/1000: Sitagliptin 100 mg and metformin hydrochloride 1000 mg

Dosage Forms: Canada Note: Refer also to Dosage Forms. Excipient information presented when available (limited, particularly for generics); consult specific product labeling.

Tablet, oral:

Janumet 50/850: Sitagliptin 50 mg and metformin hydrochloride 850 mg

Sitagliptin and Simvastatin
(sit a GLIP tin & sim va STAT in)

Brand Names: US Juvisync™ [DSC]

Index Terms Simvastatin and Sitagliptin; Sitagliptin Phosphate and Simvastatin

Pharmacologic Category Antidiabetic Agent, Dipeptidyl Peptidase IV (DPP-IV) Inhibitor; Antilipemic Agent, HMG-CoA Reductase Inhibitor

Use For use when treatment with both sitagliptin and simvastatin is appropriate:

Sitagliptin: Management of type 2 diabetes mellitus (non-insulin dependent, NIDDM) as an adjunct to diet and exercise as monotherapy or in combination therapy with other antidiabetic agents

Simvastatin: Used with dietary therapy for the following:

Secondary prevention of cardiovascular events in hypercholesterolemic patients with established coronary heart disease (CHD) or at high risk for CHD: To reduce cardiovascular morbidity (myocardial infarction, coronary/noncoronary revascularization procedures) and mortality; to reduce the risk of stroke

Hyperlipidemias: To reduce elevations in total cholesterol (total-C), LDL-C, apolipoprotein B, triglycerides, and VLDL-C, and to increase HDL-C in patients with primary hypercholesterolemia (elevations of 1 or more components are present in Fredrickson type IIa, IIb, III, and IV hyperlipidemias); treatment of homozygous familial hypercholesterolemia

Primary and secondary prevention of atherosclerotic cardiovascular disease (ASCVD) according to the American College of Cardiology/American Heart Association: To reduce the risk of ASCVD in patients with clinical ASCVD (eg, coronary heart disease, stroke/TIA, or peripheral arterial disease presumed to be of atherosclerotic origin) who are greater than 75 years of age or not a candidate for high-intensity statin therapy; in patients without clinical ASCVD if LDL-C is 190 mg/dL or greater and not a candidate for high-intensity statin therapy; in patients without clinical ASCVD who have type 1 or type 2 diabetes and are between 40 and 75 years of age; in patients with an estimated 10-year ASCVD risk 7.5% or greater and who are between 40 and 75 years of age (Stone, 2013). Specific recommendations from the Kidney Disease: Improving Global Outcomes (KDIGO) organization have also been released for patients with chronic kidney disease (KDIGO [Tonelli, 2013]).

Medication Guide Available Yes

◀ **Dosing**

Adult Hyperlipidemia and type 2 diabetes: Oral: Initial dose: Sitagliptin 100 mg and simvastatin 40 mg once daily. **Note:** Patients already taking simvastatin <40 mg daily (with or without sitagliptin 100 mg daily) can be converted to the comparable equivalent of the combination product. Dose adjustments should be made at intervals of ≥4 weeks.

Concomitant use with insulin and/or insulin secretagogues (eg, sulfonylureas): Reduced dose of insulin and/or insulin secretagogues may be needed.

Dosage adjustment for simvastatin with concomitant medications:

Amiodarone, amlodipine, or ranolazine: Simvastatin dose should **not** exceed 20 mg daily

Diltiazem, dronedarone, or verapamil: Simvastatin dose should **not** exceed 10 mg daily

Lomitapide: Reduce simvastatin dose by 50% when initiating lomitapide. Simvastatin dose should not exceed 20 mg daily (or 40 mg daily for those who previously tolerated simvastatin 80 mg daily for ≥1 year without evidence of muscle toxicity)

Dosage adjustment for simvastatin in Chinese patients on niacin doses ≥1 g/day: Use caution with simvastatin doses of 40 mg daily because of an increased risk of myopathy

Renal Impairment Renal function may be estimated using Cockcroft-Gault formula for dosage adjustment purposes.

CrCl ≥50 mL/minute: No dosage adjustment necessary.

CrCl ≥30 to <50 mL/minute (approximate SCr of >1.7 to ≤3.0 mg/dL [males] or >1.5 to ≤2.5 mg/dL [females]): Initial: Sitagliptin 50 mg and simvastatin 40 mg once daily. **Note:** Patients already taking simvastatin <40 mg daily (with or without sitagliptin 50 mg daily) can be converted to the comparable equivalent of the combination product.

CrCl <30 mL/minute (approximate SCr of >3.0 mg/dL [males] or >2.5 mg/dL [females]): Use is not recommended.

End-stage renal disease (ESRD): Use is not recommended.

Hepatic Impairment Use is contraindicated.

Additional Information Complete prescribing information should be consulted for additional detail.

Dosage Forms Excipient information presented when available (limited, particularly for generics); consult specific product labeling.

Tablet, oral:

Juvisync 50/10: Sitagliptin 50 mg and simvastatin 10 mg [DSC]

Juvisync 50/20: Sitagliptin 50 mg and simvastatin 20 mg [DSC]

Juvisync 50/40: Sitagliptin 50 mg and simvastatin 40 mg [DSC]

Juvisync 100/10: Sitagliptin 100 mg and simvastatin 10 mg [DSC]

Juvisync 100/20: Sitagliptin 100 mg and simvastatin 20 mg [DSC]

Juvisync 100/40: Sitagliptin 100 mg and simvastatin 40 mg [DSC]

Smallpox Vaccine (SMAL poks vak SEEN)

Brand Names: US ACAM2000

Index Terms APSV; Dryvax; Live Smallpox Vaccine; Vaccinia Vaccine; WetVax

Pharmacologic Category Vaccine; Vaccine, Live (Viral)

Additional Appendix Information

Immunization Administration Recommendations *on page 1974*

Immunization Schedules *on page 1979*

Use Smallpox disease prevention: Active immunization against smallpox disease in persons determined to be at high risk for smallpox infection.

The Advisory Committee on Immunization Practices (ACIP) recommends routine vaccination for the following (CDC/ACIP [Rotz, 2001]):

• Laboratory workers at risk of exposure from cultures or contaminated animals which may be a source of vaccinia or related Orthopoxviruses capable of causing infections in humans (eg, monkeypox, cowpox, variola, vaccinia).

• Consideration may also be given for vaccination of healthcare workers having contact with clinical specimens, contaminated material, or patients receiving vaccinia or recombinant vaccinia viruses.

In a pre-event vaccination program, the ACIP recommends vaccination for the following (CDC/ACIP [Wharton, 2003]):

• Persons designated by authorities (smallpox response teams) to investigate and follow-up on initial smallpox cases with the likelihood of direct patient contact

• Hospital based health care teams who provide patient care for smallpox patients.

• Persons responsible for administering smallpox vaccine

For post-event vaccination, the ACIP recommends vaccination for the following (CDC [Petersen, 2015]):

• Persons directly exposed to an accidental or intentional release of the virus

• Household family members of a patient with confirmed, probable or suspected smallpox or others spending ≥3 hours in the household since the onset of fever

• Nonhousehold members with ≥3 hours of close contact (<6.5 feet or <2 meters) with a confirmed or suspected smallpox patient with a rash.

• Persons considered at high risk for smallpox infection (including healthcare workers) as defined by public health authorities

Prescribing and Access Restrictions ACAM2000 is deemed to have an approved REMS program. Smallpox vaccine is not available for general public use. Supplies are owned by the US federal government and are included in the Strategic National Stockpile. In August 2007, the FDA licensed the present ACAM2000 formulation of smallpox vaccine. This approval allows the vaccine to be distributed and administered in the event of a smallpox release. Most of the current vaccinations are administered by the US military. Additionally, laboratory workers who may be at risk of exposure may require vaccination. Bioterrorism experts have proposed immunization of first responders (including police, fire, and emergency workers), but these plans have not yet been implemented.

Medication Guide Available Yes

Dosing

Adult & Geriatric Primary vaccination and revaccination: Percutaneous: Not for IM, intradermal, IV, or SubQ injection: Vaccination by scarification (multiple-puncture technique) only: **Note:** A trace of blood should appear at vaccination site after 15 to 20 seconds; if no trace of blood is visible, an additional 3 insertions should be made using the same needle, without reinserting the needle into the vaccine bottle.

Use a single drop of vaccine suspension and 15 needle punctures (using the same bifurcated needle) into the superficial skin; if the patient does not have a major cutaneous reaction after the first dose (by day 6 to 8), a second dose (revaccination) from another vial or vaccine lot may be administered. If there is not a reaction to the second dose, consult the CDC or the state or local health department for further guidance

Note: According to the manufacturer, revaccination is recommended every 3 years for patients at a continued high risk for smallpox infection. The ACIP recommends routine nonemergency revaccination every 3 to 10 years, depending on type of exposure (CDC/ACIP [Rotz, 2001]). Additional information can be obtained from the Department of Defense and the CDC.

Pediatric Primary vaccination and revaccination: Children and Adolescents <16 years (in emergency conditions only) and Adolescents ≥16 years: Percutaneous: Refer to adult dosing.

Renal Impairment There are no dosage adjustments provided in the manufacturer's labeling.

Hepatic Impairment There are no dosage adjustments provided in the manufacturer's labeling.

Additional Information Complete prescribing information should be consulted for additional detail.

Dosage Forms Excipient information presented when available (limited, particularly for generics); consult specific product labeling. [DSC] = Discontinued product

Injection, powder for reconstitution [purified monkey cell source]:

ACAM2000: 1-5 x 10^8 plaque-forming units per mL [contains polymyxin B, neomycin (trace amounts) and human albumin; packed with diluent, tuberculin syringes for reconstitution, and 100 bifurcated needles for administration]

◆ SMX-TMP *see* Sulfamethoxazole and Trimethoprim *on page 1710*

◆ SMZ-TMP *see* Sulfamethoxazole and Trimethoprim *on page 1710*

◆ Snake Antivenin F(ab')2 (Equine) *see* Crotalidae Immune F(ab')₂ (Equine) *on page 452*

◆ Snake Antivenom F(ab')2 (Equine) *see* Crotalidae Immune F(ab')₂ (Equine) *on page 452*

◆ (+)-(S)-N-Methyl-γ-(1-naphthyloxy)-2-thiophenepropyl-amine Hydrochloride *see* DULoxetine *on page 610*

◆ Sochlor [OTC] *see* Sodium Chloride *on page 1671*

◆ Sodium 2-Mercaptoethane Sulfonate *see* Mesna *on page 1154*

◆ Sodium 4-Hydroxybutyrate *see* Sodium Oxybate *on page 1676*

◆ Sodium L-Triiodothyronine *see* Liothyronine *on page 1083*

Sodium Acetate (SOW dee um AS e tate)

Pharmacologic Category Electrolyte Supplement, Parenteral

Use Sodium source in large volume IV fluids to prevent or correct hyponatremia in patients with restricted intake; used to counter acidosis through conversion to bicarbonate

Dosing

Adult & Geriatric

Note: Sodium acetate is metabolized to bicarbonate on an equimolar basis outside the liver; administer in large volume IV fluids as a sodium source. Refer to Sodium Bicarbonate monograph.

Maintenance electrolyte requirements of sodium in parenteral nutrition solutions:
Daily requirements: 3-4 mEq/kg/24 hours or 25-40 mEq/1000 kcal/24 hours
Maximum: 100-150 mEq/24 hours

Pediatric Maintenance electrolyte requirements of sodium in parenteral nutrition solutions: IV: 3-4 mEq/kg/24 hours

Renal Impairment No dosage adjustment provided in manufacturer's labeling. Use with caution.

Hepatic Impairment No dosage adjustment provided in manufacturer's labeling. Use with caution.

Additional Information Complete prescribing information should be consulted for additional detail.

Dosage Forms Excipient information presented when available (limited, particularly for generics); consult specific product labeling.

Solution, Intravenous, as anhydrous:
Generic: 2 mEq/mL (20 mL, 50 mL, 100 mL); 4 mEq/mL (50 mL, 100 mL)

◆ Sodium Acid Carbonate *see* Sodium Bicarbonate *on page 1669*

◆ Sodium Acid Phosphate and Methenamine *see* Methenamine and Sodium Acid Phosphate *on page 1166*

◆ Sodium Artesunate *see* Artesunate *on page 154*

◆ Sodium Benzoate and Caffeine *see* Caffeine *on page 280*

◆ Sodium Benzoate and Sodium Phenylacetate *see* Sodium Phenylacetate and Sodium Benzoate *on page 1676*

Sodium Bicarbonate (SOW dee um bye KAR bun ate)

Brand Names: US Neut

Index Terms Baking Soda; NaHCO₃; Sodium Acid Carbonate; Sodium Hydrogen Carbonate

Pharmacologic Category Alkalinizing Agent; Antacid; Electrolyte Supplement, Oral; Electrolyte Supplement, Parenteral

Use

Management of metabolic acidosis; gastric hyperacidity; as an alkalinization agent for the urine; treatment of hyperkalemia; management of overdose of certain drugs, including tricyclic antidepressants and aspirin

Neutralizing additive (dental use): Improves onset of analgesia and reduces injection site pain by adjusting lidocaine with epinephrine solution to a more physiologic pH.

Pregnancy Considerations Animal reproduction studies have not been conducted. The use of sodium bicarbonate in pregnant women for the management of cardiac arrest and metabolic acidosis is the same as in nonpregnant women (Campbell, 2009; Vanden Hoek, 2010). Antacids containing sodium bicarbonate should not be used during pregnancy due to their potential to cause metabolic alkalosis and fluid overload (Mahadevan, 2007).

Breast-Feeding Considerations Sodium is found in breast milk (IOM, 2004).

Contraindications

Alkalosis, hypernatremia, severe pulmonary edema, hypocalcemia, unknown abdominal pain

Neutralizing additive (dental use): Not for use as a systemic alkalizer

Warnings/Precautions Rapid administration in neonates, infants, and children <2 years of age has led to hypernatremia, decreased CSF pressure, and intracranial hemorrhage. **Use of IV NaHCO₃ should be reserved for documented metabolic acidosis and for hyperkalemia-induced cardiac arrest.** Routine use in cardiac arrest is not recommended. Vesicant (at concentrations ≥8.4%); ensure proper catheter or needle position prior to and during infusion; avoid extravasation (tissue necrosis may occur due to hypertonicity). May cause sodium retention especially if renal function is impaired; not to be used in treatment of peptic ulcer; use with caution in patients with HF, edema, cirrhosis, or renal failure. Not the antacid of choice for the elderly because of sodium content and potential for systemic alkalosis.

Adverse Reactions Frequency not defined.

Cardiovascular: Cerebral hemorrhage, CHF (aggravated), edema

Central nervous system: Tetany

Gastrointestinal: Belching, flatulence (with oral), gastric distension

Endocrine & metabolic: Hypernatremia, hyperosmolality, hypocalcemia, hypokalemia, increased affinity of hemoglobin for oxygen-reduced pH in myocardial tissue necrosis when extravasated, intracranial acidosis, metabolic alkalosis, milk-alkali syndrome (especially with renal dysfunction)

Respiratory: Pulmonary edema

Drug Interactions

Metabolism/Transport Effects None known.

Avoid Concomitant Use There are no known interactions where it is recommended to avoid concomitant use.

Increased Effect/Toxicity

Sodium Bicarbonate may increase the levels/effects of: Alpha-/Beta-Agonists (Indirect-Acting); Amphetamines; Calcium Polystyrene Sulfonate; Dexmethylphenidate; Flecainide; Mecamylamine; Memantine; Methylphenidate; QuiNIDine; QuiNINE

The levels/effects of Sodium Bicarbonate may be increased by: AcetaZOLAMIDE

Decreased Effect

Sodium Bicarbonate may decrease the levels/effects of: Antipsychotic Agents (Phenothiazines); Atazanavir; Bisacodyl; Bismuth Subcitrate; Bosutinib; Captopril; Cefditoren; Cefpodoxime; Cefuroxime; Chloroquine; Corticosteroids (Oral); Cysteamine (Systemic); Dabigatran Etexilate; Dabrafenib; Dasatinib; Delavirdine; Elvitegravir; Erlotinib; Flecainide; Fosinopril; Gabapentin; Gefitinib; HMG-CoA Reductase Inhibitors; Hyoscyamine; Iron Salts; Isoniazid; Itraconazole; Ketoconazole (Systemic); Ledipasvir; Lithium; Mesalamine; Methenamine; Multivitamins/Minerals (with ADEK, Folate, Iron); Nilotinib; PAZOPanib; PenicillAMINE; Phosphate Supplements; Potassium Acid Phosphate; Rilpivirine; Riociguat; Sotalol; Sulpiride; Tetracycline Derivatives; Trientine

◀

Preparation for Administration

Prevention of contrast-induced nephropathy (off-label use): Remove 154 mL from 1000 mL bag of D_5W; replace with 154 mL of 8.4% sodium bicarbonate; resultant concentration is 154 mEq/L (Merten, 2004); more practically, institutions may remove 150 mL from 1000 mL bag of D_5W and replace with 150 mL of 8.4% sodium bicarbonate; resultant concentration is 150 mEq/L

Neutralizing additive (dental use): Add specified volume of 8.4% sodium bicarbonate directly with lidocaine and epinephrine injection and mix; use immediately after mixing.

Storage/Stability

Store injection at room temperature. Protect from heat and from freezing. Use only clear solutions.

Neutralizing additive (dental use): Store at 20°C to 25°C (68°F to 77°F).

Mechanism of Action

Dissociates to provide bicarbonate ion which neutralizes hydrogen ion concentration and raises blood and urinary pH

Neutralizing additive (dental use): Increases pH of lidocaine and epinephrine solution to improve tolerability and increase tissue uptake

Pharmacodynamics/Kinetics

Onset of action: Oral: Rapid; IV: 15 minutes

Duration: Oral: 8-10 minutes; IV: 1-2 hours

Absorption: Oral: Well absorbed

Excretion: Urine (<1%)

Dosing

Adult & Geriatric

Cardiac arrest (ACLS, 2010): IV: Initial: 1 mEq/kg/dose; repeat doses should be guided by arterial blood gases **Routine use of NaHCO₃ is not recommended.** May be considered in the setting of prolonged cardiac arrest only after adequate alveolar ventilation has been established and effective cardiac compressions. **Note:** In some cardiac arrest situations (eg, metabolic acidosis, hyperkalemia, or tricyclic antidepressant overdose), sodium bicarbonate may be beneficial.

Metabolic acidosis: IV: Dosage should be based on the following formula if blood gases and pH measurements are available:

$HCO_3^-(mEq) = 0.5$ x weight (kg) x [24 - serum HCO_3^- (mEq/L)] **or** $HCO_3^-(mEq) = 0.5$ x weight (kg) x [desired increase in serum $HCO_3^-(mEq/L)$]

Administer ½ dose initially, then remaining ½ dose over the next 24 hours; monitor pH, serum HCO_3^-, and clinical status. **Note:** These equations provide an estimated replacement dose. The underlying cause and degree of acidosis may result in the need for larger or smaller replacement doses. In most cases, the initial goal of therapy is to target a pH of ~7.2 and a plasma bicarbonate level of ~10 mEq/L to prevent overalkalinization.

Note: If acid-base status is not available: 2-5 mEq/kg IV infusion over 4-8 hours; subsequent doses should be based on patient's acid-base status

Hyperkalemia (ACLS, 2010): IV: 50 mEq over 5 minutes (as appropriate, consider methods of enhancing potassium removal/excretion)

Chronic renal failure: Oral: Initiate when plasma HCO_3^- <15 mEq/L Start with 20-36 mEq/day in divided doses, titrate to bicarbonate level of 18-20 mEq/L

Renal tubular acidosis: Oral:

Distal: 0.5-2 mEq/kg/day in 4-5 divided doses

Proximal: 5-10 mEq/kg/day; maintenance: Increase as required to maintain serum bicarbonate in the normal range

Urine alkalinization: Oral: Initial: 48 mEq (4 g), then 12-24 mEq (1-2 g) every 4 hours; dose should be titrated to desired urinary pH; doses up to 16 g/day (200 mEq) in patients <60 years and 8 g (100 mEq) in patients >60 years

Antacid: Oral: 325 mg to 2 g 1-4 times/day

Neutralize lidocaine with epinephrine dental anesthetic: Neutralizing additive: Mix 10 parts anesthetic (lidocaine with epinephrine) to 1 part 8.4% sodium bicarbonate

Add 0.18 mL sodium bicarbonate to 1.8 mL cartridge of lidocaine 2% with epinephrine 1:50,000 or 1:100,000

Add 2 mL sodium bicarbonate to 20 mL vial of lidocaine 2% with epinephrine 1:100,000

Add 3 mL sodium bicarbonate to 30 mL vial of lidocaine 2% with epinephrine 1:100,000

Add 5 mL sodium bicarbonate to 50 mL vial of lidocaine 2% with epinephrine 1:100,000

Prevention of contrast-induced nephropathy (off-label use): IV infusion: 154 mEq/L sodium bicarbonate in D_5W solution: 3 mL/kg/hour for 1 hour immediately before contrast injection, then 1mL/kg/hour during contrast exposure and for 6 hours after procedure

To prepare solution, remove 154 mL from 1000 mL bag of D_5W; replace with 154 mL of 8.4% sodium bicarbonate; resultant concentration is 154 mEq/L (Merten, 2004); more practically, institutions may remove 150 mL from 1000 mL bag of D_5W and replace with 150 mL of 8.4% sodium bicarbonate; resultant concentration is 150 mEq/L

Pediatric

Cardiac arrest (PALS, 2010): IV, I.O.: Infants and Children: 1 mEq/kg/dose; repeat doses should be guided by arterial blood gases; children <2 years of age should receive 4.2% (0.5 mEq/mL) solution. **Note:** If I.O. route is used for administration and is subsequently used to obtain blood samples for acid-base analysis, results will be inaccurate.

Routine use of NaHCO₃ is not recommended. May be considered in the setting of prolonged cardiac arrest only after adequate alveolar ventilation has been established and effective cardiac compressions. **Note:** In some cardiac arrest situations (eg, metabolic acidosis, hyperkalemia, or tricyclic antidepressant overdose), sodium bicarbonate may be beneficial.

Metabolic acidosis: IV: Infants and Children: Dosage should be based on the following formula if blood gases and pH measurements are available:

$HCO_3^-(mEq) = 0.5$ x weight (kg) x [24 - serum HCO_3^- (mEq/L)] **or** $HCO_3^-(mEq) = 0.5$ x weight (kg) x [desired increase in serum $HCO_3^-(mEq/L)$]

Administer ½ dose initially, then remaining ½ dose over the next 24 hours; monitor pH, serum HCO_3^-, and clinical status. **Note:** These equations provide an estimated replacement dose. The underlying cause and degree of acidosis may result in the need for larger or smaller replacement doses. In most cases, the initial goal of therapy is to target a pH of ~7.2 and a plasma bicarbonate level of ~10 mEq/L to prevent overalkalinization.

Note: If acid-base status is not available: Dose for older Children: 2-5 mEq/kg IV infusion over 4-8 hours; subsequent doses should be based on patient's acid-base status.

Chronic renal failure: Oral: Children: Initiate when plasma HCO_3^- <15 mEq/L: 1-3 mEq/kg/day

Renal tubular acidosis, distal: Oral: Children: 2-3 mEq/kg/day

Renal tubular acidosis, proximal: Children: Initial: 5-10 mEq/kg/day; maintenance: Increase as required to maintain serum bicarbonate in the normal range

Neutralize lidocaine with epinephrine dental anesthetic: Children and Adolescents: Neutralizing additive: Refer to adult dosing.

Urine alkalinization: Oral: Children: 1-10 mEq (84-840 mg)/kg/day in divided doses every 4-6 hours; dose should be titrated to desired urinary pH.

Dietary Considerations Some products may contain sodium. Oral product should be taken 1-3 hours after meals.

Administration For IV administration to infants, use the 0.5 mEq/mL solution or dilute the 1 mEq/mL solution 1:1 with **sterile water**; for direct IV infusion in emergencies, administer slowly (maximum rate in infants: 10 mEq/minute); for infusion, dilute to a maximum concentration of 0.5 mEq/mL in dextrose solution and infuse over 2 hours (maximum rate of administration: 1 mEq/kg/hour).

Vesicant (at concentrations ≥8.4%); ensure proper needle or catheter placement prior to and during IV infusion. Avoid extravasation.

Extravasation management: If extravasation occurs, stop infusion immediately and disconnect (leave needle/cannula in place); gently aspirate extravasated solution (do **NOT** flush the line); initiate hyaluronidase antidote; remove needle/cannula; apply dry cold compresses (Hurst, 2004); elevate extremity.

Hyaluronidase: SubQ: Inject four to five separate 0.2 mL injections of 15 units/mL around area of extravasation (Hurst, 2004).

Oral product should be administered 1-3 hours after meals.

Infiltration (dental use; Onpharma): Add specified volume of 8.4% sodium bicarbonate directly with lidocaine and epinephrine injection and mix; use immediately after mixing.

Dosage Forms Considerations

Sodium bicarbonate solution 4.2% [42 mg/mL] provides 0.5 mEq/mL each of sodium and bicarbonate

Sodium bicarbonate solution 7.5% [75 mg/mL] provides 0.9 mEq/mL each of sodium and bicarbonate

Sodium bicarbonate solution 8.4% [84 mg/mL] provides 1 mEq/mL each of sodium and bicarbonate

Dosage Forms Excipient information presented when available (limited, particularly for generics); consult specific product labeling. [DSC] = Discontinued product
Powder, Does not apply:
Generic: (1 g, 100 g, 454 g [DSC], 500 g, 2270 g [DSC], 2500 g, 10000 g, 12000 g [DSC])
Powder, Oral:
Generic: (1 g, 120 g, 454 g, 500 g, 1000 g, 2500 g, 12000 g, 25000 g, 45000 g)
Solution, Intravenous:
Neut: 4% (5 mL)
Generic: 4.2% (5 mL, 10 mL); 7.5% (50 mL); 8.4% (10 mL, 50 mL)
Tablet, Oral:
Generic: 325 mg, 650 mg

♦ Sodium Bicarbonate and Omeprazole see Omeprazole and Sodium Bicarbonate on page 1333

Sodium Chloride (SOW dee um KLOR ide)

Brand Names: US 4-Way Saline [OTC]; Afrin Saline Nasal Mist [OTC]; Allclenz [OTC] [DSC]; Altachlore [OTC]; Altamist Spray [OTC]; Atrapro Dermal Spray; Ayr Nasal Mist Allergy/Sinus [OTC]; Ayr Saline Nasal Drops [OTC]; Ayr Saline Nasal Gel [OTC]; Ayr Saline Nasal Neti Rinse [OTC]; Ayr Saline Nasal No-Drip [OTC]; AYR Saline Nasal Rinse [OTC]; Ayr Saline Nasal [OTC]; Ayr [OTC]; Baby Ayr Saline [OTC]; Broncho Saline [OTC]; Deep Sea Nasal Spray [OTC]; DiaB Klenz [OTC]; Elta Dermal Wound Cleanser [OTC]; Entsol Nasal Wash [OTC]; Entsol Nasal [OTC]; Entsol [OTC]; Humist [OTC]; HyperSal; Little Noses Decongestant [OTC] [DSC]; MicroKlenz Wound Cleanser [OTC]; Muro 128 [OTC]; Na-Zone [OTC]; Nasal Moist [OTC]; Nebusal; Ocean Complete Sinus Rinse [OTC]; Ocean Complete [OTC] [DSC]; Ocean for Kids [OTC]; Ocean Nasal Moisturizer [OTC]; Ocean Nasal Spray [OTC]; Ocean Ultra Moisturizing [OTC] [DSC]; Ocean Ultra Saline Mist [OTC]; PeleVerus [OTC]; Pretz Irrigation [OTC]; Pretz [OTC]; PulmoSal; RadiaKlenz [OTC]; Remedy 4-in-1 Body Cleanser [OTC]; Rhinaris [OTC]; Safe Wash [OTC]; Saline Flush ZR; Saline Mist Spray [OTC]; Saljet Rinse [OTC]; Saljet [OTC]; Sea Soft Nasal Mist [OTC]; Sea-Clens Wound Cleanser [OTC]; Sochlor [OTC]; Sodium Chloride Thermoject Sys; SwabFlush Saline Flush; Ultra-Klenz [OTC]; Wound Wash Saline [OTC]

Index Terms Hypertonic Saline; NaCl; Normal Saline; Saline; Salt

Pharmacologic Category Electrolyte Supplement, Parenteral; Genitourinary Irrigant; Irrigant; Lubricant, Ocular; Sodium Salt

Use
Parenteral: Restores sodium ion in patients with restricted oral intake (especially hyponatremia states or low salt syndrome).
Concentrated sodium chloride: Additive for parenteral fluid therapy
Hypertonic sodium chloride: For severe hyponatremia and hypochloremia
Hypotonic sodium chloride: Hydrating solution
Normal saline: Restores water/sodium losses
Ophthalmic: Reduces corneal edema
Inhalation: Restores moisture to pulmonary system; loosens and thins congestion caused by colds or allergies; diluent for bronchodilator solutions that require dilution before inhalation
Intranasal: Restores moisture to nasal membranes
Irrigation: Wound cleansing, irrigation, and flushing

Pregnancy Considerations Animal reproduction studies have not been conducted. Sodium requirements do not change during pregnancy (IOM, 2004). Nasal saline rinses may be used for the treatment of pregnancy rhinitis (Wallace, 2008).

Breast-Feeding Considerations Sodium is found in breast milk. Sodium requirements do not change during lactation (IOM, 2004).

Contraindications Hypersensitivity to sodium chloride or any component of the formulation; hypertonic uterus, hypernatremia, fluid retention

Warnings/Precautions The use of hypotonic saline solutions (eg, 0.225% sodium chloride) may result in hemolysis if administered rapidly and for prolonged periods. If hypotonic saline solutions become necessary, administration as $D_5W/0.2\%$ NaCl or 0.45% NaCl is recommended for most patients (eg, those without hyperglycemia). Use with caution in patients with HF, renal insufficiency, liver cirrhosis, hypertension, edema.

Administration of low sodium or sodium-free IV solutions may result in significant hyponatremia or water intoxication; monitor serum sodium concentration closely. In the treatment of acute hypernatremia (ie, development over a couple of hours), serum sodium concentration should be corrected no faster than 1-2 mEq/L per hour. If patient has been chronically hypernatremic, correct serum sodium no faster than 0.5 mEq/L per hour and by no more than 10-12 mEq/L in a given 24-hour period; use extreme caution since rapid correction may result in cerebral edema, herniation, coma, and death (Adrogue, 2000; Kraft, 2005).

When treating hyponatremia, rate of correction is dependent upon whether or not it is acute or chronic. Sodium toxicity (eg, osmotic demyelination syndrome) is almost exclusively related to how fast a sodium deficit is corrected; both rate and magnitude are extremely important. For patients with acute (<24 hours) or chronic (>48 hours), severe (<120 mEq/L) hyponatremia, a serum sodium concentration increase of 4-6 mEq/L within a 24-hour period is sufficient for most patients. In chronic severe hyponatremia, overcorrection risks iatrogenic osmotic demyelination syndrome. For patients with severe symptoms or other need for urgent correction, may increase by 4-6 mEq/L within the first 6 hours and postpone any further correction until the next day at a correction rate of 4-6 mEq/L per day. Choice of infusate sodium concentration is dependent upon the severity of the hyponatremia with more concentrated solutions (eg, 3% NaCl) for more severe cases; monitor serum sodium closely during administration (Sterns, 2013).

Benzyl alcohol and derivatives: Bacteriostatic sodium chloride contains benzyl alcohol; large amounts of benzyl alcohol (≥99 mg/kg/day) have been associated with a potentially fatal toxicity ("gasping syndrome") in neonates; the "gasping syndrome" consists of metabolic acidosis, respiratory distress, gasping respirations, CNS dysfunction (including convulsions, intracranial hemorrhage), hypotension, and cardiovascular collapse (AAP ["Inactive" 1997]; CDC, 1982); some data suggests that benzoate displaces bilirubin from protein binding sites (Ahlfors, 2001); avoid or use dosage forms containing benzyl alcohol with caution in neonates. See manufacturer's labeling.

Wound Wash Saline is for single-patient use only.

Irrigants: For external use only; not for parenteral use. Do not use during electrosurgical procedures. Irrigating fluids may be absorbed into systemic circulation; monitor for fluid or solute overload.

Concentrated solutions of sodium chloride (>1%) are vesicants; ensure proper needle or catheter placement prior to and during infusion; avoid extravasation.

Adverse Reactions Frequency not defined.
Cardiovascular: Congestive heart failure, transient hypotension (especially with adult administration of 23.4% NaCl)
Central nervous system: Central pontine myelinolysis (due to rapid correction of hyponatremia)
Endocrine & metabolic: Dilution of serum electrolytes, extravasation, hypernatremia, hypervolemia, hypokalemia, overhydration
Gastrointestinal: Nausea, vomiting (oral use)
Local: Thrombosis, phlebitis, extravasation
Respiratory: Bronchospasm (inhalation with hypertonic solutions), pulmonary edema

Drug Interactions
Metabolism/Transport Effects None known.
Avoid Concomitant Use
Avoid concomitant use of Sodium Chloride with any of the following: Tolvaptan
Increased Effect/Toxicity
Sodium Chloride may increase the levels/effects of: Tolvaptan
Decreased Effect
Sodium Chloride may decrease the levels/effects of: Lithium

Storage/Stability Store injection at room temperature; do not freeze. Protect from heat. Use only clear solutions.

Mechanism of Action Principal extracellular cation; functions in fluid and electrolyte balance, osmotic pressure control, and water distribution

Pharmacodynamics/Kinetics
Absorption: Oral: Rapid
Distribution: Widely distributed
Excretion: Primarily urine; also sweat, tears, saliva

Dosing
Adult & Geriatric
Refractory elevated ICP due to various etiologies (eg, subarachnoid hemorrhage, trauma, neoplasm), transtentorial herniation syndromes (off-label use): IV: Hypertonic saline: 23.4% (30-60 mL) given over 2-20 minutes administered via central venous access only (Koenig, 2008; Suarez, 1998; Ware, 2005)

Severe sepsis, initial fluid resuscitation (off-label use): IV: Normal saline (0.9% NaCl): Minimum of 30 mL/kg. **Note:** Administer within 3 hours of sepsis recognition for hypotension or lactate ≥4 mmol/L (≥36 mg/dL). Some patients may require more rapid administration and/or greater amount of fluid for complete resuscitation (Dellinger, 2013).

Subarachnoid hemorrhage with hyponatremia (ie, ≤135 mEq/L) to enhance cerebral perfusion (off-label use): IV: Hypertonic saline: 3% sodium chloride/acetate (50:50 mixture) 100-200 mL/hour administered via central venous catheter; titrate to clinical response up to a maximum serum sodium between 150-160 mEq/L (achieved at a rate of 0.5-1 mEq/L/hour) (Suarez, 1999)

Traumatic brain injury with elevated ICP (off-label use): IV: Hypertonic saline: **Note:** Optimal dose has not been established; due to insufficient evidence, the Brain Trauma Foundation guidelines (Bratton, 2007) do not make specific recommendations on the use of hypertonic saline for the treatment of traumatic intracranial hypertension. Clinical trials are small; few are prospective. **Some concentrations may not be commercially available; administer via central venous catheter;** protocols include:

3%: 300 mL administered over 20 minutes when ICP values exceed 20 mm Hg (Huang, 2006)

7.2%: 1.5 mL/kg administered over 15 minutes when ICP values exceed 15 mm Hg (Munar, 2000)

7.5%: 2 mL/kg administered over 20 minutes when ICP values exceed 25 mm Hg (Vialet, 2003)

23.4%: 30 mL administered over 2 minutes (Ware, 2005) **or** over >30 minutes when ICP values exceed 20 mm Hg (Kerwin, 2009)

GU irrigant: Irrigation: 1-3 L/day by intermittent irrigation

Replacement: IV: Determined by laboratory determinations mEq

Hyponatremia: IV: To correct acute (<24 hours) or chronic (>48 hours), severe (<120 mEq/L) hyponatremia: In general, a serum sodium concentration increase of 4-6 mEq/L within a 24-hour period is sufficient to improve most symptoms of hyponatremia. In chronic severe hyponatremia, overcorrection risks iatrogenic osmotic demyelination syndrome. For patients with severe symptoms or other need for urgent correction, one approach is to increase serum sodium concentration by 4-6 mEq/L within the first 6 hours and postpone any further correction until the next day at a correction rate of 4-6 mEq/L per day. Choice of sodium correction fluid concentration is dependent upon the severity of the hyponatremia with more concentrated solutions (eg, 3% NaCl) for more severe cases; monitor serum sodium closely during administration (Sterns, 2013).

Chloride maintenance electrolyte requirement in parenteral nutrition: IV: As needed to maintain acid-base balance with parenteral nutrition; use equal amounts of chloride and acetate to maintain balance and adjust ratio based on individual patient needs (Mirtallo, 2004).

Sodium maintenance electrolyte requirement in parenteral nutrition: IV: 1-2 mEq/kg/24 hours; customize amounts based on individual patient needs (Mirtallo, 2004).

Ophthalmic:

Ointment: Apply once daily or more often

Solution: Instill 1-2 drops into affected eye(s) every 3-4 hours

Bronchodilator diluent: Inhalation: 1-3 sprays (1-3 mL) to dilute bronchodilator solution in nebulizer before administration

Nasal congestion: Intranasal: 2-3 sprays in each nostril as needed

Irrigation: Spray affected area

Pediatric

Hyponatremia: IV: Children: Hypertonic solutions (>0.9%) should only be used for the initial treatment of acute serious symptomatic hyponatremia or increased intracranial pressure in the setting of traumatic brain injury.

Maintenance: 3-4 mEq/kg/day; maximum: 100-150 mEq/day; dosage varies widely depending on clinical condition

Replacement: Determined by laboratory determinations mEq

Sodium deficiency (mEq/kg) = [% dehydration (L/kg)/100 x 70 (mEq/L)] + [0.6 (L/kg) x (140 - serum sodium) (mEq/L)]

Hypovolemic septic shock, initial fluid resuscitation (off-label use): IV: Normal saline (0.9% NaCl): Up to 20 mL/kg/dose over 5-10 minutes; titrate to hypotension reversal, increasing urine output, and attainment of normal capillary refill, peripheral pulses, and level of consciousness (Dellinger, 2013)

Increased intracranial pressure (off-label use): Hypertonic saline (3%): 0.1-1 mL/kg/hour continuous infusion titrated to maintain ICP <20 mm Hg (Addleson, 2003)

Children ≥2 years:

Intranasal: Refer to adult dosing.

Irrigation: Refer to adult dosing.

Inhalation: Refer to adult dosing.

Administration

Irrigation solution: Do not warm >66°C (150°F); not for IV use. Wound Wash Saline: Before use, expel a short stream into air to clear nozzle.

IV: >2% solutions: Administration through a central line is recommended due to high osmolarity and tonicity (Mortimer, 2006). Consult individual institutional policies and procedures.

Vesicant at higher concentrations (>1%); ensure proper needle or catheter placement prior to and during infusion; avoid extravasation.

Extravasation management: If extravasation occurs, stop infusion immediately and disconnect (leave cannula/needle in place); gently aspirate extravasated solution (do **NOT** flush the line); remove needle/cannula; elevate extremity. Apply dry warm compresses (Hastings-Tolsma, 1993).

Monitoring Parameters Serum sodium, potassium, chloride, and bicarbonate concentrations; I & O, weight

Reference Range Serum/plasma sodium concentration:

Neonates:

Full-term: 133-142 mEq/L

Premature: 132-140 mEq/L

Children ≥2 months to Adults: 135-145 mEq/L

Additional Information

Normal saline (0.9%) = 154 mEq/L; 3% NaCl = 513 mEq/L; 5% NaCl = 856 mEq/L

Tablet 1g = 17.1 mEq

Dosage Forms Considerations 1 g sodium chloride = elemental sodium 393.3 mg = 17.1 mEq sodium = sodium 17.1 mmol

Dosage Forms Excipient information presented when available (limited, particularly for generics); consult specific product labeling. [DSC] = Discontinued product

Aerosol Solution, Inhalation:

Broncho Saline: 0.9% (90 mL, 240 mL)

Aerosol Solution, Nasal [preservative free]:

Ocean Complete: (177 mL [DSC]) [drug free]

Ocean Complete Sinus Rinse: (177 mL) [drug free]

Gel, Nasal:

Ayr Saline Nasal: (14.1 g) [contains aloe barbadensis, brilliant blue fcf (fd&c blue #1), methylparaben, propylparaben, soybean oil]

Ayr Saline Nasal No-Drip: (22 mL) [contains aloe barbadensis, benzalkonium chloride, benzyl alcohol, soybean oil]

Entsol Nasal: (20 g)

Ocean Nasal Moisturizer: (14 g) [drug free; contains methylparaben, propylparaben, trolamine (triethanolamine)]

Ocean Ultra Moisturizing: (14 g [DSC]) [contains methylparaben, propylparaben, trolamine (triethanolamine)]

Rhinaris: 0.2% (28.4 g) [contains benzalkonium chloride, propylene glycol]

Liquid, External:

Allclenz: (360 mL [DSC])

Atrapro Dermal Spray: (236 mL)

DiaB Klenz: (240 mL)

Elta Dermal Wound Cleanser: (240 mL)

MicroKlenz Wound Cleanser: (240 mL)

PeleVerus: 0.25% (240 mL) [contains edetate sodium (tetrasodium), methylparaben]

RadiaKlenz: (240 mL)

Remedy 4-in-1 Body Cleanser: 0.5% (236 mL)

Sea-Clens Wound Cleanser: (178 mL, 355 mL)

Ultra-Klenz: (240 mL, 360 mL)

Nebulization Solution, Inhalation:

Generic: 0.9% (3 mL)

Nebulization Solution, Inhalation [preservative free]:

HyperSal: 3.5% (4 mL) [latex free]

HyperSal: 7% (4 mL)

Nebusal: 3% (4 mL); 6% (4 mL)

PulmoSal: 7% (4 mL)

Generic: 0.9% (3 mL, 5 mL, 15 mL); 3% (4 mL, 15 mL); 7% (4 mL); 10% (4 mL, 15 mL)

Ointment, Ophthalmic:
Altachlore: 5% (3.5 g)
Muro 128: 5% (3.5 g)
Generic: 5% (3.5 g)
Packet, Nasal [preservative free]:
Ayr Saline Nasal Neti Rinse: 1.57 g (40 ea) [iodine free]
AYR Saline Nasal Rinse: 1.57 g (50 ea, 51 ea, 100 ea) [iodine free]
Solution, External:
Saljet: 0.9% (30 mL)
Wound Wash Saline: 0.9% (210 mL)
Solution, External [preservative free]:
Safe Wash: 0.9% (210 mL) [drug free, latex free]
Saljet Rinse: 0.9% (30 mL)
Solution, Injection:
Sodium Chloride Thermoject Sys: 0.9% (10 mL)
Generic: 0.9% (2 mL, 2.5 mL, 3 mL, 5 mL, 10 mL, 20 mL, 30 mL [DSC], 100 mL); 14.6% (20 mL, 40 mL); 23.4% (20 mL [DSC], 250 mL [DSC])
Solution, Injection [preservative free]:
Generic: 0.9% (1 mL, 2 mL, 2.5 mL, 3 mL, 5 mL, 10 mL, 20 mL, 50 mL)
Solution, Intravenous:
SwabFlush Saline Flush: 0.9% (10 mL)
Generic: 0.45% (25 mL, 50 mL, 100 mL, 250 mL, 500 mL, 1000 mL); 0.9% (2.5 mL, 3 mL, 5 mL [DSC], 10 mL, 25 mL, 50 mL, 100 mL, 150 mL, 250 mL, 500 mL, 1000 mL); 3% (500 mL); 5% (500 mL); 23.4% (30 mL, 100 mL, 200 mL, 250 mL)
Solution, Intravenous [preservative free]:
Saline Flush ZR: 0.9% (2.5 mL, 5 mL, 10 mL) [latex free]
Generic: 0.9% (1 mL, 2 mL, 2.5 mL, 3 mL, 5 mL, 10 mL, 50 mL, 100 mL, 125 mL, 500 mL, 1000 mL)
Solution, Irrigation:
Generic: 0.9% (250 mL, 500 mL, 1000 mL, 1500 mL, 2000 mL, 3000 mL, 4000 mL, 5000 mL)
Solution, Nasal:
4-Way Saline: (29.6 mL)
Afrin Saline Nasal Mist: 0.65% (30 mL, 45 mL)
Altamist Spray: 0.65% (45 mL, 60 mL)
Ayr: 0.65% (50 mL)
Ayr Nasal Mist Allergy/Sinus: 2.65% (50 mL) [contains benzalkonium chloride]
Ayr Saline Nasal Drops: 0.65% (50 mL)
Baby Ayr Saline: 0.65% (30 mL)
Deep Sea Nasal Spray: 0.65% (44 mL) [contains benzalkonium chloride]
Entsol: (30 mL)
Humist: 0.65% (45 mL)
Na-Zone: 0.65% (59 mL)
Nasal Moist: 0.65% (15 mL, 45 mL)
Ocean for Kids: 0.65% (37.5 mL) [alcohol free, drug free; contains benzalkonium chloride]
Ocean for Kids: 0.65% (37.5 mL) [drug free; contains benzalkonium chloride]
Ocean Nasal Spray: 0.65% (45 mL, 66 mL, 104 mL, 480 mL) [contains benzalkonium chloride]
Pretz: (50 mL, 946 mL)
Pretz Irrigation: (237 mL)
Rhinaris: 0.2% (30 mL) [contains benzalkonium chloride, propylene glycol]
Rhinaris: 0.2% (30 mL [DSC]) [drug free, odorless; contains benzalkonium chloride, propylene glycol]
Saline Mist Spray: 0.65% (45 mL) [contains benzalkonium chloride]
Sea Soft Nasal Mist: 0.65% (45 mL)
Generic: 0.65% (44 mL, 45 mL)
Solution, Nasal [preservative free]:
Entsol Nasal: 3% (100 mL) [drug free]
Entsol Nasal: (100 mL [DSC])
Entsol Nasal Wash: (237 mL)
Ocean Ultra Saline Mist: (90 mL) [drug free]
Solution, Ophthalmic:
Altachlore: 5% (15 mL, 30 mL)
Muro 128: 2% (15 mL); 5% (15 mL, 30 mL)
Sochlor: 5% (15 mL)
Generic: 5% (15 mL)
Solution, Nasal, as hydrochloride:
Little Noses Decongestant: 0.125% (15 mL [DSC]) [alcohol free; contains benzalkonium chloride, polyethylene glycol]
Swab, Nasal:
Ayr Saline Nasal Gel: (20 ea) [contains methylparaben, propylparaben, soybean oil, trolamine (triethanolamine)]
Tablet, Oral:
Generic: 1 g

◆ Sodium Chloride Thermoject Sys *see* Sodium Chloride *on page 1671*

Sodium Chondroitin Sulfate and Sodium Hyaluronate
(SOW de um kon DROY tin SUL fate & SOW de um hye al yoor ON ate)

Brand Names: US DisCoVisc; Viscoat
Index Terms Chondroitin Sulfate and Sodium Hyaluronate; Sodium Hyaluronate and Chondroitin Sulfate
Pharmacologic Category Ophthalmic Agent, Viscoelastic

Use Surgical aid: An ophthalmic surgical aid in anterior segment procedures, including cataract extraction and intraocular lens implantation
Dosing
Adult & Geriatric Surgical aid: Intraocular: Inject (using a 27-gauge cannula) into anterior chamber during surgery; may be injected into the anterior chamber prior to or following removal of crystalline lens. See directions for use in manufacturer's labeling.
Renal Impairment There are no dosage adjustments provided in the manufacturer's labeling.
Hepatic Impairment There are no dosage adjustments provided in the manufacturer's labeling.
Additional Information Complete prescribing information should be consulted for additional detail.
Dosage Forms Excipient information presented when available (limited, particularly for generics); consult specific product labeling.
Injection, solution, intraocular:
DisCoVisc: Sodium chondroitin sulfate ≤4% and sodium hyaluronate ≤1.7% (1 mL) [provided in a kit which also contains 27-gauge cannula and cannula locking ring]
Viscoat: Sodium chondroitin sulfate ≤4% and sodium hyaluronate ≤3% (0.5 mL, 0.75 mL) [packaged with 27-gauge cannula and cannula locking ring]

Sodium Citrate and Citric Acid
(SOW dee um SIT rate & SI trik AS id)

Brand Names: US Cytra-2; Oracit®; Shohl's Solution (Modified); Virtrate-2
Brand Names: Canada PMS-Dicitrate
Index Terms Bicitra; Citric Acid and Sodium Citrate; Modified Shohl's Solution
Pharmacologic Category Alkalinizing Agent, Oral
Use
Acidosis: Treatment of metabolic acidosis or acidosis in certain renal tubular disorders
Gastric acid buffer: Buffer agent to neutralize gastric acidity
Systemic alkalinizer: Alkalinizing agent in conditions where long-term maintenance of alkaline urine is desirable
Dosing
Adult & Geriatric
Acidosis or systemic alkalization: Oral: 10 to 30 mL 4 times daily
Gastric acid buffer: Oral: 15 mL as a single dose
Pediatric
Acidosis or systemic alkalization:
Manufacturer's recommendation:
Children ≥2 years and Adolescents: Oral: 5 to 15 mL 4 times daily.
Alternative dosing: **Note:** 1 mL of oral solution contains 1 mEq of bicarbonate.
Infants and Children (off label dosing): Oral: 2 to 3 mEq bicarbonate/kg/**day** in 3 to 4 divided doses (Kliegman, 2007)
Gastric acid buffer: Children and Adolescents: Oral: 15 mL as a single dose
Renal Impairment Use is contraindicated in patients with anuria, severe renal impairment, oliguria or azotemia.
Hepatic Impairment There are no dosage adjustments provided in the manufacturer's labeling; use with caution.
Additional Information Complete prescribing information should be consulted for additional detail.
Dosage Forms Considerations Each mL provides 1 mEq sodium, and is equivalent to 1 mEq bicarbonate
Dosage Forms Excipient information presented when available (limited, particularly for generics); consult specific product labeling.
Solution, oral:
Cytra-2: Sodium citrate 500 mg and citric acid 334 mg per 5 mL (480 mL) [alcohol free, dye free, sugar free; contains propylene glycol and sodium benzoate; grape flavor]
Oracit®: Sodium citrate 490 mg and citric acid 640 mg per 5 mL (15 mL, 30 mL, 500 mL, 3840 mL)
Shohl's Solution (Modified): Sodium citrate 500 mg and citric acid 300 mg per 5 mL (480 mL) [contains alcohol]

Virtrate-2: Sodium citrate 500 mg and citric acid 334 mg per 5 mL (480 mL) [sugar free; contains propylene glycol and sodium benzoate; grape flavor]

Generic: Sodium citrate 500 mg and citric acid 334 mg per 5 mL (480 mL)

♦ Sodium Citrate, Citric Acid, and Potassium Citrate see Citric Acid, Sodium Citrate, and Potassium Citrate on page 400

♦ Sodium Diuril see Chlorothiazide on page 376

♦ Sodium Edecrin see Ethacrynic Acid on page 699

♦ Sodium Etidronate see Etidronate on page 713

♦ Sodium Ferric Gluconate see Ferric Gluconate on page 760

♦ Sodium Ferric Gluconate Complex see Ferric Gluconate on page 760

♦ Sodium Fluorescein see Fluorescein on page 782

♦ Sodium Fluoride see Fluoride on page 782

Sodium Glycerophosphate Pentahydrate
(SOE dee um glis er oh FOS fate pen ta HYE drate)

Brand Names: US Glycophos

Pharmacologic Category Electrolyte Supplement, Parenteral

Use Supplement in intravenous nutrition to meet the requirements of phosphate

Dosing

Adult & Geriatric Note: When converting from inorganic phosphate products (ie, sodium phosphate and potassium phosphate), maintain the same mmol amount of phosphate. Doses are listed as mmol of phosphate. Sodium glycerophosphate pentahydrate 306.1 mg = sodium glycerophosphate 216 mg = phosphate 1 **mmol**. Sodium glycerophosphate pentahydrate will provide 2 mEq of sodium for every 1 mmol of phosphate delivered.

Phosphate replacement, parenteral nutrition: Manufacturer's labeling: IV: 10-20 mmol per day admixed within parenteral nutrition solution. Dosage should be individualized.

Phosphate repletion, general (off-label use):

Caution: With orders for IV phosphate, there is considerable confusion associated with the use of millimoles (mmol) versus milliequivalents (mEq) to express the phosphate requirement. The most reliable method of ordering IV phosphate is by millimoles.

Acute treatment of hypophosphatemia: IV: It is difficult to provide concrete guidelines for the treatment of severe hypophosphatemia because the extent of total body deficits and response to therapy are difficult to predict. Aggressive doses of phosphate may result in a transient serum elevation followed by redistribution into intracellular compartments or bone tissue. It is recommended that repletion of severe hypophosphatemia be done IV because large doses of oral phosphate may cause diarrhea and intestinal absorption may be unreliable. Intermittent IV infusion should be reserved for severe depletion situations; requires continuous cardiac monitoring. Guidelines differ based on degree of illness, need/use of TPN, and severity of hypophosphatemia. Obese patients and/or severe renal impairment were excluded from phosphate supplement trials. **Note:** 1 mmol phosphate = 31 mg phosphorus; 1 mg phosphorus = 0.032 mmol phosphate.

Critically-ill adult patients receiving concurrent enteral/ parenteral nutrition (Brown, 2006; Clark, 1995): **Note:** Round doses to the nearest 7.5 mmol for ease of preparation. If administering with phosphate-containing parenteral nutrition, do not exceed 15 mmol/L within parenteral nutrition. May use adjusted body weight for patients weighing >130% of ideal body weight (and BMI <40 kg/m^2) by using [IBW + 0.25 (ABW-IBW)]:

Low dose, serum phosphorus level 2.3-3 mg/dL (0.74-0.96 mmol/L): 0.16-0.32 mmol/kg over 4-6 hours

Intermediate dose, serum phosphorus level 1.6-2.2 mg/dL (0.51-0.71 mmol/L): 0.32-0.64 mmol/kg over 4-6 hours

High dose, serum phosphorus <1.5 mg/dL (<0.5 mmol/L): 0.64-1 mmol/kg over 8-12 hours

Parenteral nutrition: IV: 10-15 mmol/1000 kcal (Hicks, 2001) **or** 20-40 mmol/24 hours (Mirtallo, 2004 [ASPEN guidelines])

Pediatric Note: When converting from inorganic phosphate products (ie, sodium phosphate and potassium phosphate), maintain the same mmol amount of phosphate. Doses are listed as mmol of phosphate. Sodium glycerophosphate pentahydrate 306.1 mg = sodium glycerophosphate 216 mg = phosphate 1 **mmol**. Sodium glycerophosphate pentahydrate will provide 2 mEq of sodium for every 1 mmol of phosphate delivered.

Phosphate replacement, parenteral nutrition: Manufacturer's labeling: IV: Infants: 1-1.5 mmol/kg per day admixed within parenteral nutrition solution. Dosage should be individualized.

Phosphate repletion, general (off-label use):

Caution: With orders for IV phosphate, there is considerable confusion associated with the use of millimoles (mmol) versus milliequivalents (mEq) to express the phosphate requirement. The most reliable method of ordering IV phosphate is by millimoles.

Acute treatment of hypophosphatemia: IV: It is difficult to provide concrete guidelines for the treatment of severe hypophosphatemia because the extent of total body deficits and response to therapy are difficult to predict. Aggressive doses of phosphate may result in a transient serum elevation followed by redistribution into intracellular compartments or bone tissue. It is recommended that repletion of severe hypophosphatemia be done IV because large doses of oral phosphate may cause diarrhea and intestinal absorption may be unreliable. Intermittent IV infusion should be reserved for severe depletion situations; requires continuous cardiac monitoring. Guidelines differ based on degree of illness, need/use of TPN, and severity of hypophosphatemia. Obese patients and/or severe renal impairment were excluded from phosphate supplement trials. **Note:** 1 mmol phosphate = 31 mg phosphorus; 1 mg phosphorus = 0.032 mmol phosphate.

There are no prospective studies of parenteral phosphate replacement in children. **The following weight-based guidelines for adult dosing may be cautiously employed in pediatric patients.** Guidelines differ based on degree of illness, use of TPN, and severity of hypophosphatemia.

General replacement guidelines (Lentz, 1978):

Low dose, serum phosphorus losses are recent and uncomplicated: 0.08 mmol/kg over 6 hours

Intermediate dose, serum phosphorus level 0.5-1 mg/dL (0.16-0.32 mmol/L): 0.16-0.24 mmol/kg over 6 hours

Note: The initial dose may be increased by 25% to 50% if the patient is symptomatic secondary to hypophosphatemia, and lowered by 25% to 50% if the patient is hypercalcemic.

Critically-ill adult patients receiving concurrent enteral/ parenteral nutrition (Brown, 2006; Clark, 1995): **Note:** Round doses to the nearest 7.5 mmol for ease of preparation. If administering with phosphate-containing parenteral nutrition, do not exceed 15 mmol/L within parenteral nutrition. May use adjusted body weight for patients weighing >130% of ideal body weight (and BMI <40 kg/m^2) by using [IBW + 0.25 (ABW-IBW)]:

Low dose, serum phosphorus level 2.3-3 mg/dL (0.74-0.96 mmol/L): 0.16-0.32 mmol/kg over 4-6 hours

Intermediate dose, serum phosphorus level 1.6-2.2 mg/dL (0.51-0.71 mmol/L): 0.32-0.64 mmol/kg over 4-6 hours

High dose, serum phosphorus <1.5 mg/dL (<0.5 mmol/L): 0.64-1 mmol/kg over 8-12 hours

Parenteral nutrition: IV:

Infants and Children: 0.5-2 mmol/kg/24 hours (Mirtallo, 2004 [ASPEN guidelines])

Children >50 kg and Adolescents: 10-40 mmol/24 hours (Mirtallo, 2004 [ASPEN guidelines])

Renal Impairment No dosage adjustment provided in manufacturer's labeling (has not been studied); use with caution since phosphate excretion is primarily renal.

Hepatic Impairment No dosage adjustment provided in manufacturer's labeling (has not been studied); however, phosphate excretion is primarily renal

Additional Information Complete prescribing information should be consulted for additional detail.

Dosage Forms Excipient information presented when available (limited, particularly for generics); consult specific product labeling.

Solution, Intravenous:

Glycophos: 1 mmol/mL (20 mL)

Sodium Hypochlorite
(SOW dee um hye poe KLOR ite)

Brand Names: US Anasept; Di-Dak-Sol [OTC]; H-Chlor 12 [OTC]; HySept [OTC]

Index Terms Modified Dakin's Solution; Sodium Hypochlorite Solution

Pharmacologic Category Disinfectant, Antibacterial (Topical)

Use Antiseptic: Treatment and prevention of skin and tissue infections; treatment of cuts, abrasions, and skin ulcers; use pre- and postsurgery.

Anasept only:

OTC use: Cleansing and removal of dirt, debris, and foreign material from skin abrasions, lacerations, minor irritations, cuts, exit sites, and intact skin (cleanser), or management of conditions (gel).

Professional use: Cleansing of foreign materials (including microorganisms) from wounds (liquid) or management of wounds (gel) such as stage I to IV pressure ulcers, diabetic foot ulcers, postsurgical wounds, first- and second degree burns, and grafted and donor sites.

Dosing

Adult & Geriatric

Antiseptic: Topical:

Gel:

Indwelling catheter care: Apply sufficient amount to completely cover skin area around the indwelling catheter.

Ostomy care: Apply a thin layer.

Skin care: Apply a thin layer; repeat as needed.

Wound care: Apply thick layer (¼ to ½ inch) to entire wound bed; apply a thin layer to periwound skin area.

Liquid:

Skin cleansing: Apply to site.

Wound cleansing: Apply once daily. May be repeated up to a total of twice daily.

Solution:

Lightly to moderately exudative wounds: Apply once daily.

Highly exudative or contaminated wounds: Apply twice daily.

Renal Impairment There are no dosage adjustments provided in the manufacturer's labeling.

Hepatic Impairment There are no dosage adjustments provided in the manufacturer's labeling.

Additional Information Complete prescribing information should be consulted for additional detail.

Dosage Forms Excipient information presented when available (limited, particularly for generics); consult specific product labeling.

Liquid, External:

Anasept: 0.057% (237 mL)

Solution, External:

Di-Dak-Sol: 0.0125% (473 mL)

H-Chlor 12: 0.125% (473 mL)

HySept: 0.25% (473 mL); 0.5% (473 mL)

Generic: 0.125% (473 mL); 0.25% (473 mL); 0.5% (473 mL)

Sodium Nitrite (SOW dee um NYE trite)

Pharmacologic Category Antidote

Use Cyanide poisoning: Treatment of acute, life-threatening cyanide poisoning in combination with sodium thiosulfate. Consider consultation with a poison control center at 1-800-222-1222.

Dosing

Adult

Cyanide poisoning: IV: **Note:** Given in conjunction with sodium thiosulfate. Administer sodium nitrite first, followed immediately by the administration of sodium thiosulfate: 300 mg (10 mL of a 3% solution); may repeat at one-half the original dose if symptoms of cyanide toxicity return. Sodium nitrite is generally discontinued for methemoglobin levels >30%.

Alternatively, in patients who are unable to tolerate significant methemoglobinemia (eg, patients with comorbidities that compromise oxygen delivery, such as heart disease, lung disease), dosing may be based on hemoglobin levels (when rapid bedside testing is available) to prevent fatal methemoglobinemia; see table (Berlin, 1970):

Hemoglobin Level (g/dL)	Dose of 3% Sodium Nitrite Solution (maximum dose: 10 mL)
7	0.19 mL/kg
8	0.22 mL/kg
9	0.25 mL/kg
10	0.27 mL/kg
11	0.3 mL/kg
12	0.33 mL/kg
13	0.36 mL/kg
14	0.39 mL/kg

Note: Monitor the patient for 24-48 hours; if symptoms return, repeat sodium nitrite and sodium thiosulfate at one-half the original dose.

Geriatric Refer to adult dosing. Use caution due to the likelihood of decreased renal function.

Pediatric

Cyanide poisoning: IV: 6 mg/kg (0.2 mL/kg or 6-8 mL/m² of a 3% solution); maximum dose: 300 mg (10 mL of a 3% solution); may repeat at one-half the original dose if symptoms of cyanide toxicity return. **Note:** Given in conjunction with sodium thiosulfate. Administer sodium nitrite first, followed immediately by the administration of sodium thiosulfate. Sodium nitrite is generally discontinued for methemoglobin levels >30%.

Alternatively, in patients who are unable to tolerate significant methemoglobinemia (eg, patients with comorbidities that compromise oxygen delivery, such as heart disease, lung disease): Refer to adult dosing.

Note: Monitor the patient for 24-48 hours; if symptoms return, repeat sodium nitrite and sodium thiosulfate at one-half the original dose.

Renal Impairment No dosage adjustment provided in the manufacturer's labeling; however, renal elimination of sodium nitrite is significant and risk of adverse effects may be increased in patients with renal impairment.

Hepatic Impairment No dosage adjustment provided in manufacturer's labeling (has not been studied).

Additional Information Complete prescribing information should be consulted for additional detail.

Dosage Forms Excipient information presented when available (limited, particularly for generics); consult specific product labeling.

Solution, Intravenous:

Generic: 30 mg/mL (10 mL)

Sodium Nitrite and Sodium Thiosulfate
(SOW dee um NYE trite & SOW dee um thye oh SUL fate)

Brand Names: US Nithiodote

Index Terms Sodium Thiosulfate and Sodium Nitrite

Pharmacologic Category Antidote

Use Cyanide poisoning: Treatment of acute, life-threatening cyanide poisoning. Consider consultation with a poison control center at 1-800-222-1222.

Dosing

Adult Cyanide poisoning: IV: **Note:** Administer sodium nitrite first, followed immediately by the administration of sodium thiosulfate.

Sodium nitrite: 300 mg (10 mL of a 3% solution); may repeat at one-half the original dose if symptoms of cyanide toxicity return

Alternatively, in patients who are unable to tolerate significant methemoglobinemia (eg, patients with comorbidities that compromise oxygen delivery, such as heart disease, lung disease), dosing may be based on hemoglobin levels (when rapid bedside testing is available) to prevent fatal methemoglobinemia; see table (Berlin, 1970):

Hemoglobin Level (g/dL)	Dose of 3% Sodium Nitrite Solution (maximum dose: 10 mL)
7	0.19 mL/kg
8	0.22 mL/kg
9	0.25 mL/kg
10	0.27 mL/kg
11	0.3 mL/kg
12	0.33 mL/kg
13	0.36 mL/kg
14	0.39 mL/kg

Sodium thiosulfate: 12.5 g (50 mL of a 25% solution); may repeat at one-half the original dose if symptoms of cyanide toxicity return

Note: Monitor the patient for 24-48 hours; if symptoms return, repeat both sodium nitrite and sodium thiosulfate at one-half the original doses.

Geriatric Refer to adult dosing; use with caution due to the likelihood of decreased renal function.

Pediatric Cyanide poisoning: IV: **Note:** Administer sodium nitrite first, followed immediately by the administration of sodium thiosulfate.

Sodium nitrite: 6 mg/kg (0.2 mL/kg or 6-8 mL/m² of a 3% solution); maximum dose: 300 mg (10 mL of a 3% solution); may repeat at one-half the original dose if symptoms of cyanide toxicity return

Alternatively, in patients who are unable to tolerate significant methemoglobinemia (eg, patients with comorbidities that compromise oxygen delivery, such as heart disease, lung disease): Refer to adult dosing.

Sodium thiosulfate: 250 mg/kg (1 mL/kg or ~30-40 mL/m² of a 25% solution) or 500 mg/kg (2 mL/kg of a 25% solution) (Howland, 2011); maximum dose: 12.5 g (50 mL of a 25% solution); may repeat at one-half the original dose if symptoms of cyanide toxicity return

Note: Monitor the patient for 24-48 hours; if symptoms return, repeat both sodium nitrite and sodium thiosulfate at one-half the original doses.

Renal Impairment No dosage adjustment provided in manufacturer's labeling; however, renal elimination of sodium nitrite and sodium thiosulfate is significant and risk of adverse effects may be increased in patients with renal impairment.

Hepatic Impairment No dosage adjustment provided in the manufacturer's labeling (has not been studied).

Additional Information Complete prescribing information should be consulted for additional detail.

Dosage Forms Excipient information presented when available (limited, particularly for generics); consult specific product labeling.

Injection, solution [combination package]:
Nithiodote: Sodium nitrite 300 mg/10 mL (10 mL) and sodium thiosulfate 12.5 g/50 mL (50 mL)

◆ Sodium Nitroferricyanide *see* Nitroprusside *on page 1291*

◆ Sodium Nitroprusside *see* Nitroprusside *on page 1291*

Sodium Oxybate (SOW dee um ox i BATE)

Brand Names: US Xyrem
Brand Names: Canada Xyrem
Index Terms 4-Hydroxybutyrate; Gamma Hydroxybutyric Acid; GHB; Oxybate; Sodium 4-Hydroxybutyrate
Pharmacologic Category Central Nervous System Depressant
Use Excessive daytime sleepiness/cataplexy: Treatment of cataplexy and excessive daytime sleepiness in patients with narcolepsy
Prescribing and Access Restrictions Sodium oxybate is deemed to have an approved REMS program. As a requirement of the REMS program, access to this medication is restricted. Sodium oxybate oral solution will be available only to prescribers and patients enrolled in the Xyrem REMS Program and dispensed to the patient only by the central pharmacy that is specially certified (http://www.xyremrems.com or 1-866-997-3688). Prior to dispensing the first prescription, prescribers will be sent educational materials to be reviewed with the patient and enrollment forms for the postmarketing surveillance

program. Patients must be seen at least every 3 months; prescriptions can be written for a maximum of 3 months (the first prescription may only be written for a 1-month supply).
Medication Guide Available Yes
Dosing
Adult Excessive daytime sleepiness/cataplexy: Oral: Initial: 2.25 g at bedtime after the patient is in bed, and 2.25 g 2.5 to 4 hours later (4.5 g per night). Titrate to effect; usual effective dosage range: 6 to 9 g per night.
Dose titration:
U.S. labeling: Increase dose by 1.5 g per night (0.75 g per dose) in weekly intervals (maximum dose: 9 g per night)
Canadian labeling: Increase dose by 1.5 g per night (0.75 g per dose) at 2-week intervals (maximum dose: 9 g per night). Dosage may be decreased using the same titration schedule.
Dosage adjustment for concomitant therapy: Patients stabilized on sodium oxybate should have dose reduced by at least 20% with the addition of divalproex sodium. The sodium oxybate starting dose should be reduced for patients already taking divalproex sodium. Adjust dose as necessary.
Geriatric Refer to adult dosing. Use with caution; initiate at lower dosage range. Limited studies available in patients >65 years.
Renal Impairment There are no dosage adjustments provided in manufacturer's labeling (has not been studied).
Hepatic Impairment Initial: ~1.13 g at bedtime after the patient is in bed and ~1.13 g 2.5 to 4 hours later (2.25 g per night)
Additional Information Complete prescribing information should be consulted for additional detail.
Dosage Forms Excipient information presented when available (limited, particularly for generics); consult specific product labeling.
Solution, Oral:
Xyrem: 500 mg/mL (180 mL)
Controlled Substance C-I (illicit use); C-III (medical use)

Sodium Phenylacetate and Sodium Benzoate
(SOW dee um fen il AS e tate & SOW dee um BENZ oh ate)

Brand Names: US Ammonul
Index Terms NAPA and NABZ; Sodium Benzoate and Sodium Phenylacetate
Pharmacologic Category Antidote; Urea Cycle Disorder (UCD) Treatment Agent
Use Hyperammonemia: Adjunct to treatment of acute hyperammonemia and associated encephalopathy in patients with urea cycle enzyme deficiencies
Dosing
Adult & Geriatric Note: Administer as a loading dose over 90 to 120 minutes, followed by an equivalent maintenance infusion given over 24 hours. Initiate therapy as soon as the diagnosis of hyperammonemia is made; hyperammonemic coma in neonates should be aggressively treated while the diagnosis is pursued. Dosage is based on weight for neonates, infants, and young children and body surface area for older children, adolescents, and adults. Therapy should continue until ammonia levels are in normal range or patient can tolerate oral nutrition and medications. Repeat loading doses are not recommended due to neurotoxicity associated with prolonged plasma levels of phenylacetate. Antiemetics may be administered during infusion to aid control of infusion-associated nausea and vomiting.
Hyperammonemia, acute (urea cycle disorders): IV: 55 mL/m² (provides sodium phenylacetate 5.5 g/m² and sodium benzoate 5.5 g/m²) coadministered with arginine; consider conjunctive use of hemodialysis in patients with severe hyperammonemia or refractory to sodium phenylacetate/sodium benzoate.
Pediatric Note: Administer as a loading dose over 90 to 120 minutes, followed by an equivalent maintenance infusion given over 24 hours. Initiate therapy as soon as the diagnosis of hyperammonemia is made; hyperammonemic coma in neonates should be aggressively treated while the diagnosis is pursued. Dosage is based on weight for neonates, infants, and young children and body surface area for older children, adolescents, and adults. Therapy should continue until ammonia levels are in normal range or patient can tolerate oral nutrition and medications. Repeat loading doses are not recommended due to neurotoxicity associated with prolonged plasma levels of phenylacetate. Antiemetics may be administered during infusion to aid control of infusion-associated nausea and vomiting.

Hyperammonemia, acute (urea cycle disorders):
Neonates, Infants, and Children ≤20 kg: IV: 2.5 mL/kg (provides sodium phenylacetate 250 mg/kg and sodium benzoate 250 mg/kg) coadministered with arginine; consider conjunctive use of hemodialysis in patients with severe hyperammonemia or refractory to sodium phenylacetate/sodium benzoate.
Children >20 kg and Adolescents: Refer to adult dosing.

Renal Impairment There are no dosage adjustments provided in the manufacturer's labeling; however, the drug metabolites and ammonia are excreted by the kidneys. Use with caution; monitor closely.

Hepatic Impairment There are no dosage adjustments provided in the manufacturer's labeling. Use with caution.

Additional Information Complete prescribing information should be consulted for additional detail.

Dosage Forms Excipient information presented when available (limited, particularly for generics); consult specific product labeling.
Injection, solution [concentrate]:
Ammonul: Sodium phenylacetate 100 mg and sodium benzoate 100 mg per 1 mL (50 mL)

Sodium Phenylbutyrate
(SOW dee um fen il BYOO ti rate)

Brand Names: US Buphenyl
Brand Names: Canada Pheburane
Index Terms Ammonapse
Pharmacologic Category Urea Cycle Disorder (UCD) Treatment Agent
Use Adjunctive therapy in the chronic management of patients with urea cycle disorder involving deficiencies of carbamoylphosphate synthetase, ornithine transcarbamylase, or argininosuccinic acid synthetase
Dosing
Adult & Geriatric Management of urea cycle disorders: Powder or tablet: Oral: 9.9-13 g/m²/day, administered in equally divided amounts with each meal or feeding, 3-6 times daily (maximum dose: 20 g/day)
Pediatric Oral: **Management of urea cycle disorders:**
Children <20 kg: Powder: 450-600 mg/kg/day, administered in equally divided amounts with each meal or feeding, 3-6 times daily (maximum dose: 20 g/day)
Children ≥20 kg: Powder or tablet: Refer to adult dosing.
Renal Impairment No dosage adjustment provided in manufacturer's labeling. Use with caution.
Hepatic Impairment No dosage adjustment provided in manufacturer's labeling. Use with caution.
Additional Information Complete prescribing information should be consulted for additional detail.
Dosage Forms Considerations Powder products: 1 level teaspoon provides 3 g sodium phenylbutyrate, 1 level tablespoon provides 8.6 g sodium phenylbutyrate. Measurers provided with the product.
Dosage Forms Excipient information presented when available (limited, particularly for generics); consult specific product labeling.
Powder, Oral:
Buphenyl: (250 g) [contains sodium 125 mg/g]
Generic: (250 g)
Tablet, Oral:
Buphenyl: 500 mg [contains sodium 62 mg/tablet]

◆ *Sodium Phosphate and Potassium Phosphate see* Potassium Phosphate and Sodium Phosphate *on page 1484*

◆ *Sodium Phosphate Monobasic, Methenamine, Methylene Blue, Phenyl Salicylate, and Hyoscyamine see* Methenamine, Sodium Phosphate Monobasic, Phenyl Salicylate, Methylene Blue, and Hyoscyamine *on page 1166*

Sodium Phosphates (SOW dee um FOS fates)

Brand Names: US Fleet Enema Extra [OTC]; Fleet Enema [OTC]; Fleet Pedia-Lax Enema [OTC]; LaCrosse Complete [OTC]; OsmoPrep
Brand Names: Canada Fleet Enema
Index Terms Phosphates, Sodium
Pharmacologic Category Cathartic; Electrolyte Supplement, Parenteral; Laxative; Bowel Evacuant
Use
Oral solution, rectal: Short-term treatment of constipation
Oral tablets: Bowel cleansing prior to colonoscopy
IV: Source of phosphate in large volume IV fluids and parenteral nutrition; treatment and prevention of hypophosphatemia
Pregnancy Considerations Reproduction studies have not been conducted with these products. Use with caution in pregnant women.

Breast-Feeding Considerations Phosphorus, sodium, and potassium are normal constituents of human milk.
Medication Guide Available Yes
Contraindications Hypersensitivity to sodium phosphate salts or any component of the formulation; additional contraindications vary by product:
Intravenous preparation: Diseases with hyperphosphatemia, hypocalcemia, or hypernatremia
Tablets: Acute phosphate nephropathy (biopsy proven), bowel obstruction, bowel perforation, gastric bypass or stapling surgery, toxic colitis, toxic megacolon
OTC labeling (Oral Solution): When used for self-medication: Dehydration, heart failure, renal impairment, electrolyte abnormalities; use for bowel cleansing, use in children <5 years

Warnings/Precautions [US Boxed Warning]: Acute phosphate nephropathy (APN) has been reported (rarely) with use of oral products as a colon cleanser prior to colonoscopy. Some cases have resulted in permanent renal impairment (some requiring dialysis). Risk factors for acute phosphate nephropathy may include increased age (>55 years of age), preexisting renal dysfunction, bowel obstruction, active colitis, or dehydration, and the use of medicines that affect renal perfusion or function (eg, ACE inhibitors, angiotensin receptor blockers, diuretics, and possibly NSAIDs), although some cases have been reported in patients without apparent risk factors. Other preventive measures may include avoid exceeding maximum recommended doses and concurrent use of other laxatives containing sodium phosphate; encourage patients to adequately hydrate before, during, and after use; obtain baseline and postprocedure labs in patients at risk; consider hospitalization and intravenous hydration during bowel cleansing for patients unable to hydrate themselves (eg, frail patients). Use is contraindicated in patients with acute phosphate nephropathy (biopsy proven). APN has also been reported (rarely) following the use of sodium phosphate enemas. This has been primarily observed in elderly patients with and without preexisting renal impairment and with those receiving standard or doses exceeding usual doses (Ori 2012).

Use with caution in patients with impaired renal dysfunction, preexisting electrolyte imbalances, risk of electrolyte disturbance (hypocalcemia, hyperphosphatemia, hypernatremia), or dehydration. If using as a bowel evacuant, correct electrolyte abnormalities before administration. Use caution in patients with unstable angina, history of myocardial infarction arrhythmia, cardiomyopathy; use caution in patients with or at risk for arrhythmias (eg, cardiomyopathy, prolonged QT interval, history of uncontrolled arrhythmias, recent MI) or with concurrent use of other QT-prolonging medications; pre-/postdose ECGs should be considered in high-risk patients.

Use caution in inflammatory bowel disease or severe active ulcerative colitis; may induce colonic aphthous ulceration and ischemic colitis (some requiring hospitalization). Use caution in patients with any of the following: Gastric retention or hypomotility, ileus, severe, chronic constipation, colitis. Use is contraindicated in patients with bowel obstruction (including pseudo) or perforation, congenital megacolon, gastric bypass or bariatric surgery, toxic colitis, or toxic megacolon. Use caution in patients with impaired gag reflex and those prone to regurgitation or aspiration.

Use with caution in patients with a history of seizures and those at higher risk of seizures. Ensure adequate clear liquid intake prior to and during bowel evacuation regimens; inadequate fluid intake may lead to dehydration. Other oral medications may not be well absorbed when given during bowel evacuation because of rapid intestinal peristalsis. Use with caution in debilitated patients; consider each patient's ability to hydrate properly. Use with caution in geriatric patients. Laxatives and purgatives have the potential for abuse by bulimia nervosa patients.

Enemas and oral solution are available in pediatric and adult sizes; prescribe by "volume" not by "bottle."

Rare but potentially serious adverse effects (including death) may occur when exceeding recommended doses of over-the-counter (OTC) sodium phosphate preparations to treat constipation. Severe dehydration and alterations in serum electrolytes (eg, calcium, sodium, phosphate) leading to renal/cardiac adverse effects have been reported, mostly when single maximum doses were exceeded or when more than 1 dose was taken per day. Patients should be advised to adhere to the product labeling and not exceed maximum recommended doses. Health care providers should use caution when recommending doses for oral sodium phosphate preparations for children younger

than 5 years of age. Rectal preparations should never be administered to children younger than 2 years of age (FDA Drug Safety Communication, 2014).

Aluminum: The parenteral product may contain aluminum; toxic aluminum concentrations may be seen with high doses, prolonged use, or renal dysfunction. Premature neonates are at higher risk due to immature renal function and aluminum intake from other parenteral sources. Parenteral aluminum exposure of >4 to 5 mcg/kg/day is associated with CNS and bone toxicity; tissue loading may occur at lower doses (Federal Register, 2002). See manufacturer's labeling.

Benzyl alcohol and derivatives: Some dosage forms may contain sodium benzoate/benzoic acid; benzoic acid (benzoate) is a metabolite of benzyl alcohol; large amounts of benzyl alcohol (≥99 mg/kg/day) have been associated with a potentially fatal toxicity ("gasping syndrome") in neonates; the "gasping syndrome" consists of metabolic acidosis, respiratory distress, gasping respirations, CNS dysfunction (including convulsions, intracranial hemorrhage), hypotension, and cardiovascular collapse (AAP ["Inactive" 1997]; CDC, 1982); some data suggests that benzoate displaces bilirubin from protein binding sites (Ahlfors, 2001); avoid or use dosage forms containing benzyl alcohol derivative with caution in neonates. See manufacturer's labeling.

Adverse Reactions Frequency not always defined.

Central nervous system: Dizziness, headache

Gastrointestinal: Bloating (31% to 47%), nausea (26% to 35%), abdominal pain (23% to 30%), vomiting (4% to 7%), mucosal bleeding, superficial mucosal ulcerations

Endocrine & metabolic: Hyperphosphatemia (≤96%), hypocalcemia (on colonoscopy day; 47%), hypophosphatemia (2-3 days postcolonoscopy; 34%), hypokalemia (on colonoscopy day; 28%), hypernatremia

Postmarketing and/or case reports (Limited to important or life-threatening): Acute phosphate nephropathy, anaphylaxis, bronchospasm, calcium nephrolithiasis, cardiac arrhythmia, dehydration, dysphagia, dyspnea, facial edema, increased blood urea nitrogen, increased serum creatinine, ischemic colitis, lip edema, paresthesia, pharyngeal edema, pruritus, rectal bleeding, renal failure, renal insufficiency, renal tubular necrosis, seizure, skin rash, tightness in throat, tongue edema, urticaria

Drug Interactions

Metabolism/Transport Effects None known.

Avoid Concomitant Use There are no known interactions where it is recommended to avoid concomitant use.

Increased Effect/Toxicity

Sodium Phosphates may increase the levels/effects of: Nonsteroidal Anti-Inflammatory Agents

The levels/effects of Sodium Phosphates may be increased by: ACE Inhibitors; Angiotensin II Receptor Blockers; Diuretics; Tricyclic Antidepressants

Decreased Effect

The levels/effects of Sodium Phosphates may be decreased by: Antacids; Calcium Salts; Iron Salts; Magnesium Salts; Multivitamins/Minerals (with ADEK, Folate, Iron); Sucralfate

Preparation for Administration Solution for injection: In general, the dose, concentration of infusion, and rate of administration may be dependent on patient condition and specific institution policy. Intermittent infusion doses are typically prepared in 100-250 mL of NS or D_5W (usual concentration range: 0.15-0.6 mmol/mL). Observe the vial for the presence of crystals. Do not use vial if crystals are present. **Note:** Due to the potential for solution crystallization, American Regent, Inc recommends the use of a 5 micron filter when preparing IV sodium phosphate containing solutions (Important Drug Safety Information, American Regent, 2013); a similar recommendation has not been noted by other manufacturers.

Storage/Stability

Enema: Store at room temperature.

Oral solution: Store at room temperature.

Solution for injection: Store intact vials at 20°C to 25°C (68°F to 77°F); excursions permitted between 15°C and 30°C (59°F and 86°F).

Tablet: Store at 25°C (77°F); excursions permitted between 15°C and 30°C (59°F and 86°F).

Mechanism of Action As a laxative, exerts osmotic effect in the small intestine by drawing water into the lumen of the gut, producing distention and promoting peristalsis and evacuation of the bowel; phosphorous participates in bone deposition, calcium metabolism, utilization of B complex vitamins, and as a buffer in acid-base equilibrium

Pharmacodynamics/Kinetics

Onset of action: Cathartic: 3-6 hours; Rectal: 2-5 minutes

Absorption: Oral: ~1% to 20%

Excretion: Urine

Dosing

Adult Note: If phosphate repletion is required and a phosphate product is not available at your institution, consider the use of sodium glycerophosphate pentahydrate (Glycophos) as a suitable substitute. Concentration and dosing are different from FDA-approved products; use caution when switching between products. Refer to Sodium Glycerophosphate Pentahydrate monograph.

Caution: With orders for IV phosphate, there is considerable confusion associated with the use of millimoles (mmol) versus milliequivalents (mEq) to express the phosphate requirement. The most reliable method of ordering IV phosphate is by millimoles, then specifying the potassium or sodium salt. Intravenous doses listed as mmol of phosphate.

Acute treatment of hypophosphatemia: IV: It is difficult to provide concrete guidelines for the treatment of severe hypophosphatemia because the extent of total body deficits and response to therapy are difficult to predict. Aggressive doses of phosphate may result in a transient serum elevation followed by redistribution into intracellular compartments or bone tissue. It is recommended that repletion of severe hypophosphatemia be done IV because large doses of oral phosphate may cause diarrhea and intestinal absorption may be unreliable. Intermittent IV infusion should be reserved for severe depletion situations; requires continuous cardiac monitoring. Guidelines differ based on degree of illness, need/use of TPN, and severity of hypophosphatemia. If hypokalemia exists (some clinicians recommend threshold of <4 mmol/L), consider phosphate replacement strategy with potassium (eg, potassium phosphates). Obese patients and/or severe renal impairment were excluded from phosphate supplement trials. **Note:** 1 mmol phosphate = 31 mg phosphorus; 1 mg phosphorus = 0.032 mmol phosphate.

General replacement guidelines (Lentz, 1978):

Low dose, serum phosphorus losses are recent and uncomplicated: 0.08 mmol/kg over 6 hours

Intermediate dose, serum phosphorus level 0.5-1 mg/dL (0.16-0.32 mmol/L): 0.16-0.24 mmol/kg over 6 hours

Note: The initial dose may be increased by 25% to 50% if the patient is symptomatic secondary to hypophosphatemia and lowered by 25% to 50% if the patient is hypercalcemic.

Critically-ill adult patients receiving concurrent enteral/parenteral nutrition (Brown, 2006; Clark, 1995): **Note:** Round doses to the nearest 7.5 mmol for ease of preparation. If administering with phosphate-containing parenteral nutrition, do not exceed 15 mmol/L within parenteral nutrition. May use adjusted body weight for patients weighing >130% of ideal body weight (and BMI <40 kg/m^2) by using [IBW + 0.25 (ABW-IBW)]:

Low dose, serum phosphorus level 2.3-3 mg/dL (0.74-0.96 mmol/L): 0.16-0.32 mmol/kg over 4-6 hours

Intermediate dose, serum phosphorus level 1.6-2.2 mg/dL (0.51-0.71 mmol/L): 0.32-0.64 mmol/kg over 4-6 hours

High dose, serum phosphorus <1.5 mg/dL (<0.5 mmol/L): 0.64-1 mmol/kg over 8-12 hours

Parenteral nutrition: IV: 10-15 mmol/1000 kcal (Hicks, 2001) or 20-40 mmol/24 hours (Mirtallo, 2004 [ASPEN guidelines])

Laxative (Fleet): Rectal: Contents of one 4.5 oz enema as a single dose

Laxative: Oral solution: 15 mL as a single dose; maximum single daily dose: 45 mL

Bowel cleansing prior to colonoscopy: Oral tablets: **Note:** Do not use additional agents, especially other sodium phosphate products.

OsmoPrep: A total of 32 tablets and 2 quarts of clear liquids (8 ounces of clear liquids with each dose) divided as follows:

Evening before colonoscopy: 4 tablets every 15 minutes for 5 doses (total of 20 tablets)

3-5 hours prior to colonoscopy: 4 tablets every 15 minutes for 3 doses (total of 12 tablets)

Geriatric Use with caution due to increased risk of renal impairment in the elderly. Refer to adult dosing.

Pediatric Note: If phosphate repletion is required and a phosphate product is not available at your institution, consider the use of sodium glycerophosphate pentahydrate (Glycophos) as a suitable substitute. Concentration and dosing are different from FDA-approved products; use caution when switching between products. Refer to Sodium Glycerophosphate Pentahydrate monograph.

Caution: With orders for IV phosphate, there is considerable confusion associated with the use of millimoles (mmol) versus milliequivalents (mEq) to express the phosphate requirement. The most reliable method of ordering IV phosphate is by millimoles, then specifying the potassium or sodium salt. Intravenous doses listed as mmol of phosphate.

Acute treatment of hypophosphatemia: IV: It is difficult to provide concrete guidelines for the treatment of severe hypophosphatemia because the extent of total body deficits and response to therapy are difficult to predict. Aggressive doses of phosphate may result in a transient serum elevation followed by redistribution into intracellular compartments or bone tissue. It is recommended that repletion of severe hypophosphatemia be done IV because large doses of oral phosphate may cause diarrhea and intestinal absorption may be unreliable. Intermittent IV infusion should be reserved for severe depletion situations; requires continuous cardiac monitoring. Guidelines differ based on degree of illness, need/use of TPN, and severity of hypophosphatemia. If hypokalemia exists (some clinicians recommend threshold of <4 mmol/L), consider phosphate replacement strategy with potassium (eg, potassium phosphates). Obese patients and/or severe renal impairment were excluded from phosphate supplement trials.

There are no prospective studies of parenteral phosphate replacement in children. The following weight-based guidelines for adult dosing may be cautiously employed in pediatric patients. Guidelines differ based on degree of illness, use of TPN, and severity of hypophosphatemia. **Note:** 1 mmol phosphate = 31 mg phosphorus; 1 mg phosphorus = 0.032 mmol phosphate.
General replacement guidelines (Lentz, 1978):
Low dose, serum phosphorus losses are recent and uncomplicated: 0.08 mmol/kg over 6 hours
Intermediate dose, serum phosphorus level 0.5-1 mg/dL (0.16-0.32 mmol/L): 0.16-0.24 mmol/kg over 6 hours
Note: The initial dose may be increased by 25% to 50% if the patient is symptomatic secondary to hypophosphatemia and lowered by 25% to 50% if the patient is hypercalcemic.
Critically-ill adult patients receiving concurrent enteral/parenteral nutrition (Brown, 2006; Clark 1995): **Note:** Round doses to the nearest 7.5 mmol for ease of preparation. If administering with phosphate-containing parenteral nutrition, do not exceed 15 mmol/L within parenteral nutrition. May use adjusted body weight for patients weighing >130% of ideal body weight (and BMI <40 kg/m^2) by using [IBW + 0.25 (ABW-IBW)]:
Low dose, serum phosphorus level 2.3-3 mg/dL (0.74-0.96 mmol/L): 0.16-0.32 mmol/kg over 4-6 hours
Intermediate dose, serum phosphorus level 1.6-2.2 mg/dL (0.51-0.71 mmol/L): 0.32-0.64 mmol/kg over 4-6 hours
High dose, serum phosphorus <1.5 mg/dL (<0.5 mmol/L): 0.64-1 mmol/kg over 8-12 hours

Parenteral nutrition: IV:
Infants and Children: 0.5-2 mmol/kg/24 hours (Mirtallo, 2004 [ASPEN guidelines])
Children >50 kg and Adolescents: 10-40 mmol/24 hours (Mirtallo, 2004 [ASPEN guidelines])

Laxative (Fleet): Rectal:
Children 2-4 years: One-half contents of one 2.25 oz pediatric enema
Children 5-11 years: Contents of one 2.25 oz pediatric enema
Children ≥12 years: Refer to adult dosing.

Laxative: Oral solution:
Children 5-9 years: 7.5 mL as a single dose; maximum single daily dose: 7.5 mL
Children 10-11 years: 15 mL as a single dose; maximum single daily dose: 15 mL
Children ≥12 years: Refer to adult dosing.

Renal Impairment No dosage adjustment provided in manufacturer's labeling. Use with caution; ionized inorganic phosphate is excreted by the kidneys. Oral solution is contraindicated in patients with kidney disease.

Hepatic Impairment No dosage adjustment provided in manufacturer's labeling.

Dietary Considerations Bowel cleansing: Should be taken on an empty stomach with clear liquids; a clear liquid diet should be used for 12 hours prior to and during tablet administration. Clear liquids may include water, flavored water, pulp-free lemonade, ginger ale, or apple juice; purple or red colored liquids should be avoided. Some products may contain phenylalanine and/or sodium.

Administration
Administer by intermittent IV infusion; do **not** administer IV push. Must be diluted prior to parenteral administration. In general, the dose, concentration of infusion, and rate of administration may be dependent on patient condition and specific institution policy. For adult patients with severe symptomatic hypophosphatemia (ie, <1.5 mg/dL), may administer at rates up to 15 mmol/hour (Charron, 2003; Rosen, 1995). In patients with renal dysfunction and/or less severe hypophosphatemia, slower administration rates (eg, over 4 to 6 hours) or oral repletion is recommended. **Note:** Due to the potential for solution crystallization, American Regent, Inc recommends the use of a 0.22 micron in-line filter for IV administration (1.2 micron filter if admixture contains lipids) (Important Drug Safety Information, American Regent, 2013); a similar recommendation has not been noted by other manufacturers.
Bowel cleansing (oral tablets): Have patient drink 8 ounces of clear liquids with each dose of sodium phosphate; have patient rehydrate before and after colonoscopy. Clear liquids may include water, flavored water, pulp-free lemonade, ginger ale, or apple juice; purple or red colored liquids should be avoided.
Constipation (oral solution): Take on an empty stomach; dilute dose with 8 ounces cool water, then follow dose with 8 ounces water; **do not repeat dose within 24 hours**

Monitoring Parameters
IV: Serum calcium, sodium and phosphorus levels; renal function; after IV phosphate repletion, repeat serum phosphorus level should be checked 2-4 hours later
Oral: Bowel cleansing: Baseline and postprocedure labs (electrolytes, calcium, phosphorus, BUN, creatinine) in patients at risk for acute renal nephropathy, seizure, or who have a history of electrolyte abnormality; ECG in patients with risks for prolonged QT or arrhythmias. Ensure euvolemia before initiating bowel preparation.

Reference Range Note: Reference ranges may vary depending on the laboratory
Serum calcium: 8.4-10.2 mg/dL
Serum phosphorus: Both low and high ends of the normal range are higher in children than in adults.
Infants: 4.5-7.5 mg/dL (1.45-2.42 mmol/L)
Children: ~4.0-6.0 mg/dL (1.29-1.94 mmol/L)
Adults: 2.5-4.5 mg/dL (0.81-1.45 mmol/L)

Additional Information Phosphate salts may precipitate when mixed with calcium salts; solubility is improved in amino acid parenteral nutrition solutions; check with a pharmacist to determine compatibility.

Dosage Forms Considerations
Sodium 4 mEq is equivalent to sodium 92 mg
Phosphorous 3 mmol is equivalent to phosphorus 93 mg

Dosage Forms Excipient information presented when available (limited, particularly for generics); consult specific product labeling.
Injection, solution [concentrate; preservative free]: Phosphorus 3 mmol and sodium 4 mEq per 1 mL (5 mL, 15 mL, 50 mL) [equivalent to phosphorus 93 mg and sodium 92 mg per 1 mL; source of electrolytes: monobasic and dibasic sodium phosphate]
Solution, oral: Monobasic sodium phosphate monohydrate 2.4 g and dibasic sodium phosphate heptahydrate 0.9 g per 5 mL (45 mL) [sugar free; contains sodium 556 mg/5 mL, sodium benzoate; ginger-lemon flavor]
Solution, rectal [enema]: Monobasic sodium phosphate monohydrate 19 g and dibasic sodium phosphate heptahydrate 7 g per 118 mL delivered dose (133 mL)
Fleet Enema: Monobasic sodium phosphate monohydrate 19 g and dibasic sodium phosphate heptahydrate 7 g per 118 mL delivered dose (133 mL) [contains sodium 4.4 g/118 mL]
Fleet Enema Extra: Monobasic sodium phosphate monohydrate 19 g and dibasic sodium phosphate heptahydrate 7 g per 197 mL delivered dose (230 mL) [contains sodium 4.4 g/197 mL]
Fleet Pedia-Lax™ Enema: Monobasic sodium phosphate monohydrate 9.5 g and dibasic sodium phosphate heptahydrate 3.5 g per 59 mL delivered dose (66 mL) [contains sodium 2.2 g/59 mL]
LaCrosse Complete: Monobasic sodium phosphate monohydrate 19 g and dibasic sodium phosphate heptahydrate 7 g per 118 mL delivered dose (133 mL) [contains sodium 4.4 g/118 mL]
Tablet, oral [scored]:
OsmoPrep: Monobasic sodium phosphate monohydrate 1.102 g and dibasic sodium phosphate anhydrous 0.398 g [sodium phosphate 1.5 g per tablet; gluten free]

Sodium Picosulfate, Magnesium Oxide, and Citric Acid

(SOW dee um pye ko SUL fate mag NEE zhum OKS ide & SI trik AS id)

Brand Names: US Prepopik™

Brand Names: Canada Oral Purgative; Pico-Salax®; Picodan; Picoflo; Purg-Odan™

Index Terms Citric Acid, Sodium Picosulfate, and Magnesium Oxide; DA-1773; Magnesium Oxide, Sodium Picosulfate, and Citric Acid; Prepopik™; Sodium Picosulphate, Magnesium Oxide, and Citric Acid

Pharmacologic Category Laxative, Osmotic; Laxative, Stimulant

Use Bowel cleansing prior to colonoscopy

Canadian labeling: Additional uses (not in U.S. labeling): Bowel cleansing prior to x-ray examination, endoscopy, or surgery

Medication Guide Available Yes

Dosing

Adult & Geriatric Bowel cleansing: Oral:

Prepopik™:

Split-dose regimen (preferred): 150 mL (5 oz) the evening before the colonoscopy (5 PM-9 PM), followed by a second 150 mL (5 oz) dose ~5 hours before the colonoscopy.

Day-before regimen (alternative): 150 mL (5 oz) in the early evening before the colonoscopy (4 PM-6 PM), followed by a second 150 mL (5 oz) dose 6 hours later (10 PM-12 AM) the night before the colonoscopy.

Purg-Odan™ (Canadian availability): One sachet (mixed and dissolved in water) in the morning (8 AM) the day prior to the procedure followed by a second dose of one sachet in the afternoon (2 PM-4 PM) on the day prior to the procedure.

Pico-Salax® (Canadian availability):

Early colonoscopy (before 12 PM): One sachet (mixed and dissolved in water) in the evening (5 PM) the day prior to the procedure, followed by a second dose of one sachet 5 hours later (10 PM) the night before the procedure

Late colonoscopy (after 12 PM): One sachet (mixed and dissolved in water) in the late evening (7 PM) the day prior to the procedure, followed by a second dose of one sachet in the morning (6 AM) on the day of the procedure

Pediatric Bowel cleansing: Oral:

Purg-Odan™ (Canadian availability): Oral:

Children 1-5 years: One-fourth (1/4) of one sachet (mixed and dissolved in water) in the morning (8 AM) the day prior to the procedure, followed by a second dose of one-fourth (1/4) of one sachet in the afternoon (2 PM-4 PM) on the day prior to the procedure.

Children 6-12 years: One-half (1/2) of one sachet (mixed and dissolved in water) in the morning (8 AM) the day prior to the procedure, followed by a second dose of one-half (1/2) of one sachet in the afternoon (2 PM-4 PM) on the day prior to the procedure.

Pico-Salax® (Canadian availability): Oral:

Children 1-5 years: One-fourth (1/4) of one sachet (mixed and dissolved in water) in the evening (6 PM) the day prior to the procedure, followed by a second dose of one-fourth (1/4) of one sachet in the morning (8 AM) on the day of the procedure

Children 6-12 years: One-half (1/2) of one sachet (mixed and dissolved in water) in the evening (6 PM) the day prior to the procedure, followed by a second dose of one-half (1/2) of one sachet in the morning (8 AM) on the day of the procedure

Additional Information Complete prescribing information should be consulted for additional detail.

Dosage Forms Excipient information presented when available (limited, particularly for generics); consult specific product labeling.

Powder for solution, oral [kit]:

Prepopik™: Sodium picosulfate 10 mg, magnesium oxide 3.5 g, and citric acid 12 g per packet (2s) [orange flavor]

Dosage Forms: Canada Excipient information presented when available (limited, particularly for generics); consult specific product labeling.

Powder for solution, oral [kit]:

Pico-Salax®: Sodium picosulphate 10 mg, magnesium oxide 3.5 g, and citric acid 12 g per sachet (1s, 2s) [orange or cranberry flavor]

Purg-Odan™: Sodium picosulphate 10 mg, magnesium oxide 3.5 g, and citric acid 12 g per sachet (1s, 2s) [orange flavor]

◆ Sodium Picosulphate, Magnesium Oxide, and Citric Acid *see* Sodium Picosulfate, Magnesium Oxide, and Citric Acid *on page 1680*

Sodium Polystyrene Sulfonate

(SOW dee um pol ee STYE reen SUL fon ate)

Brand Names: US Kalexate; Kayexalate; Kionex; SPS

Brand Names: Canada Kayexalate®; PMS-Sodium Polystyrene Sulfonate

Pharmacologic Category Antidote

Use Treatment of hyperkalemia

Pregnancy Considerations Animal reproduction studies have not been conducted. There are no adequate and well-controlled studies in pregnant women. Use during pregnancy only if benefits outweigh the risks.

Breast-Feeding Considerations It is not known if sodium polystyrene sulfonate is excreted in breast milk. The manufacturer recommends that caution be exercised when administering sodium polystyrene sulfonate to nursing women.

Contraindications Hypersensitivity to sodium polystyrene sulfonate or any component of the formulation; hypokalemia; obstructive bowel disease; neonates with reduced gut motility (postoperatively or drug-induced); oral administration in neonates

Additional contraindications: Sodium polystyrene sulfonate suspension (**with** sorbitol): Rectal administration in neonates (particularly in premature infants); any postoperative patient until normal bowel function resumes

Warnings/Precautions Intestinal necrosis (including fatalities) and other serious gastrointestinal events (eg, bleeding, ischemic colitis, perforation) have been reported, especially when administered with sorbitol. Increased risk may be associated with a history of intestinal disease or surgery, hypovolemia, prematurity, and renal insufficiency or failure; use with sorbitol is not recommended. Avoid use in any postoperative patient until normal bowel function resumes or in patients at risk for constipation or impaction; discontinue use if constipation occurs. Oral or rectal administration of sorbitol-containing sodium polystyrene sulfonate suspensions is contraindicated in neonates (particularly with prematurity). Use with caution in patients with severe HF, hypertension, or edema; sodium load may exacerbate condition. Effective lowering of serum potassium from sodium polystyrene sulfonate may take hours to days after administration; consider alternative measures (eg, dialysis) or concomitant therapy (eg, IV sodium bicarbonate) in situations where rapid correction of severe hyperkalemia is required. Severe hypokalemia may occur; frequent monitoring of serum potassium is recommended within each 24-hour period; ECG monitoring may be appropriate in select patients. In addition to serum potassium-lowering effects, cation-exchange resins may also affect other cation concentrations possibly resulting in decreased serum magnesium and calcium. Large oral doses may cause fecal impaction (especially in elderly).

Concomitant administration of oral sodium polystyrene sulfonate with nonabsorbable cation-donating antacids or laxatives (eg, magnesium hydroxide) may result in systemic alkalosis and may diminish ability to reduce serum potassium concentrations; use with such agents is not recommended. In addition, intestinal obstruction has been reported with concomitant administration of aluminum hydroxide due to concretion formation. Enema will reduce the serum potassium faster than oral administration, but the oral route will result in a greater reduction over several hours. Oral administration in neonates and use in neonates with reduced gut motility (postoperatively or drug-induced) is contraindicated. Oral or rectal administration of sorbitol-containing sodium polystyrene sulfonate suspensions in neonates (particularly with prematurity) is also contraindicated due to propylene glycol content and risk of intestinal necrosis and digestive hemorrhage. Use sodium polystyrene sulfonate (**without** sorbitol) with caution in premature or low-birth-weight infants. Use with caution in children when administering rectally; excessive dosage or inadequate dilution may result in fecal impaction. Propylene glycol: Some dosage forms may contain propylene glycol; large amounts are potentially toxic and have been associated hyperosmolality, lactic acidosis, seizures, and respiratory depression; use caution (AAP, 1997; Zar, 2007).

Adverse Reactions

Frequency not defined:

Endocrine & metabolic: Hypernatremia, hypocalcemia, hypokalemia, hypomagnesemia, sodium retention

Gastrointestinal: Anorexia, constipation, diarrhea, fecal impaction, intestinal necrosis (rare), intestinal obstruction (due to concretions in association with aluminum hydroxide), nausea, vomiting

<1% (Limited to important or life-threatening): Acute bronchitis (rare; associated with inhalation of particles), concretions, gastrointestinal bleeding, gastrointestinal ulceration, intestinal perforation, ischemic colitis

Drug Interactions

Metabolism/Transport Effects None known.

Avoid Concomitant Use

Avoid concomitant use of Sodium Polystyrene Sulfonate with any of the following: Laxatives (Magnesium Containing); Meloxicam; Sorbitol

Increased Effect/Toxicity

Sodium Polystyrene Sulfonate may increase the levels/effects of: Aluminum Hydroxide; Digoxin

The levels/effects of Sodium Polystyrene Sulfonate may be increased by: Antacids; Laxatives (Magnesium Containing); Meloxicam; Sorbitol

Decreased Effect

Sodium Polystyrene Sulfonate may decrease the levels/effects of: Lithium; Thyroid Products

Food Interactions Some liquids may contain potassium: Management: Do not mix in orange juice or in any fruit juice known to contain potassium.

Storage/Stability Store at 25°C (77°F); excursions permitted to 15°C to 30°C (59°F to 86°F). Store repackaged product in refrigerator and use within 14 days. Freshly prepared suspensions should be used within 24 hours. Do not heat resin suspension.

Mechanism of Action Removes potassium by exchanging sodium ions for potassium ions in the intestine (especially the large intestine) before the resin is passed from the body; exchange capacity is 1 mEq/g *in vivo*, and *in vitro* capacity is 3.1 mEq/g, therefore, a wide range of exchange capacity exists such that close monitoring of serum electrolytes is necessary

Pharmacodynamics/Kinetics

Onset of action: 2-24 hours

Absorption: None

Excretion: Completely feces (primarily as potassium polystyrene sulfonate)

Dosing

Adult & Geriatric Hyperkalemia:

Oral: 15 g 1-4 times/day

Rectal: 30-50 g every 6 hours

Pediatric Hyperkalemia:

Oral: Children: 1 g/kg/dose every 6 hours

Rectal: Children: 1 g/kg/dose every 2-6 hours (in small children and infants, employ lower doses by using the practical exchange ratio of 1 mEq K⁺/g of resin as the basis for calculation)

Renal Impairment No dosage adjustment provided in manufacturer's labeling. Use with caution; risks of gastrointestinal adverse effects are greater in patients with renal insufficiency or failure.

Hepatic Impairment No dosage adjustment provided in manufacturer's labeling.

Dietary Considerations Do **not** mix in orange juice or in any fruit juice known to contain potassium. Some products may contain sodium.

Administration

Oral: Shake suspension well prior to administration. Administer orally (or via NG tube) as a suspension. **Do not mix in orange juice.** Chilling the oral mixture will increase palatability.

Powder for suspension: For each 1 g of the powdered resin, add 3-4 mL of water or syrup (amount of fluid usually ranges from 20-100 mL)

Rectal: Enema route is less effective than oral administration. Administer cleansing enema first. Each dose of the powder for suspension should be suspended in 100 mL of aqueous vehicle and administered as a warm emulsion (body temperature). The commercially available suspension should also be warmed to body temperature. During administration, the solution should be agitated gently. Retain enema in colon for at least 30-60 minutes and for several hours, if possible. Once retention time is complete, irrigate colon with a non-sodium-containing solution to remove resin.

Monitoring Parameters Serum electrolytes (potassium, sodium, calcium, magnesium); ECG in select patients

Reference Range Serum potassium: Adults: 3.5-5.2 mEq/L

Additional Information 1 g of resin binds approximately 1 mEq of potassium

Historically, sorbitol was often recommended as a cathartic agent to be administered with sodium polystyrene sulfonate (SPS) to prevent SPS-induced fecal impaction. However, SPS, particularly when used with sorbitol, has been associated with cases of intestinal necrosis and other serious GI adverse events. Due to the concern that sorbitol

may increase the risk of intestinal necrosis, concomitant use of sorbitol is no longer recommended.

Sodium polystyrene sulfonate is commercially available in a liquid suspension containing 33% sorbitol (~20 g sorbitol per 60 mL suspension).

Dosage Forms Excipient information presented when available (limited, particularly for generics); consult specific product labeling.

Powder, Oral:

Kalexate: (454 g) [sorbitol free; contains sodium 100 mg (4.1 mEq)/g]

Kayexalate: (453.6 g) [contains sodium 100 mg (4.1 mEq)/g]

Kionex: (454 g) [contains sodium 100 mg (4.1 mEq)/g]

Generic: (15 g, 453.6 g, 454 g)

Suspension, Oral:

Kionex: 15 g/60 mL (60 mL, 473 mL) [contains alcohol, usp, methylparaben, propylene glycol, propylparaben, saccharin sodium, sodium 1500 mg (65 mEq)/60 mL, sorbitol; raspberry flavor]

SPS: 15 g/60 mL (60 mL, 120 mL, 473 mL) [contains alcohol, usp, methylparaben, propylene glycol, propylparaben, saccharin sodium, sodium 1500 mg (65 mEq)/60 mL, sorbitol; cherry flavor]

Generic: 15 g/60 mL (60 mL, 480 mL, 500 mL)

Suspension, Rectal:

Generic: 30 g/120 mL (120 mL); 50 g/200 mL (200 mL)

◆ Sodium Sulamyd (Can) *see* Sulfacetamide (Ophthalmic) *on page 1707*

◆ Sodium Sulfacetamide *see* Sulfacetamide (Ophthalmic) *on page 1707*

◆ Sodium Sulfacetamide *see* Sulfacetamide (Topical) *on page 1707*

◆ Sodium Sulfacetamide and Sulfur *see* Sulfur and Sulfacetamide *on page 1716*

◆ Sodium Sulfate, Magnesium Sulfate, and Potassium Sulfate *see* Sodium Sulfate, Potassium Sulfate, and Magnesium Sulfate *on page 1681*

Sodium Sulfate, Potassium Sulfate, and Magnesium Sulfate

(SOW dee um SUL fate, poe TASS ee um SUL fate, & mag NEE zhum SUL fate)

Brand Names: US Suprep® Bowel Prep Kit

Index Terms Magnesium Sulfate, Potassium Sulfate, and Sodium Sulfate; Magnesium Sulfate, Sodium Sulfate, and Potassium Sulfate; Potassium Sulfate, Magnesium Sulfate, and Sodium Sulfate; Potassium Sulfate, Sodium Sulfate, and Magnesium Sulfate; Sodium Sulfate, Magnesium Sulfate, and Potassium Sulfate

Pharmacologic Category Laxative, Osmotic

Use Bowel cleansing prior to GI examination

Medication Guide Available Yes

Dosing

Adult & Geriatric Bowel cleansing prior to GI exam:

Oral:

Split-dose regimen: Total volume of liquid consumed over the course of treatment: 2880 mL (96 oz)

Evening before colonoscopy: Drink the entire contents of 1 bottle, diluted to a final volume of 480 mL (16 oz). Then drink 2 additional containers of water each (filled to the 16-ounce line) over the next hour, for an additional volume of 960 mL (32 oz).

Morning of the colonoscopy (10-12 hours after the evening dose): Repeat entire process with the second bottle: Drink entire contents of second bottle diluted to a final volume of 480 mL (16 oz); then drink 2 additional containers of water (each filled to the 16-ounce line) over the next hour, for an additional volume of 960 mL (32 oz). Complete at least 2 hours before the procedure.

Renal Impairment No adjustments provided in manufacturer's labeling. Use with caution, ensure adequate hydration, and consider baseline and post-colonoscopy renal function assessment.

Hepatic Impairment No dosage adjustment provided in manufacturer's labeling. However, no adjustment expected due to similar disposition to healthy patients in pharmacokinetic studies.

Additional Information Complete prescribing information should be consulted for additional detail.

Dosage Forms Excipient information presented when available (limited, particularly for generics); consult specific product labeling. [DSC] = Discontinued product

Solution, oral:

Suprep® Bowel Prep Kit: Sodium sulfate 17.5 g, potassium sulfate 3.13 g, and magnesuim sulfate 1.6 g per 180 mL (180 mL) [contains sodium benzoate]

◆ Sodium Sulfate, Potassium Sulfate, Magnesium Sulfate and PEG-Electrolyte Solution see Sodium Sulfate, Potassium Sulfate, Magnesium Sulfate, and Polyethylene Glycol-Electrolyte Solution on page 1682

◆ Sodium Sulfate, Potassium Sulfate, Magnesium Sulfate and PEG Solution see Sodium Sulfate, Potassium Sulfate, Magnesium Sulfate, and Polyethylene Glycol-Electrolyte Solution on page 1682

Sodium Sulfate, Potassium Sulfate, Magnesium Sulfate, and Polyethylene Glycol-Electrolyte Solution

(SOW dee um SUL fate, poe TASS ee um SUL fate, mag NEE zhum SUL fate, & pol i ETH i leen GLY kol ee LEK troe lite soe LOO shun)

Brand Names: US Suclear™ [DSC]

Index Terms Sodium Sulfate, Potassium Sulfate, Magnesium Sulfate and PEG Solution; Sodium Sulfate, Potassium Sulfate, Magnesium Sulfate and PEG-Electrolyte Solution

Pharmacologic Category Laxative, Osmotic

Use Bowel cleansing prior to colonoscopy

Medication Guide Available Yes

Dosing

Adult & Geriatric Bowel cleansing prior to colonoscopy: Oral: May be administered as the *split-dose (2-day) regimen* (preferred method) or the *day-before (1-day) regimen* (alternative method).

Split-dose (2-day) regimen: Total volume of liquid consumed over the course of treatment: 3440 mL (~115 oz)

Dose 1: Evening before colonoscopy (10-12 hours prior to Dose 2): Dilute the contents of the 6-ounce oral solution bottle to a final volume of 480 mL (16 oz), and drink the contents within 20 minutes. Refill container with 16 ounces of water and drink over the next 2 hours. Refill the container with the second refill of 16 oz of water, and finish drinking before bedtime (2 refills totaling 960 mL [32 oz]). Total volume of liquid consumed with Dose 1: 1440 mL (48 oz).

Dose 2: Morning of the colonoscopy (beginning at least 3.5 hours prior to colonoscopy): Drink the entire contents of the reconstituted powder which has been diluted to a final volume of 2000 mL (2 L [~67 oz]) as follows: Using the 16-ounce container provided, drink at a rate of 480 mL (16 oz) every 20 minutes (four 16-ounce containers over ~1.5 hours). Complete at least 2 hours prior to colonoscopy. Total volume of liquid consumed with Dose 2: 2000 mL (~67 oz)

Day-before (1-day) regimen: Total volume of liquid consumed over the course of treatment: 3440 mL (~115 oz)

Dose 1: Evening before colonoscopy (beginning at least 3.5 hours prior to bedtime): Drink the diluted contents of the 6-ounce oral solution bottle, which has been further diluted to a final volume of 480 mL (16 oz), preferably within 20 minutes. Refill container with 480 mL (16 oz) of water, and drink over the next 2 hours. Total volume of liquid consumed with Dose 1: 960 mL (32 oz).

Dose 2: Evening before colonoscopy (~2 hours after starting Dose 1): Drink the entire contents of the reconstituted powder which has been diluted to a final volume of 2000 mL (2 L [~67 oz]) as follows: Using the 16-ounce container provided, drink at a rate of 480 mL (16 oz) every 20 minutes (four 16-ounce containers over ~1.5 hours). Refill the container with 480 mL (16 oz) of water and finish drinking before bedtime. Total volume of liquid consumed with Dose 2: 2480 mL (~83 oz).

Renal Impairment No dosage adjustment provided in manufacturer's labeling (safety has not been adequately studied); however, use caution and ensure adequate hydration in patients with renal impairment or at risk for impairment. Moderate renal impairment (CrCl 30-49 mL/minute) resulted in a 43% higher C_{max} and a 16% lower urinary clearance of serum sulfates compared to healthy patients.

Hepatic Impairment No dosage adjustment provided in manufacturer's labeling.

Additional Information Complete prescribing information should be consulted for additional detail.

Dosage Forms Excipient information presented when available (limited, particularly for generics); consult specific product labeling.

Kit, Oral [each kit contains]:

Suclear: Powder for solution, oral: PEG 3350 210 g, sodium bicarbonate 2.86 g, sodium chloride 5.6 g, potassium chloride 0.74 g (2000 mL) [contains cherry, lemon-lime, orange, and pineapple flavor packs]

Suclear: Solution, oral: Sodium sulfate 17.5 g, potassium sulfate 3.13 g, and magnesium sulfate 1.6 g (177 mL) [contains sodium benzoate] [DSC]

Sodium Tetradecyl Sulfate

(SOW dee um tetra DEK il SUL fate)

Brand Names: US Sotradecol

Brand Names: Canada Trombovar

Pharmacologic Category Sclerosing Agent

Use Treatment of small, uncomplicated varicose veins of the lower extremities

Dosing

Adult & Geriatric Sclerosing agent: IV: Test dose: 0.5 mL given several hours prior to administration of larger dose; 0.5-2 mL (preferred maximum: 1 mL) in each vein, maximum: 10 mL per treatment session; 3% solution reserved for large varices

Renal Impairment No dosage adjustment provided in manufacturer's labeling.

Hepatic Impairment No dosage adjustment provided in manufacturer's labeling.

Additional Information Complete prescribing information should be consulted for additional detail.

Dosage Forms Excipient information presented when available (limited, particularly for generics); consult specific product labeling.

Solution, Intravenous, as sulfate:

Sotradecol: 1% (2 mL); 3% (2 mL) [contains benzyl alcohol]

Sodium Thiosulfate (SOW dee um thye oh SUL fate)

Index Terms Disodium Thiosulfate Pentahydrate; Pentahydrate; Sodium Hyposulfate; Sodium Thiosulphate; Thiosulfuric Acid Disodium Salt

Pharmacologic Category Antidote; Antidote, Extravasation

Use Cyanide poisoning: Treatment of acute, life-threatening cyanide poisoning in combination with sodium nitrite. Consider consultation with a poison control center at 1-800-222-1222.

Dosing

Adult

Cyanide poisoning: IV: **Note:** Administer in conjunction with sodium nitrite. Administer sodium nitrite first, followed immediately by the administration of sodium thiosulfate: 12.5 g (50 mL of a 25% solution); may repeat at one-half the original dose if symptoms of cyanide toxicity return

Note: Monitor the patient for 24 to 48 hours; if symptoms return, repeat both sodium nitrite and sodium thiosulfate at one-half the original doses.

Calciphylaxis (off-label use): IV: **Note:** Optimal dose is not established.

Dialysis patients: 25 g administered 3 times per week during the last hour of or after the hemodialysis session. Therapy should continue until there is complete resolution of symptoms (Ackermann 2007; Auriemma 2011; Cicone 2004; Nigwekar 2013; Subramaniam 2008).

Patients not on dialysis (normal renal function or mildly reduced GFR): 25 g administered 3 times per week (Baker 2007; Hackett 2011).

Extravasation management (off-label use):

Mechlorethamine: SubQ (off-label route): Inject 2 mL of a 1/6 M (~4%) sodium thiosulfate solution (into the extravasation site) for each mg of mechlorethamine suspected to have extravasated (Pérez Fidalgo 2012; Polovich 2009)

Cisplatin, concentrated: Inject 2 mL of a 1/6 M (~4%) sodium thiosulfate solution into existing IV line for each 100 mg of cisplatin extravasated; consider also injecting 1 mL of a 1/6 M (~4%) sodium thiosulfate solution as 0.1 mL subcutaneous injections (clockwise) into the area around the extravasation, may repeat subcutaneous injections several times over the next 3-4 hours (Ener 2004)

Bendamustine: SubQ: Bendamustine extravasation may be managed with 1/6 M (~4%) sodium thiosulfate solution in the same manner as mechlorethamine extravasation (Schulmeister 2011)

Geriatric Refer to adult dosing; use with caution due to likelihood of decreased renal function.

Pediatric Cyanide poisoning: IV: **Note:** Administer in conjunction with sodium nitrite. Administer sodium nitrite first, followed immediately by the administration of sodium thiosulfate. 250 mg/kg (1 mL/kg or ~30 to 40 mL/m^2 of a 25% solution) or 500 mg/kg (2 mL/kg of a 25% solution) (Howland 2011); maximum dose: 12.5 g (50 mL of a 25% solution); may repeat at one-half the original dose if symptoms of cyanide toxicity return

Note: Monitor the patient for 24-48 hours; if symptoms return, repeat both sodium nitrite and sodium thiosulfate at one-half the original doses.

Renal Impairment

No dosage adjustment provided in manufacturer's labeling; however, renal elimination is significant and risk of adverse effects may be increased in patients with renal impairment.

Calciphylaxis (off-label use): No dosage adjustment necessary. When used for patients not on dialysis (normal renal function or mildly reduced GFR), because sodium thiosulfate is cleared by the kidney, dose may be adjusted based on appearance of adverse effects (eg, metabolic acidosis, hypotension) (Hackett 2011; Nigwekar 2013).

Hepatic Impairment No dosage adjustment provided in the manufacturer's labeling (has not been studied).

Additional Information Complete prescribing information should be consulted for additional detail.

Dosage Forms Excipient information presented when available (limited, particularly for generics); consult specific product labeling. [DSC] = Discontinued product

Solution, Intravenous:

Generic: 10% [100 mg/mL] (10 mL [DSC]); 25% [250 mg/mL] (50 mL)

♦ Sodium Thiosulfate and Sodium Nitrite *see* Sodium Nitrite and Sodium Thiosulfate *on page 1675*

♦ Sodium Thiosulphate *see* Sodium Thiosulfate *on page 1682*

♦ Sof-Lax [OTC] *see* Docusate *on page 578*

♦ Soflax [OTC] (Can) *see* Docusate *on page 578*

♦ Soflax C [OTC] (Can) *see* Docusate *on page 578*

♦ Soflax EX [OTC] (Can) *see* Bisacodyl *on page 231*

Sofosbuvir (soe FOS bue vir)

Brand Names: US Sovaldi

Brand Names: Canada Sovaldi

Index Terms Sovaldi

Pharmacologic Category Antihepaciviral, Polymerase Inhibitor (Anti-HCV)

Use Chronic hepatitis C: Treatment of genotype 1, 2, 3, or 4 chronic hepatitis C (CHC) as a component of a combination antiviral treatment regimen.

Pregnancy Considerations Adverse events were not observed in animal reproduction studies using sofosbuvir. However, sofosbuvir is only to be used in combination with ribavirin or peginterferon alfa/ribavirin for the treatment of hepatitis C virus (HCV), therefore use is contraindicated in pregnancy. A negative pregnancy test is required before initiation and monthly thereafter. Avoid pregnancy in female patients and female partners of male patients during therapy by using two effective forms of nonhormonal contraception; continue contraceptive measures for at least 6 months after completion of therapy. Also refer to the Peginterferon Alfa and Ribavirin monographs for additional information.

If pregnancy occurs during use or within 6 months after treatment with ribavirin, report to the ribavirin pregnancy registry (800-593-2214). In addition, because sofosbuvir may be used for the treatment of HCV infection in women coinfected with HIV, inadvertent administration of sofosbuvir in women with HCV/HIV coinfection during pregnancy should also be reported to the Antiretroviral Pregnancy Registry (1-800-258-4263).

Breast-Feeding Considerations It is not known if sofosbuvir is excreted into breast milk. Due to the potential for serious adverse reactions in the nursing infant, the manufacturer recommends a decision be made whether to discontinue nursing or to discontinue the drug, taking into account the importance of treatment to the mother. Breast-feeding is not linked to the spread of hepatitis C virus; however, if nipples are cracked or bleeding, breast-feeding is not recommended (Workowski, 2010). Mothers coinfected with HIV are discouraged from breast-feeding to decrease potential transmission of HIV (DHHS [perinatal], 2012). Also refer to the Peginterferon Alfa and Ribavirin monographs for additional information.

Contraindications

All contraindications also applicable to ribavirin and peginterferon alfa including women who are pregnant or who may become pregnant and use by male partners of pregnant women.

Also refer to Peginterferon Alfa and Ribavirin monographs for individual product contraindications.

Canadian labeling: Additional contraindications (not in U.S. labeling): Hypersensitivity to sofosbuvir or any component of the formulation; males whose female partners may become pregnant

Warnings/Precautions Avoid pregnancy in females and female partners of male patients during therapy and for at least 6 months following treatment since used in combination with ribavirin for all indications; two nonhormonal forms of effective contraception must be used. Combination therapy with ribavirin is contraindicated in pregnancy; ribavirin may cause birth defects and/or death of the exposed fetus. Do not use as monotherapy; use only in combination with ribavirin (with or without peginterferon alfa depending upon the clinical indication). Alternative recommendations also use in combination with simeprevir in select patients (AASLD/IDSA, 2014). Potentially significant drug-drug interactions may exist, requiring dose or frequency adjustment, additional monitoring, and/or selection of alternative therapy, including use with potent P-gp inducers (eg, rifampin, St John's wort). Symptomatic bradycardia (some requiring pacemaker intervention) has occurred in patients receiving amiodarone and sofosbuvir in combination with simeprevir or an investigational NS5A inhibitor. Fatal cardiac arrest occurred when a patient took the ledipasvir/sofosbuvir combination product. Bradycardia generally occurred within hours to days following coadministration, however some cases have occurred 2 weeks following the initiation of sofosbuvir. The risk of bradycardia may be increased in patients taking beta blockers or patients with underlying cardiac comorbidities and/or advanced liver disease. Bradycardia generally resolves following discontinuation of sofosbuvir. Coadministration of amiodarone and sofosbuvir in combination with another direct acting antiviral (DAA) is not recommended. However, if patients have no treatment alternatives, patients should have in-patient cardiac monitoring for the first 48 hours, followed by daily outpatient or self-monitoring of heart rate for at least the first 2 weeks of treatment. Due to the long half-life of amiodarone, cardiac monitoring (as described) is also recommended if amiodarone was discontinued just prior to beginning treatment with sofosbuvir. Patients should seek medical attention immediately if they experience fainting or near-fainting, dizziness, lightheadedness, malaise, weakness, excessive tiredness, shortness of breath, chest pains, confusion or memory problems.

Adverse Reactions Adverse reactions reported with combination therapy.

>10%:

Central nervous system: Fatigue (30% to 59%), headache (24% to 36%), insomnia (15% to 25%), chills (2% to 17%), irritability (10% to 13%)

Dermatologic: Pruritus (11% to 27%), skin rash (8% to 18%)

Gastrointestinal: Nausea (22% to 34%), decreased appetite (18%), diarrhea (9% to 12%)

Hematologic & oncologic: Decreased hemoglobin (<10 g/dL: 6% to 23%; <8.5 g/dL: ≤2%), anemia (6% to 21%), neutropenia (<1% [interferon-free regimen] to 17% [interferon-containing regimen]), decreased neutrophils (≥0.5 to <0.75 times 10^9/L: <1% [interferon-free regimen] to 15%; <0.5 times 10^9/L: ≤5%)

Neuromuscular & skeletal: Weakness (5% to 21%), myalgia (6% to 14%)

Respiratory: Flu-like symptoms (6% to 16%)

Miscellaneous: Fever (4% to 18%)

1% to 10%:

Gastrointestinal: Increased serum lipase (>3 times ULN: ≤2%)

Hematologic & oncologic: Thrombocytopenia (≤1%)

Hepatic: Increased serum bilirubin (>2.5 times ULN: 3%)

Renal: Increased creatine kinase (≥10 times ULN: 1% to 2%)

<1% (Limited to important or life-threatening): Pancytopenia, severe depression, suicidal ideation

Drug Interactions

Metabolism/Transport Effects Substrate of P-glycoprotein

Avoid Concomitant Use

Avoid concomitant use of Sofosbuvir with any of the following: Amiodarone; Modafinil; OXcarbazepine; P-glycoprotein/ABCB1 Inducers; Rifabutin; Rifapentine

Increased Effect/Toxicity

Sofosbuvir may increase the levels/effects of: Amiodarone

The levels/effects of Sofosbuvir may be increased by: Lumacaftor; P-glycoprotein/ABCB1 Inhibitors; Ranolazine

Decreased Effect

The levels/effects of Sofosbuvir may be decreased by: Lumacaftor; Modafinil; OXcarbazepine; P-glycoprotein/ABCB1 Inducers; Rifabutin; Rifapentine

Storage/Stability Store below 30°C (86°F). Dispense only in original container.

◄ **Mechanism of Action** Sofosbuvir, a direct-acting antiviral agent against the hepatitis C virus, is a prodrug converted to its pharmacologically active form (GS-461203) via intracellular metabolism. It inhibits HCV NS5B RNA-dependent RNA polymerase, essential for viral replication, and acts as a chain terminator.

Pharmacodynamics/Kinetics
Protein binding: ~61% to 65%

Metabolism: Hepatic; forms pharmacologically active nucleoside (uridine) analog triphosphate GS-461203; dephosphorylation results in the formation of nucleoside inactive metabolite GS-331007

Half-life elimination: 0.4 hours

Time to peak: ~0.5 to 2 hours

Excretion: Urine (80%)

Dosing
Adult & Geriatric
Chronic hepatitis C (CHC) infection in monoinfected (HCV) or coinfected (HCV/HIV-1) patients: Oral: 400 mg daily with concomitant ribavirin and with or without peginterferon alfa (maximum: 400 mg daily). **Note:** Treatment regimen and duration based on HCV genotype and/or clinical scenario as noted below:

Treatment-naive patients:

Genotype 1:

Patients who can receive interferon: 400 mg once daily with concomitant ribavirin and peginterferon alfa for 12 weeks. **Note:** A recommended regimen (AASLD/IDSA, 2014)

Patients who cannot receive interferon:

Manufacturer's labeling: 400 mg once daily with concomitant ribavirin for 24 weeks. **Note:** A recommended regimen (AASLD/IDSA, 2014)

Alternative dosing (off-label regimen): 400 mg once daily with simeprevir and with or without ribavirin for 12 weeks. **Note:** A recommended regimen (AASLD/IDSA, 2014)

Genotype 2: 400 mg once daily with concomitant ribavirin for 12 weeks. **Note:** A recommended regimen (AASLD/IDSA, 2014)

Genotype 3:

Regardless of patient eligibility for peginterferon: *Manufacturer's labeling:* 400 mg once daily with concomitant ribavirin for 24 weeks. **Note:** A recommended regimen (AASLD/IDSA, 2014)

Patients who can receive interferon: *Alternative dosing (off-label regimen):* 400 mg once daily with concomitant ribavirin and peginterferon alfa for 12 weeks. **Note:** A recommended regimen (AASLD/IDSA, 2014)

Genotype 4:

Patients who can receive interferon: *Manufacturer's labeling:* 400 mg once daily with concomitant ribavirin and peginterferon alfa for 12 weeks. **Note:** A recommended regimen (AASLD/IDSA, 2014)

Patients who cannot receive interferon: *Alternative dosing (off-label regimen):* 400 mg once daily with concomitant ribavirin for 24 weeks. **Note:** A recommended regimen (AASLD/IDSA, 2014)

Genotype 5 or 6 (off-label use): Patients who can receive interferon: 400 mg once daily with concomitant ribavirin and peginterferon alfa for 12 weeks. **Note:** A recommended regimen (AASLD/IDSA, 2014)

Relapser patients (nonresponders to a previous regimen of ribavirin and peginterferon alfa **without** an HCV protease inhibitor):

Regardless of patient eligibility for peginterferon:

Genotype 1 (off-label regimen): 400 mg once daily with simeprevir and **with** or **without** ribavirin for 12 weeks. **Note:** A recommended regimen (AASLD/IDSA, 2014)

Relapser patients (nonresponders to a previous regimen of ribavirin and peginterferon alfa **with** or **without** an HCV protease inhibitor):

Patients who can receive interferon:

Genotype 1 (off-label regimen): 400 mg once daily for 12 weeks with ribavirin and peginterferon alfa for 12-24 weeks. **Note:** A recommended regimen (AASLD/IDSA, 2014)

Genotype 4: 400 mg once daily with concomitant ribavirin and peginterferon alfa for 12 weeks. **Note:** A recommended regimen (AASLD/IDSA, 2014)

Genotype 5 or 6 (off-label use): 400 mg once daily with concomitant ribavirin and peginterferon alfa for 12 weeks. **Note:** A recommended regimen (AASLD/IDSA, 2014)

Regardless of patient eligibility for peginterferon:

Genotype 2 (off-label regimen): 400 mg once daily with concomitant ribavirin for 12 weeks. Note: A recommended regimen; also patients with cirrhosis may benefit from a total of 16 weeks of treatment (AASLD/IDSA, 2014)

Genotype 3: 400 mg once daily with concomitant ribavirin for 24 weeks. **Note:** A recommended regimen (AASLD/IDSA, 2014)

Patients with hepatocellular carcinoma awaiting liver transplantation: 400 mg once daily with concomitant ribavirin for 48 weeks or until the time of liver transplantation, whichever occurs first

Missed dose: If a dose is missed within the calendar day it is usually taken, take as soon as possible. If the calendar day when the dose is usually taken has passed, do not take the missed dose and resume the usual dosing schedule. Do not take >400 mg daily. The Canadian labeling recommends that patients who vomit <2 hours after administration take another dose but if >2 hours, take dose at the next regularly scheduled time.

Renal Impairment
Sofosbuvir:

CrCl ≥30 mL/minute: No dosage adjustment necessary.

CrCl <30 mL/minute: There are no dosage adjustments provided in manufacturer's labeling (has not been studied). Predominant metabolite accumulates in impaired renal function.

End stage renal disease (ESRD), including those requiring intermittent hemodialysis (IHD): There are no dosage adjustments provided in manufacturer's labeling (has not been studied). Predominant metabolite accumulates in impaired renal function.

Peginterferon Alfa and Ribavirin: Refer to individual monographs.

Hepatic Impairment
Child-Pugh class A, B, or C: No dosage adjustment necessary.

Decompensated cirrhosis: There are no dosage adjustments provided in manufacturer's labeling (has not been studied).

Peginterferon Alfa and Ribavirin: Refer to individual monographs; peginterferon alfa is contraindicated in hepatic decompensation.

Adjustment for Toxicity
Sofosbuvir requires no dosage adjustment; concomitant agents should be adjusted as described below:

Patients with Genotype 1 or 4: Dose reduction dependent upon ribavirin and/or peginterferon doses; refer to individual monographs.

Patients with Genotype 2 or 3 **without** cardiac history: Hemoglobin 8.5 to <10 g/dL: Decrease ribavirin dose to 600 mg daily in divided doses (eg, 200 mg in the morning, 400 mg in the evening).

Hemoglobin <8.5 g/dL: Permanently discontinue treatment.

Patients with Genotype 2 or 3 **with** stable cardiac history:

Hemoglobin has decreased ≥2 g/dL during any 4-week period of treatment: Decrease ribavirin dose to 600 mg daily in divided doses (eg, 200 mg in the morning, 400 mg in the evening).

Hemoglobin has decreased to <12 g/dL despite 4 weeks at reduced dose: Permanently discontinue treatment.

Note: Once ribavirin has been withheld due to clinical adverse event or laboratory abnormality, an attempt to restart ribavirin at 600 mg daily (in divided doses) can be made, with a further ribavirin increase to 800 mg daily. Increasing the ribavirin dose to its original level (usually 1000-1200 mg daily) is not recommended.

Administration Administer with or without food.

Monitoring Parameters
Bilirubin, liver enzymes, and serum creatinine at baseline and periodically when clinically indicated. If used in combination with amiodarone and another direct acting antiviral (DAA) (or in patients who discontinued amiodarone just prior to initiating sofosbuvir in combination with a DAA), inpatient cardiac monitoring for the first 48 hours of coadministration, then daily outpatient or self monitoring of heart rate through at least the first 2 weeks of treatment.

Serum HCV-RNA at baseline, during treatment, at the end of treatment, during treatment follow-up, and when clinically indicated.

Pretreatment and monthly pregnancy tests up to 6 months following discontinuation of therapy for women of childbearing age.

Dosage Forms Excipient information presented when available (limited, particularly for generics); consult specific product labeling.
Tablet, Oral:
  Sovaldi: 400 mg

◆ Sofosbuvir and Ledipasvir *see* Ledipasvir and Sofosbuvir *on page 1038*
◆ Solaquin® (Can) *see* Hydroquinone *on page 893*
◆ Solaquin Forte® (Can) *see* Hydroquinone *on page 893*
◆ Solia *see* Ethinyl Estradiol and Desogestrel *on page 701*

Solifenacin (sol i FEN a sin)

Brand Names: US VESIcare
Brand Names: Canada Sandoz-Solifenacin; Teva-Solifenacin; VESIcare
Index Terms Solifenacin Succinate; YM905
Pharmacologic Category Anticholinergic Agent
Use Treatment of overactive bladder with symptoms of urinary frequency, urgency, or urge incontinence
Pregnancy Considerations Adverse events were observed in some animal reproduction studies.
Breast-Feeding Considerations It is not known if solifenacin is excreted in breast milk. The manufacturer recommends a decision be made whether to discontinue nursing or to discontinue the drug.
Contraindications Hypersensitivity to solifenacin or any component of the formulation; urinary retention; gastric retention; uncontrolled narrow-angle glaucoma.
Warnings/Precautions Cases of angioedema involving the face, lips, tongue, and/or larynx have been reported during treatment; some cases have occurred after the first dose. Immediately discontinue if tongue, hypopharynx, or larynx is involved. Anaphylactic reactions have been reported rarely with solifenacin; immediately discontinue therapy if anaphylactic reaction develops. Do not use in patients with a known or suspected hypersensitivity. Central nervous system effects have been reported (eg, headache, confusion, hallucinations, somnolence); monitor, particularly at treatment initiation or dose increase, reduce dose or discontinue if necessary. May cause drowsiness and/or blurred vision, which may impair physical or mental abilities; patients must be cautioned about performing tasks which require mental alertness (eg, operating machinery or driving). Heat prostration may occur in the presence of increased environmental temperature; use caution in hot weather and/or exercise. Use with caution in patients with bladder outflow obstruction, gastrointestinal obstructive disorders, and decreased gastrointestinal motility. Use with caution in patients with a known history of QT prolongation or other risk factors for QT prolongation (eg, concomitant use of medications known to prolong QT interval and/or electrolyte abnormalities); the risk for QT prolongation is dose-related. Use with caution in patients with controlled (treated) narrow-angle glaucoma; use is contraindicated with uncontrolled narrow-angle glaucoma. Dosage adjustment is required for patients with severe renal impairment (CrCl <30 mL/minute) or moderate (Child-Pugh class B) hepatic impairment; use is not recommended with severe hepatic impairment (Child-Pugh class C). Patients on potent CYP3A4 inhibitors require the lower dose of solifenacin. This medication is associated with potent anticholinergic properties which may be inappropriate in older adults depending on comorbidities (eg, dementia, delirium) (Beers Criteria).

Adverse Reactions
>10%: Gastrointestinal: Xerostomia (11% to 28%; dose-related), constipation (5% to 13%; dose-related)
1% to 10%:
  Cardiovascular: Edema (≤1%), hypertension (≤1%)
  Central nervous system: Fatigue (1% to 2%), depression (≤1%)
  Gastrointestinal: Dyspepsia (1% to 4%), nausea (2% to 3%), upper abdominal pain (1% to 2%)
  Genitourinary: Urinary tract infection (3% to 5%), urinary retention (≤1%)
  Ophthalmic: Blurred vision (4% to 5%), dry eye syndrome (≤2%)
  Respiratory: Cough (≤1%)
  Miscellaneous: Influenza (≤2%)
<1% (Limited to important or life-threatening): Abnormal hepatic function tests, anaphylaxis, angioedema, atrial fibrillation, confusion, delirium, erythema multiforme, exfoliative dermatitis, fecal impaction, gastroesophageal reflux disease, gastrointestinal obstruction, glaucoma, hallucination, hyperkalemia, hypersensitivity reactions, intestinal obstruction, palpitations, prolonged Q-T interval on ECG, renal insufficiency, tachycardia, torsades de pointes, voice disorder

Drug Interactions
Metabolism/Transport Effects Substrate of CYP3A4 (major); **Note:** Assignment of Major/Minor substrate status based on clinically relevant drug interaction potential
Avoid Concomitant Use
Avoid concomitant use of Solifenacin with any of the following: Aclidinium; Cimetropium; Conivaptan; Eluxadoline; Fusidic Acid (Systemic); Glucagon; Glycopyrrolate; Glycopyrrolate (Oral Inhalation); Idelalisib; Ipratropium (Oral Inhalation); Levosulpiride; Potassium Chloride; Tiotropium; Umeclidinium
Increased Effect/Toxicity
Solifenacin may increase the levels/effects of: AbobotulinumtoxinA; Analgesics (Opioid); Anticholinergic Agents; Cannabinoid-Containing Products; Cimetropium; Eluxadoline; Glucagon; Glycopyrrolate; Glycopyrrolate (Oral Inhalation); Highest Risk QTc-Prolonging Agents; Moderate Risk QTc-Prolonging Agents; OnabotulinumtoxinA; Potassium Chloride; Ramosetron; RimabotulinumtoxinB; Thiazide Diuretics; Tiotropium; Topiramate

The levels/effects of Solifenacin may be increased by: Aclidinium; Antifungal Agents (Azole Derivatives, Systemic); Aprepitant; Conivaptan; CYP3A4 Inhibitors (Moderate); CYP3A4 Inhibitors (Strong); Dasatinib; Fosaprepitant; Fusidic Acid (Systemic); Idelalisib; Ipratropium (Oral Inhalation); Ivacaftor; Luliconazole; Mianserin; Mifepristone; Mirabegron; Netupitant; Osimertinib; Palbociclib; Pramlintide; Simeprevir; Stiripentol; Umeclidinium
Decreased Effect
Solifenacin may decrease the levels/effects of: Acetylcholinesterase Inhibitors; Gastrointestinal Agents (Prokinetic); Itopride; Levosulpiride; Secretin

The levels/effects of Solifenacin may be decreased by: Acetylcholinesterase Inhibitors; Bosentan; CYP3A4 Inducers (Moderate); CYP3A4 Inducers (Strong); Dabrafenib; Deferasirox; Enzalutamide; Mitotane; Osimertinib; Siltuximab; St Johns Wort; Tocilizumab
Food Interactions Grapefruit juice may increase the serum level effects of solifenacin. Management: Monitor closely with concurrent use.
Storage/Stability Store at controlled room temperature of 25°C (77°F); excursions permitted to 15°C to 30°C (59°F to 86°F).
Mechanism of Action Inhibits muscarinic receptors resulting in decreased urinary bladder contraction, increased residual urine volume, and decreased detrusor muscle pressure.
Pharmacodynamics/Kinetics
Distribution: V_d: ~600 L
Protein binding: ~98% bound primarily to alpha$_1$-acid glycoprotein
Metabolism: Extensively hepatic; via N-oxidation and 4 R-hydroxylation, forms 1 active and 3 inactive metabolites; primary pathway for elimination is via CYP3A4
Bioavailability: ~90%
Half-life elimination: 45-68 hours following chronic dosing; prolonged in severe renal (CrCl <30 mL/minute) or moderate hepatic (Child-Pugh class B) impairment
Time to peak, plasma: 3-8 hours
Excretion: Urine (69%; <15% as unchanged drug); feces (23%)
Dosing
Adult Overactive bladder: Oral: 5 mg once daily; if tolerated, may increase to 10 mg once daily
  Dosage adjustment with concomitant CYP3A4 inhibitors: Maximum solifenacin dose: 5 mg/day
Geriatric Base dosing on renal/hepatic function.
Renal Impairment Use with caution in reduced renal function; CrCl <30 mL/minute: Maximum dose: 5 mg/day
Hepatic Impairment Use with caution in reduced hepatic function:
  Moderate (Child-Pugh class B): Maximum dose: 5 mg/day
  Severe (Child-Pugh class C): Use is not recommended
Dietary Considerations May be taken without regard to meals.
Administration Swallow tablet whole; administer with liquids; may be administered without regard to meals.
Monitoring Parameters Anticholinergic effects (eg, fixed and dilated pupils, blurred vision, tremors, or dry skin); creatinine clearance (prior to treatment for dosing adjustment); liver function
Dosage Forms Excipient information presented when available (limited, particularly for generics); consult specific product labeling.
Tablet, Oral, as succinate:
  VESIcare: 5 mg, 10 mg

◆ Solifenacin Succinate *see* Solifenacin *on page 1685*
◆ Soliris *see* Eculizumab *on page 614*

Somatropin (soe ma TROE pin)

Brand Names: US Genotropin; Genotropin MiniQuick; Humatrope; Norditropin FlexPro; Norditropin NordiFlex Pen [DSC]; Nutropin AQ NuSpin 10; Nutropin AQ NuSpin 20; Nutropin AQ NuSpin 5; Nutropin AQ Pen; Nutropin AQ [DSC]; Nutropin [DSC]; Omnitrope; Saizen; Saizen Click.-Easy; Serostim; Tev-Tropin [DSC]; Zomacton; Zorbtive

Brand Names: Canada Genotropin GoQuick; Genotropin MiniQuick; Humatrope; Norditropin Nordiflex; Norditropin Simplexx; Nutropin AQ NuSpin; Nutropin AQ Pen; Omnitrope; Saizen; Serostim

Index Terms Growth Hormone, Human; hGH; Human Growth Hormone

Pharmacologic Category Growth Hormone

Use

Children:

Treatment of growth failure due to inadequate endogenous growth hormone secretion (Genotropin, Humatrope, Norditropin, Nutropin, Nutropin AQ, Omnitrope, Saizen, Tev-Tropin, Zomacton)

Treatment of short stature associated with Turner syndrome (Genotropin, Humatrope, Norditropin, Nutropin, Nutropin AQ, Omnitrope)

Treatment of Prader-Willi syndrome (Genotropin, Omnitrope)

Treatment of growth failure associated with chronic renal insufficiency (CRI) up until the time of renal transplantation (Nutropin, Nutropin AQ)

Treatment of growth failure in children born small for gestational age who fail to manifest catch-up growth by 2 years of age (Genotropin, Omnitrope) or by 2-4 years of age (Humatrope, Norditropin)

Treatment of idiopathic short stature (nongrowth hormone-deficient short stature) defined by height standard deviation score (SDS) ≤-2.25 and growth rate not likely to attain normal adult height (Genotropin, Humatrope, Nutropin, Nutropin AQ, Omnitrope)

Treatment of short stature or growth failure associated with short stature homeobox gene (SHOX) deficiency (Humatrope)

Treatment of short stature associated with Noonan syndrome (Norditropin)

Adults:

HIV patients with wasting or cachexia with concomitant antiviral therapy (Serostim)

Replacement of endogenous growth hormone in patients with adult growth hormone deficiency who meet both of the following criteria (Genotropin, Humatrope, Norditropin, Nutropin, Nutropin AQ, Omnitrope, Saizen):

Biochemical diagnosis of adult growth hormone deficiency by means of a subnormal response to a standard growth hormone stimulation test (peak growth hormone ≤5 mcg/L). Confirmatory testing may not be required in patients with congenital/genetic growth hormone deficiency or multiple pituitary hormone deficiencies due to organic diseases.

and

Adult-onset: Patients who have adult growth hormone deficiency whether alone or with multiple hormone deficiencies (hypopituitarism) as a result of pituitary disease, hypothalamic disease, surgery, radiation therapy, or trauma

or

Childhood-onset: Patients who were growth hormone deficient during childhood, confirmed as an adult before replacement therapy is initiated

Treatment of short-bowel syndrome (Zorbtive)

Pregnancy Considerations Teratogenic effects were not observed in animal studies. Reproduction studies have not been conducted with all agents. During normal pregnancy, maternal production of endogenous growth hormone decreases as placental growth hormone production increases. Data with somatropin use during pregnancy is limited.

Breast-Feeding Considerations It is not known if somatropin is excreted in breast milk. The manufacturer recommends that caution be exercised when administering somatropin to nursing women.

Contraindications Hypersensitivity to growth hormone or any component of the formulation; growth promotion in pediatric patients with closed epiphyses; progression or recurrence of any underlying intracranial lesion or actively growing intracranial tumor; acute critical illness due to complications following open heart or abdominal surgery; multiple accidental trauma or acute respiratory failure; evidence of active malignancy; active proliferative or severe nonproliferative diabetic retinopathy; use in patients with Prader-Willi syndrome **without** growth hormone deficiency (except Genotropin) or in patients with Prader-Willi syndrome **with** growth hormone deficiency who are severely obese, have a history of upper airway obstruction or sleep apnea, or have severe respiratory impairment

Warnings/Precautions Initiation of somatropin is contraindicated with acute critical illness due to complications following open heart or abdominal surgery, multiple accidental trauma, or acute respiratory failure; mortality may be increased. The safety of continuing somatropin in patients who develop these illnesses during therapy has not been established; use with caution. Use in contraindicated with active malignancy; monitor patients with preexisting tumors or growth failure secondary to an intracranial lesion for recurrence or progression of underlying disease; discontinue therapy with evidence of recurrence. An increased risk of second neoplasm has been reported in childhood cancer survivors treated with somatropin; the most common second neoplasms were meningiomas in patients treated with radiation to the head for their first neoplasm. Patients with HIV and pediatric patients with short stature (genetic cause) have increased baseline risk of developing malignancies; consider risk/benefits prior to initiation of therapy and monitor these patients carefully. Monitor all patients for any malignant transformation of skin lesions.

Somatropin may decrease insulin sensitivity; use with caution in patients with diabetes or with risk factors for impaired glucose tolerance. Adjustment of antidiabetic medications may be necessary. Pancreatitis has been rarely reported; incidence in children (especially girls) with Turner syndrome may be greater than adults. Monitor for hypersensitivity reactions. Patients with hypoadrenalism may require increased dosages of glucocorticoids (especially cortisone acetate and prednisone) due to somatropin-mediated inhibition of 11 beta-hydroxysteroid dehydrogenase type 1; undiagnosed central hypoadrenalism may be unmasked. Excessive glucocorticoid therapy may inhibit the growth promoting effects of somatropin in children; monitor and adjust glucocorticoids carefully. Untreated/undiagnosed hypothyroidism may decrease response to therapy; monitor thyroid function test periodically and initiate/adjust thyroid replacement therapy as needed. Closely monitor other hormonal replacement treatments in patients with hypopituitarism. Obese patients may experience an increased incidence of adverse events when using a weight-based dosing regimen. Intracranial hypertension (IH) with headache, nausea, papilledema, visual changes, and/or vomiting has been reported with somatropin; funduscopic examination prior to initiation of therapy and periodically thereafter is recommended. Treatment should be discontinued in patients who develop papilledema; resuming treatment at a lower dose may be considered once IH-associated signs and symptoms have resolved. Patients with Turner syndrome, chronic renal failure and Prader-Willi syndrome may be at increased risk for IH. Progression of scoliosis may occur in children experiencing rapid growth. Patients with growth hormone deficiency may develop slipped capital epiphyses more frequently; evaluate any child with new onset of a limp or with complaints of hip or knee pain. Patients with Turner syndrome are at increased risk for otitis media and other ear/hearing disorders, cardiovascular disorders (including stroke, aortic aneurysm, hypertension), and thyroid disease, monitor carefully. Fluid retention may occur frequently in adults during use; manifestations of fluid retention (eg, edema, arthralgia, myalgia, nerve compression syndromes/paresthesias) are generally transient and dose dependent. Potentially significant drug-drug interactions may exist, requiring dose or frequency adjustment, additional monitoring, and/or selection of alternative

therapy. Products may contain m-cresol. Not for IV injection. According to the Centers for Disease Control and Prevention (CDC), pen-shaped injection devices should never be used for more than one person (even when the needle is changed) because of the risk of infection. The injection device should be clearly labeled with individual patient information to ensure that the correct pen is used (CDC, 2012).

Benzyl alcohol and derivatives: Diluent may contain benzyl alcohol; large amounts of benzyl alcohol (≥99 mg/kg/day) have been associated with a potentially fatal toxicity ("gasping syndrome") in neonates; the "gasping syndrome" consists of metabolic acidosis, respiratory distress, gasping respirations, CNS dysfunction (including convulsions, intracranial hemorrhage), hypotension, and cardiovascular collapse (AAP ["Inactive" 1997]; CDC, 1982); some data suggests that benzoate displaces bilirubin from protein binding sites (Ahlfors, 2001); avoid or use dosage forms containing benzyl alcohol with caution in neonates. See manufacturer's labeling.

Fatalities have been reported in pediatric patients with Prader-Willi syndrome following the use of growth hormone. The reported fatalities occurred in patients with one or more risk factors, including severe obesity, sleep apnea, respiratory impairment, or unidentified respiratory infection; male patients with one or more of these factors may be at greater risk. Treatment interruption is recommended in patients who show signs of upper airway obstruction, including the onset of, or increased, snoring. In addition, evaluation of and/or monitoring for sleep apnea and respiratory infections are recommended.

Patients with HIV infection should be maintained on antiretroviral therapy to prevent the potential increase in viral replication.

Avoid use in the elderly, except as hormone replacement following pituitary gland removal; use results in minimal effect on body composition and is associated with edema, arthralgia, carpal tunnel syndrome, gynecomastia, and impaired fasting glucose (Beers Criteria). Elderly may be more sensitive to the actions of somatropin; consider lower starting doses.

Safety and efficacy have not been established for the treatment of Noonan syndrome in children with significant cardiac disease. Children with epiphyseal closure who are treated for adult GHD need reassessment of therapy and dose. Administration site rotation is necessary to prevent tissue atrophy.

Adverse Reactions

Growth hormone deficiency: Adverse reactions reported with growth hormone deficiency vary greatly by age. Generally, percentages are less in pediatric patients than adults, and many of the reactions reported in adults are dose related. Percentages reported also vary by product. Below is a listing by age group; events reported more commonly overall are noted with an asterisk (*).

Children: Antibodies development, arthralgia, benign intracranial hypertension, edema, eosinophilia, glycosuria, Hb A$_{1c}$ increased, headache, hematoma, hematuria, hyperglycemia (mild), hypertriglyceridemia, hypoglycemia, hypothyroidism, injection site reaction, intracranial tumor, leg pain, lipoatrophy, leukemia, meningioma, muscle pain, papilledema, pseudotumor cerebri, psoriasis exacerbation, rash, scoliosis progression, seizure, slipped capital femoral epiphysis, weakness

Adults: Acne, ALT increased, AST increased, arthralgia*, back pain, bronchitis, carpal tunnel syndrome, chest pain, cough, depression, diabetes mellitus (type 2), diaphoresis, dizziness, edema*, fatigue, flu-like syndrome*, gastritis, glucose intolerance, glucosuria, headache*, hyperglycemia (mild), hypertension, hypoesthesia, hypothyroidism, infection, insomnia, insulin resistance, joint disorder, leg edema, muscle pain, myalgia*, nausea, pain in extremities, paresthesia*, peripheral edema*, pharyngitis, retinopathy, rhinitis, skeletal pain*, stiffness in extremities, surgical procedure, upper respiratory tract infection, weakness

Additional/postmarketing reactions observed with growth hormone deficiency: Gynecomastia, increased growth of preexisting nevi, pancreatitis

HARS: Serostim®: Limited to >10%: Edema (peripheral) (19% to 45%), arthralgia (28% to 37%), pain (extremity) (5% to 19%), hypoesthesia (9% to 15%), headache (4% to 14%), blood glucose increased (4% to 14%), paresthesia (11% to 13%), myalgia (3% to 13%)

Idiopathic short stature: Percentages reported using Humatrope® versus placebo: Myalgia (24%), scoliosis (19%), otitis media (16%), arthralgia (11%), arthrosis (11%), hyperlipidemia (8%), gynecomastia (5%), hip pain (3%), hypertension (3%). Additional adverse reactions listed as reported using other products from ISS NCGS

Cohort (frequencies <1%): Aggressiveness, benign intracranial hypertension, diabetes, edema, hair loss, headache, injection site reaction

Prader-Willi syndrome: Genotropin® (frequency not defined): Aggressiveness, arthralgia, edema, hair loss, headache, benign intracranial hypertension, myalgia; fatalities associated with use in this population have been reported

Turner syndrome: Percentages reported using Humatrope® compared to untreated patients. Additional adverse reactions reported from other products, frequency not specified: Surgical procedures (45%), otitis media (43%), ear disorders (18%), joint pain, respiratory illness, urinary tract infection

HIV patients with wasting or cachexia: Serostim® (limited to ≥5%): Musculoskeletal disorders (arthralgia, arthrosis, myalgia: 78%), peripheral edema (26%), headache (13%), nausea (9%), paresthesia (8%), edema (6%), gynecomastia (6%), hypoesthesia (5%)

Short-bowel syndrome: Zorbtive® (limited to >10%): Peripheral edema (69% to 81%), facial edema (44% to 50%), arthralgia (31% to 44%), nausea (13% to 31%), injection site pain (up to 31%), flatulence (25%), injection site reaction (19% to 25%), abdominal pain (13% to 25%), vomiting (19%), pain (6% to 19%), chest pain (up to 19%), dehydration (up to 19%), infection (up to 19%), rhinitis (up to 19%), hearing symptoms (13%), dizziness (6% to 13%), rash (6% to 13%), diaphoresis (up to 13%), generalized edema (up to 13%), malaise (up to 13%), moniliasis (up to 13%), myalgia (up to 13%)

SHOX deficiency: Humatrope®: Arthralgia (11%), gynecomastia (8%), excessive cutaneous nevi (7%), scoliosis (4%)

Small for gestational age: Genotropin®, Humatrope® (frequency not defined): Mild, transient hyperglycemia; benign intracranial hypertension (rare); central precocious puberty; jaw prominence (rare); aggravation of preexisting scoliosis (rare); injection site reactions; progression of pigmented nevi; carpal tunnel syndrome (rare) diabetes mellitus (rare); otitis media; headache; slipped capital femoral epiphysis

Drug Interactions

Metabolism/Transport Effects None known.

Avoid Concomitant Use There are no known interactions where it is recommended to avoid concomitant use.

Increased Effect/Toxicity There are no known significant interactions involving an increase in effect.

Decreased Effect

Somatropin may decrease the levels/effects of: Antidiabetic Agents; Cortisone; PredniSONE

The levels/effects of Somatropin may be decreased by: Estrogen Derivatives

Preparation for Administration

Genotropin: Reconstitute with diluent provided.

Genotropin MiniQuick: Reconstitute with diluent provided. Consult the instructions provided with the reconstitution device.

Humatrope:

Cartridge: Consult HumatroPen User Guide for complete instructions for reconstitution. **Dilute with solution provided with cartridges ONLY; do not use diluent provided with vials.**

Vial: 5 mg: Reconstitute with 1.5 to 5 mL diluent provided. Swirl gently; do not shake.

Nutropin: Vial:

5 mg: Reconstitute with 1 to 5 mL bacteriostatic water for injection. Swirl gently, do not shake.

10 mg: Reconstitute with 1 to 10 mL bacteriostatic water for injection. Swirl gently, do not shake.

Omnitrope powder: Reconstitute with provided diluent. Swirl gently; do not shake.

Saizen: Vial:

5 mg: Reconstitute with 1 to 3 mL bacteriostatic water for injection or sterile water for injection. Gently swirl; do not shake.

8.8 mg: Reconstitute with 2 to 3 mL bacteriostatic water for injection or sterile water for injection. Gently swirl; do not shake.

Serostim: Vial: Reconstitute with 0.5 to 1 mL sterile water for injection.

Tev-Tropin, Zomacton: **Note:** Only use the provided diluent for the 5 mg and 10 mg vial; diluents differ, do not interchange.

5 mg vial: Reconstitute with 1 to 5 mL of provided diluent (bacteriostatic 0.9% sodium chloride for injection [benzyl alcohol preserved]). Swirl gently; do not shake. Use preservative-free NS for injection for use in newborns. When reconstituting with NS for injection, use only one dose per vial; discard unused portion.

10 mg vial: Reconstitute with 1 mL of provided diluent (bacteriostatic water for injection [metacresol 0.33% preserved]). Use the 25-gauge mixing needle provided. Swirl gently; do not shake.

Zorbtive: 8.8 mg vial: Reconstitute with 1 to 2 mL bacteriostatic water for injection. Swirl gently.

Storage/Stability

Genotropin: Store at 2°C to 8°C (36°F to 46°F); do not freeze. Protect from light. Following reconstitution of 5.8 mg and 13.8 mg cartridge, store under refrigeration and use within 28 days.

Genotropin Miniquick: Store in refrigerator prior to dispensing, but may be stored ≤25°C (77°F) for up to 3 months after dispensing. Once reconstituted, solution must be refrigerated and used within 24 hours. Discard unused portion.

Humatrope:

Vial: Before and after reconstitution, store at 2°C to 8°C (36°F to 46°F); do not freeze. When reconstituted with provided diluent or bacteriostatic water for injection, use within 14 days. When reconstituted with sterile water for injection, use within 24 hours and discard unused portion.

Cartridge: Before and after reconstitution, store at 2°C to 8°C (36°F to 46°F); do not freeze. Following reconstitution with provided diluent, stable for 28 days under refrigeration.

Norditropin: Store at 2°C to 8°C (36°F to 46°F); do not freeze. Avoid direct light. When refrigerated, prefilled pen must be used within 4 weeks after initial injection. Orange and blue prefilled pens may also be stored up to 3 weeks at ≤25°C (77°F).

Nutropin: Before and after reconstitution, store at 2°C to 8°C (36°F to 46°F); do not freeze.

Nutropin vial: Use reconstituted vials within 14 days. When reconstituted with sterile water for injection, use immediately and discard unused portion.

Nutropin AQ formulations: Use within 28 days following initial use.

Omnitrope:

Powder for injection: Prior to reconstitution, store under refrigeration at 2°C to 8°C (36°F to 46°F); do not freeze. Protect from light. Reconstitute with provided diluent. Swirl gently; do not shake. Following reconstitution with the provided diluents, the 5.8 mg vial may be stored under refrigeration for up to 3 weeks. Store vial in carton to protect from light.

Solution: Prior to use, store under refrigeration at 2°C to 8°C (36°F to 46°F). Once the cartridge is loaded into the pen delivery system, store under refrigeration for up to 28 days after first use.

Saizen: Prior to reconstitution, store at room temperature 15°C to 30°C (59°F to 86°F). Following reconstitution with bacteriostatic water for injection, reconstituted solution should be refrigerated and used within 14 days. When reconstituted with sterile water for injection, use immediately and discard unused portion. The Saizen easy click cartridge, when reconstituted with the provided bacteriostatic water, should be stored under refrigeration and used within 21 days.

Serostim: Prior to reconstitution, store at room temperature 15°C to 30°C (59°F to 86°F). When reconstituted with sterile water for injection, use immediately and discard unused portion.

Tev-Tropin, Zomacton: Prior to reconstitution, store at 2°C to 8°C (36°F to 46°F). Following reconstitution with the provided diluents, should be refrigerated and used within 14 days (5 mg vial) or 28 days (10 mg vial); do not freeze. Some cloudiness may occur; do not use if cloudiness persists after warming to room temperature.

Zorbtive: Store unopened vials and diluent at room temperature of 15°C to 30°C (59°F to 86°F). Store reconstituted vial under refrigeration at 2°C to 8°C (36°F to 46°F) for up to 14 days; do not freeze.

Mechanism of Action Somatropin is a purified polypeptide hormones of recombinant DNA origin; somatropin contains the identical sequence of amino acids found in human growth hormone; human growth hormone assists growth of linear bone, skeletal muscle, and organs by stimulating chondrocyte proliferation and differentiation, lipolysis, protein synthesis, and hepatic glucose output; stimulates erythropoietin which increases red blood cell mass; exerts both insulin-like and diabetogenic effects; enhances the transmucosal transport of water, electrolytes, and nutrients across the gut

Pharmacodynamics/Kinetics

Duration: Maintains supraphysiologic levels for 18 to 20 hours

Absorption: IM, SubQ: Well absorbed

Distribution: ~1 L/kg

Metabolism: Hepatic and renal (~90%)

Bioavailability: SubQ: ~70% to 90%; **Note:** Variable; product-dependent

Half-life elimination: Preparation and route of administration dependent; SubQ: ~2 to 4 hours

Excretion: Urine (small amount)

Note: Patients with chronic renal failure (CRF) and end-stage renal disease ESRD) have decreased clearance compared with healthy individuals.

Dosing

Adult Note: Nutropin (lyophilized powder) has been discontinued in the US for more than 1 year.

Growth hormone deficiency: Adjust dose based on individual requirements: To minimize adverse events in older or overweight patients, reduced dosages may be necessary. During therapy, dosage should be decreased if required by the occurrence of side effects or excessive IGF-I levels.

Weight-based dosing:

Norditropin: SubQ: Initial dose ≤0.004 mg/kg/day; after 6 weeks of therapy, may increase dose up to 0.016 mg/kg/day

Nutropin, Nutropin AQ: SubQ: ≤0.006 mg/kg/day; dose may be increased up to a maximum of 0.025 mg/kg/day in patients <35 years of age, or up to a maximum of 0.0125 mg/kg/day in patients ≥35 years of age

Humatrope: SubQ: ≤0.006 mg/kg/day; dose may be increased up to a maximum of 0.0125 mg/kg/day

Genotropin, Omnitrope: SubQ: Weekly dosage: ≤0.04 mg/kg divided into equal doses 6 to 7 days per week; dose may be increased at 4- to 8-week intervals to a maximum of 0.08 mg/kg/week

Saizen: SubQ: ≤0.005 mg/kg/day; dose may be increased to not more than 0.01 mg/kg/day after 4 weeks

Non-weight-based dosing: SubQ: Initial: 0.2 mg/day (range: 0.15 to 0.3 mg/day); may increase every 1 to 2 months by 0.1 to 0.2 mg/day based on response and/or serum IGF-I levels

Dosage adjustment with estrogen supplementation (growth hormone deficiency): Larger doses of somatropin may be needed for women taking oral estrogen replacement products; dosing not affected by topical products

HIV-associated adipose redistribution syndrome (HARS) (off-label use): Serostim: SubQ: Induction: 4 mg once daily at bedtime for 12 weeks; Maintenance: 2 mg or 4 mg every other day at bedtime for 12 to 24 weeks. **Note:** Every-other-day dosing during induction has also been studied. Although a greater response was seen with daily dosing, it was associated with an increased incidence of adverse events.

HIV patients with wasting or cachexia:

Serostim: SubQ: 0.1 mg/kg once daily at bedtime (maximum: 6 mg/day). Alternately, patients at risk for side effects may be started at 0.1 mg/kg every other day. Patients who continue to lose weight after 12 weeks should be re-evaluated for opportunistic infections or other clinical events; rotate injection sites to avoid lipodystrophy. Adjust dose if needed to manage side effects.

Daily dose based on body weight:

<35 kg: 0.1 mg/kg

35 to 45 kg: 4 mg

45 to 55 kg: 5 mg

>55 kg: 6 mg

Short-bowel syndrome: *Zorbtive:* SubQ: 0.1 mg/kg once daily for 4 weeks (maximum: 8 mg/day)

Fluid retention (moderate) or arthralgias: Treat symptomatically or reduce dose by 50%

Severe toxicity: Discontinue therapy for up to 5 days; when symptoms resolve, restart at 50% of dose. If severe toxicity recurs or does not disappear within 5 days after discontinuation, permanently discontinue treatment.

Geriatric Patients ≥65 years of age may be more sensitive to the action of growth hormone and more prone to adverse effects; in general, dosing should be cautious, beginning at low end of dosing range.

Pediatric Note: Nutropin (lyophilized powder) has been discontinued in the US for more than 1 year.

Growth hormone deficiency:

Genotropin, Omnitrope: SubQ: Weekly dosage: 0.16 to 0.24 mg/kg divided into equal doses 6 to 7 days per week

Humatrope: SubQ: Weekly dosage: 0.18 to 0.3 mg/kg divided into equal doses 6 to 7 days per week

Norditropin: SubQ: 0.024 to 0.034 mg/kg/day, 6 to 7 days per week

Nutropin, Nutropin AQ: SubQ: Weekly dosage: 0.3 mg/kg divided into equal daily doses; pubertal patients: ≤0.7 mg/kg divided into equal daily doses

Tev-Tropin, Zomacton: SubQ: Up to 0.1 mg/kg/dose administered 3 days per week

Saizen: IM, SubQ: Weekly dosage: 0.18 mg/kg divided into equal daily doses **or** as 0.06 mg/kg/dose administered 3 days per week **or** as 0.03 mg/kg/dose administered 6 days per week

Note: Therapy should be discontinued when patient has reached satisfactory adult height, when epiphyses have fused, or when the patient ceases to respond. Growth of 5 cm/year or more is expected, if growth rate does not exceed 2.5 cm in a 6-month period, double the dose for the next 6 months; if there is still no satisfactory response, discontinue therapy

Chronic renal insufficiency (CRI): *Nutropin, Nutropin AQ:* SubQ: Weekly dosage: 0.35 mg/kg divided into daily injections; continue until the time of renal transplantation

Dosage recommendations in patients treated for CRI who require dialysis:

Hemodialysis: Administer dose at night prior to bedtime or at least 3 to 4 hours after hemodialysis to prevent hematoma formation from heparin

CCPD: Administer dose in the morning following dialysis

CAPD: Administer dose in the evening at the time of overnight exchange

Turner syndrome:

Genotropin, Omnitrope: SubQ: Weekly dosage: 0.33 mg/kg divided into equal doses 6 to 7 days per week

Humatrope: SubQ: Weekly dosage: 0.375 mg/kg divided into equal doses 6 to 7 days per week

Norditropin: SubQ: Up to 0.067 mg/kg/day

Nutropin, Nutropin AQ: SubQ: Weekly dosage: ≤0.375 mg/kg divided into equal doses 3 to 7 days per week

Prader-Willi syndrome: *Genotropin, Omnitrope:* SubQ: Weekly dosage: 0.24 mg/kg divided into equal doses 6 to 7 days per week

Small for gestational age:

Genotropin, Omnitrope: SubQ: Weekly dosage: 0.48 mg/kg divided into equal doses 6 to 7 days per week

Humatrope: SubQ: Weekly dosage: 0.47 mg/kg divided into equal doses 6 to 7 days per week

Norditropin: SubQ: Up to 0.067 mg/kg/day

Alternate dosing (small for gestational age): In older/early pubertal children or children with very short stature, consider initiating therapy at higher doses (0.067 mg/kg/day) and then consider reducing the dose (0.033 mg/kg/day) if substantial catch-up growth observed. In younger children (<4 years) with less severe short stature, consider initiating therapy with lower doses (0.033 mg/kg/day) and then titrating the dose upwards as needed.

Idiopathic short stature:

Genotropin, Omnitrope: SubQ: Weekly dosage: 0.47 mg/kg divided into equal doses 6 to 7 days per week

Humatrope: SubQ: Weekly dosage: 0.37 mg/kg divided into equal doses 6 to 7 days per week

Nutropin, Nutropin AQ: SubQ: Weekly dosage: Up to 0.3 mg/kg divided into equal daily doses

SHOX deficiency: *Humatrope:* SubQ: Weekly dosage: 0.35 mg/kg divided into equal doses 6 to 7 days per week

HIV patients with wasting or cachexia (off-label use): *Serostim:* SubQ: Limited data; doses of 0.04 mg/kg/day were reported in five children, 6 to 17 years of age; doses of 0.07 mg/kg/day were reported in six children, 8 to 14 years of age

Noonan syndrome: *Norditropin:* SubQ: Up to 0.066 mg/kg/day

Renal Impairment There are no dosage adjustments provided in the manufacturer's labeling (has not been studied).

Hepatic Impairment There are no dosage adjustments provided in the manufacturer's labeling (has not been studied).

Dietary Considerations

Prader-Willi syndrome: All patients should have effective weight control (use is contraindicated in severely-obese patients).

Short-bowel syndrome: Intravenous parenteral nutrition requirements may need reassessment as gastrointestinal absorption improves.

Administration Do not shake; administer SubQ or IM (not all products are approved for IM administration). Rotate administration sites to avoid tissue atrophy. When administering to newborns, do not reconstitute with a diluent that contains benzyl alcohol; sterile water for injection may be used as an alternative.

Norditropin cartridge must be administered using the corresponding color-coded NordiPen injection pen.

Omnitrope: Solution in the cartridges must be administered using the Omnitrope pen; when installing a new cartridge, prime pen prior to first use.

Humatrope: When administering for growth hormone deficiency, SubQ route is preferred

Tev-Tropin, Zomacton: Administer SubQ injections with standard sterile disposable needle or Tjet Needle-Free (Tev-Tropin) or ZOMA-Jet Needle-Free (Zomacton) injection device.

Monitoring Parameters Growth curve, Tanner staging (children), periodic thyroid function tests, bone age (annually), periodical urine testing for glucose, somatomedin C (IGF-I) levels; funduscopic examinations at initiation of therapy and periodically during treatment; serum phosphorus, alkaline phosphatase and parathyroid hormone. If growth deceleration is observed in children treated for growth hormone deficiency, and not due to other causes, evaluate for presence of antibody formation. Periodic blood glucose monitoring; strict blood glucose monitoring in patients with diabetes. Progression or recurrence of preexisting tumors or malignant transformation of skin lesions. **Note:** Practice guidelines recommend monitoring for efficacy and adverse effects every 1-2 months during dose titration and semiannually, thereafter (TES, 2006).

CRI: Progression of renal osteodystrophy

Prader-Willi syndrome: Monitor for sleep apnea, respiratory infections, snoring (onset of or increased)

Turner syndrome: Ear disorders including otitis media; cardiovascular disorders

Noonan syndrome: Prior to use, verify short stature syndrome.

Product Availability

Nutropin (lyophilized powder) has been discontinued in the US for more than 1 year.

Zomacton: Ferring Pharmaceuticals acquired Tev-Tropin from Teva Pharmaceuticals in December 2014 and received FDA approval for a name change from Tev-Tropin to Zomacton. Zomacton became commercially available in June 2015. A needle-free administration device for Zomacton, ZOMA-Jet Needle-Free, is expected to be available for the 5 mg dose and in a new 10 mg dose later in 2015.

Dosage Forms Excipient information presented when available (limited, particularly for generics); consult specific product labeling. [DSC] = Discontinued product

Solution, Subcutaneous:

Norditropin FlexPro: 5 mg/1.5 mL (1.5 mL); 10 mg/1.5 mL (1.5 mL); 15 mg/1.5 mL (1.5 mL); 30 mg/3 mL (3 mL) [contains phenol]

Norditropin NordiFlex Pen: 30 mg/3 mL (3 mL [DSC]) [contains phenol]

Nutropin AQ: 10 mg/2 mL (2 mL [DSC])

Nutropin AQ NuSpin 5: 5 mg/2 mL (2 mL) [contains phenol]

Nutropin AQ NuSpin 10: 10 mg/2 mL (2 mL) [contains phenol]

Nutropin AQ NuSpin 20: 20 mg/2 mL (2 mL) [contains phenol]

Nutropin AQ Pen: 10 mg/2 mL (2 mL)

Nutropin AQ Pen: 20 mg/2 mL (2 mL) [contains phenol]

Omnitrope: 5 mg/1.5 mL (1.5 mL) [contains benzyl alcohol]

Omnitrope: 10 mg/1.5 mL (1.5 mL) [contains phenol]

Solution Reconstituted, Injection:

Humatrope: 5 mg (1 ea)

Humatrope: 6 mg (1 ea); 12 mg (1 ea); 24 mg (1 ea) [contains glycerin, metacresol]

Saizen: 5 mg (1 ea); 8.8 mg (1 ea)

Saizen Click.Easy: 8.8 mg (1 ea)

Solution Reconstituted, Subcutaneous:

Genotropin: 5 mg (1 ea); 12 mg (1 ea) [contains metacresol]

Nutropin: 10 mg (1 ea [DSC]) [contains benzyl alcohol]

Omnitrope: 5.8 mg (1 ea)

Serostim: 4 mg (1 ea); 5 mg (1 ea); 6 mg (1 ea)

Tev-Tropin: 5 mg (1 ea [DSC])

Zomacton: 5 mg (1 ea) [contains benzyl alcohol]

Zomacton: 10 mg (1 ea) [contains metacresol]

Zorbtive: 8.8 mg (1 ea) [contains benzyl alcohol]

Solution Reconstituted, Subcutaneous [preservative free]:

Genotropin MiniQuick: 0.2 mg (1 ea); 0.4 mg (1 ea); 0.6 mg (1 ea); 0.8 mg (1 ea); 1 mg (1 ea); 1.2 mg (1 ea); 1.4 mg (1 ea); 1.6 mg (1 ea); 1.8 mg (1 ea); 2 mg (1 ea)

◆ Somatuline Autogel (Can) *see* Lanreotide *on page 1031*

◆ Somatuline Depot *see* Lanreotide *on page 1031*

◆ Somavert *see* Pegvisomant *on page 1414*

◆ Sominex [OTC] *see* DiphenhydrAMINE (Systemic) *on page 561*

Sonidegib (soe ni DEG ib)

Brand Names: US Odomzo

Index Terms Erismodegib; LDE225; NVP-LDE225; Sonidegib Phosphate

Pharmacologic Category Antineoplastic Agent, Hedgehog Pathway Inhibitor

Use Basal cell carcinoma, locally advanced: Treatment of adult patients with locally advanced basal cell carcinoma (BCC) that has recurred following surgery or radiation therapy, or those who are not candidates for surgery or radiation therapy.

Pregnancy Considerations [US Boxed Warning]: Sonidegib can cause embryo-fetal death or severe birth defects when administered to a pregnant woman. Sonidegib is embryotoxic, fetotoxic, and teratogenic in animals. Verify the pregnancy status of females of reproductive potential prior to initiating therapy. Advise females of reproductive potential to use effective contraception during treatment with sonidegib and for at least 20 months after the last dose. Advise males of the potential risk of exposure through semen and to use condoms with a pregnant partner or a female partner of reproductive potential during treatment with sonidegib and for at least 8 months after the last dose. It is not known if sonidegib is present in semen. Males with female partners of reproductive potential should use condoms even following a vasectomy. Advise male patients not to donate sperm during sonidegib treatment and for at least 8 months after the last sonidegib dose.

Health care providers should notify the manufacturer of pregnancies which may occur following exposure to sonidegib (888-669-6682).

Breast-Feeding Considerations It is not known if sonidegib is excreted in breast milk. Due to the potential for serious adverse reactions in the nursing infant, breast-feeding is not recommended by the manufacturer during therapy and for 20 months after treatment.

Medication Guide Available Yes

Contraindications There are no contraindications listed in the manufacturer's labeling.

Warnings/Precautions Hazardous agent - use appropriate precautions for handling and disposal (meets NIOSH 2014 criteria). **[US Boxed Warning]: Sonidegib can cause embryo-fetal death or severe birth defects when administered to a pregnant woman. Sonidegib is embryotoxic, fetotoxic, and teratogenic in animals. Verify the pregnancy status of females of reproductive potential prior to initiating therapy. Advise females of reproductive potential to use effective contraception during treatment with sonidegib and for at least 20 months after the last dose. Advise males of the potential risk of exposure through semen and to use condoms with a pregnant partner or a female partner of reproductive potential during treatment with sonidegib and for at least 8 months after the last dose.** It is not known if sonidegib is present in semen. Advise patients not to donate sperm during sonidegib treatment and for at least 8 months after the last sonidegib dose. Amenorrhea lasting for at least 18 months was observed in women of reproductive potential. Advise patients not to donate blood or blood products during sonidegib treatment and for at least 20 months after the last sonidegib dose.

Musculoskeletal toxicity occurred in more than two-thirds of patients treated with sonidegib (including grade 3 and 4 events). Muscle spasms, musculoskeletal pain, and myalgia were the most frequently reported musculoskeletal adverse reactions. Increased serum creatine kinase (CK) levels were also commonly observed (some events were grade 3 or 4); CK elevations were usually preceded by musculoskeletal pain and myalgia. When CK elevations were grade 2 or higher, the median time to symptom onset was ~13 weeks (range: 2 to 39 weeks), and the median time to resolution (to ≤ grade 1) was 12 days. More than one-quarter of patients required medical management for musculoskeletal toxicity (eg, magnesium supplementation, muscle relaxants, and analgesics/narcotics); several patients required intravenous hydration or hospitalization. Rhabdomyolysis was observed in 1 patient in clinical trials (at a dose higher than the FDA-approved dose). Monitor serum CK levels and serum creatinine at baseline and periodically during therapy (more frequently if muscle symptoms are reported or if clinically indicated). Advise patients to promptly report new unexplained muscle pain, tenderness, or weakness (either occurring during therapy or persisting after discontinuation). May require therapy interruption or discontinuation. Increased serum creatinine was observed in the majority of patients receiving sonidegib, although the measurement remained within the normal range in more than 75% of patients. While dosage adjustment is not required in patients with renal impairment, monitor serum creatinine at baseline and periodically, particularly if patients present with musculoskeletal toxicity. Potentially significant interactions may exist, requiring dose or frequency adjustment, additional monitoring, and/or selection of alternative therapy.

Adverse Reactions

\>10%:

Central nervous system: Fatigue (41%), headache (15%), pain (14%)

Dermatologic: Alopecia (53%)

Endocrine & metabolic: Hyperglycemia (51%), weight loss (30%), increased serum ALT (19%), increased serum AST (19%), increased amylase (16%)

Gastrointestinal: Dysgeusia (46%), increased serum lipase (43%), nausea (39%), diarrhea (32%), decreased appetite (23%), abdominal pain (18%), vomiting (11%)

Hematologic & oncologic: Anemia (32%), lymphocytopenia (28%, grades 3/4: 3%)

Neuromuscular & skeletal: Increased creatine phosphokinase (61%, grades 3/4: 8%), muscle spasm (54%; grade 3: 3%), musculoskeletal pain (32%, grade 3: 1%), myalgia (19%)

Renal: Increased serum creatinine (92%)

1% to 10%:

Dermatologic: Pruritus (10%)

<1% (Limited to important or life-threatening): Amenorrhea, rhabdomyolysis

Drug Interactions

Metabolism/Transport Effects Substrate of CYP3A4 (major); **Note:** Assignment of Major/Minor substrate status based on clinically relevant drug interaction potential; **Inhibits** BCRP

Avoid Concomitant Use

Avoid concomitant use of Sonidegib with any of the following: Conivaptan; CYP3A4 Inducers (Moderate); CYP3A4 Inducers (Strong); CYP3A4 Inhibitors (Strong); Fusidic Acid (Systemic); Idelalisib

Increased Effect/Toxicity

The levels/effects of Sonidegib may be increased by: Conivaptan; CYP3A4 Inhibitors (Moderate); CYP3A4 Inhibitors (Strong); Dasatinib; Fosaprepitant; Fusidic Acid (Systemic); Idelalisib; Ivacaftor; Luliconazole; Mifepristone; Osimertinib; Palbociclib; Simeprevir; Stiripentol

Decreased Effect

The levels/effects of Sonidegib may be decreased by: CYP3A4 Inducers (Moderate); CYP3A4 Inducers (Strong); Deferasirox; Osimertinib; Siltuximab; Tocilizumab

Food Interactions Taking sonidegib with a high-fat meal (~1,000 calories with 50% fat content) will increase systemic exposure (7- to 8-fold). Management: Do not administer with food; must be taken on an empty stomach, at least 1 hour before and 2 hours after food.

Storage/Stability Store at 25°C (77°F); excursions permitted to 15°C to 30°C (59°F to 86°F).

Mechanism of Action Basal cell cancer is associated with mutations in Hedgehog pathway components. Hedgehog regulates cell growth and differentiation in embryogenesis; while generally not active in adult tissue, Hedgehog mutations associated with basal cell cancer can activate the pathway resulting in unrestricted proliferation of skin basal cells (Von Hoff, 2009). Sonidegib is a selective Hedgehog pathway inhibitor which binds to and inhibits Smoothened homologue (SMO), the transmembrane protein involved in Hedgehog signal transduction.

Pharmacodynamics/Kinetics

Absorption: AUC_{inf} and C_{max} are increased by 7.4- to 7.8-fold, respectively, when administered with a high-fat meal (~1,000 calories with 50% fat content)

Distribution: 9,166 L

Protein binding: >97%

Metabolism: Primarily hepatic through CYP3A

Bioavailability: <10% of an oral dose is absorbed

Half-life elimination: ~28 days

Time to peak: 2 to 4 hours

Excretion: Feces (~70%); urine (30%)

Dosing

Adult & Geriatric Note: Verify pregnancy status of females of reproductive potential prior to therapy initiation. Measure serum creatine kinase (CK) levels and renal function tests in all patients prior to starting treatment.

Basal cell carcinoma, locally advanced: Oral: 200 mg once daily until disease progression or unacceptable toxicity (Migden, 2015)

Missed doses: If a dose is missed, skip the missed dose and resume dosing with the next scheduled dose.

Renal Impairment No dosage adjustment is necessary.

Hepatic Impairment

Mild impairment (total bilirubin ≤ULN and AST >ULN or total bilirubin >1 to 1.5 times ULN): No dosage adjustment is necessary.

Moderate or severe impairment: There are no dosage adjustments provided in the manufacturer's labeling (has not been studied).

Adjustment for Toxicity

Withhold treatment for any of the following (may resume at 200 mg daily upon resolution of toxicity):

Creatine kinase (CK) serum elevation between 2.5 and 10 times ULN (first occurrence) or between 2.5 and 5 times ULN (recurrent)

Musculoskeletal toxicity, severe or intolerable

Permanently discontinue therapy for:

CK serum elevation >2.5 times ULN with worsening renal function

CK serum elevation >10 times ULN

CK serum elevation >5 times ULN (recurrent)

Musculoskeletal toxicity, severe or intolerable (recurrent)

Administration Administer orally on an empty stomach at least 1 hour before or 2 hours after a meal. Hazardous agent; use appropriate precautions for handling and disposal (meets NIOSH 2014 criteria)

Monitoring Parameters Serum creatine kinase (CK) and serum creatinine (baseline, periodically during treatment, and at least weekly with musculoskeletal toxicity and CK elevations >2.5 times ULN until resolution), liver function, pregnancy status, signs/symptoms of musculoskeletal toxicity.

Dosage Forms Excipient information presented when available (limited, particularly for generics); consult specific product labeling.

Capsule, Oral:

Odomzo: 200 mg

♦ Sonidegib Phosphate *see* Sonidegib *on page 1690*

♦ Soolantra *see* Ivermectin (Topical) *on page 1006*

♦ Soothe & Cool INZO Antifungal [OTC] *see* Miconazole (Topical) *on page 1201*

♦ Soothe Redness (Can) *see* Naphazoline (Ophthalmic) *on page 1256*

SORAfenib (sor AF e nib)

Brand Names: US NexAVAR
Brand Names: Canada Nexavar
Index Terms BAY 43-9006; Sorafenib Tosylate
Pharmacologic Category Antineoplastic Agent, Tyrosine Kinase Inhibitor; Antineoplastic Agent, Vascular Endothelial Growth Factor (VEGF) Inhibitor

Use

Hepatocellular cancer: Treatment of unresectable hepatocellular cancer (HCC)

Renal cell cancer, advanced: Treatment of advanced renal cell cancer (RCC)

Thyroid cancer, differentiated: Treatment of locally recurrent or metastatic, progressive, differentiated thyroid cancer (refractory to radioactive iodine treatment)

Pregnancy Considerations Animal reproduction studies have demonstrated teratogenicity and fetal loss. Based on its mechanism of action and because sorafenib inhibits angiogenesis, a critical component of fetal development, adverse effects on pregnancy would be expected. Women of childbearing potential should be advised to avoid pregnancy. Men and women of reproductive potential should use effective birth control during treatment and for at least 2 weeks after treatment is discontinued.

Breast-Feeding Considerations It is not known if sorafenib is excreted in human milk. Due to the potential for serious adverse reactions in the nursing infant, the decision to discontinue sorafenib or to discontinue breast-feeding during therapy should take into account the benefits of treatment to the mother.

Prescribing and Access Restrictions Available from specialty pharmacies. Further information may be obtained at 1-866-639-2827 or www.nexavar-us.com.

Contraindications Known severe hypersensitivity to sorafenib or any component of the formulation; use in combination with carboplatin and paclitaxel in patients with squamous cell lung cancer

Warnings/Precautions Hazardous agent - use appropriate precautions for handling and disposal (NIOSH 2014 [group 1]). May cause hypertension (generally mild-to-moderate), especially in the first 6 weeks of treatment; monitor; use caution in patients with underlying or poorly-controlled hypertension; consider discontinuing (temporary or permanent) in patients who develop severe or persistent hypertension while on appropriate antihypertensive therapy. May cause cardiac ischemia or infarction; consider discontinuing (temporarily or permanently) in patients who develop these conditions; use in patients with unstable coronary artery disease or recent myocardial infarction has not been studied. QT prolongation has been observed; may increase the risk for ventricular arrhythmia. Avoid use in patients with congenital long QT syndrome; monitor electrolytes and ECG in patients with heart failure, bradyarrhythmias, and concurrent medications known to prolong the QT interval; correct electrolyte (calcium, magnesium, potassium) imbalances; interrupt treatment for QTc interval >500 msec or for ≥60 msec increase from baseline.

Serious bleeding events may occur (consider permanently discontinuing if serious); monitor PT/INR in patients on warfarin therapy. Fatal bleeding events have been reported. Thyroid cancer patients with tracheal, bronchial, and esophageal infiltration should be treated with local therapy prior to administering sorafenib due to the potential bleeding risk. May complicate wound healing; temporarily withhold treatment for patients undergoing major surgical procedures (the appropriate timing for reinitiation after surgical procedures has not been determined). Gastrointestinal perforation has been reported (rare); monitor patients for signs/symptoms (abdominal pain, constipation, or vomiting); discontinue treatment if gastrointestinal perforation occurs. Potentially significant drug-drug interactions may exist, requiring dose or frequency adjustment, additional monitoring, and/or selection of alternative therapy. Avoid concurrent use with strong CYP3A4 inducers (eg, carbamazepine, dexamethasone, phenobarbital, phenytoin, rifampin, St John's wort); may decrease sorafenib levels/effects. Use caution when administering sorafenib with compounds that are metabolized predominantly via UGT1A1 (eg, irinotecan). Use in combination with carboplatin and paclitaxel in patients with squamous cell lung cancer is contraindicated.

Hand-foot skin reaction and rash (generally grades 1 or 2) are the most common drug-related adverse events, and typically appear within the first 6 weeks of treatment; usually managed with topical treatment, treatment delays, and/or dose reductions. Consider permanently discontinuing with severe or persistent dermatological toxicities. The risk for hand-foot skin reaction increased with cumulative doses of sorafenib (Azad, 2009). The incidence of hand-foot syndrome is also increased in patients treated with sorafenib plus bevacizumab in comparison to those treated with sorafenib monotherapy (Azad, 2009). Severe dermatologic toxicities, including Stevens-Johnson syndrome (SJS) and toxic epidermal necrolysis (TEN) have been reported; may be life-threatening; discontinue sorafenib for suspected SJS or TEN.

Sorafenib impairs exogenous thyroid suppression; TSH level elevations were commonly observed in the thyroid cancer study; monitor TSH levels monthly and as clinically necessary, and adjust thyroid replacement as needed. Sorafenib levels in patients with mild-to-moderate hepatic impairment (Child-Pugh classes A and B) were similar to levels observed in patients without hepatic impairment; has not been studied in patients with severe hepatic impairment. In a small study of Asian patients with advanced HCC, sorafenib demonstrated efficacy with adequate tolerability in a hepatitis B-endemic area (Yau, 2009). There have been reports of sorafenib-induced hepatitis (including hepatic failure and death) which is characterized by hepatocellular liver damage and transaminase increases (significant); increased bilirubin and INR may also occur. Monitor hepatic function regularly; discontinue sorafenib for unexplained significant transaminase increases.

Adverse Reactions

>10%:

Cardiovascular: Hypertension (9% to 41%; grade 3: 3% to 4%; grade 4: <1%; grades 3/4: 10%, onset: ~3 weeks)

Central nervous system: Fatigue (37% to 46%), headache (≤10% to 17%), mouth pain (14%), voice disorder (13%), peripheral sensory neuropathy (≤13%), pain (11%)

Dermatologic: Palmar-plantar erythrodysesthesia (21% to 69%; grade 3: 6% to 8%; grades 3/4: 19%), alopecia (14% to 67%), skin rash (including desquamation; 19% to 40%; grade 3: ≤1%; grades 3/4: 5%), pruritus (14% to 20%), xeroderma (10% to 13%), erythema (≥10%)

Endocrine & metabolic: Hypoalbuminemia (≤59%), weight loss (10% to 49%), hypophosphatemia (35% to 45%; grade 3: 11% to 13%; grade 4: <1%), increased thyroid stimulating hormone level (>0.5 mU/L: 41%; due to impairment of exogenous thyroid suppression), hypocalcemia (12% to 36%), increased amylase (30% to 34% [usually transient])

Gastrointestinal: Diarrhea (43% to 68%; grade 3: 2% to 10%; grade 4: <1%), increased serum lipase (40% to 41% [usually transient]), abdominal pain (11% to 31%), decreased appetite (30%), anorexia (16% to 29%), stomatitis (24%), nausea (21% to 24%), constipation (14% to 16%), vomiting (11% to 16%)

Hematologic & oncologic: Lymphocytopenia (23% to 47%; grades 3/4: ≤13%), thrombocytopenia (12% to 46%; grades 3/4: 1% to 4%), increased INR (≤42%), neutropenia (≤18%; grades 3/4: ≤5%), hemorrhage (15% to 17%; grade 3: 2%), leukopenia

Hepatic: Increased serum ALT (59%; grades 3/4: 4%), increased serum AST (54%; grades 3/4: 2%), hepatic insufficiency (≤11%; grade 3: 2%; grade 4: 1%)

Infection: Infection

Neuromuscular & skeletal: Limb pain (15%), weakness (12%), myalgia

Respiratory: Dyspnea (≤14%), cough (≤13%)

Miscellaneous: Fever (11%)

1% to 10%:

Cardiovascular: Ischemic heart disease (including myocardial infarction; ≤3%), cardiac failure (2%, congestive), flushing

Central nervous system: Depression, glossalgia

Dermatologic: Hyperkeratosis (7%), acne vulgaris, exfoliative dermatitis, folliculitis

Endocrine & metabolic: Hypokalemia (5% to 10%), hyponatremia, hypothyroidism

Gastrointestinal: Dysgeusia (6%), dyspepsia, dysphagia, gastroesophageal reflux disease, mucositis, xerostomia

Genitourinary: Erectile dysfunction, proteinuria

Hematologic & oncologic: Squamous cell carcinoma of skin (3%; grades 3/4: 3%), anemia

Hepatic: Increased serum transaminases (transient)

Neuromuscular & skeletal: Muscle spasm (10%), arthralgia (≤10%), myalgia

Renal: Renal failure

Respiratory: Epistaxis (7%), flu-like symptoms, hoarseness, rhinorrhea

<1% (Limited to important or life-threatening): Acute renal failure, amyotrophy, anaphylaxis, angioedema, aortic dissection, cardiac arrhythmia, cardiac failure, cerebral hemorrhage, cholangitis, cholecystitis, dehydration, eczema, erythema multiforme, gastritis, gastrointestinal hemorrhage, gastrointestinal perforation, gynecomastia, hepatic failure, hepatitis, hypersensitivity reaction (skin reaction, urticaria), hypertensive crisis, hyperthyroidism, increased serum alkaline phosphatase, increased serum bilirubin, interstitial pulmonary disease (acute respiratory distress, interstitial pneumonia, lung inflammation, pneumonitis, pulmonitis, radiation pneumonitis), malignant neoplasm of skin (keratoacanthomas), nephrotic syndrome, ostealgia, osteonecrosis (jaw), pancreatitis, pleural effusion, prolonged QT interval on ECG, respiratory tract hemorrhage, reversible posterior leukoencephalopathy syndrome (RPLS), rhabdomyolysis, Stevens-Johnson syndrome, thromboembolism, toxic epidermal necrolysis (TEN), transient ischemic attacks, tumor lysis syndrome, tumor pain

Drug Interactions

Metabolism/Transport Effects Substrate of CYP3A4 (minor), UGT1A9; **Note:** Assignment of Major/Minor substrate status based on clinically relevant drug interaction potential; **Inhibits** BSEP, CYP2B6 (moderate), CYP2C8 (weak), CYP2C9 (moderate), UGT1A9

Avoid Concomitant Use

Avoid concomitant use of SORAfenib with any of the following: Amodiaquine; BCG (Intravesical); CARBOplatin; Cholic Acid; CYP3A4 Inducers (Strong); Deferiprone; Dipyrone; Natalizumab; PACLitaxel (Conventional); Pimecrolimus; St Johns Wort; Tacrolimus (Topical); Tofacitinib; Vaccines (Live)

Increased Effect/Toxicity

SORAfenib may increase the levels/effects of: Acetaminophen; Amodiaquine; Bisphosphonate Derivatives; Bosentan; BuPROPion; Cannabis; CARBOplatin; Carvedilol; Cholic Acid; CloZAPine; CYP2B6 Substrates; CYP2C9 Substrates; Deferiprone; DOCEtaxel; DOXOrubicin (Conventional); Dronabinol; Fingolimod; Fluorouracil (Systemic); Fluorouracil (Topical); Highest Risk QTc-Prolonging Agents; Irinotecan Products; Leflunomide; Moderate Risk QTc-Prolonging Agents; Natalizumab; PACLitaxel (Conventional); Propacetamol; Tetrahydrocannabinol; Tofacitinib; Vaccines (Live); Warfarin

The levels/effects of SORAfenib may be increased by: Acetaminophen; Bevacizumab; CYP3A4 Inhibitors (Strong); Denosumab; Dipyrone; Mifepristone; Pimecrolimus; Roflumilast; Tacrolimus (Topical); Trastuzumab

Decreased Effect

SORAfenib may decrease the levels/effects of: BCG (Intravesical); Coccidioides immitis Skin Test; Cyclophosphamide; Dacarbazine; Fluorouracil (Systemic); Fluorouracil (Topical); Sipuleucel-T; Vaccines (Inactivated); Vaccines (Live)

The levels/effects of SORAfenib may be decreased by: CYP3A4 Inducers (Strong); Echinacea; Neomycin; St Johns Wort

Food Interactions Bioavailability is decreased 29% with a high-fat meal (bioavailability is similar to fasting state when administered with a moderate-fat meal). Management: Administer on an empty stomach 1 hour before or 2 hours after eating.

Storage/Stability Store at 25°C (77°F); excursions are permitted between 15°C and 30°C (59°F and 86°F). Protect from moisture.

Mechanism of Action Multikinase inhibitor; inhibits tumor growth and angiogenesis by inhibiting intracellular Raf kinases (CRAF, BRAF, and mutant BRAF), and cell surface kinase receptors (VEGFR-1, VEGFR-2, VEGFR-3, PDGFR-beta, cKIT, FLT-3, RET, and RET/PTC)

Pharmacodynamics/Kinetics

Protein binding: 99.5%

Metabolism: Hepatic, via CYP3A4 (primarily oxidated to the pyridine N-oxide; active, minor) and UGT1A9 (glucuronidation)

Bioavailability: 38% to 49%; reduced by 29% when administered with a high-fat meal

Half-life elimination: 25 to 48 hours

Time to peak, plasma: ~3 hours

Excretion: Feces (77%, 51% of dose as unchanged drug); urine (19%, as metabolites)

Dosing

Adult & Geriatric Note: Interrupt treatment (temporarily) in patients undergoing major surgical procedures.

Hepatocellular cancer (HCC): Oral: 400 mg twice daily; continue until no longer clinically benefiting or until unacceptable toxicity occurs (Llovet, 2008)

Renal cell cancer (RCC), advanced: Oral: 400 mg twice daily; continue until no longer clinically benefiting or until unacceptable toxicity occurs (Escudier, 2007; Escudier, 2009)

Thyroid cancer, differentiated: Oral: 400 mg twice daily; continue until no longer clinically benefiting or until unacceptable toxicity occurs (Brose, 2013)

Angiosarcoma (off-label use): Oral: 400 mg twice daily (Maki, 2009)

Gastrointestinal stromal tumor (GIST) (off-label use): Oral: 400 mg twice daily (Wiebe, 2008)

Renal Impairment

Manufacturer's labeling: No dosage adjustment is necessary for mild, moderate, or severe impairment (not dependent on dialysis); has not been studied in dialysis patients.

The following adjustments have also been reported: Safety and pharmacokinetics were studied in varying degrees of renal dysfunction with the following empiric dose levels recommended based on patient tolerance (Miller, 2009):

Mild renal dysfunction (CrCl 40 to 59 mL/minute): 400 mg twice daily

Moderate renal dysfunction (CrCl 20 to 39 mL/minute): 200 mg twice daily

Severe renal dysfunction (CrCl <20 mL/minute): Data inadequate to define dose

Hemodialysis (any CrCl): 200 mg once daily

Hepatic Impairment

Hepatic impairment at baseline:

Manufacturer's labeling:

Mild to moderate (Child-Pugh class A and B) impairment: No dosage adjustment is necessary.

Severe impairment (Child-Pugh class C): There are no dosage adjustments provided in the manufacturer's labeling (has not been studied).

The following adjustments have also been reported: Safety and pharmacokinetics were studied in varying degrees of hepatic dysfunction with the following empiric dose levels recommended based on patient tolerance (Miller, 2009):

Mild hepatic dysfunction (bilirubin >1 to ≤1.5 times ULN and/or AST >ULN): 400 mg twice daily

Moderate hepatic dysfunction (bilirubin >1.5 to ≤3 times ULN; any AST): 200 mg twice daily

Severe hepatic dysfunction:

Bilirubin >3 to 10 x ULN (any AST): 200 mg every 3 days was **not** tolerated

Albumin <2.5 g/dL (any bilirubin and any AST): 200 mg once daily

Drug-induced liver injury during treatment: Unexplained (eg, not due to viral hepatitis or progressive underlying malignancy) significantly increased transaminases: Discontinue treatment.

Adjustment for Toxicity Temporary interruption and/or dosage reduction may be necessary for management of adverse drug reactions.

Cardiovascular toxicity:

Cardiac ischemia or infarction: Consider temporary interruption or permanent discontinuation.

Hypertension, severe or persistent (despite antihypertensive therapy): Consider temporary interruption or permanent discontinuation.

QT prolongation (QTc interval >500 msec or ≥60 msec increase from baseline): Interrupt treatment.

Gastrointestinal perforation: Permanently discontinue.

Hemorrhage requiring medical intervention: Consider permanent discontinuation.

Dermatologic toxicity: If Stevens-Johnson syndrome or toxic epidermal necrolysis is suspected, discontinue therapy.

U.S. labeling:

RCC and HCC: If dosage reductions are necessary, decrease dose to 400 mg once daily. If further reductions are needed, decrease dose to 400 mg every other day.

Grade 1 (numbness, dysesthesia, paresthesia, tingling, painless swelling, erythema, or discomfort of the hands or feet which do not disrupt normal activities): Continue sorafenib and consider symptomatic treatment with topical therapy.

Grade 2 (painful erythema and swelling of the hands or feet and/or discomfort affecting normal activities):

First occurrence: Continue sorafenib and consider symptomatic treatment with topical therapy. **Note:** If no improvement within 7 days, see dosing for second or third occurrence.

Second or third occurrence (or no improvement after 7 days of 1st occurrence): Hold treatment until resolves to grade 0-1; resume treatment with dose reduced by one dose level (400 mg daily or 400 mg every other day).

Fourth occurrence: Discontinue treatment.

Grade 3 (moist desquamation, ulceration, blistering, or severe pain of the hands or feet or severe discomfort that prevents working or performing daily activities):

First or second occurrence: Hold treatment until resolves to grade 0-1; resume treatment with dose reduced by one dose level (400 mg daily or 400 mg every other day).

Third occurrence: Discontinue treatment.

Thyroid cancer:

First dose level reduction: Reduce to 600 mg daily (in 2 divided doses, as 400 mg and 200 mg, separated by 12 hours).

Second dose level reduction: Reduce dose to 200 mg twice daily.

Third dose level reduction: Reduce dose to 200 mg once daily.

Grade 1 (numbness, dysesthesia, paresthesia, tingling, painless swelling, erythema, or discomfort of the hands or feet which do not disrupt normal activities): Continue sorafenib treatment.

Grade 2 (painful erythema and swelling of the hands or feet and/or discomfort affecting normal activities):

First occurrence: Decrease dose to 600 mg daily (in divided doses). **Note:** If no improvement within 7 days, see dosing for second occurrence.

Second occurrence (or no improvement after 7 days of the reduced dose after 1st occurrence): Hold treatment until resolved or improved to grade 1; if resumed, decrease the dose by 1 dose level.

Third occurrence: Hold treatment until resolved or improved to grade 1; if resumed, decrease the dose by 1 dose level.

Fourth occurrence: Permanently discontinue.

Grade 3 (moist desquamation, ulceration, blistering, or severe pain of the hands or feet or severe discomfort that prevents working or performing daily activities):

First occurrence: Hold treatment until resolved or improved to grade 1; if resumed, decrease by 1 dose level.

Second occurrence: Hold treatment until resolved or improved to grade 1; if resumed, decrease by 2 dose levels.

Third occurrence: Permanently discontinue.

Following improvement of grade 2 or 3 dermatologic toxicity to grade 0 or 1 after at least 28 days of a reduced dose, the sorafenib dose may be increased 1 dose level from the reduced dose (~50% of patients requiring dose reduction for dermatologic toxicity may meet the criteria for increased dosing; and half of those patients may tolerate the increased dose without recurrent grade 2 or higher dermatologic toxicity).

Canadian labeling: RCC and HCC:

Grade 1 (any occurrence): Initiate supportive treatment immediately and continue sorafenib.

Grade 2:

First occurrence: Initiate supportive treatment immediately and consider a dose reduction to 400 mg daily for 28 days. If toxicity resolves to ≤ grade 1 after 28 days with dose reduction, increase dose to 400 mg twice daily. If toxicity does not resolve to ≤ grade 1 despite dose reduction, withhold treatment for a minimum of 7 days until toxicity resolves to ≤ grade 1, then resume treatment at reduced dose of 400 mg daily for 28 days. If toxicity remains ≤ grade 1 at the reduced dose for 28 days, increase dose to 400 mg twice daily.

Second or third occurrence: Follow procedure for first occurrence; however, when resuming treatment, decrease dose to 400 mg daily (indefinitely).

Fourth occurrence: Treatment discontinuation should be considered based on clinical assessment and patient preference.

Grade 3:

First occurrence: Initiate supportive measures immediately and withhold treatment for a minimum of 7 days and until toxicity ≤ grade 1. Resume at reduced dose of 400 mg daily for 28 days. If toxicity remains ≤ grade 1 at the reduced dose for 28 days, increase dose to 400 mg twice daily.

Second occurrence: Follow procedure for first occurrence; however, when resuming treatment, decrease dose to 400 mg daily (indefinitely).

Third occurrence: Treatment discontinuation should be considered based on clinical assessment and patient preference.

Administration Administer on an empty stomach (1 hour before or 2 hours after eating).

Hazardous agent; use appropriate precautions for handling and disposal (NIOSH 2014 [group 1]).

Monitoring Parameters

CBC with differential, electrolytes (magnesium, potassium, calcium), phosphorus, lipase and amylase levels; liver function tests; blood pressure (baseline, weekly for the first 6 weeks, then periodic); monitor for hand-foot skin reaction and other dermatologic toxicities; monitor ECG in patients at risk for prolonged QT interval; signs/symptoms of bleeding; signs/symptoms of GI perforation. Additionally the Canadian labeling recommends considering monitoring of left ventricular ejection fraction at baseline and periodically during treatment.

Thyroid function testing:

Patients with differentiated thyroid cancer: Monitor TSH monthly.

Patients with RCC and HCC (Hamnvik, 2011):

Preexisting levothyroxine therapy: Obtain baseline TSH levels, then monitor every 4 weeks until levels and levothyroxine dose are stable, then monitor every 2 months

Without preexisting thyroid hormone replacement: TSH at baseline, then every 4 weeks for 4 months, then every 2 to 3 months

Additional Information Hand-foot skin reaction (HFSR) management (Lacouture, 2008): The following treatments may be used in addition to the recommended dosage modifications. Prior to treatment initiation, a pedicure is recommended to remove hyperkeratotic areas/calluses, which may predispose to HFSR; avoid vigorous exercise/ activities which may stress hands or feet. During therapy, patients should reduce exposure to hot water (may exacerbate hand-foot symptoms); avoid constrictive footwear and excessive skin friction. Patients may also wear thick cotton gloves or socks and should wear shoes with padded ▶

insoles. Grade 1 HFSR may be relieved with moisturizing creams, cotton gloves and socks (at night) and/or keratolytic creams such as urea (20% to 40%) or salicylic acid (6%). Apply topical steroid (eg, clobetasol ointment) twice daily to erythematous areas of Grade 2 HFSR; topical anesthetics (eg, lidocaine 2%) and then systemic analgesics (if appropriate) may be used for pain control. Resolution of acute erythema may result in keratotic areas which may be softened with keratolytic agents.

Dosage Forms Excipient information presented when available (limited, particularly for generics); consult specific product labeling.

Tablet, Oral:

NexAVAR: 200 mg

Extemporaneous Preparations Hazardous agent: Use appropriate precautions for handling and disposal (NIOSH 2014 [group 1]).

An oral suspension may be prepared with tablets. Place two 200 mg tablets into a glass containing 60 mL (2 oz) water; let stand 5 minutes before stirring. Stir until tablets are completely disintegrated, forming a uniform suspension. Administer within 1 hour after preparation. Stir suspension again immediately before administration. To ensure the full dose is administered, rinse glass several times with a total of 180 mL (6 oz) water and administer residue. **Note:** Brown tablet coating may initially form a thin film but has no effect on the dosing accuracy.
Nexavar data on file, Bayer Healthcare Pharmaceuticals.

◆ Sorafenib Tosylate see SORAfenib on page 1691

Sorbitol (SOR bi tole)

Pharmacologic Category Genitourinary Irrigant; Laxative, Osmotic

Use Genitourinary irrigant in transurethral prostatic resection or other transurethral resection or other transurethral surgical procedures; diuretic; humectant; sweetening agent; hyperosmotic laxative; facilitate the passage of sodium polystyrene sulfonate through the intestinal tract

Dosing

Adult & Geriatric

Hyperosmotic laxative (as single dose, at infrequent intervals):

Oral: 30-150 mL (as 70% solution)

Rectal enema: 120 mL as 25% to 30% solution

Adjunct to sodium polystyrene sulfonate: 15 mL as 70% solution orally until diarrhea occurs (10-20 mL/2 hours) or 20-100 mL as an oral vehicle for the sodium polystyrene sulfonate resin

Transurethral surgical procedures: Irrigation: Topical: 3% to 3.3% as transurethral surgical procedure irrigation

Pediatric

Hyperosmotic laxative (as single dose, at infrequent intervals):

Children 2-11 years:

Oral: 2 mL/kg (as 70% solution)

Rectal enema: 30-60 mL as 25% to 30% solution

Children >12 years: Oral, Rectal enema: Refer to adult dosing.

Additional Information Complete prescribing information should be consulted for additional detail.

Dosage Forms Excipient information presented when available (limited, particularly for generics); consult specific product labeling. [DSC] = Discontinued product

Solution, Irrigation:

Generic: 3% (3000 mL, 5000 mL [DSC]); 3.3% (2000 mL, 4000 mL)

Solution, Oral:

Generic: 70% (30 mL, 473 mL, 474 mL, 480 mL, 3840 mL)

Solution, Rectal:

Generic: 70% (473 mL)

◆ Sorbulax [OTC] see Psyllium on page 1529

◆ Sore Throat Relief [OTC] see Benzocaine on page 217

◆ Soriatane see Acitretin on page 34

◆ Sorilux see Calcipotriene on page 282

◆ Sorine see Sotalol on page 1694

Sotalol (SOE ta lole)

Brand Names: US Betapace; Betapace AF; Sorine; Sotylize

Brand Names: Canada Apo-Sotalol; CO Sotalol; Dom-Sotalol; Med-Sotalol; Mylan-Sotalol; Novo-Sotalol; Nu-Sotalol; PHL-Sotalol; PMS-Sotalol; PRO-Sotalol; ratio-Sotalol; Rhoxal-sotalol; Riva-Sotalol; Rylosol; Sandoz-Sotalol; ZYM-Sotalol

Index Terms Sotalol Hydrochloride

Pharmacologic Category Antiarrhythmic Agent, Class II; Antiarrhythmic Agent, Class III; Beta-Adrenergic Blocker, Nonselective

Additional Appendix Information

Adult ACLS Algorithms on page 1993

Use

Betapace, Sorine, Sotylize: Treatment of documented ventricular arrhythmias (ie, sustained ventricular tachycardia), that in the judgment of the health care provider are life-threatening

Betapace AF, Sotylize: Maintenance of normal sinus rhythm (delay in time to recurrence of atrial fibrillation/atrial flutter) in patients with symptomatic atrial fibrillation/atrial flutter who are currently in sinus rhythm. Manufacturer states substitutions should not be made for Betapace AF due to significant differences in labeling (ie, patient package insert and safety information)

According to the American Heart Association/American College of Cardiology/Heart Rhythm Society (AHA/ACC/HRS), sotalol is not effective for conversion of atrial fibrillation to sinus rhythm but may be used to prevent atrial fibrillation (AHA/ACC/HRS [January 2014])

Injection: Substitution for oral sotalol in those who are unable to take sotalol orally

Pregnancy Considerations Adverse events were not observed in the initial animal reproduction studies; therefore, the manufacturer classifies sotalol as pregnancy category B. Sotalol crosses the placenta and is found in amniotic fluid. In a cohort study, an increased risk of cardiovascular defects was observed following maternal use of beta-blockers during pregnancy (Lennestål 2009). Intrauterine growth restriction (IUGR), small placentas, as well as fetal/neonatal bradycardia, hypoglycemia, and/or respiratory depression have been observed following in utero exposure to beta-blockers as a class. Adequate facilities for monitoring infants at birth should be available. Untreated chronic maternal hypertension and pre-eclampsia are also associated with adverse events in the fetus, infant, and mother; however, sotalol is currently not recommended for the initial treatment of hypertension in pregnancy (ACOG 2013). Because sotalol crosses the placenta in concentrations similar to the maternal serum, it has been used for the treatment of fetal atrial flutter or fetal supraventricular tachycardia without hydrops (Sonesson 1998). The clearance of sotalol is increased during the third trimester of pregnancy, but other pharmacokinetic parameters do not significantly differ from nonpregnant values (O'Hare 1983).

Breast-Feeding Considerations Sotalol is excreted in breast milk in concentrations higher than those found in the maternal serum (O'Hare 1980). Although adverse events in nursing infants have not been observed in case reports, close monitoring for bradycardia, hypotension, respiratory distress, and hypoglycemia is advised. Due to the potential for serious adverse reactions in the nursing infant, the manufacturer recommends a decision be made whether to discontinue nursing or to discontinue the drug, taking into account the importance of treatment to the mother.

Contraindications

Hypersensitivity to sotalol or any component of the formulation; bronchial asthma; sinus bradycardia (<50 bpm during waking hours [Betapace AF, Sotylize]); second- or third-degree AV block (unless a functioning pacemaker is present); congenital or acquired long QT syndromes; cardiogenic shock; uncontrolled heart failure

Additional contraindications (Betapace AF, Sotylize, sotalol injection): Baseline QTc interval >450 msec (or JT >330 msec if QRS >100 msec); bronchospastic conditions; CrCl <40 mL/minute; serum potassium <4 mEq/L; sick sinus syndrome

Documentation of allergic cross-reactivity for beta-adrenergic blockers is limited. However, because of similarities in chemical structure and/or pharmacologic actions, the possibility of cross-sensitivity cannot be ruled out with certainty.

Warnings/Precautions [US Boxed Warning]: Sotalol can cause life-threatening ventricular tachycardia associated with QT interval prolongation (ie, torsades de pointes). Do not initiate if baseline QTc interval is >450 msec (Betapace AF, Sotylize, or sotalol injection). If QTc interval prolongs to 500 msec or exceeds 500 msec during therapy, reduce the dose, prolong the interval between doses, prolong the duration of the infusion (sotalol injection), or discontinue use (Betapace AF, Sotylize, sotalol injection). Adjust the dosing interval based on creatinine clearance (CrCl). QTc prolongation is directly related to the concentration of sotalol; reduced CrCl, female gender, and large doses increase the risk of QTc prolongation and subsequent torsades de pointes. Patients initiated or

reinitiated on sotalol or sotalol AF and patients who are converted from IV to oral administration should be placed for a minimum of 3 days (on their maintenance dose) in a facility that can provide cardiac resuscitation, continuous electrocardiographic (ECG) monitoring, and calculations of CrCl. Some experts will initiate therapy on an outpatient basis in patients if in sinus rhythm provided the QT interval and serum potassium are normal and the patient is not receiving any other QT-interval prolonging medications but require inpatient hospitalization if patient is in atrial fibrillation (AHA/ACC/HRS [January 2014]). Calculation of CrCl must occur prior to administration of the first dose. Dosage should be adjusted gradually with 3 days between dosing increments to achieve steady-state concentrations, and to allow time to monitor QT intervals. Monitor and adjust dose to prevent QTc prolongation. Potentially significant drug-drug interactions may exist, requiring dose or frequency adjustment, additional monitoring, and/or selection of alternative therapy.

[US Boxed Warning]: Adjust dosing interval based on CrCl to decrease risk of proarrhythmia; QT interval prolongation is directly related to sotalol concentration. CrCl must be calculated with dose initiation and dose increases. According to the manufacturers of sotalol injection, Betapace AF, and Sotylize, the use of sotalol is contraindicated in patients with CrCl <40 mL/minute. Correct electrolyte imbalances before initiating (especially hypokalemia and hypomagnesemia) because these conditions increase the risk of torsades de pointes. Consider preexisting conditions such as sick sinus syndrome before initiating. May cause bradycardia (including heart block) and hypotension. Dose adjustments of agents that slow AV nodal conduction may be necessary when sotalol is initiated. Use cautiously within the first 2 weeks post-MI, especially in patients with markedly impaired ventricular function (experience limited). Administer cautiously in compensated heart failure and monitor for a worsening of the condition. Use is contraindicated in patients with uncontrolled (or decompensated) heart failure. May precipitate or aggravate symptoms of arterial insufficiency in patients with PVD and Raynaud disease; use with caution and monitor for progression of arterial obstruction. Bradycardia may be observed more frequently in elderly patients (>65 years of age); dosage reductions may be necessary. In the treatment of atrial fibrillation in elderly patients, avoid antiarrhythmics as first-line treatment. In older adults, data suggests rate control may provide more benefits than risks compared to rhythm control for most patients (Beers Criteria). Beta-blocker therapy should not be withdrawn abruptly (particularly in patients with CAD), but gradually tapered to avoid acute tachycardia, hypertension, and/or ischemia. Severe exacerbation of angina, ventricular arrhythmias, and myocardial infarction (MI) have been reported following abrupt withdrawal of beta-blocker therapy. Temporary but prompt resumption of beta-blocker therapy may be indicated with worsening of angina or acute coronary insufficiency. When QTc prolongation occurs, consider weighing the risk of abrupt withdrawal of sotalol with the risk of QTc prolongation. Chronic beta-blocker therapy should not be routinely withdrawn prior to major surgery. Use cautiously in diabetics because it can mask prominent hypoglycemic symptoms. Use with caution in patients with bronchospastic disease, myasthenia gravis, or psychiatric disease. Adequate alpha-blockade is required prior to use of any beta-blocker for patients with untreated pheochromocytoma. May mask signs of hyperthyroidism (eg, tachycardia); if hyperthyroidism is suspected, carefully manage and monitor; abrupt withdrawal may exacerbate symptoms of hyperthyroidism or precipitate thyroid storm. Use caution with history of severe anaphylaxis to allergens; patients taking beta-blockers may become more sensitive to repeated challenges. Treatment of anaphylaxis (eg, epinephrine) in patients taking beta-blockers may be ineffective or promote undesirable effects.

[US Boxed Warning]: Sotalol is indicated for both the treatment of documented life-threatening ventricular arrhythmias (marketed as Betapace, Sorine, and Sotylize) and for the maintenance of normal sinus rhythm in patients with symptomatic atrial fibrillation/flutter who are currently in sinus rhythm (marketed as Betapace AF and Sotylize). Betapace should not be substituted for Betapace AF; Betapace AF is distributed with an educational insert specifically for patients with atrial fibrillation/flutter.

Adverse Reactions There is minimal clinical experience with IV sotalol; however, since exposure is similar between IV and oral sotalol, adverse reactions are expected to be similar.

>10%:
Cardiovascular: Bradycardia (dose related; 8% to 16%), chest pain (3% to 16%), palpitations (3% to 14%)
Central nervous system: Fatigue (dose related; 5% to 20%), dizziness (3% to 20%), headache (2% to 12%)
Neuromuscular & skeletal: Weakness (4% to 13%)
Respiratory: Dyspnea (dose related; 5% to 21%)
1% to 10%:
Cardiovascular: Edema (2% to 8%), ECG abnormality (2% to 7%), hypotension (3% to 6%), congestive heart failure (1% to 5%; incidence may be higher in patients with risk factors), syncope (1% to 5%), proarrhythmia (<1% to 5%), torsades de pointes (dose related; 1% to 4%), peripheral vascular disorder (1% to 3%), angina pectoris (2%), presyncope (1% to 2%), cardiovascular signs and symptoms (<1% to 2%), worsened ventricular tachycardia (1%), cerebrovascular accident (≤1%), hypertension (≤1%), vasodilation (≤1%), prolonged Q-T interval on ECG (dose related)
Central nervous system: Sleep disorder (1% to 8%), insomnia (3% to 4%), anxiety (2% to 4%), depression (1% to 4%), paresthesia (1% to 4%), sensation of cold (2% to 3%), impaired consciousness (1% to 3%), mood changes (≤1%)
Dermatologic: Hyperhidrosis (5%), skin rash (2% to 5%), diaphoresis (1% to 3%)
Endocrine & metabolic: Weight changes (1%)
Gastrointestinal: Nausea and vomiting (4% to 10%), diarrhea (2% to 7%), abdominal pain (<1% to 4%), dyspepsia (2% to 3%), abdominal distention (<1% to 3%), decreased appetite (2%), change in appetite (1% to 2%), colonic disease (1% to 2%), flatulence (<1% to 2%)
Genitourinary: Sexual disorder (≤3%), genitourinary complaint (≤1%)
Hematologic & oncologic: Hemorrhage (<1% to 2%)
Infection: Infection (1% to 2%), influenza (1% to 2%)
Local: Local pain (1% to 2%)
Neuromuscular & skeletal: Limb pain (2% to 7%), musculoskeletal pain (3% to 4%), musculoskeletal chest pain (2% to 3%), back pain (<1% to 3%)
Ophthalmic: Visual disturbance (1% to 5%)
Respiratory: Upper respiratory complaint (1% to 8%), pulmonary disease (3% to 5%), tracheobronchitis (1% to 3%), asthma (<1% to 2%)
Miscellaneous: Fever (1% to 3%), laboratory test abnormality (1% to 3%), AICD discharge (<1% to 2%)
<1% (Limited to important or life-threatening): Alopecia, eosinophilia, increased liver enzymes, leukopenia, paralysis, phlebitis, pruritus, pulmonary edema, skin photosensitivity, thrombocytopenia
Drug Interactions
Metabolism/Transport Effects None known.
Avoid Concomitant Use
Avoid concomitant use of Sotalol with any of the following: Beta2-Agonists; Ceritinib; Fingolimod; Floctafenine; Highest Risk QTc-Prolonging Agents; Ivabradine; Methacholine; Mifepristone; Moderate Risk QTc-Prolonging Agents; Propafenone; Rivastigmine
Increased Effect/Toxicity
Sotalol may increase the levels/effects of: Alpha-/Beta-Agonists (Direct-Acting); Alpha1-Blockers; Alpha2-Agonists; Amifostine; Antipsychotic Agents (Phenothiazines); Antipsychotic Agents (Second Generation [Atypical]); Bradycardia-Causing Agents; Bupivacaine; Cardiac Glycosides; Ceritinib; Cholinergic Agonists; DULoxetine; Ergot Derivatives; Grass Pollen Allergen Extract (5 Grass Extract); Highest Risk QTc-Prolonging Agents; Hypotension-Associated Agents; Insulin; Lacosamide; Levodopa; Lidocaine (Systemic); Lidocaine (Topical); Mepivacaine; Methacholine; Midodrine; Sulfonylureas

The levels/effects of Sotalol may be increased by: Acetylcholinesterase Inhibitors; Alpha2-Agonists; Anilidopiperidine Opioids; Antipsychotic Agents (Phenothiazines); Barbiturates; Blood Pressure Lowering Agents; Bretylium; Brimonidine (Topical); Calcium Channel Blockers (Nondihydropyridine); Diazoxide; Dipyridamole; Fingolimod; Floctafenine; Herbs (Hypotensive Properties); Ivabradine; Lidocaine (Topical); Mifepristone; Moderate Risk QTc-Prolonging Agents; Molsidomine; Nicorandil; NIFEdipine; Obinutuzumab; Pentoxifylline; Phosphodiesterase 5 Inhibitors; Propafenone; Prostacyclin Analogues; QTc-Prolonging Agents (Indeterminate Risk and Risk Modifying); Regorafenib; Reserpine; Rivastigmine; Ruxolitinib; Tofacitinib
Decreased Effect
Sotalol may decrease the levels/effects of: Beta2-Agonists; Theophylline Derivatives

The levels/effects of Sotalol may be decreased by: Antacids; Barbiturates; Nonsteroidal Anti-Inflammatory Agents; Rifamycin Derivatives

Food Interactions Sotalol peak serum concentrations may be decreased if taken with food. Management: Administer without regard to meals.

Preparation for Administration To prepare sotalol infusion, see manufacturer's prescribing information. Usually prepared in a volume of 100 to 250 mL; appropriate diluents are NS, D_5W, or LR.

Storage/Stability Store at ~25°C (77°F); excursions are permitted between 15°C and 30°C (59°F and 86°F). Protect injection from freezing and light.

Mechanism of Action

Beta-blocker which contains both beta-adrenoreceptor-blocking (Vaughan Williams Class II) and cardiac action potential duration prolongation (Vaughan Williams Class III) properties

Class II effects: Increased sinus cycle length, slowed heart rate, decreased AV nodal conduction, and increased AV nodal refractoriness Sotalol has both $beta_1$- and $beta_2$-receptor blocking activity. The beta-blocking effect of sotalol is a noncardioselective (half maximal at about 80 mg/day and maximal at doses of 320 to 640 mg/day). Significant beta-blockade occurs at oral doses as low as 25 mg/day.

Class III effects: Prolongation of the atrial and ventricular monophasic action potentials, and effective refractory prolongation of atrial muscle, ventricular muscle, and atrioventricular accessory pathways in both the antegrade and retrograde directions. Sotalol is a racemic mixture of d- and l-sotalol; both isomers have similar Class III antiarrhythmic effects while the l-isomer is responsible for virtually all of the beta-blocking activity. The Class III effects are seen only at oral doses ≥160 mg/day.

Pharmacodynamics/Kinetics

Onset of action:
Oral: Rapid; at 1 to 2 hours post dosing (steady-state), reductions in heart rate and cardiac index seen (Winters 1993)
IV: When administered IV over 5 minutes for ongoing VT, onset of action is ~5 to 10 minutes (Ho 1994)

Absorption: Oral: Well absorbed (Hanyok 1993); decreased ~20% by meals compared with fasting

Distribution: V_d: 1.2 to 2.4 L/kg (Hanyok 1993)

Protein binding: None

Metabolism: None

Bioavailability: Oral: 90% to 100%

Half-life elimination: Oral: Adults: 12 hours; Children: 9.5 hours; terminal half-life decreases with age <2 years (time to steady state may be ≥1 week in neonates); IV: Pharmacokinetics of the IV formulation (administered over 5 hours) are similar to the oral formulations (Somberg 2010). Half-life increases with renal dysfunction.

Time to peak, serum: Oral: 2 to 4 hours

Excretion: Urine (as unchanged drug)

Dosing

Adult & Geriatric

Baseline QTc interval and creatinine clearance must be determined prior to initiation. If CrCl ≤60 mL/minute, dosing interval adjustment is necessary. Sotalol should be initiated and doses increased in a hospital for at least 3 days with facilities for cardiac rhythm monitoring and assessment. Proarrhythmic events can occur after initiation of therapy and with each upward dosage adjustment.

Atrial fibrillation/flutter (symptomatic):
IV: Substitution for oral sotalol: **Note:** The effects of the initial IV dose must be monitored and the dose titrated either upward or downward, if needed, based on clinical effect, QTc interval, or adverse reactions.
Initial dose: 75 mg infused over 5 hours twice daily
Dose adjustment: If the initial dose does not reduce the frequency of relapse and excessive QTc prolongation does not occur, may increase to 112.5 mg twice daily. If at steady state this dose still does not control arrhythmia and QTc prolongation does not occur, may further increase dose to 150 mg twice daily.
Dose range: Usual therapeutic dose: 112.5 mg twice daily; maximum dose: 150 mg twice daily
Conversion from oral sotalol to IV sotalol:
80 mg oral equivalent to 75 mg IV
120 mg oral equivalent to 112.5 mg IV
160 mg oral equivalent to 150 mg IV
Oral: Betapace AF, Sotylize: *Initial:* 80 mg twice daily. If the initial dose does not reduce frequency of relapse and excessive QTc prolongation does not occur after 3 days, the dose may be increased to 120 mg twice daily; may further increase to a maximum dose of 160 mg twice daily if response is inadequate and QTc prolongation is not excessive.

Ventricular arrhythmias (Betapace, Sorine, Sotylize):
IV: Substitution for oral sotalol: **Note:** The effects of the initial IV dose must be monitored and the dose titrated either upward or downward, if needed, based on clinical effect, QTc interval, or adverse reactions.
Initial dose: 75 mg infused over 5 hours twice daily
Dose adjustment: If the initial dose does not reduce the frequency of relapse and excessive QTc prolongation does not occur, may increase after at least 3 days to 112.5 mg twice daily. May further increase dose every 3 days in increments of 75 mg/day.
Dose range: Usual therapeutic dose: 75 to 150 mg twice daily; maximum dose: 300 mg twice daily.
Conversion from oral sotalol to IV sotalol:
80 mg oral equivalent to 75 mg IV
120 mg oral equivalent to 112.5 mg IV
160 mg oral equivalent to 150 mg IV
Oral:
Initial dose: 80 mg twice daily; dose may be increased (in increments of 80 mg/day [Sotylize]) gradually to 160 to 320 mg daily; allow 3 days between dosing increments in order to attain steady-state plasma concentrations and to allow for monitoring of QT intervals
Usual range: Most patients respond to a total daily dose of 160 to 320 mg in 2 to 3 divided doses.
Some patients, with life-threatening refractory ventricular arrhythmias, may require total daily doses as high as 480 to 640 mg; however, these doses should only be prescribed when the potential benefit outweighs the increased risk of adverse events.
Monomorphic VT (hemodynamically stable) (off-label use): IV: 1.5 mg/kg over 5 minutes (AHA [Neumar 2010]); **Note:** Clinical trial employed standard dose of 100 mg (Ho 1994).

Pediatric Baseline QTc interval and creatinine clearance must be determined prior to initiation. If CrCl ≤60 mL/minute, dosing interval adjustment is necessary. Sotalol should be initiated and doses increased in a hospital for at least 3 days with facilities for cardiac rhythm monitoring and assessment. Proarrhythmic events can occur after initiation of therapy and with each upward dosage adjustment. **Note:** Dosing per manufacturer, based on pediatric pharmacokinetic data; wait at least 36 hours between dosage adjustments to allow monitoring of QTc intervals.

Atrial fibrillation/flutter (symptomatic): Oral: Betapace AF, Sotylize:
Infants and Children ≤2 years: Dosage should be adjusted (decreased) by plotting of the child's age on a logarithmic scale; see graph or refer to manufacturer's package labeling.
Children >2 years and Adolescents: Initial: 90 mg/m²/day in 3 divided doses; may be incrementally increased to a maximum of 180 mg/m²/day

Ventricular arrhythmias: Oral: Betapace, Sorine, Sotylize:
Infants and Children ≤2 years: Dosage should be adjusted (decreased) by plotting of the child's age on a logarithmic scale; see graph or refer to manufacturer's package labeling.
Children >2 years and Adolescents: Initial: 90 mg/m²/day in 3 divided doses; may be incrementally increased to a maximum of 180 mg/m²/day

Sotalol Age Factor Nomogram for Patients ≤2 Years of Age

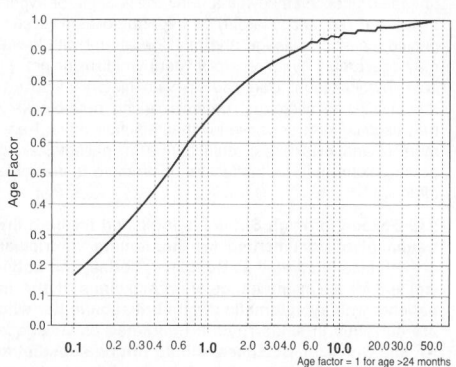

Adapted from U.S. Food and Drug Administration.
http://www.fda.gov/cder/foi/label/2001/2115s3lbl.PDF

Renal Impairment Adults: Dose escalations in renal impairment should be done after administration of at least 5 to 6 doses at appropriate intervals.

CrCl >60 mL/minute: Administer every 12 hours.

CrCl 40 to 60 mL/minute: Administer every 24 hours.

CrCl <40 mL/minute: Use is contraindicated. **Note:** The manufacturer's labeling for some products (Betapace, Sorine) recommend alternate dosing for patients with CrCl <40 mL/minute (refer to manufacturer's labeling).

Hemodialysis: Use is contraindicated in patients with CrCl <40 mL/minute. **Note:** The manufacturer's labeling for some products (Betapace, Sorine) recommend extreme caution be employed if sotalol is used in patients with renal failure undergoing hemodialysis. Multiple cases of torsades de pointes have been reported when sotalol was used even at low dosages (eg, 80 mg daily) in patients with end-stage renal disease treated with hemodialysis (Huynh-Do 1996). Hemodialysis would be expected to reduce sotalol plasma concentrations because sotalol is not bound to plasma proteins and does not undergo extensive metabolism.

Peritoneal dialysis: Use is contraindicated in patients with CrCl <40 mL/minute. Cases of torsades de pointes have been reported when sotalol was used even at low dosages (eg, 80 mg daily) in patients with end-stage renal disease treated with peritoneal dialysis (Dancey 1997; Tang 1997).

Hepatic Impairment There are no dosage adjustments provided in the manufacturer's labeling. However, dosage adjustment unlikely because sotalol is not metabolized by the liver.

Adjustment for Toxicity

QTc ≥500 msec during initiation period:

Betapace AF, Sotylize: Reduce dose, prolong the dosing interval (Sotylize), or discontinue sotalol

Sotalol injection: Reduce dose, prolong the infusion time by decreasing the infusion rate, or discontinue sotalol

QTc ≥520 msec (or JT interval ≥430 msec if the QRS >100 msec) during maintenance therapy (Betapace AF, sotalol injection): Reduce dose and carefully monitor QTc until <520 msec. If QTc interval ≥520 msec on the lowest maintenance dose, discontinue sotalol.

QTc ≥550 msec (Betapace, Sorine): Reduce dose or discontinue sotalol.

Administration

Oral: Administer without regard to meals.

IV:

Substitution for oral: Administer over 5 hours; may prolong duration of infusion if QT interval prolongs ≥500 msec.

Hemodynamically stable monomorphic VT: Administer IV push over 5 minutes; use with caution because of increased risk of adverse events (eg, bradycardia, hypotension, torsade de pointes) (ACLS 2010).

Monitoring Parameters Serum creatinine (creatinine clearance), magnesium, potassium; heart rate, blood pressure; ECG (eg, QTc interval, PR interval). If baseline QTc >450 msec (or JT interval >330 msec if QRS over 100 msec), sotalol (Betapace AF, Sotylize) is contraindicated.

Betapace AF, Sotylize; During initiation and titration period, monitor QTc interval 2 to 4 hours after each dose. If QTc interval is ≥500 msec, reduce dose, prolong the dosing interval (Sotylize), or discontinue sotalol. If the QTc interval is <500 msec after 3 days (after fifth or sixth dose if patient receiving once-daily dosing), patient may be discharged on current regimen. Monitor QTc interval periodically thereafter.

For IV use, measure QTc interval after completion of each infusion.

Consult individual institutional policies and procedures.

Test Interactions May falsely increase urinary metanephrine values when fluorimetric or photometric methods are used; does not interact with HPLC assay with solid phase extraction for determination of urinary catecholamines

Additional Information Pharmacokinetics in children are more relevant for BSA than age.

Dosage Forms Excipient information presented when available (limited, particularly for generics); consult specific product labeling.

Solution, Intravenous, as hydrochloride:

Generic: 150 mg/10 mL (10 mL)

Solution, Oral, as hydrochloride:

Sotylize: 5 mg/mL (250 mL, 480 mL) [contains sodium benzoate; grape flavor]

Tablet, Oral, as hydrochloride:

Betapace: 80 mg, 120 mg, 160 mg [scored; contains fd&c blue #2 aluminum lake]

Betapace AF: 80 mg, 120 mg, 160 mg [scored]

Sorine: 80 mg, 120 mg, 160 mg, 240 mg [scored]

Generic: 80 mg, 120 mg, 160 mg, 240 mg

Extemporaneous Preparations Note: Commercial oral solution is available (5 mg/mL)

A 5 mg/mL sotalol syrup may be made with Betapace, Sorine, or Betapace AF tablets and Simple Syrup containing sodium benzoate 0.1% (Syrup, NF). Place 120 mL Syrup, NF in a 6-ounce amber plastic (polyethylene terephthalate) prescription bottle; add five Betapace, Sorine, or Betapace AF 120 mg tablets and shake the bottle to wet the tablets. Allow tablets to hydrate for at least 2 hours, then shake intermittently over ≥2 hours until the tablets are completely disintegrated; a dispersion of fine particles (water-insoluble inactive ingredients) in syrup should be obtained. **Note:** To simplify the disintegration process, tablets can hydrate overnight; tablets may also be crushed, carefully transferred into the bottle and shaken well until a dispersion of fine particles in syrup is obtained. Label "shake well". Stable for 3 months at 15°C to 30°C (59°F to 86°F) and ambient humidity.

Betapace prescribing information, Bayer HealthCare Pharmaceuticals Inc, Wayne, NJ, 2011.

Betapace AF prescribing information, Bayer HealthCare Pharmaceuticals Inc, Wayne, NJ, 2011.

Sorine prescribing information, Upsher-Smith, Minneapolis, MN, 2012.

Spinosad (SPIN oh sad)

Brand Names: US Natroba

Index Terms NatrOVA

Pharmacologic Category Antiparasitic Agent, Topical; Pediculocide

Use Head lice: Topical treatment of head lice (*Pediculosis capitis*) infestation in adults and children ≥6 months of age

Dosing

Adult & Geriatric Head lice: Topical: Apply sufficient amount to cover dry scalp and completely cover dry hair; 120 mL may be necessary depending on the length of hair. If live lice are seen 7 days after first treatment, repeat with second application.

Pediatric Head lice: Infants ≥6 months, Children, and Adolescents: Topical: Refer to adult dosing.

Renal Impairment There are no dosage adjustments provided in the manufacturer's labeling. However, dosage adjustment unlikely due to low systemic absorption.

Hepatic Impairment There are no dosage adjustments provided in the manufacturer's labeling. However, dosage adjustment unlikely due to low systemic absorption.

Additional Information Complete prescribing information should be consulted for additional detail.

Dosage Forms Excipient information presented when available (limited, particularly for generics); consult specific product labeling.

Suspension, External:

Natroba: 0.9% (120 mL) [contains benzyl alcohol, cetearyl alcohol, fd&c yellow #6 (sunset yellow), isopropyl alcohol, propylene glycol]

Generic: 0.9% (120 mL)

Spironolactone (speer on oh LAK tone)

Brand Names: US Aldactone

Brand Names: Canada Aldactone; Teva-Spironolactone

Pharmacologic Category Antihypertensive; Diuretic, Potassium-Sparing; Mineralocorticoid (Aldosterone) Receptor Antagonists

Use Management of edema associated with excessive aldosterone excretion or with congestive heart failure (HF) unresponsive to other therapies; hypertension; primary hyperaldosteronism (establishing diagnosis, short-term preoperative treatment, and long-term maintenance therapy in selected patients); hypokalemia; cirrhosis of liver accompanied by edema or ascites; nephrotic syndrome; severe HF (NYHA class III-IV) to increase survival and reduce hospitalization when added to standard therapy

Note: The ACCF/AHA 2013 heart failure guidelines recommend the use of aldosterone antagonists, along with other guideline-directed medical therapies, to reduce morbidity and mortality in patients with HF (NYHA class III-IV) with LVEF ≤35% (Yancy 2013).

According to the Eighth Joint National Committee (JNC 8) guidelines, aldosterone antagonists are not recommended for the initial treatment of hypertension (James 2013).

According to the 2013 ACCF/AHA guidelines for the management of ST-elevation myocardial infarction (STEMI) and the guidelines for the management of unstable angina/non-STEMI, an aldosterone antagonist should be given to patients who are already on an ACE inhibitor and beta-blocker, who have an LVEF ≤40% and either symptomatic HF or diabetes mellitus (ACCF/AHA [Anderson 2013]; ACCF/AHA [O'Gara 2013]).

Pregnancy Considerations Adverse events were observed in some animal reproduction studies. The anti-androgen effects of spironolactone have been shown to cause feminization of the male fetus in animal studies. Spironolactone crosses the placenta (Regitz-Zagrosek 2011).

The treatment of heart failure is generally the same in pregnant and nonpregnant women; however, spironolactone should be avoided in the first trimester due to its antiandrogenic effects (Regitz-Zagrosek 2011). The use of mineralocorticoid receptor antagonists is not recommended to treat chronic uncomplicated hypertension in pregnant women and should generally be avoided in women of reproductive potential. When treatment for hypertension in pregnancy is needed, other agents are preferred (ACOG 2013). Use of diuretics to treat edema during normal pregnancies is not appropriate; use may be considered when edema is due to pathologic causes (as in the nonpregnant patient); monitor.

Breast-Feeding Considerations The active metabolite of spironolactone (canrenone) has been found in breast milk. Information is available from a case report following maternal use of spironolactone 25 mg twice daily throughout pregnancy, then 4 times daily after delivery. Milk and maternal serum samples were obtained 17 days after birth. Two hours after the maternal dose, canrenone concentrations were ~144 ng/mL (serum) and ~104 ng/mL (milk). When measured 14.5 hours after the dose, canrenone concentrations were ~92 ng/mL (serum) and ~47 ng/mL (milk). The authors calculated the estimated maximum amount of canrenone to the nursing infant to be ~0.2% of the maternal dose (Phelps 1977). Effects to humans are not known; however, this metabolite was found to be carcinogenic in rats. Diuretics have the potential to decrease milk volume and suppress lactation. According to the manufacturer, the decision to continue or discontinue breast-feeding during therapy should take into account the risk of exposure to the infant and the benefits of treatment to the mother; if use of spironolactone is essential, an alternative method of feeding should be used.

Contraindications

Anuria; acute renal insufficiency; significant impairment of renal excretory function; hyperkalemia; Addison's disease; concomitant use with eplerenone

Canadian labeling: Additional contraindications (not in U.S. labeling): Hypersensitivity to spironolactone or any component of the formulation; concomitant use with heparin or low molecular weight heparin

Warnings/Precautions Hazardous agent - use appropriate precautions for handling and disposal (NIOSH 2014 [group 2]).

[US Boxed Warning]: Shown to be a tumorigen in chronic toxicity animal studies. Avoid unnecessary use.

Monitor closely for hyperkalemia; increases in serum potassium are dose related and rates of hyperkalemia also increase with declining renal function. The concurrent use of larger doses of ACE inhibitors (eg, ≥ lisinopril 10 mg daily in adults) also increases the risk of hyperkalemia (ACCF/AHA [Yancy 2013]). Dose reduction or interruption of therapy may be necessary with development of hyperkalemia. Use is contraindicated in patients with hyperkalemia; use caution in conditions known to cause hyperkalemia. Risk of hyperkalemia is increased with declining renal function. Use with caution in patients with mild renal impairment; contraindicated with anuria, acute renal insufficiency, or significant impairment of renal excretory function. Potentially significant drug-drug interactions may exist, requiring dose or frequency adjustment, additional monitoring, and/or selection of alternative therapy. Somnolence and dizziness have been reported with use; advise patients to use caution when driving or operating machinery until response to initial treatment has been

determined. Concurrent use with ethanol may Increase risk of orthostasis. Excess amounts can lead to profound diuresis with fluid and electrolyte loss; close medical supervision and dose evaluation are required. Watch for and correct electrolyte disturbances; adjust dose to avoid dehydration. In cirrhosis, avoid electrolyte and acid/base imbalances that might lead to hepatic encephalopathy. Gynecomastia is related to dose and duration of therapy; typically is reversible following discontinuation of therapy but may persist (rare). Discontinue use prior to adrenal vein catheterization. When evaluating a heart failure patient for spironolactone treatment, eGFR should be >30 mL/minute/1.73 m² or creatinine should be ≤2.5 mg/dL (men) or ≤2 mg/dL (women) with no recent worsening and potassium <5 mEq/L with no history of severe hyperkalemia (ACCF/AHA [Yancy 2013]). Serum potassium levels require close monitoring and management if elevated. The manufacturer recommends to discontinue or interrupt therapy if serum potassium >5 mEq/L or serum creatinine >4 mg/dL. The ACCF/AHA recommends considering discontinuation upon the development of serum potassium >5.5 mEq/L or worsening renal function with careful evaluation of the entire medical regimen. Avoid routine triple therapy with the combined use of an ACE inhibitor, ARB, and spironolactone. Instruct patients with heart failure to discontinue use during an episode of diarrhea or dehydration or when loop diuretic therapy is interrupted (ACCF/AHA [Yancy 2013]).

In the elderly, avoid use of doses >25 mg/day in patients with heart failure or with reduced renal function (eg, CrCl <30 mL/minute or eGFR ≤30 mL/minute/1.73 m² [Yancy 2013]); risk of hyperkalemia is increased for heart failure patients receiving >25 mg/day, particularly if taking concomitant medications such as NSAIDS, ACE inhibitor, angiotensin receptor blocker, or potassium supplements (Beers Criteria).

Adverse Reactions Frequency not defined.

Cardiovascular: Vasculitis

Central nervous system: Ataxia, confusion, drowsiness, headache, lethargy

Dermatologic: Erythematous maculopapular rash, Stevens-Johnson syndrome, toxic epidermal necrolysis, urticaria

Endocrine & metabolic: Amenorrhea, gynecomastia, hyperkalemia

Gastrointestinal: Abdominal cramps, diarrhea, gastritis, gastrointestinal hemorrhage, gastrointestinal ulcer, nausea, vomiting

Genitourinary: Impotence, irregular menses, postmenopausal bleeding

Hematologic & oncologic: Agranulocytosis, malignant neoplasm of breast

Hepatic: Hepatotoxicity

Hypersensitivity: Anaphylaxis

Immunologic: DRESS syndrome

Renal: Increased blood urea nitrogen, renal failure, renal insufficiency

Miscellaneous: Fever

Drug Interactions

Metabolism/Transport Effects None known.

Avoid Concomitant Use

Avoid concomitant use of Spironolactone with any of the following: AMILoride; CycloSPORINE (Systemic); Tacrolimus (Systemic); Triamterene

Increased Effect/Toxicity

Spironolactone may increase the levels/effects of: ACE Inhibitors; Amifostine; Ammonium Chloride; Antipsychotic Agents (Second Generation [Atypical]); Cardiac Glycosides; Ciprofloxacin (Systemic); CycloSPORINE (Systemic); Digoxin; DULoxetine; Hypotension-Associated Agents; Levodopa; Neuromuscular-Blocking Agents (Nondepolarizing); Sodium Phosphates; Tacrolimus (Systemic)

The levels/effects of Spironolactone may be increased by: Alfuzosin; AMILoride; Analgesics (Opioid); Angiotensin II Receptor Blockers; AtorvaSTATin; Barbiturates; Brimonidine (Topical); Canagliflozin; Cholestyramine Resin; Diazoxide; Drospirenone; Eplerenone; Heparin; Heparin (Low Molecular Weight); Herbs (Hypotensive Properties); Molsidomine; Nicorandil; Nitrofurantoin; Nonsteroidal Anti-Inflammatory Agents; Obinutuzumab; Pentoxifylline; Phosphodiesterase 5 Inhibitors; Potassium Salts; Prostacyclin Analogues; Tolvaptan; Triamterene; Trimethoprim

Decreased Effect

Spironolactone may decrease the levels/effects of: Abiraterone Acetate; Alpha-/Beta-Agonists; Cardiac Glycosides; Mitotane; QuiNIDine

The levels/effects of Spironolactone may be decreased by: Amphetamines; Herbs (Hypertensive Properties); Methylphenidate; Nonsteroidal Anti-Inflammatory Agents; Yohimbine

Food Interactions Food increases absorption. Management: Administer with food to increase absorption and decrease GI upset.

Storage/Stability Store below 25°C (77°F).

Mechanism of Action Competes with aldosterone for receptor sites in the distal renal tubules, increasing sodium chloride and water excretion while conserving potassium and hydrogen ions; may block the effect of aldosterone on arteriolar smooth muscle as well

Pharmacodynamics/Kinetics

Duration: 2-3 days

Protein binding: >90%

Metabolism: Hepatic to multiple metabolites, including active metabolites canrenone and 7-alpha-spirolactone

Half-life elimination: Spironolactone: ~1.4 hours; Canrenone: 12-20 hours (Skluth 1990); 7-alpha-spirolactone: ~13.8 hours

Time to peak, serum: 3-4 hours (primarily as the active metabolite)

Excretion: Urine and feces

Dosing

Adult To reduce delay in onset of effect, a loading dose of 2 or 3 times the daily dose may be administered on the first day of therapy.

Ascites, due to cirrhosis (off-label dose): Initial: 100 mg once daily; titrate every 3 to 5 days as clinically indicated (usual maximum: 400 mg once daily) (Runyon 2013)

Edema: Oral: 25 to 200 mg daily in 1 to 2 divided doses

Hypokalemia: Oral: 25 to 100 mg once daily

Hypertension: Oral: Initial: The manufacturer's labeling recommends 50 to 100 mg in 1 to 2 divided doses; after 2 weeks, may adjust dose. In patients with resistant hypertension, an initial daily dose of 25 mg may also be added to other antihypertensive agents with an increase to 50 mg daily if needed (Vaclavik 2014; Williams 2015). Usual dosage range (ASH/ISH [Weber 2014]): 25 to 50 mg daily

Diagnosis of primary aldosteronism: Oral: Long test: 400 mg once daily for 3 to 4 weeks; short test: 400 mg once daily for 4 days; maintenance until surgical correction: 100 to 400 mg once daily

Heart failure, severe (NYHA class III-IV): Oral: Initial: 12.5 to 25 mg once daily; maximum daily dose: 50 mg. If 25 mg once daily not tolerated, may reduce to 25 mg every other day. The ACCF/AHA 2013 HF guidelines also recommend the use of aldosterone receptor antagonists (eg, spironolactone) in patients with NYHA class II HF and LVEF ≤35% who have a history of prior cardiovascular hospitalization or elevated plasma natriuretic peptide levels and postmyocardial infarction patients with LVEF ≤40% who develop HF symptoms or have a history of diabetes mellitus (ACCF/AHA [Yancy 2013]).

Note: Per the manufacturer, if potassium >5 mEq/L or serum creatinine >4 mg/dL, discontinue or interrupt therapy. Alternatively, the ACCF/AHA 2013 HF guidelines recommend withholding treatment if potassium >5.5 mEq/L or renal function worsens; hold doses until potassium is <5 mEq/L and consider restarting with a reduced dose after confirming resolution of hyperkalemia/renal insufficiency for at least 72 hours (ACCF/AHA [Yancy 2013]).

Acne in women (off-label use): Oral: 50 to 200 mg once daily (Goodfellow 1984; Muhlemann 1986)

Hirsutism in women (off-label use): Oral: 50 to 200 mg daily in 1 to 2 divided doses (Koulouri 2008; Martin 2008)

Geriatric

Hypertension: Oral: No initial dosage adjustment necessary (Aronow 2011).

Heart failure: Oral: Avoid using doses >25 mg daily (Beers Criteria); monitor potassium closely/use with caution.

Pediatric Administration with food increases absorption. To reduce delay in onset of effect, a loading dose of 2 or 3 times the daily dose may be administered on the first day of therapy.

Edema, hypertension (off-label use): Oral: Children 1-17 years: Initial: 1 mg/kg/day divided every 12 to 24 hours (maximum dose: 3.3 mg/kg/day, up to 100 mg daily) (NHBPEP 2004)

Renal Impairment Heart failure (ACCF/AHA [Yancy 2013]):

eGFR ≥50 mL/minute/1.73 m²: Initial dose: 12.5-25 mg once daily; Maintenance dose (after 4 weeks of treatment with potassium ≤5 mEq/L): 25 mg once or twice daily

eGFR 30-49 mL/minute/1.73 m²: Initial dose: 12.5 mg once daily or every other day; Maintenance dose (after 4 weeks of treatment with potassium ≤5 mEq/L): 12.5-25 mg once daily

eGFR <30 mL/minute/1.73 m²: Not recommended.

Note: Contraindicated in patients with anuria, acute renal insufficiency, or significant impairment of renal excretory function.

Hepatic Impairment There are no dosage adjustments provided in manufacturer's labeling.

Dietary Considerations Should be taken with food to decrease gastrointestinal irritation and to increase absorption. Excessive potassium intake (eg, salt substitutes, low-salt foods, bananas, nuts) should be avoided.

Monitoring Parameters Blood pressure, serum electrolytes (potassium, sodium), renal function, I & O ratios and daily weight throughout therapy

ACCF/AHA heart failure guideline recommendations (ACCF/AHA [Yancy 2013]): Serum potassium and renal function should be checked in 3 days after initiation, at 1 week after initiation, at least monthly for the first 3 months of therapy, and every 3 months thereafter. If adding or increasing the dose of concomitant ACE inhibitors or ARBs, a new cycle of monitoring should be done. If serum potassium increases to >5.5 mEq/L or renal function worsens, hold doses until potassium is <5 mEq/L and consider restarting with a reduced dose after confirming resolution of hyperkalemia/renal insufficiency for at least 72 hours.

Test Interactions May interfere with the radioimmunoassay for digoxin.

Additional Information Maximum diuretic effect may be delayed 2-3 days and maximum antihypertensive effects may be delayed 2-3 weeks.

Dosage Forms Excipient information presented when available (limited, particularly for generics); consult specific product labeling.

Tablet, Oral:

Aldactone: 25 mg

Aldactone: 50 mg, 100 mg [scored]

Generic: 25 mg, 50 mg, 100 mg

Extemporaneous Preparations Hazardous agent; use appropriate precautions for handling and disposal (NIOSH 2014 [group 2]).

A 1 mg/mL oral suspension may be made with tablets. Crush ten 25 mg tablets in a mortar and reduce to a fine powder. Add a small amount of purified water and soak for 5 minutes; add 50 mL 1.5% carboxymethylcellulose, 100 mL syrup NF, and mix to a uniform paste; mix while adding purified water in incremental proportions to **almost** 250 mL; transfer to a calibrated bottle, rinse mortar with purified water, and add quantity of purified water sufficient to make 250 mL. Label "shake well". Stable for 3 months at room temperature or refrigerated (Nahata 1993).

A 2.5 mg/mL oral suspension may be made with tablets. Crush twelve 25 mg tablets in a mortar and reduce to a fine powder. Add small portions of distilled water or glycerin and mix to a uniform paste; mix while adding cherry syrup to **almost** 120 mL; transfer to a calibrated bottle, rinse mortar with cherry syrup, and add quantity of cherry syrup sufficient to make 120 mL. Label "shake well" and "refrigerate". This method may also be used with twenty-four 25 mg tablets for a 5 mg/mL oral suspension. Both concentrations are stable for 28 days refrigerated (Mathur 1989).

A 25 mg/mL oral suspension may be made with tablets and either a 1:1 mixture of Ora-Sweet and Ora-Plus or a 1:1 mixture of Ora-Sweet SF and Ora-Plus. Crush one-hundred-twenty 25 mg tablets in a mortar and reduce to a fine powder. Add small portions of chosen vehicle and mix to a uniform paste; mix while adding vehicle in incremental proportions to **almost** 120 mL; transfer to a calibrated bottle, rinse mortar with vehicle, and add quantity of vehicle sufficient to make 120 mL. Store in amber bottles; label "shake well" and "refrigerate". Stable for 60 days refrigerated (Allen 1996).

Allen LV Jr and Erickson MA 3rd, "Stability of Ketoconazole, Metolazone, Metronidazole, Procainamide Hydrochloride, and Spironolactone in Extemporaneously Compounded Oral Liquids," *Am J Health Syst Pharm.* 1996, 53(17):2073-8.

Mathur LK and Wickman A, "Stability of Extemporaneously Compounded Spironolactone Suspensions," *Am J Hosp Pharm.* 1989, 46(10):2040-2.

Nahata MC, Morosco RS, and Hipple TF, "Stability of Spironolactone in an Extemporaneously Prepared Suspension at Two Temperatures," *Ann Pharmacother.* 1993, 27(10):1198-9.

♦ **SPM 927** *see* Lacosamide *on page 1021*

♦ **Sporanox** *see* Itraconazole *on page 998*

♦ **Sporanox Pulsepak** *see* Itraconazole *on page 998*

♦ **SPP100** *see* Aliskiren *on page 70*

Stavudine (STAV yoo deen)

Brand Names: US Zerit
Brand Names: Canada Zerit
Index Terms d4T
Pharmacologic Category Antiretroviral, Reverse Transcriptase Inhibitor, Nucleoside (Anti-HIV)
Use Treatment of HIV infection in combination with other antiretroviral agents
Medication Guide Available Yes
Dosing

Adult HIV infection (in combination with other antiretrovirals): Oral:
<60 kg: 30 mg every 12 hours
≥60 kg: 40 mg every 12 hours
Note: According to the Department and Health and Human Services (HHS) HIV treatment guidelines, the World Health Organization recommends 30 mg every 12 hours in all adult and adolescent patients regardless of body weight (HHS [adult] 2015).

Geriatric Older patients should be closely monitored for signs and symptoms of peripheral neuropathy. Dosage should be carefully adjusted to renal function.

Pediatric HIV infection: Oral:
Newborns (Birth to 13 days): 0.5 mg/kg every 12 hours
Children:
≥14 days and <30 kg: 1 mg/kg every 12 hours
≥30 kg: Refer to adult dosing.

Renal Impairment
Adults:
CrCl >50 mL/minute:
<60 kg: 30 mg every 12 hours
≥60 kg: 40 mg every 12 hours
CrCl 26-50 mL/minute:
<60 kg: 15 mg every 12 hours
≥60 kg: 20 mg every 12 hours
CrCl 10-25 mL/minute, hemodialysis (administer dose after hemodialysis on day of dialysis):
<60 kg: 15 mg every 24 hours
≥60 kg: 20 mg every 24 hours
Children: Specific recommendations not available. Reduction in dose or increase in dosing interval should be considered.

Hepatic Impairment There are no dosage adjustments provided in the manufacturer's labeling. Use with caution.
Additional Information Complete prescribing information should be consulted for additional detail.
Dosage Forms Excipient information presented when available (limited, particularly for generics); consult specific product labeling.
Capsule, Oral:
Zerit: 15 mg, 20 mg, 30 mg, 40 mg
Generic: 15 mg, 20 mg, 30 mg, 40 mg
Solution Reconstituted, Oral:
Zerit: 1 mg/mL (200 mL) [dye free; fruit flavor]
Generic: 1 mg/mL (200 mL)

Streptomycin (strep toe MYE sin)

Brand Names: Canada Streptomycin for Injection
Index Terms Streptomycin Sulfate
Pharmacologic Category Antibiotic, Aminoglycoside; Antitubercular Agent
Use

Tuberculosis:
Treatment of tuberculosis, in combination with other appropriate antituberculosis agents, when the primary agents (eg, isoniazid, rifampin, ethambutol, pyrazinamide) are contraindicated because of toxicity or intolerance.

Nontuberculosis infections:
Treatment of infections caused by susceptible bacteria that are not amenable to therapy with less potentially toxic agents,including sensitive *Yersinia pestis* (plague); *Francisella tularensis* (tularemia); *Brucella*; *Klebsiella granulomatis* (donovanosis, granuloma inguinale); *Haemophilus ducreyi* (chancroid); *Haemophilus influenzae* (in respiratory, endocardial, and meningeal infections, concomitantly with another antibacterial agent); *Klebsiella pneumoniae* pneumonia (concomitantly with another antibacterial agent); *Escherichia coli*, *Proteus* spp., *Enterobacter aerogenes*, *K. pneumoniae*, and *Enterococcus faecalis* in urinary tract infections; *Streptococcus viridans*; *E. faecalis* (in endocardial infections, concomitant with penicillin); and gram-negative bacillary bacteremia (concomitant with another antibacterial agent).

Pregnancy Considerations Streptomycin crosses the placenta. Streptomycin may cause fetal harm if administered to a pregnant woman. There are multiple reports of total irreversible bilateral congenital deafness in children whose mothers received streptomycin during pregnancy. Streptomycin should never be substituted as first line therapy for the treatment of tuberculosis in pregnant women (Blumberg 2003).

Breast-Feeding Considerations Streptomycin is excreted into breast milk. Due to the potential for serious adverse reactions in the nursing infant, the manufacturer recommends a decision be made whether to discontinue nursing or to discontinue the drug, taking into account the importance of treatment to the mother. As a class, aminoglycosides are expected to be poorly distributed into breast milk, limiting systemic exposure to a nursing infant. In general, modification of bowel flora may occur with any antibiotic exposure (Chung 2002).

Contraindications Hypersensitivity to streptomycin, other aminoglycosides, or any component of the formulation

Warnings/Precautions [US Boxed Warnings]: May cause neurotoxicity (eg, disturbances of vestibular and cochlear function, optic nerve dysfunction, peripheral neuritis, arachnoiditis, encephalopathy), nephrotoxicity, and/or neuromuscular blockade and respiratory paralysis; usual risk factors include preexisting renal impairment, concomitant neuro-/nephrotoxic medications, advanced age and dehydration. The drug's neurotoxicity can result in respiratory paralysis from

neuromuscular blockade, especially when the drug is given soon after anesthesia or muscle relaxants. Use with caution in patients with preexisting vertigo, tinnitus, hearing loss, neuromuscular disorders, or renal impairment; modify dosage in patients with renal impairment; ototoxicity is directly proportional to the amount of drug given and the duration of treatment; tinnitus or vertigo are indications of vestibular injury and impending bilateral irreversible damage; renal damage is usually reversible. Monitor renal function closely; peak serum concentrations should not surpass 20 to 25 mcg/mL in patients with renal impairment. Some formulations may contain metabisulfite; may cause allergic reactions in patients with sulfite sensitivity. **[US Boxed Warning]: Parenteral form should be used only where appropriate audiometric and laboratory testing facilities are available.** Prolonged use may result in fungal or bacterial superinfection, including *C. difficile*-associated diarrhea (CDAD) and pseudomembranous colitis; CDAD has been observed >2 months postantibiotic treatment. IM injections should be administered in a large muscle well within the body to avoid peripheral nerve damage and local skin reactions. Potentially significant interactions may exist, requiring dose or frequency adjustment, additional monitoring, and/or selection of alternative therapy. **[US Boxed Warning]: Avoid concomitant or sequential use with other neurotoxic and/or nephrotoxic drugs (eg, neomycin, kanamycin, gentamicin, paromomycin, polymyxin B, colistin, tobramycin, cyclosporine).**

Adverse Reactions Frequency not defined.

Cardiovascular: Hypotension

Central nervous system: Drug fever, headache, neurotoxicity, paresthesia of face

Dermatologic: Angioedema, exfoliative dermatitis, skin rash, urticaria

Gastrointestinal: Nausea, vomiting

Hematologic: Eosinophilia, hemolytic anemia, leukopenia, pancytopenia, thrombocytopenia

Neuromuscular & skeletal: Arthralgia, tremor, weakness

Ocular: Amblyopia

Otic: Ototoxicity (auditory), ototoxicity (vestibular)

Renal: Azotemia, nephrotoxicity

Respiratory: Difficulty in breathing

Miscellaneous: Anaphylaxis

Postmarketing and/or case reports: Drug reaction with eosinophilia and systemic symptoms (DRESS), toxic epidermal necrolysis

Drug Interactions

Metabolism/Transport Effects None known.

Avoid Concomitant Use

Avoid concomitant use of Streptomycin with any of the following: Bacitracin (Systemic); BCG (Intravesical); Foscarnet; Mannitol; Mannitol (Systemic); Mecamylamine

Increased Effect/Toxicity

Streptomycin may increase the levels/effects of: AbobotulinumtoxinA; Bacitracin (Systemic); Bisphosphonate Derivatives; CARBOplatin; Colistimethate; CycloSPORINE (Systemic); Mecamylamine; Neuromuscular-Blocking Agents; OnabotulinumtoxinA; RimabotulinumtoxinB; Tenofovir Products

The levels/effects of Streptomycin may be increased by: Amphotericin B; Capreomycin; Cefazedone; Cephalosporins (2nd Generation); Cephalosporins (3rd Generation); Cephalosporins (4th Generation); Cephradine; CISplatin; Foscarnet; Loop Diuretics; Mannitol; Mannitol (Systemic); Nonsteroidal Anti-Inflammatory Agents; Tenofovir Products; Vancomycin

Decreased Effect

Streptomycin may decrease the levels/effects of: BCG (Intravesical); BCG Vaccine (Immunization); Sodium Picosulfate; Typhoid Vaccine

The levels/effects of Streptomycin may be decreased by: Penicillins

Preparation for Administration

IM: Reconstitute vial with 4.2 mL, 3.2 mL, or 1.8 mL sterile water for injection (SWFI) to yield a final concentration of ~200 mg/mL, ~250 mg/mL, or ~400 mg/mL, respectively

IV: Further dilute dose to concentration of 5 to 10 mg/mL in D5W or NS (Morris 1994; Peloquin 1992; Tanoira 2014)

Storage/Stability

Store intact vials at 20°C to 25°C (68°F to 77°F). Protect from light. Reconstituted solution may be stored at room temperature for up to 1 week.

Depending upon manufacturer, reconstituted solution remains stable for 24 hours at room temperature. Exposure to light causes darkening of solution without apparent loss of potency.

Mechanism of Action Inhibits bacterial protein synthesis by binding directly to the 30S ribosomal subunits causing faulty peptide sequence to form in the protein chain

Pharmacodynamics/Kinetics

Absorption: Oral: Poorly absorbed; IM: Well absorbed

Distribution: Poorly distributed into CSF

Half-life elimination: Adults: ~5 to 6 hours

Time to peak: IM: Within 1 hour

Excretion: Urine (29% to 89% as unchanged drug)

Dosing

Adult Note: Manufacturer's labeling states for IM administration only, however, IV administration (off-label route) has been described (Morris 1994; Peloquin 1992; Tanoira 2014).

Usual dosage range: IM: 15 to 30 mg/kg/day or 1 to 2 g daily

Indication-specific dosing:

Brucellosis: IM: 1 g daily in 2 to 4 divided doses for 14 to 21 days (with doxycycline) (Skalsky 2008)

Endocarditis:

Enterococcal:

Manufacturer's labeling: IM: 1 g every 12 hours for 2 weeks, followed by 500 mg every 12 hours for 4 weeks in combination with penicillin

Alternate dosing (susceptible to penicillin, vancomycin, and streptomycin and resistant to gentamicin): IM, IV: 15 mg/kg/day in divided doses every 12 hours for 4 to 6 weeks (minimum of 6 weeks for prosthetic valves) in combination with ampicillin, penicillin, or vancomycin (Baddour 2005)

Streptococcal: IM: 1 g every 12 hours for 1 week, followed by 500 mg every 12 hours for 1 week in combination with penicillin.

***Mycobacterium avium* complex (MAC) (off-label use):** IM: Adjunct therapy (with macrolide, rifamycin, and ethambutol): 8 to 25 mg/kg 2 to 3 times weekly for first 2 to 3 months for severe disease (maximum single dose for age >50 years: 500 mg) (Griffith 2007)

***Mycobacterium avium* complex (MAC) disease, disseminated in HIV-infected patients (off-label use):** IM, IV: 1 g daily as optional adjunct therapy with ethambutol (plus clarithromycin or azithromycin) (HHS [OI adult 2015])

***Mycobacterium kansasii* disease (rifampin-resistant) (off-label use):** IM: 750 mg to 1 g daily (as part of a three-drug regimen based on susceptibilities) (Campbell 2000; Griffith 2007)

***Mycobacterium ulcerans* (Buruli ulcers) (off-label use):** IM: 15 mg/kg once daily (maximum dose: 1 g) in combination with rifampin for 8 weeks or in combination with rifampin for 4 weeks, followed by 4 weeks of rifampin and clarithromycin (WHO 2012)

Plague: IM:

Manufacturer's labeling: 1 g twice daily for a minimum of 10 days.

Alternate dosing: 30 mg/kg/day (maximum dose: 2 g) divided every 12 hours until the patient is afebrile for at least 2 to 3 days. **Note:** Full course is considered 10 days (CDC 2014; WHO 2009).

Tuberculosis:

Manufacturer's labeling: IM:

Daily therapy: 15 mg/kg/day (maximum: 1 g)

Directly observed therapy (DOT), twice weekly: 25 to 30 mg/kg (maximum: 1.5 g)

Directly observed therapy (DOT), 3 times weekly: 25 to 30 mg/kg (maximum: 1.5 g)

Alternate dosing: IM, IV: 15 mg/kg (maximum dose: 1 g) once daily for 5 to 7 days per week for 2 to 4 months, followed by 15 mg/kg (maximum dose: 1 g) 2 to 3 times weekly (ATS 2003)

Tularemia: IM:

Manufacturer's labeling: 1 to 2 g daily in divided doses every 12 hours for 7 to 14 days until the patients is afebrile for 5 to 7 days

Alternative regimen: 2 g daily in 2 divided doses for ≥10 days (WHO 2007)

Geriatric

Manufacturer's labeling: IM: Dose reductions are necessary in patients >60 years.

Endocarditis, streptococcal: 500 mg every 12 hours for 2 weeks.

Alternate dosing: Tuberculosis: >59 years: IM, IV: 10 mg/kg (maximum: 750 mg) once daily for 5 to 7 days per week for 2 to 4 months, followed by 10 mg/kg (maximum: 750 mg) 2 to 3 times weekly (ATS 2003)

Pediatric Note: Manufacturer's labeling states for IM administration only, however, IV administration (off-label route) has been described (Morris 1994; Peloquin 1992; Tanoira 2014).

Usual dosage range: Infants, Children, and Adolescents: IM: 20 to 40 mg/kg/day in divided doses every 6 to 12 hours (maximum: 1,000 mg/dose; maximum daily dose: 2,000 mg)

Indication-specific dosing: Infants, Children, and Adolescents:

Endocarditis, enterococcal (susceptible to penicillin, vancomycin, and streptomycin and resistant to gentamicin) (off-label use): IM, IV: 20 to 30 mg/kg/day in divided doses every 12 hours (maximum daily dose: 2,000 mg/day) for 4 to 6 weeks (minimum of 6 weeks for prosthetic valves) in combination with ampicillin, penicillin, or vancomycin (Baddour 2005).

Mycobacterium avium **complex (MAC) disease, disseminated in HIV-infected patients (off-label use):** Adolescents: Refer to adult dosing.

Mycobacterium ulcerans **(Buruli ulcers) (off-label use):** IM: 15 mg/kg once daily (maximum daily dose: 1,000 mg) in combination with rifampin for 8 weeks or in combination with rifampin for 4 weeks, followed by 4 weeks of rifampin and clarithromycin (WHO 2012)

Plague (off-label use): IM: 30 mg/kg/day divided every 12 hours (maximum daily dose: 2,000 mg) for 10 days or until 2 to 3 days after the temperature returns to normal (Red Book [AAP 2015]; WHO 2009)

Tularemia (off-label use): IM: 15 mg/kg twice daily (maximum daily dose: 2,000 mg) for 10 days (WHO 2007)

Tuberculosis:

Manufacturer's labeling: IM:

Daily therapy: 20 to 40 mg/kg/day (maximum: 1,000 mg daily)

Directly observed therapy (DOT), twice weekly: 25 to 30 mg/kg (maximum: 1,500 mg)

Directly observed therapy (DOT), 3 times weekly: 25 to 30 mg/kg (maximum: 1,500 mg)

Alternate dosing: IM, IV:

Infants, Children ≤40 kg, and Adolescents <15 years or ≤40 kg:

Daily therapy: 20 to 40 mg/kg/day once daily (maximum daily dose: 1,000 mg) (ATS 2003; WHO 2009). **Note:** Some clinicians suggest every 12 hour dosing may be utilized (Berenberg 1951; Bradley 2015)

Directly observed therapy (DOT), twice weekly: 20 mg/kg/dose twice weekly (maximum daily dose: 1,000 mg/dose) (ATS 2003)

Children and Adolescents >40 kg or ≥15 years: 15 mg/kg/day once daily (maximum daily dose: 1,000 mg) for 5 to 7 days per week for 2 to 4 months, followed by 15 mg/kg/day (maximum daily dose: 1,000 mg) 2 to 3 times weekly (ATS 2003)

Renal Impairment There are no dosage adjustments provided in the manufacturer's labeling; however, the following adjustments have been recommended:

Adults:

Aronoff 2007: **Note:** Recommendations are based on doses of 1 to 2 g every 6 to 12 hours (1 g once daily for tuberculosis):

CrCl >50 mL/minute: No dosage adjustment necessary.

CrCl 10 to 50 mL/minute: Administer every 24 to 72 hours.

CrCl <10 mL/minute: Administer every 72 to 96 hours.

End-stage renal disease (ESRD):

Intermittent hemodialysis (IHD): One-half the recommended dose administered after hemodialysis on dialysis days. Note: Dosing dependent on the assumption of 3 times weekly complete IHD sessions.

Peritoneal dialysis (PD): Administration via PD fluid: 20 to 40 mg/L (20 to 40 mcg/mL) of PD fluid

Continuous renal replacement therapy (CRRT): Administer every 24 to 72 hours; monitor levels. Note: Drug clearance is highly dependent on the method of renal replacement, filter type, and flow rate. Appropriate dosing requires close monitoring of pharmacologic response, signs of adverse reactions due to drug accumulation, as well as drug concentrations in relation to target trough (if appropriate).

ATS 2003:

Tuberculosis:

CrCl ≥30 mL/minute: No dosage adjustment necessary.

CrCl <30 mL/minute: 12 to 15 mg/kg/dose (maximum dose: 1 g) 2 to 3 times weekly

End-stage renal disease (ESRD) on intermittent hemodialysis (IHD): 12 to 15 mg/kg/dose (maximum dose: 1 g) 2 to 3 times weekly.

Infants, Children, and Adolescents: **Note:** Recommendations are based on doses of 20 to 40 mg/kg/dose every 24 hours (Aronoff 2007)

GFR >50 mL/minute/1.73 m^2: No dosage adjustment necessary.

GFR 30 to 50 mL/minute/1.73 m^2: 7.5 mg/kg/dose every 24 hours.

GFR 10 to 29 mL/minute/1.73 m^2: 7.5 mg/kg/dose every 48 hours.

GFR <10 mL/minute/1.73 m^2: 7.5 mg/kg/dose every 72 to 96 hours.

End-stage renal disease (ESRD):

Intermittent hemodialysis (IHD): 7.5 mg/kg/dose every 72 to 96 hours

Peritoneal dialysis (PD): Administer 7.5 mg/kg/dose every 72 to 96 hours

Continuous renal replacement therapy (CRRT): Administer 7.5 mg/kg/dose every 24 hours; monitor levels. **Note:** Drug clearance is highly dependent on the method of renal replacement, filter type, and flow rate. Appropriate dosing requires close monitoring of pharmacologic response, signs of adverse reactions due to drug accumulation, as well as drug concentrations in relation to target trough (if appropriate).

Hepatic Impairment There are no dosage adjustments provided in the manufacturer's labeling.

Administration

IM: Inject deep IM into large muscle mass; midlateral thigh muscle (preferred site for children); midlateral thigh muscle or upper outer quadrant of buttocks (adults); rotate injection sites.

IV (off-label route): After dilution in admixture, infuse over 30 to 60 minutes (Morris 1994; Peloquin 1992; Tanoira 2014)

Monitoring Parameters Baseline and periodic hearing tests (audiograms), BUN, creatinine; serum drug concentrations should be monitored in all patients

Reference Range Therapeutic: Peak: 20 to 30 mcg/mL; Trough: <5 mcg/mL (Edson 1991); Toxic: Peak: >50 mcg/mL; Trough: >10 mcg/mL

Dosage Forms Excipient information presented when available (limited, particularly for generics); consult specific product labeling.

Solution Reconstituted, Intramuscular:

Generic: 1 g (1 ea)

Succimer (SUKS si mer)

Brand Names: US Chemet
Brand Names: Canada Chemet
Index Terms DMSA
Pharmacologic Category Antidote
Use Treatment of lead poisoning in children with serum lead levels >45 mcg/dL
Dosing

Adult & Geriatric Lead poisoning (off-label use; Kosnett, 2007): For the treatment of high blood lead levels in adults, chelation therapy is recommended with blood lead levels >50 mcg/dL and significant symptoms; chelation therapy may also be indicated with blood lead levels ≥100 mcg/dL and/or symptoms.

Oral: Consider using labeled dose for children: 10 mg/kg/dose (or 350 mg/m^2/dose) every 8 hours for 5 days, followed by 10 mg/kg/dose (or 350 mg/m^2/dose) every 12 hours for 14 days; Maximum: 500 mg/dose.

Note: Treatment courses may be repeated, but 2-week intervals between courses is generally recommended.

Pediatric Lead poisoning: For the treatment of high blood lead levels in children, the CDC recommends chelation treatment when blood lead levels are >45 mcg/dL (CDC, 2002). Children with blood lead levels >70 mcg/dL or symptomatic lead poisoning should be treated with parenteral agents (AAP, 2005).

Oral: 10 mg/kg/dose (or 350 mg/m^2/dose) every 8 hours for 5 days followed by 10 mg/kg/dose (or 350 mg/m^2/dose) every 12 hours for 14 days. Maximum: 500 mg/dose.

Note: Treatment courses may be repeated, but 2-week intervals between courses is generally recommended.

Renal Impairment No dosage adjustment provided in the manufacturer's labeling; use with caution. Succimer is dialyzable; however, the lead chelates are not.

Hepatic Impairment No dosage adjustment provided in the manufacturer's labeling; has not been studied. More frequent monitoring of serum transaminases may be required in patients with a history of liver disease due to the risk of transient increases.

Adjustment for Toxicity ANC <1200 mm^3: The manufacturer recommends withholding treatment; treatment may be cautiously resumed when ANC returns to baseline or >1500/mm^3. Consultation with a medical toxicologist to determine the risk versus benefit of withholding treatment is recommended.

Additional Information Complete prescribing information should be consulted for additional detail.

Dosage Forms Excipient information presented when available (limited, particularly for generics); consult specific product labeling.

Capsule, Oral:

Chemet: 100 mg

Succinylcholine (suks in il KOE leen)

Brand Names: US Anectine; Quelicin; Quelicin-1000
Brand Names: Canada Quelicin
Index Terms Succinylcholine Chloride; Suxamethonium Chloride
Pharmacologic Category Neuromuscular Blocker Agent, Depolarizing
Use
Neuromuscular blockade: As an adjunct to general anesthesia, to facilitate tracheal intubation, and to provide skeletal muscle relaxation during surgery or mechanical ventilation.
Note: Does not relieve pain or produce sedation
Pregnancy Considerations Animal reproduction studies have not been conducted. Small amounts cross the placenta. Sensitivity to succinylcholine may be increased due to a ~24% decrease in plasma cholinesterase activity during pregnancy and several days postpartum.
Breast-Feeding Considerations It is not known if succinylcholine is excreted in breast milk. The manufacturer recommends that caution be exercised when administering succinylcholine to nursing women.
Contraindications
Hypersensitivity to succinylcholine or any component of the formulation; personal or familial history of malignant hyperthermia; skeletal muscle myopathies; acute phase of injury following major burns, multiple trauma, extensive denervation of skeletal muscle, or upper motor neuron injury.
Documentation of allergenic cross-reactivity for neuromuscular blockers is limited. However, because of similarities in chemical structure and/or pharmacologic actions, the possibility of cross-sensitivity cannot be ruled out with certainty.
Warnings/Precautions [US Boxed Warning]: Use caution in children and adolescents. Acute rhabdomyolysis with hyperkalemia, ventricular arrhythmias and cardiac arrest have been reported (rarely) in children with undiagnosed skeletal muscle myopathy (eg, Duchenne muscular dystrophy); occurs soon after administration and requires immediate treatment of hyperkalemia. Prolonged resuscitation may be required. Use in children should be reserved for emergency intubation, when immediate airway control is necessary (eg, laryngospasm, difficult airway, full stomach), or IM use when a suitable vein is inaccessible. Respiratory alkalosis, hypercalcemia, demyelinating lesions, peripheral neuropathies, denervation, muscle trauma, and diabetes mellitus may result in antagonism of neuromuscular blockade (Greenberg, 2013; Miller, 2010; Murray, 2002; Naguib, 2002). Electrolyte abnormalities (eg, severe hypocalcemia, severe hypokalemia, hypermagnesemia), neuromuscular diseases, metabolic acidosis, respiratory acidosis, Eaton-Lambert syndrome and myasthenia gravis may result in potentiation of neuromuscular blockade (Greenberg, 2013; Miller, 2010; Naguib, 2002). May increase vagal tone.

Succinylcholine is metabolized by plasma cholinesterase; use with caution (if at all) in patients suspected of being homozygous for the atypical plasma cholinesterase gene. Plasma cholinesterase activity may also be reduced by burns, anemia, decompensated heart disease, infections,

malignant tumors, myxedema, pregnancy, severe hepatic or renal dysfunction, peptic ulcer, and certain medications and chemicals.

Use with caution in patients with extensive or severe burns; risk of hyperkalemia is increased following injury. Onset of time and duration of risk are variable, but risk is generally greatest 7-10 days after injury. Resistance may occur in burn patients (≥20% of total body surface area), usually several days after the injury, and may persist for several months after wound healing (Han, 2009). May increase intraocular pressure; avoid use in patients in which an increase in IOP is undesirable (eg, narrow-angle glaucoma, penetrating eye injuries). Risk of bradycardia may be increased with second dose and may occur more in children. Occurrence may be reduced by pretreating with anticholinergic agents (eg, atropine). Use may be associated with acute onset of malignant hyperthermia; risk may be increased with concomitant administration of volatile anesthetics. Use with caution in the elderly; effects and duration are more variable.

Severe anaphylactic reactions (some life-threatening and fatal) have been reported. Cross-sensitivity with other neuromuscular-blocking agents may occur; use extreme caution in patients with previous anaphylactic reactions. May cause a transient increase in intracranial pressure (adequate anesthetic induction prior to administration of succinylcholine will minimize this effect). May increase intragastric pressure, which could result in regurgitation and possible aspiration of stomach contents. Use with caution in patients with fractures or muscle spasm; initial muscle fasciculations may cause additional trauma. Use with extreme caution in patients with preexisting hyperkalemia. Severe hyperkalemia may develop in patients with chronic abdominal infections, burn injuries, multiple trauma, extensive denervation of skeletal muscle, upper motor neuron injury, subarachnoid hemorrhage, or conditions which cause degeneration of the central and peripheral nervous system.

Maintenance of an adequate airway and respiratory support is critical. If possible, to avoid distress to the patient, do not administer before unconsciousness has been induced. Should be administered by adequately trained individuals familiar with its use. Potentially significant interactions may exist, requiring dose or frequency adjustment, additional monitoring, and/or selection of alternative therapy.

Adverse Reactions Frequency not defined.
Cardiovascular: Arrhythmias, bradycardia (higher with second dose, more frequent in children), cardiac arrest, hyper-/hypotension, tachycardia
Dermatologic: Rash
Endocrine & metabolic: Hyperkalemia
Gastrointestinal: Salivation (excessive)
Neuromuscular & skeletal: Jaw rigidity, muscle fasciculation, postoperative muscle pain, rhabdomyolysis (with possible myoglobinuric acute renal failure)
Ocular: Intraocular pressure increased
Renal: Acute renal failure (secondary to rhabdomyolysis)
Respiratory: Apnea, respiratory depression (prolonged)
Miscellaneous: Anaphylaxis, malignant hyperthermia
Postmarketing and/or case reports: Acute quadriplegic myopathy syndrome (prolonged use), myositis ossificans (prolonged use)
Drug Interactions
Metabolism/Transport Effects None known.
Avoid Concomitant Use
Avoid concomitant use of Succinylcholine with any of the following: QuiNINE
Increased Effect/Toxicity
Succinylcholine may increase the levels/effects of: Analgesics (Opioid); Cardiac Glycosides; OnabotulinumtoxinA; RimabotulinumtoxinB

The levels/effects of Succinylcholine may be increased by: AbobotulinumtoxinA; Acetylcholinesterase Inhibitors; Aminoglycosides; Bambuterol; Capreomycin; Clindamycin (Topical); Colistimethate; Cyclophosphamide; CycloSPORINE (Systemic); Echothiophate Iodide; Lincosamide Antibiotics; Lithium; Loop Diuretics; Magnesium Salts; Minocycline; Phenelzine; Polymyxin B; Procainamide; QuiNIDine; QuiNINE; Tetracycline Derivatives; Vancomycin
Decreased Effect
The levels/effects of Succinylcholine may be decreased by: Loop Diuretics
Storage/Stability Manufacturer recommends refrigeration at 2°C to 8°C (36°F to 46°F) and may be stored at room temperature for 14 days; however, additional testing has demonstrated stability for ≤6 months unrefrigerated (25°C) (Ross, 1988; Roy, 2008). Stability in polypropylene

syringes (20 mg/mL) at room temperature (25°C) is 45 days (Storms, 2003).

Mechanism of Action Acts similar to acetylcholine, produces depolarization of the motor endplate at the myoneural junction which causes sustained flaccid skeletal muscle paralysis produced by state of accommodation that develops in adjacent excitable muscle membranes

Pharmacodynamics/Kinetics

Onset of action: IM: 2 to 3 minutes; IV: Flaccid paralysis: <60 seconds

Duration: IV: 4 to 6 minutes with single administration

Metabolism: Rapidly hydrolyzed by plasma pseudocholinesterase

Excretion: Urine (~10% excreted unchanged)

Dosing

Adult & Geriatric Neuromuscular blockade: Dose to effect; doses will vary due to interpatient variability. Use carefully and/or consider dose reduction in patients with reduced plasma cholinesterase activity due to genetic abnormalities of plasma cholinesterase or when associated with other conditions (eg, electrolyte abnormalities, neuromuscular disease); prolonged neuromuscular blockade may occur.

IM: Up to 3 to 4 mg/kg, maximum total dose: 150 mg
IV:

Intubation: 0.6 mg/kg (range: 0.3 to 1.1 mg/kg)

Intubation (rapid sequence) (off-label dosing): 1 to 1.5 mg/kg (Sluga 2005; Weiss 1997)

Long surgical procedures (intermittent administration): Initial: 0.3 to 1.1 mg/kg; administer 0.04 to 0.07 mg/kg at appropriate intervals as needed.

Note: Pretreatment with atropine may reduce occurrence of bradycardia. Initial dose of succinylcholine must be increased when nondepolarizing agent pretreatment used because of the antagonism between succinylcholine and nondepolarizing neuromuscular-blocking agents (Miller, 2010).

Pediatric Neuromuscular blockade: Dose to effect; doses will vary due to interpatient variability. Use carefully and/or consider dose reduction in patients with reduced plasma cholinesterase activity due to genetic abnormalities of plasma cholinesterase or when associated with other conditions (eg, electrolyte abnormalities, neuromuscular disease); prolonged neuromuscular blockade may occur.

IM: Refer to adult dosing.
IV:

Neonates, Infants ≤6 months: Intubation: 2 to 3 mg/kg/dose

Infants >6 months and Children ≤2 years: Intubation: 1 to 2 mg/kg/dose

Older Children and Adolescents: Intubation: 1 mg/kg/dose

Note: Pretreatment with atropine may reduce occurrence of bradycardia. Initial dose of succinylcholine must be increased when nondepolarizing agent pretreatment used because of the antagonism between succinylcholine and nondepolarizing neuromuscular-blocking agents (Miller, 2010).

Renal Impairment There are no dosage adjustments provided in the manufacturer's labeling.

Hepatic Impairment There are no dosage adjustments provided in the manufacturer's labeling.

Obesity Use total body weight for obese patients (Bentley, 1982; Brunette, 2004; Rose, 2000).

Administration

IM: Administer deep IM only when IV access is not available.

IV: May be administered undiluted by rapid IV injection.

Monitoring Parameters Monitor cardiac, blood pressure, and oxygenation during administration; temperature, serum potassium and calcium, assisted ventilator status; neuromuscular function with a peripheral nerve stimulator

Dosage Forms Excipient information presented when available (limited, particularly for generics); consult specific product labeling.

Solution, Injection, as chloride:

Anectine: 20 mg/mL (10 mL) [contains methylparaben]

Quelicin: 20 mg/mL (10 mL) [contains methylparaben, propylparaben]

Quelicin-1000: 100 mg/mL (10 mL)

♦ Succinylcholine Chloride see Succinylcholine on page 1703

♦ Suclear™ [DSC] see Sodium Sulfate, Potassium Sulfate, Magnesium Sulfate, and Polyethylene Glycol-Electrolyte Solution on page 1682

♦ Sucraid see Sacrosidase on page 1630

♦ Sucraid® (Can) see Sacrosidase on page 1630

Sucralfate (soo KRAL fate)

Brand Names: US Carafate

Brand Names: Canada Apo-Sucralfate; Dom-Sucralfate; Novo-Sucralate; Nu-Sucralate; PMS-Sucralate; Sucralfate-1; Sulcrate®; Sulcrate® Suspension Plus; Teva-Sucralfate

Index Terms Aluminum Sucrose Sulfate, Basic

Pharmacologic Category Gastrointestinal Agent, Miscellaneous

Use Short-term (≤8 weeks) management of duodenal ulcers; maintenance therapy for duodenal ulcers

Dosing

Adult & Geriatric Treatment of duodenal ulcer: Oral:

Initial treatment: 1 g 4 times daily on an empty stomach for 4-8 weeks

Maintenance/prophylaxis of duodenal ulcer: 1 g twice daily

Pediatric Doses of 40-80 mg/kg/day divided every 6 hours have been used

Renal Impairment No dosage adjustment provided in manufacturer's labeling. Aluminum salt is minimally absorbed; however, may accumulate in renal impairment; use with caution in patients with chronic renal failure.

Hepatic Impairment No dosage adjustment provided in manufacturer's labeling.

Additional Information Complete prescribing information should be consulted for additional detail.

Dosage Forms Excipient information presented when available (limited, particularly for generics); consult specific product labeling.

Suspension, Oral:

Carafate: 1 g/10 mL (420 mL) [contains fd&c red #40, methylparaben; cherry flavor]

Tablet, Oral:

Carafate: 1 g [scored; contains fd&c blue #1 aluminum lake]

Generic: 1 g

♦ Sucralfate-1 (Can) see Sucralfate on page 1704

♦ Sucrets® Children's [OTC] see Dyclonine on page 613

♦ Sucrets® Maximum Strength [OTC] see Dyclonine on page 613

♦ Sucrets® Regular Strength [OTC] see Dyclonine on page 613

Sucroferric Oxyhydroxide (soo kroe FER ik ox ee hye DROX ide)

Brand Names: US Velphoro

Index Terms PA21; Polynuclear Iron (III)-Oxyhydroxide (pn-FeOOH)

Pharmacologic Category Phosphate Binder

Use Hyperphosphatemia: For control of serum phosphorus levels in patients with chronic kidney disease (CKD) receiving dialysis

Pregnancy Considerations Adverse events were not observed in most animal reproduction studies. Maternal systemic absorption of sucroferric oxyhydroxide is low

Breast-Feeding Considerations It is not known if sucroferric oxyhydroxide is excreted into breast milk; however, because maternal systemic absorption is limited, it is unlikely

Contraindications There are no contraindications listed in the manufacturer's labeling.

Warnings/Precautions Patients with significant gastrointestinal (GI) disorders or hepatic disorders, post major GI surgery, peritonitis during peritoneal dialysis, or with a history of hemochromatosis or other conditions associated with iron accumulation were not included in clinical studies; monitor effect and iron homeostasis in these patients. Chew tablets thoroughly to decrease risk of adverse GI effects; do not swallow whole. Potentially significant interactions may exist, requiring dose or frequency adjustment, additional monitoring, and/or selection of alternative therapy.

Adverse Reactions

>10%: Gastrointestinal: Diarrhea (4% to 24%), darkening of stools (12% to 16%)

1% to 10%: Gastrointestinal: Nausea (2% to 10%), dysgeusia (2%)

Drug Interactions

Metabolism/Transport Effects None known.

Avoid Concomitant Use

Avoid concomitant use of Sucroferric Oxyhydroxide with any of the following: Levothyroxine

Increased Effect/Toxicity There are no known significant interactions involving an increase in effect.

Decreased Effect
Sucroferric Oxyhydroxide may decrease the levels/ effects of: Levothyroxine; Tetracycline Derivatives

Storage/Stability Store at 25°C (77°F); excursions are permitted between 15°C and 30°C (59°F and 86°F). Protect from moisture.

Mechanism of Action Binds phosphate in the aqueous environment of the GI tract via ligand exchange between hydroxyl groups and/or water in sucroferric oxyhydroxide and dietary phosphate. Reduced dietary phosphate absorption results in reduced serum phosphorus levels and calcium-phosphorus product levels.

Pharmacodynamics/Kinetics
Absorption: Not systemically absorbed
Metabolism: Not metabolized
Excretion: Feces (as bound phosphate)

Dosing
Adult Hyperphosphatemia: Oral: Initial: 500 mg iron 3 times daily with meals. May titrate weekly (beginning 1 week after initiation) in increments or decrements of 500 mg iron per day as needed to appropriate serum phosphorus levels (≤5.5 mg/dL); usual maintenance dose: 1.5 to 2 g iron daily; doses of up to 3 g iron daily have been evaluated.

Renal Impairment There are no dosage adjustments provided in the manufacturer's labeling; however, not systemically absorbed or metabolized.

Hepatic Impairment There are no dosage adjustments provided in the manufacturer's labeling; however, not systemically absorbed or metabolized.

Administration Tablets must be chewed; do not swallow whole. Tablets may be crushed to aid with chewing and swallowing. Must administer with meals. The total daily dose should be divided among meals.

Monitoring Parameters Serum phosphorus levels

Dosage Forms Excipient information presented when available (limited, particularly for generics); consult specific product labeling.
Tablet Chewable, Oral:
Velphoro: 500 mg [berry flavor]

♦ Sudafed *see* Pseudoephedrine *on page 1527*

♦ Sudafed [OTC] *see* Pseudoephedrine *on page 1527*

♦ Sudafed 12 Hour [OTC] *see* Pseudoephedrine *on page 1527*

♦ Sudafed 24 Hour [OTC] *see* Pseudoephedrine *on page 1527*

♦ Sudafed Childrens [OTC] *see* Pseudoephedrine *on page 1527*

♦ Sudafed® Children's Cold & Cough [OTC] *see* Pseudoephedrine and Dextromethorphan *on page 1528*

♦ Sudafed® Decongestant (Can) *see* Pseudoephedrine *on page 1527*

♦ Sudafed PE Childrens [OTC] *see* Phenylephrine (Systemic) *on page 1442*

♦ Sudafed PE® Children's Cold & Cough [OTC] *see* Dextromethorphan and Phenylephrine *on page 535*

♦ Sudafed PE Maximum Strength [OTC] *see* Phenylephrine (Systemic) *on page 1442*

♦ Sudafed PE® Non-Drying Sinus [OTC] *see* Guaifenesin and Phenylephrine *on page 862*

♦ Sudafed PE Sinus/Allergy [OTC] *see* Chlorpheniramine and Phenylephrine *on page 376*

♦ Sudafed Sinus Advance (Can) *see* Pseudoephedrine and Ibuprofen *on page 1528*

♦ Sudanyl [OTC] *see* Pseudoephedrine *on page 1527*

♦ SudoGest [OTC] *see* Pseudoephedrine *on page 1527*

♦ SudoGest 12 Hour [OTC] *see* Pseudoephedrine *on page 1527*

♦ Sudogest PE [OTC] *see* Phenylephrine (Systemic) *on page 1442*

♦ SudoGest™ Sinus & Allergy [OTC] *see* Chlorpheniramine and Pseudoephedrine *on page 377*

♦ Sufenta *see* SUFentanil *on page 1705*

SUFentanil (soo FEN ta nil)

Brand Names: US Sufenta
Brand Names: Canada Sufenta; Sufentanil Citrate Injection, USP
Index Terms Sufentanil Citrate
Pharmacologic Category Analgesic, Opioid; Anilidopiperidine Opioid; General Anesthetic
Use
Epidural analgesia: For epidural administration as an analgesic combined with low-dose bupivacaine during labor and vaginal delivery.

Surgical analgesia: Analgesic adjunct for the maintenance of balanced general anesthesia in patients who are intubated and ventilated.

Surgical anesthesia: As a primary anesthetic agent for the induction and maintenance of anesthesia with 100% oxygen in patients undergoing major surgical procedures; in patients who are intubated and ventilated, such as cardiovascular surgery or neurosurgical procedures in the sitting position; to provide favorable myocardial and cerebral oxygen balance or when extended postoperative ventilation is anticipated.

Dosing
Adult
Surgical analgesia (as a component of balanced anesthesia) (surgery expected to last: 1 to 2 hours): IV: Total dose: 1 to 2 mcg/kg with N_2O/O_2; ≥75% of total dose may be administered by slow injection or infusion prior to intubation (titrate to individual response)
Maintenance:
Incremental dosing: According to the manufacturer, 10 to 25 mcg may be administered as needed when movement and/or changes in vital signs indicate surgical stress or lightening of analgesia. May also administer doses in the range of 5 to 20 mcg as needed (Barash, 2009) **or** 0.1 to 0.25 mcg/**kg** as needed (Miller, 2010). Total dose should not exceed 1 mcg/kg/hour of expected surgical time.
Continuous infusion: May also be administered as a continuous infusion with the infusion rate based on the induction dose used. Maximum infusion rate according to the manufacturer: 1 mcg/kg/hour. May also administer doses in the range of 0.3 to 0.9 mcg/kg/hour (Barash, 2009) **or** 0.5 to 1.5 mcg/kg/hour (Miller, 2010).

Surgical analgesia (as a component of balanced anesthesia) (surgery expected to last 2 to 8 hours): Total dose: 2 to 8 mcg/kg with N_2O/O_2; ≤75% of total dose may be administered by slow injection or infusion prior to intubation (titrate to individual response).
Maintenance:
Incremental dosing: According to the manufacturer, 10 to 50 mcg may be administered as needed when movement and/or changes in vital signs indicate surgical stress or lightening of analgesia. Total dose should not exceed 1 mcg/kg/hour of expected surgical time.
Continuous infusion: May also be administered as a continuous infusion with the infusion rate based on the induction dose used. Maximum infusion rate according to the manufacturer: 1 mcg/kg/hour. May also administer doses in the range of 0.3 to 0.9 mcg/kg/hour (Barash, 2009) **or** 0.5 to 1.5 mcg/kg/hour (Miller, 2010).

Surgical anesthesia: Total dose: 8 to 30 mcg/kg as a slow injection, infusion, or injection followed by infusion; titrate to individual patient response. **Note:** In patients administered high doses of sufentanil, qualified personnel and adequate facilities are necessary to manage the potential for postoperative respiratory depression.
Maintenance:
Incremental dosing: 0.5 to 10 mcg/kg as needed in anticipation of surgical stress
Continuous infusion: Base infusion rate on the induction dose so that the total dose for the procedure does not exceed 30 mcg/kg

Analgesia for labor and delivery: Epidural: 10 to 15 mcg with bupivacaine 0.125% with/without epinephrine. Dose can be repeated twice (for a total of 3 doses) at not less than 1-hour intervals until delivery.

Geriatric Dosage should be reduced. Refer to adult dosing.

Pediatric Surgical anesthesia (cardiovascular surgery): IV: Children <12 years: Induction: 10 to 25 mcg/kg with 100% O_2; maintenance: up to 25 to 50 mcg based on response to initial dose and as determined by changes in vital signs indicating surgical stress or lightening of anesthesia.

Renal Impairment There are no dosage adjustments provided in the manufacturer's labeling. Use with caution.

Hepatic Impairment There are no dosage adjustments provided in the manufacturer's labeling. Use with caution.

Obesity IV: In adult obese patients (eg, >20% above ideal body weight), use lean body weight to determine dosage.

Additional Information Complete prescribing information should be consulted for additional detail.

Dosage Forms Excipient information presented when available (limited, particularly for generics); consult specific product labeling. [DSC] = Discontinued product
Solution, Intravenous:
Generic: 50 mcg/mL (1 mL [DSC]); 100 mcg/2 mL (2 mL [DSC]); 250 mcg/5 mL (5 mL [DSC])

Solution, Intravenous [preservative free]:
Sufenta: 50 mcg/mL (1 mL); 100 mcg/2 mL (2 mL); 250 mcg/5 mL (5 mL)
Generic: 50 mcg/mL (1 mL); 100 mcg/2 mL (2 mL); 250 mcg/5 mL (5 mL)

Controlled Substance C-II

◆ Sufentanil Citrate see SUFentanil on page 1705
◆ Sufentanil Citrate Injection, USP (Can) see SUFentanil on page 1705

Sugammadex (soo GAM ma dex)

Index Terms Bridion; ORG-25969; Sugammadex Sodium
Pharmacologic Category Antidote; Selective Relaxant Binding Agent
Use
Reversal of rocuronium or vecuronium: For the reversal of neuromuscular blockade induced by rocuronium or vecuronium in adults undergoing surgery
Limitations of use: Sugammadex has not been evaluated for reversal of rocuronium or vecuronium in the intensive care unit. Do not use sugammadex for neuromuscular blockade induced by nonsteroidal neuromuscular blocking agents (eg, succinylcholine or benzylisoquinolinium compounds) or steroidal agents other than rocuronium or vecuronium.

Pregnancy Considerations Adverse events were observed in some animal reproduction studies. Limited information is available related to the use of sugammadex for the reversal of rocuronium-induced neuromuscular blockade after cesarean section (Pühringer 2010; Stourac 2013). The effects of hormonal contraception may be decreased following sugammadex administration. An additional nonhormonal contraceptive (eg, condom, spermicide) should be used for 7 days after a dose of sugammadex in women using oral or non-oral hormonal contraception.

Breast-Feeding Considerations It is not known if sugammadex is excreted into breast milk. According to the manufacturer, the decision to breastfeed after therapy should take into account the risk of exposure to the infant and the benefits of treatment to the mother.

Contraindications Hypersensitivity to sugammadex or any component of the formulation

Warnings/Precautions Marked bradycardia and bradycardia with cardiac arrest have been reported, usually within minutes after administration of sugammadex. Monitor closely for hemodynamic changes during and after reversal of neuromuscular blockade and use appropriate pharmacologic treatment (eg, atropine) if significant bradycardia occurs. Hypersensitivity reactions (including anaphylaxis) have been reported (uncommonly); symptoms include flushing, urticaria, erythematous rash as well as severe hypotension, tachycardia, oropharyngeal/tongue edema, and acute bronchospasm. May occur in patients without prior exposure to sugammadex. Recurrence of neuromuscular blockade has occurred in controlled trials, usually associated with suboptimal dosing. After initial reversal with sugammadex, continue respiratory monitoring and ensure adequate ventilator support remains accessible following extubation. Potentiation of neuromuscular blockade by other drugs used in the post-operative period should also be considered for the possibility of recurrence. Since other drugs (eg, opioids) used in the peri- and post-operative period may depress respiratory function, ventilatory support is mandatory until adequate spontaneous respiration is restored and ability to maintain a patent airway is assured. In addition, some patients experience a delayed or minimal response to recommended doses of sugammadex.

Use caution in patients with or at risk for impaired hemostasis (eg, coagulopathies, severe liver impairment, or concurrent use of anticoagulants at therapeutic doses). Dose-dependent transient increases in activated partial thromboplastin time (aPTT) and normalized prothrombin time (PT[INR]) have been observed. In clinical trials, significant effects on bleeding were not observed with low-dose sugammadex alone or in conjunction with therapeutic anticoagulation; high-risk patients and those receiving high-dose sugammadex were not adequately studied. Careful monitoring of hemostatic and coagulation parameters is recommended. Use caution with severe hepatic impairment (has not been studied) due to potential effects on hemostasis. Use is not recommended in patients with severe renal impairment (CrCl <30 mL/minute) or on dialysis. Potentially significant drug-drug interactions may exist, requiring dose or frequency adjustment, additional monitoring, and/or selection of alternative therapy. Use caution in patients with cardiovascular disease and in elderly patients; reversal time may be delayed.

Use in intensive care (ICU) setting has not been evaluated. Not indicated for reversal of neuromuscular-blocking agents other than rocuronium or vecuronium. Must be administered under supervision of experienced anesthetist familiar with its use. Signs of light anesthesia (eg, coughing, grimacing, or suckling of tracheal tube) may become apparent when neuromuscular blockade is reversed intentionally in the middle of anesthesia.

Adverse Reactions
>10%:
Cardiovascular: Hypotension (5% to 13%)
Central nervous system: Headache (10%)
Gastrointestinal: Nausea (26%), vomiting (11% to 15%)
Local: Pain at injection site (48% to 52%)
1% to 10%:
Cardiovascular: Hypertension (9%), prolonged QT interval on ECG (6%), bradycardia (5%), tachycardia (2% to 5%)
Central nervous system: Anesthesia complication (1% to 9%), chills (7%), incisional pain (4% to 6%), dizziness (3% to 6%), insomnia (5%), hypoesthesia (3%), anxiety (1% to 3%), restlessness (1% to 2%), depression (≤2%)
Dermatologic: Pruritus (3%), erythema (2%)
Endocrine & metabolic: Hypocalcemia (2%)
Gastrointestinal: Abdominal pain (4% to 6%), flatulence (3%), xerostomia (≤2%)
Hematologic & oncologic: Wound hemorrhage (2%), decreased red blood cells (1% to 2%)
Neuromuscular & skeletal: Limb pain (6%), musculoskeletal pain (2%), myalgia (2%), increased creatine phosphokinase (1% to 2%), neuromuscular blockade (≤2%; reoccurrence)
Respiratory: Cough (3% to 8%)
Miscellaneous: Fever (5% to 9%), procedural complications (8%), hysterectomy (2%)
<1%, postmarketing, and/or case reports: Anaphylaxis, atrial fibrillation, atrioventricular block, bronchospasm, cardiac arrest, dyspnea, extrasystoles, hypersensitivity, laryngospasm, pulmonary edema, respiratory arrest, ST segment changes on ECG, supraventricular tachycardia, urticaria, ventricular fibrillation, ventricular tachycardia, wheezing

Drug Interactions
Metabolism/Transport Effects None known.
Avoid Concomitant Use There are no known interactions where it is recommended to avoid concomitant use.
Increased Effect/Toxicity
Sugammadex may increase the levels/effects of: Anticoagulants
Decreased Effect
Sugammadex may decrease the levels/effects of: Contraceptives (Estrogens); Contraceptives (Progestins)

The levels/effects of Sugammadex may be decreased by: Fusidic Acid (Systemic); Toremifene

Storage/Stability Store at 25°C (77°F); excursions permitted to 15°C to 30°C (59°F to 86°F). Protect from light. When not protected from light, the vial should be used within 5 days.

Mechanism of Action Sugammadex is a modified gamma cyclodextrin which is a selective relaxant binding agent. It forms a complex with the neuromuscular-blocking agents rocuronium or vecuronium in plasma, reducing the amount of neuromuscular-blocking agent available to bind to nicotinic receptors in the neuromuscular junction. This results in the reversal of neuromuscular blockade induced by rocuronium or vecuronium.

Pharmacodynamics/Kinetics
Onset: <3 minutes
Distribution: V_d: 11 to 14 L
Protein binding: Negligible
Metabolism: Not metabolized
Half-life elimination: Effective: ~2 hours; Prolonged in renal impairment: Mild renal impairment: 4 hours; Moderate renal impairment: 6 hours; Severe renal impairment: 19 hours
Excretion: Urine (95% as unchanged drug)
Dosing
Adult & Geriatric Note: Dosing based on actual body weight.
Routine reversal of rocuronium- or vecuronium-induced blockade: IV:
Deep block (at least 1 to 2 post-tetanic counts but prior to appearance of T_2): 4 mg/kg as a single dose
Moderate block (after appearance of T_2): 2 mg/kg as a single dose

Readministration of rocuronium/vecuronium: Following sugammadex use for routine reversal, waiting times for readministration of rocuronium or vecuronium vary greatly (5 minutes to 24 hours) depending on agent, dose, and renal function (consult product labeling); if immediate neuromuscular blockade is needed, a non-steroidal neuromuscular-blocking agent may be required.

Immediate reversal of rocuronium-induced blockade:
IV: 16 mg/kg as a single dose administered soon (~3 minutes) after administration of a single dose of 1.2 mg/kg of rocuronium. **Note:** This dose of sugammadex has not been evaluated following administration of vecuronium.

Readministration of rocuronium or administration of vecuronium: Following sugammadex use for immediate reversal of rocuronium, wait 24 hours before readministering rocuronium or administering vecuronium. If more immediate neuromuscular blockade is needed, a nonsteroidal neuromuscular-blocking agent may be required.

Renal Impairment
Mild to moderate impairment: No dosage adjustment necessary.
Severe impairment: Use is not recommended.
Dialysis: Use is not recommended.

Hepatic Impairment Mild to severe impairment: There are no dosage adjustments provided in the manufacturer's labeling (has not been studied); use with caution, particularly if accompanied by coagulopathy or severe edema.

Administration IV: Administer as rapid IV push over 10 seconds; if administered in same IV line as other products, flush with saline before and after administration of sugammadex.

Monitoring Parameters Neuromuscular stimulation (eg, post-tetanic counts [PTC] and train-of-four [TOF]); hemostatic and coagulation parameters in select patients; respiratory function during recovery

Test Interactions May interfere with the serum progesterone assay; interaction may be observed for up to 30 minutes after a 16 mg/kg dose of sugammadex.

♦ Sugammadex Sodium see Sugammadex on page 1706
♦ Sulamyd see Sulfacetamide (Ophthalmic) on page 1707
♦ Sulamyd see Sulfacetamide (Topical) on page 1707
♦ Sular see Nisoldipine on page 1285
♦ Sulbactam and Ampicillin see Ampicillin and Sulbactam on page 125

Sulconazole (sul KON a zole)

Brand Names: US Exelderm
Index Terms Sulconazole Nitrate
Pharmacologic Category Antifungal Agent, Imidazole Derivative; Antifungal Agent, Topical
Use Fungal infections:
Cream: Treatment of tinea pedis (athlete's foot), tinea cruris, and tinea corporis caused by *Trichophyton rubrum*, *Trichophyton mentagrophytes*, *Epidermophyton floccosum*, and *Microsporum canis*; treatment of tinea versicolor
Solution: Treatment of tinea cruris and tinea corporis caused by *Trichophyton rubrum*, *Trichophyton mentagrophytes*, *Epidermophyton floccosum*, and *Microsporum canis*; treatment of tinea versicolor
Limitations of use: Effectiveness has not been proven in tinea pedis (athlete's foot).

Dosing
Adult & Geriatric
Tinea corporis/tinea cruris/tinea versicolor: Topical: Apply a small amount to the affected and surrounding skin areas once or twice daily for 3 weeks
Tinea pedis: Topical: Cream: Apply a small amount to the affected area twice daily for 4 weeks

Renal Impairment There are no dosage adjustments provided in the manufacturer's labeling.

Hepatic Impairment There are no dosage adjustments provided in the manufacturer's labeling.

Additional Information Complete prescribing information should be consulted for additional detail.

Dosage Forms Excipient information presented when available (limited, particularly for generics); consult specific product labeling.
Cream, External, as nitrate:
Exelderm: 1% (15 g, 30 g, 60 g) [contains cetyl alcohol, propylene glycol]
Solution, External, as nitrate:
Exelderm: 1% (30 mL) [contains propylene glycol]

♦ Sulconazole Nitrate see Sulconazole on page 1707

♦ Sulcrate® (Can) see Sucralfate on page 1704
♦ Sulcrate® Suspension Plus (Can) see Sucralfate on page 1704

Sulfacetamide (Ophthalmic) (sul fa SEE ta mide)

Brand Names: US Bleph-10
Brand Names: Canada AK Sulf Liq; Bleph 10 DPS; Diosulf; PMS-Sulfacetamide; Sodium Sulamyd
Index Terms Sodium Sulfacetamide; Sulamyd; Sulfacetamide Sodium
Pharmacologic Category Antibiotic, Ophthalmic
Use
Ocular infections:
Ophthalmic ointment and solution: Treatment of conjunctivitis and other superficial ocular infections due to susceptible microorganisms: *Escherichia coli*, *Staphylococcus aureus*, *Streptococcus pneumoniae*, *Streptococcus* (viridans group), *Haemophilus influenzae*, *Klebsiella species*, and *Enterobacter* species.
Ophthalmic solution: Treatment of trachoma as an adjunctive to systemic sulfonamide therapy
Limitations of use: Topically applied sulfonamides do not provide adequate coverage against *Neisseria* species, *Serratia marcescens* and *Pseudomonas aeruginosa*. A significant percentage of staphylococcal isolates are also completely resistant to sulfa drugs.

Dosing
Adult & Geriatric
Conjunctivitis, other superficial ocular infections:
Note: Taper dose by increasing dosage time interval as condition responds; usual duration of treatment: 7 to 10 days:
Ophthalmic solution: Instill 1 to 2 drops every 2 to 3 hours
Ophthalmic ointment: Apply ~1/2-inch ribbon every 3 to 4 hours and at bedtime
Trachoma: Ophthalmic solution: Instill 2 drops every 2 hours; must be used in conjunction with systemic therapy
Pediatric Conjunctivitis, other superficial ocular infections, or trachoma: Infants ≥2 months, Children, and Adolescents: Ophthalmic: Refer to adult dosing.

Additional Information Complete prescribing information should be consulted for additional detail.

Dosage Forms Excipient information presented when available (limited, particularly for generics); consult specific product labeling.
Ointment, Ophthalmic, as sodium:
Generic: 10% (3.5 g)
Solution, Ophthalmic, as sodium:
Bleph-10: 10% (5 mL)
Generic: 10% (5 mL, 15 mL)

Sulfacetamide (Topical) (sul fa SEE ta mide)

Brand Names: US APOP [DSC]; Klaron; Mexar Wash [DSC]; Ovace Plus; Ovace Plus Wash; Ovace Wash; Seb-Prev Wash; Seb-Prev [DSC]
Brand Names: Canada Sulfacet-R
Index Terms Sodium Sulfacetamide; Sulamyd; Sulfacetamide Sodium
Pharmacologic Category Acne Products; Antibiotic, Sulfonamide Derivative; Topical Skin Product, Acne
Use
Acne (Klaron lotion, topical suspension): Treatment of acne vulgaris.
Bacterial infections (cream, wash, Ovace Plus lotion and foam): Treatment of bacterial infections of the skin.
Scaling dermatoses (cream, shampoo, wash, Ovace Plus lotion and foam): Treatment of scaling dermatoses (seborrheic dermatitis and seborrhea sicca [dandruff]).
Dosing
Adult & Geriatric
Acne: Topical: Klaron lotion, topical suspension: Apply thin film to affected area twice daily
Bacterial infections: Topical:
Cream, Ovace Plus lotion: Apply to affected areas twice daily for 8 to 10 days.
Foam: Apply to affected areas 1 to 3 times daily
Wash: Apply to affected areas 1 to 2 times daily for 8 to 10 days.
Scaling dermatoses: Topical:
Cream, Ovace Plus lotion: Apply to affected areas twice daily for 8 to 10 days. Dosing interval may be lengthened as eruption subsides. Applications once or twice weekly, or every other week may be used for prevention. If treatment needs to be reinitiated, start therapy as a twice-daily regimen.
Foam: Apply to affected areas 1 to 3 times daily
Shampoo: Wash hair at least twice weekly.

◄

Wash:

Ovace Plus Wash Liquid, Ovace Plus Wash cleansing gel, Ovace wash: Wash affected areas twice with a 10- to 20-second interval between washings; repeat twice daily for 8 to 10 days. Dosing interval may be lengthened as eruption subsides. Applications once or twice weekly, or every other week may be used for prevention. If treatment needs to be reinitiated, start therapy as a twice-daily regimen.

SEB-Prev: Wash affected areas twice daily for 8 to 10 days. Dosing interval may be lengthened as eruption subsides. Applications once or twice weekly, or every other week may be used for prevention. If treatment needs to be reinitiated, start therapy as a twice-daily regimen.

Pediatric Acne, seborrheic dermatitis, or secondary cutaneous bacterial infections: Topical: Children ≥12 years and Adolescents: Refer to adult dosing.

Additional Information Complete prescribing information should be consulted for additional detail.

Dosage Forms Considerations APOP gel is formulated in a vehicle containing 0.5% bakuchiol, a natural compound extracted from *Psoralea corylifolia* purported to exert antimicrobial and anti-inflammatory activity, as well as reduce scarring from acne lesions.

Dosage Forms Excipient information presented when available (limited, particularly for generics); consult specific product labeling. [DSC] = Discontinued product

Cream, External, as sodium:
Ovace Plus: 10% (57 g) [contains benzyl alcohol, butylparaben, cetyl alcohol, disodium edta, ethylparaben, methylparaben, propylparaben]

Foam, External:
Ovace Plus: 9.8% (100 g) [contains benzyl alcohol, cetyl alcohol, propylene glycol]

Gel, External, as sodium:
APOP: 10% (57 g [DSC]) [contains benzyl alcohol, cetyl alcohol, disodium edta]
Ovace Plus Wash: 10% (355 mL) [contains cetearyl alcohol, edetate disodium dihydrate, methylparaben]
Generic: 10% (355 mL); 10% (355 mL)

Liquid, External, as sodium:
Mexar Wash: 10% (170 mL [DSC]) [contains methylparaben]
Ovace Plus Wash: 10% (180 mL, 473 mL) [contains cetearyl alcohol, edetate disodium, methylparaben]
Ovace Wash: 10% (180 mL, 355 mL, 480 mL) [contains edetate disodium, methylparaben]
Seb-Prev Wash: 10% (340 mL) [contains edetate disodium, methylparaben]
Generic: 10% (177 mL, 354.8 mL, 355 mL, 480 mL)

Lotion, External, as sodium:
Klaron: 10% (118 mL)
Klaron: 10% (118 mL) [contains disodium edta, methylparaben, propylene glycol, sodium metabisulfite]
Ovace Plus: 9.8% (57 g, 113 g) [contains benzyl alcohol, cetyl alcohol, disodium edta]
Seb-Prev: 10% (118 mL [DSC]) [contains methylparaben, sodium metabisulfite]
Generic: 10% (118 mL)

Pad, External, as sodium:
Generic: 10% (30 ea [DSC])

Shampoo, External, as sodium:
Ovace Plus: 10% (237 mL) [contains cetearyl alcohol, methylparaben, propylparaben]
Generic: 10% (237 mL)

Suspension, External, as sodium:
Generic: 10% (118 mL)

Sulfacetamide and Prednisolone
(sul fa SEE ta mide & pred NIS oh lone)

Brand Names: US Blephamide
Brand Names: Canada AK Cide Oph; Blephamide; Dioptimyd
Index Terms Prednisolone and Sulfacetamide
Pharmacologic Category Antibiotic/Corticosteroid, Ophthalmic
Use Inflammatory ocular conditions: Treatment of steroid-responsive inflammatory ocular conditions in which a corticosteroid is indicated and where infection is present or there is a risk of infection; chronic anterior uveitis; corneal injury from chemical, radiation or thermal burns; penetration of foreign bodies.

Dosing
Adult & Geriatric
Inflammatory ocular conditions: Ophthalmic:
Ointment: Apply ~1/2 inch ribbon to lower conjunctival sac 3 to 4 times/day and 1 to 2 times at night
Solution: Instill 2 drops every 4 hours
Suspension: Instill 2 drops every 4 hours during the day and at bedtime

Pediatric Inflammatory ocular conditions: Children ≥6 years and Adolescents: Ophthalmic: Refer to adult dosing.

Renal Impairment There are no dosage adjustments provided in the manufacturer's labeling.

Hepatic Impairment There are no dosage adjustments provided in the manufacturer's labeling.

Additional Information Complete prescribing information should be consulted for additional detail.

Dosage Forms Excipient information presented when available (limited, particularly for generics); consult specific product labeling.

Ointment, ophthalmic:
Blephamide: Sulfacetamide sodium 10% and prednisolone acetate 0.2% (3.5 g)

Solution, ophthalmic [drops]: Sulfacetamide sodium 10% and prednisolone sodium phosphate 0.25% (5 mL, 10 mL)

Suspension, ophthalmic [drops]:
Blephamide: Sulfacetamide sodium 10% and prednisolone acetate 0.2% (5 mL, 10 mL) [contains benzalkonium chloride]

◆ Sulfacetamide and Sulfur *see* Sulfur and Sulfacetamide on page 1716

◆ Sulfacetamide Sodium *see* Sulfacetamide (Ophthalmic) on page 1707

◆ Sulfacetamide Sodium *see* Sulfacetamide (Topical) on page 1707

◆ Sulfacet-R (Can) *see* Sulfacetamide (Topical) on page 1707

◆ Sulfacet-R (Can) *see* Sulfur and Sulfacetamide on page 1716

◆ SulfaCleanse 8/4 *see* Sulfur and Sulfacetamide on page 1716

SulfADIAZINE (sul fa DYE a zeen)

Pharmacologic Category Antibiotic, Sulfonamide Derivative
Use Treatment of the following conditions (per product labeling): Chancroid, trachoma, inclusion conjunctivitis, nocardiosis, urinary tract infections, toxoplasmosis encephalitis, malaria, meningococcal meningitis, acute otitis media, rheumatic fever (prophylaxis), meningitis (adjunctive)

Refer to current guidelines for appropriate use.

Pregnancy Considerations Adverse events have been observed in animal reproduction studies. Sulfadiazine crosses the placenta (Speert, 1943). Available studies and case reports have failed to show an increased risk for congenital malformations after sulfadiazine use (Heinonen, 1977); however, studies with sulfonamides as a class have shown mixed results (ACOG, 2011).

Sulfadiazine is recommended for use in pregnant women to prevent *T. gondii* infection of the fetus, for the maternal treatment of *Toxoplasmic gondii* encephalitis, and as an alternative agent for the secondary prevention of rheumatic fever (CDC, 2009; DHHS, 2013; Gerber, 2009). Sulfonamides may be used to treat other infections in pregnant women when clinically appropriate for confirmed infections caused by susceptible organisms; use during the first trimester should be limited to situations where no alternative therapies are available (ACOG, 2011). Because safer options are available for the treatment of urinary tract infections in pregnant women, use of sulfonamide-containing products >32 weeks gestation should be avoided (Lee, 2008). Due to the theoretical increased risk for hyperbilirubinemia and kernicterus, sulfadiazine is contraindicated by the manufacturer for use near term. Neonatal healthcare providers should be informed if maternal sulfonamide therapy is used near the time of delivery (DHHS, 2013).

Breast-Feeding Considerations Sulfadiazine distributes into human milk. Sulfonamides should not be used while nursing an infant with G6PD deficiency or hyperbilirubinemia (Della-Giustina, 2003). Per the manufacturer, sulfadiazine is contraindicated in nursing mothers since sulfonamides cross into the milk and may cause kernicterus in the newborn. Nondose-related effects could include modification of bowel flora.

Contraindications Hypersensitivity to any sulfa drug or any component of the formulation; infants <2 months of age unless indicated for the treatment of congenital toxoplasmosis; pregnancy (at term); breast-feeding

Warnings/Precautions Fatalities associated with severe reactions including agranulocytosis, aplastic anemia and other blood dyscrasias, hepatic necrosis, Stevens-Johnson syndrome, and toxic epidermal necrolysis have

occurred; discontinue use at first sign of rash or signs of serious adverse reactions. Use with caution in patients with allergies or asthma.

Not for the treatment of group A beta-hemolytic streptococcal infections. Prolonged use may result in fungal or bacterial superinfection, including *C. difficile*-associated diarrhea (CDAD) and pseudomembranous colitis; CDAD has been observed >2 months postantibiotic treatment. Use with caution in patients with G6PD deficiency; hemolysis may occur. Use with caution in patients with hepatic impairment. Use with caution in patients with renal impairment; dosage modification required. Maintain adequate hydration to prevent crystalluria. Sulfa antibiotics have been shown to displace bilirubin from protein binding sites which may potentially lead to hyperbilirubinemia and kernicterus in neonates and young infants; do not use in neonates; avoid use in infants <2 months unless other options are not available.

Benzyl alcohol and derivatives: Some dosage forms may contain sodium benzoate/benzoic acid; benzoic acid (benzoate) is a metabolite of benzyl alcohol; large amounts of benzyl alcohol (≥99 mg/kg/day) have been associated with a potentially fatal toxicity ("gasping syndrome") in neonates; the "gasping syndrome" consists of metabolic acidosis, respiratory distress, gasping respirations, CNS dysfunction (including convulsions, intracranial hemorrhage), hypotension, and cardiovascular collapse (AAP ["Inactive" 1997]; CDC, 1982); some data suggests that benzoate displaces bilirubin from protein binding sites (Ahlfors, 2001); avoid or use dosage forms containing benzyl alcohol derivative with caution in neonates. See manufacturer's labeling.

Sulfonamide ("sulfa") allergy: Traditionally, concerns for cross-reactivity have extended to all compounds containing the sulfonamide structure (SO_2NH_2). An expanded understanding of allergic mechanisms indicates cross-reactivity between antibiotic sulfonamides and nonantibiotic sulfonamides may not occur, or at the very least this potential is extremely low (Brackett 2004; Johnson 2005; Slatore 2004; Tornero 2004). In particular, mechanisms of cross-reaction due to antibody production (anaphylaxis) are unlikely to occur with nonantibiotic sulfonamides and antibiotic sulfonamides. A nonantibiotic sulfonamide compound which contains the arylamine structure and therefore may cross-react with antibiotic sulfonamides is sulfasalazine (Zawodniak 2010). T-cell-mediated (type IV) reactions (eg, maculopapular rash) are less understood and it is not possible to completely exclude this potential based on current insights. In cases where prior reactions were severe (Stevens-Johnson syndrome/TEN), some clinicians choose to avoid exposure to these classes.

Adverse Reactions Frequency not defined.

Cardiovascular: Allergic myocarditis, periarteritis nodosa

Central nervous system: Ataxia, chills, convulsions, depression, fever, hallucinations, headache, insomnia, vertigo

Dermatologic: Epidermal necrolysis, erythema multiforme, exfoliative dermatitis, photosensitivity, pruritus, purpura, rash, skin eruptions, Stevens-Johnson syndrome, urticaria

Endocrine & metabolic: Hypoglycemia, thyroid function disturbance

Gastrointestinal: Abdominal pain, anorexia, diarrhea, nausea, pancreatitis, stomatitis, vomiting

Genitourinary: Crystalluria, stone formation, toxic nephrosis with oliguria and anuria

Hematologic: Agranulocytopenia, aplastic anemia, hemolytic anemia, hypoprothrombinemia, leukopenia, methemoglobinemia, thrombocytopenia

Hepatic: Hepatitis

Neuromuscular & skeletal: Arthralgia, peripheral neuritis

Ocular: Conjunctival/scleral injection, periorbital edema

Otic: Tinnitus

Renal: Diuresis

Miscellaneous: Anaphylactoid reactions, lupus erythematosus, serum sickness-like reactions

Drug Interactions

Metabolism/Transport Effects Substrate of CYP2C9 (major), CYP2E1 (minor), CYP3A4 (minor); **Note:** Assignment of Major/Minor substrate status based on clinically relevant drug interaction potential; **Inhibits** CYP2C9 (strong)

Avoid Concomitant Use

Avoid concomitant use of SulfADIAZINE with any of the following: BCG (Intravesical); Mecamylamine; Methenamine; Potassium P-Aminobenzoate; Procaine

Increased Effect/Toxicity

SulfADIAZINE may increase the levels/effects of: Bosentan; Carvedilol; CycloSPORINE (Systemic); CYP2C9 Substrates; Diclofenac (Systemic); Dronabinol; Hypoglycemia-Associated Agents; Lacosamide; Mecamylamine; Methotrexate; Ospemifene; Parecoxib; Porfimer; Prilocaine; Ramelteon; Sodium Nitrite; Sulfonylureas; Tetrahydrocannabinol; Verteporfin; Vitamin K Antagonists

The levels/effects of SulfADIAZINE may be increased by: Androgens; Antidiabetic Agents; Cannabis; Ceritinib; CYP2C9 Inhibitors (Moderate); CYP2C9 Inhibitors (Strong); Dapsone (Topical); Dexketoprofen; Herbs (Hypoglycemic Properties); Lumacaftor; MAO Inhibitors; Methenamine; Mifepristone; Nitric Oxide; Pegvisomant; Quinolone Antibiotics; Salicylates; Selective Serotonin Reuptake Inhibitors

Decreased Effect

SulfADIAZINE may decrease the levels/effects of: BCG (Intravesical); BCG Vaccine (Immunization); CycloSPORINE (Systemic); Sodium Picosulfate; Typhoid Vaccine

The levels/effects of SulfADIAZINE may be decreased by: CYP2C9 Inducers (Strong); Dabrafenib; Enzalutamide; Lumacaftor; Potassium P-Aminobenzoate; Procaine; Quinolone Antibiotics

Food Interactions Vitamin C or acidifying agents (cranberry juice) may cause crystalluria. Management: Avoid large quantities of vitamin C or acidifying agents (cranberry juice).

Storage/Stability Store at controlled room temperature of 20°C to 25°C (68°F to 77°F). Protect from light.

Mechanism of Action Interferes with bacterial growth by inhibiting bacterial folic acid synthesis through competitive antagonism of PABA

Pharmacodynamics/Kinetics

Absorption: Well absorbed

Distribution: Throughout body tissues and fluids including pleural, peritoneal, synovial, and ocular fluids; throughout total body water; readily diffused into CSF

Protein binding: 38% to 48%

Metabolism: Via N-acetylation

Half-life elimination: 10 hours

Time to peak: Within 3-6 hours

Excretion: Urine (43% to 60% as unchanged drug, 15% to 40% as metabolites)

Dosing

Adult & Geriatric

General dosing guidelines: Oral: 2 to 4 g/day in 3 to 6 divided doses

Rheumatic fever prophylaxis: Oral:

<30 kg: 0.5 g/day

≥30 kg: 1 g/day

***Toxoplasma gondii* encephalitis (HIV-infected patients) (off-label dose):** Oral:

Treatment: 1,000 mg (<60 kg) or 1,500 mg (≥60 kg) every 6 hours in combination with pyrimethamine plus leucovorin calcium (preferred) or alternatively, may give 1,000 mg (<60 kg) or 1,500 mg (≥60 kg) every 6 hours in combination with atovaquone; treat for ≥6 weeks; longer duration may be necessary if clinical or radiographic disease is extensive or if response is incomplete at 6 weeks (HHS [OI adult 2015]).

Chronic maintenance therapy: 2,000 to 4,000 mg/day in 2 to 4 divided doses in combination with pyrimethamine and leucovorin calcium (preferred) or alternatively, may give 2,000 to 4,000 mg/day in 2 to 4 divided doses in combination with atovaquone; may discontinue if successfully completed initial treatment, remain asymptomatic of toxoplasmic encephalitis, and CD4 count >200 cells/mm3 for 6 months in response to ART (HHS [OI adult 2015]).

Pediatric

General dosing guidelines: Oral: Children >2 months of age: Initial: 75 mg/kg; Maintenance: 150 mg/kg/day in 4 to 6 divided doses (maximum: 6 g/24 hours)

Rheumatic fever prophylaxis: Oral: Children:

<30 kg: 0.5 g/day

≥30 kg: 1 g/day

Toxoplasmosis (HIV-exposed/-infected patients) (off-label dose): Oral:

Congenital toxoplasmosis: Infants: 100 mg/kg/day in divided doses every 12 hours for 12 months in combination with pyrimethamine plus leucovorin calcium (HHS [OI pediatric 2013])

Acquired toxoplasmosis: Infants and Children:

Acute induction therapy: 25 to 50 mg/kg/dose given 4 times/day (maximum: 1 to 1.5 g/dose) in combination with pyrimethamine and leucovorin calcium. Continue acute induction therapy for ≥6 weeks, then follow with chronic suppressive therapy (HHS [OI pediatric 2013]).

◄

Chronic maintenance therapy (prior to encephalitis): 85 to 120 mg/kg/day divided every 6 to 12 hours (maximum: 2 to 4 g/day) in combination with pyrimethamine plus leucovorin calcium (HHS [OI pediatric 2013])

Toxoplasma gondii encephalitis: Adolescents: Refer to adult dosing.

Dietary Considerations Supplemental leucovorin calcium should be administered to reverse symptoms or prevent problems due to folic acid deficiency.

Administration Administer with at least 8 ounces of water and around-the-clock to promote less variation in peak and trough serum levels. Oral sodium bicarbonate may be used to alkalinize the urine of patients unable to maintain adequate fluid intake (in order to prevent crystalluria, azotemia, oliguria) (Lerner, 1996).

Monitoring Parameters Perform culture and sensitivity testing prior to initiating therapy; frequent CBC and urinalysis during therapy; signs of serious blood disorders (sore throat, fever, pallor, purpura, jaundice); CD4+ count in HIV-exposed/-positive patients treated for toxoplasmosis; sulfonamide blood concentrations may be monitored for severe infections (target: 12-15 mg/100 mL)

Dosage Forms Excipient information presented when available (limited, particularly for generics); consult specific product labeling.

Tablet, Oral:

Generic: 500 mg

Extemporaneous Preparations A 200 mg/mL oral suspension may be made with sulfadiazine powder and sterile water. Place 50 g sulfadiazine powder in a glass mortar. Add small portions of sterile water and mix to a uniform paste; mix while incrementally adding sterile water to **almost** 250 mL; transfer to a calibrated bottle, rinse mortar with sterile water, and add sufficient quantity of sterile water to make 250 mL. Label "shake well" and "refrigerate". Stable for 3 days refrigerated. **Note:** Suspension may also be prepared by crushing one-hundred 500 mg tablets; however, it is stable for only 2 days.

Pathmanathan U, Halgrain D, Chiadmi F, et al, "Stability of Sulfadiazine Oral Liquids Prepared From Tablets and Powder," *J Pharm Pharm Sci*, 2004, 7(1):84-7.

Sulfamethoxazole and Trimethoprim
(sul fa meth OKS a zole & trye METH oh prim)

Brand Names: US Bactrim; Bactrim DS; Sulfatrim Pediatric

Brand Names: Canada Apo-Sulfatrim; Apo-Sulfatrim DS; Apo-Sulfatrim Pediatric; Protrin DF; Septra Injection; Teva-Trimel; Teva-Trimel DS; Trisulfa; Trisulfa DS; Trisulfa S

Index Terms Co-Trimoxazole; Septra; SMX-TMP; SMZ-TMP; Sulfatrim; TMP-SMX; TMP-SMZ; Trimethoprim and Sulfamethoxazole

Pharmacologic Category Antibiotic, Miscellaneous; Antibiotic, Sulfonamide Derivative

Use

Oral: Treatment of urinary tract infections due to *E. coli*, *Klebsiella* and *Enterobacter* sp, *M. morganii*, *P. mirabilis* and *P. vulgaris*; acute otitis media; acute exacerbations of chronic bronchitis due to susceptible strains of *H. influenzae* or *S. pneumoniae*; treatment and prophylaxis of *Pneumocystis* pneumonia (PCP); traveler's diarrhea due to enterotoxigenic *E. coli*; treatment of enteritis caused by *Shigella flexneri* or *Shigella sonnei*

IV: Treatment of *Pneumocystis* pneumonia (PCP); treatment of enteritis caused by *Shigella flexneri* and *Shigella sonnei*; treatment of severe or complicated urinary tract infections due to *E. coli*, *Klebsiella* and *Enterobacter* spp, *M. morganii*, *P. mirabilis*, and *P. vulgaris*

Pregnancy Considerations Adverse events have been observed in animal reproduction studies. Trimethoprim-sulfamethoxazole (TMP-SMX) crosses the placenta and distributes to amniotic fluid (Ylikorkala, 1973). An increased risk of congenital malformations (neural tube defects, cardiovascular malformations, urinary tract defects, oral clefts, club foot) following maternal use of TMP-SMX during pregnancy has been observed in some studies. Folic acid supplementation may decrease this risk (Crider 2009; Czeizel 2001; Hernandez-Diaz 2000; Hernandez-Diaz 2001; Matok 2009). Due to theoretical concerns that sulfonamides pass the placenta and may cause kernicterus in the newborn, neonatal healthcare providers should be informed if maternal sulfonamide therapy is used near the time of delivery (DHHS 2013).

The pharmacokinetics of TMP-SMX are similar to non-pregnant patients in early pregnancy (Ylikorkala, 1973). TMP-SMX is recommended for the prophylaxis or treatment of *Pneumocystis jirovecii* pneumonia (PCP), prophylaxis of *Toxoplasmic gondii* encephalitis (TE), and for the acute and chronic treatment of Q fever in pregnancy (CDC 2013; DHHS 2013). Sulfonamides may also be used to treat other infections in pregnant women when clinically appropriate; use during the first trimester should be limited to situations where no alternative therapies are available (ACOG 2011). Because safer options are available for the treatment of urinary tract infections in pregnant women, use of TMP-containing products in the first trimester and sulfonamide-containing products >32 weeks gestation should be avoided (Lee 2008).

Breast-Feeding Considerations Small amounts of TMP and SMX are transferred into breast milk. The manufacturer recommends that caution be used if administered to nursing women, especially if breast-feeding ill, jaundiced, premature, or stressed infants due to the potential risk of bilirubin displacement and kernicterus. Sulfonamides should not be used while nursing an infant with G6PD deficiency or hyperbilirubinemia (Della-Giustina, 2003). Maternal indications for TMP-SMX must also be considered prior to nursing. Nondose-related effects could include modification of bowel flora.

Contraindications

Hypersensitivity to any sulfa drug, trimethoprim, or any component of the formulation; history of drug induced-immune thrombocytopenia with use of sulfonamides or trimethoprim; megaloblastic anemia due to folate deficiency; infants <2 months of age (manufacturer's labeling), infants <4 weeks of age (CDC 2009); marked hepatic damage or severe renal disease (if patient not monitored)

Note: Although the FDA approved product labeling states this medication is contraindicated with other sulfonamide-containing drug classes, the scientific basis of this statement has been challenged. See "Warnings/Precautions" for more detail.

Warnings/Precautions Use with caution in patients with G6PD deficiency, impaired renal or hepatic function or potential folate deficiency (malnourished, chronic anticonvulsant therapy, or elderly); maintain adequate hydration to prevent crystalluria; adjust dosage in patients with renal impairment.

Fatalities associated with severe reactions including Stevens-Johnson syndrome, toxic epidermal necrolysis, hepatic necrosis, agranulocytosis, aplastic anemia, thrombocytopenia and other blood dyscrasias have been reported; discontinue use at first sign of rash or serious adverse reactions. Elderly patients appear at greater risk for more severe adverse reactions. May cause hypoglycemia, particularly in malnourished, or patients with renal or hepatic impairment. Use with caution in patients with porphyria or thyroid dysfunction. Potentially significant interactions may exist, requiring dose or frequency adjustment, additional monitoring, and/or selection of alternative therapy. Slow acetylators may be more prone to adverse reactions. Caution in patients with allergies or asthma. Incidence of adverse effects appears to be increased in patients with AIDS. Prolonged use may result in fungal or bacterial superinfection, including *C. difficile*-associated diarrhea (CDAD) and pseudomembranous colitis; CDAD has been observed >2 months postantibiotic treatment. Avoid concomitant use with leucovorin when treating *Pneumocystis jirovecii* pneumonia (PCP) in HIV patients; may increase risk of treatment failure and death.

When used for uncomplicated urinary tract infections, this combination should not be used if a single agent is effective. Additionally, sulfonamides should not be used to treat group A beta-hemolytic streptococcal infections.

May cause hyponatremia or hyperkalemia. Potential risk factors for trimethoprim-induced hypokalemia include high dosage (20 mg/kg/day of trimethoprim), renal impairment, older age, hypoaldosteronism, and concomitant use of medications causing or exacerbating hyperkalemia (Perazella, 2000). Elderly patients are at an increased risk for severe and potentially life-threatening hyperkalemia when trimethoprim is used concomitantly with spironolactone, ACE inhibitors, or ARBs (Antoniou 2010; Antoniou 2011; Antoniou 2015).

Injection vehicle may contain and sodium metabisulfite.

Benzyl alcohol and derivatives: Some dosage forms may contain benzyl alcohol; large amounts of benzyl alcohol (≥99 mg/kg/day) have been associated with a potentially fatal toxicity ("gasping syndrome") in neonates; the "gasping syndrome" consists of metabolic acidosis, respiratory distress, gasping respirations, CNS dysfunction (including convulsions, intracranial hemorrhage), hypotension, and cardiovascular collapse (AAP ["Inactive" 1997]; CDC 1982); some data suggests that benzoate displaces bilirubin from protein binding sites (Ahlfors 2001); avoid or use dosage forms containing benzyl alcohol with caution in neonates. See manufacturer's labeling.

Propylene glycol: Some dosage forms may contain propylene glycol; large amounts are potentially toxic and have been associated hyperosmolality, lactic acidosis, seizures, and respiratory depression; use caution (AAP ["Inactive" 1997]; Zar 2007).

Sulfonamide ("sulfa") allergy: Traditionally, concerns for cross-reactivity have extended to all compounds containing the sulfonamide structure (SO_2NH_2). An expanded understanding of allergic mechanisms indicates cross-reactivity between antibiotic sulfonamides and nonantibiotic sulfonamides may not occur, or at the very least this potential is extremely low (Brackett 2004; Johnson 2005; Slatore 2004; Tornero 2004). In particular, mechanisms of cross-reaction due to antibody production (anaphylaxis) are unlikely to occur with nonantibiotic sulfonamides and antibiotic sulfonamides. A nonantibiotic sulfonamide compound which contains the arylamine structure and therefore may cross-react with antibiotic sulfonamides is sulfasalazine (Zawodniak 2010). T-cell-mediated (type IV) reactions (eg, maculopapular rash) are less understood and it is not possible to completely exclude this potential based on current insights. In cases where prior reactions were severe (Stevens-Johnson syndrome/TEN), some clinicians choose to avoid exposure to these classes.

Adverse Reactions Frequency not defined:

Cardiovascular: Allergic myocarditis, periarteritis nodosa (rare)

Central nervous system: Apathy, aseptic meningitis, ataxia, chills, depression, fatigue, hallucination, headache, insomnia, nervousness, peripheral neuritis, seizure, vertigo

Dermatologic: Erythema multiforme (rare), exfoliative dermatitis (rare), pruritus, skin photosensitivity, skin rash, Stevens-Johnson syndrome (rare), toxic epidermal necrolysis (rare), urticaria

Endocrine & metabolic: Hyperkalemia (generally at high dosages), hypoglycemia (rare), hyponatremia

Gastrointestinal: Abdominal pain, anorexia, diarrhea, glottis edema, kernicterus (in neonates), nausea, pancreatitis, pseudomembranous colitis, stomatitis, vomiting

Genitourinary: Crystalluria, diuresis (rare), nephrotoxicity (in association with cyclosporine), toxic nephrosis (with anuria and oliguria)

Hematologic & oncologic: Agranulocytosis, anaphylactoid purpura (IgA vasculitis; rare), aplastic anemia, eosinophilia, hemolysis (with G6PD deficiency), hemolytic anemia, hypoprothrombinemia, leukopenia, megaloblastic anemia, methemoglobinemia, neutropenia, thrombocytopenia

Hepatic: Cholestatic jaundice, hepatotoxicity (including hepatitis, cholestasis, and hepatic necrosis), hyperbilirubinemia, increased transaminases

Hypersensitivity: Anaphylaxis, angioedema, hypersensitivity reaction, serum sickness

Neuromuscular & skeletal: Arthralgia, myalgia, rhabdomyolysis (mainly in AIDS patients), systemic lupus erythematosus (rare), weakness

Ophthalmic: Conjunctival injection, injected sclera

Otic: Tinnitus

Renal: Increased blood urea nitrogen, increased serum creatinine, interstitial nephritis, renal failure

Respiratory: Cough, dyspnea, pulmonary infiltrates

Miscellaneous: Fever

<1% (Limited to important or life-threatening): Idiopathic thrombocytopenic purpura, prolonged Q-T interval on ECG, thrombotic thrombocytopenic purpura

Drug Interactions

Metabolism/Transport Effects Refer to individual components.

Avoid Concomitant Use

Avoid concomitant use of Sulfamethoxazole and Trimethoprim with any of the following: Amodiaquine; BCG (Intravesical); Dofetilide; Leucovorin Calcium-Levoleucovorin; Mecamylamine; Methenamine; Potassium P-Aminobenzoate; Procaine

Increased Effect/Toxicity

Sulfamethoxazole and Trimethoprim may increase the levels/effects of: ACE Inhibitors; Amantadine; Amodiaquine; Angiotensin II Receptor Blockers; Antidiabetic Agents (Thiazolidinedione); AzaTHIOprine; Bosentan; Cannabis; Carvedilol; CycloSPORINE (Systemic); CYP2C8 Substrates; CYP2C9 Substrates; Dapsone (Systemic); Dapsone (Topical); Digoxin; Dofetilide; Dronabinol; Eplerenone; Fosphenytoin; Highest Risk QTc-Prolonging Agents; Hypoglycemia-Associated Agents; LamiVUDine; Mecamylamine; Memantine; Mercaptopurine; MetFORMIN; Methotrexate; Moderate Risk QTc-Prolonging Agents; Phenytoin; Porfimer; PRALAtrexate; Prilocaine; Procainamide; Repaglinide; Sodium Nitrite; Spironolactone; Sulfonylureas; Tetrahydrocannabinol; Varenicline; Verteporfin; Vitamin K Antagonists

The levels/effects of Sulfamethoxazole and Trimethoprim may be increased by: Amantadine; Androgens; Antidiabetic Agents; Ceritinib; CYP2C9 Inhibitors (Moderate); CYP2C9 Inhibitors (Strong); Dapsone (Systemic); Dexketoprofen; Herbs (Hypoglycemic Properties); MAO Inhibitors; Memantine; Methenamine; Mifepristone; Nitric Oxide; Osimertinib; Pegvisomant; Quinolone Antibiotics; Salicylates; Selective Serotonin Reuptake Inhibitors

Decreased Effect

Sulfamethoxazole and Trimethoprim may decrease the levels/effects of: BCG (Intravesical); BCG Vaccine (Immunization); CycloSPORINE (Systemic); Sodium Picosulfate; Typhoid Vaccine

The levels/effects of Sulfamethoxazole and Trimethoprim may be decreased by: Bosentan; CYP2C9 Inducers (Strong); CYP3A4 Inducers (Moderate); CYP3A4 Inducers (Strong); Dabrafenib; Deferasirox; Enzalutamide; Fosphenytoin; Leucovorin Calcium-Levoleucovorin; Mitotane; Osimertinib; Phenytoin; Potassium P-Aminobenzoate; Procaine; Quinolone Antibiotics; Siltuximab; St Johns Wort; Tocilizumab

Preparation for Administration IV: Must dilute well prior to administration (ie, 1:15 to 1:25, which equates to 5 mL of drug solution diluted in 75-125 mL base solution)

Storage/Stability

Injection: Store at room temperature; do not refrigerate. Less soluble in more alkaline pH. Protect from light. Solution must be diluted prior to administration. Following dilution, store at room temperature; do not refrigerate. Manufacturer recommended dilutions and stability of parenteral admixture at room temperature (25°C):

5 mL/125 mL D_5W; stable for 6 hours.

5 mL/100 mL D_5W; stable for 4 hours.

5 mL/75 mL D_5W; stable for 2 hours.

Studies have also confirmed limited stability in NS; detailed references should be consulted.

Suspension, tablet: Store at controlled room temperature of 15°C to 25°C (59°F to 77°F). Protect from light.

Mechanism of Action Sulfamethoxazole interferes with bacterial folic acid synthesis and growth via inhibition of dihydrofolic acid formation from para-aminobenzoic acid; trimethoprim inhibits dihydrofolic acid reduction to tetrahydrofolate resulting in sequential inhibition of enzymes of the folic acid pathway

Pharmacodynamics/Kinetics

Absorption: Oral: Rapid

Distribution: Both SMX and TMP distribute to middle ear fluid, sputum, vaginal fluid; TMP also distributes into bronchial secretions

Protein binding: SMX: ~70%, TMP: ~44%

Metabolism: Hepatic, both to multiple metabolites; SMX to hydroxy (via CYP2C9) and acetyl derivatives, and also conjugated with glucuronide; TMP to oxide and hydroxy derivatives; the free forms of both SMX and TMP are therapeutically active

Half-life elimination: Oral (mean): SMX: 10 hours, TMP: 8-10 hours; both are prolonged in renal failure

Time to peak, serum: Oral: 1-4 hours

Excretion: Both are excreted in urine as metabolites and unchanged drug

Dosing

Adult & Geriatric Dosage recommendations are based on the trimethoprim component. double-strength tablets are equivalent to sulfamethoxazole 800 mg and trimethoprim 160 mg.

General dosing guidelines:

Oral: 1 to 2 double-strength tablets (sulfamethoxazole 800 mg; trimethoprim 160 mg) every 12 to 24 hours

IV: 8 to 20 mg TMP/kg/day divided every 6 to 12 hours

Bite wounds (animal) (off-label use) (IDSA [Stevens 2014]):

Oral: One double-strength tablet twice daily; in combination with clindamycin or metronidazole

IV: 5 to 10 mg TMP/kg/day in divided doses every 6 to 12 hours in combination with clindamycin or metronidazole

Chronic bronchitis (acute): Oral: One double-strength tablet every 12 hours for 10 to 14 days

Cyclosporiasis (off-label use): Oral, IV: 160 mg TMP twice daily for 7 to 10 days. **Note:** AIDS patients: Oral: One double-strength tablet 2 to 4 times/day for 10 days, then 1 double-strength tablet 3 times/week for 10 weeks (Pape 1994; Verdier 2000).

Granuloma inguinale (donovanosis) (off-label use): Oral: One double-strength tablet every 12 hours for at least 3 weeks and until lesions have healed (CDC 2010)

Isosporiasis (*Isospora belli* infection) in HIV-infected patients (off-label use; HHS [OI adult 2015]):
Treatment: Oral, IV: 160 mg TMP 4 times/day for 10 days **or** 160 mg TMP 2 times/day for 7 to 10 days. May start with twice daily regimen and increase dose and/or duration up to 3 to 4 weeks if symptoms worsen or persist.

Chronic maintenance therapy (secondary prophylaxis) in patients with CD4 count <200 cells/mm³: Oral: 160 mg TMP 3 times/week (preferred) or alternatively, 160 mg TMP daily or 320 mg TMP 3 times/week.

Melioidosis (*Burkholderia pseudomallei*) (off-label use) (Lipsitz 2012): Oral, IV:
Severe, acute phase involving brain, prostate, bone, or joint: Administer as 2 divided doses; given with ceftazidime or a carbapenem for ≥10 days followed by eradication therapy:
Adults <40 kg: 320 mg TMP daily
Adults 40 to 60 kg: 480 mg TMP daily
Adults >60 kg: 640 mg TMP daily
Eradication therapy: Administer as 2 divided doses for ≥12 weeks:
Adults <40 kg: 320 mg TMP daily
Adults 40 to 60 kg: 480 mg TMP daily
Adults >60 kg: 640 mg TMP daily
Postexposure prophylaxis: Administer as 2 divided doses for 21 days:
Adults <40 kg: 320 mg TMP daily
Adults 40 to 60 kg: 480 mg TMP daily
Adults >60 kg: 640 mg TMP daily

Meningitis (bacterial): IV: 10 to 20 mg TMP/kg/day in divided doses every 6-12 hours:
Nocardia (off-label use): Oral, IV:
Cutaneous infections: 5 to 10 mg TMP/kg/day in 2 to 4 divided doses
Severe infections (pulmonary/cerebral): 15 mg TMP/kg/day in 2 to 4 divided doses for 3 to 4 weeks, then 10 mg TMP/kg/day in 2 to 4 divided doses. Treatment duration is controversial; an average of 7 months has been reported.
Note: Therapy for severe infection may be initiated IV and converted to oral therapy (frequently converted to approximate dosages of oral solid dosage forms: 2 DS tablets every 8 to 12 hours). Although not widely available, sulfonamide levels should be considered in patients with questionable absorption, at risk for dose-related toxicity, or those with poor therapeutic response.

Osteomyelitis due to MRSA (off-label use): Oral, IV: 3.5 to 4 mg TMP/kg/dose every 8 to 12 hours for a minimum of 8 weeks with rifampin 600 mg once daily (Liu 2011)

Pneumocystis pneumonia (PCP):
Manufacturer's labeling:
Oral:
Prophylaxis: 160 mg TMP daily
Treatment: 15 to 20 mg TMP/kg/day divided every 6 hours for 14 to 21 days
IV: Treatment: 15 to 20 mg TMP/kg/day divided every 6 to 8 hours for up to 14 days
Alternate dosing in HIV-infected patients (off-label dose; HHS [OI adult 2015]):
Primary or secondary prophylaxis: Oral: 80 or 160 mg TMP daily **or** alternatively, 160 mg TMP 3 times/week
Duration of prophylaxis: May discontinue primary or secondary prophylaxis if CD4 count increases from <200 cells/mm³ to ≥200 cells/mm³ for at least 3 months in response to ART; therapy must be restarted if CD4 count <200 cells/mm³
Treatment:
Mild to moderate: Oral: 15 to 20 mg TMP/kg/day in 3 divided doses for 21 days **or** alternatively, 320 mg TMP 3 times/day for 21 days
Moderate to severe: IV: 15 to 20 mg TMP/kg/day in 3 to 4 divided doses for 21 days; may switch to oral therapy after clinical improvement

Prosthetic joint infection (off-label use): Oral phase treatment (after completion of pathogen-specific IV therapy) following debridement and prosthesis retention or 1-stage exchange:
Total ankle, elbow, hip, or shoulder arthroplasty: 160 mg TMP 2 times daily for 3 months. **Note:** Must be used in combination with rifampin (Cordero-Ampuero 2007; Osmon 2013).
Total knee arthroplasty: Adults: 160 mg TMP 2 times daily for 6 months. **Note:** Must be used in combination with rifampin (Cordero-Ampuero 2007; Osmon 2013).

Q fever (off-label use): Oral:
Acute (in pregnant women) (CDC 2013): 160 mg TMP twice daily throughout pregnancy but not beyond 32 weeks gestation. **Note:** Discontinue therapy for the final 8 weeks of pregnancy due to hyperbilirubinemia risk
Chronic: Infectious Disease consult recommended for treatment of chronic Q fever
Sepsis: IV: 20 mg TMP/kg/day divided every 6 hours
Septic arthritis due to MRSA (off-label use): Oral, IV: 3.5 to 4 mg TMP/kg/dose every 8 to 12 hours for 3 to 4 weeks (some experts combine with rifampin) (Liu 2011)
Shigellosis: Note: Due to reported widespread resistance, empiric therapy with sulfamethoxazole and trimethoprim is not recommended (CDC-NARMS 2010; WHO 2005).
Oral: One double-strength tablet every 12 hours for 5 days
IV: 8-10 mg TMP/kg/day in divided doses every 6, 8, or 12 hours for up to 5 days
Skin/soft tissue infection due to MSSA or MRSA (off-label use): Oral: 1 to 2 double-strength tablets every 12 hours for 5 to 10 days (Lui 2011) or 7 to 14 days (IDSA [Stevens 2014]); **Note:** If beta-hemolytic *Streptococcus* spp are also suspected, a beta-lactam antibiotic should be added to the regimen (Liu 2011)
Spontaneous bacterial peritonitis (prevention) (off-label use): Oral: Long-term prophylaxis: One double-strength (trimethoprim 160 mg/sulfamethoxazole 800 mg) tablet once daily (preferred) (Lontos 2014). Daily dosing for 5 days per week has been studied (Alvarez 2005; Singh 1995), but concerns regarding bacterial resistance with intermittent dosing limit use (AASLD [Runyon 2012]). American Association for the Study of Liver Diseases (AASLD) guidelines note that intermittent dosing (ie, 5 days/week, once weekly) of antibiotics, although shown to be effective in SBP prevention, may be inferior to daily dosing due to development of bacterial resistance. Daily dosing regimens are preferred (AASLD [Runyon 2012]).
Stenotrophomonas maltophilia **(ventilator-associated pneumonia) (off-label use):** IV: Most clinicians have utilized 12 to 15 mg TMP/kg/day for the treatment of VAP caused by *Stenotrophomonas maltophilia*. Higher doses (up to 20 mg TMP/kg/day) have been mentioned for treatment of severe infection in patients with normal renal function (Looney 2009; Vartivarian 1989; Wood 2010)
Surgical site infections (trunk or extremity [away from axilla or perineum]) (off-label use): Oral: One double-strength tablet every 6 hours (IDSA [Stevens 2014])
Toxoplasma gondii **encephalitis in HIV-infected patients (off-label use; HHS [OI adult 2015]:** Oral:
Primary prophylaxis: Oral: 160 mg TMP daily (preferred) **or** 160 mg TMP 3 times/week **or** 80 mg TMP daily; primary prophylaxis is indicated for Toxoplasma IgG-positive patients with CD4 count <100 cells/mm³
Treatment (alternative to preferred therapy): Oral, IV: 5 mg/kg TMP twice daily for at least 6 weeks; longer duration may be needed if clinical or radiologic disease is extensive or response is incomplete at 6 weeks.
Chronic maintenance therapy (alternative to preferred therapy): Oral: 160 mg TMP twice daily; may discontinue when asymptomatic and CD4 count >200 cells/mm³ for 6 months in response to ART
Travelers' diarrhea: Oral: One double-strength tablet every 12 hours for 5 days
Urinary tract infection:
Oral: One double-strength tablet every 12 hours
Duration of therapy: Uncomplicated: 3 to 5 days; Complicated: 7 to 10 days
Pyelonephritis: 14 days
Prostatitis: Acute: 2 weeks; Chronic: 2 to 3 months
IV: 8 to 10 mg TMP/kg/day in divided doses every 6, 8, or 12 hours for up to 14 days with severe infections
Pediatric Recommendations are based on the trimethoprim component.
General dosing guidelines: Children >2 months: Manufacturer's labeling:
Mild-to-moderate infections: Oral: 8 mg TMP/kg/day in divided doses every 12 hours
Serious infection:
Oral: 15 to 20 mg TMP/kg/day in divided doses every 6 hours
IV: 8 to 12 mg TMP/kg/day in divided doses every 6 to 12 hours

Indication specific dosing:

Acute otitis media: Infants >2 months and Children: Oral: 8 mg TMP/kg/day in divided doses every 12 hours for 10 days. **Note:** Recommended by the American Academy of Pediatrics as an alternative agent in penicillin allergic patients at a dose of 6 to 10mg TMP/kg/day (AOM guidelines 2004).

Cyclosporiasis (off-label use): Infants >2 months and Children: Oral, IV: 5 mg TMP/kg twice daily for 7 to 10 days (*Red Book* 2009)

Isosporiasis (*Isospora belli* infection) in HIV-infected patients (off-label use): Adolescents: Refer to adult dosing.

Melioidosis (*Burkholderia pseudomallei*) (off-label use; Lipsitz 2012): Oral, IV:

Severe, acute phase involving brain, prostate, bone, or joint: Administer as 2 divided doses; given with ceftazidime or a carbapenem for ≥10 days followed by eradication therapy:
Children: 16 mg TMP/kg/day (maximum: 640 mg TMP daily)
Adolescents: Refer to adult dosing

Eradication therapy: Administer as 2 divided doses for ≥12 weeks:
Children: 16 mg TMP/kg/day (maximum: 640 mg TMP daily)
Adolescents: Refer to adult dosing

Postexposure prophylaxis: Administer as 2 divided doses for 21 days:
Children: 16 mg TMP/kg/day (maximum: 640 mg TMP daily)
Adolescents: Refer to adult dosing

***Pneumocystis* pneumonia (PCP):**
Infants >2 months and Children:
Treatment: Manufacturer's labeling:
Oral: 15 to 20 mg TMP/kg/day in divided doses every 6 hours for 14 to 21 days
IV: 15 to 20 mg TMP/kg/day in divided doses every 6 to 8 hours for up to 14 days
Prophylaxis: Oral:
Manufacturer's labeling: 150 mg TMP/m²/day in divided doses every 12 hours and administered for 3 days/week on consecutive (maximum: trimethoprim 320 mg and sulfamethoxazole 1,600 mg/day)
Alternate dosing: HIV-exposed/-infected patients: 150 mg TMP/m²/day in 2 divided doses daily (CDC 2009)
Adolescents: HV-infected patients (off-label dose; HHS [OI adult 2015]):
Primary prophylaxis: Oral: 80 to 160 mg TMP daily or alternatively, 160 mg TMP 3 times/week
Secondary prophylaxis: Oral: 80 to 160 mg TMP daily or alternatively, 160 mg TMP 3 times/week
Duration of prophylaxis: May discontinue primary or secondary prophylaxis if CD4 count increases from <200 cells/mm³ to ≥200 cells/mm³ for at least 3 months in response to ART; therapy must be restarted if CD4 count <200 cells/mm³
Treatment:
Mild-to-moderate: Oral: 15 to 20 mg TMP/kg/day in 3 divided doses for 21 days or alternatively, 320 mg TMP 3 times/day for 21 days
Moderate-to-severe: IV: 15 to 20 mg TMP/kg/day in 3 to 4 divided doses for 21 days; may switch to oral therapy after clinical improvement

Q fever (off-label use): Oral:
Acute: Infants ≥2 months and Children <8 years with mild or uncomplicated illness (if patient remains febrile past 5 days of doxycycline treatment): 4 to 20 mg TMP/kg/day in divided doses every 12 hours (maximum: trimethoprim 320 mg daily) (CDC 2013). **Note:** Some clinicians may recommend initial treatment with sulfamethoxazole and trimethoprim for children <8 years with mild or uncomplicated illness (CDC 2013; Hartzell 2008).
Chronic: Infectious Disease consult recommended for treatment of chronic Q fever (CDC 2013)

Shigellosis: Note: Due to reported widespread resistance, empiric therapy with sulfamethoxazole and trimethoprim is not recommended (CDC-NARMS 2010; WHO 2005).
Oral:
Manufacturer's labeling: 8 mg TMP/kg/day in divided doses every 12 hours for 5 days
Alternate recommendations (off-label dose): 10 mg TMP/kg/day in divided doses every 12 hours for 5 days (Ashkenazi 1993)
IV: 8 to 10 mg TMP/kg/day in divided doses every 6, 8, or 12 hours for up to 5 days

Skin/soft tissue infection due to MSSA or MRSA (off-label use): Note: If beta-hemolytic *Streptococcus* spp are also suspected, a beta-lactam antibiotic should be added to the regimen (Liu 2011)
Oral: 8 to 12 mg TMP/kg/day in divided doses every 12 hours for 5 to 10 days (IDSA [Liu 2011] or 7 to 14 days (IDSA [Stevens 2014])
IV: 8 to 12 mg TMP/kg/day in divided doses every 6 hours for 7 to 14 days (IDSA [Stevens 2014])

***Toxoplasma gondii* encephalitis in HIV-exposed/-infected patients (off-label use):**
Primary prophylaxis:
Infants ≥2 months and Children: Oral: 150 mg TMP/m²/day for 3 to 7 days of every week; total daily dose may be given in divided doses every 12 hours for 3 consecutive or alternating days, in divided doses every 12 hours every day or as a single daily dose for 3 consecutive days (HHS [OI pediatric 2013])
Adolescents: Oral: Refer to adult dosing.
Treatment (alternative to preferred therapy): Adolescents: Oral, IV: Refer to adult dosing.
Chronic maintenance therapy (alternative to preferred therapy): Adolescents: Oral: Refer to adult dosing.

Urinary tract infection: Infants >2 months and Children:
Treatment:
Oral: Manufacturer's labeling: 8 mg TMP/kg/day in divided doses every 12 hours for 10 days
IV: Manufacturer's labeling: 8 to 10 mg TMP/kg/day in divided doses every 6, 8, or 12 hours for up to 14 days with serious infections
Prophylaxis: Oral: 2 mg TMP/kg/dose daily or 5 mg TMP/kg/dose twice weekly

Renal Impairment Oral, IV:
Manufacturer's labeling: Children and Adults:
CrCl >30 mL/minute: No dosage adjustment required
CrCl 15-30 mL/minute: Administer 50% of recommended dose
CrCl <15 mL/minute: Use is not recommended
Alternate recommendations:
CrCl 15-30 mL/minute:
Treatment: Administer full daily dose (divided every 12 hours) for 24-48 hours, then decrease daily dose by 50% and administer every 24 hours (**Note:** For serious infections including *Pneumocystis jirovecii* pneumonia (PCP), full daily dose is given in divided doses every 6-8 hours for 2 days, followed by reduction to 50% daily dose divided every 12 hours) (Nahata 1995).
PCP prophylaxis: One-half single-strength tablet (40 mg trimethoprim) daily **or** 1 single-strength tablet (80 mg trimethoprim) daily or 3 times weekly (Masur 2002).
CrCl <15 mL/minute:
Treatment: Administer full daily dose every 48 hours (Nahata 1995)
PCP prophylaxis: One-half single-strength tablet (40 mg trimethoprim) daily **or** 1 single-strength tablet (80 mg trimethoprim) 3 times weekly (Masur 2002). While the guidelines do acknowledge the alternative of giving 1 single-strength tablet daily, this may be inadvisable in the uremic/ESRD patient.
GFR <10 mL/minute/1.73 m²: Children: Use is not recommended, but if required, administer 5-10 mg trimethoprim/kg every 24 hours (Aronoff 2007).
Intermittent Hemodialysis (IHD) (administer after hemodialysis on dialysis days):
Adults: 2.5-10 mg/kg trimethoprim every 24 hours or 5-20 mg/kg trimethoprim 3 times weekly after IHD. **Note:** Dosing is highly dependent upon indication for use (eg, treatment of cystitis versus treatment of PCP pneumonia (Heinz 2009).
PCP prophylaxis: One single-strength tablet (80 mg trimethoprim) after each dialysis session (Masur 2002)
Note: Dosing dependent on the assumption of 3 times/week, complete IHD sessions.
Children: Use is not recommended, but if required, administer 5-10 mg trimethoprim/kg every 24 hours (Aronoff 2007).
Peritoneal dialysis (PD):
Use CrCl <15 mL/minute dosing recommendations. Not significantly removed by PD; supplemental dosing is not required (Aronoff 2007):
GFR <10 mL/minute/1.73 m²: Children: Use is not recommended, but if required 5-10 mg TMP/kg every 24 hours.
Exit-site and tunnel infections: Oral: One single-strength tablet daily (Li 2010)

Intraperitoneal: Loading dose: TMP-SMX 320/1600 mg/L; Maintenance: TMP-SMX 80/400 mg/L (Aronoff 2007; Warady 2000)

Peritonitis: Oral: One double-strength tablet twice daily (Li 2010)

Continuous renal replacement therapy (CRRT) (Heintz 2009; Trotman 2005): Drug clearance is highly dependent on the method of renal replacement, filter type, and flow rate. Appropriate dosing requires close monitoring of pharmacologic response, signs of adverse reactions due to drug accumulation, as well as drug concentrations in relation to target trough (if appropriate). The following are general recommendations only (based on dialysate flow/ultrafiltration rates of 1-2 L/hour and minimal residual renal function) and should not supersede clinical judgment:

CVVH/CVVHD/CVVHDF: 2.5-7.5 mg/kg of TMP every 12 hours. **Note:** Dosing regimen dependent on clinical indication. Critically-ill patients with *P. jirovecii* pneumonia receiving CVVHDF may require up to 10 mg/kg every 12 hours (Heintz 2009).

Hepatic Impairment There are no dosage adjustments provided in manufacturer's labeling. Use with caution; use is contraindicated in cases of marked hepatic damage.

Dietary Considerations Should be taken with 8 oz of water. May be taken without regard to meals.

Administration

IV: Infuse diluted solution over 60-90 minutes; not for IM injection

Oral: Administer without regard to meals. Administer with at least 8 ounces of water.

Monitoring Parameters Perform culture and sensitivity testing prior to initiating therapy; CBC, serum potassium, creatinine, BUN

Test Interactions Increased creatinine (Jaffé alkaline picrate reaction); increased serum methotrexate by dihydrofolate reductase method

Dosage Forms Considerations The 5:1 ratio (SMX:TMP) remains constant in all dosage forms.

Dosage Forms Excipient information presented when available (limited, particularly for generics); consult specific product labeling.

Solution, Intravenous:

Generic: Sulfamethoxazole 80 mg and trimethoprim 16 mg per mL (5 mL, 10 mL, 30 mL)

Suspension, Oral:

Sulfatrim Pediatric: Sulfamethoxazole 200 mg and trimethoprim 40 mg per 5 mL (473 mL) [contains alcohol, usp, fd&c red #40, fd&c yellow #6 (sunset yellow), methylparaben, polysorbate 80, propylene glycol, propylparaben, saccharin sodium; cherry flavor]

Generic: Sulfamethoxazole 200 mg and trimethoprim 40 mg per 5 mL (20 mL, 473 mL)

Tablet, Oral:

Bactrim: Sulfamethoxazole 400 mg and trimethoprim 80 mg [scored; contains sodium benzoate]

Bactrim DS: Sulfamethoxazole 800 mg and trimethoprim 160 mg [scored; contains sodium benzoate]

Generic: Sulfamethoxazole 400 mg and trimethoprim 80 mg, Sulfamethoxazole 800 mg and trimethoprim 160 mg

◆ Sulfamylon *see* Mafenide *on page 1118*

Sulfanilamide (sul fa NIL a mide)

Brand Names: US AVC Vaginal

Index Terms p-amino-benzenesulfonamide

Pharmacologic Category Antifungal Agent, Vaginal

Use Vulvovaginitis: Treatment of vulvovaginitis caused by *Candida albicans*

Dosing

Adult & Geriatric Vulvovaginitis: Intravaginal: Insert one applicatorful intravaginally once or twice daily for 30 days

Renal Impairment There are no dosage adjustments provided in the manufacturer's labeling

Hepatic Impairment There are no dosage adjustments provided in the manufacturer's labeling

Additional Information Complete prescribing information should be consulted for additional detail.

Dosage Forms Excipient information presented when available (limited, particularly for generics); consult specific product labeling.

Cream, Vaginal:

AVC Vaginal: 15% (120 g) [contains methylparaben, propylene glycol, propylparaben, trolamine (triethanolamine)]

SulfaSALAzine (sul fa SAL a zeen)

Brand Names: US Azulfidine; Azulfidine EN-tabs; Sulfazine; Sulfazine EC

Brand Names: Canada Apo-Sulfasalazine; PMS-Sulfasalazine; Salazopyrin; Salazopyrin En-Tabs

Index Terms Salicylazosulfapyridine

Pharmacologic Category 5-Aminosalicylic Acid Derivative

Use

U.S. labeling:

Juvenile rheumatoid arthritis: Delayed release: Treatment of pediatric patients with polyarticular-course juvenile rheumatoid arthritis who have responded inadequately to salicylates or other nonsteroidal anti-inflammatory drugs (NSAIDs).

Rheumatoid arthritis: Delayed release: Treatment of patients with rheumatoid arthritis who have responded inadequately to salicylates or other NSAIDs.

Ulcerative colitis: Immediate and delayed release: Treatment of mild to moderate ulcerative colitis; adjunctive therapy in severe ulcerative colitis; prolongation of the remission period between acute attacks of ulcerative colitis.

Canadian labeling: Adjunctive therapy in severe ulcerative colitis, distal ulcerative colitis or proctitis, and Crohn disease; enteric coated tablets are also used for rheumatoid arthritis unsuccessfully treated with first-line therapy

Pregnancy Considerations Adverse events have not been observed in animal reproduction studies. Sulfasalazine and sulfapyridine cross the placenta; a potential for kernicterus in the newborn exists. Agranulocytosis was noted in an infant following maternal use of sulfasalazine during pregnancy. Additionally, cases of neural tube defects have been reported (causation undetermined); sulfasalazine is known to inhibit the absorption and metabolism of folic acid and may diminish the effects of folic acid supplementation. Based on available data, an increase in fetal malformations has not been observed following maternal use of sulfasalazine for the treatment of inflammatory bowel disease or ulcerative colitis. When treatment for inflammatory bowel disease is needed during pregnancy, sulfasalazine may be used, although supplementation with folic acid is recommended (Habal, 2012; Mahadevan, 2009; Mottet, 2007).

Breast-Feeding Considerations Sulfasalazine is excreted in breast milk; sulfapyridine concentrations are ~30% to 60% of the maternal serum. Bloody stools or diarrhea have been reported in nursing infants. Although sulfapyridine has poor bilirubin-displacing ability, exposure may cause kernicterus in the newborn. The manufacturer recommends that caution be used in women who are breast-feeding. Other sources consider use of sulfasalazine to be safe while breast-feeding; monitoring of the infant is recommended (Habal, 2012; Mahadevan, 2009; Mottet, 2007).

Contraindications

Hypersensitivity to sulfasalazine, sulfa drugs, salicylates, or any component of the formulation; intestinal or urinary obstruction; porphyria

Note: Although the FDA approved product labeling states this medication is contraindicated with other sulfonamide-containing drug classes, the scientific basis of this statement has been challenged. See "Warnings/Precautions" for more detail.

Canadian labeling: Additional contraindications (not in U.S. labeling): Severe renal impairment (GFR <30 mL/minute/1.73 m^2); severe hepatic impairment; use in pediatric patients <2 years of age; patients in whom acute asthmatic attacks, urticaria, rhinitis or other allergic manifestations are precipitated by acetyl salicylic acid (ASA) or other NSAIDs

Warnings/Precautions Use with extreme caution in patients with renal impairment (Canadian labeling contraindicates use in severe impairment [GFR <30 mL/minute/1.73 m^2]), impaired hepatic function (Canadian labeling contraindicates use in severe impairment), or blood dyscrasias. Fatalities associated with severe reactions including agranulocytosis, aplastic anemia, and other blood dyscrasias have occurred; discontinue use at first sign of rash or signs of serious adverse reactions. The presence of clinical signs such as sore throat, fever, pallor, or purpura may be indicative of a serious blood disorder; monitor complete blood counts frequently. Serious infections (some fatal), including sepsis and pneumonia, have been reported. Infections may be associated with agranulocytosis, neutropenia, or myelosuppression. Monitor for signs/symptoms of infection during and after sulfasalazine therapy and promptly evaluate if infection occurs; discontinue therapy for serious infections. Use cautiously in

patients with a history of recurring or chronic infections or with underlying conditions or concomitant therapy which may predispose them to infectious complications.

Use caution in patients with severe allergies or bronchial asthma. Hemolytic anemia may occur when used in patients with G6PD deficiency; use cautiously. May decrease folic acid absorption. Deaths from irreversible neuromuscular or central nervous system changes, fibrosing alveolitis, agranulocytosis, aplastic anemia, and other blood dyscrasias have been reported. In males, oligospermia (rare) and infertility has been reported. Slow acetylators may be more prone to adverse reactions. Discontinue enteric coated tablets if noted to pass without disintegrating.

Severe skin reactions (some fatal), including Stevens-Johnson syndrome (SJS), exfoliative dermatitis, and toxic epidermal necrolysis (TEN) have occurred with sulfonamides (including sulfasalazine), most commonly during the first month of treatment; discontinue use at first sign of skin rash, mucosal lesions, or any other sign of dermatologic toxicity. Severe and life-threatening hypersensitivity reactions, including drug rash with eosinophilia and systemic symptoms (DRESS) syndrome have been reported. Fever or lymphadenopathy may be present prior to rash development. Other severe hypersensitivity reactions may include internal organ involvement, such as hepatitis, nephritis, myocarditis, mononucleosis-like syndrome, hematologic abnormalities (including hematophagic histiocytosis), and/or pneumonitis including eosinophilic infiltration. Discontinue treatment for severe reactions and evaluate promptly.

Sulfonamide ("sulfa") allergy: Traditionally, concerns for cross-reactivity have extended to all compounds containing the sulfonamide structure (SO_2NH_2). An expanded understanding of allergic mechanisms indicates cross-reactivity between antibiotic sulfonamides and nonantibiotic sulfonamides may not occur, or at the very least this potential is extremely low (Brackett 2004; Johnson 2005; Slatore 2004; Tornero 2004). In particular, mechanisms of cross-reaction due to antibody production (anaphylaxis) are unlikely to occur with nonantibiotic sulfonamides and antibiotic sulfonamides. A nonantibiotic sulfonamide compound which contains the arylamine structure and therefore may cross-react with antibiotic sulfonamides is sulfasalazine (Zawodniak 2010). T-cell-mediated (type IV) reactions (eg, maculopapular rash) are less understood and it is not possible to completely exclude this potential based on current insights. In cases where prior reactions were severe (Stevens-Johnson syndrome/TEN), some clinicians choose to avoid exposure to these classes.

Adverse Reactions

>10%:

Central nervous system: Headache (RA 9%)

Dermatologic: Skin rash (RA 13%)

Gastrointestinal: Nausea (RA 19%), dyspepsia (RA 13%), anorexia, gastric distress, vomiting

Genitourinary: Oligospermia (reversible)

1% to 10%:

Central nervous system: Dizziness

Dermatologic: Pruritus (RA 4%), urticaria

Gastrointestinal: Abdominal pain (RA 8%), stomatitis (RA 4%)

Hematologic & oncologic: Leukopenia (RA 3%), thrombocytopenia (RA 1%), Heinz body anemia, hemolytic anemia

Hepatic: Abnormal hepatic function tests (RA 4%)

Respiratory: Cyanosis

Miscellaneous: Fever

<1% (limited to important or life-threatening; includes reactions reported with mesalamine or other sulfonamides): Agranulocytosis, alopecia, anaphylaxis, angioedema, aplastic anemia, arthralgia, cauda equina syndrome, cholestatic hepatitis, cholestatic jaundice, conjunctival injection, crystalluria, depression, diarrhea, DRESS syndrome, drowsiness, eosinophilia, exfoliative dermatitis, folate deficiency, fulminant hepatitis, Guillain-Barré syndrome, hallucination, hearing loss, hematologic abnormality, hematologic disease (pseudomononucleosis), hematuria, hemolytic-uremic syndrome, hepatic cirrhosis, hepatic failure, hepatic necrosis, hepatitis, hepatotoxicity (idiosyncratic) (Chalasani, 2014), hypoglycemia, hypoprothrombinemia, injected sclera, insomnia, interstitial nephritis, interstitial pulmonary disease, jaundice, Kawasaki syndrome (single case report), lupus-like syndrome, megaloblastic anemia, meningitis, methemoglobinemia, myelitis, myelodysplastic syndrome, myocarditis (allergic), nephritis, nephrolithiasis, nephrotic syndrome, neutropenia (congenital), neutropenic enterocolitis, oropharyngeal pain, pancreatitis, parapsoriasis varioliformis acuta, periarteritis nodosa, pericarditis, periorbital edema, peripheral neuropathy, pleurisy, pneumonia, pneumonitis, proteinuria, pulmonary alveolitis,

purpura, renal disease (acute), rhabdomyolysis, seizure, sepsis, serum sickness-like reaction (children with JRA have frequent and severe reaction), skin discoloration, skin photosensitivity, Stevens-Johnson syndrome, thyroid function impairment, toxic epidermal necrolysis, toxic nephrosis, urine discoloration, vasculitis

Drug Interactions

Metabolism/Transport Effects None known.

Avoid Concomitant Use There are no known interactions where it is recommended to avoid concomitant use.

Increased Effect/Toxicity

SulfaSALAzine may increase the levels/effects of: Heparin; Heparin (Low Molecular Weight); Methotrexate; Prilocaine; Sodium Nitrite; Thiopurine Analogs; Varicella Virus-Containing Vaccines

The levels/effects of SulfaSALAzine may be increased by: Dapsone (Topical); Nitric Oxide; Nonsteroidal Anti-Inflammatory Agents

Decreased Effect

SulfaSALAzine may decrease the levels/effects of: Cardiac Glycosides; Folic Acid; Methylfolate

Storage/Stability Store at 25°C (77°F); excursions permitted to 15°C to 30°C (59°F to 86°F).

Mechanism of Action 5-aminosalicylic acid (5-ASA) is the active component of sulfasalazine; the specific mechanism of action of 5-ASA is unknown; however, it is thought that it modulates local chemical mediators of the inflammatory response, especially leukotrienes, and is also postulated to be a free radical scavenger or an inhibitor of tumor necrosis factor (TNF); action appears topical rather than systemic

Pharmacodynamics/Kinetics

Absorption: ≤15% as unchanged drug from small intestine

Protein binding: Sulfasalazine: >99% to albumin; Sulfapyridine: ~70% to albumin; Acetylsulfapyridine (AcSP): ~90% to plasma proteins

Distribution: V_d: Sulfasalazine ~7.5 L

Metabolism: Via colonic intestinal flora to sulfapyridine and 5-aminosalicylic acid (5-ASA). Following absorption, sulfapyridine undergoes acetylation to form AcSP and ring hydroxylation while 5-ASA undergoes N-acetylation (non-acetylation phenotype dependent process); rate of metabolism via acetylation dependent on acetylation phenotype

Bioavailability: Sulfasalazine: <15%; Sulfapyridine: ~60%; 5-aminosalicylic acid: ~10% to 30%

Half-life elimination: Sulfasalazine: 5.7-10 hours (prolonged in elderly); Sulfapyridine: 14.8 hours (slow acetylators) and 10.4 hours (fast acetylators)

Time to peak: Sulfasalazine: 3-12 hours (mean: 6 hours); Metabolites: ~10 hours

Excretion: Primarily urine (as unchanged drug, conjugates, and acetylated metabolites); feces (small amounts)

Dosing

Adult & Geriatric

U.S. labeling:

Rheumatoid arthritis: Oral: Enteric coated tablet: Initial: 0.5 to 1 g daily; increase weekly to maintenance dose of 2 g daily in 2 divided doses; maximum: 3 g daily (if response to 2 g daily is inadequate after 12 weeks of treatment)

Ulcerative colitis: Oral:

Initial: 3 to 4 g daily in evenly divided doses at ≤8-hour intervals; may initiate therapy with 1 to 2 g daily to reduce GI intolerance. **Note:** American College of Gastroenterology guideline recommendations: Titrate to 4 to 6 g daily in 4 divided doses (Kornbluth, 2010).

Maintenance dose: 2 g daily in evenly divided doses at ≤8-hour intervals; if GI intolerance occurs reduce dosage by 50% and gradually increase to target dose after several days. If GI intolerance persists, stop drug for 5 to 7 days and reintroduce at a lower daily dose.

Crohn disease, active mild/moderate, ileocolonic or colonic disease (off-label use): Oral: 3 to 6 g daily in divided doses (Lichtenstein, 2009)

Desensitization regimen: For patients who may be sensitive to treatment, it is suggested to start with a total dose of 50 to 250 mg daily and double it every 4 to 7 days until the desired dose is achieved. Discontinue if symptoms of sensitivity occur. Do not attempt in patients with a history of agranulocytosis or those who have had a previous anaphylactoid reaction on sulfasalazine therapy

Canadian labeling:

Rheumatoid arthritis: Oral: Enteric coated tablet: Initial: 500 mg daily; increase dose weekly by 500 mg (total daily dose given in 2 divided doses) to maintenance dose of 1 g twice daily; if inadequate response to 1 g twice daily after 2 months, may increase dose to 3 g daily. Clinical improvement usually observed 1 to 2 months after initiating therapy. Concurrent use of analgesics and/or anti-inflammatory agents is recommended until therapeutic effect of sulfasalazine is observed.

Ulcerative colitis, inflammatory bowel disease, Crohn disease: Oral: **Note:** Consider dose reduction or use of enteric coated tablet in patients experiencing adverse gastrointestinal effects with uncoated tablet.

Acute attacks: Severe: 1 to 2 g 3 to 4 times daily; mild to moderate: 1 g 3 to 4 times daily

Maintenance of remission: 1 g 2 to 3 times daily; continue dose indefinitely unless patient experiences adverse effects. In the event patient condition worsens, increase dose to 1 to 2 g 3 to 4 times daily.

Pediatric

U.S. labeling:

Juvenile rheumatoid arthritis: Children ≥6 years: Oral: Enteric coated tablet: 30 to 50 mg/kg/day in 2 divided doses; Initial: Begin with 1/4 to 1/3 of expected maintenance dose; increase weekly; maximum: 2 g daily typically

Ulcerative colitis: Children ≥6 years: Oral: Initial: 40 to 60 mg/kg/day in 3 to 6 divided doses; maintenance dose: 30 mg/kg/day in 4 divided doses

Desensitization regimen: Refer to adult dosing for patients who may be sensitive to treatment.

Canadian labeling:

Ulcerative colitis, inflammatory bowel disease, Crohn disease: Oral: **Note:** Consider dose reduction or use of enteric coated tablet in patients experiencing adverse gastrointestinal effects with uncoated tablet.

Acute attacks:

Body weight 25 to <35 kg: 500 mg 3 times daily

Body weight 35 to 50 kg: 1 g 2 to 3 times daily

Maintenance of remission:

Body weight 25 to <35 kg: 500 mg 2 times daily

Body weight 35 to 50 kg: 500 mg 2 to 3 times daily

Renal Impairment There are no dosage adjustments provided in the manufacturer's labeling; use with extreme caution. Canadian labeling contraindicates use in severe impairment (GFR <30 mL/minute/1.73 m²).

Hepatic Impairment There are no dosage adjustments provided in the manufacturer's labeling; use with extreme caution. Canadian labeling contraindicates use in severe impairment.

Dietary Considerations Sulfasalazine impairs folate absorption. Adequate fluid intake is required to prevent crystalluria and stone formation.

Administration Tablets should be administered in evenly divided doses, preferably after meals. Enteric coated tablets should be swallowed whole.

Monitoring Parameters CBC with differential and liver function tests (prior to therapy, then every other week for first 3 months of therapy, followed by every month for the second 3 months, then once every 3 months thereafter or as clinically indicated); periodic urinalysis and renal/liver function tests (Canadian labeling also recommends renal function tests [including urinalysis] prior to therapy and monthly for first 3 months); stool frequency; signs of infection, dermatologic toxicity, or hypersensitivity reactions

Reference Range Sulfapyridine concentrations >50 mcg/mL are associated with increased adverse events.

Test Interactions Reports of possible interference with measurements, by liquid chromatography, of urinary normetanephrine causing a false-positive test result have been observed in patients exposed to sulfasalazine or its metabolite, mesalamine/mesalazine.

Dosage Forms Excipient information presented when available (limited, particularly for generics); consult specific product labeling.

Tablet, Oral:

Azulfidine: 500 mg [scored]

Sulfazine: 500 mg [scored]

Generic: 500 mg

Tablet Delayed Release, Oral:

Azulfidine EN-tabs: 500 mg

Sulfazine EC: 500 mg

Generic: 500 mg

Extemporaneous Preparations A 100 mg/mL oral suspension may be made with tablets. Place twenty 500 mg tablets in a mortar and add a small amount of a 1:1 mixture of Ora-Sweet® and Ora-Plus® to cover the tablets. Let soak for 20-30 minutes. Crush the tablets and mix to a uniform paste; mix while adding the vehicle in equal proportions to **almost** 100 mL; transfer to a calibrated bottle, rinse mortar with vehicle, and add sufficient quantity of vehicle to make 100 mL. Label "shake well". Stable 91 days under refrigeration or at room temperature.

Lingertat-Walsh K, Walker SE, Law S, et al, "Stability of Sulfasalazine Oral Suspension," *Can J Hosp Pharm*, 2006, 59(4):194-200.

♦ Sulfatrim *see* Sulfamethoxazole and Trimethoprim *on page 1710*

♦ Sulfatrim Pediatric *see* Sulfamethoxazole and Trimethoprim *on page 1710*

♦ Sulfazine *see* SulfaSALAzine *on page 1714*

♦ Sulfazine EC *see* SulfaSALAzine *on page 1714*

Sulfur and Sulfacetamide

(SUL fur & sul fa SEE ta mide)

Brand Names: US AVAR; AVAR LS; AVAR-e; AVAR-e Green; AVAR-e LS; BP 10-1; BP Cleansing Wash; Clarifoam EF; Claris [DSC]; Clenia [DSC]; Plexion; Prascion; Prascion FC; Prascion RA; Rosanil; Rosula Wash; SSS 10-5; SulfaCleanse 8/4; Sumadan; Sumadan XLT; Sumaxin; Sumaxin TS; Verti-sulf [DSC]; Zencia

Brand Names: Canada Sulfacet-R

Index Terms Sodium Sulfacetamide and Sulfur; Sulfacetamide and Sulfur; Sulfur and Sulfacetamide Sodium

Pharmacologic Category Acne Products; Antibiotic, Sulfonamide Derivative; Antiseborrheic Agent, Topical; Topical Skin Product, Acne

Use Aid in the treatment of acne vulgaris, acne rosacea, and seborrheic dermatitis

Dosing

Adult & Geriatric Acne vulgaris, acne rosacea, seborrheic dermatitis: Topical: Apply in a thin film 1-3 times/day. Cleansing products should be used 1-2 times/day.

Pediatric Children ≥12 years: Refer to adult dosing.

Renal Impairment Use is contraindicated.

Hepatic Impairment No dosage adjustment provided in manufacturer's labeling.

Additional Information Complete prescribing information should be consulted for additional detail.

Dosage Forms Excipient information presented when available (limited, particularly for generics); consult specific product labeling. [DSC] = Discontinued product

Cleanser, topical: Sulfur 2% and sulfacetamide sodium 10% (227 g), Sulfur 4.8% and sulfacetamide sodium 9.8% (285 g), Sulfur 5% and sulfacetamide sodium 10% (170 g, 340 g)

AVAR: Sulfur 5% and sulfacetamide sodium 10% (227 g) [contains benzyl alcohol]

AVAR LS: Sulfur 2% and sulfacetamide sodium 10% (227 g) [contains benzyl alcohol]

Plexion: Sulfur 4.8% and sulfacetamide sodium 9.8% (285 g) [contains benzyl alcohol]

Prascion: Sulfur 5% and sulfacetamide sodium 10% (170 g, 340 g)

Rosanil: Sulfur 5% and sulfacetamide sodium 10% (170 g)

Cream, topical: Sulfur 2% and sulfacetamide sodium 10% (57 g), Sulfur 4.8% and sulfacetamide sodium 9.8% (57 g), Sulfur 5% and sulfacetamide sodium 10% (28 g)

AVAR-e: Sulfur 5% and sulfacetamide sodium 10% (45 g [DSC], 57 g) [contains benzyl alcohol]

AVAR-e Green: Sulfur 5% and sulfacetamide sodium 10% (45 g [DSC], 57 g) [contains benzyl alcohol; color corrective cream]

AVAR-e LS: Sulfur 2% and sulfacetamide sodium 10% (45 g [DSC], 57 g) [contains benzyl alcohol]

Clenia: Sulfur 5% and sulfacetamide sodium 10% (28 g) [DSC]

Plexion: Sulfur 4.8% and sulfacetamide sodium 9.8% (57 g) [contains benzyl alcohol]

Prascion RA: Sulfur 5% and sulfacetamide sodium 10% (45 g) [contains benzyl alcohol and sunscreen]

SSS 10-5: Sulfur 5% and sulfacetamide sodium 10% (28 g)

Virti-sulf: Sulfur 5% and sulfacetamide sodium 10% (28 g) [DSC]

Foam, topical: Sulfur 5% and sulfacetamide sodium 10% (60 g)

AVAR: Sulfur 5% and sulfacetamide sodium 9.5% (100 g) [contains benzyl alcohol]

AVAR LS: Sulfur 2% and sulfacetamide sodium 10% (100 g) [contains benzyl alcohol]

Clarifoam EF: Sulfur 5% and sulfacetamide sodium 10% (60 g, 100 g)

SSS 10-5: Sulfur 5% and sulfacetamide sodium 10% (60 g, 100 g)

Gel, topical: Sulfur 5% and sulfacetamide sodium 10% (45 g)

Lotion, topical: Sulfur 4.8% and sulfacetamide sodium 9.8% (57 g)

Plexion: Sulfur 4.8% and sulfacetamide sodium 9.8% (57 g) [contains benzyl alcohol]

Pad, topical [cleansing cloth]: Sulfur 4% and sulfacetamide sodium 10% (60s)

Avar: Sulfur 5% and sulfacetamide sodium 9.5% (30s, 60s)

Avar LS: Sulfur 2% and sulfacetamide sodium 10% (30s, 60s)

Plexion: Sulfur 4.8% and sulfacetamide sodium 9.8% (60s) [contains benzyl alcohol]

Prascion FC: Sulfur 5% and sulfacetamide sodium 10% (30s, 60s)

Rosula: Sulfur 5% and sulfacetamide sodium 10% (30s, 60s)

Sumaxin: Sulfur 4% and sulfacetamide sodium 10% (60s) [contains aloe]

Suspension, topical: Sulfur 4% and sulfacetamide sodium 8% (473 mL), sulfur 5% and sulfacetamide sodium10% (30 g)

SulfaCleanse 8/4: Sulfur 4% and sulfacetamide sodium 8% (473 mL) [contains aloe]

Sumaxin TS: Sulfur 4% and sulfacetamide sodium 8% (473 mL) [contains aloe]

Wash, topical: Sulfur 4% and sulfacetamide sodium 9% (480 mL); Sulfur 4.5% and sulfacetamide sodium 9% (454 g)

BP 10-1: Sulfur 1% and sulfacetamide sodium 10% (170 g)

BP Cleansing Wash: Sulfur 5% and sulfacetamide sodium 10% (480 mL) [contains urea]

Clenia: Sulfur 5% and sulfacetamide sodium 10% (170 g, 340 g) [DSC]

Rosula Wash: Sulfur 4.5% and sulfacetamide sodium 10% (340.2 g)

Sumaxin: Sulfur 4% and sulfacetamide sodium 9% (473 mL) [contains aloe]

Zencia: Sulfur 4% and sulfacetamide sodium 9% (480 mL) [contains aloe]

Wash, topical [emulsion-based]:

BP Cleansing Wash: Sulfur 4% and sulfacetamide sodium 10% (473 mL) [contains urea]

Claris: Sulfur 4% and sulfacetamide sodium 10% (473 mL) [contains urea 10%] [DSC]

Sumadan: Sulfur 4.5% and sulfacetamide sodium 9% (454 g)

Sumadan XLT: Sulfur 4.5% and sulfacetamide sodium 9% (454 g) [packaged in a kit with Niseko sunscreen SPF 25]

◆ Sulfur and Sulfacetamide Sodium see Sulfur and Sulfacetamide on page 1716

Sulindac (SUL in dak)

Brand Names: US Clinoril [DSC]
Brand Names: Canada Apo-Sulin; Teva-Sulindac
Index Terms Clinoril
Pharmacologic Category Nonsteroidal Anti-inflammatory Drug (NSAID), Oral
Use Management of inflammatory diseases including osteoarthritis, rheumatoid arthritis, acute gouty arthritis, ankylosing spondylitis, acute painful shoulder (bursitis/tendonitis)
Medication Guide Available Yes
Dosing
Adult & Geriatric Note: Maximum daily dose: 400 mg
Osteoarthritis, rheumatoid arthritis, ankylosing spondylitis: 150 mg twice daily
Acute painful shoulder (bursitis/tendonitis): 200 mg twice daily; usual treatment: 7-14 days
Acute gouty arthritis: 200 mg twice daily; usual treatment: 7 days
Pediatric Dose not established
Renal Impairment No dosage adjustment provided in manufacturer's labeling. However, sulindac is not recommended with advanced renal impairment; if required, decrease dose and monitor closely.
Hepatic Impairment No dosage adjustment provided in manufacturer's labeling. However, dosage reduction may be necessary; discontinue if abnormal liver function tests occur.
Additional Information Complete prescribing information should be consulted for additional detail.
Dosage Forms Excipient information presented when available (limited, particularly for generics); consult specific product labeling. [DSC] = Discontinued product
Tablet, Oral:
Clinoril: 200 mg [DSC]
Generic: 150 mg, 200 mg

◆ Sumadan see Sulfur and Sulfacetamide on page 1716
◆ Sumadan XLT see Sulfur and Sulfacetamide on page 1716

SUMAtriptan (soo ma TRIP tan)

Brand Names: US Alsuma; Imitrex; Imitrex STATdose Refill; Imitrex STATdose System; Sumavel DosePro; Zecuity
Brand Names: Canada ACT-Sumatriptan; Apo-Sumatriptan; Ava-Sumatriptan; Dom-Sumatriptan; Imitrex DF; Imitrex Injection; Imitrex Nasal Spray; Mylan-Sumatriptan; PHL-Sumatriptan; PMS-Sumatriptan; Sandoz-Sumatriptan; Sumatriptan DF; Taro-Sumatriptan; Teva-Sumatriptan; Teva-Sumatriptan DF
Index Terms Sumatriptan Succinate
Pharmacologic Category Antimigraine Agent; Serotonin 5-HT$_{1B, 1D}$ Receptor Agonist
Use
Migraine: Intranasal, Oral, SubQ, Transdermal: Acute treatment of migraine with or without aura in adults
Cluster headache: SubQ: Acute treatment of cluster headache episodes in adults
Pregnancy Considerations Adverse events were observed in animal reproduction studies. In a study using full term healthy human placentas, limited amounts of sumatriptan were found to cross the placenta (Schenker, 1995).

An overall increased risk of major congenital malformations has not been observed following first trimester exposure to sumatriptan in several studies. Pregnancy outcome information for sumatriptan is available from a pregnancy registry sponsored by GlaxoSmithKline. As of October 2008, data was available for 558 infants/fetuses exposed to sumatriptan, and seven exposed to both sumatriptan and naratriptan. The risk of major birth defects following sumatriptan exposure was 4.6% (95% CI: 2.9-7.2) (Cunnington, 2009). The pregnancy registry was closed in January, 2012 and additional information may be obtained from the manufacturer (800-336-2176). An analysis of data collected between 1995-2008 using the Swedish Medical Birth Register reported pregnancy outcomes following 5-HT$_{1B/1D}$ agonist exposure. An increased risk of major congenital malformations was not observed following sumatriptan exposure (2229 exposed during the first trimester) (Källén, 2011). An increased risk of major congenital malformations was not observed in the prospective Norwegian Mother and Child Cohort Study. The study included women with 5-HT$_{1B/1D}$ agonist exposure between 1999-2006 (n=455); of these, 217 were exposed to sumatriptan (Nezvalová-Henriksen, 2010; Nezvalová-Henriksen, 2012).

If treatment for cluster headaches is needed during pregnancy, sumatriptan may be used (Jürgens, 2009). Other agents are preferred for the initial treatment of migraine in pregnancy (Da Silva, 2012; MacGregor, 2012; Williams, 2012); however, sumatriptan may be considered if first-line agents fail (MacGregor, 2012).

Breast-Feeding Considerations The excretion of sumatriptan into breast milk was studied in five lactating women, 10-28 weeks postpartum (mean: 22.2 weeks). Sumatriptan 6 mg SubQ was administered and maternal milk and blood samples were collected over 8 hours after the dose. Sumatriptan was detected in breast milk. Maximum concentrations in the maternal blood (mean: 80.2 mcg/L; 0.25 hours after the dose) and milk (mean: 87.2 mcg/L; 2.5 hours after the dose) were similar. However, the amount of sumatriptan an infant would be exposed to following breast-feeding is considered to be small (although the mean milk-to-plasma ratio was ~4.9, weight-adjusted doses estimates suggest breast-fed infants receive 3.5% of a maternal dose). Expressing and discarding the milk for 8-12 hours after a single dose is suggested to reduce the amount present even further (Wojnar-Horton, 1996). Breast-feeding is not recommended by some manufacturers; however, according to other sources if treatment is needed, breast-feeding does not need to be discontinued (Jürgens, 2009; MacGregor, 2012).

Contraindications Hypersensitivity to sumatriptan or any component of the formulation, including allergic contact dermatitis to the transdermal patch; ischemic heart disease or signs or symptoms of ischemic heart disease (including Prinzmetal angina, angina pectoris, myocardial infarction, silent myocardial ischemia); cerebrovascular syndromes (including strokes, transient ischemic attacks), history of hemiplegic or basilar migraine; peripheral vascular disease (including ischemic bowel disease); uncontrolled hypertension; use within 24 hours of ergotamine derivatives; use within 24 hours of another 5-HT$_1$ agonist; concurrent administration or within 2 weeks of

discontinuing an MAO type A inhibitors; Wolff-Parkinson-White syndrome or arrhythmias associated with other cardiac accessory conduction pathway disorders; severe hepatic impairment (not Sumavel)

Warnings/Precautions Anaphylactic, anaphylactoid, and hypersensitivity reactions (including angioedema) have been reported; may be life threatening or fatal. Sumatriptan is only indicated for the acute treatment of migraine or cluster headache (product dependent); not indicated for migraine or cluster headache prophylaxis, or for the treatment of hemiplegic or basilar migraine. Acute migraine agents (eg, 5-HT$_1$ agonists, opioids, ergotamine, or a combination of the agents) used for 10 or more days per month may lead to worsening of headaches (medication overuse headache); withdrawal treatment may be necessary in the setting of overuse. May cause CNS depression, such as dizziness, weakness, or drowsiness, which may impair physical or mental abilities; patients must be cautioned about performing tasks which require mental alertness (eg, operating machinery or driving). If a patient does not respond to the first dose, the diagnosis of migraine or cluster headache should be reconsidered; rule out underlying neurologic disease in patients with atypical headache and in patients with no prior history of migraine or cluster headache. Cardiac events (coronary artery vasospasm, transient ischemia, myocardial infarction, ventricular tachycardia/fibrillation, cardiac arrest and death), cerebral/subarachnoid hemorrhage, and stroke have been reported with 5-HT$_1$ agonist administration (some occurring within a few hours of administration). Discontinue sumatriptan if these events occur. Patients who experience sensations of chest pain/pressure/tightness or symptoms suggestive of angina following dosing should be evaluated for coronary artery disease or Prinzmetal's angina before receiving additional doses; if dosing is resumed and similar symptoms recur, monitor with ECG. Perform a cardiovascular evaluation in 5-HT$_1$ agonists-naive patients who have risk factors for CAD prior to initiation of therapy. Patients with suspected CAD should have cardiovascular evaluation to rule out CAD before considering use; if cardiovascular evaluation is "satisfactory," first dose should be given in the health care provider's office (consider ECG monitoring). Periodic evaluation of cardiovascular status should be done in these patients during intermittent long-term use.

Significant elevation in blood pressure, including hypertensive crisis, has been reported on rare occasions in patients with and without a history of hypertension; use is contraindicated in patients with uncontrolled hypertension. Peripheral vascular ischemia, GI vascular ischemia and infarction, splenic infarction, and Raynaud syndrome been reported with 5-HT$_1$ agonists. Transient and permanent blindness and significant partial vision loss have been very rarely reported. Use with caution in patients with a history of seizure disorder or in patients with a lowered seizure threshold; seizures have been reported after sumatriptan administration in patients with or without a history of seizures. Use the oral formulation with caution (and with dosage limitations) in patients with mild to moderate hepatic impairment where treatment is necessary and advisable. Presystemic clearance of orally administered sumatriptan is reduced in hepatic impairment, leading to increased plasma concentrations; dosage reduction of the oral product is recommended. Non-oral routes of administration (intranasal, subcutaneous) do not undergo similar hepatic first-pass metabolism and are not expected to result in significantly altered pharmacokinetics in patients with hepatic impairment. Use of the oral, intranasal, transdermal, or Imitrex injectable is contraindicated in severe hepatic impairment; Sumavel is not recommended in severe hepatic impairment. Allergic contact dermatitis may occur with use of transdermal patch; erythematous plaque and/or erythemato-vesicular or erythemato-bullous eruptions may develop. Erythema alone is common and not by itself an indication of sensitization. Discontinue use if allergic contact dermatitis is suspected. Patients sensitized from use of transdermal system may develop systemic sensitization or other systemic reactions if sumatriptan-containing products are taken by other routes (oral, subcutaneous); if treatment with sumatriptan by other routes is required, first dose should be taken under close medical supervision. Do not apply transdermal patch in areas near or over electrically-active implantable or body-worn medical devices (eg, implantable cardiac pacemaker, body-worn insulin pump, implantable deep brain stimulator); patch contains metal parts and must be removed before magnetic resonance imaging (MRI) procedures.

Potentially significant drug-drug interactions may exist, requiring dose or frequency adjustment, additional monitoring, and/or selection of alternative therapy. Serotonin syndrome may occur with 5-HT$_1$ agonists, particularly when used concomitantly with other serotonergic drugs; symptoms (eg, mental status changes, tachycardia, hyperthermia, nausea, vomiting, diarrhea, hyperreflexia, incoordination) typically occur minutes to hours after initiation/dose increase of a serotonergic drug. Discontinue use if serotonin syndrome is suspected. Use with caution in the elderly; perform a cardiovascular evaluation prior to initiation of therapy in elderly patients with cardiovascular risk factors (eg, diabetes, hypertension, smoking, obesity, strong family history of coronary artery disease) and periodically during intermittent long-term use.

Adverse Reactions

Injection:
>10%:
Central nervous system: Paresthesia (5% to 14%), dizziness (12%), localized warm feeling (11%)
Local: Injection site reaction (≤86%; includes bleeding, bruising, swelling, and erythema)

1% to 10%:
Cardiovascular: Flushing (7%), chest discomfort (2% to 5%)
Central nervous system: Burning sensation (7%), feeling of heaviness (7%), pressure sensation (7%), feeling of tightness (5%), drowsiness (3%), feeling strange (2%), headache (2%), tight feeling in head (2%), nasal cavity pain (≤2%), anxiety (1%), cold sensation (1%), malaise (1%)
Dermatologic: Diaphoresis (2%)
Gastrointestinal: Nausea and vomiting (4%), sore throat (3%), abdominal distress (1%), dysphagia (1%)
Neuromuscular & skeletal: Neck pain (5%), numbness (5%), weakness (5%), jaw pain (2%), myalgia (2%), muscle cramps (1%)
Ophthalmic: Visual disturbance (1%)
Respiratory: Nasal signs and symptoms (2%), sinus discomfort (≤2%), bronchospasm (1%)

Nasal spray:
>10%: Gastrointestinal: Unpleasant taste (13% to 24%), nausea (11% to 13%), vomiting (11% to 13%)
1% to 10%:
Central nervous system: Dizziness (1% to 2%)
Gastrointestinal: Sore throat (1% to 2%)
Respiratory: Nasal signs and symptoms (2% to 4%)

Tablet:
1% to 10%:
Cardiovascular: Hot and cold flashes (2% to 3%, placebo 2%), chest pain (1% to 2%), palpitations (1%), syncope (1%)
Central nervous system: Paresthesia (3% to 5%), malaise (2% to 3%), sensation of pressure (neck/throat/jaw: 2% to 3%; nonspecified: 1% to 3%, placebo 2%), pain (nonspecified; 1% to 2%, placebo 1%), vertigo (<1% to 2%), dizziness (>1%), drowsiness (>1%), headache (>1%), migraine (>1%), sleepiness (>1%), burning sensation (1%), hyperacusis (1%), numbness (1%)
Gastrointestinal: Nausea (>1%), reduced salivation (>1%), vomiting (>1%), diarrhea (1%)
Genitourinary: Hematuria (1%)
Hematologic & oncologic: Hemolytic anemia (1%), hemorrhage (ear: 1%; nose/throat: 1%)
Hypersensitivity: Hypersensitivity reaction (1%)
Neuromuscular & skeletal: Myalgia (1%)
Otic: Hearing loss (1%), tinnitus (1%)
Respiratory: Allergic rhinitis (1%), dyspnea (1%), rhinitis (1%), sinusitis (1%), upper respiratory tract inflammation (1%)

Transdermal system:
>10%: Local: Localized pain (26%)
1% to 10%:
Central nervous system: Localized warm feeling (6%), feeling abnormal (paresthesia, warm/cold sensation: 2%), sensation of pressure (chest/neck/throat/jaw: 2%)
Dermatologic: Skin discoloration (application site: 3% to 5%), allergic contact dermatitis (4%), skin vesicle (application site: 3%)
Hematologic & oncologic: Bruise (application site: 1% to 2%)
Local: Localized pruritus (8%), localized irritation (4%)
<1%: Skin erosion (application site)

Route unspecified: <1%: (Limited to important or life-threatening): Abdominal aortic aneurysm, abnormal hepatic function tests, accommodation disturbance, acute renal failure, anemia, cardiac arrhythmia, cardiomyopathy, cerebrovascular accident, colonic ischemia, coronary artery vasospasm, cyanosis, deafness, dystonic reaction, giant-cell arteritis, hallucination, hematuria, hemorrhage (nose/throat), hypersensitivity reaction, increased intracranial pressure, increased thyroid stimulating hormone level, intestinal obstruction, myocardial

infarction, optic neuropathy (ischemic), pancytopenia, Prinzmetal angina, psychomotor disturbance, pulmonary embolism, Raynaud's phenomenon, retinal blood vessel occlusion (artery), seizure, serotonin syndrome, skin photosensitivity, subarachnoid hemorrhage, thrombosis, vasculitis

Drug Interactions

Metabolism/Transport Effects None known.

Avoid Concomitant Use

Avoid concomitant use of SUMAtriptan with any of the following: Dapoxetine; Ergot Derivatives; MAO Inhibitors

Increased Effect/Toxicity

SUMAtriptan may increase the levels/effects of: Antipsychotic Agents; Droxidopa; Ergot Derivatives; Metoclopramide; Serotonin Modulators

The levels/effects of SUMAtriptan may be increased by: Antiemetics (5HT3 Antagonists); Antipsychotic Agents; Dapoxetine; Ergot Derivatives; MAO Inhibitors; Metaxalone

Decreased Effect There are no known significant interactions involving a decrease in effect.

Storage/Stability

Alsuma: Store at 25°C (77°F); excursions are permitted between 15°C and 30°C (59°F and 86°F); do not refrigerate. Protect from light.

Imitrex injectable, tablet, intranasal: Store at 2°C to 30°C (36°F to 86°F). Protect from light.

Sumavel DosePro: Store at 20°C to 25°C (68°F to 77°F); excursions are permitted between 15°C and 30°C (59°F and 86°F); do not freeze. Protect from light.

Zecuity: Store at 20°C to 25°C (68°F to 77°F); excursions are permitted between 15°C and 30°C (59°F and 86°F); do not refrigerate or freeze.

Mechanism of Action Selective agonist for serotonin (5-HT$_{1B}$ and 5-HT$_{1D}$ receptors) on intracranial blood vessels and sensory nerves of the trigeminal system; causes vasoconstriction and reduces neurogenic inflammation associated with antidromic neuronal transmission correlating with relief of migraine

Pharmacodynamics/Kinetics

Onset of action: Oral: ~30 minutes; Intranasal: ~15 to 30 minutes; SubQ: ~10 minutes

Distribution: V$_d$: 2.4 L/kg

Protein binding: 14% to 21%

Metabolism: Hepatic, primarily via MAO-A isoenzyme; extensive first-pass metabolism following oral administration

Bioavailability: Intranasal: 17% (compared to SubQ); Oral: 15%; SubQ: 97% ± 16%

Half-life elimination: ~2 to 3 hours

Time to peak, serum: Oral: 2 to 2.5 hours; SubQ: 12 minutes (range: 4 to 20 minutes); Transdermal patch: ~1 hour

Excretion:

Intranasal: Urine (42% of total dose as indole acetic acid metabolite; 3% of total dose as unchanged drug)

Oral: Urine (~60% of total dose, mostly as indole acetic acid metabolite; 3% of total dose as unchanged drug); feces (~40%)

SubQ: Urine (38% of total dose as indole acetic acid metabolite; 22% of total dose as unchanged drug)

Transdermal patch: Urine (69% of total dose as indole acetic acid metabolite; 11% of total dose as unchanged drug)

Dosing

Adult & Geriatric

Migraine:

Oral: A single dose of 25 mg, 50 mg, or 100 mg (taken with fluids). If a satisfactory response has not been obtained at 2 hours, a second dose may be administered. Results from clinical trials show that initial doses of 50 mg and 100 mg are more effective than doses of 25 mg, and that 100 mg doses do not provide a greater effect than 50 mg and may have increased incidence of side effects. Although doses of up to 300 mg/day have been studied, the total daily dose should not exceed 200 mg. The safety of treating an average of >4 headaches in a 30-day period have not been established.

Intranasal: A single dose of 5 mg, 10 mg, or 20 mg administered in one nostril. A 10 mg dose may be achieved by administering a single 5 mg dose in each nostril. If headache returns, the dose may be repeated once after 2 hours, not to exceed a total daily dose of 40 mg. In clinical trials, a greater number of patients responded to initial doses of 20 mg versus 5 mg. The safety of treating an average of >4 headaches in a 30-day period has not been established.

SubQ: Initial: Alsuma: 6 mg; Imitrex: 6 mg, if side effects are dose limiting, use lower doses 1 to 5 mg; Sumavel: 6 mg, if side effects are dose limiting, use 4 mg. May repeat if needed ≥1 hour after initial dose (maximum: 6 mg per dose; two 6 mg injections per 24-hour period; or maximum cumulative dose of 12 mg in 24 hours, separated by at least 1 hour). However, controlled clinical trials have failed to document a benefit with administration of a second 6 mg dose in nonresponders.

Transdermal: Initial: Apply one patch (provides 6.5 mg per 4 hour); a second patch may be applied no sooner than 2 hours after activation of the first patch (maximum: 2 patches per 24-hour period). The safety of using >4 transdermal systems in 1 month has not been established.

Cluster headache: SubQ: Initial: 6 mg; may repeat if needed ≥1 hour after initial dose (maximum: 6 mg per dose; two 6 mg injections per 24-hour period)

Renal Impairment There are no dosage adjustments provided in the manufacturer's labeling (has not been studied). However, dosage adjustment not expected due to extensive metabolism to inactive agents.

Hepatic Impairment

Mild to moderate hepatic impairment:

Oral: Bioavailability of oral sumatriptan is increased with liver disease. If treatment is needed, do not exceed single doses of 50 mg.

Intranasal: There are no dosage adjustments provided in the manufacturer's labeling (has not been studied). However, because the spray does not undergo first-pass metabolism, levels would not be expected to be altered.

Subcutaneous: No dosage adjustment necessary.

Transdermal patch: There are no dosage adjustments provided in the manufacturer's labeling (has not been studied).

Severe hepatic impairment: Oral, intranasal, subcutaneous (Alsuma and Imitrex injection), and transdermal formulations are contraindicated in severe hepatic impairment. Sumavel is not recommended in severe hepatic impairment.

Administration Administer as soon as symptoms appear.

Intranasal: Each nasal spray unit is preloaded with 1 dose; **do not** test the spray unit before use; remove unit from plastic pack when ready to use; while sitting down, gently blow nose to clear nasal passages; keep head upright and close one nostril gently with index finger; hold container with other hand, with thumb supporting bottom and index and middle fingers on either side of nozzle; insert nozzle into nostril about 1/2 inch; close mouth; take a breath through nose while releasing spray into nostril by pressing firmly on blue plunger; remove nozzle from nostril; keep head level for 10 to 20 seconds and gently breathe in through nose and out through mouth; **do not breathe deeply**

SubQ: Not for IM or IV use. Needle penetrates 1/4 inch of skin; use in areas of the body with adequate skin and subcutaneous thickness (lateral thigh or upper arm).

Needleless administration (Sumavel DosePro): Administer to the abdomen (>2 inches from the navel) or thigh; not for IM or IV administration. Do not administer to other areas of the body (eg, arm). Device is for single use only, discard after use; do not use if the tip of the device is tilted or broken.

Transdermal: Apply transdermal system to dry intact, non-irritated skin on the upper arm or thigh on a site that is relatively hair free and without scars, tattoos, abrasions, or other skin conditions (ie, generalized skin irritation, eczema, psoriasis, melanoma, contact dermatitis); secure with medical tape if needed. Do not apply to a previous application site until the site remains erythema free for at least 3 days. After application, the activation button must be pushed, and the red light emitting diode (LED) will turn on; the system will stop operating when dosing is completed and the LED will turn off, signaling that the system can be removed; if the LED turns off before 4 hours, dosing has stopped and the system can be removed. If headache relief is incomplete, a second system can be applied to a different site, if >2 hours have elapsed since the first system was applied. Patient should not swim, bathe, or shower while wearing patch. After use, fold the system so the adhesive side sticks to itself and discard away from children and pets. The system contains lithium-manganese dioxide batteries; dispose in accordance with state and local regulations.

Monitoring Parameters Headache severity, blood pressure, signs/symptoms suggestive of angina; perform a cardiovascular evaluation prior to initiation of therapy in 5-HT$_1$ agonist-naive patients who have multiple cardiovascular risk factors (eg, increased age, diabetes, hypertension, smoking, obesity, strong family history of CAD); ▶

monitor ECG with first dose in patients with multiple cardiovascular risk factors who have a negative cardiovascular evaluation and consider periodic cardiovascular evaluation in such patients during intermittent long-term use.

Dosage Forms Excipient information presented when available (limited, particularly for generics); consult specific product labeling. [DSC] = Discontinued product

Patch, Transdermal, as succinate [strength expressed as base]:

Zecuity: 6.5 mg/4 hr (1 ea) [contains basic butylated methacrylate coploymer, methylparaben]

Solution, Nasal:

Imitrex: 5 mg/actuation (1 ea); 20 mg/actuation (1 ea)

Generic: 5 mg/actuation (1 ea); 20 mg/actuation (1 ea)

Solution, Subcutaneous, as succinate [strength expressed as base]:

Alsuma: 6 mg/0.5 mL (0.5 mL)

Imitrex: 6 mg/0.5 mL (0.5 mL)

Imitrex STATdose Refill: 4 mg/0.5 mL (0.5 mL)

Imitrex STATdose System: 4 mg/0.5 mL (0.5 mL)

Generic: 4 mg/0.5 mL (0.5 mL); 6 mg/0.5 mL (0.5 mL)

Solution, Subcutaneous, as succinate [strength expressed as base, preservative free]:

Generic: 6 mg/0.5 mL (0.5 mL)

Solution Auto-injector, Subcutaneous, as succinate [strength expressed as base]:

Imitrex STATdose System: 6 mg/0.5 mL (0.5 mL)

Generic: 6 mg/0.5 mL (0.5 mL)

Solution Cartridge, Subcutaneous, as succinate [strength expressed as base]:

Imitrex STATdose Refill: 6 mg/0.5 mL (0.5 mL)

Generic: 4 mg/0.5 mL (0.5 mL [DSC]); 6 mg/0.5 mL (0.5 mL [DSC])

Solution Jet-injector, Subcutaneous, as succinate [strength expressed as base]:

Sumavel DosePro: 4 mg/0.5 mL (0.5 mL); 6 mg/0.5 mL (0.5 mL)

Solution Prefilled Syringe, Subcutaneous, as succinate [strength expressed as base]:

Generic: 6 mg/0.5 mL (0.5 mL [DSC])

Solution Prefilled Syringe, Subcutaneous, as succinate [strength expressed as base, preservative free]:

Generic: 6 mg/0.5 mL (0.5 mL)

Tablet, Oral, as succinate [strength expressed as base]:

Imitrex: 25 mg, 50 mg, 100 mg

Generic: 25 mg, 50 mg, 100 mg

Extemporaneous Preparations A 5 mg/mL oral liquid preparation made from tablets and one of three different vehicles (Ora-Sweet®, Ora-Sweet® SF, or Syrpalta® syrups). **Note:** Ora-Plus® Suspending Vehicle is used with Ora-Sweet® or Ora-Sweet® SF to facilitate dispersion of the tablets (Ora-Plus® is not necessary if Syrpalta® is the vehicle). Crush nine 100 mg tablets in a mortar and reduce to a fine powder. Add 40 mL of Ora-Plus® in 5 mL increments and mix thoroughly between each addition; rinse mortar and pestle 5 times with 10 mL of Ora-Plus®, pouring into bottle each time, and add quantity of appropriate syrup (Ora-Sweet® or Ora-Sweet® SF) sufficient to make 180 mL. Store in amber glass bottles in the dark; label "shake well", "refrigerate", and "protect from light". Stable for 21 days refrigerated.

Fish DN, Beall HD, Goodwin SD, et al, "Stability of Sumatriptan Succinate in Extemporaneously Prepared Oral Liquids," *Am J Health Syst Pharm,* 1997, 54(14):1619-22.

Sumatriptan and Naproxen
(soo ma TRIP tan & na PROKS en)

Brand Names: US Treximet

Index Terms Naproxen and Sumatriptan; Naproxen Sodium and Sumatriptan; Naproxen Sodium and Sumatriptan Succinate; Sumatriptan Succinate and Naproxen; Sumatriptan Succinate and Naproxen Sodium

Pharmacologic Category Antimigraine Agent; Nonsteroidal Anti-inflammatory Drug (NSAID), Oral; Serotonin 5-HT$_{1B, 1D}$ Receptor Agonist

Use Migraine headache: Acute treatment of migraine attacks with or without aura in adults and pediatric patients ≥12 years

Medication Guide Available Yes

Dosing

Adult & Geriatric Note: Use care when prescribing; there are 2 different Treximet tablet strengths available.

Migraine headache: Oral: Sumatriptan 85 mg/naproxen 500 mg. If a satisfactory response has not been obtained at 2 hours, a second dose may be administered (maximum: sumatriptan 170 mg/naproxen 1,000 mg in 24 hours). **Note:** The safety of treating an average of >5 migraine headaches in a 30-day period has not been established.

Pediatric Note: Use care when prescribing; there are 2 different Treximet tablet strengths available.

Migraine headache: Children and Adolescents ≥12 to 17 years: Sumatriptan 10 mg/naproxen 60 mg; maximum: sumatriptan 85 mg/naproxen 500 mg (adult dose) in 24 hours. **Note:** The safety of treating an average of >2 migraine headaches in a 30-day period has not been established.

Renal Impairment

CrCl ≥30 mL/minute: There are no dosage adjustments provided in the manufacturer's labeling (has not been studied); use with caution and monitor renal function.

CrCl <30 mL/minute: Use not recommended.

Hepatic Impairment

Mild to moderate impairment: Sumatriptan 10 mg/naproxen 60 mg in 24 hours.

Severe impairment: Use is contraindicated.

Additional Information Complete prescribing information should be consulted for additional detail.

Product Availability Treximet (sumatriptan 10 mg and naproxen sodium 60 mg) tablets: FDA approved May 2015; availability anticipated later in 2015.

Dosage Forms Excipient information presented when available (limited, particularly for generics); consult specific product labeling.

Tablet, Oral:

Treximet 10/60: Sumatriptran 10 mg and naproxen sodium 60 mg [contains sodium ~20 mg/tablet]

Treximet 85/500: Sumatriptan 85 mg and naproxen sodium 500 mg [contains sodium ~60 mg/tablet]

◆ Sumatriptan DF (Can) *see* SUMAtriptan *on page 1717*

◆ Sumatriptan Succinate *see* SUMAtriptan *on page 1717*

◆ Sumatriptan Succinate and Naproxen *see* Sumatriptan and Naproxen *on page 1720*

◆ Sumatriptan Succinate and Naproxen Sodium *see* Sumatriptan and Naproxen *on page 1720*

◆ Sumavel DosePro *see* SUMAtriptan *on page 1717*

◆ Sumaxin *see* Sulfur and Sulfacetamide *on page 1716*

◆ Sumaxin TS *see* Sulfur and Sulfacetamide *on page 1716*

SUNItinib (su NIT e nib)

Brand Names: US Sutent

Brand Names: Canada Sutent

Index Terms SU011248; SU11248; Sunitinib Malate

Pharmacologic Category Antineoplastic Agent, Tyrosine Kinase Inhibitor; Antineoplastic Agent, Vascular Endothelial Growth Factor (VEGF) Inhibitor; Vascular Endothelial Growth Factor (VEGF) Inhibitor

Use

Gastrointestinal stromal tumor: Treatment of gastrointestinal stromal tumor (GIST) after disease progression on or intolerance to imatinib

Pancreatic neuroendocrine tumors, advanced: Treatment of progressive, well-differentiated pancreatic neuroendocrine tumors in patients with unresectable locally advanced or metastatic disease

Renal cell carcinoma, advanced: Treatment of advanced renal cell carcinoma

Pregnancy Considerations Animal reproduction studies have demonstrated teratogenicity, embryotoxicity, and fetal loss. Because sunitinib inhibits angiogenesis, a critical component of fetal development, adverse effects on pregnancy would be expected. Women of childbearing potential should be advised to avoid pregnancy if receiving sunitinib.

Breast-Feeding Considerations It is not known if sunitinib is excreted in human milk. Due to the potential for serious adverse reactions in the nursing infant, the decision to discontinue breast-feeding or discontinue sunitinib should take into account the benefits of treatment to the mother.

Medication Guide Available Yes

Contraindications There are no contraindications listed in the manufacturer's US labeling.

Canadian labeling: Hypersensitivity to sunitinib or any component of the formulation; pregnancy

Warnings/Precautions Hazardous agent - use appropriate precautions for handling and disposal (NIOSH 2014 [group 1]). **[U.S. Boxed Warning]: Hepatotoxicity, which may be severe and/or fatal, has been observed in clinical trials and in postmarketing surveillance.** Signs of liver failure include jaundice, elevated transaminases, and/or hyperbilirubinemia, in conjunction with encephalopathy, coagulopathy and/or renal failure. Monitor liver function tests at baseline, with each treatment cycle, and if clinically indicated. Withhold treatment for grade 3 or 4 hepatotoxicity; discontinue if hepatotoxicity does not resolve. Do not reinitiate in patients with severe changes in liver function tests or other signs/symptoms of liver failure. Sunitinib has not been studied in patients with

ALT or AST >2.5 times ULN (or >5 times ULN if due to liver metastases).

Cardiovascular events (some fatal), including heart failure, cardiomyopathy, myocardial ischemia and myocardial infarction (MI) have been reported. Use with caution in patients at risk for cardiovascular events. May cause a decrease in left ventricular ejection fraction (LVEF), including some grade 3 reductions. Obtain LVEF evaluation prior to treatment. Discontinue with clinical signs and symptoms of heart failure. Interrupt therapy and/or decrease dose with LVEF <50% and >20% reduction from baseline in patients without clinical heart failure signs/symptoms. Patients with cardiac events (MI, bypass grafts, symptomatic heart failure, cerebrovascular accident, transient ischemic attack, and pulmonary embolism) within the previous 12 months were excluded from clinical trials and it is not known if the risk for left ventricular dysfunction is increased in patient with these conditions; assess risks versus benefits; monitor for clinical signs/symptoms of heart failure, in addition to baseline, also obtain periodic LVEF evaluation.

May cause hypertension; monitor and control with antihypertensives if needed; interrupt therapy until hypertension is controlled for severe hypertension. Use caution and closely monitor in patients with underlying or poorly controlled hypertension. Potentially significant drug-drug interactions may exist, requiring dose or frequency adjustment, additional monitoring, and/or selection of alternative therapy.

Hemorrhagic events have been reported including epistaxis, rectal, gingival, upper GI, urinary tract, genital, brain, wound bleeding, tumor-related, and hemoptysis/pulmonary hemorrhage; may be serious and/or fatal. Proteinuria and nephrotic syndrome have been reported; some cases have led to renal failure and fatal outcomes. Monitor for new onset or worsening proteinuria with baseline and periodic urinalysis and follow up with 24-hour urine protein if clinically indicated. If urine protein is ≥3 g/24 hours, interrupt treatment and reduce the dose. Discontinue treatment in patients with nephrotic syndrome or persistent urine protein ≥3 g/24 hours despite dose reductions. The safety of continuing treatment with sunitinib in patients with moderate to severe proteinuria has not been evaluated. Thrombotic microangiopathy (including thrombotic thrombocytopenic purpura and hemolytic uremic syndrome), sometimes leading to renal failure or fatality, has been reported with sunitinib, both as monotherapy and in combination with bevacizumab. Discontinue if thrombotic microangiopathy develops; effects may be reversible after discontinuation. Impaired wound healing has been reported with sunitinib; temporarily withhold treatment for patients undergoing major surgical procedures; the optimal time to resume treatment after a procedure has not been determined. Serious and fatal GI complications, including GI perforation, have occurred (rarely). Pancreatitis has been observed in RCC patients; discontinue sunitinib if symptoms are present. Thyroid dysfunction (eg, hypothyroidism, hyperthyroidism, and thyroiditis) may occur; the risk for hypothyroidism appears to increase with therapy duration; hyperthyroidism, sometimes followed by hypothyroidism has also been reported; monitor thyroid function at baseline. Patients not receiving thyroid hormone replacement therapy at sunitinib initiation should be monitored (TSH) every 4 weeks for 4 months and then every 2 to 3 months; those already receiving levothyroxine prior to initiating sunitinib should have TSH monitored every 4 weeks until levels and levothyroxine dose are stable, then monitor every 2 months (Hamnvik, 2011). Adrenal function abnormalities have been reported; monitor for adrenal insufficiency in patients with stress such as trauma, severe infection, or who are undergoing surgery. Symptomatic hypoglycemia has been associated with sunitinib; may result in loss of consciousness or require hospitalization. Hypoglycemia occurred infrequently in patients with renal cell cancer and gastrointestinal stromal tumors (GIST); however, the incidence is higher (~10%) in patients with pancreatic neuroendocrine tumors (PNET); preexisting glucose homeostasis abnormalities were not always present in hypoglycemic patients with PNET. Blood glucose decreases may be worse in patients with diabetes. Monitor blood glucose levels regularly during and following discontinuation of treatment. Dose modifications of antidiabetic medications may be necessary to minimize the risk of hypoglycemia.

Severe cutaneous reactions, including erythema multiforme (EM), Stevens-Johnson syndrome (SJS), and toxic epidermal necrolysis (TEN) have been reported (some fatal); if signs/symptoms of EM, SJS, or TEN (progressive skin rash, often with blisters or mucosal lesions) are present, discontinue sunitinib. Do not restart treatment if SJS or TEN are suspected. Necrotizing fasciitis (with fatalities) has been reported, including perineum necrotizing fasciitis and fasciitis secondary to fistula formation. Discontinue sunitinib in patients who develop necrotizing fasciitis. Sunitinib may cause skin and/or hair depigmentation or discoloration. Hand-foot skin reaction (HFSR) observed with tyrosine kinase inhibitors (TKIs) is distinct from hand-foot syndrome (palmar-plantar erythrodysesthesia) associated with traditional chemotherapy agents; HFSR due to TKIs is localized with defined hyperkeratotic lesions; symptoms include burning, dysesthesia, paresthesia, or tingling on the palms/soles, and generally occur within the first 2 to 4 weeks of treatment; pressure and flexor areas may develop blisters (callus-like), dry/cracked skin, edema, erythema, desquamation, or hyperkeratosis (Appleby, 2011). The following treatments may be used in addition to the recommended dosage modifications (Lacouture, 2008). Prior to treatment initiation, a pedicure is recommended to remove hyperkeratotic areas/calluses, which may predispose to HFSR; avoid vigorous exercise/activities that may stress hands or feet. During therapy, patients should reduce exposure to hot water (may exacerbate hand-foot symptoms); avoid constrictive footwear and excessive skin friction. Patients may also wear thick cotton gloves or socks and should wear shoes with padded insoles. Grade 1 HFSR may be relieved with moisturizing creams, cotton gloves and socks (at night) and/or keratolytic creams such as urea (20% to 40%) or salicylic acid (6%). Apply topical steroid (eg, clobetasol ointment) twice daily to erythematous areas of grade 2 HFSR; topical anesthetics (eg, lidocaine 2%) and then systemic analgesics (if appropriate) may be used for pain control. Resolution of acute erythema may result in keratotic areas which may be softened with keratolytic agents. Reversible posterior leukoencephalopathy syndrome (RPLS) has been reported (rarely, some fatal); symptoms include confusion, headache, hypertension, lethargy, seizure, blindness and/or other vision, or neurologic disturbances; interrupt treatment and begin hypertension management. Tumor lysis syndrome (TLS), including fatalities, has been reported, predominantly in patients with RCC or GIST; risk for TLS is higher in patients with a high tumor burden prior to treatment; monitor closely; correct clinically significant dehydration and treat high uric acid levels prior to initiation of treatment. An increased incidence of fatigue, thyroid dysfunction and treatment-induced hypertension was reported in patients with renal insufficiency (CrCl ≤60 mL/minute) who received sunitinib for the treatment of renal cell cancer (Gupta, 2011). Osteonecrosis of the jaw (ONJ) has been observed with sunitinib; concurrent bisphosphonate use or dental disease may increase the risk for ONJ. If possible, avoid invasive dental procedures in patients with current or prior bisphosphonate use. Consider a dental exam and appropriate prophylactic dentistry prior to treatment initiation Dosing schedules vary by indication; some treatment regimens are continuous daily dosing; other treatment schedules are daily dosing for 4 weeks of a 6-week cycle (4 weeks on, 2 weeks off).

Adverse Reactions

>10%:

Cardiovascular: Hypertension (27% to 34%, GIST: 8% to 15%; grade 3: 10% to 13%, GIST: 4%), decreased left ventricular ejection fraction (RCC: 16% to 27%, grade 3: 3% to 7%; GIST: 11%, grade 3: 1%), peripheral edema (RCC: 24%), chest pain (RCC: 13%), severe hypertension (4% to 10%; >200 mmHg systolic or 110 mmHg diastolic)

Central nervous system: Fatigue (RCC: 62%, pNET: 33%), glossalgia (pNET: ≤48%; RCC: 11%), mouth pain (pNET: ≤48%; RCC: 6% to 14%), headache (18% to 23%), insomnia (15% to 18%), chills (RCC: 14%), depression (RCC: 11%), dizziness (RCC: 11%)

Dermatologic: Skin discoloration (≤25% to 30%; yellow color), hair discoloration (20% to 29%; GIST: 7%), palmar-plantar erythrodysesthesia (23% to 29%, GIST: 14%; grades 3/4: 4% to 8%), xeroderma (15% to 23%), skin rash (14% to 18%; RCC: 29%), alopecia (5% to 14%), erythema (RCC: 12%), pruritus (RCC: 12%)

Endocrine & metabolic: Increased uric acid (RCC: 46%), decreased serum calcium (34% to 42%), decreased serum albumin (pNET: 41%, RCC: 28%), decreased serum phosphate (31% to 36%), increased serum glucose (RCC: 23%), decreased serum potassium (12% to 21%), decreased serum sodium (RCC: 20%), decreased serum magnesium (pNET: 19%), increased serum potassium (16% to 18%), hypothyroidism (4% to 7%; RCC: 16%), increased serum calcium (RCC: 13%), increased serum sodium (10% to 13%)

Gastrointestinal: Diarrhea (59% to 66%; GIST: 40%), nausea (RCC: 58%; pNET: 45%), increased serum lipase (17% to 25%; RCC: 56%; grades 3/4: 5% to 18%), anorexia (RCC: 48%; GIST: 33%), mucositis (47% to 48%, GIST: 29%; includes aphthous stomatitis, dry mucous membranes, gingival pain, gingivitis, glossitis, oral discomfort, oral mucosal ulcer, stomatitis, tongue ulceration), dysgeusia (21%; RCC: 47%), vomiting (34% to 39%), abdominal pain (30% to 39%), increased serum amylase (17% to 20%; RCC: 35%; grades 3/4: 4% to 6%), dyspepsia (RCC: 34%; pNET: 15%), constipation (20% to 23%), weight loss (16%), flatulence (RCC: 14%), xerostomia (RCC: 13%), gastroesophageal reflux disease (RCC: 12%)

Hematologic & oncologic: Decreased hemoglobin (RCC: 79%, pNET: 65%, GIST: 26%; grades 3/4: ≤8%), leukocyte disorder (decreased leukocytes; RCC: 78%; grades 3/4: 8%), decreased neutrophils (71% to 77%, GIST: 53%; grades 3/4: 10% to 17%), abnormal absolute lymphocyte count (decreased; RCC: 68%, pNET: 56%, GIST: 38%; grades 3/4: RCC: 18%, pNET: 7%), decreased platelet count (60% to 68%, GIST: 38%, GIST and RCC: grades 3/4: 5% to 9%), hemorrhage (18% to 22%; RCC: 37%; RCC and GIST, grades 3/4: 3% to 4%; includes hematemesis, hematochezia, hematoma, hemoptysis, melena, metrorrhagia)

Hepatic: Increased serum AST (pNET: 72%, RCC: 56%, GIST: ≤39%; grades 3/4: ≤2% to 5%), increased serum ALT (pNET: 61%; RCC: 51%; GIST: ≤39%; grades 3/4: ≤2% to 4%), increased serum alkaline phosphatase (RCC: 46%; GIST: 24%; grades 3/4: 2% to 4%), increased serum bilirubin (16% to 20%; pNET: 37%; RCC and GIST, grades 3/4: 1%), increased indirect serum bilirubin (RCC and GIST: 10% to 13%; grades 3/4: ≤1%)

Neuromuscular & skeletal: Increased creatine phosphokinase (RCC: 49%), limb pain (RCC: 40%; GIST: ≤14%), weakness (22% to 34%), arthralgia (RCC: 30%; pNET: 15%), back pain (RCC: 28%), myalgia (GIST: ≤14%)

Renal: Increased serum creatinine (RCC: 70%; GIST: 12%)

Respiratory: Cough (RCC: 27%), dyspnea (RCC: 26%), epistaxis (pNET: 20%), nasopharyngitis (RCC: 14%), oropharyngeal pain (RCC: 14%), upper respiratory tract infection (RCC: 11%)

Miscellaneous: Fever (RCC: 22%)

1% to 10%:

Cardiovascular: Deep vein thrombosis (≤3%), pulmonary embolism (≤3%)

Endocrine & metabolic: Hypoglycemia (2%; pNET: 10%)

Gastrointestinal: Hemorrhoids (RCC: 10%), pancreatitis (1%)

Respiratory: Flu-like symptoms (RCC: 5%)

<1% (Limited to important or life-threatening): Acute renal failure, adrenocortical insufficiency, arterial thrombosis (includes cerebral infarction, cerebrovascular accident, transient ischemic attack), cardiac failure, cardiomyopathy, cerebral hemorrhage, cholecystitis (particularly acalculous), erythema multiforme, esophagitis, fistula (sometimes associated with tumor necrosis and/or regression), fulminant necrotizing fasciitis (including of the perineum), gastrointestinal hemorrhage, gastrointestinal perforation, hemolytic uremic syndrome, hepatic failure, hepatotoxicity, hypersensitivity (includes angioedema), hyperthyroidism, ischemic heart disease, myocardial infarction, nephrotic syndrome, neutropenic infection, osteonecrosis of the jaw, preeclampsia (proteinuria and reversible hypertension) (Gallucci 2013; Patel 2008), prolonged Q-T interval on ECG (dose dependent), proteinuria, pulmonary hemorrhage, pyoderma gangrenosum (including positive dechallenges), renal insufficiency, respiratory tract hemorrhage, respiratory tract infection (may be serious), reversible posterior leukoencephalopathy syndrome, rhabdomyolysis (with/without acute renal failure), seizure, sepsis, skin infection (may be serious), Stevens-Johnson syndrome, thrombotic thrombocytopenic purpura, thyroiditis (Feldt 2012), torsades de pointes, toxic epidermal necrolysis, tumor hemorrhage, tumor lysis syndrome, urinary tract hemorrhage, urinary tract infection (may be serious), ventricular arrhythmia, wound healing impairment

Drug Interactions

Metabolism/Transport Effects Substrate of CYP3A4 (major); **Note:** Assignment of Major/Minor substrate status based on clinically relevant drug interaction potential; **Inhibits** BCRP, P-glycoprotein

Avoid Concomitant Use

Avoid concomitant use of SUNItinib with any of the following: BCG (Intravesical); Bevacizumab; Bosutinib; Conivaptan; Fusidic Acid (Systemic); Idelalisib; Natalizumab; PAZOPanib; Pimecrolimus; Silodosin; St Johns Wort; Tacrolimus (Topical); Temsirolimus; Tofacitinib; Topotecan; Vaccines (Live); VinCRIStine (Liposomal)

Increased Effect/Toxicity

SUNItinib may increase the levels/effects of: Afatinib; Bevacizumab; Bisphosphonate Derivatives; Bosutinib; Brentuximab Vedotin; Colchicine; Dabigatran Etexilate; DOXOrubicin (Conventional); Edoxaban; Everolimus; Fingolimod; Highest Risk QTc-Prolonging Agents; Hypoglycemia-Associated Agents; Ledipasvir; Leflunomide; Moderate Risk QTc-Prolonging Agents; Naloxegol; Natalizumab; PAZOPanib; P-glycoprotein/ABCB1 Substrates; Prucalopride; Ranolazine; Rifaximin; Silodosin; Tofacitinib; Topotecan; Vaccines (Live); VinCRIStine (Liposomal)

The levels/effects of SUNItinib may be increased by: Androgens; Antidiabetic Agents; Antifungal Agents (Azole Derivatives, Systemic); Aprepitant; Bevacizumab; Conivaptan; CYP3A4 Inhibitors (Moderate); CYP3A4 Inhibitors (Strong); Dasatinib; Denosumab; Fosaprepitant; Fusidic Acid (Systemic); Herbs (Hypoglycemic Properties); Idelalisib; Ivacaftor; Luliconazole; MAO Inhibitors; Mifepristone; Netupitant; Osimertinib; Palbociclib; Pegvisomant; Pimecrolimus; Quinolone Antibiotics; Roflumilast; Salicylates; Selective Serotonin Reuptake Inhibitors; Simeprevir; Stiripentol; Tacrolimus (Topical); Temsirolimus; Trastuzumab

Decreased Effect

SUNItinib may decrease the levels/effects of: BCG (Intravesical); Coccidioides immitis Skin Test; Sipuleucel-T; Vaccines (Inactivated); Vaccines (Live)

The levels/effects of SUNItinib may be decreased by: Bosentan; CYP3A4 Inducers (Moderate); CYP3A4 Inducers (Strong); Dabrafenib; Deferasirox; Dexamethasone (Systemic); Echinacea; Enzalutamide; Mitotane; Osimertinib; Quinolone Antibiotics; Siltuximab; St Johns Wort; Tocilizumab

Food Interactions Grapefruit juice may increase the levels/effects of sunitinib. Food has no effect on the bioavailability of sunitinib. Management: Avoid grapefruit juice.

Storage/Stability Store at 25°C (77°F); excursions are permitted between 15°C to 30°C (59°F to 86°F).

Mechanism of Action Exhibits antitumor and antiangiogenic properties by inhibiting multiple receptor tyrosine kinases, including platelet-derived growth factors (PDGFRα and PDGFRβ), vascular endothelial growth factors (VEGFR1, VEGFR2, and VEGFR3), FMS-like tyrosine kinase-3 (FLT3), colony-stimulating factor type 1 (CSF-1R), and glial cell-line-derived neurotrophic factor receptor (RET).

Pharmacodynamics/Kinetics

Distribution: V_d/F: 2230 L

Protein binding: Sunitinib: 95%; SU12662: 90%

Metabolism: Hepatic; primarily metabolized by CYP3A4 to the N-desethyl metabolite SU12662 (active)

Half-life elimination: Terminal: Sunitinib: 40 to 60 hours; SU12662: 80 to 110 hours

Time to peak, plasma: 6 to 12 hours

Excretion: Feces (61%); urine (16%)

Dosing

Adult & Geriatric Note: Dosage modifications should be done in increments or decrements of 12.5 mg; individualize based on safety and tolerability.

Gastrointestinal stromal tumor (GIST): Oral: 50 mg once daily for 4 weeks of a 6-week treatment cycle (4 weeks on, 2 weeks off)

GIST off-label dosing: Oral: 37.5 mg once daily, continuous daily dosing (George, 2009, *EJC*)

Pancreatic neuroendocrine tumors, advanced (PNET): Oral: 37.5 mg once daily, continuous daily dosing (maximum daily dose used in clinical trials: 50 mg)

Renal cell cancer, advanced (RCC): Oral: 50 mg once daily for 4 weeks of a 6-week treatment cycle (4 weeks on, 2 weeks off)

Soft tissue sarcoma, non-GIST (off-label use): Oral: 37.5 mg once daily, continuous daily dosing (George, 2009, *JCO*)

Thyroid cancer, refractory (off-label use): Oral: 50 mg once daily for 4 weeks of a 6-week treatment cycle (4 weeks on, 2 weeks off) (Cohen, 2008; Ravaud, 2008)

Dosage adjustment with concurrent CYP3A4 inhibitor: Avoid concomitant administration with strong CYP3A4 inhibitors (eg, clarithromycin, erythromycin, itraconazole, ketoconazole, nefazodone, protease inhibitors, telithromycin, voriconazole); if concomitant administration with a strong CYP3A4 inhibitor cannot be avoided, consider a dose reduction to a minimum of 37.5 mg/day (GIST, RCC) or 25 mg/day (PNET).

Dosage adjustment with concurrent CYP3A4 inducer: Avoid concomitant administration with strong CYP3A4 inducers (eg, carbamazepine, dexamethasone, phenobarbital, phenytoin, rifampin, St John's wort); if concomitant administration with a strong CYP3A4 inducer cannot be avoided, consider a dosage increase (with careful monitoring for toxicity) to a maximum of 87.5 mg/day (GIST, RCC) or 62.5 mg/day (PNET).

Renal Impairment

Mild, moderate, or severe impairment: No initial adjustment required; subsequent adjustments may be needed based on safety and tolerance.

ESRD on hemodialysis: No initial adjustment required; subsequent dosage **increases** (up to twofold) may be required due to reduced (47%) exposure

Hepatic Impairment

Preexisting hepatic impairment: No adjustment is necessary with mild-to-moderate (Child-Pugh class A or B) hepatic impairment; not studied in patients with severe (Child-Pugh class C) hepatic impairment. Studies excluded patients with ALT or AST >2.5 x ULN, or if due to liver metastases, ALT or AST >5 x ULN.

Hepatotoxicity during treatment: Hepatic adverse events ≥ grade 3 or 4: Withhold treatment; discontinue if hepatotoxicity does not resolve. Do not reinitiate in patients with severe changes in liver function tests or other signs/symptoms of liver failure.

Adjustment for Toxicity Dosage modifications should be done in increments or decrements of 12.5 mg; individualize based on safety and tolerability.

Cardiac toxicity:

Ejection fraction <50% and >20% below baseline without evidence of CHF: Interrupt treatment and/or reduce dose.

LV dysfunction with CHF clinical manifestations: Discontinue treatment.

Dermatologic toxicity:

Signs/symptoms of erythema multiforme (EM), Stevens-Johnson syndrome (SJS), and toxic epidermal necrolysis (TEN), including progressive skin rash, often with blisters or mucosal lesions: Discontinue sunitinib; do not restart treatment if SJS or TEN are suspected.

Necrotizing fasciitis: Discontinue sunitinib.

Hypertension, severe: Temporarily interrupt treatment until hypertension is controlled.

Nephrotic syndrome: Discontinue treatment.

Pancreatitis: Discontinue treatment.

Proteinuria:

Urine protein ≥3 g/24 hours: Interrupt treatment and reduce the dose.

Persistent urine protein ≥3 g/24 hours despite dose reductions: Discontinue treatment.

Reversible posterior leukoencephalopathy (RPLS): Temporarily withhold treatment; after resolution, may resume with discretion.

Thrombotic microangiopathy: Discontinue treatment.

Dietary Considerations Avoid grapefruit juice.

Administration May be administered with or without food. Hazardous agent; use appropriate precautions for handling and disposal (NIOSH 2014 [group 1]). Avoid contact with broken or leaking capsules; if contact occurs, wash immediately with soap and water. If it is necessary to manipulate the capsules (eg, to prepare an oral suspension), it is recommended to double glove, wear a protective gown, and prepare in a controlled device (NIOSH, 2014).

Monitoring Parameters LVEF, baseline (and periodic with cardiac risk factors), ECG (12-lead; baseline and periodic), blood pressure; adrenal function CBC with differential and platelets (prior to each treatment cycle), liver function tests (baseline, with each cycle and if clinically indicated), serum chemistries including magnesium, phosphate, and potassium (prior to each treatment cycle), blood glucose levels (regularly during and following discontinuation of treatment), urinalysis (for proteinuria development or worsening); consider dental exam prior to treatment initiation; symptoms of hypothyroidism, hyperthyroidism, or thyroiditis; signs/symptoms of hypoglycemia

Thyroid function testing (Hamnvik, 2011):

Preexisting levothyroxine therapy: Obtain baseline TSH levels, then monitor every 4 weeks until levels and levothyroxine dose are stable, then monitor every 2 months

Without preexisting thyroid hormone replacement: TSH at baseline, then every 4 weeks for 4 months, then every 2-3 months

Dosage Forms Excipient information presented when available (limited, particularly for generics); consult specific product labeling.

Capsule, Oral:

Sutent: 12.5 mg, 25 mg, 37.5 mg, 50 mg

Extemporaneous Preparations Hazardous agent: Use appropriate precautions for handling and disposal (NIOSH 2014 [group 1]). When manipulating capsules, NIOSH recommends double gloving, a protective gown, and preparation in a controlled device; if not prepared in a controlled device, respiratory and eye protection as well as ventilated engineering controls are recommended (NIOSH, 2014).

A 10 mg/mL sunitinib oral suspension may be made with capsules and a 1:1 mixture of Ora-Sweet and Ora-Plus. Empty the contents of three 50 mg sunitinib capsules into a mortar; add small portions of vehicle and mix to a uniform paste. Mix while adding vehicle in incremental proportions to 15 mL. Transfer to amber plastic bottle and label "shake well". This suspension maintains an average concentration of 96% to 106% (of the original concentration) at room temperature or refrigerated for up to 60 days in plastic amber prescription bottles.

Navid F, Christensen R, Minkin P, et al, "Stability of Sunitinib in Oral Suspension," *Ann Pharmacother*, 2008, 42(7):962-6.

Suvorexant (soo voe REX ant)

Brand Names: US Belsomra

Index Terms MK4305

Pharmacologic Category Hypnotic, Miscellaneous; Orexin Receptor Antagonist

Use Insomnia: Treatment of insomnia characterized by difficulties with sleep onset and/or sleep maintenance.

Pregnancy Considerations Adverse events have been observed in some animal reproduction studies.

Breast-Feeding Considerations It is not known if suvorexant is excreted into breast milk. The manufacturer recommends that caution be used if administered to a nursing woman.

Medication Guide Available Yes

Contraindications Narcolepsy

Warnings/Precautions Hypnotics have been associated with abnormal thinking and behavior changes (eg, amnesia, anxiety, hallucinations). May cause CNS depression impairing physical and mental capabilities; patients must be cautioned about performing tasks which require mental alertness (operating machinery or driving). Suvorexant should only be administered when the patient is able to stay in bed a full night (≥7 hours) before being active again. Discontinue or decrease the dose in patients who drive if daytime somnolence occurs. Sleep paralysis (inability to move or speak for up to several minutes during sleep-wake transitions), hypnagogic/hypnopompic hallucinations, and mild cataplexy may occur. Cataplexy symptoms may include periods of leg weakness lasting from seconds to a few minutes, can occur both at night and during the day, and may not be associated with a triggering event (eg, laughter, surprise). An increased risk for hazardous sleep-related activities such as sleep-driving; cooking and eating food, making phone calls, or having sex while asleep have also been noted. Discontinue treatment in patients who report any sleep-related episodes. Potentially significant interactions may exist, requiring dose or frequency adjustment, additional monitoring, and/or selection of alternative therapy.

Symptomatic treatment of insomnia should be initiated only after careful evaluation of potential causes of sleep disturbance. Failure of sleep disturbance to resolve after 7 to 10 days may indicate psychiatric and/or medical illness.

Use with caution in patients with depression; worsening of depression, including suicide or suicidal ideation has been reported with the use of hypnotics. Intentional overdose may be an issue in this population. The minimum dose that will effectively treat the individual patient should be used. Prescriptions should be written for the smallest quantity consistent with good patient care. Use with caution in patients with a history of drug dependence. Risk of abuse is increased with prolonged use of suvorexant, in patients with a history of drug abuse, or those who use suvorexant in combination with alcohol or other abused drugs. Use with caution in patients with respiratory compromise, COPD, or sleep apnea. Use is not recommended in patients with severe hepatic impairment (has not been studied). Exposure is increased in females compared to males and in obese compared to nonobese patients. Consider the increased risk of exposure-related adverse effects, particularly in obese females, before increasing the dose.

Adverse Reactions Frequency not always defined.

Central nervous system: Drowsiness (2% to 12%; dose dependent and more common in females), headache (7%; more common in females), dizziness (3%), abnormal dreams (2%; more common in females), abnormality in thinking, amnesia, anxiety, behavioral changes, central nervous system depression, drug abuse, drug dependence, exacerbation of depression, hallucination, hypnagogic hallucinations, sleep driving, suicidal ideation

Endocrine & metabolic: Increased serum cholesterol

Gastrointestinal: Diarrhea (2%), xerostomia (2%; more common in females)

Neuromuscular & skeletal: Lower extremity weakness, sleep paralysis

Respiratory: Cough (2%; more common in females), upper respiratory tract infection (2%; more common in females)

Drug Interactions

Metabolism/Transport Effects Substrate of CYP2C19 (minor), CYP3A4 (major); **Note:** Assignment of Major/Minor substrate status based on clinically relevant drug interaction potential

Avoid Concomitant Use

Avoid concomitant use of Suvorexant with any of the following: Alcohol (Ethyl); Azelastine (Nasal); Conivaptan; CYP3A4 Inducers (Strong); CYP3A4 Inhibitors (Strong); Fusidic Acid (Systemic); Idelalisib; Orphenadrine; Paraldehyde; Sodium Oxybate; Thalidomide

Increased Effect/Toxicity

Suvorexant may increase the levels/effects of: Azelastine (Nasal); Buprenorphine; Hydrocodone; Methotrimeprazine; Metyrosine; Orphenadrine; Paraldehyde; Pramipexole; ROPINIRole; Rotigotine; Selective Serotonin Reuptake Inhibitors; Sodium Oxybate; Thalidomide; Zolpidem

The levels/effects of Suvorexant may be increased by: Alcohol (Ethyl); Brimonidine (Topical); Cannabis; CNS Depressants; Conivaptan; CYP3A4 Inhibitors (Moderate); CYP3A4 Inhibitors (Strong); Dasatinib; Dronabinol; Droperidol; Fosaprepitant; Fusidic Acid (Systemic); Idelalisib; Ivacaftor; Kava Kava; Luliconazole; Magnesium Sulfate; Methotrimeprazine; Mifepristone; Minocycline; Nabilone; Osimertinib; Palbociclib; Perampanel; Rufinamide; Simeprevir; Stiripentol; Tapentadol; Tetrahydrocannabinol

Decreased Effect

The levels/effects of Suvorexant may be decreased by: Bosentan; CYP3A4 Inducers (Moderate); CYP3A4 Inducers (Strong); Dabrafenib; Deferasirox; Osimertinib; Siltuximab; St Johns Wort; Tocilizumab

Storage/Stability Store at 20°C to 25°C (68°F to 77°F); excursions are permitted between 15°C and 30°C (59°F and 86°F). Protect from light and moisture.

Mechanism of Action Suvorexant blocks the binding of wake-promoting neuropeptides orexin A and orexin B to receptors OX1R and OX2R, which is thought to suppress wake drive. Antagonism of orexin receptors may also underlie potential adverse effects such as signs of narcolepsy/cataplexy.

Pharmacodynamics/Kinetics

Onset of action: ~30 minutes

Absorption: Decreased at higher doses

Distribution: V_d: ~49 L

Protein binding: >99%

Metabolism: Primarily hepatic by CYP3A with a minor contribution from CYP2C19; the hydroxy-suvorexant metabolite is inactive.

Bioavailability: 82%

Half-life elimination: ~12 hours

Half-life terminal: ~15 hours (healthy subjects, range: 10 to 22 hours), ~19 hours (moderate hepatic disease, range: 11 to 49 hours)

Time to peak: 2 hours (range: 30 minutes to 6 hours); Delayed ~1.5 hours when administered with a meal

Excretion: Feces (~66%); urine (~23%)

Dosing

Adult & Geriatric

Insomnia: Oral: **Note:** Use the lowest effective dose for the patient. Usual dose: 10 mg once daily within 30 minutes of bedtime; may increase to a maximum of 20 mg once daily if the 10 mg dose is well tolerated but not effective. Maximum daily dose: 20 mg

Dosage adjustment for concomitant therapy:

Moderate CYP3A inhibitors (eg, amprenavir, aprepitant, atazanavir, ciprofloxacin, diltiazem, erythromycin, fluconazole, fosamprenavir, grapefruit juice, imatinib, verapamil): Usual dose: 5 mg once daily; maximum daily dose: 10 mg

Strong CYP3A inhibitors (eg, ketoconazole, itraconazole, posaconazole, clarithromycin, nefazodone, ritonavir, saquinavir, nelfinavir, indinavir, boceprevir, telaprevir, telithromycin, conivaptan): Use of suvorexant is not recommended.

CNS depressants: Dosage adjustment of suvorexant and/or the other CNS depressant may be necessary.

Renal Impairment No dosage adjustment necessary.

Hepatic Impairment

Mild or moderate impairment: No dosage adjustment necessary.

Severe impairment: Use is not recommended (has not been studied).

Obesity Consider the increased risk of exposure-related adverse effects in obese women before increasing the dose.

Dietary Considerations For faster sleep onset, do no administer with (or immediately after) a meal.

Administration Oral: Administer within 30 minutes of bedtime with at least 7 hours remaining before planned time of awakening. Onset is delayed with food; do not administer with or immediately after a meal.

Monitoring Parameters Daytime alertness; respiratory rate; behavior profile; tolerance, abuse, dependence

Dosage Forms Excipient information presented when available (limited, particularly for generics); consult specific product labeling.

Tablet, Oral:

Belsomra: 5 mg

Belsomra: 10 mg [contains fd&c blue #1 aluminum lake]

Belsomra: 15 mg, 20 mg

Controlled Substance C-IV

Tacrolimus (Systemic) (ta KROE li mus)

Brand Names: US Astagraf XL; Envarsus XR; Hecoria
[DSC]; Prograf

Brand Names: Canada Advagraf; Prograf; Sandoz-
Tacrolimus

Index Terms FK506

Pharmacologic Category Calcineurin Inhibitor; Immunosuppressant Agent

Use Organ rejection prophylaxis:

US labeling:

Astagraf XL: Prevention of organ rejection in kidney
transplant recipients

Envarsus XR: Prevention of organ rejection in kidney
transplant recipients converted from tacrolimus immediate-release formulation

Hecoria and Prograf: Prevention of organ rejection in
heart, kidney, and liver transplant recipients

Canadian labeling:

Advagraf: Prevention of organ rejection in kidney and
liver transplant recipients

Prograf: Prevention of organ rejection in heart, kidney, or
liver transplant recipients; treatment of refractory rejection in kidney or liver transplant recipients; treatment of
active rheumatoid arthritis in adult patients nonresponsive to disease-modifying antirheumatic drug (DMARD)
therapy or when DMARD therapy is inappropriate

Pregnancy Considerations Adverse events were
observed in animal reproduction studies. Tacrolimus
crosses the human placenta and is measurable in the cord
blood, amniotic fluid, and newborn serum. Tacrolimus
concentrations in the placenta may be higher than the
maternal serum (Jain 1997). Infants with lower birth
weights have been found to have higher tacrolimus concentrations (Bramham 2013). Transient neonatal hyperkalemia and renal dysfunction have been reported.

Tacrolimus pharmacokinetics are altered during pregnancy. Whole blood concentrations decrease as pregnancy progresses; however, unbound concentrations
increase. Measuring unbound concentrations may be preferred, especially in women with anemia or hypoalbuminemia. If unbound concentration measurement is not
available, interpretation of whole blood concentrations
should account for RBC count and serum albumin concentration (Hebert 2013; Zheng 2012).

In general, women who have had a kidney transplant
should be instructed that fertility will be restored following
the transplant but that pregnancy should be avoided for ~2
years. Tacrolimus may be used as an immunosuppressant
during pregnancy. The risk of infection, hypertension, and
pre-eclampsia may be increased in pregnant women who
have had a kidney transplant (EPBG 2002).

The National Transplantation Pregnancy Registry (NTPR)
is a registry which follows pregnancies which occur in
maternal transplant recipients or those fathered by male
transplant recipients. The NTPR encourages reporting of
pregnancies following solid organ transplant by contacting
them at 877-955-6877.

Breast-Feeding Considerations Tacrolimus is excreted
into breast milk; concentrations are variable and lower than
that of the maternal serum. The low bioavailability of
tacrolimus following oral absorption may also decrease
the amount of exposure to a nursing infant (Bramham
2013; French 2003; Gardiner 2006). In one study, tacrolimus serum concentrations in the infants did not differ
between those who were bottle fed or breast-fed (all
infants were exposed to tacrolimus throughout pregnancy)
(Bramham 2013). Available information suggests that
tacrolimus exposure to the nursing infant is ≤0.5% of the
weight-adjusted maternal dose (Bramham 2013; French
2003; Gardiner 2006). The manufacturer recommends that
nursing be discontinued, taking into consideration the
importance of the drug to the mother.

Medication Guide Available Yes

Contraindications Hypersensitivity to tacrolimus, polyoxyl
60 hydrogenated castor oil (HCO-60), or any other component of the formulation.

Warnings/Precautions Hazardous agent - use appropriate precautions for handling and disposal (NIOSH 2014
[group 2]).

**[US Boxed Warning]: Risk of developing infections
(including bacterial, viral [including CMV], fungal,
and protozoal infections [including opportunistic
infections]) is increased.** Latent viral infections may be
activated, including BK virus (associated with polyoma
virus-associated nephropathy [PVAN]) and JC virus (associated with progressive multifocal leukoencephalopathy
[PML]); may result in serious adverse effects. Immunosuppression increases the risk for CMV viremia and/or CMV
disease; the risk of CMV disease is increased for patients
who are CMV-seronegative prior to transplant and receive
a graft from a CMV-seropositive donor. Consider reduction
in immunosuppression if PVAN, PML, CMV viremia and/or
CMV disease occurs. **[US Boxed Warning]: Immunosuppressive therapy may result in the development of
lymphoma and other malignancies (predominantly
skin malignancies).** The risk for new-onset diabetes and
insulin-dependent post-transplant diabetes mellitus
(PTDM) is increased with tacrolimus use after transplantation, including in patients without pretransplant history of
diabetes mellitus; insulin dependence may be reversible;
monitor blood glucose frequently; risk is increased in
African-American and Hispanic kidney transplant patients.
Nephrotoxicity (acute or chronic) occur when used in high
doses, in patients with impaired renal function, or with
other nephrotoxic drugs (eg, sirolimus, cyclosporine). Monitor renal function and consider dosage reduction in nephrotoxicity occurs. Neurotoxicity may occur especially when
used in high doses; tremor headache, coma and delirium
have been reported and are associated with serum concentrations. Seizures may also occur. Posterior reversible
encephalopathy syndrome (PRES) has been reported;
symptoms (altered mental status, headache, hypertension,
seizures, and visual disturbances) are reversible with dose
reduction or discontinuation of therapy; stabilize blood
pressure and reduce dose with suspected or confirmed
PRES diagnosis.

Pure red cell aplasia (PRCA) has been reported in patients
receiving tacrolimus. Use with caution in patients with risk
factors for PRCA including parvovirus B19 infection,
underlying disease, or use of concomitant medications
associated with PRCA (eg, mycophenolate). Discontinuation of therapy should be considered with diagnosis of
PRCA. Monitoring of serum concentrations (trough for oral
therapy) is essential to prevent organ rejection and reduce
drug-related toxicity. Use caution in renal or hepatic dysfunction, dosing adjustments may be required. Delay initiation of therapy in kidney transplant patients if
postoperative oliguria occurs; begin therapy no sooner
than 6 hours and within 24 hours post-transplant, but
may be delayed until renal function has recovered. Mild-
to-severe hyperkalemia may occur; monitor serum potassium levels. Hypertension may commonly occur; antihypertensive treatment may be necessary; avoid use of
potassium-sparing diuretics due to risk of hyperkalemia;
concurrent use of calcium channel blockers may require
tacrolimus dosage adjustment. Gastrointestinal perforation
may occur; all reported cases were considered to be a
complication of transplant surgery or accompanied by
infection, diverticulum, or malignant neoplasm. Myocardial
hypertrophy has been reported (rare). Prolongation of the
QT/QTc and torsade de pointes may occur; avoid use in
patients with congenital long QT syndrome. Consider
obtaining electrocardiograms and monitoring electrolytes
(magnesium, potassium, calcium) periodically during treatment in patients with congestive heart failure, bradyarrhythmias, those taking certain antiarrhythmic
medications or other medicinal products that lead to QT
prolongation, and those with electrolyte disturbances such
as hypokalemia, hypocalcemia, or hypomagnesemia.
Potentially significant drug-drug/drug-food interactions
may exist, requiring dose or frequency adjustment, additional monitoring, and/or selection of alternative therapy. In

liver transplantation, the tacrolimus dose and target range should be reduced to minimize the risk of nephrotoxicity when used in combination with everolimus. Extended release tacrolimus in combination with sirolimus is not recommended in renal transplant patients; the safety and efficacy of immediate release tacrolimus in combination with sirolimus has not been established in this patient population. Concomitant use was associated with increased mortality, graft loss, and hepatic artery thrombosis in liver transplant patients, as well as increased risk of renal impairment, wound healing complications, and PTDM in heart transplant recipients.

Immediate release and extended release capsules are NOT interchangeable or substitutable. The extended release formulation is a once daily preparation; and immediate release is intended for twice daily administration. Serious adverse events, including organ rejection may occur if inadvertently substituted. **[US Boxed Warning]: Astagraf XL was associated with increased mortality in female liver transplant recipients; the use of extended release tacrolimus is not recommended in liver transplantation.** Mortality at 12 months was 18% in females who received extended release tacrolimus compared to 8% for females who received regular release tacrolimus. Each mL of injection contains polyoxyl 60 hydrogenated castor oil (HCO-60) (200 mg) and dehydrated alcohol USP 80% v/v.

Hypersensitivity reactions, including anaphylaxis, have been reported with tacrolimus injection. Tacrolimus injection contains polyoxyl 60 hydrogenated castor oil (HCO-60), a castor oil derivative. HCO-60 is a solubilizer similar to polyoxyethylated castor oil (also known as polyoxyl 35 castor oil or Cremophor EL); polyoxyethylated castor oil is associated with hypersensitivity reactions (Nicolai 2012). Tacrolimus intravenous (IV) use should be limited to patients unable to take oral capsules. Monitor patient for a minimum of 30 minutes after initiation of infusion and then at frequent intervals; discontinue infusion if anaphylaxis occurs. Patients should be transitioned from IV to oral tacrolimus as soon as the patient can tolerate oral administration. Patients should not be immunized with live vaccines during or shortly after treatment and should avoid close contact with recently vaccinated (live vaccine) individuals. Oral formulations contain lactose; the Canadian labeling does not recommend use of these products in patients who may be lactose intolerant (eg, Lapp lactase deficiency, glucose-galactose malabsorption, galactose intolerance). **[US Boxed Warning]: Should be administered under the supervision of a physician experienced in immunosuppressive therapy and organ transplantation in a facility appropriate for monitoring and managing therapy.**

Adverse Reactions As reported for kidney, liver, and heart transplantation:

≥15%:

Cardiovascular: Hypertension (13% to 89%), peripheral edema (11% to 36%), chest pain (19%), edema (<15% to 18%), pericardial effusion (heart transplant 15%; Astagraf XL <15%)

Central nervous system: Headache (10% to 64%), insomnia (9% to 64%), pain (24% to 63%), paresthesia (<15% to 40%), dizziness (<15% to 19%), fatigue (2% to 16%)

Dermatologic: Pruritus (<15% to 36%), skin rash (10% to 24%)

Endocrine & metabolic: Diabetes mellitus (post-transplant; kidney transplant 20% to 75%; heart transplant 13% to 22%; liver transplant 11% to 18%), hyperglycemia (16% to 70%), hypertriglyceridemia (65%), hypoglycemia (<15% to 61%), hypercholesterolemia (<15% to 57%), hypophosphatemia (5% to 49%), hypomagnesemia (3% to 48%), hyperkalemia (13% to 45%), hyperlipidemia (7% to 34%), hypokalemia (13% to 29%)

Gastrointestinal: Diarrhea (25% to 72%), abdominal pain (29% to 59%; Astagraf XL <15%), nausea (13% to 46%), constipation (14% to 40%), anorexia (7% to 34%), vomiting (13% to 29%), dyspepsia (18% to 28%; Astagraf XL <15%)

Genitourinary: Urinary tract infection (1% to 34%), oliguria (<15% to 19%)

Hematologic & oncologic: Anemia (5% to 50%; hemoglobin <10 g/dL 65%), leukopenia (11% to 48%), leukocytosis (8% to 32%), thrombocytopenia (14% to 24%)

Hepatic: Abnormal hepatic function tests (6% to 36%), ascites (7% to 27%)

Infection: Infection (15% to 45%), bacterial infection (8% to 41%), cytomegalovirus disease (heart transplant 32%; kidney transplant 6% to 12%), serious infection (19% to 24%)

Local: Postoperative wound complication (kidney transplant 28%)

Neuromuscular & skeletal: Tremor (15% to 56%; heart transplant 15%), weakness (11% to 52%), back pain (17% to 30%), arthralgia (25%; Astagraf XL <15%)

Renal: Renal function abnormality (36% to 56%), increased serum creatinine (16% to 45%), increased blood urea nitrogen (12% to 30%)

Respiratory: Pleural effusion (30% to 36%), respiratory tract infection (22% to 34%), dyspnea (5% to 29%), atelectasis (5% to 28%), cough (<15% to 18%), bronchitis (17%)

Miscellaneous: Fever (19% to 48%), postoperative pain (kidney transplant 29%), graft complications (kidney transplant 14% to 24%)

<15%:

Cardiovascular: Angina pectoris, atrial fibrillation, atrial flutter, bradycardia, cardiac arrest, cardiac arrhythmia, cardiac failure, cardiorespiratory arrest, cerebral infarction, cerebral ischemia, decreased heart rate, deep vein thrombophlebitis, deep vein thrombosis, ECG abnormality (QRS or ST segment or T wave), flushing, hemorrhagic stroke, hypertrophic cardiomyopathy, hypotension, ischemic heart disease, myocardial infarction, orthostatic hypotension, peripheral vascular disease, phlebitis, syncope, tachycardia, thrombosis, vasodilatation, ventricular premature contractions

Central nervous system: Abnormal dreams, abnormality in thinking, agitation, amnesia, anxiety, aphasia, ataxia, brain disease, carpal tunnel syndrome, chills, confusion, convulsions, depression, drowsiness, emotional lability, excessive crying, falling, flaccid paralysis, hallucination, hypertonia, hypoesthesia, mental status changes, mood elevation, myasthenia, myoclonus, nervousness, neurotoxicity, nightmares, paresis, peripheral neuropathy, psychosis, seizure, vertigo, voice disorder, writing difficulty

Dermatologic: Acne vulgaris, alopecia, bruise, cellulitis, condyloma acuminatum, dermal ulcer, dermatitis (including fungal), dermatological reaction, diaphoresis, exfoliative dermatitis, hypotrichosis, skin discoloration, skin photosensitivity

Endocrine & metabolic: Acidosis, albuminuria, alkalosis, anasarca, Cushing's syndrome, decreased serum bicarbonate, decreased serum iron, dehydration, gout, hirsutism, hypercalcemia, hyperphosphatemia, hyperuricemia, hypervolemia, hypocalcemia, hyponatremia, increased gamma-glutamyl transferase, increased lactate dehydrogenase, weight changes

Gastrointestinal: Gastroenteritis (2% to 7%), aphthous stomatitis, cholangitis, colitis, delayed gastric emptying, duodenitis, dysphagia, enlargement of abdomen, esophagitis (including ulcerative), flatulence, gastric ulcer, gastritis, gastroesophageal reflux disease, gastrointestinal hemorrhage, gastrointestinal perforation, hernia, hiccups, increased appetite, intestinal obstruction, oral candidiasis, pancreatic disease (pseudocyst), pancreatitis (including hemorrhagic and necrotizing), peritonitis, rectal disease, stomach cramps, stomatitis

Genitourinary: Anuria, bladder spasm, cystitis, dysuria, hematuria, nocturia, proteinuria, toxic nephrosis, urinary frequency, urinary incontinence, urinary retention, urinary urgency, vaginitis

Hematologic & oncologic: Blood coagulation disorder, decreased prothrombin time, hemolytic anemia, hemorrhage, hypochromic anemia, hypoproteinemia, increased hematocrit, increased INR, Kaposi's sarcoma, malignant neoplasm of bladder, malignant neoplasm of thyroid (papillary), neutropenia, pancytopenia, polycythemia, skin neoplasm

Hepatic: Cholestatic jaundice, hepatic injury, hepatitis (including acute, chronic, and granulomatous), hyperbilirubinemia, increased liver enzymes, increased serum alkaline phosphatase, jaundice

Hypersensitivity: Hypersensitivity reaction

Infection: Polyoma virus infection (≤5%), abscess, Epstein Barr virus infection, herpes simplex infection, sepsis, tinea versicolor

Local: Localized phlebitis

Neuromuscular & skeletal: Arthropathy, leg cramps, muscle spasm, muscle weakness of the extremities, myalgia, neuropathy (including compression), osteopenia, osteoporosis

Ophthalmic: Amblyopia, blurred vision, conjunctivitis, visual disturbance

Otic: Hearing loss, otalgia, otitis externa, otitis media, tinnitus

Renal: Acute renal failure, hydronephrosis, renal disease (BK nephropathy), renal tubular necrosis

Respiratory: Allergic rhinitis, asthma, emphysema, flu-like symptoms, pharyngitis, pneumonia, pneumothorax, pulmonary disease, pulmonary edema, pulmonary infiltrates, respiratory depression, respiratory failure, rhinitis, sinusitis

Miscellaneous: Wound healing impairment

Postmarketing and/or case reports (limited to important or life-threatening): Adult respiratory distress syndrome, agranulocytosis, anaphylactoid reaction, anaphylaxis, angioedema, basal cell carcinoma, biliary tract disease (stenosis), blindness, cerebrovascular accident, coma, deafness, decreased serum fibrinogen, delirium, disseminated intravascular coagulation, dysarthria, graft versus host disease (acute and chronic), hemiparesis, hemolytic-uremic syndrome, hemorrhagic cystitis, hepatic cirrhosis, hepatic failure, hepatic necrosis, hepatic veno-occlusive disease, hepatosplenic T-cell lymphomas, hepatotoxicity, hyperpigmentation, interstitial pulmonary disease, leukemia, leukoencephalopathy, liver steatosis, lymphoproliferative disorder (post-transplant or related to EBV), malignant melanoma, multi-organ failure, mutism, optic atrophy, osteomyelitis, photophobia, polyarthritis, progressive multifocal leukoencephalopathy (PML), prolonged partial thromboplastin time, prolonged Q-T interval on ECG, pulmonary hypertension, pure red cell aplasia, quadriplegia, reversible posterior leukoencephalopathy syndrome, rhabdomyolysis, septicemia, squamous cell carcinoma, status epilepticus, Stevens-Johnson syndrome, supraventricular extrasystole, supraventricular tachycardia, thrombocytopenic purpura, thrombotic thrombocytopenic purpura, torsades de pointes, toxic epidermal necrolysis, venous thrombosis, ventricular fibrillation

Note: Calcineurin inhibitor-induced hemolytic uremic syndrome/thrombotic thrombocytopenic purpura/thrombotic microangiopathy (HUS/TTP/TMA) have been reported (with concurrent sirolimus).

Drug Interactions
Metabolism/Transport Effects Substrate of CYP3A4 (major), P-glycoprotein; **Note:** Assignment of Major/Minor substrate status based on clinically relevant drug interaction potential; **Inhibits** P-glycoprotein

Avoid Concomitant Use
Avoid concomitant use of Tacrolimus (Systemic) with any of the following: BCG (Intravesical); Bosutinib; Conivaptan; Crizotinib; CycloSPORINE (Systemic); Deferiprone; Dipyrone; Enzalutamide; Eplerenone; Foscarnet; Fusidic Acid (Systemic); Grapefruit Juice; Idelalisib; Mifepristone; Natalizumab; Nelfinavir; PAZOPanib; Pimecrolimus; Potassium-Sparing Diuretics; Silodosin; Sirolimus; Tacrolimus (Topical); Temsirolimus; Tofacitinib; Topotecan; Vaccines (Live); VinCRIStine (Liposomal)

Increased Effect/Toxicity
Tacrolimus (Systemic) may increase the levels/effects of: Afatinib; Bosutinib; Brentuximab Vedotin; CloZAPine; Colchicine; CycloSPORINE (Systemic); Dabigatran Etexilate; Deferiprone; DOXOrubicin (Conventional); Dronedarone; Edoxaban; Everolimus; Fenofibrate and Derivatives; Fingolimod; Fosphenytoin; Highest Risk QTc-Prolonging Agents; Ledipasvir; Leflunomide; Moderate Risk QTc-Prolonging Agents; Naloxegol; Natalizumab; PAZOPanib; P-glycoprotein/ABCB1 Substrates; Phenytoin; Prucalopride; Rifaximin; Silodosin; Sirolimus; Temsirolimus; Tofacitinib; Topotecan; Vaccines (Live); VinCRIStine (Liposomal)

The levels/effects of Tacrolimus (Systemic) may be increased by: Alcohol (Ethyl); Antidepressants (Serotonin Reuptake Inhibitor/Antagonist); Aprepitant; Boceprevir; Calcium Channel Blockers (Dihydropyridine); Calcium Channel Blockers (Nondihydropyridine); Chloramphenicol; Clotrimazole (Oral); Clotrimazole (Topical); Conivaptan; Crizotinib; CycloSPORINE (Systemic); CYP3A4 Inhibitors (Moderate); CYP3A4 Inhibitors (Strong); Danazol; Dasatinib; Denosumab; Dipyrone; Dronedarone; Efonidipine; Eplerenone; Ertapenem; Fluconazole; Fosaprepitant; Foscarnet; Fusidic Acid (Systemic); Grapefruit Juice; Idelalisib; Itraconazole; Ivacaftor; Ketoconazole (Systemic); Levofloxacin (Systemic); Luliconazole; Macrolide Antibiotics; Mifepristone; Nelfinavir; Netupitant; Nonsteroidal Anti-Inflammatory Agents; Ombitasvir, Paritaprevir, and Ritonavir; Ombitasvir, Paritaprevir, Ritonavir, and Dasabuvir; Osimertinib; Palbociclib; P-glycoprotein/ABCB1 Inhibitors; Pimecrolimus; Posaconazole; Potassium-Sparing Diuretics; Protease Inhibitors; Proton Pump Inhibitors; Ranolazine; Ritonavir; Roflumilast; Schisandra; Sirolimus; Stiripentol; Tacrolimus (Topical); Telaprevir; Temsirolimus; Trastuzumab; Voriconazole

Decreased Effect
Tacrolimus (Systemic) may decrease the levels/effects of: Antidiabetic Agents; BCG (Intravesical); Coccidioides immitis Skin Test; Sipuleucel-T; Vaccines (Inactivated); Vaccines (Live)

The levels/effects of Tacrolimus (Systemic) may be decreased by: Bosentan; Caspofungin; Cinacalcet; CYP3A4 Inducers (Moderate); CYP3A4 Inducers (Strong); Dabrafenib; Deferasirox; Echinacea; Efavirenz; Enzalutamide; Fosphenytoin; Mitotane; Osimertinib; P-glycoprotein/ABCB1 Inducers; Phenytoin; Rifamycin Derivatives; Sevelamer; Siltuximab; Sirolimus; St Johns Wort; Temsirolimus; Tocilizumab

Food Interactions
Ethanol: Alcohol may increase the rate of release of extended-release tacrolimus and adversely affect tacrolimus safety and/or efficacy. Management: Avoid alcohol.
Food: Food decreases rate and extent of absorption. High-fat meals have most pronounced effect (37% and 25% decrease in AUC, respectively, and 77% and 25% decrease in C_{max}, respectively, for immediately release and extended release formulations). Grapefruit juice, a CYP3A4 inhibitor, may increase serum level and/or toxicity of tacrolimus. Management: Administer with or without food (immediate release), but be consistent. Administer extended release on an empty stomach. Avoid concurrent use of grapefruit juice.

Preparation for Administration Hazardous agent; use appropriate precautions for handling and disposal (NIOSH 2014 [group 2]).

Injection: Dilute with 5% dextrose injection or 0.9% sodium chloride injection to a final concentration between 0.004 mg/mL and 0.02 mg/mL.

Storage/Stability
Injection: Prior to dilution, store at 5°C to 25°C (41°F to 77°F). Following dilution, stable for 24 hours in D_5W or NS in glass or polyethylene containers. Do not store in polyvinyl chloride containers since the polyoxyl 60 hydrogenated castor oil injectable vehicle may leach phthalates from polyvinyl chloride containers.
Capsule, tablet:
   Astagraf XL, Envarsus XR, Prograf: Store at 25°C (77°F); excursions permitted between 15°C and 30°C (59°F and 86°F).
   Hecoria: Store at 20°C to 25°C (68°F to 77°F).

Mechanism of Action Suppresses cellular immunity (inhibits T-lymphocyte activation), by binding to an intracellular protein, FKBP-12 and complexes with calcineurin dependent proteins to inhibit calcineurin phosphatase activity

Pharmacodynamics/Kinetics
Absorption: Better in resected patients with a closed stoma; unlike cyclosporine, clamping of the T-tube in liver transplant patients does not alter trough concentrations or AUC; Oral: Incomplete and variable; the rate and extent of absorption is decreased by food (particularly a high-fat meal). Oral absorption may be variable in stem cell transplant patients with mucositis due to the conditioning regimen.
Distribution: V_d: Children: 0.5 to 4.7 L/kg; Adults: 0.55 to 2.47 L/kg
Protein binding: ~99% primarily to albumin and alpha$_1$-acid glycoprotein
Metabolism: Extensively hepatic via CYP3A4 to eight possible metabolites (major metabolite, 31-demethyl tacrolimus, shows same activity as tacrolimus *in vitro*)
Bioavailability: Oral: Children: 7% to 55%; Adults: 7% to 32%; Absolute: Unknown
Half-life elimination:
   Immediate release: Variable, 23 to 46 hours in healthy volunteers; 2.1 to 36 hours in transplant patients
   Extended release: 23 to 41 hours
Time to peak: 0.5 to 6 hours
Excretion: Feces (~93%); urine (<1% as unchanged drug)

Dosing
Adult & Geriatric
   Prevention of organ rejection in transplant recipients: Note: The initial postoperative dose of tacrolimus (immediate release) should begin no sooner than 6 hours after liver and heart transplant and within 24 hours of kidney transplant (but may be delayed until renal function has recovered); titrate to target trough concentrations. Adjunctive therapy with corticosteroids is recommended early post-transplant. IV route should only be used in patients not able to take oral medications and continued only until oral medication can be tolerated; anaphylaxis has been reported with IV administration. If switching from IV to oral, the oral dose should be started 8 to 12 hours after stopping the infusion.

   Liver transplant:
      Oral:
         Immediate release: Initial: 0.1 to 0.15 mg/kg/day in 2 divided doses, given every 12 hours (titrate to target trough concentrations)

Extended release: Canadian labeling (Advagraf): 0.1 to 0.2 mg/kg once daily in combination with corticosteroids; initiate within 12 to 18 hours of transplantation. Titrate to target trough concentrations.

Conversion from immediate release to extended release: Patients stable on immediate release tacrolimus may be converted to extended release by initiating extended-release treatment in a 1:1 ratio (mg:mg) using previously established total daily dose of immediate-release product. Administer once daily.

IV: Initial: 0.03 to 0.05 mg/kg/day as a continuous infusion

Heart transplant: Use in combination with azathioprine or mycophenolate mofetil is recommended.

Oral: Immediate release: Initial: 0.075 mg/kg/day in 2 divided doses, given every 12 hours (titrate to target trough concentrations)

IV: Initial: 0.01 mg/kg/day as a continuous infusion

Kidney transplant: Use in combination with azathioprine or mycophenolate mofetil is recommended. **Note:** African-American patients may require larger doses to attain trough concentration.

Oral:

US labeling:

Immediate release (Hecoria, Prograf): Initial: 0.2 mg/kg/day in combination with azathioprine or 0.1 mg/kg/day in combination with mycophenolate mofetil; titrate to target trough concentrations. Administer in 2 divided doses, given every 12 hours.

Extended release (Astagraf XL):

With basiliximab induction (prior to or within 48 hours of transplant completion): 0.15 mg/kg once daily (in combination with corticosteroids and mycophenolate); titrate to target trough concentrations

Without basiliximab induction: Preoperative dose (administer within 12 hours prior to reperfusion): 0.1 mg/kg

Without basiliximab induction: Postoperative dosing (administer at least 4 hours after preoperative dose and within 12 hours of reperfusion): 0.2 mg/kg once daily (in combination with corticosteroids and mycophenolate); titrate to target trough concentrations

Conversion from IV to extended release: Administer the first oral extended release dose 8 to 12 hours after discontinuation of IV tacrolimus

Conversion from immediate release to extended release: Initiate extended release treatment in a 1:1 ratio (mg:mg) using previously established total daily dose of immediate release (Van Hooff 2012). Administer once daily.

Extended release (Envarsus XR): Conversion from immediate release to extended release: Initiate extended-release treatment with a once-daily dose that is 80% of the total daily dose of the immediate-release tacrolimus

Canadian labeling:

Immediate release (Prograf): Initial: 0.2 to 0.3 mg/kg/day in 2 divided doses, given every 12 hours in combination with corticosteroids and other immunosuppressive agents; titrate to target trough concentrations

Extended release (Advagraf): Initial: 0.15 to 0.2 mg/kg once daily; titrate to target trough concentrations. Administer in combination with corticosteroids and mycophenolate mofetil (MMF) in de novo kidney transplant recipients. Antibody induction therapy should also be used.

Conversion from immediate release to extended release: Initiate extended release treatment in a 1:1 ratio (mg:mg) using previously established total daily dose of immediate release. Administer once daily.

IV: Initial: 0.03 to 0.05 mg/kg/day as a continuous infusion

Graft-versus-host disease (GVHD) (off-label use):

Prevention:

Oral: Convert from IV to immediate release oral dose (1:4 ratio): Multiply total daily IV dose times 4 and administer in 2 divided oral doses per day, every 12 hours (Uberti 1999; Yanik 2000).

IV: Initial: 0.03 mg/kg/day (based on lean body weight) as continuous infusion. Treatment should begin at least 24 hours prior to stem cell infusion and continued only until oral medication can be tolerated (Przepiorka 1999; Yanik 2000).

Treatment:

Oral: Immediate release: 0.06 mg/kg twice daily (Furlong 2000; Przepiorka 1999)

IV: Initial: 0.03 mg/kg/day (based on lean body weight) as continuous infusion (Furlong 2000; Przepiorka 1999)

Lung transplant (off-label use): Usually used in a combination regimen that contains a corticosteroid and either azathioprine or mycophenolate (Snell 2013).

Oral, nasogastric: Immediate release: 0.05 to 0.3 mg/kg/day in 2 divided doses, given every 12 hours (usual dose: 0.05 mg/kg every 12 hours); titrate to target trough concentrations (Treede 2001; Treede 2012; Zuckermann 2003). May also be administered sublingually at ~50% of the oral/NG dose (Doligalski 2014; Watkins 2012).

Note: May convert from twice-daily dosing to once-daily dosing (on a mg per mg basis) using the extended-release formulation (Astagraf XL [US] or Advagraf [Canada]) in stable lung transplant recipients (Mendez 2014).

IV: 0.01 to 0.05 mg/kg over 24 hours as a continuous IV infusion; titrate to target trough concentrations (Treede 2001; Treede 2012; Zuckermann 2003). For patients receiving the initial dose of tacrolimus intravenously, may begin immediately after transplantation, or up to 2 days postoperatively depending on renal function and hemodynamic stability (Treede 2001; Treede 2012; Witt 2013; Zuckermann 2003). When patient is able to take oral medication, may switch to an oral maintenance regimen (typically transitioned after extubation).

Rheumatoid arthritis: Canadian labeling (not in US labeling): Oral: Immediate release: 3 mg once daily; carefully monitor serum creatinine during therapy

Pediatric

Liver transplant:

Oral: Immediate release: Initial: 0.15-0.20 mg/kg/day in 2 divided doses, given every 12 hours (titrate to target trough concentrations)

IV: Initial: 0.03-0.05 mg/kg/day as a continuous infusion

Note: The initial postoperative dose of tacrolimus should begin no sooner than 6 hours after liver and heart transplant and within 24 hours of kidney transplant (but may be delayed until renal function has recovered). Adjunctive therapy with corticosteroids is recommended early post-transplant. IV route should only be used in patients not able to take oral medications and continued only until oral medication can be tolerated; anaphylaxis has been reported with IV administration. If switching from IV to oral, the oral dose should be started 8-12 hours after stopping the infusion. Patients without preexisting renal or hepatic dysfunction have required (and tolerated) higher doses than adults to achieve similar blood concentrations. It is recommended that therapy be initiated at the **high end** of the recommended adult IV and oral dosing ranges; dosage adjustments may be required.

Prevention of graft-vs-host disease (GVHD) (off-label use): Oral, IV: Refer to adult dosing.

Renal Impairment Evidence suggests that lower doses should be used; patients should receive doses at the lowest value of the recommended IV and oral dosing ranges; further reductions in dose below these ranges may be required. May also require dose reductions due to nephrotoxicity.

Kidney transplant: Tacrolimus therapy in patients with postoperative oliguria should begin no sooner than 6 hours and within 24 hours (immediate release) or 48 hours (extended release) post-transplant, but may be delayed until renal function displays evidence of recovery.

Hemodialysis: Not removed by hemodialysis; supplemental dose is not necessary.

Peritoneal dialysis: Significant drug removal is unlikely based on physiochemical characteristics.

Hepatic Impairment Use of tacrolimus in liver transplant recipients experiencing post-transplant hepatic impairment may be associated with increased risk of developing renal insufficiency related to high whole blood levels of tacrolimus. The presence of moderate-to-severe hepatic dysfunction (serum bilirubin >2 mg/dL; Child-Pugh score ≥10) appears to affect the metabolism of tacrolimus. The half-life of the drug was prolonged and the clearance reduced after IV administration. The bioavailability of tacrolimus was also increased after oral administration. The higher plasma concentrations as determined by ELISA, in patients with severe hepatic dysfunction are probably due to the accumulation of metabolites of lower activity. These patients should be monitored closely and dosage adjustments should be considered. Some evidence indicates that lower doses could be used in these patients.

Dietary Considerations Capsule: Administer immediate release with or without food; be consistent with timing and composition of meals, food decreases bioavailability. Administer extended release on an empty stomach 1 hour before or 2 hours after a meal. Avoid grapefruit and grapefruit juice. Avoid alcohol.

Administration

IV: If IV administration is necessary, administer by continuous infusion only. Do not use PVC tubing when administering diluted solutions. Tacrolimus is usually intended to be administered as a continuous infusion over 24 hours. Do not mix with solutions with a pH ≥9 (eg, acyclovir or ganciclovir) due to chemical degradation of tacrolimus (use different ports in multilumen lines). Do not alter dose with concurrent T-tube clamping. Adsorption of the drug to PVC tubing may become clinically significant with low concentrations.

Oral:

Immediate release: Administer with or without food; be consistent with timing and composition of meals if GI intolerance occurs and administration with food becomes necessary (per manufacturer). If dosed once daily, administer in the morning. If dosed twice daily, doses should be 12 hours apart. If the morning and evening doses differ, the larger dose (differences are never >0.5-1 mg) should be given in the morning. If dosed 3 times daily, separate doses by 8 hours.

Combination therapy with everolimus for liver transplantation: Administer tacrolimus at the same time as everolimus.

Extended release: Administer on an empty stomach at least 1 hour before or 2 hours after a meal. Advagraf [Canadian product] labeling suggests that the capsule may be taken with food if necessary but should be administered consistently with or without food. Swallow whole, do not chew, crush, or divide. Take once daily in the morning at a consistent time each day. Missed doses may be taken up to 14 hours (15 hours for Envarsus XR) after scheduled time; if >14 hours (>15 hours for Enbarsus XR), resume at next regularly scheduled time; do not double a dose to make up for a missed dose.

Nasogastric tube: In patients unable to swallow capsules, contents of immediate release capsule(s) may be mixed with water and flushed through a nasogastric tube; clamp nasogastric tube for 30 to 60 minutes after administration (Taylor 2001).

Sublingual: In patients unable to swallow capsules, tacrolimus may be administered sublingually (at a reduced dose) by opening the immediate-release capsules and placing the contents of the capsule(s) under the tongue allowing contents to completely dissolve; avoid food, beverages, or mechanical suctioning for at least 30 minutes after administration (Doligalski 2014; Watkins 2012).

Hazardous agent; use appropriate precautions for handling and disposal (NIOSH 2014 [group 2]). Avoid contact with broken capsules. If it is necessary to manipulate capsules (eg, to open capsules or prepare an oral suspension), it is recommended to double glove, wear a protective gown, and prepare in a controlled device (NIOSH 2014).

Monitoring Parameters Renal function, hepatic function, serum electrolytes (calcium, magnesium, potassium), glucose and blood pressure, measure 3 times/week for first few weeks, then gradually decrease frequency as patient stabilizes. Whole blood concentrations should be used for monitoring (trough for oral therapy); frequency varies depending on transplant type, time since transplantation, and clinical situation. Signs/symptoms of anaphylactic reactions during IV infusion should also be monitored. Patients should be monitored for hypersensitivity during the first 30 minutes of the infusion, and frequently thereafter. Monitor for QT prolongation; consider echocardiographic evaluation in patients who develop renal failure, electrolyte abnormalities, or clinical manifestations of ventricular dysfunction.

Tacrolimus serum levels may be falsely elevated in infected liver transplant patients due to interference from β-galactosidase antibodies.

Reference Range

Heart transplant: Typical whole blood trough concentrations:

Months 1 to 3: 10 to 20 ng/mL

Months ≥4: 5 to 15 ng/mL

Kidney transplant: Whole blood trough concentrations:

Immediate release:

In combination with azathioprine:

Months 1 to 3: 7 to 20 ng/mL

Months 4 to 12: 5 to 15 ng/mL

In combination with mycophenolate mofetil/IL-2 receptor antagonist (eg, daclizumab): Months 1 to 12: 4 to 11 ng/mL

Extended release:

With basiliximab induction:

Days 1 to 60: 5 to 17 ng/mL

Month 3 to 12: 4 to 12 ng/mL

Without induction:

Days 1 to 60: 6 to 20 ng/mL

Month 3 to 12: 6 to 14 ng/mL

Liver transplant: Whole blood trough concentrations:

U.S. labeling: Months 1 to 12: 5 to 20 ng/mL

Canadian labeling: Months 1 to 2: 5 to 20 ng/mL; Months 3 to 12: 5 to 15 ng/mL

Recommended therapeutic ranges when administered in combination with everolimus for liver transplant (Zortress product labeling 2013): By 3 weeks after first everolimus dose and through month 12 post-transplant: 3 to 5 ng/mL

Lung transplant (off-label use): Whole blood trough concentrations: 5 to 15 ng/mL (ACCP [Baughman 2012])

Prevention of graft-versus-host disease (off-label use): 10 to 20 ng/mL (Uberti 1999) although some institutions use a lower limit of 5 ng/mL and an upper limit of 15 ng/mL (Przepiorka 1999; Yanik 2000)

Dosage Forms Considerations Prograf injection contains polyoxyl 60 hydrogenated castor oil (HCO-60)

Dosage Forms Excipient information presented when available (limited, particularly for generics); consult specific product labeling. [DSC] = Discontinued product

Capsule, Oral:

Hecoria: 0.5 mg [DSC], 1 mg [DSC], 5 mg [DSC]

Prograf: 0.5 mg, 1 mg, 5 mg

Generic: 0.5 mg, 1 mg, 5 mg

Capsule Extended Release 24 Hour, Oral:

Astagraf XL: 0.5 mg, 1 mg, 5 mg

Solution, Intravenous:

Prograf: 5 mg/mL (1 mL) [contains alcohol, usp, cremophor el]

Tablet Extended Release 24 Hour, Oral:

Envarsus XR: 0.75 mg, 1 mg, 4 mg

Dosage Forms: Canada Note: Also refer to Dosage Forms

Excipient information presented when available (limited, particularly for generics); consult specific product labeling.

Capsule Extended Release 24 Hour, Oral:

Advagraf: 0.5 mg, 1 mg, 3 mg, 5 mg

Extemporaneous Preparations Hazardous agent; use appropriate precautions for handling and disposal (NIOSH 2014 [group 2]). When manipulating capsules, NIOSH recommends double gloving, a protective gown, and preparation in a controlled device; if not prepared in a controlled device, respiratory and eye protection as well as ventilated engineering controls are recommended (NIOSH 2014).

A 0.5 mg/mL tacrolimus oral suspension may be made with immediate release capsules and a 1:1 mixture of Ora-Plus and Simple Syrup, N.F. Mix the contents of six 5 mg tacrolimus capsules with quantity of vehicle sufficient to make 60 mL. Store in glass or plastic amber prescription bottles; label "shake well". Stable for 56 days at room temperature (Esquivel 1996; Foster 1996).

A 1 mg/mL tacrolimus oral suspension may be made with immediate release capsules, sterile water, Ora-Plus, and Ora-Sweet. Pour the contents of six 5 mg capsules into a plastic amber prescription bottle. Add ~5 mL of sterile water and agitate bottle until drug disperses into a slurry. Add equal parts Ora-Plus and Ora-Sweet in sufficient quantity to make 30 mL. Store in plastic amber prescription bottles; label "shake well". Stable for 4 months at room temperature (Elefante 2006).

Elefante A, Muindi J, West K, et al, "Long-Term Stability of a Patient-Convenient 1 mg/mL Suspension of Tacrolimus for Accurate Maintenance of Stable Therapeutic Levels," *Bone Marrow Transplant.* 2006, 37(8):781-4.

Esquivel C, So S, McDiarmid S, Andrews W, and Colombani PM, "Suggested Guidelines for the Use of Tacrolimus in Pediatric Liver Transplant Patients," *Transplantation,* 1996, 61(5):847-8.

Foster JA, Jacobson PA, Johnson CE, et al, "Stability of Tacrolimus in an Extemporaneously Compounded Oral Liquid (Abstract of Meeting Presentation)," *American Society of Health-System Pharmacists Annual Meeting,* 1996, 53:P-52(E).

Tacrolimus (Topical) (ta KROE li mus)

Brand Names: US Protopic

Brand Names: Canada Protopic®

Pharmacologic Category Calcineurin Inhibitor; Immunosuppressant Agent; Topical Skin Product

Use Moderate-to-severe atopic dermatitis in immunocompetent patients not responsive to conventional therapy or when conventional therapy is not appropriate

◀ *Canadian labeling: Additional use (not in U.S. labeling):* Maintenance therapy to prevent flares and extend flare-free intervals in patients with moderate-to-severe atopic dermatitis who are responsive to initial therapy and experiencing ≥5 flares per year

Medication Guide Available Yes

Dosing

Adult & Geriatric Atopic dermatitis (moderate-to-severe): Topical:

Treatment: Apply thin layer of 0.03% or 0.1% ointment to affected area twice daily; rub in gently and completely. Discontinue use when symptoms have cleared. If no improvement within 6 weeks, patients should be re-examined to confirm diagnosis.

Maintenance therapy (Canadian labeling; not in U.S. labeling): Apply one application (thin layer of 0.03% or 0.1% ointment) to areas usually affected twice a week, allowing 2-3 days between applications (eg, one application on Monday and Thursday). Re-evaluate after 12 months. Safety of maintenance therapy >12 months has not been established.

Note: Patients experiencing flares should resume twice daily treatment.

Pediatric Moderate-to-severe atopic dermatitis: Topical:

Treatment:

Children ≥2-15 years: Apply thin layer of 0.03% ointment to affected area twice daily; rub in gently and completely. Discontinue use when symptoms have cleared. If no improvement within 6 weeks, patients should be re-examined to confirm diagnosis.

Children >15 years: Refer to adult dosing.

Maintenance therapy (Canadian labeling; not in U.S. labeling):

Children ≥2-15 years: Apply one application (thin layer of 0.03% ointment) to areas usually affected twice a week, allowing 2-3 days between applications (eg, one application on Monday and Thursday). Re-evaluate after 12 months. Safety of maintenance therapy >12 months has not been established.

Children >15 years: Refer to adult dosing.

Note: Patients experiencing flares should resume twice daily treatment.

Additional Information Complete prescribing information should be consulted for additional detail.

Dosage Forms Excipient information presented when available (limited, particularly for generics); consult specific product labeling.

Ointment, External:

Protopic: 0.03% (30 g, 60 g, 100 g); 0.1% (30 g, 60 g, 100 g)

Generic: 0.03% (30 g, 60 g, 100 g); 0.1% (30 g, 60 g, 100 g)

◆ **Tactupump (Can)** see Adapalene and Benzoyl Peroxide on page 44

◆ **Tactupump Plus (Can)** see Adapalene and Benzoyl Peroxide on page 44

Tadalafil (tah DA la fil)

Brand Names: US Adcirca; Cialis

Brand Names: Canada Adcirca; Apo-Tadalafil PAH; Cialis

Index Terms GF196960

Pharmacologic Category Phosphodiesterase-5 Enzyme Inhibitor

Use

Benign prostatic hyperplasia (Cialis only): Treatment of the signs and symptoms of benign prostatic hyperplasia (BPH).

Erectile dysfunction (Cialis only): Treatment of erectile dysfunction.

Erectile dysfunction and benign prostatic hyperplasia (Cialis only): Treatment of erectile dysfunction and the signs and symptoms of BPH.

Pulmonary arterial hypertension (Adcirca only): Treatment of pulmonary arterial hypertension (World Health Organization group 1) to improve exercise ability. Studies establishing effectiveness included predominantly patients with New York Heart Association (NYHA) functional class II to III symptoms and etiologies of idiopathic or heritable pulmonary arterial hypertension (61%) or pulmonary arterial hypertension associated with connective tissue diseases (23%).

Pregnancy Considerations Teratogenic events were not reported in animal reproduction studies. Postnatal development and pup survival was decreased at some doses. There are no adequate and well-controlled studies in pregnant women. Less than 0.0005% is found in the semen of healthy males.

Breast-Feeding Considerations It is not known if tadalafil is excreted in breast milk. The manufacturer recommends that caution be exercised when administering tadalafil to nursing women.

Contraindications

Serious hypersensitivity to tadalafil or any component of the formulation; concurrent use of organic nitrate (regularly and/or intermittently) or guanylate cyclase stimulators (eg, riociguat).

Canadian labeling: Additional contraindications (not in US labeling): Previous episode of nonarteritic anterior ischemic optic neuropathy

Warnings/Precautions There is a degree of cardiac risk associated with sexual activity; therefore, physicians should consider the cardiovascular status of their patients prior to initiation. Use is not recommended in patients with hypotension (<90/50 mm Hg), uncontrolled hypertension (>170/100 mm Hg), NYHA class II-IV heart failure within the last 6 months, uncontrolled arrhythmias, stroke within the last 6 months, MI within the last 3 months, unstable angina or angina during sexual intercourse; safety and efficacy have not been evaluated in these patients. Safety and efficacy in PAH have not been evaluated in patients with clinically significant aortic and/or mitral valve disease, life-threatening arrhythmias, hypotension (<90/50 mm Hg), uncontrolled hypertension, significant left ventricular dysfunction, pericardial constriction, restrictive or congestive cardiomyopathy, symptomatic coronary artery disease. Use caution in patients with left ventricular outflow obstruction (eg, aortic stenosis, hypertrophic obstructive cardiomyopathy); may be more sensitive to vasodilator effects. Patients experiencing anginal chest pain after tadalafil administration should seek immediate medical attention.

Pulmonary vasodilators may exacerbate the cardiovascular status in patients with pulmonary veno-occlusive disease (PVOD); use is not recommended. In patients with unrecognized PVOD, signs of pulmonary edema should prompt investigation into this diagnosis. Use with caution in patients with mild to moderate hepatic impairment; dosage adjustment/limitation is needed. Use is not recommended in patients with severe hepatic impairment or cirrhosis. Use with caution in patients with renal impairment; dosage adjustment/limitation is needed. Use caution in patients with bleeding disorders or peptic ulcer disease due to effect on platelets (bleeding).

When used to treat BPH or erectile dysfunction, potential underlying causes of BPH or erectile dysfunction should be evaluated prior to treatment. Use with caution in patients with anatomical deformation of the penis (angulation, cavernosal fibrosis, or Peyronie's disease), or who have conditions which may predispose them to priapism (sickle cell anemia, multiple myeloma, leukemia). Priapism, painful erection >6 hours in duration has been reported (rarely). Instruct patients to seek immediate medical attention if erection persists >4 hours. Potentially significant drug-drug interactions may exist, requiring dose or frequency adjustment, additional monitoring, and/or selection of alternative therapy. Concomitant use (regularly/intermittently) with all forms of nitrates is contraindicated. Nitrate-mediated vasodilation is markedly exaggerated and prolonged in the presence of PDE-5 inhibitors. When tadalafil is used for BPH, erectile dysfunction, or PAH and nitrate administration is medically necessary (eg, chest pain refractory to other treatments) following the use of tadalafil, at least 48 hours should elapse after the tadalafil dose and nitrate administration. When used for PAH, per the manufacturer, nitrate may be administered within 48 hours of tadalafil. For both situations, administration of nitrates should only be done under close medical supervision with hemodynamic monitoring.

Rare cases of nonarteritic anterior ischemic optic neuropathy (NAION) have been reported; patients who have already experienced NAION are at an increased risk of recurrence. Other risk factors for NAION include heart disease, diabetes, hypertension, smoking, age >50 years, or history of certain eye problems. Use with caution in these patients only when the benefits outweigh the risks. The Canadian labeling contraindicates use in patients with previous episodes of NAION. Sudden decrease or loss of hearing has been reported rarely; hearing changes may be accompanied by tinnitus and dizziness. A direct relationship between therapy and vision or hearing loss has not been determined. Instruct patients to seek medical assistance for sudden loss of vision in one or both eyes, sudden decrease in hearing, or sudden loss of hearing.

Patients with genetic retinal disorders (eg, retinitis pigmentosa) were not evaluated in clinical trials; use is not recommended.

Adverse Reactions Based upon usual doses for either indication. For erectile dysfunction, similar adverse events are reported with once-daily versus intermittent dosing, but are generally lower than with doses used intermittently.

>10%:
Cardiovascular: Flushing (1% to 13%; dose related)
Central nervous system: Headache (3% to 42%; dose related)
Gastrointestinal: Dyspepsia (1% to 13%), nausea (10% to 11%)
Neuromuscular & skeletal: Myalgia (1% to 14%; dose related), back pain (2% to 12%), extremity pain (1% to 11%)
Respiratory: Respiratory tract infection (3% to 13%), nasopharyngitis (2% to 13%)

2% to 10%:
Cardiovascular: Hypertension (1% to 3%)
Gastrointestinal: Gastroenteritis (viral; 3% to 5%), GERD (1% to 3%), abdominal pain (1% to 2%), diarrhea (1% to 2%)
Genitourinary: Urinary tract infection (≤2%)
Respiratory: Nasal congestion (≤9%), cough (2% to 4%), bronchitis (≤2%)
Miscellaneous: Flu-like syndrome (2% to 5%)

<2% (Limited to important or life-threatening): Amnesia (transient global), angina pectoris, arthralgia, basal cell carcinoma (Loeb 2015), blurred vision, chest pain, color vision decreased, conjunctival hyperemia, conjunctivitis, diaphoresis, dizziness, dysphagia, dyspnea, epistaxis, esophagitis, exfoliative dermatitis, eye pain, eyelid swelling, facial edema, fatigue, gastritis, GGTP increased, hearing decreased, hearing loss, hepatic enzymes increased, hypoesthesia, hypotension, insomnia, lacrimation, melanoma (Loeb 2015), migraine, MI, neck pain, nonarteritic ischemic optic neuropathy (NAION), orthostatic hypotension, pain, palpitation, paresthesia, pharyngitis, priapism, pruritus, rash, retinal artery occlusion, retinal vein occlusion, seizure, somnolence, spontaneous penile erection, Stevens-Johnson syndrome, stroke, sudden cardiac death, syncope, tachycardia, tinnitus, urticaria, vertigo, visual field loss, vomiting, weakness, xerostomia

Drug Interactions

Metabolism/Transport Effects Substrate of CYP3A4 (major); **Note:** Assignment of Major/Minor substrate status based on clinically relevant drug interaction potential

Avoid Concomitant Use
Avoid concomitant use of Tadalafil with any of the following: Alprostadil; Amyl Nitrite; Conivaptan; Dapoxetine; Fusidic Acid (Systemic); Idelalisib; Molsidomine; Phosphodiesterase 5 Inhibitors; Riociguat; Tipranavir; Vasodilators (Organic Nitrates)

Increased Effect/Toxicity
Tadalafil may increase the levels/effects of: Alpha1-Blockers; Alprostadil; Amyl Nitrite; Blood Pressure Lowering Agents; Bosentan; Phosphodiesterase 5 Inhibitors; Riociguat; Vasodilators (Organic Nitrates)

The levels/effects of Tadalafil may be increased by: Alcohol (Ethyl); Aprepitant; Boceprevir; Cobicistat; Conivaptan; CYP3A4 Inhibitors (Moderate); CYP3A4 Inhibitors (Strong); Dapoxetine; Dasatinib; Fluconazole; Fosaprepitant; Fusidic Acid (Systemic); Idelalisib; Itraconazole; Ivacaftor; Ketoconazole (Systemic); Lorcaserin; Luliconazole; Mifepristone; Molsidomine; Netupitant; Osimertinib; Palbociclib; Posaconazole; Ritonavir; Sapropterin; Simeprevir; Stiripentol; Telaprevir; Tipranavir; Voriconazole

Decreased Effect
The levels/effects of Tadalafil may be decreased by: Bosentan; CYP3A4 Inducers (Strong); Etravirine; Osimertinib

Food Interactions Rate and extent of absorption are not affected by food. Grapefruit juice may increase serum levels/toxicity of tadalafil. Management: Use of grapefruit juice should be limited or avoided.

Storage/Stability Store at 25°C (77°F); excursions permitted to 15°C to 30°C (59°F to 86°F).

Mechanism of Action
BPH: Exact mechanism unknown; effects likely due to PDE-5 mediated reduction in smooth muscle and endothelial cell proliferation, decreased nerve activity, and increased smooth muscle relaxation and tissue perfusion of the prostate and bladder
Erectile dysfunction: Does not directly cause penile erections, but affects the response to sexual stimulation. The physiologic mechanism of erection of the penis involves release of nitric oxide (NO) in the corpus cavernosum during sexual stimulation. NO then activates the enzyme guanylate cyclase, which results in increased levels of cyclic guanosine monophosphate (cGMP), producing smooth muscle relaxation and inflow of blood to the corpus cavernosum. Tadalafil enhances the effect of NO by inhibiting phosphodiesterase type 5 (PDE-5), which is responsible for degradation of cGMP in the corpus cavernosum; when sexual stimulation causes local release of NO, inhibition of PDE-5 by tadalafil causes increased levels of cGMP in the corpus cavernosum, resulting in smooth muscle relaxation and inflow of blood to the corpus cavernosum. At recommended doses, it has no effect in the absence of sexual stimulation.
PAH: Inhibits phosphodiesterase type 5 (PDE-5) in smooth muscle of pulmonary vasculature where PDE-5 is responsible for the degradation of cyclic guanosine monophosphate (cGMP). Increased cGMP concentration results in pulmonary vasculature relaxation; vasodilation in the pulmonary bed and the systemic circulation (to a lesser degree) may occur.

Pharmacodynamics/Kinetics
Onset of action: Within 1 hour
Peak effect (pulmonary artery vasodilation): 75 to 90 minutes (Ghofrani 2004)
Duration: Erectile dysfunction: Up to 36 hours
Distribution: V_d: 63 to 77 L
Protein binding: 94%
Metabolism: Hepatic, via CYP3A4 to metabolites (inactive)
Half-life elimination: 15 to 17.5 hours; Pulmonary hypertension (not receiving bosentan): 35 hours
Time to peak, plasma: ~2 hours (range: 30 minutes to 6 hours)
Excretion: Feces (~61%, predominantly as metabolites); urine (~36%, predominantly as metabolites)

Dosing

Adult

Benign prostatic hyperplasia (with or without concomitant erectile dysfunction) (Cialis): Oral: 5 mg once daily. **Note:** When tadalafil is used with finasteride to initiate BPH therapy, the recommended duration of therapy is ≤26 weeks.
Dosing adjustment with concomitant medications:
Alpha₁-blockers: Not recommended for use in combination with alpha-blockers for the treatment of BPH.
CYP3A4 inhibitors (strong):
US labeling: 2.5 mg once daily; maximum: 2.5 mg once daily
Canadian labeling: No initial dosage adjustment necessary; may decrease dose to 2.5 mg once daily based on tolerability.

Erectile dysfunction (Cialis):
As-needed dosing: 10 mg (U.S. labeling) or 20 mg (Canadian labeling) at least 30 minutes prior to anticipated sexual activity as one single dose and not more than once daily. Dose may be adjusted based on tolerability (dosing range: 5 to 20 mg [US labeling] or 10 to 20 mg [Canadian labeling]). **Note:** Erectile function may be improved for up to 36 hours following a single dose.
Once-daily dosing: 2.5 mg once daily (U.S. labeling) or 5 mg once daily (Canadian labeling) at approximately the same time daily without regard to timing of sexual activity. Dose may be adjusted based on tolerability (dosage range: 2.5 to 5 mg/day).
Dosing adjustment with concomitant medications:
Oral:
U.S. labeling: Alpha₁-blockers: Patients should be stable on alpha-blocker therapy prior to initiating tadalafil treatment, and tadalafil should be initiated at the lowest recommended dose.
Canadian labeling: Nonselective alpha-blockers (eg, doxazosin): As-needed dosing: 10 mg at least 30 minutes prior to anticipated sexual activity
CYP3A4 inhibitors (strong):
As-needed dosing:
U.S. labeling: Maximum: 10 mg, not more frequently than every 72 hours
Canadian labeling: 10 mg, not more frequently than every 48 hours (maximum: 3 doses/week); may increase to 20 mg if lower dose is tolerated but ineffective. Discontinue use if 10 mg dose is not tolerated.
Once-daily dosing:
U.S. labeling: Maximum: 2.5 mg once daily
Canadian labeling: 2.5 to 5 mg once daily

Pulmonary arterial hypertension (Adcirca): Oral: 40 mg once daily
Dosing adjustment with concomitant medications:
Concurrent use with ritonavir:
Initiation of tadalafil in patients currently receiving ritonavir for at least 1 week: Initiate tadalafil at 20 mg once daily; increase to 40 mg once daily based on individual tolerability.

Initiation of ritonavir in patients currently receiving tadalafil: Discontinue tadalafil at least 24 hours prior to the initiation of ritonavir. After at least 1 week of ritonavir, resume tadalafil at 20 mg once daily; increase to 40 mg once daily based on individual tolerability.

Geriatric Refer to adult dosing. No dose adjustment for patients >65 years of age in the absence of renal or hepatic impairment.

Renal Impairment

Benign prostatic hyperplasia (with or without concomitant erectile dysfunction) (Cialis):
CrCl ≥51 mL/minute: No dosage adjustment necessary.
CrCl 30 to 50 mL/minute: Initial: 2.5 mg once daily; maximum: 5 mg once daily.
CrCl <30 mL/minute: Use not recommended.
ESRD requiring hemodialysis: Use not recommended.

Erectile dysfunction (Cialis):
As-needed use:
U.S. labeling:
CrCl ≥51 mL/minute: No dosage adjustment necessary.
CrCl 30 to 50 mL/minute: Initial: 5 mg once daily; maximum: 10 mg (not more frequently than every 48 hours).
CrCl <30 mL/minute: Maximum: 5 mg (not more frequently than every 72 hours).
ESRD requiring hemodialysis: Maximum: 5 mg (not more frequently than every 72 hours).
Canadian labeling:
CrCl >80 mL/minute: No dosage adjustment necessary.
CrCl ≥31 to 80 mL/minute: 10 mg, not more frequently than every 48 hours (maximum: 3 doses/week); may increase to 20 mg if lower dose is tolerated but ineffective. Discontinue use if 10 mg dose is not tolerated.
CrCl <30 mL/minute: There are no dosage adjustments provided in the manufacturer's labeling. Use with caution; has not been adequately studied.
ESRD requiring hemodialysis: There are no dosage adjustments provided in the manufacturer's labeling. Use with caution; has not been adequately studied.
Once-daily use:
CrCl ≥31 mL/minute: No dosage adjustment necessary.
CrCl <30 mL/minute: Use not recommended.
ESRD requiring hemodialysis: Use not recommended.

Pulmonary arterial hypertension (Adcirca):
CrCl 31 to 80 mL/minute: Initial: 20 mg once daily; increase to 40 mg once daily based on individual tolerability.
CrCl ≤30 mL/minute: Avoid use due to increased tadalafil exposure, limited clinical experience, and lack of ability to influence clearance by dialysis.
ESRD requiring hemodialysis: Avoid use due to increased tadalafil exposure, limited clinical experience, and lack of ability to influence clearance by dialysis.

Hepatic Impairment

Benign prostatic hyperplasia (with or without concomitant erectile dysfunction) (Cialis):
Mild to moderate hepatic impairment (Child-Pugh class A or B): Use with caution; the use of tadalafil for once-daily use has not been extensively evaluated in patients with hepatic impairment.
Severe hepatic impairment (Child-Pugh class C): Use is not recommended.

Erectile dysfunction (Cialis):
As-needed use:
U.S. labeling:
Mild to moderate impairment (Child-Pugh class A or B): Use with caution; dose should not exceed 10 mg once daily. The use of tadalafil once per day has not been evaluated extensively in patients with hepatic impairment.
Severe impairment (Child-Pugh class C): Use is not recommended.
Canadian labeling:
Mild to moderate impairment (Child-Pugh class A or B): 10 mg, not more frequently than every 48 hours (maximum: 3 doses/week); may increase to 20 mg if lower dose is tolerated but ineffective. Discontinue use if 10 mg dose is not tolerated.
Severe impairment (Child-Pugh class C): There are no dosage adjustments provided in the manufacturer's labeling. Use with caution; has not been adequately studied.

Once-daily use:
U.S. labeling:
Mild to moderate impairment (Child-Pugh class A or B): Use with caution; the use of tadalafil for once-daily use has not been extensively evaluated in patients with hepatic impairment.
Severe impairment (Child-Pugh class C): Use is not recommended.
Canadian labeling:
Mild to moderate impairment (Child-Pugh class A or B): No dosage adjustment necessary.
Severe impairment (Child-Pugh class C): Use is not recommended.

Pulmonary arterial hypertension (Adcirca):
Mild to moderate hepatic impairment (Child-Pugh class A or B): Use with caution; consider initial dose of 20 mg once daily.
Severe hepatic impairment (Child-Pugh class C): Avoid use; has not been studied in patients with severe hepatic cirrhosis.

Administration May be administered with or without food.
Adcirca: Administer daily dose all at once; dividing doses throughout the day is not advised.
Cialis: When used on an as-needed basis, should be taken at least 30 minutes prior to sexual activity. When used on a once-daily basis, should be taken at the same time each day, without regard to timing of sexual activity.

Monitoring Parameters Blood pressure, response and adverse effects; urine flow, PSA

Dosage Forms Excipient information presented when available (limited, particularly for generics); consult specific product labeling.
Tablet, Oral:
Adcirca: 20 mg
Cialis: 2.5 mg, 5 mg, 10 mg, 20 mg

Extemporaneous Preparations A 5 mg/mL tadalafil oral suspension may be made with tablets in a 1:1 mixture of Ora-Plus® and Ora-Sweet®. Crush fifteen 20 mg tadalafil tablets in a glass mortar and reduce to a fine powder. Prepare the vehicle by mixing 30 mL of Ora-Plus® and 30 mL of Ora-Sweet®; stir vigorously. Add 30 mL of the vehicle in geometric proportions to the powder and mix to form a smooth suspension. Transfer the mixture to a 2 ounce amber plastic prescription bottle. Rinse mortar with a quantity of the vehicle sufficient to make a final volume of 60 mL. Label "shake well." Stable for 91 days when stored in amber plastic prescription bottles at room temperature.
Pettit RS, Johnson CE, and Caruthers RL, "Stability of an Extemporaneously Prepared Tadalafil Suspension," *Am J Health Syst Pharm*, 2012, 69(7):592-4.

Talc (Sterile) (talk STARE il)

Brand Names: US Sclerosol Intrapleural; Sterile Talc Powder

Index Terms Intrapleural Talc; Sterile Talc; Talc; Talc for Pleurodesis

Pharmacologic Category Sclerosing Agent

Use Pleural effusion, malignant: Sclerosing agent to decrease or prevent the recurrence of malignant pleural effusion in symptomatic patients (following maximal drainage of pleural effusion)

Dosing

Adult Pleural effusion, malignant:
Intrapleural aerosol: 4 to 8 g (1 to 2 cans) as a single dose
Intrapleural suspension: 5 g

Renal Impairment There are no dosage adjustments provided in the manufacturer's labeling.

Hepatic Impairment There are no dosage adjustments provided in the manufacturer's labeling.

Additional Information Complete prescribing information should be consulted for additional detail.

Dosage Forms Excipient information presented when available (limited, particularly for generics); consult specific product labeling.
Aerosol Powder, Intrapleural:
Sclerosol Intrapleural: 4 g (30 g) [contains dichlorodifluoromethane]
Suspension Reconstituted, Intrapleural:
Sterile Talc Powder: 5 g (1 ea)

Taliglucerase Alfa (tal i GLOO ser ase AL fa)

Brand Names: US Elelyso
Brand Names: Canada Elelyso
Pharmacologic Category Enzyme
Use
Gaucher disease: Treatment of adult and pediatric patients with a confirmed diagnosis of type 1 Gaucher disease.
Canadian labeling: Additional use (not in US labeling): Treatment of hematologic manifestations in pediatric patients 2 to 17 years of age with a confirmed diagnosis of type 3 Gaucher disease (limited data)
Prescribing and Access Restrictions Product access is restricted to the Gaucher Personal Support (GPS) program. Healthcare providers and patients may obtain additional information by contacting the GPS program at 855-353-5976.
Dosing
Adult & Geriatric Note: Pretreatment with antihistamines and/or corticosteroids can be considered for prevention of subsequent infusion reactions in patients with an infusion reaction requiring symptomatic treatment; during clinical studies, patients were not routinely premedicated prior to infusion.

US labeling:
Gaucher disease (type 1): IV: 60 units/kg every 2 weeks; dosing is individualized based on disease severity.
Conversion from imiglucerase: Initiate taliglucerase alfa using the patient's same previous imiglucerase dose and administer every 2 weeks. **Note:** Conversion to taliglucerase alfa is based on a single study of patients stabilized on a biweekly imiglucerase dose for ≥6 months.
Canadian labeling: **Gaucher disease (type 1):** IV: 30 to 60 units/kg every 2 weeks; dosing is individualized based on disease severity (better clinical response has been observed with 60 unit/kg dose).

Pediatric Note: Pretreatment with antihistamines, antipyretics, and/or corticosteroids can be considered for prevention of subsequent infusion reactions in patients with an infusion reaction requiring symptomatic treatment; during clinical studies, patients were not routinely premedicated prior to infusion.

US labeling: **Gaucher disease (type 1):** Children ≥4 years and Adolescents: Refer to adult dosing.
Canadian labeling:
Gaucher disease (type 1): Children ≥2 years and Adolescents: Refer to adult dosing.
Gaucher disease (type 3): Children ≥2 years and Adolescents: IV: 30 to 60 units/kg every 2 weeks; dosing is individualized based on disease severity (data are extremely limited; in a small clinical trial of pediatric patients [N=11], 2 were identified as having type 3 Gaucher disease [Zimran 2015]).
Renal Impairment There are no dosage adjustments provided in the manufacturer's labeling.
Hepatic Impairment There are no dosage adjustments provided in the manufacturer's labeling.
Additional Information Complete prescribing information should be consulted for additional detail.
Dosage Forms Excipient information presented when available (limited, particularly for generics); consult specific product labeling.
Solution Reconstituted, Intravenous [preservative free]:
Elelyso: 200 units (1 ea) [contains polysorbate 80]

◆ Talwin *see* Pentazocine *on page 1425*
◆ Tambocor *see* Flecainide *on page 772*
◆ Tambocor [DSC] *see* Flecainide *on page 772*
◆ Tamiflu *see* Oseltamivir *on page 1342*

Tamoxifen (ta MOKS i fen)

Brand Names: US Soltamox
Brand Names: Canada Apo-Tamox; Mylan-Tamoxifen; Nolvadex-D; PMS-Tamoxifen; Teva-Tamoxifen
Index Terms ICI-46474; Nolvadex; Tamoxifen Citras; Tamoxifen Citrate

Pharmacologic Category Antineoplastic Agent, Estrogen Receptor Antagonist; Selective Estrogen Receptor Modulator (SERM)
Use Treatment of metastatic (female and male) breast cancer; adjuvant treatment of breast cancer after primary treatment with surgery and radiation; reduce risk of invasive breast cancer in women with ductal carcinoma *in situ* (DCIS) after surgery and radiation; reduce the incidence of breast cancer in women at high risk
Pregnancy Considerations Animal reproduction studies have demonstrated fetal adverse effects and fetal loss. There have been reports of vaginal bleeding, birth defects and fetal loss in pregnant women. Tamoxifen use during pregnancy may have a potential long term risk to the fetus of a DES-like syndrome. For sexually-active women of childbearing age, initiate during menstruation (negative β-hCG immediately prior to initiation in women with irregular cycles). Tamoxifen may induce ovulation. Barrier or non-hormonal contraceptives are recommended. Pregnancy should be avoided during treatment and for 2 months after treatment has been discontinued.
Breast-Feeding Considerations It is not known if tamoxifen is excreted in breast milk, however, it has been shown to inhibit lactation. Due to the potential for adverse reactions, women taking tamoxifen should not breast-feed.
Medication Guide Available Yes
Contraindications Hypersensitivity to tamoxifen or any component of the formulation; concurrent warfarin therapy or history of deep vein thrombosis or pulmonary embolism (when tamoxifen is used for breast cancer risk reduction in women at high risk for breast cancer or with ductal carcinoma *in situ* [DCIS])
Warnings/Precautions Hazardous agent - use appropriate precautions for handling and disposal (NIOSH 2014 [group 1]). **[U.S. Boxed Warning]: Serious and life-threatening events (some fatal), including stroke, pulmonary emboli, and uterine or endometrial malignancies, have occurred at an incidence greater than placebo during use for breast cancer risk reduction in women at high-risk for breast cancer and in women with ductal carcinoma *in situ* (DCIS). In women already diagnosed with breast cancer, the benefits of tamoxifen treatment outweigh risks; evaluate risks versus benefits (and discuss with patients) when used for breast cancer risk reduction.** An increased incidence of thromboembolic events, including DVT and pulmonary embolism, has been associated with use for breast cancer; risk is increased with concomitant chemotherapy; use with caution in individuals with a history of thromboembolic events. Thrombocytopenia and/or leukopenia may occur; neutropenia and pancytopenia have been reported rarely. Although the relationship to tamoxifen therapy is uncertain, rare hemorrhagic episodes have occurred in patients with significant thrombocytopenia. Use with caution in patients with hyperlipidemias; infrequent postmarketing cases of hyperlipidemias have been reported. Decreased visual acuity, retinal vein thrombosis, retinopathy, corneal changes, color perception changes, and increased incidence of cataracts (and the need for cataract surgery), have been reported. Hypercalcemia has occurred in some patients with bone metastasis, usually within a few weeks of therapy initiation; institute appropriate hypercalcemia management; discontinue if severe. Local disease flare and increased bone and tumor pain may occur in patients with metastatic breast cancer; may be associated with (good) tumor response.

Potentially significant drug-drug interactions may exist, requiring dose or frequency adjustment, additional monitoring, and/or selection of alternative therapy. Decreased efficacy and an increased risk of breast cancer recurrence has been reported with concurrent moderate or strong CYP2D6 inhibitors (Aubert, 2009; Dezentje, 2009). Concomitant use with select SSRIs may result in decreased tamoxifen efficacy. Strong CYP2D6 inhibitors (eg, fluoxetine, paroxetine) and moderate CYP2D6 inhibitors (eg, sertraline) are reported to interfere with transformation to the active metabolite endoxifen; when possible, select alternative medications with minimal or no impact on endoxifen levels (NCCN Breast Cancer Risk Reduction Guidelines v.1.2013; Sideras, 2010). Weak CYP2D6 inhibitors (eg, venlafaxine, citalopram) have minimal effect on the conversion to endoxifen (Jin, 2005; NCCN Breast Cancer Risk Reduction Guidelines v.1.2013); escitalopram is also a weak CYP2D6 inhibitor. In a retrospective analysis of breast cancer patients taking tamoxifen and SSRIs, concomitant use of paroxetine and tamoxifen was associated with an increased risk of death due to breast cancer (Kelly, 2010). Lower plasma concentrations of endoxifen have been observed in patients associated with reduced CYP2D6 activity (Jin, 2005; Schroth, 2009) and may be associated with reduced efficacy, although data is

conflicting. Routine CYP2D6 testing is not recommended at this time in order to determine optimal endocrine therapy (NCCN Breast Cancer Guidelines v.2.2013; Visvanathan, 2009).

Tamoxifen use may be associated with changes in bone mineral density (BMD) and the effects may be dependent upon menstrual status. In postmenopausal women, tamoxifen use is associated with a protective effect on bone mineral density (BMD), preventing loss of BMD which lasts over the 5-year treatment period. In premenopausal women, a decline (from baseline) in BMD mineral density has been observed in women who continued to menstruate; may be associated with an increased risk of fractures. Liver abnormalities such as cholestasis, fatty liver, hepatitis, and hepatic necrosis have occurred. Hepatocellular carcinomas have been reported in some studies; relationship to treatment is unclear. Tamoxifen is associated with an increased incidence of uterine or endometrial cancers. Endometrial hyperplasia, polyps, endometriosis, uterine fibroids, and ovarian cysts have occurred. Monitor and promptly evaluate any report of abnormal vaginal bleeding. Amenorrhea and menstrual irregularities have been reported with tamoxifen use.

Adverse Reactions

>10%:
Cardiovascular: Vasodilation (41%), flushing (33%), hypertension (11%), peripheral edema (11%)
Central nervous system: Mood changes (12% to 18%), pain (3% to 16%), depression (2% to 12%)
Dermatologic: Skin changes (6% to 19%), rash (13%)
Endocrine & metabolic: Hot flashes (3% to 80%), fluid retention (32%), altered menses (13% to 25%), amenorrhea (16%)
Gastrointestinal: Nausea (5% to 26%), weight loss (23%), vomiting (12%)
Genitourinary: Vaginal discharge (13% to 55%), vaginal bleeding (2% to 23%)
Neuromuscular & skeletal: Weakness (18%), arthritis (14%), arthralgia (11%)
Respiratory: Pharyngitis (14%)
Miscellaneous: Lymphedema (11%)
1% to 10%:
Cardiovascular: Chest pain (5%), venous thrombotic events (5%), edema (4%), cardiovascular ischemia (3%), angina (2%), deep venous thrombus (≤2%), MI (1%)
Central nervous system: Insomnia (9%), dizziness (8%), headache (8%), anxiety (6%), fatigue (4%)
Dermatologic: Alopecia (≤5%)
Endocrine & metabolic: Oligomenorrhea (9%), breast pain (6%), menstrual disorder (6%), breast neoplasm (5%), hypercholesterolemia (4%)
Gastrointestinal: Abdominal pain (9%), weight gain (9%), constipation (4% to 8%), diarrhea (7%), dyspepsia (6%), throat irritation (oral solution 5%), abdominal cramps (1%), anorexia (1%)
Genitourinary: Urinary tract infection (10%), leukorrhea (9%), vaginal hemorrhage (6%), vaginitis (5%), vulvovaginitis (5%), ovarian cyst (3%)
Hematologic: Thrombocytopenia (≤10%), anemia (5%)
Hepatic: AST increased (5%), serum bilirubin increased (2%)
Neuromuscular & skeletal: Back pain (10%), bone pain (6% to 10%), osteoporosis (7%), fracture (7%), arthrosis (5%), joint disorder (5%), myalgia (5%), paresthesia (5%), musculoskeletal pain (3%)
Ocular: Cataract (7%)
Renal: Serum creatinine increased (≤2%)
Respiratory: Cough (4% to 9%), dyspnea (8%), bronchitis (5%), sinusitis (5%)
Miscellaneous: Infection/sepsis (≤9%), diaphoresis (6%), flu-like syndrome (6%), cyst (5%), neoplasm (5%), allergic reaction (3%)
<1 or frequency not defined (limited to important or life-threatening): Angioedema, bullous pemphigoid, cholestasis, corneal changes, endometrial cancer, endometrial hyperplasia, endometrial polyps, endometriosis, erythema multiforme, fatty liver, hepatic necrosis, hepatitis, hypercalcemia, hyperlipidemia, hypersensitivity reactions, hypertriglyceridemia, impotence (males), interstitial pneumonitis, loss of libido (males), pancreatitis, phlebitis, pruritus vulvae, pulmonary embolism, retinal vein thrombosis, retinopathy, second primary tumors, Stevens-Johnson syndrome, stroke; tumor pain and local disease flare (including increase in lesion size and erythema) during treatment of metastatic breast cancer (generally resolves with continuation); uterine fibroids, vaginal dryness, visual color perception changes

Drug Interactions

Metabolism/Transport Effects Substrate of CYP2A6 (minor), CYP2B6 (minor), CYP2C9 (major), CYP2D6 (major), CYP2E1 (minor), CYP3A4 (major); **Note:** Assignment of Major/Minor substrate status based on clinically relevant drug interaction potential; **Inhibits** CYP2B6 (weak), CYP2C8 (moderate), CYP2C9 (weak), P-glycoprotein

Avoid Concomitant Use
Avoid concomitant use of Tamoxifen with any of the following: Amodiaquine; Bosutinib; Conivaptan; CYP2D6 Inhibitors (Strong); Fusidic Acid (Systemic); Idelalisib; Ospemifene; PAZOPanib; Silodosin; Topotecan; VinCRIStine (Liposomal); Vitamin K Antagonists

Increased Effect/Toxicity
Tamoxifen may increase the levels/effects of: Afatinib; Amodiaquine; Bosutinib; Brentuximab Vedotin; Colchicine; CYP2C8 Substrates; Dabigatran Etexilate; DOXOrubicin (Conventional); Edoxaban; Everolimus; Highest Risk QTc-Prolonging Agents; Ledipasvir; Mipomersen; Moderate Risk QTc-Prolonging Agents; Naloxegol; Ospemifene; PAZOPanib; P-glycoprotein/ABCB1 Substrates; Prucalopride; Ranolazine; Rifaximin; Silodosin; Topotecan; VinCRIStine (Liposomal); Vitamin K Antagonists

The levels/effects of Tamoxifen may be increased by: Abiraterone Acetate; Conivaptan; CYP2C9 Inhibitors (Moderate); CYP2C9 Inhibitors (Strong); CYP3A4 Inhibitors (Moderate); CYP3A4 Inhibitors (Strong); Dasatinib; Fosaprepitant; Fusidic Acid (Systemic); Idelalisib; Ivacaftor; Luliconazole; Mifepristone; Netupitant; Osimertinib; Palbociclib; Panobinostat; Peginterferon Alfa-2b; Simeprevir

Decreased Effect
Tamoxifen may decrease the levels/effects of: Anastrozole; Letrozole; Ospemifene

The levels/effects of Tamoxifen may be decreased by: Bexarotene (Systemic); Bosentan; CYP2C9 Inducers (Strong); CYP2D6 Inhibitors (Moderate); CYP2D6 Inhibitors (Strong); CYP3A4 Inducers (Moderate); CYP3A4 Inducers (Strong); Dabrafenib; Deferasirox; Enzalutamide; Mitotane; Osimertinib; Peginterferon Alfa-2b; Rifamycin Derivatives; Siltuximab; St Johns Wort; Tocilizumab

Food Interactions Grapefruit juice may decrease the metabolism of tamoxifen. Management: Avoid grapefruit juice.

Storage/Stability
Oral solution: Store at ≤25°C (77°F); do not freeze or refrigerate. Protect from light. Discard opened bottle after 3 months.
Tablets: Store at 20°C to 25°C (68°F to 77°F). Protect from light.

Mechanism of Action Competitively binds to estrogen receptors on tumors and other tissue targets, producing a nuclear complex that decreases DNA synthesis and inhibits estrogen effects; nonsteroidal agent with potent antiestrogenic properties which compete with estrogen for binding sites in breast and other tissues; cells accumulate in the G_0 and G_1 phases; therefore, tamoxifen is cytostatic rather than cytocidal.

Pharmacodynamics/Kinetics
Absorption: Well absorbed
Distribution: High concentrations found in uterus, endometrial and breast tissue
Protein binding: 99%
Metabolism: Hepatic; via CYP2D6 to 4-hydroxytamoxifen and via CYP3A4/5 to N-desmethyl-tamoxifen. Each is then further metabolized into endoxifen (4-hydroxy-tamoxifen via CYP3A4/5 and N-desmethyl-tamoxifen via CYP2D6); both 4-hydroxy-tamoxifen and endoxifen are 30- to 100-fold more potent than tamoxifen
Half-life elimination: Tamoxifen: ~5-7 days; N-desmethyl tamoxifen: ~14 days
Time to peak, serum: ~5 hours
Excretion: Feces (26% to 51%); urine (9% to 13%)

Dosing
Adult & Geriatric Note: For the treatment of breast cancer, patients receiving both tamoxifen and chemotherapy should receive treatment sequentially, with tamoxifen following completion of chemotherapy.
Breast cancer treatment: Oral:
Adjuvant therapy (females): 20 mg once daily for 5 years
Premenopausal women: Duration of treatment is 5 years (Burstein, 2010; NCCN Breast Cancer guidelines v.2.2013)

Postmenopausal women: Duration of tamoxifen treatment is 2-3 years followed by an aromatase inhibitor (AI) to complete 5 years; may take tamoxifen for the full 5 years (if contraindications or intolerance to AI) or extended therapy: 4.5-6 years of tamoxifen followed by 5 years of an AI (Burstein, 2010; NCCN Breast Cancer guidelines v.2.2013)

ER-positive early breast cancer: Extended duration: Duration of treatment of 10 years demonstrated a reduced risk of recurrence and mortality (Davies, 2012)

Metastatic (males and females): 20-40 mg daily (doses >20 mg should be given in 2 divided doses). **Note:** Although the FDA-approved labeling recommends dosing up to 40 mg daily, clinical benefit has not been demonstrated with doses above 20 mg daily (Bratherton, 1984).

Ductal carcinoma in situ (DCIS) (females), to reduce the risk for invasive breast cancer: 20 mg once daily for 5 years

Breast cancer risk reduction (pre- and postmenopausal high-risk females): Oral: 20 mg once daily for 5 years

Endometrial carcinoma, recurrent, metastatic, or high-risk (endometrioid histologies only) (off-label use): Oral:

Monotherapy: 20 mg twice daily until disease progression or unacceptable toxicity (Thigpen, 2001)

Combination therapy: 20 mg twice daily for 3 weeks (alternating with megestrol acetate every 3 weeks); continue alternating until disease progression or unacceptable toxicity) (Fiorica, 2004)

Induction of ovulation (off-label use): Oral: 20 mg once daily (range: 20-80 mg once daily) for 5 days (Steiner, 2005)

Ovarian cancer, advanced and/or recurrent (off-label use): Oral: 20 mg twice daily (Hatch, 1991; Markman, 1996)

Paget's disease of the breast (risk reduction; with DCIS or without associated cancer): Oral: 20 mg once daily for 5 years (NCCN Breast Cancer Guidelines, v.2.2013)

Dosage adjustment for DVT, pulmonary embolism, cerebrovascular accident, or prolonged immobilization: Discontinue tamoxifen (NCCN Breast Cancer Risk Reduction Guidelines, v.1.2013)

Pediatric Females: Precocious puberty secondary to McCune-Albright syndrome (off-label use): Oral: A dose of 20 mg daily has been reported in patients 2-10 years of age; safety and efficacy have not been established for treatment of longer than 1 year duration (Eugster, 2003)

Renal Impairment No dosage adjustment provided in manufacturer's labeling.

Chronic dialysis: No dosage adjustment necessary (Janus, 2013).

Hepatic Impairment No dosage adjustment provided in manufacturer's labeling (has not been studied).

Dietary Considerations Tablets and oral solution may be taken with or without food. Avoid grapefruit and grapefruit juice.

Administration Administer tablets or oral solution orally with or without food. Use supplied dosing cup for oral solution.

Hazardous agent; use appropriate precautions for handling and disposal (NIOSH 2014 [group 1]).

Monitoring Parameters CBC with platelets, serum calcium, LFTs; triglycerides and cholesterol (in patients with preexisting hyperlipidemias); INR and PT (in patients on vitamin K antagonists); abnormal vaginal bleeding; breast and gynecologic exams (baseline and routine), mammogram (baseline and routine); signs/symptoms of DVT (leg swelling, tenderness) or PE (shortness of breath); ophthalmic exam (if vision problem or cataracts); bone mineral density (premenopausal women)

Test Interactions T_4 elevations (which may be explained by increases in thyroid-binding globulin) have been reported; not accompanied by clinical hyperthyroidism

Additional Information Estrogen receptor status may predict if adjuvant treatment with tamoxifen is of benefit. In metastatic breast cancer, patients with estrogen receptor positive tumors are more likely to benefit from tamoxifen treatment. With tamoxifen use to reduce the incidence of breast cancer in high risk-women, high risk is defined as women ≥35 years of age with a 5 year NCI Gail model predicted risk of breast cancer ≥1.67%.

Oncology Comment: The American Society of Clinical Oncology (ASCO) guidelines for adjuvant endocrine therapy in postmenopausal women with HR-positive breast cancer (Burstein, 2010) recommend considering aromatase inhibitor (AI) therapy at some point in the treatment

course (primary, sequentially, or extended). Optimal duration at this time is not known; however, treatment with an AI should not exceed 5 years in primary and extended therapies, and 2-3 years if followed by tamoxifen in sequential therapy (total of 5 years). If initial therapy with AI has been discontinued before the 5 years, consideration should be taken to receive tamoxifen for a total of 5 years. The optimal time to switch to an AI is also not known; but data supports switching after 2-3 years of tamoxifen (sequential) or after 5 years of tamoxifen (extended). If patient becomes intolerant or has poor adherence, consideration should be made to switch to another AI or initiate tamoxifen.

Recent data suggest that continuing tamoxifen for 10 years (rather than stopping after 5 years of therapy) may provide a further reduction in breast cancer recurrence and mortality in women with early stage disease (Davies, 2012). The Adjuvant Tamoxifen: Longer Against Shorter (ATLAS) trial randomized 6846 patients with estrogen receptor positive disease to continue tamoxifen for a total of 10 years of treatment or to stop after 5 years. Breast cancer recurrence was observed in 617 patients in the 10-year arm versus 711 recurrences in the 5-year arm (p=0.002). Breast cancer mortality was significantly reduced with 10 years of tamoxifen therapy versus 5 years (331 deaths vs 397 deaths, respectively; p=0.01) (Davies, 2012).

The adjuvant endocrine therapy of choice is tamoxifen for men with breast cancer and for pre- or perimenopausal women at diagnosis. CYP2D6 genotyping is not recommended, however, due to the potential for drug-drug interactions use caution and consider avoiding concomitant therapy with tamoxifen and known CYP2D6 inhibitors.

Dosage Forms Excipient information presented when available (limited, particularly for generics); consult specific product labeling.

Solution, Oral:

Soltamox: 10 mg/5 mL (150 mL) [sugar free; contains alcohol, usp, propylene glycol; licorice-aniseed flavor]

Tablet, Oral:

Generic: 10 mg, 20 mg

Extemporaneous Preparations Hazardous agent: Use appropriate precautions for handling and disposal (NIOSH 2014 [group 1]).

A 0.5 mg/mL oral suspension may be prepared with tablets. Place two 10 mg tablets into 40 mL purified water and let stand ~2-5 minutes. Stir until tablets are completely disintegrated (dispersion time for each 10 mg tablet is ~2-5 minutes). Administer immediately after preparation. To ensure the full dose is administered, rinse glass several times with water and administer residue.

Lam MS, "Extemporaneous Compounding of Oral Liquid Dosage Formulations and Alternative Drug Delivery Methods for Anticancer Drugs," *Pharmacotherapy*, 2011, 31(2):164-92.

◆ Tamoxifen Citras see Tamoxifen on page 1733

◆ Tamoxifen Citrate see Tamoxifen on page 1733

Tamsulosin (tam SOO loe sin)

Brand Names: US Flomax

Brand Names: Canada Apo-Tamsulosin CR; Flomax CR; Mylan-Tamsulosin; ratio-Tamsulosin; Sandoz-Tamsulosin; Tamsulosin CR; Teva-Tamsulosin; Teva-Tamsulosin CR

Index Terms Tamsulosin Hydrochloride

Pharmacologic Category Alpha₁ Blocker

Use

Benign prostatic hyperplasia: Treatment of signs and symptoms of benign prostatic hyperplasia (BPH)

Limitations of use: Not indicated for the treatment of hypertension.

Pregnancy Considerations Adverse events were not observed in animal reproduction studies. For pregnant women with kidney stones, other treatments such as stents or ureteroscopy, are recommended if stone removal is needed (Preminger, 2007; Tan, 2013).

Contraindications Hypersensitivity to tamsulosin or any component of the formulation

Warnings/Precautions Not intended for use as an antihypertensive drug. May cause significant orthostatic hypotension and syncope, especially with first dose; anticipate a similar effect if therapy is interrupted for a few days, if dosage is rapidly increased, or if another antihypertensive drug (particularly vasodilators) or a PDE-5 inhibitor (eg, sildenafil, tadalafil, vardenafil) is introduced. "First-dose" orthostatic hypotension may occur 4 to 8 hours after dosing; may be dose related. Patients should be cautioned about performing hazardous tasks, driving, or operating heavy machinery when starting new therapy or adjusting dosage upward. Discontinue if symptoms of angina occur or worsen. Rule out prostatic carcinoma with screening

before beginning therapy with tamsulosin and then screen at regular intervals.

Intraoperative floppy iris syndrome (IFIS) is characterized by a combination of flaccid iris that billows with intraoperative currents, progressive intraoperative miosis despite dilation, and potential iris prolapse. IFIS has been observed in cataract and glaucoma surgery patients who were on or were previously treated with alpha₁-blockers, particularly with tamsulosin use (Abdel-Aziz, 2009); in some cases, patients had discontinued the alpha₁-blocker 5 weeks to 9 months prior to the surgery. The benefit of discontinuing alpha-blocker therapy prior to cataract or glaucoma surgery has not been established. IFIS may increase the risk of ocular complications during and after surgery. May require modifications to surgical technique; instruct patients to inform ophthalmologist of current or previous alpha₁-blocker use when considering eye surgery. Initiation of tamsulosin therapy in patients with planned cataract or glaucoma surgery is not recommended. Priapism has been associated with use (rarely). Rarely, patients with a sulfa allergy have also developed an allergic reaction to tamsulosin; avoid use when previous reaction has been severe or life-threatening. Potentially significant drug-drug interactions may exist, requiring dose or frequency adjustment, additional monitoring, and/or selection of alternative therapy.

Adverse Reactions

>10%:

Cardiovascular: Orthostatic hypotension (first dose: 6% to 19%; symptomatic orthostatic hypotension (chronic therapy) <1%)

Central nervous system: Headache (19% to 21%), dizziness (15% to 17%)

Genitourinary: Ejaculation failure (8% to 18%)

Infection: Infection (9% to 11%)

Respiratory: Rhinitis (13% to 18%)

1% to 10%:

Central nervous system: Drowsiness (3% to 4%), insomnia (1% to 2%), vertigo (≤1%)

Endocrine & metabolic: Loss of libido (2%)

Gastrointestinal: Diarrhea (6%), nausea (4%)

Neuromuscular & skeletal: Weakness (8% to 9%), back pain (7% to 8%)

Ophthalmic: Blurred vision (≤2%)

Respiratory: Pharyngitis (6%), cough (3% to 5%), sinusitis (4%)

<1% (Limited to important or life-threatening): Epistaxis, exfoliative dermatitis, hypersensitivity reaction, hypotension, intraoperative floppy iris syndrome, palpitations, priapism, syncope

Drug Interactions

Metabolism/Transport Effects Substrate of CYP2D6 (minor), CYP3A4 (major); **Note:** Assignment of Major/Minor substrate status based on clinically relevant drug interaction potential

Avoid Concomitant Use

Avoid concomitant use of Tamsulosin with any of the following: Alpha1-Blockers; Conivaptan; CYP3A4 Inhibitors (Strong); Fusidic Acid (Systemic); Idelalisib

Increased Effect/Toxicity

Tamsulosin may increase the levels/effects of: Alpha1-Blockers; Amifostine; Antipsychotic Agents (Second Generation [Atypical]); Calcium Channel Blockers; DULoxetine; Hypotension-Associated Agents; Levodopa

The levels/effects of Tamsulosin may be increased by: Aprepitant; Barbiturates; Beta-Blockers; Blood Pressure Lowering Agents; Brimonidine (Topical); Cimetidine; Conivaptan; CYP2D6 Inhibitors (Strong); CYP3A4 Inhibitors (Moderate); CYP3A4 Inhibitors (Strong); Dapoxetine; Dasatinib; Diazoxide; Fosaprepitant; Fusidic Acid (Systemic); Herbs (Hypotensive Properties); Idelalisib; Ivacaftor; Luliconazole; Mifepristone; Molsidomine; Netupitant; Nicorandil; Obinutuzumab; Osimertinib; Palbociclib; Pentoxifylline; Phosphodiesterase 5 Inhibitors; Prostacyclin Analogues; Simeprevir; Stiripentol

Decreased Effect

Tamsulosin may decrease the levels/effects of: Alpha-/Beta-Agonists; Alpha1-Agonists

The levels/effects of Tamsulosin may be decreased by: Bosentan; CYP3A4 Inducers (Moderate); CYP3A4 Inducers (Strong); Dabrafenib; Deferasirox; Enzalutamide; Mitotane; Osimertinib; Siltuximab; St Johns Wort; Tocilizumab

Food Interactions Fasting increases bioavailability by 30% and peak concentration 40% to 70%. Management: Administer 30 minutes after the same meal each day.

Storage/Stability Store at 25°C (77°F); excursions are permitted between 15°C and 30°C (59°F and 86°F).

Mechanism of Action Tamsulosin is an antagonist of alpha₁A-adrenoreceptors in the prostate. Smooth muscle

tone in the prostate is mediated by alpha₁A-adrenoreceptors; blocking them leads to relaxation of smooth muscle in the bladder neck and prostate causing an improvement of urine flow and decreased symptoms of BPH. Approximately 75% of the alpha₁-receptors in the prostate are of the alpha₁A subtype.

Pharmacodynamics/Kinetics

Absorption: >90%

Distribution: V_d: 16 L

Protein binding: 94% to 99%, primarily to alpha₁ acid glycoprotein (AAG)

Metabolism: Hepatic (extensive) via CYP3A4 and 2D6; metabolites undergo extensive conjugation to glucuronide or sulfate

Bioavailability: Fasting: 30% increase

Steady-state: By the fifth day of once-daily dosing

Half-life elimination: Healthy volunteers: 9 to 13 hours; Target population: 14 to 15 hours

Time to peak: Fasting: 4 to 5 hours; With food: 6 to 7 hours

Excretion: Urine (76%, <10% as unchanged drug); feces (21%)

Dosing

Adult & Geriatric

Benign prostatic hyperplasia (BPH): Males: Oral: 0.4 mg once daily ~30 minutes after the same meal each day; dose may be increased after 2 to 4 weeks to 0.8 mg once daily in patients who fail to respond. If therapy is discontinued or interrupted for several days, restart with 0.4 mg once daily.

Bladder outlet obstruction symptoms (off-label use): Oral: 0.4 mg once daily (Rossi, 2001)

Ureteral calculi (distal) expulsion (off-label use): Oral: 0.4 mg once daily, discontinue after successful expulsion (average time to expulsion was 1 to 2 weeks) (Agrawal, 2009; Ahmed, 2010). **Note:** Patients with stones >10 mm were excluded from studies.

Renal Impairment

CrCl ≥10 mL/minute: No dosage adjustment necessary.

CrCl <10 mL/minute: There are no dosage adjustments provided in the manufacturer's labeling (has not been studied).

Hepatic Impairment

Mild-to-moderate impairment: No dosage adjustment is necessary.

Severe impairment: There are no dosage adjustments provided in the manufacturer's labeling (has not been studied).

Administration Administer 30 minutes after the same mealtime each day. Capsules should be swallowed whole; do not crush, chew, or open.

Monitoring Parameters Blood pressure; urinary symptoms

Dosage Forms Excipient information presented when available (limited, particularly for generics); consult specific product labeling.

Capsule, Oral, as hydrochloride:

Flomax: 0.4 mg [contains fd&c blue #2 (indigotine)]

Generic: 0.4 mg

Tapentadol (ta PEN ta dol)

Brand Names: US Nucynta; Nucynta ER

Brand Names: Canada Nucynta ER; Nucynta IR

Index Terms CG5503; Tapentadol Hydrochloride

Pharmacologic Category Analgesic, Opioid

Use Pain:

Immediate release formulations: Management of moderate-to-severe acute pain in adults

Extended release formulation:

U.S. labeling: Pain or neuropathic pain associated with diabetic peripheral neuropathy (DPN) severe enough to require daily, around-the-clock, long-term opioid analgesia and for which alternative treatments are inadequate.

Canadian labeling: Relief of moderate to moderately severe pain in patients who require continuous treatment for several days or more.

Limitations of use: Because of the risks of addiction, abuse, and misuse with opioids, even at recommended doses, and because of the greater risks of overdose and death with extended-release opioid formulations, reserve tapentadol ER for use in patients for whom alternative treatment options (eg, nonopioid analgesics, immediate-release opioids) are ineffective, not tolerated, or would be otherwise inadequate to provide sufficient management of pain. Tapentadol ER is not indicated as an as-needed analgesic.

Pregnancy Considerations Adverse events were observed in animal reproduction studies. Opioids cross the placenta. Tapentadol is not recommended for use during labor and delivery and if exposure occurs the neonate should be monitored for respiratory depression. Use in pregnant women is contraindicated in the Canadian labeling.

U.S. Boxed Warning]: Prolonged maternal use of opioids during pregnancy can cause neonatal withdrawal syndrome in the newborn which may be life-threatening if not recognized and treated according to protocols developed by neonatology experts. If prolonged opioid therapy is required in a pregnant woman, ensure treatment is available and warn patient of risk to the neonate. If chronic opioid exposure occurs in pregnancy, adverse events in the newborn (including withdrawal) may occur; monitoring of the neonate is recommended. The minimum effective dose should be used if opioids are needed (Chou, 2009). Neonatal abstinence syndrome following opioid exposure may present with autonomic (eg, fever, temperature instability), gastrointestinal (eg, diarrhea, vomiting, poor feeding/weight gain), or neurologic (eg, high-pitched crying, increased muscle tone, irritability, seizure, tremor) symptoms (Dow, 2012; Hudak, 2012).

Long-term opioid use may cause secondary hypogonadism, which may lead to sexual dysfunction or infertility (Brennan, 2013).

Breast-Feeding Considerations Limited information is available on the excretion of tapentadol in human milk; however, data suggests it may be excreted in human milk. The possibility of sedation or respiratory depression in the nursing infant should be considered; withdrawal may occur when maternal therapy is stopped. Due to the potential for serious adverse reactions in the nursing infant, the U.S. manufacturer recommends a decision be made whether to discontinue nursing or to discontinue the drug, taking into account the importance of treatment to the mother. Use while breast-feeding is contraindicated in the Canadian labeling.

Medication Guide Available Yes

Contraindications

Hypersensitivity to tapentadol or any component of the formulation; significant respiratory depression; acute or severe asthma or hypercapnia in unmonitored settings or in absence of resuscitative equipment or ventilatory support; known or suspected paralytic ileus; use with or within 14 days of MAO inhibitors

Canadian labeling: Additional contraindications (not in U.S. labeling): Hypersensitivity to opioids; acute respiratory depression; cor pulmonale; obstructive airway; gastrointestinal obstruction or any disease/condition that affects bowel transit (eg, ileus of any type, strictures); severe renal impairment (CrCl <30 mL/minute); severe hepatic impairment (Child-Pugh class C); mild, intermittent, or short-duration pain that can be managed with alternative pain medication; management of perioperative pain (extended-release tablets); acute alcoholism, delirium tremens, and seizure disorders; severe CNS depression, increased cerebrospinal or intracranial pressure or head injury; pregnancy; breast-feeding; use during labor/delivery

Warnings/Precautions Use with caution and monitor for respiratory depression in patients with significant chronic obstructive pulmonary disease or cor pulmonale, and patients having a substantially decreased respiratory reserve, hypoxia, hypercarbia, or preexisting respiratory depression, particularly when initiating therapy and titrating with tapentadol; even therapeutic doses may decrease respiratory drive to the point of apnea. Consider the use of alternative nonopioid analgesics in these patients. Use with caution in debilitated or cachectic patients; there is a greater potential for critical respiratory depression, even at therapeutic dosages. Use with extreme caution in patients with head injury, intracranial lesions, or elevated intracranial pressure (ICP); exaggerated elevation of ICP may occur. Use caution in patients with a history of seizures or conditions predisposing patients to seizures; patients with a history of seizures were excluded in clinical trials of tapentadol. Tramadol, an analgesic with similar pharmacologic properties to tapentadol, has been associated with

seizures, particularly in patients with predisposing factors. May cause severe hypotension; use with caution in patients with risk factors (eg, hypovolemia, concomitant use of other hypotensive agents). Avoid use in patients with circulatory shock. Potentially life-threatening serotonin syndrome (SS) has occurred with concomitant use of tapentadol and serotonergic agents (eg, SSRIs, SNRIs, triptans, TCAs, fentanyl, lithium, tramadol, buspirone, St John's wort, tryptophan) or agents that impair metabolism of serotonin (eg, MAO inhibitors intended to treat psychiatric disorders, other MAO inhibitors [ie, linezolid and intravenous methylene blue]). Monitor patients closely for signs of SS such as mental status changes (eg, agitation, hallucinations, delirium, coma); autonomic instability (eg, tachycardia, labile blood pressure, diaphoresis); neuromuscular changes (eg, tremor, rigidity, myoclonus); GI symptoms (eg, nausea, vomiting, diarrhea); and/or seizures. Discontinue treatment (and any concomitant serotonergic agent) immediately if signs/symptoms arise.

Opioids may obscure diagnosis or clinical course of patients with acute abdominal conditions. May cause CNS depression, which may impair physical or mental abilities; patients must be cautioned about performing tasks which require mental alertness (eg, operating machinery or driving). Effects may be potentiated when used with other CNS depressants (eg, sedatives, anxiolytics, hypnotics, neuroleptics, other opioids). Potentially significant drug-drug interactions may exist, requiring dose or frequency adjustment, additional monitoring, and/or selection of alternative therapy.

Use with caution in patients with adrenal insufficiency (including Addison's disease), patients with biliary tract dysfunction or acute pancreatitis (opioids may cause spasm of the sphincter of Oddi), patients with CNS depression (avoid use in patients with impaired consciousness or coma as these patients are susceptible to intracranial effects of CO_2 retention), patients with hypothyroidism, prostatic hyperplasia and/or urinary stricture. Use opioids with caution in the elderly; consider decreasing initial dose. May have a greater potential for critical respiratory depression. Serum concentrations are increased in hepatic impairment; use with caution in patients with moderate hepatic impairment (dosage adjustment required). Not recommended for use in severe hepatic impairment (not studied). Use with caution in patients with mild-to-moderate renal impairment; no dosage adjustments recommended. Not recommended for use in severe renal impairment (not studied). Canadian labeling contraindicates use of the extended-release formulation for perioperative pain relief and also recommends withholding its use for at least 48 hours prior to surgery and during the immediate postoperative period. May resume therapy after the patient recovers from the postoperative period; dosage adjustment may be necessary to provide adequate pain relief (Nucynta ER Canadian product monograph, 2014).

Prolonged use increases risk of abuse, addiction, and withdrawal symptoms. An opioid-containing regimen should be tailored to each patient's needs with respect to degree of tolerance for opioids (naïve versus chronic user), age, weight, and medical condition. Concurrent use of mixed agonist/antagonist analgesics (eg, pentazocine, nalbuphine, butorphanol) or partial agonist (eg, buprenorphine) analgesics may precipitate withdrawal symptoms and/or reduced analgesic efficacy in patients following prolonged therapy with mu opioid agonists. Taper dose gradually when discontinuing. In order to avoid dosing errors, include the dose in mL and mg when writing prescriptions. Instruct patients to always use the enclosed calibrated oral syringe to ensure the dose is measured and administered accurately.

Extended release tablets:

[U.S. Boxed Warning]: May cause serious, life-threatening, or fatal respiratory depression. Monitor closely for respiratory depression, especially during initiation or dose escalation. Patients should swallow tablets whole; crushing, chewing, or dissolving can cause rapid release and a potentially fatal dose. Carbon dioxide retention from opioid-induced respiratory depression can exacerbate the sedating effects of opioids. Therapy should only be prescribed by healthcare professionals familiar with the use of potent opioids for chronic pain. **[U.S. Boxed Warning]: Accidental ingestion of even one dose, especially in children, can result in a fatal overdose of tapentadol.**

[U.S. Boxed Warning]: Patients should not consume alcoholic beverages or medication containing ethanol while taking tapentadol ER; ethanol may increase tapentadol plasma levels resulting in a potentially fatal overdose.

[U.S. Boxed Warning]: Prolonged maternal use of opioids during pregnancy can cause neonatal withdrawal syndrome in the newborn which may be life-threatening if not recognized and treated according to protocols developed by neonatology experts. If prolonged opioid therapy is required in a pregnant woman, ensure treatment is available and warn patient of risk to the neonate. Signs and symptoms include irritability, hyperactivity and abnormal sleep pattern, high pitched cry, tremor, vomiting, diarrhea and failure to gain weight. Onset, duration and severity depend on the drug used, duration of use, maternal dose, and rate of drug elimination by the newborn.

[U.S. Boxed Warning]: Users are exposed to the risks of addiction, abuse, and misuse, potentially leading to overdose and death. Assess each patient's risk prior to prescribing; monitor all patients regularly for development of these behaviors or conditions. Risk of opioid abuse is increased in patients with a history or family history of alcohol or drug abuse or mental illness.

Adverse Reactions

Immediate release:

>10%:

Central nervous system: Dizziness (24%), drowsiness (15%)

Gastrointestinal: Nausea (30%), vomiting (18%)

1% to 10%:

Central nervous system: Fatigue (3%), insomnia (2%), abnormal dreams (1%), anxiety (1%), confusion (1%), lethargy (1%)

Dermatologic: Pruritus (3% to 5%), hyperhidrosis (3%), skin rash (1%)

Endocrine & metabolic: Hot flash (1%)

Gastrointestinal: Constipation (8%), xerostomia (4%), decreased appetite (2%), dyspepsia (2%)

Genitourinary: Urinary tract infection (1%)

Neuromuscular & skeletal: Arthralgia (1%), tremor (1%)

Respiratory: Nasopharyngitis (1%), upper respiratory tract infection (1%)

Extended release:

>10%:

Central nervous system: Dizziness (17% to 18%), headache (10% to 15%), drowsiness (12% to 14%)

Gastrointestinal: Nausea (21% to 27%), constipation (13% to 17%), vomiting (8% to 12%)

1% to 10%:

Cardiovascular: Hypotension (1%)

Central nervous system: Fatigue (9%), anxiety (2% to 5%), insomnia (4%), irritability (2%), lethargy (2%), abnormal dreams (1% to 2%), vertigo (1% to 2%), chills (1%), depression (1%), hypoesthesia (1%), lack of concentration (1%), nervousness (1%), sedation (1%), withdrawal syndrome (1%)

Dermatologic: Pruritus (1% to 8%), hyperhidrosis (3% to 5%), skin rash (1%)

Endocrine & metabolic: Hot flash (2% to 3%)

Gastrointestinal: Diarrhea (7%), xerostomia (7%), decreased appetite (2% to 6%), dyspepsia (1% to 3%), abdominal distress (1%)

Genitourinary: Erectile dysfunction (1%)

Neuromuscular & skeletal: Tremor (1% to 3%), weakness (2%)

Ophthalmic: Blurred vision (1%)

Respiratory: Dyspnea (1%)

Immediate and/or extended release:<1% (Limited to important or life-threatening): Abnormality in thinking, altered mental status, anaphylaxis, angioedema, ataxia, decreased blood pressure, delayed gastric emptying, disorientation, drug withdrawal, dysarthria, euphoria, hallucination, hypersensitivity, hypogonadism (Brennan, 2013; Debono, 2011), impaired consciousness, intoxicated feeling, memory impairment, panic attack, pollakiuria, presyncope, respiratory depression, seizure, syncope, urinary hesitation, visual disturbance

Drug Interactions

Metabolism/Transport Effects Substrate of CYP2C9 (minor), CYP2D6 (minor); **Note:** Assignment of Major/Minor substrate status based on clinically relevant drug interaction potential

Avoid Concomitant Use

Avoid concomitant use of Tapentadol with any of the following: Alcohol (Ethyl); Azelastine (Nasal); Dapoxetine; Eluxadoline; MAO Inhibitors; Mixed Agonist / Antagonist Opioids; Orphenadrine; Paraldehyde; Thalidomide

Increased Effect/Toxicity

Tapentadol may increase the levels/effects of: Alvimopan; Azelastine (Nasal); CNS Depressants; Desmopressin; Diuretics; Eluxadoline; Hydrocodone; MAO Inhibitors; Methotrimeprazine; Metoclopramide; Metyrosine; Orphenadrine; Paraldehyde; Pramipexole;

Ramosetron; ROPINIRole; Rotigotine; Serotonin Modulators; Suvorexant; Thalidomide; Zolpidem

The levels/effects of Tapentadol may be increased by: Alcohol (Ethyl); Amphetamines; Anticholinergic Agents; Brimonidine (Topical); Cannabis; Dapoxetine; Dronabinol; Droperidol; Kava Kava; Magnesium Sulfate; Methotrimeprazine; Minocycline; Nabilone; Perampanel; Rufinamide; Sodium Oxybate; Succinylcholine; Tetrahydrocannabinol

Decreased Effect

Tapentadol may decrease the levels/effects of: Pegvisomant

The levels/effects of Tapentadol may be decreased by: Ammonium Chloride; Antiemetics (5HT3 Antagonists); Mixed Agonist / Antagonist Opioids; Naltrexone

Food Interactions

Ethanol: Concomitant use with alcohol can increase the bioavailability of extended release tablets. Management: Avoid use of alcohol during therapy.

Food: When administered after a high fat/calorie meal, the AUC and C_{max} increased by 25% and 16%, respectively. Management: May administer without regard to meals.

Storage/Stability Store at room temperature up to 25°C (77°F); excursions are permitted between 15°C and 30°C (59°F and 86°F). Protect tablets from moisture.

Mechanism of Action Binds to μ-opiate receptors in the CNS causing inhibition of ascending pain pathways, altering the perception of and response to pain; also inhibits the reuptake of norepinephrine, which also modifies the ascending pain pathway

Pharmacodynamics/Kinetics

Absorption: Rapid and complete

Distribution: V_d: IV: 442-638 L

Protein binding: ~20%

Metabolism: Extensive metabolism, including first pass metabolism; metabolized primarily via phase 2 glucuronidation to glucuronides (major metabolite: tapentadol-O-glucuronide); minimal phase 1 oxidative metabolism; also metabolized to a lesser degree by CYP2C9, CYP2C19, and CYP2D6; all metabolites pharmacologically inactive

Bioavailability: ~32%

Half-life elimination: Immediate release: ~4 hours; Long acting formulations: ~5-6 hours

Time to peak, plasma: Immediate release: 1.25 hours; Long acting formulations: 3-6 hours

Excretion: Urine (99%: 70% conjugated metabolites; 3% unchanged drug)

Dosing

Adult Dose and dosage intervals should be individualized according to pain severity with respect to patient's previous experience with similar opioid analgesics. In patients receiving extended release tapentadol, immediate-release opioid or nonopioid medication may be used for rescue relief of breakthrough pain and during dosage adjustments. The Canadian labeling does not recommend use of fentanyl as rescue medication. To reduce the risk of withdrawal symptoms, it is recommended to taper the dose when discontinuing therapy.

Acute moderate-severe pain: Oral: *Immediate release tablets and solution:* Day 1: 50 to 100 mg (2.5 to 5 mL) every 4 to 6 hours as needed; may administer a second dose ≥1 hour after the initial dose (maximum dose on first day: 700 mg daily); Day 2 and subsequent dosing: 50 to 100 mg (2.5 to 5 mL) every 4 to 6 hours as needed (maximum: 600 mg daily)

Chronic pain (U.S. and Canadian labeling), neuropathic pain associated with diabetic peripheral neuropathy (U.S. labeling): Oral: *Extended release:*

Opioid naive (use as the first opioid analgesic or use in patients who are **not** opioid tolerant): Initial: 50 mg twice daily (recommended interval: every 12 hours) **Note:** Opioid tolerance is defined as: Patients already taking at least 60 mg of oral morphine daily, 25 mcg of transdermal fentanyl per hour, 30 mg of oral oxycodone daily, 8 mg oral hydromorphone daily, 25 mg oral oxymorphone daily, or an equivalent dose of another opioid for at least 1 week.

Conversion from other oral opioids to extended release tapentadol: Discontinue all other around-the-clock opioids when extended release tapentadol is initiated. Substantial interpatient variability exists in relative potency. Therefore, it is safer to underestimate a patient's daily oral tapentadol requirement and provide breakthrough pain relief with rescue medication (eg, immediate release opioid) than to overestimate requirements. In general, begin with a dose that is 50% of the estimated daily tapentadol requirement and use immediate release rescue medications to supplement dose. Per the Canadian product labeling, comparable pain relief was observed between

tapentadol ER and oxycodone CR at a dose ratio of 5:1 in clinical studies.

Conversion from tapentadol immediate release to extended release: Convert using same total daily dose but divide into 2 equal doses and administer twice daily (recommended interval: ~12 hours) (maximum dose: 500 mg daily).

Conversion from methadone to extended release tapentadol: Close monitoring is required when converting methadone to another opioid. Ratio between methadone and other opioid agonists varies widely according to previous dose exposure. Methadone has a long half-life and can accumulate in the plasma.

Dose titration: Titrate in increments of 50 mg no more frequently than twice daily every 3 days to effective dose (therapeutic range: 100 to 250 mg twice daily) (maximum dose: 500 mg daily).

Discontinuation of therapy: Gradually titrate dose downward to prevent withdrawal signs/symptoms. Do not abruptly discontinue.

Geriatric Initial: Consider initiating at lower range of dosing. Refer to adult dosing.

Renal Impairment

CrCl ≥30 mL/minute: No dosage adjustment necessary.

CrCl <30 mL/minute: Use not recommended (not studied); use is contraindicated in the Canadian labeling.

Hepatic Impairment

Mild impairment (Child-Pugh class A): No dosage adjustment necessary.

Moderate impairment (Child-Pugh class B):

Immediate release tablets and solution: Initial: 50 mg every 8 hours or longer (maximum: 3 doses/24 hours). Further treatment for maintenance of analgesia may be achieved by either shortening or lengthening the dosing interval.

Extended release: Initial: 50 mg every 24 hours or longer; maximum: 100 mg once daily

Severe impairment (Child-Pugh class C): Use not recommended (not studied); use is contraindicated in the Canadian labeling.

Dietary Considerations May be taken without regard to meals.

Administration Administer orally with or without food.

Tablets: Long acting formulations must be swallowed whole and should **not** be split, crushed, broken, chewed, or dissolved; patients should be instructed to swallow 1 tablet at a time, immediately after placing in mouth. The Canadian labeling recommends that immediate release tablets be swallowed whole.

Oral solution: Always use the enclosed calibrated oral syringe to ensure the dose is measured and administered accurately.

Monitoring Parameters Respiratory and cardiovascular status, blood pressure, heart rate; signs of misuse, abuse, or addiction; signs or symptoms of hypogonadism or hypoadrenalism (Brennan, 2013)

Extended release tablets: Monitor for respiratory depression for 72 hours of initiating dose.

Dosage Forms Excipient information presented when available (limited, particularly for generics); consult specific product labeling.

Tablet, Oral:

Nucynta: 50 mg, 75 mg, 100 mg

Tablet Extended Release 12 Hour, Oral:

Nucynta ER: 50 mg

Nucynta ER: 100 mg, 150 mg [contains fd&c blue #2 aluminum lake]

Nucynta ER: 200 mg, 250 mg [scored; contains fd&c blue #2 aluminum lake]

Dosage Forms: Canada Excipient information presented when available (limited, particularly for generics); consult specific product labeling.

Tablet, Oral:

Nucynta IR: 50 mg, 75 mg, 100 mg

Tablet, Controlled Release, Oral:

Nucynta ER: 50 mg, 100 mg, 150 mg, 200 mg, 250 mg

Controlled Substance C-II

Tasimelteon (tas i MEL tee on)

Brand Names: US Hetlioz

Index Terms VEC-162

Pharmacologic Category Hypnotic, Miscellaneous; Melatonin Receptor Agonist

Use Non-24-hour sleep-wake disorder: Treatment of non-24-hour sleep-wake disorder (non-24). **Note:** Efficacy was established in totally blind patients with non-24-hour sleep-wake disorder.

Pregnancy Considerations Adverse events were observed in some animal reproduction studies.

Breast-Feeding Considerations It is not known if tasimelteon is excreted into breast milk. The manufacturer recommends that caution be used if administered to a breast-feeding woman.

Contraindications There are no contraindications listed in the manufacturer's labeling.

Warnings/Precautions May cause CNS depression impairing physical and mental capabilities; patients must be cautioned about performing tasks, which require mental alertness (operating machinery or driving). Use is not recommended in patients with severe hepatic impairment. Smoking causes induction of CYP1A2 levels; tasimelteon exposure is decreased in smokers compared to non-smokers that may reduce tasimelteon efficacy. Use with caution in the elderly; exposure is increased; may increase the risk of adverse events. Potentially significant drug-drug interactions may exist, requiring dose or frequency adjustment, additional monitoring, and/or selection of alternative therapy.

Adverse Reactions

>10%: Central nervous system: Headache (17%)

1% to 10%:

Central nervous system: Abnormal dreams (10%)

Genitourinary: Urinary tract infection (7%)

Hepatic: Increased serum ALT (10%)

Respiratory: Upper respiratory tract infection (7%)

Drug Interactions

Metabolism/Transport Effects Substrate of CYP1A2 (major), CYP3A4 (major); **Note:** Assignment of Major/Minor substrate status based on clinically relevant drug interaction potential

Avoid Concomitant Use

Avoid concomitant use of Tasimelteon with any of the following: Azelastine (Nasal); CYP1A2 Inhibitors (Strong); CYP3A4 Inducers (Strong); Orphenadrine; Paraldehyde; Sodium Oxybate; Thalidomide

Increased Effect/Toxicity

Tasimelteon may increase the levels/effects of: Alcohol (Ethyl); Azelastine (Nasal); Buprenorphine; CNS Depressants; Hydrocodone; Methotrimeprazine; Metyrosine; Mirtazapine; Orphenadrine; Paraldehyde; Pramipexole; ROPINIRole; Rotigotine; Selective Serotonin Reuptake Inhibitors; Sodium Oxybate; Suvorexant; Thalidomide; Zolpidem

The levels/effects of Tasimelteon may be increased by: Abiraterone Acetate; Brimonidine (Topical); Cannabis; CYP1A2 Inhibitors (Moderate); CYP1A2 Inhibitors (Strong); CYP3A4 Inhibitors (Strong); Deferasirox; Doxylamine; Dronabinol; Droperidol; HydrOXYzine; Kava Kava; Magnesium Sulfate; Methotrimeprazine; Minocycline; Nabilone; Osimertinib; Peginterferon Alfa-2b; Perampanel; Rufinamide; Tapentadol; Tetrahydrocannabinol; Vemurafenib

Decreased Effect

The levels/effects of Tasimelteon may be decreased by: Bosentan; Cannabis; CYP3A4 Inducers (Moderate); CYP3A4 Inducers (Strong); Cyproterone; Dabrafenib; Deferasirox; Osimertinib; Siltuximab; St Johns Wort; Teriflunomide; Tocilizumab

Storage/Stability Store at 25°C (77°F); excursions are permitted between 15°C and 30°C (59°F and 86°F). Protect from light and moisture.

Mechanism of Action Agonist of melatonin receptors MT_1 and MT_2 (greater affinity for the MT_2 receptor than the MT_1 receptor). Agonism of MT_1 is thought to preferentially induce sleepiness, while MT_2 receptor activation preferentially influences regulation of circadian rhythms.

Pharmacodynamics/Kinetics

Onset: Effect may take weeks or months (due to individual differences in circadian rhythms)

Absorption: High-fat meals delayed T_{max} and maximum serum concentration was reduced by 44%

Protein binding: ~90%

Distribution: V_d: ~59 to 126 L

Metabolism: Hepatic (extensive); oxidative metabolism primarily through CYP1A2 and CYP3A4. Phenolic glucuronidation is the major phase II metabolic route.

Bioavailability: ~38%

Half-life elimination: ~1 to 2 hours

Time to peak: Fasting: ~0.5 to 3 hours (increased by ~1.75 hours with a high-fat meal)

Excretion: Urine (80%; <1% as unchanged drug); feces (~4%)

Dosing

Adult Note: Effect may not occur for weeks or months due to differences in circadian rhythms.

Non-24-hour sleep-wake disorder: Adults: Oral: 20 mg once daily at the same time each night before bedtime.

Renal Impairment No dosage adjustment necessary.

Hepatic Impairment

Mild or moderate impairment: No dosage adjustment necessary.

Severe impairment: There are no dosage adjustments provided in manufacturer's labeling (has not been studied). Use is not recommended.

Dietary Considerations Avoid or limit ethanol.

Administration Administer orally without food. Should be taken at the same time every night before bedtime. Swallow capsule whole. After administration, activities should be limited to preparing for sleep. If the dose cannot be taken at approximately the same time on a given night, that dose should be skipped.

Dosage Forms Excipient information presented when available (limited, particularly for generics); consult specific product labeling.

Capsule, Oral:

Hetlioz: 20 mg [contains brilliant blue fcf (fd&c blue #1), fd&c yellow #6 (sunset yellow)]

◆ Tasmar *see* Tolcapone *on page 1807*

Tavaborole (ta va BOR ole)

Brand Names: US Kerydin

Pharmacologic Category Antifungal Agent, Topical

Use Onychomycosis: Topical treatment of onychomycosis of the toenail(s) due to *Trichophyton rubrum* and *Trichophyton mentagrophytes*

Dosing

Adult & Geriatric Onychomycosis: Topical: Apply to affected toenail(s) once daily for 48 weeks.

Renal Impairment There are no dosage adjustments provided in the manufacturer's labeling. However, dosage adjustment unlikely due to low systemic absorption.

Hepatic Impairment There are no dosage adjustments provided in the manufacturer's labeling. However, dosage adjustment unlikely due to low systemic absorption.

Additional Information Complete prescribing information should be consulted for additional detail.

Dosage Forms Excipient information presented when available (limited, particularly for generics); consult specific product labeling.

Solution, External:

Kerydin: 5% (4 mL, 10 mL) [contains edetate calcium disodium, propylene glycol]

◆ Tavist Allergy [OTC] *see* Clemastine *on page 404*

◆ Tavist ND *see* Loratadine *on page 1101*

◆ Taxol *see* PACLitaxel (Conventional) *on page 1369*

◆ Taxotere *see* DOCEtaxel *on page 573*

Tazarotene (taz AR oh teen)

Brand Names: US Avage; Fabior; Tazorac

Brand Names: Canada Tazorac

Pharmacologic Category Acne Products; Keratolytic Agent; Topical Skin Product, Acne

Use

Acne (Fabior, Tazorac 0.1% cream, Tazorac 0.1% gel): Topical treatment of acne vulgaris in patients 12 years and older.

Psoriasis:

Tazorac 0.05% and 0.1% cream: Topical treatment of plaque psoriasis in patients 18 years and older.

Tazorac 0.05% and 0.1% gel: Topical treatment of stable plaque psoriasis of up to 20% body surface area involvement in patients 12 years and older.

Wrinkling, hyper- and hypopigmentation, lentigines (Avage): Adjunctive agent for use in the mitigation (palliation) of facial fine wrinkling, facial mottled hyper- and hypopigmentation, and benign facial lentigines in patients 17 years and older who use comprehensive skin care and sunlight avoidance programs.

Limitations of use: Does not eliminate or prevent wrinkles, repair sun-damaged skin, reverse photoaging, or restore more youthful or younger skin. Has not demonstrated a mitigating effect on significant signs of chronic sunlight exposure such as coarse or deep wrinkling, tactile roughness, telangiectasia, skin laxity, keratinocytic atypia, melanocytic atypia, or dermal elastosis. Safety and effectiveness for the prevention or treatment of actinic keratoses, skin neoplasms, or lentigo maligna has not been established. Use for greater than 52 weeks has not been established.

Dosing

Adult & Geriatric Note: In patients experiencing excessive pruritus, burning, skin redness, or peeling, discontinue until integrity of the skin is restored, or reduce dosing to an interval the patient is able to tolerate.

Acne: Topical:

Fabior: Apply a small amount to affected area once daily in the evening.

Tazorac cream/gel 0.1%: Apply a thin film (2 mg/cm²) to affected area once daily in the evening.

Palliation of fine facial wrinkles, facial mottled hyper-/hypopigmentation, benign facial lentigines: Topical: Avage: Apply a pea-sized amount to entire face once daily at bedtime.

Psoriasis: Topical: Tazorac cream/gel: Initial: 0.05%: Apply once daily to psoriatic lesions using enough (2 mg/cm²) to cover only the lesion with a thin film. May increase strength to 0.1% if tolerated and necessary.

Pediatric Note: In patients experiencing excessive pruritus, burning, skin redness, or peeling, discontinue until integrity of the skin is restored, or reduce dosing to an interval the patient is able to tolerate.

Acne: Children ≥12 years and Adolescents: Refer to adult dosing.

Psoriasis: Children ≥12 years and Adolescents: Topical: Tazorac gel: Refer to adult dosing.

Palliation of fine facial wrinkles, facial mottled hyper-/hypopigmentation, benign facial lentigines: Adolescents ≥17 years: Topical: Avage: Refer to adult dosing.

Additional Information Complete prescribing information should be consulted for additional detail.

Dosage Forms Excipient information presented when available (limited, particularly for generics); consult specific product labeling.

Cream, External:

Avage: 0.1% (30 g) [contains benzyl alcohol]

Tazorac: 0.05% (30 g, 60 g); 0.1% (30 g, 60 g) [contains benzyl alcohol]

Foam, External:

Fabior: 0.1% (50 g, 100 g)

Gel, External:

Tazorac: 0.05% (30 g, 100 g); 0.1% (30 g, 100 g) [contains benzyl alcohol]

- Tazicef see CefTAZidime on page 345
- Tazidime see CefTAZidime on page 345
- Tazobactam and Ceftolozane see Ceftolozane and Tazobactam on page 348
- Tazobactam and Piperacillin see Piperacillin and Tazobactam on page 1456
- Tazocin (Can) see Piperacillin and Tazobactam on page 1456
- Tazorac see Tazarotene on page 1740
- Taztia XT see Diltiazem on page 553
- TBC see Trypsin, Balsam Peru, and Castor Oil on page 1849
- Tbo-Filgrastim see Filgrastim on page 766
- TB Skin Test see Tuberculin Tests on page 1850
- 3TC see LamiVUDine on page 1024
- 3TC, Abacavir, and Zidovudine see Abacavir, Lamivudine, and Zidovudine on page 18
- T-Cell Growth Factor see Aldesleukin on page 60
- TCGF see Aldesleukin on page 60
- TCN see Tetracycline on page 1773
- Td see Diphtheria and Tetanus Toxoid on page 565
- TD-6424 see Telavancin on page 1745
- Td Adsorbed (Can) see Diphtheria and Tetanus Toxoid on page 565
- Tdap see Diphtheria and Tetanus Toxoids, and Acellular Pertussis Vaccine on page 567
- TDF see Tenofovir Disoproxil Fumarate on page 1756
- T-DM1 see Ado-Trastuzumab Emtansine on page 47
- Tebrazid™ (Can) see Pyrazinamide on page 1530
- Tecfidera see Dimethyl Fumarate on page 557
- Technivie see Ombitasvir, Paritaprevir, and Ritonavir on page 1327
- Tecnu First Aid [OTC] see Lidocaine (Topical) on page 1074
- Tecta (Can) see Pantoprazole on page 1390

Tedizolid (ted eye ZOE lid)

Brand Names: US Sivextro
Index Terms DA-7157; DA-7158; DA-7218; Tedizolid Phosphate; Torezolid; TR-700; TR-701 FA
Pharmacologic Category Antibiotic, Oxazolidinone
Use Acute bacterial skin and skin structure infections: Treatment of adult patients with acute bacterial skin and skin structure infections (ABSSSI) caused by susceptible isolates of the following gram-positive microorganisms: Staphylococcus aureus (including methicillin-resistant [MRSA] and methicillin-susceptible [MSSA] isolates), Streptococcus pyogenes, Streptococcus agalactiae, Streptococcus anginosus group (including Streptococcus anginosus, Streptococcus intermedius, and Streptococcus constellatus), and Enterococccus faecalis
Pregnancy Considerations Adverse events were observed in animal reproduction studies.
Breast-Feeding Considerations It is not known if tedizolid is excreted into breast milk. The manufacturer recommends that caution be used if administered to a nursing woman.
Contraindications There are no contraindications listed in the manufacturer's labeling.
Warnings/Precautions Not recommended for use in patients with neutrophil counts <1000 cells/mm³. Alternative therapies should be considered when treating patients with neutropenia and ABSSI. Prolonged use may result in fungal or bacterial superinfection, including C. difficile-associated diarrhea (CDAD) and pseudomembranous colitis; CDAD has been observed >2 months postantibiotic treatment.
Adverse Reactions
1% to 10%:
Cardiovascular: Flushing (<2%), hypertension (<2%), palpitations (<2%), tachycardia (<2%)
Central nervous system: Headache (6%), dizziness (2%), facial paralysis (<2%), hypoesthesia (<2%), insomnia (<2%), paresthesia (<2%), peripheral neuropathy (1%)
Dermatologic: Dermatitis (<2%), pruritus (<2%), urticaria (<2%)
Gastrointestinal: Nausea (8%), diarrhea (4%), vomiting (3%), oral candidiasis (<2%), pseudomembranous colitis (<2%)
Hematologic & oncologic: Decreased hemoglobin (males <10.1 g/dL; females <9 g/dL: 3%), decreased platelet count (<112,000/mm³: 2%), anemia (<2%), decreased white blood cell count (<2%)
Hepatic: Increased serum transaminases (<2%)

Hypersensitivity: Hypersensitivity (<2%)
Infection: Fungal infection (vulvovaginal: <2%)
Ophthalmic: Asthenopia (<2%), blurred vision (<2%), visual impairment (<2%), vitreous opacity (<2%)
Miscellaneous: Infusion related reaction (<2%)
<1% (Limited to important or life-threatening): Clostridium difficile associated diarrhea, decrease in absolute neutrophil count (<800/mm³), optic neuropathy
Drug Interactions
Metabolism/Transport Effects Inhibits Monoamine Oxidase
Avoid Concomitant Use
Avoid concomitant use of Tedizolid with any of the following: Alcohol (Ethyl); Anilidopiperidine Opioids; Apraclonidine; AtoMOXetine; Atropine (Ophthalmic); BCG (Intravesical); Bezafibrate; Buprenorphine; BuPROPion; BusPIRone; CarBAMazepine; Cyclobenzaprine; Cyproheptadine; Dapoxetine; Deferiprone; Dextromethorphan; Diethylpropion; Dipyrone; EPINEPHrine (Oral Inhalation); HYDROmorphone; Isometheptene; Levonordefrin; Linezolid; Maprotiline; Meperidine; Mequitazine; Methyldopa; Methylene Blue; Methylphenidate; Mianserin; Moclobemide; Morphine (Liposomal); Morphine (Systemic); Oxymorphone; Pholcodine; Pizotifen; Serotonin 5-HT1D Receptor Agonists; Tapentadol; Tetrabenazine; Tetrahydrozoline (Nasal); Tianeptine
Increased Effect/Toxicity
Tedizolid may increase the levels/effects of: Antipsychotic Agents; Apraclonidine; AtoMOXetine; Atropine (Ophthalmic); Betahistine; Bezafibrate; Blood Glucose Lowering Agents; Brimonidine (Ophthalmic); Brimonidine (Topical); BuPROPion; CloZAPine; Cyproheptadine; Deferiprone; Dextromethorphan; Diethylpropion; Domperidone; EPINEPHrine (Oral Inhalation); EPINEPHrine (Systemic); Hydrocodone; HYDROmorphone; Isometheptene; Levonordefrin; Linezolid; Lithium; Meperidine; Mequitazine; Methadone; Methyldopa; Methylene Blue; Methylphenidate; Metoclopramide; Mianserin; Moclobemide; Morphine (Liposomal); Morphine (Systemic); OxyCODONE; Pizotifen; Reserpine; Serotonin 5-HT1D Receptor Agonists; Serotonin Modulators; Sympathomimetics; Tetrahydrozoline (Nasal)

The levels/effects of Tedizolid may be increased by: Alcohol (Ethyl); Anilidopiperidine Opioids; Antiemetics (5HT3 Antagonists); Antipsychotic Agents; Buprenorphine; BusPIRone; CarBAMazepine; COMT Inhibitors; Cyclobenzaprine; Dapoxetine; Dipyrone; Levodopa; Maprotiline; Metaxalone; Oxymorphone; Pholcodine; Tapentadol; Tetrabenazine; Tianeptine; TraMADol
Decreased Effect
Tedizolid may decrease the levels/effects of: BCG (Intravesical); BCG Vaccine (Immunization); Domperidone; Sodium Picosulfate; Typhoid Vaccine

The levels/effects of Tedizolid may be decreased by: Cyproheptadine; Domperidone
Preparation for Administration Reconstitute with 4 mL SWFI. Do **NOT** shake. Gently swirl the contents and let the vial stand until the cake has completely dissolved and any foam disperses. If necessary, invert the vial to dissolve any remaining powder and swirl gently to prevent foaming. The reconstituted solution is clear and colorless to pale-yellow in color; Tilt the upright vial and insert a syringe into the bottom corner of the vial and remove 4 mL of the reconstituted solution. Do **NOT** invert the vial during extraction. The reconstituted solution must be further diluted in 250 mL of NS only. Invert the bag gently to mix. Do not shake the bag (may cause foaming).
Storage/Stability Store at 20°C to 25°C (68°F to 77°F); excursions are permitted between 15°C and 30°C (59°F and 86°F) The total storage time of the reconstituted solution should not exceed 24 hours at either room temperature or under refrigeration at 2°C to 8°C (36°F to 46°F).
Mechanism of Action After conversion from the prodrug, tedizolid phosphate, tedizolid binds to the 50S bacterial ribosomal subunit. This prevents the formation of a functional 70S initiation complex that is essential for the bacterial translation process and subsequently inhibits protein synthesis. Tedizolid is bacteriostatic against enterococci, staphylococci, and streptococci (Kisgen, 2014).
Pharmacodynamics/Kinetics
Absorption: Oral: Well absorbed
Distribution: V_{dss}: 67 to 80 L
Protein binding: 70% to 90%
Metabolism: Tedizolid phosphate is converted by phosphatases to tedizolid (active, parent drug); no other significant circulating metabolites.
Bioavailability: Oral: ~91%
Half-life elimination: ~12 hours
Time to peak: Oral: ~3 hours; IV: 1 to 1.5 hours

Excretion: Feces (82%) and urine (18%), both as inactive sulfate conjugates. Less than 3% excreted in feces or urine as parent drug.

Dosing

Adult & Geriatric

Usual dosage range: Oral, IV: 200 mg once daily

Acute bacterial skin and skin structure infections: Oral, IV: 200 mg once daily for 6 days

Missed doses: Administer as soon as possible any time up to 8 hours prior to the next scheduled dose; if less than 8 hours remain before the next dose, wait until the next scheduled dose.

Renal Impairment No dosage adjustment necessary.

Hepatic Impairment No dosage adjustment necessary.

Usual Infusion Concentrations: Adult 200 mg in 250 mL (concentration: 0.8 mg/mL) of NS only

Administration

Oral: Administer with or without food.

Intravenous: Administer as an IV infusion over 1 hour; do not administer as an IV push or bolus. Not for intra-arterial, IM, intrathecal, intraperitoneal, or subcutaneous administration. If the same IV line is to be used for sequential infusion of other drugs or solutions, the line should be flushed with NS before and after tedizolid infusion.

Monitoring Parameters Baseline complete blood count (CBC) with differential

Dosage Forms Excipient information presented when available (limited, particularly for generics); consult specific product labeling.

Solution Reconstituted, Intravenous, as phosphate [preservative free]:

Sivextro: 200 mg (10 ea)

Tablet, Oral, as phosphate:

Sivextro: 200 mg

◆ Tedizolid Phosphate *see* Tedizolid *on page 1741*

Teduglutide (te due GLOO tide)

Brand Names: US Gattex

Index Terms ALX-0600; Teduglutide Recombinant; Teduglutide [rDNA origin]

Pharmacologic Category Glucagon-Like Peptide-2 (GLP-2) Analog

Use Short bowel syndrome: Treatment of short bowel syndrome in adults who are dependent on parenteral support.

Pregnancy Considerations Adverse events were not observed in animal reproduction studies.

Breast-Feeding Considerations It is not known if teduglutide is excreted into breast milk. Due to the potential for serious adverse reactions in the nursing infant, a decision should be made whether to discontinue nursing or to discontinue the drug, taking into account the importance of treatment to the mother.

Medication Guide Available Yes

Contraindications

There are no contraindications listed in the manufacturer's labeling.

Canadian labeling: Additional contraindications (not in US labeling): Hypersensitivity to teduglutide or any component of the formulation; active gastrointestinal (GI) malignancy (GI tract, hepatobiliary, pancreatic); history of GI tract malignancies (including the hepatobiliary system) within the last 5 years.

Warnings/Precautions Teduglutide may increase the risk of hyperplastic changes, including neoplasia. In patients at increased risk for malignancy, consider treatment only if benefits outweigh the risks. Discontinue treatment in patients with active gastrointestinal malignancy (GI tract, hepatobiliary, pancreatic); evaluate risk versus benefit in patients with active non-GI malignancy. Monitor for small bowel neoplasia; remove any benign neoplasm. Development of colorectal polyps has occurred. Preform a baseline colonoscopy of the entire colon with polyp removal ≤6 months prior to initiation of therapy. Follow-up colonoscopy (or alternative imaging) should be performed at 1 year and at least every 5 years, thereafter. Discontinue teduglutide in patients who develop colorectal cancer.

May increase heart rate; use with caution in patients with cardiac conditions that may be worsened by increased heart rate (eg, ischemic heart disease, tachyarrhythmias) (Canadian labeling). Intestinal and stomal obstructions have been reported; temporarily discontinue treatment in patients that develop obstruction. Teduglutide may be resumed (if clinically indicated) once the obstruction is resolved. Increased fluid absorption and subsequent fluid overload/congestive heart failure has been reported; consider modification of parenteral support in patients who develop fluid overload, especially in patients with underlying cardiovascular disease; if significant cardiac deterioration develops, reassess the need for continued teduglutide treatment. Cholecystitis, cholangitis, cholelithiasis, and pancreatitis have been reported; monitor serum bilirubin, alkaline phosphatase, lipase, and amylase ≤6 month prior to initiation of therapy and at least every 6 months for duration of therapy; if clinically meaningful changes are detected, perform gallbladder/biliary tract/ pancreatic imaging and reassess the need for continued teduglutide treatment.

Teduglutide may increase absorption of oral medications; monitor therapy of medications with a narrow therapeutic index. Treatment discontinuation may result in fluid and electrolyte imbalance; carefully monitor fluid/electrolyte status.

Adverse Reactions

>10%:

Central nervous system: Headache (16%)

Endocrine & metabolic: Hypervolemia (12%)

Gastrointestinal: Abdominal pain (30% to 38%), nausea (18% to 25%), abdominal distension (14% to 20%), vomiting (12%)

Immunologic: Antibody development (3% to 48%; 3% at month 3, 18% at month 6, 25% at month 12, 31% at month 24, and 48% at month 30)

Local: Injection site reaction (12% to 22%)

Respiratory: Upper respiratory tract infection (12% to 26%)

Miscellaneous: Intestinal stoma complication (42%)

1% to 10%:

Central nervous system: Disturbed sleep (5%)

Dermatologic: Dermal hemorrhage (5%)

Hypersensitivity: Hypersensitivity reaction (8%)

Gastrointestinal: Flatulence (9%), change in appetite (7%), intestinal obstruction (4%), intestinal polyps (2%)

Respiratory: Cough (5%)

<1% (Limited to important or life-threatening): Cardiac arrest, cardiac failure, cerebral hemorrhage, cholecystitis, cholelithiasis, cholestasis, congestive heart failure, gallbladder perforation, malignant neoplasm, pancreatic pseudocyst, pancreatitis

Drug Interactions

Metabolism/Transport Effects None known.

Avoid Concomitant Use There are no known interactions where it is recommended to avoid concomitant use.

Increased Effect/Toxicity

Teduglutide may increase the levels/effects of: Benzodiazepines

Decreased Effect There are no known significant interactions involving a decrease in effect.

Preparation for Administration Reconstitute each vial with 0.5 mL of preservative-free SWFI (provided in syringe); let stand for 30 seconds and then roll vial between palms for 15 seconds. Do not shake. Allow vial to stand for an additional ~2 minutes; if undissolved material remains, roll between palms again. If particles are not dissolved after second attempt, discard vial. Once reconstituted, each vial provides 3.8 mg/0.38 mL (concentration is 10 mg/mL).

Storage/Stability Prior to dispensing, store intact vials refrigerated at 2°C to 8°C (36°F to 46°F); do not freeze. The carton of ancillary supplies should be stored at 25°C (77°F). After dispensing, store vials at 25°C (77°F); once dispensed, vials must be used within 90 days. Once reconstituted, store at ≤25°C (77°F); do not shake or freeze; use within 3 hours. Discard any unused portion.

Mechanism of Action Teduglutide is an analog of glucagon-like peptide-2 (GLP-2), which is secreted in the distal intestine. Endogenous GLP-2 increases intestinal and portal blood flow while inhibiting gastric acid secretion, thereby reducing intestinal losses and improving intestinal absorption. Teduglutide binds and activates GLP-2 receptors, resulting in release of mediators including insulin-like growth factor (IGF)-1, nitric oxide and keratinocyte growth factor (KGF).

Pharmacodynamics/Kinetics

Distribution: 0.1 L/kg

Metabolism: Similar to endogenous catabolism of GLP-2 but slower due to a single amino acid substitution (Ferrone, 2006)

Bioavailability: SubQ: 88%

Half-life elimination: ~2 hours (healthy patients); 1.3 hours (short bowel syndrome patients)

Time to peak, plasma: 3 to 5 hours

Excretion: Urine

Dosing

Adult & Geriatric Short bowel syndrome: SubQ: 0.05 mg/kg once daily

Missed doses: If a dose is missed, take as soon as possible on that day; do **NOT** take 2 doses on the same day.

Renal Impairment

CrCl ≥50 mL/minute: No dosage adjustment necessary.

CrCl <50 mL/minute: Administer 50% of the usual dose.

ESRD: Administer 50% of the usual dose.

Hepatic Impairment

Mild-to-moderate impairment (Child-Pugh class B): No dosage adjustment necessary.

Severe impairment: There are no dosage adjustments provided in the manufacturer's labeling (has not been studied).

Administration SubQ: Rotate injection site between thighs, upper arms, and quadrants of the abdomen. Do not administer IM or IV

Monitoring Parameters Serum bilirubin, alkaline phosphatase, lipase and amylase (baseline [within 6 months prior to initiation] and every 6 months thereafter); colonoscopy of entire colon and removal of polyps (baseline [within 6 months prior to initiation], 1 year, and ≤5 years thereafter if no polyps found); monitor fluid status in patients with cardiovascular disease; signs/symptoms of intestinal obstruction; signs/symptoms suggestive of gall bladder disease or pancreatitis; monitor fluid and electrolyte balance following therapy discontinuation

Dosage Forms Excipient information presented when available (limited, particularly for generics); consult specific product labeling.

Kit, Subcutaneous [preservative free]:

Gattex: 5 mg

◆ Teduglutide [rDNA origin] see Teduglutide on page 1742

◆ Teduglutide Recombinant see Teduglutide on page 1742

◆ Teflaro see Ceftaroline Fosamil on page 344

◆ Tegaderm CHG Dressing [OTC] see Chlorhexidine Gluconate on page 373

◆ TEGretol see CarBAMazepine on page 303

◆ Tegretol (Can) see CarBAMazepine on page 303

◆ TEGretol-XR see CarBAMazepine on page 303

◆ TEI-6720 see Febuxostat on page 743

◆ Tekturna see Aliskiren on page 70

◆ Tekturna HCT see Aliskiren and Hydrochlorothiazide on page 72

Telaprevir (tel A pre vir)

Brand Names: US Incivek [DSC]

Brand Names: Canada Incivek [DSC]

Index Terms LY570310; MP-424; MP424; VRT111950; VX-950; VX950

Pharmacologic Category Antihepaciviral, Protease Inhibitor (Anti-HCV)

Use Chronic hepatitis C: Treatment of genotype 1 chronic hepatitis C (in combination with peginterferon alfa and ribavirin) in adult patients with compensated liver disease (including cirrhosis) who are treatment naive or who have received previous interferon-based treatment, including null or partial responders, and treatment relapsers.

Pregnancy Considerations Adverse events were not observed in telaprevir animal developmental studies; however, telaprevir must not be used as monotherapy (must be used in combination with peginterferon alfa and ribavirin). Significant ribavirin teratogenic effects have been observed in all animal studies at ~0.01 times the maximum recommended daily human dose. Use of ribavirin is contraindicated in pregnancy. In addition, animal studies with interferons have demonstrated abortifacient effects. Negative pregnancy test is required before initiation and monthly thereafter. Hormonal contraceptive measures may not be effective in patients taking telaprevir or for 2 weeks after discontinuing therapy. Avoid pregnancy in female patients and female partners of male patients during therapy by using two effective nonhormonal forms of contraception; continue contraceptive measures for at least 6 months after completion of therapy. If patient or female partner becomes pregnant during treatment, she should be counseled about potential risks of exposure. If pregnancy occurs during use or within 6 months after treatment, report to the ribavirin pregnancy registry (800-593-2214).

Breast-Feeding Considerations It is not known if telaprevir or ribavirin are excreted into breast milk. The manufacturer recommends that breast-feeding be discontinued prior to the initiation of treatment.

Medication Guide Available Yes

Contraindications

Combination treatment with ribavirin: Pregnancy; male partners of pregnant women

Coadministration with alfuzosin, cisapride, ergot derivatives (eg, dihydroergotamine, ergonovine, ergotamine, methylergonovine), lovastatin, midazolam (oral), pimozide, sildenafil/tadalafil (when used for treatment of pulmonary arterial hypertension), simvastatin, triazolam, rifampin, St John's wort, carbamazepine, phenobarbital, phenytoin

Canadian labeling: Additional contraindications (not in U.S. labeling): Hypersensitivity to telaprevir or any component of the formulation; coadministration with amiodarone, astemizole (not available in Canada), eletriptan, eplerenone, flecainide, propafenone, quinidine, terfenadine (not available in Canada), vardenafil

Also refer to Peginterferon Alfa and Ribavirin monographs for individual product contraindications.

Warnings/Precautions [U.S. Boxed Warning] Serious skin reactions (some fatal) including Stevens-Johnson syndrome (SJS), drug reaction with eosinophilia and systemic symptoms (DRESS), and toxic epidermal necrolysis (TEN), have been reported with telaprevir combination therapy. Fatal cases have been reported in patients with progressive rash and systemic symptoms who received ongoing therapy after diagnoses of serious skin reactions. Discontinue telaprevir, peginterferon alfa, and ribavirin immediately for serious skin reactions (including rash with systemic symptoms or a progressive severe rash) and refer for immediate medical care. Rash has been typically observed within first 4 weeks of therapy initiation but may occur at any time. Severe rashes (other than DRESS, SJS) are generalized, bullous, vesicular or ulcerative; may also have an eczematous appearance. Discontinue telaprevir (may continue peginterferon alfa and ribavirin) for severe rash or for mild-to-moderate rash that progresses; if no improvement in rash within 1 week of stopping telaprevir, interruption or discontinuation of peginterferon alfa and/or ribavirin should be considered (or sooner if clinically indicated). May use oral antihistamines/topical corticosteroids for rash treatment; do not use systemic corticosteroids. Do not restart telaprevir if discontinued due to any skin reaction.

Telaprevir-containing regimens are not recommended for treatment-naive patients or for prior relapse patients nonresponsive to peginterferon/ribavirin regimens with or without an HCV protease inhibitor (AASLD/IDSA, 2014).

Prerenal azotemia (with or without acute renal failure) and uric acid nephropathy have been reported. Assess serum electrolytes, creatinine, and uric acid pretreatment, at weeks 2, 4, 8, and 12, and when clinically indicated. Maintain adequate hydration. Anemia has been reported with peginterferon alfa and ribavirin; addition of telaprevir is associated with further hemoglobin decreases. Low hemoglobin levels were measured during the first 4 weeks of treatment, and the lowest at the end of telaprevir treatment (week 12). Dose modifications of ribavirin were needed more often in patients also taking telaprevir. Assess hematologic parameters (CBC with differential and platelet count) pretreatment, at weeks 2, 4, 8, and 12, and when clinically indicated. May require ribavirin dose reduction, interruption or discontinuation of treatment; if ribavirin dose reductions are inadequate, may consider discontinuing telaprevir. Do not reduce telaprevir dose. If ribavirin is discontinued, telaprevir must also be discontinued. Do not restart telaprevir if ribavirin therapy is reinitiated.

Avoid pregnancy in female patients and female partners of male patients, during therapy, and for at least 6 months after treatment; two forms of nonhormonal contraception should be used. Hormonal contraceptives may not be effective in patients taking telaprevir or for two weeks after discontinuing therapy. Safety and efficacy have not been established in patients who have uncompensated cirrhosis, received liver transplants, or who have failed to respond to other NS3/4A inhibitors (including repeated courses of telaprevir). Monotherapy is not effective for chronic hepatitis C infection. Not recommended in moderate or severe hepatic impairment (Child-Pugh class B or C) or decompensated hepatic disease. Potentially significant drug-drug interactions may exist, requiring dose or frequency adjustments, additional monitoring, and/or selection of alternative therapy.

Adverse Reactions

>10%:

Central nervous system: Fatigue (56%)

Dermatologic: Rash (56%), pruritus (47%)

Endocrine and Metabolic: Hyperuricemia (<12.1 mg/dL: 66%; ≥12.1 mg/dL: 7%)

Gastrointestinal: Nausea (39%), diarrhea (26%), vomiting (13%), hemorrhoids (12%), anorectal discomfort (11%)

Hematologic: Anemia (36%), lymphopenia (15%)

Hepatic: Hyperbilirubinemia (<2.6 x ULN: 37%; ≥2.6 x ULN: 4%)

1% to 10%:
Gastrointestinal: Abnormal taste (10%), anal pruritus (6%)
Hematologic: Thrombocytopenia (3%)
<1% (Limited to important or life-threatening): Drug reaction with eosinophilia and systemic symptoms (DRESS), erythema multiforme, prerenal azotemia (with or without acute renal failure/insufficiency), Stevens-Johnson syndrome, toxic epidermal necrolysis, uric acid nephropathy

Drug Interactions

Metabolism/Transport Effects Substrate of CYP3A4 (major), P-glycoprotein; **Note:** Assignment of Major/Minor substrate status based on clinically relevant drug interaction potential; **Inhibits** CYP3A4 (strong), P-glycoprotein, SLCO1B1

Avoid Concomitant Use

Avoid concomitant use of Telaprevir with any of the following: Ado-Trastuzumab Emtansine; Alfuzosin; Aprepitant; Astemizole; AtorvaSTATin; Avanafil; Axitinib; Barnidipine; Bosutinib; Bromocriptine; Cabozantinib; CarBAMazepine; Ceritinib; Cisapride; Cobicistat; Cobimetinib; Conivaptan; Crizotinib; CYP3A4 Inducers (Strong); Dabrafenib; Dapoxetine; Darunavir; Dihydroergotamine; Domperidone; Dronedarone; Eletriptan; Eplerenone; Ergoloid Mesylates; Ergonovine; Ergotamine; Everolimus; Flibanserin; Fosamprenavir; Fosphenytoin; Fusidic Acid (Systemic); Halofantrine; Ibrutinib; Idelalisib; Irinotecan Products; Isavuconazonium Sulfate; Ivabradine; Lapatinib; Lercanidipine; Lomitapide; Lopinavir; Lovastatin; Lurasidone; Macitentan; Methylergonovine; Midazolam; Naloxegol; Nilotinib; NiMODipine; Nisoldipine; Olaparib; Osimertinib; Palbociclib; PAZOPanib; PHENobarbital; Phenytoin; Pimozide; Ranolazine; Red Yeast Rice; Regorafenib; Rifabutin; Rifampin; Rivaroxaban; Salmeterol; Sildenafil; Silodosin; Simeprevir; Simvastatin; Sonidegib; St Johns Wort; Suvorexant; Tamsulosin; Terfenadine; Ticagrelor; Tipranavir; Tolvaptan; Topotecan; Toremifene; Trabectedin; Triazolam; Ulipristal; Vemurafenib; VinCRIStine (Liposomal); Vorapaxar

Increased Effect/Toxicity

Telaprevir may increase the levels/effects of: Ado-Trastuzumab Emtansine; Afatinib; Alfuzosin; Alitretinoin (Systemic); Almotriptan; Alosetron; ALPRAZolam; Amiodarone; Apixaban; Aprepitant; ARIPiprazole; ARIPiprazole Lauroxil; Astemizole; Atazanavir; AtorvaSTATin; Avanafil; Axitinib; Barnidipine; Bedaquiline; Bepridil; Bortezomib; Bosentan; Bosutinib; Brentuximab Vedotin; Brexpiprazole; Brinzolamide; Bromocriptine; Budesonide (Nasal); Budesonide (Oral Inhalation); Budesonide (Systemic); Budesonide (Topical); Buprenorphine; Cabazitaxel; Cabozantinib; Cannabis; CarBAMazepine; Cariprazine; Ceritinib; Cilostazol; Cisapride; Clarithromycin; Cobimetinib; Colchicine; Conivaptan; Corticosteroids (Orally Inhaled); Corticosteroids (Systemic); Crizotinib; CycloSPORINE (Systemic); CYP3A4 Substrates; Dabigatran Etexilate; Dabrafenib; Daclatasvir; Dapoxetine; Dasatinib; Digoxin; Dihydroergotamine; Dofetilide; Domperidone; DOXOrubicin (Conventional); Dronabinol; Dronedarone; Dutasteride; Edoxaban; Eletriptan; Eliglustat; Eplerenone; Ergoloid Mesylates; Ergonovine; Ergotamine; Erlotinib; Erythromycin (Systemic); Estazolam; Etizolam; Everolimus; FentaNYL; Fesoterodine; Flecainide; Flibanserin; Fluticasone (Nasal); Fluticasone (Oral Inhalation); Fluvastatin; Fosphenytoin; Gefitinib; GuanFACINE; Halofantrine; Hydrocodone; Ibrutinib; Iloperidone; Imatinib; Imidafenacin; Irinotecan Products; Isavuconazonium Sulfate; Itraconazole; Ivabradine; Ivacaftor; Ixabepilone; Ketoconazole (Systemic); Lacosamide; Lapatinib; Ledipasvir; Lercanidipine; Levobupivacaine; Levomilnacipran; Lidocaine (Systemic); Lomitapide; Lovastatin; Lumefantrine; Lurasidone; Macitentan; Maraviroc; Methylergonovine; MethylPREDNISolone; Midazolam; Mifepristone; Naloxegol; Nilotinib; NiMODipine; Nintedanib; Nisoldipine; Olaparib; Osimertinib; Ospemifene; Oxybutynin; OxyCODONE; Palbociclib; Panobinostat; Paricalcitol; PAZOPanib; P-glycoprotein/ABCB1 Substrates; Phenytoin; Pimecrolimus; Pimozide; Pitavastatin; PONATinib; Posaconazole; Pranlukast; Pravastatin; Propafenone; Prucalopride; QUEtiapine; QuiNIDine; Ramelteon; Ranolazine; Red Yeast Rice; Regorafenib; Repaglinide; Retapamulin; Rifabutin; Rifaximin; Rilpivirine; Rivaroxaban; RomiDEPsin; Rosuvastatin; Ruxolitinib; Salmeterol; Saxagliptin; Sildenafil; Silodosin; Simeprevir; Simvastatin; Sirolimus; Sonidegib; SORAfenib; Suvorexant; Tacrolimus (Systemic); Tadalafil; Tamsulosin; Tasimelteon; Telithromycin; Tenofovir Disoproxil Fumarate; Terfenadine; Tetrahydrocannabinol; Ticagrelor; Tofacitinib; Tolterodine; Tolvaptan; Topotecan; Toremifene; Trabectedin; TraMADol; TraZODone; Triazolam; Ulipristal; Vardenafil; Vemurafenib; Vilazodone; VinCRIStine (Liposomal); Vindesine; Vinorelbine; Vorapaxar; Voriconazole; Warfarin; Zopiclone; Zuclopenthixol

The levels/effects of Telaprevir may be increased by: Clarithromycin; Cobicistat; Conivaptan; CYP3A4 Inhibitors (Moderate); CYP3A4 Inhibitors (Strong); Erythromycin (Systemic); Fusidic Acid (Systemic); Idelalisib; Itraconazole; Ketoconazole (Systemic); Luliconazole; Mifepristone; Netupitant; P-glycoprotein/ABCB1 Inhibitors; Posaconazole; Ritonavir; Stiripentol; Telithromycin; Voriconazole

Decreased Effect

Telaprevir may decrease the levels/effects of: Contraceptives (Estrogens); Contraceptives (Progestins); Darunavir; Efavirenz; Escitalopram; Fosamprenavir; Ifosfamide; Methadone; Prasugrel; Ticagrelor; Voriconazole; Warfarin; Zolpidem

The levels/effects of Telaprevir may be decreased by: Atazanavir; Bosentan; CarBAMazepine; Corticosteroids (Systemic); CYP3A4 Inducers (Moderate); CYP3A4 Inducers (Strong); Darunavir; Deferasirox; Efavirenz; Etravirine; Fosamprenavir; Fosphenytoin; Lopinavir; PHENobarbital; Phenytoin; Rifabutin; Rifampin; Ritonavir; Siltuximab; St Johns Wort; Tipranavir; Tocilizumab

Storage/Stability Store at 25°C (77°F); excursions permitted to 15°C to 30°C (59°F to 86°F).

Mechanism of Action Binds reversibly to nonstructural protein 3 (NS 3) serine protease and inhibits replication of the hepatitis C virus. Considered a direct-acting antiviral treatment for HCV, also called a specifically targeted antiviral therapy for HCV (STAT-C).

Pharmacodynamics/Kinetics Note: Telaprevir total exposure ($AUC_{24h,ss}$) was similar regardless of whether the total daily dose of 2250 mg was administered as 750 mg every 8 hours or 1125 mg twice daily.

Absorption: Food (not low fat) enhances absorption
Distribution: V_d: ~252 L
Protein binding: 59% to 76%
Metabolism: Primarily hepatic to less active (30x) and inactive metabolites. Some oxidative CYP3A4 metabolism.
Half-life elimination: Plasma: Adults: ~4-5 hours (single dose); steady state: ~9-11 hours
Time to peak, serum: 4-5 hours
Excretion: Feces (82%); urine (1%)

Dosing

Adult & Geriatric Treatment of chronic hepatitis C (CHC): Oral: 1125 mg twice daily (in combination with peginterferon alfa and ribavirin).

Treatment-naive or prior relapse patients: **Note:** Relapse includes patients with an undetectable HCV-RNA upon completion of treatment (non-telaprevir based regimen) but with detectable HCV-RNA during the follow up period.

Weeks 1-12: Triple therapy: Telaprevir 1125 mg twice daily in combination with peginterferon alfa and ribavirin

Weeks 13-23 (based on HCV-RNA results at weeks 4 and 12):

HCV-RNA **undetectable** (level less than ~10-15 units/mL) at both weeks 4 and 12 (eRVR): Dual therapy: Peginterferon alfa with concomitant ribavirin only (through week 24)

HCV-RNA **detectable** (level greater than ~10-15 units/mL but ≤1000 units/mL) at week 4 and/or week 12: Dual therapy: Peginterferon alfa and ribavirin only (through week 48 discussed below)

HCV-RNA **detectable** (level >1000 units/mL) at week 4 or week 12 (treatment futility): Discontinue telaprevir, peginterferon alfa and ribavirin at week 12

Weeks ≥24 (based on HCV-RNA results at week 24):

HCV-RNA **detectable** (level greater than ~10-15 units/mL but ≤1000 units/mL) at week 4 and/or week 12: Peginterferon alfa with concomitant ribavirin only (through week 48)

HCV-RNA **detectable** (level greater than ~10-15 units/mL) at week 24 (treatment futility): Discontinue peginterferon alfa and concomitant ribavirin

Treatment-naive patients with cirrhosis, compensated:

Weeks 1-12: Triple therapy: Telaprevir 1125 mg twice daily in combination with peginterferon alfa and ribavirin

Weeks 13-24 (based on HCV-RNA results at weeks 4 and 12):

HCV-RNA **undetectable** at both weeks 4 and 12 (eRVR): Dual therapy: Peginterferon alfa and ribavirin only (through week 48 discussed below)

HCV-RNA **detectable** (level greater than ~10-15 units/mL but ≤1000 units/mL) at week 4 and/or week 12: Dual therapy: Peginterferon alfa and ribavirin only (through week 48 discussed below)

HCV-RNA **detectable** (level >1000 units/mL) at week 4 or week 12 (treatment futility): Discontinue telaprevir, peginterferon alfa and ribavirin at week 12

Weeks ≥24 (based on HCV-RNA results at week 24):

HCV-RNA **undetectable** at week 24: Peginterferon alfa with concomitant ribavirin only (through week 48)

HCV-RNA **detectable** (level greater than ~10-15 units/mL) at week 24 (treatment futility): Discontinue peginterferon alfa and ribavirin

Previously-treated patients (partial response or null responders): **Note:** Previously treated does not include prior treatment with telaprevir. Partial response includes patients with a >2-$\log_{10}$ HCV-RNA decrease by week 12 but a nonsustained virologic response thereafter. Null response includes patients with a <2-$\log_{10}$ HCV-RNA decrease at week 12.

Weeks 1-12: Triple therapy: Telaprevir 1125 mg twice daily with peginterferon alfa and ribavirin

Weeks 13-48 (based on HCV-RNA results at weeks 4 and 12):

HCV-RNA **undetectable** (level less than ~10-15 units/mL) or detectable (level ≤1000 units/mL) at both weeks 4 and 12: Dual therapy: Peginterferon alfa and ribavirin only (through week 48)

HCV-RNA **detectable** (level >1000 units/mL) at week 4 or week 12: Discontinue telaprevir, peginterferon alfa, and ribavirin at week 12

HCV-RNA **detectable** (level greater than ~10-15 units/mL) at week 24: Discontinue peginterferon alfa and concomitant ribavirin

Missed dose: If a dose is missed within 6 hours of the time it is usually taken, take as soon as possible. If more than 6 hours have passed since the dose is usually taken, do not take the missed dose and the patient should resume the usual schedule.

Renal Impairment

Telaprevir: No dosage adjustment necessary. Not studied in patients with CrCl ≤50 mL/minute or in hemodialysis.

Peginterferon Alfa and Ribavirin: Refer to individual monographs.

Hepatic Impairment

Telaprevir:

Mild (Child-Pugh class A) impairment: No dosage adjustment necessary.

Moderate or severe impairment (Child-Pugh class B or C): Use is not recommended in patients with decompensated liver disease or with moderate or severe hepatic impairment (has not been studied).

Peginterferon Alfa and Ribavirin: Refer to individual monographs.

Dietary Considerations
Take with a meal (not low fat).

Administration
Administer with a meal (not low fat) within 30 minutes prior to each dose. Doses should be taken approximately every 10-14 hours. Administer concurrently with peginterferon alfa and ribavirin. Maintain adequate fluid intake/hydration. Swallow tablets whole; do not chew, crush, break, cut, or dissolve the tablets. If a dose is missed within 6 hours of the time it is usually taken, take as soon as possible. If more than 6 hours have passed since the dose is usually taken, the missed dose should not be taken and the patient should resume the usual schedule.

Monitoring Parameters

CBC with differential and platelet count, serum electrolytes, serum creatinine, TSH, bilirubin, liver enzymes, and uric acid at baseline and weeks 2, 4, 8 and 12, then periodically (and when clinically indicated)

Serum HCV-RNA at baseline, weeks 4, 8, 12 and 24, end of treatment, during treatment follow up, and when clinically indicated

Pretreatment and monthly pregnancy test up to 6 months following discontinuation of therapy for women of child-bearing age

Hydration status, including fluid intake/output, urine output, signs/symptoms of dehydration

Reference Range

Treatment futility: HCV-RNA ≥1000 units/mL at treatment week 4 or 12 or confirmed, detectable HCV-RNA at treatment week 24

Rapid virologic response (RVR): Absence of detectable HCV-RNA after 4 weeks of treatment

Extended rapid virologic response (eRVR): Absence of detectable HCV-RNA after 4 and 12 weeks of treatment

Early virologic response (EVR): Absence of detectable HCV-RNA after 12 weeks of treatment

Sustained virologic response (SVR): Absence of HCV-RNA in the serum 32-78 weeks after completion of a 24 week treatment course or 56-78 weeks after a 48 week treatment course.

Additional Information In clinical studies of treatment-naive patients, a sustained virologic response (SVR) of ~75% (~65% in African-Americans) was observed with peginterferon alfa, ribavirin, and telaprevir versus 46% with peginterferon and ribavirin alone. Adherence to 3 times/day dosing is needed; resistance is increased and efficacy is affected when dosed every 12 hours.

Dosage Forms Excipient information presented when available (limited, particularly for generics); consult specific product labeling. [DSC] = Discontinued product

Tablet, Oral:

Incivek: 375 mg [DSC] [contains fd&c blue #2 (indigotine), fd&c red #40]

Telavancin (tel a VAN sin)

Brand Names: US Vibativ

Index Terms TD-6424; Telavancin Hydrochloride

Pharmacologic Category Glycopeptide

Use

Complicated skin and skin structure infections: Treatment of complicated skin and skin structure infections caused by susceptible gram-positive organisms including methicillin-susceptible or -resistant *Staphylococcus aureus*, vancomycin-susceptible *Enterococcus faecalis*, and *Streptococcus pyogenes*, *Streptococcus agalactiae*, or *Streptococcus anginosus* group

Hospital-acquired and ventilator-associated bacterial pneumonia (HABP/VABP): Treatment of HABP/VABP caused by susceptible isolates of *Staphylococcus aureus* when alternative treatments are not appropriate

Pregnancy Considerations [U.S. Boxed Warning]: Based on animal data, adverse developmental outcomes have been observed. Prior to use, women of childbearing potential should have a serum pregnancy test. Use of telavancin is not recommended during pregnancy unless the potential benefit to the mother outweighs the possible risk to the fetus. Telavancin crosses the placenta (Nanovskaya, 2012). In women of childbearing potential, effective contraception should be used during therapy.

Healthcare providers are encouraged to enroll women exposed to telavancin during pregnancy in the Vibativ Pregnancy Registry 855-633-8479).

Breast-Feeding Considerations It is not known if telavancin is excreted in breast milk. The manufacturer recommends that caution be exercised when administering telavancin to nursing women.

Medication Guide Available Yes

Contraindications Hypersensitivity to telavancin or any component of the formulation; concomitant use of intravenous unfractionated heparin

Warnings/Precautions Hazardous agent - use appropriate precautions for handling and disposal (NIOSH 2014 [group 3]). **[U.S. Boxed Warning]: Based on animal data, adverse developmental outcomes have been observed. Prior to use, women of childbearing potential should have a serum pregnancy test. Use of telavancin is not recommended during pregnancy unless the potential benefit outweighs the risk to the fetus. [U.S. Boxed Warning]: New-onset or worsening renal impairment has occurred. Monitor renal function prior to, during (at least every 48 to 72 hours; more frequently if indicated), and following therapy in all patients.** May cause nephrotoxicity; usual risk factors include concomitant nephrotoxic medications or baseline comorbidities associated with decreased renal function (eg, baseline renal dysfunction, diabetes, hypertension, or heart failure). **[U.S. Boxed Warning]: In clinical studies, patients with preexisting moderate-to-severe renal impairment (CrCl ≤50 mL/minute) treated for hospital-acquired/ventilator-associated bacterial pneumonia (HABP/VABP) had increased (all cause) mortality versus vancomycin. Use in HABP/VABP only when benefit outweighs risk.** Serious hypersensitivity reactions, including anaphylaxis, have been reported after first or subsequent doses; some have been fatal. Discontinue if hypersensitivity or rash occurs. Telavancin is a semisynthetic derivative of vancomycin; cross-reactivity rates are unknown. Use with caution in patients with known vancomycin hypersensitivity.

May prolong QTc interval; avoid use in patients with a history of QTc prolongation, uncompensated heart failure, severe left ventricular hypertrophy, or concurrent administration of other medications known to prolong the QT interval. Clinical studies indicate mean maximal QTc prolongation of 12 to 15 msec at the end of 10 mg/kg infusion. Contains solubilizer cyclodextrin (hydroxypropyl-beta-cyclodextrin) which may accumulate in patients with renal dysfunction, although the clinical significance of this finding

is uncertain (Luke, 2010). Prolonged use may result in fungal or bacterial superinfection, including *C. difficile*-associated diarrhea (CDAD) and pseudomembranous colitis; CDAD has been observed >2 months postantibiotic treatment. Potentially significant drug-drug interactions may exist, requiring dose or frequency adjustment, additional monitoring, and/or selection of alternative therapy.

May interfere with tests used to monitor coagulation (eg, prothrombin time, INR, activated partial thromboplastin time, activated clotting time, coagulation based factor Xa tests) when samples drawn ≤18 hours after drug administration. Blood samples should be collected as close to the next dose of telavancin as possible or a non-phospholipid dependent coagulation test (eg, bleeding time, factor Xa [chromogenic assay], platelet aggregation study, thrombin time) should be used. Consider selecting an alternative anticoagulant not requiring aPTT monitoring; concomitant use of telavancin with IV unfractionated heparin is contraindicated. Rapid IV administration may result in flushing, rash, urticaria, and/or pruritus; slowing or stopping the infusion may alleviate these symptoms. In the elderly, lower doses are often required secondary to age-related decreases in renal function.

Adverse Reactions

>10%:

Central nervous system: Insomnia (13%), psychiatric disturbance (12%), headache (11%)

Gastrointestinal: Metallic taste (33%), nausea (5% to 27%), vomiting (5% to 14%)

Genitourinary: Proteinuria (13%)

Renal: Increased serum creatinine (8% to 16%)

1% to 10%:

Central nervous system: Dizziness (6%), paresthesia (5%), local pain (4%), rigors (4%)

Dermatologic: Pruritus (3% to 6%), skin rash (4%), localized erythema (3%)

Endocrine & metabolic: Albuminuria (micro) (7%), hypokalemia (7%)

Gastrointestinal: Diarrhea (7%), decreased appetite (3%), abdominal pain (2%)

Genitourinary: Acute renal failure (5%)

Hematologic & oncologic: Thrombocytopenia (7%)

Renal: Renal insufficiency (3%)

Respiratory: Dyspnea (8%)

<1% (Limited to important or life-threatening): *Clostridium difficile* associated diarrhea, hearing loss (transient), hypersensitivity reaction, nephrotoxicity, prolonged Q-T interval on ECG, urticaria

Drug Interactions

Metabolism/Transport Effects None known.

Avoid Concomitant Use

Avoid concomitant use of Telavancin with any of the following: BCG (Intravesical); Heparin; Highest Risk QTc-Prolonging Agents; Ivabradine; Mifepristone

Increased Effect/Toxicity

Telavancin may increase the levels/effects of: Highest Risk QTc-Prolonging Agents; Moderate Risk QTc-Prolonging Agents

The levels/effects of Telavancin may be increased by: Ivabradine; Mifepristone; QTc-Prolonging Agents (Indeterminate Risk and Risk Modifying)

Decreased Effect

Telavancin may decrease the levels/effects of: BCG (Intravesical); BCG Vaccine (Immunization); Heparin; Sodium Picosulfate; Typhoid Vaccine

Preparation for Administration Hazardous agent; use appropriate precautions for handling and disposal (NIOSH 2014 [group 3]).

Reconstitute 250 mg vial with 15 mL of D$_5$W, NS, or SWFI to yield 15 mg/mL (total volume of ~17 mL). Reconstitute 750 mg vial with 45 mL of of D$_5$W, NS, or SWFI to yield 15 mg/mL (total volume of ~50 mL). Allow vacuum to pull the diluent into the vial; discard vial if this did not occur. Reconstitution generally takes <2 minutes, although may take up to 20 minutes. Do not shake the vial or final solution for infusion. Prior to administration, dilute dose in 100-250 mL D$_5$W, LR, or NS to a final concentration of 0.6-8 mg/mL.

Storage/Stability Store intact vials at 2°C to 8°C (35°F to 46°F); excursions permitted up to 25°C (77°F); avoid excess heat. **Note:** Vials contain no bacteriostatic agent. Reconstituted solution in the vial should be used within 12 hours at room temperature or 7 days refrigerated; solutions admixed for infusion are stable at room temperature for 12 hours or under refrigeration for 7 days. Total time in vial **plus** time in infusion bag should not exceed 12 hours at room temperature or 7 days if refrigerated at 2°C to 8°C (35°F to 46°F). Solutions admixed for infusion can also be stored at -30°C to -10°C (-22°F to 14°F) for ≤32 days.

Mechanism of Action Exerts concentration-dependent bactericidal activity; inhibits bacterial cell wall synthesis by blocking polymerization and cross-linking of peptidoglycan by binding to D-Ala-D-Ala portion of cell wall. Unlike vancomycin, additional mechanism involves disruption of membrane potential and changes cell permeability due to presence of lipophilic side chain moiety.

Pharmacodynamics/Kinetics

Distribution: V$_{ss}$: 0.13 L/kg

Protein binding: ~90%; primarily to albumin

Half-life elimination: 6.6-9.6 hours

Excretion: Urine (~76%); feces (<1%)

Dosing

Adult & Geriatric

Complicated skin and skin structure infection: IV: 10 mg/kg every 24 hours for 1-2 weeks

Hospital-acquired and ventilator-associated bacterial pneumonia (HABP/VABP): IV: 10 mg/kg every 24 hours for 1-3 weeks

Renal Impairment Note: Renal function may be estimated using the Cockcroft-Gault formula for dosage adjustment purposes.

CrCl >50 mL/minute: No dosage adjustment necessary

CrCl 30-50 mL/minute: 7.5 mg/kg every 24 hours

CrCl 10 to <30 mL/minute: 10 mg/kg every 48 hours

CrCl <10 mL/minute: No dosage adjustment provided in manufacturer's labeling (has not been studied).

ESRD and hemodialysis patients: No dosage adjustment provided in manufacturer's labeling (has not been studied).

Hepatic Impairment

Mild-to-moderate hepatic impairment (Child-Pugh class A or B): No dosage adjustment necessary.

Severe hepatic impairment (Child-Pugh class C): No dosage adjustment provided in manufacturer's labeling (has not been studied).

Administration Administer IV over 60 minutes. Other medications should not be infused simultaneously through the same IV line. When the same intravenous line is used for sequential infusion of other medications, flush line with D$_5$W, LR, or NS before and after infusing telavancin.

Red-man syndrome may occur if the infusion is too rapid. It is not an allergic reaction, but may be characterized by hypotension and/or a maculopapular rash appearing on the face, neck, trunk, and/or upper extremities. If this should occur, discontinuing or slowing the infusion rate may eliminate these reactions.

Hazardous agent; use appropriate precautions for handling and disposal (NIOSH 2014 [group 3]).

Monitoring Parameters Renal function (prior to start, every 48-72 hours; more frequently if indicated, and following therapy), pregnancy test

Test Interactions

Interferes with the following coagulation assessments when using samples drawn 18 hours or less after telavancin administration (causes artificially increased clotting times): PT, INR, aPTT, ACT, Xa (coagulation based assay). Collect blood samples for these coagulation tests as close as possible prior to administration of the next dose of telavancin, use a non-phospholipid dependent coagulation test (eg, bleeding time, factor Xa [chromogenic assay], platelet aggregation study, thrombin time), or select an alternative anticoagulant not requiring aPTT monitoring; concomitant use of telavancin and IV unfractionated heparin is contraindicated.

Interferes with urine protein via qualitative dipstick and quantitative dye methods.

Dosage Forms Excipient information presented when available (limited, particularly for generics); consult specific product labeling.

Solution Reconstituted, Intravenous [preservative free]:

Vibativ: 250 mg (1 ea); 750 mg (1 ea)

◆ Telavancin Hydrochloride see Telavancin *on page 1745*

Telithromycin (tel ith roe MYE sin)

Brand Names: US Ketek

Index Terms HMR 3647

Pharmacologic Category Antibiotic, Ketolide

Use Community-acquired pneumonia: Treatment of mild to moderate community-acquired pneumonia (CAP) due to *Streptococcus pneumoniae* (including multidrug-resistant isolates), *Haemophilus influenzae*, *Moraxella catarrhalis*, *Chlamydophila* (also known as *Chlamydia*) *pneumoniae*, or *Mycoplasma pneumoniae* in patients 18 years and older.

Medication Guide Available Yes

Dosing

Adult & Geriatric Community-acquired pneumonia (CAP): Oral: 800 mg once daily for 7-10 days

Renal Impairment
CrCl ≥30 mL/minute: No dosage adjustment necessary
CrCl <30 mL/minute: 600 mg once daily
CrCl <30 mL/minute and concomitant hepatic impairment: 400 mg once daily
Hemodialysis: 600 mg once daily; administer after dialysis on dialysis days

Hepatic Impairment No dosage adjustment necessary, unless concurrent renal impairment (eg, CrCl <30 mL/minute) is present.

Additional Information Complete prescribing information should be consulted for additional detail.

Dosage Forms Excipient information presented when available (limited, particularly for generics); consult specific product labeling.
Tablet, Oral:
Ketek: 300 mg, 400 mg

Telmisartan (tel mi SAR tan)

Brand Names: US Micardis
Brand Names: Canada ACT Telmisartan; Micardis; Mylan-Telmisartan; PMS-Telmisartan; Ran-Telmisartan; Sandoz-Telmisartan; Teva-Telmisartan
Pharmacologic Category Angiotensin II Receptor Blocker; Antihypertensive

Use
Cardiovascular risk reduction: Cardiovascular risk reduction in patients ≥55 years of age unable to take ACE inhibitors and who are at high risk of major cardiovascular events (eg, MI, stroke, death)
Hypertension: For the treatment of hypertension, alone or in combination with other antihypertensive agents

Guideline recommendations:
Hypertension: The 2014 guideline for the management of high blood pressure in adults (Eighth Joint National Committee [JNC 8; James, 2013]) recommends initiation of pharmacologic treatment to lower blood pressure for the following patients:
• Patients ≥60 years of age with systolic blood pressure (SBP) ≥150 mm Hg or diastolic blood pressure (DBP) ≥90 mm Hg. Goal of therapy is SBP <150 mm Hg and DBP <90 mm Hg.
• Patients <60 years of age with SBP ≥140 mm Hg or DBP ≥90 mm Hg. Goal of therapy is SBP <140 mm Hg and DBP <90 mm Hg.
• Patients ≥18 years of age with diabetes and SBP ≥140 mm Hg or DBP ≥90 mm Hg. Goal of therapy is SBP <140 mm Hg and DBP <90 mm Hg.
• Patients ≥18 years of age with chronic kidney disease (CKD) and SBP ≥140 mm Hg or DBP ≥90 mm Hg. Goal of therapy is SBP <140 mm Hg and DBP <90 mm Hg.
Chronic kidney disease (CKD) and hypertension: Regardless of race or diabetes status, the use of an ACE inhibitor (ACEI) or angiotensin receptor blocker (ARB) as initial therapy is recommended to improve kidney outcomes. In the general nonblack population (without CKD), including those with diabetes, initial antihypertensive treatment should consist of a thiazide-type diuretic, calcium channel blocker, ACEI, or ARB. In the general black population (without CKD), including those with diabetes, initial antihypertensive treatment should consist of a thiazide-type diuretic or a calcium channel blocker instead of an ACEI or ARB.
Coronary artery disease and hypertension: The American Heart Association, American College of Cardiology and American Society of Hypertension (AHA/ACC/ASH) 2015 scientific statement for the treatment of hypertension in patients with coronary artery disease (CAD) recommends the use of an ARB (or ACE inhibitor) as part of a regimen in patients with hypertension and chronic stable angina if there is prior MI, LV systolic dysfunction, diabetes mellitus, or CKD. A BP target of <140/90 mm Hg is reasonable for the secondary prevention of cardiovascular events. A lower target BP (<130/80 mm Hg) may be appropriate in some individuals with CAD, previous MI, stroke or transient ischemic attack, or CAD risk equivalents (AHA/ACC/ASH [Rosendorff 2015]).

Pregnancy Considerations [U.S. Boxed Warning]: Drugs that act on the renin-angiotensin system can cause injury and death to the developing fetus. Discontinue as soon as possible once pregnancy is detected. The use of drugs which act on the renin-angiotensin system are associated with oligohydramnios. Oligohydramnios, due to decreased fetal renal function, may lead to fetal lung hypoplasia and skeletal malformations. Use is also associated with anuria, hypotension, renal failure, skull hypoplasia, and death in the fetus/neonate. The exposed fetus should be monitored for fetal growth, amniotic fluid volume, and organ formation. Infants exposed *in utero* should be monitored for hyperkalemia, hypotension, and oliguria (exchange transfusions or dialysis may be needed). These adverse events are generally associated with maternal use in the second and third trimesters.

Untreated chronic maternal hypertension is also associated with adverse events in the fetus, infant, and mother. The use of angiotensin II receptor blockers is not recommended to treat chronic uncomplicated hypertension in pregnant women and should generally be avoided in women of reproductive potential (ACOG, 2013).

Breast-Feeding Considerations It is not known if telmisartan is excreted in breast milk. Due to the potential for serious adverse reactions in the nursing infant, a decision should be made whether to discontinue nursing or to discontinue the drug, taking into account the importance of treatment to the mother. The Canadian labeling contraindicates use in nursing women.

Contraindications Known hypersensitivity (eg, anaphylaxis, angioedema) to telmisartan or any component of the formulation; concurrent use of aliskiren in patients with diabetes

Canadian labeling: Additional contraindications: Concomitant use with aliskiren in patients with moderate-to-severe renal impairment (GFR <60 mL/min/1.73 m^2); pregnancy; breast-feeding; fructose intolerance

Warnings/Precautions [U.S. Boxed Warning]: Drugs that act on the renin-angiotensin system can cause injury and death to the developing fetus. Discontinue as soon as possible once pregnancy is detected. May cause hyperkalemia; avoid potassium supplementation unless specifically required by healthcare provider. Avoid use or use a smaller dose in patients who are volume depleted; correct depletion first. May be associated with deterioration of renal function and/or increases in serum creatinine, particularly in patients with low renal blood flow (eg, renal artery stenosis, heart failure) whose glomerular filtration rate (GFR) is dependent on efferent arteriolar vasoconstriction by angiotensin II. Use with caution in unstented unilateral/bilateral renal artery stenosis. When unstented bilateral renal artery stenosis is present, use is generally avoided due to the elevated risk of deterioration in renal function unless possible benefits outweigh risks. Use with caution with preexisting renal insufficiency; significant aortic/mitral stenosis. Potentially significant drug-drug interactions may exist, requiring dose or frequency adjustment, additional monitoring, and/or selection of alternative therapy. Use with caution in patients who have biliary obstructive disorders or hepatic dysfunction. In surgical patients on chronic angiotensin receptor blocker (ARB) therapy, intraoperative hypotension may occur with induction and maintenance of general anesthesia. Product contains sorbitol. The Canadian labeling contraindicates use in fructose intolerant patients.

Angioedema has been reported rarely with some angiotensin II receptor antagonists (ARBs) and may occur at any time during treatment (especially following first dose). It may involve the head and neck (potentially compromising airway) or the intestine (presenting with abdominal pain). Patients with idiopathic or hereditary angioedema or previous angioedema associated with ACE-inhibitor therapy may be at an increased risk. Prolonged frequent monitoring may be required, especially if tongue, glottis, or larynx are involved, as they are associated with airway obstruction. Patients with a history of airway surgery may have a higher risk of airway obstruction. Discontinue therapy immediately if angioedema occurs. Aggressive early management is critical. Intramuscular (IM) administration of epinephrine may be necessary. Do not readminister to patients who have had angioedema with ARBs.

Adverse Reactions May be associated with worsening of renal function in patients dependent on renin-angiotensin-aldosterone system.

1% to 10%:
Cardiovascular: Intermittent claudication (7%; placebo 6%), chest pain (≥1%), hypertension (≥1%), peripheral edema (≥1%)
Central nervous system: Dizziness (≥1%), fatigue (≥1%), headache (≥1%), pain (≥1%)
Dermatologic: Skin ulcer (3%; placebo 2%)
Gastrointestinal: Diarrhea (3%), abdominal pain (≥1%), dyspepsia (≥1%), nausea (≥1%)
Genitourinary: Urinary tract infection (≥1%)
Neuromuscular & skeletal: Back pain (3%), myalgia (≥1%)
Respiratory: Upper respiratory infection (7%), sinusitis (3%), cough (≥1%), pharyngitis (1%)
<1% (Limited to important or life-threatening): Abnormal ECG, abscess, allergic reaction, anaphylaxis, anemia,

angina, angioedema, arthritis, asthma, atrial fibrillation, bradycardia, cerebrovascular disorder, CHF, conjunctivitis, creatinine kinase increased, depression, diabetes mellitus, eczema, edema, epistaxis, erectile dysfunction, fixed drug eruption, fungal infection, gastroenteritis, gout, hepatic dysfunction, hypercholesterolemia, hyperkalemia, hypersensitivity, hypoglycemia (diabetic patients), hypotension, impotence, insomnia, MI, migraine, neoplasm, orthostatic hypotension (more frequent in dialysis patients), otitis media, renal failure, rhabdomyolysis, reflux, serum creatinine increased, syncope, tachycardia, tendon pain, thrombocytopenia, uric acid increased

Drug Interactions

Metabolism/Transport Effects Inhibits CYP2C19 (weak)

Avoid Concomitant Use

Avoid concomitant use of Telmisartan with any of the following: Ramipril

Increased Effect/Toxicity

Telmisartan may increase the levels/effects of: ACE Inhibitors; Amifostine; Antipsychotic Agents (Second Generation [Atypical]); Cardiac Glycosides; Ciprofloxacin (Systemic); CycloSPORINE (Systemic); Drospirenone; DULoxetine; Hypotension-Associated Agents; Levodopa; Lithium; Nonsteroidal Anti-Inflammatory Agents; Potassium-Sparing Diuretics; Ramipril; Sodium Phosphates

The levels/effects of Telmisartan may be increased by: Alfuzosin; Aliskiren; Barbiturates; Brimonidine (Topical); Canagliflozin; Dapoxetine; Diazoxide; Eplerenone; Heparin; Heparin (Low Molecular Weight); Herbs (Hypotensive Properties); Molsidomine; Nicorandil; Obinutuzumab; Pentoxifylline; Phosphodiesterase 5 Inhibitors; Potassium Salts; Prostacyclin Analogues; Tolvaptan; Trimethoprim

Decreased Effect

The levels/effects of Telmisartan may be decreased by: Amphetamines; Herbs (Hypertensive Properties); Methylphenidate; Nonsteroidal Anti-Inflammatory Agents; Yohimbine

Storage/Stability Store at 25°C (77°F); excursions are permitted between 15°C and 30°C (59°F and 86°F). Tablets should not be removed from blisters until immediately before administration.

Mechanism of Action Angiotensin II acts as a vasoconstrictor. In addition to causing direct vasoconstriction, angiotensin II also stimulates the release of aldosterone. Once aldosterone is released, sodium as well as water is reabsorbed. The end result is an elevation in blood pressure. Telmisartan is a nonpeptide AT1 angiotensin II receptor antagonist. This binding prevents angiotensin II from binding to the receptor thereby blocking the vasoconstriction and the aldosterone secreting effects of angiotensin II.

Pharmacodynamics/Kinetics Orally active, not a prodrug

Onset of action: 1 to 2 hours

Duration: Up to 24 hours

Distribution: V_d: 500 L

Protein binding: >99.5%; primarily to albumin and alpha$_1$-acid glycoprotein

Metabolism: Hepatic via conjugation to inactive metabolites; not metabolized via CYP

Bioavailability (dose dependent): 42% to 58%; Hepatic impairment: Approaches 100%

Half-life elimination: Terminal: 24 hours

Time to peak, plasma: 0.5 to 1 hours

Excretion: Feces (97%)

Clearance: Total body: 800 mL/minute

Dosing

Adult & Geriatric

Hypertension: Oral: Initial: 40 mg once daily; usual dosage range (ASH/ISH [Weber, 2014]): 40 to 80 mg daily. Patients with volume depletion should be initiated on the lower dosage range with close supervision

Cardiovascular risk reduction: Oral: 80 mg once daily. **Note:** It is unknown whether doses <80 mg daily are associated with a reduction in risk of cardiovascular morbidity or mortality.

Renal Impairment No dosage adjustment necessary; hemodialysis patients are more susceptible to orthostatic hypotension

Hepatic Impairment Initiate therapy with low dose; titrate slowly and monitor closely.

Canadian labeling: Recommended initial dose: 40 mg daily

Dietary Considerations May be taken without regard to meals. Product contains sorbitol.

Administration May be administered without regard to meals.

Monitoring Parameters Blood pressure; electrolytes, serum creatinine, BUN

Dosage Forms Excipient information presented when available (limited, particularly for generics); consult specific product labeling.

Tablet, Oral:

Micardis: 20 mg, 40 mg, 80 mg

Generic: 20 mg, 40 mg, 80 mg

Telmisartan and Amlodipine

(tel mi SAR tan & am LOE di peen)

Brand Names: US Twynsta

Brand Names: Canada Twynsta

Index Terms Amlodipine and Telmisartan; Amlodipine Besylate and Telmisartan

Pharmacologic Category Angiotensin II Receptor Blocker; Antianginal Agent; Antihypertensive; Calcium Channel Blocker; Calcium Channel Blocker, Dihydropyridine

Use Hypertension:

U.S. labeling: Treatment of hypertension, including initial treatment in patients who will require multiple antihypertensives for adequate control

Canadian labeling: Treatment of mild-to-moderate hypertension in patients whom combination therapy is appropriate; not indicated for initial therapy

Dosing

Adult Dose is individualized; combination product may be substituted for individual components in patients currently maintained on both agents separately or in patients not adequately controlled with monotherapy (using one of the agents or an agent within the same antihypertensive class). May also be used as initial therapy in patients who are likely to need >1 antihypertensive to control blood pressure. **Note:** Use as initial therapy is not an approved indication in the Canadian labeling.

Hypertension: Oral:

Initial therapy (antihypertensive naive): Telmisartan 40 mg/amlodipine 5 mg once daily; dose may be increased after 2 weeks of therapy. Patients requiring larger blood pressure reductions may be started on telmisartan 80 mg/amlodipine 5 mg once daily. Maximum recommended dose: Telmisartan 80 mg/day, amlodipine 10 mg/day

Add-on/replacement therapy: Telmisartan 40-80 mg and amlodipine 5-10 mg once daily depending upon previous doses, current control, and goals of therapy; dose may be titrated after 2 weeks of therapy. Maximum recommended dose: Telmisartan 80 mg/day; amlodipine 10 mg/day

Geriatric Not recommended for initial therapy in patients ≥75 years of age. For add-on/replacement therapy, initiate amlodipine therapy at 2.5 mg once daily and titrate slowly. **Note:** Use of individual agents may be necessary if the appropriate combination dose is not available. **Note:** Use as initial therapy is not an approved indication in the Canadian labeling.

Renal Impairment No dosage adjustment necessary; titrate slowly in severe impairment.

Hepatic Impairment Not recommended for initial therapy. For add-on/replacement therapy, initiate amlodipine at 2.5 mg once daily with low-dose telmisartan and titrate slowly; **Note:** Use of individual agents is necessary as the appropriate combination dose is not available. Upon titration to therapeutic dose, may initiate combination dose if available. Canadian labeling contraindicates use in severe hepatic impairment or with biliary obstructive disorders.

Additional Information Complete prescribing information should be consulted for additional detail.

Dosage Forms Excipient information presented when available (limited, particularly for generics); consult specific product labeling.

Tablet, oral:

Twynsta® 40/5: Telmisartan 40 mg and amlodipine 5 mg

Twynsta® 40/10: Telmisartan 40 mg and amlodipine 10 mg

Twynsta® 80/5: Telmisartan 80 mg and amlodipine 5 mg

Twynsta® 80/10: Telmisartan 80 mg and amlodipine 10 mg

Generic: Telmisartan 40 mg and amlodipine 5 mg; telmisartan 40 mg and amlodipine 10 mg; telmisartan 80 mg and amlodipine 5 mg; telmisartan 80 mg and amlodipine 10 mg

Telmisartan and Hydrochlorothiazide

(tel mi SAR tan & hye droe klor oh THYE a zide)

Brand Names: US Micardis HCT

Brand Names: Canada ACH-Telmisartan HCTZ; ACT Telmisartan/HCT; Micardis Plus; Mylan-Telmisartan HCTZ; PMS-Telmisartan HCTZ; RAN-Telmisartan HCTZ; Sandoz-

Telmisartan HCT; Telmisartan HCTZ; Teva-Telmisartan HCTZ

Index Terms Hydrochlorothiazide and Telmisartan

Pharmacologic Category Angiotensin II Receptor Blocker; Antihypertensive; Diuretic, Thiazide

Use Hypertension: Treatment of hypertension; **Note:** A fixed-dose combination product should not be used for initial therapy

Dosing

Adult

Hypertension: Oral:

Replacement therapy: Combination product can be substituted for individual titrated agents.

Initiation of combination therapy when monotherapy has failed to achieve desired effects:

Patients currently on telmisartan:

U.S. labeling: Initial dose if blood pressure is not currently controlled on monotherapy of telmisartan 80 mg: Telmisartan 80 mg/hydrochlorothiazide 12.5 mg once daily; manufacturer labeling suggests that dose may be titrated up to telmisartan 160 mg/hydrochlorothiazide 25 mg if needed; however, in mild to moderate hypertension, doses of telmisartan >80 mg were not associated with a greater reduction in blood pressure (Smith, 2000).

Canadian labeling: If blood pressure is not currently controlled on monotherapy of telmisartan 80 mg: Telmisartan 80 mg/hydrochlorothiazide 12.5 mg once daily; may titrate up to telmisartan 80 mg/hydrochlorothiazide 25 mg if needed.

Patients currently on hydrochlorothiazide:

U.S. labeling: Initial dose if blood pressure is not currently controlled on monotherapy of 25 mg once daily: Telmisartan 80 mg/hydrochlorothiazide 12.5 mg once daily or telmisartan 80 mg/hydrochlorothiazide 25 mg once daily; manufacturer labeling suggests that dose may be titrated up to telmisartan 160 mg/hydrochlorothiazide 25 mg if blood pressure remains uncontrolled after 2-4 weeks of therapy. In mild to moderate hypertension, doses of telmisartan >80 mg were not associated with a greater reduction in blood pressure (Smith, 2000). Patients who develop hypokalemia while on hydrochlorothiazide 25 mg may be switched to telmisartan 80 mg/hydrochlorothiazide 12.5 mg.

Canadian labeling: Specific dosing recommendations for the combination product are not provided by the manufacturer. When possible, discontinue the diuretic 2-3 days prior to initiation of telmisartan monotherapy. If diuretic therapy is necessary, use of individual agents may be necessary to allow for dose titration.

Geriatric Refer to adult dosing. Monitor renal function.

Renal Impairment

CrCl >30 mL/minute: No dosage adjustment necessary.

CrCl ≤30 mL/minute: Not recommended.

Hepatic Impairment

Mild to moderate hepatic impairment or biliary obstructive disorders: Initial: Telmisartan 40 mg/hydrochlorothiazide 12.5 mg.

Severe hepatic impairment: Not recommended.

Additional Information Complete prescribing information should be consulted for additional detail.

Dosage Forms Excipient information presented when available (limited, particularly for generics); consult specific product labeling.

Tablet, oral:

Micardis® HCT:

40/12.5: Telmisartan 40 mg and hydrochlorothiazide 12.5 mg

80/12.5: Telmisartan 80 mg and hydrochlorothiazide 12.5 mg

80/25: Telmisartan 80 mg and hydrochlorothiazide 25 mg

Generic:

40/12.5: Telmisartan 40 mg and hydrochlorothiazide 12.5 mg

80/12.5: Telmisartan 80 mg and hydrochlorothiazide 12.5 mg

80/25: Telmisartan 80 mg and hydrochlorothiazide 25 mg

Dosage Forms: Canada Excipient information presented when available (limited, particularly for generics); consult specific product labeling.

Tablet, oral:

Micardis Plus:

80/12.5: Telmisartan 80 mg and hydrochlorothiazide 12.5 mg

80/25: Telmisartan 80 mg and hydrochlorothiazide 25 mg

◆ Telmisartan HCTZ (Can) *see* Telmisartan and Hydrochlorothiazide *on page 1748*

◆ Telzir (Can) *see* Fosamprenavir *on page 811*

Temazepam (te MAZ e pam)

Brand Names: US Restoril

Brand Names: Canada Apo-Temazepam; Dom-Temazepam; PHL-Temazepam; PMS-Temazepam; Restoril; Temazepam-15; Temazepam-30; Teva-Temazepam

Pharmacologic Category Benzodiazepine

Use Insomnia: Short-term treatment of insomnia

Medication Guide Available Yes

Dosing

Adult Insomnia: Oral: Usual dose: 15-30 mg at bedtime; some patients may respond to 7.5 mg in transient insomnia

Geriatric Insomnia: Oral:

U.S. labeling: Initial: 7.5 mg in elderly or debilitated patients at bedtime.

Canadian labeling: Initial: 15 mg in elderly or debilitated patients at bedtime.

Renal Impairment No dosage adjustment provided in manufacturer's labeling.

Hepatic Impairment No dosage adjustment provided in manufacturer's labeling.

Additional Information Complete prescribing information should be consulted for additional detail.

Dosage Forms Excipient information presented when available (limited, particularly for generics); consult specific product labeling.

Capsule, Oral:

Restoril: 7.5 mg, 15 mg, 22.5 mg, 30 mg [contains brilliant blue fcf (fd&c blue #1)]

Generic: 7.5 mg, 15 mg, 22.5 mg, 30 mg

Dosage Forms: Canada Excipient information presented when available (limited, particularly for generics); consult specific product labeling.

Capsule, Oral:

Restoril: 15 mg, 30 mg

Controlled Substance C-IV

◆ Temazepam-15 (Can) *see* Temazepam *on page 1749*

◆ Temazepam-30 (Can) *see* Temazepam *on page 1749*

◆ Temodal (Can) *see* Temozolomide *on page 1749*

◆ Temodar *see* Temozolomide *on page 1749*

◆ Temovate *see* Clobetasol *on page 412*

◆ Temovate E *see* Clobetasol *on page 412*

Temozolomide (te moe ZOE loe mide)

Brand Names: US Temodar

Brand Names: Canada ACH-Temozolomide; ACT Temozolomide; Temodal

Index Terms SCH 52365; TMZ

Pharmacologic Category Antineoplastic Agent, Alkylating Agent (Triazene)

Use

Anaplastic astrocytoma: Treatment of refractory anaplastic astrocytoma (refractory to a regimen containing a nitrosourea and procarbazine)

Glioblastoma multiforme: Treatment of newly-diagnosed glioblastoma multiforme (initially in combination with radiotherapy, then as maintenance treatment)

Canadian labeling: Treatment of newly-diagnosed glioblastoma multiforme (initially in combination with radiotherapy, then as maintenance treatment), treatment of recurrent or progressive glioblastoma multiforme or anaplastic astrocytoma

Pregnancy Considerations Adverse events were observed in animal reproduction studies. May cause fetal harm when administered to pregnant women. Male and female patients should avoid pregnancy while receiving temozolomide. The Canadian labeling recommends that male and female patients also avoid pregnancy for 6 months after discontinuation of therapy.

Breast-Feeding Considerations It is not known if temozolomide is excreted in breast milk. Due to the potential for serious adverse reactions in the nursing infant, the manufacturer recommends a decision be made whether to discontinue nursing or to discontinue the drug, taking into account the importance of treatment to the mother.

Contraindications

Hypersensitivity (eg, allergic reaction, anaphylaxis, urticaria, Stevens-Johnson syndrome, toxic epidermal necrolysis) to temozolomide or any component of the formulation; hypersensitivity to dacarbazine (both drugs are metabolized to MTIC)

Canadian labeling: Additional contraindications (not in U.S. labeling): Not recommended in patients with severe myelosuppression

Warnings/Precautions Hazardous agent - use appropriate precautions for handling and disposal (NIOSH 2014 [group 1]). *Pneumocystis jirovecii* pneumonia (PCP) may occur; risk is increased in those receiving steroids or longer dosing regimens; monitor all patients for development of PCP (particularly if also receiving corticosteroids); PCP prophylaxis is required in patients receiving radiotherapy in combination with the 42-day temozolomide regimen. Myelosuppression may occur; may require treatment interruption, dose reduction, and/or discontinuation; monitor blood counts; an increased incidence has been reported in geriatric and female patients. Prolonged pancytopenia resulting in aplastic anemia has been reported (may be fatal); concurrent use of temozolomide with medications associated with aplastic anemia (eg, carbamazepine, co-trimoxazole, phenytoin) may obscure assessment for development of aplastic anemia. ANC should be ≥1,500/mm^3 and platelets ≥100,000/mm^3 prior to treatment. Rare cases of myelodysplastic syndrome and secondary malignancies, including acute myeloid leukemia, have been reported. Use caution in patients with severe hepatic or renal impairment; has not been studied in dialysis patients. Hepatotoxicity has been reported; may be severe or fatal. Monitor liver function tests at baseline, halfway through the first cycle, prior to each subsequent cycle, and at ~2 to 4 weeks after the last dose. Post-marketing reports of hepatotoxicity have included liver function abnormalities, hepatitis, hepatic failure, cholestasis, hepatitis cholestasis, jaundice, cholelithiasis, hepatic steatosis, hepatic necrosis, hepatic lesion, and hepatic encephalopathy (Sarganas 2012).

Temozolomide is associated with a moderate emetic potential (Dupuis 2011; Roila 2010); antiemetics are recommended to prevent nausea and vomiting. Increased MGMT (O-6-methylguanine-DNA methyltransferase) activity/levels within tumor tissue is associated with temozolomide resistance. Glioblastoma patients with decreased levels (due to methylated MGMT promoter) may be more likely to benefit from the combination of radiation therapy and temozolomide (Hegi 2008; Stupp 2009). Determination of MGMT status may be predictive for response to alkylating agents. Potentially significant drug-drug interactions may exist, requiring dose or frequency adjustment, additional monitoring, and/or selection of alternative therapy. Bioequivalence has only been established when IV temozolomide is administered over 90 minutes; shorter or longer infusion times may result in suboptimal dosing.

Polysorbate 80: Some dosage forms may contain polysorbate 80 (also known as Tweens). Hypersensitivity reactions, usually a delayed reaction, have been reported following exposure to pharmaceutical products containing polysorbate 80 in certain individuals (Isaksson 2002; Lucente 2000; Shelley 1995). Thrombocytopenia, ascites, pulmonary deterioration, and renal and hepatic failure have been reported in premature neonates after receiving parenteral products containing polysorbate 80 (Alade 1986; CDC 1984). See manufacturer's labeling.

Adverse Reactions

>10%:

Cardiovascular: Peripheral edema (11%)

Central nervous system: Fatigue (34% to 61%), headache (23% to 41%), convulsions (6% to 23%), hemiparesis (18%), dizziness (5% to 12%), ataxia (8% to 11%)

Dermatologic: Alopecia (55%), skin rash (8% to 13%)

Gastrointestinal: Nausea (49% to 53%; grades 3/4: 1% to 10%), vomiting (29% to 42%; grades 3/4: 2% to 6%), constipation (22% to 33%), anorexia (9% to 27%), diarrhea (10% to 16%)

Hematologic & oncologic: Lymphocytopenia (grades 3/4: 55%), thrombocytopenia (grades 3/4: adults: 4% to 19%; children: 25%), neutropenia (grades 3/4: adults: 8% to 14%; children: 20%), leukopenia (grades 3/4: 11%)

Infection: Viral infection (11%)

Neuromuscular & skeletal: Weakness (7% to 13%)

Miscellaneous: Fever (13%)

1% to 10%:

Central nervous system: Amnesia (10%), insomnia (4% to 10%), drowsiness (9%), paresthesia (9%), paresis (8%), anxiety (7%), memory impairment (7%), abnormal gait (6%), depression (6%), confusion (5%)

Dermatologic: Pruritus (5% to 8%), xeroderma (5%), erythema (1%)

Endocrine & metabolic: Hypercorticoidism (8%), weight gain (5%)

Gastrointestinal: Stomatitis (9%), abdominal pain (5% to 9%), dysphagia (7%), dysgeusia (5%)

Genitourinary: Urinary incontinence (8%), urinary tract infection (8%), mastalgia (females 6%), urinary frequency (6%)

Hematologic & oncologic: Anemia (grades 3/4: 4%)

Hypersensitivity: Hypersensitivity reaction (≤3%)

Neuromuscular & skeletal: Back pain (8%), arthralgia (6%), myalgia (5%)

Ophthalmic: Blurred vision (5% to 8%), diplopia (5%), visual disturbance (visual deficit/vision changes 5%)

Respiratory: Pharyngitis (8%), upper respiratory tract infection (8%), cough (5% to 8%), sinusitis (6%), dyspnea (5%)

Miscellaneous: Radiation injury (2% maintenance phase after radiotherapy)

<1% (Limited to important or life-threatening): Alveolitis, anaphylaxis, aplastic anemia, cytomegalovirus disease (primary and reactivation), diabetes insipidus, emotional lability, erythema multiforme, febrile neutropenia, flu-like symptoms, hallucination, hematoma, hemorrhage, hepatitis, hepatitis B (reactivation), hepatotoxicity, herpes simplex infection, herpes zoster, hyperbilirubinemia, hyperglycemia, hypersensitivity pneumonitis, hypokalemia, metastases (including myeloid leukemia), myelodysplastic syndrome, opportunistic infection (including pneumocystosis), oral candidiasis, pancytopenia (may be prolonged), peripheral neuropathy, petechia, pneumonitis, pulmonary fibrosis, Stevens-Johnson syndrome

Drug Interactions

Metabolism/Transport Effects None known.

Avoid Concomitant Use

Avoid concomitant use of Temozolomide with any of the following: BCG (Intravesical); Deferiprone; Dipyrone; Natalizumab; Pimecrolimus; Tacrolimus (Topical); Tofacitinib; Vaccines (Live)

Increased Effect/Toxicity

Temozolomide may increase the levels/effects of: CloZAPine; Deferiprone; Fingolimod; Leflunomide; Natalizumab; Tofacitinib; Vaccines (Live)

The levels/effects of Temozolomide may be increased by: Denosumab; Dipyrone; Pimecrolimus; Roflumilast; Tacrolimus (Topical); Trastuzumab; Valproate Products

Decreased Effect

Temozolomide may decrease the levels/effects of: BCG (Intravesical); Coccidioides immitis Skin Test; Sipuleucel-T; Vaccines (Inactivated); Vaccines (Live)

The levels/effects of Temozolomide may be decreased by: Echinacea

Food Interactions Food reduces rate and extent of absorption. Management: Administer consistently either with food or without food (was administered in studies under fasting and nonfasting conditions).

Preparation for Administration Hazardous agent; use appropriate precautions for handling and disposal (NIOSH 2014 [group 1]). Bring to room temperature prior to reconstitution. Reconstitute each 100 mg vial with 41 mL sterile water for injection to a final concentration of 2.5 mg/mL. Swirl gently; do not shake. Place dose without further dilution into a 250 mL empty sterile infusion bag. Infusion must be completed within 14 hours of reconstitution.

Storage/Stability

Capsule: Store at room temperature of 25°C (77°F); excursions permitted to 15°C to 30°C (59°F to 86°F).

Injection: Store intact vials refrigerated at 2°C to 8°C (36°F to 46°F). Reconstituted vials may be stored for up to 14 hours at room temperature of 25°C (77°F); infusion must be completed within 14 hours of reconstitution.

Mechanism of Action Temozolomide is a prodrug which is rapidly and nonenzymatically converted to the active alkylating metabolite MTIC [(methyl-triazene-1-yl)-imidazole-4-carboxamide]; this conversion is spontaneous, nonenzymatic, and occurs under physiologic conditions in all tissues to which it distributes. The cytotoxic effects of MTIC are manifested through alkylation (methylation) of DNA at the O^6, N^7 guanine positions which lead to DNA double strand breaks and apoptosis. Non-cell cycle specific.

Pharmacodynamics/Kinetics

Absorption: Oral: Rapid and complete

Distribution: V_d: Parent drug: 0.4 L/kg; penetrates blood-brain barrier; CSF levels are ~35% to 39% of plasma levels (Yung 1999)

Protein binding: 15%

Metabolism: Prodrug, hydrolyzed to the active form, MTIC; MTIC is eventually eliminated as CO_2 and 5-aminoimidazole-4-carboxamide (AIC), a natural constituent in urine; CYP isoenzymes play only a minor role in metabolism (of temozolomide and MTIC)

Bioavailability: Oral: 100% (on a mg-per-mg basis, IV temozolomide, infused over 90 minutes, is bioequivalent to an oral dose)

Half-life elimination: Mean: Parent drug: 1.8 hours

Time to peak: Oral: Empty stomach: 1 hour; with food (high-fat meal): 2.25 hours

Excretion: Urine (~38%; parent drug 6%); feces <1%

Dosing

Adult Note: Temozolomide is associated with a moderate emetic potential (Roila 2010); antiemetics are recommended to prevent nausea and vomiting. Prior to dosing, ANC should be ≥1,500/mm³ and platelets ≥100,000/mm³.

Anaplastic astrocytoma (refractory): Oral, IV: Initial dose: 150 mg/m² once daily for 5 consecutive days of a 28-day treatment cycle. If ANC ≥1,500/mm³ and platelets ≥100,000/mm³, on day 1 of subsequent cycles, may increase to 200 mg/m² once daily for 5 consecutive days of a 28-day treatment cycle. May continue until disease progression.

Dosage modification for toxicity:

ANC <1,000/mm³ or platelets <50,000/mm³ on day 22 or day 29 (day 1 of next cycle): Postpone therapy until ANC >1,500/mm³ and platelets >100,000/mm³; reduce dose by 50 mg/m²/day (but not below 100 mg/m²) for subsequent cycle

ANC 1,000 to 1,500/mm³ or platelets 50,000-100,000/mm³ on day 22 or day 29 (day 1 of next cycle): Postpone therapy until ANC >1,500/mm³ and platelets >100,000/mm³; maintain initial dose

Glioblastoma multiforme (newly diagnosed, high-grade glioma): Oral, IV:

Concomitant phase: 75 mg/m² once daily for 42 days with focal radiotherapy (60 Gy administered in 30 fractions). **Note:** PCP prophylaxis is required during concomitant phase and should continue in patients who develop lymphocytopenia until lymphocyte recovery to ≤ grade 1. Obtain weekly CBC.

Continue at 75 mg/m² once daily throughout the 42-day concomitant phase (up to 49 days) as long as ANC ≥1,500/mm³, platelet count ≥100,000/mm³, and nonhematologic toxicity ≤ grade 1 (excludes alopecia, nausea/vomiting)

Dosage modification for toxicity:

ANC ≥500/mm³ but <1,500/mm³ or platelet count ≥10,000/mm³ but <100,000/mm³ or grade 2 nonhematologic toxicity (excludes alopecia, nausea/vomiting): Interrupt therapy

ANC <500/mm³ or platelet count <10,000/mm³ or grade 3/4 nonhematologic toxicity (excludes alopecia, nausea/vomiting): Discontinue therapy

Maintenance phase (consists of 6 treatment cycles):

Begin 4 weeks after concomitant phase completion. **Note:** Each subsequent cycle is 28 days (consisting of 5 days of drug treatment followed by 23 days without treatment). Draw CBC on day 22 (or within 48 hours of day 22); hold next cycle and do weekly CBC until ANC >1,500/mm³ and platelet count >100,000/mm³; dosing modification should be based on lowest blood counts and worst nonhematologic toxicity during the previous cycle.

Cycle 1: 150 mg/m² once daily for 5 days of a 28-day treatment cycle

Cycles 2 to 6: May increase to 200 mg/m² once daily for 5 days; repeat every 28 days (if ANC ≥1,500/mm³, platelets ≥100,000/mm³ and nonhematologic toxicities for cycle 1 are ≤ grade 2 [excludes alopecia, nausea/vomiting]); **Note:** If dose was not escalated at the onset of cycle 2, do not increase for cycles 3 to 6)

Dosage modification (during maintenance phase) for toxicity:

ANC <1,000/mm³, platelet count <50,000/mm³, or grade 3 nonhematologic toxicity (excludes alopecia, nausea/vomiting) during previous cycle: Decrease dose by 1 dose level (by 50 mg/m²/day for 5 days), unless dose has already been lowered to 100 mg/m²/day, then discontinue therapy.

If dose reduction <100 mg/m²/day is required or grade 4 nonhematologic toxicity (excludes alopecia, nausea/vomiting), or if the same grade 3 nonhematologic toxicity occurs after dose reduction: Discontinue therapy

Glioblastoma multiforme (recurrent glioma): *Canadian labeling (off-label use in the U.S.):* 200 mg/m² once daily for 5 days every 28 days; if previously treated with chemotherapy, initiate at 150 mg/m² once daily for 5 days every 28 days and increase to 200 mg/m² once daily for 5 days every 28 days with cycle 2 if no hematologic toxicity (Brada 2001; Yung 2000)

Cutaneous T-cell lymphoma, advanced (mycosis fungoides [MF] and Sézary syndrome [SS]; off-label use): Oral: 200 mg/m² once daily for 5 days every 28 days for up to 1 year (Querfeld 2011)

Ewing's sarcoma, recurrent or progressive (off-label use): Oral: 100 mg/m²/dose days 1 to 5 every 21 days (in combination with irinotecan) (Casey 2009). Additional data may be necessary to further define the role of temozolomide in this condition

Melanoma, advanced or metastatic (off-label use): Oral: 200 mg/m² once daily for 5 days every 28 days (for up to 12 cycles). For subsequent cycles reduce dose to 75% of the original dose for grade 3/4 hematologic toxicity and reduce the dose to 50% of the original dose for grade 3/4 nonhematologic toxicity (Middleton 2000).

Neuroendocrine tumors, advanced (off-label use): Oral: 150 mg/m² once daily for 7 days every 14 days (in combination with thalidomide) until disease progression (Kulke 2006) **or** 200 mg/m² once daily (at bedtime) days 10 to 14 of a 28-day treatment cycle (in combination with capecitabine) (Strosberg 2011)

Primary CNS lymphoma, refractory (off-label use): Oral: 150 mg/m² once daily for 5 days every 28 days, initially in combination with rituximab (for 4 cycles), followed by temozolomide monotherapy: 150 mg/m² once daily for 5 days every 28 days for 8 cycles (Wong 2004) **or** 150 mg/m² once daily on days 1 to 7 and 15 to 21 every 28 days (initially in combination with rituximab for 1 or 2 cycles), followed by temozolomide maintenance monotherapy: 150 mg/m² once daily for 5 days every 28 days (Enting 2004). However, additional data may be necessary to further define the role of temozolomide in this condition.

Soft tissue sarcoma (off-label use): Oral:

Soft tissue sarcoma, metastatic or unresectable: 75 mg/m² once daily for 6 weeks (Garcia del Muro 2005)

Hemangiopericytoma/solitary fibrous tumor: 150 mg/m² once daily days 1 to 7 and days 15 to 21 of a 28-day treatment cycle (in combination with bevacizumab) (Park 2011). Additional data may be necessary to further define the role of temozolomide in this condition

Geriatric Refer to adult dosing. **Note:** Patients ≥70 years of age in the anaplastic astrocytoma study had a higher incidence of grade 4 neutropenia and thrombocytopenia in the first cycle of therapy than patients <70 years of age.

Pediatric Note: Temozolomide is associated with a moderate emetic potential (Dupuis 2011); antiemetics are recommended to prevent nausea and vomiting.

Ewing's sarcoma, recurrent or progressive (off-label use): Children and Adolescents: Oral: Refer to adult dosing.

Neuroblastoma, relapsed or refractory (off-label use):

Children and Adolescents: Oral: 100 mg/m²/dose days 1 to 5 every 21 days (in combination with irinotecan) for up to 6 cycles (Bagatell 2011)

Children ≥6 months and Adolescents: Oral: 150 mg/m²/dose days 1 to 5 every 28 days (in combination with topotecan) until disease progression or unacceptable toxicity (Di Giannatale 2014)

Renal Impairment Oral:

CrCl ≥36 mL/minute/m²: There are no dosage adjustments provided in the manufacturer's labeling; however, dosage adjustment is not likely needed as no effect on temozolomide clearance was demonstrated.

Severe renal impairment (CrCl <36 mL/minute/m²): There are no dosage adjustments provided in the manufacturer's labeling; use with caution (has not been studied).

Dialysis patients: There are no dosage adjustments provided in the manufacturer's labeling (has not been studied).

Hepatic Impairment

Mild to moderate impairment: There are no dosage adjustments provided in the manufacturer's labeling; however, pharmacokinetics are similar to patients with normal hepatic function.

Severe hepatic impairment: There are no dosage adjustments provided in the manufacturer's labeling; use with caution (has not been studied).

Obesity *ASCO Guidelines for appropriate chemotherapy dosing in obese adults with cancer:* Utilize patient's actual body weight (full weight) for calculation of body surface area- or weight-based dosing, particularly when the intent of therapy is curative; manage regimen-related toxicities in the same manner as for nonobese patients; if a dose reduction is utilized due to toxicity, consider resumption of full weight-based dosing with subsequent cycles, especially if cause of toxicity (eg, hepatic or renal impairment) is resolved (Griggs 2012).

Dietary Considerations The incidence of nausea/vomiting is decreased when taken on an empty stomach. Take capsules consistently either with food or without food (absorption is affected by food). The Canadian labeling recommends taking capsules on an empty stomach one hour before a meal.

Administration Temozolomide is associated with a moderate emetic potential (Dupuis 2011; Roila 2010); antiemetics are recommended to prevent nausea and vomiting. Oral:

US labeling: Swallow capsules whole with a glass of water. Absorption is affected by food; therefore, administer consistently either with food or without food (was administered in studies under fasting and nonfasting conditions). May administer on an empty stomach and/or at bedtime to reduce nausea and vomiting. Do not repeat dose if vomiting occurs after dose is administered; wait until the next scheduled dose. Do not open or chew capsules; avoid contact with skin or mucous membranes if capsules are accidentally opened or damaged.

Canadian labeling: Administer on an empty stomach at least one hour before a meal. Swallow capsules whole with a glass of water. Do not repeat dose if vomiting occurs after dose is administered; wait until the next scheduled dose. Do not open or chew capsules; avoid contact with skin or mucous membranes if capsules are accidentally opened or damaged.

IV: Infuse over 90 minutes. Flush line before and after administration. May be administered through the same IV line as sodium chloride 0.9%; do not administer other medications through the same IV line.

Hazardous agent; use appropriate precautions for handling and disposal (NIOSH 2014 [group 1]). NIOSH recommends single gloving for administration of intact capsules. Although the manufacturer does not recommend opening capsules, if necessary to manipulate the capsules (eg, to prepare an oral suspension), it is recommended to double glove, wear a protective gown, and prepare in a controlled device (NIOSH 2014).

Monitoring Parameters CBC with differential and platelets (prior to each cycle; weekly during glioma concomitant phase treatment; at or within 48 hours of day 22 and weekly until ANC >1,500/mm^3 and platelets >100,000/mm^3 for glioma maintenance and astrocytoma treatment). Monitor liver function tests at baseline, halfway through the first cycle, prior to each subsequent cycle, and at ~2 to 4 weeks after the last dose. The Canadian labeling additionally recommends HBV screening at baseline (all patients) and monitoring for hepatitis or HBV reactivation during therapy and for several months after discontinuation (patients with evidence of current or prior HBV infection).

Dosage Forms Excipient information presented when available (limited, particularly for generics); consult specific product labeling.

Capsule, Oral:

Temodar: 5 mg [contains fd&c blue #2 (indigotine)]

Temodar: 20 mg, 100 mg

Temodar: 140 mg [contains fd&c blue #2 (indigotine)]

Temodar: 180 mg, 250 mg

Generic: 5 mg, 20 mg, 100 mg, 140 mg, 180 mg, 250 mg

Solution Reconstituted, Intravenous:

Temodar: 100 mg (1 ea) [pyrogen free; contains polysorbate 80]

Extemporaneous Preparations Hazardous agent: Use appropriate precautions for handling and disposal (NIOSH 2014 [group 1]). When manipulating capsules, NIOSH recommends double gloving, a protective gown, and preparation in a controlled device; if not prepared in a controlled device, respiratory and eye protection as well as ventilated engineering controls are recommended (NIOSH 2014).

A 10 mg/mL temozolomide oral suspension may be compounded in a vertical flow hood. Mix the contents of ten 100 mg capsules and 500 mg of povidone K-30 powder in a glass mortar; add 25 mg anhydrous citric acid dissolved in 1.5 mL purified water and mix to a uniform paste; mix while adding 50 mL Ora-Plus in incremental proportions.

Transfer to an amber plastic bottle, rinse mortar 4 times with small portions of either Ora-Sweet or Ora-Sweet SF, and add quantity of Ora-Sweet or Ora-Sweet SF sufficient to make 100 mL. Store in plastic amber prescription bottles; label "shake well" and "refrigerate". Note the beyond-use date. Stable for 7 days at room temperature or 60 days refrigerated (preferred).

Trissel LA, Yanping Z, and Koontz SE, "Temozolomide Stability in Extemporaneously Compounded Oral Suspension," *Int J Pharm Compound*, 2006, 10(5):396-9.

◆ **Tempra (Can)** *see* Acetaminophen *on page 25*

Temsirolimus (tem sir OH li mus)

Brand Names: US Torisel

Brand Names: Canada Torisel

Index Terms CCI-779

Pharmacologic Category Antineoplastic Agent, mTOR Kinase Inhibitor

Use Renal cell carcinoma, advanced: Treatment of advanced renal cell carcinoma (RCC)

Pregnancy Considerations Adverse events have been observed in animal reproduction studies. Based on its mechanism of action, temsirolimus may cause fetal harm if administered to a pregnant woman. Women of child-bearing potential should be advised to avoid pregnancy. Men and women should use effective birth control during temsirolimus treatment, and continue for 3 months after temsirolimus discontinuation.

Breast-Feeding Considerations It is not known if temsirolimus is excreted in breast milk. Due to the potential for serious adverse reactions in the nursing infant, a decision should be made to discontinue breast-feeding or to discontinue temsirolimus, taking into account the importance of treatment to the mother.

Contraindications Bilirubin >1.5 times the upper limit of normal (ULN)

Canadian labeling: Additional contraindications (not in U.S. labeling): History of anaphylaxis after exposure to temsirolimus, sirolimus, or any component of the formulation

Warnings/Precautions Hazardous agent - use appropriate precautions for handling and disposal (NIOSH 2014 [group 1]).

Hypersensitivity/infusion reactions (eg, anaphylaxis, apnea, dyspnea, flushing, loss of consciousness, hypotension, and/or chest pain) have been reported. Infusion reaction may occur during the initial infusion (early in infusion) or with subsequent infusions. Premedicate with an antihistamine (H$_1$ antagonist) prior to infusion; monitor throughout infusion (appropriate supportive care should be available); interrupt infusion for hypersensitivity reaction and observe patient for 30-60 minutes. With discretion, treatment may be resumed at a slower infusion rate; administer an H$_1$ antagonist (if not given as premedication) and/or an IV H$_2$ antagonist ~30 minutes prior to resuming infusion. For severe infusion reactions, assess risk versus benefit of continued treatment. Use with caution in patients with hypersensitivity temsirolimus, sirolimus (a metabolite), or polysorbate 80. Angioneurotic edema has been reported; concurrent use with other drugs known to cause angioedema (eg, ACE inhibitors) may increase risk.

Temsirolimus is predominantly cleared by the liver; use with caution and reduce dose in patients with mild hepatic impairment (bilirubin >1 to 1.5 x ULN or AST >ULN with bilirubin ≤ULN). Toxicities were increased in patients with baseline bilirubin >1.5 x ULN. Use is contraindicated in patients with moderate-to-severe hepatic impairment (bilirubin >1.5 x ULN).

Potentially significant interactions may exist, requiring dose or frequency adjustment, additional monitoring, and/or selection of alternative therapy. Avoid concomitant use with strong CYP3A4 inhibitors and strong CYP3A4 inducers; consider alternative agents that avoid or lessen the potential for CYP-mediated interactions. Patients should not be immunized with live, viral vaccines during or shortly after treatment and should avoid close contact with recently vaccinated (live vaccine) individuals. Patients who are receiving anticoagulant therapy or those with CNS tumors/metastases may be at increased risk for developing intracerebral bleeding (may be fatal). Combination therapy with temsirolimus and sunitinib has resulted in dose-limiting toxicities, including grade 3 or 4 rash, gout, and/or cellulitis.

Some dosage forms may contain polysorbate 80 (also known as Tweens). Hypersensitivity reactions, usually a delayed reaction, have been reported following exposure to pharmaceutical products containing polysorbate 80 in certain individuals (Isaksson, 2002; Lucente 2000; Shelley, 1995). Thrombocytopenia, ascites, pulmonary

deterioration, and renal and hepatic failure have been reported in premature neonates after receiving parenteral products containing polysorbate 80 (Alade, 1986; CDC, 1984). See manufacturer's labeling.

Increases in serum glucose commonly occur during treatment; initiation or alteration of insulin and/or oral hypoglycemic therapy may be required; monitor serum glucose before and during treatment; use with caution in patients with diabetes. Use with caution in patients with hyperlipidemia; may increase serum lipids (cholesterol and triglycerides); initiation or dosage adjustment of antihyperlipidemic agents may be required; monitor cholesterol/triglyceride panel at baseline and periodically during treatment. Treatment may result in immunosuppression, may increase risk of opportunistic infections and/or sepsis. Pneumocystis jiroveci pneumonia (PCP) has been reported; some cases were fatal. Development of PCP may be associated with the use of concomitant corticosteroids or other immunosuppressive agents; consider PCP prophylaxis in patients receiving concomitant immunosuppressive or corticosteroid therapy. Interstitial lung disease (ILD), sometimes fatal, has been reported; symptoms include dyspnea, cough, hypoxia, and/or fever, although asymptomatic or mild cases may present; promptly evaluate worsening respiratory symptoms. If symptoms develop, consider withholding temsirolimus until symptom recovery and radiographic improvement occur. Consider empiric treatment with corticosteroids and/or antibiotic therapy; baseline chest radiographic assessment (CT scan or x-ray) is recommended; follow periodically, even in the absence of clinical pulmonary symptoms. Cases of bowel perforation (fatal) have occurred (usually presenting with abdominal pain, bloody stools, diarrhea, fever, or metabolic acidosis); promptly evaluate any new or worsening abdominal pain or bloody stools. Temsirolimus may be associated with impaired wound healing; use caution in the perioperative period. Cases of acute renal failure with rapid progression have been reported (unrelated to disease progression), including cases unresponsive to dialysis. An increased incidence of rash, infection and dose interruptions have been reported in patients with renal insufficiency (CrCl ≤60 mL/minute) who received mTOR inhibitors for the treatment of renal cell cancer (Gupta, 2011). Elderly patients may be more likely to experience adverse reactions, including diarrhea, edema, and pneumonia.

Adverse Reactions
>10%:
Cardiovascular: Edema (35%), chest pain (16%)
Central nervous system: Pain (28%), headache (15%), insomnia (12%)
Dermatologic: Skin rash (47%), pruritus (19%), nail disease (14%), xeroderma (11%)
Endocrine & metabolic: Increased serum glucose (89%; grades 3/4: 16%), increased serum cholesterol (87%; grades 3/4: 2%), hypertriglyceridemia (83%; grades 3/4: 44%), hypophosphatemia (49%; grades 3/4: 18%), hyperglycemia (26%), hyperlipidemia (≥30%), hypokalemia (21%; grades 3/4: 5%), weight loss (19%)
Gastrointestinal: Mucositis (41%), nausea (37%), anorexia (32%), diarrhea (27%), abdominal pain (21%; grades 3/4: 4%), constipation (20%), dysgeusia (20%), stomatitis (20%), vomiting (19%)
Genitourinary: Urinary tract infection (15%)
Hematologic & oncologic: Decreased hemoglobin (94%; grades 3/4: 20%), lymphocytopenia (53%; grades 3/4: 16%), thrombocytopenia (40%; grades 3/4: 1%; dose-limiting toxicity), decreased white blood cell count (32%; grades 3/4: 1%), anemia (≥30%), decreased neutrophils (19%; grades 3/4: 5%)
Hepatic: Increased serum alkaline phosphatase (68%; grades 3/4: 3%), increased serum AST (38%; grades 3/4: 2%)
Infection: Infection (20%; grades 3/4: 3%; includes abscess, bronchitis, cellulitis, herpes simplex, herpes zoster)
Neuromuscular & skeletal: Weakness (51%), back pain (20%), arthralgia (18%)
Renal: Increased serum creatinine (57%; grades 3/4: 3%)
Respiratory: Dyspnea (28%), cough (26%), epistaxis (12%), pharyngitis (12%)
Miscellaneous: Fever (24%; grades 3/4: 1%)
1% to 10%:
Cardiovascular: Hypertension (7%), venous thromboembolism (2%; includes deep vein thrombosis and pulmonary embolism), pericardial effusion (1%), thrombophlebitis (1%)
Central nervous system: Chills (8%), depression (4%), convulsions (1%)
Dermatologic: Acne vulgaris (10%)
Endocrine & metabolic: Diabetes mellitus (5%)
Gastrointestinal: Gastrointestinal hemorrhage (1%)

Hematologic & oncologic: Rectal hemorrhage (1%)
Hepatic: Hyperbilirubinemia (8%)
Infection: Sepsis (1%), wound infection (1%)
Neuromuscular & skeletal: Myalgia (8%)
Ophthalmic: Conjunctivitis (8%; including lacrimation disorder)
Respiratory: Rhinitis (10%), pneumonia (8%), upper respiratory tract infection (7%), pleural effusion (4%)
Miscellaneous: Wound healing impairment (1%)
<1% (Limited to important or life-threatening): Acute renal failure, angioedema, cholecystitis, cholelithiasis, causalgia, decreased glucose tolerance, extravasation reactions (with pain, swelling, warmth, erythema), hypersensitivity reaction, interstitial pulmonary disease, intestinal perforation, pancreatitis, pneumonitis, rhabdomyolysis, seizure, Stevens-Johnson syndrome

Drug Interactions
Metabolism/Transport Effects Substrate of CYP3A4 (major), P-glycoprotein; **Note:** Assignment of Major/Minor substrate status based on clinically relevant drug interaction potential; **Inhibits** CYP2D6 (weak)

Avoid Concomitant Use
Avoid concomitant use of Temsirolimus with any of the following: BCG (Intravesical); Conivaptan; Deferiprone; Dipyrone; Fusidic Acid (Systemic); Idelalisib; Natalizumab; Pimecrolimus; SUNItinib; Tacrolimus (Systemic); Tacrolimus (Topical); Tofacitinib; Vaccines (Live)

Increased Effect/Toxicity
Temsirolimus may increase the levels/effects of: ACE Inhibitors; ARIPiprazole; CloZAPine; CycloSPORINE (Systemic); Deferiprone; Fingolimod; Leflunomide; Natalizumab; SUNItinib; Tacrolimus (Systemic); Tacrolimus (Topical); Tofacitinib; Vaccines (Live)

The levels/effects of Temsirolimus may be increased by: Aprepitant; Conivaptan; CYP3A4 Inhibitors (Moderate); CYP3A4 Inhibitors (Strong); Dasatinib; Denosumab; Dipyrone; Fluconazole; Fosaprepitant; Fusidic Acid (Systemic); Idelalisib; Itraconazole; Ivacaftor; Ketoconazole (Systemic); Luliconazole; Macrolide Antibiotics; Mifepristone; Netupitant; Osimertinib; Palbociclib; P-glycoprotein/ABCB1 Inhibitors; Pimecrolimus; Posaconazole; Protease Inhibitors; Ranolazine; Roflumilast; Simeprevir; Stiripentol; Tacrolimus (Systemic); Tacrolimus (Topical); Trastuzumab

Decreased Effect
Temsirolimus may decrease the levels/effects of: Antidiabetic Agents; BCG (Intravesical); Coccidioides immitis Skin Test; Sipuleucel-T; Tacrolimus (Systemic); Vaccines (Inactivated); Vaccines (Live)

The levels/effects of Temsirolimus may be decreased by: Bosentan; CarBAMazepine; CYP3A4 Inducers (Moderate); CYP3A4 Inducers (Strong); Dabrafenib; Deferasirox; Echinacea; Enzalutamide; Fosphenytoin; Mitotane; Osimertinib; P-glycoprotein/ABCB1 Inducers; Phenytoin; Rifamycin Derivatives; Siltuximab; St Johns Wort; Tocilizumab

Food Interactions Grapefruit and grapefruit juice may increase the levels/effects of sirolimus. Management: Avoid grapefruit and grapefruit juice.

Preparation for Administration Hazardous agent; use appropriate precautions for handling and disposal (NIOSH 2014 [group 1]). Preparation requires a two-step dilution process (do not add undiluted temsirolimus to aqueous solution; addition to aqueous solution prior to step 1 will result in precipitation). Step 1: Total amount in undiluted vial is 30 mg/1.2 mL (25 mg/mL concentration); contains overfill. Vials should initially be diluted with 1.8 mL of provided diluent to a concentration of 10 mg/mL. Once diluted with provided diluent, mix by inverting vial. Step 2: After allowing air bubbles to subside, the intended dose should be withdrawn from the 10 mg/mL diluted vial (ie, 2.5 mL for a 25 mg dose) and further diluted in 250 mL of NS in a non-DEHP/non-PVC container (glass, polyolefin, or polypropylene). Mix by inverting bottle or bag; avoid excessive shaking (may result in foaming).

Storage/Stability Store intact vials refrigerated at 2°C to 8°C (36°F to 46°F). Diluted solution in the vial (10 mg/mL) is stable for 24 hours at room temperature (below 25°C [77°F]). Solutions diluted for infusion (in NS) must be infused within 6 hours of preparation. Protect from light during storage, preparation, and handling.

Mechanism of Action Temsirolimus and its active metabolite, sirolimus, are targeted inhibitors of mTOR (mechanistic target of rapamycin) kinase activity. Temsirolimus (and sirolimus) bind to FKBP-12, an intracellular protein, to form a complex which inhibits mTOR signaling, halting the cell cycle at the G1 phase in tumor cells. Inhibition of mTOR blocks downstream phosphorylation of p70S6k and S6 ribosomal proteins. In renal cell carcinoma, mTOR inhibition also exhibits anti-angiogenesis activity by

reducing levels of HIF-1 and HIF-2 alpha (hypoxia inducible factors) and vascular endothelial growth factor (VEGF).

Pharmacodynamics/Kinetics

Distribution: V_{dss}: 172 L

Metabolism: Hepatic; via CYP3A4 to sirolimus (primary active metabolite) and 4 minor metabolites

Half-life elimination: Temsirolimus: ~17 hours; Sirolimus: ~55 hours

Time to peak, plasma: Temsirolimus: At end of infusion; Sirolimus: 0.5 to 2 hours after temsirolimus infusion

Excretion: Feces (78%); urine (<5%)

Dosing

Adult & Geriatric Note: For infusion reaction prophylaxis, premedicate with an H_1 antagonist (eg, diphenhydramine 25 to 50 mg IV) ~30 minutes prior to infusion.

Renal cell cancer (RCC), advanced: IV: 25 mg once weekly; continue until disease progression or unacceptable toxicity

Dosage adjustment for concomitant CYP3A4 inhibitors/inducers:

CYP3A4 inhibitors: Avoid concomitant administration with strong CYP3A4 inhibitors (eg, clarithromycin, itraconazole, ketoconazole, nefazodone, protease inhibitors, telithromycin, voriconazole); if concomitant administration with a strong CYP3A4 inhibitor cannot be avoided, consider a dose reduction to 12.5 mg once weekly. When a strong CYP3A4 inhibitor is discontinued; allow ~1 week to elapse prior to adjusting the temsirolimus upward to the dose used prior to initiation of the CYP3A4 inhibitor.

CYP3A4 inducers: Avoid concomitant administration with strong CYP3A4 inducers (eg, carbamazepine, dexamethasone, phenobarbital, phenytoin, rifabutin, rifampin, St John's wort); if concomitant administration with a strong CYP3A4 inducer cannot be avoided, consider adjusting temsirolimus dose up to 50 mg once weekly. If the strong CYP3A4 enzyme inducer is discontinued, reduce the temsirolimus to the dose used prior to initiation of the CYP3A4 inducer.

Renal Impairment No dosage adjustment necessary.

Hemodialysis: There are no dosage adjustments provided in the manufacturer's labeling (has not been studied).

Hepatic Impairment

Mild hepatic impairment (bilirubin >1 to 1.5 x ULN or AST >ULN with bilirubin ≤ULN): Reduce dose to 15 mg once weekly.

Moderate-to-severe hepatic impairment (bilirubin >1.5 x ULN): Use is contraindicated.

Adjustment for Toxicity

Hematologic toxicity: ANC <1000/mm^3 or platelets <75,000/mm^3: Withhold treatment until resolves and reinitiate treatment with the dose reduced by 5 mg weekly; minimum dose: 15 mg weekly if adjustment for toxicity is needed.

Nonhematologic toxicity: Any toxicity ≥ grade 3: Withhold treatment until resolves to ≤ grade 2; reinitiate treatment with the dose reduced by 5 mg weekly; minimum dose: 15 mg weekly if adjustment for toxicity is needed.

Infusion/hypersensitivity reaction: Interrupt infusion and observe for 30 to 60 minutes; treatment may be resumed with discretion at a slower infusion rate (up to 60 minutes); administer an H_1 antagonist (if not given as premedication) and/or an IV H_2 antagonist 30 minutes prior to resuming infusion.

Interstitial lung disease: Consider withholding treatment for clinically significant respiratory symptoms until after recovery of symptoms or radiographic improvement.

Dietary Considerations Avoid grapefruit juice (may increase the levels of the major metabolite, sirolimus).

Administration Infuse over 30 to 60 minutes via an infusion pump (preferred). Use polyethylene-lined non-DEHP administration tubing. Administer through an inline polyethersulfone filter ≤5 micron; if set does not contain an inline filter, a polyethersulfone end filter (0.2 to 5 micron) should be added (do not use both an inline and an end filter). Premedicate with an H_1 antagonist (eg, diphenhydramine 25 to 50 mg IV) ~30 minutes prior to infusion. Monitor during infusion; interrupt infusion for hypersensitivity/infusion reaction; monitor for 30 to 60 minutes; may reinitiate at a reduced infusion rate (over 60 minutes) with discretion, 30 minutes after administration of a histamine H_1 antagonist and/or a histamine H_2 antagonist (eg, famotidine or ranitidine). Administration should be completed within 6 hours of admixture.

Hazardous agent; use appropriate precautions for handling and disposal (NIOSH 2014 [group 1]).

Monitoring Parameters CBC with differential and platelets (weekly), serum chemistries including glucose (baseline and every other week), serum cholesterol and triglycerides (baseline and periodic), liver function (baseline and periodic), renal function tests (baseline and periodic)

Monitor for infusion reactions; infection; symptoms of ILD (or radiographic changes), symptoms of hyperglycemia (excessive thirst, polyuria); symptoms of bowel perforation

Dosage Forms Excipient information presented when available (limited, particularly for generics); consult specific product labeling.

Solution, Intravenous:

Torisel: 25 mg/mL (1 mL) [contains alcohol, usp, polyethylene glycol, polysorbate 80, propylene glycol]

Tenecteplase (ten EK te plase)

Brand Names: US TNKase

Brand Names: Canada TNKase®

Pharmacologic Category Thrombolytic Agent

Use Management of ST-elevation myocardial infarction (STEMI) for the lysis of thrombi in the coronary vasculature to restore perfusion and reduce mortality.

Recommended criteria for treatment of STEMI (ACCF/AHA; O'Gara, 2013): Ischemic symptoms within 12 hours of treatment or evidence of ongoing ischemia 12-24 hours after symptom onset with a large area of myocardium at risk or hemodynamic instability.

STEMI ECG definition: New ST-segment elevation at the J point in at least 2 contiguous leads of ≥2 mm (0.2 mV) in men or ≥1.5 mm (0.15 mV) in women in leads V_2-V_3 and/or of ≥1 mm (0.1 mV) in other contiguous precordial leads or limb leads on ECG. New or presumably new left bundle branch block (LBBB) may interfere with ST-elevation analysis and should not be considered diagnostic in isolation.

At non-PCI-capable hospitals, the ACCF/AHA recommends thrombolytic therapy administration when the anticipated first medical contact (FMC)-to-device time at a PCI-capable hospital is >120 minutes due to unavoidable delays.

Pregnancy Considerations Adverse events have been observed in some animal reproduction studies. The risk of bleeding may be increased in pregnant women. Administer to pregnant women only if the potential benefits justify the risk to the fetus.

Breast-Feeding Considerations It is not known if tenecteplase is excreted in breast milk. The manufacturer recommends that caution be exercised when administering tenecteplase to nursing women.

Contraindications Active internal bleeding; history of cerebrovascular accident; recent (ie, within 2 months) intracranial/intraspinal surgery or trauma; intracranial neoplasm; arteriovenous malformation or aneurysm; bleeding diathesis; severe uncontrolled hypertension

Additional contraindications (ACCF/AHA; O'Gara, 2013): Ischemic stroke within 3 months; prior intracranial hemorrhage; active bleeding (excluding menses); suspected aortic dissection; significant closed head or facial trauma within 3 months

Warnings/Precautions Use with caution in patients receiving oral anticoagulants; increased risk of bleeding. Adjunctive use of parenteral anticoagulants (eg, enoxaparin, heparin, or fondaparinux) is recommended to improve vessel patency and prevent reocclusion and may also contribute to bleeding; monitor for bleeding (ACCF/AHA; O'Gara, 2013). Stop antiplatelet agents and heparin if serious bleeding occurs. Avoid IM injections and nonessential handling of the patient for a few hours after administration. Monitor for bleeding complications. Venipunctures should be performed carefully and only when necessary. If arterial puncture is necessary, then use an upper extremity that can be easily compressed manually. For the following conditions, the risk of bleeding is higher with use of tenecteplase and the use of tenecteplase should be weighed against the benefits: Recent major surgery, cerebrovascular disease, recent GI or GU bleed, recent trauma, uncontrolled hypertension (systolic BP >180 mm Hg and/or diastolic BP >110 mm Hg), suspected left heart thrombus, acute pericarditis, subacute bacterial endocarditis, hemostatic defects, severe hepatic dysfunction, hemorrhagic diabetic retinopathy or other hemorrhagic ophthalmic conditions, pregnancy, septic thrombophlebitis or occluded arteriovenous cannula at seriously infected site, advanced age, anticoagulants, recent administration of GP IIb/IIIa inhibitors. Use with caution in patients with advanced age; increased risk of bleeding. Mortality and rate of intracranial hemorrhage increases with increasing age >65 years of age; the risks and benefits of use should be weighed carefully in the elderly. Coronary thrombolysis may result in reperfusion arrhythmias. Caution with readministration of tenecteplase.

Adverse Reactions As with all drugs which may affect hemostasis, bleeding is the major adverse effect associated with tenecteplase. Hemorrhage may occur at virtually any site. Risk is dependent on multiple variables, including the dosage administered, concurrent use of multiple agents which alter hemostasis, and patient predisposition. Rapid lysis of coronary artery thrombi by thrombolytic agents may be associated with reperfusion-related arterial and/or ventricular arrhythmia.

>10%:
Local: Hematoma (12% minor)
Hematologic: Bleeding (22% minor: ASSENT-2 trial)
1% to 10%:
Central nervous system: Stroke (2%)
Gastrointestinal: Epistaxis (2% minor), GI hemorrhage (1% major, 2% minor)
Genitourinary: GU bleeding (4% minor)
Hematologic: Bleeding (5% major; ASSENT-2 trial)
Local: Bleeding at catheter puncture site (4% minor), hematoma (2% major)
Respiratory: Pharyngeal (3% minor)
<1% (Limited to important or life-threatening): Anaphylaxis, angioedema, bleeding at catheter puncture site (<1% major), cholesterol embolism (clinical features may include livedo reticularis, "purple toe" syndrome, acute renal failure, gangrenous digits, hypertension, pancreatitis, MI, cerebral infarction, spinal cord infarction, retinal artery occlusion, bowel infarction, rhabdomyolysis), GU bleeding (<1% major), intracranial hemorrhage (0.9%), laryngeal edema, rash, respiratory tract bleeding, retroperitoneal bleeding, urticaria
Additional cardiovascular events associated with use in MI: Arrhythmia, AV block, cardiac arrest, cardiac tamponade, cardiogenic shock, embolism, electromechanical dissociation, fever, heart failure, hypotension, mitral regurgitation, myocardial reinfarction, myocardial rupture, nausea, pericardial effusion, pericarditis, pulmonary edema, recurrent myocardial ischemia, thrombosis, vomiting

Drug Interactions
Metabolism/Transport Effects None known.
Avoid Concomitant Use There are no known interactions where it is recommended to avoid concomitant use.
Increased Effect/Toxicity
Tenecteplase may increase the levels/effects of: Anticoagulants; Dabigatran Etexilate; Prostacyclin Analogues

The levels/effects of Tenecteplase may be increased by: Agents with Antiplatelet Properties; Herbs (Anticoagulant/Antiplatelet Properties); Limaprost; Salicylates
Decreased Effect
The levels/effects of Tenecteplase may be decreased by: Aprotinin

Preparation for Administration Tenecteplase should be reconstituted using the supplied 10 mL syringe with Twin-Pak™ Dual Cannula Device and 10 mL sterile water for injection. Do not shake when reconstituting. Slight foaming is normal and will dissipate if left standing for several minutes. The reconstituted solution is 5 mg/mL. Any unused solution should be discarded. If reconstituted and not used immediately, store in refrigerator and use within 8 hours.

Storage/Stability Store under refrigeration of 2°C to 8°C (36°F to 46°F) or at room temperature; do not exceed 30°C (86°F). If reconstituted and not used immediately, store in refrigerator and use within 8 hours.

Mechanism of Action Promotes initiation of fibrinolysis by binding to fibrin and converting plasminogen to plasmin. Tenecteplase is essentially alteplase with the exception of 3 point mutations and is more fibrin specific, more resistant to plasminogen activator inhibitor -1 (PAI-1), with a longer duration of action compared to alteplase. Produced by recombinant DNA technology using a mammalian cell line (Chinese hamster ovary cells).

Pharmacodynamics/Kinetics
Distribution: V_d is weight related and approximates plasma volume
Metabolism: Primarily hepatic
Half-life elimination: Biphasic: Initial: 20-24 minutes; Terminal: 90-130 minutes
Excretion: Clearance: Plasma: 99-119 mL/minute
Dosing
Adult
STEMI: IV: The recommended total dose should not exceed 50 mg and is based on weight. Administer as a single bolus over 5 seconds:
<60 kg: 30 mg
≥60 to <70 kg: 35 mg
≥70 to <80 kg: 40 mg
≥80 to <90 kg: 45 mg
≥90 kg: 50 mg

Note: Thrombolytic should be administered within 30 minutes of hospital arrival. Generally, there is only a small trend for benefit of therapy after a delay of 12 to 24 hours from symptom onset, but thrombolysis may be considered for selected patients with ongoing ischemic pain and extensive ST elevation; however, primary PCI is preferred in these patients. Administer concurrent aspirin, clopidogrel, and anticoagulant therapy (ie, unfractionated heparin, enoxaparin, or fondaparinux) with tenecteplase (O'Gara, 2013).

Geriatric Refer to adult dosing. Although dosage adjustments are not recommended, the elderly have a higher incidence of morbidity and mortality with the use of tenecteplase.

Renal Impairment No dosage adjustment necessary.
Hepatic Impairment
Mild to moderate impairment: No dosage adjustment provided in manufacturer's labeling.
Severe impairment: No dosage adjustment provided in manufacturer's labeling; weigh the risk of bleeding against the benefits with tenecteplase especially in those with a coagulopathy.

Administration Tenecteplase is **incompatible** with dextrose solutions. Dextrose-containing lines must be flushed with a saline solution before and after administration. Administer as a single IV bolus over 5 seconds. Avoid IM injections and nonessential handling of patient.

Monitoring Parameters CBC, aPTT, signs and symptoms of bleeding, ECG monitoring

Test Interactions Altered results of coagulation and fibrinolytic activity tests

Dosage Forms Excipient information presented when available (limited, particularly for generics); consult specific product labeling.
Kit, Intravenous:
TNKase: 50 mg

◆ Tenex *see* GuanFACINE *on page 865*

Teniposide (ten i POE side)

Brand Names: US Vumon [DSC]
Brand Names: Canada Vumon
Index Terms EPT; PTG; VM-26
Pharmacologic Category Antineoplastic Agent, Podophyllotoxin Derivative; Antineoplastic Agent, Topoisomerase II Inhibitor
Use Acute lymphoblastic leukemia, refractory: Treatment of refractory childhood acute lymphoblastic leukemia (ALL) in combination with other chemotherapy
Dosing
Adult Note: Patients with Down syndrome and leukemia may be more sensitive to the myelosuppressive effects; administer the first course at half the usual dose and adjust dose in subsequent cycles upward based on degree of toxicities (myelosuppression and mucositis) in the previous course(s).
Acute lymphoblastic leukemia (ALL) consolidation treatment (off-label use; combination chemotherapy): IV: 165 mg/m²/dose days 1, 4, 8, and 11 of alternating consolidation cycles (Linker, 1991)
Pediatric Note: Patients with Down syndrome and leukemia may be more sensitive to the myelosuppressive effects; administer the first course at half the usual dose and adjust dose in subsequent cycles upward based on degree of toxicities (myelosuppression and mucositis) in the previous course(s).

Acute lymphoblastic leukemia (ALL), refractory (combination chemotherapy): IV: 165 mg/m² twice weekly for 8 to 9 doses (in combination with cytarabine) or 250 mg/m² weekly for 4 to 8 weeks (in combination with vincristine and prednisone)
Renal Impairment There are no specific dosage adjustments provided in the manufacturer's labeling (has not been studied). However, dosage adjustment may be necessary in patients with significant renal impairment.
Hepatic Impairment There are no specific dosage adjustments provided in the manufacturer's labeling (has not been studied). However, dosage adjustment may be necessary in patients with significant hepatic impairment.
Additional Information Complete prescribing information should be consulted for additional detail.
Dosage Forms Considerations Injectable solution may contain alcohol, benzyl alcohol, or polyoxyl 35/polyoxyethylated castor oil (Cremophor EL)

Dosage Forms Excipient information presented when available (limited, particularly for generics); consult specific product labeling. [DSC] = Discontinued product

Solution, Intravenous:

Vumon: 10 mg/mL (5 mL [DSC]) [contains alcohol, usp, benzyl alcohol, cremophor el, dimethylacetamide]

Generic: 10 mg/mL (5 mL)

◆ Tenivac *see* Diphtheria and Tetanus Toxoid *on page 565*

◆ Tenofovir Alafenamide, Elvitegravir, Cobicistat, and Emtricitabine *see* Elvitegravir, Cobicistat, Emtricitabine, and Tenofovir Alafenamide *on page 632*

Tenofovir Disoproxil Fumarate
(ten OF oh vir dye soe PROX il FUE ma rate)

Brand Names: US Viread
Brand Names: Canada Viread
Index Terms PMPA; TDF
Pharmacologic Category Antihepadnaviral, Reverse Transcriptase Inhibitor, Nucleotide (Anti-HBV); Antiretroviral, Reverse Transcriptase Inhibitor, Nucleotide (Anti-HIV)

Use

Chronic hepatitis B: Treatment of chronic hepatitis B virus (HBV) in patients ≥12 years of age

HIV infection: In combination with other antiretroviral agents for the treatment of HIV-1 infection in adults and pediatric patients ≥2 years of age

Pregnancy Considerations Adverse events were observed in some animal reproduction studies. Tenofovir has a high level of transfer across the human placenta. Intrauterine growth has not been affected in human studies, but one study found lower length and head circumference. Clinical studies in children have shown bone demineralization with chronic use. No increased risk of overall birth defects has been observed following first trimester exposure according to data collected by the antiretroviral pregnancy registry. Limited data indicate decreased maternal bioavailability during the third trimester; dose adjustments are not needed. Cases of lactic acidosis/hepatic steatosis syndrome related to mitochondrial toxicity have been reported in pregnant women with prolonged use of nucleoside analogues. It is not known if pregnancy itself potentiates this known side effect; however, women may be at increased risk of lactic acidosis and liver damage. In addition, these adverse events are similar to other rare but life-threatening syndromes which occur during pregnancy (eg, HELLP syndrome). Hepatic enzymes and electrolytes should be monitored in women receiving nucleoside analogues and clinicians should watch for early signs of the syndrome. In addition, mitochondrial dysfunction may develop in infants following *in utero* exposure. Renal function should also be monitored. The DHHS Perinatal HIV Guidelines consider tenofovir in combination with either emtricitabine or lamivudine to be a preferred NRTI backbone for use in antiretroviral-naive pregnant women. The DHHS Perinatal HIV Guidelines consider emtricitabine plus tenofovir, or lamivudine plus tenofovir as recommended dual NRTI/NtRTI backbones for HIV/HBV coinfected pregnant women. Hepatitis B flare may occur if tenofovir is discontinued postpartum.

Regardless of CD4 count or HIV RNA copy number, all HIV-infected pregnant women should receive a combination antiretroviral (ARV) drug regimen. A combination of antepartum, intrapartum, and infant ARV prophylaxis is recommended. ARV therapy should be started as soon as possible in women with symptomatic infection. Although earlier initiation may be more effective in reducing the perinatal transmission of HIV, also consider maternal conditions (eg, nausea and vomiting) and the potential risks of first trimester fetal exposure for specific agents. A scheduled cesarean delivery at 38 weeks' gestation is recommended for all women with HIV RNA >1000 copies/mL or unknown concentrations near delivery in order to decrease transmission. If ARV therapy must be interrupted for <24 hours during the peripartum period, stop then restart all medications simultaneously in order to decrease the chance of developing resistance. Long-term follow-up is recommended for all infants exposed to ARV medications. In couples who want to conceive, the HIV-infected partner should attain maximum viral suppression prior to conception.

Health care providers are encouraged to enroll pregnant women exposed to antiretroviral medications in the Antiretroviral Pregnancy Registry (1-800-258-4263 or www.-APRegistry.com). Health care providers caring for HIV-infected women and their infants may contact the National Perinatal HIV Hotline (888-448-8765) for clinical consultation (HHS [perinatal] 2014).

Breast-Feeding Considerations Tenofovir is excreted in breast milk. Maternal or infant antiretroviral therapy does not completely eliminate the risk of postnatal HIV transmission. In addition, multiclass-resistant virus has been detected in breast-feeding infants despite maternal therapy. Therefore, in the United States, where formula is accessible, affordable, safe, and sustainable, and the risk of infant mortality due to diarrhea and respiratory infections is low, complete avoidance of breast-feeding by HIV-infected women is recommended to decrease potential transmission of HIV (HHS [perinatal] 2014).

Contraindications

U.S. labeling: There are no contraindications listed in the manufacturer's labeling.

Canadian labeling: Hypersensitivity to tenofovir or any component of the formulation; concurrent use with fixed-dose combination products that contain tenofovir (Truvada, Atripla, Complera, or Stribild); concurrent use with adefovir (Hepsera)

Warnings/Precautions [U.S Boxed Warning]: Lactic acidosis and severe hepatomegaly with steatosis have been reported with tenofovir and other nucleoside analogues, including fatal cases; use with caution in patients with risk factors for liver disease (risk may be increased in obese patients or prolonged nucleoside exposure) and suspend treatment in any patient who develops clinical or laboratory findings suggestive of lactic acidosis (transaminase elevation may/may not accompany hepatomegaly and steatosis). May cause redistribution of fat (eg, buffalo hump, peripheral wasting with increased abdominal girth, cushingoid appearance). Immune reconstitution syndrome may develop resulting in the occurrence of an inflammatory response to an indolent or residual opportunistic infection during initial HIV treatment or activation of autoimmune disorders (eg, Graves' disease, polymyositis, Guillain-Barré syndrome) later in therapy; further evaluation and treatment may be required. Use caution in hepatic impairment; limited data supporting treatment of chronic hepatitis B in patients with decompensated liver disease; observe for increased adverse reactions, including renal dysfunction.

In clinical trials, use has been associated with decreases in bone mineral density in HIV-1 infected adults and increases in bone metabolism markers. Serum parathyroid hormone and 1,25 vitamin D levels were also higher. Decreases in bone mineral density have also been observed in clinical trials of HIV-1 infected pediatric patients. Observations in chronic hepatitis B infected pediatric patients (aged 12-18 years) were similar. Consider monitoring of bone density in adult and pediatric patients with a history of pathologic fractures or with other risk factors for bone loss or osteoporosis. Consider calcium and vitamin D supplementation for all patients; effect of supplementation has not been studied but may be beneficial. Long-term bone health and fracture risk unknown. Skeletal growth (height) appears to be unaffected in tenofovir-treated children and adolescents.

May cause osteomalacia with proximal renal tubulopathy. Bone pain, extremity pain, fractures, arthralgias, weakness and muscle pain have been reported. In patients at risk for renal dysfunction, persistent or worsening bone or muscle symptoms should be evaluated for hypophosphatemia and osteomalacia.

Do not use as monotherapy in treatment of HIV. Clinical trials in HIV-infected patients whose regimens contained only three nucleoside reverse transcriptase inhibitors (NRTI) show less efficacy, early virologic failure and high rates of resistance substitutions. Use three NRTI regimens with caution and monitor response carefully. Triple drug regimens with two NRTIs in combination with a non-nucleoside reverse transcriptase inhibitor or a HIV-1 protease inhibitor are usually more effective. Treatment of HIV in patients with unrecognized/untreated hepatitis B virus (HBV) may lead to rapid HBV resistance. Patients should be tested for presence of chronic hepatitis B infection prior to initiation of therapy. In patients coinfected with HIV and HBV, an appropriate antiretroviral combination should be selected due to HIV resistance potential; these patients should receive tenofovir dosed for HIV therapy.

Tenofovir is predominately eliminated renally; use caution in renal impairment. May cause acute renal failure or Fanconi syndrome; use caution with other nephrotoxic agents (including high dose or multiple NSAID use or those which compete for active tubular secretion). Acute renal failure has occurred in HIV-infected patients with risk factors for renal impairment who were on a stable tenofovir regimen to which a high dose or multiple NSAID therapy was added. Consider alternatives to NSAIDS in patients taking tenofovir and at risk for renal impairment. Calculate creatinine clearance prior to initiation of therapy and

monitor renal function (including recalculation of creatinine clearance and serum phosphorus) during therapy. Dosage adjustment required in patients with CrCl <50 mL/minute. IDSA guidelines recommend avoiding tenofovir in HIV patients with preexisting kidney disease (CrCl <50 mL/minute and not on hemodialysis or GFR <60 mL/minute/1.73 m²) when other effective HIV treatment options exist because data suggest risk of chronic kidney disease (CKD) is increased (IDSA [Lucas 2014]). IDSA guidelines also recommend discontinuing tenofovir (and substituting with alternative antiretroviral therapy) in HIV-infected patients who develop a decline in GFR (a >25% decrease in GFR from baseline and to a level of <60 mL/minute/1.73 m²) during use, particularly in presence of proximal tubular dysfunction (eg, euglycemic glycosuria, increased urinary phosphorus excretion and hypophosphatemia, proteinuria [new onset or worsening]) (IDSA [Lucas 2014]). Use caution in patients with low body weight, or concurrent medications which increase tenofovir levels. Use caution in the elderly; dosage adjustment based on renal function may be required. Pancreatitis has been reported; use with caution in patients with a prior history or risk factors for pancreatitis. Discontinue if pancreatitis is suspected.

[U.S. Boxed Warning]: If treating HBV, acute exacerbation of hepatitis B may occur upon discontinuation. Monitor liver function closely for several months after discontinuing treatment; reinitiation of antihepatitis B therapy may be required. Treatment of HBV in patients with unrecognized/untreated HIV may lead to HIV resistance; patients should be tested for presence of HIV infection prior to initiating therapy. Do not use as monotherapy in treatment of HIV. Treatment of HIV in patients with unrecognized/untreated HBV may lead to rapid HBV resistance. Patients should be tested for presence of chronic hepatitis B prior to initiation of therapy. Potentially significant drug-drug interactions may exist, requiring dose or frequency adjustment, additional monitoring, and/or selection of alternative therapy. Do not use concurrently with adefovir or tenofovir combination products.

Adverse Reactions Includes data from both treatment-naive and treatment-experienced HIV patients and in chronic hepatitis B.

>10%:
Central nervous system: Insomnia (3% to 18%), headache (5% to 14%), pain (12% to 13%), dizziness (8% to 13%), depression (4% to 11%)
Dermatologic: Skin rash (includes maculopapular, pustular, or vesiculobullous rash; pruritus; or urticaria: 5% to 18%), pruritus (16%)
Endocrine & metabolic: Hypercholesterolemia (19% to 22%), increased serum triglycerides (1% to 4%)
Gastrointestinal: Abdominal pain (4% to 22%), nausea (8% to 20%), diarrhea (9% to 16%), vomiting (2% to 13%)
Neuromuscular & skeletal: Decreased bone mineral density (28%; ≥5% at spine or ≥7% at hip), increased creatine phosphokinase (2% to 12%), weakness (6% to 11%)
Miscellaneous: Fever (4% to 11%)
1% to 10%:
Cardiovascular: Chest pain (3%)
Central nervous system: Fatigue (9%), anxiety (6%), peripheral neuropathy (1% to 5%)
Dermatologic: Diaphoresis (3%)
Endocrine & metabolic: Weight loss (2% to 4%), glycosuria (grades 3/4: ≤3%), hyperglycemia (grades 3/4: 2% to 3%), lipodystrophy (1%)
Gastrointestinal: Increased serum amylase (grades 3/4: 4% to 9%), anorexia (3% to 4%), dyspepsia (3% to 4%), flatulence (3% to 4%)
Genitourinary: Hematuria (≤ grades 3/4: 3% to 7%)
Hematologic & oncologic: Neutropenia (3%)
Hepatic: Increased serum ALT (2% to 10%), increased serum AST (3% to 5%), increased serum transaminases (2% to 5%), increased serum alkaline phosphatase (1%)
Neuromuscular & skeletal: Back pain (4% to 9%), arthralgia (5%), myalgia (4%)
Renal: Increased serum creatinine (9%), renal failure (7%)
Respiratory: Sinusitis (8%), upper respiratory tract infection (8%), nasopharyngitis (5%), pneumonia (2% to 5%)
Postmarketing and/or case reports: Angioedema, exacerbation of hepatitis B (following discontinuation), Fanconi's syndrome, hepatitis, hypersensitivity reaction, hypokalemia, hypophosphatemia, immune reconstitution syndrome, increased gamma-glutamyl transferase, interstitial nephritis, lactic acidosis, myopathy, nephrogenic diabetes insipidus, nephrotoxicity, osteomalacia, pancreatitis, polyuria, proteinuria, proximal tubular

nephropathy, renal insufficiency, renal tubular necrosis, rhabdomyolysis, severe hepatomegaly with steatosis

Drug Interactions
Metabolism/Transport Effects Substrate of BCRP, P-glycoprotein; **Inhibits** CYP1A2 (weak)

Avoid Concomitant Use
Avoid concomitant use of Tenofovir Disoproxil Fumarate with any of the following: Adefovir; Didanosine

Increased Effect/Toxicity
Tenofovir Disoproxil Fumarate may increase the levels/effects of: Acyclovir-Valacyclovir; Adefovir; Aminoglycosides; Cidofovir; Darunavir; Didanosine; Ganciclovir-Valganciclovir; TiZANidine

The levels/effects of Tenofovir Disoproxil Fumarate may be increased by: Acyclovir-Valacyclovir; Adefovir; Aminoglycosides; Atazanavir; Cidofovir; Cobicistat; Darunavir; Diclofenac (Systemic); Ganciclovir-Valganciclovir; Ledipasvir; Lopinavir; Nonsteroidal Anti-Inflammatory Agents; Simeprevir; Telaprevir

Decreased Effect
Tenofovir Disoproxil Fumarate may decrease the levels/effects of: Atazanavir; Didanosine; Simeprevir; Tipranavir

The levels/effects of Tenofovir Disoproxil Fumarate may be decreased by: Adefovir; Tipranavir

Food Interactions Fatty meals may increase the bioavailability of tenofovir. Management: May administer with or without food.

Storage/Stability Store at 25°C (77°F); excursions are permitted between 15°C and 30°C (59°F and 86°F). Dispense only in original container.

Mechanism of Action Tenofovir disoproxil fumarate (TDF), a nucleotide reverse transcriptase inhibitor, is an analog of adenosine 5'-monophosphate; it interferes with the HIV viral RNA dependent DNA polymerase resulting in inhibition of viral replication. TDF is first converted intracellularly by hydrolysis to tenofovir and subsequently phosphorylated to the active tenofovir diphosphate. Tenofovir inhibits replication of HBV by inhibiting HBV polymerase.

Pharmacodynamics/Kinetics
Distribution: V_d: 1.2-1.3 L/kg
Protein binding: <7% to serum proteins
Metabolism: Tenofovir disoproxil fumarate (TDF) is converted intracellularly by hydrolysis (by non-CYP enzymes) to tenofovir, then phosphorylated to the active tenofovir diphosphate
Bioavailability: ~25% (fasting); increases ~40% with high-fat meal
Half-life elimination: ~17 hours
Time to peak, serum: Fasting: 36-84 minutes; With high-fat meal: 96-144 minutes
Excretion: Urine (70% to 80%) via filtration and active secretion, primarily as unchanged tenofovir

Dosing
Adult & Geriatric
Hepatitis B infection: Oral: 300 mg once daily
Note: Tenofovir is recommended for first-line treatment of HBV (Lok 2009). Concurrent use with adefovir and/or tenofovir combination products should be avoided.
Treatment duration (AASLD practice guidelines 2009):
Note: Patients not achieving <2 log decrease in serum HBV DNA after at least 6 months of therapy should either receive additional treatment or be switched to an alternative therapy (Lok, 2009).
Hepatitis Be antigen (HBeAg) positive chronic hepatitis: Treat ≥1 year until HBeAg seroconversion and undetectable serum HBV DNA; continue therapy for ≥6 months after HBeAg seroconversion
HBeAg negative chronic hepatitis: Treat >1 year until hepatitis B surface antigen (HBsAg) clearance
Decompensated liver disease: Lifelong treatment is recommended
HIV infection: Oral: 300 mg once daily (in combination with other antiretrovirals). **Note:** Tenofovir is a component of recommended initial regimens in treatment-naive patients (when coadministered with emtricitabine plus dolutegravir, with emtricitabine plus darunavir/ritonavir, or with emtricitabine plus raltegravir; lamivudine may be substituted for emtricitabine in any of these regimens) and is a component of a recommended initial regimen in treatment-naive patients with pre-ART CrCl >70 mL/minute (when coadministered with emtricitabine plus elvitegravir/cobicistat) (HHS [adult] 2015).

Pediatric
Hepatitis B infection: Oral: Children ≥12 years (and ≥35 kg) and Adolescents: Refer to adult dosing. **Note:** Canadian labeling does not approve of use in patients <18 years of age.

HIV infection: Oral:

Children 2 to <12 years: 8 mg/kg once daily (maximum: 300 mg once daily) (in combination with other antiretrovirals). **Note:** Canadian labeling does not approve of use in children <12 years of age.

Dosing recommendations based on body weight if using the **oral powder: Note:** One level scoop of powder = 40 mg tenofovir

10 to <12 kg: 80 mg once daily
12 to <14 kg: 100 mg once daily
14 to <17 kg: 120 mg once daily
17 to <19 kg: 140 mg once daily
19 to <22 kg: 160 mg once daily
22 to <24 kg: 180 mg once daily
24 to <27 kg: 200 mg once daily
27 to <29 kg: 220 mg once daily
29 to <32 kg: 240 mg once daily
32 to <34 kg: 260 mg once daily
34 to <35 kg: 280 mg once daily
≥35 kg: 300 mg once daily

Dosing recommendations based on body weight if using the **oral tablets:**

17 to <22 kg: 150 mg once daily
22 to <28 kg: 200 mg once daily
28 to <35 kg: 250 mg once daily
≥35 kg: 300 mg once daily

Children ≥12 years (and ≥35 kg) and Adolescents: Refer to adult dosing. **Note:** Tenofovir is a component of recommended initial regimens in adolescent treatment-naive patients (when coadministered with emtricitabine plus dolutegravir, with emtricitabine plus darunavir/ritonavir, or with emtricitabine plus raltegravir; lamivudine may be substituted for emtricitabine in any of these regimens) and is a component of a recommended initial regimen in adolescent treatment-naive patients with pre-ART CrCl >70 mL/minute (when coadministered with emtricitabine plus elvitegravir/cobicistat) (HHS [adult] 2015).

Renal Impairment

Adults: **Note:** Use of powder formulation has not been evaluated in renal impairment.

Manufacturer's labeling:

CrCl ≥50 mL/minute: No dosage adjustment necessary.
CrCl 30-49 mL/minute: 300 mg every 48 hours
CrCl 10-29 mL/minute: 300 mg every 72-96 hours
CrCl <10 mL/minute without hemodialysis: No dosage adjustment provided in manufacturer's labeling; has not been studied.
Hemodialysis: 300 mg following dialysis every 7 days or after a total of ~12 hours of dialysis (usually once weekly assuming 3 dialysis sessions lasting about 4 hours each).

Alternate recommendations (IDSA [Lucas 2014]):
CrCl <50 mL/minute (and not on hemodialysis) or GFR <60 mL/minute/1.73 m^2: Avoid use
Peritoneal dialysis: Use with caution; dose reduction recommended (no specific adjustment provided)

Children: No dosage adjustment provided in manufacturer's labeling (has not been studied).

Hepatic Impairment No dosage adjustment necessary.

Dietary Considerations Consider calcium and vitamin D supplementation.

Administration Tablets may be administered without regard to meals. Powder should be mixed with 2-4 ounces of soft food (applesauce, baby food, yogurt) and swallowed immediately (avoids bitter taste); do not mix in liquid (powder may float on top of the liquid even after stirring). Measure powder using only the supplied dosing scoop.

Monitoring Parameters

Patients with HIV: CBC with differential, reticulocyte count, creatine kinase, CD4 count, HIV RNA plasma levels, serum phosphorus; serum creatinine (prior to initiation and as clinically indicated during therapy), urine glucose and urine protein (in patients at risk for renal impairment or who experienced renal impairment while taking adefovir), hepatic function tests, bone density (patients with a history of bone fracture or have risk factors for bone loss); testing for HBV is recommended prior to the initiation of antiretroviral therapy; weight (children)

Patients with HBV: HIV status (prior to initiation of therapy); serum phosphorus; serum creatinine (prior to initiation and as clinically indicated during therapy), urine glucose and urine protein (in patients at risk for renal impairment or who experienced renal impairment while taking adefovir); bone density (patients with a history of bone fracture or have risk factors for bone loss); HBV DNA (every 3-6 months during therapy); HBeAg and anti-HBe; LFTs every 3 months during therapy and for several months following discontinuation of tenofovir; signs/symptoms of HBV relapse/exacerbation following discontinuation of therapy

Patients with HIV and HBV coinfection should be monitored for several months following tenofovir discontinuation.

Dosage Forms Excipient information presented when available (limited, particularly for generics); consult specific product labeling.

Powder, Oral, as disoproxil fumarate:
Viread: 40 mg/g (60 g)
Tablet, Oral, as disoproxil fumarate:
Viread: 150 mg, 200 mg, 250 mg
Viread: 300 mg [contains fd&c blue #2 aluminum lake]

Dosage Forms: Canada Refer to Dosage Forms. **Note:** Oral powder for reconstitution is not available in Canada.

◆ Tenofovir Disoproxil Fumarate and Emtricitabine *see* Emtricitabine and Tenofovir Disoproxil Fumarate *on page 635*

◆ Tenofovir Disoproxil Fumarate, Efavirenz, and Emtricitabine *see* Efavirenz, Emtricitabine, and Tenofovir Disoproxil Fumarate *on page 621*

◆ Tenofovir Disoproxil Fumarate, Elvitegravir, Cobicistat, and Emtricitabine *see* Elvitegravir, Cobicistat, Emtricitabine, and Tenofovir Disoproxil Fumarate *on page 632*

◆ Tenofovir Disoproxil Fumarate, Emtricitabine, and Rilpivirine *see* Emtricitabine, Rilpivirine, and Tenofovir Disoproxil Fumarate *on page 636*

◆ Tenofovir Disoproxil Fumarate, Rilpivirine, and Emtricitabine *see* Emtricitabine, Rilpivirine, and Tenofovir Disoproxil Fumarate *on page 636*

◆ Tenormin *see* Atenolol *on page 166*

◆ Tensilon (Can) *see* Edrophonium *on page 618*

◆ Tenuate *see* Diethylpropion *on page 546*

◆ Tenuate Dospan *see* Diethylpropion *on page 546*

◆ Terazol 3 *see* Terconazole *on page 1763*

◆ Terazol 7 *see* Terconazole *on page 1763*

Terazosin (ter AY zoe sin)

Brand Names: Canada Apo-Terazosin; Dom-Terazosin; Hytrin; Nu-Terazosin; PHL-Terazosin; PMS-Terazosin; ratio-Terazosin; Teva-Terazosin

Index Terms Hytrin

Pharmacologic Category Alpha$_1$ Blocker; Antihypertensive

Use

Hypertension: Management of mild-to-moderate hypertension; alone or in combination with other agents such as diuretics or beta-blockers

Note: The 2014 guideline for the management of high blood pressure in adults (Eighth Joint National Committee [JNC 8]) does **not** recommend the use of terazosin in the treatment of hypertension (JNC8 [James, 2013]).

Benign prostate hyperplasia: Benign prostate hyperplasia (BPH)

Pregnancy Considerations Teratogenic effects have not been observed in animal studies. Decreased fetal weight and increased risk of fetal mortality were noted in some animal reproduction studies. There are no adequate and well-controlled studies in pregnant women. Use only if benefit outweighs risk.

Untreated chronic maternal hypertension is associated with adverse events in the fetus, infant, and mother. If treatment for hypertension during pregnancy is needed, other agents are generally preferred (ACOG, 2013).

Breast-Feeding Considerations It is not known if terazosin is excreted in breast milk. The manufacturer recommends that caution be exercised when administering terazosin to nursing women.

Contraindications Hypersensitivity to terazosin or any component of the formulation

Warnings/Precautions Can cause significant orthostatic hypotension and syncope, especially with first dose; anticipate a similar effect if therapy is interrupted for a few days, if dosage is rapidly increased, or if another antihypertensive drug (particularly vasodilators) or a PDE-5 inhibitor is introduced. Discontinue if symptoms of angina occur or worsen. Patients should be cautioned about performing hazardous tasks when starting new therapy or adjusting dosage upward. Prostate cancer should be ruled out before starting for BPH. Intraoperative floppy iris syndrome has been observed in cataract surgery patients who were on or were previously treated with alpha$_1$-blockers. Causality has not been established and there appears to be no benefit in discontinuing alpha-blocker therapy prior to surgery. Priapism has been associated with use (rarely). In the elderly, avoid use as an antihypertensive due to high risk of orthostatic hypotension; alternative agents preferred due to a more favorable risk/benefit profile (Beers Criteria).

Adverse Reactions

>10%:

Central nervous system: Dizziness (9% to 19%)

Neuromuscular & skeletal: Muscle weakness (7% to 11%)

1% to 10%:

Cardiovascular: Peripheral edema (1% to 6%), orthostatic hypotension (1% to 4%), palpitation (≤4%), tachycardia (≤2%), syncope (≤1%)

Central nervous system: Somnolence (4% to 5%), vertigo (1%)

Gastrointestinal: Nausea (2% to 4%), weight gain (≤1%)

Genitourinary: Impotence (≤2%), libido decreased (≤1%)

Neuromuscular & skeletal: Extremity pain (≤4%), paresthesia (≤3%), back pain (≤2%)

Ocular: Blurred vision (≤2%)

Respiratory: Nasal congestion (2% to 6%), dyspnea (2% to 3%), sinusitis (≤3%)

<1% (Limited to important or life-threatening): Abdominal pain, abnormal vision, allergic reactions, anaphylaxis, anxiety, arrhythmia, arthralgia, arthritis, atrial fibrillation, bronchitis, chest pain, conjunctivitis, constipation, cough, diaphoresis, diarrhea, dyspepsia, epistaxis, facial edema, fever, flatulence, flu-like syndrome, gout, insomnia, intraoperative floppy iris syndrome (IFIS), joint disorder, myalgia, neck pain, pharyngitis, polyuria, priapism, pruritus, rash, rhinitis, shoulder pain, thrombocytopenia, tinnitus, urinary incontinence, urinary tract infection, vasodilation, vomiting, xerostomia

Drug Interactions

Metabolism/Transport Effects None known.

Avoid Concomitant Use

Avoid concomitant use of Terazosin with any of the following: Alpha1-Blockers

Increased Effect/Toxicity

Terazosin may increase the levels/effects of: Alpha1-Blockers; Amifostine; Antipsychotic Agents (Second Generation [Atypical]); Calcium Channel Blockers; DULoxetine; Hypotension-Associated Agents; Levodopa

The levels/effects of Terazosin may be increased by: Barbiturates; Beta-Blockers; Brimonidine (Topical); Dapoxetine; Diazoxide; Herbs (Hypotensive Properties); Molsidomine; Nicorandil; Obinutuzumab; Pentoxifylline; Phosphodiesterase 5 Inhibitors; Prostacyclin Analogues

Decreased Effect

Terazosin may decrease the levels/effects of: Alpha-/Beta-Agonists; Alpha1-Agonists

The levels/effects of Terazosin may be decreased by: Amphetamines; Herbs (Hypertensive Properties); Methylphenidate; Yohimbine

Storage/Stability Store at 20°C to 25°C (68°F to 77°F); protect from light and moisture.

Mechanism of Action Alpha$_1$-specific blocking agent with minimal alpha$_2$ effects; this allows peripheral postsynaptic blockade, with the resultant decrease in arterial tone, while preserving the negative feedback loop which is mediated by the peripheral presynaptic alpha$_2$-receptors; terazosin relaxes the smooth muscle of the bladder neck, thus reducing bladder outlet obstruction

Pharmacodynamics/Kinetics

Onset of action: 1-2 hours

Absorption: Rapid and complete

Protein binding: 90% to 95%

Metabolism: Hepatic; minimal first-pass

Half-life elimination: ~12 hours

Time to peak, serum: ~1 hour

Excretion: Feces (~60%, ~20% as unchanged drug); urine (~40%, ~10% as unchanged drug)

Dosing

Adult Note: If drug is discontinued for greater than several days, consider beginning with initial dose and retitrate as needed.

Hypertension: Oral: Initial: 1 mg at bedtime; slowly increase dose to achieve desired blood pressure, up to 20 mg/day; usual dosage range (ASH/ISH [Weber, 2014]: 1-2 mg daily. **Note:** Dosage may be given on a twice daily regimen if response is diminished at 24 hours and hypotension is observed at 2-4 hours following a dose.

Benign prostatic hyperplasia: Oral: Initial: 1 mg at bedtime; thereafter, titrate upwards, if needed, over several weeks, balancing therapeutic benefit with terazosin-induced postural hypotension; most patients require 10 mg day; if no response after 4-6 weeks of 10 mg/day, may increase to 20 mg/day

Dosage adjustment with concurrent medication:

Concurrent use with a diuretic or other antihypertensive agent (especially verapamil): Dosage reduction may be needed when adding

Concurrent use with PDE-5 inhibitors: Initiate PDE-5 inhibitor therapy at the lowest dose due to additive orthostatic and blood pressure lowering effects

Geriatric Refer to adult dosing. In the management of hypertension, consider lower initial doses (eg, immediate release: 0.5 mg once daily) and titrate to response (Aronow, 2011).

Pediatric Hypertension (off-label use): Oral: Initial: 1 mg once daily; gradually increase dose as necessary, up to maximum of 20 mg/day

Renal Impairment No dosage adjustment necessary. Hemodialysis: No supplemental dose necessary.

Hepatic Impairment No dosage adjustment provided in manufacturer's labeling.

Dietary Considerations May be taken without regard to meals at the same time each day.

Administration Administer without regard to meals at the same time each day.

Monitoring Parameters Standing and sitting/supine blood pressure, especially following the initial dose at 2-4 hours following the dose and thereafter at the trough point to ensure adequate control throughout the dosing interval; urinary symptoms

Dosage Forms Excipient information presented when available (limited, particularly for generics); consult specific product labeling.

Capsule, Oral:

Generic: 1 mg, 2 mg, 5 mg, 10 mg

Dosage Forms: Canada Excipient information presented when available (limited, particularly for generics); consult specific product labeling.

Tablet, Oral: 1 mg, 2 mg, 5 mg, 10 mg

Terbinafine (Systemic) (TER bin a feen)

Brand Names: US LamISIL; Terbinex

Brand Names: Canada Apo-Terbinafine; Auro-Terbinafine; CO Terbinafine; Dom-Terbinafine; GD-Terbinafine; JAMP-Terbinafine; Lamisil; Mylan-Terbinafine; PHL-Terbinafine; PMS-Terbinafine; Q-Terbinafine; Riva-Terbinafine; Sandoz-Terbinafine; Teva-Terbinafine

Index Terms Terbinafine Hydrochloride

Pharmacologic Category Antifungal Agent, Oral

Use

Onychomycosis (tablets only): Treatment of onychomycosis of the toenail or fingernail caused by dermatophytes (tinea unguium).

Tinea capitis (granules only): Treatment of tinea capitis in patients 4 years and older.

Canadian labeling: Additional use (not in U.S. labeling): Severe tineal skin infections (tinea cruris and tinea pedis) unresponsive to topical therapy

Pregnancy Considerations Adverse events were not observed in animal reproduction studies. Avoid use in pregnancy since treatment of onychomycosis is postponable.

Breast-Feeding Considerations Terbinafine is excreted in breast milk; the milk/plasma ratio is 7:1. Breast-feeding is not recommended by the manufacturer.

Contraindications Hypersensitivity to terbinafine or any component of the formulation

Warnings/Precautions Due to potential toxicity, confirmation of diagnostic testing of nail or skin specimens prior to treatment of onychomycosis or dermatomycosis is recommended. Use caution in patients sensitive to allylamine antifungals (eg, naftifine, butenafine); cross sensitivity to terbinafine may exist. Transient decreases in absolute lymphocyte counts were observed in clinical trials; severe neutropenia (reversible upon discontinuation) has also been reported. Monitor CBC in patients with preexisting immunosuppression if therapy is to continue >6 weeks and discontinue therapy if ANC ≤1000/mm^3.

Serious skin and hypersensitivity reactions (eg, Stevens-Johnson syndrome, toxic epidermal necrolysis, erythema multiforme, exfoliative dermatitis, bullous dermatitis, drug reaction with eosinophilia and systemic symptoms [DRESS] syndrome) have occurred. If progressive skin rash or signs and symptoms of a hypersensitivity reaction occur, discontinue treatment. Cases of hepatic failure, some leading to liver transplant or death, have been reported; not recommended for use in patients with active or chronic liver disease. If clinical evidence of liver injury develops (eg, nausea, anorexia, fatigue, vomiting, right upper abdominal pain, jaundice, dark urine, pale stools), assess hepatic function immediately; discontinue therapy in cases of elevated liver function tests. Use with caution in patients with renal dysfunction (CrCl ≤50 mL/minute) (per Canadian labeling, not recommended for use); clearance is reduced by ~50%.

Disturbances of taste and/or smell may occur; resolution may be delayed (eg, >1 year) following discontinuation of therapy or in some cases, disturbance may be permanent. Discontinue therapy in patients with symptoms of taste or smell disturbance.

Adverse Reactions Adverse events listed for tablets unless otherwise specified. Granules were studied in patients 4-12 years of age.

>10%: Central nervous system: Headache (13%; granules 7%)

1% to 10%:

Dermatologic: Skin rash (6%; granules 2%), pruritus (3%; granules 1%), urticaria (1%)

Gastrointestinal: Diarrhea (6%; granules 3%), vomiting (<1%; granules 5%), dyspepsia (4%), dysgeusia (may be severe and result in weight loss and depression; 3%), nausea (3%; granules 2%), abdominal pain (2%; granules 2% to 4%), flatulence (2%), sore throat (granules 2%), toothache (granules 1%)

Hepatic: Liver enzyme disorder (3%)

Infection: Influenza (granules 2%)

Ophthalmic: Visual disturbance (1%)

Respiratory: Nasopharyngitis (granules 10%), cough (granules 6%), upper respiratory tract infection (granules 5%), nasal congestion (granules 2%), rhinorrhea (granules 2%)

Miscellaneous: Fever (granules 7%)

<1% (Limited to important or life-threatening): Acute generalized exanthematous pustulosis, acute pancreatitis, agranulocytosis, alopecia, altered sense of smell, anaphylaxis, angioedema, depression, DRESS syndrome, exacerbation of psoriasis, exacerbation of systemic lupus erythematosus, hepatic disease, hepatic failure, hypersensitivity reaction, pancytopenia, rhabdomyolysis, severe neutropenia, Stevens-Johnson syndrome, thrombocytopenia, toxic epidermal necrolysis, vasculitis, visual field loss

Drug Interactions

Metabolism/Transport Effects Substrate of CYP1A2 (minor), CYP2C19 (minor), CYP2C9 (minor), CYP3A4 (minor); **Note:** Assignment of Major/Minor substrate status based on clinically relevant drug interaction potential; **Inhibits** CYP2D6 (strong)

Avoid Concomitant Use

Avoid concomitant use of Terbinafine (Systemic) with any of the following: Mequitazine; Pimozide; Saccharomyces boulardii; Tamoxifen; Thioridazine

Increased Effect/Toxicity

Terbinafine (Systemic) may increase the levels/effects of: Amitriptyline; ARIPiprazole; ARIPiprazole Lauroxil; AtoMOXetine; Brexpiprazole; CYP2D6 Substrates; Dapoxetine; Desipramine; DOXOrubicin (Conventional); DULoxetine; Eliglustat; Fesoterodine; Iloperidone; Imipramine; Mequitazine; Metoprolol; Nebivolol; Nortriptyline; Pimozide; Propafenone; Tamsulosin; Tetrabenazine; Thioridazine; TraMADol; Vortioxetine

Decreased Effect

Terbinafine (Systemic) may decrease the levels/effects of: Codeine; Hydrocodone; Iloperidone; Saccharomyces boulardii; Tamoxifen; TraMADol

The levels/effects of Terbinafine (Systemic) may be decreased by: Rifampin

Storage/Stability

Granules: Store at 25°C (77°F); excursions permitted between 15°C to 30°C (59°F to 86°F).

Tablet: Store below 25°C (77°F). Protect from light.

Mechanism of Action Synthetic allylamine derivative which inhibits squalene epoxidase, a key enzyme in sterol biosynthesis in fungi. This results in a deficiency in ergosterol within the fungal cell wall and results in fungal cell death.

Pharmacodynamics/Kinetics

Absorption: >70%

Distribution: Distributed to sebum and skin predominantly

Protein binding: Plasma: >99%

Metabolism: Hepatic predominantly via CYP1A2, 3A4, 2C8, 2C9, and 2C19 to inactive metabolites

Bioavailability: ~40%; Children 36% to 64%

Half-life elimination: Terminal half-life: 200-400 hours; very slow release of drug from skin and adipose tissues occurs; effective half-life: ~36 hours; Children: 27-31 hours

Time to peak, plasma: Within 2 hours

Excretion: Urine (~70%)

Dosing

Adult

U.S. labeling: Oral:

Onychomycosis: Tablet: Fingernail: 250 mg once daily for 6 weeks; Toenail: 250 mg once daily for 12 weeks

Missed doses: If a dose is missed, take as soon as remembered, unless it is less than 4 hours before the next dose is due.

Tinea capitis (patients >35 kg): Granules: 250 mg once daily for 6 weeks

Canadian labeling: Oral: Tablet: **Note:** Mycologic cure may precede complete resolution of symptoms by several weeks (skin infections) or by several months (onychomycosis).

Onychomycosis (finger or toenail): 250 mg/day in 1-2 divided doses for 6 weeks to 3 months (≥6 months may be necessary in some patients with infections of the big toenail)

Tinea corporis, tinea cruris: 250 mg/day in 1-2 divided doses for 2-4 weeks

Tinea pedis (interdigital and plantar/moccasin type): 250 mg/day in 1-2 divided doses for 2-6 weeks

Sporotrichosis, lymphocutaneous and cutaneous (off-label use): Oral: 500 mg twice daily as alternative therapy; treat for 2-4 weeks after resolution of all lesions (usual duration: 3-6 months) (Kauffman, 2007)

Geriatric Use with caution; refer to adult dosing.

Pediatric

Tinea capitis: Oral: Granules: Children ≥4 years and Adolescents:

<25 kg: 125 mg once daily for 6 weeks

25-35 kg: 187.5 mg once daily for 6 weeks

>35 kg: 250 mg once daily for 6 weeks

Onychomycosis (off-label use; Gupta, 1997): Oral: Tablet: Children and Adolescents:

10-20 kg: 62.5 mg once daily for 6 weeks (fingernails) **or** 12 weeks (toenails)

20-40 kg: 125 mg once daily for 6 weeks (fingernails) **or** 12 weeks (toenails)

>40 kg: 250 mg once daily for 6 weeks (fingernails) **or** 12 weeks (toenails)

Renal Impairment

U.S. labeling: No dosage adjustment provided in manufacturer's labeling (has not been studied); however, clearance is decreased 50% in patients with CrCl ≤50 mL/minute.

Canadian labeling: Use is not recommended in patients with CrCl ≤50 mL/minute.

Hepatic Impairment Use is not recommended in chronic or active hepatic disease.

Administration Administer tablets without regard to meals. Administer granules with food; sprinkle granules on a spoonful of pudding or other soft, nonacidic food (eg, mashed potatoes); swallow entire spoonful without chewing; do not mix granules with applesauce or other fruit-based foods.

Monitoring Parameters AST/ALT prior to initiation, repeat if used >6 weeks; CBC; taste and/or smell disturbances

Dosage Forms Considerations Terbinex Kit contains terbinafine 250 mg tablets and hydroxypropyl-chitosan 1% nail lacquer

Dosage Forms Excipient information presented when available (limited, particularly for generics); consult specific product labeling.

Kit, Combination:

Terbinex: 250 mg & 1%

Packet, Oral:

LamISIL: 125 mg (1 ea, 14 ea); 187.5 mg (1 ea, 14 ea) [contains polyethylene glycol]

Tablet, Oral:

LamISIL: 250 mg

Generic: 250 mg

Dosage Forms: Canada Excipient information presented when available (limited, particularly for generics); consult specific product labeling.

Tablet, oral:

LamISIL: 125 mg [contains lactose]

Extemporaneous Preparations A 25 mg/mL oral suspension may be made using tablets. Crush twenty 250 mg tablets and reduce to a fine powder. Add small amount of a 1:1 mixture of Ora-Sweet® and Ora-Plus® and mix to a uniform paste; mix while adding the vehicle in geometric proportions to **almost** 200 mL; transfer to a calibrated bottle, rinse mortar with vehicle, and add quantity of vehicle sufficient to make 200 mL. Label "shake well" and "refrigerate". Stable 42 days.

Nahata MC, Pai VB, and Hipple TF, *Pediatric Drug Formulations*, 5th ed, Cincinnati, OH: Harvey Whitney Books Co, 2004.

Terbinafine (Topical) (TER bin a feen)

Brand Names: US LamISIL Advanced [OTC]; LamISIL Jock Itch [OTC]; LamISIL AT Spray [OTC]; LamISIL AT [OTC]; LamISIL Spray

Brand Names: Canada Lamisil

Index Terms Terbinafine Hydrochloride

Pharmacologic Category Antifungal Agent, Topical

Use Antifungal for the treatment of tinea pedis (athlete's foot), tinea cruris (jock itch), and tinea corporis (ringworm) [OTC/Canadian prescription formulations]; cutaneous candidiasis and tinea versicolor [Canadian prescription formulations]

Dosing

Adult & Geriatric

Tinea pedis: Topical:

Cream: Apply between the toes to affected area once or twice daily for at least 1 week [OTC/Canadian prescription formulations]; apply on the bottom or sides of feet twice daily for 2 weeks [OTC formulations]

Gel: Apply to affected area once daily for at least 1 week [OTC formulations]

Solution: Apply to affected area once daily for at least 1 week [OTC/Canadian prescription formulations]

Tinea corporis, Tinea cruris: Topical:

Cream: Apply to affected area once daily for 1 week [OTC/Canadian prescription formulations]

Gel: Apply to affected area once daily for 1 week [OTC formulations]

Solution: Apply to affected area once daily for 1 week [OTC/Canadian prescription formulations]

Cutaneous candidiasis: Apply to affected area once or twice daily for 1-2 weeks [Canadian prescription formulation]

Tinea versicolor: Topical:

Cream: Apply to affected area once or twice daily for 1-2 weeks [Canadian prescription formulation]

Solution: Apply to affected area twice daily for 1 week [Canadian prescription formulation]

Pediatric

Tinea pedis: Children ≥12 years and Adolescents: Topical:

Cream: Apply between the toes to affected area twice daily for at least 1 week [OTC formulations]; apply on the bottom or sides of feet twice daily for 2 weeks [OTC formulations]

Gel, Solution: Refer to adult dosing.

Tinea corporis, Tinea cruris: Children ≥12 years and Adolescents: Refer to adult dosing.

Additional Information Complete prescribing information should be consulted for additional detail.

Dosage Forms Excipient information presented when available (limited, particularly for generics); consult specific product labeling.

Cream, External, as hydrochloride:

LamISIL AT: 1% (12 g, 24 g, 30 g, 36 g, 42 g) [contains benzyl alcohol, cetyl alcohol]

LamISIL AT Jock Itch: 1% (12 g) [contains benzyl alcohol, cetyl alcohol]

Generic: 1% (12 g, 15 g, 24 g, 30 g)

Gel, External:

LamISIL Advanced: 1% (12 g) [contains alcohol, usp]

Solution, External, as hydrochloride:

LamISIL AT Spray: 1% (30 mL, 125 mL) [contains alcohol, usp, propylene glycol]

LamISIL Spray: 1% (30 mL) [contains alcohol, usp]

Dosage Forms: Canada Excipient information presented when available (limited, particularly for generics); consult specific product labeling.

Cream, topical, as hydrochloride: 1% (12 g, 24 g)

Lamisil®: 1% (15 g, 30 g)

Solution, topical, as hydrochloride [spray]:

Lamisil®: 1% (30 mL)

◆ Terbinafine Hydrochloride *see* Terbinafine (Systemic) *on page 1759*

◆ Terbinafine Hydrochloride *see* Terbinafine (Topical) *on page 1760*

◆ Terbinex *see* Terbinafine (Systemic) *on page 1759*

Terbutaline (ter BYOO ta leen)

Brand Names: Canada Bricanyl Turbuhaler

Index Terms Brethaire; Brethine; Bricanyl; Terbutaline Sulfate

Pharmacologic Category Antidote, Extravasation; Beta₂ Agonist

Use Asthma/Bronchospasm: Bronchodilator in reversible airway obstruction and bronchial asthma

Pregnancy Considerations Adverse events have been observed in animal reproduction studies. Terbutaline crosses the placenta; umbilical cord concentrations are ~11% to 48% of maternal blood levels.

Uncontrolled asthma is associated with adverse events on pregnancy (increased risk of perinatal mortality, preeclampsia, preterm birth, low birth weight infants). Terbutaline is not recommended for the treatment of asthma during pregnancy; inhaled beta₂-receptor agonists are preferred (NAEPP 2005).

[U.S. Boxed Warning]: Terbutaline is not FDA approved for and should not be used for prolonged tocolysis (>48 to 72 hours). Use for maintenance tocolysis should not be done in the outpatient setting. Adverse events observed in pregnant women include arrhythmias, increased heart rate, hyperglycemia (transient), hypokalemia, myocardial ischemia, and pulmonary edema. Heart rate may be increased in the fetus and hypoglycemia may occur in the neonate. Terbutaline has been used in the management of preterm labor. Tocolytics may be used for the short-term (48 hour) prolongation of pregnancy to allow for the administration of antenatal steroids and should not be used prior to fetal viability or when the risks of use to the fetus or mother are greater than the risk of preterm birth (ACOG 2012).

Breast-Feeding Considerations Terbutaline is excreted in breast milk; concentrations are similar to or higher than those in the maternal plasma. Based on information from four cases, exposure to the breast-fed infant would be <1% of the weight-adjusted maternal dose. Adverse events were not observed in nursing infants (Boréus 1982; Lönnerholm 1982). The manufacturer recommends that terbutaline be used in breast-feeding women only if the potential benefit to the mother outweighs the possible risk to the infant. The use of beta₂-receptor agonists are not considered a contraindication to breast-feeding (NAEPP 2005).

Contraindications

Hypersensitivity to terbutaline, sympathomimetic amines, or any component of the formulation

Injection: Additional contraindications: Prolonged (>72 hours) prevention or management of preterm labor

Oral: Additional contraindications: Prevention or treatment of preterm labor

Bricanyl Turbuhaler [Canadian product]: Hypersensitivity to sympathomimetic amines; history of tachyarrhythmias; as tocolytic in patients at risk of premature labor or threatened abortion.

Warnings/Precautions [US Boxed Warning]: Terbutaline is not FDA approved for and should not be used for prolonged tocolysis (>48 to 72 hours). Use for maintenance tocolysis should not be done in the outpatient setting. Adverse events observed in pregnant women include arrhythmias, increased heart rate, hyperglycemia (transient), hypokalemia, myocardial ischemia, and pulmonary edema. Heart rate may be increased in the fetus and hypoglycemia may occur in the neonate. Oral terbutaline is contraindicated for acute or chronic use in the management of preterm labor. Use of Bricanyl Turbuhaler [Canadian product] as a tocolytic in patients at risk of premature labor or threatened abortion is contraindicated.

Use caution in patients with cardiovascular disease (arrhythmia or hypertension or HF). Use of Bricanyl Turbuhaler [Canadian product] in patients with a history of tachyarrhythmias is contraindicated. Use with caution in convulsive disorders, diabetes, glaucoma, hyperthyroidism, or hypokalemia. Beta-agonists may cause elevation in blood pressure, heart rate, and result in CNS stimulation/excitation. Beta₂-agonists may increase risk of arrhythmia, increase serum glucose, or decrease serum potassium. Use with caution in patients with hypokalemia or taking concomitant drugs that cause hypokalemia.

When used as a bronchodilator, optimize anti-inflammatory treatment before initiating maintenance treatment with terbutaline. Do not use as a component of chronic therapy without an anti-inflammatory agent. Only the mildest form of asthma (Step 1 and/or exercise-induced) would not require concurrent use based upon asthma guidelines. Patient must be instructed to seek medical attention in cases where acute symptoms are not relieved or a previous level of response is diminished. The need to increase frequency of use may indicate deterioration of asthma, and treatment must not be delayed.

Immediate hypersensitivity reactions (urticaria, angioedema, rash, bronchospasm) have been reported. Do not exceed recommended dose; serious adverse events including fatalities, have been associated with excessive use of inhaled sympathomimetics. Rarely, paradoxical bronchospasm may occur with use of inhaled bronchodilating agents; this should be distinguished from inadequate response. Potentially significant drug-drug interactions may exist, requiring dose or frequency adjustment, additional monitoring, and/or selection of alternative therapy.

Adverse Reactions

>10%:

Central nervous system: Nervousness, restlessness

Endocrine & metabolic: Serum glucose increased, serum potassium decreased

Neuromuscular & skeletal: Trembling

1% to 10%:

Cardiovascular: Tachycardia, hypertension, pounding heartbeat

Central nervous system: Dizziness, lightheadedness, drowsiness, headache, insomnia

Gastrointestinal: Dry mouth, nausea, vomiting, bad taste in mouth

Neuromuscular & skeletal: Muscle cramps, weakness

Miscellaneous: Diaphoresis

<1% (Limited to important or life-threatening): Arrhythmia, cardiac arrest (preterm labor), chest pain, hyperglycemia (preterm labor), hypokalemia (preterm labor), hypotension (preterm labor), paradoxical bronchospasm, myocardial infarction (preterm labor), myocardial ischemia (preterm labor), pulmonary edema (preterm labor)

Drug Interactions

Metabolism/Transport Effects None known.

Avoid Concomitant Use

Avoid concomitant use of Terbutaline with any of the following: Beta-Blockers (Nonselective); Iobenguane I 123; Loxapine

Increased Effect/Toxicity

Terbutaline may increase the levels/effects of: Atosiban; Doxofylline; Highest Risk QTc-Prolonging Agents; Loop Diuretics; Loxapine; Moderate Risk QTc-Prolonging Agents; Sympathomimetics; Thiazide Diuretics

The levels/effects of Terbutaline may be increased by: AtoMOXetine; Cannabinoid-Containing Products; Linezolid; MAO Inhibitors; Mifepristone; Tedizolid; Tricyclic Antidepressants

Decreased Effect

Terbutaline may decrease the levels/effects of: Iobenguane I 123

The levels/effects of Terbutaline may be decreased by: Beta-Blockers (Beta1 Selective); Beta-Blockers (Nonselective); Betahistine

Preparation for Administration For extravasation management (off-label use): Using vial for injection, dilute 1 mg with 9 mL (total volume: 10 mL) (large extravasation site) **or** 1 mg with 1 mL (total volume: 2 mL) (small/distal extravasation site) of 0.9% sodium chloride (Stier 1999).

Storage/Stability Store injection at room temperature; do not freeze. Protect from heat and light. Use only clear solutions. Store powder for inhalation (Bricanyl® Turbuhaler [Canadian availability]) at room temperature between 15°C and 30°C (58°F and 86°F).

Mechanism of Action Relaxes bronchial and uterine smooth muscle by action on beta$_2$-receptors with less effect on heart rate

Pharmacodynamics/Kinetics

Onset of action: Oral: 30 to 45 minutes; SubQ: 6 to 15 minute; Inhalation: 5 minutes (maximum effect: 15 to 60 minutes)

Duration: Inhalation: 4 to 7 hours

Protein binding: 25%

Metabolism: Hepatic to inactive sulfate conjugates

Bioavailability: SubQ doses are more bioavailable than oral

Half-life elimination: 11 to 16 hours

Excretion: Urine; feces

Dosing

Adult & Geriatric

Asthma/bronchospasm:

Oral: 5 mg/dose every 6 hours 3 times/day; if side effects occur, reduce dose to 2.5 mg every 6 hours; not to exceed 15 mg in 24 hours.

SubQ:

Manufacturer's labeling: 0.25 mg/dose; may repeat in 15 to 30 minutes (maximum: 0.5 mg/4-hour period)

Off-label dose: 0.25 mg/dose; may repeat every 20 minutes for 3 doses (maximum: 0.75 mg/1-hour period) (NAEPP 2007)

Inhalation: Bricanyl Turbuhaler [Canadian product]: One inhalation; if not effective after 5 minutes may repeat dose. If second dose is not effective, consult healthcare provider immediately. Additional doses may be administered however >6 inhalations in a 24 hour period should not be needed. **Note:** If adequate relief is not obtained with previously effective dose, or if effects of inhalation last <3 hours, patient should be reassessed promptly; may indicate worsening asthma.

Extravasation management, sympathomimetic vasoconstrictors (off-label use; based on limited case reports): SubQ:

Large extravasations: Infiltrate extravasation area using a solution of 1 mg diluted in 9 mL (total volume: 10 mL) of 0.9% sodium chloride; volume of terbutaline solution administered varied from 3 to 10 mL (Stier 1999).

Small/distal extravasations: Infiltrate extravasation area using a solution of 1 mg diluted in 1 mL (total volume: 2 mL) of 0.9% sodium chloride; volume of terbutaline solution administered varied from 0.5 to 1 mL (Stier 1999).

Premature labor (acute; short-term [≤72 hours] tocolysis; off-label use):

IV: 2.5 to 5 mcg/minute; increased gradually every 20 to 30 minutes by 2.5 to 5 mcg/minute; effective maximum dosages from 17.5 to 30 mcg/minute have been used with caution. Duration of infusion is at least 12 hours (Travis 1993).

SubQ: 0.25 mg every 20 minutes to 3 hours; hold for pulse >120 beats per minute. Terbutaline has not been approved for and should not be used for prolonged tocolysis (beyond 48 to 72 hours) (ACOG 2012; Hearne 2000).

Pediatric

Asthma/bronchospasm:

Oral: Children and Adolescents:

<12 years: Initial: 0.05 mg/kg/dose 3 times/day, increased gradually as required; maximum: 0.15 mg/kg/dose 3 to 4 times/day or a total of 5 mg/24 hours

12 to 15 years: 2.5 mg every 6 hours 3 times/day; not to exceed 7.5 mg in 24 hours

>15 years: 5 mg/dose every 6 hours 3 times/day; if side effects occur, reduce dose to 2.5 mg every 6 hours; not to exceed 15 mg in 24 hours

SubQ: Children and Adolescents:

<12 years: 0.005 to 0.01 mg/kg/dose to a maximum of 0.4 mg/dose every 15 to 20 minutes for 3 doses; may repeat every 2 to 6 hours as needed

≥12 years: Refer to adult dosing.

Inhalation: Bricanyl Turbuhaler [Canadian product]: Children ≥6 years and Adolescents: Refer to adult dosing.

Renal Impairment There are no dosage adjustments provided in the manufacturer's labeling.

Hepatic Impairment There are no dosage adjustments provided in the manufacturer's labeling.

Administration

IV: Use infusion pump.

Oral: Administer around-the-clock to promote less variation in peak and trough serum levels

Inhalation: Bricanyl Turbuhaler [Canadian product]: After removing lid, patient should hold inhaler upright and turn blue grip as far as it will go in one direction then turn it back to original position. Clicking sound indicates that inhaler is ready for use. Patient should exhale fully but not into the inhaler and then place mouthpiece gently between teeth, close lips around inhaler and inhale deeply. Inhaler should be removed from mouth prior to exhaling. Instruct patients to rinse mouth with water after each inhalation as some medication may stick to the inside of the mouth and throat. If inhaler is dropped or shaken, or if patient exhales into the inhaler after a dose is loaded, the dose will be lost and a new dose should be loaded and inhaled. Outside of mouthpiece should be cleaned once weekly with a dry tissue. Instruct patient to keep inhaler dry. First appearance of red mark in dose indicator (window underneath mouthpiece) indicates that 20 doses remain. When red mark reaches bottom of dose indicator no doses remain and Turbuhaler should be discarded.

SubQ: Extravasation management, sympathomimetic vasopressors (off-label use): Stop vesicant infusion immediately and disconnect IV line (leave needle/cannula in place); gently aspirate extravasated solution from the IV line (do **NOT** flush the line); remove needle/cannula; elevate extremity. Infiltrate extravasation area with terbutaline solution 1 mg diluted with 9 mL (large extravasation site) **or** 1 mg diluted with 1 mL (small/distal extravasation site) of 0.9% sodium chloride into extravasation site (Stier 1999).

Monitoring Parameters Serum potassium, glucose; intake/output; heart rate, blood pressure, respiratory rate; chest pain, shortness of breath; monitor for signs and symptoms of pulmonary edema (when used as a tocolytic); monitor FEV$_1$, peak flow, and/or other pulmonary function tests (when used as bronchodilator). If used for extravasation management, monitor and document extravasation site.

Dosage Forms Excipient information presented when available (limited, particularly for generics); consult specific product labeling.

Solution, Injection, as sulfate:

Generic: 1 mg/mL (1 mL)

Tablet, Oral, as sulfate:

Generic: 2.5 mg, 5 mg

Dosage Forms: Canada Excipient information presented when available (limited, particularly for generics); consult specific product labeling.

Powder for oral inhalation:

Bricanyl Turbuhaler: 500 mcg/actuation [100 or 200 metered actuations]

Extemporaneous Preparations A 1 mg/mL oral suspension may be made with tablets. Crush twenty-four 5 mg tablets in a mortar and reduce to a fine powder. Add 5 mL purified water USP and mix to a uniform paste; mix while adding simple syrup, NF in incremental proportions to almost 120 mL; transfer to a calibrated bottle, rinse mortar with vehicle, and add quantity of simple syrup, NF sufficient to make 120 mL. Label "shake well" and "refrigerate". Stable for 30 days.

Nahata MC, Pai VB, and Hipple TF, *Pediatric Drug Formulations*, 5th ed, Cincinnati, OH: Harvey Whitney Books Co, 2004.

◆ Terbutaline Sulfate *see* Terbutaline *on page 1761*

Terconazole (ter KONE a zole)

Brand Names: US Terazol 3; Terazol 7; Zazole
Brand Names: Canada Taro-Terconazole; Terazol 7
Index Terms Triaconazole
Pharmacologic Category Antifungal Agent, Azole Derivative; Antifungal Agent, Vaginal
Use Candidiasis: For the local treatment of vulvovaginal candidiasis (moniliasis). As terconazole is effective only for vulvovaginitis caused by the genus *Candida*, the diagnosis should be confirmed by KOH smears or cultures.
Dosing
Adult & Geriatric Vulvovaginal candidiasis: Intravaginal:

Vaginal cream 0.4%: Insert 1 applicatorful intravaginally at bedtime for 7 consecutive days.

Vaginal cream 0.8%: Insert 1 applicatorful intravaginally at bedtime for 3 consecutive days.

Vaginal suppository: Insert 1 suppository intravaginally at bedtime for 3 consecutive days.

Additional Information Complete prescribing information should be consulted for additional detail.
Dosage Forms Excipient information presented when available (limited, particularly for generics); consult specific product labeling. [DSC] = Discontinued product

Cream, Vaginal:

Terazol 7: 0.4% (45 g) [contains cetyl alcohol, polysorbate 80, propylene glycol]

Terazol 3: 0.8% (20 g) [contains cetyl alcohol, polysorbate 80, propylene glycol]

Zazole: 0.4% (45 g); 0.8% (20 g)

Generic: 0.4% (45 g); 0.8% (20 g)

Suppository, Vaginal:

Terazol 3: 80 mg (3 ea [DSC])

Zazole: 80 mg (3 ea)

Generic: 80 mg (3 ea)

Teriflunomide (ter i FLOO noh mide)

Brand Names: US Aubagio
Brand Names: Canada Aubagio
Index Terms A771726; HMR1726
Pharmacologic Category Pyrimidine Synthesis Inhibitor
Use Multiple sclerosis: Treatment of patients with relapsing forms of multiple sclerosis.
Pregnancy Considerations Adverse events have been observed in animal reproduction studies conducted using doses lower than the expected human exposure. **[US Boxed Warning]: Based on animal data, teriflunomide may cause major birth defects if used in pregnant women. Teriflunomide is contraindicated in pregnant women or women of childbearing potential who are not using reliable contraception. Pregnancy must be avoided during therapy or prior to completing the accelerated elimination treatment protocol.** Pregnancy must be excluded prior to initiating treatment. Women of childbearing potential should not receive therapy until pregnancy has been excluded, they have been counseled concerning fetal risk, and reliable contraceptive measures have been confirmed. Following treatment, pregnancy should be avoided until undetectable serum concentrations (<0.02 mg/L) are verified. This may be accomplished by the use of an enhanced drug elimination procedure using cholestyramine or activated charcoal powder. If pregnancy occurs during treatment, discontinue therapy and initiate the accelerated elimination procedure. Pregnant women exposed to teriflunomide should be registered with the pregnancy registry (800-745-4447, option 2). Teriflunomide is also found in semen. Males and their female partners should use reliable contraception during therapy. Males taking teriflunomide who wish to father a child should consider discontinuing therapy and using the accelerated elimination procedure to decrease the potential risk of fetal exposure. (**Note:** Without use of the accelerated elimination procedure, teriflunomide may remain in the serum for up to 2 years)

Breast-Feeding Considerations It is not known whether teriflunomide is secreted in human milk. Because the potential for serious adverse reactions exists in the nursing infant, a decision should be made whether to discontinue nursing or discontinue the drug, taking into account the importance of the drug to the mother.

Medication Guide Available Yes
Contraindications

Severe hepatic impairment; concomitant use with leflunomide; women of childbearing age who will not use contraception reliably; pregnancy

Canadian labeling: Additional contraindications (not in US labeling): Hypersensitivity to teriflunomide, leflunomide or any component of the formulation; immunodeficiency states (eg, AIDS); impaired bone marrow function or significant anemias, leucopenia, neutropenia, or thrombocytopenia; serious active infections

Warnings/Precautions Hazardous agent; use appropriate precautions for handling and disposal (meets NIOSH 2014 criteria). **[US Boxed Warning]: Use of leflunomide has been associated with reports of hepatotoxicity, hepatic failure, and death, therefore, a similar risk is expected with teriflunomide. Patients with preexisting liver disease (acute or chronic liver disease or ALT >2 x ULN) may be at an increased risk of developing elevated transaminases during therapy; use is contraindicated in patients with severe impairment. Use in patients with concurrent exposure to potentially hepatotoxic drugs may increase the risk of hepatotoxicity. Obtain transaminase and bilirubin levels within 6 months prior to initiation of treatment. Monitor ALT levels at least monthly for first 6 months during therapy; if hepatotoxicity is likely teriflunomide-induced, start drug elimination procedures (eg, cholestyramine, activated charcoal) and monitor liver function tests weekly until normalized. Discontinuation of therapy may be considered if transaminases increase >3 x ULN.** Due to the potential risk of hepatotoxicity, the Canadian labeling recommends that patients avoid the use of ethanol during therapy.

Use of leflunomide has been associated with interstitial lung disease; discontinue in patients who develop new onset or worsening of pulmonary symptoms. Drug elimination procedures should be considered (eg, cholestyramine, activated charcoal) if evidence of interstitial lung disease; fatal outcomes have been reported. May increase susceptibility to infection, including opportunistic pathogens. Severe infections, sepsis, and fatalities have been reported with leflunomide. One case of fatal sepsis has been reported with teriflunomide. Not recommended in patients with severe immunodeficiency, bone marrow dysplasia, or severe, uncontrolled infections. Caution should be exercised when considering the use in patients with a history of new/recurrent infections, with conditions that predispose them to infections, or with chronic, latent, or localized infections. Patients who develop a new infection while undergoing treatment should be monitored closely; consider suspension or discontinuation of therapy and drug elimination procedures if infection is serious.

Use may affect defenses against malignancies; impact on the development and course of malignancies is not fully defined. As compared to the general population, an increased risk of lymphoma has been noted in clinical trials with use of some immunosuppressive medications. Use with caution in patients with a prior history of significant hematologic abnormalities; avoid use with bone marrow dysplasia. Neutropenia, leukopenia, and thrombocytopenia have been reported in clinical trials. Use of leflunomide has been associated with rare pancytopenia, agranulocytosis, and thrombocytopenia, therefore, a similar risk may be expected with teriflunomide. Monitoring of hematologic function is required; discontinue if evidence of bone marrow suppression and begin drug elimination procedures (eg, cholestyramine, activated charcoal). If coadministered with other potential immunosuppressive agents or switching from teriflunomide to another known immunosuppressant, increased monitoring for hematological adverse effects is necessary. Rare cases of dermatologic reactions (including Stevens-Johnson syndrome and toxic epidermal necrolysis) have been reported with leflunomide, therefore patients taking teriflunomide may also be at risk; discontinue if evidence of severe dermatologic reaction occurs, and begin drug elimination procedures (eg, cholestyramine or activated charcoal). Cases of peripheral neuropathy (including polyneuropathy and mononeuropathy) have been reported; use with caution in patients >60 years of age, receiving concomitant neurotoxic medications, or

patients with diabetes; discontinue if evidence of peripheral neuropathy occurs and begin drug elimination procedures (eg, cholestyramine, activated charcoal).

Transient acute renal failure, most likely due to acute uric acid nephropathy has been reported. Increases in blood pressure have been reported; monitor at initiation of therapy and periodically thereafter. Very rare cases of pancreatitis have been reported (Aubagio Canadian product monograph 2015); discontinue therapy in patients with symptoms of acute pancreatitis suspected to be drug-induced and begin accelerated drug elimination procedures (eg, cholestyramine, activated charcoal).

Safety has not been established in patients with latent tuberculosis infection. Patients should be screened for tuberculosis and if necessary, treated prior to initiating therapy. Potentially significant drug-drug interactions may exist, requiring dose or frequency adjustment, additional monitoring, and/or selection of alternative therapy. Patients should be brought up to date with all immunizations before initiating therapy. Live vaccines should not be given concurrently; there is no data available concerning secondary transmission of live vaccines in patients receiving therapy. Due to variations in clearance, it may take up to 2 years to reach low levels of teriflunomide metabolite serum concentrations. A drug elimination procedure using cholestyramine or activated charcoal is recommended when a more rapid elimination is needed. If a response to teriflunomide had already been observed, the use of a rapid elimination procedure may result in the return of disease activity. **[US Boxed Warning]: Based on animal data, teriflunomide may cause major birth defects if used in pregnant women. Teriflunomide is contraindicated in pregnant women or women of childbearing potential who are not using reliable contraception. Pregnancy must be avoided during therapy or prior to completing the accelerated elimination treatment protocol.**

Adverse Reactions
>10%:
Central nervous system: Headache (16% to 22%)
Dermatologic: Alopecia (10% to 13%)
Endocrine & metabolic: Hypophosphatemia (4% to 18%)
Gastrointestinal: Diarrhea (13% to 18%), nausea (8% to 14%)
Hematologic & oncologic: Neutropenia (2% to 16%), lymphocytopenia (7% to 12%)
Hepatic: Increased serum ALT (6% to 15%)
Infection: Influenza (12%)
1% to 10%:
Cardiovascular: Hypertension (3% to 4%), palpitations (2% to 3%)
Central nervous system: Paresthesia (8% to 10%), anxiety (3% to 4%), sciatica (3%), burning sensation (2% to 3%)
Dermatologic: Pruritus (3% to 4%), acne vulgaris (3%)
Endocrine & metabolic: Increased gamma-glutamyl transferase (3% to 5%), weight loss (2% to 3%), hyperkalemia (1%)
Gastrointestinal: Abdominal pain (5% to 6%), viral gastroenteritis (2% to 4%), abdominal distension (1% to 2%)
Genitourinary: Cystitis (2% to 4%)
Hematologic & oncologic: Decreased platelet count (10%), leukopenia (1% to 2%)
Hepatic: Increased serum AST (2% to 3%)
Hypersensitivity: Seasonal allergy (2% to 3%)
Infection: Herpes simplex infection (4%), serious infection (3%)
Neuromuscular & skeletal: Arthralgia (6% to 8%), musculoskeletal pain (4% to 5%), myalgia (3% to 4%), carpal tunnel syndrome (1% to 3%), peripheral neuropathy (1% to 2%)
Ophthalmic: Blurred vision (3%), conjunctivitis (3%)
Renal: Renal failure (transient, 1%)
Respiratory: Upper respiratory tract infection (9%), bronchitis (8%), sinusitis (6%)
<1% (Limited to important or life-threatening): Cytomegalovirus disease (reactivation), jaundice, increased serum creatinine, infection, myocardial infarction

Drug Interactions
Metabolism/Transport Effects Substrate of BCRP; **Inhibits** BCRP, CYP2C8 (moderate), SLCO1B1, SLCO1B3; **Induces** CYP1A2 (weak/moderate)
Avoid Concomitant Use
Avoid concomitant use of Teriflunomide with any of the following: Amodiaquine; BCG (Intravesical); Leflunomide; Natalizumab; PAZOPanib; Pimecrolimus; Tacrolimus (Topical); Tofacitinib; Vaccines (Live)
Increased Effect/Toxicity
Teriflunomide may increase the levels/effects of: Amodiaquine; BCRP/ABCG2 Substrates; CYP2C8 Substrates; Fingolimod; Natalizumab; OAT3 Substrates; OATP1B1/SLCO1B1 Substrates; PAZOPanib;

Repaglinide; Rosuvastatin; Tofacitinib; Topotecan; Vaccines (Live)

The levels/effects of Teriflunomide may be increased by: Denosumab; Leflunomide; Pimecrolimus; Roflumilast; Tacrolimus (Topical); Trastuzumab
Decreased Effect
Teriflunomide may decrease the levels/effects of: BCG (Intravesical); Caffeine and Caffeine Containing Products; Coccidioides immitis Skin Test; CYP1A2 Substrates; Sipuleucel-T; Vaccines (Inactivated); Vaccines (Live); Warfarin

The levels/effects of Teriflunomide may be decreased by: Bile Acid Sequestrants; Charcoal, Activated; Echinacea
Food Interactions
Ethanol may potentiate the hepatotoxicity of teriflunomide. Management: Avoid the use of ethanol during therapy.
Storage/Stability Store at 20°C to 25°C (68°F to 77°F); excursions permitted to 15°C to 30°C (59°F to 86°F).
Mechanism of Action Teriflunomide is an immunomodulatory agent that inhibits pyrimidine synthesis, resulting in antiproliferative and anti-inflammatory effects. It may reduce the number of activated lymphocytes in the CNS.
Pharmacodynamics/Kinetics
Distribution: V_d: IV: 11 L
Protein binding: >99%
Metabolism: Primarily by hydrolysis to minor metabolites; secondary pathways include oxidation, conjugation, and N-acetylation
Half-life elimination: Median: 18-19 days; enterohepatic recycling appears to contribute to the long half-life of this agent, since activated charcoal and cholestyramine substantially reduce plasma half-life
Time to peak, plasma: 1-4 hours
Excretion: Feces (~38%); urine (~23%)
Dosing
Adult
Multiple sclerosis: Adults: Oral:
US labeling: 7 mg or 14 mg once daily
Canadian labeling: 14 mg once daily
Renal Impairment
Mild, moderate, or severe impairment: No dosage adjustment necessary.
Severe impairment requiring dialysis: Data from a small pharmacokinetic study (n=5) suggest that hemodialysis removes a negligible amount of teriflunomide (Bergner, 2013); the Canadian labeling recommends avoiding use in this patient population.
Hepatic Impairment
Mild to moderate impairment: No dosage adjustment necessary.
Severe impairment: Use is contraindicated (has not been studied).
Adjustment for Toxicity
ALT elevations >3 times ULN: Discontinue teriflunomide and initiate cholestyramine or activated charcoal to enhance elimination

Drug elimination procedure: To achieve nondetectable serum concentrations (<0.02 mg/L) of teriflunomide administer either of the following:
Cholestyramine: 8 g every 8 hours for 11 days. If not tolerated, may decrease to 4 g every 8 hours for 11 days. The 11 days do not need to be consecutive unless plasma concentrations need to be lowered rapidly.
or
Activated charcoal: 50 g every 12 hours for 11 days. The 11 days do not need to be consecutive unless plasma concentrations need to be lowered rapidly.
Note: Both treatments have successfully lead to >98% decrease in teriflunomide concentrations.
Dietary Considerations May be taken with or without food.
Administration Administer without regard to meals. Hazardous agent; use appropriate precautions for handling and disposal (meets NIOSH 2014 criteria).
Monitoring Parameters CBC within 6 months of initiation and periodically thereafter based on signs/symptoms of infection; serum creatinine; serum transaminase and bilirubin within 6 months of initiation of therapy and monthly during the initial 6 months of treatment. In addition, monitor for signs/symptoms of severe infection, abnormalities in hepatic function tests, symptoms of hepatotoxicity, and blood pressure (baseline and periodically thereafter). Monitor hepatic function tests weekly until normalized in patients with suspected teriflunomide-induced hepatotoxicity. Screen for tuberculosis and pregnancy prior to therapy.

Dosage Forms Excipient information presented when available (limited, particularly for generics); consult specific product labeling.
Tablet, Oral:
Aubagio: 7 mg
Aubagio: 14 mg [contains fd&c blue #2 aluminum lake]
Dosage Forms: Canada Excipient information presented when available (limited, particularly for generics); consult specific product labeling.
Tablet, Oral:
Aubagio: 14 mg

Teriparatide (ter i PAR a tide)

Brand Names: US Forteo
Brand Names: Canada Forteo
Index Terms Parathyroid Hormone (1-34); Recombinant Human Parathyroid Hormone (1-34); rhPTH(1-34)
Pharmacologic Category Parathyroid Hormone Analog
Use
Glucocorticoid-induced osteoporosis: Treatment of men and women with osteoporosis associated with sustained systemic glucocorticoid therapy (daily dosage equivalent to prednisone 5 mg or more) at high risk for fracture.
Osteoporosis in men: To increase bone mass in men with primary or hypogonadal osteoporosis who are at high risk for fracture.
Osteoporosis in postmenopausal women: Treatment of postmenopausal women with osteoporosis who are at high risk for fracture.
Pregnancy Considerations Adverse events were observed in animal studies; the effect on human fetal development has not been studied. Teriparatide is not indicated for use in pregnant or premenopausal women.
Breast-Feeding Considerations It is not known if teriparatide is excreted in breast milk. According to the manufacturer, the decision to discontinue teriparatide or discontinue breast-feeding should take into account the exposure to the infant and the benefits of treatment to the mother.
Medication Guide Available Yes
Contraindications
Hypersensitivity to teriparatide or any component of the formulation
Canadian labeling: Additional contraindications (not in US labeling): Preexisting hypercalcemia; severe renal impairment; metabolic bone diseases other than primary osteoporosis (including hyperparathyroidism and Paget's disease of the bone); unexplained elevations of alkaline phosphatase; prior external beam or implant radiation therapy involving the skeleton; bone metastases or history of skeletal malignancies; pregnancy; breast-feeding mothers; pediatric patients or young adults with open epiphysis
Warnings/Precautions [US Boxed Warning]: In animal studies, teriparatide has been associated with an increase in osteosarcoma; risk was dependent on both dose and duration. Avoid use in patients with an increased risk of osteosarcoma (including Paget disease, prior radiation, unexplained elevation of alkaline phosphatase, prior external beam or implant radiation therapy involving the skeleton, or in patients with open epiphyses). Do not use in patients with bone metastases, a history of skeletal metastases, hyperparathyroidism, or preexisting hypercalcemia. Not for use in patients with metabolic bone disease other than osteoporosis. A voluntary patient registry has been established to collect information regarding osteosarcoma; patients are encouraged to enroll. Registry information may be obtained at www.forteoregistry.rti.org or by calling 866-382-6813.

May cause orthostatic hypotension. Transient orthostatic hypotension usually occurs within 4 hours of dosing and within the first several doses. Use with caution in patients with active or recent urolithiasis because of risk of exacerbation. Use in severe renal impairment is contraindicated in the Canadian labeling.

Use of teriparatide for longer than 2 years is not recommended. Appropriate use in men and women with glucocorticoid-induced osteoporosis: For use in men and women at high risk of fracture, which is defined as a history of osteoporotic fracture or multiple risk factors for fracture. May also be used in patients who have failed or are intolerant to other available osteoporosis therapy. Appropriate use in men with osteoporosis: For use in men at high risk for fracture, which is defined as a history of osteoporotic fracture or multiple risk factors for fracture. May also be used in men who have failed or are intolerant to previous osteoporosis therapy. Appropriate use in postmenopausal osteoporosis: For use in women at high risk for fracture, which is defined as a history of osteoporotic fracture or multiple risk factors for fracture. May also be used in women who have failed or are intolerant of previous osteoporosis therapy. In postmenopausal women with osteoporosis, teriparatide reduces the risk of vertebral and nonvertebral fractures.

According to the Centers for Disease Control and Prevention (CDC), pen-shaped injection devices should never be used for more than one person (even when the needle is changed) because of the risk of infection. The injection device should be clearly labeled with individual patient information to ensure that the correct pen is used (CDC, 2012). Potentially significant drug-drug interactions may exist, requiring dose or frequency adjustment, additional monitoring, and/or selection of alternative therapy.
Adverse Reactions
>10%: Endocrine & metabolic: Hypercalcemia (transient increases noted 4 to 6 hours postdose [women 11%; men 6%])
1% to 10%:
Cardiovascular: Orthostatic hypotension (5%; transient), angina pectoris (3%), syncope (3%)
Central nervous system: Dizziness (8%), headache (8%), insomnia (5%), anxiety (4%), depression (4%), vertigo (4%)
Endocrine & metabolic: Hyperuricemia (3%)
Gastrointestinal: Nausea (9% to 14%), gastritis (7%), dyspepsia (5%), vomiting (3%)
Immunologic: Antibody development (3% of women in long-term treatment; hypersensitivity reactions or decreased efficacy were not associated in preclinical trials)
Infection: Herpes zoster (3%)
Neuromuscular & skeletal: Arthralgia (10%), weakness (9%), leg cramps (3%)
Respiratory: Rhinitis (10%), pharyngitis (6%), dyspnea (4% to 6%), pneumonia (3% to 6%)
<1% (Limited to important or life-threatening): Allergic reactions, anaphylaxis, angioedema, chest pain, dyspnea (acute), facial edema, hypercalcemia (>13 mg/dL), injection site reactions (bruising, pain, swelling), mouth edema, muscle spasm, osteosarcoma, urticaria
Drug Interactions
Metabolism/Transport Effects None known.
Avoid Concomitant Use There are no known interactions where it is recommended to avoid concomitant use.
Increased Effect/Toxicity There are no known significant interactions involving an increase in effect.
Decreased Effect There are no known significant interactions involving a decrease in effect.
Storage/Stability Store refrigerated at 2°C to 8°C (36°F to 46°F); do not freeze (discard if freezing occurs). Protect from light. Discard pen 28 days after first injection, even if it still contains some unused solution. Do not use if solution is cloudy, colored, or contains solid particles.
Mechanism of Action Teriparatide is a recombinant formulation of endogenous parathyroid hormone (PTH), containing a 34-amino-acid sequence which is identical to the N-terminal portion of this hormone. The pharmacologic activity of teriparatide, which is similar to the physiologic activity of PTH, includes stimulating osteoblast function, increasing gastrointestinal calcium absorption, and increasing renal tubular reabsorption of calcium. Treatment with teriparatide results in increased bone mineral density, bone mass, and strength. In postmenopausal women, teriparatide has been shown to decrease osteoporosis-related fractures.
Pharmacodynamics/Kinetics
Distribution: V_d: ~0.12 L/kg
Metabolism: Hepatic (nonspecific proteolysis)
Bioavailability: 95%
Half-life elimination: IV: 5 minutes; SubQ: ~1 hour
Time to peak, serum: ~30 minutes
Excretion: Urine (as metabolites)
Dosing
Adult & Geriatric Osteoporosis (men, postmenopausal women, glucocorticoid induced): SubQ: 20 mcg once daily; **Note:** Initial administration should occur under circumstances in which the patient may sit or lie down, in the event of orthostasis.
Renal Impairment No dosage adjustment necessary. Use in severe renal impairment is contraindicated in the Canadian labeling.
Hepatic Impairment There is no dosage adjustment provided in the manufacturer's labeling (has not been studied).

◀ **Dietary Considerations** Ensure adequate calcium and vitamin D intake; if dietary intake is inadequate, dietary supplementation is recommended. Women and men should consume:

Calcium: 1,000 mg/day (men: 50 to 70 years) **or** 1,200 mg/day (women ≥51 years and men ≥71 years) (IOM, 2011; NOF [Cosman 2014])

Vitamin D: 800 to 1,000 int. units/day (men and women ≥50 years) (NOF [Cosman 2014]). Recommended Dietary Allowance (RDA): 600 int. units/day (men and women ≤70 years) **or** 800 int. units/day (men and women ≥71 years) (IOM, 2011).

Administration Inject subcutaneously into the thigh or abdominal wall. Administer without regard to meals or time of day. May administer dose immediately following removal from the refrigerator. Initial administration should occur under circumstances in which the patient may sit or lie down, in the event of orthostasis. Each teriparatide delivery device can be used for up to 28 days after the first injection. **Note:** The 3 mL prefilled pen (Canadian availability; not available in US) must be primed prior to each dose.

Monitoring Parameters Orthostatic hypotension; urinary calcium (patients with suspected active urolithiasis or preexisting hypercalciuria); bone mineral density (BMD) should be evaluated 1 to 2 years after initiating therapy and every 2 years thereafter (NOF [Cosman 2014]); annual measurements of height and weight, assessment of chronic back pain; serum calcium and 25(OH)D; consider measuring biochemical markers of bone turnover

Reference Range

Calcium (total): Adults: 9.0 to 11.0 mg/dL (2.05 to 2.54 mmol/L), may slightly decrease with aging

Phosphorus: 2.5 to 4.5 mg/dL (0.81 to 1.45 mmol/L)

Vitamin D: There is no clear consensus on a reference range for total serum 25(OH)D concentrations or the validity of this level as it relates clinically to bone health. In addition, there is significant variability in the reporting of serum 25(OH)D levels as a result of different assay types in use; however, the following ranges have been suggested:

Adults (IOM, 2011): Sufficient levels in practically all persons: ≥20 ng/mL (50 nmol/L); concern for risk of toxicity: >50 ng/mL (125 nmol/L)

Osteoporosis patients (NOF [Cosman 2014]): Recommended level to reach and maintain: ~30 ng/mL (75 nmol/L)

Test Interactions Transiently increases serum calcium; maximal effect 4 to 6 hours postdose; generally returns to baseline ~16 hours postdose

Additional Information Teriparatide was formerly marketed as a diagnostic agent (Perithar™); that agent was withdrawn from the market in 1997. Teriparatide (Forteo®) is manufactured through recombinant DNA technology using a strain of *E. coli*.

Patients are encouraged to enroll in the Forteo® Patient Registry which is designed to monitor the potential risk of osteosarcoma and teriparatide treatment. Enrollment information may be found at www.forteoregistry.rti.org or by calling 1-866-382-6813.

Dosage Forms Excipient information presented when available (limited, particularly for generics); consult specific product labeling.

Solution, Subcutaneous:

Forteo: 600 mcg/2.4 mL (2.4 mL) [contains metacresol]

Dosage Forms: Canada Excipient information presented when available (limited, particularly for generics); consult specific product labeling.

Injection, solution:

Forteo: 250 mcg/mL (3 mL) [delivers teriparatide 20 mcg/dose]

◆ Tersi *see* Selenium Sulfide *on page 1647*

Tesamorelin (tes a moe REL in)

Brand Names: US Egrifta

Index Terms Tesamorelin Acetate; TH9507

Pharmacologic Category Growth Hormone Releasing Factor

Use HIV-associated lipodystrophy: Reduction of excess abdominal fat in HIV-infected patients with lipodystrophy

Prescribing and Access Restrictions In order to prescribe Egrifta, healthcare providers must call the Axis Center at 1-877-714-2947. Egrifta is only available through specialty pharmacy distribution.

Dosing

Adult & Geriatric HIV-associated lipodystrophy: SubQ: 2 mg once daily

---

Renal Impairment There are no dosage adjustments provided in the manufacturer's labeling (has not been studied).

Hepatic Impairment There are no dosage adjustments provided in the manufacturer's labeling (has not been studied).

Adjustment for Toxicity Consider discontinuing with persistent elevations of IGF-1 (eg, >3 standard deviation scores). Discontinue if symptoms of hypersensitivity occur.

Additional Information Complete prescribing information should be consulted for additional detail.

Dosage Forms Excipient information presented when available (limited, particularly for generics); consult specific product labeling.

Solution Reconstituted, Subcutaneous [preservative free]:

Egrifta: 1 mg (1 ea); 2 mg (1 ea)

◆ Tesamorelin Acetate *see* Tesamorelin *on page 1766*

◆ TESPA *see* Thiotepa *on page 1783*

◆ Tessalon [DSC] *see* Benzonatate *on page 218*

◆ Tessalon Perles *see* Benzonatate *on page 218*

◆ Testim *see* Testosterone *on page 1766*

◆ Testopel *see* Testosterone *on page 1766*

Testosterone (tes TOS ter one)

Brand Names: US Androderm; AndroGel; AndroGel Pump; Aveed; Axiron; Depo-Testosterone; First-Testosterone; First-Testosterone MC; Fortesta; Natesto; Striant; Testim; Testopel; Vogelxo; Vogelxo Pump

Brand Names: Canada Andriol; Androderm; AndroGel; Axiron; Delatestryl; Depo-Testosterone; PMS-Testosterone; Taro-Testosterone; Testim

Index Terms Delatestryl; Testosterone Cypionate; Testosterone Enanthate; Testosterone Undecanoate

Pharmacologic Category Androgen

Use

Breast cancer, metastatic: Injection (enanthate): Secondary treatment in women with advancing inoperable metastatic (skeletal) mammary cancer who are 1 to 5 years postmenopausal. Use may be considered in premenopausal women with breast cancer who have benefited from oophorectomy and have a hormone-responsive tumor.

Delayed puberty: Injection (enanthate); pellet: Androgen replacement in carefully selected males with delayed puberty. Generally observed in males with a familial pattern of delayed puberty; not secondary to a pathological disorder.

Hypogonadism, hypogonadotropic (congenital or acquired): Buccal; Gel (nasal, transdermal); Injection (cypionate, enanthate, undecanoate); Patch (transdermal); Pellet; Solution (transdermal): Gonadotropin or luteinizing hormone-releasing hormone deficiency, or pituitary-hypothalamic injury from tumors, trauma, or radiation. Generally observed in men with low serum testosterone and gonadotropins in the normal or low range.

Hypogonadism, primary (congenital or acquired): Buccal; Gel (nasal, transdermal); Injection (cypionate, enanthate, undecanoate); Patch (transdermal); Pellet; Solution (transdermal): Treatment of testicular failure due to cryptorchidism, bilateral torsion, orchitis, vanishing testis syndrome, orchiectomy, Klinefelter syndrome, chemotherapy, or toxic damage from alcohol or heavy metals. Generally observed in men with low serum testosterone and gonadotropins (follicle-stimulating hormone, luteinizing hormone) above the normal range.

Replacement therapy (capsule [Canadian product]): Testosterone replacement in adult males for conditions associated with a deficiency or absence of endogenous testosterone.

Limitations of use: In adult males, testosterone is indicated as replacement therapy in conditions associated with a deficiency or absence of endogenous testosterone. Use in age-related hypogonadism (or late-onset hypogonadism) has not been established.

Pregnancy Considerations Use is contraindicated in pregnant women or women who may become pregnant. Exposure to a fetus may cause virilization of varying degrees. Because of the potential for secondary exposure, all children and women should avoid skin-to-skin contact to areas where testosterone has been applied topically on another person.

Some products contain benzyl alcohol, which can cross the placenta.

Large doses of testosterone may suppress spermatogenesis. Treatment of hypogonadotropic hypogonadism is not recommended for men desiring fertility (Bhasin 2010).

Breast-Feeding Considerations Testosterone is excreted into breast milk. Most products are contraindicated while breast-feeding.

Distribution of testosterone in breast milk was evaluated following use of the subcutaneous pellet in a nursing woman. Prior to therapy, milk concentrations of testosterone were 96 pg/mL. Following SubQ implantation of the 100 mg pellet, milk samples ranged from 88 pg/mL (day 2) to 100 pg/mL (day 7 [morning]). Reported maternal serum samples ranged from <100 pg/mL (baseline), 2830 pg/mL (day 2), and 1,480 pg/mL (day 7 [morning]). Adverse events were not observed in the nursing male infant after 7 months of continuous maternal therapy (Glaser 2009).

Because of the potential for secondary exposure, all children and women should avoid skin-to-skin contact to areas where testosterone has been applied topically on another person.

High levels of endogenous maternal testosterone, such as those caused by certain ovarian cysts, suppress milk production. Maternal serum testosterone levels generally fall following pregnancy and return to normal once breast-feeding is stopped (Betzold 2004; Hoover 2002).

Medication Guide Available Yes

Contraindications

Breast cancer (males); prostate cancer (known or suspected); pregnant women or women who may become pregnant

Androderm, Androgel, Axiron, Fortesta, Natesto, Striant, Testim, Vogelxo: Additional contradiction: Breast-feeding women

Andriol [Canadian product]: Additional contraindications: Hypersensitivity to any component of the formulation; use in women

Aveed: Additional contraindications: Hypersensitivity to testosterone undecanoate, castor oil, benzyl benzoate; breast-feeding women

Depo-Testosterone: Additional contraindications: Hypersensitivity to testosterone cypionate, serious cardiac, hepatic, or renal disease

Testosterone enanthate: Additional contraindications: Hypersensitivity to any component of the formulation

Documentation of allergenic cross-reactivity for androgens is limited. However, because of similarities in chemical structure and/or pharmacologic actions, the possibility of cross-sensitivity cannot be ruled out with certainty.

Warnings/Precautions Hazardous agent; use appropriate precautions for handling and disposal (NIOSH 2014 [group 3]).

When used to treat delayed male puberty, perform radiographic examination of the hand and wrist every 6 months to determine the rate of bone maturation. May cause hypercalcemia in patients with prolonged immobilization or cancer. May accelerate bone maturation (without producing compensating gain in linear growth) and premature closure of the epiphysis in children. May alter serum lipid profile; use caution with history of MI or coronary artery disease. Androgens may worsen BPH. Use caution in elderly patients or patients with other demographic factors which may increase the risk of prostatic carcinoma; careful monitoring is required. Discontinue therapy if urethral obstruction develops in patients with BPH (use lower dose if restarted). Withhold therapy pending urological evaluation in patients with palpable prostate nodule or induration, PSA >4 ng/mL, or PSA >3 ng/mL in men at high risk of prostate cancer (Bhasin 2010). Venous thromboembolic events including deep vein thrombosis (DVT) and pulmonary embolism (PE) have been reported with testosterone products. Evaluate patients with symptoms of pain, edema, warmth and erythema in the lower extremity for DVT and those with acute shortness of breath for PE. Discontinue therapy if a venous thromboembolism is suspected. Use with caution in patients with diseases that may be exacerbated by fluid retention including cardiac, hepatic, or renal dysfunction; testosterone may cause fluid retention. Treatment of androgen deficiency syndromes is not recommended for men with uncontrolled or poorly controlled heart failure (Bhasin 2010). May cause gynecomastia, which may persist in patients treated for hypogonadism. Large doses may suppress spermatogenesis. During treatment for metastatic breast cancer, women should be monitored for signs of virilization; discontinue if mild virilization is present to prevent irreversible symptoms.

May be inappropriate in the elderly due to potential risk of cardiac problems and contraindication for use in men with prostate cancer; in general, avoid use in older adults except in the setting of moderate-to-severe hypogonadism

(Beers Criteria). In addition, elderly patients may be at greater risk for prostatic hyperplasia, prostate cancer, fluid retention, and transaminase elevations.

Prolonged use of high doses of oral androgens has been associated with serious hepatic effects (peliosis hepatis, hepatic neoplasms, cholestatic hepatitis, jaundice). Prolonged use of intramuscular testosterone enanthate has been associated with multiple hepatic adenomas. Discontinue therapy if signs or symptoms of hepatic dysfunction (such as jaundice) develop. Long term use (>10 years) of parenteral testosterone for male hypogonadism may increase the risk of breast cancer (Medras 2006).

May potentiate sleep apnea in some male patients especially those with risk factors (eg, obesity or chronic lung disease). May increase hematocrit requiring dose adjustment or discontinuation; discontinue therapy if hematocrit exceeds 54%; may reinitiate at lower dose (Bhasin 2010). Oligospermia may occur after prolonged administration or excessive dosage; discontinue therapy if this occurs, if restarted, a lower dose should be used. Priapism or excessive sexual stimulation may occur; discontinue therapy if this occurs, if restarted, a lower dose should be used.

Testosterone undecanoate injection: **[US Boxed Warning]: Serious pulmonary oil microembolism (POME) reactions and anaphylaxis have been reported with testosterone undecanoate injection. Reactions include anaphylaxis, chest pain, urge to cough, dizziness, dyspnea, throat tightening, and syncope; may be life threatening. Reactions may occur after any injection during the course of therapy, including the first dose. Patients must be monitored for 30 minutes after injection. Due to the risk of serious POME reactions, Aveed is only available through the Aveed REMS program.** To minimize risk of adverse reactions, inject deeply into gluteal muscle.

[US Boxed Warning]: Virilization in children has been reported following contact with unwashed or unclothed application sites of men using topical testosterone. Patients should strictly adhere to instructions for use in order to prevent secondary exposure. Children and women should avoid contact with application sites of men using topical products. Symptoms of virilization generally regress following removal of exposure; however, in some children, enlarged genitalia and bone age did not fully return to age appropriate normal. Signs of inappropriate virilization in women or children following secondary exposure to topical testosterone should be brought to the attention of a healthcare provider. Topical testosterone products (gels and solution) may have different doses, strengths, or application instructions that may result in different systemic exposure; these products are not interchangeable. Use of the intranasal gel is not recommended in patients with sinus disease, mucosal inflammatory disorders (eg, Sjogren syndrome), or with a history of nasal disorders, nasal or sinus surgery, nasal fracture within the previous 6 months, or nasal fracture that caused a deviated anterior nasal septum. Safety and efficacy have not been established in males with a BMI >35 kg/m². Transdermal patch may contain conducting metal (eg, aluminum); remove patch prior to MRI. Gels, solution, transdermal, and buccal system have not been evaluated in males <18 years; safety and efficacy of testosterone cypionate injection have not been established in males <12 years. Some products may contain castor oil. Use of Axiron in males with BMI >35 kg/m² has not been established. Anabolic steroids may be abused; abuse may be associated with adverse physical and psychological effects. Dependance may occur when used outside of approved dosage/indications.

Available studies are inconclusive regarding the risk of developing major adverse cardiovascular events (MACE) such as nonfatal MI, stroke, or cardiovascular death following testosterone use. Studies have suggested an increased risk of cardiovascular events among groups of men prescribed testosterone therapy (Basaria 2010; Finkle 2014; Vigen 2013). The Endocrine Society suggests it may be prudent to avoid testosterone therapy in men who have experienced a cardiovascular event (eg, MI, stroke, acute coronary syndrome) in the past six months (The Endocrine Society 2014). Evaluate patients for cardiovascular risk factors prior to initiating therapy and monitor closely during therapy for cardiovascular events.

Benzyl alcohol and derivatives: Some dosage forms may contain benzyl alcohol; large amounts of benzyl alcohol (≥99 mg/kg/day) have been associated with a potentially fatal toxicity ("gasping syndrome") in neonates; the "gasping syndrome" consists of metabolic acidosis, respiratory distress, gasping respirations, CNS dysfunction (including

convulsions, intracranial hemorrhage), hypotension, and cardiovascular collapse (AAP ["Inactive" 1997]; CDC 1982); some data suggests that benzoate displaces bilirubin from protein binding sites (Ahlfors 2001); avoid or use dosage forms containing benzyl alcohol with caution in neonates. See manufacturer's labeling. Testosterone cypionate should not be used interchangeably with testosterone propionate due to differences in duration of action. Potentially significant interactions may exist, requiring dose or frequency adjustment, additional monitoring, and/ or selection of alternative therapy.

Adverse Reactions Frequency not always defined.

Cardiovascular: Hypertension (≥3%), increased blood pressure (1%), decreased blood pressure, deep vein thrombosis, edema, vasodilatation

Central nervous system: Headache (1% to ≥3%), fatigue (2%), irritability (2%), insomnia (≤2%), mood swings (≤2%), aggressive behavior (1%), taste disorder (1%), altered sense of smell (≤1%), abnormal dreams, amnesia, anxiety, chills, depression, dizziness, emotional lability, excitement, hostility, malaise, nervousness, outbursts of anger, paresthesia, seizure, sleep apnea, suicidal ideation

Dermatologic: Acne vulgaris (5%), hyperhidrosis (1%), alopecia, contact dermatitis, diaphoresis, erythema, folliculitis, hair discoloration, pruritus, seborrhea, skin rash, xeroderma

Endocrine & metabolic: Increased plasma estradiol concentration (3%), weight gain (1%), gynecomastia (≤1%), hot flash (≤1%), change in libido, decreased gonadotropin, fluid retention, hirsutism (increase in pubic hair growth), hypercalcemia, hyperchloremia, hypercholesterolemia, hyperglycemia, hyperkalemia, hyperlipidemia, hypernatremia, hypoglycemia, hypokalemia, inorganic phosphate retention, menstrual disease (including amenorrhea)

Gastrointestinal: Diarrhea (≥3%), gastroesophageal reflux disease, gastrointestinal hemorrhage, gastrointestinal irritation, increased appetite, nausea, vomiting

Following buccal administration (most common): Dysgeusia, gingival pain, gingival swelling, mouth irritation (including gums), unpleasant taste

Genitourinary: Prostate specific antigen increase (5% to 11%), prostatitis (≥3%), ejaculatory disorder (1%), prostate induration (1%), spontaneous erections (≤1%), benign prostatic hypertrophy, difficulty in micturition, hematuria, impotence, irritable bladder, mastalgia, oligospermia, priapism, testicular atrophy, urinary tract infection, virilization

Hepatic: Abnormal hepatic function tests, cholestatic hepatitis, cholestatic jaundice, hepatic insufficiency, hepatic necrosis, hepatocellular neoplasms, increased serum bilirubin, peliosis hepatis

Hematologic & oncologic: Increased hematocrit (1% to 3%), increased hemoglobin (2%), malignant neoplasm of prostate (1%), anemia, clotting factors suppression, hemorrhage, leukopenia, polycythemia, prostate carcinoma

Hypersensitivity: Anaphylactoid reaction, hypersensitivity reaction (including pulmonary oil microembolism)

Local: Pain at injection site (5%), erythema at injection site (1%), application site reaction (gel, solution), inflammation at injection site

Transdermal system: Application site pruritus (17% to 37%), application site vesicles (including burn-like blisters under system; 6% to 12%), application site erythema (≤7%), local allergic contact dermatitis (4%), application site burning (3%), application site induration (3%), local skin exfoliation (<3%)

Neuromuscular & skeletal: Arthralgia (≥3%), back pain (≥3%), abnormal bone growth (accelerated), hemarthrosis, hyperkinesia, weakness

Ophthalmic: Increased lacrimation

Renal: Increased serum creatinine, polyuria

Respiratory: Bronchitis (≥3%), nasopharyngitis (≥3%), sinusitis (≥3%), upper respiratory tract infection (≥3%), dyspnea

<1% (Limited to important or life-threatening): Injection, gel: Abnormal erythropoiesis, abscess at injection site, anaphylaxis, androgenetic alopecia, asthma, cardiac arrest, cardiac failure, cerebrovascular accident, chronic obstructive pulmonary disease, cognitive dysfunction, diabetes mellitus, epididymitis, hearing loss (sudden), hematoma at injection site, hepatotoxicity (idiosyncratic) (Chalasani, 2014), hyperparathyroidism, hypersensitivity angiitis, increased intraocular pressure, Korsakoff's psychosis (nonalcoholic), migraine, myocardial infarction, personality disorder, prolonged prothrombin time, prostatic intraepithelial neoplasia, reversible ischemic neurological deficit, spermatocele, systemic lupus erythematosus, tachycardia, thrombocytopenia, thrombosis, urinary incontinence, venous insufficiency,

vesicobullous rash, virilization (of children, following secondary exposure to topical gel [advanced bone age, aggressive behavior, enlargement of clitoris requiring surgery, enlargement of penis, increased erections, increased libido, pubic hair development]), vitreous detachment

Drug Interactions

Metabolism/Transport Effects Substrate of CYP2B6 (minor), CYP2C19 (minor), CYP2C9 (minor), CYP3A4 (minor); **Note:** Assignment of Major/Minor substrate status based on clinically relevant drug interaction potential

Avoid Concomitant Use

Avoid concomitant use of Testosterone with any of the following: Dehydroepiandrosterone

Increased Effect/Toxicity

Testosterone may increase the levels/effects of: Blood Glucose Lowering Agents; C1 inhibitors; CycloSPORINE (Systemic); Vitamin K Antagonists

The levels/effects of Testosterone may be increased by: Corticosteroids (Systemic); Dehydroepiandrosterone

Decreased Effect There are no known significant interactions involving a decrease in effect.

Preparation for Administration Injection:

Testosterone enanthate, testosterone cypionate: Warm to room temperature; shaking vial will help redissolve crystals that have formed after storage.

Testosterone undecanoate: Inject 3 mL of air through the gray rubber stopper into the vial to create positive pressure, and then withdraw 3 mL of solution (750 mg) from the vial. Expel any air bubbles from the syringe and change the syringe needle to a new IM needle. **Discard unused portion.**

Storage/Stability

Andriol [Canadian product]: Store between 15°C and 30°C; protect from light and moisture; do not refrigerate.

Androderm: Store at 20°C to 25°C (68°F to 77°F). Do not store outside of pouch. Excessive heat may cause system to burst.

AndroGel 1%, Axiron: Store at 25°C (77°F); excursions are permitted between 15°C and 30°C (59°F and 86°F).

AndroGel 1.62%, Natesto, Testim, Vogelxo: Store at 20°C and 25°C (68°F to 77°F); excursions are permitted between 15°C and 30°C (59°F and 86°F).

Aveed: Store at 25°C (77°F); excursions are permitted between 15°C and 30°C (59°F and 86°F) Store in original container.

Depo-Testosterone: Store at 20°C to 25°C (68°F to 77°F). Protect from light.

Fortesta: Store at 20°C to 25°C (68°F to 77°F); excursions are permitted between 15°C and 30°C (59°F and 86°F). Do not freeze.

Striant: Store at 20°C to 25°C (68°F to 77°F). Protect from heat and moisture.

Testopel: Store in a cool location.

Testosterone enanthate injection: Store at 20°C to 25°C (68°F to 77°F).

Mechanism of Action Principal endogenous androgen responsible for promoting the growth and development of the male sex organs and maintaining secondary sex characteristics in androgen-deficient males

Pharmacodynamics/Kinetics

Duration (route and ester dependent): IM: Cypionate and enanthate esters: 2 to 4 weeks; Undecanoate: 10 weeks; Transdermal gel: 24 hours

Absorption: Transdermal gel: ~10% of applied dose

Protein binding: 98%; bound to sex hormone-binding globulin (40%) and albumin

Metabolism: Hepatic; forms metabolites, including dihydrotestosterone (DHT) and estradiol (both active)

Bioavailability: Oral capsule [Canadian product]: ~7%

Half-life elimination: Variable: 10 to 100 minutes; Testosterone cypionate: ~8 days

Time to peak: IM undecanoate: 7 days (median; range: 4 to 42 days); Intranasal: ~40 minutes; Transdermal system: 8 hours (range: 4 to 12 hours); Buccal system: 10 to 12 hours; Oral capsule [Canadian product]: 4 to 5 hours

Excretion: Urine (90%; oral capsule [Canadian product]: 45% to 48%); feces (6%)

Dosing

Adult & Geriatric

Breast cancer (females): *IM (testosterone enanthate):* 200 to 400 mg every 2 to 4 weeks

Delayed puberty (males):

IM (testosterone enanthate): 50 to 200 mg every 2 to 4 weeks for a limited duration (eg, 4 to 6 months)

Pellet (for subcutaneous implantation): 150 to 450 mg every 3 to 6 months. Dosing is generally at the lower range for a limited duration (eg, 4 to 6 months).

Hypogonadism (primary) or hypogonadism (hypogo-nadotropic) (males):

IM (testosterone enanthate or testosterone cypionate): 50 to 400 mg every 2 to 4 weeks (FDA-approved dosing range); 75 to 100 mg/week or 150 to 200 mg every 2 weeks (Bhasin 2010)

IM (Testosterone undecanoate): Initial dose: 750 mg, followed by 750 mg administered 4 weeks later, then 750 mg administered every 10 weeks thereafter.

Intranasal: Testosterone gel: Natesto: 11 mg (2 pump actuations; 1 actuation per nostril) administered intranasally 3 times daily (6 to 8 hours apart). Total daily dose: 33 mg

Dose adjustment based on testosterone levels:

Less than normal range: Consider alternative treatment if consistently <300 ng/mL

Greater than normal range: Discontinue if consistently >1050 ng/mL

Pellet (for subcutaneous implantation): 150 to 450 mg every 3 to 6 months

Topical:

Buccal: 30 mg twice daily (every 12 hours) applied to the gum region above the incisor tooth. Discontinue if serum testosterone concentrations are consistently outside of the normal range.

Gel:

AndroGel 1%: 50 mg applied once daily in the morning to the shoulder and upper arms, or abdomen. Dosage range: 50 to 100 mg daily.

Dose adjustment based on testosterone levels:

Less than normal range: Increase dose from 50 mg to 75 mg or from 75 mg to 100 mg once daily

Greater than normal range: Decrease dose. Discontinue if consistently above normal at 50 mg daily

AndroGel 1.62%: 40.5 mg applied once daily in the morning to the shoulder and upper arms. Dosage range: 20.25 mg to 81 mg daily.

Dose adjustment based on testosterone levels:

>750 ng/dL: Decrease dose by 20.25 mg daily

≥350 ng/dL to ≤750 ng/dL: Maintain current dose

<350 ng/dL: Increase dose by 20.25 mg daily

Fortesta: 40 mg once daily in the morning. Apply to the thighs. Dosing range: 10 to 70 mg daily

Dose adjustment based on serum testosterone levels:

≥2500 ng/dL: Decrease dose by 20 mg daily

≥1250 to <2500 ng/dL: Decrease dose by 10 mg daily

≥500 and <1250 ng/dL: Maintain current dose

<500 ng/dL: Increase dose by 10 mg daily

Testim: 50 mg applied once daily (preferably in the morning) to the shoulder and upper arms. If testosterone concentrations are less than the normal range, dosage may be increased from 50 mg to 100 mg once daily.

Vogelxo: 50 mg applied once daily to the shoulder and/or upper arms. Dosage may be increased to a maximum of 100 mg daily.

Dose adjustment based on testosterone levels:

Less than normal range: Increase dose from 50 mg to 100 mg once daily

Solution (Axiron): 60 mg once daily (dosage range: 30 to 120 mg daily). Apply to the axilla at the same time each morning.

Dose adjustment based on serum testosterone levels:

>1050 ng/dL: Decrease 60 mg daily dose to 30 mg daily; if levels >1050 ng/dL persist after dose reduction, discontinue therapy

<300 ng/dL: Increase 60 mg daily dose to 90 mg daily, or increase 90 mg daily dose to 120 mg daily

Transdermal system (Androderm):

Initial: 4 mg daily (as one 4 mg/day patch; do **not** use two 2 mg/day patches)

Dose adjustment based on testosterone levels:

>930 ng/dL: Decrease dose to 2 mg daily

400 to 930 ng/dL: Continue 4 mg daily

<400 ng/dL: Increase dose to 6 mg daily(as one 4 mg/day and one 2 mg/day patch)

Dosing conversion: The 2.5 mg/day and the 5 mg/day patches have been discontinued in the US; patients may be switched from the 2.5 mg/day patch, 5 mg/day patch, or the combination (ie, 7.5 mg/day) as follows:

From 2.5 mg/day patch to 2 mg/day patch

From 5 mg/day patch to 4 mg/day patch

From 7.5 mg daily (one 2.5 mg/day and one 5 mg/day patch) to 6 mg daily (one 2 mg/day and one 4 mg/day patch)

Note: Patch change should occur at the next scheduled dosing. Measure early morning testosterone concentrations ~2 weeks after switching therapy.

Replacement therapy (males): *Oral capsule (Andriol [Canadian product]):* Initial: 120 to 160 mg daily in 2 divided doses for 2 to 3 weeks; adjust according to individual response and/or testosterone levels; usual maintenance dose: 40 to 120 mg daily (in divided doses)

Pediatric

Delayed puberty (adolescent males):

IM (testosterone enanthate): Refer to adult dosing.

Pellet (for subcutaneous implantation): Refer to adult dosing.

Hypogonadism (primary) or hypogonadism (hypogo-nadotropic) (adolescent males):

IM (testosterone enanthate or testosterone cypionate): Refer to adult dosing.

Pellet (for subcutaneous implantation): Refer to adult dosing.

Renal Impairment There are no dosage adjustments provided in manufacturer's labeling (has not been studied). May enhance edema formation. Testosterone cypionate is contraindicated in serious renal disease.

Hepatic Impairment There are no dosage adjustments provided in manufacturer's labeling (has not been studied). May enhance edema formation. Testosterone cypionate is contraindicated in serious hepatic disease.

Dietary Considerations Food and beverages have not been found to interfere with buccal system; ensure system is in place following eating, drinking, or brushing teeth.

Administration

IM: Administer by deep IM injection into the gluteal muscle. Testosterone undecanoate: Inject into the gluteus medius; alternate injection between left and right buttock. Avoid intravascular injection, may lead to pulmonary oil microembolism; avoid the superior gluteal arteries and sciatic nerve.

Intranasal gel (Natesto): Administer intranasally 3 times daily, 6 to 8 hours apart, preferably at the same time each day. Prime pump prior to first use by inverting then depressing pump 10 times (discard this portion of product into sink). Blow nose prior to application. To administer the dose, insert actuator into nostril until pump reaches base of nose; tilt so the tip is in contact with the lateral wall of nostril. Depress slowly until pump stops, then remove from nose while wiping tip to transfer gel to lateral side of nostril. Following administration, press on the nostrils at a point just below the bridge of the nose and lightly massage. Refrain from blowing nose or sniffing for 1 hour after administration. If gel gets on hands, wash with warm soap and water. Temporarily discontinue with episodes of severe rhinitis; if severe rhinitis symptoms persist consider an alternative therapy.

Oral, buccal application (Striant): One mucoadhesive for buccal application (buccal system) should be applied to a comfortable area above the incisor tooth twice daily. Gently push the curved side against the upper gum. Hold buccal system firmly in place by pushing down on outside of the upper lip for 30 seconds to ensure adhesion. The buccal system should adhere to gum until it is removed. Rotate to alternate sides of mouth with each application. If the buccal system falls out, replace with a new system. If the system falls out within the first 8 hours of dosing, replace with a new buccal system and continue for a total of 12 hours from the placement of the first system. If the system falls out of position after 8 hours of dosing, a new buccal system should be applied and it may remain in place for 12 hours, then continue with the next regularly scheduled dosing. System will soften and mold to shape of gum as it absorbs moisture from mouth. Do not chew or swallow the buccal system. The buccal system will not dissolve; gently remove by sliding downwards from gum; avoid scratching gum. Remove prior to routine morning and evening oral care, prior to application of new system.

Oral, capsule (Andriol [Canadian product]): Administer with meals. Should be swallowed whole; do not crush or chew.

Subcutaneous implant (Testopel): Using strict sterile technique, must be surgically implanted.

Transdermal patch (Androderm): Apply to skin immediately upon removal from the protective pouch. Apply at the same time each night to clean, dry area of skin on the back, abdomen, upper arms, or thigh. Do not apply to bony areas or parts of the body that are subject to prolonged pressure while sleeping or sitting. Do not apply to oily, damaged or irritated skin. Do not apply to the scrotum. Rotate administration sites, allowing 7 days between applying to the same site. Avoid showering, washing the site, or swimming for ≥3 hours after application. Following patch removal, mild skin irritation may be

treated with OTC hydrocortisone cream. A small amount of triamcinolone acetonide 0.1% cream may be applied under the system to decrease irritation; do not use ointment (triamcinolone ointment decreases testosterone absorption). Dispose of any used or unused patches by folding adhesive ends together, replace in pouch or sealed container and discard properly in trash away from children and pets.

Topical gel and solution: Alcohol-based gels and solutions are flammable; avoid fire, flames, or smoking until dry. Testosterone may be transferred to another person following skin-to-skin contact with the application site. Strict adherence to application instructions is needed in order to decrease secondary exposure. Thoroughly wash hands after application and cover application site with clothing (ie, shirt) once gel or solution has dried, or clean application site thoroughly with soap and water prior to contact in order to minimize transfer. In addition to skin-to-skin contact, secondary exposure has also been reported following exposure to secondary items (eg, towel, shirt, sheets). If secondary exposure occurs, the other person should thoroughly wash the skin with soap and water as soon as possible. The application sites and doses of these products are not interchangeable.

AndroGel 1%: Apply at the same time each morning to clean, dry, intact skin to an area of the shoulder, upper arms, and/or abdomen that will be covered by a short sleeve t-shirt. Do not apply to other parts of the body such as the genitals, chest, back, axillae, or knees. Upon opening the packet(s), the entire contents should be squeezed into the palm of the hand and immediately applied to the application site(s). Alternatively, a portion may be squeezed onto palm of hand and applied, repeating the process at the same or other site until entire packet has been applied. Avoid swimming, showering or washing the application site for ≥5 hours following application. Cover application site with clothing (eg, t-shirt) once the gel has dried. When using the multidose pump, prime pump 3 times (and discard this portion of product) prior to initial use. Each actuation delivers 12.5 mg of testosterone (4 actuations = 50 mg; 6 actuations = 75 mg; 8 actuations = 100 mg). When using the pump, the gel may be delivered into the palm of the hand prior to application or applied directly to the application site.

AndroGel 1.62%: Apply at the same time each morning to clean, dry, intact skin to an area of the shoulder and upper arms that will be covered by a short sleeve t-shirt. Do not apply to other parts of the body such as the abdomen, genitals, chest, axillae, or knees. Upon opening the packet(s), the entire contents should be squeezed into the palm of the hand and immediately applied to the application site(s). Alternatively, a portion may be squeezed onto palm of hand and applied, repeating the process at the same or other site until entire packet has been applied. Avoid swimming, showering or washing the application site for ≥2 hours following application. Cover application site with clothing (eg, t-shirt) once the gel has dried. When using the multidose pump, prime pump 3 times (and discard this portion of product) prior to initial use. Each actuation delivers 20.25 mg of testosterone (2 actuations = 40.5 mg; 3 actuations = 60.75 mg; 4 actuations = 81 mg). When using the pump, the gel may be delivered into the palm of the hand prior to application or applied directly to the application site.

Axiron: Apply using the applicator to clean, dry, intact skin on an area of the axilla at the same time each morning. Do not apply to other parts of the body (eg, abdomen, genitals, shoulders, upper arms). Avoid washing the site or swimming for 2 hours after application. Prior to first use, prime the applicator pump by depressing it 3 times (discard this portion of the product). After priming, position the nozzle over the applicator cup and depress pump fully one time; ensure liquid enters cup. Each pump actuation delivers testosterone 30 mg. No more than 30 mg (one pump) should be added to the cup at one time. The total dose should be divided between axilla (example, 30 mg/day: apply to one axilla only; 60 mg/day: apply 30 mg to each axilla; 90 mg/day: apply 30 mg to each axilla, allow to dry, then apply an additional 30 mg to one axilla; etc). To apply dose, keep applicator upright and wipe into the axilla; if solution runs or drips, use cup to wipe. Do not rub into skin with fingers or hand. If more than one 30 mg dose is needed, repeat process. Apply roll-on or stick antiperspirants or deodorants prior to testosterone. Once application site is dry, cover with clothing. After use, rinse applicator under running water and pat dry with a tissue.

Fortesta: Apply to clean dry intact skin once daily in the morning to skin of front and inner thighs. Do not apply to genitals or other parts of the body. Use one finger to rub gel evenly onto skin of each thigh. Avoid showering, washing the site, or swimming for ≥2 hours after application. Prior to first dose, prime the pump by holding canister upright and fully depressing the pump 8 times (discard this portion of the product). Each pump actuation delivers testosterone 10 mg. The total dose should be divided between thighs (example, 10 mg/day: apply 10 mg to one thigh only; 20 mg/day: apply 10 mg to each thigh; 30 mg/day: apply 20 mg to one thigh and 10 mg to the other thigh; etc). Once application site is dry, cover with clothing.

Testim: Apply once daily (preferably in the morning) to clean, dry, intact skin to an area of the shoulder and upper arms that will be covered by a short sleeve t-shirt. Do not apply to the genitals or abdomen. Upon opening the tube, the entire contents should be squeezed into the palm of the hand and immediately applied to the application site(s). Avoid swimming, showering or washing the application site for ≥2 hours following application. Cover application site with clothing (eg, t-shirt) once the gel has dried.

Vogelxo: Apply once daily at the same time each morning to clean dry intact skin to an area of the shoulder and upper arms that will be covered by a short sleeve t-shirt. Do not apply to the genitals or to the abdomen. Upon opening the tube or packet, the entire contents should be squeezed into the palm of the hand and immediately applied to the application site(s). If two doses (testosterone 100 mg) are needed, apply one dose (50 mg) to upper arm and or/shoulder, then apply the second dose (50 mg) to the opposite upper arm and/or shoulder. Avoid showering, washing the site, or swimming for at least 2 hours following application. Cover application site with clothing (eg, t-shirt) once the gel has dried. When using the multidose pump, prime pump 3 times by fully depressing the pump mechanism (actuation) and discard this portion of product. Each actuation delivers testosterone 12.5 mg (4 actuations = 50 mg; 8 actuations = 100 mg).

Hazardous agent; use appropriate precautions for handling and disposal (NIOSH 2014 [group 3]).

Monitoring Parameters Periodic liver function tests, lipid panel, hemoglobin and hematocrit (prior to therapy, at 3 to 6 months, then annually); radiologic examination of wrist and hand every 6 months (when using in prepubertal children). Withhold initial treatment with hematocrit >50% (discontinue therapy if hematocrit exceeds 54% [Bhasin 2010]), hyperviscosity, untreated obstructive sleep apnea, or uncontrolled severe heart failure. Monitor urine and serum calcium and signs of virilization in women treated for breast cancer. Serum glucose (may be decreased by testosterone, monitor patients with diabetes). Evaluate males for response to treatment and adverse events 3 to 6 months after initiation and then annually; monitor for cardiovascular events closely during therapy. Confirm hypogonadism (prior to therapy) by measuring morning serum testosterone on at least 2 separate days.

Aveed: Monitor for 30 minutes after injection; appropriate treatment should be available in the event of a serous POME reaction or anaphylaxis.

Bone mineral density: Monitor after 1 to 2 years of therapy in hypogonadal men with osteoporosis or low trauma fracture (Bhasin 2010)

PSA: In men >40 years of age with baseline PSA >0.6 ng/mL, PSA and prostate exam (prior to therapy, at 3 to 6 months, then as based on current guidelines). Withhold treatment pending urological evaluation in patients with palpable prostate nodule or induration or PSA >4 ng/mL or if PSA >3 ng/mL in men at high risk of prostate cancer (Bhasin 2010).

Do not treat with severe untreated BPH with IPSS symptom score >19.

Serum testosterone: After initial dose titration (if applicable), monitor 3 to 6 months after initiating treatment, then annually.

Injection:

Testosterone enanthate or cypionate: Measure midway between injections. Adjust dose or frequency if testosterone concentration is <400 ng/dL or >700 ng/dL (Bhasin 2010).

Testosterone undecanoate: Measure just prior to each subsequent injection and adjust dosing interval to maintain serum testosterone in mid-normal range (Bhasin 2010).

AndroGel 1%, Testim: Morning serum testosterone levels ~14 days after start of therapy or dose adjustments

AndroGel 1.62%: Morning serum testosterone levels after 14 and 28 days of starting therapy or dose adjustments and periodically thereafter

Androderm: Morning serum testosterone levels (following application the previous evening) ~14 days after start of therapy or dose adjustments

Axiron: Serum testosterone levels can be measured 2 to 8 hours after application and after 14 days of starting therapy or dose adjustments

Fortesta: Serum testosterone levels can be measured 2 hours after application and after 14 and 35 days of starting therapy or dose adjustments

Natesto: Measure total serum testosterone periodically, beginning 1 month after initiating therapy. Discontinue therapy if if the total serum testosterone consistently exceed 1050 ng/dL. If total serum testosterone is consistently <300 ng/dL consider an alternative therapy.

Striant: Examine application area of gums; total serum testosterone 4 to 12 weeks after initiating treatment, prior to morning dose. Discontinue therapy if the total serum testosterone are consistently outside of the normal range (300 to 1050 ng/dL).

Testopel: Measure at the end of the dosing interval (Bhasin 2010)

Vogelxo: Measure serum testosterone ~14 days after initiation of therapy, in the morning, prior to application

Reference Range The lower limit of the normal free testosterone range varies by laboratory (Bhasin 2010).

Test Interactions Testosterone may decrease thyroxine-binding globulin, resulting in decreased total T_4 and increased resin uptake of T_3 and T_4; free thyroid hormone levels are not changed.

Dosage Forms Considerations First-Testosterone MC cream and First-Testosterone ointment are compounding kits. Refer to manufacturer's labeling for compounding instructions.

Dosage Forms Excipient information presented when available (limited, particularly for generics); consult specific product labeling.

Cream, Transdermal:
  First-Testosterone MC: 2% (60 g) [contains benzyl alcohol, sesame oil]
Gel, Nasal:
  Natesto: 5.5 mg/actuation (7.32 g)
Gel, Transdermal:
  AndroGel: 25 mg/2.5 g (1%) (2.5 g); 50 mg/5 g (1%) (5 g); 20.25 mg/1.25 g (1.62%) (1.25 g); 40.5 mg/2.5 g (1.62%) (2.5 g) [contains alcohol, usp]
  AndroGel Pump: 12.5 mg/actuation (1%) (75 g); 20.25 mg/actuation (1.62%) (75 g) [contains alcohol, usp]
  Fortesta: 10 mg/actuation (2%) (60 g) [odorless; contains propylene glycol, trolamine (triethanolamine)]
  Testim: 50 mg/5 g (1%) (5 g) [contains alcohol, usp, propylene glycol, tromethamine]
  Vogelxo: 50 mg/5 g (1%) (5 g) [contains alcohol, usp, tromethamine]
  Vogelxo Pump: 12.5 mg/actuation (1%) (75 g) [contains alcohol, usp, tromethamine]
  Generic: 25 mg/2.5 g (1%) (2.5 g); 50 mg/5 g (1%) (5 g); 10 mg/actuation (2%) (60 g); 12.5 mg/actuation (1%) (75 g); 50 MG/5GM (1%) (5 g)
Miscellaneous, Buccal:
  Striant: 30 mg (60 ea)
Ointment, Transdermal:
  First-Testosterone: 2% (60 g) [contains benzyl alcohol, butylated hydroxytoluene (bht), petrolatum, sesame oil]
Patch 24 Hour, Transdermal:
  Androderm: 2 mg/24 hr (1 ea, 60 ea); 4 mg/24 hr (1 ea, 30 ea)
Pellet, Implant:
  Testopel: 75 mg (10 ea, 100 ea)
Pellet, Implant [preservative free]:
  Generic: 12.5 mg (1 ea); 25 mg (1 ea); 37.5 mg (1 ea); 50 mg (1 ea)
Solution, Transdermal:
  Axiron: 30 mg/actuation (90 mL) [contains isopropyl alcohol]

Solution, Intramuscular, as cypionate:
  Depo-Testosterone: 100 mg/mL (10 mL); 200 mg/mL (1 mL, 10 mL) [contains benzyl alcohol, benzyl benzoate]
  Generic: 100 mg/mL (10 mL); 200 mg/mL (1 mL, 10 mL)
Solution, Intramuscular, as enanthate:
  Generic: 200 mg/mL (5 mL)
Solution, Intramuscular, as undecanoate:
  Aveed: 750 mg/3 mL (3 mL) [contains benzyl benzoate, castor oil (ricine oil)]

Dosage Forms: Canada Excipient information presented when available (limited, particularly for generics); consult specific product labeling.
Capsule, gelatin, as undecanoate:
  Andriol: 40 mg (10s)

Controlled Substance C-III

♦ **Testosterone Cypionate** see Testosterone on page 1766

♦ **Testosterone Enanthate** see Testosterone on page 1766

♦ **Testosterone Undecanoate** see Testosterone on page 1766

♦ **Testred** see MethylTESTOSTERone on page 1188

♦ **Tetanus and Diphtheria Toxoid** see Diphtheria and Tetanus Toxoid on page 565

Tetanus Immune Globulin (Human)
(TET a nus i MYUN GLOB yoo lin HYU man)

Brand Names: US HyperTET S/D
Brand Names: Canada HyperTET S/D
Index Terms TIG
Pharmacologic Category Blood Product Derivative; Immune Globulin
Additional Appendix Information
Immunization Administration Recommendations on page 1974
Immunization Schedules on page 1979
Use
Tetanus prophylaxis: For prophylaxis against tetanus following injury in patients whose immunization is incomplete or uncertain
Tetanus treatment: Treatment of active tetanus

The Advisory Committee on Immunization Practices (ACIP) recommends passive immunization with TIG for the following:
• Persons with a wound that is not clean or minor and who have received ≤2 or an unknown number of adsorbed tetanus toxoid doses (CDC 55[RR3] 2006; CDC 55[RR17] 2006).
• Persons who are wounded in bombings or similar mass casualty events if no reliable history of completed primary vaccination with tetanus exists. In case of shortage, use should be reserved for persons ≥60 years of age and immigrants from regions other than Europe or North America (CDC 57[RR6] 2008).
Dosing
Adult & Geriatric
Tetanus, prophylaxis: IM: 250 units
Tetanus, treatment: IM: 3,000 to 6,000 units. Infiltration of part of the dose around the wound is recommended (MMWR 2015; Red Book [AAP 2015]). Some experts recommend a lower 500 unit dose which appears to be as effective as higher doses and may cause less discomfort (Red Book [AAP 2015]; WHO 2010).

Tetanus prophylaxis in wound management: IM: Tetanus prophylaxis in patients with wounds should based on if the wound is clean or contaminated and the immunization status of the patient. Would management includes proper use of tetanus toxoid and/or tetanus immune globulin (TIG), wound cleaning, and (if required) surgical debridement and the proper use of antibiotics. Patients with an uncertain or incomplete tetanus immunization status should have additional follow up to ensure a series is completed. Patients with a history of Arthus reaction following a previous dose of a tetanus toxoid-containing vaccine should not receive a tetanus toxoid-containing vaccine until >10 years after the most recent dose even if they have a wound that is neither clean nor minor. See table on next page.

Tetanus Prophylaxis in Wound Management

History of Tetanus Immunization Doses	Clean, Minor Wounds		All Other Wounds[1]	
	Tetanus Toxoid[2]	TIG	Tetanus Toxoid[2]	TIG
Uncertain or <3 doses	Yes	No	Yes	Yes
3 or more doses	No[3]	No	No[4]	No

[1]Such as, but not limited to, wounds contaminated with dirt, feces, soil, and saliva; puncture wounds; wounds from crushing, tears, burns, and frostbite.

[2]Tetanus toxoid in this chart refers to a tetanus toxoid-containing vaccine. For children <7 years of age, DTaP (DT, if pertussis vaccine contraindicated) is preferred to tetanus toxoid alone. For children ≥7 years and Adults, Td preferred to tetanus toxoid alone; Tdap may be preferred if the patient has not previously been vaccinated with Tdap.

[3]Yes, if ≥10 years since last dose.

[4]Yes, if ≥5 years since last dose.

Adapted from CDC "Pink Book," " Epidemiology and Prevention of Vaccine-Preventable Diseases, Tetanus" (available at http://www.cdc.gov/vaccines/pubs/pinkbook/index.html) and *MMWR* 2006, 55(RR-17).

Abbreviations: **DT** = Diphtheria and Tetanus Toxoids (formulation for age ≤6 years); **DTaP** = Diphtheria and Tetanus Toxoids, and Acellular Pertussis (formulation for age ≤6 years; Daptacel, Infanrix); **Td** = Diphtheria and Tetanus Toxoids (formulation for age ≥7 years; Decavac,Tenivac); **TT**= Tetanus Toxoid (adsorbed [formulation for age ≥7 years]); **Tdap** = Diphtheria and Tetanus Toxoids, and Acellular Pertussis (Adacel or Boostrix [formulations for age ≥7 years]); **TIG** = Tetanus Immune Globulin

Pediatric

Tetanus, prophylaxis:
Infants and Children <7 years: IM: 4 units/kg; some recommend administering 250 units (*Red Book* [AAP 2015])
Children ≥7 years and Adolescents: Refer to adult dosing.

Tetanus, treatment: Refer to adult dosing.

Tetanus prophylaxis in wound management: Refer to adult dosing.

Renal Impairment There are no dosage adjustments provided in the manufacturer's labeling.

Hepatic Impairment There are no dosage adjustments provided in the manufacturer's labeling.

Additional Information Complete prescribing information should be consulted for additional detail.

Dosage Forms Excipient information presented when available (limited, particularly for generics); consult specific product labeling.
Injectable, Intramuscular:
HyperTET S/D: 250 units/mL (1 ea)

◆ Tetanus Toxoid *see* Diphtheria and Tetanus Toxoids, Acellular Pertussis, Poliovirus and *Haemophilus* b Conjugate Vaccine *on page 567*

◆ Tetanus Toxoid, Reduced Diphtheria Toxoid, and Acellular Pertussis, Adsorbed *see* Diphtheria and Tetanus Toxoids, and Acellular Pertussis Vaccine *on page 567*

◆ Tetcaine *see* Tetracaine (Ophthalmic) *on page 1772*

Tetrabenazine (tet ra BEN a zeen)

Brand Names: US Xenazine
Brand Names: Canada Nitoman; PMS-Tetrabenazine
Pharmacologic Category Central Monoamine-Depleting Agent
Use Chorea associated with Huntington disease: Treatment of chorea associated with Huntington disease
Canadian labeling: Treatment of hyperkinetic movement disorders, including Huntington chorea, hemiballismus, senile chorea, Tourette syndrome, and tardive dyskinesia
Prescribing and Access Restrictions Xenazine is available only through specialty pharmacies. For more information regarding the procurement of Xenazine, healthcare providers, patients, and caregivers may contact the Xenazine Information Center (XIC) at 1-888-882-6013 or at:
Health care providers: http://www.xenazineusa.com/HCP/PrescribingXenazine/Default.aspx
Patients and caregivers: http://www.xenazineusa.com/AboutXenazine/Getting-Your-Prescription.aspx
Medication Guide Available Yes
Dosing
Adult Dose should be individualized; titrate slowly
Chorea associated with Huntington disease: Oral:
Initial: 12.5 mg once daily in the morning, may increase to 12.5 mg twice daily after 1 week. Dosage may be increased by 12.5 mg daily at weekly intervals; daily doses >37.5 mg should be divided into 3 doses (maximum single dose: 25 mg)

Patients requiring doses >50 mg/day: Genotype for CYP2D6:
Extensive/intermediate metabolizers: Maximum: 100 mg/day; 37.5 mg/dose
Poor metabolizers: Maximum: 50 mg/day; 25 mg/dose
Concomitant use with strong CYP2D6 inhibitors (eg, fluoxetine, paroxetine, quinidine): Maximum: 50 mg/day; 25 mg dose.
Note: If treatment is interrupted for >5 days, retitration is recommended. If treatment is interrupted for <5 days resume at previous maintenance dose.

Canadian labeling: Hyperkinetic movement disorders: Initial: 12.5 mg 2 to 3 times daily; may be increased by 12.5 mg daily at weekly intervals; should be titrated slowly to maximal tolerated and effective dose (dose is individualized)
Usual maximum tolerated dosage: 25 mg 3 times/day; maximum recommended dose: 200 mg/day
Note: If there is no improvement at the maximum tolerated dose after 7 days, improvement is unlikely.

Geriatric Canadian labeling: Elderly and/or debilitated patients: Consider initiation at lower doses; must be titrated slowly to individualize dosage.

Renal Impairment There are no dosage adjustments provided in the manufacturer's labeling (has not been studied).

Hepatic Impairment Use is contraindicated.

Adjustment for Toxicity For toxicity/adverse reaction, including akathisia, restlessness, parkinsonism, insomnia, depression, suicidality, anxiety, sedation (intolerable): Suspend upward dosage titration and reduce dose; consider discontinuing if adverse reaction does not resolve (may be discontinued without tapering).

Additional Information Complete prescribing information should be consulted for additional detail.

Dosage Forms Excipient information presented when available (limited, particularly for generics); consult specific product labeling.
Tablet, Oral:
Xenazine: 12.5 mg
Xenazine: 25 mg [scored]
Generic: 12.5 mg, 25 mg

Dosage Forms: Canada Excipient information presented when available (limited, particularly for generics); consult specific product labeling.
Tablet:
Nitoman: 25 mg

Tetracaine (Systemic) (TET ra kane)

Brand Names: US Pontocaine [DSC]
Brand Names: Canada Pontocaine
Index Terms Amethocaine Hydrochloride; Tetracaine Hydrochloride
Pharmacologic Category Local Anesthetic
Use Spinal anesthesia
Dosing
Adult & Geriatric Spinal anesthesia: Injection: **Note:** Dosage varies with the anesthetic procedure, the degree of anesthesia required, and the individual patient response; it is administered by subarachnoid injection for spinal anesthesia.
Perineal anesthesia: 5 mg
Perineal and lower extremities: 10 mg
Anesthesia extending up to costal margin: 15 mg; doses up to 20 mg may be given, but are reserved for exceptional cases
Low spinal anesthesia (saddle block): 2-5 mg
Renal Impairment No dosage adjustment provided in manufacturer's labeling.
Hepatic Impairment No dosage adjustment provided in manufacturer's labeling.
Additional Information Complete prescribing information should be consulted for additional detail.
Dosage Forms Excipient information presented when available (limited, particularly for generics); consult specific product labeling. [DSC] = Discontinued product
Solution, Injection, as hydrochloride [preservative free]:
Pontocaine: 1% (2 mL [DSC])
Generic: 1% (2 mL)
Solution Reconstituted, Injection, as hydrochloride:
Pontocaine: 20 mg (1 ea [DSC])

Tetracaine (Ophthalmic) (TET ra kane)

Brand Names: US Altacaine; Tetcaine; TetraVisc; Tetra-Visc Forte
Index Terms Amethocaine Hydrochloride; Tetracaine Hydrochloride

Pharmacologic Category Local Anesthetic

Use Local anesthesia for various ophthalmic procedures of short duration (eg, tonometry, gonioscopy); minor ophthalmic surgical procedures (eg, removal of corneal foreign bodies, suture removal); and for various diagnostic purposes (eg, conjunctival scrapings)

Dosing

Adult & Geriatric

Short-term (nonsurgical procedures) anesthesia: Ophthalmic: Instill 1-2 drops into affected eye just prior to evaluation

Minor surgical procedures: Ophthalmic: Instill 1-2 drops into affected eye every 5-10 minutes for up to 3 doses

Prolonged surgical procedures: Ophthalmic: Instill 1-2 drops into affected eye every 5-10 minutes for up to 5 doses

Renal Impairment No dosage adjustment provided in manufacturer's labeling.

Hepatic Impairment No dosage adjustment provided in manufacturer's labeling.

Additional Information Complete prescribing information should be consulted for additional detail.

Dosage Forms Excipient information presented when available (limited, particularly for generics); consult specific product labeling.

Solution, Ophthalmic, as hydrochloride:

Altacaine: 0.5% (1 ea, 15 mL, 30 mL)

Tetcaine: 0.5% (15 mL) [contains chlorobutanol (chlorobutol), edetate disodium]

TetraVisc: 0.5% (1 ea, 5 mL) [contains benzalkonium chloride]

TetraVisc Forte: 0.5% (1 ea, 5 mL) [contains benzalkonium chloride, edetate disodium]

Generic: 0.5% (1 mL, 2 mL, 15 mL)

Tetracaine (Topical) (TET ra kane)

Brand Names: US Pontocaine [DSC]

Brand Names: Canada Ametop; Pontocaine

Index Terms Amethocaine Hydrochloride; Tetracaine Hydrochloride

Pharmacologic Category Local Anesthetic

Use Applied to nose and throat for diagnostic procedures

Dosing

Adult & Geriatric Topical mucous membranes (rhinolaryngology): Used as a 0.25% or 0.5% solution by direct application or nebulization; total dose should not exceed 20 mg

Additional Information Complete prescribing information should be consulted for additional detail.

Dosage Forms Excipient information presented when available (limited, particularly for generics); consult specific product labeling. [DSC] = Discontinued product

Solution, Mouth/Throat, as hydrochloride:

Pontocaine: 2% (118 mL [DSC])

♦ Tetracaine and Lidocaine *see* Lidocaine and Tetracaine *on page 1077*

♦ Tetracaine, Benzocaine, and Butamben *see* Benzocaine, Butamben, and Tetracaine *on page 218*

♦ Tetracaine Hydrochloride *see* Tetracaine (Ophthalmic) *on page 1772*

♦ Tetracaine Hydrochloride *see* Tetracaine (Systemic) *on page 1772*

♦ Tetracaine Hydrochloride *see* Tetracaine (Topical) *on page 1773*

♦ Tetracosactide *see* Cosyntropin *on page 449*

♦ Tetracosactrin *see* Cosyntropin *on page 449*

Tetracycline (tet ra SYE kleen)

Brand Names: Canada Apo-Tetra; Nu-Tetra

Index Terms Achromycin; TCN; Tetracycline Hydrochloride

Pharmacologic Category Antibiotic, Tetracycline Derivative

Use

Acute intestinal amebiasis: Adjunctive therapy in acute intestinal amebiasis caused by *Entamoeba histolytica*.

Acne: Adjunctive therapy for the treatment of severe acne.

Actinomycosis: Treatment of actinomycosis caused by *Actinomyces* species when penicillin is contraindicated.

Anthrax: Treatment of anthrax due to *Bacillus anthracis* when penicillin is contraindicated.

Campylobacter: Treatment of infections caused by *Campylobacter fetus*.

Cholera: Treatment of cholera caused by *Vibrio cholerae*.

Clostridium: Treatment of infections caused by *Clostridium* spp. when penicillin is contraindicated.

Gram-negative infections: Treatment of infections caused by *Escherichia coli*, *Enterobacter aerogenes*, *Shigella* spp., *Acinetobacter* spp., *Klebsiella* spp., and *Bacteroides* spp.

Listeriosis: Treatment of listeriosis due to *Listeria monocytogenes* when penicillin is contraindicated.

Ophthalmic infections: Treatment of inclusion conjunctivitis or trachoma caused by *Chlamydia trachomatis*.

Relapsing fever: Treatment of relapsing fever due to *Borrelia* spp.

Respiratory tract infection: Treatment of respiratory tract infections caused by *Haemophilus influenzae* (upper respiratory tract only), *Klebsiella* spp. (lower respiratory tract only), *Mycoplasma pneumoniae* (lower respiratory tract only), *Streptococcus pneumoniae*, or *Streptococcus pyogenes*.

Rickettsial infections: Treatment of Rocky Mountain spotted fever, typhus group infections, Q fever, and rickettsialpox caused by *Rickettsiae*.

Sexually transmitted diseases: Treatment of lymphogranuloma venereum or uncomplicated urethral, endocervical, or rectal infections caused by *C. trachomatis*; chancroid caused by *Haemophilus ducreyi*; granuloma inguinale (donovanosis) caused by *Klebsiella granulomatis*; syphilis caused by *Treponema pallidum*, when penicillin is contraindicated.

Limitations of use: Tetracycline is not a recommended alternative for uncomplicated gonorrhea according to the Centers for Disease Control and Prevention (CDC) sexually transmitted diseases guidelines (CDC [Workowski 2015]).

Skin and skin structure infections: Treatment of skin and skin structure infections caused by *Staphylococcus aureus* or *S. pyogenes*.

Urinary tract infections: Treatment of urinary tract infections caused by susceptible gram-negative organisms (eg, *E. coli*, *Klebsiella* spp.).

Vincent infection: Treatment of Vincent infection caused by *Fusobacterium fusiforme* when penicillin is contraindicated.

Yaws: Treatment of yaws caused by *Treponema pertenue* when penicillin is contraindicated.

Zoonotic infections: Treatment of psittacosis (ornithosis) due to *Chlamydophila psittaci*; plague due to *Yersinia pestis*; tularemia due to *Francisella tularensis*; brucellosis due to *Brucella* spp. (in conjunction with an aminoglycoside); bartonellosis due to *Bartonella bacilliformis*.

Dosing

Adult & Geriatric

Usual dosage range: Oral: 250 to 500 mg every 6 to 12 hours

Acne: Oral: Initial dose: 1 g daily in divided doses; reduce gradually to 125 to 500 mg/day once improvement is noted (alternate day or intermittent therapy may be adequate in some patients).

***Helicobacter pylori* eradication (off-label use):** 500 mg 4 times daily for 10 to 14 days, in combination with bismuth subsalicylate, metronidazole, and either ranitidine or a proton pump inhibitor (Chey 2007)

Malaria, severe, treatment (off-label use): Oral: 250 mg 4 times daily for 7 days with quinidine gluconate. **Note:** Quinidine gluconate duration is region specific; consult CDC for current recommendations (CDC 2013).

Malaria, uncomplicated, treatment (off-label use): Oral: 250 mg 4 times daily for 7 days with quinine sulfate. **Note:** Quinine sulfate duration is region specific; consult CDC for current recommendations (CDC 2013).

Periodontitis (off-label use): Oral: 250 mg every 6 hours until improvement (usually 10 days)

Syphilis, penicillin-allergic patients: Note: Data to support the use of alternatives to penicillin are limited in primary and secondary syphilis and are not well documented in the treatment of latent syphilis (CDC [Workowski 2015])

Early syphilis (primary or secondary infection): 500 mg 4 times daily for 14 days.

Latent syphilis (late or of unknown duration): 500 mg 4 times daily for 28 days.

Tularemia (mild to moderate): Oral: 500 mg 4 times daily for at least 14 days (IDSA [Stevens 2014])

Vibrio cholerae: Oral: 500 mg 4 times daily for 3 days (Seas 1996)

Pediatric Usual dosage range: Children >8 years and Adolescents: Oral: 25 to 50 mg/kg/day in divided doses every 6 hours

Malaria, severe, treatment (off-label use): Children ≥8 years and Adolescents: Oral: 25 mg/kg/day in divided doses every 6 hours (maximum dose: 250 mg every 6 hours) for 7 days with quinidine gluconate. **Note:** Quinidine gluconate duration is region specific; consult CDC for current recommendations (CDC 2013).

Malaria, uncomplicated, treatment (off-label use): Children ≥8 years and Adolescents: Oral: 25 mg/kg/day in divided doses every 6 hours (maximum dose: 250 mg every 6 hours) for 7 days with quinine sulfate. **Note:** Quinine sulfate duration is region specific; consult CDC for current recommendations (CDC 2013).

Renal Impairment

Adults:

Manufacturer's labeling: There are dosage adjustments provided in the manufacturer's labeling; decrease dose and/or extend dosing interval.

Alternative dosing (Aronoff 2007): Note: Renally adjusted dose recommendations are based on doses of 250 mg to 500 mg twice daily to 4 times daily.

GFR >50 mL/minute: Administer recommended dose based on indication every 8 to 12 hours.

GFR 10 to 50 mL/minute: Administer recommended dose based on indication every 12 to 24 hours.

GFR <10 mL/minute: Administer recommended dose based on indication every 24 hours.

Children >8 years and Adolescents: There are dosage adjustments provided in the manufacturer's labeling; decrease dose and/or extend dosing interval.

Hepatic Impairment There are no dosage adjustments provided in the manufacturer's labeling.

Additional Information Complete prescribing information should be consulted for additional detail.

Dosage Forms Excipient information presented when available (limited, particularly for generics); consult specific product labeling.

Capsule, Oral, as hydrochloride:

Generic: 250 mg, 500 mg

Tetrastarch (TET ra starch)

Brand Names: US Voluven

Brand Names: Canada Volulyte; Voluven

Index Terms Etherified Starch; HES; HES 130/0.4; Hydroxyethyl Starch

Pharmacologic Category Plasma Volume Expander, Colloid

Use Blood volume expander used in treatment and prevention of hypovolemia

Dosing

Adult & Geriatric Plasma volume expansion: IV infusion: May administer up to 50 mL/kg/day (or up to 3500 mL per day in a 70 kg patient); may administer repetitively over several days. **Note:** With severe dehydration, administer crystalloid first. Daily dose and rate of infusion dependent on amount of blood lost, on maintenance or restoration of hemodynamics, and on amount of hemodilution. Titrate to individual colloid needs, hemodynamics, and hydration status. Do not use in the critically ill including patients with sepsis, those with preexisting renal dysfunction or receiving dialysis, those with preexisting bleeding disorders or those with intracranial bleeding.

Pediatric Plasma volume expansion: IV infusion: **Note:** With severe dehydration, administer crystalloid first. Daily dose and rate of infusion dependent on amount of blood lost, on maintenance or restoration of hemodynamics, and on amount of hemodilution. Titrate to individual colloid needs, hemodynamics, and hydration status. Do not use in the critically ill including patients with sepsis, those with preexisting renal dysfunction or receiving dialysis, those with preexisting bleeding disorders or those with intracranial bleeding.

Children ≤12 years and Adolescents: May administer up to 50 mL/kg/day (or up to 3500 mL per day in a 70 kg patient); may administer repetitively over several days.

Mean daily dose ± SD in pediatric clinical trials:

Children <2 years: 16 ± 9 mL/kg

Children 2-12 years: 36 ± 11 mL/kg

Renal Impairment Avoid use in patients with preexisting renal dysfunction. Use is contraindicated in oliguric/anuric renal failure unrelated to hypovolemia or patients receiving dialysis. Discontinue use at the first sign of renal injury.

Hepatic Impairment No dosage adjustment provided in manufacturer's labeling; use is contraindicated in severe liver disease.

Additional Information Complete prescribing information should be consulted for additional detail.

Dosage Forms Excipient information presented when available (limited, particularly for generics); consult specific product labeling.

Solution, Intravenous:

Voluven: 6% (500 mL) [dehp free, latex free, pvc free]

Dosage Forms: Canada

Excipient information presented when available (limited, particularly for generics); consult specific product labeling.

Infusion, premixed in isotonic electrolyte solution:

Volulyte: 6% (250 mL, 500 mL)

Thalidomide (tha LI doe mide)

Brand Names: US Thalomid
Brand Names: Canada Thalomid
Pharmacologic Category Angiogenesis Inhibitor; Antineoplastic Agent; Immunomodulator, Systemic
Use

US labeling:

Erythema nodosum leprosum: Acute treatment of cutaneous manifestations of moderate to severe erythema nodosum leprosum; maintenance treatment for prevention and suppression of cutaneous manifestations of erythema nodosum leprosum recurrence
Limitation of use: Thalidomide is not indicated as monotherapy for erythema nodosum leprosum treatment in the presence of moderate to severe neuritis.

Multiple myeloma: Treatment of newly diagnosed multiple myeloma (in combination with dexamethasone)

Canadian labeling: **Multiple myeloma:** Treatment of patients ≥65 years of age with previously untreated multiple myeloma (in combination with melphalan and prednisone)

Pregnancy Considerations [US Boxed Warning]: Thalidomide may cause severe birth defects or embryo-fetal death if taken during pregnancy. Thalidomide cannot be used in women who are pregnant or may become pregnant during therapy as even a single dose may cause severe birth defects. In order to decrease the risk of fetal exposure, thalidomide is available only through a special restricted distribution program (Thalomid REMS). Reproduction studies in animals and data from pregnant women have shown evidence of fetal abnormalities; use is contraindicated in women who are or may become pregnant. Anomalies observed in humans include amelia, phocomelia, bone defects, ear and eye abnormalities, facial palsy, congenital heart defects, urinary and genital tract malformations; mortality in ~40% of infants at or shortly after birth has also been reported.

Women of reproductive potential must avoid pregnancy 4 weeks prior to therapy, during therapy, during therapy interruptions, and for ≥4 weeks after therapy is discontinued. Two forms of effective contraception or total abstinence from heterosexual intercourse must be used by females who are not infertile or who have not had a hysterectomy. A negative pregnancy test (sensitivity of at least 50 milliunits/mL) 10 to 14 days prior to therapy, within 24 hours prior to beginning therapy, weekly during the first 4 weeks, and every 4 weeks (every 2 weeks for women with irregular menstrual cycles) thereafter is required for women of childbearing potential. Thalidomide must be immediately discontinued for a missed period, abnormal pregnancy test or abnormal menstrual bleeding; refer patient to a reproductive toxicity specialist if pregnancy occurs during treatment.

Females of reproductive potential (including health care workers and caregivers) must also avoid contact with thalidomide capsules.

Thalidomide is also present in the semen of males. Males (even those vasectomized) must use a latex or synthetic condom during any sexual contact with women of childbearing potential and for up to 28 days following discontinuation of therapy. Males taking thalidomide must not donate sperm.

The parent or legal guardian for patients between 12 to 18 years of age must agree to ensure compliance with the required guidelines.

If pregnancy occurs during treatment, thalidomide must be immediately discontinued and the patient referred to a reproductive toxicity specialist. Any suspected fetal exposure to thalidomide must be reported to the FDA via the MedWatch program (1-800-FDA-1088) and to Celgene Corporation (1-888-423-5436). In Canada, thalidomide is available only through a restricted-distribution program called RevAid (1-888-738-2431).

Breast-Feeding Considerations It is not known if thalidomide is excreted in breast milk. Due to the potential for serious adverse reactions in the infant, a decision should be made to discontinue nursing or discontinue treatment with thalidomide, taking into account the importance of treatment to the mother. Use in breast-feeding women is contraindicated in the Canadian labeling.

Prescribing and Access Restrictions US: As a requirement of the REMS program, access to this medication is restricted. Thalidomide is approved for marketing only under a special distribution program, the Thalomid REMS (https://www.celgeneriskmanagement.com or 1-888-423-5436), which has been approved by the FDA. Prescribers, patients, and pharmacies must be certified with the program to prescribe or dispense thalidomide. No more than a 4-week supply should be dispensed. Blister packs should be dispensed intact (do not repackage capsules). Prescriptions must be filled within 7 days (for females of reproductive potential) or within 30 days (for all other patients) after authorization number obtained. Subsequent prescriptions may be filled only if fewer than 7 days of therapy remain on the previous prescription. A new prescription is required for further dispensing (a telephone prescription may not be accepted.) Pregnancy testing is required for females of childbearing potential.

Canada: Access to thalidomide is restricted through a controlled distribution program called RevAid. Only physicians and pharmacists enrolled in this program are authorized to prescribe or dispense thalidomide. Patients must be enrolled in the program by their physicians. Further information is available at www.RevAid.ca or by calling 1-888-738-2431.

Medication Guide Available Yes
Contraindications
Hypersensitivity to thalidomide or any component of the formulation; pregnancy
Canadian labeling: Additional contraindications (not in US labeling): Hypersensitivity to lenalidomide or pomalidomide; both females at risk of becoming pregnant and male patients who are unable to follow or comply with conditions for use (refer to manufacturer labeling); breast-feeding

Warnings/Precautions Hazardous agent - use appropriate precautions for handling and disposal (NIOSH 2014 [group 2]). Avoid exposure to nonintact capsules and body fluids of patients receiving thalidomide. If exposure occurs, wash area with soap and water. Wear gloves to prevent cutaneous exposure.

[US Boxed Warning]: Thalidomide use for the treatment of multiple myeloma is associated with an increased risk for venous thromboembolism (VTE), including deep vein thrombosis (DVT) and pulmonary embolism (PE); the risk is increased when used in combination with standard chemotherapy agents, including dexamethasone. In one controlled study, the incidence of VTE was 22.5% in patients receiving thalidomide in combination with dexamethasone, compared to 4.9% for dexamethasone alone. Monitor for signs and symptoms of thromboembolism (shortness of breath, chest pain, or arm or leg swelling) and instruct patients to seek prompt medical attention with development of these symptoms. Consider thromboprophylaxis based on risk factors. Ischemic heart disease, including MI and stroke, also occurred at a higher rate (compared to placebo) in myeloma patients receiving thalidomide plus dexamethasone who had not received prior treatment. Assess individual risk factors for thromboembolism and consider thromboprophylaxis. The American Society of Clinical Oncology guidelines for VTE prophylaxis and treatment recommend thromboprophylaxis for patients receiving thalidomide in combination with chemotherapy and/or dexamethasone; either aspirin or low molecular weight heparin (LMWH) are recommended for lower risk patient and LMWH is recommended for higher risk patients (Lyman 2013). Anticoagulant prophylaxis should be individualized and selected based on the venous thromboembolism risk of the combination treatment regimen, using the safest and easiest to administer (Palumbo 2008). The Canadian labeling recommends anticoagulant prophylaxis for at least the first 5 months of thalidomide-based therapy. Monitor for signs/symptoms of thromboembolism and advise patients to seek immediate care if symptoms (shortness of breath, chest pain, arm/leg swelling) develop. Other medications that are also associated with thromboembolism should be used with caution.

May cause leukopenia and neutropenia; avoid initiating therapy if ANC <750/mm^3. Persistent neutropenia may require treatment interruption. Thrombocytopenia (including grades 3 and 4) has been reported; may require dose reduction, treatment delay, or discontinuation. Monitor for signs and symptoms of bleeding (including petechiae, epistaxis, and gastrointestinal bleeding), especially if concomitant medication may increase the risk of bleeding. Monitor CBC with differential and platelets. Anemia has also been observed. May cause bradycardia; use with caution when administering concomitantly with medications that may also decrease heart rate. May require thalidomide dose reduction or discontinuation. Stevens-Johnson syndrome (SJS) and toxic epidermal necrolysis (TEN) have been reported (may be fatal); withhold therapy and evaluate if skin rash occurs; permanently discontinue if rash is exfoliative, purpuric, bullous or if SJS or TEN is suspected. Hypersensitivity, including erythematous macular rash, possibly associated with fever, tachycardia and hypotension has been reported. May require treatment interruption for severe reactions; discontinue if recurs with rechallenge. Abnormal liver function tests have been reported. Hepatotoxicity (including some serious and fatal cases of hepatic injury) has been observed usually within the first 2 months of treatment (Thalomid Canadian labeling 2015); most events resolved without intervention after discontinuing thalidomide.

Increased incidence of second primary malignancies (SPMs), including acute myeloid leukemia (AML) and myelodysplastic syndrome (MDS), has been observed in previously untreated multiple myeloma patients receiving thalidomide in combination with melphalan, and prednisone. In addition to AML and MDS, solid tumors have been reported with thalidomide maintenance treatment for multiple myeloma (Usmani, 2012). Carefully evaluate patients for SPMs prior to and during treatment and manage as clinically indicated.

Thalidomide is commonly associated with peripheral neuropathy; may be irreversible. Neuropathy generally occurs following chronic use (over months), but may occur with short-term use; onset may be delayed. Use caution with other medications that may also cause peripheral neuropathy. Monitor for signs/symptoms of neuropathy monthly for the first 3 months of therapy and regularly thereafter. Electrophysiological testing may be considered at baseline and every 6 months to detect asymptomatic neuropathy.

To limit further damage, immediately discontinue (if clinically appropriate) in patients who develop neuropathy. Reinitiate therapy only if neuropathy returns to baseline; may require dosage reduction or permanent discontinuation. Seizures (including grand mal convulsions) have been reported in postmarketing data; monitor closely for clinical changes indicating potential seizure activity in patients with a history of seizures, concurrent therapy with drugs that alter seizure threshold, or conditions that predispose to seizures. May cause dizziness, drowsiness, and/or somnolence; caution patients about performing tasks that require mental alertness (eg, operating machinery or driving). Avoid ethanol and concomitant medications that may exacerbate these symptoms; dose reductions may be necessary for excessive drowsiness or somnolence. May cause orthostatic hypotension; use with caution in patients who would not tolerate transient hypotensive episodes. When arising from a recumbent position, advise patients to sit upright for a few minutes prior to standing. Constipation may commonly occur. May require treatment interruption or dosage reduction. Certain adverse reactions (constipation, fatigue, weakness, nausea, hypokalemia, hyperglycemia, DVT, pulmonary embolism, atrial fibrillation) are more likely in elderly patients. In studies conducted prior to the use of highly active antiretroviral therapy, thalidomide use was associated with increased viral loads in HIV infected patients. Monitor viral load after the 1st and 3rd months of therapy and every 3 months thereafter. Patients with a high tumor burden may be at risk for tumor lysis syndrome; monitor closely; institute appropriate management for hyperuricemia.

Potentially significant drug-drug interactions may exist, requiring dose or frequency adjustment, additional monitoring, and/or selection of alternative therapy. Patients should not donate blood during thalidomide treatment and for 1 month after therapy discontinuation

[US Boxed Warning]: Thalidomide may cause severe birth defects or embryo-fetal death if taken during pregnancy. Thalidomide cannot be used in women who are pregnant or may become pregnant during therapy as even a single dose may cause severe birth defects. In order to decrease the risk of fetal exposure, thalidomide is available only through a special restricted distribution program (Thalomid REMS). Use is contraindicated in women who are or may become pregnant. Pregnancy must be excluded prior to therapy initiation with 2 negative pregnancy tests. Women of reproductive potential must avoid pregnancy 4 weeks prior to therapy, during therapy, during therapy interruptions, and for ≥4 weeks after therapy is discontinued; two reliable methods of birth control, or abstinence from heterosexual intercourse, must be used. Males taking thalidomide (even those vasectomized) must use a latex or synthetic condom during any sexual contact with women of childbearing potential and for up to 28 days following discontinuation of therapy. Males taking thalidomide must not donate sperm. Some forms of contraception may not be appropriate in certain patients. An intrauterine device (IUD) or implantable contraceptive may increase the risk of infection or bleeding; estrogen containing products may increase the risk of thromboembolism.

Due to the embryo-fetal risk, thalidomide is only available through a restricted program under the Thalomid REMS program. Prescribers and pharmacies must be certified with the program to prescribe or dispense thalidomide. Patients must sign an agreement and comply with the REMS program requirements.

Adverse Reactions

>10%:

Cardiovascular: Edema (57%), thrombosis/embolism (23%; grade 3: 13%, grade 4: 9%), hypotension (16%)

Central nervous system: Fatigue (79%; grade 3: 14%, grade 4: 3%), somnolence (36% to 38%), dizziness (4% to 20%), sensory neuropathy (54%), confusion (28%), anxiety/agitation (9% to 26%), fever (19% to 23%), motor neuropathy (22%), headache (13% to 19%)

Dermatologic: Rash/desquamation (21% to 30%; grade 3: 4%), dry skin (21%), maculopapular rash (4% to 19%), acne (3% to 11%)

Endocrine & metabolic: Hypocalcemia (72%)

Gastrointestinal: Constipation (3% to 55%), nausea (4% to 28%), anorexia (3% to 28%), weight loss (23%), weight gain (22%), diarrhea (4% to 19%), oral moniliasis (4% to 11%)

Hematologic: Leukopenia (17% to 35%), neutropenia (31%), anemia (6% to 13%), lymphadenopathy (6% to 13%)

Hepatic: AST increased (3% to 25%), bilirubin increased (14%)

Neuromuscular & skeletal: Muscle weakness (40%), tremor (4% to 26%), weakness (6% to 22%), myalgia (17%), paresthesia (6% to 16%), arthralgia (13%)

Renal: Hematuria (11%)

Respiratory: Dyspnea (42%)

Miscellaneous: Diaphoresis (13%)

1% to 10%:

Cardiovascular: Peripheral edema (3% to 8%), facial edema (4%)

Central nervous system: Insomnia (9%), nervousness (3% to 9%), malaise (8%), vertigo (8%), pain (3% to 8%)

Dermatologic: Dermatitis (fungal 4% to 9%), pruritus (3% to 8%), nail disorder (3% to 4%)

Endocrine & metabolic: Hyperlipemia (6% to 9%)

Gastrointestinal: Xerostomia (8% to 9%), flatulence (8%), tooth pain (4%)

Genitourinary: Impotence (3% to 8%)

Hepatic: LFTs abnormal (9%)

Neuromuscular & skeletal: Neuropathy (8%), back pain (4% to 6%), neck pain (4%), neck rigidity (4%)

Renal: Albuminuria (3% to 8%)

Respiratory: Pharyngitis (4% to 8%), rhinitis (4%), sinusitis (3% to 8%)

Miscellaneous: Infection (6% to 8%)

Postmarketing and/or case reports (limited to important or life-threatening): Acute renal failure, alkaline phosphatase increased, ALT increased, amenorrhea, angioedema, aphthous stomatitis, arrhythmia, atrial fibrillation, bile duct obstruction, bradycardia, BUN increased, carpal tunnel, cerebral vascular accident, CML, creatinine clearance decreased, creatinine increased, deafness, depression, diplopia, dysesthesia, ECG abnormalities, enuresis, eosinophilia, epistaxis, erythema multiforme, erythema nodosum, erythroleukemia, exfoliative dermatitis, febrile neutropenia, foot drop, galactorrhea, granulocytopenia, gynecomastia, hearing loss, hepatomegaly, Hodgkin's disease, hypercalcemia, hyper-/hypokalemia, hypersensitivity, hypertension, hyper-/hypothyroidism, hypersensitivity, hyperuricemia, hypomagnesemia, hyponatremia, hypoproteinemia, intestinal obstruction, intestinal perforation, interstitial pneumonitis, LDH increased, lethargy, leukocytosis, loss of consciousness, lymphedema, lymphopenia, mental status changes, metrorrhagia, MI, myxedema, nystagmus, oliguria, orthostatic hypotension, pancytopenia, paresthesia, petechiae, peripheral neuritis, photosensitivity, pleural effusion, prothrombin time changes, psychosis, pulmonary embolus, pulmonary hypertension, purpura, Raynaud's syndrome, renal failure, secondary malignancy (AML, MDS, solid tumors), seizure, sepsis, septic shock, sexual dysfunction, sick sinus syndrome, status epilepticus, Stevens-Johnson syndrome, stomach ulcer, stupor, suicide attempt, syncope, tachycardia, thrombocytopenia, toxic epidermal necrolysis, transient ischemic attack, tumor lysis syndrome, urticaria

Drug Interactions

Metabolism/Transport Effects None known.

Avoid Concomitant Use

Avoid concomitant use of Thalidomide with any of the following: Abatacept; Anakinra; Azelastine (Nasal); BCG (Intravesical); Canakinumab; Certolizumab Pegol; CNS Depressants; Deferiprone; Dipyrone; Natalizumab; Orphenadrine; Paraldehyde; Pimecrolimus; Rilonacept; Tacrolimus (Topical); Tocilizumab; Tofacitinib; Vaccines (Live); Vedolizumab

Increased Effect/Toxicity

Thalidomide may increase the levels/effects of: Abatacept; Alcohol (Ethyl); Amifostine; Anakinra; Azelastine (Nasal); Bisphosphonate Derivatives; Canakinumab; Certolizumab Pegol; Deferiprone; DULoxetine; Fingolimod; Hypotension-Associated Agents; Leflunomide; Levodopa; Metyrosine; Natalizumab; Orphenadrine; Pamidronate; Paraldehyde; Pramipexole; Rilonacept; ROPINIRole; Rotigotine; Selective Serotonin Reuptake Inhibitors; Tofacitinib; Vaccines (Live); Vedolizumab; Zoledronic Acid

The levels/effects of Thalidomide may be increased by: Alfuzosin; Blood Pressure Lowering Agents; Brimonidine (Topical); Cannabis; CNS Depressants; Contraceptives (Estrogens); Contraceptives (Progestins); Denosumab; Dexamethasone (Systemic); Diazoxide; Dipyrone; Dronabinol; Erythropoiesis-Stimulating Agents; Estrogen Derivatives; Herbs (Hypotensive Properties); Kava Kava; Magnesium Sulfate; Minocycline; Molsidomine; Nabilone; Nicorandil; Obinutuzumab; Pentoxifylline; Phosphodiesterase 5 Inhibitors; Pimecrolimus; Prostacyclin Analogues; Roflumilast; Rufinamide; Tacrolimus (Topical); Tetrahydrocannabinol; Tocilizumab; Trastuzumab

Decreased Effect

Thalidomide may decrease the levels/effects of: BCG (Intravesical); Coccidioides immitis Skin Test; Sipuleucel-T; Vaccines (Inactivated); Vaccines (Live)

The levels/effects of Thalidomide may be decreased by: Echinacea

Storage/Stability Store at 20°C to 25°C (68°F to 77°F); excursions are permitted between 15°C and 30°C (59°F and 86°F). Protect from light. Keep in original package.

Mechanism of Action Immunomodulatory and antiangiogenic characteristics; immunologic effects may vary based on conditions; may suppress excessive tumor necrosis factor-alpha production in patients with ENL, yet may increase plasma tumor necrosis factor-alpha levels in HIV-positive patients. In multiple myeloma, thalidomide is associated with an increase in natural killer cells and increased levels of interleukin-2 and interferon gamma. Other proposed mechanisms of action include suppression of angiogenesis, prevention of free-radical-mediated DNA damage, increased cell mediated cytotoxic effects, and altered expression of cellular adhesion molecules.

Pharmacodynamics/Kinetics

Absorption: Slow, good

Protein binding: 55% to 66%

Metabolism: Minimal (unchanged drug is the predominant circulating component)

Half-life elimination: 5.5 to 7.3 hours

Time to peak, plasma: ~2 to 5 hours

Excretion: Urine (92%; <4% of the dose as unchanged drug); feces (<2%)

Dosing

Adult & Geriatric

Erythema nodosum leprosum, acute cutaneous: Oral: Initial: 100 to 300 mg once daily at bedtime, continue until signs/symptoms subside (usually ~2 weeks), then taper off in 50 mg decrements every 2 to 4 weeks. For severe cases with moderate to severe neuritis, corticosteroids may be initiated with thalidomide (taper off and discontinue corticosteroids when neuritis improves).

Patients weighing <50 kg: Initiate at lower end of the dosing range

Severe cutaneous reaction or patients previously requiring high doses: May be initiated at up to 400 mg once daily at bedtime or in divided doses

Erythema nodosum leprosum, maintenance (prevention/suppression, or with flares during tapering attempts): Oral: Maintain on the minimum dosage necessary to control the reaction; efforts to taper off should be attempted every 3 to 6 months, in decrements of 50 mg every 2 to 4 weeks.

Multiple myeloma, newly diagnosed: Oral:

US labeling: 200 mg once daily at bedtime (in combination with dexamethasone)

Canadian labeling: Adults ≥65 years: 200 mg once daily; maximum: 12 six-week cycles (in combination with melphalan and prednisone)

Multiple myeloma (off-label dosing):

In combination with bortezomib and dexamethasone (off-label combination): Induction therapy: 100 mg once daily for the first 14 days, then 200 mg once daily for 3 (21-day) cycles (Cavo, 2010) or 100 mg once daily for up to 8 (21-day) cycles (Kaufman, 2010)

In combination with melphalan and prednisone (off-label combination in US): 200 to 400 mg once daily (Facon, 2007) or 100 mg once daily (Palumbo, 2008)

Multiple myeloma, maintenance (following autologous stem cell transplant; off-label use): Oral: 200 mg once daily starting 3 to 6 months after transplant; continue until disease progression or unacceptable toxicity (Brinker, 2006) or 100 mg once daily starting 42 to 60 days following transplant; increase to 200 mg once daily after 2 weeks if tolerated; continue for up to 12 months (in combination with prednisolone) (Spencer, 2009)

Multiple myeloma, salvage therapy: Initial: 200 mg once daily at bedtime; may increase daily dose by 200 mg every 2 weeks for 6 weeks (if tolerated) to a maximum of 800 mg once daily at bedtime (Singhal, 1999) or 100 mg once daily (in combination with dexamethasone) (Palumbo, 2001) or 200 mg once daily (in combination with bortezomib and dexamethasone) for 1 year (Garderet, 2012) or 400 mg once daily at bedtime (in combination with dexamethasone, cisplatin, doxorubicin, cyclophosphamide and etoposide) (Lee, 2003)

AIDS-related aphthous stomatitis (off-label use): Oral: 200 mg once daily at bedtime for up to 8 weeks, if no response, then 200 mg twice daily for 4 weeks (Jacobson, 1997)

Chronic graft-versus-host disease (refractory), treatment (off-label second-line use; optimum dose not determined): Oral: Initial: 100 mg once daily at bedtime, with dose escalation up to 400 mg daily in 3 to 4 divided doses (Wolff, 2010) **or** Initial: 50 to 100 mg 3 times daily; maximum dose: 600 to 1,200 mg daily (Kulkarni, 2003) **or** 200 mg 4 times daily (dose adjusted to goal thalidomide concentration of ≥5 mcg/mL 2 hours postdose) (Vogelsang, 1992) **or** 100 to 300 mg 4 times daily (Parker, 1995)

Systemic light chain amyloidosis (off-label use): Oral: 200 mg once daily (starting dose 50 to 100 mg once daily; titrate at 4-week intervals) in combination with cyclophosphamide and dexamethasone (Wechalekar, 2007)

Waldenström macroglobulinemia (off-label use): Oral: ≤200 mg once daily for up to 52 weeks (in combination with rituximab) (Treon, 2008)

Pediatric

Erythema nodosum leprosum, acute cutaneous: Children ≥12 years: Oral: Refer to adult dosing.

Erythema nodosum leprosum, maintenance (prevention/suppression, or with flares during tapering attempts): Children ≥12 years: Oral: Refer to adult dosing.

Chronic graft-versus-host disease (refractory), treatment (off-label second-line use; limited data): Children ≥3 years: Oral: 3 mg/kg 4 times daily (dose adjusted to goal thalidomide concentration of ≥5 mcg/mL 2 hours postdose) (Vogelsang 1992) **or** Initial: 3 to 6 mg/kg/day in 2 to 4 divided doses; target dose 12 mg/kg/day; Maximum daily dose: 800 mg (Rovelli, 1998)

Renal Impairment No dosage adjustment necessary for patients with renal impairment and on dialysis (per manufacturer). In a study of 6 patients with end-stage renal disease on dialysis, although clearance was increased by dialysis, a supplemental dose was not needed (Eriksson, 2003).

Multiple myeloma: An evaluation of 29 newly diagnosed myeloma patients with renal failure (serum creatinine ≥2 mg/dL) treated with thalidomide and dexamethasone (some also received cyclophosphamide) found that toxicities and efficacy were similar to patients with normal renal function (Seol, 2010). A study evaluating induction therapy with thalidomide and dexamethasone in 31 newly diagnosed myeloma patients with renal failure (CrCl <50 mL/minute), including 16 patients with severe renal impairment (CrCl <30 mL/minute) and 7 patients on chronic hemodialysis found that toxicities were similar to patients without renal impairment and that thalidomide and dexamethasone could be administered safely (Tosi, 2009).

Hepatic Impairment There are no dosage adjustments provided in the manufacturer's labeling (has not been studied). However, thalidomide does not appear to undergo significant hepatic metabolism.

Adjustment for Toxicity

ANC ≤750/mm^3: Withhold treatment if clinically appropriate

Grade 3 or 4 adverse reactions: Consider dose reduction, delay or discontinuation (based on clinical judgment).

Multiple myeloma:

US labeling: Constipation, oversedation, peripheral neuropathy: Temporarily withhold or continue with a reduced dose

Canadian labeling:

ANC <1,500/mm^3: Withhold melphalan and prednisone for 1 week; resume melphalan and prednisone after 1 week if ANC >1,500/mm^3 **or** if ANC 1,000 to 1,500/mm^3 reduce melphalan dose by 50% **or** if ANC <1,000/mm^3 adjust chemotherapy dose based on clinical status of patient.

Constipation, oversedation: Temporarily withhold thalidomide treatment or continue with a reduced dose

Peripheral neuropathy, Grade 1 (paresthesia, weakness and/or loss of reflexes) without loss of function): Evaluate patient and consider dose reduction with worsening of symptoms; symptom improvement may not follow dose reduction, however.

Peripheral neuropathy, Grade 2 (interferes with function but not with daily activities), Grade 3 (interferes with daily activities), or Grade 4 (disabling neuropathy): Discontinue thalidomide treatment

Thromboembolic events: Withhold therapy and initiate standard anticoagulant treatment; may resume thalidomide therapy at original dose following stabilization of patient and resolution of thromboembolic event; maintain anticoagulant treatment for duration of thalidomide therapy

Off-label dosage adjustment (Richardson, 2012):

Peripheral neuropathy:

Grade 1: Reduce dose by 50%

Grade 2: Temporarily interrupt therapy; once resolved to ≤ grade 1, resume therapy with a 50% dosage reduction (if clinically appropriate)

Grade 3 or higher: Discontinue therapy

Administration Oral: Swallow capsules whole with water. Do not open or crush capsules. Avoid extensive handling of capsules; capsules should remain in blister pack until ingestion.

US labeling: Administer orally, preferably at bedtime once daily, at least 1 hour after the evening meal. Doses >400 mg/day may be given in divided doses at least 1 hour after meals.

Canadian labeling: Administer orally as a single dose at the same time each day (preferably at bedtime to decrease somnolence); may be taken without regard to meals.

Missed doses: For missed doses, if <12 hours patient may receive dose; if >12 hours wait until next dose due.

Hazardous agent; use appropriate precautions for handling and disposal (NIOSH 2014 [group 2]). Wear gloves to prevent cutaneous exposure. If exposed to the powder content from broken capsules or body fluids from patients receiving thalidomide, the exposed area should be washed with soap and water. Although the manufacturer does not recommend opening the capsules, if it is necessary to manipulate the capsules (eg, to prepare an oral suspension), it is recommended to double glove, wear a protective gown, and prepare in a controlled device (NIOSH 2014).

Monitoring Parameters CBC with differential, platelets; thyroid function tests (TSH at baseline then every 2 to 3 months during thalidomide treatment [Hamnvik 2011]). Hepatic function tests (periodic; particularly with preexisting hepatic dysfunction or concomitant use of drugs associated with hepatotoxicity). In HIV-seropositive patients: viral load after 1 and 3 months, then every 3 months. Pregnancy testing (sensitivity of at least 50 milliunits/mL) is required within 24 hours prior to initiation of therapy, weekly during the first 4 weeks, then every 4 weeks in women with regular menstrual cycles or every 2 weeks in women with irregular menstrual cycles. Signs of neuropathy monthly for the first 3 months, then periodically during treatment; consider monitoring of sensory nerve application potential amplitudes (at baseline and every 6 months) to detect asymptomatic neuropathy. Monitor for signs and symptoms of thromboembolism (shortness of breath, chest pain, arm/leg swelling), tumor lysis syndrome, bradycardia and syncope; monitor for clinical changes indicating potential seizure activity (in patients with a history of seizure).

Reference Range Graft-vs-host disease: Therapeutic plasma thalidomide levels are 5 to 8 mcg/mL, although it has been suggested that lower plasma levels (0.5 to 1.5 mcg/mL) may be therapeutic; peak serum thalidomide level after a 200 mg dose: 1.8 mcg/mL

Dosage Forms Excipient information presented when available (limited, particularly for generics); consult specific product labeling.

Capsule, Oral:

Thalomid: 50 mg, 100 mg

Thalomid: 150 mg, 200 mg [contains fd&c blue #2 (indigotine)]

Extemporaneous Preparations Hazardous agent; use appropriate precautions for handling and disposal (NIOSH 2014 [group 2]). When manipulating capsules, NIOSH recommends double gloving, a protective gown, and preparation in a controlled device; if not prepared in a controlled device, respiratory and eye protection, as well as ventilated engineering controls, are recommended (NIOSH, 2014).

A 20 mg/mL oral suspension may be prepared with capsules and a 1:1 mixture of Ora-Sweet and Ora-Plus. Empty the contents of twelve 100 mg capsules into a glass mortar. Add small portions of the vehicle and mix to a uniform paste; mix while adding the vehicle in incremental proportions to almost 60 mL; transfer to an amber calibrated bottle, rinse mortar with vehicle, and add quantity of vehicle sufficient to make 60 mL. Label "shake well," "protect from light," and "refrigerate". Stable for 35 days refrigerated.

Kraft S, Johnson CE, and Tyler RP, "Stability of an Extemporaneously Prepared Thalidomide Suspension," *Am J Health Syst Pharm*, 2011, 69(1):56-8.

◆ Thalitone [DSC] *see* Chlorthalidone *on page 380*

◆ Thalomid *see* Thalidomide *on page 1776*

◆ Tham *see* Tromethamine *on page 1848*

◆ THC *see* Dronabinol *on page 606*

Theophylline (thee OFF i lin)

Brand Names: US Elixophyllin; Theo-24; Theochron
Brand Names: Canada Apo-Theo LA®; Novo-Theophyl SR; PMS-Theophylline; Pulmophylline; ratio-Theo-Bronc; Teva-Theophylline SR; Theo ER; Theolair; Uniphyl
Index Terms Theo-Dur; Theobid Duracaps; TheoCap; Theophylline Anhydrous; Uniphyl
Pharmacologic Category Phosphodiesterase Enzyme Inhibitor, Nonselective
Use
Treatment of symptoms and reversible airway obstruction due to chronic asthma, or other chronic lung diseases
Guideline recommendations:
Asthma: The 2015 Global Initiative for Asthma Guidelines (GINA) and the 2007 National Heart, Lung and Blood Institute Asthma Guidelines do not recommend oral theophylline as a long-term control medication for asthma in children ≤5 years of age. Additionally, GINA guidelines do not recommend oral theophylline for asthma in children 6 to 11 years of age. Oral theophylline is a potential alternative option (not preferred) in adolescents and adults as a long-term control medication in mild asthma or as an add-on long-term control medication in moderate to severe asthma; however, a stepwise approach using inhaled corticosteroids (+/-inhaled long-acting beta agonists depending on asthma severity) is preferred to theophylline due to efficacy concerns and potential for adverse events (GINA 2015). Both guidelines recommend against theophylline for the treatment of asthma exacerbations due to poor efficacy and safety concerns (GINA 2015; NAEPP 2007).
COPD: The Global Initiative for Chronic Obstructive Lung Disease Guidelines (2013) suggest that while higher doses of slow release formulations of theophylline have been proven to be effective for use in COPD, it is not a preferred agent due to its potential for toxicity.
Pregnancy Considerations Teratogenic effects were observed in animal reproduction studies. Theophylline crosses the placenta; adverse effects may be seen in the newborn. Use is generally safe when used at the recommended doses (serum concentrations 5-12 mcg/mL) however maternal adverse events may be increased and efficacy may be decreased in pregnant women. Theophylline metabolism may change during pregnancy; the half-life is similar to that observed in otherwise healthy, non-smoking adults with asthma during the first and second trimesters (~8.7 hours), but may increase to 13 hours (range: 8-18 hours) during the third trimester. The volume of distribution is also increased during the third trimester. Monitor serum levels. The recommendations for the use of theophylline in pregnant women with asthma are similar to those used in nonpregnant adults (National Heart, Lung, and Blood Institute Guidelines 2004).
Breast-Feeding Considerations The concentration of theophylline in breast milk is similar to the maternal serum concentration. Irritability may be observed in the nursing infant. Serious adverse events in the infant are unlikely unless toxic serum levels are present in the mother.
Contraindications Hypersensitivity to theophylline or any component of the formulation; premixed injection may contain corn-derived dextrose and its use is contraindicated in patients with allergy to corn-related products
Warnings/Precautions If a patient develops signs and symptoms of theophylline toxicity (eg, persistent, repetitive vomiting), a serum theophylline level should be measured and subsequent doses held. Serum theophylline monitoring may be lessened as lower therapeutic ranges are established. More intense monitoring may be required during acute illness or when interacting drugs are introduced into the regimen. Use with caution in patients with peptic ulcer, hyperthyroidism, seizure disorders, and patients with tachyarrhythmias (eg, sinus tachycardia, atrial fibrillation); use may exacerbate these conditions. Theophylline-induced nonconvulsive status epilepticus has been reported (rarely) and should be considered in patients who develop CNS abnormalities. Theophylline

clearance may be decreased in patients with acute pulmonary edema, congestive heart failure, cor-pulmonale, fever, hepatic disease, acute hepatitis, cirrhosis, hypothyroidism, sepsis with multiorgan failure, and shock; clearance may also be decreased in neonates, infants <3 months of age with decreased renal function, infants <1 year of age, the elderly >60 years, and patients following cessation of smoking. Some dosage forms may contain propylene glycol; large amounts are potentially toxic and have been associated hyperosmolality, lactic acidosis, seizures, and respiratory depression; use caution (AAP, 1997; Zar 2007).
Adverse Reactions Frequency not defined. Adverse events observed at therapeutic serum levels:
Cardiovascular: Flutter, tachycardia
Central nervous system: Headache, hyperactivity (children), insomnia, restlessness, seizures, status epilepticus (nonconvulsive)
Endocrine & metabolic: Hypercalcemia (with concomitant hyperthyroid disease)
Gastrointestinal: Nausea, reflux or ulcer aggravation, vomiting
Genitourinary: Difficulty urinating (elderly males with prostatism)
Neuromuscular & skeletal: Tremor
Renal: Diuresis (transient)
Drug Interactions
Metabolism/Transport Effects Substrate of CYP1A2 (major), CYP2E1 (major), CYP3A4 (major); **Note:** Assignment of Major/Minor substrate status based on clinically relevant drug interaction potential; **Inhibits** CYP1A2 (weak)
Avoid Concomitant Use
Avoid concomitant use of Theophylline with any of the following: Conivaptan; Deferasirox; Doxofylline; Fusidic Acid (Systemic); Idelalisib; Iobenguane I 123; Riociguat; Stiripentol
Increased Effect/Toxicity
Theophylline may increase the levels/effects of: Doxofylline; Formoterol; Indacaterol; Olodaterol; Pancuronium; Riociguat; Sympathomimetics; TiZANidine

The levels/effects of Theophylline may be increased by: Abiraterone Acetate; Alcohol (Ethyl); Allopurinol; Antithyroid Agents; Aprepitant; AtoMOXetine; Cannabinoid-Containing Products; Cimetidine; Conivaptan; CYP1A2 Inhibitors (Moderate); CYP1A2 Inhibitors (Strong); CYP3A4 Inhibitors (Moderate); CYP3A4 Inhibitors (Strong); Dasatinib; Deferasirox; Disulfiram; Estrogen Derivatives; Febuxostat; FluvoxaMINE; Fosaprepitant; Fusidic Acid (Systemic); Idelalisib; Interferons; Isoniazid; Ivacaftor; Linezolid; Luliconazole; Macrolide Antibiotics; Methotrexate; Metreleptin; Mexiletine; Mifepristone; Netupitant; Osimertinib; Palbociclib; Peginterferon Alfa-2b; Pentoxifylline; Propafenone; QuiNINE; Quinolone Antibiotics; Simeprevir; Stiripentol; Tedizolid; Thiabendazole; Ticlopidine; Vemurafenib; Zafirlukast; Zileuton
Decreased Effect
Theophylline may decrease the levels/effects of: Adenosine; Benzodiazepines; CarBAMazepine; Fosphenytoin; Iobenguane I 123; Lithium; Pancuronium; Phenytoin; Regadenoson; Zafirlukast

The levels/effects of Theophylline may be decreased by: Adalimumab; Barbiturates; Beta-Blockers (Beta1 Selective); Beta-Blockers (Nonselective); Bosentan; Cannabis; CarBAMazepine; CYP1A2 Inducers (Strong); CYP3A4 Inducers (Moderate); CYP3A4 Inducers (Strong); Cyproterone; Dabrafenib; Enzalutamide; Fosphenytoin; Isoproterenol; Metreleptin; Mitotane; Osimertinib; Phenytoin; Protease Inhibitors; Siltuximab; St Johns Wort; Teriflunomide; Thyroid Products; Tocilizumab
Food Interactions
Ethanol: Ethanol may decrease theophylline clearance. Management: Avoid or limit ethanol.
Food: Food does not appreciably affect the absorption of liquid, fast-release products, and most sustained release products; however, food may induce a sudden release (dose-dumping) of once-daily sustained release products resulting in an increase in serum drug levels and potential toxicity. Changes in diet may affect the elimination of theophylline; charbroiled foods may increase elimination, reducing half-life by 50%. Management: Should be taken with water 1 hour before or 2 hours after meals. Avoid extremes of dietary protein and carbohydrate intake.
Storage/Stability Tablet, premixed infusion, solution: Store at controlled room temperature of 25°C (77°F).
Mechanism of Action Causes bronchodilatation, diuresis, CNS and cardiac stimulation, and gastric acid secretion by blocking phosphodiesterase which increases tissue concentrations of cyclic adenine monophosphate (cAMP) which in turn promotes catecholamine stimulation of lipolysis, glycogenolysis, and gluconeogenesis and induces release of epinephrine from adrenal medulla cells

Pharmacodynamics/Kinetics

Absorption: Oral: Dosage form dependent

Distribution: 0.45 L/kg (range: 0.3-0.7 L/kg) based on ideal body weight; distributes poorly into body fat; V_d may increase in premature neonates, patients with hepatic cirrhosis, acidemia (uncorrected), the elderly

Metabolism: Children >1 year and Adults: Hepatic; involves CYP1A2, 2E1 and 3A4; forms active metabolites (caffeine and 3-methylxanthine)

Protein binding: 40%, primarily to albumin

Half-life elimination: Highly variable and dependent upon age, liver function, cardiac function, lung disease, and smoking history

Premature infants, postnatal age 3-15 days: 30 hours (range: 17-43 hours)

Premature infants, postnatal age 25-57 days: 20 hours (range: 9.4-30.6 hours)

Children 6-17 years: 3.7 hours (range: 1.5-5.9 hours)

Adults 16-60 years with asthma, nonsmoking, otherwise healthy: 8.7 hours (range: 6.1-12.8 hours)

Time to peak, serum:

Oral: Liquid: 1 hour

IV: Within 30 minutes

Excretion: Urine

Neonates: 50% as unchanged theophylline

Children >3 months and Adults: ~10% as unchanged theophylline

Dosing

Adult Doses should be individualized based on steady-state serum concentrations and ideal body weight.

Acute symptoms: Manufacturer's labeling:

Loading dose: Oral, IV:

Asthma exacerbations: The treatment of asthma exacerbations with theophylline is not supported or recommended by current clinical practice guidelines (GINA 2015; NAEPP 2007).

COPD treatment: Theophylline is currently considered second-line intravenous therapy in the emergency department or hospital setting when there is inadequate or insufficient response to short acting bronchodilators (Global Initiative for COPD Guidelines 2013).

If no theophylline received within the previous 24 hours: 4.6 mg/kg loading dose (~5.8 mg/kg hydrous aminophylline) IV or 5 mg/kg orally. Loading dose intended to achieve a serum level of approximately 10 mcg/mL; loading doses should be given intravenously (preferred) or with a rapidly absorbed oral product (not an extended-release product). **Note:** On the average, for every 1 mg/kg theophylline given, blood levels will rise 2 mcg/mL.

If theophylline has been administered in the previous 24 hours: A loading dose is not recommended without obtaining a serum theophylline concentration. The loading dose should be calculated as follows:

Dose = (desired serum theophylline concentration - measured serum theophylline concentration) (V_d)

Acute symptoms: Manufacturer's labeling:

Maintenance dose: IV: **Note:** To achieve a target concentration of 10 mcg/mL unless otherwise noted. Lower initial doses may be required in patients with reduced theophylline clearance. Dosage should be adjusted according to serum level measurements during the first 12- to 24-hour period.

Adults 16-60 years (otherwise healthy, nonsmokers): 0.4 mg/kg/hour; maximum: 900 mg/day unless serum levels indicate need for larger dose

Adults >60 years: 0.3 mg/kg/hour; maximum: 400 mg/day unless serum levels indicate need for larger dose

Treatment of chronic conditions: With newer guidelines suggesting lower therapeutic theophylline ranges, it is unlikely that doses larger than >10 mg/kg/day will be required in children ≥1 year of age.

Oral solution: Initial dose: 300 mg/day administered in divided doses every 6-8 hours; Maintenance: 400-600 mg/day (maximum: 600 mg/day)

Oral extended release formulations: Initial dose: 300-400 mg once daily; Maintenance: 400-600 mg once daily (maximum: 600 mg/day)

Dosage adjustment after serum theophylline measurement: Asthma: Within normal limits: Adults: 5-15 mcg/mL: Maintain dosage if tolerated. Recheck serum theophylline concentration at 24-hour intervals (for acute IV dosing) or at 6- to 12-month intervals (for oral dosing). Finer adjustments in dosage may be needed for some patients. If levels ≥15 mcg/mL, consider 10% dose reduction to improve safety margin.

Note: Recheck serum theophylline levels after 3 days when using oral dosing, or after 12 hours (children) or 24 hours (adults) when dosing intravenously. Patients maintained with oral therapy may be reassessed at 6- to 12-month intervals.

Geriatric

Acute symptoms: Adults >60 years:

Loading dose: Oral, IV: Refer to adult dosing.

Maintenance dose: IV: 0.3 mg/kg/hour; maximum 400 mg/day unless serum levels indicate need for larger dose

Chronic conditions: Oral: Adults >60 years: Do not exceed a dose of 400 mg/day

Cardiac decompensation, cor pulmonale, hepatic dysfunction, sepsis with multiorgan failure, shock: Refer to adult dosing.

Pediatric Doses should be individualized based on steady-state serum concentrations and ideal body weight.

Acute symptoms: Manufacturer's labeling:

Loading dose: Oral, IV:

Asthma exacerbations: The treatment of asthma exacerbations with theophylline is not supported or recommended by current clinical practice guidelines (GINA 2015; NAEPP 2007).

If no theophylline received within the previous 24 hours: 4.6 mg/kg loading dose (~5.8 mg/kg hydrous aminophylline) IV or 5 mg/kg orally. Loading dose intended to achieve a serum level of approximately 10 mcg/mL; loading doses should be given intravenously (preferred) or with a rapidly absorbed oral product (not an extended-release product). **Note:** On the average, for every 1 mg/kg theophylline given, blood levels will rise 2 mcg/mL.

If theophylline has been administered in the previous 24 hours: A loading dose is not recommended without obtaining a serum theophylline concentration. The loading dose should be calculated as follows:

Dose = (desired serum theophylline concentration - measured serum theophylline concentration) (V_d)

Acute symptoms: Manufacturer's labeling:

Maintenance dose: IV: **Note:** To achieve a target concentration of 10 mcg/mL unless otherwise noted. Lower initial doses may be required in patients with reduced theophylline clearance. Dosage should be adjusted according to serum level measurements during the first 12- to 24-hour period.

Infants 6-52 weeks: mg/kg/hour = (0.008) (age in weeks) + 0.21

Children 1-9 years: 0.8 mg/kg/hour

Children 9-12 years: 0.7 mg/kg/hour

Adolescents 12-16 years (cigarette or marijuana smokers): 0.7 mg/kg/hour

Adolescents 12-16 years (nonsmokers): 0.5 mg/kg/hour; maximum: 900 mg/day unless serum levels indicate need for larger dose

Treatment of chronic conditions: With newer guidelines suggesting lower therapeutic theophylline ranges, it is unlikely that doses larger than >10 mg/kg/day will be required in children ≥1 year of age.

Oral solution:

Infants <1 year: **Note:** Doses should be adjusted to maintain the peak steady state serum concentrations. The time to reach steady state will vary based on age and the presence of risk factors which may affect theophylline clearance.

Full-term Infants and Infants <26 weeks: Total daily dose (mg)= [(0.2 x age in weeks) +5] x (weight in kg); divide dose into 3 equal amounts and administer at 8-hour intervals

Full-term Infants and Infants ≥26 weeks and <52 weeks: Total daily dose (mg) = [(0.2 x age in weeks) +5] x (weight in kg); divide dose into 4 equal amounts and administer at 6-hour intervals

Children ≥1 year and <45 kg: Initial dose: 10-14 mg/kg/day (maximum: 300 mg/day) administered in divided doses every 4-6 hours; Maintenance: Up to 20 mg/kg/day (maximum: 600 mg/day)

Children >45 kg: Refer to adult dosing.

Oral extended release formulations:

Children ≥1 year and <45 kg: Initial: 10-14 mg/kg once daily (maximum: 300 mg/day); Maintenance up to 20 mg/kg/day (maximum: 600 mg/day)

Children >45 kg: Refer to adult dosing.

Dosage adjustment after serum theophylline measurement: Asthma: Within normal limits: Children: 5-10 mcg/mL: Maintain dosage if tolerated. Recheck serum theophylline concentration at 24-hour intervals (for acute IV dosing) or at 6- to 12-month intervals (for oral dosing). Finer adjustments in dosage may be needed for some patients. If levels ≥15 mcg/mL, consider 10% dose reduction to improve safety margin.

Note: Recheck serum theophylline levels after 3 days when using oral dosing, or after 12 hours (children) or 24 hours (adults) when dosing intravenously. Patients maintained with oral therapy may be reassessed at 6- to 12-month intervals.

Renal Impairment Oral: IV:

Infants 1-3 months: Consider dose reduction and frequent monitoring of serum theophylline concentrations. Infants >3 months, Children, Adolescents, and Adults: No dosage adjustment necessary.

Hepatic Impairment

Oral: Infants, Children, Adolescents, and Adults: No dosage adjustment provided in manufacturer's labeling. However, dose reduction and frequent monitoring of serum theophylline concentration are required in patients with decreased hepatic function (eg, cirrhosis, acute hepatitis, cholestasis). Maximum dose: 400 mg daily

IV: Infants, Children, Adolescents, and Adults: Initial: 0.2 mg/kg/hour; maximum daily dose: 400 mg daily unless serum concentrations indicate need for larger dose. Use with caution and monitor serum theophylline concentrations frequently.

Obesity Use ideal body weight for obese patients.

Dietary Considerations Should be taken with water 1 hour before or 2 hours after meals. Premixed injection may contain corn-derived dextrose and its use is contraindicated in patients with allergy to corn-related products.

Administration

IV: Administer loading dose over 30 minutes; follow with a continuous infusion as appropriate

Oral: Long-acting preparations should be taken with a full glass of water, swallowed whole, or cut in half if scored. Do **not** crush. Extended release capsule forms may be opened and the contents sprinkled on soft foods; do **not** chew beads.

Monitoring Parameters Monitor heart rate, CNS effects (insomnia, irritability); respiratory rate (COPD patients often have resting controlled respiratory rates in low 20s); arterial or capillary blood gases (if applicable)

Theophylline levels: Serum theophylline levels should be monitored prior to making dose increases; in the presence of signs or symptoms of toxicity; or when a new illness, worsening of a present illness, or medication changes occur that may change theophylline clearance

IV loading dose: Measure serum concentrations 30 minutes after the end of an IV loading dose

IV infusion: Measure serum concentrations one half-life after starting a continuous infusion, then every 12-24 hours

Reference Range Therapeutic levels: Asthma:

Children: 5-10 mcg/mL

Adults: 5-15 mcg/mL

Test Interactions Plasma glucose, uric acid, free fatty acids, total cholesterol, HDL, HDL/LDL ratio, and urinary free cortisol excretion may be increased by theophylline. Theophylline may decrease triiodothyronine.

Dosage Forms Excipient information presented when available (limited, particularly for generics); consult specific product labeling.

Capsule Extended Release 24 Hour, Oral:

Theo-24: 100 mg

Theo-24: 200 mg [contains fd&c yellow #10 (quinoline yellow)]

Theo-24: 300 mg [contains brilliant blue fcf (fd&c blue #1), fd&c red #40]

Theo-24: 400 mg [contains fd&c red #40]

Elixir, Oral:

Elixophyllin: 80 mg/15 mL (473 mL) [contains fd&c red #40, saccharin sodium; mixed fruit flavor]

Solution, Intravenous:

Generic: 400 mg (250 mL, 500 mL); 800 mg (500 mL)

Solution, Oral:

Generic: 80 mg/15 mL (473 mL)

Tablet Extended Release 12 Hour, Oral:

Theochron: 100 mg, 200 mg, 300 mg [scored]

Generic: 100 mg, 200 mg, 300 mg, 450 mg

Tablet Extended Release 24 Hour, Oral:

Generic: 400 mg, 600 mg

Extemporaneous Preparations Note: An alcohol-containing commercial oral solution is available (80 mg/15 mL).

A 5 mg/mL oral suspension may be made with tablets. Crush one 300 mg extended release tablet in a mortar and reduce to a fine powder. Add small portions of a 1:1 mixture of Ora-Sweet® and Ora-Plus® and mix to a uniform paste; mix while adding the vehicle in equal proportions to **almost** 60 mL; transfer to a calibrated bottle, rinse mortar with vehicle, and add sufficient quantity of vehicle to make 60 mL. Label "shake well". Stable for 90 days at room temperature.

Johnson CE, VanDeKoppel S, and Myers E, "Stability of Anhydrous Theophylline in Extemporaneously Prepared Alcohol-Free Oral Suspensions," *Am J Health-Syst Pharm,* 2005, 62(23):2518-20.

Thiamine (THYE a min)

Brand Names: Canada Betaxin

Index Terms Aneurine Hydrochloride; Thiamin; Thiamine Hydrochloride; Thiaminium Chloride Hydrochloride; Vitamin B_1

Pharmacologic Category Vitamin, Water Soluble

Use Treatment of thiamine deficiency including beriberi, Wernicke's encephalopathy, Korsakoff's syndrome, neuritis associated with pregnancy, or in alcoholic patients; dietary supplement

Dosing

Adult & Geriatric

Recommended daily intake:

≥19 years: Females: 1.1 mg; Males: 1.2 mg

Pregnancy, lactation: 1.4 mg

Parenteral nutrition supplementation: 6 mg/day; may be increased to 25-50 mg/day with history of alcohol abuse

Thiamine deficiency (beriberi): 5-30 mg/dose IM or IV 3 times/day (if critically ill); then orally 5-30 mg/day in single or divided doses 3 times/day for 1 month

Alcohol withdrawal syndrome: 100 mg/day IM or IV for several days, followed by 50-100 mg/day orally

Wernicke's encephalopathy: Treatment (manufacturer labeling): Initial: 100 mg IV, then 50-100 mg/day IM or IV until consuming a regular, balanced diet. However, larger doses may be required based on failure of lower doses to produce clinical improvement in some patients.

Alternate dosage: The Royal College of Physicians (U.K.) has recommended the use of higher doses of thiamine (in combination with other B vitamins, ascorbic acid, potassium, phosphate, and magnesium) for the management of Wernicke's encephalopathy (Thomson, 2002):

Prophylaxis: 250 mg IV once daily for 3-5 days

Treatment: Initial: 500 mg IV 3 times/day for 3 days. If response to thiamine after 3 days, continue with 250 mg IM or IV once daily for an additional 5 days or until clinical improvement.

Pediatric

Adequate Intake:

0-6 months: 0.2 mg/day

7-12 months: 0.3 mg/day

Recommended daily intake:

1-3 years: 0.5 mg

4-8 years: 0.6 mg

9-13 years: 0.9 mg

14-18 years: Females: 1 mg; Males: 1.2 mg

≥19 years: Refer to adult dosing.

Parenteral nutrition supplementation: Infants: 1.2 mg/day

Thiamine deficiency (beriberi): Children: 10-25 mg/dose IM or IV daily (if critically ill), or 10-50 mg/dose orally every day for 2 weeks, then 5-10 mg/dose orally daily for 1 month

Renal Impairment No dosage adjustment provided in manufacturer's labeling.

Hepatic Impairment No dosage adjustment provided in manufacturer's labeling.

Additional Information Complete prescribing information should be consulted for additional detail.

Dosage Forms Excipient information presented when available (limited, particularly for generics); consult specific product labeling.

Capsule, Oral, as hydrochloride:
Generic: 50 mg
Solution, Injection, as hydrochloride:
Generic: 100 mg/mL (2 mL)
Tablet, Oral, as hydrochloride:
Generic: 50 mg, 100 mg, 250 mg
Tablet, Oral, as hydrochloride [preservative free]:
Generic: 100 mg

◆ Thiamine Hydrochloride *see* Thiamine *on page 1782*
◆ Thiaminium Chloride Hydrochloride *see* Thiamine *on page 1782*

Thioguanine (thye oh GWAH neen)

Brand Names: US Tabloid
Brand Names: Canada Lanvis®
Index Terms 2-Amino-6-Mercaptopurine; 6-TG (error-prone abbreviation); 6-Thioguanine (error-prone abbreviation); TG; Tioguanine
Pharmacologic Category Antineoplastic Agent, Antimetabolite; Antineoplastic Agent, Antimetabolite (Purine Analog)
Use Treatment of acute myelogenous (nonlymphocytic) leukemia (AML)
Dosing
Pediatric Pediatric ALL (off-label use; combination therapy): Oral: Delayed intensification treatment phase: 60 mg/m²/day for 14 days (Lange, 2002; Nachman, 1998)
Renal Impairment
Adults: There are no dosage adjustments provided in manufacturer's labeling.
Children: No adjustment required (Aronoff, 2007).
Hepatic Impairment Deterioration in transaminases, alkaline phosphatase or bilirubin, toxic hepatitis, biliary stasis, clinical jaundice, evidence of hepatic sinusoidal obstruction syndrome (veno-occlusive disease), or evidence of portal hypertension: Discontinue treatment.
Additional Information Complete prescribing information should be consulted for additional detail.
Dosage Forms Excipient information presented when available (limited, particularly for generics); consult specific product labeling. [DSC] = Discontinued product
Tablet, Oral:
Tabloid: 40 mg
Tabloid: 40 mg [DSC] [scored]

◆ 6-Thioguanine (error-prone abbreviation) *see* Thioguanine *on page 1783*
◆ Thiophosphoramide *see* Thiotepa *on page 1783*
◆ Thioplex *see* Thiotepa *on page 1783*

Thioridazine (thye oh RID a zeen)

Index Terms Mellaril; Thioridazine Hydrochloride
Pharmacologic Category First Generation (Typical) Antipsychotic
Use Schizophrenia: Management of schizophrenic patients who fail to respond adequately to treatment with other antipsychotic drugs, either because of insufficient effectiveness or the inability to achieve an effective dose because of intolerable adverse effects from those medications. Before initiating treatment with thioridazine, it is strongly recommended that a patient be given at least 2 trials, each with a different antipsychotic drug product, at an adequate dose and for an adequate duration.
Dosing
Adult & Geriatric
Schizophrenia: Oral: Initial: 50 to 100 mg 3 times daily; dosage may be increased at gradual increments based on response and tolerability; usual dosage: 300 to 800 mg in 2 to 4 divided doses (APA [Lehman, 2004]); maximum: 800 mg daily
Pediatric
Schizophrenia: Oral: Initial: 0.5 mg/kg/day in 2 to 4 divided doses; dosage may be increased at gradual increments based on response and tolerability; maximum 3 mg/kg/day.
Renal Impairment There are no dosage adjustments provided in the manufacturer's labeling.
Hepatic Impairment There are no dosage adjustments provided in the manufacturer's labeling; use with caution (hepatic metabolism).

Additional Information Complete prescribing information should be consulted for additional detail.

Dosage Forms Excipient information presented when available (limited, particularly for generics); consult specific product labeling.
Tablet, Oral, as hydrochloride:
Generic: 10 mg, 25 mg, 50 mg, 100 mg

◆ Thioridazine Hydrochloride *see* Thioridazine *on page 1783*
◆ Thiosulfuric Acid Disodium Salt *see* Sodium Thiosulfate *on page 1682*

Thiotepa (thye oh TEP a)

Index Terms TESPA; Thiophosphoramide; Thioplex; Triethylenethiophosphoramide; TSPA
Pharmacologic Category Antineoplastic Agent, Alkylating Agent
Use Treatment of superficial papillary bladder cancer; palliative treatment of adenocarcinoma of breast or ovary; controlling intracavitary effusions caused by metastatic tumors
Dosing
Adult & Geriatric
Bladder cancer: Intravesical: 60 mg in 30 to 60 mL NS retained for 2 hours once weekly for 4 weeks
Ovarian, breast cancer: IV: 0.3 to 0.4 mg/kg every 1 to 4 weeks
Effusions: Intracavitary: 0.6 to 0.8 mg/kg
Leptomeningeal metastases (off-label use/route): Intrathecal: 10 mg twice a week (on days 1 and 4 each week) for 8 weeks (Grossman, 1993)
Hematopoietic stem cell transplant (HSCT) for CNS malignancy (off-label use; combination chemotherapy): IV: 250 mg/m²/day for 3 days beginning 9 days prior to transplant (Soussain, 2008) **or** 150 mg/m²/dose every 12 hours for 6 doses, followed by stem cell reinfusion 96 hours after completion of thiotepa (Abrey, 2006)
Pediatric Note: In children, thiotepa is associated with a high emetic potential at doses ≥300 mg/m²; antiemetics are recommended to prevent nausea and vomiting (Dupuis, 2011).

Hematopoietic stem cell transplant (HSCT) for CNS malignancy (off-label use; combination chemotherapy): IV: 300 mg/m²/day for 3 days beginning 8 days prior to transplant (Gilheeney, 2010) **or** 300 mg/m²/day for 3 days beginning 5 days prior to transplant (Dunkel, 2010; Grodman, 2009)
Renal Impairment There are no dosage adjustments provided in the manufacturer's labeling. Use with caution; reduced dose may be warranted. Use may be contraindicated with existing renal impairment and should be limited to cases where benefit outweighs risk.
Hepatic Impairment There are no dosage adjustments provided in the manufacturer's labeling. Use with caution; reduced dose may be warranted. Use may be contraindicated with existing hepatic impairment and should be limited to cases where benefit outweighs risk.
Obesity
*American Society of Clinical Oncology (ASCO) Guidelines for appropriate chemotherapy dosing in obese adults with cancer (**Note:** Excludes HSCT dosing):* Utilize patient's actual body weight (full weight) for calculation of body surface area- or weight-based dosing, particularly when the intent of therapy is curative; manage regimen-related toxicities in the same manner as for nonobese patients; if a dose reduction is utilized due to toxicity, consider resumption of full weight-based dosing with subsequent cycles, especially if cause of toxicity (eg, hepatic or renal impairment) is resolved (Griggs, 2012).
American Society for Blood and Marrow Transplantation (ASBMT) practice guideline committee position statement on chemotherapy dosing in obesity: Utilize actual body weight (full weight) for calculation of body surface area in thiotepa dosing for hematopoietic stem cell transplant conditioning regimens in adult patients weighing ≤120% of their ideal body weight (IBW). In patients weighing >120% IBW, utilize adjusted body weight 40% (ABW40) to calculate BSA (Bubalo, 2014). ABW40: Adjusted wt (kg) = Ideal body weight (kg) + 0.4 [actual wt (kg) - ideal body weight (kg)]
Adjustment for Toxicity IV: **Note:** Use may be contraindicated with preexisting marrow damage and should be limited to cases where benefit outweighs risk.
WBC ≤3000/mm³: Discontinue treatment
Platelets ≤150,000/mm³: Discontinue treatment
Additional Information Complete prescribing information should be consulted for additional detail.

Dosage Forms Excipient information presented when available (limited, particularly for generics); consult specific product labeling.
Solution Reconstituted, Injection:
Generic: 15 mg (1 ea)

Thiothixene (thye oh THIKS een)

Brand Names: Canada Navane
Index Terms Navane; Tiotixene
Pharmacologic Category First Generation (Typical) Antipsychotic
Use Schizophrenia: For the management of schizophrenia
Dosing
Adult Schizophrenia: Oral: Initial: Mild-to-moderate symptoms: 2 mg 3 times daily; usual dose 15 mg daily; severe symptoms: 5 mg twice daily; usual dose 20-30 mg daily. Increase dose gradually. Maximum: 60 mg daily.
Pediatric Schizophrenia: Children >12 years and Adolescents (off-label use): Refer to adult dosing.
Renal Impairment No dosage adjustment provided in manufacturer's labeling.
Hepatic Impairment No dosage adjustment provided in manufacturer's labeling.
Additional Information Complete prescribing information should be consulted for additional detail.
Dosage Forms Excipient information presented when available (limited, particularly for generics); consult specific product labeling.
Capsule, Oral:
Generic: 1 mg, 2 mg, 5 mg, 10 mg

♦ Thonzonium, Neomycin, Colistin, and Hydrocortisone see Neomycin, Colistin, Hydrocortisone, and Thonzonium on page 1266

♦ Thorazine see ChlorproMAZINE on page 379

♦ Three-Factor PCC see Factor IX Complex (Human) [(Factors II, IX, X)] on page 734

♦ Thrive [OTC] see Nicotine on page 1277

♦ Thrombate III see Antithrombin on page 135

♦ Thrombate III® (Can) see Antithrombin on page 135

♦ Thymocyte Stimulating Factor see Aldesleukin on page 60

♦ Thymoglobulin see Antithymocyte Globulin (Rabbit) on page 137

♦ Thyrogen see Thyrotropin Alfa on page 1784

Thyroid, Desiccated (THYE roid DES i kay tid)

Brand Names: US Armour Thyroid; Nature-Throid; NP Thyroid; Westhroid; Westhroid-P [DSC]; WP Thyroid
Index Terms Desiccated Thyroid; Levothyroxine and Liothyronine; Tetraiodothyronine and Triiodothyronine; Thyroid Extract; Thyroid USP
Pharmacologic Category Thyroid Product
Use Replacement or supplemental therapy in hypothyroidism; pituitary TSH suppressants (thyroid nodules, thyroiditis, multinodular goiter, thyroid cancer)
Dosing
Adult Note: The American Association of Clinical Endocrinologists does not recommend the use of desiccated thyroid for thyroid replacement therapy for hypothyroidism (Baskin, 2002). Tablet strengths may vary by manufacturer in terms of grains or mg; dosing recommendations are based on general clinical equivalencies that 1 grain = 60 mg or 65 mg; 1/2 grain = 30 mg or 32.5 mg; and 1/4 grain = 15 mg or 16.25 mg.

Hypothyroidism: Oral: Initial: 15-30 mg; increase with 15 mg increments every 2-3 weeks; use 15 mg in patients with cardiovascular disease or long-standing myxedema. Maintenance dose: Usually 60-120 mg/day; monitor TSH and clinical symptoms.
Geriatric Not recommended for use in the elderly.
Pediatric Hypothyroidism: Oral: See table. **Note:** The American Thyroid Association/American Association of Clinical Endocrinologists do not recommend the use of desiccated thyroid for thyroid replacement therapy for hypothyroidism (ATA/AACE [Garber 2012]). Tablet strengths may vary by manufacturer in terms of grains or mg; dosing recommendations are based on general clinical equivalencies that 1 grain = 60 mg or 65 mg; 1/2 grain = 30 mg or 32.5 mg; and 1/4 grain = 15 mg or 16.25 mg.

Recommended Pediatric Dosage for Congenital Hypothyroidism

Age	Daily Dose (mg)	Daily Dose/kg (mg)
0-6 mo	15-30	4.8-6
6-12 mo	30-45	3.6-4.8
1-5 y	45-60	3-3.6
6-12 y	60-90	2.4-3
>12 y	>90	1.2-1.8

Renal Impairment No dosage adjustment provided in manufacturer's labeling.
Hepatic Impairment No dosage adjustment provided in manufacturer's labeling.
Additional Information Complete prescribing information should be consulted for additional detail.
Dosage Forms Excipient information presented when available (limited, particularly for generics); consult specific product labeling. [DSC] = Discontinued product
Tablet, Oral:
Armour Thyroid: 15 mg, 30 mg, 60 mg, 90 mg, 120 mg
Armour Thyroid: 180 mg [scored]
Armour Thyroid: 240 mg
Armour Thyroid: 300 mg [scored]
Nature-Throid: 16.25 mg, 32.5 mg
Nature-Throid: 48.75 mg, 65 mg, 81.25 mg, 97.5 mg, 113.75 mg, 130 mg, 146.25 mg, 162.5 mg, 195 mg, 260 mg, 325 mg [scored]
NP Thyroid: 30 mg, 60 mg, 90 mg
Westhroid: 16.25 mg [DSC], 32.5 mg
Westhroid: 48.75 mg [DSC], 65 mg [scored]
Westhroid: 81.25 mg [DSC]
Westhroid: 97.5 mg, 113.75 mg [DSC], 130 mg, 146.25 mg [DSC], 162.5 mg [DSC], 195 mg, 260 mg [DSC], 325 mg [scored]
Westhroid-P: 16.25 mg [DSC], 32.5 mg [DSC]
Westhroid-P: 48.75 mg [DSC], 65 mg [DSC], 97.5 mg [DSC], 130 mg [DSC] [scored]
WP Thyroid: 16.25 mg, 32.5 mg
WP Thyroid: 48.75 mg, 65 mg [scored]
WP Thyroid: 81.25 mg
WP Thyroid: 97.5 mg, 113.75 mg, 130 mg [scored]

♦ Thyroid Extract see Thyroid, Desiccated on page 1784

♦ Thyroid USP see Thyroid, Desiccated on page 1784

♦ Thyrolar see Liotrix on page 1084

♦ ThyroShield [OTC] see Potassium Iodide on page 1481

Thyrotropin Alfa (thye roe TROH pin AL fa)

Brand Names: US Thyrogen
Brand Names: Canada Thyrogen
Index Terms Human Thyroid Stimulating Hormone; Recombinant Human Thyrotropin; Rh-TSH; Thyrotropin Alpha; TSH
Pharmacologic Category Diagnostic Agent
Use
Diagnostic imaging: Adjunctive diagnostic tool for serum thyroglobulin (Tg) testing (with or without radioiodine imaging) in follow up of patients with well-differentiated thyroid cancer who have previously undergone thyroidectomy.
Limitations of use: Thyrotropin alfa-stimulated Tg levels are generally lower than and do not correlate with Tg levels after thyroid hormone withdrawal; even when thyrotropin alfa-stimulated Tg testing is performed in combination with radioiodine imaging, there is a risk of missing a thyroid cancer diagnosis or of underestimating disease extent; anti-Tg antibodies may confound Tg assay and render Tg levels uninterpretable, in such cases, even with a negative or low-stage thyrotropin alfa radioiodine scan, consider further patient evaluation.
Thyroid tissue remnant ablation: Adjunctive treatment for radioiodine ablation of thyroid tissue remnants after total or near-total thyroidectomy in patients with well-differentiated thyroid cancer without evidence of metastatic disease
Limitations of use: The effect of thyrotropin alfa on long-term thyroid cancer outcomes has not been determined. Due to relatively small clinical experience, it is not possible to conclude if long-term thyroid cancer outcomes would be equivalent after thyrotropin alfa use or withholding thyroid hormone for TSH elevation prior to remnant ablation.

Dosing

Adult & Geriatric Note: Consider pretreatment with glucocorticoids for patients in whom local tumor expansion may compromise vital anatomic structures (such as trachea, CNS, or extensive macroscopic lung metastases).

Diagnostic imaging: IM: 0.9 mg, followed 24 hours later by a second 0.9 mg dose; obtain serum Tg sample 72 hours after the second thyrotropin alfa injection

Thyroid tissue remnant ablation: IM: 0.9 mg, followed 24 hours later by a second 0.9 mg dose.

Radioiodine administration should be given 24 hours following the second thyrotropin alfa injection (for diagnostic scanning and remnant ablation). Perform diagnostic scanning 48 hours after radioiodine administration (72 hours after the second thyrotropin alfa injection). Post-therapy scanning may be delayed (additional days) to allow decline of background activity.

Renal Impairment There are no dosage adjustments provided in the manufacturer's labeling; however, elimination is significantly slower in dialysis-dependent end-stage renal impairment and TSH level elevation may be prolonged.

Hepatic Impairment There are no dosage adjustments provided in the manufacturer's labeling (has not been studied).

Additional Information Complete prescribing information should be consulted for additional detail.

Dosage Forms Excipient information presented when available (limited, particularly for generics); consult specific product labeling.

Solution Reconstituted, Intramuscular:
Thyrogen: 1.1 mg (1 ea)

◆ Thyrotropin Alpha *see* Thyrotropin Alfa *on page 1784*

◆ Tiacumicin B *see* Fidaxomicin *on page 765*

TiaGABine (tye AG a been)

Brand Names: US Gabitril
Index Terms Tiagabine Hydrochloride
Pharmacologic Category Anticonvulsant, Miscellaneous
Use Partial seizures: Adjunctive therapy in adults and children ≥12 years in the treatment of partial seizures
Pregnancy Considerations Adverse events were observed in animal reproduction studies. Information specific to the use of tiagabine in pregnancy is limited (Leppik 1999; Neppe 2000). Patients exposed to tiagabine during pregnancy are encouraged to enroll themselves into the North American Antiepileptic Drug (NAAED) Pregnancy Registry by calling 1-888-233-2334. Additional information is available at www.aedpregnancyregistry.org.

Breast-Feeding Considerations It is not known if tiagabine is excreted into breast milk. Information specific to the use of tiagabine while breast-feeding is limited (Neppe, 2000). According to the manufacturer, tiagabine should be used in breast-feeding women only when the benefits outweigh the potential risks.

Medication Guide Available Yes

Contraindications Hypersensitivity to tiagabine or any component of the formulation

Warnings/Precautions Antiepileptics are associated with an increased risk of suicidal behavior/thoughts with use (regardless of indication). Monitor all patients for notable changes in behavior that might indicate suicidal thoughts or depression; notify health care provider immediately if symptoms occur. New-onset seizures and status epilepticus have been associated with tiagabine use when taken for off-label indications. Seizures have occurred with doses as low as 4 mg/day and shortly after a dosage increase, even after stable therapy. In most cases, patients were using concomitant medications (eg, antidepressants, antipsychotics, stimulants, opioids). In these instances, the discontinuation of tiagabine, followed by an evaluation for an underlying seizure disorder, is suggested. Use for unapproved indications, however, has not been proven to be safe or effective and is not recommended. Anticonvulsants should not be discontinued abruptly because of the possibility of increasing seizure frequency; therapy should be withdrawn gradually to minimize the potential of increased seizure frequency, unless safety concerns require a more rapid withdrawal.

Use with caution in patients with hepatic impairment. Evidence of residual binding of tiagabine in the retina and uvea after 3 weeks has been observed in animal studies; although not directly measured, melanin binding is suggested. Long-term (up to 1 year) toxicological studies of tiagabine in animals showed no treatment-related ophthalmoscopic changes and macro- and microscopic examinations of the eye were unremarkable. The ability of available tests to detect potentially adverse consequences, if any, of the binding of tiagabine to melanin-containing tissue is unknown, and there was no systematic monitoring for relevant ophthalmological changes during the clinical development of tiagabine. Prescribers should be aware of the possibility of long-term ophthalmologic effects. Moderately severe to incapacitating generalized weakness has been reported after administration of tiagabine. The weakness resolved in all cases after a reduction in dose or discontinuation of tiagabine. Severe reactions, including Stevens-Johnson syndrome, although rarely reported, have resulted in fatalities. Experience in patients not receiving enzyme-inducing drugs has been limited; caution should be used in treating any patient who is not receiving one of these medications (decreased dose and slower titration may be required). May cause CNS depression, which may impair physical or mental abilities; patients must be cautioned about performing tasks that require mental alertness (eg, operating machinery or driving). Potentially significant interactions may exist, requiring dose or frequency adjustment, additional monitoring, and/ or selection of alternative therapy.

Adverse Reactions

>10%:
Central nervous system: Dizziness (27% to 31%), drowsiness (18% to 21%), nervousness (10% to 14%), lack of concentration (6% to 14%)
Gastrointestinal: Nausea (11%)
Infection: Infection (19%)
Neuromuscular & skeletal: Weakness (18% to 23%), tremor (9% to 21%)
Miscellaneous: Accidental injury (21%)

1% to 10%:
Cardiovascular: Vasodilation (2%), chest pain (≥1%), edema (≥1%), hypertension (≥1%), palpitations (≥1%), peripheral edema (≥1%), syncope (≥1%), tachycardia (≥1%)
Central nervous system: Ataxia (5% to 9%), pain (5% to 7%), depression (1% to 7%), insomnia (5% to 6%), confusion (5%), status epilepticus (5%), abnormal gait (3% to 5%), hostility (2% to 5%), memory impairment (4%), paresthesia (4%), speech disturbance (4%), emotional lability (3%), chills (≥1%), depersonalization (≥1%), dysarthria (≥1%), euphoria (≥1%), hallucination (≥1%), hypertonia (≥1%), hypoesthesia (≥1%), hyporeflexia (≥1%), hypotonia (≥1%), malaise (≥1%), migraine (≥1%), myoclonus (≥1%), paranoia (≥1%), personality disorder (≥1%), stupor (≥1%), twitching (≥1%), vertigo (≥1%), agitation (1%), myasthenia (1%)
Dermatologic: Bruise (6%), skin rash (5%), pruritus (2%), alopecia (≥1%), xeroderma (≥1%)
Gastrointestinal: Diarrhea (7% to 10%), vomiting (7%), abdominal pain (5% to 7%), increased appetite (2%), gingivitis (≥1%), stomatitis (≥1%), oral mucosa ulcer (1%)
Endocrine & metabolic: Weight gain (≥1%), weight loss (≥1%)
Genitourinary: Urinary tract infection (5%), abnormal uterine bleeding (≥1%), dysmenorrhea (≥1%), dysuria (≥1%), urinary incontinence (≥1%), vaginitis (≥1%)
Hematologic & oncologic: Lymphadenopathy (≥1%)
Hypersensitivity: Hypersensitivity reaction (≥1%)
Neuromuscular & skeletal: Myalgia (5%), arthralgia (≥1%), hyperkinesia (≥1%), hypokinesia (≥1%), neck pain (≥1%)
Ophthalmic: Amblyopia (9%), nystagmus (2%), visual disturbance (≥1%)
Otic: Otalgia (≥1%), otitis media (≥1%), tinnitus (≥1%)
Respiratory: Flu-like symptoms (6% to 9%), pharyngitis (7% to 8%), increased cough (4%), bronchitis (≥1%), dyspnea (≥1%), epistaxis (≥1%), pneumonia (≥1%)
Miscellaneous: Language problems (2%), cyst (≥1%), diaphoresis (≥1%)

<1% (Limited to important or life-threatening): Abnormal electroencephalogram, abnormal erythrocytes, abnormal hepatic function tests, abnormal pap smear, abnormal stools, abscess, altered sense of smell, amenorrhea, anemia, angina pectoris, apathy, aphthous stomatitis, apnea, arthritis, asthma, benign skin neoplasm, blepharitis, blindness, brain disease, breast hypertrophy, bursitis, cellulitis, cerebral ischemia, cholecystitis, cholelithiasis, CNS neoplasm, coma, contact dermatitis, cutaneous nodule, cystitis, deafness, dehydration, delusions, dental caries, dermal ulcer, dysgeusia, dysphagia, ECG abnormality, eczema, eructation, exfoliative dermatitis, eye pain, facial edema, fecal incontinence, fibrocystic breast disease, furunculosis, gastritis, gastrointestinal hemorrhage, gingival hyperplasia, glossitis, goiter, hematuria, hemiplegia, hemoptysis, hemorrhage, hepatomegaly, hernia, herpes simplex infection, herpes zoster, hirsutism, hyperacusis, hypercholesteremia, hyperglycemia, hypermenorrhea, hyperreflexia, hyperventilation, hypoglycemia, hypokalemia, hyponatremia, hypotension,

hypothyroidism, impotence, increased libido, keratoconjunctivitis, laryngitis, leg cramps, leukopenia, maculopapular rash, mastalgia, melena, movement disorder, muscle spasm, myocardial infarction, neuritis, oral paresthesia, orthostatic hypotension, osteoarthrosis, otitis externa, pallor, paralysis, pelvic pain, periodontal abscess, peripheral neuritis, peripheral vascular disease, petechia, phlebitis, photophobia, psoriasis, psychoneurosis, psychosis, pyelonephritis, rectal hemorrhage, renal failure, salpingitis, seizure (in patients with or without underlying seizure disorder), sepsis, sialorrhea, skin carcinoma, skin discoloration, skin photosensitivity, status epilepticus, Stevens-Johnson syndrome, subcutaneous nodule, suicidal ideation, suicidal tendencies, tendinous contracture, thrombocytopenia, thrombophlebitis, urethritis, urinary retention, urinary urgency, vaginal hemorrhage, vesiculobullous dermatitis, visual field defect, voice disorder, withdrawal seizures

Drug Interactions

Metabolism/Transport Effects Substrate of CYP3A4 (major); **Note:** Assignment of Major/Minor substrate status based on clinically relevant drug interaction potential

Avoid Concomitant Use

Avoid concomitant use of TiaGABine with any of the following: Azelastine (Nasal); Conivaptan; Fusidic Acid (Systemic); Idelalisib; Orphenadrine; Paraldehyde; Thalidomide

Increased Effect/Toxicity

TiaGABine may increase the levels/effects of: Alcohol (Ethyl); Azelastine (Nasal); Buprenorphine; CNS Depressants; Hydrocodone; Methotrimeprazine; Metyrosine; Mirtazapine; Orphenadrine; Paraldehyde; Pramipexole; ROPINIRole; Rotigotine; Selective Serotonin Reuptake Inhibitors; Suvorexant; Thalidomide; Zolpidem

The levels/effects of TiaGABine may be increased by: Aprepitant; Brimonidine (Topical); Cannabis; Conivaptan; CYP3A4 Inhibitors (Moderate); CYP3A4 Inhibitors (Strong); Dasatinib; Doxylamine; Dronabinol; Droperidol; Fosaprepitant; Fusidic Acid (Systemic); HydrOXYzine; Idelalisib; Ivacaftor; Kava Kava; Luliconazole; Magnesium Sulfate; Methotrimeprazine; Mifepristone; Minocycline; Nabilone; Netupitant; Osimertinib; Palbociclib; Perampanel; Rufinamide; Simeprevir; Sodium Oxybate; Stiripentol; Tapentadol; Tetrahydrocannabinol

Decreased Effect

The levels/effects of TiaGABine may be decreased by: Bosentan; CYP3A4 Inducers (Moderate); CYP3A4 Inducers (Strong); Dabrafenib; Deferasirox; Enzalutamide; Mefloquine; Mianserin; Mitotane; Orlistat; Osimertinib; Siltuximab; St Johns Wort; Tocilizumab

Food Interactions Food reduces the rate but not the extent of absorption. Management: Administer with food.

Storage/Stability Store at controlled room temperature of 20°C to 25°C (68°F to 77°F). Protect from moisture and light.

Mechanism of Action The exact mechanism by which tiagabine exerts antiseizure activity is not definitively known; however, *in vitro* experiments demonstrate that it enhances the activity of gamma aminobutyric acid (GABA). It is thought that the binding of tiagabine to the GABA uptake carrier inhibits the uptake of GABA into presynaptic neurons, allowing an increased amount of GABA to be available to postsynaptic neurons; based on *in vitro* studies, tiagabine does not inhibit the uptake of dopamine, norepinephrine, serotonin, glutamate, or choline

Pharmacodynamics/Kinetics

Absorption: Rapid (45 minutes), well absorbed; prolonged with food

Protein binding: 96%, primarily to albumin and α_1-acid glycoprotein

Metabolism: Hepatic via CYP (primarily 3A4)

Bioavailability: Oral: Absolute: ~90%

Half-life elimination: 2 to 5 hours when administered with enzyme inducers; 7 to 9 hours when administered without enzyme inducers

Time to peak, plasma: 45 minutes

Excretion: Feces (63%); urine (25%); 2% as unchanged drug; primarily as metabolites

Dosing

Adult & Geriatric

Partial seizures (adjunct): Oral: **Note:** Do not use a loading dose, rapid titration, and/or increases with large dose increments.

Patients receiving enzyme-inducing AED regimens: Initial: 4 mg once daily for 1 week; may increase by 4 to 8 mg at weekly intervals, based on clinical response, up to 56 mg daily in 2 to 4 divided doses; usual maintenance: 32 to 56 mg/day

Patients **not** receiving enzyme-inducing AED regimens: The estimated plasma concentrations of tiagabine in patients not taking enzyme-inducing medications is twice that of patients receiving enzyme-inducing AEDs. Lower doses are required; slower titration may be necessary.

Dosage adjustment: Consider dosage adjustment when a change in enzyme-inducing status occurs due to the addition, discontinuation, or dose change of the enzyme-inducing agent. If multiple doses are missed, evaluate if retitration is clinically indicated.

Pediatric

Partial seizures: Oral: **Note:** Do not use a loading dose, rapid titration, and/or increases with large dose increments.

Patients receiving enzyme-inducing AED regimens: Children and Adolescents 12 to 18 years: Initial: 4 mg once daily for 1 week; may increase to 8 mg daily in 2 divided doses for 1 week; then may increase by 4 to 8 mg at weekly intervals, based on clinical response, up to 32 mg daily in 2 to 4 divided doses

Patients **not** receiving enzyme-inducing AED regimens: Refer to adult dosing.

Dosage adjustment: Consider dosage adjustment when a change in enzyme-inducing status occurs due to the addition, discontinuation, or dose change of the enzyme-inducing agent. If multiple doses are missed, evaluate if retitration is clinically indicated.

Renal Impairment No dosage adjustment necessary.

Hepatic Impairment There are no specific dosage adjustments provided in manufacturer's labeling. However, dosage reduction may be necessary since clearance is reduced in the setting of hepatic impairment.

Administration Oral: Administer with food.

Monitoring Parameters Seizure frequency, liver function tests (periodically), suicidality (eg, suicidal thoughts, depression, behavioral changes)

Reference Range A therapeutic range for tiagabine plasma concentrations has not been established. Because of the potential for pharmacokinetic interactions between tiagabine and drugs that induce or inhibit hepatic metabolizing enzymes, it may be useful to obtain plasma levels of tiagabine before and after changes are made in the therapeutic regimen. A tentative target trough concentration of 50 to 250 nmol/L has been suggested (Johannessen 2003; Johannessen 2006).

Dosage Forms Excipient information presented when available (limited, particularly for generics); consult specific product labeling.

Tablet, Oral, as hydrochloride:
Gabitril: 2 mg [contains fd&c yellow #6 (sunset yellow)]
Gabitril: 4 mg [contains fd&c yellow #10 (quinoline yellow)]
Gabitril: 12 mg [contains brilliant blue fcf (fd&c blue #1), fd&c yellow #10 (quinoline yellow)]
Gabitril: 16 mg [contains fd&c blue #2 (indigotine)]
Generic: 2 mg, 4 mg

Extemporaneous Preparations A 1 mg/mL tiagabine hydrochloride oral suspension may be made with tablets and a 1:1 mixture of Ora-Sweet® and Ora-Plus®. Crush ten 12 mg tablets in a mortar and reduce to a fine powder. Add small portions of the vehicle and mix to a uniform paste; mix while adding the vehicle in incremental proportions to **almost** 120 mL; transfer to a graduated cylinder; rinse mortar with vehicle, and add quantity of vehicle sufficient to make 120 mL. Label "shake well" and "refrigerate". Store in amber plastic prescription bottles; stable for 70 days at room temperature or 91 days refrigerated (preferred) (Nahata 2004).

A 1 mg/mL oral suspension may be made with tablets and a 6:1 mixture of simple syrup, NF and methylcellulose 1%. Crush ten 12 mg tablets in a mortar and reduce to a fine powder. Add 17 mL of methylcellulose 1% gel and mix to a uniform paste; mix while adding simple syrup, NF in incremental proportions to **almost** 120 mL; transfer to a graduated cylinder, rinse mortar with syrup, and add quantity of syrup sufficient to make 120 mL. Label "shake well" and "refrigerate". Store in amber plastic prescription bottles; stable for 42 days at room temperature or 91 days refrigerated (preferred) (Nahata 2004).

♦ Tiagabine Hydrochloride *see* TiaGABine *on page 1785*

♦ Tiamol (Can) *see* Fluocinonide *on page 781*

♦ Tiazac *see* Diltiazem *on page 553*

♦ Tiazac XC (Can) *see* Diltiazem *on page 553*

Ticagrelor (tye KA grel or)

Brand Names: US Brilinta
Brand Names: Canada Brilinta

Index Terms AZD6140

Pharmacologic Category Antiplatelet Agent; Antiplatelet Agent, Cyclopentyltriazolopyrimidine

Additional Appendix Information

Oral Antiplatelet Comparison Chart *on page 1963*

Use Acute coronary syndrome: Reduction of the rate of cardiovascular death, myocardial infarction (MI), and stroke in patients with acute coronary syndrome (ACS) or a history of MI. Ticagrelor also reduces the rate of stent thrombosis in patients who have been stented for treatment of ACS.

Pregnancy Considerations Fetal mortality and/or abnormalities were observed in animal studies at doses greater than maximum recommended human doses. There are no adequate and well-controlled studies in pregnant women. Use only if potential benefits outweigh potential risk to fetus. The Canadian labeling recommends women of childbearing potential use appropriate contraceptive measures.

Breast-Feeding Considerations Excretion into breast milk is unknown; use is not recommended.

Medication Guide Available Yes

Contraindications

Hypersensitivity (eg, angioedema) to ticagrelor or any component of the formulation; active pathological bleeding (eg, peptic ulcer or intracranial hemorrhage); history of intracranial hemorrhage

Canadian labeling: Additional contraindications (not in US labeling): Moderate to severe hepatic impairment; concomitant use of strong CYP3A4 inhibitors (eg, ketoconazole, clarithromycin, ritonavir, atazanavir, nefazodone)

Warnings/Precautions [US Boxed Warning]: Ticagrelor increases the risk of bleeding including significant and sometimes fatal bleeding. Use is contraindicated in patients with active pathological bleeding (eg, peptic ulcer bleeding or intracranial hemorrhage) or history of intracranial hemorrhage. Additional risk factors for bleeding include propensity to bleed (eg, recent trauma or surgery, recent or recurrent GI bleeding, active PUD, moderate to severe hepatic impairment), CABG or other surgical procedure, concomitant use of medications that increase risk of bleeding (eg, warfarin, NSAIDs), and advanced age. Bleeding should be suspected if patient becomes hypotensive after undergoing recent coronary angiography, PCI, CABG, or other surgical procedure even if overt signs of bleeding do not exist. **Where possible, manage bleeding without discontinuing ticagrelor as the risk of cardiovascular events is increased upon discontinuation.** If discontinuation of ticagrelor is necessary, resume as soon as possible after the bleeding source is identified and controlled. Hemostatic benefits of platelet transfusions are not known; may inhibit transfused platelets. Premature discontinuation of therapy will increase the risk of MI, stroke and death. If ticagrelor must be discontinued (eg, treatment of bleeding or for significant surgery), restart ticagrelor as soon as possible. Duration of therapy, in general, is determined by the type of stent placed (bare metal or drug eluting) and whether an ACS event was ongoing at the time of placement. Use with caution in patients who are at an increased risk of bradycardia (eg, second- or third-degree AV block, sick sinus syndrome) or taking other bradycardic-inducing agents (eg, beta blockers, nondihydropyridine calcium channel blockers). Ventricular pauses ≥3 seconds were noted more frequently with ticagrelor than with clopidogrel during the first week after hospitalization for ACS in a substudy of the Platelet Inhibition and Patient Outcomes (PLATO) trial; however, most ventricular pauses were asymptomatic and transient (Scirica, 2011). Dyspnea (often mild to moderate and transient) was observed more frequently in patients receiving ticagrelor than clopidogrel or aspirin alone during clinical trials; resolution of dyspnea was observed within 1 week in most patients. Ticagrelor-related dyspnea does not require specific treatment nor does it warrant therapy interruption; however, therapy should be discontinued in patients unable to tolerate ticagrelor-related dyspnea.

[US Boxed Warning]: Maintenance doses of aspirin greater than 100 mg/day reduce the efficacy of ticagrelor and should be avoided. Use of higher maintenance doses of aspirin (ie, >100 mg/day) was associated with relatively unfavorable outcomes for ticagrelor versus clopidogrel in the PLATO trial (Gaglia, 2011; Wallentin, 2009). Canadian labeling recommends a maximum maintenance aspirin dose of 150 mg/day.

[US Boxed Warning]: Avoid initiation of ticagrelor when urgent CABG surgery is planned; when possible discontinue use at least 5 days before any surgery. Discontinue 5 days before elective surgery (except in patients with cardiac stents that have not completed their full course of dual antiplatelet therapy; patient-specific situations need to be discussed with cardiologist) (ACCF/AHA [Hillis, 2011]). The ACCF/AHA STEMI guidelines recommend discontinuation for at least 24 hours prior to on-pump CABG if possible; off-pump CABG may be performed within 24 hours of ticagrelor administration if the benefits of prompt revascularization outweigh the risks of bleeding (ACCF/AHA [O'Gara, 2013]).

Use with caution in patients with moderate hepatic impairment due to limited experience. Use in severe hepatic impairment has not been studied; avoid use in these patients; Canadian labeling contraindicates use in moderate to severe hepatic impairment. Use with caution in patients with renal impairment, a history of hyperuricemia or gouty arthritis. Canadian labeling does not recommend use in patients with uric acid nephropathy. Potentially significant interactions may exist, requiring dose or frequency adjustment, additional monitoring, and/or selection of alternative therapy.

Adverse Reactions As with all drugs which may affect hemostasis, bleeding is associated with ticagrelor. Hemorrhage may occur at virtually any site. Risk is dependent on multiple variables, including the concurrent use of multiple agents which alter hemostasis and patient susceptibility.

>10%:

Endocrine & metabolic: Increased uric acid (22%)

Hematologic & oncologic: Major bleeding (4% to 12%)

Respiratory: Dyspnea (12% to ≤14%), dyspnea on exertion (2% to ≤14%)

1% to 10%:

Cardiovascular: Ventricular pause (2% to 6%), atrial fibrillation (4%), hypertension (4%), bradycardia (3%), chest pain (3%), hypotension (3%), cardiac failure (2%), peripheral edema (2%), ventricular tachycardia (2%), presyncope (≤2%), syncope (≤2%), angina pectoris (1%), palpitations (1%), sinus bradycardia (1%), ventricular premature contractions (1%)

Central nervous system: Headache (7%), dizziness (5%), noncardiac chest pain (4%), fatigue (3%), anxiety (2%), insomnia (2%), vertigo (2%), loss of consciousness (≤2%), depression (1%)

Dermatologic: Ecchymoses (2%), skin rash (2%), pruritus (1%), dermal hemorrhage

Endocrine & metabolic: Hypokalemia (2%), diabetes mellitus (1%), dyslipidemia (1%), hypercholesterolemia (1%)

Gastrointestinal: Diarrhea (4%), nausea (4%), vomiting (3%), abdominal pain (2%), constipation (2%), dyspepsia (2%), gastrointestinal hemorrhage (2%)

Genitourinary: Hematuria (2%), urinary tract infection (2%), urinary tract hemorrhage

Hematologic & oncologic: Minor bleeding (4% to 5%), bruise (4%), anemia (2%), hematoma (2%), hematoma (2%; puncture site), postprocedural hemorrhage (2%), subcutaneous hemorrhage

Neuromuscular & skeletal: Back pain (4%), arthralgia (2%), limb pain (2%), musculoskeletal chest pain (2%), musculoskeletal pain (2%), weakness (2%), myalgia (1%)

Renal: Increased serum creatinine (7% to 8%; transient; mechanism undetermined), renal failure (1%)

Respiratory: Epistaxis (1% to 6%), cough (5%), nasopharyngitis (2%), bronchitis (1%), pneumonia (1%)

Miscellaneous: Fever (3%)

<1% (Limited to important or life-threatening): Confusion, conjunctival hemorrhage, gastritis, gout, gynecomastia, hemarthrosis, hemopericardium, hemophthalmos, hemoptysis, hypersensitivity, intracranial hemorrhage (including fatalities), paresthesia, retinal hemorrhage, retroperitoneal hemorrhage, ventricular fibrillation

Drug Interactions

Metabolism/Transport Effects Substrate of CYP3A4 (major); **Note:** Assignment of Major/Minor substrate status based on clinically relevant drug interaction potential; **Inhibits** CYP2B6 (weak), CYP2C9 (moderate), CYP2D6 (weak), CYP3A4 (weak)

Avoid Concomitant Use

Avoid concomitant use of Ticagrelor with any of the following: CYP3A4 Inducers (Strong); CYP3A4 Inhibitors (Strong); Dexamethasone (Systemic); Pimozide; Urokinase

Increased Effect/Toxicity

Ticagrelor may increase the levels/effects of: Agents with Antiplatelet Properties; Anticoagulants; Apixaban; ARIPiprazole; AtorvaSTATin; Bosentan; Cannabis; Carvedilol; Collagenase (Systemic); CYP2C9 Substrates; Dabigatran Etexilate; Deoxycholic Acid; Digoxin; Dofetilide; Dronabinol; Edoxaban; Flibanserin; Hydrocodone; Ibritumomab; Lomitapide; Lovastatin; NiMODipine; Obinutuzumab; Pimozide; Rivaroxaban; Salicylates; Simvastatin; Tetrahydrocannabinol; Thrombolytic Agents; Tositumomab and Iodine I 131 Tositumomab; Urokinase

The levels/effects of Ticagrelor may be increased by: Aspirin; CycloSPORINE (Systemic); CYP3A4 Inhibitors (Strong); Dasatinib; Glucosamine; Grapefruit Juice; Herbs (Anticoagulant/Antiplatelet Properties); Ibrutinib; Limaprost; Multivitamins/Fluoride (with ADE); Multivitamins/Minerals with ADEK, Folate, Iron); Multivitamins/Minerals (with AE, No Iron); Omega-3 Fatty Acids; Osimertinib; Pentosan Polysulfate Sodium; Pentoxifylline; Prostacyclin Analogues; Tipranavir; Vitamin E; Vitamin E (Oral)

Decreased Effect

The levels/effects of Ticagrelor may be decreased by: Aspirin; Bosentan; CYP3A4 Inducers (Moderate); CYP3A4 Inducers (Strong); CYP3A4 Inhibitors (Strong); Dabrafenib; Deferasirox; Dexamethasone (Systemic); Osimertinib; Siltuximab; St Johns Wort; Tocilizumab

Storage/Stability Store at 25°C (77°F); excursions permitted to 15°C to 30°C (59°F to 86°F).

Mechanism of Action Reversibly and noncompetitively binds the adenosine diphosphate (ADP) P2Y$_{12}$ receptor on the platelet surface which prevents ADP-mediated activation of the GPIIb/IIIa receptor complex thereby reducing platelet aggregation. Due to the reversible antagonism of the P2Y$_{12}$ receptor, recovery of platelet function is likely to depend on serum concentrations of ticagrelor and its active metabolite.

Pharmacodynamics/Kinetics

Onset of inhibition of platelet aggregation (IPA): 180 mg loading dose: ~41% within 30 minutes (similar to clopidogrel 600 mg at 8 hours)

Peak effect: Time to maximal IPA: 180 mg loading dose: IPA ~88% at 2 hours post administration

Duration of IPA: 180 mg loading dose: 87% to 89% maintained from 2 to 8 hours; 24 hours after the last maintenance dose, IPA is 58% (similar to maintenance clopidogrel)

Time after discontinuation when IPA is 30%: ~56 hours; IPA 10%: ~110 hours (Gurbel, 2009). Mean IPA observed with ticagrelor at 3 days post-discontinuation was comparable to that observed with clopidogrel at 5 days post discontinuation.

Absorption: Rapid

Distribution: 88 L

Protein binding: >99% (parent drug and active metabolite)

Metabolism: Hepatic via CYP3A4/5 to active metabolite (AR-C124910XX)

Bioavailability: ~36% (range: 30% to 42%)

Half-life elimination: Parent drug: ~7 hours; active metabolite: ~9 hours

Time to peak:

Whole tablets: Parent drug: 1.5 hours (median; range: 1 to 4 hours); Active metabolite (AR-C124910XX): 2.5 hours (median; range: 1.5 to 5 hours)

Crushed tablets: Oral or nasogastric tube administration: Parent drug: ~1 hour (median; range: 1 to 4 hours); Active metabolite (AR-C124910XX): 2 hours (median; range: 1 to 8 hours). **Note:** Significantly higher concentrations of both ticagrelor and AR-C124910XX may appear at earlier time points (0.5 and 1 hour, respectively) when administered as crushed tablets (Teng 2015).

Excretion: Feces (58%); urine (26%); actual amount of parent drug and active metabolite excreted in urine was <1% of total dose administered

Dosing

Adult & Geriatric

Acute coronary syndrome: Unstable angina, non-ST-segment elevation myocardial infarction (NSTEMI), ST-segment elevation myocardial infarction (STEMI): Oral, NG: Initial: 180 mg loading dose (with a loading dose of aspirin [eg, 325 mg] if not already receiving); Maintenance: 90 mg twice daily; initiated 12 hours after initial loading dose with low-dose aspirin 75 to 100 mg/day (US labeling) or 75 to 150 mg/day (Canadian labeling) or 81 mg/day indefinitely in patients with UA/NSTEMI or STEMI as recommended by ACCF/AHA/SCAI). Continue initial therapy with ticagrelor for up to 12 months. After 12 months of initial therapy, reduce ticagrelor dose to 60 mg twice daily. Patients in the clinical trial were followed up over a period of 3 years (Bonaca, 2015).

Duration of ticagrelor (in combination with aspirin) after stent placement: **Premature interruption of therapy may result in stent thrombosis with subsequent fatal and nonfatal MI.** According to the ACCF/AHA/SCAI PCI guidelines, in patients with ACS receiving either stent type (bare metal [BMS] or drug-eluting stent [DES]) or those receiving a DES for a non-ACS indication, ticagrelor for at least 12 months is recommended (ACCF/AHA/SCAI [Levine, 2011]). The ACCF/AHA guidelines for the management of UA/NSTEMI recommend up to 12 months of ticagrelor in patients with ACS who receive a BMS (ACCF/AHA [Anderson, 2013]). A

duration >12 months may be considered in patients with DES placement. After 12 months of initial therapy, the manufacturer recommends reducing the dose of ticagrelor to 60 mg twice daily. Recent data have demonstrated that continued dual antiplatelet therapy (ticagrelor not included in clinical trial) for a total of 30 months (compared to 12 months) significantly reduced the risk of stent thrombosis and major adverse cardiovascular/cerebrovascular events but was associated with a higher risk of bleeding (Mauri, 2014). Patients receiving a BMS for a non-ACS indication should be given ticagrelor for at least 1 month and ideally up to 12 months; if patient is at increased risk of bleeding, give for a minimum of 2 weeks (ACCF/AHA/SCAI [Levine, 2011]).

Conversion from clopidogrel to ticagrelor: May initiate ticagrelor 90 mg twice daily beginning 24 hours after last clopidogrel dose (loading or maintenance). Patients who are in the acute phase of an acute coronary syndrome, especially if determined to be clopidogrel nonresponsive, may be considered for administration of ticagrelor 180 mg loading dose followed by 90 mg twice daily regardless of previous clopidogrel exposure, taking into consideration the administration of other antiplatelet agents (eg, GP IIb/IIIa inhibitors) (Gurbel, 2010; Wallentin, 2009). In one single blinded study, patients with ACS receiving ongoing clopidogrel treatment who were converted to ticagrelor *without* a loading dose did not experience a reduction in platelet inhibition compared to those who received a loading dose of ticagrelor (Caiazzo, 2014). **Note:** In general, conversion to ticagrelor results in an absolute inhibition of platelet aggregation (IPA) increase of 26.4%.

Renal Impairment No dosage adjustment necessary.

Hemodialysis: No dosage adjustments provided by the manufacturer; however, ticagrelor is not renally eliminated. Ticagrelor is not expected to be dialyzable.

Hepatic Impairment

US labeling:

Mild impairment: No dosage adjustment necessary.

Moderate impairment: There are no dosage adjustments provided in the manufacturer's labeling (has not been studied); however, undergoes hepatic metabolism; use caution.

Severe impairment: Avoid use.

Canadian labeling:

Mild impairment: No dosage adjustment necessary.

Moderate or severe impairment: Use is contraindicated.

Dietary Considerations May be taken without regard to meals.

Administration May be administered without regard to meals. Missed doses should be taken at their next regularly scheduled time. For patients unable to swallow whole, tablets may be crushed and mixed with water to create a suspension for oral or NG (CH8/Fr8 or greater according to the manufacturer) use. If suspension is administered orally, refill glass with water, stir and drink; if administered via NG tube, flush NG tube through with water after administration (Crean, 2013; Parodi, 2015). Administration of crushed tablets, while bioequivalent to administration of whole tablets, may result in increased concentrations of ticagrelor and the major active metabolite at earlier time points (Teng 2015).

Monitoring Parameters Signs of bleeding; hemoglobin and hematocrit periodically; renal function; uric acid levels (patients with gout or at risk of hyperuricemia); signs/symptoms of dyspnea; may consider platelet function testing to determine platelet inhibitory response if results of testing may alter management (ACCF/AHA [Anderson, 2013]).

Additional Information Unlike thienopyridines (eg, clopidogrel, prasugrel) which are prodrugs and require metabolic transformation to their active metabolites for their activity, ticagrelor and its active metabolite both exhibit antiplatelet activity by reversibly and noncompetitively binding to the adenosine diphosphate (ADP) P2Y$_{12}$ receptor on the platelet surface. Due to the reversible antagonism of the P2Y$_{12}$ receptor, recovery of platelet function is faster than with use of irreversible P2Y$_{12}$ receptor antagonists such as clopidogrel or prasugrel.

Dosage Forms Excipient information presented when available (limited, particularly for generics); consult specific product labeling.

Tablet, Oral:

Brilinta: 60 mg, 90 mg

Dosage Forms: Canada Excipient information presented when available (limited, particularly for generics); consult specific product labeling.

Tablet, oral:

Brilinta: 90 mg

Extemporaneous Preparations A suspension for oral administration may be prepared by crushing one or two

90 mg tablets in a mortar (for 60 seconds) and placing in a dosing cup. To ensure the full dose is received, rinse mortar with 100 mL purified water, transfer to dosing cup, and repeat rinse (Crean, 2013; Parodi, 2015).

A suspension for NG tube administration may be prepared by crushing one or two 90 mg tablets in a mortar (for 60 seconds); add 50 mL purified water to mortar and stir (for 60 seconds); transfer the suspension to a 50 mL oral enteral syringe and administer via NG tube. To ensure the full dose is received, add another 50 mL purified water to the mortar and stir for 60 seconds; using the same 50 mL oral enteral syringe, withdraw the suspension and administer entire amount via NG tube (Crean, 2013).

When stored in a PVC oral syringe for up to 2 hours, there was no degradation of the suspension detected (Crean, 2013).

◆ Tice BCG see BCG (Intravesical) on page 203
◆ TIG see Tetanus Immune Globulin (Human) on page 1771
◆ Tigan see Trimethobenzamide on page 1846

Tigecycline (tye ge SYE kleen)

Brand Names: US Tygacil
Brand Names: Canada Tygacil
Index Terms GAR-936
Pharmacologic Category Antibiotic, Glycylcycline
Use
Community-acquired bacterial pneumonia:
US labeling: Treatment of community-acquired pneumonia in patients 18 years and older caused by *Streptococcus pneumoniae* (penicillin-susceptible isolates), including cases with concurrent bacteremia, *Haemophilus influenzae* (beta-lactamase negative isolates), and *Legionella pneumophila.*
Canadian labeling: Treatment of mild or moderate community-acquired pneumonia in patients 18 years and older caused by *S. pneumoniae* (penicillin-susceptible isolates), *H. influenzae, Mycoplasma pneumoniae,* and *Chlamydia pneumoniae.*
Complicated intra-abdominal infections: Treatment of complicated intra-abdominal infections in patients 18 years and older caused by *Citrobacter freundii, Enterobacter cloacae, Escherichia coli, Klebsiella oxytoca, Klebsiella pneumoniae, Enterococcus faecalis* (vancomycin-susceptible isolates), *Staphylococcus aureus* (methicillin-susceptible and methicillin-resistant isolates [US labeling] or methicillin-susceptible isolates [Canadian labeling]), *Streptococcus anginosus* group (includes *S. anginosus, Streptococcus intermedius,* and *Streptococcus constellatus), Bacteroides fragilis, Bacteroides thetaiotaomicron, Bacteroides uniformis, Bacteroides vulgatus, Clostridium perfringens,* and *Peptostreptococcus micros.*
Complicated skin and skin structure infections: Treatment of complicated skin and skin structure infections in patients 18 years and older caused by *E. coli, E. faecalis* (vancomycin-susceptible isolates), *S. aureus* (methicillin-susceptible and methicillin-resistant isolates), *Streptococcus agalactiae, S. anginosus* group (includes *S. anginosus, S. intermedius,* and *S. constellatus*) [US labeling] or *S. anginosus* [Canadian labeling], *Streptococcus pyogenes, E. cloacae, K. pneumoniae,* and *B. fragilis.*
Pregnancy Considerations Because adverse effects were observed in animals and because of the potential for permanent tooth discoloration, tigecycline is classified pregnancy category D. Tigecycline frequently causes nausea and vomiting and, therefore, may not be ideal for use in a patient with pregnancy-related nausea.
Breast-Feeding Considerations It is not known if tigecycline is found in breast milk. The manufacturer recommends caution if giving tigecycline to a nursing woman. Nondose-related effects could include modification of bowel flora.
Contraindications
Hypersensitivity to tigecycline or any component of the formulation
Documentation of allergenic cross-reactivity for tetracyclines is limited. However, because of similarities in chemical structure and/or pharmacologic actions, the possibility of cross-sensitivity cannot be ruled out with certainty.
Canadian labeling: Additional contraindications (not in U.S. labeling): Hypersensitivity to tetracycline class of antibiotics

Warnings/Precautions [U.S. Boxed Warning]: In Phase 3 and 4 clinical trials, an increase in all-cause mortality was observed in patients treated with tigecycline compared to those treated with comparator antibiotics; cause has not been established. Use should be reserved for situations in which alternative treatments are not appropriate. In general, deaths were the result of worsening infection, complications of infection, or underlying comorbidity. May cause life-threatening anaphylaxis/anaphylactoid reactions. Due to structural similarity with tetracyclines, use caution in patients with prior hypersensitivity and/or severe adverse reactions associated with tetracycline use (Canadian labeling contraindicates use in patients with hypersensitivity to tetracyclines). Due to structural similarities with tetracyclines, may be associated with photosensitivity, pseudotumor cerebri, pancreatitis, and antianabolic effects (including increased BUN, azotemia, acidosis, and hyperphosphatemia) observed with this class. Acute pancreatitis (including fatalities) has been reported, including patients without known risk factors; discontinue use when suspected. May cause fetal harm if used during pregnancy; patients should be advised of potential risks associated with use. Permanent discoloration of the teeth may occur if used during tooth development (fetal stage through children up to 8 years of age).

Safety and efficacy in children <18 years of age have not been established due to increased mortality observed in trials of adult patients. Use only if no alternative antibiotics are available. Because of effects on tooth development (yellow-gray-brown discoloration), use in patients <8 years is not recommended.

Use caution in hepatic impairment; dosage adjustment recommended in severe hepatic impairment. Abnormal liver function tests (increased total bilirubin, prothrombin time, transaminases) have been reported. Isolated cases of significant hepatic dysfunction and hepatic failure have occurred. Closely monitor for worsening hepatic function in patients that develop abnormal liver function tests during therapy. Adverse hepatic effects may occur after drug discontinuation.

Prolonged use may result in fungal or bacterial superinfection, including *C. difficile*-associated diarrhea (CDAD) and pseudomembranous colitis; CDAD has been observed >2 months postantibiotic treatment. Use with caution if using as monotherapy for patients with intestinal perforation (in the small sample of available cases, septic shock occurred more frequently than patients treated with imipenem/cilastatin comparator). Do not use for diabetic foot infections; non-inferiority was not demonstrated in studies. Do not use for healthcare-acquired pneumonia (HAP) or ventilator-associated pneumonia (VAP); increased mortality and decreased efficacy have been reported in HAP and VAP trials.

Adverse Reactions Note: Frequencies relative to placebo are not available; some frequencies are lower than those experienced with comparator drugs.
>10%: Gastrointestinal: Nausea (26%; severe: 1%), vomiting (18%; severe: 1%), diarrhea (12%)
2% to 10%:
Cardiovascular: Localized phlebitis (3%)
Central nervous system: Headache (6%), dizziness (3%)
Dermatologic: Skin rash (3%)
Endocrine & metabolic: Hyponatremia (2%), increased amylase (3%)
Gastrointestinal: Abdominal pain (6%), dyspepsia (2%)
Hematologic & oncologic: Anemia (5%), hypoproteinemia (5%)
Hepatic: Increased serum ALT (5%), increased serum AST (4%), increased serum alkaline phosphatase (3%), hyperbilirubinemia (2%)
Infection: Infection (7%), abscess (2%)
Neuromuscular & skeletal: Weakness (3%)
Renal: Increased blood urea nitrogen (3%)
Respiratory: Pneumonia (2%)
Miscellaneous: Abnormal healing (3%)
<2% (Limited to important or life-threatening): Acute pancreatitis, allergic skin reaction, anaphylactoid reaction, anaphylaxis, anorexia, *Clostridium difficile* associated diarrhea, dysgeusia, eosinophilia, hepatic insufficiency, hepatic failure, hypocalcemia, hypoglycemia, increased INR, increased serum creatinine, increased serum transaminases, increased INR, increased serum creatinine, increased serum transaminases, prolonged partial thromboplastin time, prolonged prothrombin time, pruritus, septic shock, Stevens-Johnson syndrome, swelling at injection site, thrombocytopenia, thrombophlebitis, vaginal moniliasis, vaginitis
Drug Interactions
Metabolism/Transport Effects None known.
Avoid Concomitant Use There are no known interactions where it is recommended to avoid concomitant use. ▶

Increased Effect/Toxicity

Tigecycline may increase the levels/effects of: Warfarin

Decreased Effect There are no known significant inter-actions involving a decrease in effect.

Preparation for Administration Add 5.3 mL NS, D_5W, or LR to each 50 mg vial. Swirl gently to dissolve. Resulting solution is 10 mg/mL. Reconstituted solution must be further diluted to allow IV administration. Transfer to 100 mL IV bag for infusion (final concentration should not exceed 1 mg/mL). Reconstituted solution should be yellow-orange; discard if not this color.

Storage/Stability Prior to reconstitution, store at 20°C to 25°C (68°F to 77°F); excursions are permitted between 15°C and 30°C (59°F and 86°F). Reconstituted solution may be stored at room temperature (not to exceed 25°C [77°F]) for up to 6 hours in the vial or up to 24 hours if further diluted in a compatible IV solution. Alternatively, may be stored refrigerated at 2°C to 8°C (36°F to 46°F) for up to 48 hours following immediate transfer of the reconstituted solution into NS or D_5W.

Mechanism of Action A glycylcycline antibiotic that binds to the 30S ribosomal subunit of susceptible bacteria, thereby, inhibiting protein synthesis. Generally considered bacteriostatic; however, bactericidal activity has been demonstrated against isolates of *S. pneumoniae* and *L. pneumophila*. Tigecycline is a derivative of minocycline (9-t-butylglycylamido minocycline), and while not classified as a tetracycline, it may share some class-associated adverse effects. Tigecycline has demonstrated activity against a variety of gram-positive and -negative bacterial pathogens including methicillin-resistant staphylococci.

Pharmacodynamics/Kinetics

Distribution: V_d: 7-9 L/kg; extensive tissue distribution

Protein binding: 71% to 89%

Metabolism: Hepatic, via glucuronidation, N-acetylation, and epimerization to several metabolites, each <10% of the dose

Half-life elimination: Single dose: 27 hours; following multiple doses: 42 hours

Excretion: Feces (59%, primarily as unchanged drug); urine (33%, with 22% of the total dose as unchanged drug)

Dosing

Adult & Geriatric Note: Duration of therapy dependent on severity/site of infection and clinical status and response to therapy.

Pneumonia, community-acquired: IV: Initial: 100 mg as a single dose; Maintenance dose: 50 mg every 12 hours for 7-14 days

Intra-abdominal infections, complicated (cIAI): IV: Initial: 100 mg as a single dose; Maintenance dose: 50 mg every 12 hours for 5-14 days; **Note:** 2010 IDSA guidelines recommend a treatment duration of 4-7 days (provided source controlled) for community-acquired, mild-to-moderate IAI

Skin/skin structure infections, complicated: IV: Initial: 100 mg as a single dose; Maintenance dose: 50 mg every 12 hours for 5-14 days

Pediatric Children ≥8 years and Adolescents: Limited data available: **Note:** Use should be reserved for situations when no effective alternative therapy is available

General dosing, susceptible infection: IV: Dosing based on data from pharmacokinetic trials.

Children 8-11 years: 1.2 mg/kg/dose every 12 hours; maximum dose: 50 mg

Children ≥12 years and Adolescents: 50 mg every 12 hours

Renal Impairment No dosage adjustment necessary.

Poorly dialyzed; no supplemental dose or dosage adjustment necessary, including patients on intermittent hemodialysis, peritoneal dialysis, or continuous renal replacement therapy (eg, CVVHD).

Hepatic Impairment

Mild-to-moderate hepatic impairment (Child-Pugh class A or B): No dosage adjustment necessary.

Severe hepatic impairment (Child-Pugh class C): Initial: 100 mg single dose; Maintenance: 25 mg every 12 hours.

Administration Infuse over 30-60 minutes through dedicated line or via Y-site

Dosage Forms Excipient information presented when available (limited, particularly for generics); consult specific product labeling.

Solution Reconstituted, Intravenous:

Tygacil: 50 mg (1 ea)

◆ Tikosyn *see* Dofetilide *on page 579*

◆ Tilia Fe *see* Ethinyl Estradiol and Norethindrone *on page 708*

Timolol (Systemic) (TIM oh lol)

Brand Names: Canada Apo-Timol®; Nu-Timolol; Teva-Timolol

Index Terms Timolol Maleate

Pharmacologic Category Antihypertensive; Beta-Blocker, Nonselective

Use Treatment of hypertension and angina; to reduce mortality following myocardial infarction; prophylaxis of migraine

The 2014 guideline for the management of high blood pressure in adults (JNC 8) recommends initiation of pharmacologic treatment to lower blood pressure for the following patients (JNC8 [James, 2013]):

• Patients ≥60 years of age, with systolic blood pressure (SBP) ≥150 mm Hg or diastolic blood pressure (DBP) ≥90 mm Hg. Goal of therapy is SBP <150 mm Hg and DBP <90 mm Hg.

• Patients <60 years of age, with SBP ≥140 mm Hg or DBP ≥90 mm Hg. Goal of therapy is SBP <140 mm Hg and DBP <90 mm Hg.

• Patients ≥18 years of age with diabetes, with SBP ≥140 mm Hg or DBP ≥90 mm Hg. Goal of therapy is SBP <140 mm Hg and DBP <90 mm Hg.

• Patients ≥18 years of age with chronic kidney disease (CKD), with SBP ≥140 mm Hg or DBP ≥90 mm Hg. Goal of therapy is SBP <140 mm Hg and DBP <90 mm Hg.

In patients with chronic kidney disease (CKD), regardless of race or diabetes status, the use of an ACE inhibitor (ACEI) or angiotensin receptor blocker (ARB) as initial therapy is recommended to improve kidney outcomes. In the general nonblack population (without CKD) including those with diabetes, initial antihypertensive treatment should consist of a thiazide-type diuretic, calcium channel blocker, ACEI, or ARB. In the general black population (without CKD) including those with diabetes, initial antihypertensive treatment should consist of a thiazide-type diuretic or a calcium channel blocker **instead of** an ACEI or ARB.

Dosing

Adult & Geriatric

Hypertension: Oral: Initial: 10 mg twice daily, increase gradually every 7 days, usual dosage: 20 to 40 mg/day in 2 divided doses; maximum: 60 mg/day.

Prevention of myocardial infarction: Oral: 10 mg twice daily initiated within 1 to 4 weeks after infarction.

Migraine prophylaxis: Oral: Initial: 10 mg twice daily, increase to maximum of 30 mg/day.

Atrial fibrillation (rate control) (off-label use): Initial: 10 mg twice daily, increase at weekly intervals as tolerated to 20 mg twice daily then to a maximum of 30 mg twice daily; may use in combination with digoxin (Ribeiro, 1986).

Renal Impairment There are no specific dosage adjustments provided in manufacturer's labeling. However, timolol is primarily eliminated renally; dosage reduction may be necessary. Significant hypotension has been seen in patients with severe impairment and undergoing dialysis. Use with caution.

Hepatic Impairment There are no specific dosage adjustments provided in manufacturer's labeling. However, timolol is partially metabolized by the liver; dosage reduction may be necessary.

Additional Information Complete prescribing information should be consulted for additional detail.

Dosage Forms Excipient information presented when available (limited, particularly for generics); consult specific product labeling.

Tablet, Oral, as maleate:

Generic: 5 mg, 10 mg, 20 mg

Timolol (Ophthalmic) (TIM oh lol)

Brand Names: US Betimol; Istalol; Timoptic; Timoptic Ocudose; Timoptic-XE

Brand Names: Canada Apo-Timop; Dom-Timolol; Odan-Timol; PMS-Timolol; Sandoz-Timolol; Timolol Maleate-EX; Timoptic; Timoptic-XE

Index Terms Timolol Hemihydrate; Timolol Maleate

Pharmacologic Category Beta-Blocker, Nonselective; Ophthalmic Agent, Antiglaucoma

Use Elevated intraocular pressure: Treatment of elevated intraocular pressure (IOP) in patients with ocular hypertension or open-angle glaucoma

Dosing

Adult & Geriatric

Elevated intraocular pressure: Ophthalmic:

Gel-forming solution (Timolol GFS, Timoptic-XE): Instill 1 drop (either 0.25% or 0.5% solution) once daily

Solution: Initial: Instill 1 drop (0.25% solution) into affected eye(s) twice daily; if response is not adequate, increase to 1 drop (0.5% solution) twice daily. May decrease dose to 1 drop once daily if intraocular pressure is well controlled (maximum dose: 1 drop twice daily of 0.5% solution)

Istalol: Instill 1 drop (0.5% solution) once daily in the morning

Pediatric

Elevated intraocular pressure: Infants, Children, and Adolescents: Ophthalmic: Use lowest effective dose; the gel formulation may be preferable due to decreased systemic absorption (Coppens, 2009).

Gel-forming solution (Timolol GFS, Timoptic-XE): Instill 1 drop (either 0.25% or 0.5%) once daily into affected eye(s) (Coppens 2009; Moore 2007)

Solution: Limited data available: Initial: 0.25% solution, instill 1 drop twice daily into affected eye(s); increase to 0.5% solution if response not adequate; decrease to 1 drop once daily into affected eye(s) if controlled; maximum dose: 1 drop (0.5% solution)/dose (Hoskins 1985; Moore 2007).

Renal Impairment There are no dosage adjustments provided in the manufacturer's labeling.

Hepatic Impairment There are no dosage adjustments provided in the manufacturer's labeling.

Additional Information Complete prescribing information should be consulted for additional detail.

Dosage Forms Excipient information presented when available (limited, particularly for generics); consult specific product labeling.

Gel Forming Solution, Ophthalmic, as maleate [strength expressed as base]:

Timoptic-XE: 0.25% (5 mL); 0.5% (5 mL)

Generic: 0.25% (5 mL); 0.5% (5 mL)

Solution, Ophthalmic, as hemihydrate [strength expressed as base]:

Betimol: 0.25% (5 mL); 0.5% (5 mL, 10 mL, 15 mL) [contains benzalkonium chloride]

Solution, Ophthalmic, as maleate [strength expressed as base]:

Istalol: 0.5% (2.5 mL, 5 mL) [contains benzalkonium chloride]

Timoptic: 0.25% (5 mL); 0.5% (5 mL, 10 mL) [contains benzalkonium chloride]

Generic: 0.25% (5 mL, 10 mL, 15 mL); 0.5% (5 mL, 10 mL, 15 mL)

Solution, Ophthalmic, as maleate [strength expressed as base, preservative free]:

Timoptic Ocudose: 0.25% (60 ea); 0.5% (60 ea)

Tinzaparin (tin ZA pa rin)

Brand Names: Canada Innohep®

Index Terms Tinzaparin Sodium

Pharmacologic Category Anticoagulant; Anticoagulant, Low Molecular Weight Heparin

Use Treatment of deep vein thrombosis (DVT) and/or pulmonary embolism (PE) (except in patients with severe hemodynamic instability); prevention of venous thromboembolism (VTE) following orthopedic surgery or following general surgery in patients at high risk of VTE; prevention of clotting in indwelling intravenous lines and extracorporeal circuit during hemodialysis (in patients without high bleeding risk)

Pregnancy Considerations Teratogenic events were not observed in animal reproduction studies. Tinzaparin does not cross the human placenta. A pharmacokinetic study in pregnant women found no dose adjustment was needed during pregnancy. Vaginal bleeding was reported in ~10% of pregnant patients during tinzaparin therapy. LMWH is recommended over unfractionated heparin for the treatment of acute venous thromboembolism (VTE) in pregnant women. LMWH is also recommended over unfractionated heparin for VTE prophylaxis in pregnant women with certain risk factors. LMWH should be discontinued prior to induction of labor or a planned cesarean delivery. When choosing therapy, fetal outcomes (ie, pregnancy loss, malformations), maternal outcomes (ie, VTE, hemorrhage), burden of therapy, and maternal preference should be considered (Guyatt, 2012). Contains benzyl alcohol; use with caution in pregnant women due to association with gasping syndrome in premature infants.

Breast-Feeding Considerations Small amounts of LMWH have been detected in breast milk; however, because it has a low oral bioavailability, it is unlikely to cause adverse events in a nursing infant. Use of LMWH may be continued in breast-feeding women (Guyatt, 2012).

Contraindications Hypersensitivity to tinzaparin sodium, heparin or other low molecular weight heparins (LMWH), or any component of the formulation; active bleeding; history of confirmed or suspected immunologically mediated heparin-induced thrombocytopenia (HIT) or positive in vitro platelet-aggregation test in the presence of tinzaparin; acute or subacute endocarditis; generalized hemorrhage tendency and other conditions involving increased risks of hemorrhage (eg, severe hepatic insufficiency, imminent abortion); hemophilia or major blood clotting disorders; acute cerebral insult or hemorrhagic cerebrovascular accidents without systemic emboli; uncontrolled severe hypertension; diabetic or hemorrhagic retinopathy; injury or surgery involving the brain, spinal cord, eyes or ears; spinal/epidural anesthesia in patients requiring treatment dosages of tinzaparin; use of multidose vials containing benzyl alcohol in children <2 years of age, premature infants, and neonates

Note: Use of tinzaparin in patients with current HIT or HIT with thrombosis is **not** recommended and considered contraindicated due to high cross-reactivity to heparin-platelet factor-4 antibody (Guyatt [ACCP], 2012; Warkentin, 1999).

Warnings/Precautions Spinal or epidural hematomas, including subsequent paralysis, may occur with recent or anticipated neuraxial anesthesia (epidural or spinal) or spinal puncture in patients anticoagulated with low molecular weight heparin (LMWH) or heparinoids. Consider risk versus benefit prior to spinal procedures; risk is increased by the use of concomitant agents which may alter hemostasis, the use of indwelling epidural catheters for analgesia, a history of spinal deformity or spinal surgery, as well as traumatic or repeated epidural or spinal punctures. Avoid invasive spinal procedures for 12 hours following tinzaparin administration and withhold the next tinzaparin dose for at least 2 hours after the spinal procedure. Patient should be observed closely for signs and symptoms of neurological impairment. Not to be used interchangeably (unit for unit) with heparin or any other LMWHs.

Monitor patient closely for signs or symptoms of bleeding. Certain patients are at increased risk of bleeding. Risk factors include bacterial endocarditis; congenital or acquired bleeding disorders; active ulcerative or angiodysplastic GI diseases; severe uncontrolled hypertension; history of hemorrhagic stroke; use shortly after brain, spinal, or ophthalmologic surgery; those concomitantly treated with drugs that increase bleeding risk (eg, antiplatelet agents, anticoagulants); recent GI bleeding; thrombocytopenia or platelet defects; severe liver disease; hypertensive or diabetic retinopathy; or in patients undergoing invasive procedures. Withhold or discontinue for minor bleeding. Protamine infusion may be necessary for serious bleeding (consult Protamine monograph for dosing recommendations). Cases of thrombocytopenia including thrombocytopenia with thrombosis have occurred. Use with caution in patients with history of thrombocytopenia (drug-induced or congenital) or platelet defects; monitor platelet count closely. Use is contraindicated in patients with history of confirmed or suspected heparin-induced thrombocytopenia (HIT) or positive in vitro test for antiplatelet antibodies in the presence of tinzaparin. Discontinue therapy and consider alternative treatment if platelets are <100,000/mm^3 and/or thrombosis develops. Asymptomatic thrombocytosis has been observed with use, particularly in patients undergoing orthopedic surgery or with concurrent inflammatory process; discontinue use with increased platelet counts and evaluate the risks/necessity of further therapy. Prosthetic valve thrombosis has been

reported in patients receiving thromboprophylaxis therapy with LMWHs. Pregnant women may be at increased risk.

Use with caution in hepatic impairment; associated with transient, dose-dependent increases in AST/ALT which typically resolve within 2 to 4 weeks of therapy discontinuation. Use with caution in patients with renal insufficiency. Reduced tinzaparin clearance has been observed in patients with moderate-to-severe renal impairment; Consider dosage reduction in patients with CrCl <30 mL/minute. Use with caution in the elderly (delayed elimination may occur). Use is not recommended in patients >70 years of age with renal impairment. An increase in all-cause mortality has been observed in patients ≥70 years (mean age: >82 years) with CrCl ≤60 mL/minute treated with tinzaparin compared to unfractionated heparin for acute DVT (Leizorovicz, 2011).

Heparin can cause hyperkalemia by suppressing aldosterone production; similar reactions could occur with LMWHs. Monitor for hyperkalemia which most commonly occurs in patients with risk factors for the development of hyperkalemia (eg, renal dysfunction, concomitant use of potassium-sparing diuretics or potassium supplements, hematoma in body tissues). For subcutaneous use only; do not administer intramuscularly or intravenously. Use with caution in patients <45 kg or >120 kg; limited experience in these patients. Individualized clinical and laboratory monitoring are recommended. Derived from porcine intestinal mucosa. Some dosage forms may contain sodium metabisulfite.

Benzyl alcohol and derivatives: Some dosage forms may contain benzyl alcohol and should not be used in pregnant women. In neonates, large amounts of benzyl alcohol (≥99 mg/kg/day) have been associated with a potentially fatal toxicity ("gasping syndrome"); the "gasping syndrome" consists of metabolic acidosis, respiratory distress, gasping respirations, CNS dysfunction (including convulsions, intracranial hemorrhage), hypotension, and cardiovascular collapse (AAP ["Inactive" 1997]; CDC, 1982); some data suggests that benzoate displaces bilirubin from protein binding sites (Ahlfors, 2001); avoid or use dosage forms containing benzyl alcohol with caution in neonates. See manufacturer's labeling.

Adverse Reactions As with all anticoagulants, bleeding is the major adverse effect of tinzaparin. Hemorrhage may occur at virtually any site. Risk is dependent on multiple variables. **Note:** Incidence not always reported.

>10%:

Hepatic: ALT increased (≤13%)
Local: Injection site hematoma

1% to 10%:

Cardiovascular: Chest pain (2%), angina pectoris (≥1%), arrhythmia (≥1%), coronary thrombosis/MI (≥1%), dependent edema (≥1%), thromboembolism (≥1%)
Central nervous system: Fever (2%), headache (2%), pain (2%)
Dermatologic: Bullous eruption (≥1%), erythematous rash (≥1%), maculopapular rash (≥1%), skin necrosis (≥1%)
Gastrointestinal: Nausea (2%), abdominal pain (1%), constipation (1%), diarrhea (1%), vomiting (1%)
Genitourinary: Urinary tract infection (4%)
Hematologic: Bleeding events (major events including intracranial, retroperitoneal, or bleeding into a major prosthetic joint: ≤3%; hemorrhage site not specified (2%); other bleeding events reported at an incidence of ≥1% include anorectal bleeding, GI hemorrhage, hemarthrosis, hematemesis, hematuria, hemopericardium, injection site bleeding, melena, purpura, intra-abdominal bleeding, vaginal bleeding, wound hemorrhage), granulocytopenia (≥1%), thrombocytopenia (≥1%)
Hepatic: AST increased (9%)
Local: Injection site cellulitis (≥1%)
Neuromuscular & skeletal: Back pain (2%)
Respiratory: Epistaxis (2%), dyspnea (1%)
Miscellaneous: Allergic reaction (≥1%), neoplasm (≥1%)
<1% (Limited to important or life-threatening): Agranulocytosis, angioedema, anaphylactoid reaction, GGT increased, hemoptysis, hypoaldosteronism, hyperkalemia, LDH increased, lipase increased, metabolic acidosis, ocular hemorrhage, osteopenia, osteoporosis, priapism, pruritus, rash, spinal epidural hematoma, Stevens-Johnson syndrome, thrombocytosis, toxic epidermal necrolysis, urticaria

Drug Interactions

Metabolism/Transport Effects None known.

Avoid Concomitant Use

Avoid concomitant use of Tinzaparin with any of the following: Apixaban; Dabigatran Etexilate; Edoxaban; Hemin; Omacetaxine; Rivaroxaban; Urokinase; Vorapaxar

Increased Effect/Toxicity

Tinzaparin may increase the levels/effects of: ACE Inhibitors; Aliskiren; Angiotensin II Receptor Blockers; Anticoagulants; Canagliflozin; Collagenase (Systemic); Deferasirox; Deoxycholic Acid; Eplerenone; Ibritumomab; Nintedanib; Obinutuzumab; Omacetaxine; Palifermin; Potassium Salts; Potassium-Sparing Diuretics; Rivaroxaban; Tositumomab and Iodine I 131 Tositumomab

The levels/effects of Tinzaparin may be increased by: 5-ASA Derivatives; Agents with Antiplatelet Properties; Apixaban; Dabigatran Etexilate; Dasatinib; Edoxaban; Hemin; Herbs (Anticoagulant/Antiplatelet Properties); Ibrutinib; Limaprost; Nonsteroidal Anti-Inflammatory Agents; Omega-3 Fatty Acids; Pentosan Polysulfate Sodium; Pentoxifylline; Prostacyclin Analogues; Salicylates; Sugammadex; Thrombolytic Agents; Tibolone; Tipranavir; Urokinase; Vitamin E; Vitamin E (Oral); Vorapaxar

Decreased Effect

Tinzaparin may decrease the levels/effects of: Factor X (Human)

The levels/effects of Tinzaparin may be decreased by: Estrogen Derivatives; Progestins

Storage/Stability Store at 15°C to 25°C (59°F to 77°F).

Mechanism of Action Tinzaparin is a low molecular weight heparin (average molecular weight ranges between 5500 and 7500 daltons, distributed as <2000 daltons [<10%], 2000-8000 daltons [60% to 72%], and >8000 daltons [22% to 36%]) that binds antithrombin III, enhancing the inhibition of several clotting factors, particularly factor Xa. Tinzaparin anti-Xa activity (70-120 units/mg) is greater than anti-IIa activity (~55 units/mg) and it has a higher ratio of antifactor Xa to antifactor IIa activity compared to unfractionated heparin. Low molecular weight heparins have a small effect on the activated partial thromboplastin time.

Pharmacodynamics/Kinetics Note: Values reflective of anti-Xa activity.

Onset of action: 2-3 hours
Duration: Detectable anti-Xa activity persists for 24 hours
Absorption: Slow; absorption half-life ~3 hours after subcutaneous administration
Distribution: 4 L
Metabolism: Does not undergo hepatic metabolism
Bioavailability: SubQ: ~90%
Half-life elimination: 82 minutes; prolonged in renal impairment
Time to peak: 4-6 hours
Excretion: Urine

Dosing

Adult Note: 1 mg of tinzaparin equals 70-120 units of anti-Xa activity

DVT and/or PE treatment: SubQ: 175 anti-Xa units/kg once daily (maximum: 18,000 anti-Xa units/day). The 2012 Chest guidelines recommend starting warfarin on the first or second treatment day and continuing tinzaparin until INR is ≥2 for at least 24 hours (usually 5-7 days) (Guyatt, 2012). Body weight dosing using prefilled syringes may also be considered. Refer to manufacturer labeling for detailed dosing recommendations.

DVT prophylaxis: SubQ:

Hip replacement surgery: **Note:** The American College of Chest Physicians recommends initiation of LMWH ≥12 hours preoperatively **or** ≥12 hours postoperatively; extended duration up to 35 days suggested (Guyatt, 2012).

Preoperative regimen: 50 anti-Xa units/kg given 2 hours preoperatively followed by 50 anti-Xa units/kg once daily for 7-10 days

Postoperative regimen: 75 anti-Xa units/kg once daily, with initial dose given postoperatively and continued for 7-10 days

Knee replacement surgery: 75 anti-Xa units/kg once daily, with initial dose given postoperatively and continued for 7-10 days. **Note:** The American College of Chest Physicians recommends initiation of LMWH ≥12 hours preoperatively **or** ≥12 hours postoperatively; extended duration of up to 35 days suggested (Guyatt, 2012). Body weight dosing using prefilled syringes may also be considered. Refer to manufacturer labeling for detailed dosing recommendations.

General surgery: 3500 anti-Xa units once daily, with initial dose given 2 hours prior to surgery and then continued postoperatively for 7-10 days

Anticoagulant in extracorporeal circuit during hemo-dialysis (recommendations apply to stable patients with chronic renal failure): IV:

Dialysis session ≤4 hours (no hemorrhage risk): Initial bolus (via arterial side of circuit or IV): 4500 anti-Xa units at beginning of dialysis; typically achieves plasma concentrations of 0.5-1 anti-Xa units/mL; may give larger bolus for dialysis sessions >4 hours. For subsequent dialysis sessions, may adjust dose as necessary in increments of 500 anti-Xa units based on previous outcome.

Dialysis session ≤4 hours (hemorrhage risk): Initial bolus (IV only): 2250 anti-Xa units at beginning of dialysis (do not add to dialysis circuit). A smaller second IV dose may be administered during dialysis sessions >4 hours. For subsequent dialysis sessions, adjust dose as necessary to achieve plasma concentrations of 0.2-0.4 anti-Xa units/mL.

Geriatric Refer to adult dosing. Increased sensitivity to tinzaparin in elderly patients may be possible due to a decline in renal function. Use is not recommended in patients >70 years of age with renal impairment.

Pediatric Note: 1 mg of tinzaparin equals 70-120 units of anti-Xa activity

VTE treatment (off-label use; Monagle, 2012): SubQ: Infants, Children, and Adolescents: **Note:** May initiate a vitamin K antagonist on day 1 of tinzaparin therapy; discontinue tinzaparin on day 6 or later if INR is not >2.
Birth to 2 months: 275 anti-Xa units/kg once daily
2-12 months: 250 anti-Xa units/kg once daily
1-5 years: 240 anti-Xa units/kg once daily
5-10 years: 200 anti-Xa units/kg once daily
10-16 years: 175 anti-Xa units/kg once daily

Renal Impairment
CrCl ≥30 mL/minute: No dosage adjustment provided in manufacturer's labeling; however, primarily undergoes renal elimination. Clearance is decreased in renal impairment; use with caution.
CrCl <30 mL/minute: Manufacturer's labeling suggests that a reduction in dose be considered but does not provide specific dose recommendations. Use with caution.

Hepatic Impairment No dosage adjustment provided in manufacturer's labeling. Does not undergo hepatic metabolism; however, has been associated with transient increases in transaminase levels; use with caution.

Obesity A pharmacokinetic study confirmed that weight-based dosing (single doses of 75 or 175 units/kg) using actual body weight in heavy/obese patients between 100 and 165 kg led to achievement of similar anti-Xa activity levels compared to normal-weight patients (Hainer, 2002). However, there is limited clinical experience in patients with a BMI >40 kg/m^2.

Administration Patient should be lying down or sitting. Administer by deep SubQ injection into the lower abdomen, outer thigh, lower back, or upper arm. Injection site should be varied daily. To minimize bruising, do not rub the injection site. In hemodialysis patients, may be administered IV (patients with high or low hemorrhage risk) or added to the dialyzer circuit (patients with low hemorrhage risk).

Monitoring Parameters CBC (at baseline then twice weekly throughout therapy); renal function (use Cockcroft-Gault formula); hepatic function; potassium (baseline in patients at risk for hyperkalemia, monitor regularly if duration >7 days); stool for occult blood. Routine monitoring of anti-Xa levels is generally not recommended; however, anti-Xa levels may be beneficial in certain patients (eg, children, obese patients, patients with severe renal insufficiency receiving therapeutic doses, and possibly pregnant women receiving therapeutic doses) (Guyatt, 2012). Peak anti-Xa levels are measured 4-6 hours after administration. Monitoring of PT and/or aPTT is not of clinical benefit.

Reference Range Anti-Xa level (measured 4 hours after administration): Fixed-dose (3500 units): 0.15 anti-Xa units/mL; weight-based (75-175 units/kg): 0.34-0.70 anti-Xa units/mL; in treatment of venous thromboembolism, a target of 0.85 anti-Xa units/mL has been recommended (Garcia, 2012)

Children: Target anti-Xa level: 0.5-1 anti-Xa units/mL 4-6 hours after administration or 0.5-0.8 anti-Xa units/mL 2-6 hours after administration (Monagle, 2012)

Dosage Forms: Canada Excipient information presented when available (limited, particularly for generics); consult specific product labeling. [DSC] = Discontinued product Injection, solution, as sodium:
Innohep®: 10,000 anti-Xa units/mL (2 mL) [contains benzyl alcohol, sodium metabisulfite]
Innohep®: 20,000 anti-Xa units/mL (0.5 mL, 0.7 mL, 0.9 mL) [contains sodium metabisulfite]

Innohep®: 20,000 anti-Xa units/mL (2 mL) [contains benzyl alcohol, sodium metabisulfite]
Injection, solution, as sodium [preservative free]:
Innohep®: 10,000 anti-Xa units/mL (0.25 mL, 0.35 mL, 0.45 mL)

♦ **Tinzaparin Sodium** *see Tinzaparin on page 1791*
♦ **Tioguanine** *see Thioguanine on page 1783*
♦ **Tiotixene** *see Thiothixene on page 1784*

Tiotropium (ty oh TRO pee um)

Brand Names: US Spiriva HandiHaler; Spiriva Respimat
Brand Names: Canada Spiriva; Spiriva Respimat
Index Terms Tiotropium Bromide Monohydrate
Pharmacologic Category Anticholinergic Agent; Anticholinergic Agent, Long-Acting

Use
US labeling:
Asthma: Maintenance treatment of asthma in patients 12 years and older.
Chronic obstructive pulmonary disease: Maintenance treatment of bronchospasm associated with chronic obstructive pulmonary disease (COPD), including chronic bronchitis and emphysema; reduction of COPD exacerbations
Limitations of use: Not indicated for the relief of acute bronchospasm.

Canadian labeling:
Asthma: Add-on maintenance bronchodilator therapy in asthmatic adults who remain symptomatic despite combination therapy with an inhaled corticosteroid (equivalent to, but not limited to ≥500 mcg fluticasone or ≥800 mcg budesonide) and a long acting beta-2 agonist and who have experienced ≥1 severe exacerbations in the prior year.
Chronic obstructive pulmonary disease: Maintenance treatment of bronchospasm associated with chronic obstructive pulmonary disease (COPD), including chronic bronchitis and emphysema; reduction of COPD exacerbations
Limitations of use: Not indicated as rescue medication for relief of acute bronchospasm. Not indicated as first-line treatment or as monotherapy in asthma.

Pregnancy Considerations Adverse events have been observed in animal reproduction studies.

Breast-Feeding Considerations It is not known if tiotropium is excreted in breast milk. The manufacturer recommends that caution be exercised when administering tiotropium to nursing women.

Contraindications
Hypersensitivity to ipratropium, tiotropium, or any component of the formulation
Canadian labeling: Additional contraindications (not in US labeling): Hypersensitivity to atropine or its derivatives

Warnings/Precautions Paradoxical bronchospasm may occur with use of inhaled agents; discontinue use and consider other therapy if bronchospasm occurs. May cause dizziness and blurred vision; patients must be cautioned about performing tasks that require mental alertness (eg, operating machinery or driving).

Not indicated for the initial (rescue) treatment of acute episodes of bronchospasm. Use with caution in patients with narrow-angle glaucoma, prostatic hyperplasia, moderate-severe renal impairment, or bladder neck obstruction; avoid inadvertent instillation into the eyes. Immediate hypersensitivity reactions may occur; discontinue immediately if signs/symptoms occur. Use with caution in patients with a history of hypersensitivity to atropine. The Canadian labeling contraindicates use in patients with a history of hypersensitivity to atropine or its derivatives.

The contents of Spiriva capsules are for inhalation only via the HandiHaler device. There have been reports of incorrect administration (swallowing of the capsules). Capsule for oral inhalation contains lactose; use with caution in patients with severe milk protein allergy. The contents of Spiriva inhalation spray are for inhalation only via the Respimat inhaler. Potentially significant interactions may exist, requiring dose or frequency adjustment, additional monitoring, and/or selection of alternative therapy.

Adverse Reactions Non-postmarketing incidences listed are for powder for inhalation unless otherwise specified.
>10%:
Gastrointestinal: Xerostomia (powder and solution: 4% to 16%)
Respiratory: Upper respiratory tract infection (41% to 43%), pharyngitis (powder and solution: 7% to 16%), sinusitis (powder and solution: 3% to 11%)

1% to 10%:

Cardiovascular: Chest pain (powder and solution ≤7%), edema (dependent, 3% to 5%), angina pectoris (1% to 3%; includes exacerbation of angina pectoris), palpitations (powder and solution: ≤3%), hypertension (solution: 1% to 2%)

Central nervous system: Headache (powder and solution: 4% to 6%), depression (≤4%), insomnia (powder and solution: ≤4%), dizziness (powder and solution: ≤3%), paresthesia (1% to 3%), voice disorder (powder and solution: ≤3%)

Dermatologic: Skin rash (powder and solution: 1% to 4%), pruritus (powder and solution: ≤3%)

Endocrine & metabolic: Hypercholesterolemia (1% to 3%), hyperglycemia (1% to 3%)

Gastrointestinal: Abdominal pain (5% to 6%), dyspepsia (1% to 6%), constipation (powder and solution: 1% to 5%), omitting (1% to 4%), gastroesophageal reflux disease (powder and solution: ≤3%), gastrointestinal disease (not otherwise specified; 1% to 3%), oropharyngeal candidiasis (powder and solution:≤3%), stomatitis (includes ulcerative stomatitis; powder and solution: ≤3%), diarrhea (powder and solution: 1% to 2%)

Genitourinary: Urinary tract infection (powder and solution: 1% to 7%)

Hypersensitivity: Hypersensitivity reaction (powder and solution: ≤3%)

Infection: Candidiasis (3% to 4%), infection (1% to 4%), herpes zoster (powder and solution ≤3%)

Neuromuscular & skeletal: Arthralgia (4%), myalgia (4%), arthritis (≥3%), leg pain (1% to 3%), skeletal pain (1% to 3%)

Ophthalmic: Cataract (1% to 3%)

Respiratory: Rhinitis (powder and solution ≤6%), epistaxis (powder and solution ≤4%), cough (powder: ≥3%; solution: 1% to 2%), flu-like symptoms (≥3%), bronchitis (solution: 3%), laryngitis (powder and solution: ≤3%), allergic rhinitis (solution: 1% to 2%)

Respiratory: Rhinitis (powder and solution ≤6%), epistaxis (powder and solution ≤4%), cough (powder: ≥3%; solution: 1% to 2%), flu-like symptoms (≥3%), bronchitis (solution: 3%), laryngitis (powder and solution: ≤3%), allergic rhinitis (solution: 1% to 2%)

<1%, postmarketing, and/or case reports: Abnormal hepatic function tests, anaphylaxis, angioedema, application site irritation (powder; includes glossitis, oral mucosa ulcer, pharyngolaryngeal pain), atrial fibrillation, blurred vision, bronchospasm, dehydration, dermal ulcer, dysphagia, dysuria, gingivitis, glaucoma, glossitis, hepatic insufficiency, hoarseness, increased intraocular pressure, intestinal obstruction (includes paralytic ileus), joint swelling, limb pain, muscle spasm, mydriasis (if powder comes in contact with eyes), oropharyngeal pain, paradoxical bronchospasm, skin infection, supraventricular tachycardia, tachycardia, throat irritation, tonsillitis, urinary retention, urticaria, xeroderma

<1% (Limited to important or life-threatening): Anaphylaxis, application site irritation (powder; includes glossitis, oral mucosa ulcer, pharyngolaryngeal pain), atrial fibrillation, dermal ulcer, gingivitis, glaucoma, glossitis, hepatic insufficiency, intestinal obstruction (includes paralytic ileus), joint swelling, paradoxical bronchospasm, skin infection, supraventricular tachycardia, tachycardia, tonsillitis, urinary retention

Drug Interactions

Metabolism/Transport Effects Substrate of CYP2D6 (minor), CYP3A4 (minor); **Note:** Assignment of Major/Minor substrate status based on clinically relevant drug interaction potential

Avoid Concomitant Use

Avoid concomitant use of Tiotropium with any of the following: Aclidinium; Anticholinergic Agents; Cimetropium; Eluxadoline; Glucagon; Glycopyrrolate; Glycopyrrolate (Oral Inhalation); Ipratropium (Oral Inhalation); Levosulpiride; Loxapine; Potassium Chloride; Umeclidinium

Increased Effect/Toxicity

Tiotropium may increase the levels/effects of: AbobotulinumtoxinA; Analgesics (Opioid); Cannabinoid-Containing Products; Cimetropium; Eluxadoline; Glucagon; Glycopyrrolate; Glycopyrrolate (Oral Inhalation); Loxapine; Mirabegron; OnabotulinumtoxinA; Potassium Chloride; Ramosetron; RimabotulinumtoxinB; Thiazide Diuretics; Topiramate

The levels/effects of Tiotropium may be increased by: Aclidinium; Anticholinergic Agents; Ipratropium (Oral Inhalation); Mianserin; Pramlintide; Umeclidinium

Decreased Effect

Tiotropium may decrease the levels/effects of: Acetylcholinesterase Inhibitors; Gastrointestinal Agents (Prokinetic); Itopride; Levosulpiride; Secretin

The levels/effects of Tiotropium may be decreased by: Acetylcholinesterase Inhibitors

Storage/Stability Spiriva HandiHaler: Store at 25°C (77°F); excursions are permitted between 15°C and 30°C (59°F and 86°F). Avoid excessive temperatures and moisture. Do not store capsules in HandiHaler device. Capsules should be stored in the blister pack and only removed immediately before use. Once protective foil is peeled back and/or removed, the capsule should be used immediately; if capsule is not used immediately it should be discarded.

Spiriva Respimat: Store at 25°C (77°F); excursions are permitted between 15°C and 30°C (59°F and 86°F). Avoid freezing.

Mechanism of Action Competitively and reversibly inhibits the action of acetylcholine at type 3 muscarinic (M_3) receptors in bronchial smooth muscle causing bronchodilation

Pharmacodynamics/Kinetics

Absorption: Poorly absorbed from GI tract, systemic absorption may occur from lung

Distribution: V_d: 32 L/kg

Protein binding: 72%

Metabolism: Hepatic (minimal), via CYP2D6 and CYP3A4

Bioavailability: Following inhalation, 19.5% (dry powder inhalation) or ~33% (inhalation solution); Oral solution: 2% to 3%

Half-life elimination:

Dry powder inhalation: 5 to 6 days

Inhalation solution: Asthma: 44 hours; COPD: 25 hours

Time to peak, plasma:

Spiriva HandiHaler: 5 minutes (following inhalation)

Spiriva Respimat: 5 to 7 minutes (following inhalation)

Excretion: Urine (14% of an inhaled dose [Spiriva HandiHaler]; 18.6% of an inhaled dose (COPD) or 12.8% (asthma) [Spiriva Respimat]); feces (primarily nonabsorbed drug)

Dosing

Adult & Geriatric

Asthma::

US labeling: Oral inhalation: Spiriva Respimat (1.25 mcg/actuation): Two inhalations (2.5 mcg) once daily (maximum: 2 inhalations per 24 hours). **Note:** Maximum benefits may take up to 4 to 8 weeks of dosing.

Canadian labeling: Oral inhalation: Spiriva Respimat (2.5 mcg/actuation): Two inhalations (5 mcg) once daily (maximum: 2 inhalations per 24 hours). **Note:** Must be used in combination with an inhaled corticosteroid and a long acting beta₂-agonist.

COPD: Oral inhalation:

Spiriva HandiHaler: Contents of 1 capsule (18 mcg) inhaled once daily using HandiHaler device. **Note:** To ensure drug delivery, the contents of each capsule should be inhaled twice.

Spiriva Respimat (2.5 mcg/actuation): Two inhalations (5 mcg) once daily (maximum: 2 inhalations per 24 hours).

Pediatric Asthma: Children ≥12 years and Adolescents: Oral inhalation: Spiriva Respimat: Refer to adult dosing.

Renal Impairment No dosage adjustment necessary; use caution in moderate to severe renal impairment; monitor closely.

Hepatic Impairment No dosage adjustment necessary.

Administration For oral inhalation only.

Spiriva Handihaler: Capsule should not be swallowed. Administer once daily at the same time each day. Remove capsule from foil blister immediately before use. Place capsule in the center chamber of the HandiHaler Inhaler. Must only use the HandiHaler Inhaler. Close mouthpiece firmly until a click is heard, leaving dustcap open. The capsule is pierced by pressing and releasing the green piercing button on the side of the HandiHaler device. Exhale fully. Close lips tightly around mouthpiece; do not exhale into inhaler. Tilt head slightly back and inhale (rapidly, steadily, and deeply); the capsule vibration (rattle) may be heard within the device. Hold breath for a few seconds then repeat procedure using the same tiotropium capsule. Throw away empty capsule by tipping into a trash can without touching it; do not leave in inhaler. Keep capsules and inhaler dry.

Spiriva Respimat: Prior to first use, insert cartridge into the inhaler and prime the unit by actuating the inhaler toward the ground until an aerosol cloud is visible; repeat three more times and then the unit is primed and ready for use. If not used for more than 3 days, actuate the inhaler once to prepare the inhaler for use (Canadian labeling indicates that this process is required if the inhaler has not been used for more than 7 days). If not used for more than 21 days, actuate the inhaler until an aerosol cloud is visible and then repeat the process three more times to prepare the inhaler for use.

Monitoring Parameters FEV$_1$, peak flow (or other pulmonary function studies); anticholinergic adverse reactions (patients with CrCl ≤50 mL/min); signs and symptoms of narrow angle glaucoma and urinary retention

Dosage Forms Considerations Spiriva Respimat 4 g cartridges contain 60 metered actuations (institutional pack contains 28 metered actuations).

Dosage Forms Excipient information presented when available (limited, particularly for generics); consult specific product labeling.

Aerosol Solution, Inhalation:

Spiriva Respimat: 1.25 mcg/actuation (4 g); 2.5 mcg/actuation (4 g) [contains benzalkonium chloride, disodium edta]

Capsule, Inhalation:

Spiriva HandiHaler: 18 mcg [contains milk protein]

Tiotropium and Olodaterol
(ty oh TRO pee um & oh loe DA ter ol)

Brand Names: US Stiolto Respimat

Index Terms Tiotropium Bromide and Olodaterol

Pharmacologic Category Anticholinergic Agent; Anticholinergic Agent, Long-Acting; Beta$_2$ Agonist; Beta$_2$ Agonist, Long-Acting

Use

Chronic obstructive pulmonary disease: Maintenance treatment of airflow obstruction in patients with chronic obstructive pulmonary disease (COPD), including chronic bronchitis and/or emphysema.

Limitations of use: Not indicated to treat acute deteriorations of COPD; not indicated to treat asthma (safety and effectiveness in asthma have not been established)

Dosing

Adult & Geriatric COPD: Oral inhalation: Two inhalations once daily (maximum: 2 inhalations per day)

Renal Impairment

CrCl >60 mL/minute: No dosage adjustment necessary.

CrCl ≤60 mL/minute: No dosage adjustment necessary; monitor closely for anticholinergic adverse effects.

Hepatic Impairment No dosage adjustment necessary.

Additional Information Complete prescribing information should be consulted for additional detail.

Dosage Forms Excipient information presented when available (limited, particularly for generics); consult specific product labeling.

Aerosol Solution, Inhalation:

Stiolto Respimat: Tiotropium 2.5 mcg and olodaterol 2.5 mcg per actuation (4 g) [contains benzalkonium chloride, edetate disodium]

◆ Tiotropium Bromide and Olodaterol see Tiotropium and Olodaterol on page 1795

◆ Tiotropium Bromide Monohydrate see Tiotropium on page 1793

◆ Tipiracil and Trifluridine see Trifluridine and Tipiracil on page 1845

Tipranavir (tip RA na veer)

Brand Names: US Aptivus

Brand Names: Canada Aptivus

Index Terms PNU-140690E; TPV

Pharmacologic Category Antiretroviral, Protease Inhibitor (Anti-HIV)

Use HIV-1 infection: Treatment of HIV-1 infection in combination with ritonavir and other antiretroviral agents; limited to treatment-experienced or multiprotease inhibitor-resistant patients.

Pregnancy Considerations Adverse events were observed in some animal reproduction studies. Tipranavir crosses the human placenta. The DHHS Perinatal HIV Guidelines note there are insufficient data to recommend use during pregnancy; however, if used, tipranavir must be given with low-dose ritonavir boosting. A small increased risk of preterm birth has been associated with maternal use of protease inhibitor-based combination antiretroviral (ARV) therapy during pregnancy; however, the benefits of use generally outweigh this risk and protease inhibitors (PIs) should not be withheld if otherwise recommended. Hyperglycemia, new onset of diabetes mellitus, or diabetic ketoacidosis have been reported with PIs; it is not clear if pregnancy increases this risk.

Regardless of CD4 count or HIV RNA copy number, all HIV-infected pregnant women should receive a combination ARV drug regimen. A combination of antepartum, intrapartum, and infant ARV prophylaxis is recommended. ARV therapy should be started as soon as possible in women with symptomatic infection. Although earlier initiation may be more effective in reducing the perinatal transmission of HIV, initiation may be delayed until after 12 weeks' gestation in women who do not require immediate treatment after careful consideration of maternal conditions (eg, nausea and vomiting) and the potential risks of first trimester fetal exposure for specific agents. A scheduled cesarean delivery at 38 weeks' gestation is recommended for all women with HIV RNA >1000 copies/mL or unknown concentrations near delivery in order to decrease transmission. If ARV therapy must be interrupted for <24 hours during the peripartum period, stop then restart all medications simultaneously in order to decrease the chance of developing resistance. Long-term follow-up is recommended for all infants exposed to ARV medications. In couples who want to conceive, the HIV-infected partner should attain maximum viral suppression prior to conception.

Health care providers are encouraged to enroll pregnant women exposed to antiretroviral medications in the Antiretroviral Pregnancy Registry (1-800-258-4263 or www.APRegistry.com). Health care providers caring for HIV-infected women and their infants may contact the National Perinatal HIV Hotline (888-448-8765) for clinical consultation (HHS [perinatal] 2014).

Women receiving estrogen (as hormonal contraception or replacement therapy) may have an increased incidence of rash.

Breast-Feeding Considerations It is not known if tipranavir is excreted into breast milk. Maternal or infant antiretroviral therapy does not completely eliminate the risk of postnatal HIV transmission. In addition, multiclass-resistant virus has been detected in breast-feeding infants despite maternal therapy. Therefore, in the United States, where formula is accessible, affordable, safe, and sustainable, and the risk of infant mortality due to diarrhea and respiratory infections is low, complete avoidance of breast-feeding by HIV-infected women is recommended to decrease potential transmission of HIV (HHS [perinatal] 2014).

Contraindications

Concurrent therapy of tipranavir/ritonavir with drugs highly dependent upon CYP3A for clearance or are potent CYP3A inducers, including alfuzosin, amiodarone, bepridil, cisapride, ergot derivatives (eg, dihydroergotamine, ergonovine, ergotamine, methylergonovine), flecainide, lovastatin, midazolam (oral), pimozide, propafenone, quinidine, rifampin, sildenafil (for pulmonary arterial hypertension [eg, Revatio]), simvastatin, St John's wort, and triazolam; moderate-to-severe hepatic impairment (Child-Pugh class B or C)

Canadian labeling: Additional contraindications (not in US labeling): Hypersensitivity to tipranavir or any component of the product, concurrent therapy with colchicine, astemizole (not available in Canada), terfenadine (not available in Canada), or quetiapine.

Warnings/Precautions [US Boxed Warning]: In combination with ritonavir, clinical hepatitis and hepatic decompensation, including some fatalities, have been reported. May exacerbate preexisting hepatic dysfunction (causal relationship not established); patients with chronic hepatitis B or C coinfection have an increased risk. Assess liver function tests at baseline and frequently throughout treatment. Monitor patients closely, especially those with chronic hepatitis B or C coinfection; discontinue use if signs or symptoms of toxicity occur (eg, fatigue, malaise, anorexia, nausea, jaundice, bilirubinemia, acholic stools, liver tenderness or hepatomegaly) or if asymptomatic AST/ALT elevations >10 times ULN or AST/ALT elevations >5 to 10 times ULN concurrently with total bilirubin >2.5 times ULN occur. Treatment experienced patients with chronic hepatitis B or C coinfection or elevated transaminases are at ~2-fold risk for developing Grade 3 or 4 transaminase elevations or hepatic decompensation.

Use with caution in patients with Child-Pugh class A (mild) hepatic impairment; contraindicated in Child-Pugh class B or C (moderate-to-severe) impairment. Has been associated with a variety of skin reactions including rash (urticarial or maculopapular) and possible photosensitivity. In some cases rash was accompanied by joint pain or stiffness, throat tightness or generalized pruritus. Risk of rash increases in patients with lower CD4 counts. May be associated with fat redistribution (buffalo hump, increased abdominal girth, breast engorgement, facial atrophy). Use caution in hemophilia. With coadministered ritonavir, may increase cholesterol and/or triglycerides; hypertriglyceridemia may increase risk of pancreatitis. May cause hyperglycemia. Use with caution in patients with sulfonamide allergy. Patients may develop immune reconstitution syndrome resulting in the occurrence of an inflammatory response to an indolent or residual opportunistic infection during initial HIV treatment or activation of autoimmune

disorders (eg, Graves' disease, polymyositis, Guillain-Barré syndrome) later in therapy; further evaluation and treatment may be required.

[US Boxed Warning]: Tipranavir in combination with ritonavir has been associated with rare reports of fatal and nonfatal intracranial hemorrhage; causal relationship not established. Events often occurred in patients with medical conditions (eg, CNS lesions, head trauma, recent neurosurgery, coagulopathy, alcohol abuse) or concurrent therapy which may have influenced these events. No abnormal pattern of coagulation parameters has been observed in patients in general, or preceding intracranial hemorrhage development Tipranavir may inhibit platelet aggregation. Use with caution in patients who may be at risk for increased bleeding (trauma, surgery, other medical conditions or taking antiplatelet agents, anticoagulants, or supplemental high doses of vitamin E).

Potentially significant drug-drug interactions may exist, requiring dose or frequency adjustment, additional monitoring, and/or selection of alternative therapy.. Capsules contain dehydrated alcohol 7% w/w (0.1 g per capsule).

Adverse Reactions

>10%:

Dermatologic: Rash (children 21%; adults 3% to 10%)

Endocrine & metabolic: Hypertriglyceridemia (>400 mg/dL: 61%), hypercholesterolemia (>300 mg/dL: 22%)

Gastrointestinal: Diarrhea (15%)

Hepatic: Transaminases increased (>2.5 x ULN: 26% to 32%; grade 3/4: 10% to 20%)

Neuromuscular & skeletal: CPK increased (grade 3/4: children 11%)

2% to 10%:

Central nervous system: Fever (6% to 8%), fatigue (6%), headache (5%)

Endocrine & metabolic: Dehydration (2%)

Gastrointestinal: Nausea (5% to 9%), amylase increased (grade 3: 6% to 8%), vomiting (6%), abdominal pain (4%), diarrhea (children 4%), weight loss (2%)

Hematologic: Bleeding (children 8%), WBC decreased (grades 3: 5%), anemia (3%), neutropenia (2%)

Hepatic: ALT increased (2%, grades 3/4: 10%), AST increased (grades 3/4: 6%), GGT increased (2%)

Neuromuscular & skeletal: Myalgia (2%)

Respiratory: Cough (children 6%), dyspnea (2%), epistaxis (children 4%)

<2% (Limited to important or life-threatening): Abdominal distension, anorexia, appetite decreased, diabetes mellitus, dizziness, dyspepsia, exanthem, facial wasting, flatulence, flu-like syndrome, gastroesophageal reflux, hepatic failure, hepatic steatosis, hepatitis, hyperbilirubinemia, hyperglycemia, hypersensitivity, immune reconstitution syndrome, insomnia, intracranial hemorrhage, lipase increased, lipoatrophy, lipodystrophy (acquired), lipohypertrophy, malaise, mitochondrial toxicity, muscle cramp, neuropathy (peripheral), pancreatitis, pruritus, renal insufficiency, sleep disorder, somnolence, thrombocytopenia

Drug Interactions

Metabolism/Transport Effects Substrate of CYP3A4 (major); **Note:** Assignment of Major/Minor substrate status based on clinically relevant drug interaction potential; **Inhibits** BSEP, CYP2D6 (strong); **Induces** P-glycoprotein

Avoid Concomitant Use

Avoid concomitant use of Tipranavir with any of the following: Alfuzosin; Amiodarone; AtorvaSTATin; Bepridil; Boceprevir; Cholic Acid; Cisapride; Dabigatran Etexilate; Ergot Derivatives; Etravirine; Flecainide; Fluticasone (Nasal); Fluticasone (Oral Inhalation); Ledipasvir; Lomitapide; Lovastatin; Mequitazine; Midazolam; Pimozide; Propafenone; Protease Inhibitors; QuiNIDine; Rifampin; Salmeterol; Simeprevir; Simvastatin; Sofosbuvir; St Johns Wort; Tadalafil; Tamoxifen; Telaprevir; Thioridazine; Triazolam; VinCRIStine (Liposomal)

Increased Effect/Toxicity

Tipranavir may increase the levels/effects of: Agents with Antiplatelet Properties; Alfuzosin; ALPRAZolam; Amiodarone; Anticoagulants; ARIPiprazole; ARIPiprazole Lauroxil; AtoMOXetine; AtorvaSTATin; Bepridil; Bosentan; Brexpiprazole; Calcium Channel Blockers (Nondihydropyridine); CarBAMazepine; Cholic Acid; Cisapride; Clarithromycin; Colchicine; Contraceptives (Progestins); Cyclophosphamide; CycloSPORINE (Systemic); CYP2D6 Substrates; Dapoxetine; Digoxin; DOXOrubicin (Conventional); DULoxetine; Eliglustat; Eluxadoline; Enfuvirtide; Ergot Derivatives; Fesoterodine; Flecainide; Fluticasone (Nasal); Fluticasone (Oral Inhalation); Iloperidone; Itraconazole; Ketoconazole (Systemic); Lomitapide; Lovastatin; Meperidine; Mequitazine; Metoprolol; Midazolam; Nebivolol; Nefazodone; Pimozide;

Propafenone; Protease Inhibitors; QuiNIDine; Rifabutin; Riociguat; Rosuvastatin; Salmeterol; Sildenafil; Simeprevir; Simvastatin; Tacrolimus (Systemic); Tacrolimus (Topical); Tadalafil; Tamsulosin; Temsirolimus; Tetrabenazine; Thioridazine; TraMADol; TraZODone; Triazolam; Tricyclic Antidepressants; Vitamin E; Vitamin E (Oral); Vortioxetine

The levels/effects of Tipranavir may be increased by: Clarithromycin; CycloSPORINE (Systemic); Delavirdine; Disulfiram; Enfuvirtide; Estrogen Derivatives; Fluconazole; MetroNIDAZOLE (Systemic); MetroNIDAZOLE (Topical); Osimertinib; Simeprevir

Decreased Effect

Tipranavir may decrease the levels/effects of: Abacavir; Afatinib; Antidiabetic Agents; Boceprevir; Brentuximab Vedotin; Clarithromycin; Codeine; Dabigatran Etexilate; Delavirdine; Didanosine; Dolutegravir; DOXOrubicin (Conventional); Estrogen Derivatives; Etravirine; Fosphenytoin; Hydrocodone; Iloperidone; Ledipasvir; Linagliptin; Meperidine; Methadone; P-glycoprotein/ABCB1 Substrates; PHENobarbital; Phenytoin; Protease Inhibitors; Proton Pump Inhibitors; Raltegravir; Sofosbuvir; Tamoxifen; Telaprevir; Tenofovir Disoproxil Fumarate; Theophylline Derivatives; TraMADol; Valproate Products; VinCRIStine (Liposomal); Zidovudine

The levels/effects of Tipranavir may be decreased by: Boceprevir; Bosentan; CarBAMazepine; CYP3A4 Inducers (Moderate); CYP3A4 Inducers (Strong); Dabrafenib; Deferasirox; Enzalutamide; Fosphenytoin; Garlic; Mitotane; Osimertinib; PHENobarbital; Phenytoin; Rifampin; Siltuximab; St Johns Wort; Tenofovir Disoproxil Fumarate; Tocilizumab

Storage/Stability

Capsule: Prior to opening bottle, store at 2°C to 8°C (36°F to 46°F). After bottle is opened, may be stored at 25°C (77°F) for up to 60 days.

Oral solution: Store at 25°C (77°F); excursions permitted to 15°C to 30°C (59°F to 86°F). After bottle is open, use within 60 days. Do not refrigerate or freeze oral solution.

Mechanism of Action

Binds to the site of HIV-1 protease activity and inhibits cleavage of viral Gag-Pol polyprotein precursors into individual functional proteins required for infectious HIV. This results in the formation of immature, noninfectious viral particles.

Pharmacodynamics/Kinetics

Absorption: Incomplete (percentage not established)

Distribution: V_d: 7.7 to 10 L

Protein binding: >99% (albumin, alpha$_1$-acid glycoprotein)

Metabolism: Hepatic, via CYP3A4 (minimal when coadministered with ritonavir)

Bioavailability: Not established

Half-life elimination: Children 2 to <6 years of age: ~8 hours, 6 to <12 years of age: ~7 hours, 12 to 18 years: ~5 hours; Adults: 6 hours

Time to peak, plasma: 3 hours

Excretion: Feces (82%); urine (4%); primarily as unchanged drug (when coadministered with ritonavir)

Dosing

Adult & Geriatric HIV-1 infection: Oral: 500 mg twice daily; **Note:** Coadministration with ritonavir (200 mg twice daily) is required.

Pediatric

HIV-1 infection: Children ≥2 years and Adolescents: Oral: Canadian labeling does not approve of use in patients <18 years.

US labeling: 14 mg/kg or 375 mg/m² (maximum: 500 mg/dose) twice daily. **Note:** Coadministration with ritonavir (6 mg/kg or 150 mg/m² [maximum: 200 mg/dose] twice daily) is required.

If intolerance or toxicity develops and virus is not resistant to multiple protease inhibitors: May decrease dose to 12 mg/kg or 290 mg/m² twice daily. **Note:** Coadministration with ritonavir (5 mg/kg or 115 mg/m² twice daily) is required.

Renal Impairment There are no dosage adjustments provided in the manufacturer's labeling (has not been studied). However, dosage adjustment not expected since renal clearance is negligible. Guidelines state that dosage adjustment is not required (HHS [adult] 2015).

Hepatic Impairment

Child-Pugh class A (mild impairment): There are no dosage adjustments provided in the manufacturer's labeling; use with caution.

Child-Pugh class B or C (moderate-to-severe impairment): Use is contraindicated.

Adjustment for Toxicity

Asymptomatic patients:

AST or ALT 5 to 10 times ULN and total bilirubin >2.5 times ULN: Discontinue therapy.

AST or ALT >10 times ULN: Discontinue therapy.

Dietary Considerations Capsule contains dehydrated ethanol. Oral solution formulation contains vitamin E; additional vitamin E supplements should be avoided.

Administration Oral: Tipranavir must be coadministered with ritonavir. When using ritonavir tablets, administer with food (HHS [adult] 2015; (HHS [pediatric] 2014). When using ritonavir capsules or solution, administer with food for pediatric patients (HHS [pediatric] 2014); may be administered without regard to meals for adult patients (HHS [adult] 2015). Canadian labeling states that adults should take with food.

Monitoring Parameters Triglycerides and total cholesterol at baseline and during therapy. Liver function tests (including bilirubin) at baseline and frequently throughout therapy; patients with chronic hepatitis B or C coinfection should be monitored closely. Monitor also for symptoms of hepatotoxicity (eg, fatigue, malaise, anorexia, nausea, jaundice, bilirubinemia, acholic stools, liver tenderness or hepatomegaly) or if asymptomatic AST/ALT elevations >10 times ULN or AST/ALT elevations >5 to 10 times ULN concurrently with total bilirubin >2.5 times the ULN (discontinue if it occurs). Monitor viral load, CD4, and serum glucose as clinically indicated

Dosage Forms Excipient information presented when available (limited, particularly for generics); consult specific product labeling.

Capsule, Oral:
Aptivus: 250 mg
Solution, Oral:
Aptivus: 100 mg/mL (95 mL) [contains polyethylene glycol, propylene glycol, tocophersolan; buttermint-butter toffee flavor]

Tirofiban (tye roe FYE ban)

Brand Names: US Aggrastat
Brand Names: Canada Aggrastat
Index Terms MK383; Tirofiban Hydrochloride
Pharmacologic Category Antiplatelet Agent, Glycoprotein IIb/IIIa Inhibitor
Use Unstable angina/non-ST-elevation myocardial infarction: Decrease the rate of thrombotic cardiovascular events (combined end point of death, MI, or refractory ischemia/repeat cardiac procedure) in patients with non-ST-elevation acute coronary syndrome (unstable angina/non-ST-elevation myocardial infarction [UA/NSTEMI]).

Pregnancy Considerations Adverse events have not been observed in animal reproduction studies. Information related to use in pregnancy is limited; successful use during pregnancy has been described in a case report (Boztosun, 2008).

Breast-Feeding Considerations It is not known if tirofiban is excreted in breast milk. Due to the potential for serious adverse reactions in the nursing infant, a decision should be made whether to discontinue nursing or to discontinue the drug, taking into account the importance of treatment to the mother.

Contraindications Severe hypersensitivity reaction (ie, anaphylactic reaction) to tirofiban or any component of the formulation; history of thrombocytopenia following prior exposure to tirofiban; active internal bleeding or a history of bleeding diathesis, major surgical procedure, or severe physical trauma within the previous month

Warnings/Precautions Bleeding is the most common complication encountered during this therapy; most major bleeding occurs at the arterial access site for cardiac catheterization. Caution in patients with platelets <150,000/mm³; patients with hemorrhagic retinopathy; chronic dialysis patients; when used in combination with other drugs impacting on coagulation. Percutaneous coronary intervention: Prior to pulling the sheath, ACT should be <180 seconds or aPTT <50 seconds (ACCF/AHA/SCAI [Levine, 2011]). Use standard compression techniques after sheath removal. Watch the site closely afterwards for further bleeding. Sheath hemostasis should be achieved at least 4 hours before hospital discharge. Other trauma and vascular punctures should be minimized. Avoid obtaining vascular access through a noncompressible site (eg, subclavian or jugular vein).

Profound thrombocytopenia has been reported with use of tirofiban. If during therapy platelet count decreases to <90,000/mm³, monitor platelet counts to exclude pseudo-thrombocytopenia. If thrombocytopenia is confirmed, discontinue tirofiban and heparin if administered concurrently. Platelet counts should recover rapidly (within 1 to 5 days) after discontinuation. Previous exposure to a glycoprotein IIb/IIIa inhibitor may increase the risk of thrombocytopenia. Use is contraindicated in patients with a history of thrombocytopenia following exposure to tirofiban. Specific management guidelines for GP IIb/IIIa induced thrombocytopenia have been published (Huxtable, 2006; Llevadot, 2000).

Discontinue at least 2 to 4 hours prior to coronary artery bypass graft surgery (ACCF/AHA [Anderson, 2013]; ACCF/AHA [Hillis, 2011]). Dosage reduction of the maintenance infusion rate is necessary in patients with CrCl ≤60 mL/minute.

Adverse Reactions Bleeding is the major drug-related adverse effect. Patients received background treatment with aspirin and heparin. Adverse reactions reported are derived from both the high-dose bolus regimen **and** the dosing regimen used in studies that established the effectiveness of tirofiban. Frequency not always defined.

>10%: Hematologic & oncologic: Minor hemorrhage (TIMI criteria minor bleeding; 10.5% to 12%; transfusion required: 4% to 4.3%)

1% to 10%:
Cardiovascular: Coronary artery dissection (5%), bradycardia (4%), edema (2%), vasodepressor syncope (2%)
Central nervous system: Dizziness (3%), headache (>1%)
Dermatologic: Diaphoresis (2%)
Gastrointestinal: Nausea (>1%)
Genitourinary: Pelvic pain (6%)
Hematologic & oncologic: Major hemorrhage (TIMI criteria major bleeding: 1.4% to 2.2%; including hematoma [femoral]: 2% [Valgimigli, 2005], intracranial bleeding, GI bleeding, retroperitoneal bleeding [Aydin, 2003], GU bleeding, pulmonary alveolar hemorrhage [Guo, 2012], spinal-epidural hematoma), thrombocytopenia: <90,000/mm³ (1.5% to 1.9%), <50,000/mm³ (0.3% to 0.5%)
Neuromuscular & skeletal: Leg pain (3%)
Miscellaneous: Fever (>1%)
<1% (Limited to important or life-threatening): Anaphylaxis, hemopericardium, hypersensitivity

Drug Interactions
Metabolism/Transport Effects None known.
Avoid Concomitant Use
Avoid concomitant use of Tirofiban with any of the following: Urokinase
Increased Effect/Toxicity
Tirofiban may increase the levels/effects of: Agents with Antiplatelet Properties; Anticoagulants; Apixaban; Collagenase (Systemic); Dabigatran Etexilate; Deoxycholic Acid; Edoxaban; Ibritumomab; Obinutuzumab; Rivaroxaban; Salicylates; Thrombolytic Agents; Tositumomab and Iodine I 131 Tositumomab; Urokinase

The levels/effects of Tirofiban may be increased by: Dasatinib; Glucosamine; Herbs (Anticoagulant/Antiplatelet Properties); Ibrutinib; Limaprost; Multivitamins/Fluoride (with ADE); Multivitamins/Minerals (with ADEK, Folate, Iron); Multivitamins/Minerals (with AE, No Iron); Omega-3 Fatty Acids; Pentosan Polysulfate Sodium; Pentoxifylline; Prostacyclin Analogues; Tipranavir; Vitamin E; Vitamin E (Oral)

Decreased Effect There are no known significant interactions involving a decrease in effect.

Storage/Stability Store at 25°C (77°F); excursions are permitted between 15°C and 30°C (59°F and 86°F); do not freeze. Protect from light during storage.

Mechanism of Action A reversible antagonist of fibrinogen binding to the glycoprotein (GP) IIb/IIIa receptor, the major platelet surface receptor involved in platelet aggregation. When administered intravenously, it inhibits *ex vivo* platelet aggregation in a dose- and concentration-dependent manner. When given according to the recommended regimen, >90% inhibition is attained within 10 minutes after initiation. Platelet aggregation inhibition is reversible following cessation of the infusion.

Pharmacodynamics/Kinetics
Onset: >90% inhibition of platelet aggregation (reversible after discontinuation) seen within 10 minutes
Distribution: V_{dss}: 22 to 42 L
Protein Binding: 65% (concentration dependent)
Metabolism: Negligible
Half-life elimination: 2 hours; **Note:** In ~90% of patients, *ex vivo* platelet aggregation returns to near baseline in 4 to 8 hours after discontinuation.
Excretion: Urine (65%) and feces (25%) primarily as unchanged drug

Dosing
Adult & Geriatric
Unstable angina/non-ST-elevation myocardial infarction (UA/NSTEMI): IV: Loading dose: 25 mcg/kg administered over 5 minutes or less; Maintenance infusion: 0.15 mcg/kg/minute continued for up to 18 hours

Percutaneous coronary intervention (PCI): IV: Loading dose: 25 mcg/kg administered over 5 minutes or less at the time of PCI; Maintenance infusion: 0.15 mcg/kg/minute continued for up to 18 hours (ACCF/AHA [Anderson 2013]; ACCF/AHA/SCAI [Levine 2011]; Valgimigli 2004).

Stable ischemic heart disease (high-risk features) undergoing elective PCI (off-label use): Loading dose: 25 mcg/kg administered over 5 minutes or less at the time of PCI; Maintenance infusion: 0.15 mcg/kg/minute; was continued for up to 48 hours in the clinical trial (ACCF/AHA/SCAI [Levine 2011], Valgimigli 2004). **Note:** Reserve for patients who were not pretreated with clopidogrel or who are undergoing elective PCI with stent implantation with adequate clopidogrel pretreatment (ACCF/AHA/SCAI [Levine 2011]).

ST-elevation myocardial infarction (STEMI) undergoing primary PCI (off-label use): IV Loading dose: 25 mcg/kg administered over 5 minutes or less at the time of PCI; Maintenance infusion: 0.15 mcg/kg/minute in combination with heparin or bivalirudin in selected patients; was continued for 18-24 hours in clinical trials (ACCF/AHA [O'Gara 2013]; ACCF/AHA/SCAI [Levine 2011]; Valgimigli 2008; Van't Hof 2008)

Renal Impairment
CrCl >60 mL/minute: No dosage reduction necessary.
CrCl ≤60 mL/minute: IV Loading dose: 25 mcg/kg administered over 5 minutes or less; Maintenance infusion: 0.075 mcg/kg/minute continued for up to 18 hours.

Administration IV: Administer loading dose over 5 minutes or less, followed by a continuous infusion. **Note:** Clinical trials administered tirofiban loading dose over a period of 3 minutes (Valgimigli 2004; Valgimigli 2005; Valgimigli 2009).

Monitoring Parameters Platelet count (baseline; 6 hours after initiation and daily thereafter during therapy). Monitor platelet counts more closely in patients who have had previous exposure to glycoprotein IIb/IIa antagonists. Persistent reductions of platelet counts <90,000/mm^3 may require interruption or discontinuation of infusion; hemoglobin and hematocrit; signs of bleeding.

Standard post-PCI assessment if patient undergoes PCI (eg, monitoring vascular access site, monitoring for chest pain and signs of bleeding)

Dosage Forms Excipient information presented when available (limited, particularly for generics); consult specific product labeling.
Solution, Intravenous:
Aggrastat: 50 mcg/mL (100 mL, 250 mL)

TiZANidine (tye ZAN i deen)

Brand Names: US Zanaflex
Brand Names: Canada Apo-Tizanidine; Gen-Tizanidine; Mylan-Tizanidine; Pal-Tizanidine; Zanaflex
Index Terms Sirdalud
Pharmacologic Category Alpha$_2$-Adrenergic Agonist
Use Muscle spasticity: Management of spasticity; reserve treatment with tizanidine for daily activities and times when relief of spasticity is most important.
Pregnancy Considerations Adverse events were observed in some animal reproduction studies.
Breast-Feeding Considerations Excretion in breast milk is unknown, but expected due to lipid solubility.
Contraindications Concomitant therapy with ciprofloxacin or fluvoxamine (potent CYP1A2 inhibitors)
Warnings/Precautions Significant hypotension, syncope, and sedation may occur; use caution in patients at risk for severe hypotensive effects (eg, patients taking concurrent medications which may predispose to hypotension) or sedative effects (patients must be cautioned about performing tasks which require mental alertness [eg, operating machinery or driving]). Effects with other sedative drugs or ethanol may be potentiated. Potentially significant drug-drug interactions may exist, requiring close or frequency adjustment, additional monitoring, and/or selection of alternative therapy. Use caution in any patient with renal impairment. Clearance decreased significantly in patients with severe impairment (CrCl <25 mL/minute); dose reductions recommended. Use not recommended in patients with hepatic impairment; potential for hepatotoxicity likely

due to extensive hepatic metabolism. Monitor aminotransferases prior to and during use or if hepatic injury is suspected.

May be inappropriate in older adults depending on comorbidities (eg, dementia, delirium) due to its potent anticholinergic effects (Beers Criteria). Use with caution; clearance decreased fourfold in the elderly; may increase risk of adverse effects and/or duration of effects. Elderly with severe renal impairment (CrCl <25 mL/minute) may have clearance reduced by >50% compared to healthy elderly subjects.

Use has been associated with visual hallucinations or delusions; use caution in patients with psychiatric disorders. Consider discontinuation of therapy if hallucinations occur. Withdrawal resulting in rebound hypertension, tachycardia, and hypertonia may occur upon discontinuation; doses should be decreased slowly, particularly in patients taking concomitant narcotics or receiving high doses (20 to 28 mg daily) for prolonged periods (≥9 weeks). Food alters absorption profile relative to administration under fasting conditions. In addition, bioequivalence between capsules and tablets is altered by food; capsules and tablets are bioequivalent under fasting conditions, but not under nonfasting conditions.

Adverse Reactions Frequency percentages below reported during multiple-dose studies, unless specified otherwise.
>10%:
Cardiovascular: Hypotension (16% to 33%)
Central nervous system: Somnolence (48%), dizziness (16%)
Gastrointestinal: Xerostomia (49%)
Neuromuscular & skeletal: Weakness (41%)
1% to 10%:
Cardiovascular: Bradycardia (12% to 10%)
Central nervous system: Nervousness (3%), speech disorder (3%), visual hallucinations/delusions (3%), anxiety (1%), depression (1%), fever (1%)
Dermatologic: Rash (1%), skin ulcer (1%)
Gastrointestinal: Constipation (4%), vomiting (3%), abdominal pain (1%), diarrhea (1%), dyspepsia (1%)
Genitourinary: UTI (10%), urinary frequency (3%)
Hepatic: Liver enzymes increased (3% to 5%)
Neuromuscular & skeletal: Dyskinesia (3%), back pain (1%), myasthenia (1%), paresthesia (1%)
Ocular: Blurred vision (3%)
Respiratory: Pharyngitis (3%), rhinitis (3%)
Miscellaneous: Infection (6%), flu-like syndrome (3%), diaphoresis (1%)
<1%, frequency not defined, and postmarketing experience (limited to important or life-threatening): Abnormal dreams, abnormal thinking, abscess, adrenal insufficiency, allergic reaction, anemia, angina pectoris, arrhythmia, carcinoma (including skin), cholelithiasis, deafness, dementia, depersonalization, dyslipidemia, gastrointestinal hemorrhage, glaucoma, heart failure, hepatomegaly, hemiplegia, hepatic failure, hepatitis, hepatoma, herpes infections, hypercholesterolemia, hyperglycemia, hypokalemia, hyponatremia, hypoproteinemia, hypothyroidism, intestinal obstruction, jaundice, leukopenia, leukocytosis, MI, migraine, neuralgia, optic neuritis, orthostatic hypotension, palpitation, paralysis, psychotic-like symptoms, pulmonary embolus, purpura, respiratory acidosis, retinal hemorrhage, seizure, sepsis, suicide attempt, syncope, thrombocythemia, thrombocytopenia, ventricular extrasystoles, ventricular tachycardia, vertigo

Drug Interactions
Metabolism/Transport Effects Substrate of CYP1A2 (major); **Note:** Assignment of Major/Minor substrate status based on clinically relevant drug interaction potential
Avoid Concomitant Use
Avoid concomitant use of TiZANidine with any of the following: Azelastine (Nasal); Ceritinib; CYP1A2 Inhibitors (Moderate); CYP1A2 Inhibitors (Strong); Iobenguane I 123; Orphenadrine; Paraldehyde; Thalidomide
Increased Effect/Toxicity
TiZANidine may increase the levels/effects of: ACE Inhibitors; Alcohol (Ethyl); Amifostine; Antipsychotic Agents (Second Generation [Atypical]); Azelastine (Nasal); Beta-Blockers; Bradycardia-Causing Agents; Buprenorphine; Ceritinib; CNS Depressants; DULoxetine; Highest Risk QTc-Prolonging Agents; Hydrocodone; Hypotension-Associated Agents; Ivabradine; Lacosamide; Levodopa; Lisinopril; Methotrimeprazine; Metyrosine; Moderate Risk QTc-Prolonging Agents; Orphenadrine; Paraldehyde; Pramipexole; Rotigotine; Selective Serotonin Reuptake Inhibitors; Suvorexant; Thalidomide; Zolpidem

The levels/effects of TiZANidine may be increased by: Alfuzosin; Barbiturates; Beta-Blockers; Blood Pressure Lowering Agents; Bretylium; Brimonidine (Topical);

Cannabis; CYP1A2 Inhibitors (Moderate); CYP1A2 Inhibitors (Strong); CYP1A2 Inhibitors (Weak); Diazoxide; Doxylamine; Dronabinol; Droperidol; Herbs (Hypotensive Properties); HydrOXYzine; Magnesium Sulfate; Methotrimeprazine; Mifepristone; Minocycline; Molsidomine; Nabilone; Nicorandil; Obinutuzumab; Perampanel; Phosphodiesterase 5 Inhibitors; Prostacyclin Analogues; Rufinamide; Ruxolitinib; Sodium Oxybate; Tapentadol; Tetrahydrocannabinol; Tofacitinib

Decreased Effect

TiZANidine may decrease the levels/effects of: lobenguane I 123

The levels/effects of TiZANidine may be decreased by: Mirtazapine; Serotonin/Norepinephrine Reuptake Inhibitors; Tricyclic Antidepressants

Food Interactions The tablet and capsule dosage forms are not bioequivalent when administered with food. Food increases both the time to peak concentration and the extent of absorption for both the tablet and capsule. However, maximal concentrations of tizanidine achieved when administered with food were increased by 30% for the tablet, but decreased by 20% for the capsule. Under fed conditions, the capsule is approximately 80% bioavailable relative to the tablet. Management: Administer with or without food, but keep consistent.

Storage/Stability Store at 25°C (77°F); excursions are permitted between 15°C and 30°C (59°F and 86°F).

Mechanism of Action An alpha$_2$-adrenergic agonist agent which decreases spasticity by increasing presynaptic inhibition; effects are greatest on polysynaptic pathways; overall effect is to reduce facilitation of spinal motor neurons.

Pharmacodynamics/Kinetics

Onset: Single dose (8 mg): Peak effect: 1-2 hours

Duration: Single dose (8 mg): 3-6 hours

Absorption: Tablets and capsules are bioequivalent under fasting conditions, but not under nonfasting conditions.

Tablets administered with food: Peak plasma concentration is increased by ~30%; time to peak increased by 25 minutes; extent of absorption increased by ~30%.

Capsules administered with food: Peak plasma concentration decreased by 20%; time to peak increased by 2-3 hours; extent of absorption increased by ~10%.

Capsules opened and sprinkled on applesauce are not bioequivalent to administration of intact capsules under fasting conditions. Peak plasma concentration and AUC are increased by 15% to 20%; time to peak decreased by 15 minutes.

Distribution: IV: 2.4 L/kg

Protein binding: ~30%

Metabolism: Extensively hepatic via CYP1A2 to inactive metabolites

Bioavailability: ~40% (extensive first-pass metabolism)

Half-life elimination: ~2.5 hours

Time to peak, serum:
Fasting state: Capsule, tablet: 1 hour
Fed state: Capsule: 3-4 hours, Tablet: 1.5 hours

Excretion: Urine (60%); feces (20%)

Dosing

Adult Spasticity: Oral: Initial: 2 mg up to 3 times daily (at 6- to 8-hour intervals) as needed; may titrate to optimal effect in 2-4 mg increments per dose (with a minimum of 1-4 days between dose increases); maximum: 36 mg daily. Note: Single doses >16 mg have not been studied. *Discontinuation of therapy:* Gradually taper dose by 2-4 mg daily.

Geriatric Use with caution; clearance is decreased. Refer to adult dosing.

Renal Impairment

CrCl ≥25 mL/minute: No dosage adjustment provided in manufacturer's labeling; however, caution may be needed as creatinine clearance decreases.

CrCl <25 mL/minute: Use with caution; clearance reduced >50%. During initial dose titration, use reduced doses. If higher doses are necessary, increase dose instead of increasing dosing frequency.

Hepatic Impairment Avoid use in hepatic impairment; if used, reduce dose during initial dose titration. If higher doses are necessary, increase dose instead of increasing dosing frequency. Monitor aminotransferases.

Dietary Considerations Administration with food compared to administration in the fasting state results in clinically-significant differences in absorption and other pharmacokinetic parameters. Patients should be consistent and should not switch administration of the tablets or the capsules between the fasting and nonfasting state. In addition, switching between the capsules and the tablets in the fed state will also result in significant differences. Opening capsule contents to sprinkle on applesauce compared to swallowing intact capsules whole will also result in

significant absorption differences. Patients should be consistent with regards to administration.

Administration Capsules may be opened and contents sprinkled on food; however, extent of absorption is increased up to 20% relative to administration of the capsule under fasted conditions.

Monitoring Parameters Monitor liver function (aminotransferases) at baseline and 1 month after maximum dose achieved or if hepatic injury suspected; blood pressure; renal function

Dosage Forms Excipient information presented when available (limited, particularly for generics); consult specific product labeling.

Capsule, Oral:
Zanaflex: 2 mg, 4 mg, 6 mg
Generic: 2 mg, 4 mg, 6 mg

Tablet, Oral:
Zanaflex: 4 mg [scored]
Generic: 2 mg, 4 mg

Tobramycin (Systemic) (toe bra MYE sin)

Brand Names: Canada JAMP-Tobramycin; Tobramycin For Injection; Tobramycin For Injection, USP; Tobramycin Injection; Tobramycin Injection, USP

Index Terms Tobramycin Sulfate

Pharmacologic Category Antibiotic, Aminoglycoside

Use Treatment of documented or suspected infections caused by susceptible gram-negative bacilli, including *Pseudomonas aeruginosa*.

Pregnancy Considerations [US Boxed Warning]: Aminoglycosides may cause fetal harm if administered to a pregnant woman. Tobramycin crosses the placenta. There are several reports of total irreversible bilateral congenital deafness in children whose mothers received another aminoglycoside (streptomycin) during pregnancy. Although serious side effects to the fetus/infant have not been reported following maternal use of all aminoglycosides, a potential for harm exists.

Due to pregnancy-induced physiologic changes, some pharmacokinetic parameters of tobramycin may be altered (Bourget 1991). Tobramycin injection may be used for the management of cystic fibrosis in pregnant patients with *Pseudomonas aeruginosa* (inhalation is preferred unless risk of infection is great) (Edenborough 2008).

Breast-Feeding Considerations Tobramycin is found in breast milk following injection (Festini 2006; Uwaydah 1975).

As a class, aminoglycosides are expected to be poorly distributed into breast milk, limiting systemic exposure to a nursing infant. In general, modification of bowel flora may occur with any antibiotic exposure (Chung 2002). Based on low serum concentrations and low absorption, breast-feeding is generally considered compatible in women

using tobramycin for the management of cystic fibrosis (Edenborough 2008).

Contraindications Hypersensitivity to tobramycin, other aminoglycosides, or any component of the formulation

Warnings/Precautions [US Boxed Warning]: Aminoglycosides may cause neurotoxicity and/or nephrotoxicity; usual risk factors include preexisting renal impairment, concomitant neuro-/nephrotoxic medications, advanced age, and dehydration. Ototoxicity may be directly proportional to the amount of drug given and the duration of treatment; tinnitus or vertigo are indications of vestibular injury and impending hearing loss; renal damage is usually reversible. Tinnitus and/or hearing loss have also been reported. May cause neuromuscular blockade, respiratory failure, and prolonged respiratory paralysis, especially when given soon after anesthesia or muscle relaxants. **[US Boxed Warnings]: Aminoglycosides may cause fetal harm if administered to a pregnant woman.**

Not intended for long-term therapy due to toxic hazards associated with extended administration; use caution in preexisting renal insufficiency, vestibular or cochlear impairment, myasthenia gravis, Parkinson's disease, hypocalcemia, and conditions which depress neuromuscular transmission. Dosage modification required in patients with impaired renal function during systemic therapy. Prolonged use may result in fungal or bacterial superinfection, including *C. difficile*-associated diarrhea (CDAD) and pseudomembranous colitis; CDAD has been observed >2 months postantibiotic treatment. Solution may contain sodium metabisulfate; use caution in patients with sulfite allergy. Solution for injection may contain sodium metabisulfate; use caution in patients with sulfite allergy.

Potentially significant drug-drug interactions may exist, requiring dose or frequency adjustment, additional monitoring, and/or selection of alternative therapy.

Adverse Reactions Frequency not defined.

Central nervous system: Confusion, disorientation, dizziness, headache, lethargy, vertigo

Dermatologic: Exfoliative dermatitis, pruritus, skin rash, urticaria

Endocrine & metabolic: Decreased serum calcium, decreased serum magnesium, decreased serum potassium, decreased serum sodium, increased lactate dehydrogenase, increased nonprotein nitrogen

Gastrointestinal: Diarrhea, nausea, vomiting

Genitourinary: Casts in urine, oliguria, proteinuria

Hematologic & oncologic: Anemia, eosinophilia, granulocytopenia, leukocytosis, leukopenia, thrombocytopenia

Hepatic: Increased serum ALT, increased serum AST, increased serum bilirubin

Local: Pain at injection site

Otic: Auditory ototoxicity, hearing loss, tinnitus, vestibular ototoxicity

Renal: Increased blood urea nitrogen, increased serum creatinine

Miscellaneous: Fever

<1% (Limited to important or life-threatening): Anaphylaxis, *clostridium difficile* associated diarrhea, erythema multiforme, Stevens-Johnson syndrome, toxic epidermal necrolysis

Drug Interactions

Metabolism/Transport Effects None known.

Avoid Concomitant Use

Avoid concomitant use of Tobramycin (Systemic) with any of the following: BCG (Intravesical); Foscarnet; Mannitol; Mannitol (Systemic); Mecamylamine

Increased Effect/Toxicity

Tobramycin (Systemic) may increase the levels/effects of: AbobotulinumtoxinA; Bisphosphonate Derivatives; CARBOplatin; Colistimethate; CycloSPORINE (Systemic); Mecamylamine; Neuromuscular-Blocking Agents; OnabotulinumtoxinA; RimabotulinumtoxinB; Tenofovir Products

The levels/effects of Tobramycin (Systemic) may be increased by: Amphotericin B; Capreomycin; Cefazedone; Cephalosporins (2nd Generation); Cephalosporins (3rd Generation); Cephalosporins (4th Generation); Cephradine; CISplatin; Foscarnet; Loop Diuretics; Mannitol; Mannitol (Systemic); Nonsteroidal Anti-Inflammatory Agents; Tenofovir Products; Vancomycin

Decreased Effect

Tobramycin (Systemic) may decrease the levels/effects of: BCG (Intravesical); BCG Vaccine (Immunization); Sodium Picosulfate; Typhoid Vaccine

The levels/effects of Tobramycin (Systemic) may be decreased by: Penicillins

Preparation for Administration Solution for injection: Dilute in 50-100 mL NS or D$_5$W for IV infusion.

Storage/Stability Stable at room temperature both as the clear, colorless solution and as the dry powder. Reconstituted solutions remain stable for 24 hours at room temperature and 96 hours when refrigerated.

Mechanism of Action Interferes with bacterial protein synthesis by binding to 30S and 50S ribosomal subunits, resulting in a defective bacterial cell membrane

Pharmacodynamics/Kinetics

Absorption:

Oral: Poorly absorbed

IM: Rapid and complete

Distribution: V$_d$: 0.2 to 0.3 L/kg; Pediatrics: 0.2 to 0.7 L/kg; to extracellular fluid, including serum, abscesses, ascitic, pericardial, pleural, synovial, lymphatic, and peritoneal fluids; poor penetration into CSF, eye, bone, prostate

Protein binding: <30%

Half-life elimination:

Neonates: ≤1200 g: 11 hours; >1200 g: 2 to 9 hours

Adults: IV: 2 to 3 hours; directly dependent upon glomerular filtration rate

Adults with impaired renal function: 5 to 70 hours

Time to peak, serum: IM: 30 to 60 minutes; IV: ~30 minutes

Excretion: Normal renal function: Urine (~90% to 95%) within 24 hours

Dosing

Adult Note: Individualization is **critical** because of the low therapeutic index.

In underweight and nonobese patients, use of total body weight (TBW) instead of ideal body weight for determining the initial mg/kg/dose is widely accepted (Nicolau, 1995). Ideal body weight (IBW) also may be used to determine doses for patients who are neither underweight nor obese (Gilbert, 2009).

Initial and periodic plasma drug levels (eg, peak and trough with conventional dosing, post dose level at a prespecified time with extended-interval dosing) should be determined, particularly in critically-ill patients with serious infections or in disease states known to significantly alter aminoglycoside pharmacokinetics (eg, cystic fibrosis, burns, or major surgery).

Severe life-threatening infections: IM, IV:

Conventional: 1 to 2.5 mg/kg/dose every 8 to 12 hours; to ensure adequate peak concentrations early in therapy, higher initial dosage may be considered in selected patients when extracellular water is increased (edema, septic shock, postsurgical, and/or trauma)

Once-daily: 4 to 7 mg/kg/dose once daily; some clinicians recommend this approach for all patients with normal renal function; this dose is at least as efficacious with similar, if not less, toxicity than conventional dosing.

Brucellosis: IM, IV: 240 mg (IM) daily or 5 mg/kg (IV) daily for 7 days; either regimen recommended in combination with doxycycline

Cholangitis: IM, IV: 4 to 6 mg/kg once daily with ampicillin

CNS shunt infection: Intrathecal (off-label route): 5 to 20 mg/day (Tunkel, 2004)

Diverticulitis, complicated: IM, IV: 1.5 to 2 mg/kg every 8 hours (with ampicillin and metronidazole)

Infective endocarditis (*Pseudomonas aeruginosa*) (off-label use): IM, IV: 8 mg/kg once daily (in combination with an extended-spectrum penicillin, or ceftazidime or cefepime) for a minimum of 6 weeks; adjust doses to maintain peak concentrations of 15 to 20 mcg/mL and trough concentrations ≤2 mcg/mL (AHA/IDSA [Baddour, 2005]; Rybak, 1986)

Meningitis (*Enterococcus* or *Pseudomonas aeruginosa*): IV: 5 mg/kg/day in divided doses every 8 hours (administered with another bacteriocidal drug)

Pelvic inflammatory disease: IM, IV: Loading dose: 2 mg/kg, then 1.5 mg/kg every 8 hours **or** 4.5 mg/kg once daily

Plague *(Yersinia pestis)*: IM, IV: Treatment: 5 mg/kg/day, followed by postexposure prophylaxis with doxycycline

Pneumonia, hospital- or ventilator-associated: IM, IV: 7 mg/kg/day (with antipseudomonal beta-lactam or carbapenem)

Prophylaxis against endocarditis (dental, oral, upper respiratory procedures, GI/GU procedures): IM, IV: 1.5 mg/kg with ampicillin (50 mg/kg) 30 minutes prior to procedure. **Note:** AHA guidelines now recommend prophylaxis only in patients undergoing invasive procedures and in whom underlying cardiac conditions may predispose to a higher risk of adverse outcomes should infection occur. As of April 2007, routine prophylaxis no longer recommended by the AHA.

Tularemia: IM, IV: 5 mg/kg/day divided every 8 hours for 1 to 2 weeks

Urinary tract infection: IM, IV: 1.5 mg/kg/dose every 8 hours

Geriatric Dosage should be based on an estimate of ideal body weight.

IM, IV: 1.5 to 5 mg/kg/day in 1 to 2 divided doses

IV: Once daily or extended interval: 5 to 7 mg/kg/dose given every 24, 36, or 48 hours based on creatinine clearance

Pediatric Individualization is **critical** because of the low therapeutic index

Use of ideal body weight (IBW) for determining the mg/kg/dose appears to be more accurate than dosing on the basis of total body weight (TBW).

Usual dosage range: IM, IV:

Infants and Children <5 years: 2.5 mg/kg/dose every 8 hours

Children >5 years: 2 to 2.5 mg/kg/dose every 8 hours

CNS shunt infection: Intrathecal (off-label route): Refer to adult dosing.

Cystic fibrosis: IM, IV: 2.5 to 3.3 mg/kg every 6 to 8 hours. **Note:** Some patients may require larger or more frequent doses if serum levels document the need (eg, cystic fibrosis or febrile granulocytopenic patients).

Renal Impairment IM, IV:

Conventional dosing:

CrCl ≥60 mL/minute: Administer every 8 hours.

CrCl 40 to 60 mL/minute: Administer every 12 hours.

CrCl 20 to 40 mL/minute: Administer every 24 hours.

CrCl 10 to 20 mL/minute: Administer every 48 hours.

CrCl <10 mL/minute: Administer every 72 hours.

High-dose therapy: Interval may be extended (eg, every 48 hours) in patients with moderate renal impairment (CrCl 30 to 59 mL/minute) and/or adjusted based on serum level determinations.

Intermittent hemodialysis (IHD) (administer after hemodialysis on dialysis days) (Heintz, 2009): Dialyzable (25% to 70%; variable; dependent on filter, duration, and type of HD): IV:

Loading dose of 2 to 3 mg/kg, followed by:

Mild UTI or synergy: IV: 1 mg/kg every 48 to 72 hours; monitor levels

Moderate-to-severe UTI: IV: 1 to 1.5 mg/kg every 48 to 72 hours; monitor levels

Systemic gram-negative infection: IV: 1.5 to 2 mg/kg every 48 to 72 hours; monitor levels

Note: Dosing dependent on the assumption of 3 times/week, complete IHD sessions.

Peritoneal dialysis (PD):

Administration via peritoneal dialysis (PD) fluid:

Gram-negative infection: 4 to 8 mg/L (4 to 8 mcg/mL) of PD fluid

Gram-positive infection (ie, synergy): 3 to 4 mg/L (3 to 4 mcg/mL) of PD fluid

Administration IVPB/IM: Dose as for CrCl <10 mL/minute and follow levels

Continuous renal replacement therapy (CRRT) (Heintz, 2009; Trotman, 2005): Drug clearance is highly dependent on the method of renal replacement, filter type, and flow rate. Appropriate dosing requires close monitoring of pharmacologic response, signs of adverse reactions due to drug accumulation, as well as target drug concentrations (if appropriate). The following are general recommendations only (based on dialysate flow/ultrafiltration rates of 1 to 2 L/hour and minimal residual renal function) and should not supersede clinical judgment:

CVVH/CVVHD/CVVHDF: IV: Loading dose of 2 to 3 mg/kg, followed by:

Mild UTI or synergy: IV 1 mg/kg every 24 to 36 hours; monitor levels

Moderate-severe UTI: IV: 1 to 1.5 mg/kg every 24 to 36 hours; monitor levels

Systemic gram-negative infection: IV: 1.5 to 2.5 mg/kg every 24 to 48 hours; monitor levels

Hepatic Impairment No dosage adjustment necessary; does not undergo hepatic metabolism.

Obesity In moderate obesity (TBW/IBW ≥1.25) or greater, (eg, morbid obesity [TBW/IBW >2]), initial dosage requirement may be estimated using a dosing weight of IBW + 0.4 (TBW - IBW) (Traynor, 1995).

Dietary Considerations May require supplementation of calcium, magnesium, potassium.

Administration IV: Infuse over 30 to 60 minutes. Flush with saline before and after administration.

Some penicillins (eg, carbenicillin, ticarcillin, and piperacillin) have been shown to inactivate aminoglycosides *in vitro*. This has been observed to a greater extent with tobramycin and gentamicin, while amikacin has shown greater stability against inactivation. Concurrent use of these agents may pose a risk of reduced antibacterial efficacy in vivo, particularly in the setting of profound renal impairment. However, definitive clinical evidence is lacking. If combination penicillin/aminoglycoside therapy is desired in a patient with renal dysfunction, separation of doses (if feasible), and routine monitoring of aminoglycoside levels, CBC, and clinical response should be considered.

Monitoring Parameters

Urinalysis, urine output, BUN, serum creatinine, peak and trough plasma tobramycin levels. Levels are typically obtained after the third dose in conventional dosing. Be alert to ototoxicity; hearing should be tested before and during treatment

Some penicillin derivatives may accelerate the degradation of aminoglycosides in vitro. This may be clinically-significant for certain penicillin (ticarcillin, piperacillin, carbenicillin) and aminoglycoside (gentamicin, tobramycin) combination therapy in patients with significant renal impairment. Close monitoring of aminoglycoside levels is warranted.

Reference Range

Timing of serum samples: Draw peak 30 minutes after 30-minute infusion has been completed or 1 hour following IM injection or beginning of infusion; draw trough immediately before next dose

Therapeutic levels:

Peak:

Serious infections: 6 to 8 mcg/mL (SI: 13 to 17 micromole/L)

Life-threatening infections: 8 to 10 mcg/mL (SI: 17 to 21 micromole/L)

Urinary tract infections: 4 to 6 mcg/mL (SI: 9 to 13 micromole/L)

Infective endocarditis (*Pseudomonas aeruginosa*): 15 to 20 mcg/mL (SI: 32 to 43 micromole/L)

Trough:

Serious infections: 0.5 to 1 mcg/mL

Life-threatening infections: 1 to 2 mcg/mL

The American Thoracic Society (ATS) recommends trough levels of <1 mcg/mL for patients with hospital-acquired pneumonia.

Monitor serum creatinine and urine output; obtain drug levels after the third dose unless otherwise directed

Test Interactions Some penicillin derivatives may accelerate the degradation of aminoglycosides in vitro, leading to a potential underestimation of aminoglycoside serum concentration.

Additional Information Once-daily dosing: Higher peak serum drug concentration to MIC ratios, demonstrated aminoglycoside postantibiotic effect, decreased renal cortex drug uptake, and improved cost-time efficiency are supportive reasons for the use of once daily dosing regimens for aminoglycosides. Current research indicates these regimens to be as effective for non-life-threatening infections, with no higher incidence of nephrotoxicity, than those requiring multiple daily doses. Doses are determined by calculating the entire day's dose via usual multiple dose calculation techniques and administering this quantity as a single dose. Doses are then adjusted to maintain mean serum concentrations above the MIC(s) of the causative organism(s). (Example: 2.5 to 5 mg/kg as a single dose; expected Cp_{max}: 10 to 20 mcg/mL and Cp_{min}: <1 mcg/mL). Further research is needed for universal recommendation in all patient populations and gram-negative disease; exceptions may include those with known high clearance (eg, children, patients with cystic fibrosis, or burns who may require shorter dosage intervals) and patients with renal function impairment for whom longer than conventional dosage intervals are usually required.

Dosage Forms Excipient information presented when available (limited, particularly for generics); consult specific product labeling.

Solution, Injection:

Generic: 10 mg/mL (2 mL); 80 mg/2 mL (2 mL); 1.2 g/30 mL (30 mL); 2 g/50 mL (50 mL)

Solution, Intravenous:

Generic: 80 mg (100 mL)

Solution Reconstituted, Injection:

Generic: 1.2 g (1 ea)

Solution Reconstituted, Injection [preservative free]:

Generic: 1.2 g (1 ea)

Tobramycin (Ophthalmic) (toe bra MYE sin)

Brand Names: US Tobrex

Brand Names: Canada PMS-Tobramycin; Sandoz-Tobramycin; Tobrex®

Index Terms Tobramycin Sulfate

Pharmacologic Category Antibiotic, Aminoglycoside; Antibiotic, Ophthalmic

Use Treatment of superficial ophthalmic infections caused by susceptible bacteria

Dosing

Adult Ocular infections: Ophthalmic:

Ointment: Instill ½" (1.25 cm) 2-3 times/day; for severe infections, apply every 3-4 hours

Solution: Instill 1-2 drops every 2-4 hours; for severe infections, instill up to 2 drops every hour until improved, then reduce to less frequent intervals

Pediatric Ocular infections: Ophthalmic: Children ≥2 months: Refer to adult dosing.

Additional Information Complete prescribing information should be consulted for additional detail.

Dosage Forms Excipient information presented when available (limited, particularly for generics); consult specific product labeling.

Ointment, Ophthalmic:

Tobrex: 0.3% (3.5 g)

Solution, Ophthalmic:

Tobrex: 0.3% (5 mL)

Generic: 0.3% (5 mL)

Tobramycin (Oral Inhalation) (toe bra MYE sin)

Brand Names: US Bethkis; Kitabis Pak; Tobi; Tobi Podhaler; Tobramycin Pak

Brand Names: Canada TOBI; TOBI Podhaler

Index Terms Tobramycin Sulfate

Pharmacologic Category Antibiotic, Aminoglycoside

Use Management of cystic fibrosis patients with *Pseudomonas aeruginosa*.

Dosing

Adult

Cystic fibrosis: Inhalation:

Bethkis, Kitabis Pak, Tobi: 300 mg every 12 hours (do not administer doses <6 hours apart); administer in repeated cycles of 28 days on drug followed by 28 days off drug.

Tobi Podhaler: 112 mg (4 x 28 mg capsules) every 12 hours (do not administer doses <6 hours apart); administer in repeated cycles of 28 days on drug followed by 28 days off drug.

Pediatric

Cystic fibrosis: Children ≥6 years and Adolescents: Inhalation: Refer to adult dosing.

Renal Impairment There are no dosage adjustments provided in the manufacturer's labeling (has not been studied).

Hepatic Impairment No dosage adjustment necessary; does not undergo hepatic metabolism.

Additional Information Complete prescribing information should be consulted for additional detail.

Dosage Forms Excipient information presented when available (limited, particularly for generics); consult specific product labeling.

Capsule, Inhalation:

Tobi Podhaler: 28 mg

Nebulization Solution, Inhalation:

Tobramycin Pak: 300 mg/5 mL (5 mL) [contains sodium chloride, sodium hydroxide, sulfuric acid]

Nebulization Solution, Inhalation [preservative free]:

Bethkis: 300 mg/4 mL (4 mL)

Kitabis Pak: 300 mg/5 mL (5 mL)

Tobi: 300 mg/5 mL (5 mL)

Generic: 300 mg/5 mL (5 mL)

Dosage Forms: Canada Also refer to Dosage Forms. Excipient information presented when available (limited, particularly for generics); consult specific product labeling.

Powder, for oral inhalation [capsule]:

TOBI Podhaler: 28 mg/capsule (224s)

Tobramycin and Dexamethasone (toe bra MYE sin & deks a METH a sone)

Brand Names: US TobraDex; TobraDex ST

Brand Names: Canada Tobradex

Index Terms Dexamethasone and Tobramycin

Pharmacologic Category Antibiotic/Corticosteroid, Ophthalmic

Use Ocular inflammatory conditions: Treatment of steroid-responsive ocular inflammatory conditions (where either a superficial bacterial ocular infection or the risk of a bacterial ocular infection exists) of the palpebral and bulbar conjunctiva, cornea and anterior segment of the globe; chronic anterior uveitis; corneal injury from chemical, radiation or thermal burns; penetration of foreign bodies.

Dosing

Adult & Geriatric

Ocular inflammatory conditions: Ophthalmic:

Ointment: Apply ~½-inch ribbon in the conjunctival sac of the affected eye(s) up to 3 to 4 times daily

Suspension:

TobraDex: Instill 1 to 2 drops into the conjunctival sac of the affected eye(s) every 4 to 6 hours; may be increased to 1 to 2 drops every 2 hours for the first 24 to 48 hours, then reduce to less frequent intervals as signs and symptoms improve

TobraDex ST: Instill 1 drop into the conjunctival sac of the affected eye(s) every 4 to 6 hours; may be increased to 1 drop every 2 hours for the first 24 to 48 hours, then reduce to less frequent intervals as signs and symptoms improve

Pediatric Ocular inflammatory conditions: Children ≥2 years and Adolescents: Refer to adult dosing.

Renal Impairment There are no dosage adjustments provided in the manufacturer's labeling. However, dosage adjustment unlikely due to low systemic absorption.

Hepatic Impairment There are no dosage adjustments provided in the manufacturer's labeling. However, dosage adjustment unlikely due to low systemic absorption.

Additional Information Complete prescribing information should be consulted for additional detail.

Dosage Forms Excipient information presented when available (limited, particularly for generics); consult specific product labeling.

Ointment, ophthalmic:

TobraDex®: Tobramycin 0.3% and dexamethasone 0.1% (3.5 g) [contains chlorobutanol]

Suspension, ophthalmic: Tobramycin 0.3% and dexamethasone 0.1% (2.5 mL, 5 mL, 10 mL)

TobraDex®: Tobramycin 0.3% and dexamethasone 0.1% (2.5 mL, 5 mL, 10 mL) [contains benzalkonium chloride]

TobraDex® ST: Tobramycin 0.3% and dexamethasone 0.05% (5 mL) [contains benzalkonium chloride]

- Tobramycin and Loteprednol Etabonate *see* Loteprednol and Tobramycin *on page 1110*

- Tobramycin For Injection (Can) *see* Tobramycin (Systemic) *on page 1799*

- Tobramycin For Injection, USP (Can) *see* Tobramycin (Systemic) *on page 1799*

- Tobramycin Injection (Can) *see* Tobramycin (Systemic) *on page 1799*

- Tobramycin Injection, USP (Can) *see* Tobramycin (Systemic) *on page 1799*

- Tobramycin Pak *see* Tobramycin (Oral Inhalation) *on page 1802*

- Tobramycin Sulfate *see* Tobramycin (Ophthalmic) *on page 1801*

- Tobramycin Sulfate *see* Tobramycin (Oral Inhalation) *on page 1802*

- Tobramycin Sulfate *see* Tobramycin (Systemic) *on page 1799*

- Tobrex *see* Tobramycin (Ophthalmic) *on page 1801*

- Tobrex® (Can) *see* Tobramycin (Ophthalmic) *on page 1801*

Tocilizumab (toe si LIZ oo mab)

Brand Names: US Actemra

Brand Names: Canada Actemra

Index Terms Atlizumab; MRA; R-1569; RoActemra

Pharmacologic Category Antirheumatic, Disease Modifying; Interleukin-6 Receptor Antagonist

Use

Polyarticular juvenile idiopathic arthritis: Treatment of active polyarticular juvenile idiopathic arthritis in patients 2 years and older.

Rheumatoid arthritis: Treatment of adults with moderately to severely active rheumatoid arthritis (RA) who have had an inadequate response to one or more disease-modifying antirheumatic drugs (DMARDs).

Systemic juvenile idiopathic arthritis: Treatment of active systemic juvenile idiopathic arthritis in patients 2 years and older.

Pregnancy Considerations Adverse events have been observed in some animal reproduction studies. Monoclonal antibodies cross the placenta, with the largest amount transferred during the third trimester. A pregnancy registry has been established to monitor outcomes of women exposed to tocilizumab during pregnancy (877-311-8972).

Breast-Feeding Considerations It is not known if tocilizumab is excreted in human milk. Because many immunoglobulins are excreted in human milk and the potential for serious adverse reactions exists, a decision should be made whether to discontinue nursing or to discontinue the drug, taking into account the importance of the drug to the mother.

Medication Guide Available Yes

Contraindications

Hypersensitivity to tocilizumab or any component of the formulation

Canadian labeling: Additional contraindications (not in U.S. labeling): Active infections

Warnings/Precautions [U.S. Boxed Warning]: Serious and potentially fatal infections (including active tuberculosis, invasive fungal, bacterial, viral, protozoal, and other opportunistic infections) have been reported in patients receiving tocilizumab; infection may lead to hospitalization or death. Most of the serious infections have occurred in patients on concomitant immunosuppressive therapy. Patients should be closely monitored for signs and symptoms of infection during and after treatment. If serious infection occurs during treatment, withhold tocilizumab until infection is controlled. Prior to treatment initiation, carefully consider risk versus benefit in patients with chronic or recurrent infections, tuberculosis exposure, history of or current opportunistic infection, underlying conditions predisposing to infection, or patients residing in or with travel to areas of endemic tuberculosis or endemic mycosis, The most common serious infections occurring have included pneumonia, UTI, cellulitis, herpes zoster, gastroenteritis, diverticulitis, sepsis, and bacterial arthritis. Do not administer tocilizumab to a patient with an active infection, including localized infection. Interrupt treatment for opportunistic infection or sepsis. **[U.S. Boxed Warning]: Tuberculosis (pulmonary or extrapulmonary) has been reported in patients receiving tocilizumab;** both reactivation of latent infection and new infections have been reported. Patients should be tested for latent tuberculosis infection before and during therapy; consider treatment of latent tuberculosis prior to tocilizumab treatment. Some patients who test negative prior to therapy may develop active infection; monitor for signs and symptoms of tuberculosis during and after treatment in all patients. Patients should be evaluated for tuberculosis risk factors with a tuberculin skin test prior to starting therapy. Consider antituberculosis treatment in patients with a history of latent or active tuberculosis if adequate treatment course cannot be confirmed, and for patients with risk factors for tuberculosis despite a negative test. Rare reactivation of herpes zoster has been reported. Patients should be brought up to date with all immunizations before initiating therapy. Live vaccines should not be given concurrently; there is no data available concerning secondary transmission of infection from live vaccines in patients receiving therapy.

Use of tocilizumab may affect defenses against malignancies; impact on the development and course of malignancies is not fully defined, however, malignancies were observed in clinical trials. Use with caution in patients with preexisting or recent onset CNS demyelinating disorders; rare cases of CNS demyelinating disorders (eg, multiple sclerosis) have occurred. All patients should be monitored for signs and symptoms of demyelinating disorders. May cause hypersensitivity or anaphylaxis; anaphylactic events including fatalities have been reported with IV administration; hypersensitivity reactions have occurred in patients who were premedicated, in patients with and without a prior history of hypersensitivity, and as early as the first infusion. Medications for the treatment of hypersensitivity reactions should be available for immediate use. Patients should seek medical attention if symptoms of hypersensitivity reaction occur with subcutaneous use. Stop infusion and permanently discontinue treatment in patients who develop a hypersensitivity reaction to tocilizumab. In clinical studies, reactions requiring treatment discontinuation included generalized erythema, rash, and urticaria. Use is not recommended in patients with active hepatic disease or hepatic impairment. Monitor ALT and AST. Do not initiate treatment if ALT or AST is >1.5 times ULN. Use with caution in patients at increased risk for gastrointestinal perforation; perforation has been reported, typically secondary to diverticulitis. Monitor for new-onset abdominal symptoms; promptly evaluate if new symptoms occur.

Use may cause increases in total cholesterol, triglycerides, LDL and HDL cholesterol; monitor ~4-8 weeks after initiation, then approximately every 6 months; hyperlipidemia should be managed according to current guidelines. Neutropenia and thrombocytopenia may occur; may require treatment interruption, dose or interval modification, or discontinuation. Monitor neutrophils and platelets. Do not initiate treatment in patients with an ANC <2000/mm³ or platelet count <100,000/mm³; discontinue treatment for ANC <500/mm³ or platelet count <50,000/mm³. Monitor transaminases; treatment should be discontinued in patients who develop elevated ALT or AST >5 x ULN. Patients receiving concomitant hepatotoxic drugs (eg, methotrexate) are at an increased risk of developing elevated transaminases; elevations are typically reversible and do not result in clinically evident hepatic injury.

Potentially significant drug/drug interactions may exist, requiring dose or frequency adjustment, additional monitoring, and/or selection of alternative therapy. Concomitant use with other biological DMARDs (eg, TNF blockers, IL-1 receptor blockers, anti-CD20 monoclonal antibodies, selective costimulation modulators) has not been studied and should should be avoided. Cautious use is recommended in elderly patients due to an increased incidence of serious infections. Subcutaneous administration is only indicated for adult patients with rheumatoid arthritis. Do not use subcutaneous injection for IV infusion.

Some dosage forms may contain polysorbate 80 (also known as Tweens). Hypersensitivity reactions, usually a delayed reaction, have been reported following exposure to pharmaceutical products containing polysorbate 80 in certain individuals (Isaksson, 2002; Lucente 2000; Shelley, 1995). Thrombocytopenia, ascites, pulmonary deterioration, and renal and hepatic failure have been reported in premature neonates after receiving parenteral products containing polysorbate 80 (Alade, 1986; CDC, 1984). See manufacturer's labeling.

Adverse Reactions Incidence as reported for monotherapy, except where noted. Combination therapy refers to use in rheumatoid arthritis with nonbiological DMARDs or use in SJIA or PJIA in trials where most patients (~70% to 80%) were taking methotrexate at baseline.

>10%:

Endocrine & metabolic: Increased serum cholesterol (>240 mg/dL; 19% to 20%; >1.5-2 x ULN; combination therapy; children and adolescents <1% to 2%)

Hepatic: Increased serum ALT (≤36%; grades 3/4: <1%), increased serum AST (≤22%; grades 3/4: <1%)

Miscellaneous: Infusion-related reaction (combination therapy; 4% to 16%)

1% to 10%:

Cardiovascular: Hypertension (1% to 6%), peripheral edema (<2%)

Central nervous system: Headache (1% to 7%), dizziness (3%)

Dermatologic: Skin rash (2%), dermatological reaction (combination therapy; 1% [includes pruritus, urticaria])

Endocrine & metabolic: Increased LDL cholesterol (9% to 10%; >1.5-2 x ULN; combination therapy; children and adolescents <1% to 2%), hypothyroidism (<2%)

Gastrointestinal: Diarrhea (children and adolescents ≤5%), abdominal pain (2%), oral mucosa ulcer (2%), gastric ulcer (<2%), stomatitis (<2%), weight gain (<2%), gastritis (1%)

Hematologic & oncologic: Neutropenia (combination therapy; grade 3: 2% to 7%; grade 4: <1%), thrombocytopenia (combination therapy; 1% to 2%), leukopenia (<2%)

Hepatic: Increased serum bilirubin (<2%)

Immunologic: Antibody development (<2%)

Infection: Herpes simplex infection (<2%)

Local: Injection site reaction (SubQ: Including erythema, pruritus, pain, and hematoma; 4% to 10%)

Ophthalmic: Conjunctivitis (<2%)

Renal: Nephrolithiasis (<2%)

Respiratory: Upper respiratory tract infection (7%), nasopharyngitis (7%), bronchitis (3%), cough (<2%), dyspnea (<2%)

<1% (Limited to important or life-threatening): Anaphylaxis, anaphylactoid reaction, angioedema, aspergillosis, candidiasis, cellulitis, chronic inflammatory demyelinating polyneuropathy, cryptococcosis, diverticulitis, gastroenteritis, gastrointestinal perforation, herpes zoster, hypersensitivity, hypersensitivity pneumonitis, hypertriglyceridemia, hypotension, increased HDL cholesterol, malignant neoplasm (including breast and colon cancer), multiple sclerosis, otitis media, pneumonia, pneumocystosis, reactivation of latent Epstein-Barr virus, septic arthritis, sepsis, Stevens-Johnson syndrome, tuberculosis, urinary tract infection, varicella

Drug Interactions

Metabolism/Transport Effects None known.

Avoid Concomitant Use

Avoid concomitant use of Tocilizumab with any of the following: Abatacept; Anti-TNF Agents; BCG (Intravesical); Belimumab; Natalizumab; Pimecrolimus; Tacrolimus (Topical); Tofacitinib; Vaccines (Live)

Increased Effect/Toxicity

Tocilizumab may increase the levels/effects of: Abatacept; Anti-TNF Agents; Belimumab; Fingolimod; Leflunomide; Natalizumab; Tofacitinib; Vaccines (Live)

The levels/effects of Tocilizumab may be increased by: Denosumab; Pimecrolimus; Roflumilast; Tacrolimus (Topical); Trastuzumab

Decreased Effect

Tocilizumab may decrease the levels/effects of: BCG (Intravesical); Coccidioides immitis Skin Test; CYP3A4 Substrates; Sipuleucel-T; Vaccines (Inactivated); Vaccines (Live)

The levels/effects of Tocilizumab may be decreased by: Echinacea

Preparation for Administration IV: Prior to administration, dilute to 50 mL (children <30 kg) or 100 mL (children ≥30 kg and adults) by slowly adding to 0.9% sodium chloride. Use vials for IV to prepare infusion solutions; do **not** use prefilled SubQ syringes to prepare IV solutions. Withdraw equal volume of 0.9% sodium chloride to the volume of tocilizumab required for dose; slowly add tocilizumab dose into infusion bag or bottle. Gently invert to mix (avoid foaming). Diluted solutions may be stored under refrigeration or at room temperature for up to 24 hours (protected from light) and are compatible with polypropylene, polyethylene (PE), polyvinyl chloride (PVC), and glass infusion containers. Allow diluted solution to reach room temperature prior to infusion.

Storage/Stability Store intact vials/syringes at 2°C to 8°C (36°F to 46°F). Do not freeze. Protect vials and syringes from light (store in the original package until time of use); keep syringes dry. Solutions diluted for IV infusion may be stored at 2°C to 8°C (36°F to 46°F) or room temperature for up to 24 hours and should be protected from light. Discard unused product remaining in the vials.

Mechanism of Action Antagonist of the interleukin-6 (IL-6) receptor. Endogenous IL-6 is induced by inflammatory stimuli and mediates a variety of immunological responses. Inhibition of IL-6 receptors by tocilizumab leads to a reduction in cytokine and acute phase reactant production.

Pharmacodynamics/Kinetics

Distribution: V_{dss}: Children: 2.54-4.08 L; Adults: 6.4 L

Bioavailability: SubQ: 80%

Half life elimination:

IV: Terminal, single dose: 6.3 days (concentration-dependent; may be increased up to 16-23 days [children] or 11-13 days [adults] at steady state)

SubQ: Concentration dependent: Adults: Up to 5 days (every other week dosing) or 13 days (every week dosing)

Dosing

Adult Note: Do not initiate if ANC is <2000/mm³, platelets are <100,000/mm³ or if ALT or AST are >1.5 times ULN.

Rheumatoid arthritis: Note: Methotrexate or other *non-biologic* disease-modifying antirheumatic drugs (DMARDs) may be continued for the treatment of rheumatoid arthritis. Tocilizumab should not be used in combination with *biologic* DMARDs.

IV: Initial: 4 mg/kg every 4 weeks; may be increased to 8 mg/kg based on clinical response (maximum dose: 800 mg).

SubQ:

<100 kg: 162 mg every other week; increase to every week based on clinical response

≥100 kg: 162 mg every week

Transitioning from IV therapy to SubQ therapy: Administer the first SubQ dose instead of the next scheduled IV dose.

Pediatric Note: Do not initiate if ANC is <2000/mm³, platelets are <100,000/mm³ or if ALT or AST are >1.5 times ULN.

Polyarticular juvenile idiopathic arthritis (PJIA): Children ≥2 years: IV: **Note:** Dose adjustment should not be made based solely on a single-visit body weight measurement due to fluctuations in body weight. May be used as monotherapy or in combination with methotrexate.

<30 kg: 10 mg/kg every 4 weeks

≥30 kg: 8 mg/kg every 4 weeks

Systemic juvenile idiopathic arthritis (SJIA): Children ≥2 years: IV: **Note:** Dose adjustment should not be made based solely on a single-visit body weight measurement due to fluctuations in body weight. May be used as monotherapy or in combination with methotrexate.

<30 kg: 12 mg/kg every 2 weeks

≥30 kg: 8 mg/kg every 2 weeks

Renal Impairment

Mild renal impairment: No dosage adjustment necessary. Moderate-to-severe renal impairment: There are no dosage adjustments provided in the manufacturer's labeling (has not been studied).

Hepatic Impairment

There are no dosage adjustments provided in the manufacturer's labeling (has not been studied). Not recommended for use in patients with active hepatic disease or hepatic impairment.

Hepatotoxicity during treatment: Rheumatoid arthritis:

>1 to 3 x ULN: Adjust concomitant DMARDs as appropriate. For patients receiving IV therapy with persistent increases >1 to 3 x ULN, reduce dose to 4 mg/kg or interrupt until ALT/AST have normalized. For patients receiving SubQ therapy with persistent increases >1 to 3 x ULN, reduce injection frequency to every other week or interrupt until ALT/AST have normalized; increase frequency to every week as clinically appropriate.

>3 to 5 x ULN (confirmed with repeat testing): Interrupt until ALT/AST <3 x ULN and follow dosage adjustments recommended for liver enzyme abnormalities >1 to 3 x ULN. For persistent increases >3 x ULN, discontinue.

>5 x ULN: Discontinue.

Adjustment for Toxicity

Hypersensitivity (anaphylaxis or other clinically-significant hypersensitivity reaction): Stop immediately and discontinue permanently.

Infection (serious infection, opportunistic infection or sepsis): Interrupt treatment until the infection is controlled.

Polyarticular and systemic juvenile idiopathic arthritis: Dose reductions have not been studied; however, dose interruptions are recommended for liver enzyme abnormalities, low neutrophil counts, and low platelets similar to recommendations provided for rheumatoid arthritis. In addition, consider interrupting or discontinuing concomitant methotrexate and/or other medications and hold tocilizumab dosing until the clinical situation has been assessed.

Rheumatoid arthritis (RA):

Low absolute neutrophil counts (ANC):

ANC >1000 cells/mm³: Maintain dose.

ANC 500-1000 cells/mm³: Interrupt therapy; when ANC >1000 cells/mm³, resume IV tocilizumab at 4 mg/kg (may increase to 8 mg/kg as clinically appropriate). or resume SubQ tocilizumab at every other week dosing (increase frequency to every week as clinically appropriate).

ANC <500 cells/mm³: Discontinue.

Low platelet counts:

Platelets 50,000-100,000 cells/mm³: Interrupt therapy; when platelet count is >100,000 cells/mm³, resume IV tocilizumab at 4 mg/kg (may increase to 8 mg/kg as clinically appropriate) or resume SubQ tocilizumab at every other week dosing (increase frequency to every week as clinically appropriate).

Platelets <50,000 cells/mm³: Discontinue.

Administration

IV: Allow diluted solution for infusion to reach room temperature prior to administration; infuse over 60 minutes using a dedicated IV line. Do not infuse other agents through same IV line. Do not administer IV push or IV bolus. Do not use if opaque particles or discoloration is visible.

SubQ: Rheumatoid arthritis: When transitioning from IV administration to SubQ administration, give the first SubQ dose instead of the next scheduled IV dose. Administer the full amount in the prefilled syringe. Allow to reach room temperature prior to use. Do not use if particulate matter or discoloration is visible; solution should be clear and colorless to pale yellow. Rotate injection sites; avoid injecting into moles, scars, or tender, bruised, red, or hard skin. Prefilled syringe is available for use by patients (self-administration).

Monitoring Parameters Latent TB screening prior to therapy initiation; neutrophils, platelets, ALT/AST (prior to therapy, 4-8 weeks after start of therapy, and every 3 months thereafter [RA]); neutrophils, platelets, ALT/AST (prior to therapy, at second infusion, and every 2-4 weeks [SJIA, U.S. labeling; SJIA and PJIA, Canadian labeling] or 4-8 weeks [PJIA, U.S. labeling] thereafter); additional liver function tests (eg, bilirubin) as clinically indicated; lipid panel (prior to, at 4-8 weeks following initiation, and every ~6 months during therapy); signs and symptoms of infection (prior to, during, and after therapy); signs and symptoms of CNS demyelinating disorders

Dosage Forms Excipient information presented when available (limited, particularly for generics); consult specific product labeling.

Solution, Intravenous [preservative free]:

Actemra: 80 mg/4 mL (4 mL); 200 mg/10 mL (10 mL); 400 mg/20 mL (20 mL) [contains polysorbate 80]

Solution Prefilled Syringe, Subcutaneous [preservative free]:

Actemra: 162 mg/0.9 mL (0.9 mL) [contains polysorbate 80]

◆ **Today Sponge** [OTC] *see* Nonoxynol 9 *on page 1296*

Tofacitinib (toe fa SYE ti nib)

Brand Names: US Xeljanz
Brand Names: Canada Xeljanz
Index Terms CP-690, 550; Tofacitinib Citrate
Pharmacologic Category Antirheumatic Miscellaneous; Antirheumatic, Disease Modifying; Janus Associated Kinase Inhibitor

Use

Rheumatoid arthritis: Treatment of moderately- to severely-active rheumatoid arthritis (as monotherapy or in combination with methotrexate or other nonbiologic disease-modifying antirheumatic drugs [DMARDs]) in adults who have had an inadequate response to, or are intolerant of, methotrexate

Limitations of use: The use of tofacitinib in combination with biologic DMARDs or with potent immunosuppressants (eg, azathioprine, cyclosporine) is not recommended.

Pregnancy Considerations Adverse events have been observed in animal reproduction studies. Healthcare providers are encouraged to enroll women exposed to tofacitinib during pregnancy in the Xeljanz Pregnancy Registry (877-311-8972); patients may also enroll themselves. Canadian labeling recommends avoiding use during pregnancy.

Breast-Feeding Considerations It is not known if tofacitinib is excreted in breast milk. Due to the potential for serious adverse reactions in a nursing infant, a decision should be made to discontinue tofacitinib or to discontinue breast-feeding during therapy, taking into account the importance of treatment to the mother.

Prescribing and Access Restrictions Available through specialty/network pharmacies. Further information may be obtained from the manufacturer, Pfizer Inc, at 1-855-493-5526 or at http://www.xeljanz.com/.

Medication Guide Available Yes

Contraindications

There are no contraindications listed in the manufacturer's US labeling.

Canadian labeling: Hypersensitivity to tofacitinib or any component of the formulation.

Warnings/Precautions Hazardous agent - use appropriate precautions for handling and disposal (meets NIOSH 2014 criteria). **[US Boxed Warning]: Patients receiving tofacitinib are at increased risk for serious infections, which may result in hospitalization and/or fatality; infections often developed in patients receiving concomitant immunosuppressive agents (eg, methotrexate or corticosteroids). Active tuberculosis (pulmonary or extrapulmonary), invasive fungal (including cryptococcosis and pneumocystosis [may present as disseminated rather than local disease) and bacterial, viral or other opportunistic infections (including esophageal candidiasis, multidermatomal herpes zoster, cytomegalovirus, and BK virus) have been reported in patients receiving tofacitinib. Closely monitor patients for the development of signs/symptoms of infection during and after tofacitinib treatment. If a serious infection develops, interrupt tofacitinib until the infection is controlled. Carefully consider the risks and benefits of treatment with tofacitinib prior to initiating therapy in patients with chronic or recurrent infection.** The most common serious infections reported included pneumonia, cellulitis, urinary tract infections and herpes zoster infections, although other serious infections may occur. Reactivation of viral infections (eg, herpes zoster) was observed in clinical trials; the incidence of chronic viral hepatitis reactivation is unknown. Screen for viral hepatitis. The risk for herpes zoster is increased with tofacitinib; patients within Asian countries appear to have a higher incidence of herpes zoster cases (Winthrop, 2014). Use with caution in patients that have been exposed to tuberculosis, with a history of serious or opportunistic infection, taking concomitant immunosuppressants, with comorbid conditions that predispose them to infections (eg, diabetes), or in patients who live in or travel to/from areas of endemic mycoses (ie, blastomycosis, coccidioidomycosis, histoplasmosis). Do not initiate tofacitinib in patients with active infections, including localized infections. Use with caution in elderly patients; general incidence of infection is higher in elderly. Use with caution in Asian patients; an increased incidence of adverse reactions (eg, herpes zoster, opportunistic infections, decreased WBC, interstitial lung disease, increased transaminases) has been observed (Wollenhaupt, 2014; Xeljanz Canadian product monograph, 2014).

[US Boxed Warning]: Tuberculosis (pulmonary or extrapulmonary) has been reported in patients receiving tofacitinib. Patients should be evaluated for tuberculosis risk factors and active or latent infection (with a tuberculin skin test) before and during therapy. Treatment of latent tuberculosis should be initiated before use. Patients with initial negative tuberculin skin tests should receive continued monitoring for tuberculosis throughout treatment; active tuberculosis has developed in this population during treatment with tofacitinib. Use with caution in patients who have resided in regions where tuberculosis is endemic. Consider anti-tuberculosis therapy if an adequate course of treatment cannot be confirmed in patients with a history of latent or active tuberculosis or for patients with risk factors despite negative skin test.

[US Boxed Warning]: Lymphoma and other malignancies have been reported in patients receiving tofacitinib; Epstein Barr Virus-associated post-transplant lymphoproliferative disorder has been observed at an increased rate in renal transplant patients receiving tofacitinib and concomitant immunosuppressive medications. The most common types of malignancy observed were lung, breast, gastric, colorectal, renal cell, prostate, lymphoma, and malignant melanoma. Consider risks versus benefits prior to use in patients with a known malignancy (other than successfully treated nonmelanoma skin cancers [NMSCs]) or when continuing tofacitinib in patients who develop a new malignancy. NMSCs have been reported; patients at increased risk for skin cancer should have periodic skin examinations.

Lymphocytopenia (after an initial lymphocytosis), neutropenia (<2000 cells/mm^3), and anemia have been observed with tofacitinib therapy. Lymphocyte counts <500 cells/mm^3 were associated with increased incidence of treated and serious infections; avoid tofacitinib initiation in patients with lymphocytes <500 cells/mm^3 at baseline. Avoid use in patients with ANC <1000 cells/mm^3 at baseline; interrupt therapy if ANC is persistently between 500-1000 cells/mm^3 or if ANC <500 cells/mm^3 during treatment. Consider resuming tofacitinib when ANC ≥1000 cells/mm^3. Avoid use in patients with hemoglobin <9 g/dL; interrupt therapy if hemoglobin decreases >2 g/dL or if hemoglobin <8 g/dL. Monitor lymphocyte counts at baseline and every 3 months thereafter; ANC, platelet counts, and hemoglobin should be assessed at baseline, after 4-8 weeks of therapy, and every 3 months thereafter.

Use with caution in patients at increased risk for gastrointestinal perforation (eg, history of diverticulitis); perforations have been reported in clinical trials. Promptly evaluate new-onset abdominal symptoms in patients taking tofacitinib. Increases in lipid parameters (eg, total cholesterol, LDL, and HDL cholesterol) were observed in patients receiving tofacitinib; maximum lipid increases were typically seen within 6 weeks of initiation. Assess lipids 4-8 weeks after tofacitinib initiation and manage lipid abnormalities accordingly. Increased incidence of liver enzyme elevation was observed in patients taking tofacitinib compared to placebo. Routine liver function test monitoring is recommended; interrupt therapy if drug-induced liver injury is suspected.

A decrease in heart rate and prolonged PR interval have been reported with tofacitinib in clinical trials. Use caution in patients with baseline heart rate <60 bpm, conduction abnormalities, syncope or arrhythmia, ischemic heart disease, heart failure, or receiving concomitant therapy known to decrease heart rate or prolong the PR interval (Xeljanz Canadian product monograph, 2014). Interstitial lung disease (ILD) has been reported; patients developing ILD were receiving concomitant therapy associated with ILD (eg, methotrexate). Use with caution in patients with risk/history of ILD (Xeljanz Canadian product monograph, 2014).

Immunization status should be current before initiating therapy. Live vaccines should not be given concomitantly with tofacitinib; no data are available concerning vaccination response or secondary transmission of infection by live vaccines in patients receiving therapy.

Potentially significant drug-drug interactions may exist, requiring dose or frequency adjustment, additional monitoring, and/or selection of alternative therapy. Tofacitinib should not be administered in combination with strong immunosuppressive medications (eg, azathioprine, tacrolimus, cyclosporine) due to the risk of additive immunosuppression; such combinations have not been studied in rheumatoid arthritis. Tofacitinib should not be administered in combination with biologic DMARDs.

Use is not recommended in patients with severe hepatic impairment; dosage reduction required in patients with moderate hepatic impairment. Dosage reduction required in patients with moderate or severe renal impairment.

Adverse Reactions Percentages noted include the highest frequency regardless of dosage. Frequencies may vary for specific doses; consult prescribing information.

>10%: Infection: Infection (20% to 22%)

1% to 10%:

Cardiovascular: Hypertension (2%)

Central nervous system: Headache (4%)

Gastrointestinal: Diarrhea (4%)

Genitourinary: Urinary tract infection (2%)

Hepatic: Increased serum ALT (>3 x upper limit of normal; 1%)

Infection: Serious infection (2% to 3%)

Renal: Increased serum creatinine (<2%)

Respiratory: Upper respiratory tract infection (5%), nasopharyngitis (4%)

<1% (Limited to important or life-threatening): Abdominal pain, anemia, BK virus, cellulitis, cryptococcosis, cytomegalovirus disease, decreased heart rate, dehydration, dyspepsia, erythema, esophageal candidiasis, gastritis, hepatotoxicity, herpes zoster, increased creatine kinase, increased serum AST, interstitial pulmonary disease, liver steatosis, lymphocytopenia, malignant neoplasm, musculoskeletal pain, neutropenia, paresthesia, peripheral edema, pneumocystosis, pneumonia, prolongation P-R interval on ECG, pruritus, rhabdomyolysis, sinus congestion, skin carcinoma, skin rash, tendonitis, tuberculosis

Drug Interactions

Metabolism/Transport Effects Substrate of CYP2C19 (minor), CYP3A4 (major); **Note:** Assignment of Major/Minor substrate status based on clinically relevant drug interaction potential

Avoid Concomitant Use

Avoid concomitant use of Tofacitinib with any of the following: Abatacept; Anakinra; Anti-TNF Agents; BCG (Intravesical); Conivaptan; CYP3A4 Inducers (Strong); Deferiprone; Dipyrone; Fusidic Acid (Systemic); Idelalisib; Immunosuppressants; Natalizumab; Pimecrolimus; RiTUXimab; Tacrolimus (Topical); Tocilizumab; Vaccines (Live)

Increased Effect/Toxicity

Tofacitinib may increase the levels/effects of: Bradycardia-Causing Agents; CloZAPine; Deferiprone; Natalizumab; Vaccines (Live)

The levels/effects of Tofacitinib may be increased by: Abatacept; Anakinra; Anti-TNF Agents; Aprepitant; Conivaptan; CYP3A4 Inhibitors (Moderate); CYP3A4 Inhibitors (Strong); Denosumab; Dipyrone; Fluconazole; Fosaprepitant; Fusidic Acid (Systemic); Idelalisib; Immunosuppressants; Ivacaftor; Luliconazole; Methotrexate; Mifepristone; Netupitant; Pimecrolimus; RiTUXimab; Roflumilast; Simeprevir; Sitaxentan; Stiripentol; Tacrolimus (Topical); Tocilizumab; Trastuzumab

Decreased Effect

Tofacitinib may decrease the levels/effects of: BCG (Intravesical); Coccidioides immitis Skin Test; Sipuleucel-T; Vaccines (Inactivated); Vaccines (Live)

The levels/effects of Tofacitinib may be decreased by: Bosentan; CYP3A4 Inducers (Moderate); CYP3A4 Inducers (Strong); Dabrafenib; Deferasirox; Echinacea; St Johns Wort

Storage/Stability Store between 20°C and 25°C (68°F to 77°F).

Mechanism of Action Tofacitinib inhibits Janus kinase (JAK) enzymes, which are intracellular enzymes involved in stimulating hematopoiesis and immune cell function through a signaling pathway. In response to extracellular cytokine or growth factor signaling, JAKs activate signal transducers and activators of transcription (STATs), which regulate gene expression and intracellular activity. Inhibition of JAKs prevents cytokine- or growth factor-mediated gene expression and intracellular activity of immune cells, reduces circulating CD16/56+ natural killer cells, serum IgG, IgM, IgA, and C-reactive protein, and increases B cells.

Pharmacodynamics/Kinetics

Absorption: Oral: Rapid (74%); C_{max} is reduced by 32% when administered with high-fat meal, but AUC remains unchanged.

Distribution: V_d: 87 L

Protein binding: ~40% (predominantly to albumin)

Metabolism: Hepatic (70%): CYP3A4 and CYP2C19 to inactive metabolites

Half-life elimination: ~3 hours

Time to peak: 0.5 to 1 hour

Excretion: Primarily urine (30%) as unchanged drug

Dosing

Adult & Geriatric Rheumatoid arthritis (monotherapy or in combination with nonbiologic disease-modifying antirheumatic drugs (DMARDs)): Oral: 5 mg twice daily

Note: Tofacitinib should not be used in combination with biologic DMARDs or with strong immunosuppressants, such as azathioprine, tacrolimus, or cyclosporine. Do not initiate therapy in patients with an absolute lymphocyte count <500 cells/mm³, absolute neutrophil count <1000 cells/mm³, or hemoglobin <9 g/dL.

Dosage adjustment for strong CYP3A4 inducers (eg, rifampin): Coadministration is not recommended

Dosage adjustment for strong CYP3A4 inhibitors (eg, ketoconazole): Reduce dose to 5 mg once daily

Dosage adjustment for concomitant moderate CYP3A4 inhibitors and potent CYP2C19 inhibitors (eg, fluconazole): Reduce dose to 5 mg once daily

Renal Impairment

Mild impairment: No dosage adjustment necessary.

Moderate-to-severe impairment: Reduce dose to 5 mg once daily. **Note:** Tofacitinib has not been studied in patients with baseline CrCl <40 mL/minute.

Hepatic Impairment

Mild impairment: No dosage adjustment necessary.

Moderate impairment: Reduce dose to 5 mg once daily.

Severe impairment: Use is not recommended (has not been studied in patients with severe hepatic impairment or in patients with hepatitis B or hepatitis C viruses).

Adjustment for Toxicity

Lymphopenia (lymphocytes ≥500 cells/mm³): Maintain dose.

Lymphopenia (lymphocytes <500 cells/mm³) confirmed by repeat evaluation: Discontinue therapy.

Neutropenia (ANC >1000 cells/mm³): Maintain dose.

Neutropenia (ANC persistently between 500 to 1000 cells/mm³): Interrupt therapy; resume at 5 mg twice daily when ANC >1000 cells/mm³.

Neutropenia (ANC <500 cells/mm³) confirmed by repeat evaluation: Discontinue therapy.

Anemia (hemoglobin ≥9 g/dL **and** decrease ≤2 g/dL): Maintain dose.

Anemia (hemoglobin <8 g/dL **or** decrease >2 g/dL) confirmed by repeat evaluation: Interrupt therapy until hemoglobin values have normalized.

Administration May be taken with or without food. Hazardous agent; use appropriate precautions for handling and disposal (meets NIOSH 2014 criteria).

Monitoring Parameters Lymphocyte count (baseline and every 3 months thereafter); neutrophil/platelet counts (baseline, after 4-8 weeks, and every 3 months thereafter); hemoglobin (baseline, after 4-8 weeks, and every 3 months thereafter); lipids (4-8 weeks after therapy initiation and periodically); LFTs; viral hepatitis (prior to initiating therapy in accordance with clinical guidelines); signs/symptoms of infections (including tuberculosis) during and after therapy; abdominal symptoms; skin examinations (periodically, in patients at increased risk for skin cancer); heart rate and blood pressure at baseline and periodically thereafter.

Dosage Forms Excipient information presented when available (limited, particularly for generics); consult specific product labeling.

Tablet, Oral:

Xeljanz: 5 mg

TOLAZamide (tole AZ a mide)

Pharmacologic Category Antidiabetic Agent, Sulfonylurea

Use Adjunct to diet for the management of mild-to-moderately severe, stable, type 2 diabetes mellitus (noninsulin dependent, NIDDM)

Dosing

Adult & Geriatric

Type 2 diabetes: Oral (doses >500 mg/day should be given in 2 divided doses):

Initial: 100-250 mg/day with breakfast or the first main meal of the day

Fasting blood sugar <200 mg/dL: 100 mg/day

Fasting blood sugar >200 mg/dL: 250 mg/day

Patient is malnourished, underweight, elderly, or not eating properly: 100 mg/day

Adjustment/titration: Increase in increments of 100-250 mg/day at weekly intervals to response; maximum daily dose: 1 g (doses >1 g/day are not likely to improve control)

Conversion from insulin to tolazamide:

<20 units day = 100 mg/day

21-<40 units/day = 250 mg/day

≥40 units/day = 250 mg/day and 50% of insulin dose

Renal Impairment No dosage adjustment provided in manufacturer's labeling. However, conservative initial and maintenance doses are recommended because tolazamide is metabolized to active metabolites, which are eliminated in the urine.

Hepatic Impairment No dosage adjustment provided in manufacturer's labeling. However, conservative initial and maintenance doses and careful monitoring of blood glucose are recommended.

Additional Information Complete prescribing information should be consulted for additional detail.

Dosage Forms Excipient information presented when available (limited, particularly for generics); consult specific product labeling.
Tablet, Oral:
Generic: 250 mg, 500 mg

TOLBUTamide (tole BYOO ta mide)

Brand Names: Canada Apo-Tolbutamide®
Index Terms Orinase; Tolbutamide Sodium
Pharmacologic Category Antidiabetic Agent, Sulfonylurea
Use Adjunct to diet for the management of type 2 diabetes mellitus (noninsulin dependent, NIDDM)
Dosing
Adult Type 2 diabetes: Oral: Initial: 1-2 g/day as a single dose in the morning or in divided doses throughout the day. Maintenance dose: 0.25-3 g/day; however, a maintenance dose >2 g/day is seldom required. **Note:** Divided doses may improve gastrointestinal tolerance
Geriatric Initial: 250 mg 1-3 times/day; usual: 500-2000 mg; maximum: 3 g/day
Renal Impairment No dosage adjustment provided in manufacturer's labeling. However, conservative initial and maintenance doses are recommended.
Hemodialysis: Not dialyzable (0% to 5%)
Hepatic Impairment No dosage adjustment provided in manufacturer's labeling. However, conservative initial and maintenance doses and careful monitoring of blood glucose are recommended.
Additional Information Complete prescribing information should be consulted for additional detail.
Dosage Forms Excipient information presented when available (limited, particularly for generics); consult specific product labeling.
Tablet, Oral:
Generic: 500 mg

◆ **Tolbutamide Sodium** see TOLBUTamide on page 1807

Tolcapone (TOLE ka pone)

Brand Names: US Tasmar
Pharmacologic Category Anti-Parkinson's Agent, COMT Inhibitor
Use Adjunct to levodopa and carbidopa for the treatment of signs and symptoms of idiopathic Parkinson's disease in patients with motor fluctuations not responsive to other therapies
Prescribing and Access Restrictions A patient signed consent form acknowledging the risks of hepatic injury should be obtained by the treating physician.
Dosing
Adult & Geriatric Note: Tolcapone is only appropriate in patients receiving concomitant carbidopa and levodopa. If clinical improvement is not observed after 3 weeks of therapy (regardless of dose), tolcapone treatment should be discontinued.

Parkinson's disease: Oral: Initial: 100 mg 3 times daily; may increase as tolerated to 200 mg 3 times daily only if clinical benefit is justified (dosage associated with an increased incidence of ALT elevations). **Note:** Levodopa dose may need to be decreased upon initiation of tolcapone (average reduction in clinical trials was 30%). As many as 70% of patients receiving levodopa doses >600 mg daily required levodopa dosage reduction in clinical trials. Patients with moderate-to-severe dyskinesia prior to initiation are also more likely to require dosage reduction.
Renal Impairment
Mild-to-moderate impairment (CrCl ≥25 mL/minute): No dosage adjustment necessary.
Severe impairment (CrCl <25 mL/minute): No dosage adjustment provided in manufacturer's labeling (has not been studied). Use with caution.
Hepatic Impairment Use is contraindicated in patients with liver disease. Discontinue immediately if signs/symptoms of hepatic impairment develop.
Additional Information Complete prescribing information should be consulted for additional detail.

Dosage Forms Excipient information presented when available (limited, particularly for generics); consult specific product labeling.
Tablet, Oral:
Tasmar: 100 mg
Generic: 100 mg

◆ **Tolectin** see Tolmetin on page 1807

Tolmetin (TOLE met in)

Index Terms Tolectin; Tolmetin Sodium
Pharmacologic Category Nonsteroidal Anti-inflammatory Drug (NSAID), Oral
Use
Juvenile rheumatoid arthritis: Treatment of juvenile rheumatoid arthritis (JRA) in pediatric patients ≥2 years.
Rheumatoid/Osteoarthritis: Relief of signs and symptoms of rheumatoid and osteoarthritis, including acute flares and the long-term management of the chronic disease.
Medication Guide Available Yes
Dosing
Adult Note: Use the lowest effective dose for the shortest possible duration.
Osteoarthritis/RA: Oral: Initial: 400 mg 3 times daily; adjust dose according to patient response after 1 to 2 weeks; Maintenance: 600 mg to 1,800 mg/day in 3 divided doses (maximum: 1,800 mg/day)
Geriatric Refer to adult dosing; use with caution.
Pediatric Note: Use the lowest effective dose for the shortest possible duration.
Juvenile rheumatoid arthritis: Children ≥2 years and Adolescents: Oral: Initial: 20 mg/kg/day in 3 to 4 divided doses; Maintenance: 15 to 30 mg/kg/day in 3 to 4 divided doses (maximum: 30 mg/kg/day)
Analgesic (off-label use): Oral: Children ≥2 years and Adolescents: 5 to 7 mg/kg/dose every 6 to 8 hours (Berde 1990)
Renal Impairment There are no dosage adjustments provided in the manufacturer's labeling; not recommended in patients with advanced renal disease.
Hepatic Impairment There are no dosage adjustments provided in the manufacturer's labeling; use with caution.
Additional Information Complete prescribing information should be consulted for additional detail.
Dosage Forms Excipient information presented when available (limited, particularly for generics); consult specific product labeling.
Capsule, Oral:
Generic: 400 mg
Tablet, Oral:
Generic: 200 mg, 600 mg

◆ **Tolmetin Sodium** see Tolmetin on page 1807

Tolnaftate (tole NAF tate)

Brand Names: US Anti-Fungal [OTC]; Antifungal [OTC]; Athletes Foot Spray [OTC]; Dr Gs Clear Nail [OTC]; Fungi-Guard [OTC]; Fungoid-D [OTC]; Jock Itch Spray [OTC]; LamISIL AF Defense [OTC]; Medi-First Anti-Fungal [OTC]; Mycocide Clinical NS [OTC]; Podactin [OTC]; Tinactin Deodorant [OTC]; Tinactin Jock Itch [OTC]; Tinactin [OTC]; Tinamar [OTC] [DSC]; Tinaspore [OTC]; Tolnaftate Antifungal [OTC]
Brand Names: Canada Pitrex
Pharmacologic Category Antifungal Agent, Topical
Use Treatment of tinea pedis, tinea cruris, tinea corporis
Dosing
Adult & Geriatric Tinea infection: Topical: Wash and dry affected area; spray aerosol or apply 1-3 drops of solution or a small amount of cream, or powder and rub into the affected areas 2 times/day
Note: May use for up to 4 weeks for tinea pedis or tinea corporis, and up to 2 weeks for tinea cruris.
Pediatric Children ≥2 years: Refer to adult dosing.
Additional Information Complete prescribing information should be consulted for additional detail.
Dosage Forms Excipient information presented when available (limited, particularly for generics); consult specific product labeling. [DSC] = Discontinued product
Aerosol, External:
Athletes Foot Spray: 1% (150 g) [contains sd alcohol 40]
Tinactin: 1% (150 g)
Aerosol Powder, External:
Jock Itch Spray: 1% (130 g) [contains sd alcohol 40b]
LamISIL AF Defense: 1% (133 g)
Tinactin: 1% (133 g)
Tinactin Deodorant: 1% (133 g)

Cream, External:
Antifungal: 1% (15 g) [odorless]
Fungi-Guard: 1% (15 g)
Fungoid-D: 1% (113 g) [contains cetyl alcohol, methylparaben, propylene glycol, propylparaben, trolamine (triethanolamine)]
Medi-First Anti-Fungal: 1% (1 ea)
Tinactin: 1% (15 g, 30 g)
Tinactin Jock Itch: 1% (15 g)
Tinamar: 1% (15 g [DSC])
Tolnaftate Antifungal: 1% (114 g) [contains cetyl alcohol, methylparaben, polysorbate 80, propylene glycol, propylparaben]
Generic: 1% (15 g, 20 g, 28.3 g, 30 g)
Powder, External:
Anti-Fungal: 1% (45 g)
LamISIL AF Defense: 1% (113 g)
Podactin: 1% (45 g)
Tinactin: 1% (108 g)
Tinamar: 1% (45 g [DSC], 90 g [DSC])
Generic: 1% (45 g)
Solution, External:
Dr Gs Clear Nail: 1% (18 mL) [contains propylene glycol]
Mycocide Clinical NS: 1% (30 mL) [contains propylene glycol]
Tinamar: 1% (10 mL [DSC])
Tinaspore: 1% (10 mL)
Generic: 1% (10 mL)

◆ Tolnaftate Antifungal [OTC] *see* Tolnaftate on page 1807

◆ Toloxin (Can) *see* Digoxin on page 547

Tolterodine (tole TER oh deen)

Brand Names: US Detrol; Detrol LA
Brand Names: Canada Detrol®; Detrol® LA; Unidet®
Index Terms Tolterodine Tartrate
Pharmacologic Category Anticholinergic Agent
Use Treatment of patients with an overactive bladder with symptoms of urinary frequency, urgency, or urge incontinence
Pregnancy Considerations Teratogenic effects were observed in some animal reproduction studies.
Breast-Feeding Considerations It is not known if tolterodine is excreted in breast milk. Due to the potential for serious adverse reactions in the nursing infant, a decision should be made whether to discontinue nursing or to discontinue the drug, taking into account the importance of treatment to the mother.
Contraindications Hypersensitivity to tolterodine or fesoterodine (both are metabolized to 5-hydroxymethyl tolterodine) or any component of the formulation; urinary retention; gastric retention; uncontrolled narrow-angle glaucoma
Warnings/Precautions Cases of angioedema have been reported; some cases have occurred after a single dose. Discontinue immediately if angioedema and associated difficulty breathing, airway obstruction, or hypotension develop. May cause drowsiness, dizziness, and/or blurred vision, which may impair physical or mental abilities; patients must be cautioned about performing tasks which require mental alertness (eg, operating machinery or driving). Consider dose reduction or discontinuation if CNS effects occur. Use with caution in patients with bladder flow obstruction, may increase the risk of urinary retention. Use with caution in patients with gastrointestinal obstructive disorders (ie, pyloric stenosis), may increase the risk of gastric retention. Use with caution in patients with myasthenia gravis and controlled (treated) narrow-angle glaucoma; metabolized in the liver and excreted in the urine and feces, dosage adjustment is required for patients with renal or hepatic impairment. Tolterodine has been associated with QTc prolongation at high (supratherapeutic) doses. The manufacturer recommends caution in patients with congenital prolonged QT or in patients receiving concurrent therapy with QTc-prolonging drugs (class Ia or III antiarrhythmics). However, the mean change in QTc even at supratherapeutic dosages was less than 15 msec. Individuals who are CYP2D6 poor metabolizers or in the presence of inhibitors of CYP2D6 and CYP3A4 may be more likely to exhibit prolongation. Dosage adjustment is recommended in patients receiving CYP3A4 inhibitors (a lower dose of tolterodine is recommended). This medication is associated with potent anticholinergic properties which may be inappropriate in older adults depending on comorbidities (eg, dementia, delirium) (Beers Criteria).
Adverse Reactions As reported with immediate release tablet, unless otherwise specified

>10%: Gastrointestinal: Dry mouth (35%; extended release capsules 23%)

1% to 10%:
Cardiovascular: Chest pain (2%)
Central nervous system: Headache (7%; extended release capsules 6%); dizziness (5%; extended release capsules 2%), fatigue (4%; extended release capsules 2%), somnolence (3%; extended release capsules 3%), anxiety (extended release capsules 1%)
Dermatologic: Dry skin (1%)
Gastrointestinal: Constipation (7%; extended release capsules 6%), abdominal pain (5%; extended release capsules 4%), diarrhea (4%), dyspepsia (4%; extended release capsules 3%), weight gain (1%)
Genitourinary: Dysuria (2%; extended release capsules 1%)
Neuromuscular & skeletal: Arthralgia (2%)
Ocular: Dry eyes (3%; extended release capsules 3%), abnormal vision (2%; extended release capsules 1%)
Respiratory: Bronchitis (2%), sinusitis (extended release capsules 2%)
Miscellaneous: Flu-like syndrome (3%), infection (1%)
<1% (Limited to important or life-threatening): Anaphylaxis, angioedema, confusion, dementia aggravated, disorientation, hallucinations, memory impairment, palpitation, peripheral edema, QTc prolongation, tachycardia
Drug Interactions
Metabolism/Transport Effects Substrate of CYP2C19 (minor), CYP2C9 (minor), CYP2D6 (major), CYP3A4 (major); **Note:** Assignment of Major/Minor substrate status based on clinically relevant drug interaction potential
Avoid Concomitant Use
Avoid concomitant use of Tolterodine with any of the following: Aclidinium; Cimetropium; Conivaptan; Eluxadoline; Fusidic Acid (Systemic); Glucagon; Glycopyrrolate; Glycopyrrolate (Oral Inhalation); Idelalisib; Ipratropium (Oral Inhalation); Levosulpiride; Potassium Chloride; Tiotropium; Umeclidinium
Increased Effect/Toxicity
Tolterodine may increase the levels/effects of: AbobotulinumtoxinA; Analgesics (Opioid); Anticholinergic Agents; Cannabinoid-Containing Products; Cimetropium; Eluxadoline; Glucagon; Glycopyrrolate; Glycopyrrolate (Oral Inhalation); Highest Risk QTc-Prolonging Agents; Mirabegron; Moderate Risk QTc-Prolonging Agents; OnabotulinumtoxinA; Potassium Chloride; Ramosetron; RimabotulinumtoxinB; Thiazide Diuretics; Tiotropium; Topiramate; Warfarin

The levels/effects of Tolterodine may be increased by: Abiraterone Acetate; Aclidinium; Aprepitant; Conivaptan; CYP2D6 Inhibitors (Moderate); CYP2D6 Inhibitors (Strong); CYP3A4 Inhibitors (Moderate); CYP3A4 Inhibitors (Strong); Dasatinib; Fosaprepitant; Fusidic Acid (Systemic); Idelalisib; Ipratropium (Oral Inhalation); Ivacaftor; Luliconazole; Mianserin; Mifepristone; Netupitant; Osimertinib; Palbociclib; Panobinostat; Peginterferon Alfa-2b; Pramlintide; Simeprevir; Stiripentol; Umeclidinium; VinBLAStine
Decreased Effect
Tolterodine may decrease the levels/effects of: Acetylcholinesterase Inhibitors; Gastrointestinal Agents (Prokinetic); Itopride; Levosulpiride; Secretin

The levels/effects of Tolterodine may be decreased by: Acetylcholinesterase Inhibitors; Bosentan; CYP3A4 Inducers (Moderate); CYP3A4 Inducers (Strong); Dabrafenib; Deferasirox; Enzalutamide; Mitotane; Osimertinib; Peginterferon Alfa-2b; Siltuximab; St Johns Wort; Tocilizumab
Food Interactions Food increases bioavailability (~53% increase) of tolterodine tablets (dose adjustment not necessary); does not affect the pharmacokinetics of tolterodine extended release capsules. As a CYP3A4 inhibitor, grapefruit juice may increase the serum level and/or toxicity of tolterodine, but unlikely secondary to high oral bioavailability. Management: Monitor patients closely with concurrent grapefruit juice use.
Storage/Stability Store at 25°C (77°F); excursions permitted to 15°C to 30°C (59°F to 86°F). Protect from light.
Mechanism of Action Tolterodine is a competitive antagonist of muscarinic receptors. In animal models, tolterodine demonstrates selectivity for urinary bladder receptors over salivary receptors. Urinary bladder contraction is mediated by muscarinic receptors. Tolterodine increases residual urine volume and decreases detrusor muscle pressure.
Pharmacodynamics/Kinetics
Absorption: Immediate release tablet: Rapid; ≥77%
Distribution: IV: V_d: 113 ± 27 L
Protein binding: >96% (primarily to alpha$_1$-acid glycoprotein)
Metabolism: Extensively hepatic, primarily via CYP2D6 to 5-hydroxymethyltolterodine (active) and 3A4 usually (minor pathway). In patients with a genetic deficiency of CYP2D6, metabolism via 3A4 predominates.

Bioavailability: Immediate release tablet: Increased 53% with food

Half-life elimination:
Immediate release tablet: Extensive metabolizers: ~2 hours; Poor metabolizers: ~10 hours
Extended release capsule: Extensive metabolizers: ~7 hours; Poor metabolizers: ~18 hours

Time to peak: Immediate release tablet: 1-2 hours; Extended release capsule: 2-6 hours

Excretion: Urine (77%); feces (17%); primarily as metabolites (<1% unchanged drug) of which the active 5-hydroxymethyl metabolite accounts for 5% to 14% (<1% in poor metabolizers); as unchanged drug (<1%; <2.5% in poor metabolizers)

Dosing

Adult Treatment of overactive bladder: Oral:
Immediate release tablet: 2 mg twice daily; the dose may be lowered to 1 mg twice daily based on individual response and tolerability
Dosing adjustment in patients concurrently taking strong CYP3A4 inhibitors (eg, ketoconazole, clarithromycin, ritonavir): 1 mg twice daily
Extended release capsule: 4 mg once daily; dose may be lowered to 2 mg once daily based on individual response and tolerability
Dosing adjustment in patients concurrently taking strong CYP3A4 inhibitors (eg, ketoconazole, clarithromycin, ritonavir): 2 mg once daily

Geriatric Refer to adult dosing. Safety and efficacy in patients >64 years was found to be similar to that in younger patients; no dosage adjustment is needed based on age.

Renal Impairment
Immediate release tablet: Significantly reduced renal function (studies conducted in patients with CrCl 10-30 mL/minute): 1 mg twice daily; use with caution
Extended release capsule:
CrCl 10-30 mL/minute: 2 mg once daily
CrCl <10 mL/minute: Use is not recommended; has not been studied.

Hepatic Impairment
Immediate release tablet: Significantly reduced hepatic function: 1 mg twice daily; use with caution
Extended release capsule:
Mild-to-moderate impairment (Child-Pugh class A or B): 2 mg once daily
Severe impairment (Child-Pugh class C): Use is not recommended; has not been studied.

Administration Extended release capsule: Swallow whole; do not crush, chew, or open

Monitoring Parameters Renal function (BUN, creatinine); hepatic function

Dosage Forms Excipient information presented when available (limited, particularly for generics); consult specific product labeling.
Capsule Extended Release 24 Hour, Oral, as tartrate:
Detrol LA: 2 mg, 4 mg
Generic: 2 mg, 4 mg
Tablet, Oral, as tartrate:
Detrol: 1 mg, 2 mg
Generic: 1 mg, 2 mg

◆ Tolterodine Tartrate *see* Tolterodine *on page 1808*

Tolvaptan (tol VAP tan)

Brand Names: US Samsca
Brand Names: Canada Jinarc; Samsca
Index Terms OPC-41061
Pharmacologic Category Vasopressin Antagonist

Use
Samsca:
Hypervolemic and euvolemic hyponatremia: Treatment of clinically significant hypervolemic or euvolemic hyponatremia (serum sodium <125 mEq/L or less marked hyponatremia that is symptomatic and resistant to fluid restriction), including patients with heart failure and Syndrome of Inappropriate Antidiuretic Hormone (SIADH).
Limitations of use: Not indicated for use when urgent treatment of hyponatremia is required to prevent or treat serious neurological symptoms. It has not been established that raising serum sodium with tolvaptan provides symptomatic benefit.

Jinarc [Canadian product]:
Autosomal dominant polycystic kidney disease (ADPKD): Slow the progression of kidney enlargement in patients with ADPKD.

Limitations of use: Clinical trials evaluated ADPKD patients having a total kidney volume ≥750 mL with relatively preserved renal function (eg, estimated creatinine clearance ≥60 mL/minute, generally corresponding to a CKD-EPI eGFR ≥30 mL/minute/1.73 m^2 at the time of therapy initiation).

Prescribing and Access Restrictions Jinarc [Canadian product]: Only physicians experienced in the diagnosis and treatment of polycystic kidney disease should prescribe Jinarc. Prior to initiating therapy, a patient-prescriber agreement (PPAF) is required outlining relevant patient selection criteria for consideration, expected benefits and risks of treatment, and the need for mandatory hepatic function monitoring. Jinarc is available only through a hepatic safety monitoring and distribution program conducted and maintained by Otsuka Canada Pharmaceuticals Incorporated. All patients initiating therapy should be offered participation in the Canadian Jinarc patient outcomes registry.

Medication Guide Available Yes

Dosing
Adult
Hyponatremia: Oral:
Samsca: Initial: 15 mg once daily; after at least 24 hours, may increase to 30 mg once daily to a maximum of 60 mg once daily titrating at 24-hour intervals to desired serum sodium concentration. Avoid fluid restriction during the first 24 hours of therapy. Do not use for more than 30 days due to the risk of hepatotoxicity.
Canadian labeling: **Note:** Based on serum sodium concentrations following an initial dose of 15 mg the following dose titration is recommended (at 24-hour intervals):
Change <5 mEq/L in 24 hours and serum sodium <130 mEq/L:
Day 2: Consider titration to 30 mg once daily.
Day 3 through discontinuation: Consider titration to 60 mg once daily.
Change ≥5 mEq/L in 24 hours:
Day 2: Consider maintenance dose of 15 mg once daily.
Day 3 through discontinuation: Consider maintenance of prior current dose.
Change >8 mEq/L in 8 hours or >12 mEq/L in 24 hours: Day 2 through discontinuation: Consider withholding dose and/or increase hypotonic fluid intake; monitor sodium closely.
Serum sodium ≥140 mEq/L at any time: Discontinue therapy and consider increasing hypotonic fluid intake.

Autosomal dominant polycystic kidney disease (ADPKD): Jinarc [Canadian product]: Oral: **Note:** Prior to initiating therapy, restrict overnight fluid intake for 10 to 14 hours to assess ability to concentrate urine using urine osmolality or specific gravity (less accurate). Upon initiation of therapy fluid intake should not be restricted.
Initial: 60 mg/day in divided doses (45 mg upon wakening and 15 mg approximately 8 hours later); titrate per response and tolerability at intervals of at least 7 days to 90 mg/day (60 mg upon wakening and 30 mg approximately 8 hours later) and then to 120 mg/day (90 mg upon wakening and 30 mg approximately 8 hours later). Downward titration may be necessary based on tolerability.
Maintenance: Maintain patient on highest tolerated dose to decrease urine osmolality 200 to 300 mOsm/kg (preferable in most cases) from baseline. Urine osmolality or specific gravity should be measured before morning dose. Urine osmolality <300 mOsm/kg (corresponds to a specific gravity of 1.005) should be maintained at all times if possible. Avoid unnecessary interruptions in therapy; however if the ability to drink or accessibility to water is limited therapy should be interrupted.

Dosage adjustment with concomitant medication: Jinarc [Canadian product]:
Strong CYP3A inhibitors (eg, ketoconazole, clarithromycin, ritonavir, saquinavir): Patients receiving tolvaptan 120 mg/day or 90 mg/day: Reduce dose to 30 mg/day administered upon wakening. Patients receiving tolvaptan 60 mg/day: Reduce dose to 15 mg/day administered upon wakening. Titrate cautiously per response and tolerability. Further downward titration or discontinuation of concurrent therapy may be necessary based on tolerability.
Moderate CYP3A inhibitors (eg, erythromycin, fluconazole, verapamil): Decrease daily dose by 50% administered as split regimen with first dose upon wakening and second dose ~8 hours later (eg, 120 mg/day [90 mg + 30 mg/day] is reduced to 60 mg/day [45 mg + 15 mg/day]). When adjusting the dose

reduce the first daily dose as needed and maintain the second daily dose at 15 mg.

Geriatric Refer to adult dosing. **Note:** Jinarc [Canadian product] has not been studied in patients >65 years.

Renal Impairment

CrCl ≥10 mL/minute: No dosage adjustment necessary.

CrCl <10 mL/minute: Use not recommended (has not been studied); contraindicated in anuria (no benefit expected).

Hepatic Impairment

US labeling: Avoid use in patients with underlying liver disease, including cirrhosis.

Canadian labeling:

Jinarc:

Preexisting hepatic impairment: There are no dosage adjustments provided in the manufacturer's labeling; use with caution and monitor closely. Avoid initiation of therapy if AST/ALT >3 times ULN. Use is contraindicated in patients with clinically relevant impairment.

Dosage adjustment for toxicity (during therapy): Interrupt therapy if hepatotoxicity is suspected and promptly evaluate hepatic function; upon resolution may consider reinitiating therapy cautiously.

ALT or AST <3 times ULN: Continue therapy cautiously and monitor frequently.

Permanently discontinue for any the following: ALT or AST >8 times ULN, ALT or AST >5 times ULN for >2 weeks, ALT or AST >3 times ULN and total bilirubin >2 times ULN or INR >1.5, ALT or AST >3 times ULN with persistent symptoms of hepatic injury.

Samsca: No dosage adjustment is necessary. Use with caution and monitor closely due to risks of hepatotoxicity; discontinue use promptly if hepatotoxicity is suspected.

Additional Information Complete prescribing information should be consulted for additional detail.

Dosage Forms Excipient information presented when available (limited, particularly for generics); consult specific product labeling.

Tablet, Oral:

Samsca: 15 mg, 30 mg [contains fd&c blue #2 aluminum lake]

Dosage Forms: Canada Excipient information presented when available (limited, particularly for generics); consult specific product labeling.

Tablet, oral:

Jinarc: 15 mg, 30 mg, 45 mg, 60 mg, 90 mg

Samsca: 15 mg, 30 mg, 60 mg

Topiramate (toe PYRE a mate)

Brand Names: US Qudexy XR; Topamax; Topamax Sprinkle; Topiragen [DSC]; Trokendi XR

Brand Names: Canada Abbott-Topiramate; ACT Topiramate; Apo-Topiramate; AURO-Topiramate; Dom-Topiramate; Jamp-Topiramate; Mint-Topiramate; Mylan-Topiramate; PHL-Topiramate; PMS-Topiramate; PRO-Topiramate; RAN-Topiramate; Sandoz-Topiramate; TEVA-Topiramate; Topamax

Pharmacologic Category Anticonvulsant, Miscellaneous

Use

Epilepsy:

Monotherapy: As initial monotherapy in patients ≥2 years (immediate release and Qudexy XR) or ≥10 years (Trokendi XR) with partial-onset or primary generalized tonic-clonic seizures

Adjunctive therapy: As adjunctive therapy in patients ≥2 years (immediate release and Qudexy XR only) or ≥6 years (Trokendi XR only) with partial-onset seizures, primary generalized tonic-clonic seizures, or seizures associated with Lennox-Gastaut syndrome

Migraine (immediate release only): Prophylaxis of migraine headache in adults and adolescents ≥12 years.

Pregnancy Considerations Adverse events have been observed in animal reproduction studies. Based on limited data (n=5), topiramate was found to cross the placenta and could be detected in neonatal serum (Ohman 2002). Topiramate may cause fetal harm if administered to a pregnant woman. An increased risk of oral clefts (cleft lip and/or palate) has been observed following first trimester exposure. Data from the North American Antiepileptic Drug (NAAED) Pregnancy Registry reported that the prevalence of oral clefts was 1.2% for infants exposed to topiramate during the first trimester of pregnancy, versus 0.39% to 0.46% for infants exposed to other antiepileptic drugs and 0.12% with no exposure. Although not evaluated during pregnancy, metabolic acidosis may be induced by topiramate. In general, metabolic acidosis during pregnancy may result in adverse effects and fetal death. Pregnant women and their newborns should be monitored for metabolic acidosis. Maternal serum concentrations may decrease during the second and third trimesters of pregnancy therefore therapeutic drug monitoring should be considered in pregnant women who require therapy (Ohman 2009; Westin 2009).

Use for migraine prophylaxis is contraindicated per the Canadian labeling in pregnant women or women of childbearing potential who are not using effective contraception.

Patients exposed to topiramate during pregnancy are encouraged to enroll themselves into the AED Pregnancy Registry by calling 1-888-233-2334. Additional information is available at www.aedpregnancyregistry.org.

Breast-Feeding Considerations Topiramate is excreted into breast milk. Based on information from five nursing infants, infant plasma concentrations of topiramate have been reported as 10% to 20% of the maternal plasma concentration. The manufacturer recommends that caution be used if administered to a nursing woman.

Medication Guide Available Yes

Contraindications

Extended release: Recent alcohol use (ie, within 6 hours prior to and 6 hours after administration) (Trokendi XR only); patients with metabolic acidosis who are taking concomitant metformin

Immediate release: There are no contraindications listed in the manufacturer's labeling.

Canadian labeling (not in U.S. labeling): Hypersensitivity to topiramate or any component of the formulation or container; pregnancy and women in childbearing years not using effective contraception (migraine prophylaxis only)

Warnings/Precautions Hazardous agent – use appropriate precautions for handling and disposal (NIOSH 2014 [group 3]).

Antiepileptics are associated with an increased risk of suicidal behavior/thoughts with use (regardless of indication); patients should be monitored for signs/symptoms of depression, suicidal tendencies, and other unusual behavior changes during therapy and instructed to inform their healthcare provider immediately if symptoms occur. Use with caution in patients with hepatic, respiratory, or renal impairment. Topiramate may decrease serum bicarbonate concentrations (up to 67% of epilepsy patients and 77% of migraine patients). Risk may be increased in patients with a predisposing condition (organ dysfunction, diarrhea, ketogenic diet, status epilepticus, or concurrent treatment with other drugs which may cause acidosis). Metabolic acidosis may occur at dosages as low as 50 mg/day. Monitor serum bicarbonate as well as potential complications of chronic acidosis (nephrolithiasis, nephrocalcinosis, osteomalacia/osteoporosis, and reduced growth rates and/or weight in children). Kidney stones have been reported in both children and adults; the risk of kidney stones is about 2-4 times that of the untreated population; consider avoiding use in patients on a ketogenic diet; the risk of kidney stones may be reduced by increasing fluid intake.

Cognitive dysfunction (confusion, psychomotor slowing, difficulty with concentration/attention, difficulty with memory, speech or language problems), psychiatric disturbances (depression or mood disorders), and sedation (somnolence or fatigue) may occur with topiramate use; incidence may be related to rapid titration and higher doses. Patients must be cautioned about performing tasks which require mental alertness (eg, operating machinery or driving). Effects with other sedative drugs or ethanol may

be potentiated. Topiramate may also cause paresthesia, dizziness, and ataxia. Topiramate has been associated with acute myopia and secondary angle-closure glaucoma in adults and children, typically within 1 month of initiation; discontinue in patients with acute onset of decreased visual acuity and/or ocular pain. Visual field defects have also been reported independent of increased intraocular pressure; generally reversible upon discontinuation. Consider discontinuation if visual problems occur at any time during treatment. Hyperammonemia with or without encephalopathy may occur with or without concomitant valproate administration; valproic acid dose-dependency was observed in limited pediatric studies; use with caution in patients with inborn errors of metabolism or decreased hepatic mitochondrial activity. Hypothermia (core body temperature <35°C [95°F]) has been reported with concomitant use of topiramate and valproic acid; may occur with or without associated hyperammonemia and may develop after topiramate initiation or dosage increase; discontinuation of topiramate or valproic acid may be necessary. Topiramate may be associated with oligohydrosis and hyperthermia, most frequently in children; use caution and monitor closely during strenuous exercise, during exposure to high environmental temperature, or in patients receiving receiving other carbonic anhydrase inhibitors and drugs with anticholinergic activity. Use with caution in the elderly; dosage adjustment may be required.

The exacerbation and development of eating disorders, including anorexia nervosa and bulimia, has been reported in case reports of adolescents receiving topiramate for migraines or chronic headaches and an adult receiving topiramate for epilepsy. Prior to initiation of topiramate screen for a history of eating disorder symptoms, eating disorder risk factors (eg, history of dieting behavior), cognitive symptoms of eating disorders (eg, weigh or shape concerns, fear of gaining weight, drive for thinness), and any recent changes in social functioning including increased withdrawal or isolation. Inquire whether the patient has unrealistic or unhealthy weight goals. Evaluate exercise habits (eg, look for over-exercising or compulsive exercising above that of similarly athletic peers) and dietary intake; assess rigid patterns or avoidance of specific categories of foods and preoccupation with maintaining a "healthy diet" or experimentation with fad diets. In adolescents assess developmental weight history with growth curves. Monitor eating behaviors and weight closely in patients receiving topiramate who have eating disorder symptoms or risk factors (Lebow 2015; Rosenow 2002).

Potentially significant drug-drug interactions may exist, requiring dose or frequency adjustment, additional monitoring, and/or selection of alternative therapy. Avoid abrupt withdrawal of topiramate therapy; it should be withdrawn/tapered slowly to minimize the potential of increased seizure frequency. Doses were also gradually withdrawn in migraine prophylaxis studies.

Adverse Reactions Adverse events are reported for adult and pediatric patients for various indications and regimens. **Note:** A wide range of dosages were studied. Incidence of adverse events was frequently lower in the pediatric population studied.

Epilepsy, monotherapy:
>10%:
  Central nervous system: Paresthesia (adolescents ≥16 years and adults: 21% to 40%; children and adolescents 6 to <16 years: 2% to 16%), drowsiness (adolescents ≥16 years and adults: 9% to 15%), fatigue (14%), dizziness (adolescents ≥16 years and adults: 13% to 14%), memory impairment (adolescents ≥16 years and adults: 5% to 11%; children and adolescents 6 to <16 years: 1% to 3%), mood disorder (1% to 11%)
  Endocrine & metabolic: Decreased serum bicarbonate (children ≥6 years, adolescents, and adults: 9% to 25%), weight loss (6% to 21%)
  Gastrointestinal: Anorexia (4% to 14%), diarrhea (5% to 11%)
  Respiratory: Upper respiratory tract infection (children and adolescents 6 to <16 years: 16% to 18%)
  Miscellaneous: Fever (children and adolescents 6 to <16 years: ≤12%)
1% to 10%:
  Cardiovascular: Flushing (children and adolescents 6 to <16 years: ≤5%), chest pain (adolescents ≥16 years and adults: 1% to 2%)
  Central nervous system: Lack of concentration (7% to 10%), depression (≤9%), insomnia (adolescents ≥16 years and adults: 8% to 9%), cognitive dysfunction (≤7%), anxiety (adolescents ≥16 years and adults: 4% to 6%), hypoesthesia (adolescents ≥16 years and adults: 4% to 5%), nervousness (children and adolescents 10 to 16 years: 4% to 5%), psychomotor retardation (adolescents ≥16 years and adults: 3% to 5%),

ataxia (adolescents ≥16 years and adults: 3% to 4%), confusion (≤4%), behavioral problems (children and adolescents 6 to <16 years: ≤3%), hypertonia (adolescents ≥16 years and adults: ≤3%), vertigo (children and adolescents 6 to <16 years: ≤3%)
  Dermatologic: Alopecia (1% to 5%), pruritus (adolescents ≥16 years and adults: 1% to 4%), skin rash (1% to 4%), acne vulgaris (adolescents ≥16 years and adults: 2% to 3%)
  Endocrine & metabolic: Increased gamma-glutamyl transferase (adolescents ≥16 years and adults: 1% to 3%), intermenstrual bleeding (children and adolescents 6 to <16 years: ≤3%)
  Gastrointestinal: Dysgeusia (adolescents ≥16 years and adults: 3% to 5%), constipation (adolescents ≥16 years and adults: 1% to 4%), gastritis (adolescents ≥16 years and adults: ≤3%), xerostomia (adolescents ≥16 years and adults: 1% to 3%), gastroesophageal reflux disease (adolescents ≥16 years and adults: 1% to 2%)
  Genitourinary: Decreased libido (adolescents ≥16 years and adults: ≤3%), urinary frequency (≤3%), vaginal hemorrhage (adolescents ≥16 years and adults: ≤3%), cystitis (adolescents ≥16 years and adults: 1% to 3%), urinary incontinence (children and adolescents 6 to <16 years: 1% to 3%), dysuria (adolescents ≥16 years and adults: ≤2%), urinary tract infection (adolescents ≥16 years and adults: 1% to 2%)
  Hematologic & oncologic: Anemia (1% to 3%)
  Infection: Viral infection (3% to 9%), infection (2% to 8%)
  Neuromuscular & skeletal: Weakness (≤6%), muscle spasm (children and adolescents 6 to <16 years: ≤3%), leg pain (adolescents ≥16 years and adults: 2% to 3%)
  Renal: Nephrolithiasis (adolescents ≥16 years and adults: ≤3%)
  Respiratory: Rhinitis (2% to 7%), bronchitis (1% to 7%), sinusitis (children and adolescents 6 to <16 years: 1% to 5%), epistaxis (children and adolescents 6 to <16 years: ≤4%), dyspnea (adolescents ≥16 years and adults: 1% to 2%)

Migraine prophylaxis:
Frequency not always defined.
Central nervous system: Paresthesia (adults: 35% to 51%; children and adolescents ≥12 years: 19% to 20%; dose related), fatigue (8% to 15%; dose related), insomnia (6% to 9%), drowsiness (6% to 8%; dose related), memory impairment (adults 7%; dose related), hypoesthesia (adults 6% to 7%; dose related), dizziness (children and adolescents ≥12 years: 6%), lack of concentration (adults: 3% to 6%; children and adolescents ≥12 years: ≤2%), mood disorder (adults: 3% to 6%; dose related), anxiety (adults: 4% to 5%; dose related), headache (children and adolescents ≥12 years: 4%; adults: >1%), nervousness (4%), confusion (adults: 3%; dose related), psychomotor retardation (≤3%), agitation (adults: 2%), cognitive dysfunction (adults: 2%), exacerbation of depression (adults: 2%), ataxia (adults: 1% to 2%), pain (children and adolescents ≥12 years: >1%), sensory disturbance (adults: >1%), vertigo (adults: >1%), speech disturbance (adults: 1%; dose related)
Dermatologic: Pruritus (4%), alopecia (adults: >1%), skin rash (>1%)
Endocrine & metabolic: Decreased serum bicarbonate (23% to 39%), hyperammonemia (children and adolescents ≥12 years: 14% to 26%), weight loss (4% to 9%; dose related), menstrual disease (adults: 3%), increased thirst (adults: 2%), intermenstrual bleeding (adults: >1%), hyperchloremia, increased serum total protein, increased uric acid
Gastrointestinal: Anorexia (9% to 15%; dose related), abdominal pain (6% to 15%), dysgeusia (6% to 15%), nausea (6% to 13%), dyspepsia (adults: 4% to 5%), gastroenteritis (3%), xerostomia (adults: 3%; dose related), diarrhea (children and adolescents ≥12 years: 2%), constipation (adults: >1%), gastroesophageal reflux disease (adults: >1%), vomiting (children and adolescents ≥12 years: >1%), ageusia (adults: 1%)
Genitourinary: Urinary tract infection (4%), premature ejaculation (adults: ≤3%), genital candidiasis (adults: >1%), urinary incontinence (children and adolescents ≥12 years: >1%)
Hematologic & oncologic: Neoplasm (adults: 2%), abnormal phosphorus levels (decreased), thrombocythemia
Hypersensitivity: Hypersensitivity reaction (≤4%)
Infection: Viral infection (4% to 8%), infection (>1%)
Neuromuscular & skeletal: Arthralgia (adults: 3% to 7%), leg pain (children and adolescents ≥12 years: 2%), muscle spasm (adults: 2%; dose related), weakness (adults: 2%), back pain (children and adolescents ≥12 years: >1%), myalgia (>1%), tremor (adults: >1%)

Ophthalmic: Conjunctivitis (children and adolescents ≥12 years: 7%; adults: 2%), blurred vision (adults: 4%), visual disturbance (1% to 2%; dose related), accommodation disturbance (adults: >1%), eye pain (>1%)

Otic: Otitis media (adults: 1% to 2%)

Renal: Nephrolithiasis (adults: ≤1%; dose related), increased blood urea nitrogen, increased serum creatinine

Respiratory: Upper respiratory tract infection (children and adolescents ≥12 years: 23% to 26%; adults: 13% to 14%), sinusitis (4% to 10%), rhinitis (children and adolescents ≥12 years: 6% to 7%; adults: 2%), cough (2% to 7%), pharyngitis (5% to 6%), bronchitis (adults: 3%; children and adolescents ≥12 years: >1%), dyspnea (adults: 3%), epistaxis (2%), asthma (>1%), flu-like symptoms (children and adolescents ≥12 years: >1%), pneumonia (adults: >1%)

Miscellaneous: Accidental injury (9%), language problems (adults: 6% to 7%), fever (children and adolescents ≥12 years: 4% to 6%)

<1%, postmarketing, and/or case reports (**any indication**): Abnormal electroencephalogram, acute myopia with secondary angle-closure glaucoma, albuminuria, alcohol intolerance, angina pectoris, apraxia, atrioventricular block, bone marrow depression, brain disease, bullous rash, cerebellar syndrome, chloasma, deep vein thrombosis, dehydration, delirium, delusions, diabetes mellitus, erythema multiforme, hepatic failure, hepatitis, hyperchloremic metabolic acidosis (nonanion gap), hyperesthesia, hyperglycemia, hyperlipidemia, hypernatremia, hyperthermia, hypocalcemia, hypocholesterolemia, hypohidrosis, hyponatremia, hypotension, hypothermia (with valproic acid, with or without hyperammonemia), impotence, iritis, lymphadenopathy, lymphocytopenia, lymphocytosis, maculopathy, manic reaction, melena, neuropathy, ostealgia, pancreatitis, pancytopenia, pemphigus, phlebitis, photophobia, polycythemia, psychosis, pulmonary embolism, renal pain, scotoma, skin photosensitivity, Stevens-Johnson syndrome, stomatitis, strabismus, suicidal ideation, suicidal tendencies, tongue edema, tongue paralysis, toxic epidermal necrolysis, upper motor neuron lesion, urinary retention, urticaria, vasodilatation, vasospasm, visual field defect, xerophthalmia

Drug Interactions

Metabolism/Transport Effects Inhibits CYP2C19 (weak)

Avoid Concomitant Use

Avoid concomitant use of Topiramate with any of the following: Alcohol (Ethyl); Azelastine (Nasal); Carbonic Anhydrase Inhibitors; Orphenadrine; Paraldehyde; Thalidomide; Ulipristal

Increased Effect/Toxicity

Topiramate may increase the levels/effects of: Alpha-/Beta-Agonists (Indirect-Acting); Amitriptyline; Amphetamines; Azelastine (Nasal); Buprenorphine; Carbonic Anhydrase Inhibitors; CNS Depressants; Flecainide; Fosphenytoin; Hydrocodone; Lithium; Memantine; MetFORMIN; Methotrimeprazine; Metyrosine; Mirtazapine; Orphenadrine; Paraldehyde; Phenytoin; Pramipexole; Primidone; QuiNIDine; ROPINIRole; Rotigotine; Selective Serotonin Reuptake Inhibitors; Suvorexant; Thalidomide; Valproate Products; Zolpidem

The levels/effects of Topiramate may be increased by: Alcohol (Ethyl); Anticholinergic Agents; Brimonidine (Topical); Cannabis; Doxylamine; Dronabinol; Droperidol; HydrOXYzine; Kava Kava; Loop Diuretics; Magnesium Sulfate; Methotrimeprazine; Minocycline; Nabilone; Perampanel; Rufinamide; Salicylates; Sodium Oxybate; Tapentadol; Tetrahydrocannabinol; Thiazide Diuretics

Decreased Effect

Topiramate may decrease the levels/effects of: Contraceptives (Estrogens); Contraceptives (Progestins); Methenamine; Primidone; Ulipristal

The levels/effects of Topiramate may be decreased by: CarBAMazepine; Fosphenytoin; Mefloquine; Mianserin; Orlistat; Phenytoin

Food Interactions Ketogenic diet may increase the possibility of acidosis and/or kidney stones. Management: Monitor for symptoms of acidosis or kidney stones.

Storage/Stability

Extended release capsules: Store at 15°C to 30°C (59°F to 86°F). Protect from moisture. Protect from light.

Sprinkle capsules: Store at or below 25°C (77°F). Protect from moisture.

Tablets: Store at 15°C to 30°C (59°F to 86°F). Protect from moisture.

Mechanism of Action Anticonvulsant activity may be due to a combination of potential mechanisms: Blocks neuronal voltage-dependent sodium channels, enhances GABA(A) activity, antagonizes AMPA/kainate glutamate receptors, and weakly inhibits carbonic anhydrase.

Pharmacodynamics/Kinetics

Absorption: Good, rapid; immediate release formulation is unaffected by food. A single Trokendi XR dose with a high-fat meal increased the C_{max} by 37% and shortened the T_{max} to approximately 8 hours; this effect is significantly reduced following repeat administrations. A single Qudexy XR dose with a high-fat meal delayed the T_{max} by 4 hours.

Protein binding: 15% to 41% (inversely related to plasma concentrations)

Metabolism: Minor amounts metabolized in liver via hydroxylation, hydrolysis, and glucuronidation; there is evidence of renal tubular reabsorption; percentage of dose metabolized in liver and clearance are increased in patients receiving enzyme inducers (eg, carbamazepine, phenytoin)

Bioavailability: ~80% (immediate release)

Half-life elimination: 21 hours (immediate release); ~31 hours (Trokendi XR); ~56 hours (Qudexy XR)

Time to peak, serum: ~1 to 4 hours (immediate release); ~24 hours (Trokendi XR); ~20 hours (Qudexy XR)

Excretion: Urine (~70% as unchanged drug)

Dosing

Adult Note: Do not abruptly discontinue therapy; taper dosage gradually to prevent rebound effects. (In clinical trials, adult doses were withdrawn by decreasing in weekly intervals of 50 to 100 mg daily gradually over 2 to 8 weeks for seizure treatment, and by decreasing in weekly intervals by 25 or 50 mg daily for migraine prophylaxis.) Bioequivalence has not been demonstrated between Trokendi XR and Qudexy XR.

Epilepsy, monotherapy: Partial-onset seizure and primary generalized tonic-clonic seizure: Oral:

Immediate release: Initial: 25 mg twice daily; may increase weekly by 50 mg daily up to 100 mg twice daily (week 4 dose); thereafter, may further increase weekly by 100 mg daily up to the recommended dose of 200 mg twice daily.

Extended release: Initial: 50 mg daily for 1 week; may increase weekly by 50 mg daily up to 200 mg once daily (week 4 dose); thereafter, may further increase weekly by 100 mg daily up to the recommended dose of 400 mg once daily.

Canadian labeling: Oral: Immediate release: Initial: 25 mg once daily (in evening); may increase to 25 mg twice daily in weeks 2 or 3 and up to 50 mg twice daily by weeks 3 or 4; may further increase weekly in increments of 50 mg daily up to recommended maximum of 200 mg twice daily.

Epilepsy, adjunctive therapy: Partial-onset seizure, primary generalized tonic-clonic seizure, or Lennox-Gastaut syndrome: Oral: **Note:** Doses >1600 mg have not been studied.

Immediate release: Initial: 25 mg once or twice daily for 1 week; may increase weekly by 25 to 50 mg daily until response; usual maintenance dose: 100 to 200 mg twice daily (partial-onset seizures) or 200 mg twice daily (primary generalized tonic-clonic seizures). Doses >400 mg have not shown additional benefit for treatment of partial-onset seizures.

Extended release: Initial: 25 to 50 mg once daily for 1 week; may increase weekly by 25 to 50 mg daily until response; usual maintenance dose: 200 to 400 mg once daily (partial-onset seizures, Lennox-Gastaut syndrome) or 400 mg once daily (primary generalized tonic-clonic seizures). Doses >400 mg daily have not shown additional benefit for treatment of partial-onset seizures.

Canadian labeling: Oral: Immediate release: Initial: 25 mg once or twice daily; may increase weekly by 50 mg daily up to the recommended dose of 100 to 200 mg twice daily (maximum recommended dose: 800 mg daily; doses >400 mg daily have shown no additional benefit).

Migraine prophylaxis: Oral: Immediate release: Initial: 25 mg once daily (in evening); may increase weekly by 25 mg daily up to the recommended dose of 100 mg daily given in 2 divided doses. Increased intervals between dose adjustments may be considered. Doses >100 mg daily have shown no additional benefit.

Cluster headache prophylaxis (off-label use): Oral: Initial: 25 mg daily, titrated at weekly intervals in 25 mg increments, up to 200 mg daily (Pascual 2007)

Essential tremor (off-label use): Oral: Initial: 25 mg once daily; increase dose at weekly intervals based on response and tolerability in 25 mg increments up to 100 mg/day and then in 50 mg increments up to 400 mg/day (Ondo 2006). Alternatively, once 200 mg/day is achieved, doses may be increased weekly in 100 mg increments up to 400 mg/day (Connor 2008). For dosages ≥50 mg/day administer in 2 divided doses (Ondo 2006). Average doses in clinical trials were 292 mg/day (median: 375 mg/day) (Ondo 2006) and 215 mg/day (range: 25 to 400 mg/day) (Connor 2008).

Status epilepticus, refractory (off-label use): Oral, NG: Initial: 200 to 400 mg; maintenance: 300 to 1600 mg in 2 to 4 divided doses (NCS [Brophy 2012]). Additional data is necessary to further define the role of topiramate in this condition.

Geriatric Most older adults have creatinine clearances <70 mL/minute/1.73 m^2; obtain a serum creatinine and calculate creatinine clearance prior to initiation of therapy. An initial dose of 25 mg/day may be recommended, followed by incremental increases of 25 mg at weekly intervals until an effective dose is reached; refer to adult dosing for titration schedule.

Pediatric Note: Do not abruptly discontinue therapy; taper dosage gradually to prevent rebound effects. Bioequivalence has not been demonstrated between Trokendi XR and Qudexy XR.

Epilepsy, monotherapy: Partial-onset seizure and primary generalized tonic-clonic seizure:

Children 2 to <10 years: Oral:

Immediate release:

Initial: 25 mg once daily (in evening); may increase to 25 mg twice daily in week 2; thereafter, may increase by 25 to 50 mg daily at weekly intervals over 5 to 7 weeks up to the following minimum recommended maintenance dose:

≤11 kg: 150 mg daily in 2 divided doses
12 to 22 kg: 200 mg daily in 2 divided doses
23 to 31 kg: 200 mg daily in 2 divided doses
32 to 38 kg: 250 mg daily in 2 divided doses
≥39 kg: 250 mg daily in 2 divided doses

Maximum maintenance dose: If additional seizure control is needed and therapy is tolerated, may further increase by 25 to 50 mg daily at weekly intervals up to the following maximum recommended maintenance dose:

≤11 kg: 250 mg daily in 2 divided doses
12 to 22 kg: 300 mg daily in 2 divided doses
23 to 31 kg: 350 mg daily in 2 divided doses
32 to 38 kg: 350 mg daily in 2 divided doses
≥39 kg: 400 mg daily in 2 divided doses

Extended release (Qudexy XR only):

Initial: 25 mg once daily (in the evening); if tolerated, may increase to 50 mg once daily in week 2; thereafter, may increase by 25 to 50 mg daily at weekly intervals over 5 to 7 weeks up to the following minimum recommended maintenance dose:

≤11 kg: 150 mg once daily
12 to 31 kg: 200 mg once daily
≥32 kg: 250 mg once daily

Maximum maintenance dose: If additional seizure control is needed and therapy is tolerated, may further increase by 25 to 50 mg daily at weekly intervals up to the following maximum recommended maintenance dose:

≤11 kg: 250 mg once daily
12 to 22 kg: 300 mg once daily
23 to 38 kg: 350 mg once daily
>38 kg: 400 mg once daily

Children ≥10 years and Adolescents: Refer to adult dosing.

Canadian labeling: Children ≥6 years: Refer to adult dosing.

Epilepsy, adjunctive therapy: Partial-onset seizure, primary generalized tonic-clonic seizure, or Lennox-Gastaut syndrome:

Children 2 to <6 years: Oral:

Immediate release: Initial: 25 mg (1 to 3 mg/kg/day) once daily (in evening) for 1 week; may increase every 1 to 2 weeks in increments of 1 to 3 mg/kg/day up to the recommended dose of 5 to 9 mg/kg/day in 2 divided doses.

Extended release (Qudexy XR only): Initial: 25 mg (1 to 3 mg/kg/day) once daily (in evening) for 1 week; may increase every 1 to 2 weeks in increments of 1 to 3 mg/kg/day up to the recommended dose of 5 to 9 mg/kg once daily.

Children ≥6 years and Adolescents <17 years: Oral:

Immediate release: Initial: 25 mg (1 to 3 mg/kg/day) once daily (in evening) for 1 week; may increase every 1 to 2 weeks in increments of 1 to 3 mg/kg/day up to the recommended dose of 5 to 9 mg/kg/day in 2 divided doses.

Extended release (Qudexy XR and Trokendi XR): Initial: 25 mg (1 to 3 mg/kg/day) once daily (in evening) for 1 week; may increase every 1 to 2 weeks in increments of 1 to 3 mg/kg/day up to the recommended dose of 5 to 9 mg/kg once daily.

Adolescents ≥17 years: Refer to adult dosing.

Migraine prophylaxis: Adolescents ≥12 years: Oral: Immediate release: Refer to adult dosing.

Renal Impairment

CrCl <70 mL/minute/1.73 m^2: Administer 50% dose and titrate more slowly.

Hemodialysis: Supplemental dose may be needed during hemodialysis

Hepatic Impairment There are no dosage adjustments provided in the manufacturer's labeling. However, topiramate clearance in hepatic impairment may be reduced. Use with caution.

Administration Administer without regard to meals. Administer the immediate release formulation in divided doses. It is not recommended to crush, break, or chew immediate release tablets due to bitter taste. Swallow extended release (ER) and sprinkle capsules whole. Sprinkle capsules and Qudexy XR capsules may also be opened to sprinkle the entire contents on a small amount (~1 teaspoon) of soft food; swallow immediately and do not chew. Do not store drug/food mixture for future use. Do not sprinkle Trokendi XR capsules on food, chew, or crush. Avoid alcohol use with Trokendi XR capsules within 6 hours prior to and 6 hours after administration.

Hazardous agent; use appropriate precautions for handling and disposal (NIOSH 2014 [group 3]).

Monitoring Parameters Seizure frequency, hydration status; electrolytes (recommended monitoring includes serum bicarbonate at baseline and periodically during treatment); serum creatinine; monitor for symptoms of acute acidosis and complications of long-term acidosis (nephrolithiasis, nephrocalcinosis, osteomalacia/osteoporosis, and reduced growth rates and/or weight in children); ammonia level in patients with unexplained lethargy, vomiting, or mental status changes; intraocular pressure, symptoms of secondary angle closure glaucoma; suicidality (eg, suicidal thoughts, depression, behavioral changes); weight and eating behaviors in patients with eating disorder symptoms or risk factors

Additional Information May be associated with weight loss in some patients

Dosage Forms Excipient information presented when available (limited, particularly for generics); consult specific product labeling. [DSC] = Discontinued product

Capsule ER 24 Hour Sprinkle, Oral:

Qudexy XR: 25 mg (30 ea, 500 ea); 50 mg (30 ea, 500 ea); 100 mg (30 ea, 500 ea); 150 mg (30 ea, 500 ea); 200 mg (30 ea, 500 ea)

Generic: 25 mg (30 ea, 500 ea); 50 mg (30 ea, 500 ea); 100 mg (30 ea, 500 ea); 150 mg (30 ea, 500 ea); 200 mg (30 ea, 500 ea)

Capsule Extended Release 24 Hour, Oral:

Trokendi XR: 25 mg [contains brilliant blue fcf (fd&c blue #1), sodium benzoate]

Trokendi XR: 50 mg, 100 mg, 200 mg [contains brilliant blue fcf (fd&c blue #1), fd&c yellow #6 (sunset yellow), sodium benzoate]

Capsule Sprinkle, Oral:

Topamax Sprinkle: 15 mg, 25 mg

Generic: 15 mg, 25 mg

Tablet, Oral:

Topamax: 25 mg, 50 mg, 100 mg, 200 mg

Topiragen: 25 mg [DSC], 50 mg [DSC], 100 mg [DSC], 200 mg [DSC]

Generic: 25 mg, 50 mg, 100 mg, 200 mg

Dosage Forms: Canada Refer to Dosage Forms. **Note:** Extended release capsules not available in Canada.

Extemporaneous Preparations Hazardous agent; use appropriate precautions for handling and disposal (NIOSH 2014 [group 3]).

A 6 mg/mL topiramate oral suspension may be made with tablets and one of two different vehicles (a 1:1 mixture of Ora-Sweet and Ora-Plus, or a mixture of Simple Syrup, NF and methylcellulose 1% with parabens). Crush six 100 mg tablets in a mortar and reduce to a fine powder. Add a small amount of methylcellulose gel and mix to a uniform paste (**Note:** Use a small amount of methylcellulose gel when using the 1:1 Ora-Sweet and Ora-Plus mixture as the vehicle; use 10 mL methylcellulose 1% with parabens when using Simple Syrup, NF as the vehicle); mix while

◄ adding the chosen vehicle in incremental proportions to almost 100 mL; transfer to a graduated cylinder; rinse mortar with vehicle, and add quantity of vehicle sufficient to make 100 mL. Store in plastic prescription bottles; label "shake well" and "refrigerate". Stable for 90 days refrigerated (preferred) or at room temperature.

Nahata MC, Pai VB, and Hipple TF, *Pediatric Drug Formulations*, 5th ed, Cincinnati, OH: Harvey Whitney Books Co, 2004.

◆ Toposar *see* Etoposide *on page 714*

Topotecan (toe poe TEE kan)

Brand Names: US Hycamtin
Brand Names: Canada Hycamtin; Topotecan For Injection; Topotecan Hydrochloride For Injection
Index Terms Hycamptamine; SKF 104864; SKF 104864-A; Topotecan Hydrochloride
Pharmacologic Category Antineoplastic Agent, Camptothecin; Antineoplastic Agent, Topoisomerase I Inhibitor
Use
Cervical cancer, recurrent or resistant: Treatment of recurrent or resistant (stage IVB) cervical cancer (in combination with cisplatin) which is not amenable to curative treatment
Ovarian cancer, metastatic: Treatment of metastatic ovarian cancer (as a single agent) after disease progression on or after initial or subsequent chemotherapy
Small cell lung cancer, relapsed:
Injection: Treatment of small cell lung cancer (as a single agent) in patients with platinum-sensitive disease which has progressed at least 60 days after initiation of first-line chemotherapy
Oral: Treatment of relapsed small cell lung cancer in patients with a prior complete or partial response and who are at least 45 days from the end of first-line chemotherapy
Pregnancy Considerations Adverse effects were observed in animal reproduction studies. May cause fetal harm in pregnant women. Women of childbearing potential should use highly effective contraception to prevent pregnancy during treatment and for at least 1 month after therapy discontinuation. Males with female partners of childbearing potential should use highly effective contraception during treatment and for 3 months after therapy discontinuation. Topotecan may have both acute and long-term effects on fertility in women; fertility in males may be impaired due to effects on spermatogenesis.
Breast-Feeding Considerations It is not known if topotecan is excreted in breast milk. Due to the potential for serious adverse reactions in the nursing infant, the manufacturer recommends to discontinue breast-feeding in women who are receiving topotecan.
Contraindications
Hypersensitivity to topotecan or any component of the formulation
Canadian labeling: Additional contraindications (not in U.S. labeling): Severe renal impairment (CrCl <20 mL/minute); pregnancy; breast-feeding; severe bone marrow depression
Warnings/Precautions Hazardous agent - use appropriate precautions for handling and disposal (NIOSH 2014 [group 1]). **[US Boxed Warning]: May cause severe myelosuppression. Monitor blood counts frequently. Do NOT administer to patients with baseline neutrophils <1500/mm³ and platelets <100,000/mm³.** The dose-limiting toxicity is bone marrow suppression (primarily neutropenia); may also cause thrombocytopenia and anemia. Grade 3 and 4 events were common. Severe myelotoxicity has also been reported when used in combination with cisplatin. Neutropenia is not cumulative overtime. The median duration of neutropenia and thrombocytopenia was 7 days and 5 days, respectively. Nadir neutrophil and platelet counts occurred at a median of 15 days (when administered orally). In a clinical study comparing IV to oral topotecan, G-CSF support was administered in a higher percentage of patients receiving oral topotecan (Eckardt 2007). Bone marrow suppression may require dosage reduction and/or growth factor support. Topotecan-induced neutropenia may lead to typhlitis (neutropenic enterocolitis), including fatalities; should be considered in patients presenting with neutropenia, fever, and abdominal pain.

Diarrhea has been reported with oral topotecan; may be severe (requiring hospitalization); incidence may be higher in the elderly; educate patients on early recognition and proper management, including diet changes, increase in fluid intake, antidiarrheals, and antibiotics. The median time to onset of diarrhea (grade 2 or worse) was 9 days. The incidence of diarrhea may be higher in the elderly. Do not administer in patients with grade 3 or 4 diarrhea; reduce dose upon recovery to ≤ grade 1 toxicity. Interstitial

lung disease (ILD) (with fatalities) has been reported; discontinue use in patients with confirmed ILD diagnosis; risk factors for ILD include a history of ILD, pulmonary fibrosis, lung cancer, thoracic radiation, and the use of colony-stimulating factors or medication with pulmonary toxicity; monitor pulmonary symptoms (cough, fever, dyspnea, and/or hypoxia). Use caution in renal impairment; may require dose adjustment (use in severe renal impairment is contraindicated in the Canadian labeling). Potentially significant drug-drug interactions may exist, requiring dose or frequency adjustment, additional monitoring, and/or selection of alternative therapy. Topotecan exposure is increased when oral topotecan is used concurrently with P-glycoprotein inhibitors; avoid concurrent use. Topotecan overdoses have been reported; potential causes include omission of the leading zero and missing the decimal point when prescribing, preparing, and administering. Recommended intravenous doses should generally not exceed 4 mg in adults; verify dose prior to administration. Extravasation injuries have been reported (some severe); if extravasation occurs, discontinue infusion immediately and manage appropriately. Ensure proper needle or catheter placement prior to and during infusion. Avoid extravasation.

Adverse Reactions
>10%:
Central nervous system: Fatigue (oral: 11% to 19%)
Dermatologic: Alopecia (oral: 10% to 20%)
Gastrointestinal: Nausea (oral: 27% to 33%), anorexia (intravenous: 32%; oral: 7% to 14%), diarrhea (oral: 14% to 22%; grade 3: 4%, grade 4: ≤1%; intravenous: grades 3/4: 6%), vomiting (oral: 19% to 21%)
Hematologic & oncologic: Anemia (oral: 94% to 98%; grades 3/4: 25%; grade 3: 15% to 18%; grade 4: 7% to 10%; intravenous: grades 3/4: 37% to 42%), neutropenia (oral: 83% to 91%; grade 3: 24% to 28%; grade 4: 32% to 33%; intravenous: grade 4: 70% to 80%; nadir 12 to 15 days; duration: 7 days), thrombocytopenia (oral: 81%; grade 3: 29% to 30%; grade 4: 6% to 7%; intravenous: grade 4: 27% to 29%; nadir: 15 days; duration: 3 to 5 days), febrile neutropenia (intravenous: grade 3/4: 23% to 28%; oral: grade 4: 4%), neutropenic infection (13% to 17%)

1% to 10%:
Gastrointestinal: Abdominal pain (intravenous: grades 3/4: 5% to 6%)
Hepatic: Increased liver enzymes (intravenous: 8%; transient)
Neuromuscular & skeletal: Weakness (3% to 7%)
Respiratory: Dyspnea (intravenous: 6% to 9%)
Miscellaneous: Fever (oral: 5% to 7%), sepsis (intravenous: grades 3/4: 5%; oral: 2%)
<1% (Limited to important or life-threatening): Dermatitis (severe), extravasation, hemorrhage (severe, associated with thrombocytopenia), hypersensitivity reaction, interstitial pulmonary disease, leukopenia, myalgia, neutropenic enterocolitis, pancytopenia, paresthesia, pruritus (severe), skin rash, stomatitis, typhlitis

Drug Interactions
Metabolism/Transport Effects Substrate of BCRP
Avoid Concomitant Use
Avoid concomitant use of Topotecan with any of the following: BCG (Intravesical); Deferiprone; Dipyrone; Natalizumab; P-glycoprotein/ABCB1 Inhibitors; Pimecrolimus; Tacrolimus (Topical); Tofacitinib; Vaccines (Live)
Increased Effect/Toxicity
Topotecan may increase the levels/effects of: CloZAPine; Deferiprone; Fingolimod; Leflunomide; Natalizumab; Tofacitinib; Vaccines (Live)

The levels/effects of Topotecan may be increased by: BCRP/ABCG2 Inhibitors; Denosumab; Dipyrone; Filgrastim; P-glycoprotein/ABCB1 Inhibitors; Pimecrolimus; Platinum Derivatives; Roflumilast; Tacrolimus (Topical); Trastuzumab
Decreased Effect
Topotecan may decrease the levels/effects of: BCG (Intravesical); Coccidioides immitis Skin Test; Sipuleucel-T; Vaccines (Inactivated); Vaccines (Live)

The levels/effects of Topotecan may be decreased by: Echinacea; Fosphenytoin-Phenytoin
Preparation for Administration Hazardous agent; use appropriate precautions for handling and disposal (NIOSH 2014 [group 1]). Reconstitute lyophilized powder with 4 mL SWFI. Reconstituted lyophilized powder and solution for injection should be further diluted in D_5W or NS for infusion.

Storage/Stability

IV:

Solution for injection: Store intact vials at 2°C to 8°C (36°F to 45°F). Protect from light. Single-use vials should be discarded after initial vial entry. Stability of solutions diluted for infusion is variable; refer to specific product information for details.

Lyophilized powder: Store intact vials at 20°C to 25°C (68°F to 77°F). Protect from light. Reconstituted solution is stable for up to 28 days at 20°C to 25°C (68°F to 77°F), although the manufacturer recommends use immediately after reconstitution. Solutions diluted in D_5W or NS are stable for 24 hours at room temperature (manufacturer's labeling) or up to 7 days under refrigeration (Craig 1997). Reconstituted solution for injection (reconstituted with bacteriostatic SWFI to 1 mg/mL) for oral administration is stable for 14 days at 4°C in plastic syringes (Daw 2004).

Oral: Store at 2°C to 8°C (36°F to 46°F). Protect from light.

Mechanism of Action Binds to topoisomerase I and stabilizes the cleavable complex so that religation of the cleaved DNA strand cannot occur. This results in the accumulation of cleavable complexes and single-strand DNA breaks. Topotecan acts in S phase of the cell cycle.

Pharmacodynamics/Kinetics

Absorption: Oral: Rapid

Distribution: V_d: 25 to 75 L/m^2 (Hartmann 2006)

Protein binding: ~35%

Metabolism: Undergoes a rapid, pH-dependent hydrolysis of the lactone ring to yield a relatively inactive hydroxy acid in plasma; metabolized in the liver to N-demethylated metabolite

Bioavailability: Oral: ~40%

Half-life elimination: IV: 2 to 3 hours; renal impairment: ~5 hours; Oral: 3 to 6 hours

Time to peak, plasma: Oral: 1 to 2 hours; delayed with high-fat meal (3 to 4 hours)

Excretion:

IV: Urine (51%; ~3% as N-desmethyl topotecan); feces (18%; ~2% as N-desmethyl topotecan)

Oral: Urine (20%; 2% as N-desmethyl topotecan); feces (33%; <2% as N-desmethyl topotecan)

Dosing

Adult & Geriatric Note: Baseline neutrophil count should be ≥1500/mm^3 and platelets should be ≥100,000/mm^3 prior to treatment; for re-treatment, neutrophil count should be >1000/mm^3; platelets >100,000/mm^3 and hemoglobin ≥9 g/dL. Intravenous doses should generally not exceed 4 mg; verify dose prior to administration.

Cervical cancer, recurrent or resistant: IV: 0.75 mg/m^2/day for 3 days (in combination with cisplatin on day 1 only, [with hydration]) every 21 days

Ovarian cancer, metastatic: IV: 1.5 mg/m^2/day for 5 consecutive days every 21 days **or** (off-label dosing) 1.25 mg/m^2/day for 5 days every 21 days until disease progression or unacceptable toxicity or a maximum of 12 months (Sehouli 2011) **or** (weekly administration; off-label dosing) 4 mg/m^2 on days 1, 8, and 15 every 28 days until disease progression or unacceptable toxicity or a maximum of 12 months (Sehouli 2011)

Small cell lung cancer (SCLC), relapsed:

IV: 1.5 mg/m^2/day for 5 consecutive days every 21 days

Oral: 2.3 mg/m^2/day for 5 consecutive days every 21 days (round dose to the nearest 0.25 mg); if patient vomits after dose is administered, do not give a replacement dose.

Ewing's sarcoma, relapsed/refractory or metastatic (off-label use): IV: 0.75 mg/m^2/day for 5 consecutive days every 21 days (in combination with cyclophosphamide) (Hunold 2006; Saylors 2001)

Primary CNS lymphoma, relapsed or refractory (off-label use): IV: 1.5 mg/m^2 for 5 days every 21 days for a maximum of 10 cycles or until disease progression or unacceptable toxicity (Voloschin 2008). Additional data may be necessary to further define the role of topotecan in this condition.

Rhabdomyosarcoma, metastatic (off-label use): Adults <21 years: IV: 0.75 mg/m^2/day for 5 consecutive days every 21 days for 2 cycles (window therapy; in combination with cyclophosphamide); if objective response occurred by week 6, follow with alternating cycles of vincristine, topotecan, and cyclophosphamide (VTC) with vincristine, dactinomycin, and cyclophosphamide (VAC) (Walterhouse 2004)

Pediatric Note: Baseline neutrophil count should be ≥1500/mm^3 and platelets should be ≥100,000/mm^3 prior to treatment; for re-treatment, neutrophil count should be >1000/mm^3; platelets >100,000/mm^3 and hemoglobin ≥9 g/dL. Intravenous doses should generally not exceed 4 mg; verify dose prior to administration.

CNS malignancy, relapsed/refractory (off-label use; based on limited data): Oral: 0.8 mg/m^2/day for 21 consecutive days every 4 weeks for ≥12 cycles (Minturn 2011); additional data may be necessary to further define the role of topotecan in this condition

Ewing's sarcoma, relapsed/refractory or metastatic (off-label use): IV: 0.75 mg/m^2/day for 5 consecutive days every 21 days (in combination with cyclophosphamide) (Hunold 2006; Saylors 2001)

Neuroblastoma, relapsed/refractory (off-label use): IV: 0.75 mg/m^2/day for 5 days every 21 days (in combination with cyclophosphamide) (Ashraf 2013; London 2010) **or** 2 mg/m^2/day for 5 days every 21 days (monotherapy) (London 2010)

Rhabdomyosarcoma, metastatic (off-label use): IV: 0.75 mg/m^2/day for 5 consecutive days every 21 days for 2 cycles (window therapy; in combination with cyclophosphamide); if objective response occurred by week 6, follow with alternating cycles of vincristine, topotecan, and cyclophosphamide (VTC) with vincristine, dactinomycin, and cyclophosphamide (VAC) (Walterhouse 2004)

Renal Impairment

Manufacturer's labeling

IV (single agent topotecan):

CrCl ≥40 mL/minute: No dosage adjustment necessary.

CrCl 20 to 39 mL/minute: Reduce dose to 0.75 mg/m^2/dose

CrCl <20 mL/minute: There are no dosage adjustments provided in manufacturer's U.S. labeling (insufficient data available for dosing recommendation); use is contraindicated in the Canadian labeling.

Oral:

CrCl ≥50 mL/minute: No dosage adjustment necessary.

CrCl 30 to 49 mL/minute: Reduce dose to 1.5 mg/m^2/day; may increase after the 1st cycle by 0.4 mg/m^2/day if no severe hematologic or gastrointestinal toxicities occur.

CrCl <30 mL/minute: Reduce dose to 0.6 mg/m^2/day; may increase after the 1st cycle by 0.4 mg/m^2/day if no severe hematologic or gastrointestinal toxicities occur.

Alternate recommendations:

Aronoff 2007: IV:

Adults:

CrCl >50 mL/minute: Administer 75% of dose

CrCl 10 to 50 mL/minute: Administer 50% of dose

CrCl <10 mL/minute: Administer 25% of dose

Hemodialysis: Avoid use

Continuous ambulatory peritoneal dialysis (CAPD): Avoid use

Continuous renal replacement therapy (CRRT): 0.75 mg/m^2

Children:

CrCl 30 to 50 mL/minute: Administer 75% of dose

CrCl 10 to 29 mL/minute: Administer 50% of dose

CrCl <10 mL/minute: Administer 25% of dose

Continuous renal replacement therapy (CRRT): Administer 50% of dose

Kintzel 1995: IV:

CrCl 46 to 60 mL/minute: Administer 80% of dose

CrCl 31 to 45 mL/minute: Administer 75% of dose

CrCl ≤30 mL/minute: Administer 70% of dose

Hepatic Impairment Manufacturer's labeling:

IV:

US labeling: Bilirubin 1.7 to 15 mg/dL: There are no dosage adjustments provided in the manufacturer's labeling, although clearance is reduced up to 33%.

Canadian labeling: Bilirubin >1.5 to <10 mg/dL: No dosage adjustment is necessary (the half-life is increased slightly; usual doses are generally tolerated).

Oral: There is no dosage adjustment provided in the manufacturer's labeling; however, dosage adjustment is likely not necessary as the pharmacokinetics of topotecan do not differ significantly based on serum bilirubin, ALT, or AST.

Obesity ASCO Guidelines for appropriate chemotherapy dosing in obese adults with cancer: Utilize patient's actual body weight (full weight) for calculation of body surface area- or weight-based dosing, particularly when the intent of therapy is curative; manage regimen-related toxicities in the same manner as for nonobese patients; if a dose reduction is utilized due to toxicity, consider resumption of full weight-based dosing with subsequent cycles, especially if cause of toxicity (eg, hepatic or renal impairment) is resolved (Griggs 2012).

Adjustment for Toxicity

Cervical cancer (cisplatin may also require dosage adjustment): IV: Severe febrile neutropenia (<1000/mm^3 with temperature of ≥38°C) or platelet count <25,000/mm^3: Reduce topotecan to 0.6 mg/m^2/day for subsequent cycles (may consider G-CSF support [beginning on day 4] prior to instituting dose reduction for neutropenic fever).

If necessary, may further reduce dose to 0.45 mg/m^2/day for subsequent cycles.

Ovarian cancer: IV: Dosage adjustment for hematological effects: Severe neutropenia (<500/mm^3) or platelet count <25,000/mm^3: Reduce dose to 1.25 mg/m^2/day for subsequent cycles (may consider G-CSF support [beginning on day 6] prior to instituting dose reduction for severe neutropenia). **Note:** The Canadian labeling states that the dose may be further reduced to 1 mg/m^2/day if necessary.

Small cell lung cancer (SCLC):

IV: Dosage adjustment for hematological effects: Severe neutropenia (<500/mm^3) or platelet count <25,000/mm^3: Reduce dose to 1.25 mg/m^2/day for subsequent cycles (may consider G-CSF support [beginning on day 6] prior to instituting dose reduction for severe neutropenia). **Note:** The Canadian labeling states that the dose may be further reduced to 1 mg/m^2/day if necessary.

Oral:

Severe neutropenia (neutrophils <500/mm^3 associated with fever or infection or lasting ≥7 days) or prolonged neutropenia (neutrophils 500/mm^3 to 1000/mm^3 lasting beyond day 21) or platelets <25,000/mm^3: Reduce dose by 0.4 mg/m^2/day for subsequent cycles.

Diarrhea (grade 3 or 4): Do not administer to patients with grade 3 or 4 diarrhea. Upon recovery to ≤ grade 1 toxicity, reduce dose by 0.4 mg/m^2/day for subsequent cycles.

Administration

IV: Administer IVPB over 30 minutes. For combination chemotherapy with cisplatin, administer pretreatment hydration.

Oral: Administer without regard to meals. Swallow whole; do not open, crush, chew, or divide capsule. If vomiting occurs after dose, do not take replacement dose. For patients unable to swallow capsules whole, reconstituted topotecan solution for injection (1 mg/mL concentration) may be mixed with up to 30 mL of acidic fruit juice (eg, apple, orange, grape) immediately prior to oral administration (Daw 2004).

Hazardous agent; use appropriate precautions for handling and disposal (NIOSH 2014 [group 1]).

Monitoring Parameters CBC with differential and platelet count, renal function tests, bilirubin; monitor for symptoms of interstitial lung disease; diarrhea symptoms/hydration status

Dosage Forms Excipient information presented when available (limited, particularly for generics); consult specific product labeling.

Capsule, Oral:

Hycamtin: 0.25 mg, 1 mg

Solution, Intravenous:

Generic: 4 mg/4 mL (4 mL)

Solution, Intravenous [preservative free]:

Generic: 4 mg/4 mL (4 mL)

Solution Reconstituted, Intravenous:

Hycamtin: 4 mg (1 ea)

Generic: 4 mg (1 ea)

Solution Reconstituted, Intravenous [preservative free]:

Generic: 4 mg (1 ea)

Extemporaneous Preparations Hazardous agent; use appropriate precautions for handling and disposal (NIOSH 2014 [group 1]). When compounding an oral solution, NIOSH recommends double gloving, a protective gown, and preparation in a controlled device; if not prepared in a controlled device, respiratory and eye protection as well as ventilated engineering controls are recommended (NIOSH 2014).

For patients unable to swallow capsules whole, reconstituted topotecan solution for injection (1 mg/mL concentration) may be mixed with up to 30 mL of acidic fruit juice (eg, apple, orange, grape) immediately prior to oral administration.

Daw NC, Santana VM, Iacono LC, et al. Phase I and pharmacokinetic study of topotecan administered orally once daily for 5 days for 2 consecutive weeks to pediatric patients with refractory solid tumors. *J Clin Oncol.* 2004;22(5):829-837.

◆ Topotecan For Injection (Can) see Topotecan on page 1814

◆ Topotecan Hydrochloride see Topotecan on page 1814

◆ Topotecan Hydrochloride For Injection (Can) see Topotecan on page 1814

◆ Toprol XL see Metoprolol on page 1193

◆ Topsyn (Can) see Fluocinonide on page 781

◆ Toradol see Ketorolac (Systemic) on page 1015

◆ Toradol® (Can) see Ketorolac (Systemic) on page 1015

◆ Toradol® IM (Can) see Ketorolac (Systemic) on page 1015

◆ Torasemide see Torsemide on page 1816

Toremifene (tore EM i feen)

Brand Names: US Fareston

Brand Names: Canada Fareston

Index Terms FC1157a; Toremifene Citrate

Pharmacologic Category Antineoplastic Agent, Estrogen Receptor Antagonist; Selective Estrogen Receptor Modulator (SERM)

Use Breast cancer, metastatic: Treatment of metastatic breast cancer in postmenopausal women with estrogen receptor positive or estrogen receptor status unknown tumors

Dosing

Adult & Geriatric

Breast cancer, metastatic: Postmenopausal women: Oral: 60 mg once daily, continue until disease progression.

Soft tissue sarcoma (desmoid tumors) (off-label use): Oral: 180 mg once daily until disease progression or unacceptable toxicity (Fiore, 2011) **or** 200 mg daily; in some patients with tumor progression, the dose was increased to 400 to 600 mg daily (Brooks, 1992). Additional data may be necessary to further define the role of toremifene in this condition.

Renal Impairment There are no dosage adjustments listed in the manufacturer's labeling. However, pharmacokinetics in patients with renal impairment are similar to those in patients with normal renal function and dosage adjustment is unlikely to be necessary.

Hepatic Impairment There are no dosage adjustments provided in the manufacturer's labeling. However, hepatic impairment increases the half-life of toremifene.

Additional Information Complete prescribing information should be consulted for additional detail.

Dosage Forms Excipient information presented when available (limited, particularly for generics); consult specific product labeling.

Tablet, Oral:

Fareston: 60 mg

◆ Toremifene Citrate see Toremifene on page 1816

◆ Torezolid see Tedizolid on page 1741

◆ Torisel see Temsirolimus on page 1752

Torsemide (TORE se mide)

Brand Names: US Demadex

Index Terms Demadex; Torasemide

Pharmacologic Category Antihypertensive; Diuretic, Loop

Use

Management of edema associated with heart failure and hepatic or renal disease (including chronic renal failure); treatment of hypertension

Note: According to the Eighth Joint National Committee (JNC 8) guidelines, loop diuretics are not recommended for the initial treatment of hypertension (James, 2013). In patients with chronic kidney disease (ie, eGFR <30 mL/minute/1.73 m^2), the American Society of Hypertension/International Society of Hypertension (ASH/ISH) suggests that the use of a loop diuretic may be necessary (Weber, 2014).

Pregnancy Considerations A decrease in fetal weight, an increase in fetal resorption, and delayed fetal ossification has occurred in animal studies.

Breast-Feeding Considerations It is not known if torsemide is excreted in breast milk. The manufacturer recommends that caution be exercised when administering torsemide to nursing women.

Contraindications Hypersensitivity to torsemide, any component of the formulation, or any sulfonylurea; anuria

Warnings/Precautions Loop diuretics are potent diuretics; excess amounts can lead to profound diuresis with fluid and electrolyte loss; close medical supervision and dose evaluation are required. Potassium supplementation and/or use of potassium-sparing diuretics may be necessary to prevent hypokalemia. In contrast to thiazide diuretics, a loop diuretic can also lower serum calcium concentrations. Electrolyte disturbances can predispose

a patient to serious cardiac arrhythmias. Use with caution in patients with cirrhosis; avoid sudden changes in fluid and electrolyte balance and acid/base status which may lead to hepatic encephalopathy. Administration with an aldosterone antagonist or potassium-sparing diuretic may provide additional diuretic efficacy and maintain normokalemia. Coadministration of antihypertensives may increase the risk of hypotension.

Monitor fluid status and renal function in an attempt to prevent oliguria, azotemia, and reversible increases in BUN and creatinine; close medical supervision of aggressive diuresis required. Diuretic resistance may occur in some patients, despite higher doses of loop diuretic treatment, and can usually be overcome by intravenous administration, the use of two diuretics together (eg, furosemide and chlorothiazide), or the use of a diuretic with a positive inotropic agent. When such combinations are used, serum electrolytes need to be monitored even more closely (Cody, 1994; ACC/AHA [Yancy, 2013]; HFSA, 2010). Ototoxicity has been demonstrated following oral administration of torsemide and following rapid IV administration of other loop diuretics. Other possible risk factors may include use in renal impairment, excessive doses, and concurrent use of other ototoxins (eg, aminoglycosides). If given the morning of surgery, torsemide may render the patient volume depleted and blood pressure may be labile during general anesthesia.

Sulfonamide ("sulfa") allergy: The FDA-approved product labeling for many medications containing a sulfonamide chemical group includes a broad contraindication in patients with a prior allergic reaction to sulfonamides. There is a potential for cross-reactivity between members of a specific class (eg, two antibiotic sulfonamides). However, concerns for cross-reactivity have previously extended to all compounds containing the sulfonamide structure (SO_2NH_2). An expanded understanding of allergic mechanisms indicates cross-reactivity between antibiotic sulfonamides and nonantibiotic sulfonamides may not occur or at the very least this potential is extremely low (Brackett 2004; Johnson 2005; Slatore 2004; Tornero 2004). In particular, mechanisms of cross-reaction due to antibody production (anaphylaxis) are unlikely to occur with nonantibiotic sulfonamides. T-cell-mediated (type IV) reactions (eg, maculopapular rash) are less well understood and it is not possible to completely exclude this potential based on current insights. In cases where prior reactions were severe (Stevens-Johnson syndrome/TEN), some clinicians choose to avoid exposure to these classes.

Adverse Reactions
1% to 10%:
Cardiovascular: ECG abnormality (2%), chest pain (1%)
Central nervous system: Nervousness (1%)
Gastrointestinal: Constipation (2%), diarrhea (2%), dyspepsia (2%), nausea (2%), sore throat (2%)
Genitourinary: Excessive urination (7%)
Neuromuscular & skeletal: Arthralgia (2%), myalgia (2%), weakness (2%)
Respiratory: Rhinitis (3%), cough (2%)
<1% (Limited to important or life-threatening): Angioedema, arthritis, atrial fibrillation, esophageal hemorrhage, GI hemorrhage, hyperglycemia, hyperuricemia, hypokalemia, hyponatremia, hypotension, hypovolemia, impotence, leukopenia, pancreatitis, rash, rectal bleeding, shunt thrombosis, Stevens-Johnson syndrome, syncope, thirst, thrombocytopenia, toxic epidermal necrolysis, ventricular tachycardia, vomiting

Drug Interactions
Metabolism/Transport Effects Substrate of CYP2C8 (minor), CYP2C9 (major), SLCO1B1; **Note:** Assignment of Major/Minor substrate status based on clinically relevant drug interaction potential

Avoid Concomitant Use
Avoid concomitant use of Torsemide with any of the following: Levosulpiride; Mecamylamine

Increased Effect/Toxicity
Torsemide may increase the levels/effects of: ACE Inhibitors; Allopurinol; Amifostine; Aminoglycosides; Antipsychotic Agents (Second Generation [Atypical]); Cardiac Glycosides; Cefotiam; Ceftizoxime; CISplatin; Dofetilide; DULoxetine; Foscarnet; Hypotension-Associated Agents; Ivabradine; Levodopa; Levosulpiride; Lithium; Mecamylamine; Methotrexate; Neuromuscular-Blocking Agents; Nonsteroidal Anti-Inflammatory Agents; RisperiDONE; Salicylates; Sodium Phosphates; Tobramycin (Oral Inhalation); Topiramate; Warfarin

The levels/effects of Torsemide may be increased by: Alfuzosin; Analgesics (Opioid); Barbiturates; Beta2-Agonists; Brimonidine (Topical); Canagliflozin; Cefazedone; Cephradine; Ceritinib; Corticosteroids (Orally Inhaled); Corticosteroids (Systemic); CycloSPORINE (Systemic); CYP2C9 Inhibitors (Moderate); CYP2C9 Inhibitors (Strong); Diazoxide; Eltrombopag; Empagliflozin; Herbs (Hypotensive Properties); Licorice; Lumacaftor; Methotrexate; Mifepristone; Molsidomine; Nicorandil; Obinutuzumab; Pentoxifylline; Phosphodiesterase 5 Inhibitors; Probenecid; Prostacyclin Analogues; Teriflunomide

Decreased Effect
Torsemide may decrease the levels/effects of: Antidiabetic Agents; Lithium; Neuromuscular-Blocking Agents

The levels/effects of Torsemide may be decreased by: Amphetamines; Bile Acid Sequestrants; CYP2C9 Inducers (Strong); Dabrafenib; Enzalutamide; Herbs (Hypertensive Properties); Lumacaftor; Methotrexate; Methylphenidate; Nonsteroidal Anti-Inflammatory Agents; Probenecid; Salicylates; Yohimbine

Storage/Stability
IV: Store at 15°C to 30°C (59°F to 86°F). If torsemide is to be administered via continuous infusion, stability has been demonstrated through 24 hours at room temperature in plastic containers for the following fluids and concentrations:
200 mg torsemide (10 mg/mL) added to 250 mL D_5W, 250 mL NS or 500 mL 0.45% sodium chloride
50 mg torsemide (10 mg/mL) added to 500 mL D_5W, 500 mL NS, or 500 mL 0.45% sodium chloride
Tablets: Store at 15°C to 30°C (59°F to 86°F).

Mechanism of Action
Inhibits reabsorption of sodium and chloride in the ascending loop of Henle and distal renal tubule, interfering with the chloride-binding cotransport system, thus causing increased excretion of water, sodium, chloride, magnesium, and calcium; does not alter GFR, renal plasma flow, or acid-base balance

Pharmacodynamics/Kinetics
Onset of action: Diuresis: Oral: Within 1 hour
Peak effect: Diuresis: Oral: 1-2 hours; Antihypertensive: Oral: 4-6 weeks (up to 12 weeks)
Duration: Diuresis: Oral: ~6-8 hours
Absorption: Oral: Rapid
Distribution: V_d: 12-15 L; Cirrhosis: Approximately doubled
Protein binding: >99%
Metabolism: Hepatic (~80%) via CYP
Bioavailability: ~80%
Half-life elimination: ~3.5 hours; Cirrhosis: 7-8 hours
Time to peak, plasma: Oral: 1 hour; delayed ~30 minutes when administered with food
Excretion: Urine (~20% as unchanged drug)

Dosing
Adult & Geriatric Note: IV and oral dosing are equivalent. Dose equivalency for patients with normal renal function (approximate): Torsemide 20 mg = Bumetanide 1 mg = furosemide 40 mg = ethacrynic acid 50 mg
Edema:
Chronic renal failure: Oral, IV: Initial: 20 mg once daily; may increase gradually by doubling dose until the desired diuretic response is obtained (maximum recommended daily dose: 200 mg)
Heart failure:
Oral: Initial: 10 to 20 mg once daily; may increase gradually by doubling dose until the desired diuretic response is obtained. **Note:** ACCF/AHA 2013 guidelines for heart failure maximum recommended daily dose: 200 mg (Yancy, 2013).
IV: Initial: 10 to 20 mg; may repeat every 2 hours with double the dose as needed.
Continuous IV infusion (off-label dose): Initial: 20 mg IV load, then 5 to 20 mg/hour; repeat loading dose before increasing infusion rate. **Note:** With lower baseline creatinine clearance (eg, CrCl <25 mL/minute), the upper end of the initial infusion dosage range should be considered (ACCF/AHA [Yancy, 2013]; Brater, 1998)
Hepatic cirrhosis: Oral: Initial: 5 to 10 mg once daily; may increase gradually by doubling dose until the desired diuretic response is obtained (maximum recommended single dose: 40 mg). **Note:** Administer with an aldosterone antagonist or a potassium-sparing diuretic.
Hypertension: Oral: Initial: 5 mg once daily; may increase to 10 mg once daily after 4 to 6 weeks if adequate antihypertensive response is not apparent; if still not effective, an additional antihypertensive agent may be added. Usual dosage range (ASH/ISH [Weber, 2014]): 10 mg daily.
Renal Impairment No dosage adjustment necessary. However, higher doses may be required to achieve diuretic response.
Hepatic Impairment There are no dosage adjustments provided in manufacturer's labeling; use with caution.

Dietary Considerations May be taken without regard to meals; however, food slows the rate and reduces the extent of absorption and may reduce diuretic efficacy (Bard, 2004). May require increased intake of potassium-rich foods.

Administration

IV: Administer over ≥2 minutes; reserve IV administration for situations which require rapid onset of action

Oral: Administer without regard to meals; patients may be switched from the IV form to the oral (and vice-versa) with no change in dose

Monitoring Parameters Renal function, electrolytes, and fluid status (weight and I & O), blood pressure

Additional Information 10-20 mg torsemide is approximately equivalent to furosemide 40 mg or bumetanide 1 mg.

Dosage Forms Excipient information presented when available (limited, particularly for generics); consult specific product labeling. [DSC] = Discontinued product

Solution, Intravenous:

Generic: 20 mg/2 mL (2 mL [DSC]); 50 mg/5 mL (5 mL [DSC])

Tablet, Oral:

Demadex: 5 mg, 10 mg, 20 mg, 100 mg [DSC] [scored]

Generic: 5 mg, 10 mg, 20 mg, 100 mg

◆ Total Allergy [OTC] see DiphenhydrAMINE (Systemic) on page 561

◆ Total Allergy Medicine [OTC] see DiphenhydrAMINE (Systemic) on page 561

Total Parenteral Nutrition
(TOE tal par EN ter al noo TRISH un)

Brand Names: US Kabiven

Index Terms Hyperal; Hyperalimentation; Parenteral Nutrition; PN; TPN

Pharmacologic Category Caloric Agent; Intravenous Nutritional Therapy

Use Infusion of nutrient solutions into the bloodstream to support nutritional needs during a time when patient is unable to absorb nutrients via the gastrointestinal tract, cannot take adequate nutrition orally or enterally, or have had (or are expected to have) inadequate oral intake for 7-14 days.

Dosing

Adult & Geriatric Nutritional supplementation: IV:

Total calories: Calculate using Harris-Benedict equation or based on stress level as indicated below:

Harris-Benedict Equation (BEE):

Females: 655.1 + [(9.56 x W) + (1.85 x H) - (4.68 x A)]

Males: 66.47 + [(13.75 x W) + (5 x H) - (6.76 x A)]

Then multiply BEE x (activity factor) x (stress factor)

W = weight in kg; H = height in cm; A = age in years

Activity factor = 1.2 sedentary, 1.3 normal activity, 1.4 active, 1.5 very active

Stress factor = 1.5 for trauma, stressed, or surgical patients and underweight (to promote weight gain); 2.0 for severe burn patients

Stress level:

Normal/mild stress level: 20-25 kcal/kg/day

Moderate stress level: 25-30 kcal/kg/day

Severe stress level: 30-40 kcal/kg/day

Pregnant women in second or third trimester: Add an additional 300 kcal/day

Fluid: mL/day = 30-40 mL/kg

Carbohydrate (dextrose):

5 g/kg/day or 3.5 mg/kg/minute (maximum rate: 4-7 mg/kg/minute)

Minimum recommended amount: 400 calories/day or 100 g/day

Protein (amino acids):

Maintenance: 0.8-1 g/kg/day

Normal/mild stress level: 1-1.2 g/kg/day

Moderate stress level: 1.2-1.5 g/kg/day

Severe stress level: 1.5-2 g/kg/day

Burn patients (severe): Increase protein until significant wound healing achieved

Solid organ transplant: Perioperative: 1.5-2 g/kg/day

Renal failure:

Acute (severely malnourished or hypercatabolic): 1.5-1.8 g/kg/day

Chronic, with dialysis: 1.2-1.3 g/kg/day

Chronic, without dialysis: 0.6-0.8 g/kg/day

Continuous hemofiltration: ≥1 g/kg/day

Hepatic failure:

Acute management when other treatments have failed:

With encephalopathy: 0.6-1 g/kg/day

Without encephalopathy: 1-1.5 g/kg/day

Chronic encephalopathy: Use branch chain amino acid enriched diets only if unresponsive to pharmacotherapy

Pregnant women in second or third trimester: Add an additional 10-14 g/day

Fat:

Initial: 20% to 40% of total calories (maximum: 60% of total calories or 2.5 g/kg/day); **Note:** Monitor triglycerides while receiving intralipids.

Safe for use in pregnancy

IV lipids are safe in adults with pancreatitis if triglyceride levels <400 mg/dL

Pediatric Nutritional supplementation: Children: IV: **Note:** Give within 5-7 days if unable to meet needs orally or with enteral nutrition:

Total calories:

<6 months: 85-105 kcal/kg/day

6-12 months: 80-100 kcal/kg/day

1-7 years: 75-90 kcal/kg/day

7-12 years: 50-75 kcal/kg/day

12-18 years: 30-50 kcal/kg/day

Fluid:

2-10 kg: 100 mL/kg

>10-20 kg: 1000 mL for 10 kg plus 50 mL/kg for each kg >10

>20 kg: 1500 mL for 10 kg plus 20 mL/kg for each kg >20

Carbohydrate (dextrose): 40% to 50% of caloric intake

<1 year: Initial: 6-8 mg/kg/minute; goal: 10-14 mg/kg/minute

1-10 years: Initial: 10% to 12.5%; daily increase: 5% increments (maximum: 15 mg/kg/minute)

>10 years: Initial: 10% to 15%; daily increase: 5% increments (maximum: 8.5 mg/kg/minute)

Protein (amino acids):

1-12 months: Initial: 2-3 g/kg/day; daily increase: 1 g/kg/day (maximum: 3 g/kg/day)

1-10 years: Initial: 1-2 g/kg/day; daily increase: 1 g/kg/day (maximum: 2-2.5 g/kg/day)

>10 years: Initial: 0.8-1.5 g/kg/day; daily increase: 1 g/kg/day (maximum: 1.5-2 g/kg/day)

Fat: Initial: 1 g/kg/day; daily increase: 1 g/kg/day (maximum: 3 g/kg/day); **Note:** Monitor triglycerides while receiving intralipids.

Additional Information Complete prescribing information should be consulted for additional detail.

Dosage Forms Excipient information presented when available (limited, particularly for generics); consult specific product labeling.

Emulsion, Intravenous:

Kabiven: (1026 mL,1540 mL, 2053 mL, 2566 mL) [sulfite free; lipid chamber contains egg phospholipids (egg lecithin), soybean oil]

Perikabiven: (1440 mL,1920 mL, 2400 mL) [sulfite free; lipid chamber contains egg phospholipids (egg lecithin), soybean oil]

◆ Totect see Dexrazoxane on page 531

◆ Toujeo SoloStar see Insulin Glargine on page 956

◆ Toviaz see Fesoterodine on page 763

◆ tPA see Alteplase on page 80

◆ TPN see Total Parenteral Nutrition on page 1818

◆ TPV see Tipranavir on page 1795

◆ TR-700 see Tedizolid on page 1741

◆ TR-701 FA see Tedizolid on page 1741

◆ tRA see Tretinoin (Systemic) on page 1838

Trabectedin (tra BEK te din)

Brand Names: US Yondelis

Brand Names: Canada Yondelis

Index Terms Ecteinascidin; Ecteinascidin 743; ET-743

Pharmacologic Category Antineoplastic Agent, Miscellaneous

Use

US labeling:

Soft tissue sarcoma: Treatment of unresectable or metastatic soft tissue sarcoma (liposarcoma or leiomyosarcoma) in patients who have received a prior anthracycline-containing regimen.

Canadian labeling:

Ovarian cancer: Treatment of relapsed platinum-sensitive ovarian cancer (in combination with doxorubicin liposomal)

Soft tissue sarcoma: Treatment of metastatic soft tissue sarcoma (liposarcoma or leiomyosarcoma) after failure of prior anthracycline and ifosfamide chemotherapy

Pregnancy Considerations Animal reproduction studies have not been conducted. Based on the mechanism of action, trabectedin may cause fetal harm if administered during pregnancy. Women of reproductive potential should use effective contraception during and for at least 2 months after treatment (Canadian labeling: 3 months). Males with partners of reproductive potential should use effective contraception during and for at least 5 months following treatment. Trabectedin may cause decreased fertility in males and females. The Canadian labeling recommends that male patients who wish to father a child during or after treatment should seek advice regarding sperm cryopreservation prior to treatment initiation.

Breast-Feeding Considerations It is not known if trabectedin is excreted in human milk. Due to the potential for serious adverse reactions in the nursing infant, the manufacturer recommends discontinuing nursing during trabectedin treatment. Breast-feeding is contraindicated during and for 3 months after treatment in the Canadian labeling.

Contraindications

Hypersensitivity (including anaphylaxis) to trabectedin or any component of the formulation

Canadian labeling: Additional contraindications: Active serious or uncontrolled infection; breast-feeding

Warnings/Precautions Hazardous agent - use appropriate precautions for handling and disposal (meets NIOSH 2014 criteria). Anemia, neutropenia, and thrombocytopenia commonly occur; neutropenic fever and neutropenic sepsis (with fatalities) have been reported. The median onset for first occurrence of grade 3/4 neutropenia was 16 days (range: 8 days to ~10 months) and median time to recovery was 13 days (range: 3 days to ~2 months). Monitor neutrophil count prior to each dose and periodically throughout treatment cycle. Withhold treatment for neutrophil count <1,500/mm^3. Reduce dose (permanently) for life-threatening or prolonged severe neutropenia in the preceding cycle.

Trabectedin may cause rhabdomyolysis and musculoskeletal toxicity (some fatal). Creatine phosphokinase (CPK) elevations occurred in nearly one-third of patients receiving trabectedin; grade 3 and 4 CPK elevations, some complicated by renal failure, occurred. The median time to first occurrence of grade 3 or 4 CPK elevation was 2 months (range: 1 to 11.5 months) and the median time to complete resolution was 14 days (range: 5 to 30 days). Monitor CPK levels prior to each dose; withhold treatment for CPK levels >2.5 times upper limit of normal (ULN); discontinue permanently if rhabdomyolysis occurs.

Cardiomyopathy, including heart failure, decreased ejection fraction, diastolic dysfunction, or right ventricular dysfunction, has been observed; some events were grades 3 and 4. The median time to development of grades 3 and 4 cardiomyopathy was ~5 months (range: 1 to 15 months). Monitor left ventricular ejection fraction (LVEF) by echocardiogram or MUGA scan prior to treatment initiation and every 2 to 3 months until trabectedin is discontinued. Withhold treatment if LVEF is below the lower limit of normal (LLN); permanently discontinue for symptomatic cardiomyopathy or persistent ventricular dysfunction that does not recover to LLN within 3 weeks. Patients with a history of New York Heart Association class II, III, or IV heart failure or abnormal LVEF were excluded from the sarcoma study. Pulmonary embolism has been reported.

Hepatotoxicity (including hepatic failure) may occur with trabectedin. Grade 3 and 4 liver function test (LFT) elevations (AST, ALT, total bilirubin, or alkaline phosphatase) occurred in over one-third of patients. The median onset for grade 3/4 ALT or AST elevations was 29 days (range: 3 days to 11.5 months) and the median time to resolution was 13 days (range: 4 days to ~4 months). Drug-induced liver injury (ALT or AST elevation >3 times ULN, alkaline phosphatase <2 times ULN, and total bilirubin ≥2 times ULN) and ALT or AST elevations >8 times ULN have been reported. Monitor LFTs prior to each dose; may require treatment interruption, dose reduction, and/or discontinuation (based on severity and duration). Premedication with dexamethasone appears to reduce the frequency and severity of transaminase elevations (Yondelis Canadian labeling 2014). Trabectedin should only be used in patients with a normal bilirubin and AST or ALT ≤2.5 times ULN. Patients with bilirubin above the ULN or AST or ALT >2.5 times the ULN were excluded from the sarcoma clinical trial. Use is also not recommended in the Canadian labeling if alkaline phosphatase (nonosseous origin) >2.5 times ULN, albumin <25 g/L, or in patients with clinically relevant liver disease (eg, active chronic hepatitis). Serious hypersensitivity reactions have been reported (Yondelis Canadian labeling 2014). The Canadian labeling recommends to avoid use in patients with CrCl <30 mL/minute (single-agent therapy); use is not recommended in patients with

CrCl <60 mL/minute (combination therapy with doxorubicin liposomal); monitor renal function.

Vesicant; ensure proper needle or catheter placement prior to and during infusion. Infuse through a central line. Avoid extravasation. Extravasation of trabectedin with subsequent tissue necrosis requiring debridement has been reported; evidence of necrosis may be delayed up to 1 week after extravasation. Nausea and vomiting are common; corticosteroid premedication (eg, dexamethasone) is recommended; other antiemetics may also be needed. Constipation and diarrhea (generally mild) also commonly occur. Potentially significant drug-drug interactions may exist, requiring dose or frequency adjustment, additional monitoring, and/or selection of alternative therapy.

Adverse Reactions Note: Adverse reactions as reported for monotherapy and combination therapy with doxorubicin liposomal.

>10%:

Central nervous system: Fatigue (46% to 53%), fever (5% to 20%), headache (15% to 16%), paresthesia (monotherapy: 11%)

Dermatologic: Palmar-Plantar erythrodysesthesia (24%), alopecia (3% to 12%), skin rash (11%)

Endocrine & metabolic: Hypokalemia (5% to 42%), hypophosphatemia (34%)

Gastrointestinal: Nausea (72% to 74%; grade 3: 4% to 10%), vomiting (39% to 56%; grade 3: 2% to 12%; grade 4: <1%), anorexia (19% to 32%), constipation (18% to 32%), diarrhea (15% to 26%), abdominal pain (5% to 20%), stomatitis (20%), weight gain (monotherapy: 20%), dyspepsia (5% to 13%), mucosal inflammation (12%)

Hematologic: Anemia (27% to 97%; grade 3: 1% to 13%; grade 4: ≤6%), leukopenia (12% to 95%; grade 3: 3% to 45%; grade 4: 2% to 18%), neutropenia (49% to 92%; grade 3: 22% to 30%; grade 4: 13% to 42%), thrombocytopenia (20% to 64%; grade 3: 8% to 12%, grade 4: 2% to 11%), decreased neutrophils (12%; grade 3: 6%; grade 4: 3%)

Hepatic: Increased ALT (54% to 96%; grade 3: 37% to 46%; grade 4: 2% to 5%), increased AST (47% to 89%, grade 3: 12% to 23%; grade 4: ≤2%), increased alkaline phosphatase (28% to 61%; grade 3: 2%), hyperbilirubinemia (8% to 25%; grade 3: ≤1%)

Local: Phlebitis (monotherapy: 15%), injection/catheter site reactions (14%)

Neuromuscular & skeletal: Increased CPK (2% to 26%; grade 3: 1% to 4%, grade 4: 1% to 4%), weakness (15% to 17%), arthralgia (5% to 12%)

Renal: Increased serum creatinine (28%: grade 3: <1%; grade 4: <1%)

Respiratory: Dyspnea (5% to 15%), cough (12%)

1% to 10%:

Cardiovascular: Peripheral edema (5% to 9%), palpitation (4%), edema (3%), syncope (2%), chest pain (1%), left ventricular dysfunction (1%; grade 3: <1%)

Central nervous system: Insomnia (6% to 10%), dizziness (5%)

Dermatologic: Hyperpigmentation (6%)

Endocrine & metabolic: Dehydration (5%)

Gastrointestinal: Decreased appetite (6%), dysgeusia (5% to 8%)

Hematologic: Bleeding complications (9%), febrile neutropenia (2% to 8%, grade 3: 6%, grade 4: 2%), decreased white blood cell count (7%; grade 3: 3%), decreased hemoglobin (5%), decreased platelet count (5%; grade 3: 1%), bone marrow failure (2%), granulocytopenia (2%), pancytopenia (2%), neutropenic infection (1%; grade 3: 1%)

Hepatic: Increased serum transaminases (5%; grade 3: 2%), hepatotoxicity (2%; grade 3: 1%)

Hypersensitivity: Hypersensitivity (2%)

Local: Catheter site pain (3%), catheter site erythema (2%), catheter site inflammation (2%)

Neuromuscular & skeletal: Myalgia (5% to 10%), peripheral neuropathy (5%), musculoskeletal pain (4%)

Renal: Renal failure (2%; grade 3: 1%; grade 4: <1%)

Respiratory: Pulmonary embolism (5%), pulmonary edema (1%)

Miscellaneous: Neutropenic sepsis (1%; grade 3: <1%; grade 4: <1%)

<1% (Limited to important or life-threatening): Extravasation (with tissue necrosis, requiring debridement), prolonged QT interval on ECG, rhabdomyolysis

Drug Interactions

Metabolism/Transport Effects Substrate of CYP3A4 (major), P-glycoprotein; **Note:** Assignment of Major/Minor substrate status based on clinically relevant drug interaction potential

Avoid Concomitant Use

Avoid concomitant use of Trabectedin with any of the following: Alcohol (Ethyl); BCG (Intravesical); Conivaptan; CYP3A4 Inducers (Strong); CYP3A4 Inhibitors (Moderate); CYP3A4 Inhibitors (Strong); Deferiprone; Dipyrone; Fusidic Acid (Systemic); Idelalisib; Natalizumab; Pimecrolimus; St Johns Wort; Tacrolimus (Topical); Tofacitinib; Vaccines (Live)

Increased Effect/Toxicity

Trabectedin may increase the levels/effects of: CloZAPine; Deferiprone; Fingolimod; Leflunomide; Natalizumab; Tofacitinib; Vaccines (Live)

The levels/effects of Trabectedin may be increased by: Alcohol (Ethyl); Conivaptan; CYP3A4 Inhibitors (Moderate); CYP3A4 Inhibitors (Strong); Dasatinib; Denosumab; Dipyrone; Fosaprepitant; Fusidic Acid (Systemic); HMG-CoA Reductase Inhibitors; Idelalisib; Ivacaftor; Luliconazole; Osimertinib; Palbociclib; P-glycoprotein/ABCB1 Inhibitors; Pimecrolimus; Ranolazine; Roflumilast; Simeprevir; Stiripentol; Tacrolimus (Topical); Trastuzumab

Decreased Effect

Trabectedin may decrease the levels/effects of: BCG (Intravesical); Coccidioides immitis Skin Test; Sipuleucel-T; Vaccines (Inactivated); Vaccines (Live)

The levels/effects of Trabectedin may be decreased by: Bosentan; CYP3A4 Inducers (Moderate); CYP3A4 Inducers (Strong); Dabrafenib; Deferasirox; Echinacea; Osimertinib; P-glycoprotein/ABCB1 Inducers; Siltuximab; St Johns Wort; Tocilizumab

Food Interactions Coadministration with grapefruit or grapefruit juice may increase trabectedin plasma concentrations. Management: Avoid concomitant administration with grapefruit or grapefruit juice.

Preparation for Administration Hazardous agent; use appropriate precautions for handling and disposal (meets NIOSH 2014 criteria). Reconstitute the 1 mg vial with 20 mL SWFI resulting in a reconstituted concentration of 0.05 mg/mL. Shake until completely dissolved. Immediately after reconstitution, further dilute for infusion in 500 mL sodium chloride 0.9% or D_5W. Diluted solution is compatible in type I glass, polyvinyl chloride (PVC) and polyethylene (PE) bags and tubing, PE and polypropylene (PP) mixture bags, polyethersulfone (PES) inline filters, titanium, platinum, or plastic ports, silicone and polyurethane catheters, and pumps with PVC, PE, or PE/PP contact surfaces. Do not mix with other medications.

Storage/Stability Store intact vials at 2°C to 8°C (36°F to 46°F). Solutions diluted for infusion should be used within 30 hours of reconstitution (infusion should be completed within that 30 hours).

Mechanism of Action Trabectedin is a marine-derived compound which blocks the cell cycle at the G_2/M phase by covalently binding to the minor DNA groove, bending the helix toward the major groove and altering DNA transcription (Garcia-Carbonero 2005). Also alters DNA repair mechanism.

Pharmacodynamics/Kinetics

Distribution: V_d: >5,000 L

Protein binding: ~97%; to plasma proteins

Metabolism: Extensively hepatic; via CYP3A4

Half-life elimination: ~175 hours

Excretion: Feces (58%; only negligible amounts as unchanged drug); urine (6%; only negligible amounts as unchanged drug)

Dosing

Adult & Geriatric Note: Prior to each treatment cycle, ANC should be ≥1500/mm³, platelets ≥100,000/mm³ total bilirubin ≤ULN, and alkaline phosphatase, ALT, AST, and CPK ≤2.5 times ULN.

Premedications: Administer dexamethasone 20 mg IV 30 minutes prior to each infusion. Additional antiemetics may be necessary.

Soft tissue sarcoma, unresectable/metastatic: IV: 1.5 mg/m² continuous infusion over 24 hours once every 3 weeks, continue until disease progression or unacceptable toxicity (Demetri 2015)

Ovarian cancer, relapsed, platinum sensitive (Canadian labeling; not an approved use in the US): IV: 1.1 mg/m² over 3 hours every 3 weeks (in combination with doxorubicin liposomal), continue as long as clinical benefit is demonstrated (Monk 2010; Monk 2012; Poveda 2011)

Renal Impairment

US labeling:

CrCl ≥30 mL/minute: No dosage adjustment is necessary.

CrCl <30 mL/minute or ESRD: There is no dosage adjustment provided in the manufacturer's labeling (has not been studied).

Canadian labeling:

Mild to moderate impairment: Renal impairment should have minimal impact on pharmacokinetics/elimination.

CrCl <30 mL/minute or serum creatinine >1.5 mg/dL: Avoid use (has not been studied).

CrCl <60 mL/minute: Combination therapy with doxorubicin liposomal is not recommended (has not been studied).

Hepatic Impairment

Hepatic impairment prior to treatment:

US labeling:

Bilirubin within normal limits and AST or ALT ≤2.5 times ULN: No dosage adjustment necessary.

Bilirubin >ULN: There is no dosage adjustment provided in the manufacturer's labeling (has not been studied).

Canadian labeling: Bilirubin >ULN, alkaline phosphatase (nonosseous origin) >2.5 times ULN, ALT and AST >2.5 times ULN, albumin <25 g/L, or clinically relevant liver disease (eg, active chronic hepatitis): Use is not recommended (has not been studied).

Hepatotoxicity during treatment: US labeling:

Total bilirubin >ULN: Delay dose for up to 3 weeks and reduce the next dose by one dose level

AST or ALT >2.5 times ULN: Delay dose for up to 3 weeks

AST or ALT >5 times ULN: Reduce the next dose by one dose level

Alkaline phosphatase >2.5 times ULN: Delay dose for up to 3 weeks and reduce the next dose by one dose level

Severe liver dysfunction (bilirubin 2 times ULN and AST or ALT 3 times ULN with alkaline phosphatase <2 times ULN in prior treatment cycle): Permanently discontinue

Obesity ASCO Guidelines for appropriate chemotherapy dosing in obese adults with cancer: Utilize patient's actual body weight (full weight) for calculation of body surface area- or weight-based dosing, particularly when the intent of therapy is curative; manage regimen-related toxicities in the same manner as for nonobese patients; if a dose reduction is utilized due to toxicity, consider resumption of full weight-based dosing with subsequent cycles, especially if cause of toxicity (eg, hepatic or renal impairment) is resolved (Griggs 2012).

Adjustment for Toxicity

US labeling: Soft tissue sarcoma:

Recommended dose reduction levels (once a dose is reduced it should not be increased in subsequent cycles):

First dose reduction: 1.2 mg/m² once every 3 weeks

Second dose reduction: 1 mg/m² once every 3 weeks

Hematologic toxicity:

ANC <1,500/mm³: Delay dose for up to 3 weeks

ANC <1,000/mm³ with fever or infection or <500/mm³ lasting >5 days: Reduce the next dose by one dose level

Platelets <100,000/mm³: Delay dose for up to 3 weeks

Platelets <25,000/mm³: Reduce the next dose by one dose level

Nonhematologic toxicity:

Creatine phosphokinase: >2.5 times ULN: Delay dose for up to 3 weeks

Creatine phosphokinase: >5 times ULN: Reduce the next dose by one dose level

Decreased left ventricular ejection fraction (LVEF): Less than the lower limit of normal (LLN) or clinical evidence of cardiomyopathy: Delay dose for up to 3 weeks

Decreased LVEF: Absolute decrease of 10% or more from baseline and less than the LLN or clinical evidence of cardiomyopathy: Reduce the next dose by one dose level

Other nonhematologic toxicity: Grade 3 or 4: Delay dose for up to 3 weeks and reduce the next dose by one dose level

Adverse reactions with trabectedin administered at 1 mg/m² and requiring further dose reduction: Permanently discontinue

Persistent adverse events requiring a delay of more than 3 weeks: Permanently discontinue.

Canadian labeling:

Delay the next treatment cycle for up to 3 weeks if ANC <1,500/mm³, platelets <100,000/mm³, hemoglobin <9 g/dL, bilirubin >ULN; alkaline phosphatase (nonosseous origin), ALT, and AST >2.5 times ULN; albumin <25 g/L, creatinine clearance <30 mL/minute (single-agent therapy), serum creatinine >1.5 mg/dL or creatinine clearance <60 mL/minute (combination therapy with doxorubicin liposomal); if persists beyond 3 weeks, consider discontinuing treatment.

Reduce dose if the following occur in between cycles: ANC <500/mm^3 for >5 days or associated with fever or infection, platelets <25,000/mm^3, bilirubin >ULN, alkaline phosphatase (nonosseous origin) >2.5 times ULN, ALT or AST >2.5 times ULN (single-agent therapy) or >5 times ULN (combination therapy with doxorubicin liposomal) which has not recovered by day 21, or any other grade 3 or 4 adverse reaction (eg, nausea, vomiting, fatigue):

Ovarian cancer:

First occurrence: Reduce trabectedin dose to 0.9 mg/m^2 (also reduce doxorubicin liposomal dose)

Second occurrence: Reduce trabectedin dose to 0.75 mg/m^2 (also reduce doxorubicin liposomal dose)

Third occurrence: Consider treatment discontinuation.

Soft tissue sarcoma (liposarcoma or leiomyosarcoma):

First occurrence: Reduce trabectedin dose to 1.2 mg/m^2

Second occurrence: Reduce trabectedin dose to 1 mg/m^2

Third occurrence: Consider treatment discontinuation.

CPK >2.5 times ULN: Withhold treatment until full recovery.

Dietary Considerations Avoid grapefruit and grapefruit juice.

Administration Infuse through a central line with a 0.2 micron polyethersulfone filter. Infusion must be completed within 30 hours of reconstitution. Premedicate with a corticosteroid (eg, dexamethasone IV) 30 minutes prior to treatment; additional antiemetics may be needed.

Soft tissue sarcoma: Single-agent therapy: Infuse as a continuous infusion over 24 hours

Ovarian cancer: Canadian labeling: Combination therapy with doxorubicin liposomal: Administer doxorubicin liposomal first, flush line with D$_5$W, then follow with trabectedin infusion over 3 hours.

Vesicant; ensure proper needle or catheter placement prior to and during infusion; avoid extravasation.

Extravasation management: If extravasation occurs, stop infusion immediately and disconnect (leave cannula/needle in place); gently aspirate extravasated solution (do **NOT** flush the line); remove needle/cannula; elevate extremity.

Hazardous agent; use appropriate precautions for handling and disposal (meets NIOSH 2014 criteria).

Monitoring Parameters CBC with differential (baseline and periodically during treatment cycles); total bilirubin (prior to each cycle), ALT, AST, and alkaline phosphatase (prior to each cycle); renal function (baseline and during treatment); CPK (prior to each treatment cycle), evaluate LVEF via MUGA or echocardiogram (baseline and every 2 to 3 months); monitor infusion site for signs/symptoms of extravasation

Product Availability Yondelis: FDA approved October 2015; anticipated availability is currently unknown.

Dosage Forms Excipient information presented when available (limited, particularly for generics); consult specific product labeling.

Solution Reconstituted, Intravenous:
Yondelis: 1 mg (1 ea)

Dosage Forms: Canada Excipient information presented when available (limited, particularly for generics); consult specific product labeling.

Injection, powder for reconstitution:
Yondelis: 1 mg [contains sucrose]

◆ Tracleer see Bosentan *on page 246*

◆ Tradjenta *see* Linagliptin *on page 1078*

◆ Trajenta *see* Linagliptin *on page 1078*

◆ Tramacet (Can) *see* Acetaminophen and Tramadol *on page 29*

TraMADol (TRA ma dole)

Brand Names: US Active-Tramadol; ConZip; EnovaRX-Tramadol; Rybix ODT [DSC]; Ryzolt [DSC]; Synapryn FusePaq; Ultram; Ultram ER

Brand Names: Canada Apo-Tramadol; Durela; Ralivia; Tridural; Ultram; Zytram XL

Index Terms Ryzolt; Tramadol Hydrochloride

Pharmacologic Category Analgesic, Opioid

Use Relief of moderate to moderately-severe pain

Extended release formulations are indicated for patients requiring around-the-clock management of moderate to moderately-severe pain for an extended period of time

Pregnancy Considerations Adverse events were observed in animal reproduction studies. Tramadol has been shown to cross the human placenta when administered during labor. Postmarketing reports following tramadol use during pregnancy include neonatal seizures, withdrawal syndrome, fetal death, and stillbirth. Tramadol is not recommended for use during labor and delivery. Some Canadian products are contraindicated for use in pregnant women.

If chronic opioid exposure occurs in pregnancy, adverse events in the newborn (including withdrawal) may occur; monitoring of the neonate is recommended (Chou, 2009). Neonatal abstinence syndrome following opioid exposure may present with autonomic (eg, fever, temperature instability), gastrointestinal (eg, diarrhea, vomiting, poor feeding/weight gain), or neurologic (eg, high-pitched crying, increased muscle tone, irritability, seizure, tremor) symptoms (Dow, 2012; Hudak, 2012).

Breast-Feeding Considerations Tramadol is excreted into breast milk. Sixteen hours following a single 100 mg IV dose, the amount of tramadol found in breast milk was 0.1% of the maternal dose. Use is not recommended by the manufacturer for postdelivery analgesia in nursing mothers. Some Canadian products are contraindicated for use in nursing women. Nursing infants exposed to large doses of opioids should be monitored for apnea and sedation (Montgomery, 2012).

Contraindications Hypersensitivity to tramadol, opioids, or any component of the formulation

Additional contraindications for Ultram®, Rybix™ ODT, and Ultram® ER: Any situation where opioids are contraindicated, including acute intoxication with alcohol, hypnotics, centrally-acting analgesics, opioids, or psychotropic drugs

Additional contraindications for ConZip: Severe/acute bronchial asthma, hypercapnia, or significant respiratory depression in the absence of appropriately monitored setting and/or resuscitative equipment

Canadian product labeling:

Tramadol is contraindicated during or within 14 days following MAO inhibitor therapy

Extended release formulations: Additional contraindications:

Ralivia™, Tridural™: Severe (CrCl <30 mL/minute) renal dysfunction, severe (Child-Pugh class C) hepatic dysfunction

Durela™ and Zytram® XL: Severe (CrCl <30 mL/minute) renal dysfunction, severe (Child-Pugh class C) hepatic dysfunction; known or suspected mechanical GI obstruction or any disease/condition that affects bowel transit; mild, intermittent or short-duration pain that can be managed with other pain medication; management of peri-operative pain; obstructive airway, acute respiratory depression, cor pulmonale, delirium tremens, seizure disorder, severe CNS depression, increased cerebrospinal or intracranial pressure, head injury, breast-feeding, pregnancy; use during labor and delivery

Warnings/Precautions Rare but serious anaphylactoid reactions (including fatalities) often following initial dosing have been reported. Pruritus, hives, bronchospasm, angioedema, toxic epidermal necrolysis (TEN) and Stevens-Johnson syndrome also have been reported with use. Previous anaphylactoid reactions to opioids may increase risks for similar reactions to tramadol. Caution patients to swallow extended release tablets whole. Rapid release and absorption of tramadol from extended release tablets that are broken, crushed, or chewed may lead to a potentially lethal overdose. May cause CNS depression, which may impair physical or mental abilities; patients must be cautioned about performing tasks which require mental alertness (eg, operating machinery or driving). Effects with other sedative drugs or ethanol may be potentiated. May cause CNS depression and/or respiratory depression, particularly when combined with other CNS depressants. Use with caution and reduce dosage when administered to patients receiving other CNS depressants. An increased risk of seizures may occur in patients receiving serotonin reuptake inhibitors (SSRIs or anorectics), tricyclic antidepressants or other cyclic compounds (including cyclobenzaprine, promethazine), neuroleptics, drugs which may lower seizure threshold, or drugs which impair metabolism of tramadol (ie, CYP2D6 and 3A4 inhibitors). Patients with a history of seizures, or with a risk of seizures (head trauma, metabolic disorders, CNS infection, or malignancy, or during ethanol/drug withdrawal) are also at increased risk. Potentially significant

drug interactions may exist, requiring dose or frequency adjustment, additional monitoring, and/or selection of alternative therapy.

Elderly (particularly >75 years of age), debilitated patients and patients with chronic respiratory disorders may be at greater risk of adverse events. Use with caution in patients with increased intracranial pressure or head injury. Avoid use in patients who are suicidal or addiction prone; use with caution in patients taking tranquilizers and/or antidepressants, or those with an emotional disturbance including depression. Healthcare provider should be alert to problems of abuse, misuse, and diversion. Use caution in heavy alcohol users. Use caution in treatment of acute abdominal conditions; may mask pain. Use tramadol with caution and reduce dosage in patients with liver disease or renal dysfunction. Avoid using extended release tablets in severe hepatic impairment. Tolerance or drug dependence may result from extended use (withdrawal symptoms have been reported); abrupt discontinuation should be avoided. Tapering of dose at the time of discontinuation limits the risk of withdrawal symptoms. Some products may contain phenylalanine.

After chronic maternal exposure to opioids, neonatal withdrawal syndrome may occur in the newborn; monitor neonate closely. Signs and symptoms include irritability, hyperactivity and abnormal sleep pattern, high pitched cry, tremor, vomiting, diarrhea and failure to gain weight. Onset, duration and severity depend on the drug used, duration of use, maternal dose, and rate of drug elimination by the newborn. Opioid withdrawal syndrome in the neonate, unlike in adults, may be life-threatening and should be treated according to protocols developed by neonatology experts.

Adverse Reactions
>10%:
Cardiovascular: Flushing (8% to 16%)
Central nervous system: Dizziness (10% to 33%), headache (4% to 32%), drowsiness (7% to 25%), central nervous system stimulation (7% to 14%), insomnia (2% to 11%)
Dermatologic: Pruritus (3% to 12%)
Gastrointestinal: Constipation (9% to 46%), nausea (15% to 40%), vomiting (5% to 17%), xerostomia (3% to 13%), dyspepsia (1% to 13%)
Neuromuscular & skeletal: Weakness (4% to 12%)
1% to 10%:
Cardiovascular: Orthostatic hypotension (2% to 5%), chest pain (1% to <5%), hypertension (1% to <5%), peripheral edema (1% to <5%), vasodilation (1% to <5%)
Central nervous system: Agitation (1% to <5%), anxiety (1% to <5%), apathy (1% to <5%), ataxia (1% to <5%), chills (1% to <5%), confusion (1% to <5%), depersonalization (1% to <5%), depression (1% to <5%), euphoria (1% to <5%), hypertonia (1% to <5%), hypoesthesia (1% to <5%), lethargy (1% to <5%), malaise (<1% to <5%), nervousness (1% to <5%), pain (1% to <5%), paresthesia (1% to <5%), restlessness (1% to <5%), rigors (1% to <5%), sleep disorder (1% to <5%) withdrawal syndrome (1% to <5%), fatigue (2%), vertigo (2%)
Dermatologic: Diaphoresis (2% to 9%), dermatitis (1% to <5%), skin rash (1% to <5%)
Endocrine & metabolic: Hot flash (1% to <5%), hyperglycemia (1% to <5%), weight loss (1% to <5%)
Gastrointestinal: Diarrhea (5% to 10%), anorexia (1% to 6%), abdominal pain (1% to <5%), decreased appetite (1% to <5%), flatulence (<1% to <5%), sore throat (1% to <5%)
Genitourinary: Menopausal symptoms (1% to <5%), pelvic pain (1% to <5%), prostatic disease (1% to <5%), urine abnormality (1% to <5%), urinary tract infection (1% to <5%), urinary frequency (<1% to <5%), urinary retention (<1% to <5%)
Neuromuscular & skeletal: Arthralgia (1% to 5%), back pain (1% to <5%), increased creatine phosphokinase (1% to <5%), myalgia (1% to <5%), neck pain (1% to <5%), tremor (1% to <5%)
Ophthalmic: Blurred vision (1% to <5%), miosis (1% to <5%), visual disturbance (1% to <5%)
Respiratory: Bronchitis (1% to <5%), cough (1% to <5%), dyspnea (1% to <5%), nasopharyngitis (1% to <5%), pharyngitis (1% to <5%), respiratory congestion (1% to <5%), rhinitis (1% to <5%), rhinorrhea (1% to <5%), sinusitis (1% to <5%), sneezing (1% to <5%), upper respiratory tract infection (1% to <5%)
Miscellaneous: Accidental injury (<5%), fever (1% to <5%), flu-like syndrome (1% to <5%)

<1% (Limited to important or life-threatening): Abnormal gait, anemia, appendicitis, bradycardia, cataract, cellulitis, cholecystitis, cholelithiasis, cognitive dysfunction, deafness, dysphagia, dysuria, ECG abnormality, edema, fecal impaction, gastroenteritis, gastrointestinal hemorrhage, gout, hematuria, hepatic failure, hypersensitivity reaction, hypoglycemia, increased blood urea nitrogen, increased gamma-glutamyl transferase, increased liver enzymes, increased serum creatinine, ischemic heart disease, menstrual disease, migraine, muscle spasm, mydriasis, night sweats, otitis, palpitations, pancreatitis, peripheral ischemia, pneumonia, proteinuria, pulmonary edema, pulmonary embolism, sedation, seizure, serotonin syndrome, skin vesicle, speech disturbance, Stevens-Johnson syndrome, stomatitis, suicidal tendencies, syncope, tachycardia, thrombocytopenia

Drug Interactions
Metabolism/Transport Effects Substrate of CYP2B6 (minor), CYP2D6 (major), CYP3A4 (major); Note: Assignment of Major/Minor substrate status based on clinically relevant drug interaction potential

Avoid Concomitant Use
Avoid concomitant use of TraMADol with any of the following: Azelastine (Nasal); CarBAMazepine; Dapoxetine; Eluxadoline; Mixed Agonist / Antagonist Opioids; Orphenadrine; Paraldehyde; Thalidomide

Increased Effect/Toxicity
TraMADol may increase the levels/effects of: Alcohol (Ethyl); Alvimopan; Antipsychotic Agents; Azelastine (Nasal); CarBAMazepine; CNS Depressants; Desmopressin; Diuretics; Eluxadoline; Hydrocodone; MAO Inhibitors; Methotrimeprazine; Metoclopramide; Metyrosine; Orphenadrine; Paraldehyde; Pramipexole; Ramosetron; ROPINIRole; Rotigotine; Selective Serotonin Reuptake Inhibitors; Serotonin Modulators; Suvorexant; Thalidomide; Tricyclic Antidepressants; Vitamin K Antagonists; Zolpidem

The levels/effects of TraMADol may be increased by: Amphetamines; Anticholinergic Agents; Antipsychotic Agents; Antipsychotic Agents (Phenothiazines); Brimonidine (Topical); Cannabis; Cyclobenzaprine; CYP2D6 Inhibitors (Strong); CYP3A4 Inhibitors (Strong); Dapoxetine; Doxylamine; Dronabinol; Droperidol; HydrOXYzine; Kava Kava; Magnesium Sulfate; Metaxalone; Methotrimeprazine; Minocycline; Nabilone; Osimertinib; Perampanel; Ritonavir; Rufinamide; Selective Serotonin Reuptake Inhibitors; Sodium Oxybate; Succinylcholine; Tapentadol; Tetrahydrocannabinol; Tricyclic Antidepressants

Decreased Effect
TraMADol may decrease the levels/effects of: CarBAMazepine; Pegvisomant

The levels/effects of TraMADol may be decreased by: Ammonium Chloride; Antiemetics (5HT3 Antagonists); Bosentan; CarBAMazepine; CYP2D6 Inhibitors (Moderate); CYP2D6 Inhibitors (Strong); CYP3A4 Inducers (Moderate); CYP3A4 Inducers (Strong); Dabrafenib; Deferasirox; Enzalutamide; Mitotane; Mixed Agonist / Antagonist Opioids; Naltrexone; Osimertinib; Ritonavir; Siltuximab; St Johns Wort; Tocilizumab

Food Interactions
Immediate release tablet: Rate and extent of absorption were not significantly affected by food. Management: Administer without regard to meals.
Extended release:
ConZip™: Rate and extent of absorption were unaffected by food. Management: Administer without regard to meals.
Ultram® ER: High-fat meal reduced C_{max} and AUC, and increased T_{max} by 3 hours. Management: Administer with or without food, but keep consistent.
Orally disintegrating tablet: Food delays the time to peak serum concentration by 30 minutes; extent of absorption was not significantly affected. Management: Administer without regard to meals.

Storage/Stability
Store at 25°C (77°F); excursions permitted to 15°C to 30°C (59°F to 86°F).

Mechanism of Action
Tramadol and its active metabolite (M1) binds to μ-opiate receptors in the CNS causing inhibition of ascending pain pathways, altering the perception of and response to pain; also inhibits the reuptake of norepinephrine and serotonin, which are neurotransmitters involved in the descending inhibitory pain pathway responsible for pain relief (Grond, 2004)

Pharmacodynamics/Kinetics
Onset of action: Immediate release: ~1 hour
Duration: 9 hours
Absorption: Immediate release formulation: Rapid and complete; Extended release formulation: Delayed
Distribution: V_d: 2.5-3 L/kg
Protein binding, plasma: ~20%

Metabolism: Extensively hepatic via demethylation (mediated by CYP3A4 and CYP2B6), glucuronidation, and sulfation; has pharmacologically active metabolite formed by CYP2D6 (M1; O-desmethyl tramadol)

Bioavailability: Immediate release: 75%; Extended release: Ultram® ER: 85% to 90% (as compared to immediate release), Zytram® XL, Tridural™: 70%

Half-life elimination: Tramadol: ~6-8 hours; Active metabolite: 7-9 hours; prolonged in elderly, hepatic or renal impairment; Zytram™ XL: Apparent half-life: ~16 hours; Durela™, Ralivia™, Tridural™: ~5-9 hours

Time to peak: Immediate release: ~2 hours; Extended release: ConZip™: ~10-12 hours, Tridural™: ~4 hours; Durela™, Ultram® ER: ~12 hours

Excretion: Urine (30% as unchanged drug; 60% as metabolites)

Dosing

Adult Moderate-to-severe pain: Oral:

Immediate release: 50-100 mg every 4-6 hours (not to exceed 400 mg/day). For patients not requiring rapid onset of effect, tolerability may be improved by starting dose at 25 mg/day and titrating dose by 25 mg every 3 days, until reaching 25 mg 4 times/day. The total daily dose may then be increased by 50 mg every 3 days as tolerated, to reach dose of 50 mg 4 times/day. After titration, 50-100 mg may be given every 4-6 hours as needed up to a maximum 400 mg/day.

Orally-disintegrating tablet (Rybix™ ODT): 50-100 mg every 4-6 hours (not to exceed 400 mg/day); for patients not requiring rapid onset of effect, tolerability may be improved by starting dose at 50 mg/day and titrating dose by 50 mg every 3 days, until reaching 50 mg 4 times/day. After titration, 50-100 mg may be given every 4-6 hours as needed up to a maximum 400 mg/day.

Extended release:

U.S. labeling: ConZip™, Ultram® ER:

Patients not currently on immediate-release tramadol: 100 mg once daily; titrate every 5 days (ConZip™, Ultram® ER); maximum dose: 300 mg daily

Patients currently on immediate-release tramadol: Calculate 24-hour immediate release total dose and initiate total extended release daily dose (round dose to the next lowest 100 mg increment); titrate as tolerated to desired effect (maximum: 300 mg daily)

Canadian labeling: **Note:** Patients currently on immediate-release tramadol: When switching to extended release, initiate at the same or lowest nearest total daily tramadol dose. Not to exceed recommended maximum daily dosing.

Durela™, Ralivia™, Tridural™: Patients not currently on immediate-release tramadol or opioids: Initial: 100 mg once daily; titrate every 5 days (Durela™, Ralivia™) or every 2 days (Tridural™) as needed based on clinical response and severity of pain (maximum: 300 mg daily)

Zytram® XL: Patients not currently on immediate-release tramadol or opioids: 150 mg once daily; if pain relief is not achieved may titrate by increasing dosage incrementally, with sufficient time to evaluate effect of increased dosage; generally not more often than every 7 days (maximum: 400 mg daily)

Geriatric Elderly >65 years: Oral: Use caution and initiate at the lower end of the dosing range. Refer to adult dosing.

Elderly >75 years:

Immediate release: Do not exceed 300 mg/day; see dosing adjustments for renal and hepatic impairment.

Extended release: Use with great caution; see dosing for adults, renal, and hepatic impairment.

Pediatric Moderate-to-severe pain: Oral: Children ≥17 years: Refer to adult dosing.

Renal Impairment

Immediate release: CrCl <30 mL/minute: Administer 50-100 mg dose every 12 hours (maximum: 200 mg/day).

Extended release: Should not be used in patients with CrCl <30 mL/minute.

Hepatic Impairment

Immediate release: Cirrhosis: Recommended dose: 50 mg every 12 hours.

Extended release: Should not be used in patients with severe (Child-Pugh class C) hepatic dysfunction.

Dietary Considerations Some products may contain phenylalanine.

Administration

Immediate release: Administer without regard to meals.

Extended release: Swallow whole; do not crush, chew, or split. **Note:** Durela™, Ralivia™, and Tridural™: Canadian availability; products not available in U.S.:

ConZip™, Zytram® XL, Durela™: May administer without regard to meals.

Ultram® ER, Ralivia™, Tridural™: May administer without regard to meals, but administer in a consistent manner of either with or without meals.

Orally-disintegrating tablet: Remove from foil blister by peeling back (do not push tablet through the foil). Place tablet on tongue and allow to dissolve (may take ~1 minute); water is not needed, but may be administered with water. Do not chew, break, or split tablet.

Monitoring Parameters Pain relief, respiratory rate, blood pressure, and pulse; signs of tolerance, abuse, or suicidal ideation

Reference Range 100-300 ng/mL; however, serum level monitoring is not required

Test Interactions May interfere with urine detection of phencyclidine (false-positive).

Dosage Forms Considerations

ConZip extended release capsules are formulated as a biphasic product, providing immediate and extended release components:

100 mg: 25 mg (immediate release) and 75 mg (extended release)

200 mg: 50 mg (immediate release) and 150 mg (extended release)

300 mg: 50 mg (immediate release) and 250 mg (extended release)

EnovaRX-Tramadol and Active-Tramadol creams are compounded from kits. Refer to manufacturer's labeling for compounding instructions.

Synapryn FusePaq is a compounding kit for the preparation of an oral suspension. Refer to manufacturer's labeling for compounding instructions.

Dosage Forms Excipient information presented when available (limited, particularly for generics); consult specific product labeling. [DSC] = Discontinued product

Capsule Extended Release 24 Hour, Oral, as hydrochloride:

ConZip: 100 mg, 200 mg, 300 mg [contains fd&c blue #2 aluminum lake, fd&c yellow #10 aluminum lake]

Generic: 100 mg, 150 mg, 200 mg, 300 mg

Cream, External, as hydrochloride:

Active-Tramadol: 8% (120 g) [contains chlorocresol (chloro-m-cresol)]

EnovaRX-Tramadol: 5% (60 g, 120 g) [contains cetyl alcohol]

Suspension Reconstituted, Oral, as hydrochloride:

Synapryn FusePaq: 10 mg/mL (500 mL) [contains saccharin sodium, sodium benzoate]

Tablet, Oral, as hydrochloride:

Ultram: 50 mg [scored]

Generic: 50 mg

Tablet Dispersible, Oral, as hydrochloride:

Rybix ODT: 50 mg [DSC] [contains aspartame]

Tablet Extended Release 24 Hour, Oral, as hydrochloride:

Ryzolt: 100 mg [DSC], 200 mg [DSC], 300 mg [DSC]

Ultram ER: 100 mg, 200 mg, 300 mg

Generic: 100 mg, 200 mg, 300 mg

Dosage Forms: Canada Excipient information presented when available (limited, particularly for generics); consult specific product labeling.

Capsule Extended Release 24 Hour, Oral, as hydrochloride:

Durela: 100 mg, 200 mg, 300 mg

Tablet Extended Release 24 Hour, Oral, as hydrochloride

Ralivia: 100 mg, 200 mg, 300 mg

Tridural: 100 mg, 200 mg, 300 mg

Zytram XL: 75 mg, 150 mg, 200 mg, 300 mg, 400 mg

Controlled Substance C-IV

Extemporaneous Preparations A 5 mg/mL oral suspension may be made with tablets and either Ora-Sweet® SF or a mixture of 30 mL Ora-Plus® and 30 mL strawberry syrup. Crush six 50 mg tramadol tablets in a mortar and reduce to a fine powder. Add small portions of the chosen vehicle and mix to a uniform paste; mix while adding vehicle in incremental proportions to **almost** 60 mL; transfer to a calibrated bottle, rinse mortar with vehicle, and add quantity of vehicle sufficient to make 60 mL. Label "shake well before use". Stable for 90 days refrigerated or at room temperature.

Wagner DS, Johnson CE, Cichon-Hensley BK, et al, "Stability of Oral Liquid Preparations of Tramadol in Strawberry Syrup and a Sugar-Free Vehicle," *Am J Health Syst Pharm*, 2003, 60(12):1268-70.

♦ Tramadol Hydrochloride see TraMADol on page 1821
♦ Tramadol Hydrochloride and Acetaminophen see Acetaminophen and Tramadol on page 29

Trametinib (tra ME ti nib)

Brand Names: US Mekinist

Brand Names: Canada Mekinist

Index Terms GSK1120212; Trametinib Dimethyl Sulfoxide

Pharmacologic Category Antineoplastic Agent, MEK Inhibitor

Use

Melanoma, metastatic or unresectable: Treatment of unresectable or metastatic melanoma in patients with a BRAF V600E or BRAF V600K mutation (as detected by an approved test), either as a single-agent or in combination with dabrafenib.

Limitations of use: Trametinib as a single-agent is not indicated for use in patients who have received prior BRAF-inhibitor therapy.

Pregnancy Considerations Adverse effects were observed in animal reproduction studies. Based on its mechanism of action, trametinib would be expected to cause fetal harm if administered to a pregnant woman. Females of reproductive potential should use a highly effective contraceptive during therapy and for 4 months after treatment is complete. When trametinib is used in combination with dabrafenib, a highly effective nonhormonal contraceptive method should be used (dabrafenib may diminish efficacy of hormonal contraceptives). Fertility may also be impaired in females. Due to a risk for impaired spermatogenesis, males who may want to father a child should seek fertility/family planning counseling prior to initiating combination therapy with dabrafenib.

Breast-Feeding Considerations It is not known if trametinib is excreted into breast milk. Due to the potential for serious adverse reactions in the nursing infant, breast-feeding is not recommended by the manufacturer during treatment and for 4 months after the last dose.

Contraindications There are no contraindications listed in the manufacturer's US labeling.

Canadian labeling: Hypersensitivity to trametinib or any component of the formulation.

Warnings/Precautions Hazardous agent - use appropriate precautions for handling and disposal (meets NIOSH 2014 criteria). Cardiac events such as heart failure, left ventricular dysfunction, or decreased left ventricular ejection fraction (LVEF) were observed in clinical trials (for single-agent trametinib and when used in combination with dabrafenib; the median time to onset of cardiomyopathy for single-agent trametinib was ~2 months (range: 16 to 156 days) and ~8 months (range: ~1 to 25 months) when used in combination with dabrafenib. In some patients, cardiomyopathy developed within the first month of treatment. Assess LVEF (by echocardiogram or MUGA scan) prior to therapy initiation, at one month, and then at 2- to 3-month intervals while on therapy. Cardiac dysfunction may require treatment interruption, dosage reduction, or discontinuation; such measures resulted in resolution of cardiomyopathy in some patients. May cause hypertension; monitor blood pressure. Venous thromboembolism events (some fatal) may occur (was observed when used in combination with dabrafenib). DVT and PE occurred at an increased incidence with combination therapy. Patients should seek immediate medical attention with symptoms of DVT or PE (shortness of breath, chest pain, arm/leg swelling). Withhold trametinib for uncomplicated DVT or PE; may resume at a lower dose if improves within 3 weeks; permanently discontinue trametinib for life-threatening PE. Interstitial lung disease (ILD) and pneumonitis were observed in clinical trials; median time to initial presentation was ~5 months (range: 2 to ~6 months). Monitor for new or progressive pulmonary symptoms (eg, cough, dyspnea, hypoxia, pleural effusion, infiltrates); withhold treatment if symptoms occur; permanently discontinue with diagnosis of ILD or pneumonitis.

Dermatologic toxicity (eg, rash, dermatitis, acneiform rash, palmar-plantar erythrodysesthesia syndrome, and erythema) was commonly observed in trametinib-treated patients (either as a single-agent or when used in combination with dabrafenib); some patients required hospitalization for severe toxicity or for secondary skin infections. The median time to onset and resolution of skin toxicity for single-agent trametinib was 15 days (range: 1 to 221 days) and 48 days (range: 1 to 282 days), respectively. The median time to onset and resolution of skin toxicity for combination therapy was 2 months (range: 1 day to 22 months) and 1.2 months (range: 1 day to ~24 months), respectively. Monitor for dermatologic toxicity and signs/symptoms of secondary infections. Treatment interruption, dose reductions, and/or therapy discontinuation may be necessary. New primary cutaneous malignancies (which are associated with dabrafenib as single-agent therapy) may occur when trametinib is given in combination with dabrafenib. The incidence of basal cell carcinoma (BCC) is ~3% for combination therapy versus 6% for single-agent dabrafenib. The median time to BCC diagnosis ranged from ~3 to 24 months for patients receiving combination therapy. Cutaneous squamous cell carcinomas (SCC), including keratoacanthoma, occurred at a lower rate for combination therapy compared to single-agent dabrafenib

(3% vs 10%, respectively), with a median time to diagnosis ranging from ~2 to 17 months for combination therapy. Dermatologic exams should be performed prior to initiation of combination therapy, every 2 months while receiving combination treatment, and for up to 6 months following discontinuation.

Retinal pigment epithelial detachments (RPED) and retinal vein occlusion were seen in clinical trials (rare). Detachments were typically bilateral and multifocal and occurred in the central macular area of the retina. Retinal vein occlusion may lead to macular edema, degeneration, decreased visual function, neovascularization, and glaucoma. Promptly (within 24 hours) refer patients for ophthalmological evaluations if loss of vision or other visual disturbances occur. Ophthalmic exams (including retinal evaluation) should be performed periodically during treatment and with visual disturbances. Interrupt trametinib therapy for RPED; may resume if resolves within 3 weeks; reduce the dose or discontinue if not resolved within 3 weeks. Permanently discontinue if retinal vein occlusion develops. Uveitis and iritis have been reported when trametinib is used in combination with dabrafenib and are managed symptomatically with ophthalmic steroid and mydriatic drops (does not require alteration in trametinib therapy).

Serious febrile reactions and fever (any severity) accompanied by hypotension, rigors/chills, dehydration, or renal failure may occur when trametinib is used in combination with dabrafenib. The incidence and severity were higher with combination therapy than with single-agent dabrafenib; the median time to onset of fever was 30 days and duration was 6 days for patients receiving combination therapy. Withhold trametinib for fever >104°F (if using in combination, withhold dabrafenib for fever ≥101.3°F) or for any fever with rigors/chills, hypotension, dehydration, or renal failure (evaluate for infection); may require prophylactic antipyretics as secondary prophylaxis upon therapy resumption. Administer corticosteroids (eg, prednisone 10 mg daily or equivalent) for at least 5 days for second or subsequent episodes of pyrexia if temperature does not return to baseline within 3 days of fever onset, or for pyrexia associated with complications (eg, dehydration, hypotension, severe chills/rigors with no evidence of active infection). Hemorrhage, including symptomatic bleeding in a critical area/organ, may occur with trametinib, either as a single agent or in combination with dabrafenib. Major bleeding events (some fatal) included intracranial or gastrointestinal hemorrhage; may require treatment interruption and dosage reduction; permanently discontinue trametinib (and dabrafenib) for all grade 4 hemorrhagic events and any grade 3 event that does not improve with therapy interruption. While not reported with single-agent trametinib, hyperglycemia may occur while on combination therapy with dabrafenib; may require initiation of insulin or oral hypoglycemic agent therapy (or an increased dose if already taking); monitor serum glucose at baseline and as clinically necessary in patients with preexisting diabetes or hyperglycemia. Instruct patients to report symptoms of severe hyperglycemia (eg, polydipsia, polyuria).

Prior to initiating therapy, confirm BRAF mutation status with an approved test; approved for use in patients with BRAF V600K and BRAF V600E mutations. Current data regarding use in patients with BRAF V600K mutation is limited; compared to BRAF V600E mutation, lower response rates have been observed with BRAF V600K mutation. Data regarding other less common BRAF V600 mutations is lacking. There are case reports of noncutaneous malignancies, including pancreatic cancer (KRAS mutation-positive), colorectal cancer (recurrent NRAS mutation-positive), hand and neck cancer, and glioblastoma, with combination therapy; monitor for signs/symptoms of noncutaneous malignancies. No trametinib dosage modification is necessary for new primary cutaneous and noncutaneous malignancies; dabrafenib should be permanently discontinued if RAS mutation-positive noncutaneous malignancies develop. Serious adverse reactions (tumor promotion, hemolytic anemia), which occur with single-agent dabrafenib, may also occur when trametinib is administered in combination with dabrafenib. Potentially significant drug-drug interactions may exist, requiring dose or frequency adjustment, additional monitoring, and/or selection of alternative therapy.

Adverse Reactions

Adverse reactions reported with monotherapy:

>10%:

Cardiovascular: Hypertension (15%; grade 3/4: 12%), cardiomyopathy (7% to 11%; defined as cardiac failure, decreased left ventricular ejection fraction, or left ventricular dysfunction)

Dermatologic: Skin toxicity (87%, most commonly dermatitis acneiform rash, erythema, skin rash; severe: 12%; severe toxicity and secondary skin infection requiring hospitalization: 3%; skin rash (57%; grades 3/4: 8%), acneiform eruption (19%; grades 3/4: <1%), xeroderma (11%)

Endocrine & metabolic: Hypoalbuminemia (42%)

Gastrointestinal: Diarrhea (43%), stomatitis (15%), abdominal pain (13%)

Hematologic & oncologic: Anemia (38%; grades 3/4: 2%), lymphedema (32%; includes edema, peripheral edema; grade 3/4: 1%), hemorrhage (13%; includes epistaxis, gingival bleeding, hematochezia, rectal hemorrhage, melena, vaginal hemorrhage, hemorrhoidal hemorrhage, hematuria, conjunctival hemorrhage; grade 3/4: <1%)

Hepatic: Increased serum AST (60%), increased serum ALT (39%), increased serum alkaline phosphatase (24%)

1% to 10%:

Cardiovascular: Decreased left ventricular ejection fraction (5%, ≥20% below baseline), bradycardia

Central nervous system: Dizziness

Dermatologic: Paronychia (10%), pruritus (10%; grade 3/4: 2%), cellulitis, folliculitis, pustular rash

Gastrointestinal: Dysgeusia, xerostomia

Neuromuscular & skeletal: Rhabdomyolysis

Ophthalmic: Blurred vision, dry eye syndrome

Respiratory: Interstitial lung disease (or pneumonitis; 2%)

<1% (Limited to important or life-threatening): Palmar-plantar erythrodysesthesia, retinal detachment, retinal vein occlusion

Adverse reactions reported with dual therapy (trametinib plus dabrafenib):

>10%

Cardiovascular: Peripheral edema (28% to 31%; includes edema and lymphedema), prolonged Q-T Interval on ECG (13% QTcF increased >60 msec; 4% QTcF prolongation to >500 msec)

Central nervous system: Chills (50% to 58%; grade 3/4: 2%), fatigue (53% to 57%), headache (29% to 37%), insomnia (11% to 18%), dizziness (13% to 16%)

Dermatologic: Skin toxicity (65%; any skin toxicity), skin rash (43% to 45%; includes generalized rash, pruritic rash, erythematous rash, papular rash, vesicular rash, macular rash, maculopapular rash; grade 3/4: ≤2%), night sweats (15% to 24%), xeroderma (9% to 18%), acneiform eruption (11% to 16%), erythema (6% to 15%), pruritus (11%)

Endocrine & metabolic: Hyperglycemia (58% to 67%; grade 3/4: 5% to 6%), increased gamma-glutamyl transferase (54% to 56%), hyponatremia (48% to 55%), hypoalbuminemia (43% to 53%), hypophosphatemia (41% to 47%), hypokalemia (15% to 29%), hyperkalemia (18% to 22%), hypocalcemia (13% to 20%), hypercalcemia (15% to 19%), hypomagnesemia (2% to 18%), dehydration (6% to 11%; grade 3/4: ≤2%)

Gastrointestinal: Nausea (44% to 46%; grade 3/4: 2% to 6%), vomiting (40% to 43%), diarrhea (26% to 36%; grade 3/4: ≤2%), abdominal pain (24% to 33%), decreased appetite (22% to 30%), constipation (17% to 22%), xerostomia (11%)

Genitourinary: Urinary tract infection (6% to 13%)

Hematologic & oncologic: Leukopenia (46% to 62%; grade 3/4: 4% to 5%), lymphocytopenia (55% to 59%; grade 3/4: 19% to 22%), anemia (46% to 55%; grade 3/4: 4% to 7%), neutropenia (37% to 55%; grade 3/4: 2% to 13%), thrombocytopenia (31%; grade 3/4: 2% to 4%), hemorrhage (11% to 16%; includes brain stem hemorrhage, cerebral hemorrhage, epistaxis, eye hemorrhage, gastric hemorrhage, gingival hemorrhage, hematuria, intracranial hemorrhage, vaginal hemorrhage, vitreous hemorrhage; grade 3/4: ≤5%)

Hepatic: Increased serum alkaline phosphatase (60% to 67%), increased serum AST (54% to 60%), increased serum ALT (35% to 42%), hyperbilirubinemia (7% to 15%)

Infection: Actinic keratosis (7% to 15%)

Neuromuscular & skeletal: Arthralgia (27% to 44%), myalgia (22% to 24%), back pain (11% to 18%), limb pain (11% to 16%), muscle spasm (2% to 16%)

Renal: Increased serum creatinine (20% to 24%)

Respiratory: Cough (11% to 29%), oropharyngeal pain (7% to 13%)

Miscellaneous: Fever (57% to 71%; grade 3/4: 5% to 9%), febrile reaction (complicated with chills/rigors: 51%, accompanied by hypotension, rigors or chills: 25%, complicated with dehydration: 9%, complicated with renal failure: 4%, complicated with syncope: 4%)

1% to 10%

Cardiovascular: Cardiomyopathy (8% to 9%), hypertension

Dermatologic: Cellulitis, folliculitis, hyperhidrosis, hyperkeratosis, palmar-plantar erythrodysesthesia, paronychia, pustular rash

Gastrointestinal: Pancreatitis, stomatitis

Hematologic & oncologic: Basal cell carcinoma (9%), squamous cell carcinoma of skin (7%; including keratoacanthoma), major hemorrhage (5%; gastric or intracranial hemorrhage), cutaneous papilloma

Neuromuscular & skeletal: Weakness

Ophthalmic: Uveitis (1%), blurred vision, transient blindness

Renal: Renal failure (2% to 7%; includes acute renal failure; grade 3/4: ≤7%)

<1% (Limited to important or life-threatening): Deep vein thrombosis, pulmonary embolism

Drug combination trials:

Cardiovascular: Decreased left ventricular ejection fraction (2%; ≥20% below baseline)

Drug Interactions

Metabolism/Transport Effects Inhibits CYP2C8 (weak)

Avoid Concomitant Use

Avoid concomitant use of Trametinib with any of the following: Amodiaquine

Increased Effect/Toxicity

Trametinib may increase the levels/effects of: Amodiaquine; Dabrafenib

Decreased Effect There are no known significant interactions involving a decrease in effect.

Food Interactions Administration with a high-fat, high-calorie meal decreased AUC by 24%, C_{max} by 70%, and delayed T_{max} by ~4 hours. Management: Administer 1 hour before or 2 hours after a meal.

Storage/Stability Store refrigerated at 2°C to 8°C (36°F to 46°F); do not freeze. Dispense in original bottle; do not remove desiccant. Protect from light and moisture. Do not transfer to pill boxes.

Mechanism of Action Reversibly and selectively inhibits mitogen-activated extracellular kinase (MEK) 1 and 2 activation and kinase activity. MEK is a downstream effector of the protein kinase B-raf (BRAF); BRAF V600 mutations result in constitutive activation of the BRAF pathway (including MEK1 and MEK2). Through inhibition of MEK 1 and 2 kinase activity, trametinib causes decreased cellular proliferation, cell cycle arrest, and increased apoptosis (Kim, 2013). The combination of trametinib and dabrafenib allows for greater inhibition of the MAPK pathway, resulting in BRAF V600 melanoma cell death (Flaherty, 2012).

Pharmacodynamics/Kinetics

Absorption: Rapid; decreased with a high-fat, high-calorie meal

Distribution: 214 L

Protein binding: ~97% to plasma proteins

Metabolism: Predominantly deacetylation (via hydrolytic enzymes) alone or with mono-oxygenation or in combination with glucuronidation

Bioavailability: 72%

Half-life elimination: 4 to 5 days

Time to peak: 1.5 hours; delayed with a high-fat, high-calorie meal

Excretion: Feces (>80%); urine (<20% with <0.1% as unchanged drug)

Dosing

Adult

Melanoma, metastatic or unresectable (with BRAF V600E or BRAF V600K mutations): Oral: 2 mg once daily (either as a single-agent or in combination with dabrafenib), continue until disease progression or unacceptable toxicity

Missed doses: Do not take a missed dose within 12 hours of the next dose.

Renal Impairment

Mild to moderate impairment (GFR ≥30 mL/minute/1.73 m²): No dosage adjustment necessary.

Severe impairment (GFR <30 mL/minute/1.73 m²): No dosage adjustment provided in manufacturer's labeling (has not been studied); however, renal excretion is low and is unlikely to affect drug exposure.

Hepatic Impairment

Mild impairment (total bilirubin ≤ ULN and AST > ULN or total bilirubin >1 to 1.5 times ULN with any AST): No dosage adjustment necessary.

Moderate to severe impairment: No dosage adjustment provided in manufacturer's labeling (has not been studied).

Adjustment for Toxicity

Recommended trametinib dose reductions for toxicity:

First dose reduction: 1.5 mg once daily

Second dose reduction: 1 mg once daily

Subsequent modification (if unable to tolerate 1 mg once daily): Permanently discontinue

Note: If using combination therapy, refer to Dabrafenib monograph for recommended dabrafenib dose reductions

Cardiac:

Asymptomatic, 10% or greater absolute decrease in LVEF from baseline and LVEF is below institutional lower limits of normal (LLN) from pretreatment value: Interrupt trametinib therapy for up to 4 weeks. If LVEF improves to normal within 4 weeks following therapy interruption, resume at a lower dose level. If LVEF does not improve to normal within 4 weeks following therapy interruption, permanently discontinue trametinib.

>20% absolute decrease in LVEF from baseline and LVEF is below institutional LLN: Permanently discontinue trametinib.

Symptomatic heart failure: Permanently discontinue trametinib.

Dermatologic:

Intolerable Grade 2 skin toxicity or Grade 3 or 4 skin toxicity: Interrupt trametinib therapy for up to 3 weeks. If toxicity improves within 3 weeks, resume at a lower dose level. If toxicity does not improve within 3 weeks following therapy interruption, permanently discontinue trametinib.

New primary cutaneous malignancies: No trametinib dosage modification is necessary.

Fever: Fever >40°C (104°F) or fever (any severity) complicated by rigors, hypotension, dehydration, or renal failure: Interrupt trametinib therapy until fever resolves, then resume at the same or a lower dose level. May require prophylactic antipyretics (secondary prophylaxis) upon resumption. Administer corticosteroids (eg, prednisone 10 mg daily or equivalent) for at least 5 days for second or subsequent pyrexia if temperature does not return to baseline within 3 days of onset of fever, or for fever associated with complications (eg, dehydration, hypotension, severe chills/rigors with no evidence of active infection).

Hemorrhage:

Grade 3 hemorrhage: Interrupt trametinib therapy. If hemorrhage improves, resume at a lower dose level. If hemorrhage does not improve following therapy interruption, permanently discontinue trametinib.

Grade 4 hemorrhage: Permanently discontinue trametinib.

Ocular:

Uveitis and iritis: No trametinib dosage modification necessary.

Retinal pigment epithelial detachments (RPED): Interrupt trametinib therapy for up to 3 weeks. If improves within 3 weeks following therapy interruption, resume at the same or lower dose level. If RPED does not improve within 3 weeks following therapy interruption, reduce dose or permanently discontinue trametinib.

Recurrence of RPED (any grade) after dose reduction/therapy interruption: *Canadian labeling (not in U.S. labeling):* Permanently discontinue trametinib.

Retinal vein occlusion: Permanently discontinue trametinib.

Pulmonary: Interstitial lung disease or pneumonitis: Permanently discontinue trametinib.

Venous thromboembolism:

Uncomplicated DVT or PE: Interrupt trametinib therapy for up to 3 weeks. If improves to ≤ grade 1 within 3 weeks following therapy interruption, resume at a lower dose level. If toxicity does not improve within 3 weeks following therapy interruption, permanently discontinue trametinib.

Life-threatening PE: Permanently discontinue trametinib.

Other toxicity:

Intolerable Grade 2 adverse reaction or any Grade 3 adverse reaction: Interrupt therapy. If toxicity improves to ≤ grade 1 following therapy interruption, resume at a lower dose level. If toxicity does not improve following therapy interruption, permanently discontinue trametinib.

Grade 4 adverse reaction, first occurrence: Interrupt trametinib therapy until improves to ≤ grade 1, then resume at a lower dose level **or** permanently discontinue trametinib.

Grade 4 adverse reaction, recurrent: Permanently discontinue trametinib.

New primary noncutaneous malignancy: No trametinib dosage modification is necessary.

Administration Administer at least 1 hour before or 2 hours after a meal. Do not take a missed dose within 12 hours of the next dose. When administered in combination with dabrafenib, take the once daily trametinib dose at the same time each day with either the morning or evening dose of dabrafenib.

Hazardous agent; use appropriate precautions for handling and disposal (meets NIOSH 2014 criteria). NIOSH recommends single gloving for administration of intact tablets (NIOSH 2014).

Monitoring Parameters BRAF V600K or V600E mutation status (prior to treatment); CBC and liver function tests at baseline and periodically; assess LVEF (by echocardiogram or MUGA scan) at baseline, 1 month after therapy initiation, and then at 2- to 3-month intervals; ophthalmological evaluation periodically during treatment and with visual disturbances; monitor for signs/symptoms of pulmonary toxicity (eg, cough dyspnea, hypoxia, pleural effusion, or infiltrates); monitor for dermatologic toxicity and secondary skin infections; blood pressure; diarrhea; signs/symptoms of bleeding.

For patients receiving combination therapy with dabrafenib: Blood glucose (baseline and periodically in patients with preexisting diabetes or hyperglycemia); dermatologic exams should be performed prior to treatment initiation, every 2 months while receiving combination treatment, and for up to 6 months following therapy discontinuation. Monitor for signs/symptoms of cutaneous and noncutaneous malignancies and uveitis/iritis.

Dosage Forms Excipient information presented when available (limited, particularly for generics); consult specific product labeling.

Tablet, Oral:

Mekinist: 0.5 mg, 2 mg

◆ Trametinib Dimethyl Sulfoxide *see* Trametinib *on page 1823*

◆ Trandate *see* Labetalol *on page 1019*

◆ Trandate [DSC] *see* Labetalol *on page 1019*

Trandolapril (tran DOE la pril)

Brand Names: US Mavik

Brand Names: Canada Mavik

Pharmacologic Category Angiotensin-Converting Enzyme (ACE) Inhibitor; Antihypertensive

Use

Heart failure post myocardial infarction or left-ventricular dysfunction postmyocardial infarction (MI): Treatment of post-MI heart failure (HF) or post-MI left ventricular (LV) dysfunction

Hypertension: Treatment of hypertension alone or in combination with other antihypertensive agents

Guideline recommendations:

Hypertension: The 2014 guideline for the management of high blood pressure in adults (Eighth Joint National Committee [JNC 8]) recommends initiation of pharmacologic treatment to lower blood pressure for the following patients:

• Patients ≥60 years of age with systolic blood pressure (SBP) ≥150 mm Hg or diastolic blood pressure (DBP) ≥90 mm Hg. Goal of therapy is SBP <150 mm Hg and DBP <90 mm Hg.

• Patients <60 years of age with SBP ≥140 mm Hg or DBP is ≥90 mm Hg. Goal of therapy is SBP <140 mm Hg and DBP <90 mm Hg.

• Patients ≥18 years of age with diabetes and SBP ≥140 mm Hg or DBP ≥90 mm Hg. Goal of therapy is SBP <140 mm Hg and DBP <90 mm Hg.

• Patients ≥18 years of age with chronic kidney disease (CKD) and SBP ≥140 mm Hg or DBP ≥90 mm Hg. Goal of therapy is SBP <140 mm Hg and DBP <90 mm Hg.

Chronic kidney disease (CKD) and hypertension: Regardless of race or diabetes status, the use of an ACE inhibitor (ACEI) or angiotensin receptor blocker (ARB) as initial therapy is recommended to improve kidney outcomes. In the general nonblack population (without CKD) including those with diabetes, initial antihypertensive treatment should consist of a thiazide-type diuretic, calcium channel blocker, ACEI, or ARB. In the general black population (without CKD) including those with diabetes, initial antihypertensive treatment should consist of a thiazide-type diuretic or a calcium channel blocker **instead of** an ACEI or ARB.

Coronary artery disease (CAD) and hypertension: The American Heart Association, American College of Cardiology and American Society of Hypertension (AHA/ACC/ASH) 2015 scientific statement for the treatment of hypertension in patients with CAD recommends the use of an ACE inhibitor (or an ARB) as part of a regimen in patients with hypertension and chronic stable angina if there is prior MI, LV systolic dysfunction, diabetes mellitus, or CKD. A BP target of <140/90 mm Hg is reasonable for the secondary prevention of cardiovascular events. A lower target BP (<130/80 mm Hg) may be appropriate in some individuals with CAD, previous MI, stroke or transient ischemic attack, or CAD risk equivalents (AHA/ACC/ASH [Rosendorff 2015]).

Heart failure: The American College of Cardiology Foundation/American Heart Association (ACCF/AHA) 2013 heart failure guidelines recommend the use of ACE inhibitors, along with other guideline directed medical therapies, to prevent heart failure in patients with a reduced ejection fraction who have a history of MI (Stage B HF), to prevent heart failure in any patient with a reduced ejection fraction (Stage B HF), or to treat those with heart failure and reduced ejection fraction (Stage C HFrEF) (ACCF/AHA [Yancy 2013]).

STEMI: The 2013 ACCF/AHA guidelines for the management of patients with ST-elevation myocardial infarction (STEMI) states that an ACE inhibitor should be initiated within the first 24 hours after STEMI in patients with anterior MI, heart failure, or left ventricular ejection fraction (LVEF) of 0.4 or less. It is also reasonable to initiate an ACE inhibitor in all patients with STEMI (O'Gara 2013).

Dosing

Adult & Geriatric

Hypertension: Oral:

Patients not receiving a diuretic:

US labeling: Initial: 1 mg once daily (2 mg daily in black patients). Adjust dosage at intervals of ≥1 week according to blood pressure response; usual dosage (ASH/ISH [Weber 2014]): 2 to 8 mg daily. There is little experience with doses >8 mg daily. Patients inadequately treated with once daily dosing at 4 mg may be treated with twice daily dosing. If blood pressure is not adequately controlled with trandolapril monotherapy, a diuretic may be added.

Canadian labeling: Initial: 1 mg once daily. Adjust dosage at intervals of 2 to 4 weeks according to blood pressure response; usual maintenance dose: 1 mg to 2 mg once daily (maximum: 4 mg once daily).

Patients receiving a diuretic: Consider discontinuing diuretic therapy 2 to 3 days before initiating trandolapril if possible; if blood pressure is not controlled by trandolapril alone, diuretic therapy should be resumed; if unable to discontinue diuretic, initiate trandolapril 0.5 mg once daily and monitor closely until blood pressure is stable; titrate to response as tolerated and needed.

Post-MI heart failure or LV dysfunction: Oral:

US labeling: Initial: 1 mg once daily; titrate (as tolerated) towards target dose of 4 mg once daily. If 4 mg dose is not tolerated, patients may continue therapy with the greatest tolerated dose. The American College of Cardiology Foundation/American Heart Association guidelines recommend the use of a 0.5 mg test dose with titration up to 4 mg daily as tolerated (O'Gara 2013).

Canadian labeling: Initial (beginning ≥3 days after acute MI): 1 mg once daily; after 2 days may increase to 2 mg once daily as tolerated for 1 month and then increase to 4 mg once daily; patients unable to tolerate a dose increase may be maintained at the previously tolerated dose.

Heart failure with reduced ejection fraction (HFrEF) (off-label use): Oral: Initial: 1 mg once daily; target dose: 4 mg once daily (ACCF/AHA [Yancy 2013]).

Renal Impairment

US labeling:

CrCl ≥30 mL/minute: No dosage adjustment necessary.

CrCl <30 mL/minute: Initial: 0.5 mg once daily; titrate as tolerated to optimal response.

Canadian labeling:

CrCl ≥30 mL/minute/1.73 m^2: No dosage adjustment necessary.

CrCl <30 mL/minute/1.73 m^2: Initial: 0.5 mg once daily; titrate as tolerated (maximum: 1 mg once daily)

CrCl <10 mL/minute/1.73 m^2: Initial: 0.5 mg once daily (maximum: 0.5 mg once daily)

Hepatic Impairment

US labeling:

Mild to severe impairment: There are no dosage adjustments provided in the manufacturer's labeling.

Cirrhosis: Initial: 0.5 mg once daily; titrate as tolerated to optimal response

Canadian labeling:

Mild impairment: No dosage adjustment necessary.

Moderate to severe impairment: Initial: 0.5 mg once daily; titrate as tolerated to optimal response

Additional Information Complete prescribing information should be consulted for additional detail.

Dosage Forms Excipient information presented when available (limited, particularly for generics); consult specific product labeling.

Tablet, Oral:

Mavik: 1 mg [scored]

Mavik: 2 mg, 4 mg

Generic: 1 mg, 2 mg, 4 mg

Dosage Forms: Canada Excipient information presented when available (limited, particularly for generics); consult specific product labeling.

Capsule, Oral:

Mavik: 0.5 mg, 1 mg, 2 mg, 4 mg

Trandolapril and Verapamil (tran DOE la pril & ver AP a mil)

Brand Names: US Tarka

Brand Names: Canada Tarka

Index Terms Verapamil and Trandolapril

Pharmacologic Category Angiotensin-Converting Enzyme (ACE) Inhibitor; Antihypertensive; Calcium Channel Blocker

Use

Hypertension: Treatment of hypertension.

Limitation of use: Not indicated for initial treatment of hypertension.

Dosing

Adult Hypertension: Oral: Dose is individualized. Patients receiving trandolapril (up to 8 mg) and verapamil (up to 240 mg) in separate tablets may receive Tarka at equivalent dosages once daily.

Geriatric Refer to dosing in individual monographs.

Renal Impairment Usual regimen need not be adjusted unless patient's creatinine clearance is <30 mL/minute. Titration of individual components must be done prior to switching to combination product. The Canadian labeling contraindicates use of the combination product if CrCl <30 mL/minute or in patients receiving dialysis.

Hepatic Impairment No dosage adjustment provided in manufacturer's labeling (has not been studied). However, verapamil is hepatically metabolized; adjustment of dosage in hepatic impairment is recommended. The Canadian labeling recommends avoiding use in severe impairment and contraindicates use in cirrhosis with ascites.

Additional Information Complete prescribing information should be consulted for additional detail.

Dosage Forms Excipient information presented when available (limited, particularly for generics); consult specific product labeling.

Tablet, variable release: Trandolapril 2 mg [immediate release] and verapamil hydrochloride 180 mg [sustained release]; Trandolapril 2 mg [immediate release] and verapamil hydrochloride 240 mg [sustained release]; Trandolapril 4 mg [immediate release] and verapamil hydrochloride 240 mg [sustained release]

Tarka®:

1/240: Trandolapril 1 mg [immediate release] and verapamil hydrochloride 240 mg [sustained release]

2/180: Trandolapril 2 mg [immediate release] and verapamil hydrochloride 180 mg [sustained release]

2/240: Trandolapril 2 mg [immediate release] and verapamil hydrochloride 240 mg [sustained release]

4/240: Trandolapril 4 mg [immediate release] and verapamil hydrochloride 240 mg [sustained release]

Tranexamic Acid (tran eks AM ik AS id)

Brand Names: US Cyklokapron; Lysteda

Brand Names: Canada Cyklokapron; Tranexamic Acid Injection BP

Index Terms Cyklokapron

Pharmacologic Category Antifibrinolytic Agent; Antihemophilic Agent; Hemostatic Agent; Lysine Analog

Use

Tooth extraction in patients with hemophilia (injection): Short-term use (2 to 8 days) in hemophilia patients to reduce or prevent hemorrhage and reduce need for replacement therapy during and following tooth extraction

Cyclic heavy menstrual bleeding (oral): Treatment of cyclic heavy menstrual bleeding

Dosing

Adult & Geriatric

Elective cesarean section, blood loss reduction (off-label use): IV: 1000 mg over 5 minutes at least 10 minutes prior to skin incision (Gungorduk 2011)

Hereditary angioedema (HAE) (off-label use):

Long-term prophylaxis: Oral: 1000-1500 mg 2-3 times daily; reduce to 500 mg/dose once or twice daily when frequency of attacks reduces (Gompels 2005; Levy 2010) **or** 25 mg/kg/dose administered 2-3 times daily (Bowen 2004)

Short-term prophylaxis (eg, for dental work): Oral: 75 mg/kg/day divided 2-3 times daily for 5 days before and 2 days after the event (Bowen 2004) **or** 1000 mg 4 times daily for 48 hours before and after procedure (Gompels 2005)

Treatment of acute HAE attack: Oral, IV: 25 mg/kg/dose (maximum single dose: 1000 mg) every 3-4 hours (maximum: 75 mg/kg/day) (Bowen 2004) **or** 1000 mg 4 times daily for 48 hours (Gompels 2005)

Hip fracture surgery, blood conservation (off-label use): IV:15 mg/kg administered at the time of skin incision followed by a second dose (15 mg/kg) 3 hours later (Zufferey 2010). Additional data may be necessary to further define the role of tranexamic acid in this setting.

Menorrhagia: Oral: 1300 mg 3 times daily (3900 mg daily) for up to 5 days during monthly menstruation

Orthognathic surgery, blood loss reduction (off-label use): IV: 20 mg/kg over 15 minutes prior to incision (Choi 2009)

Perioperative blood loss reduction in *bilateral* total knee arthroplasty (off-label use): IV:

Three-dose regimen: 10 mg/kg administered as a slow IV infusion 30 minutes before tourniquet deflation for the first operation, 30 minutes before tourniquet deflation for the second operation, and 3 hours after commencement of the second dose (Kim 2014).

Two-dose regimen: 10 or 15 mg/kg administered over 10 minutes before deflation of the first tourniquet, with the second dose administered 3 hours after the first dose (MacGillivray 2011).

Perioperative blood loss reduction in *unilateral* total knee arthroplasty (off-label use): IV:

Intra- and postoperative regimen: 10 mg/kg at least 10 to 30 minutes prior to tourniquet release (deflation) and 10 mg/kg at 3 hours after the first dose (Alvarez 2008; Camarasa 2006; Maniar 2012). Instead of the second dose, a postoperative infusion may be administered at 1 mg/kg/hour for 6 hours (Alvarez 2008).

Pre- and intraoperative regimen: 10 mg/kg at least 20 minutes or immediately before tourniquet inflation and repeated at least 15 minutes prior to deflation or immediately after release of tourniquet (Lozano 2008; Maniar 2012).

Pre-, intra-, and postoperative regimen: 10 mg/kg at least 20 minutes before tourniquet inflation, repeated at least 15 minutes prior to deflation and postoperatively at 3 hours after the second dose (Maniar 2012).

Prevention of dental procedure bleeding in patients on oral anticoagulant therapy (off-label use): Oral rinse: 4.8% solution: Hold 10 mL in mouth and rinse for 2 minutes then spit out. Repeat 4 times daily for 2 days after procedure. **Note:** Patient should not eat or drink for 1 hour after using oral rinse (Carter 2003).

Prevention of perioperative bleeding associated with cardiac surgery (off-label use): IV: Loading dose of 30 mg/kg over 30 minutes (total loading dose includes a test dose administered over the first 10 minutes followed by the remainder of dose) prior to incision, followed by 16 mg/kg/hour until sternal closure; add an additional 2 mg/kg to cardiopulmonary bypass circuit (Fergusson 2008)

or

Loading dose of 10 mg/kg over 20 minutes prior to incision followed by 2 mg/kg/hour continued for 2 hours after transfer to ICU; add a prime dose of 50 mg for a 2.5 L cardiopulmonary bypass circuit; maintenance infusion adjusted for renal insufficiency (Nuttall 2008)

or

Loading dose of 10-15 mg/kg over 10 to 15 minutes, followed by 1-1.5 mg/kg/hour. The authors suggest adding 2-2.5 mg/kg to cardiopulmonary bypass circuit; however, amounts have varied widely in clinical trials (Gravlee 2008).

Prevention of perioperative bleeding associated with spinal surgery (eg, spinal fusion) (off-label use): IV: 2000 mg over 20 minutes prior to incision followed by 100 mg/hour during surgery and for 5 hours postoperatively (Elwatidy 2008) **or** 10 mg/kg prior to incision followed by 1 mg/kg/hour for the remainder of the surgery; discontinue at time of wound closure (Wong 2008)

Tooth extraction in patients with hemophilia (in combination with appropriate factor replacement therapy): IV: 10 mg/kg immediately before surgery, then 10 mg/kg/dose 3-4 times daily; may be used for 2-8 days

Total hip replacement surgery, blood conservation (off-label use): IV: 10 to 15 mg/kg (or 1000 mg) administered over 5-10 minutes immediately before the operation or 15 minutes before skin incision; the preoperative dose may be followed by 10 mg/kg administered 3 to 12 hours after the operation. Postoperative doses ranged from a 10 mg/kg IV bolus (or 1000 mg) to a 1 mg/kg/hour infusion over 10 hours (Gandhi 2013; Oremus 2014).

Note: Multiple regimens have been evaluated in varying degrees of evidence quality. The regimen listed here reflects the more commonly used dosing based on a number of prospective randomized controlled trials (Johansson 2005; McConnell 2011; Niskanen 2005; Oremus 2014). Metaanalyses have also been conducted demonstrating significant reduction in blood loss perioperatively without an increased risk of thromboembolic events (Gandhi 2013; Sukeik 2011; Zhou 2013). The use of *intra-articular* tranexamic acid (ie, 1000 mg/50 mL of NaCl 0.9% sprayed into the wound at the end of the procedure) has also been evaluated demonstrating effectiveness (Alshryda 2014a; Alshryda 2014b).

Transurethral prostatectomy, blood loss reduction (off-label use): Oral: 2000 mg 3 times daily on the operative and first postoperative day (Rannikko 2004)

Trauma-associated hemorrhage (off-label use): IV: Loading dose: 1000 mg over 10 minutes, followed by 1000 mg over the next 8 hours. **Note:** Clinical trial included patients with significant hemorrhage (SBP <90 mm Hg, heart rate >110 bpm, or both) or those at risk of significant hemorrhage. Treatment began within 8 hours of injury (CRASH-2 Trial Collaborators 2010).

Traumatic hyphema (off-label use): Oral: 25 mg/kg administered 3 times daily for 5-7 days (Rahmani, 1999; Vangsted, 1983; Varnek, 1980). **Note:** This same regimen may also be used for secondary hemorrhage after an initial traumatic hyphema event.

Pediatric

Menorrhagia: Children ≥12 years and Adolescents: Oral: 1300 mg 3 times daily (3900 mg daily) for up to 5 days during monthly menstruation

Hereditary angioedema (HAE) (off-label use): Oral:

Long-term prophylaxis: 20-40 mg/kg/day in 2-3 divided doses (maximum dose: 3000 mg daily) (Farkas 2007) **or** 50 mg/kg/day (or 1000-2000 mg daily) depending on age and size of patient; may consider alternate-day regimen or twice-weekly regimen when frequency of attacks reduces; diarrhea may be a dose-limiting side effect (Gompels 2005)

Short-term prophylaxis: 20-40 mg/kg/day in 2-3 divided doses (maximum dose: 3000 mg daily) (Farkas 2007) **or** 500 mg 4 times daily (Gompels 2005). **Note:** For short-term prophylaxis (eg, dental work), initiate 2-5 days before and continue for 2 days after the procedure (Bowen 2004; Gompels 2005).

Prevention of perioperative bleeding associated with cardiac surgery (off-label use): IV: 10 mg/kg given over 30 minutes prior to incision, 10 mg/kg while on cardiopulmonary bypass, and 10 mg/kg administered after protamine reversal (Chauhan 2004a; Chauhan 2004b)

or

Loading dose of 100 mg/kg over 15 minutes prior to incision, followed by 10 mg/kg/hour infusion (continued until ICU transport); add 100 mg/kg to pump reservoir when cardiopulmonary bypass initiated (Reid, 1997)

Prevention of perioperative bleeding associated with craniosynostosis surgery (off-label use): IV: Loading dose of 50 mg/kg over 15 minutes prior to incision, followed by 5 mg/kg/hour (Goobie 2011) **or** 15 mg/kg over 15 minutes prior to incision, followed by 10 mg/kg/hour until skin closure (Dadure 2011)

Prevention of perioperative bleeding associated with spinal surgery (eg, spinal fusion) (off-label use): Children and Adolescents: IV: 10 mg/kg given over 15 minutes prior to incision followed by 1 mg/kg/hour for the remainder of the surgery; discontinue at time of wound closure (Neilipovitz 2001; Verma 2010)

or

100 mg/kg over 15 minutes prior to incision followed by 10 mg/kg/hour until skin closure (Sethna 2005)

or

30 mg/kg over 20 minutes prior to incision followed by 1 mg/kg/hour during surgery and for 5 hours postoperatively (Elwatidy 2008)

Tooth extraction in patients with hemophilia (in combination with appropriate factor replacement therapy): Children and Adolescents: IV: Refer to adult dosing.

Traumatic hyphema (off-label use): Oral: Refer to adult dosing.

Renal Impairment

IV formulation:

Tooth extraction in patients with hemophilia:

Serum creatinine 1.36-2.83 mg/dL: Maintenance dose of 10 mg/kg/dose twice daily

Serum creatinine 2.83-5.66 mg/dL: Maintenance dose of 10 mg/kg/dose once daily

Serum creatinine >5.66 mg/dL: Maintenance dose of 10 mg/kg/dose every 48 hours **or** 5 mg/kg/dose once daily

Cardiac surgery (the following dose adjustments have been recommended [Nuttall 2008]):

Serum creatinine 1.6-3.3 mg/dL: Reduce maintenance infusion to 1.5 mg/kg/hour (based on a 25% reduction from 2 mg/kg/hour)

Serum creatinine 3.3-6.6 mg/dL: Reduce maintenance infusion to 1 mg/kg/hour (based on a 50% reduction from 2 mg/kg/hour)

Serum creatinine >6.6 mg/dL: Reduce maintenance infusion to 0.5 mg/kg/hour (based on a 75% reduction from 2 mg/kg/hour)

Oral formulation: Cyclic heavy menstrual bleeding:

Serum creatinine >1.4-2.8 mg/dL: 1300 mg twice daily (2600 mg daily) for up to 5 days

Serum creatinine 2.9-5.7 mg/dL: 1300 mg once daily for up to 5 days

Serum creatinine >5.7 mg/dL: 650 mg once daily for up to 5 days

Hepatic Impairment No dosage adjustment is necessary.

Additional Information Complete prescribing information should be consulted for additional detail.

Dosage Forms Excipient information presented when available (limited, particularly for generics); consult specific product labeling.

Solution, Intravenous:

Cyklokapron: 100 mg/mL (10 mL)

Generic: 100 mg/mL (10 mL)

Solution, Intravenous [preservative free]:

Generic: 100 mg/mL (10 mL)

Tablet, Oral:

Lysteda: 650 mg

Generic: 650 mg

Tranylcypromine (tran il SIP roe meen)

Brand Names: US Parnate

Brand Names: Canada Parnate®

Index Terms Transamine Sulphate; Tranylcypromine Sulfate

Pharmacologic Category Antidepressant, Monoamine Oxidase Inhibitor

Use Treatment of major depressive episode without melancholia

Pregnancy Considerations Adverse events were observed in animal reproduction studies.

Breast-Feeding Considerations Tranylcypromine is excreted in breast milk.

Medication Guide Available Yes

Contraindications

Cardiovascular disease (including hypertension); cerebrovascular defect; history of headache; history of hepatic disease or abnormal liver function tests; pheochromocytoma

Concurrent use of antihistamines, antihypertensives, antiparkinson drugs, bupropion, buspirone, caffeine (excessive use), CNS depressants (including ethanol and opioids), dextromethorphan, diuretics, elective surgery requiring general anesthesia (discontinue tranylcypromine ≥10 days prior to elective surgery), local vasoconstrictors, meperidine, MAO inhibitors or dibenzazepine derivatives (eg, amitriptyline, clomipramine, desipramine, imipramine, nortriptyline, protriptyline, doxepin, carbamazepine, cyclobenzaprine, amoxapine, maprotiline, trimipramine), SSRIs or SNRIs, spinal anesthesia (hypotension may be exaggerated), sympathomimetics (including amphetamines, cocaine, phenylephrine, pseudoephedrine) or related compounds (methyldopa, reserpine, levodopa, tryptophan), or foods high in tyramine content

Bupropion: At least 14 days should elapse between MAO inhibitor discontinuation and bupropion initiation.

Buspirone: At least 10 days should elapse between tranylcypromine discontinuation and buspirone initiation.

MAO inhibitors or dibenzazepine derivatives: At least 1-2 weeks should elapse between the use of another MAO inhibitor or dibenzazepine derivative and tranylcypromine use.

Meperidine: At least 2-3 weeks should elapse between MAO inhibitor discontinuation and meperidine use.

SSRIs or SNRIs: At least 2 weeks should elapse between the discontinuation of sertraline or paroxetine and the initiation of tranylcypromine. At least 5 weeks should elapse between the discontinuation of fluoxetine and the initiation of tranylcypromine. At least 1 week should elapse between discontinuation of a SNRI and the initiation of tranylcypromine. At least 2 weeks should elapse between the discontinuation of tranylcypromine and the initiation of SNRIs and SSRIs.

Warnings/Precautions Risk of suicide: [U.S. Boxed Warning]: Antidepressants increase the risk of suicidal thinking and behavior in children, adolescents, and young adults (18-24 years of age) with major depressive disorder (MDD) and other psychiatric disorders; consider risk prior to prescribing. Short-term studies did not show an increased risk in patients >24 years of age and showed a decreased risk inpatients >65 years. Closely monitor for clinical worsening, suicidality, or unusual changes in behavior such as anxiety, agitation, panic attacks, insomnia, irritability, hostility, impulsivity, akathisia, hypomania, and mania. The patient's family or caregiver should be instructed to closely observe the patient and communicate condition with healthcare provider. Such observation would generally include at least weekly face-to-face contact with patients or their family members or caregivers during the first 4 weeks of treatment, then every other week visits for the next 4 weeks, then at 12 weeks, and as clinically indicated beyond 12 weeks. Additional contact by telephone may be appropriate between face-to-face visits. A medication guide should be dispensed with each prescription. **Tranylcypromine is not FDA approved for treatment of children and adolescents.**

All patients treated with antidepressants should be observed similarly for clinical worsening and suicidality, especially during the initial few months of a course of drug therapy, or at times of dose changes, either increases or decreases. The possibility of a suicide attempt is inherent in major depression and may persist until remission occurs. Worsening depression and severe abrupt suicidality that are not part of the presenting symptoms may require discontinuation or modification of drug therapy. Use caution in high-risk patients during initiation of therapy. Prescriptions should be written for the smallest quantity consistent with good patient care.

Hypertensive crisis may occur with foods/supplements high in tyramine, tryptophan, phenylalanine, or tyrosine content; treatment with phentolamine is recommended for hypertensive crisis. Use with caution in patients who have glaucoma, hyperthyroidism, diabetes or hypotension. May cause orthostatic hypotension (especially at dosages >30 mg/day). Use with caution in patients at risk of seizures, or in patients receiving other drugs which may lower seizure threshold. Use with caution in patients with a

history of drug abuse or acute alcoholism; potential for drug dependency exists especially in patients using excessive doses. Discontinue at least 48 hours prior to myelography. May increase the risks associated with electroconvulsive therapy. Use with caution in patients with renal impairment. Do not use with other MAO inhibitors or antidepressants. Avoid products containing sympathomimetic stimulants or dextromethorphan. Concurrent use with antihypertensive agents may lead to exaggeration of hypotensive effects. Effects may be potentiated when used with other sedative drugs or ethanol. Tranylcypromine is not generally considered a first-line agent for the treatment of depression; tranylcypromine is typically used in patients who have failed to respond to other treatments. May worsen psychosis in some patients or precipitate a shift to mania or hypomania in patients with bipolar disorder. **Tranylcypromine is not FDA approved for the treatment of bipolar depression.**

Abrupt discontinuation or interruption of antidepressant therapy has been associated with a discontinuation syndrome. Symptoms arising may vary with antidepressant however commonly include nausea, vomiting, diarrhea, headaches, lightheadedness, dizziness, diminished appetite, sweating, chills, tremors, paresthesias, fatigue, somnolence, and sleep disturbances (eg, vivid dreams, insomnia). Greater risks for developing a discontinuation syndrome have been associated with antidepressants with shorter half-lives, longer durations of treatment, and abrupt discontinuation. More severe symptoms have also been associated with MAO inhibitors. For antidepressants of short or intermediate half-lives, symptoms may emerge within 2-5 days after treatment discontinuation and last 7-14 days (APA, 2010; Fava, 2006; Haddad, 2001; Shelton, 2001; Warner, 2006). According to the manufacturer, tranylcypromine use within 10 days prior to elective surgery is contraindicated. Currently, an MAO-safe anesthetic technique which excludes the use of meperidine and indirect-acting adrenergic agonists is recommended for patients requiring continued MAO inhibitor therapy (Huyse, 2006).

Adverse Reactions
Frequency not defined:
- Cardiovascular: Edema, orthostatic hypotension, palpitation, tachycardia
- Central nervous system: Agitation, anxiety, chills, dizziness, drowsiness, headache, insomnia, mania, restlessness
- Dermatologic: Alopecia (rare), rash (rare), urticaria
- Endocrine & metabolic: Sexual dysfunction (anorgasmia, ejaculatory disturbances, impotence); SIADH
- Gastrointestinal: Abdominal pain, anorexia, constipation, diarrhea, nausea, xerostomia
- Genitourinary: Urinary retention
- Hematologic: Agranulocytosis, anemia, leukopenia, thrombocytopenia
- Hepatic: Hepatitis (rare)
- Neuromuscular & skeletal: Muscle spasm, myoclonus, numbness, paresthesia, tremor, weakness
- Ocular: Blurred vision
- Otic: Tinnitus
- Miscellaneous: Diaphoresis

Postmarketing and/or case reports: Akinesia, ataxia, confusion, cystic acne, disorientation, memory loss, mouth fissures, polyuria, scleroderma (localized), urinary incontinence, urticaria, withdrawal symptoms

Drug Interactions
Metabolism/Transport Effects Inhibits CYP1A2 (moderate), CYP2A6 (strong), CYP2C19 (moderate), CYP2C8 (weak), CYP2C9 (weak), CYP2D6 (moderate), CYP2E1 (weak), Monoamine Oxidase

Avoid Concomitant Use
Avoid concomitant use of Tranylcypromine with any of the following: Aclidinium; Alcohol (Ethyl); Alpha-/Beta-Agonists (Indirect-Acting); Alpha1-Agonists; Amodiaquine; Amphetamines; Anilidopiperidine Opioids; Antidepressants (Serotonin Reuptake Inhibitor/Antagonist); Apraclonidine; Artesunate; AtoMOXetine; Atropine (Ophthalmic); Bezafibrate; Buprenorphine; BuPROPion; BusPIRone; CarBAMazepine; Cimetropium; Cyclobenzaprine; Cyproheptadine; Dapoxetine; Dexmethylphenidate; Dextromethorphan; Diethylpropion; Eluxadoline; EPINEPHrine (Oral Inhalation); Glucagon; Glycopyrrolate; Glycopyrrolate (Oral Inhalation); HYDROmorphone; Ipratropium (Oral Inhalation); Isometheptene; Levonordefrin; Levosulpiride; Linezolid; Maprotiline; Meperidine; Mequitazine; Methyldopa; Methylene Blue; Methylphenidate; Mianserin; Mirtazapine; Moclobemide; Morphine (Liposomal); Morphine (Systemic); Oxymorphone; Pholcodine; Pizotifen; Potassium Chloride; Selective Serotonin Reuptake Inhibitors; Serotonin 5-HT1D Receptor Agonists; Serotonin/Norepinephrine Reuptake Inhibitors; Tapentadol; Tegafur; Tetrabenazine;

Tetrahydrozoline (Nasal); Thioridazine; Tianeptine; Tiotropium; TiZANidine; Tricyclic Antidepressants; Tryptophan; Umeclidinium

Increased Effect/Toxicity
Tranylcypromine may increase the levels/effects of: AbobotulinumtoxinA; Agomelatine; Alpha-/Beta-Agonists (Indirect-Acting); Alpha1-Agonists; Amifostine; Amodiaquine; Amphetamines; Analgesics (Opioid); Anticholinergic Agents; Antidepressants (Serotonin Reuptake Inhibitor/Antagonist); Antipsychotic Agents; Antipsychotic Agents (Second Generation [Atypical]); Apraclonidine; ARIPiprazole; Artesunate; AtoMOXetine; Atropine (Ophthalmic); Beta2-Agonists; Betahistine; Bezafibrate; Blood Glucose Lowering Agents; Brexpiprazole; Brimonidine (Ophthalmic); Brimonidine (Topical); BuPROPion; Cannabinoid-Containing Products; Cilostazol; Cimetropium; Clemastine; CYP1A2 Substrates; CYP2A6 Substrates; CYP2C19 Substrates; CYP2D6 Substrates; Cyproheptadine; Dexmethylphenidate; Dextromethorphan; Diethylpropion; Domperidone; Doxapram; DOXOrubicin (Conventional); Doxylamine; Eliglustat; Eluxadoline; EPINEPHrine (Nasal); EPINEPHrine (Oral Inhalation); Epinephrine (Racemic); EPINEPHrine (Systemic); Fesoterodine; Glucagon; Glycopyrrolate; Glycopyrrolate (Oral Inhalation); Hydrocodone; HYDROmorphone; Hypotension-Associated Agents; Isometheptene; Levonordefrin; Linezolid; Lithium; Meperidine; Mequitazine; Methadone; Methyldopa; Methylene Blue; Methylphenidate; Metoclopramide; Metoprolol; Mianserin; Mirabegron; Mirtazapine; Moclobemide; Morphine (Liposomal); Morphine (Systemic); Nebivolol; Norepinephrine; OnabotulinumtoxinA; OxyCODONE; Pirfenidone; Pizotifen; Potassium Chloride; Ramosetron; Reserpine; RimabotulinumtoxinB; Selective Serotonin Reuptake Inhibitors; Serotonin 5-HT1D Receptor Agonists; Serotonin Modulators; Serotonin/Norepinephrine Reuptake Inhibitors; Tetrahydrozoline (Nasal); Thiazide Diuretics; Thioridazine; Tiotropium; TiZANidine; Topiramate; Tricyclic Antidepressants

The levels/effects of Tranylcypromine may be increased by: Aclidinium; Alcohol (Ethyl); Alfuzosin; Altretamine; Anilidopiperidine Opioids; Antiemetics (5HT3 Antagonists); Antipsychotic Agents; Barbiturates; Blood Pressure Lowering Agents; Brimonidine (Topical); Buprenorphine; BusPIRone; CarBAMazepine; COMT Inhibitors; Cyclobenzaprine; Dapoxetine; Diazoxide; Herbs (Hypotensive Properties); Ipratropium (Oral Inhalation); Levodopa; Maprotiline; Metaxalone; Molsidomine; Nicorandil; Obinutuzumab; Oxymorphone; Pentoxifylline; Pholcodine; Phosphodiesterase 5 Inhibitors; Pramlintide; Propafenone; Prostacyclin Analogues; Tapentadol; Tedizolid; Tetrabenazine; Tianeptine; TraMADol; Tryptophan; Umeclidinium

Decreased Effect
Tranylcypromine may decrease the levels/effects of: Acetylcholinesterase Inhibitors; Artesunate; Clopidogrel; Codeine; Domperidone; Gastrointestinal Agents (Prokinetic); Itopride; Levosulpiride; Secretin; Tamoxifen; Tegafur

The levels/effects of Tranylcypromine may be decreased by: Acetylcholinesterase Inhibitors; Cyproheptadine; Domperidone

Food Interactions Concurrent ingestion of foods rich in tyramine, dopamine, tyrosine, phenylalanine, tryptophan, or caffeine may cause sudden and severe high blood pressure (hypertensive crisis or serotonin syndrome). Beverages containing tyramine (eg, hearty red wine and beer) may increase toxic effects. Management: Avoid tyramine-containing foods (aged or matured cheese, air-dried or cured meats including sausages and salamis; fava or broad bean pods, tap/draft beers, Marmite concentrate, sauerkraut, soy sauce, and other soybean condiments). Food's freshness is also an important concern; improperly stored or spoiled food can create an environment in which tyramine concentrations may increase. Avoid foods containing dopamine, tyrosine, phenylalanine, tryptophan, or caffeine. Avoid beverages containing tyramine.

Storage/Stability Store at room temperature of 15°C to 30°C (59°F to 86°F).

Mechanism of Action Tranylcypromine is a nonhydrazine monoamine oxidase inhibitor. It increases endogenous concentrations of epinephrine, norepinephrine, dopamine, and serotonin through inhibition of the enzyme (monoamine oxidase) responsible for the breakdown of these neurotransmitters.

Pharmacodynamics/Kinetics

Onset of action: Therapeutic: 2 days to 3 weeks continued dosing

Duration: MAO inhibition may persist for up to 10 days following discontinuation

Half-life elimination: 90-190 minutes

Time to peak, serum: ~2 hours

Excretion: Urine

Dosing

Adult & Geriatric Note: 20 mg of tranylcypromine = 45 mg phenelzine = 40 mg of isocarboxazid (Sheehan 1980)

Depression: Oral: Usual effective dose: 30 mg/day in divided doses; if symptoms don't improve after 2 weeks, increase by 10 mg increments at 1- to 3-week intervals; maximum: 60 mg/day

Discontinuation of therapy: Upon discontinuation of antidepressant therapy, gradually taper the dose to minimize the incidence of withdrawal symptoms and allow for the detection of re-emerging symptoms. Evidence supporting ideal taper rates is limited. APA and NICE guidelines suggest tapering therapy over at least several weeks with consideration to the half-life of the antidepressant; antidepressants with a shorter half-life and MAO inhibitors may need to be tapered more conservatively. In addition for long-term treated patients, WFSBP guidelines recommend tapering over 4-6 months. If intolerable withdrawal symptoms occur following a dose reduction, consider resuming the previously prescribed dose and/or decrease dose at a more gradual rate (APA, 2010; Bauer, 2002; Haddad, 2001; NCCMH, 2010; Schatzberg, 2006; Shelton, 2001; Warner, 2006).

MAO inhibitor recommendations:

Switching to or from an MAO inhibitor intended to treat psychiatric disorders:

Allow 14 days to elapse between discontinuing an alternative antidepressant without long half-life metabolites (eg, TCAs, paroxetine, fluvoxamine, venlafaxine) or MAO inhibitor intended to treat psychiatric disorders and initiation of tranylcypromine.

Allow 5 weeks to elapse between discontinuing fluoxetine (with long half-life metabolites) intended to treat psychiatric disorders and initiation of tranylcypromine.

Allow at least 7-14 days days to elapse between discontinuing tranylcypromine and initiation of an alternative antidepressant or MAO inhibitor intended to treat psychiatric disorders.

Use with other MAO inhibitors (such as linezolid or IV methylene blue):

Do not initiate tranylcypromine in patients receiving linezolid or IV methylene blue; consider other interventions for psychiatric condition.

If urgent treatment with linezolid or IV methylene blue is required in a patient already receiving tranylcypromine and potential benefits outweigh potential risks, discontinue tranylcypromine promptly and administer linezolid or IV methylene blue. Monitor for serotonin syndrome for 2 weeks or until 24 hours after the last dose of linezolid or IV methylene blue, whichever comes first. May resume tranylcypromine 24 hours after the last dose of linezolid or IV methylene blue.

Renal Impairment No dosage adjustment provided in manufacturer's labeling.

Hepatic Impairment No dosage adjustment provided in manufacturer's labeling. Use is contraindicated in patients with a history of liver disease or abnormal liver function tests.

Dietary Considerations Avoid tyramine-containing foods/ beverages. Some examples include aged or matured cheese, air-dried or cured meats (including sausages and salamis), fava or broad bean pods, tap/draft beers, Marmite concentrate, sauerkraut, soy sauce and other soybean condiments. Food's freshness is also an important concern; improperly stored or spoiled food can create an environment where tyramine concentrations may increase.

Monitoring Parameters Blood glucose; blood pressure, mental status, suicide ideation (especially at the beginning of therapy or when doses are increased or decreased)

Additional Information Tranylcypromine has a more rapid onset of therapeutic effect than other MAO inhibitors, but causes more severe hypertensive reactions.

Dosage Forms Excipient information presented when available (limited, particularly for generics); consult specific product labeling.

Tablet, Oral:

Parnate: 10 mg [contains fd&c blue #2 (indigotine), fd&c red #40, fd&c yellow #6 (sunset yellow)]

Generic: 10 mg

◆ Tranylcypromine Sulfate *see* Tranylcypromine *on page 1829*

Trastuzumab (tras TU zoo mab)

Brand Names: US Herceptin

Brand Names: Canada Herceptin

Index Terms anti-c-erB-2; anti-ERB-2; Conventional Trastuzumab; MOAB HER2; rhuMAb HER2; Trastuzumab (Conventional)

Pharmacologic Category Antineoplastic Agent, Anti-HER2; Antineoplastic Agent, Monoclonal Antibody

Use

Breast cancer, adjuvant treatment: Treatment (adjuvant) of human epidermal growth receptor 2 (HER2)-overexpressing node positive or node negative (estrogen receptor/progesterone receptor negative or with 1 high risk feature) breast cancer as part of a treatment regimen consisting of doxorubicin, cyclophosphamide, and either paclitaxel or docetaxel; with docetaxel and carboplatin; or as a single agent following multimodality anthracycline-based therapy.

Breast cancer, metastatic: First-line treatment of HER2-overexpressing metastatic breast cancer (in combination with paclitaxel); single agent treatment of HER2-overexpressing breast cancer in patients who have received 1 or more chemotherapy regimens for metastatic disease.

Gastric cancer, metastatic: Treatment of HER2-overexpressing metastatic gastric or gastroesophageal junction adenocarcinoma (in combination with cisplatin and either capecitabine or 5-fluorouracil) in patients who have not received prior treatment for metastatic disease.

Pregnancy Considerations Trastuzumab inhibits HER2 protein, which has a role in embryonic development. **[US Boxed Warning]: Trastuzumab exposure during pregnancy may result in oligohydramnios and oligohydramnios sequence (pulmonary hypoplasia, skeletal malformations and neonatal death).** Oligohydramnios (reversible in some cases) has been reported with trastuzumab use alone or with combination chemotherapy. If trastuzumab exposure occurs during pregnancy, monitor for oligohydramnios. Women of reproductive potential should use effective contraception during treatment and for at least 7 months after the last trastuzumab dose. If trastuzumab is administered during pregnancy, or if a patient becomes pregnant during or within 7 months after treatment, report exposure to Genentech Adverse Events at 1-888-835-2555. Women exposed to trastuzumab during pregnancy (or within 7 months of conception) are encouraged to enroll in MotHER (the Herceptin Pregnancy Registry; 1-800-690-6720).

European Society for Medical Oncology (ESMO) guidelines for cancer during pregnancy recommend delaying treatment with trastuzumab (and other HER-2 targeted agents) until after delivery in pregnant patients with HER-2 positive disease (Peccatori 2013).

Breast-Feeding Considerations It is not known whether trastuzumab is secreted in human milk. Because many immunoglobulins are secreted in milk, and the potential for serious adverse reactions in the nursing infant exists, the decision to discontinue trastuzumab or discontinue breast-feeding during treatment should take in account the benefits of treatment to the mother. The extended half-life should also be considered for decisions regarding breast-feeding after therapy completion.

Contraindications

There are no contraindications listed in the manufacturer's US labeling.

Canadian labeling: Hypersensitivity to trastuzumab, Chinese hamster ovary (CHO) cell proteins, or any component of the formulation

Warnings/Precautions Hazardous agent - use appropriate precautions for handling and disposal (meets NIOSH 2014 criteria). **[US Boxed Warning]: Trastuzumab is associated with symptomatic and asymptomatic reductions in left ventricular ejection fraction (LVEF) and heart failure (HF); the incidence is highest in patients receiving trastuzumab with an anthracycline-containing chemotherapy regimen. Evaluate LVEF in all patients prior to and during treatment; discontinue for cardiomyopathy.** Extreme caution should be used in patients with preexisting cardiac disease or dysfunction. Prior or concurrent exposure to anthracyclines or radiation therapy significantly increases the risk of cardiomyopathy; other potential risk factors include advanced age, high or low body mass index, smoking, diabetes, hypertension, and hyper-/hypothyroidism. Patients who receive anthracyclines after completion or discontinuation of trastuzumab are at increased risk of cardiac dysfunction (anthracyclines should be avoided for at least 7 months after the last

trastuzumab dose, and then monitor cardiac function closely if anthracyclines are used. Discontinuation should be strongly considered in patients who develop a clinically significant reduction in LVEF during therapy; treatment with HF medications (eg, ACE inhibitors, beta-blockers) should be initiated. Withhold treatment for ≥16% decrease from pretreatment levels or LVEF below normal limits and ≥10% decrease from baseline (see Dosage Adjustment for Cardiotoxicity). Cardiomyopathy due to trastuzumab is generally reversible over a period of 1 to 3 months after discontinuation. Long term (8 years) follow up in the adjuvant setting (trastuzumab for 1 or 2 years administered sequentially following chemotherapy and radiation therapy) has demonstrated a low incidence of cardiac events, which were generally reversible in most patients (de Azambuja, 2014). Trastuzumab is also associated with arrhythmias, hypertension, mural thrombus formation, stroke, and even cardiac death.

[US Boxed Warning]: Serious adverse events, including hypersensitivity reaction (anaphylaxis), infusion reactions (including fatalities), and pulmonary events (including acute respiratory distress syndrome [ARDS]) have been associated with trastuzumab. Discontinue for anaphylaxis, angioedema, ARDS or interstitial pneumonitis. Most of these events occur with the first infusion; pulmonary events may occur during or within 24 hours of the first infusion; delayed reactions have occurred. Interrupt infusion for dyspnea or significant hypotension; monitor until symptoms resolve. Infusion reactions may consist of fever and chills, and may also include nausea, vomiting, pain, headache, dizziness, dyspnea, hypotension, rash, and weakness. Re-treatment of patients who experienced severe hypersensitivity reactions has been attempted (with premedication). Some patients tolerated re-treatment, while others experienced a second severe reaction. When used in combination with myelosuppressive chemotherapy, trastuzumab may increase the incidence of neutropenia (moderate-to-severe) and febrile neutropenia; the incidence of anemia may be higher when trastuzumab is added to chemotherapy. Rare cases of nephrotic syndrome with evidence of glomerulopathy have been reported, with an onset of 4 to 18 months from trastuzumab initiation; complications may include volume overload and HF. The incidence of renal impairment was increased in metastatic gastric cancer patients when trastuzumab is added to chemotherapy.

May cause serious pulmonary toxicity (dyspnea, hypoxia, interstitial pneumonitis, pulmonary infiltrates, pleural effusion, noncardiogenic pulmonary edema, pulmonary insufficiency, acute respiratory distress syndrome, and/or pulmonary fibrosis); use caution in patients with preexisting pulmonary disease or patients with extensive pulmonary tumor involvement. Establish HER2 status prior to treatment; has only been studied in patients with evidence of HER2 protein overexpression, either by validated immunohistochemistry (IHC) assay or fluorescence in situ hybridization (FISH) assay. Tests appropriate for the specific tumor type (breast or gastric) should be used to assess HER2 status. **[US Boxed Warning]: Trastuzumab exposure during pregnancy may result in oligohydramnios and oligohydramnios sequence (pulmonary hypoplasia, skeletal malformations and neonatal death).** Effective contraception is recommended in women of childbearing potential during treatment and for at least 7 months after the last trastuzumab dose. Conventional trastuzumab and ado-trastuzumab emtansine are **not** interchangeable; verify product label prior to reconstitution and administration to prevent medication errors. Dosing and treatment schedules between conventional trastuzumab (Herceptin) and ado-trastuzumab emtansine (Kadcyla) are different; confusion between the products may potentially cause harm to the patient. Potentially significant drug-drug interactions may exist, requiring dose or frequency adjustment, additional monitoring, and/or selection of alternative therapy.

Adverse Reactions Note: Percentages reported with single-agent therapy.

>10%:
Cardiovascular: Decreased left ventricular ejection fraction (4% to 22%)
Central nervous system: Pain (47%), chills (5% to 32%), headache (10% to 26%), insomnia (14%), dizziness (4% to 13%)
Dermatologic: Skin rash (4% to 18%)
Gastrointestinal: Nausea (6% to 33%), diarrhea (7% to 25%), vomiting (4% to 23%), abdominal pain (2% to 22%), anorexia (14%)
Infection: Infection (20%)
Neuromuscular & skeletal: Weakness (4% to 42%), back pain (5% to 22%)

Respiratory: Cough (5% to 26%), dyspnea (3% to 22%), rhinitis (2% to 14%), pharyngitis (12%)
Miscellaneous: Infusion related reaction (21% to 40%, chills and fever most common; severe: 1%), fever (6% to 36%)
1% to 10%:
Cardiovascular: Peripheral edema (5% to 10%), edema (8%), cardiac failure (2% to 7%; severe: <1%), tachycardia (5%), hypertension (4%), arrhythmia (3%), palpitations (3%)
Central nervous system: Paresthesia (2% to 9%), depression (6%), peripheral neuritis (2%), neuropathy (1%)
Dermatologic: Acne vulgaris (2%), nail disease (2%), pruritus (2%)
Gastrointestinal: Constipation (2%), dyspepsia (2%)
Genitourinary: Urinary tract infection (3% to 5%)
Hematologic & oncologic: Anemia (4%; grade 3: <1%), leukopenia (3%)
Hypersensitivity: Hypersensitivity reaction (3%)
Infection: Influenza (4%), herpes simplex infection (2%)
Neuromuscular & skeletal: Arthralgia (6% to 8%), ostealgia (3% to 7%), myalgia (4%), muscle spasm (3%)
Respiratory: Flu-like symptoms (2% to 10%), sinusitis (2% to 9%), nasopharyngitis (8%), upper respiratory tract infection (3%), epistaxis (2%), pharyngolaryngeal pain (2%)
Miscellaneous: Accidental injury (6%)
<1% (Limited to important or life-threatening; as a single-agent or with combination chemotherapy): Adult respiratory distress syndrome, amblyopia, anaphylaxis, apnea, ascites, asthma, ataxia, blood coagulation disorder, bronchitis, cardiogenic shock, cardiomyopathy, cellulitis, cerebrovascular accident, colitis, coma, confusion, deafness, dermal ulcer, erysipelas, esophageal ulcer, febrile neutropenia, gastroenteritis, glomerulopathy, hematemesis, hemorrhage, hemorrhagic cystitis, hepatic failure, hepatitis, herpes zoster, hydrocephalus, hydronephrosis, hypercalcemia, hypotension, hypothyroidism, hypoxia, intestinal obstruction, interstitial pneumonitis, leukemia (acute), lymphangitis, madarosis, mania, meningitis, myopathy, neutropenia, neutropenic sepsis, oligohydramnios, onychoclasis, osteonecrosis, pancreatitis, pancytopenia, paresis, paroxysmal nocturnal dyspnea, pathological fracture, pericardial effusion, pleural effusion, pneumonitis, pneumothorax, pulmonary edema (noncardiogenic), pulmonary fibrosis, pulmonary hypertension, pyelonephritis, radiation injury, renal failure, respiratory failure, seizure, sepsis, syncope, stomatitis, thyroiditis (autoimmune), ventricular dysfunction

Drug Interactions
Metabolism/Transport Effects None known.
Avoid Concomitant Use
Avoid concomitant use of Trastuzumab with any of the following: Belimumab
Increased Effect/Toxicity
Trastuzumab may increase the levels/effects of: Antineoplastic Agents (Anthracycline, Systemic); Belimumab; Immunosuppressants

The levels/effects of Trastuzumab may be increased by: PACLitaxel (Conventional)
Decreased Effect
Trastuzumab may decrease the levels/effects of: PACLitaxel (Conventional)
Preparation for Administration Hazardous agent; use appropriate precautions for handling and disposal (meets NIOSH 2014 criteria). Check vial labels to assure appropriate product is being reconstituted (conventional trastuzumab and ado-trastuzumab emtansine are different products and are **NOT** interchangeable).

Reconstitute each vial with 20 mL of bacteriostatic sterile water for injection to a concentration of 21 mg/mL. Swirl gently; do not shake. Allow vial to rest for ~5 minutes. If the patient has a known hypersensitivity to benzyl alcohol, trastuzumab may be reconstituted with sterile water for injection without preservatives, which must be used immediately. Further dilute the appropriate volume for the trastuzumab dose in 250 mL NS prior to administration. Gently invert bag to mix.

Storage/Stability Prior to reconstitution, store intact vials under refrigeration at 2°C to 8°C (36°F to 46°F). Following reconstitution with bacteriostatic water, the solution in the vial is stable refrigerated for 28 days from the date of reconstitution; do not freeze. Solutions reconstituted with sterile water for injection without preservatives must be used immediately. The solution diluted in 250 mL NS for infusion may be stored refrigerated for up to 24 hours prior to use; do not freeze.

Mechanism of Action Trastuzumab is a monoclonal antibody which binds to the extracellular domain of the human epidermal growth factor receptor 2 protein (HER-2); it mediates antibody-dependent cellular cytotoxicity by inhibiting proliferation of cells which overexpress HER-2 protein.

Pharmacodynamics/Kinetics Note: In most patients, trastuzumab concentrations will decrease to ~3% (~97% washout) by 7 months following discontinuation.

Dosing

Adult & Geriatric Note: Do **NOT** substitute conventional trastuzumab for or with ado-trastuzumab emtansine; products are different and are **NOT** interchangeable. Details concerning dosing in combination regimens should also be consulted.

Breast cancer, adjuvant treatment, HER2+: IV: **Note:** Extending adjuvant treatment beyond 1 year is not recommended

With concurrent paclitaxel or docetaxel:
Initial loading dose: 4 mg/kg infused over 90 minutes, followed by
Maintenance dose: 2 mg/kg infused over 30 minutes weekly for total of 12 weeks, followed 1 week later (when concurrent chemotherapy completed) by 6 mg/kg infused over 30 to 90 minutes every 3 weeks for total therapy duration of 52 weeks

With concurrent docetaxel/carboplatin:
Initial loading dose: 4 mg/kg infused over 90 minutes, followed by
Maintenance dose: 2 mg/kg infused over 30 minutes weekly for total of 18 weeks, followed 1 week later (when concurrent chemotherapy completed) by 6 mg/kg infused over 30 to 90 minutes every 3 weeks for total therapy duration of 52 weeks

Following completion of multi-modality anthracycline-based chemotherapy:
Initial loading dose: 8 mg/kg infused over 90 minutes, followed by
Maintenance dose: 6 mg/kg infused over 30 to 90 minutes every 3 weeks for total therapy duration of 52 weeks

Breast cancer, metastatic, HER2+ (either as a single agent or in combination with paclitaxel): IV:
Initial loading dose: 4 mg/kg infused over 90 minutes, followed by
Maintenance dose: 2 mg/kg infused over 30 minutes weekly until disease progression

Gastric cancer, metastatic, HER2+ (in combination with cisplatin and either capecitabine or fluorouracil for 6 cycles followed by trastuzumab monotherapy; Bang, 2010): IV:
Initial loading dose: 8 mg/kg infused over 90 minutes, followed by
Maintenance dose: 6 mg/kg infused over 30 to 90 minutes every 3 weeks until disease progression

Missed doses: If a dose is missed by ≤1 week, the usual maintenance dose should be administered as soon as possible (do not wait until the next planned cycle) and subsequent maintenance doses should be administered 7 or 21 days later (based on patient's maintenance dose/schedule); if a dose is missed by >1 week, then a re-loading dose (4 mg/kg if patient receives trastuzumab weekly; 8 mg/kg if on an every-3-week schedule) should be administered, followed by the usual maintenance dose administered 7 or 21 days later (based on patient's maintenance dose/schedule).

Breast cancer (early stage, locally advanced, or inflammatory), neoadjuvant treatment, HER2+ (off-label use): IV: Trastuzumab, pertuzumab, and docetaxel (in patients with operable disease who had received no prior chemotherapy): Initial: 8 mg/kg (cycle 1) followed by 6 mg/kg every 3 weeks for a total of 4 neoadjuvant cycles; postoperatively, administer 3 cycles of adjuvant FEC [fluorouracil, epirubicin, and cyclophosphamide] chemotherapy and continue trastuzumab to complete 1 year of treatment (Gianni, 2012)

Breast cancer, metastatic, HER2+ (off-label combinations): IV: **Note:** There are multiple trastuzumab-containing regimens for the treatment of HER2+ metastatic breast cancer; commonly used regimens are listed below:
Trastuzumab, pertuzumab, and docetaxel (in patients with no prior anti-HER2 therapy or chemotherapy to treat metastatic disease): Initial: 8 mg/kg followed by a maintenance dose of 6 mg/kg every 3 weeks until disease progression or unacceptable toxicity (Baselga, 2012)
Trastuzumab, pertuzumab, and weekly paclitaxel: Initial: 8 mg/kg followed by a maintenance dose of 6 mg/kg every 3 weeks until disease progression (Dang, 2015)

Trastuzumab and lapatinib (in patients with progression on prior trastuzumab containing therapy): Initial: 4 mg/kg followed by a maintenance dose of 2 mg/kg every week (Blackwell, 2010; Blackwell, 2012)
Other trastuzumab combinations: Initial: 8 mg/kg followed by a maintenance dose of 6 mg/kg every 3 weeks until disease progression or unacceptable toxicity (in combination with docetaxel **or** vinorelbine) (Andersson, 2011) **or** 4 mg/kg loading dose followed by a maintenance dose of 2 mg/kg weekly until disease progression (in combination with docetaxel) (Marty, 2005)

Renal Impairment There are no dosage adjustments provided in the manufacturer's labeling, although data suggest that the disposition of trastuzumab is not altered based on serum creatinine (up to 2 mg/dL)

Hepatic Impairment There are no dosage adjustments provided in the manufacturer's labeling.

Adjustment for Toxicity
Cardiotoxicity: LVEF ≥16% decrease from baseline or LVEF below normal limits and ≥10% decrease from baseline: Withhold treatment for at least 4 weeks and repeat LVEF every 4 weeks. May resume trastuzumab treatment if LVEF returns to normal limits within 4 to 8 weeks and remains at ≤15% decrease from baseline value. Discontinue permanently for persistent (>8 weeks) LVEF decline or for >3 incidents of treatment interruptions for cardiomyopathy.
Infusion-related events:
Mild-moderate infusion reactions: Decrease infusion rate.
Dyspnea, clinically significant hypotension: Interrupt infusion.
Severe or life-threatening infusion reactions: Discontinue.

Administration Check label to ensure appropriate product is being administered (conventional trastuzumab and ado-trastuzumab emtansine are different products and are **NOT** interchangeable).

Administered by IV infusion; loading doses are infused over 90 minutes; maintenance doses may be infused over 30 minutes if tolerated. Do not administer with D₅W. **Do not administer IV push or by rapid bolus. Do not mix with any other medications.**

Observe patients closely during the infusion for fever, chills, or other infusion-related symptoms. Treatment with acetaminophen, diphenhydramine, and/or meperidine is usually effective for managing infusion-related events.

Hazardous agent; use appropriate precautions for handling and disposal (meets NIOSH 2014 criteria).

Monitoring Parameters Assessment for HER2 overexpression and HER2 gene amplification by validated immunohistochemistry (IHC) or fluorescence *in situ* hybridization (FISH) methodology (pretherapy); test should be specific for cancer type (breast vs gastric cancer). Pregnancy test (prior to treatment). Monitor vital signs during infusion; signs and symptoms of cardiac dysfunction; LVEF (baseline, every 3 months during treatment, upon therapy completion and if component of adjuvant therapy, every 6 months for at least 2 years; if treatment is withheld for significant LVEF dysfunction, monitor LVEF at 4-week intervals); signs and symptoms of infusion reaction or pulmonary toxicity; if pregnancy inadvertently occurs during treatment, monitor amniotic fluid volume

Dosage Forms Excipient information presented when available (limited, particularly for generics); consult specific product labeling.
Solution Reconstituted, Intravenous:
Herceptin: 440 mg (1 ea) [contains benzyl alcohol, mouse protein (murine) (hamster)]

Travoprost (TRA voe prost)

Brand Names: US Travatan Z
Brand Names: Canada Apo-Travoprost Z; Sandoz-Travoprost; Teva-Travoprost Z Ophthalmic Solution; Travatan Z

Pharmacologic Category Ophthalmic Agent, Antiglaucoma; Prostaglandin, Ophthalmic

Use Elevated intraocular pressure: Reduction of elevated intraocular pressure in patients with open-angle glaucoma or ocular hypertension

Dosing

Adult & Geriatric Elevated intraocular pressure: Ophthalmic: Instill 1 drop into affected eye(s) once daily in the evening; do not exceed once-daily dosing (may decrease IOP-lowering effect).

Pediatric Elevated intraocular pressure: Adolescents ≥16 years: Ophthalmic: Refer to adult dosing. **Note:** Canadian labeling does not include an indication for use in patients <18 years.

Renal Impairment There are no dosage adjustments provided in the manufacturer's labeling. However, dosage adjustments are unlikely due to low systemic absorption.

Hepatic Impairment There are no dosage adjustments provided in the manufacturer's labeling. However, dosage adjustments are unlikely due to low systemic absorption.

Additional Information Complete prescribing information should be consulted for additional detail.

Dosage Forms Excipient information presented when available (limited, particularly for generics); consult specific product labeling.

Solution, Ophthalmic:

Travatan Z: 0.004% (2.5 mL, 5 mL) [benzalkonium free; contains cremophor el, propylene glycol]

Generic: 0.004% (2.5 mL, 5 mL)

TraZODone (TRAZ oh done)

Brand Names: US Oleptro

Brand Names: Canada Apo-Trazodone; Apo-Trazodone D; Dom-Trazodone; Mylan-Trazodone; Novo-Trazodone; Nu-Trazodone; Nu-Trazodone D; Oleptro; PHL-Trazodone; PMS-Trazodone; ratio-Trazodone; Teva-Trazodone; Trazorel; ZYM-Trazodone

Index Terms Desyrel; Trazodone Hydrochloride

Pharmacologic Category Antidepressant, Serotonin Reuptake Inhibitor/Antagonist

Use Treatment of major depressive disorder

Pregnancy Considerations Adverse effects were observed in some animal reproduction studies. When trazodone is taken during pregnancy, an increased risk of major malformations has not been observed in the limited number of pregnancies studied (Einarson, 2003; Einarson, 2009). The long-term effects of in utero trazodone exposure on infant development and behavior are not known.

The ACOG recommends that therapy with antidepressants during pregnancy be individualized; treatment of depression during pregnancy should incorporate the clinical expertise of the mental health clinician, obstetrician, primary healthcare provider, and pediatrician. According to the American Psychiatric Association (APA), the risks of medication treatment should be weighed against other treatment options and untreated depression. Consideration should be given to using agents with safety data in pregnancy. For women who discontinue antidepressant medications during pregnancy and who may be at high risk for postpartum depression, the medications can be restarted following delivery. Treatment algorithms have been developed by the ACOG and the APA for the management of depression in women prior to conception and during pregnancy (ACOG, 2008; APA, 2010; Yonkers, 2009).

Breast-Feeding Considerations Trazodone is excreted into breast milk; breast milk concentrations peak ~2 hours following administration. It is not known if the trazodone metabolite is found in breast milk (Verbeeck, 1986). The long-term effects on neurobehavior have not been studied. The manufacturer recommends that caution be exercised when administering trazodone to nursing women.

Medication Guide Available Yes

Contraindications Hypersensitivity to trazodone or any component of the formulation; use of MAO inhibitors intended to treat psychiatric disorders (concurrently or within 14 days of discontinuing either trazodone or the MAO inhibitor); initiation of trazodone in a patient receiving linezolid or intravenous methylene blue

Warnings/Precautions [U.S. Boxed Warning]: Antidepressants increase the risk of suicidal thinking and behavior in children, adolescents, and young adults (18 to 24 years of age) with major depressive disorder (MDD) and other psychiatric disorders; consider risk prior to prescribing. Short-term studies did not show an increased risk in patients >24 years of age and showed a decreased risk in patients ≥65 years of age. Closely monitor for clinical worsening, suicidality, or unusual changes in behavior, particularly during the initial 1 to 2 months of therapy or during periods of dosage adjustments (increases or decreases); the patient's family or caregiver should be instructed to closely observe the patient and communicate condition with healthcare provider. A medication guide should be dispensed with each prescription. **Trazodone is not FDA approved for use in children.**

The possibility of a suicide attempt is inherent in major depression and may persist until remission occurs. Worsening depression and severe abrupt suicidality that are not part of the presenting symptoms may require discontinuation or modification of drug therapy. The patient's family or caregiver should be alerted to monitor patients for the emergence of suicidality and associated behaviors (such as agitation, irritability, hostility, impulsivity, and hypomania) and call healthcare provider.

May worsen psychosis in some patients or precipitate a shift to mania or hypomania in patients with bipolar disorder. Patients presenting with depressive symptoms should be screened for bipolar disorder. Monotherapy in patients with bipolar disorder should be avoided. **Trazodone is not FDA approved for the treatment of bipolar depression.**

Priapism, including cases resulting in permanent dysfunction, has occurred with the use of trazodone. Instruct patient to seek medical assistance for erection lasting >4 hours; use with caution in patients who have conditions which may predispose them to priapism (eg, sickle cell anemia, multiple myeloma, leukemia). Not recommended for use in a patient during the acute recovery phase of MI. The risks of sedation, postural hypotension, and/or syncope are high relative to other antidepressants. Trazodone frequently causes sedation, which may result in impaired performance of tasks requiring alertness (eg, operating machinery or driving).

Use with caution in patients with a history of cardiovascular disease (including previous MI, stroke, tachycardia, or conduction abnormalities). Although the risk of conduction abnormalities with this agent is low relative to other antidepressants, QT prolongation (with or without torsade de pointes), ventricular tachycardia, and other arrhythmias have been observed with the use of trazodone (reports limited to immediate-release formulation); use with caution in patients with preexisting cardiac disease. May impair platelet aggregation resulting in increased risk of bleeding events (eg, epistaxis, life threatening bleeding).

Potentially life-threatening serotonin syndrome (SS) has occurred with serotonergic agents (eg, SSRIs, SNRIs), particularly when used in combination with other serotonergic agents (eg, triptans, TCAs, fentanyl, lithium, tramadol, buspirone, St John's wort, tryptophan) or agents that impair metabolism of serotonin (eg, MAO inhibitors intended to treat psychiatric disorders, other MAO inhibitors [ie, linezolid and intravenous methylene blue]). Discontinue treatment (and any concomitant serotonergic agent) immediately if signs/symptoms arise.

Serotonin syndrome (SS)/neuroleptic malignant syndrome (NMS)-like reactions may occur with trazodone when used alone, particularly if used with other serotonergic agents (eg, serotonin/norepinephrine reuptake inhibitors [SNRIs], selective serotonin reuptake inhibitors [SSRIs], or triptans), drugs that impair serotonin metabolism (eg, MAO inhibitors), or antidopaminergic agents (eg, antipsychotics). If concurrent use is clinically warranted, carefully observe patient during treatment initiation and dose increases. Do not use concurrently with serotonin precursors (eg, tryptophan).

Use caution in patients with a previous seizure disorder or condition predisposing to seizures such as brain damage, or alcoholism. Bone fractures have been associated with antidepressant treatment. Consider the possibility of a fragility fracture if an antidepressant-treated patient presents with unexplained bone pain, point tenderness, swelling, or bruising (Rabenda, 2013; Rizzoli, 2012). Use with caution in patients with hepatic or renal dysfunction and in elderly patients. May cause SIADH and hyponatremia, predominantly in the elderly; volume depletion and/or concurrent use of diuretics likely increases risk. May cause mild pupillary dilation which in susceptible individuals can lead to an episode of narrow-angle glaucoma. Consider evaluating patients who have not had an iridectomy for narrow-angle glaucoma risk factors. Potentially significant drug-drug interactions may exist, requiring dose or frequency adjustment, additional monitoring, and/or selection of alternative therapy.

Abrupt discontinuation or interruption of antidepressant therapy has been associated with a discontinuation syndrome. Symptoms arising may vary with antidepressant however commonly include nausea, vomiting, diarrhea, headaches, lightheadedness, dizziness, diminished appetite, sweating, chills, tremors, paresthesias, fatigue, somnolence, and sleep disturbances (eg, vivid dreams, insomnia). Greater risks for developing a discontinuation syndrome have been associated with antidepressants with shorter half-lives, longer durations of treatment, and abrupt discontinuation. For antidepressants of short or intermediate half-lives, symptoms may emerge within 2 to 5 days after treatment discontinuation and last 7 to 14 days (APA, 2010; Fava, 2006; Haddad, 2001; Shelton, 2001; Warner, 2006).

Adverse Reactions
>10%:

Central nervous system: Sedation (46%), headache (33%), dizziness (25%), fatigue (15%)

Gastrointestinal: Xerostomia (25%), nausea (21%)

1% to 10%:

Cardiovascular: Edema (≥1%)

Central nervous system: Agitation (≥1%), ataxia (≥1%), confusion (≥1%), disorientation (≥1%), memory impairment (≥1%), migraine (≥1%)

Dermatologic: Night sweats (≥1%)

Endocrine & metabolic: Decreased libido (2%)

Gastrointestinal: Constipation (8%), abdominal pain (≥1%), dysgeusia (≥1%), vomiting (≥1%)

Genitourinary: Ejaculatory disorder (2%), urinary urgency (≥1%)

Neuromuscular & skeletal: Back pain (5%), myalgia (≥1%), tremor (≥1%)

Ophthalmic: Blurred vision (5%), visual disturbance (≥1%)

Respiratory: Dyspnea (≥1%)

<1% (Limited to important or life-threatening): Abnormal dreams, abnormal orgasm, acne, akathisia, allergic reactions, alopecia, amylase increased, anemia, angle-closure glaucoma, anxiety, aphasia, apnea, appetite increased, arrhythmia, ataxia, atrial fibrillation, bladder pain, bradycardia, breast enlargement/engorgement, cardiac arrest, cardiospasm, cerebrovascular accident, chest pain, CHF, chills, cholestasis, clitorism, conduction block, diplopia, dry eyes, early menses, erectile dysfunction, extrapyramidal symptoms, eye pain, flushing, gait disturbance, hallucination, hearing loss (partial), hematuria, hemolytic anemia, hepatitis, hirsutism, hyperbilirubinemia, hyperhidrosis, hypersalivation, hypersensitivity, hypoesthesia, hypomania, impaired speech, impotence, insomnia, jaundice, lactation, leukocytosis, leukonychia, libido decreased, liver enzyme alteration, methemoglobinemia, MI, muscle twitching, orthostatic hypotension, palpitation, paranoia, photophobia, photosensitivity reaction, priapism, pruritus, psoriasis, psychosis, QT prolongation, rash, reflux esophagitis, retrograde ejaculation, salivation increased, seizure, SIADH, speech impairment, stupor, tachycardia, tardive dyskinesia, tinnitus, torsade de pointes, urinary frequency increased, urinary incontinence, urinary retention, urticaria, vasodilation, ventricular ectopy, ventricular tachycardia, vertigo, weakness

Drug Interactions
Metabolism/Transport Effects Substrate of CYP2D6 (minor), CYP3A4 (major); **Note:** Assignment of Major/Minor substrate status based on clinically relevant drug interaction potential; **Induces** P-glycoprotein

Avoid Concomitant Use
Avoid concomitant use of TraZODone with any of the following: Conivaptan; Dapoxetine; Fusidic Acid (Systemic); Idelalisib; Linezolid; Lopinavir; MAO Inhibitors; Methylene Blue; Saquinavir

Increased Effect/Toxicity
TraZODone may increase the levels/effects of: Antipsychotic Agents; Antipsychotic Agents (Phenothiazines); Clarithromycin; Fosphenytoin; Highest Risk QTc-Prolonging Agents; Methylene Blue; Metoclopramide; Moderate Risk QTc-Prolonging Agents; Phenytoin; Serotonin Modulators

The levels/effects of TraZODone may be increased by: Alcohol (Ethyl); Antiemetics (5HT3 Antagonists); Antipsychotic Agents; Antipsychotic Agents (Phenothiazines); Aprepitant; Atazanavir; Boceprevir; BusPIRone; Clarithromycin; Conivaptan; CYP3A4 Inhibitors (Moderate); CYP3A4 Inhibitors (Strong); Dapoxetine; Darunavir; Dasatinib; Fosamprenavir; Fosaprepitant; Fusidic Acid (Systemic); Idelalisib; Indinavir; Ivacaftor; Linezolid; Lopinavir; Luliconazole; MAO Inhibitors; Metaxalone; Mifepristone; Nelfinavir; Netupitant; Osimertinib; Palbociclib; Ritonavir; Saquinavir; Selective Serotonin Reuptake Inhibitors; Simeprevir; Stiripentol; Tedizolid; Telaprevir; Tipranavir; Venlafaxine

Decreased Effect
TraZODone may decrease the levels/effects of: Warfarin

The levels/effects of TraZODone may be decreased by: Bosentan; CYP3A4 Inducers (Moderate); CYP3A4 Inducers (Strong); Dabrafenib; Deferasirox; Enzalutamide; Fosphenytoin; Mitotane; Osimertinib; Phenytoin; Siltuximab; St Johns Wort; Tocilizumab

Food Interactions Time to peak serum levels may be increased if immediate release trazodone is taken with food. Management: Administer immediate release after meals to decrease lightheadedness and postural hypotension. Administer extended release on an empty stomach.

Storage/Stability
Immediate release tablet: Store at room temperature; avoid temperatures >40°C (>104°F). Protect from light.

Extended release tablet: Store at room temperature of 15°C to 30°C (59°F to 86°F). Protect from light.

Mechanism of Action Inhibits reuptake of serotonin, causes adrenoreceptor subsensitivity, and induces significant changes in 5-HT presynaptic receptor adrenoreceptors. Trazodone also significantly blocks histamine (H$_1$) and alpha$_1$-adrenergic receptors.

Pharmacodynamics/Kinetics
Onset of action: Therapeutic (antidepressant): Up to 6 weeks; sleep aid: 1 to 3 hours

Absorption: Well absorbed; Extended release: C$_{max}$ increases ~86% when taken shortly after ingestion of a high-fat meal compared to fasting conditions

Protein binding: 85% to 95%

Metabolism: Hepatic via CYP3A4 (extensive) to an active metabolite (mCPP)

Half-life elimination: 7 to 10 hours

Time to peak, serum:

Immediate release: 30 to 100 minutes; delayed with food (up to 2.5 hours)

Extended release: 9 hours; not significantly affected by food

Excretion: Primarily urine (<1% excreted unchanged); secondarily feces

Dosing
Adult
Depression: Oral: Initial: 150 mg daily in divided doses (may increase by 50 mg daily every 3 to 4 days); maximum dose (manufacturer's labeling): 600 mg daily (inpatients); 400 mg daily (outpatients). **Note:** Clinical practice guidelines recommend doses up to 600 mg daily without noted consideration to inpatient or outpatient status (APA 2010; Bauer 2013).

Extended release formulation: Initial: 150 mg once daily at bedtime (may increase by 75 mg daily every 3 days); maximum dose: 375 mg daily; once adequate response obtained, gradually reduce with adjustment based on therapeutic response

Note: Therapeutic effects may take up to 6 weeks. Therapy is normally maintained for 6 to 12 months after optimum response is reached to prevent recurrence of depression.

Insomnia (off-label use): 50 mg to 100 mg at bedtime (Mendelson 2005; Roth 2011). Doses up to 500 mg have been evaluated in patients with insomnia associated with depression (typical ranges of 50 to 300 mg); however, the quality of the evidence precludes definitive conclusions of efficacy (Mendelson 2005).

Discontinuation of therapy: Upon discontinuation of antidepressant therapy, gradually taper the dose to minimize the incidence of withdrawal symptoms and allow for the detection of re-emerging symptoms. Evidence supporting ideal taper rates is limited. APA and NICE guidelines suggest tapering therapy over at least several weeks with consideration to the half-life of the antidepressant; antidepressants with a shorter half-life may need to be tapered more conservatively. In addition for long-term treated patients, WFSBP guidelines recommend tapering over 4 to 6 months. If intolerable withdrawal symptoms occur following a dose reduction, consider resuming the previously prescribed dose and/or decrease dose at a more gradual rate (APA 2010; Bauer 2002; Haddad 2001; NCCMH 2010; Schatzberg 2006; Shelton 2001; Warner 2006).

MAO inhibitor recommendations:
Switching to or from an MAO inhibitor intended to treat psychiatric disorders:

Allow 14 days to elapse between discontinuing an MAO inhibitor intended to treat psychiatric disorders and initiation of trazodone.

Allow 14 days to elapse between discontinuing trazodone and initiation of an MAO inhibitor intended to treat psychiatric disorders.

Use with other MAO inhibitors (linezolid or IV methylene blue):

Do not initiate trazodone in patients receiving linezolid or IV methylene blue; consider other interventions for psychiatric condition.

If urgent treatment with linezolid or IV methylene blue is required in a patient already receiving trazodone and potential benefits outweigh potential risks, discontinue trazodone promptly and administer linezolid or IV methylene blue. Monitor for serotonin syndrome for 2 weeks or until 24 hours after the last dose of linezolid or IV methylene blue, whichever comes first. May resume trazodone 24 hours after the last dose of linezolid or IV methylene blue.

Geriatric
Immediate release: Oral: 25 to 50 mg at bedtime with 25 to 50 mg daily dose increase every 3 days for inpatients and weekly for outpatients, if tolerated; usual dose: 75 to 150 mg daily
Extended release: Refer to adult dosing. Use with caution in the elderly; clinical experience is limited.

Discontinuation of therapy: Refer to adult dosing.
MAO inhibitor recommendations: Refer to adult dosing.

Pediatric
Depression (off-label use):
Children 6 to 12 years: Initial: 1.5 to 2 mg/kg/day in divided doses; increase gradually every 3 to 4 days as needed; maximum: 6 mg/kg/day in 3 divided doses
Adolescents: Initial: 25 to 50 mg daily; increase to 100 to 150 mg daily in divided doses
Note: Once daily doses at bedtime may be considered to minimize adverse effects (Haria,1994; Rawls,1982).

Discontinuation of therapy: Refer to adult dosing.
MAO inhibitor recommendations: Refer to adult dosing.

Renal Impairment There are no dosage adjustments provided in manufacturer's labeling (has not been studied). Use with caution.

Hepatic Impairment There are no dosage adjustments provided in manufacturer's labeling (has not been studied). Use with caution.

Administration
Immediate release tablet: Dosing after meals may decrease lightheadedness and postural hypotension
Extended release tablet: Take on an empty stomach; swallow whole or as a half tablet without food. Tablet may be broken along the score line, but do not crush or chew.

Monitoring Parameters Baseline liver function prior to and periodically during therapy; suicide ideation (especially at the beginning of therapy or when doses are increased or decreased); suicide ideation (especially at the beginning of therapy or when doses are increased or decreased); signs/symptoms of serotonin syndrome

Reference Range Plasma levels do not always correlate with clinical effectiveness
Therapeutic: 0.5 to 2.5 mcg/mL
Potentially toxic: >2.5 mcg/mL
Toxic: >4 mcg/mL

Test Interactions May interfere with urine detection of amphetamine/methamphetamine (false-positive).

Dosage Forms Excipient information presented when available (limited, particularly for generics); consult specific product labeling.
Tablet, Oral, as hydrochloride:
Generic: 50 mg, 100 mg, 150 mg, 300 mg
Tablet Extended Release 24 Hour, Oral, as hydrochloride:
Oleptro: 150 mg, 300 mg [scored]

◆ Trazodone Hydrochloride *see* TraZODone *on page 1834*

◆ Trazorel (Can) *see* TraZODone *on page 1834*

◆ Treanda *see* Bendamustine *on page 213*

◆ Trelstar *see* Triptorelin *on page 1847*

◆ Trelstar Mixject *see* Triptorelin *on page 1847*

◆ Tremytoine Inj (Can) *see* Phenytoin *on page 1444*

◆ Trental *see* Pentoxifylline *on page 1427*

◆ TRENtal [DSC] *see* Pentoxifylline *on page 1427*

Treprostinil (tre PROST in il)

Brand Names: US Orenitram; Remodulin; Tyvaso; Tyvaso Refill; Tyvaso Starter
Brand Names: Canada Remodulin
Index Terms Treprostinil Sodium
Pharmacologic Category Prostacyclin; Prostaglandin; Vasodilator

Use Pulmonary arterial hypertension:
Injection: Treatment of pulmonary arterial hypertension (PAH) (WHO Group I) in patients with NYHA class II-IV symptoms to decrease exercise-associated symptoms; to diminish clinical deterioration when transitioning from epoprostenol (IV)
Inhalation: Treatment of pulmonary arterial hypertension (PAH) (WHO Group I) in patients with NYHA class III symptoms to improve exercise ability. **Note:** Nearly all controlled clinical trial experience has been with concomitant bosentan or sildenafil.
Oral: Treatment of pulmonary arterial hypertension (PAH) (WHO Group 1) in patients with WHO functional class II-III symptoms to improve exercise capacity.

Pregnancy Considerations Adverse events were observed in some animal reproduction studies. Women with pulmonary arterial hypertension (PAH) are encouraged to avoid pregnancy (McLaughlin, 2009).

Breast-Feeding Considerations It is not known if treprostinil is excreted in breast milk. The manufacturers of the injection recommend that caution be exercised when administering treprostinil to nursing women. The manufacturer of the oral product recommends that a decision be made whether to discontinue nursing or to discontinue the drug.

Contraindications
Injection/inhalation: There are no contraindications listed in the manufacturer's labeling.
Oral: Severe hepatic impairment (Child-Pugh class C).
Documentation of allergenic cross-reactivity for prostaglandins is limited. However, because of similarities in chemical structure and/or pharmacologic actions, the possibility of cross-sensitivity cannot be ruled out with certainty.

Warnings/Precautions May produce symptomatic hypotension; use with caution in patients with low systemic arterial blood pressure. Abrupt withdrawal/large dosage reductions may worsen symptoms of pulmonary arterial hypertension (PAH). If a SubQ or IV infusion is restarted within a few hours of discontinuation, the same dose rate may be used. Interruptions for longer periods may require retitration. Regardless of administration route (inhalation, IV, oral, or SubQ), treatment interruptions should be avoided. Immediate access to medication, back-up inhalation device, or pump and infusion sets is essential to prevent treatment interruptions. Chronic continuous IV infusion of treprostinil via a chronic indwelling central venous catheter has been associated with serious blood stream infections. This method of administration should be reserved for patients who are intolerant of the SubQ route or in whom the benefit outweighs the potential risks. Treprostinil injection should only be used by clinicians experienced in the treatment of PAH. Prior to initiation, patients should be carefully evaluated for ability to administer treprostinil, either as an IV/SubQ infusion or inhalation, and care for the infusion system/inhalation device. Initiation of infusion must occur in a setting where adequate personnel and equipment necessary for hemodynamic monitoring and emergency treatment is available.

Use with caution in patients with hepatic impairment. IV/SubQ: Dose reduction is recommended for the initial dose in patients with mild to moderate hepatic insufficiency; titrate dose slowly in patients with hepatic insufficiency; has not been studied in severe hepatic impairment. Oral: Dose reduction is recommended for patients with mild hepatic impairment. Avoid use in patients with moderate impairment; use is contraindicated in patients with severe impairment.

Has not been studied in renal impairment (inhalation/IV/SubQ); use with caution in renal impairment; titrate dose slowly in patients with renal insufficiency. May inhibit platelet aggregation and increases the risk of bleeding. Inhalation: Safety and efficacy have not been established in patients with underlying pulmonary disease (eg, asthma, COPD). Patients with acute pulmonary infections should be monitored closely for exacerbation or reduced efficacy. Tablets can lodge in diverticulum; use with caution in patients with diverticulosis; should not be administered with ethanol since the release of treprostinil from the tablet may occur at a faster rate than intended. Potentially significant drug-drug interactions may exist, requiring dose or frequency adjustment, additional monitoring, and/or selection of alternative therapy.

Adverse Reactions

>10%:

Cardiovascular: Flushing (11% to 15%)

Central nervous system: Headache (27% to 63%)

Dermatologic: Skin rash (14%)

Gastrointestinal: Diarrhea (25% to 30%), nausea (19% to 30%)

Local: Pain at injection site (SubQ: 85%; may improve after several months of therapy), infusion site reaction (SubQ: 83%)

Neuromuscular & skeletal: Limb pain (Oral: 14%), jaw pain (11% to 13%)

Respiratory: Cough (Inhalation: 54%), pharyngolaryngeal pain (Inhalation: 25%), throat irritation (Inhalation: 25%)

1% to 10%:

Cardiovascular: Edema (9%), syncope (Inhalation: 6%), hypotension (4%)

Central nervous system: Dizziness (9%)

Dermatologic: Pruritus (8%)

Endocrine & metabolic: Hypokalemia (Oral: 9%)

Gastrointestinal: Abdominal distress (Oral: 6%)

Respiratory: Epistaxis (Inhalation), hemoptysis, pneumonia, wheezing (Inhalation)

<1% (Limited to important or life-threatening): Angioedema, catheter infection (central venous), catheter sepsis (central venous), cellulitis, decreased platelet aggregation, hematoma, ostealgia, pain, paresthesia, swelling of extremities, thrombocytopenia, thrombophlebitis

Drug Interactions

Metabolism/Transport Effects Substrate of CYP2C8 (minor), CYP2C9 (minor); **Note:** Assignment of Major/Minor substrate status based on clinically relevant drug interaction potential

Avoid Concomitant Use There are no known interactions where it is recommended to avoid concomitant use.

Increased Effect/Toxicity

Treprostinil may increase the levels/effects of: Agents with Antiplatelet Properties; Anticoagulants; Blood Pressure Lowering Agents; Highest Risk QTc-Prolonging Agents; Moderate Risk QTc-Prolonging Agents; Nonsteroidal Anti-Inflammatory Agents; Salicylates

The levels/effects of Treprostinil may be increased by: Alcohol (Ethyl); CYP2C8 Inhibitors (Strong); Mifepristone; Thrombolytic Agents

Decreased Effect

The levels/effects of Treprostinil may be decreased by: CYP2C8 Inducers (Strong)

Preparation for Administration Injection solution: For SubQ infusion, **product should not be diluted prior to use**. For IV infusion, dilute in SWFI, NS, Remodulin sterile diluent, or Flolan sterile diluent to a final volume of either 50 mL or 100 mL (dependent on system reservoir and calculated dose).

Storage/Stability

Injection solution: Store vials at 25°C (77°F); excursions are permitted between 15°C and 30°C (59°F and 86°F). Contents of a vial should not be used past 30 days after initial needle access into the vial. Stability for up to 14 days at 37°C has been shown for IV infusion concentrations as low as 4,000 ng/mL.

Solution for inhalation: Store ampuls in foil packs at 25°C (77°F); excursions are permitted between 15°C and 30°C (59°F and 86°F). Protect from light. Once foil pack is opened, ampuls should be used within 7 days. Following transfer of solution to inhalation device, solution should remain in device for no more than 24 hours; discard unused portion.

Tablets: Store at 25°C (77°F); excursions are permitted between 15°C and 30°C (59°F and 86°F).

Mechanism of Action Treprostinil is a direct vasodilator of both pulmonary and systemic arterial vascular beds; also inhibits platelet aggregation.

Pharmacodynamics/Kinetics

Absorption: SubQ: Rapidly and completely

Distribution: 14 L/70 kg ideal body weight

Protein binding: 91% to 96%

Metabolism: Hepatic (primarily by CYP2C8); forms 5 inactive metabolites (HU1-HU5)

Bioavailability: Inhalation: 64% to 72% (dose-dependent); SubQ: 100%; Oral: ~17%

Half-life elimination: Terminal: ~4 hours

Time to peak: Oral: 4-6 hours

Excretion:

Urine (79%; 4% as unchanged drug, 64% as metabolites); feces (13%)

Oral: urine (0.19% as unchanged drug); feces (1.13% as unchanged drug)

Dosing

Adult

Pulmonary arterial hypertension (PAH):

Inhalation: **Note:** Prior to initiation, patients should be carefully evaluated for ability to administer treprostinil and care for the inhalation system and accessories required for administration. Immediate access to a back-up inhalation device, accessories, and medication is essential to prevent treatment interruptions.

Initial: 18 mcg (or 3 inhalations) every 4 hours 4 times/day; if 3 inhalations are not tolerated, reduce to 1 to 2 inhalations, then increase to 3 inhalations as tolerated

Maintenance: If tolerated, increase dose by an additional 3 inhalations at approximately 1- to 2-week intervals; target dose and maximum dose: 54 mcg (or 9 inhalations) 4 times/day

Oral: Initial: 0.25 mg every 12 hours or 0.125 mg every 8 hours; may increase dose in increments of 0.25 mg or 0.5 mg every 12 hours or 0.125 mg every 8 hours every 3 to 4 days as tolerated to achieve optimal clinical response. If dose increments are not tolerated, consider slower titration. Maximum dose is determined by tolerability. If intolerable effects occur, decrease dose in increments of 0.25 mg; avoid abrupt discontinuation. Upon discontinuation, reduce the dose in increments of 0.5 mg to 1 mg daily.

Missed doses: If a dose is missed, take the missed dose as soon as possible. If ≥2 doses are missed, restart at a lower dose and retitrate.

Dosage adjustment for concurrent use in patients receiving strong CYP2C8 inhibitors (gemfibrozil): Initiate a starting dose of 0.125 mg every 12 hours; increase in increments of 0.125 mg every 12 hours every 3 to 4 days.

Planned short-term treatment interruption: If patients are unable to continue oral treatment, a temporary infusion of subcutaneous or IV treprostinil may be considered. Divide the oral total daily dose by 5 to calculate the total daily dose (mg) of parenteral treprostinil.

SubQ (preferred) or IV infusion: **Note:** Prior to initiation, patients should be carefully evaluated for ability to administer treprostinil and care for the infusion system outside of inpatient setting. Immediate access to a back-up pump, infusion sets, and medication is essential to prevent treatment interruptions.

New to prostacyclin therapy: Initial: 1.25 ng/kg/minute; if dose cannot be tolerated due to systemic effects, reduce to 0.625 ng/kg/minute. Increase dose in increments of 1.25 ng/kg/minute per week for first 4 weeks, followed by increments of 2.5 ng/kg/minute per week for remainder of therapy. Limited experience with doses >40 ng/kg/minute. **Note:** Dose must be carefully and individually titrated (symptom improvement with minimal adverse effects). Avoid abrupt withdrawal. If infusion is restarted within a few hours of discontinuation, the same dose rate may be used. Interruptions for longer periods may require retitration.

Transitioning from epoprostenol (see table): **Note:** Transition should occur in a hospital setting to follow response (eg, walking distance, sign/symptoms of disease progression). May take 24 to 48 hours to transition. Transition is accomplished by initiating the infusion of treprostinil, and increasing it while simultaneously reducing the dose of intravenous epoprostenol. During transition, increases in PAH symptoms should be first treated with an increase in treprostinil dose. Occurrence of prostacyclin associated side effects should be treated by decreasing the dose of epoprostenol.

Transitioning From IV Epoprostenol to SubQ (Preferred) or IV Treprostinil

Step	Epoprostenol Dose	Treprostinil Dose
1	Maintain current dose	Initiate at 10% initial epoprostenol dose
2	Decrease to 80% initial dose	Increase to 30% initial epoprostenol dose
3	Decrease to 60% initial dose	Increase to 50% initial epoprostenol dose
4	Decrease to 40% initial dose	Increase to 70% initial epoprostenol dose
5	Decrease to 20% initial dose	Increase to 90% initial epoprostenol dose
6	Decrease to 5% initial dose	Increase to 110% initial epoprostenol dose
7	Discontinue epoprostenol	Maintain current dose plus additional 5% to 10% as needed

Geriatric Refer to adult dosing. Limited experience in patients ≥65 years; use caution.

Pediatric SubQ; IV infusion: Limited experience in patients ≤16 years of age.

Renal Impairment

Inhalation, SubQ infusion, IV infusion: There are no dosage adjustments provided in manufacturer's labeling (has not been studied). Use with caution and titrate slowly.

Oral: No dosage adjustment necessary.

Hemodialysis: Treprostinil is not removed by dialysis.

Hepatic Impairment

Inhalation: There are no dosage adjustments provided in manufacturer's labeling. However, hepatic impairment increases systemic exposure to treprostinil. Use with caution and titrate slowly.

Mild to moderate impairment: Initial: 0.625 ng/kg/minute (ideal body weight). Use with caution and titrate slowly.

Severe impairment: There are no dosage adjustments provided in manufacturer's labeling (has not been studied). Use with caution and titrate slowly.

Oral:

Mild impairment (Child-Pugh class A): Initial: 0.125 mg every 12 hours; increase in increments of 0.125 mg every 12 hours every 3 to 4 days.

Moderate impairment (Child-Pugh class B): Avoid use.

Severe impairment (Child-Pugh class C): Use is contraindicated by the manufacturer.

Administration Avoid treatment interruptions or rapid large dosage reductions with use of inhalation, IV, or SubQ formulations. Immediate access to medication, a back-up inhalation device, or pump and infusion sets is essential to prevent treatment interruptions.

Inhalation: Do not mix with other medications. For inhalation only via the Tyvaso Inhalation System. Prior to the first treatment session of each day, transfer the entire contents of one ampule into the medicine chamber; one ampule contains sufficient volume of medication for all 4 treatment sessions in a single day. Between each session, the device should be capped and stored upright with the remaining medication inside. At the end of each day, the medicine chamber and any remaining medication must be discarded. Avoid contact of solution with eyes or skin; wash hands after handling.

IV infusion: IV use is recommended when SubQ infusion is not tolerated or when the benefit outweighs the potential risks of an indwelling central venous catheter. Solution must be diluted in SWFI, NS, Remodulin sterile diluent, or Flolan sterile diluent prior to use and administered by continuous infusion using a central indwelling catheter and infusion pump. The ambulatory infusion pump should be small and lightweight; have occlusion/no delivery, low battery, programming error, and motor malfunction alarms; have ± 6% accuracy of the programmed rate; and be positive pressure driven. The reservoir should be made of polyvinyl chloride, polypropylene, or glass. Peripheral infusion may be used temporarily until central line is established. Infusion sets with an in-line 0.22 or 0.2 micron filter should be used for central and peripheral administration.

Oral: Administer with food. Swallow tablets whole; do not crush, split or chew; use only intact tablets.

SubQ infusion (preferred): Administer undiluted via continuous SubQ infusion using an appropriately designed infusion pump. The ambulatory infusion pump should be small and lightweight; be able to adjust infusion rates in ~0.002 mL/hour increments; have occlusion/no delivery, low battery, programming error, and motor malfunction alarms; have ± 6% accuracy of the programmed rate; and be positive pressure driven. The reservoir should be made of polyvinyl chloride, polypropylene, or glass. Proactively manage infusion-site reactions based on individual patient needs and by combining multiple strategies, including improved dosing strategies (eg, more rapid dose escalation), appropriate site selection, less frequent infusion site changes (eg, every 2 to 5 weeks [Skoro-Sajer 2007]), and analgesic care (pharmacologic and nonpharmacologic) when pain occurs. Rotate infusion site when patient experiences continued site pain, itching, erythema, drainage, or bleeding; decreased site pain and need for site changes or discontinuation due to site pain may be reduced in patients who are managed proactively in this manner (Mathier 2010; Skoro-Sajer 2008; White 2013).

Monitoring Parameters BP, dyspnea, fatigue, activity tolerance, symptoms of excessive dose (eg, headache, nausea, vomiting)

Dosage Forms Excipient information presented when available (limited, particularly for generics); consult specific product labeling.

Solution, Inhalation:
Tyvaso: 0.6 mg/mL (2.9 mL)
Tyvaso Refill: 0.6 mg/mL (2.9 mL)
Tyvaso Starter: 0.6 mg/mL (2.9 mL)

Solution, Injection:
Remodulin: 1 mg/mL (20 mL); 2.5 mg/mL (20 mL); 5 mg/mL (20 mL); 10 mg/mL (20 mL) [contains metacresol]

Tablet Extended Release, Oral:
Orenitram: 0.125 mg, 0.25 mg, 1 mg, 2.5 mg [contains fd&c blue #2 (indigotine)]

♦ Treprostinil Sodium *see* Treprostinil *on page 1836*

♦ Tresiba FlexTouch *see* Insulin Degludec *on page 954*

♦ Tretin-X *see* Tretinoin (Topical) *on page 1841*

♦ Tretinoin and Clindamycin *see* Clindamycin and Tretinoin *on page 410*

♦ Tretinoin, Fluocinolone Acetonide, and Hydroquinone *see* Fluocinolone, Hydroquinone, and Tretinoin *on page 781*

Tretinoin (Systemic) (TRET i noyn)

Brand Names: Canada Vesanoid

Index Terms *trans* Vitamin A Acid; *trans*-Retinoic Acid; All-*trans* Retinoic Acid; All-*trans* Vitamin A Acid; ATRA; Ro 5488; tRA; Tretinoinum; Vesanoid

Pharmacologic Category Antineoplastic Agent, Retinoic Acid Derivative; Retinoic Acid Derivative

Use Induction of remission in patients with acute promyelocytic leukemia (APL), French American British (FAB) classification M3 (including the M3 variant) characterized by t(15;17) translocation and/or PML/RARα gene presence

Pregnancy Considerations Adverse events were observed in animal reproduction studies. **[U.S. Boxed Warning]: High risk of teratogenicity; if treatment with tretinoin is required in women of childbearing potential, two reliable forms of contraception should be used simultaneously during and for 1 month after treatment, unless abstinence is the chosen method. Within 1 week prior to starting therapy, serum or urine pregnancy test (sensitivity at least 50 milliunits/mL) should be collected. If possible, delay therapy until results are available. Repeat pregnancy testing and contraception counseling monthly throughout the period of treatment.** Contraception must be used even when there is a history of infertility or menopause, unless a hysterectomy has been preformed. Tretinoin was detected in the serum of a neonate at birth following maternal use of standard doses during pregnancy (Takitani, 2005). Use in humans for the treatment of acute promyelocytic leukemia (APL) is limited and exposure occurred after the first trimester in most cases (Valappil, 2007). However, major fetal abnormalities and spontaneous abortions have been reported with other retinoids; some of these abnormalities were fatal. If the clinical condition of a patient presenting with APL during pregnancy warrants immediate treatment, tretinoin use should be avoided in the first trimester; treatment with tretinoin may be considered in the second and third trimester with careful fetal monitoring, including cardiac monitoring (Sanz, 2009).

Breast-Feeding Considerations It is not known if tretinoin is excreted in breast milk. Due to the potential for serious adverse reactions in the nursing infant, breast-feeding should be discontinued prior to treatment initiation.

Contraindications Hypersensitivity to tretinoin, other retinoids, parabens, or any component of the formulation

Warnings/Precautions Hazardous agent: Use appropriate precautions for handling and disposal (NIOSH 2014 [group 3]).

[U.S. Boxed Warning]: About 25% of patients with APL treated with tretinoin have experienced APL differentiation syndrome (DS) (formerly called retinoic-acid-APL [RA-APL] syndrome), which is characterized by fever, dyspnea, acute respiratory distress, weight gain, radiographic pulmonary infiltrates and pleural or pericardial effusions, edema, and hepatic, renal, and/or multiorgan failure. DS usually occurs during the first month of treatment, with some cases reported following the first dose. DS has been observed with or without concomitant leukocytosis and has occasionally been accompanied by impaired myocardial contractility and episodic hypotension; endotracheal intubation and mechanical ventilation have been required in some cases due to progressive hypoxemia, and several patients have expired with multiorgan failure. About one-half of DS cases are severe, which is associated with increased mortality. Management has not been defined, although high-dose steroids given at the first suspicion appear to reduce morbidity and mortality. Regardless of the leukocyte count, at the first signs suggestive of DS, immediately initiate steroid therapy with dexamethasone 10 mg IV every 12 hours for 3-5 days; taper off over 2 weeks. Most patients do not require termination of tretinoin therapy during treatment of DS.

[U.S. Boxed Warning]: During treatment, ~40% of patients will develop rapidly evolving leukocytosis. A high WBC at diagnosis increases the risk for further leukocytosis and may be associated with a higher risk of life-threatening complications. If signs and symptoms of the APL-DS syndrome are present together with leukocytosis, initiate treatment with high-dose steroids immediately. Consider adding full-dose chemotherapy (including an anthracycline, if not contraindicated) to the tretinoin therapy on day 1 or 2 for patients presenting with a WBC count of >5 x 10^9/L. Consider adding chemotherapy immediately in patients who presented with a WBC count of <5 x 10^9/L, yet the WBC count reaches ≥6 x 10^9/L by day 5, or ≥10 x 10^9/L by day 10, or ≥15 x 10^9/L by day 28.

[U.S. Boxed Warning]: High risk of teratogenicity; if treatment with tretinoin is required in women of child-bearing potential, two reliable forms of contraception should be used during and for 1 month after treatment. Microdosed progesterone products ("minipill") may provide inadequate pregnancy protection. Repeat pregnancy testing and contraception counseling monthly throughout the period of treatment. If possible, initiation of treatment with tretinoin should be delayed until negative pregnancy test result is confirmed.

Retinoids have been associated with pseudotumor cerebri (benign intracranial hypertension), especially in children. Concurrent use of other drugs associated with this effect (eg, tetracyclines) may increase risk. Early signs and symptoms include papilledema, headache, nausea, vomiting, visual disturbances, intracranial noises, or pulsate tinnitus.

Up to 60% of patients experienced hypercholesterolemia or hypertriglyceridemia, which were reversible upon completion of treatment. Venous thrombosis and MI have been reported in patient without risk factors for thrombosis or MI; the risk for thrombosis (arterial and venous) is increased during the first month of treatment. Use with caution with antifibrinolytic agents; thrombotic complications have been reported (rarely) with concomitant use. Elevated liver function test results occur in 50% to 60% of patients during treatment. Carefully monitor liver function test results during treatment and give consideration to a temporary withdrawal of tretinoin if test results reach >5 times the upper limit of normal. Most liver function test abnormalities will resolve without interruption of treatment or after therapy completion. May cause headache, malaise, and/or dizziness; caution patients about performing tasks which require mental alertness (eg, operating machinery or driving). Effects may be potentiated when used with other sedative drugs or ethanol. Patients with APL are at high risk and can have severe adverse reactions to tretinoin.

[U.S. Boxed Warning]: Should be administered under the supervision of an experienced cancer chemotherapy physician. Tretinoin treatment for CPL should be initiated early, discontinue if pending cytogenetic analysis does not confirm APL by t(15;17) translocation or the presence of the PML/RARα fusion protein (caused by translocation of the promyelocytic [PML] gene on chromosome 15 and retinoic acid receptor [RAR] alpha gene on chromosome 17).

Tretinoin (which is also known as all-*trans* retinoic acid, or ATRA) and isotretinoin may be confused, while both products may be used in cancer treatment, they are **not** interchangeable; verify product prior to dispensing and administration to prevent medication errors.

Adverse Reactions Most patients will experience drug-related toxicity, especially headache, fever, weakness and fatigue. These are seldom permanent or irreversible and do not typically require therapy interruption.

>10%:

Cardiovascular: Peripheral edema (52%), chest discomfort (32%), edema (29%), arrhythmias (23%), flushing (23%), hypotension (14%), hypertension (11%)

Central nervous system: Headache (86%), fever (83%), malaise (66%), pain (37%), dizziness (20%), anxiety (17%), depression (14%), insomnia (14%), confusion (11%)

Dermatologic: Skin/mucous membrane dryness (77%), rash (54%), pruritus (20%), alopecia (14%), skin changes (14%)

Endocrine & metabolic: Hypercholesterolemia and/or hypertriglyceridemia (≤60%)

Gastrointestinal: Nausea/vomiting (57%), GI hemorrhage (34%), abdominal pain (31%), mucositis (26%), diarrhea (23%), weight gain (23%), anorexia (17%), constipation (17%), weight loss (17%), dyspepsia (14%), abdominal distention (11%)

Hematologic: Hemorrhage (60%), leukocytosis (40%), disseminated intravascular coagulation (DIC) (26%)

Hepatic: Liver function tests increased (50% to 60%)

Local: Phlebitis (11%)

Neuromuscular & skeletal: Bone pain (77%), paresthesia (17%), myalgia (14%)

Ocular: Ocular disorder (17%), visual disturbances (17%)

Otic: Earache/ear fullness (23%)

Renal: Renal insufficiency (11%)

Respiratory: Upper respiratory tract disorders (63%), dyspnea (60%), respiratory insufficiency (26%), pleural effusion (20%), expiratory wheezing (14%), pneumonia (14%), rales (14%)

Miscellaneous: Shivering (63%), infections (58%), retinoic acid-acute promyelocytic leukemia syndrome differentiation syndrome (≤25%), diaphoresis (20%)

1% to 10%:

Cardiovascular: Cerebral hemorrhage (9%), cardiac failure (6%), facial edema (6%), pallor (6%), cardiac arrest (3%), cardiomyopathy (3%), heart enlarged (3%), heart murmur (3%), ischemia (3%), MI (3%), myocarditis (3%), pericarditis (3%), stroke (3%)

Central nervous system: Agitation (9%), intracranial hypertension (9%), hallucination (6%), aphasia (3%), cerebellar edema (3%), CNS depression (3%), coma (3%), dementia (3%), encephalopathy (3%), facial paralysis (3%), forgetfulness (3%), hypotaxia (3%), hypothermia (3%), light reflex absent (3%), seizure (3%), slow speech (3%), somnolence (3%), spinal cord disorder (3%), unconsciousness (3%)

Dermatologic: Cellulitis (8%)

Endocrine & metabolic: Fluid imbalance (6%), acidosis (3%)

Gastrointestinal: Hepatosplenomegaly (9%), ulcer (3%)

Genitourinary: Dysuria (9%), micturition frequency (3%), prostate enlarged (3%)

Hepatic: Ascites (3%), hepatitis (3%)

Neuromuscular & skeletal: Flank pain (9%), abnormal gait (3%), asterixis (3%), bone inflammation (3%), dysarthria (3%), hemiplegia (3%), hyporeflexia (3%), leg weakness (3%), tremor (3%)

Ocular: Visual acuity change (6%), agnosia (3%), visual field deficit (3%)

Otic: Hearing loss (6%)

Renal: Acute renal failure (3%), renal tubular necrosis (3%)

Respiratory: Lower respiratory tract disorders (9%), pulmonary infiltration (6%), bronchial asthma (3%), larynx edema (3%), pulmonary hypertension (3%)

Miscellaneous: Lymph disorder (6%)

<1% (Limited to important or life-threatening): Arterial thrombosis, basophilia, erythema nodosum, genital ulceration, hypercalcemia, hyperhistaminemia, irreversible hearing loss, myositis, organomegaly, pancreatitis, pseudotumor cerebri, renal infarct, Sweet's syndrome, thrombocytosis, vasculitis (skin), venous thrombosis

◀ **Drug Interactions**

Metabolism/Transport Effects Substrate of CYP2A6 (minor), CYP2B6 (minor), CYP2C8 (major), CYP2C9 (minor); **Note:** Assignment of Major/Minor substrate status based on clinically relevant drug interaction potential; **Inhibits** CYP2C9 (weak); **Induces** CYP2E1 (weak/moderate)

Avoid Concomitant Use

Avoid concomitant use of Tretinoin (Systemic) with any of the following: BCG (Intravesical); Multivitamins/Fluoride (with ADE); Multivitamins/Minerals (with ADEK, Folate, Iron); Multivitamins/Minerals (with AE, No Iron); Natalizumab; Pimecrolimus; Tacrolimus (Topical); Tetracycline Derivatives; Tofacitinib; Vaccines (Live); Vitamin A

Increased Effect/Toxicity

Tretinoin (Systemic) may increase the levels/effects of: Amifostine; Antifibrinolytic Agents; Antipsychotic Agents (Second Generation [Atypical]); DULoxetine; Fingolimod; Hypotension-Associated Agents; Leflunomide; Levodopa; Natalizumab; Porfimer; Tofacitinib; Vaccines (Live); Verteporfin

The levels/effects of Tretinoin (Systemic) may be increased by: Abiraterone Acetate; Alfuzosin; Barbiturates; Blood Pressure Lowering Agents; Brimonidine (Topical); CYP2C8 Inhibitors (Moderate); CYP2C8 Inhibitors (Strong); Deferasirox; Denosumab; Diazoxide; Herbs (Hypotensive Properties); Lumacaftor; Mifepristone; Molsidomine; Multivitamins/Fluoride (with ADE); Multivitamins/Minerals (with ADEK, Folate, Iron); Multivitamins/Minerals (with AE, No Iron); Nicorandil; Obinutuzumab; Pentoxifylline; Phosphodiesterase 5 Inhibitors; Pimecrolimus; Prostacyclin Analogues; Roflumilast; Tacrolimus (Topical); Tetracycline Derivatives; Trastuzumab; Vitamin A

Decreased Effect

Tretinoin (Systemic) may decrease the levels/effects of: BCG (Intravesical); Coccidioides immitis Skin Test; Contraceptives (Estrogens); Contraceptives (Progestins); Sipuleucel-T; Vaccines (Inactivated); Vaccines (Live)

The levels/effects of Tretinoin (Systemic) may be decreased by: CYP2C8 Inducers (Strong); Dabrafenib; Echinacea; Lumacaftor

Food Interactions Absorption of retinoids has been shown to be enhanced when taken with food. Management: Administer with a meal.

Storage/Stability Store capsule at 20°C to 25°C (68°F to 77°F). Protect from light.

Mechanism of Action Tretinoin appears to bind one or more nuclear receptors and decreases proliferation and induces differentiation of APL cells; initially produces maturation of primitive promyelocytes and repopulates the marrow and peripheral blood with normal hematopoietic cells to achieve complete remission

Pharmacodynamics/Kinetics

Absorption: Well absorbed

Protein binding: >95%, predominantly to albumin

Metabolism: Hepatic via CYP; primary metabolite: 4-oxo-all-*trans*-retinoic acid; displays autometabolism

Half-life elimination: Terminal: Parent drug: 0.5-2 hours

Time to peak, serum: 1-2 hours

Excretion: Urine (63%); feces (30%)

Dosing

Adult & Geriatric Details concerning dosing in combination regimens should also be consulted. **Note:** Induction treatment of APL with tretinoin should be initiated early; discontinue if pending cytogenetic analysis does not confirm t(15;17) translocation or the presence of the PML/RARα fusion protein.

Acute promyelocytic leukemia (APL): Oral:

Remission induction (in combination with an anthracycline ± cytarabine; off-label use): 45 mg/m²/day in 2 equally divided doses until complete remission or 90 days (Powell, 2010) or until complete hematologic remission (Ades, 2008; Sanz, 2008; Sanz, 2010)

Remission induction (in combination with arsenic trioxide; off-label use): 45 mg/m²/day in 2 equally divided doses until <5% blasts in marrow and no abnormal promyelocytes or up to 85 days (Estey, 2006; Ravandi, 2009)

Consolidation therapy (off-label use): 45 mg/m²/day in 2 equally divided doses for 15 days each month for 3 months (in combination with chemotherapy) (Lo-Coco, 2010; Sanz 2010) **or** 45 mg/m²/day for 14 days every 4 weeks for 7 cycles (in combination with arsenic trioxide) (Ravandi, 2009)

Maintenance therapy, intermediate- and high-risk patients (off-label use): 45 mg/m²/day in 2 equally divided doses for 15 days every 3 months for 2 years (Sanz, 2004)

Pediatric Details concerning dosing in combination regimens should also be consulted. **Note:** Induction treatment of APL with tretinoin should be initiated early; discontinue if pending cytogenetic analysis does not confirm t(15;17) translocation or the presence of the PML/RARα fusion protein.

Acute promyelocytic leukemia (APL): Oral:

Remission induction: 45 mg/m²/day in 2 equally divided doses until documentation of complete remission (CR); discontinue 30 days after CR or after 90 days of treatment, whichever occurs first

Remission induction (in combination with an anthracycline; off-label use): 25 mg/m²/day in 2 equally divided doses until complete remission or 90 days (Ortega, 2005)

Consolidation therapy, intermediate- and high-risk patients (off-label use): 25 mg/m²/day in 2 equally divided doses for 15 days each month for 3 months (Ortega, 2005)

Maintenance therapy, intermediate- and high-risk patients (off-label use): 25 mg/m²/day in 2 equally divided doses for 15 days every 3 months for 2 years (Ortega, 2005)

Renal Impairment No dosage adjustment provided in the manufacturer's labeling (has not been studied).

Hepatic Impairment No dosage adjustment provided in the manufacturer's labeling (has not been studied).

Obesity *ASCO Guidelines for appropriate chemotherapy dosing in obese adults with cancer:* Utilize patient's actual body weight (full weight) for calculation of body surface area- or weight-based dosing, particularly when the intent of therapy is curative; manage regimen-related toxicities in the same manner as for nonobese patients; if a dose reduction is utilized due to toxicity, consider resumption of full weight-based dosing with subsequent cycles, especially if cause of toxicity (eg, hepatic or renal impairment) is resolved (Griggs, 2012).

Adjustment for Toxicity

APL differentiation syndrome: Initiate dexamethasone 10 mg IV every 12 hours for 3-5 days; consider interrupting tretinoin until resolution of hypoxia

Liver function tests >5 times the upper limit of normal: Consider temporarily withholding treatment

Dietary Considerations The absorption of retinoids (as a class) is enhanced when taken with food. Capsule contains soybean oil.

Administration Administer orally with a meal; do not crush capsules.

Although the manufacturer does not recommend the use of the capsule contents to extemporaneously prepare tretinoin suspension, there are limited case reports of use in patients who are unable to swallow the capsules whole. In a patient with a nasogastric (NG) tube, tretinoin capsules were cut open, with partial aspiration of the contents into a glass syringe, the residual capsule contents were mixed with soy bean oil and aspirated into the same syringe and administered (Shaw, 1995). Tretinoin capsules have also been mixed with sterile water (~20 mL) and heated in a water bath (37°C) to melt the capsules and create an oily suspension for NG tube administration (Bargetzi, 1996). Tretinoin has also been administered sublingually by squeezing the capsule contents beneath the tongue (Kueh, 1999). Low plasma concentrations have been reported when tretinoin has been administered through a feeding tube, although patient-specific impaired absorption or a lack of excipient (eg, soybean oil) may have been a contributing factor (Takitani, 2004).

Hazardous agent - use appropriate precautions for handling and disposal (NIOSH 2014 [group 3]).

Monitoring Parameters Bone marrow cytology to confirm t(15;17) translocation or the presence of the PML/RARα fusion protein (do not withhold treatment initiation for results); monitor CBC with differential, coagulation profile, liver function test results, and triglyceride and cholesterol levels frequently; monitor closely for signs of APL differentiation syndrome (eg, monitor volume status, pulmonary status, temperature, respiration)

Dosage Forms Excipient information presented when available (limited, particularly for generics); consult specific product labeling.

Capsule, Oral:

Generic: 10 mg

Extemporaneous Preparations Hazardous agent: Use appropriate precautions for handling and disposal (NIOSH 2014 [group 3]).

Although the manufacturer does not recommend the use of the capsule contents to extemporaneously prepare a suspension of tretinoin (due to reports of low plasma levels) (Vesanoid® data on file), there are limited case reports of use in patients who are unable to swallow the capsules whole. In a patient with a nasogastric (NG) tube,

tretinoin capsules were cut open, with partial aspiration of the contents aspirated into a glass syringe. The residual capsule contents were mixed with soybean oil, aspirated into the syringe, and administered (Shaw, 1995). Tretinoin capsules have also been mixed with sterile water (~20 mL) and heated in a water bath to melt the capsules and create an oily suspension for NG tube administration (Bargetzi, 1996). Tretinoin has also been administered sublingually by squeezing the capsule contents beneath the tongue (Kueh, 1999).

Bargetzi MJ, Tichelli A, Gratwohl A, et al, "Oral All-Transretinoic Acid Administration in Intubated Patients With Acute Promyelocytic Leukemia," *Schweiz Med Wochenschr*, 1996, 126(45):1944-5.

Kueh YK, Liew PP, Ho PC, et al, "Sublingual Administration of All-*Trans*-Retinoic Acid to a Comatose Patient With Acute Promyelocytic Leukemia," *Ann Pharmacother*, 1999, 33(4):503-5.

Shaw PJ, Atkins MC, Nath CE, et al, "ATRA Administration in the Critically Ill Patient," *Leukemia*, 1995, 9(7):1288.

Vesanoid® data on file, Roche Pharmaceuticals

Tretinoin (Topical) (TRET i noyn)

Brand Names: US Atralin; Avita; Refissa; Renova; Renova Pump; Retin-A; Retin-A Micro; Retin-A Micro Pump; Tretin-X

Brand Names: Canada Retin-A; Retin-A Micro; Stieva-A; Vitamin A Acid

Index Terms *trans*-Retinoic Acid; Retinoic Acid; Vitamin A Acid

Pharmacologic Category Acne Products; Retinoic Acid Derivative; Topical Skin Product, Acne

Use

Acne vulgaris: Atralin, Avita, Retin-A, Retin-A Micro, Stieva-A [Canadian product], Tretin-X, Vitamin-A Acid [Canadian product]: Treatment of acne vulgaris.

Limitations of use (Stieva-A [Canadian product]): In most cases, use is not effective for the treatment of severe pustular and deep cystic nodular acne.

Palliation of fine wrinkles: Renova: Adjunctive treatment for mitigation (palliation) of fine wrinkles in patients who use comprehensive skin care and sun avoidance programs.

Palliation of fine wrinkles, mottled hyperpigmentation, and facial skin roughness: Refissa: Adjunctive treatment for mitigation (palliation) of fine wrinkles, mottled hyperpigmentation, and tactile roughness of facial skin in patients who do not achieve such palliation using comprehensive skin care and sun avoidance programs alone.

Dosing

Adult

Acne vulgaris: Topical:

US labeling: Apply once daily to acne lesions before bedtime or in the evening.

Canadian labeling: Initial: Apply once daily to affected area before bedtime (in clinical trials therapy lasted up to 12 weeks). May consider less frequent application or using a reduced strength during the first few weeks of treatment if needed (eg, patients with sensitive and/or fair complexion, exacerbation of acne or skin irritation). Interrupt therapy if necessary for skin irritation; may resume therapy after subsides. Discontinue therapy for persistent irritation. Maintenance: Upon satisfactory response may consider less frequent application.

Palliation of fine wrinkles (Refissa/Renova), mottled hyperpigmentation, and tactile roughness of facial skin (Refissa): Topical: Apply a pea-sized amount of cream to entire face once daily in the evening or before bedtime.

Geriatric Refer to adult dosing; safety/efficacy of Refissa has not been established in patients >50 years of age; safety/efficacy of Renova has not been established in patients >71 years of age.

Pediatric Acne vulgaris: Children ≥10 years (Atralin only) or Children ≥12 years and Adolescents: Topical: Refer to adult dosing.

Renal Impairment There are no dosage adjustments provided in the manufacturer's labeling. Stieva-A [Canadian product] labeling indicates that there are no dosage adjustments necessary.

Hepatic Impairment There are no dosage adjustments provided in the manufacturer's labeling. Stieva-A [Canadian product] labeling indicates that there are no dosage adjustments necessary.

Additional Information Complete prescribing information should be consulted for additional detail.

Dosage Forms Excipient information presented when available (limited, particularly for generics); consult specific product labeling.

Cream, External:

Avita: 0.025% (20 g, 45 g)

Refissa: 0.05% (20 g, 40 g) [contains edetate disodium, methylparaben, propylparaben]

Renova: 0.02% (40 g, 60 g) [contains benzyl alcohol, cetyl alcohol, edetate disodium, methylparaben, propylparaben]

Renova Pump: 0.02% (44 g) [contains benzyl alcohol, cetyl alcohol, edetate disodium, methylparaben, propylparaben]

Retin-A: 0.025% (20 g, 45 g); 0.05% (20 g, 45 g); 0.1% (20 g, 45 g)

Tretin-X: 0.0375% (35 g); 0.075% (35 g)

Generic: 0.025% (20 g, 45 g); 0.05% (20 g, 40 g, 45 g, 60 g)); 0.1% (20 g, 45 g)

Gel, External:

Atralin: 0.05% (45 g) [contains benzyl alcohol, butylparaben, ethylparaben, fish collagen hydrolyzates, isobutylparaben, methylparaben, propylparaben, trolamine (triethanolamine)]

Avita: 0.025% (20 g, 45 g)

Retin-A: 0.01% (15 g, 45 g); 0.025% (15 g, 45 g)

Retin-A Micro: 0.04% (20 g, 45 g); 0.1% (20 g, 45 g) [contains benzyl alcohol, disodium edta, propylene glycol, trolamine (triethanolamine)]

Retin-A Micro Pump: 0.04% (50 g); 0.08% (50 g); 0.1% (50 g) [contains benzyl alcohol, disodium edta, propylene glycol, trolamine (triethanolamine)]

Generic: 0.01% (15 g, 45 g); 0.025% (15 g, 45 g); 0.04% (20 g, 45 g, 50 g); 0.05% (45 g); 0.1% (20 g, 45 g, 50 g)

Kit, External:

Tretin-X: 0.025%, 0.05%, 0.1% [contains benzyl alcohol, cetearyl alcohol, disodium edta, fd&c red #40, methylparaben, propylparaben, tartrazine (fd&c yellow #5), trolamine (triethanolamine)]

Dosage Forms: Canada Excipient information presented when available (limited, particularly for generics); consult specific product labeling.

Cream, External:

Retin-A: 0.01% (30 g); 0.025% (30 g); 0.05% (30 g); 0.1% (30 g)

Stieva-A: 0.01%, 0.025%, 0.05%, (25 g, 45 g); 0.1% (45 g)

Gel, External:

Retin-A: 0.01% (30 g); 0.025% (30 g)

Retin-A Micro Pump: 0.04% (20 g, 45 g); 0.1% (50 g) [contains benzyl alcohol, disodium edta, propylene glycol, trolamine (triethanolamine)]

Vitamin A Acid: 0.01% (25 g); 0.025% (25 g), 0.05% (25 g) [contains isopropyl alcohol, tetrasodium edta, propylene glycol, trolamine (triethanolamine), methylparaben, propylparaben]

◆ **Tretinoinum** *see* Tretinoin (Systemic) *on page 1838*

◆ **Trexall** *see* Methotrexate *on page 1169*

◆ **Treximet** *see* Sumatriptan and Naproxen *on page 1720*

◆ **Triacetyluridine** *see* Uridine Triacetate *on page 1854*

◆ **Triaconazole** *see* Terconazole *on page 1763*

◆ **Triaderm (Can)** *see* Triamcinolone (Topical) *on page 1843*

Triamcinolone (Systemic) (trye am SIN oh lone)

Brand Names: US Aristospan Intra-Articular; Aristospan Intralesional; Kenalog; Pro-C-Dure 5; Pro-C-Dure 6

Brand Names: Canada Aristospan

Index Terms Triamcinolone Acetonide, Parenteral; Triamcinolone Hexacetonide

Pharmacologic Category Corticosteroid, Systemic

Additional Appendix Information

Corticosteroids Systemic Equivalencies *on page 1950*

Use

Intra-articular (soft tissue): Acute gouty arthritis, acute/subacute bursitis, acute tenosynovitis, epicondylitis, rheumatoid arthritis, synovitis of osteoarthritis

Intralesional: Alopecia areata, discoid lupus erythematosus, keloids, granuloma annulare lesions (localized hypertrophic, infiltrated, or inflammatory), lichen planus plaques, lichen simplex chronicus plaques, psoriatic plaques, necrobiosis lipoidica diabeticorum, cystic tumors of aponeurosis or tendon (ganglia)

Systemic: Adrenocortical insufficiency, dermatologic diseases, endocrine disorders, gastrointestinal diseases, hematologic and neoplastic disorders, nervous system disorders, nephrotic syndrome, rheumatic disorders, allergic states, respiratory diseases, systemic lupus erythematosus (SLE), and other diseases requiring anti-inflammatory or immunosuppressive effects

Dosing

Adult & Geriatric The lowest possible dose should be used to control the condition; when dose reduction is possible, the dose should be reduced gradually.

Dermatoses (steroid-responsive, including contact/atopic dermatitis): Injection:

Acetonide: Intradermal: Initial: 1 mg

Hexacetonide: Intralesional, sublesional: Up to 0.5 mg/square inch of affected skin; range: 2 to 48 mg/day

Hay fever/pollen asthma: IM: 40 to 100 mg as a single injection/season

Multiple sclerosis (acute exacerbation): IM: 160 mg daily for 1 week, followed by 64 mg every other day for 1 month

Rheumatic or arthritic disorders:

Intra-articular (or similar injection as designated):

Acetonide: Intra-articular, intrabursal, tendon sheaths: Initial: Smaller joints: 2.5 to 5 mg, larger joints: 5 to 15 mg; may require up to 10 mg for small joints and up to 40 mg for large joints; maximum dose/treatment (several joints at one time): 20 to 80 mg

Hexacetonide: Intra-articular: Average dose: 2 to 20 mg; smaller joints: 2 to 6 mg; larger joints: 10 to 20 mg. Frequency of injection into a single joint is every 3 to 4 weeks as necessary; to avoid possible joint destruction use as infrequently as possible.

IM: Acetonide: Range: 2.5 to 100 mg/day; Initial: 60 mg See table.

Triamcinolone Dosing

	Acetonide	Hexacetonide
Intrasynovial	5-40 mg	
Intralesional	1-30 mg (usually 1 mg per injection site); 10 mg/mL suspension usually used	Up to 0.5 mg/sq inch affected area
Sublesional	1-30 mg	
Systemic IM	2.5-60 mg/dose (usual adult dose: 60 mg; may repeat with 20-100 mg dose when symptoms recur)	
Intra-articular	2.5-40 mg	2-20 mg average
large joints	5-15 mg	10-20 mg
small joints	2.5-5 mg	2-6 mg
Tendon sheaths	2.5-10 mg	
Intradermal	1 mg/site	

Pediatric Rheumatic conditions: *IM (acetonide):*

Range: 2.5 to 100 mg/day

Children: Initial: 0.11 to 1.6 mg/kg/day in 3 to 4 divided doses

Children 6 to 12 years: Initial: 40 mg

Children ≥12 years: Refer to adult dosing.

Renal Impairment No dosage adjustment provided in the manufacturer's labeling; use with caution.

Hepatic Impairment No dosage adjustment provided in the manufacturer's labeling.

Additional Information Complete prescribing information should be consulted for additional detail.

Dosage Forms Excipient information presented when available (limited, particularly for generics); consult specific product labeling.

Kit, Injection, as acetonide:

Pro-C-Dure 5: 40 mg/mL (2 x 1 mL) [contains benzyl alcohol, polysorbate 80]

Pro-C-Dure 6: 40 mg/mL (3 x 1 mL) [contains benzyl alcohol, polysorbate 80]

Suspension, Injection, as acetonide:

Kenalog: 10 mg/mL (5 mL); 40 mg/mL (1 mL, 5 mL, 10 mL) [contains benzyl alcohol, polysorbate 80]

Suspension, Injection, as hexacetonide:

Aristospan Intra-Articular: 20 mg/mL (1 mL, 5 mL) [contains benzyl alcohol]

Aristospan Intralesional: 5 mg/mL (5 mL) [contains benzyl alcohol]

Triamcinolone (Nasal) (trye am SIN oh lone)

Brand Names: US Nasacort Allergy 24HR Children [OTC]; Nasacort Allergy 24HR [OTC]; Nasacort AQ; Nasal Allergy 24 Hour [OTC]

Brand Names: Canada Nasacort Allergy 24HR; Nasacort AQ

Index Terms Triamcinolone Acetonide

Pharmacologic Category Corticosteroid, Nasal

Use

Allergic rhinitis:

US labeling:

Rx: Management of seasonal and perennial allergic rhinitis in adults and children 2 years and older

OTC: For the relief of hay fever and other upper respiratory allergies (eg, nasal congestion, runny nose, sneezing, itchy nose) in adults and children 2 years and older

Canadian labeling:

Rx: Management of seasonal and perennial allergic rhinitis unresponsive to conventional treatment in children 4 to 12 years

OTC: Management of seasonal and perennial allergic rhinitis in adults and children 12 years and older

Dosing

Adult & Geriatric

Allergic rhinitis: Intranasal:

US labeling: Two sprays (110 mcg) in each nostril once daily; once symptoms controlled reduce to 1 spray (55 mcg) in each nostril once daily (maximum: 2 sprays [110 mcg] in each nostril once daily). Discontinue therapy if adequate symptomatic relief is not observed within 3 weeks (1 week for OTC use).

Canadian labeling: Two sprays (110 mcg) in each nostril once daily; once symptoms controlled reduce to 1 spray (55 mcg) in each nostril once daily (maximum: 2 sprays [110 mcg] in each nostril once daily). Discontinue therapy if significant symptomatic relief is not observed within 1 week (for OTC use)

Pediatric

Allergic rhinitis: Intranasal:

US labeling: **Note:** Discontinue therapy if adequate symptomatic relief is not observed within 3 weeks (1 week for OTC use).

Children 2 to <6 years: One spray (55 mcg) in each nostril once daily (maximum: 1 spray [55 mcg] in each nostril once daily

Children 6 to <12 years: Initial: One spray (55 mcg) in each nostril once daily; may increase to 2 sprays (110 mcg) in each nostril once daily if response not adequate; once symptoms controlled may reduce to 1 spray (55 mcg) in each nostril once daily (maximum: 2 sprays [110 mcg] in each nostril once daily)

Children ≥12 years and Adolescents: Refer to adult dosing.

Canadian labeling:

Children 4 to <12 years: Initial: One spray (55 mcg) in each nostril once daily; may increase to 2 sprays (110 mcg) in each nostril once daily if response not adequate; once symptoms controlled may reduce to 1 spray (55 mcg) in each nostril once daily (maximum: 2 sprays [110 mcg] in each nostril once daily). Discontinue therapy if significant symptomatic relief is not observed within 3 weeks.

Children ≥12 years and Adolescents: Refer to adult dosing.

Renal Impairment There are no dosage adjustments provided in the manufacturer's labeling (has not been studied).

Hepatic Impairment There are no dosage adjustments provided in the manufacturer's labeling (has not been studied).

Additional Information Complete prescribing information should be consulted for additional detail.

Dosage Forms Considerations Nasacort AQ 16.5 g bottles contain 120 sprays.

Dosage Forms Excipient information presented when available (limited, particularly for generics); consult specific product labeling.

Aerosol, Nasal, as acetonide:

Nasacort Allergy 24HR: 55 mcg/actuation (10.8 mL, 16.9 mL) [contains benzalkonium chloride, edetate disodium, polysorbate 80]

Nasacort Allergy 24HR Children: 55 mcg/actuation (10.8 mL) [contains benzalkonium chloride, edetate disodium, polysorbate 80]

Nasacort AQ: 55 mcg/actuation (16.5 g)

Nasal Allergy 24 Hour: 55 mcg/actuation (16.9 mL) [contains benzalkonium chloride, edetate disodium, polysorbate 80]

Generic: 55 mcg/actuation (16.5 g)

Triamcinolone (Ophthalmic) (trye am SIN oh lone)

Brand Names: US Triesence

Index Terms Triamcinolone acetonide

Pharmacologic Category Corticosteroid, Ophthalmic

Use

Intravitreal: Treatment of sympathetic ophthalmia, temporal arteritis, uveitis, ocular inflammatory conditions unresponsive to topical corticosteroids

Triesence™: Visualization during vitrectomy

Dosing

Adult & Geriatric

Ocular disease: Intravitreal: Initial: 4 mg as a single dose; additional doses may be given as needed

Visualization during vitrectomy: Intravitreal (Triesence™): 1-4 mg

Pediatric Ocular disease/visualization during vitrectomy: Refer to adult dosing.

Renal Impairment No dosage adjustment provided in the manufacturer's labeling.

Hepatic Impairment No dosage adjustment provided in the manufacturer's labeling.

Additional Information Complete prescribing information should be consulted for additional detail.

Dosage Forms Excipient information presented when available (limited, particularly for generics); consult specific product labeling.

Suspension, Intraocular, as acetonide:
Triesence: 40 mg/mL (1 mL) [contains polysorbate 80]

Triamcinolone (Topical) (trye am SIN oh lone)

Brand Names: US Dermasorb TA; Kenalog; Oralone; Pediaderm TA; Trianex; Triderm
Brand Names: Canada Kenalog; Oracort; Triaderm
Pharmacologic Category Corticosteroid, Topical
Additional Appendix Information
Topical Corticosteroids on page 1952

Use

Dermatoses (corticosteroid-responsive): Topical: Relief of inflammatory and pruritic manifestations of corticosteroid-responsive dermatoses.

Oral inflammatory and ulcerative lesions: Oral paste: Adjunctive treatment and temporary relief of symptoms associated with oral inflammatory and ulcerative lesions resulting from trauma

Dosing

Adult

Dermatoses (corticosteroid-responsive): Topical:
Note: Frequency of application based upon severity of condition

Cream, ointment: Apply thin film to affected areas 2 to 4 times daily

Lotion:
0.025%: Apply a thin film to affected area 3 to 4 times daily
0.1%: Apply a thin film to affected area 2 to 4 times daily

Aerosol solution: Apply to affected area 3 to 4 times daily

Oral inflammatory and ulcerative lesions: Oral paste: Press a small amount (about ¼ inch) to the lesion at bedtime; a larger quantity may be required for coverage of some lesions. For severe lesions, may be used 2 or 3 times daily after meals.

Geriatric Refer to adult dosing. Use the lowest effective dose.

Pediatric Dermatoses (corticosteroid-responsive): Children and Adolescents: Topical: **Note:** Frequency based upon severity of condition: Cream, ointment, lotion, aerosol solution: Refer to adult dosing.

Renal Impairment There are no dosage adjustments provided in the manufacturer's labeling.

Hepatic Impairment There are no dosage adjustments provided in the manufacturer's labeling.

Additional Information Complete prescribing information should be consulted for additional detail.

Dosage Forms Excipient information presented when available (limited, particularly for generics); consult specific product labeling. [DSC] = Discontinued product

Aerosol Solution, External, as acetonide:
Kenalog: 0.147 mg/g (63 g, 100 g)
Generic: 0.147 mg/g (63 g, 100 g)

Cream, External, as acetonide:
Triderm: 0.1% (28.4 g, 85.2 g) [contains propylene glycol]
Generic: 0.025% (15 g, 80 g, 454 g); 0.1% (15 g, 30 g, 80 g, 453.6 g, 454 g); 0.5% (15 g)

Kit, External, as acetonide:
Dermasorb TA: 0.1% [contains cetyl alcohol, milk protein, propylene glycol]
Pediaderm TA: 0.1% [contains cetyl alcohol, methylparaben, polysorbate 80, propylene glycol, propylparaben]

Lotion, External, as acetonide:
Generic: 0.025% (60 mL); 0.1% (60 mL)

Ointment, External, as acetonide:
Trianex: 0.05% (17 g [DSC], 85 g [DSC], 430 g)
Generic: 0.025% (15 g, 80 g, 454 g); 0.1% (15 g, 80 g, 453.6 g, 454 g); 0.5% (15 g)
Paste, Mouth/Throat, as acetonide:
Oralone: 0.1% (5 g)
Generic: 0.1% (5 g)

◆ Triamcinolone Acetonide see Triamcinolone (Nasal) on page 1842

◆ Triamcinolone acetonide see Triamcinolone (Ophthalmic) on page 1842

◆ Triamcinolone Acetonide, Parenteral see Triamcinolone (Systemic) on page 1841

◆ Triamcinolone and Nystatin see Nystatin and Triamcinolone on page 1305

◆ Triamcinolone Hexacetonide see Triamcinolone (Systemic) on page 1841

◆ Triaminic Allerchews [OTC] see Loratadine on page 1101

◆ Triaminic Childrens Allergy [OTC] [DSC] see DiphenhydrAMINE (Systemic) on page 561

◆ Triaminic® Children's Chest & Nasal Congestion [OTC] see Guaifenesin and Phenylephrine on page 862

◆ Triaminic Children's Fever Reducer Pain Reliever [OTC] see Acetaminophen on page 25

◆ Triaminic® Children's Night Time Cold & Cough [OTC] see Diphenhydramine and Phenylephrine on page 564

◆ Triaminic® Children's Softchews® Cough & Runny Nose [OTC] see Dextromethorphan and Chlorpheniramine on page 534

◆ Triaminic® Cold & Allergy (Can) see Chlorpheniramine and Pseudoephedrine on page 377

◆ Triaminic Cold/Allergy Child [OTC] see Chlorpheniramine and Phenylephrine on page 376

◆ Triaminic Cough & Congestion [OTC] see Guaifenesin and Dextromethorphan on page 861

◆ Triaminic Cough/Runny Nose [OTC] see DiphenhydrAMINE (Systemic) on page 561

◆ Triaminic® Day Time Cold & Cough [OTC] see Dextromethorphan and Phenylephrine on page 535

Triamterene (trye AM ter een)

Brand Names: US Dyrenium
Pharmacologic Category Antihypertensive; Diuretic, Potassium-Sparing
Use Edema: For the treatment of edema associated with congestive heart failure, cirrhosis of the liver and the nephrotic syndrome; also in steroid-induced edema, idiopathic edema and edema due to secondary hyperaldosteronism.

Dosing

Adult

Edema: Oral: 100 to 300 mg daily in 1 to 2 divided doses; maximum dose: 300 mg daily

Prevention of antihypertensive diuretic-induced hypokalemia (off-label use): Oral: Usual dose (ASH/ISH [Weber, 2014]): 100 mg daily

Geriatric Refer to adult dosing. In the management of hypertension, consider lower initial doses and titrate to response (Aronow, 2011).

Pediatric Hypertension (off-label use): Oral: Initial: 1 to 2 mg/kg/day in 2 divided doses; maximum: 3 to 4 mg/kg/day, up to 300 mg daily (NHLBI, 2004)

Renal Impairment

Mild-to-moderate impairment: No dosage adjustment provided in manufacturer's labeling.

Severe impairment or progressive kidney disease: Use is contraindicated.

The following adjustments have also been recommended (Aronoff, 2007); **Note:** Renal function may be estimated using the Cockcroft-Gault formula for dosage adjustment purposes: Adults:
CrCl >50 mL/minute: No dosage adjustment necessary.
CrCl ≤50 mL/minute: Use not recommended.

Hepatic Impairment

Mild-to-moderate impairment: No dosage adjustment provided in manufacturer's labeling (has not been studied).
Severe hepatic disease: Use is contraindicated.

Additional Information Complete prescribing information should be consulted for additional detail.

Dosage Forms Excipient information presented when available (limited, particularly for generics); consult specific product labeling.
Capsule, Oral:
Dyrenium: 50 mg [contains fd&c yellow #6 (sunset yellow)]
Dyrenium: 100 mg

◆ **Triamterene and Hydrochlorothiazide** see Hydrochlorothiazide and Triamterene on page 884

◆ **Trianex** see Triamcinolone (Topical) on page 1843

Triazolam (trye AY zoe lam)

Brand Names: US Halcion
Pharmacologic Category Benzodiazepine
Use Insomnia: Short-term (generally 7 to 10 days) treatment of insomnia
Medication Guide Available Yes
Dosing
Adult
Insomnia (short-term use): Usual dose: 0.25 mg at bedtime; 0.125 mg at bedtime may be sufficient in some patients, such as those with low body weight; maximum dose: 0.5 mg daily
Dental preprocedure oral sedation (off-label use): 0.25 mg 1 hour before procedure; 0.125 mg used for elderly patients or patients sensitive to sedative effects (Dionne, 2006)
Geriatric Elderly and/or debilitated patients: Insomnia (short-term use): Oral: Initial: 0.125 mg at bedtime; maximum dose: 0.25 mg daily
Renal Impairment There are no dosage adjustments provided in the manufacturer's labeling; use with caution.
Hepatic Impairment There are no dosage adjustments provided in the manufacturer's labeling; use with caution.
Additional Information Complete prescribing information should be consulted for additional detail.
Dosage Forms Excipient information presented when available (limited, particularly for generics); consult specific product labeling.
Tablet, Oral:
Halcion: 0.25 mg [scored]
Generic: 0.125 mg, 0.25 mg
Controlled Substance C-IV

◆ **Tribavirin** see Ribavirin (Oral Inhalation) on page 1578

◆ **Tribavirin** see Ribavirin (Systemic) on page 1574

◆ **Tribenzor™** see Olmesartan, Amlodipine, and Hydrochlorothiazide on page 1321

◆ **Tri-Buffered Aspirin [OTC]** see Aspirin on page 157

◆ **Tricira Lo (Can)** see Ethinyl Estradiol and Norgestimate on page 710

◆ **Tricode GF** see Guaifenesin, Pseudoephedrine, and Codeine on page 863

◆ **Tricor** see Fenofibrate and Derivatives on page 746

◆ **Tricosal** see Choline Magnesium Trisalicylate on page 382

◆ **Tri-Cyclen (Can)** see Ethinyl Estradiol and Norgestimate on page 710

◆ **Tri-Cyclen Lo (Can)** see Ethinyl Estradiol and Norgestimate on page 710

◆ **Triderm** see Triamcinolone (Topical) on page 1843

◆ **Tridesilon (Can)** see Desonide on page 523

◆ **Tridil** see Nitroglycerin on page 1289

◆ **Tridural (Can)** see TraMADol on page 1821

◆ **Trien** see Trientine on page 1844

Trientine (TRYE en teen)

Brand Names: US Syprine
Brand Names: Canada Syprine®
Index Terms 2,2,2-tetramine; Trien; Trientine Hydrochloride; Triethylene Tetramine Dihydrochloride
Pharmacologic Category Chelating Agent
Use Treatment of Wilson's disease in patients intolerant to penicillamine
Dosing
Adult & Geriatric Wilson's disease: Oral: 750-1250 mg/day in divided doses 2-4 times/day; maximum dose: 2 g/day. AASLD practice guidelines suggest typical doses of 750-1500 mg/day in 2-3 divided doses with maintenance therapy of 750-1000 mg/day (Roberts, 2008).

Pediatric Wilson's disease: Oral:
Children <12 years: 500-750 mg/day in divided doses 2-4 times/day; maximum: 1.5 g/day. AASLD practice guidelines suggest 20 mg/kg/day rounded off to the nearest 250 mg, given in 2-3 divided doses (Roberts, 2008).
Children ≥12 years: Refer to adult dosing.
Renal Impairment No dosage adjustment provided in manufacturer's labeling.
Hepatic Impairment No dosage adjustment provided in manufacturer's labeling.
Additional Information Complete prescribing information should be consulted for additional detail.
Dosage Forms Excipient information presented when available (limited, particularly for generics); consult specific product labeling.
Capsule, Oral, as hydrochloride:
Syprine: 250 mg

◆ **Trientine Hydrochloride** see Trientine on page 1844

◆ **Triesence** see Triamcinolone (Ophthalmic) on page 1842

◆ **Tri-Estarylla** see Ethinyl Estradiol and Norgestimate on page 710

◆ **Triethylene Tetramine Dihydrochloride** see Trientine on page 1844

◆ **Triethylenethiophosphoramide** see Thiotepa on page 1783

Trifluoperazine (trye floo oh PER a zeen)

Index Terms Stelazine; Trifluoperazine Hydrochloride
Pharmacologic Category First Generation (Typical) Antipsychotic
Use
Nonpsychotic anxiety: Short-term treatment of generalized nonpsychotic anxiety.
Schizophrenia: Management of schizophrenia.
Dosing
Adult
Nonpsychotic anxiety: Oral: 1 or 2 mg twice daily; titrate dose gradually based on response and tolerability; maximum: 6 mg/day; therapy for anxiety should not exceed 12 weeks; do not exceed 6 mg/day for longer than 12 weeks when treating anxiety because of risks for tardive dyskinesia
Schizophrenia: Oral: Initial: 2 to 5 mg twice daily; titrate dose gradually based on response and tolerability; usual dosage: 15 or 20 mg/day in divided doses although some patients may require up to 50 mg/day (APA [Lehman 2004])
Geriatric Refer to adult dosing. Dose selection should start at the low end of the dosage range and titration must be gradual.
Pediatric
Schizophrenia:
Children 6 to 12 years: Oral: Initial: 1 mg once or twice daily; titrate dose gradually based on response and tolerability. It is usually not necessary to exceed 15 mg/day; however, older children with severe symptoms may require higher doses.
Adolescents: Refer to adult dosing.
Renal Impairment There are no dosage adjustments provided in the manufacturer's labeling.
Hepatic Impairment There are no dosage adjustments provided in the manufacturer's labeling; use is contraindicated in patients with hepatic disease.
Additional Information Complete prescribing information should be consulted for additional detail.
Dosage Forms Excipient information presented when available (limited, particularly for generics); consult specific product labeling.
Tablet, Oral:
Generic: 1 mg, 2 mg, 5 mg, 10 mg
Dosage Forms: Canada Note: Refer also to Dosage Forms. Excipient information presented when available (limited, particularly for generics); consult specific product labeling.
Tablet, Oral: 20 mg

◆ **Trifluoperazine Hydrochloride** see Trifluoperazine on page 1844

◆ **Trifluorothymidine** see Trifluridine on page 1844

Trifluridine (trye FLURE i deen)

Brand Names: US Viroptic
Brand Names: Canada Sandoz-Trifluridine; Viroptic®
Index Terms F_3T; Trifluorothymidine
Pharmacologic Category Antiviral Agent, Ophthalmic

Use Treatment of primary keratoconjunctivitis and recurrent epithelial keratitis caused by herpes simplex virus types I and II

Dosing

Adult & Geriatric Herpes keratoconjunctivitis, keratitis: Ophthalmic: Instill 1 drop into affected eye every 2 hours while awake, to a maximum of 9 drops daily, until re-epithelialization of corneal ulcer occurs; then use 1 drop every 4 hours while awake for another 7 days (minimum daily dosage of 5 drops is recommended). Do **not** exceed 21 days of treatment; if improvement has not taken place in 7-14 days, consider another form of therapy

Pediatric Children ≥6 years and Adolescents: Ophthalmic: Refer to adult dosing.

Renal Impairment No dosage adjustment provided in manufacturer's labeling.

Hepatic Impairment No dosage adjustment provided in manufacturer's labeling.

Additional Information Complete prescribing information should be consulted for additional detail.

Dosage Forms Excipient information presented when available (limited, particularly for generics); consult specific product labeling.

Solution, Ophthalmic:

Viroptic: 1% (7.5 mL) [contains thimerosal]

Generic: 1% (7.5 mL)

Trifluridine and Tipiracil
(trye FLURE i deen & tye PIR a sil)

Brand Names: US Lonsurf

Index Terms TAS-102; Tipiracil and Trifluridine; Trifluridine and Tipiracil Hydrochloride

Pharmacologic Category Antineoplastic Agent, Antimetabolite; Antineoplastic Agent, Antimetabolite (Pyrimidine Analog); Thymidine Phosphorylase Inhibitor

Use Colorectal cancer, metastatic: Treatment of metastatic colorectal cancer in patients who have been previously treated with fluoropyrimidine-, oxaliplatin- and irinotecan-based chemotherapy, an anti-VEGF biological therapy, and if RAS wild-type, an anti-EGFR therapy.

Pregnancy Considerations Based on the mechanism of action, use of trifluridine/tipiracil would be expected to cause fetal harm when used during pregnancy. Females of reproductive potential should use effective contraception during therapy. Males who have female partners of reproductive potential should use condoms during therapy and for ≥3 months following the final dose.

Breast-Feeding Considerations It is not known if trifluridine or tipiracil are excreted in breast milk. Due to the potential for serious adverse reactions in the nursing infant, breast-feeding is not recommended by the manufacturer during therapy and for one day following the last dose.

Contraindications There are no contraindications listed in the manufacturer's labeling.

Warnings/Precautions Hazardous agent – use appropriate precautions for handling and disposal (meets NIOSH 2014 criteria). Severe and life-threatening bone marrow suppression (anemia, neutropenia, thrombocytopenia) has occurred, including a fatality related to neutropenic infection. In one clinical trial, close to 10% of patients received growth factor support. Monitor blood counts prior to the start of each cycle as well as on day 15, or more frequently if clinically necessary. May require therapy interruption and/or dose reduction. Nausea, vomiting, diarrhea, and abdominal pain have been commonly reported. Stomatitis may also occur. Advise patients to report severe gastrointestinal toxicity to their health care provider. Patients with moderate (total bilirubin >1.5 to 3 times ULN and any AST) or severe (total bilirubin >3 times ULN and any AST) were excluded from the clinical trial; use with caution in patients with moderate or severe hepatic impairment. Use with caution in patients with renal impairment; dosage adjustments due to toxicities may be necessary in patients with moderate impairment. Patients with severe renal impairment (CrCl <30 mL/minute) or end-stage renal disease (ESRD) were excluded from the clinical trial. Patients ≥65 years experienced a higher incidence of grade 3 and grade 4 neutropenia and thrombocytopenia, as well as increased grade 3 anemia compared to younger patients. Trifluridine/tipiracil is available in two tablet strengths (trifluridine 15 mg/tipiracil 6.14 mg and trifluridine 20 mg/tipiracil 8.19 mg); both tablet strengths may be necessary to provide the correct dose. Read labels carefully in order to ensure the appropriate dose is administered. Dosing is based on the trifluridine component. The manufacturer recommends rounding doses to the nearest 5 mg increment.

Adverse Reactions

>10%:

Central nervous system: Fatigue (≤52%)

Gastrointestinal: Nausea (48%), decreased appetite (39%), diarrhea (32%), vomiting (28%), abdominal pain (21%)

Hematologic & oncologic: Anemia (77%; grade 3: 18%), neutropenia (67%; grade 3: 27%; grade 4: 11%), thrombocytopenia (42%; grade 3: 5%; grade 4: 1%)

Neuromuscular & skeletal: Weakness (≤52%)

Miscellaneous: Fever (19%)

1% to 10%:

Cardiovascular: Pulmonary embolism (2%)

Dermatologic: Alopecia (7%)

Gastrointestinal: Stomatitis (8%), dysgeusia (7%)

Genitourinary: Urinary tract infection (4%)

Respiratory: Nasopharyngitis (4%)

<1% (Limited to important or life-threatening): Lung disease

Drug Interactions

Metabolism/Transport Effects None known.

Avoid Concomitant Use

Avoid concomitant use of Trifluridine and Tipiracil with any of the following: BCG (Intravesical); Deferiprone; Dipyrone; Natalizumab; Pimecrolimus; Tacrolimus (Topical); Tofacitinib; Vaccines (Live)

Increased Effect/Toxicity

Trifluridine and Tipiracil may increase the levels/effects of: CloZAPine; Deferiprone; Fingolimod; Highest Risk QTc-Prolonging Agents; Leflunomide; Moderate Risk QTc-Prolonging Agents; Natalizumab; Tofacitinib; Vaccines (Live)

The levels/effects of Trifluridine and Tipiracil may be increased by: Denosumab; Dipyrone; Mifepristone; Pimecrolimus; Roflumilast; Tacrolimus (Topical); Trastuzumab

Decreased Effect

Trifluridine and Tipiracil may decrease the levels/effects of: BCG (Intravesical); Coccidioides immitis Skin Test; Sipuleucel-T; Vaccines (Inactivated); Vaccines (Live)

The levels/effects of Trifluridine and Tipiracil may be decreased by: Echinacea

Storage/Stability Store at 20°C to 25°C (68°F to 77°F); excursions are permitted to 15°C to 30°C (59°F to 86°F). If stored outside the original bottle, discard tablets after 30 days.

Mechanism of Action Trifluridine, the active cytotoxic component of trifluridine/tipiracil, is a thymidine-based nucleic acid analogue; the triphosphate form of trifluridine is incorporated into DNA which interferes with DNA synthesis and inhibits cell proliferation. Tipiracil is a potent thymidine phosphorylase inhibitor which prevents the rapid degradation of trifluridine, allowing for increased trifluridine exposure (Mayer 2015).

Pharmacodynamics/Kinetics

Protein binding: Trifluridine: >96% (primarily to albumin); Tipiracil: <8%

Metabolism: Trifluridine and tipiracil are not metabolized by cytochrome P450 (CYP) enzymes. Trifluridine is mainly eliminated by metabolism via thymidine phosphorylase to form an inactive metabolite, 5-(trifluoromethyl) uracil (FTY)

Half-life elimination: Trifluridine: 2.1 hours (at steady state); Tipiracil: 2.4 hours (at steady state)

Time to peak, plasma: ~2 hours

Excretion: Trifluridine: Urine (<2% [as unchanged drug]; ~19% [as inactive metabolite FTY]); Tipiracil: Urine (~29% [as unchanged drug])

Dosing

Adult & Geriatric Note: Obtain blood counts prior to starting each cycle and on day 15 of each cycle. Do not initiate a cycle until ANC ≥1,500/mm^3 or febrile neutropenia is resolved, platelets are ≥75,000/mm^3, and/or grade 3 or 4 nonhematologic reactions are ≤ grade 1.

Colorectal cancer, metastatic: Oral: 35 mg/m^2 (based on the trifluridine component) twice daily on days 1 to 5 and days 8 to 12 of a 28-day cycle (maximum per dose: trifluridine 80 mg); continue until disease progression or unacceptable toxicity (Mayer 2015). The manufacturer recommends rounding each dose to the nearest 5 mg increment.

Missed dose: Do not take additional doses to make up for missed or held doses.

Renal Impairment

CrCl ≥30 mL/minute: No initial dosage adjustment is necessary. Monitor closely; patients with moderate impairment (CrCl 30 to 59 mL/minute) may experience greater toxicity and may require dose reduction during treatment.

CrCl <30 mL/minute and ESRD: There are no dosage adjustments provided in the manufacturer's labeling (has not been studied).

Hepatic Impairment

Mild impairment (total bilirubin ≤ULN and AST >ULN or total bilirubin <1 to 1.5 times ULN and any AST): No dosage adjustment necessary.

Moderate impairment (total bilirubin >1.5 to 3 times ULN and any AST) or severe impairment (total bilirubin >3 times ULN and any AST): There are no dosage adjustments provided in the manufacturer's labeling (has not been studied).

Adjustment for Toxicity A maximum of 3 dose reductions are allowed (to a minimum dose of 20 mg/m^2). Do not re-escalate dose after it has been reduced.

Hematologic toxicity:

ANC <500/mm^3 (uncomplicated or resulting in >1 week delay in the start of the next cycle) or febrile neutropenia: Interrupt therapy; following recovery to ANC ≥1,500/mm^3 or resolution of febrile neutropenia, may resume therapy with the dose reduced by 5 mg/m^2/dose from the previous dose

Platelets <50,000/mm^3 (or resulting in >1 week delay in the start of the next cycle): Interrupt therapy; following recovery to platelets ≥75,000/mm^3, may resume therapy with the dose reduced by 5 mg/m^2/dose from the previous dose

Nonhematologic toxicity: Grade 3 or 4 toxicity: Interrupt therapy until recovery to ≤ grade 1; following recovery, may resume with the dose reduced by 5 mg/m^2/dose from the previous dose (excludes dose reduction for grade 3 nausea and/or vomiting controlled by antiemetic therapy or grade 3 diarrhea responsive to antidiarrheal treatment).

Administration

Hazardous agent: Use appropriate precautions for handling and disposal (meets NIOSH 2014 criteria). Wash hands after handling tablets; caregivers should wear gloves when handling. NIOSH recommends single gloving for administration of intact tablets (NIOSH 2014).

Administer orally twice daily within 1 hour of completion of morning and evening meals.

Monitoring Parameters Complete blood counts prior to each cycle and on day 15 of each cycle (or more frequently if clinically necessary); signs/symptoms of gastrointestinal toxicity.

Dosage Forms Excipient information presented when available (limited, particularly for generics); consult specific product labeling.

Tablet, Oral:

Lonsurf: Trifluridine 15 mg and tipiracil 6.14 mg, Trifluridine 20 mg and tipiracil 8.19 mg

◆ Trifluridine and Tipiracil Hydrochloride *see* Trifluridine and Tipiracil *on page 1845*

◆ Triglide *see* Fenofibrate and Derivatives *on page 746*

◆ Trigofen [OTC] [DSC] *see* Chlorpheniramine and Phenylephrine *on page 376*

◆ Trigofen DM [OTC] *see* Chlorpheniramine, Phenylephrine, and Dextromethorphan *on page 378*

Trihexyphenidyl (trye heks ee FEN i dil)

Brand Names: Canada PMS-Trihexyphenidyl; Trihexyphenidyl

Index Terms Artane; Benzhexol Hydrochloride; Trihexyphenidyl Hydrochloride

Pharmacologic Category Anti-Parkinson's Agent, Anticholinergic; Anticholinergic Agent

Use

Drug-induced extrapyramidal disorders: Control of extrapyramidal disorders caused by CNS drugs (eg, dibenzoxazepines, phenothiazines, thioxanthenes, butyrophenones)

Parkinsonism: Treatment of all forms of parkinsonism (postencephalitic, arteriosclerotic, and idiopathic) as adjunctive therapy

Dosing

Adult

Drug-induced extrapyramidal disorders: Oral: Initial: 1 mg/day; increase as necessary to usual range: 5 to 15 mg/day in 3 to 4 divided doses

Parkinsonism: Oral: Initial: 1 mg/day, increase by 2 mg increments at intervals of 3 to 5 days; usual dose: 6 to 10 mg/day in 3 to 4 divided doses; doses of 12 to 15 mg/day may be required

Use in combination with levodopa: When trihexyphenidyl is used concomitantly with levodopa, the usual dose of each may need to be reduced. Usual range: 3 to 6 mg/day in divided doses

Geriatric Refer to adult dosing. **Note:** Conservative initial doses and gradual titration is especially important in patients >60 years of age.

Renal Impairment There are no dosage adjustments provided in the manufacturer's labeling; use with caution.

Hepatic Impairment There are no dosage adjustments provided in the manufacturer's labeling; use with caution.

Additional Information Complete prescribing information should be consulted for additional detail.

Dosage Forms Excipient information presented when available (limited, particularly for generics); consult specific product labeling.

Elixir, Oral, as hydrochloride:

Generic: 0.4 mg/mL (473 mL)

Tablet, Oral, as hydrochloride:

Generic: 2 mg, 5 mg

◆ Trihexyphenidyl Hydrochloride *see* Trihexyphenidyl *on page 1846*

◆ Trilafon *see* Perphenazine *on page 1433*

◆ Tri-Legest Fe *see* Ethinyl Estradiol and Norethindrone *on page 708*

◆ Trileptal *see* OXcarbazepine *on page 1352*

◆ Tri-Linyah *see* Ethinyl Estradiol and Norgestimate *on page 710*

◆ Trilipix *see* Fenofibrate and Derivatives *on page 746*

◆ Trilisate *see* Choline Magnesium Trisalicylate *on page 382*

◆ Tri-Lo-Estarylla *see* Ethinyl Estradiol and Norgestimate *on page 710*

◆ Tri-Lo-Sprintec *see* Ethinyl Estradiol and Norgestimate *on page 710*

◆ Tri-Luma® *see* Fluocinolone, Hydroquinone, and Tretinoin *on page 781*

◆ TriLyte *see* Polyethylene Glycol-Electrolyte Solution *on page 1466*

Trimethobenzamide (trye meth oh BEN za mide)

Brand Names: US Tigan

Brand Names: Canada Tigan

Index Terms Trimethobenzamide HCl; Trimethobenzamide Hydrochloride

Pharmacologic Category Antiemetic

Use Nausea and vomiting: Treatment of postoperative nausea and vomiting; treatment of nausea associated with gastroenteritis

Dosing

Adult

Nausea/vomiting:

Oral: 300 mg 3 or 4 times daily

IM: 200 mg 3 or 4 times daily

Geriatric According to the manufacturer, consider dosage reduction or increasing the dosing interval in elderly patients with renal impairment, although use should be avoided in this age group due to the risk of EPS adverse effects combined with lower efficacy, as compared to other antiemetics (Beers Criteria).

Renal Impairment CrCl ≤70 mL/minute/1.73 m^2: Although no specific dosage adjustment provided in the manufacturer's labeling, dosage reduction or increasing the dosing interval is recommended.

Hepatic Impairment No dosage adjustment provided in the manufacturer's labeling.

Additional Information Complete prescribing information should be consulted for additional detail.

Dosage Forms Excipient information presented when available (limited, particularly for generics); consult specific product labeling. [DSC] = Discontinued product

Capsule, Oral, as hydrochloride:

Tigan: 300 mg

Generic: 300 mg

Solution, Intramuscular, as hydrochloride:

Tigan: 100 mg/mL (2 mL)

Tigan: 100 mg/mL (20 mL) [contains phenol]

Generic: 100 mg/mL (2 mL [DSC], 20 mL [DSC])

◆ Trimethobenzamide HCl *see* Trimethobenzamide *on page 1846*

◆ Trimethobenzamide Hydrochloride *see* Trimethobenzamide *on page 1846*

Trimethoprim (trye METH oh prim)

Brand Names: US Primsol

Brand Names: Canada Apo-Trimethoprim®

Index Terms TMP

Pharmacologic Category Antibiotic, Miscellaneous

Use Treatment of urinary tract infections due to susceptible strains of *E. coli*, *P. mirabilis*, *K. pneumoniae*, *Enterobacter* spp and coagulase-negative *Staphylococcus* including *S. saprophyticus*; acute otitis media due to susceptible strains of *S. pneumoniae* and *H. influenzae* in children

Dosing

Adult & Geriatric

***Pneumocystis jirovecii* pneumonia, mild-to-moderate (off-label use) (CDC, 2009):** Oral: 15 mg/kg/day in 3 divided doses in combination with dapsone

Susceptible infections: Oral: 100 mg every 12 hours or 200 mg every 24 hours for 10 days

Urinary tract infection, uncomplicated (off-label duration): Oral:

Treatment: 100 mg every 12 hours for 3 days (Gupta, 2011)

Prophylaxis: 100 mg once daily (Kodner, 2010)

Pediatric

Susceptible infections: Children ≥2 months: Oral: 4-6 mg/kg/day in divided doses every 12 hours (dosing for UTI in Schleiss, 2007); **Note:** AAP guidelines on treatment of UTI recommend 6-12 mg trimethoprim/kg/day (in combination with sulfamethoxazole) in 2 divided doses (AAP, 1999)

Acute otitis media: Children ≥6 months: Oral: 10 mg/kg/day in divided doses every 12 hours for 10 days

Renal Impairment

CrCl 15-30 mL/minute: Administer 50 mg every 12 hours.

CrCl <15 mL/minute: Not recommended.

Moderately dialyzable (20% to 50%)

Hepatic Impairment No dosage adjustment provided in manufacturer's labeling; use with caution.

Additional Information Complete prescribing information should be consulted for additional detail.

Dosage Forms Excipient information presented when available (limited, particularly for generics); consult specific product labeling.

Solution, Oral [strength expressed as base]:

Primsol: 50 mg/5 mL (473 mL) [alcohol free, dye free]

Tablet, Oral:

Generic: 100 mg

Trimethoprim and Polymyxin B (trye METH oh prim & pol i MIKS in bee)

Brand Names: US Polytrim®

Brand Names: Canada PMS-Polytrimethoprim; Polytrim™

Index Terms Polymyxin B and Trimethoprim

Pharmacologic Category Antibiotic, Ophthalmic

Use Treatment of surface ocular bacterial conjunctivitis and blepharoconjunctivitis

Dosing

Adult & Geriatric Conjunctivitis, blepharoconjunctivitis: Ophthalmic: Instill 1 drop in affected eye(s) every 3 hours (maximum: 6 doses per day) for 7-10 days; has also been used 4 times daily for 5-7 days (Williams, 2013; The Wills Eye Manual, 2004)

Pediatric Children ≥2 months: Refer to adult dosing.

Renal Impairment No dosage adjustment provided in manufacturer's labeling.

Hepatic Impairment No dosage adjustment provided in manufacturer's labeling.

Additional Information Complete prescribing information should be consulted for additional detail.

Dosage Forms Excipient information presented when available (limited, particularly for generics); consult specific product labeling.

Solution, ophthalmic: Trimethoprim 1 mg and polymyxin B sulfate 10,000 units per 1 mL (10 mL)

Polytrim®: Trimethoprim 1 mg and polymyxin B sulfate 10,000 units per 1 mL (10 mL) [contains benzalkonium chloride]

Triprolidine and Pseudoephedrine (trye PROE li deen & soo doe e FED rin)

Brand Names: US Aprodine [OTC]; Ed A-Hist PSE [OTC]; Entre-Hist PSE; Genac; Hist-PSE; Histafed; Pediatex TD [DSC]; Trip-PSE

Brand Names: Canada Actifed

Index Terms Pseudoephedrine and Triprolidine

Pharmacologic Category Alkylamine Derivative; Alpha/Beta Agonist; Decongestant; Histamine H$_1$ Antagonist; Histamine H$_1$ Antagonist, First Generation

Use Cold, allergy symptoms: Temporary relief of nasal congestion, decongest sinus openings, runny nose, sneezing, itching of nose or throat and itchy, watery eyes due to common cold, hay fever (allergic rhinitis), or other upper respiratory allergies or sinusitis

Dosing

Adult & Geriatric

Cold, allergy symptoms: Oral:

Liquid (triprolidine 0.938 mg and pseudoephedrine 10 mg per 1 mL): 2.67 mL every 6 hours (maximum: 4 doses [10.68 mL]/24 hours)

Syrup (triprolidine 1.25 mg and pseudoephedrine 30 mg per 5 mL): 10 mL every 4 to 6 hours (maximum: 4 doses [40 mL]/24 hours)

Tablet (triprolidine 2.5 mg and pseudoephedrine 60 mg): One tablet every 4 to 6 hours (maximum: 4 doses/24 hours)

Pediatric

Cold, allergy symptoms: Oral:

Liquid (triprolidine 0.938 mg and pseudoephedrine 10 mg per 1 mL):

Children 6 to <12 years: 1.33 mL every 6 hours (maximum: 4 doses [5.32 mL]/24 hours)

Children ≥12 years and Adolescents: Refer to adult dosing.

Syrup (triprolidine 1.25 mg and pseudoephedrine 30 mg per 5 mL):

Children 6 to <12 years: 5 mL every 4 to 6 hours (maximum: 4 doses [20 mL]/24 hours)

Children ≥12 years and Adolescents: Refer to adult dosing.

Tablet (triprolidine 2.5 mg and pseudoephedrine 60 mg):

Children 6 to <12 years: One-half tablet every 4 to 6 hours (maximum: 4 doses/24 hours)

Children ≥12 years and Adolescents: Refer to adult dosing.

Renal Impairment There are no dosage adjustments provided in the manufacturer's labeling.

Hepatic Impairment There are no dosage adjustments provided in the manufacturer's labeling.

Additional Information Complete prescribing information should be consulted for additional detail.

Dosage Forms Excipient information presented when available (limited, particularly for generics); consult specific product labeling. [DSC] = Discontinued product

Liquid, oral:

Entre-Hist PSE: Triprolidine hydrochloride 0.938 mg and pseudoephedrine hydrochloride 10 mg per 1 mL (30 mL) [cotton candy flavor]

Pediatex TD: Triprolidine hydrochloride 0.938 mg and pseudoephedrine hydrochloride 10 mg per 1 mL (30 mL [DSC]) [cotton candy flavor]

Syrup, oral: Triprolidine hydrochloride 1.25 mg and pseudoephedrine hydrochloride 30 mg per 5 mL (120 mL) [DSC]

Aprodine: Triprolidine hydrochloride 1.25 mg and pseudoephedrine hydrochloride 30 mg per 5 mL (120 mL)

Tablet, oral:

Aprodine: Triprolidine hydrochloride 2.5 mg and pseudoephedrine hydrochloride 60 mg

Ed A-Hist PSE: Triprolidine hydrochloride 2.5 mg and pseudoephedrine hydrochloride 60 mg

---

Triptorelin (trip toe REL in)

Brand Names: US Trelstar; Trelstar Mixject

Brand Names: Canada Decapeptyl; Trelstar

◀

Index Terms AY-25650; CL-118,532; D-Trp(6)-LHRH; Detryptoreline; Triptorelin Embonate; Triptorelin Pamoate; Tryptoreline

Pharmacologic Category Gonadotropin Releasing Hormone Agonist

Use

Advanced prostate cancer: Palliative treatment of advanced prostate cancer

Assisted reproductive technologies: Decapeptyl [Canadian product]: Adjunctive therapy in women undergoing controlled ovarian hyperstimulation for assisted reproductive technologies (ART)

Dosing

Adult & Geriatric

Advanced prostate carcinoma: IM:
3.75 mg once every 4 weeks **or**
11.25 mg once every 12 weeks **or**
22.5 mg once every 24 weeks

Controlled ovarian hyperstimulation for assisted reproductive technologies (ART) (adjunctive therapy): *Decapeptyl [Canadian product]):* Females: SubQ: Usual dose: 0.1 mg once daily initiated on day 2 or 3 or days 21 to 23 of menstrual cycle (or 5 to 7 days prior to expected onset of menses). Dose may be adjusted according to ovarian response as measured by ovarian ultrasound with or without serum estradiol levels. Treatment is continued until follicles achieve suitable size (typically 4 to 7 weeks).

Treatment of paraphilia/hypersexuality (off-label use; Guay, 2009; Thibaut, 1993): Males:
Note: May cause an initial increase in androgen concentrations which may be treated with an antiandrogen (eg, flutamide, cyproterone) for 1 to 2 months (Guay, 2009). Avoid use in patients with osteoporosis or active pituitary pathology.
SubQ: Test dose: 1 mg (observe for hypersensitivity)
IM: 3.75 mg monthly

Renal Impairment There are no dosage adjustments provided in the manufacturer's labeling. However, renal impairment increases systemic exposure to triptorelin.

Hepatic Impairment There are no dosage adjustments provided in the manufacturer's labeling. However, hepatic impairment increases systemic exposure to triptorelin.

Additional Information Complete prescribing information should be consulted for additional detail.

Dosage Forms Excipient information presented when available (limited, particularly for generics); consult specific product labeling.
Suspension Reconstituted, Intramuscular:
Trelstar: 3.75 mg (1 ea); 11.25 mg (1 ea) [contains polysorbate 80]
Trelstar Mixject: 3.75 mg (1 ea); 11.25 mg (1 ea); 22.5 mg (1 ea) [contains polysorbate 80]

Dosage Forms: Canada Refer also to Dosage Forms. Excipient information presented when available (limited, particularly for generics); consult specific product labeling.
Injection, solution, as acetate [preservative free]:
Decapeptyl: 100 mcg/mL (equivalent to 95.6 mcg triptorelin free base) (1 mL) [prefilled syringe]

◆ Triptorelin Embonate *see* Triptorelin *on page 1847*

◆ Triptorelin Pamoate *see* Triptorelin *on page 1847*

◆ Triquilar (Can) *see* Ethinyl Estradiol and Levonorgestrel *on page 703*

◆ Tris Buffer *see* Tromethamine *on page 1848*

◆ Trisenox *see* Arsenic Trioxide *on page 154*

◆ Tris(hydroxymethyl)aminomethane *see* Tromethamine *on page 1848*

◆ Tri-Sprintec *see* Ethinyl Estradiol and Norgestimate *on page 710*

◆ Trisulfa (Can) *see* Sulfamethoxazole and Trimethoprim *on page 1710*

◆ Trisulfa DS (Can) *see* Sulfamethoxazole and Trimethoprim *on page 1710*

◆ Trisulfa S (Can) *see* Sulfamethoxazole and Trimethoprim *on page 1710*

◆ Triumeq *see* Abacavir, Dolutegravir, and Lamivudine *on page 18*

◆ Trivagizole-3 (Can) *see* Clotrimazole (Topical) *on page 428*

◆ Trivora *see* Ethinyl Estradiol and Levonorgestrel *on page 703*

◆ Trizivir *see* Abacavir, Lamivudine, and Zidovudine *on page 18*

◆ Trocaine Throat [OTC] *see* Benzocaine *on page 217*

◆ Trokendi XR *see* Topiramate *on page 1810*

◆ Trombovar (Can) *see* Sodium Tetradecyl Sulfate *on page 1682*

Tromethamine (troe METH a meen)

Brand Names: US Tham

Index Terms Tris Buffer; Tris(hydroxymethyl)aminomethane

Pharmacologic Category Alkalinizing Agent, Parenteral

Use Correction of metabolic acidosis associated with cardiac bypass surgery or cardiac arrest; to correct excess acidity of stored blood that is preserved with acid citrate dextrose (ACD); indicated in infants needing alkalinization after receiving maximum sodium bicarbonate (8-10 mEq/kg/24 hours)

Dosing

Adult & Geriatric Dose depends on buffer base deficit; when deficit is known: tromethamine (mL of 0.3 M solution) = body weight (kg) x base deficit (mEq/L) x 1.1

Metabolic acidosis with cardiac arrest:
IV: 3.6-10.8 g (111-333 mL); additional amounts may be required to control acidosis after arrest reversed
Open chest: Intraventricular: 2-6 g (62-185 mL). **Note:** Do not inject into cardiac muscle

Acidosis associated with cardiac bypass surgery: IV: Average dose: 9 mL/kg (2.7 mEq/kg); 500 mL is adequate for most adults; maximum dose: 500 mg/kg over at least 1 hour

Excess acidity of acid citrate dextrose (ACD) blood in cardiac bypass surgery: 15-77 mL of 0.3 molar solution added to each 500 mL of ACD blood

Renal Impairment No dosage adjustment provided in manufacturer's labeling. Tromethamine is substantially excreted by the kidneys; use with caution; monitor ECG and potassium levels.

Hepatic Impairment No dosage adjustment provided in manufacturer's labeling.

Additional Information Complete prescribing information should be consulted for additional detail.

Dosage Forms Excipient information presented when available (limited, particularly for generics); consult specific product labeling.
Solution, Intravenous:
Tham: 30 mEq/100 mL (500 mL)

Tropicamide (troe PIK a mide)

Brand Names: US Mydral [DSC]; Mydriacyl

Brand Names: Canada Diotrope; Mydriacyl

Index Terms Bistropamide

Pharmacologic Category Ophthalmic Agent, Mydriatic

Use Mydriasis/Cycloplegia: For mydriasis and cycloplegia in diagnostic procedures

Dosing

Adult & Geriatric Note: Individuals with heavily pigmented eyes may require higher strength or additional doses:

Cycloplegia: Ophthalmic: Instill 1 to 2 drops (1%) in the eye(s); repeat in 5 minutes. If the patient is not examined within 20 to 30 minutes, instill an additional drop to prolong effect.

Mydriasis: Ophthalmic: Instill 1 to 2 drops (0.5%) in the eye(s) 15 to 20 minutes before exam

Pediatric Cycloplegia, mydriasis: Children and Adolescents: Refer to adult dosing.

Renal Impairment There are no dosage adjustments provided in the manufacturer's labeling.

Hepatic Impairment There are no dosage adjustments provided in the manufacturer's labeling.

Additional Information Complete prescribing information should be consulted for additional detail.

Dosage Forms Excipient information presented when available (limited, particularly for generics); consult specific product labeling. [DSC] = Discontinued product
Solution, Ophthalmic:
Mydral: 0.5% (15 mL [DSC]); 1% (15 mL [DSC])
Mydriacyl: 1% (3 mL, 15 mL)
Generic: 0.5% (15 mL); 1% (2 mL, 3 mL, 15 mL)

◆ Trosec (Can) *see* Trospium *on page 1848*

Trospium (TROSE pee um)

Brand Names: US Sanctura XR [DSC]; Sanctura [DSC]

Brand Names: Canada Sanctura® XR; Trosec

Index Terms Trospium Chloride

Pharmacologic Category Anticholinergic Agent

Use Treatment of overactive bladder with symptoms of urgency, incontinence, and urinary frequency

Pregnancy Considerations Adverse events were observed in animal studies. There are no adequate or well-controlled studies in pregnant women; use only if clearly needed.

Breast-Feeding Considerations It is not known if trospium is excreted in breast milk. According to the manufacturer, the decision to continue or discontinue breast-feeding during therapy should take into account the risk of exposure to the infant and the benefits of treatment to the mother.

Contraindications Hypersensitivity to trospium or any component of the formulation; urinary retention; gastric retention; uncontrolled narrow-angle glaucoma

Warnings/Precautions Cases of angioedema involving the face, lips, tongue, and/or larynx have been reported. Immediately discontinue if tongue, hypopharynx, or larynx are involved. May cause drowsiness, confusion, dizziness, hallucinations, and/or blurred vision, which may impair physical or mental abilities; patients must be cautioned about performing tasks which require mental alertness (eg, operating machinery or driving). Effects with other sedative drugs or ethanol may be potentiated. May occur in the presence of increased environmental temperature; use caution in hot weather and/or exercise. Use with caution in patients with bladder flow obstruction, may increase the risk of urinary retention. Use with caution in patients with gastrointestinal obstructive disorders (eg, pyloric stenosis); may increase the risk of gastric retention. Use caution in patients with decreased GI motility (eg, myasthenia gravis, ulcerative colitis). Use immediate release formulation with caution in renal dysfunction; dosage adjustment is required. Use of the extended release formulation is contraindicated in patients with severe renal impairment (CrCl <30 mL/minute). Ethanol should not be ingested within 2 hours of the administration of the extended release formulation. Concurrent ethanol use may increase the incidence of drowsiness. Active tubular secretion (ATS) is a route of elimination; use caution with other medications that are eliminated by ATS (eg, procainamide, pancuronium, vancomycin, morphine, metformin, and tenofovir). Use with extreme caution in patients with controlled (treated) narrow-angle glaucoma. Use caution in patients with moderate or severe hepatic dysfunction. Use caution in Alzheimer's patients. Use caution in the elderly (≥65 years of age); increased anticholinergic side effects are seen. This medication is associated with potent anticholinergic properties which may be inappropriate in older adults depending on comorbidities (eg, dementia, delirium) (Beers Criteria).

Adverse Reactions

>10%: Gastrointestinal: Xerostomia (9% to 22%)

1% to 10%:
Cardiovascular: Tachycardia (<2%)
Central nervous system: Headache (4% to 7%), fatigue (2%)
Dermatologic: Skin rash (<2%), xeroderma
Gastrointestinal: Constipation (9% to 10%), abdominal pain (1% to 3%), dyspepsia (1% to 2%), flatulence (1% to 2%), abdominal distention (<2%), nausea (1%), dysgeusia, vomiting
Genitourinary: Urinary tract infection (1% to 7%), urinary retention (≤1%)
Infection: Influenza (2%)
Ophthalmic: Dry eye syndrome (1% to 2%), blurred vision (1%)
Respiratory: Nasopharyngitis (3%), dry nose (1%)

<1% (Limited to important or life-threatening): Anaphylaxis, angioedema, confusion, delirium, drowsiness, fecal impaction, gastritis, hallucination, heat intolerance, hypertensive crisis, inversion T wave on ECG, palpitations, rhabdomyolysis, Stevens-Johnson syndrome, supraventricular tachycardia, syncope, visual disturbance

Drug Interactions

Metabolism/Transport Effects None known.

Avoid Concomitant Use

Avoid concomitant use of Trospium with any of the following: Aclidinium; Cimetropium; Eluxadoline; Glucagon; Glycopyrrolate; Glycopyrrolate (Oral Inhalation); Ipratropium (Oral Inhalation); Levosulpiride; Potassium Chloride; Tiotropium; Umeclidinium

Increased Effect/Toxicity

Trospium may increase the levels/effects of: AbobotulinumtoxinA; Analgesics (Opioid); Anticholinergic Agents; Cannabinoid-Containing Products; Cimetropium; Eluxadoline; Glucagon; Glycopyrrolate; Glycopyrrolate (Oral Inhalation); Mirabegron; OnabotulinumtoxinA; Potassium

Chloride; Ramosetron; RimabotulinumtoxinB; Thiazide Diuretics; Tiotropium; Topiramate

The levels/effects of Trospium may be increased by: Aclidinium; Alcohol (Ethyl); Ipratropium (Oral Inhalation); Mianserin; Pramlintide; Umeclidinium

Decreased Effect

Trospium may decrease the levels/effects of: Acetylcholinesterase Inhibitors; Gastrointestinal Agents (Prokinetic); Itopride; Levosulpiride; Secretin

The levels/effects of Trospium may be decreased by: Acetylcholinesterase Inhibitors; MetFORMIN

Food Interactions

Ethanol: Ethanol may increase the peak (maximum) serum concentration of trospium when consumed within 2 hours of taking extended release trospium. Management: Avoid consuming any alcohol within 2 hours of taking a dose of extended release trospium.

Food: Administration with a fatty meal reduces the absorption and bioavailability of trospium. Management: Administer 1 hour prior to meals or an empty stomach. Administer extended release capsules in the morning with a full glass of water.

Storage/Stability Store at 20°C to 25°C (68°F to 77°F); excursions permitted between 15°C to 30°C (59°F to 86°F).

Mechanism of Action Trospium antagonizes the effects of acetylcholine on muscarinic receptors in cholinergically innervated organs. It reduces the smooth muscle tone of the bladder.

Pharmacodynamics/Kinetics

Absorption: <10%; decreased with a high-fat meal
Distribution: V_d: 395 - >600 L, primarily in plasma
Protein binding: 48% to 85% *in vitro*
Metabolism: Hypothesized to be via esterase hydrolysis and conjugation; forms metabolites
Bioavailability: Immediate release formulation: ~10% (range: 4% to 16%)
Half-life elimination: Immediate release formulation: 20 hours
Severe renal insufficiency (CrCl <30 mL/minute): ~33 hours; extended release formulation: ~35 hours
Time to peak, plasma: 5-6 hours
Excretion: Feces (85%); urine (~6%; mostly as unchanged drug) primarily via active tubular secretion

Dosing

Adult Overactive bladder: Oral:
Immediate release: 20 mg twice daily
Extended release: 60 mg once daily

Geriatric Elderly ≥75 years: Immediate release: Consider initial dose of 20 mg once daily (based on tolerability); Extended release: Refer to adult dosing.

Renal Impairment

CrCl ≥30 mL/minute: No dosage adjustment provided in manufacturer's labeling. However, renal impairment increases systemic exposure to trospium. Monitor for increased adverse effects.
CrCl <30 mL/minute:
Immediate release: 20 mg once daily at bedtime
Extended release: Use not recommended

Hepatic Impairment

Mild impairment: No dosage adjustment provided in manufacturer's labeling.
Moderate to severe impairment: No dosage adjustment provided in manufacturer's labeling; use with caution.

Dietary Considerations Take 1 hour prior to meals or on an empty stomach.

Administration Administer 1 hour prior to meals or on an empty stomach. Administer extended release capsules in the morning with a full glass of water.

Dosage Forms Excipient information presented when available (limited, particularly for generics); consult specific product labeling. [DSC] = Discontinued product
Capsule Extended Release 24 Hour, Oral, as chloride:
Sanctura XR: 60 mg [DSC]
Generic: 60 mg
Tablet, Oral, as chloride:
Sanctura: 20 mg [DSC]
Generic: 20 mg

◆ Trospium Chloride *see* Trospium *on page 1848*

◆ Trulicity *see* Dulaglutide *on page 609*

◆ Trusopt *see* Dorzolamide *on page 588*

◆ Truvada *see* Emtricitabine and Tenofovir Disoproxil Fumarate *on page 635*

Trypsin, Balsam Peru, and Castor Oil
(TRIP sin, BAL sam pe RUE, & KAS tor oyl)

Brand Names: US Granulex®; TBC; Vasolex™; Xenaderm® [DSC]

Index Terms Balsam Peru, Castor Oil, and Trypsin; Castor Oil, Trypsin, and Balsam Peru

Pharmacologic Category Protectant, Topical

Use

Granulex®: Treatment of decubitus ulcers, varicose ulcers, debridement of eschar, dehiscent wounds and sunburn; promote wound healing; reduce odor from necrotic wounds

Vasolex™, Xenaderm®: Treatment of decubitus ulcers, varicose ulcers, and dehiscent wounds; promote wound healing; reduce odor from necrotic wounds

Dosing

Adult & Geriatric Dermatologic conditions: Topical: Apply a minimum of twice daily or as often as necessary

Additional Information Complete prescribing information should be consulted for additional detail.

Dosage Forms Excipient information presented when available (limited, particularly for generics); consult specific product labeling. [DSC] = Discontinued product

Aerosol, spray, topical:

Granulex®: Trypsin 0.12 mg, balsam Peru 87 mg, and castor oil 788 mg per gram (60 g, 120 g [DSC])

TBC: Trypsin 0.1 mg, balsam Peru 72.5 mg, and castor oil 650 mg per 0.82 mL (60 g, 120 g)

Ointment, topical:

Vasolex™: Trypsin 90 USP units, balsam Peru 87 mg, and castor oil 788 mg per gram (5 g, 30 g, 60 g)

Xenaderm®: Trypsin 90 USP units, balsam Peru 87 mg, and castor oil 788 mg per gram (30 g [DSC], 60 g [DSC])

Tuberculin Tests (too BER kyoo lin tests)

Brand Names: US Aplisol; Tubersol

Index Terms Mantoux; PPD; TB Skin Test; TST; Tuberculin Purified Protein Derivative; Tuberculin Skin Test

Pharmacologic Category Diagnostic Agent

Use Skin test in diagnosis of tuberculosis

Dosing

Adult & Geriatric

Diagnosis of tuberculosis, cell-mediated immunodeficiencies: Intradermal: 0.1 mL

TST interpretation: Criteria for positive TST read at 48-72 hours (see Note below for healthcare workers):

Induration ≥5 mm: Persons with HIV infection (or risk factors for HIV infection, but unknown status), recent close contact to person with known active TB, persons with chest x-ray consistent with healed TB, persons who are immunosuppressed

Induration ≥10 mm: Persons with clinical conditions which increase risk of TB infection, recent immigrants, IV drug users, residents and employees of high-risk settings, children <4 years of age

Induration ≥15 mm: Persons who do not meet any of the above criteria (no risk factors for TB)

Note: A two-step test is recommended when testing will be performed at regular intervals (eg, for healthcare workers). If the first test is negative, a second TST should be administered 1-3 weeks after the first test was read.

TST interpretation (CDC guidelines) in a healthcare setting:

Baseline test: ≥10 mm is positive (either first or second step)

Serial testing without known exposure: Increase of ≥10 mm is positive

Known exposure:

≥5 mm is positive in patients with baseline of 0 mm

≥10 mm is positive in patients with negative baseline or previous screening result of ≥0 mm

Read test at 48-72 hours following placement. Test results with 0 mm induration or measured induration less than the defined cutoff point are considered to signify absence of infection with *M. tuberculosis*. Test results should be documented in millimeters even if classified as negative. Erythema and redness of skin are not indicative of a positive test result.

Pediatric Refer to adult dosing.

Additional Information Complete prescribing information should be consulted for additional detail.

Dosage Forms Excipient information presented when available (limited, particularly for generics); consult specific product labeling.

Solution, Intradermal:

Aplisol: 5 units/0.1 mL (1 mL, 5 mL) [latex free; contains phenol, polysorbate 80]

Tubersol: 5 units/0.1 mL (1 mL, 5 mL) [contains phenol]

- Tylenol® Severe Allergy [OTC] *see* Acetaminophen and Diphenhydramine *on page 29*
- Tylenol with Codeine #3 *see* Acetaminophen and Codeine *on page 28*
- Tylenol with Codeine #4 *see* Acetaminophen and Codeine *on page 28*
- Tylox *see* Oxycodone and Acetaminophen *on page 1361*
- Typherix (Can) *see* Typhoid Vaccine *on page 1851*
- Typhim Vi *see* Typhoid Vaccine *on page 1851*

Typhoid Vaccine (TYE foid vak SEEN)

Brand Names: US Typhim Vi; Vivotif
Brand Names: Canada Typherix; Typhim Vi; Vivotif
Index Terms Ty21a Vaccine; Typhoid Vaccine Live Oral Ty21a; Vi Vaccine; ViCPS
Pharmacologic Category Vaccine; Vaccine, Inactivated (Bacterial); Vaccine, Live (Bacterial)
Additional Appendix Information
Immunization Administration Recommendations *on page 1974*
Immunization Schedules *on page 1979*
Use Active immunization against typhoid fever caused by *Salmonella typhi*:
Oral: Immunization of adults and children >6 years of age; complete the vaccine regimen at least 1 week before potential exposure to typhoid bacteria.
Canadian labeling: Approved for use in patients ≥5 years of age.
Parenteral: Immunization of adults and children ≥2 years of age; complete the vaccine regimen at least 2 weeks before potential exposure to typhoid bacteria.
Not for routine vaccination. In the United States (CDC/ACIP [Jackson 2015]) and Canada, use should be limited to:
- Travelers to areas with a recognized risk of exposure to *S. typhi*
- Persons with intimate exposure to a household contact with *S. typhi* fever or a known carrier
- Laboratory technicians with frequent exposure to *S. typhi*
Additional Canadian recommendations: May consider administration to travelers with achlorhydria, hypochlorhydria, or receiving acid suppression therapy; anatomic or functional asplenia (Canadian Immunization Guide)
Medication Guide Available Yes
Dosing
Adult & Geriatric Immunization:
Oral:
Primary immunization: One capsule on alternate days (day 1, 3, 5, and 7) for a total of 4 doses; all doses should be complete at least 1 week prior to potential exposure
Reimmunization (with repeated or continued exposure to typhoid fever):
US labeling: Repeat full course of primary immunization every 5 years
Canadian labeling: Repeat full course of primary immunization every 7 years
IM:
Initial: 0.5 mL given at least 2 weeks prior to expected exposure
Reimmunization (with repeated or continued exposure to typhoid fever):
Typhim Vi: 0.5 mL every 2 years
Typherix (Canadian labeling; not available in US): 0.5 mL every 3 years
Pediatric Immunization:
Children ≥6 years (US labeling) or ≥5 years (Canadian labeling) and Adolescents: Oral: Refer to adult dosing.
Children ≥2 years and Adolescents: IM: Refer to adult dosing.
Renal Impairment There are no dosage adjustments provided in manufacturer's labeling.
Hepatic Impairment There are no dosage adjustments provided in manufacturer's labeling.
Additional Information Complete prescribing information should be consulted for additional detail.
Dosage Forms Excipient information presented when available (limited, particularly for generics); consult specific product labeling.
Capsule, enteric coated [live]:
Vivotif: Viable *S. typhi* Ty21a 2-6.8 x 10⁹ colony-forming units and nonviable *S. typhi* Ty21a 5-50 x 10⁹ bacterial cells [contains lactose 100-180 mg/capsule and sucrose 26-130 mg/capsule]
Injection, solution [inactivated]:
Typhim Vi: Purified Vi capsular polysaccharide 25 mcg/0.5 mL (0.5 mL, 10 mL) [derived from *S. typhi* Ty2 strain]

Dosage Forms: Canada Excipient information presented when available (limited, particularly for generics); consult specific product labeling.
Injection, solution:
Typherix: Vi capsular polysaccharide 25 mcg/0.5 mL (0.5 mL) [derived from *S. typhi* Ty2 strain]

- Typhoid Vaccine Live Oral Ty21a *see* Typhoid Vaccine *on page 1851*
- Tysabri *see* Natalizumab *on page 1261*
- Tyvaso *see* Treprostinil *on page 1836*
- Tyvaso Refill *see* Treprostinil *on page 1836*
- Tyvaso Starter *see* Treprostinil *on page 1836*
- 506U78 *see* Nelarabine *on page 1265*
- U-90152S *see* Delavirdine *on page 514*
- UCB-P071 *see* Cetirizine *on page 364*
- Uceris *see* Budesonide (Systemic) *on page 255*
- U-Cort *see* Urea and Hydrocortisone *on page 1854*
- UK-88,525 *see* Darifenacin *on page 496*
- UK-427,857 *see* Maraviroc *on page 1127*
- UK92480 *see* Sildenafil *on page 1653*
- UK109496 *see* Voriconazole *on page 1908*
- U-Kera E *see* Urea *on page 1853*
- Ulcidine (Can) *see* Famotidine *on page 741*
- Ulesfia *see* Benzyl Alcohol *on page 220*

Ulipristal (ue li PRIS tal)

Brand Names: US Ella
Brand Names: Canada Fibristal
Index Terms CDB-2914; Ulipristal Acetate
Pharmacologic Category Contraceptive; Progestin Receptor Modulator
Use
Emergency contraceptive (Ella): Prevention of pregnancy following unprotected intercourse or a known or suspected contraceptive failure. Ulipristal is not intended for routine use as a contraceptive.
Uterine fibroids (Fibristal [Canadian product]): Treatment of moderate-to-severe signs/symptoms of uterine fibroids in premenopausal adult women eligible for surgery. **Note:** Treatment is limited to 3 months.
Dosing
Adult
Emergency contraception (Ella): Oral: 30 mg as soon as possible, but within 120 hours (5 days) of unprotected intercourse or contraceptive failure
Treatment of moderate-to-severe signs/symptoms of uterine fibroids (Fibristal [Canadian product]): Females (premenopausal): Oral: 5 mg daily for 3 consecutive months. **Note:** Treatment is limited to 3 months.
Note: Not indicated for use in postmenopausal women.
Geriatric Not indicated for use in postmenopausal women.
Pediatric Emergency contraception (Ella): Oral:
Children and Adolescents (prepubertal): Not indicated for use prior to menarche.
Adolescents (postpubertal): Refer to adult dosing.
Renal Impairment
US labeling (Ella): There are no dosage adjustments provided in the manufacturer's labeling (has not been studied).
Canadian labeling (Fibristal): Use is not recommended in moderate-to-severe renal impairment unless patient is monitored closely.
Hepatic Impairment
US labeling (Ella): There are no dosage adjustments provided in the manufacturer's labeling (has not been studied).
Canadian labeling (Fibristal): Use is not recommended in hepatic impairment unless patient is monitored closely.
Additional Information Complete prescribing information should be consulted for additional detail.
Dosage Forms Excipient information presented when available (limited, particularly for generics); consult specific product labeling.
Tablet, Oral, as acetate:
Ella: 30 mg
Dosage Forms: Canada Excipient information presented when available (limited, particularly for generics); consult specific product labeling.
Tablet, Oral, as acetate:
Fibristal: 5 mg

- Ulipristal Acetate *see* Ulipristal *on page 1851*
- Uloric *see* Febuxostat *on page 743*

Umeclidinium (ue me kli DIN ee um)

Brand Names: US Incruse Ellipta
Brand Names: Canada Incruse Ellipta
Index Terms Umeclidinium Bromide
Pharmacologic Category Anticholinergic Agent; Anticholinergic Agent, Long-Acting
Use Chronic obstructive pulmonary disease: Maintenance treatment of airflow obstruction in patients with chronic obstructive pulmonary disease (COPD), including chronic bronchitis and/or emphysema
Pregnancy Considerations Adverse events were not observed in animal reproduction studies. Systemic absorption following oral inhalation is negligible.
Breast-Feeding Considerations It is not known if umeclidinium is excreted into breast milk; however, systemic absorption following oral inhalation is negligible. The manufacturer recommends a decision be made whether to discontinue nursing or to discontinue the drug, taking into account the importance of treatment to the mother.
Contraindications Hypersensitivity to umeclidinium or any component of the formulation; severe hypersensitivity to milk proteins
Warnings/Precautions Do not use for acute episodes of chronic obstructive pulmonary disease (COPD). Do not initiate in patients with significantly worsening or acutely deteriorating COPD. Do not increase the daily dose beyond the recommended dose. Paradoxical bronchospasm may occur with the use of inhaled agents, which may be life threatening; discontinue use immediately and consider other therapy if bronchospasm occurs. May worsen the symptoms of narrow angle glaucoma, prostatic hyperplasia, and/or bladder neck obstruction; use with caution. Hypersensitivity reactions, including anaphylaxis, may occur. Powder for oral inhalation contains lactose; use is contraindicated in patients with severe milk protein allergy.
Adverse Reactions
1% to 10%:
Cardiovascular: Tachycardia (1%)
Gastrointestinal: Toothache (1%), upper abdominal pain (1%)
Hematologic & oncologic: Bruise (1%)
Neuromuscular & skeletal: Arthralgia (2%), myalgia (1%)
Respiratory: Nasopharyngitis (8%), upper respiratory tract infection (5%), cough (3%), pharyngitis (1%), viral upper respiratory tract infection (1%)
<1% (Limited to important or life-threatening): Atrial fibrillation
Drug Interactions
Metabolism/Transport Effects **Substrate** of CYP2D6 (minor), P-glycoprotein; **Note:** Assignment of Major/Minor substrate status based on clinically relevant drug interaction potential
Avoid Concomitant Use
Avoid concomitant use of Umeclidinium with any of the following: Aclidinium; Anticholinergic Agents; Cimetropium; Eluxadoline; Glucagon; Glycopyrrolate; Glycopyrrolate (Oral Inhalation); Ipratropium (Oral Inhalation); Levosulpiride; Loxapine; Potassium Chloride; Tiotropium
Increased Effect/Toxicity
Umeclidinium may increase the levels/effects of: AbobotulinumtoxinA; Analgesics (Opioid); Anticholinergic Agents; Cannabinoid-Containing Products; Cimetropium; Eluxadoline; Glucagon; Glycopyrrolate; Glycopyrrolate (Oral Inhalation); Loxapine; Mirabegron; OnabotulinumtoxinA; Potassium Chloride; Ramosetron; RimabotulinumtoxinB; Thiazide Diuretics; Tiotropium; Topiramate

The levels/effects of Umeclidinium may be increased by: Aclidinium; Ipratropium (Oral Inhalation); Mianserin; Pramlintide

Decreased Effect
Umeclidinium may decrease the levels/effects of: Acetylcholinesterase Inhibitors; Gastrointestinal Agents (Prokinetic); Itopride; Levosulpiride; Secretin

The levels/effects of Umeclidinium may be decreased by: Acetylcholinesterase Inhibitors
Storage/Stability Store between 68°F and 77°F (20°C and 25°C); excursions are permitted between 59°F and 86°F (15°C and 30°C). Protect from moisture, heat or sunlight. Remove inhaler from tray immediately prior to initial use. Discard inhaler 6 weeks after opening the foil tray or after the labeled number of inhalations have reached zero, whichever comes first.
Mechanism of Action Competitively and reversibly inhibits the action of acetylcholine at type 3 muscarinic (M_3) receptors in bronchial smooth muscle causing bronchodilation.
Pharmacodynamics/Kinetics
Absorption: Lung; minimum contribution from oral absorption
Distribution: V_d: 86 L (following IV administration)
Protein binding: ~89%
Metabolism: Hepatic via CYP2D6 and is a substrate for the P-glycoprotein (P-gp) transporter.
Half-life elimination: 11 hours
Time to peak: 5 to 15 minutes
Excretion: Urine <1%; feces 92% (following oral administration)
Dosing
Adult Chronic obstructive pulmonary disease (COPD):
1 inhalation (62.5 mcg) once daily; maximum dose: 1 inhalation (62.5 mcg) once daily
Geriatric Refer to adult dosing
Renal Impairment No dosage adjustment necessary.
Hepatic Impairment
Mild to moderate hepatic impairment: No dosage adjustment necessary.
Severe hepatic impairment: There are no dosage adjustments provided in the manufacturer's labeling (has not been studied).
Administration Administer via oral inhalation once daily at the same time each day; do not use more than 1 inhalation every 24 hours. Do not shake inhaler. Remove from sealed pouch immediately prior to first use. Slide cover of mouthpiece down until a "click" is heard. Prior to inhaling the dose, exhale fully (do not exhale into the inhaler); close lips tightly around the inhaler mouthpiece and inhale (rapidly, steadily, and deeply); do not breathe through nose or block air vent with fingers. Remove inhaler and hold breath for a few seconds then breathe out slowly and gently. Only open inhaler cover when ready for administration; opening and closing the cover without inhaling the medicine will cause a dose to be lost (the lost dose will be securely held inside the inhaler, but it will no longer be available to be inhaled). Do not close inhaler cover until medication has been inhaled.
Monitoring Parameters FEV_1, peak flow, and/or other pulmonary function tests; signs and symptoms of narrow angle glaucoma and urinary retention
Dosage Forms Excipient information presented when available (limited, particularly for generics); consult specific product labeling.
Aerosol Powder Breath Activated, Inhalation:
Incruse Ellipta: 62.5 mcg/inhalation (7 ea, 30 ea) [contains lactose monohydrate]

Urea (yoor EE a)

Brand Names: US Aluvea; Aquaphilic/Carbamide [OTC]; Atrac-Tain [OTC]; Beta Care Betamide [OTC]; Carb-O-Lac HP [OTC]; Carb-O-Lac5 [OTC]; Carb-O-Philic/10 [OTC]; Carb-O-Philic/20 [OTC]; Carb-O-Philic/40 [DSC]; Carmol 10 [OTC]; Carmol 20 [OTC]; Carmol [OTC]; CEM-Urea; Cerovel; Dermal Therapy Finger Care [OTC]; Dermasorb XM; DPM [OTC]; Gordons Urea; Gordons Urea [OTC]; Gormel 10 [OTC]; Gormel [OTC]; Hydro 35; Hydro 40; Kerafoam; Kerafoam 42; Keralac; Lanaphilic/Urea [OTC]; Latrix XM; Mycocide CX Callus Exfoliator [OTC]; Nutraplus [OTC]; Rea Lo 39; Rea Lo 40 [OTC]; Rea-Lo [OTC]; Remeven; Rinnovi Nail System [DSC]; TL Urea [DSC]; U-Kera E; Ultra Mide 25 [OTC]; Umecta; Umecta Mousse; Umecta Nail Film; Umecta PD; Uramaxin; Uramaxin GT; Urea Hydrating; Urea Nail; Urea-C40; Ureacin-10 [OTC]; Ureacin-20 [OTC]; Urevaz; Utopic; X-Viate [DSC]

Index Terms Carbamide

Pharmacologic Category Keratolytic Agent; Topical Skin Product

Use Hyperkeratotic conditions: Debridement and promotion of normal healing of hyperkeratotic surface lesions, particularly where healing is retarded by local infection, necrotic tissue, fibrinous or purulent debris, or eschar; treatment of hyperkeratotic conditions, such as dry, rough skin; skin cracks and fissures; dermatitis; psoriasis; xerosis; ichthyosis; eczema; keratosis; keratoderma; corns and calluses; damaged, ingrown, and devitalized nails.

Dosing

Adult & Geriatric Hyperkeratotic conditions: Topical: Apply 1-3 times daily.

Additional Information Complete prescribing information should be consulted for additional detail.

Dosage Forms Excipient information presented when available (limited, particularly for generics); consult specific product labeling. [DSC] = Discontinued product

Cream, External:
Aluvea: 39% (227 g)
Atrac-Tain: 10% (2 g, 57 g, 142 g)
Carb-O-Lac5: Urea 20% and Ammonium Lactate 10% (236 g) [contains propylene glycol]
Carb-O-Lac HP: Urea 20% and Ammonium Lactate 10% (277 g) [contains propylene glycol]
Carb-O-Philic/10: 10% (410 g) [contains propylene glycol]
Carb-O-Philic/20: 20% (85 g) [contains propylene glycol]
Carb-O-Philic/40: 40% (85 g [DSC], 200 g [DSC]) [contains cetyl alcohol, propylene glycol, trolamine (triethanolamine)]
Carmol 20: 20% (85 g)
DPM: (170 g) [lanolin free, mineral oil free, paraben free; contains brilliant blue fcf (fd&c blue #1), propylene glycol, tartrazine (fd&c yellow #5), trolamine (triethanolamine)]
Gormel: 20% (75 g, 120 g, 480 g, 2400 g) [contains cetyl alcohol, methylparaben, propylene glycol, propylparaben, trolamine (triethanolamine)]
Keralac: 47% (142 g) [contains edetate disodium, menthol]
Mycocide CX Callus Exfoliator: 12% (100 mL) [contains methylparaben, propylene glycol, propylparaben]
Nutraplus: 10% (90 g [DSC])
Nutraplus: 10% (453 g) [odorless; contains cetearyl alcohol, methylparaben, propylene glycol, propylparaben]
Nutraplus: 10% (85 g) [odorless; contains cetyl alcohol, methylparaben, propylene glycol, propylparaben]
Rea Lo 40: 40% (28.3 g, 85 g, 198.4 g)
Rea Lo 39: 39% (227 g) [fragrance free]
Rea-Lo: 30% (227 g, 59 mL)
Remeven: 50% (142 g, 255 g) [contains disodium edta]
U-Kera E: 40% (28.35 g, 85.05 g, 198.45 g) [contains trolamine (triethanolamine)]
Uramaxin: 45% (255 g) [contains alcohol, usp, edetate disodium, menthol]
Ureacin-20: 20% (113.4 g)
Urevaz: 44% (60 g) [contains disodium edta]
Utopic: 41% (227 g) [contains cetyl alcohol, propylene glycol]

X-Viate: 40% (28.3 g [DSC], 85 g [DSC], 199 g [DSC])
Generic: 10% (85 g); 20% (85 g); 39% (226.8 g, 227 g); 40% (28 g, 28.35 g, 85 g, 85.05 g, 198 g, 198.4 g, 198.6 g); 45% (255 g); 47% (142 g); 50% (142 g, 255 g); 39% (227 g)

Emulsion, External:
Latrix XM: 45% (240 mL) [contains cetyl alcohol, disodium edta, propylene glycol, trolamine (triethanolamine)]
Umecta: 40% (120 g, 227 g) [contains trolamine (triethanolamine)]
Umecta PD: 40% (198.5 g) [contains disodium edta, glycine soja (soybean) sterol]
Generic: 50% (284 g, 300 g)

Foam, External:
Hydro 35: 35% (150 g) [contains ethylparaben, methylparaben, propylene glycol, propylparaben, trolamine (triethanolamine)]
Hydro 40: 40% (150 g) [contains ethylparaben, methylparaben, propylene glycol, propylparaben, trolamine (triethanolamine)]
Kerafoam: 30% (60 g, 100 g) [contains cetyl alcohol, methylparaben, propylene glycol, propylparaben]
Kerafoam 42: 42% (60 g, 100 g) [contains cetearyl alcohol, edetate disodium, methylparaben, propylene glycol, propylparaben]
Umecta Mousse: 40% (113.4 g) [contains soya sterol, trolamine (triethanolamine)]
Uramaxin: 20% (100 g) [contains cetyl alcohol, propylene glycol]
Urea Hydrating: 35% (150 g) [contains ethylparaben, methylparaben, propylene glycol, propylparaben, trolamine (triethanolamine)]

Gel, External:
Carb-O-Philic/40: 40% (15 g [DSC]) [contains disodium edta, trolamine (triethanolamine)]
Cerovel: 40% (25 mL)
Uramaxin: 45% (28 mL) [contains edetate disodium, menthol, propylene glycol]
Uramaxin GT: 45% (20 mL) [contains edetate disodium, menthol, propylene glycol]
Urea Nail: 45% (28 mL) [contains edetate disodium, menthol, propylene glycol]
X-Viate: 40% (15 mL [DSC]) [contains methylparaben]
Generic: 40% (15 mL)

Kit, External:
Dermasorb XM: 39% [contains ceteareth-20, cetyl alcohol, chlorocresol (chloro-m-cresol)]
Rinnovi Nail System: 50% [DSC] [contains benzalkonium chloride, disodium edta, lactic acid, propylene glycol, pyrithione zinc, trolamine (triethanolamine)]
Uramaxin GT: 45% [contains edetate disodium, menthol, propylene glycol]
Urea Nail: 40 & 0.2% [contains disodium edta, methylparaben, propylparaben, trolamine (triethanolamine)]

Lotion, External:
Atrac-Tain: 5% (118 mL, 237 mL)
Beta Care Betamide: 25% (120 mL, 480 mL)
Carmol 10: 10% (177 mL)
Cerovel: 40% (325 mL) [contains alcohol, usp, trolamine (triethanolamine)]
Dermal Therapy Finger Care: 20% (18 mL)
Gormel 10: 10% (240 mL)
Nutraplus: 10% (236 mL [DSC], 480 mL [DSC])
Nutraplus: 10% (236 mL, 473 mL) [odorless; contains methylparaben, propylparaben]
Rea Lo 40: 40% (236.6 mL) [fragrance free]
Rea-Lo: 15% (120 mL)
TL Urea: 45% (480 g [DSC]) [contains alcohol, usp, edetate disodium, menthol]
Ultra Mide 25: 25% (236 mL) [paraben free; contains cetyl alcohol, edetate sodium (tetrasodium)]
Uramaxin: 45% (480 g) [contains alcohol, usp, edetate disodium, menthol]
Urea-C40: 40% (236.6 mL)
Ureacin-10: 10% (236.56 mL)
X-Viate: 40% (237 mL [DSC]) [contains cetyl alcohol, methylparaben, propylene glycol, propylparaben, trolamine (triethanolamine)]
Generic: 10% (180 mL, 240 mL, 480 mL); 40% (226.8 g, 236.6 mL); 45% (480 g)

Ointment, External:
Aquaphilic/Carbamide: 10% (180 g, 454 g); 20% (454 g)
Gordons Urea: 22% (30 g); 40% (30 g)
Lanaphilic/Urea: 10% (454 g); 20% (454 g)
Generic: 10% (454 g [DSC]); 20% (454 g [DSC])

Shampoo, External:
Carmol: 10% (240 mL)

Solution, External:
  CEM-Urea: 45% (20 mL) [contains edetate disodium, menthol, methylparaben, propylene glycol]
Stick, External:
  Urea Nail: 50% (2.4 mL) [contains cetyl alcohol, disodium edta]
Suspension, External:
  Umecta: 40% (283.4 g) [contains trolamine (triethanolamine)]
  Umecta Nail Film: 40% (3 g, 18 mL) [contains disodium edta]
  Umecta PD: 40% (255.1 g) [contains disodium edta, glycine soja (soybean) sterol]
  Generic: 40% (283.4 g, 18 mL); 50% (284 g)

Urea and Hydrocortisone
(yoor EE a & hye droe KOR ti sone)

Brand Names: US Carmol-HC® [DSC]; U-Cort
Brand Names: Canada Ti-U-Lac® H; Uremol® HC
Index Terms Hydrocortisone and Urea
Pharmacologic Category Corticosteroid, Topical
Use Inflammation of corticosteroid-responsive dermatoses
Dosing

Adult & Geriatric Steroid-responsive dermatoses: Topical: Apply thin film and rub in well 2-4 times/day. Therapy should be discontinued when control is achieved; if no improvement is seen, reassessment of diagnosis may be necessary.

Pediatric Refer to adult dosing.

Additional Information Complete prescribing information should be consulted for additional detail.

Dosage Forms Excipient information presented when available (limited, particularly for generics); consult specific product labeling.
Cream, topical:
  Carmol-HC®: Urea 10% and hydrocortisone acetate 1% (28 g) [DSC]
  U-Cort: Urea 10% and hydrocortisone acetate 1% (28 g)

Uridine Triacetate (URE i deen trye AS e tate)

Index Terms PN401; Triacetyluridine; Vistogard; Vistonuridine; Xuriden
Pharmacologic Category Antidote; Endocrine and Metabolic Agent, Miscellaneous
Use

Hereditary orotic aciduria: Treatment of hereditary orotic aciduria

Fluoropyrimidine overdose/overexposure: Emergency treatment of fluorouracil or capecitabine overdose (regardless of the presence of symptoms) or early-onset severe or life-threatening cardiac or CNS toxicity and/or early-onset unusually severe adverse reactions (eg, GI toxicity and/or neutropenia) within 96 hours following the end of fluorouracil or capecitabine administration (in pediatrics and adults).

Limitations of use: Uridine triacetate is not recommended for nonemergent treatment of adverse reactions associated with fluorouracil or capecitabine (because it may diminish efficacy of these medications). Safety and efficacy of uridine triacetate initiated more than 96 hours following the end of fluorouracil or capecitabine administration have not been established.

Prescribing and Access Restrictions Fluorouracil accidental overdose/overexposure: Uridine triacetate (formerly called vistonuridine) is supplied for emergency use under an expanded access protocol and FDA emergency treatment provisions. Procurement information is available from Wellstat Therapeutics at 1-443-831-5626.
Dosing

Adult & Geriatric

Fluoropyrimidine overdose/overexposure: Oral: 10 g every 6 hours for 20 doses beginning as soon as possible after overdose or early-onset toxicity within 96 hours after the end of fluorouracil or capecitabine administration (Bamat, 2013; von Borstel, 2009).

Hereditary orotic aciduria: Oral: Initial: 60 mg/kg once daily; increase to 120 mg/kg (maximum: 8 g) for insufficient efficacy (eg, urine orotic acid levels remaining above normal or increasing above the usual/expected range for the patient; lab values affected by orotic acid [red or white blood cell indices] worsening; worsening disease signs/symptoms).

Uridine Triacetate Daily Dose for Hereditary Orotic Aciduria Based on Weight (kg)

Patient weight	60 mg/kg[1] dose Dose in grams (dose in teaspoons[2])	120 mg/kg[1] dose Dose in grams (dose in teaspoons[2])
≤5 kg	0.4 g (1/8 tsp)	0.8 g (1/4 tsp)
6 to 10 kg	0.4 to 0.6 g (1/4 tsp)	0.8 to 1.2 g (1/2 tsp)
11 to 15 kg	0.7 to 0.9 g (1/2 tsp)	1.4 to 1.8 g (3/4 tsp or 1 entire packet)
16 to 20 kg	1 to 1.2 g (1/2 tsp)	2 to 2.4 g (1 tsp)
21 to 25 kg	1.3 to 1.5 g (1/2 tsp)	2.6 to 3 g (1 tsp)
26 to 30 kg	1.6 to 1.8 g (3/4 tsp or 1 entire packet)	3.2 to 3.6 g (1 1/4 tsp)
31 to 35 kg	1.9 to 2.1 g (3/4 tsp or 1 entire packet)	3.8 to 4.2 g (1 1/2 tsp or 2 entire packets)
36 to 40 kg	2.2 to 2.4 g (1 tsp)	4.4 to 4.8 g (1 3/4 tsp)
41 to 45 kg	2.5 to 2.7 g (1 tsp)	5 to 5.4 g (2 tsp or 3 entire packets)
46 to 50 kg	2.8 to 3 g (1 tsp)	5.6 to 6 g (2 tsp or 3 entire packets)
51 to 55 kg	3.1 to 3.3 g (1 1/4 tsp)	6.2 to 6.6 g (2 1/4 tsp)
56 to 60 kg	3.4 to 3.6 g (1 1/4 tsp)	6.8 to 7.2 g (2 1/2 tsp)
61 to 65 kg	3.7 to 3.9 g (1 1/2 tsp or 2 entire packets)	7.4 to 7.8 g (2 1/2 tsp)
66 to 70 kg	4 to 4.2 g (1 1/2 tsp or 2 entire packets)	8 g (2 3/4 tsp or 4 entire packets)
71 to 75 kg	4.3 to 4.5 g (1 1/2 tsp or 2 entire packets)	8 g (2 3/4 tsp or 4 entire packets)
>75 kg	6 g (2 tsp or 3 entire packets)	8 g (2 3/4 tsp or 4 entire packets)

Note: One packet contains uridine triacetate 2 g.

[1] Doses rounded (by the manufacturer) by weight category to achieve approximate dose level

[2] A 2 gram uridine triacetate (Xuriden) packet contains approximately 3/4 tsp

Pediatric

Fluoropyrimidine overdose/overexposure: Oral: 6.2 g/m² (maximum: 10 g/dose) every 6 hours for 20 doses beginning as soon as possible after overdose or early-onset toxicity within 96 hours after the end of fluorouracil or capecitabine administration.

Uridine Triacetate Pediatric Daily Dose for Fluoropyrimidine Overdose/Overexposure Based on Body Surface Area (BSA; m²)

Patient BSA	Uridine Triacetate 6.2 g/m²/dose[a]	
	Dose in grams	Dose in graduated teaspoons
0.34 to 0.44 m²	2.1 to 2.7 g	1 tsp
0.45 to 0.55 m²	2.8 to 3.4 g	1 ¼ tsp
0.56 to 0.66 m²	3.5 to 4.1 g	1 ½ tsp
0.67 to 0.77 m²	4.2 to 4.8 g	1 ¾ tsp
0.78 to 0.88 m²	4.9 to 5.4 g	2 tsp
0.89 to 0.99 m²	5.5 to 6.1 g	2 ¼ tsp
1 to 1.1 m²	6.2 to 6.8 g	2 ½ tsp
1.11 to 1.21 m²	6.9 to 7.5 g	2 ¾ tsp
1.22 to 1.32 m²	7.6 to 8.1 g	3 tsp
1.33 to 1.43 m²	8.2 to 8.8 g	3 ¼ tsp
>1.44 m²	10 g	1 full packet

Note: One Vistogard packet contains uridine triacetate 10 g.

[a] Doses rounded by BSA to achieve approximate dose; each dose is administered every 6 hours for 20 doses.

Hereditary orotic aciduria: Infants, Children, and Adolescents: Oral: Refer to adult dosing.

Renal Impairment There are no dosage adjustments provided in the manufacturer's labeling.

Hepatic Impairment There are no dosage adjustments provided in the manufacturer's labeling.

Additional Information Complete prescribing information should be consulted for additional detail.

Product Availability

Vistogard: FDA approved December 2015; anticipated availability is currently unknown. Vistogard is indicated for the emergency treatment of fluorouracil or capecitabine overdose or treatment of certain severe or life-threatening toxicities within 96 hours following the end of fluorouracil or capecitabine administration. Consult prescribing information for additional information. Information pertaining to this product within the monograph is pending revision.

Xuriden: FDA approved September 2015; availability anticipated in early 2016. Xuriden is FDA approved for the treatment of hereditary orotic aciduria. Consult prescribing information for additional information.

◆ **Urimar-T** see Methenamine, Sodium Phosphate Monobasic, Phenyl Salicylate, Methylene Blue, and Hyoscyamine on page 1166

◆ **Urinary Pain Relief [OTC]** see Phenazopyridine on page 1435

◆ **Urispas** see FlavoxATE on page 772

◆ **Urispas® (Can)** see FlavoxATE on page 772

◆ **Ur N-C** see Methenamine, Sodium Phosphate Monobasic, Phenyl Salicylate, Methylene Blue, and Hyoscyamine on page 1166

◆ **Uro-L** see Methenamine, Sodium Phosphate Monobasic, Phenyl Salicylate, Methylene Blue, and Hyoscyamine on page 1166

Urofollitropin (yoor oh fol li TROE pin)

Brand Names: US Bravelle
Brand Names: Canada Bravelle
Index Terms Follicle-Stimulating Hormone, Human; FSH; hFSH
Pharmacologic Category Gonadotropin; Ovulation Stimulator
Use

Multifollicular development during ART: Development of multiple follicles with assisted reproductive technologies (ART) in women who have previously received pituitary suppression.

Limitations of use: Prior to therapy, perform a complete gynecologic exam (including demonstration of tubal patency) and endocrinologic evaluation (cause of infertility should be diagnosed prior to ART); exclude the possibility of pregnancy; evaluate the fertility status of the male partner; exclude a diagnosis of primary ovarian failure.

Ovulation induction: Ovulation induction in women who previously received GnRH agonist or antagonist for pituitary suppression.

Dosing

Adult Note: Dose should be individualized. Use the lowest dose consistent with the expectation of good results. Over the course of treatment, doses may vary depending on individual patient response.

Assisted reproductive technologies (ART): Adults: Females: SubQ: Starting on day 2 or 3 of cycle, administer 225 units once daily for the first 5 days; urofollitropin may be administered together with menotropins and the total initial dose of both products combined should not exceed 225 units (menotropins 150 units and urofollitropin 75 units; or menotropins 75 units and urofollitropin 150 units). Adjust dose after 5 days based on ultrasound monitoring of ovarian response and measurement of serum estradiol levels. Do not make additional adjustments more frequently than once every 2 days or by >75-150 units. Maximum daily dose: 450 units (of urofollitropin, or menotropins plus urofollitropin); treatment >12 days is not recommended; once adequate follicular development is evident, hCG should be administered. Withhold the hCG dose if ovarian monitoring suggests an increased risk of OHSS.

Ovulation induction: Adults: Females: IM, SubQ: Initial: 150 units once daily for 5 days in the first cycle of treatment. After 5 days, dose adjustments up to 75-150 units can be made every ≥2 days based on ultrasound monitoring of ovarian response and/or measurement of serum estradiol levels; maximum daily dose: 450 units; treatment >12 days is not recommended. If response to follitropin is appropriate, administer hCG; withhold the hCG dose if ovarian monitoring suggests an increased risk of OHSS and advise the patient to refrain from intercourse. For subsequent cycles, the starting dose and dosage adjustments should be determined based on historical ovarian response.

Renal Impairment There are no dosage adjustments provided in manufacturer's labeling (has not been studied).

Hepatic Impairment There are no dosage adjustments provided in manufacturer's labeling (has not been studied).

Additional Information Complete prescribing information should be consulted for additional detail.

Dosage Forms Excipient information presented when available (limited, particularly for generics); consult specific product labeling.
Solution Reconstituted, Injection:
Bravelle: 75 units (1 ea)

◆ **Uro-Mag [OTC]** see Magnesium Oxide on page 1121

◆ **Uromitexan (Can)** see Mesna on page 1154

◆ **Uro-MP** see Methenamine, Sodium Phosphate Monobasic, Phenyl Salicylate, Methylene Blue, and Hyoscyamine on page 1166

◆ **Urophen MB** see Methenamine, Phenyl Salicylate, Methylene Blue, Benzoic Acid, and Hyoscyamine on page 1166

◆ **Uroqid-Acid® No. 2** see Methenamine and Sodium Acid Phosphate on page 1166

◆ **Uroxatral** see Alfuzosin on page 68

◆ **Urozide (Can)** see Hydrochlorothiazide on page 881

◆ **Urso (Can)** see Ursodiol on page 1855

◆ **Urso 250** see Ursodiol on page 1855

◆ **Ursodeoxycholic Acid** see Ursodiol on page 1855

◆ **Ursodesoxycholic Acid** see Ursodiol on page 1855

Ursodiol (ur soe DYE ol)

Brand Names: US Actigall; Urso 250; Urso Forte
Brand Names: Canada Dom-Ursodiol C; PHL-Ursodiol C; PMS-Ursodiol C; Urso; Urso DS
Index Terms Ursodeoxycholic Acid; Ursodesoxycholic Acid
Pharmacologic Category Gallstone Dissolution Agent
Use

Gallstones (capsules only):
For patients with radiolucent, noncalcified gallbladder stones less than 20 mm in greatest diameter in whom elective cholecystectomy would be undertaken except for the presence of increased surgical risk caused by systemic disease, advanced age, idiosyncratic reaction to general anesthesia, or for those patients who refuse surgery. Safety for use of ursodiol beyond 24 months is not established.

For the prevention of gallstone formation in obese patients experiencing rapid weight loss.

Primary biliary cirrhosis (tablets only): For the treatment of patients with primary biliary cirrhosis (PBC).

Dosing

Adult & Geriatric

Gallstone dissolution (Actigall): Oral: 8-10 mg/kg/day in 2-3 divided doses; use beyond 24 months is not established

Gallstone prevention (Actigall): Oral: 300 mg twice daily

Primary biliary cirrhosis (Urso, Urso Forte): Oral: 13-15 mg/kg/day in 2-4 divided doses (with food)

Renal Impairment There are no dosage adjustments provided in the manufacturer's labeling.

Hepatic Impairment There are no dosage adjustments provided in the manufacturer's labeling.

Additional Information Complete prescribing information should be consulted for additional detail.

Dosage Forms Excipient information presented when available (limited, particularly for generics); consult specific product labeling.

Capsule, Oral:
Actigall: 300 mg
Generic: 300 mg

Tablet, Oral:
Urso 250: 250 mg
Urso Forte: 500 mg [scored]
Generic: 250 mg, 500 mg

◆ **Urso DS (Can)** *see* Ursodiol *on page 1855*

◆ **Urso Forte** *see* Ursodiol *on page 1855*

Ustekinumab (yoo stek in YOO mab)

Brand Names: US Stelara
Brand Names: Canada Stelara
Index Terms CNTO 1275
Pharmacologic Category Antipsoriatic Agent; Interleukin-12 Inhibitor; Interleukin-23 Inhibitor; Monoclonal Antibody

Use

Plaque psoriasis: Treatment of adults with moderate-to-severe plaque psoriasis who are candidates for phototherapy or systemic therapy

Psoriatic arthritis: Treatment of adults with active psoriatic arthritis (as monotherapy or in combination with methotrexate)

Pregnancy Considerations Adverse events were not observed in animal reproduction studies. There is limited information related to the use of ustekinumab in pregnancy (Andrulonis, 2012). In general, other agents are preferred for the treatment of plaque psoriasis in pregnant women (Hsu, 2012). Patients exposed to ustekinumab during pregnancy are encouraged to enroll in the pregnancy registry by calling 877-311-8972.

Breast-Feeding Considerations It is not known whether ustekinumab is secreted in human milk. Because many immunoglobulins are secreted in milk it is expected that ustekinumab will be present in breast milk. The U.S. labeling recommends caution be used in nursing women. The Canadian labeling recommends discontinuing nursing or discontinuing ustekinumab.

Medication Guide Available Yes

Contraindications

Clinically significant hypersensitivity to ustekinumab or any component of the formulation

Canadian labeling: Additional contraindications (not in U.S. labeling): Severe infections such as sepsis, tuberculosis, and opportunistic infections

Warnings/Precautions May increase the risk for malignancy although the impact on the development and course of malignancies is not fully defined. Rapidly appearing cutaneous squamous cell carcinomas (multiple) have been reported in patients receiving ustekinumab who were at risk for developing nonmelanoma skin cancer. Monitor all patients closely for the development of nonmelanoma skin cancer; closely follow patients >60 years of age, with a history of prolonged immunosuppression, and in patients with a history of PUVA treatment. Use with caution in patients with prior malignancy (use not studied in this population).

May increase the risk for infections or reactivation of latent infections. Serious bacterial, fungal, and viral infections have been observed with use. Avoid use in patients with clinically important active infection. Caution should be exercised when considering use in patients with a history of new/recurrent infections, with conditions that predispose them to infections (eg, diabetes or residence/travel from areas of endemic mycoses), or with chronic, latent, or localized infections, or who are genetically deficient in IL-12/IL-23 (IL-12/IL-23 genetic deficiency may predispose patients to disseminated infection). Patients who develop a new infection while undergoing treatment should be monitored closely. If a patient develops a serious infection, therapy should be discontinued or withheld until successful resolution of infection.

Do not use in patients with active tuberculosis (TB). Patients should be evaluated for latent tuberculosis infection with a tuberculin skin test prior to starting therapy. Treatment of latent TB should be initiated before ustekinumab therapy is used. Consider antituberculosis treatment in patients with a history of latent or active tuberculosis if an adequate prior treatment course cannot be confirmed. During and following treatment, monitor for signs/symptoms of active TB.

Antibody formation to ustekinumab has been observed with therapy and has been associated with decreased serum levels and therapeutic response in some patients. Hypersensitivity, including anaphylaxis and angioedema, has been reported. Discontinue immediately with signs/symptoms of hypersensitivity reaction and treat appropriately as indicated. Reversible posterior leukoencephalopathy syndrome (RPLS) has been observed (rare). RPLS symptoms include headache, seizures, confusion, and visual disturbances; may be fatal. Monitor; discontinue ustekinumab if symptoms occur and administer appropriate therapy. Use in combination with other immunosuppressive drugs during psoriasis studies has not been evaluated; use caution. Use in combination with methotrexate during psoriatic arthritis studies did not appear to affect safety or efficacy. Use in combination with phototherapy has not been studied; use caution. Patients should be brought up to date with all immunizations before initiating therapy. **Live vaccines should not be given concurrently;** inactivated or nonlive vaccines may be given concurrently, but may not elicit a proper immune response. BCG vaccines should not be given 1 year prior to, during, or 1 year following treatment. Patients >100 kg may require higher dose to achieve adequate serum levels. Use in hepatic or renal impairment has not been studied.

The packaging may contain latex. Some dosage forms may contain polysorbate 80 (also known as Tweens). Hypersensitivity reactions, usually a delayed reaction, have been reported following exposure to pharmaceutical products containing polysorbate 80 in certain individuals (Isaksson, 2002; Lucente 2000; Shelley, 1995). Thrombocytopenia, ascites, pulmonary deterioration, and renal and hepatic failure have been reported in premature neonates after receiving parenteral products containing polysorbate 80 (Alade, 1986; CDC, 1984). See manufacturer's labeling. Potentially significant interactions may exist, requiring dose or frequency adjustment, additional monitoring, and/or selection of alternative therapy.

Adverse Reactions

>10%: Infection: Infection (27% to 70%; severe infection: ≤3%)

1% to 10%:
Central nervous system: Headache (5%), fatigue (3%), dizziness (2%), depression (1%)
Dermatologic: Pruritus (2%)
Gastrointestinal: Nausea (3%)
Immunologic: Antibody development (3% to 6%)
Local: Erythema at injection site (1% to 2%)
Neuromuscular & skeletal: Arthralgia (3%), back pain (2%)
Respiratory: Pharyngolaryngeal pain (2%)

<1%, postmarketing, and/or case reports (Limited to important or life-threatening): Anaphylaxis, angina pectoris, angioedema, appendicitis, bacterial infection, bleeding at injection site, bruising at injection site, cellulitis, cerebrovascular accident, cholecystitis, dactylitis, diverticulitis, erythrodermic psoriasis, exfoliative dermatitis, fungal infection, gastroenteritis, herpes zoster, hypersensitivity reaction, hypertension, induration at injection site, irritation at injection site, itching at injection site, malignant melanoma (*in situ*), malignant neoplasm (breast, colon, head and neck, kidney, prostate, thyroid), myocardial infarction, nephrolithiasis, osteomyelitis, pain at injection site, pneumonia, pustular psoriasis, reversible posterior leukoencephalopathy syndrome, sepsis, squamous cell carcinoma of skin, swelling at injection site, urinary tract infection, viral infection

Drug Interactions

Metabolism/Transport Effects None known.

Avoid Concomitant Use

Avoid concomitant use of Ustekinumab with any of the following: BCG (Intravesical); Belimumab; InFLIXimab; Natalizumab; Pimecrolimus; Tacrolimus (Topical); Tofacitinib; Vaccines (Live)

Increased Effect/Toxicity
Ustekinumab may increase the levels/effects of: Belimumab; Fingolimod; InFLIXimab; Leflunomide; Natalizumab; Tofacitinib; Vaccines (Live)

The levels/effects of Ustekinumab may be increased by: Denosumab; Pimecrolimus; Roflumilast; Tacrolimus (Topical); Trastuzumab

Decreased Effect
Ustekinumab may decrease the levels/effects of: BCG (Intravesical); Coccidioides immitis Skin Test; Sipuleucel-T; Vaccines (Inactivated); Vaccines (Live)

The levels/effects of Ustekinumab may be decreased by: Echinacea

Storage/Stability Refrigerate at 2°C to 8°C (36°F to 46°F); do not freeze. Store vials upright. Keep the product in the original carton to protect from light until the time of use. Do not shake. Discard any unused portion.

Mechanism of Action Ustekinumab is a human monoclonal antibody that binds to and interferes with the proinflammatory cytokines, interleukin (IL)-12 and IL-23. Biological effects of IL-12 and IL-23 include natural killer (NK) cell activation, CD4+ T-cell differentiation and activation. Ustekinumab also interferes with the expression of monocyte chemotactic protein-1 (MCP-1), tumor necrosis factor-alpha (TNF-α), interferon-inducible protein-10 (IP-10), and interleukin-8 (IL-8). Significant clinical improvement in psoriasis and psoriatic arthritis patients is seen in association with reduction of these proinflammatory signalers.

Pharmacodynamics/Kinetics
Distribution: V_d (terminal elimination phase): 45 mg: 0.161 ± 0.065 L/kg; 90 mg: 0.179 ± 0.085 L/kg
Bioavailability: Absolute bioavailability: SubQ: ~57%
Half-life elimination: 10-126 days
Time to peak, plasma: 45 mg: 13.5 days; 90 mg: 7 days

Dosing
Adult & Geriatric
Plaque psoriasis: SubQ:
Initial and maintenance: **Note:** Following an interruption in therapy, re-treatment may be initiated at the initial dosing interval. Consider therapy discontinuation in any patient failing to demonstrate a response after 12 weeks of therapy.
≤100 kg: 45 mg at 0- and 4 weeks, and then every 12 weeks thereafter
>100 kg: 90 mg at 0- and 4 weeks, and then every 12 weeks thereafter. **Note:** Doses of 45 mg given to patients >100 kg were also efficacious; however, 90 mg is the recommended dose in these patients due to greater efficacy.
Note: The Canadian labeling suggests that if the response is inadequate on every-12-week therapy, may consider increasing frequency to every 8 weeks.
Psoriatic arthritis: SubQ: **Note:** When used for psoriatic arthritis, may be administered alone or in combination with methotrexate.
U.S. labeling:
Initial and maintenance: 45 mg at 0- and 4 weeks, and then every 12 weeks thereafter.
Coexistent psoriatic arthritis and moderate-to-severe plaque psoriasis in patients >100 kg: Initial and maintenance: 90 mg at 0- and 4 weeks, and then every 12 weeks thereafter.
Canadian labeling: Initial and maintenance:
≤100 kg: 45 mg at 0- and 4 weeks, and then every 12 weeks thereafter.
>100 kg: 90 mg at 0- and 4 weeks, and then every 12 weeks thereafter.
Renal Impairment There are no dosage adjustment provided in the manufacturer's labeling (has not been studied).
Hepatic Impairment There are no dosage adjustment provided in the manufacturer's labeling (has not been studied).
Administration Administer by subcutaneous injection into the top of the thigh, abdomen, upper arms, or buttocks. Rotate sites. Do not inject into tender, bruised, erythematous, or indurated skin. Avoid areas of skin where psoriasis is present. Do not use if cloudy or discolored. Discard any unused portion. Intended for use under supervision of physician; self-injection may occur after proper training.
Monitoring Parameters Tuberculosis screening (prior to initiating and periodically during therapy); CBC; ustekinumab-antibody formation; monitor for signs/symptoms of infection, reversible posterior leukoencephalopathy syndrome (RPLS), and squamous cell skin carcinoma

Dosage Forms Excipient information presented when available (limited, particularly for generics); consult specific product labeling.
Solution Prefilled Syringe, Subcutaneous [preservative free]:
Stelara: 45 mg/0.5 mL (0.5 mL); 90 mg/mL (1 mL) [contains polysorbate 80]

◆ **Ustell** see Methenamine, Sodium Phosphate Monobasic, Phenyl Salicylate, Methylene Blue, and Hyoscyamine *on page 1166*

◆ **Utibron Neohaler [DSC]** see Indacaterol and Glycopyrrolate *on page 934*

◆ **Uticap** see Methenamine, Sodium Phosphate Monobasic, Phenyl Salicylate, Methylene Blue, and Hyoscyamine *on page 1166*

◆ **Utira-C** see Methenamine, Sodium Phosphate Monobasic, Phenyl Salicylate, Methylene Blue, and Hyoscyamine *on page 1166*

◆ **Utopic** see Urea *on page 1853*

◆ **Utrona-C** see Methenamine, Sodium Phosphate Monobasic, Phenyl Salicylate, Methylene Blue, and Hyoscyamine *on page 1166*

◆ **Uvadex** see Methoxsalen (Systemic) *on page 1175*

Vaccinia Immune Globulin (Intravenous)
(vax IN ee a i MYUN GLOB yoo lin IN tra VEE nus)

Brand Names: US CNJ-016
Index Terms IV-VIG; VIG; VIGIV
Pharmacologic Category Blood Product Derivative; Immune Globulin
Use Vaccinia conditions: Treatment and/or modification of the following conditions:
- Aberrant infections induced by vaccinia virus that include its accidental implantation in eyes (except in cases of isolated keratitis), mouth, or other areas where vaccinia infection would constitute a special hazard.
- Eczema vaccinatum
- Progressive vaccinia
- Severe generalized vaccinia
- Vaccinia infections in individuals who have skin conditions such as burns, impetigo, varicella-zoster, or poison ivy; or in individuals who have eczematous skin lesions because of either the activity or extensiveness of such lesions

The Advisory Committee on Immunization Practices (ACIP) recommends the following (CDC 2009; CDC [Rotz 2001]; CDC [Wharton 2003]):
Use is recommended for:
- Inadvertent inoculation (considering severity, toxicity of affected person, and pain)
- Eczema vaccinatum
- Generalized vaccinia (severe form or if underlying illness is present)
- Progressive vaccinia
Use may be considered for:
- Severe ocular complications except isolated keratitis
Use is not recommended for:
- Inadvertent inoculation that is not severe
- Mild or limited generalized vaccinia
- Nonspecific rashes, erythema multiforme, or Stevens-Johnson syndrome
- Postvaccinial encephalitis or encephalomyelitis

Prescribing and Access Restrictions Vaccinia immune globulin is not available for general public use. All supplies are currently owned by the federal government for inclusion in the Strategic National Stockpile. The CDC Smallpox Adverse Events Clinical Consultation team will coordinate shipment. The State Health Department should be contacted first concerning severe or unexpected adverse events from smallpox vaccination.

Dosing
Adult Vaccinia treatment/modification: IV: 6,000 units/kg; may repeat dose based on severity of symptoms and response to treatment (specific data are lacking); 9,000 units/kg may be considered if patient does not respond to initial dose. Single doses up to 24,000 unit/kg were tolerated in healthy volunteers.
Pediatric Vaccinia treatment/modification: Adolescents ≥16 years: Refer to adult dosing.
Renal Impairment There are no dosage adjustments provided in the manufacturer's labeling. Use caution. In patients at risk of renal dysfunction, the rate of infusion and concentration of solution should be minimized; discontinue if renal function deteriorates.
Hepatic Impairment There are no dosage adjustments provided in manufacturer's labeling.
Additional Information Complete prescribing information should be consulted for additional detail.

Dosage Forms Excipient information presented when available (limited, particularly for generics); consult specific product labeling.

Injection, solution [preservative free; solvent-detergent treated]:

CNJ-016: ≥50,000 units/15 mL (15 mL) [contains maltose 10% and polysorbate 80 0.03%]

◆ Vaccinia Vaccine see Smallpox Vaccine on page 1668

◆ Vacuant Mini-Enema [OTC] [DSC] see Docusate on page 578

◆ Vagifem see Estradiol (Topical) on page 686

◆ Vagifem10 (Can) see Estradiol (Topical) on page 686

◆ Vagistat-3 [OTC] see Miconazole (Topical) on page 1201

ValACYclovir (val ay SYE kloe veer)

Brand Names: US Valtrex

Brand Names: Canada Apo-Valacyclovir; CO Valacyclovir; DOM-Valacyclovir; Mylan-Valacyclovir; PHL-Valacyclovir; PMS-Valacyclovir; PRO-Valacyclovir; Riva-Valacyclovir; Valtrex

Index Terms Valacyclovir Hydrochloride

Pharmacologic Category Antiviral Agent; Antiviral Agent, Oral

Use Treatment of herpes zoster (shingles) in immunocompetent patients; treatment of first-episode and recurrent genital herpes; suppression of recurrent genital herpes and reduction of transmission of genital herpes in immunocompetent patients; suppression of genital herpes in HIV-infected individuals; treatment of herpes labialis (cold sores); chickenpox in immunocompetent children

Pregnancy Considerations Adverse events were not observed in animal reproduction studies. Valacyclovir is metabolized to acyclovir. In a pharmacokinetic study, maternal acyclovir serum concentrations were higher in pregnant women receiving valacyclovir than those given acyclovir for the suppression of recurrent herpes simplex virus (HSV) infection late in pregnancy. Amniotic fluid concentrations were also higher; however, there was no evidence that fetal exposure differed between the groups (Kimberlin, 1998). Data from an acyclovir pregnancy registry has shown no increased rate of birth defects than that of the general population; however, the registry is small and the manufacturer notes that use during pregnancy is only warranted if the potential benefit to the mother justifies the risk of the fetus. Because more data is available for acyclovir, that agent is preferred for the treatment of genital herpes in pregnant women (ACOG 2000; CDC 2010); however, valacyclovir may be considered for use due to its simplified dosing schedule (DHHS 2013). Pregnant women who have a history of genital herpes recurrence, suppressive therapy is recommended starting at 36 weeks gestation (ACOG 2000; DHHS 2013).

Breast-Feeding Considerations Valacyclovir is metabolized to acyclovir; acyclovir (but not unchanged valacyclovir) can be detected in breast milk. Peak concentrations in breast milk range from 0.5-2.3 times the corresponding maternal acyclovir serum concentration. This is expected to provide a nursing infant with a dose of acyclovir equivalent to ~0.6 mg/kg/day following ingestion of valacyclovir 500 mg twice daily by the mother. The manufacturer recommends that caution be used if administered to a nursing woman. Other sources note that women with HSV infection taking valacyclovir may breast-feed as long as there are not lesions on the breast, body lesions are covered, and strict hand hygiene is practiced (ACOG 2000; Jaiyeoba 2012). Women with HSV who also have HIV infection should not breast-feed; complete avoidance of breast-feeding by HIV-infected women is recommended to decrease potential transmission of HIV (DHHS [perinatal] 2012).

Contraindications Hypersensitivity to valacyclovir, acyclovir, or any component of the formulation

Warnings/Precautions Thrombotic thrombocytopenic purpura/hemolytic uremic syndrome has occurred in immunocompromised patients (at doses of 8 g/day). Safety and efficacy have not been established for treatment/suppression of recurrent genital herpes or disseminated herpes in patients with profound immunosuppression (eg, advanced HIV with CD4 <100 cells/mm³). CNS adverse effects (including agitation, hallucinations, confusion, delirium, seizures, and encephalopathy) have been reported. Use caution in patients with renal impairment, the elderly, and/or those receiving nephrotoxic agents. Acute renal failure has been observed in patients with renal dysfunction; dose adjustment may be required. Precipitation in renal tubules may occur leading to urinary precipitation; adequately hydrate patient. For cold sores, treatment should begin at with earliest symptom (tingling, itching, burning). For genital herpes, treatment should begin as soon as possible after the first signs and symptoms (within 72 hours of onset of first diagnosis or within 24 hours of onset of recurrent episodes). For herpes zoster, treatment should begin within 72 hours of onset of rash. For chickenpox, treatment should begin with earliest sign or symptom. Use with caution in the elderly; CNS effects have been reported.

Adverse Reactions

>10%:

Central nervous system: Headache (13% to 38%)

Gastrointestinal: Nausea (5% to 15%), abdominal pain (1% to 11%)

Hepatic: ALT increased (≤14%), AST increased (2% to 16%)

Respiratory: Nasopharyngitis (≤16%)

1% to 10%:

Central nervous system: Fatigue (≤8%), depression (≤7%), fever (children 4%), dizziness (2% to 4%)

Dermatologic: Rash (≤8%)

Endocrine: Dysmenorrhea (≤1% to 8%), dehydration (children 2%)

Gastrointestinal: Vomiting (<1% to 6%), diarrhea (children 5%; adults <1%)

Hematologic: Thrombocytopenia (≤3%), mild leukopenia (≤1%)

Hepatic: Alkaline phosphatase increased (≤4%)

Neuromuscular & skeletal: Arthralgia (<1 to 6%)

Respiratory: Rhinorrhea (children 2%)

Miscellaneous: Herpes simplex (children 2%)

<1% (Limited to important or life-threatening): Acute hypersensitivity reactions (angioedema, anaphylaxis, dyspnea, pruritus, rash, urticaria); aggression, agitation, alopecia, anemia, aplastic anemia, ataxia, creatinine increased, coma, confusion, consciousness decreased, delirium, dysarthria, encephalopathy, erythema multiforme, facial edema, hallucinations (auditory and visual), hemolytic uremic syndrome (HUS), hepatitis, hypertension, leukocytoclastic vasculitis, mania, photosensitivity reaction, psychosis, renal failure, renal pain, seizure, tachycardia, thrombotic thrombocytopenic purpura (TTP), tremor, urinary precipitation, visual disturbances

Drug Interactions

Metabolism/Transport Effects None known.

Avoid Concomitant Use

Avoid concomitant use of ValACYclovir with any of the following: Foscarnet; Varicella Virus Vaccine; Zoster Vaccine

Increased Effect/Toxicity

ValACYclovir may increase the levels/effects of: Mycophenolate; Tenofovir Products; Zidovudine

The levels/effects of ValACYclovir may be increased by: Foscarnet; Mycophenolate; Tenofovir Products

Decreased Effect

ValACYclovir may decrease the levels/effects of: Talimogene Laherparepvec; Varicella Virus Vaccine; Zoster Vaccine

Storage/Stability Store at 15°C to 25°C (59°F to 77°F).

Mechanism of Action Valacyclovir is rapidly and nearly completely converted to acyclovir by intestinal and hepatic metabolism. Acyclovir is converted to acyclovir monophosphate by virus-specific thymidine kinase then further converted to acyclovir triphosphate by other cellular enzymes. Acyclovir triphosphate inhibits DNA synthesis and viral replication by competing with deoxyguanosine triphosphate for viral DNA polymerase and being incorporated into viral DNA.

Pharmacodynamics/Kinetics

Absorption: Rapid

Distribution: Acyclovir is widely distributed throughout the body including brain, kidney, lungs, liver, spleen, muscle, uterus, vagina, and CSF

Protein binding: ~14% to 18%

Metabolism: Hepatic; valacyclovir is rapidly and nearly completely converted to acyclovir and L-valine by first-pass effect; acyclovir is hepatically metabolized to a very small extent by aldehyde oxidase and by alcohol and aldehyde dehydrogenase (inactive metabolites)

Bioavailability: ~55% once converted to acyclovir

Half-life elimination: Normal renal function: Adults: Acyclovir: 2.5-3.3 hours, Valacyclovir: ~30 minutes; End-stage renal disease: Acyclovir: 14 to 20 hours; During hemodialysis: 4 hours

Excretion: Urine, primarily as acyclovir (89%); **Note:** Following oral administration of radiolabeled valacyclovir, 46% of the label is eliminated in the feces (corresponding to nonabsorbed drug), while 47% of the radiolabel is eliminated in the urine.

Dosing

Adult & Geriatric

CMV prophylaxis in allogeneic HSCT recipients (off-label use): 2 g 4 times daily

Herpes labialis (cold sores): Oral: 2 g twice daily for 1 day (separate doses by ~12 hours)

Herpes labialis (cold sores) in HIV-infected patients (off-label use): Oral: 1 g twice daily for 5 to 10 days (HHS [OI adult 2015])

Herpes zoster (shingles): Oral:
Immunocompetent patients: 1 g 3 times daily for 7 days
HIV-infected patients (off-label use): 1 g 3 times daily for 7 to 10 days; consider longer duration if lesions resolve slowly.

HSV, VZV in cancer patients (off-label use):
Prophylaxis: 500 mg 2-3 times daily
Treatment: 1 g 3 times daily

Herpes simplex virus, genital infection: Oral:
Manufacturer's labeling:
Initial episode: Immunocompetent patients: 1 g twice daily for 10 days
Recurrent episode: Immunocompetent patients: 500 mg twice daily for 3 days
Reduction of transmission: 500 mg once daily (source partner)
Suppressive therapy:
Immunocompetent patients: 1 g once daily (500 mg once daily in patients with ≤9 recurrences per year)
HIV-infected patients (CD4 ≥100 cells/mm^3): 500 mg twice daily
Alternate dosing: HIV-infected patients:
Initial or recurrent episodes (off-label use): 1 g twice daily for 5 to 14 days (HHS [OI adult 2015])
Chronic suppressive therapy: 500 mg twice daily; continue indefinitely regardless of CD4 count in patients with severe recurrences or in patients who want to minimize frequency of recurrences (HHS [OI adult 2015])

Varicella (chickenpox) in HIV-infected patients (off-label use): 1 g 3 times daily for 5 to 7 days in uncomplicated cases (HHS [OI adult 2015])

Pediatric

Herpes labialis (cold sores): Oral: Children ≥12 years and Adolescents: Refer to adult dosing.

Herpes labialis (cold sores) in HIV-infected patients (off-label use): Adolescents: Refer to adult dosing.

Herpes simplex virus, genital infection in HIV-infected patients: Adolescents (off-label population): Oral:
Initial or recurrent episodes (off-label use): 1 g twice daily for 5 to 14 days (HHS [OI adult 2015])
Chronic suppressive therapy (off-label dose): 500 mg twice daily; continue indefinitely regardless of CD4 count in patients with severe recurrences or in patients who want to minimize frequency of recurrences (HHS [OI adult 2015])

Herpes zoster (shingles) in HIV-infected patients (off-label use): Adolescents: Refer to adult dosing.

Varicella (chickenpox): Oral:
Immunocompetent patients: Children ≥2 years and Adolescents: 20 mg/kg/dose 3 times daily for 5 days (maximum: 1 g 3 times daily)
HIV-infected patients (off-label use): Adolescents: Refer to adult dosing.

Renal Impairment

Herpes zoster: Adults:
CrCl 30 to 49 mL/minute: 1 g every 12 hours
CrCl 10 to 29 mL/minute: 1 g every 24 hours
CrCl <10 mL/minute: 500 mg every 24 hours

Genital herpes: Adults:
U.S. labeling:
Initial episode:
CrCl 10 to 29 mL/minute: 1 g every 24 hours
CrCl <10 mL/minute: 500 mg every 24 hours
Recurrent episode: CrCl <29 mL/minute: 500 mg every 24 hours
Suppressive therapy: CrCl <29 mL/minute:
For usual dose of 1 g every 24 hours, decrease dose to 500 mg every 24 hours
For usual dose of 500 mg every 24 hours, decrease dose to 500 mg every 48 hours
HIV-infected patients: 500 mg every 24 hours
Canadian labeling:
Initial episode:
CrCl 10 to 29 mL/minute: 1 g every 24 hours
CrCl <10 mL/minute: 500 mg every 24 hours
Recurrent episode:
CrCl 10 to 29 mL/minute: 500 mg every 24 hours
CrCl <10 mL/minute: 500 mg every 24 hours
Suppressive therapy:
CrCl 10 to 29 mL/minute:
Immunocompetent or HIV-infected patients: 500 mg every 24 hours
Immunocompetent patients with ≤9 recurrences/year: 500 mg every 48 hours

CrCl <10 mL/minute:
Immunocompetent or HIV-infected patients: 500 mg every 24 hours
Immunocompetent patients with ≤9 recurrences/year: 500 mg every 48 hours

Herpes labialis: Adolescents and Adults (U.S. labeling) or Adults (Canadian labeling):
CrCl 30 to 49 mL/minute: 1 g every 12 hours for 2 doses
CrCl 10 to 29 mL/minute: 500 mg every 12 hours for 2 doses
CrCl <10 mL/minute: 500 mg as a single dose
Hemodialysis: Dialyzable (~33% removed during 4-hour session); administer dose postdialysis
Chronic ambulatory peritoneal dialysis/continuous arteriovenous hemofiltration dialysis: Pharmacokinetic parameters are similar to those in patients with ESRD; supplemental dose not needed following dialysis

Hepatic Impairment No dosage adjustment necessary.

Dietary Considerations May be taken with or without food.

Administration If GI upset occurs, administer with meals.

Monitoring Parameters Urinalysis, BUN, serum creatinine, liver enzymes, and CBC

Dosage Forms Excipient information presented when available (limited, particularly for generics); consult specific product labeling.
Tablet, Oral:
Valtrex: 500 mg [contains fd&c blue #2 aluminum lake]
Valtrex: 1 g [scored; contains fd&c blue #2 aluminum lake]
Generic: 500 mg, 1 g

Extemporaneous Preparations A 50 mg/mL oral suspension may be made with caplets and either Ora-Sweet® or Ora-Sweet SF®. Crush eighteen 500 mg caplets in a mortar and reduce to a fine powder. Add 5 mL portions of chosen vehicle (40 mL total) and mix to a uniform paste; transfer to a 180 mL calibrated amber glass bottle, rinse mortar with 10 mL of vehicle 5 times, and add quantity of vehicle sufficient to make 180 mL. Label "shake well" and "refrigerate". Stable for 21 days refrigerated.
Fish DN, Vidaurri VA, and Deeter RG, "Stability of Valacyclovir Hydrochloride in Extemporaneously Prepared Oral Liquids," *Am J Health Syst Pharm,* 1999, 56(19):1957-60.

◆ **Valacyclovir Hydrochloride** see ValACYclovir on page 1858

◆ **Valchlor** see Mechlorethamine (Topical) on page 1130

◆ **Valcyte** see ValGANciclovir on page 1859

◆ **23-Valent Pneumococcal Polysaccharide Vaccine** see Pneumococcal Polysaccharide Vaccine (23-Valent) on page 1464

ValGANciclovir (val gan SYE kloh veer)

Brand Names: US Valcyte
Brand Names: Canada Apo-Valganciclovir; Valcyte
Index Terms Valganciclovir Hydrochloride
Pharmacologic Category Antiviral Agent

Use

CMV disease (prophylaxis):
Prevention of CMV disease in high-risk adult patients (donor CMV seropositive/recipient CMV seronegative) undergoing kidney, heart, or kidney/pancreas transplantation
Prevention of CMV disease in high risk pediatric patients undergoing kidney transplant (age 4 months to 16 years) or heart transplant (age 1 month to 16 years)

Cytomegalovirus (CMV) retinitis (treatment): Treatment of cytomegalovirus (CMV) retinitis in patients with acquired immunodeficiency syndrome (AIDS)

Pregnancy Considerations [U.S. Boxed Warning]: May cause temporary or permanent inhibition of spermatogenesis; has the potential to cause birth defects in humans. Valganciclovir is converted to ganciclovir and shares its reproductive toxicity. Ganciclovir crosses the placenta. Based on animal data, temporary or permanent impairment of fertility may occur in males and females. Ganciclovir is also teratogenic in animals. The manufacturer recommends females of reproductive potential undergo pregnancy testing prior to therapy. Females should use effective contraception during treatment and for 30 days after; males should use barrier contraception during treatment and for 90 days after.

Adverse events following congenital CMV infection may also occur. Hearing loss, mental retardation, microcephaly, seizures, and other medical problems have been observed. The indications for treating CMV retinitis during pregnancy are the same as in non-pregnant HIV infected woman; however systemic therapy should be avoided during the first trimester when possible. Use of valganciclovir is recommended to treat maternal infection, but not

recommended for the treatment of asymptomatic maternal disease for the sole purpose of preventing infant infection. Monitoring of the fetus is recommended. Current recommendations for use of valganciclovir in HIV infected pregnant women are based on data from ganciclovir use in pregnant women following organ transplant or use late in pregnancy in non-HIV infected women [DHHS Adult OI, 2014].

Breast-Feeding Considerations It is not known if ganciclovir or valganciclovir are excreted into breast milk; breast feeding is not recommended. HIV-infected mothers are discouraged from breast-feeding to decrease the potential transmission of HIV. The manufacturer also notes the potential for hematologic toxicity or cancer to the nursing infant following exposure to ganciclovir.

Contraindications Hypersensitivity to valganciclovir, ganciclovir, or any component of the formulation

Warnings/Precautions Hazardous agent - use appropriate precautions for handling and disposal (NIOSH 2014 [group 2]).

[US Boxed Warning]: Severe leukopenia, neutropenia, anemia, thrombocytopenia, pancytopenia, bone marrow aplasia and aplastic anemia have been reported; do not use in patients with an absolute neutrophil count <500/mm^3, platelet count <25,000/mm^3, or hemoglobin <8 g/dL. Use with caution in patients with impaired renal function (dose adjustment required). Acute renal failure (ARF) may occur; ensure adequate hydration and use with caution in patients receiving concomitant nephrotoxic agents. Elderly patients with or without preexisting renal impairment may develop ARF; use with caution and adjust dose as needed. **[US Boxed Warning]: May cause temporary or permanent inhibition of spermatogenesis; has the potential to cause birth defects and cancers in humans.** Due to its teratogenic potential, females should use effective contraception during treatment and for 30 days after; males should use barrier contraception during treatment and for 90 days after. Fertility may be temporarily or permanently impaired in males and females.

Due to differences in bioavailability, valganciclovir tablets cannot be substituted for ganciclovir capsules on a one-to-one basis. The preferred dosage form for pediatric patients is the oral solution; however, valganciclovir tablets may used so long as the calculated dose is within 10% of the available tablet strength (450 mg). Not indicated for use in liver transplant patients (higher incidence of tissue-invasive CMV relative to oral ganciclovir was observed in trials). Use of valganciclovir for the treatment of congenital CMV disease has not been evaluated.

Benzyl alcohol and derivatives: Some dosage forms may contain sodium benzoate/benzoic acid; benzoic acid (benzoate) is a metabolite of benzyl alcohol; large amounts of benzyl alcohol (≥99 mg/kg/day) have been associated with a potentially fatal toxicity ("gasping syndrome") in neonates; the "gasping syndrome" consists of metabolic acidosis, respiratory distress, gasping respirations, CNS dysfunction (including convulsions, intracranial hemorrhage), hypotension, and cardiovascular collapse (AAP ["Inactive" 1997]; CDC, 1982); some data suggests that benzoate displaces bilirubin from protein binding sites (Ahlfors, 2001); avoid or use dosage forms containing benzyl alcohol derivative with caution in neonates. See manufacturer's labeling.

Adverse Reactions

>10%:
Cardiovascular: Hypertension (12% to 18%)
Central nervous system: Headache (6% to 22%), insomnia (6% to 20%)
Gastrointestinal: Diarrhea (16% to 41%), nausea (8% to 30%), vomiting (3% to 21%), abdominal pain (15%)
Hematologic: Anemia (≤31%), thrombocytopenia (≤22%), neutropenia (3% to 19%)
Immunologic: Graft rejection (24%)
Neuromuscular & skeletal: Tremor (12% to 28%)
Ophthalmic: Retinal detachment (15%)
Renal: Increased serum creatinine (S$_{cr}$ >1.5 to 2.5 mg/dL: 12% to 50%; S$_{cr}$ >2.5: 3% to 17%)
Miscellaneous: Fever (9% to 31%)

1% to 10%:
Cardiovascular: Edema (<5%), hypotension (<5%), peripheral edema (<5%)
Central nervous system: Peripheral neuropathy (9%), paresthesia (≤8%), agitation (<5%), confusion (<5%), depression (<5%), dizziness (<5%), fatigue (<5%), hallucination (<5%), pain (<5%), psychosis (<5%), seizure (<5%)
Dermatologic: Acne vulgaris (<5%), dermatitis (<5%), increased wound secretion (<5%), pruritus (<5%)

Endocrine & metabolic: Dehydration (<5%), hyperglycemia (<5%), hyperkalemia (<5%), hypocalcemia (<5%), hypokalemia (<5%), hypomagnesemia (<5%), hypophosphatemia (<5%)
Gastrointestinal: Abdominal distention (<5%), constipation (<5%), decreased appetite (<5%), dyspepsia (<5%)
Genitourinary: Dysuria (<5%), urinary tract infection (<5%)
Hematologic: Aplastic anemia (<5%), bone marrow depression (<5%), pancytopenia (<5%)
Hepatic: Ascites (<5%), hepatic insufficiency (<5%)
Hypersensitivity: Hypersensitivity reaction (<5%)
Immunologic: Organ transplant rejection (6% to 9%)
Infection: Localized infection (<5%), sepsis (<5%), wound infection (<5%)
Local: Catheter infection (3%)
Neuromuscular & skeletal: Arthralgia (<5%), back pain (<5%), limb pain (<5%), muscle cramps (<5%), weakness (<5%)
Renal: Decreased creatinine clearance (<5%), renal impairment (<5%)
Respiratory: Cough (<5%), dyspnea (<5%), nasopharyngitis (<5%), pharyngitis (<5%), pleural effusion (<5%), rhinorrhea (<5%), upper respiratory tract infection (<5%)
Miscellaneous: Postoperative complication (<5%), postoperative pain (<5%), wound dehiscence (<5%)
Postmarketing and/or case reports (Limited to important or life-threatening): Acute renal failure, anaphylaxis, bone marrow aplasia, reduced fertility (males)

Drug Interactions

Metabolism/Transport Effects None known.

Avoid Concomitant Use There are no known interactions where it is recommended to avoid concomitant use.

Increased Effect/Toxicity
ValGANciclovir may increase the levels/effects of: Imipenem; Mycophenolate; Reverse Transcriptase Inhibitors (Nucleoside); Tenofovir Products

The levels/effects of ValGANciclovir may be increased by: Mycophenolate; Probenecid; Tenofovir Products

Decreased Effect There are no known significant interactions involving a decrease in effect.

Food Interactions Coadministration with a high-fat meal increased AUC by 30%. Management: Valganciclovir should be taken with meals.

Preparation for Administration Hazardous agent; use appropriate precautions for handling and disposal (NIOSH 2014 [group 2]).

Oral solution: Reconstitute powder for oral solution with appropriate amount of water (in 2 equal portions) as specified in the manufacturer's labeling. Shake well for 1 minute after each addition. Discard any unused medication after 49 days. A reconstituted 100 mL bottle will only provide 88 mL of solution for administration.

Storage/Stability
Oral solution: Store dry powder at 25°C (77°F); excursions permitted to 15°C to 30°C (59°F to 86°F). Store oral solution at 2°C to 8°C (36°F to 46°F); do not freeze. Discard any unused medication after 49 days.
Tablet: Store at 25°C (77°F); excursions permitted to 15°C to 30°C (59°F to 86°F).

Mechanism of Action Valganciclovir is rapidly converted to ganciclovir in the body. The bioavailability of ganciclovir from valganciclovir is increased 10-fold compared to oral ganciclovir. A dose of 900 mg achieved systemic exposure of ganciclovir comparable to that achieved with the recommended doses of intravenous ganciclovir of 5 mg/kg. Ganciclovir is phosphorylated to a substrate which competitively inhibits the binding of deoxyguanosine triphosphate to DNA polymerase resulting in inhibition of viral DNA synthesis.

Pharmacodynamics/Kinetics
Absorption: Well absorbed; high-fat meal increases AUC by 30%
Distribution: V$_{dss}$: Ganciclovir: 0.7 L/kg; widely to all tissue including CSF and ocular tissue
Protein binding: Ganciclovir: 1% to 2%
Metabolism: Converted to ganciclovir by intestinal mucosal cells and hepatocytes
Bioavailability: With food: 60%
Half-life elimination: Ganciclovir: 4.08 hours; prolonged with renal impairment; Severe renal impairment: Up to 68 hours
Time to peak: Ganciclovir: 1-3 hours
Excretion: Urine (primarily as ganciclovir)

Dosing
Adult & Geriatric Note: Manufacturer recommends that adult patients should use tablet formulation, NOT the oral solution.

CMV retinitis (treatment): Oral:

Induction: 900 mg twice daily for 21 days

Maintenance: Following induction treatment, or for patients with inactive CMV retinitis who require maintenance therapy: 900 mg once daily

CMV disease (prophylaxis): 900 mg once daily beginning within 10 days of transplantation; continue therapy until 100 days (heart or kidney-pancreas transplant) or 200 days (kidney transplant) post-transplantation

Pediatric

Infants, Children, and Adolescents 1 month to 16 years:

CMV disease (prophylaxis) following heart transplantation: Oral: Dose (mg) = 7 x body surface area x creatinine clearance (see Calculation below) once daily beginning within 10 days of transplantation; continue therapy until 100 days post-transplantation. Doses should be rounded to the nearest 10 mg increment; maximum dose: 900 mg daily.

Infants, Children, and Adolescents 4 months to 16 years:

CMV disease (prophylaxis) following kidney transplantation: Oral: Dose (mg) = 7 x body surface area x creatinine clearance (see Calculation below) once daily beginning within 10 days of transplantation; continue therapy until 200 days post-transplantation. Doses should be rounded to the nearest 10 mg increment; maximum dose: 900 mg daily.

Calculation of creatinine clearance: CrCl (mL/minute/ 1.73 m^2) = [k x Height (cm)] divided by serum creatinine (mg/dL)

Note: If the calculated CrCl is >150 mL/minute/1.73 m^2, then a maximum value of 150 mL/minute/1.73 m^2 should be used to calculate the dose.

Note: Calculated using *modified* Schwartz formula where k is as follows:

Infants with low birth weight for gestational age: k = 0.33

Infants with birth weight appropriate for gestational age: k = 0.45

Children 1 to <2 years: k = 0.45

Girls 2 to 16 years: k = 0.55

Boys 2 to <13 years: k = 0.55

Boys 13 to 16 years: k = 0.7

Adolescents >16 years: Oral: Refer to adult dosing

Renal Impairment

Infants, Children, and Adolescents 1 month to 16 years: No dosage adjustment necessary; calculation for pediatric dosing adjusts for renal function.

Adolescents >16 years and Adults:

Induction dose:

CrCl ≥60 mL/minute: No dosage adjustment necessary

CrCl 40 to 59 mL/minute: 450 mg twice daily

CrCl 25 to 39 mL/minute: 450 mg once daily

CrCl 10 to 24 mL/minute: 450 mg every 2 days

CrCl <10 mL/minute:

Manufacturer labeling: Use not recommended; ganciclovir (with appropriately specified renal dosage adjustment) should be used instead of valganciclovir

Alternate dosing: HIV-1 infected persons: Consider valganciclovir solution 200 mg 3 times weekly (Lucas, 2014)

End stage renal disease (ESRD) on intermittent hemodialysis (IHD):

Manufacturer labeling: Use not recommended; ganciclovir (with appropriately specified renal dosage adjustment) should be used instead of valganciclovir.

Alternate dosing: HIV-1 infected persons: Consider valganciclovir solution 200 mg 3 times weekly (Lucas, 2014); valganciclovir is dialyzable and should be administered following dialysis.

Maintenance/prevention dose:

CrCl ≥60 mL/minute: No dosage adjustment necessary

CrCl 40 to 59 mL/minute: 450 mg once daily

CrCl 25 to 39 mL/minute: 450 mg every 2 days

CrCl 10 to 24 mL/minute: 450 mg twice weekly

CrCl <10 mL/minute:

Manufacturer labeling: Use not recommended; ganciclovir (with appropriately specified renal dosage adjustment) should be used instead of valganciclovir

Alternate dosing: HIV infected persons: Consider valganciclovir solution 100 mg 3 times weekly (Lucas, 2014)

End stage renal disease (ESRD) on intermittent hemodialysis (IHD):

Manufacturer labeling: Use not recommended; ganciclovir (with appropriately specified renal dosage adjustment) should be used instead of valganciclovir.

Alternate dosing: HIV-1 infected persons: Consider valganciclovir solution: 100 mg 3 times weekly (Lucas, 2014); valganciclovir is dialyzable and should be administered following dialysis.

Hepatic Impairment There are no dosage adjustments provided in the manufacturer labeling (has not been studied).

Dietary Considerations Should be taken with meals.

Administration Oral: Valganciclovir should be taken with meals. The preferred dosage form for pediatric patients is the oral solution; however, valganciclovir tablets may used so long as the calculated dose is within 10% of the available tablet strength (450 mg). Manufacturer recommends that adult patients should use tablet formulation, NOT the oral solution.

Due to the carcinogenic and mutagenic potential, avoid direct contact with broken or crushed tablets, powder for oral solution, and oral solution. Consideration should be given to handling and disposal according to guidelines issued for antineoplastic drugs. However, there is no consensus on the need for these precautions.

Hazardous agent; use appropriate precautions for handling and disposal (NIOSH 2014 [group 2]).

Monitoring Parameters Retinal exam (at least every 4-6 weeks) when treating CMV retinitis, CBC, platelet count, serum creatinine at baseline and periodically during therapy

Dosage Forms Excipient information presented when available (limited, particularly for generics); consult specific product labeling.

Solution Reconstituted, Oral:

Valcyte: 50 mg/mL (88 mL) [contains saccharin sodium, sodium benzoate; tutti-frutti flavor]

Tablet, Oral:

Valcyte: 450 mg

Generic: 450 mg

Extemporaneous Preparations Hazardous agent; use appropriate precautions for handling and disposal (NIOSH 2014 [group 2]).

Note: Commercial preparation is available (50 mg/mL).

A 60 mg/mL oral suspension may be with tablets and a 1:1 mixture of Ora-Sweet® and Ora-Plus®. Crush sixteen 450 mg tablets and reduce to a fine powder. Add 1 mL portions of chosen vehicle (10 mL total) and mix to a uniform paste; mix while adding the vehicle in incremental proportions to **almost** 120 mL; transfer to a calibrated amber glass bottle, rinse mortar with vehicle, and add quantity of vehicle sufficient to make 120 mL. Label "shake well" and "refrigerate". Stable for 35 days refrigerated.

Henkin CC, Griener JC, and Ten Eick AP, "Stability of Valganciclovir in Extemporaneously Compounded Liquid Formulations," *Am J Health Syst Pharm*, 2003, 60(7):687-90.

Valproic Acid and Derivatives
(val PROE ik AS id & dah RIV ah tives)

Brand Names: US Depacon; Depakene; Depakote; Depakote ER; Depakote Sprinkles; Stavzor

Brand Names: Canada Apo-Divalproex; Apo-Valproic; Depakene; Dom-Divalproex; Dom-Valproic Acid; Dom-Valproic Acid E.C.; Epival; Mylan-Divalproex; Mylan-Valproic; Novo-Valproic; PHL-Divalproex; PHL-Valproic Acid; PHL-Valproic Acid E.C.; PMS-Divalproex; PMS-Valproic Acid; PMS-Valproic Acid E.C.; ratio-Valproic; Sandoz-Valproic; Teva Divalproex

Index Terms 2-Propylpentanoic Acid; 2-Propylvaleric Acid; Dipropylacetic Acid; Divalproex Sodium; DPA; Valproate Semisodium; Valproate Sodium; Valproic Acid; Valproic Acid Derivative

Pharmacologic Category Anticonvulsant, Miscellaneous; Antimanic Agent; Histone Deacetylase Inhibitor

Use

Oral, IV: Monotherapy and adjunctive therapy in the treatment of patients with complex partial seizures; monotherapy and adjunctive therapy of simple and complex absence seizures; adjunctive therapy in patients with multiple seizure types that include absence seizures

Additional indications: Depakote, Depakote ER, Stavzor: Mania associated with bipolar disorder; migraine prophylaxis

Limitation of use: Do not administer to a woman of childbearing potential unless essential for the management of her condition.

Pregnancy Considerations Adverse events have been observed in animal reproduction studies and in human pregnancies. **[U.S. Boxed Warning]: May cause major congenital malformations, such as neural tube defects (eg, spina bifida) and decreased IQ scores following in utero exposure. Use is contraindicated in pregnant women for the prevention of migraine. Use is not recommended in women of childbearing potential for any other condition unless valproate is essential to manage her condition and alternative therapies are not appropriate. Effective contraception should be used during therapy.**

Valproic acid crosses the placenta (Harden 2009b). Neural tube defects, craniofacial defects, cardiovascular malformations, hypospadias, and limb malformations have been reported. Information from the North American Antiepileptic Drug Pregnancy Registry notes the rate of major malformations to be 9% to 11% following an average exposure to valproate monotherapy 1,000 mg/day; this is an increase in congenital malformations when compared with monotherapy with other antiepileptic drugs (AED). Based on data from the CDC National Birth Defects Prevention Network, the risk of spinal bifida is approximately 1% to 2% following valproate exposure (general population risk estimated to be 0.06% to 0.07%).

Nonteratogenic adverse effects have also been reported. Decreased IQ scores have been noted in children exposed to valproate in utero when compared to children exposed to other antiepileptic medications or no antiepileptic medications; the risk of autism spectrum disorders may also be increased. Fatal hepatic failure and hypoglycemia in infants have been noted in case reports following in utero exposure to valproic acid.

Clotting factor abnormalities (hypofibrinogenemia, thrombocytopenia, or decrease in other coagulation factors) may develop in the mother following valproate use during pregnancy; close monitoring of coagulation factors is recommended.

Current guidelines recommend complete avoidance of valproic acid and derivatives for the treatment of epilepsy in pregnant women whenever possible (Harden 2009a), especially when used for conditions not associated with permanent injury or risk of death. Effective contraception should be used during treatment. When pregnancy is being planned, consider tapering off of therapy prior to conception if appropriate; abrupt discontinuation of therapy may cause status epilepticus and lead to maternal and fetal hypoxia. Folic acid decreases the risk of neural tube defects in the general population; supplementation with folic acid should be used prior to conception and during pregnancy in all women, including those taking valproate.

A pregnancy registry is available for women who have been exposed to valproic acid. Patients may enroll themselves in the North American Antiepileptic Drug (NAAED) Pregnancy Registry by calling (888) 233-2334. Additional information is available at www.aedpregnancyregistry.org.

Breast-Feeding Considerations Valproate is excreted into breast milk. Breast milk concentrations of valproic acid have been reported as 1% to 10% of maternal concentration. The weight-adjusted dose to the infant has been calculated to be ~4% (Hagg, 2000). The manufacturer recommends that caution be used if administered to nursing women.

Medication Guide Available Yes

Contraindications Hypersensitivity to valproic acid, divalproex, derivatives, or any component of the formulation; hepatic disease or significant impairment; urea cycle disorders; pregnant women for the prevention of migraine; known mitochondrial disorders caused by mutations in mitochondrial DNA polymerase gamma (POLG; eg, Alpers-Huttenlocher syndrome [AHS]) or children <2 years of age suspected of having a POLG-related disorder

Warnings/Precautions Hazardous agent - use appropriate precautions for handling and disposal (NIOSH 2014 [groups 2 and 3]).

[U.S. Boxed Warning]: Hepatic failure resulting in fatalities has occurred in patients, usually in the initial 6 months of therapy; children <2 years of age are at considerable risk. Risk is also increased in patients with hereditary neurometabolic syndromes caused by DNA mutations of the mitochondrial DNA polymerase gamma (POLG) gene (eg, Alpers-Huttenlocher syndrome [AHS]). Other risk factors include organic brain disease, mental retardation with severe seizure disorders, congenital metabolic disorders, and patients on multiple anticonvulsants. Monitor patients closely for appearance of malaise, weakness, facial edema, anorexia, jaundice, and vomiting; discontinue immediately with signs/symptom of significant or suspected impairment. Liver function tests should be performed at baseline and at regular intervals after initiation of therapy, especially within the first 6 months. Hepatic dysfunction may progress despite discontinuing treatment. Should only be used as monotherapy and with extreme caution in children <2 years of age and/or patients at high risk for hepatotoxicity. Contraindicated with significant hepatic impairment.

[U.S. Boxed Warning]: Risk of valproate-induced acute liver failure and death is increased in patients with hereditary neurometabolic syndromes caused by DNA mutations of the mitochondrial polymerase gamma (POLG) gene (eg, Alpers-Huttenlocher syndrome [AHS]). Use is contraindicated in patients with known mitochondrial disorders caused by POLG mutations and children <2 years of age suspected of having a POLG-related disorder. Use in children ≥2 years of age suspected of having a POLG-related disorder only after other anticonvulsants have failed and with close monitoring for the development of acute liver injury. POLG mutation testing should be performed in accordance with current clinical practice.

[U.S. Boxed Warning]: Cases of life-threatening pancreatitis, occurring at the start of therapy or following years of use, have been reported in adults and children. Some cases have been hemorrhagic with rapid progression of initial symptoms to death. Promptly evaluate symptoms of abdominal pain, nausea, vomiting, and/or anorexia; should generally be discontinued if pancreatitis is diagnosed.

[U.S. Boxed Warning]: May cause major congenital malformations such as neural tube defects (eg, spina bifida) and decreased IQ scores following in utero exposure. Use is contraindicated in pregnant women for the prevention of migraine. Use is not recommended in women of childbearing potential for any other condition unless valproate is essential to manage her condition and alternative therapies are not appropriate. Effective contraception should be used during therapy.

Multiorgan hypersensitivity reactions (also known as drug reaction with eosinophilia and systemic symptoms [DRESS]): Potentially serious, sometimes fatal multiorgan hypersensitivity reactions have rarely been reported with some antiepileptic drugs including valproate therapy in adults and children; monitor for signs and symptoms of possible disparate manifestations associated with lymphatic, hepatic, renal, and/or hematologic organ systems; discontinuation and conversion to alternative therapy may be required.

May cause dose-related thrombocytopenia, inhibition of platelet aggregation, and bleeding. In some cases, platelet counts may be normalized with continued treatment; however, reduce dose or discontinue drug if patient develops evidence of hemorrhage, bruising, or a disorder of hemostasis/coagulation. Evaluate platelet counts prior to initiating therapy and periodically thereafter. In addition to platelets, valproate may be associated with a decrease in other cell lines and myelodysplasia.

Hyperammonemia and/or encephalopathy, sometimes fatal, have been reported following the initiation of valproate therapy and may be present with normal transaminase levels. Ammonia levels should be measured in patients who develop unexplained lethargy and vomiting, changes in mental status, or in patients who present with hypothermia (unintentional drop in core body temperature to <35°C/95°F). Discontinue therapy if ammonia levels are increased and evaluate for possible urea cycle disorder (UCD). Hyperammonemic encephalopathy has been reported in patients with UCD, particularly ornithine transcarbamylase deficiency. Use is contraindicated in patients with known UCD. Evaluation of UCD should be considered for the following patients prior to the start of therapy: History of unexplained encephalopathy or coma; encephalopathy associated with protein load; pregnancy or postpartum encephalopathy; unexplained mental

retardation; history of elevated plasma ammonia or glutamine; history of cyclical vomiting and lethargy; episodic extreme irritability, ataxia; low BUN or protein avoidance; family history of UCD or unexplained infant deaths (particularly male); or signs or symptoms of UCD (hyperammonemia, encephalopathy, respiratory alkalosis). Hypothermia has been reported with valproate therapy; hypothermia may or may not be associated with hyperammonemia; may also occur with concomitant topiramate therapy following topiramate initiation or dosage increase. Hyperammonemia and/or encephalopathy may also occur with concomitant topiramate therapy in patients who previously tolerated monotherapy with either medication.

In vitro studies have suggested valproate stimulates the replication of HIV and CMV viruses under experimental conditions. The clinical consequence of this is unknown, but should be considered when monitoring affected patients.

Antiepileptics are associated with an increased risk of suicidal behavior/thoughts with use (regardless of indication); patients should be monitored for signs/symptoms of depression, suicidal tendencies, and other unusual behavior changes during therapy and instructed to inform their healthcare provider immediately if symptoms occur.

Intravenous valproate is not recommended for post-traumatic seizure prophylaxis in patients with acute head trauma; study results for this indication suggested increased mortality with IV valproate use compared to IV phenytoin. Anticonvulsants should not be discontinued abruptly because of the possibility of increasing seizure frequency; valproate should be withdrawn gradually to minimize the potential of increased seizure frequency, unless safety concerns require a more rapid withdrawal. Patients treated for bipolar disorder should be monitored closely for clinical worsening or suicidality; prescriptions should be written for the smallest quantity consistent with good patient care.

Reversible and irreversible cerebral and cerebellar atrophy have been reported; motor and cognitive function should be routinely monitored to assess for signs and symptoms of brain atrophy. CNS depression may occur with valproate use. Patients must be cautioned about performing tasks which require mental alertness (operating machinery or driving). Effects with other sedative drugs or ethanol may be potentiated. Use with caution in the elderly as the elderly may be more sensitive to sedating effects and dehydration; in some elderly patients with somnolence, concomitant decreases in nutritional intake and weight loss were observed. Reduce initial dosages in elderly and closely monitor fluid status, nutritional intake, somnolence, and other adverse events. Potentially significant drug-drug interactions may exist, requiring dose or frequency adjustment, additional monitoring, and/or selection of alternative therapy.

Medication residue in stool has been reported (rarely) with oral Depakote (divalproex sodium) formulations; some reports have occurred in patients with shortened GI transit times (eg, diarrhea) or anatomic GI disorders (eg, ileostomy, colostomy). In patients reporting medication residue in stool, it is recommended to monitor valproate level and clinical condition.

Adverse Reactions

Frequency not always defined.

>10%:
Central nervous system: Headache (3% to ≤31%), drowsiness (2% to 30%), dizziness (>1% to 25%), insomnia (>1% to 15%), pain (1% to 11%), nervousness (≤11%)

Dermatologic: Alopecia (>1% to 24%)

Gastrointestinal: Nausea (3% to 48%), vomiting (1% to 27%), dyspepsia (7% to 23%), abdominal pain (1% to 23%), diarrhea (≤23%), anorexia (>1% to 12%)

Hematologic & oncologic: Thrombocytopenia (1% to 27%; dose related)

Infection: Infection (≤20%)

Neuromuscular & skeletal: Tremor (≤57%), weakness (≤27%)

Ophthalmic: Diplopia (>1% to 16%), visual disturbance (amblyopia, blurred vision ≤1% to 12%)

Respiratory: Flu-like symptoms (>1% to 12%)

Miscellaneous: Accidental injury (>1% to 11%)

1% to 10%:
Cardiovascular: Peripheral edema (>1% to 8%), chest pain (>1% to 5%), edema (>1% to 5%), facial edema (>1% to 5%), hypertension (>1% to 5%), palpitations (>1% to 5%), tachycardia (>1% to <5%), hypotension (1% to 5%), orthostatic hypotension (1% to 5%), vasodilatation (≤5%),

Central nervous system: Ataxia (>1% to 8%), amnesia (>1% to 7%), paresthesia (≤7%), emotional lability (>1% to 6%), abnormality in thinking (>1% to 6%), abnormal dreams (>1% to 5%), abnormal gait (>1% to 5%), confusion (>1% to 5%), depression (>1% to 5%), hallucination (>1% to 5%), hypertonia (>1% to 5%), speech disturbance (>1% to 5%), tardive dyskinesia (>1% to 5%), agitation (1% to 5%), catatonia (1% to 5%), chills (1% to 5%), hyper-reflexia (1% to 5%), vertigo (1% to 5%), anxiety (>1% to <5%), malaise (>1% to <5%), myasthenia (>1% to <5%), personality disorder (>1% to <5%), twitching (>1% to <5%), sleep disorder (>1%)

Dermatologic: Skin rash (>1% to 6%), maculopapular rash (>1% to 5%), pruritus (>1% to 5%), xeroderma (>1% to 5%), furunculosis (1% to 5%), seborrhea (1% to 5%), erythema nodosum (>1%), vesiculobullous dermatitis (>1%), diaphoresis

Endocrine & metabolic: Weight gain (>1% to 9%), weight loss (6%), amenorrhea (>1% to <5%), menstrual disease (>1%)

Gastrointestinal: Increased appetite (>1% to 6%), constipation (>1% to 5%), flatulence (>1% to 5%), periodontal abscess (>1% to 5%), fecal incontinence (1% to 5%), gastroenteritis (1% to 5%), glossitis (1% to 5%), stomatitis (1% to 5%), xerostomia (1% to 5%), dysgeusia (>1% to <5%), eructation (>1% to <5%), hematemesis (>1% to <5%), pancreatitis (>1% to <5%), dysphagia, gingival hemorrhage, hiccups, oral mucosa ulcer

Genitourinary: Cystitis (>1% to 5%), dysmenorrhea (>1% to 5%), dysuria (>1% to 5%), urinary incontinence (>1% to 5%), vaginal hemorrhage (>1% to 5%), urinary frequency (>1% to <5%), vaginitis (>1% to <5%)

Hematologic & oncologic: Ecchymoses (>1% to 5%), petechia (>1% to <5%), prolonged bleeding time (>1%), hypoproteinemia

Hepatic: Increased serum ALT (>1% to <5%), increased serum AST (>1% to <5%)

Infection: Viral infection (>1% to 5%), fungal infection (>1%)

Local: Pain at injection site (3%), injection site reaction (2%)

Neuromuscular & skeletal: Back pain (>1% to 8%), arthralgia (>1% to 5%), discoid lupus erythematosus (>1% to 5%), leg cramps (>1% to 5%), hypokinesia (1% to 5%), neck pain (1% to 5%), neck stiffness (1% to 5%), osteoarthritis (1% to 5%), dysarthria (>1% to <5%), myalgia (>1% to <5%)

Ophthalmic: Nystagmus (1% to 8%), conjunctivitis (1% to 5%), dry eye syndrome (1% to 5%), eye pain (1% to 5%), photophobia (>1%)

Otic: Tinnitus (1% to 7%), deafness (>1% to 5%), otitis media (>1% to <5%)

Respiratory: Pharyngitis (≤8%), bronchitis (5%), rhinitis (>1% to 5%), dyspnea (1% to 5%), cough (>1% to <5%), epistaxis (>1% to <5%), pneumonia (>1% to <5%), sinusitis (>1% to <5%)

Miscellaneous: Fever (>1% to 6%)

<1% (Limited to important and/or life-threatening): Abnormal thyroid function tests, acute porphyria, aggressive behavior, agranulocytosis, anemia, aplastic anemia, bradycardia, brain disease (rare), breast hypertrophy, cerebral atrophy (reversible or irreversible), coma (rare), decreased bone mineral density, decreased plasma carnitine concentrations, decreased platelet aggregation, dementia, eosinophilia, Fanconi-like syndrome (rare, in children), galactorrhea, hemorrhage, hepatic failure, hepatotoxicity, hostility, hyperactivity, hyperammonemia, hyperammonemic encephalopathy (in patients with UCD), hyperandrogenism, hyperglycinemia, hypersensitivity angiitis, hypersensitivity reaction, hypofibrinogenemia, hyponatremia, hypothermia, leukopenia, lymphocytosis, macrocytosis, ostealgia, osteopenia, pancytopenia, parotid gland enlargement, polycystic ovary syndrome (rare), psychosis, severe hypersensitivity (with multiorgan dysfunction), SIADH, Stevens-Johnson syndrome, suicidal ideation, suicidal tendencies, toxic epidermal necrolysis (rare), urinary tract infection

Drug Interactions

Metabolism/Transport Effects Substrate of CYP2A6 (minor), CYP2B6 (minor), CYP2C19 (minor), CYP2C9 (minor), CYP2E1 (minor); **Note:** Assignment of Major/Minor substrate status based on clinically relevant drug interaction potential; **Inhibits** CYP2C9 (weak); **Induces** CYP2A6 (weak/moderate)

Avoid Concomitant Use

Avoid concomitant use of Valproic Acid and Derivatives with any of the following: Cosyntropin; Lesinurad

Increased Effect/Toxicity

Valproic Acid and Derivatives may increase the levels/effects of: Barbiturates; CarBAMazepine; Ethosuximide; LamoTRIgine; Lesinurad; LORazepam; Minoxidil (Systemic); Paliperidone; Primidone; RisperiDONE; Rufinamide; Sodium Oxybate; Temozolomide; Tricyclic Antidepressants; Vorinostat; Zidovudine

The levels/effects of Valproic Acid and Derivatives may be increased by: ChlorproMAZINE; Cosyntropin; Felbamate; GuanFACINE; Primidone; Salicylates; Topiramate

Decreased Effect

Valproic Acid and Derivatives may decrease the levels/effects of: Fosphenytoin-Phenytoin; OLANZapine; OXcarbazepine; Urea Cycle Disorder Agents

The levels/effects of Valproic Acid and Derivatives may be decreased by: Barbiturates; CarBAMazepine; Carbapenems; Ethosuximide; Fosphenytoin-Phenytoin; Mefloquine; Methylfolate; Mianserin; Orlistat; Protease Inhibitors; Rifampin

Food Interactions Food may delay but does not affect the extent of absorption. Management: May administer with food if GI upset occurs.

Preparation for Administration Hazardous agent; use appropriate precautions for handling and disposal (NIOSH 2014 [groups 2 and 3]).

IV: Prior to administration of the injectable solution, dilute in 50 mL of a compatible diluent.

Storage/Stability

Oral capsules:

Depakene: Store at 15°C to 25°C (59°F to 77°F).

Stavzor: Store at 25°C (77°F); excursions are permitted between 15°C and 30°C (59°F and 86°F).

Oral sprinkle capsules (Depakote): Store below 25°C (77°F).

Oral solution (Depakene): Store below 30°C (86°F).

Oral tablets:

Depakote: Store below 30°C (86°F).

Depakote ER: Store tablets at 25°C (77°F); excursions are permitted between 15°C and 30°C (59°F and 86°F).

IV: Store at controlled room temperature 15°C to 30°C (59°F to 86°F). Stable in D_5W, NS, and LR for at least 24 hours when stored in glass or PVC.

Mechanism of Action Causes increased availability of gamma-aminobutyric acid (GABA), an inhibitory neurotransmitter, to brain neurons or may enhance the action of GABA or mimic its action at postsynaptic receptor sites. Divalproex sodium is a compound of sodium valproate and valproic acid; divalproex dissociates to valproate in the GI tract.

Pharmacodynamics/Kinetics

Distribution: Total valproate: 11 L/1.73 m²; free valproate 92 L/1.73 m²

Protein binding (concentration dependent): 80% to 90%; free fraction: ~10% at 40 mcg/mL and ~18.5% at 130 mcg/mL; protein binding decreased in the elderly and with hepatic or renal dysfunction

Metabolism: Extensively hepatic via glucuronide conjugation (30% to 50% of administered dose) and 40% via mitochondrial beta-oxidation; other oxidative metabolic pathways occur to a lesser extent. The relationship between dose and total valproate concentration is nonlinear; concentration does not increase proportionally with the dose, but increases to a lesser extent due to saturable plasma protein binding. The kinetics of unbound drug are linear.

Bioavailability: Depakote ER: ~90% relative to IV dose and ~89% relative to delayed release formulation

Half-life elimination (increased in neonates, elderly and those with liver disease): Children >2 months: 7-13 hours; Adults: 9-19 hours

Time to peak, serum:

Oral: Depakote tablet: ~4 hours; Depakote ER: 4-17 hours; Stavzor: 2 hours

Rectal (off-label route): 1-3 hours (Graves, 1987)

Excretion: Urine (30% to 50% as glucuronide conjugate, <3% as unchanged drug)

Note: ER tablets have 10% to 20% less fluctuation in serum concentration than delayed-release tablets. ER tablets are not bioequivalent to delayed-release tablets.

Dosing

Adult

Seizures: Note: Administer doses >250 mg/day in divided doses.

Oral:

Simple and complex absence seizure: Initial: 15 mg/kg/day; increase by 5-10 mg/kg/day at weekly intervals until therapeutic levels are achieved; maximum: 60 mg/kg/day.

Complex partial seizure: Initial: 10 to 15 mg/kg/day; increase by 5 to 10 mg/kg/day at weekly intervals until therapeutic levels are achieved; maximum: 60 mg/kg/day.

Note: Regular release and delayed release formulations are usually given in 2 to 4 divided doses per day; extended release formulation (Depakote ER) is usually given once daily. Depakote ER is not recommended for use in children <10 years of age. In patients previously maintained on regular release valproic acid therapy (Depakene) who convert to delayed release valproate tablets or capsules (Depakote, Stavzor), the same daily dose and frequency as the regular release should be used; once therapy is stabilized, the frequency of Depakote or Stavzor may be adjusted to 2 to 3 times daily.

Conversion to Depakote ER from a stable dose of Depakote: May require an increase in the total daily dose between 8% and 20% to maintain similar serum concentrations.

Conversion to monotherapy from adjunctive therapy: The concomitant antiepileptic drug (AED) can be decreased by ~25% every 2 weeks; dosage reduction of the concomitant AED may begin when valproate therapy is initiated or 1 to 2 weeks following valproate initiation.

IV: Total daily IV dose should be equivalent to the total daily dose of the oral valproate product; administer dose as a 60-minute infusion (≤20 mg/minute) with the same frequency as oral products; switch patient to oral products as soon as possible. Alternatively, rapid infusions of 1.5 to 6 mg/kg/minute have been used in clinical trials to quickly achieve therapeutic concentrations, and were generally well tolerated (Ramsay, 2003; Venkataraman, 1999; Wheless, 2004). One study reported undiluted valproic acid administered at ≤10 mg/kg/minute (dose of ≤30 mg/kg) was well tolerated (Limdi, 2007).

Mania: Oral:

Depakote tablet, Stavzor: Initial: 750 mg/day in divided doses; dose should be adjusted as rapidly as possible to desired clinical effect; maximum recommended dosage: 60 mg/kg/day

Depakote ER: Initial: 25 mg/kg/day given once daily; dose should be adjusted as rapidly as possible to desired clinical effect; maximum recommended dose: 60 mg/kg/day.

Migraine prophylaxis: Oral:

Depakote tablet, Stavzor: 250 mg twice daily; adjust dose based on patient response, up to 1,000 mg/day

Depakote ER: 500 mg once daily for 7 days, then increase to 1,000 mg once daily; adjust dose based on patient response; usual dosage range 500 to 1,000 mg/day

Diabetic neuropathy (off-label use): Oral: 500 to 1,200 mg/day (Bril, 2011)

Status epilepticus (off-label use): IV: Loading dose: 20 to 40 mg/kg administered at rate of 3 to 6 mg/kg/minute; if necessary, may give an additional dose of 20 mg/kg 10 minutes after the loading infusion (NCS [Brophy, 2012]).

Geriatric Oral, IV: Lower initial doses are recommended due to decreased elimination and increased incidences of somnolence in the elderly; no specific dosage recommendations are provided by the manufacturer. Upward titration should be done slowly and with close monitoring for adverse events (eg, sedation, dehydration, decreased nutritional intake). Safety and efficacy for use in patients >65 years have not been studied for migraine prophylaxis.

Pediatric

Seizures: Note: Administer doses >250 mg daily in divided doses.

Oral:

Simple and complex absence seizures: Refer to adult dosing. Larger maintenance doses may be required in younger children.

Complex partial seizures: Children ≥10 years: Refer to adult dosing. Larger maintenance doses may be required in younger children.

Note: Depakote ER is not recommended for use in children <10 years of age.

Conversion to Depakote ER from a stable dose of Depakote: Refer to adult dosing.

Conversion to monotherapy from adjunctive therapy: Refer to adult dosing.

IV: Refer to adult dosing.

Rectal (off-label route): Dilute syrup 1:1 with water for use as a retention enema; acute and maintenance dose: 6 to 15 mg/kg/dose (Graves, 1987)

Migraine prophylaxis: Children ≥12 years and Adolescents (Stavzor): Oral: Refer to adult dosing.

Status epilepticus (off-label use): Children and Adolescents: IV: 20 to 40 mg/kg administered at rate of 1.5 to 3 mg/kg/minute; if necessary, may give an additional dose of 20 mg/kg 10 minutes after the loading infusion (NCS [Brophy, 2012]). A continuous infusion may be initiated at 5 mg/kg/hour until a 6 hour seizure-free period then reduced at a rate of 1 mg/kg/hour every 2 hours followed by a maintenance dose of 10 mg/kg every 8 hours (Mehta, 2007).

Renal Impairment Mild to severe impairment: No dosage adjustment necessary (including patients on hemodialysis); however, due to decreased protein binding in renal impairment, monitoring only total valproate concentrations may be misleading.

Hepatic Impairment

Mild to moderate impairment: Not recommended for use in hepatic disease; clearance is decreased with liver impairment. Hepatic disease is also associated with decreased albumin concentrations and 2- to 2.6-fold increase in the unbound fraction. Free concentrations of valproate may be elevated while total concentrations appear normal, therefore, monitoring only total valproate concentrations may be misleading.

Severe impairment: Use is contraindicated.

Administration

Oral: Oral valproate products may cause GI upset; taking with food or slowly increasing the dose may decrease GI upset should it occur.

Depakote ER: Swallow whole; do not crush or chew.

Depakote Sprinkle capsules may be swallowed whole or capsule opened and sprinkled on small amount (1 teaspoonful) of soft food (eg, pudding, applesauce) to be used immediately (do not store or chew).

Depakene capsule, Stavzor: Swallow whole; do not chew.

IV: Following dilution to final concentration, manufacturer's labeling recommends administering over 60 minutes at a rate ≤20 mg/minute. Alternatively, more rapid infusion rates of 1.5-6 mg/kg/minute have been used in clinical trials to quickly achieve therapeutic concentrations, and were generally well tolerated (Ramsay, 2003; Wheless, 2004). One study reported undiluted valproic acid administered at ≤10 mg/kg/minute (dose of ≤30 mg/kg) was well tolerated (Limdi, 2007).

Neurocritical Care Society recommendations for status epilepticus (NCS [Brophy, 2012]):

Adults: Maximum administration rate of 3 to 6 mg/kg/minute for the loading dose

Children and Adolescents: Maximum administration rate of 1.5 to 3 mg/kg/minute for the loading dose

Hazardous agent - use appropriate precautions for handling and disposal (NIOSH 2014 [groups 2 and 3]).

Monitoring Parameters Liver enzymes (at baseline and frequently during therapy especially during the first 6 months), CBC with platelets (baseline and periodic intervals), PT/PTT (especially prior to surgery), serum ammonia (with symptoms of lethargy, mental status change), serum valproate levels; suicidality (eg, suicidal thoughts, depression, behavioral changes); motor and cognitive function (for signs or symptoms of brain atrophy)

Reference Range Note: In general, trough concentrations should be used to assess adequacy of therapy; peak concentrations may also be drawn if clinically necessary (eg, concentration-related toxicity). Within 2-4 days of initiation or dose adjustment, trough concentrations should be drawn just before the next dose (extended-release preparations) or before the morning dose (for immediate-release preparations). Patients with epilepsy should not delay taking their dose for >2-3 hours. Additional patient-specific factors must be taken into consideration when interpreting drug levels, including indication, age, clinical response, pregnancy status, adherence, comorbidities, adverse effects, and concomitant medications (Patsalos, 2008; Reed, 2006).

Therapeutic:

Epilepsy: 50-100 mcg/mL (SI: 350-700 micromole/L); although seizure control may improve at levels >100 mcg/mL (SI: 700 micromole/L), toxicity may occur at levels of 100-150 mcg/mL (SI: 700-1040 micromole/L)

Mania: 50-125 mcg/mL (SI: 350-875 micromole/L)

Toxic: Some laboratories may report >200 mcg/mL (SI: >1390 micromole/L) as a toxic threshold, although clinical toxicity can occur at lower concentrations. Probability of thrombocytopenia increases with total valproate levels ≥110 mcg/mL in females or ≥135 mcg/mL in males.

Epilepsy: Although seizure control may improve at levels >100 mcg/mL (SI: 700 micromole/L), toxicity may occur at levels of 100-150 mcg/mL (SI: 700-1050 micromole/L)

Mania: Clinical response seen with trough levels between 50-125 mcg/mL (SI: 350-875 micromole/L); risk of toxicity increases at levels >125 mcg/mL (SI: 875 micromole/L)

Test Interactions May cause a false-positive result for urine ketones (valproate partially eliminated as a keto-metabolite in the urine); may alter thyroid function tests

Dosage Forms Considerations

Strengths of divalproex sodium and valproate sodium products are expressed in terms of valproic acid

Dosage Forms Excipient information presented when available (limited, particularly for generics); consult specific product labeling.

Capsule, Oral, as valproic acid:
Depakene: 250 mg
Generic: 250 mg

Capsule Delayed Release, Oral, as valproic acid:
Stavzor: 125 mg, 250 mg, 500 mg [contains fd&c yellow #6 (sunset yellow)]

Capsule Delayed Release Sprinkle, Oral, as divalproex sodium:
Depakote Sprinkles: 125 mg [contains brilliant blue fcf (fd&c blue #1)]
Generic: 125 mg

Solution, Intravenous, as valproate sodium:
Depacon: 100 mg/mL (5 mL)

Solution, Intravenous, as valproate sodium [preservative free]:
Generic: 100 mg/mL (5 mL); 500 mg/5 mL (5 mL)

Solution, Oral, as valproate sodium:
Generic: 250 mg/5 mL (473 mL)

Syrup, Oral, as valproate sodium:
Depakene: 250 mg/5 mL (480 mL)
Generic: 250 mg/5 mL (5 mL, 10 mL, 473 mL)

Tablet Delayed Release, Oral, as divalproex sodium:
Depakote: 125 mg [contains brilliant blue fcf (fd&c blue #1), fd&c red #40]
Depakote: 250 mg [contains fd&c yellow #6 (sunset yellow)]
Depakote: 500 mg [contains fd&c blue #2 (indigotine)]
Generic: 125 mg, 250 mg, 500 mg

Tablet Extended Release 24 Hour, Oral, as divalproex sodium:
Depakote ER: 250 mg, 500 mg
Generic: 250 mg, 500 mg

Valrubicin (val ROO bi sin)

Brand Names: US Valstar

Brand Names: Canada Valtaxin

Index Terms N-trifluoroacetyladriamycin-14-valerate; AD32

Pharmacologic Category Antineoplastic Agent, Anthracycline; Antineoplastic Agent, Topoisomerase II Inhibitor

Use Bladder cancer: Intravesical treatment of BCG-refractory bladder carcinoma *in situ* of the urinary bladder when cystectomy would be associated with unacceptable morbidity or mortality.

Dosing

Adult & Geriatric Note: Delay for at least 2 weeks after transurethral resection and/or fulguration.

Bladder cancer: Intravesical: 800 mg once weekly (retain for 2 hours) for 6 weeks

Renal Impairment There are no dosage adjustments provided in the manufacturer's labeling. However, dosage adjustment unlikely due to low systemic absorption.

Hepatic Impairment There are no dosage adjustments provided in the manufacturer's labeling. However, dosage adjustment unlikely due to low systemic absorption.

Adjustment for Toxicity In clinical trials (Steinberg 2000), treatment was delayed for 1 week for the following adverse events: Grade 3 dysuria (not controlled with phenazopyridine), frequency/urgency lasting >24 hours, grade 2 gross hematuria (without clots) lasting >48 hours, grade 3 hematuria (with clots) lasting >48 hours. For local toxicities < grade 4 (eg, dysuria [not controlled with phenazopyridine] or severe bladder spasm), anticholinergic therapy (systemic or topical) or topical anesthesia was administered prior to subsequent instillations.

Additional Information Complete prescribing information should be consulted for additional detail.

Dosage Forms Excipient information presented when available (limited, particularly for generics); consult specific product labeling.

Solution, Intravesical [preservative free]:
Valstar: 40 mg/mL (5 mL) [contains alcohol, usp, cremophor® el]

Valsartan (val SAR tan)

Brand Names: US Diovan

Brand Names: Canada ACT Valsartan; Apo-Valsartan; Auro-Valsartan; Ava-Valsartan; Diovan; Mylan-Valsartan; PMS-Valsartan; Ran-Valsartan; Sandoz-Valsartan; Teva-Valsartan

Pharmacologic Category Angiotensin II Receptor Blocker; Antihypertensive

Use Alone or in combination with other antihypertensive agents in the treatment of primary hypertension; reduction of cardiovascular mortality in patients with left ventricular dysfunction postmyocardial infarction; treatment of heart failure (NYHA Class II-IV)

Guideline recommendations:

Hypertension: The 2014 guideline for the management of high blood pressure in adults (Eighth Joint National Committee [JNC 8; James, 2013]) recommends initiation of pharmacologic treatment to lower blood pressure for the following patients:

- Patients ≥60 years of age with systolic blood pressure (SBP) ≥150 mm Hg or diastolic blood pressure (DBP) ≥90 mm Hg. Goal of therapy is SBP <150 mm Hg and DBP <90 mm Hg.
- Patients <60 years of age with SBP ≥140 mm Hg or DBP ≥90 mm Hg. Goal of therapy is SBP <140 mm Hg and DBP <90 mm Hg.
- Patients ≥18 years of age with diabetes and SBP ≥140 mm Hg or DBP ≥90 mm Hg. Goal of therapy is SBP <140 mm Hg and DBP <90 mm Hg.
- Patients ≥18 years of age with chronic kidney disease (CKD) and SBP ≥140 mm Hg or DBP ≥90 mm Hg. Goal of therapy is SBP <140 mm Hg and DBP <90 mm Hg.

Chronic kidney disease (CKD) and hypertension: Regardless of race or diabetes status, the use of an ACE inhibitor (ACEI) or angiotensin receptor blocker (ARB) as initial therapy is recommended to improve kidney outcomes. In the general nonblack population (without CKD), including those with diabetes, initial antihypertensive treatment should consist of a thiazide-type diuretic, calcium channel blocker, ACEI, or ARB. In the general black population (without CKD), including those with diabetes, initial antihypertensive treatment should consist of a thiazide-type diuretic or a calcium channel blocker instead of an ACEI or ARB.

Coronary artery disease and hypertension: The American Heart Association, American College of Cardiology and American Society of Hypertension (AHA/ACC/ASH) 2015 scientific statement for the treatment of hypertension in patients with coronary artery disease (CAD) recommends the use of an ARB (or ACE inhibitor) as part of a regimen in patients with hypertension and chronic stable angina if there is prior MI, LV systolic dysfunction, diabetes mellitus, or CKD. A BP target of <140/90 mm Hg is reasonable for the secondary prevention of cardiovascular events. A lower target BP (<130/80 mm Hg) may be appropriate in some individuals with CAD, previous MI, stroke or transient ischemic attack, or CAD risk equivalents (AHA/ACC/ASH [Rosendorff 2015]).

Heart failure: The ACCF/AHA 2013 heart failure guidelines recommend the use of ARBs (ie, candesartan, losartan, and valsartan) in patients with HF with reduced ejection fraction who cannot tolerate ACE inhibitors (due to cough) to reduce morbidity and mortality. They also suggest that ARBs are reasonable first-line alternatives to ACE inhibitors in patients already maintained on an ARB for other indications (ACCF/AHA [Yancy 2013]).

Acute coronary syndrome (ACS): According to the ACCF/AHA guidelines for the management of ST-elevation myocardial infarction (STEMI) and guidelines for the management of unstable angina/non-ST-elevation myocardial infarction (UA/NSTEMI), an angiotensin receptor blocker should be given to patients who, after STEMI or UA/NSTEMI, have indications for (eg, clinical or radiologic signs of heart failure or LVEF ≤0.4) but are intolerant to ACE inhibitors. Valsartan is preferred in patients with STEMI (ACCF/AHA [Anderson, 2013]; ACCF/AHA [O'Gara 2013]).

Pregnancy Considerations [US Boxed Warning]: Drugs that act on the renin-angiotensin system can cause injury and death to the developing fetus. Discontinue as soon as possible once pregnancy is detected. The use of drugs which act on the renin-angiotensin system are associated with oligohydramnios. Oligohydramnios, due to decreased fetal renal function, may lead to fetal lung hypoplasia and skeletal malformations. Use is also associated with anuria, hypotension, renal failure, skull hypoplasia, and death in the fetus/neonate. in The exposed fetus should be monitored for fetal growth, amniotic fluid volume, and organ formation. Infants exposed *in utero* should be monitored for hyperkalemia, hypotension, and oliguria (exchange transfusions or dialysis may be needed). These adverse events are generally associated with maternal use in the second and third trimesters.

Untreated chronic maternal hypertension is also associated with adverse events in the fetus, infant, and mother. The use of angiotensin II receptor blockers is not recommended to treat chronic uncomplicated hypertension in pregnant women and should generally be avoided in women of reproductive potential (ACOG, 2013).

Breast-Feeding Considerations It is not known if valsartan is found in breast milk. Due to the potential for serious adverse reactions in the nursing infant, the manufacturer recommends a decision be made whether to discontinue nursing or to discontinue the drug, taking into account the importance of treatment to the mother. The Canadian labeling contraindicates use in nursing women.

Contraindications Hypersensitivity to valsartan or any component of the formulation; concomitant use with aliskiren in patients with diabetes mellitus

Canadian labeling: Additional contraindications (not in U.S. labeling): Concomitant use with aliskiren in patients with moderate-to-severe renal impairment (GFR <60 mL/minute/1.73 m^2); pregnancy; breast-feeding

Warnings/Precautions [US Boxed Warning]: Drugs that act on the renin-angiotensin system can cause injury and death to the developing fetus. Discontinue as soon as possible once pregnancy is detected. May cause hyperkalemia; avoid potassium supplementation unless specifically required by healthcare provider. During the initiation of therapy, hypotension may occur, particularly in patients with heart failure or post-MI patients. Use extreme caution with concurrent administration of potassium-sparing diuretics or potassium supplements, in patients with mild-to-moderate hepatic dysfunction (adjust dose), in those who may be sodium/water depleted (eg, on high-dose diuretics), and in the elderly; correct depletion first.

Use caution with unstented unilateral/bilateral renal artery stenosis. When unstented bilateral renal artery stenosis is present, use is generally avoided due to the elevated risk of deterioration in renal function unless possible benefits outweigh risks. Use with caution with preexisting renal insufficiency; significant aortic/mitral stenosis. May be associated with deterioration of renal function and/or increases in serum creatinine, particularly in patients with low renal blood flow (eg, renal artery stenosis, heart failure) whose glomerular filtration rate (GFR) is dependent on efferent arteriolar vasoconstriction by angiotensin II. Use caution in patients with severe renal impairment or significant hepatic dysfunction. Monitor renal function closely in patients with severe heart failure; changes in renal function should be anticipated and dosage adjustments of valsartan or concomitant medications may be needed. Potentially significant drug-drug interactions may exist, requiring dose or frequency adjustment, additional monitoring, and/or selection of alternative therapy. In surgical patients on chronic angiotensin receptor blocker (ARB) therapy, intraoperative hypotension may occur with induction and maintenance of general anesthesia.

Angioedema has been reported rarely with some angiotensin II receptor antagonists (ARBs) and may occur at any time during treatment (especially following first dose). It may involve the head and neck (potentially compromising airway) or the intestine (presenting with abdominal pain). Patients with idiopathic or hereditary angioedema or previous angioedema associated with ACE-inhibitor therapy may be at an increased risk. Prolonged frequent monitoring may be required, especially if tongue, glottis, or larynx are involved, as they are associated with airway obstruction. Patients with a history of airway surgery may have a higher risk of airway obstruction. Discontinue therapy immediately if angioedema occurs. Aggressive early management is critical. Intramuscular (IM) administration of epinephrine may be necessary. Do not readminister to patients who have had angioedema with ARBs.

Adverse Reactions

>10%:

Central nervous system: Dizziness (heart failure trials 17%)

Renal: Increased blood urea nitrogen (>50% increase; heart failure trials 17%)

1% to 10%:

Cardiovascular: Hypotension (heart failure trials 7%; MI trial 1%), orthostatic hypotension (heart failure trials 2%), syncope (up to >1%)

Central nervous system: Dizziness (hypertension trial 2% to 8%), fatigue (heart failure trials 3%; hypertension trial 2%), orthostatic dizziness (heart failure trials 2%), headache (heart failure trials >1%), vertigo (up to >1%)

Endocrine & metabolic: Increased serum potassium (>20% increase; 4% to 10%), hyperkalemia (heart failure trials 2%)

Gastrointestinal: Diarrhea (heart failure trials 5%), abdominal pain (2%), nausea (heart failure trials >1%), upper abdominal pain (heart failure trials >1%)

Hematologic & oncologic: Neutropenia (2%)

Infection: Viral infection (3%)

Neuromuscular & skeletal: Arthralgia (heart failure trials 3%), back pain (≤3%)

Ophthalmic: Blurred vision (heart failure trials >1%)

Renal: Increased serum creatinine (doubled: MI trial 4%; >50% increase: heart failure trials 4%), renal insufficiency (>1%)

Respiratory: Cough (1% to 3%)

All indications: <1% (Limited to important or life-threatening): Alopecia, anaphylaxis, anemia, angioedema, anorexia, bullous dermatitis, decreased hematocrit, decreased hemoglobin, dyspepsia, flatulence, hepatitis (rare), hypersensitivity reaction, impotence, insomnia, liver function tests increased, microcytic anemia, myalgia, palpitation, paresthesia, photosensitivity, pruritus, renal failure, rhabdomyolysis, skin rash, taste disorder, thrombocytopenia (very rare), vasculitis, xerostomia

Drug Interactions

Metabolism/Transport Effects Substrate of MRP2, SLCO1B1; **Inhibits** CYP2C9 (weak)

Avoid Concomitant Use There are no known interactions where it is recommended to avoid concomitant use.

Increased Effect/Toxicity

Valsartan may increase the levels/effects of: ACE Inhibitors; Amifostine; Antipsychotic Agents (Second Generation [Atypical]); Ciprofloxacin (Systemic); CycloSPORINE (Systemic); Drospirenone; DULoxetine; Hydrochlorothiazide; Hypotension-Associated Agents; Levodopa; Lithium; Nonsteroidal Anti-Inflammatory Agents; Potassium-Sparing Diuretics; Sodium Phosphates

The levels/effects of Valsartan may be increased by: Alfuzosin; Aliskiren; Barbiturates; Brimonidine (Topical); Canagliflozin; Dapoxetine; Diazoxide; Eltrombopag; Eplerenone; Heparin; Heparin (Low Molecular Weight); Herbs (Hypotensive Properties); Hydrochlorothiazide; Molsidomine; Nicorandil; Obinutuzumab; Pentoxifylline; Phosphodiesterase 5 Inhibitors; Potassium Salts; Prostacyclin Analogues; Teriflunomide; Tolvaptan; Trimethoprim

Decreased Effect

The levels/effects of Valsartan may be decreased by: Amphetamines; Herbs (Hypertensive Properties); Methylphenidate; Nonsteroidal Anti-Inflammatory Agents; Yohimbine

Food Interactions Food decreases the peak plasma concentration and extent of absorption by 50% and 40%, respectively. Management: Administer consistently with regard to food.

Storage/Stability Store at 25°C (77°F); excursions permitted to 15°C to 30°C (59°F to 86°F). Protect from moisture.

Mechanism of Action Valsartan produces direct antagonism of the angiotensin II (AT2) receptors, unlike the ACE inhibitors. It displaces angiotensin II from the AT1 receptor and produces its blood pressure-lowering effects by antagonizing AT1-induced vasoconstriction, aldosterone release, catecholamine release, arginine vasopressin release, water intake, and hypertrophic responses. This action results in more efficient blockade of the cardiovascular effects of angiotensin II and fewer side effects than the ACE inhibitors.

Pharmacodynamics/Kinetics

Onset of action: ~2 hours

Duration: 24 hours

Distribution: V_d: 17 L (adults)

Protein binding: 95%, primarily albumin

Metabolism: To inactive metabolite

Bioavailability: Tablet: 25% (range: 10% to 35%); suspension: ~40% (~1.6 times more than tablet)

Half-life elimination: ~6 hours

Time to peak, serum: 2 to 4 hours

Excretion: Feces (83%) and urine (13%) as unchanged drug

Dosing

Adult & Geriatric

Hypertension: Initial: 80 mg or 160 mg once daily (in patients who are not volume depleted); dose may be increased to achieve desired effect; usual dosage range (ASH/ISH [Weber, 2014]): 80 to 320 mg daily; target dose (JNC8 [James, 2013]): 160 to 320 mg daily; maximum recommended dose: 320 mg/day

Heart failure: Initial: 40 mg twice daily; titrate dose to 80 to 160 mg twice daily, as tolerated; maximum daily dose: 320 mg. The ACCF/AHA 2013 heart failure guidelines suggest initial dose of 20 to 40 mg twice daily and a target dose of 160 mg twice daily (Yancy, 2013).

Left ventricular dysfunction after MI: Initial: 20 mg twice daily; titrate dose to target of 160 mg twice daily as tolerated; may initiate ≥12 hours following MI

Pediatric Hypertension: Oral: Children 6 to 16 years: Initial: 1.3 mg/kg once daily (maximum: 40 mg/day); dose may be increased to achieve desired effect; doses >2.7 mg/kg (maximum: 160 mg) have not been studied. **Note:** Use in patients <18 years of age is not approved in the Canadian labeling.

Renal Impairment

CrCl ≥30 mL/minute: No dosage adjustment necessary.

CrCl <30 mL/minute: There are no dosage adjustments provided in the manufacturer's labeling; safety and efficacy have not been established.

Dialysis: Not significantly removed.

Hepatic Impairment

Mild-to-moderate impairment: No dosage adjustment necessary; use caution in patients with liver disease. Patients with mild-to-moderate chronic disease have twice the exposure as healthy volunteers.

Severe impairment: There are no dosage adjustments provided in the manufacturer's labeling; has not been studied

Dietary Considerations Avoid salt substitutes which contain potassium. May be taken with or without food.

Administration Administer with or without food.

Monitoring Parameters Baseline and periodic electrolyte panels, renal function, BP; in HF, serum potassium during dose escalation and periodically thereafter

2013 ACCF/AHA Heart Failure guideline recommendations: Within 1 to 2 weeks after initiation, reassess blood pressure (including postural blood pressure changes), renal function, and serum potassium; follow closely after dose changes. Patients with systolic blood pressure <80 mm Hg, low serum sodium, diabetes mellitus, and impaired renal function should be closely monitored (Yancy, 2013)

Additional Information Valsartan may have an advantage over losartan due to minimal metabolism requirements and consequent use in mild-to-moderate hepatic impairment.

Dosage Forms Excipient information presented when available (limited, particularly for generics); consult specific product labeling. [DSC] = Discontinued product

Tablet, Oral:

Diovan: 40 mg [DSC]

Diovan: 40 mg [scored]

Diovan: 80 mg, 160 mg, 320 mg

Generic: 40 mg, 80 mg, 160 mg, 320 mg

Extemporaneous Preparations A 4 mg/mL oral suspension may be made from tablets, Ora-Plus®, and Ora-Sweet® SF. Add 80 mL of Ora-Plus® to an 8-ounce amber glass bottle containing eight valsartan 80 mg tablets. Shake well for ≥2 minutes. Allow the suspension to stand for a minimum of 1 hour, then shake for ≥1 minute. Add 80 mL of Ora-Sweet SF® to the bottle and shake for ≥10 seconds. Store in amber glass prescription bottles; label "shake well". Stable for 30 days at room temperature or 75 days refrigerated.

Diovan® prescribing information, Novartis Pharmaceuticals Corp, East Hanover, NJ, 2012.

◆ Valsartan and Amlodipine *see* Amlodipine and Valsartan *on page 105*

Valsartan and Hydrochlorothiazide

(val SAR tan & hye droe klor oh THYE a zide)

Brand Names: US Diovan HCT

Brand Names: Canada Apo-Valsartan/HCTZ; Ava-Valsartan/HCT; Diovan HCT; Mylan-Valsartan HCTZ; Sandoz Valsartan HCT; Teva-Valsartan HCTZ; Valsartan-HCT; Valsartan-HCTZ

Index Terms Hydrochlorothiazide and Valsartan

Pharmacologic Category Angiotensin II Receptor Blocker; Antihypertensive; Diuretic, Thiazide

Use

U.S. labeling: Treatment of hypertension (initial, add-on, or as substitute for titrated components)

Canadian labeling: Treatment of mild-to-moderate hypertension where combination therapy is appropriate. Not indicated for initial treatment.

Dosing

Adult & Geriatric

Hypertension: Oral:

U.S. labeling: Dose is individualized; combination product may be used as initial therapy or substituted for individual components in patients currently maintained on both agents separately or in patients not adequately controlled with monotherapy (using one of the agents or an agent within same antihypertensive class).

Initial therapy: Valsartan 160 mg and hydrochlorothiazide 12.5 mg once daily; dose may be titrated after 1-2 weeks of therapy. Maximum recommended daily doses: Valsartan 320 mg; hydrochlorothiazide 25 mg.

Add-on/replacement therapy: Valsartan 80-320 mg and hydrochlorothiazide 12.5-25 mg once daily; dose may be titrated after 3-4 weeks of therapy. Maximum recommended daily dose: Valsartan 320 mg; hydrochlorothiazide 25 mg.

Canadian labeling: Dose is individualized; combination product may be used as substitute for individual components following successful titration of each component. Maximum recommended daily dose: Valsartan 320 mg; hydrochlorothiazide 25 mg. Not approved for initial therapy.

Renal Impairment

CrCl ≥30 mL/minute: No dosage adjustment necessary.

CrCl <30 mL/minute: No dosage adjustment provided in manufacturer's labeling (has not been studied). Use is contraindicated in patients with anuria (U.S. and Canadian labeling) and not recommended in severe impairment (Canadian labeling).

Hepatic Impairment

Mild-to-moderate impairment: No dosage adjustment necessary; use with caution. Patients with mild-to-moderate chronic disease have twice the exposure of valsartan as healthy volunteers.

Severe impairment: No dosage adjustment provided in manufacturer's labeling (has not been studied). The Canadian labeling does not recommend use in severe impairment.

Additional Information Complete prescribing information should be consulted for additional detail.

Dosage Forms Excipient information presented when available (limited, particularly for generics); consult specific product labeling.

Tablet, oral: 80 mg/12.5 mg: Valsartan 80 mg and hydrochlorothiazide 12.5 mg; 160 mg/12.5 mg: Valsartan 160 mg and hydrochlorothiazide 12.5 mg; 160 mg/25 mg: Valsartan 160 mg and hydrochlorothiazide 25 mg; 320 mg/12.5 mg: Valsartan 320 mg and hydrochlorothiazide 12.5 mg; 320 mg/25 mg: Valsartan 320 mg and hydrochlorothiazide 25 mg

Diovan HCT® 80 mg/12.5 mg: Valsartan 80 mg and hydrochlorothiazide 12.5 mg

Diovan HCT® 160 mg/12.5 mg: Valsartan 160 mg and hydrochlorothiazide 12.5 mg

Diovan HCT® 160 mg/25 mg: Valsartan 160 mg and hydrochlorothiazide 25 mg

Diovan HCT® 320 mg/12.5 mg: Valsartan 320 mg and hydrochlorothiazide 12.5 mg

Diovan HCT® 320 mg/25 mg: Valsartan 320 mg and hydrochlorothiazide 25 mg

---

Vancomycin (van koe MYE sin)

Brand Names: US First-Vancomycin 25; First-Vancomycin 50; Vancocin HCl; Vancomycin+SyrSpend SF PH4

Brand Names: Canada JAMP-Vancomycin; PMS-Vancomycin; Sterile Vancomycin Hydrochloride, USP; Val-Vancomycin; Vancocin; Vancomycin Hydrochloride for Injection; Vancomycin Hydrochloride for Injection, USP

Index Terms Vancocin; Vancomycin Hydrochloride

Pharmacologic Category Glycopeptide

Use

IV: Treatment of patients with infections caused by staphylococcal species and streptococcal species

Oral: Treatment of *C. difficile*-associated diarrhea and treatment of enterocolitis caused by *Staphylococcus aureus* (including methicillin-resistant strains)

Pregnancy Considerations Adverse events have not been observed in animal reproduction studies. Vancomycin crosses the placenta and can be detected in fetal serum, amniotic fluid, and cord blood (Bourget 1991; Reyes 1989). Adverse fetal effects, including sensorineural hearing loss or nephrotoxicity, have not been reported following maternal use during the second or third trimesters of pregnancy.

The pharmacokinetics of vancomycin may be altered during pregnancy and pregnant patients may need a higher dose of vancomycin. Maternal half-life is unchanged, but the volume of distribution and the total plasma clearance may be increased (Bourget 1991). Individualization of therapy through serum concentration monitoring may be warranted. Vancomycin is recommended for the treatment of mild, moderate, or severe *Clostridium difficile* infections in pregnant women (ACG [Surawicz 2013]). Vancomycin is recommended as an alternative agent to prevent the transmission of group B streptococcal (GBS) disease from mothers to newborns (ACOG 2011; CDC 2010).

Breast-Feeding Considerations Vancomycin is excreted in human milk following IV administration. If given orally to the mother, the minimal systemic absorption of the dose would limit the amount available to pass into the milk. Vancomycin is recommended for the treatment of mild, moderate, or severe *Clostridium difficile* infections in breast-feeding women (ACG [Surawicz 2013]). Due to the potential for serious adverse reactions in the nursing infant, the manufacturer recommends a decision be made whether to discontinue nursing or to discontinue the drug, taking into account the importance of treatment to the mother. Nondose-related effects could include modification of bowel flora.

Contraindications Hypersensitivity to vancomycin or any component of the formulation

Warnings/Precautions May cause nephrotoxicity although limited data suggest direct causal relationship; usual risk factors include preexisting renal impairment, concomitant nephrotoxic medications, advanced age, and dehydration (nephrotoxicity has also been reported following treatment with oral vancomycin, typically in patients >65 years of age). If multiple sequential (≥2) serum creatinine concentrations demonstrate an increase of 0.5 mg/dL or ≥50% increase from baseline (whichever is greater) in the absence of an alternative explanation, the patient should be identified as having vancomycin-induced nephrotoxicity (Rybak, 2009). Discontinue treatment if signs of nephrotoxicity occur; renal damage is usually reversible.

May cause neurotoxicity; usual risk factors include preexisting renal impairment, concomitant neuro-/nephrotoxic medications, advanced age, and dehydration. Ototoxicity, although rarely associated with monotherapy, is proportional to the amount of drug given and the duration of treatment. Tinnitus or vertigo may be indications of vestibular injury and impending bilateral irreversible damage. Discontinue treatment if signs of ototoxicity occur. Prolonged therapy (>1 week) or total doses exceeding 25 g may increase the risk of neutropenia; prompt reversal of neutropenia is expected after discontinuation of therapy. Prolonged use may result in fungal or bacterial superinfection, including *C. difficile*-associated diarrhea (CDAD) and pseudomembranous colitis; CDAD has been observed >2 months postantibiotic treatment. Use with caution in patients with renal impairment or those receiving other nephrotoxic or ototoxic drugs; dosage modification required in patients with impaired renal function (especially elderly). Accumulation may occur after multiple oral doses of vancomycin in patients with renal impairment; consider monitoring trough concentrations in this circumstance.

IV vancomycin is an irritant; ensure proper needle or catheter placement prior to and during infusion; avoid extravasation. Pain, tenderness, and necrosis may occur with extravasation. Rapid IV administration may result in hypotension, flushing, erythema, urticaria, and/or pruritus. Oral vancomycin is only indicated for the treatment of pseudomembranous colitis due to *C. difficile* and enterocolitis due to *S. aureus* and is not effective for systemic infections; parenteral vancomycin is not effective for the treatment of colitis due to *C. difficile* and enterocolitis due to *S. aureus*. Clinically significant serum concentrations have been reported in patients with inflammatory disorders of the intestinal mucosa who have taken oral vancomycin (multiple doses) for the treatment of *C. difficile*-associated diarrhea. Although use may be warranted, the risk for adverse reactions may be higher in this situation; consider monitoring serum trough concentrations, especially with

renal insufficiency, severe colitis, concurrent rectal vanco-mycin administration, and/or concomitant IV aminoglyco-sides. The Society for Healthcare Epidemiology of America (SHEA) and the Infectious Diseases Society of America (IDSA) suggest that it is appropriate to obtain trough concentrations when a patient is receiving long courses of ≥2 g/day in adults (SHEA/IDSA [Cohen, 2010]). **Note:** The SHEA, the IDSA, and the American College of Gastro-enterology (ACG) recommend the use of oral metronida-zole for initial treatment of mild to moderate *C. difficile* infection and the use of oral vancomycin for initial treat-ment of severe *C. difficile* infection (SHEA/IDSA [Cohen, 2010]; ACG [Surawicz, 2013]).

Adverse Reactions

Injection:

>10%:
 Cardiovascular: Hypotension accompanied by flushing
 Dermatologic: Erythematous rash on face and upper body (red neck or red man syndrome)

1% to 10%:
 Central nervous system: Chills, drug fever
 Hematologic: Eosinophilia, reversible neutropenia
 Local: Phlebitis

<1% (Limited to important or life-threatening): Drug rash with eosinophilia and systemic symptoms (DRESS), oto-toxicity (rare; use of other ototoxic agents may increase risk), renal failure (limited data suggesting direct relation-ship), Stevens-Johnson syndrome, thrombocytopenia, vasculitis

Oral:

>10%: Gastrointestinal: Abdominal pain, bad taste (with oral solution), nausea

1% to 10%:
 Cardiovascular: Peripheral edema
 Central nervous system: Fatigue, fever, headache
 Gastrointestinal: Diarrhea, flatulence, vomiting
 Genitourinary: Urinary tract infection
 Neuromuscular & skeletal: Back pain

<1% (Limited to important or life-threatening): Creatinine increased, interstitial nephritis, ototoxicity, renal failure, renal impairment, thrombocytopenia, vasculitis

Drug Interactions

Metabolism/Transport Effects None known.

Avoid Concomitant Use
 Avoid concomitant use of Vancomycin with any of the following: BCG (Intravesical)

Increased Effect/Toxicity
 Vancomycin may increase the levels/effects of: Amino-glycosides; Colistimethate; Neuromuscular-Blocking Agents

 The levels/effects of Vancomycin may be increased by: Nonsteroidal Anti-Inflammatory Agents; Piperacillin

Decreased Effect
 Vancomycin may decrease the levels/effects of: BCG (Intravesical); BCG Vaccine (Immunization); Sodium Picosulfate; Typhoid Vaccine

 The levels/effects of Vancomycin may be decreased by: Bile Acid Sequestrants

Preparation for Administration Injection: Reconstitute 500 mg vial with 10 mL SWFI, 750 mg vial with 15 mL SWFI, 1 g vial with 20 mL SWFI, 5 g vial with 100 mL SWFI (final concentration: 500 mg/10 mL), and 10 g vial with 95 mL SWFI (final concentration: 1 g/10 mL). The reconstituted solution must be further diluted with at least 100 mL of a compatible diluent per 500 mg of vancomycin prior to parenteral administration.

Intrathecal (off-label route): Vancomycin is available as a powder for injection and may be diluted to 1-5 mg/mL concentration in preservative free 0.9% sodium chloride for administration into the CSF.

Storage/Stability

Capsules: Store at controlled room temperature of 15°C to 30°C (59°F to 86°F).

Galaxy containers: Store Galaxy containers in a freezer capable of maintaining a temperature at or below −20°C (−4°F). The thawed solution in Galaxy plastic containers remains chemically stable for 72 hours at room temper-ature (25°C [77°F]) or for 30 days when stored under refrigeration (5°C [41°F]). Do not refreeze thawed anti-biotics.

Vials: Store at 20°C to 25°C (68°F to 77°F). After initial reconstitution with sterile water for injection, D_5W or NS, solutions are stable for 14 days if refrigerated. After further dilution with D_5W or NS, the solution may be stored in a refrigerator for 14 days without significant loss of potency. Solutions diluted with D_5W and NS, LR, D_5LR, or Normosol-M and dextrose 5% may be stored in a refrigerator for 96 hours.

Pharmacy bulk packages: Store at 20°C to 25°C (68°F to 77°F). Discard pharmacy bulk packages no later than 4 hours after initial closure puncture.

Mechanism of Action Inhibits bacterial cell wall synthesis by blocking glycopeptide polymerization through binding tightly to D-alanyl-D-alanine portion of cell wall precursor

Pharmacodynamics/Kinetics

Absorption: Oral: Poor; may be enhanced with bowel inflammation; IM: Erratic; Intraperitoneal: ~38%

Distribution: V_d: 0.4-1 L/kg; Distributes widely in body tissue and fluids, except for CSF

 Relative diffusion from blood into CSF: Good only with inflammation (exceeds usual MICs)

 Uninflamed meninges: 0-4 mcg/mL; serum concentra-tion dependent

 Inflamed meninges: 6-11 mcg/mL; serum concentration dependent

 CSF:blood level ratio: Normal meninges: Nil; Inflamed meninges: 20% to 30%

Protein binding: ~50%

Half-life elimination: Biphasic: Terminal:
 Newborns: 6-10 hours
 Infants and Children 3 months to 4 years: 4 hours
 Children >3 years: 2.2-3 hours
 Adults: 5-11 hours; significantly prolonged with renal impairment
 End-stage renal disease: 200-250 hours

Time to peak, serum: IV: Immediately after completion of infusion

Excretion: IV: Urine (80% to 90% as unchanged drug); Oral: Primarily feces

Dosing

Adult & Geriatric

Usual dosage range: Note: Initial intravenous dosing should be based on actual body weight; subsequent dosing adjusted based on serum trough vancomycin concentrations.

IV:
 Manufacturer's labeling: Usual dose: 500 mg every 6 hours **or** 1,000 mg every 12 hours
 Alternate recommendations: 15 to 20 mg/kg/dose every 8 to 12 hours (ASHP/IDSA/SIDP [Rybak, 2009]); **Note:** Dose requires adjustment in renal impairment.
 Complicated infections in seriously ill patients: A loading dose of 25 to 30 mg/kg (based on actual body weight) may be used to rapidly achieve target concentrations (ASHP/IDSA/SIDP [Rybak, 2009]).

Oral: 500 to 2,000 mg daily in divided doses every 6 hours. **Note:** Not appropriate for systemic infections due to low absorption.

Indication-specific dosing:

Bacteremia (*S. aureus* [methicillin-resistant]) (off-label use): IV: 15 to 20 mg/kg/dose (based on actual body weight) every 8 to 12 hours for 2 to 6 weeks depending on severity. A loading dose of 25 to 30 mg/kg (based on actual body weight) may be used to rapidly achieve target concentrations in seriously ill patients (ASHP/IDSA/SIDP [Rybak, 2009]; IDSA [Liu, 2011]).

Brain abscess, subdural empyema, spinal epidural abscess (*S. aureus* [methicillin-resistant]) (off-label use): IV: 15 to 20 mg/kg/dose (based on actual body weight) every 8 to 12 hours for 4 to 6 weeks (with or without rifampin). A loading dose of 25 to 30 mg/kg (based on actual body weight) may be used to rapidly achieve target concentrations in seriously ill patients (ASHP/IDSA/SIDP [Rybak, 2009]; IDSA [Liu, 2011]).

Catheter-related infections: Antibiotic lock technique (Mermel, 2009): 2 mg/mL ± 10 units heparin/mL **or** 2.5 mg/mL ± 2,500 **or** 5,000 units heparin/mL **or** 5 mg/mL ± 5,000 units heparin/mL (preferred regimen); instill into catheter port with a volume sufficient to fill the catheter (2 to 5 mL). **Note:** May use SWFI/NS or D_5W as diluents. Do not mix with any other solutions. Dwell times generally should not exceed 48 hours before renewal of lock solution. Remove lock solution prior to catheter use, then replace.

***C. difficile*-associated diarrhea (CDAD):** Oral:
 Manufacturer's labeling: 125 mg 4 times daily for 10 days
 Alternate dosing:
 HIV-infected patients: 125 mg 4 times daily for 10 to 14 days (HHS [OI adult 2015])
 Mild to moderate disease unresponsive to metronida-zole: 125 mg 4 times daily for 10 days (ACG [Sur-awicz, 2013])
 Severe disease (defined as serum albumin <3 g/dL and either WBC ≥15,000 or abdominal tenderness): 125 mg 4 times daily for 10 days (ACG [Sura-wicz, 2013])

Severe, complicated infection without abdominal distention: 125 mg 4 times daily with IV metronidazole (ACG [Surawicz, 2013])

Severe, complicated infection: 500 mg every 6 hours for 10 to 14 days with or without concurrent IV metronidazole. May consider vancomycin retention enema (in patients with complete ileus) (SHEA/IDSA [Cohen, 2010])

Severe, complicated infection with significant abdominal distention, ileus, and/or toxic colon: 500 mg 4 times daily plus rectal vancomycin in combination with IV metronidazole (ACG [Surawicz, 2013])

Recurrent, severe infection (if initial regimen did not include vancomycin): 125 mg 4 times daily for 10 days (ACG [Surawicz, 2013])

Rectal (off-label route): Retention enema:

Severe, complicated infection in patients with ileus: 500 mg every 6 hours (in 100 mL 0.9% sodium chloride) with oral vancomycin with or without concurrent IV metronidazole (SHEA/IDSA [Cohen, 2010])

Severe and complicated disease with abdominal distention, ileus, and/or toxic colon: 500 mg 4 times daily (in 500 mL NS) in combination with oral vancomycin and IV metronidazole (ACG [Surawicz, 2013])

Endocarditis:

Native valve (*Enterococcus*, vancomycin MIC ≤4 mg/L) (off-label use): IV: 15 to 20 mg/kg/dose (based on actual body weight) every 8 to 12 hours. A loading dose of 25 to 30 mg/kg (based on actual body weight) may be used to rapidly achieve target concentrations in seriously ill patients (ASHP/IDSA/SIDP [Rybak, 2009]) **or** 1,000 mg every 12 hours for 4 to 6 weeks (combine with gentamicin for 4 to 6 weeks) (BSAC [Gould, 2012]).

Native valve (*S. aureus* [methicillin-resistant]) (off-label use): IV: 15 to 20 mg/kg/dose (based on actual body weight) every 8 to 12 hours for 6 weeks. A loading dose of 25 to 30 mg/kg (based on actual body weight) may be used to rapidly achieve target concentrations in seriously ill patients (ASHP/IDSA/SIDP [Rybak, 2009]; IDSA [Liu, 2011]). **Note:** European guidelines support the entire duration of therapy to be 4 weeks and in combination with rifampin (BSAC [Gould, 2012]).

Native or prosthetic valve (streptococcal [penicillin MIC >0.5 mg/L or patient intolerant to penicillin]) (off-label use): IV: 15 to 20 mg/kg/dose (based on actual body weight) every 8 to 12 hours for 6 weeks. A loading dose of 25 to 30 mg/kg (based on actual body weight) may be used to rapidly achieve target concentrations in seriously ill patients (AHA [Baddour, 2005]; ASHP/IDSA/SIDP [Rybak, 2009]) **or** 1,000 mg every 12 hours for 4 to 6 weeks (combine with gentamicin for at least the first 2 weeks). **Note:** The longer duration of treatment (ie, 6 weeks) should be used for patients with prosthetic valve endocarditis (BSAC [Gould, 2012]).

Prosthetic valve (*Enterococcus*, vancomycin MIC ≤4 mg/L) (off-label use): IV: Adults: 15 to 20 mg/kg/dose (based on actual body weight) every 8 to 12 hours for 6 weeks. A loading dose of 25 to 30 mg/kg (based on actual body weight) may be used to rapidly achieve target concentrations in seriously ill patients (AHA [Baddour, 2005]; ASHP/IDSA/SIDP [Rybak, 2009]) **or** 1,000 mg every 12 hours for 6 weeks (combine with gentamicin for 6 weeks) (BSAC [Gould, 2012]).

Prosthetic valve (*S. aureus* [methicillin-resistant]) (off-label use): IV: 15 to 20 mg/kg/dose (based on actual body weight) every 8 to 12 hours for at least 6 weeks (combine with rifampin for the entire duration of therapy and gentamicin for the first 2 weeks). A loading dose of 25 to 30 mg/kg (based on actual body weight) may be used to rapidly achieve target concentrations in seriously ill patients (ASHP/IDSA/SIDP [Rybak, 2009]; IDSA [Liu, 2011]).

Endophthalmitis (off-label use): Intravitreal: Usual dose: 1 mg/0.1 mL NS instilled into vitreum; may repeat administration, if necessary, in 2 to 3 days, usually in combination with ceftazidime or an aminoglycoside (Kelsey, 1995). **Note:** Based on concerns for retinotoxicity, some clinicians have recommended using a lower dose of 0.2 mg/0.1mL; may repeat in 3 to 4 days, if necessary (Gan, 2001).

Enterocolitis (*S. aureus*): Oral: 500 to 2,000 mg/day in 3 to 4 divided doses for 7 to 10 days (usual dose: 125 to 500 mg every 6 hours)

Group B streptococcus (neonatal prophylaxis): IV: 1,000 mg every 12 hours until delivery. **Note:** Reserved for penicillin allergic patients at high risk for anaphylaxis if organism is resistant to clindamycin or where no susceptibility data are available (CDC, 2010).

Meningitis:

IV: 15 to 20 mg/kg/dose (based on actual body weight) every 8 to 12 hours (for empiric therapy, use in combination with a third-generation cephalosporin; for patients >50 years, include ampicillin); duration of therapy should be individualized based upon clinical response (in general, 10 to 21 days). A loading dose of 25 to 30 mg/kg (based on actual body weight) may be used to rapidly achieve target concentration in seriously ill patients (ASHP/IDSA/SIDP [Rybak, 2009]; IDSA [Tunkel, 2004]). **Note:** For PCN-resistant *Streptococcus pneumoniae* (MIC ≥2 mcg/mL), combine with a third-generation cephalosporin (IDSA [Tunkel, 2004]). For methicillin-resistant S. aureus, treat for 2 weeks (with or without rifampin) (IDSA [Liu, 2011]). Intrathecal, intraventricular (off-label route): 5 to 20 mg/day (IDSA [Tunkel, 2004])

Osteomyelitis (*S. aureus* [methicillin-resistant]) (off-label use): IV: 15 to 20 mg/kg/dose (based on actual body weight) every 8 to 12 hours for a minimum of 8 weeks (with or without rifampin). A loading dose of 25 to 30 mg/kg (based on actual body weight) may be used to rapidly achieve target concentrations in seriously ill patients (ASHP/IDSA/SIDP [Rybak, 2009]; IDSA [Liu, 2011]).

Pneumonia: IV:

Community-acquired pneumonia (CAP): S. aureus (methicillin-resistant): 15 to 20 mg/kg/dose (based on actual body weight) every 8 to 12 hours for 7 to 21 days depending on severity. A loading dose of 25 to 30 mg/kg (based on actual body weight) may be used to rapidly achieve target concentrations in seriously ill patients (ASHP/IDSA/SIDP [Rybak, 2009]; IDSA [Liu, 2011]).

Healthcare-associated pneumonia (HAP): S. aureus (methicillin-resistant): 15 to 20 mg/kg/dose (based on actual body weight) every 8 to 12 hours for 7 to 21 days depending on severity. A loading dose of 25 to 30 mg/kg (based on actual body weight) may be used to rapidly achieve target concentrations in seriously ill patients (ASHP/IDSA/SIDP [Rybak, 2009]; IDSA [Liu, 2011]).

Prophylaxis against infective endocarditis: IV:

Dental, oral, or upper respiratory tract surgery: 1,000 mg 1 hour before surgery. **Note:** AHA guidelines now recommend prophylaxis only in patients undergoing invasive procedures and in whom underlying cardiac conditions may predispose to a higher risk of adverse outcomes should infection occur

GI/GU procedure: 1,000 mg plus 1.5 mg/kg gentamicin 1 hour prior to surgery. **Note:** As of April 2007, routine prophylaxis no longer recommended by the AHA.

Prosthetic joint infection (off-label use): IV:

Enterococcus spp (penicillin-susceptible or –resistant), *Propionibacterium acnes*, streptococci (beta-hemolytic): 15 mg/kg every 12 hours for 4 to 6 weeks, followed by an oral antibiotic suppressive regimen (IDSA [Osman, 2013]).

Note: For penicillin-susceptible or -resistant *Enterococcus* spp, consider addition of an aminoglycoside; in penicillin-susceptible *Enterococcus*, beta-hemolytic streptococcus or *Propionibacterium acnes* infections, only use vancomycin if patient has penicillin allergy (IDSA [Osman, 2013]).

Staphylococci (oxacillin-susceptible or –resistant): 15 mg/kg every 12 hours for 2 to 6 weeks in combination with rifampin followed by oral antibiotic treatment and suppressive regimens (IDSA [Osman, 2013]).

Sepsis/Septic shock (empiric treatment or treatment for specific sensitive organism): IV: 15 to 20 mg/kg/dose (based on actual body weight) every 8 to 12 hours. A loading dose of 25 to 30 mg/kg (based on actual body weight) may be used to rapidly achieve target concentrations in seriously ill patients (ASHP/IDSA/SIDP [Rybak, 2009]). The Society of Critical Care Medicine recommends administration of empiric antibiotics within 1 hour of identifying severe sepsis (SCCM [Dellinger, 2013]).

Septic arthritis (*S. aureus* [methicillin-resistant]) (off-label use): IV: 15 to 20 mg/kg/dose (based on actual body weight) every 8 to 12 hours for 3 to 4 weeks. A loading dose of 25 to 30 mg/kg (based on actual body weight) may be used to rapidly achieve target concentrations in seriously ill patients (ASHP/IDSA/SIDP [Rybak, 2009]; IDSA [Liu, 2011]).

Septic thrombosis of cavernous or dural venous sinus (S. aureus [methicillin-resistant]) (off-label use): IV: 15 to 20 mg/kg/dose (based on actual body weight) every 8 to 12 hours for 4 to 6 weeks (with or without rifampin). A loading dose of 25 to 30 mg/kg (based on actual body weight) may be used to rapidly achieve target concentrations in seriously ill patients (ASHP/IDSA/SIDP [Rybak, 2009]; IDSA [Liu, 2011]).

Skin and skin structure infections (S. aureus [methicillin-resistant]) (off-label use): IV: 15 to 20 mg/kg/dose every 8 to 12 hours for 7 to 14 days (IDSA [Liu 2011; Stevens 2014]). A loading dose of 25 to 30 mg/kg (based on actual body weight) may be used to rapidly achieve target concentrations in seriously ill patients (ASHP/IDSA/SIDP [Rybak 2009]; IDSA [Liu 2011]).

Skin and soft tissue necrotizing infections due to S. aureus (resistant strains) or polymicrobial (mixed) (off-label use): IV: 15 mg/kg/dose every 12 hours. **Note:** Give in combination with piperacillin/tazobactam for empiric therapy of polymicrobial [mixed] infections. Continue until further debridement is not necessary, patient has clinically improved, and patient is afebrile for 48 to 72 hours (IDSA [Stevens, 2014]).

Surgical (perioperative) prophylaxis (off-label use): IV: 15 mg/kg within 120 minutes prior to surgical incision. May be administered in combination with other antibiotics depending upon the surgical procedure (ASHP/IDSA/SIS/SHEA [Bratzler, 2013]).

Note: For patients known to be colonized with methicillin-resistant S. aureus, a single 15 mg/kg preoperative dose may be added to other recommended agents for the specific procedure (ASHP/IDSA/SIS/SHEA [Bratzler, 2013]).

The Society of Thoracic Surgeons recommends 1,000 to 1,500 mg or 15 mg/kg over 60 minutes with completion within 1 hour of skin incision. Although not well established, a second dose of 7.5 mg/kg may be considered during cardiopulmonary bypass (STS [Engelman, 2007]).

Surgical site infections (trunk or extremity [away from axilla or perineum]) (unlabeled use): IV: 15 mg/kg/dose every 12 hours (IDSA [Stevens 2014])

Pediatric

Usual dosage range: Note: Initial IV dosing should be based on actual body weight; subsequent dosing adjusted based on serum trough vancomycin concentrations.

Infants >1 month, Children, and Adolescents: IV:
Manufacturer's labeling: 10 mg/kg/dose every 6 hours
Alternate recommendations: 15 mg/kg/dose (maximum: 2,000 mg/dose) every 6 hours (IDSA [Liu, 2011])

Indication-specific dosing:

Bacteremia (S. aureus [methicillin-resistant]) (off-label use): Children and Adolescents: IV: 15 mg/kg/dose every 6 hours for 2 to 6 weeks depending on severity (IDSA [Liu, 2011])

Brain abscess, subdural empyema, spinal epidural abscess (S. aureus [methicillin-resistant]) (off-label use): Children and Adolescents: IV: 15 mg/kg/dose every 6 hours for 4 to 6 weeks (with or without rifampin) (IDSA [Liu, 2011])

C. difficile-associated diarrhea (CDAD): Infants >1 month, Children, and Adolescents: Oral:
Manufacturer's labeling: 40 mg/kg/day in 3 to 4 divided doses for 7 to 10 days (maximum: 2,000 mg/day)
Alternate dosing: Adolescents: HIV-infected patients: 125 mg 4 times daily for 10 to 14 days (HHS [OI adult 2015])

Endocarditis:
Native valve (S. aureus [methicillin-resistant]) (off-label use): Children and Adolescents: IV: 15 mg/kg/dose every 6 hours for 6 weeks (IDSA [Liu, 2011])
Prosthetic valve (S. aureus [methicillin-resistant]) (off-label use): Children and Adolescents: IV: 15 mg/kg/dose every 6 hours for at least 2 to 6 weeks depending on source, presence of endovascular infection, and metastatic foci of infection (IDSA [Liu, 2011]).
Enterocolitis (S. aureus): Infants >1 months, Children, and Adolescents: Oral: 40 mg/kg/day in 3 to 4 divided doses for 7 to 10 days (maximum: 2,000 mg/day)
Meningitis: Infants >1 month, Children, and Adolescents:
IV: 15 mg/kg/dose every 6 hours (for empiric therapy, use in combination with a third-generation cephalosporin); duration of therapy should be individualized based upon clinical response (in general, 10 to 21 days) (IDSA [Tunkel, 2004]). For methicillin-resistant S. aureus, treat for 2 weeks (with or without rifampin) (IDSA [Liu, 2011]).
Intrathecal, intraventricular (off-label route): 5 to 20 mg/day (IDSA [Tunkel, 2004])

Osteomyelitis (S. aureus [methicillin-resistant]) (off-label use): Children and Adolescents: IV: 15 mg/kg/dose every 6 hours for 4 to 6 weeks (IDSA [Liu, 2011]).

Pneumonia:
Community-acquired pneumonia (CAP) (IDSA/PIDS, 2011): Infants >3 months, Children, and Adolescents: IV: **Note:** In children ≥5 years, a macrolide antibiotic should be added if atypical pneumonia cannot be ruled out. Also consider if community-acquired MRSA suspected.

Group A *Streptococcus* (alternative to ampicillin or penicillin in beta-lactam allergic patients): 40 to 60 mg/kg/day divided every 6 to 8 hours

Presumed bacterial (in addition to recommended antibiotic therapy), S. pneumoniae, moderate to severe infection (MICs to penicillin ≤2.0 mcg/mL) (alternative to ampicillin or penicillin): 40 to 60 mg/kg/day divided every 6 to 8 hours

S. aureus (methicillin-susceptible) (alternative to cefazolin/oxacillin): 40 to 60 mg/kg/day divided every 6 to 8 hours

S. aureus, moderate to severe infection (methicillin-resistant +/- clindamycin susceptible) (preferred): 40 to 60 mg/kg/day divided every 6 to 8 hours **or** dosing to achieve AUC/MIC >400
Alternate regimen: 60 mg/kg/day divided every 6 hours for 7 to 21 days, depending on severity (Liu, 2011)

S. pneumoniae, moderate to severe infection (MICs to penicillin ≥4.0 mcg/mL) (alternative to ceftriaxone in beta-lactam allergic patients): 40 to 60 mg/kg/day divided every 6 to 8 hours

Healthcare-associated pneumonia (HAP), S. aureus (methicillin-resistant): IV: Infants, Children, and Adolescents: 60 mg/kg/day divided every 6 hours for 7 to 21 days depending on severity (IDSA [Liu, 2011])

Prophylaxis against infective endocarditis: Children and Adolescents: IV:
Dental, oral, or upper respiratory tract surgery: 20 mg/kg/dose administered 1 hour prior to the procedure. **Note:** American Heart Association (AHA) guidelines recommend prophylaxis only in patients undergoing invasive procedures and in whom underlying cardiac conditions may predispose to a higher risk of adverse outcomes should infection occur.
GI/GU procedure: 20 mg/kg (plus gentamicin 1.5 mg/kg) administered 1 hour prior to surgery. **Note:** Routine prophylaxis no longer recommended by the AHA.

Septic arthritis (S. aureus [methicillin-resistant]) (off-label use): Children and Adolescents: IV: 15 mg/kg/dose every 6 hours for minimum of 3 to 4 weeks (IDSA [Liu, 2011])

Septic thrombosis of cavernous or dural venous sinus (S. aureus [methicillin-resistant]) (off-label use): Children and Adolescents: IV: 15 mg/kg/dose every 6 hours for 4 to 6 weeks (with or without rifampin) (IDSA [Liu, 2011])

Skin and skin structure infections (S. aureus [methicillin-resistant]) (off-label use): Children and Adolescents: IV: 10 to 15 mg/kg/dose every 6 hours for 7 to 14 days (IDSA [Liu 2011; Stevens 2014])

Skin and soft tissue necrotizing infections due to S. aureus (resistant strains) or polymicrobial (mixed) (off-label use): Children and Adolescents: IV: 15 mg/kg/dose every 6 hours. **Note:** Give in combination with piperacillin/tazobactam for empiric therapy of polymicrobial [mixed] infections. Continue until further debridement is not necessary, patient has clinically improved, and patient is afebrile for 48 to 72 hours (IDSA [Stevens 2014])

Surgical (perioperative) prophylaxis (off-label use): Children and Adolescents: IV: 15 mg/kg/dose within 120 minutes prior to surgical incision. May be administered in combination with other antibiotics depending upon the surgical procedure (ASHP/IDSA/SIS/SHEA [Bratzler, 2013]).
Note: for patients known to be colonized with methicillin-resistant S. aureus, a single 15 mg/kg preoperative dose may be added to other recommended agents for the specific procedure (ASHP/IDSA/SIS/SHEA [Bratzler, 2013]).

Renal Impairment
Oral: No dosage adjustment provided in manufacturer's labeling. However, dosage adjustment unlikely due to low systemic absorption.
IV: Vancomycin levels should be monitored in patients with any renal impairment:
CrCl >50 mL/minute: Start with 15 to 20 mg/kg/dose (usual: 750 to 1,500 mg) every 8 to 12 hours
CrCl 20 to 49 mL/minute: Start with 15 to 20 mg/kg/dose (usual: 750 to 1,500 mg) every 24 hours

CrCl <20 mL/minute: Will need longer intervals; determine by serum concentration monitoring

Note: In the critically-ill patient with renal insufficiency, the initial loading dose (25 to 30 mg/kg) should not be reduced. However, subsequent dosage adjustments should be made based on renal function and trough serum concentrations.

Poorly dialyzable by intermittent hemodialysis (0% to 5%); however, use of high-flux membranes and continuous renal replacement therapy (CRRT) increases vancomycin clearance, and generally requires replacement dosing.

Intermittent hemodialysis (IHD) (administer after hemodialysis on dialysis days): Following loading dose of 15 to 25 mg/kg, give either 500 to 1,000 mg **or** 5 to 10 mg/kg after each dialysis session (Heintz, 2009). **Note:** Dosing dependent on the assumption of 3 times/week, complete IHD sessions.

Redosing based on pre-HD concentrations:
<15 mg/L: Administer 1,000 mg after HD
10 to 25 mg/L: Administer 500 to 750 mg after HD
>25 mg/L: Hold vancomycin

Redosing based on post-HD concentrations: <10 to 15 mg/L: Administer 500 to 1,000 mg

Peritoneal dialysis (PD):
Administration via PD fluid: 15 to 30 mg/L (15 to 30 mcg/mL) of PD fluid
Systemic: Loading dose of 1,000 mg, followed by 500 to 1,000 mg every 48 to 72 hours with close monitoring of levels

Continuous renal replacement therapy (CRRT) (Heintz, 2009; Trotman, 2005): Drug clearance is highly dependent on the method of renal replacement, filter type, and flow rate. Appropriate dosing requires close monitoring of pharmacologic response, signs of adverse reactions due to drug accumulation, as well as drug concentrations in relation to target trough (if appropriate). The following are general recommendations only (based on dialysate flow/ultrafiltration rates of 1 to 2 L/hour and minimal residual renal function) and should not supersede clinical judgment:

CVVH: Loading dose of 15 to 25 mg/kg, followed by either 1,000 mg every 48 hours **or** 10 to 15 mg/kg every 24 to 48 hours
CVVHD: Loading dose of 15 to 25 mg/kg, followed by either 1,000 mg every 24 hours **or** 10 to 15 mg/kg every 24 hours
CVVHDF: Loading dose of 15 to 25 mg/kg, followed by either 1,000 mg every 24 hours **or** 7.5 to 10 mg/kg every 12 hours

Note: Consider redosing patients receiving CRRT for vancomycin concentrations <10 to 15 mg/L.

Hepatic Impairment
Oral: No dosage adjustment provided in the manufacturer's labeling. However, dosage adjustment unlikely due to low systemic absorption.
IV: No dosage adjustment provided in manufacturer's labeling. However, degrees of hepatic dysfunction do not affect the pharmacokinetics of vancomycin (Marti, 1996).

Dietary Considerations May be taken with food.

Administration
Intravenous: Administer vancomycin with a final concentration not to exceed 5 mg/mL by IV intermittent infusion over at least 60 minutes (recommended infusion period of ≥30 minutes for every 500 mg administered). Not for IM administration.

If a maculopapular rash appears on the face, neck, trunk, and/or upper extremities (red man syndrome), slow the infusion rate to over 1¹/₂ to 2 hours and increase the dilution volume. Hypotension, shock, and cardiac arrest (rare) have also been reported with too rapid of infusion. Reactions are often treated with antihistamines and steroids.

Irritant; ensure proper needle or catheter placement prior to and during infusion. Avoid extravasation.

Extravasation management: If extravasation occurs, stop infusion immediately and disconnect (leave cannula/needle in place); gently aspirate extravasated solution (do **NOT** flush the line); remove needle/cannula; elevate extremity. Apply dry cold compresses (Hurst, 2004).

Intrathecal (off-label route): Vancomycin is available as a powder for injection and may be diluted to 1 to 5 mg/mL concentration in preservative free 0.9% sodium chloride for intrathecal administration.

Intravitreal: (off-label use): Administer vancomycin intravitreally with a final concentration of 1.0 mg/0.1 mL NS (Kelsey, 1995). **Note:** Due to retinotoxicity, some clinicians recommend using a lower dose of 0.2 mg/0.1 mL NS (Gan, 2001).

Oral: Vancomycin powder for injection may be reconstituted and used for oral administration (SHEA/IDSA [Cohen, 2010]). Reconstituted powder for injection (not premixed solution) may be administered orally by diluting the reconstituted solution in 30 mL of water; common flavoring syrups may be added to improve taste. The unflavored, diluted solution may also be administered via nasogastric tube. Also see Extemporaneous Preparations.

Rectal (off-label route): May be administered as a retention enema per rectum (SHEA/IDSA [Cohen, 2010]); 500 mg in 100 to 500 mL of NS, volume may depend on length of segment being treated. If sodium chloride causes hyperchloremia could use solution with lower chloride concentration (eg, LR) (ACG [Surawicz, 2013]).

Monitoring Parameters Intravenous: Periodic renal function tests, urinalysis, WBC; serum trough vancomycin concentrations in select patients (eg, aggressive dosing, unstable renal function, concurrent nephrotoxins, prolonged courses)

Suggested frequency of trough vancomycin concentration monitoring (Rybak, 2009):
Hemodynamically stable patients: Draw trough concentrations at least once-weekly.
Hemodynamically unstable patients: Draw trough concentrations more frequently or in some instances daily.
Prolonged courses (>3-5 days): Draw at least one steady-state trough concentration; repeat as clinically appropriate.
Note: Drawing >1 trough concentration prior to the fourth dose for short course (<3 days) or lower intensity dosing (target trough concentrations <15 mcg/mL) is not recommended.

Oral/rectal therapy: Serum sample monitoring is not typically required; consider monitoring serum trough concentrations, especially with renal insufficiency, severe colitis, concurrent rectal vancomycin administration, and/or concomitant IV aminoglycosides.

Reference Range
Timing of serum samples: Draw trough just before the administration of a dose at steady-state conditions. Steady state conditions generally occur approximately after the fourth dose. Drawing peak concentrations is no longer recommended.

Therapeutic levels: Trough: ≥10 mcg/mL. For pathogens with an MIC ≤1 mcg/mL, the minimum trough concentration should be 15 mcg/mL to meet target AUC/MIC of ≥400 (see **"Note"** below). For complicated infections (eg, bacteremia, endocarditis, osteomyelitis, meningitis, and hospital-acquired pneumonia caused by *S. aureus*), trough concentrations of 15-20 mcg/mL are recommended to improve penetration and improve clinical outcomes (Liu, 2011; Rybak, 2009). The American Thoracic Society (ATS) guidelines for hospital-acquired pneumonia and the Infectious Disease Society of America (IDSA) meningitis guidelines also recommend trough concentrations of 15-20 mcg/mL.

Note: Although AUC/MIC is the preferred pharmacokinetic-pharmacodynamic parameter used to determine clinical effectiveness, trough serum concentrations may be used as a surrogate marker for AUC and are recommended as the most accurate and practical method of vancomycin monitoring (Liu, 2011; Rybak, 2009).

Toxic: >80 mcg/mL (SI: >54 micromole/L)

Additional Information Because of its long half-life, vancomycin should be dosed on an every 8- to 12-hour basis. Monitoring of trough serum concentrations is advisable in certain situations. "Red man syndrome", characterized by skin rash and hypotension, is not an allergic reaction but rather is associated with too rapid infusion of the drug. To alleviate or prevent the reaction, infuse vancomycin at a rate of ≥30 minutes for each 500 mg of drug being administered (eg, 1 g over ≥60 minutes); 1.5 g over ≥90 minutes.

Dosage Forms Considerations First-Vancomycin oral solution and Vancomycin+SyrSpend SF oral suspension are compounding kits. Refer to manufacturer's labeling for compounding instructions.

Dosage Forms Excipient information presented when available (limited, particularly for generics); consult specific product labeling.

Capsule, Oral:
Vancocin HCl: 125 mg, 250 mg [contains fd&c blue #2 (indigotine)]
Generic: 125 mg, 250 mg
Solution, Intravenous:
Generic: 500 mg/100 mL (100 mL); 750 mg/150 mL (150 mL); 1 g/200 mL (200 mL)

Solution, Oral:
First-Vancomycin 25: 25 mg/mL (150 mL, 300 mL) [contains fd&c red #40, fd&c yellow #10 (quinoline yellow), sodium benzoate; white grape flavor]
First-Vancomycin 50: 50 mg/mL (150 mL, 210 mL, 300 mL) [contains fd&c red #40, fd&c yellow #10 (quinoline yellow), sodium benzoate; white grape flavor]
Solution Reconstituted, Intravenous:
Generic: 500 mg (1 ea); 750 mg (1 ea); 1000 mg (1 ea); 5000 mg (1 ea); 10 g (1 ea)
Solution Reconstituted, Intravenous [preservative free]:
Generic: 1000 mg (1 ea); 5000 mg (1 ea); 10 g (1 ea)
Suspension, Oral:
Vancomycin+SyrSpend SF PH4: 50 mg/mL (1 ea)

Extemporaneous Preparations Note: A vancomycin (25 mg/mL or 50 mg/mL) suspension is commercially available as a compounding kit (First-Vancomycin).

Using a vial of vancomycin powder for injection (reconstituted to 50 mg/mL), add the appropriate volume for the dose to 30 mL of water and administer orally or via NG tube. For oral administration, common flavoring syrups may be added to improve taste.
Vancomycin Hydrochloride for Injection, USP (prescribing information), Schaumburg, Il, APP Pharmaceuticals, LLC, 2011.

A vancomycin 25 mg/mL solution in Ora-Sweet® and water (1:1) may be prepared by reconstituting vancomycin for injection with sterile water, then dilute with a 1:1 mixture of Ora-Sweet® and distilled water to a final concentration of 25 mg/mL; transfer to amber prescription bottle. Stable for 75 days refrigerated or for 26 days at room temperature.
Ensom MH, Decarie D, and Lakhani A, "Stability of Vancomycin 25 mg/mL in Ora-Sweet and Water in Unit-Dose Cups and Plastic Bottles at 4°C and 25°C," *Can J Hosp Pharm*, 2010, 63(5):366-72.

♦ Vancomycin Hydrochloride see Vancomycin on page 1868

♦ Vancomycin Hydrochloride for Injection (Can) see Vancomycin on page 1868

♦ Vancomycin Hydrochloride for Injection, USP (Can) see Vancomycin on page 1868

♦ Vancomycin+SyrSpend SF PH4 see Vancomycin on page 1868

♦ Vandazole see MetroNIDAZOLE (Topical) on page 1199

Vandetanib (van DET a nib)

Brand Names: US Caprelsa
Brand Names: Canada Caprelsa
Index Terms AZD6474; Zactima; ZD6474; Zictifa
Pharmacologic Category Antineoplastic Agent, Epidermal Growth Factor Receptor (EGFR) Inhibitor; Antineoplastic Agent, Tyrosine Kinase Inhibitor; Antineoplastic Agent, Vascular Endothelial Growth Factor (VEGF) Inhibitor
Use Thyroid cancer: Treatment of metastatic or unresectable locally-advanced medullary thyroid cancer (symptomatic or progressive)
Pregnancy Considerations Animal reproduction studies have demonstrated teratogenic effects and fetal loss. Because vandetanib inhibits angiogenesis, a critical component of fetal development, adverse effects on pregnancy would be expected. Women of childbearing potential should be advised to avoid pregnancy and use effective contraception during and for 4 months following treatment with vandetanib. Canadian labeling recommends that nonsterile males employ reliable contraceptive methods (barrier method in conjunction with spermicide) during and for 2 months after vandetanib treatment.
Breast-Feeding Considerations It is not known if vandetanib is excreted in human breast milk. Due to the potential for serious adverse reactions in the nursing infant, a decision should be made to discontinue vandetanib or to discontinue breast-feeding, taking into account the importance of treatment to the mother.
Prescribing and Access Restrictions As a requirement of the REMS program, access to vandetanib is restricted. Vandetanib is approved for marketing under a Food and Drug Administration (FDA) approved, risk management program, and through a restricted distribution program, the Vandetanib REMS Program (1-800-236-9933). Prescribers and pharmacies must be certified with the program to prescribe or dispense vandetanib.

In Canada, vandetanib is available only through the CAPRELSA Restricted Distribution Program. Prescribers and pharmacies must be certified with the program to prescribe or dispense vandetanib. Further information may be obtained at 1-800-668-6000.
Medication Guide Available Yes

Contraindications Congenital long QT syndrome

Canadian labeling: Additional contraindications (not in U.S. labeling): Hypersensitivity to vandetanib or any component of the formulation; persistent Fridericia-corrected QT interval (QTcF) ≥500 ms; uncorrected hypokalemia, hypomagnesemia, or hypocalcemia; uncontrolled hypertension

Warnings/Precautions Hazardous agent - use appropriate precautions for handling and disposal (NIOSH 2014 [group 1]). **[U.S. Boxed Warning]: May prolong the QT interval; torsade de pointes and sudden death have been reported. Do not use in patients with hypocalcemia, hypokalemia, hypomagnesemia, or long QT syndrome. Correct electrolyte imbalance prior to initiating therapy. Monitor electrolytes and ECG (to monitor QT interval) at baseline, at 2-4 weeks, at 8-12 weeks, and every 3 months thereafter; monitoring (at the same frequency) is required following dose reductions for QT prolongation or with dose interruptions >2 weeks. Avoid the use of QT-prolonging agents; if concomitant use with QT prolonging agents cannot be avoided, monitor ECG more frequently. Vandetanib has a long half-life (19 days), therefore, adverse reactions (including QT prolongation) may resolve slowly; monitor appropriately.** Ventricular tachycardia has also been reported. The potential for QT prolongation is dose-dependent. Do not initiate treatment unless QT interval, Fridericia-corrected QT interval (QTcF) is <450 msec. During treatment, if QTcF >500 msec, withhold vandetanib and resume at a reduced dose when QTcF is <450 msec. Do not use in patients with a history of torsade de pointes, congenital long QT syndrome, bradyarrhythmias or uncompensated heart failure. Patients with ventricular arrhythmias or recent MI were excluded from clinical trials. To reduce the risk of QT prolongation, maintain serum calcium and magnesium within normal limits and maintain serum potassium ≥4 mEq/L. Heart failure (HF) has been reported; monitor for signs and symptoms of HF; may require discontinuation (HF may not be reversible upon discontinuation). Hypertension and hypertensive crisis have been observed with vandetanib; monitor blood pressure and initiate or adjust antihypertensive therapy as needed; may require vandetanib dosage adjustment or treatment interruption; discontinue vandetanib (permanently) if blood pressure cannot be adequately controlled. Canadian labeling contraindicates use in uncontrolled hypertension.

Diarrhea has been reported with use; may cause electrolyte imbalance (closely monitor electrolytes and ECGs to detect QT prolongation resulting from dehydration); routine antidiarrheals are recommended; withhold vandetanib treatment until resolution for severe diarrhea; dose reduction is recommended when treatment is resumed. Stevens-Johnson syndrome and other serious skin reactions (including fatal) have been reported. Mild-to-moderate skin reactions, including acne, dermatitis, dry skin, palmar-plantar erythrodysesthesia syndrome, pruritus, and rash have also been reported. Withhold treatment for dermatologic toxicity of grade 3 or higher; consider a reduced dose or permanent discontinuation upon improvement in symptoms. Consider discontinuation for severe dermatologic toxicity. Mild-to-moderate toxicity has responded to corticosteroids (systemic or topical), oral antihistamines, and antibiotics (topical or systemic). Increased risk of photosensitivity is associated with use; effective sunscreen and protective clothing are recommended during and for at least 4 months after treatment discontinuation.

Reversible posterior leukoencephalopathy syndrome (RPLS) been observed with vandetanib; symptoms of RPLS include altered mental function, confusion, headache, seizure, or visual disturbances; generally associated with hypertension; consider discontinuing treatment if RPLS occurs. Serious and sometimes fatal hemorrhagic events have been reported with use; discontinue in patients with severe hemorrhage; do not administer in patients with a recent history of hemoptysis with ≥2.5 mL of red blood. Ischemic cerebrovascular events (some fatal) have been observed with vandetanib; discontinue treatment in patients with severe ischemic events (the safety of resuming treatment after an ischemic event has not been studied). Interstitial lung disease (ILD) or pneumonitis (including fatalities) has been reported with vandetanib. Patients should be advised to report any new or worsening respiratory symptoms; ILD should be suspected with nonspecific respiratory symptoms such as hypoxia, pleural effusion, cough or dyspnea. Interrupt therapy for acute or worsening pulmonary symptoms; discontinue if ILD diagnosis is confirmed.

Increased doses of thyroid replacement therapy have been required in patients with prior thyroidectomy; obtain TSH at baseline, at 2-4 weeks, 8-12 weeks, and every 3 months after vandetanib initiation; if signs and symptoms of hypothyroidism occur during treatment, evaluate thyroid hormone levels and adjust replacement therapy if needed. Dosage reduction is recommended in patients with moderate-to-severe renal impairment. Exposure is increased in patients with impaired renal function; closely monitor QT interval; has not been studied in patients with end stage renal disease requiring dialysis. Not recommended for use in patients with moderate-to-severe hepatic impairment. Potentially significant drug-drug interactions may exist, requiring dose or frequency adjustment, additional monitoring, and/or selection of alternative therapy. Due to the risk for serious treatment-related adverse events, use in patients whose disease is not progressive or symptomatic should be only be undertaken after careful consideration.

[U.S. Boxed Warning]: Vandetanib is only available through a restricted access program; prescribers and pharmacies must be certified with the restricted distribution program to prescribe and dispense vandetanib.

Adverse Reactions

>10%:

Cardiovascular: Hypertension (33%; grades 3/4: 9%), prolonged Q-T interval on ECG (14%; grades 3/4: 8%)

Central nervous system: Headache (26%; grades 3/4: 1%), fatigue (24%; grades 3/4: 6%), insomnia (13%)

Dermatologic: Skin rash (53%; grades 3/4: 5%), acne vulgaris (35%; grades 3/4: 1%), xeroderma (15%), skin photosensitivity (13%; grades 3/4: 2%), pruritus (11%; grades 3/4: 1%)

Endocrine & metabolic: Hypocalcemia (11% to 57%; grades 3/4: 2%), hypoglycemia (24%)

Gastrointestinal: Pseudomembranous colitis (57%; grades 3/4: 11%), nausea (33%; grades 3/4: 1%), abdominal pain (21%; grades 3/4: 3%), decreased appetite (21%; grades 3/4: 1% to 4%), vomiting (15%; grades 3/4: 1%), dyspepsia (11%)

Hematologic & oncologic: Leukopenia (19%), hemorrhage (13% to 14%), anemia (13%; grades 3/4: <1%)

Hepatic: Increased serum ALT (51%), increased serum bilirubin (13%)

Neuromuscular & skeletal: Weakness (15%)

Ophthalmic: Corneal changes (13%; corneal edema, corneal opacity, corneal dystrophy, iris hyperpigmentation, keratopathy, arcus lipoides, corneal deposits, acquired corneal dystrophy)

Renal: Increased serum creatinine (16%)

Respiratory: Upper respiratory tract infection (23%), cough (11%), nasopharyngitis (11%)

1% to 10%:

Cardiovascular: Cardiac failure (2%), cerebral ischemia (1%)

Central nervous system: Depression (10%; grades 3/4: 2%)

Dermatologic: Nail disease (9%; inflammation, tenderness, paronychia), alopecia (8%)

Endocrine & metabolic: Weight loss (10%), hypercalcemia (7%), hypomagnesemia (7%), hyperkalemia (6%), hypokalemia (6%), hypothyroidism (6%), hyperglycemia (5%), hypermagnesemia (3%)

Gastrointestinal: Xerostomia (9%), dysgeusia (8%)

Genitourinary: Proteinuria (10%)

Hematologic & oncologic: Neutropenia (10%; grades 3/4: <1%), thrombocytopenia (9%)

Infection: Sepsis (2%)

Neuromuscular & skeletal: Muscle spasm (6%)

Ophthalmic: Blurred vision (9%)

Respiratory: Aspiration pneumonia (2%), respiratory arrest (2%), respiratory failure (2%)

<1% (Limited to important or life-threatening): Cardiorespiratory arrest, interstitial pulmonary disease, palmar-plantar erythrodysesthesia, pancreatitis, pneumonitis, reversible posterior leukoencephalopathy syndrome, Stevens-Johnson syndrome, torsades de pointes, ventricular tachycardia

Drug Interactions

Metabolism/Transport Effects Substrate of CYP3A4 (major); **Note:** Assignment of Major/Minor substrate status based on clinically relevant drug interaction potential; **Inhibits** BCRP, P-glycoprotein

Avoid Concomitant Use

Avoid concomitant use of Vandetanib with any of the following: Bosutinib; CYP3A4 Inducers (Strong); Highest Risk QTc-Prolonging Agents; Ivabradine; Mifepristone; Moderate Risk QTc-Prolonging Agents; PAZOPanib; Silodosin; St Johns Wort; Topotecan; VinCRIStine (Liposomal)

Increased Effect/Toxicity

Vandetanib may increase the levels/effects of: Afatinib; Bisphosphonate Derivatives; Bosutinib; Brentuximab Vedotin; Colchicine; Dabigatran Etexilate; Digoxin; DOXOrubicin (Conventional); Edoxaban; Everolimus; Highest Risk QTc-Prolonging Agents; Ledipasvir; MetFORMIN; Naloxegol; PAZOPanib; P-glycoprotein/ABCB1 Substrates; Prucalopride; Rifaximin; Silodosin; Topotecan; VinCRIStine (Liposomal)

The levels/effects of Vandetanib may be increased by: Ivabradine; Mifepristone; Moderate Risk QTc-Prolonging Agents; QTc-Prolonging Agents (Indeterminate Risk and Risk Modifying)

Decreased Effect

The levels/effects of Vandetanib may be decreased by: Bosentan; CYP3A4 Inducers (Moderate); CYP3A4 Inducers (Strong); Dabrafenib; Deferasirox; Siltuximab; St Johns Wort; Tocilizumab

Storage/Stability Store at 25°C (77°F); excursions permitted to 15°C to 30°C (59°F to 86°F).

Mechanism of Action Multikinase inhibitor; inhibits tyrosine kinases including epidermal growth factor reception (EGFR), vascular endothelial growth factor (VEGF), rearranged during transfection (RET), protein tyrosine kinase 6 (BRK), TIE2, EPH kinase receptors and SRC kinase receptors, selectively blocking intracellular signaling, angiogenesis and cellular proliferation

Pharmacodynamics/Kinetics

Absorption: Slow

Protein binding: ~90%; to albumin and alpha 1-acid-glycoprotein

Distribution: V_d: ~7450 L

Metabolism: Hepatic, via CYP3A4 to N-desmethyl vandetanib and via flavin-containing monooxygenase enzymes to vandetanib-N-oxide

Bioavailability: Not affected by food

Half life, elimination: 19 days

Time to peak: 6 hours (range: 4-10 hours)

Excretion: Feces (~44%); urine (~25%)

Dosing

Adult & Geriatric Note: Do not initiate treatment unless QTcF <450 msec. Avoid concomitant use of QT-prolonging agents and strong CYP3A4 inducers. To reduce the risk of QT prolongation, maintain serum calcium and magnesium within normal limits and maintain serum potassium ≥4 mEq/L.

Medullary thyroid cancer, locally-advanced or metastatic: Oral: 300 mg once daily, continue treatment until no longer clinically benefiting or until unacceptable toxicity

Renal Impairment

CrCl ≥50 mL/minute: No dosage adjustment necessary.

CrCl <50 mL/minute: Reduce initial dose to 200 mg once daily; closely monitor QT interval.

Hepatic Impairment

Mild impairment (Child-Pugh class A): No dosage adjustment provided in manufacturer's labeling.

Moderate and severe impairment (Child-Pugh class B or C): Use is not recommended.

Adjustment for Toxicity

Toxicity ≥ grade 3: Interrupt dose until resolves or improves to grade 1, then resume at a reduced dose

Dosage reduction: Reduce from 300 mg once daily to 200 mg once daily, further reduce if needed to 100 mg once daily. For recurrent toxicities, reduce dose to 100 mg once daily after symptom improvement to ≤ grade 1 toxicity, if continued treatment is warranted.

Management of specific toxicities:

Cardiac: QTcF >500 msec: Withhold dose until QTcF returns to <450 msec, then resume at a reduced dose

Diarrhea (severe): Withhold treatment until resolution. Dose reduction is recommended when treatment is resumed. Routine antidiarrheals are recommended. Closely monitor electrolytes and ECGs to detect QT prolongation resulting from dehydration.

Heart failure: May require discontinuation.

Hemorrhage (severe): Discontinue.

Hypertension: Initiate or adjust antihypertensive therapy as needed; may require vandetanib dosage adjustment or treatment interruption; discontinue permanently if blood pressure cannot be adequately controlled.

Interstitial lung disease (ILD)/pneumonitis: Interrupt therapy for acute or worsening pulmonary symptoms. Discontinue if ILD diagnosis is confirmed.

Ischemic cerebrovascular events (severe): Discontinue treatment (safety of resuming treatment after an ischemic event has not been studied).

Reversible posterior leukoencephalopathy syndrome (RPLS): Discontinue treatment.

Skin reactions: Withhold treatment for dermatologic toxicity of grade 3 or higher. Consider a reduced dose or permanent discontinuation upon improvement in symptoms. Consider permanent discontinuation for severe dermatologic toxicity. Mild-to-moderate toxicity has responded to corticosteroids (systemic or topical), oral antihistamines, and antibiotics (topical or systemic).

Dietary Considerations May be taken with or without food.

Administration May be administered with or without food. Missed doses should be omitted if within 12 hours of the next scheduled dose. Do not crush tablet. If unable to swallow tablet whole or if nasogastric or gastrostomy tube administration is necessary, disperse one tablet in 2 ounces of water (noncarbonated only) and stir for 10 minutes to disperse (will not dissolve completely) and administer immediately. Rinse residue in glass with additional 4 ounces of water (noncarbonated only) and administer.

Hazardous agent; use appropriate precautions for handling and disposal (NIOSH 2014 [group 1]).

Monitoring Parameters Monitor electrolytes (calcium, magnesium, potassium), TSH, and ECG (QT interval) at baseline, at 2-4 weeks, at 8-12 weeks, and every 3 months thereafter; also monitor QT interval at same frequency for dose reduction due to QT interval or treatment delays >2 weeks (monitor electrolytes and ECG more frequently if diarrhea). Monitor renal function, hepatic function, blood pressure; monitor for signs and symptoms of heart failure, reversible posterior leukoencephalopathy syndrome (RPLS), pulmonary and skin toxicities

Dosage Forms Excipient information presented when available (limited, particularly for generics); consult specific product labeling. [DSC] = Discontinued product
Tablet, Oral:
  Caprelsa: 100 mg, 300 mg
  Generic: 100 mg [DSC], 300 mg [DSC]

Extemporaneous Preparations Hazardous agent: Use appropriate precautions for handling and disposal (NIOSH 2014 [group 1]).

An oral solution may be prepared using the tablet. Disperse one tablet in 2 ounces of water (noncarbonated only) and stir for 10 minutes to disperse (will not dissolve completely) and administer immediately. Rinse residue in glass with additional 4 ounces of water (noncarbonated only) and administer.

Vardenafil (var DEN a fil)

Brand Names: US Levitra; Staxyn
Brand Names: Canada Levitra; Staxyn
Index Terms Vardenafil Hydrochloride
Pharmacologic Category Phosphodiesterase-5 Enzyme Inhibitor
Use Erectile dysfunction: Treatment of erectile dysfunction (ED)
Pregnancy Considerations Teratogenic effects were not observed in animal studies; however, vardenafil is not indicated for use in women. No effects on sperm motility or morphology were observed in healthy males.
Breast-Feeding Considerations It is not known if vardenafil is excreted in breast milk. Vardenafil is not indicated for use in women.
Contraindications
Coadministration with nitrates (either regularly and/or intermittently), nitric oxide donors, or guanylate cyclase stimulators (eg, riociguat).

Canadian labeling: Additional contraindications (not in US labeling): Hypersensitivity to vardenafil or any component of the formulation; concomitant use with indinavir, ritonavir, ketoconazole or itraconazole (Levitra, Staxyn) and erythromycin or clarithromycin (Staxyn); prior episode of non-arteritic anterior ischemic optic neuropathy (NAION).

Warnings/Precautions There is a degree of cardiac risk associated with sexual activity; therefore, physicians may wish to consider the patient's cardiovascular status prior to initiating any treatment for erectile dysfunction. Use caution in patients with anatomical deformation of the penis (angulation, cavernosal fibrosis, or Peyronie's disease) and in patients who have conditions which may predispose them to priapism (sickle cell anemia, multiple myeloma, leukemia). Priapism, painful erection >6 hours in duration has been reported (rarely). Instruct patients to seek immediate medical attention if erection persists >4 hours.

Use is not recommended in patients with hypotension (<90/50 mm Hg); uncontrolled hypertension (>170/100 mm Hg); unstable angina or angina during intercourse; life-threatening arrhythmias, stroke, or MI within the last 6 months; cardiac failure or coronary artery disease causing unstable angina. Safety and efficacy have not been studied in these patients. Use caution in patients with left ventricular outflow obstruction (eg, aortic stenosis, hypertrophic cardiomyopathy with outflow tract obstruction). Use caution in the elderly or those with hepatic impairment (Child-Pugh class B); dosage adjustment is needed. Potentially significant drug-drug interactions may exist, requiring dose or frequency adjustment, additional monitoring, and/or selection of alternative therapy. Concomitant use with all forms of nitrates is contraindicated. If nitrate administration is medically necessary, it is not known when nitrates can be safely administered following the use of vardenafil; however, when a 20 mg (film-coated tablet) was administered 24 hours prior to a 0.4 mg sublingual dose of nitroglycerin, no changes in blood pressure or heart rate were detected.

Rare cases of NAION have been reported; patients who have already experienced NAION are at an increased risk of recurrence. Other risk factors for NAION include heart disease, diabetes, hypertension, smoking, age >50 years, or history of certain eye problems. Use with caution in these patients only when the benefits outweigh the risks. The Canadian labeling contraindicates use in patients with a prior episode of NAION. Sudden decrease or loss of hearing has been reported rarely; hearing changes may be accompanied by tinnitus and dizziness.

Safety and efficacy have not been studied in patients with the following conditions, therefore, use in these patients is not recommended at this time: Congenital QT prolongation, patients taking medications known to prolong the QT interval (avoid use in patients taking Class Ia or III antiarrhythmics); severe hepatic impairment (Child-Pugh class C); end-stage renal disease requiring dialysis); retinitis pigmentosa or other degenerative retinal disorders. Potential underlying causes of erectile dysfunction should be evaluated prior to treatment. Some products may contain phylalanine. Some products may contain sorbitol; do not use in patients with fructose intolerance.

Adverse Reactions
>10%:
  Cardiovascular: Flushing (8% to 11%)
  Central nervous system: Headache (14% to 15%)
2% to 10%:
  Central nervous system: Dizziness (2%)
  Gastrointestinal: Dyspepsia (3% to 4%), nausea (2%)
  Neuromuscular & skeletal: Back pain (2%), CPK increased (2%)
  Respiratory: Rhinitis (9%), nasal congestion (3%), sinusitis (3%)
  Miscellaneous: Flu-like syndrome (3%)
<2% (Limited to important or life-threatening): Abnormal ejaculation, amnesia (transient global), anaphylactic reaction, angina, angioedema, arthralgia, basal cell carcinoma (Loeb 2015), dyspnea, hearing decreased, hearing loss, hyper-/hypotension, insomnia, liver function tests abnormal, melanoma (Loeb 2015), MI, myalgia, nonarteritic ischemic optic neuropathy (NAION), orthostatic hypotension, pain, photophobia, photosensitivity, priapism, pruritus, rash, somnolence, syncope, tachycardia, tinnitus, ventricular tachyarrhythmia, vertigo, vision abnormal, visual acuity reduced, visual field defects, vision loss (temporary or permanent)
Drug Interactions
  Metabolism/Transport Effects Substrate of CYP3A4 (major); **Note:** Assignment of Major/Minor substrate status based on clinically relevant drug interaction potential

Avoid Concomitant Use

Avoid concomitant use of Vardenafil with any of the following: Alprostadil; Amyl Nitrite; Conivaptan; Dapoxetine; Fusidic Acid (Systemic); Idelalisib; Molsidomine; Phosphodiesterase 5 Inhibitors; Riociguat; Vasodilators (Organic Nitrates)

Increased Effect/Toxicity

Vardenafil may increase the levels/effects of: Alpha1-Blockers; Alprostadil; Amyl Nitrite; Blood Pressure Lowering Agents; Bosentan; Highest Risk QTc-Prolonging Agents; Moderate Risk QTc-Prolonging Agents; Phosphodiesterase 5 Inhibitors; Riociguat; Vasodilators (Organic Nitrates)

The levels/effects of Vardenafil may be increased by: Alcohol (Ethyl); Aprepitant; Boceprevir; Clarithromycin; Cobicistat; Conivaptan; CYP3A4 Inhibitors (Moderate); CYP3A4 Inhibitors (Strong); Dapoxetine; Dasatinib; Erythromycin (Systemic); Fluconazole; Fosaprepitant; Fusidic Acid (Systemic); Idelalisib; Itraconazole; Ivacaftor; Ketoconazole (Systemic); Lorcaserin; Luliconazole; Mifepristone; Molsidomine; Netupitant; Osimertinib; Palbociclib; Posaconazole; Sapropterin; Simeprevir; Stiripentol; Telaprevir; Voriconazole

Decreased Effect

The levels/effects of Vardenafil may be decreased by: Bosentan; Etravirine; Osimertinib

Food Interactions High-fat meals decrease maximum serum concentration 18% to 50%. Serum concentrations/toxicity may be increased with grapefruit juice. Management: Do not take with a high-fat meal. Avoid grapefruit juice.

Storage/Stability Store at 25°C (77°F); excursions permitted to 15°C to 30°C (59°F to 86°F). Keep oral disintegrating tablets sealed in blisterpack until ready to use.

Mechanism of Action Does not directly cause penile erections, but affects the response to sexual stimulation. The physiologic mechanism of erection of the penis involves release of nitric oxide (NO) in the corpus cavernosum during sexual stimulation. NO then activates the enzyme guanylate cyclase, which results in increased levels of cyclic guanosine monophosphate (cGMP), producing smooth muscle relaxation and inflow of blood to the corpus cavernosum. Vardenafil enhances the effect of NO by inhibiting phosphodiesterase type 5 (PDE-5), which is responsible for degradation of cGMP in the corpus cavernosum; when sexual stimulation causes local release of NO, inhibition of PDE-5 by vardenafil causes increased levels of cGMP in the corpus cavernosum, resulting in smooth muscle relaxation and inflow of blood to the corpus cavernosum; at recommended doses, it has no effect in the absence of sexual stimulation.

Pharmacodynamics/Kinetics

Onset of action: ~60 minutes

Absorption: Rapid

Distribution: V_d: 208 L

Protein binding: ~95% (parent drug and metabolite)

Metabolism: Hepatic via CYP3A4 (major), CYP2C and 3A5 (minor); forms metabolite (active)

Bioavailability: ~15%

Film-coated tablet: Elderly (≥65 years): AUC increased by 52%; Hepatic impairment (moderate, Child-Pugh class B): AUC increased by 160%

Oral disintegrating tablet: Elderly (≥65 years): AUC increased by 21% more compared to film-coated tablet. When administered with water, AUC decreases by 29%.

Half-life elimination: Terminal: Vardenafil and metabolite: 4 to 6 hours

Time to peak, plasma: 0.5 to 2 hours

Excretion: Feces (~91% to 95% as metabolites); urine (~2% to 6%)

Dosing

Adult Note: Oral disintegrating tablets should not be used interchangeably with film-coated tablets; patients requiring a dose other than 10 mg should use the film-coated tablets.

Erectile dysfunction: Oral:

Film-coated tablet (Levitra): 10 mg administered ~60 minutes prior to sexual activity; dosing range: 5 to 20 mg; taken as one single dose and not taken more than once daily; maximum 20 mg daily

Oral disintegrating tablet (Staxyn): 10 mg administered ~60 minutes prior to sexual activity; maximum: 10 mg daily

Dosing adjustment with concomitant medications:

Alpha-blocker (dose should be stable at time of vardenafil initiation):

Film-coated tablet (Levitra): Initial vardenafil dose: 5 mg taken no more than once daily; if an alpha-blocker is added to vardenafil therapy, it should be initiated at the smallest possible dose and titrated carefully. **Note:** With coadministration, the Canadian labeling recommends considering a time interval of several hours (eg, 6 hours) between dosing with alpha-blockers; separation of dosing is not required with tamsulosin.

Oral disintegrating tablet (Staxyn): Do not use to initiate therapy. Initial therapy should be with film-coated tablets at lower doses. Patients who have previously used film-coated tablets may be switched to oral disintegrating tablets as recommended by healthcare provider. With coadministration, consider a time interval between dosing (eg, 6-hour interval).

CYP3A4 inhibitors:

US labeling:

Film-coated tablet (Levitra): The dosage of vardenafil may require adjustment in patients receiving potent CYP3A4 inhibitors (eg, atazanavir, clarithromycin, erythromycin, indinavir, itraconazole, ketoconazole, ritonavir, saquinavir).

For ritonavir, a single dose of vardenafil 2.5 mg should not be exceeded in a 72-hour period.

For indinavir, saquinavir, atazanavir, ketoconazole 400 mg daily, itraconazole 400 mg daily, and clarithromycin, a single dose of vardenafil 2.5 mg should not be exceeded in a 24-hour period.

For ketoconazole 200 mg daily, itraconazole 200 mg daily, and erythromycin, a single dose of vardenafil 5 mg should not be exceeded in a 24-hour period.

Oral disintegrating tablet (Staxyn): Concurrent use not recommended with potent or moderate CYP3A4 inhibitors (atazanavir, clarithromycin, erythromycin, indinavir, itraconazole, ketoconazole, ritonavir, saquinavir)

Canadian labeling:

Film-coated tablet (Levitra): If used concurrently with erythromycin or clarithromycin, vardenafil dose should not exceed 5 mg. Concurrent use with indinavir, ritonavir, ketoconazole, or itraconazole is contraindicated.

Oral disintegrating tablet (Staxyn): Concurrent use with indinavir, ritonavir, ketoconazole, itraconazole, erythromycin or clarithromycin is contraindicated.

Geriatric Erectile dysfunction: Elderly ≥65 years: Film-coated tablet (Levitra): Oral: Consider a starting dose of 5 mg administered ~60 minutes prior to sexual activity; taken as one single dose and not taken more than once daily.

Renal Impairment

Mild, moderate, or severe impairment: No dosage adjustment necessary.

Hemodialysis: Use is not recommended.

Hepatic Impairment

Mild impairment (Child-Pugh class A):

US labeling: No dosage adjustment necessary.

Canadian labeling:

Film-coated tablet (Levitra): No dosage adjustment necessary.

Oral disintegrating tablet (Staxyn): Do not use to initiate therapy (film-coated tablets are recommended).

Moderate impairment (Child-Pugh class B):

Film-coated tablet (Levitra): Initial: 5 mg administered ~60 minutes prior to sexual activity (maximum dose: 10 mg daily); taken as one single dose and not taken more than once daily

Oral disintegrating tablet (Staxyn): Use is not recommended.

Severe impairment (Child-Pugh class C): Use is not recommended (has not been studied).

Dietary Considerations Avoid grapefruit juice. Some products may contain phenylalanine. Some products may contain sorbitol; do not use in patients with fructose intolerance.

Administration May be administered with or without food, approximately 60 minutes prior to sexual activity.

Oral disintegrating tablet should not be removed from blister pack until administered. Using dry hands, place immediately on tongue. Tablet will dissolve within seconds; do not take with liquid. Do not crush, split, or chew.

Monitoring Parameters Monitor for response, adverse reactions, blood pressure, and heart rate.

Dosage Forms Excipient information presented when available (limited, particularly for generics); consult specific product labeling.

Tablet, Oral:

Levitra: 2.5 mg, 5 mg, 10 mg, 20 mg

Tablet Dispersible, Oral:

Staxyn: 10 mg [contains aspartame; peppermint flavor]

◆ **Vardenafil Hydrochloride** *see* Vardenafil *on page 1875*

Varenicline (var EN i kleen)

Brand Names: US Chantix; Chantix Continuing Month Pak; Chantix Starting Month Pak

Brand Names: Canada Champix®

Index Terms Varenicline Tartrate

Pharmacologic Category Partial Nicotine Agonist; Smoking Cessation Aid

Use Smoking cessation: As an aid to smoking cessation treatment

Pregnancy Considerations Adverse events have been observed in animal reproduction studies.

Breast-Feeding Considerations It is not known if varenicline is excreted in breast milk. Due to the potential for serious adverse reactions in the nursing infant, the manufacturer recommends a decision be made whether to discontinue nursing or to discontinue the drug, taking into account the importance of treatment to the mother.

Medication Guide Available Yes

Contraindications Serious hypersensitivity reactions or skin reactions to varenicline or any component of the formulation

Warnings/Precautions [U.S. Boxed Warning]: Serious neuropsychiatric events (including depression, suicidal thoughts, and suicide) have been reported with use; some cases may have been complicated by symptoms of nicotine withdrawal following smoking cessation. Smoking cessation (with or without treatment) is associated with nicotine withdrawal symptoms and the exacerbation of underlying psychiatric illness; however, some of the behavioral disturbances were reported in treated patients who continued to smoke. Neuropsychiatric symptoms (eg, mood disturbances, psychosis, hostility) have occurred in patients with and without preexisting psychiatric disease; many cases resolved following therapy discontinuation although in some cases, symptoms persisted. Monitor all patients for behavioral changes and psychiatric symptoms (eg, agitation, depression, suicidal behavior, suicidal ideation); inform patients to discontinue treatment and contact their healthcare provider immediately if they experience any behavioral and/or mood changes. Patients with preexisting psychiatric illness (eg, bipolar disorder, major severe depression, schizophrenia) were not studied in premarketing clinical trials and limited safety data is available from postmarketing studies. Due to rare neuropsychiatric events, caution is warranted if treatment is initiated; worsening of psychiatric illness has been reported. **[U.S. Boxed Warning]: Before prescribing, the risks of serious neuropsychiatric events must be weighed against the immediate and long term benefits of smoking abstinence for each patient.**

Post-marketing reports of hypersensitivity reactions (including angioedema) and rare cases of serious skin reactions (including Stevens-Johnson syndrome and erythema multiforme) have been reported. Patients should be instructed to discontinue use and contact healthcare provider if signs/symptoms occur. Treatment may increase risk of cardiovascular events. A meta-analysis of 15 clinical trials, including a placebo-controlled trial in patients with stable cardiovascular disease, showed an increased incidence of major cardiovascular events (combined outcome of cardiovascular-related death, nonfatal MI, nonfatal stroke) in patients using varenicline compared with placebo. Cardiovascular events were uncommon in both the varenicline and placebo groups. These findings did not reach statistical significance, although data was consistent. Events occurred primarily in patients with known cardiovascular disease. The meta-analysis also showed a lower incidence of all-cause and cardiovascular mortality in varenicline-treated patients, although this was not statistically significant either. Seizures have been reported in patients with or without a history of seizures. Seizures generally occurred within the first month of therapy. Consider the risks against the benefits before initiating in patients with a history of seizures or other factors that can lower the seizure threshold; discontinue use if seizures occur during therapy. Dose-dependent nausea may occur; both transient and persistent nausea has been reported. Dosage reduction may be considered for intolerable nausea. May cause CNS depression, which may impair physical or mental abilities; patients must be cautioned about performing tasks which require mental alertness (eg, operating machinery or driving). There have been postmarketing reports of traffic accidents, near-miss incidents in traffic, or other accidental injuries in patients taking varenicline.

Use caution in renal dysfunction; dosage adjustment required with severe impairment. Potentially significant drug-drug interactions may exist, requiring dose or frequency adjustment, additional monitoring, and/or selection of alternative therapy. Consult drug interactions database for more detailed information.

Adverse Reactions

>10%:
Central nervous system: Headache (15% to 19%), insomnia (10% to 19%), abnormal dreams (9% to 13%), irritability (11%), suicidal ideation (11%), depression (4% to 11%)

Gastrointestinal: Nausea (16% to 40%), vomiting (5% to 11%)

1% to 10%:
Cardiovascular: Angina pectoris (4%), chest pain (3%), peripheral edema (2%), myocardial infarction (≤1%)

Central nervous system: Agitation (7%), malaise (7%), sleep disorder (5%), tension (4%), drowsiness (3%), hostility (2% to 3%), lethargy (1% to 2%), nightmares (1% to 2%)

Dermatologic: Skin rash (3%)

Gastrointestinal: Flatulence (6% to 9%), constipation (5% to 8%), dysgeusia (5% to 8%), abdominal pain (7%), diarrhea (6%), xerostomia (6%), dyspepsia (5%), increased appetite (3% to 4%), anorexia (2%), gastroesophageal reflux disease (1%)

Respiratory: Upper respiratory tract infection (5% to 7%), dyspnea (2%), rhinorrhea (≤1%)

<1% (Limited to important or life-threatening): Acute renal failure, amnesia, anemia, atrial fibrillation, Bell's palsy, cataract (subcapsular), cerebrovascular accident, conjunctivitis, cor pulmonale, coronary artery disease, decreased visual acuity, diabetes mellitus, dissociative disorder, dysarthria, dysphagia, ECG abnormality, eczema, enterocolitis, erectile dysfunction, erythema multiforme, gallbladder disease, gastrointestinal hemorrhage, homicidal ideation, hyperhidrosis, hyperlipidemia, hypersensitivity, hypoglycemia, hypokalemia, intestinal obstruction, leukocytosis, loss of consciousness, lymphadenopathy, mania, Meniere's disease, migraine, multiple sclerosis, myositis, nephrolithiasis, nocturnal amblyopia, nystagmus, ophthalmic vascular disease, oral mucosa ulcer, osteoporosis, pancreatitis, panic, photophobia, psychomotor agitation, psychomotor retardation, psychosis, pulmonary embolism, restless leg syndrome, seizure, skin photosensitivity, splenomegaly, Stevens-Johnson syndrome, syncope, tachycardia, thrombocytopenia, thrombosis, thyroid disease, transient blindness, transient ischemic attacks, urinary retention, ventricular premature contractions

Drug Interactions

Metabolism/Transport Effects Substrate of OCT2

Avoid Concomitant Use There are no known interactions where it is recommended to avoid concomitant use.

Increased Effect/Toxicity

Varenicline may increase the levels/effects of: Alcohol (Ethyl); Nicotine

The levels/effects of Varenicline may be increased by: BuPROPion; H2-Antagonists; Quinolone Antibiotics; Trimethoprim

Decreased Effect There are no known significant interactions involving a decrease in effect.

Storage/Stability Store at 25°C (77°F); excursions permitted to 15°C to 30°C (59°F to 86°F).

Mechanism of Action Partial neuronal α_4 β_2 nicotinic receptor agonist; prevents nicotine stimulation of mesolimbic dopamine system associated with nicotine addiction. Also binds to 5-HT$_3$ receptor (significance not determined) with moderate affinity. Varenicline stimulates dopamine activity but to a much smaller degree than nicotine does, resulting in decreased craving and withdrawal symptoms.

Pharmacodynamics/Kinetics

Absorption: Well absorbed; unaffected by food

Protein binding: ≤20%

Metabolism: Minimal (<10% of clearance is through metabolism)

Bioavailability: ~90%

Half-life elimination: ~24 hours

Time to peak, plasma: ~3 to 4 hours

Excretion: Urine (92% as unchanged drug)

Dosing

Adult & Geriatric Smoking cessation: Oral:
Initial:
Days 1 to 3: 0.5 mg once daily
Days 4 to 7: 0.5 mg twice daily
Maintenance (≥ Day 8):
U.S. labeling: 1 mg twice daily for 11 weeks
Canadian labeling: 0.5 to 1 mg twice daily for 11 weeks

Note: Start 1 week before target quit date. Alternatively, patients may consider setting a quit date up to 35 days after initiation of varenicline (some data suggest that an extended pretreatment regimen may result in higher abstinence rates [Hajek, 2011]). If patient successfully quits smoking at the end of the 12 weeks, may continue for another 12 weeks to help maintain success. Patients who are motivated to quit and do not succeed in stopping smoking during prior therapy, or who relapse after treatment, should be encouraged to make another attempt with varenicline once factors contributing to the failed attempt have been identified and addressed.

Renal Impairment
CrCl ≥30 mL/minute: No dosage adjustment necessary.
CrCl <30 mL/minute: Initiate: 0.5 mg once daily; maximum dose: 0.5 mg twice daily
End-stage renal disease (ESRD) (receiving hemodialysis): Maximum dose: 0.5 mg once daily

Hepatic Impairment No dosage adjustment necessary.

Adjustment for Toxicity Patients who cannot tolerate adverse events may require temporary (or permanent) reduction in dose.

Dietary Considerations Take after eating and with a full glass of water to decrease gastric upset.

Administration Administer after eating and with a full glass of water.

Monitoring Parameters Monitor for behavioral changes and psychiatric symptoms (eg, agitation, depression, suicidal behavior, suicidal ideation).

Additional Information In all studies, patients received an educational booklet on smoking cessation and received up to 10 minutes of counseling at each weekly visit. Dosing started 1 week before target quit date. Successful cessation of smoking may alter pharmacokinetic properties of other medications (eg, theophylline, warfarin, insulin).

Dosage Forms Excipient information presented when available (limited, particularly for generics); consult specific product labeling.
Tablet, Oral:
Chantix: 0.5 mg, 1 mg
Chantix Continuing Month Pak: 1 mg
Chantix Starting Month Pak: 0.5 mg x 11 & 1 mg x 42

◆ Varenicline Tartrate see Varenicline on page 1877

◆ Varicella, Measles, Mumps, and Rubella Vaccine see Measles, Mumps, Rubella, and Varicella Virus Vaccine on page 1129

Varicella Virus Vaccine
(var i SEL a VYE rus vak SEEN)

Brand Names: US Varivax
Brand Names: Canada Varilrix; Varivax III
Index Terms Chickenpox Vaccine; VAR; Varicella-Zoster Virus (VZV) Vaccine (Varicella); VZV Vaccine (Varicella)
Pharmacologic Category Vaccine; Vaccine, Live (Viral)
Additional Appendix Information
Immunization Administration Recommendations on page 1974
Immunization Schedules on page 1979
Use
Varicella prevention: For the prevention of varicella in persons 12 months and older
The Advisory Committee on Immunization Practices (ACIP) recommends vaccination for all children, adolescents, and adults who do not have evidence of immunity (CDC/ACIP [Marin, 2007]). Vaccination is especially important for:
• Healthcare personnel
• Household contacts of immunocompromised persons
• Persons living or working in environments where transmission is likely (teachers, child-care workers, residents and staff of institutional settings)
• Persons in environments where transmission has been reported
• Nonpregnant women of childbearing age
• Adolescents and adults in households with children
• International travelers
Medication Guide Available Yes
Dosing
Adult & Geriatric Varicella immunization: SubQ:
US labeling: Two doses of 0.5 mL separated by ≥4 weeks (4 to 8 weeks apart per ACIP). **Note:** The ACIP recommends that all children and adults without evidence of immunity receive 2 doses of the vaccine; those who received only 1 dose of vaccine receive a second dose (CDC/ACIP [Marin 2007]).

Canadian labeling: Two single doses 0.5 mL separated by 4 to 8 weeks (Varivax III) or ≥6 weeks (Varilrix); **Note:** The NACI recommends that adolescents (≥13 years of age) and adults (<50 years of age) who received only 1 dose of vaccine receive a second dose (NACI 2012).

Postexposure prophylaxis (healthy, previously unvaccinated individuals) (off-label use): SubQ: 0.5 mL administered ideally within 72 hours postexposure but may be used up to 120 hours (5 days) postexposure (CDC/ACIP [Marin 2007])

Pediatric Varicella immunization: SubQ:
US labeling:
Children ≥12 months: 0.5 mL; a second dose may be administered ≥3 months later
Note: The ACIP recommends the routine childhood vaccination be 2 doses, with the first dose administered at 12 to 15 months of age. The second dose should be administered at 4 to 6 years of age before school entry, but it may be administered earlier provided ≥3 months have elapsed after the first dose. Children ≥7 years and adolescents who received only 1 dose of vaccine should receive a second dose (CDC/ACIP [Marin 2007]). If the second dose was administered ≥4 weeks after the first dose, it may be considered as valid (CDC/ACIP [Strikas 2015]).
Adolescents ≥13 years: Refer to adult dosing.

Canadian labeling:
Children ≥12 months:
Varilrix: Two doses of 0.5 mL separated by ≥6 weeks
Varivax III: 0.5 mL as a single dose
Alternative recommendations (NACI, 2012): Two doses of 0.5 mL with first dose administered at 12 to 15 months of age. Separate doses by ≥3 months; however, if rapid protection is necessary, may administer second dose after ≥6 weeks.
Adolescents ≥13 years: Refer to adult dosing.

Postexposure prophylaxis (healthy, previously unvaccinated individuals) (off-label use): Children ≥12 months and Adolescents: SubQ: 0.5 mL administered ideally within 72 hours postexposure but may be used up to 120 hours (5 days) postexposure (CDC/ACIP [Marin 2007])

Renal Impairment There are no dosage adjustments provided in the manufacturer's labeling

Hepatic Impairment There are no dosage adjustments provided in the manufacturer's labeling

Additional Information Complete prescribing information should be consulted for additional detail.

Dosage Forms Excipient information presented when available (limited, particularly for generics); consult specific product labeling.
Injectable, Subcutaneous [preservative free]:
Varivax: 1350 PFU/0.5 mL (1 ea)

Dosage Forms: Canada Excipient information presented when available (limited, particularly for generics); consult specific product labeling.
Injection, powder for reconstitution [preservative free]:
Varivax III: 1350 plaque-forming units (PFU) [contains gelatin and trace amounts of neomycin; packaged with diluent]
Injection, powder for reconstitution:
Varilrix: $10^{3.3}$ plaque-forming units (PFU) [contains albumin and gelatin; packaged with diluent]

◆ Varicella Zoster see Varicella-Zoster Immune Globulin (Human) on page 1878

Varicella-Zoster Immune Globulin (Human)
(var i SEL a- ZOS ter i MYUN GLOB yoo lin HYU man)

Brand Names: US VariZIG
Brand Names: Canada VariZIG
Index Terms Varicella Zoster; VZIG
Pharmacologic Category Blood Product Derivative; Immune Globulin
Additional Appendix Information
Immunization Administration Recommendations on page 1974
Immunization Schedules on page 1979
Use
U.S. labeling: Postexposure prophylaxis of varicella in high-risk individuals. High-risk groups include:
- Immunocompromised children and adults
- Newborns of mothers with varicella shortly before or after delivery
- Premature infants
- Neonates and infants <1 year of age
- Adults without evidence of immunity
- Pregnant women

Canadian labeling: In pregnant women, for the prevention or reduction in severity of maternal infection within 4 days of exposure to the varicella zoster virus.

The Advisory Committee on Immunization Practices (ACIP) recommends varicella-zoster immune globulin (VZIG) to patients who are at high risk for severe varicella infection and complications; and who were exposed to varicella or herpes zoster; and for whom varicella vaccine is contraindicated. The decision to use VZIG should take into consideration if the patient lacks evidence of immunity; if exposure is likely to result in an infection; and if the patient is at greater risk for varicella complications than the general population. The following are patient groups for whom VZIG is recommended (CDC 2013):

- Immunocompromised patients without evidence of immunity (seronegative), including those with neoplastic disease (eg, leukemia or lymphoma); primary or acquired immunodeficiency; immunosuppressive therapy (including steroid therapy equivalent to prednisone ≥2 mg/kg or 20 mg/day)
- Newborn of mother who had onset of varicella (chickenpox) within 5 days before delivery or within 48 hours after delivery
- Hospitalized premature infants (≥28 weeks gestation) who were exposed during the neonatal period and whose mother has no evidence of immunity
- Hospitalized premature infants (<28 weeks gestation or ≤1000 g) regardless of maternal history and who were exposed during the neonatal period
- Pregnant women without evidence of immunity who have been exposed

Dosing
Adult

Postexposure prophylaxis: *U.S. labeling:* IM: Administer a single dose based on body weight. Dose may be repeated for high-risk patients with additional exposure >3 weeks after initial administration. The minimum dose is 62.5 units and the maximum dose is 625 units.

≤2 kg: 62.5 units
2.1 to 10 kg: 125 units
10.1 to 20 kg: 250 units
20.1 to 30 kg: 375 units
30.1 to 40 kg: 500 units
≥40.1 kg: 625 units

Note: Administration should begin as soon as possible (ideally within 96 hours) and within 10 days after exposure (CDC 2013). Administration should begin within 96 hours (ideally 48 hours) in hematopoietic cell transplant (HCT) recipients who are exposed to varicella or zoster or a varicella zoster vaccine vaccinee who develops a varicella-like rash (Tomblyn 2009).

Prevention or reduction of maternal infection: *Canadian labeling:* IM, IV: 12.5 units/kg (one 125 units vial per 10 kg body weight); minimum dose: 125 units; maximum dose: 625 units. Administer within 96 hours of exposure.

Geriatric Postexposure prophylaxis: IM: Refer to adult dosing.

Pediatric Postexposure prophylaxis: Infants, Children, and Adolescents: IM: Refer to adult dosing.

Renal Impairment There are no dosage adjustments provided in manufacturer's labeling.

Hepatic Impairment There are no dosage adjustments provided in manufacturer's labeling.

Additional Information Complete prescribing information should be consulted for additional detail.

Dosage Forms Excipient information presented when available (limited, particularly for generics); consult specific product labeling.

Solution, Intramuscular [preservative free]:
VariZIG: 125 units/1.2 mL (1.2 mL) [contains polysorbate 80]

Solution Reconstituted, Intramuscular [preservative free]:
VariZIG: 125 units (1 ea) [contains polysorbate 80]

Vasopressin (vay soe PRES in)

Brand Names: US Pitressin Synthetic [DSC]; Vasostrict
Brand Names: Canada Pressyn; Pressyn AR
Index Terms 8-Arginine Vasopressin; ADH; Antidiuretic Hormone; AVP
Pharmacologic Category Antidiuretic Hormone Analog; Hormone, Posterior Pituitary
Additional Appendix Information
Adult ACLS Algorithms *on page 1993*

Use

Diabetes Insipidus (Pitressin Synthetic only): Treatment of central diabetes insipidus; differential diagnosis of diabetes insipidus

Vasodilatory shock (Vasostrict only): To increase blood pressure in adults patients with vasodilatory shock (eg, postcardiotomy or sepsis) who remain hypotensive despite fluids and catecholamines

Pregnancy Considerations Animal reproduction studies have not been conducted. Vasopressin may produce tonic uterine contractions; however, doses sufficient for diabetes insipidus are not likely to produce this effect.

Breast-Feeding Considerations It is not known if vasopressin is excreted in breast milk. Oral absorption by a nursing infant is unlikely because vasopressin is rapidly destroyed in the GI tract; however, consider pumping and discarding breast milk for 1.5 hours after receiving vasopressin (Vasostrict only) to minimize potential exposure to the breast-fed infant. The manufacturer recommends that caution be exercised when administering vasopressin to nursing women.

Contraindications Hypersensitivity to vasopressin or any component of the formulation; hypersensitivity to chlorobutanol (Vasostrict only); uncorrected chronic nephritis with nitrogen retention (Pitressin Synthetic only)

Warnings/Precautions Use with caution in patients with seizure disorders, migraine, asthma, vascular disease, renal disease, cardiovascular disease, including arteriosclerosis; goiter with cardiac complications. IV administration (off-label route): Vesicant; ensure proper needle or catheter placement prior to and during infusion; extravasation may lead to severe vasoconstriction and localized tissue necrosis, gangrene of extremities, tongue, and ischemic colitis; avoid extravasation. May cause water intoxication; early signs include drowsiness, listlessness, and headache, these should be recognized to prevent coma and seizures. Elderly patients should be cautioned not to increase their fluid intake beyond that sufficient to satisfy their thirst in order to avoid water intoxication and hyponatremia; under experimental conditions, the elderly have shown to have a decreased responsiveness to vasopressin with respect to its effects on water homeostasis.

Adverse Reactions Frequency not defined.

Cardiovascular: Angina pectoris, atrial fibrillation, bradycardia, cardiac arrest, cardiac arrhythmia, ischemic heart disease, limb ischemia (distal), localized blanching, low cardiac output, myocardial infarction, right heart failure, shock, vasoconstriction (peripheral)

Central nervous system: Headache (pounding), vertigo

Dermatologic: Circumoral pallor, diaphoresis, gangrene of skin or other tissues, skin lesion (ischemic), urticaria

Endocrine & metabolic: Hyponatremia, hypovolemic shock, water intoxication

Gastrointestinal: Abdominal cramps, flatulence, mesenteric ischemia, nausea, vomiting

Hematologic & oncologic: Decreased platelet count, hemorrhage (intractable)

Hepatic: Increased serum bilirubin

Hypersensitivity: Anaphylaxis

Neuromuscular & skeletal: Tremor

Renal: Renal insufficiency

Respiratory: Bronchoconstriction

Drug Interactions

Metabolism/Transport Effects None known.

Avoid Concomitant Use There are no known interactions where it is recommended to avoid concomitant use.

Increased Effect/Toxicity There are no known significant interactions involving an increase in effect.

Decreased Effect There are no known significant interactions involving a decrease in effect.

Food Interactions Ethanol may decrease the antidiuretic effect. Management: Avoid ethanol.

Preparation for Administration Vasostrict: **Note:** Discard unused diluted solution after 18 hours at room temperature or 24 hours under refrigeration. Discard vial after 48 hours after first entry.

No fluid restriction: Final concentration vasopressin 0.1 units/mL: Reconstitute vasopressin 50 units (2.5 mL) with 500 mL NS or D_5W.

Fluid restriction: Final concentration 1 unit/mL: Reconstitute vasopressin 100 units (5 mL) with 100 mL NS or D_5W.

Storage/Stability

Store intact vials between 2°C and 8°C (36°F and 46°F). Do not freeze.

Vasostrict: May also remove intact vials from refrigeration and store at 20°C to 25°C (68°F to 77°F) for up to 12 months or manufacturer expiration date, whichever is earlier (indicate date of removal on the vial). Discard unused diluted solution after 18 hours at room temperature or 24 hours under refrigeration. Discard vial after 48 hours after first entry.

Mechanism of Action Increases cyclic adenosine monophosphate (cAMP) which increases water permeability at the renal tubule resulting in decreased urine volume and increased osmolality; causes peristalsis by directly stimulating the smooth muscle in the GI tract; direct vasoconstrictor without inotropic or chronotropic effects. In vasodilatory shock, vasopressin increases systemic vascular resistance and mean arterial blood pressure and decreases heart rate and cardiac output.

Pharmacodynamics/Kinetics

Onset of action: Nasal: 1 hour; IV: ≤15 minutes

Duration: Nasal: 3 to 8 hours; IM, SubQ: 2 to 8 hours; IV: ≤20 minutes

Metabolism: Nasal/Parenteral: Hepatic, renal (inactive metabolites)

Half-life elimination: Nasal: 15 minutes; Parenteral: 10 to 20 minutes

Excretion: Nasal: Urine; SubQ: Urine (5% as unchanged drug) after 4 hours; IV: Urine (~6% as unchanged drug)

Dosing

Adult & Geriatric

Central diabetes insipidus: Note: Dosage is highly variable; titrated based on serum and urine sodium and osmolality in addition to fluid balance and urine output. Use of vasopressin is impractical for chronic therapy.

IM, SubQ: 5 to 10 units 2 to 4 times daily as needed

Continuous IV infusion (off-label route): Continuous infusion has not been formally evaluated in the postneurosurgical adult. However, some convert IM/SubQ requirement to an hourly continuous IV infusion rate.

Vasodilatory shock: IV: **Note:** Dosage provided is empirical; titrate to lowest dose compatible with an acceptable response.

Post-cardiotomy shock: Initial: 0.03 units per minute. If the target blood pressure response is not achieved, titrate up by 0.005 units per minute at 10- to 15-minute intervals (maximum dose: 0.1 units per minute). After target blood pressure has been maintained for 8 hours without the use of catecholamines, taper by 0.005 units per minute every hour as tolerated to maintain target blood pressure.

Septic shock:

Surviving Sepsis Campaign recommendations: 0.03 units per minute added to norepinephrine to raise MAP to target or to decrease norepinephrine dose. Doses >0.03 units per minute may have more cardiovascular side effects and should only be reserved for salvage therapy (ie, failure to achieve MAP goal with other vasopressors) (SCCM [Dellinger 2013]). To prevent subsequent hypotension after withdrawal of vasopressors, vasopressin should be slowly tapered (eg, titrated down by 0.01 units per minute every 30 minutes) **after** the catecholamine(s) are discontinued until no longer required (Bauer 2010).

Manufacturer's labeling: Initial: 0.01 units per minute. If the target blood pressure response is not achieved, titrate up by 0.005 units per minute at 10- to 15-minute intervals. Maximum dose: 0.07 units per minute. After target blood pressure has been maintained for 8 hours without the use of catecholamines, taper by 0.005 units per minute every hour as tolerated to maintain target blood pressure.

Cadaveric organ donation (hormonal resuscitation) (off-label use): IV: Initial: 1 unit bolus followed by a continuous infusion of 0.5 to 4 units/hour administered to the brain-dead donor who is hemodynamically unstable requiring significant vasopressor support; titrate to SVR of 800 to 1200 dynes-sec/cm5; give concomitantly with levothyroxine or liothyronine (preferred), methylprednisolone, and continuous regular insulin infusion (Rosendale 2003a; Rosendale 2003b; Rosengard 2002; Zaroff 2002)

Central diabetes insipidus, post-traumatic (off-label use): IV: Initial: 2.5 units/hour; titrate to adequately reduce urine output (Levitt 1984)

Gastroesophageal variceal hemorrhage (off-label use): Note: Other therapies may be preferred.

Continuous IV infusion: Initial: 0.2 to 0.4 units per minute, may titrate dose as needed to a maximum dose of 0.8 units per minute; maximum duration: 24 hours at highest effective dose continuously (to reduce incidence of adverse effects). Patient should also receive IV nitroglycerin concurrently to prevent myocardial ischemic complications. Monitor closely for signs/symptoms of ischemia (myocardial, peripheral, bowel) (AASLD [Garcia-Tsao 2007]).

Pediatric

Central diabetes insipidus: Note: Dosage is highly variable; titrated based on serum and urine sodium and osmolality in addition to fluid balance and urine output. Use of vasopressin is impractical for chronic therapy.

IM, SubQ: 2.5 to 10 units 2 to 4 times daily as needed

Continuous IV infusion (off-label route): Initial: 0.0005 units/kg/hour; increase dose by 0.0005 units/kg/hour increments every 5 to 10 minutes as needed to adequately reduce urine output (maximum dose: 0.01 unit/kg/hour) (Wise-Faberowski 2004). **Note:** Although clinical trial titrated every 5 to 10 minutes, a reduced frequency of titration (eg, every 30 minutes) may be more appropriate given the half-life of vasopressin. To provide the infusion dose, the concentration used during the study was 20 units in 500 mL (0.04 units/mL) in D_5W.

GI hemorrhage (off-label use): Note: Other therapies may be preferred.

Initial IV bolus: 0.3 units/kg (maximum: 20 units) may be given

Continuous IV infusion: 0.001 to 0.01 units/kg/minute; titrate dose as needed; maximum: 0.01 units/kg/minute; if bleeding controlled for 12 to 24 hours, then taper off over 24 to 36 hours

Renal Impairment There are no dosage adjustments provided in the manufacturer's labeling.

Hepatic Impairment There are no dosage adjustments provided in the manufacturer's labeling.

Usual Infusion Concentrations: Adult IV infusion: 50 units in 500 mL (concentration: 0.1 unit/mL) **or** 100 units in 100 mL (concentration: 1 unit/mL) of D_5W or NS

Administration Pitressin Synthetic: For IM or SubQ administration (per manufacturer).

IV: May administer as IV bolus over seconds (ACLS 2010) or as a continuous IV infusion (refer to indication-specific infusion rates in dosing for detailed recommendations); when administered as a continuous IV infusion for vasodilatory shock, the use of a central venous catheter is recommended. Use extreme caution to avoid extravasation because of risk of necrosis and gangrene. In treatment of varices, infusions are often supplemented with nitroglycerin infusions to minimize cardiac effects.

Continuous IV infusion: Dilute in NS or D_5W to 0.1 to 1 unit/mL.

Vesicant; ensure proper needle or catheter placement prior to and during infusion; avoid extravasation.

Extravasation management: If extravasation occurs, stop infusion immediately and disconnect (leave cannula/needle in place); gently aspirate extravasated solution (do **NOT** flush the line); remove needle/cannula; elevate extremity. Initiate phentolamine (or alternative antidote).

Phentolamine (no longer available in the US): Dilute 5 to 10 mg in 10 to 15 mL NS and administer into extravasation site as soon as possible after extravasation (Peberdy 2010).

Alternatives to phentolamine:

Nitroglycerin topical 2% ointment (based on limited case reports in neonates/infants): Apply 4 mm/kg as a thin ribbon to the affected areas; may repeat after 8 hours if needed (Wong 1992) **or** apply a 1-inch strip on the affected site (Denkler 1989).

Terbutaline (based on limited case reports): Infiltrate extravasation area using a solution of terbutaline 1 mg diluted to 10 mL in NS (large extravasation site; administration volume varied from 3 to 10 mL) **or** 1 mg diluted in 1 mL NS (small/distal extravasation site; administration volume varied from 0.5 to 1 mL) (Stier 1999).

Intranasal (topical administration on nasal mucosa; off-label route): Administer injectable vasopressin on cotton plugs, as nasal spray, or by dropper. Should not be inhaled.

Endotracheal (off-label route): If no IV or intraosseous access, may give endotracheally. ACLS guidelines do not recommend a specific endotracheal dose; however, may be given endotracheally using the same IV dose (ACLS 2010; Wenzel 1997). Mix with 5 to 10 mL of water or normal saline, and administer down the endotracheal tube.

Monitoring Parameters Serum and urine sodium, urine specific gravity, urine and serum osmolality; urine output, fluid input and output, blood pressure, heart rate

Consult individual institutional policies and procedures.
Additional Information Vasopressin increases factor VIII levels and may be useful in hemophiliacs.
Dosage Forms Excipient information presented when available (limited, particularly for generics); consult specific product labeling. [DSC] = Discontinued product
Solution, Injection:
  Pitressin Synthetic: 20 units/mL (1 mL [DSC]) [contains chlorobutanol (chlorobutol)]
  Generic: 20 units/mL (0.5 mL [DSC], 1 mL, 10 mL [DSC])
Solution, Intravenous:
  Vasostrict: 20 units/mL (1 mL) [contains chlorobutanol (chlorobutol)]

◆ Vasostrict see Vasopressin on page 1879
◆ Vasotec see Enalapril on page 636
◆ Vazculep see Phenylephrine (Systemic) on page 1442
◆ VCF Vaginal Contraceptive [OTC] see Nonoxynol 9 on page 1296
◆ VEC-162 see Tasimelteon on page 1739
◆ Vecamyl see Mecamylamine on page 1129
◆ Vectibix see Panitumumab on page 1386
◆ Vectical see Calcitriol on page 284

Vecuronium (vek ue ROE nee um)

Brand Names: Canada Norcuron®
Index Terms Norcuron; ORG NC 45
Pharmacologic Category Neuromuscular Blocker Agent, Nondepolarizing
Use To facilitate endotracheal intubation and to relax skeletal muscles during surgery; to facilitate mechanical ventilation in ICU patients; does not relieve pain or produce sedation
Pregnancy Considerations Animal reproduction studies have not been conducted. The pharmacokinetics of vecuronium are altered during pregnancy. Use in cesarean section has been reported; umbilical venous concentrations were 11% of maternal values at delivery.
Breast-Feeding Considerations It is not known if vecuronium is excreted in breast milk. The manufacturer recommends that caution be exercised when administering vecuronium to nursing women.
Contraindications Hypersensitivity to vecuronium or any component of the formulation
Warnings/Precautions Ventilation must be supported during neuromuscular blockade. Vecuronium does not relieve pain or produce sedation; use should include appropriate anesthesia, pain control, and sedation. In patients requiring long-term administration, use of a peripheral nerve stimulator to monitor drug effects is strongly recommended. Additional doses of vecuronium or any other neuromuscular-blocking agent should be avoided unless nerve stimulation response suggests inadequate neuromuscular blockade. Certain clinical conditions may result in potentiation (dosage reduction may be necessary) or antagonism (dosage increase may be necessary) of neuromuscular blockade:
  Antagonism: Respiratory alkalosis, hypercalcemia, demyelinating lesions, peripheral neuropathies, denervation, and muscle trauma
  Potentiation: Electrolyte abnormalities (eg, severe hypocalcemia, severe hypokalemia, hypermagnesemia), neuromuscular diseases, metabolic acidosis, metabolic alkalosis, respiratory acidosis, Eaton-Lambert syndrome, and myasthenia gravis

Resistance may occur in burn patients (≥20% of total body surface area), usually several days after the injury, and may persist for several months after wound healing. Resistance may occur in patients who are immobilized. Hypothermia may prolong the duration of action. Use with caution in patients with hepatic impairment; clinical duration may be prolonged. Use with caution in patients who are anephric; clinical duration may be prolonged. Use with caution in patients who have underlying respiratory disease. Some patients may experience delayed recovery of neuromuscular function after administration (especially after prolonged use). Other factors associated with delayed recovery should be considered (eg, corticosteroid

use, disease-related conditions). Cross-sensitivity with other neuromuscular-blocking agents may occur; use extreme caution in patients with previous anaphylactic reactions. Use caution in the elderly; dosage reduction may be considered. Children 1-10 years of age may require slightly higher initial doses and slightly more frequent supplementation. **[US Boxed Warning]: Should be administered by adequately trained individuals familiar with its use.**

Benzyl alcohol and derivatives: Diluent may contain benzyl alcohol; large amounts of benzyl alcohol (≥99 mg/kg/day) have been associated with a potentially fatal toxicity ("gasping syndrome") in neonates; the "gasping syndrome" consists of metabolic acidosis, respiratory distress, gasping respirations, CNS dysfunction (including convulsions, intracranial hemorrhage), hypotension, and cardiovascular collapse (AAP ["Inactive" 1997]; CDC, 1982); some data suggests that benzoate displaces bilirubin from protein binding sites (Ahlfors, 2001); avoid or use dosage forms containing benzyl alcohol with caution in neonates. See manufacturer's labeling.
Adverse Reactions <1% (Limited to important or life-threatening): Acute quadriplegic myopathy syndrome (prolonged use), Bradycardia, circulatory collapse, edema, flushing; hypersensitivity reaction (hypotension, tachycardia, erythema, rash, urticaria); itching, myositis ossificans (prolonged use), rash
Drug Interactions
  Metabolism/Transport Effects None known.
  Avoid Concomitant Use
    Avoid concomitant use of Vecuronium with any of the following: QuiNINE
  Increased Effect/Toxicity
    Vecuronium may increase the levels/effects of: Cardiac Glycosides; Corticosteroids (Systemic); OnabotulinumtoxinA; RimabotulinumtoxinB

    The levels/effects of Vecuronium may be increased by: AbobotulinumtoxinA; Aminoglycosides; Calcium Channel Blockers; Capreomycin; Clindamycin (Topical); Colistimethate; CycloSPORINE (Systemic); Dantrolene; Fosphenytoin-Phenytoin; Inhalational Anesthetics; Ketorolac (Nasal); Ketorolac (Systemic); Lincosamide Antibiotics; Lithium; Loop Diuretics; Magnesium Salts; Minocycline; Piperacillin; Polymyxin B; Procainamide; QuiNIDine; QuiNINE; Spironolactone; Tetracycline Derivatives; Vancomycin
  Decreased Effect
    The levels/effects of Vecuronium may be decreased by: Acetylcholinesterase Inhibitors; CarBAMazepine; Fosphenytoin-Phenytoin; Loop Diuretics
Preparation for Administration Reconstitute with compatible solution for injection to final concentration of 1 mg/mL. May further dilute reconstituted vial to 0.1-0.2 mg/mL in a compatible solution for IV infusion.
Storage/Stability Store intact vials of powder for injection at room temperature 20°C to 25°C (68°F to 77°F). Vials reconstituted with bacteriostatic water for injection (BWFI) may be stored for 5 days under refrigeration or at room temperature. Vials reconstituted with other compatible diluents (nonbacteriostatic) should be stored under refrigeration and used within 24 hours.
Mechanism of Action Blocks acetylcholine from binding to receptors on motor endplate inhibiting depolarization
Pharmacodynamics/Kinetics
  Onset of action:
    Good intubation conditions: Within 2.5-3 minutes
    Maximum neuromuscular blockade: Within 3-5 minutes
  Duration: Under balanced anesthesia (time to recovery to 25% of control): 25-40 minutes; recovery 95% complete ~45-65 minutes after injection of intubating dose
  Distribution: V_d: 0.3-0.4 L/kg
  Protein binding: 60% to 80%
  Metabolism: Active metabolite: 3-desacetyl vecuronium (1/2 the activity of parent drug)
  Half-life elimination: Healthy surgical patients and renal failure patients undergoing transplant surgery: 65-75 minutes; Late pregnancy: 35-40 minutes
  Excretion: Primarily feces (40% to 75%); urine (30% as unchanged drug and metabolites)
Dosing
  Adult Dose to effect; doses will vary due to interpatient variability.
    Surgical relaxation: IV (do not administer IM):
      Tracheal intubation: IV: Initial: 0.08-0.1 mg/kg. **Note:** If intubation is performed using succinylcholine (not preferred agent in pediatric patients), the initial dose of vecuronium may be reduced to 0.04-0.06 mg/kg with inhalation anesthesia and 0.05-0.06 mg/kg with balanced anesthesia.

Obesity: For obese (≥130% of IBW) adult patients, may use ideal body weight (IBW) (Erstad, 2004; Schwartz, 1992; Weinstein, 1988); onset time may be slightly delayed using IBW.

Pretreatment/priming: Adults: 10% of intubating dose given 3-5 minutes before intubating dose

Maintenance for continued surgical relaxation (only after return of neuromuscular function): Intermittent dosing: 0.01-0.015 mg/kg **or** continuous infusion of 0.8-1.2 **mcg**/kg/**minute** (0.048-0.072 **mg**/kg/**hour**).

Note: Use lower end of the dosing range when anesthesia is maintained with an inhaled anesthetic agent, with the redosing interval guided by monitoring with a peripheral nerve stimulator.

ICU paralysis (eg, facilitate mechanical ventilation) in selected adequately sedated patients (Darrah, 1989; Greenberg, 2013; Murray, 2002; Rudis, 1997): IV: Initial bolus dose: 0.08-0.1 mg/kg, then a continuous IV infusion of 0.8-1.7 **mcg**/kg/**minute** (0.048-0.102 **mg**/kg/**hour**); monitor depth of blockade every 1-2 hours initially until stable dose, then every 8-12 hours. Usual maintenance infusion dose range: 0.8-1.2 **mcg**/kg/**minute** (0.048-0.072 **mg**/kg/**hour**).

Dosage adjustment (Rudis, 1996; Rudis, 1997): Adjust rate of administration in increments of 0.3 **mcg**/kg/**minute** (or 0.018 **mg**/kg/**hour**) or by 50% reductions of previous dose according to peripheral nerve stimulation response or desired clinical response. Discontinue infusion if neuromuscular function does not return.

Note: When possible, minimize depth and duration of paralysis. Stopping the infusion daily for some time until forced to restart based on patient condition is recommended to reduce post-paralytic complications (eg, acute quadriplegic myopathy syndrome [AQMS]) (Murray, 2002; Segredo, 1992).

Intermittent bolus dosing (Hunter, 1985): 0.1-0.2 mg/kg/dose; may be repeated when neuromuscular function returns

Control of refractory shivering in adequately sedated patients during therapeutic hypothermia after cardiac arrest (off-label use; Bernard, 2002; Nolan, 2003; Polderman, 2009): IV: 8-12 mg; redose as needed to control shivering. **Note:** Duration of action prolonged in hypothermic patients. May mask seizure activity.

Geriatric No specific guidelines available; refer to adult dosing. Dose selection should be cautious, at low end of dosage range, and titration should be slower to evaluate response.

Pediatric Dose to effect; doses will vary due to interpatient variability.

Surgical relaxation: Tracheal intubation: IV (do not administer IM): Children ≥1 year: Refer to adult dosing. **Note:** Children 1-10 years may require slightly higher initial doses and more frequent supplementation.

ICU paralysis (eg, facilitate mechanical ventilation) in selected adequately sedated patients (off-label; Martin, 1999): IV: Initial bolus dose: 0.1-0.15 mg/kg, then a continuous IV infusion of 1-2.5 **mcg**/kg/**minute** (0.06-0.15 **mg**/kg/**hour**); monitor depth of blockade using peripheral nerve stimulator every 2-3 hours initially until stable dose, then every 8-12 hours

Intermittent bolus dosing (Eldadah, 1989): 0.1 mg/kg every 1 hour as needed

Renal Impairment No dosage adjustment provided in manufacturer's labeling. However, patients with renal impairment do not experience clinically significant prolongation of neuromuscular blockade with vecuronium; however, in patients who are anephric, the clinical duration is prolonged.

Hepatic Impairment No dosage adjustment provided in manufacturer's labeling. However, dosage reduction may be necessary in patients with liver disease.

Obesity Refer to indication-specific dosing for obesity-related information (may not be available for all indications).

Usual Infusion Concentrations: Pediatric IV infusion: 0.1 mg/mL, 0.2 mg/mL, 1 mg/mL

Usual Infusion Concentrations: Adult IV infusion: 10 mg in 100 mL (concentration: 0.1 mg/mL), 20 mg in 100 mL (concentration: 0.2 mg/mL), **or** 50 mg in 50 mL (concentration: 1 mg/mL) of D_5W or NS

Administration Concentration of 1 mg/mL may be administered by rapid IV injection; may also be used for IV infusion in fluid-restricted patients.

Monitoring Parameters Blood pressure, heart rate; peripheral nerve stimulation (eg, train-of-four [TOF] count)

Additional Information Vecuronium is classified as an intermediate-duration neuromuscular-blocking agent. It produces minimal, if any, histamine release; does not relieve pain or produce sedation. It may produce cumulative effect on duration of blockade.

Dosage Forms Excipient information presented when available (limited, particularly for generics); consult specific product labeling.

Solution Reconstituted, Intravenous, as bromide:
Generic: 10 mg (1 ea); 20 mg (1 ea)
Solution Reconstituted, Intravenous, as bromide [preservative free]:
Generic: 10 mg (1 ea); 20 mg (1 ea)

Vedolizumab (ve doe LIZ ue mab)

Brand Names: US Entyvio

Pharmacologic Category Gastrointestinal Agent, Miscellaneous; Monoclonal Antibody; Monoclonal Antibody, Selective Adhesion-Molecule Inhibitor

Use

Crohn disease: Treatment of moderately to severely active Crohn disease in patients who have had an inadequate response with, lost response to, or were intolerant to inhibitors of tumor necrosis factor-alpha (TNF-alpha) blocker or immunomodulator; or had an inadequate response with, were intolerant to, or demonstrated dependence on corticosteroids.

Ulcerative colitis Treatment of moderately to severely active ulcerative colitis in patients who have had an inadequate response with, were intolerant to inhibitors of tumor necrosis factor-alpha (TNF-alpha) blocker or immunomodulator; or had an inadequate response with, were intolerant to, or demonstrated dependence on corticosteroids.

Pregnancy Considerations Adverse events have not been observed in animal reproduction studies. Monoclonal antibodies are transported across the placenta in a linear fashion as pregnancy progresses, with the largest amount transferred during the third trimester. Any adverse pregnancy effect would likely be greater during the second and third trimesters of pregnancy.

Health care providers are encouraged to enroll women exposed to vedolizumab during pregnancy in a pregnancy exposure registry. Information about the registry can be obtained by calling 1-877-825-3327.

Breast-Feeding Considerations It is not known if vedolizumab is excreted in breast milk. The manufacturer recommends that caution be exercised when administering vedolizumab to nursing women.

Medication Guide Available Yes

Contraindications Serious or severe hypersensitivity to vedolizumab or any component of the formulation

Warnings/Precautions Hypersensitivity reactions have been reported including anaphylaxis. Allergic reactions including dyspnea, bronchospasm, urticaria, flushing, rash, and increased blood pressure and heart rate have also been observed. Symptom onset may vary from during the infusion, immediately post-infusion, to several hours post-infusion. If serious reactions occur, discontinue administration immediately. Use may be associated with an increased risk for developing infections; most commonly reported infections included upper respiratory and nasal mucosa. Serious infections have also been reported in patients treated, including anal abscess, sepsis (some fatal), tuberculosis, salmonella sepsis, *Listeria* meningitis, giardiasis, and cytomegaloviral colitis. Therapy is not recommended in patients with uncontrolled, active, severe infections. If a patient develops a serious infection, consider discontinuing therapy. Use with caution in patients with a history of recurring severe infections. Screening for tuberculosis should be considered.

Integrin receptor antagonists have been associated with progressive multifocal leukoencephalopathy (PML), a rare and often fatal opportunistic infection of the central nervous system caused by the John Cunningham (JC) virus. Monitor patients for any new onset or worsening of neurological signs and symptoms including progressive weakness on one side of the body or clumsiness of limbs, disturbance of vision, and changes in thinking, memory, and orientation leading to confusion and personality changes. Symptoms may progress over days to weeks and can lead to death or severe disability in weeks to months. If PML is suspected withhold therapy and refer to a neurologist; if confirmed, discontinue therapy permanently. Elevations of transaminase and/or bilirubin have been reported in patients receiving vedolizumab. Discontinue therapy in patients with jaundice or other evidence of significant liver injury such as fatigue, anorexia, right upper abdominal discomfort, or dark urine. Patients should be

brought up to date with all immunizations according to immunization guidelines before initiating therapy. Live vaccines should not be given concurrently unless the benefits outweigh the risks; there are no data on the secondary transmission of infection by live vaccines with vedolizumab. Non-live vaccines may be given concurrently.

Adverse Reactions

>10%:

Central nervous system: Headache (12%)

Immunologic: Antibody development (4% to 13%; neutralizing: 2%)

Neuromuscular & skeletal: Arthralgia (12%)

Respiratory: Nasopharyngitis (13%)

1% to 10%:

Central nervous system: Fatigue (6%)

Dermatologic: Pruritus (3%), skin rash (3%)

Gastrointestinal: Nausea (9%)

Hepatic: Increased serum ALT (≥3 x ULN: <2%), increased serum AST (≥3 x ULN: <2%)

Infection: Influenza (4%)

Neuromuscular & skeletal: Back pain (4%), limb pain (3%)

Respiratory: Upper respiratory tract infection (7%), cough (5%), bronchitis (4%), oropharyngeal pain (3%), sinusitis (3%)

Miscellaneous: Fever (9%), infusion related reaction (4%)

<1% (Limited to important or life-threatening): Hepatitis, hypersensitivity reaction, infection (including anal abscess, sepsis, tuberculosis, salmonella sepsis, listeria meningitis, giardiasis, cytomegaloviral colitis), malignant neoplasm (excluding dysplasia and basal cell carcinoma)

Drug Interactions

Metabolism/Transport Effects None known.

Avoid Concomitant Use

Avoid concomitant use of Vedolizumab with any of the following: Anti-TNF Agents; BCG (Intravesical); Belimumab; Natalizumab; Pimecrolimus; Tacrolimus (Topical); Tofacitinib; Vaccines (Live)

Increased Effect/Toxicity

Vedolizumab may increase the levels/effects of: Belimumab; Fingolimod; Leflunomide; Natalizumab; Tofacitinib; Vaccines (Live)

The levels/effects of Vedolizumab may be increased by: Anti-TNF Agents; Denosumab; Pimecrolimus; Roflumilast; Tacrolimus (Topical); Trastuzumab

Decreased Effect

Vedolizumab may decrease the levels/effects of: BCG (Intravesical); Cholera Vaccine; Coccidioides immitis Skin Test; Sipuleucel-T; Vaccines (Inactivated); Vaccines (Live)

The levels/effects of Vedolizumab may be decreased by: Echinacea

Preparation for Administration Reconstitute at room temperature with 4.8 mL of sterile water for injection. Gently swirl vial for at least 15 seconds; do not vigorously shake or invert. Allow the solution to sit for up to 20 minutes at room temperature to allow for reconstitution and for any foam to settle; the vial can be swirled and inspected for dissolution during this time. If not fully dissolved after 20 minutes, allow another 10 minutes for dissolution. Do not use the vial if the drug product is not dissolved within 30 minutes. Solution should be clear or opalescent, colorless to light brownish yellow and free of visible particulates. Do not administer reconstituted solution showing uncharacteristic color or containing particulates.

Prior to withdrawing the reconstituted vedolizumab solution from the vial for dilution, gently invert vial 3 times. Add the 5 mL (300 mg) of reconstituted vedolizumab solution to 250 mL of sterile sodium chloride 0.9% and gently mix the infusion bag. Once reconstituted and diluted, use the infusion solution as soon as possible.

Storage/Stability Refrigerate unopened vials at 2°C to 8°C (36°F to 46°F). Retain in original package to protect from light. Following reconstitution and dilution, the infusion solution may be stored for up to 4 hours at 2°C to 8°C (36°F to 46°F). Do not freeze. Discard any unused portion.

Mechanism of Action Vedolizumab is a humanized monoclonal antibody that binds to the alpha4beta7 integrin and blocks the interaction of alpha4beta7 integrin with mucosal addressin cell adhesion molecule-1 (MAdCAM-1) and inhibits the migration of memory T-lymphocytes across the endothelium into inflamed gastrointestinal parenchymal tissue. The interaction of the alpha4beta7 integrin with MAdCAM-1 has been implicated as an important contributor to the chronic inflammation that is a hallmark of ulcerative colitis and Crohn disease.

Pharmacodynamics/Kinetics

Distribution: V_d: 5 L

Half-life elimination: 25 days (serum, at 300 mg dosage)

Dosing

Adult & Geriatric Note: Prior to initiating treatment, all patients should be brought up to date with all immunizations according to current immunization guidelines.

Crohn disease or ulcerative colitis: IV: 300 mg at 0, 2, and 6 weeks and then every 8 weeks thereafter. Discontinue therapy in patients who show no evidence of therapeutic benefit by week 14.

Renal Impairment There are no dosage adjustments provided in the manufacturer's labeling (has not been studied).

Hepatic Impairment There are no dosage adjustments provided in the manufacturer's labeling (has not been studied). Discontinue use with jaundice or signs/symptoms of hepatic injury.

Administration IV: Infuse over 30 minutes. Do not administer by IV push or bolus. Following infusion, flush with 30 mL of sterile 0.9% sodium chloride injection. Observe patients during infusion (until complete) and monitor for hypersensitivity reactions; discontinue if a reaction occurs.

Monitoring Parameters Observe patients during infusion (until complete) and monitor for hypersensitivity reactions; LFTs; tuberculosis screening according to local practice; signs/symptoms of infection; any new onset or worsening of neurological signs and symptoms

Dosage Forms Excipient information presented when available (limited, particularly for generics); consult specific product labeling.

Solution Reconstituted, Intravenous [preservative free]:

Entyvio: 300 mg (1 ea) [contains mouse protein (murine) (hamster), polysorbate 80]

Velaglucerase Alfa (vel a GLOO ser ase AL fa)

Brand Names: US Vpriv

Brand Names: Canada VPRIV

Index Terms Gene-Activated Human Acid-Beta-Glucosidase; GlcCerase

Pharmacologic Category Enzyme

Use Gaucher disease: For long-term enzyme replacement therapy for pediatric and adult patients with type 1 Gaucher disease.

Dosing

Adult & Geriatric Note: Pretreatment with antihistamines and/or corticosteroids can be considered for prevention of subsequent infusion reactions in patients with hypersensitivity reactions requiring symptomatic treatment; during clinical studies, patients were not routinely premedicated prior to infusion.

Gaucher's disease (type 1): IV: 60 units/kg administered every 2 weeks; adjust dose based upon disease activity (range: 15-60 units/kg evaluated in clinical trials)

Note: When switching from imiglucerase to velaglucerase alfa in stable patients, initiate treatment 2 weeks after the last imiglucerase dose and at the same dose.

Pediatric Note: Pretreatment with antihistamines and/or corticosteroids can be considered for prevention of subsequent infusion reactions in patients with hypersensitivity reactions requiring symptomatic treatment; during clinical studies, patients were not routinely premedicated prior to infusion.

Gaucher's disease (type 1): Children ≥4 years and Adolescents: Refer to adult dosing.

Renal Impairment No dosage adjustment provided in manufacturer's labeling.

Hepatic Impairment No dosage adjustment provided in manufacturer's labeling.

Additional Information Complete prescribing information should be consulted for additional detail.

Dosage Forms Excipient information presented when available (limited, particularly for generics); consult specific product labeling.

Solution Reconstituted, Intravenous [preservative free]:

Vpriv: 400 units (1 ea)

◆ **Veltassa** see Patiromer *on page 1403*

◆ **Veltin** see Clindamycin and Tretinoin *on page 410*

Vemurafenib (vem ue RAF e nib)

Brand Names: US Zelboraf

Brand Names: Canada Zelboraf

Index Terms BRAF(V600E) Kinase Inhibitor RO5185426; PLX4032; RG7204; RO5185426

Pharmacologic Category Antineoplastic Agent, BRAF Kinase Inhibitor

Use Melanoma, unresectable or metastatic:

US labeling: Treatment of unresectable or metastatic melanoma in patients with a BRAFV600E mutation (as detected by an approved test).

Canadian labeling: Treatment of unresectable or metastatic melanoma in patients with a BRAFV600 mutation (as identified by a validated test).

Limitations of use: Vemurafenib is not indicated in patients with wild-type BRAF melanoma.

Pregnancy Considerations Adverse effects were not demonstrated in animal reproduction studies. Based on the mechanism of action, vemurafenib may cause fetal harm if administered during pregnancy or in patients who become pregnant during treatment. Women of childbearing potential and men of reproductive potential should use adequate contraception methods during and for at least 2 months after treatment (Canadian labeling recommends during and for at least 6 months after treatment).

Breast-Feeding Considerations It is not known if vemurafenib is excreted in breast milk. Due to the potential for serious adverse reactions in the nursing infant, the manufacturer recommends a decision be made to discontinue nursing or to discontinue the drug, taking into account the importance of treatment to the mother.

Prescribing and Access Restrictions Available through specialty pharmacies. Further information may be obtained from the manufacturer, Genentech, at 1-888-249-4918, or at http://www.zelboraf.com.

Medication Guide Available Yes

Contraindications There are no contraindications listed in the manufacturer's labeling.

Canadian labeling: Hypersensitivity to vemurafenib or any component of the formulation.

Warnings/Precautions Hazardous agent - use appropriate precautions for handling and disposal (NIOSH 2014 [group 1]). Only patients with a BRAFV600 mutation-positive melanoma (including BRAFV600E) will benefit from treatment; mutation must be detected and confirmed by an approved test prior to treatment. The cobas 4800 BRAF V600 Mutation Test was used in clinical trials and is FDA-approved to detect BRAFV600E mutation.

Cutaneous squamous cell carcinomas (cuSCC), keratoacanthomas, and melanoma have been reported (at a higher rate in patients receiving vemurafenib compared to control). Cutaneous SCC generally occurs early in the treatment course (median onset: 7 to 8 weeks) and is managed with excision (while continuing vemurafenib treatment). Approximately one-third of patients experienced >1 cuSCC occurrence and the median time between occurrences was 6 weeks. Potential risk factors for cuSCC include age ≥65 years, history of skin cancer, or chronic sun exposure. Monitor for skin lesions (with dermatology evaluation) at baseline and every 2 months during treatment; consider continued monitoring for 6 months after treatment. Noncutaneous squamous cell carcinomas (SCC) of the head and neck have also been observed; monitor closely for signs/symptoms. Vemurafenib may promote malignancies correlated with RAS activation; monitor for signs/symptoms of other malignancies.

Dermatologic reactions have been observed, including case reports of Stevens-Johnson syndrome and toxic epidermal necrolysis; discontinue (permanently) for severe dermatologic toxicity. Photosensitivity ranging from mild to severe has been reported. Advise patients to avoid sun exposure and wear protective clothing and use effective UVA/UVB sunscreen and lip balm (SPF ≥30) when outdoors. Dosage modifications are recommended for intolerable photosensitivity consisting of erythema ≥10% to 30% of body surface area. Uveitis (including iritis), blurred vision, and photophobia may occur; monitor for signs and symptoms. Uveitis may be managed with corticosteroid and mydriatic eye drops. Retinal vein occlusion has been reported in clinical trials. Radiation sensitization and recall (some cases may be severe or involve cutaneous and visceral organs) have been reported in patients treated with radiation prior to, during, or after treatment with vemurafenib. Monitor closely when vemurafenib is administered concomitantly or sequentially with radiation treatment.

QT prolongation (dose-dependent) has been observed; may lead to increased risk for ventricular arrhythmia, including torsade de pointes. Monitor electrolytes (calcium, magnesium and potassium) at baseline and with dosage adjustments. Monitor ECG at baseline, 15 days after initiation, then monthly for 3 months, then every 3 months thereafter (more frequently if clinically appropriate); also monitor with dosage adjustments. Do not initiate treatment if baseline QTc >500 msec. During treatment, if QTc >500 msec, temporarily interrupt treatment; correct electrolytes and control other risk factors for QT prolongation. May reinitiate with a dose reduction once QTc falls to <500 msec. Discontinue (permanently) if, after correction of risk factors, both the QTc continues to increase >500 msec and there is >60 msec change above baseline. Do not initiate treatment in patients with electrolyte abnormalities which are not correctable, long QT syndrome, or taking concomitant medication known to prolong the QT interval.

Liver injury has been reported with use, and may cause functional impairment such as coagulopathy or other organ dysfunction. Monitor transaminases, alkaline phosphatase and bilirubin at baseline and monthly during therapy, or as clinically necessary. May require dosage reduction, therapy interruption, or discontinuation. Anaphylaxis and severe hypersensitivity may occur during treatment or upon reinitiation. Serious reactions have included generalized rash, erythema, hypotension, and drug rash with eosinophilia and systemic symptoms (DRESS syndrome). Discontinue (permanently) with severe hypersensitivity reaction. Pancreatitis has been reported (case reports), with onset generally occurring within 2 weeks of initiation (Muluneh 2013; Zelboraf Canadian product monograph 2015); exacerbation of pancreatitis has also occurred upon rechallenge. Patients with unexplained abdominal pain should be promptly evaluated for pancreatitis (eg, serum lipase and amylase; abdominal CT) as clinically indicated. Elderly patients may be at increased risk for adverse effects; in clinical trials, there was an increased incidence of cuSCC and keratoacanthoma, atrial fibrillation, peripheral edema, and nausea/decreased appetite in patients ≥65 years of age. Potentially significant drug-drug interactions may exist, requiring dose or frequency adjustment, additional monitoring, and/or selection of alternative therapy.

Adverse Reactions

>10%:

Cardiovascular: Peripheral edema (17% to 23%)

Central nervous system: Fatigue (38% to 54%; grade 3: 2% to 4%), headache (23% to 27%)

Dermatologic: Skin rash (37% to 52%; grade 3: 7% to 8%), skin photosensitivity (33% to 49%; grade 3: 3%), alopecia (36% to 45%; grade 3: 2%), pruritus (23% to 30%; grade 3: 2%), hyperkeratosis (24% to 28%; actinic: 8% to 17%; seborrheic: 10% to 14%; pilaris: ≤10%), maculopapular rash (9% to 21%; grade 3: 2% to 6%), xeroderma (16% to 19%), sunburn (10% to 14%), erythema (8% to 14%), papular rash (5% to 13%)

Gastrointestinal: Nausea (35% to 37%; grade 3: 2%), diarrhea (28% to 29%; grade 3: <1%), vomiting (18% to 26%; grade 3: 1% to 2%), decreased appetite (18% to 21%), constipation (12% to 16%), dysgeusia (11% to 14%)

Hematologic & oncologic: Cutaneous papilloma (21% to 30%), squamous cell carcinoma of skin (24%; grade 3: 22% to 24%)

Hepatic: Increased gamma-glutamyl transferase (5% to 15%)

Neuromuscular & skeletal: Arthralgia (53% to 67%; grade 3: 4% to 8%), myalgia (13% to 24%; grade 3: <1%), limb pain (9% to 18%), back pain (8% to 11%; grade 3: <1%), musculoskeletal pain (8% to 11%), weakness (2% to 11%)

Respiratory: Cough (8% to 12%)

Miscellaneous: Fever (17% to 19%)

1% to 10%:

Cardiovascular: Atrial fibrillation, hypotension, prolonged Q-T interval on ECG, retinal vein occlusion, vasculitis

Central nervous system: Cranial nerve palsy (facial), dizziness, peripheral neuropathy

Dermatologic: Erythema nodosum, folliculitis, palmar-plantar erythrodysesthesia, Stevens-Johnson syndrome, toxic epidermal necrolysis

Endocrine & metabolic: Weight loss

Hematologic & oncologic: Basal cell carcinoma, malignant melanoma (new primary), squamous cell carcinoma (oropharyngeal)

Hepatic: Increased serum alkaline phosphatase, increased serum ALT, increased serum AST, increased serum bilirubin

Hypersensitivity: Anaphylaxis, hypersensitivity
Neuromuscular & skeletal: Arthritis
Ophthalmic: Blurred vision, iritis, photophobia, uveitis
Renal: Increased serum creatinine
<1% (Limited to important or life-threatening): Chronic myelomonocytic leukemia with NRAS mutation (progression of preexisting condition), drug reaction with eosinophilia and systemic symptoms (DRESS syndrome), febrile neutropenia, hepatic failure, neutropenia, pancreatitis, panniculitis, recall skin sensitization

Drug Interactions

Metabolism/Transport Effects Substrate of BCRP, CYP3A4 (major), P-glycoprotein; **Note:** Assignment of Major/Minor substrate status based on clinically relevant drug interaction potential; **Inhibits** BCRP, CYP1A2 (moderate), CYP2D6 (weak), P-glycoprotein; **Induces** CYP3A4 (weak)

Avoid Concomitant Use

Avoid concomitant use of Vemurafenib with any of the following: Bosutinib; Conivaptan; CYP3A4 Inducers (Strong); CYP3A4 Inhibitors (Strong); Fusidic Acid (Systemic); Highest Risk QTc-Prolonging Agents; Idelalisib; Ivabradine; Mifepristone; Moderate Risk QTc-Prolonging Agents; PAZOPanib; Silodosin; TiZANidine; Topotecan; VinCRIStine (Liposomal)

Increased Effect/Toxicity

Vemurafenib may increase the levels/effects of: Afatinib; Bosutinib; Brentuximab Vedotin; Colchicine; CYP1A2 Substrates; Dabigatran Etexilate; Digoxin; DOXOrubicin (Conventional); Edoxaban; Everolimus; Highest Risk QTc-Prolonging Agents; Ledipasvir; Naloxegol; PAZOPanib; P-glycoprotein/ABCB1 Substrates; Pirfenidone; Porfimer; Prucalopride; Rifaximin; Silodosin; TiZANidine; Topotecan; Verteporfin; VinCRIStine (Liposomal); Warfarin

The levels/effects of Vemurafenib may be increased by: Aprepitant; Conivaptan; CYP3A4 Inhibitors (Moderate); CYP3A4 Inhibitors (Strong); Fosaprepitant; Fusidic Acid (Systemic); Idelalisib; Ipilimumab; Ivabradine; Ivacaftor; Luliconazole; Mifepristone; Moderate Risk QTc-Prolonging Agents; Netupitant; Palbociclib; P-glycoprotein/ABCB1 Inhibitors; QTc-Prolonging Agents (Indeterminate Risk and Risk Modifying); Simeprevir; Stiripentol

Decreased Effect

Vemurafenib may decrease the levels/effects of: ARIPiprazole; Hydrocodone; NiMODipine; Saxagliptin

The levels/effects of Vemurafenib may be decreased by: Bosentan; CYP3A4 Inducers (Moderate); CYP3A4 Inducers (Strong); Dabrafenib; Deferasirox; P-glycoprotein/ABCB1 Inducers; Siltuximab; St Johns Wort; Tocilizumab

Food Interactions Grapefruit and grapefruit juice may inhibit CYP3A4-mediated metabolism of vemurafenib. Management: Avoid concurrent use (Zelboraf Canadian product monograph 2015).

Storage/Stability Store at room temperature of 20°C to 25°C (68°F to 77°F); excursions permitted to 15°C and 30°C (59°F and 86°F). Store in the original container with the lid tightly closed.

Mechanism of Action BRAF kinase inhibitor (potent) which inhibits tumor growth in melanomas by inhibiting kinase activity of certain mutated forms of BRAF, including BRAF with V600E mutation, thereby blocking cellular proliferation in melanoma cells with the mutation. Does not have activity against cells with wild-type BRAF. BRAFV600E activating mutations are present in ~50% of melanomas; V600E mutation involves the substitution of glutamic acid for valine at amino acid 600. The cobas 4800 BRAF V600 mutation test is approved to detect BRAFV600E mutation.

Pharmacodynamics/Kinetics

Distribution: V_d: ~106 L
Protein binding: >99%, to albumin and α_1-acid glycoprotein
Half-life, elimination: 57 hours (range: 30 to 120 hours)
Time to peak: ~3 hours
Excretion: Feces (~94%); urine (~1%)

Dosing

Adult & Geriatric

US labeling: Melanoma, metastatic or unresectable (with BRAFV600E mutation): Oral: 960 mg every 12 hours; continue until disease progression or unacceptable toxicity.

Canadian labeling: Melanoma, metastatic or unresectable (with BRAFV600 mutation): Oral: 960 mg twice daily; continue until disease progression or unacceptable toxicity.

Missed doses: A missed dose may be taken up to 4 hours prior to the next scheduled dose. If it is within 4 hours of the next scheduled dose, administer the next dose at the regular schedule. If vomiting occurs after a dose is taken, do not take an additional dose; continue with the next scheduled dose.

Melanoma, metastatic or unresectable (with BRAFV600K mutation; off-label use): Oral: 960 mg every 12 hours; continue until disease progression or unacceptable toxicity (Sossman 2012).

Melanoma, metastatic or unresectable (with BRAFV600E or V600K mutations; off-label combination): Oral: 960 mg every 12 hours (in combination with cobimetinib); continue until disease progression or unacceptable toxicity (Larkin 2014).

Renal Impairment

US labeling:
Mild to moderate impairment (preexisting): No dosage adjustment necessary.
Severe impairment (preexisting): There are no dosage adjustments provided in the manufacturer's labeling (data are insufficient to determine if dosage adjustment is necessary); use with caution.
Canadian labeling: There are no dosage adjustments provided in the manufacturer's labeling.

Hepatic Impairment

Mild to moderate impairment (preexisting): No dosage adjustment necessary.
Severe impairment (preexisting): There are no dosage adjustments provided in manufacturer's labeling (data are insufficient to determine if dosage adjustment is necessary); use with caution.
Hepatotoxicity/lab abnormalities during treatment: Refer to Dosage Adjustment for Toxicity and manage with dose reduction, treatment interruption, or discontinuation.

Adjustment for Toxicity Note: Do not dose reduce below 480 mg twice daily. NCI Common Terminology Criteria for Adverse Events (CTC-AE) version 4.0 used for adverse event grades.

Grade 1 or grade 2 (tolerable) toxicity: No dosage adjustment recommended.

Grade 2 (intolerable) or grade 3 toxicity:
US labeling:
First incident: Interrupt treatment until toxicity returns to grade 0 or 1, then resume at 720 mg twice daily
Second incident: Interrupt treatment until toxicity returns to grade 0 or 1, then resume at 480 mg twice daily
Third incident: Discontinue permanently.
Canadian labeling:
First incident: Interrupt treatment until toxicity returns to grade 0 or 1, then resume at 720 mg twice daily or 480 mg twice daily if dose previously reduced.
Second incident: Interrupt treatment until toxicity returns to grade 0 or 1, then resume at 480 mg twice daily or discontinue permanently if dose previously reduced to 480 mg twice daily.
Third incident: Discontinue permanently.

Grade 4 toxicity:
First incident: Interrupt treatment until toxicity returns to grade 0 or 1, then resume at 480 mg twice daily **or** discontinue permanently
Second incident: Discontinue permanently.

Specific toxicities:
Severe hypersensitivity or severe dermatologic toxicity: Discontinue permanently.
QTc interval changes:
US labeling:
QTc >500 msec (grade ≥3): Temporarily withhold treatment, correct electrolytes and control risk factors for QT prolongation; may reinitiate with a dose reduction once QTc ≤500 msec.
QTc persistently >500 msec and >60 msec above baseline: Discontinue permanently.
Canadian labeling:
QTc >500 msec during treatment and ≤60 msec change from baseline:
First incident: Interrupt treatment until QTc <500 msec, then resume at 720 mg twice daily or 480 mg twice daily if dose previously reduced.
Second incident: Interrupt treatment until QTc <500 msec, then resume at 480 mg twice daily or discontinue permanently if dose previously reduced to 480 mg twice daily.
Third incident: Discontinue permanently.
QTc >500 msec during treatment and >60 msec above baseline: Discontinue permanently.

Dietary Considerations Avoid grapefruit and grapefruit juice.

Administration Doses should be administered orally in the morning and evening, ~12 hours apart. May be taken with or without a meal. If vomiting occurs after a dose is taken, do not take an additional dose; continue with the next scheduled dose.

Swallow whole with a glass of water; do not crush or chew. There are case reports of vemurafenib administration after crushing (Janson 2013; Khimani 2014), however vemurafenib is nearly insoluble in water and is manufactured as a microprecipitated bulk powder core (to improve solubility/bioavailability) within a film coated tablet (Shah 2013). Pharmacokinetics and efficacy of administration other than swallowing tablets whole have not been determined.

Hazardous agent; use appropriate precautions for handling and disposal (NIOSH 2014 [group 1]). NIOSH recommends single gloving for administration of intact tablets (NIOSH 2014). Although crushing of the tablets is not recommended, if it is necessary to manipulate tablets, it is recommended to double glove, wear a protective gown, and prepare in a controlled device (NIOSH 2014).

Monitoring Parameters Liver transaminases, alkaline phosphatase and bilirubin at baseline and monthly during treatment (or as clinically appropriate). Electrolytes (calcium, magnesium and potassium) at baseline and after dosage modification. ECG at baseline, 15 days after initiation, then monthly for 3 months, then every 3 months thereafter (more frequently if clinically appropriate) and with dosage adjustments. Dermatology evaluation (for new skin lesions) at baseline and every 2 months during treatment; also consider continued monitoring for 6 months after completion of treatment. Signs/symptoms of hypersensitivity reactions, uveitis, and malignancies; signs of radiation sensitization and recall.

Dosage Forms Excipient information presented when available (limited, particularly for generics); consult specific product labeling.

Tablet, Oral:
Zelboraf: 240 mg

Venlafaxine (ven la FAX een)

Brand Names: US Effexor XR
Brand Names: Canada ACT Venlafaxine XR; Apo-Venlafaxine XR; Dom-Venlafaxine XR; Effexor XR; GD-Venlafaxine XR; Mylan-Venlafaxine XR; PMS-Venlafaxine XR; Ran-Venlafaxine XR; Riva-Venlafaxine XR; Sandoz-Venlafaxine XR; Teva-Venlafaxine XR; Venlafaxine XR
Pharmacologic Category Antidepressant, Serotonin/Norepinephrine Reuptake Inhibitor
Use

Generalized anxiety disorder (extended-release capsules only): Treatment of generalized anxiety disorder (GAD)

Major depressive disorder: Treatment of major depressive disorder (MDD)

Panic disorder (extended-release capsules only): Treatment of panic disorder, with or without agoraphobia

Social anxiety disorder (extended-release capsules and tablets only): Treatment of social anxiety disorder, also known as social phobia

Pregnancy Considerations Adverse events have been observed in some animal reproduction studies. Venlafaxine and its active metabolite ODV cross the human placenta. An increased risk of teratogenic effects following venlafaxine exposure during pregnancy has not been observed, based on available data. The risk of spontaneous abortion may be increased. Neonatal seizures and neonatal abstinence syndrome have been noted in case reports following maternal use of venlafaxine during pregnancy. Nonteratogenic effects in the newborn following SSRI/SNRI exposure late in the third trimester include respiratory distress, cyanosis, apnea, seizures, temperature instability, feeding difficulty, vomiting, hypoglycemia, hyper- or hypotonia, hyper-reflexia, jitteriness, irritability, constant crying, and tremor. Symptoms may be due to the toxicity of the SNRI or a discontinuation syndrome and may be consistent with serotonin syndrome associated with treatment. The long-term effects of *in utero* SNRI/SSRI exposure on infant development and behavior are not known.

Due to pregnancy-induced physiologic changes, some pharmacokinetic parameters of venlafaxine may be altered. Women should be monitored for decreased efficacy. The ACOG recommends that therapy with SSRIs or SNRIs during pregnancy be individualized; treatment of depression during pregnancy should incorporate the clinical expertise of the mental health clinician, obstetrician, primary healthcare provider, and pediatrician. According to the American Psychiatric Association (APA), the risks of medication treatment should be weighed against other treatment options and untreated depression. For women who discontinue antidepressant medications during pregnancy and who may be at high risk for postpartum depression, the medications can be restarted following delivery. Treatment algorithms have been developed by the ACOG and the APA for the management of depression in women prior to conception and during pregnancy.

Breast-Feeding Considerations Venlafaxine and ODV are found in breast milk and the serum of nursing infants. Adverse events have not been observed; however, it is recommended to monitor the infant for adverse events if the decision to breast-feed has been made. The long-term effects on neurobehavior have not been studied, thus one should prescribe venlafaxine to a mother who is breast-feeding only when the benefits outweigh the potential risks. The manufacturer does not recommend breast-feeding during therapy.

Medication Guide Available Yes

Contraindications Hypersensitivity to venlafaxine or any component of the formulation; use of MAOIs intended to treat psychiatric disorders (concurrently or within 14 days of discontinuing the MAOI); initiation of MAOI intended to treat psychiatric disorders within 7 days of discontinuing venlafaxine; initiation in patients receiving linezolid or IV methylene blue

Warnings/Precautions [U.S. Boxed Warning]: Antidepressants increase the risk of suicidal thinking and behavior in children, adolescents, and young adults (18-24 years of age) with major depressive disorder (MDD) and other psychiatric disorders; consider risk prior to prescribing. Short-term studies did not show an increased risk in patients >24 years of age and showed a decreased risk in patients ≥65 years. Closely monitor for clinical worsening, suicidality, or unusual changes in behavior, particularly during the first few months of therapy or during periods of dosage adjustments (increases or decreases); the patient's family or caregiver should be instructed to closely observe the patient and communicate condition with healthcare provider. Reduced growth rate has been observed with venlafaxine therapy in children. A medication guide should be dispensed with each prescription.

The possibility of a suicide attempt is inherent in major depression and may persist until remission occurs. Use caution in high-risk patients. Worsening depression and severe abrupt suicidality that are not part of the presenting symptoms may require discontinuation or modification of drug therapy. The patient's family or caregiver should be alerted to monitor patients for the emergence of suicidality and associated behaviors (such as agitation, irritability, hostility, impulsivity, and hypomania) and call healthcare provider.

May precipitate a shift to mania or hypomania in patients with bipolar disorder. Patients presenting with depressive symptoms should be screened for bipolar disorder, including details regarding family history of suicide, bipolar disorder, and depression. Monotherapy in patients with bipolar disorder should be avoided. **Venlafaxine is not FDA approved for the treatment of bipolar depression.**

Potentially life-threatening serotonin syndrome (SS) has occurred with serotonergic agents (eg, SSRIs, SNRIs), particularly when used in combination with other serotonergic agents (eg, triptans, TCAs, fentanyl, lithium, tramadol, buspirone, St John's wort, tryptophan) or agents that impair metabolism of serotonin (eg, MAO inhibitors intended to treat psychiatric disorders, other MAO inhibitors [ie, linezolid and intravenous methylene blue]). Discontinue treatment (and any concomitant serotonergic agent) immediately if signs/symptoms arise.

May cause sustained increase in blood pressure or tachycardia; dose related and increases are generally modest (12-15 mm Hg diastolic). Control preexisting hypertension prior to initiation of venlafaxine. Use caution in patients with recent history of MI, unstable heart disease, cerebrovascular conditions, or hyperthyroidism; may cause increase in anxiety, nervousness, insomnia; may cause weight loss (use with caution in patients where weight loss is undesirable); may cause increases in serum cholesterol and triglycerides; monitor during long-term treatment. Use caution with hepatic or renal impairment; dosage adjustments recommended. May cause hyponatremia/SIADH, age (the elderly), volume depletion and/or concurrent use of diuretics likely increases risk. Discontinue treatment in patients with symptomatic hyponatremia.

May impair platelet aggregation resulting in increased risk of bleeding events, particularly if used concomitantly with aspirin, or NSAIDs, warfarin, or other anticoagulants. Bleeding related to SSRI or SNRI use has been reported to range from relatively minor bruising and epistaxis to life-threatening hemorrhage. Interstitial lung disease and eosinophilic pneumonia have been rarely reported; may present as progressive dyspnea, cough, and/or chest pain. Prompt evaluation and possible discontinuation of therapy may be necessary. Venlafaxine may increase the risks associated with electroconvulsive therapy. Use cautiously in patients with previous seizure disorder. The risks of cognitive or motor impairment, as well as the potential for anticholinergic effects are very low. May cause or exacerbate sexual dysfunction. Bone fractures have been associated with antidepressant treatment. Consider the possibility of a fragility fracture if an antidepressant-treated patient presents with unexplained bone pain, point tenderness, swelling, or bruising (Rabenda, 2013; Rizzoli, 2012).

Use caution in elderly patients; may cause or exacerbate syndrome of inappropriate antidiuretic hormone secretion or hyponatremia; monitor sodium closely with initiation or dosage adjustments in older adults (Beers Criteria). Use caution in patients with increased intraocular pressure or at risk of acute narrow-angle glaucoma (angle-closure glaucoma). Potentially significant drug-drug interactions may exist, requiring dose or frequency adjustment, additional monitoring, and/or selection of alternative therapy.

Abrupt discontinuation or interruption of antidepressant therapy has been associated with a discontinuation syndrome. Symptoms arising may vary with antidepressant however commonly include nausea, vomiting, diarrhea, headaches, lightheadedness, dizziness, diminished appetite, sweating, chills, tremors, paresthesias, fatigue, somnolence, and sleep disturbances (eg, vivid dreams, insomnia). Greater risks for developing a discontinuation syndrome have been associated with antidepressants with shorter half-lives, longer durations of treatment, and abrupt discontinuation. For antidepressants of short or intermediate half-lives, symptoms may emerge within 2-5 days after treatment discontinuation and last 7-14 days (APA, 2010; Fava, 2006; Haddad, 2001; Shelton, 2001; Warner, 2006).

Adverse Reactions Note: Actual frequency may be dependent upon formulation and/or indication.

>10%:
Central nervous system: Headache (38%), insomnia (15% to 24%), drowsiness (12% to 20%), dizziness (11% to 20%)
Dermatologic: Diaphoresis (10% to 14%)
Endocrine & metabolic: Weight loss (children & adolescents 18% to 47%; adults 2% to 7%)
Gastrointestinal: Nausea (21% to 35%), xerostomia (12% to 17%), anorexia (8% to 17%)
Genitourinary: Abnormal ejaculation (8% to 19%)
Neuromuscular & skeletal: Weakness (8% to 19%)

1% to 10%:
Cardiovascular: Vasodilation (3% to 4%), hypertension (dose related; 3% in patients receiving <100 mg/day, up to 13% in patients receiving >300 mg/day), palpitations (3%), chest pain (≥1%), edema (≥1%), tachycardia (≥1%)
Central nervous system: Nervousness (6% to 10%), abnormal dreams (3% to 7%), anxiety (5%), yawning (3% to 5%), agitation (3%), depression (3%), twitching (3%), anorgasmia (females: 2% to 4%; more common in males), paresthesia (2% to 3%), abnormality in thinking (≥1%), amnesia (≥1%), chills (≥1%), confusion (≥1%), depersonalization (≥1%), hypoesthesia (≥1%), migraine (≥1%), trismus (≥1%), vertigo (≥1%)
Dermatologic: Pruritus (1%), ecchymoses (≥1%)
Endocrine & metabolic: Decreased libido (3% to 8%), hypercholesterolemia (5%), orgasm abnormal (2% to 5%), albuminuria (≥1%), weight gain (≥1%), increased serum triglycerides
Gastrointestinal: Constipation (8% to 10%), diarrhea (8%), dyspepsia (7%), abdominal pain (6%), vomiting (3% to 5%), flatulence (4%), dysgeusia (≥1%), increased appetite (≥1%)
Genitourinary: Impotence (4% to 6%), urinary disorder (≥1%)
Neuromuscular & skeletal: Tremor (4% to 5%), neck pain (≥1%)
Ophthalmic: Visual disturbance (4% to 5%), accommodation disturbance (≥1%), mydriasis (≥1%)
Respiratory: Pharyngitis (7%), dyspnea (≥1%), increased cough (≥1%)
Miscellaneous: Accidental injury (4%), fever (≥1%)

<1% (Limited to important or life-threatening): Abnormal behavior, abnormal gait, abnormal healing, abortion, acne vulgaris, adjustment disorder, ageusia, agranulocytosis, alcohol abuse, alcohol intolerance, alcohol intoxication, alopecia, altered sense of smell, amenorrhea, anaphylaxis, anemia, aneurysm, angina pectoris, angle-closure glaucoma, apathy, aphasia, appendicitis, arthritis, arthropathy, asthma, atelectasis, atrophic striae, attempted suicide, bacteremia, balanitis, basophilia, bigeminy, biliary colic, bladder pain, blepharitis, bone spur, bradycardia, bruxism, buccoglossal syndrome, bundle branch block, bursitis, candidiasis, carcinoma, cardiac arrhythmia (including atrial fibrillation, supraventricular tachycardia, ventricular extrasystoles, ventricular fibrillation, ventricular tachycardia, and torsades de pointes), cardiovascular disease (mitral valve and circulatory disturbance), cataract, cellulitis, central nervous system stimulation, cerebrovascular accident, cervicitis, changes in LDH, cheilitis, chest congestion, chills, cholecystitis, cholelithiasis, chromatopsia, colitis, congenital anomalies, congestive heart failure, conjunctival edema, conjunctivitis, corneal lesion, coronary artery disease, crystalluria, cystitis, deafness, decreased pupillary reflex, deep vein thrombosis, dehydration, delirium, delusions, dementia, diabetes mellitus, diplopia, duodenitis, dysphagia, dyspnea, dysuria, eczema, electric shock-like sensation, emotional lability, endometriosis, eosinophilia, erythema multiforme, esophagitis, extrapyramidal reaction, eye pain, facial paralysis, first degree atrioventricular block, furunculosis, gastroenteritis, gastroesophageal reflux disease, gastrointestinal ulcer, gingivitis, glossitis, glycosuria, goiter, gout, granuloma, Guillain-Barré syndrome, hair discoloration, hematoma, hemochromatosis, hemorrhage (eye, GI, gum, mucocutaneous, rectal, retinal, subconjunctival, uterine, vaginal), hemorrhoids, hepatic effects (including GGT elevation; abnormalities of unspecified liver function tests; liver damage, necrosis, or failure; and fatty liver), hepatitis, homicidal ideation, hostility, hyperacidity, hyperacusis, hypercalciuria, hyperesthesia, hyperreflexia, hyperthyroidism, hypertonia, hyperuricemia, hyperventilation, hypoglycemia, hypohidrosis, hypokalemia, hypokinesia, hypomenorrhea, hyponatremia, hypophosphatemia, hyporeflexia, hypotension, hypothyroidism, hypotonia, hypoventilation, hysteria, ileitis, impulse control disorder, increased energy, increased libido, increased serum prolactin, interstitial pulmonary disease (including eosinophilic pneumonia), intestinal obstruction, keratitis, labyrinthitis, laryngismus, laryngitis, leukocytosis, leukoderma, leukopenia, leukorrhea, lichenoid dermatitis, loss of consciousness, lymphadenopathy, lymphocytosis, melena, menopause, miliaria, miosis, multiple myeloma, muscle spasm, myasthenia, nephrolithiasis, neuralgia, neuritis, neuropathy, neutropenia, night sweats, nystagmus, oliguria, onychia sicca, oral candidiasis, oral mucosa ulcer, oral paresthesia, orchitis, ostealgia, osteoporosis, osteosclerosis, otitis externa, otitis media, ovarian cyst, pancreatitis, pancytopenia, panic, papilledema, paranoia, paresis, parotitis, pathological fracture, pelvic pain, periodontitis, peripheral vascular disease, petechial rash, plantar fasciitis, pleurisy, pneumonia, polyuria, proctitis, prolonged bleeding time, prolonged erection, prostatic disease, pruritic rash, psoriasis, psychosis, psychotic depression, pulmonary embolism, purpura, pustular rash, pyelonephritis, pyuria, rectal disease, renal failure, renal function abnormality, renal pain, rhabdomyolysis, rheumatoid arthritis, rupture of tendon, salpingitis, scleritis, seborrhea, seizure, serotonin syndrome, SIADH, sialorrhea, sinus arrhythmia, skin atrophy, skin discoloration, skin hypertrophy, skin photosensitivity, sleep apnea, speech disturbance, Stevens-Johnson syndrome, stomatitis, stupor, suicidal ideation (reported at a frequency up to 2% in children/adolescents with major depressive disorder), tenosynovitis, thrombocythemia, thrombocytopenia, thyroiditis, thyroid nodule, tongue discoloration, uremia, urinary incontinence, urinary urgency, urolithiasis, urticaria, uterine spasm, uveitis, vaginal dryness, vaginitis, vesicobullous dermatitis, visual field defect, voice disorder, withdrawal syndrome, xeroderma, xerophthalmia

Drug Interactions

Metabolism/Transport Effects Substrate of CYP2C19 (minor), CYP2C9 (minor), CYP2D6 (major), CYP3A4 (major); **Note:** Assignment of Major/Minor substrate status based on clinically relevant drug interaction potential; **Inhibits** CYP2B6 (weak), CYP2D6 (weak)

Avoid Concomitant Use

Avoid concomitant use of Venlafaxine with any of the following: Conivaptan; Dapoxetine; Fusidic Acid (Systemic); Idelalisib; Iobenguane I 123; Linezolid; MAO Inhibitors; Methylene Blue; Urokinase

Increased Effect/Toxicity

Venlafaxine may increase the levels/effects of: Agents with Antiplatelet Properties; Alpha-/Beta-Agonists; Anticoagulants; Antipsychotic Agents; Apixaban; ARIPiprazole; Aspirin; Collagenase (Systemic); Dabigatran

Etexilate; Deoxycholic Acid; Edoxaban; Highest Risk QTc-Prolonging Agents; Ibritumomab; Methylene Blue; Moderate Risk QTc-Prolonging Agents; NSAID (Nonselective); Obinutuzumab; Rivaroxaban; Salicylates; Serotonin Modulators; Thrombolytic Agents; Tositumomab and Iodine I 131 Tositumomab; TraZODone; Urokinase; Vitamin K Antagonists

The levels/effects of Venlafaxine may be increased by: Abiraterone Acetate; Alcohol (Ethyl); Antiemetics (5HT3 Antagonists); Antipsychotic Agents; Aprepitant; Conivaptan; CYP2D6 Inhibitors (Moderate); CYP2D6 Inhibitors (Strong); CYP3A4 Inhibitors (Moderate); CYP3A4 Inhibitors (Strong); Dapoxetine; Dasatinib; Fosaprepitant; Fusidic Acid (Systemic); Glucosamine; Herbs (Anticoagulant/Antiplatelet Properties); Ibrutinib; Idelalisib; Ivacaftor; Limaprost; Linezolid; Luliconazole; MAO Inhibitors; Metaxalone; Metoclopramide; Mifepristone; Multivitamins/Fluoride (with ADE); Multivitamins/Minerals (with ADEK, Folate, Iron); Multivitamins/Minerals (with AE, No Iron); Netupitant; Omega-3 Fatty Acids; Osimertinib; Palbociclib; Panobinostat; Peginterferon Alfa-2b; Pentosan Polysulfate Sodium; Pentoxifylline; Propafenone; Prostacyclin Analogues; Simeprevir; Stiripentol; Tedizolid; Vitamin E; Vitamin E (Oral); Voriconazole

Decreased Effect

Venlafaxine may decrease the levels/effects of: Alpha2-Agonists; Indinavir; Iobenguane I 123; Ioflupane I 123

The levels/effects of Venlafaxine may be decreased by: Bosentan; CYP3A4 Inducers (Moderate); CYP3A4 Inducers (Strong); Dabrafenib; Deferasirox; Enzalutamide; Mitotane; Osimertinib; Peginterferon Alfa-2b; Siltuximab; St Johns Wort; Tocilizumab

Storage/Stability Store immediate-release tablets and extended-release capsules at 20°C to 25°C (68°F to 77°F). Store extended-release tablets at 25°C (77°F); excursions are permitted between 15°C and 30°C (59°F and 86°F).

Mechanism of Action Venlafaxine and its active metabolite, O-desmethylvenlafaxine (ODV), are potent inhibitors of neuronal serotonin and norepinephrine reuptake and weak inhibitors of dopamine reuptake. Venlafaxine and ODV have no significant activity for muscarinic cholinergic, H_1-histaminergic, or alpha$_2$-adrenergic receptors. Venlafaxine and ODV do not possess MAO-inhibitory activity. Venlafaxine functions like an SSRI in low doses (37.5 mg/day) and as a dual mechanism agent affecting serotonin and norepinephrine at doses above 225 mg/day (Harvey, 2000; Kelsey, 1996).

Pharmacodynamics/Kinetics

Absorption: Oral: ≥92%; extended-release has a slightly slower rate of absorption compared to immediate-release

Distribution: V_{dss}: Venlafaxine 7.5 ± 3.7 L/kg, ODV 5.7 ± 1.8 L/kg

Protein binding: Venlafaxine 27% ± 2%, ODV 30% ± 12%

Metabolism: Hepatic via CYP2D6 to active metabolite, O-desmethylvenlafaxine (ODV); other metabolites include N-desmethylvenlafaxine and N,O-didesmethylvenlafaxine

Bioavailability: Oral: ~45%

Half-life elimination: Venlafaxine: 5 ± 2 hours; ODV: 11 ± 2 hours; prolonged with cirrhosis (venlafaxine: ~30%, ODV: ~60%), renal impairment (venlafaxine: ~50%, ODV: ~40%), and during dialysis (venlafaxine: ~180%, ODV: ~142%)

Time to peak:

Immediate release: Venlafaxine: 2 hours, ODV: 3 hours

Extended release: Venlafaxine: 5.5 hours, ODV: 9 hours

Excretion: Urine (~87%; 5% of total dose as unchanged drug; 29% of total dose as unconjugated ODV; 26% of total dose as conjugated ODV; 27% of total dose as minor inactive metabolites)

Dosing

Adult

Depression: Oral:

Immediate-release tablets: Initial: 37.5 to 75 mg/day, administered in 2 or 3 divided doses; may increase in ≤75 mg/day increments at intervals of ≥4 days as tolerated; usual dosage: 75 to 225 mg/day (maximum dose: 375 mg/day) (APA 2010)

Extended-release capsules or tablets: Initial: 37.5 to 75 mg once daily; in patients who are initiated at 37.5 mg once daily, may increase to 75 mg once daily after 4 to 7 days; dose may then be increased by ≤75 mg/day increments at intervals of ≥4 days as tolerated; usual dosage: 75 to 225 mg once daily (maximum daily dose: 225 mg)

Note: Patients treated with a therapeutic dose with venlafaxine immediate release may be switched to venlafaxine extended release (ER) at the nearest equivalent dose (mg/day). Following the formulation switch individual dosage adjustments may be necessary.

Generalized anxiety disorder: Oral: *Extended-release capsules:* Initial: 37.5 to 75 mg once daily; in patients who are initiated at 37.5 mg once daily, may increase to 75 mg once daily after 4 to 7 days; may then be increased by ≤75 mg/day increments at intervals of ≥4 days as tolerated; usual dosage: 75 to 225 mg once daily (maximum daily dose: 225 mg)

Panic disorder: Oral: *Extended-release capsules:* Initial: 37.5 mg once daily for 1 week; may increase to 75 mg once daily after 7 days, may then be increased by ≤75 mg/day increments at intervals of ≥7 days; usual dosage: 75 to 225 mg once daily (maximum daily dose: 225 mg).

Social anxiety disorder: Oral: *Extended-release capsules or tablets:* 75 mg once daily; no evidence that doses >75 mg/day offer any additional benefit

Attention-deficit disorder (off-label use): Oral: Initial: Doses vary between 18.75 to 75 mg/day; may increase after 4 weeks to 150 mg/day; if tolerated, doses up to 225 mg/day have been used (Maidment 2003)

Diabetic neuropathy (off-label use): Extended release: Oral: Initial: 37.5 mg or 75 mg once daily; increase by 75 mg each week to a maximum dosage of 225 mg daily based on tolerance and effect. An adequate duration to determine effect and to accomplish titration has been documented to be 4 to 6 weeks (Bril 2011; Kadiroglu 2008; Rowbotham 2004).

Hot flashes (off-label use): Oral: Immediate-release and extended release: Dosage range studied: 37.5 to 150 mg daily; therapy usually initiated with 37.5 mg daily to minimize adverse effects; dose may remain at 37.5 mg daily or titrated by 37.5 mg per week to a dose of 75 mg or 150 mg daily administered in a single daily dose or in divided doses (AACE [Goodman 2011]; Evans 2005; Loibl 2007; Loprinzi 2000; Loprinzi 2006)

Obsessive-compulsive disorder (off-label use): Oral: Titrate to usual dosage range of 150 to 300 mg/day; however, doses up to 375 mg/day have been used; response may be seen in 4 weeks (Phelps 2005)

Post-traumatic stress disorder (PTSD) (off-label use): Oral: *Extended release formulation:* 37.5 to 300 mg/day (Bandelow 2008; Benedek 2009)

Note: When discontinuing this medication after more than 1 week of treatment, it is generally recommended that the dose be tapered. If venlafaxine is used for 6 weeks or longer, the dose should be tapered over 2 weeks when discontinuing its use.

Discontinuation of therapy: Upon discontinuation of antidepressant therapy, gradually taper the dose to minimize the incidence of withdrawal symptoms and allow for the detection of re-emerging symptoms. Evidence supporting ideal taper rates is limited. APA and NICE guidelines suggest tapering therapy over at least several weeks with consideration to the half-life of the antidepressant; antidepressants with a shorter half-life may need to be tapered more conservatively. In addition for long-term treated patients, WFSBP guidelines recommend tapering over 4 to 6 months. If intolerable withdrawal symptoms occur following a dose reduction, consider resuming the previously prescribed dose and/or decrease dose at a more gradual rate (APA 2010; Bauer 2002; Haddad 2001; NCCMH 2010; Schatzberg 2006; Shelton 2001; Warner 2006).

In clinical studies with extended-release venlafaxine, tapering was achieved by reducing the daily dose by 75 mg at 1-week intervals.

MAO inhibitor recommendations:

Switching to or from an MAO inhibitor intended to treat psychiatric disorders:

Allow 14 days to elapse between discontinuing an MAO inhibitor intended to treat psychiatric disorders and initiation of venlafaxine.

Allow 7 days to elapse between discontinuing venlafaxine and initiation of an MAO inhibitor intended to treat psychiatric disorders.

Use with other MAO inhibitors (linezolid or IV methylene blue):

Do not initiate venlafaxine in patients receiving linezolid or IV methylene blue; consider other interventions for psychiatric condition.

If urgent treatment with linezolid or IV methylene blue is required in a patient already receiving venlafaxine and potential benefits outweigh potential risks, discontinue venlafaxine promptly and administer linezolid or IV methylene blue. Monitor for SS for 7 days or until 24 hours after the last dose of linezolid or IV methylene blue, whichever comes first. May resume venlafaxine 24 hours after the last dose of linezolid or IV methylene blue.

Geriatric Refer to adult dosing. No specific recommendations for elderly; use with caution

Discontinuation of therapy: Refer to adult dosing.
MAO inhibitor recommendations: Refer to adult dosing.
Pediatric Attention-deficit/hyperactivity disorder (off-label use; Olvera, 1996): Children and Adolescents: Oral: Initial: 12.5 mg/day
Children <40 kg: Increase by 12.5 mg/week to maximum of 50 mg/day in 2 divided doses
Children ≥40 kg: Increase by 25 mg/week to maximum of 75 mg/day in 3 divided doses.
Mean dose: 60 mg or 1.4 mg/kg administered in 2 to 3 divided doses.

Discontinuation of therapy: Refer to adult dosing.
MAO inhibitor recommendations: Refer to adult dosing.
Renal Impairment
Mild to moderate impairment (CrCl 30 to 89 mL/minute): Extended release: Reduce total daily dose by 25% to 50%
Immediate release: Reduce total daily dose by 25%
Severe impairment: (CrCl <30 mL/minute): Reduce total daily dose by 50% or more
Hemodialysis: Reduce total daily dose by 50% or more
Hepatic Impairment
Mild to moderate impairment (Child-Pugh score 5 to 9): Reduce total daily dose by 50%
Severe impairment (Child-Pugh score 10 to 15) or cirrhosis: Reduce total daily dose by 50% or more
Dietary Considerations Administer with food.
Administration Administer with food.
Extended-release formulations: Administer either in the morning or in the evening at approximately the same time each day. Swallow capsule or tablet whole with fluid; do not divide, crush, chew, or place in water. Contents of capsule may be sprinkled on a spoonful of applesauce and swallowed immediately without chewing; followed with a glass of water to ensure complete swallowing of the pellets.
Monitoring Parameters Blood pressure should be regularly monitored, especially in patients with a high baseline blood pressure; may cause mean increase in heart rate of 4-9 beats/minute; cholesterol; mental status for depression, suicide ideation (especially at the beginning of therapy or when doses are increased or decreased), anxiety, social functioning, mania, panic attacks; signs/symptoms of serotonin syndrome, hyponatremia, discontinuation symptoms; height and weight should be monitored in children; intraocular pressure and mydriasis (in patients with raised ocular pressure or at risk of acute narrow angle glaucoma) (APA, 2010)
Test Interactions May interfere with urine detection of phencyclidine and amphetamine (false-positives).
Dosage Forms Excipient information presented when available (limited, particularly for generics); consult specific product labeling.
Capsule Extended Release 24 Hour, Oral:
Effexor XR: 37.5 mg, 75 mg, 150 mg
Generic: 37.5 mg, 75 mg, 150 mg
Tablet, Oral:
Generic: 25 mg, 37.5 mg, 50 mg, 75 mg, 100 mg
Tablet Extended Release 24 Hour, Oral:
Generic: 37.5 mg, 75 mg, 150 mg, 225 mg

Verapamil (ver AP a mil)

Brand Names: US Calan; Calan SR; Covera-HS [DSC]; Isoptin SR; Verelan; Verelan PM
Brand Names: Canada Apo-Verap; Apo-Verap SR; Dom-Verapamil SR; Isoptin SR; Mylan-Verapamil; Mylan-Verapamil SR; Novo-Veramil; Novo-Veramil SR; PHL-Verapamil SR; PMS-Verapamil SR; PRO-Verapamil SR; Riva-Verapamil SR; Verapamil Hydrochloride Injection, USP; Verapamil SR; Verelan

Index Terms Iproveratril Hydrochloride; Verapamil Hydrochloride
Pharmacologic Category Antianginal Agent; Antiarrhythmic Agent, Class IV; Antihypertensive; Calcium Channel Blocker; Calcium Channel Blocker, Nondihydropyridine
Use
IV: Supraventricular tachyarrhythmia (PSVT, atrial fibrillation/flutter [rate control])
Oral: Treatment of hypertension; angina pectoris (vasospastic, chronic stable, unstable) (Calan, Covera-HS); supraventricular tachyarrhythmia (PSVT, atrial fibrillation/flutter [rate control])

Guideline recommendations:
Acute coronary syndrome (ACS): The ACCF/AHA guidelines for the management of unstable angina/non-ST-elevation myocardial infarction recommend verapamil to treat hypertension or ongoing ischemia if beta-blocker therapy is ineffective or contraindicated and in the absence of left ventricular dysfunction, pulmonary congestion, or AV block (ACCF/AHA [Anderson, 2013]).
Hypertension: The 2014 guideline for the management of high blood pressure in adults (JNC 8) recommends initiation of pharmacologic treatment to lower blood pressure for the following patients (JNC 8 [James, 2013]):
• Patients ≥60 years of age with systolic blood pressure (SBP) ≥150 mm Hg or diastolic blood pressure (DBP) ≥90 mm Hg. Goal of therapy is SBP <150 mm Hg and DBP <90 mm Hg.
• Patients <60 years of age with SBP ≥140 mm Hg or DBP ≥90 mm Hg. Goal of therapy is SBP <140 mm Hg and DBP <90 mm Hg.
• Patients ≥18 years of age with diabetes with SBP ≥140 mm Hg or DBP ≥90 mm Hg. Goal of therapy is SBP <140 mm Hg and DBP <90 mm Hg.
• Patients ≥18 years of age with chronic kidney disease (CKD) with SBP ≥140 mm Hg or DBP ≥90 mm Hg. Goal of therapy is SBP <140 mm Hg and DBP <90 mm Hg.
Chronic kidney disease (CKD) and hypertension: Regardless of race or diabetes status, the use of an ACE inhibitor (ACEI) or angiotensin receptor blocker (ARB) as initial therapy is recommended to improve kidney outcomes. In the general nonblack population (without CKD) including those with diabetes, initial antihypertensive treatment should consist of a thiazide-type diuretic, calcium channel blocker, ACEI, or ARB. In the general black population (without CKD) including those with diabetes, initial antihypertensive treatment should consist of a thiazide-type diuretic or a calcium channel blocker instead of an ACEI or ARB.
Coronary artery disease (CAD) and hypertension: The American Heart Association, American College of Cardiology and American Society of Hypertension (AHA/ACC/ASH) 2015 scientific statement for the treatment of hypertension in patients with coronary artery disease (CAD) recommends that a non-dihydropyridine CCB (verapamil, diltiazem) may be used as a substitute for a beta blocker in patients who have an intolerance or contraindication to beta blockers with ongoing ischemia, hypertension and chronic stable angina, or if angina or hypertension continues to be uncontrolled while receiving standard therapies (eg, beta blocker). However, a non-dihydropyridine CCB (eg, verapamil, diltiazem) should be avoided in patients with LV dysfunction or heart failure (with reduced ejection fraction). A BP target of <140/90 mm Hg is reasonable for the secondary prevention of cardiovascular events. A lower target BP (<130/80 mm Hg) may be appropriate in some individuals with CAD, previous MI, stroke or transient ischemic attack, or CAD risk equivalents (AHA/ACC/ASH [Rosendorff 2015]).
Pregnancy Considerations Adverse events were observed in some animal reproduction studies in doses which also caused maternal toxicity. Verapamil crosses the placenta. Use during pregnancy may cause adverse fetal effects (bradycardia, heart block, hypotension) (Tan, 2001). Women with hypertrophic cardiomyopathy who are controlled with verapamil prior to pregnancy may continue therapy, but increased fetal monitoring is recommended (Gersh, 2011). Verapamil is not the preferred treatment for paroxysmal supraventricular tachycardia (PSVT) in pregnant women (Blomström-Lundqvist, 2003). Untreated chronic maternal hypertension is associated with adverse events in the fetus, infant, and mother. If treatment for hypertension during pregnancy is needed, other agents are preferred (ACOG, 2013).
Breast-Feeding Considerations Verapamil is excreted into breast milk; the estimated exposure to the nursing infant is <1% of the maternal dose. Breast-feeding is not recommended by some manufacturers.

Contraindications Hypersensitivity to verapamil or any component of the formulation; severe left ventricular dysfunction; hypotension (systolic pressure <90 mm Hg) or cardiogenic shock; sick sinus syndrome (except in patients with a functioning artificial ventricular pacemaker); second- or third-degree AV block (except in patients with a functioning artificial ventricular pacemaker); atrial flutter or fibrillation and an accessory bypass tract (Wolff-Parkinson-White [WPW] syndrome, Lown-Ganong-Levine syndrome)

IV: Additional contraindications include concurrent use of IV beta-blocking agents; ventricular tachycardia

Warnings/Precautions Avoid use in heart failure; can exacerbate condition; use is contraindicated in severe left ventricular dysfunction. Symptomatic hypotension with or without syncope can rarely occur; blood pressure must be lowered at a rate appropriate for the patient's clinical condition. Rare increases in hepatic enzymes can be observed. Can cause first-degree AV block or sinus bradycardia; use is contraindicated in patients with sick sinus syndrome, second- or third-degree AV block (except in patients with a functioning artificial pacemaker), or an accessory bypass tract (eg, WPW syndrome). Other conduction abnormalities are rare. Considered contraindicated in patients with wide complex tachycardias unless known to be supraventricular in origin; severe hypotension likely to occur upon administration (ACLS, 2010). Use caution when using verapamil together with a beta-blocker. Administration of IV verapamil and an IV beta-blocker within a few hours of each other may result in asystole and should be avoided; simultaneous administration is contraindicated. Use with other agents known to reduce SA node function and/or AV nodal conduction (eg, digoxin) or reduce sympathetic outflow (eg, clonidine) may increase the risk of serious bradycardia. Verapamil significantly increases digoxin serum concentrations; adjust digoxin dose. Use with caution in patients with HCM with outflow tract obstruction (especially those with high gradients, advanced heart failure, or sinus bradycardia); may be used in patients who cannot tolerate beta-blockade. Verapamil should not be used in those with systemic hypotension or severe dyspnea at rest (Gersh, 2011; Nishimura, 2004).

Decreased neuromuscular transmission has been reported with verapamil; use with caution in patients with attenuated neuromuscular transmission (Duchenne's muscular dystrophy, myasthenia gravis); dosage reduction may be required. Use with caution in renal impairment; monitor hemodynamics and possibly ECG if severe impairment, particularly if concomitant hepatic impairment. Use with caution in patients with hepatic impairment; dosage reduction may be required; monitor hemodynamics and possibly ECG if severe impairment. May prolong recovery from nondepolarizing neuromuscular-blocking agents. Use Covera-HS (extended-release delivery system) with caution in patients with severe GI narrowing. In patients with extremely short GI transit times (eg, <7 hours), dosage adjustment may be required; inadequate pharmacokinetic data. In neonates and young infants, avoid IV use for SVT due to severe apnea, bradycardia, hypotensive reactions, and cardiac arrest; in children, use IV with caution as myocardial depression and hypotension may occur.

Adverse Reactions
>10%:
Central nervous system: Headache (1% to 12%)
Gastrointestinal: Gingival hyperplasia (≤19%), constipation (7% to 12%)

1% to 10%:
Cardiovascular: Peripheral edema (1% to 4%), hypotension (3%), CHF/pulmonary edema (2%), AV block (1% to 2%), bradycardia (HR <50 bpm: 1%), flushing (1%)
Central nervous system: Fatigue (2% to 5%), dizziness (1% to 5%), lethargy (3%), pain (2%), sleep disturbance (1%)
Dermatologic: Rash (1% to 2%)
Gastrointestinal: Dyspepsia (3%), nausea (1% to 3%), diarrhea (2%)
Hepatic: Liver enzymes increased (1%)
Neuromuscular & skeletal: Myalgia (1%), paresthesia (1%)
Respiratory: Dyspnea (1%)
Miscellaneous: Flu-like syndrome (4%)
Oral: ≤1%: Abdominal discomfort, alopecia, angina, arthralgia, atrioventricular dissociation, blurred vision, bruising, cerebrovascular accident, chest pain, claudication, confusion, diaphoresis, ECG abnormal, equilibrium disorders, erythema multiforme, exanthema, extrapyramidal symptoms, galactorrhea/hyperprolactinemia, gastrointestinal distress, gynecomastia, hyperkeratosis, impotence, insomnia, macules, MI, muscle cramps, palpitation, psychosis, purpura (vasculitis), shakiness, somnolence, spotty menstruation, Stevens-Johnson syndrome, syncope, tinnitus, urination increased, urticaria, weakness, xerostomia

IV: <1% (Limited to important or life-threatening): Bronchi/laryngeal spasm, depression, diaphoresis, itching, muscle fatigue, respiratory failure, rotary nystagmus, seizure, sleepiness, urticaria, vertigo
Postmarketing and/or case reports: Asystole, eosinophilia, EPS, exfoliative dermatitis, GI obstruction, hair color change, paralytic ileus, Parkinsonian syndrome, pulseless electrical activity, shock, ventricular fibrillation

Drug Interactions
Metabolism/Transport Effects Substrate of CYP1A2 (minor), CYP2B6 (minor), CYP2C9 (minor), CYP2E1 (minor), CYP3A4 (major), P-glycoprotein; **Note:** Assignment of Major/Minor substrate status based on clinically relevant drug interaction potential; **Inhibits** CYP1A2 (weak), CYP2C9 (weak), CYP2D6 (weak), CYP3A4 (moderate), P-glycoprotein

Avoid Concomitant Use
Avoid concomitant use of Verapamil with any of the following: Aprepitant; Bosutinib; Ceritinib; Cobimetinib; Conivaptan; Dantrolene; Disopyramide; Dofetilide; Domperidone; Flibanserin; Fusidic Acid (Systemic); Ibrutinib; Idelalisib; Ivabradine; Lomitapide; Naloxegol; Olaparib; PAZOPanib; Pimozide; Silodosin; Simeprevir; Tolvaptan; Topotecan; Trabectedin; Ulipristal; VinCRIStine (Liposomal)

Increased Effect/Toxicity
Verapamil may increase the levels/effects of: Afatinib; Alcohol (Ethyl); Aliskiren; Amifostine; Amiodarone; Antipsychotic Agents (Second Generation [Atypical]); Apixaban; Aprepitant; ARIPiprazole; AtorvaSTATin; Atosiban; Avanafil; Beta-Blockers; Bosentan; Bosutinib; Bradycardia-Causing Agents; Brentuximab Vedotin; Brexpiprazole; Bromocriptine; Budesonide (Systemic); Budesonide (Topical); BusPIRone; Calcium Channel Blockers (Dihydropyridine); Cannabis; CarBAMazepine; Cardiac Glycosides; Ceritinib; Cilostazol; Cobimetinib; Colchicine; CycloSPORINE (Systemic); CYP3A4 Substrates; Dabigatran Etexilate; Dapoxetine; Disopyramide; Dofetilide; Domperidone; DOXOrubicin (Conventional); Dronabinol; Dronedarone; DULoxetine; Edoxaban; Eletriptan; Eliglustat; Eplerenone; Everolimus; FentaNYL; Fexofenadine; Fingolimod; Flecainide; Flibanserin; Fosphenytoin; Halofantrine; Hydrocodone; Hypotension-Associated Agents; Ibrutinib; Imatinib; Ivabradine; Ivacaftor; Lacosamide; Ledipasvir; Levodopa; Lithium; Lomitapide; Lovastatin; Lurasidone; Magnesium Salts; Midodrine; Naloxegol; Neuromuscular-Blocking Agents (Nondepolarizing); NiMODipine; Nintedanib; Nitroprusside; Olaparib; OxyCODONE; PAZOPanib; P-glycoprotein/ABCB1 Substrates; Phenytoin; Pimecrolimus; Pimozide; Propafenone; Prucalopride; QuiNIDine; Ranolazine; Red Yeast Rice; Rifaximin; RisperiDONE; Rivaroxaban; Salicylates; Salmeterol; Saxagliptin; Silodosin; Simeprevir; Simvastatin; Sonidegib; Suvorexant; Tacrolimus (Systemic); Tacrolimus (Topical); Tetrahydrocannabinol; TiZANidine; Tolvaptan; Topotecan; Trabectedin; Ulipristal; Vilazodone; VinCRIStine (Liposomal); Vindesine; Zopiclone; Zuclopenthixol

The levels/effects of Verapamil may be increased by: Alfuzosin; Alpha1-Blockers; Anilidopiperidine Opioids; Antifungal Agents (Azole Derivatives, Systemic); AtorvaSTATin; Barbiturates; Bretylium; Brimonidine (Topical); Calcium Channel Blockers (Dihydropyridine); Cimetidine; CloNIDine; Conivaptan; CycloSPORINE (Systemic); CYP3A4 Inhibitors (Moderate); CYP3A4 Inhibitors (Strong); Dantrolene; Dasatinib; Diazoxide; Dronedarone; Fluconazole; Fosaprepitant; Fusidic Acid (Systemic); Grapefruit Juice; Herbs (Hypotensive Properties); Idelalisib; Ivabradine; Luliconazole; Macrolide Antibiotics; Magnesium Salts; Mifepristone; Molsidomine; Netupitant; Nicorandil; Obinutuzumab; Osimertinib; Palbociclib; Pentoxifylline; P-glycoprotein/ABCB1 Inhibitors; Phosphodiesterase 5 Inhibitors; Prostacyclin Analogues; Protease Inhibitors; QuiNIDine; Regorafenib; Ruxolitinib; Stiripentol; Telithromycin; Tofacitinib

Decreased Effect
Verapamil may decrease the levels/effects of: Clopidogrel; Ifosfamide; MetFORMIN

The levels/effects of Verapamil may be decreased by: Amphetamines; Barbiturates; Bosentan; Calcium Salts; CarBAMazepine; CYP3A4 Inducers (Moderate); CYP3A4 Inducers (Strong); Dabrafenib; Deferasirox; Efavirenz; Enzalutamide; Herbs (Hypertensive Properties); Methylphenidate; Mitotane; Nafcillin; Osimertinib; P-glycoprotein/ABCB1 Inducers; Phenytoin; Rifamycin Derivatives; Siltuximab; St Johns Wort; Tocilizumab; Yohimbine

Food Interactions
Ethanol: Verapamil may increase ethanol levels. Management: Monitor patients and caution about increased effects.

Food: Grapefruit juice may increase the serum concentration of verapamil. Management: Avoid grapefruit juice or use with caution and monitor for effects.

Storage/Stability Store at controlled room temperature of 15°C to 30°C (59°F to 86°F). Protect from light.

Mechanism of Action Inhibits calcium ion from entering the "slow channels" or select voltage-sensitive areas of vascular smooth muscle and myocardium during depolarization; produces relaxation of coronary vascular smooth muscle and coronary vasodilation; increases myocardial oxygen delivery in patients with vasospastic angina; slows automaticity and conduction of AV node.

Pharmacodynamics/Kinetics

Onset of action: Peak effect: Oral: Immediate release: 1-2 hours; IV: 1-5 minutes

Duration: Oral: Immediate release tablets: 6-8 hours; IV: 10-20 minutes

Absorption: Well absorbed

Distribution: V_d: 3.89 L/kg (Storstein, 1984)

Protein binding: ~90%

Metabolism: Hepatic (extensive first-pass effect) via multiple CYP isoenzymes; primary metabolite is norverapamil (20% pharmacologic activity of verapamil)

Bioavailability: Oral: 20% to 35%

Half-life elimination: Infants: 4.4-6.9 hours; Adults: Single dose: 3-7 hours, Multiple doses: 4.5-12 hours; severe hepatic impairment: 14-16 hours

Time to peak, serum: Oral:

Immediate release: 1-2 hours

Extended release (Covera-HS, Verelan PM): ~11 hours, drug release delayed ~4-5 hours

Sustained release: 5.21 hours (Calan SR, Isoptin SR); 7-9 hours (Verelan)

Excretion: Urine (70% as metabolites, 3% to 4% as unchanged drug); feces (16%)

Dosing

Adult

Angina: Oral: **Note:** When switching from immediate-release to extended/sustained release formulations, the total daily dose remains the same unless formulation strength does not allow for equal conversion.

Immediate release: Initial: 80 to 120 mg 3 times daily (elderly or small stature: 40 mg 3 times daily); Usual dose range (Gibbons, 2003): 80 to 160 mg 3 times daily

Extended release (Covera-HS): Initial: 180 mg once daily at bedtime; if inadequate response, may increase dose at weekly intervals to 240 mg once daily, then 360 mg once daily, then 480 mg once daily; maximum dose: 480 mg daily

PSVT prophylaxis: Oral: Immediate release: 240 to 480 mg daily in 3 to 4 divided doses

Hypertension: Oral: **Note:** When switching from immediate-release to extended/sustained release formulations, the total daily dose remains the same unless formulation strength does not allow for equal conversion.

Immediate release: Initial: 80 mg 3 times daily; usual dose range (ASH/ISH [Weber, 2014]): 240 to 480 mg daily

Sustained release: Usual dose range (ASH/ISH [Weber, 2014]): 240 to 480 mg daily; **Note:** There is no evidence of additional benefit with doses >360 mg daily.

Calan SR, Isoptin SR: Initial: 180 mg once daily in the morning (elderly or small stature: 120 mg daily); if inadequate response, may increase dose at weekly intervals to 240 mg once daily, then 180 mg twice daily (or 240 mg in the morning followed by 120 mg in the evening); maximum dose: 240 mg twice daily.

Verelan: Initial: 180 mg once daily in the morning (elderly or small stature: 120 mg/day); if inadequate response, may increase dose at weekly intervals to 240 mg once daily, then 360 mg once daily, then 480 mg once daily; maximum dose: 480 mg daily

Extended release: Usual dosage range (ASH/ISH [Weber, 2014]): 240 to 480 mg daily

Covera-HS: Initial: 180 mg once daily at bedtime; if inadequate response, may increase dose at weekly intervals to 240 mg once daily, then 360 mg once daily, then 480 mg once daily; maximum dose: 480 mg daily

Verelan PM: Initial: 200 mg once daily at bedtime (elderly or small stature: 100 mg daily); if inadequate response, may increase dose at weekly intervals to 300 mg once daily, then 400 mg once daily; maximum dose: 400 mg daily

Atrial fibrillation (rate control):

IV: Initial: 0.075 to 0.15 mg/kg (usual dose: 5 to 10 mg) administered as a bolus over 2 minutes; if no response, may give an additional 10 mg after 15 to 30 minutes; if patient responds to the initial or repeat

bolus dose, then may begin a continuous infusion (AHA/ACC/HRS [January, 2014]; Phillips, 1997)

Continuous infusion: Initial: 5 mg/hour; titrate to goal heart rate (Barbarash, 1986; Phillips, 1997)

Oral:

Extended release (off-label use): Usual maintenance dose range: 180 to 480 mg once daily (AHA/ACC/HRS [January, 2014])

Immediate release: 240 to 480 mg daily in 3 to 4 divided doses

SVT (ACLS, 2010): IV: 2.5 to 5 mg over 2 minutes; second dose of 5 to 10 mg (~0.15 mg/kg) may be given 15 to 30 minutes after the initial dose if patient tolerates, but does not respond to initial dose; maximum total dose: 20 to 30 mg

Geriatric Refer to adult dosing.

Hypertension: Oral: **Note:** When switching from immediate release to extended or sustained release formulations, the total daily dose remains the same unless formulation strength does not allow for equal conversion.

Manufacturer's labeling:

Immediate release: Initial: 40 mg 3 times daily

Sustained release: Calan SR, Isoptin SR, Verelan: Initial: 120 mg once daily in the morning

Extended release:

Covera-HS: Initial: 180 mg once daily at bedtime

Verelan PM: Initial: 100 mg once daily at bedtime

ACCF/AHA Expert Consensus recommendations: Consider lower initial doses and titrating to response (Aronow, 2011)

Pediatric SVT: Note: Verapamil is no longer included in the Pediatric Advanced Life Support (PALS) tachyarrhythmia algorithm.

Children: 1-15 years: IV: 0.1 to 0.3 mg/kg/dose over 2 minutes; maximum: 5 mg/dose, may repeat dose in 30 minutes if inadequate response; maximum for second dose: 10 mg

Renal Impairment Manufacturer recommends caution and additional ECG monitoring in patients with renal insufficiency. The manufacturer of Verelan PM recommends an initial dose of 100 mg daily at bedtime. **Note:** A multiple dose study in adults suggests reduced renal clearance of verapamil and its metabolite (norverapamil) with advanced renal failure (Storstein, 1984). Additionally, several clinical papers report adverse effects of verapamil in patients with chronic renal failure receiving recommended doses of verapamil (Pritza, 1991; Váquez, 1996). In contrast, a number of single dose studies show no difference in verapamil (or norverapamil metabolite) disposition between chronic renal failure and control patients (Beyerlein, 1990; Hanyok, 1988; Mooy, 1985; Zachariah, 1991).

Dialysis: Not removed by hemodialysis (Mooy, 1985); supplemental dose is not necessary.

Hepatic Impairment In cirrhosis, reduce dose to 20% and 50% of normal for oral and intravenous administration, respectively, and monitor ECG (Somogyi, 1981). The manufacturer of Verelan PM recommends an initial adult dose of 100 mg/day at bedtime. The manufacturers of Calan, Calan SR, Covera-HS, Isoptin SR, and Verelan recommend giving 30% of the normal dose to patients with severe hepatic impairment.

Dietary Considerations Calan SR and Isoptin SR products may be taken with food or milk, other formulations may be administered without regard to meals; sprinkling contents of Verelan or Verelan PM capsule onto applesauce does not affect oral absorption.

Administration

Oral: Do not crush or chew sustained or extended release products.

Calan SR, Isoptin SR: Administer with food.

Verelan, Verelan PM: Capsules may be opened and the contents sprinkled on 1 tablespoonful of applesauce, then swallowed immediately without chewing. Do not subdivide contents of capsules.

IV: Rate of infusion: Over 2 minutes; over 3 minutes in older patients (ACLS, 2010)

Monitoring Parameters Monitor blood pressure and heart rate; periodic liver function tests; ECG, especially with renal and/or hepatic impairment

Consult individual institutional policies and procedures.

Test Interactions May interfere with urine detection of methadone (false-positive).

Dosage Forms Excipient information presented when available (limited, particularly for generics); consult specific product labeling. [DSC] = Discontinued product
Capsule Extended Release 24 Hour, Oral, as hydrochloride:
  Verelan: 120 mg, 180 mg [contains fd&c red #40, methylparaben, propylparaben]
  Verelan: 240 mg, 360 mg [contains brilliant blue fcf (fd&c blue #1), fd&c red #40, methylparaben, propylparaben]
  Verelan PM: 100 mg, 200 mg, 300 mg [contains brilliant blue fcf (fd&c blue #1), fd&c red #40]
  Generic: 100 mg, 120 mg, 180 mg, 200 mg, 240 mg, 300 mg, 360 mg
Solution, Intravenous, as hydrochloride:
  Generic: 2.5 mg/mL (2 mL, 4 mL)
Tablet, Oral, as hydrochloride:
  Calan: 80 mg, 120 mg [scored]
  Generic: 40 mg, 80 mg, 120 mg
Tablet Extended Release, Oral, as hydrochloride:
  Calan SR: 120 mg
  Calan SR: 180 mg [scored]
  Calan SR: 240 mg [scored; contains fd&c blue #2 aluminum lake, fd&c yellow #10 aluminum lake]
  Isoptin SR: 120 mg
  Isoptin SR: 180 mg [scored]
  Isoptin SR: 240 mg [scored; contains fd&c blue #2 aluminum lake, fd&c yellow #10 aluminum lake]
  Generic: 120 mg, 180 mg, 240 mg
Tablet Extended Release 24 Hour, Oral, as hydrochloride:
  Covera-HS: 180 mg [DSC], 240 mg [DSC]
Extemporaneous Preparations A 50 mg/mL oral suspension may be made with immediate release tablets and either a 1:1 mixture of Ora-Sweet and Ora-Plus or a 1:1 mixture of Ora-Sweet SF and Ora-Plus or cherry syrup. When using cherry syrup, dilute cherry syrup concentrate 1:4 with simple syrup, NF. Crush seventy-five verapamil hydrochloride 80 mg tablets in a mortar and reduce to a fine powder. Add small portions of chosen vehicle (40 mL total) and mix to a uniform paste; mix while adding the vehicle in incremental proportions to **almost** 120 mL; transfer to a calibrated bottle, rinse mortar with vehicle, and add quantity of vehicle sufficient to make 120 mL. Label "shake well", "refrigerate", and "protect from light". Stable for 60 days refrigerated (preferred) or at room temperature (Allen, 1996).

A 50 mg/mL oral suspension may be made with immediate release tablets, a 1:1 preparation of methylcellulose 1% and simple syrup, and purified water. Crush twenty 80 mg verapamil tablets in a mortar and reduce to a fine powder. Add 3 mL purified water USP and mix to a uniform paste; mix while adding the vehicle incremental proportions to **almost** 32 mL; transfer to a calibrated bottle, rinse mortar with vehicle, and add quantity of vehicle sufficient to make 32 mL. Label "shake well" and "refrigerate". Stable for 91 days refrigerated (preferred) or at room temperature (Nahata, 1997).
Allen LV Jr and Erickson MA 3rd, "Stability of Labetalol Hydrochloride, Metoprolol Tartrate, Verapamil Hydrochloride, and Spironolactone With Hydrochlorothiazide in Extemporaneously Compounded Oral Liquids," *Am J Health Syst Pharm*, 1996, 53(19):304-9.
Nahata MC, "Stability of Verapamil in an Extemporaneous Liquid Dosage Form," *J Appl Ther Res*, 1997,1(3):271-3.

Vigabatrin (vye GA ba trin)

Brand Names: US Sabril
Brand Names: Canada Sabril
Pharmacologic Category Anticonvulsant, Miscellaneous
Use
  US labeling:
    Infantile spasms: As monotherapy for pediatric patients 1 month to 2 years of age with infantile spasms for whom the potential benefits outweigh the potential risk of vision loss.
    Refractory complex partial seizures: As adjunctive therapy for adults and pediatric patients 10 years and older with refractory complex partial seizures who have inadequately responded to several alternative treatments and for whom the potential benefits outweigh the risk of vision loss.
  Canadian labeling:
    Infantile spasms: As monotherapy for pediatric patients 2 months to 2 years of age with infantile spasms for whom the potential benefits outweigh the risk of ophthalmologic abnormalities.
    Partial seizures with or without secondary generalization: As adjunctive therapy for adults and pediatric patients ≥2 years and older with partial seizures with or without secondary generalization who have inadequately responded to other antiepileptic drug therapy and for whom the potential benefits outweigh the risk of ophthalmologic abnormalities.
Prescribing and Access Restrictions As a requirement of the REMS program, access to this medication is restricted. Vigabatrin is only available in the U.S. under a special restricted distribution program (SHARE). Under the SHARE program, only prescribers and pharmacies registered with the program are able to prescribe and distribute vigabatrin. Vigabatrin may only be dispensed to patients who are enrolled in and meet all conditions of SHARE. Contact the SHARE program at 1-888-45-SHARE.
Medication Guide Available Yes

Dosing
Adult
US labeling:

Refractory complex partial seizures: Oral: Initial: 500 mg twice daily; increase daily dose by 500 mg increments at weekly intervals based on response and tolerability. Recommended dose: 1.5 g twice daily. **Note:** To taper, decrease dose by 1 g daily on a weekly basis.

Canadian labeling:

Partial seizures with or without secondary generalization (adjunctive treatment): Oral: Initial: 1 g/day in 1 or 2 divided doses (initial doses up to 2 g/day may be necessary for severe seizure activity); titrate daily dose in 0.5 g increments per tolerability and response; optimal range: 2 to 3 g/day (maximum dose: 3 g/day; higher doses are not associated with increased efficacy and may increase risk of adverse reactions). **Note:** To taper, decrease dose by 1 g/day once a week. Discontinue therapy if clinically meaningful improvement in seizure control is not observed within 3 months.

Geriatric Refractory complex partial seizures: Refer to adult dosing. Initiate at low end of dosage range; monitor closely for sedation and confusion.

Pediatric
US labeling:

Infantile spasms: Infants and Children 1 month to 2 years: Oral: Initial dosing: 50 mg/kg/day divided twice daily; may titrate upwards by 25 to 50 mg/kg/day increments every 3 days to a maximum of 150 mg/kg/day divided twice daily. **Note:** To taper, decrease dose by 25 to 50 mg/kg/day increments every 3 to 4 days.

Refractory complex partial seizures:

Children and Adolescents 10 to <17 years and 25 to 60 kg: Initial: 250 mg twice daily; increase daily dose by 500 mg increments at weekly intervals based on response and tolerability. Recommended dose: 1,000 mg twice daily. **Note:** To taper, decrease daily dose by one-third every week for 3 weeks.

Children ≥10 years and >60 kg and Adolescents ≥17 years: Refer to adult dosing.

Canadian labeling:

Infantile spasms: Infants and Children 2 months to 2 years: Oral solution: Initial dosing: 50 mg/kg/day divided twice daily; may titrate upwards by 25 to 50 mg/kg/day increments every 3 days to a maximum of 150 mg/kg/day. Note: To taper, decrease dose by 25 to 50 mg/kg/day increments every 3 to 4 days. Discontinue therapy if clinically meaningful improvement in seizure control is not observed within 4 weeks.

Partial seizures with or without secondary generalization (adjunctive treatment):

Children ≥2 years and Adolescents ≤16 years: Oral: Initial: 40 mg/kg/day divided twice daily; maintenance dosages based on patient weight:

10 to 15 kg: 500 to 1,000 mg daily divided twice daily

16 to 30 kg: 1,000 to 1,500 mg daily divided twice daily

31 to 50 kg: 1,500 to 3,000 mg daily divided twice daily

>50 kg: 2,000 to 3,000 mg daily divided twice daily

Adolescents ≥17 years: Refer to adult dosing.

Renal Impairment
US labeling: **Note:** Renal function may be estimated using the Schwartz equation (children 10 to <12 years) and the Cockcroft-Gault formula (children ≥12 years, adolescents, and adults):

Children (≥10 years), Adolescents, and Adults:

CrCl >50 to 80 mL/minute: Decrease dose by 25%

CrCl >30 to 50 mL/minute: Decrease dose by 50%

CrCl >10 to 30 mL/minute: Decrease dose by 75%

Canadian labeling: **Note:** Renal function may be estimated using the Cockcroft-Gault formula:

CrCl >50 to 80 mL/minute: Decrease dose by 25%

CrCl >30 to 50 mL/minute: Decrease dose by 50%

CrCl >10 to 30 mL/minute: Decrease dose by 75%

Hepatic Impairment There are no dosage adjustments provided in the manufacturer's labeling; has not been studied. However, does not undergo appreciable hepatic metabolism.

Additional Information Complete prescribing information should be consulted for additional detail.

Dosage Forms Excipient information presented when available (limited, particularly for generics); consult specific product labeling.

Packet, Oral:

Sabril: 500 mg (50 ea)

Tablet, Oral:

Sabril: 500 mg [scored]

Dosage Forms: Canada Excipient information presented when available (limited, particularly for generics); consult specific product labeling.

Powder for suspension, oral [sachets]:

Sabril: 0.5 g

◆ Vigamox *see* Moxifloxacin (Ophthalmic) *on page 1238*

◆ VIGIV *see* Vaccinia Immune Globulin (Intravenous) *on page 1857*

◆ Viibryd *see* Vilazodone *on page 1893*

◆ Viibryd Starter Pack *see* Vilazodone *on page 1893*

◆ Vilanterol and Fluticasone *see* Fluticasone and Vilanterol *on page 798*

◆ Vilanterol and Fluticasone Furoate *see* Fluticasone and Vilanterol *on page 798*

Vilazodone (vil AZ oh done)

Brand Names: US Viibryd; Viibryd Starter Pack

Index Terms EMD 68843; SB659746-A; Vilazodone Hydrochloride

Pharmacologic Category Antidepressant, Selective Serotonin Reuptake Inhibitor/5-HT$_{1A}$ Receptor Partial Agonist

Use Major depressive disorder: Treatment of major depressive disorder (MDD)

Pregnancy Considerations Adverse events have been observed in animal reproduction studies. An increased risk of teratogenic effects may be associated with maternal use of other SSRIs. However, available information is conflicting and information specific to the use of vilazodone has not been located. Nonteratogenic effects in the newborn following SSRI/SNRI exposure late in the third trimester include respiratory distress, cyanosis, apnea, seizures, temperature instability, feeding difficulty, vomiting, hypoglycemia, hypo- or hypertonia, hyper-reflexia, jitteriness, irritability, constant crying, and tremor. Symptoms may be due to the toxicity of the SSRIs/SNRIs or a discontinuation syndrome and may be consistent with serotonin syndrome associated with SSRI treatment. Persistent pulmonary hypertension of the newborn (PPHN) has also been reported with SSRI exposure. The long-term effects of *in utero* SSRI exposure on infant development and behavior are not known.

The ACOG recommends that therapy with SSRIs or SNRIs during pregnancy should be individualized; treatment of depression during pregnancy should incorporate the clinical expertise of the mental health clinician, obstetrician, primary healthcare provider, and pediatrician. According to the American Psychiatric Association (APA), the risks of medication treatment should be weighed against other treatment options and untreated depression. For women who discontinue antidepressant medications during pregnancy and who may be at high risk for postpartum depression, the medications can be restarted following delivery. Treatment algorithms have been developed by the ACOG and the APA for the management of depression in women prior to conception and during pregnancy. Consideration should be given to using an agent with some safety information in pregnant women.

Breast-Feeding Considerations It is not known if vilazodone is excreted in breast milk. According to the manufacturer, the decision to continue or discontinue breast-feeding during therapy should take into account the risk of exposure to the infant and the benefits of treatment to the mother. Maternal use of an SSRI during pregnancy may cause delayed milk secretion. Long-term effects on development and behavior have not been studied.

Medication Guide Available Yes

Contraindications Use of MAO inhibitors (concurrently or within 14 days of discontinuing either vilazodone or the MAO inhibitor), including MAO inhibitors such as linezolid or intravenous methylene blue

Warnings/Precautions [US Boxed Warning]: Antidepressants increase the risk of suicidal thinking and behavior in children, adolescents, and young adults (18 to 24 years of age) with major depressive disorder (MDD) and other psychiatric disorders; consider risk prior to prescribing. Short-term studies did not show an increased risk in patients >24 years of age and showed a decreased risk in patients ≥65 years. Closely monitor patients for clinical worsening, suicidality, or unusual changes in behavior, particularly during the initial 1 to 2 months of therapy or during periods of dosage adjustments (increases or decreases); the patient's family or caregiver should be instructed to closely observe the patient and communicate condition with healthcare provider. A medication guide concerning the use of antidepressants should be dispensed with each prescription. **Vilazodone is not FDA approved for use in children.**

The possibility of a suicide attempt is inherent in major depression and may persist until remission occurs. Use caution in high-risk patients. Worsening depression and severe abrupt suicidality that are not part of the presenting symptoms may require discontinuation or modification of drug therapy. The patient's family or caregiver should be alerted to monitor patients for the emergence of suicidality and associated behaviors (such as agitation, irritability, hostility, impulsivity, and hypomania) and call healthcare provider.

May worsen psychosis in some patients or precipitate a shift to mania or hypomania in patients with bipolar disorder. Screen patients for a personal or family history of bipolar disorder, mania, or hypermania before initiating therapy, including details regarding family history of suicide, bipolar disorder, and depression (APA 2010).

Potentially life-threatening serotonin syndrome (SS) has occurred with serotonergic agents (eg, SSRIs, SNRIs), particularly when used in combination with other serotonergic agents (eg, triptans, TCAs, fentanyl, lithium, tramadol, buspirone, St John's wort, tryptophan) or agents that impair metabolism of serotonin (eg, MAO inhibitors, including linezolid and intravenous methylene blue). Discontinue treatment (and any concomitant serotonergic agent) immediately if signs/symptoms arise. Bone fractures have been associated with antidepressant treatment. Consider the possibility of a fragility fracture if an antidepressant-treated patient presents with unexplained bone pain, point tenderness, swelling, or bruising (Rabenda 2013; Rizzoli 2012). Potentially significant drug-drug interactions may exist, requiring dose or frequency adjustment, additional monitoring, and/or selection of alternative therapy.

Use with caution in patients with seizure disorders. Use caution in elderly patients; may be potentially inappropriate in patients with a history of falls or fractures, and may cause or exacerbate syndrome of inappropriate antidiuretic hormone secretion or hyponatremia; monitor sodium closely with initiation or dosage adjustments in older adults (Beers Criteria). May cause or exacerbate sexual dysfunction. May cause mild pupillary dilation which in susceptible individuals can lead to an episode of narrow-angle glaucoma. Consider evaluating patients who have not had an iridectomy for narrow-angle glaucoma risk factors.

Abrupt discontinuation or interruption of antidepressant therapy has been associated with a discontinuation syndrome. Symptoms arising may vary with antidepressant however commonly include nausea, vomiting, diarrhea, headaches, light-headedness, dizziness, diminished appetite, sweating, chills, tremors, paresthesias, fatigue, somnolence, and sleep disturbances (eg, vivid dreams, insomnia). Greater risks for developing a discontinuation syndrome have been associated with antidepressants with shorter half-lives, longer durations of treatment, and abrupt discontinuation. For antidepressants of short or intermediate half-lives, symptoms may emerge within 2 to 5 days after treatment discontinuation and last 7 to 14 days (APA 2010; Fava 2006; Haddad 2001; Shelton 2001; Warner 2006).

Adverse Reactions
>10%:
Central nervous system: Headache (15%)
Gastrointestinal: Diarrhea (26% to 29%), nausea (22% to 24%)
1% to 10%:
Cardiovascular: Palpitations (1% to 2%)
Central nervous system: Dizziness (6% to 8%), insomnia (6% to 7%), drowsiness (4% to 5%), fatigue (4%), abnormal dreams (3%), restlessness (2% to 3%), paresthesia (2%), delayed ejaculation (1% to 2%), migraine (≥1%), sedation (>1%), panic attack (≤1%), ventricular premature contractions (≤1%)
Dermatologic: Hyperhidrosis (≤1%), night sweats (≤1%)
Endocrine & metabolic: Decreased libido (2% to 4%), weight gain (2%)
Gastrointestinal: Xerostomia (7% to 8%), abdominal pain (4% to 7%), vomiting (4% to 5%), dyspepsia (3%), flatulence (3%), increased appetite (3%), abdominal distension (2%), gastroenteritis (2%)
Genitourinary: Erectile dysfunction (≤3%), orgasm disturbance (1% to 2%)
Neuromuscular & skeletal: Arthralgia (2%), tremor (>1%)
Ophthalmic: Blurred vision (≤1%), xerophthalmia (≤1%)
<1% (Limited to important or life-threatening): Angle-closure glaucoma, hallucination, hyponatremia, mania, seizure, serotonin syndrome, suicidal tendencies

Drug Interactions
Metabolism/Transport Effects Substrate of CYP2C19 (minor), CYP2D6 (minor), CYP3A4 (major); **Note:** Assignment of Major/Minor substrate status based on clinically relevant drug interaction potential; **Inhibits** CYP2C8 (weak), CYP2D6 (weak); **Induces** CYP2C19 (weak/moderate)

Avoid Concomitant Use
Avoid concomitant use of Vilazodone with any of the following: Amodiaquine; Dapoxetine; Dosulepin; Iobenguane I 123; Linezolid; MAO Inhibitors; Methylene Blue; Pimozide; Tryptophan; Urokinase

Increased Effect/Toxicity
Vilazodone may increase the levels/effects of: Agents with Antiplatelet Properties; Amodiaquine; Anticoagulants; Antidepressants (Serotonin Reuptake Inhibitor/Antagonist); Antipsychotic Agents; Apixaban; ARIPiprazole; Aspirin; Beta-Blockers; Blood Glucose Lowering Agents; BusPIRone; CarBAMazepine; CloZAPine; Collagenase (Systemic); Dabigatran Etexilate; Deoxycholic Acid; Desmopressin; Dextromethorphan; Digoxin; Dosulepin; Edoxaban; Galantamine; Ibritumomab; Methadone; Methylene Blue; Mexiletine; NSAID (COX-2 Inhibitor); NSAID (Nonselective); Obinutuzumab; Pimozide; RisperiDONE; Rivaroxaban; Salicylates; Serotonin Modulators; Thiazide Diuretics; Thrombolytic Agents; Tositumomab and Iodine I 131 Tositumomab; TraMADol; Urokinase; Vitamin K Antagonists

The levels/effects of Vilazodone may be increased by: Alcohol (Ethyl); Analgesics (Opioid); Antiemetics (5HT3 Antagonists); Antipsychotic Agents; BusPIRone; Cimetidine; CNS Depressants; CYP3A4 Inhibitors (Moderate); CYP3A4 Inhibitors (Strong); Dapoxetine; Dasatinib; Glucosamine; Herbs (Anticoagulant/Antiplatelet Properties); Ibrutinib; Limaprost; Linezolid; Lithium; MAO Inhibitors; Metaxalone; Metoclopramide; Metyrosine; Multivitamins/Fluoride (with ADE); Multivitamins/Minerals (with ADEK, Folate, Iron); Multivitamins/Minerals (with AE, No Iron); Omega-3 Fatty Acids; Osimertinib; Pentosan Polysulfate Sodium; Pentoxifylline; Prostacyclin Analogues; Tedizolid; Tipranavir; TraMADol; Tryptophan; Vitamin E; Vitamin E (Oral)

Decreased Effect
Vilazodone may decrease the levels/effects of: Iobenguane I 123; Ioflupane I 123; Thyroid Products

The levels/effects of Vilazodone may be decreased by: Bosentan; CarBAMazepine; CYP3A4 Inducers (Moderate); CYP3A4 Inducers (Strong); Cyproheptadine; Dabrafenib; Deferasirox; Enzalutamide; Mitotane; NSAID (COX-2 Inhibitor); NSAID (Nonselective); Osimertinib; Siltuximab; St Johns Wort; Tocilizumab

Food Interactions Vilazodone concentrations in the fasted state can be decreased by ~50% compared to the fed state, and may result in a decreased effect in some patients. Management: Administer with food.

Storage/Stability Store at 25°C (77°F); excursions permitted to 15°C to 30°C (50°F to 86°F).

Mechanism of Action Vilazodone inhibits CNS neuron serotonin uptake; minimal or no effect on reuptake of norepinephrine or dopamine. It also binds selectively with high affinity to 5-HT$_{1A}$ receptors and is a 5-HT$_{1A}$ receptor partial agonist. 5-HT$_{1A}$ receptor activity may be altered in depression and anxiety.

Pharmacodynamics/Kinetics
Protein binding: ~96% to 99%
Metabolism: Extensively hepatic, via CYP3A4 (major pathway) and 2C19 and 2D6 (minor pathways)
Bioavailability: 72% (with food); blood concentrations (AUC) may be decreased ~50% in the fasted state
Half-life elimination: Terminal: ~25 hours
Time to peak, serum: 4 to 5 hours
Excretion: Urine (1% as unchanged drug); feces (2% as unchanged drug)

Dosing
Adult & Geriatric Major depressive disorder (MDD):
Oral: Initial: 10 mg once daily for 7 days, then increase to 20 mg once daily; may increase up to 40 mg once daily after a minimum of 7 days based on response and tolerability (maximum dose: 40 mg once daily)

Discontinuation of therapy: Upon discontinuation of antidepressant therapy, gradually taper the dose to minimize the incidence of withdrawal symptoms and allow for the detection of re-emerging symptoms. To discontinue therapy in patients taking 40 mg/day, taper dose to 20 mg once daily for 4 days, then 10 mg once daily for 3 days; to discontinue therapy in patients taking 20 mg/day, taper dose to 10 mg once daily for 7 days.

Evidence supporting ideal taper rates is limited. APA and NICE guidelines suggest tapering therapy over at least several weeks with consideration to the half-life of the antidepressant; antidepressants with a shorter half-life may need to be tapered more conservatively. In addition for long-term treated patients, WFSBP guidelines recommend tapering over 4 to 6 months. If intolerable withdrawal symptoms occur following a dose reduction, consider resuming the previously prescribed dose and/or decrease dose at a more gradual rate (APA 2010; Bauer 2002; Haddad 2001; NCCMH 2010; Schatzberg 2006; Shelton 2001; Warner 2006).

MAO inhibitor recommendations:
Switching to or from an MAO inhibitor intended to treat psychiatric disorders:
Allow 14 days to elapse between discontinuing an MAO inhibitor intended to treat psychiatric disorders and initiation of vilazodone.
Allow 14 days to elapse between discontinuing vilazodone and initiation of an MAO inhibitor intended to treat psychiatric disorders.
Use with other MAO inhibitors (linezolid or IV methylene blue):
Do not initiate vilazodone in patients receiving linezolid or IV methylene blue; consider other interventions for psychiatric condition.
If urgent treatment with linezolid or IV methylene blue is required in a patient already receiving vilazodone and potential benefits outweigh potential risks, discontinue vilazodone promptly and administer linezolid or IV methylene blue. Monitor for serotonin syndrome for 2 weeks or until 24 hours after the last dose of linezolid or IV methylene blue, whichever comes first. May resume vilazodone 24 hours after the last dose of linezolid or IV methylene blue.

Dosing adjustment for concomitant medications:
Strong CYP3A4 inhibitors (eg, clarithromycin, itraconazole, voriconazole): The vilazodone dose should not exceed 20 mg once daily. Readjust vilazodone to original dose when CYP3A4 inhibitor is discontinued.
Strong CYP3A4 inducers (eg, carbamazepine, phenytoin, rifampin): Based on clinical response, consider increasing the dose 2-fold when used concomitantly for >14 days. Maximum daily dose: 80 mg. If CYP3A4 inducer is discontinued, reduce vilazodone dose to original level over 7 to 14 days.
Renal Impairment No dosage adjustment necessary.
Hepatic Impairment No dosage adjustment necessary.
Dietary Considerations Take with food.
Administration Administer with food.
Monitoring Parameters Monitor patient periodically for symptom resolution, mental status for depression, suicidal ideation (especially at the beginning of therapy or when doses are increased or decreased), anxiety, social functioning, mania, panic attacks, signs/symptoms of serotonin syndrome; akathisia
Dosage Forms Excipient information presented when available (limited, particularly for generics); consult specific product labeling. [DSC] = Discontinued product
Kit, Oral, as hydrochloride:
Viibryd: 10 & 20 & 40 mg [DSC] [contains brilliant blue fcf (fd&c blue #1), fd&c red #40, fd&c yellow #6 (sunset yellow)]
Viibryd Starter Pack: 10 & 20 mg [contains fd&c red #40, fd&c yellow #6 (sunset yellow)]
Tablet, Oral, as hydrochloride:
Viibryd: 10 mg [contains fd&c red #40]
Viibryd: 20 mg [contains fd&c yellow #6 (sunset yellow)]
Viibryd: 40 mg [contains brilliant blue fcf (fd&c blue #1)]

◆ Vilazodone Hydrochloride *see* Vilazodone
   on page 1893

◆ Vimizim *see* Elosulfase Alfa *on page 625*

◆ Vimpat *see* Lacosamide *on page 1021*

VinBLAStine (vin BLAS teen)

Brand Names: Canada Vinblastine Sulphate Injection
Index Terms Velban; Vinblastine Sulfate; Vincaleukoblastine; VLB
Pharmacologic Category Antineoplastic Agent, Antimicrotubular; Antineoplastic Agent, Vinca Alkaloid
Use Treatment of Hodgkin lymphoma; lymphocytic lymphoma; histiocytic lymphoma; mycosis fungoides; testicular cancer; Kaposi sarcoma; histiocytosis X (Letterer-Siwe disease); has also been used for the treatment of refractory/resistant breast cancer and choriocarcinoma
Pregnancy Considerations Adverse effects were observed in animal reproduction studies. May cause fetal harm if administered during pregnancy. Women of

childbearing potential should avoid becoming pregnant during vinblastine treatment. Aspermia has been reported in males who have received treatment with vinblastine.
Breast-Feeding Considerations It is not known if vinblastine is excreted in breast milk. Due to the potential for serious adverse reactions in the nursing infant, a decision should be made whether to discontinue vinblastine or to discontinue breast-feeding, taking into account the importance of treatment to the mother.
Contraindications Significant granulocytopenia (unless as a result of condition being treated); presence of bacterial infection
Warnings/Precautions Hazardous agent - use appropriate precautions for handling and disposal (NIOSH 2014 [group 1]). Avoid eye contamination (exposure may cause severe irritation). **[US Boxed Warning]: For IV use only. Intrathecal administration may result in death.** To prevent administration errors, the Institute for Safe Medication Practices (ISMP) Targeted Medication Safety Best Practices for Hospitals initiative strongly recommends dispensing vinblastine diluted in a minibag (ISMP, 2014). **If not dispensed in a minibag, affix an auxiliary label stating "For intravenous use only - fatal if given by other routes" and also place in an overwrap labeled "Do not remove covering until moment of injection."** Vinblastine should **NOT** be prepared during the preparation of any intrathecal medications. After preparation, keep vinblastine in a location **away** from the separate storage location recommended for intrathecal medications. Vinblastine should **NOT** be delivered to the patient at the same time with any medications intended for central nervous system administration.

[US Boxed Warning]: Vinblastine is a vesicant; ensure proper needle or catheter placement prior to and during infusion. Avoid extravasation. Extravasation may cause significant irritation. Individuals administering should be experienced in vinblastine administration. If extravasation occurs, discontinue immediately and initiate appropriate extravasation management, including local injection of hyaluronidase and moderate heat application to the affected area. Use a separate vein to complete administration.

Leukopenia commonly occurs; granulocytopenia may be severe with higher doses. The leukocyte nadir generally occurs 5 to 10 days after administration; recovery typically occurs 7 to 14 days later. Monitor for infections if WBC <2,000/mm^3. Leukopenia may be more pronounced in cachectic patients and patients with skin ulceration and may be less pronounced with lower doses used for maintenance therapy. Leukocytes and platelets may fall considerably with moderate doses when marrow is infiltrated with malignant cells (further use in this situation is not recommended). Thrombocytopenia and anemia may occur rarely.

May rarely cause disabling neurotoxicity; usually reversible. Seizures and severe and permanent CNS damage has occurred with higher then recommended doses and/or when administered more frequently than recommended. Acute shortness of breath and severe bronchospasm have been reported, most often in association with concurrent administration of mitomycin; may occur within minutes to several hours following vinblastine administration or up to 14 days following mitomycin administration; use caution in patients with preexisting pulmonary disease. Use with caution in patients with hepatic impairment; toxicity may be increased; may require dosage modification. Use with caution in patients with ischemic heart disease. Stomatitis may occur (rare); may be disabling, but is usually reversible.

Potentially significant drug-drug interactions may exist, requiring dose or frequency adjustment, additional monitoring, and/or selection of alternative therapy. **[US Boxed Warning]: Should be administered under the supervision of an experienced cancer chemotherapy physician.**

Benzyl alcohol and derivatives: Some dosage forms may contain benzyl alcohol; large amounts of benzyl alcohol (≥99 mg/kg/day) have been associated with a potentially fatal toxicity ("gasping syndrome") in neonates; the "gasping syndrome" consists of metabolic acidosis, respiratory distress, gasping respirations, CNS dysfunction (including convulsions, intracranial hemorrhage), hypotension, and cardiovascular collapse (AAP ["Inactive" 1997]; CDC, 1982); some data suggests that benzoate displaces bilirubin from protein binding sites (Ahlfors, 2001); avoid or use dosage forms containing benzyl alcohol with caution in neonates. See manufacturer's labeling.

◄ **Adverse Reactions** Frequency not defined.
Common:
Cardiovascular: Hypertension
Central nervous system: Malaise
Dermatologic: Alopecia
Gastrointestinal: Constipation
Hematologic: Myelosuppression, leukopenia/granulocytopenia (nadir: 5-10 days; recovery: 7-14 days; dose-limiting toxicity)
Neuromuscular & skeletal: Bone pain, jaw pain, tumor pain
Less common:
Cardiovascular: Angina, cerebrovascular accident, coronary ischemia, ECG abnormalities, limb ischemia, MI, myocardial ischemia, Raynaud's phenomenon
Central nervous system: Depression, dizziness, headache, neurotoxicity (duration: >24 hours), seizure, vertigo
Dermatologic: Dermatitis, photosensitivity (rare), rash, skin blistering
Endocrine & metabolic: Aspermia, hyperuricemia, SIADH
Gastrointestinal: Abdominal pain, anorexia, diarrhea, gastrointestinal bleeding, hemorrhagic enterocolitis, ileus, metallic taste, nausea (mild), paralytic ileus, rectal bleeding, stomatitis, toxic megacolon, vomiting (mild)
Genitourinary: Urinary retention
Hematologic: Anemia, thrombocytopenia (recovery within a few days), thrombotic thrombocytopenic purpura
Local: Cellulitis (with extravasation), irritation, phlebitis (with extravasation), radiation recall
Neuromuscular & skeletal: Deep tendon reflex loss, myalgia, paresthesia, peripheral neuritis, weakness
Ocular: Nystagmus
Otic: Auditory damage, deafness, vestibular damage
Renal: Hemolytic uremic syndrome
Respiratory: Bronchospasm, dyspnea, pharyngitis

Drug Interactions
Metabolism/Transport Effects Substrate of CYP2D6 (minor), CYP3A4 (major), P-glycoprotein; **Note:** Assignment of Major/Minor substrate status based on clinically relevant drug interaction potential; **Inhibits** CYP2D6 (weak); **Induces** P-glycoprotein

Avoid Concomitant Use
Avoid concomitant use of VinBLAStine with any of the following: BCG (Intravesical); Conivaptan; Dabigatran Etexilate; Deferiprone; Dipyrone; Fusidic Acid (Systemic); Idelalisib; Ledipasvir; Natalizumab; Pimecrolimus; Sofosbuvir; Tacrolimus (Topical); Tofacitinib; Vaccines (Live); VinCRIStine (Liposomal)

Increased Effect/Toxicity
VinBLAStine may increase the levels/effects of: ARIPiprazole; CloZAPine; Deferiprone; Fingolimod; Leflunomide; MitoMYcin (Systemic); Natalizumab; Tofacitinib; Tolterodine; Vaccines (Live)

The levels/effects of VinBLAStine may be increased by: Aprepitant; Conivaptan; CYP3A4 Inhibitors (Moderate); CYP3A4 Inhibitors (Strong); Dasatinib; Denosumab; Dipyrone; Fosaprepitant; Fusidic Acid (Systemic); Idelalisib; Itraconazole; Ivacaftor; Lopinavir; Luliconazole; Macrolide Antibiotics; Mifepristone; Netupitant; Osimertinib; Palbociclib; P-glycoprotein/ABCB1 Inhibitors; Pimecrolimus; Posaconazole; Ranolazine; Ritonavir; Roflumilast; Simeprevir; Stiripentol; Tacrolimus (Topical); Trastuzumab; Voriconazole

Decreased Effect
VinBLAStine may decrease the levels/effects of: Afatinib; BCG (Intravesical); Brentuximab Vedotin; Coccidioides immitis Skin Test; Dabigatran Etexilate; DOXOrubicin (Conventional); Ledipasvir; Linagliptin; P-glycoprotein/ABCB1 Substrates; Sipuleucel-T; Sofosbuvir; Vaccines (Inactivated); Vaccines (Live); VinCRIStine (Liposomal)

The levels/effects of VinBLAStine may be decreased by: Bosentan; CYP3A4 Inducers (Moderate); CYP3A4 Inducers (Strong); Dabrafenib; Deferasirox; Echinacea; Enzalutamide; Mitotane; Osimertinib; P-glycoprotein/ABCB1 Inducers; Siltuximab; St Johns Wort; Tocilizumab

Preparation for Administration Hazardous agent; use appropriate precautions for handling and disposal (NIOSH 2014 [group 1]). For infusion, may dilute in 25 to 50 mL NS or D_5W; dilution in larger volumes (≥100 mL) of IV fluids is not recommended. **Note:** In order to prevent inadvertent intrathecal administration, the Institute for Safe Medication Practices (ISMP) strongly recommends dispensing vinblastine in a minibag (**NOT** in a syringe).

Storage/Stability Note: Dispense in an overwrap which bears the statement "Do not remove covering until the moment of injection. Fatal if given intrathecally. For IV use only." If dispensing in a syringe (minibag is preferred) should be labeled: "Fatal if given intrathecally. For IV use only."

Store intact vials under refrigeration at 2°C to 8°C (36°F to 46°F). Protect from light.

Mechanism of Action Vinblastine binds to tubulin and inhibits microtubule formation, therefore, arresting the cell at metaphase by disrupting the formation of the mitotic spindle; it is specific for the M and S phases. Vinblastine may also interfere with nucleic acid and protein synthesis by blocking glutamic acid utilization.

Pharmacodynamics/Kinetics
Metabolism: Hepatic (via CYP3A) to active metabolite
Half-life elimination: Terminal: ~25 hours
Excretion: Feces (30% to 36%); urine (12% to 17%)

Dosing
Adult & Geriatric Note: Frequency and duration of therapy may vary by indication, concomitant combination chemotherapy and hematologic response. **For IV use only.** In order to prevent inadvertent intrathecal administration, the Institute for Safe Medication Practices (ISMP) strongly recommends dispensing vinblastine in a minibag (**NOT** a syringe).

Hodgkin lymphoma, lymphocytic lymphoma, histiocytic lymphoma, mycosis fungoides, testicular cancer, Kaposi sarcoma, histiocytosis X (Letterer-Siwe disease): *Manufacturer's labeling:* IV: 3.7 mg/m²; adjust dose every 7 days (based on white blood cell response) up to 5.5 mg/m² (second dose); 7.4 mg/m² (third dose); 9.25 mg/m² (fourth dose); and 11.1 mg/m² (fifth dose); do not administer more frequently than every 7 days. Usual dosage range: 5.5 to 7.4 mg/m² every 7 days; Maximum dose: 18.5 mg/m²; dosage adjustment goal is to reduce white blood cell count to ~3,000/mm³

Off-label and/or indication-specific dosing:
Hodgkin lymphoma (off-label dosing): IV:
ABVD regimen: 6 mg/m² days 1 and 15 of a 28-day cycle (in combination with doxorubicin, bleomycin, and dacarbazine) for 2 cycles (early/favorable disease) or for 4 cycles (unfavorable disease) (Eich, 2010; Engert, 2007)
Stanford V regimen: 6 mg/m² weeks 1, 3, 5, 7, 9, and 11 (in combination with doxorubicin, mechlorethamine, vincristine, bleomycin, etoposide, and prednisone) (Bartlett, 1995; Horning, 2002)

Testicular cancer (off-label dosing): VelP regimen: IV: 0.11 mg/kg daily for 2 days every 21 days (in combination with ifosfamide, cisplatin, and mesna) for 4 cycles (Loehrer, 1988; Loehrer, 1988 [correction]; Loehrer, 1998)

Bladder cancer (off-label use): IV:
Metastatic disease:
Dose-dense MVAC regimen: 3 mg/m² day 2 every 14 days (in combination with methotrexate, doxorubicin, and cisplatin) until disease progression or unacceptable toxicity (Sternberg, 2001; Sternberg, 2006)
MVAC regimen: 3 mg/m² days 2, 15, and 22 every 28 days (in combination with methotrexate, doxorubicin, and cisplatin) for up to 6 cycles (von der Maase, 2000) **or** 3 mg/m² days 2, 15, and 22 every 28 days (in combination with methotrexate, doxorubicin, and cisplatin) until disease progression or unacceptable toxicity (Sternberg, 2001; Sternberg, 2006) **or** 3 mg/m² days 1, 15, and 22 every 28 days (in combination with methotrexate, doxorubicin, and cisplatin) for up to 6 cycles (Bamias, 2004)
Neoadjuvant treatment:
MVAC regimen: 3 mg/m² days 2, 15, and 22 every 28 days (in combination with methotrexate, doxorubicin, and cisplatin) for 3 cycles (Grossman, 2003)
CMV regimen: 4 mg/m² days 1 and 8 every 21 days (in combination with methotrexate, cisplatin, and leucovorin) for 3 cycles (Griffiths, 2011)

Melanoma, metastatic (off-label use): IV:
CVD regimen: 2 mg/m² days 1 to 4 and 22 to 25 of a 6-week treatment cycle (in combination with cisplatin and dacarbazine); may repeat if tumor response (Eton, 2002)
CVD + immunotherapy regimen: 1.5 mg/m² days 1 to 4 and 22 to 25 of a 6-week treatment cycle (in combination with cisplatin, dacarbazine, aldesleukin, and interferon alfa-2b); may repeat if tumor response (Eton, 2002)

Non-small cell lung cancer (off-label use): IV:
Adjuvant treatment after complete resection: 4 mg/m² days 1, 8, 15, 22, and 29, then every 2 weeks (in combination with cisplatin) until last cisplatin dose (Arriagada, 2004)
Concurrent radiation: 5 mg/m² days 1, 8, 15, 22, and 29 (in combination with cisplatin and concurrent radiation therapy) (Curran, 2011)

Soft tissue sarcoma (desmoid tumors, aggressive fibromatosis), advanced (off-label use): IV: 6 mg/m² every 7 to 10 days (dose usually rounded to 10 mg) in combination with methotrexate for 1 year (Azzarelli, 2001).

Pediatric Note: Frequency and duration of therapy may vary by indication, concomitant combination chemotherapy and hematologic response. **For IV use only.** In order to prevent inadvertent intrathecal administration, the Institute for Safe Medication Practices (ISMP) strongly recommends dispensing vinblastine in a minibag (**NOT** a syringe).

Hodgkin lymphoma: IV: Initial dose: 6 mg/m²; do not administer more frequently than every 7 days **or** ABVD regimen (off-label dosing): IV: 6 mg/m² days 1 and 15 of a 28-day cycle (in combination with doxorubicin, bleomycin, and dacarbazine) for 6 cycles (Hutchinson, 1998).

Letterer-Siwe disease: IV: Initial dose: 6.5 mg/m²; do not administer more frequently than every 7 days

Testicular cancer: IV: Initial dose: 3 mg/m²; do not administer more frequently than every 7 days

Renal Impairment No dosage adjustment necessary.

Hepatic Impairment

The manufacturer's labeling recommends the following adjustment: Serum bilirubin >3 mg/dL: Administer 50% of dose

The following adjustments have also been recommended (Floyd, 2006; Superfin, 2007):

Serum bilirubin 1.5 to 3 mg/dL or transaminases 2 to 3 times ULN: Administer 50% of dose

Serum bilirubin >3 times ULN: Avoid use.

Obesity *ASCO Guidelines for appropriate chemotherapy dosing in obese adults with cancer:* Utilize patient's actual body weight (full weight) for calculation of body surface area- or weight-based dosing, particularly when the intent of therapy is curative; manage regimen-related toxicities in the same manner as for nonobese patients; if a dose reduction is utilized due to toxicity, consider resumption of full weight-based dosing with subsequent cycles, especially if cause of toxicity (eg, hepatic or renal impairment) is resolved (Griggs, 2012).

Administration In order to prevent inadvertent intrathecal administration, the Institute for Safe Medication Practices (ISMP) strongly recommends dispensing vinblastine in a minibag (NOT in a syringe). For IV administration only. **Fatal if given intrathecally.** The preferred administration is as a short infusion in a 25 to 50 mL minibag. If administration via a minibag is not possible, may also be administered as an undiluted 1-minute infusion into a free flowing IV line to prevent venous irritation/extravasation. Prolonged administration times (≥30 to 60 minutes) and/or increased administration volumes may increase the risk of vein irritation and extravasation.

Vesicant; ensure proper needle or catheter placement prior to and during infusion. Avoid extravasation.

Extravasation management: If extravasation occurs, stop infusion immediately and disconnect (leave cannula/needle in place); gently aspirate extravasated solution (do **NOT** flush the line); initiate hyaluronidase antidote; remove needle/cannula; apply dry warm compresses for 20 minutes 4 times a day for 1-2 days; elevate extremity (Perez Fidalgo, 2012). Remaining portion of the vinblastine dose should be infused through a separate vein.

Hyaluronidase: If needle/cannula still in place, administer 1-6 mL hyaluronidase (150 units/mL) into the existing IV line; the usual dose is 1 mL hyaluronidase for each 1 mL of extravasated drug (Perez Fidalgo, 2012; Schulmeister, 2011). If needle/cannula was removed, inject 1-6 mL (150 units/mL) subcutaneously in a clockwise manner using 1 mL for each 1 mL of drug extravasated (Schulmeister, 2011) **or** administer 1 mL (150 units/mL) as 5 separate 0.2 mL injections (using a 25-gauge needle) subcutaneously into the extravasation site (Polovich, 2009).

Hazardous agent; use appropriate precautions for handling and disposal (NIOSH 2014 [group 1]).

Monitoring Parameters CBC with differential and platelet count, serum uric acid, hepatic function tests

Dosage Forms Excipient information presented when available (limited, particularly for generics); consult specific product labeling.

Solution, Intravenous, as sulfate:
Generic: 1 mg/mL (10 mL)

Solution Reconstituted, Intravenous, as sulfate:
Generic: 10 mg (1 ea)

◆ Vinblastine Sulfate *see* VinBLAStine *on page* 1895

◆ Vinblastine Sulphate Injection (Can) *see* VinBLAStine *on page* 1895

◆ Vincaleukoblastine *see* VinBLAStine *on page* 1895

◆ Vincasar PFS *see* VinCRIStine *on page* 1897

VinCRIStine (vin KRIS teen)

Brand Names: US Vincasar PFS

Brand Names: Canada Vincristine Sulfate Injection; Vincristine Sulfate Injection USP

Index Terms Conventional Vincristine; Leurocristine Sulfate; Oncovin; Vincristine (Conventional); Vincristine Sulfate

Pharmacologic Category Antineoplastic Agent, Antimicrotubular; Antineoplastic Agent, Vinca Alkaloid

Use Treatment of acute lymphocytic leukemia (ALL), Hodgkin lymphoma, non-Hodgkin lymphomas, Wilms' tumor, neuroblastoma, rhabdomyosarcoma

Pregnancy Considerations Animal reproduction studies have demonstrated teratogenicity and fetal loss. May cause fetal harm if administered during pregnancy. Women of childbearing potential should avoid becoming pregnant during treatment.

Breast-Feeding Considerations It is not known if vincristine is excreted in breast milk. Due to the potential for serious adverse reactions in the nursing infant, the decision to discontinue vincristine or to discontinue breast-feeding should take into account the benefits of treatment to the mother.

Contraindications Patients with the demyelinating form of Charcot-Marie-Tooth syndrome

Warnings/Precautions Hazardous agent - use appropriate precautions for handling and disposal (NIOSH 2014 [group 1]); avoid eye contamination.

[U.S. Boxed Warning]: For IV administration only; inadvertent intrathecal administration usually results in death. To prevent administration errors, the Institute for Safe Medication Practices (ISMP) Targeted Medication Safety Best Practices for Hospitals initiative and the World Health Organization strongly recommend dispensing vincristine diluted in a minibag (ISMP, 2014; WHO, 2007), **if not dispensed in a minibag, affix an auxiliary label stating "For intravenous use only - fatal if given by other routes" and also place in an overwrap labeled "Do not remove covering until moment of injection."** Vincristine should **NOT** be prepared during the preparation of any intrathecal medications. After preparation, keep vincristine in a location **away** from the separate storage location recommended for intrathecal medications. Vincristine should **NOT** be delivered to the patient at the same time with any medications intended for central nervous system administration.

[U.S. Boxed Warning]: Vincristine is a vesicant; ensure proper needle or catheter placement prior to and during infusion. Avoid extravasation. Individuals administering should be experienced in vincristine administration. Extravasation may cause significant irritation. If extravasation occurs, discontinue immediately and initiate appropriate extravasation management, including local injection of hyaluronidase and moderate heat application to the affected area. Use a separate vein to complete administration.

Neurotoxicity, including alterations in mental status such as depression, confusion, or insomnia may occur; neurologic effects are dose-limiting (may require dosage reduction) and may be additive with those of other neurotoxic agents and spinal cord irradiation. Use with caution in patients with preexisting neuromuscular disease and/or with concomitant neurotoxic agents. Constipation, paralytic ileus, intestinal necrosis and/or perforation may occur; constipation may present as upper colon impaction with an empty rectum (may require flat film of abdomen for diagnosis); generally responds to high enemas and laxatives. All patients should be on a prophylactic bowel management regimen.

Potentially significant drug-drug interactions may exist, requiring dose or frequency adjustment, additional monitoring, and/or selection of alternative therapy. Acute shortness of breath and severe bronchospasm have been reported with vinca alkaloids, usually when used in combination with mitomycin. Onset may be several minutes to hours after vincristine administration and up to 2 weeks after mitomycin. Progressive dyspnea may occur. Permanently discontinue vincristine if pulmonary dysfunction occurs.

Use with caution in patients with hepatic impairment; dosage modification should occur. May be associated with hepatic sinusoidal obstruction syndrome (SOS; formerly called veno-occlusive disease), increased risk in children <3 years of age; use with caution in hepatobiliary dysfunction. Monitor for signs or symptoms of hepatic SOS,

including bilirubin >1.4 mg/dL, unexplained weight gain, ascites, hepatomegaly, or unexplained right upper quadrant pain (Arndt, 2004). Acute uric acid nephropathy has been reported with vincristine. Use with caution in the elderly; may cause or exacerbate syndrome of inappropriate antidiuretic hormone secretion or hyponatremia; monitor sodium closely with initiation or dosage adjustments in older adults (Beers Criteria).

Adverse Reactions Frequency not defined.

Cardiovascular: Edema, hyper-/hypotension, MI, myocardial ischemia

Central nervous system: Ataxia, coma, cranial nerve dysfunction (auditory damage, extraocular muscle impairment, laryngeal muscle impairment, paralysis, paresis, vestibular damage, vocal cord paralysis), dizziness, fever, headache, neurotoxicity (dose-related), neuropathic pain (common), seizure, vertigo

Dermatologic toxicity: Alopecia (common), rash

Endocrine & metabolic: Hyperuricemia, parotid pain, SIADH (rare)

Gastrointestinal: Abdominal cramps, abdominal pain, anorexia, constipation (common), diarrhea, intestinal necrosis, intestinal perforation, nausea, oral ulcers, paralytic ileus, vomiting, weight loss

Genitourinary: Bladder atony, dysuria, polyuria, urinary retention

Hematologic: Anemia (mild), leukopenia (mild), thrombocytopenia (mild), thrombotic thrombocytopenic purpura

Hepatic: Hepatic sinusoidal obstruction syndrome (SOS), veno-occlusive liver disease)

Local: Phlebitis, tissue irritation/necrosis (if infiltrated)

Neuromuscular & skeletal: Back pain, bone pain, deep tendon reflex loss, difficulty walking, foot drop, gait changes, jaw pain, limb pain, motor difficulties, muscle wasting, myalgia, paralysis, paresthesia, peripheral neuropathy (common), sensorimotor dysfunction, sensory loss

Ocular: Cortical blindness (transient), nystagmus, optic atrophy with blindness

Otic: Deafness

Renal: Acute uric acid nephropathy, hemolytic uremic syndrome

Respiratory: Bronchospasm, dyspnea, pharyngeal pain

Miscellaneous: Allergic reactions (rare), anaphylaxis (rare), hypersensitivity (rare)

Drug Interactions

Metabolism/Transport Effects Substrate of CYP3A4 (major), P-glycoprotein; **Note:** Assignment of Major/Minor substrate status based on clinically relevant drug interaction potential

Avoid Concomitant Use

Avoid concomitant use of VinCRIStine with any of the following: BCG (Intravesical); Conivaptan; Fusidic Acid (Systemic); Idelalisib; Natalizumab; Pimecrolimus; Tacrolimus (Topical); Tofacitinib; Vaccines (Live)

Increased Effect/Toxicity

VinCRIStine may increase the levels/effects of: Fingolimod; Leflunomide; MitoMYcin (Systemic); Natalizumab; Tofacitinib; Vaccines (Live)

The levels/effects of VinCRIStine may be increased by: Aprepitant; Conivaptan; CYP3A4 Inhibitors (Moderate); CYP3A4 Inhibitors (Strong); Dasatinib; Denosumab; Fosaprepitant; Fusidic Acid (Systemic); Idelalisib; Itraconazole; Ivacaftor; Lopinavir; Luliconazole; Macrolide Antibiotics; Mifepristone; Netupitant; NIFEdipine; Osimertinib; Palbociclib; P-glycoprotein/ABCB1 Inhibitors; Pimecrolimus; Posaconazole; Ranolazine; Ritonavir; Roflumilast; Simeprevir; Stiripentol; Tacrolimus (Topical); Teniposide; Trastuzumab; Voriconazole

Decreased Effect

VinCRIStine may decrease the levels/effects of: BCG (Intravesical); Coccidioides immitis Skin Test; Fosphenytoin; Phenytoin; Sipuleucel-T; Vaccines (Inactivated); Vaccines (Live)

The levels/effects of VinCRIStine may be decreased by: Bosentan; CYP3A4 Inducers (Moderate); CYP3A4 Inducers (Strong); Dabrafenib; Deferasirox; Echinacea; Enzalutamide; Fosphenytoin; Mitotane; Osimertinib; P-glycoprotein/ABCB1 Inducers; Phenytoin; Siltuximab; St Johns Wort; Tocilizumab

Preparation for Administration Hazardous agent; use appropriate precautions for handling and disposal (NIOSH 2014 [group 1]).

Solutions for IV infusion may be mixed in NS or D_5W. **Note:** In order to prevent inadvertent intrathecal administration the World Health Organization (WHO) and the Institute for Safe Medication Practices (ISMP) strongly recommend dispensing vincristine in a minibag (**NOT** in a syringe). Vincristine should **NOT** be prepared during the preparation of any intrathecal medications. If dispensing

vincristine in a syringe, affix an auxiliary label stating **"For intravenous use only - fatal if given by other routes"** to the syringe, and the syringe must also be packaged in the manufacturer-provided overwrap which bears the statement **"Do not remove covering until the moment of injection. For intravenous use only. Fatal if given intrathecally."**

Storage/Stability Store intact vials refrigerated at 2°C to 8°C (36°F to 46°F). Protect from light.

IV solution: Diluted in 25 to 50 mL NS or D_5W, stable for 7 days under refrigeration, or 2 days at room temperature. In ambulatory pumps, solution is stable for 7 days at room temperature. After preparation, keep vincristine in a location away from the separate storage location recommended for intrathecal medications.

Mechanism of Action Binds to tubulin and inhibits microtubule formation, therefore, arresting the cell at metaphase by disrupting the formation of the mitotic spindle; it is specific for the M and S phases. Vincristine may also interfere with nucleic acid and protein synthesis by blocking glutamic acid utilization.

Pharmacodynamics/Kinetics

Distribution: Rapidly removed from bloodstream and tightly bound to tissues; penetrates blood-brain barrier poorly

Metabolism: Extensively hepatic, via CYP3A4

Half-life elimination: Terminal: 85 hours (range: 19-155 hours)

Excretion: Feces (~80%); urine (10% to 20%; <1% as unchanged drug)

Dosing

Adult & Geriatric Note: Doses may be capped at a maximum of 2 mg/dose. Dosing and frequency may vary by protocol and/or treatment phase; refer to specific protocol. In order to prevent inadvertent intrathecal administration, the World Health Organization (WHO) and the Institute for Safe Medication Practices (ISMP) strongly recommend dispensing vincristine in a minibag (**NOT** a syringe).

Doses in the manufacturer's U.S. labeling: IV: 1.4 mg/m²/dose; frequency may vary based on protocol

Additional dosing in combination therapy; indication-specific and/or off-label dosing:

Acute lymphocytic leukemia (ALL): IV:

Hyper-CVAD regimen: 2 mg/dose days 4 and 11 during odd-numbered cycles (cycles 1, 3, 5, 7) of an 8-cycle phase, followed by maintenance treatment (if needed) of 2 mg monthly for 2 years (Kantarjian, 2004)

CALBG 8811 regimen: Induction phase: 2 mg/dose days 1, 8, 15, and 22 (4-week treatment cycle); Early intensification phase: 2 mg/dose days 15, and 22 (4-week treatment cycle, repeat once); Late intensification phase: 2 mg/dose days 1, 8, 15 (8-week treatment cycle); Maintenance phase: 2 mg/dose day 1 every 4 weeks until 24 months from diagnosis (Larson, 1995)

Central nervous system tumors: IV: PCV regimen: 1.4 mg/m²/dose (maximum dose: 2 mg) on days 8 and 29 of a 6-week treatment cycle for a total of 6 cycles (van de Bent, 2006) **or** 1.4 mg/m²/dose (no maximum dose) on days 8 and 29 of a 6-week treatment cycle for up to 4 cycles (Cairncross, 2006)

Hodgkin lymphoma: IV:

BEACOPP regimen: 1.4 mg/m²/dose (maximum dose: 2 mg) on day 8 of a 21-day treatment cycle (Diehl, 2003)

Stanford-V regimen: 1.4 mg/m²/dose (maximum dose: 2 mg) in weeks 2, 4, 6, 8, 10, and 12 (Horning, 2000; Horning, 2002)

Non-Hodgkin lymphoma: IV:

Burkitt lymphoma:

CODOX-M/IVAC: Cycles 1 and 3 (CODOX-M): 1.5 mg/m² (no maximum dose) days 1 and 8 of cycle 1 and days 1, 8, and 15 of cycle 3 (Magrath, 1996) **or** 1.5 mg/m² (maximum dose: 2 mg) days 1 and 8 of cycles 1 and 3 (Mead 2002; Mead 2008); CODOX-M is in combination with cyclophosphamide, doxorubicin, methotrexate, and CNS prophylaxis and alternates with IVAC (etoposide, ifosfamide, mesna, cytarabine, and CNS prophylaxis) for a total of 4 cycles

Hyper-CVAD: 2 mg (flat dose) days 4 and 11 of courses 1, 3, 5, and 7 (in combination with cyclophosphamide, doxorubicin, and dexamethasone) and alternates with even courses 2, 4, 6, and 8 (methotrexate and cytarabine) (Thomas, 2006)

Follicular lymphoma: CVP regimen: 1.4 mg/m²/dose (maximum dose: 2 mg) on day 1 of a 21-day treatment cycle (in combination with cyclophosphamide and prednisone) for 8 cycles (Marcus, 2005)

Large B-cell lymphoma:
CHOP regimen: 1.4 mg/m^2/dose (maximum dose: 2 mg) on day 1 of a 21-day treatment cycle for 8 cycles (Coiffier, 2002)
EPOCH regimen: 0.4 mg/m^2/day continuous infusion for 4 days (over 96 hours) (total 1.6 mg/m^2/cycle; dose not usually capped) of a 21-day treatment cycle (Wilson, 2002)

Ewing's sarcoma (off-label use): IV: VAC/IE regimen: VAC: 2 mg/m^2 (maximum dose: 2 mg) on day 1 of a 21-day treatment cycle (in combination with doxorubicin and cyclophosphamide), alternates with IE (ifosfamide and etoposide) for a total of 17 cycles (Grier, 2003)

Gestational trophoblastic tumors, high-risk (off-label use): IV: EMA/CO regimen: 1 mg/m^2 on day 8 of 2-week treatment cycle (in combination with etoposide methotrexate, dactinomycin, and cyclophosphamide), continue for at least 2 treatment cycles after a normal hCG level (Escobar, 2003)

Multiple myeloma (off-label use): IV:
DVD regimen: 1.4 mg/m^2/dose (maximum dose: 2 mg) on day 1 of a 28-day treatment cycle (Rifkin, 2006)
VAD regimen: 0.4 mg/day continuous infusion for 4 days (over 96 hours) (total 1.6 mg/cycle) of a 28-day treatment cycle (Rifkin, 2006)

Ovarian cancer (off-label use): IV: VAC regimen: 1.5 mg/m^2/dose (maximum dose: 2 mg) weekly for 8-12 weeks (Slayton, 1985)

Small cell lung cancer (off-label use): IV: CAV regimen: 1.4 mg/m^2/dose day 1 of a 21-day treatment cycle (Hong, 1989) **or** 2 mg/dose on day 1 of a 21-day treatment cycle (von Pawel, 1999)

Thymoma, advanced (off-label use): IV: ADOC regimen: 0.6 mg/m^2 on day 3 every 3 weeks (in combination with cisplatin, doxorubicin, and cyclophosphamide) (Fornasiero, 1991)

Pediatric Note: Doses may be capped at a maximum of 2 mg/dose. Dosing and frequency may vary by protocol and/or treatment phase; refer to specific protocol. In order to prevent inadvertent intrathecal administration, the World Health Organization (WHO) and the Institute for Safe Medication Practices (ISMP) strongly recommend dispensing vincristine in a minibag (**NOT** in a syringe).
Doses in the manufacturer's U.S. labeling: IV:
Children ≤10 kg: 0.05 mg/kg/dose once weekly
Children >10 kg: 1.5-2 mg/m^2/dose; frequency may vary based on protocol

Additional dosing in combination therapy; indication-specific and/or off-label dosing:

Acute lymphocytic lymphoma (ALL): IV: Induction phase: 1.5 mg/m^2/dose days 0, 7, 14, and 21; Consolidation phase: 1.5 mg/m^2/dose days 0, 28, and 56; Delayed intensification phase: 1.5 mg/m^2/dose days 0, 7, and 14; Maintenance phase: 1.5 mg/m^2/dose days 0, 28, and 56 (Bostrom, 2003) **or** Induction phase: 1.5 mg/m^2/dose days 0, 7, 14, and 21; Consolidation phase: 1.5 mg/m^2/dose days 0, 28, and 56; Interim maintenance phases: 1.5 mg/m^2/dose days 0 and 28; Delayed intensification phase: 1.5 mg/m^2/dose days 0, 7, and 14; Maintenance phase: 1.5 mg/m^2/dose every 4 weeks (Avramis, 2002)

Burkitt lymphoma and B-cell ALL: IV: 1.5 mg/m^2 (maximum dose: 2 mg) on days 4 and 11 of initial phase cycle (initial phase is in combination with cyclophosphamide, doxorubicin, and CNS prophylaxis; alternates with secondary phase) for a total of 4 cycles of each phase (Bowman, 1996) **or** 1.5 mg/m^2 (maximum dose: 2 mg) on day 1 of cycle AA (in combination with dexamethasone, ifosfamide, methotrexate, cytarabine, etoposide and CNS prophylaxis) and on day 1 of cycle BB (in combination with dexamethasone, cyclophosphamide, methotrexate, doxorubicin, and CNS prophylaxis) (Reiter, 1999)

Ewing's sarcoma (off-label use): IV: 2 mg/m^2/dose (maximum dose: 2 mg) on day 1 of a 21-day cycle, administer either every cycle or during odd-numbered cycles (Grier, 2003) **or** 0.67 mg/m^2/day continuous infusion days 1, 2, and 3 (total 2 mg/m^2/cycle; maximum dose/cycle: 2 mg) during cycles 1, 2, 3, and 6 (Kolb, 2003)

Hodgkin lymphoma: IV: BEACOPP regimen: 2 mg/m^2/dose (maximum dose: 2 mg) on day 7 of a 21-day treatment cycle (Kelly, 2002)

Neuroblastoma: IV:
CE-CAdO regimen: 1.5 mg/m^2 (maximum dose: 2 mg) days 1 and 5 every 21 days for 2 cycles (Rubie, 1998) **or** 0.05 mg/kg days 1 and 5 for 2 cycles (Rubie, 2001)
CAV-P/VP regimen (off-label dosing): 0.033 mg/kg/day continuous infusion days 1, 2, and 3, then 1.5 mg/m^2 bolus day 9 of courses 1, 2, 4, and 6 (Kushner, 1994)

Retinoblastoma (off-label use): IV:
Children: 0.05 mg/kg on day 1 every 21 days (in combination with carboplatin) for 8 cycles (Rodriguez-Galindo, 2003)
or
Children ≤36 months: 0.05 mg/kg on day 0 every 28 days (in combination with carboplatin and etoposide) for 6 cycles (Freidman, 2000)
or
Children >36 months: 1.5 mg/m^2 (maximum dose: 2 mg) on day 0 every 28 days (in combination with carboplatin and etoposide) for 6 cycles (Friedman, 2000)

Rhabdomyosarcoma: IV:
VA regimen: 1.5 mg/m^2/dose (maximum dose: 2 mg) weeks 1-8, weeks 13-20, and weeks 25-32 (Crist, 2001)
VAC regimen: 1.5 mg/m^2/dose (maximum dose: 2 mg) weeks 0-12, week 16, weeks 20-25; Continuation therapy: Weeks 29-34, and weeks 38-43 (Crist, 2001)

Wilms' tumor: IV:
Children <1 year: 0.75 mg/m^2/dose weekly for 10-11 weeks, then every 3 weeks for 15 additional weeks (total 25-26 weeks) (Pritchard, 1995)
Children ≥1 year: 1.5 mg/m^2/dose weekly for 10-11 weeks, then every 3 weeks for 15 additional weeks (total 25-26 weeks) (Pritchard, 1995)
or
Children ≤30 kg: 0.05 mg/kg/dose (maximum dose: 2 mg) weeks 1, 2, 4, 5, 6, 7, 8, 10, and 11, followed by 0.067 mg/kg/dose (maximum dose: 2 mg) weeks 12, 13, 18, and 24 (Green, 2007)
Children >30 kg: 1.5 mg/m^2/dose (maximum dose: 2 mg) weeks 1, 2, 4, 5, 6, 7, 8, 10, and 11, followed by 2 mg/m^2/dose (maximum dose: 2 mg) weeks 12, 13, 18, and 24 (Green, 2007)

Renal Impairment No dosage adjustment necessary (Kintzel, 1995).

Hepatic Impairment The manufacturer's labeling recommends the following adjustment: Serum bilirubin >3 mg/dL: Administer 50% of normal dose.
The following adjustments have also been recommended:
Floyd, 2006: Serum bilirubin 1.5-3 mg/dL or transaminases 2-3 times ULN or alkaline phosphatase increased: Administer 50% of dose.
Superfin, 2007:
Serum bilirubin 1.5-3 mg/dL: Administer 50% of dose.
Serum bilirubin >3 mg/dL: Avoid use.

Obesity ASCO Guidelines for appropriate chemotherapy dosing in obese adults with cancer: Dose should be capped at a maximum of 2 mg due to neurotoxicity concerns (Griggs, 2012)

Administration For IV administration only. FATAL IF GIVEN INTRATHECALLY.

In order to prevent inadvertent intrathecal administration, the World Health Organization (WHO) and the Institute for Safe Medication Practices (ISMP) strongly recommend dispensing vincristine in a minibag (**NOT** in a syringe). Vincristine should **NOT** be delivered to the patient at the same time with any medications intended for central nervous system administration.

IV: Preferred administration is as a short 5- to 10-minute infusion in a 25 to 50 mL minibag. If administration via minibag is not possible, may also be administered as a slow (1-minute) push. Some protocols utilize a 24-hour continuous infusion.

Vesicant; ensure proper needle or catheter placement prior to and during infusion. Avoid extravasation.

Extravasation management: If extravasation occurs, stop infusion immediately and disconnect (leave cannula/needle in place); gently aspirate extravasated solution (do **NOT** flush the line); initiate hyaluronidase antidote; remove needle/cannula; apply dry warm compresses for 20 minutes 4 times a day for 1 to 2 days; elevate (Perez Fidalgo, 2012). Remaining portion of the vincristine dose should be infused through a separate vein.
Hyaluronidase: If needle/cannula still in place, administer 1 to 6 mL hyaluronidase (150 units/mL) into the existing IV line; the usual dose is 1 mL hyaluronidase for each 1 mL of extravasated drug (Perez Fidalgo, 2012; Schulmeister, 2011). If needle/cannula was removed, inject 1 to 6 mL (150 units/mL) subcutaneously in a clockwise manner using 1 mL for each 1 mL of drug extravasated (Schulmeister, 2011) **or** administer 1 mL (150 units/mL) as 5 separate 0.2 mL injections (using a 25-gauge needle) subcutaneously into the extravasation site (Polovich, 2009).

Hazardous agent; use appropriate precautions for handling and disposal (NIOSH 2014 [group 1]).

Monitoring Parameters Serum electrolytes (sodium), hepatic function tests, CBC with differential, serum uric acid; monitor infusion site; neurologic examination, monitor for constipation/ileus and for signs/symptoms of peripheral neuropathy

Dosage Forms Excipient information presented when available (limited, particularly for generics); consult specific product labeling.

Solution, Intravenous, as sulfate:
Vincasar PFS: 1 mg/mL (1 mL, 2 mL)

Solution, Intravenous, as sulfate [preservative free]:
Generic: 1 mg/mL (1 mL, 2 mL)

VinCRIStine (Liposomal)
(vin KRIS teen lye po SO mal)

Brand Names: US Marqibo

Index Terms Liposomal Vincristine; Liposome Vincristine; Vincristine Liposome; Vincristine Sulfate Liposome; VSLI

Pharmacologic Category Antineoplastic Agent, Antimicrotubular; Antineoplastic Agent, Vinca Alkaloid

Use Treatment of relapsed Philadelphia chromosome-negative (Ph-) acute lymphoblastic leukemia (ALL) in adult patients whose disease has progressed after two or more antileukemic therapies

Pregnancy Considerations Adverse events (fetal malformations, decreased fetal weight, and fetal loss) were observed in animal reproduction studies at doses less than the recommended human dose. Given the mechanism of action, adverse fetal events would be expected to occur with use in pregnant women. Women of childbearing potential should avoid becoming pregnant during therapy.

Breast-Feeding Considerations Due to the potential for adverse reactions in the nursing infant, the decision to discontinue breast-feeding or to discontinue liposomal vincristine should take into account the benefits of treatment to the mother.

Contraindications Hypersensitivity to vincristine, liposomal vincristine, or any component of the formulation; patients with Charcot-Marie-Tooth syndrome or other demyelinating conditions; administration via the intrathecal route

Warnings/Precautions Hazardous agent - use appropriate precautions for handling and disposal (NIOSH 2014 [group 1]). **[US Boxed Warning]: For IV administration only. Intrathecal administration is contraindicated; inadvertent intrathecal administration has resulted in death.** Liposomal vincristine should **NOT** be prepared during the preparation of any intrathecal medications. After preparation, keep liposomal vincristine in a location **away** from the separate storage location recommended for intrathecal medications. Liposomal vincristine should **NOT** be delivered to the patient at the same time with any medications intended for central nervous system administration.

[US Boxed Warning]: Vincristine LIPOSOME and conventional vincristine are NOT interchangeable. Dosing differs between formulations; verify intended product and dose prior to preparation and administration to avoid overdoses. Avoid extravasation of liposomal vincristine (conventional vincristine is a vesicant). Only individuals experienced with vesicant administration should administer liposomal vincristine. Check for proper needle placement; if extravasation occurs, discontinue liposomal vincristine infusion immediately and institute appropriate extravasation management procedures.

Grade 3 and greater neutropenia, anemia, and thrombocytopenia were observed in clinical trials. Monitor blood counts closely and adjust dose or withhold therapy if necessary. Constipation, ileus, bowel obstruction, and colonic pseudo-obstruction have occurred with liposomal vincristine. Patients should be initiated on a prophylactic bowel regimen including a stool softener, dietary fiber, and hydration; laxative treatments may be considered. Severe fatigue was noted in clinical trials; treatment delay, dosage adjustment, or discontinuation may be necessary.

Neuropathies (sensory and motor) are common and cumulative. Neuropathy symptoms may include paresthesia, hyper-/hypoesthesia, hyporeflexia or areflexia, neuralgia, jaw pain, cranial neuropathy, ileus, arthralgia, myalgia, muscle spasm, and/or weakness. Evaluate neurologic status of patients closely prior to liposomal vincristine administration; neurologic toxicity risk is greater when given to patients with preexisting neuromuscular conditions or when used concomitantly with other neurotoxic agents. Treatment delay, dosage adjustment, and/or discontinuation may be necessary. Tumor lysis syndrome

may occur as a consequence of therapy; monitor closely for signs and symptoms and manage accordingly.

Hepatotoxicity (including fatal cases) and increased AST have been reported. Monitor hepatic function tests; reduce dose or interrupt therapy if necessary. Use caution in patients with hepatic impairment; liposomal vincristine has not been studied in patients with severe hepatic impairment. In a study in a limited number of melanoma patients with moderate (Child-Pugh class B) hepatic impairment secondary to liver metastases, C_{max} and AUC were comparable to those in patients with normal hepatic function; patients with hepatic impairment received a dose of 1 mg/m^2 every 2 weeks versus 2 mg/m^2 in subjects with normal hepatic function (Bedikian, 2011). Potentially significant drug-drug interactions may exist, requiring dose or frequency adjustment, additional monitoring, and/or selection of alternative therapy. Avoid concomitant therapy with strong CYP3A4 or P-glycoprotein (P-gp) inducers or inhibitors. Use with caution in the elderly patient population; conventional vincristine may cause or exacerbate hyponatremia or syndrome of inappropriate antidiuretic hormone secretion; monitor sodium closely with therapy initiation or dosage adjustments (Beers Criteria).

Adverse Reactions
>10%:
Central nervous system: Fever (43%), fatigue (41%), insomnia (32%)

Gastrointestinal: Constipation (57%), nausea (52%), diarrhea (37%), appetite decreased (33%)

Hematologic: Neutropenic fever (38%; grades 3/4: 31%), anemia (34%; grades 3/4: 17%), neutropenia (grades 3/4: 18%), thrombocytopenia (grades 3/4: 17%)

Hepatic: AST increased (grades 3/4: 6% to 11%)

Neuromuscular & skeletal: Peripheral neuropathy (39%; grades 3/4: 17%)

1% to 10%:
Cardiovascular: Cardiac arrest (grades 3/4: 6%), hypotension (grades 3/4: 6%)

Central nervous system: Pain (grades 3/4: 8%), mental status changes (grades 3/4: 4%)

Gastrointestinal: Abdominal pain (grades 3/4: 8%), ileus (grades 3/4: 6%)

Neuromuscular & skeletal: Weakness (grades 3/4: 5%), muscle weakness (grades 3/4: 1%)

Respiratory: Pneumonia (grades 3/4: 8%), respiratory distress (grades 3/4: 6%), respiratory failure (grades 3/4: 5%)

Miscellaneous: Septic shock (grades 3/4: 6%), staphylococcal bacteremia (grades 3/4: 6%)

Drug Interactions

Metabolism/Transport Effects Substrate of CYP3A4 (major), P-glycoprotein; **Note:** Assignment of Major/Minor substrate status based on clinically relevant drug interaction potential

Avoid Concomitant Use
Avoid concomitant use of VinCRIStine (Liposomal) with any of the following: BCG (Intravesical); Conivaptan; CYP3A4 Inducers (Strong); CYP3A4 Inhibitors (Strong); Deferiprone; Dexamethasone (Systemic); Dipyrone; Fusidic Acid (Systemic); Idelalisib; Natalizumab; P-glycoprotein/ABCB1 Inducers; P-glycoprotein/ABCB1 Inhibitors; Pimecrolimus; St Johns Wort; Tacrolimus (Topical); Tofacitinib; Vaccines (Live)

Increased Effect/Toxicity
VinCRIStine (Liposomal) may increase the levels/effects of: CloZAPine; Deferiprone; Fingolimod; Leflunomide; MitoMYcin (Systemic); Natalizumab; Tofacitinib; Vaccines (Live)

The levels/effects of VinCRIStine (Liposomal) may be increased by: Aprepitant; Conivaptan; CYP3A4 Inhibitors (Moderate); CYP3A4 Inhibitors (Strong); Dasatinib; Denosumab; Dipyrone; Fosaprepitant; Fusidic Acid (Systemic); Idelalisib; Luliconazole; Macrolide Antibiotics; Mifepristone; Netupitant; NIFEdipine; Osimertinib; Palbociclib; P-glycoprotein/ABCB1 Inhibitors; Pimecrolimus; Roflumilast; Stiripentol; Tacrolimus (Topical); Teniposide; Trastuzumab

Decreased Effect
VinCRIStine (Liposomal) may decrease the levels/effects of: BCG (Intravesical); Coccidioides immitis Skin Test; Sipuleucel-T; Vaccines (Inactivated); Vaccines (Live)

The levels/effects of VinCRIStine (Liposomal) may be decreased by: Bosentan; CYP3A4 Inducers (Moderate); CYP3A4 Inducers (Strong); Dabrafenib; Deferasirox; Dexamethasone (Systemic); Echinacea; Osimertinib; P-glycoprotein/ABCB1 Inducers; Siltuximab; St Johns Wort; Tocilizumab

Preparation for Administration Hazardous agent; use appropriate precautions for handling and disposal (NIOSH 2014 [group 1]). Vincristine liposome preparation requires 60-90 minutes of dedicated time utilizing the manufacturer supplied kit. Do not reuse kit components with future doses.

1). Outside the sterile area, fill a water bath to a depth of at least 8 cm (3.2 inches); water should be heated to and maintained at **63°C to 67°C** (145.4°F to 152.6°F) for the entire procedure (use calibrated thermometer to monitor temperature). Maintain water depth of at least 8 cm (3.2 inches) throughout process. Water bath must remain outside the sterile area.

2). In a biological safety cabinet, vent the sodium phosphate vial with a sterile venting needle (with a 0.2 micron filter or other suitable venting device). Venting needle should always be kept above liquid level. Remove 1 mL of sphingomyelin/cholesterol liposome injection and inject into the sodium phosphate vial. Withdraw 5 mL of vincristine sulfate injection and inject into the sodium phosphate vial. Remove the venting needle and gently invert the sodium phosphate vial 5 times to mix (do **not** shake). Place flotation ring on the sodium phosphate vial.

3). Confirm the water bath is maintained between **63°C to 67°C** (145.4°F to 152.6°F). Outside the sterile area, place constituted sodium phosphate vial in the water bath for 10 minutes. Record constitution start and stop time, as well as starting and ending water temperature. After 10 minutes, remove the vial (with tongs), remove flotation ring, then dry the vial, affix vial overlabel, and gently invert 5 times to mix (do **not** shake). Allow the vial to equilibrate for at least 30 minutes at room temperature of 15°C to 30°C (59°F to 86°F), but for no longer than 12 hours. Once prepared, vincristine sulfate liposome concentration is 5 mg/31 mL (0.16 mg/mL).

4). Return vial to biologic safety cabinet. Calculate patient's vincristine liposome dose (based on actual BSA); remove corresponding volume from 100 mL NS or D$_5$W infusion bag. Inject vincristine liposome dose into the infusion bag (final volume of 100 mL). Do not use if a precipitate or other foreign matter is present in the vial or infusion bag. The amount contained in each vial may exceed the prescribed dose; use care with dosage and volume calculations. Discard unused portion of the vial. After preparation, keep liposomal vincristine in a location away from the separate storage location recommended for intrathecal medications.

Storage/Stability Store intact kit (containing vincristine vial, sphingomyelin/cholesterol liposome vial, and sodium phosphate vial) refrigerated at 2°C to 8°C (36°F to 46°F); do not freeze. Use appropriate precautions for handling and disposal. Once prepared, liposomal vincristine is stable for no more than 12 hours at room temperature. After preparation, keep liposomal vincristine in a location away from the separate storage location recommended for intrathecal medications.

Mechanism of Action Vincristine is a cell cycle specific agent which binds to tubulin, leading to microtubule depolymerization and cellular apoptosis. The liposomal formulation increases the half-life, allowing for enhanced cytotoxic activity in tumor cells.

Pharmacodynamics/Kinetics
Distribution: V$_{dss}$: 2.7 L (Bedikian, 2006)
Metabolism: Primarily hepatic
Half-life elimination: 45 hours (urinary half-life); dependent on rate of vincristine release from sphingosome (Bedikian, 2006)
Excretion: Feces (69%); urine (<8%)

Dosing
Adult & Geriatric Note: Vincristine liposomal and conventional vincristine are **NOT** interchangeable. Dosing differs between formulations; verify intended product and dose prior to preparation and administration. The liposomal vincristine dose is based on actual body surface area (BSA) and was not capped in studies (O'Brien, 2009; Rodriguez, 2009; Silverman, 2010).

Acute lymphoblastic leukemia (ALL; Philadelphia chromosome-negative), relapsed: IV: 2.25 mg/m^2 once every 7 days

Renal Impairment No dosage adjustment provided in manufacturer's labeling (has not been studied); however, liposomal vincristine is minimally excreted by the kidney and like the conventional formulation, likely does not require dosage adjustment in renal impairment.

Hepatic Impairment
Moderate impairment (Child-Pugh class B): In a study in a limited number of melanoma patients with moderate (Child-Pugh class B) hepatic impairment secondary to liver metastases, C$_{max}$ and AUC were comparable to those in patients with normal hepatic function; patients with hepatic impairment received a dose of 1 mg/m^2

every 2 weeks versus 2 mg/m^2 in subjects with normal hepatic function (Bedikian, 2011).
Severe impairment (Child-Pugh class C): No dosage adjustment provided in manufacturer's labeling (has not been studied).
Hepatotoxicity during treatment: Reduce dose or interrupt treatment.

Adjustment for Toxicity
Fatigue, severe: Consider dose delay, reduction, or therapy discontinuation.
Hematologic toxicity: Grade 3 or 4 neutropenia, thrombocytopenia, or anemia: Consider dose reduction or modification.
Hepatic toxicity: Reduce dose or interrupt treatment.
Peripheral neuropathy:
Grade 3 or persistent grade 2 toxicity: Interrupt therapy until recovery to grade 1 or 2, then reduce dose to 2 mg/m^2. If grade 3 toxicity persists or if grade 4 toxicity occurs, discontinue liposomal vincristine.
Persistent grade 2 toxicity after first dose reduction to 2 mg/m^2: Interrupt therapy for up to 7 days until recovery to grade 1, then reduce dose to 1.825 mg/m^2. If neuropathy increases to grade 3 or 4, discontinue liposomal vincristine.
Persistent grade 2 toxicity after second dose reduction to 1.825 mg/m^2: Interrupt therapy for up to 7 days until recovery to grade 1, then reduce dose to 1.5 mg/m^2. If neuropathy increases to grade 3 or 4, discontinue liposomal vincristine.
Preexisting neuropathy, severe: Assess treatment benefit versus risk.

Administration Conventional vincristine is a vesicant. Limited information is available regarding liposomal vincristine extravasation, but may cause inflammation if extravasated; avoid extravasation. **For IV administration only. FATAL IF GIVEN INTRATHECALLY.** Liposomal vincristine should **NOT** be delivered to the patient at the same time as any medications intended for central nervous system administration.

IV: Infuse over 1 hour. Do not administer IV push or bolus; do not use with in-line filters. Infusion must be completed within 12 hours of preparation.

Hazardous agent; use appropriate precautions for handling and disposal (NIOSH 2014 [group 1]).

Monitoring Parameters CBC with differential and platelets; hepatic function; signs/symptoms of peripheral neuropathy or other neurologic toxicities; sodium (in elderly patients; conventional vincristine may cause or exacerbate hyponatremia or syndrome of inappropriate antidiuretic hormone secretion); signs/symptoms of tumor lysis syndrome; symptoms of constipation; monitor infusion site for extravasation

Additional Information The liposomal formulation of vincristine consists of vincristine encapsulated in sphingosomes, which are composed of sphingomyelin and cholesterol (Bedikian, 2006).

Dosage Forms Excipient information presented when available (limited, particularly for generics); consult specific product labeling.
Suspension, Intravenous, as sulfate:
Marqibo: 5 mg/31 mL (1 ea)

Vinorelbine (vi NOR el been)

Brand Names: US Navelbine
Brand Names: Canada Navelbine; Vinorelbine Injection, USP; Vinorelbine Tartrate for Injection
Index Terms Dihydroxydeoxynorvinkaleukoblastine; Vinorelbine Tartrate
Pharmacologic Category Antineoplastic Agent, Antimicrotubular; Antineoplastic Agent, Vinca Alkaloid
Use Treatment of non-small cell lung cancer (NSCLC)

Pregnancy Considerations Animal reproduction studies have demonstrated embryotoxicity, fetotoxicity, decreased fetal weight, and delayed ossification. May cause fetal harm if administered during pregnancy. Women of child-bearing potential should avoid becoming pregnant during vinorelbine treatment.

Breast-Feeding Considerations It is not known if vinorelbine is excreted in breast milk. Due to the potential for serious adverse reactions in the nursing infant, breast-feeding should be discontinued during treatment.

Contraindications Pretreatment granulocyte counts <1000/mm³

Warnings/Precautions Hazardous agent - use appropriate precautions for handling and disposal (NIOSH 2014 [group 1]). **[U.S. Boxed Warning]: For IV use only; intrathecal administration of other vinca alkaloids has resulted in death. If dispensed in a syringe, should be labeled "for intravenous use only - fatal if given intrathecally". [U.S. Boxed Warning]: Vesicant; ensure proper needle or catheter placement prior to and during infusion. Avoid extravasation. Extravasation may cause local tissue necrosis and/or thrombophlebitis. [U.S. Boxed Warning]: Severe granulocytopenia may occur with treatment (may lead to infection); granulocyte counts should be ≥1000 cells/mm³ prior to treatment initiation; dosage adjustment may be required based on blood counts (monitor blood counts prior to each dose).** Granulocytopenia is a dose-limiting toxicity; nadir is generally 7-10 days after administration and recovery occurs within the following 7-14 days. Monitor closely for infections and/or fever in patients with severe granulocytopenia. Use with extreme caution in patients with compromised marrow reserve due to prior chemotherapy or radiation therapy.

Fatal cases of interstitial pulmonary changes and ARDS have been reported (with single-agent therapy (mean onset of symptoms: 1 week); promptly evaluate changes in baseline pulmonary symptoms or any new onset pulmonary symptoms (eg, dyspnea, cough, hypoxia). Acute shortness of breath and severe bronchospasm have been reported with vinca alkaloids; usually associated with the concurrent administration of mitomycin.

Vinorelbine should **NOT** be prepared during the preparation of any intrathecal medications. After preparation, keep vinorelbine in a location **away** from the separate storage location recommended for intrathecal medications. Elimination is predominantly hepatic; while there is no evidence that toxicity is enhanced in patients with elevated transaminases, use with caution in patients with severe hepatic injury or impairment; dosage modification required for elevated total bilirubin. May cause new onset or worsening of preexisting neuropathy; use with caution in patients with neuropathy; monitor for new or worsening sign/symptoms of neuropathy; dosage adjustment required. May cause severe constipation (grade 3-4), paralytic ileus, intestinal obstruction, necrosis, and/or perforation; some events were fatal. Oral vinorelbine (not available in the U.S.) is associated with a moderate antiemetic potential; antiemetics are recommended to prevent nausea/vomiting (Dupuis, 2011; Roila, 2010); IV vinorelbine has a minimal emetic potential (Dupuis, 2011; Roila, 2010). Potentially significant drug-drug interactions may exist, requiring dose or frequency adjustment, additional monitoring, and/or selection of alternative therapy. May have radiosensitizing effects with prior or concurrent radiation therapy; radiation recall reactions may occur in patients who have received prior radiation therapy. Avoid eye contamination (exposure may cause severe irritation). **[U.S. Boxed Warning]: Should be administered under the supervision of an experienced cancer chemotherapy physician.**

Adverse Reactions Note: Reported with single-agent therapy.

>10%:
Central nervous system: Fatigue (27%)
Dermatologic: Alopecia (12% to 30%)
Gastrointestinal: Nausea (31% to 44%; grade 3: 1% to 2%), constipation (35%; grade 3: 3%), vomiting (20% to 31%; grade 3: 1% to 2%), diarrhea (12% to 17%)
Hematologic: Leukopenia (83% to 92%; grade 4: 6% to 15%), granulocytopenia (90%; grade 4: 36%; nadir: 7-10 days; recovery 14-21 days), neutropenia (85%; grade 4: 28%), anemia (83%; grades 3/4: 9%)
Hepatic: AST increased (67%; grade 3: 5%; grade 4: 1%), total bilirubin increased (5% to 13%; grade 3: 4%; grade 4: 3%)
Local: Injection site reaction (22% to 28%; includes erythema, vein discoloration), injection site pain (16%)
Neuromuscular & skeletal: Weakness (36%), peripheral neuropathy (25%; grade 3: 1%; grade 4: <1%)
Renal: Creatinine increased (13%)

1% to 10%:
Cardiovascular: Chest pain (5%)
Dermatologic: Rash (<5%)
Gastrointestinal: Paralytic ileus (1%)
Hematologic: Neutropenic fever/sepsis (8%; grade 4: 4%), thrombocytopenia (3% to 5%; grades 3/4: 1%)
Local: Phlebitis (7% to 10%)
Neuromuscular & skeletal: Loss of deep tendon reflexes (<5%), myalgia (<5%), arthralgia (<5%), jaw pain (<5%)
Otic: Ototoxicity (≤1%)
Respiratory: Dyspnea (7%)
<1% (Limited to important or life-threatening): Abdominal pain, allergic reactions, anaphylaxis, angioedema, back pain, DVT, dysphagia, esophagitis, flushing, gait instability, headache, hemolytic uremic syndrome, hemorrhagic cystitis, hyper-/hypotension, hyponatremia, intestinal necrosis, intestinal obstruction, intestinal perforation, interstitial pulmonary changes, local rash, local urticaria, MI (rare), mucositis, muscle weakness, myocardial ischemia, pancreatitis, paralytic ileus, pneumonia, pruritus, pulmonary edema, pulmonary embolus, radiation recall (dermatitis, esophagitis), skin blistering, syndrome of inappropriate ADH secretion, tachycardia, thromboembolic events, thrombotic thrombocytopenic purpura, tumor pain, urticaria, vasodilation

Drug Interactions

Metabolism/Transport Effects Substrate of CYP2D6 (minor), CYP3A4 (minor); **Note:** Assignment of Major/Minor substrate status based on clinically relevant drug interaction potential; **Inhibits** CYP2D6 (weak)

Avoid Concomitant Use
Avoid concomitant use of Vinorelbine with any of the following: BCG (Intravesical); Deferiprone; Dipyrone; Natalizumab; Pimecrolimus; Tacrolimus (Topical); Tofacitinib; Vaccines (Live)

Increased Effect/Toxicity
Vinorelbine may increase the levels/effects of: ARIPiprazole; CloZAPine; Deferiprone; Fingolimod; Leflunomide; MitoMYcin (Systemic); Natalizumab; Tofacitinib; Vaccines (Live)

The levels/effects of Vinorelbine may be increased by: CISplatin; CYP3A4 Inhibitors (Strong); Denosumab; Dipyrone; Gefitinib; Macrolide Antibiotics; PACLitaxel (Conventional); PACLitaxel (Protein Bound); Pimecrolimus; Posaconazole; Roflumilast; Tacrolimus (Topical); Trastuzumab; Voriconazole

Decreased Effect
Vinorelbine may decrease the levels/effects of: BCG (Intravesical); Coccidioides immitis Skin Test; Sipuleucel-T; Vaccines (Inactivated); Vaccines (Live)

The levels/effects of Vinorelbine may be decreased by: Echinacea

Preparation for Administration Hazardous agent; use appropriate precautions for handling and disposal (NIOSH 2014 [group 1]). Dilute in D₅W or NS to a final concentration of 1.5-3 mg/mL (for syringe) or D₅W, NS, ½NS, D₅½NS, LR, or Ringer's to a final concentration of 0.5-2 mg/mL (for IV bag). Vinorelbine should **NOT** be prepared during the preparation of any intrathecal medications.

Storage/Stability Store intact vials refrigerated at 2°C to 8°C (36°F to 46°F); do not freeze. Protect from light. Intact vials are stable at room temperature of 25°C (77°F) for up to 72 hours. Solutions diluted for infusion in polypropylene syringes or polyvinyl chloride bags are stable for 24 hours at 5°C to 30°C (41°F to 86°F). After preparation, keep vinorelbine in a location **away** from the separate storage location recommended for intrathecal medications.

Mechanism of Action Semisynthetic vinca alkaloid which binds to tubulin and inhibits microtubule formation, therefore, arresting the cell at metaphase by disrupting the formation of the mitotic spindle; it is specific for the M and S phases. Vinorelbine may also interfere with nucleic acid and protein synthesis by blocking glutamic acid utilization.

Pharmacodynamics/Kinetics
Distribution: V_d: 25-40 L/kg; binds extensively to human platelets and lymphocytes (80% to 91%)
Protein binding: 80% to 91%
Metabolism: Extensively hepatic, via CYP3A4, to two metabolites, deacetylvinorelbine (active) and vinorelbine N-oxide
Half-life elimination: Triphasic: Terminal: 28-44 hours
Excretion: Feces (46%); urine (18%, 10% to 12% as unchanged drug)

Dosing

Adult & Geriatric
Non-small cell lung cancer (NSCLC): IV:
Single-agent therapy: 30 mg/m² every 7 days until disease progression or unacceptable toxicity

Combination therapy: 25-30 mg/m² every 7 days (in combination with cisplatin)

Off-label dosing: 25 mg/m² days 1 and 8 every 21 days (in combination with cisplatin and cetuximab) for up to 6 cycles (Pirker, 2009) **or** 25-30 mg/m² days 1, 8, and 15 every 28 days (in combination with gemcitabine) for 6 cycles **or** until disease progression or unacceptable toxicity (Herbst, 2002; Greco, 2007)

Breast cancer, metastatic (off-label use): IV: 25 mg/m² every 7 days (as a single agent) until disease progression or unacceptable toxicity (Zelek, 2001) **or** 30 mg/m² every 7 days (as a single agent); after 13 weeks, may administer every 14 days for patient convenience, continue until disease progression or unacceptable toxicity (Vogel, 1999) **or** 25 mg/m² every 7 days (in combination with trastuzumab) until disease progression or unacceptable toxicity (Burstein, 2001; Burstein 2007) **or** 30 or 35 mg/m² days 1 and 8 every 21 days (in combination with trastuzumab) until disease progression or unacceptable toxicity (Andersson, 2011)

Cervical cancer (off-label use): IV: 30 mg/m² days 1 and 8 of a of a 21-day treatment cycle (Muggia, 2004; Muggia, 2005)

Hodgkin lymphoma, relapsed or refractory (off-label use): IV:

GVD regimen: 15 mg/m² (post-transplant patients) or 20 mg/m² (transplant-naïve patients) on days 1 and 8 of a 21-day cycle (in combination with gemcitabine and doxorubicin liposomal) for 2 to 6 cycles (Bartlett, 2007)

IGEV regimen: 20 mg/m² on day 1 of a 21-day cycle (in combination with ifosfamide, mesna, gemcitabine, and prednisolone) for 4 cycles (Santoro, 2007)

Malignant pleural mesothelioma (off-label use): IV: 30 mg/m² (maximum dose: 60 mg) every 7 days per 6-week treatment cycle, continue until disease progression (Stebbing, 2009) **or** 30 mg/m² (maximum dose: 60 mg) every 7 days for 6 weeks, off 2 weeks, then repeat cycle (Muers, 2008)

Ovarian cancer, relapsed (off-label use): IV: 25 mg/m² every 7 days (Bajetta, 1996) **or** 30 mg/m² days 1 and 8 of a 21-day treatment cycle (Rothenberg, 2004) until disease progression or unacceptable toxicity

Salivary gland cancer, recurrent (off-label use): IV: 25 mg/m² on days 1 and 8 of a 21-day cycle (in combination with cisplatin) for a minimum of 3 cycles and for up to 6 cycles (Airoldi, 2001) **or** 30 mg/m² every 7 days (monotherapy) for a minimum of 9 weeks and for up to 6 cycles (Airoldi, 2001)

Small cell lung cancer, refractory (off-label use): IV: 25 or 30 mg/m² every 7 days until disease progression or unacceptable toxicity (Furuse, 1996; Jessem, 1993)

Soft tissue sarcoma, advanced (off-label use): IV: 25 mg/m² days 1 and 8 of a 21-day treatment cycle (in combination with gemcitabine) until disease progression or unacceptable toxicity (Dileo, 2007)

Renal Impairment

Renal insufficiency: No dosage adjustment necessary.

Hemodialysis: Initial: IV: Reduce dose to 20 mg/m²/week; administer either after dialysis (on dialysis days) or on nondialysis days (Janus, 2010)

Hepatic Impairment Note: In patients with concurrent hematologic toxicity and hepatic impairment, administer the lower of the doses determined from the adjustment recommendations.

Administer with caution in patients with hepatic insufficiency. In patients who develop hyperbilirubinemia during treatment with vinorelbine, the dose should be adjusted for total bilirubin as follows:

Serum bilirubin ≤2 mg/dL: Administer 100% of dose

Serum bilirubin 2.1-3 mg/dL: Administer 50% of dose (Ecklund, 2005; Floyd, 2006; Superfin, 2006)

Serum bilirubin >3 mg/dL: Administer 25% of dose (Ecklund, 2005; Floyd, 2006; Superfin, 2006)

Patients (breast cancer) with extensive liver metastases (>75% of liver volume): Administer 50% of dose (Ecklund, 2005; Superfin, 2006)

Obesity *ASCO Guidelines for appropriate chemotherapy dosing in obese adults with cancer:* Utilize patient's actual body weight (full weight) for calculation of body surface area- or weight-based dosing, particularly when the intent of therapy is curative; manage regimen-related toxicities in the same manner as for nonobese patients; if a dose reduction is utilized due to toxicity, consider resumption of full weight-based dosing with subsequent cycles, especially if cause of toxicity (eg, hepatic or renal impairment) is resolved (Griggs, 2012).

Adjustment for Toxicity Note: In patients with concurrent hematologic toxicity and hepatic impairment, administer the lower of the doses determined from the adjustment recommendations.

Dosage adjustment in hematological toxicity (based on granulocyte counts):

Granulocytes ≥1500 cells/mm³ on day of treatment: Administer 100% of starting dose.

Granulocytes 1000-1499 cells/mm³ on day of treatment: Administer 50% of starting dose.

Granulocytes <1000 cells/mm³ on day of treatment: Do not administer. Repeat granulocyte count in 1 week. If 3 consecutive doses are held because granulocyte count is <1000 cells/mm³, discontinue vinorelbine.

Adjustment: For patients who, during treatment, have experienced fever or sepsis while granulocytopenic or had 2 consecutive weekly doses held due to granulocytopenia, subsequent doses of vinorelbine should be:

75% of starting dose for granulocytes ≥1500 cells/mm³

37.5% of starting dose for granulocytes 1000-1499 cells/mm³

Dosage adjustment for neurotoxicity: Neurotoxicity ≥ grade 2: Discontinue treatment

Dosage adjustment for other adverse events: Severe adverse events: Reduce dose or discontinue treatment

Administration For IV use only; **FATAL IF GIVEN INTRATHECALLY.** Administer as a direct intravenous push or rapid bolus, over 6-10 minutes (up to 30 minutes). Longer infusions may increase the risk of pain and phlebitis. Intravenous doses should be followed by at least 75-125 mL of saline or D_5W to reduce the incidence of phlebitis and inflammation.

Vesicant; ensure proper needle or catheter position prior to administration. Avoid extravasation.

Extravasation management: If extravasation occurs, stop infusion immediately and disconnect (leave cannula/needle in place); gently aspirate extravasated solution (do **NOT** flush the line); initiate hyaluronidase antidote; remove needle/cannula; apply dry warm compresses for 20 minutes 4 times a day for 1-2 days; elevate extremity (Perez Fidalgo, 2012). Remaining portion of the vinorelbine dose should be infused through a separate vein.

Hyaluronidase: If needle/cannula still in place, administer 1-6 mL hyaluronidase (150 units/mL) into the existing IV line; the usual dose is 1 mL hyaluronidase for each 1 mL of extravasated drug (Perez Fidalgo, 2012; Schulmeister, 2011). If needle/cannula was removed, inject 1-6 mL (150 units/mL) subcutaneously in a clockwise manner using 1mL for each 1 mL of drug extravasated (Schulmeister, 2011) **or** administer 1 mL (150 units/mL) as 5 separate 0.2 mL injections (using a 25-gauge needle) subcutaneously into the extravasation site (Polovich, 2009).

Hazardous agent; use appropriate precautions for handling and disposal (NIOSH 2014 [group 1]).

Monitoring Parameters CBC with differential and platelet count (prior to each dose, and after treatment), hepatic function tests; monitor for new-onset pulmonary symptoms (or worsening from baseline); monitor for neuropathy (new or worsening symptoms; monitor infusion site; monitor for signs symptoms of constipation/ileus

Dosage Forms Excipient information presented when available (limited, particularly for generics); consult specific product labeling.

Solution, Intravenous:

Navelbine: 10 mg/mL (1 mL); 50 mg/5 mL (5 mL)

Generic: 10 mg/mL (1 mL); 50 mg/5 mL (5 mL)

Solution, Intravenous [preservative free]:

Generic: 10 mg/mL (1 mL); 50 mg/5 mL (5 mL)

◆ **Vinorelbine Injection, USP (Can)** *see* Vinorelbine *on page 1901*

◆ **Vinorelbine Tartrate** *see* Vinorelbine *on page 1901*

◆ **Vinorelbine Tartrate for Injection (Can)** *see* Vinorelbine *on page 1901*

◆ **Viokace** *see* Pancrelipase *on page 1384*

◆ **Viokase (Can)** *see* Pancrelipase *on page 1384*

◆ **Viorele** *see* Ethinyl Estradiol and Desogestrel *on page 701*

◆ **Viosterol** *see* Ergocalciferol *on page 663*

◆ **Viracept** *see* Nelfinavir *on page 1266*

◆ **Viramune** *see* Nevirapine *on page 1270*

◆ **Viramune XR** *see* Nevirapine *on page 1270*

◆ **Virazole** *see* Ribavirin (Oral Inhalation) *on page 1578*

◆ **Virdec [OTC] [DSC]** *see* Chlorpheniramine and Phenylephrine *on page 376*

◆ **Virdec DM [OTC] [DSC]** *see* Chlorpheniramine, Phenylephrine, and Dextromethorphan *on page 378*

◆ **Viread** *see* Tenofovir Disoproxil Fumarate *on page 1756*

- Viroptic see Trifluridine on page 1844
- Viroptic® (Can) see Trifluridine on page 1844
- Virt-Gard see Folic Acid, Cyanocobalamin, and Pyridoxine on page 805
- Virt-Phos 250 Neutral see Potassium Phosphate and Sodium Phosphate on page 1484
- Virtrate-2 see Sodium Citrate and Citric Acid on page 1673
- Virtrate-3 see Citric Acid, Sodium Citrate, and Potassium Citrate on page 400
- Virtrate-K see Potassium Citrate and Citric Acid on page 1481
- Virtussin A/C see Guaifenesin and Codeine on page 861
- Virtussin DAC see Guaifenesin, Pseudoephedrine, and Codeine on page 863
- Virt-Vite see Folic Acid, Cyanocobalamin, and Pyridoxine on page 805
- Virt-Vite Forte see Folic Acid, Cyanocobalamin, and Pyridoxine on page 805
- Viscoat see Sodium Chondroitin Sulfate and Sodium Hyaluronate on page 1673
- Viscous Lidocaine see Lidocaine (Topical) on page 1074
- Visine-A [OTC] see Naphazoline and Pheniramine on page 1256
- Visine Advanced Allergy (Can) see Naphazoline and Pheniramine on page 1256
- Visken (Can) see Pindolol on page 1454

Vismodegib (vis moe DEG ib)

Brand Names: US Erivedge
Brand Names: Canada Erivedge
Index Terms GDC-0449; Hedgehog Antagonist GDC-0449
Pharmacologic Category Antineoplastic Agent, Hedgehog Pathway Inhibitor
Use Basal cell carcinoma, metastatic or locally advanced: Treatment of metastatic basal cell carcinoma, or locally-advanced basal cell carcinoma that has recurred following surgery or in patients who are not candidates for surgery, and not candidates for radiation therapy

Pregnancy Considerations [US Boxed Warning]: May result in severe birth defects or embryo-fetal death. Teratogenic effects (severe midline defects, missing digits, and other irreversible malformations), embryotoxic, and fetotoxic events were observed in animal reproduction studies when administered in doses less than the normal human dose. Based on its mechanism of action adverse effects on pregnancy would be expected. [US Boxed Warning]: Verify pregnancy status (in females of reproductive potential) within 7 days prior to initiating treatment and advise patients (female and male) of the risk of birth defects, the need for contraception and risk of exposure through semen and to use condoms with a pregnant partner or a female partner of childbearing potential. In females of childbearing potential, obtain pregnancy test within 7 days prior to treatment initiation; after the negative pregnancy test, initiate highly effective contraception prior to the first vismodegib dose and continue during and for 7 months after treatment. During treatment (including treatment interruptions) and for 3 months after treatment, male patients should not donate sperm and should use condoms with spermicide (even after vasectomy) if their partner is of childbearing potential.

Women exposed to vismodegib during pregnancy (directly or via seminal fluid) are encouraged to participate in the Erivedge Pregnancy Pharmacovigilance program by contacting the Genentech Adverse Event Line (1-888-835-2555). Pregnancies occurring during or within 7 months after treatment should be reported to the Genentech Adverse Event Line.

The Canadian labeling recommends that females of childbearing potential use 2 simultaneous forms of effective contraception beginning at least 4 weeks prior to treatment initiation, during treatment (including treatment interruptions), and for 24 months after discontinuation. Pregnancy testing should be performed within 7 days prior to treatment initiation, monthly during treatment (including treatment interruptions) and for 24 months after discontinuation. For females of child bearing potential, a new prescription is required each month to allow for monthly pregnancy testing. Any suspected exposure (directly or via seminal fluid) during pregnancy should be immediately reported to the Erivedge Pregnancy Prevention Program (EPPP) at 1-888-748-8926.

Breast-Feeding Considerations It is not known if vismodegib is excreted in breast milk. Due to the potential for serious adverse reactions in the nursing infant, breast-feeding is not recommended by the manufacturer during therapy and for 7 months after treatment. The Canadian labeling contraindicates use in women who are nursing and recommends that women abstain from nursing for 24 months after discontinuation of therapy.

Prescribing and Access Restrictions
U.S.: Available at specialty pharmacies through the Erivedge Access Solutions program. Further information may be obtained from the manufacturer, Genentech, at 1-888-249-4918, or at www.ErivedgeAccessSolutions.com

Canada: Available through a controlled distribution program called Erivedge Pregnancy Prevention Program (EPPP). Registration with the program is required for participating prescribers and pharmacies. Patients must also be registered with the program and meet all necessary requirements to receive vismodegib. Consult product monograph for detailed information regarding program requirements. Further information may also be obtained at 1-888-748-8926 or at www.erivedge.ca.

Medication Guide Available Yes
Contraindications
US labeling: There are no contraindications listed in the manufacturer's labeling.
Canadian labeling: Hypersensitivity to vismodegib or any component of the formulation; pregnancy or females at risk of becoming pregnant; breast-feeding; male patients or female patients of childbearing potential who do not comply with the Erivedge Pregnancy Prevention Program; children and adolescents <18 years of age.

Warnings/Precautions Hazardous agent - use appropriate precautions for handling and disposal (meets NIOSH 2014 criteria). **[U.S. Boxed Warnings]: May result in severe birth defects or embryo-fetal death. Teratogenic effects (severe midline defects, missing digits, and other irreversible malformations), embryotoxic, and fetotoxic events were observed in animal reproduction studies. Verify pregnancy status (in females of reproductive potential) within 7 days prior to initiating treatment and advise patients (female and male) of the risk of birth defects, the need for contraception and risk of exposure through semen and to use condoms with a pregnant partner or a female partner of childbearing potential.** Amenorrhea was observed in women of reproductive potential; it is unknown if this is reversible.

Cardiac events (eg, cardiac failure, atrial fibrillation, left ventricular dysfunction, restrictive cardiomyopathy, myocardial infarction) have been observed during treatment. All events ≥ grade 3 occurred in patients with a history of significant cardiac disease. Cases of cutaneous squamous cell cancer (cuSCC) have been reported. Patients with advanced basal cell carcinoma are at risk for developing cuSCC; monitor during treatment. Vismodegib is associated with a moderate emetic potential; antiemetics may be needed to prevent nausea and vomiting. Diarrhea, constipation, abdominal pain, and decreased appetite may also occur.

Vismodegib metabolism is primarily hepatic. Elevated liver function tests (ALT, AST, total bilirubin, and alkaline phosphatase) have been observed; cases of cholestasis, hepatitis, and hepatocellular injury have also been reported. Monitor liver function tests; may require treatment interruption or discontinuation (Erivedge Canadian product monograph, 2015). Population pharmacokinetic analyses demonstrate that creatinine clearance (range: 30 to 80 mL/minute) does not have a clinically meaningful effect on systemic exposure; urinary excretion is <5%.

Advise patients not to donate blood or blood products during vismodegib treatment and for at least 7 months after the last vismodegib dose. The Canadian labeling recommends patients not donate blood or blood products during treatment (including treatment interruptions) and for 24 months after discontinuation. Vismodegib is present in semen, although the amount of drug in semen that may cause embryotoxicity and/or fetotoxicity is not known. Advise patients not to donate sperm during vismodegib treatment and for 3 months after the last vismodegib dose. In a study of vismodegib in patients with basal cell nevus syndrome (not an approved use), with discontinuation of vismodegib treatment, taste alteration and muscle cramps abated within 1 month, and scalp and body hair began to regrow within 3 months (Tang 2012). Potentially significant drug-drug interactions may exist, requiring dose or frequency adjustment, additional monitoring, and/or selection of alternative therapy.

Adverse Reactions

>10%:
Central nervous system: Fatigue (40%)
Dermatologic: Alopecia (64%)
Endocrine & metabolic: Amenorrhea (30%)
Gastrointestinal: Dysgeusia (55%), weight loss (45%), nausea (30%), diarrhea (29%), decreased appetite (25%), constipation (21%), vomiting (14%), ageusia (11%)
Neuromuscular & skeletal: Muscle spasm (72%), arthralgia (16%)
1% to 10%:
Endocrine & metabolic: Hyponatremia (grade 3: 4%), hypokalemia (grade 3: 1%)
Renal: Azotemia (grade 3: 2%)
<1% (Limited to important or life-threatening): Cholestasis, hepatic injury, hepatitis, rhabdomyolysis

Drug Interactions

Metabolism/Transport Effects Substrate of CYP2C9 (minor), CYP3A4 (minor), P-glycoprotein; **Note:** Assignment of Major/Minor substrate status based on clinically relevant drug interaction potential; **Inhibits** BCRP, CYP2C19 (weak), CYP2C9 (weak)
Avoid Concomitant Use There are no known interactions where it is recommended to avoid concomitant use.
Increased Effect/Toxicity There are no known significant interactions involving an increase in effect.
Decreased Effect There are no known significant interactions involving a decrease in effect.
Storage/Stability Store at 20°C to 25°C (68°F to 77°F); excursions permitted to 15°C to 30°C (59°F to 86°F).
Mechanism of Action Basal cell cancer is associated with mutations in Hedgehog pathway components. Hedgehog regulates cell growth and differentiation in embryogenesis; while generally not active in adult tissue, Hedgehog mutations associated with basal cell cancer can activate the pathway resulting in unrestricted proliferation of skin basal cells. Vismodegib is a selective Hedgehog pathway inhibitor which binds to and inhibits Smoothened homologue (SMO), the transmembrane protein involved in Hedgehog signal transduction.

Pharmacodynamics/Kinetics

Distribution: V_d: 16.4 to 26.6 L
Males: In a small pharmacokinetic study, the average vismodegib concentration in semen was 6.5% of the average steady state plasma concentration on day 8
Protein binding: >99%; primarily to serum albumin and alpha$_1$ acid glycoprotein (AAG)
Metabolism: Metabolized by oxidation, glucuronidation, and pyridine ring cleavage, although >98% of circulating components are as the parent drug
Bioavailability: ~32%
Half-life, elimination: Continuous daily dosing: ~4 days; Single dose: ~12 days
Time to peak: ~2.4 days (Graham, 2011)
Excretion: Feces (82%); urine (4%)

Dosing

Adult Note: Vismodegib is associated with a moderate emetic potential; antiemetics may be needed to prevent nausea and vomiting.

Basal cell carcinoma, metastatic or locally advanced:
Oral: 150 mg once daily until disease progression or unacceptable toxicity.
Missed doses: If a dose is missed, do not make up; resume dosing with the next scheduled dose.
Renal Impairment No dosage adjustment necessary.
Hepatic Impairment No dosage adjustment necessary.
Adjustment for Toxicity In clinical trials, no dosage reductions were allowed for toxicities, however, treatment interruptions up to 4 to 8 weeks were allowed for toxicity recovery (Basset-Seguin 2015; Sekulik 2012).
Administration Oral: May be taken with or without food. Swallow capsules whole; do not open or crush. Vismodegib is associated with a moderate emetic potential; antiemetics may be needed to prevent nausea and vomiting. Hazardous agent; use appropriate precautions for handling and disposal (meets NIOSH 2014 criteria).
Monitoring Parameters Pregnancy test within 1 week prior to treatment initiation.

Canadian labeling: Pregnancy testing (minimum sensitivity of 25 milliunits/mL) within 1 week prior to treatment initiation, monthly during treatment (including during treatment interruptions), and for 24 months after discontinuation; CBC with differential and comprehensive metabolic panel at baseline and every 4 weeks thereafter; liver function tests; skin examination routinely during therapy.

Dosage Forms Excipient information presented when available (limited, particularly for generics); consult specific product labeling.
Capsule, Oral:
Erivedge: 150 mg

◆ Vistaril *see* HydrOXYzine *on page 898*
◆ Vistide *see* Cidofovir *on page 384*
◆ Vistogard *see* Uridine Triacetate *on page 1854*
◆ Vistonuridine *see* Uridine Triacetate *on page 1854*
◆ VIT 45 *see* Ferric Carboxymaltose *on page 759*
◆ Vita-C [OTC] *see* Ascorbic Acid *on page 155*
◆ Vitamin C *see* Ascorbic Acid *on page 155*
◆ Vitamin D₃ and Alendronate *see* Alendronate and Cholecalciferol *on page 68*
◆ Vitamin D and Calcium Carbonate *see* Calcium and Vitamin D *on page 286*

Vitamin A (VYE ta min aye)

Brand Names: US A-25 [OTC]; AFirm 1X [OTC]; AFirm 2X [OTC]; AFirm 3X [OTC]; Aquasol A; Gordons-Vite A [OTC]; Vitamin A Fish [OTC]
Index Terms Oleovitamin A
Pharmacologic Category Vitamin, Fat Soluble
Use Treatment and prevention of vitamin A deficiency; parenteral (IM) route is indicated when oral administration is not feasible or when absorption is insufficient (malabsorption syndrome); dietary supplement (OTC)

Dosing

Adult & Geriatric
Dietary Reference Intake for vitamin A (presented as retinol activity equivalent [RAE]) (IOM, 2000): Oral:
Recommended dietary allowance (RDA):
Males: 900 mcg/day (3000 units/day)
Females: 700 mcg/day (2330 units/day)
Pregnant females ≥19 years: 770 mcg/day (2560 units/day)
Lactating females ≥19 years: 1300 mcg/day (4330 units/day)
Deficiency (manufacturer recommendation): IM:
Note: IM route is indicated when oral administration is not feasible or when absorption is insufficient (malabsorption syndrome): 100,000 units/day for 3 days, followed by 50,000 units/day for 2 weeks
Note: Follow-up therapy with an oral therapeutic multivitamin (containing additional vitamin A) is recommended: Oral: 10,000-20,000 units/day for 2 months
High-dose supplementation in patients at high risk for deficiency (off-label dose) (eg, persons living in developing areas of the world where deficiency is a public health problem, especially persons with severe infectious disease or malnutrition): Oral:
Adults: 200,000 units/dose every 6 months (WHO, 2008)
Pregnant females: Maximum 10,000 units daily or 25,000 units once weekly. Administer for a minimum of 12 weeks during pregnancy or until delivery (WHO, 2008; WHO, 2011c)
Postpartum females: 200,000 units at delivery or within 8 weeks of delivery (WHO, 2008)
Treatment of xerophthalmia (off-label use): Oral:
Adults (except females of reproductive age): 200,000 units once daily for 2 days; repeat with single dose after 2 weeks (WHO, 2008)
Females of reproductive age (WHO, 1997; WHO, 2008):
With night blindness or Bitot's spots (less severe xerophthalmia): 5000-10,000 units daily (maximum 10,000 units/day) or ≤25,000 units once weekly for ≥4 weeks
Severe xerophthalmia: Refer to adult dosing.
Pediatric
Dietary Reference Intake for vitamin A (presented as retinol activity equivalent [RAE]) (IOM, 2000): Oral:
Adequate intake (AI):
1-6 months: 400 mcg/day (1330 units/day)
7-12 months: 500 mcg/day (1670 units/day)
Recommended dietary allowance (RDA):
1-3 years: 300 mcg/day (1000 units/day)
4-8 years: 400 mcg/day (1330 units/day)
9-13 years: 600 mcg/day (2000 units/day)
Males >13 years: 900 mcg/day (3000 units/day)
Females >13 years: 700 mcg/day (2330 units/day)
Pregnant females 14-18 years: 750 mcg/day (2500 units/day)
Lactating females 14-18 years: 1200 mcg/day (4000 units/day)

Deficiency (manufacturer recommendation): IM:
Note: IM route is indicated when oral administration is not feasible or when absorption is insufficient (malabsorption syndrome):
Infants: 7500-15,000 units/day for 10 days
Children 1-8 years: 17,500-35,000 units/day for 10 days
Children >8 years: Refer to adult dosing.
Note: Follow-up therapy with an oral therapeutic multivitamin (containing additional vitamin A) is recommended: Oral:
Low Birth Weight Infants: Additional vitamin A is recommended; however, no dosage amount has been established.
Children ≤8 years: 5000-10,000 units/day for 2 months
Children >8 years: Refer to adult dosing.
High-dose supplementation in patients at high risk for deficiency (off-label dose) (eg, persons living in developing areas of the world where deficiency is a public health problem, especially persons with severe infectious disease or malnutrition): Oral:
Infants <6 months: Not recommended (WHO, 2011a)
Infants 6-12 months: 100,000 units/dose; repeat every 4-6 months, but do not readminister within 30 days of previous dose (WHO, 1997; WHO, 2010)
Children >1 year: 200,000 units/dose; repeat every 4-6 months, but do not readminister within 30 days of previous dose (WHO, 1997; WHO, 2010)
Treatment of measles (off-label use) (WHO, 2004; WHO, 2010): Oral: **Note:** Repeat with single dose in 2-4 weeks if severe malnutrition exists or ophthalmic evidence of a vitamin deficiency is present:
Infants <6 months: 50,000 units once daily for 2 days
Infants 6-11 months: 100,000 units once daily for 2 days
Children >11 months to 5 years: 200,000 units once daily for 2 days
Treatment of xerophthalmia (off-label use): Oral:
Infants <6 months: 50,000 units once daily for 2 days; repeat with single dose after 2 weeks (WHO, 2010)
Infants 6-12 months: 100,000 units once daily for 2 days; repeat with single dose after 2 weeks (WHO, 2010)
Children >1 year (except females of reproductive age): 200,000 units once daily for 2 days; repeat with single dose after 2 weeks (WHO, 2008)
Females of reproductive age: Refer to adult dosing.
Additional Information Complete prescribing information should be consulted for additional detail.
Dosage Forms Excipient information presented when available (limited, particularly for generics); consult specific product labeling.
Capsule, Oral:
A-25: 25,000 units
Vitamin A Fish: 7500 units
Generic: 10,000 units
Capsule, Oral [preservative free]:
A-25: 25,000 units [dye free]
Generic: 8000 units
Cream, External:
AFirm 1X: 0.15% (30 g) [fragrance free; contains benzyl alcohol, cetyl alcohol, disodium edta, methylparaben, peg-10 soya sterol, trolamine (triethanolamine)]
AFirm 2X: 0.3% (30 g) [fragrance free; contains benzyl alcohol, cetyl alcohol, disodium edta, methylparaben, peg-10 soya sterol, trolamine (triethanolamine)]
AFirm 3X: 0.6% (30 g) [fragrance free; contains benzyl alcohol, cetyl alcohol, disodium edta, methylparaben, peg-10 soya sterol, trolamine (triethanolamine)]
Gordons-Vite A: 100,000 units/g (75 g, 120 g, 480 g, 2400 g)
Lotion, External:
Gordons-Vite A: 100,000 units (120 mL, 4000 mL)
Solution, Intramuscular:
Aquasol A: 50,000 units/mL (2 mL) [contains chlorobutanol (chlorobutol)]
Tablet, Oral:
Generic: 10,000 units, 15,000 units, Vitamin A 10000 units and beta carotene 1000 units

◆ Vitamin A Acid see Tretinoin (Topical) on page 1841

Vitamin A and Vitamin D (Systemic)
(VYE ta min aye & VYE ta min dee)

Brand Names: US A&D Jr. [OTC]; D-Natural-5 [OTC]
Index Terms Cod Liver Oil
Pharmacologic Category Vitamin, Fat Soluble
Use Dietary supplement
Dosing
Adult & Geriatric Dietary supplement: Oral: One tablet or capsule once daily.
Additional Information Complete prescribing information should be consulted for additional detail.

Dosage Forms Excipient information presented when available (limited, particularly for generics); consult specific product labeling.
Capsule, softgel, oral: Vitamin A 1250 units and vitamin D 130 units, Vitamin A 1250 units and vitamin D 135 units, Vitamin A 5,000 units and vitamin D 400 units, Vitamin A 10,000 units and vitamin D 400 units, Vitamin A 25,000 units and vitamin D 1000 units
A&D Jr.: Vitamin A 10,000 units and vitamin D 400 units [contains soybean oil]
D-Natural-5: Vitamin A 10,000 units and vitamin D 5000 units
Oil, oral: Vitamin A 5000 units and vitamin D 500 units per 5 mL (120 mL, 473 mL)
Tablet, oral: Vitamin A 10,000 units and vitamin D 400 units

Vitamin A and Vitamin D (Topical)
(VYE ta min aye & VYE ta min dee)

Brand Names: US A+D® Original [OTC]; Baza® Clear [OTC]; Sween Cream® [OTC]
Index Terms Cod Liver Oil
Pharmacologic Category Topical Skin Product
Use Temporary relief of discomfort due to chapped skin or lips, cuts and scrapes, diaper rash, or minor burns
Dosing
Adult & Geriatric Skin protectant: Topical: Apply to affected areas as needed.
Pediatric
Diaper rash: Topical: Apply with each diaper change and any time prolonged exposure to wet diapers may occur (ie, at bedtime).
Skin protectant: Topical: Refer to adult dosing.
Additional Information Complete prescribing information should be consulted for additional detail.
Dosage Forms Excipient information presented when available (limited, particularly for generics); consult specific product labeling.
Cream, topical:
Sween Cream®: (57 g, 142 g)
Cream, topical [original formula]:
Sween Cream®: (2 g, 14 g, 85 g, 184 g, 339 g)
Ointment, topical: (5 g, 60 g, 120 g, 454 g)
A+D® Original: (42.5 g); (120 g); (454 g) [in lanolin-petrolatum base]
Baza® Clear: (50 g, 142 g, 227 g) [in petrolatum base]

◆ Vitamin A Fish [OTC] see Vitamin A on page 1905
◆ Vitamin B₁ see Thiamine on page 1782
◆ Vitamin B₂ see Riboflavin on page 1579
◆ Vitamin B₃ see Niacin on page 1273
◆ Vitamin B₃ see Niacinamide on page 1274
◆ Vitamin B₆ see Pyridoxine on page 1533
◆ Vitamin B₁₂ see Cyanocobalamin on page 453
◆ Vitamin B₁₂ₐ see Hydroxocobalamin on page 894
◆ Vitamin D2 see Ergocalciferol on page 663

Vitamin E (VYE ta min ee)

Brand Names: US Alph-E [OTC]; Alph-E-Mixed 1000 [OTC]; Alph-E-Mixed [OTC]; Aquasol E [OTC]; Aquavit-E [OTC]; Aqueous Vitamin E [OTC]; E-400 [OTC]; E-400-Clear [OTC]; E-400-Mixed [OTC]; E-Max-1000 [OTC]; E-Pherol [OTC]; Formula E 400 [OTC]; Gordons-Vite E [OTC]; Natural Vitamin E Moisturizing [OTC]; Natural Vitamin E [OTC]; Nutr-E-Sol [OTC]; Vita-Plus E [OTC]; Vitamin E Beauty [OTC]; Vitamin E/D-Alpha Natural [OTC] [DSC]; Vitec [OTC]; Xtra-Care [OTC]
Index Terms d-Alpha Tocopherol; dl-Alpha Tocopherol
Pharmacologic Category Vitamin, Fat Soluble
Use Dietary supplement
Note: According to the 2014 USPSTF recommendations for the primary prevention of cardiovascular disease and cancer, the use of vitamin E supplements are not recommended (Moyer, 2014).
Dosing
Adult & Geriatric Vitamin E may be expressed as alpha-tocopherol equivalents (ATE), which refer to the biologically-active (R) stereoisomer content.
Recommended daily allowance (RDA) (IOM, 2000):
Oral: 15 mg; upper limit of intake should not exceed 1000 mg/day
Pregnant female:
≤18 years: 15 mg; upper level of intake should not exceed 800 mg/day
19-50 years: 15 mg; upper level of intake should not exceed 1000 mg/day

Lactating female:
≤18 years: 19 mg; upper level of intake should not exceed 800 mg/day
19-50 years: 19 mg; upper level of intake should not exceed 1000 mg/day
Vitamin E deficiency: Oral: 60-75 units/day
Superficial dermatologic irritation: Topical: Apply a thin layer over affected area.

Pediatric Vitamin E may be expressed as alpha-tocopherol equivalents (ATE), which refer to the biologically-active (R) stereoisomer content.
Adequate intake (AI): Oral (IOM, 2000): Infants (RDA not established):
1-6 months: 4 mg
7-12 months: 5 mg
Recommended daily allowance (RDA): Oral (IOM, 2000): Children:
1-3 years: 6 mg; upper limit of intake should not exceed 200 mg/day
4-8 years: 7 mg; upper limit of intake should not exceed 300 mg/day
9-13 years: 11 mg; upper limit of intake should not exceed 600 mg/day
14-18 years: 15 mg; upper limit of intake should not exceed 800 mg/day

Vitamin E deficiency: Oral: Children (with malabsorption syndrome): 1 unit/kg/day of water miscible vitamin E (to raise plasma tocopherol concentrations to the normal range within 2 months and to maintain normal plasma concentrations)
Cystic fibrosis supplementation (Borowitz 2002): Oral:
1-12 months: 40-50 units/day
1-3 years: 80-150 units/day
4-8 years: 100-200 units/day
>8 years: 200-400 units/day

Additional Information Complete prescribing information should be consulted for additional detail.
Dosage Forms Excipient information presented when available (limited, particularly for generics); consult specific product labeling. [DSC] = Discontinued product
Capsule, Oral:
Alph-E: 400 units
Alph-E-Mixed: 200 units
Alph-E-Mixed 1000: 1000 units
Alph-E-Mixed: 400 units [corn free, milk free, sugar free, wheat free, yeast free]
Formula E 400: 400 units
Vita-Plus E: 400 units
Vitamin E/D-Alpha Natural: 400 units [DSC]
Generic: 100 units, 200 units, 400 units, 600 units [DSC], 1000 units
Capsule, Oral [preservative free]:
E-400: 400 units [corn free, gluten free, milk derivatives/products, no artificial color(s), no artificial flavor(s), sodium free, soy free, starch free, sugar free, yeast free]
E-400-Clear: 400 units [dye free]
E-400-Mixed: 400 units [dye free]
E-Max-1000: 1000 units [dye free]
Generic: 100 units, 400 units
Cream, External:
Gordons-Vite E: 1500 units/30 g (15 g, 75 g, 480 g, 2400 g)
Generic: 1000 units (112 g)
Gel, External:
Natural Vitamin E Moisturizing: (237 mL) [contains methylparaben, polyethylene glycol]
Liquid, External:
Generic: 920 units/mL (28.5 mL, 57 mL, 114 mL)
Liquid, Oral:
Nutr-E-Sol: 400 units/15 mL (473 mL) [color free, starch free, sugar free]
Lotion, External:
Vitec: (113 g)
Xtra-Care: (2 mL, 59 mL, 118 mL, 237 mL, 621 mL, 1000 mL, 3840 mL)
Oil, External:
Vitamin E Beauty: 24,000 units/52 mL (52 mL); 49,000 units/52 mL (52 mL)
Solution, Oral:
Aquasol E: 15 units/0.3 mL (12 mL, 30 mL) [contains polysorbate 80, propylene glycol, saccharin]
Aquavit-E: 15 units/0.3 mL (30 mL) [butterscotch flavor]
Aqueous Vitamin E: 15 units/0.3 mL (30 mL) [anise-butterscotch flavor]
Generic: 15 units/0.3 mL (12 mL)

Tablet, Oral:
E-Pherol: 400 units
Natural Vitamin E: 200 units, 400 units [animal products free, gelatin free, gluten free, kosher certified, lactose free, no artificial color(s), no artificial flavor(s), starch free, sugar free, yeast free]
Generic: 100 units, 200 units, 400 units

Vorapaxar (vor a PAX ar)

Brand Names: US Zontivity
Index Terms SCH530348; Vorapaxar Sulfate
Pharmacologic Category Antiplatelet Agent; Protease-Activated Receptor-1 (PAR-1) Antagonist
Additional Appendix Information
Oral Antiplatelet Comparison Chart *on page 1963*
Use History of myocardial infarction or established peripheral arterial disease: To reduce thrombotic cardiovascular events (cardiovascular death, MI, stroke, urgent coronary revascularization) in patients with a history of myocardial infarction (MI) or with peripheral arterial disease (PAD)
Pregnancy Considerations Adverse events have not been observed in animal reproduction studies.
Breast-Feeding Considerations It is not known if vorapaxar is excreted in breast milk. Breast-feeding is not recommended by the manufacturer.
Medication Guide Available Yes
Contraindications History of stroke, transient ischemic attack (TIA), or intracranial hemorrhage (ICH); active pathological bleeding (eg, ICH, peptic ulcer bleeding)
Warnings/Precautions [US Boxed Warning]: Use is contraindicated in patients with history of stroke, TIA, or ICH; or active pathological bleeding. Vorapaxar increases the risk of bleeding, including ICH and fatal

bleeding. The risk of bleeding is proportional to the patient's underlying bleeding risk. General risk factors for bleeding include older age, low body weight, reduced renal or hepatic function, history of bleeding disorders, and concomitant use of medications known to increase the risk of bleeding (eg, anticoagulants, NSAIDS, selective serotonin reuptake inhibitors [SSRIs], serotonin norepinephrine reuptake inhibitors [SNRIs]); avoid use with warfarin or other anticoagulants. **Note:** No specific antidote exists for vorapaxar reversal. Significant inhibition of platelet aggregation remains 4 weeks after discontinuation.

Due to increased risk of bleeding, use is not recommended in patients with severe hepatic impairment; use with caution in patients with mild or moderate hepatic impairment and in patients with renal impairment. Potentially significant interactions may exist, requiring dose or frequency adjustment, additional monitoring, and/or selection of alternative therapy.

Adverse Reactions

>10%:

Hematologic and oncologic: Hemorrhage (any GUSTO [Global Utilization of Streptokinase and Tissue Plasminogen Activator for Occluded Arteries] bleeding [severe, moderate, mild]): 25%), major hemorrhage, life-threatening (13%; clinically significant bleeding, including any bleeding requiring medical attention such as intracranial hemorrhage, or clinically significant overt signs of hemorrhage associated with a drop in hemoglobin of ≥3 g/dL [or when hemoglobin is unavailable, an absolute drop in hematocrit of ≥15% or a fall in hematocrit of 9% to <15%])

1% to 10%:

Central nervous system: Depression (2%)

Dermatologic: Skin rash (2%, includes cutaneous eruptions and exanthemas)

Endocrine & metabolic: Iron deficiency (<2%)

Gastrointestinal: Gastrointestinal hemorrhage (4%)

Hematologic and oncologic: Anemia (5%), major hemorrhage (GUSTO bleeding category "moderate or severe": 3%; GUSTO bleeding category "severe": 1%)

Ophthalmic: Retinopathy (<2%)

<1% (Limited to important or life-threatening): Hemorrhagic death, intracranial hemorrhage

Drug Interactions

Metabolism/Transport Effects Substrate of CYP2J2 (minor), CYP3A4 (minor); **Note:** Assignment of Major/Minor substrate status based on clinically relevant drug interaction potential; **Inhibits** P-glycoprotein

Avoid Concomitant Use

Avoid concomitant use of Vorapaxar with any of the following: Anticoagulants; CYP3A4 Inducers (Strong); CYP3A4 Inhibitors (Strong); St Johns Wort; Urokinase

Increased Effect/Toxicity

Vorapaxar may increase the levels/effects of: Agents with Antiplatelet Properties; Anticoagulants; Collagenase (Systemic); Deoxycholic Acid; Ibritumomab; Obinutuzumab; Salicylates; Thrombolytic Agents; Tositumomab and Iodine I 131 Tositumomab; Urokinase

The levels/effects of Vorapaxar may be increased by: CYP3A4 Inhibitors (Strong); Dasatinib; Glucosamine; Herbs (Anticoagulant/Antiplatelet Properties); Ibrutinib; Limaprost; Multivitamins/Fluoride (with ADE); Multivitamins/Minerals (with ADEK, Folate, Iron); Multivitamins/Minerals (with AE, No Iron); Omega-3 Fatty Acids; Pentosan Polysulfate Sodium; Pentoxifylline; Prostacyclin Analogues; Tipranavir; Vitamin E; Vitamin E (Oral)

Decreased Effect

The levels/effects of Vorapaxar may be decreased by: CYP3A4 Inducers (Strong); St Johns Wort

Storage/Stability Store at 20°C to 25°C (68°F to 77°F); excursions are permitted between 15°C and 30°C (59°F and 86°F). Store in the original package; protect from moisture. Keep the desiccant in the bottle.

Mechanism of Action Vorapaxar, an antagonist of the protease-activated receptor-1 (PAR-1) expressed on platelets, inhibits thrombin-induced and thrombin receptor agonist peptide (TRAP)-induced platelet aggregation. Due to the very long half-life, vorapaxar is effectively irreversible. Vorapaxar reversibly binds to the PAR-1 receptor with a long receptor dissociation half-life of approximately 20 hours; additionally, vorapaxar displays significant inhibition of platelet aggregation that remains for up to 4 weeks after discontinuation due to the very long elimination half-life (Ueno 2010).

Pharmacodynamics/Kinetics

Onset of action: ≥80% inhibition of TRAP-induced platelet aggregation within 1 week

Duration: Dose and concentration dependent; with the recommended dosing, inhibition of TRAP-induced platelet aggregation at a level of 50% can be expected 4 weeks after discontinuation

Absorption: Rapidly absorbed (Kosoglou, 2012)

Distribution: ~424 L

Protein binding: ≥99% to albumin

Metabolism: Hepatic via CYP3A4 and CYP2J2. Major active metabolite: M20 (accounts for ~20% of exposure to vorapaxar)

Bioavailability: ~100%

Half-life elimination: Effective half-life: 3 to 4 days; Terminal elimination half-life (vorapaxar and active metabolite): ~8 days (range: 5 to 13 days)

Time to peak: 1 to 2 hours

Excretion: Primarily in the form of metabolites through feces (58%); urine (25%)

Dosing

Adult & Geriatric History of myocardial infarction (MI) or established peripheral arterial disease (PAD): Oral: 2.08 mg once daily in combination with aspirin and/or clopidogrel. **Note:** No experience with use of vorapaxar as monotherapy or with antiplatelet agents other than aspirin and clopidogrel.

Renal Impairment No dosage adjustment necessary.

Hepatic Impairment

Mild to moderate impairment: No dosage adjustment necessary.

Severe impairment: Use is not recommended.

Administration Administer with or without food.

Monitoring Parameters Signs of bleeding; hemoglobin and hematocrit periodically

Dosage Forms Excipient information presented when available (limited, particularly for generics); consult specific product labeling.

Tablet, Oral:

Zontivity: 2.08 mg

◆ Vorapaxar Sulfate *see* Vorapaxar *on page 1907*

◆ Voraxaze *see* Glucarpidase *on page 847*

Voriconazole (vor i KOE na zole)

Brand Names: US Vfend; Vfend IV

Brand Names: Canada Apo-Voriconazole; Sandoz-Voriconazole; Teva-Voriconazole; VFEND; VFEND For Injection; Voriconazole For Injection

Index Terms UK109496

Pharmacologic Category Antifungal Agent, Oral; Antifungal Agent, Parenteral

Use Treatment of fungal infections: Treatment of invasive aspergillosis; treatment of esophageal candidiasis; treatment of candidemia (in non-neutropenic patients); treatment of disseminated *Candida* infections of the skin and abdomen, kidney, bladder wall and wounds; treatment of serious fungal infections caused by *Scedosporium apiospermum* and *Fusarium* spp (including *Fusarium solani*) in patients intolerant of, or refractory to, other therapy in children >12 years of age, adolescents and adults

Pregnancy Considerations Voriconazole can cause fetal harm when administered to a pregnant woman. Voriconazole was teratogenic and embryotoxic in animal studies, and lowered plasma estradiol in animal models. Women of childbearing potential should use effective contraception during treatment. Should be used in pregnant woman only if benefit to mother justifies potential risk to the fetus.

Breast-Feeding Considerations It is not known if voriconazole is excreted in breast milk. Due to the potential for serious adverse reactions in the nursing infant, the manufacturer recommends a decision be made whether to discontinue nursing or to discontinue the drug, taking into account the importance of treatment to the mother.

Contraindications Hypersensitivity to voriconazole or any component of the formulation; coadministration with astemizole, barbiturates (long acting), carbamazepine, cisapride, efavirenz (≥400 mg daily), ergot derivatives (ergotamine and dihydroergotamine), pimozide, quinidine, rifampin, rifabutin, ritonavir (≥800 mg daily; also avoid low dose [eg, 200 mg daily] dosing if possible), sirolimus, St John's wort, terfenadine

Documentation of allergenic cross-reactivity for imidazole antifungals is limited. However, because of similarities in chemical structure and/or pharmacologic actions, the possibility of cross-sensitivity cannot be ruled out with certainty.

Warnings/Precautions Hazardous agent - use appropriate precautions for handling and disposal (NIOSH 2014 [group 3]).

Visual changes, including blurred vision, changes in visual acuity, color perception, and photophobia, are commonly associated with treatment; postmarketing cases of optic neuritis and papilledema (lasting >1 month) have also been reported. Patients should be warned to avoid tasks which depend on vision, including operating machinery or driving. Changes are reversible on discontinuation following brief exposure/treatment regimens (≤28 days).

Serious (and rarely fatal) hepatic reactions (eg, hepatitis, cholestasis, fulminant failure) have been observed with voriconazole. In lung transplant recipients, median time to hepatic toxicity was 14 days with the majority occurring within 30 days of therapy initiation (Luong 2012). Use with caution in patients with serious underlying medical conditions (eg, hematologic malignancy); hepatic reactions have occurred in patients with no identifiable underlying risk factors. Liver dysfunction is usually reversible upon therapy discontinuation. Monitor serum transaminase and bilirubin at baseline and at least weekly for the first month of treatment. Monitoring frequency can then be reduced to monthly during continued use if no abnormalities are noted. If marked elevations occur compared to baseline, discontinue unless benefit/risk of treatment justifies continued use.

Voriconazole tablets contain lactose; avoid administration in hereditary galactose intolerance, Lapp lactase deficiency, or glucose-galactose malabsorption. Suspension contains sucrose; use caution with fructose intolerance, sucrase-isomaltase deficiency, or glucose-galactose malabsorption. Avoid/limit use of intravenous formulation in patients with moderate to severe renal impairment (CrCl <50 mL/minute); injection contains excipient cyclodextrin (sulfobutyl ether beta-cyclodextrin [SBECD]), which may accumulate, although the clinical significance of this finding is uncertain (Luke 2010); consider using oral voriconazole in these patients unless benefit of injection outweighs the risk. If injection is used in patients CrCl <50 mL/minute, monitor serum creatinine closely; if increases occur, consider changing therapy to oral voriconazole.

Anaphylactoid-type reactions (eg, flushing, fever, sweating, tachycardia, chest tightness, dyspnea, nausea, pruritus, rash) may occur with IV infusion. Consider discontinuation of infusion should these reactions occur. Acute renal failure has been observed in severely ill patients; use with caution in patients receiving concomitant nephrotoxic medications. Evaluate renal function (particularly serum creatinine) at baseline and periodically during therapy.

Potentially significant drug-drug interactions may exist, requiring dose or frequency adjustment, additional monitoring, and/or selection of alternative therapy. QT interval prolongation has been associated with voriconazole use; rare cases of arrhythmia (including torsade de pointes), cardiac arrest, and sudden death have been reported, usually in seriously ill patients with comorbidities and/or risk factors (eg, prior cardiotoxic chemotherapy, cardiomyopathy [especially with concomitant heart failure], electrolyte imbalance, or concomitant QTc-prolonging drugs). Also use with caution in patients with potentially proarrhythmic conditions (eg, congenital or acquired QT syndrome, sinus bradycardia, or preexisting symptomatic arrhythmias); correct electrolyte abnormalities (eg, hypokalemia, hypomagnesemia, hypocalcemia) prior to initiating and during therapy. Do not infuse concomitantly with blood products or short-term concentrated electrolyte solutions, even if the two infusions are running in separate intravenous lines (or cannulas).

Rare cases of malignancy (melanoma, squamous cell carcinoma [SCC]) have been reported in patients with prior onset of severe photosensitivity reactions or exposure to standard dose long-term voriconazole therapy (in lung transplant recipients, SCC increased by ~6% per 60 days with a 28% absolute risk increase at 5 years [Singer 2012]). Other serious exfoliative cutaneous reactions, including Stevens-Johnson syndrome, have also been reported. Patients, including children, should avoid exposure to direct sunlight and should use protective clothing and high SPF sunscreen; may cause photosensitivity, especially with long-term use. If phototoxic reactions occur, referral to a dermatologist and voriconazole discontinuation should be considered. If therapy is continued, dermatologic evaluation should be performed on a systematic and regular basis to allow early detection and management of premalignant lesions. Pediatric patients are at particular risk for phototoxicity; stringent photoprotective measures are necessary in children due to the risk of squamous cell carcinoma. In children experiencing photoaging injuries (eg, lentigines or ephelides), avoidance of sun and dermatologic follow-up are warranted even after treatment is discontinued. Discontinue use in patients who develop an exfoliative cutaneous reaction or a skin lesion consistent with squamous cell carcinoma or melanoma. Periodic total body skin examinations should be performed, particularly with prolonged use. Fluorosis and/or periostitis may occur during long-term therapy. If patient develops skeletal pain and radiologic findings of fluorosis or periostitis, discontinue therapy.

Voriconazole demonstrates nonlinear pharmacokinetics. Dose modifications may result in unpredictable changes in serum concentrations and contribute to toxicity. It is important to note that cutoff trough threshold values ranged widely among studies; however, an upper limit of <5.0 mg/L would be reasonable for most disease states (see CDC recommendations for *Exserohilum rostratum* in Reference Range) (CDC 2012). In patients >14 years of age or 12-14 years and weighing >50 kg, data suggest that pharmacokinetics are similar to adults (Friberg 2012). In patients <12 years of age, the full pharmacokinetic profile for voriconazole is not completely defined, and for patients <2 years, the data are sparse. In children 2 to <12 years, current data suggests voriconazole undergoes a high degree of variability in exposure with linear elimination at lower doses and nonlinear elimination at higher doses; therefore, to achieve similar AUC as adults, increased dosage is necessary in children (Friberg 2012; Karlsson 2009; Walsh 2004).

Correct electrolyte abnormalities (eg, hypokalemia, hypomagnesemia, hypocalcemia) prior to initiating and during therapy. Monitor pancreatic function in patients (children and adults) at risk for acute pancreatitis (eg, recent chemotherapy or hematopoietic stem cell transplantation). Pancreatitis has occurred in pediatric patients.

Benzyl alcohol and derivatives: Some dosage forms may contain sodium benzoate/benzoic acid; benzoic acid (benzoate) is a metabolite of benzyl alcohol; large amounts of benzyl alcohol (≥99 mg/kg/day) have been associated with a potentially fatal toxicity ("gasping syndrome") in neonates; the "gasping syndrome" consists of metabolic acidosis, respiratory distress, gasping respirations, CNS dysfunction (including convulsions, intracranial hemorrhage), hypotension, and cardiovascular collapse (AAP ["Inactive" 1997]; CDC 1982); some data suggests that benzoate displaces bilirubin from protein binding sites (Ahlfors 2001); avoid or use dosage forms containing benzyl alcohol derivative with caution in neonates. See manufacturer's labeling.

Adverse Reactions
>10%:
Central nervous system: Hallucination (2% to 12%; auditory and/or visual and likely serum concentration-dependent)
Ophthalmic: Visual disturbance (19%)
Renal: Increased serum creatinine (1% to 21%)
2% to 10%:
Cardiovascular: Tachycardia (≤2%)
Central nervous system: Chills (≤4%), headache (≤3%)
Dermatologic: Skin rash (≤7%)
Endocrine & metabolic: Hypokalemia (≤2%)
Gastrointestinal: Nausea (1% to 5%), vomiting (1% to 4%)
Hepatic: Increased serum alkaline phosphatase (4% to 5%), increased serum AST (2% to 4%), increased serum ALT (2% to 3%), cholestatic jaundice (1% to 2%)
Ophthalmic: Photophobia (2%)
Miscellaneous: Fever (≤6%)
<2%, postmarketing, and/or case reports (limited to important or life-threatening): Acute renal failure, adrenocortical insufficiency, agranulocytosis, alopecia, anaphylactoid reaction, anemia (aplastic, hemolytic, macrocytic, megaloblastic, or microcytic), angioedema, anorexia, anuria, arthritis, ascites, ataxia, atrial arrhythmia, atrial fibrillation, atrioventricular block, bacterial infection, bigeminy, blighted ovum, bone marrow depression, bradycardia, brain disease, bundle branch block, cardiac arrest, cardiac failure, cardiomegaly, cardiomyopathy, cellulitis, cerebral edema, cerebral hemorrhage, cerebral ischemia, cerebrovascular accident, chest pain, cholecystitis, cholelithiasis, cholestasis, chromatopsia, color blindness, coma, confusion, convulsions, corneal opacity, cyanosis, deafness, deep vein thrombophlebitis, deep vein thrombosis, delirium, dementia, dental fluorosis, depersonalization, depression, diabetes insipidus, diarrhea, discoid lupus erythematosus, disseminated intravascular coagulation, drowsiness, duodenal ulcer (active), duodenitis, dyspnea, eczema, edema, encephalitis, endocarditis, eosinophilia, erythema multiforme, esophageal ulcer, exfoliative dermatitis, extrapyramidal

reaction, extrasystoles, fixed drug eruption, fungal infection, gastric ulcer, gastrointestinal hemorrhage, glucose tolerance decreased, graft versus host disease, Guillain-Barre syndrome, hematemesis, hemorrhagic cystitis, hepatic coma, hepatic failure, hepatitis, hepatomegaly, herpes simplex infection, hydronephrosis, hyperbilirubinemia, hypercholesterolemia, hyper-/hypocalcemia, hyper-/hypoglycemia, hyper-/hypomagnesemia, hyper-/hyponatremia, hyper-/hypotension, hyper-/hypothyroidism, hyperkalemia, hypersensitivity reaction, hyperuricemia, hypophosphatemia, hypoxia, impotence, increased blood urea nitrogen, increased gamma-glutamyl transferase, increased lactate dehydrogenase, increased susceptibility to infection, intestinal perforation, intracranial hypertension, jaundice, leukopenia, lymphadenopathy, lymphangitis, maculopapular rash, malignant melanoma, melanosis, multi-organ failure, myasthenia, myocardial infarction, myopathy, nephritis, nephrosis, neuropathy, nocturnal amblyopia, nodal arrhythmia, nodule, nystagmus, oculogyric crisis, optic atrophy, optic neuritis, orthostatic hypotension, osteomalacia, osteonecrosis, osteoporosis, otitis externa, palpitations, pancreatitis, pancytopenia, papilledema, paresthesia, perforated duodenal ulcer, periosteal disease, peripheral edema, peritonitis, petechia, pleural effusion, pneumonia, prolonged bleeding time, prolonged QT interval on ECG, pruritus, pseudomembranous colitis, pseudoporphyria, psoriasis, psychosis, pulmonary edema, pulmonary embolism, purpura, rectal hemorrhage, renal insufficiency, renal tubular necrosis, respiratory distress syndrome, respiratory tract infection, retinal hemorrhage, retinitis, seizure, sepsis, skin discoloration, skin photosensitivity, splenomegaly, squamous cell carcinoma, Stevens-Johnson syndrome, subconjunctival hemorrhage, substernal pain, suicidal ideation, supraventricular extrasystole, supraventricular tachycardia, syncope, thrombocytopenia, thrombophlebitis, thrombotic thrombocytopenic purpura, tongue edema, tonic-clonic seizures, torsades de pointes, toxic epidermal necrolysis, uremia, urinary incontinence, urinary retention, urinary tract infection, urticaria, uterine hemorrhage, uveitis, vaginal hemorrhage, vasodilation, ventricular arrhythmia, ventricular fibrillation, ventricular tachycardia, visual field defect

Drug Interactions

Metabolism/Transport Effects Substrate of CYP2C19 (major), CYP2C9 (major), CYP3A4 (minor); **Note:** Assignment of Major/Minor substrate status based on clinically relevant drug interaction potential; **Inhibits** CYP2C19 (moderate), CYP2C9 (moderate), CYP3A4 (strong)

Avoid Concomitant Use

Avoid concomitant use of Voriconazole with any of the following: Ado-Trastuzumab Emtansine; Alfuzosin; Aprepitant; Astemizole; Atazanavir; Avanafil; Axitinib; Barbiturates; Barnidipine; Bosutinib; Bromocriptine; Cabozantinib; CarBAMazepine; Ceritinib; Cisapride; Cobimetinib; Conivaptan; Crizotinib; Dabrafenib; Dapoxetine; Darunavir; Dihydroergotamine; Dofetilide; Domperidone; Dronedarone; Eletriptan; Eplerenone; Ergoloid Mesylates; Ergonovine; Ergotamine; Everolimus; Flibanserin; Fluconazole; Halofantrine; Ibrutinib; Irinotecan Products; Isavuconazonium Sulfate; Ivabradine; Lapatinib; Lercanidipine; Lomitapide; Lopinavir; Lovastatin; Lumacaftor; Lurasidone; Macitentan; Methylergonovine; Naloxegol; Nilotinib; NiMODipine; Nisoldipine; Olaparib; Osimertinib; Palbociclib; Pimozide; QuiNIDine; Ranolazine; Red Yeast Rice; Regorafenib; Rifamycin Derivatives; Ritonavir; Saccharomyces boulardii; Salmeterol; Silodosin; Simeprevir; Simvastatin; Sirolimus; Sonidegib; St Johns Wort; Suvorexant; Tamsulosin; Terfenadine; Ticagrelor; Tolvaptan; Toremifene; Trabectedin; Uliprisatl; Vemurafenib; VinCRIStine (Liposomal); Vorapaxar

Increased Effect/Toxicity

Voriconazole may increase the levels/effects of: Ado-Trastuzumab Emtansine; Alfuzosin; Alitretinoin (Systemic); Almotriptan; Alosetron; Antineoplastic Agents (Vinca Alkaloids); Apixaban; Aprepitant; ARIPiprazole; ARIPiprazole Lauroxil; Astemizole; AtorvaSTATin; Avanafil; Axitinib; Barnidipine; Bedaquiline; Boceprevir; Bortezomib; Bosentan; Bosutinib; Brentuximab Vedotin; Brexpiprazole; Brinzolamide; Bromocriptine; Budesonide (Nasal); Budesonide (Oral Inhalation); Budesonide (Systemic); Budesonide (Topical); BusPIRone; Busulfan; Cabazitaxel; Cabozantinib; Calcium Channel Blockers; Cannabis; Cariprazine; Carvedilol; Ceritinib; Cilostazol; Cisapride; Citalopram; Cobicistat; Cobimetinib; Colchicine; Conivaptan; Contraceptives (Estrogens); Contraceptives (Progestins); Corticosteroids (Orally Inhaled); Corticosteroids (Systemic); Crizotinib; CycloSPORINE (Systemic); CYP2C19 Substrates; CYP2C9 Substrates; CYP3A4 Substrates; Dabrafenib; Daclatasvir; Dapoxetine; Dasatinib; Diclofenac (Systemic); Diclofenac (Topical); Dienogest; Dihydroergotamine; DOCEtaxel; Dofetilide; Domperidone; DOXOrubicin (Conventional); Dronabinol; Dronedarone; Drospirenone; Dutasteride; Efavirenz; Eletriptan; Eliglustat; Elvitegravir; Eplerenone; Ergoloid Mesylates; Ergonovine; Ergotamine; Erlotinib; Estazolam; Etizolam; Etravirine; Everolimus; FentaNYL; Fesoterodine; Flibanserin; Fluticasone (Nasal); Fluticasone (Oral Inhalation); Fosamprenavir; Fosphenytoin; Gefitinib; GuanFACINE; Halofantrine; Highest Risk QTc-Prolonging Agents; Hydrocodone; Ibrutinib; Ibuprofen; Idelalisib; Iloperidone; Imatinib; Imidafenacin; Irinotecan Products; Isavuconazonium Sulfate; Ivabradine; Ivacaftor; Ixabepilone; Lacosamide; Lapatinib; Lercanidipine; Levobupivacaine; Levomilnacipran; Lomitapide; Losartan; Lovastatin; Lurasidone; Macitentan; Maraviroc; MedroxyPROGESTERone; Meloxicam; Methadone; Methylergonovine; MethylPREDNISolone; Mifepristone; Moderate Risk QTc-Prolonging Agents; Naloxegol; Nelfinavir; Nilotinib; NiMODipine; Nisoldipine; Olaparib; Osimertinib; Ospemifene; Oxybutynin; OxyCODONE; Palbociclib; Panobinostat; Parecoxib; Paricalcitol; PAZOPanib; Phenytoin; Pimecrolimus; Pimozide; PONATinib; Porfimer; Pranlukast; PrednisoLONE (Systemic); PredniSONE; Propafenone; Proton Pump Inhibitors; QUEtiapine; QuiNIDine; Ramelteon; Ranolazine; Red Yeast Rice; Regorafenib; Repaglinide; Retapamulin; Reverse Transcriptase Inhibitors (Non-Nucleoside); Rifamycin Derivatives; Rilpivirine; RomiDEPsin; Ruxolitinib; Salmeterol; Saxagliptin; Sildenafil; Silodosin; Simeprevir; Simvastatin; Sirolimus; Solifenacin; Sonidegib; SORAfenib; Sulfonylureas; SUNItinib; Suvorexant; Tacrolimus (Systemic); Tacrolimus (Topical); Tadalafil; Tamsulosin; Tasimelteon; Telaprevir; Terfenadine; Tetrahydrocannabinol; Ticagrelor; Tofacitinib; Tolterodine; Tolvaptan; Toremifene; Trabectedin; TraMADol; Uliprisatl; Vardenafil; Vemurafenib; Venlafaxine; Verteporfin; Vilazodone; VinCRIStine (Liposomal); Vitamin K Antagonists; Vorapaxar; Zolpidem; Zopiclone; Zuclopenthixol

The levels/effects of Voriconazole may be increased by: Atazanavir; Boceprevir; Chloramphenicol; Cobicistat; Contraceptives (Estrogens); Contraceptives (Progestins); CYP2C19 Inhibitors (Moderate); CYP2C19 Inhibitors (Strong); CYP2C9 Inhibitors (Moderate); CYP2C9 Inhibitors (Strong); Etravirine; Fluconazole; Fosamprenavir; Luliconazole; Mifepristone; Proton Pump Inhibitors; Telaprevir

Decreased Effect

Voriconazole may decrease the levels/effects of: Amphotericin B; Atazanavir; Clopidogrel; Ifosfamide; Prasugrel; Saccharomyces boulardii; Ticagrelor

The levels/effects of Voriconazole may be decreased by: Antihepaciviral Combination Products; Atazanavir; Barbiturates; CarBAMazepine; CYP2C9 Inducers (Strong); Darunavir; Didanosine; Efavirenz; Enzalutamide; Etravirine; Fosphenytoin; Lopinavir; Lumacaftor; Phenytoin; Reverse Transcriptase Inhibitors (Non-Nucleoside); Rifamycin Derivatives; Ritonavir; St Johns Wort; Sucralfate; Telaprevir

Food Interactions Food may decrease voriconazole absorption. Management: Oral voriconazole should be taken 1 hour before or 1 hour after a meal. Maintain adequate hydration unless instructed to restrict fluid intake.

Preparation for Administration

Powder for injection: Reconstitute 200 mg vial with 19 mL of sterile water for injection (use of automated syringe is not recommended). Resultant solution (20 mL) has a concentration of 10 mg/mL. Prior to infusion, must dilute to <5 mg/mL with NS, LR, D_5WLR, $D_5W^{1/2}NS$, D_5W, D_5W with KCl 20 mEq, 1/2NS, or D_5WNS. Do not dilute with 4.2% sodium bicarbonate infusion.

Powder for oral suspension: Add 46 mL of water to the bottle to make 40 mg/mL suspension. Shake vigorously for ~1 minute. Do not refrigerate or freeze.

Hazardous agent - use appropriate precautions for handling and disposal (NIOSH 2014 [group 3]).

Storage/Stability

Powder for injection: Store vials between 15°C to 30°C (59°F to 86°F). Reconstituted solutions are stable for up to 24 hours under refrigeration at 2°C to 8°C (36°F to 46°F).

Powder for oral suspension: Store at 2°C to 8°C (36°F to 46°F). Reconstituted oral suspension is stable for up to 14 days if stored at 15°C to 30°C (59°F to 86°F). Do not refrigerate or freeze.

Tablets: Store at 15°C to 30°C (59°F to 86°F).

Mechanism of Action Interferes with fungal cytochrome P450 activity (selectively inhibits 14-alpha-lanosterol demethylation), decreasing ergosterol synthesis (principal sterol in fungal cell membrane) and inhibiting fungal cell membrane formation.

Pharmacodynamics/Kinetics

Absorption: Well absorbed after oral administration; multiple doses administered with high-fat meals demonstrate decreased C_{max} and AUC

Distribution: V_d: 4.6 L/kg

Protein binding: 58%

Metabolism: Hepatic, via CYP2C19 (major pathway) and CYP2C9 and CYP3A4 (less significant); saturable (may demonstrate nonlinearity); the N-oxide major metabolite has minimal antifungal activity

Bioavailability: 96%

Half-life elimination: Variable, dose-dependent. **Note:** Steady-state trough concentrations are achieved within 1 day when an IV loading dose is administered and 5 days if no loading dose is used.

Time to peak: Oral: 1 to 2 hours

Excretion: Urine (<2% as unchanged drug)

Dosing

Adult & Geriatric Note: Actual body weight should be used for all weight-based dosing calculations.

Aspergillosis, invasive, including disseminated and extrapulmonary infection: Duration of therapy should be a minimum of 6-12 weeks or throughout period of immunosuppression (Walsh 2008); duration of therapy in HIV-positive patients should be until resolution of infection and CD4 count >200 cells/mm³ (HHS [OI adult 2015]):

IV:

Initial: 6 mg/kg every 12 hours for 2 doses
Maintenance dose: 4 mg/kg every 12 hours

Oral: Maintenance dose:

Manufacturer's labeling: **Note:** If patient has inadequate clinical response, titrate in 50 mg/dose increments for weight <40 kg and 100 mg/dose increments for weight ≥40 kg.
Weight <40 kg: 100 mg every 12 hours
Weight ≥40 kg: 200 mg every 12 hours
IDSA recommendations (Walsh 2008): May consider oral therapy in place of IV with dosing of 4 mg/kg (rounded up to convenient tablet dosage form) every 12 hours; however, IV administration is preferred in serious infections since comparative efficacy with the oral formulation has not been established.

Candidemia in non-neutropenic patients and disseminated Candida infections in skin, and infections in abdomen, kidney, bladder wall and wounds: Treatment should continue for a minimum of 14 days following resolution of symptoms or following last positive culture, whichever is longer.

IV:

Initial: 6 mg/kg every 12 hours for 2 doses
Maintenance: 3 to 4 mg/kg every 12 hours

Oral:

Manufacturer's labeling: Maintenance dose: **Note:** If patient has inadequate clinical response, titrate in 50 mg/dose increments for weight <40 kg and 100 mg/dose increments for weight ≥40 kg
Weight <40 kg: 100 mg every 12 hours
Weight ≥40 kg: 200 mg every 12 hours
Alternate recommendations (Pappas 2009):
Initial: 400 mg every 12 hours for 2 doses
Maintenance: 200 mg every 12 hours

Coccidioidomycosis in HIV-infected patients (alternative to preferred therapy) (off-label use; HHS [OI adult 2015]): Oral:

Mild infections (eg, focal pneumonia): 200 mg twice daily; patients who complete initial therapy should be considered for lifelong suppressive therapy.
Chronic suppressive therapy: 200 mg twice daily

Esophageal candidiasis:

Manufacturer's labeling: Oral: Treatment should continue for a minimum of 14 days, and for at least 7 days following resolution of symptoms. **Note:** If patient has inadequate clinical response, titrate in 50 mg/dose increments for weight <40 kg and 100 mg/dose increments for weight ≥40 kg
Weight <40 kg: 100 mg every 12 hours; maximum: 300 mg daily
Weight ≥40 kg: 200 mg every 12 hours; maximum: 600 mg daily
Alternative dosing: HIV-positive patients (alternative to preferred therapy): Oral, IV: 200 mg twice daily for 14 to 21 days (HHS [OI adult 2015])

Scedosporiosis, fusariosis:

IV:

Initial: 6 mg/kg every 12 hours for 2 doses
Maintenance dose: 4 mg/kg every 12 hours for >7 days

Oral: Maintenance dose: **Note:** If patient has inadequate clinical response, titrate in 50 mg/dose increments for weight <40 kg and 100 mg/dose increments for weight ≥40 kg.

Weight <40 kg: 100 mg every 12 hours.
Weight ≥40 kg: 200 mg every 12 hours.

Endophthalmitis, fungal (off-label use; Pappas 2009):
IV: 6 mg/kg every 12 hours for 2 doses, then 3 to 4 mg/kg every 12 hours.

Infection prophylaxis in graft-versus-host disease (GVHD) (high-risk patients) (off-label use; Maertens 2011; Tomblyn 2009; Wingard 2010): Note: The optimal duration of prophylaxis in GVHD has not been determined.
Oral: Weight >40 kg: 200 mg every 12 hours
IV: Weight >40 kg: 4 mg/kg every 12 hours

Infection prophylaxis in standard- or high-risk patients with allogeneic hematopoietic stem cell transplant (HSCT) or certain autologous HSCT (off-label use; Castagna 2012; Maertens 2011; Tomblyn 2009; Wingard 2010): Note: Begin prophylaxis at the start of chemotherapy or the day of transplantation. The ASBMT recommends continuing prophylaxis until engraftment (ie, 30 days) or for 7 days after the ANC reaches >1000 cells/mm³ (Tomblyn 2009). The IDSA recommends anti-mold prophylaxis in allograft HSCT patients "through the neutropenic period and beyond," based on a demonstrated survival advantage in patients receiving prophylaxis for 75 days post-HSCT, or until cessation of immunosuppressive therapy (Freifeld 2011).
Oral: Weight >40 kg: 200 mg every 12 hours
IV: Weight >40 kg: 4 mg/kg every 12 hours.

Meningitis (secondary to contaminated [eg, *Exserohilum rostratum*] steroid products) (off-label use) (CDC [parameningeal] 2012; Kauffman 2013): Note: Consult an infectious disease specialist and current CDC guidelines for specific treatment recommendations. Therapy duration is ≥3 months; trough serum concentrations must be maintained between 2 to 5 mcg/mL.
IV: 6 mg/kg every 12 hours. If patient does not improve or has severe disease, consider adding amphotericin B (liposomal).
Oral (only in mild disease in adherent patients whose trough concentrations/response to therapy can be closely monitored): 6 mg/kg every 12 hours (CDC [parameningeal] 2012).

Osteoarticular infection involving the spine, discitis, epidural abscess or vertebral osteomyelitis (secondary to contaminated [eg, *Exserohilum rostratum*] steroid products) (off-label use) (CDC [osteoarticular] 2012; Kauffman 2013): IV: 6 mg/kg every 12 hours for ≥3 months. **Note:** Consult an infectious disease specialist and current CDC guidelines for specific treatment recommendations. Trough serum concentrations must be maintained between 2 to 5 mcg/mL. If patient has severe disease, consider adding amphotericin B (liposomal). Patients may be switched to oral therapy if condition has improved or stabilized.

Osteoarticular infection not involving the spine (secondary to contaminated [eg, *Exserohilum rostratum*] steroid products) (off-label use) (CDC [osteoarticular] 2012; Kauffman 2013): Note: Consult an infectious disease specialist and current CDC guidelines for specific treatment recommendations. Therapy duration is ≥3 months. Trough serum concentrations must be maintained between 2 to 5 mcg/mL.
IV: 6 mg/kg every 12 hours for 2 doses, then 4 mg/kg every 12 hours. If patient has severe disease, consider adding amphotericin B (liposomal)
Oral (only in mild disease in adherent patients whose trough concentrations/response to therapy can be closely monitored): 6 mg/kg every 12 hours for 2 doses, then 4 mg/kg every 12 hours

***Penicillium marneffei* infection in HIV-infected patients (off-label use; HHS [OI adult 2015]):**
Acute infection in severely ill patients: 6 mg/kg IV every 12 hours for 2 doses, then 4 mg/kg IV every 12 hours for at least 3 days, followed by 200 mg orally twice daily for a maximum of 12 weeks; follow with itraconazole chronic maintenance therapy
Mild disease: Oral: 400 mg twice daily for 2 doses, then 200 mg twice daily for a maximum of 12 weeks; follow with itraconazole chronic maintenance therapy

Dosage adjustment in patients with inadequate response:
IV: Maintenance dose may be increased from 3 mg/kg every 12 hours to 4 mg/kg every 12 hours, depending upon condition.
Oral: Maintenance dose may be increased from 200 mg every 12 hours to 300 mg every 12 hours in patients weighing ≥40 kg (or to 150 mg every 12 hours in patients <40 kg), depending upon condition.

Dosage adjustment in patients unable to tolerate treatment:

IV: Maintenance dose may be reduced from 4 mg/kg every 12 hours to 3 mg/kg every 12 hours, depending upon condition.

Oral: Maintenance dose may be reduced in 50 mg decrements to a minimum dosage of 200 mg every 12 hours in patients weighing ≥40 kg (or to 100 mg every 12 hours in patients <40 kg), depending upon condition.

Dosage adjustment in patients receiving concomitant CYP450 enzyme inducers or substrates:

Efavirenz: Oral: Increase maintenance dose of voriconazole to 400 mg every 12 hours and reduce efavirenz dose to 300 mg once daily; upon discontinuation of voriconazole, return to the initial dose of efavirenz.

Phenytoin:

IV: Increase voriconazole maintenance dose to 5 mg/kg every 12 hours.

Oral: Increase voriconazole maintenance dose to 400 mg every 12 hours in patients ≥40 kg (200 mg every 12 hours in patients <40 kg).

Pediatric Note: Actual body weight should be used for all weight-based dosing calculations.

Aspergillosis, invasive including disseminated and extrapulmonary infection treatment (off-label use):

Children >2 to <12 years (<40 kg): Duration of therapy should be a minimum of 6 to 12 weeks or throughout period of immunosuppression (Walsh 2008):

IV: **Note:** Data suggest higher doses (mg/kg) are required; consider using a loading dose: 9 mg/kg/dose every 12 hours for 2 doses on day 1, followed by a maintenance dose: 8 to 9 mg/kg/dose every 12 hours; maximum dose: 350 mg. Monitoring of concentrations may be warranted (Driscoll 2011; *Red Book* [AAP 2012]).

Non-HIV-exposed/-positive (Walsh 2008): 5 to 7 mg/kg/dose every 12 hours; see **Note** regarding higher dose recommendations

HIV-exposed/-positive (CDC 2009): See **Note** regarding higher dose recommendations.

Initial: 6 to 8 mg/kg/dose (maximum: 400 mg/dose) every 12 hours for 2 doses on day 1

Maintenance: 7 mg/kg/dose (maximum: 200 mg/dose) every 12 hours; change to oral administration when able; duration of therapy (IV and oral combined): ≥12 weeks but should be individualized

Oral suspension: May consider oral therapy once the patient is stable

Non-HIV-exposed/-positive (Red Book [AAP 2012]): 9 mg/kg every 12 hours

HIV-exposed/-positive (CDC 2009): **Note:** Data suggest higher doses (mg/kg) are required (9 mg/kg every 12 hours) (*Red Book* [AAP 2012])

Initial: 8 mg/kg/dose (maximum: 400 mg/dose) every 12 hours for 2 doses on day 1

Maintenance: 7 mg/kg/dose (maximum: 200 mg/dose) every 12 hours

Children ≥12 years and Adolescents: Refer to adult dosing.

Candidiasis or other serious fungal infection, treatment (off-label use; Driscoll 2011; *Red Book* [AAP 2012]):

Children >2 to <12 years: IV: Loading dose: 9 mg/kg/dose every 12 hours for 2 doses on day 1, followed by a maintenance dose: 8 to 9 mg/kg/dose every 12 hours; maximum dose: 350 mg

Children ≥12 years and Adolescents: Refer to adult dosing.

Catheter-related bloodstream infections due to *Malassezia furfur* (off-label use; Mermel 2009):

Children >2 to <12 years: IV: **Note:** Recent data suggest higher doses (mg/kg) than described in the guideline may be required (Driscoll 2011):

Initial: 6 mg/kg every 12 hours for 2 doses.

Maintenance: 4 mg/kg every 12 hours.

Children ≥12 years and Adolescents: Refer to adult dosing.

Coccidioidomycosis in HIV-infected patients (alternative to preferred therapy) (off-label use; HHS [OI adult 2015]): Adolescents: Oral: Refer to adult dosing.

Esophageal candidiasis:

Manufacturer's labeling: Children ≥12 years and Adolescents: Refer to adult dosing.

Alternative dosing: HIV-infected patients (alternative to preferred therapy): Adolescents: Refer to adult dosing.

Infection prophylaxis in graft-versus-host disease (GVHD) (off-label use; Tombyln 2009; Wingard 2010):

Children >2 to <12 years: **Note:** The optimal duration of prophylaxis in GVHD has not been determined.

IV: 4 mg/kg every 12 hours (maximum dose not to exceed weight-based oral dose)

Oral:

Weight <20 kg: 50 mg every 12 hours

Weight ≥20 kg: 100 mg every 12 hours

Children ≥12 years and Adolescents: Refer to adult dosing.

Infection prophylaxis in standard- or high-risk patients with allogeneic hematopoietic stem cell transplant (HSCT) or certain autologous HSCT (off-label use): Adolescents (>40 kg): Refer to adult dosing.

***Penicillium marneffei* infection in HIV-infected patients (off-label use; HHS [OI adult 2015]):** Refer to adult dosing.

Renal Impairment

IV:

CrCl ≥50 mL/minute: There are no dosage adjustments provided in the manufacturer's labeling.

CrCl <50 mL/minute: There are no specific dosage adjustments provided in the manufacturer's labeling. Due to accumulation of the intravenous vehicle (cyclodextrin), the manufacturer recommends the use of oral voriconazole in these patients unless an assessment of the benefit:risk justifies the use of IV voriconazole; if IV therapy is used, closely monitor serum creatinine and change to oral voriconazole when possible. IV therapy has been used in select patients with CrCl <50 mL/minute using varying doses (median duration of treatment 7 to 10 days) (Neofytos 2012; Oude Lashof 2012).

Oral:

Mild to severe impairment: No dosage adjustment necessary.

Dialysis: Poorly dialyzed; no supplemental dose or dosage adjustment necessary, including patients on intermittent hemodialysis (IHD) with thrice weekly sessions or peritoneal dialysis.

Continuous renal replacement therapy (CRRT) (Heintz 2009): Drug clearance is highly dependent on the method of renal replacement, filter type, and flow rate. Appropriate dosing requires close monitoring of pharmacologic response, signs of adverse reactions due to drug accumulation, as well as drug concentrations in relation to target trough (if appropriate). The following are general recommendations only (based on dialysate flow/ultrafiltration rates of 1 to 2 L/hour and minimal residual renal function) and should not supersede clinical judgment:

CVVH, CVVHD, and CVVHDF: Loading dose of 400 mg every 12 hours for 2 doses, followed by 200 mg every 12 hours.

Hepatic Impairment

Mild to moderate impairment (Child-Pugh class A or B): Following standard loading dose, reduce maintenance dosage by 50%

Severe impairment (Child-Pugh class C): There are no dosage adjustments provided in the manufacturer's labeling (has not been studied). Should only be used if benefit outweighs risk; monitor closely for toxicity

Administration

Oral: Administer 1 hour before or 1 hour after a meal. Shake oral suspension for approximately 10 seconds before each use. Enteral tube feedings may decrease oral absorption; may hold tube feedings for 1 hour before and 1 hour after a voriconazole dose (Williams 2012).

IV: Infuse over 1 to 2 hours (rate not to exceed 3 mg/kg/hour). Do not administer as an IV bolus injection. Do not infuse **concomitantly** into same line or cannula with other drug infusions. Do not infuse **concomitantly** in separate drug lines or cannulas with concentrated electrolyte solutions or blood products. May be infused simultaneously with nonconcentrated electrolytes or TPN through a separate IV line. If TPN is infused through a multiple lumen catheter, use a different port than used for voriconazole.

Hazardous agent - use appropriate precautions for handling and disposal (NIOSH 2014 [group 3]).

Monitoring Parameters Hepatic function at initiation, weekly during the first month and monthly during course of treatment; renal function; serum electrolytes (particularly calcium, magnesium and potassium) prior to initiation and during therapy; visual function (visual acuity, visual field and color perception) if treatment course continues >28 days; phototoxic reactions (especially in pediatric patients); monitor trough serum concentrations on day 5 of therapy and weekly thereafter for 4 to 6 weeks or when dosing adjustments are made; for infections other than

meningitis or osteoarticular infections, may consider obtaining voriconazole trough level to assure therapeutics serum concentrations, in patients failing therapy or in those exhibiting signs of toxicity; pancreatic function (in patients at risk for acute pancreatitis); total body skin examination yearly (more frequently if lesions noted)

Trough recommendations in adult patients:
Meningitis or osteoarticular infections for *Exserohilum rostratum* (CDC 2012): 2 to 5 mcg/mL
Other infections (Dolton 2012; Hamada 2012; Mitsani 2012; Park 2012):
Efficacy: >1.0 mcg/mL
Toxicity: <4.0 mcg/mL
Therapeutic range in adult patients (CDC 2012; Dolton 2012; Hamada 2012; Mitsani 2012; Park 2012; Tomblyn 2009): 1 to 5 mcg/mL

Refer to Additional Information for detailed discussion of these data and data in pediatric patients.

Reference Range Note: Refer to Additional Information section for detailed discussion of these data and data in pediatric patients.

Trough recommendations in adult patients:
Meningitis or osteoarticular infections for *Exserohilum rostratum* (CDC 2012): 2 to 5 mcg/mL
Other infections (Dolton 2012; Hamada 2012; Mitsani 2012; Park 2012):
Efficacy: >1.0 mcg/mL
Toxicity: <4.0 mcg/mL
Therapeutic range in adult patients (CDC 2012; Dolton 2012; Hamada 2012; Mitsani 2012; Park 2012; Tomblyn 2009): 1 to 5 mcg/mL

Additional Information The rationale supporting proposed therapeutic drug monitoring for voriconazole includes variable and unpredictable pharmacokinetics and drug toxicities. The metabolism of voriconazole is greatly influenced by hepatic enzyme saturation and genetic polymorphisms in the CYP2C19 isoenzyme system. These factors result in a nonlinear pharmacokinetic profile and wide inter-subject variability and poor dose-concentration relationship. Several studies have been published that have attempted to use therapeutic drug monitoring to decrease trough variability among patients receiving voriconazole. In one study, only 50% of patients achieved voriconazole trough concentrations within the target trough range without dose adjustments; the authors adjusted the dose of voriconazole to achieve a range of 1.0 to 5.5 mcg/mL (Park 2012). Regarding the utility of therapeutic drug monitoring and treatment outcomes, several recent studies have reported a relationship between voriconazole trough concentrations and clinical success (Dolton 2012; Hamada 2012; Mitsani 2012; Park 2012; Soler-Palacin 2012). Although there is variability among studies regarding the cutoff trough value associated with improved outcomes, it does appear that the probability of a positive outcome has been strongest when the voriconazole trough concentration is >1.0 mcg/mL. For toxicity, the strongest correlations have been made between voriconazole trough concentrations and neurological and dermatological adverse events (Dolton 2012; Hamada 2012; Mitsani 2012; Park 2012; Soler-Palacin 2012). In these reports, the authors generally noted increased toxicity when trough concentrations exceeded threshold values. There are much less data supporting the existence between a cutoff threshold and hepatotoxicity. It is important to note that cutoff trough values ranged widely among studies; however, an upper limit <5.0 mcg/mL would be reasonable for most infections based on the available literature (see CDC recommendations for *Exserohilum rostratum* which follow).

Another controversy is determining in which patients drug levels should be obtained. Most clinical laboratories do not perform on-site drug analysis for voriconazole. Therefore, the utility of routine drug levels may be limited in the acute management of patients. Therapeutic drug monitoring of voriconazole troughs may be reasonable if a patient is not responding to therapy or if they are being placed on long-term prophylaxis or treatment. In response to the outbreak of infections secondary to contaminated (eg, *Exserohilum rostratum*) steroid products, the CDC has recommended that trough serum concentrations for treatment of *Exserohilum rostratum* must be maintained between 2 to 5 mcg/mL (CDC 2012).

Trough recommendations in adult patients:
Meningitis or osteoarticular infections for *Exserohilum rostratum* (CDC 2012): 2 to 5 mcg/mL
Other infections (Dolton 2012; Hamada 2012; Mitsani 2012; Park 2012):
Efficacy: >1.0 mcg/mL
Toxicity: <4.0 mcg/mL

Therapeutic range in adult patients (CDC 2012; Dolton 2012; Hamada 2012; Mitsani 2012; Park 2012; Tomblyn 2009): 1 to 5 mcg/mL
In children, plasma voriconazole levels vary widely; in older children, voriconazole pharmacokinetics trend toward nonlinear relationships. In one study, the median doses to achieve therapeutic levels for children <5 years of age and for children >5 years of age were 38 mg/kg/day and 15 mg/kg/day, respectively (Soler-Palacin 2012). Trough concentration recommendations for children have not been determined.

Dosage Forms Excipient information presented when available (limited, particularly for generics); consult specific product labeling.
Solution Reconstituted, Intravenous:
Generic: 200 mg (1 ea)
Solution Reconstituted, Intravenous [preservative free]:
Vfend IV: 200 mg (1 ea) [latex free]
Vfend IV: 200 mg (1 ea)
Suspension Reconstituted, Oral:
Vfend: 40 mg/mL (75 mL) [contains sodium benzoate; orange flavor]
Generic: 40 mg/mL (75 mL)
Tablet, Oral:
Vfend: 50 mg, 200 mg
Generic: 50 mg, 200 mg

◆ Voriconazole For Injection (Can) *see* Voriconazole on page 1908

Vorinostat (vor IN oh stat)

Brand Names: US Zolinza
Brand Names: Canada Zolinza
Index Terms SAHA; Suberoylanilide Hydroxamic Acid
Pharmacologic Category Antineoplastic Agent, Histone Deacetylase (HDAC) Inhibitor
Use Cutaneous T-cell lymphoma: Treatment of cutaneous manifestations of cutaneous T-cell lymphoma (CTCL) with progressive, persistent, or recurrent disease on or following 2 systemic treatments
Pregnancy Considerations Adverse events were observed in animal reproduction studies. Based on the mechanism of action, may cause fetal harm if administered during pregnancy. Inform patient of potential hazard if used during pregnancy or if pregnancy occurs during treatment.
Breast-Feeding Considerations It is not known if vorinostat is excreted in breast milk. Due to the potential for serious adverse reactions in the nursing infant, the decision to discontinue vorinostat or to discontinue breast-feeding should take into account the benefits of treatment to the mother.
Contraindications There are no contraindications in the manufacturer's U.S. labeling.

Canadian labeling: Hypersensitivity to vorinostat or any component of the formulation; severe hepatic impairment (total bilirubin ≥3 times ULN)
Warnings/Precautions Hazardous agent - use appropriate precautions for handling and disposal (NIOSH 2014 [group 1]). Pulmonary embolism and deep vein thrombosis (DVT) have been reported; monitor for signs/symptoms; use caution in patients with a history of thrombotic events. Dose-related thrombocytopenia and/or anemia may occur; may require dosage adjustments or discontinuation; monitor blood counts (every 2 weeks for 2 months, then monthly). Gastrointestinal bleeding due to severe thrombocytopenia has been reported in patients receiving vorinostat in combination with other histone deacetylase inhibitors (eg, valproic acid); monitor platelet counts more frequently in patients receiving concomitant histone deacetylase inhibitor therapy. QTc prolongation has been observed; baseline and periodic ECGs were done in clinical trials (Duvic, 2007; Olsen, 2007). Correct electrolyte abnormalities prior to treatment and monitor and correct potassium, calcium, and magnesium levels during therapy. Use caution in patients with a history of QTc prolongation or with medications known to prolong the QT interval. May cause hyperglycemia (may be severe); monitor serum glucose and use with caution in diabetics; may require diet and/or therapy modifications. Nausea, vomiting, and diarrhea may occur; antiemetics and anti-diarrheals may be required; control preexisting nausea, vomiting, and diarrhea prior to treatment initiation; replace fluids and electrolytes to avoid dehydration. Adverse anastomotic healing events have occurred in patients recovering from bowel surgery; use with caution in the perioperative period in patients requiring bowel surgery. May cause dizziness or fatigue; caution patients about performing tasks which require mental alertness (eg, operating machinery or driving). Use with caution in patients with hepatic impairment; dose reductions are ▶

recommended (elimination is predominantly hepatic). The Canadian labeling does not recommend use in patients with moderate hepatic impairment (total bilirubin 1.5 to 3 times ULN) and contraindicates use in severe hepatic impairment (bilirubin ≥3 times ULN). Potentially significant drug-drug interactions may exist, requiring dose or frequency adjustment, additional monitoring, and/or selection of alternative therapy.

Adverse Reactions

>10%:

Cardiovascular: Peripheral edema (13%)

Central nervous system: Fatigue (52%), chills (16%), dizziness (15%), headache (12%), fever (11%)

Dermatologic: Alopecia (19%), pruritus (12%)

Endocrine & metabolic: Hyperglycemia (8% to 69%; grade 3: 5%), dehydration (1% to 16%)

Gastrointestinal: Diarrhea (52%), nausea (41%), taste alteration (28%), anorexia (24%), weight loss (21%), xerostomia (16%), constipation (15%), vomiting (15%), appetite decreased (14%)

Hematologic: Thrombocytopenia (26%; grades 3/4: 6%), anemia (14%; grades 3/4: 2%)

Neuromuscular & skeletal: Muscle spasm (20%)

Renal: Proteinuria (51%), creatinine increased (16% to 47%)

Respiratory: Cough (11%), upper respiratory infection (11%)

1% to 10%:

Cardiovascular: QTc prolongation (3% to 4%)

Dermatologic: Squamous cell carcinoma (4%)

Respiratory: Pulmonary embolism (5%)

<1% (Limited to important or life-threatening): Abdominal pain, angioneurotic edema, blurred vision, chest pain, cholecystitis, deafness, diverticulitis, dysphagia, DVT, enterococcal infection, exfoliative dermatitis, gastrointestinal bleeding, gastrointestinal hemorrhage, Guillain-Barré syndrome, hemoptysis, hypertension, hypokalemia, hyponatremia, infection, lethargy, leukopenia, MI, neutropenia, pneumonia, renal failure, sepsis, spinal cord injury, streptococcal bacteremia, stroke (ischemic), syncope, T-cell lymphoma, tumor hemorrhage, ureteric obstruction, ureteropelvic junction obstruction, urinary retention, vasculitis, weakness

Drug Interactions

Metabolism/Transport Effects None known.

Avoid Concomitant Use

Avoid concomitant use of Vorinostat with any of the following: BCG (Intravesical); Deferiprone; Dipyrone

Increased Effect/Toxicity

Vorinostat may increase the levels/effects of: CloZAPine; Deferiprone; Highest Risk QTc-Prolonging Agents; Moderate Risk QTc-Prolonging Agents; Vitamin K Antagonists

The levels/effects of Vorinostat may be increased by: Dipyrone; Mifepristone; Valproate Products

Decreased Effect

Vorinostat may decrease the levels/effects of: Antidiabetic Agents; BCG (Intravesical)

Storage/Stability Store at 20°C to 25°C (68°F to 77°F); excursions permitted to 15°C to 30°C (59°F to 86°F).

Mechanism of Action Inhibits histone deacetylase enzymes, HDAC1, HDAC2, HDAC3, and HDAC6, which catalyze acetyl group removal from protein lysine residues (including histones and transcription factors). Histone deacetylase inhibition results in accumulation of acetyl groups, which alters chromatin structure and transcription factor activation; cell growth is terminated and apoptosis occurs.

Pharmacodynamics/Kinetics

Protein binding: ~71%

Metabolism: Glucuronidated and hydrolyzed (followed by beta-oxidation) to inactive metabolites

Bioavailability: Fasting: ~43%

Half-life elimination: ~2 hours

Time to peak, plasma: With high-fat meal: ~4 hours (range: 2 to 10 hours)

Excretion: Urine: 52% (~52% as inactive metabolites; <1% as unchanged drug)

Dosing

Adult & Geriatric Cutaneous T-cell lymphoma (CTCL): Oral: 400 mg once daily until disease progression or unacceptable toxicity

Renal Impairment There are no dosage adjustments provided in the manufacturer's labeling (has not been studied). However, based on the minimal renal elimination, adjustment not expected. Use with caution.

Hepatic Impairment

U.S. labeling: Initial:

Mild-to-moderate impairment (total bilirubin 1-3 times ULN **or** AST >ULN): 300 mg once daily

Severe impairment (total bilirubin >3 times ULN): There are no dosage adjustments provided in the manufacturer's labeling (evidence is insufficient for a starting dose recommendation). Doses of 100 to 200 mg once daily were studied in a limited number of patients with severe impairment (Ramalingam, 2010); according to the manufacturer, the maximum dose used was 200 mg once daily.

Canadian labeling:

Mild impairment (total bilirubin >1 to 1.5 times ULN or total bilirubin ≤ULN and AST >ULN): 300 mg once daily

Moderate impairment (total bilirubin 1.5-3 times ULN): Use is not recommended

Severe impairment (total bilirubin ≥3 times ULN): Use is contraindicated

Adjustment for Toxicity

U.S. labeling: Intolerance: Reduce dose to 300 mg once daily; if needed, may further reduce to 300 mg daily for 5 consecutive days per week

Canadian labeling: Grade 3 or 4 toxicity: Interrupt therapy until resolves to ≤ grade 1 (excluding grade 3 anemia and thrombocytopenia). Upon recovery, may reduce dose to 300 mg once daily. If necessary, may further reduce dose to 300 mg once daily for 5 consecutive days per week.

Additionally, in clinical trials, **dose reductions** were instituted for the following adverse events: Increased serum creatinine, decreased appetite, hypokalemia, leukopenia, nausea, neutropenia, thrombocytopenia, and vomiting. Vorinostat was **discontinued** for the following adverse events: Anemia, angioneurotic edema, weakness, chest pain, exfoliative dermatitis, DVT, ischemic stroke, lethargy, pulmonary embolism, and spinal cord injury. Baseline

Treatment was withheld in clinical trials for grade 4 anemia or thrombocytopenia or other grade 3 or 4 drug related toxicity, until resolved to ≤ grade 1. Treatment was reinitiated with dose reduction (Olsen, 2007).

Administration Administer with food. Do not open, crush, break, or chew capsules. Maintain adequate hydration (≥2 L/day fluids) during treatment.

Hazardous agent; use appropriate precautions for handling and disposal (NIOSH 2014 [group 1]). Avoid direct skin or mucous membrane contact with crushed or broken capsules and/or capsule contents.

Monitoring Parameters CBC with differential and serum chemistries, including calcium, magnesium, potassium, glucose and creatinine (baseline, then every 2 weeks for 2 months, then monthly, or as clinically necessary), hepatic function, INR (if on concomitant warfarin therapy), fluid status, signs/symptoms of thromboembolism. Baseline and periodic ECGs were done in clinical trials (and are recommended in the Canadian labeling).

Dosage Forms Excipient information presented when available (limited, particularly for generics); consult specific product labeling.

Capsule, Oral:

Zolinza: 100 mg

Extemporaneous Preparations Hazardous agent: Use appropriate precautions for handling and disposal (NIOSH 2014 [group 1]).

Although not recommended by the manufacturer, a 50 mg/mL oral suspension may be prepared with capsules. Add 20 mL Ora-Plus® into a glass bottle (≥4 oz). Add the contents of twenty 100 mg capsules and shake thoroughly to disperse (may take up to 3 minutes). Add 20 mL Ora-Sweet® and shake to disperse. Label "shake well". Stable for 14 days at room temperature.

Fouladi M, Park JR, Stewart CF, et al, "Pediatric Phase I Trial and Pharmacokinetic Study of Vorinostat: A Children's Oncology Group Phase I Consortium Report," *J Clin Oncol*, 2010, 28(22):3623-9.

Vortioxetine (vor tye OX e teen)

Brand Names: US Brintellix

Brand Names: Canada Trintellix

Index Terms Lu AA21004; Vortioxetine Hydrobromide

Pharmacologic Category Antidepressant, Selective Serotonin Reuptake Inhibitor; Serotonin 5-HT$_{1A}$ Receptor Agonist; Serotonin 5-HT$_3$ Receptor Antagonist

Use Major depressive disorder: Treatment of major depressive disorder (MDD)

Pregnancy Considerations Adverse events were observed in animal reproduction studies. Nonteratogenic effects in the newborn following SSRI/SNRI exposure late in the third trimester include respiratory distress, cyanosis, apnea, seizures, temperature instability, feeding difficulty, vomiting, hypoglycemia, hypo- or hypertonia, hyperreflexia, jitteriness, irritability, constant crying, and tremor. Symptoms may be due to the toxicity of the SSRIs/SNRIs

or a discontinuation syndrome and may be consistent with serotonin syndrome associated with SSRI treatment. Persistent pulmonary hypertension of the newborn (PPHN) has also been reported with SSRI exposure.

The ACOG recommends that therapy with SSRIs or SNRIs during pregnancy be individualized; treatment of depression during pregnancy should incorporate the clinical expertise of the mental health clinician, obstetrician, primary healthcare provider, and pediatrician (ACOG, 2008). According to the American Psychiatric Association (APA), the risks of medication treatment should be weighed against other treatment options and untreated depression. For women who discontinue antidepressant medications during pregnancy and who may be at high risk for postpartum depression, the medications can be restarted following delivery (APA, 2010). Treatment algorithms have been developed by the ACOG and the APA for the management of depression in women prior to conception and during pregnancy (Yonkers, 2009).

Breast-Feeding Considerations It is not known if vortioxetine is excreted into breast milk. Due to the potential for serious adverse reactions in the nursing infant, the manufacturer recommends a decision be made whether to discontinue nursing or to discontinue the drug, taking into account the importance of treatment to the mother.

Medication Guide Available Yes

Contraindications Hypersensitivity to vortioxetine or any component of the formulation; use of MAO inhibitors intended to treat psychiatric disorders (concurrently or within 21 days of discontinuing vortioxetine or within 14 days of discontinuing the MAO inhibitor); initiation of vortioxetine in a patient receiving linezolid or intravenous methylene blue

Warnings/Precautions [U.S. Boxed Warning]: Antidepressants increase the risk of suicidal thinking and behavior in children, adolescents, and young adults (18 to 24 years of age) with major depressive disorder (MDD) and other psychiatric disorders; consider risk prior to prescribing. Short-term studies did not show an increased risk in patients >24 years of age and showed a decreased risk in patients ≥65 years. Closely monitor patients for clinical worsening, suicidality, or unusual changes in behavior, particularly during the initial 1 to 2 months of therapy or during periods of dosage adjustments (increases or decreases); the patient's family or caregiver should be instructed to closely observe the patient and communicate condition with healthcare provider. A medication guide concerning the use of antidepressants should be dispensed with each prescription. **Vortioxetine is not approved for use in children.**

The possibility of a suicide attempt is inherent in major depression and may persist until remission occurs. Use caution in high-risk patients. Worsening depression and severe abrupt suicidality that are not part of the presenting symptoms may require discontinuation or modification of drug therapy. The patient's family or caregiver should be alerted to monitor patients for the emergence of suicidality and associated behaviors (such as agitation, irritability, hostility, aggressiveness, impulsivity, and hypomania) and call healthcare provider.

May worsen psychosis in some patients or precipitate a mixed/manic episode in patients at risk for bipolar disorder. Use with caution in patients with a family history of bipolar disorder, mania, or hypomania. Patients presenting with depressive symptoms should be screened for bipolar disorder. **Vortioxetine is not FDA approved for the treatment of bipolar depression.**

Potentially life-threatening serotonin syndrome (SS) has occurred with serotonergic antidepressants (eg, SSRIs, SNRIs), particularly when used in combination with other serotonergic agents (eg, triptans, TCAs, fentanyl, lithium, tramadol, buspirone, St John's wort, tryptophan) or agents that impair metabolism of serotonin (eg, MAO inhibitors intended to treat psychiatric disorders, other MAO inhibitors [ie, linezolid and intravenous methylene blue]). Discontinue treatment (and any concomitant serotonergic agent) immediately if signs/symptoms arise.

May impair platelet aggregation resulting in increased risk of bleeding events, particularly if used concomitantly with aspirin, NSAIDs, warfarin or other anticoagulants. Bleeding related to antidepressant use has been reported to range from relatively minor bruising and epistaxis to life-threatening hemorrhage. May cause hyponatremia/SIADH (elderly at increased risk); volume depletion (diuretics may increase risk) may occur. Bone fractures have been associated with antidepressant treatment. Consider the possibility of a fragility fracture if an antidepressant-treated patient presents with unexplained bone pain, point tenderness, swelling, or bruising (Rabenda, 2013; Rizzoli, 2012).

Use caution in elderly patients; may be potentially inappropriate in patients with a history of falls or fractures, and may cause or exacerbate syndrome of inappropriate antidiuretic hormone secretion or hyponatremia; monitor sodium closely with initiation or dosage adjustments in older adults (Beers Criteria). May cause mild pupillary dilation which in susceptible individuals can lead to an episode of narrow-angle glaucoma. Consider evaluating patients who have not had an iridectomy for narrow-angle glaucoma risk factors. May cause CNS depression, which may impair physical or mental abilities; patients must be cautioned about performing tasks that require mental alertness (eg, operating machinery or driving). Angioedema has been reported. Use with caution in patients with seizure disorders; seizures (rare) have been reported in patients without a prior history of seizures. Potentially significant drug-drug interactions may exist, requiring dose or frequency adjustment, additional monitoring, and/or selection of alternative therapy. Use is not recommended in severe hepatic impairment.

Abrupt discontinuation or interruption of antidepressant therapy has been associated with a discontinuation syndrome. Symptoms arising may vary with antidepressant however commonly include nausea, vomiting, diarrhea, headaches, lightheadedness, dizziness, diminished appetite, sweating, chills, tremors, paresthesias, fatigue, somnolence, and sleep disturbances (eg, vivid dreams, insomnia). Greater risks for developing a discontinuation syndrome have been associated with antidepressants with shorter half-lives, longer durations of treatment, and abrupt discontinuation. For antidepressants of short or intermediate half-lives, symptoms may emerge within 2 to 5 days after treatment discontinuation and last 7 to 14 days (APA, 2010; Fava, 2006; Haddad, 2001; Shelton, 2001; Warner, 2006).

Adverse Reactions

>10%:
- Central nervous system: Female sexual disorder (self-reporting: 1% to 2%; Arizona Sexual Experience Scale: 22% to 34%), male sexual disorder (self-reporting: 3% to 5%; Arizona Sexual Experience Scale: 16% to 29%)
- Gastrointestinal: Nausea (dose-related, females >males, 21% to 32%; commonly occurs within the first week of treatment, then decreases in frequency but can persist in some patients)

1% to 10%:
- Central nervous system: Dizziness (8% to 9%), abnormal dreams (2% to 3%)
- Dermatologic: Pruritus (2% to 3%)
- Gastrointestinal: Diarrhea (7% to 10%), xerostomia (7% to 8%), constipation (5% to 6%), vomiting (3% to 6%), flatulence (2% to 3%)

<1% (Limited to important or life-threatening): Angle-closure glaucoma, hypomania, hyponatremia, mania, seizure, serotonin syndrome, withdrawal syndrome

Drug Interactions

Metabolism/Transport Effects Substrate of CYP2A6 (minor), CYP2B6 (minor), CYP2C19 (minor), CYP2C8 (minor), CYP2C9 (minor), CYP2D6 (major), CYP3A4 (major); **Note:** Assignment of Major/Minor substrate status based on clinically relevant drug interaction potential

Avoid Concomitant Use

Avoid concomitant use of Vortioxetine with any of the following: Dapoxetine; Dosulepin; Iobenguane I 123; Linezolid; MAO Inhibitors; Methylene Blue; Pimozide; Tryptophan; Urokinase

Increased Effect/Toxicity

Vortioxetine may increase the levels/effects of: Agents with Antiplatelet Properties; Anticoagulants; Antidepressants (Serotonin Reuptake Inhibitor/Antagonist); Antipsychotic Agents; Apixaban; Aspirin; Beta-Blockers; Blood Glucose Lowering Agents; BusPIRone; CarBAMazepine; CloZAPine; Collagenase (Systemic); Dabigatran Etexilate; Deoxycholic Acid; Desmopressin; Dextromethorphan; Dosulepin; Edoxaban; Galantamine; Ibritumomab; Methadone; Methylene Blue; Mexiletine; NSAID (COX-2 Inhibitor); NSAID (Nonselective); Obinutuzumab; Pimozide; RisperiDONE; Rivaroxaban; Salicylates; Serotonin Modulators; Thiazide Diuretics; Thrombolytic Agents; Tositumomab and Iodine I 131 Tositumomab; TraMADol; Urokinase; Vitamin K Antagonists

The levels/effects of Vortioxetine may be increased by: Abiraterone Acetate; Alcohol (Ethyl); Analgesics (Opioid); Antiemetics (5HT3 Antagonists); Antipsychotic Agents; BuPROPion; BusPIRone; Cimetidine; CNS Depressants; Cobicistat; CYP2D6 Inhibitors (Moderate); CYP2D6 Inhibitors (Strong); Dapoxetine; Darunavir; Dasatinib; Glucosamine; Herbs (Anticoagulant/Antiplatelet Properties); Ibrutinib; Limaprost; Linezolid; Lithium; MAO Inhibitors; Metaxalone; Metoclopramide; Metyrosine; Multivitamins/Fluoride (with ADE); Multivitamins/Minerals

(with ADEK, Folate, Iron); Multivitamins/Minerals (with AE, No Iron); Omega-3 Fatty Acids; Osimertinib; Panobinostat; Peginterferon Alfa-2b; Pentosan Polysulfate Sodium; Pentoxifylline; Prostacyclin Analogues; Tedizolid; TraMADol; Tryptophan; Vitamin E; Vitamin E (Oral)

Decreased Effect

Vortioxetine may decrease the levels/effects of: Iobenguane I 123; Ioflupane I 123; Thyroid Products

The levels/effects of Vortioxetine may be decreased by: Bosentan; CarBAMazepine; CYP3A4 Inducers (Moderate); CYP3A4 Inducers (Strong); Cyproheptadine; Dabrafenib; Deferasirox; Enzalutamide; Mitotane; NSAID (COX-2 Inhibitor); NSAID (Nonselective); Osimertinib; Peginterferon Alfa-2b; Siltuximab; St Johns Wort; Tocilizumab

Storage/Stability Store at 25°C (77°F); excursions are permitted between 15°C and 30°C (59°F and 86°F).

Mechanism of Action Inhibits reuptake of serotonin (5-HT); also has agonist activity at the 5-HT$_{1A}$ receptor and antagonist activity at the 5-HT$_3$ receptor.

Pharmacodynamics/Kinetics

Absorption: Not affected by food
Distribution: V$_d$: 2600 L
Protein binding: 98%
Metabolism: Hepatic primarily through oxidation via CYP450 isoenzymes, primarily CYP2D6, and subsequent glucuronic acid conjugation to an inactive carboxylic acid metabolite
Bioavailability: 75%
Half-life elimination: ~66 hours
Time to peak: 7-11 hours
Excretion: Urine (59%); feces (26%)

Dosing

Adult

Major depressive disorder: Oral: Initial: 10 mg once daily; increase to 20 mg once daily as tolerated; consider 5 mg once daily for patients who do not tolerate higher doses. Maintenance: 5-20 mg once daily.

Dosage adjustment for CYP2D6 poor metabolizers: Maximum dose: 10 mg once daily.
Dosage adjustment for concomitant therapy with strong CYP2D6 inhibitors: Reduce total daily dose by one half when a strong CYP2D6 inhibitor (eg, bupropion, fluoxetine, paroxetine, or quinidine) is coadministered. Increase dose to original level when the CYP2D6 inhibitor is discontinued.

Consider increasing the dose when a strong CYP inducer (eg, rifampin, carbamazepine, phenytoin) is coadministered for >14 days. Maximum dose should not exceed three times the original dose. Reduce the dose to the original level within 14 days of discontinuing the CYP inducer.

Discontinuation of therapy: Upon discontinuation of antidepressant therapy, gradually taper the dose to minimize the incidence of withdrawal symptoms and allow for the detection of re-emerging symptoms. Evidence supporting ideal taper rates is limited. APA and NICE guidelines suggest tapering therapy over at least several weeks with consideration to the half-life of the antidepressant; antidepressants with a shorter half-life may need to be tapered more conservatively. In addition for long-term treated patients, WFSBP guidelines recommend tapering over 4-6 months. If intolerable withdrawal symptoms occur following a dose reduction, consider resuming the previously prescribed dose and/or decrease dose at a more gradual rate (APA, 2010; Bauer, 2002; Haddad, 2001; NCCMH, 2010; Schatzberg, 2006; Shelton, 2001; Warner, 2006).

Vortioxetine doses of 15 mg once daily or more are recommended by the manufacturer to be decreased to 10 mg once daily for one week before full discontinuation to prevent withdrawal symptoms.

MAO inhibitor recommendations:

Switching to or from an MAO inhibitor intended to treat psychiatric disorders:
Allow 14 days to elapse between discontinuing an MAO inhibitor intended to treat psychiatric disorders and initiation of vortioxetine.
Allow 21 days to elapse between discontinuing vortioxetine and initiation of an MAO inhibitor intended to treat psychiatric disorders.
Use with other MAO inhibitors (linezolid or IV methylene blue):
Do not initiate vortioxetine in patients receiving linezolid or IV methylene blue; consider other interventions for psychiatric condition.
If urgent treatment with linezolid or IV methylene blue is required in a patient already receiving vortioxetine and potential benefits outweigh potential risks, discontinue vortioxetine promptly and administer linezolid or IV methylene blue. Monitor for serotonin syndrome for 21 days or until 24 hours after the last dose of linezolid or IV methylene blue, whichever comes first. May resume vortioxetine 24 hours after the last dose of linezolid or IV methylene blue.

Geriatric

Major depressive disorder:
U.S. labeling: Refer to adult dosing.
Canadian labeling: Oral: Initial: 5 mg once daily; may increase to 10 mg once daily as tolerated. Use caution with doses >10 mg daily (maximum: 20 mg daily).

Renal Impairment No dosage adjustment necessary.

Hepatic Impairment
Mild-to-moderate impairment: No dosage adjustment necessary.
Severe impairment: Use not recommended (has not been studied).

Administration Administer without regard to meals.

Monitoring Parameters Mental status for depression, suicidal ideation (especially at the beginning of therapy or when doses are increased or decreased), anxiety, social functioning, mania, panic attacks; akathisia; signs/symptoms of serotonin syndrome and/or hyponatremia; hepatic function (baseline).

Dosage Forms Excipient information presented when available (limited, particularly for generics); consult specific product labeling.
Tablet, Oral:
Brintellix: 5 mg, 10 mg, 20 mg

Dosage Forms: Canada Excipient information presented when available (limited, particularly for generics); consult specific product labeling.
Tablet, Oral:
Trintellix: 5 mg, 10 mg, 20 mg

Warfarin (WAR far in)

Brand Names: US Coumadin; Jantoven
Brand Names: Canada Apo-Warfarin; Coumadin; Mylan-Warfarin; Novo-Warfarin; Taro-Warfarin
Index Terms Warfarin Sodium
Pharmacologic Category Anticoagulant; Anticoagulant, Vitamin K Antagonist

Additional Appendix Information

Oral Anticoagulant Comparison Chart *on page 1957*
Reversal of Oral Anticoagulants *on page 1959*

Use

Prophylaxis and treatment of thromboembolic disorders (eg, venous, pulmonary) and embolic complications arising from atrial fibrillation or cardiac valve replacement:

Nonvalvular AF or atrial flutter: The 2014 American Heart Association/American College of Cardiology/Heart Rhythm Society guidelines for the management of AF recommend oral anticoagulation for patients with nonvalvular AF or atrial flutter with prior stroke, TIA, or a CHA_2DS_2-VASc score ≥2. In patients with AF or atrial flutter of ≥48 hours duration or when the duration is unknown, anticoagulation with warfarin is recommended for at least 3 weeks prior to and 4 weeks after cardioversion regardless of the CHA_2DS_2-VASc score and method used to restore sinus rhythm (AHA/ACC [January, 2014]).

Valvular AF: The 2014 American Heart Association/American Stroke Association (AHA/ASA) guidelines for the primary prevention of stroke recommend chronic oral anticoagulation with warfarin for patients with valvular atrial fibrillation at high risk for stroke, defined as a CHA2DS2-VASc score of ≥2, and acceptably low risk for hemorrhagic complications (AHA/ASA [Meschia, 2014]).

Mechanical prosthetic cardiac valves: The 2014 American Heart Association/American Stroke Association (AHA/ASA) guidelines for the primary prevention of stroke recommend warfarin and low-dose aspirin in the patients who have received an aortic mechanical prosthetic valve (with or without risk factors) or any mitral mechanical prosthetic valve. Target INRs vary depending on valve position and/or risk factors (AHA/ASA [Meschia, 2014]).

Adjunct to reduce risk of systemic embolism (eg, recurrent MI, stroke) after myocardial infarction:
According to the American College of Cardiology/American Heart Association (ACCF/AHA) guidelines for the management of patients with ST-elevation myocardial infarction (STEMI), warfarin should be administered to patients with STEMI and AF and a $CHADS_2$ score of 2 or more, mechanical valve, venous thromboembolism, or hypercoagulable disorder. Use is reasonable in patients with STEMI and asymptomatic LV mural thrombi and may be considered in patients with STEMI and anterior apical akinesis or dyskinesis (O'Gara, 2013).

Pregnancy Considerations Warfarin crosses the placenta; concentrations in the fetal plasma are similar to maternal values. Teratogenic effects have been reported following first trimester exposure and may include coumarin embryopathy (nasal hypoplasia and/or stippled epiphyses; limb hypoplasia may also be present). Adverse CNS events to the fetus have also been observed following exposure during any trimester and may include CNS abnormalities (including ventral midline dysplasia, dorsal midline dysplasia). Spontaneous abortion, fetal hemorrhage, and fetal death may also occur. Use is contraindicated during pregnancy (or in women of reproductive potential) except in women with mechanical heart valves who are at high risk for thromboembolism; use is also contraindicated in women with threatened abortion, eclampsia, or preeclampsia. Frequent pregnancy tests are recommended for women who are planning to become pregnant and adjusted-dose heparin or low molecular weight heparin (LMWH) should be substituted as soon as pregnancy is confirmed or adjusted-dose heparin or LMWH should be used instead of warfarin prior to conception.

In pregnant women with high-risk mechanical heart valves, the benefits of warfarin therapy should be discussed with the risks of available treatments (ACCP [Bates, 2012]; AHA/ACC [Nishimura, 2014]); when possible avoid warfarin use during the first trimester (ACCP [Bates, 2012]) and close to delivery (ACCP [Bates, 2012]; AHA/ACC [Nishimura, 2014]). Use of warfarin during the first trimester may be considered if the therapeutic INR can be achieved with a dose ≤5 mg/day (AHA/ACC [Nishimura, 2014]). Adjusted-dose LMWH or adjusted-dose heparin may be used throughout pregnancy or until week 13 of gestation when therapy can be changed to warfarin. LMWH or heparin should be resumed close to delivery. In women who are at a very high risk for thromboembolism (older generation mechanical prosthesis in mitral position or history of thromboembolism), warfarin can be used throughout pregnancy and replaced with LMWH or heparin near term; the use of low-dose aspirin is also recommended (ACCP [Bates, 2012] AHA/ACC [Nishimura, 2014]). Women who require long-term anticoagulation with warfarin and who are considering pregnancy, LMWH

substitution should be done prior to conception when possible. If anti-Xa monitoring cannot be done, do not use LMWH therapy in pregnant patients with a mechanical prosthetic valve (AHA/ACC [Nishimura, 2014]). When choosing therapy, fetal outcomes (ie, pregnancy loss, malformations), maternal outcomes (ie, VTE, hemorrhage), burden of therapy, and maternal preference should be considered (ACCP [Bates, 2012]).

Breast-Feeding Considerations Breast-feeding women may be treated with warfarin. Based on available data, warfarin does not pass into breast milk. Women who are breast-feeding should be carefully monitored to avoid excessive anticoagulation. According to the American College of Chest Physicians (ACCP), warfarin may be used in lactating women who wish to breast-feed their infants (Bates, 2012). Monitor nursing infants for bruising or bleeding (per manufacturer).

Medication Guide Available Yes

Contraindications Hypersensitivity to warfarin or any component of the formulation; hemorrhagic tendencies (eg, patients bleeding from the GI, respiratory, or GU tract; cerebral aneurysm; cerebrovascular hemorrhage; dissecting aortic aneurysm; spinal puncture and other diagnostic or therapeutic procedures with potential for significant bleeding; history of bleeding diathesis); recent or potential surgery of the eye or CNS; major regional lumbar block anesthesia or traumatic surgery resulting in large, open surfaces; blood dyscrasias; severe uncontrolled or malignant hypertension; pericarditis or pericardial effusion; bacterial endocarditis; unsupervised patients with conditions associated with a high potential for noncompliance; eclampsia/pre-eclampsia, threatened abortion, pregnancy (except in women with mechanical heart valves at high risk for thromboembolism)

Warnings/Precautions Hazardous agent; use appropriate precautions for handling and disposal (NIOSH 2014 [group 3]).

Use care in the selection of patients appropriate for this treatment. Ensure patient cooperation especially from the alcoholic, illicit drug user, demented, or psychotic patient; ability to comply with routine laboratory monitoring is essential. Use with caution in trauma, acute infection, moderate-severe renal insufficiency, prolonged dietary insufficiencies, moderate-severe hypertension, polycythemia vera, vasculitis, open wound, active TB, any disruption in normal GI flora, history of PUD, anaphylactic disorders, indwelling catheters, severe diabetes, and menstruating and postpartum women. Use with caution in patients with thyroid disease; warfarin responsiveness may increase (Ageno, 2012). Use with caution in protein C deficiency. Use with caution in patients with heparin-induced thrombocytopenia and DVT. Warfarin monotherapy is contraindicated in the initial treatment of active HIT. Reduced liver function, regardless of etiology, may impair synthesis of coagulation factors leading to increased warfarin sensitivity.

[U.S. Boxed Warning]: May cause major or fatal bleeding. Risk factors for bleeding include high intensity anticoagulation (INR >4), age (>65 years), variable INRs, history of GI bleeding, hypertension, cerebrovascular disease, serious heart disease, anemia, malignancy, trauma, renal insufficiency, drug-drug interactions, long duration of therapy, or known genetic deficiency in CYP2C9 activity. Patient must be instructed to report bleeding, accidents, or falls. Unrecognized bleeding sites (eg, colon cancer) may be uncovered by anticoagulation. Patient must also report any new or discontinued medications, herbal or alternative products used, or significant changes in smoking or dietary habits. Necrosis or gangrene of the skin and other tissue can occur, usually in conjunction with protein C or S deficiency. Consider alternative therapies if anticoagulation is necessary. Warfarin therapy may release atheromatous plaque emboli; symptoms depend on site of embolization, most commonly kidneys, pancreas, liver, and spleen. In some cases may lead to necrosis or death. "Purple toes syndrome," due to cholesterol microembolization, may rarely occur. The elderly may be more sensitive to anticoagulant therapy.

Presence of the CYP2C9*2 or *3 allele and/or polymorphism of the vitamin K oxidoreductase (VKORC1) gene may increase the risk of bleeding. Lower doses may be required in these patients; genetic testing may help determine appropriate dosing.

When temporary interruption is necessary before surgery, discontinue for approximately 5 days before surgery; when there is adequate hemostasis, may reinstitute warfarin therapy ~12-24 hours after surgery (evening of or next morning). Decision to safely continue warfarin therapy through the procedure and whether or not bridging of anticoagulation is necessary is dependent upon risk of ▶

perioperative bleeding and risk of thromboembolism, respectively. If risk of thromboembolism is elevated, consider bridging warfarin therapy with an alternative anticoagulant (eg, unfractionated heparin, LMWH) (Guyatt, 2012).

Adverse Reactions Bleeding is the major adverse effect of warfarin. Hemorrhage may occur at virtually any site. Risk is dependent on multiple variables, including the intensity of anticoagulation and patient susceptibility.

Cardiovascular: Vasculitis

Central nervous system: Signs/symptoms of bleeding (eg, dizziness, fatigue, fever, headache, lethargy, malaise, pain)

Dermatologic: Alopecia, bullous eruptions, dermatitis, rash, pruritus, urticaria

Gastrointestinal: Abdominal pain, diarrhea, flatulence, gastrointestinal bleeding, nausea, taste disturbance, vomiting

Genitourinary: Hematuria

Hematologic: Anemia, retroperitoneal hematoma, unrecognized bleeding sites (eg, colon cancer) may be uncovered by anticoagulation

Hepatic: Hepatitis (including cholestatic hepatitis), transaminases increased

Neuromuscular & skeletal: Osteoporosis (potential association with long-term use), paralysis, paresthesia, weakness

Respiratory: Respiratory tract bleeding, tracheobronchial calcification

Miscellaneous: Anaphylactic reaction, hypersensitivity/allergic reactions, skin necrosis, gangrene, "purple toes" syndrome

Drug Interactions

Metabolism/Transport Effects Substrate of CYP1A2 (minor), CYP2C19 (minor), CYP2C9 (major), CYP3A4 (minor); **Note:** Assignment of Major/Minor substrate status based on clinically relevant drug interaction potential; **Inhibits** CYP2C19 (weak), CYP2C9 (weak)

Avoid Concomitant Use

Avoid concomitant use of Warfarin with any of the following: Apixaban; Dabigatran Etexilate; Edoxaban; Enzalutamide; Hemin; Omacetaxine; Rivaroxaban; Streptokinase; Tamoxifen; Urokinase; Vorapaxar

Increased Effect/Toxicity

Warfarin may increase the levels/effects of: Anticoagulants; Collagenase (Systemic); Deferasirox; Deoxycholic Acid; Ethotoin; Fosphenytoin; Ibritumomab; Nintedanib; Obinutuzumab; Omacetaxine; Phenytoin; Regorafenib; Rivaroxaban; Sulfonylureas; Tositumomab and Iodine I 131 Tositumomab

The levels/effects of Warfarin may be increased by: Acetaminophen; Agents with Antiplatelet Properties; Allopurinol; Amiodarone; Androgens; Apixaban; Atazanavir; Benzbromarone; Bicalutamide; Boceprevir; Capecitabine; Cephalosporins; Ceritinib; Chloral Hydrate; Chloramphenicol; Chondroitin Sulfate; Cimetidine; Clopidogrel; Cloxacillin; Cobicistat; Corticosteroids (Systemic); Cranberry; CYP2C9 Inhibitors (Moderate); CYP2C9 Inhibitors (Strong); Dabigatran Etexilate; Dasatinib; Desvenlafaxine; Dexmethylphenidate; Disulfiram; Dronedarone; Econazole; Edoxaban; Efavirenz; Erlotinib; Erythromycin (Ophthalmic); Esomeprazole; Ethacrynic Acid; Ethotoin; Etoposide; Etoposide Phosphate; Exenatide; Fenofibrate and Derivatives; Fenugreek; Fibric Acid Derivatives; Fluconazole; Fluorouracil (Systemic); Fluorouracil (Topical); Fosamprenavir; Fosphenytoin; Fusidic Acid (Systemic); Gefitinib; Gemcitabine; Ginkgo Biloba; Glucagon; Glucosamine; Green Tea; Hemin; Herbs (Anticoagulant/Antiplatelet Properties); HMG-CoA Reductase Inhibitors; Ibrutinib; Ifosfamide; Imatinib; Itraconazole; Ivermectin (Systemic); Ketoconazole (Systemic); Lansoprazole; Leflunomide; LevOCARNitine; Levomilnacipran; Limaprost; Lomitapide; Lumacaftor; Macrolide Antibiotics; Methylphenidate; Metreleptin; MetroNIDAZOLE (Systemic); Miconazole (Oral); Miconazole (Topical); Mifepristone; Milnacipran; Mirtazapine; Multivitamins/Fluoride (with ADE); Multivitamins/Minerals (with ADEK, Folate, Iron); Multivitamins/Minerals (with AE, No Iron); Nelfinavir; Neomycin; Nonsteroidal Anti-Inflammatory Agents; NSAID (COX-2 Inhibitor); NSAID (Nonselective); Omega-3 Fatty Acids; Omeprazole; Oritavancin; Orlistat; Penicillins; Pentosan Polysulfate Sodium; Pentoxifylline; Phenytoin; Posaconazole; Proguanil; Propacetamol; Propafenone; Prostacyclin Analogues; QuiNIDine; QuiNINE; Quinolone Antibiotics; Ranitidine; RomiDEPsin; Salicylates; Saquinavir; Selective Serotonin Reuptake Inhibitors; Sitaxentan; SORAfenib; Streptokinase; Sugammadex; Sulfinpyrazone; Sulfonamide Derivatives; Sulfonylureas; Tamoxifen; Tegafur; Telaprevir; Tetracycline Derivatives; Thrombolytic Agents; Thyroid Products; Tibolone; Tigecycline; Tipranavir; Tolterodine;

Toremifene; Torsemide; TraMADol; Tranilast (Systemic); Tricyclic Antidepressants; Urokinase; Vemurafenib; Venlafaxine; Vitamin E; Vitamin E (Oral); Vorapaxar; Voriconazole; Vorinostat; Zafirlukast; Zileuton

Decreased Effect

The levels/effects of Warfarin may be decreased by: Adalimumab; Alcohol (Ethyl); Antithyroid Agents; Aprepitant; AzaTHIOprine; Barbiturates; Bile Acid Sequestrants; Boceprevir; Bosentan; CarBAMazepine; Cloxacillin; Coenzyme Q-10; Contraceptives (Estrogens); Contraceptives (Progestins); CYP2C9 Inducers (Strong); Dabrafenib; Darunavir; Dicloxacillin; Efavirenz; Enzalutamide; Eslicarbazepine; Estrogen Derivatives; Flucloxacillin [Floxacillin]; Fosaprepitant; Ginseng (American); Glutethimide; Green Tea; Griseofulvin; Leflunomide; Lixisenatide; Lopinavir; Lumacaftor; Mercaptopurine; Metreleptin; Multivitamins/Minerals (with ADEK, Folate, Iron); Nafcillin; Nelfinavir; Phytonadione; Progestins; Rifamycin Derivatives; Ritonavir; St Johns Wort; Sucralfate; Telaprevir; Teriflunomide; Tranilast (Systemic); TraZODone

Food Interactions

Ethanol: Acute ethanol ingestion (binge drinking) decreases the metabolism of oral anticoagulants and increases PT/INR. Chronic daily ethanol use increases the metabolism of oral anticoagulants and decreases PT/INR. Management: Avoid ethanol.

Food: The anticoagulant effects of warfarin may be decreased if taken with foods rich in vitamin K. Vitamin E may increase warfarin effect. Cranberry juice may increase warfarin effect. Management: Maintain a consistent diet; consult prescriber before making changes in diet. Take warfarin at the same time each day.

Preparation for Administration Reconstitute with 2.7 mL of sterile water for injection (yields 2 mg/mL solution).

Hazardous agent; use appropriate precautions for handling and disposal (NIOSH 2014 [group 3]).

Storage/Stability

Injection: Prior to reconstitution, store at 15°C to 30°C (59°F to 86°F). Following reconstitution with 2.7 mL of sterile water (yields 2 mg/mL solution), stable for 4 hours at 15°C to 30°C (59°F to 86°F). Protect from light.

Tablet: Store at 15°C to 30°C (59°F to 86°F). Protect from light.

Mechanism of Action Hepatic synthesis of coagulation factors II (half-life 42 to 72 hours), VII (half-life 4 to 6 hours), IX, and X (half-life 27 to 48 hours), as well as proteins C and S, requires the presence of vitamin K. These clotting factors are biologically activated by the addition of carboxyl groups to key glutamic acid residues within the proteins' structure. In the process, "active" vitamin K is oxidatively converted to an "inactive" form, which is then subsequently reactivated by vitamin K epoxide reductase complex 1 (VKORC1). Warfarin competitively inhibits the subunit 1 of the multi-unit VKOR complex, thus depleting functional vitamin K reserves and hence reduces synthesis of active clotting factors.

Pharmacodynamics/Kinetics

Onset of action: Anticoagulation: Oral: 24-72 hours

Peak effect: Full therapeutic effect: 5-7 days; INR may increase in 36-72 hours

Duration: 2-5 days

Absorption: Oral: Rapid, complete

Distribution: 0.14 L/kg

Protein binding: 99%

Metabolism: Hepatic, primarily via CYP2C9; minor pathways include CYP2C8, 2C18, 2C19, 1A2, and 3A4

Genomic variants: Approximately 37% reduced clearance of S-warfarin in patients heterozygous for 2C9 (*1/*2 or *1/*3), and ~70% reduced in patients homozygous for reduced function alleles (*2/*2, *2/*3, or *3/*3)

Half-life elimination: 20-60 hours; Mean: 40 hours; highly variable among individuals

Time to peak, plasma: Oral: ~4 hours

Excretion: Urine (92%, primarily as metabolites)

Dosing

Adult Note: Coumadin injection has been discontinued in the US for more than 1 year.

Note: Labeling identifies genetic factors which may increase patient sensitivity to warfarin. Specifically, genetic variations in the proteins CYP2C9 and VKORC1, responsible for warfarin's primary metabolism and pharmacodynamic activity, respectively, have been identified as predisposing factors associated with decreased dose requirement and increased bleeding risk. Genotyping tests are available, and may provide guidance on initiation of anticoagulant therapy. The American College of Chest Physicians recommends against the use of routine pharmacogenomic testing to guide dosing (Guyatt, 2012). For management of elevated INRs as a result of warfarin therapy, see Additional Information for guidance.

Prevention/treatment of thrombosis/embolism:

IV (administer as a slow bolus injection): 2-5 mg/day

Oral: Initial dosing must be individualized. Consider the patient (hepatic function, cardiac function, age, nutritional status, concurrent therapy, risk of bleeding) in addition to prior dose response (if available) and the clinical situation. Start 2-5 mg once daily for 2 days **or** for healthy individuals, 10 mg once daily for 2 days; lower doses (eg, 5 mg once daily) recommended for patients with confirmed HIT once platelet recovery has occurred (Guyatt, 2012). In patients with acute venous thromboembolism, initiation may begin on the first or second day of low molecular weight heparin or unfractionated heparin therapy (Guyatt, 2012). Adjust dose according to INR results; usual maintenance dose ranges from 2-10 mg daily (individual patients may require loading and maintenance doses outside these general guidelines).

Note: Lower starting doses may be required for patients with hepatic impairment, poor nutrition, CHF, elderly, high risk of bleeding, or patients who are debilitated, or those with reduced function genomic variants of the catabolic enzymes CYP2C9 (*2 or *3 alleles) or VKORC1 (-1639 polymorphism); see table. Higher initial doses may be reasonable in selected patients (ie, receiving enzyme-inducing agents and with low risk of bleeding). Overlapping a parenteral anticoagulant and warfarin therapy by at least 5 days is necessary in treatment of DVT/PE even if the INR is therapeutic earlier. Although an elevation in INR (due to factor VII depletion) may be seen early (within the first 24-48 hours) in warfarin therapy, it does not represent adequate anticoagulation. Factors II and X must also be depleted which takes considerably longer (ACCP [Guyatt, 2012]).

Range[1] of Expected Therapeutic Maintenance Dose Based on CYP2C9[2] and VKORC1[3] Genotypes

VKORC1	CYP2C9					
	*1/*1	*1/*2	*1/*3	*2/*2	*2/*3	*3/*3
GG	5-7 mg	5-7 mg	3-4 mg	3-4 mg	3-4 mg	0.5-2 mg
AG	5-7 mg	3-4 mg	3-4 mg	3-4 mg	0.5-2 mg	0.5-2 mg
AA	3-4 mg	3-4 mg	0.5-2 mg	0.5-2 mg	0.5-2 mg	0.5-2 mg

Note: Must also take into account other patient related factors when determining initial dose (eg, age, body weight, concomitant medications, comorbidities). The American College of Chest Physicians recommends against the use of routine pharmacogenomic testing to guide dosing (Guyatt, 2012).

[1]Ranges derived from multiple published clinical studies.

[2]Patients with CYP2C9 *1/*3, *2/*2, *2/*3, and *3/*3 alleles may take up to 4 weeks to achieve maximum INR with a given dose regimen.

[3]VKORC1 -1639G>A (rs 9923231) variant is used in this table; other VKORC1 variants may also be important determinants of dose.

Geriatric Oral: Initial dose ≤5 mg. Usual maintenance dose: 2-5 mg/day. The elderly tend to require lower dosages to produce a therapeutic level of anticoagulation (due to changes in the pattern of warfarin metabolism).

Pediatric Note: Coumadin injection has been discontinued in the US for more than 1 year.

Note: Labeling identifies genetic factors which may increase patient sensitivity to warfarin. Specifically, genetic variations in the proteins CYP2C9 and VKORC1, responsible for warfarin's primary metabolism and pharmacodynamic activity, respectively, have been identified as predisposing factors associated with decreased dose requirement and increased bleeding risk. Genotyping tests are available, and may provide guidance on initiation of anticoagulant therapy. The American College of Chest Physicians recommends against the use of routine pharmacogenomic testing to guide dosing (Guyatt, 2012). For management of elevated INRs as a result of warfarin therapy, see Additional Information for guidance.

Prevention/treatment of thrombosis: Oral: Infants and Children (off-label use): Initial loading dose (if baseline INR is 1-1.3): 0.2 mg/kg (maximum: 10 mg/dose); adjust dose based on INR (reported ranges to maintain INR of 2-3: 0.09-0.33 mg/kg/day). Infants <12 months of age may require doses at or near the high end of this range; consistent anticoagulation may be difficult to maintain in children <5 years of age (Monagle, 2012).

Renal Impairment No dosage adjustment necessary. However, patients with renal failure have an increased risk of bleeding complications; monitor closely.

Hepatic Impairment No dosage adjustment provided in manufacturer's labeling. However, the response to oral anticoagulants may be markedly enhanced in obstructive jaundice, hepatitis, and cirrhosis. INR should be closely monitored.

Dietary Considerations Foods high in vitamin K (eg, leafy green vegetables) inhibit anticoagulant effect. The list of usual foods with high vitamin K content is well known, however, some unique ones include green tea (*Camellia sinensis*), chewing tobacco, a variety of oils (canola, corn, olive, peanut, safflower, sesame seed, soybean, and sunflower) (Booth, 1999; Kuykendall, 2004; Nutescu, 2011). Snack foods containing Olestra have 80 mcg of vitamin K added to each ounce (Harrell, 1999). Some natural products may contain hidden sources of vitamin K (Nutescu, 2006). Avoid drastic changes in diet (eg, intake of large amounts of alfalfa, asparagus, broccoli, Brussels sprouts, cabbage, cauliflower, green teas, kale, lettuce, spinach, turnip greens, watercress) which decrease efficacy of warfarin. A balanced diet with a consistent intake of vitamin K is essential. The recommended dietary allowance for vitamin K in adults is 75 to 120 mcg/day (USDA Dietary Reference Intake).

Administration

Oral: Administer with or without food. Take at the same time each day.

IV: Administer as a slow bolus injection over 1-2 minutes; avoid all IM injections

Hazardous agent; use appropriate precautions for handling and disposal (NIOSH 2014 [group 3]).

Monitoring Parameters Prothrombin time, hematocrit; INR (frequency varies depending on INR stability); may consider genotyping of CYP2C9 and VKORC1 prior to initiation of therapy, if available

Reference Range

INR = patient prothrombin time/mean normal prothrombin time

ISI = international sensitivity index

INR should be increased by 2-3.5 times depending upon indication. An INR >4 does not generally add additional therapeutic benefit and is associated with increased risk of bleeding. **Note:** To prevent gastrointestinal bleeding events in patients receiving the combination of warfarin, aspirin, and clopidogrel, an INR of 2-2.5 is recommended unless condition requires a higher INR target (eg, certain mechanical heart valves) (Bhatt, 2008).

Adult Target INR Ranges Based Upon Indication

Indication	Targeted INR	Targeted INR Range
Cardiac		
Anterior myocardial infarction with LV thrombus or high risk for LV thrombus (EF<40%, anteroapical wall motion abnormality)[1,2,3]	2.5	2-3
Atrial fibrillation (nonvalvular)[4] or atrial flutter	2.5	2-3
LV systolic dysfunction (without established CAD) (eg, Takotsubo cardiomyopathy) with an LV thrombus	2.5	2-3
Valvular		
Carbomedics or St. Jude Medical bileaflet or Medtronic Hall tilting disk mechanical aortic valve in normal sinus rhythm and normal LA size[5]	2.5	2-3
Bileaflet or tilting disk mechanical mitral valve[5]	3	2.5-3.5
Caged ball or caged disk mechanical valve[5]	3	2.5-3.5
Mechanical aortic valve[6,7,8]	2.5	2-3
Mechanical aortic valve (with risk factors[6,9]), mechanical mitral valve[6], **or** mechanical valves in both the aortic and mitral positions[6]	3	2.5-3.5
Bioprosthetic mitral valve[10]	2.5	2-3
Rheumatic mitral valve disease (particularly mitral stenosis) and normal sinus rhythm (LA diameter >5.5 cm), AF, previous systemic embolism, or LA thrombus	2.5	2-3
Thromboembolism Treatment		
Venous thromboembolism[11]	2.5	2-3
Thromboprophylaxis		
Idiopathic pulmonary artery hypertension (IPAH)[12]	2	1.5-2.5
Antiphospholipid syndrome (no other risk factors)	2.5	2-3
Antiphospholipid syndrome and recurrent thromboembolism	2.5	2-3
Total hip or knee replacement or hip fracture surgery[13]	2.5	2-3

(continued)

Adult Target INR Ranges Based Upon Indication
(continued)

Indication	Targeted INR	Targeted INR Range
Other Indications		
Ischemic stroke due to AF[14]	2.5	2-3
Cryptogenic stroke (recurrent) and either patent foramen ovale (PFO) or atrial septal aneurysm	2.5	2-3

Note: Unless otherwise noted, all recommendations derived from "Antithrombotic Therapy and Prevention of Thrombosis, 9th ed: American College of Chest Physicians Evidence-Based Clinical Practice Guidelines."

[1]If coronary stent placed, triple therapy (warfarin, low-dose aspirin, and clopidogrel) is recommended for 1 month (bare-metal stent) or 3-6 months (drug-eluting stent) followed by discontinuation of warfarin and use of dual antiplatelet therapy (eg, aspirin and clopidogrel) for up to 12 months.

[2]If coronary stent **not** placed, maintain anticoagulation (in combination with low-dose aspirin) for 3 months followed by discontinuation of warfarin and use of dual antiplatelet therapy (eg, aspirin and clopidogrel) for up to 12 months.

[3]The ACCF/AHA guidelines for the management of STEMI, suggest that a lower INR range of 2-2.5 might be considered in patients with STEMI receiving dual antiplatelet therapy (O'Gara, 2013).

[4]Recommended for those patients with nonvalvular AF or atrial flutter with prior stroke, TIA, or a CHA$_2$DS$_2$-VASc score ≥2 (AHA/ACC/HRS [January, 2014]).

[5]Recommendation from Stein, 2001.

[6]If at low risk of bleeding, combine with aspirin 81 mg/day.

[7]The AHA/ASA recommends use in patients with bileaflet mechanical or current-generation, single-tilting-disk prostheses (AHA/ASA [Meschia, 2014]).

[8]The On-X prosthetic aortic valve requires an initial INR of 2 to 3 for 3 months after valve insertion followed by an INR of 1.5 to 2 indefinitely. Unless contraindicated, continuous use of concurrent aspirin 75 to 100 mg daily is also recommended.

[9]Risk factors defined by the AHA/ASA include atrial fibrillation, previous thromboembolism, left ventricular dysfunction, and hypercoagulable condition (AHA/ASA [Meschia, 2014]).

[10]Maintain anticoagulation for 3 months after valve insertion then switch to aspirin 81 mg/day if no other indications for warfarin exist or clinically reassess need for warfarin in patients with prior history of systemic embolism.

[11]Treat for 3 months in patients with provoked VTE due to transient reversible risk factor. Treat for a minimum of 3 months in patients with unprovoked VTE and evaluate for extended anticoagulant therapy (ie, >3 months of therapy without a scheduled stop date). Other risk groups (eg, cancer) may require extended anticoagulant therapy.

[12]Recommendation from the ACCF/AHA 2009 Expert Consensus Document on Pulmonary Hypertension (McLaughlin, 2009)

[13]Continue for at least 10 to 14 days; up to 35 days after surgery is suggested.

[14]Instead of adjusted dose warfarin, the use of dabigatran has been suggested. In either case, oral anticoagulation should be initiated within 1 to 2 weeks after stroke onset or earlier in patients at low bleeding risk; bridging with aspirin may be required.

Warfarin levels are not used for monitoring degree of anticoagulation. They may be useful if a patient with unexplained coagulopathy is using the drug surreptitiously or if it is unclear whether clinical resistance is due to true drug resistance or lack of drug intake.

Normal prothrombin time (PT): 10.9 to 12.9 seconds. Healthy premature newborns have prolonged coagulation test screening results (eg, PT, aPTT, TT) which return to normal adult values at approximately 6 months of age. Healthy prematures, however, do not develop spontaneous hemorrhage or thrombotic complications because of a balance between procoagulants and inhibitors.

Additional Information

Pharmacogenomic Testing: The American College of Chest Physicians recommends against the use of routine pharmacogenomic testing to guide dosing (Guyatt, 2012). However, prospective genotyping is available, and may provide guidance on initiation of anticoagulant therapy. Commercial testing with PGxPredict™: WARFARIN is available from PGxHealth™ (Division of Clinical Data, Inc, New Haven, CT). The test genotypes patients for presence of the CYP2C9*2 or *3 alleles and the VKORC1 -1639G>A polymorphism. The results of the test allow patients to be phenotyped as extensive, intermediate, or poor metabolizers (CYP2C9) and as low, intermediate, or high warfarin sensitivity (VKORC1). Ordering information is available at 888-592-7327 or warfarininfo@pgxhealth.com.

Management of Elevated INR:

If INR above therapeutic range to <4.5 (no evidence of bleeding): Lower or hold next dose and monitor frequently; when INR approaches desired range, resume dosing with a lower dose (Patriquin, 2011).

If INR 4.5-10 (no evidence of bleeding): The 2012 ACCP guidelines recommend against routine vitamin K administration in this setting (Guyatt, 2012). Previously, the 2008 ACCP guidelines recommended if no risk factors for bleeding exist, to omit next 1 or 2 doses, monitor INR more frequently, and resume with an appropriately adjusted dose when INR in desired range; may consider administering vitamin K orally 1-2.5 mg if other risk factors for bleeding exist (Hirsh, 2008). Others have

recommended consideration of vitamin K 1 mg orally or 0.5 mg IV (Patriquin, 2011).

If INR >10 (no evidence of bleeding): The 2012 ACCP guidelines recommend administration of oral vitamin K (dose not specified) in this setting (Guyatt, 2012). Previously, the 2008 ACCP guidelines recommended to hold warfarin, administer vitamin K orally 2.5-5 mg, expect INR to be reduced within 24-48 hours, monitor INR more frequently and give additional vitamin K at an appropriate dose if necessary; resume warfarin at an appropriately adjusted dose when INR is in desired range (Hirsh, 2008). Others have recommended consideration of vitamin K 2-2.5 mg orally or 0.5-1 mg IV (Patriquin, 2011).

If minor bleeding at any INR elevation: Hold warfarin, may administer vitamin K orally 2.5-5 mg, monitor INR more frequently, may repeat dose after 24 hours if INR correction incomplete; resume warfarin at an appropriately adjusted dose when INR is in desired range (Patriquin, 2011).

If major bleeding at any INR elevation: The 2012 ACCP guidelines recommend administration of four-factor prothrombin complex concentrate (PCC) and IV vitamin K 5-10 mg in this setting (Guyatt, 2012). Four-factor PCCs include Beriplex P/N, Cofact, Kcentra (available in U.S.), or Octaplex (available in Canada). Previously, the 2008 ACCP guidelines recommended to hold warfarin, administer vitamin K 10 mg by slow IV infusion and supplement with PCC depending on the urgency of the situation; IV vitamin K may be repeated every 12 hours (Hirsh, 2008).

Note: Use of high doses of vitamin K (eg, 10-15 mg) may cause warfarin resistance for ≥1 week. During this period of resistance, heparin or low-molecular-weight heparin (LMWH) may be given until INR responds.

Product Availability Coumadin injection has been discontinued in the US for more than 1 year.

Dosage Forms Excipient information presented when available (limited, particularly for generics); consult specific product labeling. [DSC] = Discontinued product

Solution Reconstituted, Intravenous, as sodium:
Coumadin: 5 mg (1 ea [DSC])

Tablet, Oral, as sodium:
Coumadin: 1 mg [scored]
Coumadin: 2 mg [scored; contains fd&c blue #2 aluminum lake, fd&c red #40 aluminum lake]
Coumadin: 2.5 mg [scored; contains fd&c blue #1 aluminum lake, fd&c yellow #10 aluminum lake]
Coumadin: 3 mg [DSC] [contains fd&c blue #2 aluminum lake, fd&c red #40 aluminum lake, fd&c yellow #6 aluminum lake]
Coumadin: 3 mg [scored; contains fd&c blue #2 aluminum lake, fd&c red #40 aluminum lake, fd&c yellow #6 aluminum lake]
Coumadin: 4 mg [DSC] [contains fd&c blue #1 aluminum lake]
Coumadin: 4 mg [scored; contains fd&c blue #1 aluminum lake]
Coumadin: 5 mg [scored; contains fd&c yellow #6 aluminum lake]
Coumadin: 6 mg [scored; contains fd&c blue #1 aluminum lake, fd&c yellow #6 aluminum lake]
Coumadin: 7.5 mg [scored; contains fd&c yellow #10 aluminum lake, fd&c yellow #6 aluminum lake]
Coumadin: 10 mg [scored; dye free]
Jantoven: 1 mg [scored; contains fd&c red #40 aluminum lake]
Jantoven: 2 mg [scored; contains fd&c blue #2 aluminum lake, fd&c red #40 aluminum lake]
Jantoven: 2.5 mg [scored; contains fd&c blue #1 aluminum lake, fd&c yellow #10 aluminum lake]
Jantoven: 3 mg [scored]
Jantoven: 4 mg [scored; contains fd&c blue #1 aluminum lake]
Jantoven: 5 mg [scored; contains fd&c yellow #6 aluminum lake]
Jantoven: 6 mg [scored; contains fd&c blue #1 aluminum lake]
Jantoven: 7.5 mg [scored; contains fd&c yellow #10 aluminum lake, fd&c yellow #6 aluminum lake]
Jantoven: 10 mg [scored]
Generic: 1 mg, 2 mg, 2.5 mg, 3 mg, 4 mg, 5 mg, 6 mg, 7.5 mg, 10 mg

Wheat Dextrin (weet DEKS trin)

Brand Names: US Benefiber Drink Mix [OTC]; Benefiber For Children [OTC]; Benefiber Plus Calcium [OTC]; Benefiber [OTC]

Index Terms Dextrin; Resistant Dextrin; Resistant Maltodextrin

Pharmacologic Category Fiber Supplement; Laxative, Bulk-Producing

Use OTC labeling: Dietary fiber supplement

Dosing

Adult & Geriatric General dosing guidelines; consult specific product labeling.

Adequate intake for total fiber: Oral: **Note:** The definition of "fiber" varies; however, the soluble fiber in wheat dextrin is only one type of fiber which makes up the daily recommended intake of total fiber.

Adults 19-50 years: Males: 38 g/day; Females: 25 g/day

Adults ≥51 years: Males: 30 g/day; Females: 21 g/day

Pregnancy: 28 g/day

Lactation: 29 g/day

Pediatric General dosing guidelines; consult specific product labeling.

Adequate intake for total fiber: Oral: **Note:** The definition of "fiber" varies; however, the soluble fiber in wheat dextrin is only one type of fiber which makes up the daily recommended intake of total fiber.

Children 1-3 years: 19 g/day

Children 4-8 years: 25 g/day

Children 9-13 years: Males: 31 g/day; Females: 26 g/day

Children 14-18 years: Males: 38 g/day; Females: 26 g/day

Additional Information Complete prescribing information should be consulted for additional detail.

Dosage Forms Excipient information presented when available (limited, particularly for generics); consult specific product labeling. [DSC] = Discontinued product

Packet, Oral:

Benefiber Drink Mix: (28 ea, 34 ea [DSC]) [flavor free, gluten free, grit free, sugar free]

Benefiber Drink Mix: (8 ea) [sugar free; contains aspartame; raspberry tea flavor]

Benefiber Drink Mix: (8 ea, 24 ea) [sugar free; contains aspartame, fd&c red #40; cherry pomegranate flavor]

Benefiber Drink Mix: (16 ea, 24 ea) [sugar free; contains aspartame, fd&c red #40; kiwi strawberry flavor]

Benefiber Drink Mix: (16 ea) [sugar free; contains aspartame, fd&c yellow #6 (sunset yellow), soybean oil, tartrazine (fd&c yellow #5); citrus punch flavor]

Powder, Oral:

Benefiber: (80 g, 155 g, 245 g, 350 g, 477 g, 730 g) [gluten free, grit free, sugar free]

Benefiber: (161 g [DSC]) [grit free, sugar free; contains aspartame, fd&c red #40, fd&c yellow #6 (sunset yellow), lactose]

Benefiber: (267 g, 529 g) [grit free, sugar free; contains aspartame, fd&c red #40, fd&c yellow #6 (sunset yellow), lactose; orange flavor]

Benefiber For Children: (155 g) [grit free, sugar free; unflavored flavor]

Benefiber Plus Calcium: (423.8 g) [gluten free, grit free, sugar free]

Benefiber Plus Calcium: (305 g) [gluten free, grit free, sugar free; contains aspartame, fd&c red #40, fd&c yellow #6 (sunset yellow); orange flavor]

Tablet, Oral:

Benefiber:

Tablet Chewable, Oral:

Benefiber: [scored; gluten free, sugar free; contains aspartame, fd&c blue #1 aluminum lake, fd&c red #40 aluminum lake, fd&c yellow #6 aluminum lake; assorted fruit flavor]

Benefiber: [scored; gluten free, sugar free; contains aspartame, fd&c yellow #6 aluminum lake; orange cream flavor]

Benefiber Plus Calcium: [scored; sugar free; contains aspartame, fd&c blue #1 aluminum lake, fd&c red #40 aluminum lake, soybeans (glycine max); wild berry flavor]

- ◆ Xylocaine® MPF With Epinephrine *see* Lidocaine and Epinephrine *on page 1075*
- ◆ Xylocaine Viscous *see* Lidocaine (Topical) *on page 1074*
- ◆ Xylocaine® With Epinephrine *see* Lidocaine and Epinephrine *on page 1075*
- ◆ Xylocard (Can) *see* Lidocaine (Systemic) *on page 1072*
- ◆ Xylon *see* Hydrocodone and Ibuprofen *on page 885*
- ◆ Xyntha *see* Antihemophilic Factor (Recombinant) *on page 132*
- ◆ Xyntha Solofuse *see* Antihemophilic Factor (Recombinant) *on page 132*
- ◆ Xyrem *see* Sodium Oxybate *on page 1676*
- ◆ Xyzal *see* Levocetirizine *on page 1059*
- ◆ Yasmin *see* Ethinyl Estradiol and Drospirenone *on page 702*
- ◆ Yaz *see* Ethinyl Estradiol and Drospirenone *on page 702*
- ◆ Yaz Plus (Can) *see* Ethinyl Estradiol, Drospirenone, and Levomefolate *on page 712*

Yellow Fever Vaccine (YEL oh FEE ver vak SEEN)

Brand Names: US YF-VAX
Brand Names: Canada YF-VAX
Pharmacologic Category Vaccine; Vaccine, Live (Viral)
Additional Appendix Information
Immunization Administration Recommendations *on page 1974*
Immunization Schedules *on page 1979*
Use Yellow fever prevention: Active immunization against yellow fever virus, primarily among persons traveling to or living in areas where yellow fever infection exists and laboratory workers who may be exposed to the virus; vaccination may also be required for some international travelers

The Advisory Committee on Immunization Practices (ACIP) (CDC/ACIP [Staples 2010]) recommends vaccination for:
- Persons traveling to or living in areas at risk for yellow fever transmission
- Persons traveling to countries which require vaccination for international travel
- Laboratory personnel who may be exposed to the yellow fever virus or concentrated preparations of the vaccine

Although the vaccine is approved for use in children ≥9 months, the CDC recommends use in children as young as 6 months under unusual circumstances (eg, travel to an area where exposure is unavoidable) (CDC/ACIP [Staples 2010]).
Medication Guide Available Yes
Dosing
Adult
Immunization: SubQ: One dose (0.5 mL) ≥10 days before travel; Booster: See **"Note"**.
Note: Based on currently available data, the World Health Organization (WHO) and CDC/ACIP have determined that vaccine failure is rare and booster doses are generally not needed. A single dose of the vaccine is adequate for most travelers. The World Health Assembly plans to remove the 10-year booster dose requirement from the International Health Regulations by June 2016 (WHO 2014). However, additional dose(s) are recommended for certain patient populations with conditions at the time of their initial dose that may limit immune response (pregnant women, hematopoietic stem cell transplant recipients, HIV patients). A booster dose may also be given (≥10 years after last dose) to those who may be at increased risk for yellow fever disease (eg, certain laboratory workers [depending on antibody titers] and travelers to endemic locations for prolonged periods (CDC/ACIP [Staples 2015]; WHO 2013).
Geriatric Refer to adult dosing. Monitor closely due to an increased incidence of serious adverse events in patients ≥60 years of age, particularly in patients receiving their first dose. The ACIP guidelines note that if travel is unavoidable, the decision to vaccinate travelers ≥60 years should be made after weighing the risks vs benefits (CDC/ACIP [Staples 2010]).
Pediatric
Immunization: SubQ:
Infants 6 months to <9 months (off-label use): One dose (0.5 mL) ≥10 days before travel; Booster: See **"Note"**. (CDC/ACIP [Staples 2010]).

Infants ≥9 months (per manufacturer), Children, and Adolescents: One dose (0.5 mL) ≥10 days before travel; Booster: See **"Note"**.
Note: Based on currently available data, the World Health Organization (WHO) and CDC/ACIP have determined that vaccine failure is rare and booster doses are generally not needed. A single dose of the vaccine is adequate for most travelers. The World Health Assembly plans to remove the 10-year booster dose requirement from the International Health Regulations by June 2016 (WHO 2014). However, additional dose(s) are recommended for certain patient populations with conditions at the time of their initial dose that may limit immune response (pregnant women, hematopoietic stem cell transplant recipients, HIV patients). A booster dose may also be given (≥10 years after last dose) to those who may be at increased risk for yellow fever disease (eg, certain laboratory workers [depending on antibody titers] and travelers to endemic locations for prolonged periods (CDC/ACIP [Staples 2015]; WHO 2013).
Renal Impairment There are no dosage adjustments provided in the manufacturer's labeling.
Hepatic Impairment There are no dosage adjustments provided in the manufacturer's labeling.
Additional Information Complete prescribing information should be consulted for additional detail.
Dosage Forms Excipient information presented when available (limited, particularly for generics); consult specific product labeling.
Injection, powder for reconstitution [17D-204 strain]:
YF-VAX: ≥4.74 log_{10} plaque-forming units (PFU) per 0.5 mL dose [single-dose or 5-dose vial; produced in chicken embryos; contains gelatin; packaged with diluent; vial stopper contains latex]

- ◆ Yervoy *see* Ipilimumab *on page 975*
- ◆ YF-VAX *see* Yellow Fever Vaccine *on page 1922*
- ◆ YM087 *see* Conivaptan *on page 446*
- ◆ YM-178 *see* Mirabegron *on page 1215*
- ◆ YM905 *see* Solifenacin *on page 1685*
- ◆ YM-08310 *see* Amifostine *on page 90*
- ◆ Yodoxin *see* Iodoquinol *on page 974*
- ◆ Yondelis *see* Trabectedin *on page 1818*
- ◆ Z4942 *see* Ifosfamide *on page 913*
- ◆ Zactima *see* Vandetanib *on page 1873*
- ◆ Zaditor [OTC] *see* Ketotifen (Ophthalmic) *on page 1018*
- ◆ Zaditor (Can) *see* Ketotifen (Ophthalmic) *on page 1018*

Zafirlukast (za FIR loo kast)

Brand Names: US Accolate
Brand Names: Canada Accolate
Index Terms ICI-204,219
Pharmacologic Category Leukotriene-Receptor Antagonist
Use Asthma: Prophylaxis and chronic treatment of asthma in adults and children 5 years and older.
Pregnancy Considerations Adverse events were not observed in animal reproduction studies except with doses that were also maternally toxic. Based on limited data, an increased risk of teratogenic effects has not been observed with zafirlukast use in pregnancy (Bakhireva, 2007). Uncontrolled asthma is associated with adverse events on pregnancy (increased risk of perinatal mortality, pre-eclampsia, preterm birth, low birth weight infants). Zafirlukast may be considered for use in women who had a favorable response prior to becoming pregnant; however, initiating a leukotriene receptor antagonist during pregnancy is an alternative (but not preferred) treatment option for mild persistent asthma (NAEPP, 2005).
Breast-Feeding Considerations Zafirlukast is excreted into breast milk. In women receiving zafirlukast 40 mg twice daily, maternal serum concentrations were 225 ng/mL and breast milk concentrations were 50 ng/mL. Due to the potential for adverse reactions in the nursing infant, breast-feeding is not recommended by the manufacturer.
Contraindications Hypersensitivity to zafirlukast or any component of the formulation; hepatic impairment (including hepatic cirrhosis)

Canadian labeling: Additional contraindications (not in U.S. labeling): Patients in whom zafirlukast was discontinued due to treatment related hepatotoxicity
Warnings/Precautions Zafirlukast is not approved for use in the reversal of bronchospasm in acute asthma attacks, including status asthmaticus. Therapy with zafirlukast can be continued during acute exacerbations of asthma.

Hepatic adverse events (including hepatitis, hyperbilirubinemia, and hepatic failure) have been reported; female patients may be at greater risk. Periodic testing of liver function may be considered (early detection coupled with therapy discontinuation is generally believed to improve the likelihood of recovery). Advise patients to be alert for and to immediately report symptoms (eg, anorexia, right upper quadrant abdominal pain, nausea). If hepatic dysfunction is suspected (due to clinical signs/symptoms), discontinue use immediately and measure liver function tests (particularly ALT); resolution observed in most but not all cases upon discontinuation of therapy. Do not resume or restart if hepatic function studies indicate dysfunction. Use in patients with hepatic impairment (including hepatic cirrhosis) is contraindicated. Postmarketing reports of behavioral changes (ie, depression, insomnia) have been noted. Instruct patients to report neuropsychiatric symptoms/events during therapy.

Monitor INR closely with concomitant warfarin use. Rare cases of eosinophilic vasculitis (Churg-Strauss) have been reported in patients receiving zafirlukast (usually, but not always, associated with reduction in concurrent steroid dosage). No causal relationship established. Monitor for eosinophilic vasculitis, rash, pulmonary symptoms, cardiac symptoms, or neuropathy.

Clearance is decreased in elderly patients; C_{max} and AUC are increased approximately two- to threefold in adults ≥65 years compared to younger adults; however, no dosage adjustments are recommended in this age group. An increased proportion of zafirlukast patients >55 years of age reported infections as compared to placebo-treated patients. These infections were mostly mild or moderate in intensity and predominantly affected the respiratory tract. Infections occurred equally in both sexes, were dose-proportional to total milligrams of zafirlukast exposure, and were associated with coadministration of inhaled corticosteroids.

Adverse Reactions Incidence reported in children ≥12 years and adults unless otherwise specified.
>10%: Central nervous system: Headache (13%; children 5-11 years: 5%)
1% to 10%:
Central nervous system: Dizziness (2%), pain (2%), fever (2%)
Gastrointestinal: Nausea (3%), diarrhea (3%), abdominal pain (2%; children 5-11 years: 3%), vomiting (2%), dyspepsia (1%)
Hepatic: ALT increased (2%)
Neuromuscular & skeletal: Back pain (2%), myalgia (2%), weakness (2%)
Miscellaneous: Infection (4%)
<1% (Limited to important or life-threatening): Agranulocytosis, angioedema, arthralgia, bleeding, bruising, depression, edema, eosinophilia (systemic), eosinophilic pneumonia, hepatic failure, hepatitis, hyperbilirubinemia, hypersensitivity reactions, insomnia, malaise, pruritus, rash, urticaria, vasculitis with clinical features of Churg-Strauss syndrome (rare)

Drug Interactions
Metabolism/Transport Effects Substrate of CYP2C9 (major); **Note:** Assignment of Major/Minor substrate status based on clinically relevant drug interaction potential; **Inhibits** CYP1A2 (weak), CYP2C19 (weak), CYP2C8 (weak), CYP2C9 (moderate), CYP2D6 (weak)

Avoid Concomitant Use
Avoid concomitant use of Zafirlukast with any of the following: Amodiaquine; Loxapine
Increased Effect/Toxicity
Zafirlukast may increase the levels/effects of: Amodiaquine; ARIPiprazole; Bosentan; Cannabis; Carvedilol; CYP2C9 Substrates; Dronabinol; Loxapine; Tetrahydrocannabinol; Theophylline Derivatives; TiZANidine; Vitamin K Antagonists

The levels/effects of Zafirlukast may be increased by: Ceritinib; CYP2C9 Inhibitors (Moderate); CYP2C9 Inhibitors (Strong); Lumacaftor; Mifepristone

Decreased Effect
The levels/effects of Zafirlukast may be decreased by: CYP2C9 Inducers (Strong); Dabrafenib; Enzalutamide; Erythromycin (Systemic); Lumacaftor; Theophylline Derivatives

Food Interactions Food decreases bioavailability of zafirlukast by 40%. Management: Take on an empty stomach 1 hour before or 2 hours after meals.

Storage/Stability Store tablets at controlled room temperature of 20°C to 25°C (68°F to 77°F). Protect from light and moisture; dispense in original airtight container.

Mechanism of Action Zafirlukast is a selectively and competitive leukotriene-receptor antagonist (LTRA) of leukotriene D4 and E4 (LTD4 and LTE4), components of slow-reacting substance of anaphylaxis (SRSA). Cysteinyl leukotriene production and receptor occupation have been correlated with the pathophysiology of asthma, including airway edema, smooth muscle constriction, and altered cellular activity associated with the inflammatory process, which contribute to the signs and symptoms of asthma.

Pharmacodynamics/Kinetics
Distribution: V_{dss}: ~70 L
Protein binding: >99%, primarily to albumin
Metabolism: Extensively hepatic via CYP2C9
Bioavailability: Reduced 40% with food
Half-life elimination: ~10 hours
Time to peak, serum: 3 hours
Excretion: Feces (~90%); Urine (~10%)

Dosing
Adult & Geriatric
Asthma: Oral: 20 mg twice daily
Chronic urticaria (off-label use): Oral: 20 mg twice daily (Bagenstose, 2004)
Pediatric Asthma: Oral:
US labeling:
Children 5 to 11 years: 10 mg twice daily
Children ≥12 years: Refer to adult dosing.
Canadian labeling: Children ≥12 years: Refer to adult dosing.
Renal Impairment No dosage adjustment necessary.
Hepatic Impairment Use is contraindicated.
Dietary Considerations Should be taken on an empty stomach (1 hour before or 2 hours after meals).
Administration Oral: Administer at least 1 hour before or 2 hours after a meal.
Monitoring Parameters Monitor for improvements in air flow; monitor closely for sign/symptoms of hepatic injury; periodic monitoring of LFTs may be considered (not proved to prevent serious injury, but early detection may enhance recovery)
Dosage Forms Excipient information presented when available (limited, particularly for generics); consult specific product labeling.
Tablet, Oral:
Accolate: 10 mg, 20 mg
Generic: 10 mg, 20 mg

Zaleplon (ZAL e plon)

Brand Names: US Sonata
Pharmacologic Category Hypnotic, Miscellaneous
Use Insomnia: Short-term treatment of insomnia.
Medication Guide Available Yes
Dosing
Adult
Insomnia: Oral: Usual dosage 10 mg immediately before bedtime (range: 5 to 20 mg); 5 mg may be sufficient for certain low weight patients (maximum dose: 20 mg daily). Has been used for up to 5 weeks of treatment in controlled trial setting.
Debilitated patients: Oral: Usual dosage 5 mg immediately before bedtime (maximum dose: 10 mg daily)
Concomitant therapy: 5 mg initially should be given to patients concomitantly taking cimetidine.
Geriatric Insomnia: Oral: Usual dosage 5 mg immediately before bedtime (maximum dose: 10 mg daily).
Renal Impairment
Mild to moderate impairment: No dosage adjustment necessary.
Severe impairment: There are no dosage adjustments provided in the manufacturer's labeling (has not been studied).
Hepatic Impairment
Mild to moderate impairment: 5 mg immediately before bedtime
Severe impairment: Use is not recommended.
Additional Information Complete prescribing information should be consulted for additional detail.
Dosage Forms Excipient information presented when available (limited, particularly for generics); consult specific product labeling.
Capsule, Oral:
Sonata: 5 mg, 10 mg [contains tartrazine (fd&c yellow #5)]
Generic: 5 mg, 10 mg
Controlled Substance C-IV

◆ Zaltrap see Ziv-Aflibercept (Systemic) on page 1933
◆ Zamicet see Hydrocodone and Acetaminophen on page 884

◆ Zamine (Can) *see* Ethinyl Estradiol and Drospirenone on page 702

◆ Zanaflex *see* TiZANidine *on page 1798*

Zanamivir (za NA mi veer)

Brand Names: US Relenza Diskhaler
Brand Names: Canada Relenza
Pharmacologic Category Antiviral Agent; Neuraminidase Inhibitor
Use Influenza:

Prophylaxis: Prophylaxis of influenza in adults and pediatric patients 5 years and older (US labeling) or 7 years and older (Canadian labeling).

Treatment: Treatment of uncomplicated acute illness caused by influenza A and B virus in adults and pediatric patients 7 years and older who have been symptomatic for no more than 2 days.

The Advisory Committee on Immunization Practices (ACIP) recommends that **treatment** be considered for the following:

• Persons with severe, complicated or progressive illness
• Hospitalized persons
• Persons at higher risk for influenza complications:
  - Children <2 years of age (highest risk in children <6 months of age)
  - Adults ≥65 years of age
  - Persons with chronic disorders of the pulmonary (including asthma) or cardiovascular systems (except hypertension)
  - Persons with chronic metabolic diseases (including diabetes mellitus, hepatic disease, renal dysfunction, hematologic disorders (including sickle cell disease), or immunosuppression (including immunosuppression caused by medications or HIV)
  - Persons with neurologic/neuromuscular conditions (including conditions such as spinal cord injuries, seizure disorders, cerebral palsy, stroke, mental retardation, moderate to severe developmental delay, or muscular dystrophy) which may compromise respiratory function, the handling of respiratory secretions, or that can increase the risk of aspiration
  - Pregnant or postpartum women (≤2 weeks after delivery)
  - Persons <19 years of age on long-term aspirin therapy
  - American Indians and Alaskan Natives
  - Persons who are morbidly obese (BMI ≥40)
  - Residents of nursing homes or other chronic care facilities
• Use may also be considered for previously healthy, nonhigh-risk outpatients with confirmed or suspected influenza based on clinical judgment when treatment can be started within 48 hours of illness onset.

The ACIP recommends that **prophylaxis** be considered for the following:

• Postexposure prophylaxis may be considered for family or close contacts of suspected or confirmed cases, who are at higher risk of influenza complications, and who have not been vaccinated against the circulating strain at the time of the exposure.
• Postexposure prophylaxis may be considered for unvaccinated healthcare workers who had occupational exposure without protective equipment.
• Pre-exposure prophylaxis should only be used for persons at very high risk of influenza complications who cannot be otherwise protected at times of high risk for exposure.
• Prophylaxis should also be administered to all eligible residents of institutions that house patients at high risk when needed to control outbreaks.

Pregnancy Considerations Adverse events have not been observed in animal reproduction studies. An increased risk of adverse neonatal or maternal outcomes has not been observed following use of zanamivir during pregnancy. Untreated influenza infection is associated with an increased risk of adverse events to the fetus and an increased risk of complications or death to the mother. Neuraminidase inhibitors are currently recommended for the treatment or prophylaxis of influenza in pregnant women and women up to 2 weeks postpartum (CDC 60 [1] 2011; CDC March 13 2014; January 2015).

Breast-Feeding Considerations It is not known if zanamivir is excreted in breast milk. The manufacturer recommends that caution be exercised when administering zanamivir to nursing women. Influenza may cause serious illness in postpartum women and prompt evaluation for febrile respiratory illnesses is recommended (Louie 2011).

Prescribing and Access Restrictions Zanamivir *aqueous solution* intended for intravenous (IV) administration is **not** currently approved for use. Data on safety and efficacy via this route of administration are limited. However, limited supplies of zanamivir aqueous solution may be made available through the Zanamivir Compassionate Use Program for qualifying patients for the treatment of serious influenza illness. For information, contact the GlaxoSmithKline Clinical Support Help Desk at 1-866-341-9160 or gskclinicalsupportHD@gsk.com.

Contraindications Hypersensitivity to zanamivir or any component of the formulation (contains milk proteins)

Warnings/Precautions Allergic-like reactions, including anaphylaxis, oropharyngeal edema, and serious skin rashes have been reported. Rare occurrences of neuropsychiatric events (including confusion, delirium, hallucinations, seizure, and/or self-injury) have been reported, primarily in pediatric patients; may be abrupt in onset. Direct causation is difficult to establish influenza infection may also be associated with behavioral and neurologic changes. Patients must be instructed in the use of the delivery system. Antiviral treatment should begin within 48 hours of symptom onset. However, the CDC recommends that treatment may still be beneficial and should be started in hospitalized patients with severe, complicated or progressive illness if >48 hours. Treatment should not be delayed while awaiting results of laboratory tests for influenza (CDC 2015). Nonhospitalized persons who are not at high risk for developing severe or complicated illness and who have a mild disease are not likely to benefit if treatment is started >48 hours after symptom onset. Nonhospitalized persons who are already beginning to recover do not need treatment (CDC 2011). Effectiveness has not been established in patients with significant underlying medical conditions or for prophylaxis of influenza in nursing home patients (per manufacturer). The CDC recommends zanamivir be used to control institutional outbreaks of influenza when circulating strains are suspected of being resistant to oseltamivir (refer to current guidelines) (CDC 2011). Not recommended for use in patients with underlying respiratory disease, such as asthma or COPD, due to lack of efficacy in influenza treatment and risk of serious bronchospasm. If zanamivir is prescribed in such patients, closely monitor respiratory function. Bronchospasm, including serious cases and some with fatal outcomes, and decreased lung function have been reported in patients with and without airway disease; discontinue with bronchospasm or decreased lung function. For a patient with an underlying airway disease where a medical decision has been made to use zanamivir, a fast-acting bronchodilator should be made available. Not a substitute for annual flu vaccination; has not been shown to reduce risk of transmission of influenza to others. Consider primary or concomitant bacterial infections. Safety and efficacy of repeated courses have not been established. Powder for oral inhalation contains lactose; use contraindicated in patients allergic to milk proteins. The inhalation powder should only be administered via inhalation using the provided Diskhaler delivery device. The commercially available formulation is a lactose-containing powder and is **not** intended to be solubilized or administered via any nebulizer/mechanical ventilator; inappropriate administration has resulted in death.

Adverse Reactions Most adverse reactions occurred at a frequency which was less than or equal to the control (lactose vehicle).

>10%:
Central nervous system: Headache (prophylaxis 13% to 24%; treatment 2%)
Gastrointestinal: Throat/tonsil discomfort/pain (prophylaxis 8% to 19%)
Respiratory: Nasal signs and symptoms (prophylaxis 12% to 20%; treatment 2%), cough (prophylaxis 7% to 17%; treatment ≤2%)
Miscellaneous: Viral infection (prophylaxis 3% to 13%)
1% to 10%:
Central nervous system: Fever/chills (prophylaxis 5% to 9%; treatment <1.5%), fatigue (prophylaxis 5% to 8%; treatment <1.5%), malaise (prophylaxis 5% to 8%; treatment <1.5%), dizziness (treatment 1% to 2%)
Dermatologic: Urticaria (treatment <1.5%)
Gastrointestinal: Anorexia/appetite decreased (prophylaxis 2% to 4%), appetite increased (prophylaxis 2% to 4%), nausea (prophylaxis 1% to 2%; treatment ≤3%), diarrhea (prophylaxis 2%; treatment 2% to 3%), vomiting (prophylaxis 1% to 2%; treatment 1% to 2%), abdominal pain (treatment <1.5%)
Neuromuscular & skeletal: Muscle pain (prophylaxis 3% to 8%), musculoskeletal pain (prophylaxis 6%), arthralgia/articular rheumatism (prophylaxis 2%), arthralgia (treatment <1.5%), myalgia (treatment <1.5%)
Respiratory: Infection (ear/nose/throat; prophylaxis 2%; treatment 1% to 5%), sinusitis (treatment 3%), bronchitis (treatment 2%), nasal inflammation (prophylaxis 1%)

<1% (Limited to important or life-threatening): Allergic or allergic-like reaction (including oropharyngeal edema), arrhythmia, bronchospasm, consciousness altered, delusions, dyspnea, hallucinations, neuropsychiatric events (self-injury, confusion, delirium), nightmares, rash (including serious cutaneous reactions [eg, erythema multiforme, Stevens-Johnson syndrome, toxic epidermal necrolysis]), seizure, syncope

Drug Interactions
Metabolism/Transport Effects None known.
Avoid Concomitant Use There are no known interactions where it is recommended to avoid concomitant use.
Increased Effect/Toxicity There are no known significant interactions involving an increase in effect.
Decreased Effect
Zanamivir may decrease the levels/effects of: Influenza Virus Vaccine (Live/Attenuated)

Storage/Stability Store at 25°C (77°F); excursions permitted to 15°C to 30°C (59°F to 86°F). Do not puncture blister until taking a dose using the Diskhaler.

Mechanism of Action Zanamivir inhibits influenza virus neuraminidase enzymes, potentially altering virus particle aggregation and release.

Pharmacodynamics/Kinetics
Absorption: Inhalation: Systemic: ~4% to 17%
Protein binding, plasma: <10%
Metabolism: None
Half-life elimination, serum: 2.5 to 5.1 hours; Mild to moderate renal impairment: 4.7 hours; Severe renal impairment: 18.5 hours
Time to peak, plasma: 1 to 2 hours
Excretion: Urine (as unchanged drug); feces (unabsorbed drug)

Dosing
Adult & Geriatric Influenza: Oral inhalation:
Manufacturer's labeling:
Prophylaxis, household setting: Two inhalations (10 mg) once daily for 10 days. Begin within 36 hours following onset of signs or symptoms of index case.
Prophylaxis, community outbreak: Two inhalations (10 mg) once daily for 28 days. Begin within 5 days of outbreak.
Treatment: Two inhalations (10 mg) twice daily for 5 days. Doses on first day should be separated by at least 2 hours; on subsequent days, doses should be spaced by ~12 hours. Begin within 2 days of signs or symptoms. Longer treatment may be considered for patients who remain severely ill after 5 days (CDC 2015).
Alternate dosing:
Prophylaxis (household exposure): Two inhalations (10 mg) once daily for 7 days after last known exposure (CDC 2015)
Prophylaxis (institutional outbreak): Two inhalations (10 mg) once daily; continue for ≥2 weeks and until ~7 days after identification of illness onset in the last patient (CDC 2015). Zanamivir is to be used to control institutional outbreaks of influenza when circulating strains are suspected of being resistant to oseltamivir (CDC 2011).
Prophylaxis (community outbreak): Two inhalations (10 mg) once daily; continue until influenza activity in community subsides or immunity obtained from immunization; up to 28 days has been well tolerated (CDC 2011; CDC 2015)

Missed dose: If a dose is missed, administer as soon as possible unless it is ≤2 hours before the next scheduled dose. Then, continue administration at the previous schedule; do not administer a double dose.

Pediatric Influenza: Oral inhalation:
Manufacturer's labeling:
Prophylaxis, household setting: Children ≥5 years (US labeling) or ≥7 years (Canadian labeling) and Adolescents: Refer to adult dosing.
Prophylaxis, community outbreak: Adolescents: Refer to adult dosing.
Treatment: Children ≥7 years and Adolescents: Refer to adult dosing.
Alternate dosing:
Prophylaxis (household exposure): Children ≥5 years and Adolescents: Refer to adult dosing.
Prophylaxis (institutional outbreak): Children ≥5 years and Adolescents: Refer to adult dosing.
Prophylaxis (community outbreak): Children ≥5 years and Adolescents: Refer to adult dosing.

Missed dose: If a dose is missed, administer as soon as possible unless it is ≤2 hours before the next scheduled dose. Then, continue administration at the previous schedule; do not administer a double dose.

Renal Impairment No dosage adjustment necessary; however, the potential for drug accumulation should be considered.
Hepatic Impairment There are no dosage adjustments provided in the manufacturer's labeling (has not been studied.)
Administration Oral inhalation: Must be used with Diskhaler delivery device. The foil blister disk containing zanamivir inhalation powder should not be manipulated, solubilized, or administered via a nebulizer. Patients scheduled to use an inhaled bronchodilator at the same time as zanamivir should use their bronchodilator prior to zanamivir. With the exception of the initial dose when used for treatment, administer at approximately the same time each day.
Additional Information Majority of patients included in clinical trials were infected with influenza A, however, a number of patients with influenza B infections were also enrolled. Patients with lower temperature or less severe symptoms appeared to derive less benefit from therapy. No consistent treatment benefit was demonstrated in patients with chronic underlying medical conditions.

The absence of symptoms does not rule out viral influenza infection and clinical judgment should guide the decision for therapy. Treatment should not be delayed while waiting for the results of diagnostic tests. Treatment should be considered for high-risk patients with symptoms despite a negative rapid influenza test when the illness cannot be contributed to another cause. Use of zanamivir is not a substitute for vaccination (when available); susceptibility to influenza infection returns once therapy is discontinued.

Dosage Forms Excipient information presented when available (limited, particularly for generics); consult specific product labeling.
Aerosol Powder Breath Activated, Inhalation:
Relenza Diskhaler: 5 mg/blister (20 ea) [contains lactose]

Ziconotide (zi KOE no tide)

Brand Names: US Prialt

Pharmacologic Category Analgesic, Nonopioid; Calcium Channel Blocker, N-Type

Use Management of severe chronic pain in patients requiring intrathecal therapy and who are intolerant or refractory to other therapies

Dosing

Adult Chronic pain: Intrathecal: Initial dose: ≤2.4 mcg/day (0.1 mcg/hour)

Dose may be titrated by ≤2.4 mcg/day (0.1 mcg/hour) at intervals ≤2-3 times/week to a maximum dose of 19.2 mcg/day (0.8 mcg/hour) by day 21; average dose at day 21: 6.9 mcg/day (0.29 mcg/hour). A faster titration should be used only if the urgent need for analgesia outweighs the possible risk to patient safety.

Geriatric Refer to adult dosing. Use with caution.

Renal Impairment No dosage adjustment provided in manufacturer's labeling (has not been studied).

Hepatic Impairment No dosage adjustment provided in manufacturer's labeling (has not been studied).

Adjustment for Toxicity

Cognitive impairment: Reduce dose or discontinue. Effects are generally reversible within 3-15 days of discontinuation.

Reduced level of consciousness: Discontinue until event resolves.

CK elevation with neuromuscular symptoms: Consider dose reduction or discontinuation.

Additional Information Complete prescribing information should be consulted for additional detail.

Dosage Forms Excipient information presented when available (limited, particularly for generics); consult specific product labeling.

Solution, Intrathecal, as acetate [preservative free]:

Prialt: 500 mcg/20 mL (20 mL); 100 mcg/mL (1 mL); 500 mcg/5 mL (5 mL)

Zidovudine (zye DOE vyoo deen)

Brand Names: US Retrovir

Brand Names: Canada Apo-Zidovudine; AZT; Novo-AZT; Retrovir; Retrovir (AZT)

Index Terms Azidothymidine; AZT (error-prone abbreviation); Compound S; ZDV

Pharmacologic Category Antiretroviral, Reverse Transcriptase Inhibitor, Nucleoside (Anti-HIV)

Use

HIV-1 infection: Treatment of HIV-1 infection in combination with at least two other antiretroviral agents.

Perinatal HIV-1 transmission: Prevention of perinatal HIV-1 transmission

Pregnancy Considerations Adverse events have been observed in some animal reproduction studies. Zidovudine has a high level of transfer across the human placenta and the placenta also metabolizes zidovudine to the active metabolite. No increased risk of overall birth defects has been observed following first trimester exposure according to data collected by the antiretroviral pregnancy registry. The pharmacokinetics of zidovudine are not significantly altered in pregnancy and dosing adjustment is not needed. The HHS Perinatal HIV Guidelines consider zidovudine in combination with lamivudine to be a preferred NRTI backbone for use in antiretroviral-naive pregnant women. Zidovudine should be administered IV near delivery regardless of antepartum regimen or mode of delivery in women with HIV RNA >1000 copies/mL or unknown HIV RNA status.

Cases of lactic acidosis/hepatic steatosis syndrome related to mitochondrial toxicity have been reported in pregnant women with prolonged use of nucleoside analogues. It is not known if pregnancy itself potentiates this known side effect; however, women may be at increased risk of lactic acidosis and liver damage. In addition, these adverse events are similar to other rare but life-threatening syndromes which occur during pregnancy (eg, HELLP syndrome). Hepatic enzymes and electrolytes should be monitored in women receiving nucleoside analogues and clinicians should watch for early signs of the syndrome. In addition, mitochondrial dysfunction may develop in infants following in utero exposure.

Regardless of CD4 count or HIV RNA copy number, all HIV-infected pregnant women should receive a combination antiretroviral (ARV) drug regimen. A combination of antepartum, intrapartum, and infant ARV prophylaxis is recommended. ARV therapy should be started as soon as possible in women with symptomatic infection. Although earlier initiation may be more effective in reducing the perinatal transmission of HIV, initiation may be delayed until after 12 weeks' gestation in women who do not require immediate treatment after careful consideration of maternal conditions (eg, nausea and vomiting) and the potential risks of first trimester fetal exposure for specific agents. A scheduled cesarean delivery at 38 weeks' gestation is recommended for all women with HIV RNA >1000 copies/mL or unknown concentrations near delivery in order to decrease transmission. If ARV therapy must be interrupted for <24 hours during the peripartum period, stop then restart all medications simultaneously in order to decrease the chance of developing resistance. Long-term follow-up is recommended for all infants exposed to ARV medications. In couples who want to conceive, the HIV-infected partner should attain maximum viral suppression prior to conception.

Health care providers are encouraged to enroll pregnant women exposed to antiretroviral medications in the Antiretroviral Pregnancy Registry (1-800-258-4263 or www.APRegistry.com). Health care providers caring for HIV-infected women and their infants may contact the National Perinatal HIV Hotline (888-448-8765) for clinical consultation (HHS [perinatal], 2014).

Breast-Feeding Considerations Zidovudine is excreted into breast milk. Concentrations of zidovudine in breast milk are similar to those in the maternal serum. Maternal or infant antiretroviral therapy does not completely eliminate the risk of postnatal HIV transmission. In addition, multiclass-resistant virus has been detected in breast-feeding infants despite maternal therapy. Therefore, in the United States, where formula is accessible, affordable, safe, and sustainable, and the risk of infant mortality due to diarrhea and respiratory infections is low, complete avoidance of breast-feeding by HIV-infected women is recommended to decrease potential transmission of HIV (HHS [perinatal], 2014).

Contraindications

Potentially life-threatening hypersensitivity to zidovudine or any component of the formulation

Canadian labeling: Additional contraindications (not in U.S. labeling): Neutrophil count <750/mm^3 or hemoglobin <7.5 g/dL (4.65 mmol/L)

Warnings/Precautions Hazardous agent - use appropriate precautions for handling and disposal (NIOSH 2014 [group 2]).

[US Boxed Warning]: Hematologic toxicity, including neutropenia and severe anemia have been reported with use, especially with advanced HIV-1 disease. Toxicity may be related to duration of use and prior bone marrow reserve. Hemoglobin reduction may occur as early as 2 to 4 weeks; neutropenia usually occurs after 6 to 8 weeks. Pancytopenia has been reported (usually reversible). Use with caution in patients with bone marrow compromise (granulocytes <1,000 cells/mm^3 or hemoglobin <9.5 mg/dL); dose interruption may be required in patients who develop anemia or neutropenia. **[US Boxed Warning]: Lactic acidosis and severe hepatomegaly with steatosis have been reported, including fatal cases.** Risks may be increased with liver disease, obesity, pregnancy, prolonged exposure, or in females. Suspend treatment with zidovudine in any patient who develops clinical or laboratory findings suggestive of lactic acidosis (transaminase elevation may/may not accompany

hepatomegaly and steatosis). Use caution in combination with interferon alfa with or without ribavirin in HIV/HCV coinfected patients; monitor closely for hepatic decompensation, anemia, or neutropenia; dose reduction or discontinuation of interferon and/or ribavirin may be required if toxicity evident.

Zidovudine newborn prophylaxis may affect diagnostic virologic assays in HIV-exposed infants. If a virologic assay result is negative while the infant is receiving combination antiretroviral prophylaxis, repeat virologic testing should be considered 2 to 4 weeks after cessation of antiretroviral prophylaxis (HHS [pediatric], 2014).

[US Boxed Warning]: Prolonged use has been associated with symptomatic myopathy and myositis. Pathological changes observed are similar to that produced by HIV-1 disease. May cause redistribution of fat (eg, buffalo hump, peripheral wasting with increased abdominal girth, cushingoid appearance). Immune reconstitution syndrome may develop resulting in the occurrence of an inflammatory response to an indolent or residual opportunistic infection during initial HIV treatment or activation of autoimmune disorders (eg, Graves disease, polymyositis, Guillain-Barré syndrome) later in therapy; further evaluation and treatment may be required. Hematologic toxicity may be increased due to increased serum concentrations in patients with severe hepatic impairment. Use with caution in patients with severe renal impairment; dosage adjustment recommended. Reduce dose in patients with severe renal impairment. Potentially significant interactions may exist, requiring dose or frequency adjustment, additional monitoring, and/or selection of alternative therapy. Latex is used in injection vial stopper and may cause allergic reactions in latex-sensitive individuals.

Benzyl alcohol and derivatives: Some dosage forms may contain sodium benzoate/benzoic acid; benzoic acid (benzoate) is a metabolite of benzyl alcohol; large amounts of benzyl alcohol (≥99 mg/kg/day) have been associated with a potentially fatal toxicity ("gasping syndrome") in neonates; the "gasping syndrome" consists of metabolic acidosis, respiratory distress, gasping respirations, CNS dysfunction (including convulsions, intracranial hemorrhage), hypotension, and cardiovascular collapse (AAP ["Inactive" 1997]; CDC, 1982); some data suggests that benzoate displaces bilirubin from protein binding sites (Ahlfors, 2001); avoid or use dosage forms containing benzyl alcohol derivative with caution in neonates. See manufacturer's labeling.

Adverse Reactions Note: Percentages noted with adults unless otherwise stated.

>10%:
Central nervous system: Headache (63%), malaise (53%), fever (children 25%)
Dermatologic: Rash (children 12%)
Gastrointestinal: Nausea (adults 51%; children 8%), anorexia (20%), vomiting (adults 17%; children 8%)
Hematologic: Macrocytosis (children >50%), anemia (neonates 22%; children 4%; adults 1%; onset 2-4 weeks)
Hepatic: Hepatomegaly (children 11%)
Respiratory: Cough (children 15%)

1% to 10%:
Cardiovascular: ECG abnormality (children <6%), edema (children <6%), heart failure (children <6%), left ventricular dilation (children <6%)
Central nervous system: Irritability (children <6%), nervousness (children <6%), chills (≥5%), fatigue (≥5%), insomnia (≥5%)
Gastrointestinal: Diarrhea (children 8%), constipation (6%), weight loss (children <6%), abdominal cramps (≥5%), abdominal pain (≥5%), dyspepsia (≥5%)
Genitourinary: Hematuria (children <6%)
Hematologic: Neutropenia (children 8%), granulocytopenia (2%; onset 6-8 weeks), thrombocytopenia (children 1%)
Hepatic: Transaminases increased (1% to 3%)
Neuromuscular & skeletal: Weakness (9%), arthralgia (≥5%), musculoskeletal pain (≥5%), myalgia (≥5%), neuropathy (≥5%)
Otic: Discharge/erythema/pain/swelling (7%)
Postmarketing and/or case reports: Allergic reactions, amblyopia, anaphylaxis, angioedema, anxiety, aplastic anemia, back pain, body fat redistribution, cardiomyopathy, confusion, CPK increased, depression, diabetes, dizziness, dyslipidemias, dyspnea, gynecomastia, hearing loss, hemolytic anemia, hepatitis, hepatomegaly with steatosis, immune reconstitution syndrome, insulin resistance, jaundice, lactic acidosis, LDH increased, leukopenia, loss of mental acuity, lymphadenopathy, macular edema, mania, myopathy, myositis, oral mucosa pigmentation, pancreatitis, pancytopenia with marrow hypoplasia, paresthesia, photophobia, pruritus, pure red cell aplasia, rhabdomyolysis, seizure, skin/nail pigmentation changes (blue), Stevens-Johnson syndrome, syncope, taste perversion, toxic epidermal necrolysis, tremor, urticaria, vertigo

Drug Interactions

Metabolism/Transport Effects Substrate of CYP2A6 (minor), CYP2C19 (minor), CYP2C9 (minor), CYP3A4 (minor), OAT3; **Note:** Assignment of Major/Minor substrate status based on clinically relevant drug interaction potential

Avoid Concomitant Use
Avoid concomitant use of Zidovudine with any of the following: Amodiaquine; BCG (Intravesical); Deferiprone; Dipyrone; Stavudine

Increased Effect/Toxicity
Zidovudine may increase the levels/effects of: Amodiaquine; CloZAPine; Deferiprone; Ribavirin (Oral Inhalation); Ribavirin (Systemic)

The levels/effects of Zidovudine may be increased by: Acyclovir-Valacyclovir; Clarithromycin; Dexketoprofen; Dipyrone; DOXOrubicin (Conventional); DOXOrubicin (Liposomal); Fluconazole; Ganciclovir-Valganciclovir; Interferons; Methadone; Probenecid; Raltegravir; Teriflunomide; Valproate Products

Decreased Effect
Zidovudine may decrease the levels/effects of: BCG (Intravesical); Stavudine

The levels/effects of Zidovudine may be decreased by: Clarithromycin; DOXOrubicin (Conventional); DOXOrubicin (Liposomal); Protease Inhibitors; Rifamycin Derivatives

Preparation for Administration Hazardous agent; use appropriate precautions for handling and disposal (NIOSH 2014 [group 2]).

Solution for injection should be removed from the vial and diluted with D_5W to a concentration ≤4 mg/mL.

Storage/Stability
IV: Store undiluted vials at 15°C to 25°C (59°F to 77°F). Protect from light. When diluted, solution is physically and chemically stable for 24 hours at room temperature and 48 hours if refrigerated. Attempt to administer diluted solution within 8 hours if stored at room temperature or 24 hours if refrigerated to minimize potential for microbial-contaminated solutions (vials are single-use and do not contain preservative).
Tablets, capsules, syrup: Store at 15°C to 25°C (59°F to 77°F). Protect capsules from moisture.

Mechanism of Action Zidovudine is a thymidine analog which interferes with the HIV viral RNA-dependent DNA polymerase resulting in inhibition of viral replication; nucleoside reverse transcriptase inhibitor

Pharmacodynamics/Kinetics
Distribution: Significant penetration into the CSF
V_d: 1 to 2.2 L/kg
Relative diffusion from blood into CSF: Adequate with or without inflammation (exceeds usual MICs)
CSF:blood level ratio: Normal meninges: ~60%
Protein binding: 25% to 38%
Metabolism: Hepatic via glucuronidation to inactive metabolites, including GZDV; extensive first-pass effect
Bioavailability: 54% to 74%
Half-life elimination: Terminal: 0.5 to 3 hours
Time to peak, serum: 30 to 90 minutes
Excretion:
Oral: Urine (72% to 74% as metabolites, 14% to 18% as unchanged drug)
IV: Urine (45% to 60% as metabolites, 18% to 29% as unchanged drug)

Dosing
Adult & Geriatric Note: Patients should receive IV therapy only until oral therapy can be administered.

Prevention of maternal-fetal HIV transmission: Dose adjustment not required in pregnant women. Begin oral therapy with usual recommended dose based on current treatment guidelines. Zidovudine should be administered by continuous IV infusion near delivery regardless of antepartum regimen or mode of delivery in women with HIV RNA >1,000 copies/mL or unknown HIV RNA status. If oral zidovudine was part of the antepartum regimen, discontinue during intrapartum IV infusion. Other antiretroviral agents should be continued orally. Zidovudine IV is not required in women receiving combination antiretroviral therapy who have HIV RNA <1000 copies/mL near delivery and there are no concerns related to adherence with the regimen (HHS [perinatal], 2014).

During labor and delivery, administer zidovudine IV at 2 mg/kg as loading dose followed by a continuous IV infusion of 1 mg/kg/hour until delivery. For scheduled cesarean delivery, begin IV zidovudine 3 hours before surgery.

Treatment of HIV infection:
Oral:
US labeling: 300 mg twice daily
Canadian labeling: 300 mg twice daily or 200 mg 3 times daily
IV:
US labeling: 1 mg/kg/dose administered every 4 hours around-the-clock (5 to 6 doses daily)
Canadian labeling: 1 to 2 mg/kg/dose administered every 4 hours around-the-clock (6 doses daily)

Postexposure prophylaxis (off-label use): Oral: 300 mg twice daily or 200 mg 3 times daily in combination with lamivudine or emtricitabine. A third agent may be added for high-risk exposures. Therapy should be started within hours of exposure and continued for 4 weeks (CDC, 2005).

Pediatric Note: Patients should receive IV therapy only until oral therapy can be administered.

Prevention of perinatal HIV transmission (in neonates): Note: Start as soon as possible after birth, preferably within 6 to 12 hours of delivery. Continue dose from birth through 6 weeks of age (a 4-week course may be considered if the mother received ART therapy during pregnancy consistent with viral suppression and there are no concerns related to adherence with the regimen). Use zidovudine in combination with nevirapine in select situations (eg, infants born to mothers with only intrapartum therapy or no therapy) (HHS [perinatal], 2014).
Oral:
Manufacturer's labeling: Full-term infants: 2 mg/kg every 6 hours
Alternative dosing (HHS [perinatal], 2014):
Infants ≥35 weeks: 4 mg/kg/dose twice daily
Infants ≥30 weeks and <35 weeks gestation at birth: 2 mg/kg/dose every 12 hours; at 15 days of age, advance to 3 mg/kg/dose every 12 hours
Infants <30 weeks gestation at birth: 2 mg/kg/dose every 12 hours; at 4 weeks of age, advance to 3 mg/kg/dose every 12 hours
IV (infants unable to receive oral dosing): Start as soon as possible after birth, preferably within 6 to 12 hours of delivery; continue dose from birth through 6 weeks of age (HHS [perinatal], 2014):
Manufacturer's labeling: 1.5 mg/kg/dose every 6 hours
Alternate dosing (HHS [perinatal], 2014):
Infants ≥35 weeks: 3 mg/kg/dose every 12 hours
Infants ≥30 weeks and <35 weeks gestation at birth: 1.5 mg/kg/dose every 12 hours; at 15 days of age, advance to 2.3 mg/kg/dose every 12 hours
Infants <30 weeks gestation at birth: 1.5 mg/kg/dose every 12 hours; at 4 weeks of age, advance to 2.3 mg/kg/dose every 12 hours

Treatment of HIV infection:
Infants, Children, and Adolescents 4 weeks to <18 years:
Oral: Dose should be calculated by body weight (in kg) or body surface area and should not exceed the recommended adult dose. **Note:** Doses calculated by body weight may not be the same as those calculated by body surface area.
Dosing based on body surface area: 240 mg/m^2 twice daily (maximum: 300 mg twice daily) **or** 160 mg/m^2/dose 3 times daily (maximum: 200 mg 3 times daily)
Dosing based on weight (**Note:** 3 times daily dose is approved but rarely used in clinical practice):
4 to <9 kg: 12 mg/kg/dose twice daily **or** 8 mg/kg/dose 3 times daily
≥9 to <30 kg: 9 mg/kg/dose twice daily **or** 6 mg/kg/dose 3 times daily
≥30 kg: 300 mg twice daily **or** 200 mg 3 times daily
Infants ≥3 months and Children (Canadian labeling): IV intermittent infusion: 120 mg/m^2/dose every 6 hours
Adolescents ≥30 kg (Canadian labeling): IV intermittent infusion: 1 to 2 mg/kg/dose every 4 hours around-the-clock (6 doses daily)

Renal Impairment
CrCl ≥15 mL/minute: No dosage adjustment necessary.
CrCl <15 mL/minute
Oral:
Manufacturer's labeling: 100 mg every 6 to 8 hours
Alternate dosing: 100 mg 3 times daily or 300 mg once daily (HHS [adult] 2015)

IV: 1 mg/kg every 6 to 8 hours
ESRD on intermittent hemodialysis (IHD) (administer dose after dialysis on dialysis days):
Oral:
Manufacturer's labeling: 100 mg every 6 to 8 hours
Alternate dosing: 100 mg 3 times daily or 300 mg once daily (HHS [adult] 2015)
IV: 1 mg/kg every 6 to 8 hours
Peritoneal dialysis (PD):
Oral: 100 mg every 6 to 8 hours
IV: 1 mg/kg every 6 to 8 hours
Continuous renal replacement therapy (CRRT): No adjustment needed (Aronoff, 2007)

Hepatic Impairment There are no specific dosage adjustments provided in the manufacturer's labeling (has not been studied). However, adjustment may be necessary due to extensive hepatic metabolism.

Adjustment for Toxicity Consider dose interruption for significant anemia (hemoglobin <7.5 g/dL or >25% reduction from baseline) and/or neutropenia (granulocyte count <750 cells/mm^3 or >50% reduction from baseline) until evidence of recovery. Anemia associated with chronic zidovudine may warrant dose reduction.

Administration
Oral: Administer around-the-clock to promote less variation in peak and trough serum levels; may be administered without regard to meals
IV: Avoid rapid infusion or bolus injection. Do not administer IM
US labeling:
Neonates: Infuse over 30 minutes
Adults: Infuse over 1 hour; in pregnant women, infuse loading dose over 1 hour followed by continuous infusion
Canadian labeling:
Neonates: Infuse over 30 minutes
Infants ≥3 months, Children, Adolescents, and Adults: Infuse over 1 hour; in pregnant women, infuse loading dose over 1 hour followed by continuous infusion

Hazardous agent; use appropriate precautions for handling and disposal (NIOSH 2014 [group 2]).

Monitoring Parameters
Monitor viral load (2 to 8 weeks after initiation/modification of therapy, and then every 3 to 6 months); CBC with differential (every 3 to 6 months); liver function tests (every 6 to 12 months); lipids, glucose (yearly if normal); observe for appearance of opportunistic infections [DHHS (adult), 2014])
Monitor CD4 count every 3 to 6 months; every 6 to 12 months once clinically stable. For patients who have been on ART for at least 2 years with consistent viral suppression, CD4 count frequency may be reduced to every 12 months for CD4 count 300 to 500 cells/mm^3 and is considered optional for CD4 count >500 cells/mm^3. Resume more frequent CD4 count monitoring in patients with viral rebound, new HIV-associated clinical symptoms, or when there are conditions or a new therapy that may reduce CD4 cell count (DHHS [adult], 2014]).

Additional Information Potential compliance problems, frequency of administration, and adverse effects should be discussed with patients before initiating therapy to help prevent the emergence of resistance.

Dosage Forms Excipient information presented when available (limited, particularly for generics); consult specific product labeling. [DSC] = Discontinued product
Capsule, Oral:
Retrovir: 100 mg [contains soybean lecithin]
Generic: 100 mg
Solution, Intravenous [preservative free]:
Retrovir: 10 mg/mL (20 mL)
Syrup, Oral:
Retrovir: 50 mg/5 mL (240 mL) [contains sodium benzoate; strawberry flavor]
Generic: 50 mg/5 mL (240 mL)
Tablet, Oral:
Retrovir: 300 mg [DSC]
Generic: 300 mg

◆ Zidovudine, Abacavir, and Lamivudine *see* Abacavir, Lamivudine, and Zidovudine *on page 18*

◆ Zidovudine and Lamivudine *see* Lamivudine and Zidovudine *on page 1026*

◆ Zilactin [OTC] *see* Benzyl Alcohol *on page 220*

◆ Zilactin-B® (Can) *see* Benzocaine *on page 217*

◆ Zilactin Baby [OTC] *see* Benzocaine *on page 217*

◆ Zilactin Baby® (Can) *see* Benzocaine *on page 217*

Zileuton (zye LOO ton)

Brand Names: US Zyflo; Zyflo CR

Pharmacologic Category 5-Lipoxygenase Inhibitor
Use Prophylaxis and chronic treatment of asthma
Dosing
Adult & Geriatric Asthma: Oral:
Immediate release: 600 mg 4 times/day
Extended release: 1200 mg twice daily
Pediatric Asthma: Oral: Children ≥12 years: Refer to adult dosing.
Renal Impairment No dosage adjustment necessary.
Hepatic Impairment Contraindicated with hepatic impairment.
Additional Information Complete prescribing information should be consulted for additional detail.
Dosage Forms Excipient information presented when available (limited, particularly for generics); consult specific product labeling.
Tablet, Oral:
Zyflo: 600 mg [scored]
Tablet Extended Release 12 Hour, Oral:
Zyflo CR: 600 mg

- ◆ Zinacef see Cefuroxime on page 353
- ◆ Zinacef in Sterile Water see Cefuroxime on page 353
- ◆ Zinc 15 [OTC] see Zinc Sulfate on page 1929
- ◆ Zinc-220 [OTC] see Zinc Sulfate on page 1929

Zinc Acetate (zink AS e tate)

Brand Names: US Galzin
Pharmacologic Category Trace Element
Use Maintenance treatment of Wilson's disease following initial chelation therapy
Dosing
Adult & Geriatric Wilson's disease: Oral: Dose expressed in mg elemental zinc:
Males and nonpregnant females: 150 mg/day in 3 divided doses
Pregnant females: 75 mg/day in 3 divided doses; may increase to 150 mg/day in 3 divided doses if inadequate response to lower dose
Pediatric Wilson's disease: Oral: Dose expressed in mg elemental zinc:
Children ≥10 years: 75 mg/day in 3 divided doses; may increase to 150 mg/day in 3 divided doses if inadequate response to lower dose
American Association for the Study of Liver Diseases (AASLD) practice guideline recommendations (Roberts, 2008):
Children <50 kg and >5 years: 75 mg/day in 3 divided doses
Children >50 kg: 150 mg/day in 3 divided doses
Renal Impairment No dosage adjustment provided in manufacturer's labeling.
Hepatic Impairment No dosage adjustment provided in manufacturer's labeling.
Additional Information Complete prescribing information should be consulted for additional detail.
Dosage Forms Considerations Strength of Galzin capsule is expressed as elemental zinc
Dosage Forms Excipient information presented when available (limited, particularly for generics); consult specific product labeling.
Capsule, Oral:
Galzin: 25 mg, 50 mg

- ◆ Zincate [DSC] see Zinc Sulfate on page 1929

Zinc Chloride (zink KLOR ide)

Pharmacologic Category Trace Element
Use Cofactor for replacement therapy to different enzymes; helps maintain normal growth rates, normal skin hydration, and senses of taste and smell
Dosing
Adult & Geriatric
Nutritional supplement: IV:
Stable with fluid loss from small bowel: 12.2 mg zinc/L TPN or 17.1 mg zinc/kg (added to 1000 mL IV fluids) of stool or ileostomy output
Metabolically stable: 2.5-4 mg/day, add 2 mg/day for acute catabolic states
Note: Clinical response may not occur for up to 6-8 weeks.
Pediatric
Nutritional supplement: IV: Added to IV solutions:
Premature Infants <1500 g, up to 3 kg: 300 mcg/kg/day
Infants (full term) and Children ≤5 years: 100 mcg/kg/day
Renal Impairment No dosage adjustment provided in manufacturer's labeling. However, dosage adjustment may be necessary in severe impairment since zinc is

primarily renally excreted. Additionally, aluminum accumulation may occur in the setting of renal impairment.
Hepatic Impairment No dosage adjustment provided in manufacturer's labeling.
Additional Information Complete prescribing information should be consulted for additional detail.
Dosage Forms Considerations Strength of zinc chloride injection is expressed as elemental zinc
Dosage Forms Excipient information presented when available (limited, particularly for generics); consult specific product labeling.
Solution, Intravenous:
Generic: 1 mg/mL (10 mL)

Zinc Gelatin (zink JEL ah tin)

Brand Names: US Gelucast®
Index Terms Dome Paste Bandage; Unna's Boot; Unna's Paste; Zinc Gelatin Boot
Pharmacologic Category Topical Skin Product
Use As a protectant and to support varicosities and similar lesions of the lower limbs
Dosing
Adult & Geriatric Protectant: Topical: Apply externally as an occlusive boot
Additional Information Complete prescribing information should be consulted for additional detail.
Dosage Forms Excipient information presented when available (limited, particularly for generics); consult specific product labeling.
Bandage: 3" x 10 yards; 4" x 10 yards

- ◆ Zinc Gelatin Boot see Zinc Gelatin on page 1929
- ◆ Zincofax® (Can) see Zinc Oxide on page 1929

Zinc Oxide (zink OKS ide)

Brand Names: US Ammens® Original Medicated [OTC]; Ammens® Shower Fresh [OTC]; Balmex® [OTC]; Boudreaux's® Butt Paste [OTC]; Critic-Aid Skin Care® [OTC]; Desitin Maximum Strength Original [OTC]; Desitin Rapid Relief [OTC]; Dr. Smith's Diaper Rash [OTC]; Elta Seal Moisture Barrier [OTC]; Pharmabase Barrier [OTC]
Brand Names: Canada Zincofax®
Index Terms Base Ointment; Lassar's Zinc Paste
Pharmacologic Category Topical Skin Product
Use Protective coating for mild skin irritations and abrasions; soothing and protective ointment to promote healing of chapped skin, diaper rash
Dosing
Adult & Geriatric Protectant: Topical: Apply as required to affected areas several times daily
Pediatric Protectant: Topical: Apply as required to affected areas several times daily
Additional Information Complete prescribing information should be consulted for additional detail.
Dosage Forms Excipient information presented when available (limited, particularly for generics); consult specific product labeling.
Cream, topical:
Balmex®: 11.3% (60 g, 120 g, 480 g) [contains aloe, benzoic acid, soybean oil, and vitamin E]
Desitin Rapid Relief: 13% (57 g, 113 g)
Elta Seal Moisture Barrier: 6% (114 g)
Cream, topical [stick]:
Balmex®: 11.3% (56 g) [contains aloe, benzoic acid, soybean oil, and vitamin E]
Ointment, topical: 20% (30 g, 60 g, 454 g); 40% (120 g)
Dr. Smith's Diaper Rash: 10% (57 g, 85 g, 27 g)
Pharmabase Barrier: 9.38% (500 g)
Paste, topical:
Boudreaux's® Butt Paste: 16% (30 g, 60 g, 120 g, 480 g) [contains castor oil, boric acid, mineral oil, and Peruvian balsam]
Desitin Maximum Strength Original: 40% (28 g, 57 g, 85 g, 120 g, 113 g, 454 g) [contains cod liver oil and lanolin]
Critic-Aid Skin Care®: 20% (71 g, 170 g)
Powder, topical:
Ammens® Original Medicated: 9.1% (312 g)
Ammens® Shower Fresh: 9.1% (312 g)

Zinc Sulfate (zink SUL fate)

Brand Names: US Eye-Sed [OTC]; Orazinc [OTC]; Zinc 15 [OTC]; Zinc-220 [OTC]; Zincate [DSC]
Brand Names: Canada Anuzinc; Rivasol
Index Terms ZnSO$_4$ (error-prone abbreviation)
Pharmacologic Category Trace Element

Use Zinc supplement (oral and parenteral); may improve wound healing in those who are deficient

Dosing

Adult & Geriatric

Recommended daily allowance (RDA): Oral (dose expressed as elemental zinc): Adults ≥19 years:
Males: 11 mg/day
Females: 8 mg/day
Pregnancy: 11 mg/day
Lactation: 12 mg/day

Parenteral TPN: IV:
Acute metabolic states: 4.5-6 mg/day
Metabolically stable: 2.5-4 mg/day
Replacement for small bowel fluid loss (metabolically stable): An additional 12.2 mg zinc/L of fluid lost, or an additional 17.1 mg zinc per kg of stool or ileostomy output

Pediatric

Adequate intake (AI): Oral (dose expressed as elemental zinc): 1-6 months: 2.0 mg/day

Recommended daily allowance (RDA): Oral (dose expressed as elemental zinc):
7-12 months: 3 mg/day
1-3 years: 3 mg/day
4-8 years: 5 mg/day
9-13 years: 8 mg/day
14-18 years:
Males: 11 mg/day
Females: 9 mg/day
Pregnancy: 12 mg/day
Lactation: 13 mg/day

Parenteral TPN: IV:
Infants (premature, birth weight <1500 g up to 3 kg): 300 mcg/kg/day
Infants (full term) and Children ≤5 years: 100 mcg/kg/day

Additional Information Complete prescribing information should be consulted for additional detail.

Dosage Forms Considerations

Strength of zinc sulfate injection is expressed as elemental zinc

Oral zinc sulfate is approximately 23% elemental zinc

Dosage Forms Excipient information presented when available (limited, particularly for generics); consult specific product labeling. [DSC] = Discontinued product

Capsule, Oral:
Orazinc: 220 mg
Zinc-220: 220 mg
Zincate: 220 mg [DSC]
Generic: 220 mg
Solution, Intravenous:
Generic: 1 mg/mL (10 mL [DSC]); 5 mg/mL (5 mL)
Solution, Ophthalmic:
Eye-Sed: 0.217% (15 mL) [contains benzalkonium chloride, boric acid]
Tablet, Oral:
Orazinc: 110 mg
Zinc 15: 66 mg
Generic: 220 mg
Tablet, Oral [preservative free]:
Generic: 220 mg

Ziprasidone (zi PRAS i done)

Brand Names: US Geodon

Brand Names: Canada Zeldox

Index Terms Zeldox; Ziprasidone Hydrochloride; Ziprasidone Mesylate

Pharmacologic Category Second Generation (Atypical) Antipsychotic

Use Treatment of schizophrenia; treatment of acute manic or mixed episodes associated with bipolar disorder with or without psychosis; maintenance treatment of bipolar disorder as an adjunct to lithium or valproate; acute agitation in patients with schizophrenia

Pregnancy Considerations Adverse events were observed in animal reproduction studies. Antipsychotic use during the third trimester of pregnancy has a risk for abnormal muscle movements (extrapyramidal symptoms [EPS]) and/or withdrawal symptoms in newborns following delivery. Symptoms in the newborn may include agitation, feeding disorder, hypertonia, hypotonia, respiratory distress, somnolence, and tremor; these effects may be self-limiting or require hospitalization. Ziprasidone may cause hyperprolactinemia, which may decrease reproductive function in both males and females.

The ACOG recommends that therapy during pregnancy be individualized; treatment with psychiatric medications during pregnancy should incorporate the clinical expertise of the mental health clinician, obstetrician, primary healthcare provider, and pediatrician. Safety data related to atypical antipsychotics during pregnancy is limited and routine use is not recommended. However, if a woman is inadvertently exposed to an atypical antipsychotic while pregnant, continuing therapy may be preferable to switching to a typical antipsychotic that the fetus has not yet been exposed to; consider risk:benefit (ACOG, 2008).

Healthcare providers are encouraged to enroll women 18-45 years of age exposed to ziprasidone during pregnancy in the Atypical Antipsychotics Pregnancy Registry (1-866-961-2388 or http://www.womensmentalhealth.org/pregnancyregistry).

Breast-Feeding Considerations It is not known if ziprasidone is excreted into breast milk. Breast-feeding is not recommended by the manufacturer.

Contraindications Hypersensitivity to ziprasidone or any component of the formulation; history of (or current) prolonged QT; congenital long QT syndrome; recent myocardial infarction; uncompensated heart failure; concurrent use of other QTc-prolonging agents including arsenic trioxide, chlorpromazine, class Ia antiarrhythmics (eg, disopyramide, quinidine, procainamide), class III antiarrhythmics (eg, amiodarone, dofetilide, ibutilide, sotalol), dolasetron, droperidol, gatifloxacin, halofantrine, levomethadyl, mefloquine, mesoridazine, moxifloxacin, pentamidine, pimozide, probucol, sparfloxacin, tacrolimus, and thioridazine

Warnings/Precautions Hazardous agent - use appropriate precautions for handling and disposal (NIOSH 2014 [group 3]). **[US Boxed Warning]: Elderly patients with dementia-related behavioral disorders treated with antipsychotics are at an increased risk of death compared to placebo.** Most deaths appeared to be either cardiovascular (eg, heart failure, sudden death) or infectious (eg, pneumonia) in nature. Use with caution in dementia with Lewy bodies; antipsychotics may worsen dementia symptoms and patients with dementia with Lewy bodies are more sensitive to the extrapyramidal side effects (APA [Rabins, 2007]). Ziprasidone is not approved for the treatment of dementia-related psychosis.

May result in QTc prolongation (dose related), which has been associated with the development of malignant ventricular arrhythmias (torsade de pointes) and sudden death. Note contraindications related to this effect. Observed prolongation was greater than with other atypical antipsychotic agents (risperidone, olanzapine, quetiapine), but less than with thioridazine. Correct electrolyte disturbances, especially hypokalemia or hypomagnesemia, prior to use and throughout therapy. Use caution in patients with bradycardia. Discontinue in patients found to have persistent QTc intervals >500 msec. Patients with symptoms of dizziness, palpitations, or syncope should receive further cardiac evaluation. May cause orthostatic hypotension. Use is contraindicated in patients with recent acute myocardial infarction (MI), QT prolongation, or uncompensated heart failure. Avoid use in patients with a history of cardiac arrhythmias; use with caution in patients with history of MI or unstable heart disease. Dyslipidemia has been reported with atypical antipsychotics; risk profile may differ between agents.

Leukopenia, neutropenia, and agranulocytosis (sometimes fatal) have been reported in clinical trials and postmarketing reports with antipsychotic use; presence of risk factors (eg, preexisting low WBC or history of drug-induced leuko-/neutropenia) should prompt periodic blood count assessment. Discontinue therapy at first signs of blood dyscrasias or if absolute neutrophil count <1,000/mm^3. Cases of dermatologic reactions (including Stevens-Johnson syndrome and drug reaction with eosinophilia and systemic symptoms [DRESS]) have been reported; may be fatal. Symptoms of DRESS include a combination of 3 or more of the following: severe skin eruption (rash or exfoliative dermatitis), fever, lymphadenopathy, eosinophilia and one or more systemic complications (eg, hepatitis, nephritis, pneumonitis, myocarditis, and pericarditis). Discontinue use if DRESS or other severe cutaneous reactions are suspected.

May cause extrapyramidal symptoms (EPS). Risk of dystonia (and probably other EPS) may be greater with increased doses, use of conventional antipsychotics, males, and younger patients. Impaired core body temperature regulation may occur; caution with strenuous exercise, heat exposure, dehydration, and concomitant medication possessing anticholinergic effects; not reported in premarketing trials of ziprasidone. Antipsychotic use may also be associated with neuroleptic malignant

syndrome (NMS). Use with caution in patients at risk of seizures.

Atypical antipsychotics have been associated with development of hyperglycemia. There is limited documentation with ziprasidone and specific risk associated with this agent is not known. Use caution in patients with diabetes or other disorders of glucose regulation; monitor for worsening of glucose control. May increase prolactin levels; clinical significance of hyperprolactinemia in patients with breast cancer or other prolactin-dependent tumors is unknown.

Use in elderly patients with dementia is associated with an increased risk of mortality and cerebrovascular accidents; avoid antipsychotic use for behavioral problems associated with dementia unless alternative nonpharmacologic therapies have failed and patient may harm self or others. In addition, use may cause or exacerbate syndrome of inappropriate antidiuretic hormone secretion or hyponatremia; monitor sodium closely with initiation or dosage adjustments in older adults (Beers Criteria).

Cognitive and/or motor impairment (sedation) is common with ziprasidone. CNS effects may be potentiated when used with other sedative drugs or ethanol. Use with caution in disorders where CNS depression is a feature. Use with caution in Parkinson disease; antipsychotics may aggravate the motor disturbances of Parkinson disease (APA [Rabins, 2007]). Antipsychotic use has been associated with esophageal dysmotility and aspiration; use with caution in patients at risk of pneumonia (ie, Alzheimer's disease). Use caution in hepatic impairment. Ziprasidone has been associated with a fairly high incidence of rash (5%). Significant weight gain has been observed with antipsychotic therapy; incidence varies with product. Monitor waist circumference and BMI. Rare cases of priapism have been reported. Use the intramuscular formulation with caution in patients with renal impairment; formulation contains cyclodextrin, an excipient which may accumulate in renal insufficiency, although the clinical significance of this finding is uncertain (Luke, 2010).

The possibility of a suicide attempt is inherent in psychotic illness or bipolar disorder; use caution in high-risk patients during initiation of therapy. Prescriptions should be written for the smallest quantity consistent with good patient care.

Adverse Reactions Frequencies represent oral administration unless otherwise indicated. **Note:** Although minor QTc prolongation (mean: 10 msec at 160 mg/day) may occur more frequently (incidence not specified), clinically relevant prolongation (>500 msec) was rare (0.06%) and less than placebo (0.23%).

>10%:

Central nervous system: Drowsiness (oral and IM: 8% to 31%; may be dose-related), extrapyramidal reaction (oral: 1% to 31%), headache (oral and IM: 5% to 18%), dizziness (oral and IM: 3% to 16%; includes lightheadedness; may be dose-related)

Gastrointestinal: Nausea (oral and IM: 8% to 12%)

1% to 10%:

Cardiovascular: Orthostatic hypotension (IM: ≤5%, oral: ≥1%; may be dose-related), chest pain (3%), hypertension (oral and IM: 1% to 3%), tachycardia (1% to 2%), bradycardia (oral and IM: ≤2%), facial edema (≥1%), angina pectoris (≤1%), peripheral edema (≤1%)

Central nervous system: Akathisia (oral: 8% to 10%; IM: ≤2%), anxiety (oral: 5%; may be dose-related), hypoesthesia (1% to 2%), agitation (oral: ≥1%, IM: ≤2%), personality disorder (IM: ≤2%), speech disturbance (oral and IM: ≤2%), amnesia (≥1%), ataxia (≥1%), chills (≥1%), confusion (≥1%), delirium (≥1%), dystonia (≥1%; may be dose-related), falling (≥1%), flank pain (≥1%), hostility (≥1%), hypothermia (≥1%), vertigo (≥1%), withdrawal syndrome (≥1%), anorgasmia (≤1%), atrial fibrillation (≤1%), male sexual disorder (≤1%), paralysis (≤1%), insomnia

Dermatologic: Skin rash (1% to 5%; may be dose-related), fungal dermatitis (1% to 2%), diaphoresis (IM: ≤2%), furunculosis (IM: ≤2%), skin photosensitivity (≥1%), alopecia (≤1%), contact dermatitis (≤1%), ecchymoses (≤1%), eczema (≤1%), exfoliative dermatitis (≤1%), maculopapular rash (≤1%), urticaria (≤1%), vesiculobullous dermatitis (≤1%)

Endocrine & metabolic: Weight gain (4% to 16%), albuminuria (≤1%), amenorrhea (≤1%), dehydration (≤1%), glycosuria (≤1%), hypercholesterolemia (≤1%), hyperglycemia (≤1%), hypermenorrhea (≤1%), hypokalemia (≤1%), increased lactate dehydrogenase (≤1%), increased thirst (≤1%)

Gastrointestinal: Constipation (oral: 9%, IM: ≤2%), dyspepsia (oral: 8%, IM: 2% to 3%), vomiting (oral and IM: 1% to 5%), xerostomia (oral: 4% to 5%; may be dose-related), diarrhea (oral and IM: ≤5%), sialorrhea (4%; may be dose-related), abdominal pain (oral and IM: ≤2%), anorexia (oral and IM: ≤2%; may be dose-related), dysmenorrhea (IM: ≤2%), dysphagia (≤2%), buccoglossal syndrome (≥1%)

Genitourinary: Hematuria (≤1%), impotence (≤1%), lactation (female: ≤1%), priapism (IM: ≤1%), urinary retention (≤1%)

Hematologic & oncologic: Rectal hemorrhage (oral and IM: ≤2%), anemia (≤1%), eosinophilia (≤1%), leukocytosis (≤1%), leukopenia (≤1%), lymphadenopathy (≤1%)

Hepatic: Increased serum alkaline phosphatase (≤1%), increased serum transaminases (≤1%)

Hypersensitivity: Tongue edema (≤3%)

Local: Pain at injection site (IM: 7% to 8%)

Neuromuscular & skeletal: Weakness (oral: 5% to 6%; may be dose-related), myalgia (1% to 2%), paresthesia (oral and IM: ≤2%), abnormal gait (≥1%), akinesia (≥1%), choreoathetosis (≥1%), dysarthria (≥1%), dyskinesia (≥1%), hyperkinesia (≥1%), hypokinesia (≥1%), hypotonia (≥1%), neuropathy (≥1%), tremor (≥1%; may be dose-related), twitching (≥1%), cogwheel rigidity (oral: ≥1%), hypertonia (≥1%), increased creatine phosphokinase (≤1%), tenosynovitis (≤1%)

Ophthalmic: Visual disturbance (3% to 6%; may be dose-related), diplopia (≥1%), oculogyric crisis (≥1%), blepharitis (≤1%), cataract (≤1%), conjunctivitis (≤1%), photophobia (≤1%), xerophthalmia (≤1%)

Otic: Tinnitus (≤1%)

Renal: Polyuria (≤1%)

Respiratory: Respiratory tract infection (8%), rhinitis (oral: 4%), cough (3%), pharyngitis (3%), dyspnea (1% to 2%), flu-like symptoms (oral: ≥1%), epistaxis (≤1%), pneumonia (≤1%)

Miscellaneous: Accidental injury (4%), fever (≥1%), motor vehicle accident (≥1%)

<1% (Limited to important or life-threatening): Agranulocytosis, basophilia, bundle branch block, cardiomegaly, cerebral infarction, cerebrovascular accident, cholestatic jaundice, decreased glucose tolerance, deep vein thrombophlebitis, diabetic coma, DRESS syndrome, ejaculatory disorder, facial droop, fecal impaction, female sexual disorder, first degree atrioventricular block, galactorrhea, gingival hemorrhage, granulocytopenia, gynecomastia, hematemesis, hemophthalmos, hemoptysis, hepatitis, hepatomegaly, hyperchloremia, hyperkalemia, hyperreflexia, hypersensitivity reaction (including allergic dermatitis, orofacial edema), hyperthyroidism, hyperuricemia, hypocalcemia, hypochloremia, hypocholesterolemia, hypochromic anemia, hypoglycemia, hypomagnesemia, hypomania, hyponatremia, hypoproteinemia, hypothyroidism, increased blood urea nitrogen, increased gamma-glutamyl transferase, increased monocytes, increased serum creatinine, increased serum prolactin, jaundice, keratitis, keratoconjunctivitis, ketosis, laryngismus, liver steatosis, lymphedema, lymphocytosis, mania, melena, myocarditis, myoclonus, myopathy, neuroleptic malignant syndrome, neutropenia, nocturia, nystagmus, oliguria, opisthotonos, oral kouplakisa, oral paresthesia, phlebitis, polycythemia, prolonged Q-T interval on ECG, pulmonary embolism, respiratory alkalosis, seizure, serotonin syndrome (with or without serotonergic medications), Stevens-Johnson syndrome, syncope, tardive dyskinesia, thrombocythemia, thrombocytopenia, thrombophlebitis, thyroiditis, torsade de pointes, torticollis, trismus, urinary incontinence, vaginal hemorrhage, visual field defect

Drug Interactions

Metabolism/Transport Effects Substrate of CYP1A2 (minor), CYP3A4 (minor); **Note:** Assignment of Major/Minor substrate status based on clinically relevant drug interaction potential; **Inhibits** CYP2D6 (weak)

Avoid Concomitant Use

Avoid concomitant use of Ziprasidone with any of the following: Amisulpride; Azelastine (Nasal); FLUoxetine; Highest Risk QTc-Prolonging Agents; Ivabradine; Metoclopramide; Mifepristone; Moderate Risk QTc-Prolonging Agents; Orphenadrine; Paraldehyde; Sulpiride; Thalidomide

Increased Effect/Toxicity

Ziprasidone may increase the levels/effects of: Alcohol (Ethyl); Amisulpride; Azelastine (Nasal); CNS Depressants; FLUoxetine; Highest Risk QTc-Prolonging Agents; Hydrocodone; Methotrimeprazine; Methylphenidate; Metyrosine; Orphenadrine; Paraldehyde; Selective Serotonin Reuptake Inhibitors; Serotonin Modulators; Sulpiride; Suvorexant; Thalidomide; Zolpidem

The levels/effects of Ziprasidone may be increased by: Acetylcholinesterase Inhibitors (Central); Blood Pressure Lowering Agents; Brimonidine (Topical); Cannabis; Doxylamine; Dronabinol; FLUoxetine; Ivabradine; Kava Kava; Magnesium Sulfate; Methotrimeprazine; Methylphenidate; Metoclopramide; Metyrosine; Mifepristone; Minocycline; Moderate Risk QTc-Prolonging Agents; Nabilone; Perampanel; QTc-Prolonging Agents (Indeterminate Risk and Risk Modifying); Rufinamide; Serotonin Modulators; Sodium Oxybate; Tapentadol; Tetrahydrocannabinol

Decreased Effect

Ziprasidone may decrease the levels/effects of: Amphetamines; Antidiabetic Agents; Anti-Parkinson's Agents (Dopamine Agonist); Quinagolide

The levels/effects of Ziprasidone may be decreased by: CarBAMazepine

Food Interactions Administration with a meal containing at least 500 calories increases serum levels ~80%. Management: Administer with a meal containing at least 500 calories (Lincoln, 2010).

Preparation for Administration Hazardous agent; use appropriate precautions for handling and disposal (NIOSH 2014 [group 3]).

Each vial should be reconstituted with 1.2 mL SWFI. Shake vigorously; will form a pale, pink solution containing 20 mg/mL ziprasidone.

Storage/Stability

Capsule: Store at 25°C (77°F); excursion permitted to 15°C to 30°C (59°F to 86°F).

Vials for injection: Store at 25°C (77°F); excursion permitted to 15°C to 30°C (59°F to 86°F). Protect from light. Following reconstitution, injection may be stored at room temperature up to 24 hours or under refrigeration for up to 7 days. Protect from light.

Mechanism of Action Ziprasidone is a benzylisothiazolylpiperazine antipsychotic. The exact mechanism of action is unknown. However, *in vitro* radioligand studies show that ziprasidone has high affinity for D_2, D_3, $5-HT_{2A}$, $5-HT_{1A}$, $5-HT_{2C}$, $5-HT_{1D}$, and alpha$_1$-adrenergic; moderate affinity for histamine H_1 receptors; and no appreciable affinity for alpha$_2$-adrenergic receptors, beta-adrenergic, $5-HT_3$, $5-HT_4$, cholinergic, mu, sigma, or benzodiazepine receptors. Ziprasidone functions as an antagonist at the D_2, $5-HT_{2A}$, and $5-HT_{1D}$ receptors and as an agonist at the $5-HT_{1A}$ receptor. Ziprasidone moderately inhibits the reuptake of serotonin and norepinephrine.

Pharmacodynamics/Kinetics

Absorption: Well absorbed; administration with 500-calorie meals increases serum levels ~80% (Lincoln, 2010).

Distribution: V_d: 1.5 L/kg

Protein binding: >99%, primarily to albumin and alpha-1 acid glycoprotein

Metabolism: Extensively hepatic, primarily chemical and enzymatic reductions via glutathione and aldehyde oxidase, respectively; less than 1/3 of total metabolism via CYP3A4 and CYP1A2 (minor)

Bioavailability: Oral (with food): 60%; IM: 100%

Half-life elimination: Oral: Mean terminal half-life: 7 hours; IM: Mean half-life: 2 to 5 hours

Time to peak: Oral: 6 to 8 hours; IM: ≤60 minutes

Excretion: Feces (~66%; <4% of total dose as unchanged drug); urine (~20%; <1% of total dose as unchanged drug)

Dosing

Adult

Bipolar disorder (acute and maintenance as adjuncts to lithium or valproate): Oral: Initial: 40 mg twice daily; may increase to 60 or 80 mg twice daily on second day of treatment; subsequently adjust dose based on response and tolerability. Usual dosage: 40 to 80 mg twice daily.

Schizophrenia: Initial: 20 mg twice daily (US labeling) or 20 to 40 mg twice daily (Canadian labeling). Increase dose based on response and tolerability no more frequently than every 2 days; ordinarily patients should be observed for improvement over several weeks before adjusting the dose. Usual dosage: 40 to 100 mg twice daily. **Note:** Dosages up to 320 mg per day appear safe; however, there is no data suggesting improved efficacy at higher doses (APA 2004).

Acute agitation (schizophrenia): IM: 10 mg every 2 hours **or** 20 mg every 4 hours (maximum: 40 mg daily). Oral therapy should replace IM administration as soon as possible.

Major depressive disorder (adjunct to antidepressants) (off-label use): Oral: Initial: 20 mg twice daily; may increase dose by 20 mg twice daily at weekly increments up to 80 mg twice daily based on response and tolerability. Average daily dose was 98 mg/day in the clinical trial (Papakostas 2015).

Geriatric No dosage adjustment is recommended; consider initiating at a low end of the dosage range, with slower titration.

Renal Impairment

Oral: No dosage adjustment necessary.

IM: Cyclodextrin, an excipient in the IM formulation, is cleared by renal filtration; use with caution.

Ziprasidone is not removed by hemodialysis.

Hepatic Impairment

US labeling: There are no dosage adjustments provided in the manufacturer's labeling; however, drug undergoes extensive hepatic metabolism and systemic exposure may be increased. Use with caution.

Canadian labeling: Manufacturer labeling suggests that dose reductions should be considered but does not provide specific dosing recommendations.

Dietary Considerations Capsule: Take with food.

Administration

Oral: Administer with a meal containing at least 500 calories (Lincoln, 2010).

Injection: For IM administration only.

Hazardous agent; use appropriate precautions for handling and disposal (NIOSH 2014 [group 3]).

Monitoring Parameters Mental status; vital signs (as clinically indicated); blood pressure (baseline; repeat 3 months after antipsychotic initiation, then yearly); ECG (as clinically indicated); weight, height, BMI, waist circumference (baseline; repeat at 4, 8, and 12 weeks after initiating or changing therapy, then quarterly; consider switching to a different antipsychotic for a weight gain ≥5% of initial weight); CBC (as clinically indicated; monitor frequently during the first few months of therapy in patients with preexisting low WBC or history of drug-induced leukopenia/neutropenia); electrolytes (annually and as clinically indicated; perform baseline potassium and magnesium measurements in patients at risk for electrolyte disturbances and periodically monitor if diuretics are initiated during ziprasidone treatment); liver function (annually and as clinically indicated); personal and family history of obesity, diabetes, dyslipidemia, hypertension, or cardiovascular disease (baseline; repeat annually); fasting plasma glucose level/HbA$_{1c}$ (baseline; repeat 3 months after starting antipsychotic, then yearly); fasting lipid panel (baseline; repeat 3 months after initiation of antipsychotic; if LDL level is normal repeat at 2-5 year intervals or more frequently if clinical indicated); changes in menstruation, libido, development of galactorrhea, erectile and ejaculatory function (at each visit for the first 12 weeks after the antipsychotic is initiated or until the dose is stable, then yearly); abnormal involuntary movements or parkinsonian signs (baseline; repeat weekly until dose stabilized for at least 2 weeks after introduction and for 2 weeks after any significant dose increase); tardive dyskinesia (every 12 months; high-risk patients every 6 months); ocular examination (yearly in patients >40 years; every 2 years in younger patients) (ADA, 2004; Lehman, 2004; Marder, 2004).

Additional Information The increased potential to prolong QTc, as compared to other available antipsychotic agents, should be considered in the evaluation of available alternatives.

Dosage Forms Excipient information presented when available (limited, particularly for generics); consult specific product labeling.

Capsule, Oral, as hydrochloride:
Geodon: 20 mg, 40 mg, 60 mg, 80 mg
Generic: 20 mg, 40 mg, 60 mg, 80 mg

Solution Reconstituted, Intramuscular, as mesylate [strength expressed as base]:
Geodon: 20 mg (1 ea)

Dosage Forms: Canada Excipient information presented when available (limited, particularly for generics); consult specific product labeling.

Capsule, Oral, as hydrochloride:
Zeldox: 20 mg, 40 mg, 60 mg, 80 mg

Extemporaneous Preparations Hazardous agent: Use appropriate precautions for handling and disposal (NIOSH 2014 [group 3]).

A 2.5 mg/mL oral solution may be made with the injection. Use 8 vials of the 20 mg injectable powder. Add 1.2 mL of distilled water to each vial to make a 20 mg/mL solution. Once dissolved, transfer 7.5 mL to a calibrated bottle and add quantity of vehicle (Ora-Sweet®) sufficient to make 60 mL. Label "shake well" and "refrigerate". Stable for 14 days at room temperature or 42 days refrigerated (preferred).

Green K and Parish RC, "Stability of Ziprasidone Mesylate in an Extemporaneously Compounded Oral Solution," *J Pediatr Pharmacol Ther*, 2010, 15:138-41.

◆ Ziprasidone Hydrochloride *see* Ziprasidone on page 1930

Ziv-Aflibercept (Systemic) (ziv a FLIB er sept)

Brand Names: US Zaltrap

Index Terms Aflibercept I.V.; Vascular Endothelial Growth Factor Trap; VEGF Trap; VEGF Trap R1R2

Pharmacologic Category Antineoplastic Agent; Vascular Endothelial Growth Factor (VEGF) Inhibitor

Use Colorectal cancer, metastatic: Treatment of metastatic colorectal cancer (in combination with fluorouracil, leucovorin, and irinotecan [FOLFIRI]) in patients who are resistant to or have progressed on an oxaliplatin-based regimen

Pregnancy Considerations Adverse events were observed in animal reproduction studies with doses providing systemic exposure equivalent to ~30% of a human dose. The incidence of fetal malformations increased with increasing doses. Patients (male and female) should use effective contraception during therapy and for at least 3 months following treatment.

Breast-Feeding Considerations It is not known if ziv-aflibercept is excreted into breast milk. Due to the potential for serious adverse reactions in the nursing infant, the manufacturer recommends a decision to be made whether to discontinue nursing or to discontinue aflibercept, taking into account the importance of treatment to the mother.

Contraindications There are no contraindications listed in the manufacturer's labeling.

Warnings/Precautions The risk for hemorrhage is increased with ziv-aflibercept. **[U.S. Boxed Warning]: Severe and occasionally fatal hemorrhage, including gastrointestinal (GI) bleeding, has been reported with ziv-aflibercept/FOLFIRI. Monitor for signs and symptoms of GI and other severe bleeding events; do not administer to patients with severe hemorrhage;** discontinue if severe hemorrhage develops. Hemorrhagic events have also included hematuria, postprocedural hemorrhage, intracranial hemorrhage, and pulmonary hemorrhage/hemoptysis.

[U.S. Boxed Warning]: Severe or fatal GI perforation is a possibility; discontinue ziv-aflibercept if GI perforation occurs; monitor for signs/symptoms of GI perforation. The risk for GI and non-GI fistulas is increased with ziv-aflibercept; fistula sites have included anal, enterovesical, enterocutaneous, colovaginal and intestinal; discontinue in patients who develop fistula. Severe diarrhea and dehydration have been reported; the incidence of diarrhea is increased in patients ≥65 years of age; monitor elderly patients closely for diarrhea.

Proteinuria, nephrotic syndrome, and thrombotic microangiopathy (TMA) have been associated with ziv-aflibercept. Evaluate for proteinuria during treatment with urine dipstick and/or urinary protein creatinine ratio (UPCR); if dipstick ≥2+ for protein or UPCR >1, obtain 24-hour urine collection. Withhold ziv-aflibercept for proteinuria ≥2 g per 24 hours; for recurrent proteinuria, withhold treatment until <2 g per 24 hours and then resume with permanent dose reduction. Discontinue treatment for nephrotic syndrome or TMA.

The risk for grades 3/4 hypertension is increased; onset is generally within the first 2 treatment cycles. Monitor blood pressure every 2 weeks (more frequently if clinically indicated); treat with appropriate antihypertensive therapy (may require adjustment of existing antihypertensives); temporarily withhold treatment with uncontrolled hypertension; may reinitiate with permanent dose reduction when controlled. Discontinue for hypertensive crisis or encephalopathy. Patients with NYHA class III or IV heart failure were excluded from clinical trials.

[U.S. Boxed Warning]: Severely compromised wound healing may occur with ziv-aflibercept/FOLFIRI. Discontinue ziv-aflibercept with compromised wound healing. Withhold ziv-aflibercept at least 4 weeks prior to elective surgery. Do not resume ziv-aflibercept treatment until at least 4 weeks after major surgery AND until the surgical wound is completely healed. For minor surgeries (eg, central venous access port placement, biopsy, or tooth extraction), ziv-aflibercept may be resumed or initiated as soon as the surgical wound is fully healed.

A higher incidence of neutropenia and complications due to neutropenia (neutropenic fever and infection) occurred in patients receiving ziv-aflibercept; leukopenia and thrombocytopenia were also observed in clinical trials; monitor CBC with differential (baseline and prior to each cycle); delay treatment until ANC is ≥1,500/mm³. Cases of reversible posterior leukoencephalopathy syndrome (RPLS) have been reported; confirm diagnosis with MRI; discontinue ziv-aflibercept if verified; symptoms generally resolve or improve within days, although persistent neurologic symptoms and death have been reported. Arterial thrombotic events (ATE), including transient ischemic attack, cerebrovascular accidents, and angina have occurred. Discontinue ziv-aflibercept in patients who experience ATEs. Certain adverse events, such as diarrhea, dizziness, weakness, weight loss, and dehydration, occurred at a higher incidence in elderly compared to younger adults; monitor closely during treatment.

Adverse Reactions Note: Reactions reported in combination therapy with fluorouracil, leucovorin, and irinotecan (FOLFIRI).

>10%:

Cardiovascular: Hypertension (41%; grades 3/4: 19%)

Central nervous system: Fatigue (48%), dysphonia (25%), headache (22%)

Dermatologic: Palmar-plantar erythrodysesthesia (11%)

Gastrointestinal: Diarrhea (69%), stomatitis (50%), appetite decreased (32%), weight loss (32%), abdominal pain (27%), upper abdominal pain (11%)

Hematologic: Leukopenia (78%; grades 3/4: 16%), neutropenia (67%; grades 3/4: 37%), thrombocytopenia (48%; grades 3/4: 3%), bleeding (38%; grades 3/4: 3%)

Hepatic: AST increased (62%), ALT increased (50%)

Neuromuscular & skeletal: Weakness (18%)

Renal: Proteinuria (62%; grades 3/4: 8%), creatinine increased (23%)

Respiratory: Epistaxis (28%), dyspnea (12%)

Miscellaneous: Infection (46%)

1% to 10%:

Cardiovascular: Venous thromboembolic events (9%), arterial thromboembolic events (3%; grades 3/4: 2%)

Central nervous system: Reversible posterior encephalopathy syndrome (RPLS) (1%)

Dermatologic: Hyperpigmentation (8%)

Endocrine & metabolic: Dehydration (9%)

Gastrointestinal: Hemorrhoids (6%), proctalgia (5%), rectal hemorrhage (5%), gastrointestinal perforation (1%)

Genitourinary: Urinary tract infection (9%)

Hematologic: Neutropenic fever (grades 3/4: 4%), neutropenic infection/sepsis (grades 3/4: 2%)

Renal: Nephrotic syndrome (1%)

Respiratory: Oropharyngeal pain (8%), rhinorrhea (6%), pulmonary embolism (5%)

Miscellaneous: Antibody formation (3%), fistula formation (2%; grades 3/4: <1%)

<1% (Limited to important or life-threatening): Hypersensitivity reactions, thrombotic microangiopathy, wound healing impaired

Drug Interactions

Metabolism/Transport Effects None known.

Avoid Concomitant Use

Avoid concomitant use of Ziv-Aflibercept (Systemic) with any of the following: BCG (Intravesical); Deferiprone; Dipyrone

Increased Effect/Toxicity

Ziv-Aflibercept (Systemic) may increase the levels/effects of: Bisphosphonate Derivatives; CloZAPine; Deferiprone

The levels/effects of Ziv-Aflibercept (Systemic) may be increased by: Dipyrone

Decreased Effect

Ziv-Aflibercept (Systemic) may decrease the levels/effects of: BCG (Intravesical)

Preparation for Administration Prior to infusion, dilute in D₅W or NS to a final concentration of 0.6-8 mg/mL. Use polyvinyl chloride (PVC) infusion bags containing DEHP or polyolefin bags. After initial vial puncture, do not re-enter; discard any unused portion of the vial. Do not mix with other medications.

Storage/Stability

Store intact vials refrigerated at 2°C to 8°C (36°F to 46°F). Protect from light (store in original outer carton).

Solutions diluted for infusion may be stored in refrigerator for up to 24 hours, or at 20°C to 25°C (68°F to 77°F) for up to 8 hours.

Mechanism of Action Also known as VEGF-trap, ziv-aflibercept is a recombinant fusion protein which is comprised of portions of binding domains for vascular endothelial growth factor (VEGF) receptors 1 and 2, attached to the Fc portion of human IgG1. Ziv-aflibercept acts as a decoy receptor for VEGF-A, VEGF-B, and placental growth factor (PlGF) which prevent VEGF receptor binding/activation to their receptors (an action critical to angiogenesis), thus leading to antiangiogenesis and tumor regression.

Pharmacodynamics/Kinetics Half-life elimination: ~6 days (range: 4 to 7 days)

Dosing

Adult & Geriatric Colorectal cancer, metastatic: IV: 4 mg/kg every 2 weeks (in combination with fluorouracil, leucovorin, and irinotecan [FOLFIRI]), continue until disease progression or unacceptable toxicity

Renal Impairment There are no dosage adjustments provided in the manufacturer's labeling; however, need for adjustment is not likely because exposure in patients with mild, moderate, and severe impairment was similar to that of patients with normal renal function.

Hepatic Impairment

Mild (total bilirubin >1 to 1.5 times ULN) to moderate (total bilirubin >1.5 to 3 times ULN) impairment: There are no dosage adjustments provided in the manufacturer's labeling; however, need for adjustment is not likely because exposure was similar to that of patients with normal hepatic function.

Severe impairment (total bilirubin >3 times ULN): There are no dosage adjustments provided in the manufacturer's labeling (no data available).

Adjustment for Toxicity

Arterial thrombotic events: Discontinue treatment.

Fistula formation: Discontinue treatment.

Gastrointestinal perforation: Discontinue treatment.

Hemorrhage, severe: Discontinue treatment.

Hypertension:

Recurrent or severe hypertension: Temporarily withhold treatment until controlled and then resume with a permanent dose reduction to 2 mg/kg every 2 weeks.

Hypertensive crisis or hypertensive encephalopathy: Discontinue treatment.

Neutropenia: Temporarily withhold treatment until ANC is ≥1500/mm³.

Renal effects:

Proteinuria (≥2 g/24 hours): Temporarily withhold treatment until proteinuria <2 g/24 hours and then resume at previous dose.

Recurrent proteinuria: Temporarily withhold treatment until proteinuria <2 g/24 hours and then resume with a permanent dose reduction to 2 mg/kg every 2 weeks.

Nephrotic syndrome or thrombotic microangiopathy: Discontinue treatment

Reversible posterior leukoencephalopathy syndrome (RPLS): Discontinue treatment.

Surgery/wound healing impairment:

Elective surgery: Temporarily withhold treatment for at least 4 weeks prior to elective surgery; do not resume until at least 4 weeks after major surgery AND until wound is fully healed; for minor surgery (eg, biopsy, central venous port placement, tooth extraction), may be resumed after wound is fully healed.

Wound healing impaired: Discontinue treatment.

Note: For toxicities related to FOLFIRI, refer to individual Fluorouracil or Irinotecan monographs.

Administration IV: Infuse over 1 hour. Do not administer as an IV push or bolus. Administer prior to any FOLFIRI component. Do not administer other medications through the same intravenous line.

Infuse via a 0.2 micron polyethersulfone filter; do not use filters made of polyvinylidene fluoride (PVDF) or nylon. Administer with one of the following types of infusion sets: Polyvinyl chloride (PVC) containing DEHP, DEHP-free PVC containing trioctyl-trimellitate (TOTM), polypropylene, polyethylene lined PVC, or polyurethane.

Monitoring Parameters CBC with differential (baseline and prior to each cycle); urine protein (dipstick analysis and/or urinary protein creatinine ratio [UPCR], obtain 24-hour urine collection if dipstick ≥2+ for protein or UPCR >1); blood pressure (every 2 weeks; more frequently if clinically indicated); monitor for signs/symptoms of hemorrhage or GI perforation; monitor elderly patients closely for diarrhea and/or dehydration. Monitor wounds for healing impairment.

Dosage Forms Excipient information presented when available (limited, particularly for generics); consult specific product labeling.

Solution, Intravenous [preservative free]:

Zaltrap: 100 mg/4 mL (4 mL); 200 mg/8 mL (8 mL) [contains mouse protein (murine) (hamster)]

Zoledronic Acid (zoe le DRON ik AS id)

Brand Names: US Reclast; Zometa

Brand Names: Canada Aclasta; Taro-Zoledronic Acid; Taro-Zoledronic Acid Concentrate; Zoledronic Acid Injection; Zoledronic Acid for Injection; Zoledronic Acid Z; Zometa Concentrate

Index Terms CGP-42446; Zol 446; Zoledronate

Pharmacologic Category Bisphosphonate Derivative

Use

Glucocorticoid-induced osteoporosis (Reclast, Aclasta [Canadian product]): Treatment and prevention of glucocorticoid-induced osteoporosis in men and women who are initiating or continuing systemic glucocorticoids in a daily dose equivalent to 7.5 mg or more of prednisone and who are expected to remain on glucocorticoids for at least 12 months.

Hypercalcemia of malignancy (Zometa): Treatment of hypercalcemia (albumin-corrected serum calcium ≥12 mg/dL) of malignancy.

Multiple myeloma and bone metastases from solid tumors (Zometa): Treatment of patients with multiple myeloma and patients with documented bone metastases from solid tumors, in conjunction with standard antineoplastic therapy.

Osteoporosis in men (Reclast, Aclasta [Canadian product]): To increase bone mass in men with osteoporosis.

Paget disease of bone (Reclast, Aclasta [Canadian product]): Treatment of Paget disease of bone in men and women. **Note:** In patients without contraindications, zoledronic acid is recommended as the treatment of choice per Endocrine Society guidelines (Singer, 2014).

Postmenopausal osteoporosis (Reclast, Aclasta [Canadian product]): Treatment and prevention of osteoporosis in postmenopausal women.

Pregnancy Considerations Adverse events were observed in animal reproduction studies. It is not known if bisphosphonates cross the placenta, but fetal exposure is expected (Djkanovic, 2008; Stathopoulos, 2011). Bisphosphonates are incorporated into the bone matrix and gradually released over time. The amount available in the systemic circulation varies by dose and duration of therapy. Theoretically, there may be a risk of fetal harm when pregnancy follows the completion of therapy; however, available data have not shown that exposure to bisphosphonates during pregnancy significantly increases the risk of adverse fetal events (Djkanovic, 2008; Levy, 2009; Stathopoulos, 2011). Until additional data is available, most sources recommend discontinuing bisphosphonate therapy in women of reproductive potential as early as possible prior to a planned pregnancy; use in premenopausal women should be reserved for special circumstances when rapid bone loss is occurring (Bhalla, 2010; Pereira, 2012; Stathopoulos, 2011). Because hypocalcemia has been described following *in utero* bisphosphonate exposure, exposed infants should be monitored for hypocalcemia after birth (Djkanovic, 2008; Stathopoulos, 2011). Use in pregnant women is contraindicated per the Canadian labeling.

Breast-Feeding Considerations It is not known if zoledronic acid is excreted into breast milk. Due to the potential for serious adverse reactions in the nursing infant, the U.S. manufacturer recommends a decision be made whether to discontinue nursing or to discontinue the drug, taking into account the importance of treatment to the mother. Use in nursing women is contraindicated per the Canadian labeling.

Medication Guide Available Yes

Contraindications

U.S. labeling:

Hypersensitivity to zoledronic acid or any component of the formulation; hypocalcemia (Reclast only); CrCl <35 mL/minute and in those with evidence of acute renal impairment (Reclast only).

Documentation of allergenic cross-reactivity for bisphosphonates is limited. However, because of similarities in chemical structure and/or pharmacologic actions, the possibility of cross-sensitivity cannot be ruled out with certainty.

Canadian labeling:

All indications: Hypersensitivity to zoledronic acid or other bisphosphonates, or any component of the formulation; uncorrected hypocalcemia at the time of infusion; pregnancy, breast-feeding

Nononcology uses: Additional contraindications: Use in patients with CrCl <35 mL/minute and use in patients with evidence of acute renal impairment due to an increased risk of renal failure

Warnings/Precautions Hazardous agent - use appropriate precautions for handling and disposal (NIOSH 2014 [group 3]).

Osteonecrosis of the jaw (ONJ) has been reported in patients receiving bisphosphonates. Risk factors include invasive dental procedures (eg, tooth extraction, dental implants, boney surgery); a diagnosis of cancer, with concomitant chemotherapy (including antiangiogenesis treatment), radiotherapy, or corticosteroids; poor oral hygiene, ill-fitting dentures; and comorbid disorders (anemia, coagulopathy, infection, preexisting dental disease). Most reported cases occurred after IV bisphosphonate therapy; however, cases have been reported following oral therapy. A dental exam and preventive dentistry should be performed prior to placing patients with risk factors on chronic bisphosphonate therapy. The manufacturer's labeling states that there are no data to suggest whether discontinuing bisphosphonates in patients requiring invasive dental procedures reduces the risk of ONJ. However, other experts suggest that there is no evidence that discontinuing therapy reduces the risk of developing ONJ (Assael, 2009). The risk:benefit must be assessed by the treating physician and/or dentist/surgeon prior to any invasive dental procedure. Patients developing ONJ while on bisphosphonates should receive care by an oral surgeon.

Atypical, low-energy, or low-trauma femur fractures have been reported in patients receiving bisphosphonates. The fractures include subtrochanteric femur (bone just below the hip joint) and diaphyseal femur (long segment of the thigh bone). Some patients experience prodromal pain weeks or months before the fracture occurs. It is unclear if bisphosphonate therapy is the cause for these fractures; atypical femur fractures have also been reported in patients not taking bisphosphonates, and in patients receiving glucocorticoids. Patients receiving long-term (>3 to 5 years) bisphosphonate therapy may be at an increased risk. Patients presenting with thigh or groin pain with a history of receiving bisphosphonates should be evaluated for femur fracture. Consider interrupting bisphosphonate therapy in patients who develop a femoral shaft fracture; assess for fracture in the contralateral limb.

Infrequently, severe (and occasionally debilitating) musculoskeletal (bone, joint, and/or muscle) pain have been reported during bisphosphonate treatment. The onset of pain ranged from a single day to several months. Consider discontinuing therapy in patients who experience severe symptoms; symptoms usually resolve upon discontinuation. Some patients experienced recurrence when rechallenged with same drug or another bisphosphonate; avoid use in patients with a history of these symptoms in association with bisphosphonate therapy.

Hypocalcemia (including severe and life-threatening cases) has been reported with use; patients with Paget disease may be at significant risk for hypocalcemia after treatment with zoledronic acid (because pretreatment rate of bone turnover may be elevated); severe and life-threatening hypocalcemia has also been reported with oncology-related uses. Measure serum calcium prior to treatment initiation. Correct preexisting hypocalcemia before initiation of therapy in patients with Paget disease, osteoporosis, or oncology indications. Use with caution with other medications known to cause hypocalcemia (severe hypocalcemia may develop). Ensure adequate calcium and vitamin D supplementation during therapy. Use caution in patients with disturbances of calcium and mineral metabolism (eg, hypoparathyroidism, thyroid/parathyroid, surgery, malabsorption syndromes, excision of small intestine).

Nononcology indications: Use is contraindicated in patients with CrCl <35 mL/minute and in patients with evidence of acute renal impairment due to an increased risk of renal failure. Obtain serum creatinine and calculate creatinine clearance (using actual body weight) with the Cockcroft-Gault formula prior to each administration. In the management of osteoporosis, reevaluate the need for continued therapy periodically; the optimal duration of treatment has not yet been determined. Consider discontinuing after 3 to 5 years of use in patients at low risk for fracture; following discontinuation, reevaluate fracture risk periodically.

Oncology indications: Use caution in mild to moderate renal dysfunction; dosage adjustment required. In cancer patients, renal toxicity has been reported with doses >4 mg or infusions administered over 15 minutes. Risk factors for renal deterioration include preexisting renal insufficiency and repeated doses of zoledronic acid and other bisphosphonates. Dehydration and the use of other nephrotoxic drugs which may contribute to renal deterioration should be identified and managed. Use is not recommended in patients with severe renal impairment (serum creatinine >3 mg/dL or CrCl <30 mL/minute) and bone metastases (limited data); use in patients with hypercalcemia of malignancy and severe renal impairment (serum creatinine >4.5 mg/dL for hypercalcemia of malignancy) should only be done if the benefits outweigh the risks. Diuretics should not be used before correcting hypovolemia. Renal deterioration, resulting in renal failure and dialysis has occurred in patients treated with zoledronic acid after single and multiple infusions at recommended doses of 4 mg over 15 minutes. Assess renal function prior to treatment and withhold for renal deterioration [increase in serum creatinine of 0.5 mg/dL (if baseline level normal) or increase of 1 mg/dL (if baseline level abnormal)]; treatment should be withheld until renal function returns to within 10% of baseline.

Adequate hydration is required during treatment (urine output ~2 L/day); avoid overhydration, especially in patients with heart failure. Preexisting renal compromise, severe dehydration, and concurrent use with diuretics or other nephrotoxic drugs may increase the risk for renal impairment. Single and multiple infusions in patients with both normal and impaired renal function have been associated with renal deterioration, resulting in renal failure and dialysis or death (rare). Patients with underlying moderate to severe renal impairment, increased age, concurrent use of nephrotoxic or diuretic medications, or severe dehydration prior to or after zoledronic acid administration may have an increased risk of acute renal impairment or renal failure. Others with increased risk include patients with renal impairment or dehydration secondary to fever, sepsis, gastrointestinal losses, or diuretic use. If history or physical exam suggests dehydration, treatment should not be given until the patient is normovolemic. Transient increases in serum creatinine may be more pronounced in patients with impaired renal function; consider monitoring creatinine clearance in at-risk patients taking other renally eliminated drugs.

Conjunctivitis, uveitis, episcleritis, iritis, scleritis, and orbital inflammation have been reported (infrequently) with use; further ophthalmic evaluation (and possibly therapy discontinuation) may be necessary in patients with complicated infection. Use caution in patients with aspirin-sensitive asthma (may cause bronchoconstriction) and elderly patients (because decreased renal function occurs more commonly in elderly patients). Rare cases of urticaria and angioedema and very rare cases of anaphylactic reactions/shock have been reported. Do not administer Zometa and Reclast (Aclasta [Canadian product]) to the same patient for different indications.

Breast cancer (metastatic): The American Society of Clinical Oncology (ASCO) updated guidelines on the role of bone-modifying agents (BMAs) in the prevention and treatment of skeletal-related events for metastatic breast cancer patients (Van Poznak, 2011). The guidelines recommend initiating a BMA (denosumab, pamidronate, zoledronic acid) in patients with metastatic breast cancer to the bone. There is currently no literature indicating the superiority of one particular BMA. Optimal duration is not yet defined; however, the guidelines recommend continuing therapy until substantial decline in patient's performance status. The ASCO guidelines are in alignment with prescribing information for dosing, renal dose adjustments, infusion times, prevention and management of osteonecrosis of the jaw, and monitoring of laboratory parameter recommendations. BMAs are not the first-line therapy for pain. BMAs are to be used as adjunctive therapy for cancer-related bone pain associated with bone metastasis, demonstrating a modest pain control benefit. BMAs should

be used in conjunction with agents such as NSAIDS, opioid and nonopioid analgesics, corticosteroids, radiation/surgery, and interventional procedures.

Multiple myeloma: The American Society of Clinical Oncology (ASCO) has published guidelines on bisphosphonate use for prevention and treatment of bone disease in multiple myeloma (Kyle, 2007). Bisphosphonate (pamidronate or zoledronic acid) use is recommended in multiple myeloma patients with lytic bone destruction or compression spine fracture from osteopenia. Bisphosphonates may also be considered in patients with pain secondary to osteolytic disease, adjunct therapy to stabilize fractures or impending fractures, and for multiple myeloma patients with osteopenia but no radiographic evidence of lytic bone disease. Bisphosphonates are not recommended in patients with solitary plasmacytoma, smoldering (asymptomatic) or indolent myeloma, or monoclonal gammopathy of undetermined significance. The guidelines recommend monthly treatment for a period of 2 years. At that time, consider discontinuing in responsive and stable patients, and reinitiate if a new-onset skeletal-related event occurs. The ASCO guidelines are in alignment with prescribing information for dosing, renal dose adjustments, infusion times, prevention and management of osteonecrosis of the jaw, and monitoring of laboratory parameter recommendations. According to the guidelines, in patients with a serum creatinine >3 mg/dL or CrCl <30 mL/minute or extensive bone disease, an alternative bisphosphonate (pamidronate) should be used. Monitor for albuminuria every 3 to 6 months; in patients with unexplained albuminuria >500 mg/24 hours, withhold the dose until level returns to baseline, then recheck every 3 to 4 weeks. Upon reinitiation, the guidelines recommend considering increasing the zoledronic acid infusion time to at least 30 minutes; however, one study has demonstrated that extending the infusion to 30 minutes did not change the safety profile (Berenson, 2011).

Adverse Reactions Note: An acute reaction (eg, arthralgia, fever, flu-like symptoms, myalgia) may occur within the first 3 days following infusion in up to 44% of patients; usually resolves within 3-4 days of onset, although may take up to 14 days to resolve. The incidence may be decreased with acetaminophen (prior to infusion and for 72 hours postinfusion).

Oncology indications:
>10%:
Cardiovascular: Lower extremity edema (5% to 21%), hypotension (11%)
Central nervous system: Fatigue (39%), headache (5% to 19%), dizziness (18%), insomnia (15% to 16%), anxiety (11% to 14%), depression (14%), agitation (13%), confusion (7% to 13%), hypoesthesia (12%), rigors (11%)
Dermatologic: Alopecia (12%), dermatitis (11%)
Endocrine & metabolic: Dehydration (5% to 14%), hypophosphatemia (13%), hypokalemia (12%), hypomagnesemia (11%)
Gastrointestinal: Nausea (29% to 46%), vomiting (14% to 32%), constipation (27% to 31%), diarrhea (17% to 24%), anorexia (9% to 22%), abdominal pain (14% to 16%), weight loss (16%), decreased appetite (13%)
Genitourinary: Urinary tract infection (12% to 14%)
Hematologic & oncologic: Anemia (22% to 33%), progression of cancer (16% to 20%), neutropenia (12%)
Infection: Candidiasis (12%)
Neuromuscular & skeletal: Ostealgia (55%), weakness (5% to 24%), myalgia (23%), arthralgia (5% to 21%), back pain (15%), paresthesia (15%), limb pain (14%), skeletal pain (12%)
Renal: Renal insufficiency (8% to 17%; up to 40% in patients with abnormal baseline creatinine)
Respiratory: Dyspnea (22% to 27%), cough (12% to 22%)
Miscellaneous: Fever (32% to 44%)
1% to 10%:
Cardiovascular: Chest pain (5% to 10%)
Central nervous system: Somnolence (5% to 10%)
Endocrine & metabolic: Hypocalcemia (5% to 10%; grades 3/4: ≤1%), hypermagnesemia (grade 3: 2%)
Gastrointestinal: Dyspepsia (10%), dysphagia (5% to 10%), mucositis (5% to 10%), stomatitis (8%), sore throat (8%)
Hematologic & oncologic: Granulocytopenia (5% to 10%), pancytopenia (5% to 10%), thrombocytopenia (5% to 10%)
Infection: Infection (nonspecific; 5% to 10%)
Renal: Increased serum creatinine (grades 3/4: ≤2%)
Respiratory: Upper respiratory tract infection (10%)

Nononcology indications:
>10%:
Cardiovascular: Hypertension (5% to 13%)
Central nervous system: Pain (2% to 24%), fever (9% to 22%), headache (4% to 20%), chills (2% to 18%), fatigue (2% to 18%)
Endocrine & metabolic: Hypocalcemia (≤3%; Paget's disease 21%)
Gastrointestinal: Nausea (5% to 18%)
Immunologic: Infusion related reaction (4% to 25%)
Neuromuscular & skeletal: Arthralgia (9% to 27%), myalgia (5% to 23%), back pain (4% to 18%), limb pain (3% to 16%), musculoskeletal pain (≤12%)
Respiratory: Flu-like symptoms (1% to 11%)
1% to 10%:
Cardiovascular: Chest pain (1% to 8%), peripheral edema (3% to 6%), atrial fibrillation (1% to 3%), palpitations (≤3%)
Central nervous system: Dizziness (2% to 9%), rigors (8%), malaise (1% to 7%), hypoesthesia (≤6%), lethargy (3% to 5%), vertigo (1% to 4%), paresthesia (2%), hyperthermia (≤2%)
Dermatologic: Skin rash (2% to 3%), hyperhidrosis (≤3%)
Gastrointestinal: Abdominal pain (1% to 9%), diarrhea (5% to 8%), vomiting (2% to 8%), constipation (6% to 7%), dyspepsia (2% to 7%), abdominal discomfort (1% to 2%), anorexia (1% to 2%)
Hematologic & oncologic: Change in serum protein (C-reactive protein increased; ≤5%)
Neuromuscular & skeletal: Ostealgia (3% to 9%), arthritis (2% to 9%), shoulder pain (≤7%), neck pain (1% to 7%), weakness (2% to 6%), muscle spasm (2% to 6%), stiffness (1% to 5%), jaw pain (2% to 4%), joint swelling (≤3%)
Ophthalmic: Eye pain (≤2%)
Renal: Increased serum creatinine (2%)
Respiratory: Dyspnea (5% to 7%)

All indications: <1% (Limited to important or life-threatening): Acute renal failure (requiring hospitalization/dialysis), arthralgia (sometimes severe and/or incapacitating), bradycardia, femur fracture (diaphyseal or subtrochanteric), hematuria, hyperesthesia, hyperparathyroidism, hypersensitivity, injection site reaction (eg, itching, pain, redness), interstitial lung disease, iritis, myalgia (sometimes severe and/or incapacitating), osteonecrosis (primarily of the jaws), periorbital swelling, scleritis, Stevens-Johnson syndrome, toxic epidermal necrolysis

Drug Interactions
Metabolism/Transport Effects None known.
Avoid Concomitant Use There are no known interactions where it is recommended to avoid concomitant use.
Increased Effect/Toxicity
Zoledronic Acid may increase the levels/effects of: Deferasirox

The levels/effects of Zoledronic Acid may be increased by: Aminoglycosides; Calcitonin; Nonsteroidal Anti-Inflammatory Agents; Systemic Angiogenesis Inhibitors; Thalidomide
Decreased Effect
The levels/effects of Zoledronic Acid may be decreased by: Proton Pump Inhibitors

Preparation for Administration Hazardous agent; use appropriate precautions for handling and disposal (NIOSH 2014 [group 3]).
Solution for injection:
Reclast, Aclasta [Canadian product]: No further preparation is necessary.
Zometa concentrate vials: Further dilute in 100 mL NS or D₅W prior to administration.
Zometa ready-to-use bottles: No further preparation is necessary. If reduced doses are required for patients with renal impairment, withdraw the appropriate volume of solution and replace with an equal amount of NS or D₅W.

Storage/Stability Solution for injection:
Aclasta [Canadian product]: Store at room temperature of 15°C to 30°C (59°F to 86°F). Keep sealed in original package until administration.
Reclast: Store at room temperature of 25°C (77°F); excursions permitted to 15°C to 30°C (59°F to 86°F). After opening, stable for 24 hours at 2°C to 8°C (36°F to 46°F). If refrigerated, allow the refrigerated solution to reach room temperature before administration.
Zometa: Store concentrate vials and ready-to-use bottles at 25°C (77°F); excursions permitted to 15°C to 30°C (59°F to 86°F). Diluted solutions for infusion which are not used immediately after preparation should be refrigerated at 2°C to 8°C (36°F to 46°F). Infusion of solution must be completed within 24 hours of preparation. The ready-to-use bottles are for single use only; if any

preparation is necessary (preparing reduced dosage for patients with renal impairment), the prepared, diluted solution may be refrigerated at 2°C to 8°C (36°F to 46°F) if not used immediately. Infusion of solution must be completed within 24 hours of preparation. The previously withdrawn volume from the ready-to-use solution should be discarded; do not store or reuse.

Mechanism of Action A bisphosphonate which inhibits bone resorption via actions on osteoclasts or on osteoclast precursors; inhibits osteoclastic activity and skeletal calcium release induced by tumors. Decreases serum calcium and phosphorus, and increases their elimination. In osteoporosis, zoledronic acid inhibits osteoclast-mediated resorption, therefore reducing bone turnover.

Pharmacodynamics/Kinetics

Distribution: Binds to bone

Protein binding: 23% to 53%

Metabolism: Primarily eliminated intact via the kidney; metabolism not likely

Half-life elimination: Triphasic; Terminal: 146 hours

Excretion: Urine (39% ± 16% as unchanged drug) within 24 hours; feces (<3%)

Dosing

Adult & Geriatric Note: Acetaminophen administration after the infusion may reduce symptoms of acute-phase reactions. Patients treated for multiple myeloma and Paget disease should receive a daily calcium and vitamin D supplement, and patients with osteoporosis should receive calcium and vitamin D supplementation if dietary intake is inadequate.

Hypercalcemia of malignancy (albumin-corrected serum calcium ≥12 mg/dL) (Zometa): IV: 4 mg (maximum) given as a single dose. Wait at least 7 days before considering re-treatment.

Multiple myeloma or metastatic bone lesions from solid tumors (Zometa): IV: 4 mg once every 3 to 4 weeks

Osteoporosis, glucocorticoid-induced, treatment and prevention (Reclast, Aclasta [Canadian product]): IV: 5 mg once a year

Osteoporosis, prevention: IV:

Reclast: 5 mg once every 2 years

Aclasta [Canadian product]: 5 mg as a single (one-time) dose

Osteoporosis, treatment (Reclast, Aclasta [Canadian product]): IV: 5 mg once a year; consider discontinuing after 3 to 5 years of use in patients at low risk for fracture

Paget disease: IV:

Reclast, Aclasta [Canadian product]: 5 mg as a single dose.

Re-treatment:

Reclast: Data concerning retreatment is not available; retreatment may be considered for relapse (increase in alkaline phosphatase) if appropriate, for inadequate response, or in patients who are symptomatic.

Aclasta [Canadian product]: Data concerning retreatment is limited; retreatment with 5 mg (single dose) may be considered for relapse after an interval of at least 1 year from initial treatment.

The Endocrine Society guidelines suggest re-treatment is seldom required within 5 years (Singer, 2014).

Prevention of aromatase inhibitor-induced bone loss in breast cancer (off-label use): IV: 4 mg once every 6 months for 5 years (Brufsky, 2012)

Prevention of androgen deprivation-induced bone loss in nonmetastatic prostate cancer (off-label use): IV: 4 mg once every 3 months for 1 year (Smith, 2003) or 4 mg every 12 months (Michaelson, 2007)

Renal Impairment Note: Prior to each dose, obtain serum creatinine and calculate the creatinine clearance using the Cockcroft-Gault formula.

Nononcology uses: Note: Use actual body weight in the Cockcroft-Gault formula when calculating clearance for nononcology uses.

CrCl ≥35 mL/minute: No dosage adjustment is necessary.

CrCl <35 mL/minute: Use is contraindicated.

Oncology uses:

Multiple myeloma and bone metastases:

CrCl >60 mL/minute: 4 mg (no dosage adjustment is necessary)

CrCl 50 to 60 mL/minute: Reduce dose to 3.5 mg

CrCl 40 to 49 mL/minute: Reduce dose to 3.3 mg

CrCl 30 to 39 mL/minute: Reduce dose to 3 mg

CrCl <30 mL/minute: Use is not recommended.

Hypercalcemia of malignancy:

Mild to moderate impairment: No dosage adjustment is necessary.

Severe impairment (serum creatinine >4.5 mg/dL):

U.S. labeling: Evaluate risk versus benefit

Canadian labeling: Use is not recommended.

Dosage adjustment for renal toxicity (during treatment):

Hypercalcemia of malignancy: Evidence of renal deterioration: Evaluate risk versus benefit.

Multiple myeloma and bone metastases: Evidence of renal deterioration: Withhold dose until renal function returns to within 10% of baseline; renal deterioration defined as follows:

Normal baseline creatinine: Increase of 0.5 mg/dL

Abnormal baseline creatinine: Increase of 1 mg/dL

Reinitiate therapy at the same dose administered prior to treatment interruption.

Multiple myeloma: Albuminuria >500 mg/24 hours (unexplained): Withhold dose until return to baseline, then reevaluate every 3 to 4 weeks; consider reinitiating with a longer infusion time of at least 30 minutes (Kyle, 2007).

Hepatic Impairment There are no dosage adjustments provided in the manufacturer's labeling (has not been studied); however, zoledronic acid is not metabolized hepatically.

Dietary Considerations

Multiple myeloma or metastatic bone lesions from solid tumors: Take daily calcium supplement (500 mg) and daily multivitamin (with 400 units vitamin D).

Osteoporosis: Ensure adequate calcium and vitamin D intake; if dietary intake is inadequate, dietary supplementation is recommended. Women and men should consume:

Calcium: 1,000 mg/day (men: 50 to 70 years) **or** 1200 mg/day (women ≥51 years and men ≥71 years) (IOM, 2011; NOF [Cosman 2014])

Vitamin D: 800 to 1,000 int. units/day (men and women ≥50 years) (NOF, 2014). Recommended Dietary Allowance (RDA): 600 int. units/day (men and women ≤70 years) **or** 800 int. units/day (men and women ≥71 years) (IOM, 2011).

Paget disease: Take elemental calcium 1500 mg/day (750 mg twice daily or 500 mg 3 times/day) and vitamin D 800 units/day, particularly during the first 2 weeks after administration.

Administration

If refrigerated, allow solution to reach room temperature before administration. Infuse over at least 15 minutes. Flush IV line with 10 mL NS flush following infusion. Infuse in a line separate from other medications. Patients must be appropriately hydrated prior to treatment. Acetaminophen after administration may reduce the incidence of acute reaction (eg, arthralgia, fever, flu-like symptoms, myalgia).

Multiple myeloma: If treatment is withheld for unexplained albuminuria, consider increasing the infusion time to at least 30 minutes upon reinitiation (Kyle, 2007).

Hazardous agent; use appropriate precautions for handling and disposal (NIOSH 2014 [group 3]).

Monitoring Parameters Prior to initiation of therapy, dental exam and preventive dentistry for patients at risk for osteonecrosis, including all cancer patients

Nononcology uses: Serum creatinine prior to each dose, especially in patients with risk factors, calculate creatinine clearance before each treatment (consider interim monitoring in patients at risk for acute renal failure), evaluate fluid status and adequately hydrate patients prior to and following administration.

Osteoporosis: Bone mineral density (BMD) should be evaluated 1 to 2 years after initiating therapy and every 2 years thereafter (NOF [Cosman 2014]); in patients with combined zoledronic acid and glucocorticoid treatment, BMD should be made at initiation of therapy and repeated after 6 to 12 months; serum calcium and 25 (OH)D; annual measurements of height and weight, assessment of chronic back pain; serum calcium and 25(OH)D; phosphorus and magnesium; may consider monitoring biochemical markers of bone turnover

Paget disease: Alkaline phosphatase at 6 to 12 weeks for initial response to treatment (when bone turnover will have shown a substantial decline) and potentially at 6 months (maximal suppression of high bone turnover); following treatment completion, monitor at ~1- to 2-year intervals (Singer, 2014); monitoring more specific biochemical markers of bone turnover (eg, serum P1NP, NTX, serum beta-CTx) is generally only warranted in patients with Paget disease who have abnormal liver or biliary tract function or when early assessment of response to treatment is needed (eg, spinal compression, very active disease) (Singer, 2014); serum calcium and 25(OH)D; phosphorus and magnesium; symptoms of hypocalcemia, pain

Oncology uses: Serum creatinine prior to each dose; serum electrolytes, phosphate, magnesium, and hemoglobin/hematocrit should be evaluated regularly. Monitor serum calcium to assess response and avoid overtreatment. In patients with multiple myeloma, monitor urine every 3 to 6 months for albuminuria.

Reference Range

Calcium (total): Adults: 9 to 11 mg/dL (2.05 to 2.54 mmol/L), may slightly decrease with aging

Phosphorus: 2.5 to 4.5 mg/dL (0.81 to 1.45 mmol/L)

Vitamin D: There is no clear consensus on a reference range for total serum 25(OH)D concentrations or the validity of this level as it relates clinically to bone health. In addition, there is significant variability in the reporting of serum 25(OH)D levels as a result of different assay types in use; however, the following ranges have been suggested:

Adults (IOM, 2011): Sufficient levels in practically all persons: ≥20 ng/mL (50 nmol/L); concern for risk of toxicity: >50 ng/mL (125 nmol/L)

Osteoporosis patients (NOF [Cosman 2014]): Recommended level to reach and maintain: ~30 ng/mL (75 nmol/L)

Test Interactions Bisphosphonates may interfere with diagnostic imaging agents such as technetium-99m-diphosphonate in bone scans.

Dosage Forms Excipient information presented when available (limited, particularly for generics); consult specific product labeling.

Concentrate, Intravenous:
Zometa: 4 mg/5 mL (5 mL)
Generic: 4 mg/5 mL (5 mL)
Concentrate, Intravenous [preservative free]:
Generic: 4 mg/5 mL (5 mL)
Solution, Intravenous:
Reclast: 5 mg/100 mL (100 mL)
Zometa: 4 mg/100 mL (100 mL)
Generic: 5 mg/100 mL (100 mL)
Solution, Intravenous [preservative free]:
Generic: 4 mg/100 mL (100 mL); 5 mg/100 mL (100 mL)
Solution Reconstituted, Intravenous:
Generic: 4 mg (1 ea)

Dosage Forms: Canada Excipient information presented when available (limited, particularly for generics); consult specific product labeling.

Concentrate, Intravenous:
Zometa: 4 mg/5 mL (5 mL)
Infusion, Solution [premixed]:
Aclasta: 5 mg/100 mL (100 mL)

♦ Zoledronic Acid for Injection (Can) see Zoledronic Acid on page 1934

♦ Zoledronic Acid Injection (Can) see Zoledronic Acid on page 1934

♦ Zoledronic Acid Z (Can) see Zoledronic Acid on page 1934

♦ Zolinza see Vorinostat on page 1913

ZOLMitriptan (zohl mi TRIP tan)

Brand Names: US Zomig; Zomig ZMT
Brand Names: Canada Dom-Zolmitriptan; JAMP-Zolmitriptan; JAMP-Zolmitriptan ODT; Mar-Zolmitriptan; Mint-Zolmitriptan; Mint-Zolmitriptan ODT; Mylan-Zolmitriptan; Mylan-Zolmitriptan ODT; NAT-Zolmitriptan; PMS-Zolmitriptan; PMS-Zolmitriptan ODT; Riva-Zolmitriptan; Sandoz-Zolmitriptan; Sandoz-Zolmitriptan ODT; Septa-Zolmitriptan ODT; Teva-Zolmitriptan; Teva-Zolmitriptan OD; Zolmitriptan ODT; Zomig; Zomig Nasal Spray; Zomig Rapimelt
Index Terms 311C90
Pharmacologic Category Antimigraine Agent; Serotonin 5-HT$_{1B, 1D}$ Receptor Agonist
Use Migraines:
Nasal inhalation: Acute treatment of migraine with or without aura in adults and pediatric patients ≥12 years.
Oral: Acute treatment of migraine with or without aura in adults.

Pregnancy Considerations Adverse events were observed in animal reproduction studies. Information related to zolmitriptan use in pregnancy is limited (Källén, 2011; Nezvalová-Henriksen, 2010; Nezvalová-Henriksen, 2012). Until additional information is available, other agents are preferred for the initial treatment of migraine in pregnancy (Da Silva, 2012; MacGregor, 2012; Williams, 2012).

Breast-Feeding Considerations It is not known if zolmitriptan is excreted in breast milk. Due to the potential for serious adverse reactions in the nursing infant, the decision to continue or discontinue breast-feeding during therapy should take into account the risk of exposure to the infant and the benefits of treatment to the mother.

Contraindications

Ischemic coronary artery disease (angina pectoris, history of myocardial infarction [MI], or documented silent ischemia); coronary artery vasospasm, including Prinzmetal variant angina, or other significant underlying cardiovascular disease; Wolff-Parkinson-White syndrome or arrhythmias associated with other cardiac accessory conduction pathway disorders; peripheral vascular disease; ischemic bowel disease; uncontrolled hypertension; recent use (within 24 hours) of treatment with another 5-HT$_1$ agonist, or an ergotamine-containing or ergot-type medication like dihydroergotamine or methysergide; history of stroke, transient ischemic attack, or history of hemiplegic or basilar migraine; coadministration of monoamine oxidase A (MAO A) inhibitors or use of zolmitriptan within 2 weeks of discontinuation of MAO A inhibitor therapy; hypersensitivity to zolmitriptan or any component of the formulation.

Documentation of allergic cross-reactivity for triptans is limited. However, because of similarities in chemical structure and/or pharmacologic actions, the possibility of cross-sensitivity cannot be ruled out with certainty.

Warnings/Precautions Zolmitriptan is indicated only in patient populations with a clear diagnosis of migraine. If a patient does not respond to the first dose, the diagnosis of migraine should be reconsidered; rule out underlying neurologic disease in patients with atypical headache and in patients with no prior history of migraine. Not indicated for migraine prophylaxis (may be used off-label for menstrual migraine prophylaxis) or for the treatment of cluster headache. Acute migraine agents (eg, triptans, opioids, ergotamine, or a combination of the agents) used for 10 or more days per month may lead to worsening of headaches (medication overuse headache); withdrawal treatment may be necessary in the setting of overuse. The safety of treating >3 headaches (oral) or >4 headaches (nasal inhalation) during a 30 day period has not been established. Not for prophylactic treatment of migraine headaches. Cardiac events (coronary artery vasospasm, transient ischemia, myocardial infarction, ventricular tachycardia/fibrillation, cardiac arrest, and death) have been reported within a few hours of 5-HT$_1$ agonist administration; use in contraindicated in patients with ischemic or vasospastic coronary artery disease. Patients who experience sensations of chest pain/pressure/tightness or symptoms suggestive of angina following dosing should be evaluated for coronary artery disease or Prinzmetal's angina before receiving additional doses; if dosing is resumed and similar symptoms recur, monitor with ECG. Patients with Prinzmetal's variant angina, Wolff-Parkinson-White Syndrome or arrhythmias associated with other cardiac accessory conduction pathway disorders should not receive zolmitriptan. Should not be given to patients who have risk factors for CAD (eg, hypertension, hypercholesterolemia, smoker, obesity, diabetes, strong family history of CAD, menopause, male >40 years of age) without adequate cardiac evaluation. Patients with suspected CAD should have cardiovascular evaluation to rule out CAD before considering zolmitriptan's use; if cardiovascular evaluation negative, first dose would be safest if given in the healthcare provider's office (consider ECG monitoring). Periodic evaluation of those without cardiovascular disease, but with continued risk factors, should be done. Significant elevation in blood pressure, including hypertensive crisis, has been reported in patients with and without a history of hypertension. Use is contraindicated in patients with uncontrolled hypertension. Peripheral vascular ischemia, gastrointestinal vascular ischemia, and infarction (presenting with abdominal pain and bloody diarrhea, splenic infarction, and Raynaud's syndrome have been reported with 5-HT$_1$ agonists. In patients who experience signs or symptoms suggestive of a vasospastic reaction following use of a 5-HT$_1$ agonist, rule out a vasospastic reaction before receiving additional doses. Cerebral/subarachnoid hemorrhage and stroke have been reported with 5-HT$_1$ agonist administration and some have resulted in fatalities. Do not administer to patients with a history of stroke or TIA; discontinue use if a cerebrovascular event occurs. Rarely, partial vision loss and blindness (transient and permanent) have been reported with 5-HT$_1$ agonists. Use with caution in patients with hepatic impairment. Zomig-ZMT tablets contain phenylalanine. Symptoms of agitation, confusion, hallucinations, labile blood pressure, hyper-reflexia, incoordination, myoclonus, shivering, and tachycardia (serotonin syndrome) may occur with concomitant proserotonergic drugs (eg, SSRIs, SNRIs, TCAs, MAO inhibitors, or triptans) or agents which reduce zolmitriptan's metabolism. Potentially significant interactions may exist, requiring dose or frequency adjustment, additional monitoring, and/or selection of alternative therapy. Elderly patients are more likely to have underlying cardiovascular disease and hepatic or renal impairment;

use with caution. Cardiovascular evaluation is recommended for elderly patients with other cardiovascular risk factors prior to initiation of therapy. Zomig-ZMT tablets contain phenylalanine.

Adverse Reactions

>10%: Gastrointestinal: Unpleasant taste (nasal: adults: 17% to 21%; children & adolescents: 6% to 10%)

1% to 10%:

Cardiovascular: Chest pain (oral: 2% to 4%), chest pressure (nasal: 1% to <2%), facial edema (nasal: 1% to <2%), palpitations (nasal: 1% to <2%), cardiac arrhythmia (≤1%), hypertension (≤1%), syncope (≤1%), tachycardia (≤1%)

Central nervous system: Dizziness (adults: 6% to 10%; children & adolescents: 2%), paresthesia (5% to 10%), drowsiness (4% to 8%), local alterations in temperature sensations (oral: 5% to 7%), sensation of pressure (oral: 2% to 5%), hyperesthesia (nasal: 1% to 5%), (1% to 5%), flushing sensation (nasal: 4%), pain (nasal: 2% to 4%), vertigo (oral: 2%), chills (nasal: 1% to <2%), depersonalization (nasal: 1% <2%), headache (1% to <2%), agitation (≤1%), amnesia (≤1%), anxiety (≤1%), depression (≤1%), emotional lability (oral: ≤1%), insomnia (≤1%), nervousness (nasal: ≤1%)

Dermatologic: Diaphoresis (oral: 2% to 3%), pruritus (≤1%), skin rash (≤1%), urticaria (≤1%)

Gastrointestinal: Nausea (adults: 4% to 9%; children & adolescents: 2%), xerostomia (2% to 5%), dyspepsia (oral: 2% to 3%), dysphagia (1% to 2%), abdominal pain (nasal: 1% to <2%), vomiting (1% to <2%)

Genitourinary: Urinary frequency (oral: ≤1%), urinary urgency (≤1%)

Hypersensitivity: Hypersensitivity reaction (≤1%)

Local: Local pain (4% to 10%; neck/throat/jaw), application site irritation (nasal: 3%)

Neuromuscular & skeletal: Weakness (oral: 5% to 9%; nasal: 3%), arthralgia (nasal: 1% to <2%), myalgia (nasal: 1% to <2%)

Otic: Tinnitus (≤1%)

Renal: Polyuria (≤1%)

Respiratory: Nasal discomfort (nasal: 3%), constriction of the pharynx (nasal: 2%), pressure on pharynx (nasal: 1% to <2%), bronchitis (nasal: ≤1%), cough (nasal: ≤1%), dyspnea (nasal: ≤1%), epistaxis (nasal: ≤1%), laryngeal edema (nasal: ≤1%), pharyngitis (nasal: ≤1%), rhinitis (nasal: ≤1%), sinusitis (nasal: ≤1%)

<1% (Limited to important or life-threatening): Amblyopia, anaphylactoid reaction, anaphylaxis, angina pectoris, ataxia, atrial fibrillation, bradycardia, breast carcinoma, breast neoplasm, cerebral ischemia, confusion, convulsions, coronary artery vasospasm, cyanosis, erythema multiforme, fibrocystic breast disease, gastrointestinal carcinoma, gastrointestinal infarction, gastrointestinal necrosis, genitourinary neoplasm, hallucination, hepatic neoplasm, hypertensive crisis, hyperthyroidism, infection, intestinal obstruction, ischemic colitis, ischemic heart disease, mania, myocardial infarction, neoplasm, pneumonia, psychosis, pyelonephritis, seizure, serotonin syndrome, sialadenitis, skin neoplasm, splenic infarction, tardive dyskinesia, urinary tract infection, uterine fibroid enlargement, vaginitis, vasodilatation, ventricular fibrillation, ventricular tachycardia, visual field defect

Drug Interactions

Metabolism/Transport Effects Substrate of CYP1A2 (minor); **Note:** Assignment of Major/Minor substrate status based on clinically relevant drug interaction potential

Avoid Concomitant Use

Avoid concomitant use of ZOLMitriptan with any of the following: Dapoxetine; Ergot Derivatives; MAO Inhibitors

Increased Effect/Toxicity

ZOLMitriptan may increase the levels/effects of: Antipsychotic Agents; Droxidopa; Ergot Derivatives; Metoclopramide; Serotonin Modulators

The levels/effects of ZOLMitriptan may be increased by: Antiemetics (5HT3 Antagonists); Antipsychotic Agents; Cimetidine; Dapoxetine; Ergot Derivatives; MAO Inhibitors; Metaxalone; Propranolol

Decreased Effect There are no known significant interactions involving a decrease in effect.

Storage/Stability Store at 20°C to 25°C (68°F to 77°F). Protect tablets from light and moisture.

Mechanism of Action Selective agonist for serotonin (5-HT$_{1B}$ and 5-HT$_{1D}$ receptors) in cranial arteries and sensory nerves of the trigeminal system; causes vasoconstriction and reduces inflammation associated with antidromic neuronal transmission correlating with relief of migraine

Pharmacodynamics/Kinetics

Absorption: Well absorbed

Distribution: V_d: Oral: 7 L/kg; Nasal spray: 8.4 L/kg

Protein binding: 25%

Metabolism: Converted to an active N-desmethyl metabolite (2-6 times more potent than zolmitriptan at 5-HT$_{1B}$ and 5-HT$_{1D}$ receptors)

Bioavailability: 40% (not impacted by food); mean bioavailability of nasal spray compared with oral tablet: 102%

Half-life elimination: 3 hours

Time to peak, serum: Tablet: 1.5 hours; Orally-disintegrating tablet and nasal spray: 3 hours

Excretion: Urine (~60% to 65% total dose; 8% of total dose as unchanged drug; 4% of total dose as N-desmethyl metabolite); feces (30%)

Dosing

Adult

Migraine:

Initial dose: **Note:** Administer at the onset of migraine headache.

Nasal inhalation: 2.5 mg (maximum single dose: 5 mg)

Oral:

Tablet: 1.25 to 2.5 mg (maximum single dose: 5 mg)

Orally disintegrating tablet: 2.5 mg (maximum single dose: 5 mg)

Second dose (either nasal inhalation or oral): May repeat in 2 hours if the migraine headache has not resolved or returns after transient improvement (maximum daily dose: 10 mg)

Menstrual migraine, prophylaxis (off-label use): Oral: 2.5 mg 2 to 3 times daily starting 2 days prior to the expected onset of menses and continued through to 5 days after the onset of menses (7 days total) (Tuchman 2008)

Dosage adjustment for concomitant therapy with cimetidine: Maximum single dose: 2.5 mg (maximum daily dose: 5 mg)

Geriatric Refer to adult dosing. Initiate therapy at the low end of the dosing range.

Pediatric Migraine: Children ≥12 years and Adolescents: Nasal inhalation: Refer to adult dosing.

Renal Impairment No dosage adjustment provided in manufacturer's labeling; however, zolmitriptan clearance is reduced in patients with severe renal impairment (CrCl 5 to 25 mL/minute).

Hepatic Impairment

Oral:

Tablet:

Mild impairment: There is no dosage adjustment provided in the manufacturer's labeling.

Moderate to severe impairment: Initial: 1.25 mg (maximum daily dose: 5 mg in severe impairment)

Orally disintegrating tablet:

Mild impairment: There is no dosage adjustment provided in the manufacturer's labeling.

Moderate to severe impairment: Use is not recommended.

Nasal inhalation:

Mild impairment: No dosage adjustment necessary.

Moderate to severe: Use is not recommended.

Dietary Considerations Some products may contain phenylalanine.

Administration Administer as soon as migraine headache starts.

Tablet: May be broken in half to achieve a smaller initial dose.

Orally-disintegrating tablet: Must be taken whole; do not break, crush, or chew. Place on tongue and allow to dissolve. Administration with liquid is not required.

Nasal spray: Blow nose gently prior to use. After removing protective cap, instill device into nostril. Block opposite nostril; breathe in gently through nose while pressing plunger of spray device. Breathe gently through mouth for 5-10 seconds.

Monitoring Parameters Headache severity, signs/symptoms suggestive of angina; blood pressure; ECG with first dose in patients with likelihood of unrecognized coronary disease, such as patients with significant hypertension, hypercholesterolemia, obese patients, patients with diabetes, smokers with other risk factors or strong family history of coronary artery disease

Dosage Forms Excipient information presented when available (limited, particularly for generics); consult specific product labeling. [DSC] = Discontinued product

Solution, Nasal:

Zomig: 2.5 mg (6 ea); 5 mg (6 ea)

Tablet, Oral:

Zomig: 2.5 mg [DSC]

Zomig: 2.5 mg [scored]

Zomig: 5 mg

Generic: 2.5 mg, 5 mg

Tablet Dispersible, Oral:
Zomig ZMT: 2.5 mg [DSC] [contains aspartame]
Zomig ZMT: 2.5 mg [contains aspartame; orange flavor]
Zomig ZMT: 5 mg [DSC] [contains aspartame]
Zomig ZMT: 5 mg [contains aspartame; orange flavor]
Generic: 2.5 mg, 5 mg

◆ Zolmitriptan ODT (Can) see ZOLMitriptan on page 1938
◆ Zoloft see Sertraline on page 1649

Zolpidem (zole PI dem)

Brand Names: US Ambien; Ambien CR; Edluar; Inter-
mezzo; Zolpimist
Brand Names: Canada Sublinox
Index Terms Zolpidem Tartrate
Pharmacologic Category Hypnotic, Miscellaneous
Use Insomnia:
Ambien, Edluar, Zolpimist: Short-term treatment of insomnia with difficulty of sleep onset
Ambien CR: Treatment of insomnia with difficulty of sleep
onset and/or sleep maintenance
Intermezzo: "As needed" treatment of insomnia when
middle-of-the-night awakening is followed by difficulty
returning to sleep and the patient has ≥4 hours of sleep
time remaining
Sublinox [Canadian product]: Short-term treatment of
insomnia (with difficulty of sleep onset, frequent awakenings, and/or early awakenings)
Pregnancy Considerations Adverse events were
observed in some animal reproduction studies. Zolpidem
crosses the placenta (Juric, 2009). Severe neonatal respiratory depression has been reported when zolpidem was
used at the end of pregnancy, especially when used
concurrently with other CNS depressants. Children born
of mothers taking sedative/hypnotics may be at risk for
withdrawal; neonatal flaccidity has been reported in infants
following maternal use of sedative/hypnotics during pregnancy. Additional adverse effects to the fetus/newborn
have been noted in some studies (Wang, 2010; Wikner,
2011).
Breast-Feeding Considerations Zolpidem is excreted in
breast milk. The manufacturer recommends that caution
be exercised when administering zolpidem to nursing
women.
Medication Guide Available Yes
Contraindications
Hypersensitivity to zolpidem or any component of the
formulation
Canadian labeling: Additional contraindications (not in U.S.
labeling): Significant obstructive sleep apnea syndrome
and acute and/or severe impairment of respiratory function; myasthenia gravis; severe hepatic impairment; personal or family history of sleepwalking
Warnings/Precautions Should be used only after evaluation of potential causes of sleep disturbance. Failure of
sleep disturbance to resolve after 7-10 days may indicate
the need for psychiatric and/or medical illness reevaluation. Hypnotics/sedatives have been associated with
abnormal thinking and behavior changes including
decreased inhibition, aggression, bizarre behavior, agitation, visual and auditory hallucinations, and depersonalization. These changes may occur unpredictably and may
indicate previously unrecognized psychiatric disorders;
evaluate appropriately. Sedative/hypnotics may produce
withdrawal symptoms following abrupt discontinuation.
Use with caution in patients with depression; worsening
of depression, including suicide or suicidal ideation has
been reported with the use of hypnotics. Intentional overdose may be an issue in this population. The minimum
dose that will effectively treat the individual patient should
be used. Prescriptions should be written for the smallest
quantity consistent with good patient care. May cause
CNS depression impairing physical and mental capabilities; patients must be cautioned about performing tasks
which require mental alertness (operating machinery or
driving). Drowsiness and a decreased level of consciousness may lead to falls and severe injuries; hip fractures
and intracranial hemorrhage have been reported. Zolpidem should only be administered when the patient is able
to stay in bed a full night (7 to 8 hours) before being active
again. Intermezzo should be taken in bed if patient awakes
in the middle of the night (ie, if ≥4 hours left before waking)
and there is difficulty in returning to sleep.

Potentially significant drug-drug interactions may exist,
requiring dose or frequency adjustment, additional monitoring, and/or selection of alternative therapy.

Use caution in patients with myasthenia gravis (contraindicated in the Canadian labeling). Avoid use in patients
with sleep apnea or a history of sedative-hypnotic abuse.

Postmarketing studies have indicated that the use of
hypnotic/sedative agents (including zolpidem) for sleep
has been associated with hypersensitivity reactions including anaphylaxis as well as angioedema. Do not rechallenge patient if such reactions occur. An increased risk for
hazardous sleep-related activities such as sleep-driving;
cooking and eating food, making phone calls or having sex
while asleep have also been noted; amnesia, anxiety, and
other neuropsychiatric symptoms may also occur. Discontinue treatment in patients who report any sleep-related
episodes. Canadian labeling recommends avoiding use in
patients with disorders (eg, restless legs syndrome, periodic limb movement disorder, sleep apnea) that may
disrupt sleep and cause frequent awakenings, potentially
increasing the risk of complex sleep-related behaviors.
Use with caution in patients with a history of drug dependence. Risk of abuse is increased in patients with a history
or family history of alcohol or drug abuse or mental illness.

Use caution with respiratory disease (Canadian labeling
contraindicates use with acute and/or severe impairment
of respiratory function). Use caution with hepatic impairment (Canadian labeling contraindicates use in severe
impairment); dose adjustment required. Because of the
rapid onset of action, administer immediately prior to bedtime, after the patient has gone to bed and is having
difficulty falling asleep, or during the middle of the night
when at least 4 hours are left before waking (Intermezzo).

Use caution in the elderly; dose adjustment recommended.
Closely monitor elderly or debilitated patients for impaired
cognitive and/or motor performance, confusion, and potential for falling. Avoid chronic use (>90 days) in older adults;
adverse events, including delirium, falls, fractures, have
been observed with nonbenzodiazepine hypnotic use in
the elderly similar to events observed with benzodiazepines. Data suggests improvements in sleep duration and
latency are minimal (Beers Criteria).

Dosage adjustment is recommended for females; pharmacokinetic studies involving zolpidem showed a significant
increase in maximum concentration and exposure in
females compared to males at the same dose. When
studied for the unapproved use of insomnia associated
with ADHD in children, a higher incidence (~7%) of hallucinations was reported. In addition, sleep latency did not
decrease compared to placebo.

Some dosage forms may contain polysorbate 80 (also
known as Tweens). Hypersensitivity reactions, usually a
delayed reaction, have been reported following exposure
to pharmaceutical products containing polysorbate 80 in
certain individuals (Isaksson, 2002; Lucente 2000; Shelley,
1995). Thrombocytopenia, ascites, pulmonary deterioration, and renal and hepatic failure have been reported in
premature neonates after receiving parenteral products
containing polysorbate 80 (Alade, 1986; CDC, 1984).
See manufacturer's labeling.
Adverse Reactions Actual frequency may be dosage
form, dose, and/or age dependent
>10%: Central nervous system: Headache (3% to 19%),
drowsiness (2% to 15%), dizziness (5% to 12%)
1% to 10%:
Cardiovascular: Chest discomfort, increased blood pressure, palpitations
Central nervous system: Fatigue (1%), abnormal dreams,
amnesia, anxiety, apathy, ataxia, burning sensation,
confusion, depersonalization, depression, disinhibition,
disorientation, drugged feeling, eating disorder (binge
eating), emotional lability, equilibrium disturbance,
euphoria, hallucination, hypoesthesia, increased body
temperature, insomnia, lack of concentration, lethargy,
memory impairment, paresthesia, psychomotor retardation, sleep disorder, stress, vertigo
Dermatologic: Skin rash, urticaria, wrinkling of skin
Endocrine & metabolic: Hypermenorrhea
Gastrointestinal: Abdominal distress, abdominal tenderness, change in appetite, constipation, diarrhea, dyspepsia, flatulence, frequent bowel movements,
gastroenteritis, gastroesophageal reflux disease, hiccups, nausea, vomiting, xerostomia
Genitourinary: Dysuria, urinary tract infection, vaginal
dryness
Hypersensitivity: Hypersensitivity reaction
Neuromuscular & skeletal: Arthralgia, back pain, muscle
cramps, muscle spasm, myalgia, neck pain, tremor,
weakness
Ophthalmic: Accommodation disturbance, asthenopia,
blurred vision, diplopia, eye redness, visual disturbance
(including altered depth perception)
Otic: Labyrinthitis, tinnitus
Respiratory: Dry throat, flu-like symptoms, lower respiratory tract infection, pharyngitis, sinusitis, throat irritation,
upper respiratory tract infection

Miscellaneous: Fever

<1% (Limited to important or life-threatening): Abnormal hepatic function tests, acute renal failure, aggressive behavior, anaphylaxis, anemia, angina pectoris, angioedema, anorexia, arteritis, arthritis, breast fibroadenosis, breast neoplasm, bronchitis, cardiac arrhythmia, cerebrovascular disease, circulatory shock, cognitive dysfunction, corneal ulcer, delusions, dementia, dermatitis, drug tolerance, dysarthria, dysphagia, edema, extrasystoles, glaucoma, hepatic insufficiency, hyperbilirubinemia, hyperglycemia, hyperlipidemia, hypertension, hypotension, hysteria, illusion, impotence, leukopenia, lymphadenopathy, migraine, myocardial infarction, neuralgia, neuritis, neuropathy, orthostatic hypotension, panic disorder, personality disorder, psychoneurosis, pulmonary edema, pulmonary embolism, pyelonephritis, respiratory depression, restless leg syndrome, rhinitis, scleritis, somnambulism, syncope, tachycardia, tenesmus, tetany, thrombosis, urinary incontinence, vaginitis, ventricular tachycardia

Drug Interactions

Metabolism/Transport Effects Substrate of CYP1A2 (minor), CYP2C19 (minor), CYP2C9 (minor), CYP2D6 (minor), CYP3A4 (major); **Note:** Assignment of Major/Minor substrate status based on clinically relevant drug interaction potential

Avoid Concomitant Use

Avoid concomitant use of Zolpidem with any of the following: Azelastine (Nasal); Orphenadrine; Paraldehyde; Sodium Oxybate; Thalidomide

Increased Effect/Toxicity

Zolpidem may increase the levels/effects of: Alcohol (Ethyl); Azelastine (Nasal); Buprenorphine; CarBAMazepine; Hydrocodone; Methotrimeprazine; Metyrosine; Orphenadrine; Paraldehyde; Pramipexole; ROPINIRole; Rotigotine; Selective Serotonin Reuptake Inhibitors; Sodium Oxybate; Suvorexant; Thalidomide

The levels/effects of Zolpidem may be increased by: Antifungal Agents (Azole Derivatives, Systemic); Brimonidine (Topical); Cannabis; CNS Depressants; Dronabinol; Droperidol; FluvoxaMINE; Kava Kava; Ketoconazole (Systemic); Magnesium Sulfate; Methotrimeprazine; Minocycline; Nabilone; Osimertinib; Perampanel; Ritonavir; Rufinamide; Tapentadol; Tetrahydrocannabinol

Decreased Effect

The levels/effects of Zolpidem may be decreased by: Bosentan; CarBAMazepine; CYP3A4 Inducers (Moderate); CYP3A4 Inducers (Strong); Dabrafenib; Deferasirox; Enzalutamide; Flumazenil; Mitotane; Osimertinib; Rifamycin Derivatives; Siltuximab; St Johns Wort; Telaprevir; Tocilizumab

Food Interactions Maximum plasma concentration and bioavailability are decreased with food; time to peak plasma concentration is increased; half-life remains unchanged. Grapefruit juice may decrease the metabolism of zolpidem. Management: Do not administer with (or immediately after) a meal. Avoid grapefruit juice.

Storage/Stability

Ambien, Edluar, Intermezzo: Store at 20°C to 25°C (68°F to 77°F). Protect sublingual tablets from light and moisture.

Ambien CR: Store at 15°C to 25°C (59°F to 77°F); limited excursions permitted up to 30°C (86°F).

Zolpimist: Store upright at 25°C (77°F); excursions are permitted to 15°C to 30°C (59°F to 86°F). Do not freeze. Avoid prolonged exposure to temperatures >30°C (86°F).

Sublinox [Canadian product]: Store at 15°C to 30°C (59°F to 86°F); protect from light and moisture.

Mechanism of Action Zolpidem, an imidazopyridine hypnotic that is structurally dissimilar to benzodiazepines, enhances the activity of the inhibitory neurotransmitter, γ-aminobutyric acid (GABA), via selective agonism at the benzodiazepine-1 (BZ$_1$) receptor; the result is increased chloride conductance, neuronal hyperpolarization, inhibition of the action potential, and a decrease in neuronal excitability leading to sedative and hypnotic effects. Because of its selectivity for the BZ$_1$ receptor site over the BZ$_2$ receptor site, zolpidem exhibits minimal anxiolytic, myorelaxant, and anticonvulsant properties (effects largely attributed to agonism at the BZ$_2$ receptor site).

Pharmacodynamics/Kinetics

Onset of action: Immediate release: 30 minutes

Duration: Immediate release: 6-8 hours

Absorption: Rapid; C$_{max}$ and AUC is increased by ~45% in females compared to male subjects

Distribution: V$_d$: 0.54 L/kg after an IV dose (Holm, 2000)

Protein binding: ~93%

Metabolism: Hepatic methylation and hydroxylation via CYP3A4 (~60%), CYP2C9 (~22%), CYP1A2 (~14%), CYP2D6 (~3%), and CYP2C19 (~3%) to 3 inactive metabolites (Holm, 2000)

Bioavailability: Immediate-release tablet: 70% (Holm, 2000)

Half-life elimination:

Immediate release, Extended release: ~2.5 hours (range: 1.4-4.5 hours); Cirrhosis: Up to 9.9 hours; Elderly: Prolonged up to 32%

Spray: ~3 hours (range: 1.7-8.4)

Sublingual tablet (Edluar, Intermezzo): ~3 hours (range: 1.4-6.7 hours)

Time to peak, plasma:

Immediate release: 1.6 hours; 2.2 hours with food

Extended release: 1.5 hours; 4 hours with food

Spray: ~0.9 hours

Sublingual tablet: Edluar: ~1.4 hours, ~1.8 hours with food; Intermezzo: 0.6-1.3 hours, ~3 hours with food

Excretion: Urine (48% to 67%, primarily as metabolites); feces (29% to 42%, primarily as metabolites)

Dosing

Adult Insomnia: Oral: **Note:** The lowest effective dose should be used; higher doses may be more likely to impair next morning activities.

Immediate release tablet, spray: 5 mg (females) or 5 to 10 mg (males) immediately before bedtime; maximum dose: 10 mg daily

Extended release tablet: 6.25 mg (females) or 6.25 to 12.5 mg (males) immediately before bedtime; maximum dose: 12.5 mg daily

Sublingual tablet:

Edluar, Sublinox [Canadian product]: 5 mg (females) or 5 to 10 mg (males) immediately before bedtime; if 5 mg dose is ineffective may increase to 10 mg (maximum dose: 10 mg daily)

Intermezzo: **Note:** Take in bed only if ≥4 hours left before waking and there is difficulty in returning to sleep

Females: 1.75 mg once per night as needed (maximum: 1.75 mg/night)

Males: 3.5 mg once per night as needed (maximum: 3.5 mg/night)

Dosage adjustment with concomitant CNS depressants: Females and males: 1.75 mg once per night as needed; dose adjustment of concomitant CNS depressant(s) may be necessary.

Debilitated:

Immediate release tablet, spray: 5 mg immediately before bedtime

Sublingual tablet:

Edluar, Sublinox [Canadian product]: 5 mg immediately before bedtime

Extended release tablet: 6.25 mg immediately before bedtime

Geriatric Oral:

Immediate release tablet, spray: 5 mg immediately before bedtime

Sublingual tablet:

Edluar, Sublinox [Canadian product]: 5 mg immediately before bedtime

Intermezzo: Females and males: 1.75 mg once per night as needed (maximum: 1.75 mg/night). **Note:** Take in bed only if ≥4 hours left before waking and there is difficulty in returning to sleep.

Extended release tablet: 6.25 mg immediately before bedtime

Renal Impairment No dosage adjustment necessary. Use with caution and monitor patients with renal impairment closely.

Hemodialysis: Not dialyzable

Hepatic Impairment

U.S. labeling:

Immediate release tablet, spray: 5 mg immediately before bedtime

Extended release tablet: 6.25 mg immediately before bedtime

Sublingual tablet:

Edluar: 5 mg immediately before bedtime

Intermezzo: Females and males: 1.75 mg once per night as needed. **Note:** Take in bed only if ≥4 hours left before waking and there is difficulty in returning to sleep.

Canadian labeling: Sublingual tablet: Sublinox:

Mild-to-moderate impairment: 5 mg immediately before bedtime

Severe impairment: Use is contraindicated.

Dietary Considerations For faster sleep onset, do not administer with (or immediately after) a meal.

Administration Ingest immediately before bedtime due to rapid onset of action. Regardless of dosage form, do not administer with or immediately after a meal. Intermezzo should be taken in bed if patient awakes in the middle of the night (ie, if ≥4 hours left before waking) and there is difficulty in returning to sleep.

Ambien CR tablets should be swallowed whole; do not divide, crush, or chew.

Edluar, Intermezzo, or Sublinox [Canadian product] sublingual tablets should be placed under the tongue and allowed to disintegrate; do not swallow or administer Edluar or Sublinox with water.

Zolpimist oral spray should be sprayed directly into the mouth over the tongue. Prior to initial use, pump should be primed by spraying 5 times. If pump is not used for at least 14 days, reprime pump with 1 spray.

Monitoring Parameters Daytime alertness; fall risk, respiratory rate; behavior profile; tolerance, abuse, and dependence; reevaluate if insomnia persists after 7 to 10 days of use.

Test Interactions Increased aminotransferase [ALT/AST], bilirubin (S); decreased RAI uptake

Additional Information Causes fewer disturbances in sleep stages as compared to benzodiazepines. Time spent in sleep stages 3 and 4 are maintained; zolpidem decreases sleep latency; should not be prescribed in quantities exceeding a 1-month supply.

Dosage Forms Excipient information presented when available (limited, particularly for generics); consult specific product labeling.

Solution, Oral, as tartrate:
Zolpimist: 5 mg/actuation (7.7 mL) [contains benzoic acid, propylene glycol; cherry flavor]
Tablet, Oral, as tartrate:
Ambien: 5 mg [contains fd&c red #40, polysorbate 80]
Ambien: 10 mg
Generic: 5 mg, 10 mg
Tablet Extended Release, Oral, as tartrate:
Ambien CR: 6.25 mg
Ambien CR: 12.5 mg [contains fd&c blue #2 (indigotine)]
Generic: 6.25 mg, 12.5 mg
Tablet Sublingual, Sublingual, as tartrate:
Edluar: 5 mg, 10 mg [contains saccharin sodium]
Intermezzo: 1.75 mg, 3.5 mg

Dosage Forms: Canada Excipient information presented when available (limited, particularly for generics); consult specific product labeling.

Tablet, Sublingual, as tartrate:
Sublinox: 5 mg, 10 mg

Controlled Substance C-IV

Zonisamide (zoe NIS a mide)

Brand Names: US Zonegran
Pharmacologic Category Anticonvulsant, Miscellaneous
Use Partial seizures: Adjunct treatment of partial seizures in adolescents >16 years of age and adults with epilepsy

Pregnancy Considerations Teratogenic effects were observed in animal reproduction studies. Zonisamide crosses the placenta and can be detected in the newborn following delivery (Kawada 2002; Shimoyama 1999). Information related to pregnancy outcomes following maternal use of zonisamide is limited (Hernández-Díaz 2014; Kanemoto 2007; Kondo 1996; Ohtahara 2007). Metabolic acidosis is an adverse effect of zonisamide therapy; newborns exposed to zonisamide in utero should be monitored for transient metabolic acidosis after birth and pregnant women taking zonisamide should be monitored and treated as nonpregnant patients. In general, maternal polytherapy with antiepileptic drugs may increase the risk of congenital malformations; monotherapy with the lowest effective dose is recommended. Newborns of women taking antiepileptic medications may be at an increased risk of adverse events (Harden and Meader 2009).

Zonisamide clearance may increase during pregnancy, requiring dosage adjustment (Oles 2008; Reisinger

2013). Women of childbearing potential are advised to use effective contraception during therapy. Until additional data is available, other agents may be preferred for the treatment of epilepsy in pregnant women (Ohtahara 2007).

Patients exposed to zonisamide during pregnancy are encouraged to enroll themselves into the NAAED Pregnancy Registry by calling 1-888-233-2334. Additional information is available at http://www.aedpregnancyregistry.org.

Breast-Feeding Considerations Zonisamide is excreted into breast milk in concentrations similar to those in the maternal plasma and can be detected in the plasma of a nursing infant (Ando 2013; Kawada 2002; Shimoyama 1999). Due to the potential for serious adverse reactions in the nursing infant, the manufacturer recommends a decision be made whether to discontinue nursing or to discontinue the drug, taking into account the importance of treatment to the mother.

Medication Guide Available Yes

Contraindications

Hypersensitivity to zonisamide, sulfonamides, or any component of the formulation

Note: Although the FDA approved product labeling states this medication is contraindicated with other sulfonamide-containing drug classes, the scientific basis of this statement has been challenged. See "Warnings/Precautions" for more detail.

Warnings/Precautions Hazardous agent - use appropriate precautions for handling and disposal (NIOSH 2014 [group 3]).

Use may be associated with the development of metabolic acidosis (generally dose-dependent) in certain patients; predisposing conditions/therapies include renal disease, severe respiratory disease, diarrhea, status epilepticus, ketogenic diet, and other medications. Metabolic acidosis can occur at doses as low as 25 mg daily. Pediatric patients may also be at an increased risk for and may have more severe metabolic acidosis. Serum bicarbonate should be monitored in all patients prior to and during use; if metabolic acidosis occurs, consider decreasing the dose or tapering the dose to discontinue. If use continued despite acidosis, alkali treatment should be considered. Untreated metabolic acidosis may increase the risk of developing nephrolithiasis, nephrocalcinosis, osteomalacia (or rickets in children), or osteoporosis; pediatric patients may also have decreased growth rates.

Pooled analysis of trials involving various antiepileptics (regardless of indication) showed an increased risk of suicidal thoughts/behavior (incidence rate: 0.43% treated patients compared to 0.24% of patients receiving placebo); risk observed as early as 1 week after initiation and continued through duration of trials (most trials ≤24 weeks). Monitor all patients for notable changes in behavior that might indicate suicidal thoughts or depression; notify healthcare provider immediately if symptoms occur.

Discontinue zonisamide in patients who develop acute renal failure or a significant sustained increase in creatinine/BUN concentration. Kidney stones have been reported. Do not use in patients with renal impairment (GFR <50 mL/minute); use with caution in patients with hepatic impairment. Use with caution in patients with hepatic impairment.

Significant CNS effects include psychiatric symptoms (eg, depression, psychosis), psychomotor slowing (eg, difficulty with concentration, speech or language problems), and fatigue or somnolence; may occur within the first month of treatment, most commonly at doses of ≥300 mg/day. May cause sedation, which may impair physical or mental abilities; patients must be cautioned about performing tasks which require mental alertness (eg, operating machinery or driving). Anticonvulsants should not be discontinued abruptly because of the possibility of increasing seizure frequency; therapy should be withdrawn gradually to minimize the potential of increased seizure frequency, unless safety concerns require a more rapid withdrawal.

Decreased sweating (oligohydrosis) and hyperthermia requiring hospitalization have been reported in children; use with caution when used in combination with other drugs that may predispose patients to heat-related disorders (eg, anticholinergics). Potentially significant interactions may exist, requiring dose or frequency adjustment, additional monitoring, and/or selection of alternative therapy. Consult drug interactions database for more detailed information.

Sulfonamide ("sulfa") allergy: The FDA-approved product labeling for many medications containing a sulfonamide chemical group includes a broad contraindication in patients with a prior allergic reaction to sulfonamides.

There is a potential for cross-reactivity between members of a specific class (eg, two antibiotic sulfonamides). However, concerns for cross-reactivity have previously extended to all compounds containing the sulfonamide structure (SO_2NH_2). An expanded understanding of allergic mechanisms indicates cross-reactivity between antibiotic sulfonamides and nonantibiotic sulfonamides may not occur or at the very least this potential is extremely low (Brackett 2004; Johnson 2005; Slatore 2004; Tornero 2004). In particular, mechanisms of cross-reaction due to antibody production (anaphylaxis) are unlikely to occur with nonantibiotic sulfonamides. T-cell-mediated (type IV) reactions (eg, maculopapular rash) are less well understood and it is not possible to completely exclude this potential based on current insights. In cases where prior reactions were severe (Stevens-Johnson syndrome/TEN), some clinicians choose to avoid exposure to these classes.

Adverse Reactions Frequency not always defined. Frequencies noted in patients receiving other anticonvulsants:

>10%:
Central nervous system: Drowsiness (17%), dizziness (13%)
Gastrointestinal: Anorexia (13%)

1% to 10%:
Cardiovascular: Facial edema (1%)
Central nervous system: Headache (10%), agitation (9%), irritability (9%), fatigue (7% to 8%), tiredness (7%), confusion (6%), depression (6%), insomnia (6%), lack of concentration (6%), memory impairment (6%), ataxia (≥1% to 6%), speech disturbance (5%), decreased mental acuity (4%), anxiety (3%), nervousness (2%), schizophreniform disorder (2%), speech disturbance (2%), convulsions (≥1%), hyperesthesia (≥1%), seizure (1%), status epilepticus (1%), hypotonia (≤1%), hyperthermia
Dermatologic: Skin rash (1% to 3%), bruising (2%), pruritus (≥1%), hypohidrosis (children), Stevens-Johnson syndrome, toxic epidermal necrolysis
Endrocrine & metabolic: Metabolic acidosis
Gastrointestinal: Nausea (9%), abdominal pain (6%), diarrhea (5%), dyspepsia (3%), weight loss (3%), constipation (2%), dysgeusia (2%), xerostomia (2%), vomiting (≥1%)
Hematologic & oncologic: Agranulocytosis, aplastic anemia
Neuromuscular & skeletal: Paresthesia (4%), abnormal gait (≥1%), tremor (≥1%), weakness (≥1%)
Ophthalmic: Diplopia (6%), nystagmus (4%), amblyopia (≥1%)
Otic: Tinnitus (≥1%)
Renal: Nephrolithiasis (4%, children 3% to 8%), increased blood urea nitrogen
Respiratory: Rhinitis (2%), increased cough (≥1%), pharyngitis (≥1%)
Miscellaneous: Flu-like syndrome (4%), accidental injury (≥1%)

<1% (Limited to important or life threatening): Alopecia, amenorrhea, apnea, arthritis, atrial fibrillation, bladder calculus, bradycardia, brain disease, cardiac failure, cerebrovascular accident, cholangitis, cholecystitis, cholestatic jaundice, colitis, deafness, duodenitis, fecal incontinence, gastrointestinal ulcer, gingivitis, glaucoma, hematemesis, hematuria, hemoptysis, hirsutism, hypermenorrhea, hypersensitivity reaction, hypertension, hypoglycemia, hyponatremia, hypotension, immunodeficiency, impotence, iritis, leukopenia, lupus erythematosus, lymphadenopathy, mastitis, neuropathy, oculogyric crisis, pancreatitis, photophobia, psychomotor disturbance, pulmonary embolism, rectal hemorrhage, stroke, suicidal behavior, suicidal ideation, syncope, thrombocytopenia, thrombophlebitis, urinary incontinence, ventricular premature contractions

Drug Interactions
Metabolism/Transport Effects Substrate of CYP2C19 (minor), CYP3A4 (major); **Note:** Assignment of Major/Minor substrate status based on clinically relevant drug interaction potential

Avoid Concomitant Use
Avoid concomitant use of Zonisamide with any of the following: Azelastine (Nasal); Carbonic Anhydrase Inhibitors; Orphenadrine; Paraldehyde; Thalidomide

Increased Effect/Toxicity
Zonisamide may increase the levels/effects of: Alcohol (Ethyl); Alpha-/Beta-Agonists (Indirect-Acting); Amphetamines; Azelastine (Nasal); Buprenorphine; Carbonic Anhydrase Inhibitors; CNS Depressants; Flecainide; Hydrocodone; Memantine; MetFORMIN; Methotrimeprazine; Metyrosine; Mirtazapine; Orphenadrine; Paraldehyde; Pramipexole; QuiNIDine; ROPINIRole; Rotigotine; Selective Serotonin Reuptake Inhibitors; Suvorexant; Thalidomide; Zolpidem

The levels/effects of Zonisamide may be increased by: Brimonidine (Topical); Cannabis; Doxylamine; Dronabinol; Droperidol; HydrOXYzine; Kava Kava; Magnesium Sulfate; Methotrimeprazine; Minocycline; Nabilone; Osimertinib; Perampanel; Rufinamide; Salicylates; Sodium Oxybate; Tapentadol; Tetrahydrocannabinol

Decreased Effect
Zonisamide may decrease the levels/effects of: Lithium; Methenamine

The levels/effects of Zonisamide may be decreased by: Bosentan; CYP3A4 Inducers (Moderate); CYP3A4 Inducers (Strong); Dabrafenib; Deferasirox; Enzalutamide; Fosphenytoin; Mefloquine; Mianserin; Mitotane; Orlistat; Osimertinib; PHENobarbital; Phenytoin; Siltuximab; St Johns Wort; Tocilizumab

Food Interactions Food delays time to maximum concentration, but does not affect bioavailability. Management: Administer without regard to meals.

Storage/Stability Store at 25°C (77°F) excursions are permitted between 15°C and 30°C (59°F and 86°F). Protect from moisture and light.

Mechanism of Action Stabilizes neuronal membranes and suppresses neuronal hypersynchronization through action at sodium and calcium channels; does not affect GABA activity.

Pharmacodynamics/Kinetics
Distribution: V_d: 1.45 L/kg
Protein binding: 40%
Metabolism: Hepatic via CYP3A4; forms N-acetyl zonisamide and 2-sulfamoylacetyl phenol (SMAP)
Half-life elimination: Plasma: ~63 hours
Time to peak: 2 to 6 hours
Excretion: Urine (62%, 35% as unchanged drug, 65% as metabolites); feces (3%)

Dosing
Adult
Adjunctive treatment of partial seizures: Oral: Initial: 100 mg/day. Dose may be increased to 200 mg/day after 2 weeks. Further dosage increases to 300 mg and 400 mg/day can then be made with a minimum of 2 weeks between adjustments, in order to reach steady state at each dosage level. Doses of up to 600 mg/day have been studied, however, there is no evidence of increased response with doses >400 mg/day. **Note:** Doses of 300 mg/day and higher are associated with increased side effects.

Geriatric Data from clinical trials is insufficient for patients older than 65. Begin dosing at the low end of the dosing range.

Pediatric Adolescents >16 years: Refer to adult dosing.

Renal Impairment
GFR ≥50 mL/minute: There are no dosage adjustments provided in the manufacturer's labeling. However, slower titration and frequent monitoring are indicated in patients with renal disease; use with caution.
GFR <50 mL/minute: Use is not recommended. Marked renal impairment (CrCl <20 mL/minute) was associated with a 35% increase in AUC.

Hepatic Impairment There are no dosage adjustments provided in the manufacturer's labeling (has not been studied). However, slower titration and frequent monitoring are indicated in patients with hepatic impairment; use with caution.

Administration Capsules should be swallowed whole. Administer once or twice daily with or without food. Hazardous agent; use appropriate precautions for handling and disposal (NIOSH 2014 [group 3]).

Monitoring Parameters Metabolic profile, specifically BUN, serum creatinine; serum bicarbonate (prior to initiation and periodically during therapy); suicidality (eg, suicidal thoughts, depression, behavioral changes); decreased sweating, elevated body temperature especially in warm or hot weather (particularly in pediatric patients)

Dosage Forms Excipient information presented when available (limited, particularly for generics); consult specific product labeling.
Capsule, Oral:
Zonegran: 25 mg, 100 mg
Zonegran: 100 mg [contains fd&c red #40, fd&c yellow #6 (sunset yellow)]
Generic: 25 mg, 50 mg, 100 mg

Extemporaneous Preparations Hazardous agent; use appropriate precautions during preparation and disposal (NIOSH 2014 [group 3]).

A 10 mg/mL suspension may be made using capsules and either simple syrup or methylcellulose 0.5%. Empty contents of ten 100 mg capsules into glass mortar. Reduce to a fine powder and add a small amount of Simple Syrup, NF and mix to a uniform paste; mix while adding the chosen vehicle in incremental proportions to **almost** 100 mL; transfer to an amber calibrated plastic bottle, rinse mortar

with vehicle, and add quantity of vehicle sufficient to make 100 mL. Label "shake well" and "refrigerate". When using simple syrup vehicle, stable 28 days at room temperature or refrigerated (preferred). When using methylcellulose vehicle, stable 7 days at room temperature or 28 days refrigerated. **Note:** Although no visual evidence of microbial growth was observed, storage under refrigeration would be recommended to minimize microbial contamination.

Abobo CV, Wei B, and Liang D, "Stability of Zonisamide in Extemporaneously Compounded Oral Suspensions," *Am J Health Syst Pharm*, 2009, 66(12):1105-9.

♦ *Zontivity* see Vorapaxar *on page 1907*

♦ *Zorbtive* see Somatropin *on page 1686*

♦ *Zortress* see Everolimus *on page 719*

♦ *Zorvolex* see Diclofenac (Systemic) *on page 540*

♦ *Zostavax* see Zoster Vaccine *on page 1944*

Zoster Vaccine (ZOS ter vak SEEN)

Brand Names: US Zostavax
Brand Names: Canada Zostavax
Index Terms Herpes Zoster Vaccine; HZV; Shingles Vaccine; VZV Vaccine (Zoster)
Pharmacologic Category Vaccine; Vaccine, Live (Viral)
Additional Appendix Information
Immunization Administration Recommendations *on page 1974*
Immunization Schedules *on page 1979*
Use
Herpes zoster prevention: Prevention of herpes zoster (shingles) in patients ≥50 years of age
The Advisory Committee on Immunization Practices (ACIP) recommends:
Routine vaccination of **all patients ≥60 years of age, including** patients who report a previous episode of zoster; patients with chronic medical conditions (eg, chronic renal failure, diabetes mellitus, rheumatoid arthritis, chronic pulmonary disease) unless those conditions are contraindications; and residents of nursing homes and other long-term care facilities ≥60 years of age without contraindications (CDC/ACIP [Harpaz, 2008]).

Limitations of use: Not indicated for treatment of zoster or postherpetic neuralgia (PHN); not indicated for prophylaxis of primary varicella infection (chickenpox).
Medication Guide Available Yes
Dosing
Adult & Geriatric Shingles prevention:
Manufacturer labeling: Adults ≥50 years: SubQ: 0.65 mL administered as a single dose
ACIP recommendation: Adults ≥60 years: SubQ: 0.65 mL administered as a single dose; there are no data to support readministration of the vaccine (CDC/ACIP [Harpaz, 2008])
Renal Impairment There are no dosage adjustments provided in the manufacturer's labeling.
Hepatic Impairment There are no dosage adjustments provided in the manufacturer's labeling.
Additional Information Complete prescribing information should be consulted for additional detail.
Dosage Forms Considerations Zostavax contains porcine gelatin
Dosage Forms Excipient information presented when available (limited, particularly for generics); consult specific product labeling.
Solution Reconstituted, Subcutaneous [preservative free]:
Zostavax: 19,400 units/0.65 mL (1 ea)

♦ *Zosyn* see Piperacillin and Tazobactam *on page 1456*

♦ *Zovia* see Ethinyl Estradiol and Ethynodiol Diacetate *on page 702*

♦ *Zovirax* see Acyclovir (Systemic) *on page 37*

♦ *Zovirax* see Acyclovir (Topical) *on page 41*

♦ *Z-Pak* see Azithromycin (Systemic) *on page 190*

♦ *Zubsolv* see Buprenorphine and Naloxone *on page 267*

♦ *Zuplenz* see Ondansetron *on page 1335*

♦ *Zyban* see BuPROPion *on page 269*

♦ *Zyclara* see Imiquimod *on page 926*

♦ *Zyclara Pump* see Imiquimod *on page 926*

♦ *Zydelig* see Idelalisib *on page 911*

♦ *Zydone [DSC]* see Hydrocodone and Acetaminophen *on page 884*

♦ *Zyflo* see Zileuton *on page 1928*

♦ *Zyflo CR* see Zileuton *on page 1928*

♦ *Zykadia* see Ceritinib *on page 360*

♦ *Zylet* see Loteprednol and Tobramycin *on page 1110*

♦ *Zyloprim* see Allopurinol *on page 73*

♦ *Zymar (Can)* see Gatifloxacin *on page 829*

♦ *Zymaxid* see Gatifloxacin *on page 829*

♦ *ZYM-Cholestyramine-Light (Can)* see Cholestyramine Resin *on page 381*

♦ *ZYM-Cholestyramine-Regular (Can)* see Cholestyramine Resin *on page 381*

♦ *ZYM-Clonazepam (Can)* see ClonazePAM *on page 419*

♦ *ZYM-Cyclobenzaprine (Can)* see Cyclobenzaprine *on page 454*

♦ *ZYM-Fluoxetine (Can)* see FLUoxetine *on page 786*

♦ *ZYM-Mirtazapine (Can)* see Mirtazapine *on page 1216*

♦ *ZYM-Sotalol (Can)* see Sotalol *on page 1694*

♦ *ZYM-Trazodone (Can)* see TraZODone *on page 1834*

♦ *Zyncof [OTC]* see Guaifenesin and Dextromethorphan *on page 861*

♦ *Zypram [DSC]* see Pramoxine and Hydrocortisone *on page 1489*

♦ *ZyPREXA* see OLANZapine *on page 1314*

♦ *Zyprexa (Can)* see OLANZapine *on page 1314*

♦ *Zyprexa Intramuscular (Can)* see OLANZapine *on page 1314*

♦ *ZyPREXA Relprevv* see OLANZapine *on page 1314*

♦ *Zyprexa Zydis* see OLANZapine *on page 1314*

♦ *ZyPREXA Zydis* see OLANZapine *on page 1314*

♦ *ZyrTEC Allergy [OTC]* see Cetirizine *on page 364*

♦ *ZyrTEC Allergy Childrens [OTC]* see Cetirizine *on page 364*

♦ *ZyrTEC Childrens Allergy [OTC]* see Cetirizine *on page 364*

♦ *ZyrTEC Childrens Hives Relief [OTC]* see Cetirizine *on page 364*

♦ *ZyrTEC Hives Relief [OTC]* see Cetirizine *on page 364*

♦ *ZyrTEC Itchy Eye [OTC]* see Ketotifen (Ophthalmic) *on page 1018*

♦ *Zytiga* see Abiraterone Acetate *on page 21*

♦ *Zytram XL (Can)* see TraMADol *on page 1821*

♦ *Zyvox* see Linezolid *on page 1080*

♦ *Zyvoxam (Can)* see Linezolid *on page 1080*

♦ *ZzzQuil [OTC]* see DiphenhydrAMINE (Systemic) *on page 561*

APPENDIX TABLE OF CONTENTS

ASSESSMENT OF LIVER FUNCTION

Child-Pugh Score

Component	Score Given for Observed Findings		
	1	2	3
Encephalopathy grade[1]	None	1 to 2	3 to 4
Ascites	None	Mild or controlled by diuretics	Moderate or refractory despite diuretics
Albumin (g/dL)	>3.5	2.8 to 3.5	<2.8
Total bilirubin (mg/dL)	<2 (<34 micromoles/L)	2 to 3 (34 to 50 micromoles/L)	>3 (>50 micromoles/L)
or			
Modified total bilirubin[2]	<4	4 to 7	>7
Prothrombin time (seconds prolonged)	<4	4 to 6	>6
or			
INR	<1.7	1.7 to 2.3	>2.3

[1]**Encephalopathy Grades**
Grade 0: Normal consciousness, personality, neurological examination, electroencephalogram
Grade 1: Restless, sleep disturbed, irritable/agitated, tremor, impaired handwriting, 5 cps waves
Grade 2: Lethargic, time-disoriented, inappropriate, asterixis, ataxia, slow triphasic waves
Grade 3: Somnolent, stuporous, place-disoriented, hyperactive reflexes, rigidity, slower waves
Grade 4: Unrousable coma, no personality/behavior, decerebrate, slow 2 to 3 cps delta activity

Alternative Encephalopathy Grades
Grade 1: Mild confusion, anxiety, restlessness, fine tremor, slowed coordination
Grade 2: Drowsiness, disorientation, asterixis
Grade 3: Somnolent but rousable, marked confusion, incomprehensible speech, incontinent, hyperventilation
Grade 4: Coma, decerebrate posturing, flaccidity

[2]Modified total bilirubin used to score patients who have Gilbert syndrome or who are taking indinavir.

CHILD-PUGH CLASSIFICATION

Class A (mild hepatic impairment): Score 5 to 6
Class B (moderate hepatic impairment): Score 7 to 9
Class C (severe hepatic impairment): Score 10 to 15

REFERENCES

Centers for Disease Control and Prevention (CDC). Report of the NIH panel to define principles of therapy of HIV infection and guidelines for the use of antiretroviral agents in HIV-infected adults and adolescents. March 2004. Available at http://www.aidsinfo.nih.gov
US Department of Health and Human Services Food and Drug Administration. Guidance for industry, pharmacokinetics in patients with impaired hepatic function: study design, data analysis, and impact on dosing and labeling. May 2003. Available at http://www.fda.gov/OHRMS/DOCKETS/98fr/99D-5047-GDL00002.pdf

RENAL FUNCTION ESTIMATION IN ADULT PATIENTS

Evaluation of a patient's renal function often includes the use of equations to estimate glomerular filtration rate (GFR) (eg, estimated GFR [eGFR] creatinine clearance [CrCl]) using an endogenous filtration marker (eg, serum creatinine) and other patient variables. For example, the Cockcroft-Gault equation estimates renal function by calculating CrCl and is typically used to steer medication dosing. Equations which calculate eGFR are primarily used to categorize chronic kidney disease (CKD) staging and monitor progression. The rate of creatinine clearance does not always accurately represent GFR; creatinine may be cleared by other renal mechanisms in addition to glomerular filtration and serum creatinine concentrations may be affected by nonrenal factors (eg, age, gender, race, body habitus, illness, diet). In addition, these equations were developed based on studies in limited populations and may either over- or underestimate the renal function of a specific patient.

Nevertheless, most clinicians estimate renal function using CrCl as an indicator of actual renal function for the purpose of adjusting medication doses. For medications that require dose adjustment for renal impairment, utilization of eGFR (ie, Modification of Diet in Renal Disease [MDRD]) may overestimate renal function by up to 40% which may result in supratherapeutic medication doses (Hermsen 2009). These equations should only be used in the clinical context of patient-specific factors noted during the physical exam/work-up. The 2012 National Kidney Foundation (NKF)-Kidney Disease Improving Global Outcomes (KDIGO) CKD guidelines state that drug dosing should be based on an e-GFR which is **not** adjusted for body surface area (BSA) (ie, reported in units of mL/minute per 1.73 m^2) since the effect of eGFR adjusted for BSA compared to eGFR without adjustments for BSA has not been extensively studied. **Decisions regarding drug therapy and doses must be based on clinical judgment.**

RENAL FUNCTION ESTIMATION EQUATIONS

Commonly used equations to estimate renal function utilizing the endogenous filtration marker serum creatinine include the Cockcroft-Gault, Jelliffe, four-variable Modification of Diet in Renal Disease (MDRD), six-variable MDRD (aka, MDRD extended), and Chronic Kidney Disease Epidemiology Collaboration (CKD-EPI). All of these equations, except for the CKD-EPI, were originally developed using a serum creatinine assay measured by the alkaline picrate-based (Jaffe) method. Many substances, including proteins, can interfere with the accuracy of this assay and overestimate serum creatinine concentration. The NKF and The National Kidney Disease Education Program (NDKEP) advocated for a universal creatinine assay, in order to ensure an accurate estimate of renal function in patients. As a result, a more specific enzymatic assay with an isotope dilution mass spectrometry (IDMS)-traceable international standard was developed. Compared to the older methods, IDMS-traceable assays may report lower serum creatinine values and may, therefore, overestimate renal function when used in the original equations not re-expressed for use with a standardized serum creatinine assay (eg, Cockcroft-Gault, Jelliffe, original MDRD). Updated four-variable MDRD and six-variable MDRD equations based on serum creatinine measured by the IDMS-traceable method has been proposed for adults (Levey 2006); the Cockcroft-Gault and Jelliffe equations have not been re-expressed and may overestimate renal function when used with a serum creatinine measured by the IDMS-traceable method. However, at this point, all laboratories should be using creatinine methods calibrated to be IDMS traceable.

The CKD-EPI creatinine equation, published in 2009, uses the same four variables as the four-variable MDRD (serum creatinine, age, sex, and race), but allows for more precision when estimating higher GFR values (eg, eGFR >60 mL/minute per 1.73 m^2) as compared to the MDRD equation. The NKDEP has not made a recommendation on the general implementation of the CKD-EPI equation but does suggest that laboratories which report numeric values for eGFR >60 mL/minute per 1.73 m^2 should consider the use of CKD-EPI. The NKD-KDIGO 2012 CKD guidelines recommend that clinicians use a creatinine-derived equation for the evaluation and management of CKD and specifically recommend that clinical laboratories use the 2009 CKD-EPI equation when reporting eGFR in adults.

The following factors may contribute to an inaccurate estimation of renal function (Stevens 2006):

- Increased creatinine generation (may underestimate renal function):
  - Black patients
  - Muscular body habitus
  - Ingestion of cooked meats
- Decreased creatinine generation (may overestimate renal function):
  - Increased age
  - Female patients
  - Hispanic patients
  - Asian patients
  - Amputees
  - Malnutrition, inflammation, or deconditioning (eg, cancer, severe cardiovascular disease, hospitalized patients)
  - Neuromuscular disease
  - Vegetarian diet
- Rapidly changing serum creatinine (either up or down): In patients with rapidly rising serum creatinines (ie, increasing by >0.5 to 0.7 mg/dL/day), it is best to assume that the patient's renal function is severely impaired

Use extreme caution when estimating renal function in the following patient populations:

- Low body weight (actual body weight < ideal body weight)
- Liver transplant
- Elderly patients (>90 years of age)
- Dehydration
- Recent kidney transplantation (serum creatinine values may decrease rapidly and can lead to renal function under-estimation; conversely, delayed graft function may be present)

Note: In most situations, the use of the patient's ideal body weight (IBW) is recommended for estimating renal function, except when the patient's actual body weight (ABW) is less than ideal. Use of actual body weight (ABW) in obese patients (and possibly patients with ascites) may significantly overestimate renal function. Some clinicians prefer to use an adjusted body weight in such cases [eg, IBW + 0.4 (ABW - IBW)]; the adjustment factor may vary based on practitioner and/or institutional preference.

IDMS-traceable methods

Method 1: MDRD equation[1]:

$$eGFR = 175 \times (Creatinine)^{-1.154} \times (Age)^{-0.203} \times (Gender) \times (Race)$$
where:

eGFR = estimated GFR; calculated in mL/minute per 1.73 m²
Creatinine is input in mg/dL
Age is input in years
Gender: Females: Gender = 0.742; Males: Gender = 1
Race: Black: Race = 1.212; White or other: Race = 1

Method 2: MDRD Extended equation:

$$eGFR = 161.5 \times (Creatinine)^{-0.999} \times (Age)^{-0.176} \times (SUN)^{-0.170} \times (Albumin)^{0.318} \times (Gender) \times (Race)$$
where:

eGFR = estimated GFR; calculated in mL/minute per 1.73 m²
Creatinine is input in mg/dL
Age is input in years
SUN = Serum Urea Nitrogen; input in mg/dL
Albumin = Serum Albumin; input in g/dL
Gender: Females: Gender = 0.762; Males: Gender = 1
Race: Black: Race = 1.18; White or other: Race = 1

Method 3: CKD-EPI equation[2]:

$$eGFR = 141 \times (Creatinine/k)^{Exp} \times (0.993)^{Age} \times (Gender) \times (Race)$$
where:

eGFR = estimated GFR; calculated in mL/minute per 1.73 m²
(Creatinine/k):
  Creatinine is input in mg/dL
  k: Females: k = 0.7; Males: k = 0.9
  Exp:
    When (Creatinine/k) is ≤1: Females: Exp = -0.329; Males: Exp = -0.411
    When (Creatinine/k) is >1: Exp = -1.209
Age is input in years
Gender: Females: Gender = 1.018; Males: Gender = 1
Race: Black: Race = 1.159; White or other: Race = 1

Alkaline picrate-based (Jaffe) methods

Note: These equations have not been updated for use with serum creatinine methods traceable to IDMS. Use with IDMS-traceable serum creatinine methods may overestimate renal function; use with caution.

Method 1: MDRD equation:

$$eGFR = 186 \times (Creatinine)^{-1.154} \times (Age)^{-0.203} \times (Gender) \times (Race)$$
where:

eGFR = estimated GFR; calculated in mL/minute per 1.73 m²
Creatinine is input in mg/dL
Age is input in years
Gender: Females: Gender = 0.742; Males: Gender = 1
Race: Black: Race = 1.212; White or other: Race = 1

Method 2: MDRD Extended equation:

$$eGFR = 170 \times (Creatinine)^{-0.999} \times (Age)^{-0.176} \times (SUN)^{-0.170} \times (Albumin)^{0.318} \times (Gender) \times (Race)$$
where:

eGFR = estimated GFR; calculated in mL/minute per 1.73 m²
Creatinine is input in mg/dL
Age is input in years
SUN = Serum Urea Nitrogen; input in mg/dL
Albumin = Serum Albumin; input in g/dL
Gender: Females: Gender = 0.762; Males: Gender = 1
Race: Black: Race = 1.18; White or other: Race = 1

Method 3: Cockroft-Gault equation[3]

Males: CrCl = [(140 - Age) × Weight] / (72 × Creatinine)
Females: CrCl = {[(140 - Age) × Weight] / (72 × Creatinine)} × 0.85
where:

CrCl = creatinine clearance; calculated in mL/minute
Age is input in years
Weight is input in kg
Creatinine is input in mg/dL

Method 4: Jelliffe equation

Males: CrCl = {98 - [0.8 × (Age - 20)]} / (Creatinine)
Females: CrCl = Use above equation, then multiply result by 0.9
where:

CrCl = creatinine clearance; calculated in mL/minute per 1.73 m²
Age is input in years
Creatinine is input in mg/dL

FOOTNOTES

[1]Preferred equation for CKD staging National Kidney Disease Education Program
[2]Recommended equation for the reporting of eGFR by the NKD-KDIGO guidelines
[3]Equation typically used for adjusting medication doses

REFERENCES

Cockcroft DW, Gault MH. Prediction of creatinine clearance from serum creatinine. *Nephron.* 1976;16(1):31-41.

Dowling TC, Matzke GR, Murphy JE, Burckart GJ. Evaluation of renal drug dosing: prescribing information and clinical pharmacist approaches. *Pharmacotherapy.* 2010;30(8):776-786.

Hermsen ED, Maiefski M, Florescu MC, Qiu F, Rupp ME. Comparison of the modification of diet in renal disease and Cockcroft-Gault equations for dosing antimicrobials. *Pharmacotherapy.* 2009;29(6):649-655.

Jelliffe RW. Letter: creatinine clearance: bedside estimate. *Ann Intern Med.* 1973;79(4):604-605.

Kidney disease: improving global outcomes (KDIGO) CKD work group. KDIGO 2012 clinical practice guidelines for the evaluation and management of chronic kidney disease. *Kidney Inter.* 2013;3:1-150. http://www.kdigo.org/clinical_practice_guidelines/pdf/CKD/KDIGO_2012_CKD_GL.pdf

Levey AS, Bosch JP, Lewis JB, Greene T, Rogers N, Roth D. A more accurate method to estimate glomerular filtration rate from serum creatinine: a new prediction equation. Modification of diet in renal disease study group. *Ann Intern Med.* 1999;16;130(6):461-470.

Levey AS, Coresh J, Greene T, et al. Using standardized serum creatinine values in the modification of diet in renal disease study equation for estimating glomerular filtration rate. *Ann Intern Med.* 2006;145(4):247-254.

Levey AS, Stevens LA, Schmid CH, et al. A new equation to estimate glomerular filtration rate. *Ann Intern Med.* 2009;150(9):604-612.

National Kidney Disease Education Program. GFR calculators. http://www.nkdep.nih.gov/professionals/gfr_calculators. Accessed April 24, 2013.

Stevens LA, Coresh J, Greene T, Levey AS. Assessing kidney function – measured and estimated glomerular filtration rate. *N Engl J Med.* 2006;354 (23):2473-2483.

CORTICOSTEROIDS SYSTEMIC EQUIVALENCIES

Glucocorticoid	Approximate Equivalent Dose (mg)	Routes of Administration	Relative Anti-inflammatory Potency	Relative Mineralocorticoid Potency	Protein Binding (%)	Half-life Plasma (min)
		Short-Acting				
Cortisone	25	PO, IM	0.8	0.8	90	30
Hydrocortisone	20	IM, IV	1	1	90	90
		Intermediate-Acting				
MethylPREDNISolone[1]	4	PO, IM, IV	5	0	—	180
PrednisoLONE	5	PO, IM, IV, intra-articular, intradermal, soft tissue injection	4	0.8	90 to 95	200
PredniSONE	5	PO	4	0.8	<50	120 to 180
Triamcinolone[1]	4	IM, intra-articular, intradermal, intrasynovial, soft tissue injection	5	0	—	300
		Long-Acting				
Betamethasone	0.75	PO, IM, intra-articular, intradermal, intrasynovial, soft tissue injection	25	0	64	100 to 300
Dexamethasone	0.75	PO, IM, IV, intra-articular, intradermal, soft tissue injection	25 to 30	0	—	100 to 300
		Mineralocorticoids				
Fludrocortisone	—	PO	10	125	42	200

[1]May contain propylene glycol as an excipient in injectable forms

Asare K. Diagnosis and treatment of adrenal insufficiency in the critically ill patient. *Pharmacotherapy.* 2007;27(11):1512-1528.

Frey BM, Frey FJ. Clinical pharmacokinetics of prednisone and prednisolone. *Clin Pharmacokinet.* 1990;19(2):126-146.

INHALED CORTICOSTEROIDS

Estimated Comparative Daily Dosage

Children ≥12 Years of Age and Adults

Drug	Low Daily Dose	Medium Daily Dose	High Daily Dose
Beclomethasone aerosol solution inhalation	80 to 240 mcg	>240 to 480 mcg	>480 mcg
Budesonide aerosol powder breath-activated inhalation	180 to 600 mcg	>600 to 1,200 mcg	>1,200 mcg
Ciclesonide HFA	160 to 320 mcg	>320 to 640 mcg	>640 mcg
Flunisolide aerosol solution inhalation	320 mcg	>320 to 640 mcg	>640 mcg
Fluticasone HFA	88 to 264 mcg	>264 to 440 mcg	>440 mcg
Fluticasone aerosol powder breath-activated inhalation	100 to 300 mcg	>300 to 500 mcg	>500 mcg
Mometasone aerosol powder breath-activated inhalation	200 mcg	400 mcg	>400 mcg

HFA = hydrofluoroalkane

Children <12 Years of Age

Drug	Low Daily Dose	Medium Daily Dose	High Daily Dose
Beclomethasone inhalation	0 to 4 years: NA 5 to 11 years: 80 to 160 mcg	0 to 4 years: NA 5 to 11 years: >160 to 320 mcg	0 to 4 years: NA 5 to 11 years: >320 mcg
Budesonide aerosol powder breath-activated inhalation	0 to 4 years: NA 5 to 11 years: 180 to 400 mcg	0 to 4 years: NA 5 to 11 years: >400 to 800 mcg	0 to 4 years: NA 5 to 11 years: >800 mcg
Budesonide nebulized	0 to 4 years: 0.25 to 0.5 mg 5 to 11 years: 0.5 mg	0 to 4 years: >0.5 to 1 mg 5 to 11 years: 1 mg	0 to 4 years: >1 mg 5 to 11 years: 2 mg
Ciclesonide HFA	0 to 4 years: NA 5 to 11 years: 80 to 160 mcg	0 to 4 years: NA 5 to 11 years: >160 to 320 mcg	0 to 4 years: NA 5 to 11 years: >320 mcg
Flunisolide aerosol solution inhalation	0 to 4 years: NA 5 to 11 years: 160 mcg	0 to 4 years: NA 5 to 11 years: 320 mcg	0 to 4 years: NA 5 to 11 years: ≥640 mcg
Fluticasone HFA	0 to 4 years: 176 mcg 5 to 11 years: 88 to 176 mcg	0 to 11 years: >176 to 352 mcg	0 to 11 years: >352 mcg
Fluticasone aerosol powder breath-activated inhalation	0 to 4 years: NA 5 to 11 years: 100 to 200 mcg	0 to 4 years: NA 5 to 11 years: >200 to 400 mcg	0 to 4 years: NA 5 to 11 years: >400 mcg
Mometasone aerosol powder breath-activated inhalation	NA	NA	NA

HFA = hydrofluoroalkane, NA = not approved for use in this age group or no data available

REFERENCE

Expert Panel Report 3. Guidelines for the diagnosis and management of asthma. *Clinical Practice Guidelines*, National Institutes of Health, National Heart, Lung, and Blood Institute, NIH Publication No. 08-4051. Available at http://www.nhlbi.nih.gov/guidelines/asthma/asthgdln.htm

TOPICAL CORTICOSTEROIDS

GUIDELINES FOR SELECTION AND USE OF TOPICAL CORTICOSTEROIDS

The quantity prescribed and the frequency of refills should be monitored to reduce the risk of adrenal suppression. In general, short courses of high-potency agents are preferable to prolonged use of low potency. After control is achieved, control should be maintained with a low potency preparation.

1. Low- to medium-potency agents are usually effective for treating thin, acute, inflammatory skin lesions; whereas, high or super-potent agents are often required for treating chronic, hyperkeratotic, or lichenified lesions.

2. Since the stratum corneum is thin on the face and intertriginous areas, low-potency agents are preferred but a higher potency agent may be used for 2 weeks.

3. Because the palms and soles have a thick stratum corneum, high or super-potent agents are frequently required.

4. Low potency agents are preferred for infants and elderly patients. Infants have a high body surface area to weight ratio; elderly patients have thin, fragile skin.

5. The vehicle in which the topical corticosteroid is formulated influences the absorption and potency of the drug. Ointment bases are preferred for thick, lichenified lesions; they enhance penetration of the drug. Creams are preferred for acute and subacute dermatoses; they may be used on moist skin areas or intertriginous areas. Solutions, gels, and sprays are preferred for the scalp or for areas where a nonoil-based vehicle is needed.

6. In general, super-potent agents should not be used for longer than 2 to 3 weeks unless the lesion is limited to a small body area. Medium- to high-potency agents usually cause only rare adverse effects when treatment is limited to 3 months or less, and use on the face and intertriginous areas are avoided. If long-term treatment is needed, intermittent vs continued treatment is recommended.

7. Most preparations are applied once or twice daily. More frequent application may be necessary for the palms or soles because the preparation is easily removed by normal activity and penetration is poor due to a thick stratum corneum. Every-other-day or weekend-only application may be effective for treating some chronic conditions.

Relative Potency of Selected Topical Corticosteroids

	Steroid	Dosage Form
Very High Potency		
0.05%	Betamethasone dipropionate, augmented	Gel, lotion, ointment
0.05%	Clobetasol propionate	Cream, foam, gel, lotion, ointment, shampoo, spray
0.05%	Diflorasone diacetate	Ointment
0.05%	Halobetasol propionate	Cream, ointment
High Potency		
0.1%	Amcinonide	Cream, ointment, lotion
0.05%	Betamethasone dipropionate, augmented	Cream
0.05%	Betamethasone dipropionate	Cream, ointment
0.1%	Betamethasone valerate	Ointment
0.05%	Desoximetasone	Gel
0.25%	Desoximetasone	Cream, ointment
0.05%	Diflorasone diacetate	Cream, ointment
0.05%	Fluocinonide	Cream, ointment, gel
0.1%	Halcinonide	Cream, ointment
0.5%	Triamcinolone acetonide	Cream, spray
Intermediate Potency		
0.05%	Betamethasone dipropionate	Lotion
0.1%	Betamethasone valerate	Cream
0.1%	Clocortolone pivalate	Cream
0.05%	Desoximetasone	Cream
0.1%	Diflucortolone	Cream, oily cream, ointment
0.02%	Flumethasone pivalate	Cream
0.025%	Fluocinolone acetonide	Cream, ointment
0.05%	Flurandrenolide	Cream, ointment, lotion, tape
0.005%	Fluticasone propionate	Ointment
0.05%	Fluticasone propionate	Cream, lotion
0.1%	Hydrocortisone butyrate[1]	Ointment, solution
0.2%	Hydrocortisone valerate[1]	Cream, ointment
0.1%	Mometasone furoate[1]	Cream, ointment, lotion
0.1%	Prednicarbate	Cream, ointment
0.025%	Triamcinolone acetonide	Cream, ointment, lotion
0.1%	Triamcinolone acetonide	Cream, ointment, lotion
Low Potency		
0.05%	Alclometasone dipropionate[1]	Cream, ointment
0.05%	Desonide	Cream, ointment
0.01%	Fluocinolone acetonide	Cream, solution
0.5%	Hydrocortisone[1]	Cream, ointment, lotion
0.5%	Hydrocortisone acetate[1]	Cream, ointment
1%	Hydrocortisone acetate[1]	Cream, ointment
1%	Hydrocortisone[1]	Cream, ointment, lotion, solution
2.5%	Hydrocortisone[1]	Cream, ointment, lotion

[1]Not fluorinated

IMMUNE GLOBULIN PRODUCT COMPARISON

Brand Name	Concentration	pH	Initial Rate IV	Initial Rate SubQ[1]	Max Rate IV[2]	Max Rate SubQ[1]	IgA Content (mcg/mL)	Osmolarity/Osmolality (mOsmol/kg)	Comments
Bivigam	10%	4 to 4.6	0.3 mL/kg/h	–	3.6 mL/kg/h	–	≤200	Not available	Contains polysorbate 80
Carimune NF[3]	3%	6.4 to 6.8	1 mL/kg/h	–	6 mL/kg/h	–	Trace[4]	192 to 498[5]	Contains sucrose
Carimune NF[3]	12%	6.4 to 6.8	0.24 mL/kg/h	–	1.5 mL/kg/h	–	Trace[4]	768 to 1074[5]	Contains sucrose
Flebogamma DIF	5%	5 to 6	0.6 mL/kg/h	–	6 mL/kg/h	–	<50	240 to 370	
Flebogamma DIF	10%	5 to 6	0.6 mL/kg/h	–	4.8 mL/kg/h	–	<100	240 to 370	
GamaSTAN S/D	15% to 18%	6.4 to 7.2	–	–	–	–	Not available	Not available	For IM use
Gammagard S/D	5%	6.4 to 7.2	0.5 mL/kg/h	–	4 mL/kg/h	–	≤1[6]	636	Contains polysorbate 80
Gammagard S/D	10%	6.4 to 7.2	0.5 mL/kg/h	–	8 mL/kg/h	–	≤2[6]	1,250	Contains polysorbate 80
Gammagard Liquid	10%	4.6 to 5.1	0.5 mL/kg/h	<40 kg: 15 mL/h/site with a maximum of 8 sites; ≥40 kg: 20 mL/h/site with a maximum of 8 sites	5 mL/kg/h (MMN only)	<40 kg: 20 mL/h/site with a maximum of 8 sites; **total rate: 160 mL/h**; ≥40 kg: 30 mL/h/site with a maximum of 8 sites; **total rate: 240 mL/h**	37	240 to 300	
Gammaked	10%	4 to 4.5	0.6 mL/kg/h; 1.2 mL/kg/h (CIDP only)	20 mL/h/site with a maximum of 8 sites	4.8 mL/kg/h	Not determined	46	258	
Gammaplex	5%	4.8 to 5	0.6 mL/kg/h	–	4.8 mL/kg/h	–	<10	420 to 500	Contains polysorbate 80
Gamunex-C	10%	4 to 4.5	0.6 mL/kg/h; 1.2 mL/kg/h (CIDP only)	20 mL/h/site with a maximum of 8 sites	4.8 mL/kg/h	Not determined	46	258	
Hizentra	20%	4.6 to 5.2	–	15 mL/h/site with a maximum of 4 sites	–	Up to 25 mL/h/site with a maximum of 4 sites; **total rate: 50 mL/h**	≤50	380	Contains L-proline and polysorbate 80
HyQvia	10%	4.6 to 5.1	–	*First 2 infusions:* <40 kg: 5 mL/h for 5 to 15 min; 10 mL/h for 5 to 15 min; 20 mL/h for 5 to 15 min; 40 mL/h for 5 to 15 min; then 80 mL/h for remainder of infusion; ≥40 kg: 10 mL/h for 5 to 15 min; 30 mL/h for 5 to 15 min; 60 mL/h for 5 to 15 min; 120 mL/h for 5 to 15 min; then 240 mL/h for remainder of infusion. *Next 2 or 3 infusions:* <40 kg: 10 mL/h for 5 to 15 min; 20 mL/h for 5 to 15 min; 40 mL/h for 5 to 15 min; 80 mL/h for 5 to 15 min; then 160 mL/h for remainder of infusion; ≥40 kg: 10 mL/h for 5 to 15 min; 30 mL/h for 5 to 15 min; 120 mL/h for 5 to 15 min; 240 mL/h for 5 to 15 min; then 300 mL/h for remainder of infusion	–	<40 kg: 160 mL/h; ≥40 kg: 300 mL/h	37	240 to 300	Supplied with hyaluronidase (human recombinant)

| Brand Name | Concentration | pH | Initial Rate | | Max Rate | | IgA Content (mcg/mL) | Osmolarity/Osmolality (mOsmol/kg) | Comments |
			IV	SubQ[1]	IV[2]	SubQ[1]			
Octagam	5%	5.1 to 6	0.6 mL/kg/h	–	4 mL/kg/h	–	≤200	310 to 380	Contains maltose
Octagam	10%	4.5 to 5	0.6 mL/kg/h	–	7.2 mL/kg/h	–	106	310 to 380	Sucrose-free
Privigen	10%	4.6 to 5	0.3 mL/kg/h	–	2.4 mL/kg/h (ITP) 4.8 mL/kg/h	–	≤25	240 to 440	Contains L-proline

CIDP = chronic inflammatory demyelinating polyneuropathy, ITP = immune (idiopathic) thrombocytopenic purpura, MMN = multifocal motor neuropathy

[1]Subcutaneous administration **only** for the treatment of primary humoral immunodeficiency (PI)

[2]Lower infusion rates should be used in patients at risk for renal dysfunction or thrombotic complications; see specific product information for details.

[3]Other concentrations may be prepared; see product information for additional details.

[4]Per product information; other sources list IgA content as 1,000 to 2,000 mcg/mL for 6% solution (Siegel J. Immune globulins: therapeutic, pharmaceutical, cost, and administration considerations. *Pharm Prac News*. 2013).

[5]Osmolarity depends on concentration and diluent used; see product information for details.

[6]Data presented is based on the maximum concentration that can be prepared. The 5% solution with IgA content <2.2 mcg/mL has been discontinued. The lower IgA product (ie, IgA <1 mcg/mL for the 5% prepared solution) is available by special request; contact manufacturer or see specific product information for details.

OPIOID CONVERSION TABLE AND MORPHINE EQUIVALENT DOSE TABLE

Opioid Conversion Table

This table serves as a general guide to opioid conversion. Utilization of a direct conversion without a detailed patient and medication assessment is not recommended and may result in over- or underdosing. Chronic administration may alter pharmacokinetics and change the parenteral:oral ratio.

Opioid Analgesics – Initial Oral Dosing Commonly Used for Severe Pain

Drug	Equianalgesic Dose (mg)		Initial Oral Dose	
	Oral[1]	Parenteral[2]	Children[3] (mg/kg)	Adults (mg)
Buprenorphine	—	0.4	—	—
Butorphanol	—	2	—	—
FentaNYL	—	0.1	—	—
HYDROmorphone	7.5	1.5	0.06	4 to 8
Levorphanol	Acute: 4 Chronic: 1	Acute: 2 Chronic: 1	0.04	2 to 4
Meperidine[4]	300	75	Not recommended	
Methadone[5]	See Guidelines for Conversion to Oral Methadone in Adults	Variable	0.2	5 to 10
Morphine	30	10	0.3	15 to 30
Nalbuphine	—	10	—	—
OxyCODONE	20	—	0.2	10 to 20
Oxymorphone	10	1	—	5 to 10
Pentazocine	50	30	—	—

Guidelines for Conversion to Oral Methadone in Adults[5]

Oral Morphine Dose or Equivalent (mg/day)	Oral Morphine:Oral Methadone (Conversion Ratio)
<90	4:1
90 to 300	8:1
>300	12:1

[1]Elderly patients: Starting dose should be lower for this population group.

[2]Standard parenteral doses (IM) for acute pain in adults; can be used to convert doses for IV infusions and repeated small IV boluses. For single IV boluses, use half the IM dose.

[3]The pharmacokinetics of opioids in children and infants >6 months old are similar to adults, but infants <6 months old, especially premature or physically compromised ones, are at risk of apnea.

[4]Not recommended for routine use

[5]Conversion of higher doses may be guided by the following (consult a pain or palliative care specialist if unfamiliar with methadone prescribing): As the total daily chronic dose of morphine increases, the equianalgesic dose ratio (morphine:methadone) changes (American Pain Society 2008). Total daily dose should be divided by 3; delivered every 8 hours. Methadone is significantly more potent with repetitive dosing (due to its active metabolite). Begin methadone at lower doses and gradually titrate. Applicability to pediatric patients is unknown.

Morphine Equivalent Dose Table

This table should only be used to determine the morphine equivalent dose and **should NOT be used to determine doses when converting a patient from one opioid to another**.

Drug	Morphine Equivalent Dose (MED) Conversion Factor
Buprenorphine patch[1]	12.6
Buprenorphine tablet or film	10
Butorphanol	7
Codeine	0.15
Dihydrocodeine	0.25
FentaNYL buccal or sublingual tablet, lozenge, or troche[2]	0.13
FentaNYL film or oral spray[3]	0.18
FentaNYL nasal spray[4]	0.16
FentaNYL patch[5]	7.2
Hydrocodone	1
HYDROmorphone	4
Levorphanol tartrate	11
Meperidine hydrochloride	0.1
Methadone	3
Morphine	1
Nalbuphine	1

OPIOID CONVERSION TABLE AND MORPHINE EQUIVALENT DOSE TABLE

Drug	Morphine Equivalent Dose (MED) Conversion Factor
Opium	1
OxyCODONE	1.5
Oxymorphone	3
Pentazocine	0.37
Tapentadol	0.4
TraMADol	0.1

[1]The MED conversion factor for buprenorphine patches is based on the assumption that 1 mg of parenteral buprenorphine is equivalent to 75 mg of oral morphine, that one patch delivers the dispensed mcg/hr over a 24-hour day, and that the patch remains in place for 7 days.

[2]The MED conversion factor for fentanyl buccal tablets, sublingual tablets, lozenges, and troches is 0.13. This conversion factor should be multiplied by the number of mcg in a given lozenge/troche.

[3]The MED conversion factor for fentanyl film and oral spray is 0.18. This reflects a 40% greater bioavailability for films compared to lozenges and tablets and 38% greater bioavailability for oral sprays compared to lozenges and tablets.

[4]The MED conversion factor for fentanyl nasal spray is 0.16, which reflects a 20% greater bioavailability for sprays compared to lozenges and tablets.

[5]The MED conversion factor for fentanyl patches is based on the assumption that 1 mg of parenteral fentanyl is equivalent to 100 mg of oral morphine, that one patch delivers the dispensed mcg/hour over a 24-hour day, and that the patch remains in place for 72 hours.

This table is derived from the Department of Health and Human Services (DHHS) Centers for Medicare and Medicaid Services (CMS) "Opioid Morphine Equivalent Conversion Factors" table. Available at https://www.cms.gov/Medicare/Prescription-Drug-Coverage/PrescriptionDrugCovContra/Downloads/Opioid-Morphine-EQ-Conversion-Factors-March-2015.pdf

REFERENCES

Department of Health and Human Services (DHHS) Centers for Medicare and Medicaid Services (CMS). Opioid morphine equivalent conversion factors. March 2015. Available at https://www.cms.gov/Medicare/Prescription-Drug-Coverage/PrescriptionDrugCovContra/Downloads/Opioid-Morphine-EQ-Conversion-Factors-March-2015.pdf

National Cancer Institute. Pain (PDQ). Last modified May 7, 2009. Available at http://www.cancer.gov/cancertopics/pdq/supportivecare/pain/Health-Professional/page1

National Comprehensive Cancer Network (NCCN). Clinical practice guidelines in oncology: adult cancer pain. Version 1, 2009. Available at http://www.nccn.org/professionals/physician_gls/PDF/pain.pdf

Patanwala AE, Duby J, Waters D, Erstad BL. Opioid conversions in acute care. *Ann Pharmacother.* 2007;41(2):255-266.

Principles of Analgesic Use in the Treatment of Acute Pain and Cancer Pain. 6th ed. Glenview, IL: American Pain Society; 2008.

ORAL ANTICOAGULANT COMPARISON CHART

Medication	Mechanism of Action	Metabolism	Monitoring Parameters	Pharmacotherapy Pearls	Reversal Strategies[1]	Preoperative/Preprocedure Management (General Guide)
Warfarin	Inhibits formation of vitamin K-dependent clotting factors II, VII, IX, X, and proteins C and S	CYP2C9 CYP1A2 CYP3A4 CYP2C19	PT/INR (individualized; depends on INR stability)	CYP1A2, 3A4, 2C9, and 2C19 drug interactions and vitamin K-containing food interactions Full therapeutic effect usually seen within 5 to 7 days Half-life is ~40 hours	Vitamin K (route and dose will depend on clinical situation and INR) For major bleeding (at any INR): Consider PCC with vitamin K ± FFP	Hold at least 5 days before surgery; depending on urgency of surgery/procedure, may administer low-dose IV or oral vitamin K Minor dental and minor dermatological procedures or cataract surgery: Continue warfarin (with hemostatic agent [dental] or local hemostasis [dermatological]); may also discontinue use 2 to 3 days prior to dental procedures. Patients with prior stroke undergoing dental procedures should routinely continue warfarin.
Dabigatran (Pradaxa)	Directly inhibits thrombin	Hepatic glucuronidation P-gp substrate	Routine lab monitoring not required; aPTT, ECT (if available), TT (most sensitive) may be used to detect presence of dabigatran Renal function	Compliance issues (BID dosing) Specific conversions to/from warfarin, parenteral anticoagulants Renal dosing adjustment required; per ACCP, contraindicated with CrCl ≤30 mL/minute Use with caution in patients ≥80 years of age Dose reduction or avoidance required if used with dronedarone, ketoconazole, P-gp inhibitors P-gp drug interactions Half-life is 12 to 17 hours; considerably prolonged with severe renal impairment	Idarucizumab Dabigatran is ~60% dialyzable Activated charcoal may be used if ingestion occurred <2 hours prior to presentation	CrCl ≥50 mL/minute: Hold 1 to 2 days before surgery CrCl <50 mL/minute: Hold 3 to 5 days before surgery May consider holding for >5 days in patients undergoing major surgery, spinal puncture, or insertion of a spinal or epidural catheter or port
Edoxaban (Savaysa)	Directly inhibits factor Xa	CYP3A4 (minor) Hydrolysis (minimal) P-gp substrate	Routine lab monitoring not required	Specific conversions to/from warfarin, parenteral anticoagulants DVT/PE: Dose reduction necessary for patients <60 kg, concomitant P-gp inhibitor, or if CrCl 15 to 50 mL/min. Not recommended if CrCl <15 mL/min NVAF: **Do not use if CrCl >95 mL/min.** Dose reduction necessary if CrCl 15 to 50 mL/min. Not recommended if CrCl <15 mL/min	No specific antidote Edoxaban is **not** dialyzable	Discontinue at least 24 hours prior to elective surgery or invasive procedures

Medication	Mechanism of Action	Metabolism	Monitoring Parameters	Pharmacotherapy Pearls	Reversal Strategies[1]	Preoperative/Preprocedure Management (General Guide)
Rivaroxaban (Xarelto)	Directly inhibits factor Xa	CYP3A4 CYP3A5 CYP2J2 P-gp substrate	Routine lab monitoring not required; may use PT to detect presence of rivaroxaban. Renal and hepatic function	Administer doses ≥15 mg/day with food. Dosing frequency depends on indication. Specific conversions to/from warfarin, parenteral anticoagulants. Renal dosing adjustment required. Avoid in moderate or severe hepatic impairment. CYP3A4 and P-gp drug interactions. Half-life is 5 to 9 hours; slightly prolonged with renal impairment	No specific antidote; for major bleeding, may consider PCC, activated PCC (ie, FEIBA NF), or recombinant factor VIIa[3]. Rivaroxaban is **not** dialyzable	Hold at least 24 hours before surgery; longer duration of treatment cessation may be necessary based on individual patient situation and physician clinical judgment
Apixaban (Eliquis)	Directly inhibits factor Xa	CYP3A4 P-gp substrate	Routine lab monitoring not required; PT, INR, and aPTT may be used to detect presence of apixaban	Compliance issues (BID dosing). Specific conversions to/from warfarin, parenteral anticoagulants. Renal dosing adjustment required (NVAF); the AHA/ASA recommends to avoid use with CrCl <25 mL/minute. Not recommended in patients with severe liver impairment. CYP3A4 and P-gp drug interactions. Half-life is ~8 to 15 hours; slightly prolonged with renal impairment	No specific antidote; for major bleeding, may consider PCC, activated PCC (ie, FEIBA NF), or recombinant factor VIIa. Apixaban is **not** dialyzable. Activated charcoal may be used if ingestion occurred within 2 to 6 hours of presentation	Hold at least 24 to 48 hours, depending on risk or location of bleeding, before elective surgery or invasive procedures.

Abbreviations: ACCP = American College of Chest Physicians, AHA/ASA = American Heart Association/American Stroke Association, aPTT = activated partial thromboplastin time, BID = twice daily, DVT = deep venous thrombosis, ECT = ecarin clotting time, FFP = fresh frozen plasma, INR = international normalized ratio, NVAF = nonvalvular atrial fibrillation, PCC = prothrombin complex concentrate, PE = pulmonary embolism, P-gp = P-glycoprotein, PT = prothrombin time, TT = thrombin time.

Note: Recommendations listed reflect only the US labeling or US clinical practice guidelines.

[1]Management of anticoagulant-associated bleeding requires careful consideration of the indication for anticoagulant therapy and bleeding extent (eg, epistaxis vs intracranial hemorrhage); minor bleeding may only require local hemostasis.

[2]The use of rFVIIa in healthy subjects treated with another direct thrombin inhibitor, melagatran (not FDA-approved), did not reverse the anticoagulant effects of melagatran.

[3]The evidence in support of these reversal strategies is limited; an exception to this may be the use of a 4-factor PCC for rivaroxaban reversal. The only available 4-factor PCC currently in the US is Kcentra. Other 4-factor PCCs **not** available in the US include Beriplex P/N, Cofact, and Octaplex. Bebulin VH and Profilnine SD **do not** contain adequate levels of factor VII and are considered 3-factor PCCs.

Armstrong MJ, Gronseth G, Anderson DC, et al. Summary of evidence-based guideline: periprocedural management of antithrombotic medications in patients with ischemic cerebrovascular disease: report of the Guideline Development Subcommittee of the American Academy of Neurology. *Neurology.* 2013;80(22):2065-2069.

Furie KL, Goldstein LB, Albers GW, et al. Oral antithrombotic agents for the prevention of stroke in nonvalvular atrial fibrillation: a science advisory for health care professionals from the American Heart Association/American Stroke Association. *Stroke.* 2012;43 (12):3442-3453.

Guyatt GH, Akl EA, Crowther M, et al. Executive summary: antithrombotic therapy and prevention of thrombosis, 9th ed: American College of Chest Physicians evidence-based clinical practice guidelines. *Chest.* 2012;141(2 Suppl):7S-47S.

Kaatz S, Kouides PA, Garcia DA, et al. Guidance on the emergent reversal of oral thrombin and factor Xa inhibitors. *Am J Hematol.* 2012;87(Suppl 1):S141-S145.

Levi M, Eerenberg E, Kamphuisen PW. Bleeding risk and reversal strategies for old and new anticoagulants and antiplatelet agents. *J Thromb Haemost.* 2011;9(9):1705-1712.

Poulsen BK, Grove EL, Husted SE. New oral anticoagulants: a review of the literature with particular emphasis on patients with impaired renal function. *Drugs.* 2012;72(13):1739-1753.

Wolzt M, Levi M, Sarich TC, et al. Effect of recombinant factor VIIa on melagatran-induced inhibition of thrombin generation and platelet activation in healthy volunteers. *Thromb Haemost.* 2004;91(6):1090-1096.

REVERSAL OF ORAL ANTICOAGULANTS

Both oral and parenteral anticoagulants have established use in the prevention and treatment of a variety of thrombotic conditions (eg, acute coronary syndrome, venous thromboembolism, stroke). Although much has been done to prevent bleeding events associated with these agents, hemorrhagic events still continue to occur. Therefore, a thorough understanding of how best to reverse these agents when bleeding does occur is imperative. Information in this area is surfacing rapidly and recommendations may be changing. Refer to the most recent literature or guidelines for more detail and guidance. Reversal of parenteral anticoagulants, such as heparin and low molecular weight heparin (LMWH), and management of bleeding associated with these agents is established and beyond the focus of this piece.

For many years, vitamin K antagonists (eg, warfarin, acenocoumarol) were the only effective oral anticoagulants available. Recently, newer oral anticoagulants have been developed and are now marketed for prevention of stroke in patients with nonvalvular atrial fibrillation and prevention and treatment of venous thromboembolism. These include dabigatran, apixaban, and rivaroxaban. Dabigatran is an oral direct thrombin inhibitor. Apixaban, edoxaban, and rivaroxaban are both oral factor Xa inhibitors.

VITAMIN K ANTAGONIST-INDUCED BLEEDING

Warfarin is the more commonly used vitamin K antagonist (VKA) in North America. The management of bleeding and reversal of other VKAs is the same. Therefore, the term VKA will be used here. VKAs interfere with the cyclic interconversion of vitamin K and vitamin K epoxide, ultimately resulting in lowered production of effective factors II, VII, IX, and X. VKAs also inhibit the production of proteins C, S, and Z which may result in procoagulation. The half-life of racemic warfarin ranges from 36 to 42 hours. Other VKAs, such as acenocoumarol, have significantly shorter half-lives. Warfarin, due to metabolism via the cytochrome P450 enzyme system (specifically CYP2C9, CYP3A4, CYP1A2, and CYP2C19), is subject to a number of drug-drug interactions which may occur by inhibiting these isoenzymes, leading to reduced metabolism and elevated warfarin concentrations. Intensity of anticoagulation with VKAs can predict the incidence of bleeding events. When the INR is greater than 5, the incidence of bleeding increases dramatically; patient factors also play a major role in risk of bleeding (eg, prior history of bleeding, advanced age, renal insufficiency) (Ageno 2012).

Patients with elevated INR may not need reversal unless undergoing an invasive procedure. If the invasive procedure is elective, the procedure should be delayed until INR is acceptable for the procedure. In general, for patients with an INR of 6 to 10, up to ~2.5 days may elapse before the INR reduces to <4 (Patel 2000). Some patients may require bridging with a parenteral anticoagulant during this time to prevent thrombosis.

Patients who are bleeding may require reversal with vitamin K (or phytonadione). Rapid reversal is necessary if the bleeding is life-threatening. In this case, the use of intravenous vitamin K and either fresh frozen plasma (FFP), prothrombin complex concentrates (PCC), or recombinant factor VIIa (rFVIIa) becomes imperative. Currently, the American College of Chest Physicians recommends an intravenous vitamin K dose of 5 to 10 mg administered slowly. Due to the occurrence of anaphylactoid reaction with rapid intravenous administration with vitamin K, intravenous vitamin K should always be diluted in a minimum of 50 mL of a compatible solution and infused over at least 20 minutes (Ageno 2012). Reduction of INR with intravenous administration usually begins within 2 hours of administration. Subcutaneous administration of vitamin K is not recommended due to slower resolution of elevated INR.

The choice as to which coagulation factor (FFP, PCC, or rFVIIa) to use in addition to intravenous vitamin K for the patient who has life-threatening bleeding has not been established. Advantages and disadvantages exist with all the coagulation factors. Regardless of which one is chosen, the target INR for the patient with a life-threatening bleed is typically <1.5. FFP contains all of the factors inhibited by warfarin (factors II, VII, IX, and X) and would be an ideal agent to use for reversal. However, high volumes of FFP may be problematic in patients who are sensitive to rapid fluid shifts (eg, heart failure). FFP also has the disadvantages of possible allergic reaction, transfusion-related lung injury (TRALI), transmission of infection, and prolonged preparation time due to frozen storage. A solvent-detergent treated plasma substitute (OctaplaseLG) is available and has been shown to not cause TRALI and other side effects seen with FFP. PCCs, although more costly compared to FFP, are advantageous in that they have a lower infusion volume, lower transmission rate of infection, can be administered rapidly with rapid reversal of VKA-associated coagulopathy, do not require cross-matching, and are associated with less complications. Currently, the American College of Chest Physicians recommends the use of four-factor PCCs over FFP and rFVIIa. The only available four-factor PCC in the US is Kcentra (known as Beriplex P/N or Confidex outside the US). Other four-factor PCCs not available in the US include Cofact, Kanokad, and Octaplex. Bebulin and Profilnine do not contain adequate levels of factor VII and are considered three-factor PCCs (see table on next page).

Composition of Prothrombin Complex Concentrates

Prothrombin Complex Concentrate	Factor II	Factor VII	Factor IX	Factor X	Heparin	Human Antithrombin III	Protein C	Protein S	Protein Z
"Three-Factor (minimal factor VII component) PCCs"									
Bebulin	24 to 38 IU/mL	<5 IU/mL	24 to 38 IU/mL	24 to 38 IU/mL	<0.15 IU/IU FIX	–	–	–	–
Profilnine	NMT 150 units per 100 FIX units	NMT 35 units per 100 FIX units	100 units	NMT 100 units per 100 FIX units	–	–	–	–	–
"Four-Factor PCCs"									
Cofact[a]	14 to 35 IU/mL	7 to 20 IU/mL	25 IU/mL	14 to 35 IU/mL	–	<0.6 IU/mL	11 to 39 IU/mL	1 to 8 IU/mL	–
Kanokad[a]	14 to 35 IU/mL	7 to 20 IU/mL	25 IU/mL	14 to 35 IU/mL	–	–	–	–	–
Kcentra (known as Beriplex P/N or Confidex outside the US)	19 to 40 IU/mL	10 to 25 IU/mL	20 to 31 IU/mL	25 to 51 IU/mL	0.4 to 2 IU/mL	0.2 to 1.5 IU/mL	21 to 41 IU/mL	12 to 34 IU/mL	–
Octaplex[a]	14 to 38 IU/mL	9 to 24 IU/mL	25 IU/mL	18 to 30 IU/mL	5 to 12.5 IU/mL		13 to 31 IU/mL	12 to 32 IU/mL	–
"Activated PCC"									
FEIBA NF	1.3 IU/IU[b]	0.9 IU/IU	1.4 IU/IU[b]	1.1 IU/IU[b]	–		1.1 IU/IU	–	

FIX = Factor IX, NMT = not more than

[a]Not available in the US

[b]Mainly nonactivated form

The use of rFVIIa gained some interest; however, it has not been shown to be superior to PCC or FFP and is the most expensive agent of the three. The combination of rFVIIa and three-factor PCC (along with intravenous vitamin K) has been used with some success (Sarode 2012); however, the combination cannot be recommended at this time.

DABIGATRAN-INDUCED BLEEDING

Dabigatran is an oral direct thrombin inhibitor with an elimination half-life of 12 to 17 hours. Dabigatran is 80% excreted in the urine as unchanged drug and therefore elimination half-life is prolonged in patients with renal impairment (up to 28 hours with severe impairment). Dabigatran is hepatically metabolized via glucuronidation to active acylglucuronide isomers. Although not a substrate for CYP450, dabigatran is a substrate of P-glycoprotein (P-gp). Therefore, P-gp inhibitors may increase dabigatran concentrations, resulting in a higher risk of bleeding events.

Unlike its parenteral counterparts (eg, argatroban), dabigatran has a specific reversal agent. Idarucizumab (Praxbind), a monoclonal antibody fragment, was recently approved for the reversal of the anticoagulant effects of dabigatran. Idarucizumab was evaluated in a phase 3 clinical trial for use in patients who either had overt, uncontrollable, or life-threatening bleeding or required surgery or other invasive procedure that could not be delayed for at least 8 hours and hemostasis was required. Idarucizumab was shown to completely reverse the anticoagulant effect of dabigatran (Pollack 2015). The dose of idarucizumab was devised based upon the highest range of dabigatran concentrations measured within the RE-LY trial (Pollack 2015; Reilly 2014). Although the duration of effect typically lasts at least 24 hours, coagulation parameters (eg, aPTT, TT, ecarin clotting time [not routinely available]) reelevated in a limited number of patients between 12 and 24 hours after administration; some patients experienced reelevation as early as 1 to 4 hours after administration which may have been due to high initial baseline dabigatran concentrations (Pollack 2015). Although the INR may be elevated with dabigatran use, vitamin K is not effective for dabigatran-induced bleeding. In addition, the aPTT rises as dabigatran concentrations increase; however, the use of protamine will not reverse these effects on the aPTT. Activated charcoal should be administered if oral intake was recent (ie, within a couple of hours of presentation). Hemodialysis, although this may be impractical, has been shown to remove 62% to 68% over 2 to 4 hours (Stangier 2010). Prior to the availability of idarucizumab, multiple case reports with various types of dabigatran-induced hemorrhages showed successful achievement of hemostasis using aPCC (ie, FEIBA) and the use of a four-factor PCC (Cofact; not available in the US) has been shown to be ineffective for dabigatran reversal (Dager 2013; Eerenberg 2011; Faust 2014; Kiraly 2013; Neyens 2014; Schulman 2014). Clinicians should be aware that there is no standardized laboratory assay to monitor the reversal strategy chosen.

ORAL FACTOR XA INHIBITOR-INDUCED BLEEDING

Apixaban, edoxaban, and rivaroxaban are oral factor Xa inhibitors. Apixaban has an elimination half-life of 8 to 15 hours and is metabolized to a minor degree via the cytochrome P450 system (specifically CYP1A2, CYP2C19, CYP2C8, CYP2C9, and CYP3A4) and is a P-gp substrate. Apixaban is also partially excreted (~27%) as unchanged drug in the urine. Edoxaban has an elimination half-life of 10 to 14 hours, is metabolized minimally (hydrolysis, conjugation, and oxidation by CYP3A4), is a substrate for P-gp, and is excreted (~50%) as unchanged drug in the urine. Rivaroxaban has an elimination half-life of 5 to 9 hours and is excreted (~36%) as unchanged drug in the urine. Rivaroxaban is hepatically metabolized via CYP3A4/5 and CYP2J2 and is a substrate of P-gp as well.

The use of rFVIIa has been shown to decrease the bleeding time in animal models; however, it does not reverse the anticoagulant effect of rivaroxaban. The use of rFVIIa has not been formally evaluated in humans treated with apixaban, edoxaban, or rivaroxaban. The use of a four-factor PCC (Cofact; not available in the US) has been shown to reverse the anticoagulant effect of rivaroxaban in humans (Eerenberg 2011). A more recent in vitro comparison of the 3 procoagulants (aPCC [FEIBA], 4-factor PCC [Beriplex P/N], and rFVIIa [NovoSeven]) for the reversal of rivaroxaban demonstrated that rFVIIa and aPCC were more effective at reversing the effects of rivaroxaban on the PT, clotting time, and thrombin generation lag time; however, the reversal effect reached a plateau with a maximal effect of ~50% (Perzborn 2014). Although this information is helpful, the lack of in vivo human data still does not allow an overall formal recommendation to be made for rapid reversal with these agents in bleeding patients. However, based on the limited data, some have suggested the use of a 4-factor PCC (eg, Kcentra) as the first-line reversal agent for oral factor Xa inhibitors (Nutescu 2013). For life-threatening bleeding, the EHRA suggests the use of a 4-factor PCC; aPCC may be considered as first-line if a 4-factor PCC is unavailable (EHRA [Heidbuchel 2013]). As with dabigatran, there is no standardized laboratory assay to monitor the reversal strategy chosen for oral factor Xa inhibitors.

CONCLUSION

The approach to the bleeding patient receiving oral anticoagulation is challenging. While idarucizumab is now available for reversal of dabigatran anticoagulation, data supporting other specific reversal agents is somewhat lacking beyond the known antidotes used for specific therapies (eg, warfarin). Research in this area is expanding the knowledge; however, much research is still needed to further define specific approaches to patients receiving newer oral anticoagulants. Reversal agents for some of these new oral anticoagulants are being developed, such as the recombinant antidote andexanet alfa (PRT064445) for factor Xa inhibitors or ciraparantag (PER977) which is a water soluble molecule for direct inhibitors of factor Xa and IIa, as well as heparin-based anticoagulants. Ciraparantag has also been reported to reverse the effects of all anticoagulants except VKAs and argatroban. Andexanet alfa has demonstrated reversal of factor Xa inhibitors (ie, apixaban, betrixaban, and rivaroxaban) within minutes of administration and ciraparantag within 10 to 30 minutes (Das 2015; Lu 2013). These reveral agents may become available in the near future.

REFERENCES

Ageno W, Gallus AS, Wittkowsky A, et al. Oral anticoagulant therapy: antithrombotic therapy and prevention of thrombosis, 9th ed: American College of Chest Physicians evidence-based clinical practice guidelines. *Chest*. 2012;141(2 Suppl):e44S-e88S.

Baron TH, Kamath PS, McBane RD. Management of antithrombotic therapy in patients undergoing invasive procedures. *N Engl J Med*. 2013;368 (22):2113-2124.

Bauer KA. Reversal of antithrombotic agents. *Am J Hematol*. 2012;87(Suppl 1):S119-S126.

Bechtel BF, Nunez TC, Lyon JA, Cotton BA, Barrett TW. Treatments for reversing warfarin anticoagulation in patients with acute intracranial hemorrhage: a structured literature review. *Int J Emerg Med*. 2011;4(1):40.

Dager WE. Developing a management plan for oral anticoagulant reversal. *Am J Health Syst Pharm*. 2013;70(10 Suppl 1):S21-S31.

Dager WE, Gosselin RC, Kitchen S, Dwyre D. Dabigatran effects on the international normalized ratio, activated partial thromboplastin time, thrombin time, and fibrinogen: a multicenter, in vitro study. *Ann Pharmacother*. 2012;46(12):1627-1636.

Dager WE, Gosselin RC, Roberts AJ. Reversing dabigatran in life-threatening bleeding occurring during cardiac ablation with factor eight inhibitor bypassing activity. *Crit Care Med*. 2013;41(5):e42-e46

Das A, Liu D. Novel antidotes for target specific oral anticoagulants. *Exp Hematol Oncol*. 2015;4:25.

Dumkow LE, Voss JR, Peters M, Jennings DL. Reversal of dabigatran-induced bleeding with a prothrombin complex concentrate and fresh frozen plasma. *Am J Health Syst Pharm*. 2012;69(19):1646-1650.

Dzik WS. Reversal of drug-induced anticoagulation: old solutions and new problems. *Transfusion*. 2012;52(Suppl 1):45S-55S.

Eerenberg ES, Kamphuisen PW, Sijpkens MK, Meijers JC, Buller HR, Levi M. Reversal of rivaroxaban and dabigatran by prothrombin complex concentrate: a randomized, placebo-controlled, crossover study in healthy subjects. *Circulation*. 2011;124(14):1573-1579.

Faust AC, Peterson EJ. Management of dabigatran-associated intracerebral and intraventricular hemorrhage: a case report. *J Emerg Med*. 2014;46 (4):525-529.

Goldstein JN, Refaai MA, Milling TJ Jr, et al. Four-factor prothrombin complex concentrate versus plasma for rapid vitamin K antagonist reversal in patients needing urgent surgical or invasive interventions: a phase 3b, open-label, non-inferiority, randomised trial [published online February 25, 2015]. *Lancet*.

Heidbuchel H, Verhamme P, Alings M, et al. European Heart Rhythm Association Practical Guide on the use of new oral anticoagulants in patients with non-valvular atrial fibrillation. *Europace*. 2013;15(5):625-651.

Holbrook A, Schulman S, Witt DM, et al. Evidence-based management of anticoagulant therapy: antithrombotic therapy and prevention of thrombosis, 9th ed: American College of Chest Physicians evidence-based clinical practice guidelines. *Chest*. 2012;141(2 Suppl):e152S-e184S.

Kaatz S, Kouides PA, Garcia DA, et al. Guidance on the emergent reversal of oral thrombin and factor Xa inhibitors. *Am J Hematol*. 2012;87(Suppl 1): S141-S145.

Kalus JS. Pharmacologic interventions for reversing the effects of oral anticoagulants. *Am J Health Syst Pharm*. 2013;70(10 Suppl 1):S12-S21.

Kiraly A, Lyden A, Periyanayagam U, Chan J, Pang PS. Management of hemorrhage complicated by novel oral anticoagulants in the emergency department: case report from the northwestern emergency medicine residency. *Am J Ther*. 2013;20(3):300-306.

Lu G, DeGuzman FR, Hollenbach SJ, et al. A specific antidote for reversal of anticoagulation by direct and indirect inhibitors of coagulation factor Xa. *Nat Med*. 2013;19(4):446-451.

Marlu R, Hodaj E, Paris A, Albaladejo P, Cracowski JL, Pernod G. Effect of non-specific reversal agents on anticoagulant activity of dabigatran and rivaroxaban: a randomised crossover *ex vivo* study in healthy volunteers. *Thromb Haemost*. 2012;108(2):217-224.

Miesbach W, Seifried E. New direct oral anticoagulants – current therapeutic options and treatment recommendations for bleeding complications. *Thromb Haemost*. 2012;108(4):625-632.

Miyares MA, Davis K. Newer oral anticoagulants: a review of laboratory monitoring options and reversal agents in the hemorrhagic patient. *Am J Health Syst Pharm*. 2012;69(17):1473-1484.

Neyens R, Bohm N, Cearley M, Andrews C, Chalela J. Dabigatran-associated subdural hemorrhage: using thromboelastography (TEG®) to guide decision-making. *J Thromb Thrombolysis*. 2014;37(2):80-83.

Nitzki-George D, Wozniak I, Caprini JA. Current state of knowledge on oral anticoagulant reversal using procoagulant factors. *Ann Pharmacother*. 2013;47(6):841-855.

Nutescu EA, Dager WE, Kalus JS, Lewin JJ 3rd, Cipolle MD. Management of bleeding and reversal strategies for oral anticoagulants: clinical practice considerations. *Am J Health Syst Pharm*. 2013;70(21):1914-1929.

Ortel TL. Perioperative management of patients on chronic antithrombotic therapy. *Hematology Am Soc Hematol Educ Program*. 2012;2012:529-535.

Patel RJ, Witt DM, Saseen JJ, Tillman DJ, Wilkinson DS. Randomized, placebo-controlled trial of oral phytonadione for excessive anticoagulation. *Pharmacotherapy*. 2000;20(10):1159-1166.

Patriquin C, Crowther M. Treatment of warfarin-associated coagulopathy with vitamin K. *Expert Rev Hematol*. 2011;4(6):657-665.

Perzborn E, Heitmeier S, Laux V, Buchmüller A. Reversal of rivaroxaban-induced anticoagulation with prothrombin complex concentrate, activated prothrombin complex concentrate and recombinant activated factor VII in vitro. *Thromb Res*. 2014;133(4):671-681.

Pollack CV Jr, Reilly PA, Eikelboom J, et al. Idarucizumab for dabigatran reversal [published online June 22, 2015]. *N Engl J Med*.

Reilly PA, Lehr T, Haertter S, et al. The effect of dabigatran plasma concentrations and patient characteristics on the frequency of ischemic stroke and major bleeding in atrial fibrillation patients: the RE-LY Trial (Randomized Evaluation of Long-Term Anticoagulation Therapy). *J Am Coll Cardiol*. 2014;63(4):321-328.

Sarode R, Matevosyan K, Bhagat R, Rutherford C, Madden C, Beshay JE. Rapid warfarin reversal: a 3-factor prothrombin complex concentrate and recombinant factor VIIa cocktail for intracerebral hemorrhage. *J Neurosurg*. 2012;116(3):491-497.

Sarode R, Milling TJ Jr, Refaai MA, et al. Efficacy and safety of a four-factor prothrombin complex concentrate (4F-PCC) in patients on vitamin K antagonists presenting with major bleeding: a randomized, plasma-controlled, phase IIIb study. *Circulation*. 2013.

Schulman S, Ritchie B, Goy JK, Nahirniak S, Almutawa M, Ghanny S. Activated prothrombin complex concentrate for dabigatran-associated bleeding. *Br J Haematol*. 2014;164(2):308-310.

Siegal DM, Crowther MA. Acute management of bleeding in patients on novel oral anticoagulants. *Eur Heart J*. 2013;34(7):489-498b.

Stangier J, Rathgen K, Stähle H, Mazur D. Influence of renal impairment on the pharmacokinetics and pharmacodynamics of oral dabigatran etexilate: an open-label, parallel-group, single-centre study. *Clin Pharmacokinet*. 2010;49(4):259-268.

van Ryn J, Stangier J, Haertter S, et al. Dabigatran etexilate – a novel, reversible, oral direct thrombin inhibitor: interpretation of coagulation assays and reversal of anticoagulant activity. *Thromb Haemost*. 2010;103(6):1116-1127.

Wanek MR, Horn ET, Elapavaluru S, Baroody SC, Sokos G. Safe use of hemodialysis for dabigatran removal before cardiac surgery. *Ann Pharmacother*. 2012;46(9):e21.

Weitz JI, Eikelboom JW, Samama MM; American College of Chest Physicians. New antithrombotic drugs: antithrombotic therapy and prevention of thrombosis, 9th ed: American College of Chest Physicians evidence-based clinical practice guidelines. *Chest*. 2012;141(2 Suppl):e120S-e151S.

Weitz JI, Quinlan DJ, Eikelboom JW. Periprocedural management and approach to bleeding in patients taking dabigatran. *Circulation*. 2012;126(20):2428-2432.

ORAL ANTIPLATELET COMPARISON CHART

Medication	Mechanism of Action	Reversible Platelet Inhibition	Prodrug	Metabolism	Pharmacotherapy Pearls	Reversal Strategies[1]	Preoperative/Preprocedure Management (General Guide)
Aspirin	Inhibits cyclooxygenase-1 and 2	No	No	CYP2C9	Chronic NSAID use can compromise antiplatelet effects Monitor for GI ulceration	No specific antidote Consider platelet transfusion ± DDAVP Normal platelet function returns within 7 to 10 days after discontinuation	Hold 7 to 10 days before surgery May be continued through surgery for CABG or noncardiac surgery in patients with moderate to high cardiac risk Minor dental or dermatological procedures or cataract surgery: Continue through procedure. AAN recommends continuation when undergoing any dental procedure for patients taking aspirin for ischemic stroke prevention.
Cilostazol (Pletal)	Inhibits platelet phosphodiesterase III	Yes	No	CYP3A4 CYP2C19 CYP1A2 CYP2D6	Administer before or 2 hours after meals Contraindicated in patients with heart failure of any severity CYP3A4 and 2C19 drug interactions	No specific antidote Normal platelet function returns within 4 days after discontinuation	Hold 2 to 3 days before surgery
Clopidogrel (Plavix)	Inhibits P2Y$_{12}$ component of ADP receptors	No	Yes	CYP2C19 CYP3A4	CYP2C19 inhibitors may reduce concentrations of active metabolite CYP2C19 polymorphisms may affect clopidogrel efficacy	No specific antidote Consider platelet transfusion ± DDAVP Normal platelet function returns within 7 to 10 days after discontinuation	Hold 5 to 10 days before surgery[2]
Prasugrel (Effient)	Inhibits P2Y$_{12}$ component of ADP receptors	No	Yes	CYP3A4 CYP2B6	Reduce maintenance dose to 5 mg in patients <60 kg Contraindicated in patients with history of stroke, TIA Not recommended in patients ≥75 years of age	No specific antidote Consider platelet transfusion ± DDAVP Normal platelet function returns within 5 to 9 days after discontinuation	Hold 5 to 7 days before surgery[2]
Ticagrelor (Brilinta)	Inhibits P2Y$_{12}$ component of ADP receptors	Yes	No	CYP3A4 CYP3A5	Used in combination with aspirin; daily maintenance aspirin dose should not exceed 81 mg CYP3A4 drug interactions BID dosing Monitor closely for dyspnea, bradyarrhythmia (including ventricular pauses)	No specific antidote Consider aminocaproic acid, tranexamic acid, recombinant factor VIIa Normal platelet function returns within 3 to 5 days after discontinuation	Hold at least 5 days before surgery[2]

Medication	Mechanism of Action	Reversible Platelet Inhibition	Prodrug	Metabolism	Pharmacotherapy Pearls	Reversal Strategies[1]	Preoperative/Preprocedure Management (General Guide)
Ticlopidine	Inhibits P2Y[12] component of ADP receptors	No	Yes	CYP3A4	Black Box warning on hematologic toxicities (aplastic anemia, TTP) Frequent CBC monitoring required BID dosing	No specific antidote Consider platelet transfusion ± DDAVP Normal platelet function returns within 5 to 10 days after discontinuation	Hold 10 to 14 days before surgery
Vorapaxar	Inhibits PAR-1	Yes[3]	No	CYP3A4 CYP2J2	Use in combination with aspirin and/or clopidogrel Contraindicated in patients with history of stroke, TIA, or ICH Extremely long effective half-life of 3 to 5 days	No specific antidote Significant inhibition of platelet aggregation remains 4 weeks after discontinuation	No recommendation can be made

[1]Management of antiplatelet-associated bleeding requires careful consideration of the indication for antiplatelet therapy and bleeding extent (eg, epistaxis vs intracranial hemorrhage); minor bleeding may only require local hemostasis.

[2]When urgent CABG is necessary, the ACCF/AHA CABG guidelines recommend discontinuation for at least 24 hours prior to surgery (Hillis 2011).

[3]Due to the very long half-life, vorapaxar is effectively irreversible.

Armstrong MJ, Gronseth G, Anderson DC, et al. Summary of evidence-based guideline: periprocedural management of antithrombotic medications in patients with ischemic cerebrovascular disease: report of the Guideline Development Subcommittee of the American Academy of Neurology. *Neurology.* 2013;80(22):2065-2069.

Hillis LD, Smith PK, Anderson JL, et al. 2011 ACCF/AHA guideline for coronary artery bypass graft surgery: executive summary: a report of the American College of Cardiology Foundation/American Heart Association task force on practice guidelines. *Circulation.* 2011;124(23):2610-2642.

Levi M, Eerenberg E, Kamphuisen PW. Bleeding risk and reversal strategies for old and new anticoagulants and antiplatelet agents. *J Thromb Haemost.* 2011;9(9):1705-1712.

Patrono C, Andreotti F, Arnesen H, et al. Antiplatelet agents for the treatment and prevention of atherothrombosis. *Eur Heart J.* 2011;32(23):2922-2932.

PERITONEAL DIALYSIS SOLUTIONS

	Product and Distributor	Icodextrin (g/liter)	Dextrose (g/liter)	Sodium (mEq/Liter)	Calcium (mEq/Liter)	Magnesium (mEq/Liter)	Chloride (mEq/Liter)	Lactate (mEq/Liter)	Osmolarity (mOsm/liter)	How Supplied
Rx	Delflex low magnesium, low calcium with 1.5% dextrose (Fresenius)	0	15	132	2.5	0.5	95	40	344	In 1,000; 1,500; 2,000; 2,500; 3,000; and 500 mL
Rx	Dianeal low calcium with 1.5% dextrose (Baxter)									Preservative-free / In 2,000; 2,500; 3,000; 5,000; and 6,000 mL AMBU-FLEX II and AMBU-FLEX III containers / and / 1,500; 2,000; 2,500; and 3,000 mL UltraBag containers
Rx	Delflex low magnesium with 1.5% dextrose (Baxter)	0	15	132	3.5	0.5	96	40	346	In 1,000; 1,500; 2,000; 2,500; 3,000; and 5,000 mL
Rx	Dianeal PD-2 with 1.5% dextrose (Baxter)									Preservative-free / In 1,000; 2,000; 2,500; 3,000; 5,000; and 6,000 mL AMBU-FLEX II and AMBU-FLEX III containers / and / 250 and 500 mL AMBU-FLEX III containers / and / 1,500; 2,000; 2,500; and 3,000 mL UltraBag containers
Rx	Delflex standard with 1.5% dextrose (Baxter)	0	15	132	3.5	1.5	102	35	347	In 1,000; 1,500; 2,000; 2,500; 3,000; and 5,000 mL
Rx	Delflex low magnesium, low calcium with 2.5% dextrose (Baxter)	0	25	132	2.5	0.5	95	40	394	In 1,000; 1,500; 2,500; 3,000; and 5,000 mL
Rx	Dianeal low calcium with 2.5% dextrose (Baxter)	0	25	132	2.5	0.5	95	40	395	Preservative-free / In 2,000; 2,500; 3,000; 5,000; and 6,000 mL AMBU-FLEX II and AMBU-FLEX III containers / and / 1,500; 2,000; 2,500; and 3,000 mL UltraBag containers
Rx	Delflex low magnesium with 2.5% dextrose (Baxter)	0	25	132	3.5	0.5	96	0	396	In 1,000; 1,500; 2,000; 2,500; 3,000; and 5,000 mL
Rx	Dianeal PD-2 with 2.5% dextrose (Baxter)									Preservative-free / In 1,000; 2,000; 2,500; 3,000; 5,000; and 6,000 mL AMBU-FLEX II and AMBU-FLEX III containers / and / 500 mL AMBU-FLEX III containers / and / 1,500; 2,000; 2,500; and 3,000 mL UltraBag containers
Rx	Delflex standard with 2.5% dextrose (Baxter)	0	25	132	3.5	1.5	102	35	398	In 1,000; 1,500; 2,000; 2,500; 3,000; and 5,000 mL

	Product and Distributor	Icodextrin (g/liter)	Dextrose (g/liter)	Sodium (mEq/Liter)	Calcium (mEq/Liter)	Magnesium (mEq/Liter)	Chloride (mEq/Liter)	Lactate (mEq/Liter)	Osmolarity (mOsm/liter)	How Supplied
Rx	Delflex low magnesium, low calcium with 4.25% dextrose (Baxter)	0	42.5	132	2.5	0.5	95	40	483	In 1,000; 1,500; 2,500; 3,000; and 5,000 mL
Rx	Dianeal low calcium with 4.25% dextrose (Baxter)									Preservative-free In 2,000; 2,500; 3,000; 5,000; and 6,000 mL *AMBU-FLEX II* and *AMBU-FLEX III* containers and 1,500; 2,000; 2,500; and 3,000 mL *UltraBag* containers
Rx	Delflex low magnesium with 4.25% dextrose (Baxter)	0	42.5	132	3.5	0.5	96	40	485	In 1,000; 1,500; 2,000; 2,500; 3,000; and 5,000 mL
Rx	Dianeal PD-2 with 4.25% dextrose (Baxter)									Preservative-free In 1,000; 2,000; 2,500; 3,000; 5,000; and 6,000 mL *AMBU-FLEX II* and *AMBU-FLEX III* containers and 500 mL *AMBU-FLEX III* containers and 1,500; 2,000; 2,500; and 3,000 mL *UltraBag* containers
Rx	Delflex standard with 5.25% dextrose (Baxter)	0	42.5	132	3.5	1.5	102	35	486	In 1,000; 1,500; 2,000; 2,500; 3,000; and 5,000 mL
Rx	Extraneal (Baxter)	75	0	132	3.5	0.5	96	40	282 to 286	In 1,500; 2,000; and 2,500 mL *UltraBag* containers and 2,000 and 2,500 mL *AMBU-FLEX II* containers and 1,500; 2,000; and 2,500 mL *AMBU-FLEX III* containers

CYTOCHROME P450 ENZYMES: SUBSTRATES, INHIBITORS, AND INDUCERS

INTRODUCTION

Most drugs are eliminated from the body, at least in part, by being chemically altered to less lipid-soluble products (ie, metabolized), and thus are more likely to be excreted via the kidneys or the bile. Phase I metabolism includes drug hydrolysis, oxidation, and reduction, and results in drugs that are more polar in their chemical structure, while Phase II metabolism involves the attachment of an additional molecule onto the drug (or partially metabolized drug) in order to create an inactive and/or more water soluble compound. Phase II processes include (primarily) glucuronidation, sulfation, glutathione conjugation, acetylation, and methylation.

Virtually any of the Phase I and II enzymes can be inhibited by some xenobiotic or drug. Some of the Phase I and II enzymes can be induced. Inhibition of the activity of metabolic enzymes will result in increased concentrations of the substrate (drug), whereas induction of the activity of metabolic enzymes will result in decreased concentrations of the substrate. For example, the well-documented enzyme-inducing effects of phenobarbital may include a combination of Phase I and II enzymes. Phase II glucuronidation may be increased via induced UDP-glucuronosyltransferase (UGT) activity, whereas Phase I oxidation may be increased via induced cytochrome P450 (CYP) activity. However, for most drugs, the primary route of metabolism (and the primary focus of drug-drug interaction) is Phase I oxidation.

CYP enzymes may be responsible for the metabolism (at least partial metabolism) of ~75% of all drugs, with the CYP3A subfamily responsible for nearly half of this activity. Found throughout plant, animal, and bacterial species, CYP enzymes represent a superfamily of xenobiotic metabolizing proteins. There have been several hundred CYP enzymes identified in nature, each of which has been assigned to a family (1, 2, 3, etc), subfamily (A, B, C, etc), and given a specific enzyme number (1, 2, 3, etc) according to the similarity in amino acid sequence that it shares with other enzymes. Of these many enzymes, only a few are found in humans, and even fewer appear to be involved in the metabolism of xenobiotics (eg, drugs). The key human enzyme subfamilies include CYP1A, CYP2A, CYP2B, CYP2C, CYP2D, CYP2E, and CYP3A. However, the number of distinct isozymes (eg, CYP2C9) found to be functionally active in humans, as well as, the number of genetically variant forms of these isozymes (eg, CYP2C9*2) in individuals continues to expand.

CYP enzymes are found in the endoplasmic reticulum of cells in a variety of human tissues (eg, skin, kidneys, brain, lungs), but their predominant sites of concentration and activity are the liver and intestine. Though the abundance of CYP enzymes throughout the body is relatively equally distributed among the various subfamilies, the relative contribution to drug metabolism is (in decreasing order of magnitude) CYP3A4 (nearly 50%), CYP2D6 (nearly 25%), CYP2C8/9 (nearly 15%), then CYP1A2, CYP2C19, CYP2A6, and CYP2E1. Owing to their potential for numerous drug-drug interactions, those drugs that are identified in preclinical studies as substrates of CYP3A enzymes are often given a lower priority for continued research and development in favor of drugs that appear to be less affected by (or less likely to affect) this enzyme subfamily.

Each enzyme subfamily possesses unique selectivity toward potential substrates. For example, CYP1A2 preferentially binds medium-sized, planar, lipophilic molecules, while CYP2D6 preferentially binds molecules that possess a basic nitrogen atom. Some CYP subfamilies exhibit polymorphism (ie, genetic variation that results in a modified enzyme with small changes in amino acid sequences that may manifest differing catalytic properties). The best described polymorphisms involve CYP2C9, CYP2C19, and CYP2D6. Individuals possessing "wild type" genes exhibit normal functioning CYP capacity. Others, however, possess genetic variants that leave the person with a subnormal level of catalytic potential (so called "poor metabolizers"). Poor metabolizers would be more likely to experience toxicity from drugs metabolized by the affected enzymes (or less effects if the enzyme is responsible for converting a prodrug to it's active form as in the case of codeine). The percentage of people classified as poor metabolizers varies by enzyme and population group. As an example, ~7% of white patients and only about 1% of Asian patients appear to be CYP2D6 poor metabolizers.

CYP enzymes can be both inhibited and induced by other drugs, leading to increased or decreased serum concentrations (along with the associated effects), respectively. Induction occurs when a drug causes an increase in the amount of smooth endoplasmic reticulum, secondary to increasing the amount of the affected CYP enzymes in the tissues. This "revving up" of the CYP enzyme system may take several days to reach peak activity, and likewise, may take several days, even months, to return to normal following discontinuation of the inducing agent.

CYP inhibition occurs via several potential mechanisms. Most commonly, a CYP inhibitor competitively (and reversibly) binds to the active site on the enzyme, thus preventing the substrate from binding to the same site, and preventing the substrate from being metabolized. The affinity of an inhibitor for an enzyme may be expressed by an inhibition constant (Ki) or IC50 (defined as the concentration of the inhibitor required to cause 50% inhibition under a given set of conditions). In addition to reversible competition for an enzyme site, drugs may inhibit enzyme activity by binding to sites on the enzyme other than that to which the substrate would bind, and thereby cause a change in the functionality or physical structure of the enzyme. A drug may also bind to the enzyme in an irreversible (ie, "suicide") fashion. In such a case, it is not the concentration of drug at the enzyme site that is important (constantly binding and releasing), but the number of molecules available for binding (once bound, always bound).

Although an inhibitor or inducer may be known to affect a variety of CYP subfamilies, it may only inhibit one or two in a clinically important fashion. Likewise, although a substrate is known to be at least partially metabolized by a variety of CYP enzymes, only one or two enzymes may contribute significantly enough to its overall metabolism to warrant concern when used with potential inducers or inhibitors. Therefore, when attempting to predict the level of risk of using two drugs that may affect each other via altered CYP function, it is important to identify the relative effectiveness of the inhibiting/inducing drug on the CYP subfamilies that significantly contribute to the metabolism of the substrate. The contribution of a specific CYP pathway to substrate metabolism should be considered not only in light of other known CYP pathways, but also other nonoxidative pathways for substrate metabolism (eg, glucuronidation) and transporter proteins (eg, P-glycoprotein) that may affect the presentation of a substrate to a metabolic pathway.

HOW TO USE THIS TABLE

The following table provides a clinically relevant perspective on drugs that are affected by, or affect, cytochrome P450 (CYP) enzymes. Not all human, drug-metabolizing CYP enzymes are specifically (or separately) included in the table. Some enzymes have been excluded because they do not appear to significantly contribute to the metabolism of marketed drugs (eg, CYP2C18). In the case of CYP3A4, the industry routinely uses this single enzyme designation to represent all enzymes in the CYP3A subfamily. CYP3A7 is present in fetal livers. It is effectively absent from adult livers. CYP3A4 (adult) and CYP3A7 (fetal) appear to share similar properties in their respective hosts. The impact of CYP3A7 in fetal and neonatal drug interactions has not been investigated.

An enzyme that appears to play a clinically significant (major) role in a drug's metabolism is indicated by "S". A clinically significant designation is the result of a two-phase review. The first phase considered the contribution of each CYP enzyme to the overall metabolism of the drug. The enzyme pathway was considered potentially clinically relevant if it was responsible for at least 30% of the metabolism of the drug. If so, the drug was subjected to a second phase. The second phase considered the clinical relevance of a substrate's concentration being increased twofold, or decreased by one-half (such as might be observed if combined with an effective CYP inhibitor or inducer, respectively). If either of these changes was considered to present a clinically significant concern, the CYP pathway for the drug was designated "major." If neither change would appear to present a clinically significant concern, or if the CYP enzyme was responsible for a smaller portion of the overall metabolism (ie, <30%), then no association between the enzyme and the drug will appear in the table.

CYTOCHROME P450 ENZYMES: SUBSTRATES, INHIBITORS, AND INDUCERS

Enzymes that are strongly or moderately inhibited by a drug are indicated by "↓". Enzymes that are weakly inhibited are not identified in the table. The designations are the result of a review of published clinical reports, available Ki data, and assessments published by other experts in the field. As it pertains to Ki values set in a ratio with achievable serum drug concentrations ([I]) under normal dosing conditions, the following parameters were employed: [I]/Ki ≥1 = strong; [I]/Ki 0.1 to 1 = moderate; [I]/Ki <0.1 = weak.

Enzymes that appear to be effectively induced by a drug are indicated by "↑". This designation is the result of a review of published clinical reports and assessments published by experts in the field.

In general, clinically significant interactions are more likely to occur between substrates ("S") and either inhibitors or inducers of the same enzyme(s), which have been indicated by "↓" and "↑", respectively. However, these assessments possess a degree of subjectivity, at times based on limited indications regarding the significance of CYP effects of particular agents. An attempt has been made to balance a conservative, clinically-sensitive presentation of the data with a desire to avoid the numbing effect of a "beware of everything" approach. It is important to note that information related to CYP metabolism of drugs is expanding at a rapid pace, and thus, the contents of this table should only be considered to represent a "snapshot" of the information available at the time of publication.

SELECTED READINGS

Bjornsson TD, Callaghan JT, Einolf HJ, et al. The conduct of in vitro and in vivo drug-drug interaction studies: a PhRMA perspective. *J Clin Pharmacol.* 2003;43(5):443-469.

Drug-Drug Interactions. Rodrigues AD, ed. New York, NY: Marcel Dekker, Inc; 2002.

Metabolic Drug Interactions. Levy RH, Thummel KE, Trager WF, et al, eds. Philadelphia, PA: Lippincott Williams & Wilkins; 2000.

Michalets EL. Update: clinically significant cytochrome P-450 drug interactions. *Pharmacotherapy.* 1998;18(1):84-112.

Thummel KE, Wilkinson GR. In vitro and in vivo drug interactions involving human CYP3A. *Annu Rev Pharmacol Toxicol.* 1998;38:389-430.

Zhang Y, Benet LZ. The gut as a barrier to drug absorption: combined role of cytochrome P450 3A and P-Glycoprotein. *Clin Pharmacokinet.* 2001;40 (3):159-168.

SELECTED WEBSITES

http://www.cypalleles.ki.se/
http://www.fda.gov/Drugs/DevelopmentApprovalProcess/DevelopmentResources/DrugInteractionsLabeling/ucm080499.htm

CYP: Substrates, Inhibitors, Inducers

S = substrate; ↓ = inhibitor; ↑ = inducer

Drug	1A2	2A6	2B6	2C8	2C9	2C19	2D6	2E1	3A4
Acenocoumarol	S				S				
Alfentanil									S
Alfuzosin									S
Alosetron	S								
ALPRAZolam									S
Ambrisentan						S			S
Aminophylline	S								
Amiodarone		↓		S	↓		↓		S, ↓
Amitriptyline							S		
AmLODIPine	↓								S
Amobarbital		↑							
Amoxapine							S		
Aprepitant									S, ↓
ARIPiprazole							S		S
Armodafinil						↓			S, ↑
Atazanavir									S, ↓
Atomoxetine							S		
Atorvastatin									S
Benzphetamine									S
Betaxolol	S						S		
Bisoprolol									S
Bortezomib						S, ↓			S
Bosentan					S, ↑				S, ↑
Bromazepam									S
Bromocriptine									S
Budesonide									S
Buprenorphine									S
BuPROPion			S						
BusPIRone									S
Busulfan									S
Caffeine	S								↓
Captopril							S		
CarBAMazepine	↑		↑	↑	↑	↑			S, ↑
Carisoprodol						S			
Carvedilol					S		S		
Celecoxib				↓	S				
ChlordiazePOXIDE									S
Chloroquine							S, ↓		S
Chlorpheniramine									S
ChlorproMAZINE							S, ↓		
Chlorzoxazone								S	
Ciclesonide									S

CYP: Substrates, Inhibitors, Inducers (continued)

Drug	1A2	2A6	2B6	2C8	2C9	2C19	2D6	2E1	3A4
Cilostazol									S
Cimetidine	↓					↓	↓		↓
Cinacalcet							↓		
Ciprofloxacin	↓								
Cisapride									S
Citalopram						S			S
Clarithromycin									S, ↓
Clobazam						S			S
ClomiPRAMINE	S					S	S, ↓		
ClonazePAM									S
Clorazepate									S
Clotrimazole									↓
CloZAPine	S						↓		
Cobicistat									S, ↓
Cocaine							↓		S
Codeine[1]							S		
Colchicine									S
Conivaptan									S, ↓
Cyclobenzaprine	S								
Cyclophosphamide[2]			S						S
CycloSPORINE									S, ↓
Dacarbazine	S							S	
Dantrolene									S
Dapsone					S				S
Darifenacin							↓		S
Darunavir									S
Dasabuvir				S					
Dasatinib									S
Delavirdine					↓	↓	↓		S, ↓
Desipramine		↓	↓				S, ↓		↓
Desogestrel						S			
Dexamethasone									S, ↑
Dexlansoprazole						S, ↓			S
Dexmedetomidine		S					↓		
Dextromethorphan							S		
Diazepam						S			S
Diclofenac	↓								
Dihydroergotamine									S
Diltiazem									S, ↓
DiphenhydrAMINE							↓		
Disopyramide									S
Disulfiram								↓	
DOCEtaxel									S
Doxepin							S		
DOXOrubicin			↓				S		S
Doxycycline									↓
DULoxetine	S						S, ↓		
Efavirenz[3]			S		↓	↓			S, ↓, ↑
Eletriptan									S
Eplerenone									S
Ergoloid mesylates									S
Ergonovine									S
Ergotamine									S
Erlotinib									S
Erythromycin									S, ↓
Escitalopram						S			S
Esomeprazole						S, ↓			S
Estradiol	S								S
Estrogens, conjugated A/synthetic	S								S
Estrogens, conjugated equine	S								S
Estrogens, esterified	S								S
Estropipate	S								S
Eszopiclone									S
Ethinyl estradiol									S
Ethosuximide									S
Etoposide									S
	1A2	2A6	2B6	2C8	2C9	2C19	2D6	2E1	3A4

CYP: Substrates, Inhibitors, Inducers *(continued)*

Drug	1A2	2A6	2B6	2C8	2C9	2C19	2D6	2E1	3A4
Exemestane									S
Felbamate									S
Felodipine				↓					S
FentaNYL									S
Flecainide							S		
Fluconazole					↓	↓			↓
Flunisolide									S
FLUoxetine	↓				S	↓	S, ↓		
FluPHENAZine							S		
Flurazepam									S
Flurbiprofen					↓				
Flutamide	S								S
Fluticasone									S
Fluvastatin					S, ↓				
FluvoxaMINE	S, ↓					↓	S		
Fosamprenavir (as amprenavir)									S, ↓
Fosaprepitant									S, ↓
Fosphenytoin (as phenytoin)			↑	↑	S, ↑	S, ↑			↑
Fospropofol	↓		S		S	↓			↓
Gefitinib									S
Gemfibrozil	↓			↓	↓	↓			
Glimepiride					S				
GlipiZIDE					S				
Guanabenz	S								
Haloperidol							S, ↓		S, ↓
Halothane								S	
Ibuprofen					↓				
Ifosfamide[4]		S				S			S
Imatinib							↓		S, ↓
Imipramine						S	S, ↓		
Indinavir									S, ↓
Indomethacin					↓				
Irbesartan				↓	↓				
Irinotecan			S						S
Isoflurane								S	
Isoniazid		↓				↓	↓	S, ↓	
Isosorbide dinitrate									S
Isosorbide mononitrate									S
Isradipine									S
Itraconazole									S, ↓
Ixabepilone									S
Ketamine			S		S				S
Ketoconazole	↓	↓			↓	↓	↓		S, ↓
Lansoprazole						S, ↓			S
Lapatinib									S
Letrozole		↓							
Levonorgestrel									S
Lidocaine							S, ↓		S, ↓
Lomustine							S		
Lopinavir									S
Loratadine							↓		
Losartan				↓	S, ↓				S
Lovastatin									S
Maprotiline							S		
Maraviroc									S
MedroxyPROGESTERone									S
Mefenamic acid					↓				
Mefloquine									S
Mephobarbital						S			
Mestranol[5]					S				S
Methadone							↓		S
Methamphetamine							S		
Methoxsalen	↓	↓							
Methsuximide						S			
Methylergonovine									S
MethylPREDNISolone									S

CYP: Substrates, Inhibitors, Inducers (continued)

Drug	1A2	2A6	2B6	2C8	2C9	2C19	2D6	2E1	3A4
Metoprolol							S		
MetroNIDAZOLE									↓
Mexiletine	S, ↓						S		
Miconazole	↓	↓			↓	↓	↓	↓	S, ↓
Midazolam									S
Mirtazapine	S						S		S
Moclobemide						S	S		
Modafinil						↓			S
Montelukast					S				S
Nafcillin									↑
Nateglinide					S				S
Nebivolol							S		
Nefazodone							S		S, ↓
Nelfinavir						S			S, ↓
Nevirapine			↑						S, ↑
NiCARdipine					↓	↓	↓		S, ↓
NIFEdipine	↓								S
Nilotinib									S
Nilutamide						S			
NiMODipine									S
Nisoldipine									S
Norethindrone									S
Norfloxacin	↓								↓
Norgestrel									S
Nortriptyline							S		
Ofloxacin	↓								
OLANZapine	S								
Omeprazole					↓	S, ↓			S
Ondansetron									S
OXcarbazepine									↑
PACLitaxel				S	S				S
Pantoprazole						S, ↓			
Paricalcitol									S
Paritaprevir									S
PARoxetine			↓				S, ↓		
PAZOPanib									S
Pentamidine						S			
PENTobarbital		↑							↑
Perphenazine							S		
PHENobarbital	↑	↑	↑	↑	↑	S			↑
Phenytoin			↑	↑	S, ↑	S, ↑			↑
Pimozide	S								S
Pindolol							S		
Pioglitazone				S, ↓					
Piroxicam					↓				
Posaconazole									↓
Primaquine	↓								S
Primidone	↑		↑	↑	↑				↑
Procainamide							S		
Progesterone						S			S
Promethazine			S				S		
Propafenone							S		
Propofol	↓		S		S	↓			↓
Propranolol	S						S		
Protriptyline							S		
Pyrimethamine					↓				
Quazepam							S		S
QUEtiapine									S
QuiNIDine							↓		S, ↓
QuiNINE				↓	↓		↓		S
RABEprazole				↓		S, ↓			S
Ramelteon	S								
Ranolazine							↓		S
Rasagiline	S								
Repaglinide				S					S
Rifabutin									S, ↑

◀ **CYP: Substrates, Inhibitors, Inducers** *(continued)*

Drug	1A2	2A6	2B6	2C8	2C9	2C19	2D6	2E1	3A4
Rifampin	↑	↑	↑	↑	↑	↑			↑
Rifapentine				↑	↑				↑
Riluzole	S								
RisperiDONE							S		
Ritonavir				↓			S, ↓		S, ↓
ROPINIRole	S								
Ropivacaine	S								
Rosiglitazone				S, ↓					
Salmeterol									S
Saquinavir									S, ↓
Secobarbital		↑		↑	↑				
Selegiline			S						
Sertraline			↓			S, ↓	S, ↓		↓
Sevoflurane								S	
Sibutramine									S
Sildenafil									S
Simvastatin									S
Sirolimus									S
Sitaxsentan				↓	↓				↓
Solifenacin									S
SORAfenib			↓	↓	↓				
Spiramycin									S
SUFentanil									S
SulfADIAZINE					S, ↓				
Sulfamethoxazole					S, ↓				
SUNItinib									S
Tacrine	S								
Tacrolimus									S
Tadalafil									S
Tamoxifen				↓	S		S		S
Tamsulosin							S		S
Telithromycin									S, ↓
Temsirolimus									S
Teniposide									S
Terbinafine							↓		
Tetracycline									S, ↓
Theophylline	S							S	S
Thiabendazole	↓								
Thioridazine							S, ↓		
Thiotepa			↓						
Thiothixene	S								
TiaGABine									S
Ticlopidine						↓	↓		S
Timolol							S		
Tinidazole									S
Tipranavir									S
TiZANidine	S								
TOLBUTamide					S, ↓				
Tolterodine							S		S
Toremifene									S
Torsemide					S				
TraMADol[1]							S		S
Tranylcypromine	↓	↓				↓	↓		
TraZODone									S
Tretinoin				S					
Triazolam									S
Trifluoperazine	S								
Trimethoprim				↓	S, ↓				
Trimipramine						S	S		S
Vardenafil									S
Venlafaxine							S		S
Verapamil									S, ↓
VinBLAStine									S
VinCRIStine									S
Vinorelbine									S
Voriconazole					S	S			↓

CYP: Substrates, Inhibitors, Inducers (continued)

Drug	1A2	2A6	2B6	2C8	2C9	2C19	2D6	2E1	3A4
Warfarin					S, ↓				
Zafirlukast					S, ↓				
Zileuton	↓								
Zolpidem									S
Zonisamide									S
Zopiclone					S				S
Zuclopenthixol							S		

[1]This opioid analgesic is bioactivated in vivo via CYP2D6. Inhibiting this enzyme would decrease the effects of the analgesic. The active metabolite might also affect, or be affected by, CYP enzymes.

[2]Cyclophosphamide is bioactivated in vivo to acrolein via CYP2B6 and 3A4. Inhibiting these enzymes would decrease the effects of cyclophosphamide.

[3]Data have shown both induction (in vivo) and inhibition (in vitro) of CYP3A4.

[4]Ifosfamide is bioactivated in vivo to acrolein via CYP3A4. Inhibiting this enzyme would decrease the effects of ifosfamide.

[5]Mestranol is bioactivated in vivo to ethinyl estradiol via CYP2C8/9. See Ethinyl Estradiol for additional CYP information.

IMMUNIZATION ADMINISTRATION RECOMMENDATIONS

The following tables are taken from the General Recommendations on Immunization 2011:

- Guidelines for Spacing of Live and Inactivated Antigens
- Guidelines for Administering Antibody-Containing Products and Vaccines
- Recommended Intervals Between Administration of Antibody-Containing Products and Measles- or Varicella-Containing Vaccine, by Product and Indication for Vaccination
- Vaccination of persons with Primary and Secondary Immunodeficiencies
- Needle length and Injection Site of IM injections

Guidelines for Spacing of Live and Inactivated Antigens

Antigen Combination	Recommended Minimum Interval Between Doses
Two or more inactivated[1]	May be administered simultaneously or at any interval between doses
Inactivated and live	May be administered simultaneously or at any interval between doses
Two or more live injectable[2]	28 days minimum interval, if not administered simultaneously

[1]Certain experts suggest a 28-day interval between tetanus toxoid, reduced diphtheria toxoid, and reduced acellular pertussis (Tdap) vaccine and tetravalent meningococcal conjugate vaccine if they are not administered simultaneously.

[2]Live oral vaccines (eg, Ty21a typhoid vaccine and rotavirus vaccine) may be administered simultaneously or at any interval before or after inactivated or live injectable vaccines.

Adapted from American Academy of Pediatrics. Pertussis. Pickering LK, Baker CJ, Kimberlin DW, et al, eds. *Red Book*: 2009 Report of the Committee on Infectious Diseases. 28th ed. Elk Grove Village, IL: American Academy of Pediatrics; 2009;22.

Guidelines for Administering Antibody-Containing Products[1] and Vaccines

Simultaneous Administration (during the same office visit)

Products Administered	Recommended Minimum Interval Between Doses
Antibody-containing products and inactivated antigen	Can be administered simultaneously at different anatomic sites or at any time interval between doses.
Antibody-containing products and live antigen	Should **not** be administered simultaneously.[2] If simultaneous administration of measles-containing vaccine or varicella vaccine is unavoidable, administer at different sites and revaccinate or test for seroconversion after the recommended interval.

Nonsimultaneous Administration

Products Administered		Recommended Minimum Interval Between Doses
Administered first	Administered second	
Antibody-containing products	Inactivated antigen	No interval necessary
Inactivated antigen	Antibody-containing products	No interval necessary
Antibody-containing products	Live antigen	Dose-related[2,3]
Live antigen	Antibody-containing products	2 weeks[2]

[1]Blood products containing substantial amounts of immune globulin include intramuscular and intravenous immune globulin, specific hyperimmune globulin (eg, hepatitis B immune globulin, tetanus immune globulin, varicella zoster immune globulin, and rabies immune globulin), whole blood, packed red blood cells, plasma, and platelet products.

[2]Yellow fever vaccine, rotavirus vaccine, oral Ty21a typhoid vaccine, live-attenuated influenza vaccine, and zoster vaccine are exceptions to these recommendations. These live-attenuated vaccines can be administered at any time before, after, or simultaneously with an antibody-containing product.

[3]The duration of interference of antibody-containing products with the immune response to the measles component of measles-containing vaccine, and possibly varicella vaccine, is dose-related.

Recommended Intervals Between Administration of Antibody-Containing Products and Measles- or Varicella-Containing Vaccine, by Product and Indication for Vaccination

Product/Indication	Dose (mg IgG/kg) and Route[1]	Recommended Interval Before Measles- or Varicella-Containing Vaccine[2] Administration (mo)
Tetanus IG	IM: 250 units (10 mg IgG/kg)	3
Hepatitis A IG		
Contact prophylaxis	IM: 0.02 mL/kg (3.3 mg IgG/kg)	3
International travel	IM: 0.06 mL/kg (10 mg IgG/kg)	3
Hepatitis B IG	IM: 0.06 mL/kg (10 mg IgG/kg)	3
Rabies IG	IM: 20 int. units/kg (22 mg IgG/kg)	4
Varicella IG	IM: 125 units/10 kg (60 to 200 mg IgG/kg) (maximum: 625 units)	5
Measles prophylaxis IG		
Standard (ie, nonimmunocompromised) contact	IM: 0.25 mL/kg (40 mg IgG/kg)	5
Immunocompromised contact	IM: 0.50 mL/kg (80 mg IgG/kg)	6
Blood transfusion		
Red blood cells (RBCs), washed	IV: 10 mL/kg (negligible IgG/kg)	None
RBCs, adenine-saline added	IV: 10 mL/kg (10 mg IgG/kg)	3
Packed RBCs (hematocrit 65%)[3]	IV: 10 mL/kg (60 mg IgG/kg)	6
Whole blood cells (hematocrit 35% to 50%)[3]	IV: 10 mL/kg (80 to 100 mg IgG/kg)	6
Plasma/platelet products	IV: 10 mL/kg (160 mg IgG/kg)	7
Cytomegalovirus intravenous immune globulin (IGIV)	150 mg/kg maximum	6

Recommended Intervals Between Administration of Antibody-Containing Products and Measles- or Varicella-Containing Vaccine, by Product and Indication for Vaccination (continued)

Product/Indication	Dose (mg IgG/kg) and Route[1]	Recommended Interval Before Measles- or Varicella-Containing Vaccine[2] Administration (mo)
IGIV		
Replacement therapy for immune deficiencies[4]	IV: 300 to 400 mg/kg[4]	8
Immune thrombocytopenic purpura treatment	IV: 400 mg/kg	8
Postexposure varicella prophylaxis[5]	IV: 400 mg/kg	8
Immune thrombocytopenic purpura treatment	IV: 1,000 mg/kg	10
Kawasaki disease	IV: 2 g/kg	11
Monoclonal antibody to respiratory syncytial virus F protein (Synagis [Medimmune])[6]	IM: 15 mg/kg	None

HIV = human immunodeficiency virus, IG = immune globulin, IgG = immune globulin G, IGIV = intravenous immune globulin, mg IgG/kg = milligrams of immune globulin G per kilogram of body weight, IM = intramuscular, IV = intravenous, RBCs = red blood cells

[1] This table is not intended for determining the correct indications and dosages for using antibody-containing products. Unvaccinated persons might not be fully protected against measles during the entire recommended interval, and additional doses of IG or measles vaccine might be indicated after measles exposure. Concentrations of measles antibody in an IG preparation can vary by manufacturer's lot. Rates of antibody clearance after receipt of an IG preparation also might vary. Recommended intervals are extrapolated from an estimated half-life of 30 days for passively acquired antibody and an observed interference with the immune response to measles vaccine for 5 months after a dose of 80 mg IgG/kg.

[2] Does not include zoster vaccine. Zoster vaccine may be given with antibody-containing blood products.

[3] Assumes a serum IgG concentration of 16 mg/mL.

[4] Measles and varicella vaccinations are recommended for children with asymptomatic or mildly symptomatic HIV infection but are contraindicated for persons with severe immunosuppression from HIV or any other immunosuppressive disorder.

[5] The investigational product VariZIG, similar to licensed varicella-zoster IG (VZIG), is a purified human IG preparation made from plasma containing high levels of anti-varicella antibodies (IgG). The interval between VariZIG and varicella vaccine (Var or MMRV) is 5 months.

[6] Contains antibody only to respiratory syncytial virus

Vaccination of Persons With Primary and Secondary Immunodeficiencies

Category	Specific Immunodeficiency	Contraindicated Vaccines[1] Primary	Risk-Specific Recommended Vaccines[1]	Effectiveness and Comments
B-lymphocyte (humoral)	Severe antibody deficiencies (eg, X-linked agammaglobulinemia and common variable immunodeficiency)	Oral poliovirus (OPV)[2] Smallpox Live-attenuated influenza vaccine (LAIV) BCG Ty21a (live oral typhoid) Yellow fever	Pneumococcal Consider measles and varicella vaccination	The effectiveness of any vaccine is uncertain if it depends only on the humoral response (eg, PPSV or MPSV4) IGIV interferes with the immune response to measles vaccine and possibly varicella vaccine
	Less severe antibody deficiencies (eg, selective IgA deficiency and IgG subclass deficiency)	OPV[2] BCG Yellow Fever Other live-vaccines appear to be safe	Pneumococcal	All vaccines likely effective; immune response may be attenuated
T-lymphocyte (cell-mediated and humoral)	Complete defects (eg, severe combined immunodeficiency [SCID] disease, complete DiGeorge syndrome)	All live vaccines[3,4,5]	Pneumococcal	Vaccines might be ineffective
	Partial defects (eg, most patients with DiGeorge syndrome, Wiskott-Aldrich syndrome, ataxia-telangiectasia)	All live vaccines[3,4,5]	Pneumococcal Meningococcal Hib (if not administered in infancy)	Effectiveness of any vaccine depends on degree of immune suppression
Complement	Persistent complement, properdin, or factor B deficiency	None	Pneumococcal Meningococcal	All routine vaccines likely effective
Phagocytic function	Chronic granulomatous disease, leukocyte adhesion defect, and myeloperoxidase deficiency	Live bacterial vaccines[3]	Pneumococcal[6]	All inactivated vaccines safe and likely effective; live viral vaccines likely safe and effective

Vaccination of Persons With Primary and Secondary Immunodeficiencies *(continued)*

Category	Specific Immunodeficiency	Contraindicated Vaccines[1] Secondary	Risk-Specific Recommended Vaccines[1]	Effectiveness and Comments
	HIV/AIDS	OPV[2] Smallpox BCG LAIV Withhold MMR and varicella in severely immunocompromised persons Yellow fever vaccine might have a contraindication or a precaution depending on clinical parameters of immune function[9]	Pneumococcal Consider Hib (if not administered in infancy) and meningococcal vaccination.	MMR, varicella, rotavirus, and all inactivated vaccines, including inactivated influenza, might be effective[7]
	Malignant neoplasm, transplantation, immunosuppressive or radiation therapy	Live viral and bacterial, depending on immune status[3,4]	Pneumococcal	Effectiveness of any vaccine depends on degree of immune suppression
	Asplenia	None	Pneumococcal Meningococcal Hib (if not administered in infancy)	All routine vaccines likely effective
	Chronic renal disease	LAIV	Pneumococcal Hepatitis B[8]	All routine vaccines likely effective

AIDS = acquired immunodeficiency syndrome; BCG = bacille Calmette-Guerin; Hib = *Haemophilus influenzae* type b; HIV = human immunodeficiency virus; IG = immunoglobulin; IGIV = immune globulin intravenous; LAIV = live, attenuated influenza vaccine; MMR = measles, mumps, and rubella; MPSV4 = quadrivalent meningococcal polysaccharide vaccine; OPV = oral poliovirus vaccine (live); PPSV = pneumococcal polysaccharide vaccine; TIV = trivalent inactivated influenza vaccine

[1] Other vaccines that are universally or routinely recommended should be administered if not contraindicated.

[2] OPV is no longer available in the United States.

[3] Live bacterial vaccines: BCG and oral Ty21a *Salmonella typhi* vaccine

[4] Live viral vaccines: MMR, MMRV, OPV, LAIV, yellow fever, zoster, rotavirus, varicella, and vaccinia (smallpox). Smallpox vaccine is not recommended for children or the general public.

[5] Regarding T-lymphocyte immunodeficiency as a contraindication for rotavirus vaccine, data exist only for severe combined immunodeficiency.

[6] Pneumococcal vaccine is not indicated for children with chronic granulomatous disease beyond age-based universal recommendations for PCV. Children with chronic granulomatous disease are not at increased risk for pneumococcal disease.

[7] HIV-infected children should receive IG after exposure to measles and may receive varicella and measles vaccine if CD4+ lymphocyte count is ≥15%.

[8] Indicated based on the risk from dialysis-based bloodborne transmission

[9] Symptomatic HIV infection or CD4+ T-lymphocyte count of <200/mm³ or <15% of total lymphocytes for children aged <6 years is a contraindication to yellow fever vaccine administration. Asymptomatic HIV infection with CD4+ T-lymphocyte count of 200 to 499/mm³ for persons aged ≥6 years or 15% to 24% of total lymphocytes for children aged <6 years is a precaution for yellow fever vaccine administration. Details of yellow fever vaccine recommendations are available from the CDC. (CDC. Yellow fever vaccine: recommendations of the Advisory Committee on Immunization Practices [ACIP]. *MMWR Recomm Rep.* 2010;59[No. RR-7].)

Adapted from American Academy of Pediatrics. Passive immunization. Pickering LK, Baker CJ, Kimberline DW, et al. eds. *Red Book*: 2009 Report of the Committee on Infectious Diseases. 28th ed. Elk Grove Village, IL: American Academy of Pediatrics; 2009;74-75.

◀ **Needle Length and Injection Site of IM for Children ≤18 years of age (by age) and Adults ≥19 years of age (by sex and weight)**

Age Group	Needle Length	Injection Site
Children (birth to 18 y)		
Neonates[1]	5/8" (16 mm)[2]	Anterolateral thigh
Infant 1 to 12 mo	1" (25 mm)	Anterolateral thigh
Toddler 1 to 2 y	1 to 1¼" (25 to 32 mm)	Anterolateral thigh[3]
	5/8[2] to 1" (16 to 25 mm)	Deltoid muscle of the arm
Children 3 to 18 y	5/8[2] to 1" (16 to 25 mm)	Deltoid muscle of the arm[3]
	1 to 1¼" (25 to 32 mm)	Anterolateral thigh
Adults ≥19 y		
Men and women <60 kg (130 lb)	1" (25 mm)[4]	Deltoid muscle of the arm
Men and women 60 to 70 kg (130 to 152 lb)	1" (25 mm)	
Men 70 to 118 kg (152 to 260 lb)	1 to 1½" (25 to 38 mm)	
Women 70 to 90 kg (152 to 200 lb)		
Men >118 kg (260 lb)	1½" (38 mm)	
Women >90 kg (200 lb)		

IM = intramuscular

[1] First 28 days of life

[2] If skin is stretched tightly and subcutaneous tissues are not bunched

[3] Preferred site

[4] Some experts recommend a 5/8" needle for men and women who weigh <60 kg.

Adapted from Poland GA, Borrud A, Jacobsen RM, et al. Determination of deltoid fat pad thickness: implications for needle length in adult immunization. *JAMA.* 1997;277:1709-1711.

REFERENCE

Centers for Disease Control and Prevention (CDC). Recommendations of the Advisory Committee on Immunization Practices (ACIP): general recommendations on immunization. *MMWR Recomm Rep.* 2011;60(2):1-61.

IMMUNIZATION SCHEDULES

Recommended Immunization Schedule for Persons 0 to 18 Years of Age — United States, 2015[*]

Vaccine	Birth	1 mo	2 mos	4 mos	6 mos	9 mos	12 mos	15 mos	18 mos	19–23 mos	2–3 yrs	4–6 yrs	7–10 yrs	11–12 yrs	13–15 yrs	16–18 yrs
Hepatitis B[1] (HepB)	1st dose	2nd dose			3rd dose											
Rotavirus[2] (RV) RV-1 (2-dose series); RV-5 (3-dose series)			1st dose	2nd dose	see footnote 2											
Diphtheria, tetanus & acellular pertussis[3] (DTaP: <7 yrs)			1st dose	2nd dose	3rd dose		4th dose					5th dose				
Tetanus, diphtheria & acellular pertussis[4] (Tdap: ≥ 7 yrs)														(Tdap)		
Haemophilus influenzae type b[5] (Hib)			1st dose	2nd dose	see footnote 5		3rd or 4th dose, see footnote 5									
Pneumococcal conjugate[6] (PCV13)			1st dose	2nd dose	3rd dose		4th dose									
Pneumococcal polysaccharide[6] (PPSV23)																
Inactivated poliovirus[7] (IPV) (<18 years)			1st dose	2nd dose	3rd dose							4th dose				
Influenza[8] (IIV; LAIV) 2 doses for some: see footnote 8					Annual vaccination (IIV only) 1 or 2 doses							Annual vaccination (LAIV or IIV) 1 or 2 doses		Annual vaccination (LAIV or IIV) 1 dose only		
Measles, mumps, rubella[9] (MMR)						see footnote 9	1st dose					2nd dose				
Varicella[10] (VAR)							1st dose					2nd dose				
Hepatitis A[11] (Hep A)							2 dose series, see footnote 11									
Human papillomavirus[12] (HPV2: females only; HPV4: males and females)														(3 dose series)		
Meningococcal[13] (Hib-MenCY ≥ 6 wks; MenACWY-D ≥ 9 mos; MenACWY-CRM ≥ 2 mos.)						see footnote 13								1st dose		booster

Legend:
- Range of recommended ages for all children.
- Range of recommended ages for catch-up immunization.
- Range of recommended ages for certain high-risk groups.
- Range of recommended ages during which catch-up is encouraged and for certain high-risk groups.
- Not routinely recommended.

NOTE: The recommendations in the tables must be read along with the following footnotes.

[*] This schedule includes recommendations in effect as of January 1, 2015. Any dose not administered at the recommended age should be administered at a subsequent visit, when indicated and feasible. The use of a combination vaccine generally is preferred over separate injections of its equivalent component vaccines. Vaccination providers should consult the relevant Advisory Committee on Immunization Practices (ACIP) statement for detailed recommendations, available online at http://www.cdc.gov/vaccines/hcp/acip-recs/index.html. Clinically significant adverse events that follow vaccination should be reported to the Vaccine Adverse Event Reporting System (VAERS) online (http://www.vaers.hhs.gov/) or by telephone (800-822-7967).Suspected cases of vaccine-preventable diseases should be reported to the state or local health department. Additional information, including precautions and contraindications for vaccination, is available from CDC online (http://www.cdc.gov/vaccines/recs/vac-admin/contraindications.htm) or by telephone (800-CDC-INFO [800-232-4636]). This schedule is approved by the Advisory Committee on Immunization Practices (http://www.cdc.gov/vaccines/acip), the American Academy of Pediatrics (http://www.aap.org), the American Academy of Family Physicians (http://www.aafp.org), and the American College of Obstetricians and Gynecologists (http://www.acog.org).

Catch-up Immunization Schedule for Persons 4 Months to 18 Years of Age Who Start Late or Who Are >1 Month Behind – United States, 2015

This table provides catch-up schedules and minimum intervals between doses for children whose vaccinations have been delayed. A vaccine series does not need to be restarted, regardless of the time that has elapsed between doses. Use the section appropriate for the child's age. Always use this table in conjunction with the previous "Recommended immunization schedule for persons aged 0 through 18 years" and the footnotes that follow.

Vaccine	Minimum Age for Dose 1	Minimum Interval Between Doses			
		Dose 1 to Dose 2	Dose 2 to Dose 3	Dose 3 to Dose 4	Dose 4 to Dose 5
Catch-up Schedule for Persons 4 Months to 6 Years of Age					
Hepatitis B[1]	Birth	4 weeks	8 weeks and ≥16 weeks after first dose; minimum age for final dose is 24 weeks		
Rotavirus[2]	6 weeks	4 weeks	4 weeks[2]		
Diphtheria, tetanus, and acellular pertussis[3]	6 weeks	4 weeks	4 weeks	6 months	6 months[3]
Haemophilus influenzae type b[5]	6 weeks	**4 weeks** if first dose was administered before the 1st birthday **8 weeks** (as final dose) if first dose was administered at 12 to 14 months of age **No further doses needed** if first dose was administered at ≥15 months of age	**4 weeks[5]** if currently <12 months of age **and** first dose was administered at <7 months of age **and** at least 1 previous dose was PRP-T (ActHib, Pentacel) or unknown **8 weeks** and 12 to 59 months of age (as final dose)[5] if currently <12 months of age **and** first dose was administered at 7 to 11 months of age **or** if currently 12 to 59 months of age **and** first dose was administered before the 1st birthday **and** second dose was administered at <15 months of age **or** if both doses were PRP-OMP (PredvaxHIB, Comvax) and were administered before the 1st birthday **No further doses needed** if previous dose was administered at ≥15 months of age	**8 weeks** (as final dose) This dose is only necessary for children 12 to 59 months of age who received 3 doses before the 1st birthday	

Vaccine	Minimum Age for Dose 1	Minimum Interval Between Doses			
		Dose 1 to Dose 2	Dose 2 to Dose 3	Dose 3 to Dose 4	Dose 4 to Dose 5
Pneumococcal[6]	6 weeks	**4 weeks** if first dose was administered before the 1st birthday **8 weeks** (as final dose for healthy children) if first dose was administered at or after the 1st birthday **No further doses needed** for healthy children if first dose was administered at ≥24 months of age	**4 weeks** if currently <12 months of age and previous dose was given at <7 months of age **8 weeks** (as final dose for healthy children) if previous dose was given at 7 to 11 months of age (wait until >12 months of age) **or** if currently ≥12 months of age and at least 1 dose was given before 12 months of age **No further doses needed** for healthy children if previous dose was administered at ≥24 months of age	**8 weeks** (as final dose) This dose is only necessary for children 12 to 59 months of age who received 3 doses before 12 months of age or for children at high risk who received 3 doses at any age	
Inactivated poliovirus[7]	6 weeks	**4 weeks**[7]	**4 weeks**[7]	**6 months**[7] minimum 4 years of age for final dose	
Meningococcal[13]	6 weeks	**8 weeks**[13]	See footnote 13	See footnote 13	
Measles, mumps, rubella[9]	12 months	**4 weeks**			
Varicella[10]	12 months	**3 months**			
Hepatitis A[11]	12 months	**6 months**			
Catch-up Schedule for Persons 7 to 18 Years of Age					
Tetanus, diphtheria; tetanus, diphtheria, and acellular pertussis[4]	7 years[4]	**4 weeks**	**4 weeks** if first dose of DTaP/DT was administered before the 1st birthday **6 months** (as final dose) if first dose of DTaP/DT administered at or after the 1st birthday	**6 months** if first dose of DTaP/DT was administered before the 1st birthday	
Human papillomavirus[12]	9 years	Routine dosing intervals are recommended[12]			
Hepatitis A[11]	N/A	**6 months**			
Hepatitis B[1]	N/A	**4 weeks**	8 weeks and ≥16 weeks after first dose		
Inactivated poliovirus[7]	N/A	**4 weeks**	**4 weeks**[7]	**6 months**[7]	
Meningococcal[13]	N/A	**8 weeks**[13]			
Measles, mumps, rubella[9]	N/A	**4 weeks**			
Varicella[10]	N/A	**3 months** if <13 years of age **4 weeks** if ≥13 years of age			

Footnotes to Recommended Immunization Schedule for Persons 0 to 18 Years of Age and the Catch-up Immunization Schedule – United States, 2015

Note: For further guidance on the use of the vaccines mentioned below, see http://www.cdc.gov/vaccines/hcp/acip-recs/index.html. For vaccine recommendations for persons ≥19 years of age, see the adult immunization schedule.

[1]**Hepatitis B (HepB) vaccine** (Minimum age: Birth)

Routine vaccination:

At birth:

- Administer monovalent HepB vaccine to all newborns before hospital discharge.

- For infants born to hepatitis B surface antigen (HBsAg)-positive mothers, administer HepB vaccine and 0.5 mL of hepatitis B immune globulin (HBIG) within 12 hours of birth. These infants should be tested for HBsAg and antibody to HBsAg (anti-HBs) 1 to 2 months after completion of the HepB series at 9 to 18 months of age (preferably at the next well-child visit).

- If the mother's HBsAg status is unknown, within 12 hours of birth, administer HepB vaccine to all infants regardless of birth weight. For infants weighing <2,000 grams, administer HBIG in addition to HepB vaccine within 12 hours of birth. Determine the mother's HBsAg status as soon as possible and if she is HBsAg-positive, also administer HBIG for infants weighing ≥2,000 grams as soon as possible but no later than 7 days of age.

Doses following the birth dose:

- The second dose should be administered at 1 or 2 months of age. Monovalent HepB vaccine should be used for doses administered before 6 weeks of age.

- Infants who did not receive a birth dose should receive 3 doses of a HepB-containing vaccine on a schedule of 0, 1 to 2 months, and 6 months of age starting as soon as feasible. See the previous "Catch-up Immunization Schedule".

- Administer the second dose 1 to 2 months after the first dose (minimum interval of 4 weeks); administer the third dose ≥8 weeks after the second dose **and** ≥16 weeks after the **first** dose. The final (third or fourth) dose in the HepB vaccine series should be administered **no earlier than 24 weeks of age**.

- Administration of a total of 4 doses of HepB vaccine is permitted when a combination vaccine containing HepB is administered after the birth dose.

Catch-up vaccination:

- Unvaccinated persons should complete a 3-dose series.

- A 2-dose series (doses separated by at least 4 months) of adult formulation Recombivax HB is licensed for use in children 11 to 15 years of age.

- For other catch-up guidance, see the previous "Catch-up Immunization Schedule".

[2]**Rotavirus (RV) vaccine** *(Minimum age: 6 weeks for both RV-1 [Rotarix] and RV-5 [RotaTeq])*
Routine vaccination:

- Administer a series of RV vaccine to all infants as follows:

  - If Rotarix is used, administer a 2-dose series at 2 and 4 months of age.

  - If RotaTeq is used, administer a 3-dose series at ages 2, 4, and 6 months of age.

  - If any dose in the series was RotaTeq or vaccine product is unknown for any dose in the series, a total of 3 doses of RV vaccine should be administered.

Catch-up vaccination:

- The maximum age for the first dose in the series is 14 weeks, 6 days; vaccination should not be initiated for infants ≥15 weeks, 0 days of age.

- The maximum age for the final dose in the series is 8 months, 0 days.

- For other catch-up guidance, see the previous "Catch-up Immunization Schedule".

[3]**Diphtheria and tetanus toxoids and acellular pertussis (DTaP) vaccine** *(Minimum age: 6 weeks; exception: DTaP-IPV [Kinrix]: 4 years)*
Routine vaccination:

- Administer a 5-dose series of DTaP vaccine at 2, 4, 6, and 15 to 18 months of age, and at 4 to 6 years of age. The fourth dose may be administered as early as 12 months of age, provided at least 6 months have elapsed since the third dose. However, the fourth dose of DTaP need not be repeated if it was administered ≥4 months after the third dose of DTaP.

Catch-up vaccination:

- The fifth dose of DTaP vaccine is not necessary if the fourth dose was administered at ≥4 years of age.

- For other catch-up guidance, see the previous "Catch-up Immunization Schedule".

[4]**Tetanus and diphtheria toxoids and acellular pertussis (Tdap) vaccine** *(Minimum age: 10 years for Adacel and Boostrix)*
Routine vaccination:

- Administer 1 dose of Tdap vaccine to all adolescents 11 to 12 years of age.

- Tdap can be administered regardless of the interval since the last tetanus and diphtheria toxoid-containing vaccine.

- Administer 1 dose of Tdap vaccine to pregnant adolescents during each pregnancy (preferred during 27 to 36 weeks gestation), regardless of time since prior Td or Tdap vaccination.

Catch-up vaccination:

- Persons ≥7 years of age who are not fully immunized with DTaP vaccine should receive Tdap vaccine as 1 dose (preferably the first) in the catch-up series; if additional doses are needed, use Td vaccine. For children 7 to 10 years of age who receive a dose of Tdap as part of the catch-up series, an adolescent Tdap vaccine dose at 11 to 12 years of age should **not** be administered. Td should be administered instead 10 years after the Tdap dose.

- Persons 11 to 18 years of age who have not received Tdap vaccine should receive a dose, followed by tetanus and diphtheria toxoid (Td) booster doses every 10 years thereafter.

- Inadvertent doses of DTaP vaccine:

  - If administered inadvertently to a child 7 to 10 years of age, the dose may count as part of the catch-up series. This dose can count as the adolescent Tdap dose or the child can later receive a Tdap booster dose at 11 to 12 years of age.

  - If administered inadvertently to an adolescent 11 to 18 years of age, the dose should be counted as the adolescent Tdap booster.

- For other catch-up guidance, see the previous "Catch-up Immunization Schedule".

[5]**Haemophilus influenzae type b conjugate vaccine (Hib)** *(Minimum age: 6 weeks for PRP-T [ActHIB, DTaP-IPV/Hib (Pentacel), and Hib-MenCY (MenHibrix)], PRP-OMP [PedvaxHIB or COMVAX], 12 months for PRP-T [Hiberix])*
Routine vaccination:

- Administer a 2- or 3-dose Hib vaccine primary series and a booster dose (dose 3 or 4 depending on vaccine used in primary series) at 12 to 15 months of age to complete a full Hib vaccine series.

- The primary series with ActHIB, MenHibrix, or Pentacel consists of 3 doses and should be administered at 2, 4, and 6 months of age. The primary series with PedvaxHib or COMVAX consists of 2 doses and should be administered at 2 and 4 months of age; a dose at 6 months of age is not indicated.

- One booster dose (dose 3 or 4 depending on vaccine used in primary series) of any Hib vaccine should be administered at 12 to 15 months of age. An exception is Hiberix vaccine. Hiberix should only be used for the booster (final) dose in children 12 months to 4 years of age who have received at least 1 prior dose of Hib-containing vaccine.

- For recommendations on the use of MenHibrix in patients at increased risk for meningococcal disease, please refer to the meningococcal vaccine footnotes and also to *MMWR*. 2014;63(RR01);1-13. Available at http://www.cdc.gov/mmwr/pdf/rr/rr6301.pdf.

Catch-up vaccination:

- If dose 1 was administered at 12 to 14 months of age, administer a second (final) dose at least 8 weeks after dose 1, regardless of Hib vaccine used in the primary series.

- If the first 2 doses were PRP-OMP (PedvaxHIB or COMVAX) and were administered before the 1st birthday, the third (and final) dose should be administered at 12 to 59 months of age and at least 8 weeks after the second dose.

- If the first dose was administered at 7 to 11 months of age, administer the second dose ≥4 weeks later and a third (and final) dose at 12 to 15 months of age or 8 weeks after the second dose, whichever is later.

- If the first dose is administered before the first birthday and the second dose is administered at <15 months of age, a third (and final) dose should be given 8 weeks later.

- For unvaccinated children ≥15 months of age, administer only 1 dose.

- For other catch-up guidance, see the previous "Catch-up Immunization Schedule". For catch-up guidance related to MenHibrix, please see the meningococcal vaccine footnotes and also *MMWR*. 2014;63(RR01);1-13. Available at http://www.cdc.gov/mmwr/pdf/rr/rr6301.pdf.

Vaccination of persons with high-risk conditions:

- Children 12 to 59 months of age who are at increased risk for Hib disease, including chemotherapy recipients and those with anatomic or functional asplenia (including sickle cell disease), human immunodeficiency virus (HIV) infection, immunoglobulin deficiency, or early component complement deficiency, who have received either no doses or only 1 dose of Hib vaccine before 12 months of age, should receive 2 additional doses of Hib vaccine 8 weeks apart; children who received ≥2 doses of Hib vaccine before 12 months of age should receive 1 additional dose.

- For patients <5 years of age undergoing chemotherapy or radiation treatment who received a Hib vaccine dose(s) within 14 days of starting therapy or during therapy, repeat the dose(s) ≥3 months following therapy completion.

- Recipients of hematopoietic stem cell transplant (HSCT) should be revaccinated with a 3-dose regimen of Hib vaccine starting 6 to 12 months after successful transplant, regardless of vaccination history; doses should be administered ≥4 weeks apart.

- A single dose of any Hib-containing vaccine should be administered to unimmunized* children and adolescents ≥15 months of age undergoing an elective splenectomy; if possible, vaccine should be administered ≥14 days before the procedure.

- Hib vaccine is not routinely recommended for patients ≥5 years of age. However, 1 dose of Hib vaccine should be administered to unimmunized* persons ≥5 years of age who have anatomic or functional asplenia (including sickle cell disease) and unvaccinated persons 5 to 18 years of age with human immunodeficiency virus (HIV) infection.

*Patients who have not received a primary series and booster dose or ≥1 dose of Hib vaccine after 14 months of age are considered unimmunized.

[6]**Pneumococcal vaccines** (*Minimum age: 6 weeks for PCV13, 2 years for PPSV23*)

Routine vaccination with PCV13:

- Administer a 4-dose series of PCV13 vaccine at 2, 4, 6, and 12 to 15 months of age.

- For children 14 to 59 months of age who have received an age-appropriate series of 7-valent PCV (PCV7), administer a single supplemental dose of 13-valent PCV (PCV13).

Catch-up vaccination with PCV13:

- Administer 1 dose of PCV13 to all healthy children 24 to 59 months of age who are not completely vaccinated for their age.

- For other catch-up guidance, see the previous "Catch-up Immunization Schedule".

Vaccination of persons with high-risk conditions with PCV13 and PPSV23:

- All recommended PCV13 doses should be administered prior to PPSV23 vaccination if possible.

- For children 2 to 5 years of age with any of the following conditions: Chronic heart disease (particularly cyanotic congenital heart disease and cardiac failure); chronic lung disease (including asthma if treated with high-dose oral corticosteroid therapy); diabetes mellitus; cerebrospinal fluid leak; cochlear implant; sickle cell disease and other hemoglobuinopathies; anatomic or functional asplenia; HIV infection; chronic renal failure; nephrotic syndrome; diseases associated with treatment with immunosuppressive drugs or radiation therapy, including malignant neoplasms, leukemias, lymphomas, and Hodgkin disease; solid organ transplantation; or congenital immunodeficiency:

  1. Administer 1 dose of PCV13 if any incomplete schedule of 3 doses of PCV (PCV7 and/or PCV13) were received previously.

  2. Administer 2 doses of PCV13 ≥8 weeks apart if unvaccinated or any incomplete schedule of <3 doses of PCV (PCV7 and/or PCV13) were received previously.

  3. Administer 1 supplemental dose of PCV13 if 4 doses of PCV7 or other age-appropriate complete PCV7 series was received previously.

  4. The minimum interval between doses of PCV (PCV7 or PCV13) is 8 weeks.

  5. For children with no history of PPSV23 vaccination, administer PPSV23 ≥8 weeks after the most recent dose of PCV13.

- For children 6 to 18 years of age who have cerebrospinal fluid leak; cochlear implant; sickle cell disease and other hemoglobinopathies; anatomic or functional asplenia; congenital or acquired immunodeficiencies; HIV infection; chronic renal failure; nephrotic syndrome; diseases associated with treatment with immunosuppressive drugs or radiation therapy, including malignant neoplasms, leukemias, lymphomas, and Hodgkin disease; generalized malignancy; solid organ transplantation; or multiple myeloma:

  1. If neither PCV13 nor PPSV23 has been received previously, administer 1 dose of PCV13 now and 1 dose of PPSV23 ≥8 weeks later.

  2. If PCV13 has been received previously but PPSV23 has not, administer 1 dose of PPSV23 ≥8 weeks after the most recent dose of PCV13.

  3. If PPSV23 has been received but PCV13 has not, administer 1 dose of PCV13 ≥8 weeks after the most recent dose of PPSV23.

- For children 6 to 18 years of age with chronic heart disease (particularly cyanotic congenital heart disease and cardiac failure), chronic lung disease (including asthma if treated with high-dose oral corticosteroid therapy), diabetes mellitus, alcoholism, or chronic liver disease, who have not received PPSV23, administer 1 dose of PPSV23. If PCV13 has been received previously, then PPSV23 should be administered ≥8 weeks after any prior PCV13 dose.

- A single revaccination with PPSV23 should be administered 5 years after the first dose to children with sickle cell disease or other hemoglobinopathies; anatomic or functional asplenia; congenital or acquired immunodeficiencies; HIV infection; chronic renal failure; nephrotic syndrome; diseases associated with treatment with immunosuppressive drugs or radiation therapy, including malignant neoplasms, leukemias, lymphomas, and Hodgkin disease; generalized malignancy; solid organ transplantation; or multiple myeloma.

[7]**Inactivated poliovirus vaccine (IPV)** (*Minimum age: 6 weeks*)

Routine vaccination:

- Administer a 4-dose series of IPV at 2, 4, and 6 to 18 months of age and at 4 to 6 years of age. The final dose in the series should be administered on or after the fourth birthday and ≥6 months after the previous dose.

Catch-up vaccination:

- In the first 6 months of life, minimum age and minimum intervals are only recommended if the person is at risk for imminent exposure to circulating poliovirus (ie, travel to a polio-endemic region or during an outbreak).

- If ≥4 doses are administered before 4 years of age, an additional dose should be administered at 4 to 6 years of age and ≥6 months after the previous dose.

- A fourth dose is not necessary if the third dose was administered at ≥4 years of age and ≥6 months after the previous dose.

- If both OPV and IPV were administered as part of a series, a total of 4 doses should be administered, regardless of the child's current age. IPV is not routinely recommended for US residents ≥18 years of age.

- For other catch-up guidance, see the previous "Catch-up Immunization Schedule".

[8]**Influenza vaccines** (*Minimum age: 6 months for inactivated influenza vaccine [IIV]; 2 years for live, attenuated influenza vaccine [LAIV]*)

Routine vaccination:

- Administer influenza vaccine annually to all children beginning at 6 months of age. For most healthy, nonpregnant persons 2 to 49 years of age, either LAIV or IIV may be used. However, LAIV should **not** be administered to some persons, including 1) persons who have experienced severe allergic reactions to LAIV, any of its components, or to a previous dose of any other influenza vaccine; 2) children 2 to 17 years of age receiving aspirin or aspirin-containing products; 3) persons who are allergic to eggs; 4) pregnant women; 5) immunosuppressed persons; 6) children 2 to 4 years of age with asthma or who had wheezing in the past 12 months; or 7) persons who have taken influenza antiviral medicatons in the previous 48 hours. For all other contraindications and precautions to the use of LAIV, see *MMWR*. 2014;63(32);691-697. Available at http://www.cdc.gov/mmwr/pdf/wk/mm6332.pdf.

For children 6 months to 8 years of age:

- For the 2014 to 2015 season, administer 2 doses (separated by ≥4 weeks) to children who are receiving influenza vaccine for the first time. Some children in this age group who have been vaccinated previously will also need 2 doses. For additional guidance, follow dosing guidelines in the 2014 to 2015 ACIP influenza vaccine recommendations. See *MMWR*. 2014;63(32);691-697. Available at http://www.cdc.gov/mmwr/pdf/wk/mm6332.pdf.

- For the 2015 to 2016 season, follow dosing guidelines in the 2015 ACIP influenza vaccine recommendations.

For persons ≥9 years of age:

- Administer 1 dose.

[9]**Measles, mumps, and rubella (MMR) vaccine** (*Minimum age: 12 months for routine vaccination*)

Routine vaccination:

- Administer a 2-dose series of MMR vaccine at 12 to 15 months of age and 4 to 6 years of age. The second dose may be administered before 4 years of age, provided at least 4 weeks have elapsed since the first dose.

- Administer 1 dose of MMR vaccine to infants 6 to 11 months of age before departure from the United States for international travel. These children should be revaccinated with 2 doses of MMR vaccine, the first at 12 to 15 months of age (12 months if the child remains in an area where disease risk is high) and the second dose ≥4 weeks later.

- Administer 2 doses of MMR vaccine to children ≥12 months of age before departure from the United States for international travel. The first dose should be administered at ≥12 months of age and the second dose ≥4 weeks later.

Catch-up vaccination:

- Ensure that all school-aged children and adolescents have had 2 doses of MMR vaccine; the minimum interval between the 2 doses is 4 weeks.

[10]**Varicella (VAR) vaccine** (*Minimum age: 12 months*)

Routine vaccination:

- Administer a 2-dose series of VAR vaccine at 12 to 15 months of age and 4 to 6 years of age. The second dose may be administered before 4 years of age, provided at least 3 months have elapsed since the first dose. If the second dose was administered ≥4 weeks after the first dose, it can be accepted as valid.

Catch-up vaccination:

- Ensure that all persons 7 to 18 years of age without evidence of immunity (see *MMWR*. 2007;56[No. RR-4]. Available at http://www.cdc.gov/mmwr/pdf/rr/rr5604.pdf) have 2 doses of varicella vaccine. For children 7 to 12 years of age, the recommended minimum interval between doses is 3 months (if the second dose was administered ≥4 weeks after the first dose, it can be accepted as valid); for persons ≥13 years of age, the minimum interval between doses is 4 weeks.

[11]**Hepatitis A (HepA) vaccine** (*Minimum age: 12 months*)

Routine vaccination:

- Initiate the 2-dose HepA vaccine series at 12 to 23 months of age; separate the 2 doses by 6 to 18 months.

- Children who have received 1 dose of HepA vaccine before 24 months of age should receive a second dose 6 to 18 months after the first dose.

- For any person ≥2 years of age who has not already received the HepA vaccine series, 2 doses of HepA vaccine separated by 6 to 18 months may be administered if immunity against hepatitis A virus infection is desired.

Catch-up vaccination:

- The minimum interval between the 2 doses is 6 months.

Special populations:

- Administer 2 doses of HepA vaccine ≥6 months apart to previously unvaccinated persons who live in areas where vaccination programs target older children or who are at increased risk for infection. This includes persons traveling to or working in countries that have high or intermediate endemicity of infection; men having sex with men; users of injection and noninjection illicit drugs; persons who work with HAV-infected primates or with HAV in a research laboratory; persons with clotting-factor disorders; persons with chronic liver disease; and persons who anticipate close, personal contact (eg, household or regular babysitting) with an international adoptee during the first 60 days after arrival in the United States from a country with high or intermediate endemicity. The first dose should be administered as soon as the adoption is planned, ideally ≥2 weeks before the arrival of the adoptee.

[12]**Human papillomavirus (HPV) vaccines** (*Minimum age: 9 years for HPV2 [Cervarix] and HPV4 [Gardasil]*)

Routine vaccination:

- Administer a 3-dose series of HPV vaccine on a schedule of 0, 1 to 2, and 6 months to all adolescents 11 to 12 years of age. Either HPV4 or HPV2 may be used for females and only HPV4 may be used for males.

- The vaccine series can be started beginning at 9 years of age.

- Administer the second dose 1 to 2 months after the first dose (minimum interval of 4 weeks) and administer the third dose 24 weeks after the first dose and 16 weeks after the second dose (minimum interval of 12 weeks).

Catch-up vaccination:

- Administer the vaccine series to females (either HPV2 or HPV4) and males (HPV4) at 13 to 18 years of age if not previously vaccinated.

- Use recommended routine dosing intervals (see above) for vaccine series catch-up.

[13]**Meningococcal conjugate vaccines** (*Minimum age: 6 weeks for Hib-MenCY [MenHibrix], 9 months for MenACWY-D [Menactra], 2 months for MenACWY-CRM [Menveo]*)

Routine vaccination:

- Administer a single dose of Menactra or Menveo vaccine at 11 to 12 years of age with a booster dose at 16 years of age.

- Adolescents 11 to 18 years of age with human immunodeficiency virus (HIV) infection should receive a 2-dose primary series of Menactra or Menveo with ≥8 weeks between doses.

- For children 2 months to 18 years of age with high-risk conditions, see below.

Catch-up vaccination:

- Administer Menactra or Menveo vaccine at 13 to 18 years of age if not previously vaccinated.

- If the first dose is administered at 13 to 15 years of age, a booster dose should be administered at 16 to 18 years of age with a minimum interval of ≥8 weeks between doses.

- If the first dose is administered at ≥16 years of age, a booster dose is not needed.

- For other catch-up guidance, see the previous "Catch-up Immunization Schedule".

Vaccination of persons with high-risk conditions and other persons at increased risk of disease:

- Children with anatomic or functional asplenia (including sickle cell disease):

  1. Menveo

     – *Children who initiate vaccination at 8 weeks to 6 months of age:* Administer doses at 2, 4, 6, and 12 months of age

     – *Unvaccinated children 7 to 23 months of age:* Administer 2 doses, with the second dose ≥12 weeks after the first dose **and** after the first birthday

     – *Children ≥24 months who have not received a complete series:* Administer 2 primary doses ≥8 weeks apart

  2. MenHibrix

     – *Children 6 weeks to 18 months of age:* Administer doses at 2, 4, 6, and 12 to 15 months of age.

     – If the first dose of MenHibrix is given ≥12 months of age, a total of 2 doses should be given ≥8 weeks apart to ensure protection against serogroups C and Y meningococcal disease.

  3. Menactra

     – *Children ≥24 months who have not received a complete series:* Administer 2 primary doses ≥8 weeks apart. If Menactra is administered to a child with asplenia (including sickle cell disease), do not administer Menactra until 2 years of age and ≥4 weeks after the completion of all PCV13 doses.

- Children with persistent complement component deficiency:

  1. Menveo

     – *Children who initiate vaccination at 8 weeks to 6 months of age:* Administer doses at 2, 4, 6, and 12 months of age.

     – *Unvaccinated children 7 to 23 months of age:* Administer 2 doses, with the second dose ≥12 weeks after the first dose **and** after the first birthday.

     – *Children ≥24 months of age who have not received a complete series:* Administer 2 primary doses ≥8 weeks apart.

  2. MenHibrix

     – *Children 6 weeks to 18 months:* Administer doses at 2, 4, 6, and 12 to 15 months of age.

     – If the first dose of MenHibrix is given at ≥12 months of age, a total of 2 doses should be given ≥8 weeks apart to ensure protection against serogroups C and Y meningococcal disease.

  3. Menactra

     – *Children 9 to 23 months of age:* Administer 2 primary doses ≥12 weeks apart.

     – *Children ≥24 months of age who have not received a complete series:* Administer 2 primary doses ≥8 weeks apart.

- For children who travel to or reside in countries in which meningococcal disease is hyperendemic or epidemic, including countries in the African meningitis belt or the Hajj, administer an age-appropriate formulation and series of Menactra or Menveo for protection against serogroups A and W meningococcal disease. Prior receipt of MenHibrix is not sufficient for children traveling to the meningitis belt or the Hajj because it does not contain serogroups A or W.

- For children at risk during a community outbreak attributable to a vaccine serogroup, administer or complete an age- and formulation-appropriate series of MenHibrix, Menactra, or Menveo.

- For booster doses among persons with high-risk conditions, refer to MMWR. 2013;62(RR02);1-22. Available at http://www.cdc.gov/mmwr/preview/mmwrhtml/rr6202a1.htm

For other catch-up recommendations for these persons and complete information on the use of meningococcal vaccines, including guidance related to vaccination of persons at increased risk of infection, see MMWR. 2013;62(RR02);1-22. Available at http://www.cdc.gov/mmwr/preview/mmwrhtml/rr6202a1.htm

This schedule is approved by the Advisory Committee on Immunization Practices (**http://www.cdc.gov/vaccines/acip/index.-html**), the American Academy of Pediatrics (**http://www.aap.org**), the American Academy of Family Physicians (**http://www.aafp.org**), and the American College of Obstetricians and Gynecologists (**http://www.acog.org**).

REFERENCE

Centers for Disease Control and Prevention (CDC). Advisory Committee on Immunization Practices (ACIP) recommended immunization schedules for persons aged 0 through 18 years and adults aged 19 years and older – United States, 2015. Available at http://www.cdc.gov/vaccines/schedules/hcp/child-adolescent.html

Recommended Adult Immunization Schedule by Vaccine and Age Group[1] — United States, 2015

Vaccine	19 to 21 years	22 to 26 years	27 to 49 years	50 to 59 years	60 to 64 years	≥ 65 years
Influenza[2,*]	1 dose annually					
Tetanus, diphtheria, pertussis (Td/Tdap)[3,*]	Substitute 1-time dose of Tdap for Td booster; then boost with Td every 10 y					
Varicella[4,*]	2 doses					
Human papillomavirus (HPV) female[5,*]	3 doses					
Human papillomavirus (HPV) male[5,*]	3 doses					
Zoster[6]					1 dose	
Measles, mumps, rubella (MMR)[7,*]	1 or 2 doses					
Pneumococcal 13-valent conjugate (PCV13)[8,*]					1-time dose	
Pneumococcal polysaccharide (PPSV23)[8]	1 or 2 doses					1 dose
Meningococcal[9,*]	1 or more doses					
Hepatitis A[10,*]	2 doses					
Hepatitis B[11,*]	3 doses					
Haemophilus influenzae type b (Hib)[12,*]	1 or 3 doses					

*Covered by the Vaccine Injury Compensation Program.

For all persons in this category who meet the age requirements and who lack documentation of vaccination or have no evidence of previous infection; zoster vaccine recommended regardless of prior episode of zoster.

Recommended if some other risk factor is present (eg, on the basis of medical, occupational, lifestyle, or other indication).

No recommendation.

NOTE: The recommendations in the tables must be read along with the following footnotes.

Vaccines That Might Be Indicated for Adults Based on Medical and Other Indications[1]

Vaccine	Pregnancy	Immunocompromising conditions (excluding human immunodeficiency virus [HIV])[4,6,7,8,13]	HIV infection CD4+ T lymphocyte count[4,6,7,8,13] < 200 cells/µL	HIV infection CD4+ T lymphocyte count[4,6,7,8,13] ≥ 200 cells/µL	Men who have sex with men (MSM)	Kidney failure, end-stage renal disease, receipt of hemodialysis	Heart disease, chronic lung disease, chronic alcoholism	Asplenia (including elective splenectomy and persistent complement component deficiencies)[8,12]	Chronic liver disease	Diabetes	Healthcare personnel
Influenza[2,*]	1 dose IIV annually				1 dose IIV or LAIV annually	1 dose IIV annually					1 dose IIV or LAIV annually
Tetanus, diphtheria, pertussis (Td/Tdap)[3,*]	1 dose Tdap each pregnancy	Substitute 1-time dose of Tdap for Td booster; then boost with Td every 10 years									
Varicella[4,*]	Contraindicated				2 doses						
Human papillomavirus (HPV) female[5,*]	3 doses through age 26 yrs				3 doses through age 26 yrs						
Human papillomavirus (HPV) male[5,*]	3 doses through age 26 yrs				3 doses through age 21 yrs						
Zoster[6]	Contraindicated				1 dose						
Measles, mumps, rubella (MMR)[7,*]	Contraindicated				1 or 2 doses						
Pneumococcal 13-valent conjugate (PCV13)[8,*]					1 dose						
Pneumococcal polysaccharide (PPSV23)[8]					1 or 2 doses						
Meningococcal[9,*]	1 or more doses										
Hepatitis A[10,*]	2 doses										
Hepatitis B[11,*]	3 doses										
Haemophilus influenzae type b (Hib)[12,*]	post-HSCT recipients only	1 or 3 doses									

*Covered by the Vaccine Injury Compensation Program.

For all persons in this category who meet the age requirements and who lack documentation of vaccination or have no evidence of previous infection; zoster vaccine recommended regardless of prior episode of zoster.

Recommended if some other risk factor is present (eg, on the basis of medical, occupational, lifestyle, or other indication).

No recommendation.

NOTE: The recommendations in the tables must be read along with the following footnotes.

Footnotes to Recommended Adult Immunization Schedule – United States, 2015

[1]Additional information

- Additional guidance for the use of the vaccines described in this supplement is available at http://www.cdc.gov/vaccines/hcp/acip-recs/index.html.

- Information on vaccination recommendations when vaccination status is unknown and other general immunization information can be found in the General Recommendations on Immunization at http://www.cdc.gov/mmwr/preview/mmwrhtml/rr6002a1.htm.

- Information on travel vaccine requirements and recommendations (eg, for hepatitis A and B, meningococcal, other vaccines) is available at http://wwwnc.cdc.gov/travel/destinations/list.

- Additional information and resources regarding vaccination of pregnant women can be found at http://www.cdc.gov/vaccines/adults/rec-vac/pregnant.html.

[2]Influenza vaccination

- Annual vaccination against influenza is recommended for all persons ≥6 months of age.

- Persons ≥6 months of age, including pregnant women and persons with hives-only allergy to eggs, can receive the inactivated influenza vaccine (IIV). An age-appropriate IIV formulation should be used.

- Adults ≥18 years of age can receive the recombinant influenza vaccine (RIV) (FluBlok). RIV does not contain any egg protein and can be given to age-appropriate persons with egg allergy of any severity.

- Healthy, nonpregnant persons 2 to 49 years of age without high-risk medical conditions can receive either intranasally administered live, attenuated influenza vaccine (LAIV) (FluMist) or IIV.

- Health care personnel who care for severely immunocompromised persons who require care in a protected environment should receive IIV or RIV; health care personnel who receive LAIV should avoid providing care for severely immunosuppressed persons for 7 days after vaccination.

- The intramuscularly or intradermally administered IIV are options for adults 18 to 64 years of age.

- Adults ≥65 years of age can receive the standard-dose IIV or the high-dose IIV (Fluzone High-Dose).

- A list of currently available influenza vaccines can be found at http://www.cdc.gov/flu/protect/vaccine/vaccines.htm.

[3]Tetanus, diphtheria, and acellular pertussis (Td/Tdap) vaccination

- Administer 1 dose of Tdap vaccine to pregnant women during each pregnancy (preferably during 27 to 36 weeks' gestation), regardless of interval since prior Td or Tdap vaccination.

- Persons ≥11 years of age who have not received Tdap vaccine or for whom vaccine status is unknown should receive a dose of Tdap, followed by tetanus and diphtheria toxoids (Td) booster doses every 10 years thereafter. Tdap can be administered regardless of interval since the most recent tetanus or diphtheria-toxoid-containing vaccine.

- Adults with an unknown or incomplete history of completing a 3-dose primary vaccination series with Td-containing vaccines should begin or complete a primary vaccination series, including a Tdap dose.

- For unvaccinated adults, administer the first 2 doses ≥4 weeks apart and the third dose 6 to 12 months after the second.

- For incompletely vaccinated adults (ie, <3 doses), administer remaining doses.

- Refer to the ACIP statement for recommendations for administering Td/Tdap as prophylaxis in wound management (see footnote 1).

[4]Varicella vaccination

- All adults without evidence of immunity to varicella (as defined below) should receive 2 doses of single-antigen varicella vaccine or a second dose if they have received only 1 dose.

- Vaccination should be emphasized for those who have close contact with persons at high risk for severe disease (eg, health care personnel and family contacts of persons with immunocompromising conditions) or who are at high risk for exposure or transmission (eg, teachers; child care employees; residents and staff members of institutional settings, including correctional institutions; college students; military personnel; adolescents and adults living in households with children; nonpregnant women of childbearing age; international travelers).

- Pregnant women should be assessed for evidence of varicella immunity. Women who do not have evidence of immunity should receive the first dose of varicella vaccine upon completion or termination of pregnancy and before discharge from the health care facility. The second dose should be administered 4 to 8 weeks after the first dose.

- Evidence of immunity to varicella in adults includes any of the following:

  - Documentation of 2 doses of varicella vaccine ≥4 weeks apart

  - US-born before 1980, except health care personnel and pregnant women

  - History of varicella based on diagnosis or verification of varicella disease by a health care provider

  - History of herpes zoster based on diagnosis or verification of herpes zoster disease by a health care provider, or

  - Laboratory evidence of immunity or laboratory confirmation of disease

[5]Human papillomavirus (HPV) vaccination

- Two vaccines are licensed for use in females, bivalent HPV vaccine (HPV2) and quadrivalent HPV vaccine (HPV4), and one HPV vaccine for use in males, HPV4.

- For females, either HPV4 or HPV2 is recommended in a 3-dose series for routine vaccination at 11 or 12 years of age, and for those 13 to 26 years of age, if not previously vaccinated.

- For males, HPV4 is recommended in a 3-dose series for routine vaccination at 11 or 12 years of age, and for those 13 to 21 years of age, if not previously vaccinated. Males 22 to 26 years of age may be vaccinated.

- HPV4 is recommended for men who have sex with men through 26 years of age for those who did not get any or all doses when they were younger.

- Vaccination is recommended for immunocompromised persons (including those with HIV infection) through 26 years of age for those who did not get any or all doses when they were younger.

- A complete series for either HPV4 or HPV2 consists of 3 doses. The second dose should be administered 4 to 8 weeks (minimum interval of 4 weeks) after the first dose; the third dose should be administered 24 weeks after the first dose and 16 weeks after the second dose (minimum interval of ≥12 weeks).

- HPV vaccines are not recommended for use in pregnant women. However, pregnancy testing is not needed before vaccination. If a woman is found to be pregnant after initiating the vaccination series, no intervention is needed; the remainder of the 3-dose series should be delayed until completion or termination of pregnancy.

[6]Zoster vaccination

- A single dose of zoster vaccine is recommended for adults ≥60 years of age, regardless of whether they report a prior episode of herpes zoster. Although the vaccine is licensed by the US Food and Drug Administration for use among and can be administered to persons ≥50 years of age, ACIP recommends that vaccination begin at 60 years of age.

- Persons ≥60 years of age with chronic medical conditions may be vaccinated, unless their condition constitutes a contraindication, such as pregnancy or severe immunodeficiency.

[7]Measles, mumps, rubella (MMR) vaccination

- Adults born before 1957 generally are considered immune to measles and mumps. All adults born in 1957 or later should have documentation of ≥1 dose of MMR vaccine, unless they have a medical contraindication to the vaccine or laboratory evidence of immunity to each of the three diseases. Documentation of provider-diagnosed disease is not considered acceptable evidence of immunity for measles, mumps, or rubella.

- **Measles component:**
  - A routine second dose of MMR vaccine, administered a minimum of 28 days after the first dose, is recommended for adults who:
    - Are students in postsecondary educational institutions
    - Work in a health care facility, or
    - Plan to travel internationally
  - Persons who received inactivated (killed) measles vaccine or measles vaccine of unknown type during 1963 to 1967 should be revaccinated with 2 doses of MMR vaccine.

- **Mumps component:**
  - A routine second dose of MMR vaccine, administered a minimum of 28 days after the first dose, is recommended for adults who:
    - Are students in a postsecondary educational institution
    - Work in a health care facility, or
    - Plan to travel internationally
  - Persons vaccinated before 1979 with either killed mumps vaccine or mumps vaccine of unknown type who are at high risk for mumps infection (eg, persons who are working in a health care facility) should be considered for revaccination with 2 doses of MMR vaccine.

- **Rubella component:** For women of childbearing age, regardless of birth year, rubella immunity should be determined. If there is no evidence of immunity, women who are not pregnant should be vaccinated. Pregnant women who do not have evidence of immunity should receive MMR vaccine upon completion or termination of pregnancy and before discharge from the health care facility.

- **Health care personnel born before 1957:** For unvaccinated health care personnel born before 1957 who lack laboratory evidence of measles, mumps, and/or rubella immunity or laboratory confirmation of disease, health care facilities should consider vaccinating personnel with 2 doses of MMR vaccine at the appropriate interval for measles and mumps or 1 dose of MMR vaccine for rubella.

[8]**Pneumococcal (13-valent pneumococcal conjugate vaccine [PCV13] and 23-valent pneumococcal polysaccharide vaccine [PPSV23]) vaccination**

- General information
  - When indicated, only a single dose of PCV13 is recommended for adults.
  - No additional dose of PPSV23 is indicated for adults vaccinated with PPSV23 at ≥65 years of age.
  - When both PCV13 and PPSV23 are indicated, PCV13 should be administered first; PCV13 and PPSV23 should not be administered during the same visit.
  - When indicated, PCV13 and PPSV23 should be administered to adults whose pneumococcal vaccination history is incomplete or unknown.

- Adults ≥65 years of age who:
  - Have not received PCV13 or PPSV23: Administer PCV13, followed by PPSV23 in 6 to 12 months.
  - Have not received PCV13 but have received a dose of PPSV23 at ≥65 years of age: Administer PCV13 ≥1 year after the dose of PPSV23 received at ≥65 years of age.
  - Have not received PCV13 but have received ≥1 doses of PPSV23 before 65 years of age: Administer PCV13 ≥1 year after the most recent dose of PPSV23; administer a dose of PPSV23 6 to 12 months after PCV13, or as soon as possible if this time window has passed, and ≥5 years after the most recent dose of PPSV23.
  - Have received PCV13 but not PPSV23 before 65 years of age: Administer PPSV23 6 to 12 months after PCV13 or as soon as possible if this time window has passed.
  - Have received PCV13 and ≥1 doses of PPSV23 before 65 years of age: Administer PPSV23 6 to 12 months after PCV13, or as soon as possible if this time window has passed, and ≥5 years after the most recent dose of PPSV23.

- Adults 19 to 64 years of age with immunocompromising conditions or anatomical or functional asplenia (defined below) who:
  - Have not received PCV13 or PPSV23: Administer PCV13, followed by PPSV23 ≥8 weeks after PCV13; administer a second dose of PPSV23 ≥5 years after the first dose of PPSV23.
  - Have not received PCV13 but have received 1 dose of PPSV23: Administer PCV13 ≥1 year after the PPSV23; administer a second dose of PPSV23 ≥8 weeks after PCV13 and ≥5 years after the first dose of PPSV23.
  - Have not received PCV13 but have received 2 doses of PPSV23: Administer PCV13 ≥1 year after the most recent dose of PPSV23.
  - Have received PCV13 but not PPSV23: Administer PPSV23 ≥8 weeks after PCV13; administer a second dose of PPSV23 ≥5 years after the first dose of PPSV23.
  - Have received PCV13 and 1 dose of PPSV23: Administer a second dose of PPSV23 ≥5 years after the first dose of PPSV23.

- Adults 19 to 64 years with cerebrospinal fluid leaks or cochlear implants: Administer PCV13, followed by PPSV23 ≥8 weeks after PCV13.

- Adults 19 to 64 years of age with chronic heart disease (including congestive heart failure and cardiomyopathies, excluding hypertension), chronic lung disease (including chronic obstructive lung disease, emphysema, and asthma), chronic liver disease (including cirrhosis), alcoholism, or diabetes mellitus: Administer PPSV23.

- Adults 19 to 64 years of age who smoke cigarettes or reside in nursing home or long-term care facilities: Administer PPSV23.

- Routine pneumococcal vaccination is not recommended for America Indian/Alaska Native or other adults, unless they have the indications as above; however, public health authorities may consider recommending the use of pneumococcal vaccines for American Indians/Alaska Natives or other adults who live in areas with increased risk for invasive pneumococcal disease.

- Immunocomopromising conditions that are indications for pneumococcal vaccination are: Congenital or acquired immunodeficiency (including B- or T-lymphocyte deficiency, complement deficiencies, and phagocytic disorders, excluding chronic granulomatous disease), HIV infection, chronic renal failure, nephrotic syndrome, leukemia, lymphoma, Hodgkin disease, generalized malignancy, multiple myeloma, solid organ transplant, and iatrogenic immunosuppression (including long-term systemic corticosteroids and radiation therapy).

- Anatomical or functional asplenia that are indications for pneumococcal vaccination are: Sickle cell disease and other hemoglobinopathies, congenital or acquired asplenia, splenic dysfunction, and splenectomy. Administer pneumococcal vaccines ≥2 weeks before immunosuppresssive therapy or an elective splenectomy, and as soon as possible to adults who are newly diagnosed with asymptomatic or symptomatic HIV infection.

[9]Meningococcal vaccination

- Administer 2 doses of quadrivalent meningococcal conjugate vaccine (MenACWY [Menactra, Menveo]) ≥2 months apart to adults of all ages with anatomical or functional asplenia or persistent complement component deficiencies. HIV infection is not an indication for routine vaccination with MenACWY. If an HIV-infected person of any age is vaccinated, 2 doses of MenACWY should be administered ≥2 months apart.

- Administer a single dose of meningococcal vaccine to microbiologists routinely exposed to isolates of *Neisseria meningitidis*, military recruits, persons at risk during an outbreak attributable to a vaccine serogroup, and persons who travel to or live in countries in which meningococcal disease is hyperendemic or epidemic.

- First-year college students ≤21 years of age who are living in residence halls should be vaccinated if they have not received a dose on or after their 16th birthday.

- MenACWY is preferred for adults with any of the preceding indications who are ≤55 years of age, as well as for adults ≥56 years of age: a) who were vaccinated previously with MenACWY and are recommended for revaccination, or b) for whom multiple doses are anticipated. Meningococcal polysaccharide vaccine (MPSV4 [Menomune]) is preferred for adults ≥56 years of age who have not received MenACWY previously and who require a single dose only (eg, travelers).

- Revaccination with MenACWY every 5 years is recommended for adults previously vaccinated with MenACWY or MPSV4 who remain at increased risk for infection (eg, adults with anatomic or functional asplenia, persistent complement component deficiencies, or microbiologists).

[10]Hepatitis A vaccination

- Vaccinate any person seeking protection from hepatitis A virus (HAV) infection and persons with any of the following indications:

  – Men who have sex with men and persons who use injection or noninjection illicit drugs

  – Persons working with HAV-infected primates or with HAV in a research laboratory setting

  – Persons with chronic liver disease and persons who receive clotting factor concentrates

  – Persons traveling to or working in countries that have high or intermediate endemicity of hepatitis A, and

  – Unvaccinated persons who anticipate close personal contatct (eg, household, regular babysitting) with an international adoptee during the first 60 days after arrival in the United States from a country with high or intermediate endemicity (see footnote 1 for more information on travel recommendations). The first dose of the 2-dose hepatitis A vaccine series should be administered as soon as adoption is planned, ideally ≥2 weeks before the arrival of the adoptee.

- Single-antigen vaccine formulations should be administered in a 2-dose schedule at either 0 and 6 to 12 months (Havrix) or 0 and 6 to 18 months (Vaqta). If the combined hepatitis A and hepatitis B vaccine (Twinrix) is used, administer 3 doses at 0, 1, and 6 months; alternatively, a 4-dose schedule may be used, administered on days 0, 7, and 21 to 30, followed by a booster dose at month 12.

[11]Hepatitis B vaccination

- Vaccinate persons with any of the following indications and any person seeking protection from hepatitis B virus (HBV) infection:

  – Sexually active persons who are not in a long-term, mutually monogamous relationship (eg, persons with >1 sex partner during the previous 6 months), persons seeking evaluation or treatment for a sexually transmitted disease (STD), current or recent injection drug users, and men who have sex with men

  – Health care personnel and public safety workers who are potentially exposed to blood or other infectious body fluids

  – Persons with diabetes who are <60 years of age as soon as feasible after diagnosis; persons with diabetes who are ≥60 years of age at the discretion of the treating clinician, based on the likelihood of acquiring HBV infection, including the risk posed by an increased need for assisted blood glucose monitoring in long-term care facilities, the likelihood of experiencing chronic sequelae if infected with HBV, and the likelihood of immune response to vaccination

  – Persons with end-stage renal disease, including patients receiving hemodialysis, persons with HIV infection, and persons with chronic liver disease

  – Household contacts and sex partners of hepatitis B surface antigen-positive persons, clients and staff members of institutions for persons with developmental disabilities, and international travelers to countries with high or intermediate prevalence of chronic HBV infection, and

  – All adults in the following settings: STD treatment facilities, HIV testing and treatment facilities, facilities providing drug-abuse treatment and prevention services, health care settings targeting services to injection drug users or men who have sex with men, correctional facilities, end-stage renal disease programs and facilities for chronic hemodialysis patients, and institutions and nonresidential day care facilities for persons with developmental disabilities

- Administer missing doses to complete a 3-dose series of hepatitis B vaccine to those persons not vaccinated or not completely vaccinated. The second dose should be administered 1 month after the first dose; the third dose should be given ≥2 months after the second dose (and ≥4 months after the first dose). If the combined hepatitis A and hepatitis B vaccine (Twinrix) is used, give 3 doses at 0, 1, and 6 months; alternatively, a 4-dose Twinrix schedule, administered on days 0, 7, and 21 to 30, followed by a booster dose at month 12, may be used.

- Adult patients receiving hemodialysis or with other immunocompromising conditions should receive 1 dose of 40 mcg/mL (Recombivax HB) administered on a 3-dose schedule at 0, 1, and 6 months, or 2 doses of 20 mcg/mL (Engerix-B) administered simultaneously on a 4-dose schedule at 0, 1, 2, and 6 months.

[12]*Haemophilus influenzae* type b (Hib) vaccination

- One dose of Hib vaccine should be administered to persons who have anatomical or functional asplenia or sickle cell disease or to those who are undergoing elective splenectomy if they have not previously received Hib vaccine. Hib vaccination ≥14 days before splenectomy is suggested.

- Receipients of a hematopoietic stem cell transplant (HSCT) should be vaccinated with a 3-dose regimen 6 to 12 months after a successful transplant, regardless of vaccination history; ≥4 weeks should separate doses.

- Hib vaccine is not recommended for adults with HIV infection since their risk for Hib infection is low.

[13]Immunocompromising conditions

- Inactivated vaccines generally are acceptable (eg, pneumococcal, meningococcal, inactivated influenza vaccine) and live vaccines generally are avoided in persons with immune deficiencies or immunocompromising conditions. Information on specific conditions is available at http://www.cdc.gov/vaccines/hcp/acip-recs/index.html.

REFERENCE

Centers for Disease Control and Prevention (CDC). Advisory Committee on Immunization Practices (ACIP) recommended immunization schedules for persons aged 0 through 18 years and adults aged 19 years and older – United States, 2014. Available at http://www.cdc.gov/vaccines/schedules/hcp/adult.html

PEDIATRIC ALS (PALS) ALGORITHMS

Pediatric Bradycardia
With a Pulse and Poor Perfusion

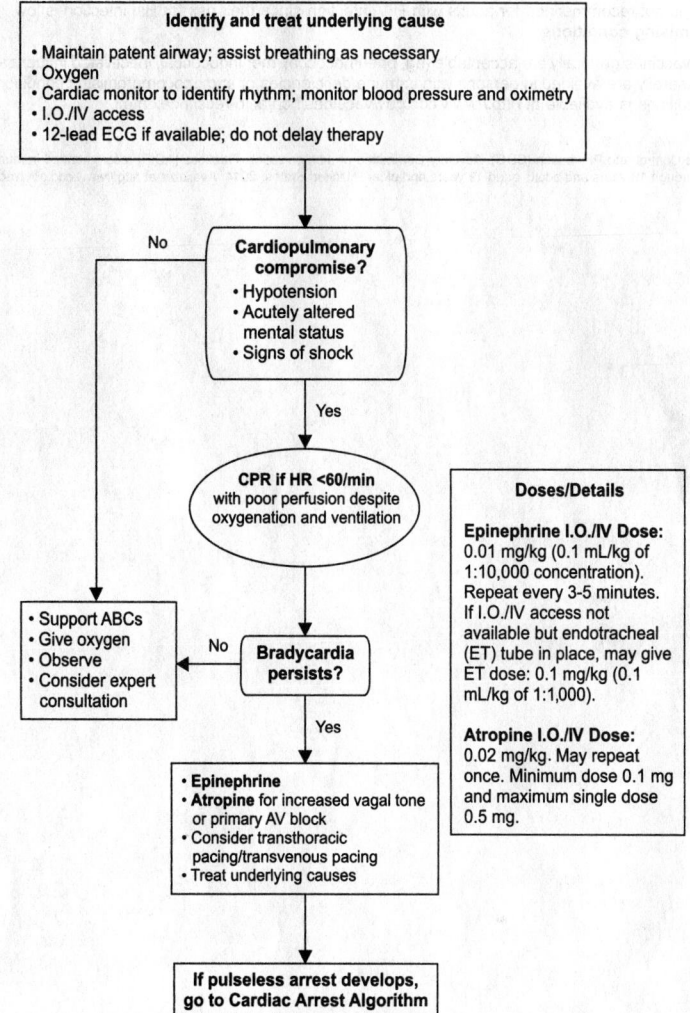

Identify and treat underlying cause

- Maintain patent airway; assist breathing as necessary
- Oxygen
- Cardiac monitor to identify rhythm; monitor blood pressure and oximetry
- I.O./IV access
- 12-lead ECG if available; do not delay therapy

No →

Cardiopulmonary compromise?
- Hypotension
- Acutely altered mental status
- Signs of shock

Yes ↓

CPR if HR <60/min with poor perfusion despite oxygenation and ventilation

- Support ABCs
- Give oxygen
- Observe
- Consider expert consultation

← No — **Bradycardia persists?**

Yes ↓

- **Epinephrine**
- **Atropine** for increased vagal tone or primary AV block
- Consider transthoracic pacing/transvenous pacing
- Treat underlying causes

If pulseless arrest develops, go to Cardiac Arrest Algorithm

Doses/Details

Epinephrine I.O./IV Dose:
0.01 mg/kg (0.1 mL/kg of 1:10,000 concentration). Repeat every 3-5 minutes. If I.O./IV access not available but endotracheal (ET) tube in place, may give ET dose: 0.1 mg/kg (0.1 mL/kg of 1:1,000).

Atropine I.O./IV Dose:
0.02 mg/kg. May repeat once. Minimum dose 0.1 mg and maximum single dose 0.5 mg.

Pediatric Cardiac Arrest Algorithm

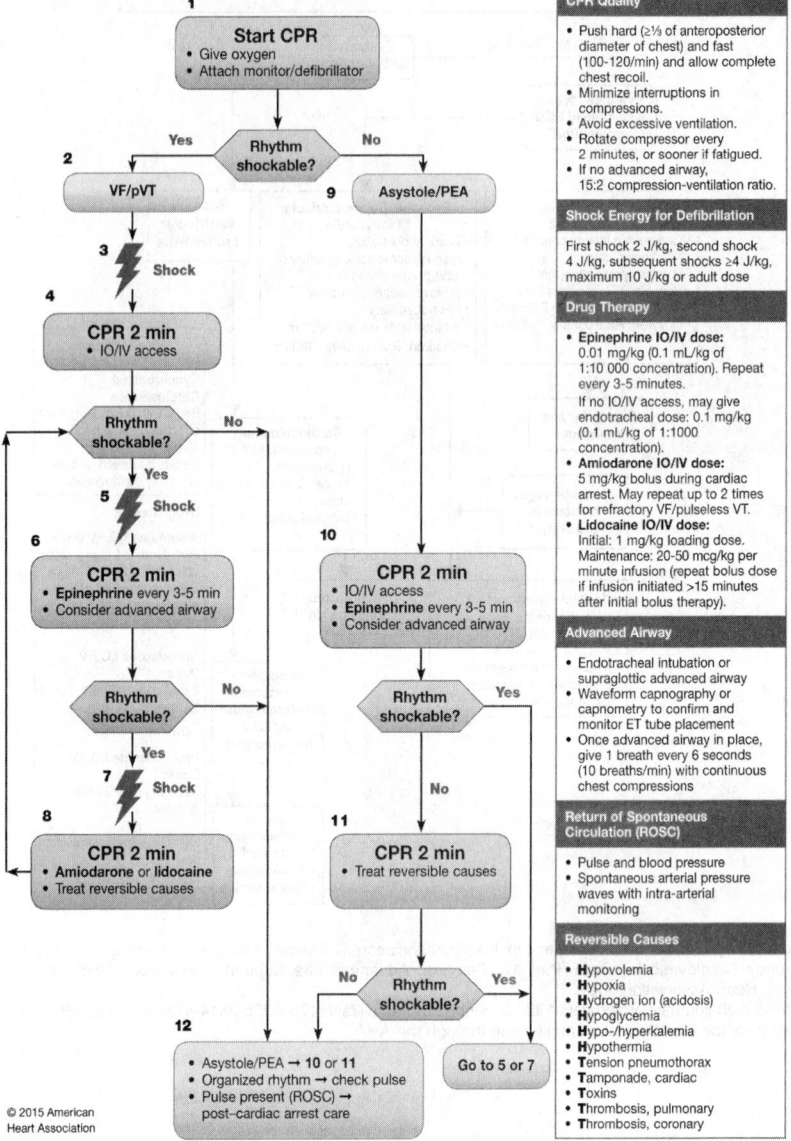

CPR Quality

- Push hard (≥⅓ of anteroposterior diameter of chest) and fast (100-120/min) and allow complete chest recoil.
- Minimize interruptions in compressions.
- Avoid excessive ventilation.
- Rotate compressor every 2 minutes, or sooner if fatigued.
- If no advanced airway, 15:2 compression-ventilation ratio.

Shock Energy for Defibrillation

First shock 2 J/kg, second shock 4 J/kg, subsequent shocks ≥4 J/kg, maximum 10 J/kg or adult dose

Drug Therapy

- **Epinephrine IO/IV dose:** 0.01 mg/kg (0.1 mL/kg of 1:10 000 concentration). Repeat every 3-5 minutes. If no IO/IV access, may give endotracheal dose: 0.1 mg/kg (0.1 mL/kg of 1:1000 concentration).
- **Amiodarone IO/IV dose:** 5 mg/kg bolus during cardiac arrest. May repeat up to 2 times for refractory VF/pulseless VT.
- **Lidocaine IO/IV dose:** Initial: 1 mg/kg loading dose. Maintenance: 20-50 mcg/kg per minute infusion (repeat bolus dose if infusion initiated >15 minutes after initial bolus therapy).

Advanced Airway

- Endotracheal intubation or supraglottic advanced airway
- Waveform capnography or capnometry to confirm and monitor ET tube placement
- Once advanced airway in place, give 1 breath every 6 seconds (10 breaths/min) with continuous chest compressions

Return of Spontaneous Circulation (ROSC)

- Pulse and blood pressure
- Spontaneous arterial pressure waves with intra-arterial monitoring

Reversible Causes

- **H**ypovolemia
- **H**ypoxia
- **H**ydrogen ion (acidosis)
- **H**ypoglycemia
- **H**ypo-/hyperkalemia
- **H**ypothermia
- **T**ension pneumothorax
- **T**amponade, cardiac
- **T**oxins
- **T**hrombosis, pulmonary
- **T**hrombosis, coronary

© 2015 American Heart Association

Pediatric Tachycardia
With a Pulse and Poor Perfusion

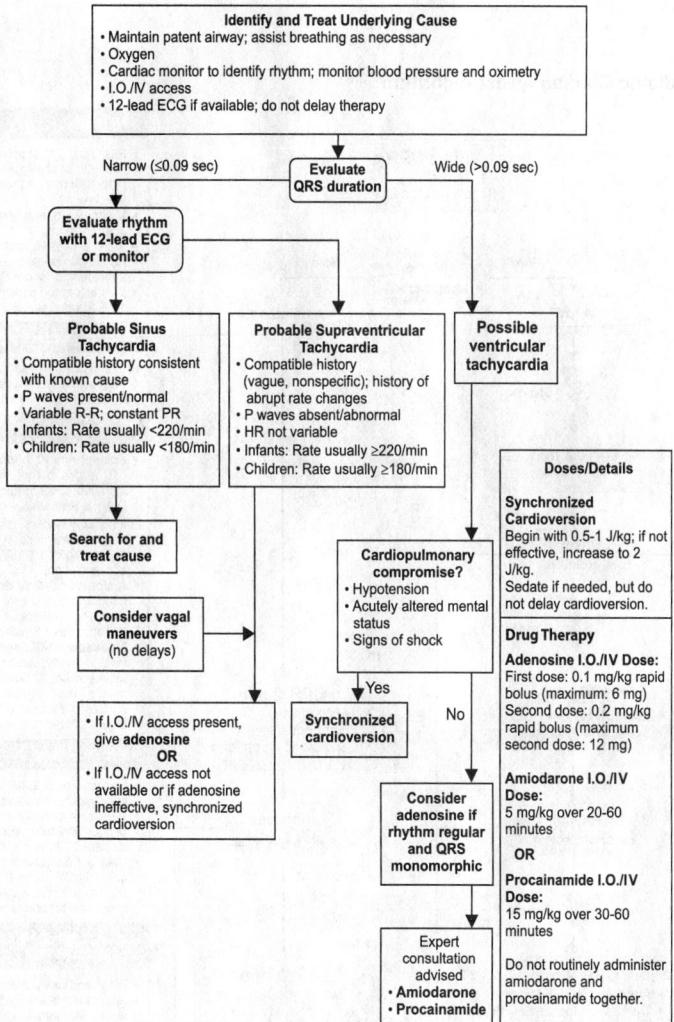

Identify and Treat Underlying Cause
- Maintain patent airway; assist breathing as necessary
- Oxygen
- Cardiac monitor to identify rhythm; monitor blood pressure and oximetry
- I.O./IV access
- 12-lead ECG if available; do not delay therapy

Narrow (≤0.09 sec) — **Evaluate QRS duration** — Wide (>0.09 sec)

Evaluate rhythm with 12-lead ECG or monitor

Probable Sinus Tachycardia
- Compatible history consistent with known cause
- P waves present/normal
- Variable R-R; constant PR
- Infants: Rate usually <220/min
- Children: Rate usually <180/min

Probable Supraventricular Tachycardia
- Compatible history (vague, nonspecific); history of abrupt rate changes
- P waves absent/abnormal
- HR not variable
- Infants: Rate usually ≥220/min
- Children: Rate usually ≥180/min

Possible ventricular tachycardia

Search for and treat cause

Consider vagal maneuvers (no delays)

Cardiopulmonary compromise?
- Hypotension
- Acutely altered mental status
- Signs of shock

Yes → **Synchronized cardioversion**

No

- If I.O./IV access present, give **adenosine**
  OR
- If I.O./IV access not available or if adenosine ineffective, synchronized cardioversion

Consider adenosine if rhythm regular and QRS monomorphic

Expert consultation advised
- **Amiodarone**
- **Procainamide**

Doses/Details

Synchronized Cardioversion
Begin with 0.5-1 J/kg; if not effective, increase to 2 J/kg.
Sedate if needed, but do not delay cardioversion.

Drug Therapy

Adenosine I.O./IV Dose:
First dose: 0.1 mg/kg rapid bolus (maximum: 6 mg)
Second dose: 0.2 mg/kg rapid bolus (maximum second dose: 12 mg)

Amiodarone I.O./IV Dose:
5 mg/kg over 20-60 minutes

  OR

Procainamide I.O./IV Dose:
15 mg/kg over 30-60 minutes

Do not routinely administer amiodarone and procainamide together.

Reprinted with permission: 2015 American Heart Association Guidelines Update for Cardiopulmonary Resuscitation and Emergency Cardiovascular Care. Part 12: Pediatric Advanced Life Support. *Circulation.* 2015;132:S526-S542. ©2015 American Heart Association, Inc.
See http://circ.ahajournals.org/content/132/18_suppl_2/S526.full?sid=175c323b-2814-4138-affd-4fa0155e634c.
All requests to use this information must come through the AHA.

ADULT ACLS ALGORITHMS

Adult Bradycardia
(With Pulse)

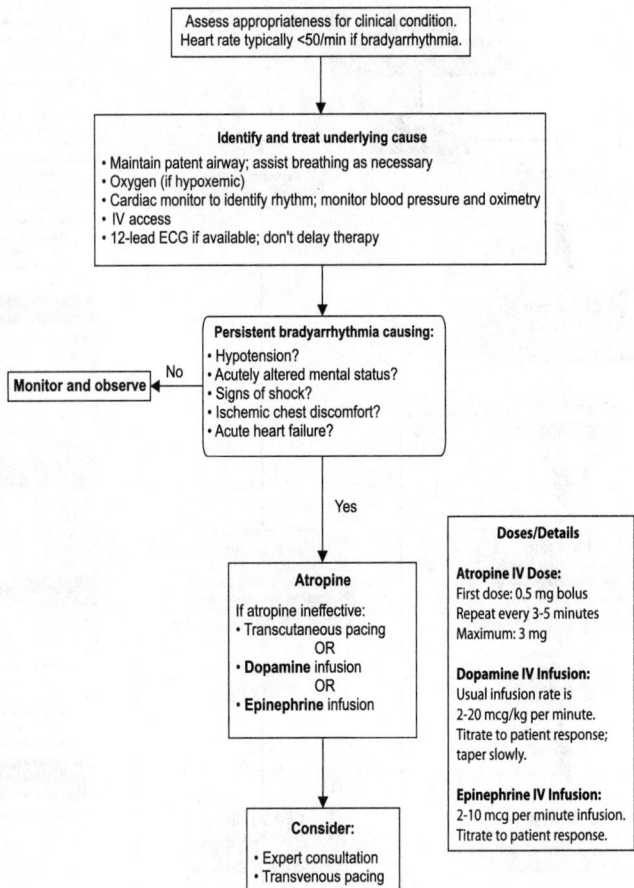

Assess appropriateness for clinical condition.
Heart rate typically <50/min if bradyarrhythmia.

Identify and treat underlying cause
- Maintain patent airway; assist breathing as necessary
- Oxygen (if hypoxemic)
- Cardiac monitor to identify rhythm; monitor blood pressure and oximetry
- IV access
- 12-lead ECG if available; don't delay therapy

Persistent bradyarrhythmia causing:
- Hypotension?
- Acutely altered mental status?
- Signs of shock?
- Ischemic chest discomfort?
- Acute heart failure?

No → **Monitor and observe**

Yes

Atropine

If atropine ineffective:
- Transcutaneous pacing
  OR
- **Dopamine** infusion
  OR
- **Epinephrine** infusion

Consider:
- Expert consultation
- Transvenous pacing

Doses/Details

Atropine IV Dose:
First dose: 0.5 mg bolus
Repeat every 3-5 minutes
Maximum: 3 mg

Dopamine IV Infusion:
Usual infusion rate is
2-20 mcg/kg per minute.
Titrate to patient response;
taper slowly.

Epinephrine IV Infusion:
2-10 mcg per minute infusion.
Titrate to patient response.

Adult Cardiac Arrest Algorithm

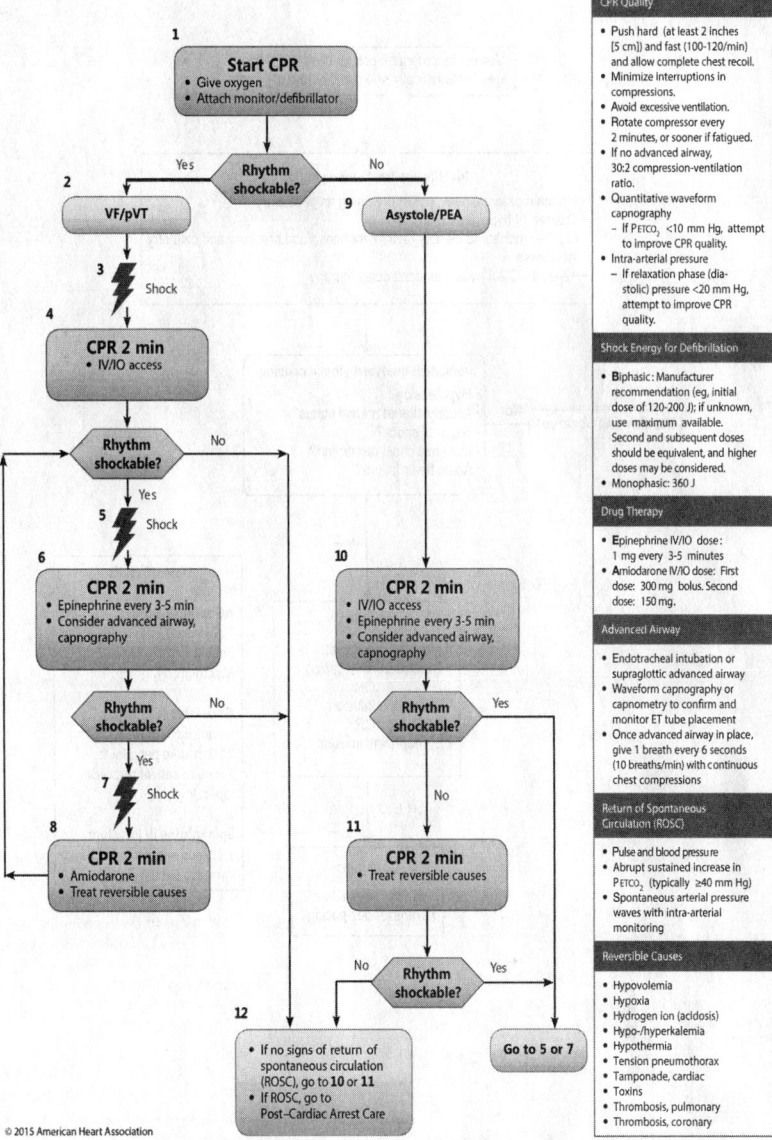

CPR Quality

- Push hard (at least 2 inches [5 cm]) and fast (100-120/min) and allow complete chest recoil.
- Minimize interruptions in compressions.
- Avoid excessive ventilation.
- Rotate compressor every 2 minutes, or sooner if fatigued.
- If no advanced airway, 30:2 compression-ventilation ratio.
- Quantitative waveform capnography
  - If PETCO$_2$ <10 mm Hg, attempt to improve CPR quality.
- Intra-arterial pressure
  - If relaxation phase (diastolic) pressure <20 mm Hg, attempt to improve CPR quality.

Shock Energy for Defibrillation

- **B**iphasic: Manufacturer recommendation (eg, initial dose of 120-200 J); if unknown, use maximum available. Second and subsequent doses should be equivalent, and higher doses may be considered.
- Monophasic: 360 J

Drug Therapy

- **E**pinephrine IV/IO dose: 1 mg every 3-5 minutes
- **A**miodarone IV/IO dose: First dose: 300 mg bolus. Second dose: 150 mg.

Advanced Airway

- Endotracheal intubation or supraglottic advanced airway
- Waveform capnography or capnometry to confirm and monitor ET tube placement
- Once advanced airway in place, give 1 breath every 6 seconds (10 breaths/min) with continuous chest compressions

Return of Spontaneous Circulation (ROSC)

- Pulse and blood pressure
- Abrupt sustained increase in PETCO$_2$ (typically ≥40 mm Hg)
- Spontaneous arterial pressure waves with intra-arterial monitoring

Reversible Causes

- Hypovolemia
- Hypoxia
- Hydrogen ion (acidosis)
- Hypo-/hyperkalemia
- Hypothermia
- Tension pneumothorax
- Tamponade, cardiac
- Toxins
- Thrombosis, pulmonary
- Thrombosis, coronary

© 2015 American Heart Association

CPR Quality

- Push hard (≥2 inches [5 cm]) and fast (≥100/min) and allow complete chest recoil
- Minimize interruptions in compressions
- Avoid excessive ventilation
- Rotate compressor every 2 minutes
- If no advanced airway, 30:2 compression-ventilation ratio
- Quantitative waveform capnography
  - If PETCO$_2$ <10 mm Hg, attempt to improve CPR quality
- Intra-arterial pressure
  - If relaxation phase (diastolic) pressure <20 mm Hg, attempt to improve CPR quality

Return of Spontaneous Circulation (ROSC)

- Pulse and blood pressure
- Abrupt sustained increase in $PETCO_2$ (typically ≥40 mm Hg)
- Spontaneous arterial pressure waves with intra-arterial monitoring

Shock Energy

- **Biphasic:** Manufacturer recommendation (120 to 200 J); if unknown, use maximum available.
  Second and subsequent doses should be equivalent, and higher doses may be considered.
- **Monophasic:** 360 J

Drug Therapy

- Epinephrine IV/I.O. Dose: 1 mg every 3 to 5 minutes
- Vasopressin IV/I.O. Dose: 40 units can replace first or second dose of epinephrine
- Amiodarone IV/I.O. Dose: First dose: 300 mg bolus; Second dose: 150 mg

Advanced Airway

- Supraglottic advanced airway or endotracheal intubation
- Waveform capnography to confirm and monitor ET tube placement
- 8 to 10 breaths per minute with continuous chest compressions

Reversible Causes

– **H**ypovolemia; **H**ypoxia; **H**ydrogen ion (acidosis); **H**ypo-/hyperkalemia; **H**ypothermia
– **T**ension pneumothorax; **T**amponade, cardiac; **T**oxins; **T**hrombosis, pulmonary; **T**hrombosis, coronary

Adult Tachycardia
(With Pulse)

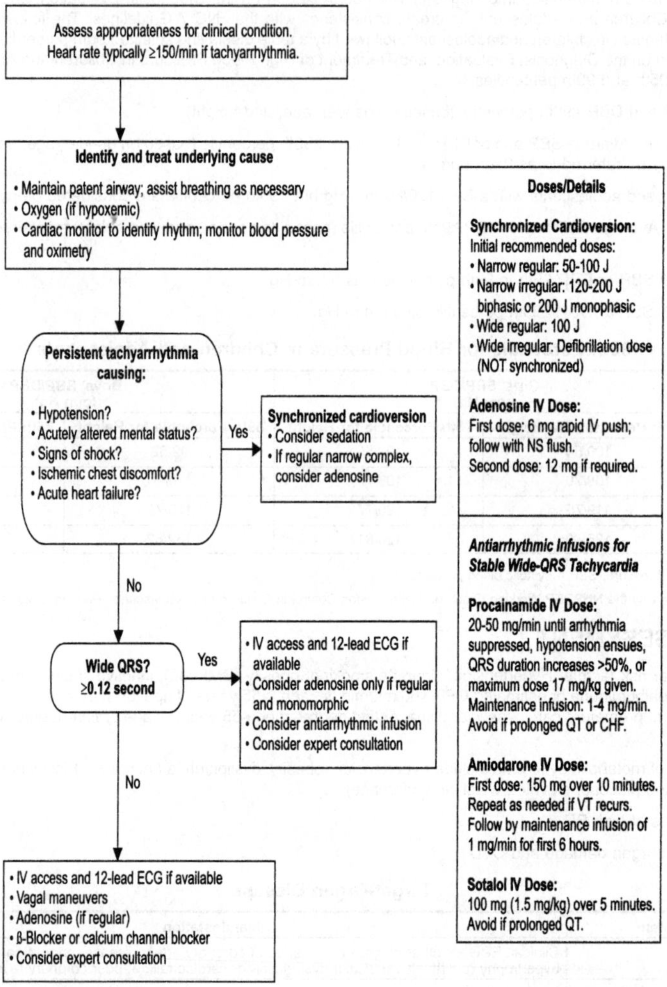

Reprinted with permission: 2015 American Heart Association Guidelines Update for Cardiopulmonary Resuscitation and Emergency Cardiovascular Care. Part 7: Adult Advanced Cardiovascular Life Support. *Circulation.* 2015;132:S444-S464. ©2015 American Heart Association, Inc.
See http://circ.ahajournals.org/content/132/18_suppl_2/S444.full?sid=d3835425-1ef7-4363-9ebe-3179f3ca0538.
All requests to use this information must go through the AHA.

HYPERTENSION

In general, the optimal blood pressure (BP) for nonelderly adults is <120/80 mm Hg. Consistent systolic blood pressure (SBP) ≥140 mm Hg or a diastolic blood pressure (DBP) ≥90 mm Hg defines hypertension in many cases. The definition of hypertension can change slightly depending on the guidelines being referenced and individual comorbidities present. Hypertension affects ~33% of the US population (67 million cases). Of those patients on antihypertensive medication, only 47% have adequately controlled blood pressure. Controlling systolic hypertension has been much more difficult than controlling diastolic hypertension. Educating patients on lifestyle management, cardiovascular risk reduction, and drug therapy aids in improving the morbidity and mortality of patients with hypertension.

The 2014 Evidence-Based Guideline for the Management of High Blood Pressure in Adults, a report created by the Eighth Joint National Committee (JNC 8), is an excellent reference and guide for the treatment of hypertension (James 2014). While JNC 8 does not reference stages of hypertension, other guidelines still recognize this staging system, including the Clinical Practice Guidelines for the Management of Hypertension in the Community, published by the American Society of Hypertension and the International Society of Hypertension (ASH/ISH). Of note, although these guidelines were endorsed by ASH, they should be considered more as an expert opinion piece. For adults, hypertension may be classified by stages (see following table).

Blood Pressure Classification in Adults

Category	Systolic (mm Hg)		Diastolic (mm Hg)
Normal	<120	and	<80
Prehypertension	120 to 139	or	80 to 89
Hypertension			
Stage 1	140 to 159	or	90 to 99
Stage 2	≥160	or	≥100

Adapted from Weber MA, Schiffrin EL, White WB, et al. Clinical practice guidelines for the management of hypertension in the community: a statement by the American Society of Hypertension and the International Society of Hypertension. *J Clin Hypertens (Greenwich)*. 2014;16(1):14-26.

Blood Pressure Classification in Children

The National High Blood Pressure Education Program (NHBPEP) Working Group on Hypertension Control in Children and Adolescents categorized hypertension into stages in The Fourth Report on the Diagnosis, Evaluation, and Treatment of High Blood Pressure in Children and Adolescents to create consistency with the JNC 7 Guidelines. The following are the staging categories of hypertension in children and adolescents, followed by a table displaying selected 90th percentile information. Refer to The Fourth Report on the Diagnosis, Evaluation, and Treatment of High Blood Pressure in Children and Adolescents for more information on the 95th and 99th percentiles.

- Normal: SBP and DBP <90th percentile (based on gender, age, and height)

- Prehypertension: Average SBP and/or DBP levels that are ≥90th percentile (based on gender, age, and height) but <95th percentile; may be referred to as "high normal"

  – Children and adolescents with a BP ≥120/80 mm Hg but <95th percentile are considered prehypertensive

- Hypertension: Average SBP and/or DBP ≥95th percentile (based on gender, age, and height) measured on three separate occasions

  – Stage 1: SBP or DBP 95th to 99th percentile plus 5 mm Hg

  – Stage 2: SBP or DBP >99th percentile plus 5 mm Hg

90th Percentile for Blood Pressure in Children and Adolescents

Age (y)	Girls' SBP/DBP (mm Hg)		Boys' SBP/DBP (mm Hg)	
	50th Percentile for Height	75th Percentile for Height	50th Percentile for Height	75th Percentile for Height
1	100/54	101/55	99/52	100/53
6	108/70	109/70	110/70	111/71
12	119/76	120/77	120/76	121/77
17	125/80	126/81	132/82	134/83

DBP = diastolic blood pressure, SBP = systolic blood pressure

Adapted from the report by the NHBPEP Working Group on Hypertension Control in Children and Adolescents. *Pediatrics*. 2004;114(2):555-576.

PATIENT ASSESSMENT

- Cardiovascular risk factors: Hypertension, cigarette smoking, obesity (BMI ≥30), inactive lifestyle, dyslipidemia, diabetes mellitus, microalbuminuria or estimated GFR <60 mL/minute, age (>55 years of age for men, >65 years of age for women), family history of premature cardiovascular disease (first-degree men <55 years of age or first-degree women <65 years of age)

- Components of metabolic syndrome include hypertension, obesity, dyslipidemia (increased triglycerides, reduced HDL-C, elevated fasting glucose, elevated waist circumference)

- Identify causes of high BP

- Assess target-organ damage and CVD

Target-Organ Disease

Organ System	Manifestation
Cardiac	Clinical, ECG, or other diagnostic evidence of coronary artery disease; prior MI, angina; left ventricular hypertrophy (LVH); left ventricular dysfunction or cardiac failure; prior coronary revascularization
Cerebrovascular	Transient ischemic attack or stroke
Peripheral vascular	Aneurysm, peripheral arterial disease
Renal	Elevated serum creatinine; proteinuria; microalbuminuria; chronic kidney disease
Ocular	Retinal hemorrhages or exudates, with or without papilledema; retinopathy

BLOOD PRESSURE MEASUREMENT

At an office visit, patients should be seated quietly for ≥5 minutes in a chair with feet on the floor and arm supported at heart level. At least two measurements should be obtained. Patients should be given their results and their goal BP.

Ambulatory BP monitoring is useful in evaluating "white coat hypertension" (no end-organ damage), drug resistance, hypotensive symptoms, episodic hypertension, and autonomic dysfunction. Ambulatory BP monitoring correlates better with end-organ damage than office measurements.

Having patients monitor their own BP helps to improve compliance and provides information on response to therapeutic interventions.

Management of Blood Pressure According to the JNC 8 Guidelines

Patient Classification[1]	Age (y)	Blood Pressure Goal[2] (mm Hg)	Considerations for Preferred Initial Therapy[2]
General population (without diabetes or CKD)	<60	SBP <140 and DBP <90	Nonblack: Thiazide-type diuretic, ACEI, ARB, or CCB (alone or in combination if necessary[3])
	≥60	SBP <150 and DBP <90	Black: Thiazide-type diuretic or CCB (alone or in combination if necessary)
Patients with diabetes (without CKD)	≥18	SBP <140 and DBP <90	Nonblack: Thiazide-type diuretic, ACEI, ARB, or CCB (alone or in combination if necessary[3])
			Black: Thiazide-type diuretic or CCB (alone or in combination if necessary)
Patients with CKD (regardless of diabetes status)	≥18	SBP <140 and DBP <90	All races: ACEI or ARB (alone or in combination with another drug class[3])

ACEI = angiotension-converting enzyme inhibitor, ARB = angiotension receptor block, CCB = calcium channel blocker, CKD = chronic kidney disease, DBP = diastolic blood pressure, SBP = systolic blood pressure

[1]For individuals with hypertension, implement lifestyle interventions and continue throughout therapy.

[2]Refer to JNC 8 guidelines for strength of recommendations.

[3]ACEIs and ARBs are not recommended to be used together.

Note: Recommendations are not intended for individuals <18 years of age.

Adapted from James PA, Oparil S, Carter BL, et al. 2014 evidence-based guideline for the management of high blood pressure in adults: report from the panel members appointed to the Eighth Joint National Committee (JNC 8). *JAMA.* 2014;311(5):507-520.

ACHIEVING BLOOD PRESSURE CONTROL

Treatment of hypertension should be individualized. Keep in mind slight variations exist between different hypertension guidelines in regards to both the treatment goals for specific patient populations and the level of evidence provided to support the given recommendations. For instance, elderly patients 65 to 79 years of age should achieve a goal SBP ≤140 mm Hg if tolerated for uncomplicated hypertension according to the ACCF/AHA 2011 Expert Consensus Document on Hypertension in the Elderly. Additionally, for patients ≥80 years of age, a goal SBP of ≤140 mm Hg should be achieved; if not tolerated, 140 to 145 mm Hg is acceptable (Aronow 2011). In comparison, the JNC 8 guidelines recommend a blood pressure goal of <150/90 mm Hg for individuals ≥60 years of age without comorbidities. Refer to the table below for additional information regarding blood pressure goals for various patient populations.

More recently, the SPRINT trial, which enrolled older patients (ie, >50 years) without diabetes at risk for cardiovascular events demonstrated a reduction in fatal and nonfatal major cardiovascular events and death from any cause when an intensive blood pressure reduction (SBP target of <120 mmHg) was employed compared to standard blood pressure management (SBP target of <140 mmHg). Automated oscillometric blood pressure (AOBP) measurements were used instead of manual auscultatory blood pressure measurements within the study. AOBP measurements are typically lower than manual auscultatory blood pressure measurements, so clinicians may need to adjust blood pressure goals based on the type of blood pressure measurement used (eg, SBP target of 125 to 135 mmHg if using standard manual auscultatory measurements). Patients should be monitored more closely for adverse events (eg, hypotension, electrolyte abnormalities) when targeting these lower blood pressures (SPRINT Research Group 2015).

Patient Classification	Guideline	Age (y)	Blood Pressure Goal[1] (mm Hg)
General population (without diabetes or CKD)	AHA/ACC/CDC	≥18	<140/90[2]
	ASH/ISH	<80	<140/90
	ASH/ISH	≥80	<150/90
	JNC 8	≥60	<150/90
	JNC 8	≥18	<140/90
Patients with diabetes (without CKD)	AACE	≥18	<130/80
	ADA	≥18	<140/80[3]
	ASH/ISH	≥18	<140/90
	JNC 8	≥18	<140/90
Patients with CKD (regardless of diabetes status)	JNC 8	≥18	<140/90
Patients with CKD and albuminuria	ASH/ISH	≥18	<130/80

AACE = American Association of Clinical Endocrinologists, ADA = American Diabetes Association, AHA/ACC/CDC = American Heart Association/American College of Cardiology/Centers for Disease Control and Prevention, ASH/ISH = American Society of Hypertension/International Society of Hypertension, JNC 8 = Eighth Joint National Committee

[1]Refer to cited guidelines for strength of recommendations and/or supportive evidence.

[2]Lower targets may be necessary for patients based on disease states and individual factors but are not specified by the AHA/ACC/CDC.

[3]Lower BP targets may be appropriate (eg, younger patients) per the ADA.

Note: Recommendations are not intended for individuals <18 years of age.

Considerations:

- Special consideration for starting combination therapy should be made in each patient.

- According to the JNC 8 guidelines, there are three strategies for dosing antihypertensive medications:

  - Initiate antihypertensive therapy with a single medication and titrate this medication to the maximum dose before adding on a second medication if further blood pressure reduction is desired.

  - Initiate antihypertensive therapy with a single medication and add a second medication prior to maximizing the dose of the initial medication if further blood pressure reduction is desired.

  - Initiate antihypertensive therapy with two medications simultaneously.

- Most patients with hypertension will require two or more drugs to achieve BP goal.

- Consider initiating therapy with two drugs simultaneously when SBP >160 mm Hg and/or DBP >100 mm Hg, or if BP is >20 mm Hg/10 mm Hg above goal.

- Low-dose aspirin therapy should be considered when BP is controlled; use in uncontrolled hypertension can increase risk of hemorrhagic stroke.

- Lifestyle modification and risk reduction should always be reviewed and reinforced.

MONITORING THERAPY

Generally, monthly follow-up is recommended until BP control is reached.

More frequent monitoring is required for those patients with Stage 2 hypertension or those with complications.

Serum potassium and serum creatinine should be monitored at least twice yearly.

When BP is at goal and stable, follow-up can be maintained every 3 to 6 months. Treat other cardiovascular risk factors if present.

Specific Therapies for Concomitant Disease States[1]

Indication	Drug Therapy
Atrial tachyarrhythmias	Beta-blocker, CCB (non-DHP)
Chronic kidney disease	
GFR <60 mL/minute per 1.73 m^2 or albuminuria	ACEI or ARB
GFR <30 mL/minute per 1.73 m^2	ACEI or ARB, loop diuretic
Diabetes	Thiazide diuretic, beta-blocker, ACEI, ARB, CCB
Nephropathy	ACEI, ARB
Essential tremor	Beta-blocker (noncardioselective)
Heart failure	
Ventricular dysfunction (asymptomatic)	ACEI or ARB, beta-blocker
Ventricular dysfunction (symptomatic)	ACEI or ARB, beta-blocker, aldosterone blocker, loop diuretic
Hypertensive women who are pregnant	Methyldopa, beta-blocker, vasodilator (eg, hydrALAZINE)
Ischemic heart disease	
Angina	Beta-blocker, CCB (long-acting)
Acute coronary syndromes	Beta-blocker, ACEI, nitroglycerin
Migraine	Beta-blocker (noncardioselective), CCB (long-acting, non-DHP)
Osteoporosis	Thiazide diuretic
Perioperative hypertension	Beta-blocker
Prostatism (BPH)	Alpha-adrenergic blocking agent (eg, prazosin)
Raynaud syndrome	CCB (DHP)
Thyrotoxicosis	Beta-blocker

ACEI = angiotensin-converting enzyme inhibitor, ARB = angiotensin receptor blocker, CCB = calcium channel blocker, DHP = dihydropyridine, GFR = glomeruler filtration rate

[1]For additional considerations and specific therapies for hypertension in elderly patients, see ACCF/AHA 2011 Expert Consensus Document on Hypertension in the Elderly (Aronow 2011).

May Have Unfavorable Effects on Comorbid Conditions

Condition	Drug Therapy to Avoid
Idiopathic or hereditary angioedema	ACEI
Bronchospastic disease	Beta-blocker
Gout	Thiazide diuretic
Heart block (second or third degree)	Beta-blocker, non-DHP CCB
Hyponatremia	Thiazide diuretic
Potassium >5 mEq/L before treatment	Potassium sparing diuretic, aldosterone antagonist

ACEI = angiotensin-converting enzyme inhibitor, ARB = angiotensin receptor blocker, CCB = calcium channel blocker, DHP = dihydropyridine

HYPERTENSIVE EMERGENCIES AND URGENCIES

General Treatment Principles in the Treatment of Hypertensive Emergencies

Principle	Considerations
Admit the patient to the hospital, preferably in the ICU. Monitor vital signs appropriately.	Establish IV access and place patient on a cardiac monitor. Place a femoral intra-arterial line and pulmonary arterial catheter, if indicated, to assess cardiopulmonary function and intravascular volume status.
Perform rapid but thorough history and physical examination.	Determine cause of, or precipitating factors to, hypertensive crisis if possible (remember to obtain a medication history, including Rx, OTC, and illicit drugs). Obtain details regarding any prior history of hypertension (severity, duration, treatment), as well as other coexisting illnesses. Assess the extent of hypertensive end organ damage. Determine if a hypertensive urgency or emergency exists.
Determine goal blood pressure based on premorbid level, duration, severity and rapidity of increase of blood pressure, concomitant medical conditions, race, and age.	Acute decreases in blood pressure to normal or subnormal levels during the initial treatment period may reduce perfusion to the brain, heart, and kidneys, and must be avoided, except in specific instances (ie, dissecting aortic aneurysm). Gradually establish a normal (or reasonable) blood pressure over the next 1 to 2 weeks.
Select an appropriate antihypertensive regimen depending on the individual patient and clinical setting.	Initiate a controlled decrease in blood pressure. Avoid concomitant administration of multiple agents that may cause precipitous falls in blood pressure. Select the agent with the best hemodynamic profile based on the primary treatment goal. Avoid diuretics and sodium restriction during the initial treatment period, unless there is a clear clinical indication (ie, CHF, pulmonary edema). Avoid sedating antihypertensives in patients with hypertensive encephalopathy, CVA, or other CNS disorders in whom mental status must be monitored. Use caution with direct vasodilating agents that induce reflex tachycardia or increase cardiac output in patients with coronary heart disease, history of angina or myocardial infarction, or dissecting aortic aneurysm. Preferably choose an agent that does not adversely affect glomerular filtration rate or renal blood flow and also agents that have favorable effects on cerebral blood flow and its autoregulation, especially for patients with hypertensive encephalopathy or CVAs. Select the most efficacious agent with the fewest adverse effects based on the underlying cause of the hypertensive crisis and other individual patient factors.
Initiate a chronic antihypertensive regimen after the patient's blood pressure is stabilized	Begin oral antihypertensive therapy once goal blood pressure is achieved before gradually tapering parenteral medications. Select the best oral regimen based on cost, ease of administration, adverse effect profile, and concomitant medical conditions.

Oral Agents Used in the Treatment of Hypertensive Urgencies

Drug	Dose	Onset	Cautions
Captopril[1]	PO: 25 mg; repeat as required	15 to 30 min	Hypotension, renal failure in bilateral renal artery stenosis
CloNIDine[1]	PO: 0.1 to 0.2 mg; repeat every hour as needed to a total dose of 0.6 mg	30 to 60 min	Hypotension, drowsiness, dry mouth
Labetalol	PO: 200 to 400 mg; repeat every 2 to 3 h	30 min to 2 h	Bronchoconstriction, heart block, orthostatic hypotension

[1]There is no clearly defined clinical advantage in the use of sublingual over oral routes of administration with these agents.

Recommendations for the Use of Intravenous Antihypertensive Drugs in Selected Hypertensive Emergencies

Condition	Agent(s) of Choice	Agent(s) to Avoid or Use With Caution	General Treatment Principles
Hypertensive encephalopathy	Nitroprusside, labetalol	Methyldopa, reserpine	Avoid drugs with CNS-sedating effects.
Acute intracranial or subarachnoid hemorrhage	NiCARdipine, nitroprusside	Beta-blocker	Careful titration with a short-acting agent.
Cerebral infarction	NiCARdipine, nitroprusside, labetalol	Beta-blocker, minoxidil	Careful titration with a short-acting agent. Avoid agents that may decrease cerebral blood flow.
Head trauma	Esmolol, labetalol	Methyldopa, reserpine, nitroprusside, nitroglycerin, hydrALAZINE	Avoid drugs with CNS-sedating effects or those that may increase intracranial pressure.
Acute myocardial infarction, myocardial ischemia	Nitroglycerin, labetalol	HydrALAZINE, minoxidil	Avoid drugs which cause reflex tachycardia and increased myocardial oxygen consumption.
Acute pulmonary edema	Nitroprusside, nitroglycerin, loop diuretics	Beta-blocker (labetalol), minoxidil, methyldopa	Avoid drugs which may cause sodium and water retention and edema exacerbation.
Renal dysfunction	HydrALAZINE, calcium channel blocker	Nitroprusside, ACE inhibitors, beta-blocker (labetalol)	Avoid drugs with increased toxicity in renal failure and those that may cause decreased renal blood flow.
Eclampsia	HydrALAZINE, labetalol, NIFEdipine, nitroprusside[1]	Diuretics	Avoid drugs that may cause adverse fetal effects, compromise placental circulation, or decrease cardiac output.
Pheochromocytoma	Phentolamine, nitroprusside, beta-blocker (esmolol) only after alpha blockade (phentolamine)	Beta-blocker in the absence of alpha blockade, methyldopa, minoxidil	Use drugs of proven efficacy and specificity. Unopposed beta-blockade may exacerbate hypertension.
Dissecting aortic aneurysm	Nitroprusside and beta-blockade	HydrALAZINE, minoxidil	Avoid drugs which may increase cardiac output.
Postoperative hypertension	Nitroprusside, niCARdipine, labetalol, clevidipine		Avoid drugs which may exacerbate postoperative ileus.

[1]Reserve nitroprusside for eclamptic patients with life-threatening hypertension unresponsive to other agents due to the potential risk to the fetus (cyanide and thiocyanate metabolites may cross the placenta).

Selected Intravenous Agents for Hypertensive Emergencies

Drug	Dose	Onset of Action	Duration of Action	Adverse Effects[1]	Special Indications
Vasodilators					
Sodium nitroprusside	0.25 to 10 mcg/kg/min as IV infusion[2] (maximum infusion rate: 10 mcg/kg/min; max rate should **not** last >10 min)	Immediate	1 to 2 min	Nausea, vomiting, muscle twitching, sweating, thiocyanate and cyanide intoxication	Most hypertensive emergencies; caution with high intracranial pressure or azotemia
NiCARdipine hydrochloride	IV: 5 to 15 mg/h	5 to 10 min	≤8 h	Tachycardia, headache, flushing, local phlebitis	Most hypertensive emergencies, except acute heart failure; caution with coronary ischemia
Clevidipine butyrate	IV: 1 to 2 mg/h	2 to 4 min	5 to 15 min	Atrial fibrillation, nausea, insomnia, fever	Most hypertensive emergencies; caution with lipid disorder
Fenoldopam mesylate	Initial: 0.03 to 0.1 mcg/kg/min as IV infusion (maximum infusion rate: 1.6 mcg/kg/min)	10 min	1 h	Tachycardia, headache, nausea, flushing	Most hypertensive emergencies; caution with glaucoma
Nitroglycerin	5 to 400 mcg/min as IV infusion	Immediate	3 to 5 min	Headache, vomiting, methemoglobinemia, tolerance with prolonged use	Coronary ischemia
Enalaprilat	IV: 1.25 to 5 mg every 6 hours	≤15 min	6 h	Precipitous fall in pressure in high-renin states; response variable	Acute left ventricular failure; avoid in acute myocardial infarction
HydrALAZINE hydrochloride	IM/IV: 10 to 20 mg every 4 to 6 h as needed	IM: 20 to 30 min IV: 10 to 20 min	1 to 4 h	Tachycardia, flushing, headache, vomiting, aggravation of angina	Eclampsia
Adrenergic Inhibitors					
Labetalol hydrochloride	IV bolus: 20 to 80 mg every 10 min; 0.5 to 2 mg/min as IV infusion	2 to 5 min	2 to 18 h (dose dependent)	Vomiting, scalp tingling, burning in throat, dizziness, nausea, heart block, orthostatic hypotension	Most hypertensive emergencies, except acute heart failure
Esmolol hydrochloride	Infusion range: 50 to 300 mcg/kg/min	2 to 10 min	10 to 30 min	Hypotension, nausea	Aortic dissection, perioperative
Phentolamine	IV: 5 to 15 mg	1 to 2 min	10 to 30 min	Tachycardia, flushing, headache	Catecholamine excess

[1]Hypotension may occur with all agents.
[2]Require special delivery system

REFERENCES

Guidelines

1999 World Health Organization-International Society of Hypertension guidelines for the management of hypertension. Guidelines subcommittee. *J Hypertens.* 1999;17(2):151-183.

American College of Obstetricians and Gynecologists, Task Force on Hypertension in Pregnancy. Hypertension in pregnancy. Report of the American College of Obstetricians and Gynecologists' Task Force on Hypertension in Pregnancy. *Obstet Gynecol.* 2013;122(5):1122-1131.

American Diabetes Association. Standards of medical care in diabetes – 2013. *Diabetes Care.* 2013;36(Suppl 1):11-66.

Aronow WS, Fleg JL, Pepine CJ, et al. ACCF/AHA 2011 expert consensus document on hypertension in the elderly: a report of the American College of Cardiology Foundation Task Force on Clinical Expert Consensus Documents. *Circulation.* 2011;123(21):2434-2506.

Chobanian AV, Bakris GL, Black HR, et al. The seventh report of the Joint National Committee on Prevention, Detection, Evaluation, and Treatment of High Blood Pressure: the JNC 7 report. *JAMA.* 2003;289(19):2560-2572.

Go AS, Bauman MA, Coleman King SM, et al. An effective approach to high blood pressure control: a science advisory from the American Heart Association, the American College of Cardiology, and the Centers for Disease Control and Prevention. *J Am Coll Cardiol.* 2014;63(12):1230-1238.

Grundy SM, Cleeman JI, Daniels SR, et al. Diagnosis and management of the metabolic syndrome: an American Heart Association/National Heart, Lung, and Blood Institute Scientific Statement. *Circulation.* 2005;112(17):2735-2752.

Handelsman Y, Mechanick JI, Blonde L, et al. American Association of Clinical Endocrinologists Medical Guidelines for Clinical Practice for developing a diabetes mellitus comprehensive care plan. *Endocr Pract.* 2011;17(Suppl 2):1-53.

James PA, Oparil S, Carter BL, et al. 2014 evidence-based guideline for the management of high blood pressure in adults: report from the panel members appointed to the Eighth Joint National Committee (JNC 8). *JAMA.* 2014;311(5):507-520.

Marik PE, Varon J. Hypertensive crises: challenges and management. *Chest.* 2007;131(6):1949-1962.

National High Blood Pressure Education Program Working Group. 1995 update of the working group reports on chronic renal failure and renovascular hypertension. *Arch Intern Med.* 1996;156(17):1938-1947.

National High Blood Pressure Education Program Working Group on High Blood Pressure in Children and Adolescents. The fourth report on the diagnosis, evaluation, and treatment of high blood pressure in children and adolescents. *Pediatrics.* 2004;114(2 Suppl 4th Report):555-576.

Stone NJ, Robinson J, Lichtenstein AH, et al. 2013 ACC/AHA guideline on the treatment of blood cholesterol to reduce atherosclerotic cardiovascular risk in adults: a report of the American College of Cardiology/American Heart Association Task Force on Practice Guidelines [published online Nov. 12, 2013]. *Circulation.* Available at http://circ.ahajournals.org/content/early/2013/11/11/01.cir.0000437738.63853.7a

The sixth report of the National Committee on Detection, Evaluation, and Treatment of High Blood Pressure (JNC-VI). *Arch Intern Med.* 1997;157 (21):2413-2446.

Weber MA, Schiffrin EL, White WB, et al. Clinical practice guidelines for the management of hypertension in the community: a statement by the American Society of Hypertension and the International Society of Hypertension. *J Clin Hypertens (Greenwich).* 2014;16(1):14-26.

Others

Appel LJ, Moore TJ, Obarzanek E, et al. A clinical trial of the effect of dietary patterns on blood pressure. The DASH Collaborative Research Group. *N Engl J Med.* 1997;336(16):1117-1124.

Centers for Disease Control and Prevention (CDC). High blood pressure. Available at http://www.cdc.gov/bloodpressure/

Epstein M, Bakris G. Newer approaches to antihypertensive therapy: use of fixed-dose combination therapy. *Arch Intern Med.* 1996;156(17):1969-1978.

Estacio RO, Schrier RW. Antihypertensive therapy in type II diabetes: implications of the appropriate blood pressure control in diabetes (ABCD) trial. *Am J Cardiol.* 1998;82(9B):9R-14R.

Flack JM, Neaton J, Grimm RJ, et al. Blood pressure and mortality among men with prior myocardial infarction. The Multiple Risk Factor Intervention Trial Research Group. *Circulation.* 1995;92(9):2437-2445.

Frishman WH, Bryzinski BS, Coulson LR, et al. A multifactorial trial design to assess combination therapy in hypertension: treatment with bisoprolol and hydrochlorothiazide. *Arch Intern Med.* 1994;154(13):1461-1468.

Furberg CD, Psaty BM, Meyer JV. Nifedipine: dose-related increase in mortality in patients with coronary heart disease. *Circulation.* 1995;92 (5):1326-1331.

Glynn RJ, Brock DB, Harris T, et al. Use of antihypertensive drugs and trends in blood pressure in the elderly. *Arch Intern Med.* 1995;155:1855-1860.

Gradman AH, Cutler NR, Davis PJ, et al. Combined enalapril and felodipine extended release (ER) for systemic hypertension. The enalapril-felodipine ER factorial study group. *Am J Cardiol.* 1997;79(4):431-435.

Grimm RH Jr, Flack JM, Grandits GA, et al. Long-term effects on plasma lipids of diet and drugs to treat hypertension. The treatment of mild hypertension study (TOMHS) research group. *JAMA.* 1996;275(20):1549-1556.

Grimm RH Jr, Grandits GA, Cutler JA, et al. Relationships of quality-of-life measures to long-term lifestyle and drug treatment in the treatment of mild hypertension study. The TOMHS research group. *Arch Intern Med.* 1997;157(6):638-648.

Grossman E, Messerli FH, Grodzicki T, et al. Should a moratorium be placed on sublingual nifedipine capsules given for hypertensive emergencies and pseudoemergencies? *JAMA.* 1996;276(16):1328-1331.

Hansson L, Zanchetti A, Carruthers SG, et al. Effects of intensive blood pressure lowering and low-dose aspirin in patients with hypertension: principal results of the hypertension optimal treatment (HOT) randomized trial. HOT study group. *Lancet.* 1998;351(9118):1755-1762.

Kaplan NM, Gifford RW Jr. Choice of initial therapy for hypertension. *JAMA.* 1996;275(20):1577-1580.

Kasiske BL, Ma JZ, Kalil RSN, et al. Effects of antihypertensive therapy in serum lipids. *Ann Intern Med.* 1995;122(2):133-141.

Kostis JB, Davis BR, Cutler J, et al. Prevention of heart failure by antihypertensive drug treatment in older persons with isolated systolic hypertension. SHEP Cooperative Research Group. *JAMA.* 1997;278(3):212-216.

Lazarus JM, Bourgoignie JJ, Buckalew VM, et al. Achievement and safety of a low blood pressure goal in chronic renal disease: the modification of diet in renal disease study group. *Hypertension.* 1997;29(2):641-650.

Lindheimer MD. Hypertension in pregnancy. *Hypertension.* 1993;22(1):127-137.

Makin A, Lip GY, Silverman S, Beevers DG. Peripheral vascular disease and hypertension: a forgotten association? *J Hum Hypertens.* 2001;15 (7):447-454.

Materson BJ, Reda DJ, Cushman WC, et al. Single-drug therapy for hypertension in men: a comparison of six antihypertensive agents with placebo. The Department of Veterans Affairs Cooperative Study Group on Antihypertensive Agents. *N Engl J Med.* 1993;328(13):914-921.

Messerli FH, Williams B, Ritz E. Essential hypertension. *Lancet.* 2007;370(9587):591-603.

Michel T, Hoffman BB. Chapter 27. Treatment of myocardial ischemia and hypertension. *Goodman & Gilman's The Pharmacological Basis of Therapeutics.* 12th ed. Brunton LL, Chabner BA, Knollmann BC, eds. New York: McGraw-Hill; 2011. Available at http://0-accesspharmacy.mhmedical.com.polar.onu.edu/content.aspx?bookid=374&Sectionid=41266234. Accessed March 17, 2014.

Miller NH, Hill M, Kottke T, et al. The multi-level compliance challenge: recommendations for a call to action; a statement for healthcare professionals. *Circulation.* 1997;95(4):1085-1090.

Mustafa R, Ahmed S, Gupta A, Venuto RC. A comprehensive review of hypertension in pregnancy. *J Pregnancy.* 2012;2012:105918.

Neaton JD, Grim RH, Prineas RJ, et al. Treatment of mild hypertension study. Final results. Treatment of mild hypertension study research group. *JAMA.* 1993;270(6):713-724.

Neaton JD, Wentworth D. Serum cholesterol, blood pressure, cigarette smoking, and death from coronary heart disease: overall findings and differences by age for 316,099 white men. The Multiple Risk Factor Intervention Trial Research Group. *Arch Intern Med.* 1992;152(1):56-64.

Nitropress [prescribing information]. Lake Forest, IL: Hospira, Inc.; December 2013.

Oparil S, Levine JH, Zuschke CA, et al. Effects of candesartan cilexetil in patients with severe systemic hypertension. *Am J Cardiol.* 1999;84(3):289-293.

Peacock WF, Varon J, Garrison N, et al. IV clevidipine for hypertension: safety, efficacy, and transition to oral therapy. *Ann Emerg Med.* 2007;50(3 Suppl):S8-S9.

Perloff D, Grim C, Flack J, et al. Human blood pressure determination by sphygmomanometry. *Circulation.* 1993;88(5 Pt 1):2460-2467.

Perry HM Jr, Bingham S, Horney A, et al. Antihypertensive efficacy of treatment regimens used in veterans administration hypertension clinics. Department of Veterans Affairs Cooperative Study Group on Antihypertensive Agents. *Hypertension.* 1998;31(3):771-779.

Preston RA, Materson BJ, Reda DJ, et al. Age-race subgroup compared with renin profile as predictors of blood pressure response to antihypertensive therapy. *JAMA.* 1998;280(13):1168-1172.

Psaty BM, Smith NL, Siscovick DS, et al. Health outcomes associated with antihypertensive therapies used as first-line agents. A systemic review and meta-analysis. *JAMA.* 1997;277(9):739-745.

Radevski IV, Valtchanova SP, Candy GP, et al. Comparison of acebutolol with and without hydrochlorothiazide versus carvedilol with and without hydrochlorothiazide in black patients with mild to moderate systemic hypertension. *Am J Cardiol.* 1999;84(1):70-75.

Rhoney D, Peacock WF. Intravenous therapy for hypertensive emergencies, part 1. *Am J Health Syst Pharm.* 2009;66(15):1343-1352.

Saseen JJ, Maclaughlin EJ. Chapter 19. Hypertension. *Pharmacotherapy: A Pathophysiologic Approach.* 8th ed. DiPiro JT, Talbert RL, Yee GC, Matzke GR, Wells BG, Posey L, eds. New York: McGraw-Hill; 2011. Available at http://0-accesspharmacy.mhmedical.com.polar.onu.edu/content.aspx?bookid=462&Sectionid=41100786. Accessed March 13, 2014.

Setaro JF, Black HR. Refractory hypertension. *N Engl J Med.* 1992;327(8):543-547.

SHEP Cooperative Research Group. Prevention of stroke by antihypertensive drug treatment in older persons with isolated systolic hypertension: final results of the Systolic Hypertension in the Elderly Program (SHEP). *JAMA.* 1991;265(24):3255-3264.

Sibai BM. Treatment of hypertension in pregnant women. *N Engl J Med.* 1996;335(4):257-265.

Singla N, Warltier DC, Gandhi SD, et al. Treatment of acute postoperative hypertension in cardiac surgery patients: an efficacy study of clevidipine assessing its postoperative antihypertensive effect in cardiac surgery-2 (ESCAPE-2), a randomized, double-blind, placebo-controlled trial. *Anesth Analg.* 2008;107(1):59-67.

Sowers JR. Comorbidity of hypertension and diabetes: the fosinopril versus amlodipine cardiovascular events trial. *Am J Cardiol.* 1998;82(9B):15R-19R.

SPRINT Research Group, Wright JT Jr, Williamson JD, et al. A randomized trial of intensive versus standard blood-pressure control. *N Engl J Med.* 2015;373(22):2103-2116.

Sternberg H, Rosenthal T, Shamiss A, et al. Altered circadian rhythm of blood pressure in shift workers. *J Hum Hypertens.* 1995;9(5):349-353.

The Hypertension Prevention Trial: three-year effects of dietary changes on blood pressure. Hypertension Prevention Trial Research Group. *Arch Intern Med.* 1990;150(1):153-162.

Trials of Hypertension Prevention Collaborative Research Group. Effects of weight loss and sodium reduction intervention on blood pressure and hypertension incidence in overweight people with high-normal blood pressure: the trials of hypertension prevention, phase II. *Arch Intern Med.* 1997;157(6):657-667.

Tuomilehto J, Rastenyte D, Birkenhager WH, et al. Effects of calcium channel blockade in older patients with diabetes and systolic hypertension. *N Engl J Med.* 1999;340(9):677-684.

Varon J. Treatment of acute severe hypertension: current and newer agents. *Drugs.* 2008;68(3):283-297.

Veelken R, Schmieder RE. Overview of alpha-1 adrenoceptor antagonism and recent advances in hypertensive therapy. *Am J Hypertens.* 1996;9 (11):139S-149S.

White WB, Black HR, Weber MA, et al. Comparison of effects of controlled onset extended release verapamil at bedtime and nifedipine gastrointestinal therapeutic system on arising on early morning blood pressure, heart rate, and the heart rate-blood pressure product. *Am J Cardiol.* 1998;81 (4):424-431.

ORAL DOSAGES THAT SHOULD NOT BE CRUSHED

There are a variety of reasons for crushing tablets or capsule contents prior to administering to the patient. Patients may have nasogastric tubes which do not permit the administration of tablets or capsules, an oral solution for a particular medication may not be available from the manufacturer or readily prepared by pharmacy, patients may have difficulty swallowing capsules or tablets, or mixing of powdered medication with food or drink may make the drug more palatable.

Generally, medications which should not be crushed fall into one of the following categories:

- **Extended Release Products:** The formulation of some tablets is specialized as to allow the medication within it to be slowly released into the body. This may be accomplished by centering the drug within the core of the tablet, with a subsequent shedding of multiple layers around the core. Wax melts in the GI tract, releasing drug contained within the wax matrix (eg, OxyCONTIN). Capsules may contain beads which have multiple layers which are slowly dissolved with time.

    Common Abbreviations for Extended Release Products

CD	Controlled dose
CR	Controlled release
CRT	Controlled release tablet
LA	Long-acting
SR	Sustained release
TR	Timed release
TD	Time delay
SA	Sustained action
XL	Extended release
XR	Extended release

- **Medications Which Are Irritating to the Stomach:** Tablets which are irritating to the stomach may be enteric-coated which delays release of the drug until the time when it reaches the small intestine. Enteric-coated aspirin is an example of this.

- **Foul-Tasting Medication:** Some drugs are quite unpleasant to taste so the manufacturer coats the tablet in a sugar coating to increase its palatability. By crushing the tablet, this sugar coating is lost and the patient tastes the unpleasant tasting medication.

- **Sublingual Medication:** Medication intended for use under the tongue should not be crushed. While it appears to be obvious, it is not always easy to determine if a medication is to be used sublingually. Sublingual medications should indicate on the package that they are intended for sublingual use.

- **Effervescent Tablets:** These are tablets which, when dropped into a liquid, quickly dissolve to yield a solution. Many effervescent tablets, when crushed, lose their ability to quickly dissolve.

- **Potentially Hazardous Substances:** Certain drugs, including antineoplastic agents, hormonal agents, some antivirals, some bioengineered agents, and other miscellaneous drugs, are considered potentially hazardous when used in humans based on their characteristics. Examples of these characteristics include carcinogenicity, teratogenicity, reproductive toxicity, organ toxicity at low doses, genotoxicity, or new drugs with structural and toxicity profiles similar to existing hazardous drugs. Exposure to these substances can result in adverse effects and should be avoided. Crushing or breaking a tablet or opening a capsule of a potentially hazardous substance may increase the risk of exposure to the substance through skin contact, inhalation, or accidental ingestion. The extent of exposure, potency, and toxicity of the hazardous substance determines the health risk. Institutions have policies and procedures to follow when handling any potentially hazardous substance. **Note:** All potentially hazardous substances may not be represented in this table. Refer to institution-specific guidelines for precautions to observe when handling hazardous substances.

RECOMMENDATIONS

1. It is not advisable to crush certain medications.

2. Consult individual monographs prior to crushing capsule or tablet.

3. If crushing a tablet or capsule is contraindicated, consult with your pharmacist to determine whether an oral solution exists or can be compounded.

ORAL DOSAGES THAT SHOULD NOT BE CRUSHED

Drug Product	Dosage Form	Dosage Reasons/Comments
Absorica (ISOtretinoin)	Capsule	Mucous membrane irritant; teratogenic potential
Accutane (ISOtretinoin)	Capsule	Mucous membrane irritant; teratogenic potential
Aciphex (RABEabeprazole)	Tablet	Extended release
Aciphex Sprinkle (RABEprazole)	Capsule	Slow release. Capsule may be opened and contents sprinkled on soft food (eg, applesauce, fruit- or vegetable-based baby food, yogurt) or emptied into a small amount of liquid (eg, infant formula, apple juice, pediatric electrolyte solution). Granules should not be chewed or crushed.
Actiq (FentaNYL)	Lozenge	Slow release. This lollipop delivery system requires the patient to dissolve it slowly.
Actoplus Met XR (Pioglitazone and Metformin)	Tablet	Variable release
Actonel (Risedronate)	Tablet	Irritant. Chewed, crushed, or sucked tablets may cause oropharyngeal irritation.
Adalat CC (NIFEdipine)	Tablet	Extended release
Adderall XR (Dextroamphetamine and Amphetamine)	Capsule	Extended release[1]
Adenovirus (Types 4, 7) Vaccine	Tablet	Teratogenic potential; enteric-coated; do not disrupt tablet to avoid releasing live adenovirus in upper respiratory tract
Advicor (Niacin and Lovastatin)	Tablet	Variable release
Afeditab CR (NIFEdipine)	Tablet	Extended release
Afinitor (Everolimus)	Tablet	Mucous membrane irritant; teratogenic potential; hazardous substance[11]
Aggrenox (Aspirin and Dipyridamole)	Capsule	Extended release. Capsule may be opened; contents include an aspirin tablet that may be chewed and dipyridamole pellets that may be sprinkled on applesauce.
Alavert Allergy and Sinus D-12 (Loratadine and Pseudoephedrine)	Tablet	Extended release
Allegra-D (Fexofenadine and Pseudoephedrine)	Tablet	Extended release
ALPRAZolam ER	Tablet	Extended release
Altoprev (Lovastatin)	Tablet	Extended release
Ambien CR (Zolpidem)	Tablet	Extended release
Amitiza (Lubiprostone)	Capsule	Manufacturer recommendation
Amnesteem (ISOtretinoin)	Capsule	Mucous membrane irritant; teratogenic potential
Ampyra (Dalfampridine)	Tablet	Extended release
Amrix (Cyclobenzaprine)	Capsule	Extended release
Aplenzin (BuPROPion)	Tablet	Extended release
Apriso (Mesalamine)	Capsule	Extended release[1]; maintain pH at ≤6
Aptivus (Tipranavir)	Capsule	Taste. Oil emulsion within spheres
Aricept 23 mg (Donepezil)	Tablet	Film-coated; chewing or crushing may increase rate of absorption
Arava (Leflunomide)	Tablet	Teratogenic potential; hazardous substance[11]
Arthrotec (Diclofenac and Misoprostol)	Tablet	Delayed release; enteric-coated
Asacol (Mesalamine)	Tablet	Slow release
Aspirin enteric-coated	Capsule, tablet	Delayed release; enteric-coated
Astagraf XL (Tacrolimus)	Capsule	Extended release
Atelvia (Risedronate)	Tablet	Extended release; tablet coating is an important part of the delayed release
Augmentin XR (Amoxicillin and Clavulanate)	Tablet	Extended release[2, 8]
AVINza (Morphine)	Capsule	Slow release[1] (not pudding)
Avodart (Dutasteride)	Capsule	Capsule should not be handled by pregnant women due to teratogenic potential[10]; hazardous substance[11]
Azulfidine EN-tabs (SulfaSALAzine)	Tablet	Delayed release
Bayer Aspirin EC (Aspirin)	Caplet	Enteric-coated
Bayer Aspirin, Low Adult 81 mg (Aspirin)	Tablet	Enteric-coated
Bayer Aspirin, Regular Strength 325 mg (Aspirin)	Caplet	Enteric-coated
Benzonatate	Capsule	Swallow whole; pharmacologic action may cause choking if chewed or opened and swallowed
Biaxin XL (Clarithromycin)	Tablet	Extended release
Biltricide (Praziquantel)	Tablet	Taste[8]
Bisac-Evac (Bisacodyl)	Tablet	Enteric-coated[3]
Bisacodyl	Tablet	Enteric-coated[3]
Boniva (Ibandronate)	Tablet	Irritant. Chewed, crushed, or sucked tablets may cause oropharyngeal irritation.
Bosulif (Bosutinib)	Tablet	Hazardous substance[11]
Budeprion SR (BuPROPion)	Tablet	Extended release
Buproban (BuPROPion)	Tablet	Extended release
BuPROPion SR	Tablet	Extended release

Drug Product	Dosage Form	Dosage Reasons/Comments
Calan SR (Verapamil)	Tablet	Extended release[8]
Campral (Acamprosate)	Tablet	Delayed release; enteric-coated
Caprelsa (Vandetanib)	Tablet	Teratogenic potential; hazardous substance[11]
Carbatrol (CarBAMazepine)	Capsule	Extended release[1]
Cardene SR (NiCARdipine)	Capsule	Extended release
Cardizem (Diltiazem)	Tablet	Not described as slow release but releases drug over 3 hours.
Cardizem CD (Diltiazem)	Capsule	Extended release
Cardizem LA (Diltiazem)	Tablet	Extended release
Cardura XL (Doxazosin)	Tablet	Extended release
Cartia XT (Diltiazem)	Capsule	Extended release
Casodex (Bicalutamide)	Tablet	Teratogenic potential; hazardous substance[11]
CeeNU (Lomustine)	Capsule	Teratogenic potential; hazardous substance[11]
Cefaclor extended release	Tablet	Extended release
Ceftin (Cefuroxime)	Tablet	Taste[2]. Use suspension for children.
Cefuroxime	Tablet	Taste[2]. Use suspension for children.
CellCept (Mycophenolate)	Capsule, tablet	Teratogenic potential; hazardous substance[9,11]
Charcoal Plus DS (Charcoal, Activated)	Tablet	Enteric-coated
Chlor-Trimeton 12-Hour (Chlorpheniramine)	Tablet	Extended release[2]
Cipro XR (Ciprofloxacin)	Tablet	Extended release[2]
Claravis (ISOtretinoin)	Capsule	Mucous membrane irritant; teratogenic potential
Claritin-D 12-Hour (Loratadine and Pseudoephedrine)	Tablet	Extended release[2]
Claritin-D 24-Hour (Loratadine and Pseudoephedrine)	Tablet	Extended release[2]
Colace (Docusate)	Capsule	Taste[5]
Colestid (Colestipol)	Tablet	Slow release
Cometriq (Cabozantinib)	Capsule	Teratogenic potential; hazardous substance[11]
Commit (Nicotine)	Lozenge	Integrity compromised by chewing or crushing
Concerta (Methylphenidate)	Tablet	Extended release
Contrave (Naltrexone and Bupropion)	Tablet	Extended release
ConZip (TraMADol)	Capsule	Variable release; tablet disruption may cause overdose
Coreg CR (Carvedilol)	Capsule	Extended release[1]; may add contents to chilled applesauce
Cotazym-S (Pancrelipase)	Capsule	Enteric-coated[1]
Covera-HS (Verapamil)	Tablet	Extended release
Creon (Pancrelipase)	Capsule	Extended release[1]; enteric-coated contents
Crixivan (Indinavir)	Capsule	Taste. Capsule may be opened and mixed with fruit puree (eg, banana).
Cyclophosphamide	Capsule, tablet	Hazardous substance[11]; manufacturer recommendation
Cymbalta (DULoxetine)	Capsule	Enteric-coated[1]; may add contents to apple juice or applesauce but not chocolate
Depakene (Valproic Acid)	Capsule	Slow release; mucous membrane irritant[2]; hazardous substance[11]
Depakote (Divalproex)	Tablet	Delayed release; hazardous substance[11]
Depakote ER (Divalproex)	Tablet	Extended release; hazardous substance[11]
Depakote Sprinkles (Divalproex)	Capsule	Extended release[1]
Detrol LA (Tolterodine)	Capsule	Extended release
Dexedrine (Dextroamphetamine)	Capsule	Extended release
Dexilant (Dexlansoprazole)	Capsule	Delayed release[1]
Diacomit (Stiripentol)	Capsule	Manufacturer recommendation[12]
Diamox Sequels (AcetaZOLAMIDE)	Capsule	Extended release
Dibenzyline (Phenoxybenzamine)	Capsule	Hazardous substance[11]
Diclegis (Doxylamine and Pyridoxine)	Tablet	Delayed release; manufacturer recommendation
Dilacor XR (Diltiazem)	Capsule	Extended release
Dilantin (Phenytoin)	Capsule	Extended release; manufacturer recommendation[12]
Dilatrate-SR (Isosorbide Dinitrate)	Capsule	Extended release
Dilt-XR (Diltiazem)	Capsule	Extended release
Diltia XT (Diltiazem)	Capsule	Extended release
Ditropan XL (Oxybutynin)	Tablet	Extended release
Divalproex ER	Tablet	Extended release
Donnatal Extentab (Hyoscyamine, Atropine, Scopolamine, and Phenobarbital)	Tablet	Extended release[2]
Drisdol (Ergocalciferol)	Capsule	Liquid filled[4]
Droxia (Hydroxyurea)	Capsule	May be opened; wear gloves to handle; hazardous substance[11]
Duavee (Estrogens [Conjugated/Equine] and Bazedoxifene)	Tablet	Manufacturer recommendation; hazardous substance[11]
Dulcolax (Bisacodyl)	Capsule	Liquid-filled

ORAL DOSAGES THAT SHOULD NOT BE CRUSHED

Drug Product	Dosage Form	Dosage Reasons/Comments
Dulcolax (Bisacodyl)	Tablet	Enteric-coated[3]
EC-Naprosyn (Naproxen)	Tablet	Delayed release; enteric-coated
Ecotrin Adult Low Strength (Aspirin)	Tablet	Enteric-coated
Ecotrin Maximum Strength (Aspirin)	Tablet	Enteric-coated
Ecotrin Regular Strength (Aspirin)	Tablet	Enteric-coated
E.E.S. (Erythromycin)	Tablet	Enteric-coated[2]
Effer-K (Potassium Bicarbonate and Potassium Citrate)	Tablet	Effervescent tablet[6]
Effervescent Potassium	Tablet	Effervescent tablet[6]
Effexor XR (Venlafaxine)	Capsule	Extended release
Elepsia XR	Tablet	Extended release
Embeda (Morphine and Naltrexone)	Capsule	Extended release[1]; do not give via NG tube
E-Mycin (Erythromycin)	Tablet	Enteric-coated
Enablex (Darifenacin)	Tablet	Slow release
Entocort EC (Budesonide)	Capsule	Extended release; enteric-coated[1]
Envarsus XR (Tacrolimus)	Tablet	Extended release
Epanova (Omega-3 Fatty Acids)	Capsule	Manufacturer recommendation
Equetro (CarBAMazepine)	Capsule	Extended release[1]
Ergomar (Ergotamine)	Tablet	Sublingual form[7]
Erivedge (Vismodegib)	Capsule	Teratogenic potential[11]
Eryc (Erythromycin)	Capsule	Enteric-coated
Ery-Tab (Erythromycin)	Tablet	Delayed release; enteric-coated
Erythromycin Stearate	Tablet	Enteric-coated
Erythromycin Base	Tablet	Enteric-coated
Erythromycin Delayed Release	Capsule	Enteric-coated pellets[1]
Etoposide	Capsule	Hazardous substance[11]
Evista (Raloxifene)	Tablet	Taste; teratogenic potential[10]; hazardous substance[11]
Exalgo (HYDROmorphone)	Tablet	Extended release; breaking, chewing, crushing, or dissolving before ingestion or injecting increases the risk of overdose
Exjade (Deferasirox)	Tablet	Do not chew or swallow whole; do not give as tablets meant to be given as a liquid
Fareston (Toremifene)	Tablet	Teratogenic potential; hazardous substance[11]
Farydak (Panobinostat)	Capsule	Manufacturer recommendation; hazardous substance[11]
Feldene (Piroxicam)	Capsule	Mucous membrane irritant
FentaNYL	Lozenge	Slow release; lollipop delivery system requires the patient to slowly dissolve in mouth
Fentora (FentaNYL)	Tablet	Buccal tablet; swallowing whole or crushing may reduce effectiveness
Feosol (Ferrous Sulfate)	Tablet	Enteric-coated[2]
Fergon (Ferrous Gluconate)	Tablet	Enteric-coated
Ferro-Sequels (Ferrous Fumarate)	Tablet	Slow release
Fetzima (Levomilnacipran)	Capsule	Extended release
Flagyl ER (MetroNIDAZOLE)	Tablet	Extended release
Fleet Laxative (Bisacodyl)	Tablet	Enteric-coated[3]
Flomax (Tamsulosin)	Capsule	Slow release
Fludara (Fludarabine)	Tablet	Teratogenic potential; hazardous substance[11]
Focalin XR (Dexmethylphenidate)	Capsule	Extended release[1]
Forfivo XL (BuPROPion)	Capsule	Extended release
Fortamet (MetFORMIN)	Tablet	Extended release
Fosamax (Alendronate)	Tablet	Mucous membrane irritant
Fosamax Plus D (Alendronate and Cholecalciferol)	Tablet	Mucous membrane irritant
Fulyzaq (Crofelemer)	Tablet	Delayed release
Galzin (Zinc Acetate)	Capsule	Manufacturer recommendation[12]; possible gastric irritation
Gengraf (CycloSPORINE)	Capsule	Teratogenic potential; hazardous substance[11]
Geodon (Ziprasidone)	Capsule	Hazardous substance[11]
Gleevec (Imatinib)	Tablet	Taste[8]. May be dissolved in water or apple juice; hazardous substance[11]
GlipiZIDE XL	Tablet	Extended release
Glucophage XR (MetFORMIN)	Tablet	Extended release
Glucotrol XL (GlipiZIDE)	Tablet	Extended release
Glumetza (MetFORMIN)	Tablet	Extended release
Gralise (Gabapentin)	Tablet	Extended release
Halfprin (Aspirin)	Tablet	Enteric-coated
Hetlioz (Tasimelteon)	Capsule	Manufacturer recommendation
Hexalen (Altretamine)	Capsule	Teratogenic potential; hazardous substance[11]
Horizant (Gabapentin)	Tablet	Extended release

Drug Product	Dosage Form	Dosage Reasons/Comments
Hycamtin (Topotecan)	Capsule	Teratogenic potential; hazardous substance[11]
Hydrea (Hydroxyurea)	Capsule	Can be opened and mixed with water; wear gloves to handle; hazardous substance[11]
Hydromorph Contin (HYDROmorphone)	Capsule	Controlled release
Ibrance (Palbociclib)	Capsule	Manufacturer recommendation; hazardous substance[11]
Iclusig (PONATinib)	Tablet	Teratogenic potential; hazardous substance[11]
Imbruvica (Ibrutinib)	Capsule	Teratogenic potential; hazardous substance[11]
Imdur (Isosorbide Mononitrate)	Tablet	Extended release[8]
Inderal LA (Propranolol)	Capsule	Extended release
Indomethacin SR	Capsule	Slow release[1,2]
Inlyta (Axitinib)	Tablet	Teratogenic potential; hazardous substance[11]
InnoPran XL (Propranolol)	Capsule	Extended release
Intelence (Etravirine)	Tablet	Tablet should be swallowed whole and not crushed; tablet may be dispersed in water
Intermezzo (Zolpidem)	Tablet	Sublingual form[7]
Intuniv (GuanFACINE)	Tablet	Extended release
Invega (Paliperidone)	Tablet	Extended release
IsoDitrate (Isosorbide Dinitrate)	Tablet	Extended release
Isoptin SR (Verapamil)	Tablet	Extended release[8]
Isosorbide Dinitrate Sublingual	Tablet	Sublingual form[7]
ISOtretinoin	Capsule	Mucous membrane irritant
Jalyn (Dutasteride and Tamsulosin)	Capsule	Capsule should not be handled by pregnant women due to teratogenic potential[10]; hazardous substance[9,11]
Janumet XR (Sitagliptin and Metformin)	Tablet	Extended release
Jurnista (HYDROmorphone)	Tablet	Extended release
Juxtapid (Lomitapide)	Capsule	Manufacturer recommendation
Kadian (Morphine)	Capsule	Extended release[1]. Do not give via NG tubes; may add contents to applesauce without crushing.
Kaletra (Lopinavir and Ritonavir)	Tablet	Film-coated; pregnant women or women who may become pregnant should not handle crushed or broken tablets; active ingredients surrounded by wax matrix to prevent health care exposure
Kapidex (Dexlansoprazole)	Capsule	Delayed release[1]
Kapvay (CloNIDine)	Tablet	Extended release
Kazano (Alogliptin and Metformin)	Tablet	Not scored; manufacturer recommendation[12]
K-Dur (Potassium Chloride)	Tablet	Slow release
Keppra (LevETIRAcetam)	Tablet	Taste[2]
Keppra XR (LevETIRAcetam)	Tablet	Extended release[2]
Ketek (Telithromycin)	Tablet	Slow release
Khedezla (Desvenlafaxine)	Tablet	Extended release
Klor-Con (Potassium Chloride)	Tablet	Extended release[2]
Klor-Con M (Potassium Chloride)	Tablet	Slow release[2]; some strengths are scored; to make liquid, place tablet in 120 mL of water; disperse 2 minutes; stir
K-Lyte/Cl (Potassium Bicarbonate and Potassium Chloride)	Tablet	Effervescent tablet[6]
Kombiglyze XR (Saxagliptin and Metformin)	Tablet	Extended release; tablet matrix may remain in stool
K-Tab (Potassium Chloride)	Tablet	Extended release[2]
LaMICtal XR (LamoTRIgine)	Tablet	Extended release
Lescol XL (Fluvastatin)	Tablet	Extended release
Letairis (Ambrisentan)	Tablet	Film-coated; slow release; hazardous substance[11]
Leukeran (Chlorambucil)	Tablet	Teratogenic potential; hazardous substance[11]
Levbid (Hyoscyamine)	Tablet	Extended release[8]
Lialda (Mesalamine)	Tablet	Delayed release, enteric-coated
Lipitor (AtorvaSTATin)	Tablet	Manufacturer recommendation[12]
Lithium Carbonate XR	Tablet	Extended release
Lithobid (Lithium)	Tablet	Extended release
Lovaza (Omega-3 Fatty Acids)	Capsule	Contents of capsule may erode walls of styrofoam or plastic materials
Luvox CR (FluvoxaMINE)	Capsule	Extended release
Lynparza (Olaparib)	Capsule	Teratogenic potential; hazardous substance[11]; manufacturer recommendation
Lysodren (Mitotane)	Tablet	Hazardous substance[11]
Mag-Tab SR (Magnesium L-Lactate)	Tablet	Extended release
Matulane (Procarbazine)	Capsule	Teratogenic potential; hazardous substance[11]
Maxiphen DM (Guaifenesin, Dextromethorphan, and Phenylephrine)	Tablet	Slow release[8]
Mestinon ER (Pyridostigmine)	Tablet	Extended release[2]
Metadate CD (Methylphenidate)	Capsule	Extended release[1]
Metadate ER (Methylphenidate)	Tablet	Extended release

ORAL DOSAGES THAT SHOULD NOT BE CRUSHED

Drug Product	Dosage Form	Dosage Reasons/Comments
Metoprolol ER	Tablet	Extended release
MicroK Extencaps (Potassium Chloride)	Capsule	Extended release[1,2]
Minocin (Minocycline)	Capsule	Slow release
Mirapex ER (Pramipexole)	Tablet	Extended release
Morphine Sulfate Extended Release	Tablet	Extended release
Motrin (Ibuprofen)	Tablet	Taste[5]
Moxatag (Amoxicillin)	Tablet	Extended release
MS Contin (Morphine)	Tablet	Extended release[2]
Mucinex (GuaiFENesin)	Tablet	Slow release
Mucinex DM (GuaiFENesin)	Tablet	Slow release[2]
Multaq (Dronedarone)	Tablet	Hazardous substance[11]
Myfortic (Mycophenolate)	Tablet	Delayed release; teratogenic potential; hazardous substance[11]
Myorisan (ISOtretinoin)	Capsule	Mucous membrane irritant; teratogenic potential
Myrbetriq (Mirabegron)	Tablet	Extended release
Namenda XR (Memantine)	Capsule	Extended release[1]
Naprelan (Naproxen)	Tablet	Extended release
Neoral (CycloSPORINE)	Capsule	Teratogenic potential; hazardous substance[11]
NexIUM (Esomeprazole)	Capsule	Delayed release[1]
Niaspan (Niacin)	Tablet	Extended release
Nicotinic Acid (Niacinamide)	Capsule, Tablet	Slow release[8]
Nifediac CC (NIFEdipine)	Tablet	Extended release
Nifedical XL (NIFEdipine)	Tablet	Extended release
NIFEdipine ER	Tablet	Extended release
Ninlaro (Ixazomib)	Capsule	Hazardous substance[11]; manufacturer recommendation
Nitrostat (Nitroglycerin)	Tablet	Sublingual route[7]
Norpace CR (Disopyramide)	Capsule	Extended release; form within a special capsule
Norvir (Ritonavir)	Tablet	Crushing tablets has resulted in decreased bioavailability of drug[2]
Noxafil (Posaconazole)	Tablet	Delayed release
Nucynta ER (Tapentadol)	Tablet	Extended release; tablet disruption may cause a potentially fatal overdose
Ofev (Nintedanib)	Capsule	Taste; hazardous substance[11]
Oleptro (TraZODone)	Tablet	Extended release[8]
Omtryg (Omega-3 Fatty Acids)	Capsule	Manufacturer recommendation
Onglyza (Saxagliptin)	Tablet	Film-coated
Opana ER (Oxymorphone)	Tablet	Extended release; tablet disruption may cause a potentially fatal overdose
Opsumit (Macitentan)	Tablet	Teratogenic potential; hazardous substance[11]
Oracea (Doxycycline)	Capsule	Delayed release
Oramorph SR (Morphine)	Tablet	Extended release[2]
Oravig (Miconazole)	Tablet	Buccal tablet
Orphenadrine Citrate ER	Tablet	Extended release
Oseni (Alogliptin and Pioglitazone)	Tablet	Manufacturer recommendation[12]
Otezla (Apremilast)	Tablet	Manufacturer recommendation
Oxtellar XR (OXcarbazepine)	Tablet	Extended release
OxyCONTIN (OxyCODONE)	Tablet	Extended release; surrounded by wax matrix; tablet disruption may cause a potentially fatal overdose
Oxymorphone ER	Tablet	Extended release
Pancrease MT (Pancrelipase)	Capsule	Enteric-coated[1]
Pancreaze (Pancrelipase)	Capsule	Slow-release[1]; enteric-coated contents
Pancrelipase	Capsule	Slow-release[1]; enteric-coated contents
Paxil CR (PARoxetine)	Tablet	Extended release
Pentasa (Mesalamine)	Capsule	Slow release[1]
Pertzye (Pancrelipase)	Capsule	Slow-release[1]; enteric-coated contents
Pexeva (PARoxetine)	Tablet	Film-coated
Phenytek (Phenytoin)	Capsule	Extended release; manufacturer recommendation[12]
Plendil (Felodipine)	Tablet	Extended release
Pomalyst (Pomalidomide)	Capsule	Teratogenic potential; hazardous substance[11]; health care workers should avoid contact with capsule contents/body fluids
Pradaxa (Dabigatran)	Capsule	Bioavailability increases by 75% when the pellets are taken without the capsule shell
Prevacid (Lansoprazole)	Capsule	Delayed release[1]
Prevacid (Lansoprazole)	Suspension	Slow release. Contains enteric-coated granules. Not for use in NG tubes; mix with water only
Prevacid SoluTab (Lansoprazole)	Tablet	Orally disintegrating. Do not swallow; dissolve in water only and dispense via dosing syringe or NG tube.
Prezcobix (Darunavir and Cobicistat)	Tablet	Film-coated

Drug Product	Dosage Form	Dosage Reasons/Comments
PriLOSEC (Omeprazole)	Capsule	Delayed release
PriLOSEC OTC (Omeprazole)	Tablet	Delayed release
Pristiq (Desvenlafaxine)	Tablet	Extended release
Procardia XL (NIFEdipine)	Tablet	Extended release
Procysbi (Cysteamine)	Capsule	Delayed release[1]
Prolopa (Benserazide and Levodopa)	Capsule	Manufacturer recommendation
Promacta (eltrombopag)	Tablet	Manufacturer recommendation
Propecia (Finasteride)	Tablet	Women who are, or may become, pregnant should not handle crushed or broken tablets due to teratogenic potential[10]; hazardous substance[11]
Proscar (Finasteride)	Tablet	Women who are, or may become, pregnant should not handle crushed or broken tablets due to teratogenic potential[10]; hazardous substance[11]
Protonix (Pantoprazole)	Tablet	Slow release
PROzac Weekly (FLUoxetine)	Capsule	Enteric-coated
Purinethol (Mercaptopurine)	Tablet	Teratogenic potential[10]; hazardous substance[11]
Pytest (Carbon 14 Urea)	Capsule	Hazardous substance[11]
Qudexy XR (Topiramate)	Capsule	Extended release
QuiNIDine ER	Tablet	Extended release[8]; enteric-coated
Ranexa (Ranolazine)	Tablet	Slow release
Rapamune (Sirolimus)	Tablet	Hazardous substance[11]; pharmacokinetic NanoCrystal technology may be affected[2]
Rayos (PredniSONE)	Tablet	Delayed release; release is dependent upon intact coating
Razadyne ER (Galantamine)	Capsule	Extended release
Renagel (Sevelamer)	Tablet	Expands in liquid if broken/crushed.
Renvela (Sevelamer)	Tablet	Enteric-coated[2]; expands in liquid if broken or crushed
Requip XL (ROPINIRole)	Tablet	Extended release
Rescriptor (Delavirdine)	Tablet	If unable to swallow, may dissolve 100 mg tablets in water and drink; 200 mg tablets must be swallowed whole
Revlimid (Lenalidomide)	Capsule	Teratogenic potential; hazardous substance[11]; health care workers should avoid contact with capsule contents/body fluids
RisperDAL M-Tab (RisperiDONE)	Tablet	Orally disintegrating. Do not chew or break tablet; after dissolving under tongue, tablet may be swallowed
Ritalin LA (Methylphenidate)	Capsule	Extended release[1]
Ritalin-SR (Methylphenidate)	Tablet	Extended release
Rytary (Carbidopa and Levodopa)	Capsule	Extended release[1]
Rythmol SR (Propafenone)	Capsule	Extended release
Ryzolt (TraMADol)	Tablet	Extended release; tablet disruption may cause overdose
SandIMMUNE (CycloSPORINE)	Capsule	Teratogenic potential; hazardous substance[11]
Saphris (Asenapine)	Tablet	Sublingual form[7]
Sensipar (Cinacalcet)	Tablet	Tablets are not scored and cutting may cause inaccurate dosage
SEROquel XR (QUEtiapine)	Tablet	Extended release
Simcor (Niacin and Simvastatin)	Tablet	Tablet contains extended release niacin
Sinemet CR (Carbidopa and Levodopa)	Tablet	Extended release[8]
Sitavig (Acyclovir)	Tablet	Buccal tablet; swallowing whole or crushing eliminates or reduces effectiveness
Slo-Niacin (Niacin)	Tablet	Slow release[8]
Slow-Mag (Magnesium Chloride)	Tablet	Delayed release
Solodyn (Minocycline)	Tablet	Extended release
Somnote (Chloral Hydrate)	Capsule	Liquid filled
Soriatane (Acitretin)	Capsule	Teratogenic potential; hazardous substance[11]
Sprycel (Dasatinib)	Tablet	Film-coated. Active ingredients are surrounded by a wax matrix to prevent health care exposure. Women who are, or may become pregnant, should not handle crushed or broken tablets; teratogenic potential; hazardous substance[11]
Stalevo (Levodopa, Carbidopa, and Entacapone)	Tablet	Manufacturer recommendation
Stavzor (Valproic Acid)	Capsule	Delayed release; hazardous substance[11]
Stivarga (Regorafenib)	Tablet	Manufacturer recommendation; teratogenic potential; hazardous substance[11]
Strattera (AtoMOXetine)	Capsule	Capsule contents can cause ocular irritation.
Sudafed 12-Hour (Pseudoephedrine)	Capsule	Extended release[2]
Sudafed 24-Hour (Pseudoephedrine)	Capsule	Extended release[2]
Sulfazine EC (SulfaSALAzine)	Tablet	Delayed release, enteric-coated
Sular (Nisoldipine)	Tablet	Extended release
Sustiva (Efavirenz)	Tablet	Tablets should not be broken (capsules should be used if dosage adjustment needed)
Symax Duotab (Hyoscyamine)	Tablet	Controlled release
Symax SR (Hyoscyamine)	Tablet	Extended release
Syprine (Trientine)	Capsule	Potential risk of contact dermatitis

ORAL DOSAGES THAT SHOULD NOT BE CRUSHED

Drug Product	Dosage Form	Dosage Reasons/Comments
Tabloid (Thioguanine)	Tablet	Teratogenic potential; hazardous substance[11]
Tafinlar (Dabrafenib)	Capsule	Teratogenic potential; hazardous substance[11]
Tamoxifen	Tablet	Teratogenic potential; hazardous substance[11]
Tasigna (Nilotinib)	Capsule	Hazardous substance[11]; altering capsule may lead to high blood levels, increasing the risk of toxicity
Taztia XT (Diltiazem)	Capsule	Extended release[1]
Tecfidera (Dimethyl Fumarate)	Capsule	Manufacturer recommendation; delayed release; irritant
TEGretol-XR (CarBAMazepine)	Tablet	Extended release[2]
Temodar (Temozolomide)	Capsule	Teratogenic potential; hazardous substance[11]. **Note:** If capsules are accidentally opened or damaged, rigorous precautions should be taken to avoid inhalation or contact of contents with the skin or mucous membranes.
Tessalon Perles (Benzonatate)	Capsule	Swallow whole; pharmacologic action may cause choking if chewed or opened and swallowed.
Tetracycline	Capsule	Hazardous substance[11]
Thalomid (Thalidomide)	Capsule	Teratogenic potential; hazardous substance[11]
Theo-24 (Theophylline)	Capsule	Extended release[1]; contains beads that dissolve through GI tract
Theochron (Theophylline)	Tablet	Extended release
Theophylline ER	Tablet	Extended release
Tiazac (Diltiazem)	Capsule	Extended release[1]
Topamax (Topiramate)	Capsule	Taste[1]
Topamax (Topiramate)	Tablet	Taste
Toprol XL (Metoprolol)	Tablet	Extended release[8]
Toviaz (Fesoterodine)	Tablet	Extended release
Tracleer (Bosentan)	Tablet	Teratogenic potential; hazardous substance[10,11]; women who are or may be pregnant should not handle crushed or broken tablets
TRENtal (Pentoxifylline)	Tablet	Extended release
Treximet (Sumatriptan and Naproxen)	Tablet	Unique formulation enhances rapid drug absorption
TriLipix (Fenofibrate)	Capsule	Extended release
Trokendi XR (Topiramate)	Capsule	Extended release
Tylenol Arthritis Pain (Acetaminophen)	Caplet	Controlled release
Tylenol 8 Hour (Acetaminophen)	Caplet	Extended release
Uceris (Budesonide)	Tablet	Extended release; coating on tablet designed to break down at pH of ≥7
Ultram ER (TraMADol)	Tablet	Extended release. Tablet disruption my cause a potentially fatal overdose.
Ultresa (Pancrelipase)	Capsule	Delayed release; enteric-coated contents
Ultrase (Pancrelipase)	Capsule	Enteric-coated[1]
Ultrase MT (Pancrelipase)	Capsule	Enteric-coated[1]
Uniphyl (Theophylline)	Tablet	Slow release
Urocit-K (Potassium Citrate)	Tablet	Wax-coated; prevents upper GI release
Uroxatral (Alfuzosin)	Tablet	Extended release
Valcyte (ValGANciclovir)	Tablet	Irritant potential[2]; teratogenic potential; hazardous substance[11]
Vascepa (Omega-3 Fatty Acids)	Capsule	Manufacturer recommendation
Venlafaxine ER	Tablet	Extended release
Verapamil SR	Tablet	Extended release[8]
Verelan (Verapamil)	Capsule	Sustained release[1]
Verelan PM (Verapamil)	Capsule	Extended release[1]
Vesanoid (Tretinoin)	Capsule	Teratogenic potential; hazardous substance[11]
VESIcare (Solifenacin)	Tablet	Film-coated
Videx EC (Didanosine)	Capsule	Delayed release
Vimovo (Naproxen and Esomeprazole)	Tablet	Delayed release
Viokace (Pancrelipase)	Tablet	Mucous membrane irritant
Viramune XR (Nevirapine)	Tablet	Extended release[2]
Voltaren-XR (Diclofenac)	Tablet	Extended release
VoSpire ER (Albuterol)	Tablet	Extended release
Votrient (PAZOPanib)	Tablet	Crushing significantly increases AUC and T_{max}; hazardous substance[11]; crushed or broken tablets may cause dangerous skin problems
Wellbutrin (BuPROPion)	Tablet	Film-coated
Wellbutrin SR (BuPROPion)	Tablet	Extended release
Wellbutrin XL (BuPROPion)	Tablet	Extended release
Xalkori (Crizotinib)	Capsule	Teratogenic potential; hazardous substance[11]
Xanax XR (ALPRAZolam)	Tablet	Extended release
Xeloda (Capecitabine)	Tablet	Teratogenic potential; hazardous substance[11].
Xigduo XR (Dapagliflozin and Metformin)	Tablet	Extended release
Xtandi (Enzalutamide)	Capsule	Teratogenic potential; hazardous substance[11]

Drug Product	Dosage Form	Dosage Reasons/Comments
Zegerid OTC (Omeprazole and Sodium Bbicarbonate)	Capsule	Delayed release[2]
Zelboraf (Vemurafenib)	Tablet	Manufacturer recommendation (based on tablet properties); teratogenic potential; hazardous substance[11]
Zenatane (ISOtretinoin)	Capsule	Mucous membrane irritant; teratogenic potential
Zenpep (Pancrelipase)	Capsule	Delayed release[1]; enteric-coated contents
Zohydro ER (HYDROcodone)	Capsule	Extended release; capsule disruption may cause a potentially fatal overdose
Zolinza (Vorinostat)	Capsule	Irritant; avoid contact with skin or mucous membranes; use gloves to handle; teratogenic potential; hazardous substance[11]
Zomig-ZMT (ZOLMitriptan)	Tablet	Oral-disintegrating form[7]
Zonatuss (Benzonatate)	Capsule	Swallow whole; pharmacologic action may cause choking if chewed or opened and swallowed
Zortress (Everolimus)	Tablet	Mucous membrane irritant; teratogenic potential; hazardous substance[11]
Zyban (BuPROPion)	Tablet	Slow release
Zydelig (Idelalisib)	Tablet	Manufacturer recommendation
Zyflo CR (Zileuton)	Tablet	Extended release
ZyrTEC-D Allergy & Congestion (Cetirizine and Pseudoephedrine)	Tablet	Extended release
Zytiga (Abiraterone)	Tablet	Teratogenic potential; hazardous substance[11]; women who are or may be pregnant should wear gloves if handling tablets

[1]Capsule may be opened and the contents taken without crushing or chewing; soft food, such as applesauce or pudding, may facilitate administration; contents may generally be administered via nasogastric tube using an appropriate fluid, provided entire contents are washed down the tube.

[2]Liquid dosage forms of the product are available; however, dose, frequency of administration, and manufacturers may differ from that of the solid dosage form.

[3]Antacids and/or milk may prematurely dissolve the coating of the tablet.

[4]Capsule may be opened and the liquid contents removed for administration.

[5]The taste of this product in a liquid form would likely be unacceptable to the patient; administration via nasogastric tube should be acceptable.

[6]Effervescent tablets must be dissolved in the amount of diluent recommended by the manufacturer.

[7]Tablets are made to disintegrate under (or on) the tongue.

[8]Tablet is scored and may be broken in half without affecting release characteristics.

[9]Skin contact may enhance tumor production; avoid direct contact.

[10]Prescribing information recommends that women who are, or may become, pregnant should not handle medication, especially if crushed or broken; avoid direct contact.

[11]Potentially hazardous or hazardous substance; refer to institution-specific guidelines for precautions to observe when handling this substance.

[12]Altering (eg, chewing, crushing, splitting, opening) the dosage form has not been studied, according to the manufacturer.

REFERENCES

Mitchell JF. Oral dosage forms that should not be crushed. Available at http://www.ismp.org/tools/DoNotCrush.pdf. Accessed November 11, 2011.

US Department of Health and Human Services; Centers for Disease Control and Prevention; National Institute for Occupational Safety and Health. NIOSH list of antineoplastic and other hazardous drugs in the healthcare settings 2014. Available at http://www.cdc.gov/niosh/docs/2014-138/pdfs/2014-138.pdf. Updated September 2014. Accessed February 6, 2015.

PHARMACOLOGIC CATEGORY INDEX

NOTES

NOTES

NOTES

NOTES

NOTES

NOTES

NOTES

NOTES

Other Lexicomp Offerings

Drug Information Handbook with International Trade Names Index

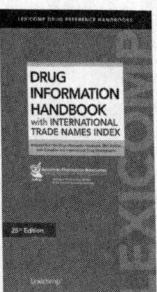

The *Drug Information Handbook with International Trade Names Index* includes the content of our *Drug Information Handbook*, plus international drug monographs for use worldwide! This easy-to-use reference is compiled especially for the pharmacist, physician, or other healthcare professional seeking quick access to extensive drug information.

Geriatric Dosage Handbook

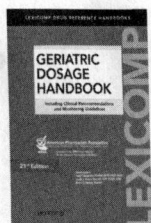

Designed for healthcare professionals managing geriatric patients.

Includes: Detailed adult and geriatric dosing; special geriatric considerations; up to 40 key fields of information in each monograph, including medication safety issues; extensive information on drug interactions, as well as dosing for patients with renal/hepatic impairment.

Drug Information Handbook for Advanced Practice Nursing

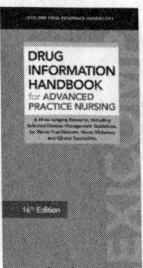

Designed to assist the advanced practice nurse with prescribing, monitoring and educating patients.

Includes: Over 4800 generic and brand names cross-referenced by page number; generic drug names and cross-references highlighted in RED; labeled and investigational indications; adult, geriatric, and pediatric dosing; and up to 75 fields of information per monograph.

Drug Information Handbook for Nursing

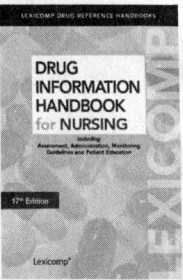

Designed for registered professional nurses and upper-division nursing students requiring dosing, administration, monitoring and patient education information. Includes: Over 4800 generic and brand name drugs, cross-referenced by page number; drug names and specific nursing fields highlighted in RED for easy reference; Nursing Actions field includes Physical Assessment and Patient Education guidelines.

Pediatric & Neonatal Dosage Handbook

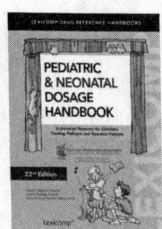

This book is designed for healthcare professionals requiring quick access to relevant pediatric drug information. Each monograph contains multiple fields of content, including usual dosage by age group, indication, and route of administration. Drug interactions, adverse reactions, extemporaneous preparations, pharmacodynamics/pharmacokinetics data, and medication safety issues are also covered.

Pediatric & Neonatal Dosage Handbook with International Trade Names Index

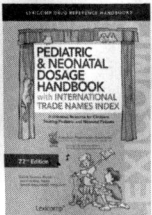

The *Pediatric & Neonatal Dosage Handbook with International Trade Names Index* is the trusted pediatric drug resource of medical professionals worldwide. The international edition contains the content of the Lexicomp *Pediatric & Neonatal Dosage Handbook*, plus an International Trade Names Index including trade names from over 100 countries.

Drug Information Handbook for Oncology

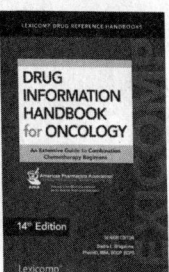

Designed for oncology professionals requiring information on combination chemotherapy regimens and dosing protocols.

Includes: Monographs containing warnings, adverse reaction profiles, drug interactions, dosing for specific indications, vesicant, emetic potential, combination regimens, and more; where applicable, a special Combination Chemotherapy field links to specific oncology monographs; Special Topics such as Cancer Treatment Related Complications, Bone Marrow Transplantation, and Drug Development.

To order, call Customer Service at 1-866-397-3433 or visit www.wolterskluwerCDI.co
Outside of the U.S., call +1-330-650-6506 or visit www.wolterskluwerCDI.com.

Other Lexicomp Offerings

Lexicomp® Online

Wolters Kluwer Clinical Drug Information applications – including Lexicomp – are used in 25 of the 27 hospitals achieving Honor Roll status as ranked by U.S. News & World Report's Best Hospitals 2015-2016 and Best Children's Hospitals 2015-2016.

Lexicomp Online integrates industry-leading databases and enhanced searching technology, delivering time-sensitive clinical information at the point of care. Our easy-to-use interface and concise information reduce the need to navigate through multiple pages or make unnecessary mouse clicks.

Lexicomp Online includes multiple databases and modules covering the following topic areas:

- Core Drug Information with Specialty Fields
- Pediatrics and Geriatrics
- Interaction Analysis
- Pharmacogenomics
- Infectious Diseases
- Laboratory Tests and Diagnostic Procedures
- Natural Products
- Patient Education
- Drug Identification
- Calculations
- IV Compatibility: King® Guide to Parenteral Admixtures™
- Toxicology

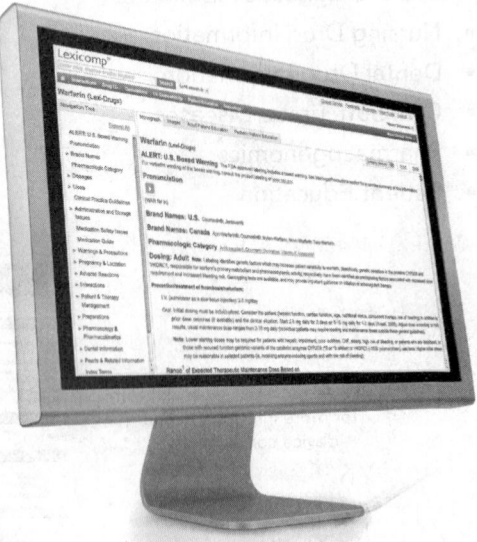

Register for a FREE 45-day trial

Visit www.wolterskluwerCDI.com/lcotrial

Academic and institutional licenses available.

For more information on Lexicomp offerings,
visit our website at www.wolterskluwerCDI.com
or call 1-855-633-0577 (or +1 330-650-6506 if outside the U.S.).

Lexicomp® Mobile Apps

Apps for smartphones and tablets

Wolters Kluwer Clinical Drug Information takes pride in creating quality drug information for use at the point of care. Our content is not subject to third-party recommendations, but based on the contributions of our respected authors and editors, internal clinical team, and thousands of professionals within the healthcare industry who continually review and validate our data.

With our Lexicomp Mobile Apps, you can be confident you are accessing timely, relevant drug information for mobile devices. All updates are included with your annual subscription.

Lexicomp Mobile Apps databases include:

- Adult Drug Information
- Pediatric & Neonatal Drug Information
- Pediatric Drug Information (Spanish Version)
- Drug Interactions
- Natural Products
- Toxicolgy
- Household Products
- Infectious Diseases
- Lab & Diagnostic Procedures
- Nursing Drug Information
- Dental Drug Information
- Oral Soft Tissue Diseases
- Pharmacogenomics
- Patient Education

- Drug ID
- Medical Calculators
- IV Compatibility*
- Drug Allergy & Idiosyncratic Reactions
- Pregnancy & Lactation
- The 5-Minute Clinical Consult
- The 5-Minute Pediatric Consult
- AHFS DI® Essentials™
- Stedman's Medical Dictionary for the Health Professions and Nursing
- Stedman's Medical Abbreviations

* I V compatibility information © copyright King Guide Publications, Inc.

Visit www.wolterskluwerCDI.com for more information and device compatibility!

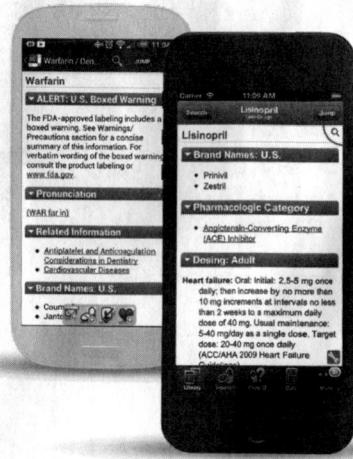

To order, call Customer Service at 1-866-397-3433 or visit www.wolterskluwerCDI.com.
Outside of the U.S., call +1-330-650-6506 or visit www.wolterskluwerCDI.com.

NOTICE

This data is intended to serve the user as a handy reference and not as a complete drug information resource. It does not include information on every therapeutic agent available. The publication covers over 1,600 commonly used drugs and is specifically designed to present important aspects of drug data in a more concise format than is typically found in medical literature or product material supplied by manufacturers.

The nature of drug information is that it is constantly evolving because of ongoing research and clinical experience and is often subject to interpretation. While great care has been taken to ensure the accuracy of the information and recommendations presented, the reader is advised that the authors, editors, reviewers, contributors, and publishers cannot be responsible for the continued currency of the information or for any errors, omissions, or the application of this information, or for any consequences arising therefrom. Therefore, the author(s) and/or the publisher shall have no liability to any person or entity with regard to claims, loss, or damage caused, or alleged to be caused, directly or indirectly, by the use of information contained herein. Because of the dynamic nature of drug information, readers are advised that decisions regarding drug therapy must be based on the independent judgment of the clinician, changing information about a drug (eg, as reflected in the literature and manufacturer's most current product information), and changing medical practices. Therefore, this data is designed to be used in conjunction with other necessary information and is not designed to be solely relied upon by any user. The user of this data hereby and forever releases the authors and publishers of this data from any and all liability of any kind that might arise out of the use of this data. The editors are not responsible for any inaccuracy of quotation or for any false or misleading implication that may arise due to the text or formulas as used or due to the quotation of revisions no longer official.

Certain of the authors, editors, and contributors have written this book in their private capacities. No official support or endorsement by any federal or state agency or pharmaceutical company is intended or inferred.

The publishers have made every effort to trace any third party copyright holders, if any, for borrowed material. If they have inadvertently overlooked any, they will be pleased to make the necessary arrangements at the first opportunity.

If you have any suggestions or questions regarding any information presented in this data, please contact our drug information pharmacists at (855) 633-0577. Book revisions are available at our website at http://www.wolterskluwercdi.com/clinical-notices/revisions/.

© 2016 Wolters Kluwer Clinical Drug Information, Inc. and its affiliates and/or licensors. All rights reserved

© 1993 to 2015, 1st to 24th Editions, Wolters Kluwer Clinical Drug Information, Inc. and its affiliates and/or licensors. All rights reserved

Printed in the United States. No part of this publication may be reproduced, stored in a retrieval system, used as a source of information for transcription into a hospital information system or electronic health or medical record, or transmitted in any form or by any means, electronic, mechanical, photocopying, recording or otherwise, without the prior written permission of the publisher. Should you or your institution have a need for this information in a format we protect, we have solutions for you. Please contact our office at the number above.

This manual was produced using LIMS — a complete publishing service of Wolters Kluwer Clinical Drug Information, Inc.

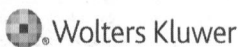

Lexicomp®

ISBN 978-1-59195-353-1 (North American Edition)

Wolters Kluwer

W9-DBQ-721

DRUG INFORMATION HANDBOOK

A Clinically Relevant Resource for All Healthcare Professionals

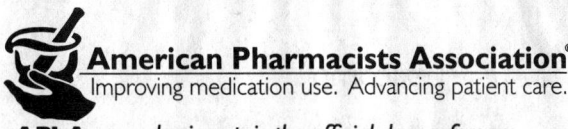

American Pharmacists Association®
Improving medication use. Advancing patient care.

APhA   *Lexicomp is the official drug reference for the American Pharmacists Association*

25th Edition

Lexicomp®